Contents

VOLUME 1

How to Use the *Medical Device Register*
Advertiser Index

VOLUME 2

How to Use the *Medical Device Register*
Advertiser Index

How to Use the Medical Device Register®

The *Medical Device Register* is the most comprehensive directory resource to the North American medical device market. This brief overview of the content and organization of the *MDR* is designed to help you unlock the full potential of the vast array of data contained within these pages.

Despite its size, the *Medical Device Register* is designed for clarity and ease of use. The two-volume directory is divided into five sections.

VOLUME 1

Section I. The **Keyword Index** cross-references the medical device product names in the *MDR* by their associated attributes and applications.

Section II. The **Product Directory** is the core of the *MDR,* listing all manufacturers of each medical device, along with available product descriptions, specifications, and prices.

VOLUME 2

Section I. The **Manufacturer Profiles** section is the reverse of the Product Directory, listing all products available from each manufacturer, together with detailed information about each company.

Section II. The **Geographical Index** identifies manufacturers by geographic location.

Section III. The **Trade Name Index** identifies manufacturers of brand-name products.

These five sections are arranged in logical order of use. What follows is a more-detailed look at the features of each section.

VOLUME 1

Keyword Index

The Keyword Index lists device names under each of their component words. Thus, the user can find any FDA/*MDR* standard medical device name by looking up any of the words that appear in it. This allows you to find a device even if you don't know the exact wording of the standard name.

SAMPLE

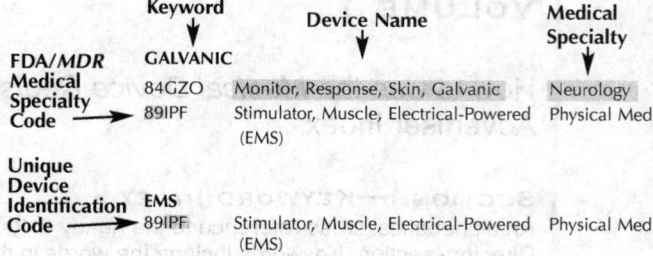

To the left of each device name in the Keyword Index is a 5-character code. This is the unique FDA/*MDR* code for each medical device and some manufacturer services. The code consists of 2 digits that identify the product's medical specialty area, and three alpha characters that identify the specific device. Together, these 5 characters supply a unique identifier for each medical device. This coding system is employed by FDA in processes for device regulation, manufacturer registration and listing, new-product approval, and product recall and risk notification. The codes are included in the *Medical Device Register* for use in inventory, filing, and ordering systems, and provide an interface compatible with current and future FDA data.

Across from the device name, the Keyword Index also shows the medical specialty area to which the device has been assigned. This information helps to confirm that you have found the correct device. It is also useful in accessing device-related FDA information, which is organized by medical specialty. However, a device's use is not necessarily limited to its officially designated specialty area. Although each device is assigned to a particular specialty's panel of experts for regulatory purposes, it may be used in other medical specialties as well. There are 19 medical specialties, corresponding to the FDA's 19 expert panels.

Due to space limitations, some medical specialty names are abbreviated in the *MDR*. The full FDA panel names, the versions used in *MDR*, and the 2-digit numeric codes, are as follows:

Medical Products

Anesth/Pul Med (73)................Anesthesiology and
Pulmonary Medicine
Cardiovascular (74) ....Cardiovascular

33RD EDITION

MEDICAL DEVICE REGISTER®

THE OFFICIAL DIRECTORY OF MEDICAL MANUFACTURERS

Produced By UBM Canon, LLC

2013

VOLUME 2

MANUFACTURER PROFILES

GEOGRAPHICAL INDEX

TRADE NAME INDEX

PARENT-SUBSIDIARY INDEX

GREY HOUSE PUBLISHING

Medical Device Register®

CHIEF EXECUTIVE OFFICER
Sally Shankland

EXECUTIVE VICE PRESIDENT/MANAGING DIRECTOR
Steve Corrick

PRODUCTION DIRECTOR
Jeff Tade

DATABASE ADMINISTRATOR
Thanh Nguyen

VICE PRESIDENT OF OPERATIONS, PUBLISHING
Roger Burg

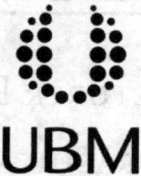

ISBN 13: 978-1-59237-880-7 ISSN: 0278-808X

UBM
Canon

Grey House
Publishing

4919 Route 22, PO Box 56, Amenia NY 12501
518-789-8700 • 800-562-2139 • FAX 845-373-6390
www.greyhouse.com • e-mail: books@greyhouse.com
Manufactured in Canada

In Vitro Diagnostic Products

Once you have found the correct FDA/*MDR* standard medical device name in the Keyword Index, you can turn to the corresponding entry in the Product Directory to identify manufacturers of the device.

Product Directory

This is the heart of the *MDR,* listing every manufacturer of each device or service. It is organized alphabetically by product or service name. If you cannot find a product in this section, it is probably because the FDA/*MDR* standard name is worded differently than the name you are looking for. Check the Keyword Index for the official FDA/*MDR* wording of the name, then turn to the corresponding entry in the Product Directory.

Alongside each device name in the Product Directory is the medical specialty area to which it's assigned, plus its unique 5-character FDA/*MDR* code. This information is followed by each of the product's manufacturers listed alphabetically, including manufacturer name, address, and telephone number.

Whenever possible, toll-free numbers are listed so that users can obtain additional product information at no cost.

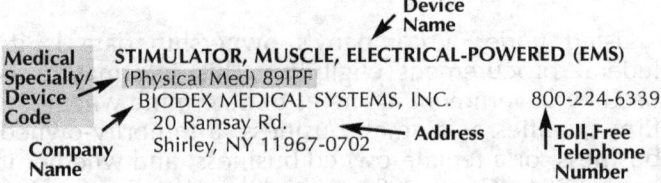

Each manufacturer's listing also includes, when available, the product's specifications and list price. The price given is based on the manufacturer's list price to hospitals for the quantity and features shown in the specs. (Actual prices vary based on quantity, special features, availability, and other factors, so you should always check with each prospective supplier before making a purchase.)

Product specifications include a variety of information. In general, the data will help you identify those manufacturers most likely to meet your needs.

Additional information on each supplier can be found in the Manufacturer Profiles section.

VOLUME 2

Manufacturer Profiles

This section contains in-depth information on all manufacturers. Entries are in alphabetical order by company name. Each name is accompanied by the manufacturer's address, telephone number, and fax number. When available, a toll-free number is included.

Beneath the company's name and address appears a 7-digit number. This is the manufacturer's unique FDA number. Like the 5-character FDA/*MDR* product code found in the Product Directory section, this number is part of FDA's system of medical device regulation, including establishment registration, manufacturing plant inspection, product approval, and product recall notification. The numbers are included in the *Medical Device Register* to help users maintain compatibility of internal data processing and filing systems with FDA.

Under the FDA number, you'll find the company's Web-site and e-mail addresses, followed by its medical-product sales volume, annual revenue, year founded, number of employees, and size of sales and marketing staffs. If the company produces CE-marked products or has a quality system in place, this is indicated as well. For publicly traded companies, stock symbols and the exchange on which the stock is traded are also reported.

Listed under a company's ownership data is its federal procurement eligibility. This information is used by government agencies to determine whether a firm qualifies as a small business, a minority-owned business, or a female-owned business, and whether it has a GSA (General Services Administration) or VA (Veterans Administration) contract.

The next field of information concerns a manufacturer's method of distributing its products. The main alternatives and their explanations are as follows:

- "Manufacturer Direct"—These companies manufacture most of their own products, and are interested in selling directly to the end user. Their products may also be available through distributors, but they would prefer to have new customers contact them directly, to be served either by the manufacturer's own employees or by a distributor assigned by the manufacturer.

- "Manufacturer through Distributor"—These companies also manufacture most of their own products, but generally prefer not to deal directly with end users. Unless negotiating a volume discount, new end users interested in these manufacturers' products should contact a local medical products distributor.

- "Exclusive Distributor"—While these companies may manufacture some of their own products, they are primarily distributors. Furthermore, each is the exclusive distributor of the products listed in its entry. End users should contact these firms directly for information on the devices they supply.

Additional distribution options can be selected by firms serving as OEMs, by those providing primarily manufacturing services, and by importers or exporters.

Also included in each manufacturer's profile are the names of several key executives, enabling you to more easily contact the appropriate individual or department for further information or quotations.

This information is followed by an alphabetical list of all medical products supplied by the company. These are the same product names under which the manufacturer is listed in the Product Directory. Across from each name is the medical specialty area associated with the product. This summary product information gives an overview of the manufacturer—how

many products it offers, which medical specialties it services, and which specific products it supplies.

At the end of the company's listing are the names of any subsidiaries also listed in the *MDR*. If you cannot locate a product under the parent company's name, you should check under those of any subsidiaries. This list of subsidiaries can also be a useful indication of the total capability of the company, and may be helpful in negotiating corporate discounts based on purchases from several divisions.

Please note that complete information on each product is not contained in this section; you must turn to the appropriate entry in the Product Directory section to obtain such information, if it has been supplied. This more-detailed information in the Product Directory may clarify what the company actually offers in a given category.

Geographical Index

This index cross-references the companies presented in the Manufacturer Profiles section by their geographic location. You can use this index to identify local manufacturers or to coordinate visits to manufacturers in a particular area. Companies are listed alphabetically by state, and then by city or municipality within the state. Canadian and Mexican manufacturers are listed alphabetically by company name at the end of the section.

Trade Name Index

If you are looking for the supplier of a specific trade-named product, and the trade name is different from the manufacturer's name, the Trade Name Index is the fastest way of identifying the company.

Trade names, with the corresponding manufacturer names, are listed alphabetically. Additional information on each supplier can be found in the Manufacturer Profiles section.

Advertiser Index

A notation of a product category and page number indicates an enhanced listing in that category or display ad near the category.

SECTION I

MANUFACTURER PROFILES

PURPOSE OF THIS SECTION

Provides additional information on particular manufacturers.

FEATURES

◆ North American medical device manufacturers, exclusive distributors, and original equipment manufacturers (OEMs) are outlined in detail in this section, with contact information that includes street address, phone and fax numbers, FDA number, e-mail address, and Web site URL.

◆ For each manufacturer, the FDA/*MDR* standard product or service category names and medical specialty areas under which that company appears in the Product Directory (Volume 1, Section III) are listed here. (For descriptive information about a product, consult the manufacturer's listing under the particular product name in the Product Directory.)

◆ Company ownership is listed, along with any subsidiaries in the *MDR*.

◆ The relative size of each manufacturer can be approximated from number of employees, number of sales and marketing staff, annual medical product sales volume, and annual revenue. Public companies trading on a stock exchange are noted, and stock symbols provided. If the company produces CE-marked products or has a quality system in place, this is indicated as well.

◆ Key executives are identified, along with their titles.

◆ How the company distributes its products, and whether it actually manufactures its own products or is an exclusive distributor or importer, is also noted.

◆ Federal procurement eligibility is identified for each company, whether as a small business, woman-owned business, minority-owned business, GSA contractor, or VA contractor.

◆ Advertisers offer additional information on their companies and products through display ads and enhanced listings.

Health Resources from Grey House Publishing

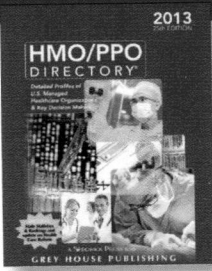

The HMO/PPO Directory

This comprehensive directory details more information about more managed health care organizations than ever before. Over 1,100 HMOs, PPOs and affiliated companies are listed, arranged alphabetically by state. Detailed listings include Key Contact Information, Drug Benefits, Enrollment, Geographical Areas served, Affiliated Physicians & Hospitals, Federal Qualifications, Status, Year Founded, Managed Care Partners, Employer References, Fees & Payment Information and more. *The HMO/PPO Directory* provides the most comprehensive information on the most companies available on the market place today.

600 pages; Softcover ISBN 978-1-59237-876-0, $325.00
Online & Directory Combo: $800.00
Online Database (Single User): $650.00

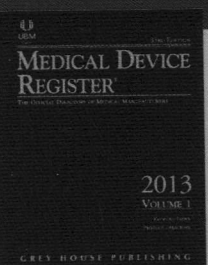

Medical Device Register

Offers fast access to over 13,000 companies - and more than 65,000 products. Volume I: Products, provides the essential information you need when purchasing or specifying medical supplies on every medical device, supply, and diagnostic available in the US. Listings provide FDA codes, Federal Procurement Eligibility, Contact information, Prices and Product Specifications. Volume 2: Suppliers, details the most complete and important data about Suppliers, Manufacturers and Distributors, with Key Executives, Contact Information along with their medical products and specialties. *Medical Device Register* is your only one-stop source for locating suppliers and products; looking for new manufacturers or hard-to-find medical devices; comparing products; know who's selling what and who to buy from cost effectively.

3,000 pages; Two Volumes; Softcover ISBN 978-1-59237-880-7, $350.00
Online Database & Print Combo, $699.00

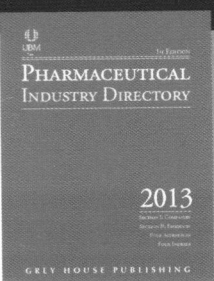

Pharmaceutical Industry Directory

This resource compiles critical information on the multi-billion dollar worldwide Pharmaceutical Industry. Coverage begins with company profiles of 5,000 Pharmaceutical Companies worldwide, with complete contact information, company description, key personnel, areas of clinical development, annual revenue, healthcare revenue, annual research and development expenditure, and number of employees. Each profile also includes a detailed list of the company's prescription drugs in development and brands on the market, over 20,000 in total. An excellent tool for research, portfolio evaluation, new business development, and competitive analyses. This new directory will be a must-have resource for professionals in the pharmaceutical and biotech industries along with public library, university and medical reference collections.

1,000 pages; Softcover ISBN 978-1-61925-174-8, $350.00
Online & Directory Combo: $950.00 | Online Database (Single User): $750.00

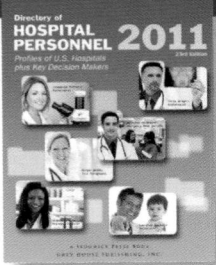

The Directory of Hospital Personnel

The Directory of Hospital Personnel is the best resource you can have at your fingertips when researching or marketing a product or service to the hospital market. A "Who's Who" of the hospital universe, this directory puts you in touch with over 150,000 key decision-makers. Every hospital in the U.S. is profiled, listed alphabetically by city within state. *The Directory of Hospital Personnel* is the only complete source for key hospital decision-makers by name. Whether you want to define or restructure sales territories... locate hospitals with the purchasing power to accept your proposals... or find information on which insurance plans are accepted, *The Directory of Hospital Personnel* gives you the information you need — easily, efficiently, effectively and accurately.

2,500 pages; Softcover ISBN 978-1-59237-856-2, $325.00
Online & Directory Combo: $800.00 | Online Database (Single User): $650.00

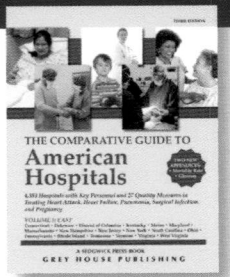

The Comparative Guide to American Hospitals

This new third edition compares and ranks all of the nation's hospitals by 49 measures of quality in the treatment of heart attack, heart failure, pneumonia, surgical procedures, pregnancy care and, new to this edition, children's asthma care, medical imaging and patient satisfaction. Each profile includes the raw percentage for that hospital, the state and US averages and data on the top hospital. Most importantly, The Comparative Guide to American Hospitals provides easy-to-use Regional State by State Statistical Summary Tables for each of the data elements to allow the user to quickly locate hospitals with the best level of service. Plus, a new 30-Day Mortality Chart, Glossary of Terms and Regional Hospital Profile Index make this a must-have source. This new, expanded edition will be a must for the reference collection at all public, medical and academic libraries.

2,000 pages; Four Volume Set; Softcover ISBN 978-1-59237-838-8, $350.00

(800) 562-2139 • www.greyhouse.com

MANUFACTURER PROFILES

A & E MEDICAL CORP.
See Alto Development Corp.

A & M INSTRUMENTS, INC.   770-772-6404
3565 Trotter Dr., Alpharetta, GA 30004
FDA Number: 1035766
Instrument, Diamond, Dental   Dental And Oral

A A BIOMEDICAL
See In Vivo Metric

A A KINDER CO., INC.
See Quad Med

A MAJOR DIFFERENCE, INC.   877-315-8638
2950 S. Jamaica Ct., Suite 300, Aurora, CO 80014   303-755-0112
FDA Number: n/a   *Fax:* 303-755-3022
Web site: www.amajordifference.com
Ownership: Private
Produces/Sells CE-marked Devices: N
Lamp, Non-heating, For Adjunctive Use In Pain Therapy   Physical Med

A PLUS DENTAL LAB   215-996-4177
1700 Horizon Drive, --suite 104, Chalfont, PA 18914
FDA Number: 3006191485
Alloy, Precious Metal, For Clinical Use   Dental And Oral
Denture, Plastic, Teeth   Dental And Oral
Material, Impression   Dental And Oral
Metal, Base   Dental And Oral
Teeth, Porcelain   Dental And Oral

A PLUS INTERNATIONAL, INC   909-591-5168
5138 Eucalyptus Ave., Chino, CA 91710
FDA Number: 2083545
Accessories, Apparel, Surgical   Surgery
Fiber, Absorbent   General
Linen, Bed   General
Sponge, External   Surgery
Sponge, Gauze   Dental And Oral

A&A ORTHOPEDICS, INCORPORATED   757-224-0177
12250 Sw 129th Court, Bldg. 01, Miami, FL 33186
FDA Number: 1042714
Band, Support, Pelvic   Physical Med
Bandage, Elastic   General
Belt, Traction, Pelvic, Orthopedic   Orthopedics
Binder, Abdominal   General
Cane   Physical Med
Crutch   Physical Med
Halter, Head, Traction   Physical Med
Joint, Knee, External Brace   Physical Med
Orthosis, Cervical-Thoracic, Rigid   Physical Med
Orthosis, Limb Brace   Physical Med
Orthosis, Lumbosacral   Physical Med
Orthosis, Rib Fracture, Soft   Physical Med
Protector, Skin Pressure   General
Restraint, Protective (Body)   General
Screen, Tangent, Felt (Campimeter)   Ophthalmology
Shoe, Cast   Physical Med
Sling, Arm, Overhead Supported   Physical Med
Splint, Clavicle   Physical Med
Splint, Hand, And Component   Physical Med
Splint, Traction   Orthopedics
Tips And Pads, Cane, Crutch And Walker   Physical Med
Traction Unit, Non-Powered   Orthopedics

A&D MEDICAL   800-726-7099
1756 Automation Parkway, San Jose, CA 95131   408-263-5333
FDA Number: 2082313   *Fax:* 408-263-0119
E-mail: support@lifesourceonline.com
Web site: www.lifesourceonline.com
Annual Revenue: $25-$50 Million
Year Founded: 1977
Total Employees: 60   *Marketing Staff:* 5   *Sales Staff:* 5
Ownership: Private
Traded On: Tokyo
Quality System Registration Information: ISO9000; ISO9001
Produces/Sells CE-marked Devices: Y
Federal Procurement Eligibility: Small Business
Distribution: Manufacturer Direct, Manufacturer Through Distributor, Manufacturer Through Manufacturer Reps, OEM, Importer, Exporter
General Admin.: Teruhisa Moriya/President, Chief Executive Officer
       Christy Mar/Vice President Human Resources
       Gary Halick/Vice President, General Manager
Mktg./Adv.: Sarah Schiltz/Director Marketing
       Jerry Wang/Director Product Development
       Tony Cao/Manager Market Research
Production: Frank Marrone/Manager Materials
Finance: Fred Lau/Controller
Balance, Analytical   Chemistry
Balance, Macro (0.1 mg Accuracy)   Chemistry
Balance, Semimicro (0.01 mg Accuracy)   Chemistry
Cuff, Blood Pressure   Cardiovascular
Monitor, Blood Pressure, Indirect (Arterial)   Cardiovascular
Scale, Laboratory   Chemistry
Sphygmomanometer, Electronic, Manual   General
Stethoscope, Electronic (Auscultoscope)   Cardiovascular
Stethoscope, Manual   Cardiovascular
Thermometer, Electronic   General

A&H PRODUCTS, INC.   918-835-8081
6946 East 13th Street, Tulsa, OK 74112
FDA Number: n/a   *Fax:* 918-459-9077
E-mail: secysvc@swbell.net
Medical Products Sales Volume: $1,400,000
Annual Revenue: $1-$5 Million
Year Founded: 1975
Total Employees: 2
Ownership: Private
Produces/Sells CE-marked Devices: N
Federal Procurement Eligibility: Small Business, Female Owned
Distribution: Manufacturer Through Manufacturer Reps, OEM
General Admin.: J. G. Glenn/President
       Bob Martin/Secretary
Mktg./Adv.: C. R. Mighton/Vice President Marketing
       Randy Swearengin/Vice President Marketing & Sales
Research: Ralph Hale/Vice President Research & Development
Finance: Arden Glenn/Treasurer
Generator, Aerosol   Ear/Nose/Throat
Nebulizer, Non-Heated   Anesthesiology
Vectorcardiograph   Cardiovascular
Ventilator, Pressure Cycled (IPPB Machine)   Anesthesiology
Medical Product Subsidiaries (Listed Separately)
All American Mold Laboratories, Inc.
Ao Sunwear Usa

A-1 ENGINEERING 1 877 929-9920

9450 7th St. Ste. J, -
Rancho Cucamonga, CA 91730
FDA Number: 3007008050 *Fax:* (909) 466-9726
E-mail: tony@a-1engineeringusa.com
Web site: a-1engineeringusa.com
Ownership: Private
Produces/Sells CE-marked Devices: N

Massager, Therapeutic	Physical Med

A-BEC MOBILITY INC.

See Sunrise Medical, Inc.

A-DEC, INC. 800-547-1883

2601 Crestview Dr., Newberg, OR 97132-9257 503-538-9471
FDA Number: 3015729 *Fax:* 503-538-5911
E-mail: domestic@a-dec.com and international_cs@a-dec.com
Web site: www.a-dec.com
Ownership: Private
Produces/Sells CE-marked Devices: N

Amalgamator, Dental, AC-Powered	Dental And Oral
Chair, Dental (With Unit)	Dental And Oral
Controller, Foot, Handpiece And Cord	Dental And Oral
Handpiece, Air-Powered, Dental	Dental And Oral
Light, Fiberoptic, Dental	Dental And Oral
Light, Surgical Operating, Dental	Dental And Oral
Operative Dental Treatment Unit	Dental And Oral
Pump, Suction Operatory	Dental And Oral
Scaler, Ultrasonic	Dental And Oral
Sterilizer, Steam (Autoclave)	General

A-M SYSTEMS, INC. 800-426-1306

131 Business Park Loop, Sequim, WA 98382 360-683-8300
FDA Number: 3020614 *Fax:* 360-683-3525
E-mail: sales@a-msystems.com
Web site: www.a-msystems.com
Medical Products Sales Volume: $1,300,000
Year Founded: 1976
Total Employees: 20
Ownership: Private
Produces/Sells CE-marked Devices: N
Federal Procurement Eligibility: Small Business
Distribution: Manufacturer Direct, Manufacturer Through Distributor, OEM
Mktg./Adv.: David Green/Manager Product Development & Sales
Production: Mr. Robert Thompson/Manager Quality Assurance

Absorbent, Carbon-Dioxide	Anesthesiology
Adapter, Tube, Tracheal	Anesthesiology
Bag, Breathing	Anesthesiology
Calibrator, Respiratory Therapy Unit	Anesthesiology
Cannula, Nasal, Oxygen	Anesthesiology
Clip, Nose	Anesthesiology
Filter, Bacterial, Breathing Circuit	Anesthesiology
Filter, Ventilator	Anesthesiology
Mask, Gas, Anesthesia	Anesthesiology
Mask, Oxygen, Aerosol Administration	Anesthesiology
Mouthpiece, Breathing	Anesthesiology
Nebulizer, Medicinal	Ear/Nose/Throat
Paper, Chart, Record, Medical	General
Spirometer, Diagnostic (Respirometer)	Anesthesiology
Syringe, Calibration Testing, Spirometer	Anesthesiology
Tube, Aspirating, Flexible, Connecting	Anesthesiology
Tube, Autoclaving	General
Tubing, Connecting	General
Tubing, Corrugated	General
Tubing, Flexible, Medical Gas, Low-Pressure	Anesthesiology
Tubing, Other	General
Tubing, Ventilator	Anesthesiology

A-T SURGICAL MANUFACTURING CO., INC. 800-225-2023

115 Clemente St., Holyoke, MA 01040-5644 413-532-4551
FDA Number: n/a *Fax:* (413) 532-0826
E-mail: at@A-Tsurgical.com
Web site: www.a-tsurgical.com
Annual Revenue: $1-$5 Million
Ownership: Private
Produces/Sells CE-marked Devices: N
Federal Procurement Eligibility: Small Business
Distribution: Manufacturer Through Distributor

Bandage, Elastic	General
Bedrail	General
Belt, Electrode	Cardiovascular
Belt, Rib (Support)	Orthopedics
Binder, Abdominal	General
Binder, Abdominal, OB/GYN	Obstetrics/Gynecology
Binder, Chest	General
Brace, Joint, Ankle (External)	Physical Med
Clothing, Protective	General
Collar, Cervical Neck	Orthopedics
Diaper, Adult	General
Holder, Catheter	Gastroenterology/Urology

A-T SURGICAL MANUFACTURING CO., INC. 800-225-2023
(cont'd)

Immobilizer, Knee	Orthopedics
Joint, Knee, External Brace	Physical Med
Legging, Compression, Non-Inflatable	General
Orthosis, Other	Physical Med
Pack, Hot Or Cold, Reusable	Physical Med
Pad, Incontinence (Underpad)	General
Pad, Pressure, Foam Convoluted	General
Sling, Arm	Physical Med
Stocking, Support (Anti-Embolic)	General
Support, Abdominal	Physical Med
Support, Ankle	Orthopedics
Support, Back	Orthopedics
Support, Elbow	Orthopedics
Support, Hot/Cold Pack	Physical Med
Support, Knee	Physical Med
Support, Leg	Physical Med
Support, Scrotal	Gastroenterology/Urology
Support, Scrotal, Therapeutic	General
Support, Thigh	Physical Med
Support, Wrist	Physical Med
Truss, Hernia (Belt)	Gastroenterology/Urology
Truss, Umbilical	Gastroenterology/Urology
Wristlet, Patient Return	Gastroenterology/Urology

A. J. P. SCIENTIFIC, INC. 973-472-7200

82 Industrial East, Clifton, NJ 07012
FDA Number: 2250039

Stain, Aniline Blue	Pathology
Stain, Carbol Fuchsin	Pathology
Stain, Congo Red	Pathology
Stain, Fetal Hemoglobin	Hematology
Stain, Giemsa	Pathology
Stain, Grams Iodine	Pathology
Stain, Heinz Body	Hematology
Stain, Hematoxylin, Harris's	Pathology
Stain, Hematoxylin, Mayer's	Pathology
Stain, Iron	Pathology
Stain, Methylene Blue	Pathology
Stain, Mucicarmine	Pathology
Stain, Nile Blue	Pathology
Stain, Nuclear Fast Red	Pathology
Stain, Papanicolau	Pathology
Stain, Phosphotungstic Acid Hematoxylin	Pathology
Stain, Reagent, Schiff	Pathology
Stain, Reticulocyte	Hematology
Stain, Safranin	Pathology
Stain, Sudan Black B	Pathology
Stain, Toluidine Blue	Pathology
Stain, Weigert's Iron Hematoxylin	Pathology
Stain, Wright's	Pathology

A. LUNT DESIGN, INC. 866-872-5868

5755 Big Tree Rd., PO Box 247, 716-662-0781
Orchard Park, NY 14127
FDA Number: n/a *Fax:* 716-662-0784
Web site: www.alunt.com
Annual Revenue: $0-$1 Million
Year Founded: 1975
Ownership: Private
Produces/Sells CE-marked Devices: N
Federal Procurement Eligibility: Small Business, Female Owned
Distribution: Manufacturer Direct, Manufacturer Through Distributor

Gown, Patient, Disposable	General

A. TITAN INSTRUMENTS, INC. 877-284-8261

97 Main St., Hamburg, NY 14075 716-648-9272
FDA Number: 2531684 *Fax:* 716-648-9296
Ownership: Private
Produces/Sells CE-marked Devices: N

Accessories, Retractor, Dental	Dental And Oral
Carver, Dental Amalgam, Operative	Dental And Oral
Carver, Wax, Dental	Dental And Oral
Curette, Surgical, Dental	Dental And Oral
Elevator, Surgical, Dental	Dental And Oral
Excavator, Dental, Operative	Dental And Oral
Filling, Instrument Plastic, Dental	Dental And Oral
Forceps, Dressing, Dental	Dental And Oral
Forceps, Tooth Extractor, Surgical	Dental And Oral
Gauge, Depth, Instrument, Dental	Dental And Oral
Handle, Instrument, Dental	Dental And Oral
Scissors, Surgical Tissue, Dental (Oral)	Dental And Oral
Suture, Dental	Dental And Oral

A.C.E. MEDICAL COMPANY

See Depuy Ace, A Johnson & Johnson Company

A.G.A. ELECTRONICS CORP. 305-592-1860

7209 N.w. 41st St., Miami, FL 33166
FDA Number: 1056645

A.G.A. ELECTRONICS CORP.   305-592-1860 *(cont'd)*
Ownership: Private
Produces/Sells CE-marked Devices: N
Gown, Examination   General

A.H. ROBINS
See Pfizer / Wyeth Consumer Healthcare Inc.

A.J. ANTUNES & CO.   800-253-2991
180 Kehoe Blvd., Carol Stream, IL 60188   630-784-1000
FDA Number: n/a   Fax: 630-784-1650
Web site: www.ajantunes.com
Ownership: Private
Produces/Sells CE-marked Devices: N
Purifier, Water   Chemistry

A.M. BICKFORD, INC.   800-795-3062
12318 Big Tree Rd., Wales Center, NY 14169   716-652-1590
FDA Number: 1316061   Fax: 716-652-2046
E-mail: customerservice@ambickford.com
Web site: www.ambickford.com
Ownership: Private
Produces/Sells CE-marked Devices: N
Federal Procurement Eligibility: Small Business
Distribution: Exclusive Distributor
Analyzer, Gas, Anesthetic   Anesthesiology
Analyzer, Gas, Oxygen, Continuous Monitor   Anesthesiology

A.M. SURGICAL, INC.   800-437-9653
290 East Main Street, Suite 200, Smithtown, NY 11787
FDA Number: 2437731   Fax: 631-980-4369
E-mail: info@amsurgical.com
Web site: www.amsurgical.com
Year Founded: 1995
Ownership: Private
Produces/Sells CE-marked Devices: N
Accessories, Arthroscope   Orthopedics
Appliance, Fix., Nail/Blade/Plate Comb., Multiple Component   Orthopedics
Cannula, Surgical, General & Plastic Surgery   Surgery
Elevator, Surgical, General & Plastic Surgery   Surgery
Knife, Other   Surgery
Orthopedic Manual Surgical Instrument   Orthopedics
Rasp, Surgical, General & Plastic Surgery   Surgery
Table, Operating Room, Mechanical   Surgery

A.M.G. MEDICAL, INC.   888-396-1213
8505 Dalton Rd., Montreal, QUE H4T-IV5 Canada   514-737-5251
FDA Number: 8022077   Fax: 514-737-6572
E-mail: ben@amgmedical.com
Web site: www.amgmedical.com
Medical Products Sales Volume: $20,000,000
Annual Revenue: $10-$25 Million
Total Employees: 90
Ownership: Private
Produces/Sells CE-marked Devices: N
Distribution: Exclusive Distributor, Importer
General Admin.: Allan Goldenberg/Chairman
Ben Topor/President, Chief Executive Officer
Mktg./Adv.: Danny Meyers/Director Marketing
Andre Renaud/Manager National Sales
Production: Ken Levesque/Manager Regulatory Affairs
Cane   Physical Med
Cover, Mattress   General
Lancet, Blood   General
Stethoscope, Manual   Cardiovascular
Strip, Adhesive   Surgery
Swabs, Alcohol   General
Syringe, Insulin   General
Traction Unit, Non-Powered   Orthopedics

A.M.O. PUERTO RICO MANUFACTURING, INC   787-826-2727
Road 402N Industrial Zone, PO Box 1408, Anasco, PR 00610
FDA Number: 2648035   Fax: 787-826-2915
Web site: www.amo-inc.com
Ownership: Private
Produces/Sells CE-marked Devices: N
Cutter, Vitreous Aspiration, AC-Powered   Ophthalmology
Cutter, Vitreous Aspiration, Battery-Powered   Ophthalmology
Guide, Intraocular Lens   Ophthalmology
Irrigator, Ocular Surgery   Ophthalmology
Keratome, AC-Powered   Ophthalmology
Laser, Surgical   Surgery
Lens, Intraocular   Ophthalmology
Lens, Intraocular, Multifocal   Ophthalmology
Phacofragmentation Unit   Ophthalmology

A.R.C. DISTRIBUTORS   800-296-8724
PO Box 599, Centreville, MD 21617   443-262-9671
FDA Number: n/a   Fax: 443-262-9673
E-mail: arcdist599@aol.com

A.R.C. DISTRIBUTORS   800-296-8724 *(cont'd)*
Web site: www.arcdistributors.com
Medical Products Sales Volume: $300,000
Annual Revenue: $0-$1 Million
Year Founded: 1989
Total Employees: 2   Marketing Staff: 2   Sales Staff: 2
Ownership: Private
Produces/Sells CE-marked Devices: N
Federal Procurement Eligibility: Small Business
Distribution: Manufacturer Through Distributor, Manufacturer Through Manufacturer Reps, Exclusive Distributor
General Admin.: Robert Reinbold/President, Chief Executive Officer
Mktg./Adv.: Cindy Houser/Manager National Sales
Accessories, Wheelchair   Physical Med
Attachment, Bag (Crutch, Walker, Wheelchair)   Physical Med
Attachment, Oxygen Canister/IV Pole, Wheelchair   General
Bag, Plastic   General
Cart, Other   General
Cart, Patient (Stretcher)   Anesthesiology
Chair, Geriatric   General
Chair, Geriatric, Wheeled   General
Chair, Other   General
Chair, Shower   General
Commode Seat   General
Component, Other   General
Lift, Wheelchair   General
Patient Transfer Unit   General
Stretcher, Hydraulic   General
Stretcher, Transfer   Surgery
System, Transport, In-House   General
Table, Overbed   General
Walker, Mechanical   Physical Med
Wheelchair, Manual   Physical Med
Wheelchair, Powered   Physical Med
Wheelchair, Special Grade   Physical Med

A.R.C. OF OTSEGO COUNTY
See Arc/Otsego

A.T.I., AIREX DIV.
See Magister Corporation

AAA POWER SYSTEMS
See Online Power, Inc.

AADCO MEDICAL, INC.   800-225-9014
2279 Vermont Rte. 66, Randolph, VT 05060-0410   802-728-3400
FDA Number: 1225473   Fax: 802-728-3107
E-mail: info@aadcomed.com
Web site: www.aadcomed.com
Ownership: Private
Produces/Sells CE-marked Devices: N
General Admin.: Robert Marchione/President, Chief Executive Officer
Apron, Lead, Dental   Dental And Oral
Barrier, Control Panel, X-Ray, Moveable   Radiology
Curtain, Protective, Radiographic   Radiology
Cushion, Table, Surgical   Surgery
Examination Device, AC-Powered   General
Glove, Protective, Radiographic   Radiology
Scanner, Computed Tomography, X-Ray, Special Procedure   Radiology
Shield, Gonadal   Radiology
Shield, Ophthalmic, Radiological   Radiology
Shield, Protective, Personnel   Radiology
Shield, Vial   Radiology
Shield, X-Ray, Leaded   Dental And Oral

AAEON ELECTRONICS, INC.   888-223-6687
3 Crown Plaza, Hazlet, NJ 07730-2441   732-203-9300
FDA Number: n/a   Fax: 732-203-9311
E-mail: sales@aaeon.com
Web site: www.aaeon.com
Medical Products Sales Volume: $16,700,000
Annual Revenue: $10-$25 Million
Year Founded: 1995
Total Employees: 33   Marketing Staff: 2   Sales Staff: 5
Ownership: AAEON Technology, Inc.
Quality System Registration Information: ISO9001
Produces/Sells CE-marked Devices: Y
Federal Procurement Eligibility: Small Business
Distribution: Manufacturer Direct, Manufacturer Through Distributor, Manufacturer Through Manufacturer Reps, OEM, Service Direct, Exporter
General Admin.: Steve Hsu/General Manager
Yuhmin Hwang/President
Mktg./Adv.: Fred Fischer/Director Marketing
Fred Fischer/Manager Market Research
Paul Yang/Manager National Sales
Paul Yang/Manager Sales Training
Steve Hsu/Vice President Marketing & Sales
Computer, Nuclear Medicine   Radiology

AAERO SWISS, INC.   800-394-5808
22347 La Palma Ave, Yorba Linda, CA 92887   714-692-0558
FDA Number: n/a   *Fax:* 714-692-0523
Medical Products Sales Volume: $2,000,000
Annual Revenue: $1-$5 Million
Total Employees: 35   *Marketing Staff:* 1   *Sales Staff:* 1
Ownership: Private
Quality System Registration Information: ISO9002
Produces/Sells CE-marked Devices: N
Federal Procurement Eligibility: Small Business
Distribution: Manufacturer Direct
General Admin.: Donald L. Jones/President
            Vera F. Jones/Vice President Human Resources
   Contract Manufacturing   General

AAF INTERNATIONAL   800-477-1214
10300 Ormsby Park Place, Louisville, KY 40223   888-223-2003
FDA Number: n/a   *Fax:* 888-223-6500
E-mail: aaf_mid_states@aafintl.com
Web site: www.aafintl.com
Annual Revenue: $0-$1 Million
Year Founded: 1921
Total Employees: 2600
Ownership: MCQUAY
Quality System Registration Information: ISO9001
Produces/Sells CE-marked Devices: N
Distribution: Manufacturer Direct, Manufacturer Through Manufacturer Reps
   Filter, Air   General

AALBA DENT, INC.   707-864-3334
400 Watt Dr., Fairfield, CA 94534
FDA Number: 2916734
   Alloy, Precious Metal, For Clinical Use   Dental And Oral

AALBORG INSTRUMENTS & CONTROLS, INC.   800-866-3837
20 Corporate Drive, Orangeburg, NY 10962   845-770-3000
FDA Number: n/a   *Fax:* 845-770-3010
E-mail: info@aalborg.com
Web site: www.aalborg.com
Medical Products Sales Volume: $3,900,000
Annual Revenue: $1-$5 Million
Year Founded: 1972
Total Employees: 47
Ownership: Private
Quality System Registration Information: ISO9001
Produces/Sells CE-marked Devices: Y
Federal Procurement Eligibility: Small Business
Distribution: Manufacturer Direct, Manufacturer Through Distributor, OEM, Exporter
Mktg./Adv.: Jason McCluskey/Sales Associate
Finance: Michael Muir/Business Specialist
   Flowmeter, Gas (Oxygen), Calibrated   Anesthesiology

AALTO SCIENTIFIC LTD.   760-431-7922
1959 Kellogg Ave., Carlsbad, CA 92008
FDA Number: 2022832   *Fax:* 760-431-6942
E-mail: kjones@aaltoscientific.com
Web site: www.aaltoscientific.com
Annual Revenue: $1-$5 Million
Year Founded: 1979
Total Employees: 20   *Marketing Staff:* 2   *Sales Staff:* 2
Ownership: Private
Quality System Registration Information: ISO9001
Produces/Sells CE-marked Devices: N
Distribution: OEM
General Admin.: Steve Mauro/President
Mktg./Adv.: Molly Tackabery/Director International Marketing
            Kevin Jones/Director Marketing & Sales
Research: Robert A. Reynolds/Vice President Research & Development
   Antigen, Antiserum, Control, Protein, Complement   Immunology
   Control, Alcohol   Toxicology
   Control, Analyte (Assayed And Unassayed)   Chemistry
   Control, Drug Mixture   Toxicology
   Control, Electrolyte (Assayed And Unassayed)   Chemistry
   Control, Enzyme (Assayed And Unassayed)   Chemistry
   Control, Multi Analyte, All Kinds (Assayed And Unassayed)   Chemistry
   Hematology Quality Control Mixture   Hematology
   Material, Raw, Production   General
   Test, Qualitative And Quantitative Factor Deficiency   Hematology

AARON MEDICAL INDUSTRIES, INC.
   See Bovie Medical Corp.

AAXON SERVICES
   See Wilkinson Hi-Rise

AB SCIEX   1 877-740-2129
110 Marsh Road, Foster City, CA 94404
FDA Number: n/a   *Fax:* 1 650-638-5884

AB SCIEX   1 877-740-2129 *(cont'd)*
E-mail: Support@absciex.com
Web site: www.absciex.com
Ownership: Private
Produces/Sells CE-marked Devices: N
General Admin.: Andy Boorn/Chief Operating Officer
            Mr. Rainer Blair/President
Mktg./Adv.: Anthony Pertrucci/Manager Communications
Production: Mr. Doug Onesko/Vice President Operations
Research: Mr. Gordon Logan/Senior Vice President Research & Development
   Mass Spectrometer, Clinical Use   Toxicology

ABARE ENT., INC.   478-994-3807
44 W. Chambers St., Forsyth, GA 31029
FDA Number: n/a
Ownership: Private
Produces/Sells CE-marked Devices: N
   Pack, Hot Or Cold, Reusable   Physical Med

ABATEMENT TECHNOLOGIES, INC.   800-634-9091
605 Satellite Blvd, Ste 300, Suwanee, GA 30024
FDA Number: 1064851   *Fax:* 678-889-4201
E-mail: dwillyard@abatement.com
Web site: www.abatement.com
Year Founded: 1985
Total Employees: 120   *Marketing Staff:* 4   *Sales Staff:* 10
Ownership: Private
Produces/Sells CE-marked Devices: N
Distribution: Manufacturer Direct
General Admin.: David Shagott/President
Mktg./Adv.: David Willyard/Vice President Sales
   Equipment, Cleaning, Air   General
   Equipment, Filtering, Air, ETO   General

ABAXIS, INC.   800-822-2947
3240 Whipple Road, Union City, CA 94587   510-675-6500
FDA Number: 2939693   *Fax:* 510-441-6150
E-mail: abaxis@abaxis.com
Web site: www.abaxis.com
Annual Revenue: $25-$50 Million
Year Founded: 1989
Total Employees: 265
Ownership: Public
Stock Symbol: ABAX
Traded On: NASDAQ
Quality System Registration Information: ISO9001
Produces/Sells CE-marked Devices: N
Federal Procurement Eligibility: Small Business
Distribution: Manufacturer Through Distributor, Manufacturer Through Manufacturer Reps
General Admin.: Mr. Donald Wood/Chief Operating Officer
            Clint Severson/President, Chief Executive Officer
            Vladimir Ostoich/Vice President Government Affairs
Research: Kenneth Aron/Vice President Development
Finance: Al Santa Ines/Vice President Finance
   Analyzer, Chemistry, Centrifuge   Chemistry
   Analyzer, Chemistry, Desk-Top   Chemistry
   Analyzer, Chemistry, Electrolyte   Chemistry
   Analyzer, Chemistry, Enzyme   Chemistry
   Analyzer, Chemistry, Photometric, Bichromatic   Chemistry
   Chromatographic, Inorganic Phosphorus   Chemistry
   NAD Reduction/NADH Oxidation, Lactate Dehydrogenase Chemistry
   Photometric Method, Magnesium   Chemistry
   Saccharogenic, Amylase   Chemistry
   Tetraphenyl Borate, Colorimetry, Potassium   Chemistry
   Urease, Photometric, Urea Nitrogen   Chemistry

ABB CONCISE OPTICAL GROUP LLC   800-852-8089
12301 NW 39th Street, Coral Springs, FL 33065
FDA Number: n/a   *Fax:* 954-733-1788
Web site: www.abboptical.com
Annual Revenue: $0-$1 Million
Year Founded: 1989
Ownership: Abb Concise Optical Group Llc
Produces/Sells CE-marked Devices: N
Federal Procurement Eligibility: Small Business
Distribution: Manufacturer Direct
General Admin.: Angel Alvarez/Chief Executive Officer
            Lynda Baker/Executive Vice President
            Brad Weinbrum/President
Finance: Cindy Pelletier/Chief Financial Officer
   Lens, Spectacle/Eyeglasses, Custom (Prescription)   Ophthalmology
Medical Product Subsidiaries (Listed Separately)
   Abb Concise Optical Group Llc

ABB OPTICALS
   See Abb Concise Optical Group Llc

MANUFACTURER PROFILES

ABBAS' GRACE
52 Meadow Ln., Manchester, NH 03109 **603-624-9559**
FDA Number: 1223948
Fax: 603-624-7597
E-mail: karen.dupuis@moorecenter.org
Ownership: Private
Produces/Sells CE-marked Devices: N
Utensil, Food — Physical Med

ABBEON CAL, INC.
123 Gray Avenue, Santa Barbara, CA 93101-1809 **800-922-0977** **805-966-0810**
FDA Number: n/a
Fax: 805-966-7659
Web site: www.Abbeon.com
Medical Products Sales Volume: $2,100,000
Annual Revenue: $1-$5 Million
Year Founded: 1946
Total Employees: 8   Marketing Staff: 2   Sales Staff: 3
Ownership: Private
Quality System Registration Information: ISO9001
Produces/Sells CE-marked Devices: N
Federal Procurement Eligibility: Small Business
Distribution: Exclusive Distributor, Importer
General Admin.: A. J. Wertheim/President
Production: Karen Burrows/Manager Operations
　　　　E. H. Alcorn/Vice President Production
Hygrometer (Humidity Indicator) — Anesthesiology

ABBEY COLOR, INC.
400 East Tioga St., Philadelphia, PA 19134 **877-922-2399** **215-739-9960**
FDA Number: 2518563
Fax: 215-739-9963
E-mail: sales@abbeycolor.com
Web site: www.abbeycolor.com
Ownership: Private
Produces/Sells CE-marked Devices: N
Stain, Dye Powder — Pathology

ABBEYMOOR MEDICAL INC.
501 East Soo Street, Parkers Prairie, MN 56361 **888-528-9073** **218-338-6700**
FDA Number: 3005249627
Fax: 218-338-6710
E-mail: customerservice@abbeymoormedical.com
Web site: www.abbeymoormedical.com
Ownership: Private
Produces/Sells CE-marked Devices: N
Stent, Other — Obstetrics/Gynecology

ABBOTT ASSOCIATES
620 West Avenue, Milford, CT 06461 **203-878-2370**
FDA Number: 1220616
Fax: 203-878-5065
E-mail: info@goabbott.com
Web site: www.goabbott.com
Medical Products Sales Volume: $1,500,000
Annual Revenue: $1-$5 Million
Year Founded: 1991
Total Employees: 15
Ownership: Private
Quality System Registration Information: ISO9002
Produces/Sells CE-marked Devices: N
Federal Procurement Eligibility: Small Business
Distribution: OEM
General Admin.: John R. Winfield/Chief Executive Officer
Cabinet, Other — General
Drape, Surgical — Surgery
Fiber, Absorbent — General
Protector, Surgical Instrument — Surgery
Washer/Disinfector — General
Wrap, Sterilization — General

ABBOTT DIABETES CARE INC.
1360 South Loop Rd., Alameda, CA 94502 **510-749-5400**
FDA Number: 2954323
Fax: 510-749-5401
E-mail: 888-522-5226
Web site: www.abbott.com
Year Founded: 1888
Ownership: Abbott Laboratories
Stock Symbol: ABT
Traded On: NYSE
Produces/Sells CE-marked Devices: N
General Admin.: Mr. Miles D. White/Chief Executive Officer, Chairman
　　　　Ms. Laura J. Schumacher/Executive Vice President
Production: Mr. Richard W. Ashley/Executive Vice President Development
Finance: Mr. Thomas C. Freyman/Executive Vice President Finance
Glucose Dehydrogenase, Glucose — Chemistry
Infusion Pump, Insulin — General
System, Test, Blood Glucose, Over-The-Counter — Chemistry

ABBOTT DIAGNOSTICS
See Abbott Hematology, Diagnostics Div.

ABBOTT DIAGNOSTICS DIV.
1921 Hurd Dr., Irving, TX 75038 **847-937-7988**
FDA Number: 1628664
Fax: 972-518-6000
E-mail: abbottlink.administration@abbott.com
Web site: www.abbottdiagnostics.com
Ownership: Abbott Laboratories
Stock Symbol: ABT
Traded On: NYSE
Produces/Sells CE-marked Devices: N
General Admin.: Mr. Edward L. Michael/Executive Vice President
　　　　Mr. Scott Luce/Vice President
Mktg./Adv.: Mr. Don Patton/Vice President Commercial Operations
　　　　Mr. Jaime Contreras/Vice President Commercial Operations
Production: Mr. Jeff Binder/Vice President Operations
Analyzer, Chemistry, Photometric, Discrete — Chemistry
Counter, Cell, Differential Classifier, Automated — Hematology
Densitometer/Scanner (Integrating, Reflectance, TLC, Radio) — Chemistry
Equipment, Laboratory, Gen. Purpose (Specific Medical Use) — Chemistry
Fluorometer, Chemistry — Chemistry
Incubator/Water Bath, Microbiology — Microbiology
Pipetting And Diluting System, Automated — Chemistry
Software, Blood Bank (Stand-Alone Products) — Hematology

ABBOTT DIAGNOSTICS DIV.
820 Mission St., South Pasadena, CA 91030 **626-440-0700**
FDA Number: 2018433
E-mail: abbottlink.administration@abbott.com
Web site: www.abbottdiagnostics.com
Ownership: Abbott Laboratories
Stock Symbol: ABT
Traded On: NYSE
Produces/Sells CE-marked Devices: N
General Admin.: Mr. Edward L. Michael/Executive Vice President
　　　　Mr. Scott Luce/Vice President
Mktg./Adv.: Mr. Don Patton/Vice President Commercial Operations
　　　　Ms. Jaime Contreras/Vice President Commercial Operations
Production: Mr. Jeff Binder/Vice President Operations
Analyzer, Chemistry, Photometric, Discrete — Chemistry
Antigen, Antiserum, Control, Complement C3 — Immunology
Antigen, Antiserum, Control, Complement C4 — Immunology
Antigen, Antiserum, Control, Haptoglobin — Immunology
Antigen, Antiserum, Control, IGA — Immunology
Antigen, Antiserum, Control, IGG — Immunology
Antigen, Antiserum, Control, IGM — Immunology
Antigen, Antiserum, Control, Prealbumin — Immunology
Antigen, Antiserum, Control, Transferrin — Immunology
Azo-Dye, Calcium — Chemistry
Bilirubin (Total and Unbound) Neonate Test System — Chemistry
Catalytic Method, Amylase — Chemistry
Colorimetric Method, Gamma-Glutamyl Transpeptidase — Chemistry
Coulometric Method, Carbon-Dioxide — Chemistry
Dye-Binding, Albumin, Bromcresol, Green — Chemistry
Dye-Binding, Albumin, Bromcresol, Purple — Chemistry
Enzymatic Esterase-Oxidase, Cholesterol — Chemistry
Enzymatic Method, Ammonia — Chemistry
Enzymatic Method, Lactic Acid — Chemistry
Enzyme Immunoassay, Barbiturate — Toxicology
Enzyme Immunoassay, Benzodiazepine — Toxicology
Enzyme Immunoassay, Cannabinoids — Toxicology
Enzyme Immunoassay, Carbamazepine — Toxicology
Enzyme Immunoassay, Cocaine And Cocaine Metabolites — Toxicology
Enzyme Immunoassay, Diphenylhydantoin — Toxicology
Enzyme Immunoassay, Methadone — Toxicology
Enzyme Immunoassay, Opiates — Toxicology
Enzyme Immunoassay, Phencyclidine — Toxicology
Enzyme Immunoassay, Phenobarbital — Toxicology
Enzyme Immunoassay, Propoxyphene — Toxicology
Enzyme Immunoassay, Theophylline — Toxicology
Ferrozine (Colorimetric) Iron Binding Capacity — Chemistry
Gas Chromatography, Methamphetamine — Toxicology
Hexokinase, Glucose — Chemistry
LDL & VLDL Precipitation, Cholesterol Via Esterase-Oxidase — Chemistry
Lipase Hydrolysis/Glycerol Kinase Enzyme, Triglycerides — Chemistry
NAD Reduction/NADH Oxidation, CPK Or Isoenzymes — Chemistry
NAD Reduction/NADH Oxidation, Lactate Dehydrogenase — Chemistry
NADH Oxidation/NAD Reduction, AST/SGOT — Chemistry
Naphthyl Phosphate, Acid Phosphatase — Chemistry
Nitrophenylphosphate, Alkaline Phosphatase Or Isoenzymes — Chemistry
Phosphorus Reagent (Test System) — Chemistry
Photometric Method, Magnesium — Chemistry
Reagent, Bilirubin (Total Or Direct Test System) — Chemistry
Reagent, Creatinine (Test System) — Chemistry
Reagent, Iron (Test System) — Chemistry
Reagent, NAD-NADH, Alcohol Enzyme Method — Toxicology
SGPT, Ultraviolet — Chemistry
System, Test, Lipoprotein(a) — Chemistry
Test, C-Reactive Protein — Immunology
Test, Rheumatoid Factor — Immunology
Turbidimetric Method, Protein Or Albumin (Urinary) — Chemistry
Turbidimetric, Total Protein — Chemistry

ABBOTT DIAGNOSTICS DIV.　626-440-0700 *(cont'd)*

Urease And Glutamic Dehydrogenase, Urea Nitrogen	Chemistry
Uricase (U.V.), Uric Acid	Chemistry

ABBOTT DIAGNOSTICS INTL, BIOTECHNOLOGY LTD　787-846-3500

Road #2 KM. 58.0 , PO Box 278, Cruce Davila, Barceloneta, PR 00617
FDA Number: 2623532
E-mail: globalcitizenship@abbott.com
Web site: www.abbott.com
Ownership: Abbott Laboratories
Stock Symbol: ABT
Traded On: NYSE
Produces/Sells CE-marked Devices: N
General Admin.: Mr. Miles D. White/Chief Executive Officer, Chairman
　　　Mr. Edward L. Michael/Executive Vice President
　　　Mr. Stephen R. Fussell/Senior Vice President Human Resources
Production: Mr. Richard W. Ashley/Executive Vice President Development
Finance: Mr. Thomas C. Freyman/Executive Vice President Finance

Antigen, Antiserum, Control, Ferritin	Immunology
Assay, Serum, Cyclosporine and Metabolites, TDX	Toxicology
Colorimetric Method, CPK Or Isoenzymes	Chemistry
Enzyme Immunoassay, Benzodiazepine	Toxicology
Enzyme Immunoassay, Carbamazepine	Toxicology
Enzyme Immunoassay, Digoxin	Toxicology
Enzyme Immunoassay, Non-Radiolabeled, Total Thyroxine	Chemistry
Fluorescence Polarization Immunoassay, Diphenylhydantoin	Toxicology
Fluorescence Polarization Immunoassay, Phenobarbital	Toxicology
Fluorescence Polarization Immunoassay, Theophylline	Toxicology
Fluorescence Polarization, Immunoassay, Cyclosporine	Chemistry
Fluorometer, Chemistry	Chemistry
Kit, Administration, Intravenous	General
Needle, Catheter	Surgery
Nitroprusside, Ketones (Urinary, Non-Quantitative)	Chemistry
Radioassay, Intrinsic Factor Blocking Antibody	Chemistry
Radioimmunoassay, Estradiol	Chemistry
Radioimmunoassay, Ferritin	Microbiology
Radioimmunoassay, Follicle Stimulating Hormone	Chemistry
Radioimmunoassay, Free Thyroxine	Chemistry
Radioimmunoassay, Luteinizing Hormone	Chemistry
Radioimmunoassay, Prolactin (Lactogen)	Chemistry
Radioimmunoassay, Thyroid Stimulating Hormone	Chemistry
Radioimmunoassay, Total Triiodothyronine	Chemistry
Radioimmunoassay, Vitamin B12	Chemistry
Test, C-Reactive Protein, FITC	Immunology
Test, Neural Tube Defect, Alpha-Fetoprotein (AFP)	Immunology
U.V. Method, CPK Isoenzymes	Chemistry

ABBOTT HEMATOLOGY, DIAGNOSTICS DIV.　800-323-9100　408-982-480

5440 Patrick Henry Dr., Santa Clara, CA 95054　*Fax:* 408-982-4864
FDA Number: 2919069
Web site: www.abbott.us
Total Employees: 72000
Ownership: Abbott Laboratories
Stock Symbol: ABT
Traded On: NYSE
Quality System Registration Information: ISO9001
Produces/Sells CE-marked Devices: Y
Distribution: Manufacturer Direct
General Admin.: Miles D. White/Chief Executive Officer, Chairman

Antigen, Streptococcus SPP.	Microbiology
Antisera, Fluorescent, Chlamydia SPP.	Microbiology
Computer, Hematology Analyzer	Hematology
Control, Cell Counter, Normal And Abnormal	Hematology
Counter, Cell	Microbiology
Fluorometer, Toxicology	Toxicology
Immunofluorescence Equipment	Immunology
Kit, Pregnancy Test	Obstetrics/Gynecology
Spectrophotometer, Fluorescence	Chemistry
Spectrophotometer, U.V./Visible	Chemistry
Spectrophotometer, Ultraviolet	Chemistry
Spectrophotometer, Visible	Chemistry
Test, Syphilis (RPR or VDRL)	Microbiology

ABBOTT LABORATORIES　800-223-2064　847-937-6100

100 Abbott Park Rd., Abbott Park, IL 60064-3500　*Fax:* 847-935-3969
FDA Number: 1415939
E-mail: globalcitizenship@abbott.com
Web site: www.abbott.com
Annual Revenue: More than $1 Billion
Year Founded: 1888
Total Employees: 68697
Ownership: Public
Stock Symbol: ABT
Traded On: NYSE
Produces/Sells CE-marked Devices: N
General Admin.: Mr. Miles D. White/Chief Executive Officer, Chairman

ABBOTT LABORATORIES　800-223-2064 *(cont'd)*

Mr. Thomas C. Freyman/Chief Financial Officer, Executive Vice President
　　　Mr. Edward L. Michael/Executive Vice President
　　　Mr. John M. Capek/Executive Vice President
　　　Mr. Richard W. Ashley/Executive Vice President

Cabinet, Table And Tray, Anesthesia	Anesthesiology
Enzyme Immunoassay, Barbiturate	Toxicology
Enzyme Immunoassay, Methadone	Toxicology
Enzyme Immunoassay, Opiates	Toxicology
Enzyme Immunoassay, Primidone	Toxicology
Fluorescence Polarization Immunoassay, Tobramycin	Toxicology
Glove, Surgical	General
Hepatitis B Test (B Core, BE Antigen & Antibody, B Core IGM)	Microbiology
Pump, Infusion	General
Pump, Infusion, Patient Controlled Analgesia (PCA)	General
Radioimmunoassay, Free Thyroxine	Chemistry
Radioimmunoassay, Luteinizing Hormone	Chemistry
Radioimmunoassay, Prolactin (Lactogen)	Chemistry
Radioimmunoassay, Total Thyroxine	Chemistry
Radioimmunoassay, Total Triiodothyronine	Chemistry

Medical Product Subsidiaries (Listed Separately)
Abbott Diabetes Care Inc.
Abbott Diagnostics Div.
Abbott Diagnostics Intl, Biotechnology Ltd
Abbott Hematology, Diagnostics Div.
Abbott Laboratories
Abbott Molecular, Inc.
Abbott Point Of Care Inc.
Abbott Spine, Inc.
Abbott Vascular Inc.
Abbott Vascular, Cardiac Therapies
Abbott Vascular, Cardiac Therapies-P.R
Abbott Vascular, Vascular Solutions
Abbott West Distribution Center

ABBOTT LABORATORIES　800-624-7677　614-624-7677

1033 Kingsmill Pkwy., Columbus, OH 43229　*Fax:* 614-227-3244
FDA Number: 1527460
Web site: www.ross.com
Total Employees: 5000
Ownership: Abbott Laboratories
Stock Symbol: ABT
Traded On: NYSE
Produces/Sells CE-marked Devices: N
Distribution: Manufacturer Direct
General Admin.: Miles White/Chief Executive Officer
　　　Joy Amundson/President
Mktg./Adv.: Robert D. Clegg/Manager Business
　　　Matthew Fisher/Vice President Marketing
　　　Gregory Lindberg/Vice President Sales
Production: Robert Barnett/Director Operations

Bag, Enteral Feeding	General
Catheter, Jejunostomy	Gastroenterology/Urology
Catheter, Malecot (Gastrostomy Tube)	Gastroenterology/Urology
Infusion Pump, Enteral	General
Kit, Administration, Enteral	Gastroenterology/Urology
Kit, Gastrostomy, Endoscopic, Percutaneous	Gastroenterology/Urology
Kit, Laparoscopy	Gastroenterology/Urology
Nipple, Feeding	General
Pump, Food (Enteral Feeding)	General
Pump, Infusion	General
Pump, Infusion, Ambulatory	General
Tube, Feeding	General
Tube, Gastro-Enterostomy	Gastroenterology/Urology
Tube, Gastrointestinal	Gastroenterology/Urology
Tube, Gastrointestinal Decompression, Baker Jejunostomy	Gastroenterology/Urology
Tube, Nasogastric	Anesthesiology

ABBOTT LABORATORIES

See Abbott Diagnostics Div.

ABBOTT LABORATORIES　847-937-2388

6480 busch blvd., Columbus, OH 43229
FDA Number: 1528738
Ownership: Abbott Laboratories
Stock Symbol: ABT
Traded On: NYSE
Produces/Sells CE-marked Devices: N

Tube, Gastrointestinal	Gastroenterology/Urology

ABBOTT LABORATORIES

See Abbott Diagnostics Div.

ABBOTT LABORATORIES　847-937-2388

U.S. 41/Martin Luther King Dr, North Chicago, IL 60064
FDA Number: 1451914
Ownership: Abbott Laboratories
Stock Symbol: ABT
Traded On: NYSE

ABBOTT LABORATORIES 847-937-2388 *(cont'd)*
Produces/Sells CE-marked Devices: N
Analyzer, Chemistry, Photometric, Discrete	Chemistry

ABBOTT LABORATORIES ASHLAND
See Hospira

ABBOTT LABS - FAULTLESS
See Hospira

ABBOTT MEDICAL OPTICS INC. 866-427-8477
1700 East St. Andrew Pl., Santa Ana, CA 92705 714-247-8200
FDA Number: 2020664
Web site: www.amo-inc.com
Annual Revenue: More than $1 Billion
Ownership: ABBOTT LABORATORIES
Stock Symbol: ABT
Traded On: NYSE
Produces/Sells CE-marked Devices: N
Acid, Hyaluoronic	Dental And Oral
Cannula, Ophthalmic	Ophthalmology
Cleaner, Lens, Contact	Ophthalmology
Cutter, Vitreous Aspiration, AC-Powered	Ophthalmology
Fluid, Intraocular	Ophthalmology
Fluidic, Phacoemulsification/fragmentation	Ophthalmology
Folders and Injectors, Intraocular Lens (IOL)	Ophthalmology
Guide, Intraocular Lens	Ophthalmology
Irrigator, Ocular Surgery	Ophthalmology
Keratome, AC-Powered	Ophthalmology
Knife, Ophthalmic	Ophthalmology
Lens, Contact, Gas-Permeable	Ophthalmology
Lens, Intraocular	Ophthalmology
Lens, Intraocular, Multifocal	Ophthalmology
Needle, Suture, Ophthalmic	Ophthalmology
Phacofragmentation Unit	Ophthalmology

ABBOTT MOLECULAR, INC. 847-937-6100
1300 E. Touhy Ave., Des Plaines, IL 60018
FDA Number: 3005248192
Web site: www.abbott.com
Year Founded: 1888
Ownership: Abbott Laboratories
Stock Symbol: ABT
Traded On: NYSE
Produces/Sells CE-marked Devices: N
General Admin.: Mr. Miles D. White/Chief Executive Officer, Chairman
Mktg./Adv.: Mr. Timothy Stenzel/Director Media
Production: Mr. Richard W. Ashley/Executive Vice President Development
Research: Mr. John Robinson/Senior Director Research & Development
Finance: Mr. Thomas C. Freyman/Executive Vice President Finance
Antigen, Tumor Marker, Bladder (Basement Membrane Complexes)	Immunology
Assay, Hybridization And/or Nucleic Acid Amplification For Detection Of Hepatitis C Rna, Hepatitis C Virus	Microbiology
Concentrator, Clinical Sample	Chemistry
Cultured Animal And Human Cells	Pathology
DNA-Probe, Chromosome, Human	Hematology
DNA-Probe, Nucleic Acid Amplification, Chlamydia	Microbiology
General Purpose Microbiology Diagnostic Device	Microbiology
Hepatitis B Test (B Core, BE Antigen & Antibody, B Core IGM)	Microbiology
Kit, Screening, Urine	Microbiology
Monitor, Test, Hiv-1	Hematology
Neisseria, DNA Reagents	Microbiology
Pipetting And Diluting System, Automated	Chemistry
Stainer, Tissue, Automated	Pathology
System, Automated Scanning Microscope And Image Analysis For Fluorescence In Situ Hybridization (fish) Assays	Immunology
Table, Slide Warming	Pathology

ABBOTT POINT OF CARE INC. 609-443-9300
104 Windsor Center Dr., East Windsor, NJ 08520
FDA Number: 2245578 Fax: 609-443-9310
Web site: www.abbottpointofcare.com
Ownership: Abbott Laboratories
Stock Symbol: ABT
Traded On: NYSE
Produces/Sells CE-marked Devices: N
General Admin.: Mr. Greg Arnsdorff/President
Medical Admin.: Mr. Thomas Bugliosi/Director Medical Div.
Activated Whole Blood Clotting Time	Hematology
Biosensor, Immunoassay, Cpk Or Isoenzymes	Chemistry
Computer, Chemistry Analyzer	Chemistry
Control, Analyte (Assayed And Unassayed)	Chemistry
Control, Coagulation, Plasma	Hematology
Control, Multi Analyte, All Kinds (Assayed And Unassayed)	Chemistry
Electrode, Blood pH	Chemistry
Electrode, Ion Specific, Calcium	Chemistry
Electrode, Ion Specific, Chloride	Chemistry
Electrode, Ion Specific, Potassium	Chemistry
Electrode, Ion Specific, Sodium	Chemistry
Electrode, Ion Specific, Urea Nitrogen	Chemistry
Enzymatic Method, Lactic Acid	Chemistry

ABBOTT POINT OF CARE INC. 609-443-9300 *(cont'd)*
Enzymatic Method, Troponin Subunit	Chemistry
Hematocrit, Manual	Hematology
Ion Electrode Based Enzymatic, Creatinine	Chemistry
Prothrombin Time	Hematology
Reagent, Glucose (Test System)	Chemistry
Test, Natriuretic Peptide	Chemistry
Tube, Capillary Blood Collection	Hematology
pH Rate Measurement, Carbon-Dioxide	Chemistry

ABBOTT SPINE, INC. 847-937-6100
12708 Riata Vista Circle, Suite B-100, Austin, TX 78727
FDA Number: 1649384
E-mail: info@abbottspine.com
Web site: http://us.abbottspine.com
Ownership: Abbott Laboratories
Produces/Sells CE-marked Devices: N
General Admin.: Christy Wistar/Director
Mr. Scott Schaffner/President
Mktg./Adv.: Mr. Kelly Carper Erickson/Manager Communications
Appliance, Fixation, Spinal Interlaminal	Orthopedics
Appliance, Fixation, Spinal Intervertebral Body	Orthopedics
Awl	Orthopedics
Biopsy Instrument	Gastroenterology/Urology
Bit, Drill	Orthopedics
Caliper	Orthopedics
Cannula, Surgical, General & Plastic Surgery	Surgery
Cerclage, Fixation	Orthopedics
Compression Instrument	Orthopedics
Curette	Orthopedics
Device, Spinal Vertebral Body Replacement	Orthopedics
Dispenser, Cement	Orthopedics
Driver, Surgical, Pin	Surgery
Forceps	Orthopedics
Gauge, Depth	Orthopedics
Guide, Surgical, Instrument	Surgery
Impactor	Orthopedics
Instrument, Bending (Contouring)	Orthopedics
Mallet, Bone	Orthopedics
Orthosis, Fixation, Pedicle, Spinal	Orthopedics
Orthosis, Fixation, Spinal, Spondylolisthesis	Orthopedics
Orthosis, Spinal Pedicle Fixation, For Degenerative Disc Disease	Orthopedics
Osteotome (Orthopedic)	Surgery
Osteotome, Manual (Plastic Surgery)	Surgery
Plate, Fixation, Bone	Orthopedics
Prosthesis, Hip, Cement Restrictor	Orthopedics
Rasp, Bone	Orthopedics
Retainer, Surgical	Surgery
Retractor, Self-Retaining, Neurology	Cns/Neurology
Retractor, Surgical	Surgery
Rongeur, Rib	Orthopedics
Screw, Fixation, Bone	Orthopedics
Screwdriver	Orthopedics
Surgical Instrument, Non-Powered, Neurosurgical	Cns/Neurology
Tamp	Orthopedics
Tap, Bone	Orthopedics
Template	Orthopedics
Tray, Surgical Instrument	Surgery
Twister, Wire	Orthopedics
Wrench	Orthopedics

ABBOTT VASCULAR INC. 800-227-9902
400 Saginaw Drive, 650-474-3000
Redwood City, CA 94063
FDA Number: 2953144 Fax: 650-474-3010
E-mail: vi.customercare@av.abbott.com
Web site: www.abbottvascular.com
Year Founded: 1888
Ownership: Abbott Laboratories
Stock Symbol: ABT
Traded On: NYSE
Produces/Sells CE-marked Devices: N
General Admin.: Mr. Miles D. White/Chief Executive Officer, Chairman
Mr. Edward L. Michael/Executive Vice President
Mr. Robert B. Hance/Executive Vice President
Production: Mr. Richard W. Ashley/Executive Vice President Development
Finance: Mr. Thomas C. Freyman/Executive Vice President Finance
Catheter, Biliary	Gastroenterology/Urology
Clip, Implantable	Surgery
Device, Hemostasis, Vascular	Cardiovascular
Dressing, Other	General
Instrument, Manual, General Surgical	Surgery
Introducer, Catheter	Cardiovascular
Surgical Instrument, Cardiovascular	Cardiovascular
Suture, Non-Absorbable, Synthetic, Polypropylene	Surgery

ABBOTT VASCULAR, CARDIAC THERAPIES 800-227-9902
26531 Ynez Rd., Mailing P.O. Box 9018, 847-937-7988
Temecula, CA 92589
FDA Number: 2024168 Fax: 800-601-8874

ABBOTT VASCULAR, CARDIAC THERAPIES   800-227-9902
(cont'd)
E-mail: vi.customercare@av.abbott.com
Web site: www.abbottvascular.com
Year Founded: 1888
Ownership: Abbott Laboratories
Stock Symbol: ABT
Traded On: NYSE
Produces/Sells CE-marked Devices: N
General Admin.: Mr. Miles D. White/Chief Executive Officer, Chairman
    Mr. Edward L. Michael/Executive Vice President
    Mr. Robert B. Hance/Executive Vice President
Production: Mr. Richard W. Ashley/Executive Vice President Development
Finance: Mr. Thomas C. Freyman/Executive Vice President Finance

Adapter, Stopcock, Manifold, Cardiopulmonary Bypass	Cardiovascular
Catheter, Angioplasty, Coronary, Transluminal, Percut. Oper.	Cardiovascular
Catheter, Angioplasty, Transluminal, Peripheral	Cardiovascular
Catheter, Biliary	Gastroenterology/Urology
Catheter, Coronary, Atherectomy	Cardiovascular
Catheter, Intravascular, Diagnostic	Cardiovascular
Catheter, Percutaneous	Cardiovascular
Catheter, Peripheral, Atherectomy	Cardiovascular
Guidewire, Catheter	Cardiovascular
Introducer, Catheter	Cardiovascular
Motor, Surgical Instrument, AC-Powered	Surgery
Stent, Cardiovascular	Cardiovascular
Syringe, Balloon Inflation	Cardiovascular
System, Retroperfusion, Artery, Coronary	Cardiovascular

ABBOTT VASCULAR, CARDIAC THERAPIES   847-937-2388
30590 Cochise Circle, Murrieta, CA 92563
FDA Number: 3006169760
Ownership: Abbott Laboratories
Stock Symbol: ABT
Traded On: NYSE
Produces/Sells CE-marked Devices: N

Adapter, Stopcock, Manifold, Cardiopulmonary Bypass	Cardiovascular
Catheter, Intravascular, Diagnostic	Cardiovascular
Catheter, Percutaneous	Cardiovascular
Guidewire, Catheter	Cardiovascular
Injector, Syringe	General
Introducer, Catheter	Cardiovascular
Syringe, Balloon Inflation	Cardiovascular

ABBOTT VASCULAR, CARDIAC THERAPIES   800-227-9902
3200 Lakeside Dr., Santa Clara, CA 95054-2807   **408-845-3000**
FDA Number: 2939561   Fax: 408-845-3333
E-mail: vi.customercare@av.abbott.com
Web site: www.abbottvascular.com
Year Founded: 1888
Ownership: ABBOTT LABORATORIES
Stock Symbol: ABT
Traded On: NYSE
Produces/Sells CE-marked Devices: N
General Admin.: Mr. Miles D. White/Chief Executive Officer, Chairman
    Ms. Laura J. Schumacher/Executive Vice President
    Mr. Robert B. Hance/Senior Vice President
Production: Mr. Richard W. Ashley/Executive Vice President Development
Finance: Mr. Thomas C. Freyman/Executive Vice President Finance

Catheter, Angioplasty, Coronary, Transluminal, Percut. Oper.	Cardiovascular
Catheter, Angioplasty, Transluminal, Peripheral	Cardiovascular
Catheter, Biliary	Gastroenterology/Urology
Catheter, Intravascular, Diagnostic	Cardiovascular
Catheter, Percutaneous	Cardiovascular
Stent, Cardiovascular	Cardiovascular

ABBOTT VASCULAR, CARDIAC THERAPIES-P.R   847-937-2388
Km 58.0, Carretera 2, Cruce Davilla, Barceloneta, PR 00617
FDA Number: 3005737652
Ownership: Abbott Laboratories
Stock Symbol: ABT
Traded On: NYSE
Produces/Sells CE-marked Devices: N

Guidewire, Catheter	Cardiovascular

ABBOTT VASCULAR, VASCULAR SOLUTIONS   800-227-9902
26531 Ynez Rd., Temecula, CA 92589   **847-937-6100**
FDA Number: 3004742046   Fax: 800-601-8874
E-mail: vi.customercare@av.abbott.com
Web site: www.abbottvascular.com
Ownership: Abbott Laboratories
Stock Symbol: ABT
Traded On: NYSE
Produces/Sells CE-marked Devices: N
General Admin.: Mr. Miles D. White/Chief Executive Officer, Chairman
    Mr. Edward L. Michael/Executive Vice President
    Mr. Robert B. Hance/Executive Vice President
Production: Mr. Richard W. Ashley/Executive Vice President Development

ABBOTT VASCULAR, VASCULAR SOLUTIONS   800-227-9902
(cont'd)
Finance: Mr. Thomas C. Freyman/Executive Vice President Finance

Catheter, Angioplasty, Transluminal, Peripheral	Cardiovascular
Catheter, Biliary	Gastroenterology/Urology
Catheter, Carotid, Temporary, For Embolization Capture	Cardiovascular
Catheter, Percutaneous	Cardiovascular
Device, Coronary Saphenous Vein Bypass Graft, Temporary, For Embolization Protection	Cardiovascular
Guidewire, Catheter	Cardiovascular
Stent, Intracranial Neurovascular	Cns/Neurology
Stent, Superficial Femoral Artery	Cardiovascular

ABBOTT VASCULAR, VASCULAR SOLUTIONS   847-937-2388
3200 Lakeside Dr, Santa Clara, CA 95054
FDA Number: 2399561
Ownership: Abbott Laboratories
Produces/Sells CE-marked Devices: N

Catheter, Angioplasty, Coronary, Transluminal, Percut. Oper.	Cardiovascular
Catheter, Angioplasty, Transluminal, Peripheral	Cardiovascular
Catheter, Biliary	Gastroenterology/Urology
Catheter, Carotid, Temporary, For Embolization Capture	Cardiovascular
Catheter, Percutaneous	Cardiovascular
Guidewire, Catheter	Cardiovascular
Stent, Cardiovascular	Cardiovascular
Stent, Coronary, Drug-eluting	Cardiovascular

ABBOTT WEST DISTRIBUTION CENTER   847-937-2388
42301 Zevo Drive, Temecula, CA 92590
FDA Number: 3006604866
Ownership: Abbott Laboratories
Stock Symbol: ABT
Traded On: NYSE
Produces/Sells CE-marked Devices: N

Stent, Coronary, Drug-eluting	Cardiovascular

ABC HEALTH SOLUTIONS LLC   877-631-4551
14008 Se 238th Lane, Kent, WA 98042   **253-631-8270**
FDA Number: 3004424059   Fax: 253-639-2467
E-mail: farabloc@abchealthsolutions.biz
Web site: www.abchealthsolutions.biz
Ownership: Private
Produces/Sells CE-marked Devices: N

Cover, Limb	Physical Med

ABC MEDICAL ENTERPRISES
See Ability Building Center, Inc.

ABEL DENTAL LAB   952-541-9622
2 West Main Street, National City Bank Building,
Uniontown, PA 15401
FDA Number: 3004142474
Ownership: Private
Produces/Sells CE-marked Devices: N

Base, Denture, Relining, Repairing, Rebasing, Resin	Dental And Oral
Crown, Preformed	Dental And Oral
Device, Anti-Snoring	Ear/Nose/Throat
Device, Repositioning, Jaw	Dental And Oral
Mouthguard	Dental And Oral

ABELNET INC   800-463-5685
91 Station St., Unit 1, Ajax, ONT L1S 3H2 Canada   **416-686-4129**
FDA Number: n/a   Fax: 416-686-6895
E-mail: tashcan@aol.com
Web site: www.ablenetinc.com
Year Founded: 1978
Total Employees: 7
Ownership: Private
Produces/Sells CE-marked Devices: N
Distribution: Manufacturer Direct, Exporter

ABI ANALYTICAL
See Applied Biosystems

ABILITATIONS   800-850-8602
PO BOX 922668, Norcross, GA 30010   **770-449-5700**
FDA Number: n/a   Fax: 800-845-1535
E-mail: orders@sportime.com
Web site: www.abilitations.com
Medical Products Sales Volume: $1,300,000
Annual Revenue: $10-$25 Million
Total Employees: 120   Marketing Staff: 12   Sales Staff: 22
Ownership: Private
Produces/Sells CE-marked Devices: N
Federal Procurement Eligibility: Small Business
Distribution: Manufacturer Direct
General Admin.: Peter Savitz/Chief Executive Officer
Mktg./Adv.: Ilana Danneman/Director Marketing
    Duane Puckett/Vice President Sales

ABILITIES   800-850-8602 *(cont'd)*
Equipment, Therapy, Handicapped/Physical   Physical Med

ABILITY BUILDING CENTER, INC.   507-281-6262
1911 14th Street NW, P.O. Box 6938, Rochester, MN 55903-6938
FDA Number: n/a   Fax: 507-281-6270
Web site: www.abcinc.org
Medical Products Sales Volume: $5,000,000
Annual Revenue: $1-$5 Million
Year Founded: 1956
Ownership: Private
Produces/Sells CE-marked Devices: N
Distribution: Manufacturer Direct
General Admin.: Larry Erickson/Assistant Director
     Steve Hill/Executive Director
     Steve Kann/President
     Dr. Thomas Bergquist/Vice President
Finance: Dick Quinn/Treasurer
   Collector, Specimen   Microbiology
   Gown, Operating Room, Disposable   Surgery

ABIOMED, INC.   800-422-8666
22 Cherry Hill Dr., Danvers, MA 01923-2579   978-777-5410
FDA Number: 1220648   Fax: 978-777-8411
E-mail: marketing@abiomed.com
Web site: www.abiomed.com
Annual Revenue: $10-$25 Million
Year Founded: 1981
Total Employees: 310   *Marketing Staff:* 10   *Sales Staff:* 40
Ownership: Public
Stock Symbol: ABMD
Traded On: NASDAQ
Quality System Registration Information: ISO9001
Produces/Sells CE-marked Devices: Y
Federal Procurement Eligibility: Small Business
Distribution: Manufacturer Direct, Manufacturer Through Distributor, Manufacturer Through Manufacturer Reps, Service Direct, Exclusive Distributor
General Admin.: Mr. David Weber/Chief Operating Officer
     Dr. Thorsten Siess/Chief Technology Officer
     Mr. Michael R. Minogue/President, Chief Executive Officer, Chairman
Medical Admin.: Mr. Andrew Greenfield/Vice President Health Care
Mktg./Adv.: Mr. Michael Howley/Vice President International Marketing
Production: Mr. William Bolt/Senior Vice President Quality Assurance
Finance: Mr. Robert Bowen/Chief Financial Officer
   Balloon, Intra-Aortic (With Control System)   Cardiovascular
   Cannula, Catheter   Cardiovascular
   Catheter, Intravascular, Diagnostic   Cardiovascular
   Catheter, Vascular, Cardiopulmonary Bypass   Cardiovascular
   Circulatory Assist Unit, Cardiac   Cardiovascular
   Condenser, Heat And Moisture (Artificial Nose)   Anesthesiology
   Controller, Pump Speed, Cardiopulmonary Bypass   Cardiovascular
   Gauge, Depth, Instrument, Dental   Dental And Oral
   Heart, Artificial   Cardiovascular
   Instrument, Dental, Manual   Dental And Oral
   Pump, Blood, Cardiopulmonary Bypass, Non-Roller Type   Cardiovascular

ABLATION FRONTIERS, INC.   760-438-4868
6354 Corte Del Abeto, Carlsbad, CA 92011
FDA Number: 3005915191   Fax: 760-438-4964
Web site: www.ablationfrontiers.com
Year Founded: 2004
Ownership: MEDTRONIC, INC.
Produces/Sells CE-marked Devices: Y

ABLE 2 PRODUCTS CO., INC.   800-641-4098
804 East Highway 248, P.O. Box 543,   417-847-4791
Cassville, MO 65625
FDA Number: n/a   Fax: 800-526-1240
E-mail: sales@able2products.com
Web site: www.able2products.com
Medical Products Sales Volume: $4,500,000
Year Founded: 1972
Total Employees: 100
Ownership: Private
Produces/Sells CE-marked Devices: N
Federal Procurement Eligibility: Small Business
Distribution: Manufacturer Through Distributor
   Communication Equipment   General
   Communication System, Emergency Alert, Personal   General
   Component, Electrical   General
   Light Source, Flash   Chemistry
   Light, Other   General
   Receptacle, Electrical   General

ABLE WALKER, LTD.   604-576-8488
16-2350 Beta Ave, Burnaby V5C 5M8 Canada
FDA Number: 8022287

ABLE WALKER, LTD.   604-576-8488 *(cont'd)*
Walker, Mechanical   Physical Med

ABLENET INC.   800-322-0956
2808 Fairview Avenue North,   651-294-2200
Roseville, MN 55113
FDA Number: n/a   Fax: 651-294-2259
Web site: http://www.ablenetinc.com
Ownership: Private
Produces/Sells CE-marked Devices: N

ABRACAIR, LLC   502-445-9471
204 N.17th Street, Louisville, KY 40203
FDA Number: n/a
Ownership: Private
Produces/Sells CE-marked Devices: N
   Purifier, Air, Ultraviolet   General

ABRASIVE TECHNOLOGY, INC.   740-548-4100
8400 Green Meadows Dr., Lewis Center, OH 43035
FDA Number: 1525838   Fax: 740-548-7617
Web site: www.abrasive-tech.com
Ownership: Private
Produces/Sells CE-marked Devices: N
   Agent, Polishing, Abrasive, Oral Cavity   Dental And Oral
   Burr, Surgical, General & Plastic Surgery   Surgery
   Cup, Prophylaxis   Dental And Oral
   Disk, Abrasive   Dental And Oral
   Drill, Dental, Intraoral   Dental And Oral
   File, Pulp Canal, Endodontic   Dental And Oral
   Guard, Disk   Dental And Oral
   Instrument, Diamond, Dental   Dental And Oral
   Matrix, Dental   Dental And Oral
   Pick, Massaging   Dental And Oral
   Point, Abrasive   Dental And Oral
   Post, Root Canal   Dental And Oral
   Reamer, Pulp Canal, Endodontic   Dental And Oral
   Strip, Polishing Agent   Dental And Oral

ABSOLUTE AIR CLEANERS & PURIFIERS, INC.   888-578-7324
401 Meadow Rd., Durango, CO 81303   970-259-3998
FDA Number: n/a   Fax: 970-259-3557
E-mail: info@aircleaners.com
Web site: www.aircleaners.com
Year Founded: 1989
Ownership: Private
Produces/Sells CE-marked Devices: N
Federal Procurement Eligibility: Small Business
Distribution: Manufacturer Direct
General Admin.: Barry Cohen/Owner
   Controller, Temperature, Humidifier   General
   Humidifier, Heat/Moisture Exchange   Anesthesiology
   Purifier, Air, Ultraviolet   General

ABSOLUTE X-RAY CORP.   845-638-8080
205 North Little Tor Rd., New City, NY 10956
FDA Number: n/a   Fax: 845-638-8082
E-mail: absolutexr@aol.com
Web site: www.ewen-parker.com
Ownership: Private
Produces/Sells CE-marked Devices: N
   Radiographic/Fluoroscopic Unit, Image-Intensified   Radiology

ABSORB-PLUS TEXTILES INC.   514-345-9770
1075 rue Hickson, Verdun, QC H4G 2L3 Canada
FDA Number: n/a
Total Employees: 100
Ownership: CITY LAUNDRY INC.
Produces/Sells CE-marked Devices: N
Distribution: Manufacturer Direct, Exporter

ABSORPTION SYSTEMS   610-280-7300
436 Creamery Way, Exton, PA 19341
FDA Number: n/a   Fax: 610-280-9667
Web site: www.absorption.com
Year Founded: 1996
Ownership: Private
Produces/Sells CE-marked Devices: N
General Admin.: Dr. Ismael J. Hidalgo/Chief Scientific Officer
     Patrick M. Dentinger/President, Chief Executive Officer
Mktg./Adv.: Dr. Chris Bode/Vice President Corporate Development
Production: Dr. Vinko Rutar/Director Quality Assurance
     Dr. Sid Bhoopathy/Vice President Operations
Research: Mr. Albert Owen/Vice President Scientific Affairs
Finance: Mr. Patrick Carr, Jr/Chief Financial Officer
   Assay, Porphyrin, Spectrophotometry, Lithium   Toxicology
   Mass Spectrometer, Clinical Use   Toxicology

AC HEALTHCARE SUPPLY, INC.
905-448-4706
116-51 230th St., Cambria Heights, NY 11411
FDA Number: 3003936589
Ownership: Private
Produces/Sells CE-marked Devices: N

Airway, Oropharyngeal, Anesthesia	Anesthesiology
Bag, Urinary Collection, Ureterostomy	Gastroenterology/Urology
Bag, Urine Collection, Leg, For External Use, Non-sterile	Gastroenterology/Urology
Bandage, Liquid	Surgery
Bottle, Blow (Exerciser)	Anesthesiology
Brush, Scrub, Operating Room	Surgery
Cannula, Injection	Gastroenterology/Urology
Cannula, Ophthalmic	Ophthalmology
Catheter, Infusion	Surgery
Catheter, Irrigation	Surgery
Catheter, Rectal, Ileostomy, Continent	Gastroenterology/Urology
Catheter, Suction (Tracheal Aspirating Tube)	Anesthesiology
Chair, Geriatric	General
Component, Cast	Orthopedics
Container, Specimen, Urine, Drugs Of Abuse, Over The Counter	Chemistry
Forceps, Biopsy, Gynecological	Obstetrics/Gynecology
Garment, Protective, For Incontinence	Gastroenterology/Urology
Glove, Patient Examination, Vinyl	General
Holder, Catheter	Gastroenterology/Urology
Infusion Stand	General
Kit, Pregnancy Test, Over The Counter, HCG	Chemistry
Kit, Wound Dressing	Surgery
Mask, Gas, Anesthesia	Anesthesiology
Mask, Oxygen, Aerosol Administration	Anesthesiology
Mask, Oxygen, Low Concentration, Venturi	Anesthesiology
Mask, Oxygen, Non-Rebreathing	Anesthesiology
Mask, Scavenging	Anesthesiology
Occluder, Umbilical	General
Pad, Medicated, Adhesive, Non-Electric	General
Solution, Saline(wound Dressing)	Surgery
Speculum, Vaginal, Non-Metal	Obstetrics/Gynecology
Stabilizer, Vein	General
Stopcock	General
Strap, Head, Gas Mask	Anesthesiology
Tourniquet, Non-Pneumatic, Surgical	Surgery
Tourniquet, Pneumatic	Surgery

ACADEMY SAVANT
800-472-8268
714-870-7880
PO Box 3670, Fullerton, CA 92834
Fax: 714-526-7400
FDA Number: n/a
E-mail: info@academysavant.com
Web site: www.academysavant.com
Medical Products Sales Volume: $500,000
Annual Revenue: $0-$1 Million
Year Founded: 1977
Total Employees: 5   *Sales Staff:* 4
Ownership: Private
Produces/Sells CE-marked Devices: N
Federal Procurement Eligibility: Small Business, Minority Owned
Distribution: Manufacturer Direct, Manufacturer Through Distributor, Manufacturer Through Manufacturer Reps, Exporter
General Admin.: Rabin D. Lai/President

Computer Software	General

ACADENTAL
888-585-0678
913-384-7390
9204 Bond Street, Overland Park, KS 66214
Fax: 913-538-6095
FDA Number: n/a
E-mail: sales@acadental.com
Ownership: Private
Produces/Sells CE-marked Devices: N

Cleanser, Root Canal	Dental And Oral

ACART EQUIPMENT LTD.
800-551-0560
905-625-5540
1020 Brevik Place, Unit 3,
Mississauga, ONT L4W-4 Canada
Fax: 905-625-0151
FDA Number: n/a
E-mail: dick_flynn@acartequipment.com
Web site: www.acart.ca
Year Founded: 1981
Total Employees: 10
Ownership: Private
Produces/Sells CE-marked Devices: N
Distribution: Manufacturer Direct, Exclusive Distributor

ACCELER8
800-810-9897
303-863-8088
7000 North Broadway, Building 3-307,
Denver, CO 80221
Fax: 303-863-1218
FDA Number: n/a
Web site: http://www.accelr8.com
Ownership: Private
Produces/Sells CE-marked Devices: N
General Admin.: Mr. Thomas Geimer/Chief Executive Officer, Chairman
Mr. David Howson/President

ACCELERATED CARE PLUS CORP.
800-350-1100
775-685-4000
4850 Joule Street, Suite A-1, Reno, NV 89502
Fax: 775-685-4013
FDA Number: 1911273
E-mail: customerservice@acplus.com
Web site: www.acplus.com
Ownership: Private
Produces/Sells CE-marked Devices: N

Assembly, Knee/Shank/Ankle/Foot, External	Physical Med
Assembly, Thigh/Knee/Shank/Ankle/Foot, External	Physical Med
Belt, Traction, Pelvic, Orthopedic	Orthopedics
Binder, Abdominal	General
Brace, Joint, Ankle (External)	Physical Med
Component, Exercise	Physical Med
Diathermy, Shortwave	Physical Med
Exerciser, Powered	Anesthesiology
Halter, Head, Traction	Physical Med
Halter, Head, Traction, Orthopedic	Orthopedics
Joint, Hip, External Brace	Physical Med
Lamp, Infrared	Physical Med
Orthosis, Abdominal	Physical Med
Orthosis, Cervical-Thoracic, Rigid	Physical Med
Orthosis, Limb Brace	Physical Med
Orthosis, Lumbar	Physical Med
Orthosis, Lumbosacral	Physical Med
Orthosis, Rib Fracture, Soft	Physical Med
Orthosis, Sacroiliac, Soft	Physical Med
Orthosis, Thoracic	Physical Med
Sling, Arm	Physical Med
Splint, Clavicle	Physical Med
Splint, Hand, And Component	Physical Med
Stimulator, Nerve, Transcutaneous (Pain Relief, TENS)	Cns/Neurology
Truss, Umbilical	Gastroenterology/Urology

ACCELERATED REHAB DESIGNS, INC.
888-397-4063
32025 Industrial Park Dr, Pinehurst, TX 77362
FDA Number: n/a
Ownership: Private
Produces/Sells CE-marked Devices: N

Wheelchair, Powered	Physical Med

ACCELLENT
See Accellent El Paso

ACCELLENT EL PASO
915-771-9112
31C Butterfield Trail, El Paso, TX 79906
Fax: 915-771-9107
FDA Number: 2431982
E-mail: info@accellent.com
Web site: www.accellent.com
Medical Products Sales Volume: $474,100,000
Annual Revenue: $100-$500 Million
Ownership: Accellent Inc.
Quality System Registration Information: ISO9001; ISO9002; ISO9003
Produces/Sells CE-marked Devices: Y
Distribution: OEM
General Admin.: Mr. Kenneth Freeman/Chairman
Mr. Jeremy Friedman/Chief Financial Officer, Executive Vice President
Mr. Jeremy Farina/Chief Technology Officer, Executive Vice President
Mr. Donald Spence/President, Chief Executive Officer

Arthroscope	Orthopedics
Contract Manufacturing	General
Electrosurgical Unit, Gastroenterology	Gastroenterology/Urology
Electrosurgical Unit, Neurological	Cns/Neurology
Forceps, Biopsy, Non-Electric	Gastroenterology/Urology
Insert, Tubal Occlusion	Obstetrics/Gynecology
Kit, Administration, Intravenous	General
Separator, Blood Cell/Plasma, Therapeutic	Gastroenterology/Urology
Snare, Flexible	Gastroenterology/Urology
Transfer Unit, IV Fluid	General
Tube, Feeding	General
Warmer, Infusion Fluid, Thermal	General

ACCELLENT ENDOSCOPY
909-982-1025
2052 West 11th St., Upland, CA 91786
Fax: 909-949-0539
FDA Number: 2027487
E-mail: info@accellent.com
Web site: www.accellent.com
Medical Products Sales Volume: $10,000,000
Ownership: Accellent Inc.
Quality System Registration Information: ISO9003
Produces/Sells CE-marked Devices: N
Federal Procurement Eligibility: Small Business
Distribution: Manufacturer Direct
General Admin.: Robert E. Kirby/President, Chief Executive Officer

Molding, Custom	General
Pin, Fixation, Smooth	Orthopedics

ACCELLENT INC.
100 Fordham Road, Wilmington, MA 01887   **866-899-1392**   **978-570-6900**
FDA Number: 1218882   Fax: 978-657-0878
E-mail: info@accellent.com
Web site: www.accellent.com
Annual Revenue: $100-$500 Million
Ownership: Valcor Engineering Corporation
Produces/Sells CE-marked Devices: N
Federal Procurement Eligibility: Small Business
Distribution: OEM, Service Direct
General Admin.: Jeremy A. Friedman/Chief Financial Officer, Executive Vice President
         Jeffrey M. Farina/Chief Technology Officer, Executive Vice President
         Kenneth W. Freeman/Executive Chairman
         Donald J. Spence/President, Chief Executive Officer
         William E. Howell/Vice President Chief Information Officer

Electrosurgical Unit, Cutting & Coagulation Device	Surgery
Phacofragmentation Unit	Ophthalmology
Service, Modification, Product	General
Surgical Instrument, Orthopedic, AC-Powered Motor	Orthopedics
Tubing, Replacement, Phacofragmentation Unit	Ophthalmology

Medical Product Subsidiaries (Listed Separately)
Accellent El Paso
Accellent Endoscopy
Accellent Inc.

ACCELLENT INC.
200 South Yorkshire St., Salem, VA 24153   **866-899-1392**   **540-389-7860**
FDA Number: n/a   Fax: 540-389-7857
E-mail: info@accellent.com
Web site: www.accellent.com
Medical Products Sales Volume: $16,000,000
Annual Revenue: $10-$25 Million
Ownership: UTI CORP.
Quality System Registration Information: ISO9002
Produces/Sells CE-marked Devices: N
Federal Procurement Eligibility: Small Business
Distribution: Manufacturer Direct
General Admin.: Robert E. Kirby/President, Chief Executive Officer

Electrode, Pacemaker, Transthoracic	Cardiovascular

ACCELLENT INC.
45 Lexington Dr., Laconia, NH 03246   **603-528-1211**
FDA Number: 1221485   Fax: 603-528-8489
E-mail: info@accellent.com
Web site: www.accellent.com
Ownership: Accellent Inc.
Produces/Sells CE-marked Devices: N
General Admin.: Robert E. Kirby/President, Chief Executive Officer

Electrosurgical Unit, Cutting & Coagulation Device	Surgery

ACCELLENT INC.
5000 Independence St., Arvada, CO 80002   **303-424-7300**
FDA Number: n/a   Fax: 303-424-6700
E-mail: info@accellent.com
Web site: www.accellent.com
Medical Products Sales Volume: $200,000
Ownership: Accellent Inc.
Quality System Registration Information: ISO9002
Produces/Sells CE-marked Devices: N
Distribution: OEM
Mktg./Adv.: Rick Riddle/Director Sales
Production: Tim Weaver/Director Operations

Guide, Wire, Angiographic (And Accessories)	Cns/Neurology
Guidewire	Cardiovascular
Guidewire, Catheter	Cardiovascular
Guidewire, Catheter, Radiological	Radiology
Lead, Pacemaker (Catheter)	Cardiovascular
Lead, Pacemaker, Implantable Endocardial	Cardiovascular
Lead, Pacemaker, Implantable Myocardial	Cardiovascular
Lead, Pacemaker, Temporary Endocardial	Cardiovascular
Lead, Pacemaker, Temporary Myocardial	Cardiovascular
Service, Device Coating, Protective	General
Stylet, Catheter	Cardiovascular
Stylet, Catheter, Gastro-Urology	Gastroenterology/Urology
Stylet, Intravenous	General
Stylet, Needle	General
Stylet, Surgical	Surgery
Stylet, Tracheal Tube	Anesthesiology
Stylet, Ureteral	Gastroenterology/Urology
Wire, Orthodontic	Dental And Oral

ACCENT PLASTICS
1925 Elise Circle, Corona, CA 92879   **951-273-7777**
FDA Number: 3000299546

Filter, Bacterial, Breathing Circuit	Anesthesiology

ACCESS ANALYTICAL SYSTEM
    See Cas Medical Systems, Inc.

ACCESS ANALYTICAL SYSTEMS
    See Idexx Laboratories, Inc.

ACCESS BATTERY AND POWER SYSTEMS, L.L.C.
    See Access Battery Inc.

ACCESS BATTERY INC.
Division of Alpha Source, Inc.   **800-654-9845**   **414-760-2222**
12104 W. Carmen Avenue
Milwaukee, WI 53225
FDA Number: 2246349   Fax: 888-654-9840
E-mail: Customer.Service@AlphaSource.com
Web site: www.alphasource.com
Medical Products Sales Volume: $3,000,000
Annual Revenue: $1-$5 Million
Year Founded: 1974
Total Employees: 25   *Marketing Staff:* 2   *Sales Staff:* 5
Ownership: Alpha Source, Inc.
Quality System Registration Information: ISO9002
Produces/Sells CE-marked Devices: Y
Federal Procurement Eligibility: Small Business, Female Owned, GSA Contract, VA Contract
Distribution: Manufacturer Direct, Manufacturer Through Distributor, Manufacturer Through Manufacturer Reps, Importer
General Admin.: John Lawrence/Chief Executive Officer
Mktg./Adv.: Ms. Karen Perkins/Regional Marketing Manager
         Mr. Charles Volwaller/Vice President Sales
Production: Alex Henderson/Director Quality Assurance & Regulatory Affairs

Analyzer, Battery	General
Battery	General
Battery, Mobile Radiographic Unit	Radiology
Box, Battery, Rechargeable (Endoscopic)	Gastroenterology/Urology
Charger, Battery	General
Power Systems, Uninterruptible (UPS)	General

ACCESS BIO INCORPORATE
65 Clyde Rd., Suite A, Somerset, NJ 08873   **732-873-4040**
FDA Number: 3003966368   Fax: 732-873-4043
E-mail: info@accessbio.net
Web site: www.accessbio.net
Ownership: Private
Produces/Sells CE-marked Devices: N

Antigen, Antiserum, Control, Albumin	Immunology
Antigen, Streptococcus SPP.	Microbiology
Antiserum, Leptospira SPP.	Microbiology
Enzymatic Method, Troponin Subunit	Chemistry
Fibrin Split Products	Hematology
Kit, Mycobacteria Identification	Microbiology
Kit, Pregnancy Test, Over The Counter, HCG	Chemistry
Kit, Test, Malaria	Toxicology
Lancet, Blood	General
Radioimmunoassay, Luteinizing Hormone	Chemistry
Reagent, Glucose (Test System)	Chemistry
Rickettsia Serological Reagents, Other	Microbiology
System, Test, Blood Glucose, Over-The-Counter	Chemistry
Test, C-Reactive Protein	Immunology

ACCESS BRIDGES
610 Nason St., Santa Rosa, CA 95404   **707-546-7671**
FDA Number: 3005497876
Ownership: Private
Produces/Sells CE-marked Devices: N

Lift, Bath, Non-AC-Powered	General

ACCESS BUSINESS GROUP LLC
7575 East Fulton St., Ada, MI 49355   **616-787-4964**
FDA Number: 1811250

Bandage, Adhesive	Surgery
Container, Specimen Mailer And Storage, Temperature Control	Pathology

ACCESS BUSINESS SYSTEMS
    See Idexx Laboratories, Inc.

ACCESS GENETICS
7550 Market Place Dr.,   **888-250-4407**
Minneapolis, MN 55344   **952-942-0671**
FDA Number: 3005310466   Fax: 952-942-0703
E-mail: skelley@access-genetics.com
Web site: www.access-genetics.com
Ownership: Private
Produces/Sells CE-marked Devices: N
General Admin.: Mr. George Hoedeman/Chief Executive Officer
         Dr. Ronald McGlennen/President
Mktg./Adv.: Mr. Scott Kelley/Vice President Marketing & Sales
Production: Mr. Aaron Franks/Vice President Operations
Finance: Mr. Paul Hoedeman/Chief Financial Officer
IS: Mr. Robert Schuldt/Vice President Technology

Fluorometer	Immunology

ACCESS GENETICS 888-250-4407 *(cont'd)*
Reagents, Specific, Analyte — Hematology
System, Communication, Image, Digital — Radiology

ACCESS LLC 800-973-0355
11 West End Rd., Totowa, NJ 07512
FDA Number: 2531854
Ownership: Private
Produces/Sells CE-marked Devices: N
Catheter, Peritoneal — Surgery

ACCESS MEDICAL SYSTEMS
See Idexx Laboratories, Inc.

ACCESS MOBILITY, INC. 800-336-1147
5240 Elmwood Ave., Indianapolis, IN 46203 317-784-2255
FDA Number: n/a *Fax:* 317-784-6391
Web site: www.accesstoday.com
Annual Revenue: $1-$5 Million
Year Founded: 1971
Ownership: Private
Produces/Sells CE-marked Devices: N
Federal Procurement Eligibility: Small Business
Distribution: Exclusive Distributor
Cane — Physical Med
Chair, Shower — General
Commode (Toilet) — General
Crutch — Physical Med
Scooter (Motorized 3-Wheeled Vehicle) — Physical Med
Walker, Mechanical — Physical Med
Wheelchair, Manual — Physical Med
Wheelchair, Powered — Physical Med

ACCESS NOW LLC 800-351-8375
1337 Burns Avenue, Iowa City, IA 52240 319-351-8375
FDA Number: 3003645159 *Fax:* 319-248-2674
E-mail: accnowjh@aol.com
Web site: www.myaccnow.info
Medical Products Sales Volume: $1,500,000
Annual Revenue: $1-$5 Million
Year Founded: 2000
Total Employees: 8
Ownership: Private
Produces/Sells CE-marked Devices: N
Federal Procurement Eligibility: Small Business, Female Owned
Distribution: Manufacturer Through Distributor, Exporter
Stretcher, Hand-Carried — General

ACCESS OPTICS LLC 918-294-1234
2001 North Willow Ave., Broken Arrow, OK 74012
FDA Number: 3004902874
Eyepiece, Lens, Non-Prescription, Endoscopic — Gastroenterology/Urology

ACCESS RADIOLOGY CORPORATION
See Emed Technologies

ACCESS SCIENTIFIC INC. 866-608-8333
12526 High Bluff Drive, Suite 360, 858-259-8333
San Diego, CA 92130
FDA Number: 3006537552 *Fax:* 858-259-5298
E-mail: info@the-wand.com
Web site: http://www.the-wand.com
Ownership: Private
Produces/Sells CE-marked Devices: N
General Admin.: Dr. Steve Bierman/Chief Executive Officer
Mr. Richard Pluth/Chief Operating Officer, Vice President
Mr. Bill Bold/President
Production: Mr. Albert Misajon/Vice President Quality Assurance & Regulatory Affairs
Introducer, Catheter — Cardiovascular

ACCESS, LIFTS & MOBILITY SYSTEMS, INC. (972) 285-3487
301 Clary Dr., Mesquite, TX 75149-3023
FDA Number: n/a *Fax:* 972-285-3387
Annual Revenue: $0-$1 Million
Total Employees: 4 *Marketing Staff:* 2 *Sales Staff:* 3
Ownership: Private
Produces/Sells CE-marked Devices: N
Federal Procurement Eligibility: Small Business, Minority Owned, Female Owned
Distribution: Manufacturer Through Distributor
General Admin.: Ron Costa/Office Manager
Sarah Costa/President
Mktg./Adv.: Mike Davidson/Manager Sales
Finance: Jimmie Williams/Treasurer
Pack, Hot Or Cold, Water Circulating — Physical Med

ACCESS/GOD LOVES YOU
See Access Battery Inc.

ACCESSCLOSURE, INC. 877-700-6969
645 Clyde Ave., Mountain View, CA 94043 650-903-1000
FDA Number: 3004939290 *Fax:* 650-903-1018
E-mail: customerservice@accessclosure.com
Web site: http://www.accessclosure.com
Year Founded: 2002
Ownership: Private
Produces/Sells CE-marked Devices: N
General Admin.: Mr. Jim Fortune/Chief Operating Officer
Mr. Greg Casciaro/President, Chief Executive Officer
Mktg./Adv.: Mr. Michael Devine/Executive Vice President Marketing & Sales
Production: Ms. Susan Aloyan/Vice President Quality Assurance & Regulatory Affairs
Research: Mr. Andy Uchida/Vice President Research & Development
Finance: Mr. John Buckley/Chief Financial Officer
Device, Hemostasis, Vascular — Cardiovascular
Tourniquet, Non-Pneumatic, Surgical — Surgery

ACCESSIBILITY PRODUCTS, INC.
See Access Mobility, Inc.

ACCESSIBLE DESIGNS, INC. 210-341-0008
401 Isom Rd., Suite 520, San Antonio, TX 78216
FDA Number: 3004365003 *Fax:* 210-341-0009
E-mail: cs@adirides.com
Web site: www.accessibledesigns.com
Ownership: Private
Produces/Sells CE-marked Devices: N
Accessories, Wheelchair — Physical Med
Component, Wheelchair — Physical Med

ACCLAIM MEDICAL MANUFACTURING LLC 856-303-2363
1100 Taylors Lane, Unit 9, Cinnaminson, NJ 08077
FDA Number: 3004111714
E-mail: contact@acclaim-dme.com
Web site: www.acclaimdme.com
Ownership: Private
Produces/Sells CE-marked Devices: N
Mattress, Air Flotation — General

ACCLARENT, INC. 877-775-2789
1525-B O'brien Dr., Menlo Park, CA 94025 650-687-5888
FDA Number: 3005172759 *Fax:* 650-687-5889
E-mail: acclarent@acclarent.com
Web site: www.acclarent.com
Year Founded: 2004
Ownership: Private
Produces/Sells CE-marked Devices: N
General Admin.: Greg Garfield/Chief Operating Officer
William Facteau/President, Chief Executive Officer
Medical Admin.: Andre Cheng/Vice President Medical Affairs
Mktg./Adv.: Karen Long/Vice President Marketing
Patrick Fabian/Vice President National Sales
Robert Wood/Vice President Strategic Planning
Production: James Zuegel/Vice President Operations
Mark Bishop/Vice President Quality Assurance & Quality Control
Su-Mien Chong/Vice President Regulatory & Clinical Affairs
Research: John Chang/Vice President Research & Development
Finance: George Harter/Chief Financial Officer
Accessories, Bronchoscope — Ear/Nose/Throat
Cannula, Sinus — Ear/Nose/Throat
ENT Manual Surgical Instrument — Ear/Nose/Throat
Forceps, ENT — Ear/Nose/Throat
Iontophoresis Device, Dental — Dental And Oral
Nasopharyngoscope (Flexible Or Rigid) — Ear/Nose/Throat
Tube, Tympanostomy — Ear/Nose/Throat

ACCOMMODATA CORPORATION 216-732-8888
20950 Edgecliff Road, Euclid, OH 44123
FDA Number: 3005031572
E-mail: info@accommodata.com
Web site: www.accommodata.com
Ownership: Private
Produces/Sells CE-marked Devices: N
Projector, Ophthalmic — Ophthalmology

ACCOR, INC. 216-381-2951
1375 Yellowstone Rd., Cleveland Heights, OH 44121
FDA Number: 1525394
Matrix, Dental — Dental And Oral

ACCRO FURNITURE INDUSTRIES 204-654-1114
305 McKay Ave, Winnipeg, MB R2G 0N5 Canada
FDA Number: n/a *Fax:* 204-654-2792
Web site: www.furniturewest.ca
Ownership: ACME CHROME FURNITURE LTD.
Produces/Sells CE-marked Devices: N
Distribution: Manufacturer Direct, Exporter

MANUFACTURER PROFILES

ACCU SCAN INSTRUMENTS, INC.   800-822-1344
5098 Trabue Road, Columbus, OH 43228-9563   **614-878-6644**
FDA Number: n/a   *Fax:* 866-650-8265
E-mail: sales@accuscan-usa.com
Web site: www.accuscan-usa.com
Annual Revenue: $0-$1 Million
Year Founded: 1996
Total Employees: 9   *Marketing Staff:* 1   *Sales Staff:* 3
Ownership: Private
Produces/Sells CE-marked Devices: Y
Federal Procurement Eligibility: Small Business, Minority Owned
Distribution: Manufacturer Direct, OEM, Service Direct, Exclusive Distributor, Exporter
General Admin.: R. H. Mandalaywala/President
Mktg./Adv.: M. E. Ocasio/Manager Advertising

Foodservice Product/Equipment	General
Sensor, Oxygen	Anesthesiology
Treadmill, Mechanical	Physical Med
Unit, Therapy, Behavior	General

ACCU-GLASS LLC   800-325-4796
10765 Trenton Avenue, St. Louis, MO 63132   **314-423-0300**
FDA Number: n/a   *Fax:* 314-423-0413
E-mail: info@accu-glass.com
Web site: www.accu-glass.com
Year Founded: 1960
Ownership: Private
Quality System Registration Information: ISO9001; ISO9002
Produces/Sells CE-marked Devices: Y
Distribution: OEM

Component, Other	General
Pipette Tip	Chemistry
Pipette, Micro	Chemistry
Tube, Blood Collection	Chemistry
Tube, Blood Microcollection	Chemistry
Tube, Capillary	Chemistry
Tube, Capillary Blood Collection	Hematology
Tubing, Other	General

ACCU-LINE PRODUCTS, INC.   800-363-7740
379 Iyannough Rd. (Rear Building),   **508-771-8022**
Hyannis, MA 02601
FDA Number: 1220372
E-mail: acculine@acculine.com   *Fax:* 508-771-8022
Web site: www.acculine.com
Medical Products Sales Volume: $3,000,000
Annual Revenue: $1-$5 Million
Year Founded: 1982
Total Employees: 10
Ownership: Private
Produces/Sells CE-marked Devices: N
Federal Procurement Eligibility: Small Business, Female Owned
Distribution: Manufacturer Direct, Exporter
General Admin.: Karleen Laviana/President
Production: Nancy E. Donnelly/General Manager Production
     James Laviana/Manager Materials

Label/Tag, Sterile	Surgery
Marker, Skin	Surgery
Pen, Marking, Surgical	Ophthalmology
Tape, Measuring, Ruler And Caliper	Surgery

ACCU-MEASURE, LLC   800-866-2727
P.O. Box 4411,   **303-799-4721**
Greenwood Village, CO 80155
FDA Number: 1722637
E-mail: info@accufitness.com   *Fax:* 303-799-4778
Web site: www.accumeasurefitness.com
Ownership: Private
Produces/Sells CE-marked Devices: N

Caliper	Orthopedics

ACCU-MED SERVICES   800-777-9141
300 Technecenter Drive, Milford, OH 45150   **513-831-1207**
FDA Number: n/a   *Fax:* 513-831-1370
E-mail: sales@accu-med.com
Web site: www.accu-med.com
Year Founded: 1984
Total Employees: 165   *Marketing Staff:* 3   *Sales Staff:* 10
Ownership: OMNICARE INC.
Produces/Sells CE-marked Devices: N
Distribution: Manufacturer Direct
General Admin.: William Oakley/Chief Financial Officer, Vice President Operations
     David Turner/President
Research: Greg Roberts/Vice President Product Development

Computer Software	General
Computer Software, Hospital/Nursing Management	General

ACCU-MED SERVICES   800-777-9141 *(cont'd)*
Computer, Patient Data Management   General

ACCU-MED TECHNOLOGIES, INC.   718-244-5330
150 Bud-mil Dr., Buffalo, NY 14206
FDA Number: 1320538

Orthosis, Limb Brace	Physical Med
Orthosis, Lumbar	Physical Med

ACCU-SCOPE, INC.   631-864-1000
73 mall dr, commack, NY 11725
FDA Number: 2435594
E-mail: info@accu-scope.com   *Fax:* 631-543-8900
Web site: www.accu-scope.com
Ownership: Private
Quality System Registration Information: ISO9001
Produces/Sells CE-marked Devices: Y
Federal Procurement Eligibility: Small Business
Distribution: Manufacturer Through Distributor
General Admin.: Jay Berliner/President, Chief Executive Officer
Mktg./Adv.: Brian Taub/Manager National Sales

Microscope	Hematology
Microscope, Inverted Stage, Tissue Culture	Pathology
Microscope, Laboratory, Optical	Microbiology
Microscope, Light	Pathology
Microscope, Phase Contrast	Pathology
Microscope, Tissue Culture	Microbiology
Oil, Immersion	Hematology
Stage, Microscope	Pathology
Television Monitor, Microscope	General

ACCUECH, LLC   800-749-9910
2641 La Mirada Drive, Vista, CA 92081   **760-599-6555**
FDA Number: 2031919
E-mail: info@accutech-llc.com
Web site: www.accutech-llc.com
Ownership: Private
Produces/Sells CE-marked Devices: N

Campylobacter Pylori	Microbiology
Enzymatic Esterase-Oxidase, Cholesterol	Chemistry
Enzyme Immunoassay, Theophylline	Toxicology
LDL & VLDL Precipitation, Cholesterol Via Esterase-Oxidase	Chemistry

ACCUGENICS
See Biomerieux Inc.

ACCUMED INTERNATIONAL
See Trek Diagnostic Systems

ACCUMED SYSTEMS, INC.   734-930-0461
6109 Jackson Road, Ann Arbor, MI 48103
FDA Number: 1833799
E-mail: info@accumedsystemsinc.com   *Fax:* 734-930-0479
Web site: www.accumedsystemsinc.com
Medical Products Sales Volume: $100,000
Annual Revenue: $0-$1 Million
Year Founded: 1991
Total Employees: 5
Ownership: Private
Quality System Registration Information: ISO9003
Produces/Sells CE-marked Devices: Y
Federal Procurement Eligibility: Small Business
Distribution: Manufacturer Direct

Orthosis, Limb Brace	Physical Med
Surgical Instrument, Cardiovascular	Cardiovascular
Tourniquet, Non-Pneumatic, Surgical	Surgery

ACCUMEDIX, INC.   847-548-8499
888 E. Belvidere Rd. Suite 212, Grayslake, IL 60030
FDA Number: 1424785
Ownership: Private
Produces/Sells CE-marked Devices: N

Burr, Dental	Dental And Oral
Implant, Endosseous	Dental And Oral

ACCUMETRICS, INC.   888-919-9333
3985 Sorrento Valley Blvd., San Diego, CA 92121   **858-643-1600**
FDA Number: 2031760
E-mail: support@accumetrics.com   *Fax:* 858-875-0603
Web site: www.accumetrics.com
Ownership: Private
Produces/Sells CE-marked Devices: N
General Admin.: Mr. Timothy Still/President, Chief Executive Officer
Mktg./Adv.: Ms. Dianah Schmidt/Executive Director Marketing & Sales
     Mr. Ad de Waard/Vice President International Marketing & Sales
     Mr. Andrew Chrisholm/Vice President Sales
Production: Mr. William Dippel/Executive Vice President Operations
     Mr. Jeff Dahlen/Vice President Regulatory & Clinical Affairs

ACCUMETRICS, INC.   888-919-9333 (cont'd)
Finance: Mr. Gregory Tibbitts/Chief Financial Officer
Analyzer, Platelet Aggregation, Automated   Hematology

ACCUMIN DIAGNOSTICS, INC.   212-659-0711
750 Lexington Ave., 20th Floor, New York, NY 10022
FDA Number: 2087480
Ownership: Private
Produces/Sells CE-marked Devices: N
Turbidimetric Method, Protein Or Albumin (Urinary)   Chemistry

ACCUPAC, INC.   215-256-7011
1501 Industrial Blvd., Mainland, PA 19451
FDA Number: 2518467
Cleaner, Denture   Dental And Oral

ACCURATE CHEMICAL & SCIENTIFIC CORP.   800-645-6264
300 Shames Dr., Westbury, NY 11590-1736   516-333-2221
FDA Number: 2429411   *Fax:* 516-997-4948
E-mail: info@accuratechemical.com
Web site: www.accuratechemical.com
Annual Revenue: $1-$5 Million
Year Founded: 1974
Total Employees: 20   *Marketing Staff:* 1   *Sales Staff:* 1
Ownership: Private
Produces/Sells CE-marked Devices: N
Federal Procurement Eligibility: Small Business, GSA Contract
Distribution: Manufacturer Direct, OEM, Exclusive Distributor
General Admin.: R Rosenberg/President
Analyzer, Chemistry, ELISA   Chemistry
Antibody, Monoclonal   Microbiology
Antigen, Antiserum, Control, IGA   Immunology
Antigen, Antiserum, Control, Transferrin   Immunology
Standard, Carbohydrate   Chemistry
Standard, Lipid   Chemistry

ACCURATE METERING SYSTEMS, INC.   270-737-6666AõÉ
1651 Wilkening Rd., Schaumburg, IL 60173
FDA Number: n/a
Annual Revenue: $0-$1 Million
Ownership: Private
Produces/Sells CE-marked Devices: Y
Distribution: Manufacturer Direct
Gauge, Gas Pressure, Cylinder/Pipeline   Anesthesiology

ACCURATE SET, INC.   973-824-0810
1199 Broad St., Newark, NJ 07114-1834
FDA Number: 2240725   *Fax:* 1 973 565 0087
E-mail: accurateset@aol.com
Annual Revenue: $0-$1 Million
Ownership: Private
Produces/Sells CE-marked Devices: N
Federal Procurement Eligibility: Small Business, Minority Owned
Distribution: Manufacturer Direct, Manufacturer Through Distributor, Exporter
Agent, Polishing, Abrasive, Oral Cavity   Dental And Oral
Crown And Bridge, Temporary, Resin   Dental And Oral
Foil, Dental   Dental And Oral
Material, Acrylic, Dental   Dental And Oral
Material, Impression   Dental And Oral
Material, Impression Tray, Resin   Dental And Oral
Syringe, Restorative And Impression Material   Dental And Oral
Tray, Impression   Dental And Oral

ACCURAY INCORPORATED   888-522-3740
1310 Chesapeake Terrace,   408-716-4600
Sunnyvale, CA 94089
FDA Number: 3005738050
Web site: www.accuray.com   *Fax:* 408-716-4601
Ownership: Private
Produces/Sells CE-marked Devices: N
General Admin.: Mr. Derek Bertocci/Chief Financial Officer, Senior Vice President
     Mr. Chris Raanes/Chief Operating Officer, Senior Vice President
     Eun Thomson/President, Chief Executive Officer
Accelerator, Linear, Medical   Radiology
System, Planning, Radiation Therapy Treatment   Radiology

ACCURAY, INC.   888-522-3740
1310 Chesapeake Terrace,   408-716-4600
Sunnyvale, CA 94089
FDA Number: 2950679   *Fax:* 408-716-4601
Web site: www.accuray.com
Year Founded: 1990
Total Employees: 487
Ownership: Public
Stock Symbol: ARAY
Traded On: NASDAQ
Produces/Sells CE-marked Devices: Y
General Admin.: Mr. Derek Bertocci/Chief Financial Officer, Executive Vice President

ACCURAY, INC.   888-522-3740 (cont'd)
     Mr. Chris Raanes/Chief Operating Officer, Senior Vice President
     Dr. Euan Thomson/President, Chief Executive Officer
Mktg./Adv.: Mr. Eric Pauwels/Senior Vice President Marketing
Accelerator, Linear, Medical   Radiology
System, Planning, Radiation Therapy Treatment   Radiology

ACCURI CYTOMETERS INC.   734-994-8000
173 Parkland Plaza, Ann Arbor, MI 48103
FDA Number: n/a   *Fax:* 734-994-8002
Web site: http://www.accuricytometers.com
Ownership: Private
Produces/Sells CE-marked Devices: N
General Admin.: Mr. Steve Chipchase/Chief Operating Officer
     Mr. Collin Rich/Chief Technology Officer
     Mr. Jeffrey Williams/President, Chief Executive Officer
Mktg./Adv.: Mr. Jack Ball/Commercial Director
Finance: Mr. John Dahler/Chief Financial Officer

ACCUSYNC MEDICAL RESEARCH CORP.   203-877-1610
132 Research Dr., Milford, CT 06460
FDA Number: 1219392   *Fax:* 203-877-8972
Ownership: Private
Produces/Sells CE-marked Devices: N
Electrocardiograph, Single Channel   Cardiovascular
Monitor, Cardiac (Cardiotachometer & Rate Alarm)   Cardiovascular
Synchronizer, Electrocardiograph, Nuclear   Radiology

ACCUTOME ULTRASOUND, INC.   800-889-0200
3222 Phoenixville Pike, Malvern, PA 19355   610-889-0200
FDA Number: 1226360   *Fax:* 610-889-3233
E-mail: info@accutome.com
Web site: www.accutome.com
Ownership: Private
Produces/Sells CE-marked Devices: N
Adaptometer (Biophotometer)   Ophthalmology
Lamp, Slit, Biomicroscope, AC-Powered   Ophthalmology
Scanner, Ultrasonic (Pulsed Echo)   Radiology
Shell, Scleral   Ophthalmology
Stimulator, Photic, Evoked Response   Cns/Neurology
Tonometer, AC-Powered   Ophthalmology
Transducer, Ultrasonic, Diagnostic   Radiology

ACCUTOME, INC.   800-979-2020
3222 Phoenixville Pike, Malvern, PA 19355   610-889-0200
FDA Number: 2521877   *Fax:* 610-889-3233
E-mail: info@accutome.com
Web site: www.accutome.com
Ownership: Private
Produces/Sells CE-marked Devices: N
Adaptometer (Biophotometer)   Ophthalmology
Caliper, Ophthalmic   Ophthalmology
Cannula, Ophthalmic   Ophthalmology
Chart, Visual Acuity   Ophthalmology
Curette, Ophthalmic   Ophthalmology
Depressor, Orbital   Ophthalmology
Dilator, Lacrimal   Ophthalmology
Forceps, Ophthalmic   Ophthalmology
Gauge, Measuring   Ear/Nose/Throat
Holder, Needle   Gastroenterology/Urology
Hook, Ophthalmic   Ophthalmology
Instrument, Microsurgical   Cns/Neurology
Knife, Ophthalmic   Ophthalmology
Knife, Surgical   Dental And Oral
Marker, Ocular   Ophthalmology
Microscope, Operating, AC-Powered, Ophthalmic   Ophthalmology
Needle, Suture, Reusable   Surgery
Perimeter, Manual   Ophthalmology
Probe   Orthopedics
Ring, Ophthalmic (Flieringa)   Ophthalmology
Scanner, Ultrasonic (Pulsed Echo)   Radiology
Scissors, Ophthalmic   Ophthalmology
Spatula, Ophthalmic   Ophthalmology
Speculum, Ophthalmic   Ophthalmology
Spoon, Ophthalmic   Ophthalmology
Sterilizer, Steam (Autoclave)   General
Strip, Fluorescein   Ophthalmology
Suture, Absorbable, Synthetic, Polyglycolic Acid   Surgery
Suture, Non-Absorbable, Silk   Surgery
Suture, Non-Absorbable, Synthetic, Polyamide   Surgery
Suture, Non-Absorbable, Synthetic, Polyethylene   Surgery
Tray, Surgical Instrument   Surgery

ACCUTRON, INC.   800-531-2221
1733 W. Parkside Lane, Phoenix, AZ 85027-2622   623-780-2020
FDA Number: n/a   *Fax:* 623-780-0444
E-mail: info@accutron-inc.com
Web site: www.accutron-inc.com
Medical Products Sales Volume: $4,300,000
Annual Revenue: $5-$10 Million

ACCUTRON, INC.   800-531-2221 *(cont'd)*
Total Employees: 30   *Marketing Staff:* 1   *Sales Staff:* 17
Ownership: Private
Quality System Registration Information: ISO9001
Produces/Sells CE-marked Devices: Y
Federal Procurement Eligibility: Small Business
Distribution: Manufacturer Through Distributor
General Admin.: Richard Blasdell/Chief Executive Officer
     Julia Vaughn/President
     Jon Blasdell/Vice President
Mktg./Adv.: Collene Schute-Fitzpatric/Director Marketing
   Gas-Machine, Analgesia   Anesthesiology

ACCUVEIN LLC   816-997-9400
40 Goose Hill Road, Cold Spring Harbor, NY 11724
FDA Number: 3007121351
E-mail: info@accuvein.com   *Fax:* 631-270-3960
Web site: http://accuvein.com
Ownership: Private
Produces/Sells CE-marked Devices: N
Distribution: Manufacturer Through Manufacturer Reps
   Locator, Vein, Liquid Crystal   General

ACE HEARING LABORATORY, LLC   877-452-2044
2304 S.E. 14th St., Bentonville, AR 72712   **479-273-6006**
FDA Number: 1650902
E-mail: questions@acehearing.com
Web site: www.acehearing.com
Ownership: Private
Produces/Sells CE-marked Devices: N
General Admin.: Mr. Dow Chandler/Owner
   Hearing-Aid   Ear/Nose/Throat

ACE HOSE & RUBBER COMPANY   888-223-4673
1333 South Jefferson St.,   **312-829-4673**
Chicago, IL 60607
FDA Number: 9310001
E-mail: brubehrs@acehose.com   *Fax:* 312-850-4673
Web site: www.acehose.com
Medical Products Sales Volume: $600,000
Annual Revenue: $0-$1 Million
Year Founded: 1943
Total Employees: 3   *Marketing Staff:* 1   *Sales Staff:* 2
Ownership: Private
Produces/Sells CE-marked Devices: N
Federal Procurement Eligibility: Small Business
Distribution: Manufacturer Direct, Manufacturer Through Distributor, Manufacturer Through Manufacturer Reps, Exclusive Distributor, Importer
General Admin.: Bruce Behrstock/President
Mktg./Adv.: Bruce Behrstock/President Marketing
   Floor Mat   General
   Floor Mat, Antibacterial   General
   Silicone Sheeting   General
   Tubing, Latex   General
   Tubing, Polyvinyl Chloride   General
   Tubing, Silicone   General

ACE LITE STEP COMPANY
   See Ace Hose & Rubber Company

ACE MEDICAL MANUFACTURING
   See Depuy Ace, A Johnson & Johnson Company

ACE ORTHOPEDIC MANUFACTURING
   See Depuy Ace, A Johnson & Johnson Company

ACE SURGICAL SUPPLY CO., INC.   800-441-3100
1034 Pearl St., Brockton, MA 02301   **508-588-3100**
FDA Number: n/a   *Fax:* 508-583-3140
E-mail: info@acesurgical.com
Web site: www.acesurgical.com
Annual Revenue: $10-$25 Million
Total Employees: 50   *Marketing Staff:* 5   *Sales Staff:* 10
Ownership: Private
Quality System Registration Information: ISO9001
Produces/Sells CE-marked Devices: Y
Federal Procurement Eligibility: Small Business
Distribution: Manufacturer Direct, Manufacturer Through Manufacturer Reps
General Admin.: J. Edward Carchidi/President, Chief Executive Officer
Mktg./Adv.: Christopher Carchidi/Director Marketing
     J. Edward Carchidi/Director Product Development
Production: Cindy Betters/Director Quality Assurance
     Craig Carchidi/Manager Regulatory Affairs
   Accessories, Apparel, Surgical   Surgery
   Blade, Scalpel   Surgery
   Burr, Dental   Dental And Oral
   Chisel, Osteotome, Surgical   Dental And Oral
   Drill, Bone, Powered   Dental And Oral
   Gauge, Depth, Instrument, Dental   Dental And Oral
   Graft, Bone   Orthopedics

ACE SURGICAL SUPPLY CO., INC.   800-441-3100 *(cont'd)*
   Implant, Endosseous   Dental And Oral
   Instrument, Dental, Manual   Dental And Oral
   Kit, Irrigation, Oral   Ear/Nose/Throat
   Motor, Surgical Instrument, Pneumatic-Powered   Surgery
   Plate, Bone, Orthodontic   Dental And Oral
   Punch, Surgical   Surgery
   Restraint, Wheelchair   General
   Saw, Powered, And Accessories   Cns/Neurology
   Screw, Fixation, Intraosseous   Dental And Oral
   Syringe, Irrigating   General
   Tube, Transfer   General
   Tubing, Fluid Delivery   General
   Wire, Orthodontic   Dental And Oral

ACEME TECHNOLOGIES INT'L.   916-549-2170
278 Howe Avenue, Suite B, Sacramento, CA 95825
FDA Number: 2953739
Ownership: Private
Produces/Sells CE-marked Devices: N
   Scooter (Motorized 3-Wheeled Vehicle)   Physical Med

ACERNA INC.   905-472-5747
19 Bryant Road, Markham, ONT L3P-5Y7 Canada
FDA Number: n/a   *Fax:* 905-472-2322
E-mail: info@acerna.ca
Web site: www.acerna.ca
Year Founded: 1995
Total Employees: 10
Ownership: Private
Produces/Sells CE-marked Devices: N

ACHESON COLLOIDS COMPANY   800-255-1908
1600 Washington Avenue, Port Huron, MI 48060   **810-984-5581**
FDA Number: n/a   *Fax:* 810-984-1446
E-mail: acphcust@ici.com
Web site: www.achesonindustries.com
Medical Products Sales Volume: $13,700,000
Annual Revenue: $100-$500 Million
Year Founded: 1908
Total Employees: 241   *Sales Staff:* 10
Ownership: ICI
Quality System Registration Information: ISO9001; ISO9002
Produces/Sells CE-marked Devices: N
Federal Procurement Eligibility: Small Business
Distribution: Manufacturer Direct, Manufacturer Through Distributor, Manufacturer Through Manufacturer Reps, Importer, Exporter
General Admin.: Derick Whyte/General Manager
Mktg./Adv.: Mike Gnaegy/Director Sales
   Lubricant, Instrument   General

ACHIEVE HEALTHCARE TECHNOLOGIES   800-869-1322
7690 Golden Triangle Drive,   **952-995-9800**
Eden Prairie, MN 55344
FDA Number: n/a   *Fax:* 952-995-9735
E-mail: info@achievehealthcare.com
Web site: www.achievehealthcare.com
Medical Products Sales Volume: $18,000,000
Annual Revenue: $10-$25 Million
Year Founded: 1994
Total Employees: 180   *Marketing Staff:* 10   *Sales Staff:* 18
Ownership: Private
Produces/Sells CE-marked Devices: N
Federal Procurement Eligibility: Small Business
Distribution: Manufacturer Direct
General Admin.: Reef Gillum/Chairman
     Larry Garatoni/Chief Executive Officer
     Rich Giddings/President
     Dawna Bowman/Vice President Human Resources
Mktg./Adv.: Zoe Bolton/Vice President Marketing
   Computer Software   General

ACHILLES USA, INC.   425-353-7000
1407 80th St. S.W., Everett, WA 98203
FDA Number: n/a   *Fax:* 425-347-5785
Web site: www.achillesusa.com
Annual Revenue: $50-$100 Million
Ownership: ACHILLES
Quality System Registration Information: ISO9001
Produces/Sells CE-marked Devices: N
Distribution: Manufacturer Direct
   Bag, Blood, Collection   Hematology
   Bag, Drainage (Incontinence)   Gastroenterology/Urology
   Bracelet, Identification   General
   Component, Plastic   General
   Cover, Mattress   General
   Pack, Cold   General

ACHILLES USA, INC. 425-353-7000 *(cont'd)*
Unit, Pad, Heating, Portable — Physical Med

ACI 913-384-7390
5830 Woodson, Suite 3, Mission, KS 66202
FDA Number: 3005863177
Ownership: Private
Produces/Sells CE-marked Devices: N
Base, Denture, Relining, Repairing, Rebasing, Resin — Dental And Oral

ACI MEDICAL, INC. 800-667-9451
1857 Diamond St., San Marcos, CA 92078-5129 760-744-4400
Fax: 760-744-4401
FDA Number: 2027046
E-mail: info@acimedical.com
Web site: www.acimedical.com
Year Founded: 1984
Total Employees: 25
Ownership: Private
Produces/Sells CE-marked Devices: N
Federal Procurement Eligibility: Small Business
Distribution: Manufacturer Direct, Manufacturer Through Manufacturer Reps, OEM
General Admin.: Edward J. Arkans/President
Mktg./Adv.: Don Kjartanson/Manager Marketing
Component, Electronic — General
Component, Plastic — General
Compression Instrument — Orthopedics
Legging, Compression, Inflatable, Sequential — Cardiovascular
Molding, Custom — General
Plethysmograph, Photo-Electric, Pneumatic Or Hydraulic — Cardiovascular
Service, Engineering/Design — General
Sleeve, Compressible Limb — Cardiovascular
Stent, Other — Obstetrics/Gynecology

ACIST MEDICAL SYSTEMS, INC. 888-667-6648
7905 Fuller Road, Eden Prairie, MN 55344 952-995-9300
Fax: 952-941-4648
FDA Number: 2134243
Total Employees: 220
Ownership: Private
Produces/Sells CE-marked Devices: N
Cable — Physical Med
Injector, Angiographic (Cardiac Catheterization) — Cardiovascular
Injector, Contrast Medium, Automatic — Radiology
Injector, Syringe — General
Plethysmograph, Impedance — Cardiovascular
Pump, Infusion — General
Tubing, Fluid Delivery — General

ACK LABORATORIES, INC. 908-707-9244
540 Stony Brook Dr., Bridgewater, NJ 08807
FDA Number: 2431311
Stimulator, Electro/Acupuncture — Anesthesiology

ACKERMAN NUCLEAR
See Nuclear Pharmacy Services

ACME OF PRECISION SURGICAL CO., INC. 973-373-6797
485 South 21st St., Irvington, NJ 07111
Fax: 973-373-1267
FDA Number: 2240230
Ownership: Private
Produces/Sells CE-marked Devices: N
Saw, Nasal — Ear/Nose/Throat
Scissors, Collar And Crown — Dental And Oral
Scissors, Disposable — General
Scissors, Episiotomy — Obstetrics/Gynecology
Scissors, Nasal — Ear/Nose/Throat
Scissors, Surgical Tissue, Dental (Oral) — Dental And Oral
Scissors, Wire Cutting, ENT — Ear/Nose/Throat

ACME-MONACO CORP. 860-224-1349
75 Winchell Drive, New Britain, CT 06052-1017
Fax: 860-827-9982
FDA Number: 1293141
E-mail: acmecorp@acmemonaco.com
Web site: www.acmemonaco.com
Medical Products Sales Volume: $8,300,000
Annual Revenue: $10-$25 Million
Year Founded: 1947
Total Employees: 180   Marketing Staff: 1   Sales Staff: 7
Ownership: Private
Quality System Registration Information: ISO9001
Produces/Sells CE-marked Devices: Y
Federal Procurement Eligibility: Small Business
Distribution: OEM
General Admin.: Michael Karabin/Chief Executive Officer, Chairman
Roger Karabin/President
Production: Richard Ohidy/Manager Regulatory Affairs
Bruce Bull/Vice President Operations
Clamp, Wire, Orthodontic — Dental And Oral
Contract Manufacturing — General
Guide, Wire, Angiographic (And Accessories) — Cns/Neurology
Guidewire — Cardiovascular

ACME-MONACO CORP. 860-224-1349 *(cont'd)*
Guidewire, Catheter — Cardiovascular
Guidewire, Catheter, Radiological — Radiology
Handle, Instrument, Dental — Dental And Oral
Spring, Orthodontic — Dental And Oral
Stylet, Catheter — Cardiovascular
Wire, Orthodontic — Dental And Oral
Medical Product Subsidiaries (Listed Separately)
Acme-Monaco Corp.

ACON LABORATORIES, INC. 858-535-2030
10125 Mesa Rim Road., San Diego, CA 92121
Fax: 858-535-2035
FDA Number: 2531491
E-mail: info@aconlabs.com
Web site: www.aconlabs.com
Medical Products Sales Volume: $6,700,000
Year Founded: 1996
Total Employees: 70
Ownership: Private
Quality System Registration Information: ISO9001
Produces/Sells CE-marked Devices: Y
Federal Procurement Eligibility: Small Business
Distribution: Manufacturer Direct, Manufacturer Through Distributor, Manufacturer Through Manufacturer Reps, OEM, Service Direct, Exclusive Distributor, Importer, Exporter
General Admin.: James Lin/Chief Executive Officer
Jixun Lin, MD, PhD/Director
Kit, Pregnancy Test — Obstetrics/Gynecology
Kit, Pregnancy Test, Over The Counter, HCG — Chemistry
Monitor, Blood Glucose (Test) — Gastroenterology/Urology
Strip, Test — Chemistry
System, Identification, Hepatitis B Antigen — Hematology
System, Test, Drugs of Abuse — Chemistry
Test System, Nicotine, Cotinine, Metabolites — Toxicology
Test, Antibody, Acquired Immune Deficiency Syndrome (AIDS) — Hematology
Test, Ethyl Alcohol — Toxicology
Test, Fertility Monitoring — Obstetrics/Gynecology
Test, Infectious Mononucleosis — Immunology

ACOR ORTHOPAEDIC, INC. 216-662-4500
18530 South Miles Pkwy., Cleveland, OH 44128-4238
FDA Number: 1527888
Web site: www.acor.com
Medical Products Sales Volume: $10,000,000
Annual Revenue: $5-$10 Million
Ownership: Private
Produces/Sells CE-marked Devices: N
Federal Procurement Eligibility: Small Business
Distribution: Manufacturer Direct, Manufacturer Through Manufacturer Reps
Accessories, Fixation, Orthopedic — Orthopedics
Brace, Joint, Ankle (External) — Physical Med
Cover, Limb — Physical Med
Custom Prosthesis — Orthopedics
Insoles, Medical — General
Orthosis, Corrective Shoe — Physical Med
Shoe, Orthopedic — Orthopedics

ACORDA THERAPEUTICS, INC 914-347-4300
15 Skyline Drive, Hawthorne, NY 10532
Fax: 914-347-4560
FDA Number: n/a
E-mail: info@acorda.com
Ownership: Private
Produces/Sells CE-marked Devices: N
General Admin.: Mr. Andrew Blight/Chief Scientific Officer
Ms. Jane Wasman/Executive Vice President
Mr. Ron Cohen/President, Chief Executive Officer
Ms. Tierney Saccavino/Senior Vice President
Ms. Denise Duca/Senior Vice President Human Resources
Medical Admin.: Mr. Thomas Wessel/Chief Medical Officer
Mktg./Adv.: Ms. Elizabeth Keating/Vice President Marketing
Mr. Kerry Clem/Vice President Sales
Production: Ms. Lauren Sabella/Executive Vice President Development
Research: Mr. Anthony Caggiano/Vice President Research & Development
Finance: Mr. David Lawrence/Chief Financial Officer
Ms. Jennifer Burstein/Vice President Finance

ACORN ENGINEERING CO.
See Whitehall Manufacturing

ACORN INTERNATIONAL GROUP, INC. 770-9931777
923 Spring Glen Place, Suwanee, GA 30024
FDA Number: 1066696
Ownership: Private
Stock Symbol: HB
Traded On: NYSE
Produces/Sells CE-marked Devices: N

ACP CHEMICALS INC. 800-363-9861
4601 blvd. Des Grandes Prairies, 514-327-0323
St-Leonard, QUE H1R-1 Canada
FDA Number: n/a *Fax:* 514-327-8474
E-mail: sales@acpchem.com
Web site: www.acpchem.com
Year Founded: 1986
Total Employees: 50
Ownership: Private
Produces/Sells CE-marked Devices: N
Distribution: Manufacturer Direct, Exclusive Distributor

ACRA CUT, INC. 800-227-2288
989 Main St., Acton, MA 01720 978-263-0250
FDA Number: 1220724 *Fax:* 978-263-4102
Web site: www.acracut.com
Ownership: Private
Produces/Sells CE-marked Devices: N
Accessories, Powered Drill Cns/Neurology
Applier, Surgical, Clip Surgery
Clip, Scalp Cns/Neurology
Drill, Powered Compound (With Burr, Trephine & Accessories) Cns/Neurology
Instrument, Clip Removal Cns/Neurology
Surgical Instrument, Disposable Surgery
Surgical Instrument, Non-Powered, Neurosurgical Cns/Neurology

ACRO ASSOCIATES 800-672-2276
1990 Olivera Rd., Suite A, Concord, CA 94520 925-676-8828
FDA Number: n/a *Fax:* 925-680-8113
E-mail: info@acroassociates.com
Web site: www.acroassociates.com
Medical Products Sales Volume: $4,000,000
Annual Revenue: $1-$5 Million
Year Founded: 1976
Total Employees: 30 *Marketing Staff:* 2 *Sales Staff:* 2
Ownership: Private
Produces/Sells CE-marked Devices: N
Federal Procurement Eligibility: Small Business
Distribution: Manufacturer Direct, OEM, Exporter
General Admin.: Mr. Al Huntley/Chief Executive Officer, Vice President
Mr. Russell Ziegler/President
Mktg./Adv.: Mr. Winston Wong/Vice President Marketing & Sales
Production: Ms. Rondi Davison/Customer Service Representative
Mr. Blaik Musolf/Director Engineering
Occluder, Cardiovascular Cardiovascular
Valve, Laboratory Chemistry

ACRO BIOTECH LLC. 909-466-6892
9500 7th Street Unit M, Cucamonga, CA 91730
FDA Number: 3005360469
Enzyme Immunoassay, Amphetamine Toxicology
Enzyme Immunoassay, Benzodiazepine Toxicology
Enzyme Immunoassay, Cannabinoids Toxicology
Enzyme Immunoassay, Cocaine And Cocaine Metabolites Toxicology
Enzyme Immunoassay, Opiates Toxicology
Enzyme Immunoassay, Phencyclidine Toxicology
Thin Layer Chromatography, Metamphetamine Toxicology

ACROMETRIX 707-746-8888
6058 Egret Ct., Benicia, CA 94510
FDA Number: 2954316
Ownership: Private
Produces/Sells CE-marked Devices: N
Control, Analyte (Assayed And Unassayed) Chemistry
Control, Multi Analyte (Assayed And Unassayed) Chemistry

ACRYDERM, INC.
See Acrymed, Inc.

ACRYMED, INC. 503-624-9830
9560 SW Nimbus Avenue, Beaverton, OR 97008
FDA Number: 3029160 *Fax:* 503-639-0846
E-mail: kjacque@acrymed.com
Web site: www.acrymed.com
Annual Revenue: $1-$5 Million
Year Founded: 2000
Total Employees: 25 *Marketing Staff:* 2 *Sales Staff:* 1
Ownership: Private
Quality System Registration Information: ISO9001
Produces/Sells CE-marked Devices: Y
Federal Procurement Eligibility: Small Business
Distribution: OEM, Exclusive Distributor
General Admin.: Dr. Bruce L. Gibbins/Chief Technology Officer
Production: Kasey Griffin/Director Quality Control & Regulatory Affairs
Finance: Jack D. McMaken/President
Dressing, Germicidal General
Dressing, Other General
Dressing, Wound and Burn, Hydrogel Surgery
Dressing, Wound and Burn, Interactive Surgery

ACRYMED, INC. 503-624-9830 *(cont'd)*
Medical Disinfectants/Cleaners for Instruments General

ACS
See Applied Cardiac Systems, Inc.

ACS
See Polymer Laboratories, Now A Part Of Varian, Inc.

ACT
See Medin Corporation

ACT ELECTRONICS, INC. 978-567-4024
2 Cabot Rd., Hudson, MA 01749
FDA Number: 3003982025
Ownership: Private
Produces/Sells CE-marked Devices: N

ACT-AEROMED COPAN TECHNOLOGIES LLC. 951-549-8793
85 Commerce Street, Glastonbury, CT 06033
FDA Number: 3005981426
Equipment, Laboratory, Gen. Purpose (Specific Medical Use) Chemistry
Pipette, Micro Chemistry

ACTALL CORP. 800-598-1745
3925 Monaco Parkway, Unit D, 303-226-4799
Denver, CO 80207
FDA Number: n/a *Fax:* 303-650-4523
E-mail: sales@actallsp.com
Web site: www.actall.com
Medical Products Sales Volume: $700,000
Annual Revenue: $1-$5 Million
Year Founded: 1991
Total Employees: 8 *Marketing Staff:* 2 *Sales Staff:* 3
Ownership: Private
Produces/Sells CE-marked Devices: N
Federal Procurement Eligibility: Small Business
Distribution: Manufacturer Through Manufacturer Reps
General Admin.: Erven Tallman/Chief Executive Officer
Ari Shore/Vice President
Communication System, Emergency Alert, Personal General
Computer Equipment General

ACTAVIS MID ATLANTIC LLC 704-735-5700
1877 Kawai Rd., Lincolnton, NC 28092
FDA Number: 1053439
Web site: www.actavis.com
Ownership: Private
Produces/Sells CE-marked Devices: N
Condom Obstetrics/Gynecology
Lubricant, Patient General

ACTEON INC. 800-289-6367
124 Gaither Drive, Suite 140, 856-222-9988
Mount Laurel, NJ 08054
FDA Number: 2243757 *Fax:* 856-222-4726
E-mail: info@us.acteongroup.com
Web site: www.acteongroup.com
Annual Revenue: $50-$100 Million
Year Founded: 1946
Total Employees: 661
Ownership: ACTEON GROUP
Quality System Registration Information: ISO9001
Produces/Sells CE-marked Devices: Y
Distribution: Manufacturer Direct, Manufacturer Through Distributor, OEM
General Admin.: Mr. Haye Hinrichs/Vice President
Mktg./Adv.: Mr. Wyatt Wilson/Manager National Sales
Production: Mr. Rick Rosati/Director Quality Assurance
Curette, Endodontic Dental And Oral
Endodontic Instrument Dental And Oral
Locator, Apex, Root Dental And Oral
Preparer, Root Canal, Endodontic Dental And Oral
Reamer, Pulp Canal, Endodontic Dental And Oral
Scaler, Ultrasonic Dental And Oral
Spreader, Pulp Canal Filling Material, Endodontic Dental And Oral
Sterilizer, Bulk, Steam & Ethylene-Oxide General

ACTION AFRICA - ARTIQUE REFRIGERATION 520-762-9293
16335 S. Houghton Rd. #115, Corona De Tucson, AZ 85641
FDA Number: n/a
Ownership: Private
Produces/Sells CE-marked Devices: N
Freezer, Blood Storage Hematology

ACTION BAG CO. 800-490-8830
1001 Entry Dr., Bensenville, IL 60106 630-496-6203
FDA Number: n/a *Fax:* 630-766-2063
E-mail: info@actionbag.com
Web site: www.actionbag.com/healthcare
Annual Revenue: $5-$10 Million
Year Founded: 1980

ACTION BAG CO.   800-490-8830 *(cont'd)*
Total Employees: 37   Marketing Staff: 3   Sales Staff: 7
Ownership: Private
Produces/Sells CE-marked Devices: N
Federal Procurement Eligibility: Small Business, Female Owned
Distribution: Manufacturer Direct, Manufacturer Through Distributor, Manufacturer Through Manufacturer Reps, Importer
General Admin.: Nancy Cwynar/President, Chief Executive Officer
Mktg./Adv.: Jaimey Alumbaugh/Director Marketing
     Diane Sabel/Sales Representative
     John Mattes/Sales Representative

Accessories, Wheelchair	Physical Med
Aid, Control, Environmental, Controlled, Breath	Physical Med
Bag, Plastic	General

ACTION LLC   757-491-4175
1112 Jensen Dr., #103, Virginia Beach, VA 23451
FDA Number: 3004466924   Fax: 757-491-4872
E-mail: sales@actionsurgical.com
Web site: www.actionsurgical.com
Ownership: Private
Produces/Sells CE-marked Devices: N

Cleaner, Ultrasonic, Medical Instrument	General

ACTION PRODUCTS, INC.   800-228-7763
954 Sweeney Drive,   301-797-1414
Hagerstown, MD 21740
FDA Number: 1181047   Fax: 301-733-2073
E-mail: service@actionproducts.com
Web site: www.actionproducts.com
Medical Products Sales Volume: $13,000,000
Annual Revenue: $10-$25 Million
Year Founded: 1970
Total Employees: 150   Marketing Staff: 3   Sales Staff: 5
Ownership: Private
Quality System Registration Information: ISO9000
Produces/Sells CE-marked Devices: Y
Federal Procurement Eligibility: VA Contract
Distribution: Manufacturer Through Manufacturer Reps, OEM, Exporter
General Admin.: Robert T. McKnight/President
Mktg./Adv.: C. P. McElroy/Vice President International Sales
     Michael Bredal/Vice President Sales
Production: D. M. Laing/Vice President Operations

Cushion, Flotation	Physical Med
Cushion, Wheelchair (Pad)	Physical Med
Exerciser, Passive, Non-Measuring (CPM Machine)	Physical Med
Insoles, Medical	General
Mattress, Non-Powered Flotation Therapy	Physical Med
Phantom, Anthropomorphic, Radiographic	Radiology
Protector, Heel	General

ACTION TOP END, DIV. OF INVACARE CORPORATION
See Invacare Top End Sports And Recreation Products

ACTIVA BRAND PRODUCTS INC.   800-991-4464
105 Industrial Cres,   902-566-3229
Summerside, PEI C1N-5 Canada
FDA Number: 8022064   Fax: 902-436-3219
E-mail: distributors@advantajet.com
Web site: www.advantajet.com
Medical Products Sales Volume: $9,000,000
Year Founded: 1985
Total Employees: 6   Marketing Staff: 2   Sales Staff: 2
Ownership: Symmetricom, Inc.
Produces/Sells CE-marked Devices: N
Distribution: Manufacturer Direct, Manufacturer Through Manufacturer Reps

ACTIVAIR DIV.
See Duracell Usa

ACTIVANT SOLUTIONS INC.   800-776-7438
19 West College Avenue, Yardley, CO 19067   215-493-8900
FDA Number: n/a   Fax: 215-321-8001
E-mail: kim.meiser@activant.com
Web site: www.turns.com
Medical Products Sales Volume: $266,000,000
Year Founded: 1972
Total Employees: 2100   Sales Staff: 6
Ownership: Private
Produces/Sells CE-marked Devices: N
Distribution: Service Direct
General Admin.: Marsha Golgart/Executive Vice President
     Brad Smith/President
Mktg./Adv.: Mr. John Hebebrand/Manager National Sales

Computer Software	General
Computer, Bar Code	General

ACTIVATOR METHODS INTERNATIONAL, LTD   800-598-0224
2950 North 7th St., Suite 200, Phoenix, AZ 85014   602-224-0220
FDA Number: 2182433   Fax: 602-224-0230
E-mail: info@activator.com
Web site: www.activator.com
Medical Products Sales Volume: $1,600,000
Year Founded: 1985
Total Employees: 11
Ownership: Private
Produces/Sells CE-marked Devices: N
Federal Procurement Eligibility: Small Business

Stimulator, Electro-Analgesic	Cns/Neurology

ACTIVE ANKLE SYSTEMS, INC.   812-258-0663
233 Quartermaster Ct., Jeffersonville, IN 47130
FDA Number: 1530896

Brace, Joint, Ankle (External)	Physical Med

ACTIVE CORPORATION   207-326-9100
PO Box 1000, 15 Main Street, Castine, ME 04421-1000
FDA Number: 1226553   Fax: 208-326-9191
E-mail: support@activecenter.com
Web site: www.activecenter.com
Annual Revenue: $0-$1 Million
Year Founded: 1999
Ownership: Private
Produces/Sells CE-marked Devices: N
Federal Procurement Eligibility: Small Business
Distribution: Manufacturer Direct

Electrocardiograph, Single Channel	Cardiovascular

ACTIVEAID, INC.   800-533-5330
101 Activeaid Rd.,   507-644-2951
Redwood Falls, MN 56283
FDA Number: 2126684   Fax: 507-644-2468
E-mail: barb@activeaid.com
Web site: www.activeaid.com
Year Founded: 1965
Total Employees: 45   Marketing Staff: 2   Sales Staff: 39
Ownership: Private
Produces/Sells CE-marked Devices: N
Federal Procurement Eligibility: Small Business
Distribution: Manufacturer Through Distributor
General Admin.: Charles Nearing/Chief Operating Officer, Vice President
     Mark Oja/President, Chief Executive Officer
Mktg./Adv.: Tom Jasina/Manager National Sales
Production: Barbara Panitzke/Director Customer Services
     Jerry Mathis/Manager Materials
     Jeff Gunderson/Manufacturing Engineer

Attachment, Commode, Wheelchair	Physical Med
Bars, Parallel, Powered	Physical Med
Bathtub, Portable	General
Belt, Support, Pelvic	Physical Med
Chair, Adjustable, Mechanical	Physical Med
Chair, Bath	General
Chair, Shower	General
Commode (Toilet)	General
Component, Exercise	Physical Med
Cushion, Wheelchair (Pad)	Physical Med
Stretcher, Hand-Carried	General
Table, Physical Therapy	Physical Med

ACUDERM INC.   800-327-0015
5370 NW 35th Terrace, Suite 106,   954-733-6935
Fort Lauderdale, FL 33309
FDA Number: 1035236   Fax: 954-486-3602
E-mail: cust-service@acuderm.com
Web site: www.acuderm.com
Medical Products Sales Volume: $5,700,000
Annual Revenue: $5-$10 Million
Year Founded: 1983
Total Employees: 72   Marketing Staff: 2   Sales Staff: 6
Ownership: Private
Quality System Registration Information: ISO9002
Produces/Sells CE-marked Devices: Y
Federal Procurement Eligibility: Small Business, GSA Contract, VA Contract
Distribution: Manufacturer Direct, Manufacturer Through Distributor, OEM, Exporter
General Admin.: Charles R. Yeh/President, Chief Executive Officer
Mktg./Adv.: Dina Callari/Director Marketing
     Nancy Rivera/Manager National Sales
Production: Cedric Patterson/Director Quality Assurance

Cautery, Radiofrequency, AC-Powered	Ophthalmology
Cautery, Thermal, Battery-Powered	Ophthalmology
Culture Media, Selective And Non-Differential	Microbiology
Curette, Surgical	Surgery
Exhaust System, Surgical	Surgery
General Use Surgical Scissors	Surgery

ACUDERM INC.   800-327-0015 *(cont'd)*
Kit, Surgical (General)	Surgery
Kit, Surgical Instrument, Disposable	Surgery
Punch, Biopsy, Surgical	Dental And Oral
Punch, Surgical	Surgery
Reagent, General Purpose	Pathology
Surgical Instrument, Manual (General Use)	Surgery

ACUFEX MICROSURGICAL, INC.
See Smith & Nephew, Inc., Endoscopy Division

ACULUX, INC.   239-643-8023
4424 Corporate Square, Naples, FL 34104
FDA Number: 1064426
Ownership: Private
Produces/Sells CE-marked Devices: N
Lamp, Operating Room	General
Light, Surgical, Endoscopic	Surgery

ACUMAR TECHNOLOGY
See Lafayette Instrument Company

ACUMED INSTRUMENTS CORP.   800-234-5045
5662 Calle Real #406,   **805 683 1133**
Santa Barbara, CA 91377
FDA Number: 2083124
E-mail: acumed@earthlink.net   *Fax:* 805 683 1199
Web site: www.e-acumed.com
Year Founded: 1985
Ownership: Private
Produces/Sells CE-marked Devices: N
Federal Procurement Eligibility: Small Business
Distribution: Manufacturer Direct
Burr	Ear/Nose/Throat
Drill, Middle Ear Surgery	Ear/Nose/Throat

ACUMED LLC   888-627-9957
5885 Nw Cornelius Pass Rd.,   **503-627-9957**
Hillsboro, OR 97124
FDA Number: 3025141
Ownership: Private
Produces/Sells CE-marked Devices: N
Bolt, Nut, Washer	Orthopedics
Cerclage, Fixation	Orthopedics
Component, Traction, Invasive	Orthopedics
Fastener, Fixation, Non-Biodegradable, Soft Tissue	Orthopedics
Pin, Fixation, Smooth	Orthopedics
Pin, Fixation, Threaded	Orthopedics
Plate, Bone, Orthodontic	Dental And Oral
Plate, Fixation, Bone	Orthopedics
Prosthesis, Elbow, Hemi-, Radial, Polymer	Orthopedics
Prosthesis, Shoulder, Hemi-, Humeral	Orthopedics
Rod, Fixation, Intramedullary	Orthopedics
Screw, Fixation, Bone	Orthopedics
Staple, Fixation, Bone	Orthopedics
Surgical Instrument, Orthopedic, Battery-Powered	Surgery
Traction Unit, Non-Powered	Orthopedics

ACUMED MEDICAL SUPPLIES LTD.   800-567-7246
44 Royal York Road,   **416-253-6060**
Toronto, ONT M8V-2 Canada
FDA Number: 3002669614
E-mail: sales@acumedmedical.com   *Fax:* 416-253-1911
Web site: www.acumedmedical.com
Year Founded: 1989
Total Employees: 10
Ownership: Private
Produces/Sells CE-marked Devices: N
Distribution: Exclusive Distributor, Importer

ACUMEDIA MANUFACTURERS, INC.   800-783-3212
620 Lesher Place, Lansing, MI 48912   **517-372-9200**
FDA Number: 1120041   *Fax:* 517-372-0108
E-mail: acumedia@neogen.com
Web site: www.neogen.com
Medical Products Sales Volume: $1,000,000
Annual Revenue: $5-$10 Million
Year Founded: 1982
Total Employees: 30   *Marketing Staff:* 2   *Sales Staff:* 4
Ownership: Private
Produces/Sells CE-marked Devices: N
Federal Procurement Eligibility: Small Business
Distribution: Manufacturer Direct, Manufacturer Through Distributor, OEM, Service Direct, Exporter
General Admin.: Mr. John George/Regional Manager
    Ms. Anne Havens/Regional Manager
Mktg./Adv.: Mr. Bob Bidlingmeyer/Director National Sales
    Mr. John Simlar/Manager Marketing
    Mr. Tony Maltese/Vice President Business Development
Production: Ms. Jessica Courter/Customer Service Representative

ACUMEDIA MANUFACTURERS, INC.   800-783-3212 *(cont'd)*
    Ms. Mari-Sue Ratliff/Director Quality Assurance
    Mr. Ken Kodilla/Vice President Manufacturing
Research: Ms. Christine Cooper/Manager Research
Culture Media, Enriched	Microbiology

ACUMEN MEDICAL, INC.   408-530-1810
275 Santa Ana Court, Sunnyvale, CA 94085
FDA Number: 3004857433
Ownership: Private
Produces/Sells CE-marked Devices: N
Catheter, Percutaneous	Cardiovascular
Introducer, Catheter	Cardiovascular

ACUNETX, INC.   877-370-0477
2301 W. 205th St., Suite 102, Torrance, CA 90501   **310-328-0477**
FDA Number: n/a   *Fax:* 310-328-0697
E-mail: contact@acunetx.com
Web site: www.acunetx.com
Year Founded: 2005
Ownership: Private
Stock Symbol: ANTX
Traded On: OTC Bulletin
Produces/Sells CE-marked Devices: N
General Admin.: Ronald A. Waldorf/President, Chief Executive Officer
Production: Douglas E. MacCarthy/Senior Vice President Operations

ACUO TECHNOLOGIES   952-905-3440
8009 34th Avenue South, Suite 900, Bloomington, MN 55425
FDA Number: 3003616184   *Fax:* 952-905-3441
Ownership: Private
Produces/Sells CE-marked Devices: N
Device, Storage, Image, Digital	Radiology

ACUSON, INC.
See Siemens Medical Solutions Usa, Inc.

ACUSTEP, INC.   866-465-2500
2775 A Arnold Ave., Salina, KS 67401   **785-826-2500**
FDA Number: 3004201339   *Fax:* 785-826-4984
E-mail: info@acustep.com
Web site: www.acustep.com
Ownership: Private
Produces/Sells CE-marked Devices: N
Orthosis, Limb Brace	Physical Med
Pressure Measurement, System, Intermittent	Physical Med

ACUTE INNOVATIONS LLC   866-623-4137
21421 Nw Jacobson Rd., Suite 700,   **503-627-9957**
Hillsboro, OR 97124
FDA Number: 3005670412
E-mail: customerservice@acuteinnovations.com
Web site: www.acuteinnovations.com
Ownership: Private
Produces/Sells CE-marked Devices: N
Appliance, Fix., Nail/Blade/Plate Comb., Multiple Component	Orthopedics
Cerclage, Fixation	Orthopedics
Plate, Fixation, Bone	Orthopedics
Screw, Fixation, Bone	Orthopedics

ACUTUS MEDICAL, INC   858-673-1621
11225 West Bernardo Court, Suite 102, San Diego, CA 92127
FDA Number: n/a   *Fax:* 858-673-2274
Web site: www.acutusmedical.com
Ownership: Private
Produces/Sells CE-marked Devices: N
General Admin.: Mr. Graydon Beatty/Chief Technology Officer
    Mr. Randy Werneth/President, Chief Executive Officer
Research: Mr. Alan Baumel/Vice President Research & Development

AD-TECH MEDICAL INSTRUMENT CORP.   800-776-1555
1901 William St, Racine, WI 53404   **262-634-1555**
FDA Number: 2183456   *Fax:* 262-634-5668
E-mail: sales@adtechmedical.com
Web site: www.adtechmedical.com
Medical Products Sales Volume: $1,500,000
Year Founded: 1983
Total Employees: 20   *Marketing Staff:* 6   *Sales Staff:* 6
Ownership: Private
Quality System Registration Information: ISO9001
Produces/Sells CE-marked Devices: Y
Federal Procurement Eligibility: Small Business
Distribution: Manufacturer Direct, Manufacturer Through Distributor, Manufacturer Through Manufacturer Reps, OEM
General Admin.: John F. Ziobro/Chief Operating Officer
    David A. Putz/President, Chief Executive Officer
Mktg./Adv.: Lisa Theama/Director Marketing
Production: Kathy Schwarz/Vice President Manufacturing

AD-TECH MEDICAL INSTRUMENT CORP. 800-776-1555 *(cont'd)*
Finance: Mary Mac Donald/Treasurer

Cable/Lead, EEG	Cns/Neurology
Device, Measurement, Velocity, Conduction, Nerve	Cns/Neurology
Electrode, Cortical	Cns/Neurology
Electrode, Depth	Cns/Neurology
Electrode, Neurological	Cns/Neurology
Electrode, Other	General
Needle, Other	General
Stimulator, Electrical, Evoked Response	Cns/Neurology

ADA TECHNOLOGIES, INC. 800-232-0296
8100 Shaffer Parkway, Suite 130, 303-874-8276
Littleton, CO 80127
FDA Number: 3004794241 Fax: 303-792-5633
Ownership: Private
Produces/Sells CE-marked Devices: N

Hook, External Limb Component, Mechanical	Physical Med

ADAC MULTI MODALITY
See Atlas Medical Technologies

ADAMATION, INC. 800-225-3075
87 Adams St., PO Box 95037, Newton, MA 02458 617-244-7500
FDA Number: n/a Fax: 617-244-4609
E-mail: info@adamationinc.com
Web site: www.adamationinc.com
Annual Revenue: $5-$10 Million
Year Founded: 1957
Total Employees: 48 *Marketing Staff:* 1 *Sales Staff:* 6
Ownership: Private
Federal Procurement Eligibility: Small Business, GSA Contract
Distribution: Manufacturer Direct
General Admin.: Hurbert A. Perry/Chief Executive Officer
William E. Ward/President
Mktg./Adv.: Fred Ferris/Director National Accounts

Conveyor, Tray	General
Foodservice Product/Equipment	General

ADAPT-ABILITY, INC. 314-432-1101
9355 Dielman Industrial Dr., St. Louis, MO 63132
FDA Number: n/a Fax: 314-432-0780
Web site: www.adapt-ability.org
Year Founded: 1986
Ownership: Private
Produces/Sells CE-marked Devices: N
Distribution: Service Direct

Service, Maintenance/Repair	General

ADAPTATIONS
See RDL Supply

ADAPTIVE ENGINEERING LTD. 800-448-4652
419 34th Ave. SE, Calgary, ALB T2G-1V1 Canada 403-243-9400
FDA Number: n/a Fax: 403-243-9455
E-mail: lifts@adaptive.ab.ca
Web site: www.adaptivelifts.com
Year Founded: 1978
Total Employees: 50
Ownership: Private
Produces/Sells CE-marked Devices: N
Distribution: Manufacturer Direct, Exporter

ADAPTIVE MEDICAL CONCEPTS, INC. 800-443-7863
1378 Bellefontaine Ave., Lima, OH 45804 419-224-5410
FDA Number: n/a Fax: 419-222-6566
E-mail: info@adaptivemedicalconcepts.com
Web site: www.AdaptiveMedicalConcepts.com
Annual Revenue: $1-$5 Million
Ownership: Private
Produces/Sells CE-marked Devices: N
Federal Procurement Eligibility: Small Business
Distribution: Manufacturer Through Distributor

Accessories, Wheelchair	Physical Med
Contract Manufacturing	General
Restraint, Protective (Body)	General

ADAPTIVE SWITCH LABORATORIES, INC. 800-626-8698
125 Spur 191, Suite C, Spicewood, TX 78669 830-798-0005
FDA Number: 1645143 Fax: 830-798-6221
E-mail: info@asl-inc.com
Web site: www.asl-inc.com
Year Founded: 1992
Ownership: Invacare Corporation
Produces/Sells CE-marked Devices: N
General Admin.: Mr. Rucker Ashmore/President
Lisa Rotelli/Vice President
Mktg./Adv.: Mr. Byron Guisbert/Director Education
Production: Mr. James Pham/Chief Engineer

ADAPTIVE SWITCH LABORATORIES, INC. 800-626-8698 *(cont'd)*
Mr. Trey Cozby/Director Operations
Finance: Codie Ealey/Manager Finance
IS: Joe Cervantez/Technical Manager

Component, Wheelchair	Physical Med

ADAPTO STEEL PRODUCTS
See Rem Systems

ADAPTO STORAGE PRODUCTS
See Rem Systems

ADAR INTERNATIONAL INC. 800-510-9286
3350 Riverwood Parkway SE, Suite 1900, 770-980-9286
Atlanta, GA 30339
FDA Number: 3004521578
E-mail: info@adarinternational.com
Web site: www.adarinternational.com
Ownership: Private
Produces/Sells CE-marked Devices: N

Crown, Preformed	Dental And Oral

ADD-ON HEALTH SYSTEMS
See Accu-Med Services

ADDEN FURNITURE, INC. 800-625-3876
26 Jackson St., Lowell, MA 01852-2102 978-454-7848
FDA Number: 1225533 Fax: 978-453-1449
E-mail: lkane@addenfurniture.com
Web site: www.addenfurniture.com
Medical Products Sales Volume: $25,000,000
Annual Revenue: $25-$50 Million
Year Founded: 2005
Total Employees: 200 *Marketing Staff:* 5 *Sales Staff:* 48
Ownership: Private
Federal Procurement Eligibility: Small Business, GSA Contract
Distribution: Manufacturer Direct, Manufacturer Through Manufacturer Reps
General Admin.: Gary Garmon/President
Mktg./Adv.: Linda Kane/Director Marketing
Jerry Gorby/Director Sales
Trey Stormer/Director Sales
Thomas Hurd/Vice President Marketing & Sales

Bed, Electric	General
Bedrail	General
Cabinet, Bedside	General
Chair, Geriatric	General
Chair, Other	General
Furniture, General	General
Furniture, Patient Room	General

ADDENT, INC. 203-778-0200
43 Miry Brook Road, Danbury, CT 06810
FDA Number: 3003694926 Fax: 203-792-2275
E-mail: info@addent.com
Web site: www.addent.com
Medical Products Sales Volume: $800,000
Annual Revenue: $0-$1 Million
Total Employees: 12 *Marketing Staff:* 2 *Sales Staff:* 22
Ownership: Private
Produces/Sells CE-marked Devices: Y
Federal Procurement Eligibility: Small Business
Distribution: Manufacturer Through Distributor, Exporter
General Admin.: Dr. Joshua Friedman/President
Mktg./Adv.: Joanne Gallagher/Managing Director Marketing & Sales
Andrine Haughton/Sales Associate

Contouring, Instrument, Matrix, Operative	Dental And Oral
Detector, Caries	Dental And Oral
Screen, Intensifying, Radiographic, Dental	Dental And Oral
Tooth Bonding Agent, Resin Restoration	Dental And Oral
Warmer, Anesthesia Tube	Dental And Oral

ADDITION TECHNOLOGY, INC. 847-297-8419
155 Moffett Park Drive,, Suite B-1, Sunnyvale, CA 94089
FDA Number: 2953726 Fax: 408-541-1411
Ownership: Private
Produces/Sells CE-marked Devices: N

Catheter, Percutaneous	Cardiovascular
Forceps, Ophthalmic	Ophthalmology
Implant, Corneal	Ophthalmology
Marker, Ocular	Ophthalmology
Rongeur, Lacrimal Sac	Ophthalmology
Spatula, Ophthalmic	Ophthalmology

ADDITION TECHNOLOGY, INC. 847-297-8419
950 Lee St., Ste. 210, Des Plaines, IL 60016
FDA Number: 3005344923 Fax: 847-297-8678
E-mail: intacs@intacs-ati.com
Web site: www.IntacsFor Keratoconus.com
Annual Revenue: $10-$25 Million
Year Founded: 2001
Ownership: Private

ADDITION TECHNOLOGY, INC.   847-297-8419 *(cont'd)*
Quality System Registration Information: ISO9001; ISO9002
Produces/Sells CE-marked Devices: Y
Federal Procurement Eligibility: Small Business
Distribution: Manufacturer Direct
General Admin.: William M. Flynn/Chief Executive Officer
      Arthur E. Brodie/Vice President International Operations
Mktg./Adv.: Brian Regan/Vice President Marketing & Sales
Finance: Tony Faoro/Vice President Finance

Implant, Corneal	Ophthalmology
Keratoprosthesis, Non-Custom	Ophthalmology

ADDTO, INC.   773-278-0294
816 N. Kostner Ave., Chicago, IL 60651-3423
FDA Number: 1419727
E-mail: Sales@addtoinc.com   *Fax:* 773-342-8329
Annual Revenue: $0-$1 Million
Year Founded: 1972
Total Employees: 5   *Marketing Staff:* 2   *Sales Staff:* 2
Ownership: Private
Produces/Sells CE-marked Devices: N
Federal Procurement Eligibility: Small Business, Female Owned
Distribution: Manufacturer Through Distributor
General Admin.: Patricia E. Voller/President

Adapter, Catheter	Surgery
Cushion, Ring, Inflatable	General
Plug, Catheter	Gastroenterology/Urology

ADELBERG LABORATORIES INC.   818-784-1141
16821 Oak View Dr., Encino, CA 91436
FDA Number: n/a   *Fax:* 818-986-9587
E-mail: adelbergk@aol.com
Web site: www.adelberglaboratories.com
Ownership: Private
Quality System Registration Information: ISO9002
Produces/Sells CE-marked Devices: Y
Distribution: Manufacturer Direct
General Admin.: Marvin Adelberg/President
      Ken Adelberg/Vice President

Clamp, Other	Surgery

ADELPHIA MEDICAL INC.   410-742-7104
1525 Edgemore Ave., Ste. 1, Salisbury, MD 21801
FDA Number: 3003908365
Ownership: Private
Produces/Sells CE-marked Devices: N

Dressing, Wound, Hydrogel W/out Drug And/or Biologic	Surgery
Dressing, Wound, Hydrophilic	Surgery
Fiber, Absorbent	General

ADENNA INC.   888-323-3662
11932 Baker Place, Santa Fe Springs, CA 90670   562-777-8026
FDA Number: 2086048   *Fax:* 562-777-8905
E-mail: info@adenna.com
Web site: www.adenna.com
Year Founded: 1997
Ownership: Private
Quality System Registration Information: ISO9001; ISO9002
Produces/Sells CE-marked Devices: Y
Federal Procurement Eligibility: Small Business, Minority Owned, GSA Contract, VA Contract
Distribution: Manufacturer Through Distributor, Manufacturer Through Manufacturer Reps
General Admin.: Maxwell Lee/President, Chief Executive Officer
      Charles Chang/Vice President, General Manager
Mktg./Adv.: Ms. Leslie McDonald/Director Marketing & Communications
      Kevin Toshima/Manager National Sales

Dress, Scrub, Disposable	Surgery
Glove, Patient Examination, Latex	General
Glove, Patient Examination, Specialty	General
Glove, Patient Examination, Vinyl	General
Gown, Operating Room, Disposable	Surgery
Gown, Patient, Disposable	General
Mask, Face	General

ADEPT MEDICAL CONCEPTS   949-635-9238
**29816 Avenida De Las Banderas,
Rancho Santa Margarita, CA 92688**
FDA Number: 3005506125
Ownership: Private
Produces/Sells CE-marked Devices: N

Laser, Surgical	Surgery

ADEPT-MED INTERNATIONAL, INC.   800-222-8445
665 Pleasant Valley Rd.,   530-621-1220
Diamond Springs, CA 95619
FDA Number: 2918699
E-mail: adeptmed@aol.com   *Fax:* 530-621-1310

ADEPT-MED INTERNATIONAL, INC.   800-222-8445 *(cont'd)*
Web site: www.adeptmed.com
Medical Products Sales Volume: $2,000,000
Annual Revenue: $1-$5 Million
Year Founded: 1973
Total Employees: 10
Ownership: Private
Produces/Sells CE-marked Devices: N
Federal Procurement Eligibility: Small Business
Distribution: Manufacturer Direct, Manufacturer Through Distributor
General Admin.: Tim Quigley/President, Chief Executive Officer
      Chris Quigley/Vice President, General Manager
Production: Chris Quigley/Director Quality Assurance

Extractor, Metal, Magnetic	Surgery
Prosthesis, Breast, Non-Inflatable, Internal	Surgery
Retainer, Surgical	Surgery
Retainer, Visceral	Surgery
Retractor, Non-Self-Retaining	Gastroenterology/Urology
Speculum, Vaginal, Non-Metal	Obstetrics/Gynecology

ADEX MEDICAL, INC.   800-873-4776
6101 Quail Valley Court, Riverside, CA 92507   909-653-9122
FDA Number: n/a   *Fax:* 909-653-9133
E-mail: info@adexmed.com
Web site: www.adexmed.com
Medical Products Sales Volume: $2,100,000
Annual Revenue: $5-$10 Million
Year Founded: 1996
Total Employees: 25   *Marketing Staff:* 2   *Sales Staff:* 20
Ownership: Private
Produces/Sells CE-marked Devices: N
Federal Procurement Eligibility: Small Business, Minority Owned
Distribution: Manufacturer Direct, Manufacturer Through Distributor, OEM, Importer, Exporter
General Admin.: Mr. Michael M. Ghafouri/Chief Executive Officer

Cover, Head, Surgical	Surgery
Cover, Shoe, Operating Room	Surgery
Depressor, Tongue	General
Gauze, Absorbable	Surgery
Glove, Patient Examination	General
Glove, Patient Examination, Poly	General
Glove, Surgical	General
Glove, Surgical, Powder-Free	Surgery
Glove, Utility	General
Goggles, Protective, Eye	Ophthalmology
Gown, Examination	General
Gown, Other	General
Mask, Face	General
Mask, Surgical	Surgery

ADHESIVE ENGINEERING & SUPPLY, INC.
See Extreme Adhesives, Inc.

ADHEZION BIOMEDICAL, LLC   610-431-2398
506 Pine Mountain Rd., Hudson, NC 28638
FDA Number: 3006385287

Bandage, Liquid	Surgery

ADI MEDICAL DIVISION OF ASIA DYNAMICS (GROUP) INC.   877-647-7699
1565 South Shields Drive, Waukegan, IL 60085   847-688-9968
FDA Number: 1451019   *Fax:* 847-688-9768
E-mail: adimedical@msn.com
Web site: www.adimedical.com
Medical Products Sales Volume: $400,000
Annual Revenue: $1-$5 Million
Year Founded: 1987
Total Employees: 9   *Marketing Staff:* 2   *Sales Staff:* 2
Ownership: Private
Produces/Sells CE-marked Devices: N
Federal Procurement Eligibility: Small Business, Minority Owned, Female Owned
Distribution: Manufacturer Through Distributor, Importer, Exporter
General Admin.: Mr. Joe Zhu/Chief Executive Officer
      Mrs. Ling Liu/President

Apron, Laboratory	Chemistry
Bag, Body	General
Bag, Plastic	General
Brush, Other	General
Gauze, Non-Absorbable, X-Ray Detectable (Internal Sponge)	Surgery
Glove, Other	General
Glove, Patient Examination	General
Glove, Patient Examination, Latex	General
Glove, Patient Examination, Vinyl	General
Glove, Surgical, Plastic Surgery	Surgery
Gown, Examination	General
Gown, Isolation, Surgical	Surgery
Gown, Patient	Surgery
Sponge, Gauze	Dental And Oral
Sponge, Laparotomy	Surgery

ADI MEDICAL DIVISION OF ASIA DYNAMICS
877-647-7699
(cont'd)

Tourniquet	General
Tourniquet, Non-Pneumatic, Surgical	Surgery
Towel, Surgical	Surgery

ADINSTRUMENTS
888-965-6040
1949 Landings Dr., Mountain View, CA 94043 · **650-965-9292**
FDA Number: n/a · *Fax:* 650-965-9293
E-mail: info@adinstruments.com
Web site: www.adinstruments.com
Annual Revenue: $0-$1 Million
Ownership: Private
Produces/Sells CE-marked Devices: Y
Federal Procurement Eligibility: Small Business
Distribution: Manufacturer Direct, OEM
General Admin.: Graham Milliken/President, Chief Executive Officer

Recorder, Chart, Laboratory	Chemistry

ADIT/ELECTRON TUBES
800-521-8382
100 Forge Way, Unit F, Rockaway, NJ 07866 · **973-586-9594**
FDA Number: n/a · *Fax:* 973-586-9771
E-mail: sales@electrontubes.com
Web site: www.electrontubes.com
Medical Products Sales Volume: $8,500,000
Annual Revenue: $5-$10 Million
Year Founded: 1994
Total Employees: 10 · *Marketing Staff:* 2 · *Sales Staff:* 4
Ownership: Private
Quality System Registration Information: ISO9001
Produces/Sells CE-marked Devices: Y
Federal Procurement Eligibility: Small Business
Distribution: Manufacturer Through Distributor
General Admin.: Louis A. Evangelist/President
Mktg./Adv.: Mike R. Avery/Manager Sales
Mr. Paul Davison/Manager Sales

Component, Electrical	General
Counter, Cell Or Particle, Automated	Hematology
Counter, Scintillation, Liquid, Toxicology	Toxicology

ADIVAMED
703-729-8836
44141 Bristow Circle, Ashburn, VA 20147-3310
FDA Number: n/a · *Fax:* 703-729-4255
E-mail: sales@adivamed.com
Web site: www.adivamed.com
Year Founded: 2001
Ownership: Private
Produces/Sells CE-marked Devices: N
Federal Procurement Eligibility: Small Business, Female Owned
Distribution: Manufacturer Direct, Exclusive Distributor, Importer, Exporter
General Admin.: Mrs. Pamela Cresine/Managing Director
Mktg./Adv.: Mr. Charles Cresine/Manager General Sales

Aspirator, Liposuction	Surgery
Insufflator, Laparoscopic	Obstetrics/Gynecology

ADJUST N' REST
See Elite Mattress Manufacturing

ADJUSTABLE FIXTURE CO.
800-558-2628
3726 N. Booth St., Milwaukee, WI 53212-1698 · **414-964-2626**
FDA Number: 7000409 · *Fax:* 414-964-2944
E-mail: mjlights@adjustablefixture.com
Web site: www.adjustablefixture.com
Medical Products Sales Volume: $600,000
Annual Revenue: $0-$1 Million
Year Founded: 1911
Total Employees: 10
Ownership: Private
Produces/Sells CE-marked Devices: N
Federal Procurement Eligibility: Small Business, GSA Contract
Distribution: Manufacturer Direct, Manufacturer Through Distributor
Mktg./Adv.: Mike Schumaker/President, Director Marketing
Research: Barb Varney/Product Development Technician

Lamp, Examination (Light)	General
Lamp, Other	General

ADJUSTO EQUIPMENT COMPANY
See Biofit Engineered Products

ADLER INSTRUMENT CO.
866-382-3537
6191 Atlantic Blvd., Norcross, GA 30071-1306 · **770-263-0203**
FDA Number: 1031981 · *Fax:* 770-441-0260
E-mail: info@adlerinstrumentsmedics.com
Web site: www.adlerinstrument.com
Medical Products Sales Volume: $20,000,000
Annual Revenue: $25-$50 Million
Year Founded: 1980
Total Employees: 42 · *Marketing Staff:* 2 · *Sales Staff:* 18
Ownership: Private

ADLER INSTRUMENT CO.
866-382-3537 *(cont'd)*
Produces/Sells CE-marked Devices: N
Federal Procurement Eligibility: Small Business
Distribution: Exclusive Distributor
General Admin.: Eddie Davis/President
Mktg./Adv.: Ron Gonyea/Vice President Sales
Production: Mani Farsinejad/Manager Materials

Scissors, Plastic Surgery (Dissecting)	Surgery
Service, Maintenance/Repair	General
Surgical Instrument, Cardiovascular	Cardiovascular
Surgical Instrument, Obstetric/Gynecologic	Obstetrics/Gynecology

ADLIB, INC.
714-895-9529
5142 Bolsa Ave., Suite 106, Huntington Beach, CA 92649
FDA Number: 2026913
Ownership: Private
Produces/Sells CE-marked Devices: N

Accessories, Wheelchair	Physical Med
Adaptor, Recreational	Physical Med
Utensil, Food	Physical Med
Utensil, Handicapped Aid	Physical Med

ADM TRONICS UNLIMITED, INC.
201-767-6040
224 Pegasus Avenue, Northvale, NJ 07647-1908
FDA Number: 2243374 · *Fax:* 201-784-0620
E-mail: sales@admtronics.com
Web site: www.admtronics.com
Medical Products Sales Volume: $1,500,000
Annual Revenue: $1-$5 Million
Year Founded: 1969
Total Employees: 2
Ownership: Public
Stock Symbol: ADMT
Traded On: OTC Bulletin
Produces/Sells CE-marked Devices: Y
Federal Procurement Eligibility: Small Business
Distribution: Manufacturer Through Distributor, Manufacturer Through Manufacturer Reps, Exporter
General Admin.: Andre Dimino/President
Production: Vincent DiMino/Vice President Manufacturing

Diathermy, Shortwave, Pulsed	Physical Med
Unit, Therapy, Tinnitus	Ear/Nose/Throat

ADOLFSON & PETERSON, INC
612-544-1561
6701 W. 23rd Street, Minneapolis, MN 55426
FDA Number: n/a · *Fax:* 952-525-2333
E-mail: APinfo@_a-p.com
Web site: www.adolfsonpeterson.com
Medical Products Sales Volume: $76,000,000
Annual Revenue: $25-$50 Million
Year Founded: 1946
Total Employees: 200
Ownership: ADOLFSON & PETERSON
Produces/Sells CE-marked Devices: N
Federal Procurement Eligibility: Small Business
Distribution: Service Direct
General Admin.: Michael Peterson/President

Service, Engineering/Design	General

ADR ULTRASOUND
See Phillips Ultrasound

ADROIT MEDICAL SYSTEMS, INC.
800-267-6077
1146 Carding Machine Road, Loudon, TN 37774 · **865-458-8600**
FDA Number: 1055823 · *Fax:* 865-458-0880
E-mail: adroitmed@aol.com
Web site: www.adroitmedical.com
Medical Products Sales Volume: $30,000,000
Annual Revenue: $25-$50 Million
Year Founded: 1991
Total Employees: 85 · *Marketing Staff:* 6 · *Sales Staff:* 30
Ownership: Private
Quality System Registration Information: ISO9001
Produces/Sells CE-marked Devices: Y
Federal Procurement Eligibility: Small Business, Female Owned, GSA Contract, VA Contract
Distribution: Manufacturer Direct, Manufacturer Through Distributor, Manufacturer Through Manufacturer Reps, OEM, Exporter
General Admin.: C. E. Gammons/President
Mktg./Adv.: Max Renfro/Senior Vice President Sales
Scott E. Gammons/Vice President Marketing
Production: Ms. Kelley Patten/Manager Regulatory Affairs

Device, Hyperthermia (Blanket, Plumbing & Heat Exchanger)	Cardiovascular
Fluidized Therapy, Unit, Dry Heat	Physical Med
Hypo/Hyperthermia Blanket	General
Hypothermia Unit (Blanket, Plumbing & Heat Exchanger)	Anesthesiology
Pack, Hot Or Cold, Water Circulating	Physical Med
Warmer, Blood, Non-Electromagnetic Radiation	Anesthesiology

ADS, INC.
See American Dental Supply, Inc.

ADTECH SYSTEMS RESEARCH, INC
1342 N. Fairfield Rd., Dayton, OH 45432   **937-426-3329**
FDA Number: 3004635141
Fax: 937-426-8087
Ownership: Private
Produces/Sells CE-marked Devices: N
Crutch — Physical Med

ADVA-LITE, INC.
7340 Bryan Dairy Road, Largo, FL 33777   **727-546-5483**
FDA Number: 1036051
Fax: 727-544-5316
E-mail: advalite@advalite.com
Web site: www.advalite.com
Medical Products Sales Volume: $15,100,000
Year Founded: 1963
Total Employees: 130   *Marketing Staff:* 2   *Sales Staff:* 14
Ownership: Private
Produces/Sells CE-marked Devices: N
Federal Procurement Eligibility: Small Business, GSA Contract
Light Source, Incandescent, Diagnostic — Gastroenterology/Urology
Light, Examination, Battery-Powered — General

ADVANCE MEDICAL DESIGNS, INC.
1241 Atlanta Industrial Drive,   **800-221-3679**
Marietta, GA 30066   **770-422-3125**
FDA Number: 1037885   *Fax:* 770-429-2471
E-mail: sales@a-m-d-inc.com
Web site: www.advancemedicaldesigns.com
Year Founded: 1984
Total Employees: 70   *Marketing Staff:* 7   *Sales Staff:* 25
Ownership: Private
Quality System Registration Information: ISO9001
Produces/Sells CE-marked Devices: Y
Federal Procurement Eligibility: Small Business
Distribution: Manufacturer Direct, Manufacturer Through Distributor, Manufacturer Through Manufacturer Reps, OEM, Exporter
General Admin.: Anthony Cottone/President, Chief Executive Officer
Mktg./Adv.: Tim Morris/Director Product Development
    Tim Morris/Manager International & National Sales
    Wayne Allison/Manager National Sales
    Harry Bickelman/Vice President Sales
Production: Mr. William Slevin/Manager Quality Assurance
    Alex Hill/Vice President Operations
Finance: Tammie Brock/Controller
Container, IV — General
Contract Manufacturing, Product, Disposable — General
Cover, Camera — Surgery
Cover, Other — General
Drape, Surgical — Surgery
Drape, Surgical, Disposable — Surgery
Syringe, Piston — General

ADVANCE SCIENTIFIC, INC.
163 Research Lane, Millersburg,, PA 17061   **1.800.724.4158**
717.692.2104
FDA Number: n/a
E-mail: sales@advancedscientifics.com
Web site: www.advancedscientifics.com
Medical Products Sales Volume: $100,000
Annual Revenue: $0-$1 Million
Total Employees: 3   *Marketing Staff:* 1   *Sales Staff:* 1
Ownership: Private
Produces/Sells CE-marked Devices: N
Federal Procurement Eligibility: Small Business, Minority Owned, Female Owned
Distribution: Manufacturer Direct, Service Direct
General Admin.: Paul F. Crosby/President, Chief Executive Officer
    Angeles San Miguel/Secretary, Treasurer
    Julianne Crosby/Vice President
Colorimetry, Salicylate — Toxicology
Cyanomethemoglobin — Hematology
Diluent, Blood Cell — Hematology
Fluid, Red Cell Diluting — Hematology
Fluid, White Cell Diluting — Hematology
Formaldehyde (Formalin, Formol) — Pathology
Formalin, Neutral Buffered — Pathology
Reagent, Other — General
Solution, Pathology, Lugol's — Pathology
Stain, Carbol Fuchsin — Pathology
Stain, Crystal Violet, Histology — Pathology
Stain, Grams Iodine — Pathology
Stain, Methylene Blue — Pathology
Stain, Methylene Blue, New — Hematology
Stain, Other — Pathology
Stain, Safranin — Pathology
Stain, Wright's — Pathology
Sulfophosphovanillin, Colorimetry, Total Lipids — Chemistry

ADVANCE TABCO
200 Heartland Blvd., Edgewood, NY 11717   **800-645-3166**
FDA Number: n/a   *Fax:* 631-242-6900
E-mail: customer@advancetabco.com
Web site: www.advancetabco.com
Ownership: Private
Produces/Sells CE-marked Devices: N
Federal Procurement Eligibility: Small Business, Female Owned
Distribution: Manufacturer Through Distributor
Cleanroom Equipment — General
Material, Metallic-Stainless Steel, Tantalum, Platinum — Ear/Nose/Throat
Sink, Hospital — General
Tray, Surgical — Surgery

ADVANCE TECH INTERNATIONAL
See Lead-Lok, Inc.

ADVANCED AESTHETIC SOLUTIONS
631-D Keeaumoku St., Honolulu, HI 96814   **1-808-941-1629**
FDA Number: 3005430381   *Fax:* 1-808-946-5675
Web site: www.advancedaesthicsolutions.com
Ownership: Private
Produces/Sells CE-marked Devices: N
Teeth, Artificial, Posterior With Metal Insert — Dental And Oral

ADVANCED AIR TECHNOLOGIES, INC.
300 Sleeseman Drive, Corunna, MI 48817   **800-295-6583**
989-743-5544
FDA Number: n/a   *Fax:* 989-743-5624
E-mail: sales@advairtech.com
Web site: www.aat.cc
Medical Products Sales Volume: $1,500,000
Annual Revenue: $1-$5 Million
Year Founded: 1988
Total Employees: 9   *Marketing Staff:* 1   *Sales Staff:* 2
Ownership: Private
Produces/Sells CE-marked Devices: N
Federal Procurement Eligibility: Small Business
Distribution: Manufacturer Direct, Manufacturer Through Manufacturer Reps
Mktg./Adv.: Marvin Biondi/Director Marketing
Production: Gina Nicolli/Engineer
    Jerry Dedic/Manager Operations
Equipment, Control, Pollution — General

ADVANCED AMERICAN BIOTECHNOLOGY (AAB) 714-870-0290
1166 E. Valencia Dr., Unit 6C, Fullerton, CA 92631-5237
FDA Number: 9200129   *Fax:* 714-870-6385
E-mail: aab@ix.netcom.com
Web site: www.aabi.com
Annual Revenue: $1-$5 Million
Total Employees: 9   *Marketing Staff:* 2   *Sales Staff:* 5
Ownership: Private
Produces/Sells CE-marked Devices: Y
Federal Procurement Eligibility: Small Business, Minority Owned
Distribution: Manufacturer Direct, Manufacturer Through Manufacturer Reps, Importer, Exporter
General Admin.: R. A. Zeineh/President, Chief Executive Officer
    Gary Davis/Vice President Human Resources
Mktg./Adv.: Minhal Yousif/Director Marketing
    Bob Stephenhagen/Manager Advertising
    Guity Ettefagh/Manager Advertising
    Hong Boui/Manager International Marketing & Sales
    Helen Sale/Vice President Marketing & Sales
Production: R. A. Zeineh/Vice President Manufacturing
Research: Eric Fisher/Vice President Research & Development
Analyzer, Ultraviolet — Chemistry
Camera, Video — General
Computer Software — General
Computer, Radiographic Image Analysis — Radiology
Counter, Colony — Microbiology
Densitometer — Cardiovascular
Densitometer, Laboratory — Chemistry
Densitometer, Radiographic — Radiology
Densitometer/Scanner (Integrating, Reflectance, TLC, Radio) — Chemistry
Equipment, Test, Western Blot — Microbiology
Laser, Laboratory — Chemistry
Scanner, Color — Dental And Oral
Scanner, Ultraviolet — Chemistry
Viewer/Analyzer, 35mm Angio — Radiology

ADVANCED BACK TECHNOLOGIES, INC.
89 Cabot Ct., Ste. F, Hauppauge, NY 11788   **631-231-0076**
FDA Number: 3004755153
Ownership: Private
Produces/Sells CE-marked Devices: N
Equipment, Traction, Powered — Physical Med
Table, Physical Therapy — Physical Med

ADVANCED BATTERY SYSTEMS, INC.
800-227-7090
1300 19th St., Suite 170, East Moline, IL 61244 **309-755-7775**
FDA Number: n/a
Fax: 309-755-7774
E-mail: customerservice@advancedbattery.com
Web site: www.advancedbattery.com
Medical Products Sales Volume: $2,000,000
Annual Revenue: $1-$5 Million
Year Founded: 1990
Total Employees: 10   *Sales Staff:* 4
Ownership: Private
Federal Procurement Eligibility: Small Business
General Admin.: Jason Miller/President, Chief Executive Officer
  Battery, Mobile Radiographic Unit | Radiology

ADVANCED BIO PROSTHETIC SURFACES, LTD
210-696-5300
4778 Research Dr., San Antonio, TX 78240
FDA Number: 3003883634
Ownership: Private
Produces/Sells CE-marked Devices: N
  Stent, Cardiovascular | Cardiovascular

ADVANCED BIO-SURFACES, INC.
952-912-5400
5909 Baker Road, Suite 550, Minnetonka, MN 55345
FDA Number: 3002675394
Ownership: Private
Produces/Sells CE-marked Devices: N
  Extractor, Nail | Orthopedics
  Motor, Surgical Instrument, Pneumatic-Powered | Surgery
  Orthopedic Manual Surgical Instrument | Orthopedics
  Prosthesis, Knee, Hemi-, Tibial Resurfacing, Uncemented | Orthopedics

ADVANCED BIOHEALING INC.
858-754-3863
10933 N. Torrey Pines Road, Suite 200, La Jolla, CA 92037
FDA Number: 2028403
  Dressing, Wound and Burn, Interactive | Surgery

ADVANCED BIOMATERIAL SYSTEMS, INC.
877-257-9040
100 Passaic Ave., Chatham, NJ 07928 **973-635-9040**
FDA Number: 2248163
Fax: 973-635-9878
Web site: www.advbiomat.com
Ownership: Private
Produces/Sells CE-marked Devices: N
  Bone Cement | Orthopedics
  Dispenser, Cement | Orthopedics
  Filler, Bone Cement (for Vertebroplasty) | Orthopedics
  Metacrylate, Methyl, Cranioplasty | Cns/Neurology
  Mixing Equipment, Cement | Orthopedics
  Orthopedic Manual Surgical Instrument | Orthopedics
  Surgical Instrument, Non-Powered, Neurosurgical | Cns/Neurology

ADVANCED BIOMEDICAL DEVICES, INC. (ABD, INC.)
978-470-1177
Dundee Park, Bldg. 17, Door 6, P.O. Box 2087, Andover, MA 01810
FDA Number: 1222263
Fax: 978-470-2270
E-mail: info@abd-inc.com
Web site: www.abd-inc.com
Year Founded: 1987
Total Employees: 3
Ownership: Private
Produces/Sells CE-marked Devices: N
Federal Procurement Eligibility: Small Business
Distribution: Manufacturer Direct, Manufacturer Through Distributor, Manufacturer Through Manufacturer Reps, OEM, Exclusive Distributor, Exporter
General Admin.: Robert E. Winters/President
  Cardiac Output Unit, Other | Cardiovascular
  Contract Manufacturing | General
  Contract Packaging | General
  Guidewire, Catheter | Cardiovascular
  Injector, Indicator | Cardiovascular
  Injector, Thermal Dilution | Cardiovascular
  Regulator, Pressure, Gas Cylinder | Anesthesiology

ADVANCED BIONICS CORP.
800-678-2575
25129 Rye Canyon Loop, **661-362-1400**
Santa Clarita, CA 91355
FDA Number: n/a
Fax: 661-362-1500
E-mail: info@advancedbionics.com
Web site: www.bionicear.com
Medical Products Sales Volume: $38,100,000
Year Founded: 1993
Total Employees: 500   *Marketing Staff:* 18   *Sales Staff:* 20
Ownership: Private
Quality System Registration Information: ISO9001
Produces/Sells CE-marked Devices: N
Distribution: Manufacturer Direct, Exporter
General Admin.: Alfred E. Mann/Chief Executive Officer
  Rob Hall/Director Human Resources

ADVANCED BIONICS CORP.
800-678-2575 *(cont'd)*
  Jeffrey Greiner/President, Chief Executive Officer
  Bob Paulson/Senior Vice President, General Manager
Mktg./Adv.: Douglas Lynch/Director Marketing
  Thomas Walsh/Manager Business Development
  Sid Bernstein/Vice President Marketing & Sales
Production: Tom Santogrossi/Vice President Manufacturing
  Kay Adair/Vice President Quality Assurance & Regulatory Affairs
Research: Mary Joe Osberger/Director Clinical Research
  Van Harrison/Vice President Research & Development
  Prosthesis, Cochlear | Ear/Nose/Throat

ADVANCED BIONICS CORP.
800-678-2575
28515 Westinghouse Place, Valencia, CA 91355 **661-362-1400**
FDA Number: 3006139571
Fax: 661-362-1500
E-mail: info@advancedbionics.com
Web site: www.advancedbionics.com
Year Founded: 1993
Ownership: Private
Produces/Sells CE-marked Devices: N
  Implant, Cochlear | Ear/Nose/Throat

ADVANCED BIOPHOTONICS INC.
631-244-8244
125 Wilbur Place, Ste. 120, Bohemia, NY 11716
FDA Number: n/a
Ownership: Private
Produces/Sells CE-marked Devices: N
  Telethermographic System (Adjunctive Use) | Radiology

ADVANCED BIOSENSOR, INC.
  See Braemar, Inc

ADVANCED BIOTECHNOLOGIES, INC.
800-426-0764
9108 Guilford Rd., Rivers Park II, **410-792-9779**
Columbia, MD 21046
FDA Number: n/a
Fax: 301-497-9773
E-mail: ewhitman@abionline.com
Web site: www.abionline.com
Annual Revenue: $1-$5 Million
Total Employees: 29   *Marketing Staff:* 2   *Sales Staff:* 2
Ownership: Private
Produces/Sells CE-marked Devices: N
Federal Procurement Eligibility: Small Business
Distribution: Manufacturer Direct, Service Direct
General Admin.: Esther M. Whitman/Executive Vice President
  James E. Whitman, Jr./President, Chief Executive Officer
  Esther M. Whitman/Vice President Human Resources
  Esther M. Whitman/Vice President, General Manager
Mktg./Adv.: Esther M. Whitman/Manager Advertising
  Dr. James E. Whitman/Manager Contract Sales
  Michael Handy/Manager National Sales
Production: Rosalind Friedman/Manager Regulatory Affairs
Research: James E. Whitman, Jr./Director Research
  Antigen, Antiserum, Control, Lymphocyte Typing | Immunology
  Antigen, Antiserum, Control, Whole Human Serum | Immunology
  Antiserum, Serratia Marcesans | Microbiology
  Contract R&D, Diagnostics | General
  Culture Media, General Nutrient Broth | Microbiology
  Culture Media, Selective And Differential | Microbiology
  Culture Media, Supplements | Microbiology

ADVANCED CARDIAC THERAPEUTICS INC.
877-876-5994
1278 Glenneyre, Suite 139, Laguna Beach, CA 92651
FDA Number: n/a
Fax: 949-861-6340
E-mail: info@actmed.net
Web site: http://www.actmed.net
Year Founded: 2007
Ownership: Private
Produces/Sells CE-marked Devices: N
Mktg./Adv.: Mr. Darren Spencer/Director Clinical Support & Sales

ADVANCED CARDIOVASCULAR SYSTEMS, INC.
  See Boston Scientific Corp.

ADVANCED CELL DIAGNOSTICS INC.
510-576-8800
26229 Eden Landing Road, Hayward, CA 94545
FDA Number: n/a
Fax: 510-576-8801
Web site: www.acdbio.com
Ownership: Private
Produces/Sells CE-marked Devices: N
General Admin.: Dr. Steve Chen/Chief Operating Officer
  Dr. Xiao-Jun Ma/Chief Scientific Officer
  Dr. Yuling Luo/President, Chief Executive Officer
Mktg./Adv.: Dr. Christopher Bunker/Senior Director Business Development

ADVANCED CHEMICAL SENSORS INC.
561-338-3116
3201 N Dixie Hwy Suite 3, Boca Raton, FL 33431-6037
FDA Number: n/a
Fax: 561-338-5737
E-mail: acsbadges@gmail.com

ADVANCED CHEMICAL SENSORS INC.   561-338-3116 *(cont'd)*

Web site: www.acsbadges.com
Medical Products Sales Volume: $300,000
Annual Revenue: $1-$5 Million
Year Founded: 1976
Total Employees: 5   *Marketing Staff:* 2   *Sales Staff:* 2
Ownership: Private
Produces/Sells CE-marked Devices: Y
Federal Procurement Eligibility: Small Business, GSA Contract
Distribution: Manufacturer Direct, Manufacturer Through Manufacturer Reps, Exporter
General Admin.: Laurence D. Locker/President

Analyzer, Ethylene-Oxide	General
Analyzer, Gas, Carbon-Dioxide, Gaseous Phase (Capnograph)	Anesthesiology
Analyzer, Gas, Carbon-Monoxide, Gaseous Phase	Anesthesiology
Analyzer, Gas, Nitrous-Oxide, Gaseous Phase	Anesthesiology
Analyzer, Gas, Oxygen, Gaseous Phase	Anesthesiology
Analyzer, Mercury	Chemistry
Formaldehyde (Formalin, Formol)	Pathology
Glutaraldehyde (Fixative)	Pathology
Methyl Metacrylate	Cns/Neurology

ADVANCED CHEMICAL TECHNOLOGY, INC.   863-687-9603
1706 South Combee Rd., Lakeland, FL 33803
FDA Number: 1058329
Ownership: Private
Produces/Sells CE-marked Devices: N

Glove, Surgical, Plastic Surgery	Surgery

ADVANCED CIRCULATORY SYSTEMS, INC.   866-737-7763
1905 County Road C West, Roseville, MN 55113   651-403-5600
FDA Number: 3003477173
E-mail: info@advancedcirculatory.com
Web site: www.advancedcirculatory.com
Ownership: Private
Produces/Sells CE-marked Devices: N

Compressor, Cardiac, External	Cardiovascular
Exerciser, Non-Measuring	Physical Med
Mask, Oxygen, Non-Rebreathing	Anesthesiology
Massager, Powered Inflatable Tube	Physical Med
Strap, Head, Gas Mask	Anesthesiology

ADVANCED CONCEPT INNOVATIONS LLC   863-577-8055
4100 S. Frontage Rd., Lakeland, FL 33815
FDA Number: 3006015326
E-mail: info@advancedconceptinnovations.com
Web site: www.advancedconceptinnovations.com
Ownership: Private
Produces/Sells CE-marked Devices: N

Cerclage, Fixation	Orthopedics
Prosthesis, Knee, Patellofemorotibial, Semi-Constrained	Orthopedics
Tape, Measuring, Ruler And Caliper	Surgery

ADVANCED DENTAL SYSTEMS   480-991-4081
5001 East Desert Jewel Dr., Paradise Valley, AZ 85253
FDA Number: 2031713
Ownership: Private
Produces/Sells CE-marked Devices: N

Illuminator, Fiberoptic, Surgical Field	Cns/Neurology
Light, Surgical, Fiberoptic	Surgery

ADVANCED DERMAL SYSTEMS LLC   847-451-0145
9109 Medill, Franklin Park, IL 60131
FDA Number: 3005359152
Ownership: Private
Produces/Sells CE-marked Devices: N

Brush, Dermabrasion	Surgery

ADVANCED DIAGNOSTICS, INC. (ADI)   800-724-4003
801 Montrose Avenue,   908-754-4880
South Plainfield, NJ 07080
FDA Number: n/a   *Fax:* 908-754-5181
E-mail: cs@inamco.com
Web site: www.inamco.com
Annual Revenue: $1-$5 Million
Year Founded: 1987
Total Employees: 34   *Marketing Staff:* 4   *Sales Staff:* 4
Ownership: Private
Produces/Sells CE-marked Devices: Y
Federal Procurement Eligibility: Small Business, Minority Owned
Distribution: Manufacturer Through Distributor, Exporter
General Admin.: VARGES GEORGE/Chief Executive Officer, Chairman
           Dr. DHARAM CHOUHAN/President

Kit, Pregnancy Test, Over The Counter, HCG	Chemistry
Test, Rheumatoid Factor	Immunology

ADVANCED ELECTRONICS SYSTEMS, INC.   800-345-1280
2005 Lincoln Way E.,   717-263-5681
Chambersburg, PA 17201
FDA Number: n/a   *Fax:* 717-263-1040
E-mail: stediwatt@comcast.net
Web site: www.stediwatt.com
Medical Products Sales Volume: $400,000
Annual Revenue: $0-$1 Million
Year Founded: 1974
Total Employees: 14   *Marketing Staff:* 2   *Sales Staff:* 2
Ownership: Private
Produces/Sells CE-marked Devices: N
Federal Procurement Eligibility: Small Business
Distribution: Manufacturer Through Manufacturer Reps
General Admin.: Richard Diller/Chief Executive Officer

Power Systems, Uninterruptible (UPS)	General

ADVANCED ENDOSCOPY DEVICES, INC.   818-227-2720
22134 Sherman Way, Canoga Park, CA 91303
FDA Number: 2085947   *Fax:* 818-227-2724
E-mail: sales@aed.md
Web site: www.aed.md
Medical Products Sales Volume: $1,500,000
Annual Revenue: $1-$5 Million
Year Founded: 1985
Total Employees: 15   *Marketing Staff:* 2   *Sales Staff:* 5
Ownership: Private
Produces/Sells CE-marked Devices: Y
Federal Procurement Eligibility: Small Business, Minority Owned, Female Owned, GSA Contract, VA Contract
Distribution: Manufacturer Through Distributor, OEM, Service Direct, Importer, Exporter
General Admin.: John Dawoodje/Chief Executive Officer

Arthroscope	Orthopedics
Cable, Fiberoptic	General
Cystoscope	Gastroenterology/Urology
Endoscope	Gastroenterology/Urology
Endoscope, Rigid	Surgery
Forceps, Endoscopic	Gastroenterology/Urology
Forceps, Grasping, Flexible Endoscopic	Gastroenterology/Urology
Laparoscope, General & Plastic Surgery	Surgery
Light, Surgical, Endoscopic	Surgery
Rhinoscope	Ear/Nose/Throat
Service, Maintenance/Repair	General
Service, Repair, Endoscopic	General

ADVANCED HEALTH CARE PRODUCTS INC.   800-265-9830
205 St. George St. N, Unit 6,   705-875-1155
Lindsay, ONT K9V-5 Canada
FDA Number: n/a   *Fax:* 705-878-1156
E-mail: info@advancedhealthcare.ca
Web site: www.advancedhealthcare.ca
Year Founded: 1991
Total Employees: 10
Ownership: Private
Produces/Sells CE-marked Devices: N
Distribution: Exclusive Distributor

ADVANCED HYPERBARIC TECHNOLOGIES, INC.   800-327-4325
124 Colts Neck Rd., Farmingdale, NJ 07727
FDA Number: 2249605
Ownership: Private
Produces/Sells CE-marked Devices: N

Chamber, Oxygen, Topical, Extremity	Surgery

ADVANCED IMAGE ENHANCEMENT, INC.   508-344-3097
306 Valentine St, Fall River, MA 02720
FDA Number: 3005916315

Image Processing System	Radiology

ADVANCED IMAGING RESEARCH, INC.   216-426-1461
4700 Lakeside Ave., Suite 400, Cleveland, OH 44114
FDA Number: 3004036149

Coil, Magnetic Resonance, Specialty	Radiology

ADVANCED IMAGING TECHNOLOGIES, INC.   509-375-3100
2400 Stevens Drive Suite B, Richland, WA 99354
FDA Number: 3023871

Holograph, Fetal, Acoustical	Obstetrics/Gynecology

ADVANCED INFUSION, INC.   909-305-9857
466 West Arrow Hwy., Unit H, San Dimas, CA 91773
FDA Number: 2031920

Pump, Infusion, Elastomeric	General

ADVANCED INPUT SYSTEMS   800-444-5923
600 W. Wilbur Ave., Coeur D'Alene, ID 83815   208-765-8000
FDA Number: n/a   *Fax:* 208-292-2275
E-mail: sales@advanced-input.com

ADVANCED INPUT SYSTEMS   800-444-5923 *(cont'd)*
Web site: www.advanced-input.com
Annual Revenue: $50-$100 Million
Year Founded: 1979
Total Employees: 350
Ownership: Private
Quality System Registration Information: ISO9001
Produces/Sells CE-marked Devices: Y
Distribution: Manufacturer Direct, Manufacturer Through Manufacturer Reps
General Admin.: Francis Brastrup/Manager Human Resources
      Brad Lawrence/President, Chief Executive Officer
Mktg./Adv.: Mr. Randy Noland/Director Marketing
Production: Mike Johnson/Director Manufacturing & Operations
      Randy Nell/Director Quality Assurance
      James R. Tsalidas/Vice President Product Engineering Development
Finance: Al Yost/Director Finance
Cleanroom Equipment	General

ADVANCED INSTRUMENT DEVELOPMENT, INC.   800-243-9729
2545 Curtiss Street, Downers Grove, IL 60515   **708-343-7777**
FDA Number: 1483291   Fax: 708-343-7795
E-mail: sales@aidxray.com
Web site: www.aidxray.com
Medical Products Sales Volume: $3,500,000
Annual Revenue: $1-$5 Million
Year Founded: 1969
Total Employees: 35   Marketing Staff: 1
Ownership: Private
Quality System Registration Information: ISO9001
Produces/Sells CE-marked Devices: Y
Federal Procurement Eligibility: Small Business
Distribution: Manufacturer Direct, Manufacturer Through Distributor, OEM, Service Direct, Exporter
General Admin.: Alice Packard/Corporate Secretary
      Edward F. Polic/President
      Mark Gadbois/Vice President
Mktg./Adv.: Jim Taylor/Director Product Development
Production: Bruce Packard/Vice President Production

Generator, Diagnostic X-Ray, High Voltage, 3-Phase	Radiology
Phototimer, Radiographic Mobile	Radiology
Power Systems, Uninterruptible (UPS)	General
Radiographic Unit, Diagnostic	Radiology
Timer, Radiographic	Radiology

ADVANCED INSTRUMENTS INC.   800-225-4034
Two Technology Way,   **781-320-9000**
Norwood, MA 02062
FDA Number: 1217058   Fax: 781-320-8181
E-mail: info@aicompanies.com
Web site: www.aicompanies.com
Medical Products Sales Volume: $7,000,000
Annual Revenue: $10-$25 Million
Total Employees: 90
Ownership: Private
Quality System Registration Information: ISO9001
Produces/Sells CE-marked Devices: Y
Federal Procurement Eligibility: Small Business, Female Owned
Distribution: Manufacturer Direct, Manufacturer Through Distributor, Manufacturer Through Manufacturer Reps, Exporter
General Admin.: John Coughlin/President, Chief Executive Officer
      Phyllis Weeton/Vice President Human Resources
      John Ryder/Vice President, General Manager
Mktg./Adv.: Kristen Vuotto/Director Marketing
      Rick Zampa/Manager International & National Sales
      Fred Ferola/Manager National Sales
      Pete Emond/Vice President Business Development
      John Ryder/Vice President Sales
Production: Bud Downs/Director Quality Assurance
      Lee Eckhart/Vice President Manufacturing
Research: Eileen Garry/Vice President Research & Development

Bilirubinometer	Chemistry
Counter, Colony, Automated	Microbiology
Osmometer	Chemistry
Reagent, Bilirubin (Total Or Direct Test System)	Chemistry
Standard/Control, All Types	Chemistry

ADVANCED LIVING SYSTEMS
See Promatura Group, Llc

ADVANCED MAGNETICS, INC.   617-576-1915
61 Mooney St., Cambridge, MA 02138
FDA Number: n/a
Web site: www.advancedmagnetics.com
Medical Products Sales Volume: $600,444
Annual Revenue: $1-$5 Million
Ownership: Private
Produces/Sells CE-marked Devices: N
Federal Procurement Eligibility: Small Business

ADVANCED MAGNETICS, INC.   617-576-1915 *(cont'd)*
Distribution: Manufacturer Through Distributor

Magnet, Permanent, MRI (Magnetic Resonance Imaging)	Radiology
Media, Radiographic Injectable Contrast	Radiology

ADVANCED MATERIALS, INC.   310-537-5444
20211 South Susana Rd., Rancho Dominguez, CA 90221
FDA Number: 2020678
Ownership: Private
Produces/Sells CE-marked Devices: N

Bag, Ice	General
Holder, Catheter	Gastroenterology/Urology

ADVANCED MECHANICAL TECHNOLOGY, INC. (AMTI)   800-422-AMTI
176 Waltham St., Watertown, MA 02472   **617-926-6700**
FDA Number: 9200022   Fax: 617-926-5045
E-mail: support@amtimail.com
Web site: www.amtiweb.com
Medical Products Sales Volume: $6,000,000
Annual Revenue: $5-$10 Million
Year Founded: 1976
Total Employees: 28   Marketing Staff: 2   Sales Staff: 5
Ownership: Private
Quality System Registration Information: ISO9001
Produces/Sells CE-marked Devices: Y
Federal Procurement Eligibility: Small Business
Distribution: Manufacturer Direct, Manufacturer Through Manufacturer Reps, Service Direct, Exporter
General Admin.: Andrew Vasilakis/President, Chief Executive Officer
      Forest Carignan/Vice President
Mktg./Adv.: Forest Carignan/Director Product Development
      Gary Blanchard/Manager International & National Sales
Production: Gary Blanchard/Manager Production
Research: Forest Carignan/Vice President Research & Development

Analyzer, Distribution, Weight, Podiatric	Orthopedics
Analyzer, Gait	Orthopedics
Analyzer, Motion	General
Balance, Analytical	Chemistry
Computer, Diagnostic, Pre-Programmed, Single-Function	Cardiovascular
Dynamometer, Other	Cns/Neurology
Platform, Force-Measuring	Physical Med

ADVANCED MEDICAL DESIGN INTERNATIONAL LLC   407-992-6694
1802 N. Alafaya Trail, Suite 132, Alafaya, FL 32826
FDA Number: 3007074235   Fax: 407-306-6129
E-mail: info@amdintl.com
Web site: http://amdintl.com
Ownership: Private
Stock Symbol: EYE
Traded On: NYSE
Produces/Sells CE-marked Devices: N

ADVANCED MEDICAL DEVICES, INC.   416-833-6681
15 Keele Street South Unit 2, Po Box 520,
King City L7B 1 Canada
FDA Number: 8043468
Ownership: Shanghai Zhijiang Biotechnology Co.,Ltd

Speculum, Vaginal, Non-Metal	Obstetrics/Gynecology

ADVANCED MEDICAL INNOVATIONS, INC.   888-367-2641
9410 De Soto Avenue,, Building J,   **818-701-7180**
Chatsworth, CA 91311, CA 91311
FDA Number: 2028390   Fax: 818-701-9708
E-mail: sales@amiwelisten.com
Web site: www.amiwelisten.com
Medical Products Sales Volume: $650,000
Annual Revenue: $1-$5 Million
Year Founded: 1995
Total Employees: 7
Ownership: American Medical Manufacturing, Inc
Quality System Registration Information: ISO9002
Produces/Sells CE-marked Devices: Y
Federal Procurement Eligibility: Small Business
Distribution: Manufacturer Direct, Manufacturer Through Distributor, Manufacturer Through Manufacturer Reps, OEM, Exporter
General Admin.: Mike Hoftman/President, Chief Executive Officer
Mktg./Adv.: Nir Hoftman/Director Product Development
      Jacky Hoftman/Manager Advertising
      Mike Hoftman/Manager Contract Sales
      Mike Hoftman/Manager International & National Sales
      Shardel Doherty/Manager National Sales
Production: Gil Hoftman/Director Quality Assurance & Regulatory Affairs
      Jacky Hoftman/Manager Materials

Accessories, Light, Surgical	Surgery
Accessories, Operating Room, Table	Surgery

ADVANCED MEDICAL INNOVATIONS, INC. 888-367-2641 *(cont'd)*

Blade, Scalpel	Surgery
Container, Sterilization (Tray)	General
Counter, Needle	Surgery
Counter, Sponge, Surgical	Surgery
Counter, Surgical Instrument	Surgery
Dilator, Vaginal	Obstetrics/Gynecology
Drape, Surgical Instrument, Magnetic	Surgery
Infusion Stand	General
Instrument, Passing, Suture, Laparoscopic	Surgery
Kit, Instruments and Accessories, Surgical	Surgery
Kit, Irrigation, Sterile	Gastroenterology/Urology
Tip, Suction Tube (Yankauer, Poole, Etc.)	Surgery
Tray, Sterilization, Instrument	Surgery
Waste Disposal Unit, Surgical Instrument (Sharps)	Surgery

ADVANCED MEDICAL INSTRUMENTS, INC. 918-250-0566
3061 West Albany, Broken Arrow, OK 74012
FDA Number: 1627304
Ownership: ADVANCED MEDICAL OPTICS, INC.
Stock Symbol: EYE
Traded On: NYSE
Produces/Sells CE-marked Devices: N

Cuff, Blood Pressure	Cardiovascular
Monitor, Blood Pressure, Indirect, Semi-Automatic	Cardiovascular
Oximeter, Intracardiac	Cardiovascular

ADVANCED MEDICAL OPTICS, INC.
See Abbott Medical Optics Inc.

ADVANCED MEDICAL SCIENCE & TECHNOLOGY, LLC 410-472-9209
410 Buedel Court, Sparks, Maryland, MD 21152
FDA Number: 3006235941   *Fax:* 410-472-9219
E-mail: info@advancedmedicals.com
Web site: www.advancedmedicals.com
Ownership: Private
Stock Symbol: EYE
Traded On: NYSE
Produces/Sells CE-marked Devices: N

Detergent	Hematology
Headlamp, Operating, Battery-Operated	Ophthalmology
Immunohistochemistry Reagents And Kits	Pathology

ADVANCED MEDICAL SUPPORT 888-800-7283 / 561-624-2845
10180 Riverside Dr, Suite 9,
N Palm Beach, FL 33410
FDA Number: 3006700079   *Fax:* 877-625-5386
E-mail: info@mydiabetic.net
Web site: www.advancedmedicalsupport.com
Ownership: Private
Stock Symbol: EYE
Traded On: NYSE
Produces/Sells CE-marked Devices: N

ADVANCED MEDICAL SYSTEMS, INC. 440-466-8005
101 N. Eagle St., Geneva, OH 44041
FDA Number: n/a
Medical Products Sales Volume: $3,500,000
Annual Revenue: $1-$5 Million
Ownership: Private
Produces/Sells CE-marked Devices: N
Federal Procurement Eligibility: Small Business

Radiographic/Fluoroscopic Unit, Fixed	Radiology
Radiographic/Fluoroscopic Unit, Special Procedure	Radiology
Radiotherapy Treatment Planning Unit	Radiology
Simulator, Radiotherapy	Radiology
Source, Teletherapy, Radionuclide	Radiology
Table, Radiographic, Non-Tilting, Powered	Radiology
Therapeutic X-Ray System	Radiology

ADVANCED MEDICAL TECHNOLOGIES, INC. 508-790-8700
101 Waterside Dr, Centerville, MA 02632
FDA Number: 3003948910
Ownership: Private
Stock Symbol: EYE
Traded On: NYSE
Produces/Sells CE-marked Devices: N

Lamp, Infrared	Physical Med

ADVANCED MEDICAL, INC 215-443-5424
935 Horsham Rd., Horsham, PA 19044
FDA Number: 2529402
Ownership: ADVANCED MEDICAL OPTICS, INC.
Stock Symbol: EYE
Traded On: NYSE
Produces/Sells CE-marked Devices: N

ADVANCED MEDITECH INTERNATIONAL 800-635-2452 / 718-672-7150
86-38 53rd Ave., Ste. 100, Flushing, NY 11373
FDA Number: n/a   *Fax:* 718-672-8501
E-mail: info@ameditech.com
Web site: www.ameditech.com
Annual Revenue: $1-$5 Million
Ownership: Private
Produces/Sells CE-marked Devices: N
Federal Procurement Eligibility: Small Business

Knife, Ophthalmic	Ophthalmology
Material, Training, Audiovisual	General
Stimulator, Nerve Locating	Cns/Neurology
Stylet, Tracheal Tube	Anesthesiology

ADVANCED MICRODERM, INC. 630-980-3300
904 S. Roselle Rd., #302, Schaumburg, IL 60193
FDA Number: 3005761517

Brush, Dermabrasion	Surgery

ADVANCED MOBILITY PRODUCTS LTD. 800-665-4442 / 604-293-0002
Suite 101-8620 Glenlyon Pky,,
BURNABY, BC V5J 0 Canada
FDA Number: n/a   *Fax:* 604-293-0005
E-mail: mainlandservice@advancedmobility.ca
Web site: www.advancedmobility.ca
Year Founded: 1987
Total Employees: 10
Ownership: Private
Produces/Sells CE-marked Devices: N
Distribution: Service Direct, Exclusive Distributor

ADVANCED MOBILITY SYSTEMS CORP. 800-661-6716 / 613-384-7460
621 Justus Dr., Kingston, ONT K7M-4H5 Canada
FDA Number: n/a   *Fax:* 613-634-3990
E-mail: info@amstilt.com
Web site: www.amstilt.com
Year Founded: 1988
Total Employees: 10
Ownership: Private
Produces/Sells CE-marked Devices: N
Distribution: Manufacturer Direct, Exclusive Distributor

ADVANCED MONITORED CAREGIVING 201-727-1703
111 John St. Suite 250, Manhattan, NY 10038
FDA Number: 3005439460

Transmitter/Receiver System, Physiological, Telephone	Cardiovascular

ADVANCED MONOBLOC
See Ccl Containers

ADVANCED MOTION MEASUREMENT, LLC 602-263-8657
1202 East Maryland Ave.,, Suite 1j, Phoenix, AZ 85014
FDA Number: n/a   *Fax:* 602-227-2326
Web site: www.amm3d.com
Ownership: Private
Produces/Sells CE-marked Devices: N
General Admin.: Mr. Phillip Cheetham/President, CTO
Mktg./Adv.: Mr. Stephen Cheethman/Vice President Sales

Examination Device, AC-Powered	General
Goniometer, AC-powered	Orthopedics

ADVANCED NEUROMODULATION SYSTEMS
See St. Jude Medical Neuromodulation Division

ADVANCED OCULAR PROSTHETICS INC. 412-787-7277
1111 Oakdale Rd., Suite 5, Oakdale, PA 15071
FDA Number: n/a
Web site: www.aopeyes.com
Ownership: Private
Produces/Sells CE-marked Devices: N

Conformer, Ophthalmic	Ophthalmology
Eye, Artificial, Non-Custom	Ophthalmology
Shell, Scleral	Ophthalmology

ADVANCED ORTHOGONAL EQUIPMENT, INCORPORATED 757-224-0177
2201 62nd Avenue North, Saint Petersburg, FL 33702
FDA Number: 3006315109

Plunger-Like Joint Manipulator	Physical Med

ADVANCED ORTHOPAEDIC SOLUTIONS, INC. 866-229-7686 / 310-533-9966
386 Beech Ave., Unit B6, Torrance, CA 90501
FDA Number: 2032480   *Fax:* 310-533-9876
E-mail: info@aosortho.com
Web site: www.aosortho.com
Ownership: Private
Produces/Sells CE-marked Devices: N

Orthopedic Manual Surgical Instrument	Orthopedics
Rod, Fixation, Intramedullary	Orthopedics

ADVANCED ORTHOPAEDIC SOLUTIONS, INC. 866-229-7686
(cont'd)
Rod, Fixation, Intramedullary And Accessories, Metallic And Non-collapsible
Orthopedics
Screw, Fixation, Bone, Non-Spinal, Metallic — Orthopedics

ADVANCED ORTHOPEDIC TECHNOLOGIES
See Novacare Orthodics

ADVANCED POLYMERS, INC. 603-327-0600
29 Northwestern Drive, Salem, NH 03079-2838
FDA Number: n/a — *Fax:* 603-327-0601
E-mail: sales@advpoly.com
Web site: www.advpoly.com
Medical Products Sales Volume: $3,900,000
Annual Revenue: $1-$5 Million
Year Founded: 1989
Total Employees: 49 — *Marketing Staff:* 1 — *Sales Staff:* 4
Ownership: Private
Quality System Registration Information: ISO9001
Produces/Sells CE-marked Devices: N
Federal Procurement Eligibility: Small Business
Distribution: Manufacturer Direct, Manufacturer Through Manufacturer Reps, OEM
General Admin.: Mark A. Saab/President
Mktg./Adv.: Ray Pellerin/Manager National Sales
Production: Ilidia Porto/Director Quality Assurance
Balloon, Angioplasty, Coronary, Heated — Cardiovascular
Catheter, Balloon, Dilatation, Vessel — Gastroenterology/Urology
Contract Assembly — General
Contract Manufacturing — General
Service, Engineering/Design — General
Tubing, Other — General

ADVANCED RADIATION MEASUREMENTS, INC. 772-340-3279
601 N.E. Emerson St., Port St. Lucie, FL 34983
FDA Number: 1058180 — *Fax:* 772-871-5595
E-mail: armx2000@aol.com
Web site: armx2000.com
Ownership: Private
Quality System Registration Information: ISO9000
Produces/Sells CE-marked Devices: Y
Federal Procurement Eligibility: Small Business
Distribution: Manufacturer Direct
Accelerator, Linear, Medical — Radiology

ADVANCED RADIATION THERAPY, LLC 978-663-7300
9 Linnell Circle, Billerica, MA 01821
FDA Number: 3006126834
Ownership: Private
Produces/Sells CE-marked Devices: N
Applicator, Radionuclide, Manual — Radiology
Applicator, Radionuclide, Remote-Controlled — Radiology

ADVANCED REFRACTIVE TECHNOLOGIES 949-940-1300
1062 Calle Negocio, Suite D, San Clemente, CA 92673
FDA Number: 2032816 — *Fax:* 949-940-1301
E-mail: admin@advancedrefractive.com
Web site: www.advancedrefractive.com
Ownership: Private
Produces/Sells CE-marked Devices: N
Keratome, Water Jet — Ophthalmology

ADVANCED RENAL TECHNOLOGIES, INC. 425-453-8777
40 Lake Bellevue, Suite 100, Suite 100, Bellevue, WA 98005
FDA Number: 3032665 — *Fax:* 425-451-9438
E-mail: info@advrenaltech.com
Web site: www.advrenaltech.com
Medical Products Sales Volume: $280,000
Year Founded: 1992
Total Employees: 2
Ownership: Private
Produces/Sells CE-marked Devices: N
Federal Procurement Eligibility: Small Business
Concentrate, Dialysis, Hemodialysis (Liquid or Powder) — Gastroenterology/Urology

ADVANCED RESEARCH TECHNOLOGIES INC. (ART) 888-278-7888
2300 Alfred Nobel, Technoparc MontrAcal, 514-832-0777
Montreal, QUE H4S-2 Canada
FDA Number: n/a — *Fax:* 514-832-0778
E-mail: info@art.ca
Web site: www.art.ca
Year Founded: 1993
Total Employees: 50
Ownership: Private
Produces/Sells CE-marked Devices: N
Distribution: Manufacturer Direct

ADVANCED SPINE TECHNOLOGY, INC. 415-241-2400
457 Mariposa St., San Francisco, CA 94107
FDA Number: 2950169
Ownership: Private
Produces/Sells CE-marked Devices: N
Appliance, Fixation, Spinal Intervertebral Body — Orthopedics
Chisel, Surgical, Manual — Surgery
Implant, Fixation Device, Spinal — Orthopedics
Microtome, Freezing Attachment — Pathology
Orthopedic Manual Surgical Instrument — Orthopedics
Orthosis, Fixation, Pedicle, Spinal — Orthopedics
Orthosis, Fixation, Spinal, Spondylolisthesis — Orthopedics
Radiographic Unit, Diagnostic, Photofluorographic — Radiology

ADVANCED STENT TECHNOLOGIES 508-650-8798
6900 Koll Center Pkwy., #415, Pleasanton, CA 94566
FDA Number: n/a
Web site: www.bostonscientific.com
Ownership: BOSTON SCIENTIFIC CORPORATION
Produces/Sells CE-marked Devices: N
Stent, Cardiovascular — Cardiovascular

ADVANCED STERILIZATION PRODUCTS 800-595-0200
33 Technology Dr., Irvine, CA 92618 949-581-5799
FDA Number: 2084725 — *Fax:* 949-450-6800
E-mail: aspservices@aspus.jnj.com
Web site: www.sterrad.com
Ownership: Johnson & Johnson
Quality System Registration Information: ISO9001
Produces/Sells CE-marked Devices: Y
Distribution: Manufacturer Direct, Manufacturer Through Distributor
General Admin.: David Powell/President
Mktg./Adv.: Karen Borg/Vice President Marketing & Sales
Production: Ross Krogh/Vice President Quality Assurance
Truc H. Le/Vice President Quality Assurance
Mizanu Kebede/Vice President Regulatory & Clinical Affairs
John Friend/Vice President Regulatory Affairs
Finance: Mike Meyers/Vice President Finance
IS: Terry D. Larkins/Director Tech. Services
Medical Disinfectants/Cleaners for Instruments — General
Pack, Sterilization Wrapper (Bag And Accessories) — Surgery
Sterilization Process Indicator, Physical/Chemical — General
Sterilizer, Vapor — General

ADVANCED SURGI-PHARM INC. 800-661-5432
850 Halpern Ave., Dorval, QUE H9P-1G1 Canada 514-631-7988
FDA Number: n/a — *Fax:* 514-631-9083
E-mail: info@surgmed.com
Web site: www.surgmed.com
Year Founded: 1991
Total Employees: 50
Ownership: Private
Produces/Sells CE-marked Devices: N
Distribution: Exclusive Distributor, Importer

ADVANCED TECHNOLOGY LABORATORIES, INC.
See Phillips Ultrasound

ADVANCED THERAPY PRODUCTS, INC. 800-548-4550
P.O. Box 3420, Glen Allen, VA 23058-3420
FDA Number: n/a — *Fax:* 804-747-0676
E-mail: info@atpwork.com
Web site: www.atpwork.com
Ownership: Private
Produces/Sells CE-marked Devices: N
Component, Exercise — Physical Med

ADVANCED URETHANE TECHNOLOGIES, INC. 630-293-0780
1750 West Downs Dr., West Chicago, IL 60185
FDA Number: 3003484742
Mattress, Non-Powered Flotation Therapy — Physical Med

ADVANCED VISION SCIENCE 800-235-5781
5743 Thornwood Drive, Goleta, CA 93117-3801 805-683-3851
FDA Number: 2020277 — *Fax:* 805-964-3065
E-mail: contactus@avsiol.com
Web site: www.advancedvisionscience.com
Medical Products Sales Volume: $5,000,000
Annual Revenue: $0-$1 Million
Year Founded: 1998
Total Employees: 40
Ownership: Private
Quality System Registration Information: ISO9001; ISO9002
Produces/Sells CE-marked Devices: Y
Federal Procurement Eligibility: Small Business, GSA Contract, VA Contract
Distribution: Manufacturer Through Distributor, Manufacturer Through
Manufacturer Reps, Importer, Exporter
Mktg./Adv.: Karen Krebaum/Manager Marketing & Sales
Production: Margaret Aldred/Vice President Product Development & Operations

ADVANCED VISION SCIENCE
800-235-5781 *(cont'd)*
Finance: Barbara Nunez/Controller
Hook, Ophthalmic — Ophthalmology

ADVANCED WOUND SYSTEMS, LLC.
541-867-4726
1530 Dunwoody Village Pkwy #115, Atlanta, GA 30350
FDA Number: 3004471916
Ownership: Private
Produces/Sells CE-marked Devices: N
Bandage, Adhesive — Surgery

ADVANSOURCE BIOMATERIALS CORP.
978-657-0075
229 Andover St., Wilmington, MA 01887
FDA Number: n/a *Fax:* 978-657-0074
E-mail: info@advbiomaterials.com
Web site: www.advbiomaterials.com
Medical Products Sales Volume: $3,207,000
Annual Revenue: $1-$5 Million
Year Founded: 1993
Total Employees: 22 *Marketing Staff:* 2 *Sales Staff:* 1
Ownership: Public
Stock Symbol: ASB
Traded On: NYSE
Produces/Sells CE-marked Devices: N
Federal Procurement Eligibility: Small Business
Distribution: Manufacturer Direct
General Admin.: Michael Adams/President, Chief Executive Officer
Research: Andrew Reed/Vice President Science & Technology
Elastomer, Other — General
Polymer, Synthetic, Other — General
System, Delivery, Drug, Non-invasive — General

ADVANTAGE BAG CO.
800-556-6307
22633 Ellinwood Dr., Torrance, CA 90505 **310-540-8197**
FDA Number: n/a *Fax:* 310-316-2561
E-mail: advantagebag@verizon.net
Web site: www.advantagebag.com
Annual Revenue: $0-$1 Million
Total Employees: 6
Ownership: Private
Produces/Sells CE-marked Devices: N
Federal Procurement Eligibility: Small Business, Female Owned
Distribution: Manufacturer Direct
General Admin.: Deborah V. Frane/Chief Executive Officer
Accessories, Wheelchair — Physical Med
Attachment, Bag (Crutch, Walker, Wheelchair) — Physical Med

ADVANTAGE MEDICAL ELECTRONICS, INC.
954-345-9800
10630 Wiles Road, Coral Springs, FL 33076
FDA Number: 1063285
Cable/Lead, ECG, With Transducer And Electrode — Cardiovascular

ADVANTAGE MEDICAL SYSTEMS, INC.
800-810-1262
2876 South Wheeling Way, Aurora, CO 80014 **303-750-2996**
FDA Number: 1724493 *Fax:* 303-750-9560
E-mail: sales@advantagemedical.info
Ownership: Private
Produces/Sells CE-marked Devices: N
Marker, Skin — Surgery
Stool, Operating Room, Adjustable — Surgery
Table, Operating Room, AC-Powered — Surgery

ADVANTIS MEDICAL
888-625-4497
2121 Southtech Dr., Ste 600, **317-859-2300**
Greenwood, IN 46143
FDA Number: n/a *Fax:* 317-859-2350
E-mail: jspencer@advantismedical.com
Web site: www.advantismedical.com
Medical Products Sales Volume: $1,600,000
Annual Revenue: $10-$25 Million
Year Founded: 1996
Total Employees: 110 *Marketing Staff:* 2 *Sales Staff:* 5
Ownership: Avalign Technologies
Quality System Registration Information: ISO9000
Produces/Sells CE-marked Devices: Y
Federal Procurement Eligibility: Small Business, GSA Contract
Distribution: Manufacturer Direct, Manufacturer Through Distributor, Manufacturer Through Manufacturer Reps, OEM, Exporter
General Admin.: James B. Spencer/President
Mktg./Adv: Carol Meguschar/Manager International & National Sales
Production: John Oliver/Director Manufacturing
Don Cobb/Vice President Manufacturing
Chris Dennis/Vice President Quality Assurance
Research: Jeffrey Leath/Vice President Engineering
Tray, Sterilization, Instrument — Surgery
Medical Product Subsidiaries (Listed Separately)
Nemcomed

ADVENTURE MEDICAL KITS
800-324-3517
7700 Edgewater Drive, Suite 526, **510-261-7414**
Oakland, CA 94624
FDA Number: 2952362 *Fax:* 510-878-2049
E-mail: questions@adventuremedicalkits.com
Web site: www.adventuremedicalkits.com
Ownership: Private
Produces/Sells CE-marked Devices: N
Dressing, Wound and Burn, Hydrogel — Surgery
Kit, First Aid — Surgery
Protector, Skin Pressure — General

ADVENTURES IN COLOR TECHNOLOGY
303-271-9644
1800 Jackson St., Suite 214, Golden, CO 80403
FDA Number: 1722370
Lenses, Soft Contact, Daily Wear — Ophthalmology

AE
See C.D. Denison Orthopaedic Appliance Corp.

AEARO CANADA LTD.
617-371-4200
7115 Tomken Rd, Mississauga L5S 1R7 Canada
FDA Number: 9680923
Sunglasses (Including Photosensitive) — Ophthalmology

AEARO COMPANY
800-678-4163
5457 West 79th Street, Indianapolis, IN 46268 **317-692-6666**
FDA Number: 1218952 *Fax:* 317-692-6772
E-mail: jim_gray@aearo.com
Web site: www.aearo.com
Medical Products Sales Volume: $100,000,000
Total Employees: 570 *Sales Staff:* 60
Ownership: Private
Quality System Registration Information: ISO9001
Produces/Sells CE-marked Devices: N
Distribution: Manufacturer Direct, Manufacturer Through Distributor, Manufacturer Through Manufacturer Reps, Exporter
General Admin.: Roland Cyr/Chairman
Jim Bernhardt/Senior Vice President
Eyeglasses, Safety — Ophthalmology
Mask, Face — General
Protector, Hearing (Insert) — Ear/Nose/Throat
Ventilator, Other — Anesthesiology

AEARO COMPANY
508-764-5713
90 Mechanic St., Southbridge, MA 01550
FDA Number: 3000131652
Ownership: Private
Produces/Sells CE-marked Devices: N

AEC, INC.
847-273-7700
1100 Woodfield Rd., Suite 588, Schaumburg, IL 60173
FDA Number: n/a *Fax:* 847-273-7804
Web site: www.aecinternet.com
Annual Revenue: $0-$1 Million
Ownership: Private
Produces/Sells CE-marked Devices: N
Distribution: Manufacturer Through Manufacturer Reps, Importer, Exporter
System, Cooling, Laser — Surgery
Medical Product Subsidiaries (Listed Separately)
Carver Inc.

AEGIS FLOORSYSTEMS
972-788-2233
14286 Gillis Road, Dallas, TX 75244
FDA Number: n/a *Fax:* 972-490-7144
E-mail: office@aegisfloors.com
Web site: http://www.aegisfloors.com/
Medical Products Sales Volume: $1,100,000
Annual Revenue: $1-$5 Million
Year Founded: 1993
Total Employees: 11 *Marketing Staff:* 3 *Sales Staff:* 3
Ownership: Private
Produces/Sells CE-marked Devices: N
Federal Procurement Eligibility: Small Business
Distribution: Manufacturer Direct, Service Direct
General Admin.: Renee Haney/Office Manager
Floor Mat — General
Flooring — General

AEGIS MEDICAL
203-838-9081
10 Wall St., Norwalk, CT 06850
FDA Number: n/a *Fax:* 203-855-9945
E-mail: aegisworld@att.net
Medical Products Sales Volume: $14,000,000
Annual Revenue: $10-$25 Million
Total Employees: 10
Ownership: Private
Produces/Sells CE-marked Devices: N
Distribution: Exclusive Distributor, Exporter

AEGIS MEDICAL   203-838-9081 *(cont'd)*
General Admin.: Abhay Singh/President, Chief Executive Officer
Mktg./Adv.: David Luster/Manager International Marketing & Sales

Accessories, Operating Room, Table	Surgery
Cast	Orthopedics
Dressing, Other	General
Glove, Surgical	General
Gown, Operating Room, Disposable	Surgery
Splint, Other	Orthopedics
Suture, Other	Surgery

AEGIS MEDICAL, INC.
See Caire, Inc.

AEI TECHNOLOGIES INC.   800-793-7751
300 William Pitt Way, Pittsburgh, PA 15238   630-548-3545
FDA Number: 3004055954   *Fax:* 630-548-3546
E-mail: info@aeitechnologies.com
Web site: www.aeitechnologies.com
Ownership: Private
Produces/Sells CE-marked Devices: N

Analyzer, Gas, Carbon-Dioxide, Gaseous Phase (Capnograph)	Anesthesiology
Analyzer, Gas, Oxygen, Gaseous Phase	Anesthesiology
Computer, Oxygen-Uptake	Anesthesiology

AEIOMED, INC.   612-455-0550
1313 5th Street Se, Ste 205, Minneapolis, MN 55414
FDA Number: 3004961637
Ownership: Private
Produces/Sells CE-marked Devices: N

Ventilator, Non-Continuous (Respirator)	Anesthesiology

AERIS THERAPEUTICS, INC.   781-937-0110
10k Gill Street, Woburn, MA 01801
FDA Number: 3003882569

ENT Drug Applicator	Ear/Nose/Throat

AERO ALL GAS CO.   800-255-4277
3150 Main Street, Hartford, CT 06120   860-278-2376 Ex
FDA Number: n/a   *Fax:* 860-527-2376
Web site: aeroallgas.com
Medical Products Sales Volume: $5,200,000
Annual Revenue: $5-$10 Million
Year Founded: 1941
Ownership: Private
Produces/Sells CE-marked Devices: N
Federal Procurement Eligibility: Small Business
Distribution: Manufacturer Direct, Manufacturer Through Manufacturer Reps, Service Direct

Gas Mixtures, Medical	General

AERO CONTACT LENS, INC.   269-345-3202
2958 Business One Drive, Kalamazoo, MI 49048
FDA Number: n/a
Ownership: Private
Produces/Sells CE-marked Devices: N

Clamp, Eyelid, Ophthalmic	Ophthalmology
Lens, Contact (Other Material)	Ophthalmology
Lenses, Soft Contact, Daily Wear	Ophthalmology

AERO INNOVATIVE RESEARCH, INC.   316-755-3477
500 W. Clay St, Valley Center, KS 67147
FDA Number: 3005837475

Wheelchair, Manual	Physical Med

AERO MEDICAL PRODUCTS CO., INC.   262-335-8000
2230 Stone Bridge Road, West Bend, WI 53095
FDA Number: 2133448   *Fax:* 262-335-8008
E-mail: marketing@medicalaircraft.com
Web site: www.medicalaircraft.com
Ownership: Private
Produces/Sells CE-marked Devices: N

Transport, Patient, Powered	Physical Med

AERODYNE CONTROLS CORP.
See Aerodyne Controls, Inc., A Circor International Company

AERODYNE CONTROLS, DIVISION OF CIRCLE SEAL CORPORATION
See Aerodyne Controls, Inc., A Circor International Company

AERODYNE CONTROLS, INC., A CIRCOR   631-737-1900
INTERNATIONAL COMPANY
30 Haynes Ct., Ronkonkoma, NY 11779-7220
FDA Number: n/a   *Fax:* 631-737-1912
E-mail: sales@circoraerospace.com
Web site: www.aerodyne-contols.com
Medical Products Sales Volume: $5,000,000
Annual Revenue: $50-$100 Million
Total Employees: 55   *Marketing Staff:* 2   *Sales Staff:* 6
Ownership: Thermo Fisher Scientific

AERODYNE CONTROLS, INC., A CIRCOR   631-737-1900 *(cont'd)*
Quality System Registration Information: ISO9001; ISO9002
Produces/Sells CE-marked Devices: N
Distribution: Manufacturer Direct
General Admin.: Michael G. Ryan/Vice President, General Manager
Production: Hugh O'Brien/Director Engineering

Regulator, Oxygen, Mechanical	General
Regulator, Pressure, Gas Cylinder	Anesthesiology
Regulator, Vacuum	General
Valve, Non-Rebreathing	Anesthesiology
Valve, Other	Chemistry

AERODYNE ULBRICH ALLOYS
See Ulbrich Stainless Steels & Special Metals

AEROS INSTRUMENTS
See Ohio Medical Corp.

AEROSCOUT   706-867-0140
1300 Island Drive, Suite 202, Redwood City, CA 94065
FDA Number: 3006784706
Ownership: Private
Produces/Sells CE-marked Devices: N

Regulator, Temperature	Chemistry

AEROSOL AND LIQUID PACKAGING, INC.   410-342-6100
715 S. Haven St., Baltimore, MD 21224
FDA Number: 1120890   *Fax:* 410-675-1636
E-mail: info@alpackaging.com
Web site: www.alpackaging.com
Ownership: Private
Produces/Sells CE-marked Devices: N

Pack, Hot Or Cold, Disposable	Physical Med

AEROSOL MONITORING & ANALYSIS, INC.   410-684-3327
1331 A Ashton Road, P.O. Box 646, Hanover, MD 21076
FDA Number: n/a   *Fax:* 410-684-3384
Web site: www.amatraining.com
Annual Revenue: $1-$5 Million
Year Founded: 1981
Ownership: Private
Produces/Sells CE-marked Devices: N
Federal Procurement Eligibility: Small Business
Distribution: Manufacturer Direct

Equipment/Service, Quality Control	General

AEROSURGICAL LTD.   650-530-0032
2995 Woodside Road, Suite 400, Woodside, CA 94062
FDA Number: n/a
Web site: http://aerosurgical.com
Ownership: Private
Produces/Sells CE-marked Devices: N
General Admin.: Dr. Conor Duffy/Chief Scientific Officer
     Mr. Nevan Elam/President, Chief Executive Officer
Medical Admin.: Dr. Anthony Senagore/Chief Medical Officer

AERSCHER DIAGNOSTICS   410-778-1144
353 High St., Chestertown, MD 21620
FDA Number: 1123776

Reagent, Guaiac	Hematology

AES CLEAN TECHNOLOGY, INC.   888-237-2532
422 Stump Road, Montgomeryville, PA 18936   215-393-6810
FDA Number: n/a   *Fax:* 215-393-6819
E-mail: sales@aesclean.com
Web site: www.aesclean.com
Medical Products Sales Volume: $29,000,000
Year Founded: 1986
Total Employees: 40
Ownership: Private
Produces/Sells CE-marked Devices: N
Federal Procurement Eligibility: Small Business
Mktg./Adv.: Ralph J. Melfi/Manager National Sales

Cleanroom Equipment	General
Environmental Control System, Powered	Physical Med
Hood, Isolation, Laminar Air Flow	General
Laminar Air Flow Unit	General
Laminar Air Flow Unit, Fixed (Air Curtain)	Chemistry
Laminar Air Flow Unit, Mobile	Chemistry

AESCULAP IMPLANT SYSTEMS INC.   1-800-234-9179
3773 Corporate Pky., Center Valley, PA 18034   610-984-9081
FDA Number: 2916714   *Fax:* 610-984-9096
E-mail: info@aesculap.com
Web site: www.aesculapusa.com
Medical Products Sales Volume: $4,500,000
Year Founded: 1977
Total Employees: 116
Ownership: Aesculap Ag & Co. Kg
Produces/Sells CE-marked Devices: N

AESCULAP IMPLANT SYSTEMS INC.   1-800-234-9179 *(cont'd)*

Federal Procurement Eligibility: Small Business, GSA Contract, VA Contract
Distribution: Manufacturer Direct, OEM, Service Direct, Exclusive Distributor, Importer
General Admin.: Denise Torcivia/Director Human Resources
          Dirk Kuyper/President
Mktg./Adv.: Yale Graves/Director Marketing
          Steve Mackay/Director National Sales
          Mark Longenbach/Manager Marketing Communications
          Gary Fredericks/Vice President Corporate Accounts
          David Derminio/Vice President Marketing
          Oliver Burckhardt/Vice President Marketing
          Steve Annunziato/Vice President Marketing
Production: Joyce Kilroy/Director Quality Assurance & Regulatory Affairs
          Brian Ranft/Vice President Operations
Finance: Mark Kilroy/Director Finance

Accessories, Cleaning, Endoscopic	Gastroenterology/Urology
Accessories, Electrical Power (Electrocautery)	Surgery
Adenotome	Ear/Nose/Throat
Airway, Nasopharyngeal (Breathing Tube)	Anesthesiology
Applicator, ENT	Ear/Nose/Throat
Applier, Aneurysm Clip	Cns/Neurology
Applier, Clip, Laparoscopic	Surgery
Applier, Surgical, Clip	Surgery
Atomizer And Tip, ENT	Ear/Nose/Throat
Biopsy Device, Endomyocardial	Cardiovascular
Biopsy Instrument	Gastroenterology/Urology
Biopsy Instrument, Mechanical, Gastrointestinal	Gastroenterology/Urology
Biopsy Instrument, Suction	Gastroenterology/Urology
Bistoury, Tracheal	Ear/Nose/Throat
Blade, Saw, Surgical, Cardiovascular	Cardiovascular
Block, Bite, ENT	Ear/Nose/Throat
Block, Bite, Intubation	Anesthesiology
Burr, Dental	Dental And Oral
Cannula, Ear	Ear/Nose/Throat
Cannula, Injection	Gastroenterology/Urology
Cannula, Sinus	Ear/Nose/Throat
Cannula, Suprapubic, With Trocar	Gastroenterology/Urology
Carrier, Sponge, Endoscopic	Gastroenterology/Urology
Carver, Dental Amalgam, Operative	Dental And Oral
Chisel, Bone, Surgical	Dental And Oral
Chisel, Middle Ear	Ear/Nose/Throat
Clamp, Penile	Gastroenterology/Urology
Clamp, Vascular	Cardiovascular
Clip, Aneurysm (Intracranial)	Cns/Neurology
Clip, Implantable	Surgery
Clip, Vascular	Cardiovascular
Clip, Vena Cava	Cardiovascular
Coagulator/Cutter, Endoscopic, Bipolar	Obstetrics/Gynecology
Coagulator/Cutter, Endoscopic, Unipolar	Obstetrics/Gynecology
Computer Software	General
Controller, Foot, Handpiece And Cord	Dental And Oral
Crimper, Wire, ENT	Ear/Nose/Throat
Curette, Adenoid	Ear/Nose/Throat
Curette, Ear	Ear/Nose/Throat
Curette, Endodontic	Dental And Oral
Curette, Ethmoid	Ear/Nose/Throat
Curette, Nasal	Ear/Nose/Throat
Curette, Operative	Dental And Oral
Curette, Periodontic	Dental And Oral
Curette, Surgical	Surgery
Curette, Surgical, Dental	Dental And Oral
Cutter, Operative	Dental And Oral
Depressor, Tongue	General
Depressor, Tongue, ENT, Metal	Ear/Nose/Throat
Dermatome	Surgery
Device, Locking, Clamp, Intestinal	Gastroenterology/Urology
Dilator, Catheter, Ureteral	Gastroenterology/Urology
Dilator, Rectal	Gastroenterology/Urology
Dilator, Tracheal	Ear/Nose/Throat
Dilator, Urethral, Mechanical	Gastroenterology/Urology
Dilator, Vessel, Surgical	Cardiovascular
Disk, Abrasive	Dental And Oral
Drill, Bone, Powered	Dental And Oral
Drill, Cranial	Cns/Neurology
Drill, Dental, Intraoral	Dental And Oral
Driver, Wire, And Bone Drill, Manual	Dental And Oral
Electrosurgical Unit, Cutting & Coagulation Device	Surgery
Elevator, ENT	Ear/Nose/Throat
Elevator, Surgical, Dental	Dental And Oral
Endoscope	Gastroenterology/Urology
Endoscope, Neurological	Cns/Neurology
Excavator, Dental, Operative	Dental And Oral
Excavator, Ear	Ear/Nose/Throat
File, Bone, Surgical	Dental And Oral
File, Margin Finishing, Operative	Dental And Oral
Forceps, Articulation Paper	Dental And Oral
Forceps, Biopsy, Bronchoscope (Rigid)	Anesthesiology
Forceps, Biopsy, Gynecological	Obstetrics/Gynecology
Forceps, Biopsy, Non-Electric	Gastroenterology/Urology
Forceps, Disconnect	Gastroenterology/Urology

AESCULAP IMPLANT SYSTEMS INC.   1-800-234-9179 *(cont'd)*

Forceps, Dressing, Dental	Dental And Oral
Forceps, ENT	Ear/Nose/Throat
Forceps, General & Plastic Surgery	Surgery
Forceps, Obstetrical	Obstetrics/Gynecology
Forceps, Rongeur, Surgical	Dental And Oral
Forceps, Tooth Extractor, Surgical	Dental And Oral
Forceps, Tube Introduction	Anesthesiology
Forceps, Wire Closure, ENT	Ear/Nose/Throat
Fork, Tuning, ENT	Ear/Nose/Throat
Gag, Mouth	Ear/Nose/Throat
Gauge, Depth, Instrument, Dental	Dental And Oral
General Use Surgical Scissors	Surgery
Gouge, Nasal	Ear/Nose/Throat
Gouge, Surgical, General & Plastic Surgery	Surgery
Guide, Surgical, Instrument	Surgery
Guide, Surgical, Needle	Surgery
Guillotine, Tonsil	Ear/Nose/Throat
Handle, Instrument, Dental	Dental And Oral
Handpiece, Belt and/or Gear Driven, Dental	Dental And Oral
Handpiece, Direct Drive, AC-Powered	Dental And Oral
Hemostat, Surgical	Dental And Oral
Hoe, Periodontic	Dental And Oral
Holder, Catheter	Gastroenterology/Urology
Holder, Ear Speculum	Ear/Nose/Throat
Holder, Needle	Gastroenterology/Urology
Holder, Speculum, ENT	Ear/Nose/Throat
Hook, Gastro-Urology	Gastroenterology/Urology
Hook, Microsurgical Ear	Ear/Nose/Throat
Hook, Surgical, General & Plastic Surgery	Surgery
Hook, Tonsil Suturing	Ear/Nose/Throat
Hook, Tracheal, ENT	Ear/Nose/Throat
Instrument, Diamond, Dental	Dental And Oral
Instrument, Manual, General Surgical	Surgery
Irrigator, Sinus	Ear/Nose/Throat
Knife, Amputation	Surgery
Knife, Ear	Ear/Nose/Throat
Knife, Laryngeal	Ear/Nose/Throat
Knife, Margin Finishing, Operative	Dental And Oral
Knife, Myringotomy	Ear/Nose/Throat
Knife, Nasal	Ear/Nose/Throat
Knife, Periodontic	Dental And Oral
Knife, Surgical	Dental And Oral
Knife, Tonsil	Ear/Nose/Throat
Laparoscope, General & Plastic Surgery	Surgery
Laparoscope, Gynecologic	Obstetrics/Gynecology
Ligator, Hemorrhoidal	Gastroenterology/Urology
Marker, Periodontic	Dental And Oral
Mirror, ENT	Ear/Nose/Throat
Mirror, Endoscopic	Surgery
Mirror, Laryngeal	Ear/Nose/Throat
Mirror, Mouth	Dental And Oral
Mobilizer, ENT	Ear/Nose/Throat
Needle, Aspiration And Injection, Reusable	Surgery
Needle, Insufflation, Laparoscopic	Surgery
Nipper, Malleus	Ear/Nose/Throat
Obturator, Endoscopic	Gastroenterology/Urology
Osteotome (Orthopedic)	Surgery
Otoscope	Ear/Nose/Throat
Perforator, Antrum	Ear/Nose/Throat
Pick, Microsurgical Ear	Ear/Nose/Throat
Pin, Retentive And Splinting	Dental And Oral
Plate, Bone, Orthodontic	Dental And Oral
Pliers, Operative	Dental And Oral
Pliers, Orthodontic	Dental And Oral
Plugger, Root Canal, Endodontic	Dental And Oral
Point, Abrasive	Dental And Oral
Probe, Gastrointestinal	Gastroenterology/Urology
Probe, Periodontic	Dental And Oral
Probe, Sinus	Ear/Nose/Throat
Punch, Adenoid	Ear/Nose/Throat
Punch, Antrum	Ear/Nose/Throat
Punch, Attic	Ear/Nose/Throat
Punch, Biopsy	Gastroenterology/Urology
Punch, Catheter	Gastroenterology/Urology
Punch, Ethmoid	Ear/Nose/Throat
Punch, Nasal	Ear/Nose/Throat
Punch, Tonsil	Ear/Nose/Throat
Rasp, Ear	Ear/Nose/Throat
Rasp, Frontal-Sinus	Ear/Nose/Throat
Rasp, Nasal	Ear/Nose/Throat
Rasp, Surgical, General & Plastic Surgery	Surgery
Reamer, Pulp Canal, Endodontic	Dental And Oral
Retractor, ENT (Thoracic)	Ear/Nose/Throat
Retractor, Non-Self-Retaining	Gastroenterology/Urology
Retractor, Self-Retaining	Gastroenterology/Urology
Retractor, Surgical	Surgery
Retractor, Vaginal	Obstetrics/Gynecology
Ring, Crimp	Gastroenterology/Urology
Rod, Measuring Ear	Ear/Nose/Throat
Saw, Bone Cutting, Micro	Orthopedics
Saw, Electric	Cardiovascular

AESCULAP IMPLANT SYSTEMS INC.   1-800-234-9179 *(cont'd)*

Saw, Manual, And Accessories	Surgery
Saw, Nasal	Ear/Nose/Throat
Saw, Other	Surgery
Scaler, Periodontic	Dental And Oral
Scaler, Rotary	Dental And Oral
Scalpel, One-Piece (Knife)	Surgery
Scissors, Ear	Ear/Nose/Throat
Scissors, Laparoscopy	Surgery
Scissors, Nasal	Ear/Nose/Throat
Scissors, Surgical Tissue, Dental (Oral)	Dental And Oral
Scissors, Wire Cutting, ENT	Ear/Nose/Throat
Scoop, Common Duct	Gastroenterology/Urology
Screw, Fixation, Bone	Orthopedics
Service, Maintenance/Repair	General
Service, Repair, Endoscopic	General
Snare, Ear	Ear/Nose/Throat
Snare, Nasal	Ear/Nose/Throat
Snare, Rigid Self-Opening	Gastroenterology/Urology
Snare, Tonsil	Ear/Nose/Throat
Sound, Urethral, Metal Or Plastic	Gastroenterology/Urology
Sound, Uterine	Obstetrics/Gynecology
Spatula, Surgical, General & Plastic Surgery	Surgery
Speculum, Ear	Ear/Nose/Throat
Speculum, Rectal	Gastroenterology/Urology
Spirometer, Diagnostic (Respirometer)	Anesthesiology
Spoon, Ear	Ear/Nose/Throat
Spreader, Bladder Neck	Gastroenterology/Urology
Spreader, Pulp Canal Filling Material, Endodontic	Dental And Oral
Staple, Implantable	Surgery
Stripper, Vein, External	Cardiovascular
Stripper, Vein, Reusable	Surgery
Stylet, Surgical	Surgery
Stylet, Tracheal Tube	Anesthesiology
Stylet, Ureteral	Gastroenterology/Urology
Surgical Instrument, Manual (General Use)	Surgery
Syringe, Ear	Ear/Nose/Throat
Syringe, Irrigating, Dental	Dental And Oral
Syringe, Periodontic, Endodontic	Dental And Oral
Syringe, Restorative And Impression Material	Dental And Oral
Tape, Measuring, Ruler And Caliper	Surgery
Tip, Suction	Anesthesiology
Tonsillectome	Ear/Nose/Throat
Tray, Surgical Instrument	Surgery
Trocar, ENT	Ear/Nose/Throat
Trocar, Gastro-Urology	Gastroenterology/Urology
Trocar, Laryngeal	Ear/Nose/Throat
Trocar, Sinus	Ear/Nose/Throat
Trocar, Tracheal	Ear/Nose/Throat
Tube, Ear Suction	Ear/Nose/Throat
Tube, Tonsil Suction	Ear/Nose/Throat
Tube, Tracheal (Endotracheal)	Anesthesiology
Wire, Orthodontic	Dental And Oral
Wrap, Sterilization	General

AESCULAP IMPLANT SYSTEMS, INC.   610-984-9074
9999 Hamilton Blvd., Bldg 8, Breiningsville, PA 18031
FDA Number: 3005739625

Appliance, Fixation, Spinal Interlaminal	Orthopedics
Orthopedic Manual Surgical Instrument	Orthopedics
Orthosis, Fixation, Pedicle, Spinal	Orthopedics
Orthosis, Fixation, Spinal, Spondylolisthesis	Orthopedics

AESCULAP, INC   650-543-3100
1810 Embarcadero Road, Suite B, Palo Alto, CA 94303
FDA Number: 3006138307
Ownership: Private
Produces/Sells CE-marked Devices: N

Electrosurgical Unit, Cutting & Coagulation Device	Surgery
Insufflator, Laparoscopic	Obstetrics/Gynecology

AESCULAP, INC.
See Aesculap Implant Systems Inc.

AESTHERA CORPORATION   925-737-2100
6634 Owens Dr., Pleasanton, CA 94588
FDA Number: 3005036462
Ownership: Private
Produces/Sells CE-marked Devices: N

Laser, Surgical	Surgery

AESTHETIC AND RECONSTRUCTIVE   866-853-6800
TECHNOLOGIES, INC.
3545 Airway Dr., Suite 106, Reno, NV 89511   775-853-6800
FDA Number: 3003897287   Fax: 775-853-6805
E-mail: customer.service@aartinc.net
Web site: www.aartinc.net
Ownership: Private
Produces/Sells CE-marked Devices: N

Elastomer, Silicone Block	Surgery
Implant, Muscle, Pectoralis	Surgery

AESTHETIC AND RECONSTRUCTIVE   866-853-6800 *(cont'd)*

Malar Implant	Surgery
Prosthesis, Chin, Internal	Surgery
Prosthesis, Nose, Internal	Surgery

AESTHETIC CONCERNS PROSTHETICS, INC.
See Touch Bionics

AESTHETIC INNOVATIONS, INC.   615-269-9166
1704a Gayle Ln., Nashville, TN 37212
FDA Number: 3003868429
Ownership: Private
Produces/Sells CE-marked Devices: N

Massager, Therapeutic	Physical Med

AESTHETIC TECHNOLOGIES, INC.   303-469-0965
14828 West 6th Avenue, Unit B9, Golden, CO 80401
FDA Number: n/a   Fax: 303-469-1748
E-mail: info@atimed.com
Web site: www.parisianpeel.com
Medical Products Sales Volume: $300,000
Year Founded: 1998
Total Employees: 3
Ownership: Private
Produces/Sells CE-marked Devices: N
Federal Procurement Eligibility: Small Business
General Admin.: Mr. James Snyder/Chief Executive Officer
   Mr. Allan Danto/President
Mktg./Adv.: Mr. Doug McBurney/Manager National Sales

Dermabrasion Unit	Surgery
Lotion, Skin Care	General
Motor, Surgical Instrument, AC-Powered	Surgery
Table, Ultrasound	General

AET SPECIALTY NETS AND NONWOVENS
See Delstar Technologies, Inc.

AETHLON MEDICAL INC.   858-459-7800-30
8910 University Center Lane., Suite 660, San Diego, CA 92122
FDA Number: 3002820472
Web site: www.aethlonmedical.com
Ownership: Public
Stock Symbol: AEMD
Traded On: OTC Bulletin
Produces/Sells CE-marked Devices: N
General Admin.: James A. Joyce/Chief Executive Officer, Chairman
   Dr. Richard H. Tullis/Chief Scientific Officer, Vice President
   Mr. Rod Kenley/President
Mktg./Adv.: Ms. John Salvador/Director Communications
Finance: Jim Frakes/Senior Vice President Finance

Hemoperfusion System, Sorbent	Gastroenterology/Urology

AETHON INC.   412-322-2975
100 Business Center Drive, Pittsburgh, PA 15205
FDA Number: n/a
E-mail: mswaney@aethon.com
Ownership: Private
Produces/Sells CE-marked Devices: N
General Admin.: Mr. Spencer Allen/Chief Technology Officer
   Mr. Aldo Zini/President, Chief Executive Officer
Mktg./Adv.: Mr. Peter Seiff/Senior Vice President Business Development
   Mr. Joe Gentile/Vice President Sales
Production: Mr. Kevin Newton/Vice President Operations
Finance: Mr. Robert Reilly/Chief Financial Officer

AETNA FOOT PRODUCTS/DIV. OF AETNA FELT   800-390-3668
CORPORATION
2401 W. Emaus Ave., Allentown, PA 18103-7234   610-791-5250
FDA Number: 2529848   Fax: 610-791-5357
E-mail: info.podiatry@aetnafelt.com
Web site: www.aetnafootproducts.com
Total Employees: 45   *Marketing Staff:* 3   *Sales Staff:* 3
Ownership: Private
Quality System Registration Information: ISO9000
Produces/Sells CE-marked Devices: N
Federal Procurement Eligibility: Small Business
Distribution: Manufacturer Direct, Manufacturer Through Distributor, Importer, Exporter
General Admin.: Gina Kostic/Office Manager
   Wilfred W. Weppler/President, Chief Executive Officer
Mktg./Adv.: Toni Tackette/Division Manager
   Arnie Weiner/National Sales Representative
Production: Mr. Scott Hoffman/Vice President Manufacturing

Cushion, Foot	Orthopedics
Felt	Surgery
Foam, Plastic	General
Moleskin	General
Shield, Bunion	Orthopedics

MANUFACTURER PROFILES

AETREX WORLDWIDE, INC
414 Alfred Avenue, Teaneck, NJ 07666
800-526-2739
201-833-2700
Fax: 201-833-1485
FDA Number: 2243810
E-mail: info@aetrex.com
Web site: www.aetrex.com
Medical Products Sales Volume: $9,500,000
Annual Revenue: $25-$50 Million
Year Founded: 1946
Total Employees: 130　　*Marketing Staff:* 10　　*Sales Staff:* 25
Ownership: Private
Produces/Sells CE-marked Devices: Y
Federal Procurement Eligibility: Small Business, VA Contract
Distribution: Manufacturer Direct, Manufacturer Through Distributor, Manufacturer Through Manufacturer Reps, OEM, Importer, Exporter
General Admin.: Richard Schwartz/Chief Executive Officer
　　　　　Evan Schwartz/Chief Operating Officer
　　　　　Larry Schwartz/President
Mktg./Adv.: Richard Schnaittacher/Vice President Sales

Cushion, Foot	Orthopedics
Equipment, Molding	General
Material, Raw, Production	General
Orthosis, Other	Physical Med
Pad, Pressure, Foam (Elbow, Heel)	General
Service, Parts, Repair	General
Support, Foot	Orthopedics

AEV
See American Emergency Vehicles

AEVERL MEDICAL, LLC
6045 Circle Of Light, Gainesville, GA 30506
770-983-1369
FDA Number: 3004889973
Ownership: Private
Produces/Sells CE-marked Devices: N

Pressure Measurement, System, Intermittent	Physical Med

AFASSCO, INC.
2244 Park Pl., Suite C, Minden, NV 89423
800-441-6774
775-783-3555
Fax: 800-232-7726
FDA Number: 7000410
E-mail: afassco@intercomm.com
Web site: www.afassco.com
Medical Products Sales Volume: $500,000,000
Annual Revenue: $1-$5 Million
Year Founded: 1970
Ownership: Private
Quality System Registration Information: ISO9002
Produces/Sells CE-marked Devices: Y
Federal Procurement Eligibility: Small Business, Female Owned
Distribution: Manufacturer Through Distributor, Exclusive Distributor, Exporter
General Admin.: Don Schumaker/Chief Executive Officer, Chairman
Mktg./Adv.: Rick Bell/Director Product Development

Bag, Ice	General
Bandage, Adhesive	Surgery
Bandage, Compression	General
Bandage, Gauze	General
Cup, Eye	Ophthalmology
Dressing, Wound and Burn, Hydrogel	Surgery
Finger Cot	General
Fountain, Eye Wash	Chemistry
Kit, Burn	General
Kit, Emergency, Insect Sting	General
Kit, First Aid	Surgery
Mask, Other	General
Pad, Eye	Ophthalmology
Scissors, Bandage/Gauze/Plaster	General
Solution, Antibacterial Cleaner	General
Splint, Extremity, Inflatable, External	Surgery
Swabs, Alcohol	General
Swabs, Antiseptic	General
Tweezers	General

AFC INDUSTRIES, INC.
13-16 133rd Place, College Point, NY 11356
718-747-0237
FDA Number: 3006268923

Holder, Radiographic Cassette, Wall-Mounted	Radiology

AFFILIATED HOSPITAL PRODUCTS INC./PERRY
See Ansell Healthcare Products, Inc.

AFFINITY BIOLOGICALS, INC.
1395 Sandhill Dr.,
Ancaster, ONT L9G-4 Canada
800-903-6020
905-304-9896
Fax: 905-304-9897
FDA Number: 3003485232
E-mail: info@affinitybiologicals.com
Web site: www.affinitybiologicals.com
Total Employees: 14
Ownership: Private
Quality System Registration Information: ISO9001
Produces/Sells CE-marked Devices: N

AFFINITY BIOLOGICALS, INC.
800-903-6020 *(cont'd)*
Distribution: OEM, Exclusive Distributor

AFFINITY MEDICAL TECHNOLOGIES LLC
1732 Reynolds Avenue, Irvine, CA 92614
949-477-9495
Fax: 949-477-9499
FDA Number: 2031044
E-mail: customercare@affinitymed.com
Web site: www.affinitymed.com
Medical Products Sales Volume: $2,800,000
Annual Revenue: $5-$10 Million
Year Founded: 1997
Total Employees: 30
Ownership: Private
Quality System Registration Information: ISO9001
Produces/Sells CE-marked Devices: Y
Federal Procurement Eligibility: Small Business
Distribution: OEM
General Admin.: Mary Phillipp/Chief Executive Officer
Mktg./Adv.: Mr. Hank Mancini/Manager Business Development
　　　　　Mr. Jim Itkin/Sales Manager
Production: Mr. Bob Frank/Director Engineering
　　　　　Mr. Kevin Kom/Manager Manufacturing
　　　　　Ms. Cindy Oldynski/Manager Quality Assurance

Cable/Lead, ECG, With Transducer And Electrode	Cardiovascular
Electrode, Electrocardiograph	Cardiovascular
Molding, Custom	General

AFFINITY MEDICAL TECHNOLOGY, LLC.
3545 Harbor Lane N.,, Plymouth, MN 55447
763-744-0412
FDA Number: n/a
Ownership: Private
Produces/Sells CE-marked Devices: N

Hearing-Aid	Ear/Nose/Throat
Hearing-Aid, Plate, Face	Ear/Nose/Throat

AFFYMETRIX
See Affymetrix, Inc.

AFFYMETRIX, INC.
3420 Central Expy., Santa Clara, CA 95051
888-DNA-CHIP
408-731-5000
Fax: 408-731-5380
FDA Number: 3003314809
E-mail: sales@affymetrix.com
Web site: www.affymetrix.com
Year Founded: 1991
Total Employees: 1100
Ownership: Public
Stock Symbol: AFFX
Traded On: NASDAQ
Produces/Sells CE-marked Devices: Y
General Admin.: Mr. Timothy Barabe/Chief Financial Officer, Executive Vice President
　　　　　Dr. Andrew Last/Executive Vice President
　　　　　Mr. John Runkel, Jr./General Counsel
　　　　　Kevin King/President, Chief Executive Officer

DNA-Probe, Reagent	Microbiology
Instrumentation For Clinical Multiplex Test Systems	Chemistry
Test, Cancer Detection, DNA-Probe	Immunology

Medical Product Subsidiaries (Listed Separately)
Usb Corporation

AFFYMETRIX, INC.
890 Embarcadero Dr., West Sacramento, CA 95605
916-376-1309
FDA Number: 3003314809
Ownership: AFFYMETRIX, INC.
Produces/Sells CE-marked Devices: N

Instrumentation For Clinical Multiplex Test Systems	Chemistry

AFP IMAGING CORP.
250 Clearbrook Road, Elmsford, NY 10523-1315
800-592-6666
914-592-6100
Fax: 914-592-6148
FDA Number: 2431643
E-mail: marketing@afpimaging.com
Web site: www.afpimaging.com
Medical Products Sales Volume: $23,000,000
Annual Revenue: $10-$25 Million
Year Founded: 1978
Total Employees: 83　　*Marketing Staff:* 3　　*Sales Staff:* 5
Ownership: Public
Stock Symbol: AFPC
Traded On: NASDAQ
Quality System Registration Information: ISO9001
Produces/Sells CE-marked Devices: N
Federal Procurement Eligibility: Small Business, GSA Contract, VA Contract
Distribution: Manufacturer Through Distributor, Exporter
General Admin.: Mr. David Vozick/Chairman
　　　　　Donald Rabinovitch/President, Chief Executive Officer
　　　　　Aida McKinney/Vice President Admin.
Mktg./Adv.: Kay-Ann Mitto/Coord. Marketing Communications
Production: Marc Irving/Vice President Manufacturing & Production

Camera, Multi Format	Radiology

AFP IMAGING CORP.   800-592-6666 (cont'd)

Camera, Multi-Image	Radiology
Holder, Radiographic Cassette, Wall-Mounted	Radiology
Image Intensification System	Radiology
Processor, Radiographic Film, Automatic	Radiology
Processor, Radiographic Film, Automatic, Dental	Dental And Oral
Radiographic Unit, Digital	Radiology
Radiographic/Fluoroscopic Unit, Angiographic, Digital	Radiology
Tube, X-Ray	Radiology

Medical Product Subsidiaries (Listed Separately)
Ansell Healthcare, Inc.

AFTON MEDICAL LLC   877-300-6288

5576 Bighorn Dr, Carson City, NV 89701
FDA Number: 3008588979   *Fax:* 877-452-5809
E-mail: info@aftonmedical.com
Web site: www.aftonmedical.com
Ownership: Private
Produces/Sells CE-marked Devices: N

Cannula, Nasal, Oxygen	Anesthesiology
Humidifier, Non-Direct Patient Interface (Home-Use)	Anesthesiology
Mask, Oxygen, Aerosol Administration	Anesthesiology
Mask, Oxygen, Low Concentration, Venturi	Anesthesiology
Mask, Oxygen, Non-Rebreathing	Anesthesiology
Nebulizer, Medicinal, Non-Ventilatory (Atomizer)	Anesthesiology
Tubing, Flexible, Medical Gas, Low-Pressure	Anesthesiology

AG INDUSTRIES   800-875-3138
     636-349-4466

3637 Scarlett Oak Blvd., St. Louis, MO 63122
FDA Number: 3004874794   *Fax:* 636-349-7069
E-mail: agindustries@worldnet.att.net
Web site: www.agindustries.com
Medical Products Sales Volume: $200,000
Annual Revenue: $1-$5 Million
Year Founded: 1983
Total Employees: 2   *Marketing Staff:* 2   *Sales Staff:* 2
Ownership: Home Health Medical Equipment
Quality System Registration Information: ISO9002
Produces/Sells CE-marked Devices: Y
Federal Procurement Eligibility: Small Business
Distribution: Manufacturer Direct, Manufacturer Through Distributor, OEM, Exclusive Distributor, Exporter
General Admin.: Harry Amann/President, Chief Executive Officer
Production: Mike Amann/Manager Regulatory Affairs

Ultrafiltration Equipment	Chemistry

AGA GAS, INC.
See Lifegas Llc

AGA HEALTHCARE
See Lifegas Llc

AGA LINDE HEALTHCARE P.R. INC.   787-622-7900

GPO Box 364727, Tres Monjitas, PO Box 363868,
San Juan, PR 00936
FDA Number: 2647548   *Fax:* 787-620-8267
E-mail: linda.cesareo@pr.aga.com
Web site: www.linde.com
Medical Products Sales Volume: $9,000,000
Annual Revenue: $5-$10 Million
Total Employees: 125   *Marketing Staff:* 4   *Sales Staff:* 20
Ownership: Lifegas Llc
Distribution: Manufacturer Direct, Exclusive Distributor
General Admin.: Oracio Lavanoleira/Chief Executive Officer
     Guillermo Witte/President
     Alejandro Suarez/Vice President Human Resources
Mktg./Adv.: Felix Venegas/Director Product Development
     Angel Torano/Director Sales
     Lisandra Gutierrez/Manager Communications
     Fredick Miranda/Manager Contract Sales
Production: Karen Velez/Manager Materials
     Luis Martinez/Manager Regulatory Affairs
     Juan Ugalde/Vice President Manufacturing

Alarm, Central Gas System	Anesthesiology
Calibrator, Blood Gas	General
Calibrator, Gas, Pressure	Anesthesiology
Column, Life Support (Electrical/Gas)	General
Cylinder, Carbon-Dioxide	Surgery
Cylinder, Compressed Gas, With Valve	Anesthesiology
Cylinder, Oxygen	Anesthesiology
Fitting, Quick Connect (Gas Connector)	General
Flowmeter, Gas (Oxygen), Calibrated	Anesthesiology
Gas Mixtures, Laboratory	General
Gas Mixtures, Medical	General
Gas Mixtures, Sterilization	General
Gas-Machine, Anesthesia	Anesthesiology
Gauge, Gas Pressure, Cylinder/Pipeline	Anesthesiology
Manifold, Gas	Chemistry
Mask, Gas, Anesthesia	Anesthesiology
Monitor, Blood Pressure, Invasive (Arterial), Anesthesia	Anesthesiology

AGA LINDE HEALTHCARE P.R. INC.   787-622-7900 (cont'd)

Monitor, ECG, Anesthesia	Anesthesiology
Monitor, EEG	Cns/Neurology
Monitor, Hemodynamic	Anesthesiology
Monitor, Oxygen	General
Monitor, Oxygen (Ventilatory) W/Wo Alarm	Anesthesiology
Monitor, Oxygen, Cutan. (Not for Infant or Under Gas Anest.)	Anesthesiology
Monitor, Ventilation	Anesthesiology
Oxygen	Anesthesiology
Regulator, Anesthesia	Anesthesiology
Regulator, Pressure, Gas Cylinder	Anesthesiology
Scavenger, Gas, Anesthesia Unit	Anesthesiology
Sterilizer, Ethylene-Oxide Gas	General
System, Pipeline, Gas	General
Vaporizer, Anesthesia, Non-Heated	Anesthesiology
Ventilator, Anesthesia Unit	Anesthesiology

AGAMATRIX   603-328-6000

10 Maor Parkway, Salem, NH 03079
FDA Number: 3004637226

Reagent, Glucose (Test System)	Chemistry

AGELESS PROCESSING TECHNOLOGIES   801-942-9250

20-707 S. Sierra Ave., Sandy, UT 84092
FDA Number: n/a   *Fax:* 801-942-9251
E-mail: apt2brad@aol.com
Annual Revenue: $0-$1 Million
Total Employees: 3
Ownership: Private
Produces/Sells CE-marked Devices: N
Federal Procurement Eligibility: Small Business
General Admin.: Karl J. Hemmerich/President
Production: James A. Stubstad/Process Engineer

Service, Consulting	General

AGENDIA INC.   888-321-2732

22 Morgan, Irvine, CA 92618
FDA Number: 3007297853   *Fax:* 888-669-3292
E-mail: customercare@agendia.com
Web site: www.agendia.com
Year Founded: 2003
Ownership: Private
Produces/Sells CE-marked Devices: N
General Admin.: Dr. Bernhard Sixt/Chief Executive Officer
     Dr. RenAc Bernards/Chief Scientific Officer
Medical Admin.: Dr. Richard Bender/Chief Medical Officer
Mktg./Adv.: Mr. Alan Carter/Vice President Business Development
     Mr. Daniel Forche/Vice President Marketing & Sales
Research: Dr. Laura van 't Veer/Director Research
Finance: Mr. Kurt Schmidt/Chief Financial Officer

Classifier, Prognostic, Recurrence Risk Assessment, Rna Gene Expression, Breast Cancer	Immunology

AGFA CORP.   800-581-2432
     201-440-2500

100 Challenger Rd.,
Ridgefield Park, NJ 07660
FDA Number: 9200027   *Fax:* 201-440-1512
Web site: www.agfa.com/en/he/index.jsp
Medical Products Sales Volume: $100,000,000
Total Employees: 300
Ownership: BAYER AG, GERMANY
Produces/Sells CE-marked Devices: N
Distribution: Manufacturer Direct, Manufacturer Through Manufacturer Reps, Importer, Exporter
General Admin.: Vishal Wanchoo/Vice President
Mktg./Adv.: Vishal Wanchoo/Vice President Marketing
     John Scarano/Vice President Sales

Cassette, Radiographic Film	Radiology
Computer, Radiographic Image Analysis	Radiology
Film, X-Ray	Radiology
Monitor, Ultrasonic, Non-Fetal	Radiology
Radiographic Picture Archiving/Communication System (PACS)	Radiology
Recorder, Radiographic Video Tape	Radiology

AGFA CORPORATION   877-777-2432
     864-421-1600

PO Box 19048, 10 South Academy Street,
Greenville, SC 29602
FDA Number: 9616389   *Fax:* 864-421-1612
E-mail: agfahealth@agfahealth.com
Web site: www.agfa.com
Year Founded: 1867
Total Employees: 170
Ownership: Agfa Gevaert N.V.
Stock Symbol: AGEB
Traded On: Brussels
Quality System Registration Information: ISO9001; ISO9002
Produces/Sells CE-marked Devices: N
Federal Procurement Eligibility: Small Business, GSA Contract, VA Contract

AGFA CORPORATION   877-777-2432 (cont'd)

Distribution: Manufacturer Through Distributor, Manufacturer Through
Manufacturer Reps
General Admin.: Bob Pryor/President
Mktg./Adv.: Rick Philo/Director National Accounts
        JeanE Bartlett/Manager Advertising & Communications
        Tom Boon/Vice President Sales
Production: Dawn Lezzer/Director Quality Assurance & Regulatory Affairs

Camera, Multi Format	Radiology
Cassette, Radiographic Film	Radiology
Changer, Radiographic Film/Cassette	Radiology
Device, Storage, Image, Digital	Radiology
Film, X-Ray, Dental, Extraoral	Dental And Oral
Film, X-Ray, Special Purpose	Radiology
Image Digitizer	Radiology
Image Processing System	Radiology
Imager, X-Ray, Electrostatic	Radiology
Processor, Cine Film	Radiology
Processor, Radiographic Film, Automatic	Radiology
Radiographic Unit, Diagnostic	Radiology
Screen, Intensifying, Radiographic, Dental	Dental And Oral
System, Communication, Image, Digital	Radiology
System, Marking, Film, Radiographic	Radiology
Unit, Imaging, Thermal	Radiology

AGFA DIV. OF BAYER CORP.

See Agfa Corp.

AGFA DIV., MILES, INC.

See Agfa Corp.

AGFA HEALTHCARE CORP.   864-421-1815
1 Crosswind Rd., Misquamicut, RI 02891

FDA Number: 1225058

Analyzer, ECG	Cardiovascular
Computer, Diagnostic, Programmable	Cardiovascular
Device, Storage, Image, Digital	Cardiovascular
Electrocardiograph, Single Channel	Cardiovascular
Image Digitizer	Radiology
Image Processing System	Radiology
Radiographic/Fluoroscopic Unit, Angiographic	Radiology
System, Communication, Image, Digital	Radiology

AGFA HEALTHCARE CORP.   864-421-1815
1636 Bushy Park Rd., Goose Creek, SC 29445

FDA Number: 1065979
Ownership: Private
Produces/Sells CE-marked Devices: N

Film, X-Ray, Special Purpose	Radiology

AGFA HEALTHCARE CORP.   864-421-1815
580 Gotham Parkway, Carlstadt, NJ 07072

FDA Number: 2249582

Device, Storage, Image, Digital	Radiology
Image Digitizer	Radiology
Image Processing System	Radiology
• System, Communication, Image, Digital	Radiology

AGFA MATRIX DIVISION

See Agfa Corp.

AGFA MEDICAL IMAGING   877-753-2432
77 Belfield Road,   416-241-1110
Toronto, ONT M9W-1 Canada

FDA Number: n/a   *Fax:* 416-614-2260
E-mail: esther.cohen.ec1@ca.agfa.com
Web site: www.agfamedical.com
Year Founded: 1996
Total Employees: 50
Ownership: Private
Produces/Sells CE-marked Devices: N
Distribution: Manufacturer Direct, Service Direct

AGFA MEDICAL IMAGING

See Agfa Corporation

AGGRESSIVE SOLUTIONS, INC.   972-242-2164
1735 N. I-35 E., Carrollton, TX 75006

FDA Number: 1650905
Ownership: Private
Produces/Sells CE-marked Devices: N

Bed, Electric	General
Bed, Patient Rotation, Powered	Physical Med
Mattress, Air Flotation	General
Table, Physical Medicine, Powered	Physical Med

AGILE MFG., INC   800-476-7436
720 Industrial Park Road, Anderson, MO 64831   417-845-6065

FDA Number: n/a   *Fax:* 417-845-6069
E-mail: sales@agilemfg.net
Web site: www.shenmfg.com
Medical Products Sales Volume: $5,200,000

AGILE MFG., INC   800-476-7436 (cont'd)

Annual Revenue: $10-$25 Million
Year Founded: 1924
Total Employees: 67
Ownership: Private
Produces/Sells CE-marked Devices: Y
Federal Procurement Eligibility: Small Business
Distribution: Manufacturer Through Distributor
General Admin.: L. Gerald Strite/President
Mktg./Adv.: Susan Olson/Director Advertising
        David Laurenz/Manager National Sales
        David Laurenz/Vice President Marketing

Incinerator	General

AGILE RADIOLOGICAL TECHNOLOGIES   877-985-9877
11180 Reed Hartman Hwy, Cincinnati, OH 45242   513-985-9877

FDA Number: 3004503085
E-mail: ray_support@techosoft.com
Web site: www.agilert.com
Ownership: Private
Produces/Sells CE-marked Devices: N

Accessory - Film Dosimetry System	Radiology

AGILENT TECHNOLOGIES

See Agilent Technologies, Inc.

AGILENT TECHNOLOGIES CANADA INC.   1 877 424-4536
6705 Millcreek Drive, Unit 5,   1 877 894-4414
Mississauga, ONT L5N 5 Canada

FDA Number: n/a   *Fax:* 1 905 282-6300
E-mail: cag_sales-na@agilent.com
Web site: www.agilent.com
Year Founded: 1961
Total Employees: 100
Ownership: Agilent Technologies
Produces/Sells CE-marked Devices: N
Distribution: Manufacturer Direct, Service Direct, Exclusive Distributor

AGILENT TECHNOLOGIES, INC.   877-424-4536
5301 Stevens Creek Blvd.,   408-345-8886
Santa Clara, CA 95051

FDA Number: 2026835   *Fax:* 408-345-8474
E-mail: contact_us@agilent.com
Web site: www.agilent.com
Total Employees: 800
Ownership: Agilent Technologies, Inc.
Stock Symbol: A
Traded On: NYSE
Quality System Registration Information: ISO9001
Produces/Sells CE-marked Devices: Y
Distribution: Manufacturer Direct, Manufacturer Through Manufacturer Reps
General Admin.: Mr. Didier Hirsch/Chief Financial Officer, Senior Vice President
        Dr. Darlene Solomon/Chief Technology Officer
        Mr. Ron Nersesian/Executive Vice President
        William (Bill) Sullivan/President, Chief Executive Officer
Mktg./Adv.: Ms. Shiela Barr Robertson/Vice President Corporate Development

Chromatography Equipment, Gas	Chemistry
Chromatography Equipment, Ion Exchange	Toxicology
Chromatography Equipment, Liquid	Chemistry
Computer, Chemistry Analyzer	Chemistry
Enzyme Immunoassay, Amphetamine	Toxicology
Enzyme Immunoassay, Barbiturate	Toxicology
Enzyme Immunoassay, Benzodiazepine	Toxicology
Enzyme Immunoassay, Cannabinoids	Toxicology
Enzyme Immunoassay, Cocaine And Cocaine Metabolites	Toxicology
Enzyme Immunoassay, Opiates	Toxicology
Enzyme Immunoassay, Phencyclidine	Toxicology
Fluorometry, Morphine	Toxicology
Gas Chromatography, Methamphetamine	Toxicology
Instrumentation, High Pressure Liquid Chromatography	Toxicology
Radioimmunoassay, Tricyclic Antidepressant Drugs	Toxicology
Reagent, NAD-NADH, Alcohol Enzyme Method	Toxicology
Resins, Ion Exchange, Liquid Chromatography	Toxicology
Test, Tetrahydrocannabinol	Toxicology
Thin Layer Chromatography, Metamphetamine	Toxicology
Thin Layer Chromatography, Morphine	Toxicology

Medical Product Subsidiaries (Listed Separately)
Agilent Technologies, Inc.
Stratagene
Varian Inc

AGION TECHNOLOGIES INC.   781-224-7100
60 Audubon Rd., Wakefield, MA 01880

FDA Number: n/a   *Fax:* 781-246-3340
E-mail: sales@agion-tech.com
Web site: www.agion-tech.com; www.agion-promo.com
Year Founded: 1997
Total Employees: 35   *Marketing Staff:* 4   *Sales Staff:* 10
Ownership: Private

AGION TECHNOLOGIES INC.   781-224-7100 *(cont'd)*
Produces/Sells CE-marked Devices: N
General Admin.: Stuart Patterson/President, Chief Executive Officer
  Test, Equipment, Sterilization   General

AGL WELDING SUPPLY CO., INC.   973-478-5000
600 Route 46, Clifton, NJ 07015
FDA Number: 2221310
  Gas, Calibrated (Specified Concentration)   Anesthesiology

AGP-MEDICAL, LLC.   860-416-0590
539 North Main Street, Suffield, CT 06078
FDA Number: 3006145905
  Orthosis, Limb Brace   Physical Med

AGR INTERNATIONAL, INC.   724-482-2163
615 Whitestown Road, PO Box 149, Butler, PA 16003
FDA Number: n/a   *Fax:* 724-482-2767
E-mail: agrsales@agrintl.com
Web site: www.agrintl.com
Annual Revenue: $25-$50 Million
Year Founded: 1936
Total Employees: 20   *Marketing Staff:* 6   *Sales Staff:* 10
Ownership: Private
Produces/Sells CE-marked Devices: Y
Federal Procurement Eligibility: Small Business
Distribution: Manufacturer Direct, OEM, Exporter
General Admin.: Henry Dimmick/Chief Executive Officer
            Ray Speicher/Regional Manager
Mktg./Adv.: Ron Puvak/Director Product Development
            David Dineff/Director Product Marketing
  Reader, Bar Code   General

AGUSTA AEROSPACE CORPORATION   888-AGUSTA-2
3050 Red Lion Road, Philadelphia, PA 19114   215-281-1400
FDA Number: n/a   *Fax:* 215-281-0447
E-mail: alexander.frederickson@agustawestland.com
Web site: www.agustausa.com
Medical Products Sales Volume: $216,700,000
Annual Revenue: $50-$100 Million
Year Founded: 1980
Total Employees: 90   *Marketing Staff:* 2   *Sales Staff:* 7
Ownership: Private
Traded On: Milan
Produces/Sells CE-marked Devices: N
Federal Procurement Eligibility: Small Business
Distribution: Manufacturer Direct
General Admin.: Dr. Robert J. Budica/President, Chief Executive Officer
Mktg./Adv.: Robert Cleland/Director Marketing & Sales
            Massimo Pugnali/Vice President Business Development
Production: John Corney/Manager Materials
            Paolo Ferreri/Vice President Customer Service
Finance: Vincent Genovese/Vice President Finance
  Ambulance, Air   General

AHLSTROM FILTRATION LLC   717-486-3438
122 West Butler Street, Mount Holly Spgs, PA 17065
FDA Number: 3000159329
Ownership: Private
Produces/Sells CE-marked Devices: N

AHLSTROM WINDSOR LOCKS LLC   860-654-8300
2 Elm St., Windsor Locks, CT 06096-2335
FDA Number: 1218934   *Fax:* 860-654-8301
E-mail: ellen.miles@ahlstrom.com
Web site: www.ahlstrom.com
Annual Revenue: More than $1 Billion
Year Founded: 1852
Total Employees: 6500
Ownership: Ahlstrom Dexter
Traded On: Helsinki
Quality System Registration Information: ISO9000; ISO9001
Produces/Sells CE-marked Devices: N
Distribution: Manufacturer Direct
General Admin.: William Cox/Vice President Human Resources
Mktg./Adv.: Jorge Crespo/Director International Sales
            Annelien Achkoyan/Manager Marketing Admin.
            David Vickers/Manager Product Marketing
            Ellen Miles/Marketing & Communications Officer
            Steven Brouillard/National Accounts Representative
Production: J. Michael Joyce/Manager Regulatory Affairs
            Andrew Uhl/Vice President Manufacturing
  Accessories, Apparel, Surgical   Surgery
  Wrap, Sterilization   General

AHNAFIELD CORP.   800-636-8060
2444 Production Dr., Indianapolis, IN 46241   317-241-2444
FDA Number: n/a

AHNAFIELD CORP.   800-636-8060 *(cont'd)*
Web site: www.ahnafield.com
Annual Revenue: $5-$10 Million
Year Founded: 1968
Ownership: Private
Produces/Sells CE-marked Devices: N
Federal Procurement Eligibility: Small Business
Distribution: Manufacturer Through Distributor, Service Direct, Exporter
General Admin.: Bruce Ahnafield/President
Mktg./Adv.: Joe Grooms/Manager International & National Sales
Production: Jeff Ahnafield/Vice President Manufacturing
  Equipment, Therapy, Handicapped/Physical   Physical Med
  Vehicle, Handicapped   Physical Med
Medical Product Subsidiaries (Listed Separately)
  Haveco Corp.

AHP MEDICAL INC.
  See Ansell Healthcare Products, Inc.

AHPC HOLDINGS INC.   630-407-0242
80 Internationale Boulevard, Unit A,
Glendale Heights, IL 60139
FDA Number: n/a
Ownership: Private
Stock Symbol: GLOV
Traded On: OTC Bulletin
Produces/Sells CE-marked Devices: N

AIGNER INDEX, INC.   800-242-3919
218 MacArthur Avenue,   845-562-4510
New Windsor, NY 12553
FDA Number: n/a   *Fax:* 845-562-2638
E-mail: holdex@frontiernet.net
Web site: www.aignerindex.com
Medical Products Sales Volume: $1,000,000
Annual Revenue: $1-$5 Million
Year Founded: 1998
Total Employees: 11   *Marketing Staff:* 3   *Sales Staff:* 3
Ownership: Private
Produces/Sells CE-marked Devices: N
Federal Procurement Eligibility: Small Business, GSA Contract
Distribution: Manufacturer Direct, Manufacturer Through Manufacturer Reps, OEM, Exporter
General Admin.: Mark Aigner/President
Mktg./Adv.: Frank Ceriello/Manager National Sales
Production: David Ibbetson/Manager Production
  Label, Device   General

AIM DENTAL LABORATORY   800-238-3500
15 Parkville Ave, Brooklyn, NY 11230-1010   718-871-3900
FDA Number: n/a   *Fax:* (718) 854-4324
E-mail: mail@aimdentallab.com
Web site: www.aimdentallab.com
Medical Products Sales Volume: $5,000,000
Ownership: Private
Produces/Sells CE-marked Devices: N
Distribution: Manufacturer Direct
  Kit, Dental Prophylaxis   Dental And Oral

AIM INSTRUMENTATION LTD.   1-800-444-9386
5232 Irmin Street,   604-438-3033
Burnaby, BC V5J-1 Canada
FDA Number: n/a   *Fax:* 604-438-7755
E-mail: aim@aiminstrumentation.com
Web site: www.info-hwy.com/aim
Year Founded: 1974
Total Employees: 10
Ownership: Private
Produces/Sells CE-marked Devices: N
Distribution: Service Direct, Exclusive Distributor

AIM INSTRUMENTATION ONTARIO INC.   1-800-871-9967
3170 Ridgeway Drive, Unit 9,   905-608-2169
Mississauga, ONT LRL-5 Canada
FDA Number: n/a   *Fax:* 905-608-2339
Web site: http://aimtechnologies.ca
Year Founded: 1995
Total Employees: 10
Ownership: Private
Produces/Sells CE-marked Devices: N
Distribution: Service Direct, Exclusive Distributor

AIM INTERNATIONAL, INC.   858-618-2799
16955 Via Del Campo, Suite 260, San Diego, CA 92127
FDA Number: 2087409
Ownership: Private
Produces/Sells CE-marked Devices: N

AIM INTERNATIONAL, INC.
858-618-2799 *(cont'd)*
Sunglasses (Including Photosensitive)
Ophthalmology

AIM SAFE AIR PRODUCTS LTD.
604-244-7272
170-13151 Vanier Pl, Richmond V6V 2J1 Canada
FDA Number: 9613742
Analyzer, Gas, Carbon-Monoxide, Gaseous Phase
Anesthesiology

AIMES MEDICAL EQUIPMENT RENTAL & PROPS
718-993-4400
2417 Third Ave., Bronx, NY 10451
FDA Number: n/a
Fax: 718-993-4260
E-mail: info@aimesmed.com
Web site: www.aimesmed.com
Medical Products Sales Volume: $500,000
Annual Revenue: $0-$1 Million
Ownership: Private
Produces/Sells CE-marked Devices: N
Federal Procurement Eligibility: Small Business
Distribution: Service Direct
Service, Used Equipment
General

AIMSCO, DELTA HI-TECH, INC.
800-378-0909
3762 S. 150 E., Salt Lake City, UT 84115
801-263-0975
FDA Number: n/a
Fax: 801-263-9487
E-mail: AIMSCO@deltahitech.net
Medical Products Sales Volume: $1,500,000
Annual Revenue: $1-$5 Million
Year Founded: 1994
Total Employees: 5   *Marketing Staff:* 1   *Sales Staff:* 6
Ownership: Private
Quality System Registration Information: ISO9000; ISO9002
Produces/Sells CE-marked Devices: N
Federal Procurement Eligibility: Small Business
Distribution: Manufacturer Through Distributor, Manufacturer Through Manufacturer Reps, Exporter
General Admin.: Glade N. James/President, Chief Executive Officer
       Kim Frank/Vice President
       Jan J. Frank/Vice President, General Manager
Finance: Tammy Smith/Controller
Lancet, Blood
General
Syringe, Insulin
General

AIMTRONICS CORP.
604-946-9666
100 Schneider Rd, Kanata K2K 1Y2 Canada
FDA Number: 9616831
Reagent, Glucose (Test System)
Chemistry

AINGUARD
See Airguard

AIONEX, INC.
615-851-4477
104 Space Park North, Goodlettsville, TN 37072
FDA Number: 3005627440
Fax: 615-851-5644
E-mail: info@aionex.com
Web site: http://aionex.com
Ownership: Private
Produces/Sells CE-marked Devices: N
Communication System, Powered
Physical Med
Environmental Control System, Powered
Physical Med
Monitor, Bed Patient
General

AIPHONE CORPORATION
425-455-0510
1700 130th Avenue NE, Bellevue, WA 98005
FDA Number: n/a
Fax: 425-455-0071
E-mail: sales@aiphone.com
Web site: www.aiphone.com
Medical Products Sales Volume: $29,500,000
Annual Revenue: $10-$25 Million
Year Founded: 1970
Total Employees: 65   *Marketing Staff:* 4   *Sales Staff:* 20
Ownership: Private
Quality System Registration Information: ISO9001; ISO9002
Produces/Sells CE-marked Devices: N
Federal Procurement Eligibility: Small Business, GSA Contract
Distribution: Manufacturer Through Distributor
General Admin.: Tak Kanie/President
Mktg./Adv.: John Mosebar/Manager Marketing & Business Development
       Joy Duffield/Manager Sales Training
       Harry Quanz/Vice President Marketing
Communication Equipment
General
Communication System, Emergency Alert, Personal
General
Nurse Call System
General

AIPHONE INTERCOM SYSTEMS
See Aiphone Corporation

AIR A MED, INC.
800-625-4963
2049 Beacon Manor Dr., Fort Myers, FL 33907
239-936-5590
FDA Number: 3004096515
Fax: 239-936-6211
E-mail: rdemaria@gmail.com

AIR A MED, INC.
800-625-4963 *(cont'd)*
Web site: www.airamed.com
Ownership: Private
Produces/Sells CE-marked Devices: N
Brace, Joint, Ankle (External)
Physical Med
Orthosis, Cervical
Physical Med
Splint, Hand, And Component
Physical Med

AIR CONTROL, INC.
252-492-2300
237 Raleigh Rd., Henderson, NC 27536-1738
FDA Number: 9200030
Fax: 252-492-9225
E-mail: sales@aircontrol-line.com
Web site: www.aircontrol-inc.com
Annual Revenue: $1-$5 Million
Year Founded: 1959
Total Employees: 25   *Marketing Staff:* 4   *Sales Staff:* 4
Ownership: Private
Produces/Sells CE-marked Devices: N
Federal Procurement Eligibility: Small Business
Distribution: Manufacturer Direct, Manufacturer Through Manufacturer Reps, Exporter
General Admin.: K. C. Dixon/Chief Executive Officer
Production: Irvin Wade/Manager Engineering
Box, Glove
Microbiology
Cleanroom Equipment
General
Hood, Fume, Chemical
Chemistry
Hood, Isolation, Laminar Air Flow
General
Laminar Air Flow Unit
General
Laminar Air Flow Unit, Fixed (Air Curtain)
Chemistry
Laminar Air Flow Unit, Mobile
Chemistry

AIR DIMENSIONS, INC.
800-650-3267
1371 W. Newport Center Dr.,
954-428-7333
Deerfield Beach, FL 33442
FDA Number: n/a
Fax: 954-360-0987
E-mail: info@airdimensions.com
Web site: www.airdimensions.com
Medical Products Sales Volume: $3,500,000
Annual Revenue: $5-$10 Million
Year Founded: 1971
Total Employees: 18   *Marketing Staff:* 2   *Sales Staff:* 3
Ownership: Private
Produces/Sells CE-marked Devices: Y
Federal Procurement Eligibility: Small Business
Distribution: Manufacturer Direct, Manufacturer Through Distributor, Manufacturer Through Manufacturer Reps, OEM
General Admin.: Thomas English/President
       David English/Vice President Human Resources
Mktg./Adv.: Greg English/Vice President Marketing & Sales
Production: Dave English/Vice President Manufacturing
Pump, Vacuum, Central
Anesthesiology

AIR FORCE, INC.
616-399-8511
933 Butternut Dr., Holland, MI 49424
FDA Number: 1836348
Fax: 616-399-4044
E-mail: info@dentalairforce.com
Web site: www.dentalairforce.com
Ownership: Private
Produces/Sells CE-marked Devices: N
Irrigator, Oral
Dental And Oral
Toothbrush, Powered
Dental And Oral

AIR LIFT UNLIMITED INC.
800-776-6771
1212 Kerr Gulch, Evergreen, CO 80439-9522
303-526-4700
FDA Number: n/a
Fax: 303-526-4774
E-mail: info@airlift.com
Web site: www.airlift.com
Medical Products Sales Volume: $4,000,000
Annual Revenue: $1-$5 Million
Year Founded: 2004
Total Employees: 12   *Marketing Staff:* 3   *Sales Staff:* 2
Ownership: Private
Produces/Sells CE-marked Devices: N
Federal Procurement Eligibility: Small Business
Distribution: Manufacturer Direct, Manufacturer Through Distributor, Manufacturer Through Manufacturer Reps, OEM, Exporter
General Admin.: Mike Moore/Chairman
       Gray Behrhorst/President, Chief Executive Officer
Mktg./Adv.: Susan Nelson/Director Sales
       Kris Phillips/Manager Sales Admin.
Production: Etta Debenham/Supervisor Warehouse Operations
Research: Ann Moore/Vice President Research & Development
Finance: Laura Borg/Vice President Finance, Controller
Bag, Medical, Physician
General
Carrier, Container, Oxygen, Portable
General
Case, Protection, Equipment
General

AIR LINK INTERNATIONAL
800-388-8237
1189-A, North Grove St., Anaheim, CA 92806   **714-632-3020**
FDA Number: n/a   *Fax:* 714-632-3621
E-mail: sales@airlinkint.com
Web site: www.airlinkint.com
Medical Products Sales Volume: $2,000,000
Year Founded: 1980
Total Employees: 14   *Marketing Staff:* 1   *Sales Staff:* 3
Ownership: Private
Produces/Sells CE-marked Devices: N
Federal Procurement Eligibility: Small Business
Distribution: Manufacturer Direct, Manufacturer Through Distributor, Manufacturer Through Manufacturer Reps, OEM, Service Direct, Exclusive Distributor, Exporter
General Admin.: Frank Marchette/President, Chief Executive Officer
  Delivery System, Pneumatic Tube   General

AIR LIQUIDE AMERICA CORPORATION
800-820-2522
1311 New Savannah Rd., Ste. 1800,   **713-868-0333**
Houston, TX 77056
FDA Number: n/a   *Fax:* 713-888-0210
Annual Revenue: $0-$1 Million
Ownership: Private
Produces/Sells CE-marked Devices: N
Distribution: Manufacturer Direct, Manufacturer Through Distributor, Importer, Exporter
General Admin.: Pierre Dufour/President, Chief Executive Officer
Mktg./Adv.: Kathy Donnovan/Vice President Marketing
                Joe Hirsch/Vice President Marketing & Sales
Production: Gary Marshall/Vice President Manufacturing
Research: Gary Prezvendowski/Vice President Research & Development
  Cylinder, Gas (Empty)   Anesthesiology

AIR LIQUIDE AMERICA CORPORATION, CAMBRIDGE DIV.
800-638-1197
821 Chesapeake Dr., Cambridge, MD 21613
FDA Number: n/a
Web site: www.airliquide.com
Annual Revenue: More than $1 Billion
Year Founded: 1902
Total Employees: 43000
Ownership: Public
Quality System Registration Information: ISO9002
Produces/Sells CE-marked Devices: Y
Distribution: Manufacturer Through Distributor, Manufacturer Through Manufacturer Reps, OEM, Exclusive Distributor, Importer
General Admin.: Benoit Potier/Chief Executive Officer, Chairman
        Jean-Pierre Duprieu/Senior Vice President
        Klaus Schmieder/Senior Vice President
        Pierre Dufour/Senior Vice President
        Guy Salzgeber/Vice President
        Ron Labarre/Vice President
        Augustin de Roubin/Vice President Human Resources
Medical Admin.: Jean-Marc de Royere/Senior Vice President Health Care
Research: Francois Darchis/Senior Vice President Research & Development
Finance: Fabienne Lecorvaisier/Vice President Finance
  Control, Blood Gas   Chemistry
  Gas Mixtures, Medical   General
  Gas, Calibrated (Specified Concentration)   Anesthesiology
  Regulator, Anesthesia   Anesthesiology

AIR LIQUIDE AMERICA SPECIALTY GASES LLC
713-402-2152
1311 New Savannah Rd., Augusta, GA 30901
FDA Number: 1037763
Ownership: Private
Produces/Sells CE-marked Devices: N
  Gas, Calibrated (Specified Concentration)   Anesthesiology
  Gas, Laser Generating   Surgery
  Generator, Gas, Microbiology   Microbiology

AIR LIQUIDE HEALTHCARE AMERICA CORPORATION
713-402-2152
12460 Arrow Route, rancho cucamonga, CA 91739
FDA Number: 2020902
Ownership: Private
Produces/Sells CE-marked Devices: N
  Gas, Calibrated (Specified Concentration)   Anesthesiology
  Gas, Laser Generating   Surgery

AIR LIQUIDE HEALTHCARE AMERICA CORPORATION
877-855-9533
2700 Post Oak Blvd., Houston, TX 77056   **713-402-2152**
FDA Number: 3003764448
Ownership: Private
Produces/Sells CE-marked Devices: N
  Control, Blood Gas   Chemistry
  Control, Multi Analyte, All Kinds (Assayed And Unassayed)   Chemistry
  Cylinder, Compressed Gas, With Valve   Anesthesiology

AIR LIQUIDE HEALTHCARE AMERICA
877-855-9533 *(cont'd)*
  Kit, Identification, Anaerobic   Microbiology
  Laser, Surgical   Surgery

AIR MOVEMENT TECHNOLOGIES, INC.
800-317-9582
320 Gateway Park Dr., N. Syracuse, NY 13212
FDA Number: 3004767172   *Fax:* 315-452-1973
E-mail: sales@emeraldresources.com
Web site: www.emeraldresources.com
Ownership: Private
Produces/Sells CE-marked Devices: N
  Accessories, Wheelchair   Physical Med
  Patient Transfer Unit, Powered   General
  Sling, Overhead Suspension, Wheelchair   Physical Med
  Transfer Device, Patient, Manual   General

AIR PRODUCTS AND CHEMICALS, INC.
800-654-4567
7201 Hamilton Blvd., Allentown, PA 18195-1501   **610-481-4911**
FDA Number: 2518141   *Fax:* 800-880-5204
E-mail: info@airproducts.com
Web site: www.airproducts.com
Medical Products Sales Volume: $8,800,000,000
Annual Revenue: More than $100 Million
Year Founded: 1940
Total Employees: 3800
Ownership: Public
Stock Symbol: APD
Traded On: NYSE
Quality System Registration Information: ISO9002
Produces/Sells CE-marked Devices: N
Distribution: Service Direct
General Admin.: Paul Zecchini/General Manager
        H. A. Wagner/President, Chairman, Chief Executive Officer
        J. P. Jones/President, Chief Operating Officer
Mktg./Adv.: Debbie Wilson/Manager Advertising
        Tracy MacGown/Manager Marketing
  Cart, Gas Cylinder (Carrier)   Anesthesiology
  Flowmeter, Gas (Oxygen), Calibrated   Anesthesiology
  Gas Mixtures, Laboratory   General
  Gas Mixtures, Magnetic Resonance Imaging   Radiology
  Gas Mixtures, Medical   General
  Gas, Calibrated (Specified Concentration)   Anesthesiology
  Manifold, Gas   Chemistry
  Oxygen   Anesthesiology
  Regulator, Pressure, Gas Cylinder   Anesthesiology
  Stand, Gas Cylinder   Anesthesiology

AIR QUALITY ENGINEERING, INC.
800-328-0787
7140 Northland Drive No.,   **763-531-9823**
Minneapolis, MN 55428
FDA Number: n/a   *Fax:* 763-531-9900
E-mail: info@air-quality.com
Web site: www.air-quality-eng.com
Medical Products Sales Volume: $3,900,000
Annual Revenue: $5-$10 Million
Year Founded: 1973
Total Employees: 50   *Marketing Staff:* 3   *Sales Staff:* 19
Ownership: Private
Produces/Sells CE-marked Devices: N
Federal Procurement Eligibility: Small Business, Female Owned
Distribution: Manufacturer Direct, Exporter
General Admin.: Heidi Oas/President, Chief Executive Officer
Mktg./Adv.: Ira Golden/Director Sales
  Equipment, Cleaning, Air   General
  Equipment, Control, Pollution   General
  Filter, Air   General

AIR SCENT INTERNATIONAL
  See Surco Products

AIR SCIENCE USA
800-306-0656
120 6th St., Fort Myers, FL 33907   **239-489-0024**
FDA Number: n/a   *Fax:* 800-306-0677
E-mail: info@airscience.com
Web site: www.airscience.com
Ownership: Private
Produces/Sells CE-marked Devices: N
  Hood, Fume   Toxicology

AIR TECHNIQUES INTERNATIONAL
410-363-9696
11403 Cronridge Drive, Owings Mills, MD 21117-2247
FDA Number: n/a   *Fax:* 410-363-9695
E-mail: info@atitest.com
Web site: www.atitest.com
Medical Products Sales Volume: $12,500,000
Year Founded: 1961
Total Employees: 56   *Marketing Staff:* 5   *Sales Staff:* 5
Ownership: HAMILTON ASSOCIATES, INC.
Quality System Registration Information: ISO9000; ISO9001

AIR TECHNIQUES INTERNATIONAL 410-363-9696 (cont'd)
Produces/Sells CE-marked Devices: Y
Federal Procurement Eligibility: Small Business, GSA Contract
Distribution: Manufacturer Direct, Manufacturer Through Distributor, OEM, Service Direct, Exporter
General Admin.: Eric Hanson/President
　　　　David Crosby/Vice President
Mktg./Adv.: R. Vijaykumar/Director Marketing
　　　　R. Vijaykumar/Director Product Development
　　　　R. Vijaykumar/Manager Sales
　　　　Ruth Lanahan/Marketing Representative
Production: Tim McDiarmid/Manager Production

Diluter	Chemistry
Generator, Aerosol	Ear/Nose/Throat
Photometer	Chemistry
Sampler, Air	General
Service, Maintenance/Repair	General
Test, Equipment, Sterilization	General

AIR TECHNIQUES, INC. 800-247-8324
1295 Walt Whitman Rd., Melville, NY 11747 516-433-7676
FDA Number: 2428225 *Fax:* 516-433-7684
E-mail: info@airtechniques.com
Web site: http://www.airtechniques.com
Annual Revenue: $50-$100 Million
Year Founded: 1962
Total Employees: 260 *Marketing Staff:* 6 *Sales Staff:* 32
Ownership: Private
Quality System Registration Information: ISO9001
Produces/Sells CE-marked Devices: Y
Distribution: Manufacturer Through Distributor, Manufacturer Through Manufacturer Reps
General Admin.: Louis E. Brooks/Chairman, Chief Executive Officer
　　　　Jeffrey Goldstein/Chief Financial Officer, Vice President
　　　　Frank Bader/President, Chief Operating Officer
　　　　Mark S. Brooks/Vice President
Mktg./Adv.: Kent Searl/Vice President Sales
Production: Joseph Carey/Director Quality Assurance

Airbrush	Dental And Oral
Colposcope	Obstetrics/Gynecology
Compressor, Air, Portable	Anesthesiology
Laser, Fluorescence Caries Detection	Dental And Oral
Light, Fiberoptic, Dental	Dental And Oral
Operative Dental Treatment Unit	Dental And Oral
Processor, Radiographic Film, Automatic	Radiology
Solution, Instrument Cleaner	General
Source, Heat, Bleaching, Teeth, Dental	Dental And Oral
Unit, Operative Dental, Accessories	Dental And Oral

AIR-TITE OF VIRGINIA, INC.
See Air-Tite Products Co., Inc.

AIR-TITE PRODUCTS CO., INC. 800-231-7762
565 Central Drive, Suite 101, 757-340-2501
Virginia Beach, VA 23454
FDA Number: 1121649 *Fax:* 757-340-2912
E-mail: atinfo@air-tite.com
Web site: www.air-tite.com
Medical Products Sales Volume: $1,600,000
Annual Revenue: $5-$10 Million
Year Founded: 1926
Total Employees: 10 *Marketing Staff:* 2 *Sales Staff:* 4
Ownership: Private
Quality System Registration Information: ISO9001
Produces/Sells CE-marked Devices: Y
Federal Procurement Eligibility: Small Business
Distribution: Manufacturer Through Distributor, Exclusive Distributor, Importer, Exporter
General Admin.: William Westendorf/President
Mktg./Adv.: Mr. Samual Gassel/Associate Director Marketing
　　　　Paul E. Oberdorfer/Vice President Business Development

Cap, Tip, Syringe	General
Catheter, Intravenous	Cardiovascular
Material, Training, Audiovisual	General
Needle, Hypodermic	General
Needle, Other	General
Syringe, Dental	Dental And Oral
Syringe, Drug, Luer-Lock	Dental And Oral
Syringe, Laboratory	Chemistry
Syringe, Piston	General

AIRBORNE AMBULANCE SERVICE
See National Air Ambulance

AIRCAST LLC 800-321-9549
1430 Decision St., Vista, CA 92081 760-727-1280
FDA Number: 2242894 *Fax:* 760-734-3595
E-mail: USInq@Aircast.com
Web site: www.aircast.com

AIRCAST LLC 800-321-9549 (cont'd)
Medical Products Sales Volume: $413,100,000
Year Founded: 2001
Total Employees: 3000
Ownership: Private
Stock Symbol: DJO
Traded On: NYSE
Produces/Sells CE-marked Devices: Y
Distribution: Manufacturer Through Manufacturer Reps, Exporter
General Admin.: Thomas A. Crowley/President, Chief Operating Officer
　　　　Michelle Romanenko/Vice President Human Resources
Mktg./Adv.: Dennis Mattessich/Director Marketing
　　　　Kathy Wozniak/Manager Contract Sales
　　　　Mary Kuh/Manager Sales Training
Production: Carol Babrowsky/Director Art
　　　　Steve Kenney/Director Quality Assurance
　　　　Fabian McCarthy/Vice President Manufacturing

Compression Instrument	Orthopedics
Orthosis, Limb Brace	Physical Med
Orthosis, Other	Physical Med
Support, Ankle	Orthopedics
Support, Arm	Physical Med
Support, Knee	Physical Med
Support, Leg	Physical Med

AIRCO GAS AND GEAR
See Boc Gases

AIRCO MEDICAL & INDUSTRIAL GASES
See Boc Gases

AIRCO WELDING PRODUCTS
See Concoa

AIRERX HEALTHCARE, LLC 615-244-3327
1843 Airlane Drive, Nashville, TN 37210
FDA Number: 3005988718

Cushion, Wheelchair (Pad)	Physical Med

AIREX, INC. 425-222-3665
13704 SE 17th St., Bellevue, WA 98050
FDA Number: n/a *Fax:* 425-880-4980
E-mail: bill.haslebacher@airexinc.com
Web site: www.airexinc.com
Annual Revenue: $0-$1 Million
Year Founded: 1994
Total Employees: 7 *Marketing Staff:* 1 *Sales Staff:* 2
Ownership: Private
Produces/Sells CE-marked Devices: N
Federal Procurement Eligibility: Small Business, GSA Contract
Distribution: Manufacturer Through Distributor, Manufacturer Through Manufacturer Reps, OEM, Exporter

Aid, Control, Environmental, Controlled, Breath	Physical Med
Air Handling Apparatus, Enclosure	Surgery
Air Handling, Apparatus, Bench	Surgery
Cleanroom Equipment	General
Filter, Bacterial, Breathing Circuit	Anesthesiology

AIREX/ALUSUISSE COMPOSITES, INC.
See Magister Corporation

AIRGAS CANADA INC. 800-661-1221
Bay 133, 3016 10th Ave., N.E., 403-272-6605
Calgary, AB AB T2 Canada
FDA Number: n/a *Fax:* 403-248-0701
Web site: www.airgas.com
Year Founded: 1982
Total Employees: 14000
Ownership: Airgas, Inc.
Stock Symbol: ARG
Traded On: NYSE
Produces/Sells CE-marked Devices: N
Distribution: Service Direct, Exclusive Distributor

AIRGAS EAST
See Airgas East, Inc.

AIRGAS EAST, INC 866-718-0685
1 Plank St., Billerica, MA 01821
FDA Number: 1217333
Web site: www.airgas.com
Year Founded: 1982
Total Employees: 14000
Ownership: AIRGAS, INC.
Stock Symbol: ARG
Traded On: NYSE
Produces/Sells CE-marked Devices: N
General Admin.: Peter McCausland/Chief Executive Officer, Chairman

Box, Glove	Microbiology
Calibrator, Gas, Volume	Anesthesiology
Gas, Laser Generating	Surgery

AIRGAS EAST, INC   866-718-0685 *(cont'd)*
Incubator/Water Bath, Microbiology   Microbiology

AIRGAS EAST, INC.   800-562-3815
140 Harding Ave., Bellmawr, NJ 08031
FDA Number: 2250062
Web site: www.airgas.com
Year Founded: 1982
Total Employees: 14000
Ownership: AIRGAS, INC.
Stock Symbol: ARG
Traded On: NYSE
Produces/Sells CE-marked Devices: N
General Admin.: Peter McCausland/Chief Executive Officer, Chairman
   Gas, Calibrated (Specified Concentration)   Anesthesiology

AIRGAS EAST, INC.   800-562-3815
27 Northwestern Drive, Salem, NH 03079
FDA Number: 1250022
E-mail: eBusinessEast@airgas.com
Web site: www.airgas.com
Medical Products Sales Volume: $122,000,000
Annual Revenue: More than $1 Billion
Year Founded: 1982
Total Employees: 14000
Ownership: Airgas, Inc.
Stock Symbol: ARG
Traded On: NYSE
Produces/Sells CE-marked Devices: N
Distribution: Manufacturer Direct, Exclusive Distributor
General Admin.: Peter McCausland/Chief Executive Officer, Chairman
   Box, Glove   Microbiology
   Calibrator, Blood Gas   General
   Gas Mixtures, Medical   General
   Incubator/Water Bath, Microbiology   Microbiology

AIRGAS EAST, INC.   800-562-3815
608 Nursery Rd., Linthicum Heights, MD 21090
FDA Number: 1111563
Web site: www.airgas.com
Year Founded: 1982
Total Employees: 14000
Ownership: AIRGAS, INC.
Stock Symbol: ARG
Traded On: NYSE
Produces/Sells CE-marked Devices: N
General Admin.: Peter McCausland/Chief Executive Officer, Chairman
   Gas, Calibrated (Specified Concentration)   Anesthesiology

AIRGAS EAST, INC.   800-562-3815
90 Research Rd., Hingham, MA 02043
FDA Number: 1218433
Web site: www.airgas.com
Year Founded: 1982
Total Employees: 14000
Ownership: AIRGAS, INC.
Stock Symbol: ARG
Traded On: NYSE
Produces/Sells CE-marked Devices: N
General Admin.: Peter McCausland/Chief Executive Officer, Chairman
   Gas, Calibrated (Specified Concentration)   Anesthesiology

AIRGAS GASPRO INC.   808-842-2282
2305 Kamehameha Hwy., Honolulu, HI 96819
FDA Number: 2919021
Web site: www.airgas.com
Year Founded: 1982
Total Employees: 14000
Ownership: AIRGAS, INC.
Stock Symbol: ARG
Traded On: NYSE
Produces/Sells CE-marked Devices: N
General Admin.: Peter McCausland/Chief Executive Officer, Chairman
   Box, Glove   Microbiology
   Gas, Calibrated (Specified Concentration)   Anesthesiology
   Incubator/Water Bath, Microbiology   Microbiology

AIRGAS GREAT LAKES, INC.   517-894-4101
5018 Empire Way, Lansing, MI 48917
FDA Number: 1835566
Web site: www.airgas.com
Year Founded: 1982
Total Employees: 14000
Ownership: AIRGAS, INC.
Stock Symbol: ARG
Traded On: NYSE
Produces/Sells CE-marked Devices: N
General Admin.: Peter McCausland/Chief Executive Officer, Chairman

AIRGAS GREAT LAKES, INC.   517-894-4101 *(cont'd)*
   Box, Glove   Microbiology
   Gas, Calibrated (Specified Concentration)   Anesthesiology
   Incubator/Water Bath, Microbiology   Microbiology
   Laser, Surgical   Surgery

AIRGAS INTERMOUNTAIN, INC.   801-288-5015
3415 South 7oo West, Salt Lake City, UT 84119
FDA Number: 1717226   Fax: 801- 288-5050
Web site: www.airgas.com
Year Founded: 1982
Total Employees: 14000
Ownership: AIRGAS, INC.
Stock Symbol: ARG
Traded On: NYSE
Produces/Sells CE-marked Devices: N
General Admin.: Peter McCausland/Chief Executive Officer, Chairman
   Box, Glove   Microbiology
   Gas, Calibrated (Specified Concentration)   Anesthesiology
   Incubator/Water Bath, Microbiology   Microbiology
   Laser, Surgical   Surgery

AIRGAS NORPAC   360-944-4091
3411 North Columbia Blvd., Portland, OR 97217
FDA Number: 3024515
Web site: www.airgas.com
Year Founded: 1982
Total Employees: 14000
Ownership: AIRGAS, INC.
Stock Symbol: ARG
Traded On: NYSE
Produces/Sells CE-marked Devices: N
General Admin.: Peter McCausland/Chief Executive Officer, Chairman
   Box, Glove   Microbiology
   Gas, Calibrated (Specified Concentration)   Anesthesiology
   Generator, Gas, Microbiology   Microbiology
   Incubator/Water Bath, Microbiology   Microbiology

AIRGAS SOUTH, INC.   770-590-6200
1311 Fulton Industrial Blvd., N.W., Suite C, Atlanta, GA 30336
FDA Number: 1033831
Web site: www.airgas.com
Year Founded: 1982
Total Employees: 14000
Ownership: AIRGAS, INC.
Stock Symbol: ARG
Traded On: NYSE
Produces/Sells CE-marked Devices: N
General Admin.: Peter McCausland/Chief Executive Officer, Chairman
   Box, Glove   Microbiology
   Disc, Strip And Reagent, Microorganism Differentiation   Microbiology
   Gas, Calibrated (Specified Concentration)   Anesthesiology

AIRGAS SOUTH, INC.   770-590-6200
1620 Tampa East Blvd., Tampa, FL 33619
FDA Number: 1056791
Web site: www.airgas.com
Year Founded: 1982
Total Employees: 14000
Ownership: AIRGAS, INC.
Stock Symbol: ARG
Traded On: NYSE
Produces/Sells CE-marked Devices: N
General Admin.: Peter McCausland/Chief Executive Officer, Chairman
   Box, Glove   Microbiology
   Gas, Calibrated (Specified Concentration)   Anesthesiology
   Incubator/Water Bath, Microbiology   Microbiology

AIRGAS SOUTH, INC.   770-590-6200
3605 Presidential Pkwy., Atlanta, GA 30340
FDA Number: 1012886
Web site: www.airgas.com
Year Founded: 1982
Total Employees: 14000
Ownership: AIRGAS, INC.
Stock Symbol: ARG
Traded On: NYSE
Produces/Sells CE-marked Devices: N
General Admin.: Peter McCausland/Chief Executive Officer, Chairman
   Box, Glove   Microbiology
   Disc, Strip And Reagent, Microorganism Differentiation   Microbiology
   Gas, Calibrated (Specified Concentration)   Anesthesiology
   Incubator/Water Bath, Microbiology   Microbiology

AIRGAS SOUTH, INC.   770-590-6200
4551 North Access Rd., Chattanooga, TN 37415
FDA Number: 1022618
Web site: www.airgas.com
Year Founded: 1982

AIRGAS SOUTH, INC.   770-590-6200 *(cont'd)*
Total Employees: 14000
Ownership: AIRGAS, INC.
Stock Symbol: ARG
Traded On: NYSE
Produces/Sells CE-marked Devices: N
General Admin.: Peter McCausland/Chief Executive Officer, Chairman
Gas, Calibrated (Specified Concentration)   Anesthesiology

AIRGAS SOUTH, INC.   251-653-2500
5480 Hamilton Blvd., Theodore, AL 36582
FDA Number: 1036958
Web site: www.airgas.com
Year Founded: 1982
Total Employees: 14000
Ownership: AIRGAS, INC.
Stock Symbol: ARG
Traded On: NYSE
Produces/Sells CE-marked Devices: N
General Admin.: Peter McCausland/Chief Executive Officer, Chairman
Box, Glove   Microbiology
Calibrator, Gas, Volume   Anesthesiology
Disc, Strip And Reagent, Microorganism Differentiation   Microbiology
Gas, Calibrated (Specified Concentration)   Anesthesiology
Generator, Gas, Microbiology   Microbiology
Incubator/Water Bath, Microbiology   Microbiology
Laser, Surgical   Surgery

AIRGAS SOUTH, INC.   770-590-6200
5837 W. Fifth St., Jacksonville, FL 32254
FDA Number: 1015630
Web site: www.airgas.com
Year Founded: 1982
Total Employees: 14000
Ownership: AIRGAS, INC.
Stock Symbol: ARG
Traded On: NYSE
Produces/Sells CE-marked Devices: N
General Admin.: Peter McCausland/Chief Executive Officer, Chairman
Box, Glove   Microbiology
Gas, Calibrated (Specified Concentration)   Anesthesiology

AIRGAS SOUTH, INC.   770-590-6200
7280 NW 58th St., Miami, FL 33166
FDA Number: 1025636
Web site: www.airgas.com
Year Founded: 1982
Total Employees: 14000
Ownership: AIRGAS, INC.
Stock Symbol: ARG
Traded On: NYSE
Produces/Sells CE-marked Devices: N
General Admin.: Peter McCausland/Chief Executive Officer, Chairman
Gas, Calibrated (Specified Concentration)   Anesthesiology

AIRGAS SOUTH, INC.
See Linde Gas North America Llc

AIRGAS SPECIALTY GASES   913-495-3621
9851 Widmer Rd., Lenexa, KS 66215
FDA Number: 3005575471
Web site: www.airgas.com
Year Founded: 1982
Total Employees: 14000
Ownership: AIRGAS, INC.
Stock Symbol: ARG
Traded On: NYSE
Produces/Sells CE-marked Devices: N
General Admin.: Peter McCausland/Chief Executive Officer, Chairman
Gas, Calibrated (Specified Concentration)   Anesthesiology

AIRGAS SPECIALTY GASES, INC.   773-785-3000
12722 South Wentworth Ave., Roseland, IL 60628
FDA Number: 1415141
Web site: www.airgas.com
Year Founded: 1982
Total Employees: 14000
Ownership: AIRGAS, INC.
Stock Symbol: ARG
Traded On: NYSE
Produces/Sells CE-marked Devices: N
General Admin.: Peter McCausland/Chief Executive Officer, Chairman
Gas, Calibrated (Specified Concentration)   Anesthesiology

AIRGAS WEST, INC.   310-505-9897
11711 South Alameda, Los Angeles, CA 90059
FDA Number: 2027603
Web site: www.airgas.com
Year Founded: 1982

AIRGAS WEST, INC.   310-505-9897 *(cont'd)*
Total Employees: 14000
Ownership: AIRGAS, INC.
Stock Symbol: ARG
Traded On: NYSE
Produces/Sells CE-marked Devices: N
General Admin.: Peter McCausland/Chief Executive Officer, Chairman
Box, Glove   Microbiology
Electrode, Ion Specific, Calcium   Chemistry
Electrode, Ion Specific, Potassium   Chemistry
Electrode, Ion Specific, Sodium   Chemistry
Gas, Calibrated (Specified Concentration)   Anesthesiology
Incubator/Water Bath, Microbiology   Microbiology

AIRGAS WEST, INC.   310-505-9897
191 South Kettering Dr., Ontario, CA 91761
FDA Number: 2029250
Web site: www.airgas.com
Year Founded: 1982
Total Employees: 14000
Ownership: AIRGAS, INC.
Stock Symbol: ARG
Traded On: NYSE
Produces/Sells CE-marked Devices: N
General Admin.: Peter McCausland/Chief Executive Officer, Chairman
Analyzer, Gas, Carbon-Dioxide, Gaseous Phase (Capnograph)   Anesthesiology
Box, Glove   Microbiology
Control, Blood Gas   Chemistry
Electrode, Ion Specific, Calcium   Chemistry
Electrode, Ion Specific, Potassium   Chemistry
Electrode, Ion Specific, Sodium   Chemistry
Gas, Calibrated (Specified Concentration)   Anesthesiology
Incubator/Water Bath, Microbiology   Microbiology

AIRGAS, INC.   610-687-5253
259 North Radnor-Chester Rd., Randor, PA 19087-5283
FDA Number: n/a   Fax: 610-687-1052
Web site: www.airgas.com
Year Founded: 1982
Total Employees: 14000
Ownership: Public
Stock Symbol: ARG
Traded On: NYSE
Produces/Sells CE-marked Devices: N
Distribution: Exclusive Distributor
General Admin.: Peter McCausand/Chief Executive Officer, Chairman
Gas Mixtures, Medical   General
Oxygen   Anesthesiology
Medical Product Subsidiaries (Listed Separately)
Airgas Canada Inc.
Airgas East, Inc.

AIRGAS, NORTHERN CALIFORNIA AND NEVADA   916-379-1050
20725 Corsair Blvd., Hayward, CA 94545
FDA Number: 3004676353
Web site: www.airgas.com
Year Founded: 1982
Total Employees: 14000
Ownership: AIRGAS, INC.
Stock Symbol: ARG
Traded On: NYSE
Produces/Sells CE-marked Devices: N
General Admin.: Peter McCausland/Chief Executive Officer, Chairman
Box, Glove   Microbiology
Gas, Calibrated (Specified Concentration)   Anesthesiology
Incubator/Water Bath, Microbiology   Microbiology

AIRGAS, NORTHERN CALIFORNIA AND NEVADA   916-379-1050
443 Hobson St., San Jose, CA 95110
FDA Number: 3004676353
Web site: www.airgas.com
Year Founded: 1982
Total Employees: 14000
Ownership: AIRGAS, INC.
Stock Symbol: ARG
Traded On: NYSE
Produces/Sells CE-marked Devices: N
General Admin.: Peter McCausland/Chief Executive Officer, Chairman
Box, Glove   Microbiology
Gas, Calibrated (Specified Concentration)   Anesthesiology
Incubator/Water Bath, Microbiology   Microbiology

AIRGAS-MID AMERICA, INC.   800-292-4404
3500 Bernard, Saint Louis, MO 63103
FDA Number: 1946773
Web site: www.airgas.com
Year Founded: 1982
Total Employees: 14000
Ownership: AIRGAS, INC.

AIRGAS-MID AMERICA, INC.   800-292-4404 *(cont'd)*
Stock Symbol: ARG
Traded On: NYSE
Produces/Sells CE-marked Devices: N
General Admin.: Peter McCausland/Chief Executive Officer, Chairman
Box, Glove	Microbiology
Gas, Calibrated (Specified Concentration)	Anesthesiology
Generator, Gas, Microbiology	Microbiology

AIRGAS-MID SOUTH, INC.   918-582-0885
9101 Bond St., Overland Park, KS 66214
FDA Number: 1912755
Web site: www.airgas.com
Year Founded: 1982
Total Employees: 14000
Ownership: Private
Stock Symbol: ARG
Traded On: NYSE
Produces/Sells CE-marked Devices: N
General Admin.: Peter McCausland/Chief Executive Officer, Chairman
Gas, Calibrated (Specified Concentration)	Anesthesiology

AIRGAS-MID SOUTH, INC.   918-582-0885
9741 E 56th St N, Tulsa, OK 74110
FDA Number: 1645341
Web site: www.airgas.com
Year Founded: 1982
Total Employees: 14000
Ownership: AIRGAS, INC.
Stock Symbol: ARG
Traded On: NYSE
Produces/Sells CE-marked Devices: N
General Admin.: Peter McCausland/Chief Executive Officer, Chairman
Box, Glove	Microbiology
Gas, Calibrated (Specified Concentration)	Anesthesiology
Gas, Laser Generating	Surgery
Incubator/Water Bath, Microbiology	Microbiology

AIRGAS-NORTH CENTRAL, INC.   630-231-9260
1601 nicholas blvd., elk grove village, IL 60007
FDA Number: 3004931173   Fax: 630-231-7768
E-mail: NOC.Web.Service@Airgas.com
Web site: www.airgas.com
Year Founded: 1982
Total Employees: 14000
Ownership: AIRGAS, INC.
Stock Symbol: ARG
Traded On: NYSE
Produces/Sells CE-marked Devices: N
General Admin.: Peter McCausland/Chief Executive Officer, Chairman
Box, Glove	Microbiology
Gas, Calibrated (Specified Concentration)	Anesthesiology
Gas, Laser Generating	Surgery
Incubator/Water Bath, Microbiology	Microbiology

AIRGAS-SOUTHWEST, INC.   800-985-0986
21 Waterway, Suite 550,   **361-288-0587**
The Woodlands, TX 77380
FDA Number: n/a
E-mail: sws.eBusiness.team@airgas.com
Web site: www.airgas.com
Year Founded: 1982
Total Employees: 14000
Ownership: AIRGAS, INC.
Stock Symbol: ARG
Traded On: NYSE
Produces/Sells CE-marked Devices: N
General Admin.: Peter McCausland/Chief Executive Officer, Chairman
     Mr. Robert McLaughlin/Chief Financial Officer, Senior Vice President
     Mr. Robert Dougherty/Chief Information Officer
     Mr. Michael Molinini/Chief Operating Officer, Executive Vice President
     Mr. Robert Young Jr./General Counsel
     Mr. Dwight Wilson/Senior Vice President Human Resources
Mktg./Adv.: Leslie Graff/Senior Vice President Corporate Development
Electrode, Blood pH	Chemistry
Gas, Calibrated (Specified Concentration)	Anesthesiology
Laser, Carbon-Dioxide, Microsurgical, ENT	Ear/Nose/Throat
Laser, Gastroenterology/Urology	Gastroenterology/Urology
Laser, Ophthalmic	Ophthalmology
Liquid Chromatography, Salicylate	Toxicology
Suture, Non-Absorbable, Synthetic, Polyester	Surgery
Transport System, Anaerobic	Microbiology

AIRGAS-SOUTHWEST, INC.   361-288-0587
2615 Joe Field Rd., Dallas, TX 75229
FDA Number: 1627104

AIRGAS-SOUTHWEST, INC.   361-288-0587 *(cont'd)*
Web site: www.airgas.com
Year Founded: 1982
Total Employees: 14000
Ownership: AIRGAS, INC.
Stock Symbol: ARG
Traded On: NYSE
Produces/Sells CE-marked Devices: N
General Admin.: Peter McCausland/Chief Executive Officer, Chairman
Box, Glove	Microbiology
Gas, Calibrated (Specified Concentration)	Anesthesiology
Gas, Laser Generating	Surgery
Incubator/Water Bath, Microbiology	Microbiology

AIRGUARD   800-999-3458
100 River Ridge Circle, Jeffersonville, IN 47130   **502-969-2304 Ex**
FDA Number: 9330047   Fax: 1-800-784-3458
E-mail: mailbag@airguard.com
Web site: www.airguard.com
Medical Products Sales Volume: $5,000,000
Year Founded: 1964
Ownership: CLARCOR FILTRATION PRODUCTS GROUP
Quality System Registration Information: ISO9001
Produces/Sells CE-marked Devices: N
General Admin.: Jeff Tumm/President, Chief Executive Officer
     Jeff Nally/Vice President Human Resources
Mktg./Adv.: Gary Heilmann/Director Marketing
     Rick Kraus/Director National Accounts
     Joe Hovekamp/Director National Sales
     Monroe Britt/Director Product Development
     Jim Crum/Manager International Sales
     Joe Havecamp/Vice President Sales
Production: Wayne Lindsey/Director Quality Assurance
     Phil Cluskey/Manager Materials
Filter, Air	General
Filter, Bacteriological, Laboratory	Chemistry

AIRISTAR TECHNOLOGIES, L.L.C.   800-755-8006
2330 Ernie Krueger Circle, Waukegan, IL 60087   **847-775-8018**
FDA Number: n/a   Fax: 847-775-8019
E-mail: info@airistar.com
Web site: www.airistar.com
Medical Products Sales Volume: $500,000
Year Founded: 2003
Total Employees: 6   *Marketing Staff:* 3   *Sales Staff:* 6
Ownership: Private
Produces/Sells CE-marked Devices: N
Federal Procurement Eligibility: Small Business, GSA Contract
Distribution: Manufacturer Direct, Manufacturer Through Distributor, Manufacturer Through Manufacturer Reps
General Admin.: Mr. Roy Kibbe/President
Mktg./Adv.: Ms. Connie Wilson/Manager Marketing
     Mr. John Warling/Manager Sales
     Mr. Sean Burke/Marketing Communications Specialist
Filter, Air	General

AIRKEM PROFESSIONAL PRODUCTS DIV.
See Ecolab Inc.

AIRON CORPORATION   888-448-1238
751 North Drive, Unit 6, Melbourne, FL 32934   **321-821-9433**
FDA Number: 3003697063   Fax: 321-821-9443
E-mail: info@pneuton.com
Web site: www.pneuton.com
Year Founded: 1997
Total Employees: 7   *Marketing Staff:* 2   *Sales Staff:* 2
Ownership: Private
Quality System Registration Information: ISO9001
Produces/Sells CE-marked Devices: Y
Federal Procurement Eligibility: Small Business, GSA Contract, VA Contract
Distribution: Manufacturer Direct, Manufacturer Through Distributor, Manufacturer Through Manufacturer Reps, OEM
General Admin.: Eric Gjerde/President, Chief Executive Officer
Attachment, Breathing, Positive End Expiratory Pressure	Anesthesiology
Ventilator, Continuous (Respirator)	Anesthesiology
Ventilator, Emergency, Powered (Resuscitator)	Anesthesiology

AIRPAL PATIENT TRANSFER SYSTEMS INC.   800-633-4725
5456 Northwood Drive, Center Valley, PA 18034   **610-282-3553**
FDA Number: n/a   Fax: 610-282-3599
E-mail: info@airpal.com
Web site: www.airpal.com
Annual Revenue: $1-$5 Million
Total Employees: 8   *Marketing Staff:* 25
Ownership: Private
Produces/Sells CE-marked Devices: Y
Federal Procurement Eligibility: Small Business

AIRPAL PATIENT TRANSFER SYSTEMS INC.   800-633-4725
(cont'd)
Distribution: Manufacturer Direct, Manufacturer Through Distributor, Manufacturer Through Manufacturer Reps, Exporter
General Admin.: James E. Weedling/President
      Robert E. Weedling/President, Chief Executive Officer, Chairman
Patient Transfer Unit   General

AIRPOT CORPORATION   800-848-7681
35 Lois St., Norwalk, CT 06851   **203-846-2021**
FDA Number: n/a   *Fax:* 203-849-0539
E-mail: service@airpot.com
Web site: www.airpot.com
Ownership: Private
Produces/Sells CE-marked Devices: N
Distribution: Manufacturer Direct
General Admin.: Eda Webb/Office Manager
      Mark Gaberman/President
Research: Tom Lee/Vice President Engineering
Cylinder, Gas (Empty)   Anesthesiology

AIRSEP CORP.   800-874-0202
401 Creekside Dr., Buffalo, NY 14228-2070   **716-691-0202**
FDA Number: n/a   *Fax:* 716-691-0707
E-mail: marketing@airsep.com
Annual Revenue: $5-$10 Million
Total Employees: 500
Ownership: Private
Produces/Sells CE-marked Devices: N
Federal Procurement Eligibility: Small Business, Minority Owned
Distribution: Manufacturer Direct, Manufacturer Through Distributor, Manufacturer Through Manufacturer Reps, Exporter
General Admin.: Ravinder Bansal/Chairman, Chief Executive Officer
      Joni Hyrick/Director Human Resources
      Joseph Priest/President, Chief Operating Officer
      Edward Vrana/Senior Vice President
Mktg./Adv.: Miriam Shapiro/Director Marketing
      Frederick B. Morgan/Manager Marketing Operations
      Robert Jacobson/Vice President National Sales
Production: Evelyn Trubits/Manager Customer Services
      Greg Dziomba/Manager Quality Assurance
      Peter Weisenborn/Vice President Manufacturing
Analyzer, Gas, Oxygen, Sampling   Anesthesiology
Calibrator, Gas, Pressure   Anesthesiology
Concentrator, Oxygen   Anesthesiology
Conserver, Oxygen   Anesthesiology
Generator, Oxygen, Portable   Anesthesiology
Nebulizer, Direct Patient Interface   Anesthesiology
Oximeter, Whole Blood   Hematology

AIRSTRIP TECHNOLOGIES, LP   877-258-5869
335 E Sonterra Blvd Suite 200,   **210-805-0444**
San Antonio, TX 78258
FDA Number: 3006104191
E-mail: info@airstriptech.com
Web site: www.airstriptech.com
Ownership: Private
Produces/Sells CE-marked Devices: N
Monitor, Perinatal   Obstetrics/Gynecology
Monitor, Physiological, Patient(without Arrhythmia Detection Or Alarms)   Cardiovascular

AIRTECH INDUSTRIES, INC.   540-949-6565
412 Ohio St., Waynesboro, VA 22980
FDA Number: 1124848
Ownership: Private
Produces/Sells CE-marked Devices: N
Handpiece, Contra- And Right-Angle Attachment, Dental   Dental And Oral

AIRWAY CAM TECHNOLOGIES, INC.   877-EPIGLOTTIS
205 Spruce Tree Rd., Radnor, PA 19087   **610-341-9560**
FDA Number: 2436864   *Fax:* 610-341-1866
E-mail: info@airwaycam.com
Web site: www.airwaycam.com
Ownership: Private
Produces/Sells CE-marked Devices: N
Accessories, Surgical Camera   Surgery

AIRWAY DIVISION OF SURGICAL APPLIANCE INDUSTRIES, INC.   800-888-0458
3960 Rosslyn Dr., Cincinnati, OH 45209-1110   **513-271-4594**
FDA Number: 7000414   *Fax:* 800-309-9055
E-mail: gfaught@saibrands.com
Web site: www.airwaymast.com
Total Employees: 150
Ownership: Truform Orthotics & Prosthetics
Produces/Sells CE-marked Devices: N
Distribution: Manufacturer Direct, Exclusive Distributor

AIRWAY DIVISION OF SURGICAL APPLIANCE   800-888-0458
(cont'd)
General Admin.: L. Thomas Applegate/President
Mktg./Adv.: Patrick Spenlau/Vice President Marketing
      Ginny Faught/Vice President Sales
Brassiere, Maternity   Obstetrics/Gynecology
Joint, Knee, External Brace   Physical Med
Prosthesis, Breast, External   Surgery
Support, Abdominal   Physical Med
Medical Product Subsidiaries (Listed Separately)
Pcp Champion

AIRWAY MANAGEMENT INC.   866-264-7667
6116 North Central Expressway, Suite 605,   **214-369-0978**
Dallas, TX 75206
FDA Number: 3003496134
E-mail: contactami@amisleep.com   *Fax:* 214-691-3151
Web site: www.amisleep.com
Ownership: Private
Produces/Sells CE-marked Devices: N
Device, Anti-Snoring   Ear/Nose/Throat
Gauge, Depth, Instrument, Dental   Dental And Oral
Material, Impression Tray, Resin   Dental And Oral
Positioner, Tooth, Preformed   Dental And Oral
Restraint, Patient, Conductive   Anesthesiology
Ventilator, Non-Continuous (Respirator)   Anesthesiology

AIRWAY SURGICAL APPLIANCES LTD.   800-267-3476
189 Colonnaide Rd.,   **613-723-4790**
Nepean, ONT K2E-7 Canada
FDA Number: n/a   *Fax:* 613-723-8091
E-mail: schell@airwaysurgical.ca
Year Founded: 1895
Total Employees: 100
Ownership: SURGICAL APPLIANCE INDUSTRIES, INC.
Produces/Sells CE-marked Devices: N
Distribution: Manufacturer Direct, Exclusive Distributor, Exporter

AIRWAY SURGICAL CO.
See Airway Division Of Surgical Appliance Industries, Inc.

AIRX LABORATORIES   800-444-8900
1640 Delmar Dr., P.O. Box 37,   **610-534-8900**
Folcroft, PA 19032
FDA Number: n/a   *Fax:* 610-534-8912
E-mail: sales@airxinfo.com
Web site: www.airxinfo.com
Medical Products Sales Volume: $4,000,000
Annual Revenue: $5-$10 Million
Ownership: THE BULLEN COMPANIES, INC.
Produces/Sells CE-marked Devices: N
Federal Procurement Eligibility: Small Business
Distribution: Manufacturer Through Distributor, Manufacturer Through Manufacturer Reps
Disinfector, Liquid   General
Sanitizer   General
Solution, Antibacterial Cleaner   General

AISLING INDUSTRIES   760-353-4000
621 East Heil Ave., El Centro, CA 92243
FDA Number: n/a   *Fax:* 760-352-7581
E-mail: crescencio@aislinginc.com
Web site: www.aislinginc.com
Medical Products Sales Volume: $3,500,000
Annual Revenue: $1-$5 Million
Total Employees: 250
Ownership: Private
Produces/Sells CE-marked Devices: N
Federal Procurement Eligibility: Small Business
Distribution: Manufacturer Direct
General Admin.: Michael J. Logue/President
Mktg./Adv.: Sergio Quiroz/Project Manager
Production: Crescencio Coronel/Production Supervisor
Component, Electronic   General
Stethoscope, Esophageal   Anesthesiology

AIT DENTAL, INC.   800-762-1765
1226 International Drive, Eau Claire, WI 54701   **715-832-7271**
FDA Number: n/a   *Fax:* 715-832-0093
E-mail: info@aitdental.com
Web site: www.aitdental.com
Ownership: Private
Produces/Sells CE-marked Devices: N
Distribution: Manufacturer Direct
General Admin.: Brian Sholder/President
Floss, Dental   Dental And Oral

AIV, INC. (FORMERLY AMERICAN IV)
7485 Shipley Avenue, Harmans, MD 21077
800-990-2911
410-787-1300
FDA Number: 1121996
Fax: 410-787-1337
E-mail: aivsales@aiv-inc.com
Web site: www.aiv-inc.com
Ownership: Private
Produces/Sells CE-marked Devices: Y
Federal Procurement Eligibility: Small Business
Distribution: Manufacturer Direct, Service Direct, Exporter
Mktg./Adv.: Mr. James Huggins/Director Business Development
Mr. Kenneth Eshenbaugh/Director Marketing
Mr. David Lyons/Director Sales
Mr. Richard Stacey/Vice President Marketing & Sales
Production: Dr. John Taylor/Director Engineering
Mr. Tim Malkus/Director Production
Mr. Greg Falk/Director Quality Assurance & Regulatory Affairs
Finance: Mrs. Paula Doyle/Controller

Accessories, Pump, Infusion	General
Adapter, Cable, Equipment	General
Cable, Electrode	Physical Med
Charger, Battery	General
Monitor, Bed Patient	General
Oximeter, Finger	General
Oximeter, Pulse	General
Oximeter, Tissue Saturation	Cardiovascular
Pump, Infusion	General
Pump, Infusion, Ambulatory	General
Pump, Infusion, Patient Controlled Analgesia (PCA)	General
Pump, Infusion, Syringe	General
Service, Maintenance/Repair	General
Service, Parts, Repair	General
Thermometer, Electronic	General
Transducer, Pressure, Intrauterine	Obstetrics/Gynecology
Transducer, Ultrasonic, Intravaginal	Obstetrics/Gynecology
Transducer, Ultrasonic, Obstetrical	Obstetrics/Gynecology

AK SPECIALTY VEHICLES
See Oshkosh Specialty Vehicles

AK, LTD.
18412 N.E. Halsey, Portland, OR 97230
503-669-0986
FDA Number: n/a
Fax: 503-661-4340
E-mail: info@akltd.com
Web site: www.akltd.com
Medical Products Sales Volume: $1,000,000
Annual Revenue: $0-$1 Million
Year Founded: 1987
Total Employees: 13 *Marketing Staff:* 1 *Sales Staff:* 1
Ownership: Private
Produces/Sells CE-marked Devices: N
Federal Procurement Eligibility: Small Business, Female Owned
Distribution: Manufacturer Direct, Manufacturer Through Distributor, Manufacturer Through Manufacturer Reps
General Admin.: Carol Sparks/President, Chief Executive Officer
Mktg./Adv.: Michele Sparks/Director Marketing
Michele Sparks/Manager National Sales

Dispenser, Other	General
Shield, Protective, Personnel	Radiology

AKCESS MEDICAL PRODUCTS, INC.
See Angiodynamics, Inc.

AKERS BIOSCIENCES, INC.
201 Grove Road, Thorofare, NJ 08086
800-451-8378
856-848-2116
FDA Number: 2247413
Fax: 856-848-0269
E-mail: info@akersbiosciences.com
Web site: www.akerslaboratories.com
Medical Products Sales Volume: $1,000,000
Annual Revenue: $10-$25 Million
Year Founded: 1989
Total Employees: 38 *Marketing Staff:* 5 *Sales Staff:* 5
Ownership: Private
Stock Symbol: AKR
Traded On: London
Produces/Sells CE-marked Devices: N
Federal Procurement Eligibility: Small Business, GSA Contract, VA Contract
Distribution: Manufacturer Direct, Manufacturer Through Distributor, Manufacturer Through Manufacturer Reps, OEM, Exclusive Distributor, Exporter
General Admin.: Raymond Akers/President, Chief Executive Officer
Mktg./Adv.: Fred Ryan/Senior Vice President Marketing & Sales
Dr. Frank Goodman/Vice President Business Development
Joe Perrone/Vice President International Marketing & Sales
Joseph P. Koz/Vice President Strategic & Gov. Sales
Production: Barbara Bagley/Director Quality Assurance
Budd Webb/Manager Materials
Donald H. Russell/Vice President Material Science
Research: Lee Meyers/Vice President Research & Development

Analyzer, Alcohol	Toxicology
Antigen, Prostate-Specific (PSA), Management, Cancer	Immunology

AKERS BIOSCIENCES, INC.
800-451-8378 *(cont'd)*

Chlamydia Trachomatis	Microbiology
Contract R&D, Diagnostics	General
Enzyme Linked Immunoabsorbent Assay, Cytomegalovirus	Microbiology
LDL & VLDL Precipitation, Cholesterol Via Esterase-Oxidase	Chemistry
Oxidase Test Device for Gonorrhea	Microbiology
Reagent, Virus, General	Pathology
Strip, Test	Chemistry
System, Identification, Hepatitis B Antigen	Hematology
System, Test, Blood Glucose, Over-The-Counter	Chemistry
System, Test, Drugs of Abuse	Chemistry
Test, Antibody, Acquired Immune Deficiency Syndrome (AIDS)	Hematology
Test, Disease, Lyme	Immunology
Test, Infectious Mononucleosis	Immunology
Test, Leukocyte Typing	Hematology
Test, Rheumatoid Factor	Immunology
Test, Syphilis (RPR or VDRL)	Microbiology

AKONNI BIOSYSTEMS
400 Sagner Ave, Suite 300, Frederick, MD 21701
301-698-0101
FDA Number: n/a
Fax: 301-698-0202
E-mail: info@akonni.com
Web site: http://www.akonni.com
Ownership: Private
Produces/Sells CE-marked Devices: N
General Admin.: Mr. Charles Daitch/Chief Executive Officer
Mr. Darrell Chandler/Chief Scientific Officer
Medical Admin.: Dr. George Rudy/Chief Medical Officer
Mktg./Adv.: Dr. Kevin Banks/Vice President Marketing & Sales
Production: Mr. Erik Black/Vice President Manufacturing
Mr. Jon Davis/Vice President Operations
Research: Mr. Phil Belgrader/Vice President Research & Development
IS: Ms. Jennifer Reynolds/Vice President Technology

AKORN, INC.
2500 Millbrook Drive, Buffalo Grove, IL 60089
800-535-7155
847-279-6179
FDA Number: 1419498
Fax: 800-943-3694
E-mail: customer.service@akorn.com
Web site: www.akorn.com
Medical Products Sales Volume: $71,300,000
Annual Revenue: $50-$100 Million
Year Founded: 1971
Total Employees: 327 *Marketing Staff:* 5 *Sales Staff:* 30
Ownership: CTC, Inc.
Stock Symbol: AKRX
Traded On: NASDAQ
Produces/Sells CE-marked Devices: N
Federal Procurement Eligibility: Small Business
Distribution: Manufacturer Direct
General Admin.: Mr. Neill Shanahan/Vice President Human Resources
Mktg./Adv.: Mr. Rick Coulon/Director Sales
Ms. Carla Hertel/Manager Product Marketing
Production: Mr. Brian Kunz/Director Materials Management
Mr. Shahid Ahmed/Senior Vice President Regulatory Affairs
Research: Dr. Abu Alam/Vice President Research & Development

Cannula, Ophthalmic	Ophthalmology
Container, Sterilization (Tray)	General
Forceps, Ophthalmic	Ophthalmology
Holder, Needle	Gastroenterology/Urology
Hook, Ophthalmic	Ophthalmology
Instrument, Microsurgical	Cns/Neurology
Keratometer	Ophthalmology
Knife, Cataract	Ophthalmology
Knife, Ophthalmic	Ophthalmology
Microscope	Hematology
Needle, Ophthalmic	Ophthalmology
Pack, Custom/Special Procedure	General
Scissors, Iris	Ophthalmology
Service, Parts, Repair	General
Spatula, Ophthalmic	Ophthalmology
Spatula, Other	Surgery
Spreader, Other	Surgery
Surgical Instrument, Radial Keratotomy	Ophthalmology

AKRIBEIA, INC.
1251 Washington St., Huntsville, AL 35801
256-564-7450
FDA Number: n/a
Ownership: Private
Produces/Sells CE-marked Devices: N

Block, Beam Shaping, Radionuclide	Radiology

AKRO-MILS, INC.
1293 S. Main St., Akron, OH 44301
800-253-2467
330-253-5592
FDA Number: n/a
Fax: 330-761-6348
E-mail: sales@po.akro-mils.com
Web site: www.akro-mils.com
Medical Products Sales Volume: $780,000,000
Year Founded: 1947
Total Employees: 5000 *Marketing Staff:* 7 *Sales Staff:* 15

AKRO-MILS, INC.
800-253-2467 (cont'd)
Ownership: Private
Quality System Registration Information: ISO9001; ISO9002
Produces/Sells CE-marked Devices: Y
Distribution: Manufacturer Through Distributor, OEM, Exporter
General Admin.: Dave Grider/General Manager
Mktg./Adv.: Jesse Prentiss/Advertising Assistant
       Joe Dluzyn/Manager Sales
       Doug Popek/Marketing Specialist
Production: Peter Dunlap/Manager Production Admin.

Bin, Storage	General
Cabinet Casework, Modular	General
Cabinet, Laboratory	Chemistry
Cabinet, Medicine	General
Cart, Other	General
System, Delivery, Drug, Unit-Dose	General

AKTINA MEDICAL PHYSICS CORP.
(888) 433-3380
360 Route 9W North, Congers, NY 10920
845-268-0101
FDA Number: 2436865
    Fax: 845-268-1700
E-mail: info@aktina.com
Web site: www.aktina.com
Ownership: Private
Produces/Sells CE-marked Devices: N

Accelerator, Linear, Medical	Radiology
Block, Beam Shaping, Radionuclide	Radiology
Couch, Radiation Therapy, Powered	Radiology
Holder, Radiographic Cassette, Wall-Mounted	Radiology
Monitor, Patient Position, Light Beam	Radiology
Phantom, Anthropomorphic, Radiographic	Radiology
Simulator, Radiotherapy, Special Purpose	Radiology

AL'S MERCHANDISE, INC.
562-690-0139
3652 South Norwich Place, Rowland Heights, CA 91748
FDA Number: 2087076
Ownership: Private
Produces/Sells CE-marked Devices: N

Pad, Menstrual, Unscented	Obstetrics/Gynecology

ALABAMA TISSUE CENTER, INC.
500 22nd Street South, Suite 102, Birmingham, AL 35233
FDA Number: n/a
Medical Admin.: Dr. Devin Eckhoff/Medical Director

Allograft, Heart Valve	Cardiovascular
Valve, Heart, Tissue	Cardiovascular

ALADDIN SYNERGETICS, INC.
800-888-8018
250 E Main Street, Hendersonville, TN 37075
615-537-3600
FDA Number: n/a
    Fax: 888-812-9956
E-mail: info@aladdin-atr.com
Web site: www.aladdintemprite.com
Ownership: Aladdin Industries Pty. Ltd.
Produces/Sells CE-marked Devices: N
Distribution: Manufacturer Direct, OEM, Exclusive Distributor, Exporter
Mktg./Adv.: Marty Rothschild/Vice President Marketing

Cart, Foodservice	General
Foodservice Product/Equipment	General

ALADDIN TEMP-RITE CANADA INC.
1-800-387-3994
740 Gana Court,
1-800-387-3994
Mississauga, ONT L5S-1 Canada
FDA Number: n/a
    Fax: (888) 812-9956
E-mail: info@aladdin-atr.com
Web site: www.aladdintemprite.com
Year Founded: 1973
Total Employees: 25
Ownership: ALADDIN TEMP-RITE LLC
Produces/Sells CE-marked Devices: N
Distribution: Service Direct, Exclusive Distributor

ALAMAR BIOSCIENCES
See Trek Diagnostic Systems

ALAN'S WHEELCHAIRS & REPAIRS
800-693-4344
109 South Harbor Blvd.,, Suite B,
714-870-9840
Fullerton, CA 92832
FDA Number: n/a
    Fax: 714-870-9839
E-mail: alanswheelchairs@hotmail.com
Web site: www.alanswheelchairs.com
Annual Revenue: $0-$1 Million
Total Employees: 4
Ownership: Private
Produces/Sells CE-marked Devices: N
Federal Procurement Eligibility: Small Business
Distribution: Service Direct
General Admin.: Douglas Alan Ensor/President, Chief Executive Officer
Mktg./Adv.: Dave Bechtel/Managing Director Marketing & Sales

Chair, Geriatric, Wheeled	General
Scooter (Motorized 3-Wheeled Vehicle)	Physical Med

ALAN'S WHEELCHAIRS & REPAIRS
800-693-4344 (cont'd)

Service, Maintenance/Repair	General
Wheelchair, Manual	Physical Med
Wheelchair, Powered	Physical Med

ALARA INC.
800-410-2525
47505 Seabridge Drive, Fremont, CA 94538
510-315-5200
FDA Number: 2953719
    Fax: 510-315-5201
E-mail: info@alara.com
Web site: www.alara.com
Year Founded: 1994
Ownership: Private
Produces/Sells CE-marked Devices: Y
Federal Procurement Eligibility: Small Business
Distribution: Manufacturer Direct, Manufacturer Through Distributor, Manufacturer Through Manufacturer Reps, OEM, Exclusive Distributor, Exporter
General Admin.: Mr. David Butler/Chief Operating Officer, Chief Financial Officer
    Mr. Christopher Mitchell/Chief Scientific Officer
    Mr. James Walker/President, Chief Executive Officer
Production: Mr. Kuldip Ahluwalia/Vice President Manufacturing & Sales
    Mrs. Diane King/Vice President Regulatory Affairs
Research: Mr. Bjarne Christensen/Vice President Engineering

Densitometer, Bone, Single Photon	Radiology
Imager, X-Ray, Solid State (Flat Panel/Digital)	Radiology
Radiographic Unit, Diagnostic, Dental (X-Ray)	Dental And Oral
Radiographic Unit, Digital	Radiology

ALARIS MEDICAL SYSTEMS, INC
800-854-7128
10221 Wateridge Circle,
858-458-7000
San Diego, CA 92121
FDA Number: 9200561
    Fax: 858-458-7760
Web site: www.alarismed.com
Medical Products Sales Volume: $600,000
Annual Revenue: $500 Million-$1 Billion
Year Founded: 1967
Total Employees: 7   Marketing Staff: 40   Sales Staff: 300
Ownership: Private
Produces/Sells CE-marked Devices: N
Federal Procurement Eligibility: Small Business
Distribution: Exporter
General Admin.: Stuart Rickerson/Vice President, General Counsel
    Frederic Denerolle/Vice President, General Manager
    Jake Phillip/Vice President, General Manager
Production: Sally Grigoriev/Vice President Operations
    William Murphy/Vice President Quality Assurance
Finance: Rob Mathews/Vice President, Controller

System, Infusion, Administration, Drug, Implantable	General

ALARM ELECTRONICS MFG. CO. INC.
800-444-3365
44 All Healing Springs Rd.,
828-632-3365
Taylorsville, NC 28681
FDA Number: 1000384710
    Fax: 828-632-7382
E-mail: info1@alarmelectronics.com
Web site: www.alarmelectronics.com
Ownership: Private
Produces/Sells CE-marked Devices: N

Environmental Control System, Powered	Physical Med

ALASKA NATIVE TRIBAL HEALTH CONSORTIUM
855-882-6842
4000 Ambassador Drive, Anchorage, AK 99508
907-729-1900
FDA Number: 3003601651
    Fax: 907-729-1901
Web site: www.anthc.org
Ownership: Private
Produces/Sells CE-marked Devices: N
General Admin.: Mr. Andy Teuber/President, Chairman
    Ms. Emily Hughes/Secretary
    Ms. Evelyn Beeter/Vice Chairman
Finance: Mr. Charles Clement/Treasurer

Computer and Software, Medical	General
Image Processing System	Radiology

ALATECH HEALTHCARE, LLC.
334-886-9337
595 E.lawrence Harris Hwy., Slocomb, AL 36375
FDA Number: 2320742
Ownership: Private
Produces/Sells CE-marked Devices: N

Condom	Obstetrics/Gynecology

ALBA HEALTH CARE DIV.
See Albahealth Llc

ALBAHEALTH LLC
800-262-2404
425 N. Gateway Avenue, Rockwood, TN 37854
865-354-0410
FDA Number: 1043612
    Fax: 865-354-1541
E-mail: info@alba1.com
Web site: www.albahealth.com
Medical Products Sales Volume: $40,000,000
Annual Revenue: $25-$50 Million

ALBAHEALTH LLC   800-262-2404 *(cont'd)*

Year Founded: 1902
Total Employees: 250   Marketing Staff: 5   Sales Staff: 23
Ownership: Private
Produces/Sells CE-marked Devices: Y
Distribution: Manufacturer Through Distributor
General Admin.: William Ott/President
Mktg./Adv.: Jon Hermanson/Director Product Development
    Jennifer Woody/Market Manager
    Keith Fox/Vice President Natl Accounts & Sales
Production: Steve Anderson/Director Manufacturing & Operations
    Marty Davidson/Director Planning
    Kathy Griffin/Manager Quality Assurance & Regulatory Affairs
Finance: Ed Byrd/Controller
Purchasing: David Watts/Manager Purchasing

Bandage, Cast	Physical Med
Bandage, Elastic	General
Dressing, Non-Adherent	General
Dressing, Other	General
Pad, Pressure, Foam (Elbow, Heel)	General
Retainer, Bandage (Elastic Net)	General
Slippers	General
Stockinette	Orthopedics
Stockinette, Cast	Orthopedics
Stocking, Support (Anti-Embolic)	General

Medical Product Subsidiaries (Listed Separately)
Encompass Group, Llc

ALBERT INTERNATIONAL, INC.   800-789-0729

989 Athens Street S.e., Gainesville, GA 30501   **770-287-7424**
FDA Number: 1037752   Fax: 770-287-7525
Web site: www.albertinternational.net
Medical Products Sales Volume: $1,500,000
Annual Revenue: $1-$5 Million
Ownership: Hohlkoerper Gmbh & Co. Kg, Albert
Produces/Sells CE-marked Devices: N
Federal Procurement Eligibility: Small Business
Distribution: Manufacturer Direct, Manufacturer Through Manufacturer Reps

Aspirator, Nasal	Ear/Nose/Throat
Douche, Vaginal	Obstetrics/Gynecology
Inflator, Cuff	General
Pump, Alternating Pressure Pad	General
Pump, Breast, Non-Powered	Obstetrics/Gynecology
Spreader, Cuff	Anesthesiology
Suction Apparatus, Single Patient, Portable, Non-Powered	Surgery
Syringe, Bulb	General
Syringe, Ear	Ear/Nose/Throat
Syringe, Irrigating	General
Syringe, Other	General
Transfer Device, Patient, Manual	General

ALBUQUERQUE EYE PROSTHETICS, INC.   505-884-2927

4117 Montgomery N.e., Albuquerque, NM 87109
FDA Number: 1722825

Eye, Artificial, Non-Custom	Ophthalmology

ALC, INC.   262-502-4665

N114 W19049 Clinton Drive, Germantown, WI 53022
FDA Number: 2183636

Chair, Position, Electric	Physical Med
Scooter (Motorized 3-Wheeled Vehicle)	Physical Med

ALCERAM TECH INC   516-849-3666

57 2ND ST, Ronkonkoma, NY 11779-5352
FDA Number: n/a   Fax: 516-609-8328
E-mail: alceram@optonline.net
Web site: www.alceram.com
Annual Revenue: $5-$10 Million
Total Employees: 40   Marketing Staff: 2   Sales Staff: 3
Ownership: Private
Quality System Registration Information: ISO9001; ISO9002
Produces/Sells CE-marked Devices: Y
Federal Procurement Eligibility: Small Business
Distribution: Manufacturer Direct, OEM
General Admin.: Norman Nager/President, Chief Executive Officer

Component, Ceramic	General
Contract Manufacturing	General
Lens, Surgical, Laser	Ophthalmology
Post, Root Canal	Dental And Oral
Probe, Ophthalmic	Ophthalmology
Prosthesis, Hip, Semi-constrained, Metal/Ceramic/Ceramic/Metal, Cemented Or Uncemented	Orthopedics

ALCOHOL COUNTERMEASURE SYSTEMS CORP.   416-619-3500

60 International Boulevard, Toronto, ONTAR M9W 6J2 Canada
FDA Number: n/a   Fax: 416-619-3501
E-mail: info@acs-corp.com
Web site: www.acs-corp.com

ALCOHOL COUNTERMEASURE   416-619-3500 *(cont'd)*

Year Founded: 1976
Total Employees: 100
Ownership: Private
Produces/Sells CE-marked Devices: Y
Distribution: Manufacturer Direct, Manufacturer Through Distributor, Service Direct, Exporter

ALCOHOL COUNTERMEASURE SYSTEMS, INC.   303-366-5699

1670 Jasper St., Suite G, Aurora, CO 80011
FDA Number: 3003483691   Fax: 303-366-5996
E-mail: info@acs-corp.com
Web site: www.acs-corp.com
Annual Revenue: $0-$1 Million
Year Founded: 1976
Total Employees: 3   Marketing Staff: 1   Sales Staff: 3
Ownership: Alcohol Countermeasure Systems Corp.
Produces/Sells CE-marked Devices: Y
Federal Procurement Eligibility: Small Business, GSA Contract
Distribution: Manufacturer Direct, Manufacturer Through Distributor, Manufacturer Through Manufacturer Reps
General Admin.: Mr. Felix J.E. Comeau/Chief Executive Officer, Chairman
Production: Christopher Wilson/Director Medical Product Testing

Analyzer, Alcohol	Toxicology

ALCON CANADA, INC.   800-268-4574

2665 Meadowpine Blvd.,   **905-826-6700**
Mississauga, ONT L5N-8 Canada
FDA Number: n/a   Fax: 905-567-0592
E-mail: david.baldwin@alconlabs.com
Web site: www.alcon.ca
Year Founded: 1959
Total Employees: 200
Ownership: NESTLE SA
Quality System Registration Information: ISO9002
Produces/Sells CE-marked Devices: N
Distribution: Exclusive Distributor, Exporter

ALCON LABORATORIES INC./CONTACT LENS DIV

See Ciba Vision Corporation

ALCON LABORATORIES, INC.

See Alcon Research, Ltd.

ALCON MANUFACTURING, LTD.   949-753-1393

15800 Alton Parkway, Irvine, CA 92618
FDA Number: 2028159
Web site: www.alcon.com
Ownership: Alcon Research, Ltd.
Stock Symbol: ACL
Traded On: NYSE
Produces/Sells CE-marked Devices: N

Fiberoptic Light Source & Carrier	Ear/Nose/Throat
Laser, Surgical	Surgery

ALCON MANUFACTURING, LTD.   304-736-5230

6065 Kyle Lane, Huntington, WV 25702-9795
FDA Number: 1119421   Fax: 304-523-1323
Web site: www.alcon.com
Ownership: Alcon Research, Ltd.
Stock Symbol: ACL
Traded On: NYSE
Produces/Sells CE-marked Devices: N
Distribution: Manufacturer Direct
General Admin.: Harold Camp/General Manager
Purchasing: Larry Sumpter/Manager Purchasing

Guide, Intraocular Lens	Ophthalmology
Lens, Intraocular	Ophthalmology
Lens, Intraocular, Multifocal	Ophthalmology

ALCON MANUFACTURING, LTD.

See Alcon Manufacturing, Ltd.

ALCON MANUFACTURING, LTD.   713-668-9100

9965 Buffalo Speedway, Houston, TX 77054-1309
FDA Number: 1644019
Web site: www.alcon.com
Ownership: Alcon Research, Ltd.
Stock Symbol: ACL
Traded On: NYSE
Produces/Sells CE-marked Devices: N

Light, Surgical, Fiberoptic	Surgery
Phacofragmentation Unit	Ophthalmology

ALCON RESEARCH, LTD

See Alcon Manufacturing, Ltd.

ALCON RESEARCH, LTD

See Alcon Manufacturing, Ltd.

ALCON RESEARCH, LTD.
6201 South Fwy., Fort Worth, TX 76134-2001
800-862-5266
817-293-0450
FDA Number: 1610287
Fax: 800-241-0677
E-mail: mary.dulle@alconlabs.com
Web site: www.alconlabs.com
Year Founded: 1945
Total Employees: 15000   *Sales Staff:* 400
Ownership: Private
Stock Symbol: ACL
Traded On: NYSE
Quality System Registration Information: ISO9000
Produces/Sells CE-marked Devices: Y
Distribution: Manufacturer Direct, Manufacturer Through Distributor, Manufacturer Through Manufacturer Reps, Exporter
General Admin.: Allen Baker/Executive Vice President
　　　　Tim Sear/President, Chief Executive Officer
　　　　Jack Walters/Vice President Human Resources
　　　　Barry Caldwell/Vice President, General Manager
　　　　Blaise McGoey/Vice President, General Manager
Mktg./Adv.: Darryl Dubbs/Director Sales Training
　　　　Rick Johnson/Manager Market Research
　　　　Bill Barton/Vice President Marketing
　　　　Scott Manning/Vice President Marketing
　　　　Bill Weir/Vice President Sales
　　　　Norb Walter/Vice President Sales
Production: Andre Bens/Vice President Manufacturing
　　　　Merrill Barden/Vice President Materials & Development
　　　　Bill Lenzie/Vice President Quality Assurance
　　　　Bill Hubregs/Vice President Regulatory Affairs
Research: Gerald Cagle/Vice President Research & Development

Accessories, Solution, Lens, Contact	Ophthalmology
Case, Contact Lens	Ophthalmology
Cautery, Thermal, Battery-Powered	Ophthalmology
Cleaner, Lens, Contact	Ophthalmology
Cryosurgical Unit	Surgery
Cutter, Vitreous Infusion Suction	Ophthalmology
Drape, Patient, Ophthalmic	Ophthalmology
Drape, Surgical, Disposable	Surgery
Electrocautery Unit, Battery-Powered	Surgery
Extractor, Metal, Magnetic	Surgery
Fluid, Intraocular	Ophthalmology
Forceps, Ophthalmic	Ophthalmology
Gonioscope (Prism)	Ophthalmology
Knife, Scalpel	Surgery
Laser, Argon, Surgical	Surgery
Laser, Combination	General
Laser, Dye	General
Laser, Nd:YAG, Surgical	Surgery
Laser, Ophthalmic	Ophthalmology
Lens, Contact(rigid Gas Permeable)-extended Wear	Ophthalmology
Needle, Suture, Disposable	Surgery
Pack, Custom/Special Procedure	General
Phacoemulsification System	Ophthalmology
Regulator, Pressure, Gas Cylinder	Anesthesiology
Shield, Corneal, Collagen	Ophthalmology
Shield, Eye, Ophthalmic	Ophthalmology
Sterilizer, Soft Lens, Thermal, AC-Powered	Ophthalmology
Strip, Schirmer	Ophthalmology
Suture, Non-Absorbable, Synthetic, Polyamide	Surgery
Suture, Non-Absorbable, Synthetic, Polyester	Surgery
Suture, Silk	Surgery
Syringe, Piston	General
System, Laser, Excimer, Ophthalmic	Ophthalmology
Tray, Surgical	Surgery
Tray, Surgical Instrument	Surgery

Medical Product Subsidiaries (Listed Separately)
　Alcon Canada, Inc.
　Alcon Manufacturing, Ltd.

ALCON SURGICAL, BELLEVUE DIV.
See Alcon Research, Ltd.

ALCON SURGICAL, INC., HUNTINGTON DIV.
See Alcon Manufacturing, Ltd.

ALCOPRO
2547 Sutherland Ave., Knoxville, TN 37919
800-227-9890
865-525-4900
FDA Number: n/a
Fax: 865-525-4935
E-mail: alcopro@alcopro.com
Web site: www.alcopro.com
Medical Products Sales Volume: $2,000,000
Annual Revenue: $1-$5 Million
Year Founded: 1982
Ownership: Private
Produces/Sells CE-marked Devices: N
Federal Procurement Eligibility: Small Business
Distribution: Manufacturer Direct

Analyzer, Alcohol	Toxicology
System, Test, Drugs of Abuse	Chemistry

ALCOTT CHROMATOGRAPHY, INC.
See GP Instruments

ALDAGEN, INC
919-484-2571
2810 Meridian Parkway, Suite 148, Durham, NC 27713
FDA Number: 3003388296
Fax: 919-484-8792
E-mail: info@aldagen.com
Web site: www.aldagen.com
Ownership: Private
Produces/Sells CE-marked Devices: N

Counter, Cell	Microbiology
Counter, Cell, Differential Classifier, Automated	Hematology
Stimulator, Cranial, Magnetic Pulse (for Psychotherapy)	Cns/Neurology

ALDEN MEDICAL LLC
413-747-9717
360 Cold Spring Ave., West Springfield, MA 01089
FDA Number: 1221361
Fax: 413-747-9721
E-mail: info@aldenmedical.com
Ownership: Private
Produces/Sells CE-marked Devices: N

Calibrator, Secondary, Clinical Chemistry	Chemistry
Dialysate Delivery System, Central Multiple Patient	Gastroenterology/Urology
Dialyzer Reprocessing System	Gastroenterology/Urology
Medical Disinfectants/Cleaners for Instruments	General
Solution-Test, Standard-Conductivity, Dialysis	Gastroenterology/Urology
Sterilant, Medical Device	General
Sterilization Process Indicator, Physical/Chemical	General

ALDEN OPTICAL LABS, INC.
716-937-9181
13295 Broadway, Alden, NY 14004-1324
FDA Number: 1315522
Fax: 716-937-3303
E-mail: info@aldenoptical.com
Web site: www.aldenoptical.com
Annual Revenue: $0-$1 Million
Year Founded: 1969
Ownership: Private
Produces/Sells CE-marked Devices: N
Federal Procurement Eligibility: Small Business
Distribution: Manufacturer Direct

Lens, Contact (Other Material)	Ophthalmology
Lens, Contact, Polymethylmethacrylate, Diagnostic	Ophthalmology

ALDERON BIOSCIENCES, INC.
919-544-8220
2810 Meridian Pkwy, Suite 152, Durham, NC 27713
FDA Number: n/a
Fax: 919-544-9808
E-mail: info@alderonbiosciences.com
Web site: www.alderonbiosciences.com
Medical Products Sales Volume: $14,000,000
Annual Revenue: $0-$1 Million
Total Employees: 12
Ownership: Private
Produces/Sells CE-marked Devices: N
Federal Procurement Eligibility: Small Business
Distribution: Manufacturer Direct
General Admin.: Robert Henkens/President, Chief Executive Officer

Detector, Strain	General
Monitor, Biological (Contamination Testing)	General

ALERCHEK, INC.
877-282-9542
203 Anderson St., Portland, ME 04101
207-775-2574
FDA Number: 1221106
Fax: 207-775-0594
Web site: www.alerchek.com
Medical Products Sales Volume: $500,000
Annual Revenue: $0-$1 Million
Year Founded: 1986
Total Employees: 4   *Marketing Staff:* 1
Ownership: Private
Produces/Sells CE-marked Devices: N
Federal Procurement Eligibility: Small Business
Distribution: Manufacturer Through Distributor, OEM, Service Direct
General Admin.: Wayne M Henry/Chief Executive Officer

Antigen, Antiserum, Control, IGE	Immunology
FC, Rhodamine, Antigen, Antiserum, Control	Immunology
Test, Allergy	Immunology

ALERE MEDICAL, INC.
775-829-8885
595 Double Eagle Court, Suite 1000, Reno, NV 89521
FDA Number: 2953203
Fax: 775-829-8637
E-mail: sales@alere.com
Web site: www.alere.com
Medical Products Sales Volume: $45,500,000
Year Founded: 1996
Total Employees: 150
Ownership: Alere, Inc.
Produces/Sells CE-marked Devices: N
Federal Procurement Eligibility: Small Business
General Admin.: Dr. Ronald D. Geraty/Chief Executive Officer
　　　　Dr. Gordon K. Norman/Executive Vice President
　　　　Dr. Timothy J. Moore/Executive Vice President

ALERE MEDICAL, INC.   775-829-8885 *(cont'd)*
Mr. Douglas Albro/Executive Vice President
Mr. Jon E. Tropsa/Executive Vice President
Mktg./Adv.: Dale Kubasak/Senior Vice President Marketing & Sales
Production: Marti Benjamin/Vice President Operations
Finance: Wayne Krachun/Chief Financial Officer
  Monitor, Heart Rate, Other   Cardiovascular

ALERE, INC.   781-647-3900
51 Sawyer Road, Suite 200, Waltham, MA 02453
FDA Number: 1223440   *Fax:* 781-647-3939
Web site: www.invernessmedical.com
Annual Revenue: $100-$500 Million
Total Employees: 5153
Ownership: Public
Stock Symbol: IMA
Traded On: NYSE
Produces/Sells CE-marked Devices: Y
General Admin.: Mr. Ron Zwanziger/Chief Executive Officer, Chairman
             Dr. David Scott/Chief Scientific Officer
             Mr. Paul T. Hempel/Senior Vice President
Research: Dr. Jerry McAleer/Vice President Research & Development
Finance: David Teitel/Chief Financial Officer
             Mr. Jon Russell/Vice President Finance
Medical Product Subsidiaries (Listed Separately)
  Alere Medical, Inc.
  Biosite Incorporated
  Cholestech Corp.
  Diamics, Inc.
  Hemosense, Inc.
  Innovacon, Inc.
  Inverness Medical
  Inverness Medical Inc.
  Inverness Medical Innovations North America, Inc
  Inverness Medical Professional Diagnostics-San Die
  QUALITY ASSURED SERVICES DBA ALERE HOME MONITORING PRODUCTS
  Redwood Toxicology Laboratories, Inc.

ALERO, INC.   951-273-7890
1550 Consumer Circle, Corona, CA 92880
FDA Number: 2020201
Ownership: Private
Produces/Sells CE-marked Devices: N
  Circuit, Breathing (W Connector, Adapter, Y Piece)   Anesthesiology
  Laryngoscope, Rigid   Anesthesiology

ALERT CARE, INC.   800-826-7444
98 Main Street, #209, Tiburon, CA 49420   415-381-9009
FDA Number: 9002510   *Fax:* 415-381-9039
E-mail: support@alertcareinc.com
Web site: www.alertcareinc.com
Medical Products Sales Volume: $225,000
Annual Revenue: $0-$1 Million
Year Founded: 1984
Total Employees: 3   *Marketing Staff:* 1   *Sales Staff:* 2
Ownership: Private
Quality System Registration Information: ISO9000
Produces/Sells CE-marked Devices: Y
Federal Procurement Eligibility: Small Business
Distribution: Service Direct
General Admin.: Tom J. Cowley/President
Production: Brice Butler/Customer Service Representative
            Candace Cowley/Director Manufacturing & Quality Assurance
IS: John Cowley/Director Systems Integration
  Monitor, Bed Patient   General
  Slippers   General

ALERT-ALL CORP.   800-253-7825
164 Orlan Road, New Holland, PA 17557
FDA Number: n/a   *Fax:* 800-445-7253
E-mail: Sales@Alertall.com
Web site: www.alertall.com
Annual Revenue: $1-$5 Million
Year Founded: 1974
Ownership: Private
Produces/Sells CE-marked Devices: N
Federal Procurement Eligibility: Small Business
Distribution: Manufacturer Direct, Exclusive Distributor
  Training Aid   Orthopedics

ALEX ORTHOPEDIC, INC.   800-544-2539
PO Box 201442, Arlington, TX 76006-1442   972-641-9680
FDA Number: 1641302   *Fax:* 972-641-9681
E-mail: info@alexorthopedic.com
Web site: www.alexorthopedic.com
Medical Products Sales Volume: $1,500,000
Year Founded: 1986
Total Employees: 20

ALEX ORTHOPEDIC, INC.   800-544-2539 *(cont'd)*
Ownership: Private
Produces/Sells CE-marked Devices: N
Federal Procurement Eligibility: Small Business
Distribution: Manufacturer Through Distributor, Manufacturer Through Manufacturer Reps
General Admin.: Ebrahim Lavi/President, Chief Executive Officer
Mktg./Adv.: Linda Lavi/Vice President Marketing
            Janet Pederson/Vice President Sales

Attachment, Commode, Wheelchair	Physical Med
Bandage, Elastic	General
Bed, Adjustable Hospital	General
Belt, Rib (Support)	Orthopedics
Cane	Physical Med
Collar, Cervical Neck	Orthopedics
Crutch	Physical Med
Cushion, Other	General
Cushion, Wheelchair (Pad)	Physical Med
Pad, Pressure, Foam Convoluted	General
Pillow, Cervical	Orthopedics
Sling, Arm	Physical Med
Support, Ankle	Orthopedics
Support, Back	Orthopedics
Support, Knee	Physical Med
Support, Wrist	Physical Med
Wheelchair, Manual	Physical Med

ALEXANDRIA RESEARCH TECHNOLOGIES, LLC   952-949-2235
13755 First Avenue North, Suite 100, Plymouth, MN 55441
FDA Number: 3004594167
Ownership: Private
Produces/Sells CE-marked Devices: N
  Motor, Surgical Instrument, Pneumatic-Powered   Surgery
  Orthopedic Manual Surgical Instrument   Orthopedics
  Prosthesis, Knee, Femorotibial, Semi-Constrained   Orthopedics

ALFA AESAR JOHNSON MATTHEY
  See Alfa Aesar, A Johnson Matthey Company

ALFA AESAR, A JOHNSON MATTHEY COMPANY   800-343-0660
26 Parkridge Road, Ward Hill, MA 01835-8099   978-521-6300
FDA Number: 2543453   *Fax:* 978-521-6350
E-mail: info@alfa.com
Web site: www.alfa.com
Annual Revenue: $10-$25 Million
Year Founded: 1963
Total Employees: 110
Ownership: Johnson Matthey, Inc.
Quality System Registration Information: ISO9002
Produces/Sells CE-marked Devices: N
Federal Procurement Eligibility: Small Business
Distribution: Manufacturer Direct
General Admin.: Barry Singelais/Director, General Manager
Mktg./Adv.: John Shirley/Director Marketing & Sales
            Gwilym Clarke/Director Sales
  Loop, Inoculating   Microbiology
  Stirrer   Chemistry

ALFA IMPORT AND EXPORT   905-457-9941
13 Halldorson Trail, Brampton L6W 4M4 Canada
FDA Number: 9680628
  Lens, Spectacle/Eyeglasses, Non-Custom   Ophthalmology

ALFA LAVAL INC   866-253-2528
955 Mearns Road, Warminster, PA 18974-0556   215-443-4000
FDA Number: 7000334   *Fax:* 215-443-4234
E-mail: customerservice.usa@alfalaval.com
Web site: www.alfalaval.us
Annual Revenue: $100-$500 Million
Total Employees: 500   *Marketing Staff:* 20   *Sales Staff:* 20
Ownership: Public
Stock Symbol: ALFA
Traded On: Stockholm
Produces/Sells CE-marked Devices: N
Distribution: Manufacturer Direct
General Admin.: Alessandro Terenghi/President
Mktg./Adv.: Mr. Chip Bressette/Vice President Communications
            Mr. Brent Smith/Vice President, Manager Business
            Mr. John Atanasio/Vice President, Manager Business
            Mr. Michael Kahler/Vice President, Manager Business
  Centrifuge, Continuous Flow   Chemistry
  Centrifuge, Explosion-Proof   Chemistry
  Centrifuge, General (Up to 5,000 rpm)   Pathology
  Centrifuge, Refrigerated   Pathology
  Filter, Membrane   Chemistry

ALFA LAVAL INC.
866-253-2528
804-222-5300

5400 International Trade Drive,
Richmond, VA 23231
FDA Number: n/a
Fax: 804-236-3276
E-mail: customerservice.usa@alfalaval.com
Web site: www.alfalaval.us
Medical Products Sales Volume: $323,180,000
Year Founded: 1997
Total Employees: 632
Ownership: Public
Traded On: Stockholm
Quality System Registration Information: ISO9000; ISO9001
Produces/Sells CE-marked Devices: N
Distribution: Manufacturer Through Distributor, Manufacturer Through Manufacturer Reps, OEM, Exclusive Distributor
General Admin.: Kirk Spitzer/President

Blender/Mixer	Chemistry

ALFA MEDICAL EQUIPMENT
800-801-9934
516-489-3855

59 Madison Avenue, Hempstead, NY 11550
FDA Number: 2436866
Fax: 516-489-9364
E-mail: email@sterilizers.com
Web site: www.sterilizers.com
Medical Products Sales Volume: $5,000,000
Annual Revenue: $1-$5 Million
Year Founded: 1987
Total Employees: 26   *Marketing Staff:* 3   *Sales Staff:* 3
Ownership: Private
Produces/Sells CE-marked Devices: N
Federal Procurement Eligibility: Small Business
Distribution: Manufacturer Direct, Manufacturer Through Distributor, Manufacturer Through Manufacturer Reps, Exclusive Distributor, Exporter
General Admin.: Shlomo Savyon/President
   Chuck Fishelson/Vice President, General Manager

Sterilizer, Steam (Autoclave), Dental	Dental And Oral

ALFA SCIENTIFIC DESIGNS, INC.
877-204-5071
858-513-3888

13200 Gregg Street, Poway, CA 92064
FDA Number: 2060833
Fax: 858-513-8388
E-mail: sales@alfascientific.com
Web site: www.alfascientific.com
Annual Revenue: $1-$5 Million
Year Founded: 1996
Total Employees: 50   *Marketing Staff:* 1   *Sales Staff:* 3
Ownership: Private
Quality System Registration Information: ISO9001
Produces/Sells CE-marked Devices: Y
Federal Procurement Eligibility: Small Business, Minority Owned, Female Owned
Distribution: Manufacturer Through Distributor, Manufacturer Through Manufacturer Reps, OEM, Exclusive Distributor, Exporter
General Admin.: Dr. Chai Bunyagidj/Chief Operating Officer
   Dr. Naishu Wang/President, Chief Executive Officer
   Mr. Jim McMenemy/Vice President
Production: Ms. Sun Dugan/Director Quality Assurance & Regulatory Affairs

Antigen, Prostate-Specific (PSA), Management, Cancer	Immunology
Campylobacter Pylori	Microbiology
Enzyme Immunoassay, Amphetamine	Toxicology
Enzyme Immunoassay, Cannabinoids	Toxicology
Enzyme Immunoassay, Cocaine And Cocaine Metabolites	Toxicology
Enzyme Immunoassay, Opiates	Toxicology
Radioimmunoassay, Human Chorionic Gonadotropin	Chemistry
Radioimmunoassay, Luteinizing Hormone	Chemistry

ALFA WASSERMANN, INC.
800-220-4488
973-882-8630

4 Henderson Drive, West Caldwell, NJ 07006
FDA Number: 2247288
Fax: 973-276-0383
E-mail: info@alfawassermannus.com
Web site: www.alfawassermannus.com
Medical Products Sales Volume: $27,000,000
Year Founded: 1960
Total Employees: 160   *Marketing Staff:* 3   *Sales Staff:* 15
Ownership: ALFA WASSERMAN GROUP, MILAN
Quality System Registration Information: ISO9001
Produces/Sells CE-marked Devices: Y
Federal Procurement Eligibility: Small Business
Distribution: Manufacturer Direct, Manufacturer Through Distributor, OEM, Importer, Exporter
General Admin.: Ira Nordlicht/Chief Executive Officer
   Adrienne Choma/Chief Operating Officer
   Barbara Burkepile/Director Human Resources
Mktg./Adv.: Frank West/Manager National Sales
   Carol Pino/Vice President International Marketing
Production: Wilhelm Wang/Director Quality Assurance & Regulatory Affairs
   Dennis Gershowitz/Director Services
   Patrick Livesey/Manager Materials
Finance: Joseph Vaughn/Vice President Finance

Analyzer, Chemistry, Electrolyte	Chemistry

ALFA WASSERMANN, INC.
800-220-4488 *(cont'd)*

Analyzer, Chemistry, Multi-Channel, Programmable	Chemistry
Analyzer, Chemistry, Photometric, Discrete	Chemistry
Electrode, Ion Specific, Sodium	Chemistry
Enzyme Immunoassay, Digoxin	Toxicology
Multi Analyte Mixture, Calibrator	Chemistry
Reagent, General Purpose	Pathology

ALFA-LAVAL SHARPLES
See Alfa Laval Inc

ALFRED UEDA
307-789-2088

145 Uplands Cir., Corte Madera, CA 94925
FDA Number: 2954924
Ownership: Private
Produces/Sells CE-marked Devices: N

Plunger-Like Joint Manipulator	Physical Med

ALGEN SCALE CORP.
800-836-8445
631-342-1975

68 Enter Lane, Islandia, NY 11749
FDA Number: 9200261
Fax: 631-342-1977
E-mail: info@algen.com
Web site: www.algen.com
Medical Products Sales Volume: $820,000
Annual Revenue: $0-$1 Million
Year Founded: 1984
Total Employees: 6   *Marketing Staff:* 3   *Sales Staff:* 3
Ownership: Private
Quality System Registration Information: ISO9000
Federal Procurement Eligibility: Small Business
Distribution: Manufacturer Direct, Manufacturer Through Distributor, Service Direct, Exclusive Distributor, Exporter
General Admin.: Irving Aigen/Chief Executive Officer
   Randall Aigen/President
   Jeffrey Aigen/Vice President

Balance, Electronic	Chemistry
Balance, Mechanical	Chemistry
Scale, Autopsy	Pathology
Scale, Chair	General
Scale, Infant	General
Scale, Laboratory	Chemistry
Scale, Platform, Wheelchair	Physical Med
Scale, Stand-On	General

ALGER EQUIPMENT COMPANY, INC.
800-320-1043
512-267-0383

320 Flightline, Lago Vista, TX 78645
FDA Number: 1625370
Fax: 512-267-0452
E-mail: jdalger@algercompany.com
Web site: www.algercompany.com
Medical Products Sales Volume: $100,000
Annual Revenue: $0-$1 Million
Year Founded: 1967
Total Employees: 3   *Marketing Staff:* 2   *Sales Staff:* 2
Ownership: Private
Quality System Registration Information: ISO9001
Produces/Sells CE-marked Devices: N
Federal Procurement Eligibility: Small Business
Distribution: Manufacturer Direct, OEM
General Admin.: John Alger/Chief Operating Officer
   David W. Alger/President, Chief Executive Officer

Brush, Ophthalmic	Ophthalmology

ALGOR, INC.
800-48-ALGOR
412-967-2700

150 Beta Dr., Pittsburgh, PA 15238-2932
FDA Number: n/a
Fax: 412-967-2781
E-mail: info.algor@autodesk.com
Web site: www.algor.com
Ownership: Autodesk, Inc.
Quality System Registration Information: ISO9001
Produces/Sells CE-marked Devices: N
Federal Procurement Eligibility: Small Business
Distribution: Manufacturer Direct

Computer Software	General

ALGOTEK INSTRUMENTS, INC.
See Natus Medical Inc.

ALICIA DIAGNOSTICS, INC.
407-365-8498

1274 Alafaya Trail, Oviedo, FL 32765
FDA Number: n/a
Fax: 407-366-9876
E-mail: info@aliciadiagnostics.com
Web site: http://aliciadiagnostics.com
Annual Revenue: $25-$50 Million
Ownership: Private
Quality System Registration Information: ISO9003
Produces/Sells CE-marked Devices: N
Distribution: Manufacturer Direct, Manufacturer Through Distributor, OEM, Importer, Exporter

Counter, Cell Or Particle, Automated	Hematology

ALICIA DIAGNOSTICS, INC. 407-365-8498 *(cont'd)*
Counter, Cell, Differential Classifier, Automated — Hematology

ALIGN PHARMACEUTICALS 908-834-0960
200 Connell Drive, Suite 1500, Berkeley Heights, NJ 07922
FDA Number: 3005755624 *Fax:* 866-725-4464
E-mail: info@alignpharma.com
Web site: www.alignpharma.com
Ownership: Private
Stock Symbol: ALGN
Traded On: NASDAQ
Produces/Sells CE-marked Devices: N

ALIGN TECHNOLOGY
See Align Technology, Inc.

ALIGN TECHNOLOGY, INC. 408-470-1000
2560 orchard parkway, san jose, CA 95131
FDA Number: 2953749 *Fax:* 408-470-1010
Web site: www.aligntech.com
Year Founded: 1997
Ownership: Public
Stock Symbol: ALGN
Traded On: NASDAQ
Produces/Sells CE-marked Devices: N
General Admin.: David E Collins/Director
    George J Morrow/Director
    Greg J Santora/Director
    Joseph Lacob/Director
    Thomas M Prescott/President, Chief Executive Officer

Adhesive, Bracket And Conditioner, Resin	Dental And Oral
Aligner, Sequential	Dental And Oral
Band, Elastic, Orthodontic	Dental And Oral
Bracket, Plastic, Orthodontic	Dental And Oral
Burr, Dental	Dental And Oral
Cleaner, Denture	Dental And Oral
Cleaner, Denture, Mechanical	Dental And Oral
Disk, Abrasive	Dental And Oral
Drill, Dental, Intraoral	Dental And Oral
Gauge, Depth, Instrument, Dental	Dental And Oral
Instrument, Diamond, Dental	Dental And Oral
Maintainer, Space Preformed, Orthodontic	Dental And Oral
Material, Impression	Dental And Oral
Pliers, Orthodontic	Dental And Oral
Point, Abrasive	Dental And Oral
Positioner, Tooth, Preformed	Dental And Oral
Strip, Polishing Agent	Dental And Oral
Tray, Impression	Dental And Oral
Wheel, Polishing Agent	Dental And Oral

ALIMED, INC. 800-225-2610
297 High St., Dedham, MA 02026-2844 781-329-2900
FDA Number: 1218386 *Fax:* 781-329-8392
E-mail: info@alimed.com
Web site: www.alimed.com
Annual Revenue: $50-$100 Million
Year Founded: 1970
Total Employees: 180 *Marketing Staff:* 9 *Sales Staff:* 3
Ownership: Private
Produces/Sells CE-marked Devices: Y
Federal Procurement Eligibility: Small Business
Distribution: Manufacturer Direct, Manufacturer Through Distributor, Manufacturer Through Manufacturer Reps, OEM, Importer, Exporter
General Admin.: Julian H. Cherubini/President, Chief Executive Officer, Chief Financial Officer
    Jonathan Bretz/Senior Vice President
    Richard Clement/Vice President, General Manager
Mktg./Adv.: Philip Dominici/Director Marketing
    Steve Austin/Director National Accounts
Production: Jonathan Bretz/Manager Regulatory Affairs

Accessories, Cart, Multipurpose	General
Accessories, Operating Room, Table	Surgery
Accessories, Walker	General
Accessories, Wheelchair	Physical Med
Anatomical Training Model	General
Apron, Laboratory	Chemistry
Apron, Lead, Radiographic	Radiology
Apron, Surgical	Surgery
Arm Rest	Physical Med
Armrest, Wheelchair	Physical Med
Attachment, Narrowing, Wheelchair	Physical Med
Bag, Breathing	Anesthesiology
Bandage, Elastic	General
Barrier, Control Panel, X-Ray, Moveable	Radiology
Bars, Parallel, Exercise	Physical Med
Bars, Parallel, Powered	Physical Med
Bars, Parallel, Walking	Physical Med
Basin, Emesis	General
Basin, Wash	General
Bassinet (Infant Bed)	General

ALIMED, INC. 800-225-2610 *(cont'd)*

Bath, Hydro-Massage (Whirlpool)	Physical Med
Bath, Paraffin	Physical Med
Bed, Obese	General
Bedrail	General
Belt, Abdominal	Gastroenterology/Urology
Belt, Support, Pelvic	Physical Med
Belt, Wheelchair	Physical Med
Binder, Chest	General
Board, Arm	Anesthesiology
Brace, Joint, Ankle (External)	Physical Med
Brake, Extension, Wheelchair	Physical Med
Brush, Scrub, Operating Room	Surgery
Cabinet, Instrument	General
Cabinet, Table And Tray, Anesthesia	Anesthesiology
Caliper	Orthopedics
Caliper, Skinfold	General
Cane	Physical Med
Cannula, Arterial	Cardiovascular
Cart, Gas Cylinder (Carrier)	Anesthesiology
Cart, Instrument	Surgery
Cart, Laundry	General
Cart, Supply	General
Chair, Shower	General
Chair, Surgical, Non-Electrical	Surgery
Chart, Anatomical Training	General
Coat, Laboratory	General
Collar, Cervical Neck	Orthopedics
Commode Seat	General
Compression Instrument	Orthopedics
Container, Sterilization (Tray)	General
Contract Manufacturing, Product, Durable	General
Counter, Radiation	Radiology
Cover, Barrier, Protective	General
Cover, Camera	Surgery
Cover, Cast	General
Cover, Film, X-Ray	Radiology
Crutch	Physical Med
Cuff, Blood Pressure	Cardiovascular
Cuff, Pusher, Wheelchair	Physical Med
Cushion, Foot	Orthopedics
Cushion, Ring, Inflatable	General
Cushion, Wheelchair (Pad)	Physical Med
Cutter, Cast	Orthopedics
Cutter, Cast, AC-Powered	Orthopedics
Densitometer	Cardiovascular
Densitometer, Radiographic	Radiology
Densitometer, Radiography, Digital, Quantitative	Radiology
Device, Anti-Tip, Wheelchair	Physical Med
Dressing, Gel	General
Dynamometer, Grip-Strength (Squeeze)	Anesthesiology
Elastomer, Silicone Rubber	General
Electrode, Gel	Cardiovascular
Electrode, TENS	Cns/Neurology
Envelope, Film, X-Ray	Radiology
Equipment, Traction, Powered	Physical Med
Exercise Stair	Physical Med
Exerciser, Bicycle	Physical Med
Exerciser, Chest	Physical Med
Exerciser, Hand	Physical Med
Exerciser, Leg And Ankle	Physical Med
Exerciser, Shoulder	Physical Med
Exerciser, Wrist	Physical Med
Eyeglasses, Safety	Ophthalmology
File, Callous	Surgery
Filter, Radiographic	Radiology
Finger Cot	General
Floor Mat	General
Footrest, Wheelchair	Physical Med
Gel, Electrode, Stimulator	Cns/Neurology
Gel, Ultrasonic Transmission	General
Glove, Patient Examination, Latex	General
Glove, Patient Examination, Vinyl	General
Glove, Utility	General
Goggles, Protective, Eye	Ophthalmology
Goniometer, Mechanical	Physical Med
Goniometer, Non-Powered	Orthopedics
Goniometer, Orthopedic	Orthopedics
Grid, Radiographic	Radiology
Halter, Head, Traction	Physical Med
Halter, Head, Traction, Orthopedic	Orthopedics
Holder, Head, Radiographic	Radiology
Holder, Leg, Arthroscopy	Orthopedics
Holder, Medical Chart	General
Illuminator, Radiographic Film	Radiology
Image Processing System	Radiology
Immobilizer, Ankle	Orthopedics
Immobilizer, Elbow	Orthopedics
Immobilizer, Knee	Orthopedics
Immobilizer, Shoulder	Orthopedics
Immobilizer, Upper Body	Orthopedics
Immobilizer, Wrist/Hand	Orthopedics

MANUFACTURER PROFILES

ALIMED, INC.   800-225-2610 *(cont'd)*

Infusion Stand	General
Insoles, Medical	General
Joint, Hip, External Brace	Physical Med
Lancet, Blood	General
Laryngoscope	Ear/Nose/Throat
Laundry Hamper	General
Legging, Compression, Non-Inflatable	General
Lift, Patient	General
Liner, Glove	General
Lotion, Skin Care	General
Loupe, Binocular, Low Power	Ophthalmology
Magnifier, Operating	Surgery
Mask, Face	General
Massager, Therapeutic	Physical Med
Mattress, Bed	General
Media, Gastroenterographic Contrast (Barium Sulfate)	Radiology
Meter, Patient Height	General
Mirror, Laryngeal	Ear/Nose/Throat
Mirror, Posture	Physical Med
Mirror, Speech	Ear/Nose/Throat
Orthosis, Corrective Shoe	Physical Med
Orthosis, Limb Brace	Physical Med
Orthosis, Lumbar	Physical Med
Otoscope	Ear/Nose/Throat
Pack, Cold	General
Pad, Pressure, Foam (Elbow, Heel)	General
Pad, Pressure, Gel, Operating Table	General
Padding, Cast/Splint	General
Paper, Chart, Record, Medical	General
Patient Transfer Unit	General
Pillow	General
Positioner, Socket	Orthopedics
Positioner, Spine, Surgical	Orthopedics
Protector, Finger	Orthopedics
Protector, Heel	General
Pump, Inflator	General
Rack, Glove, Operating Room	Surgery
Rail, Bath	General
Rail, Commode	General
Ramp, Wheelchair	General
Restraint, Patient, Conductive	Anesthesiology
Restraint, Protective (Body)	General
Restraint, Wheelchair	General
Rowing Unit	Physical Med
Sand Bag	Radiology
Scale, Infant	General
Scale, Laboratory	Chemistry
Scale, Platform, Wheelchair	Physical Med
Scale, Stand-On	General
Scissors, Bandage/Gauze/Plaster	General
Screen, Anesthesia	Anesthesiology
Separator, Toe	Orthopedics
Shield, Breast	Obstetrics/Gynecology
Shield, Eye, Ophthalmic	Ophthalmology
Shield, Syringe	General
Shoe, Cast	Physical Med
Shoe, Orthopedic	Orthopedics
Sleeve, Compressible Limb	Cardiovascular
Sling, Arm	Physical Med
Soap	General
Sock, Stump Cover	General
Sphygmomanometer, Aneroid (Arterial Pressure)	General
Splint, Abduction, Congenital Hip Dislocation	Physical Med
Splint, Abduction, Shoulder	Orthopedics
Splint, Extremity, Inflatable, External	Surgery
Splint, Hand, And Component	Physical Med
Splint, Temporary Training	Physical Med
Spreader, Plaster (Cast)	Orthopedics
Stand, Operating Room Instrument (Mayo)	Surgery
Stimulator, Muscle, Diagnostic	Physical Med
Storage Unit, X-Ray Film	Radiology
Strap, Clavicle	Orthopedics
Strap, Restraining	General
Stretcher, Wheeled (Mobile)	General
Support, Abdominal	Physical Med
Support, Ankle	Orthopedics
Support, Arch	Physical Med
Support, Arm	Physical Med
Support, Back	Orthopedics
Support, Elbow	Orthopedics
Support, Foot	Orthopedics
Support, Hand	Orthopedics
Support, Head And Trunk, Wheelchair	Physical Med
Support, Knee	Physical Med
Support, Leg	Physical Med
Support, Patient Position	Anesthesiology
Support, Patient Position, Radiographic	Radiology
Support, Wrist	Physical Med
Table, Examination/Treatment	General
Table, Instrument, Surgical	Surgery
Table, Overbed	General

ALIMED, INC.   800-225-2610 *(cont'd)*

Table, Traction	Orthopedics
Thermometer, Electronic	General
Tie Gun, Dialysis	Gastroenterology/Urology
Tip, Enema	General
Tips And Pads, Cane, Crutch And Walker	Physical Med
Tourniquet	General
Towel/Towelette, Paper	General
Traction Unit, Powered, Mobile	Orthopedics
Traction Unit, Static, Bed	Orthopedics
Transfer Aid	Physical Med
Transfer Device, Patient, Manual	General
Tray, Sterilization, Instrument	Surgery
Tray, Wheelchair	Physical Med
Treadmill, Powered	Physical Med
Utensil, Handicapped Aid	Physical Med
Vibrator, Battery-Powered	Physical Med
Volumeter	Chemistry
Warmer, Blanket	General
Waste Receptacle, Kick Bucket	General

ALIVIO CORPORATION   231-275-1345
20429 Honor Hwy., Interlochen, MI 49643
FDA Number: 3004976979
Ownership: Private
Produces/Sells CE-marked Devices: N

Stimulator, Nerve, Transcutaneous (Pain Relief, TENS)	Cns/Neurology
Stimulator, Neuromuscular, External Functional	Cns/Neurology

ALKALINE CORP.   732-531-7830
20 Meridian Road #9, Eatontown, NJ 07724
FDA Number: 2248704   *Fax:* 732-531-7830
E-mail: alkaline@allergyhelp.com
Web site: www.allergyhelp.com
Medical Products Sales Volume: $4,500,000
Annual Revenue: $1-$5 Million
Total Employees: 18   *Marketing Staff:* 7   *Sales Staff:* 7
Ownership: Private
Quality System Registration Information: ISO9002
Produces/Sells CE-marked Devices: Y
Federal Procurement Eligibility: Small Business, Minority Owned
Distribution: Manufacturer Direct
General Admin.: Isidore Bale/President

Delivery System, Allergen And Vaccine	General

ALKCO LIGHTING CO.   847-451-0700
11500 W. Melrose Avenue, Franklin Park, IL 60131-8139
FDA Number: n/a   *Fax:* 847-451-7512
E-mail: jferinga@alkco-lighting.com
Web site: www.alkco.com
Annual Revenue: $10-$25 Million
Year Founded: 1946
Total Employees: 125   *Marketing Staff:* 1   *Sales Staff:* 5
Ownership: Jji Lighting Group
Produces/Sells CE-marked Devices: N
Federal Procurement Eligibility: Small Business
Distribution: Manufacturer Through Distributor
Mktg./Adv.: Mr. Jim Feringa/Sales Specialist
         Ms. Gedra Mereckis/Vice President Sales
Finance: John Wolf/Vice President Finance & Operations

Illuminator, Radiographic Film	Radiology
Lamp, Surgical	Surgery
Light, Other	General
Light, Overbed	General
Light, Surgical, Ceiling Mounted	Surgery

ALKCO MANUFACTURING CO.
See Alkco Lighting Co.

ALKO DIAGNOSTIC CORPORATION
See Thermo Fisher Scientific Inc.

ALL AMERICAN MOLD LABORATORIES, INC.   800-654-3245
                                   405-677-2700
**2120 South Prospect Ave.,
Oklahoma City, OK 73129**
FDA Number: 1625405   *Fax:* 405-677-3900
E-mail: info@allamericanmold.com
Web site: www.allamericanmold.com
Ownership: Private
Produces/Sells CE-marked Devices: N

Hearing-Aid	Ear/Nose/Throat
Kit, Earmold Impression	Ear/Nose/Throat

ALL PRO EXERCISE PRODUCTS, INC.   800-735-9287
PO BOX 8268, Longboat Key, FL 34228
FDA Number: n/a   *Fax:* 941-387-7901
E-mail: support@allproweights.com
Web site: www.allproweights.com
Ownership: Private
Produces/Sells CE-marked Devices: N

Belt, Abdominal	Gastroenterology/Urology

ALL PRO EXERCISE PRODUCTS, INC.   800-735-9287 *(cont'd)*

Component, Exercise	Physical Med
Exerciser, Arm	Physical Med
Exerciser, Chest	Physical Med
Exerciser, Hand	Physical Med
Exerciser, Leg And Ankle	Physical Med
Exerciser, Other	Physical Med
Exerciser, Shoulder	Physical Med
Exerciser, Wrist	Physical Med

ALL STAR ORTHODONTICS, LLC   866-314-0804
4570 Progress Dr., Columbus, IN 47201   **812-314-0804**
FDA Number: 3004182778   *Fax: 812-314-0805*
E-mail: JeffF@AllStarOrthodontics.com
Web site: www.allstarorthodontics.com
Ownership: Private
Produces/Sells CE-marked Devices: N

Adhesive, Bracket And Conditioner, Resin	Dental And Oral
Band, Elastic, Orthodontic	Dental And Oral
Catheter, Intravascular, Therapeutic, Short-term Less Than 30 Days	General
Retainer, Screw Expansion, Orthodontic	Dental And Oral
Wire, Orthodontic	Dental And Oral

ALL-CRAFT WELLMAN PRODUCTS, INC.   800-340-3899
4839 E. 345th St., Willoughby, OH 44094-4606   **440-946-9646**
FDA Number: 1528078   *Fax: 440-946-9648*
E-mail: info@all-craftwellman.com
Web site: www.all-craftwellman.com
Medical Products Sales Volume: $500,000
Annual Revenue: $0-$1 Million
Year Founded: 1948
Total Employees: 15   *Marketing Staff: 1*   *Sales Staff: 1*
Ownership: Private
Produces/Sells CE-marked Devices: N
Federal Procurement Eligibility: Small Business
Distribution: Manufacturer Through Distributor, Manufacturer Through Manufacturer Reps
General Admin.: Gil Wellman/President, Chief Executive Officer
Mktg./Adv.: Gil Wellman/Manager Sales
Production: Ms. Sally Lebowitz/Customer Service Representative

Marker, X-Ray	Radiology

ALL-TRONICS MEDICAL SYSTEMS   800-ALL-TRON
3289 E. 55th St., Cleveland, OH 44127-1501   **216-429-3000**
FDA Number: n/a   *Fax: 216-429-3004*
E-mail: denalthar@aol.com
Web site: http://all-tronics.net
Annual Revenue: $1-$5 Million
Year Founded: 1975
Total Employees: 20   *Marketing Staff: 2*   *Sales Staff: 3*
Ownership: Private
Produces/Sells CE-marked Devices: N
Federal Procurement Eligibility: Small Business
Distribution: Manufacturer Direct, Manufacturer Through Distributor, OEM, Exporter
General Admin.: Dennis Althar/President

Recorder, Videotape/Videodisc	General
Transmitter, Image & Data, Radiographic	Radiology

ALLDENTE INTL., INC.   416-944-0086
600-94 Cumberland St, Toronto M5R 1A3 Canada
FDA Number: 9681438

Cleaner, Denture, Mechanical	Dental And Oral

ALLEGHENY PLASTICS, INC.   800-933-4123
1224 Freedom Rd.,   **724-776-0100**
Cranberry Township, PA 16066
FDA Number: 2522800   *Fax: 724-776-2909*
Web site: www.printedplastics.com
Ownership: Private
Produces/Sells CE-marked Devices: N

Chart, Visual Acuity	Ophthalmology
Rack, Skiascopic	Ophthalmology

ALLEGIANCE GROUP, INC.   805-569-1694
4025 Lago Dr., Santa Barbara, CA 93110
FDA Number: 2029187
Ownership: Private
Produces/Sells CE-marked Devices: N

Fixation Device, Tracheal Tube	Anesthesiology

ALLEGIANCE HEALTHCARE CANADA INC.
See Cardinal Health

ALLEGRO BIODIESEL CORPORATION   800-949-4762
6245 Bristol Parkway, Suite 263,   **310-670-2093**
Culver City, CA 90230
FDA Number: 2183953
E-mail: info@allegrobio.com   *Fax: 310-670-4107*

ALLEGRO BIODIESEL CORPORATION   800-949-4762 *(cont'd)*
Web site: www.allegrobiodiesel.com
Medical Products Sales Volume: $1,800,000
Annual Revenue: $1-$5 Million
Year Founded: 1990
Total Employees: 14   *Marketing Staff: 2*
Ownership: Public
Stock Symbol: ABDS
Traded On: OTC Bulletin
Quality System Registration Information: ISO9001
Produces/Sells CE-marked Devices: Y
Federal Procurement Eligibility: Small Business, GSA Contract
Distribution: Exclusive Distributor
Finance: Larry Betterley/Chief Financial Officer

Analyzer, Blood Gas pH	Anesthesiology
Monitor, Blood Gas, Real-Time	Cardiovascular
Monitor, Oxygen, Brain	Cns/Neurology

ALLEN CODING
See Thermo Fisher Scientific - Checkweighing, Metal And X-Ray Detection

ALLEN DATAGRAPH SYSTEMS, INC.   800-258-6360
56 Kendall Pond Road, Derry, NH 03038   **603-216-6344**
FDA Number: n/a   *Fax: 603-216-6345*
E-mail: info@allendatagraph.com
Web site: www.allendatagraph.com
Medical Products Sales Volume: $4,000,000
Annual Revenue: $1-$5 Million
Year Founded: 1980
Total Employees: 31   *Marketing Staff: 2*   *Sales Staff: 3*
Ownership: Private
Produces/Sells CE-marked Devices: N
Federal Procurement Eligibility: Small Business, Female Owned
Distribution: Manufacturer Direct, Manufacturer Through Distributor, OEM, Exporter
General Admin.: Michael Elliott/President, Chief Executive Officer
Mktg./Adv.: Michael Elliot/Coord. Marketing & Sales
     Debby Elliott/Director Marketing
     Tim Croker/Vice President Sales

Printer, Image, Video	General
Recorder, Chart, Laboratory	Chemistry

ALLEN MEDICAL INSTRUMENTS CORP.   949-646-3215
177 Riverside Avenue, Suite F - 602,
Newport Beach, CA 92663
FDA Number: 2020479   *Fax: 949-646-5908*
E-mail: allenmedical@yahoo.com
Web site: www.allenstethoscopes.com
Medical Products Sales Volume: $400,000
Year Founded: 1960
Total Employees: 3   *Marketing Staff: 1*   *Sales Staff: 1*
Ownership: Private
Produces/Sells CE-marked Devices: N
Federal Procurement Eligibility: Small Business, Female Owned
Distribution: Manufacturer Direct, Manufacturer Through Distributor, Exporter
General Admin.: Judith Allen/General Manager
     Derek R. Allen/President, Chief Executive Officer

Amnioscope, Transabdominal (Fetoscope)	Obstetrics/Gynecology
Stethoscope, Fetal	Obstetrics/Gynecology
Stethoscope, Mechanical	General

ALLEN MEDICAL SYSTEMS, INC.   800-433-5774
1 Post Office Square, Acton, MA 01720   **978-263-5401**
FDA Number: 1221538   *Fax: 978-263-8846*
E-mail: customerservice@allenmedical.com
Web site: www.allenmedical.com
Ownership: Hill-Rom Holdings, Inc.
Produces/Sells CE-marked Devices: Y
Distribution: Manufacturer Direct, Manufacturer Through Manufacturer Reps, OEM, Exporter
Mktg./Adv.: Mr. Fred Newey/Director Business Development
     Ms. Erin Herbst/Director Marketing
     Mr. Tom Skripps/Director New Product Development
     Mr. Mark Cole/Director Sales
Production: Mr. Bill McGowan/Director Manufacturing & Operations

Accessories, Cardiopulmonary Bypass	Cardiovascular
Accessories, Cart, Multipurpose	General
Accessories, Fixation, Orthopedic	Orthopedics
Accessories, Operating Room, Table	Surgery
Collector, Urine	Gastroenterology/Urology
Gel, Support	Immunology
Infusion Stand	General
Patient Transfer Unit	General
Positioner, Socket	Orthopedics
Positioner, Spine, Surgical	Orthopedics
Protector, Skin Pressure	General
Stirrup	Gastroenterology/Urology
Support, Patient Position	Anesthesiology

ALLEN MEDICAL SYSTEMS, INC.   **800-433-5774** *(cont'd)*
Traction Unit, Non-Powered   Orthopedics

ALLEN MEDICAL SYSTEMS, INC.
See Taga Medical Technologies

ALLERDERM LABORATORIES, INC.   **800-365-6868**
3400 E. McDowell Rd., Phoenix, AZ 85008
FDA Number: 2918720
E-mail: info@allerderm.com   *Fax:* 800-926-4568
Web site: www.allerderm.com
Annual Revenue: $5-$10 Million
Year Founded: 1979
Ownership: Private
Produces/Sells CE-marked Devices: N
Federal Procurement Eligibility: Small Business
Distribution: Manufacturer Direct, Exclusive Distributor, Importer, Exporter
   Dressing, Gel   General
   Elastomer, Silicone (Scar Management)   Surgery
   Glove, Other   General
   Glove, Patient Examination   General
   Glove, Patient Examination, Vinyl   General
   Liner, Glove   General
   Lotion, Skin Care   General
   Silicone Sheeting   General
   Sock, Protective, Skin   General
   Tape, Adhesive, Hypoallergenic   General
   Test, Allergy   Immunology

ALLERGAN   **800-366-6554**
2525 Dupont Dr., Irvine, CA 92623   **949-752-4500**
FDA Number: 2011068   *Fax:* 714-246-4214
Web site: www.Allergan.com
Medical Products Sales Volume: $55,000,000
Total Employees: 4700   *Marketing Staff:* 274   *Sales Staff:* 813
Ownership: Public
Stock Symbol: AGN
Traded On: NYSE
Quality System Registration Information: ISO9000
Produces/Sells CE-marked Devices: N
Distribution: Manufacturer Direct, Manufacturer Through Manufacturer Reps
General Admin.: Mr. David Pyott/Chairman, Chief Executive Officer
      Ms. F. Michael Ball/President
Research: Mr. Scott Whitcup/Senior Vice President Research & Development
Finance: Mr. Jeffrey Edwards/Chief Financial Officer, Vice President Finance
   Acid, Hyaluronic   Dental And Oral
   Applicator (Laryngo-Tracheal), Topical Anesthesia   Anesthesiology
   Cleaner, Lens, Contact   Ophthalmology
   Contract Manufacturing, Product, Disposable   General
   Cutter, Vitreous Aspiration, AC-Powered   Ophthalmology
   Extractor, Cataract   Ophthalmology
   Implant, Scleral   Ophthalmology
   Kit, Irrigation, Eye   Ophthalmology
   Lamp, Slit   Ophthalmology
   Laser, Argon, Surgical   Surgery
   Laser, Nd:YAG, Surgical   Surgery
   Laser, Ophthalmic   Ophthalmology
   Laser, Surgical   Surgery
   Lens, Intraocular   Ophthalmology
   Lens, Intraocular, Anterior Chamber   Ophthalmology
   Lens, Intraocular, Posterior Chamber   Ophthalmology
   Lens, Other   Ophthalmology
   Phacoemulsification System   Ophthalmology
   Refractometer, Ophthalmic   Ophthalmology
   Scissors, Corneal   Ophthalmology
   Stool, Operating Room, Adjustable   Surgery
   Table, Ophthalmic, Instrument, Manual   Ophthalmology
   Table, Ophthalmic, Instrument, Powered   Ophthalmology
   Tissue, Corneal   Ophthalmology
   Tray, Custom/Special Procedure   General
   Viscoelastic Surgical Aid   Ophthalmology

ALLERGAN   **800-624-4261**
71 S. Los Carneros Rd., Goleta, CA 93117   **805-683-6761**
FDA Number: 2024601   *Fax:* 805-692-5432
Web site: www.inamedcorp.com
Medical Products Sales Volume: $252,000,000
Total Employees: 990   *Marketing Staff:* 15   *Sales Staff:* 36
Ownership: Public
Stock Symbol: IMDC
Traded On: NASDAQ
Quality System Registration Information: ISO9002
Produces/Sells CE-marked Devices: Y
Federal Procurement Eligibility: Small Business
Distribution: Manufacturer Direct, Exporter
General Admin.: Richard Babbit/Chief Executive Officer
      Scott Eschbach/President
Mktg./Adv.: David Barella/Executive Vice President Marketing & Sales
Production: Sal Alongi/Vice President Operations
   Brassiere, Surgical   Surgery

ALLERGAN   **800-624-4261** *(cont'd)*
   Component, Silicone   General
   Custom Prosthesis   Orthopedics
   Drape, Surgical   Surgery
   Elastomer, Silicone Rubber   General
   Expander, Skin, Inflatable   Surgery
   Prosthesis, Breast, Inflatable, Internal   Surgery
   Prosthesis, Chin, Internal   Surgery
   Prosthesis, Nasal, Dorsal   Surgery
   Prosthesis, Rhinoplasty   Surgery

ALLERGAN INC.   **800-668-6424**
85 Enterprise Boulevard   **905-940-1660**
85 Enterprise Boulevard
Markham, ONT L6G 0 Canada
FDA Number: n/a
E-mail: strouthos_polydor@allergan.com   *Fax:* 905-940-1902
Web site: http://www.allergan.ca
Year Founded: 1966
Total Employees: 10
Ownership: Allergan, Inc.
Produces/Sells CE-marked Devices: N
Distribution: Manufacturer Direct

ALLERGAN SALES, LLC   **714-246-4388**
8301 Mars Dr., Waco, TX 76712
FDA Number: 1643525
Ownership: Private
Produces/Sells CE-marked Devices: N
   Cleaner, Lens, Contact   Ophthalmology

ALLERGAN SURGICAL
See Innovative Surgical Products, Inc.

ALLESEE ORTHODONTIC APPLIANCES   **714-516-7484**
13931 Spring St., Sturtevant, WI 53177
FDA Number: 2184045
Ownership: Sybron Dental Specialties, Inc.
Produces/Sells CE-marked Devices: N
   Aligner, Sequential   Dental And Oral
   Positioner, Socket   Orthopedics
   Positioner, Tooth, Preformed   Dental And Oral
   Retainer, Screw Expansion, Orthodontic   Dental And Oral

ALLESEE ORTHODONTIC APPLIANCES   **714-516-7400**
(CALEXICO)
341 E. First St., Calexico, CA 92231
FDA Number: 3004674232
Ownership: Sybron Dental Specialties, Inc.
Produces/Sells CE-marked Devices: N
   Aligner, Sequential   Dental And Oral
   Positioner, Tooth, Preformed   Dental And Oral
   Retainer, Screw Expansion, Orthodontic   Dental And Oral

ALLESEE ORTHODONTIC APPLIANCES, INC. -   **949-255-8766**
CONNECTICUT
6 Niblick Rd., Enfield, CT 06082
FDA Number: 3004869383
Ownership: Sybron Dental Specialties, Inc.
Produces/Sells CE-marked Devices: N
   Aligner, Sequential   Dental And Oral
   Positioner, Tooth, Preformed   Dental And Oral
   Retainer, Screw Expansion, Orthodontic   Dental And Oral

ALLEZ MEDICAL APPLICATIONS, INC.   **714-641-2098**
2141 S. Standard Avenue, Santa Ana, CA 92707
FDA Number: n/a   *Fax:* 714-557-5361
Web site: www.allezmedical.com
Ownership: Private
Produces/Sells CE-marked Devices: N
   Guide, Surgical, Needle   Surgery
   Probe   Orthopedics

ALLEZ SPINE, LLC
See Phygen, LLC

ALLFOAM INDUSTRIES LTD.   **604-277-7710**
12391 #5 Road, Richmond, BC V7A-4E9 Canada
FDA Number: n/a   *Fax:* 604-277-7752
E-mail: info@allfoam.bc.ca
Web site: www.allfoam.bc.ca
Total Employees: 15   *Marketing Staff:* 2   *Sales Staff:* 3
Ownership: Private
Produces/Sells CE-marked Devices: N
Distribution: Service Direct, Exporter

ALLGOOD PRODUCTS INC.
See Nurse Assist ,Inc.

ALLIANCE H. INC DENTECH EQUIPMENT 360-988-7080
901 W. Front Street, Sumas, WA 98295
FDA Number: n/a   *Fax:* 360-988-4050
E-mail: sales@dentechcorp.com
Web site: www.dentechcorp.com
Year Founded: 1971
Total Employees: 100   *Sales Staff:* 18
Ownership: ASH TEMPLE LTD.
Quality System Registration Information: ISO9002
Produces/Sells CE-marked Devices: Y
Federal Procurement Eligibility: Small Business, VA Contract
Distribution: Manufacturer Through Distributor
General Admin.: Steve White/President
Mktg./Adv.: Paul Coughlin/Manager International Sales
    Steve White/Vice President Marketing & Sales
Production: Dave Skipp/Director Engineering
    Gary Duling/Director Quality Assurance
    Gary Villette/Senior Engineer

Chair, Dental	Dental And Oral
Light, Dental	Dental And Oral
Operative Dental Treatment Unit	Dental And Oral

ALLIANCE HEARING SYSTEMS 828-286-9399
431 South Main St., Suite #6, Rutherfordton, NC 28139
FDA Number: 3006098331
Ownership: Private
Produces/Sells CE-marked Devices: N

Hearing-Aid	Ear/Nose/Throat

ALLIANCE LAUNDRY SYSTEMS LLC
See Unimac

ALLIANCE MEDICAL INC. 888-639-1264
7800 Cote de Liesse,   **514-344-3030**
St-Laurent, QUE H4T-1 Canada
FDA Number: n/a   *Fax:* 514-344-3131
E-mail: nackad@alliancemedical.ca
Web site: www.worldexport.com/alliancemedical/
Year Founded: 1989
Total Employees: 50
Ownership: Private
Produces/Sells CE-marked Devices: N
Distribution: Manufacturer Direct, Exporter

ALLIANCE MEDICAL PRODUCTS, INC. 949-768-4690
9342 Jeronimo Rd., Irvine, CA 92618
FDA Number: 2027189   *Fax:* 949-454-4441
Web site: http://www.amp-us.com
Ownership: Private
Produces/Sells CE-marked Devices: N

ALLIANCE PHARMACEUTICAL CORP. 858-410-5200
4660 La Jolla Village Drive, Suite 825, San Diego, CA 92122
FDA Number: n/a   *Fax:* 858-410-5201
E-mail: corpcom@allp.com
Web site: www.allp.com
Annual Revenue: $0-$1 Million
Total Employees: 1
Ownership: Public
Stock Symbol: ALLP
Traded On: OTC Bulletin
Produces/Sells CE-marked Devices: N
Federal Procurement Eligibility: Small Business
Distribution: Manufacturer Direct
General Admin.: Duane J. Roth/Chief Executive Officer, Chairman
    B. Jack DeFranco/President, Chief Financial Officer

Contract Manufacturing, Pharmaceuticals/Chemicals	General
Contract R&D, Diagnostics	General

ALLIANCE PRECISION PLASTICS 585-426-5310
1220 Lee Road, Rochester, NY 14606
FDA Number: 1319480   *Fax:* 585-425-5081
E-mail: dbrhel@allianceppc.com
Web site: www.allianceppc.com
Year Founded: 1959
Total Employees: 300   *Sales Staff:* 10
Ownership: Private
Quality System Registration Information: ISO9001
Produces/Sells CE-marked Devices: N
Distribution: Manufacturer Direct
General Admin.: David Hanna/Business Manager

Mirror, Mouth	Dental And Oral
Speculum, Vaginal, Non-Metal, Fiberoptic	Obstetrics/Gynecology

ALLIANCE PROSTHETICS & ORTHOTICS, INC. 562-921-0353
14535 Valley View Ave., Ste U, Santa Fe Spgs, CA 90670
FDA Number: 3004621012
Ownership: Private
Produces/Sells CE-marked Devices: N

ALLIANCE PROSTHETICS & ORTHOTICS, INC. 562-921-0353
(cont'd)

Cushion, Wheelchair (Pad)	Physical Med

ALLIANCE SUPPLY CORP.
See Clean Esd Products, Inc.

ALLIANCE TECH MEDICAL, INC. 800-848-8923
5305 Mission Circle, P.O. Box 6024,   **817-326-6357**
Granbury, TX 76049
FDA Number: 3004476631   *Fax:* 817-326-2182
E-mail: info@alliancetechmedical.com
Web site: www.alliancetechmedical.com
Ownership: Private
Produces/Sells CE-marked Devices: N

Filter, Bacterial, Breathing Circuit	Anesthesiology
Mouthpiece, Breathing	Anesthesiology

ALLIANT HEALTHCARE PRODUCTS 269-629-0300
8850 M89, Richland, MI 49083
FDA Number: 3004986960

Airway, Nasopharyngeal (Breathing Tube)	Anesthesiology
Carrier, Ligature	Surgery
Catheter, Vascular, Cardiopulmonary Bypass	Cardiovascular
Valve, CPB Check, Retrograde, In-Line	Anesthesiology

ALLIED BIOMEDICAL 800-276-1322
PO Box 392, Ventura, CA 93003   **805-289-1665**
FDA Number: 62392   *Fax:* 805-289-1670
E-mail: info@alliedbiomedical.com
Web site: www.alliedbiomedical.com
Medical Products Sales Volume: $500,000
Annual Revenue: $0-$1 Million
Total Employees: 6   *Marketing Staff:* 1   *Sales Staff:* 1
Ownership: Implantech Associates, Inc.
Quality System Registration Information: ISO9001
Produces/Sells CE-marked Devices: Y
Federal Procurement Eligibility: Small Business
Distribution: Manufacturer Direct, Manufacturer Through Distributor, Manufacturer Through Manufacturer Reps, Exporter

Elastomer, Silicone (Scar Management)	Surgery
Elastomer, Silicone Block	Surgery
Implant, Muscle, Pectoralis	Surgery
Malar Implant	Surgery
Prosthesis, Chin, Internal	Surgery
Prosthesis, Nose, Internal	Surgery
Silicone Sheeting	General
Tubing, Silicone	General

ALLIED BIOMEDICAL CORPORATION
See Allied Biomedical

ALLIED DIAGNOSTIC IMAGING RESOURCES, INC. 800.262.9333
5440 Oakbrook Parkway, Norcross, GA 30093-2294
FDA Number: n/a   *Fax:* 201.995.2443
Web site: www.cpacimaging.com
Medical Products Sales Volume: $20,000,000
Ownership: Cpac Equipment, Inc.
Produces/Sells CE-marked Devices: N
Federal Procurement Eligibility: Small Business
Distribution: Manufacturer Through Distributor, Exporter

Blender/Mixer	Chemistry
Chemical, Film Processor	Radiology
Processor, Radiographic Film, Automatic	Radiology
Processor, Radiographic Film, Automatic, Dental	Dental And Oral

ALLIED HEALTH & SCIENTIFIC PRODUCTS
See Fisher Scientific Co., Llc.

ALLIED HEALTHCARE PRODUCTS, INC. 800-444-3954
1720 Sublette Ave., St. Louis, MO 63110-1927   **314-771-2400**
FDA Number: 1924066   *Fax:* 314-771-0650
Web site: http://www.alliedhpi.com/
Annual Revenue: $5-$10 Million
Total Employees: 900   *Marketing Staff:* 10   *Sales Staff:* 90
Ownership: Public
Stock Symbol: AHPI
Traded On: NASDAQ
Produces/Sells CE-marked Devices: Y
Distribution: Manufacturer Through Distributor
General Admin.: Uma Aggarwal/President, Chief Executive Officer
    Ted Atwood/Vice President Human Resources
Mktg./Adv.: Joan Wyatt/Coord. Marketing
    Phil Strasser/Director National Accounts
    Peter Gonzalez/Manager Product Marketing
    Dave Grabowski/Vice President International Marketing & Sales
Production: Vernon Trimble/Director Regulatory Affairs
    Gabe Kohn/Vice President Operations

Absorbent, Carbon-Dioxide	Anesthesiology

ALLIED HEALTHCARE PRODUCTS, INC.   800-444-3954 *(cont'd)*

Alarm, Central Gas System	Anesthesiology
Aspirator, Emergency Suction	General
Aspirator, Low Volume (Gastric Suction)	Gastroenterology/Urology
Aspirator, Surgical	Surgery
Aspirator, Thoracic (Suction Unit)	Cardiovascular
Aspirator, Tracheal	Ear/Nose/Throat
Attachment, Breathing, Positive End Expiratory Pressure	Anesthesiology
Board, Spine	Orthopedics
Bottle, Collection, Vacuum (Aspirator)	General
Cabinet, Table And Tray, Anesthesia	Anesthesiology
Calibrator, Gas, Pressure	Anesthesiology
Calibrator, Gas, Volume	Anesthesiology
Canister, Oxygen	Anesthesiology
Canister, Suction	Cardiovascular
Cannula, Nasal, Oxygen	Anesthesiology
Catheter, Nasal, Oxygen (Tube)	Anesthesiology
Clamp, Circumcision	Obstetrics/Gynecology
Clip, Nose	Anesthesiology
Column, Life Support (Electrical/Gas)	General
Compressor, Air, Portable	Anesthesiology
Concentrator, Oxygen	Anesthesiology
Connector, Airway (Extension)	Anesthesiology
Console, Patient Service	General
Curette, Uterine	Obstetrics/Gynecology
Cylinder, Oxygen	Anesthesiology
Drain, Thoracic, Water Seal	Anesthesiology
Dressing, Wound and Burn, Occlusive	Surgery
Dryer, Respiratory/Anesthesia Equipment	General
Filter, Bacterial, Breathing Circuit	Anesthesiology
Fitting, Quick Connect (Gas Connector)	General
Flowmeter, Back-Pressure Compensated, Thorpe Tube	Anesthesiology
Flowmeter, Gas (Oxygen), Calibrated	Anesthesiology
Headwall System (Patient Room)	General
Holder, Gas Cylinder	Anesthesiology
Hood, Oxygen, Infant	General
Humidifier, Non-Heated	Anesthesiology
Kit, Burn	General
Kit, Suction, Airway (Tracheal)	Anesthesiology
Light, Overbed	General
Mask, Face	General
Mask, Oxygen, Low Concentration, Venturi	Anesthesiology
Mask, Oxygen, Non-Rebreathing	Anesthesiology
Mask, Oxygen, Partial Rebreathing	General
Nebulizer, Direct Patient Interface	Anesthesiology
Nebulizer, Medicinal	Ear/Nose/Throat
Nebulizer, Non-Heated	Anesthesiology
Nebulizer, Ultrasonic	Anesthesiology
Pump, Abortion, Vacuum, Central System	Obstetrics/Gynecology
Pump, Aspiration, Portable	Anesthesiology
Pump, Breast, Powered	Obstetrics/Gynecology
Pump, Nebulizer, Electric	Ear/Nose/Throat
Pump, Suction Operatory	Dental And Oral
Pump, Vacuum, Central	Anesthesiology
Regulator, Oxygen, Mechanical	General
Regulator, Pressure, Gas Cylinder	Anesthesiology
Regulator, Suction, Thoracic	Anesthesiology
Regulator, Suction, Tracheal (Nasal, Oral)	Ear/Nose/Throat
Resuscitator, Cardiopulmonary	Cardiovascular
Resuscitator, Emergency Oxygen	Dental And Oral
Resuscitator, Emergency, Protective, Infection	Anesthesiology
Resuscitator, Pulmonary, Gas	General
Resuscitator, Pulmonary, Manual (Demand Valve)	General
Spirometer, Diagnostic (Respirometer)	Anesthesiology
Stand, Gas Cylinder	Anesthesiology
Suction Apparatus, Ward Use, Portable, AC-Powered	Surgery
Suit, Pneumatic Counterpressure (Anti-Shock)	Cardiovascular
Support, Breathing Tube	Anesthesiology
Tent, Mist	General
Tent, Oxygen (Canopy)	Anesthesiology
Tent, Oxygen, Electric	Anesthesiology
Timer, Flow	Anesthesiology
Transducer, Gas Flow	Anesthesiology
Trousers, Anti-Shock	Anesthesiology
Tube, Aspirating, Flexible, Connecting	Anesthesiology
Tube, Connecting	General
Tubing, Flexible, Medical Gas, Low-Pressure	Anesthesiology
Tubing, Non-Invasive	Surgery
Ventilator, Emergency, Manual (Resuscitator)	Anesthesiology
Ventilator, Emergency, Powered (Resuscitator)	Anesthesiology
Ventilator, Neonatal Respirator	General

ALLIED HEALTHCARE PRODUCTS, INC.   800-444-3954
1720 Sublette Avenue, St. Louis, MO 63110   **314-771-2400**
FDA Number: 1314798
E-mail: CustomerService@alliedhpi.com
Web site: www.alliedhpi.com
Year Founded: 1958
Ownership: ALLIED HEALTHCARE PRODUCTS, INC.
Stock Symbol: AHPI
Traded On: NASDAQ

ALLIED HEALTHCARE PRODUCTS, INC.   800-444-3954 *(cont'd)*
Produces/Sells CE-marked Devices: N

Absorbent, Carbon-Dioxide	Anesthesiology

ALLIED INSTRUMENTATION LABORATORY
See Instrumentation Laboratory Company

ALLIED MEDCO, INC.   631-447-0093
25 Corporate Dr., Holtsville, NY 11742
FDA Number: n/a
Medical Products Sales Volume: $1,500,000
Annual Revenue: $1-$5 Million
Ownership: Private
Produces/Sells CE-marked Devices: N
Federal Procurement Eligibility: Small Business

Bed, Electric	General
Canister, Liquid Oxygen, Portable	Anesthesiology

ALLIED MINDS, INC.   617-419-1800
33 Arch Street, 32nd Floor, Boston, MA 02110
FDA Number: n/a   *Fax:* 617-419-1813
Web site: www.alliedminds.com
Ownership: Private
Produces/Sells CE-marked Devices: N
General Admin.: Mr. Marc Eichenberger/Chief Operating Officer
     Mr. Jeff Caputo/Director
     Mr. John Serafini/Director
     Mr. Omar Amirana/Director
     Mr. Roger Yang/Director
     Mr. Vincent Chun/Vice President
Finance: Mr. Mark Pritchard/President

ALLIED PHOTO PRODUCTS CO., INC.
See Allied Diagnostic Imaging Resources, Inc.

ALLIED SIGNAL BURDICK & JACKSON
See Honeywell Burdick & Jackson

ALLMAN PRODUCTS   800-223-6889
21101 Itasca St., Chatsworth, CA 91311   **818-715-0093**
FDA Number: n/a   *Fax:* 818-715-9629
E-mail: customerservice@allmanproducts.com
Web site: www.allmanproducts.com
Annual Revenue: $1-$5 Million
Year Founded: 1984
Total Employees: 15   *Sales Staff:* 15
Ownership: Private
Produces/Sells CE-marked Devices: N
Federal Procurement Eligibility: Small Business
Distribution: Manufacturer Direct, Manufacturer Through Distributor, Manufacturer Through Manufacturer Reps, OEM
General Admin.: Lawry Goldberg/President, Chief Executive Officer

Chair, Bath	General
Cover, Mattress	General
Cover, Mattress, Waterproof	General
Cushion, Foot	Orthopedics
Cushion, Other	General
Cushion, Wheelchair (Pad)	Physical Med
Diaper, Adult	General
Gown, Patient	Surgery
Linen, Bed	General
Pad, Incontinence (Underpad)	General
Pad, Pressure, Foam Convoluted	General
Pillow, Cervical	Orthopedics
Support, Back	Orthopedics
Walker, Mechanical	Physical Med

ALLODEX SYSTEMS   888-820-5836
19940 Dinner Key Dr., PO Box # 3252,   **561-477-3154**
Sarasota, FL 34230
FDA Number: 3003527637   *Fax:* 561-477-3690
Ownership: Private
Produces/Sells CE-marked Devices: N

Bracket, Metal, Orthodontic	Dental And Oral

ALLOR MEDICAL, INC.
See Medi-Dyne Healthcare Products, L.L.C.

ALLOSOURCE   888-873-8330
6278 South Troy Circle, Centennial, CO 80111   **720-873-0213**
FDA Number: 3000215346   *Fax:* 720-873-0212
E-mail: info@allosource.org
Web site: www.allosource.org
Annual Revenue: $50-$100 Million
Year Founded: 1994
Total Employees: 200   *Marketing Staff:* 2   *Sales Staff:* 20
Ownership: Private
Produces/Sells CE-marked Devices: N
Federal Procurement Eligibility: Small Business
Distribution: Manufacturer Direct, Manufacturer Through Distributor, Manufacturer Through Manufacturer Reps

ALLOSOURCE — 888-873-8330 (cont'd)
General Admin.: Tom Cycyota/President, Chief Executive Officer
Mr. J. Kevin Cmunt/Vice President
Production: Bob Brook/Vice President Operations
Donna Sin/Vice President Quality Assurance & Regulatory Affairs
Research: Simon Bogdansky/Vice President Research & Development
| Filler, Bone Void, Osteoinduction | Physical Med |
| Service, Tissue Bank | General |

ALLPRO IMAGING — 888-862-4050
1295 Walt Whitman Road, Melville, NY 11747 — 516-433-7676
FDA Number: n/a — *Fax:* 516-433-7683
E-mail: mail@allproimaging.com
Web site: http://www.allproimaging.com
Ownership: Private
Produces/Sells CE-marked Devices: N

ALLPRO, INC. — 800-243-2285
6930 West 116th Ave., Suite 10, P.o. Box 733, — 423-587-2199
Broomfield, CO 80020
FDA Number: 1721890 — *Fax:* 303-466-8965
E-mail: info@allprodental.com
Web site: www.allprodental.com
Ownership: Private
Produces/Sells CE-marked Devices: N
| Cup, Prophylaxis | Dental And Oral |

ALLSCRIPTS-MISYS HEALTHCARE SOLUTIONS — 919-847-8102
222 Merchandise Mart Plaza, Suite 2024, Chicago, IL 60654
FDA Number: n/a — *Fax:* 919-846-1555
Web site: www.allscripts.com
Medical Products Sales Volume: $192,000,000
Year Founded: 1979
Total Employees: 6000
Ownership: Public
Stock Symbol: MDRX
Traded On: NASDAQ
Produces/Sells CE-marked Devices: Y
Distribution: Manufacturer Direct
| Computer Software | General |
| Computer and Software, Medical | General |

ALLSPORT DYNAMICS, INC. — 800-594-5350
2724 S.E. Stallings Dr., — 936-569-1003
Nacogdoches, TX 75961
FDA Number: 1651603 — *Fax:* 936-569-1439
E-mail: gawhite@allsportdynamics.com
Web site: www.allsportdynamics.com
Medical Products Sales Volume: $1
Annual Revenue: $0-$1 Million
Year Founded: 1990
Total Employees: 16 — *Marketing Staff:* 4 — *Sales Staff:* 3
Ownership: Private
Stock Symbol: N/A
Produces/Sells CE-marked Devices: Y
Federal Procurement Eligibility: Small Business
Distribution: Manufacturer Through Distributor
General Admin.: Jeff Brewer/President, Chief Executive Officer
Mktg./Adv.: Gary A. White/Vice President Sales
Production: Brad Jacobson/Vice President Manufacturing
Research: Mr. Joey Michelle/Vice President, Director Research & Development
| Brace, Joint, Ankle (External) | Physical Med |

ALLSTEEL INC. — 800-624-9212
2210 Second Ave., Muscatine, IA 52761 — 319-262-4800
FDA Number: n/a — *Fax:* 563-262-4566
Web site: www.allsteeloffice.com
Medical Products Sales Volume: $75,000,000
Annual Revenue: $50-$100 Million
Total Employees: 5000
Ownership: Private
Produces/Sells CE-marked Devices: N
Distribution: Manufacturer Direct, Manufacturer Through Distributor, Manufacturer Through Manufacturer Reps
General Admin.: Eric Jungbluth/President
Mktg./Adv.: Tim Smith/Vice President Communications
Julie Zielinski/Vice President Marketing
Martin Scaglione/Vice President Sales
| Furniture, General | General |

ALLTEC INTEGRATED MANUFACTURING,INC. — 805-595-3500
4330 Santa Fe Road, San Luis Obispo, CA 93401
FDA Number: 3005598300 — *Fax:* 805-595-1024
E-mail: inforequest@alltecmfg.com
Web site: www.alltecmfg.com
Ownership: Private
Produces/Sells CE-marked Devices: N

ALLTEC INTEGRATED MANUFACTURING,INC. — 805-595-3500
(cont'd)
Accessories, Retractor, Dental	Dental And Oral
Syringe Unit, Air And/Or Water	Dental And Oral
Tray, Impression	Dental And Oral

ALLTECH ASSOCIATES, INC. — 847-282-2090
17434 Mojave Street, Hesperia, CA 92345
FDA Number: 3005269799
Ownership: Private
Produces/Sells CE-marked Devices: N
Adsorbents, Ion Exchange	Toxicology
Adsorbents, Liquid Chromatography	Toxicology
Column, Liquid Chromatography	Toxicology

ALLVETSUSA:ATTN:US-IT.NET — 954-560-4257
500 South Australian Ave., Suite 510,
West Palm Beach, FL 33401
FDA Number: n/a
Ownership: Private
Produces/Sells CE-marked Devices: N
| Stimulator, Nerve, Transcutaneous (Pain Relief, TENS) | Cns/Neurology |

ALMAT, INC. — 423-928-6861
215 East Watauga Avenue, Johnson City, TN 37601
FDA Number: 1046557 — *Fax:* 423-928-6861
E-mail: wtmathes@chartertn.net
Medical Products Sales Volume: $200,000
Year Founded: 1972
Total Employees: 2
Ownership: Private
Produces/Sells CE-marked Devices: N
Federal Procurement Eligibility: Small Business
Distribution: Exclusive Distributor
| Balloon, Middle Ear | Ear/Nose/Throat |

ALMEDIC LTD. — 514-337-4942
4900 Boulevard Cote Vertu, St-Laurent, QUE H4S-1J9 Canada
FDA Number: n/a — *Fax:* 514-337-4945
E-mail: info@almedic.com
Web site: www.almedic.com
Year Founded: 1952
Ownership: Private
Produces/Sells CE-marked Devices: N
Distribution: Importer

ALMEN LABORATORIES, INC. — 760-806-0040
1672 Gil Way, Vista, CA 92084
FDA Number: 3006947420 — *Fax:* 760) 806-7577
Ownership: Private
Produces/Sells CE-marked Devices: N
| Infusion System, Radionuclide | Radiology |

ALMORE INTERNATIONAL, INC. — 503-643-6633
PO Box 25214, Portland, OR 97298
FDA Number: 3018986 — *Fax:* 503-643-9748
E-mail: info@almore.com
Web site: www.almore.com
Medical Products Sales Volume: $500,000
Annual Revenue: $1-$5 Million
Year Founded: 1946
Total Employees: 9 — *Marketing Staff:* 1 — *Sales Staff:* 4
Ownership: Private
Produces/Sells CE-marked Devices: Y
Federal Procurement Eligibility: Small Business
Distribution: Manufacturer Direct, Importer, Exporter
General Admin.: Davy Dupon/President, Chief Executive Officer
Michele Dupon/Secretary, Treasurer
Applicator, Rapid Wax, Dental	Dental And Oral
Articulators	Dental And Oral
Base, Denture, Relining, Repairing, Rebasing, Resin	Dental And Oral
Bath, Water (Constant Temperature)	Chemistry
Brush, Dental Plate (Denture)	Dental And Oral
Carver, Wax, Dental	Dental And Oral
Chamber, Anaerobic	Microbiology
Contouring, Instrument, Matrix, Operative	Dental And Oral
Endodontic Instrument	Dental And Oral
Face Bow	Dental And Oral
Floss, Dental	Dental And Oral
Foil, Dental	Dental And Oral
Forceps, Articulation Paper	Dental And Oral
Handle, Instrument, Dental	Dental And Oral
Instrument, Dental, Manual	Dental And Oral
Kit, Identification, Anaerobic	Microbiology
Loupe, Binocular, Low Power	Ophthalmology
Marker, Periodontic	Dental And Oral
Material, Acrylic, Dental	Dental And Oral
Paper, Articulation	Dental And Oral
Remover, Crown	Dental And Oral

ALMORE INTERNATIONAL, INC. 503-643-6633 *(cont'd)*
Source, Heat, Bleaching, Teeth, Dental	Dental And Oral
Strip, Adhesive	Surgery
Strip, Polishing Agent	Dental And Oral
Washer/Sterilizer	General
Wax, Dental	Dental And Oral
Wedges	Dental And Oral
Wheel, Polishing Agent	Dental And Oral

ALMOST U 800-626-6007
91 Market St., Suite 23, 845-297-1604
Wappingers Falls, NY 12590
FDA Number: n/a   *Fax:* 845-297-1634
E-mail: info@almostu.com
Web site: www.almostu.com
Annual Revenue: $0-$1 Million
Ownership: Private
Produces/Sells CE-marked Devices: N
Federal Procurement Eligibility: Small Business
Distribution: Manufacturer Through Distributor, Importer
Pad, Breast	Obstetrics/Gynecology

ALNOR INSTRUMENT CO.
See Tsi Inc.

ALOKA (US HEADQUARTERS) 800 872-5652
10 Fairfield Blvd., Wallingford, CT 06492-7502 203-269-5088
FDA Number: 1222669   *Fax:* 203-269-6075
E-mail: mail@aloka.com
Web site: http://www.aloka.com/home.asp
Ownership: Aloka Co., Ltd.
Quality System Registration Information: ISO9001
Produces/Sells CE-marked Devices: Y
Federal Procurement Eligibility: VA Contract
Distribution: Manufacturer Direct
General Admin.: Mr. David Famiglietti/Chief Operating Officer
Mr. Hideyuki Honda/General Manager
Mktg./Adv.: Mr. Randy Baraso/Manager Business Development
Production: Mr. Richard Cehovsky/Manager Quality Assurance & Regulatory Affairs
Probe, Detector, Flow, Blood, Laparoscopy, Ultrasonic	Surgery
Scanner, Ultrasonic (Pulsed Doppler)	Radiology
Scanner, Ultrasonic (Pulsed Echo)	Radiology
Scanner, Ultrasonic, Obstetrical/Gynecological	Obstetrics/Gynecology
Scanner, Ultrasonic, Other	Radiology
System, Imaging, Laparoscopy, Ultrasonic	Radiology
Transducer, Ultrasonic	Cardiovascular
Transducer, Ultrasonic, Diagnostic	Radiology

ALPAIR INC.
See Tapcon, Inc.

ALPHA BIOSCIENCES, INC. 877-825-7428
3651 Clipper Mill Road, 410-882-7646
Baltimore, MD 21211
FDA Number: 1125797   *Fax:* 410-467-5088
E-mail: info@alphabiosciences.com
Web site: www.Alphabiosciences.com
Medical Products Sales Volume: $700,000
Year Founded: 2000
Total Employees: 11
Ownership: Private
Produces/Sells CE-marked Devices: N
Federal Procurement Eligibility: Small Business
Distribution: Manufacturer Direct, Manufacturer Through Manufacturer Reps, Exporter
Culture Media, Amino Acid Assay	Microbiology
Culture Media, Enriched	Microbiology
Culture Media, Non-Propagating Transport	Microbiology
Culture Media, Non-Selective And Differential	Microbiology
Culture Media, Non-Selective And Non-Differential	Microbiology
Culture Media, Selective And Non-Differential	Microbiology
Test, Reagent, Biochemical, Neisseria Gonorrhoeae	Microbiology

ALPHA CARDIAC SYSTEMS, INC.
See Cardiac Services, Inc.

ALPHA COMMUNICATIONS 800-666-4800
42 Central Drive, Farmingdale, NY 11735-1202 631-777-5500
FDA Number: n/a   *Fax:* 631-777-5599
E-mail: info@alpha-comm.com
Web site: www.alpha-comm.com
Ownership: Private
Produces/Sells CE-marked Devices: N
Distribution: Manufacturer Through Distributor, Manufacturer Through Manufacturer Reps, Importer
General Admin.: Mark S. Goldberg/President
Madelyn R. Goldberg/Vice President, General Manager
Communication System, Emergency Alert, Personal	General
Communication System, Room Status	General

ALPHA COMMUNICATIONS 800-666-4800 *(cont'd)*
Nurse Call System	General

ALPHA INDUSTRIES, INC. 727-443-2673
701 N Martin L King Jr Ave, Clearwater, FL 33757
FDA Number: 1048379
Annual Revenue: $0-$1 Million
Ownership: Private
Produces/Sells CE-marked Devices: N
Federal Procurement Eligibility: Small Business
Distribution: Manufacturer Direct, Manufacturer Through Distributor
Clamp, Other	Surgery
Clamp, Umbilical	Obstetrics/Gynecology
Clamp, Vascular	Cardiovascular
Clip, Towel	Surgery
Container, Surgical Instrument	Surgery
Forceps, Dressing	Surgery
Forceps, Epilation	Surgery
Forceps, Hemostatic	Surgery
Forceps, Sponge	Surgery
Forceps, Tube Introduction	Anesthesiology
Surgical Instrument, Disposable	Surgery

ALPHA MEDICAL BRACE, L.L.C. 866-547-3897
303 Church St., Rock Hill, SC 29730
FDA Number: 1062254   *Fax:* 803-366-2230
E-mail: info@alphabrace.com
Web site: www.alphamedicalproducts.com
Ownership: Private
Produces/Sells CE-marked Devices: N
Bandage, Elastic	General
Belt, Support, Pelvic	Physical Med
Brace, Joint, Ankle (External)	Physical Med
Joint, Knee, External Brace	Physical Med

ALPHA MEDICAL INSTRUMENTS LLC 949-460-0944
23455 Madero, Suite B, Mission Viejo, CA 92691
FDA Number: 3003289723   *Fax:* 949-460-0904
E-mail: info@alphamedicalinstruments.com
Web site: www.alphamedicalinstruments.com
Ownership: Private
Produces/Sells CE-marked Devices: N
Adapter, Stopcock, Manifold, Cardiopulmonary Bypass	Cardiovascular
Catheter, Electrode Recording, Or Probe	Cardiovascular
Catheter, Flow Directed	Cardiovascular
Catheter, Intravascular, Diagnostic	Cardiovascular
Electrode, Pacemaker, Temporary	Cardiovascular
Introducer, Catheter	Cardiovascular

ALPHA MEDICAL PRODUCTS, INC. 800-714-2574
1827 E. Chapman Ave., Orange, CA 92867
FDA Number: n/a   *Fax:* 714-516-2221
E-mail: alphausa@alphamedical.com
Web site: www.alphamedical.com
Ownership: Private
Produces/Sells CE-marked Devices: N
Distribution: Exclusive Distributor
Component, Other	General
Lift, Wheelchair	General
Scooter (Motorized 3-Wheeled Vehicle)	Physical Med
Sling, Arm	Physical Med
Support, Ankle	Orthopedics
Support, Back	Orthopedics
Support, Knee	Physical Med
Support, Wrist	Physical Med
Walker, Mechanical	Physical Med
Wheelchair, Manual	Physical Med
Wheelchair, Powered	Physical Med

ALPHA OMEGA MFG. INC. 936-687-4993
110 Main Street, P.o. Box 387, Grapeland, TX 75844
FDA Number: 1645404
Ownership: Private
Produces/Sells CE-marked Devices: N
Controller, Temperature, Cardiopulmonary Bypass	Cardiovascular

ALPHA OPTICS, LLC 212-431-9190
54-08 46th St., Maspeth, NY 11378
FDA Number: n/a
Ownership: Private
Produces/Sells CE-marked Devices: N
Frame, Spectacle (Eyeglasses)	Ophthalmology
Sunglasses (Including Photosensitive)	Ophthalmology

ALPHA PRO TECH, INC. 800-749-1363
60 Centurian Drive, Suite 112, 520-281-0127
Markham, ONT L3R 9 Canada
FDA Number: n/a
E-mail: sales@alphaprotech.com
Web site: www.alphaprotech.com

ALPHA PRO TECH, INC. 800-749-1363 (cont'd)
Year Founded: 1993
Total Employees: 142
Ownership: Public
Stock Symbol: APT
Traded On: AMEX
Produces/Sells CE-marked Devices: Y
Federal Procurement Eligibility: Small Business
Distribution: Manufacturer Direct, Manufacturer Through Distributor, Exporter

ALPHA SCIENTIFIC CORP. 800-242-5989
287 Great Valley Pkwy., Malvern, PA 19355
FDA Number: 2530788   Fax: 800-841-2629
Web site: www.alpha-scientific.com
Ownership: Private
Produces/Sells CE-marked Devices: N
Basin, Emesis	General
Labware, Blood Collection	Chemistry
Pipette, Micro	Chemistry
Supplies, Blood Bank	Hematology

ALPHA SCIENTIFIC CORPORATION 800-242-5989
293 Great Valley Parkway, Malvern, PA 19355   610-647-7000
FDA Number: n/a   Fax: 610-647-7496
E-mail: sales@alpha-scientific.com
Web site: www.alpha-scientific.com
Medical Products Sales Volume: $3,000,000
Annual Revenue: $1-$5 Million
Total Employees: 10
Ownership: Private
Produces/Sells CE-marked Devices: N
Federal Procurement Eligibility: Small Business, GSA Contract
Distribution: Manufacturer Direct, OEM
General Admin.: Marshall Levine/Chairman
                David Levine/President
                Daniel Levine/Vice President
Dispenser, Other	General

ALPHA SCIENTIFIC MEDICAL, INC. 909-802-7000
1751 Yeager Ave., La Verne, CA 91750
FDA Number: 2086013
Ownership: Private
Produces/Sells CE-marked Devices: N
Disc, Strip And Reagent, Microorganism Differentiation	Microbiology

ALPHA TECHNOLOGIES INC.
See CAREFUSION 211, INC..

ALPHA-OMEGA SERVICES, INC. 562-804-0604
1282 Big Woods-stark Rd., Edgerly (vinton), LA 70668
FDA Number: 3003660614
Ownership: Private
Produces/Sells CE-marked Devices: N
Applicator, Radionuclide, Remote-Controlled	Radiology
Source, Brachytherapy, Radionuclide	Radiology

ALPHA-OMEGA SERVICES, INC. 800-346-7894
9156 Rose St., Bellflower, CA 90706-6420   562-804-0604
FDA Number: 2022694   Fax: 562-804-0610
E-mail: sales@alpha-omegaserv.com
Web site: www.alpha-omegaserv.com
Medical Products Sales Volume: $1,800,000
Annual Revenue: $1-$5 Million
Year Founded: 1973
Total Employees: 16   Marketing Staff: 1   Sales Staff: 1
Ownership: Private
Produces/Sells CE-marked Devices: N
Federal Procurement Eligibility: Small Business
Distribution: Manufacturer Direct
General Admin.: Bruce Hedger/President
                Troy Hedger/Vice President, General Manager
Mktg./Adv.: David G. Erwin/Director Marketing & Sales
Production: Mr. Bob Robnett/Director Quality Assurance & Regulatory Affairs
                Cary Hedger/Manager Production & RA
Applicator, Radionuclide, Manual	Radiology
Seed, Isotope, Gold, Titanium, Platinum	Radiology
Source, Teletherapy, Radionuclide	Radiology
Source, Wire, Radioactive Iridium	Radiology

ALPHA-OMEGA-ENGINEERING CORP.
See Caire, Inc.

ALPHA-TEC SYSTEMS, INC. 800-221-6058
12019 N.E. 99th St., #1780, Vancouver, WA 98682   360-260-2779
FDA Number: 2025606   Fax: 360-260-3277
E-mail: Laurie@AlphaTecSystems.com
Web site: www.alphatecsystems.com
Medical Products Sales Volume: $3,500,000
Total Employees: 35
Ownership: Private

ALPHA-TEC SYSTEMS, INC. 800-221-6058 (cont'd)
Produces/Sells CE-marked Devices: N
Federal Procurement Eligibility: Small Business
Distribution: Manufacturer Direct
Adhesive, Albumin Based	Pathology
Clearing Agent	Pathology
Concentrator, Clinical Sample	Chemistry
Container, Specimen Mailer And Storage	Pathology
Fixative, Metallic Containing	Pathology
Reagent, General Purpose	Pathology
Solution, Formalin/Sodium Acetate	Pathology
Stain, Auramine O	Pathology
Stain, Carbol Fuchsin	Pathology
Stain, Microbiological	Microbiology

ALPHACHEM LIMITED 1-888-338-2995
2485 Milltower Court, 905-821-2995
Mississauga, ONT L5N 5 Canada
FDA Number: n/a   Fax: 905-821-2660
Year Founded: 1991
Ownership: Private
Produces/Sells CE-marked Devices: N
Distribution: Exclusive Distributor

ALPHAGAZ DIV.
See Air Liquide America Corporation, Cambridge Div.

ALPHAMEDICS INC.
See Biomerieux Inc.

ALPHAPROTECH, INC. 229-242-1931
1287 West Fairway Dr., Nogales, AZ 85621
FDA Number: 2022409
Ownership: Private
Produces/Sells CE-marked Devices: N
Accessories, Apparel, Surgical	Surgery
Cap, Surgical	Surgery
Cover, Cast	General
Cover, Shoe, Operating Room	Surgery
Gown, Examination	General
Mask, Surgical	Surgery
Shield, Eye, Ophthalmic	Ophthalmology
Shoe And Shoe Cover, Conductive	Anesthesiology

ALPHAPROTECH, INC. 229-333-9741
236 North 2200 West, Salt Lake City, UT 84116
FDA Number: 1721663
E-mail: rvogelman@alphaprotech.com
Web site: www.alphaprotech.com
Ownership: Private
Produces/Sells CE-marked Devices: N
Mask, Surgical	Surgery

ALPHAPROTECH, INC. 520-281-0127
323 s blanchard st, Valdosta, GA 31601
FDA Number: 1061152
Ownership: Private
Produces/Sells CE-marked Devices: N
Cover, Shoe, Operating Room	Surgery

ALPHATEC SPINE, INC. 800-922-1356
5818 El Camino Real, Carlsbad, CA 92008   760-431-9286
FDA Number: 2027467   Fax: 800-431-9722
E-mail: service@alphatecspine.com
Web site: www.alphatecspine.com
Ownership: Public
Stock Symbol: ATEC
Traded On: NASDAQ
Produces/Sells CE-marked Devices: N
General Admin.: Mr. Michael O'Neill/Chief Financial Officer, Vice President
                Mr. Patrick Ryan/Chief Operating Officer
                Mr. Dirk Kuyper/President, Chief Executive Officer
                Mr. Ebun Garner/Senior Vice President, General Counsel,
Secretary
Appliance, Fixation, Spinal Interlaminal	Orthopedics
Appliance, Fixation, Spinal Intervertebral Body	Orthopedics
Bit, Drill	Orthopedics
Contractor, Surgical	Surgery
Device, Spinal Vertebral Body Replacement	Orthopedics
Dissector, Surgical, General & Plastic Surgery	Surgery
Fixation Appliance, Multiple Component	Orthopedics
Gauge, Depth	Orthopedics
Handle, Scalpel	Surgery
Knife, Orthopedic	Orthopedics
Nail, Fixation, Bone	Orthopedics
Needle, Aspiration And Injection, Disposable	Surgery
Orthosis, Fixation, Pedicle, Spinal	Orthopedics
Orthosis, Fixation, Spinal, Spondylolisthesis	Orthopedics
Pin, Fixation, Threaded	Orthopedics
Plate, Fixation, Bone	Orthopedics
Reamer	Orthopedics

ALPHATEC SPINE, INC.   800-922-1356 *(cont'd)*

Retractor	Orthopedics
Rod, Fixation, Intramedullary	Orthopedics
Rongeur, Other	Surgery
Screw, Fixation, Bone	Orthopedics
Tongs, Skull, Traction	Cns/Neurology

ALPHATEK   708-345-0500
2600 S. 25th Ave., Broadview, IL 60155
FDA Number: 1419225   *Fax:* 708-345-3090
E-mail: alphatek@ameritech.net
Web site: www.alphatekcorp.com
Annual Revenue: $1-$5 Million
Total Employees: 15
Ownership: Private
Produces/Sells CE-marked Devices: N
Federal Procurement Eligibility: Small Business
Distribution: Manufacturer Through Distributor
General Admin.: Paul Kupsco/President
Finance: William Flaherty/Manager Finance

Processor, Radiographic Film, Automatic	Radiology

ALPINE DENTAL LABORATORY, INC.   800-884-5047
1220 North 500 West, Lehi, UT 84043-1117   801-766-2200
FDA Number: n/a   *Fax:* 801-766-4577
E-mail: info@alpinedental.com
Web site: www.alpinedental.com
Ownership: Private
Produces/Sells CE-marked Devices: N
Federal Procurement Eligibility: Small Business
Distribution: Manufacturer Direct

Crown And Bridge, Temporary, Resin	Dental And Oral
Crown, Preformed	Dental And Oral
Denture, Preformed	Dental And Oral
Frame, Rubber Dam	Dental And Oral
Material, Acrylic, Dental	Dental And Oral

ALPINE GROUP
See Pacifica Gloves

ALRAND, INC./BOCA DENTAL SUPPLY, INC.   800-5004908
3401 North Federal Hwy., Suite 203,   561-338-9679
Boca Raton, FL 33431
FDA Number: 1055953   *Fax:* 561-750-0535
E-mail: dlgaviria@hotmail.com
Web site: www.bocadentalsupplyinc.com
Year Founded: 10
Total Employees: 2
Ownership: Private
Quality System Registration Information: ISO9000
Produces/Sells CE-marked Devices: N
Federal Procurement Eligibility: Small Business
Distribution: Exporter

Articulators	Dental And Oral
Handpiece, Air-Powered, Dental	Dental And Oral
Tray, Impression	Dental And Oral

ALSCO INDUSTRIES, INC.   508-347-1199
174 Charlton Rd, Po Box 1168, Sturbridge, MA 01566
FDA Number: 1226210
E-mail: inquiry@alscoindustries.com
Web site: www.alscoindustries.com
Ownership: Private
Produces/Sells CE-marked Devices: N

Floss, Dental	Dental And Oral

ALSIUS CORP.   949-453-0150
15770 Laguna Canyon, Suite 150, Irvine, CA 92618
FDA Number: 2032474   *Fax:* 949-453-9702
E-mail: info@alsius.com
Web site: www.alsius.com
Ownership: Public
Stock Symbol: ALUS
Traded On: NASDAQ
Produces/Sells CE-marked Devices: N
General Admin.: William Worthen/President, Chief Executive Officer
Mktg./Adv.: Suzanne Winter/Vice President International Marketing & Sales
Production: Mike Amell/Vice President Manufacturing
    John Riolo/Vice President Quality Assurance & Regulatory Affairs
Research: Lynn Shimada/Director Research & Development
Finance: Greg Tibbitts/Chief Financial Officer

Catheter, Intravascular, Therapeutic, Short-term Less Than 30 Days	General
Controller, Temperature, Cardiopulmonary Bypass	Cardiovascular
System, Hypothermia, Intravenous, Cooling	Cns/Neurology

ALSONS CORP.   800-421-0001
3010 West Mechanic St., P.O. Box 282,   517-439-1411
Hillsdale, MI 49242
FDA Number: n/a   *Fax:* 517-439-9644

ALSONS CORP.   800-421-0001 *(cont'd)*
E-mail: info@alsons.com
Web site: www.alsons.com
Year Founded: 1958
Ownership: Private
Produces/Sells CE-marked Devices: N
Distribution: Manufacturer Through Distributor, Manufacturer Through Manufacturer Reps

Chair, Bath	General
Chair, Seat Lifting (Standing Aid)	General
Chair, Shower	General
Component, Metal, Other	General
Contract Manufacturing	General
Contract Manufacturing, Product, Durable	General
Massager, Therapeutic	Physical Med

ALSOP ENGINEERING CO.
See Ertelalsop

ALT BIOSCIENCE,LLC   859-231-3061
235 Bolivar St., Lexington, KY 40508
FDA Number: 3005621521
Web site: www.altbioscience.com
Ownership: Private
Produces/Sells CE-marked Devices: N

Colorimeter, General Use	Chemistry
Equipment, Laboratory, Gen. Purpose (Specific Medical Use)	Chemistry
Reagent, General Purpose	Pathology

ALT, INC.
See Altimate Medical, Inc.

ALTA DIAGNOSTICS   800-359-9691
2560 Business Parkway, Suite C,   775-267-3001
Minden, NV 89423
FDA Number: 2084170   *Fax:* 775-267-1142
E-mail: sales@altadiagnostics.com
Web site: www.altadiagnostics.com
Medical Products Sales Volume: $1,000,000
Annual Revenue: $1-$5 Million
Ownership: Private
Produces/Sells CE-marked Devices: N
Federal Procurement Eligibility: Small Business
Distribution: Exclusive Distributor
General Admin.: Don Feeley/President

Antigen, Antiserum, Control, Spinal Fluid, Total	Immunology
Control, Urinalysis (Assayed And Unassayed)	Chemistry
Reagent, Other	General
Standard/Control, All Types	Chemistry

ALTAIR INSTRUMENTS, INC.   805-388-8503
330 North Wood Road, Suite J, Camarillo, CA 93010
FDA Number: 2024148   *Fax:* 805-388-9503
E-mail: info@newapeel.com
Web site: www.newapeel.com
Medical Products Sales Volume: $4,250,000
Annual Revenue: $0-$1 Million
Year Founded: 1982
Total Employees: 6
Ownership: Private
Produces/Sells CE-marked Devices: N
Federal Procurement Eligibility: Small Business, Female Owned
Distribution: Manufacturer Direct
General Admin.: Marlys O. Waldron/President
Production: Steve Waldron/Vice President Manufacturing
Research: Steve Waldron/Vice President Research & Development

Dermabrasion Unit	Surgery
Drill, Bone, Powered	Dental And Oral
Instrument, Microsurgical	Cns/Neurology
Saw, Electric	Cardiovascular

ALTAIRE PHARMACEUTICALS, INC.   631-722-5988
311 West Ln., Aquebogue, NY 11931
FDA Number: 2335740
Ownership: Private
Produces/Sells CE-marked Devices: N

Accessories, Solution, Lens, Contact	Ophthalmology

ALTANA, INC.   800-231-0206
60 Baylis Road, Melville, NY 11747   631-454-7677
FDA Number: 2432435   *Fax:* 631-454-6389
E-mail: hr@altanainc.com
Web site: www.altanainc.com
Medical Products Sales Volume: $438,840,000
Annual Revenue: $100-$500 Million
Year Founded: 1963
Total Employees: 575   *Sales Staff:* 150
Ownership: Private
Stock Symbol: AAA
Traded On: NYSE

ALTANA, INC. 800-231-0206 (cont'd)
Produces/Sells CE-marked Devices: Y
Federal Procurement Eligibility: VA Contract
Distribution: Manufacturer Through Distributor, Importer, Exporter
General Admin.: Paul McGarty/Chief Executive Officer
David Klaum/Senior Vice President
Mindy Kirsch/Vice President Human Resources
Mktg./Adv.: Charles Moore/Vice President Business Development
Production: Helen Corso/Vice President Manufacturing & Operations
Iltifat Hasan/Vice President Quality Assurance & Quality Control
Research: Robert Anderson/Vice President Scientific Affairs
Finance: Art Dulik/Senior Vice President Finance

Lubricant, Instrument	General
Lubricant, Patient	General

Medical Product Subsidiaries (Listed Separately)
Fougera

ALTECH CORPORATION 908-806-9400
35 Royal Road, Flemington, NJ 08822-6001
FDA Number: n/a Fax: 908-806-9490
E-mail: altech@altechcorp.com
Web site: www.altechcorp.com
Medical Products Sales Volume: $9,900,000
Annual Revenue: $10-$25 Million
Year Founded: 1986
Total Employees: 45 Marketing Staff: 3 Sales Staff: 4
Ownership: Private
Quality System Registration Information: ISO9001
Produces/Sells CE-marked Devices: Y
Federal Procurement Eligibility: Small Business
Distribution: Manufacturer Direct, Manufacturer Through Distributor, Manufacturer Through Manufacturer Reps, Exclusive Distributor
General Admin.: Dan Schuster/General Manager
Mario Meise/President

Cabinet, Instrument	General
Cabinet, Laboratory	Chemistry
Cabinet, Other	General
Component, Electrical	General

ALTEK CORP. 301-572-2555
12210 Plum Orchard Drive, Silver Spring, MD 20904-7802
FDA Number: n/a Fax: 301-572-2510
E-mail: info@altek.com
Web site: www.altek.com
Medical Products Sales Volume: $780,000
Annual Revenue: $5-$10 Million
Year Founded: 1970
Total Employees: 10 Marketing Staff: 1 Sales Staff: 2
Ownership: Private
Federal Procurement Eligibility: Small Business, GSA Contract
Distribution: Manufacturer Through Distributor, Service Direct, Exclusive Distributor, Exporter
General Admin.: E. A. Cameron/President, Chief Executive Officer
Mktg./Adv.: Sonja Tustice/Director Marketing
Andre Kruppa/Director National Accounts

Radiographic Unit, Digital	Radiology
Table, Radiographic, Non-Tilting, Powered	Radiology
Table, Radiographic, Stationary Top	Radiology
Table, Radiographic, Tilting	Radiology
Table, Urological, Radiographic	Gastroenterology/Urology

ALTERNATIVE PRODUCTS 904-378-9081
5351 Ramona Blvd., Suite 7, 8, Jacksonville, FL 32205
FDA Number: 3003619764
Ownership: Private
Produces/Sells CE-marked Devices: N

Accessories, Wheelchair	Physical Med
Cushion, Flotation	Physical Med
Cushion, Wheelchair (Pad)	Physical Med
Mattress, Non-Powered Flotation Therapy	Physical Med
Support, Head And Trunk, Wheelchair	Physical Med

ALTIMATE MEDICAL, INC. 800-342-8968
P.O. Box 180, 262 West 1st St., 507-697-6393
Morton, MN 56270
FDA Number: 2183634 Fax: 507-697-6900
E-mail: info@easystand.com
Web site: www.easystand.com
Year Founded: 1987
Total Employees: 40 Marketing Staff: 4 Sales Staff: 5
Ownership: Invacare Corporation
Quality System Registration Information: ISO9001
Produces/Sells CE-marked Devices: N
Federal Procurement Eligibility: Small Business
Distribution: Manufacturer Through Distributor, Manufacturer Through Manufacturer Reps
Mktg./Adv.: Jackie Kaufenberg/Manager Marketing
Peter Wankelman/Manager Sales Training

ALTIMATE MEDICAL, INC. 800-342-8968 (cont'd)
Mark Schmitt/Vice President Marketing & Sales
Production: Stacey Frank/Director Quality Assurance
Mike Bavier/Vice President Manufacturing

Chair, Seat Lifting (Standing Aid)	General

ALTMAN MFG. CO, INC. 630-963-0031
1990 Ohio St., Lisle, IL 60532
FDA Number: n/a Fax: 630-963-0089
E-mail: altman@altmanmfg.com
Web site: www.altmanmfg.com
Medical Products Sales Volume: $890,000
Annual Revenue: $1-$5 Million
Year Founded: 1942
Total Employees: 10 Marketing Staff: 1 Sales Staff: 1
Ownership: Private
Produces/Sells CE-marked Devices: N
Federal Procurement Eligibility: Small Business
Distribution: OEM
General Admin.: Paul C. Altman/President
Mktg./Adv.: Mr. Brian A. Altman/Vice President Sales
Research: Paul W. Altman/Vice President Research & Development

Equipment, Molding	General

ALTO DEVELOPMENT CORP. 732-938-2266
5206 Asbury Road, Farmingdale, NJ 07727-3516
FDA Number: 2242056 Fax: 732-938-2399
E-mail: ttw@alto.com
Web site: www.aemedical.com
Medical Products Sales Volume: $4,800,000
Annual Revenue: $5-$10 Million
Year Founded: 1968
Total Employees: 60 Marketing Staff: 3 Sales Staff: 3
Ownership: Private
Quality System Registration Information: ISO9001
Produces/Sells CE-marked Devices: N
Federal Procurement Eligibility: Small Business, VA Contract
Distribution: Manufacturer Direct, Manufacturer Through Distributor, Manufacturer Through Manufacturer Reps, OEM
General Admin.: Tim Wojciechowicz/President
Mktg./Adv.: Edward Degler/Vice President Marketing

Adapter, Lead, Pacemaker	Cardiovascular
Cable, Electrosurgical Unit	Surgery
Clip, Other	Surgery
Electrosurgical Unit, Cutting & Coagulation Device	Surgery
Lead, Pacemaker, Implantable Endocardial	Cardiovascular
Retractor, Surgical	Surgery
Suture, Other	Surgery
Tip, Suction Tube (Yankauer, Poole, Etc.)	Surgery
Tip, Suction, Electrosurgical	Surgery

ALTOONA MEDICAL SUPPLY 800-442-8367
705 2nd Ave. S.W., Altoona, IA 50009-1726
FDA Number: 1929357 Fax: 515-967-6809
E-mail: dr.don@altoonamedicalsupply.com
Web site: www.altoonamedicalsupply.com
Medical Products Sales Volume: $750,000
Annual Revenue: $0-$1 Million
Year Founded: 1980
Ownership: Private
Produces/Sells CE-marked Devices: N
Federal Procurement Eligibility: Small Business
Distribution: Manufacturer Direct
General Admin.: Donald A. Mackenzie/Chief Executive Officer

Stimulator, Nerve, Transcutaneous (Pain Relief, TENS)	Cns/Neurology
Stimulator, Neuromuscular, External Functional	Cns/Neurology

ALTRON, INC. 763-427-7735
6700 Bunker Lake Blvd. N.W., Minneapolis, MN 55303-5852
FDA Number: 2183673 Fax: 763-427-3773
E-mail: sales@altronmfg.com
Web site: www.altronmfg.com
Medical Products Sales Volume: $9,100,000
Annual Revenue: $25-$50 Million
Year Founded: 1974
Total Employees: 175 Marketing Staff: 4 Sales Staff: 4
Ownership: Private
Quality System Registration Information: ISO9002; ISO9003
Produces/Sells CE-marked Devices: N
Federal Procurement Eligibility: Small Business
Distribution: Manufacturer Direct, Manufacturer Through Manufacturer Reps, OEM
General Admin.: Alan C. Phillips/President, Chief Executive Officer
Mktg./Adv.: Alan Phillips/Manager Sales
Production: Dave Griffin/Manager Materials
Ken Saari/Managing Engineer
Wendy Baker/Vice President Quality Assurance & Quality Control

Contract Assembly	General

ALTRON, INC. 763-427-7735 *(cont'd)*
Pump, Infusion General

ALUCOBOND TECHNOLOGIES, INC., AIREX DIV.
See Magister Corporation

ALUMIRAMP, INC. 800-800-3864
855 E. Chicago Road, Quincy, MI 49082-9450 517-639-8777
FDA Number: 3004865511 Fax: 517-639-4314
E-mail: sales@alumiramp.com
Web site: www.alumiramp.com
Medical Products Sales Volume: $2,000,000
Annual Revenue: $1-$5 Million
Year Founded: 1986
Total Employees: 10 Marketing Staff: 3 Sales Staff: 3
Ownership: Private
Produces/Sells CE-marked Devices: N
Federal Procurement Eligibility: Small Business, Female Owned
Distribution: Manufacturer Direct, Manufacturer Through Manufacturer Reps, OEM
General Admin.: Linda Burke/President
Mktg./Adv.: Doug Cannon/Sales Associate
 Omar Perez/Sales Associate
 Aid, Living, Handicapped General
 Ramp, Wheelchair General

ALUSUISSE COMPOSITES, INC./AIREX DIV.
See Magister Corporation

ALUWAX DENTAL PRODUCTS CO. 616-895-4385
5260 Edgewater Drive, Allendale, MI 49401
FDA Number: n/a Fax: 616-895-5060
E-mail: plgemmen@altelco.net
Web site: www.aluwaxdental.com
Annual Revenue: $0-$1 Million
Total Employees: 5
Ownership: Private
Produces/Sells CE-marked Devices: Y
Federal Procurement Eligibility: Small Business
Distribution: Manufacturer Through Distributor, Exporter
General Admin.: Patrick Gemmen/President
Mktg./Adv.: Patrick Gemmen/Vice President Marketing
 Material, Impression Dental And Oral
 Tray, Impression Dental And Oral
 Wax, Dental Dental And Oral

ALVEY WASHING EQUIPMENT CO. 800-677-0076
4600 N. Mason-Montgomery Rd., 513-923-5665
Mason, OH 45040
FDA Number: n/a Fax: 513-923-5694
E-mail: sales@alveywashing.com
Web site: www.alveywashing.com
Annual Revenue: $1-$5 Million
Ownership: Private
Produces/Sells CE-marked Devices: N
Federal Procurement Eligibility: Small Business
Distribution: Manufacturer Direct, Manufacturer Through Manufacturer Reps, Service Direct
 Washer, Cart General
 Washer, Labware Chemistry
 Washer, Pipette Chemistry
 Washer, Utensil General
 Washer/Sterilizer General

AM2 PAT INC. 919-552-9689
455 W. Depot Street, Angier, NC 27501
FDA Number: 1063652
Ownership: Private
Produces/Sells CE-marked Devices: N
 Syringe, Piston General

AMA OPTICS, INC. 877-744-3937
314 West San Marino Dr., 305-538-4124
Miami Beach, FL 33139
FDA Number: 3004571972
Ownership: Private
Produces/Sells CE-marked Devices: N
 Chart, Visual Acuity Ophthalmology
 Clip, Lens, Trial, Ophthalmic Ophthalmology
 Frame, Trial, Ophthalmic Ophthalmology
 Lens, Set, Trial, Ophthalmic Ophthalmology
 Stereoscope, Battery-Powered Ophthalmology

AMANO PIONEER ECLIPSE CORP. 800-334-2246
1 Eclipse Road, PO Box 909, Sparta, NC 28675 336-372-8080
FDA Number: n/a Fax: 336-372-2895
E-mail: sales@pioneer-eclipse.com
Web site: www.pioneer-eclipse.com
Medical Products Sales Volume: $22,000,000
Year Founded: 1974

AMANO PIONEER ECLIPSE CORP. 800-334-2246 *(cont'd)*
Total Employees: 110 Marketing Staff: 20 Sales Staff: 20
Ownership: AMANO (JAPAN)
Produces/Sells CE-marked Devices: Y
Federal Procurement Eligibility: Small Business
Distribution: Manufacturer Direct, Manufacturer Through Distributor, Exclusive Distributor, Importer, Exporter
General Admin.: Yoshio Misumi/President, Chief Executive Officer
Research: Jack Wolfe/Manager Research & Development
 Housekeeping Equipment General

AMBASSADOR MEDICAL 888-499-4554
14470 Bergen Blvd., Suite 500, 877-237-3022
Noblesville, IN 46060
FDA Number: 3002183074 Fax: 414-908-9253
Web site: www.ambassadormedical.com
Year Founded: 1979
Total Employees: 35
Ownership: Ge Healthcare
Produces/Sells CE-marked Devices: N
General Admin.: Jim Kollai/General Manager
Mktg./Adv.: Christine Wright/Director Marketing
 Rob Hargis/Manager Sales
 Scanner, Ultrasonic (Pulsed Doppler) Radiology
 Scanner, Ultrasonic (Pulsed Echo) Radiology
 Transducer, Ultrasonic, Diagnostic Radiology

AMBCO ELECTRONICS 800-345-1079
15052 Redhill Avenue,, Suite D, 714-259-7930
Tustin, CA 92780
FDA Number: 2011951 Fax: 714-259-1688
E-mail: info@ambco.com
Web site: www.ambco.com
Medical Products Sales Volume: $800,000
Annual Revenue: $0-$1 Million
Year Founded: 1941
Total Employees: 5 Sales Staff: 4
Ownership: Private
Produces/Sells CE-marked Devices: N
Federal Procurement Eligibility: Small Business, GSA Contract
Distribution: Manufacturer Direct, Manufacturer Through Distributor, OEM, Service Direct
General Admin.: George C. Koutures/President
 Maria Koutures/Secretary, Treasurer
Production: Kevin Green/Manager Manufacturing
 Audiometer Ear/Nose/Throat
 Calibrator, Audiometer Ear/Nose/Throat

AMBIDERM, S.A. DE C.V. 800-800-8008
Carr. A Bosques De San Isidro 1136 36-338-077
Col. Bosques De San Isidro
Zapopan, Jalisco 45147 Mexico
FDA Number: n/a Fax: 36-560-381
E-mail: ambiderm@orbinet.com.mx
Web site: www.ambiderm.com.mx
Total Employees: 25 Marketing Staff: 1 Sales Staff: 8
Ownership: Private
Produces/Sells CE-marked Devices: N
Distribution: Manufacturer Through Distributor, Exclusive Distributor, Importer, Exporter

AMBIT CORPORATION 770-534-4150
1636 Oakbrook Industrial Dr., Gainesville, GA 30507
FDA Number: n/a
E-mail: tim@ambit3d.net
Web site: www.ambit3d.net
Ownership: Private
Produces/Sells CE-marked Devices: N
 Hearing-Aid Ear/Nose/Throat

AMBRY GENETICS 866-262-7943
100 Columbia, #200, Aliso Viejo, CA 92656 949-900-5500
FDA Number: n/a Fax: 949-900-5501
Web site: http://www.ambrygen.com
Year Founded: 2000
Ownership: Private
Produces/Sells CE-marked Devices: N
General Admin.: Mr. Charles Dunlop/Chairman, Chief Executive Officer
 Dr. Anja Kammesheidt/Chief Scientific Officer
Mktg./Adv.: Mr. Ardy Arianpour/Vice President Business Development
Finance: Mr. Charles Caporale/Chief Financial Officer
 Instrumentation For Clinical Multiplex Test Systems Chemistry

AMBU A/S 800-262-8462
6740 Baymeadow Dr., Glen Burnie, MD 21060 410-768-6464
FDA Number: 9610691 Fax: 800-262-8673
Web site: www.AmbuUSA.com

AMBU A/S   800-262-8462 *(cont'd)*

Ownership: Private
Produces/Sells CE-marked Devices: N

Airway, Oropharyngeal, Anesthesia	Anesthesiology
Attachment, Breathing, Positive End Expiratory Pressure	Anesthesiology
Bandage, Adhesive	Surgery
Bottle, Collection, Vacuum (Aspirator)	General
Electrode, Cutaneous	Cns/Neurology
Electrode, Electrocardiograph	Cardiovascular
Electrode, Needle	Cns/Neurology
Electrode, Needle, Diagnostic Electromyograph	Physical Med
Fixation Device, Tracheal Tube	Anesthesiology
Mask, Gas, Anesthesia	Anesthesiology
Mask, Oxygen, Aerosol Administration	Anesthesiology
Mask, Oxygen, Non-Rebreathing	General
Mattress, Air Flotation	Anesthesiology
Monitor, Airway Pressure (Gauge/Alarm)	Anesthesiology
Orthosis, Cervical	Physical Med
Pump, Aspiration, Portable	Anesthesiology
Suction Apparatus, Single Patient, Portable, Non-Powered	Surgery
Support, Patient Position	Anesthesiology
Tube, Tracheal (Endotracheal)	Anesthesiology
Valve, Non-Rebreathing	Anesthesiology
Ventilator, Emergency, Manual (Resuscitator)	Anesthesiology
Ventilator, Emergency, Powered (Resuscitator)	Anesthesiology

AMBU, INC.   800-262-8462
6740 Baymeadow Drive, Glen Burnie, MD 21060   410-768-6464

FDA Number: 1220828   *Fax:* 800-262-8673
E-mail: MLC@ambu.com
Web site: www.ambu.com
Annual Revenue: $25-$50 Million
Total Employees: 55   *Marketing Staff:* 2   *Sales Staff:* 20
Ownership: Private
Quality System Registration Information: ISO9001
Produces/Sells CE-marked Devices: Y
Federal Procurement Eligibility: Small Business
Distribution: Manufacturer Direct, Manufacturer Through Distributor
General Admin.: Frank Homa/President, Chief Executive Officer
     Allan Jensen/Regional Manager
     Mark Matula/Regional Manager
     Neal Harpstrite/Regional Manager
     Trent Starkes/Regional Manager
Mktg./Adv.: Michele Creech/Marketing Assistant
     John Schmitz/Vice President Business Development
     Michael Allain/Vice President Sales
Production: Sanjay Parikh/Manager Quality Assurance & Regulatory Affairs
Finance: Robert Campbell/Chief Financial Officer
     Phyllis Straus/Controller

Airway, Oropharyngeal, Anesthesia	Anesthesiology
Aspirator, Emergency Suction	General
Attachment, Breathing, Positive End Expiratory Pressure	Anesthesiology
Cart, Emergency, Cardiopulmonary Resuscitation (Crash)	Anesthesiology
Collar, Extrication	General
Continuous Positive Airway Pressure Unit (CPAP, CPPB)	Anesthesiology
Electrode, Cutaneous	Cns/Neurology
Electrode, Needle	Cns/Neurology
Electrode, TENS	Cns/Neurology
Kit, Emergency, Cardiopulmonary Resuscitation	General
Mask, Gas, Anesthesia	Anesthesiology
Mask, Oxygen, Non-Rebreathing	Anesthesiology
Orthosis, Cervical	Physical Med
Pump, Aspiration, Portable	Anesthesiology
Resuscitator, Emergency Oxygen	Dental And Oral
Resuscitator, Emergency, Protective, Infection	Anesthesiology
Resuscitator, Pulmonary, Manual (Demand Valve)	General
Training Manikin, CPR (Resuscitation)	General
Training Manikin, Other	General
Valve, Positive End Expiratory Pressure (PEEP)	Anesthesiology
Ventilator, Emergency, Manual (Resuscitator)	Anesthesiology
Ventilator, Volume (Critical Care)	Anesthesiology

AMBULATORY FOOTWEAR INC.   800-461-8588
6 Osler Court, Dundas, ONT L9H-2P9 Canada   905-628-5778

FDA Number: n/a   *Fax:* 905-628-3789
E-mail: pwatson@ambulatoryfootwear.com
Web site: www.ambulatoryfootwear.com
Year Founded: 1988
Total Employees: 25
Ownership: Private
Produces/Sells CE-marked Devices: N
Distribution: Manufacturer Direct

AMBUTECH INC.   800-561-3340
34 DeBaets St., Winnipeg R2J-3S9 Canada   204-663-3340

FDA Number: n/a   *Fax:* 1-800-267-5059
E-mail: orders@ambutech.com
Web site: www.ambutech.com
Year Founded: 1984

AMBUTECH INC.   800-561-3340 *(cont'd)*

Total Employees: 10   *Marketing Staff:* 2   *Sales Staff:* 2
Ownership: MELET PLASTICS INC.
Quality System Registration Information: ISO9002
Produces/Sells CE-marked Devices: Y
Federal Procurement Eligibility: Small Business
Distribution: Manufacturer Direct, Manufacturer Through Distributor, Service Direct, Exporter

AMC/INFOTRONICS
     See Clear Stream Media

AMCARE SURGICAL   416-781-4494
1584 Bathurst St., Toronto, ONT M5P-3H3 Canada

FDA Number: n/a   *Fax:* 416-656-9802
E-mail: info@amcaresurgical.com
Web site: www.amcaresurgical.com
Year Founded: 1985
Total Employees: 10
Ownership: Private
Produces/Sells CE-marked Devices: N
Distribution: Exclusive Distributor

AMCI MEDICAL SYSTEMS, LLC   713-522-4865
1617 W. Alabama St., Houston, TX 77006

FDA Number: 3006131435
Ownership: Private
Produces/Sells CE-marked Devices: N

System, X-Ray, Mobile	Radiology

AMCO INTERNATIONAL MANUFACTURING & DESIGN, INC.   303-646-3583
10 Conselyea Street, Brooklyn, NY 11211

FDA Number: 3005906887

Batteries, Rechargeable, Class Ii Devices	Cardiovascular

AMCOR FLEXIBLES, INC.   608-249-0404
4101 Lien Rd., Madison, WI 53704

FDA Number: 2183283   *Fax:* 608-249-4175
Total Employees: 35000
Ownership: Private
Produces/Sells CE-marked Devices: N
General Admin.: Mr. Ken MacKenzie/Chief Executive Officer, General Manager

Packaging Material	General
Wrap, Sterilization	General

AMD TECHNOLOGIES INC.   800-423-3535
218 Bronwood Avenue, Los Angeles, CA 90049   310-471-8900

FDA Number: n/a   *Fax:* 310-471-8900
E-mail: info@ams4illuminators.com
Web site: www.digitalams.com
Medical Products Sales Volume: $6,000,000
Annual Revenue: $5-$10 Million
Year Founded: 1954
Total Employees: 30   *Marketing Staff:* 2   *Sales Staff:* 10
Ownership: Private
Stock Symbol: AMMD
Traded On: NASDAQ
Produces/Sells CE-marked Devices: Y
Federal Procurement Eligibility: Small Business
Distribution: Manufacturer Direct, Manufacturer Through Distributor, Manufacturer Through Manufacturer Reps, OEM, Importer, Exporter
General Admin.: Daniel Giesberg/President, Chief Executive Officer
Mktg./Adv.: Mrs. Tracy Brown/Manager Export Sales
     Mr. J. Greg Perry/Vice President Marketing & Sales
Production: Gerry Lomonaco/Director Manufacturing

Duplicator, X-Ray Film	Radiology
Illuminator, Radiographic Film	Radiology
Mask, X-Ray Shield	Radiology
Radiographic Picture Archiving/Communication System (PACS)	Radiology
Shield, X-Ray	Radiology
Shield, X-Ray, Throat	Radiology
Storage Unit, X-Ray Film	Radiology
Tester, Radiology Quality Assurance	Radiology

AMD-RITMED, INC.   800-445-0340
295 Firetower Road, Tonawanda, NY 14150   716-695-0258

FDA Number: 1319092   *Fax:* 716-695-3827
E-mail: amdsales@amdritmed.com
Web site: www.amdritmed.com
Medical Products Sales Volume: $260,000
Annual Revenue: $10-$25 Million
Total Employees: 2   *Marketing Staff:* 3   *Sales Staff:* 20
Ownership: Private
Quality System Registration Information: ISO9002
Produces/Sells CE-marked Devices: Y
Federal Procurement Eligibility: Small Business, VA Contract
Distribution: Manufacturer Direct, Manufacturer Through Distributor, Manufacturer Through Manufacturer Reps, Service Direct, Importer, Exporter

AMD-RITMED, INC.   800-445-0340 *(cont'd)*
General Admin.: Ms. Tammy Chase/General Manager
    Mr. Ian Levine/President
Mktg./Adv.: Mr. Scott Woolford/Manager National Sales
Production: Luc Trepanier/Director Quality Assurance & Regulatory Affairs

Accessories, Apparel, Surgical	Surgery
Bag, Drainage, Ostomy (With Adhesive)	General
Ball, Cotton	General
Bandage, Gauze	General
Bandage, Other	General
Binder, Perineal	General
Cleaner, Electrosurgical Tip	Surgery
Counter, Sponge, Surgical	Surgery
Gauze, Absorbable	Surgery
Mask, Surgical	Surgery
Packing, Surgical	Surgery
Sponge, Dissector	Pathology
Sponge, Gauze	Dental And Oral
Sponge, Laparotomy	Surgery
Sponge, Neuro	Cns/Neurology
Sponge, Ophthalmic	Ophthalmology
Sponge, Other	General
Sponge, Scrub	Surgery
Swabs, Cotton	General
Towel, Surgical	Surgery
Waste Disposal Unit, Sharps	General

AMDEN CORP.   949-581-9988
2533 North Carson Street, Carson City, NV 89706
FDA Number: 2951277

Floss, Dental	Dental And Oral
Scraper, Tongue	Dental And Oral
Toothbrush, Manual	Dental And Oral
Toothbrush, Powered	Dental And Oral

AMDL, INC.
See Radient Pharmaceuticals

AMED LTD.
See Myoderm

AMEDICA BIOTECH, INC.   888-206-9919
28301 Industrial Blvd Suite K,   510-785-5980
Hayward, CA 94545
FDA Number: 3003897257   *Fax:* 510-785-5973
E-mail: info@amedicabiotech.com
Web site: www.amedicabiotech.com
Ownership: Private
Produces/Sells CE-marked Devices: N

Chromatography, Thin Layer, Tricyclic Antidepressant Drugs	Toxicology
Enzyme Immunoassay, Amphetamine	Toxicology
Enzyme Immunoassay, Barbiturate	Toxicology
Enzyme Immunoassay, Benzodiazepine	Toxicology
Enzyme Immunoassay, Cannabinoids	Toxicology
Enzyme Immunoassay, Cocaine And Cocaine Metabolites	Toxicology
Enzyme Immunoassay, Methadone	Toxicology
Enzyme Immunoassay, Opiates	Toxicology
Enzyme Immunoassay, Phencyclidine	Toxicology
Enzyme Immunoassay, Propoxyphene	Toxicology
Gas Chromatography, Methamphetamine	Toxicology
Thin Layer Chromatography, Metamphetamine	Toxicology

AMEDICA CORPORATION   801-839-3500
1885 West 2100 South, Salt Lake City, UT 84119
FDA Number: 3005032068   *Fax:* 801-839-3605
E-mail: information@amedicacorp.com
Web site: http://www.amedicacorp.com
Ownership: Private
Produces/Sells CE-marked Devices: N
General Admin.: Mr. Ben Shappley/Chief Executive Officer
Mktg./Adv.: Mr. Steve Zeiger/Director Marketing
    Mr. Ken Eakin/Vice President Sales
Production: Mr. Robert Wolfarth/Director Quality Assurance & Product Development
    Mr. Bryan McEntire/Vice President Operations
    Mr. Jonathan Stupka/Vice President Operations
Finance: Mr. Reyn Gallacher/Chief Financial Officer, Vice President Finance

Appliance, Fix., Nail/Blade/Plate Comb., Multiple Component	Orthopedics
Appliance, Fixation, Spinal Interlaminal	Orthopedics
Appliance, Fixation, Spinal Intervertebral Body	Orthopedics
Device, Spinal Vertebral Body Replacement	Orthopedics
Intervertebral Fusion Device With Bone Graft, Cervical	Orthopedics
Orthopedic Manual Surgical Instrument	Orthopedics
Orthosis, Fixation, Pedicle, Spinal	Orthopedics
Orthosis, Pedicle Screw Spinal System, Spondylosis And Facet Degeneration	Orthopedics
Orthosis, Spinal Pedicle Fixation, For Degenerative Disc Disease	Orthopedics

Medical Product Subsidiaries (Listed Separately)
Us Spine Inc.

AMEDITECH, INC.   800-635-2452
10340 Camino Santa Fe, Suite F,   718-352-2981
San Diego, CA 92121
FDA Number: 2032598   *Fax:* 718-352-2984
E-mail: info@ameditech.com
Web site: www.ameditech.com
Ownership: Private
Produces/Sells CE-marked Devices: N

Enzyme Immunoassay, Amphetamine	Toxicology
Enzyme Immunoassay, Cannabinoids	Toxicology
Enzyme Immunoassay, Cocaine And Cocaine Metabolites	Toxicology
Enzyme Immunoassay, Opiates	Toxicology
Enzyme Immunoassay, Phencyclidine	Toxicology
Gas Chromatography, Methamphetamine	Toxicology
Radioimmunoassay, Human Chorionic Gonadotropin	Chemistry

AMEDITECH, INC.
See Freedom Meditech, Inc.

AMELIFE LLC   302-476-2631
702 West Street, Ste 101, Wilmington, DE 19801
FDA Number: 3006791146
E-mail: usasales@ame-life.com
Web site: www.ame-life.com
Ownership: Private
Produces/Sells CE-marked Devices: N

Bed, Hydraulic	General
Light, Surgical Operating, Dental	Dental And Oral
Monitor, Bed Patient	General
Stretcher, Hand-Carried	General
Stretcher, Patient Restraint	General
Stretcher, Wheeled (Mobile)	General
Suction Apparatus, Operating Room, Wall Vacuum-Powered	Surgery
Table, Operating Room, Mechanical	Surgery
Table, Surgical, Electrical	Surgery

AMERCARE PRODUCTS, INC.   425-489-9575
17661 128th Place N.E., Seattle, WA 98165
FDA Number: 3031684   *Fax:* 425-486-3875
E-mail: amercare@worldnet.att.net
Web site: www.amercareproducts.com
Ownership: Private
Produces/Sells CE-marked Devices: N
Federal Procurement Eligibility: Small Business, Minority Owned, Female Owned

Toothbrush, Manual	Dental And Oral

AMERET LLC   913-888-5248
9025 Rosehill, Lenexa, KS 66215
FDA Number: 3006278426

Exerciser, Non-Measuring	Physical Med

AMERICA GREEN DENT., MFG.   323-265-7000
3432 E. 14th St., Commerce, CA 90023
FDA Number: 2086153
Ownership: Private
Produces/Sells CE-marked Devices: N

Metal, Base	Dental And Oral
Scaler, Ultrasonic	Dental And Oral

AMERICA HEARS, INC.   215-788-0330
806 Beaver St., Bristol, PA 19007
FDA Number: 2523532

Hearing-Aid	Ear/Nose/Throat
Hearing-Aid, Plate, Face	Ear/Nose/Throat

AMERICAN AIR FILTER
See Aaf International

AMERICAN ASSOCIATED COMPANIES, INC.   800-849-7060
120 Carnigie Place, Suite 202,   770-719-4330
Fayetteville, GA 30214
FDA Number: n/a   *Fax:* 770-719-7577
E-mail: salesorder@aaco.com
Web site: www.aaco.com
Annual Revenue: $1-$5 Million
Year Founded: 1911
Ownership: Private
Produces/Sells CE-marked Devices: N
Federal Procurement Eligibility: Small Business
Distribution: Manufacturer Direct, Manufacturer Through Distributor, Exclusive Distributor, Importer

Diaper, Adult	General
Pad, Incontinence (Underpad)	General

AMERICAN AUTOCLAVE CO.   800 421 5161
7819 Riverside Drive, Sumner, WA 98390-8104   253-863-5000
FDA Number: n/a   *Fax:* 253-863-1770
E-mail: info@americanautoclave.com
Web site: www.americanautoclave.com
Year Founded: 1968

AMERICAN AUTOCLAVE CO.
800 421 5161 *(cont'd)*

Ownership: Private
Produces/Sells CE-marked Devices: N
Federal Procurement Eligibility: Small Business
Distribution: OEM

Cleaner, Bedpan (Sterilizer)	General
Service, Parts, Repair	General
Service, Used Equipment	General
Service, Waste Management	General
Sterilizer, Laboratory	Microbiology
Sterilizer, Steam (Autoclave)	General
Sterilizer, Steam (Autoclave), Surgical	Surgery
Sterilizer, Vapor	General
Sterilizer/Compactor	General
Washer, Labware	Chemistry
Washer/Sterilizer	General
Waste Disposal Unit, Syringe	General
Waste Receptacle, Contaminated	General

AMERICAN BANTEX CORP.
800-633-4839

1815 Rollins Rd., Burlingame, CA 94010
FDA Number: 2938471   *Fax:* 650-697-3596
E-mail: sales@americanbantex.com
Web site: www.americanbantex.com
Medical Products Sales Volume: $8,000,000
Annual Revenue: $10-$25 Million
Ownership: Private
Quality System Registration Information: ISO9002
Produces/Sells CE-marked Devices: Y
Federal Procurement Eligibility: Small Business
Distribution: Manufacturer Direct, Manufacturer Through Distributor, Manufacturer Through Manufacturer Reps, OEM, Importer, Exporter

Bedpan	General
Commode Seat	General
Counter, Cell	Microbiology
Counter, Colony	Microbiology
Glove, Patient Examination, Latex	General
Kit, Pregnancy Test	Obstetrics/Gynecology
Pump, Alternating Pressure Pad	General
Sphygmomanometer, Electronic, Manual	General
Thermometer, Electronic	General
Wheelchair, Manual	Physical Med

AMERICAN BIDET CO.
877-981-1111
954-981-1111

1801 Polk St # 1500, P.O. Box - # 1500,
Hollywood, FL 33022
FDA Number: n/a   *Fax:* 954-983-3333
E-mail: info@bidet.com
Web site: www.bidet.com
Medical Products Sales Volume: $1,000,000
Annual Revenue: $1-$5 Million
Year Founded: 1964
Ownership: Private
Produces/Sells CE-marked Devices: N
Federal Procurement Eligibility: Small Business
Distribution: Manufacturer Direct, Manufacturer Through Distributor

Commode (Toilet)	General

AMERICAN BIO MEDICA CORP.
800-227-1243
518-758-8158

122 Smith Rd., Kinderhook, NY 12106
FDA Number: 1320738   *Fax:* 518-758-8171
E-mail: info@abmc.com
Web site: http://www.abmc.com
Ownership: Private
Quality System Registration Information: ISO9000
Produces/Sells CE-marked Devices: N
Distribution: Manufacturer Direct, Manufacturer Through Distributor
General Admin.: Mr. Stan Cipkowski/Chief Executive Officer
    Mr. Stefan Parker/Chief Financial Officer, Executive Vice President
    Mr. Martin Gould/Chief Technology Officer, Executive Vice President
    Ms. Melissa Waterhouse/Vice President, Corporate Secretary
Mktg./Adv.: Mr. Todd Bailey/Vice President Marketing & Sales
Production: Mr. Douglas Casterlin/Executive Vice President Operations

Enzyme Immunoassay, Amphetamine	Toxicology
Enzyme Immunoassay, Barbiturate	Toxicology
Enzyme Immunoassay, Benzodiazepine	Toxicology
Enzyme Immunoassay, Cannabinoids	Toxicology
Enzyme Immunoassay, Cocaine And Cocaine Metabolites	Toxicology
Enzyme Immunoassay, Methadone	Toxicology
Enzyme Immunoassay, Opiates	Toxicology
Enzyme Immunoassay, Phencyclidine	Toxicology
Gas Chromatography, Methamphetamine	Toxicology
Radioimmunoassay, Tricyclic Antidepressant Drugs	Toxicology

AMERICAN BIO MEDICA CORP.
800-227-1243
518-758-8158

603 Heron Dr., Unit 3,
Logan Township, NJ 08085
FDA Number: 2249781   *Fax:* 518-758-8171
E-mail: info@abmc.com
Web site: www.abmc.com
Ownership: Private
Produces/Sells CE-marked Devices: N

Antigen, Antiserum, Control, Transferrin	Immunology
Antigen, Antiserum, Control, Transferrin, FITC	Immunology
Antigen, Antiserum, Control, Transferrin, Rhodamine	Immunology
Enzyme Immunoassay, Amphetamine	Toxicology
Enzyme Immunoassay, Barbiturate	Toxicology
Enzyme Immunoassay, Benzodiazepine	Toxicology
Enzyme Immunoassay, Cannabinoids	Toxicology
Enzyme Immunoassay, Cocaine And Cocaine Metabolites	Toxicology
Enzyme Immunoassay, Methadone	Toxicology
Enzyme Immunoassay, Opiates	Toxicology
Enzyme Immunoassay, Phencyclidine	Toxicology
Enzyme Immunoassay, Propoxyphene	Toxicology
Fluorometer	Immunology
Gas Chromatography, Methamphetamine	Toxicology
High Pressure Liquid Chromatography, Barbiturate	Toxicology
Liquid Chromatography, Morphine	Toxicology
Radioimmunoassay, Phencyclidine	Toxicology
Radioimmunoassay, Tricyclic Antidepressant Drugs	Toxicology
Test Paper, Cholinesterase	Toxicology
Thin Layer Chromatography, Metamphetamine	Toxicology
Thin Layer Chromatography, Salicylate	Toxicology

AMERICAN BIO-MEDICAL SERVICE CORPORATION (ABMSC)
800-755-9055

Sales, Service and Refurbishing Center   **909-599-5800**
631 West Covina Blvd.
San Dimas, CA 91773
FDA Number: 3004550027   *Fax:* 909-599-1177
E-mail: salesdept@abmsc.com
Web site: www.abmsc.com/
Medical Products Sales Volume: $3,100,000
Annual Revenue: $1-$5 Million
Year Founded: 1998
Total Employees: 15   *Marketing Staff:* 1   *Sales Staff:* 3
Ownership: Private
Produces/Sells CE-marked Devices: N
Federal Procurement Eligibility: Small Business
Distribution: Service Direct, Exclusive Distributor
General Admin.: Mr. Yale Mizrahi/Chief Executive Officer, Chairman
    Robert C. Atlis/President
Production: Michael E. Altis/Vice President Operations

Analyzer, Patient, Multiple Function (Surgery)	Surgery
Electrosurgical Unit, General Purpose (ESU)	Surgery
Gas-Machine, Anesthesia	Anesthesiology
Light, Other	General
Service, Engineering/Design	General
Sterilizer, Steam (Autoclave)	General
Table, Operating Room, Mechanical	Surgery

AMERICAN BIOCLINICAL INC.
See Oxis International, Inc.

AMERICAN BIOLOGICAL TECHNOLOGIES INC.
See Consolidated Technologies, Inc.

AMERICAN BIOMATERIALS CORP.
See Integra Lifesciences Holdings Corp.

AMERICAN BIOMED INSTRUMENTS, INC.
718-235-8900

11 Wyona St., Brooklyn, NY 11207
FDA Number: n/a   *Fax:* 718-235-8915
E-mail: amebiomed@aol.com
Web site: www.americanbiomed.net
Medical Products Sales Volume: $2,000,000
Annual Revenue: $1-$5 Million
Year Founded: 1978
Ownership: Private
Produces/Sells CE-marked Devices: N
Federal Procurement Eligibility: Small Business, Minority Owned
Distribution: Manufacturer Through Distributor, Manufacturer Through Manufacturer Reps, Importer, Exporter

Bed, Electric	General
Bed, Manual	General
Capacitor, Defibrillator	General
Chair, Dental	Dental And Oral
Concentrator, Oxygen	Anesthesiology
Dental Laboratory Equipment	Dental And Oral
Equipment, Ultrasound, Doppler, Evaluation, Fetal	Obstetrics/Gynecology
Monitor, Bed Patient	General
Monitor, EEG	Cns/Neurology
Sterilizer, Steam (Autoclave)	General
Table, Examination/Treatment	General

AMERICAN BIOMED INSTRUMENTS, INC. 718-235-8900 *(cont'd)*

Ventilator, Continuous (Respirator)	Anesthesiology
Wheelchair, Manual	Physical Med
Wheelchair, Powered	Physical Med

AMERICAN BIOMEDICAL, INC. 918-437-3009
11333 E. Pine St., Suite 60, Tulsa, OK 74116
FDA Number: 1645302
Fax: 918-272-3996
Annual Revenue: $0-$1 Million
Year Founded: 1991
Ownership: Private
Produces/Sells CE-marked Devices: N
Federal Procurement Eligibility: Small Business
Distribution: OEM

Kit, Quality Control	Microbiology

AMERICAN BIONETICS COMPANY
See Biogenex Laboratories

AMERICAN BIOPRODUCTS CO.
See Diagnostica Stago, Inc.

AMERICAN BIOSURGICAL 770-416-1992
1850-B Beaver Ridge Circle, Norcross, GA 30071
FDA Number: 1061133
Fax: 770-416-1946
E-mail: info@americanbiosurgical.com
Web site: www.americanbiosurgical.com
Medical Products Sales Volume: $10,000,000
Annual Revenue: $5-$10 Million
Year Founded: 1995
Total Employees: 10   *Marketing Staff:* 3   *Sales Staff:* 3
Ownership: Private
Quality System Registration Information: ISO9002
Produces/Sells CE-marked Devices: N
Federal Procurement Eligibility: Small Business
Distribution: Manufacturer Direct, Manufacturer Through Distributor, OEM
General Admin.: Michael Socoloff/President, Chief Executive Officer

Cable, Electric	General
Electrosurgical Unit, Cutting & Coagulation Device	Surgery

AMERICAN BREAST CARE LP 770-933-3444
2150 Newmarket Pkwy, Suite 112, Marietta, GA 30067
FDA Number: 3004134970
E-mail: info@americanbreastcare.com
Web site: www.americanbreastcare.com
Ownership: Private
Produces/Sells CE-marked Devices: N

Prosthesis, Breast, External, No Adhesive	Surgery

AMERICAN CATHETER CORP. 800-345-6714
     352-245-4816
13047 S. Hwy 475, Ocala, FL 34480
FDA Number: 1000151187
Fax: 352-347-6532
E-mail: americancatheter@earthlink.net
Web site: www.internationalmedical.com
Year Founded: 1986
Total Employees: 35
Ownership: International Medical, Inc.
Produces/Sells CE-marked Devices: N
Distribution: Manufacturer Direct, Manufacturer Through Distributor, Manufacturer Through Manufacturer Reps, OEM, Exporter
General Admin.: Peter Wettermann/Chief Executive Officer
     Paul A. Duddy/General Manager

Brush, Cytology	General
Catheter, Cholangiography	Surgery
Catheter, Suction, With Tip	General
Electrode, Other	General
Equipment, Suction/Irrigation, Laparoscopic	Surgery
Forceps, Biopsy	Surgery
Forceps, Biopsy, Bronchoscope (Rigid)	Anesthesiology
Irrigator, Suction	General
Monitor, Pressure, Intrauterine	Obstetrics/Gynecology
Snare, Polyp	Surgery

AMERICAN COIL SPRING CO. 231-726-4021
1041 E. Keating Avenue, Muskegon, MI 49442-5996
FDA Number: 1824197
Fax: 231-726-2206
E-mail: info@americancoil.com
Web site: www.americancoil.com
Medical Products Sales Volume: $7,500,000
Annual Revenue: $10-$25 Million
Year Founded: 1923
Total Employees: 100   *Marketing Staff:* 1   *Sales Staff:* 5
Ownership: Private
Quality System Registration Information: ISO9002
Produces/Sells CE-marked Devices: N
Federal Procurement Eligibility: Small Business
Distribution: Manufacturer Direct
General Admin.: Ms. Sherry White/Director Human Resources
Mktg./Adv.: Mr. Mike Hosko/Manager International & National Sales
     Mr. Tim Zwit/Vice President Sales

AMERICAN COIL SPRING CO. 231-726-4021 *(cont'd)*
Production: Ms. Annette Ream/Customer Service Representative
     Ms. Rhonda Paterra/Director Quality Assurance
     Mr. John Lundholm/Vice President Manufacturing & Engineering

Component, Metal, Other	General

AMERICAN COMB CORP. 973-523-6551
22 Kentucky Ave., Paterson, NJ 07503
FDA Number: 2248574

Detector/Remover, Lice	General

AMERICAN CONTACT LENS INC. 858-487-8684
15970 Bernardo Center Drive, San Diego, CA 92127
FDA Number: 2030467
Fax: 800-959-4448
E-mail: info@americancontactlens.com
Web site: www.biocurve.com
Medical Products Sales Volume: $670,000
Total Employees: 8
Ownership: Private
Produces/Sells CE-marked Devices: N
Federal Procurement Eligibility: Small Business

Lens, Contact (Other Material)	Ophthalmology

AMERICAN CONTAINER TECHNOLOGIES, INC.
See Medin Corporation

AMERICAN COPAK CORP. 818-576-1000
9175 Eton Ave., Chatsworth, CA 91311
FDA Number: n/a
Fax: 818-882-1637
E-mail: sales@americancopak.com
Web site: www.americancopak.com
Annual Revenue: $1-$5 Million
Ownership: Private
Produces/Sells CE-marked Devices: N
Federal Procurement Eligibility: Small Business
Distribution: Manufacturer Direct

Contract Packaging	General

AMERICAN DENT-ALL INC. 877-864-6294
     818-662-0618
5140 San Fernando Road, Glendale, CA 91204
FDA Number: 2031991
Fax: 818-662-0619
E-mail: info@dentall.us
Web site: www.dentall.us
Medical Products Sales Volume: $1,000,000
Annual Revenue: $0-$1 Million
Year Founded: 1996
Total Employees: 5
Ownership: Private
Quality System Registration Information: ISO9000
Produces/Sells CE-marked Devices: Y
Federal Procurement Eligibility: Small Business
Distribution: Manufacturer Direct, Importer, Exporter
Mktg./Adv.: Mr. Varoush Hacopians/General Manager, Manager International Marketing and Sales

Metal, Base	Dental And Oral

AMERICAN DENTAL CENTER OF PROVO 801-375-8200
777 North 500 West, Ste. 201b, Provo, UT 84601
FDA Number: n/a
Ownership: Private
Produces/Sells CE-marked Devices: N

Crown, Preformed	Dental And Oral
Denture, Plastic, Teeth	Dental And Oral

AMERICAN DENTAL DESIGNS INC. 215-643-3232
717 Bethlehem Pike, Montgomery ville, PA 18936
FDA Number: 3005713604
Fax: 215-646-3832
E-mail: amedentaldesi@comcast.net
Web site: www.americandentaldesigns.com
Ownership: Private
Produces/Sells CE-marked Devices: N

Alloy, Precious Metal, For Clinical Use	Dental And Oral
Articulators	Dental And Oral
Denture, Plastic, Teeth	Dental And Oral
Teeth, Porcelain	Dental And Oral

AMERICAN DENTAL PRODUCTS, INC. 800-846-7120
603-b Country Club Dr., Bensenville, IL 60106-1329
FDA Number: 1424367
Ownership: Private
Produces/Sells CE-marked Devices: N

Adhesive, Bracket And Conditioner, Resin	Dental And Oral
Base, Denture, Relining, Repairing, Rebasing, Resin	Dental And Oral
Cement, Dental	Dental And Oral
Detector, Caries	Dental And Oral
Material, Impression	Dental And Oral
Material, Tooth Shade, Resin	Dental And Oral
Sealant, Pit And Fissure, And Conditioner, Resin	Dental And Oral
Tooth Bonding Agent, Resin Restoration	Dental And Oral

AMERICAN DENTAL SUPPLY, INC.
800-558-5925
610-252-1464
1075 N. Gilmore Street,
Allentown, PA 18109
FDA Number: n/a   *Fax:* 610-252-2822
E-mail: custserv@americandentalsupply.net
Web site: www.americandentalinc.com
Ownership: Life Guard
Produces/Sells CE-marked Devices: Y
Federal Procurement Eligibility: Small Business, Female Owned
Distribution: Manufacturer Through Distributor
General Admin.: Pat McAuliffe/General Manager
    Les Hochhauser/Vice President
Mktg./Adv.: Julie Hochhauser/Director Marketing
    Bobbi Cesari/Sales Manager
    Julie Borger/Sales Representative
Dental Laboratory Equipment   Dental And Oral

AMERICAN DIAGNOSTIC CORPORATION (ADC)
800-232-2670
631-273-9600
55 Commerce Dr., Hauppauge, NY 11788
FDA Number: n/a   *Fax:* 631-273-9659
E-mail: info@adctoday.com
Web site: www.adctoday.com
Year Founded: 1984
Total Employees: 150   *Marketing Staff:* 2   *Sales Staff:* 55
Ownership: Private
Produces/Sells CE-marked Devices: Y
Federal Procurement Eligibility: Small Business
Distribution: Manufacturer Through Distributor
General Admin.: Mr. Andrew Galambos/Manager Human Resources
    Marc Blitstein/President
Mktg./Adv.: Mr. Peter Cirino/Director Creative Services
    Mr. Steve Kelly/Manager National Sales
Production: Mr. Mike Falco/Head Quality Assurance

Bulb, Inflation	General
Cover, Thermometer	General
Device, Assist, CPR	Anesthesiology
Hammer, Percussion	Cns/Neurology
Lamp, Other	General
Laryngoscope	Ear/Nose/Throat
Ophthalmoscope, Direct	Ophthalmology
Otoscope	Ear/Nose/Throat
Penlight, Battery-Powered	Ophthalmology
Sphygmomanometer, Aneroid (Arterial Pressure)	General
Sphygmomanometer, Electronic, Automatic	General
Sphygmomanometer, Electronic, Manual	General
Sphygmomanometer, Mercury (Arterial Pressure)	General
Stethoscope, Manual	Cardiovascular
Thermometer, Electronic	General
Tourniquet	General

AMERICAN DIAGNOSTIC MEDICINE, INC.
800-262-9645
630-834-7100
960 Industrial Drive, Suite 7, Elmhurst, IL 60126
FDA Number: n/a   *Fax:* 630-834-7115
E-mail: schroeder@admaccess.com
Web site: www.admaccess.com
Medical Products Sales Volume: $14,300,000
Annual Revenue: $25-$50 Million
Year Founded: 1984
Total Employees: 100   *Marketing Staff:* 1   *Sales Staff:* 5
Ownership: Private
Produces/Sells CE-marked Devices: N
Federal Procurement Eligibility: Small Business
Distribution: Manufacturer Direct
General Admin.: Christopher Richard/President
Mktg./Adv.: Andrea Schroeder/Admin. Sales
Camera, Multi-Image   Radiology

AMERICAN DIAGNOSTICA, INC.
888-234-4435
203-602-7777
500 West Avenue, Stamford, CT 06902-6360
FDA Number: 1220602   *Fax:* 203-602-2221
E-mail: sales@amdiag.com
Web site: www.americandiagnostica.com
Medical Products Sales Volume: $6,500,000
Annual Revenue: $5-$10 Million
Year Founded: 1982
Total Employees: 35   *Marketing Staff:* 5   *Sales Staff:* 2
Ownership: Private
Produces/Sells CE-marked Devices: N
Federal Procurement Eligibility: Small Business, Female Owned
Distribution: Manufacturer Direct
General Admin.: Richard Hart/President

Antibody, Monoclonal	Microbiology
Antigen, Antiserum, Control, Other	Immunology
Control, Coagulation, Plasma	Hematology
Enzyme Immunoassay, Other	Chemistry
Immunoassay, Other	Toxicology
Kit, Breast Cancer Detection	Obstetrics/Gynecology
Reagent, Russel Viper Venom	Hematology

AMERICAN DIAGNOSTICA, INC.
888-234-4435 *(cont'd)*

Test, Cancer Detection, Other	Hematology
Whole Blood Hemoglobin Determination	Hematology

AMERICAN DISPOSABLES, INC.
413-967-6201
6 East Main St., Ware, MA 01082
FDA Number: n/a
Ownership: Private
Produces/Sells CE-marked Devices: N
Garment, Protective, For Incontinence   Gastroenterology/Urology

AMERICAN DIVERSIFIED DENTAL SYSTEMS
800-637-2330
949-330-0140
22991 La Cadena Drive,
Laguna Hills, CA 92653
FDA Number: n/a   *Fax:* 949-330-0145
E-mail: info@mdsadds.com
Web site: www.mdsadds.com
Year Founded: 1975
Total Employees: 25
Ownership: Mds Products, Inc.
Produces/Sells CE-marked Devices: N
Federal Procurement Eligibility: Small Business
Distribution: Manufacturer Direct, Manufacturer Through Distributor

Adhesive, Dental	Dental And Oral
Airbrush	Dental And Oral
Articulators	Dental And Oral
Crown, Preformed	Dental And Oral
Dental Laboratory Equipment	Dental And Oral
Disk, Abrasive	Dental And Oral
Mask, Analgesia	Dental And Oral
Resinous Compound	Dental And Oral
Ring, Dental (Casting)	Dental And Oral
Solution, Cement Dissolving	Dental And Oral
Wax, Dental	Dental And Oral

AMERICAN DRYER CORP.
508-678-9000
88 Currant Road, Fall River, MA 02720-4781
FDA Number: n/a   *Fax:* 508-678-9447
E-mail: sales@amdry.com
Web site: www.amdry.com
Medical Products Sales Volume: $21,800,000
Year Founded: 1965
Total Employees: 280   *Marketing Staff:* 3   *Sales Staff:* 7
Ownership: Private
Quality System Registration Information: ISO9000
Produces/Sells CE-marked Devices: N
Federal Procurement Eligibility: Small Business, GSA Contract
Distribution: Manufacturer Through Distributor, OEM, Exclusive Distributor
General Admin.: Dennis Slutsky/President
Mktg./Adv.: Mauricio Lima/Manager International Marketing & Sales
    Tony Regan/Vice President Sales
Laundry Equipment   General

AMERICAN DRYER, INC.
800-485-7003
734-421-2400
12932 Farmington Road, Livonia, MI 48150-4201
FDA Number: n/a   *Fax:* 734-421-5580
E-mail: sales@americandryer.com
Web site: www.americandryer.com
Medical Products Sales Volume: $1,900,000
Annual Revenue: $1-$5 Million
Year Founded: 1952
Total Employees: 12   *Marketing Staff:* 1   *Sales Staff:* 1
Ownership: Private
Produces/Sells CE-marked Devices: N
Federal Procurement Eligibility: Small Business, GSA Contract
Distribution: Manufacturer Direct, Manufacturer Through Distributor, Manufacturer Through Manufacturer Reps
General Admin.: Daniel L. Rabahy/President, Chief Executive Officer
Mktg./Adv.: Susan R. Ebbing/Manager International & National Sales
Drying Unit   Chemistry

AMERICAN EAGLE INSTRUMENTS, INC.
800-551-5172
406-549-7451
6575 Butler Creek Rd., Missoula, MT 59808
FDA Number: 3027615   *Fax:* 406-549-7452
E-mail: customerservice@am-eagle.com
Web site: www.am-eagle.com
Ownership: Private
Produces/Sells CE-marked Devices: N

Band, Elastic, Orthodontic	Dental And Oral
Carver, Dental Amalgam, Operative	Dental And Oral
Carver, Wax, Dental	Dental And Oral
Cleaner, Ultrasonic, Medical Instrument	General
Curette, Periodontic	Dental And Oral
Handle, Instrument, Dental	Dental And Oral
Instrument, Manual, General Surgical	Surgery
Mirror, Mouth	Dental And Oral
Plugger, Root Canal, Endodontic	Dental And Oral
Preparer, Root Canal, Endodontic	Dental And Oral
Remover, Crown	Dental And Oral

AMERICAN EAGLE INSTRUMENTS, INC.   800-551-5172 *(cont'd)*
Retractor, All Types   Dental And Oral
Scaler, Ultrasonic   Dental And Oral

AMERICAN ECHO, INC.
See Medical Positioning, Inc.

AMERICAN ELECTROMEDICS CORP.
See Maico Diagnostics

AMERICAN EMERGENCY VEHICLES   800-374-9749
165 American Way, Jefferson, NC 28640   **336-982-9824**
FDA Number: n/a   Fax: 336-982-9826
E-mail: info@aev.com
Web site: www.aev.com
Annual Revenue: $50-$100 Million
Total Employees: 300   *Marketing Staff:* 8   *Sales Staff:* 8
Ownership: Private
Produces/Sells CE-marked Devices: N
Federal Procurement Eligibility: Small Business
Distribution: Manufacturer Through Distributor
General Admin.: Mark S. Van Arnam/President, Chief Executive Officer
Mktg./Adv.: Jeff Dreyer/Manager Product Development
Production: Vicki Sansbury/Coord. Production
     Steve Dillard/Manager Materials
     Randy Hanson/Vice President Manufacturing
Ambulance   General
Wheelchair, Standup   Physical Med

AMERICAN EXCELSIOR CO.   800-777-7645
850 Ave. H East, Arlington, TX 76011   **817-640-1555**
FDA Number: n/a   Fax: 817-640-3570
E-mail: marketing66@earthlink.net
Web site: www.amerexcel.com
Total Employees: 800   *Marketing Staff:* 2   *Sales Staff:* 50
Ownership: Private
Produces/Sells CE-marked Devices: N
Distribution: Manufacturer Direct
General Admin.: R. L. Gregenson/President, Chief Executive Officer
Mktg./Adv.: K. E. Starrett/Director Marketing
     Emilio Zusizarreta/Director Product Development
     Ray Clymore/Manager Contract Sales
     Paul Finazzo/Vice President Sales
Production: John Martin/Director Quality Assurance
Packaging Equipment   General

AMERICAN FIBER & FINISHING, INC.   800-522-2438
Po Box 2488, Albemarle, NC 28002   **704-983-6102**
FDA Number: 1221254   Fax: 704-985-1352
E-mail: sales@affinc.com
Web site: affinc.com
Year Founded: 1986
Total Employees: 175   *Sales Staff:* 5
Ownership: Private
Produces/Sells CE-marked Devices: N
Federal Procurement Eligibility: Small Business
Production: Mr. Larry Hatley/Quality Control, Product Engineer
Applicator, Tipped, Absorbent, Non-Sterile   General
Fiber, Absorbent   General
Sponge, External   Surgery

AMERICAN FLUOROSEAL CORP.   800-360-1050
431-A East Diamond Avenue,   **301-990-1407**
Gaithersburg, MD 20877
FDA Number: 1122024   Fax: 301-990-1472
E-mail: info@americanfluoroseal.com
Web site: www.americanfluoroseal.com
Medical Products Sales Volume: $1,400,000
Year Founded: 1986
Total Employees: 6
Ownership: Private
Produces/Sells CE-marked Devices: Y
Federal Procurement Eligibility: Small Business
Distribution: Manufacturer Direct
General Admin.: Toni L. Wade/Administrator
     Herb Cullis/President, Chief Executive Officer
     Kerry E. English/Vice President
Production: Jean. Broussard/Manager Manufacturing
Bag, Plastic   General
Container, Cryobiological Storage   Microbiology
Contract Manufacturing   General

AMERICAN GAS & CHEMICAL CO., LTD.   800-288-3647
220 Pegasus Ave., Northvale, NJ 07647-1904   **201-767-7300**
FDA Number: n/a   Fax: 201-767-1741
E-mail: contact@amgas.com
Web site: www.amgas.com
Annual Revenue: $5-$10 Million
Total Employees: 30   *Marketing Staff:* 2   *Sales Staff:* 8

AMERICAN GAS & CHEMICAL CO., LTD.   800-288-3647 *(cont'd)*
Ownership: Private
Quality System Registration Information: ISO9000
Produces/Sells CE-marked Devices: N
Federal Procurement Eligibility: Small Business
Distribution: Manufacturer Direct, Manufacturer Through Distributor
General Admin.: G. Anderson/Chief Executive Officer
Mktg./Adv.: M. Kershaw/Manager Marketing
Production: S. Bruce/Manager Production
Detector, Ethylene-Oxide Leakage   General
Monitor, Gas, Atmospheric, Environmental   General

AMERICAN HAIR REMOVAL SYSTEM, INC.   800-446-2477
42320 Cr 653, Paw Paw, MI 49079   **269-655-0005**
FDA Number: 1067004   Fax: 269-655-0005
E-mail: web22@americanhairremovalsystem.com
Web site: www.americanhairremovalsystem.com
Year Founded: 1980
Ownership: Private
Produces/Sells CE-marked Devices: Y
Federal Procurement Eligibility: Small Business
Distribution: Manufacturer Direct
Epilator, High-Frequency, Tweezer Type   Surgery

AMERICAN HAND PROSTHETICS, INC.   212-213-3700
73 Skillman Ave., Brooklyn, NY 11211
FDA Number: 3005193502
Ownership: Private
Produces/Sells CE-marked Devices: N
Prosthesis Alignment Device   Physical Med

AMERICAN HEALTH CARE APPAREL LTD.   800-252-0584
302 Town Center Blvd., Easton, PA 18040   **610-250-0584**
FDA Number: n/a   Fax: 800-262-0584
E-mail: american@enter.net
Web site: www.clothesforseniors.com
Annual Revenue: $1-$5 Million
Year Founded: 1985
Total Employees: 40   *Sales Staff:* 25
Ownership: Private
Produces/Sells CE-marked Devices: N
Federal Procurement Eligibility: Small Business
Distribution: Exclusive Distributor
General Admin.: Howard Gordon/President, Chief Executive Officer
     Joseph Zelienka/Vice President, General Manager
Accessories, Apparel, Surgical   Surgery
Gown, Patient   Surgery

AMERICAN HEALTH CARE SYSTEMS, INC.   504-831-4867
3350 Ridgelake Ave., Suite 255, Metairie, LA 70002
FDA Number: 2319391
Ownership: Private
Produces/Sells CE-marked Devices: N
Hemoperfusion System, Sorbent   Gastroenterology/Urology

AMERICAN HEALTH MONITORING, INC.
See Pioneer Medical Systems

AMERICAN HEALTH PRODUCTS CORPORATION
See American Health Products Corporation

AMERICAN HEALTH SYSTEMS   800-234-6655
PO Box 26688, Greenville, SC 29616-1688   **864-234-0496**
FDA Number: n/a   Fax: 864-234-0499
E-mail: cs@4ultraform.com
Web site: www.4ultraform.com
Annual Revenue: $5-$10 Million
Year Founded: 1989
Ownership: Private
Produces/Sells CE-marked Devices: N
Federal Procurement Eligibility: Small Business, Minority Owned, Female Owned
Distribution: Manufacturer Direct, Manufacturer Through Distributor, OEM
General Admin.: Don Bolt/Chief Executive Officer
     Tammy Yeargin/Vice President
Cover, Mattress   General
Cushion, Wheelchair (Pad)   Physical Med
Mattress, Bed   General
Mattress, Reduction, Pressure   General
Pad, Pressure, Foam Convoluted   General

AMERICAN HEALTHCARE   888-567-7733
6 Lincoln Avenue, Scarborough, ME 04074
FDA Number: 1225594   Fax: 207-883-8224
Web site: www.americanhealthcareinc.com
Year Founded: 1997
Ownership: Private
Produces/Sells CE-marked Devices: N
Federal Procurement Eligibility: Small Business
Distribution: Manufacturer Direct, Manufacturer Through Distributor, OEM
General Admin.: Jeffrey R. Lord/President

AMERICAN HEALTHCARE — 888-567-7733 (cont'd)
Regulator, Oxygen, Mechanical — General
Regulator, Pressure, Gas Cylinder — Anesthesiology

AMERICAN HEALTHCARE PRODUCTS, INC. — 888-784-1888 / 626-588-2788
1068 Westminster Avenue,
Alhambra, CA 91803
FDA Number: 2084709 — Fax: 626-588-2089
E-mail: sales@uniseal.net
Web site: www.uniseal.net
Medical Products Sales Volume: $5,500,000
Annual Revenue: $10-$25 Million
Year Founded: 1991
Total Employees: 25 — Marketing Staff: 3 — Sales Staff: 12
Ownership: Private
Quality System Registration Information: ISO9001; ISO9002
Produces/Sells CE-marked Devices: Y
Federal Procurement Eligibility: Small Business, Minority Owned
Distribution: Manufacturer Direct, Manufacturer Through Distributor, Manufacturer Through Manufacturer Reps, OEM, Service Direct, Importer
General Admin.: Tony Djie/President
Glove, Patient Examination, Latex — General

AMERICAN HEARING LABORATORY — 972-394-4370
3740 Josey Lane, Suite 125, Carrollton, TX 75007
FDA Number: 1644066
Hearing-Aid — Ear/Nose/Throat

AMERICAN HEARING SYSTEMS INC. — 763-404-1122
8001 East Bloomington Freeway, Bloomington, MN 55420
FDA Number: 2132742
Ownership: Private
Produces/Sells CE-marked Devices: N
Hearing-Aid — Ear/Nose/Throat
Hearing-Aid, Plate, Face — Ear/Nose/Throat

AMERICAN HOLOGRAPHIC, INC.
See Headwall Photonics, Inc.

AMERICAN HOME PATIENT CENTER, INC.
See American Homepatient

AMERICAN HOME PRODUCTS CORPORATION
See Pfizer / Wyeth Consumer Healthcare Inc.

AMERICAN HOMEPATIENT — 800-890-7271
5200 Maryland Way, Suite 400, Brentwood, TN 37027
FDA Number: n/a
Web site: www.ahom.com
Annual Revenue: $0-$1 Million
Ownership: Private
Quality System Registration Information: ISO9000
Produces/Sells CE-marked Devices: N
Distribution: Exclusive Distributor
Bed, Adjustable Hospital — General
Concentrator, Oxygen — Anesthesiology
Service, Consulting — General
Tube, Feeding — General
Wheelchair, Powered — Physical Med

AMERICAN IMEX — 800-521-8286 / 949-553-8885
16520 Aston St., Irvine, CA 92606
FDA Number: 2083018 — Fax: 949-852-1245
E-mail: info@americanimex.com
Web site: www.americanimex.com
Medical Products Sales Volume: $1,300,000
Annual Revenue: $1-$5 Million
Year Founded: 1984
Total Employees: 15 — Marketing Staff: 4 — Sales Staff: 51
Ownership: Private
Quality System Registration Information: ISO9000; ISO9001; ISO9002; ISO9003
Produces/Sells CE-marked Devices: Y
Federal Procurement Eligibility: Small Business, Minority Owned, Female Owned, VA Contract
Distribution: Manufacturer Direct, Manufacturer Through Distributor, Manufacturer Through Manufacturer Reps, OEM, Exclusive Distributor, Importer, Exporter
General Admin.: Joan F. Fong/President, Chief Executive Officer
Mktg./Adv.: Alex Fong/Director Marketing & Advertising
　　　　　Alex Fong/Manager Contracts
　　　　　Joe Fong/Manager International & National Sales
　　　　　John Schwartz/Manager Sales
　　　　　Joe Fong/Vice President Marketing & Sales
Production: Alex Fong/Manager Regulatory Affairs
Research: Joe Fong/Vice President Research & Development
Biofeedback Device — Cns/Neurology
Electrode, Neuromuscular Stimulator — Cns/Neurology
Exerciser, Other — Physical Med
Perineometer — Obstetrics/Gynecology
Stimulator, Muscle, Electrical-Powered (EMS) — Physical Med
Stimulator, Nerve, Transcutaneous (Pain Relief, TENS) — Cns/Neurology

AMERICAN IMEX — 800-521-8286 (cont'd)
Stimulator, Neuromuscular, External Functional — Cns/Neurology

AMERICAN INNOTEK, INC. — 800-366-3941 / 760-741-6600
2320 Meyers Ave., Escondido, CA 92029
FDA Number: 2031866 — Fax: 760-741-6622
E-mail: info@americaninnotek.com
Web site: www.americaninnotek.com
Ownership: Private
Produces/Sells CE-marked Devices: N
Bag, Leg — Gastroenterology/Urology

AMERICAN INNOVATIONS, INC. — 800-223-3913 / 215-249-1840
123 N. Main St., Dublin, PA 18917-2107
FDA Number: n/a — Fax: 215-249-1842
E-mail: sales@amer-innov.com
Web site: www.amer-innov.com
Medical Products Sales Volume: $700,000
Year Founded: 1991
Total Employees: 7 — Marketing Staff: 3 — Sales Staff: 3
Ownership: Private
Produces/Sells CE-marked Devices: N
Federal Procurement Eligibility: Small Business, GSA Contract
Distribution: Manufacturer Direct, Manufacturer Through Distributor, Manufacturer Through Manufacturer Reps, Service Direct
General Admin.: Karl J. Douglass/President, Chief Executive Officer
Mktg./Adv.: Kelly Pagnani/Manager International & National Sales
Production: Scott Pruyn/Vice President Manufacturing
Accessories, Cart, Multipurpose — General
Accessories, Walker — General
Accessories, Wheelchair — Physical Med
Bedrail — General
Crutch — Physical Med
Walker, Mechanical — Physical Med

AMERICAN INSTRUMENT CO.
See Thermo Spectronic

AMERICAN INTERNATIONAL
See Aimes Medical Equipment Rental & Props

AMERICAN INTERNATIONAL CHEMICAL — 800-238-0001 / 508-270-1800
135 Newbury St, Framingham, MA 01701
FDA Number: n/a — Fax: 508-872-1566
E-mail: info@aicma.com
Web site: www.aicma.com
Annual Revenue: $0-$1 Million
Ownership: Private
Quality System Registration Information: ISO9002
Produces/Sells CE-marked Devices: N
Federal Procurement Eligibility: Small Business
Distribution: Manufacturer Through Distributor, Exclusive Distributor
Antigen, Antiserum, Control, Albumin — Immunology

AMERICAN INTERNATIONAL MEDICAL SUPPLY CO
See Aimsco, Delta Hi-Tech, Inc.

AMERICAN LABOR — 800-424-0443 / 919-286-0726
3329 Durham-Chapel Hill Blvd, Suite 200,
Durham, NC 27715
FDA Number: 1036547 — Fax: 919-286-3956
E-mail: operations@americanlabor.org
Web site: www.americanlabor.org
Medical Products Sales Volume: $1,200,000
Annual Revenue: $1-$5 Million
Year Founded: 1984
Total Employees: 6 — Marketing Staff: 1 — Sales Staff: 2
Ownership: Private
Quality System Registration Information: ISO9001
Produces/Sells CE-marked Devices: Y
Federal Procurement Eligibility: Small Business
Distribution: Manufacturer Direct, Manufacturer Through Distributor, Manufacturer Through Manufacturer Reps, OEM, Service Direct, Exclusive Distributor, Importer, Exporter
General Admin.: Michael W. Shiflett/President, Chief Executive Officer
Aggregometer, Platelet, Thrombokinetogram — Hematology
Analyzer, Coagulation — Hematology
Analyzer, Coagulation, Automated — Hematology
Analyzer, Coagulation, Manual — Hematology

AMERICAN LABORATORIES, INC. — 402-339-2494
4410 South 102nd Street, Omaha, NE 68127
FDA Number: n/a — Fax: 402-339-0801
E-mail: info@americanlaboratories.com
Web site: www.americanlaboratories.com
Medical Products Sales Volume: $8,000,000
Annual Revenue: $10-$25 Million
Year Founded: 1967
Ownership: Private
Produces/Sells CE-marked Devices: N

AMERICAN LABORATORIES, INC. 402-339-2494 (cont'd)
Federal Procurement Eligibility: Small Business
Distribution: Manufacturer Direct, Manufacturer Through Distributor
General Admin.: Kenny Soejoto/Chief Operating Officer
Jeff Jackson/President, Chief Executive Officer
Janet Giwoyna/Vice President Admin.
Mktg./Adv.: Rod Schake/Vice President Sales
Production: Vern Maly/Vice President Production
Thomas Langdon/Vice President Quality Assurance
Allen Asherin/Vice President Regulatory Affairs

Contract Manufacturing, Pharmaceuticals/Chemicals	General
Culture Media, General Nutrient Broth	Microbiology
Hemoglobin	Cardiovascular
Lipase-Esterase, Enzymatic, Photometric, Lipase	Chemistry

AMERICAN LABORATORY PRODUCTS CO. 800-592-5726
26-G Keewaydin Drive, Salem, NH 03079 603-893-8914
FDA Number: 1222302 *Fax:* 603-898-6854
E-mail: cs@alpco.com
Web site: www.alpco.com
Annual Revenue: $1-$5 Million
Year Founded: 1990
Ownership: Private
Produces/Sells CE-marked Devices: N
Federal Procurement Eligibility: Small Business, Female Owned
Distribution: Exclusive Distributor, Importer

Analyzer, Chemistry, ELISA	Chemistry
Anti-DNA Antibody (Enzyme-Labeled), Antigen, Control	Immunology
Enzyme Linked Immunoabsorbent Assay, Rubella	Microbiology
Extractable Antinuclear Antibody (Rnp/Sm), Antigen/Control	Immunology
Radioassay, Angiotensin Converting Enzyme	Chemistry
Radioimmunoassay, ACTH	Chemistry
Radioimmunoassay, Angiotensin I And Renin	Chemistry
Radioimmunoassay, Vitamin B12	Chemistry
Test, Thyroid Autoantibody	Immunology

AMERICAN LASERS, INC. 626-300-9330
300 East Main St., Alhambra, CA 91801
FDA Number: 3005515823

Laser, Surgical	Surgery

AMERICAN MAMMOGRAPHICS, INC. 800-626-4301
5113 Highway 58, Suite 321, 423-624-9530
Chattanooga, TN 37416
FDA Number: 1054188 *Fax:* 423-893-0156
E-mail: mammospot@aol.com
Web site: www.americanmammographics.com
Ownership: Private
Produces/Sells CE-marked Devices: N

Radiographic Unit, Diagnostic, Mammographic	Radiology

AMERICAN MASSAGE PRODUCTS, INC. 716-934-2648
341 Central Ave., Silver Creek, NY 14136
FDA Number: 1310651
Ownership: Private
Produces/Sells CE-marked Devices: N

Chair, Adjustable, Mechanical	Physical Med
Chair, Blood Donor	General
Massager, Therapeutic	Physical Med

AMERICAN MASTERTECH SCIENTIFIC, INC. 209-368-4031
1330 Thurman St., Lodi, CA 95240
FDA Number: 2939235

Adhesive, Albumin Based	Pathology
Agent, Chelating, Decalcification	Pathology
Aniline Acid Fuchsin	Pathology
Clearing Agent	Pathology
Diastase	Pathology
Fixative, Acid Containing	Pathology
Fixative, Alcohol Containing	Pathology
Fixative, Formalin Containing	Pathology
Fixative, Metallic Containing	Pathology
Fluid, Bouin's	Pathology
Formaldehyde (Formalin, Formol)	Pathology
Formalin, Neutral Buffered	Pathology
Fuchsin, Basic	Pathology
Gelatin For Specimen Adhesion	Pathology
Hematoxylin Weigert's	Pathology
Iron Chloride-Weigert	Pathology
Media, Mounting	Pathology
Mercuric Chloride Formulations For Tissue	Pathology
Muller's Colloidal Iron	Pathology
Paraffin, All Formulations	Pathology
Periodic Acid	Pathology
Preservative, Cytological	Pathology
Slide, Microscope	Pathology
Solution, Pathology, Carnoy's	Pathology
Solution, Pathology, Decalcifier, Acid Containing	Pathology
Solution, Pathology, Zenker's	Pathology
Stain, Acid Fuchsin	Pathology

AMERICAN MASTERTECH SCIENTIFIC, INC. 209-368-4031
(cont'd)

Stain, Alcian Blue	Pathology
Stain, Aldehyde Fuchsin	Pathology
Stain, Alizarin Red	Pathology
Stain, Ammoniacal Silver Hydroxide Silver Nitrate	Pathology
Stain, Aniline Blue	Pathology
Stain, Biebrich Scarlet	Pathology
Stain, Bismarck Brown Y	Pathology
Stain, Carbol Fuchsin	Pathology
Stain, Carmine	Pathology
Stain, Congo Red	Pathology
Stain, Cresyl Violet Acetate	Pathology
Stain, Crystal Violet, Histology	Pathology
Stain, Dye Solution	Pathology
Stain, Eosin Y	Pathology
Stain, Fast Green	Pathology
Stain, Giemsa	Pathology
Stain, Gold Chloride	Pathology
Stain, Grams Iodine	Pathology
Stain, Hematoxylin	Pathology
Stain, Hematoxylin, Harris's	Pathology
Stain, Hematoxylin, Mayer's	Pathology
Stain, Iron	Pathology
Stain, Jenner Stain	Pathology
Stain, Light Green	Pathology
Stain, Luxol Fast Blue	Pathology
Stain, Malachite Green	Pathology
Stain, Metanil Yellow	Pathology
Stain, Methenamine Silver	Pathology
Stain, Methyl Green	Pathology
Stain, Methylene Blue	Pathology
Stain, Mucicarmine	Pathology
Stain, Papanicolau	Pathology
Stain, Reagent, Schiff	Pathology
Stain, Weigert's Iron Hematoxylin	Pathology

AMERICAN MEDICAL & DENTAL CORP.
See Acteon Inc.

AMERICAN MEDICAL ALERT CORP. 800-286-2622
3265 Lawson Blvd., Oceanside, NY 11572 516-536-5850
FDA Number: 3008846626 *Fax:* 516-536-5276
E-mail: info@amac.com
Web site: www.amac.com
Medical Products Sales Volume: $30,800,000
Annual Revenue: $25-$50 Million
Year Founded: 1981
Total Employees: 52 *Marketing Staff:* 5 *Sales Staff:* 11
Ownership: Public
Stock Symbol: AMAC
Traded On: NASDAQ
Produces/Sells CE-marked Devices: Y
Federal Procurement Eligibility: Small Business
Distribution: Manufacturer Direct, Manufacturer Through Distributor, Manufacturer Through Manufacturer Reps, Service Direct
General Admin.: Fred Siegel/Executive Vice President
Mr. Jack Rhian/President, Chief Executive Officer
Mktg./Adv.: Randi Baldwin/Senior Vice President Marketing & Business Development
Finance: Mr. Richard Rallo/Chief Financial Officer

Communication System, Emergency Alert, Personal	General
Dispenser, Other	General
Equipment, Building Security	General

AMERICAN MEDICAL BIO CARE, INC. 800-676-1434
1201 Dove St., #520, Newport Beach, CA 92660 949-477-5795
FDA Number: 2032711 *Fax:* 949-477-5799
E-mail: support@medicalbiocare.com
Web site: www.medicalbiocare.com
Medical Products Sales Volume: $1,000,000
Year Founded: 1989
Total Employees: 5
Ownership: Private
Produces/Sells CE-marked Devices: N
Federal Procurement Eligibility: Small Business

Laser, Surgical	Surgery

AMERICAN MEDICAL COMMUNICATIONS/INFOTRONICS
See Clear Stream Media

AMERICAN MEDICAL DIAGNOSTICS, INC. 703-938-6500
4031 University Drive, Suite 200, Fairfax, VA 22030
FDA Number: 3004167631
Ownership: Private
Stock Symbol: AMMD
Traded On: NASDAQ
Produces/Sells CE-marked Devices: N

Computer, Chemistry Analyzer	Chemistry

AMERICAN MEDICAL DISPOSABLES
See Amd-Ritmed, Inc.

AMERICAN MEDICAL ENDOSCOPY   305-436-0599
3020 Nw 82nd Ave., Miami, FL 33122
FDA Number: 3004361445
E-mail: info@endoscopia.com   *Fax:* 1.305.436.0399
Web site: www.endoscopia.com
Ownership: Private
Stock Symbol: AMMD
Traded On: NASDAQ
Produces/Sells CE-marked Devices: N

AMERICAN MEDICAL EQUIPMENT
See B. Braun Medical Inc., Renal Therapies Div.

AMERICAN MEDICAL INDUSTRIES   605-428-5501
330 E. 3rd Street, Suite 2, Dell Rapids, SD 57022-1918
FDA Number: 1423563
E-mail: info@thepillcrusherguys.com   *Fax:* 605-428-5502
Web site: www.pillcrusherguys.com
Medical Products Sales Volume: $2,500,000
Year Founded: 1984
Total Employees: 10   *Marketing Staff:* 3   *Sales Staff:* 5
Ownership: Private
Produces/Sells CE-marked Devices: N
Federal Procurement Eligibility: Small Business
Distribution: Manufacturer Direct, Manufacturer Through Distributor
General Admin.: James Fiocchi/Chief Executive Officer
    Daniel J. Anderson/Executive Vice President, Director

Crusher, Pill	General
Cutter, Pill	General
Device, Inflation, Middle Ear	Ear/Nose/Throat
Dispenser, Other	General
Kit, Irrigation, Wound	General
Monitor, Medication	General

AMERICAN MEDICAL INDUSTRIES, INC.
See AMERICAN MEDICAL ENDOSCOPY

AMERICAN MEDICAL INSTRUMENTS, INC.
See Tegra Medical Inc.

AMERICAN MEDICAL LINK, INC.   908-359-9328
5 Homestead Road, Bldg. 5, Units 1 & 2,
Hillsborough, NJ 08844
FDA Number: n/a
E-mail: amedlinc@aol.com   *Fax:* 908-359-9388
Annual Revenue: $25-$50 Million
Year Founded: 1996
Total Employees: 10   *Marketing Staff:* 2   *Sales Staff:* 5
Ownership: Private
Produces/Sells CE-marked Devices: N
Federal Procurement Eligibility: Small Business, Minority Owned
Distribution: Service Direct, Exclusive Distributor, Importer, Exporter
General Admin.: Nisar Khokhar/President
Mktg./Adv.: Masoud Tehami/Vice President Marketing

Service, Import/Export	General

AMERICAN MEDICAL MANUFACTURING, INC.
See Advanced Medical Innovations, Inc.

AMERICAN MEDICAL MFG., INC.   800-426-6476
                                    818-701-7171
9410 Desoto Ave., Unit J, Chatsworth, CA 91311
FDA Number: 2028390
E-mail: sales@amiwelisten.com   *Fax:* 818-701-9708
Web site: http://www.amiwelisten.com
Year Founded: 1990
Ownership: Private
Produces/Sells CE-marked Devices: N
Distribution: Manufacturer Direct, Manufacturer Through Distributor, OEM

Infusion Stand	General
Tray, Surgical Instrument	Surgery

AMERICAN MEDICAL PRODUCTS, INC.   800-279-1999
                                    480-967-0384
713 South Darrow Drive, Tempe, AZ 85281-3313
FDA Number: 2031441
E-mail: oxyears@aol.com   *Fax:* 480-829-7587
Web site: www.oxyears.com
Medical Products Sales Volume: $100,000
Year Founded: 1985
Total Employees: 1
Ownership: Private
Produces/Sells CE-marked Devices: N
Federal Procurement Eligibility: Small Business
Distribution: Manufacturer Direct, Manufacturer Through Distributor

Cannula, Nasal, Oxygen	Anesthesiology

AMERICAN MEDICAL SALES, INC.
See AMD Technologies Inc.

AMERICAN MEDICAL SOFTWARE   800-423-8836
Post Office Box 236,   618-692-1300
Edwardsville, IL 62025
FDA Number: n/a
E-mail: sales@americanmedical.com   *Fax:* 618-692-1809
Web site: www.americanmedical.com
Medical Products Sales Volume: $2,000,000
Annual Revenue: $1-$5 Million
Year Founded: 1984
Total Employees: 12   *Marketing Staff:* 2   *Sales Staff:* 4
Ownership: Private
Produces/Sells CE-marked Devices: N
Federal Procurement Eligibility: Small Business
Distribution: Manufacturer Direct, Manufacturer Through Manufacturer Reps
General Admin.: W. David Scott/President
Mktg./Adv.: Bob Bridgman/Director Marketing
    Tina Stotler/Director Sales

Computer Equipment	General
Computer and Software, Medical	General
Computer, Patient Data Management	General

AMERICAN MEDICAL SPECIALTIES, INC.   800-808-2877
10650 77th St., Suite 405, Largo, FL 33777   727-561-9400
FDA Number: 1058412
E-mail: placeorder@ammeds.com   *Fax:* 727-561-9022
Web site: www.ammeds.com
Medical Products Sales Volume: $500,000
Annual Revenue: $1-$5 Million
Year Founded: 1992
Total Employees: 7   *Marketing Staff:* 2   *Sales Staff:* 3
Ownership: Private
Stock Symbol: AMMD
Traded On: NASDAQ
Produces/Sells CE-marked Devices: N
Federal Procurement Eligibility: Small Business, Female Owned
Distribution: Manufacturer Direct, Manufacturer Through Distributor, Manufacturer Through Manufacturer Reps, Service Direct, Exporter
General Admin.: Mrs. Diane Simmons/Chief Executive
Mktg./Adv.: Mrs. April Verrier/Sales Associate
    Mrs. Lisa Allison/Sales Associate

Bit, Drill	Orthopedics
Bit, Surgical	Surgery
Blade, Bone Cutting	Orthopedics
Blade, Saw, Cast Cutting	Orthopedics
Blade, Saw, Surgical, Cardiovascular	Cardiovascular
Blade, Surgical, Saw, General & Plastic Surgery	Surgery
Burr	Ear/Nose/Throat
Burr, Cranial	Cns/Neurology
Burr, Orthopedic	Orthopedics
Burr, Other	Surgery
Burr, Podiatric	Orthopedics
Burr, Surgical, General & Plastic Surgery	Surgery
Pin, Fixation, Smooth	Orthopedics
Pin, Fixation, Threaded	Orthopedics

AMERICAN MEDICAL SUPPLIES AND EQUIPMENT   888-592-3469
8361 NW 36th Street, Miami, FL 33166   305-592-3422
FDA Number: n/a
Web site: www.amerimed.com
Annual Revenue: $0-$1 Million
Year Founded: 1983
Ownership: Private
Produces/Sells CE-marked Devices: N
Federal Procurement Eligibility: Small Business
Distribution: Manufacturer Direct, Manufacturer Through Distributor

Equipment, Therapy, Handicapped/Physical	Physical Med
Lamp, Operating Room	General
Thermometer, Electronic	General

AMERICAN MEDICAL SYSTEMS, INC.   800-328-3881
10700 Bren Road W., Minnetonka, MN 55343   952-930-6000
FDA Number: 2183959
Web site: www.visitams.com   *Fax:* 952-930-6373
Medical Products Sales Volume: $358,300,000
Year Founded: 1972
Total Employees: 1095
Ownership: Public
Stock Symbol: AMMD
Traded On: NASDAQ
Quality System Registration Information: ISO9001
Produces/Sells CE-marked Devices: Y
Distribution: Manufacturer Through Distributor, Manufacturer Through Manufacturer Reps
General Admin.: Mr. Mark A. Heggestad/Chief Financial Officer, Executive Vice President

AMERICAN MEDICAL SYSTEMS, INC.   800-328-3881 *(cont'd)*
Mr. Maxamilian Flore/Chief Technology Officer, Senior Vice
President
　　　　Mr. Anthony P. Tony Bihl/President, Chief Executive Officer
Mktg./Adv.: Mr. Richard Staples/Vice President U.S. Sales

Catheter, Urethral	Gastroenterology/Urology
Device, Incontinence, Fecal, Implanted	Gastroenterology/Urology
Device, Incontinence, Mechanical/Hydraulic	Gastroenterology/Urology
Mesh, Surgical, Polymeric	Surgery
Prosthesis, Penile	Gastroenterology/Urology
Prosthesis, Penis, Inflatable	Surgery
Prosthesis, Testicle	Gastroenterology/Urology
Prosthesis, Urethral Sphincter	Gastroenterology/Urology
Screw, Fixation, Bone	Orthopedics
Stent, Ureteral	Gastroenterology/Urology
Stent, Urethral, Bulbous, Permanent/Semi-Permanent	Gastroenterology/Urology
Stent, Urethral, Prostatic, Permanent/Semi-Permanent	Gastroenterology/Urology

Medical Product Subsidiaries (Listed Separately)
Ams Innovative Center-San Jose

AMERICAN MEDICAL TECHNOLOGIES, INC.   361-289-1145
5655 Bear Lane, Corpus Christi, TX 78405
FDA Number: 1833683　　　　　　　　*Fax:* 361-289-5554
E-mail: info@americanmedicaltech.com
Web site: www.americanmedicaltech.com
Medical Products Sales Volume: $2,800,000
Annual Revenue: $5-$10 Million
Year Founded: 1989
Total Employees: 15　　　*Marketing Staff:* 1　　　*Sales Staff:* 5
Ownership: Fisher Scientific
Stock Symbol: ADLI
Traded On: NASDAQ
Quality System Registration Information: ISO9001
Produces/Sells CE-marked Devices: Y
Federal Procurement Eligibility: Small Business
Distribution: Manufacturer Direct, Manufacturer Through Distributor, Service Direct
General Admin.: Ms. Angie DeLeon/Executive Assistant
　　　　　Mr. Roger Dartt/President, Chief Executive Officer
Production: Mr. Stefan Krisch/Director Operations
Finance: Ms. Barbara Woody/Controller

Airbrush	Dental And Oral
Camera, Other	General
Material, Tooth Shade, Resin	Dental And Oral

AMERICAN MICRO PRODUCTS, INC.   800-479-2193
4288 Armstrong Blvd., Batavia, OH 45103-1600   **513-732-2674**
FDA Number: 9044017　　　　　　　　*Fax:* 513-732-3535
E-mail: precise@american-micro.com
Web site: www.american-micro.com
Medical Products Sales Volume: $3,000,000
Annual Revenue: $10-$25 Million
Year Founded: 1957
Total Employees: 200　　　*Marketing Staff:* 4　　　*Sales Staff:* 5
Ownership: Private
Quality System Registration Information: ISO9002
Produces/Sells CE-marked Devices: N
Federal Procurement Eligibility: Small Business
Distribution: Manufacturer Direct
General Admin.: Stephen Kappers/President
Mktg./Adv.: J.W. Childs/Director National Accounts
　　　　　Brian Collins/Manager Contract Sales
Production: Boyd Arnett/Director Quality Assurance
　　　　　Jennifer Milligan/Manager Materials
Research: Rene A. Paroz/Vice President Product Development

Alloy, Precious Metal, For Clinical Use	Dental And Oral
Component, Metal, Other	General

AMERICAN MICRO-MED CORP.
See X-Ray Support, Inc

AMERICAN NATIONAL RED CROSS HEADQUARTERS   202-303-5640
2025 E Street Nw, Washington, DC 20006
FDA Number: 1124939

Software, Blood Bank (Stand-Alone Products)	Hematology

AMERICAN OF MARTINSVILLE   276-632-2061
128 East. Church St., Martinsville, VA 24115-5071
FDA Number: n/a　　　　　　　　*Fax:* 276-632-4707
E-mail: aom@americanofmartinsville.com
Web site: www.americanofmartinsville.com
Medical Products Sales Volume: $100,000,000
Annual Revenue: $50-$100 Million
Year Founded: 1906
Ownership: Private
Produces/Sells CE-marked Devices: Y
Federal Procurement Eligibility: Minority Owned
Distribution: Manufacturer Direct, Exporter

Bed, Electric	General

AMERICAN OF MARTINSVILLE   276-632-2061 *(cont'd)*
Furniture, Patient Room　　　　　　　　　General

AMERICAN OMNI MEDICAL, INC.
See Quest Medical, Inc.

AMERICAN OPTICAL CORP.
See Aearo Company

AMERICAN OPTICAL LENS MEX S. DE R.L. DE C.V.   408-735-1982
Calle 2, Orienta #133,, C.d. Industrial Mesa De Otay, Tijuana, B.c. Mexico
FDA Number: 9611737

Lens, Spectacle/Eyeglasses, Non-Custom	Ophthalmology

AMERICAN OPTICAL SCIENTIFIC INSTRUMENTS
See Leica Microsystems, Inc., Educational & Analytical Division

AMERICAN OPTICAL, SOFT CONTACT LENS DIV.
See Ciba Vision Corporation

AMERICAN OPTISURGICAL INC.   800-576-1266
25501 Arctic Ocean Dr., Lake Forest, CA 92630   **949-580-1266**
FDA Number: 2085033　　　　　　　　*Fax:* 949-580-1270
E-mail: info@optisurgical.com
Web site: www.optisurgical.com
Medical Products Sales Volume: $2,600,000
Annual Revenue: $1-$5 Million
Year Founded: 1992
Total Employees: 18　　　*Marketing Staff:* 3　　　*Sales Staff:* 5
Ownership: American Optisurgical Inc.
Quality System Registration Information: ISO9000; ISO9001
Produces/Sells CE-marked Devices: Y
Federal Procurement Eligibility: Small Business, GSA Contract, VA Contract
Distribution: Manufacturer Direct, OEM, Service Direct
General Admin.: Terri Lachman/Executive Admin.
　　　　　Herbert Cameron/President, Chief Executive Officer
　　　　　Jeanne Cameron/Vice President, General Manager
Mktg./Adv.: Tate Parham/Director Product Development
　　　　　Connie Gaetano/Manager International & National Sales
Production: Craig Brittain/Director Quality Control & Regulatory Affairs
Purchasing: Donna Farley/Purchasing Agent

Phacoemulsification System	Ophthalmology

Medical Product Subsidiaries (Listed Separately)
American Optisurgical Inc.

AMERICAN ORTHODONTICS CORP.   800-558-7687
1714 Cambridge Avenue, Sheboygan, WI 53081   **920-457-5051**
FDA Number: 2126683　　　　　　　　*Fax:* 920-457-1485
E-mail: amo@americanortho.com
Web site: www.americanortho.com
Annual Revenue: $50-$100 Million
Year Founded: 1968
Total Employees: 350　　　*Marketing Staff:* 3　　　*Sales Staff:* 36
Ownership: Private
Quality System Registration Information: ISO9001; ISO9002
Produces/Sells CE-marked Devices: Y
Federal Procurement Eligibility: Small Business
Distribution: Manufacturer Direct, Manufacturer Through Distributor, Manufacturer Through Manufacturer Reps, OEM, Service Direct, Exclusive Distributor, Importer, Exporter
General Admin.: Dan Merkel/Chief Executive Officer
　　　　　Rich Iverson/President
Research: Lee Tuneberg/Vice President Research & Development
Finance: Gregory D. Greske/Treasurer

Band, Elastic, Orthodontic	Dental And Oral
Band, Material, Orthodontic	Dental And Oral
Band, Preformed, Orthodontic	Dental And Oral
Bracket, Metal, Orthodontic	Dental And Oral
Bracket, Plastic, Orthodontic	Dental And Oral
Computer Software	General
Headgear, Extraoral, Orthodontic	Dental And Oral
Spring, Orthodontic	Dental And Oral
Tube, Orthodontic	Dental And Oral
Tucker, Ligature, Orthodontic	Dental And Oral
Wire, Orthodontic	Dental And Oral

AMERICAN ORTHOPEDIC
See Bsn Medical, Inc

AMERICAN ORTHOPEDIC SUPPLY CO., INC.   205-274-7137
37017 State Hwy. 79, Cleveland, AL 35049
FDA Number: n/a
Ownership: Private
Produces/Sells CE-marked Devices: N

Belt, Traction, Pelvic, Orthopedic	Orthopedics
Brace, Joint, Ankle (External)	Physical Med
Halter, Head, Traction, Orthopedic	Orthopedics
Joint, Hip, External Brace	Physical Med
Joint, Knee, External Brace	Physical Med

AMERICAN ORTHOPEDIC SUPPLY CO., INC. 205-274-7137
(cont'd)

Orthosis, Abdominal	Physical Med
Orthosis, Cervical	Physical Med
Orthosis, Lumbosacral	Physical Med
Orthosis, Rib Fracture, Soft	Physical Med
Orthosis, Sacroiliac, Soft	Physical Med
Orthosis, Thoracic	Physical Med
Orthosis, Truncal/Limb	Physical Med
Sling, Arm	Physical Med
Splint, Clavicle	Physical Med
Splint, Hand, And Component	Physical Med
Support, Arm	Physical Med

AMERICAN OVERSEAS AGENCY
See Metronix

AMERICAN PACEMAKER CORPORATION
See Pace Medical, Inc.

AMERICAN PACIFIC PLASTIC 714-891-3191
FABRICATORS, INC.
7274 Lampson Ave., Garden Grove, CA 92841
FDA Number: 2032003   Fax: 714-891-6770
E-mail: sales@appf.com
Web site: www.appf.comÉ_Z
Ownership: Private
Produces/Sells CE-marked Devices: N

Accessories, Operating Room, Table	Surgery

AMERICAN POWER CONVERSION 800-788-2208
132 Fairgrounds Road, West Kingston, RI 02892   401-789-5735
FDA Number: n/a   Fax: 401-788-2739
E-mail: public.relations@apcc.com
Web site: www.apcc.com
Medical Products Sales Volume: $1,970,000,000
Total Employees: 1400
Ownership: Private
Stock Symbol: APCC
Traded On: NASDAQ
Quality System Registration Information: ISO9002
Produces/Sells CE-marked Devices: N
Distribution: Manufacturer Through Distributor, OEM, Exporter
General Admin.: Mr. Jim Simonelli/Chief Technology Officer, Senior Vice President
    Mr. Laurent Vernery/President, Chief Executive Officer
Mktg./Adv.: Ms. Leanne Cunnold/Senior Vice President Business Development
    Mr. Chris Hanley/Senior Vice President Marketing & Sales
Research: Neil Rasmussen/Vice President Research & Development & Engineering
Finance: Ms. Karen Miranda/Chief Financial Officer

Power Systems, Uninterruptible (UPS)	General

AMERICAN PRINTING HOUSE FOR THE 800-223-1839
BLIND, INC.
PO Box 6085, Louisville, KY 40206-0085   502-895-2405
FDA Number: n/a   Fax: 502-899-2274
E-mail: info@aph.org
Web site: www.aph.org
Medical Products Sales Volume: $17,300,000
Annual Revenue: $10-$25 Million
Year Founded: 1858
Total Employees: 300
Ownership: Private
Produces/Sells CE-marked Devices: N
Federal Procurement Eligibility: Small Business
Distribution: Manufacturer Direct
General Admin.: Tuck Tinsley/President
Mktg./Adv.: Jan Carroll/Manager Contract Sales
    Tony Grantz/Manager International & National Sales
Production: Jack Decker/Vice President Production
Finance: Bill Beavin/Vice President Finance
Purchasing: David Manteuffel/Buyer

Utensil, Handicapped Aid	Physical Med
Vision Aid, Braille	General
Vision Aid, Image Intensification, Battery-Powered	Ophthalmology

AMERICAN QUALEX, INC. 800-772-1776
920-A Calle Negocio, San Clemente, CA 92673   949-492-8298
FDA Number: n/a   Fax: 949-492-6790
E-mail: info@americanqualex.com
Web site: www.americanqualex.com
Medical Products Sales Volume: $700,000
Annual Revenue: $0-$1 Million
Year Founded: 1981
Total Employees: 10   Sales Staff: 2
Ownership: Private
Produces/Sells CE-marked Devices: N
Federal Procurement Eligibility: Small Business
Distribution: Manufacturer Direct, OEM, Service Direct, Exclusive Distributor

AMERICAN QUALEX, INC. 800-772-1776 *(cont'd)*
General Admin.: Dan R. Moothart/President
Mktg./Adv.: Stephanie Carlan/Director Marketing & Sales

Antibody, Monoclonal	Microbiology
Antibody, Other	General
Antibody, Polyclonal	Microbiology
Azo-Dyes, Colorimetric, Bilirubin And Conjugates	Chemistry
Reagent, Virus, General	Pathology

AMERICAN QUALITY MFG., INC. 888-999-7577
400 Shearer Blvd, Cocoa, FL 32922   321-633-4446
FDA Number: 1061957   Fax: 866-237-4208
Web site: www.tanningonline.com
Ownership: Private
Produces/Sells CE-marked Devices: N

Booth, Sun Tan	Physical Med

AMERICAN RADIOSURGERY, INC. 858-451-6173
16776 Bernardo Center Dr #203, San Diego, CA 92128
FDA Number: 3005505123   Fax: 858-487-0662
E-mail: info@americanradiosurgery.net
Web site: www.americanradiosurgery.ne
Ownership: Private
Produces/Sells CE-marked Devices: N

System, Planning, Radiation Therapy Treatment	Radiology
Teletherapy System, Radionuclide	Radiology

AMERICAN RED CROSS DIAGNOSTIC 202-303-5640
MANUFACTURING DIVISI
9319 Gaither Rd., Gaithersburg, MD 20877
FDA Number: 1177732

Diluent, Blood Cell	Hematology
Medium, Lymphocyte Separation	Hematology
Solution, Stabilized Enzyme	Hematology

AMERICAN RESEARCH PRODUCTS COMPANY
See Amresco Inc.

AMERICAN SAFETY EQUIPMENT CORP.
See Micro-Aire Surgical Instruments, Inc.

AMERICAN SAFETY RAZOR CO. 800-445-9284
One Razor Blade Lane, Verona, VA 24482   540-248-8000
FDA Number: 1119522   Fax: 540-248-7122
E-mail: asr@personna.com
Web site: www.personna.com
Ownership: Private
Produces/Sells CE-marked Devices: N

Blade, Scalpel	Surgery
Instrument, Manual, General Surgical	Surgery
Scalpel, One-Piece (Knife)	Surgery
Strip, Adhesive	Surgery
Surgical, Razor	Surgery

AMERICAN SCIENTIFIC RESOURCES, INC. 847-386-1384
1112 Weston Rd., Unit 278, Weston, FL 33326
FDA Number: 1321249
E-mail: nlq@americansci.com
Web site: www.americansci.com
Ownership: Public
Stock Symbol: ASFX
Traded On: OTC Bulletin
Produces/Sells CE-marked Devices: N

Dispenser, Medication, Liquid	General
Meter, Peak Flow, Spirometry	Anesthesiology
Needle, Hypodermic, Single Lumen With Syringe	General
Thermometer, Electronic	General

Medical Product Subsidiaries (Listed Separately)
Ulster Scientific, Inc.

AMERICAN SEATING 616-732-6600
401 American Seating Ctr. NW, Grand Rapids, MI 49504
FDA Number: n/a
E-mail: website@amseco.com
Web site: www.americanseating.com
Annual Revenue: $0-$1 Million
Year Founded: 1886
Ownership: Private
Produces/Sells CE-marked Devices: N
Distribution: Manufacturer Through Distributor

Cabinet Casework, Laboratory	Chemistry
Cabinet, Laboratory	Chemistry
Furniture, General	General

AMERICAN SILK SUTURES, INC. 781-592-7200
82 Sanderson Avenue, Lynn, MA 01902
FDA Number: 1221144   Fax: 781-595-5460
E-mail: neurosp@quik.com
Medical Products Sales Volume: $3,100,000
Year Founded: 1985

AMERICAN SILK SUTURES, INC. 781-592-7200 *(cont'd)*
Total Employees: 38   Marketing Staff: 46   Sales Staff: 148
Ownership: American Silk Sutures, Inc
Produces/Sells CE-marked Devices: Y
Federal Procurement Eligibility: Small Business
Distribution: Manufacturer Direct, Manufacturer Through Distributor, Exclusive Distributor, Exporter

Sponge, External	Surgery
Sponge, External, Neurological	Cns/Neurology

AMERICAN SPECIALTIES, INC. 914-476-9000
441 Saw Mill River Road, Yonkers, NY 10701-4913
FDA Number: 9330010   Fax: 914-476-0688
E-mail: info@americanspecialties.com
Web site: www.americanspecialties.com
Annual Revenue: $10-$25 Million
Year Founded: 1961
Total Employees: 300   Marketing Staff: 2   Sales Staff: 15
Ownership: Private
Produces/Sells CE-marked Devices: N
Distribution: Manufacturer Through Distributor, Manufacturer Through Manufacturer Reps
General Admin.: Peter Rolla/President
    Charles La Barbera/Vice President, General Manager
Mktg./Adv.: Gene Pane/Vice President Marketing
    Gilbert Pesavento/Vice President Sales

Basin, Wash	General
Dispenser, Soap	General
Rack, Bedpan	General
Rail, Bath	General
Rail, Commode	General
Rail, Wall Side	General
Sink, Hospital	General

AMERICAN SPINE CENTER LTD., CLINI-LASE 618-233-6824
100 Mascoutah Avenue, Belleville, IL 62220
FDA Number: 3004464236   Fax: 1-618-233-6825
E-mail: Info@Clini-Lase.com
Web site: www.clini-lase.com
Ownership: Private
Produces/Sells CE-marked Devices: N

AMERICAN SPRAYTECH, L.L.C. 908-725-6060
205 Meister Ave., North Branch, NJ 08876
FDA Number: 3004380247   Fax: 908-725-1932
E-mail: postmaster@americanspraytech.com
Web site: www.americanspraytech.com
Ownership: Private
Produces/Sells CE-marked Devices: N

Bandage, Liquid	Surgery
Fixative, Alcohol Containing	Pathology
Lavage Unit, Water Jet	General

AMERICAN STAIR-GLIDE DIVISION
See Thyssenkrupp Access Corp.

AMERICAN SURGICAL INSTRUMENT CORP. 800-628-2879
26 Plaza Drive, Westmont, IL 60559-1124   630-986-8032
FDA Number: 1420491   Fax: 630-986-0065
E-mail: info@asico.com
Web site: www.asico.com
Medical Products Sales Volume: $800,000
Year Founded: 1983
Total Employees: 15   Marketing Staff: 1   Sales Staff: 23
Ownership: Private
Produces/Sells CE-marked Devices: N
Federal Procurement Eligibility: Small Business
Distribution: Manufacturer Direct, Manufacturer Through Distributor, Manufacturer Through Manufacturer Reps
General Admin.: Ravi Nallakrishnan/Chief Executive Officer
    Radha Nallakrishnan/Vice President, General Manager

Cannula, Ophthalmic	Ophthalmology
Forceps	Orthopedics
Forceps, Biopsy, Bronchoscope (Non-Rigid)	Anesthesiology
Forceps, Ophthalmic	Ophthalmology
Sharpener, Instrument, Surgical	Surgery
Tray, Sterilization, Instrument	Surgery
Waste Disposal Unit, Sharps	General

AMERICAN TELECARE, INC. 800-323-6667
15159 Technology Drive,   952-897-0000
Eden Prairie, MN 55344
FDA Number: ÿ2132780   Fax: 952-944-2247
E-mail: info@americantelecare.com
Web site: www.americantelecare.com
Medical Products Sales Volume: $5,900,000
Total Employees: 40   Marketing Staff: 2   Sales Staff: 10
Ownership: Private
Produces/Sells CE-marked Devices: N

AMERICAN TELECARE, INC. 800-323-6667 *(cont'd)*
Federal Procurement Eligibility: Small Business
Distribution: Manufacturer Direct
General Admin.: Dr. Randall Moore/Chief Executive Officer
Mktg./Adv.: Michael Chappuis/Senior Vice President Business Development
    Larry Diamond/Senior Vice President Sales
Production: Michael Chappuis/Vice President Manufacturing & Engineering
Finance: George Boyadjis/Chief Financial Officer

Medical Radiographic Personal Monitoring Device	Radiology
Stethoscope, Electronic (Auscultoscope)	Cardiovascular

AMERICAN TENTE CASTERS INC.
See Tente Casters, Inc.

AMERICAN THERMAL INSTRUMENTS, INC. 937-429-2114
2400 E. River Road, Dayton, OH 45439
FDA Number: 1526410

Telethermographic System	Radiology
Thermometer, Chemical Color Change	General

AMERICAN TOOTH INDUSTRIES 800-235-4639
1200 Stellar Dr., Oxnard, CA 93033-2404   805-487-9868
FDA Number: 2020523   Fax: 805-483-8482
E-mail: info@americantooth.com
Web site: www.americantooth.com
Total Employees: 76   Marketing Staff: 5   Sales Staff: 21
Ownership: Private
Quality System Registration Information: ISO9001
Produces/Sells CE-marked Devices: Y
Federal Procurement Eligibility: Small Business, GSA Contract, VA Contract
Distribution: Manufacturer Direct, Manufacturer Through Manufacturer Reps, OEM, Exclusive Distributor
General Admin.: Minda Darimbang/Manager Human Resources
    Bruno Pozzi/President, Chief Executive Officer
Production: Kathleen Norton/Manager Operations

Base, Denture, Relining, Repairing, Rebasing, Resin	Dental And Oral
Crown And Bridge, Temporary, Resin	Dental And Oral
Denture, Plastic, Teeth	Dental And Oral
Material, Tooth Shade, Resin	Dental And Oral
Powder, Porcelain	Dental And Oral
Teeth, Artificial, Backing And Facing	Dental And Oral
Tray, Impression	Dental And Oral

AMERICAN TRACK ROADSTERS, INC. 303-986-9300
1500 W. Hampden Ave., Unit 4 - G., Englewood, CO 80110
FDA Number: n/a   Fax: 303-986-9301
E-mail: greg@atrackroadster.com
Web site: www.atrackroadster.com
Ownership: Private
Produces/Sells CE-marked Devices: N

Component, Wheelchair	Physical Med
Wheelchair, Manual	Physical Med

AMERICAN TYPE CULTURE COLLECTION
See Atcc

AMERICAN VITAL TECHNOLOGIES
See Pace Tech, Inc.

AMERICAN WECO CORPORATION
See Medi Usa

AMERICAN WEIGHTS AND MEASURES
See American Medical Systems, Inc.

AMERICAN WELLNESS FOUNDATION 713-622-8499
5311 Kirby Drive Suite 100, Houston, TX 77055
FDA Number: n/a   Fax: 877-806-7737
Ownership: Private
Produces/Sells CE-marked Devices: N

Kit, Enema (For Cleaning Purposes)	Gastroenterology/Urology

AMERICAN WHITE CROSS - HOUSTON 609-514-4744
15200 I-45 North, Houston, TX 77090
FDA Number: 1625371
Ownership: Private
Produces/Sells CE-marked Devices: N

Bandage, Adhesive	Surgery
Dissector, Surgical, General & Plastic Surgery	Surgery
Dissector, Tonsil	Ear/Nose/Throat
Dressing, Other	General
Dressing, Wound, Hydrophilic	Surgery
Floss, Dental	Dental And Oral
Gauze, Non-Absorbable, X-Ray Detectable (Internal Sponge)	Surgery
Gauze/sponge, Nonresorbable For External Use	Surgery
Pad, Eye	Ophthalmology
Sponge, Gauze	Dental And Oral

AMERICAN ZETTLER, INC.
See Zettler Systems, Inc.

AMERICAN-DANISH OTICON CORP.
See Oticon, Inc.

AMERICHEM PHARMACEUTICAL CORP.   305-591-0100
2862 N. W. 79th Ave., Miami, FL 33122
FDA Number: n/a   Fax: 305-591-9223
E-mail: apc@americhempharm.com
Web site: www.americhempharm.com
Year Founded: 1982
Ownership: Private
Produces/Sells CE-marked Devices: N
Federal Procurement Eligibility: Small Business, Minority Owned
Distribution: Manufacturer Direct
General Admin.: Iliana Lloret/President
   Punch, Biopsy   Gastroenterology/Urology

AMERICOMP, INC.   800-458-1782
2901 W. Lawrence Avenue, Chicago, IL 60625   773-353-4047
FDA Number: n/a   Fax: 773-583-1751
E-mail: grego@summitindustries.net
Web site: www.americompus.net
Annual Revenue: $1-$5 Million
Year Founded: 1987
Total Employees: 25   Marketing Staff: 1   Sales Staff: 2
Ownership: Private
Produces/Sells CE-marked Devices: N
Federal Procurement Eligibility: Small Business
Distribution: Manufacturer Through Distributor
General Admin.: Gregory Oravec/President, General Manager
Aligner, Beam, X-Ray (Collimator)	Dental And Oral
Apron, Lead, Radiographic	Radiology
Cassette, Radiographic Film	Radiology
Collimator, Radiographic, Manual	Radiology
Generator, Diagnostic X-Ray, High Voltage, 3-Phase	Radiology
Generator, Diagnostic X-Ray, High Voltage, Single Phase	Radiology
Grid, Radiographic	Radiology
Hanger, X-Ray Tube	Radiology
Holder, X-Ray Film Cassette, Vertical	Radiology
Illuminator, Radiographic Film	Radiology
Radiographic Unit, Diagnostic	Radiology
Safelight, X-Ray	Radiology
System, Marking, Film, Radiographic	Radiology
Table, Radiographic	Radiology
Tube, X-Ray	Radiology

AMERICORP FINANCIAL, INC.   800-233-1574
877 S. Adams Road, Birmingham, MI 48009-7029   248-723-4500
FDA Number: n/a   Fax: 248-723-4501
E-mail: tom.dunigan@eAmericorp.com
Web site: www.eamericorp.com
Total Employees: 500   Marketing Staff: 23   Sales Staff: 23
Ownership: Private
Produces/Sells CE-marked Devices: N
Federal Procurement Eligibility: Small Business
Distribution: Service Direct
General Admin.: Thomas X. Dunigan/President, Chief Executive Officer
   Ardis Cortez/Vice President
   Service, Equipment Leasing   General

AMERICUS FORM & FUNCTION   440-237-0200
12316 York Rd., North Royalton, OH 44133
FDA Number: 3005636967
Ownership: Private
Produces/Sells CE-marked Devices: N
   Crown, Preformed   Dental And Oral

AMERIDERM LABORATORIES, LTD.   973-279-5100
13 Kentucky Avenue, Paterson, NJ 07503
FDA Number: 2249150
   Dressing, Wound, Hydrogel W/out Drug And/or Biologic   Surgery

AMERIFLO CORP.   866-573-1658
478 Gradle Drive, Carmel Industrial Park,   317-844-2019
Carmel, IN 46032
FDA Number: 1835956   Fax: 317-844-7150
E-mail: info@ameriflo.com
Web site: www.ameriflo.net
Total Employees: 50
Ownership: Private
Quality System Registration Information: ISO9001
Produces/Sells CE-marked Devices: N
Federal Procurement Eligibility: Small Business, GSA Contract
Distribution: Manufacturer Direct, Manufacturer Through Distributor, OEM
   Regulator, Pressure, Gas Cylinder   Anesthesiology

AMERIPAC, INC.   214-660-6633
4399 Cambridge Road, Fort Worth, TX 75050
FDA Number: 1648141
Ownership: Private
Produces/Sells CE-marked Devices: N

AMERIPAC, INC.   214-660-6633 (cont'd)
   Adhesive, Denture, Karaya   Dental And Oral

AMERITEK USA, INC.   425-379-2580
125 130 St. Se,, Everett, WA 98208
FDA Number: 3025672   Fax: 425-379-2624
E-mail: info@ameritek.org
Web site: www.ameritek.org
Ownership: Merit Medical Systems, Inc.
Produces/Sells CE-marked Devices: N
Alpha-Fetoprotein RIA Test System	Immunology
Antigen, Antiserum, Control, Carcinoembryonic Antigen	Immunology
Antigen, Antiserum, Control, Ferritin	Immunology
Antigen, Antiserum, Control, IGE	Immunology
Antigen, Antiserum, Control, Myoglobin	Immunology
Antigen, CF, Toxoplasma Gondii	Microbiology
Antigen, Streptococcus SPP.	Microbiology
Antiserum, Fluorescent, Mycobacterium Tuberculosis	Microbiology
Antiserum, Streptococcus SPP.	Microbiology
Azo-Dyes, Colorimetric, Bilirubin And Conjugates	Chemistry
Campylobacter Pylori	Microbiology
Chlamydia, DNA Reagents	Microbiology
Chromatographic Derivative, Total Lipids	Chemistry
Colorimetric, Occult Blood in Urine	Hematology
Diazo (Colorimetric), Nitrite (Urinary, Non-Quantitative)	Chemistry
Diazonium Colorimetry, Urobilinogen (Urinary, Non-Quant.)	Chemistry
Disc, Strip And Reagent, Microorganism Differentiation	Microbiology
Enzymatic Method, Glucose (Urinary, Non-Quantitative)	Chemistry
Enzymatic Method, Troponin Subunit	Chemistry
Enzyme Immunoassay, Amphetamine	Toxicology
Enzyme Immunoassay, Cannabinoids	Toxicology
Enzyme Immunoassay, Cocaine And Cocaine Metabolites	Toxicology
Enzyme Immunoassay, Opiates	Toxicology
Enzyme Linked Immunoabsorbent Assay, Rubella	Microbiology
Gas Chromatography, Amphetamine	Toxicology
Gas Chromatography, Methamphetamine	Toxicology
Gas Chromatography, Morphine	Toxicology
Indicator Method, Protein Or Albumin (Urinary, Non-Quant.)	Chemistry
Indicator, pH, Dye (Urinary, Non-Quantitative)	Chemistry
Kit, Pregnancy Test, Over The Counter, HCG	Chemistry
Kit, Test, Malaria	Toxicology
Kit, Test, Multiple, Drugs Of Abuse, Over The Counter	Toxicology
Nitroprusside, Ketones (Urinary, Non-Quantitative)	Chemistry
Radioimmunoassay, Human Chorionic Gonadotropin	Chemistry
Radioimmunoassay, Luteinizing Hormone	Chemistry
Radioimmunoassay, Thyroid Stimulating Hormone	Chemistry
Reagent, Occult Blood	Hematology
Refractometer	Chemistry
System, Test, Drugs of Abuse	Chemistry
Test System, Nicotine, Cotinine, Metabolites	Toxicology
Test, Human Chorionic Gonadotropin, Serum	Immunology
Test, Infectious Mononucleosis	Immunology
Test, Prostate Specific Antigen, Free, (noncomplexed) To Distinguish Prostate Cancer From Benign Conditions	Immunology
Test, Rheumatoid Factor	Immunology
Test, Syphilis, Treponemal	Hematology
Test, Tetrahydrocannabinol	Toxicology
Test, Urea (Breath or Blood)	Microbiology
Test, Urine Leukocyte	Hematology
pH Paper, Obstetric	Obstetrics/Gynecology

AMERIVAC USA INC.   877-851-6600
1207 Pennsylvania Ave., Linden, NJ 07036
FDA Number: 3005417006   Fax: 877-851-6601
E-mail: info@AmeriVacUSA.com
Web site: www.amerivacusa.com
Ownership: Private
Produces/Sells CE-marked Devices: N
Bottle, Collection, Vacuum (Aspirator)	General
Condenser, Heat And Moisture (Artificial Nose)	Anesthesiology
Connector, Airway (Extension)	Anesthesiology
Mask, Oxygen, Aerosol Administration	Anesthesiology
Tubing, Non-Invasive	Surgery

AMERIWATER   937-461-8833
1303 Stanley Ave., Dayton, OH 45404
FDA Number: 1530185
Purification System, Water	Gastroenterology/Urology
Tank, Holding, Dialysis	Gastroenterology/Urology

AMERSHAN LIFE SCIENCE, USB SPECIALTY BIOCHEMS. DIV
   See Usb Corporation

AMES DIV.
   See Siemens Healthcare Diagnostics Inc.

AMES SUPPLIES, INC.
   See Aimes Medical Equipment Rental & Props

AMEST CORP.   949-766-9692
30394 Esperanza, Rancho Santa Margarita, CA 92688
FDA Number: 2032782   Fax: 949-766-9693
E-mail: Info@AmestCorp.COM

AMEST CORP.
949-766-9692 *(cont'd)*
Web site: www.amestcorp.com
Ownership: Private
Produces/Sells CE-marked Devices: N
Lamp, Infrared — Physical Med

AMETEK
727-536-7831
8600 Somerset Dr., Largo, FL 33773
FDA Number: 1055867
Ownership: Private
Produces/Sells CE-marked Devices: N
Dynamometer, AC-Powered — Orthopedics
Dynamometer, Non-Powered — Orthopedics

AMETEK SOLIDSTATE CONTROLS
800-635-7300
875 Dearborn Dr., Columbus, OH 43085
614-846-7500
FDA Number: n/a
Fax: 614-885-3990
Web site: www.solidstatecontrolsinc.com
Year Founded: 1962
Ownership: Private
Produces/Sells CE-marked Devices: N
Federal Procurement Eligibility: Female Owned
Distribution: Manufacturer Through Manufacturer Reps, Importer, Exporter
Power Systems, Uninterruptible (UPS) — General

AMF BIOLOGICAL
See Consolidated Technologies, Inc.

AMF BIOLOGICAL AND DIAGNOSTICS CO.
See Consolidated Technologies, Inc.

AMF SUPPORT SURFACES, INC.
See Tridien Medical

AMG MEDICAL INC.
800-361-2210
8505 Dalton Rd., Montreal, QUE H4T-1V5 Canada
514-737-5251
FDA Number: n/a
Fax: 514-737-6572
E-mail: info@amgmedical.com
Web site: www.amgmedical.com
Year Founded: 1975
Total Employees: 100
Ownership: Private
Produces/Sells CE-marked Devices: N
Distribution: Exclusive Distributor, Importer

AMG, LLC
317-329-4000
4030 Guion Ln., Indianapolis, IN 46268
FDA Number: 1833787
Regulator, Pressure, Gas Cylinder — Anesthesiology

AMGEN
See Amgen Inc.

AMGEN
See R & D Systems, Inc.

AMGEN INC.
206-265-7000
1201 Amgen Court West, Seattle, WA 98119-3105
FDA Number: n/a
Web site: www.amgen.com
Medical Products Sales Volume: $710,000,000
Year Founded: 1980
Total Employees: 17000
Ownership: AMGEN INC.
Produces/Sells CE-marked Devices: Y
Distribution: Manufacturer Direct, Manufacturer Through Distributor
General Admin.: Robert Bradway/Chief Financial Officer, Executive Vice President
Kevin Sharer/President, Chief Executive Officer, Chairman
Antibody, Monoclonal — Microbiology
Antigen, Antiserum, Control, Lymphocyte Typing — Immunology
Radioimmunoassay, Other — Chemistry

AMGEN INC.
800-28-AMGEN
One Amgen Center Drive,
805-447-1000
Thousand Oaks, CA 91320
FDA Number: n/a
Fax: 805-447-1010
E-mail: NewProducts@Amgen.com
Web site: www.amgen.com
Year Founded: 1980
Total Employees: 17000
Ownership: Public
Stock Symbol: AMGN
Traded On: NASDAQ
Produces/Sells CE-marked Devices: N
Distribution: Service Direct
General Admin.: Robert Bradway/Chief Financial Officer, Executive Vice President
Kevin Sharer/President, Chief Executive Officer, Chairman
Brian McNamee/Senior Vice President Human Resources
Tom Flanagan/Senior Vice President, Chief Information Officer
Production: Fabrizio Bonanni/Executive Vice President Operations

AMGEN INC.
800-28-AMGEN *(cont'd)*
Research: Roger M. Perlmutter/Executive Vice President Research & Development
Contract R&D, Diagnostics — General

AMI DENTAL, INC.
800-969-0405
9000 S.W. Freeway, Ste. 328, Houston, TX 77074
713-777-3422
FDA Number: n/a
Fax: 713-777-9209
Medical Products Sales Volume: $1,550,000
Annual Revenue: $1-$5 Million
Ownership: Private
Produces/Sells CE-marked Devices: N
Federal Procurement Eligibility: Small Business, Minority Owned, Female Owned
Distribution: Manufacturer Through Manufacturer Reps, Service Direct, Importer, Exporter
Dental Laboratory Equipment — Dental And Oral
Instrument, Microsurgical — Cns/Neurology

AMI, INC.
800-248-4031
1101 Noank Ledyard Road, Mystic, CT 06355
860-536-3735
FDA Number: 1221884
Fax: 860-536-4362
E-mail: sales@aquamassage.com
Web site: www.amiaqua.com
Medical Products Sales Volume: $8,000,000
Annual Revenue: $5-$10 Million
Year Founded: 1988
Total Employees: 31
Ownership: Private
Produces/Sells CE-marked Devices: Y
Federal Procurement Eligibility: Small Business, GSA Contract
Distribution: Manufacturer Direct, Manufacturer Through Manufacturer Reps, Exporter
General Admin.: David Cote/President
Mktg./Adv.: Lee Cote/Manager Advertising
Dow Cote/Manager National Sales
Massager, Therapeutic — Physical Med

AMICAS, INC.
800-490-8465
20 Guest St., Suite 200, Brighton, MA 02135
617-779-7878
FDA Number: 1225690
Fax: 617-779-7879
E-mail: info@amicas.com
Web site: www.amicas.com
Medical Products Sales Volume: $6,900,000
Annual Revenue: $10-$25 Million
Year Founded: 1997
Total Employees: 70 — Marketing Staff: 4 — Sales Staff: 10
Ownership: Private
Produces/Sells CE-marked Devices: N
General Admin.: Mr. Hamid Tabatabaie/Chief Executive Officer
Mktg./Adv.: Ms. Margaret Turano/Director Marketing
Mr. Rick Lifsitz/Director Product Development
Mr. Mark Hilborn/Vice President Business Development
Ms. Margaret Turano/Vice President Business Development
Mr. John Ariatti/Vice President Sales
Radiographic Picture Archiving/Communication System (PACS) — Radiology
System, Communication, Image, Digital — Radiology

AMICAS, INC.
386.253.6222
325 Bill France Blvd., Daytona Beach, FL 32114
FDA Number: 3005631014
Fax: 386.257.6742
Ownership: Private
Produces/Sells CE-marked Devices: N

AMICI, INC.
610-948-7100
518 Vincent St., Spring City, PA 19475-1621
FDA Number: 2522920
Fax: 610-948-2018
E-mail: info@amici-inc.com
Web site: www.amici-inc.com
Medical Products Sales Volume: $1,300,000
Annual Revenue: $1-$5 Million
Year Founded: 1978
Total Employees: 8
Ownership: Private
Produces/Sells CE-marked Devices: N
Federal Procurement Eligibility: Small Business, GSA Contract
Distribution: Manufacturer Direct, Manufacturer Through Distributor, Manufacturer Through Manufacturer Reps, OEM, Exporter
General Admin.: Michael Bono/President, Chief Executive Officer
Production: Joy Young/Manager Regulatory Affairs
Clip, Nose — Anesthesiology
Contract Manufacturing — General
Filter, Bacterial, Breathing Circuit — Anesthesiology
Mask, Other — General
Mouthpiece, Breathing — Anesthesiology
Nebulizer, Direct Patient Interface — Anesthesiology
Rebreathing System, Radionuclide — Radiology

AMICO CORPORATION
85 Fulton Way,
Richmond Hill, ONT L4B 2 Canada
887-323-3209
905-764-0800
FDA Number: 9611562
Fax: 905-764-0862
E-mail: sales@amico.com
Web site: www.amico.com
Year Founded: 1976
Total Employees: 25
Ownership: Private
Quality System Registration Information: ISO9000
Produces/Sells CE-marked Devices: N
Distribution: Manufacturer Direct, Manufacturer Through Distributor, OEM, Exporter

AMIGO MOBILITY INTERNATIONAL
6693 Dixie Hwy., Bridgeport, MI 48722-9725
800-248-9131
FDA Number: 1821729
Fax: 800-334-7274
E-mail: info@myamigo.com
Web site: www.myamigo.com
Medical Products Sales Volume: $4,100,000
Annual Revenue: $5-$10 Million
Year Founded: 1968
Total Employees: 75   Marketing Staff: 3   Sales Staff: 3
Ownership: Private
Produces/Sells CE-marked Devices: Y
Federal Procurement Eligibility: Small Business, GSA Contract, VA Contract
Distribution: Manufacturer Through Distributor, Manufacturer Through Manufacturer Reps, Exporter
Mktg./Adv.: Fran Hetzner/Manager Marketing & Advertising

Lift, Wheelchair	General
Scooter (Motorized 3-Wheeled Vehicle)	Physical Med

AMKO MANUFACTURING CO.
See Premier Dental Products Co.

AMKUS RESCUE SYSTEMS
2700 Wisconsin Ave, Downers Grove, IL 60515
800-59-AMKUS
630-515-1800
FDA Number: n/a
Fax: 630-515-8866
Web site: www.amkus.com
Medical Products Sales Volume: $6,500,000
Annual Revenue: $5-$10 Million
Year Founded: 1973
Ownership: Private
Quality System Registration Information: ISO9001
Produces/Sells CE-marked Devices: N
Federal Procurement Eligibility: Small Business
Distribution: Manufacturer Direct, Manufacturer Through Distributor

Extrication Equipment	General
Rescue Equipment	General

AMMCORP. RECORDS MANAGEMENT
See X-Ray Support, Inc

AMMEX CORP.
8220 South 212 St., Kent, WA 98032
800-274-7354
425-251-4000
FDA Number: 3023862
Fax: 425-251-8656
E-mail: shop@ammex.com
Web site: www.ammex.com
Annual Revenue: $25-$50 Million
Year Founded: 1988
Total Employees: 120
Ownership: Private
Produces/Sells CE-marked Devices: N
Distribution: Manufacturer Direct, Manufacturer Through Distributor, Importer
General Admin.: Fred Crosetto/Chief Executive Officer

Glove, Patient Examination, Latex	General
Glove, Patient Examination, Poly	General
Glove, Patient Examination, Vinyl	General

AMNION ISOMET
See Sorin Group Usa

AMNIS CORPORATION
2505 Third Avenue, Suite 210,
Seattle, WA 98121
800-730-7147
206-374-7000
FDA Number: n/a
Fax: 206-576-6895
E-mail: info@amnis.com
Web site: https://www.amnis.com
Year Founded: 1999
Ownership: Private
Produces/Sells CE-marked Devices: N
General Admin.: Dr. David Basiji/Chief Executive Officer
    Mr. William Ortyn/President, Chief Operating Officer
Mktg./Adv.: Mr. Christopher Doman/Vice President Sales
Production: Mr. Jon Roudebush/Director Manufacturing
Research: Mr. David Perry/Vice President Engineering
Finance: Mr. Patrick McDermott/Chief Financial Officer
IS: Ms. Cathleen Zimmerman/Vice President Software

AMO MANUFACTURING USA, LLC
510 Cottonwood Drive, Milpitas, CA 95035
714-247-8656
FDA Number: 3006695864
Ownership: Private
Produces/Sells CE-marked Devices: N

Keratome, AC-Powered	Ophthalmology
Lamp, Slit, Biomicroscope, AC-Powered	Ophthalmology
Laser, Excimer, Surgical	Surgery
Lens, Surgical, Laser	Ophthalmology
Phacofragmentation Unit	Ophthalmology
Refractometer, Ophthalmic	Ophthalmology

AMO WAVEFRONT SCIENCES LLC
14820 Central Ave. S.e., Albuquerque, NM 87123
714-247-8656
FDA Number: 3001030050

Aberrometer, Ophthalmic	Ophthalmology
Refractometer, Ophthalmic	Ophthalmology

AMOENA
1701 Barret Lakes Blvd., Suite 410,
Kennesaw, GA 30144
800-726-6362
770-281-8300
FDA Number: 1000641183
Fax: 800-723-3464
E-mail: info@amoena.com
Web site: www.us.amoena.com
Medical Products Sales Volume: $28,000,000
Year Founded: 1977
Total Employees: 60   Marketing Staff: 10   Sales Staff: 50
Ownership: Coloplast Manufacturing Us, Llc
Produces/Sells CE-marked Devices: Y
Federal Procurement Eligibility: Small Business
Distribution: Manufacturer Direct, Service Direct, Importer, Exporter
General Admin.: Jens Stovgaard/President
    Julianne Prowse/Vice President, General Manager

Prosthesis, Breast, External	Surgery

AMOENA CORP.
See Amoena

AMORFIX LIFE SCIENCES LTD.
3403 American Drive, Mississauga, ONTAR L4V 1T4 Canada
416-847-6898
FDA Number: n/a
Fax: 416-847-6899
E-mail: info@amorfix.com
Web site: www.amorfix.com
Ownership: Public
Stock Symbol: AMF
Traded On: Toronto
Produces/Sells CE-marked Devices: N

AMP ORTHOPEDICS
1520 4th Avenue, Suite 500, Seattle, WA 98101
206-812-9494
FDA Number: n/a
Fax: 206-812-9484
E-mail: info@amportho.com
Web site: www.amportho.com
Ownership: Private
Produces/Sells CE-marked Devices: N
General Admin.: Mr. Eric Dremel/President, Chief Executive Officer
Medical Admin.: Mr. Anthony Robins/Chief Medical Officer
    Ms. Ekta Wilcox/Director Clinical Affairs
Mktg./Adv.: Mr. Peter Coffaro/Director Marketing & Sales

AMPAC FLEXIBLES
5305 Parkdale Dr., Minneapolis, MN 55416
952-693-2475
FDA Number: 2134710
Ownership: Private
Produces/Sells CE-marked Devices: N

Container, Specimen, All Types	General

AMPRONIX, INC.
15 Whatney, Irvine, CA 92620
800-400-7972
949-273-8000
FDA Number: n/a
Fax: 949-273-8020
E-mail: Info@Ampronix.com
Web site: www.Ampronix.com
Year Founded: 1982
Ownership: Private
Quality System Registration Information: ISO9001
Produces/Sells CE-marked Devices: N
Distribution: Service Direct, Exclusive Distributor

Computer and Software, Medical	General

AMRAD
2901 W. Lawrence Avenue, Chicago, IL 60625
888-772-6723
773-353-4000
FDA Number: n/a
Fax: 773-588-3424
E-mail: grego@SummitIndustries.net
Web site: www.amradxray.net
Medical Products Sales Volume: $9,900,000
Year Founded: 1984
Total Employees: 72
Ownership: Private
Produces/Sells CE-marked Devices: N

AMRAD
888-772-6723 *(cont'd)*
Federal Procurement Eligibility: Small Business, GSA Contract
Distribution: Manufacturer Through Distributor
Mktg./Adv.: Gregory Oravec/Manager Product Development

Collimator, Radiographic, Manual	Radiology
Generator, Diagnostic X-Ray, High Voltage, 3-Phase	Radiology
Generator, Diagnostic X-Ray, High Voltage, Single Phase	Radiology
Hanger, X-Ray Tube	Radiology
Radiographic Unit, Diagnostic	Radiology
Table, Radiographic	Radiology

AMREL / AMERICAN RELIANCE, INC.
800-654-9838
11801 Goldring Road, Arcadia, CA 91006-5880
FDA Number: n/a
Fax: 626-358-3838
E-mail: ariinfo@amrel.com
Web site: www.amrel.com
Year Founded: 1985
Total Employees: 100   *Marketing Staff:* 4   *Sales Staff:* 8
Ownership: Private
Produces/Sells CE-marked Devices: N
Federal Procurement Eligibility: Small Business, GSA Contract
Distribution: Manufacturer Direct, Manufacturer Through Manufacturer Reps
Mktg./Adv.: Mr. Kevin Reilly/Manager Sales
   Ms. Ariel Phillips/Media Planner

Computer Equipment	General

AMRESCO INC.
800-366-1313
30175 Solon Industrial Pkwy., Solon, OH 44139
440-349-1313
FDA Number: 1550222
Fax: 440-349-3255
E-mail: info@amersco-inc.com
Web site: www.amresco-inc.com
Year Founded: 1976
Total Employees: 100   *Marketing Staff:* 2   *Sales Staff:* 20
Ownership: Private
Quality System Registration Information: ISO9001
Produces/Sells CE-marked Devices: N
Federal Procurement Eligibility: Small Business
Distribution: Manufacturer Direct, Manufacturer Through Distributor, Manufacturer Through Manufacturer Reps, OEM, Exporter
General Admin.: Judi Sandbrook/Manager Human Resources
   David A. Camiener/President, Owner
   Jo Soukup/Vice President, General Manager
Mktg./Adv.: Suzanne Prichett/Coord. Marketing
   Milita Matousek/Director Product Development

2, 4-dinitrophenylhydrazine, Lactate Dehydrogenase	Chemistry
Analyzer, Chemistry, Sequential Multiple, Continuous Flow	Chemistry
Antibody, Polyclonal	Microbiology
Clearing Agent	Pathology
Colorimetric Method, Triglycerides	Chemistry
Contract Manufacturing, Pharmaceuticals/Chemicals	General
Contract Manufacturing, Reagent	General
Contract R&D, Diagnostics	General
Enzymatic Esterase-Oxidase, Cholesterol	Chemistry
L-Glutamylnitroanilide/Glycylglycine, Ggtp	Chemistry
Nitrophenylphosphate, Alkaline Phosphatase Or Isoenzymes	Chemistry
Reagent, Albumin, Colorimetric	Chemistry
Reagent, Bilirubin (Total Or Direct Test System)	Chemistry
Reagent, Blood Urea Nitrogen (BUN)	Chemistry
Reagent, Calcium (Test System)	Chemistry
Reagent, Cholesterol (Total Test System)	Chemistry
Reagent, Creatinine (Test System)	Chemistry
Reagent, General Purpose	Pathology
Reagent, Glucose (Test System)	Chemistry
Reagent, Iron (Test System)	Chemistry
Reagent, Kinase, Phosphate, Creatine	Chemistry
Urease And Glutamic Dehydrogenase, Urea Nitrogen	Chemistry
Uricase (Colorimetric), Uric Acid	Chemistry

AMREX ELECTROTHERAPY EQUIPMENT
800-221-9069
641 E. Walnut St., Carson, CA 90746
310-527-6868
FDA Number: 2011115
Fax: 310-366-7343
E-mail: amrex@amrex-zetron.com
Web site: http://www.amrexusa.com
Medical Products Sales Volume: $3,000,000
Annual Revenue: $1-$5 Million
Year Founded: 1935
Total Employees: 35
Ownership: Private
Produces/Sells CE-marked Devices: N
Federal Procurement Eligibility: Small Business, Minority Owned
Distribution: Manufacturer Through Distributor, OEM, Importer, Exporter
General Admin.: George Bell/President, Chief Executive Officer

Diathermy, Shortwave	Physical Med
Diathermy, Ultrasonic (Physical Therapy)	Physical Med
Stimulator, Muscle, Electrical-Powered (EMS)	Physical Med
Stimulator, Nerve, Transcutaneous (Pain Relief, TENS)	Cns/Neurology
Stimulator, Ultrasound, Muscle	Physical Med

AMREX-ZETRON INC.
See Amrex Electrotherapy Equipment

AMS INDUSTRIES
510-667-0673
14680 Doolittel Drive, San Leandro, CA 94577
FDA Number: 2939125
Fax: 510-667-9956
E-mail: garyb@fittingimage.com
Web site: www.fittingimage.com
Annual Revenue: $10-$25 Million
Year Founded: 1983
Total Employees: 400   *Sales Staff:* 2
Ownership: Private
Produces/Sells CE-marked Devices: N
Federal Procurement Eligibility: Small Business
Distribution: Manufacturer Direct, Exporter

Floss, Dental	Dental And Oral

AMS INNOVATIVE CENTER-SAN JOSE
800-356-7600
3070 Orchard Drive, San Jose, CA 95134-2011
408-943-0636
FDA Number: 2937094
Fax: 408-428-0512
E-mail: staffing@laserscope.com
Web site: www.laserscope.com
Medical Products Sales Volume: $29,500,000
Annual Revenue: $100-$500 Million
Year Founded: 1984
Total Employees: 120   *Marketing Staff:* 5   *Sales Staff:* 20
Ownership: American Medical Systems, Inc.
Quality System Registration Information: ISO9001
Produces/Sells CE-marked Devices: Y
Federal Procurement Eligibility: Small Business
Distribution: Manufacturer Direct, Manufacturer Through Distributor, Manufacturer Through Manufacturer Reps, Service Direct, Importer, Exporter
General Admin.: Eric Reuter/Chief Executive Officer, Chairman
   Dennis LaLumandiere/Chief Financial Officer, Secretary
   Marcia Harris/Director Human Resources
Mktg./Adv.: Kerrick Securda/Manager International Development
   Kim Alt/Manager Marketing & Communications
   Robert Mann/Manager National Sales
Production: Leslie Fitzgerald/Manager Customer Services
   Van Frazier/Manager Regulatory Affairs
Research: Ken Arnold/Vice President Research & Development

Accessories, Photographic, Endoscopic	Gastroenterology/Urology
Camera, Video, Multi-Image	General
Cart, Equipment, Video	General
Electrosurgical Equipment, General Purpose	Surgery
Endoscope And Accessories, AC-Powered	Surgery
Endoscope, Rigid	Surgery
Equipment/Accessories, Laser, Laparoscopy	Surgery
Forceps, Endoscopic	Gastroenterology/Urology
Forceps, Grasping, Atraumatic	Surgery
Forceps, Grasping, Traumatic	Surgery
Headlamp, Operating, AC-Powered	Ophthalmology
Illuminator, Fiberoptic (For Endoscope)	Gastroenterology/Urology
Insufflator, Hysteroscopic	Obstetrics/Gynecology
Lamp, Operating Room	General
Laser, Dye	General
Monitor, Video, Endoscope	General
Needle, Insufflation, Laparoscopic	Surgery
Probe, Electrocauterization, Multi-Use	Surgery
Probe, Electrocauterization, Single-Use	Surgery
Resuscitator, Cardiac, Mechanical, Compressor	Anesthesiology
Scissors with Removable Tips, Laparoscopy	Surgery
Table, Operating Room, AC-Powered	Surgery
Trocar, Abdominal	Gastroenterology/Urology

AMSAN
800-327-3528
1930 Energy Park Drive, Suite 260,
651-646-7933
St. Paul, MN 55108
FDA Number: n/a
Fax: 651-645-6395
E-mail: bkservice@amsan.com
Web site: www.brissman-kennedy.com
Annual Revenue: $1-$5 Million
Year Founded: 1997
Ownership: Private
Produces/Sells CE-marked Devices: N
Federal Procurement Eligibility: Small Business
Distribution: Exclusive Distributor
Mktg./Adv.: Derek Pedlar/Vice President Sales

Disinfector, Liquid	General
Lotion, Skin Care	General
Soap	General
Solution, Antibacterial Cleaner	General

AMSINO INTERNATIONAL, INC.
800-MD-AMSINO
855 Towne Center Drive, Pomona, CA 91767
909-626-5888
FDA Number: 2085175
Fax: 909-626-3888
E-mail: info@amsino.com
Web site: www.amsino.com
Medical Products Sales Volume: $39,030,000

AMSINO INTERNATIONAL, INC. 800-MD-AMSINO *(cont'd)*
Annual Revenue: $25-$50 Million
Year Founded: 1993
Total Employees: 500   Marketing Staff: 2   Sales Staff: 10
Ownership: Private
Quality System Registration Information: ISO9001
Produces/Sells CE-marked Devices: Y
Federal Procurement Eligibility: Minority Owned
Distribution: Manufacturer Through Distributor, Manufacturer Through Manufacturer Reps, OEM
General Admin.: Dr. Richard Lee/President, Chief Executive Officer
Production: Mr. Shiya Han/Chief Engineer
   Mr. Kevin Tang/Senior Vice President Operations
   Mr. Tahua Yang/Vice President Engineering & Product Development
   Eric Zou/Vice President Operations
   Mr. Gang Chen/Vice President Quality Assurance & Regulatory Affairs
Finance: Mr. Peter Sun/Chief Financial Officer

Applicator, ENT	Ear/Nose/Throat
Catheter, Suction (Tracheal Aspirating Tube)	Anesthesiology
Depressor, Tongue, ENT, Wood	Ear/Nose/Throat
Kit, Administration, Intravenous	General
Kit, Feeding, Adult (Enteral)	General
Kit, Feeding, Pediatric (Enteral)	General
Kit, Irrigation, Sterile	Gastroenterology/Urology
Kit, Urinary Drainage Collection	Gastroenterology/Urology
Needle, Intravenous	General
Spatula, Cervical, Cytology	Obstetrics/Gynecology
Speculum, Vaginal, Non-Metal	Obstetrics/Gynecology
Spoon, Medicine	General
Syringe, Irrigating	General
Syringe, Irrigating, Sterile	General
Thermometer, Mercury	General

AMSINO MEDICAL USA 866-482-1345
5209 Linbar Dr., Suite 640, Nashville, TN 37211 615-332-9959
FDA Number: 1057300
Ownership: Private
Produces/Sells CE-marked Devices: N

Catheter, Intravascular, Therapeutic, Short-term Less Than 30 Days	General

AMTAB MANUFACTURING CO. 800-878-2257
652 N. Highland Ave, Aurora, IL 60622-6050 630-301-7600
FDA Number: n/a   Fax: 630-896-7945
E-mail: info@amtab.com
Web site: www.amtab.com
Annual Revenue: $0-$1 Million
Year Founded: 1958
Ownership: Private
Produces/Sells CE-marked Devices: N
Federal Procurement Eligibility: Small Business
Distribution: Manufacturer Direct

Office Equipment	General
Table, Other	General

AMUNEAL MANUFACTURING CORP. 800-755-9843
4737 Darrah St., Philadelphia, PA 19124 215-535-3000
FDA Number: n/a   Fax: 215-743-1715
E-mail: info@amuneal.com
Web site: www.amuneal.com
Annual Revenue: $5-$10 Million
Year Founded: 1965
Ownership: Private
Produces/Sells CE-marked Devices: N
Federal Procurement Eligibility: Small Business
Distribution: Manufacturer Direct

Shield, Magnetic Field	Radiology

AMVEX CORPORATION 866-462-6839
25b east pearce street, Suite 21, 905-764-7736
Richmond Hill, ONTAR L4B2M Canada
FDA Number: 9617620   Fax: 905-764-7743
E-mail: salessupport@amvex.com
Web site: www.amvex.com
Year Founded: 1999
Total Employees: 40
Ownership: Ohio Medical Corp.
Quality System Registration Information: ISO9001
Produces/Sells CE-marked Devices: Y
Distribution: Manufacturer Through Distributor, OEM

AMYLIOR INC. 888-453-0311
6 Antoine-Henault, 514-453-0311
Notre-Dame Ile-Perrot, QUE J7V-7 Canada
FDA Number: n/a   Fax: 514-453-0268
E-mail: info@amysystems.com
Web site: www.amysystems.com
Year Founded: 1997
Total Employees: 10

AMYLIOR INC. 888-453-0311 *(cont'd)*
Ownership: Private
Produces/Sells CE-marked Devices: N
Distribution: Manufacturer Direct, Exporter

AMYSYSTEMS 1-450-424-0288
1650, chicoine, Dorion, QC J7V 8P2 Canada
FDA Number: 9615410   Fax: 877-501-8458
E-mail: info@amysystems.com
Web site: www.amysystems.com
Year Founded: 1997
Total Employees: 20   Marketing Staff: 1   Sales Staff: 14
Ownership: Amylior Inc.
Produces/Sells CE-marked Devices: N
Distribution: Manufacturer Through Manufacturer Reps

ANACAPA TECHNOLOGIES, INC. 909-394-7795
301 E. Arrow Hwy, Ste. 106, San Dimas, CA 91773
FDA Number: 3003693789

Dressing, Other	General

ANACHEMIA CANADA INC. 800-361-0209
255 Norman St., Lachine, QUE H8R-1A3 Canada 514-489-5711
FDA Number: n/a   Fax: 514-363-5281
E-mail: info@anachemia.com
Web site: www.anachemia.com
Year Founded: 1942
Ownership: Private
Produces/Sells CE-marked Devices: N
Distribution: Manufacturer Direct, Exclusive Distributor

ANAEROBE SYSTEMS 408-782-7557
15906 Concord Circle, Morgan Hill, CA 95037
FDA Number: 2916932

Culture Media, General Nutrient Broth	Microbiology
Culture Media, Multiple Biochemical Test	Microbiology
Culture Media, Non-Selective And Differential	Microbiology
Culture Media, Non-Selective And Non-Differential	Microbiology
Culture Media, Selective And Non-Differential	Microbiology
Culture Media, Single Biochemical Test	Microbiology

ANALEX CORP.
See Qinetiq North America

ANALOG DEVICES, INC. 800-262-5643
One Technology Way, P. O. Box 9106, 781-329-4700
Norwood, MA 02062
FDA Number: n/a
Web site: www.analog.com
Annual Revenue: $10-$25 Million
Ownership: Public
Stock Symbol: ADI
Traded On: NYSE
Quality System Registration Information: ISO9000; ISO9001
Produces/Sells CE-marked Devices: Y
Distribution: Manufacturer Direct, Manufacturer Through Distributor, Manufacturer Through Manufacturer Reps
General Admin.: Ray Stata/Chairman
   Peter Forte/Chief Information Officer
   Jerald G. Fishman/President, Chief Executive Officer
Finance: David A. Zinsner/Chief Financial Officer, Vice President Finance

Accelerometer	Chemistry

ANALOGIC CORPORATION 978-326-4000
8 Centennial Drive, Peabody, MA 01960-7902
FDA Number: 1220672   Fax: 978-977-6809
E-mail: proberts@analogic.com
Web site: www.analogic.com
Medical Products Sales Volume: $351,440,000
Year Founded: 1969
Total Employees: 1000
Ownership: Public
Stock Symbol: ALOG
Traded On: NASDAQ
Quality System Registration Information: ISO9000
Produces/Sells CE-marked Devices: Y
Distribution: Manufacturer Through Distributor, Manufacturer Through Manufacturer Reps, OEM, Exporter
General Admin.: John A. Tarello/Chairman
   Bernard M. Gordon/Executive Chairman
   Jim Green/President, Chief Executive Officer
   John W. Kirby/Vice President Human Resources
Mktg./Adv.: Paul M. Roberts/Director Communications

Camera, Other	General
Computer Equipment	General
Computer, Nuclear Medicine	Radiology
Computer, Radiographic Image Analysis	Radiology
Detector, Arrhythmia Alarm	Cardiovascular
Echocardiograph (Ultrasonic Scanner)	Cardiovascular

ANALOGIC CORPORATION   978-326-4000 *(cont'd)*
Monitor, Fetal, Ultrasonic, Heart Sound	Obstetrics/Gynecology
Monitor, Perinatal	Obstetrics/Gynecology
Plethysmograph, Impedance	Cardiovascular
Scanner, Computed Tomography, X-Ray, Special Procedure	Radiology

ANALOX INSTRUMENTS USA, INC.   978-582-9368
104 Sunset Lane, P.O. BOX 208, Lunenburg, MA 01462-0208
FDA Number: 1225584   *Fax:* 978-582-9588
E-mail: info@analoxusa.com
Web site: www.analox.com
Annual Revenue: $10-$25 Million
Ownership: Analox Instruments Ltd.
Quality System Registration Information: ISO9001; ISO9002
Produces/Sells CE-marked Devices: Y
Distribution: Service Direct
Analyzer, Alcohol	Toxicology
Analyzer, Chemistry, Micro	Chemistry

ANALYSER/INDUSTRIES, USA
See Lw Scientific

ANALYTIC BIO-CHEMISTRIES LABORATORY   757-224-0177
1680-d Loretta Ave., Feasterville, PA 19053
FDA Number: 2530087
Computer and Software, Medical	General

ANALYTIC ENDODONTICS
See Sybronendo

ANALYTIC TECHNOLOGY
See Sybronendo

ANALYTICAL & RESEARCH CHEMICALS, INC.
See Analytical Scientific, Ltd.

ANALYTICAL CONTROL SYSTEMS, INC.   317-841-0458
9058 Technology Drive, Fishers, IN 46038
FDA Number: 1825740   *Fax:* 317-841-3186
E-mail: info@analyticalcontrols.com
Web site: www.analyticalcontrols.com
Medical Products Sales Volume: $1,100,000
Annual Revenue: $1-$5 Million
Year Founded: 1978
Total Employees: 9
Ownership: Private
Produces/Sells CE-marked Devices: N
Federal Procurement Eligibility: Small Business
Distribution: Manufacturer Direct, Manufacturer Through Distributor, OEM
General Admin.: Pauline Bonderman/Executive Vice President
       Dean Bonderman/President
Activated Whole Blood Clotting Time	Hematology
Control, Analyte (Assayed And Unassayed)	Chemistry
Control, Coagulation, Plasma	Hematology
Control, Multi Analyte, All Kinds (Assayed And Unassayed)	Chemistry
Hemoglobin, Resistant, Alkali	Hematology
Partial Thromboplastin Time, Reagent, Control	Hematology
Reagent, Other	General
Reagent, Quality Control	General
Reagent, Thromboplastin, With Control	Hematology
Standard/Control, Hemoglobin, Normal/Abnormal	Hematology
Thromboplastin, Activated Partial	Hematology

ANALYTICAL INDUSTRIES, INC.   909-392-6900
2855 Metropolitan Pl., Pomona, CA 91767
FDA Number: 2032134   *Fax:* 909-392-3665
E-mail: info@aii1.com
Web site: www.aii1.com
Medical Products Sales Volume: $4,400,000
Year Founded: 1994
Total Employees: 45
Ownership: Private
Quality System Registration Information: ISO9001
Produces/Sells CE-marked Devices: Y
Federal Procurement Eligibility: Small Business
Distribution: Manufacturer Through Distributor, OEM
General Admin.: Frank Gregus/President
Mktg./Adv.: Fernando Murillo/Manager Sales
       Patrick J. Prindible/Vice President Marketing
Research: Mohammad Razaq/Vice President Research & Development
Analyzer, Gas, Oxygen, Gaseous Phase	Anesthesiology

ANALYTICAL INSTRUMENT SYSTEMS, INC.   908-788-7022
P.O. Box 458, Flemington, NJ 08822-0458
FDA Number: n/a   *Fax:* 908-788-5617
E-mail: ais@aishome.com
Web site: www.aishome.com
Ownership: Private
Produces/Sells CE-marked Devices: N
Analyzer, Chemistry, Electrolyte	Chemistry
Cabinet Casework, Laboratory	Chemistry
Equipment, Marking, Electrochemical	General

ANALYTICAL INSTRUMENT SYSTEMS, INC.   908-788-7022
(cont'd)
Spectrophotometer, U.V./Visible	Chemistry

ANALYTICAL MEASUREMENTS, INC.   800-635-5580
100 Hoffman Place, Hillside, NJ 07205-1009   973-399-1444
FDA Number: n/a   *Fax:* 973-399-1446
E-mail: phmeter@bellatlantic.net
Web site: www.analyticalmeasurements.com
Medical Products Sales Volume: $300,000
Annual Revenue: $0-$1 Million
Year Founded: 2000
Total Employees: 4
Ownership: Private
Produces/Sells CE-marked Devices: N
Federal Procurement Eligibility: Small Business
Distribution: Manufacturer Direct, OEM, Service Direct, Exporter
General Admin.: W. Richard Adey/President
Controller, pH	Chemistry
Electrode, Laboratory pH	Chemistry
Electrode, pH	Gastroenterology/Urology
Meter, pH, General Use	Toxicology
Meter, pH, Portable	Chemistry
Monitor, pH	Anesthesiology
Solution, pH Buffer	Chemistry
pH Rate Measurement, Carbon-Dioxide	Chemistry

ANALYTICAL SCIENTIFIC, LTD.   800-364-4848
11049 Bandera Rd., San Antonio, TX 78250   210-684-7373
FDA Number: 1626304   *Fax:* 210-520-3344
E-mail: paul@analyticalsci.com
Web site: www.analyticalsci.com
Medical Products Sales Volume: $2,500,000
Annual Revenue: $1-$5 Million
Year Founded: 1970
Ownership: Private
Produces/Sells CE-marked Devices: N
Federal Procurement Eligibility: Small Business
Distribution: Manufacturer Direct, Manufacturer Through Distributor, Manufacturer Through Manufacturer Reps
General Admin.: George Aldrich/Manager
Complexone, Cresolphthalein, Calcium	Chemistry
Diacetyl-Monoxime, Urea Nitrogen	Chemistry
Dye-Binding, Albumin, Bromcresol, Green	Chemistry
Enzymatic Esterase-Oxidase, Cholesterol	Chemistry
Indophenol, Berthelot, Urea Nitrogen	Chemistry
Orthotoluidine, Glucose	Chemistry
Phosphorus Reagent (Test System)	Chemistry
Phosphotungstate Reduction, Uric Acid	Chemistry
Reagent, Bilirubin (Total Or Direct Test System)	Chemistry
Reagent, Chloride (Test System)	Chemistry
Reagent, Cholesterol (Total Test System)	Chemistry
Reagent, Glucose (Test System)	Chemistry
Reagent, Protein, Total	Chemistry
SGOT, Ultraviolet	Chemistry
Tetrazolium Int Dye-Diaphorase, Lactate Dehydrogenase	Chemistry
Thymolphthalein Monophosphate, Alkaline Phosphatase	Chemistry

ANALYTICAL SPECTRAL DEVICES, INC.   303-444-6522
2555 55th Street, Suite A, Boulder, CO 80301
FDA Number: n/a   *Fax:* 303-444-6825
E-mail: info@asdi.com
Web site: www.asdi.com
Medical Products Sales Volume: $8,200,000
Annual Revenue: $5-$10 Million
Year Founded: 1990
Total Employees: 40   *Marketing Staff:* 1   *Sales Staff:* 4
Ownership: Private
Produces/Sells CE-marked Devices: Y
Federal Procurement Eligibility: Small Business, GSA Contract
Distribution: Manufacturer Direct, Manufacturer Through Manufacturer Reps, OEM, Importer, Exporter
General Admin.: Mr. Brian Curtiss/Chief Technology Officer
       Mr. David Rzasa/President, Chief Executive Officer
Mktg./Adv.: Mr. Michael Lands/Director Marketing & Product Development
       Amanda Griffin/Manager Communications
       Tom Brown/Manager International Marketing & Sales
Research: Dr. Alexander F. H. Goetz/Chief Scientist
       Mr. Bob Faus/Vice President Engineering
Analyzer, Chemistry, Desk-Top	Chemistry
Photometer	Chemistry
Photometer, Reflectance	Chemistry
Spectrometer, Infrared	Chemistry
Spectrophotometer, Infrared	Chemistry
Spectrophotometer, Visible	Chemistry

ANALYTICHEM INTERNATIONAL INC.
See Varian Sample Preparation Products

ANALYTICON INSTRUMENTS CORP.   973-379-6771
99 Morrison Ave, P.O. Box 92, Springfield, NJ 07081
FDA Number: n/a   *Fax:* 973-379-6795
E-mail: info@analyticon.com
Web site: www.analyticon.com
Year Founded: 1988
Ownership: Private
Produces/Sells CE-marked Devices: N
Distribution: Exclusive Distributor, Importer

Buret	Chemistry
Meter, Conductivity	Chemistry
Titrator	Chemistry

ANAOTROS CORP.
See Ge Medical Systems Information Technologies

ANATECH ANATOMICAL TECHNOLOGIES INC.   800-667-3442
205-5920 No. 6 Road,   604-273-2836
Richmond, BC V6V-1 Canada
FDA Number: n/a   *Fax:* 604-270-4512
E-mail: info@anatechinc.com
Web site: www.anatechinc.com
Year Founded: 1985
Total Employees: 25
Ownership: Private
Produces/Sells CE-marked Devices: N

ANATECH, LTD.   800-262-8324
1020 Harts Lake Rd.,   269-964-6450
Battle Creek, MI 49015
FDA Number: 1831338   *Fax:* 269-964-8084
E-mail: email@anatechltdusa.com
Web site: www.anatechltdusa.com
Medical Products Sales Volume: $1,699,000
Annual Revenue: $1-$5 Million
Total Employees: 8
Ownership: Private
Produces/Sells CE-marked Devices: N
Federal Procurement Eligibility: Small Business, Female Owned
Distribution: Manufacturer Direct
General Admin.: Ada Feldman/Chief Executive Officer
Production: Art Nunley/Vice President Manufacturing
Finance: Elizabeth K. Dapson/Chief Financial Officer
IS: Delia Wolfe/Vice President Tech. Services

Clearing Agent	Pathology
Fixative, Alcohol Containing	Pathology
Formaldehyde (Formalin, Formol)	Pathology
Formalin, Neutral Buffered	Pathology
Mounting Media, Oil Soluble	Pathology
Soap	General
Stain, Alcian Blue	Pathology
Stain, Chemical Solution	Pathology
Stain, Dye Solution	Pathology
Stain, Eosin Y	Pathology
Stain, Hematoxylin	Pathology

ANATOMIC CONCEPTS, INC.   951-549-6800
1691 Delilah Street, Corona, CA 92879
FDA Number: 2023231

Cover, Mattress	General
Cushion, Wheelchair (Pad)	Physical Med
Mattress, Non-Powered Flotation Therapy	Physical Med
Protector, Skin Pressure	General
Stretcher, Hand-Carried	General

ANATOMICAL CHART CO.   800-621-7500
4711 Golf Road, Suite 650, Skokie, IL 60076   847-679-4700
FDA Number: n/a   *Fax:* 847-674-0211
E-mail: service@anatomical.com
Web site: www.anatomical.com
Medical Products Sales Volume: $25,000,000
Annual Revenue: $25-$50 Million
Ownership: Private
Produces/Sells CE-marked Devices: N
Federal Procurement Eligibility: Small Business
Distribution: Manufacturer Direct

Anatomical Training Model	General
Chart, Anatomical Training	General
Training Aid	Orthopedics

ANATOMICAL CONCEPTS, INC.   800-837-3888
1399 E. Western Reserve Road,   330-757-3569
Poland, OH 44514
FDA Number: 1530087   *Fax:* 800-657-7236
E-mail: theprafo@aol.com
Web site: www.prafo.net
Medical Products Sales Volume: $1,100,000
Year Founded: 1990
Total Employees: 15   *Marketing Staff:* 1   *Sales Staff:* 2

ANATOMICAL CONCEPTS, INC.   800-837-3888 *(cont'd)*
Ownership: Private
Produces/Sells CE-marked Devices: Y
Federal Procurement Eligibility: Small Business
Distribution: Manufacturer Direct
General Admin.: Mr. Richard J. Siegel/General Manager
       Mr. William W DeToro/President
Mktg./Adv.: Mr. Michael P. Banks/Director Sales

Brace, Joint, Ankle (External)	Physical Med

ANCARE CORP.   800-645-6379
2647 Grand Avenue, PO BOX 814,   516-781-0755
Bellmore, NY 11710
FDA Number: n/a   *Fax:* 516-781-4937
E-mail: info@ancare.com
Web site: www.ancare.com
Annual Revenue: $5-$10 Million
Year Founded: 1965
Ownership: Private
Produces/Sells CE-marked Devices: Y
Federal Procurement Eligibility: Small Business
Distribution: Manufacturer Direct, Exclusive Distributor
General Admin.: Mitch Kanarek/President
Mktg./Adv.: John H. Munster/National Sales Manager
       Brian Gallagher/Vice President Sales

Cage, Animal	Microbiology
Contract Manufacturing, Product, Durable	General

ANCHOR PRODUCTS COMPANY   800-323-5134
52 Official Rd., Addison, IL 60101-4519   630-543-9124
FDA Number: 1416891   *Fax:* 630-543-9131
E-mail: info@anchorsurgical.com
Web site: www.anchorsurgical.com
Year Founded: 1925
Ownership: Private
Quality System Registration Information: ISO9002
Produces/Sells CE-marked Devices: Y
Federal Procurement Eligibility: Small Business
Distribution: Manufacturer Direct, Manufacturer Through Distributor, OEM, Exporter

Biopsy Instrument	Gastroenterology/Urology
Counter, Needle	Surgery
Knife, Myringotomy	Ear/Nose/Throat
Needle, Biopsy, Mammary	Obstetrics/Gynecology
Needle, Suture, Disposable	Surgery
Needle, Suture, Reusable	Surgery
Rack, Surgical Instrument	Surgery

AND, INC.
See Purdy Electronics Corp.

ANDERMAC, INC.   800-824 0214
2626 Live Oak Hwy., Yuba City, CA 95991-8810
FDA Number: 2910744
E-mail: info@hygenique.com
Web site: www.hygenique.com
Medical Products Sales Volume: $2,000,000
Annual Revenue: $1-$5 Million
Ownership: Private
Quality System Registration Information: ISO9000
Produces/Sells CE-marked Devices: Y
Federal Procurement Eligibility: Small Business
Distribution: Manufacturer Direct, Manufacturer Through Distributor, Manufacturer Through Manufacturer Reps

Bath, Sitz, Physical Medicine	Physical Med
Bed, Patient Rotation, Powered	Physical Med
Kit, Irrigation, Perineal	Gastroenterology/Urology
Kit, Irrigation, Wound	General
Lift, Patient	General
Mirror, General & Plastic Surgery	Surgery
Scale, Bed	General

Medical Product Subsidiaries (Listed Separately)
Hygiene Specialties, Inc./Andermac, Inc.

ANDERSEN INSTRUMENTS, INC.
See Thermo Fisher Scientific

ANDERSEN PRODUCTS, INC.,   800-523-1276
Health Science Park, 3202 Caroline Drive,   336-376-3000
Haw River, NC 27258
FDA Number: 1053825   *Fax:* 336-376-8153
E-mail: mailbox@anpro.com
Web site: www.anpro.com
Annual Revenue: $5-$10 Million
Year Founded: 1958
Total Employees: 40   *Marketing Staff:* 4   *Sales Staff:* 10
Ownership: Private
Produces/Sells CE-marked Devices: Y
Federal Procurement Eligibility: Small Business

ANDERSEN PRODUCTS, INC.,   800-523-1276 (cont'd)

Distribution: Manufacturer Direct, Manufacturer Through Distributor, Manufacturer Through Manufacturer Reps, OEM, Exporter
General Admin.: Dr. H.W. Anderson/Chief Executive Officer
Mktg./Adv.: Mr. A.E. (Ted) May/General Manager Marketing & Sales

Aspirator, Low Volume (Gastric Suction)	Gastroenterology/Urology
Aspirator, Thoracic (Suction Unit)	Cardiovascular
Aspirator, Wound Suction Pump	General
Cabinet, Aerator, Ethylene-Oxide Gas	General
Cartridge, Ethylene-Oxide	General
Contract Laboratory	General
Contract Manufacturing	General
Contract Manufacturing, Product, Disposable	General
Contract Packaging	General
Contract Sterilization	General
Detector, Ethylene-Oxide Leakage	General
Dosimeter, Ethylene-Oxide	General
Drain, Suction, Closed	Surgery
Drain, Sump	Gastroenterology/Urology
Equipment, Control, Pollution	General
Kit, Wound Drainage	General
Monitor, Contamination, Environmental, Personal	General
Monitor, Gas, Atmospheric, Environmental	General
Pack, Sterilization Wrapper (Bag And Accessories)	Surgery
Packaging, Sterilization	General
Recovery Equipment, Gas	General
Sterilant, Medical Device	General
Sterilization Process Indicator, Biological	General
Sterilization Process Indicator, Chemical	General
Sterilizer, Ethylene-Oxide Gas	General
Sterilizer, Ethylene-Oxide, Bulk	General
Sterilizer, Ethylene-Oxide, Table Top	General
Test, Equipment, Sterilization	General
Tube, Double Lumen For Intestinal Decompression	Gastroenterology/Urology
Tube, Drainage	Gastroenterology/Urology
Tube, Gastrointestinal	Gastroenterology/Urology
Tube, Gastrointestinal Decompression, Cantor	Gastroenterology/Urology
Tube, Gastrointestinal Decompression, Miller-Abbott	Gastroenterology/Urology
Tube, Nasogastric	Anesthesiology
Tubing, Radiopaque	General
Wrap, Sterilization	General

ANDERSON EYE PROSTHETICS   801-262-6711
164 East 5900 South, #101-b, Murray, UT 84107
FDA Number: n/a
Ownership: Private
Produces/Sells CE-marked Devices: N

Eye, Artificial, Non-Custom	Ophthalmology

ANDERSON MOULDS, INC.   209-943-1145
3131 E. Anita St., Stockton, CA 95205
FDA Number: 3006162763

Cup, Prophylaxis	Dental And Oral

ANDERSON, W.E., DIV. DWYER INSTRUMENTS, INC.   800-872-9141

102 Highway 212, Michigan City, IN 46361   **219-879-8000**
FDA Number: n/a   Fax: 219-872-9057
E-mail: info@dwyer-inst.com
Web site: www.dwyer-inst.com
Medical Products Sales Volume: $68,900,000
Annual Revenue: $50-$100 Million
Year Founded: 1931
Total Employees: 200
Ownership: Private
Quality System Registration Information: ISO9000
Produces/Sells CE-marked Devices: N
Federal Procurement Eligibility: Small Business
Distribution: Manufacturer Direct, OEM, Exporter
General Admin.: Ed Clark/Chief Executive Officer
    Steve Clark/President
Mktg./Adv.: Kris Vallarano/Admin. Advertising
    Mark Fisher/Director Marketing & Sales

Tester, Conductivity, Floor And Equipment	General
Tester, Conductivity, Shoe And Gown	General

ANDONIAN CRYOGENICS, INC.   800-446-3533
90 Hatch St., New Bedford, MA 02745
FDA Number: n/a   Fax: 508-990-0337
E-mail: info@andoniancryogenics.com
Web site: www.andoniancryogenics.com
Medical Products Sales Volume: $2,000,000
Ownership: Private
Produces/Sells CE-marked Devices: N
Federal Procurement Eligibility: Small Business
Distribution: Manufacturer Direct

Calibrator, Gas, Pressure	Anesthesiology
Canister, Liquid Oxygen, Portable	Anesthesiology
Container, Liquid Nitrogen	Anesthesiology

ANDONIAN CRYOGENICS, INC.   800-446-3533 (cont'd)

Container, Liquid Oxygen	Anesthesiology
Manifold, Gas	Chemistry
Regulator, Pressure, Gas Cylinder	Anesthesiology
Service, Maintenance/Repair	General
Valve, Other	Chemistry

ANDOVER COATED PRODUCTS, INC.
See Andover Healthcare Inc.

ANDOVER HEALTHCARE INC.   800-432-6686
9 Fanaras Dr., Salisbury, MA 01952   **978-465-0044**
FDA Number: 1220799
Web site: www.andovercoated.com
Medical Products Sales Volume: $20,000,000
Annual Revenue: $10-$25 Million
Year Founded: 1976
Ownership: Private
Quality System Registration Information: ISO9002
Produces/Sells CE-marked Devices: Y
Federal Procurement Eligibility: Small Business
Distribution: Manufacturer Through Distributor

Bandage, Adhesive	Surgery
Bandage, Elastic	General
Moleskin	General
Tape, Cotton	General

ANDREW J. DIAMOND, M.D.   770-933-8214
551 Hackney Dr., Marietta, GA 30067
FDA Number: 3004822514
Ownership: Private
Produces/Sells CE-marked Devices: N

Splint, Nasal	Ear/Nose/Throat

ANDROMED INC.   888-877-8477
5003 Levy St, St-Laurent, QUE H4R 2N9 Canada   **514-336-0043**
FDA Number: n/a   Fax: 514-336-9337
E-mail: andromed@andromed.com
Web site: www.andromed.com
Year Founded: 1997
Total Employees: 50
Ownership: Private
Produces/Sells CE-marked Devices: N
Distribution: Manufacturer Direct, Exclusive Distributor, Exporter

ANDROS, INC.   510-837-3500
870 Harbour Way South, Richmond, CA 94804-3613
FDA Number: 2936805   Fax: 510-837-3600
E-mail: info@andros.com
Web site: www.andros.com
Medical Products Sales Volume: $10,000,000
Annual Revenue: $25-$50 Million
Year Founded: 1968
Total Employees: 85   Marketing Staff: 3   Sales Staff: 7
Ownership: LumaSense Technologies Inc.
Quality System Registration Information: ISO9000; ISO9001
Produces/Sells CE-marked Devices: Y
Federal Procurement Eligibility: Small Business, GSA Contract
Distribution: OEM, Service Direct
General Admin.: John Frank/Chief Executive
Mktg./Adv.: Ms. Heidi Hughes/Director Marketing & Sales
Production: Peter Chu/Director Quality Assurance
    Mr. Seb Nardecchia/Vice President Operations
Research: Ken Christensen/Vice President Research & Development
Finance: Ms. Cindee Beechwood/Chief Financial Officer

Analyzer, Gas, Anesthetic	Anesthesiology
Analyzer, Gas, Carbon-Dioxide, Gaseous Phase (Capnograph)	Anesthesiology
Analyzer, Gas, Nitrous-Oxide, Gaseous Phase	Anesthesiology

ANDWIN SCIENTIFIC   800-497-3113
6636 Variel Ave., Woodland Hills, CA 91303   **818-999-2828**
FDA Number: 2027344   Fax: 818-999-0111
E-mail: web@andwin.com
Web site: www.andwin.com
Annual Revenue: $10-$25 Million
Ownership: Private
Quality System Registration Information: ISO9001
Produces/Sells CE-marked Devices: N
Federal Procurement Eligibility: Female Owned
Distribution: OEM

Collector, Specimen	Microbiology
Kit, Pap Smear	Obstetrics/Gynecology

ANECARE LABORATORIES, INC.   801-977-8877
3487 West 2100 South #100, Salt Lake City, UT 84119
FDA Number: 3005724505

Rebreathing Unit	Anesthesiology

ANESTHESIA ASSOCIATES, INC.   760-744-6561
460 Enterprise St., San Marcos, CA 92078-4363
FDA Number: 2022648   *Fax:* 760-744-0054
E-mail: SolutionsMDR@AincA.com
Web site: www.AincA.com
Medical Products Sales Volume: $600,000
Year Founded: 1958
Total Employees: 7
Ownership: Private
Produces/Sells CE-marked Devices: N
Federal Procurement Eligibility: Small Business, VA Contract
Distribution: Manufacturer Through Distributor, Manufacturer Through
Manufacturer Reps, OEM
General Admin.: George Jackson/President
           Donald Rowean/Vice President
Production: R. Lockwood Williams/Vice President Operations

Absorber, Carbon-Dioxide	Anesthesiology
Airway, Nasopharyngeal (Breathing Tube)	Anesthesiology
Airway, Oropharyngeal, Anesthesia	Anesthesiology
Catheter, Nasopharyngeal	Ear/Nose/Throat
Circuit, Breathing (W Connector, Adapter, Y Piece)	Anesthesiology
Circuit, Breathing, Ventilator	Anesthesiology
Cuff, Blood Pressure	Cardiovascular
Cuff, Tracheal Tube, Inflatable	Anesthesiology
Fitting, Luer	General
Forceps, General & Plastic Surgery	Surgery
Laryngoscope	Ear/Nose/Throat
Mask, Gas, Anesthesia	Anesthesiology
Resuscitator, Pulmonary, Manual (Demand Valve)	General
Scavenger, Gas, Anesthesia Unit	Anesthesiology
Spirometer, Diagnostic (Respirometer)	Anesthesiology
Stimulator, Peripheral Nerve, Blockade Monitor	Anesthesiology
Stylet, Tracheal Tube	Anesthesiology
Tubing, Conductive	General

ANESTHESIA EQUIPMENT SUPPLY, INC.   253-631-8008
24301 Roberts Dr., Black Diamond, WA 98010
FDA Number: 3022477

Airway, Oropharyngeal, Anesthesia	Anesthesiology
Gas-Machine, Anesthesia	Anesthesiology

ANESTHESIA RESPIRATORY TECHNOLOGY
See Artec Environmental Monitoring

ANESTHETIC VAPORIZER SERVICES   716-759-8490
10185 Main St., Clarence, NY 14031-2044
FDA Number: 1317847
Ownership: Private
Produces/Sells CE-marked Devices: N

Vaporizer, Anesthesia, Non-Heated	Anesthesiology

ANGEION CORPORATION   651-484-4874
350 Oak Grove Pkwy, Saint Paul, MN 55127
FDA Number: n/a   *Fax:* 651-484-4874
E-mail: investor@angeion.com
Web site: http://www.angeion.com
Year Founded: 1986
Ownership: Private
Produces/Sells CE-marked Devices: N
General Admin.: Mr. William Kullback/Chief Financial Officer, Senior Vice President
           Mr. Philip Smith/President, Chief Executive Officer
Mktg./Adv.: Mr. Terrance Kaspen/Senior Vice President Marketing & Business
Development
Production: Mr. Timothy Fitzgerald/Senior Vice President Operations

ANGEL MEDICAL SYSTEMS   800-763-5099
1163 Shrewsbury Avenue, Suite E,   **732-542-5551**
Shrewsbury, NJ 07702
FDA Number: n/a   *Fax:* 732-542-5560
E-mail: info@angel-med.com
Web site: http://www.angel-med.com
Ownership: Private
Produces/Sells CE-marked Devices: N
General Admin.: Mr. Robert Fischell/Chairman
           Mr. David Fischell/Chief Executive Officer
           Mr. Jonothan Harwood/Chief Operating Officer
           Mr. Mario Azevedo/Vice President
Finance: Mr. Andrew Taylor/Chief Financial Officer

ANGELICA IMAGE APPAREL   800-222-3112
700 Rosedale Avenue, St. Louis, MO 63112   **314-889-1111**
FDA Number: 1925239   *Fax:* 314-889-1146
E-mail: sales@angelica.com
Web site: www.angelica.com
Medical Products Sales Volume: $77,000,000
Year Founded: 1986
Total Employees: 5400
Ownership: ANGELICA CORPORATION
Produces/Sells CE-marked Devices: N

ANGELICA IMAGE APPAREL   800-222-3112 *(cont'd)*
Distribution: Manufacturer Direct, Manufacturer Through Distributor
General Admin.: Charles D. Molloy/President
           Melva Ruff-Pete/Vice President Human Resources
Mktg./Adv.: Ken Underhill/Director Marketing
           Lawrence Newman/Vice President Sales
Production: Michelle Westbrook/Vice President Product Development &
Operations

Accessories, Apparel, Surgical	Surgery
Bag, Laundry, Operating Room	General
Cap, Surgical	Surgery
Cover, Head, Surgical	Surgery
Drape, Surgical	Surgery
Dress, Scrub, Reusable	Surgery
Dress, Surgical	Surgery
Gown, Isolation, Surgical	Surgery
Gown, Operating Room, Reusable	Surgery
Gown, Other	General
Gown, Patient	Surgery
Gown, Patient, Reusable	General
Gown, Surgical	Surgery
Hood, Surgical	Surgery
Suit, Scrub, Reusable	Surgery
Suit, Surgical	Surgery
Wrapper, Surgical Instrument (Sterile)	General

ANGELICA UNIFORM GROUP
See Angelica Image Apparel

ANGELUS MEDICAL & OPTICAL CO., INC.   310-769-6060
13007 S. Western Avenue, Gardena, CA 90249-1919
FDA Number: 2014286   *Fax:* 310-769-1999
E-mail: angelusmed.@msn.com
Web site: www.angelusmedical.com
Medical Products Sales Volume: $1,500,000
Annual Revenue: $1-$5 Million
Year Founded: 1946
Total Employees: 10   *Sales Staff:* 4
Ownership: Private
Produces/Sells CE-marked Devices: N
Federal Procurement Eligibility: Small Business
Distribution: Service Direct
General Admin.: Richard D. Coryell/President
Mktg./Adv.: Laura Coryell/Manager Sales
           Michael McHugh/Vice President Business Development
           Laura Coryell/Vice President Marketing
           Richard D. Coryell/Vice President Sales
Finance: Michael McHugh/Controller

Service, Equipment Leasing	General
Service, Used Equipment	General

ANGIODYNAMICS, INC.   518-795-1400
14 Plaza Drive, Latham, NY 12110
FDA Number: 1319211   *Fax:* 518-795-1401
E-mail: info@angiodynamics.com
Web site: www.angiodynamics.com
Annual Revenue: $25-$50 Million
Year Founded: 1988
Ownership: Public
Stock Symbol: ANGO
Traded On: NASDAQ
Produces/Sells CE-marked Devices: Y
Federal Procurement Eligibility: Small Business
Distribution: Manufacturer Direct
General Admin.: Jan Keltjens/President, Chief Executive Officer
           Mr. Shawn McCarthy/Senior Vice President
Mktg./Adv.: Ms. Lynda Wallace/Senior Vice President Business Development
Production: Mr. Harold Mapes/Senior Vice President Operations
Research: Mr. William Appling/Senior Vice President Research
Finance: Joseph Gersuk/Chief Financial Officer

Adapter, Stopcock, Manifold, Cardiopulmonary Bypass	Cardiovascular
Cannula, Catheter	Cardiovascular
Catheter, Angiographic	Cns/Neurology
Catheter, Irrigation	Surgery
Guide, Catheter	Cardiovascular
Guidewire, Catheter	Cardiovascular
Injector And Syringe, Angiographic, Balloon Inflation, Reprocessed	Cardiovascular
Introducer, Catheter	Cardiovascular
Laser, Surgical	Surgery
Retention Device, Suture	Surgery
Trocar, Cardiovascular	Cardiovascular

Medical Product Subsidiaries (Listed Separately)
Angiodynamics, Inc.
Oncobionic

ANGIODYNAMICS, INC.   1 518-795-1400
14 Plaza Drive, Latham, NY 12110
FDA Number: 3008319439
E-mail: info@angiodynamics.com
Web site: www.angiodynamics.com   *Fax:* 1 518-795-1401

ANGIODYNAMICS, INC. 1 518-795-1400 *(cont'd)*
Year Founded: 1988
Ownership: Angiodynamics, Inc.
Stock Symbol: ANGO
Traded On: NASDAQ
Produces/Sells CE-marked Devices: N
General Admin.: Mr. D. Joseph Gersuk/Chief Financial Officer, Executive Vice President
  Mr. Eamonn P. Hobbs/President, Chief Executive Officer
Mktg./Adv.: Mr. Sean C. Morris/Vice President Market Development
Production: Mr. Harold C. Mapes/Vice President Operations
Catheter, Intravascular, Diagnostic	Cardiovascular
Catheter, Percutaneous	Cardiovascular
Trocar, Cardiovascular	Cardiovascular

ANGIODYNAMICS, INC. 510-771-0400
46421 Landing Parkway, Fremont, CA 94538
FDA Number: 2952363
Web site: www.angiodynamics.com
Year Founded: 1994
Total Employees: 80   *Marketing Staff:* 5   *Sales Staff:* 32
Ownership: Angiodynamics, Inc.
Traded On: NASDAQ
Quality System Registration Information: ISO9001
Produces/Sells CE-marked Devices: Y
Federal Procurement Eligibility: Small Business
Distribution: Manufacturer Direct, Manufacturer Through Distributor
Accessories, Catheter	Surgery
Electrosurgical Unit, Cutting & Coagulation Device	Surgery
Generator, Radiofrequency Lesion	Cns/Neurology
Probe, Electrosurgery, Endoscopy	Surgery

ANGIODYNAMICS, INC. 800-472-5221
One Horizon Way, Manchester, GA 31816 706-846-3126
FDA Number: 1056436   *Fax:* 706-846-3146
E-mail: info@angiodynamics.com
Web site: www.angiodynamics.com
Annual Revenue: $25-$50 Million
Year Founded: 1990
Total Employees: 151   *Marketing Staff:* 4   *Sales Staff:* 75
Ownership: Angiodynamics, Inc.
Stock Symbol: ANGO
Traded On: NASDAQ
Quality System Registration Information: ISO9001
Produces/Sells CE-marked Devices: Y
Federal Procurement Eligibility: Small Business
Distribution: Manufacturer Direct, Manufacturer Through Distributor, Manufacturer Through Manufacturer Reps, OEM, Exporter
Accessories, AV Shunt	Gastroenterology/Urology
Accessories, Catheter	Surgery
Accessories, Catheter, G-U	Gastroenterology/Urology
Adapter, AV Shunt Or Fistula	Gastroenterology/Urology
Cannula, AV Shunt	Gastroenterology/Urology
Catheter, Arterial	Cardiovascular
Catheter, Central Venous	General
Catheter, Femoral	Gastroenterology/Urology
Catheter, Hemodialysis	Gastroenterology/Urology
Catheter, Hemodialysis, Single-Needle	Gastroenterology/Urology
Catheter, Intravascular, Therapeutic, Long-term Greater Than 30 Days	General
Catheter, Multiple Lumen	Surgery
Catheter, Other	Gastroenterology/Urology
Catheter, Peritoneal	Surgery
Catheter, Peritoneal, Indwelling, Long-Term	Gastroenterology/Urology
Catheter, Subclavian	Cardiovascular
Catheter, Tenckhoff	Gastroenterology/Urology
Catheter, Vascular, Long-Term	Cardiovascular
Guidewire, Catheter	Cardiovascular
Introducer, Catheter	Cardiovascular
Port, Vascular Access	Cardiovascular
Shunt, Arteriovenous	Gastroenterology/Urology
Stylet, Catheter, Gastro-Urology	Gastroenterology/Urology

ANGIOMEDICS INC.
See Boston Scientific Corp.

ANGIOSCORE, INC. 877-264-4692
5055 Brandin Court, Fremont, CA 94538 510-933-7900
FDA Number: 3005462046   *Fax:* 510-933-7901
Web site: www.angioscore.com
Year Founded: 2003
Ownership: Private
Produces/Sells CE-marked Devices: Y
General Admin.: James Andrews/Chief Financial Officer, Vice President
  Thomas Trotter/President, Chief Executive Officer
Medical Admin.: Dr. Gary Gershony/Chief Medical Officer
Mktg./Adv.: Michael Gioffredi/Vice President Marketing & Sales
Production: Mr. Samuel Omaleki/Vice President Manufacturing
  Karin Gastineau/Vice President Quality Assurance & Regulatory Affairs
Research: Mr. Peter Johansson/Vice President Research & Development

ANGIOSCORE, INC. 877-264-4692 *(cont'd)*
Catheter, Angioplasty, Transluminal, Peripheral	Cardiovascular
Catheter, Percutaneous	Cardiovascular

ANGIOSCORE, INC. 877-264-4692
5055 Brandin Court, fremont, CA 94538 510-933-7914
FDA Number: 3005462046   *Fax:* 510-933-7901
Ownership: Private
Produces/Sells CE-marked Devices: N
General Admin.: Mr. Thomas Trotter/President, Chief Executive Officer
  Mr. James Andrews/Senior Vice President
Medical Admin.: Dr. Gary Gershony/Chief Medical Officer
Mktg./Adv.: Mr. Peter Johansson/Senior Vice President Marketing
Production: Mr. Samuel Omaleki/Vice President Manufacturing
  Mr. Kent Jones/Vice President Quality Control & Regulatory Affairs
Catheter, Angioplasty, Peripheral, Ultrasonic	Cardiovascular
Catheter, Percutaneous	Cardiovascular

ANGIOSYSTEMS, INC. 800-441-4256
7 Hopkins Pl., Ducktown, TN 37326 423-496-3221
FDA Number: 1037577   *Fax:* 423-496-3050
E-mail: jessica@angiosystems.net
Web site: www.angiosystems.net
Annual Revenue: $1-$5 Million
Total Employees: 65
Ownership: Private
Produces/Sells CE-marked Devices: N
Federal Procurement Eligibility: Small Business, Minority Owned, Female Owned
Distribution: Manufacturer Direct, Manufacturer Through Distributor, Manufacturer Through Manufacturer Reps, OEM, Exporter
General Admin.: David L. Hopkins/President, Chief Executive Officer
Production: Marci L. Hopkins/Director Quality Assurance
  Sidney McEachern/Vice President Manufacturing
Purchasing: Teri McEachern/Director Purchasing
Drape, Surgical	Surgery
Dressing, Other	General
Packaging Material	General
Shield, Protective, Personnel	Radiology
Tray, Custom/Special Procedure	General

ANGIOTEC DIV.
See Andros, Inc.

ANGIOTECH 800-424-6779
241 West Palatine Road, Wheeling, IL 60090 847-637-3333
FDA Number: 1417485   *Fax:* 847-637-3334
E-mail: info@manan.com
Web site: www.angiotech.com
Medical Products Sales Volume: $93,500,000
Annual Revenue: $50-$100 Million
Year Founded: 1965
Total Employees: 1112   *Marketing Staff:* 1   *Sales Staff:* 2
Ownership: MARMON GROUP, INC., THE
Stock Symbol: ANPI
Traded On: NASDAQ
Quality System Registration Information: ISO9001
Produces/Sells CE-marked Devices: N
Federal Procurement Eligibility: Small Business
Distribution: Manufacturer Direct
General Admin.: Werner Mittermeier/President, Chief Executive Officer
Mktg./Adv.: Wayne Black/Manager Marketing & Sales
Production: Robie Paladugu/Director Regulatory Affairs
  Gary Price/Manager Production
Research: John Pavect/Vice President Engineering
Device, Biopsy, Percutaneous	Surgery
Kit, Biopsy Needle	Gastroenterology/Urology
Needle, Biopsy, Mammary	Obstetrics/Gynecology
Needle, Catheter	Surgery

ANGIOTECH PHARMACEUTICALS, INC. 604-221-7676
1618 Station Street, Vancouver, BC V6A 1B6 Canada
FDA Number: n/a   *Fax:* 604-221-2330
E-mail: info@angio.com
Web site: www.angiotech.com
Year Founded: 1992
Ownership: Public
Stock Symbol: ANPI
Traded On: NASDAQ
Quality System Registration Information: ISO9001
Produces/Sells CE-marked Devices: Y
Federal Procurement Eligibility: Small Business
Distribution: Manufacturer Direct, Manufacturer Through Distributor, Manufacturer Through Manufacturer Reps, OEM, Service Direct

ANGUIL ENVIRONMENTAL SYSTEMS, INC. 800-488-0230
8855 N. 55th St., Milwaukee, WI 53223 414-365-6400
FDA Number: n/a   *Fax:* 414-365-6410
E-mail: info@anguil.com

ANGUIL ENVIRONMENTAL SYSTEMS, INC. 800-488-0230 (cont'd)
Web site: www.anguil.com
Medical Products Sales Volume: $22,000,000
Annual Revenue: $10-$25 Million
Year Founded: 1978
Total Employees: 47
Ownership: Private
Produces/Sells CE-marked Devices: N
Federal Procurement Eligibility: Small Business
Distribution: Manufacturer Through Manufacturer Reps
General Admin.: Gene Anguil/Chief Executive Officer
        Sandi Sutton/Manager Human Resources
Mktg./Adv.: Kate Simmons/Manager Marketing & Advertising
        Deborah Anguil/Vice President Business Development
        Chris Anguil/Vice President, Manager Sales
Production: Don Bock/Manufacturing Engineer

Environmental Control System, Powered	Physical Med
Equipment, Control, Pollution	General

ANHOLT TECHNOLOGIES, INC.   610-268-2758
440 Church Rd., Avondale, PA 19311
FDA Number: 3005216036

Table, Radiographic, Stationary Top	Radiology

ANIKA THERAPEUTICS   781-457-9000
32 Wiggins Avenue, Bedford, MA 01730
FDA Number: 1223628   *Fax:* 781-305-9720
E-mail: contact@anikatherapeutics.com
Web site: www.anikatherapeutics.com
Medical Products Sales Volume: $26,800,000
Annual Revenue: $25-$50 Million
Year Founded: 1993
Total Employees: 50   *Marketing Staff:* 2
Ownership: Public
Stock Symbol: ANIK
Traded On: NASDAQ
Quality System Registration Information: ISO9001
Produces/Sells CE-marked Devices: Y
Federal Procurement Eligibility: Small Business
Distribution: Manufacturer Through Distributor
General Admin.: Frank Luppino/Chief Operating Officer
        Charles H. Sherwood/President, Chief Executive Officer
Mktg./Adv.: Mr. Thomas Chambers/Vice President Marketing & Sales
Production: Ms. Irina Kulinets/Vice President Regulatory & Clinical Affairs
Finance: Mr. Kevin Quinlan/Chief Financial Officer

Acid, Hyaluronic	Dental And Oral

ANIMAS CORP.   877-767-7373
200 Lawrence Drive, West Chester, PA 19380   610-644-8990
FDA Number: 2531779   *Fax:* 610-644-8717
E-mail: comments@animascorp.com
Web site: www.animascorp.com
Year Founded: 1996
Total Employees: 300
Ownership: Johnson & Johnson
Quality System Registration Information: ISO9001
Produces/Sells CE-marked Devices: Y
Federal Procurement Eligibility: Small Business

Infusion Pump, Insulin	General

ANISSA'S FUN PATCHES   423-234-3404
P.O. Box 455, Chuckey, TN 37641
FDA Number: 3003897845   *Fax:* 423-234-3404
E-mail: anissasfunpatch@mounet.com
Web site: www.anissasfunpatches.com
Medical Products Sales Volume: $13,000
Annual Revenue: $0-$1 Million
Year Founded: 2002
Total Employees: 1
Ownership: Private
Produces/Sells CE-marked Devices: N
Federal Procurement Eligibility: Female Owned
Distribution: Manufacturer Direct

Shield, Eye, Ophthalmic	Ophthalmology

ANJON, LLC   904-730-9373
4801 Dawin Rd., Jacksonville, FL 32207
FDA Number: 1066368   *Fax:* 904-730-8681
E-mail: sales@anjoninc.com
Ownership: Private
Produces/Sells CE-marked Devices: N

Component, Traction, Invasive	Orthopedics

ANKO PRODUCTS, INC., MITYFLEX DIV.   800-446-2656
3007 29th Avenue E., Bradenton, FL 34208   941-749-1960
FDA Number: n/a   *Fax:* 941-748-2307
E-mail: sales@ankoproducts.com
Web site: www.ankoproducts.com

ANKO PRODUCTS, INC., MITYFLEX DIV.   800-446-2656 (cont'd)
Medical Products Sales Volume: $4,900,000
Annual Revenue: $5-$10 Million
Year Founded: 1980
Total Employees: 50   *Marketing Staff:* 2   *Sales Staff:* 4
Ownership: Private
Quality System Registration Information: ISO9002
Produces/Sells CE-marked Devices: N
Federal Procurement Eligibility: Small Business
Distribution: Manufacturer Direct, Manufacturer Through Distributor, Manufacturer Through Manufacturer Reps, OEM
Mktg./Adv.: Tom Collentine/Director Marketing & Sales

Pump, Vacuum, Central	Anesthesiology

ANN ARBOR DIGITAL DEVICES   734-834-5156
699 Skynob Court, Ann Arbor, MI 48105
FDA Number: 3004978314   *Fax:* 734-475-3114
E-mail: sales@a2dxray.com
Web site: www.a2d2xray.com
Ownership: Private
Produces/Sells CE-marked Devices: N

Digital Image, Storage And Communications, Non-diagnostic, Laboratory Information System	Chemistry

ANNA-DOTE, INC.   800-346-6132
40 Pullam Drive,   724-346-6132
West Middlesex, PA 16159
FDA Number: 2529294   *Fax:* 724-346-6132
Web site: www.anna-dote.com
Year Founded: 1989
Ownership: Private
Produces/Sells CE-marked Devices: N
Federal Procurement Eligibility: Small Business
Distribution: Manufacturer Direct
General Admin.: Frank Draskovic/President

Support, Patient Position	Anesthesiology

ANNEX MEDICAL, INC.   952-942-7576
6018 Blue Circle Dr., Minnetonka, MN 55343-9104
FDA Number: 2183873   *Fax:* 952-942-7590
E-mail: contact@annexmedical.com
Web site: www.annexmedical.com
Year Founded: 1988
Ownership: Private
Quality System Registration Information: ISO9001
Produces/Sells CE-marked Devices: Y
Federal Procurement Eligibility: Small Business
Distribution: OEM
General Admin.: Stuart Lind/President
        Eugene Karels/Vice President, General Manager

Brush, Cytology, Endoscopic	Gastroenterology/Urology
Dislodger, Stone, Basket, Ureteral, Metal	Gastroenterology/Urology
Dislodger, Stone, Flexible	Gastroenterology/Urology
Forceps, Biopsy, Non-Electric	Gastroenterology/Urology
Snare, Flexible	Gastroenterology/Urology

ANODIA SYSTEMS   866.246.2548
109 Larrimore Lane, Danville, KY 40422
FDA Number: 3003917473   *Fax:* 866.926.8246
E-mail: info@mintakleen.com
Web site: www.anodiasystems.com
Ownership: Private
Produces/Sells CE-marked Devices: N

Handpiece, Air-Powered, Dental	Dental And Oral
Operative Dental Treatment Unit	Dental And Oral

ANODYNE MEDICAL TECHNOLOGIES, INC   340-772-2846
Rr2 Box 9905, Industrial Park, Bldg 2, Kingshill, VI 00850
FDA Number: 3005535230
Ownership: Private
Produces/Sells CE-marked Devices: N

Lamp, Infrared	Physical Med

ANODYNE THERAPY, LLC   800-521-6664
14105 McCormick Drive, Tampa, FL 33626   813-645-2855
FDA Number: 1055581   *Fax:* 813-342-4417
Web site: www.anodynetherapy.com
Ownership: Private
Produces/Sells CE-marked Devices: N

Bandage, Compression	General
Binder, Medical, Therapeutic	General
Brace, Joint, Ankle (External)	Physical Med
Joint, Knee, External Brace	Physical Med
Lamp, Infrared	Physical Med
Orthosis, Limb Brace	Physical Med
Orthosis, Lumbar	Physical Med
Pad, Heating, Powered	Physical Med
Splint, Extremity, Non-Inflatable, External	Surgery

ANODYNE THERAPY, LLC 800-521-6664 *(cont'd)*
Support, Head And Trunk, Wheelchair Physical Med

ANOMERIC, INC. 225-268-3052
755 Delgado Dr., Baton Rouge, LA 70808
FDA Number: 2320429
Ownership: Private
Produces/Sells CE-marked Devices: N
Stain, Microbiological Microbiology

ANOVA IMPLANT SOLUTIONS LLC 615-457-3311
2 Maryland Farms, Suite 120, Brentwood, TN 37027
FDA Number: 300881728
E-mail: customerservice@anovaimplants.com
Web site: http://www.anovaimplants.com
Ownership: Private
Produces/Sells CE-marked Devices: N
General Admin.: Mr. Walter Spires/Chief Executive Officer

ANSCULETTE
See Cardionics, Inc.

ANSELL EDMONT INDUSTRIAL
See Ansell Protective Products

ANSELL HEALTHCARE PRODUCTS, INC. 732-345-5400
200 Schulz Dr., Red Bank, NJ 07701
FDA Number: 1529100
E-mail: info@ansellhealthcare.com
Web site: www.ansellhealthcare.com
Medical Products Sales Volume: $700,000,000
Total Employees: 11000
Ownership: Life Guard
Traded On: Sydney
Quality System Registration Information: ISO9001; ISO9002
Produces/Sells CE-marked Devices: N
Distribution: Manufacturer Direct, Manufacturer Through Distributor
General Admin.: Scott Papier/Senior Vice President
Mktg./Adv.: Patty Taylor/Vice President Market Development
  Scott Clausen/Vice President Sales
Production: Scott Lewkowitz/Director Customer Services
Research: Michael Zedalis/Senior Vice President Scientific Affairs
Catheter, Hemostatic Gastroenterology/Urology
Drain, Penrose Gastroenterology/Urology
Glove, Other General
Glove, Patient Examination General
Glove, Protective, Radiographic Radiology
Glove, Surgical General
Glove, Surgical, Hypoallergenic General
Glove, Surgical, Plastic Surgery Surgery
Glove, Surgical, Powder-Free Surgery
Glove, Utility General
Tubing, Other General

ANSELL HEALTHCARE, INC. 800-952-9916
200 Schulz Drive, Red Bank, NJ 07701 732-345-5400
FDA Number: 1019632 *Fax:* 732-219-5114
E-mail: info@ansellhealthcare.com
Web site: www.ansellhealthcare.com
Medical Products Sales Volume: $18,200,000
Year Founded: 1999
Total Employees: 240 *Marketing Staff:* 30 *Sales Staff:* 30
Ownership: Afp Imaging Corp.
Stock Symbol: ANN
Traded On: NASDAQ
Quality System Registration Information: ISO9001
Produces/Sells CE-marked Devices: Y
Federal Procurement Eligibility: Small Business
Distribution: Manufacturer Direct
General Admin.: Douglas Tough/Chief Executive Officer
  William Reed/Vice President, General Manager
Mktg./Adv.: Carol Carrozza/Manager Product Development
  Carol Carrozza/Vice President Marketing
  Kerry Hoffman/Vice President Sales
Production: Rainer Wolf/Vice President Manufacturing
  Lon McIlvain/Vice President Regulatory Affairs
  Dr. Michael Zedalis/Vice President Technology & Product Development
Research: Michael Zedalis/Vice President Research & Development
Condom Obstetrics/Gynecology

ANSELL PERRY
See Ansell Healthcare Products, Inc.

ANSELL PERRY INC. 800-363-8340
105 rue Lauder, 450-266-1850
Cowansville, QUE J2K-2 Canada
FDA Number: n/a *Fax:* 450-266-6150
E-mail: serviceclientcanada@ansell.com
Web site: www.ansellhealthcare.com
Year Founded: 1987

ANSELL PERRY INC. 800-363-8340 *(cont'd)*
Total Employees: 25
Ownership: PACIFIC DUNLOP LTD.
Produces/Sells CE-marked Devices: N
Distribution: Manufacturer Direct, Exclusive Distributor, Exporter

ANSELL PROTECTIVE PRODUCTS 800-800-0444
200 Schultz Drive, Red Bank, NJ 07701 732-345-5400
FDA Number: 1529100 *Fax:* 800-800-0445
E-mail: anselltek@ansell.com
Web site: www.ansellpro.com
Medical Products Sales Volume: $145,100,000
Annual Revenue: $500 Million-$1 Billion
Year Founded: 1905
Total Employees: 300 *Sales Staff:* 40
Ownership: Private
Produces/Sells CE-marked Devices: Y
Federal Procurement Eligibility: Small Business
Distribution: Manufacturer Through Distributor
General Admin.: Doug Tough/President
Mktg./Adv.: Robert Gaither/Vice President Marketing & Sales
Glove, Other General

ANSELL, INC.
See Ansell Healthcare, Inc.

ANSEN CORPORATION 315-393-3573
100 Chimney Point Dr., Ogd, NY 13669
FDA Number: 3003867964
Defibrillator, External, Automatic Cardiovascular

ANSOFT CORP. 412-261-3200
225 West Station Square Drive, Suite 200,
Pittsburgh, PA 15219
FDA Number: n/a *Fax:* 412-471-9427
E-mail: info@ansoft.com
Web site: www.ansoft.com
Medical Products Sales Volume: $89,100,000
Annual Revenue: $25-$50 Million
Year Founded: 1989
Total Employees: 300
Ownership: ANSYS, INC.
Stock Symbol: ANST
Traded On: NASDAQ
Quality System Registration Information: ISO9000
Produces/Sells CE-marked Devices: N
Federal Procurement Eligibility: Small Business
Distribution: Manufacturer Direct, Manufacturer Through Manufacturer Reps
General Admin.: Nick Csendes/Chief Executive Officer
  Jennifer Osgood/Human Resources Representative
Mktg./Adv.: John Arnold/Marketing Representative
  Sherry Hess/Vice President Marketing
  Tom Flynn/Vice President Sales
Finance: Mr. Tom Miller/Chief Financial Officer
Computer Equipment General

ANSPACH EFFORT INC. 800-327-6887
4500 Riverside Dr., 561-627-1080
Palm Beach Gardens, FL 33410
FDA Number: 1045834 *Fax:* 561-627-1265
Web site: www.anspach.com
Ownership: Private
Produces/Sells CE-marked Devices: N
Accessories, Powered Drill Cns/Neurology
Catheter, Suction, With Tip General
Drill, Surgical, ENT (Electric Or Pneumatic) Ear/Nose/Throat
Extractor, Nail Orthopedics
Fastener, Fixation, Non-Biodegradable, Soft Tissue Orthopedics
Instrument, Surgical, Powered, Pneumatic Orthopedics
Motor, Drill, Electric Cns/Neurology
Motor, Drill, Pneumatic Cns/Neurology
Retractor, Surgical Surgery

ANSPACH EFFORT, INC. 800-327-6887
4500 Riverside Dr., 561-627-1080
Palm Beach Gardens, FL 33410
FDA Number: 1045834 *Fax:* 561-625-9110
E-mail: info@anspach.com
Web site: www.anspach.com
Total Employees: 200 *Marketing Staff:* 5 *Sales Staff:* 10
Ownership: Private
Quality System Registration Information: ISO9000
Produces/Sells CE-marked Devices: Y
Federal Procurement Eligibility: Small Business
Distribution: Manufacturer Through Manufacturer Reps, Exporter
General Admin.: William Wachter/Chief Executive Officer
Mktg./Adv.: Heidi Rothschild/Manager Advertising
  Clement Fong/Manager International Marketing & Sales

ANSPACH EFFORT, INC.   800-327-6887 *(cont'd)*
Mr. Charles E. McGarrity/President, Director Sales
Production: Bruce Hayes/Director Quality Assurance & Regulatory Affairs
Research: Eddy DelRio/Vice President Research & Development

Cannula, Ear	Ear/Nose/Throat
Catheter, Suction, With Tip	General
Container, Sterilization (Tray)	General
Drill, Manual (With Burr, Trephine & Accessories)	Cns/Neurology
Instrument, Surgical, Powered, Pneumatic	Orthopedics
Manifold, Gas	Chemistry
Motor, Drill, Electric	Cns/Neurology
Motor, Drill, Pneumatic	Cns/Neurology
Retractor, Other	Surgery
Surgical Instrument, Disposable	Surgery
Tip, Suction Tube (Yankauer, Poole, Etc.)	Surgery
Tray, Surgical Instrument	Surgery

ANTARES PHARMA, INC.   800-328-3074
Princeton Crossroads Corporate Center   **609-359-3020**
250 Phillips Boulevard, Suite 290
Ewing, NJ 08618
FDA Number: 2182861   *Fax:* 609-359-3015
E-mail: info@antarespharma.com
Web site: www.antarespharma.com
Medical Products Sales Volume: $4,300,000
Annual Revenue: $1-$5 Million
Year Founded: 2001
Total Employees: 24
Ownership: Public
Stock Symbol: AIS
Traded On: AMEX
Quality System Registration Information: ISO9001
Produces/Sells CE-marked Devices: Y
Federal Procurement Eligibility: Small Business
Distribution: Manufacturer Direct, Manufacturer Through Distributor, Exporter
General Admin.: Dr. Dario Carrara/Managing Director
    Dr. Paul Wotton/President, Chief Executive Officer
    Dr. Peter Sadowski/Senior Vice President, General Manager
    Dr. Peter Sadowski/Vice President
Mktg./Adv.: Mike Kasprick/Director Business Development
    Dr. Kaushik Dave/Senior Vice President Product Development
Finance: Robert Apple/Chief Financial Officer, Senior Vice President Finance

Injector, Fluid, Non-Electric	General
System, Delivery, Drug, Non-invasive	General

ANTEK HEALTHWARE, INC.   800-359-0911
228 Business Center Drive,   **410-517-0330**
Reisterstown, MD 21136
FDA Number: n/a   *Fax:* 410-517-0331
E-mail: dbinfo7@antekhealthware.com
Web site: www.antekhealthware.com
Medical Products Sales Volume: $3,500,000
Annual Revenue: $5-$10 Million
Year Founded: 1987
Total Employees: 60   *Marketing Staff:* 5   *Sales Staff:* 10
Ownership: Private
Produces/Sells CE-marked Devices: N
Federal Procurement Eligibility: Small Business
Distribution: Manufacturer Direct, Manufacturer Through Distributor, Manufacturer Through Manufacturer Reps, OEM
General Admin.: Mr. Jim Milligan/President
Mktg./Adv.: Paul Taylor/Director Marketing & Sales
    Mr. Paul Taylor/Vice President Marketing & Sales
Research: Mr. Dan Schipper/Vice President Development

Computer and Software, Medical	General

ANTEK INSTRUMENTS, INC.   281-580-0339
300 Bammel Westfield Road, Houston, TX 77090-3533
FDA Number: 7000027   *Fax:* 281-580-0719
E-mail: sales@antekhou.com
Web site: www.paclp.com
Medical Products Sales Volume: $1,500,000
Annual Revenue: $10-$25 Million
Year Founded: 1967
Total Employees: 15   *Marketing Staff:* 10   *Sales Staff:* 8
Ownership: Private
Produces/Sells CE-marked Devices: Y
Federal Procurement Eligibility: Small Business
Distribution: Manufacturer Direct, Manufacturer Through Manufacturer Reps, Exporter
General Admin.: Randy L. Wreyford/Chief Operating Officer
    Donald Wreyford/President
    John Crnko/Vice President, General Manager
Mktg./Adv.: Becky Wreyford/Manager Advertising
    Roy G. Rodriguez/Manager International & National Sales
    Rudy Haas/Manager Sales Training
Production: Roy Rodriguez/Manager Regulatory Affairs

ANTEK INSTRUMENTS, INC.   281-580-0339 *(cont'd)*

Analyzer, Chemistry, Desk-Top	Chemistry
Analyzer, Protein	Chemistry
Chromatography Equipment, Gas	Chemistry
Chromatography, Liquid, Performance, High	Toxicology

ANTHEROS LLC   804-353-6464
1403 Mactavish Ave., Richmond, VA 23230
FDA Number: 3006356709
Ownership: Private
Produces/Sells CE-marked Devices: N

Medical Disinfectants/Cleaners for Instruments	General

ANTHRO CORPORATION   800-325-3841
10450 S.W. Manhasset Dr., Tualatin, OR 97062   **503-691-2556**
FDA Number: n/a   *Fax:* 800-325-0045
E-mail: nichole.stutzman@anthro.com
Web site: www.anthro.com
Total Employees: 93   *Marketing Staff:* 8   *Sales Staff:* 22
Ownership: Private
Produces/Sells CE-marked Devices: N
Federal Procurement Eligibility: Small Business
Distribution: Manufacturer Direct, OEM, Exporter
General Admin.: Shoaib Tareen/President, Chief Executive Officer
Mktg./Adv.: Jeff McCaffrey/Director Product Development
    Cathy Filgas/Vice President Marketing & Sales
Purchasing: Abood El-khal/Manager Purchasing

Cart, Equipment, Video	General
Cart, Multipurpose	General
Computer Equipment	General
Office Product	General

ANTIBODIES, INC.   800-824-8540
PO Box 1560, Davis, CA 95617-1560   **530-758-4400**
FDA Number: 2914537   *Fax:* 530-758-6307
E-mail: antibodyco@antibodiesinc.com
Web site: www.antibodiesinc.com
Medical Products Sales Volume: $1,000,000
Annual Revenue: $1-$5 Million
Total Employees: 16   *Marketing Staff:* 1   *Sales Staff:* 2
Ownership: Private
Stock Symbol: N/A
Quality System Registration Information: ISO9001
Produces/Sells CE-marked Devices: N
Federal Procurement Eligibility: Small Business, GSA Contract
Distribution: Manufacturer Direct, Manufacturer Through Distributor, OEM, Service Direct, Exporter
General Admin.: Mr. Mike Smith/General Manager
    Mr. Richard Krogsrud/President, Chief Executive Officer
Production: Ms. Jannel Teshera/Director Quality Assurance
    Mr. Mike Smith/Manager Facilities

2nd Antibody (Species Specific Anti-Animal Gamma Globulin)	Immunology
Anti-DNA Antibody, Antigen and Control	Immunology
Anti-Human Serum, Manual	Hematology
Antibody, Antinuclear, Indirect Immunofluorescent, Antigen	Immunology
Antibody, Monoclonal	Microbiology
Antibody, Other	General
Antigen, Antiserum, Control, Albumin	Immunology
Antigen, Antiserum, Control, Albumin, FITC	Immunology
Antigen, Antiserum, Control, Gamma Globulin	Immunology
Antigen, Antiserum, Control, Gamma Globulin, FITC	Immunology
Antigen, Antiserum, Control, IGA	Immunology
Antigen, Antiserum, Control, IGA, FITC	Immunology
Antigen, Antiserum, Control, IGE	Immunology
Antigen, Antiserum, Control, IGE, FITC	Immunology
Antigen, Antiserum, Control, IGG (FAB Fragment Specific)	Immunology
Antigen, Antiserum, Control, IGG (Fc Fragment Specific)	Immunology
Antigen, Antiserum, Control, IGG (Gamma Chain Specific)	Immunology
Antigen, Antiserum, Control, IGG, FITC	Immunology
Antigen, Antiserum, Control, IGG, Peroxidase	Immunology
Antigen, Antiserum, Control, IGM	Immunology
Antigen, Antiserum, Control, IGM (Mu Chain Specific)	Immunology
Antigen, Antiserum, Control, IGM, FITC	Immunology
Antigen, Antiserum, Control, Other	Immunology
Antigen, Streptococcus SPP.	Microbiology
Antinuclear Antibody, Antigen, Control	Immunology
Antiserum, Fluorescent, Groups, Streptococcus SPP.	Microbiology
Antiserum, Fluorescent, Streptococcus Pneumoniae	Microbiology
Antiserum, Streptococcus Pneumoniae	Microbiology
Antiserum, Streptococcus SPP.	Microbiology
Contract Assembly	General
Contract Manufacturing	General
Contract Manufacturing, Reagent	General
Contract R&D, Diagnostics	General
Detector, Centromere	Pathology
FC, Antigen, Antiserum, Control	Immunology
FC, FITC, Antigen, Antiserum, Control	Immunology
Giardia Spp.	Microbiology
Serum, Animal	Pathology

ANTIBODIES, INC.   800-824-8540 *(cont'd)*
Serum, Biological, General   Toxicology

ANTON PAAR USA   800-722-7556
10215 Timber Ridge Drive, Ashland, VA 23005   804-550-1051
FDA Number: n/a   *Fax:* 804-550-1057
E-mail: info.us@anton-paar.com
Web site: www.anton-paar.com
Medical Products Sales Volume: $200,000
Annual Revenue: $5-$10 Million
Ownership: Private
Quality System Registration Information: ISO9001
Produces/Sells CE-marked Devices: Y
Federal Procurement Eligibility: Small Business
Distribution: Exclusive Distributor
  Equipment, Laboratory, Gen. Purpose (Specific Medical Use)   Chemistry

ANTON/BAUER - CUSTOM POWER SYSTEMS   800-422-3473
14 Progress Drive, Shelton, CT 06484   203-929-1100
FDA Number: n/a   *Fax:* 203-929-9935
E-mail: Americas@antonbauer.com
Web site: www.antonbauer.com/cps
Medical Products Sales Volume: $11,000,000
Annual Revenue: $10-$25 Million
Year Founded: 1970
Total Employees: 100
Ownership: Vitec Group
Produces/Sells CE-marked Devices: Y
Federal Procurement Eligibility: Small Business
Distribution: Manufacturer Direct, OEM
General Admin.: Mr. Alex DeSorbo/President
Research: Mr. Greg Prentiss/Manager Development
  Battery   General
  Battery, Rechargeable, Replacement for Class III Device   Cardiovascular
  Charger, Battery   General

ANULEX TECHNOLOGIES, INC   877-326-8539
5600 Rowland Road, Suite 280,   952-224-4000
Minnetonka, MN 55343
FDA Number: 3005501497   *Fax:* 952-224-4040
E-mail: CustomerService@anulex.com
Web site: http://www.anulex.com
Ownership: Private
Produces/Sells CE-marked Devices: N
General Admin.: Mr. P. Richard Lunsford/Chief Executive Officer
Mktg./Adv.: Mr. Matt Meyer/Vice President Marketing & Sales
Production: Mr. Vic Fabano/Vice President Operations
        Mr. Tim Miller/Vice President Regulatory & Clinical Affairs
Research: Mr. Ishmael Bentley/Director Research & Development
        Mr. Steven Griffith/Vice President Scientific Affairs
Finance: Mr. David Noel/Chief Financial Officer, Vice President Finance
  Fastener, Fixation, Non-Biodegradable, Soft Tissue   Orthopedics
  Instrument, Manual, General Surgical   Surgery
  Mesh, Surgical, Polymeric   Surgery
  Suture, Non-Absorbable, Synthetic, Polyethylene   Surgery

AO EYEWEAR, INC.   800-777-1173
529 Ashland Ave., Suite 3, P.o. Box 1064,   508-764-3214
Southbridge, MA 01550
FDA Number: 1222179   *Fax:* 508-764-6853
E-mail: orders@aoeyewear.com
Web site: www.aoeyewear.com
Ownership: Private
Produces/Sells CE-marked Devices: N
  Frame, Spectacle (Eyeglasses)   Ophthalmology
  Sunglasses (Including Photosensitive)   Ophthalmology

AO REICHERT SCIENTIFIC INSTRUMENTS
See Leica Microsystems, Inc., Educational & Analytical Division

AOA
See Aoa

AOA/PRO
See Aoa

AOSS MEDICAL SUPPLY, INC.   318-325-8290
4971 Central Ave., Monroe, LA 71203
FDA Number: 2319162
  Tray, Start/Stop (Including Contents), Dialysis   Gastroenterology/Urology

APC INDUSTRIES   323-255-7101
3030 Fletcher Dr., Glassell, CA 90065
FDA Number: 2015816
Ownership: Private
Produces/Sells CE-marked Devices: N
  Floss, Dental   Dental And Oral
  Remover, Crown   Dental And Oral

APCO SPECIALTIES INC.
See Atlantic Mills, Inc.

APDYNE MEDICAL COMPANY   800-457-6853
1049 South Vine St., Denver, CO 80209-4622   303-698-4802
FDA Number: 2183861   *Fax:* 303-698-4804
E-mail: sales@apdyne.com
Web site: www.apdyne.com
Medical Products Sales Volume: $1,000,000
Annual Revenue: $1-$5 Million
Year Founded: 1989
Total Employees: 6   *Marketing Staff:* 1   *Sales Staff:* 2
Ownership: Private
Produces/Sells CE-marked Devices: N
Federal Procurement Eligibility: Small Business
Distribution: Manufacturer Direct
General Admin.: Richard A. Erickson/President, Chief Executive Officer
  Applicator, ENT   Ear/Nose/Throat
  Cuff, Tracheostomy Tube   Ear/Nose/Throat

APEC, INC.   800-746-8421
2740 North 49th St., #6, Lincoln, NE 68504   402-464-1964
FDA Number: 1933207   *Fax:* 800-746-8421
E-mail: info@apecsports.com
Web site: www.apecsports.com
Medical Products Sales Volume: $200,000
Annual Revenue: $0-$1 Million
Year Founded: 1993
Total Employees: 2   *Marketing Staff:* 2   *Sales Staff:* 2
Ownership: Private
Produces/Sells CE-marked Devices: N
Federal Procurement Eligibility: Small Business, VA Contract
Distribution: Manufacturer Direct, Manufacturer Through Manufacturer Reps,
Exclusive Distributor, Exporter
Mktg./Adv.: Mr. John H. Bacon/President, Director Sales
  Exerciser, Non-Measuring   Physical Med

APERIO TECHNOLOGIES INC.   866-478-4111
1360 Park Center Dr., Vista, CA 92081   866-478-4111
FDA Number: 3006791373   *Fax:* 760-539-1116
E-mail: info@aperio.com
Web site: www.aperio.com
Year Founded: 1999
Total Employees: 130
Ownership: Private
Produces/Sells CE-marked Devices: N
General Admin.: Dirk Soenksen/Chief Executive Officer
        Keith Hagen/Chief Operating Officer
        Ole Eichhorn/Chief Technology Officer
Medical Admin.: Dr. Jared Schwartz/Chief Medical Officer
Mktg./Adv.: Martin Stuart/Senior Vice President Marketing & Sales
        Kevin Whitely/Vice President Customer Relations
Production: Anne Brumme/Vice President Operations
Research: Gregory Crandall/Vice President Engineering
Finance: Richard Middelberg/Chief Financial Officer
  Automated Digital Image Manual Interpretation Microscope   Hematology
  Microscope, Automated, Image Analysis, Immunohistochemistry, Operator Intervention,
  Nuclear Intensity & Percent Positivity   Hematology
  Microscope, Automated, Image Analysis, Operator Intervention   Hematology

APERION BIOLOGICS   210-858-7070
11969 Starcrest Drive, San Antonio, TX 78247
FDA Number: n/a   *Fax:* 210-495-0239
Web site: http://aperionbiologics.com
Ownership: Private
Produces/Sells CE-marked Devices: N
General Admin.: Mr. Daniel Lee/Chief Executive Officer
        Dr. Russell Kronengold/Chief Scientific Officer
Production: Mr. Richard Robinson/Vice President Operations
        Mr. Lance Johnson/Vice President Quality Systems
Finance: Mr. David Cocke/Chief Financial Officer

APEX ENGINEERING PRODUCTS CORP.   800-451-6291
1241 Shoreline Drive, Aurora, IL 60504   630-820-8888
FDA Number: n/a   *Fax:* 630-820-8886
Web site: www.rdo-apex.com
Medical Products Sales Volume: $120,000
Annual Revenue: $0-$1 Million
Year Founded: 1966
Ownership: Private
Quality System Registration Information: ISO9001
Produces/Sells CE-marked Devices: N
Federal Procurement Eligibility: Small Business
Distribution: Manufacturer Direct
  Solution, Pathology, Decalcifier, Acid Containing   Pathology

APEX MEDICAL CORP.   903-314-1217
6406 Prestige Lane, Texarkana, TX 75503
FDA Number: 3005044422
Ownership: Private
Produces/Sells CE-marked Devices: N
Brush, Dermabrasion   Surgery

APEX MEDICAL CORP.
See Carex Health Brands

APEX MEDICAL TECHNOLOGIES, INC.   800-345-3208
10064 Mesa Ridge Ct., Suite 202,   858-535-0012
San Diego, CA 92121
FDA Number: 2025773
E-mail: adepaul@apexmedtech.com   Fax: 858-535-9715
Web site: www.apexmedtech.com
Annual Revenue: $1-$5 Million
Year Founded: 1985
Total Employees: 15
Ownership: Private
Produces/Sells CE-marked Devices: N
Federal Procurement Eligibility: Small Business
Distribution: Manufacturer Direct, Manufacturer Through Distributor, OEM
General Admin.: Mark McGlothlin/President, Chief Executive Officer
      Alice DePaul/Vice President
Production: Loraine McNulty/Manager Quality Assurance & Regulatory Affairs
Component, Other   General
Condom   Obstetrics/Gynecology
Container, Specimen, All Types   General
Contract Manufacturing   General
Dam, Rubber   Dental And Oral
Pump, Infusion, Elastomeric   General

APEX PLASTICS   800-467-4640
570 S Main St, Brookfield, MO 64628   660-258-7283
FDA Number: 3006801417   Fax: 660-258-7283
E-mail: dneff@apexplastics.com
Web site: www.apexplastics.com
Ownership: Private
Produces/Sells CE-marked Devices: N
Container, Specimen, Urine, Drugs Of Abuse, Over The Counter   Chemistry

APEX-CAREX HEALTHCARE PRODUCTS
See Carex Health Brands

APHERESIS TECHNOLOGIES, INC.   800-749-9284
PO Box 2081, Palm Harbor, FL 34682-2081   727-787-5616
FDA Number: 1052750   Fax: 727-784-0866
E-mail: SueHoward@IJ.net
Web site: www.apheresis.com
Medical Products Sales Volume: $700,000
Year Founded: 1990
Total Employees: 5
Ownership: Private
Quality System Registration Information: ISO9001
Produces/Sells CE-marked Devices: N
Federal Procurement Eligibility: Small Business, Female Owned
Distribution: Exclusive Distributor
Accessories, Blood Circuit, Hemodialysis   Gastroenterology/Urology
Filter, Blood, Dialysis   Gastroenterology/Urology
Kit, Tubing, Blood, Anti-Regurgitation   Gastroenterology/Urology
Pump, Blood, Extra-Luminal   Gastroenterology/Urology
Tube, Dialysate   Gastroenterology/Urology

APHERMA CORP.   408-524-1634
440 N. Wolfe Road, Sunnyvale, CA 94085
FDA Number: 3004009080
E-mail: Info@apherma.com   Fax: 408-524-1635
Web site: www.apherma.com
Medical Products Sales Volume: $3,900,000
Year Founded: 2000
Total Employees: 45
Ownership: Private
Produces/Sells CE-marked Devices: N
Federal Procurement Eligibility: Small Business
Hearing-Aid   Ear/Nose/Throat

APLICARE, INC.   800-760-3236
550 Research Parkway, Meriden, CT 06450   203-630-0500
FDA Number: 1220701   Fax: 203-630-4876
E-mail: customerservice@aplicare.com
Web site: www.aplicare.com
Year Founded: 1983
Ownership: Private
Produces/Sells CE-marked Devices: N
General Admin.: Bruce Wilson/Chief Executive Officer
      Brian Herrman/Director
      Philip Hamrock/President
Bandage, Liquid   Surgery

APLICARE, INC.   800-760-3236 (cont'd)
Kit, Administration, Intravenous   General
Kit, Wound Dressing   Surgery
Pad, Alcohol   General

APLIX, INC.   704-588-1920
12300 Steele Creek Road, Charlotte, NC 28273
FDA Number: n/a   Fax: 704-588-1941
E-mail: hygiene@aplixinc.com
Web site: www.aplix.com
Annual Revenue: $0-$1 Million
Year Founded: 1958
Ownership: APLIX S.A.
Produces/Sells CE-marked Devices: Y
Federal Procurement Eligibility: Small Business
Distribution: OEM
Exerciser, Other   Physical Med
Holder, Catheter   Gastroenterology/Urology
Pad, Pressure, Foam (Elbow, Heel)   General
Strap, Restraining   General

APM/STERNGOLD
See Sterngold

APOGEE MEDICAL, LLC   919-570-9605
90 Weathers St., Youngsville, NC 27596
FDA Number: 1055889   Fax: 707-516-1949
Web site: www.apogeemedical.com
Ownership: Private
Produces/Sells CE-marked Devices: N
Catheter, Urethral   Gastroenterology/Urology
Catheter, Urological   Gastroenterology/Urology
Ring Drape Retention, Internal (Wound Protector)   Surgery

APOLLO CORPORATION   800-247-5490
PO Box 219, Somerset, WI 54025   715-247-5625
FDA Number: 2182947   Fax: 715-247-3424
E-mail: apollosales@apollobath.com
Web site: www.apollobath.com
Annual Revenue: $1-$5 Million
Year Founded: 1978
Total Employees: 25
Ownership: Private
Produces/Sells CE-marked Devices: N
Federal Procurement Eligibility: Small Business
Distribution: Manufacturer Through Distributor, Manufacturer Through Manufacturer Reps
General Admin.: Greg Soderberg/Chief Executive Officer
      Adrian Sween/President
Mktg./Adv.: Nikki McMartin/Manager Marketing & Sales
      Norm Kruse/Vice President Sales
Production: Jerry Teigen/Director Quality Assurance
Bath, Hydro-Massage (Whirlpool)   Physical Med
Shield, Protective, Personnel   Radiology

APOLLO ENDOSURGERY, INC.   877-ENDO-130
7000 Bee Caves Road, Suite 350,   512-328-9990
Austin, TX 78746
FDA Number: 3006722112   Fax: 512-328-9994
E-mail: info@ApolloEndo.com
Web site: http://www.apolloendo.com
Year Founded: 2006
Ownership: Private
Produces/Sells CE-marked Devices: N
General Admin.: Mr. Dennis McWilliams/Chief Executive Officer
Mktg./Adv.: Mr. J. Lee Putman/Vice President Marketing & Sales
Production: Mr. Greg Mathison/Vice President Regulatory Affairs
Finance: Ms. Kery Farrell/Vice President Finance
Endoscopic Tissue Approximation Device   Gastroenterology/Urology
Forceps, Biopsy, Electric   Gastroenterology/Urology
Instrument, Knot Tying, Suture, Laparoscopic   Surgery
Unit, Electrosurgical, Endoscopic (with Or Without Accessories), Reprocessed   Gastroenterology/Urology

APOLLO MEDICAL LTD./MEDICHAIR   877-693-3330
381 Somerset St.,   506-634-7488
Saint John, NB E2K-2 Canada
FDA Number: n/a   Fax: 506-634-7404
E-mail: apollo@nb.sympatico.ca
Web site: www.medichair.com
Year Founded: 1982
Total Employees: 10
Ownership: Private
Produces/Sells CE-marked Devices: N
Distribution: Service Direct, Exclusive Distributor

APOLLO PHYSICAL THERAPY PRODUCTS LLC   650-306-9208
702 Marshall Street, Suite 312, Redwood City, CA 94063
FDA Number: 3006462253

APOLLO PHYSICAL THERAPY PRODUCTS LLC 650-306-9208
(cont'd)
Ownership: Private
Produces/Sells CE-marked Devices: N
Lamp, Infrared — Physical Med

APOLLO RESEARCH CORPORATION 800-418-1718
2300 Walden Avenue, Suite 200, 716-206-2300
Buffalo, NY 14225
FDA Number: n/a Fax: 716-206-2302
E-mail: sales@apolloresearchcorp.com
Web site: www.apolloresearchcorp.com
Annual Revenue: $0-$1 Million
Total Employees: 4 *Marketing Staff:* 1 *Sales Staff:* 1
Ownership: Private
Produces/Sells CE-marked Devices: N
Federal Procurement Eligibility: Small Business
Distribution: Manufacturer Direct, OEM
General Admin.: F. R. Thornton/President
Mktg./Adv.: Dave Jaros/Director Marketing
Accelerometer — Chemistry
Scale, Bed — General
Transducer, Blood Pressure — General
Transducer, Force — General
Transducer, Miniature Pressure — Physical Med

APOLLO SUNTAN SUPPLIES
See Megasun

APOTEX SCIENTIFIC, INC.
See Arlington Scientific, Inc. Asi

APOTHACARE 800-736-8456
PO Box 2226, Everett, WA 98213-0226 425-954-4358
FDA Number: n/a Fax: 425-967-3058
E-mail: sales@apothacare.com
Web site: www.apothacare.com
Annual Revenue: $0-$1 Million
Total Employees: 25 *Marketing Staff:* 2 *Sales Staff:* 3
Ownership: Private
Produces/Sells CE-marked Devices: N
Federal Procurement Eligibility: Small Business, Female Owned
Distribution: Manufacturer Direct
General Admin.: Tami Meritt/Chief Executive Officer
Mktg./Adv.: Bobbi Meritt/Vice President Sales
Computer Software, Home Healthcare — General

APOTHECARY PRODUCTS, INC. 800-328-2742
11750 12th Avenue S., 888-770-8767
Burnsville, MN 55337
FDA Number: 1831949 Fax: 800-328-1584
E-mail: customerservice@apothecaryproducts.com
Web site: www.apothecaryproducts.com
Medical Products Sales Volume: $29,500,000
Annual Revenue: $25-$50 Million
Year Founded: 1975
Total Employees: 130 *Marketing Staff:* 8 *Sales Staff:* 36
Ownership: Private
Produces/Sells CE-marked Devices: N
Federal Procurement Eligibility: Small Business
Distribution: Manufacturer Direct, Manufacturer Through Distributor, Manufacturer Through Manufacturer Reps, Exporter
General Admin.: Terry Noble/Chief Executive Officer
John Creel/President
Mktg./Adv.: Ms. Kelly Schwab/Director Marketing
Robert Priebe/Director Product Development
Kerry Creel/Manager Advertising
David Polfliet/Vice President National Sales
Production: David Kramer/Vice President Manufacturing
Finance: Ron Barq/Controller
Care Kit, Baby — General
Connector, Shunt — Gastroenterology/Urology
Container, Medication, Graduated Liquid — General
Detector/Remover, Lice — General
Dispenser, Medication, Liquid — General
Dropper, Medicine — General
Identification, Alert, Medical — General
Packaging System, Unit-Dose — General
Plug, Ear — Ear/Nose/Throat
Protector, Finger — Orthopedics
Splint, Other — Orthopedics
Spoon, Medicine — General
Supplementary Nitroglycerin Container — General
Tubing, Fluid Delivery — General
Vial, Medication — General

APP PHARMACEUTICALS, LLC 888-391-6300
1501 E. Woodfield Rd., Suite 300e, 847-969-2700
Schaumburg, IL 60173
FDA Number: 3002733956 Fax: 800-743-7082
E-mail: customerservice@APPpharma.com
Web site: www.apppharma.com
Ownership: Private
Produces/Sells CE-marked Devices: N
Container, IV — General
Heparin — Pathology
Set, Administration, Intravenous, Needle-Free — General
Transfer Unit, IV Fluid — General

APP PHARMACEUTICALS, LLC (708) 345-6170
2020 N. Ruby St., Melrose Park, IL 60160
FDA Number: 1450022 Fax: (708) 450-7563
Ownership: Private
Produces/Sells CE-marked Devices: N
Container, IV — General
Heparin — Pathology
Kit, Administration, Intravenous — General
Transfer Unit, IV Fluid — General

APP PHARMACEUTICALS, LLC 847-330-3953
3159 Staley Rd., Grand Island, NY 14072
FDA Number: 1321116
E-mail: contactus@APPpharma.com
Web site: www.apppharma.com
Ownership: Private
Produces/Sells CE-marked Devices: N
Container, IV — General
Heparin — Pathology
Set, Administration, Intravenous, Needle-Free — General
Transfer Unit, IV Fluid — General

APPAREL MED 425-359-6510
4902 112th St. Se, Everett, WA 98208
FDA Number: 3005765599
Support, Hernia — Gastroenterology/Urology

APPLE CONVERTING, INC. 607-337-4474
65 Hale St., Norwich, NY 13815
FDA Number: 1320248 Fax: 607-337-4499
E-mail: appleconvsales@netscape.net
Web site: www.appleconverting.com
Annual Revenue: $5-$10 Million
Year Founded: 1980
Total Employees: 55 *Marketing Staff:* 2 *Sales Staff:* 5
Ownership: Private
Produces/Sells CE-marked Devices: N
Federal Procurement Eligibility: Small Business
Distribution: Manufacturer Direct
General Admin.: Michael Manno/President, Chief Executive Officer
Mktg./Adv.: Tom Moore/Director Product Development
Fred DiLorenzo/Vice President Sales
Production: Stuart Hughes/Director Quality Assurance
Labeling Equipment — General
Packaging Equipment — General

APPLE MEDICAL CORP. 508-357-2700
28 Lord Rd., Unit 135, Marlboro, MA 01752
FDA Number: 1221923
Ownership: Private
Produces/Sells CE-marked Devices: N
Cannula, Manipulator/Injector, Uterine — Obstetrics/Gynecology
Catheter, Light, Fiberoptic, Glass, Ureteral — Gastroenterology/Urology
Catheter, Urological — Gastroenterology/Urology
Curette, Suction, Endometrial — Obstetrics/Gynecology
Device, Incontinence, Occlusion, Urethral — Gastroenterology/Urology
Electrocautery Unit, Gynecologic — Obstetrics/Gynecology
Electrode, Electrosurgical, Return (Ground, Dispersive) — Surgery
Electrosurgical Unit, Cutting & Coagulation Device — Surgery
Forceps, Biopsy, Gynecological — Obstetrics/Gynecology
Hysteroscope — Obstetrics/Gynecology
Instrument, Passing, Ligature, Knot Tying — Cns/Neurology
Laparoscope, General & Plastic Surgery — Surgery
Laparoscope, Gynecologic — Obstetrics/Gynecology
Needle, Pneumoperitoneum, Spring Loaded — Gastroenterology/Urology
Probe, Rectal, Non-Powered — Gastroenterology/Urology
Retractor — Orthopedics
Surgical Instrument, Obstetric/Gynecologic — Obstetrics/Gynecology
Surgical Instrument, Obstetric/Gynecologic, General — Obstetrics/Gynecology
Tray, Surgical Instrument — Surgery
Trocar, Other — General

APPLICATION TECHNOLOGY
See Surco Products

APPLIED AI SYSTEMS INC.
800-895-1122
1.613.839.6161
112 John Cavanaugh Drive,
Carp, ONT K0A 1 Canada
FDA Number: n/a   *Fax:* 1.613.836.5567
E-mail: info@AAI.ca
Web site: www.aai.ca
Year Founded: 1983
Total Employees: 25
Ownership: Private
Produces/Sells CE-marked Devices: N
Distribution: Exclusive Distributor, Exporter

APPLIED BIOMEDICAL CORP.
See Abiomed, Inc.

APPLIED BIOSYSTEMS
See Kratos Analytical Inc.

APPLIED BIOSYSTEMS
800-345-5724
650-638-5800
850 Lincoln Centre Drive, Foster City, CA 94404
FDA Number: n/a   *Fax:* 650-638-5884
Web site: www.appliedbiosystems.com
Annual Revenue: $0-$1 Million
Year Founded: 1981
Total Employees: 4806
Ownership: LIFE TECHNOLOGIES CORPORATION
Produces/Sells CE-marked Devices: N
Distribution: Manufacturer Direct
General Admin.: Tony L. White/Chief Executive Officer, Chairman
     Paul S. Johnson/President
     Mark P. Stevenson/President, Chief Executive Officer
     Dennis L. Winger/Senior Vice President
     William B. Sawch/Vice President, General Counsel
     Michael Hunkapiller/Vice President, General Manager
Mktg./Adv.: Patrick Carroll/Vice President Sales
Research: John Reed/Vice President Research & Development

Analyzer, Amino Acid	Microbiology
Analyzer, Peptide & Protein Sequence	Chemistry
Extractor, Plasma	Hematology
Genetic Engineering	Microbiology
Separator, Protein	Chemistry
Synthesizer, DNA	Chemistry
Synthesizer, Peptide & Protein	Chemistry
Synthesizer, Polynucleotide	Chemistry

Medical Product Subsidiaries (Listed Separately)
Tropix Inc.

APPLIED BIOSYSTEMS, DIVISION OF PERKIN-ELMER CORP.
See Applied Biosystems

APPLIED BIOTECH PRODUCTS, INC.
See Venoscope, Llc

APPLIED BIOTECHNOLOGY, INC.
See Oncogene Research Products

APPLIED CARDIAC SYSTEMS, INC.
800-423-2929
949-855-9366
22912 El Pacifico Dr.,
Laguna Hills, CA 92653
FDA Number: 2024089   *Fax:* 949-581-1009
Web site: www.acsholter.com
Annual Revenue: $10-$25 Million
Year Founded: 1981
Ownership: Private
Produces/Sells CE-marked Devices: Y
Federal Procurement Eligibility: Small Business
Distribution: Manufacturer Direct

Echocardiograph (Ultrasonic Scanner)	Cardiovascular
Recorder, Magnetic Tape/Disc	Cardiovascular

APPLIED CHROMATOGRAPHY SYSTEMS LTD.
See Polymer Laboratories, Now A Part Of Varian, Inc.

APPLIED DENTAL, INC.
888-841-8481
408-541-1393
544 E.Weddell Drive, Suite 9,
Sunnyvale, CA 94089
FDA Number: 2954705   *Fax:* 408-427-9009
E-mail: email@applied-dental.com
Web site: www.applied-dental.com
Annual Revenue: $0-$1 Million
Ownership: Private
Produces/Sells CE-marked Devices: N
Federal Procurement Eligibility: Minority Owned
Distribution: Manufacturer Direct, Manufacturer Through Distributor, Exclusive
Distributor

Absorber, Saliva, Paper	Dental And Oral
Applicator, Tipped, Absorbent, Sterile	General
Cord, Retraction	Dental And Oral
Explorer, Operative	Dental And Oral
Floss, Dental	Dental And Oral
Gown, Examination	General

APPLIED DENTAL, INC.
888-841-8481 *(cont'd)*

Handle, Instrument, Dental	Dental And Oral
Mirror, Mouth	Dental And Oral
Probe, Periodontic	Dental And Oral
Scraper, Tongue	Dental And Oral
Syringe, Restorative And Impression Material	Dental And Oral
Toothbrush, Manual	Dental And Oral

APPLIED EXTRUSION TECHNOLOGY - SPECIALTY
See Delstar Technologies, Inc.

APPLIED FIBEROPTICS
See Optim Incorporated

APPLIED IMAGING CORPORATION
See Leica Microsystems (San Jose) Corporation

APPLIED LABORATORIES, INC.
812-372-2607
3240 N. Indianapolis Road, P.O. Box 2127,
Columbus, IN 47202
FDA Number: n/a   *Fax:* 812-372-2631
E-mail: sales@appliedlabs.com
Web site: www.appliedlabs.com
Medical Products Sales Volume: $10,000,000
Annual Revenue: $5-$10 Million
Year Founded: 1984
Ownership: Private
Produces/Sells CE-marked Devices: N
Distribution: Manufacturer Direct

Contract Manufacturing, Pharmaceuticals/Chemicals	General

APPLIED MEDICAL RESOURCE CORPORATION   949-713-8000
22872 Avenida Empresa, Rancho Santa Margarita, CA 92688
FDA Number: 2027111   *Fax:* 949-713-8200
Web site: www.appliedmedical.com
Annual Revenue: $100-$500 Million
Year Founded: 1987
Ownership: Private
Produces/Sells CE-marked Devices: Y
Distribution: Manufacturer Direct, Manufacturer Through Distributor, Manufacturer
Through Manufacturer Reps, OEM

Accessories, Catheter, G-U	Gastroenterology/Urology
Angioscope	Cardiovascular
Catheter, Biliary	Gastroenterology/Urology
Catheter, Cholangiography	Surgery
Catheter, Embolectomy (Fogarty Type)	Cardiovascular
Catheter, Irrigation	Surgery
Catheter, Occlusion	Cardiovascular
Catheter, Other	Gastroenterology/Urology
Catheter, Thrombectomy	Cardiovascular
Catheter, Ureteral, Gastro-Urology	Gastroenterology/Urology
Catheter, Ureteral, General & Plastic Surgery	Surgery
Clamp, Aorta	Cardiovascular
Clamp, Bulldog	Surgery
Clamp, Other	Surgery
Clamp, Peripheral Vascular	Cardiovascular
Clamp, Surgical, General & Plastic Surgery	Surgery
Clamp, Vascular	Cardiovascular
Clip, Instrument	Surgery
Clip, Vascular	Cardiovascular
Computer, Diagnostic, Pre-Programmed, Single-Function	Cardiovascular
Cover, Laparoscope	Surgery
Equipment, Extruding/Molding	General
Injector, Syringe	General
Laparoscope, General & Plastic Surgery	Surgery
Molding, Custom	General
Needle, Insufflation, Laparoscopic	Surgery
Pad, Clamp	Surgery
Sleeve, Trocar	Surgery
Stent, Ureteral	Gastroenterology/Urology
Surgical Instrument, Cardiovascular	Cardiovascular
Surgical Instrument, G-U, Manual	Gastroenterology/Urology
Thermoforming, Extrusion, Custom	General
Trocar, Gastro-Urology	Gastroenterology/Urology
Trocar, Other	General
Tubing, Multi-Lumen	General
Tubing, Other	General
Tubing, Plastic	General
Ureteroscope	Gastroenterology/Urology
Valvulotome	Cardiovascular
Warmer, Endoscope	Surgery

APPLIED MEDICAL SYSTEMS, INC.
617-577-1604
581 Boylston Street, Suite 500, Boston, MA 02116
FDA Number: n/a   *Fax:* 617-577-8111
Annual Revenue: $0-$1 Million
Total Employees: 10
Ownership: Private
Produces/Sells CE-marked Devices: N
Federal Procurement Eligibility: Small Business, Female Owned
Distribution: Service Direct
General Admin.: Yasmeen Husain/President

APPLIED MEDICAL SYSTEMS, INC.   617-577-1604 *(cont'd)*
Service, Consulting   General

APPLIED MEDICAL TECHNOLOGY, INC.   800-869-7382
8000 Katherine Boulevard,   440-717-4000
Brecksville, OH 44141
FDA Number: 1526012   Fax: 440-717-4200
E-mail: info@appliedmedical.net
Web site: www.appliedmedical.net
Medical Products Sales Volume: $2,200,000
Annual Revenue: $5-$10 Million
Ownership: Private
Quality System Registration Information: ISO9001
Produces/Sells CE-marked Devices: Y
Federal Procurement Eligibility: Small Business
Distribution: Manufacturer Direct, Manufacturer Through Distributor, OEM, Exporter

Cannula, Other	General
Catheter, Nasal, Oxygen (Tube)	Anesthesiology
Contract Manufacturing, Product, Durable	General
Contract R&D, Equipment	General
Fixation Device, Tracheal Tube	Anesthesiology
Laparoscope, General & Plastic Surgery	Surgery
Retractor, Manual	Cns/Neurology
Retractor, Self-Retaining	Gastroenterology/Urology
System, Evacuation, Smoke, Laser	Surgery
Tube, Gastrointestinal	Gastroenterology/Urology

APPLIED NEUROSCIENCE, INC.   727-244-0240
228 176th Terrace Drive, Saint Petersburg, FL 33708
FDA Number: 3004577596   Fax: 727-392-1436
E-mail: qeeg@appliedneuroscience.com
Web site: www.appliedneuroscience.com
Year Founded: 1987
Ownership: Private
Produces/Sells CE-marked Devices: N
General Admin.: Dr. Robert Thatcher/Director
   Medical Admin.: Dr. Carl Biver/Director Chemistry
IS: Mr. Duane North/Manager Computer Operations

Analyzer, Spectrum, EEG Signal	Cns/Neurology
Echoencephalograph (Ultrasonic Scanner)	Cns/Neurology

APPLIED PRECISION INC.   425-557-1000
1040 12th Avenue Northwest, Issaquah, WA 98027
FDA Number: n/a   Fax: 425-557-1055
Web site: http://www.appliedprecision.com
Year Founded: 1968
Ownership: Private
Produces/Sells CE-marked Devices: N
Distribution: OEM

APPLIED PROSTHETIC TECHNOLOGY
See Habley Medical Technology Corp.

APPLIED SCIENCE LABORATORIES   781-275-4000
175 Middlesex Tpke., Bedford, MA 01730
FDA Number: 1218984   Fax: 781-275-3388
E-mail: asl@a-s-l.com
Web site: www.a-s-l.com
Medical Products Sales Volume: $2,000,000
Annual Revenue: $1-$5 Million
Year Founded: 1984
Total Employees: 25   Marketing Staff: 4   Sales Staff: 4
Ownership: Private
Produces/Sells CE-marked Devices: N
Federal Procurement Eligibility: Small Business
Distribution: Manufacturer Direct, Manufacturer Through Manufacturer Reps
General Admin.: Marzena Sadowski/Office Manager
   Robert Sinclair/President
Mktg./Adv.: Virginia Salem/Director Marketing & Sales
   Robert Baer/Vice President Marketing
Research: Josh Borah/Vice President Engineering

Monitor, Eye Movement	Ophthalmology
Pupillometer, AC-Powered	Ophthalmology

APPLIED SCIENCE, INC.   866-436-6356
983 Golden Gate Terrace,   530-273-8299
Grass Valley, CA 95945
FDA Number: 2951275   Fax: 530-273-8399
E-mail: sales@applied-science.com
Web site: www.applied-science.com
Medical Products Sales Volume: $1,200,000
Annual Revenue: $1-$5 Million
Ownership: Private
Produces/Sells CE-marked Devices: N
Federal Procurement Eligibility: Small Business
Distribution: Manufacturer Direct, Manufacturer Through Manufacturer Reps

Mixer/Scale, Blood	Hematology

APPLIED SPINE TECHNOLOGIES, INC.   203-503-0280
300 George Street, Suite 511, New Haven, CT 06511
FDA Number: 3005258318   Fax: 203-503-0282
E-mail: clinicaltrial@appliedspine.com
Web site: www.appliedspine.com
Ownership: Private
Produces/Sells CE-marked Devices: N
General Admin.: Craig Corrance/President, Chief Executive Officer
Production: Michele Lucey/Vice President Regulatory Affairs
Research: Dr. Bruce Robie/Vice President Research & Development
Finance: Terry Brennan/Chief Financial Officer

Orthosis, Fixation, Spinal, Spondylolisthesis	Orthopedics
Orthosis, Spinal Pedicle Fixation, For Degenerative Disc Disease	Orthopedics

APPLIED SURGICAL, LLC   205-259-2050
300 Riverchase Parkway East, Birmingham, AL 35244
FDA Number: 3005654398   Fax: 205-259-2051
E-mail: info@appliedsurgicalsolutions.com
Web site: www.appliedsurgicalsolutions.com
Ownership: Private
Produces/Sells CE-marked Devices: N

Electrosurgical Unit, Cutting & Coagulation Device	Surgery

APPLIED TECHNOLOGY CORP.
See Tidi Products, Llc

APPLIED TEST SYSTEMS, INC.   800-441-0215
154 East Brook Lane, Butler, PA 16002   724-283-1212
FDA Number: n/a   Fax: 724-283-6570
E-mail: sales@atspa.com
Web site: www.atspa.com
Medical Products Sales Volume: $4,300,000
Annual Revenue: $5-$10 Million
Year Founded: 1965
Total Employees: 46   Marketing Staff: 2   Sales Staff: 10
Ownership: Private
Produces/Sells CE-marked Devices: N
Federal Procurement Eligibility: Small Business
Distribution: Manufacturer Direct, Manufacturer Through Distributor, Manufacturer Through Manufacturer Reps, OEM, Exporter
General Admin.: F. R. Ganassi/President, Chief Executive Officer
   Mr. Don Olson/Vice President
Mktg./Adv.: Jennifer Van Gorder/Director Marketing
   Mr. Denny King/Manager Sales
   Ms. Patty McGee/Sales Associate
   Ms. Paula Fry/Sales Associate
Production: Mr. Ed Cartwright/Chief Engineering Officer
Purchasing: Ms. Theresa Graham/Purchasing Agent

Equipment, Laboratory, Gen. Purpose (Specific Medical Use)	Chemistry
Oven	Chemistry

APPLIED THERAPEUTICS, INC.   877-682-2777
3104 Cherry Palm Drive Suite 220,   813-623-1400
Tampa, FL 33619
FDA Number: 1064611   Fax: 813-623-3737
E-mail: info@arthocare.com
Web site: www.rapidrhino.com
Medical Products Sales Volume: $500,000
Year Founded: 1993
Total Employees: 16   Sales Staff: 22
Ownership: Private
Stock Symbol: ARTC
Traded On: NASDAQ
Quality System Registration Information: ISO9001
Produces/Sells CE-marked Devices: Y
Federal Procurement Eligibility: Small Business
Distribution: Manufacturer Direct
General Admin.: Mr. John Kennedy/Chief Executive Officer
   Mr. Richard Stieff/Office Manager
Mktg./Adv.: Mr. Dennis Feldman/Vice President, Manager Sales
Production: Mrs. Yvonne Corbitt/Customer Service Representative
   Mr. Jim Savaglio/Product Manager

Balloon, Epistaxis (Nasal)	Ear/Nose/Throat
Splint, Septal, Intranasal	Ear/Nose/Throat

APPLIED UROLOGY, INC.
See Applied Medical Resource Corporation

APPLIED VASCULAR DEVICES, INC.
See Applied Medical Resource Corporation

APPROPRIATE TECHNICAL RESOURCES, INC.   800-827-5931
9157 Whiskey Bottom Road, PO Box 460,   301-470-1267
Laurel, MD 20723
FDA Number: 1228216   Fax: 410-792-2837
E-mail: info@atrbiotech.com
Web site: www.atrbiotech.com
Medical Products Sales Volume: $5,000,000
Annual Revenue: $0-$1 Million

APPROPRIATE TECHNICAL RESOURCES, INC. 800-827-5931
(cont'd)
Year Founded: 1980
Total Employees: 20   Marketing Staff: 2   Sales Staff: 6
Ownership: Private
Produces/Sells CE-marked Devices: N
Federal Procurement Eligibility: Small Business, GSA Contract
Distribution: Manufacturer Through Distributor, Exclusive Distributor, Importer, Exporter
General Admin.: Stephen Mitchell/President
       LuAnn Basciano/Vice President
Mktg./Adv.: Denise Connors/Manager Accounts

Cart, Other	General
Centrifuge, General (Up to 5,000 rpm)	Pathology
Fermentation Equipment	Microbiology
Freeze Drying Equipment	Chemistry
Incubator, Aerobic	Microbiology
Service, Maintenance/Repair	General
Shaker/Stirrer	Chemistry

APPROVED MEDICAL SYSTEMS 951-353-2453
7101 Jurupa Ave - Unit 4, Riverside, CA 92504
FDA Number: n/a   Fax: 951-353-2485
E-mail: appmedsys@aol.com
Annual Revenue: $0-$1 Million
Year Founded: 1984
Total Employees: 30   Marketing Staff: 2   Sales Staff: 10
Ownership: Approved Medical Systems
Produces/Sells CE-marked Devices: N
Federal Procurement Eligibility: Small Business, Minority Owned
Distribution: Manufacturer Through Distributor, Manufacturer Through Manufacturer Reps, OEM
General Admin.: Neal Patel/President, Chief Executive Officer
Mktg./Adv.: Tom Lowry/Manager Contract Sales
       Cary Maleeny/Manager Sales
       Tim Dunn/Manager Sales

Bag, Laundry, Infection Control	General
Bag, Specimen, Laparoscopic	Surgery
Cart, Housekeeping	General
Cart, Isolation	General
Cart, Laundry	General
Cart, Waste	General
Laundry Hamper	General
Liner, Laundry Hamper	General

Medical Product Subsidiaries (Listed Separately)
   Approved Medical Systems

APREX, A DIVISION OF AARDEX
See Aprex, A Division Of Aardex

APREX, DIVISION OF APRIA HEALTHCARE
See Aprex, A Division Of Aardex

APTEC - NRC, INC.
See Canberra

APTIS MEDICAL, LLC. 502-523-6738
3602 Glenview Ave, Glenview, KY 40025
FDA Number: 3004521401   Fax: 502-425-7422
E-mail: info@aptismedical.com
Web site: www.aptismedical.com
Ownership: Private
Produces/Sells CE-marked Devices: N

Bit, Drill	Orthopedics
Gauge, Depth	Orthopedics
Guide, Surgical, Instrument	Surgery
Impactor	Orthopedics
Prosthesis, Wrist, Hemi-, Ulnar	Orthopedics
Screwdriver	Orthopedics
Template	Orthopedics
Tray, Surgical	Surgery

APTIV SOLUTIONS INC. 703-483-6400
1925 Isaac Newtown Square, Suite 100, Reston, VA 20190
FDA Number: n/a   Fax: 703-435-4031
Web site: www.aptivsolutions.com
Ownership: Private
Produces/Sells CE-marked Devices: N
General Admin.: Mr. Michael McKelvey/Chief Operating Officer
       Mr. Patrick Donelly/President, Chief Executive Officer
   Medical Admin.: Dr. Gene Resnick/Chief Medical Officer
Mktg./Adv.: Mr. Peter Gonze/Executive Vice President Business Development
       Dr. Phil Birch/Senior Vice President Corporate Development
Production: Ms. Carolyn Belcher/Senior Vice President Regulatory Affairs
Finance: Mr. Matthew Bond/Chief Financial Officer

APTUS ENDOSYSTEMS INC. 877-292-7887
777 N. Pastoria Avenue,   408-530-9050
Sunnyvale, CA 94085
FDA Number: 3008493192   Fax: 408-530-9051
E-mail: info@aptusendo.com

APTUS ENDOSYSTEMS INC. 877-292-7887 *(cont'd)*
Web site: www.aptusendosystems.com
Year Founded: 2002
Ownership: Private
Produces/Sells CE-marked Devices: N
General Admin.: Mr. Lee Bolduc/Chief Technology Officer
       Mr. Jeff Elkins/President, Chief Executive Officer
Production: Mr. Tedd Hinton/Director Manufacturing
       Mr. Burt Goodson/Director Regulatory Affairs
Finance: Mr. Dan Georgia/Director Finance

System, Treatment, Aortic Aneurysm, Endovascular Graft	Cardiovascular

APW EDER INDUSTRIES, INC. 414-761-0400
2250 W. South Branch Blvd., Oak Creek, WI 53154-4907
FDA Number: n/a   Fax: 414-761-0582
E-mail: mike.hoffmann@ederindustries.com
Web site: www.ederindustries.com
Annual Revenue: $10-$25 Million
Total Employees: 200   Sales Staff: 3
Ownership: Applied Power, Inc.
Quality System Registration Information: ISO9000
Produces/Sells CE-marked Devices: N
Federal Procurement Eligibility: Small Business
Distribution: Manufacturer Direct, Manufacturer Through Distributor, Manufacturer Through Manufacturer Reps, OEM, Service Direct
Production: Bryan Cell/Plant Manager
Research: Roger Rossman/Vice President Engineering

Contract Manufacturing	General

AQUA BATH CO., INC. 800-232-2284
921 Cherokee Avenue, Nashville, TN 37207   615-227-0017
FDA Number: 1057441   Fax: 615-227-9446
E-mail: sales.info@aquabath.com
Web site: www.aquabath.com
Medical Products Sales Volume: $2,600,000
Annual Revenue: $5-$10 Million
Year Founded: 1993
Total Employees: 35   Marketing Staff: 2   Sales Staff: 35
Ownership: Private
Produces/Sells CE-marked Devices: N
Federal Procurement Eligibility: Small Business
Distribution: Manufacturer Through Distributor, Manufacturer Through Manufacturer Reps
Mktg./Adv.: Michael S. Marcinek/Director Marketing
       Michael S. Marcinek/Vice President Sales
Production: Lola Ladd/Director Quality Assurance
Finance: Wendol Thorpe/Chief Financial Officer
IS: Joe Parchem/Technical Director

Bathtub	General

AQUA GLASS CORPORATION 800-632-0911
320 Industrial Park Rd.,   731-632-0911
Adamsville, TN 38310
FDA Number: n/a   Fax: 731-632-1557
Web site: www.aquaglass.com
Medical Products Sales Volume: $15,000,000
Total Employees: 1100   Marketing Staff: 9   Sales Staff: 5
Ownership: Mascon
Produces/Sells CE-marked Devices: N
Distribution: Manufacturer Through Distributor
General Admin.: Robert Ball/President
       Steve Simon/Vice President Human Resources
Mktg./Adv.: Steve Breymaier/Vice President Marketing

Bathtub	General
Chair, Shower	General
Equipment, Therapy, Handicapped/Physical	Physical Med

AQUA MASSAGE INTERNATIONAL, INC.
See Ami, Inc.

AQUA PRODUCTS COMPANY, INC. 800-849-4264
14301 C.R. Koon Hwy, Newberry, SC 29108   803-321-0246
FDA Number: n/a   Fax: 803-321-1980
E-mail: apc@aquaproducts.us
Web site: www.aquaproducts.us
Medical Products Sales Volume: $2,300,000
Annual Revenue: $1-$5 Million
Year Founded: 1993
Total Employees: 15   Marketing Staff: 2   Sales Staff: 25
Ownership: Private
Produces/Sells CE-marked Devices: N
Federal Procurement Eligibility: Small Business, GSA Contract
Distribution: Manufacturer Through Distributor, OEM, Exporter
General Admin.: John W. Seppamaki/President, Chief Executive Officer
Mktg./Adv.: J.R. Seppamaki/Manager Sales
       Mr. Bruce Connelly/Manager Sales
Production: Scott Bayer/Vice President Manufacturing

Air Handling Apparatus, Enclosure	Surgery

AQUA PRODUCTS COMPANY, INC.   800-849-4264 (cont'd)
Chilling Unit   Physical Med
Water, Therapy, Respiratory   Microbiology

AQUA WATER TREATMENT, INC.   850-939-9055
8195 East Bay Blvd., Navarre, FL 32566
FDA Number: 3004055604
Ownership: Private
Produces/Sells CE-marked Devices: N
Purification System, Water   Gastroenterology/Urology

AQUA-CEL CORP.   888-254-HEAT
17137 Sparkleberry St,   714-962-2776
Fountain Valley, CA 92708
FDA Number: 2025519
E-mail: aqua-cel@aqua-cel.com   Fax: 714-962-2776
Web site: www.aqua-cel.com
Medical Products Sales Volume: $300,000
Annual Revenue: $0-$1 Million
Year Founded: 1985
Total Employees: 3   Marketing Staff: 1   Sales Staff: 1
Ownership: Private
Produces/Sells CE-marked Devices: N
Federal Procurement Eligibility: Small Business
Distribution: Manufacturer Through Distributor
General Admin.: Robert E. Shaw/President, Chief Executive Officer
Bottle, Hot/Cold Water   General
Pack, Hot Or Cold, Reusable   Physical Med

AQUACHECK SYSTEMS, INC.
See Continental Hydrodyne Systems, Inc.

AQUATEC
See Clarke Health Care Products, Inc.

AQUATIC ACCESS, INC.   800-325-5438
1921 Production Drive, Louisville, KY 40223   502-425-5817
FDA Number: n/a   Fax: 502-425-9607
E-mail: info@AquaticAccess.com
Web site: www.AquaticAccess.com
Year Founded: 1986
Total Employees: 20   Marketing Staff: 1   Sales Staff: 1
Ownership: Private
Produces/Sells CE-marked Devices: N
Federal Procurement Eligibility: Small Business, Female Owned
Distribution: Manufacturer Direct, Manufacturer Through Distributor, Exporter
Lift, Patient   General

AQUEDUCT MEDICAL INCORPORATED   415-896-0134
665 Third St., Suite 20, San Francisco, CA 94107
FDA Number: 3004597813
Pack, Hot Or Cold, Water Circulating   Physical Med

AQUILA CORPORATION   866-782-9658
3827 Creekside Lane, Holmen, WI 54636   608-782-0031
FDA Number: 2134750   Fax: 608-782-0488
E-mail: aquila@aquilacorp.com
Web site: www.aquilacorp.com
Annual Revenue: $1-$5 Million
Year Founded: 1999
Total Employees: 7   Marketing Staff: 1   Sales Staff: 3
Ownership: Private
Produces/Sells CE-marked Devices: N
Federal Procurement Eligibility: Small Business
Distribution: Manufacturer Direct, Manufacturer Through Distributor, Manufacturer Through Manufacturer Reps
Component, Wheelchair   Physical Med

AR CUSTOM MEDICAL PRODUCTS, LTD.   516-242-7501
19A West Industry Court, Deer Park, NY 11729
FDA Number: 2434489
Web site: http://www.arcustommedical.com
Ownership: Private
Produces/Sells CE-marked Devices: N
Cradle, Patient, Radiographic   Radiology
Device, Limiting, Beam, Diagnostic, X-Ray   Radiology
Generator, Diagnostic X-Ray, High Voltage, Single Phase   Radiology
Radiographic Unit, Diagnostic, Mammographic   Radiology

AR WORLDWIDE   800-933-8181
160 School House Road,   215-723-8181
Souderton, PA 18964
FDA Number: n/a   Fax: 866-859-0582
E-mail: info@ar-worldwide.com
Web site: www.ar-worldwide.com
Medical Products Sales Volume: $10,000,000
Year Founded: 2001
Total Employees: 40   Marketing Staff: 5   Sales Staff: 10
Ownership: Private

AR WORLDWIDE   800-933-8181 (cont'd)
Stock Symbol: CNSI
Traded On: NYSE
Quality System Registration Information: ISO9001
Produces/Sells CE-marked Devices: Y
Federal Procurement Eligibility: Small Business
Distribution: Manufacturer Direct, Manufacturer Through Distributor, Manufacturer Through Manufacturer Reps, OEM, Exclusive Distributor
General Admin.: Ethel Shepherd/Corporate Administrator
   Donald Shepherd/President, Chief Executive Officer
Mktg./Adv.: Richard Rogers/Vice President Marketing
   Kenneth Shepherd/Vice President Sales
Production: James Maginn/Vice President Manufacturing
Finance: Harry Parke/Vice President Finance, Controller
Equipment/Service, Quality Control   General

ARACLEAN SERVICES
See Aramark Clean Room Services

ARADIGM CORP.   510-265-9000
3929 Point Eden Way, Hayward, CA 94545
FDA Number: 2953680
Nebulizer, Medicinal, Non-Ventilatory (Atomizer)   Anesthesiology

ARAGON SURGICAL INC.
See Aesculap, Inc

ARAGONA MEDICAL, INC.   201-664-8822
184 Rivervale Rd., River Vale, NJ 07675
FDA Number: 2246642   Fax: 201-664-5994
E-mail: mail@aragonamedical.com
Web site: www.aragonamedical.com
Annual Revenue: $0-$1 Million
Year Founded: 1987
Ownership: Private
Quality System Registration Information: ISO9001
Produces/Sells CE-marked Devices: Y
Federal Procurement Eligibility: Small Business
Distribution: Manufacturer Direct, Manufacturer Through Distributor, Manufacturer Through Manufacturer Reps, Service Direct, Importer, Exporter
General Admin.: Mr. Mikael Ugander/Chief Executive Officer
Heating Unit, Powered   Physical Med
Hypo/Hyperthermia Unit, Mobile   General
Hypothermia Unit   General
Lamp, Infrared   Physical Med
Warmer, Radiant, Adult   General
Warmer, Radiant, Infant   General

ARAMARK CLEAN ROOM SERVICES   800-759-0102
7650 Grant St., Hinsdale, IL 60521   630-929-6170
FDA Number: n/a
E-mail: cleanroomservices@uniform.aramark.com
Web site: www.aramark-cleanroom.com
Annual Revenue: $50-$100 Million
Year Founded: 1978
Ownership: Private
Produces/Sells CE-marked Devices: N
Distribution: Service Direct
Germ-Free Apparatus   Microbiology

ARC CHEMICAL DIV.
See Arc Specialty Products, Balchem Corporation

ARC HOME HEALTH PRODUCTS   800-278-8595
PO Box186, Windsor, CT 06095   860-681-3005
FDA Number: n/a   Fax: 607-643-0292
E-mail: info@archhp.com
Web site: www.archhp.com
Medical Products Sales Volume: $1,500,000
Total Employees: 8   Marketing Staff: 2   Sales Staff: 2
Ownership: Private
Produces/Sells CE-marked Devices: N
General Admin.: Marci Brunswick/Vice President, General Manager
Diaper, Adult   General
Garment, Protective, For Incontinence   Gastroenterology/Urology
Pad, Incontinence (Underpad)   General
Pant, Incontinence   General

ARC MEDICAL, INC.   800-950-ARC1 (2
4296 Cowan Road, Tucker, GA 30084   404-373-8311
FDA Number: 2247040   Fax: 404-373-8385
E-mail: arcinfo@arcmedical.com
Web site: www.arcmedical.com
Annual Revenue: $1-$5 Million
Year Founded: 1990
Total Employees: 10   Sales Staff: 51
Ownership: Private
Quality System Registration Information: ISO9000; ISO9001; ISO9002; ISO9003
Produces/Sells CE-marked Devices: Y
Federal Procurement Eligibility: Small Business

ARC MEDICAL, INC. 800-950-ARC1 (2 (cont'd)
Distribution: Manufacturer Through Manufacturer Reps, Exclusive Distributor, Importer
General Admin.: Hal Norris/Chief Executive Officer

Airway, Oropharyngeal, Anesthesia	Anesthesiology
Condenser, Heat And Moisture (Artificial Nose)	Anesthesiology
Filter, Bacterial, Breathing Circuit	Anesthesiology
Humidifier, Heat/Moisture Exchange	Anesthesiology

ARC SPECIALTY PRODUCTS
See Arc Specialty Products, Balchem Corporation

ARC SPECIALTY PRODUCTS, BALCHEM 845-326-560
CORPORATION
52 Sunrise Park Road, PO Box 600, New Hampton, NY 10958
FDA Number: 3003936696 Fax: 845-326-5742
Web site: www.balchem.com
Annual Revenue: $100-$500 Million
Year Founded: 1967
Total Employees: 332
Ownership: BALCHEM CORP.
Produces/Sells CE-marked Devices: N
Federal Procurement Eligibility: Small Business
Distribution: Manufacturer Direct

Gas Mixtures, Sterilization	General
Sterilizer, Ethylene-Oxide Gas	General

ARC SURGICAL LLC. 503-627-9957
21300 Nw Jacobson Rd., Hillsboro, OR 97124
FDA Number: 3004623378
Ownership: Private
Produces/Sells CE-marked Devices: N

Screw, Fixation, Bone	Orthopedics
Traction Unit, Non-Powered	Orthopedics

ARC/OTSEGO 607-432-8595
35 Academy Street, PO Box 490, Oneonta, NY 13820-1046
FDA Number: 1319400 Fax: 607-433-8430
E-mail: info@arcotsego.org
Web site: www.arcotsego.org
Annual Revenue: $1-$5 Million
Year Founded: 1965
Total Employees: 30 Marketing Staff: 1 Sales Staff: 1
Ownership: Private
Produces/Sells CE-marked Devices: N
Federal Procurement Eligibility: Small Business
Distribution: Manufacturer Through Distributor
General Admin.: Joe Judd/Chief Executive Officer
Mktg./Adv.: Bill Brown/Director Marketing & Sales
Kevin Scott/Manager Contract Sales
Production: Doug Moubray/Vice President Manufacturing

Contract Packaging	General
Gown, Patient, Disposable	General

ARCADIA MEDICAL CORPORATION 219-779-9431
1140 Millennium Drive, crown point, IN 46307
FDA Number: 3004590970 Fax: 847-620-2502
E-mail: info@arcadiamedical.com
Web site: www.arcadiamedical.com
Medical Products Sales Volume: $500,000
Annual Revenue: $0-$1 Million
Year Founded: 2001
Total Employees: 1 Marketing Staff: 1 Sales Staff: 1
Ownership: Private
Produces/Sells CE-marked Devices: Y
Federal Procurement Eligibility: Small Business
Distribution: Exclusive Distributor

Balloon, Epistaxis (Nasal)	Ear/Nose/Throat
Tube, Tracheal (Endotracheal)	Anesthesiology
Tube, Tracheostomy (W/Wo Connector)	Anesthesiology

ARCADIA RESOURCES INC. 800-733-8427
9229 Delegates Row, Suite 260, 317-569-8234
Indianapolis, IN 46240
FDA Number: n/a Fax: 317-575-6195
E-mail: info@arcadiaservices.com
Web site: http://arcadiaresourcesinc.com
Ownership: Public
Stock Symbol: KAD
Traded On: AMEX
Produces/Sells CE-marked Devices: N
General Admin.: Steve Zeller/Chief Operating Officer
Marvin R. Richardson/President, Chief Executive Officer
Finance: Matthew R. Middendorf/Chief Financial Officer

ARCAPCO, INC. 626-966-4556
754 Arrow Grand Circle, Covina, CA 91722
FDA Number: n/a
Medical Products Sales Volume: $700,000

ARCAPCO, INC. 626-966-4556 (cont'd)
Annual Revenue: $0-$1 Million
Ownership: Private
Produces/Sells CE-marked Devices: N
Federal Procurement Eligibility: Small Business
Distribution: Manufacturer Direct

Crown, Preformed	Dental And Oral
Matrix, Dental	Dental And Oral
Retainer, Matrix	Dental And Oral

ARCH-EEZ INSTITUTE
See Back Solution, The

ARCHITECTURAL SIGNING INC.
See Asi-Modulex

ARCHTEK, INC. 303-763-8916
12105 West Cedar Dr., Lakewood, CO 80228
FDA Number: 1723435

Tray, Fluoride, Disposable	Dental And Oral

ARCMATE MFG. CORP. 888-637-1926
637 S. Vinewood St., Escondido, CA 92029 760-489-1140
FDA Number: 3307221 Fax: 760-746-1926
E-mail: btraber@arcmate.com
Web site: www.arcmate.com
Medical Products Sales Volume: $940,000
Annual Revenue: $1-$5 Million
Year Founded: 1996
Total Employees: 12 Marketing Staff: 2 Sales Staff: 2
Ownership: Private
Produces/Sells CE-marked Devices: N
Federal Procurement Eligibility: Small Business
Distribution: Manufacturer Through Distributor, Exporter
Mktg./Adv.: Bob Traber/Vice President Marketing & Sales

Accessories, Wheelchair	Physical Med
Reacher (Handicapped)	General

ARCO MEDICAL PRODUCTS
See Cook Inc.

ARCOA INDUSTRIES
See Arcmate Mfg. Corp.

ARCOMA NORTH AMERICA, INC. 464-707-0690
23151 Alcalde Drive, Suite C-8, Laguna Hills, CA 92653
FDA Number: 3005998708
Ownership: Private
Produces/Sells CE-marked Devices: N

Table, Radiographic, Tilting	Radiology

ARCTURUS BIOSCIENCE, INC.
See Aviaradx, Inc.

ARCUS MEDICAL LLC 877-272-8763
4324 Barringer Dr . Suite 104, 704-332-3424
Charlotte, NC 28217
FDA Number: 3004578739 Fax: 704-332-3425
E-mail: info@arcusmedical.com
Web site: www.arcusmedical.com
Ownership: Private
Produces/Sells CE-marked Devices: N

Bag, Urine Collection, Leg, For External Use, Non-sterile	Gastroenterology/Urology
Bedpan	General
Garment, Protective, For Incontinence	Gastroenterology/Urology
System, Urine Drainage, Closed, For Non-indwelling Catheter, Non-sterile	Gastroenterology/Urology

ARDIAN INC. 650-417-6555
1380 Shorebird Way, Mountain View, CA 94043
FDA Number: 3006227845 Fax: 650-417-6599
E-mail: info@ardian.com
Web site: http://www.ardian.com
Year Founded: 2003
Ownership: MEDTRONIC, INC.
Produces/Sells CE-marked Devices: N
General Admin.: Mr. Andrew Cleeland/President, Chief Executive Officer
Medical Admin.: Dr. Paul Sobotka/Chief Medical Officer
Mr. Craig Straley/Vice President Clinical Affairs
Mktg./Adv.: Mr. Gregory Bakan/Vice President Marketing & Sales
Production: Dr. Scott Wilson/Vice President Quality Assurance & Regulatory Affairs
Research: Ms. Denise Zarins/Vice President Research & Development
Finance: Mr. Timothy Kahlenberg/Chief Financial Officer

Generator, Radiofrequency Lesion	Cns/Neurology
Probe, Radiofrequency Lesion	Cns/Neurology

ARDUS MEDICAL, INC. 800-878-1388
11297 Grooms Rd., Cincinnati, OH 45242 513-469-7867
FDA Number: n/a Fax: 513-469-2329
E-mail: sales@ardusmedical.com
Web site: www.ardusmedical.com
Year Founded: 1994

ARDUS MEDICAL, INC.
800-878-1388 (cont'd)

Total Employees: 45   *Marketing Staff:* 1   *Sales Staff:* 12
Ownership: AMI Holdings, Inc
Produces/Sells CE-marked Devices: Y
Federal Procurement Eligibility: Small Business
General Admin.: Jeff Smith/Chief Operating Officer
    Troy Powell/President, Chief Executive Officer
Production: Mr. Joe Stem/Director Operations
Finance: Mr. Chris Karl/Controller

Defibrillator, Battery-Powered	Cardiovascular
Infusion Pump, Enteral	General
Pump, Infusion, Patient Controlled Analgesia (PCA)	General

AREEDA ASSOC., LTD.
323-653-5515

1160 Glen Arbor Ave., Los Angeles, CA 90041
FDA Number: n/a
Ownership: Private
Produces/Sells CE-marked Devices: N

Computer and Software, Medical	General
Scanner, Emission Computed Tomography	Radiology

ARGEN CORP.
800-375-9077
1-800-255-5524

5855 Oberlin Dr., San Diego, CA 92121
FDA Number: 2433919   *Fax:* 858-626-8686
E-mail: argeninfo@argen.com
Web site: www.argen.com
Total Employees: 98   *Marketing Staff:* 10   *Sales Staff:* 38
Ownership: Private
Quality System Registration Information: ISO9001
Produces/Sells CE-marked Devices: Y
Federal Procurement Eligibility: Small Business
Distribution: Manufacturer Direct, Manufacturer Through Distributor, Manufacturer Through Manufacturer Reps, OEM
General Admin.: Anton Woolf/Chief Executive Officer
    Jacqueline Woolf/President, Chief Operating Officer
Mktg./Adv.: Selwyn Moss/Senior Vice President International & National Sales
Production: Jan Larman/Director Customer Services
Finance: Neil Weinstein/Chief Financial Officer
IS: Paul Cascone/Senior Vice President Technology

Alloy, Gold Based, For Clinical Use	Dental And Oral
Alloy, Precious Metal, For Clinical Use	Dental And Oral
Attachment, Precision	Dental And Oral
Powder, Porcelain	Dental And Oral

ARGENTUM MEDICAL LLC
708-927-9398

424 Stamp Creek Rd., Suite F, Salem, SC 29676
FDA Number: 1065238
Ownership: Private
Produces/Sells CE-marked Devices: N
General Admin.: Mr. Greg Silver/Chairman, Chief Executive Officer
    Mr. Ori Hadomi/Chief Executive Officer
    Mr. Eli Zehavi/Chief Operating Officer
    Mr. Moshe Shoham/Chief Technology Officer
Mktg./Adv.: Dr. Doron Dinstein/Vice President Marketing
    Mr. Avi Posen/Vice President Sales
    Mr. Christopher Sells/Vice President U.S. Sales
Production: Mr. Darren Reeves/Director Quality Assurance
Finance: Ms. Sharon Levita/Chief Financial Officer

Bandage, Adhesive	Surgery
Bandage, Liquid	Surgery
Dressing, Other	General

ARGON MEDICAL DEVICES INC.
903-675-9321

1445 Flat Creek Rd., Athens, TX 75751
FDA Number: 1625425   *Fax:* 903-677-9396
Web site: http://www.argonmedical.com
Ownership: Private
Produces/Sells CE-marked Devices: N
General Admin.: Mr. George Leondis/President
Mktg./Adv.: Mr. Christian Chilcott/Director Marketing & Sales
    Mark Landon/Senior Vice President Sales
Production: Mr. Bill Morgan/Vice President Operations
    Mr. Greg Justice/Vice President Quality Assurance & Regulatory Affairs
Finance: Ms. Sharon McNally/Vice President Finance

Adapter, Stopcock, Manifold, Cardiopulmonary Bypass	Cardiovascular
Basin, Emesis	General
Biopsy Device, Endomyocardial	Cardiovascular
Blade, Scalpel	Surgery
Cannula, Catheter	Cardiovascular
Catheter, Continuous Flush	Cardiovascular
Catheter, Flow Directed	Cardiovascular
Catheter, Intravascular, Diagnostic	Cardiovascular
Catheter, Intravascular, Therapeutic, Short-term Less Than 30 Days	General
Catheter, Multiple Lumen	Surgery
Catheter, Percutaneous	Cardiovascular
Catheter, Peritoneal Dialysis, Single-Use	Gastroenterology/Urology
Catheter, Urological	Gastroenterology/Urology
Clamp, Surgical, General & Plastic Surgery	Surgery

ARGON MEDICAL DEVICES INC.
903-675-9321 (cont'd)

Clamp, Vascular	Cardiovascular
Dilator, Vessel, Percutaneous Catheterization	Cardiovascular
Electrode, Needle	Cns/Neurology
Electrosurgical Unit, Cutting & Coagulation Device	Surgery
Filter, Intravascular, Cardiovascular	Cardiovascular
Guide, Surgical, Needle	Surgery
Guidewire, Catheter	Cardiovascular
Injector, Angiographic (Cardiac Catheterization)	Cardiovascular
Introducer, Catheter	Cardiovascular
Kit, Administration, Intravenous	General
Kit, Sampling, Arterial Blood	Anesthesiology
Monitor, Infusion, Gravity Flow	General
Needle, Biopsy, Cardiovascular	Cardiovascular
Needle, Hypodermic, Single Lumen With Syringe	General
Stethoscope, Electronic (Auscultoscope)	Cardiovascular
Sudan IV	Pathology
Syringe, Balloon Inflation	Cardiovascular
Syringe, Piston	General
Transducer, Blood Pressure, Extravascular	Cardiovascular
Transducer, Pressure, Intrauterine	Obstetrics/Gynecology
Tray, Start/Stop (Including Contents), Dialysis	Gastroenterology/Urology

Medical Product Subsidiaries (Listed Separately)
  Clinical Innovations, Inc.

ARGOSY
800-328-6105
612-942-9232

10300 W. 70th St., Eden Prairie, MN 55344-3445
FDA Number: n/a   *Fax:* 612-942-0503
E-mail: ron.scicluna@argosyhearing.com
Web site: www.argosyhearing.com
Medical Products Sales Volume: $21,000,000
Annual Revenue: $10-$25 Million
Total Employees: 225   *Marketing Staff:* 4   *Sales Staff:* 12
Ownership: Unitron Industries Ltd.
Quality System Registration Information: ISO9001
Federal Procurement Eligibility: VA Contract
Distribution: Manufacturer Through Distributor, Exporter
General Admin.: Gary Maas/President
Mktg./Adv.: Roxann Bonta/Director Marketing
    Penny Hinderaker/Manager Communications
Production: Jerald Maas/Vice President Manufacturing
Research: Ron Scicluna/Director Research & Development

Hearing-Aid	Ear/Nose/Throat

ARGOSY ELECTRONICS
See Argosy

ARGUS-HAZCO
800-332-0435
937-824-4400

6501 Centerville Business Pkwy., Dayton, OH 45459
FDA Number: n/a   *Fax:* 937-824-4444
E-mail: info@hazcoservices.com
Web site: www.argus-hazco.com
Total Employees: 19   *Marketing Staff:* 3   *Sales Staff:* 10
Ownership: Private
Produces/Sells CE-marked Devices: N
Federal Procurement Eligibility: Small Business
Distribution: Manufacturer Through Distributor, Service Direct
General Admin.: Ralph Miller/Vice President, General Manager
Production: Jerry Wright/Director Quality Assurance

Clothing, Protective	General
Safety Equipment, Laboratory	Chemistry
Security Equipment/Supplies	General

ARGYLE
See Covidien Lp

ARI
770-227-8222

2523 South Mcdonough Rd., Orchard Hill, GA 30266
FDA Number: 1037559

Refrigerant, Topical (Vapocoolant)	Physical Med

ARIBEX, INC.
801-226-5522

744 South 400 East, Orem, UT 84097
FDA Number: 3005417494

Radiographic Unit, Diagnostic, Dental, Extraoral	Dental And Oral

ARISTA SURGICAL CO.
See Arista Surgical Supply Co. Inc.

ARISTA SURGICAL SUPPLY CO. INC.
800-223-1984
781-329-2900

297 High Street, Dedham, MA 02026
FDA Number: n/a   *Fax:* 800-437-2966
E-mail: arista@alimed.com
Web site: www.aristasurgical.com
Medical Products Sales Volume: $300,000
Annual Revenue: $1-$5 Million
Year Founded: 1946
Total Employees: 2   *Marketing Staff:* 3   *Sales Staff:* 5
Ownership: Private
Produces/Sells CE-marked Devices: N

ARISTA SURGICAL SUPPLY CO. INC.   800-223-1984 *(cont'd)*
Federal Procurement Eligibility: Small Business
Distribution: Exclusive Distributor
General Admin.: Stephen R. Howard/General Manager
       Irving Horowitz/President, Chief Executive Officer
       Estelle Horowitz/Vice President

Blade, Scalpel	Surgery
Forceps	Orthopedics
General Use Surgical Scissors	Surgery
Handle, Knife Blade	Surgery
Retractor, All Types	Dental And Oral
Scalpel, One-Piece (Knife)	Surgery
Suture, Other	Surgery

ARISTO IMPORT CO., INC.   800-352-6304
85 Hunt Rd., Orangeburg, NY 10962-2596   845-359-0720
FDA Number: n/a   *Fax:* 845-359-0020
E-mail: aristoinc@aol.com
Web site: www.aristoimports.com
Medical Products Sales Volume: $1,000,000
Annual Revenue: $0-$1 Million
Year Founded: 1920
Ownership: Private
Produces/Sells CE-marked Devices: N
Federal Procurement Eligibility: Small Business
Distribution: Manufacturer Direct, Manufacturer Through Distributor, Manufacturer
Through Manufacturer Reps, Exporter

Clock, Elapsed Time	General
Counter, Differential Hand Tally	Hematology
Monitor, Blood Pressure, Indirect, Automatic	Cardiovascular
Monitor, Pulse Rate	Anesthesiology
Timeclock	General
Timer, Diagnostic Use	General

ARISTOTLE CORP.   203-358-8000
96 Cummings Point Road, Stamford, CT 06902
FDA Number: n/a
E-mail: wsmith@ihc-geneve.com
Web site: www.aristotlecorp.net
Year Founded: 1986
Total Employees: 800
Ownership: Public
Stock Symbol: ARTL
Traded On: NASDAQ
Produces/Sells CE-marked Devices: N
General Admin.: Edward Netter/Chairman
       Dean T Johnson/Chief Financial Officer, Vice President
       John L Lahey/President
       Steven B Lapin/President, Chief Operating Officer
       H William Smith/Vice President, General Counsel

ARIZANT HEALTHCARE INC.   800-733-7775
10393 W. 70th St., Eden Prairie, MN 55344-3446   952-947-1200
FDA Number: 3004542876
E-mail: webmail@arizant.com   *Fax:* 952-947-1400
Web site: www.arizanthealthcare.com
Medical Products Sales Volume: $9,600,000
Annual Revenue: $50-$100 Million
Year Founded: 1987
Total Employees: 131   *Marketing Staff:* 10   *Sales Staff:* 40
Ownership: Private
Quality System Registration Information: ISO9001
Produces/Sells CE-marked Devices: Y
Federal Procurement Eligibility: Small Business
Distribution: Manufacturer Direct, Manufacturer Through Distributor
General Admin.: John Thomas/President, Chief Executive Officer, Chairman
Mktg./Adv.: Teri Woodwick Sides/Director Marketing
       Jack Stabler/Director National Accounts
       Jami Collins/Manager Marketing Communications
       Doug Hall/Vice President Sales
Production: David Westlin/Director Quality Assurance & Regulatory Affairs
       Rick Schultz/Vice President Manufacturing
Research: Gary Maharaj/Vice President Research & Development
Finance: Preston Luman/Chief Financial Officer

Gown, Patient	Surgery
Hypo/Hyperthermia Blanket	General
Hypothermia Unit	General
Warmer, Infusion Fluid, Thermal	General

ARIZONA DEVICE MANUFACTURING   763-505-0874
2350 West Medtronic Way, Tempe, AZ 85281
FDA Number: 2032545
Ownership: Medtronic, Inc.
Produces/Sells CE-marked Devices: N

Defibrillator, Implantable, Automatic	Cardiovascular
Electrode, pH	Gastroenterology/Urology
Pacemaker, Heart, Implantable, Programmable	Cardiovascular

ARIZONA DEVICE MANUFACTURING   763-505-0874 *(cont'd)*
Recorder, Event, Implantable Cardiac, (without Arrhythmia Detection)   Cardiovascular

ARIZONA DME, INC.
See Arizona Dme--Durable Medical Equipment, Inc.

ARIZONA DME--DURABLE MEDICAL   888-665-2568
EQUIPMENT, INC.
PO BOX 15413, Scottsdale, AZ 85267   480-946-8070
FDA Number: n/a   *Fax:* 480-946-5246
E-mail: inquiries@azdme.com
Web site: www.arizonadme.com
Medical Products Sales Volume: $1,000,000
Annual Revenue: $0-$1 Million
Year Founded: 1998
Ownership: Private
Produces/Sells CE-marked Devices: N
Federal Procurement Eligibility: Small Business
Distribution: Exclusive Distributor

Electrode, TENS	Cns/Neurology
Equipment, Traction, Powered	Physical Med
Gel, Electrode, TENS	Physical Med
Stimulator, Muscle, Electrical-Powered (EMS)	Physical Med
Stimulator, Nerve, Transcutaneous (Pain Relief, TENS)	Cns/Neurology
Tips And Pads, Cane, Crutch And Walker	Physical Med
Wheelchair, Manual	Physical Med

ARIZONA INDUSTRIES FOR THE BLIND   602-269-5131
Dept. Economic Security, 3013 W. Linclon St.,
Phoenix, AZ 85009
FDA Number: n/a   *Fax:* 602-269-9462
E-mail: leslieanderson@azdes.gov
Web site: www.azdes.gov/aib
Medical Products Sales Volume: $5,000,000
Year Founded: 1947
Total Employees: 120   *Marketing Staff:* 2   *Sales Staff:* 2
Ownership: Private
Quality System Registration Information: ISO9002
Produces/Sells CE-marked Devices: N
Federal Procurement Eligibility: Small Business
Distribution: Manufacturer Direct, Manufacturer Through Distributor, OEM, Service
Direct
General Admin.: Richard Monaco/General Manager
Mktg./Adv.: Mr. Les Anderson/Admin. Marketing & Sales
Production: Ms. Dana Clayton/Customer Service Representative

Stretcher, Hand-Carried	General
Table, Surgical, Manual	General

ARJO CANADA, INC.   800-665-4831
1575 South Gateway Rd., Unit C,   905-238-7880
Mississauga, ONT L4W-5 Canada
FDA Number: n/a   *Fax:* 905-238-7881
E-mail: info@arjo.ca
Web site: www.arjo.com
Medical Products Sales Volume: $14,000,000
Year Founded: 1969
Total Employees: 50   *Marketing Staff:* 3   *Sales Staff:* 20
Ownership: Huntleigh Healthcare Plc
Produces/Sells CE-marked Devices: N
Distribution: Manufacturer Direct, Exclusive Distributor

ARJO WIGGINS MEDICAL, INC.   843-388-8080
1301 Charleston Regional Pwky, #500, Charleston, SC 29492
FDA Number: 1053306   *Fax:* 843-388-8070
E-mail: northamerica@arjomedical.com
Web site: www.medical.arjowiggins.com
Medical Products Sales Volume: $2,800,000,000
Annual Revenue: More than $1 Billion
Total Employees: 8000
Ownership: Arjo Wiggins SA
Quality System Registration Information: ISO9002
Produces/Sells CE-marked Devices: Y
Federal Procurement Eligibility: GSA Contract
Distribution: Manufacturer Direct, OEM
General Admin.: Kim Golden/Office Manager
       David F. Darby/President
Production: Barbara Lehnert/Director Quality Assurance

Packaging Equipment	General
Packaging, Sterilization	General

ARJO, INC.
See ArjoHuntleigh

ARJOHUNTLEIGH   800-323-1245
2349 West Lake Street, Suite 250,   800-323-1245
Roselle, IL 60172
FDA Number: 1419652   *Fax:* 888-389-2756
E-mail: info@arjousa.com
Web site: www.arjo.com

ARJOHUNTLEIGH   800-323-1245 *(cont'd)*

Annual Revenue: $100-$500 Million
Year Founded: 40
Total Employees: 200   Marketing Staff: 2   Sales Staff: 65
Ownership: GETINGE AB
Quality System Registration Information: ISO9001
Produces/Sells CE-marked Devices: N
Distribution: Manufacturer Direct, OEM, Service Direct
General Admin.: Mrs. Joan Santana/Human Resources Associate
    Mr. Mark Harwood/President
Mktg./Adv.: Mrs. Amy McCaw/Manager National Marketing
    Mrs. Alexis LaSalvia/Marketing Coordinator
    Mr. Keith Arnold/Vice President National Accounts
IS: Mr. Eric Schmidt/Manager Information Systems

Bath, Hydro-Massage (Whirlpool)	Physical Med
Bath, Sitz, Physical Medicine	Physical Med
Bathtub	General
Bathtub, Portable	General
Chair, Adjustable, Mechanical	Physical Med
Chair, Bath	General
Chair, Other	General
Chair, Seat Lifting (Standing Aid)	General
Chair, Shower	General
Chair, With Casters	Physical Med
Equipment, Therapy, Handicapped/Physical	Physical Med
Lift, Bath, Non-AC-Powered	General
Lift, Patient	General
Patient Transfer Unit	General
Patient Transfer Unit, Powered	General
Scale, Bed	General
Scale, Chair	General
Shower, Emergency	Chemistry
Solution, Antibacterial Cleaner	General
Stretcher, Hydraulic	General
Stretcher, Wheeled (Mobile)	General
Tank, Full Body (Bath)	General
Transfer Aid	Physical Med
Transfer Device, Patient, Manual	General
Transport, Patient, Powered	Physical Med
Walker, Mechanical	Physical Med

Medical Product Subsidiaries (Listed Separately)
  Arjo Canada, Inc.
  ArjoHuntleigh
  Bhm Medical, Inc.
  Maquet, Inc.

ARK BIO-MEDICAL CANADA CORP.   800-661-004

**Dartrey Estate De L'ile, #671 Rustico Rd. Route 7,
Miltonvale Park, WINSL CIE 1 Canada**
FDA Number: 8022266   Fax: 902-892-5644
E-mail: arkbio@pei.aibn.com
Web site: www.arkbio.ca
Year Founded: 1989
Ownership: Private
Produces/Sells CE-marked Devices: N
Distribution: Manufacturer Direct, Exporter

ARK SERVICES CORPORATION   708-371-3674

6118 W. 123 St., Palos Heights, IL 60463
FDA Number: n/a   Fax: 708-371-2926
E-mail: ark@arksvc.com
Web site: www.arksvc.com
Year Founded: 1980
Ownership: Private
Produces/Sells CE-marked Devices: N
Federal Procurement Eligibility: Small Business
Distribution: Manufacturer Direct, OEM, Service Direct
General Admin.: Allan R. Kishpaugh/President

Packaging Equipment	General
Production Equipment	General
Service, Consulting	General

ARK THERAPEUTIC SERVICES, INC.   803-438-9779

Po Box 340, 862 A Hwy. 1 South, Lugoff, SC 29078
FDA Number: 3004039409   Fax: 803-438-9724
E-mail: info@arktherapeutic.com
Web site: www.arktherapeutic.com
Ownership: Private
Produces/Sells CE-marked Devices: N

Massager, Therapeutic	Physical Med
Massager, Therapeutic, Manual	Physical Med
Ring, Teething, Non-Fluid-Filled	Dental And Oral

ARKON SAFETY EQUIPMENT, INC.   514-351-8240

10550 Boul Parkway, Anjou H1J 2K4 Canada
FDA Number: 9615400

Kit, First Aid	Surgery

ARKRAY FACTORY USA, INC.   952-646-3168

5182 West 76th St., Minneapolis, MN 55439
FDA Number: 1832816
Ownership: Private
Produces/Sells CE-marked Devices: N

Analyzer, Chemistry, Urinalysis	Chemistry
Azo-Dyes, Colorimetric, Bilirubin And Conjugates	Chemistry
Catheter, Intravascular, Therapeutic, Short-term Less Than 30 Days	General
Colorimetric, Occult Blood in Urine	Hematology
Computer, Chemistry Analyzer	Chemistry
Control, Analyte (Assayed And Unassayed)	Chemistry
Diazo (Colorimetric), Nitrite (Urinary, Non-Quantitative)	Chemistry
Diazonium Colorimetry, Urobilinogen (Urinary, Non-Quant.)	Chemistry
Enzymatic Method, Glucose (Urinary, Non-Quantitative)	Chemistry
Glucose Dehydrogenase, Glucose	Chemistry
Indicator Method, Protein Or Albumin (Urinary, Non-Quant.)	Chemistry
Indicator, pH, Dye (Urinary, Non-Quantitative)	Chemistry
Kit, Administration, Intravenous	General
Lancet, Blood	General
Nitroprusside, Ketones (Urinary, Non-Quantitative)	Chemistry
Reagent, Glucose (Test System)	Chemistry
Scalpel, One-Piece (Knife)	Surgery
Syringe, Antistick	General
System, Test, Blood Glucose, Over-The-Counter	Chemistry
Test, Urine Leukocyte	Hematology
Vapor Pressure, Osmolality Of Serum & Urine	Chemistry

ARKRAY USA   800-818-8877
    952-646-3200

5198 W 76th St., Edina, MN 55439
FDA Number: n/a   Fax: 952-646-3210
E-mail: info@arkrayusa.com
Web site: www.arkrayusa.com
Annual Revenue: $50-$100 Million
Total Employees: 130   Marketing Staff: 6   Sales Staff: 27
Ownership: Private
Quality System Registration Information: ISO9001
Produces/Sells CE-marked Devices: Y
Federal Procurement Eligibility: Small Business, GSA Contract
Distribution: Manufacturer Through Distributor, OEM, Exclusive Distributor
General Admin.: Mr. John McCrea/President
Mktg./Adv.: Ms. Michelle Dumonceaux/Manager Marketing
    Sarah Zook/Marketing Coordinator
    Mr. Jonathan Chapman/President Marketing & Sales
    Mr. Susumu Akatsu/Vice President Marketing
Production: Mr. Tom Speikers/Director Quality Assurance & Regulatory Affairs
Finance: Mr. Craig Brosseau/Vice President Finance

Analyzer, Chemistry, Urinalysis	Chemistry
Analyzer, Sedimentation Rate, Erythrocyte	Hematology
Azo-Dyes, Colorimetric, Bilirubin And Conjugates	Chemistry
Control, Analyte (Assayed And Unassayed)	Chemistry
Control, Urinalysis (Assayed And Unassayed)	Chemistry
Lancet, Blood	General
Reagent, Glucose (Test System)	Chemistry
System, Test, Blood Glucose, Over-The-Counter	Chemistry

ARLINGTON MACHINE & TOOL CO.   973-276-1377

90 New Dutch Lane, Fairfield, NJ 07004
FDA Number: n/a   Fax: 973-276-1378
Web site: www.arlingtonmachine.com
Medical Products Sales Volume: $9,700,000
Annual Revenue: $10-$25 Million
Year Founded: 1963
Ownership: Private
Quality System Registration Information: ISO9001
Produces/Sells CE-marked Devices: N
Federal Procurement Eligibility: Small Business
Distribution: Manufacturer Direct

Production Equipment	General

ARLINGTON SCIENTIFIC, INC. ASI   800-654-0146
    801-489-8911

1840 N. Technology Dr., Springville, UT 84663
FDA Number: 1641328   Fax: 801-489-5552
E-mail: info@arlingtonscientific.com
Web site: www.arlingtonscientific.com
Annual Revenue: $1-$5 Million
Year Founded: 1985
Total Employees: 30   Marketing Staff: 1   Sales Staff: 5
Ownership: Private
Produces/Sells CE-marked Devices: Y
Federal Procurement Eligibility: Small Business
Distribution: Manufacturer Direct, Manufacturer Through Distributor, Exporter
General Admin.: Ben Card/President, Chief Executive Officer
    Ben Card/President, Owner
Mktg./Adv.: Ms. Debbie Card/Director National Accounts
    Mr. Ben Card/Manager Marketing Development
    Mr. Oscar Martinez/Manager Materials & Sales
Production: Ms. Christin Smith/Director Quality Assurance & Regulatory Affairs

Assay, Agglutination, Latex, Rubella	Microbiology
Chair, Blood Donor	General

ARLINGTON SCIENTIFIC, INC. ASI
800-654-0146 *(cont'd)*

Curette, Nasal	Ear/Nose/Throat
Enzyme Immunoassay, Amphetamine	Toxicology
Enzyme Immunoassay, Barbiturate	Toxicology
Enzyme Immunoassay, Benzodiazepine	Toxicology
Enzyme Immunoassay, Cannabinoids	Toxicology
Enzyme Immunoassay, Cocaine And Cocaine Metabolites	Toxicology
Enzyme Immunoassay, Methadone	Toxicology
Enzyme Immunoassay, Opiates	Toxicology
Enzyme Immunoassay, Phencyclidine	Toxicology
Kit, Pregnancy Test, Over The Counter, HCG	Chemistry
Kit, Screening, Staphylococcus Aureus	Microbiology
Radioimmunoassay, Human Chorionic Gonadotropin	Chemistry
Reagent, Antistreptolysin-Titer/Streptolysin O	Microbiology
Reagent, Streptolysin O/Antistreptolysin-Titer	Microbiology
Rubella, Other Assays	Microbiology
Table, Blood Donor	Hematology
Test, C-Reactive Protein	Immunology
Test, Infectious Mononucleosis	Immunology
Test, Radio-Allergen Absorbent (RAST)	Immunology
Test, Rheumatoid Factor	Immunology
Test, Sickle Cell	Hematology
Test, Syphilis (RPR or VDRL)	Microbiology
Test, Systemic Lupus Erythematosus	Immunology
Thin Layer Chromatography, Metamphetamine	Toxicology
U.V. Spectrometry, Tricyclic Antidepressant Drugs	Toxicology

ARLON ENGINEERED COATED PRODUCTS
800-232-7181
6110 E. Rittiman Road, San Antonio, TX 78218 **210-798-1900**
FDA Number: 2024432 Fax: 210-798-1920
E-mail: answers@arlon.com
Web site: www.arlon.com
Annual Revenue: $50-$100 Million
Year Founded: 1958
Total Employees: 35
Ownership: BAIRNCO
Quality System Registration Information: ISO9000; ISO9001
Produces/Sells CE-marked Devices: N
Federal Procurement Eligibility: Small Business
Distribution: Manufacturer Direct, Manufacturer Through Distributor, Exporter
General Admin.: Mr. Kevin Stevens/Vice President, General Manager
Mktg./Adv.: Troy Williams/Market Research Analyst
Production: Jeffrey Birkes/Product Manager

Catheter, Other	Gastroenterology/Urology
Contract Manufacturing	General
Tape, Adhesive	General

ARMAR INTERNATIONAL INC.
514-636-6737
850 Lakeshore Drive, Ste. N4, Dorval, QUE H9S-5T9 Canada
FDA Number: n/a Fax: 514-636-0177
E-mail: armar@videotron.ca
Web site: www.armarinternational.com
Year Founded: 1984
Total Employees: 10
Ownership: Private
Produces/Sells CE-marked Devices: N

ARMEDICA MFG. CORP.
800-701-5122
212 Bell Rd., PO Box 880, Greenwood, AR 72936 **479-996-2612**
FDA Number: 1649977 Fax: 479-996-3051
E-mail: staff@armedicamfg.com
Web site: www.armedicamfg.com
Ownership: Private
Produces/Sells CE-marked Devices: N

Table, Physical Medicine, Powered	Physical Med
Table, Physical Therapy	Physical Med

ARMIN POLY-VERSION, INC.
201-451-0600
49 Fisk Street, Jersey City, NJ 07305
FDA Number: n/a Fax: 201-451-5712
Web site: http://poly-version.com/
Annual Revenue: $10-$25 Million
Year Founded: 1966
Total Employees: 5 Marketing Staff: 1 Sales Staff: 2
Ownership: Private
Produces/Sells CE-marked Devices: N
Distribution: Manufacturer Through Distributor
Mktg./Adv.: Milton Cohen/Manager Accounts

Glove, Other	General
Glove, Utility	General

ARMM, INC.
714-848-8190
17744 Sampson Lane, Huntington Beach, CA 92647
FDA Number: 2028523 Fax: 714-848-6141
E-mail: info@armminc.com
Web site: www.armminc.com
Medical Products Sales Volume: $5,200,000
Year Founded: 1992
Total Employees: 55

ARMM, INC.
714-848-8190 *(cont'd)*
Ownership: Private
Produces/Sells CE-marked Devices: Y
Federal Procurement Eligibility: Small Business
Distribution: Manufacturer Direct, Manufacturer Through Distributor, Manufacturer Through Manufacturer Reps, OEM, Service Direct, Importer, Exporter
General Admin.: Roger Wood/President

Catheter, Continuous Irrigation	Surgery
Catheter, Irrigation	Surgery
Catheter, Multiple Lumen	Surgery
Catheter, Pericardium Drainage	Cardiovascular
Contract Assembly	General
Contract Manufacturing	General
Contract Manufacturing, Product, Disposable	General
Contract Packaging	General
Contract Sterilization	General
Drain, Suction, Closed	Surgery
Drain, Sump	Gastroenterology/Urology
Drain, Thoracic (Chest)	Anesthesiology
Filter, Aspirator	Surgery
Filter, Gas	Anesthesiology
Irrigator, Suction	General
Probe, Suction, Irrigator/Aspirator, Laparoscopic	Surgery
Tray, Surgical	Surgery
Tube, Drainage	Gastroenterology/Urology
Tube, Suction	General
Tubing, Flexible, Medical Gas, Low-Pressure	Anesthesiology
Tubing, Irrigation	Surgery
Tubing, Other	General
Tubing, Plastic	General
Tubing, Polyvinyl Chloride	General
Tubing, Silicone	General
Tubing, Vinyl	General

ARMOR SPORTS HOLDINGS, LLC
520-623-9800
2030 N. Forbes Blvd., #106, Tucson, AZ 85745
FDA Number: 3005207657
Ownership: Private
Produces/Sells CE-marked Devices: N

Orthosis, Limb Brace	Physical Med

ARMOUR BIOCHEMICAL
See Serologicals Corp

ARMOUR PHARMACEUTICAL CO.
See Csl Behring

ARMOUR PHARMACEUTICAL COMP./BIOCHEMICAL
See Serologicals Corp

ARMSTRONG INDUSTRIES, INC.
972-547-1400
7290 Virginia Pkwy, Ste 3000, Mckinney, TX 75071
FDA Number: 1643748
Ownership: Private
Produces/Sells CE-marked Devices: N

Stimulator, Muscle, Electrical-Powered (EMS)	Physical Med
Stimulator, Nerve, Transcutaneous (Pain Relief, TENS)	Cns/Neurology

ARMSTRONG MEDICAL INDUSTRIES, INC.
800-323-4220
575 Knightsbridge Pkwy., **847-913-0101**
Lincolnshire, IL 60069
FDA Number: 9200082 Fax: 847-913-0138
E-mail: csr@armstrongmedical.com
Web site: www.armstrongmedical.com
Year Founded: 1957
Total Employees: 95 Marketing Staff: 2 Sales Staff: 41
Ownership: Private
Produces/Sells CE-marked Devices: N
Federal Procurement Eligibility: Small Business
Distribution: Manufacturer Direct, Importer, Exporter
General Admin.: Warren G. Armstrong/President, Chief Executive Officer
    James W. Armstrong/Vice President, General Manager
Mktg./Adv.: Corinne Walker/Manager Advertising
Production: Corinne Walker/Director Art

Accessories, Cart, Multipurpose	General
Airway, Esophageal (Obturator)	Anesthesiology
Airway, Nasopharyngeal (Breathing Tube)	Anesthesiology
Anatomical Training Model	General
Attachment, Breathing, Positive End Expiratory Pressure	Anesthesiology
Balloon, Epistaxis (Nasal)	Ear/Nose/Throat
Bin, Storage	General
Blanket, Rescue	General
Block, Bite, Intubation	Anesthesiology
Board, Cardiac Compression	Cardiovascular
Board, Spine	Orthopedics
Cabinet Casework, Modular	General
Cabinet, Narcotic Control	General
Carrier, Container, Oxygen, Portable	General
Cart, Anesthetist's	Anesthesiology
Cart, Dressing	General
Cart, Emergency, Cardiopulmonary Resuscitation (Crash)	Anesthesiology
Cart, Instrument	Surgery

MANUFACTURER PROFILES

ARMSTRONG MEDICAL INDUSTRIES, INC. 800-323-4220 *(cont'd)*

Cart, Instrument/Equipment, Laparoscopy	Surgery
Cart, Isolation	General
Cart, Medicine	General
Cart, Monitor	General
Cart, Multipurpose	General
Cart, Supply	General
Cart, Supply, Operating Room	Surgery
Changer, Tube, Endotracheal	Anesthesiology
Chart, Anatomical Training	General
Collar, Cervical Neck	Orthopedics
Collar, Extrication	General
Compress, Cold	General
Compress, Moist Heat	Physical Med
Cuff, Blood Pressure	Cardiovascular
Cushion, Other	General
Cylinder, Oxygen	Anesthesiology
Device, Assist, CPR	Anesthesiology
Encapsulator, Fluid	General
Endoscope	Gastroenterology/Urology
Extrication Equipment	General
Fitting, Quick Connect (Gas Connector)	General
Glove, Patient Examination, Latex	General
Glove, Surgical, Hypoallergenic	General
Glove, Surgical, Powder-Free	General
Goggles, Protective, Eye	Ophthalmology
Gown, Isolation, Surgical	Surgery
Holder, Catheter	Gastroenterology/Urology
Holder, Medical Chart	General
Immobilizer, Cervical	Orthopedics
Infuser, Pressure (Blood Pump)	General
Infusion Stand	General
Kit, Emergency, Cardiopulmonary Resuscitation	General
Kit, First Aid	Surgery
Kit, Irrigation, Eye	Ophthalmology
Kit, Labor and Delivery	Obstetrics/Gynecology
Kit, Quality Control	Microbiology
Kit, Suction, Airway (Tracheal)	Anesthesiology
Kit, Tracheotomy	Anesthesiology
Laryngoscope	Ear/Nose/Throat
Mask, Face	General
Material, Training, Audiovisual	General
Meter, Peak Flow, Spirometry	Anesthesiology
Ophthalmoscope, Battery-Powered	Ophthalmology
Otoscope	Ear/Nose/Throat
Oximeter, Pulse	General
Pad, Defibrillator Paddle	Cardiovascular
Patient Transfer Unit	General
Penlight, Battery-Powered	Ophthalmology
Pressure Infusor, IV Container	General
Pump, Infusion, Ambulatory	General
Receptacle, Electrical	General
Regulator, Oxygen, Mechanical	General
Rescue Equipment	General
Resuscitator, Emergency, Protective, Infection	Anesthesiology
Resuscitator, Pulmonary, Manual (Demand Valve)	General
Scale, Stand-On	General
Screen, Bedside	General
Simulator, ECG	Cardiovascular
Solution, Antimicrobial	Microbiology
Sphygmomanometer, Electronic, Automatic	General
Sphygmomanometer, Electronic, Manual	General
Splint, Extremity, Inflatable, External	Surgery
Splint, Traction	Orthopedics
Stethoscope, Amplified	General
Stethoscope, Mechanical	General
Stool, Anesthetist's	Anesthesiology
Strap, Restraining	General
Stretcher, Basket, Portable	General
Stretcher, Collapsible	General
Stretcher, Emergency, Other	General
Stretcher, Hand-Carried	General
Stretcher, Transfer	Surgery
Stretcher, Wheeled (Mobile)	General
Stretcher, Wheeled, Mechanical	Physical Med
Stylet, Tracheal Tube	Anesthesiology
Suction Apparatus, Operating Room, Wall Vacuum-Powered	Surgery
Suit, Pneumatic Counterpressure (Anti-Shock)	Cardiovascular
Thermometer, Infrared	General
Thermometer, Mercury	General
Thermometer, Tympanic	Ear/Nose/Throat
Tourniquet	General
Trainer, Auditory	Ear/Nose/Throat
Training Aid	Orthopedics
Training Aid, Arrhythmia Recognition	Cardiovascular
Training Manikin, CPR (Resuscitation)	General
Training Manikin, Intravenous Arm	General
Training Manikin, Other	General
Training Manikin, Wound Moulage	General
Transfer Device, Patient, Manual	General
Tray, Custom/Special Procedure	General
Trousers, Anti-Shock	Anesthesiology

ARMSTRONG MEDICAL INDUSTRIES, INC. 800-323-4220 *(cont'd)*

Valve, Positive End Expiratory Pressure (PEEP)	Anesthesiology
Waste Disposal Unit, Sharps	General
Waste Receptacle, Kick Bucket	General
Wheelchair, Manual	Physical Med

ARNDORFER MEDICAL SPECIALTIES   414-425-1661
5656 Grove Terrace, Greendale, WI 53129
FDA Number: 2182418

Catheter, Multiple Lumen	Surgery
Pump, Infusion	General

ARNEL HEALTHCARE, INC.   516-783-1939
1523 Dewey Ave., Bellmore, NY 11710
FDA Number: 2438157

Burr, Dental	Dental And Oral
Matrix, Dental	Dental And Oral

ARNEL, INC.   516-486-7098
73 High St., Hempstead, NY 11550
FDA Number: 2433194
Ownership: Private
Produces/Sells CE-marked Devices: N

Capsule, Dental, Amalgam	Dental And Oral
Matrix, Dental	Dental And Oral

ARNOLD TUBER INDUSTRIES   716-648-3363
97 Main Street, Hamburg, NY 14075
FDA Number: 3003988575
Ownership: Private
Produces/Sells CE-marked Devices: N

Burr, Dental	Dental And Oral
Carver, Wax, Dental	Dental And Oral
Chisel, Bone, Surgical	Dental And Oral
Curette, Periodontic	Dental And Oral
Curette, Surgical, Dental	Dental And Oral
Drill, Dental, Intraoral	Dental And Oral
Elevator, Surgical, Dental	Dental And Oral
Forceps, Rongeur, Surgical	Dental And Oral
Forceps, Tooth Extractor, Surgical	Dental And Oral
Knife, Periodontic	Dental And Oral
Plugger, Root Canal, Endodontic	Dental And Oral
Probe, Periodontic	Dental And Oral
Scaler, Periodontic	Dental And Oral
Syringe, Cartridge	Dental And Oral
Tray, Impression	Dental And Oral

AROSURGICAL INSTRUMENTS CORP.   800-776-1751
220 Newport Center Dr., Ste.11101,   888-430-7888
Newport Beach, CA 92660
FDA Number: n/a   *Fax:* 888-430-7889
E-mail: service@arosurgical.com
Web site: www.arosurgical.com
Year Founded: 1992
Ownership: Private
Produces/Sells CE-marked Devices: N
Federal Procurement Eligibility: Small Business
Distribution: Manufacturer Direct

Clip, Instrument	Surgery
Dilator, Other	Surgery
Forceps, General & Plastic Surgery	Surgery
Holder, Needle, Other	Surgery
Instrument, Microsurgical	Cns/Neurology
Scissors, Plastic Surgery (Dissecting)	Surgery
Suture, Non-Absorbable	Surgery
Suture, Other	Surgery

ARRHYTHMIA RESEARCH TECHNOLOGY, INC.   978-345-0181
25 Sawyer Passway, Fitchburg, MA 01420
FDA Number: n/a   *Fax:* 978-342-0168
E-mail: info@arthrt.com
Web site: www.arthrt.com
Medical Products Sales Volume: $19,300,000
Annual Revenue: $10-$25 Million
Year Founded: 1981
Total Employees: 12   *Marketing Staff:* 1   *Sales Staff:* 2
Ownership: Private
Stock Symbol: HRT
Traded On: AMEX
Quality System Registration Information: ISO9001
Produces/Sells CE-marked Devices: Y
Federal Procurement Eligibility: Small Business
Distribution: Manufacturer Direct, Manufacturer Through Distributor, OEM, Exporter
General Admin.: James E. Rouse/President
Mktg./Adv.: Frederick W. Lane/Director Product Development
       Mark R. LaViolette/Vice President Sales

Computer Software	General

ARRK CREATIVE NETWORK CORP.
See ARRK Product Development Group

ARRK PRODUCT DEVELOPMENT GROUP   800-735-2775
8880 Rehco Rd., San Diego, CA 92121   **858-552-1587**
FDA Number: n/a
E-mail: contactus@arrk.com
Web site: www.arrk.com
Year Founded: 1948
Ownership: ARRK CORPORATION
Quality System Registration Information: ISO9002
Produces/Sells CE-marked Devices: N
General Admin.: Toshihro Araki/Chairman
        Eiji Uchiya/President

Contract R&D, Equipment	General
Service, Engineering/Design	General

ARROW INDUSTRIES LLC   701-886-7722
530 5th Street, Neche, ND 58265-4033
FDA Number: 3004594175
Ownership: Private
Produces/Sells CE-marked Devices: N
General Admin.: Mr. Robert Symington/Owner

Operative Dental Treatment Unit	Dental And Oral

ARROW INTERNACIONAL DE MEXICO, S.A.   610-378-0131
DE C.V.

Modulo 1, Circuito 5, Parque Industrias De America, Col. Panamericana, Chihuahua Mexico
FDA Number: 9680794

Catheter, Embolectomy (Fogarty Type)	Cardiovascular
Catheter, Intravascular, Therapeutic, Long-term Greater Than 30 Days	General
Catheter, Intravascular, Therapeutic, Short-term Less Than 30 Days	General
Guidewire, Catheter	Cardiovascular
Introducer, Catheter	Cardiovascular
Kit, Administration, Intravenous	General

ARROW INTERNATIONAL, INC.   800-523-8446
2 Berry Dr, Mount Holly, NJ 08060   **610-655-8522**
FDA Number: 2242445
Web site: www.arrowintl.com
Year Founded: 1975
Ownership: Teleflex Medical
Produces/Sells CE-marked Devices: N
General Admin.: Mr. Carl G. Anderson/Chief Executive Officer, Chairman
        Mr. Jim Fitzpatrick/Vice President
        Mr. Rick Eagle/Vice President
Production: Mr. Kenneth E. Imler/Senior Vice President Regulatory Affairs
Finance: Mr. Frederick J. Hirt/Chief Financial Officer

Accessories, Catheter	Surgery
Catheter, Biliary	Gastroenterology/Urology
Catheter, Electrode Recording, Or Probe	Cardiovascular
Catheter, Embolectomy (Fogarty Type)	Cardiovascular
Catheter, Flow Directed	Cardiovascular
Catheter, Hemodialysis	Gastroenterology/Urology
Catheter, Intravascular, Diagnostic	Cardiovascular
Catheter, Intravascular, Therapeutic, Long-term Greater Than 30 Days	General
Catheter, Intravascular, Therapeutic, Short-term Less Than 30 Days	General
Catheter, Irrigation	Surgery
Catheter, Percutaneous	Cardiovascular
Catheter, Peripheral, Atherectomy	Cardiovascular
Catheter, Suction, With Tip	General
Computer, Diagnostic, Pre-Programmed, Single-Function	Cardiovascular
Drape, Surgical	Surgery
Electrode, Pacemaker, Temporary	Cardiovascular
Guidewire, Catheter	Cardiovascular
Introducer, Catheter	Cardiovascular
Kit, Administration, Intravenous	General
Kit, Anesthesia, Conduction	Anesthesiology
Kit, Anesthesia, Epidural	Anesthesiology
Kit, Anesthesia, Spinal	Anesthesiology
Port & Catheter, Infusion, Implanted, Subcut., Intraperit.	General
Port & Catheter, Infusion, Implanted, Subcutaneous, Intraspinal	General
Prosthesis, Elbow, Constrained	Orthopedics
Set, Administration, Intravenous, Needle-Free	General
Stopcock	General

ARROW INTERNATIONAL, INC.   800-523-8446
2400 Bernville Rd., Reading, PA 19605   **610-655-8522**
                                   Fax: 610-655-8566
FDA Number: 2518433
Web site: www.arrowintl.com
Medical Products Sales Volume: $342,000,000
Year Founded: 1975
Total Employees: 3250
Ownership: Teleflex Medical
Quality System Registration Information: ISO9000
Produces/Sells CE-marked Devices: Y
Distribution: Manufacturer Direct
General Admin.: Mr. Carl G. Anderson/Chief Executive Officer, Chairman

ARROW INTERNATIONAL, INC.   800-523-8446 *(cont'd)*
    Paul L. Frankhouser/Executive Vice President
    Philip Fleck/President, Chief Operating Officer
    Mr. Jim Fitzpatrick/Vice President
    Mr. Rick Eagle/Vice President
Mktg./Adv.: Jane Wenot/Manager Contract Sales
    Rick Yanchuleff/Manager Corporate Communications
    Chris Mennone/Manager International Sales
    Maria Jacoby/Manager Sales Training
Production: Nancy Martin/Manager Customer Services
    Mr. Kenneth E. Imler/Senior Vice President Regulatory Affairs
Finance: Mr. Frederick J. Hirt/Chief Financial Officer

Balloon, Intra-Aortic (With Control System)	Cardiovascular
Catheter, Arterial	Cardiovascular
Catheter, Balloon (Foley Type)	Surgery
Catheter, Cardiovascular, Balloon Type	Cardiovascular
Catheter, Central Venous	General
Catheter, Cholangiography	Surgery
Catheter, Conduction, Anesthesia	Anesthesiology
Catheter, Epidural	Obstetrics/Gynecology
Catheter, Infusion	Surgery
Catheter, Intra-Aortic Balloon	Cardiovascular
Catheter, Intravascular, Diagnostic	Cardiovascular
Catheter, Multiple Lumen	Surgery
Catheter, Other	Gastroenterology/Urology
Catheter, Percutaneous	Cardiovascular
Catheter, Subclavian	Cardiovascular
Guidewire, Catheter	Cardiovascular
Introducer, Catheter	Cardiovascular
Kit, Anesthesia, Conduction	Anesthesiology
Kit, Quality Control	Microbiology
Needle, Conduction, Anesthesia (W/Wo Introducer)	Anesthesiology
Port, Vascular Access	Cardiovascular
Pump, Infusion, Implantable, General	General
Radioimmunoassay, Digoxin (3-H)	Toxicology
System, Delivery, Drug, Unit-Dose	General
Trocar, Gallbladder	Gastroenterology/Urology
Warmer, Blood and Plasma	Hematology

Medical Product Subsidiaries (Listed Separately)
   Arrow Medical Products, Ltd.

ARROW INTERNATIONAL, INC.   800-523-8446
312 Commerce Pl, Asheboro, NC 27203   **610-655-8522**
                                   Fax: 610-655-8566
FDA Number: 1036844
Web site: www.arrowintl.com
Year Founded: 1975
Ownership: Teleflex Medical
Produces/Sells CE-marked Devices: N

Catheter, Intravascular, Diagnostic	Cardiovascular
Catheter, Percutaneous	Cardiovascular
Guidewire, Catheter	Cardiovascular
Kit, Anesthesia, Conduction	Anesthesiology
Needle, Conduction, Anesthesia (W/Wo Introducer)	Anesthesiology

ARROW INTERNATIONAL, INC.   800-523-8446
9 Plymouth St., Everett, MA 02149   **610-655-8522**
FDA Number: 1219856
Web site: www.arrowintl.com
Year Founded: 1975
Ownership: Teleflex Medical
Produces/Sells CE-marked Devices: N
General Admin.: Mr. Carl G. Anderson/Chief Executive Officer, Chairman
        Mr. Jim Fitzpatrick/Vice President
        Mr. Rick Eagle/Vice President
Production: Mr. Kenneth E. Imler/Senior Vice President Regulatory Affairs
Finance: Mr. Frederick J. Hirt/Chief Financial Officer

Balloon, Intra-Aortic (With Control System)	Cardiovascular
Flowmeter, Blood, Intravenous	Cardiovascular

ARROW INTL., INC
See Arrow International, Inc.

ARROW MEDICAL PRODUCTS, LTD.   800-387-7819
2300 Bristol Circle Unit 1,   **905-829-9473**
Oakville, ONT L6H-5 Canada
FDA Number: n/a   Fax: 905-829-9414
E-mail: paul_williams@arrowintl.com
Web site: www.arrowintl.com
Year Founded: 1985
Total Employees: 10   *Sales Staff:* 6
Ownership: Arrow International, Inc.
Produces/Sells CE-marked Devices: Y
Distribution: Exclusive Distributor, Exporter

ARROW PRECISION PRODUCTS, INC.
See Precision Medical Products, Inc.

ARROWHEAD ATHLETICS
220 Andover St., PO Box 4264,
Andover, MA 01810
FDA Number: 1221539
E-mail: wnugent@shawsheencc.com
Web site: www.aatape.com
Medical Products Sales Volume: $12,000,000
Annual Revenue: $1-$5 Million
Year Founded: 1984
Total Employees: 50
Ownership: SHAWSHEEN RUBBER CO.
Quality System Registration Information: ISO9001
Produces/Sells CE-marked Devices: Y
Federal Procurement Eligibility: Small Business
Distribution: Manufacturer Direct, Manufacturer Through Distributor
General Admin.: Walter Nugent/General Manager
Denis Kelley/President
Mktg./Adv.: Walter Nugent/Vice President Marketing

800-225-1516
978-470-1760
Fax: 978-475-8603

Tape, Orthopedic	Orthopedics

ARS ENTERPRISES
12900 Lakeland Road,
Santa Fe Springs, CA 90670
FDA Number: n/a
E-mail: info@arsenterprises.com
Web site: www.arsenterprises.com
Medical Products Sales Volume: $1,540,000
Annual Revenue: $1-$5 Million
Year Founded: 1971
Total Employees: 15
Ownership: Private
Produces/Sells CE-marked Devices: N
Federal Procurement Eligibility: Small Business
Distribution: Manufacturer Direct, Manufacturer Through Distributor, Manufacturer Through Manufacturer Reps, OEM, Service Direct
General Admin.: Glenn Caster/Chief Executive Officer
Mktg./Adv.: Glenn Caster/Director Marketing & Sales
Production: John Batton/Director Operations

800-735-9277
562-946-3505
Fax: 562-946-4120

Equipment, Control, Pollution	General
Recovery Equipment, Water	General
Sterilizer, Ethylene-Oxide Gas	General
Sterilizer, Steam (Autoclave)	General

ART OPTICAL CONTACT LENS, INC.
3175 Three Mile Road NW, PO Box 1848,
Grand Rapids, MI 49501
FDA Number: 1835957
Web site: www.artoptical.com
Medical Products Sales Volume: $5,600,000
Year Founded: 1931
Total Employees: 110
Ownership: Private
Quality System Registration Information: ISO9001
Federal Procurement Eligibility: Small Business
General Admin.: Thomas E. Anastor/President

800-253-9364
800-566-8001
Fax: 800-648-2272

Lens, Contact (Other Material)	Ophthalmology

ART-CRAFT OPTICAL CO., INC.
See Artcraft New York

ARTCRAFT NEW YORK
57 Goodway Drive South, Rochester, NY 14623
FDA Number: n/a
E-mail: aco@artcraftoptical.com
Web site: www.artcraftnewyork.com
Medical Products Sales Volume: $8,200,000
Year Founded: 1918
Total Employees: 135
Ownership: Private
Produces/Sells CE-marked Devices: N
Federal Procurement Eligibility: Small Business
Distribution: Manufacturer Through Distributor, OEM, Importer
General Admin.: C. Thomas Eagle/President, Chief Executive Officer
Linda Cooley/Vice President Human Resources
Mktg./Adv.: Mike Franz/Vice President Marketing & Sales
Production: Norm Radziwon/Vice President Manufacturing

800-828-8288
585-546-6640
Fax: 585-546-5133

Frame, Spectacle (Eyeglasses)	Ophthalmology

ARTCRAFT PACKAGING CORP.
212 Lions Estate Dr., Jonesburg, MO 63351
FDA Number: 1926956

314-488-5566

Tubing, Non-Invasive	Surgery

ARTEC ENVIRONMENTAL MONITORING
8047 Castleton Road, Indianapolis, IN 46250
FDA Number: n/a
Web site: www.artecenvironmental.com
Medical Products Sales Volume: $1,500,000

800-727-8321
317-577-7000

ARTEC ENVIRONMENTAL MONITORING *(cont'd)*
Annual Revenue: $1-$5 Million
Year Founded: 1981
Ownership: Private
Produces/Sells CE-marked Devices: N
Federal Procurement Eligibility: Small Business
Distribution: Service Direct

800-727-8321 *(cont'd)*

Monitor, Gas, Atmospheric, Environmental	General

ARTEFACTOS DE VIDRIO S.A. DE C.V.
Canela, Granjas Mexico 346, Ciudad De Mexico 08400 Mexico
FDA Number: 8030676

Tube, Vacuum Sample, With Anticoagulant	Hematology

ARTEGRAFT, INC.
220 N. Center Drive, North Brunswick, NJ 08902
FDA Number: 2247686
E-mail: info@artegraft.com
Web site: www.artegraft.com
Medical Products Sales Volume: $3,000,000
Annual Revenue: $1-$5 Million
Year Founded: 1993
Total Employees: 8
Ownership: Private
Produces/Sells CE-marked Devices: N
Federal Procurement Eligibility: Small Business
Distribution: Manufacturer Direct, Manufacturer Through Distributor, Manufacturer Through Manufacturer Reps, Service Direct, Exclusive Distributor
General Admin.: Richard A. Gibson/President, Chief Executive Officer

800-631-5264
732-422-8333
Fax: 732-422-8647

Catheter, Embolectomy (Fogarty Type)	Cardiovascular
Graft, Arterial, Biological	Cardiovascular
Graft, Bovine	Surgery
Graft, Vascular, Biological	Cardiovascular
Graft, Vascular, Biological, Hemodialysis Access	Gastroenterology/Urology
Introducer, Catheter	Cardiovascular
Prosthesis, Arterial Graft, Bovine Carotid Artery	Surgery
Prosthesis, Vascular Graft, Of 6mm And Greater Diameter	Cardiovascular
Tissue Graft of 6mm and Greater	Cardiovascular
Vascular Access Graft	Gastroenterology/Urology

ARTEL, INC.
25 Bradley Dr., Westbrook, ME 04092
FDA Number: 1221020

207-854-0860

Colorimeter, General Use	Chemistry

ARTHREX CALIFORNIA, INC.
20509 Earlgate St., Walnut, CA 91789
FDA Number: 2028919
Web site: www.arthrex.com
Ownership: Private
Produces/Sells CE-marked Devices: N

800-933-7001
239-643-5553
Fax: 800-643-9310

Forceps	Orthopedics
Orthopedic Manual Surgical Instrument	Orthopedics
Passer	Orthopedics
Probe	Orthopedics
Punch, Surgical	Surgery
Scissors, Orthopedic	Orthopedics

ARTHREX MANUFACTURING
1958 Trade Center Way, Naples, FL 34109
FDA Number: 3006448784
Ownership: Private
Produces/Sells CE-marked Devices: N

239-643-5553

Accessories, Arthroscopic	Orthopedics
Accessories, Operating Room, Table	Surgery
Bit, Drill	Orthopedics
Blade, Surgical, Saw, General & Plastic Surgery	Surgery
Bolt, Nut, Washer	Orthopedics
Burr, Surgical, General & Plastic Surgery	Surgery
Electrosurgical Unit, Cutting & Coagulation Device	Surgery
Fastener, Fixation, Non-Biodegradable, Soft Tissue	Orthopedics
Instrument, Manual, General Surgical	Surgery
Orthopedic Manual Surgical Instrument	Orthopedics
Pin, Fixation, Smooth	Orthopedics
Screw, Fixation, Bone	Orthopedics
Syringe, Piston	General
Traction Unit, Non-Powered	Orthopedics

ARTHREX, INC.
1370 Creekside Blvd., Naples, FL 34108
FDA Number: 1220246
Web site: www.arthrex.com
Year Founded: 1984
Ownership: Private
Produces/Sells CE-marked Devices: N

800-933-7001
239-643-5553
Fax: 800-643-9310

Accessories, Arthroscopic	Orthopedics
Accessories, Operating Room, Table	Surgery
Applier, Cerclage	Orthopedics
Arthroscope	Orthopedics
Bandage, Adhesive	Surgery

ARTHREX, INC.   800-933-7001 (cont'd)

Bit, Drill	Orthopedics
Blade, Surgical, Saw, General & Plastic Surgery	Surgery
Bolt, Nut, Washer	Orthopedics
Burr, Surgical, General & Plastic Surgery	Surgery
Caliper	Orthopedics
Camera, Cine, Endoscopic (Without Audio)	Surgery
Cerclage, Fixation	Orthopedics
Component, Traction, Non-Invasive	Orthopedics
Cutter, Orthopedic	Orthopedics
Dressing, Burn, Porcine	Surgery
Electrosurgical Unit, Cutting & Coagulation Device	Surgery
Fastener, Fixation, Biodegradable, Soft Tissue	Orthopedics
Fastener, Fixation, Non-Biodegradable, Soft Tissue	Orthopedics
Filler, Calcium Sulfate Preformed Pellets	Orthopedics
Finger Cot	General
Gauge, Depth	Orthopedics
Guide, Drill, Ligament	Orthopedics
Instrument, Manual, General Surgical	Surgery
Instrument, Surgical, Powered, Pneumatic	Orthopedics
Light, Surgical, Fiberoptic	Surgery
Lubricant, Patient	General
Motor, Surgical Instrument, AC-Powered	Surgery
Orthopedic Manual Surgical Instrument	Orthopedics
Pin, Fixation, Smooth	Orthopedics
Plate, Fixation, Bone	Orthopedics
Prosthesis, Shoulder, Hemi-, Humeral	Orthopedics
Prosthesis, Shoulder, Semi-Constrained, Metal/Polymer Cem.	Orthopedics
Prosthesis, Toe, Hemi-, Phalangeal	Orthopedics
Protractor	General
Pump, Infusion	Orthopedics
Reamer	Orthopedics
Retention Device, Suture	Surgery
Saw, Powered, And Accessories	Cns/Neurology
Screw, Fixation, Bone	Orthopedics
Staple, Absorbable	Orthopedics
Staple, Fixation, Bone	Orthopedics
Surgical Instrument, Orthopedic, AC-Powered Motor	Orthopedics
Surgical Instrument, Orthopedic, Battery-Powered	Surgery
Suture, Non-Absorbable, Silk	Surgery
Suture, Non-Absorbable, Synthetic, Polyester	Surgery
Suture, Non-Absorbable, Synthetic, Polyethylene	Surgery
Syringe, Piston	General
Traction Unit, Non-Powered	Orthopedics
Tray, Surgical Instrument	Surgery

ARTHRO KINETICS INC.   49-711-30511070
8 Faneuil Hall, 3rd Floor, Boston, MA 02109
FDA Number: 3005953245
Ownership: Private
Produces/Sells CE-marked Devices: N

Arthroscope	Orthopedics

ARTHROCARE CORP.   800-797-6520   408-736-0224
680 Vaqueros Avenue, Sunnyvale, CA 94085
FDA Number: 2951580   *Fax:* 888-994-2782
E-mail: info@arthocare.com
Web site: www.arthrocare.com
Medical Products Sales Volume: $520,000
Year Founded: 1993
Total Employees: 16
Ownership: Arthrocare Corp.
Stock Symbol: ARTC
Traded On: NASDAQ
Quality System Registration Information: ISO9001
Produces/Sells CE-marked Devices: Y
Federal Procurement Eligibility: Small Business
Distribution: Manufacturer Direct, Manufacturer Through Distributor, Manufacturer Through Manufacturer Reps
General Admin.: Michael Baker/President, Chief Executive Officer
Mktg./Adv.: Ross Beam/Vice President Sales
Production: Richard Christensen/Senior Vice President Operations
Finance: Michael Gluk/Senior Vice President Finance

Balloon, Epistaxis (Nasal)	Ear/Nose/Throat
Guide, Surgical, Instrument	Surgery
Needle, Suture, Disposable	Surgery
Retractor	Orthopedics
Splint, Septal, Intranasal	Ear/Nose/Throat
Suture, Non-Absorbable, Synthetic, Polyamide	Surgery
Tray, Surgical Instrument	Surgery

ARTHROCARE CORP.   800-797-6520   512-391-3900
7000 W. William Cannon Drive, Building 1, Austin, TX 78735
FDA Number: 2951580   *Fax:* 512-391-3901
E-mail: info@arthocare.com
Web site: www.arthrocare.com
Year Founded: 1993
Total Employees: 881

ARTHROCARE CORP.   800-797-6520 (cont'd)
Ownership: Private
Stock Symbol: ARTC
Traded On: NASDAQ
Produces/Sells CE-marked Devices: N
General Admin.: Mr. Todd Newton/Chief Financial Officer, Senior Vice President
    Dr. Jean Wolozsko/Chief Technology Officer, Senior Vice President
    Mr. David Fitzgerald/President, Chief Executive Officer
Mktg./Adv.: Mr. Ron Underwood/Vice President Corporate Development
    Mr. Ross Beam/Vice President Marketing & Sales
Production: Mr. Richard Christensen/Senior Vice President Operations
    Mr. Bruce Prothro/Vice President Quality Assurance & Regulatory Affairs

Applier, Surgical, Clip	Surgery
Balloon, Epistaxis (Nasal)	Ear/Nose/Throat
Bit, Drill	Orthopedics
Brace, Joint, Ankle (External)	Physical Med
Cannula, Surgical, General & Plastic Surgery	Surgery
Dispenser, Medication, Liquid	General
Drape, Adhesive, Aerosol	Surgery
Electrosurgical Unit, Cutting & Coagulation Device	Surgery
Fastener, Fixation, Non-Biodegradable, Soft Tissue	Orthopedics
Guide, Surgical, Instrument	Surgery
Instrument, Bending (Contouring)	Orthopedics
Instrument, Manual, General Surgical	Surgery
Kit, Surgical Instrument, Disposable	Surgery
Needle, Suture, Disposable	Surgery
Orthopedic Manual Surgical Instrument	Orthopedics
Osteotome, Manual (Plastic Surgery)	Surgery
Passer	Orthopedics
Retractor	Orthopedics
Screw, Fixation, Bone	Orthopedics
Splint, Septal, Intranasal	Ear/Nose/Throat
Suture, Non-Absorbable, Synthetic, Polyamide	Surgery
Tray, Surgical Instrument	Surgery

Medical Product Subsidiaries (Listed Separately)
Arthrocare Corp.

ARTHRON, INC.   800-758-5633   615-377-6595
1605 Ash Grove Ct., PO Box 1627, Brentwood, TN 37024
FDA Number: 1057427   *Fax:* 615-371-5405
E-mail: arthron@comcast.net
Web site: www.sportsinjuries.com
Medical Products Sales Volume: $100,000
Year Founded: 1992
Total Employees: 1
Ownership: Private
Produces/Sells CE-marked Devices: N
Federal Procurement Eligibility: Small Business
Distribution: Manufacturer Direct, Importer

Orthosis, Limb Brace	Physical Med
Sling, Arm	Physical Med

ARTHRONET MEDICAL, INC.   949-254-3343
520 Broadway, Ste. 350, Santa Monica, CA 90401
FDA Number: n/a
Web site: www.arthronet.com
Medical Products Sales Volume: $500,500
Annual Revenue: $0-$1 Million
Year Founded: 1999
Total Employees: 2   *Marketing Staff:* 1   *Sales Staff:* 1
Ownership: Private
Quality System Registration Information: ISO9001
Produces/Sells CE-marked Devices: Y
Federal Procurement Eligibility: Small Business
Distribution: Manufacturer Direct, OEM, Exclusive Distributor
General Admin.: Carolina Schaber/President

Arthroscope	Orthopedics
Instrument, Bending (Contouring)	Orthopedics

ARTHROPLASTICS, INC.   440-247-5131
34 West Washington St., P.o. Box 332, Chagrin Falls, OH 44022
FDA Number: 1528129
Ownership: Private
Produces/Sells CE-marked Devices: N

Arthroscope	Orthopedics

ARTHROSURFACE, INC.   508-520-3003
28 Forge Parkway, Franklin, MA 02038
FDA Number: 3004154314   *Fax:* 508-528-4604
E-mail: info@arthrosurface.com
Web site: http://arthrosurface.com
Ownership: Private
Produces/Sells CE-marked Devices: N
General Admin.: Mr. Steven Ek/Chief Operating Officer
    Mr. Steven Tallarida/President
Mktg./Adv.: Mr. Lester Fehr/Vice President Marketing & Sales

MANUFACTURER PROFILES

ARTHROSURFACE, INC. 508-520-3003 *(cont'd)*
Production: Ms. Dawn Wilson/Vice President Quality Assurance & Regulatory Affairs
  Finance: Mr. Chris Laplante/Director Finance
    Mr. Anthony Moretti/Vice President Admin., Finance

Orthopedic Manual Surgical Instrument	Orthopedics
Prosthesis, Hip, Femoral, Resurfacing	Orthopedics
Prosthesis, Knee, Patellofemoral, Semi-Constrained	Orthopedics
Prosthesis, Shoulder, Hemi-, Humeral	Orthopedics
Prosthesis, Toe, Hemi-, Phalangeal	Orthopedics

ARTHROWAVE MEDICAL TECHNOLOGIES, LLC 410-472-0360
53 Loveton Circle, Suite 207, Glencoe, MD 21152
FDA Number: 3003920777
Ownership: Private
Produces/Sells CE-marked Devices: N

Stimulator, Nerve, Transcutaneous (Pain Relief, TENS)	Cns/Neurology

ARTHUR FINNIESTON CLINIC 305-817-1604
2480 W. 82 Street #8, Hialeah, FL 33016
FDA Number: n/a   *Fax:* 305-823-8304
Annual Revenue: $0-$1 Million
Year Founded: 1928
Total Employees: 7
Ownership: Private
Produces/Sells CE-marked Devices: N
Federal Procurement Eligibility: Small Business
Distribution: Manufacturer Direct
General Admin.: Geri Kish/Administrator
    Mr. Alan Finnieston/President, Owner

Orthosis, Limb Brace	Physical Med
Prosthesis, Arm	Orthopedics

ARTHUR BLANK & CO., INC. 800-776-7333
225 Rivermoor St., Boston, MA 02132-4920 617-325-9600
FDA Number: n/a   *Fax:* 617-327-1235
E-mail: abco@abco.com
Web site: www.arthurblank.com
Medical Products Sales Volume: $32,400,000
Annual Revenue: $25-$50 Million
Year Founded: 1934
Total Employees: 210   *Marketing Staff:* 3   *Sales Staff:* 8
Ownership: Private
Produces/Sells CE-marked Devices: N
Federal Procurement Eligibility: Small Business
Distribution: Manufacturer Through Distributor
General Admin.: Stuart Blank/President, Chief Executive Officer
Mktg./Adv.: Mr. Eric Domschine/Market Manager
Production: Joe Mandile/Manager Materials

Card, Identification	General
Sign, Hospital	General

ARTICULOS HIGIENICOS S.A. DE C.V. 52 55 58997980
Av. TransformaciA3n #4, Parque Ind. Cuamatla, Cuautitlan Izcalli, EDO D 54730 Mexico
FDA Number: 9681529   *Fax:* 52 55 58703272
E-mail: export@arthig.com.mx
Web site: www.articuloshigienicos.com
Year Founded: 1982
Total Employees: 355   *Marketing Staff:* 3   *Sales Staff:* 39
Ownership: Private
Quality System Registration Information: ISO9001
Produces/Sells CE-marked Devices: Y
Distribution: Manufacturer Direct, Manufacturer Through Distributor

ARTIFICIAL KIDNEY SERVICE
See G.E.M. Water Systems, Int'L., Llc

ARTISAN DENTAL LABORATORY 800-222-6721
2532 S.E. Hawthorne Blvd., Portland, OR 97214 503-238-6006
FDA Number: n/a   *Fax:* 503-231-3684
E-mail: info@artisandental.com
Web site: www.artisandental.com
Ownership: Private
Produces/Sells CE-marked Devices: N
Federal Procurement Eligibility: Small Business
Distribution: Manufacturer Direct, Service Direct
General Admin.: Karl Koch/Owner, Chairman
    Justan Koch/President
Mktg./Adv.: Jeff Scarvie/Director Sales

Crown And Bridge, Temporary, Resin	Dental And Oral
Crown, Preformed	Dental And Oral
Denture, Preformed	Dental And Oral

ARTISAN-DAHLIN DENTAL LABORATORIES
See Artisan Dental Laboratory

ARTISTIC DENTAL LAB, INCORPORATED 757-224-0177
1500 Crescent Drive, Suite 204, Carrollton, TX 75006
FDA Number: 3006226458

ARTISTIC DENTAL LAB, INCORPORATED 757-224-0177 *(cont'd)*
  Crown, Preformed   Dental And Oral

ARTROMICK 800-848-6462
4800 Hilton Corporate Dr., Columbus, OH 43232 614-864-9966
FDA Number: n/a   *Fax:* 614-864-9937
E-mail: info@capsasolutions.com
Medical Products Sales Volume: $6,000,000
Total Employees: 45   *Marketing Staff:* 5   *Sales Staff:* 7
Ownership: Private
Produces/Sells CE-marked Devices: N
Federal Procurement Eligibility: Small Business
Distribution: Manufacturer Direct, Manufacturer Through Distributor, Manufacturer Through Manufacturer Reps
General Admin.: William E. Heimann/President, Chief Executive Officer
Mktg./Adv.: Patrick R. Stewart/Director National Accounts
    Perry W. Larson/Director National Accounts
    Chuck Land/Vice President Sales
Production: John E. Johnson/Vice President Manufacturing

Cart, Medicine	General
System, Delivery, Drug, Unit-Dose	General

ARTROMICK INTERNATIONAL, INC. 800-848-6462
4800 Hilton Corporate Drive, 614-864-9966
Columbus, OH 43232
FDA Number: 9310008   *Fax:* 614-864-9937
E-mail: info@artromick.com
Web site: www.artromick.com
Annual Revenue: $25-$50 Million
Year Founded: 1972
Total Employees: 150   *Marketing Staff:* 4   *Sales Staff:* 18
Ownership: Private
Produces/Sells CE-marked Devices: Y
Federal Procurement Eligibility: Small Business, GSA Contract, VA Contract
Distribution: Manufacturer Direct, Exporter
General Admin.: Paul Guth/President, Chief Operating Officer
Mktg./Adv.: Dan Jones/Director International Sales
    Todd Ross/Director Marketing
    Tom Burns/Vice President Sales

Cart, Medicine	General
Cart, Other	General
System, Delivery, Drug, Unit-Dose	General

ARTROMICK MEDICART, LLC
See Artromick International, Inc.

ARTRONICS 864-859-4755
464 Sweetbriar Way, Easley, SC 29640
FDA Number: n/a
Ownership: Private
Produces/Sells CE-marked Devices: N

Monitor, Temperature, Neurosurgery, Direct Contact, Powered	Cns/Neurology

ARTVENTIVE MEDICAL GROUP INC. 760-471-7700
1797 Playa Vista, San Marcos, CA 92078
FDA Number: n/a   *Fax:* 650-240-1706
Web site: http://www.artventivemedical.com
Ownership: Private
Produces/Sells CE-marked Devices: N
General Admin.: Dr. Leon Rudakov/Chief Executive Officer
    Mr. Jim Graham/President, Chairman

ARW OPTICAL CORP. 910-452-7373
6631 B. Amsterdam Way, Wilmington, NC 28405
FDA Number: n/a   *Fax:* 910-452-6326
E-mail: sales@arwoptical.com
Web site: www.arwoptical.com
Medical Products Sales Volume: $500,000
Annual Revenue: $0-$1 Million
Year Founded: 1980
Total Employees: 10
Ownership: Private
Produces/Sells CE-marked Devices: N
Federal Procurement Eligibility: Small Business
Distribution: Manufacturer Direct
General Admin.: Gunter Wolff/President
    Roger Wolff/Vice President, General Manager

Lens, Other	Ophthalmology
Prism, Endoscopic	Surgery

ARZCO MEDICAL SYSTEMS, INC.
See Cardio Command, Inc.

ARZOL CHEMICAL CO. 603-352-5242
12 Norway Ave., Ste. 2, Keene, NH 03431
FDA Number: n/a   *Fax:* 603-352-1528
Web site: http://www.arzol.com
Medical Products Sales Volume: $225,000
Annual Revenue: $0-$1 Million

ARZOL CHEMICAL CO.　603-352-5242 (cont'd)
Total Employees: 3
Ownership: Private
Produces/Sells CE-marked Devices: N
Federal Procurement Eligibility: Small Business
Distribution: Manufacturer Direct, Manufacturer Through Distributor
General Admin.: William Hollister/President
Applicator, Other .... General

AS SOFTWARE, INC.　800-613-4441
560 Sylvan Ave., Englewood Cliffs, NJ 07632　201-541-1900
FDA Number: 3005207094　*Fax:* 201-541-1199
E-mail: info@as-software.com
Web site: www.as-software.com
Ownership: Private
Produces/Sells CE-marked Devices: N
Image Processing System .... Radiology

ASANTE SOLUTIONS INC.　408-716-5600
1012 Stewart Drive, Sunnyvale, CA 94085
FDA Number: n/a
Web site: http://www.asantesolutions.com
Year Founded: 2007
Ownership: Private
Produces/Sells CE-marked Devices: N
General Admin.: Mr. Phil Hopper/President, Chief Executive Officer
Mktg./Adv.: Mr. Mark Estes/Director Marketing
Production: Mr. Ian Felix/Vice President Operations
　Ms. Naghmeh Nouri/Vice President Quality Assurance & Regulatory Affairs
Research: Dr. Wenkang Qi/Vice President Research & Development

ASCENSION ORTHOPEDICS, INC.　877-370-5001
8700 Cameron Road, Austin, TX 78754　512-836-5001
FDA Number: 1651501　*Fax:* 512-836-6933
E-mail: customerservice@ascensionortho.com
Web site: http://www.ascensionortho.com
Year Founded: 1996
Ownership: Private
Produces/Sells CE-marked Devices: N
General Admin.: Mr. Jerry Klawitter/Chief Scientific Officer
　Mr. Guy Mayer/President, Chief Executive Officer
　Mr. Cliff Seliga/Senior Vice President International Marketing Operations
Mktg./Adv.: Mr. Bill Warrender/Senior Vice President Sales
Research: Mr. Clive Scott/Senior Vice President Research & Development
Finance: Mr. Bob Johnston/Chief Financial Officer
Prosthesis, Elbow, Hemi-, Radial, Polymer .... Orthopedics
Prosthesis, Finger, Constrained, Polymer .... Orthopedics
Prosthesis, Shoulder, Hemi-, Humeral .... Orthopedics
Prosthesis, Toe, Hemi-, Phalangeal .... Orthopedics
Prosthesis, Wrist, Carpal Trapezium .... Orthopedics
Screw, Fixation, Bone .... Orthopedics

ASCENT HEALTHCARE SOLUTIONS　480-763-5300
10232 South 51st St., Phoenix, AZ 85044
FDA Number: 2090040
Ownership: Private
Produces/Sells CE-marked Devices: N
Accessories, Arthroscopic .... Orthopedics
Arthroscope .... Orthopedics
Bit, Drill .... Orthopedics
Blade, Saw, Surgical, Cardiovascular .... Cardiovascular
Blade, Surgical, Saw, General & Plastic Surgery ... Surgery
Bur, Diamond Coated, Reprocessed .... Dental And Oral
Bur, Ent, Diamond Coated, Single Use, Reprocessed ... Ear/Nose/Throat
Burr, Orthopedic .... Orthopedics
Burr, Surgical, General & Plastic Surgery .... Surgery
Catheter, Mapping, Intracardiac, Reprocessed ..... Cardiovascular
Catheter, Percutaneous .... Cardiovascular
Catheter, Recording, Electrode, Reprocessed ...... Cardiovascular
Catheter, Steerable, Reprocessed .... Cardiovascular
Chisel (Osteotome) .... Surgery
Component, Traction, Invasive .... Orthopedics
Countersink .... Orthopedics
Cuff, Blood Pressure .... Cardiovascular
Curette, Surgical .... Surgery
Device, Stabilizer, Heart .... Cardiovascular
Drills, Burrs, Trephines And Accessories (manual), Reprocessed ... Cns/Neurology
Electrosurgical Unit, Cutting & Coagulation Device ... Surgery
Fixation Appliance, Multiple Component .... Orthopedics
Fixation Appliance, Single Component .... Orthopedics
General Use Surgical Scissors .... Surgery
Gouge, Surgical, General & Plastic Surgery .... Surgery
Hook, Surgical, General & Plastic Surgery .... Surgery
Instrument, Diamond, Dental, Reprocessed .... Dental And Oral
Knife, Orthopedic .... Orthopedics
Laparoscope, General & Plastic Surgery, Reprocessed ... Gastroenterology/Urology
Microdebrider, Ent, High Speed, Single Use, Reprocessed ... Ear/Nose/Throat

ASCENT HEALTHCARE SOLUTIONS　480-763-5300 (cont'd)
Needle, Phacoemulsification, Reprocessed .... Ophthalmology
Orthopedic Manual Surgical Instrument .... Orthopedics
Rasp, Surgical, General & Plastic Surgery .... Surgery
Reamer .... Orthopedics
Rongeur, Rib .... Orthopedics
Saw, Powered, And Accessories .... Cns/Neurology
Sleeve, Compressible Limb .... Cardiovascular
Surgical Instrument, Cardiovascular .... Cardiovascular
Surgical Instrument, Disposable .... Surgery
System, Catheter Control, Reprocessed .... Cardiovascular
Tap, Bone .... Orthopedics
Tourniquet, Pneumatic .... Surgery
Trephine, Bone .... Orthopedics

ASCON MEDICAL INSTRUMENTS
See American Surgical Instrument Corp.

ASD
See Analytical Spectral Devices, Inc.

ASEPTICO, INC.　866-244-2954
8333 216th St. SE, Woodinville, WA 98072　425-487-3157
FDA Number: 3017604
Web site: www.aseptico.com
Medical Products Sales Volume: $5,000,000
Annual Revenue: $5-$10 Million
Year Founded: 1975
Ownership: Private
Quality System Registration Information: ISO9001
Produces/Sells CE-marked Devices: Y
Federal Procurement Eligibility: Small Business
Distribution: Manufacturer Direct, OEM
Chair, Dental .... Dental And Oral
Dam, Rubber .... Dental And Oral
Drill, Oral Surgery .... Dental And Oral
Eyeglasses, Safety .... Ophthalmology
Gutta Percha .... Dental And Oral
Handpiece, Direct Drive, AC-Powered .... Dental And Oral
Light, Surgical Headlight .... Dental And Oral
Light, Surgical, Floor Standing .... Surgery
Locator, Apex, Root .... Dental And Oral
Mask, Face .... General
Operative Dental Treatment Unit .... Dental And Oral
Scaler, Ultrasonic .... Dental And Oral

ASH ACCESS TECHNOLOGY INC.　765-742-4813
INOK Business Center, 3601 Sagamore Pwy. N., Suite B, Lafayette, IN 47904
FDA Number: 1831663　*Fax:* 765-742-4823
E-mail: web06@ashaccess.com
Web site: www.ashaccess.com
Year Founded: 2003
Ownership: Private
Produces/Sells CE-marked Devices: N
General Admin.: Robert Truitt/President, Chief Executive Officer
Mktg./Adv.: Daniel Olson/Director Marketing & Business Development
　Carmine Durham/Vice President Corporate Development
Production: Ken Brown/Director Manufacturing & Engineering
　Alvaro Guillem/Vice President Quality Assurance
Research: Stephen Ash/Director Research & Development
　Roland Winger/Vice President Clinical Development
Finance: Nels Bergmark/Treasurer
Catheter, Hemodialysis, Implanted .... Gastroenterology/Urology

ASHAWAY LINE & TWINE MANUFACTURING CO.　800-556-7260
24 Laurel St., P.O. Box 549, Ashaway, RI 02804　401-377-2221
FDA Number: 1210802　*Fax:* 401-377-9091
E-mail: sales@ashawayusa.com
Web site: www.ashawayusa.com
Medical Products Sales Volume: $3,200,000
Year Founded: 1824
Ownership: Private
Produces/Sells CE-marked Devices: N
Federal Procurement Eligibility: Small Business, Female Owned
Distribution: Manufacturer Direct
Suture, Laparoscopy .... Surgery
Suture, Non-Absorbable .... Surgery
Suture, Non-Absorbable, Silk .... Surgery
Suture, Non-Absorbable, Synthetic, Polyamide .... Surgery
Suture, Non-Absorbable, Synthetic, Polyester ..... Surgery

ASHEBORO ELASTICS CORP.　336-629-2626
150 North Park Street, PO Box 1143, Asheboro, NC 27203
FDA Number: n/a　*Fax:* 336-629-3782
Web site: www.asheboroelastics.com
Medical Products Sales Volume: $320,000,000
Ownership: Private
Produces/Sells CE-marked Devices: N

ASHEBORO ELASTICS CORP.
336-629-2626 *(cont'd)*
Distribution: Manufacturer Direct, Manufacturer Through Manufacturer Reps, OEM, Service Direct, Exporter
General Admin.: Jane Crisco/Chairman
  Jeff Crisco/Vice President
  John Crisco/Vice President
  Rick Grier/Vice President
  Bandage, Elastic .... General

ASHLAR HOLDINGS, LLC
573-785-8766
1908 Greenwood Drive Suite B, Poplar Bluff, MO 63901
FDA Number: 3006280816
Ownership: Private
Produces/Sells CE-marked Devices: N
  Adapter, Catheter, Ureteral .... Gastroenterology/Urology
  Cystometer, Electrical Recording .... Gastroenterology/Urology

ASHLEY EMERGENCY VEHICLES
See American Emergency Vehicles

ASHTON PUMPMATIC, INC.
800-395-1012
937-297-0741
858 Distribution Drive, Dayton, OH 45434
FDA Number: 1525728   *Fax:* 937-297-0742
E-mail: ashton@ashtongroup.com
Web site: www.ashton-pumpmatic.com
Medical Products Sales Volume: $400,000
Annual Revenue: $0-$1 Million
Year Founded: 1979
Total Employees: 6   *Marketing Staff:* 2   *Sales Staff:* 2
Ownership: Private
Produces/Sells CE-marked Devices: N
Federal Procurement Eligibility: Small Business
Distribution: Manufacturer Through Distributor
General Admin.: Richard E. Kelch/Chief Executive Officer
  John R. Kelch/President
Mktg./Adv.: James Martin/Director Marketing
  Dispenser, Pipette .... Chemistry

ASI INSTRUMENTS, INC.
800-531-1105
586-756-1222
12900 E. Ten Mile Road, Warren, MI 48089
FDA Number: n/a   *Fax:* 586-756-9737
E-mail: sales@asi-instruments.com
Web site: www.asi-instruments.com
Annual Revenue: $0-$1 Million
Total Employees: 7
Ownership: Private
Produces/Sells CE-marked Devices: Y
Federal Procurement Eligibility: Small Business
Distribution: Manufacturer Direct, Manufacturer Through Distributor
General Admin.: Chris Chiodo/President, Chief Executive Officer
  Equipment, Laboratory, Gen. Purpose (Specific Medical Use) ...... Chemistry
  Pipette .... Chemistry
  Pipette, Micro .... Chemistry

ASI MEDICAL EQUIPMENT, LTD.
800-527-0443
972-242-2164
1735 North Interstate 35 East,
Carrollton, TX 75006
FDA Number: n/a   *Fax:* 972-245-0103
E-mail: asimedical@excite.com
Medical Products Sales Volume: $5,000,000
Annual Revenue: $1-$5 Million
Total Employees: 25   *Marketing Staff:* 3   *Sales Staff:* 3
Ownership: Private
Produces/Sells CE-marked Devices: N
Federal Procurement Eligibility: Small Business
Distribution: Manufacturer Direct, Manufacturer Through Distributor, Manufacturer Through Manufacturer Reps, OEM, Importer, Exporter
General Admin.: Byron Hasty/Chairman, Chief Financial Officer
  Byron Hasty/President, Chief Executive Officer
  Dawn Hasty/Vice President Human Resources
  Mike Barta/Vice President, General Manager
Mktg./Adv.: Billy Davis/Director Marketing
  Byron Hasty/Director Product Development
  Byron Hasty/Vice President Marketing & Sales
Production: Mike Barta/Director Quality Assurance
Research: Byron Hasty/Vice President Research & Development
  Bed, Air Fluidized .... Physical Med
  Bed, Electric .... General
  Bed, Hydraulic .... General
  Bed, Manual .... General
  Bed, Scanning, Nuclear/Fluoroscopic .... Radiology
  Cover, Mattress .... General
  Mattress, Air Flotation .... General
  Mattress, Bed .... General
  Scale, Bed .... General
  Table, Radiographic, Tilting .... Radiology
  Transducer, Miniature Pressure .... Physical Med

ASI MEDICAL, INC.
800-566-9953
303-766-3646
14550 East Easter Ave., Suite 700,
Englewood, CO 80112
FDA Number: 1722638   *Fax:* 303-766-8584
E-mail: sales@asimedical.net
Web site: www.asimedical.ne
Ownership: Private
Produces/Sells CE-marked Devices: N
  Airbrush .... Dental And Oral
  Operative Dental Treatment Unit .... Dental And Oral

ASI-MODULEX
800-274-7732
214-352-9140
3860 W. Northwest Hwy., Suite 350,
Dallas, TX 75220
FDA Number: 1648184   *Fax:* 214-352-9741
E-mail: info@asimodulex.com
Web site: www.asimodulex.com
Year Founded: 1965
Total Employees: 25
Ownership: Private
Quality System Registration Information: ISO9001; ISO9003
Produces/Sells CE-marked Devices: N
Federal Procurement Eligibility: Small Business, GSA Contract
Distribution: Manufacturer Direct
Mktg./Adv.: Mr. Peter Wyro/Director Corporate Marketing
  Sign, Hospital .... General

ASICO
See American Surgical Instrument Corp.

ASO CORPORATION
941-379-0300
300 Sarasota Center Blvd., Sarasota, FL 34240
FDA Number: 1038758   *Fax:* 941-378-9040
E-mail: asocorp@asocorp.com
Web site: www.asocorp.com
Total Employees: 250   *Marketing Staff:* 4   *Sales Staff:* 15
Ownership: Private
Quality System Registration Information: ISO9001
Produces/Sells CE-marked Devices: Y
Distribution: Manufacturer Direct, Manufacturer Through Distributor, Manufacturer Through Manufacturer Reps, Service Direct, Exclusive Distributor, Importer, Exporter
General Admin.: John D. Macaskill/President, Chief Executive Officer
Mktg./Adv.: Susan Heck/Director Marketing
  Tami Calleia/Manager Sales Admin.
  John C. Pellegrino/Senior Vice President Marketing & Sales
  Mark Bolling/Vice President Sales
Production: Ron Van Ostenbridge/Vice President Manufacturing
  Joan Rubendall/Vice President Quality Assurance & Regulatory Affairs
Finance: Luis Arce/Vice President Finance, Human Resources
  Bandage, Adhesive .... Surgery
  Bandage, Liquid .... Surgery
  Dressing, Wound, Occlusive .... Surgery
  Gauze Roll .... Surgery
  Sponge, External .... Surgery
  Strip, Adhesive .... Surgery

ASO LLC
941-379-0300
12120 Esther Lama Dr., Suite 112, El Paso, TX 79936
FDA Number: 1648694
  Bandage, Adhesive .... Surgery
  Bandage, Elastic .... General
  Gauze/sponge, Nonresorbable For External Use .... Surgery
  Sponge, External .... Surgery
  Sponge, Gauze .... Dental And Oral
  Strip, Adhesive .... Surgery

ASPECT MEDICAL SYSTEMS, INC.
617-559-7000
1 Upland Road, Norwood, MA 02062
FDA Number: 1221611   *Fax:* 617-559-7400
E-mail: bis_info@aspectms.com
Web site: www.aspectmedical.com
Year Founded: 1987
Ownership: Public
Stock Symbol: ASPM
Traded On: NASDAQ
Produces/Sells CE-marked Devices: Y
General Admin.: Nassib Chamoun/Chief Executive Officer, Chairman
  Medical Admin.: Scott Kelley/Vice President Medical Affairs
Mktg./Adv.: William Floyd/Executive Vice President International Marketing & Sales
Production: John Coolidge/Vice President Manufacturing & Operations
  Paul Manberg/Vice President Quality Assurance & Regulatory Affairs
Research: Marc Davidson/Vice President Engineering
  Electroencephalograph .... Cns/Neurology

ASPECT MEDICAL SYSTEMS, INC.
617-559-7000
141 Needham St., Newton, MA 02464
FDA Number: n/a   *Fax:* 617-559-7400
E-mail: bis_info@aspectms.com

ASPECT MEDICAL SYSTEMS, INC.   617-559-7000 (cont'd)
Web site: www.aspectms.com
Year Founded: 1987
Total Employees: 288
Ownership: Public
Stock Symbol: ASPM
Traded On: NASDAQ
Quality System Registration Information: ISO9001
Produces/Sells CE-marked Devices: Y
Distribution: Manufacturer Direct
General Admin.: Nassib Chamoun/Chief Executive Officer
Mktg./Adv.: Jean Nelson/Vice President Marketing
   Steve Kane/Vice President Sales
Research: Paul Manberg/Vice President Clinical Research
   Phil Devlin/Vice President Research & Development
Finance: Neal Armstrong/Vice President Finance

Analyzer, Gas, Anesthetic	Anesthesiology
Electrode, Other	General
Electroencephalograph	Cns/Neurology
Monitor, ECG, Anesthesia	Anesthesiology
Monitor, EEG	Cns/Neurology

ASPEN HOME HEALTHCARE PRODUCTS LTD.   800-272-8851
11044 82nd Ave., Suite 120,   **780-439-6367**
Edmonton, ALB T6G-0 Canada
FDA Number: n/a   *Fax:* 780-439-5846
E-mail: lmadsen@planet.eon.net
Web site: www.aspen-health.com
Year Founded: 1986
Total Employees: 25
Ownership: DANACO VENTURES LTD.
Produces/Sells CE-marked Devices: N

ASPEN LABORATORIES INC.
See Conmed Corporation

ASPEN MEDICAL PRODUCTS   800-295-2776
6481 Oak Canyon, Irvine, CA 92618   **949-681-0200**
FDA Number: 2030775   *Fax:* 949-681-0300
E-mail: service@aspenmp.com
Web site: www.aspenmp.com
Ownership: Private
Produces/Sells CE-marked Devices: N

Orthosis, Cervical	Physical Med
Orthosis, Lumbar	Physical Med
Orthosis, Thoracic	Physical Med
Protector, Skin Pressure	General

ASPEN SEATING, LLC   866-781-1633
4211 S. Natches Ct., Suite G,   **303-781-1633**
Sheridan, CO 80110
FDA Number: 3004518501   *Fax:* 303-781-1722
Web site: www.ridedesigns.com
Ownership: Private
Produces/Sells CE-marked Devices: N

Cushion, Wheelchair (Pad)	Physical Med

ASPEN SURGICAL   800-328-7958
6945 South Belt Drive SE, Caledonia, MI 49316   **888-364-7004**
FDA Number: 1836161   *Fax:* 888-364-5381
E-mail: customerservice@aspensurgical.com
Web site: www.aspensurgical.com
Annual Revenue: $10-$25 Million
Year Founded: 1978
Total Employees: 3   *Marketing Staff:* 2   *Sales Staff:* 24
Ownership: Private
Stock Symbol: STEN
Traded On: NASDAQ
Quality System Registration Information: ISO9002
Produces/Sells CE-marked Devices: Y
Federal Procurement Eligibility: Small Business, GSA Contract, VA Contract
Distribution: Manufacturer Direct, Manufacturer Through Distributor, Exporter
General Admin.: Bill Corrigan/Manager Plant
   Ken brimmer/President
Mktg./Adv.: Bill Maass/Executive Vice President Marketing
   Jess Carsello/Executive Vice President Sales
   Robbin Metz/Manager Advertising
   Kevin Dey/Manager International & National Sales
Production: Jim Lannan/Director Quality Assurance
   James Lannan/Manager Regulatory Affairs
Finance: Mark Buckrey/Chief Financial Officer

Drain, Suction, Closed	Surgery
Kit, Wound Drainage	General
Kit, Wound Drainage, Closed	Cns/Neurology
Suction Apparatus, Single Patient, Portable, Non-Powered	Surgery
Suction Apparatus, Ward Use, Portable, AC-Powered	Surgery

ASPEN SURGICAL PUERTO RICO CORP.   201-847-4298
Rd. 183, Km. 20.3, Las Piedras, PR 00771
FDA Number: 2649798
Ownership: Private
Produces/Sells CE-marked Devices: N

Blade, Scalpel	Surgery
Handle, Scalpel	Surgery
Lancet, Blood	General
Scalpel, One-Piece (Knife)	Surgery
Surgical Instrument, Disposable	Surgery

ASPIRE BIOTECH, INC.   719-522-9800
4755 Forge Road Suite 120,, Colorado Springs, CO 80907
FDA Number: 3003994148   *Fax:* 719-522-9805
Ownership: Private
Produces/Sells CE-marked Devices: N

Protectant, Skin	Surgery

ASPYRA, INC.   800-437-9000
26115-A Mureau Road, Calabasas, CA 91302   **818-880-6700**
FDA Number: 2085063   *Fax:* 818-880-4398
E-mail: coinfo@aspyra.com
Web site: www.aspyra.com
Medical Products Sales Volume: $12,700,000
Year Founded: 1978
Total Employees: 101   *Marketing Staff:* 3   *Sales Staff:* 5
Ownership: Public
Stock Symbol: APY
Traded On: AMEX
Produces/Sells CE-marked Devices: N
Federal Procurement Eligibility: Small Business
Distribution: Manufacturer Direct
General Admin.: Rodney W. Schutt/Chief Executive Officer
   Ademola Lawal/Chief Operating Officer
Mktg./Adv.: Robert Pruter/Senior Vice President Marketing & Sales
   James R. Helms/Vice President Strategic Development
Finance: Anahita Villafane/Chief Financial Officer

Computer Software	General

Medical Product Subsidiaries (Listed Separately)
 Aspyra, Inc.

ASPYRA, INC.   904-854-2107
8649 Baypine Rd., Jacksonville, FL 32256
FDA Number: 1063008
Ownership: Aspyra, Inc.

Device, Storage, Image, Digital	Radiology
Image Processing System	Radiology

ASSAY TECHNOLOGY INC   800-833-1258
1252 Quarry Lane, Pleasanton, CA 94566-4756   **925-461-8880**
FDA Number: n/a   *Fax:* 925-461-7149
E-mail: askassy@assaytech.com
Web site: www.assaytech.com
Medical Products Sales Volume: $2,500,000
Annual Revenue: $1-$5 Million
Year Founded: 1980
Total Employees: 28   *Marketing Staff:* 1   *Sales Staff:* 3
Ownership: Private
Produces/Sells CE-marked Devices: N
Federal Procurement Eligibility: Small Business
Distribution: Manufacturer Direct, Manufacturer Through Distributor
General Admin.: Charles Manning/President, Chief Executive Officer
Mktg./Adv.: Rena Kirkpatrick/Director Marketing & Sales

Dosimeter, Ethylene-Oxide	General
Dosimeter, Nitrous-Oxide	Anesthesiology
Monitor, Contamination, Environmental, Personal	General
Sampler, Air	General

ASSISTANCE PRODUCTS LP   972-240-4279
3710 S. Country Club Rd., Garland, TX 75043
FDA Number: 3004365000
Ownership: Private
Produces/Sells CE-marked Devices: N

Accessories, Wheelchair	Physical Med

ASSISTED ACCESS-NFSS, INC.   800-950-9655
822 PRESTON COURT,   **847-265-8022**
LAKE VILLA, IL 60046
FDA Number: n/a   *Fax:* 847-265-8044
E-mail: assistedaccess-nfss@comcast.net
Web site: www.nfss.com
Medical Products Sales Volume: $100,000
Annual Revenue: $0-$1 Million
Total Employees: 2   *Marketing Staff:* 2   *Sales Staff:* 2
Ownership: Private
Produces/Sells CE-marked Devices: N
Federal Procurement Eligibility: Small Business, Female Owned
Distribution: Exclusive Distributor

ASSISTED ACCESS-NFSS, INC.   800-950-9655 *(cont'd)*
General Admin.: Diana Tischler/President, Owner
Michael J Tischler/Vice President

Adaptor, Dressing	Physical Med
Cane	Physical Med
Cane, Safety Walk	Physical Med
Communication System, Powered	Physical Med
Reading System, Closed-Circuit Television	Ophthalmology
Security Equipment/Supplies	General
Service, Maintenance/Repair	General
Stretcher, Orthopedic	Orthopedics
Telephone Equipment	General
Telephone, Handicapped Use	Physical Med
Tips And Pads, Cane, Crutch And Walker	Physical Med
Utensil, Handicapped Aid	Physical Med

ASSISTIVE LISTENING DEVICE SYSTEMS   800-665-2537
11220 Voyager Way, Unit 2,   604-244-0269
Richmond, BC V6X-3 Canada
FDA Number: n/a   *Fax:* 604-270-6308
E-mail: info@alds.com
Web site: www.alds.com
Year Founded: 1991
Total Employees: 10
Ownership: Private
Produces/Sells CE-marked Devices: N
Distribution: Manufacturer Direct, Service Direct, Exclusive Distributor, Exporter

ASSISTIVE TECHNOLOGY, INC.   800-793-9227
333 Elm Street, Suite 115, Dedham, MA 02026   781-461-8200
FDA Number: 2032609   *Fax:* 781-461-8213
E-mail: customercare@assistivetech.com
Web site: www.assistivetech.com
Medical Products Sales Volume: $4,700,000
Year Founded: 1999
Total Employees: 48
Ownership: Private
Produces/Sells CE-marked Devices: Y
Federal Procurement Eligibility: Small Business
General Admin.: Mr. James Lewis/President, Chief Executive Officer
Mktg./Adv.: Mr. John Standal/Director Sales

Aid, Control, Environmental, Controlled, Breath	Physical Med
Communication Equipment	General
Telephone, Handicapped Use	Physical Med

ASSOCIATED BAG COMPANY   800-926-6100
400 W. Boden St., Milwaukee, WI 53207
FDA Number: n/a
E-mail: customerservice@associatedbag.com
Web site: www.associatedbag.com
Year Founded: 1938
Ownership: Private
Produces/Sells CE-marked Devices: N
Federal Procurement Eligibility: Small Business
Distribution: Exclusive Distributor
General Admin.: Herb Rubenstein/President

Bag, Garbage	General
Bag, Laundry, Infection Control	General
Bag, Laundry, Operating Room	General
Bag, Plastic	General
Cover, Head, Surgical	Surgery
Foodservice Product/Equipment	General
Glove, Other	General
Glove, Surgical, Powder-Free	Surgery
Gown, Other	General
Holder, Medical Chart	General
Kit, Admission (Patient Utensil)	General
Liner, Kick Bucket	General
Sealer, Packaging	General
Towel/Towelette, Paper	General
Waste Disposal Unit, Sharps	General

ASSOCIATED CONTACTS, INC.   941-921-1200
2036 Bispham Rd., Sarasota, FL 34231
FDA Number: 1045055
Ownership: Private
Produces/Sells CE-marked Devices: N

Lens, Contact, Polymethylmethacrylate	Ophthalmology

ASSOCIATED DESIGN AND MANUFACTURING CO.   800-837-8257
8245-K Backlick Road, Lorton, VA 22079   571-642-0222
FDA Number: 9001589   *Fax:* 571-642-0213
E-mail: sales@associateddesign.com
Web site: www.associateddesign.com
Medical Products Sales Volume: $900,000
Annual Revenue: $0-$1 Million
Year Founded: 1965

ASSOCIATED DESIGN AND   800-837-8257 *(cont'd)*
Total Employees: 14   *Marketing Staff:* 2   *Sales Staff:* 2
Ownership: Private
Produces/Sells CE-marked Devices: N
Federal Procurement Eligibility: Small Business
Distribution: Manufacturer Direct, Exporter
General Admin.: Theodore Varouxis/President
Mktg./Adv.: Pamela A. Varouxis/Vice President Marketing & Sales
Production: Alexander Varouxis/Vice President Manufacturing
Research: Barry Howard/Vice President Research & Development

Contract Manufacturing	General
Service, Engineering/Design	General
Stereotaxy Equipment	Cns/Neurology

ASSOCIATED ENVIRONMENTAL SYSTEMS   978-772-0022
31 Willow Road, Ayer, MA 01432-1512
FDA Number: 7000037   *Fax:* 978-772-0088
E-mail: Sales@AssociatedEnvironmental-BMA.com
Web site: www.bmaonline.net
Medical Products Sales Volume: $2,400,000
Annual Revenue: $1-$5 Million
Year Founded: 1974
Total Employees: 18
Ownership: Private
Produces/Sells CE-marked Devices: N
Federal Procurement Eligibility: Small Business
Distribution: Manufacturer Direct
General Admin.: William M. Bryant/President

Chamber, Environmental, Platelet Storage	Hematology
Oven	Chemistry

ASSOCIATED HEALTH SYSTEMS INC.   1.877.451.6720
#12 3691 Viking Way,   604-276-8012
Richmond, BC V6V-2 Canada
FDA Number: n/a   *Fax:* 604-590-9393
E-mail: ahsbc@sprint.ca
Year Founded: 1990
Total Employees: 25
Ownership: Private
Produces/Sells CE-marked Devices: N
Distribution: Manufacturer Direct, Exclusive Distributor

ASSOCIATED PRODUCTION SERVICES, INC.   215-364-0211
365 Andrews Rd., Trevose, PA 19053
FDA Number: 2523101
E-mail: mreed@apspackage.com
Web site: www.apspackage.com
Ownership: Private
Produces/Sells CE-marked Devices: N

Glove, Patient Examination, Latex	General

ASSOCIATES OF CAPE COD, INC.   508-540-3444
124 Bernard E. Saint Jean Drive, E Falmouth, MA 02536
FDA Number: 1219145
Ownership: Private
Produces/Sells CE-marked Devices: N

Antigen, Invasive Fungal Pathogens	Microbiology

ASTA DYNAMICS, ADI MEDICAL DIVISION
See Adi Medical Division Of Asia Dynamics (Group) Inc.

ASTELLAS PHARMA US, INC.   800-888-7704
3 Parkway N., Deerfield, IL 60015-2548   800-695-4321
FDA Number: 9003924   *Fax:* 847-317-7296
E-mail: corporate.communications@us.astellas.com
Web site: www.astellas.us
Medical Products Sales Volume: $101,600,000
Annual Revenue: $0-$1 Million
Year Founded: 2005
Total Employees: 500   *Marketing Staff:* 40   *Sales Staff:* 135
Ownership: FUJISAWA PHARMACEUTICAL COMPANY
Federal Procurement Eligibility: Small Business, GSA Contract, VA Contract
Distribution: Manufacturer Direct, Manufacturer Through Manufacturer Reps, Service Direct, Importer
General Admin.: N. Maeda/President
Mktg./Adv.: Dan Lewis/Director Marketing
T. Shea/Director National Accounts
Mr. Vogt/Manager Business Development
Ms. G. Aprill/Manager International Marketing & Sales
Pat Tyrell/Manager Market Research
Maribeth Landwehr/Public Relations Specialist
Rick White/Vice President Marketing
Production: D. Baker/Manager Regulatory Affairs
S. Trippie/Vice President Manufacturing
Research: D. Wagenknecht/Vice President Research & Development

Dressing, Non-Adherent	General
General Medical Device	General

ASTELLAS PHARMA US, INC.
800-888-7704 *(cont'd)*
Solution, Nutrition, Parenteral — Gastroenterology/Urology

ASTHMATX, INC.
1-877-810-6060
888 Ross Dr., Suite 100, Sunnyvale, CA 94089 — **408-419-0100**
FDA Number: 3006139571 — *Fax:* 408-419-0101
Web site: www.asthmatx.com
Ownership: Boston Scientific Corporation
Produces/Sells CE-marked Devices: N
General Admin.: Mr. Glen French/Chief Executive Officer

Bronchoscope, Non-Rigid	Ear/Nose/Throat
Bronchoscope, Rigid	Ear/Nose/Throat
Electrosurgical Unit, Cutting & Coagulation Device	Surgery

ASTORIA-PACIFIC, INC.
800-536-3111
PO Box 830, Clakamas, OR 97015 — **503-657-3010**
FDA Number: 3050015 — *Fax:* 503-655-7367
E-mail: sales@astoria-pacific.com
Web site: www.astoria-pacific.com
Medical Products Sales Volume: $5,700,000
Year Founded: 1990
Total Employees: 38
Ownership: Private
Produces/Sells CE-marked Devices: Y
Federal Procurement Eligibility: Small Business

1-Nitroso-2-Naphthol (Fluorometric), Free Tyrosine	Chemistry
Analyzer, Chemistry, Fluorescence Immunoassay	Chemistry
Analyzer, Chemistry, Sequential Multiple, Continuous Flow	Chemistry
Enzymatic Method, Galactose	Chemistry
Fluorescent Proc. (Qual.), Galactose-1-Phosphate Uridyl	Chemistry
Ninhydrin And L-Leucyl-L-Alanine (Fluorimetric)	Chemistry

ASTRA TECH INC
800-531-3481
590 Lincoln Street, Waltham, MA 02451
FDA Number: 1222802 — *Fax:* 781-890-6808
E-mail: customerservice.us@astratech.com
Web site: http://www.astratechdental.us
Ownership: Private
Produces/Sells CE-marked Devices: N

Implant, Endosseous	Dental And Oral

ASTRA-ZENECA, INC., LUXTRAK BUSINESS GROUP
See AstraZeneca Pharmaceuticals LP

ASTRAL DIAGNOSTICS, INC.
856-224-0900
1224 Forest Pkwy., West Deptford, NJ 08066
FDA Number: 2247035

Stain, Microbiological	Microbiology
Stain, Romanowsky	Hematology

ASTRALITE CORPORATION
800-345-7703
PO Box 689, Somerset, CA 95684 — **530-333-7556**
FDA Number: n/a — *Fax:* 775-890-2487
Web site: http://www.astralitecorp.com
Medical Products Sales Volume: $80,000
Annual Revenue: $0-$1 Million
Ownership: Private
Produces/Sells CE-marked Devices: N
Federal Procurement Eligibility: Small Business
Distribution: Manufacturer Direct, Manufacturer Through Distributor, OEM
General Admin.: Dorian Swartz/President

Battery	General
Laryngoscope, Rigid	Anesthesiology
Light, Other	General
Otoscope	Ear/Nose/Throat
Power System, Isolated	General
Speculum, Other	General
Speculum, Vaginal, Non-Metal	Obstetrics/Gynecology

ASTRAZENECA PHARMACEUTICALS LP
302-886-3000
1800 Concord Pike, P.O. Box 15437, Wilmington, DE 19850-5437
FDA Number: n/a — *Fax:* 302-886-2972
Web site: www.astrazeneca-us.com
Annual Revenue: $0-$1 Million
Ownership: Astrazeneca
Produces/Sells CE-marked Devices: N
Distribution: Manufacturer Direct, Manufacturer Through Manufacturer Reps

Component, Other	General

Medical Product Subsidiaries (Listed Separately)
Aurora Medical Supplies, Inc.

ASTRO SEAL, INC.
951-787-6670
827-B Palmyrita Avenue, Riverside, CA 92507-1820
FDA Number: 1527105 — *Fax:* 951-787-6677
E-mail: sales@astroseal.com
Web site: www.astroseal.com
Medical Products Sales Volume: $1,900,000
Annual Revenue: $1-$5 Million
Year Founded: 1964
Total Employees: 34 — *Sales Staff:* 1

ASTRO SEAL, INC.
951-787-6670 *(cont'd)*
Ownership: Private
Produces/Sells CE-marked Devices: N
Federal Procurement Eligibility: Small Business
Distribution: Manufacturer Direct
General Admin.: Mike Hammer/President, Chief Executive Officer
Production: Ryan Jones/Engineer
   Karen Upfold/Manager Operations
   Mike Hammer/Manager Quality Assurance

Connector, Tubing, Blood	Cardiovascular
Contract Manufacturing	General
Contract R&D, Equipment	General

ASTRO-MED, INC.
800-343-4039
600 E. Greenwich Avenue, — **401-828-4000**
West Warwick, RI 02893
FDA Number: 1221766 — *Fax:* 401-822-2430
E-mail: mtgroup@astromed.com
Web site: www.astro-med.com
Medical Products Sales Volume: $65,500,000
Annual Revenue: $50-$100 Million
Year Founded: 1969
Total Employees: 250 — *Marketing Staff:* 10 — *Sales Staff:* 30
Ownership: Public
Stock Symbol: ALOT
Traded On: NASDAQ
Quality System Registration Information: ISO9001; ISO9003
Produces/Sells CE-marked Devices: Y
Federal Procurement Eligibility: Small Business, GSA Contract, VA Contract
Distribution: Manufacturer Direct
General Admin.: Albert Ondis/Chief Executive Officer
   Everett V. Pizzuti/President
Mktg./Adv.: Steve London/Manager Advertising
   Tina Pollard/Manager Marketing
Production: Steve Petrarca/Vice President Manufacturing
Finance: Joseph O'Connell/Chief Financial Officer

Labeling Equipment	General
Paper, Chart, Record, Medical	General
Recorder, Chart, Laboratory	Chemistry
Recorder, Paper Chart	Cardiovascular
Service, Printing	General

Medical Product Subsidiaries (Listed Separately)
Grass Technologies, An Astro-Med, Inc. Product Gro

ASTRON DENTAL CORPORATION
800-323-4144
815 Oakwood Rd. Unit G, Lake Zurich, IL 60047 — **847-726-8787**
FDA Number: 1483306 — *Fax:* 847-726-8793
E-mail: doug@astrondental.com
Web site: www.astrondental.com
Ownership: Private
Produces/Sells CE-marked Devices: N
General Admin.: Mr. Douglas Muller/President, Chief Executive Officer
Mktg./Adv.: Mr. Robert Muller/Senior Vice President Sales

Base, Denture, Relining, Repairing, Rebasing, Resin	Dental And Oral
Cleaner, Denture, Mechanical	Dental And Oral
Crown And Bridge, Temporary, Resin	Dental And Oral
Kit, Denture Repair, OTC	Dental And Oral
Lamp, Infrared	Physical Med
Material, Investment	Dental And Oral
Teeth, Artificial, Backing And Facing	Dental And Oral
Wax, Dental	Dental And Oral

ASTRON INTERNATIONAL INC.
239-435-0136
3410 Westview Dr., Naples, FL 34104
FDA Number: 1828978
Ownership: Private
Produces/Sells CE-marked Devices: N

Bar, Prism, Ophthalmic	Ophthalmology
Lens, Maddox	Ophthalmology
Measurer, Stereopsis	Ophthalmology
Prism, Rotary, Ophthalmic	Ophthalmology
Shield, Eye, Ophthalmic	Ophthalmology

ASURAGEN, INC.
877-777-1874
2150 Woodward St., Suite 100, Austin, TX 78744 — **512-681-5200**
FDA Number: 3003436513 — *Fax:* 512-681-5201
E-mail: orders@asuragen.com
Web site: www.asuragen.com
Year Founded: 1989
Ownership: Private
Produces/Sells CE-marked Devices: N
General Admin.: Dr. Matt Winkler/Chief Executive Officer
   Dr. Rollie Carson/President
Medical Admin.: Mr. Luc Van Hove/Senior Director Clinical Affairs
Finance: Ms. Lynne Hohlfeld/Chief Financial Officer

Reagent, General Purpose	Pathology
Reagents, Specific, Analyte	Hematology

MANUFACTURER PROFILES

ATC TECHNOLOGIES, INC.   781-939-0725
30-B Upton Drive, Wilmington, MA 01887
FDA Number: n/a   *Fax:* 781-939-0726
Web site: http://www.atctechnologiesinc.com
Medical Products Sales Volume: $3,000,000
Annual Revenue: $1-$5 Million
Year Founded: 1997
Total Employees: 25   *Marketing Staff:* 1   *Sales Staff:* 1
Ownership: Private
Quality System Registration Information: ISO9000
Produces/Sells CE-marked Devices: N
Federal Procurement Eligibility: Small Business
Distribution: Manufacturer Direct, Manufacturer Through Distributor, Manufacturer Through Manufacturer Reps, OEM
General Admin.: John J. Triggs/Chief Executive Officer
            Paul C. Kierce/President
Mktg./Adv.: Kenneth Freeman/Vice President Business Development
            Mike Warner/Vice President Marketing & Sales
Production: Mike Goddard/Director Operations

Biopsy Device, Endomyocardial	Cardiovascular
Cannula, Aspirating	Cardiovascular
Contract Manufacturing	General
Electrode, Electrosurgery, Laparoscopic	Surgery
Forceps, Biopsy	Surgery
Forceps, Endoscopic	Gastroenterology/Urology
Probe, Suction, Irrigator/Aspirator, Laparoscopic	Surgery
Tubing, Other	General

ATCC   800-638-6597   703-365-2700
10801 University Blvd., PO Box 1549, Manassas, VA 20108
FDA Number: n/a   *Fax:* 703-365-2750
E-mail: sales@atcc.org
Web site: www.atcc.org
Medical Products Sales Volume: $57,600,000
Annual Revenue: $10-$25 Million
Year Founded: 1925
Total Employees: 255   *Marketing Staff:* 15
Produces/Sells CE-marked Devices: N
Federal Procurement Eligibility: Small Business, GSA Contract
Distribution: Manufacturer Direct
General Admin.: Gulano Ghugnoli/Chief Information Officer
            Raymond Cypress/President, Chief Executive Officer
            Nancy Wysocki/Vice President Human Resources
Production: Phil Baird/Manager Materials
            Sylvia Fudge/Manager Regulatory Affairs
Finance: Robert Berkson/Chief Financial Officer

Culture Media, Selective And Differential	Microbiology

ATD-AMERICAN CO.   800-523-2300   215-576-1000
135 Greenwood Ave., Wyncote, PA 19095-1337
FDA Number: n/a   *Fax:* 215-576-1827
E-mail: website@atd.com
Web site: www.atd.com
Annual Revenue: $50-$100 Million
Ownership: Private
Produces/Sells CE-marked Devices: N
Federal Procurement Eligibility: Small Business, Female Owned
Distribution: Manufacturer Direct, Manufacturer Through Distributor, OEM, Service Direct, Exclusive Distributor

Bag, Laundry, Infection Control	General
Bag, Laundry, Operating Room	General
Bed, Manual	General
Belt, Sanitary	Obstetrics/Gynecology
Bib	General
Brassiere, Maternity	Obstetrics/Gynecology
Cap, Surgical	Surgery
Cart, Equipment, Video	General
Cart, Laundry	General
Cart, Supply	General
Chair, Other	General
Clothing, Protective	General
Coat, Laboratory	General
Cover, Head, Surgical	Surgery
Cover, Mattress	General
Cover, Mattress, Waterproof	General
Cover, Shoe, Non-Conductive	General
Curtain, Cubicle	General
Curtain, Shower	General
Diaper, Adult	General
Diaper, Pediatric	General
Drape, Patient, Ophthalmic	Ophthalmology
Drape, Surgical	Surgery
Drape, Surgical, Disposable	Surgery
Drape, Surgical, ENT	Ear/Nose/Throat
Drape, Surgical, Reusable	Surgery
Dress, Scrub, Disposable	Surgery
Equipment, Building Security	General
Floor Mat	General

ATD-AMERICAN CO.   800-523-2300 (cont'd)

Floor Mat, Antibacterial	General
Furniture, General	General
Furniture, Patient Room	General
Garment, Protective, For Incontinence	Gastroenterology/Urology
Gown, Examination	General
Gown, Operating Room, Disposable	Surgery
Gown, Other	General
Gown, Patient	Surgery
Gown, Patient, Disposable	General
Gown, Patient, Reusable	General
Gown, Surgical	Surgery
Hood, Surgical	Surgery
Infusion Stand	General
Kit, Admission (Patient Utensil)	General
Laundry Hamper	General
Linen	General
Linen, Bed	General
Liner, Laundry Hamper	General
Mask, Surgical	Surgery
Mattress, Bed	General
Office Equipment	General
Office Product	General
Pack, Sterilization Wrapper (Bag And Accessories)	Surgery
Pack, Surgical (Drape)	Surgery
Pad, Incontinence (Underpad)	General
Pillow	General
Restraint, Protective (Body)	General
Scale, Stand-On	General
Security Equipment/Supplies	General
Sheet, Drape	Surgery
Sheet, Drape, Disposable	Surgery
Sheet, Examination Table, Disposable	General
Sheet, Operating Room	Surgery
Sheet, Operating Room, Disposable	Surgery
Sheeting, Examination Table	General
Sign, Hospital	General
Table, Examination/Treatment	General
Table, Other	General
Toothbrush, Manual	Dental And Oral
Towel, Surgical	Surgery
Towel/Towelette, Paper	General
Waste Receptacle, General Purpose	General
Wrap, Sterilization	General
Wrapper, Surgical Instrument (Sterile)	General

ATEK MEDICAL   800-253-1540   616-643-5200
620 Watson St, Grand Rapids, MI 49504-6393
FDA Number: 1419629   *Fax:* 616-643-1044
E-mail: sales@atekmedical.com
Web site: www.atekmedical.com
Medical Products Sales Volume: $14,700,000
Year Founded: 1979
Total Employees: 180   *Marketing Staff:* 1   *Sales Staff:* 2
Ownership: Vention Medical
Quality System Registration Information: ISO9002
Produces/Sells CE-marked Devices: N
Federal Procurement Eligibility: Small Business, Female Owned
General Admin.: Ms. Christy Orris/Chief Executive Officer
            Ms. Chris Oleksy/President
            Ms. Jackie Bach/Vice President
            Scott Fetzer/Vice President, General Manager

Accessories, Cardiopulmonary Bypass	Cardiovascular
Adapter, Stopcock, Manifold, Cardiopulmonary Bypass	Cardiovascular
Cannula, Catheter	Cardiovascular
Cannula, Injection	Gastroenterology/Urology
Catheter, Multiple Lumen	Surgery
Catheter, Vascular, Cardiopulmonary Bypass	Cardiovascular
Electrosurgical Unit, Cutting & Coagulation Device	Surgery
Gauge, Pressure, Coronary, Cardiopulmonary Bypass	Cardiovascular
Introducer, Catheter	Cardiovascular
Lavage Unit, Water Jet	General
Retractor, Surgical	Surgery
Sucker, Cardiotomy Return, Cardiopulmonary Bypass	Cardiovascular
Surgical Instrument, Cardiovascular	Cardiovascular

ATHENA CONTROLS, INC.   800-782-6776   610-828-2490
5145 Campus Drive, Plymouth Meeting, PA 19462
FDA Number: n/a   *Fax:* 610-828-7084
E-mail: sales@athenacontrols.com
Web site: www.athenacontrols.com
Medical Products Sales Volume: $9,000,000
Annual Revenue: $5-$10 Million
Year Founded: 1965
Total Employees: 60
Ownership: INDUCTOTHERM INDUSTRIES, INC.
Produces/Sells CE-marked Devices: Y
Federal Procurement Eligibility: Small Business

ATHENA CONTROLS, INC.   800-782-6776 *(cont'd)*
Distribution: Manufacturer Through Distributor, Manufacturer Through Manufacturer Reps, Exporter
General Admin.: Joseph Sroka/President, Chief Executive Officer
Mktg./Adv.: Doug Crowell/Manager International & National Sales
Production: Bob Bleau/Director Quality Assurance
  Production Equipment   General

ATHENA FEMININE TECHNOLOGIES, INC   866-308-4436
179 Moraga Way, Orinda, CA 94563   925-254-6090
FDA Number: 300452462   *Fax:* 925-254-5396
E-mail: info@athenaft.com
Web site: www.athenaft.com
Total Employees: 3
Ownership: Private
Quality System Registration Information: ISO9000; ISO9001
Produces/Sells CE-marked Devices: Y
Distribution: Manufacturer Through Distributor
General Admin.: Mr. George Sarkis/Chief Executive Officer
      Ms. Barbara Sarkis/Chief Information Officer
Finance: Mr. Steven Kerkstra/Chief Financial Officer
  Exerciser, Other   Physical Med
  Stimulator, Electrical, For Incontinence   Gastroenterology/Urology
  Stimulator, Electrical, Muscle   Physical Med
  Stimulator, Muscle, Electrical-Powered (EMS)   Physical Med
  Stimulator, Muscle, Vaginal   Obstetrics/Gynecology

ATHENA TECHNOLOGY, INC.   314-344-0010
13705 Shoreline Court East, Earth City, MO 63045
FDA Number: 2029402
Web site: www.ydnt.com
Ownership: Young Innovations, Inc.
Stock Symbol: YDNT
Traded On: NASDAQ
Produces/Sells CE-marked Devices: N
  Handpiece, Air-Powered, Dental   Dental And Oral

ATHEROTECH   800-719-9807
201 London Parkway, Birmingham, AL 35211
FDA Number: n/a
Web site: www.atherotech.com
Ownership: Private
Produces/Sells CE-marked Devices: N
General Admin.: Mr. Robert Shufflebarger/Chief Operating Officer
      Mr. Michael Mullen/President, Chief Executive Officer
Medical Admin.: Dr. Michael Cobble/Chief Medical Officer
Mktg./Adv.: Mr. Scott Rezek/Commercial Director
      Mr. Rod VanWagoner/Vice President Sales
Production: Mr. Patrick Mize/Vice President Regulatory Affairs
Research: Ms. Jennifer Mason/Vice President Clinicial Development

ATI ORION
See Orion Research, Inc.

ATL ULTRASOUND
See Phillips Ultrasound

ATLAN-TOL INDUSTRIES INC.
See Astro-Med, Inc.

ATLANTA INTERNATIONAL   800-251-9864
1979 Parker Court, Suites D And E,   865-362-6022
Stone Mountain, GA 30087
FDA Number: 1066659
E-mail: customerservice@deroyal.com
Web site: www.deroyal.com
Year Founded: 1973
Ownership: DEROYAL INDUSTRIES, INC.
Produces/Sells CE-marked Devices: N
  Orthosis, Lumbosacral   Physical Med

ATLANTA ORTHODONTICS   800-535-7166
1247 Zonolite Road N.E., Atlanta, GA 30306-2005   404-875-6837
FDA Number: n/a   *Fax:* 404-875-6837
E-mail: atlantaortho@bellsouth.net
Medical Products Sales Volume: $100,000
Annual Revenue: $0-$1 Million
Year Founded: 1969
Total Employees: 2
Ownership: Private
Produces/Sells CE-marked Devices: Y
Federal Procurement Eligibility: Small Business
Distribution: Manufacturer Direct
General Admin.: James J. Reeve/Owner
  Lock, Wire, And Ligature, Intraoral   Dental And Oral
  Wire, Orthodontic   Dental And Oral

ATLANTA THERMOPLASTIC PRODUCTS, INC.
See Crespac Inc.

ATLANTIC ALLOY HEALTH & EQUIPMENT CORP.
See Atlantic Medco, Inc.

ATLANTIC AMBULANCE BUILDERS
See National Ambulance Builders, Inc.

ATLANTIC FOOTCARE
See ATLANTIC FOOTCARE

ATLANTIC MEDCO, INC.   800-203-8444
166 Bloomfield Avenue, Verona, NJ 07044   973-571-9002
FDA Number: 2246818   *Fax:* 973-571-9004
E-mail: stcharlesm@cs.com
Web site: www.stcharlesatlanticmedco.com
Medical Products Sales Volume: $3,000,000
Year Founded: 1947
Total Employees: 260   *Marketing Staff:* 6   *Sales Staff:* 12
Ownership: Private
Produces/Sells CE-marked Devices: N
Federal Procurement Eligibility: Small Business, Female Owned
Distribution: Manufacturer Direct, Manufacturer Through Distributor, Manufacturer Through Manufacturer Reps, Exporter
General Admin.: Barbara Mancuso/Chief Executive Officer
      Len Mancuso/General Manager
Mktg./Adv.: Ben Fortese/Director Marketing
      Len Mancuso/Director Marketing
  Bassinet (Infant Bed)   General
  Bed, Pediatric (Crib)   General
  Cabinet Casework, Modular   General
  Cabinet, Instrument   General
  Cabinet, Medicine   General
  Cabinet, Narcotic Control   General
  Cabinet, Other   General
  Cabinet, Warming   General
  Cart, Anesthetist's   Anesthesiology
  Cart, Laundry   General
  Cart, Medicine   General
  Cart, Multipurpose   General
  Cart, Other   General
  Cart, Supply   General
  Cover, Cart   General
  Stretcher, Wheeled (Mobile)   General
  Table, Examination/Treatment   General

ATLANTIC MEDICAL SPECIALTIES   888-487-5568
3620 Horizon Drive, King of Prussia, PA 19406   610-270-8909
FDA Number: n/a   *Fax:* 610-270-0647
E-mail: crowleyjack@hotmail.com
Web site: www.atlanticmedicalspecialties.com
Medical Products Sales Volume: $700,000
Annual Revenue: $10-$25 Million
Year Founded: 1984
Total Employees: 5   *Sales Staff:* 5
Ownership: Private
Produces/Sells CE-marked Devices: N
Federal Procurement Eligibility: Small Business
Distribution: Manufacturer Through Manufacturer Reps
General Admin.: Jack Crowley/Chief Executive Officer
  Water, Therapy, Respiratory   Microbiology

ATLANTIC MILLS, INC.   800-242-7374
1295 Towbin Ave., Lakewood, NJ 08701   732-363-9281
FDA Number: n/a   *Fax:* 732-363-4302
E-mail: sales@atlanticmill.com
Web site: www.atlanticmills.com
Medical Products Sales Volume: $500,000
Annual Revenue: $0-$1 Million
Total Employees: 23   *Sales Staff:* 5
Ownership: Private
Produces/Sells CE-marked Devices: N
Federal Procurement Eligibility: Small Business
Distribution: Manufacturer Through Distributor
General Admin.: Lesley Ward/General Manager
      William Vogel/President
Mktg./Adv.: Lesley Ward/Manager Marketing
  Mitt/Washcloth, Patient   General

ATLANTIC OPTICAL CO., INC.   800-423-5175
20801 Nordhoff Street, Chatsworth, CA 91311   818-407-1890
FDA Number: 2026552   *Fax:* 818-407-1895
E-mail: lbi@atlanticoptical.com
Web site: www.atlanticoptical.com
Medical Products Sales Volume: $7,600,000
Annual Revenue: $25-$50 Million
Year Founded: 1950
Total Employees: 80   *Marketing Staff:* 2   *Sales Staff:* 19
Ownership: Private
Produces/Sells CE-marked Devices: Y
Federal Procurement Eligibility: Small Business
Distribution: Manufacturer Direct

ATLANTIC OPTICAL CO., INC.　　800-423-5175 *(cont'd)*
General Admin.: Keith Lehrer/Executive Vice President
　　　　Sheldon Lehrer/President, Chief Executive Officer
　　　　Robert Perry/Vice President, General Manager
Mktg./Adv.: Janet Axelrad/Director Marketing
　　　　Robert Perry/Director National Accounts
　　　　Michael Schaus/Director Product Development

Frame, Spectacle (Eyeglasses)	Ophthalmology
Sunglasses (Including Photosensitive)	Ophthalmology

ATLANTIC RIM BRACE MFG. CORP.　　800-233-0356
25B Front St. Suite 5a, Nashua, NH 03064　　**603-886-8130**
FDA Number: n/a　　　　　　　　*Fax:* 603-881-4380
E-mail: sales@spinalbraces.com
Web site: www.spinalbraces.com
Ownership: Private
Produces/Sells CE-marked Devices: N

Orthosis, Truncal/Limb	Physical Med

ATLANTIC SURGICAL COMPANY INC.
See Torbot Group, Inc.

ATLANTIC ULTRAVIOLET CORP.　　631-273-0500
375 Marcus Blvd., Hauppauge, NY 11788
FDA Number: n/a　　　　　　　　*Fax:* 631-273-0771
E-mail: info@ultraviolet.com
Web site: www.ultraviolet.com
Medical Products Sales Volume: $7,500,000
Annual Revenue: $5-$10 Million
Year Founded: 1963
Total Employees: 38　　　*Marketing Staff:* 4　　　*Sales Staff:* 5
Ownership: Private
Produces/Sells CE-marked Devices: N
Federal Procurement Eligibility: Small Business
Distribution: Manufacturer Direct, Manufacturer Through Manufacturer Reps, OEM
General Admin.: Hilary Boehme/President
Mktg./Adv.: Arlene Metzroth/Manager International Marketing & Sales
Production: Eric Boehme/Manager Materials
Finance: Ann M. Wysocki/Controller

Filter, Air	General
Lamp, Ultraviolet, Germicidal	General
Lamp, Ultraviolet, Physical Medicine	Physical Med
Purification System, Water, Ultraviolet	Chemistry
Purifier, Air, Ultraviolet	General
Sterilizer, Ultraviolet	General

ATLANTIS LUMINESCENT PRODUCTS, LLC　　318-894-9490
1405 Pinhook Rd., Suite 205, Lafayette, LA 70503
FDA Number: n/a
Ownership: Private
Produces/Sells CE-marked Devices: N

Lamp, Infrared	Physical Med

ATLAS LABORATORIES CO. LTD.　　204-775-2707
757 Sargent Ave, Winnipeg, MB R3E 0B3 Canada
FDA Number: n/a　　　　　　　　*Fax:* 204-783-9664
Total Employees: 4　　　*Marketing Staff:* 1　　　*Sales Staff:* 1
Ownership: Private
Produces/Sells CE-marked Devices: N
Federal Procurement Eligibility: Small Business, Minority Owned
Distribution: Manufacturer Direct

ATLAS MEDICAL TECHNOLOGIES　　909-923-7887
1137 E. Philadelphia St., Ontario, CA 91761
FDA Number: 9045342　　　　　*Fax:* 909-923-7944
E-mail: info@atlasmedtec.com
Web site: www.atlasmedtec.com
Medical Products Sales Volume: $7,000,000
Annual Revenue: $5-$10 Million
Year Founded: 1992
Total Employees: 23　　　*Marketing Staff:* 2　　　*Sales Staff:* 4
Ownership: Private
Produces/Sells CE-marked Devices: N
Federal Procurement Eligibility: Small Business
Distribution: Manufacturer Direct, Manufacturer Through Distributor, Manufacturer Through Manufacturer Reps, Service Direct, Importer, Exporter
General Admin.: Walter Spinner/General Manager
　　　　Rick Stockton/President, Chief Executive Officer
Mktg./Adv.: Mr. Glenn Tokushige/National Accounts Representative
　　　　Mr. John Stockton/Sales Associate
　　　　Gail Spinner/Sales Representative
　　　　Mr. Dave Archibald/Sales Representative
　　　　Mr. Ron Brewer/Sales Representative

Camera, Multi Format	Radiology
Camera, Multi-Image	Radiology
Housing, X-Ray Tube, Diagnostic	Radiology
Housing, X-Ray Tube, Therapeutic	Radiology
Image Processing System	Radiology
Magnet, Permanent, MRI (Magnetic Resonance Imaging)	Radiology

ATLAS MEDICAL TECHNOLOGIES　　909-923-7887 *(cont'd)*

Magnet, Superconducting, MRI (Magnetic Resonance Imaging)	Radiology
Scanner, Computed Tomography, X-Ray, Full Body	Radiology
Scanner, Computed Tomography, X-Ray, Head	Radiology
Scanner, Computed Tomography, X-Ray, Special Procedure	Radiology
Scanner, Magnetic Resonance (NMR/MRI)	Radiology
Scanner, Positron Emission Tomography (PET)	Radiology
Service, Maintenance/Repair	General
Service, Used Equipment	General
Simulator, Radiotherapy	Radiology
Simulator, Radiotherapy, Special Purpose	Radiology
Tube, X-Ray	Radiology

ATLAS SPINE INC.　　561-741-1108
1555 Jupiter Park Dr., Ste. 4, Jupiter, FL 33458
FDA Number: 3003855635

Appliance, Fixation, Spinal Intervertebral Body	Orthopedics
Device, Spinal Vertebral Body Replacement	Orthopedics
Orthopedic Manual Surgical Instrument	Orthopedics

ATOMIC PRODUCTS CORP.
See Biodex Medical Systems, Inc.

ATRICURE, INC.　　888.347.6403
6217 Centre Park Drive,　　**513.755.4100**
West Chester, OH 45069
FDA Number: 3003502395
E-mail: customerservice@atricure.com　　*Fax:* 513.755.4567
Web site: http://atricure.com
Year Founded: 2000
Ownership: Public
Stock Symbol: ATRC
Traded On: NASDAQ
Produces/Sells CE-marked Devices: N
General Admin.: Mr. David Drachman/Chief Executive Officer
　　　　Ms. Julie Piton/Chief Financial Officer, Vice President
Mktg./Adv.: Mr. Stewart Strong/Vice President Sales
Production: Mr. Salvatore Privitera/Vice President Engineering & Product Development
　　　　Mr. Frederick Preiss/Vice President Operations
　　　　Mr. James Lucky/Vice President Regulatory Affairs

Dissector, Surgical, General & Plastic Surgery	Surgery
Electrosurgical Unit, Cutting & Coagulation Device	Surgery
Guide, Surgical, Instrument	Surgery
Retractor, Surgical	Surgery

ATRICURE, INC.　　888.347.6403
6217Centre Park Dr.,　　**513.755.4100**
West Chester, OH 45069
FDA Number: 3003502395
E-mail: customerservice@atricure.com　　*Fax:* 513.755.4567
Web site: www.enablemedical.com
Annual Revenue: $1-$5 Million
Total Employees: 50　　　*Marketing Staff:* 1　　　*Sales Staff:* 2
Ownership: Private
Quality System Registration Information: ISO9000
Produces/Sells CE-marked Devices: Y
Federal Procurement Eligibility: Small Business
Distribution: Manufacturer Direct, Manufacturer Through Distributor, OEM
General Admin.: Michael D. Hooven/President, Chief Executive Officer
　　　　Susan Spies/Vice President Human Resources
Mktg./Adv.: Jim Chaldekas/Vice President Marketing & Business Development
Production: Greg Drach/Director Operations
　　　　Mark Friedman/Manager Regulatory Affairs
Research: Jon Sherman/Vice President Engineering
Finance: Annette Gerding/Director Accounting

Clip, Implantable	Surgery
Cryosurgical Unit	Surgery
Dissector, Surgical, General & Plastic Surgery	Surgery
Electrosurgical Unit, Cutting & Coagulation Device	Surgery
Guide, Surgical, Instrument	Surgery
Lamp, Surgical	Surgery
Remover, Tissue	Surgery
Stand, Instrument, AC-Powered, Ophthalmic	Ophthalmology

ATRION CORP.　　972-390-9800
One Allentown Parkway, Allen, TX 75002-4211
FDA Number: n/a　　　　　　　　*Fax:* 972-396-7581
E-mail: ir-info@atrioncorp.com
Web site: www.atrioncorp.com
Ownership: Private
Stock Symbol: ATRI
Traded On: NASDAQ
Produces/Sells CE-marked Devices: N
General Admin.: Emile A. Battat/Chief Executive Officer, Chairman
　　　　Jeffery Strickland/Chief Financial Officer, Vice President
　　　　David A. Battat/President, Chief Operating Officer

ATRION MEDICAL PRODUCTS, INC. — 800-343-9334
1426 Curt Francis Rd., Arab, AL 35016 — **256-586-1580**
FDA Number: 1043729 — Fax: 256-586-8529
E-mail: info@atrionmedical.com
Web site: www.atrionmedical.com
Year Founded: 1968
Total Employees: 160
Ownership: Private
Quality System Registration Information: ISO9001
Produces/Sells CE-marked Devices: Y
Distribution: Manufacturer Direct, Manufacturer Through Distributor, OEM, Exporter
General Admin.: Vandy Cruise/President
Mktg./Adv.: Hollie Bradford/Director Business Development
    Thomas Kinney/Director Marketing
Production: Sheila Minor/Director Materials Management
    Dan Clark/Vice President Quality Assurance & Regulatory Affairs
Research: Rowland Kanner/Vice President Research & Development

Biopsy Instrument	Gastroenterology/Urology
Case, Contact Lens	Ophthalmology
Catheter, Balloon, Dilatation, Vessel	Gastroenterology/Urology
Closure, Other	General
Contract Manufacturing	General
Contract Packaging	General
Contract R&D, Diagnostics	General
Dilator, Urethral	Gastroenterology/Urology
Dispenser, Other	General
Evacuator, Oral Cavity	Dental And Oral
Injector, Angiographic (Cardiac Catheterization)	Cardiovascular
Injector, Syringe	General
Kit, Biopsy Needle	Gastroenterology/Urology
Kit, Surgical (General)	Surgery
Lancet, Blood	General
Lavage Unit	Gastroenterology/Urology
Molding, Custom	General
Needle, Hypodermic, Single Lumen With Syringe	General
Operative Dental Treatment Unit	Dental And Oral
Service, Engineering/Design	General
Sterilizer, Soft Lens, Thermal, AC-Powered	Ophthalmology
Surgical Instrument, Cardiovascular	Cardiovascular
Syringe, Balloon Inflation	Cardiovascular

Medical Product Subsidiaries (Listed Separately)
  Halkey-Roberts Corp.
  Quest Medical, Inc.

ATRIUM MEDICAL CORP. — 800-528-7486
5 Wentworth Dr., Hudson, NH 03051 — **603-880-1433**
FDA Number: 1219977 — Fax: 603-880-6718
E-mail: webmaster@atriummed.com
Web site: www.atriummed.com
Annual Revenue: $50-$100 Million
Year Founded: 1981
Total Employees: 425
Ownership: GETINGE AB
Quality System Registration Information: ISO9000; ISO9001; ISO9002
Produces/Sells CE-marked Devices: Y
Distribution: Manufacturer Direct, Manufacturer Through Distributor, Manufacturer Through Manufacturer Reps, Service Direct, Exporter
General Admin.: Steve Herweck/Chief Executive Officer, Chairman
    Ted Karwoski/Chief Operating Officer, Vice President Operations
    Trevor Carlton/President
Mktg./Adv.: Steve Vail/Vice President Global Marketing
    Dennis Giampietro/Vice President Sales
Finance: Paul Leleivre/Chief Financial Officer, Vice President Finance

Autotransfusion Unit (Blood)	Anesthesiology
Bag, Blood	Hematology
Catheter, Angioplasty, Coronary, Transluminal, Percut. Oper.	Cardiovascular
Catheter, Angioplasty, Transluminal, Peripheral	Cardiovascular
Catheter, Cardiovascular	Surgery
Catheter, Other	Gastroenterology/Urology
Drain, Thoracic (Chest)	Anesthesiology
Drain, Thoracic, Water Seal	Anesthesiology
Graft, Vascular, Synthetic/Biological Composite	Cardiovascular
Kit, Chest Drainage (Thoracentesis Tray)	General
Kit, Incision And Drainage	Surgery
Kit, Wound Drainage	General
Mesh, Surgical, Polymeric	Surgery
Prosthesis, PTFE/Carbon-Fiber	Surgery
Prosthesis, Vascular Graft, Of 6mm And Greater Diameter	Cardiovascular
Stent, Cardiovascular	Cardiovascular
Stent, Vascular	Cardiovascular
Trocar, Thoracic	Cardiovascular

ATS LABORATORIES, INC. — 203-579-2700
404 Knowlton St., Bridgeport, CT 06608-1814
FDA Number: 1221229 — Fax: 203-333-2681
E-mail: atslaboratories@yahoo.com
Web site: www.atslabs.com
Medical Products Sales Volume: $300,000

ATS LABORATORIES, INC. — 203-579-2700 *(cont'd)*
Annual Revenue: $0-$1 Million
Year Founded: 1978
Total Employees: 5 — Marketing Staff: 2 — Sales Staff: 2
Ownership: Private
Produces/Sells CE-marked Devices: Y
Federal Procurement Eligibility: Small Business
Distribution: Manufacturer Direct, Manufacturer Through Distributor, OEM, Exporter
General Admin.: Ms. Lynda A. Hammond/President, General Manager
IS: Robert Spaulding/Senior Vice President Tech. Affairs

Equipment/Service, Quality Control	General
Phantom, Ultrasound	Radiology

ATS MEDICAL, INC. — 949-380-9333
20412 James Bay Circle, Lake Forest, CA 92630
FDA Number: 2031780
Ownership: ATS Medical, Inc.
Produces/Sells CE-marked Devices: N

Holder, Heart Valve Prosthesis	Cardiovascular
Sizer, Heart Valve Prosthesis	Cardiovascular
Valve, Heart, Tissue	Cardiovascular

ATS MEDICAL, INC. — 800-399-1381
3905 Annapolis Lane, Suite 105, — **763-553-7736**
Minneapolis, MN 55447
FDA Number: 2134151 — Fax: 763-557-2244
E-mail: info@atsmedical.com
Web site: www.atsmedical.com
Annual Revenue: $25-$50 Million
Year Founded: 1991
Ownership: Public
Stock Symbol: ATSI
Traded On: NASDAQ
Quality System Registration Information: ISO9001
Produces/Sells CE-marked Devices: Y
Federal Procurement Eligibility: Small Business
Distribution: Manufacturer Direct, Manufacturer Through Distributor, Manufacturer Through Manufacturer Reps
General Admin.: Michael Dale/President, Chief Executive Officer
  Medical Admin.: Dr. James Cox/Medical Director
Mktg./Adv.: Thad Coffindaffer/Vice President Sales
Production: Craig Swandal/Vice President Operations
    Astrid Berthe/Vice President Regulatory Affairs
Research: David Elizondo/Vice President Research & Development
Finance: Michael Kramer/Chief Financial Officer

Holder, Heart Valve Prosthesis	Cardiovascular
Prosthesis, Cardiac Valve	Cardiovascular
Sizer, Heart Valve Prosthesis	Cardiovascular
Surgical Device, For Ablation Of Cardiac Tissue	Surgery
Surgical Instrument, Cardiovascular	Cardiovascular
Valve, Heart, Mechanical	Cardiovascular

Medical Product Subsidiaries (Listed Separately)
  Ats Medical, Inc.

ATS SCIENTIFIC INC. — 800-661-6700
4030 Mainway Drive, — **905-332-1251**
Burlington, ONT L7M-4 Canada
FDA Number: n/a — Fax: 905-332-1394
E-mail: sales@ats-scientific.com
Web site: www.ats-scientific.com
Year Founded: 1989
Ownership: Private
Produces/Sells CE-marked Devices: N
Distribution: Exclusive Distributor

ATTACHMENTS INTERNATIONAL, INC. — 800-999-3003
824 Cowan Rd., Burlingame, CA 94010 — **650-340-0393**
FDA Number: 2917088 — Fax: 650-340-8423
Web site: www.attachments.com
Annual Revenue: $0-$1 Million
Ownership: Sybron Dental Specialties, Inc.
Produces/Sells CE-marked Devices: N
Distribution: Manufacturer Direct, Manufacturer Through Distributor, Importer, Exporter
General Admin.: Peter Staubli/President
Mktg./Adv.: Karen Lane/Vice President Marketing & Sales

Accessories, Implant, Dental, Endosseous	Dental And Oral
Attachment, Precision	Dental And Oral
Dental Laboratory Equipment	Dental And Oral
Implant, Endosseous	Dental And Oral

ATTENDS HEALTHCARE PRODUCTS — 252-752-1100
1029 Old Creek Road, Greenville, NC 27834
FDA Number: 1041732
Ownership: Private
Produces/Sells CE-marked Devices: N

Garment, Protective, For Incontinence	Gastroenterology/Urology

ATTENDS HEALTHCARE PRODUCTS   **252-752-1100** *(cont'd)*
Linen, Bed   General

ATTENDS HEALTHCARE PRODUCTS   **252-752-1100**
2321 Arrow Highway, La Verne, CA 91750
FDA Number: 2022431
Garment, Protective, For Incontinence   Gastroenterology/Urology
Linen, Bed   General

ATTOSTAR LLC   **952-920-6755**
7600 West 27th Street, Suite 234, Saint Louis Park, MN 55426
FDA Number: 3005517154
Reagents, Specific, Analyte   Hematology

ATWATER CAREY, LTD.
See Wisconsin Pharmacal Co. Llc

ATWORK CORPORATION
See Per-Se Technologies

ATZEN/UNIVERSAL COMPANIES, INC.   **800-558-5571**
18260 Oak Park Drive, Abingdon, VA 24210
FDA Number: 2951001   *Fax:* 800-237-7199
E-mail: info@atzen.com
Web site: www.atzen.com
Medical Products Sales Volume: $15,900,000
Year Founded: 1999
Total Employees: 81
Ownership: Universal Companies, Inc.
Produces/Sells CE-marked Devices: N
Federal Procurement Eligibility: Small Business, Female Owned
Distribution: Manufacturer Direct, Manufacturer Through Distributor
General Admin.: Marti Morenings/Chief Executive Officer
     Gary McConnell/President
Massager, Therapeutic   Physical Med

AUBREY GROUP   **949-581-0188**
6 Cromwell, Suite 100, Irvine, CA 92618
FDA Number: 3004673969   *Fax:* 949-581-0177
E-mail: info@aubreygroup.com
Web site: http://www.aubreygroup.com
Year Founded: 1994
Ownership: Private
Produces/Sells CE-marked Devices: N
General Admin.: Mr. Tom Allen/Chief Executive Officer
     Mr. Chuck Bower/President
Mktg./Adv.: Mr. Robert Lucero/Vice President Business Development
Production: Mr. Keith Sather/Vice President Manufacturing
Accessories, Electrical Power (Electrocautery)   Surgery
Electrosurgical, Cutting & Coagulation Accessories, Laparoscopic & Endoscopic,
Reprocessed   Surgery

AUDIFON USA INC.   **800-776-0222**
403 Chairman Ct, Suite 1, P.O. Box 531700,   **386-668-8812**
Debary, FL 32713
FDA Number: 3005384855   *Fax:* 386-753-9564
E-mail: contact.usa@audifon.com
Web site: www.audifon-usa.com
Medical Products Sales Volume: $2,500,000
Annual Revenue: $1-$5 Million
Ownership: Private
Produces/Sells CE-marked Devices: N
Distribution: Manufacturer Direct, Manufacturer Through Distributor
Hearing-Aid   Ear/Nose/Throat
Masker, Tinnitus   Ear/Nose/Throat

AUDINA HEARING INSTRUMENTS, INC.   **800-223-7700**
165 E. Wildmere Ave., Longwood, FL 32750
FDA Number: 1052698
Web site: www.audina.net
Annual Revenue: $0-$1 Million
Year Founded: 1990
Ownership: Private
Quality System Registration Information: ISO9001
Produces/Sells CE-marked Devices: N
Federal Procurement Eligibility: Small Business
Distribution: Manufacturer Direct
General Admin.: Frank Robilotta/Co-Owner, Executive Vice President
     Marc McLarnon/Co-Owner, President
     Paul Bryant/Vice President, General Manager
Hearing-Aid   Ear/Nose/Throat
Hearing-Aid, Plate, Face   Ear/Nose/Throat
IV Start Kit   Surgery

AUDIO   **207-893-2920**
885 Roosevelt Trail, Windham, ME 04062
FDA Number: 2529110
Ownership: Private
Produces/Sells CE-marked Devices: N

AUDIO   **207-893-2920** *(cont'd)*
Hearing-Aid   Ear/Nose/Throat

AUDIO CONTROLE INC.   **800-567-2711**
250 King St. East,   **819-569-9986**
Sherbrooke, QUE J1G-1 Canada
FDA Number: n/a   *Fax:* 819-823-6696
E-mail: aci@audiocontrole.com
Web site: www.audiocontrole.com
Year Founded: 1980
Total Employees: 50
Ownership: Private
Produces/Sells CE-marked Devices: N
Distribution: Manufacturer Direct, Service Direct, Exclusive Distributor

AUDIO HEARING AID SERVICE   **330-364-6637**
617 Wabash Ave., N.w., New Philadelphia, OH 44663
FDA Number: 1527534
Ownership: Private
Produces/Sells CE-marked Devices: N
Hearing-Aid   Ear/Nose/Throat

AUDIOLOGICAL ENGINEERING CORP.   **800-283-4601**
9 Preston Road, Somerville, MA 02143-4242   **617-623-5562**
FDA Number: 1220580   *Fax:* 617-666-5228
E-mail: info@tactaid.com
Web site: www.tactaid.com
Medical Products Sales Volume: $400,000
Annual Revenue: $0-$1 Million
Year Founded: 1982
Total Employees: 4   *Marketing Staff:* 1
Ownership: Private
Produces/Sells CE-marked Devices: Y
Federal Procurement Eligibility: Small Business
Distribution: Manufacturer Direct, Manufacturer Through Distributor
General Admin.: David Franklin/Chief Executive Officer
     Loretta Franklin/President
Finance: Anya Olson/Treasurer
Tactile Hearing-Aid   Ear/Nose/Throat

AUDIOLOGY PRODUCTS   **877-218-6358**
c/o Pak It Rite, 126 North Wenatchee Avenue,   **509-662-7143**
Wenatchee, WA 98801
FDA Number: 3029918   *Fax:* 509-663-3506
E-mail: ullrich@crcwnet.com
Web site: www.audiologyproducts.com
Medical Products Sales Volume: $4,500,000
Ownership: Private
Produces/Sells CE-marked Devices: N
Cushion, Earphone (For Audiometric Testing)   Ear/Nose/Throat

AUDIOPHONICS
See Luminaud, Inc.

AUDIOTRONICS
See Dotronix, Inc.

AUGMENIX INC.   **781-895-3235**
204 Second Ave., Lower Level, Waltham, MA 02451
FDA Number: n/a   *Fax:* 781-895-3236
E-mail: info@augmenix.com
Web site: http://www.augmenix.com
Year Founded: 2008
Ownership: Private
Produces/Sells CE-marked Devices: N
General Admin.: Mr. Brad Poff/General Manager

AUGUSTA MEDICAL SYSTEMS, LLC   **800-827-8382**
1027 Broad St., Augusta, GA 30901   **706-821-3600**
FDA Number: 1065838   *Fax:* 706-821-3630
E-mail: info@augustams.com
Web site: www.augustams.com
Annual Revenue: $5-$10 Million
Total Employees: 70   *Marketing Staff:* 1   *Sales Staff:* 25
Ownership: Private
Produces/Sells CE-marked Devices: Y
Federal Procurement Eligibility: Small Business
Distribution: Manufacturer Direct, Manufacturer Through Manufacturer Reps,
Service Direct, Exclusive Distributor, Importer, Exporter
General Admin.: Michael Osbon/President, Chief Executive Officer
Mktg./Adv.: Mr. Louis Svehla/Vice President Marketing & Advertising
Impotence Device, Mechanical/Hydraulic   Gastroenterology/Urology

AULIE DEVICES, INC.   **541-548-7355**
3615 Northwest Way, P.O. Box 786, Redmond, OR 97756
FDA Number: 3028191   *Fax:* 541-548-7355
E-mail: aaulie@coinet.com
Ownership: Private
Produces/Sells CE-marked Devices: N

AULIE DEVICES, INC.   541-548-7355 *(cont'd)*
     Joint, Knee, External Limb Component   Physical Med

AURA INDUSTRIES, INC.   800-551-2872
     545 8th Avenue, #5W, New York, NY 10018-4352   212-290-9190
     FDA Number: n/a   *Fax:* 212-290-9191
     E-mail: info@aura-inc.com
     Web site: www.aura-inc.com
     Medical Products Sales Volume: $100,000
     Annual Revenue: $0-$1 Million
     Year Founded: 1983
     Total Employees: 2   *Marketing Staff:* 1
     Ownership: Private
     Produces/Sells CE-marked Devices: Y
     Federal Procurement Eligibility: Small Business, Female Owned
     Distribution: Manufacturer Direct, Manufacturer Through Distributor, Manufacturer Through Manufacturer Reps, Exporter
     General Admin.: H. Joshua/General Manager
                 J. Joshua/President
     Mktg./Adv.: H. Joshua/Director Product Development
     Research: Henry Joshua/Vice President Research & Development
     Accessories, Chromatography (Gas, Gel, Liquid, Thin Layer)   Chemistry
     Equipment, Analysis, Photochemical   Chemistry
     Extraction/Chromatography, Ninhydrin, Hydroxyproline   Chemistry

AURA LENS PRODUCTS, INC.   800-281-2872
     51 8th St. N., PO Box 763, St. Cloud,,   320-253-0919
     Sauk Rapids, MN 56379
     FDA Number: n/a   *Fax:* 320-253-1239
     E-mail: sales@auralens.com
     Web site: www.auralens.com
     Medical Products Sales Volume: $180,000
     Annual Revenue: $0-$1 Million
     Year Founded: 1975
     Total Employees: 5   *Marketing Staff:* 1   *Sales Staff:* 1
     Ownership: Private
     Produces/Sells CE-marked Devices: N
     Federal Procurement Eligibility: Small Business
     Distribution: Manufacturer Direct, Manufacturer Through Distributor, Manufacturer Through Manufacturer Reps, Importer, Exporter
     General Admin.: Michael Aurelius/President
     Accessories, Laser   General
     Eyeglasses   Ophthalmology
     Eyeglasses, Safety   Ophthalmology
     Mask, Face   General
     Safety Equipment, Laboratory   Chemistry
     Shield, Ophthalmic, Radiological   Radiology

AURADONICS INCORPORATED   856-764-8866
     439 St. Mihiel Dr., Riverside, NJ 08075
     FDA Number: 2247665   *Fax:* 856 764-8660
     E-mail: nancy@auradonics.com
     Web site: www.auradonics.com/
     Medical Products Sales Volume: $1,400,000
     Year Founded: 1989
     Total Employees: 12   *Marketing Staff:* 1
     Ownership: Private
     Produces/Sells CE-marked Devices: Y
     Distribution: Manufacturer Direct, Manufacturer Through Distributor
     General Admin.: John Ianieri/President
                 Nancy Ianieri/Vice President
     Band, Elastic, Orthodontic   Dental And Oral
     Bracket, Metal, Orthodontic   Dental And Oral

AURIDENT, INC.   800-422-7373
     P.O. Box 7200, 610 South State College Blvd.,   714-523-5544
     Fullerton, CA 92631
     FDA Number: 2023817   *Fax:* 714-870-0608
     E-mail: info@aurident.com
     Web site: www.aurident.com
     Ownership: Private
     Produces/Sells CE-marked Devices: N
     Alloy, Gold Based, For Clinical Use   Dental And Oral
     Alloy, Precious Metal, For Clinical Use   Dental And Oral
     Teeth, Porcelain   Dental And Oral

AURIUM RESEARCH CORP.
     See Argen Corp.

AURORA BIOMED INC.   800-883-2918
     1001 East Pender St.,   604-215-8700
     Vancouver, BC V6A-1 Canada
     FDA Number: n/a   *Fax:* 604-215-9700
     E-mail: info@aurora-instr.com
     Web site: www.aurora-instr.com
     Year Founded: 1990
     Ownership: Private
     Produces/Sells CE-marked Devices: N

AURORA BIOMED INC.   800-883-2918 *(cont'd)*
     Distribution: Manufacturer Direct, Exclusive Distributor, Exporter

AURORA IMAGING TECHNOLOGY, INC.   877-975-7530
     39 High St., North Andover, MA 01845
     FDA Number: 1225267
     E-mail: info@auroramri.com
     Web site: www.auroramri.com
     Ownership: Private
     Produces/Sells CE-marked Devices: N
     Nuclear Magnetic Resonance Imaging System   Radiology

AURUM CERAMIC DENTAL LABORATORIES LLP   800-423-6509
     1320 North Howard St.,   509-326-5885
     Spokane, WA 99201
     FDA Number: 3031799
     E-mail: aurumspokane@aurumgroup.com
     Web site: www.aurumgroup.com
     Ownership: Private
     Produces/Sells CE-marked Devices: N
     Crown, Preformed   Dental And Oral
     Positioner, Tooth, Preformed   Dental And Oral
     Retainer, Screw Expansion, Orthodontic   Dental And Oral
     Teeth, Artificial, Posterior With Metal Insert   Dental And Oral
     Tray, Impression   Dental And Oral

AUSHON BIOSYSTEMS, INC.   978-436-6400
     43 Manning Rd, Billerica, MA 01821
     FDA Number: n/a   *Fax:* 978-667-3970
     E-mail: info@aushon.com
     Web site: http://www.aushon.com/
     Ownership: Private
     Produces/Sells CE-marked Devices: N
     General Admin.: Mr. Joseph Blanchard/Chief Operating Officer
                 Mr. Peter Honkanen/President, Chief Executive Officer
     Production: Mr. Kevin Oliver/Vice President Manufacturing & Engineering
     Research: Dr. Christine Burns/Vice President Research & Development
     Finance: Mr. Ken Titlebaum/Chief Financial Officer
     Test, DNA-Probe, Other   Microbiology

AUSONICS CORP., THE
     See Instrumentarium Imaging, Inc.

AUSTENAL, INC.
     See Dentsply Prosthetics

AUSTIN AIR SYSTEMS LIMITED   716-856-3700
     500 Elk Street, Buffalo, NY 14210
     FDA Number: 42983   *Fax:* 716-856-6023
     E-mail: info@austinair.com
     Web site: www.austinair.com
     Year Founded: 1990
     Ownership: Private
     Produces/Sells CE-marked Devices: N
     Distribution: Manufacturer Direct, Manufacturer Through Distributor, Manufacturer Through Manufacturer Reps, Exporter
     General Admin.: Richard Taylor/President
     Mktg./Adv.: David Fuller/Manager Sales
     Equipment, Cleaning, Air   General

AUSTIN MEDICAL PRODUCTS, INC.   800-223-9310
     66 Eastern Ave., P.O. Box 1830, Conway, NH 03818
     FDA Number: 1220581
     E-mail: info@ampatch.com
     Web site: www.ampatch.com
     Annual Revenue: $0-$1 Million
     Year Founded: 1982
     Total Employees: 5
     Ownership: Private
     Produces/Sells CE-marked Devices: N
     Federal Procurement Eligibility: Small Business
     Distribution: Manufacturer Direct
     General Admin.: William C. Brown/President
     Protector, Ostomy   Gastroenterology/Urology

AUSTIN OCULAR PROSTHETICS CENTER, LLC   512-452-3100
     711 W 38th Street Suite G1a, Austin, TX 78705
     FDA Number: 3007067162
     Ownership: Private
     Produces/Sells CE-marked Devices: N
     Conformer, Ophthalmic   Ophthalmology
     Eye, Artificial, Non-Custom   Ophthalmology
     Shell, Scleral   Ophthalmology

AUTH CO.
     See Pacific Electronics

AUTH-FLORENCE
     See Pacific Electronics

MANUFACTURER PROFILES

AUTO CONTROL MEDICAL INC.   800-461-0991
6695 Millcreek Dr., Unit 5,   **905-814-6350**
Mississauga, ONT L5N-5 Canada
FDA Number: n/a   Fax: 905-814-6355
E-mail: info@autocontrol.com
Web site: www.autocontrol.com
Year Founded: 1993
Total Employees: 50
Ownership: Private
Produces/Sells CE-marked Devices: N
Distribution: Exclusive Distributor

AUTOGENESIS, INC.   888-325-2017
8700 Old Harford Road, Baltimore, MD 21218   **410-665-2017**
FDA Number: 3026254   Fax: 410-665-1616
E-mail: james.r.edw@gmail.com
Web site: www.autogenesisinfo.com
Annual Revenue: $0-$1 Million
Year Founded: 1989
Total Employees: 2
Ownership: Private
Produces/Sells CE-marked Devices: N
Federal Procurement Eligibility: Small Business
Distribution: Manufacturer Direct
General Admin.: James Edwards/President, Chief Executive Officer

Appliance, Fix., Nail/Blade/Plate Comb., Multiple Component	Orthopedics
Component, Traction, Invasive	Orthopedics
Stimulator, Osteogenesis, Electric, Non-Invasive	Orthopedics

AUTOGENOMICS, INCORPORATED   760-477-2251
2890 Scott St, Vista, CA 92081
FDA Number: 3005406097   Fax: 760-477-2252
E-mail: info@autogenomics.com
Web site: www.autogenomics.com
Year Founded: 1999
Ownership: Private
Produces/Sells CE-marked Devices: N
General Admin.: Nanibhushan Dattagupta/Chief Scientific Officer
     Fareed Kureshy/President, Chief Executive Officer, Chairman
Mktg./Adv.: Ramanath Vairavan/Senior Vice President Marketing & Sales
     Raymond Earl/Vice President Sales
Production: Saeed Kureshy/Vice President Operations
     Evelyn Lopez/Vice President Regulatory Affairs
Finance: Thomas Hennessey/Chief Financial Officer
     Jeffrey Irwin/Director Finance
IS: Shelley Singh/Vice President Systems

Instrumentation For Clinical Multiplex Test Systems	Chemistry
Reagents, Specific, Analyte	Hematology
Test, Factor Ii G20210a Mutations, Genomic Dna Pcr	Hematology
Test, Factor V Leiden Mutations, Genomic Dna Pcr	Hematology

AUTOLAB DIV.
See Spectra-Physics Lazors

AUTOMATED HEALTHCARE, INC.
See Mckesson

AUTOMATED IMAGING ASSOCIATION   800-994-6099
900 Victors Way, PO Box 3724,   **734-994-6088**
Ann Arbor, MI 48106
FDA Number: n/a   Fax: 734-994-3338
E-mail: info@machinevisiononline.org
Web site: www.machinevisiononline.org
Medical Products Sales Volume: $700,000
Year Founded: 1984
Total Employees: 12
Ownership: Private
Produces/Sells CE-marked Devices: N
Federal Procurement Eligibility: Small Business
General Admin.: Jeffrey A. Burnstein/Executive Director
Mktg./Adv.: Dana Whalls/Manager Marketing

Service, Consulting	General

AUTOMATED MEDICAL PRODUCTS CORP.   800-832-4567
P.O. Box 2508, Edison, NJ 08818-2508   **732-602-7717**
FDA Number: 2431453   Fax: 732-602-7706
E-mail: jbrown@ironintern.com
Web site: www.ironintern.com
Medical Products Sales Volume: $900,000
Annual Revenue: $0-$1 Million
Year Founded: 1977
Total Employees: 7   Marketing Staff: 4   Sales Staff: 15
Ownership: Private
Quality System Registration Information: ISO9002
Produces/Sells CE-marked Devices: Y
Federal Procurement Eligibility: Small Business
Distribution: Exclusive Distributor
General Admin.: Jerry M. Brown/Chief Executive Officer

AUTOMATED MEDICAL PRODUCTS CORP. 800-832-4567 *(cont'd)*
Janice Polites/President

Cable, Fiberoptic	General
Dilator, Fascia, Umbilical	Surgery
Holder, Instrument, Laparoscopic	Surgery
Holder, Laparoscope	Obstetrics/Gynecology
Holder, Retractor	Surgery
Hook, Gastro-Urology	Gastroenterology/Urology
Laparoscope, General & Plastic Surgery	Surgery
Retractor	Orthopedics
Retractor, Fan-Type, Laparoscopy	Surgery
Retractor, Fiberoptic	Gastroenterology/Urology
Retractor, Laparoscopy, Other	Surgery
Retractor, Manual	Cns/Neurology
Retractor, Other	Surgery
Retractor, Self-Retaining	Gastroenterology/Urology
Retractor, Surgical	Surgery
Retractor, Vaginal	Obstetrics/Gynecology
Surgical Instrument, Manual (General Use)	Surgery

AUTOMATIC FILM PROCESSOR CORP.
See Afp Imaging Corp.

AUTOMATIC LIQUID PACKAGING INC.
See Weiler Engineering, Inc.

AUTOMOBILITY MANUFACTURING CORPORATION   800-470-7067
1444 Lorne St., Regina S4R-2K4 Canada   **306-791-9840**
FDA Number: n/a   Fax: 306-525-0282
E-mail: automobility@net1fx.com
Web site: www.handcontrolscorp.com
Year Founded: 1991
Total Employees: 10
Ownership: Private
Produces/Sells CE-marked Devices: N
Distribution: Manufacturer Direct, Exclusive Distributor, Importer, Exporter

AUTOVAGE   412-653-5888
1631 Citation Dr., South Park, PA 15129
FDA Number: 2521802
Ownership: Private
Produces/Sells CE-marked Devices: N

Catheter, Irrigation	Surgery
Tube, Gastrointestinal	Gastroenterology/Urology

AVADA EYEWEAR INC.   800-844-2034
5605 Florida Mining Blvd. Bldg. 200, Suite 210,   **904-260-6361**
Jacksonville, FL 32257
FDA Number: 1063179   Fax: 800-299-0034
E-mail: customerservice@avadaeyewear.com
Web site: www.avadaeyewear.com
Medical Products Sales Volume: $160,000
Year Founded: 1994
Total Employees: 3
Ownership: Private
Produces/Sells CE-marked Devices: N
Federal Procurement Eligibility: Small Business
Distribution: Manufacturer Through Manufacturer Reps

Frame, Spectacle (Eyeglasses)	Ophthalmology

AVAIL MEDICAL PRODUCTS   858-635-2206
5950 Nancy Ridge Dr, Ste 500, San Diego, CA 92121
FDA Number: 2024124
Ownership: Avail Medical Products, Inc.

Container, IV	General
Transfer Unit, IV Fluid	General

AVAIL MEDICAL PRODUCTS, INC.   858-635-2206
1225 N. 28th Avenue, Suite 500, Dallas, TX 75261
FDA Number: 1629295
Ownership: Avail Medical Products, Inc.
Produces/Sells CE-marked Devices: N

Bag, Collection, Urine, Newborn	General
Drape, Surgical	Surgery
Endoscope	Gastroenterology/Urology
Mesh, Surgical, Polymeric	Surgery
Suction Apparatus, Ward Use, Portable, AC-Powered	Surgery

AVAIL MEDICAL PRODUCTS, INC.   858-635-2206
1900 Carnegie Ave., --, Santa Ana, CA 92705
FDA Number: 2025848
Ownership: Avail Medical Products, Inc.
Produces/Sells CE-marked Devices: N

Stapler, Surgical	Surgery

AVAIL MEDICAL PRODUCTS-ASHEVILLE   858-635-2206
3161 Sweeten Creek Road, Asheville, NC 28803
FDA Number: 1066958
Ownership: Avail Medical Products, Inc.

AVAIL MEDICAL PRODUCTS-ASHEVILLE 858-635-2206 *(cont'd)*
Produces/Sells CE-marked Devices: N
  Mouthpiece, Breathing   Anesthesiology

AVALON LABORATORIES
See Avalon Laboratories, Inc.

AVALON LABORATORIES, INC. 866-938-6613
2610 E Homestead Place, 310-761-8660
Rancho Dominguez, CA 90220
FDA Number: 2032228   *Fax:* 310-761-8665
E-mail: info@avalonlabs.com
Web site: www.avalonlabs.com
Annual Revenue: $10-$25 Million
Year Founded: 1990
Ownership: Private
Produces/Sells CE-marked Devices: Y
Distribution: Manufacturer Direct, Manufacturer Through Distributor, OEM, Importer, Exporter
  Cannula, Aortic   Cardiovascular
  Cannula, Coronary Artery   Cardiovascular
  Cannula, Venous   Cardiovascular
  Tube, Bronchial (W/Wo Connector)   Anesthesiology
  Tube, Tracheal (Endotracheal)   Anesthesiology

AVALON SOFTWARE, INC.
See I.F.S. Industrial & Financial Systems

AVANT MEDICAL CORP. 858-202-1560
10225 Barnes Canyon Rd.,, Suite A113, San Diego, CA 92121
FDA Number: n/a
Ownership: Private
Produces/Sells CE-marked Devices: N
  Injector, Fluid, Non-Electric   General

AVANTEC VASCULAR CORP. 408-329-5425
605 W. W. California Ave, Sunnyvale, CA 94086
FDA Number: 3003524171   *Fax:* 408-329-5499
E-mail: marketing@avantecvascular.com
Web site: www.avantecvascular.com
Ownership: Private
Produces/Sells CE-marked Devices: N
  Catheter, Angioplasty, Coronary, Transluminal, Percut. Oper.   Cardiovascular
  Guidewire, Catheter   Cardiovascular
  Stent, Cardiovascular   Cardiovascular

AVANTI POLAR LIPIDS, INC. 800-227-0651
700 Industrial Park Drive, Alabaster, AL 35007 205-663-2494
FDA Number: 1036868   *Fax:* 205-663-0756
E-mail: info@avantilipids.com
Web site: www.avantilipids.com
Medical Products Sales Volume: $4,600,000
Annual Revenue: $5-$10 Million
Year Founded: 1969
Total Employees: 53   *Marketing Staff:* 1   *Sales Staff:* 5
Ownership: Private
Produces/Sells CE-marked Devices: N
Federal Procurement Eligibility: Small Business
Distribution: Manufacturer Direct
General Admin.: Walter Shaw/President
Mktg./Adv.: Malcolm Fifer/Director Marketing
       Stephen Burgess/Director Product Development
       Rowena Shaw/Vice President Marketing
Production: Rowena Shaw/Vice President Manufacturing
  Standard, Lipid   Chemistry

AVANTIS MEDICAL SYSTEMS, INC. 408-733-1901
263 Santa Ana Ct., Sunnyvale, CA 94085
FDA Number: 3006315255
Web site: http://www.avantismedical.com
Year Founded: 2004
Ownership: Private
Produces/Sells CE-marked Devices: N
General Admin.: Mr. Scott Dodson/President, Chief Executive Officer
 Medical Admin.: Dr. Jack Higgins/Chief Medical Officer
Mktg./Adv.: Mr. Doug Gielow/Vice President Marketing & Sales
Production: Mr. John Reed/Senior Vice President Manufacturing
Research: Mr. Chad Roue/Vice President Research & Development
Finance: Mr. Dan George/Chief Financial Officer
  Biopsy Instrument   Gastroenterology/Urology
  Colonoscope, Gastro-Urology   Gastroenterology/Urology
  Endoscope   Gastroenterology/Urology
  Gastroscope, Gastro-Urology   Gastroenterology/Urology

AVANTOR PERFORMANCE MATERIALS 800-243-3768
222 Red School Lane, Phillipsburg, NJ 08865
FDA Number: n/a   *Fax:* 908-859-9318
E-mail: sales@chemical.net
Web site: http://www.avantormaterials.com
Year Founded: 1995

AVANTOR PERFORMANCE MATERIALS 800-243-3768 *(cont'd)*
Ownership: COVIDIEN LTD.
Stock Symbol: COV
Traded On: NYSE
Produces/Sells CE-marked Devices: N
General Admin.: Mr. Jean-Marc Gilson/Chief Executive Officer
       Mr. Robert Harrer/Chief Financial Officer, Executive Vice President
       Mr. Rajiv Gupta/Executive Chairman
       Mr. Robert Ferguson/Executive Vice President
Production: Mr. Brian Wilson/Executive Vice President Operations
  Celloidin   Pathology
  Collodion   Pathology
  Container, Embedding   Pathology
  Fixative, Alcohol Containing   Pathology
  Formaldehyde (Formalin, Formol)   Pathology
  Formalin, Neutral Buffered   Pathology
  Fuchsin, Basic   Pathology
  Preservative, Cytological   Pathology
  Reagent, General Purpose   Pathology
  Solution, Pathology, Decalcifier, Acid Containing   Pathology
  Stain, Acid Fuchsin   Pathology
  Stain, Aniline Blue   Pathology
  Stain, Auramine O   Pathology
  Stain, Carmine   Pathology
  Stain, Congo Red   Pathology
  Stain, Crystal Violet, Histology   Pathology
  Stain, Eosin B   Pathology
  Stain, Eosin Y   Pathology
  Stain, Erythrosin B   Pathology
  Stain, Fast Green   Pathology
  Stain, Giemsa   Pathology
  Stain, Hematoxylin   Pathology
  Stain, Indigocarmine   Pathology
  Stain, Light Green   Pathology
  Stain, Malachite Green   Pathology
  Stain, Methylene Blue   Pathology
  Stain, Microbiological   Microbiology
  Stain, Neutral Red   Pathology
  Stain, Orange G   Pathology
  Stain, Phloxine B   Pathology
  Stain, Reagent, Schiff   Pathology
  Stain, Rose Bengal   Pathology
  Stain, Safranin   Pathology
  Stain, Wright's   Pathology
  Sudan IV   Pathology

AVANTOR PERFORMANCE MATERIALS, INC. 800-582-2537
7001 Martin Luther King Blvd, Paris, KY 40361
FDA Number: 1045125
E-mail: info@avantormaterials.com
Web site: http://www.avantormaterials.com
Year Founded: 1995
Ownership: COVIDIEN LTD.
Stock Symbol: COV
Traded On: NYSE
Produces/Sells CE-marked Devices: N
  Collodion   Pathology
  Container, Embedding   Pathology
  Preservative, Cytological   Pathology
  Stain, Carmine   Pathology
  Stain, Congo Red   Pathology
  Stain, Eosin Y   Pathology
  Stain, Erythrosin B   Pathology
  Stain, Fast Green   Pathology
  Stain, Giemsa   Pathology
  Stain, Hematoxylin   Pathology
  Stain, Indigocarmine   Pathology
  Stain, Light Green   Pathology
  Stain, Malachite Green   Pathology
  Stain, Microbiological   Microbiology
  Stain, Neutral Red   Pathology
  Stain, Orange G   Pathology
  Stain, Wright's   Pathology

AVAZZIA, INC. 214-575-2820
13140 Coit Rd., Suite 515, Dallas, TX 75240
FDA Number: 3004839404   *Fax:* 214-575-2824
E-mail: info@avazzia.com
Web site: www.avazzia.com
Ownership: Private
Produces/Sells CE-marked Devices: N
  Binder, Medical, Therapeutic   General
  Biofeedback Device   Cns/Neurology
  Electrode, Cutaneous   Cns/Neurology
  Massager, Therapeutic   Physical Med
  Stimulator, Incontinence (Non-Implantable), Electrical   Gastroenterology/Urology
  Stimulator, Nerve, Transcutaneous (Pain Relief, TENS)   Cns/Neurology

AVCOR HEALTH CARE PRODUCTS, INC.　　800-282-6748
One Southfield Square, 1520 Everman Pkwy.,
Fort Worth, TX 76140
FDA Number: 1649245
E-mail: custservice@avcorhealth.com
Web site: www.avcorhealth.com
Ownership: Private
Quality System Registration Information: ISO9000
Produces/Sells CE-marked Devices: N
Federal Procurement Eligibility: Small Business
Distribution: Manufacturer Through Distributor, Manufacturer Through
Manufacturer Reps, Exporter

Bag, Ice	General
Bandage, Elastic	General
Fiber, Absorbent	General
Tourniquet	General

AVD　　503-223-2333
2326 NW Everett St., Portland, OR 97210
FDA Number: 3032534　　　　*Fax:* 503-223-8585
E-mail: info@compressar.com
Web site: www.semlertechnologies.com
Medical Products Sales Volume: $2,400,000
Year Founded: 1998
Total Employees: 10
Ownership: Private
Produces/Sells CE-marked Devices: Y
Federal Procurement Eligibility: Small Business
Distribution: Manufacturer Direct, Manufacturer Through Distributor

Device, Hemostasis, Vascular	Cardiovascular

AVECOR CARDIOVASCULAR, INC.
See Medtronic Perfusion Systems

AVEDRO, INC.　　781-768-3400
230 Third Avenue, Waltham, MA 02451
FDA Number: 300785105　　　*Fax:* 781-768-3401
Web site: www.avedro.com
Ownership: Private
Produces/Sells CE-marked Devices: N
General Admin.: Dr. David Muller/President, Chief Executive Officer
Mktg./Adv.: Mr. Steve Binn/Director Marketing
Production: Mr. Evan Sherr/Vice President Operations
Research: Dr. Howard Loree/Chief Scientist
　　　　Dr. Ronald Scharff/Vice President Engineering
Finance: Rhonda Bracey/Chief Financial Officer

Cautery, Radiofrequency, AC-Powered	Ophthalmology
Shield, Eye, Ophthalmic	Ophthalmology

AVENT AMERICA, INC.
See Philips Avent

AVENT S.A. DE C.V.　　602-748-6900
Camino De Libramiento, Km. 1.5, Nogales, Sonora Mexico
FDA Number: 9611594

Bandage, Adhesive	Surgery
Gown, Isolation, Surgical	Surgery
Gown, Surgical	Surgery
Pack, Sterilization Wrapper (Bag And Accessories)	Surgery

AVENT S.A. DE C.V.　　770-587-8393
Carretera Intl., Salida Norte, Magdalena, Sonora Mexico
FDA Number: 8030647

Gown, Surgical	Surgery
Suit, Surgical	Surgery

AVENTRIC TECHNOLOGIES　　800-228-3343
1551 E. Lincoln Ave., Suite 166, Madison Heights, MI 48071
FDA Number: n/a　　　　*Fax:* 248-542-1248
Web site: www.aventric.com
Medical Products Sales Volume: $1,000,000
Annual Revenue: $1-$5 Million
Ownership: Private
Produces/Sells CE-marked Devices: N
Federal Procurement Eligibility: Small Business
Distribution: Exclusive Distributor

Component, Electronic	General
Recorder, Long-Term, ECG, Portable (Holter Monitor)	Cardiovascular
Service, Maintenance/Repair	General

AVERY BIOMEDICAL DEVICES, INC.　　631-864-1600
61 Mall Dr., Commack, NY 11725-5703
FDA Number: 2427696
Ownership: Private
Produces/Sells CE-marked Devices: N
General Admin.: Linda Towler/Chief Executive Officer

Stimulator, Cerebral, Implantable	Cns/Neurology
Stimulator, Diaphragmatic/Phrenic Nerve, Implantable	Cns/Neurology
Stimulator, Intracerebral/Subcortical, Implantable	Cns/Neurology
Stimulator, Nerve, Transcutaneous (Pain Relief, TENS)	Cns/Neurology

AVERY BIOMEDICAL DEVICES, INC.　　631-864-1600 *(cont'd)*

Stimulator, Peripheral Nerve, Implantable (Pain Relief)	Cns/Neurology
Stimulator, Spinal Cord, Implantable (Pain Relief)	Cns/Neurology
Stimulator, Spinal Cord, Implantable, Bladder Evacuator	Cns/Neurology

AVERY DENNISON CORPORATION　　626-304-2000
150 North Orange Grove Boulevard, Pasadena, CA 91103-3596
FDA Number: n/a　　　　*Fax:* 626-304-2192
E-mail: feedback@averydennison.com
Web site: www.averydennison.com
Medical Products Sales Volume: $5,000,000
Year Founded: 1935
Ownership: Public
Stock Symbol: AVY
Traded On: NYSE
Quality System Registration Information: ISO9000
Produces/Sells CE-marked Devices: N
Distribution: Manufacturer Direct, Manufacturer Through Distributor, Service Direct,
Exclusive Distributor
General Admin.: Mr. Mitchell Butler/Chief Executive Officer
　　　　Mr. Richard Hoffman/Chief Information Officer
　　　　Mr. David Edwards/Chief Technology Officer
　　　　Dean Scarborough/President, Chief Executive Officer

Adhesive, Prosthesis, External	Surgery
Computer, Bar Code	General
Contract Manufacturing	General
Label, Bar Code	General
Label, Device	General
Labeling Equipment	General
Printer, Bar Code	General

AVERY DENNISON MEDICAL
See Avery Dennison Corporation

AVESTIN INC.　　888-283-7846
2450 Don Reid Dr., Ottawa, ONT K1H-8P5 Canada　　613-736-0019
FDA Number: n/a　　　　*Fax:* 613-736-8086
E-mail: avestin@avestin.com
Web site: www.avestin.com
Year Founded: 1988
Ownership: Private
Produces/Sells CE-marked Devices: N
Distribution: Exporter

AVEX INDUSTRIES, LTD.　　518-747-3310
27 Allen St., Hudson Falls, NY 12839
FDA Number: n/a
Ownership: Private
Produces/Sells CE-marked Devices: N

Booth, Sun Tan	Physical Med
Light, Ultraviolet, Dermatologic	Surgery

AVI BIOPHARMA, INC.　　503-227-0554
4575 SW Research Way, Suite 200, Corvallis, OR 97333
FDA Number: n/a　　　　*Fax:* 503-227-0751
E-mail: avi@avibio.com
Web site: www.avibio.com
Medical Products Sales Volume: $120,000
Annual Revenue: $0-$1 Million
Year Founded: 1980
Total Employees: 120
Ownership: Public
Stock Symbol: AVII
Traded On: NASDAQ
Produces/Sells CE-marked Devices: N
Federal Procurement Eligibility: Small Business
General Admin.: Denis R. Burger/Chief Executive Officer
　　　　Mr. Alan P. Timmins/President
Production: Dr. Dwight D. Weller/Senior Vice President Manufacturing
Research: Dr. David H. Mason, Jr./Senior Vice President Clinical Research
　　　　Dr. Patrick L. Iversen/Senior Vice President Research & Development
Finance: Mr. Mark M. Webber/Chief Financial Officer

Genetic Engineering	Microbiology

AVI-ADVANCED VISUAL INSTRUMENTS INC.　　212-262-7878
321 West 44th St., Suite 902, New York, NY 10036
FDA Number: 3005669220

Frame, Trial, Ophthalmic	Ophthalmology
Lens, Contact, Polymethylmethacrylate, Diagnostic	Ophthalmology
Microscope, Operating, Non-Electric, Ophthalmic	Ophthalmology

AVIARADX, INC.　　877-886-6739
9640 Towne Centre Dr, Ste. 200,　　858-587-5870
San Diego, CA 92121
FDA Number: n/a　　　　*Fax:* 858-587-5874
E-mail: molecular@biotheranostics.com
Ownership: Private
Produces/Sells CE-marked Devices: N

Equipment, Laboratory, Gen. Purpose (Specific Medical Use)	Chemistry

AVIARADX, INC. 877-886-6739 *(cont'd)*
Reagent, General Purpose Pathology

AVICENNA LASER TECHNOLOGY, INC. 888-AVI-LASER
1209 N. Flagler Dr., West Palm Beach, FL 33401 561-722-1153
FDA Number: 3004108999 Fax: 561-478-1758
E-mail: info@avicennalaser.com
Web site: www.avicennalaser.com
Ownership: Private
Produces/Sells CE-marked Devices: N
General Admin.: Mrs. Bruce Coren/Chairman, Chief Executive Officer
Lamp, Infrared Physical Med

AVICON INC.
See Alcon Research, Ltd.

AVID MEDICAL 800-886-0584
9000 Westmont Drive 888-564-7153
Stonehouse Commerce Park
Toano, VA 23168
FDA Number: 1047429 Fax: 757-566-8707
E-mail: avidoem@avidmedical.com
Web site: www.avidmedical.com
Medical Products Sales Volume: $53,400,000
Annual Revenue: $50-$100 Million
Year Founded: 1997
Total Employees: 355   Marketing Staff: 2   Sales Staff: 1
Ownership: Private
Quality System Registration Information: ISO9001
Produces/Sells CE-marked Devices: N
Federal Procurement Eligibility: Small Business, GSA Contract
Distribution: Manufacturer Direct, Service Direct, Importer, Exporter
General Admin.: Mr. Michael Sahady/Chief Executive Officer
            Mr. Rick Setian/President, Chief Operating Officer
            Joe Harms/Vice President, General Manager
Mktg./Adv.: Scott Henderson/Director Product Development
Production: Mr. Robert Dalby/Manager Product Support
            Mr. Larry Bogues/Manager Quality Assurance & Quality Control
            Larry Bogues/Manager Regulatory Affairs
Chamber, Decompression, Abdominal Obstetrics/Gynecology
Kit, Biopsy Needle Gastroenterology/Urology
Needle, Conduction, Anesthesia (W/Wo Introducer) Anesthesiology
Needle, Gastro-Urology Gastroenterology/Urology
Needle, Hypodermic, Single Lumen With Syringe General
Needle, Spinal, Short-Term General

AVID PRODUCTS 888-575-AVID
Aquidneck Industrial Park 401-846-1300
72 Johnny Cake Hill Rd.
Middletown, RI 02842
FDA Number: n/a Fax: 401-849-1060
E-mail: sales@avidproducts.com
Web site: www.avidcareproducts.com
Medical Products Sales Volume: $9,000,000
Year Founded: 1962
Ownership: Private
Quality System Registration Information: ISO9002
Produces/Sells CE-marked Devices: Y
Distribution: Importer, Exporter
General Admin.: Mr. Frank T. Vollaro/President
            Ms. Linda Gibeau/Vice President Human Resources
            Mr. Thomas G. Mockler/Vice President, General Manager
Mktg./Adv.: Ms. Erin Moriarity/Sales Representative
Production: Mr. Preston James/Vice President Manufacturing
Mask, Other General
Pillow General
Television, Patient Room General

AVIDA HEALTHWEAR INC. 800-361-9811
87 Northline Rd., Toronto, ONT M4B-3E9 Canada 416-751-5874
FDA Number: n/a Fax: 416-751-5875
E-mail: avida@sprint.ca
Web site: www.avidahealthwear.com
Year Founded: 1983
Total Employees: 100
Ownership: Private
Produces/Sells CE-marked Devices: N
Distribution: Manufacturer Direct, Exclusive Distributor

AVINGER INC. 650-363-2400
400 Chesapeake, Redwood City, CA 94063
FDA Number: 3007498664 Fax: 650-363-2401
E-mail: info@avinger.com
Web site: www.avinger.com
Ownership: Private
Produces/Sells CE-marked Devices: N
Mktg./Adv.: Mr. John Simpson/Vice President Commercial Operations
Production: Ms. Susan Hale/Director Quality Assurance

AVINGER INC. 650-363-2400 *(cont'd)*
Catheter, Percutaneous Cardiovascular

AVIV BIOMEDICAL, INC. 732-370-1300
750 Vassar Avenue, Lakewood, NJ 08701-6907
FDA Number: 2243455 Fax: 732-370-1303
E-mail: info@avivbiomedical.com
Web site: www.avivbiomedical.com
Annual Revenue: $1-$5 Million
Year Founded: 1971
Total Employees: 12
Ownership: Private
Produces/Sells CE-marked Devices: Y
Federal Procurement Eligibility: Small Business, GSA Contract
Distribution: Manufacturer Direct, Manufacturer Through Manufacturer Reps,
Service Direct, Exporter
General Admin.: Jack Aviv/President, Chief Executive Officer
Mktg./Adv.: Flo Aviv/Manager Business
Fluorometer, Toxicology Toxicology
Protoporphyrin Zinc Method, Fluorometric, Lead Toxicology
Protoporphyrin, Fluorometric, Lead Toxicology

AVNET, INC. 480-643-2000
2211 S. 47th St., Phoenix, AZ 85034
FDA Number: n/a
Ownership: Private
Produces/Sells CE-marked Devices: N
Device, Storage, Image, Digital Radiology
Image Processing System Radiology

AVON-ISI 888-ISI-SAFE
922 Hurricane Shoals Road, 678-495-3700
Lawrenceville, GA 30043
FDA Number: n/a Fax: 678-495-3875
E-mail: customer_service@avon-rubber.com
Web site: www.intsafety.com
Medical Products Sales Volume: $5,800,000
Annual Revenue: $10-$25 Million
Year Founded: 1980
Total Employees: 80   Marketing Staff: 5   Sales Staff: 6
Ownership: Private
Quality System Registration Information: ISO9001
Produces/Sells CE-marked Devices: N
Federal Procurement Eligibility: Small Business
Distribution: Manufacturer Through Distributor, Manufacturer Through
Manufacturer Reps, OEM, Service Direct, Exporter
General Admin.: Donald Dawson/President
Mktg./Adv.: Mike Vezmar/Manager National Marketing & Sales
Ventilator, Other Anesthesiology

AVONDALE BADGE CO 800-874-2551
4114 Herschel St., Suite 101, 904-384-8580
Jacksonville, FL 32210
FDA Number: 895797 Fax: 904-384-8422
E-mail: info@avondalebadge.com
Web site: www.avondalebadge.com
Annual Revenue: $0-$1 Million
Year Founded: 1979
Ownership: Private
Produces/Sells CE-marked Devices: N
Federal Procurement Eligibility: Minority Owned, Female Owned
Distribution: Manufacturer Direct
General Admin.: Nancy Rosenbloom/President, Chief Executive Officer
Bracelet, Identification General
Card, Identification General

AVONDALE DIV.
See Agilent Technologies, Inc.

AVOTEC, INC. 800-272-2238
603 N.W. Buck Hendry Way, Stuart, FL 34994 772-692-0750
FDA Number: 1055916 Fax: 772-692-0788
E-mail: avotec@avotecinc.com
Web site: www.avotec.org
Medical Products Sales Volume: $2,000,000
Annual Revenue: $1-$5 Million
Year Founded: 1990
Total Employees: 20   Marketing Staff: 1   Sales Staff: 1
Ownership: Private
Quality System Registration Information: ISO9001
Produces/Sells CE-marked Devices: Y
Federal Procurement Eligibility: Small Business
Distribution: Manufacturer Direct, Manufacturer Through Distributor, OEM,
Exclusive Distributor, Exporter
General Admin.: Paul Bullwinkel/President
Mktg./Adv.: James Schmidt/Vice President Marketing & Sales
Nuclear Magnetic Resonance Imaging System Radiology

AVOTEC, INC.   800-272-2238 *(cont'd)*
Transmitter, Image & Data, Radiographic   Radiology

AVOX SYSTEMS   866-278-3237
225 Erie Street, Lancaster, NY 14086-9502
FDA Number: n/a   Fax: 716-686-1553
Web site: www.avoxsys.com
Annual Revenue: $1-$5 Million
Ownership: Private
Quality System Registration Information: ISO9002
Produces/Sells CE-marked Devices: N
Distribution: Manufacturer Through Distributor, Manufacturer Through
Manufacturer Reps, OEM, Service Direct

Alarm, Central Gas System	Anesthesiology
Canister, Oxygen	Anesthesiology
Forceps, Biopsy	Surgery
Kit, Administration, Oxygen	Anesthesiology
Kit, First Aid	Surgery
Mask, Gas, Anesthesia	Anesthesiology
Mask, Oxygen, Aerosol Administration	Anesthesiology
Regulator, Oxygen, Mechanical	General
Regulator, Pressure, Gas Cylinder	Anesthesiology
Resuscitator, Emergency Oxygen	Dental And Oral
Solution, Instrument, Laparoscopic, Anti-Fog	General
Splint, Extremity, Non-Inflatable, External	Surgery
Stretcher, Transfer	Surgery
Tourniquet, Non-Pneumatic, Surgical	Surgery

AVREO, INC.   800-354-0680
4050 Azalea Road, Charleston, SC 29406
FDA Number: 2320618   Fax: 843-571-5996
E-mail: greg@cmsimaging.com
Web site: www.austinair.com
Ownership: Private
Produces/Sells CE-marked Devices: N
Distribution: Manufacturer Direct, Manufacturer Through Distributor

Computer and Software, Medical	General
Image Processing System	Radiology

AVRY'S ORTHOTIC FACILITY, INC.   330-746-5385
1441 Wick Ave., Youngstown, OH 44505
FDA Number: 1522343
Ownership: Private
Produces/Sells CE-marked Devices: N

Orthosis, Limb Brace	Physical Med
Orthosis, Lumbosacral	Physical Med
Orthosis, Thoracic	Physical Med

AW JUSTMAN BRUSH COMPANY
See Justman Brush Co.

AWARENESS TECHNOLOGY, INC.   722-283-6540
1935 S.W. Martin Hwy., Palm City, FL 34990
FDA Number: 1036223   Fax: 722-283-8020
E-mail: info@awaretech.com
Web site: www.awaretech.com
Medical Products Sales Volume: $17,000,000
Annual Revenue: $10-$25 Million
Year Founded: 1982
Total Employees: 125   *Marketing Staff:* 3   *Sales Staff:* 5
Ownership: Private
Produces/Sells CE-marked Devices: Y
Federal Procurement Eligibility: Small Business
Distribution: Manufacturer Direct, Manufacturer Through Distributor, OEM,
Exclusive Distributor, Exporter
General Admin.: Mary Freeman/President, Chief Executive Officer
Mktg./Adv.: Mary Freeman/Director Marketing
     Gary Freeman/Director Product Development
     Chris Schneider/Manager International & National Sales
Production: Steve Andrus/Director Quality Assurance

Colorimeter, General Use	Chemistry
Control, Multi Analyte, All Kinds (Assayed And Unassayed)	Chemistry
Microplate	General
Photometer	Chemistry
Pipetting And Diluting System, Automated	Chemistry
Reader, Microplate	General
Service, Engineering/Design	General
Washer, Microplate	General

AWI INDUSTRIES (USA), INC.   909-597-0808
14502 Central Avenue, Chino, CA 91710
FDA Number: n/a   Fax: 909-597-0082
E-mail: info@awi-industries.com
Web site: www.awi-industries.com
Medical Products Sales Volume: $200,000
Annual Revenue: $0-$1 Million
Year Founded: 1989
Total Employees: 8   *Marketing Staff:* 2   *Sales Staff:* 3
Ownership: Private
Quality System Registration Information: ISO9000; ISO9001; ISO9002

AWI INDUSTRIES (USA), INC.   909-597-0808 *(cont'd)*
Produces/Sells CE-marked Devices: Y
Federal Procurement Eligibility: Small Business, Minority Owned
Distribution: Manufacturer Direct, OEM, Importer, Exporter
General Admin.: Steve Y. Yim/President, Chief Executive Officer
Mktg./Adv.: Eric Yim/Director Marketing
     Stephen Woo/Manager Contract Sales

Accessories, Laser	General
Glove, Patient Examination	General
Lens, Fresnel, Flexible, Diagnostic	Ophthalmology

AXCAN PHARMA INC.   800-950-8085
22 Inverness Center Parkway,   800-472-2634
Birmingham, AL 35242
FDA Number: 1055059
E-mail: custser@axca.com   Fax: 205-991-8426
Web site: www.axcan.com
Medical Products Sales Volume: $292,320,000
Year Founded: 1982
Total Employees: 439
Ownership: Axcan Pharma Inc.
Stock Symbol: AXCA
Traded On: NASDAQ
Produces/Sells CE-marked Devices: Y
Federal Procurement Eligibility: Small Business
General Admin.: David W. Mims/Chief Executive Officer
     John H. Bischofberger/Vice President, General Manager

Cystic Fibrosis System	Gastroenterology/Urology
General Medical Device	General
Trap, Mucus	Anesthesiology

AXCESOR, INC.   1-888-717-1471
2260 Dakota Drive, Grafton, WI 53024   262-375-7530
FDA Number: 2134752   Fax: 262-375-7539
E-mail: solutions@axcesor.com
Web site: www.axcesor.com
Ownership: Private
Produces/Sells CE-marked Devices: N

Blade, Surgical, Saw, General & Plastic Surgery	Surgery
Extractor, Vacuum, Fetal	Obstetrics/Gynecology
Surgical Instrument, Orthopedic, AC-Powered Motor	Orthopedics

AXELA INC.   1-866-923-3363
50 Ronson Dr., Suite 105,   416-798-1625
Toronto, ON M9W 1 Canada
FDA Number: n/a   Fax: 416-798-8635
E-mail: dotlabinfo@axela.com
Web site: www.axelabiosensors.com
Ownership: Private
Produces/Sells CE-marked Devices: N

AXELGAARD MANUFACTURING COMPANY, LTD.   760-728-3430
520 industrial way, Fallbrook, CA 92028-2852
FDA Number: 2025066   Fax: 760-723-2356
E-mail: support@axelgaard.com
Web site: www.axelgaard.com
Medical Products Sales Volume: $16,900,000
Year Founded: 1985
Total Employees: 125
Ownership: Private
Quality System Registration Information: ISO9001
Produces/Sells CE-marked Devices: Y
Federal Procurement Eligibility: Small Business, GSA Contract
Distribution: OEM
General Admin.: Jens Axelgaard/Chief Executive Officer
     Dan P. Jeffery/President
Mktg./Adv.: Don Nelson/Vice President Sales
Production: Lynn Russell/Product Manager

Electrode, Neuromuscular Stimulator	Cns/Neurology
Electrode, TENS	Cns/Neurology

AXIOM ANALYTICAL, INC.   949-757-9300
1451 Edinger Ave, Suite A, Tustin, CA 92780
FDA Number: n/a   Fax: 949-757-9306
E-mail: info@goaxiom.com
Web site: www.goaxiom.com
Annual Revenue: $1-$5 Million
Year Founded: 1988
Ownership: Private
Produces/Sells CE-marked Devices: N
Federal Procurement Eligibility: Small Business
Distribution: Manufacturer Through Distributor, Exporter
General Admin.: Walter Doyle/President, Chief Executive Officer

Contract Laboratory	General
Probe, Other	General

AXIOM MEDICAL, INC.
800-221-8569
19320 Van Ness Ave., Torrance, CA 90501
310-533-9020
FDA Number: 2020735
Fax: 310-533-8127
E-mail: Sales@AxiomMed.com
Web site: www.AxiomMed.com
Annual Revenue: $5-$10 Million
Year Founded: 1976
Total Employees: 40   *Marketing Staff:* 2   *Sales Staff:* 3
Ownership: Private
Quality System Registration Information: ISO9001
Produces/Sells CE-marked Devices: Y
Federal Procurement Eligibility: Small Business, Female Owned, VA Contract
Distribution: Manufacturer Direct, Manufacturer Through Distributor, Manufacturer Through Manufacturer Reps, OEM, Exporter
General Admin.: E. Walker/General Manager
     J. R. Walker/President
Mktg./Adv.: V. De Silva/Manager National Sales
Production: D. Paul/Director Manufacturing & Operations

Bottle, Collection, Vacuum (Aspirator)	General
Catheter, Balloon (Foley Type)	Surgery
Catheter, Conduction, Anesthesia	Anesthesiology
Catheter, Irrigation	Surgery
Catheter, Other	Gastroenterology/Urology
Catheter, Pediatric, General & Plastic Surgery	Surgery
Catheter, Pericardium Drainage	Cardiovascular
Catheter, Ureteral, Gastro-Urology	Gastroenterology/Urology
Catheter, Urinary	Gastroenterology/Urology
Catheter, Urinary, Irrigation	Gastroenterology/Urology
Cover, Clamp	Surgery
Drain, Suction, Closed	Surgery
Drain, Sump	Gastroenterology/Urology
Drain, Thoracic (Chest)	Anesthesiology
Instrument Guard	Surgery
Kit, Wound Drainage	General
Kit, Wound Drainage, Closed	Cns/Neurology
Loop, Vascular	Cardiovascular
Pump, Infusion	General
Retractor, Surgical	Surgery
Sponge, External, Synthetic	Surgery
Trocar, Thoracic	Cardiovascular
Tubing, Multi-Lumen	General
Tubing, Other	General
Tubing, Silicone	General

AXIOM WORLDWIDE, INC.
813-969-2414
9423 Corporate Lake Dr., Tampa, FL 33634-2359
FDA Number: n/a
E-mail: axiom@axiomworldwide.com
Web site: www.axiomworldwide.com
Ownership: Private
Produces/Sells CE-marked Devices: N

Equipment, Traction, Powered	Physical Med

AXIOMED SPINE CORPORATION
216-587-5566
5350 Transportation Blvd., Suite 18,
Garfield Heights, OH 44125
FDA Number: 3007746840
Fax: 216-587-3388
Web site: http://www.axiomed.com
Ownership: Private
Produces/Sells CE-marked Devices: N
General Admin.: Mr. James Kuras/Chief Operating Officer
     Mr. Patrick McBrayer/President, Chief Executive Officer
Production: Mr. Neal Defibaugh/Vice President Regulatory & Clinical Affairs

Prosthesis, Interarticular Disc (Interpositional Implant)	Dental And Oral

AXIS DENTAL
800-355-5063
800 West Sandy Lake Rd., Suite 100, Coppell, TX 75019
FDA Number: 1645240
Web site: www.axisdental.com
Annual Revenue: $5-$10 Million
Year Founded: 1995
Ownership: Private
Quality System Registration Information: ISO9001
Produces/Sells CE-marked Devices: N
Distribution: Manufacturer Through Distributor
General Admin.: Wayne Brown/Chief Financial Officer, Vice President
     Perry Lowe/President, Chief Executive Officer

Cutter, Operative	Dental And Oral
Instrument, Diamond, Dental	Dental And Oral
Wheel, Polishing Agent	Dental And Oral

AXOGEN INC.
888-296-4361
13859 Progress Blvd., Suite 100,
386-462-6800
Alachua, FL 32615
FDA Number: n/a
Fax: 386-462-6801
E-mail: Customerservice@AxoGenInc.com
Web site: www.axogeninc.com
Year Founded: 2002

AXOGEN INC.
888-296-4361 *(cont'd)*
Ownership: Private
Produces/Sells CE-marked Devices: N
General Admin.: Ms. Karen Zaderej/Chief Executive Officer
     Mr. John Engels/Vice President
Mktg./Adv.: Ms. Monica Tarver/Director Marketing
     Mr. Jerry Chang/Director Product Development
     Mr. Brad Hedger/Vice President Sales
Production: Mr. Mike Donovan/Director Operations
     Mr. Mark Friedman/Vice President Quality Assurance & Regulatory Affairs
Research: Mr. Erick DeVinney/Director Clinical Research
     Ms. Marlo Tan Walpole/Director Tech. Development
Finance: Mr. Gregory Freitag/Chief Financial Officer
     Mr. David Hansen/Corporate Controller

Cuff, Nerve	Cns/Neurology

AXON SYSTEMS, INC.
800-888-2966
80-5 Davids Drive, Hauppauge, NY 11788
631-436-5112
FDA Number: 2434986
Fax: 631-436-5141
E-mail: info@axonsystems.com
Web site: www.axonsystems.com
Total Employees: 21   *Marketing Staff:* 3   *Sales Staff:* 6
Ownership: Private
Produces/Sells CE-marked Devices: Y
Federal Procurement Eligibility: Small Business
Distribution: Manufacturer Direct, Manufacturer Through Manufacturer Reps, Exporter
Mktg./Adv.: Jann Rasmussen/Vice President Marketing & Sales
Production: Howard Bailin/Vice President Operations

Computer, Patient Monitor	Anesthesiology
Electrode, Cutaneous	Cns/Neurology
Electrode, Needle	Cns/Neurology
Electrode, Other	General
Electroencephalograph	Cns/Neurology
Electromyograph, Diagnostic	Physical Med
Monitor, EEG, Surgery	Surgery
Monitor, EMG	Anesthesiology
Scanner, Ultrasonic (Pulsed Doppler)	Radiology
Stimulator, Electrical, Evoked Response	Cns/Neurology
Stimulator, Nerve Locating	Cns/Neurology
Stimulator, Photic, Evoked Response	Cns/Neurology
Transducer, Ultrasonic, Diagnostic	Radiology

AZMEC, INC.
877-862-9632
519 N. Smith Rd, Unit 110,
951-582-0153
Corona, CA 92880
FDA Number: 3004127034
Fax: 951-582-0135
E-mail: info@azmecinc.coml
Web site: azmecinc.com
Year Founded: 2003
Ownership: Private
Produces/Sells CE-marked Devices: N
Federal Procurement Eligibility: Minority Owned
Distribution: Manufacturer Direct, Manufacturer Through Distributor, Manufacturer Through Manufacturer Reps

Binder, Abdominal	General
Orthosis, Cervical	Physical Med
Orthosis, Limb Brace	Physical Med
Orthosis, Lumbosacral	Physical Med
Orthosis, Rib Fracture, Soft	Physical Med
Protector, Skin Pressure	General

AZOG, INC.
908-213-2900
1011 Us Hwy 22, Bldg. D Unit 4, BOX 6, Phillipsburg, NJ 08865
FDA Number: 3003788056
Fax: 908-213-2901
Ownership: Private
Produces/Sells CE-marked Devices: N

Kit, Pregnancy Test, Over The Counter, HCG	Chemistry
Test, Human Chorionic Gonadotropin, Serum	Immunology

AZONIX CORPORATION
800-967-5558
900 Middlesex Turnpike, Building 6,
978-670-6300
Billerica, MA 01821
FDA Number: n/a
Fax: 978-670-8855
E-mail: cs@azonix.com
Web site: www.azonix.com
Annual Revenue: $0-$1 Million
Year Founded: 1981
Ownership: CRANE CO.
Produces/Sells CE-marked Devices: N
Federal Procurement Eligibility: Small Business

Thermometer, Electronic	General

AZTEC HEART, INC.
530-533-7069
332 Canyon Highlands Dr, Oroville, CA 95966
FDA Number: 3003855399
Ownership: Private

AZTEC HEART, INC.   530-533-7069 *(cont'd)*
Produces/Sells CE-marked Devices: N
Band, Support, Pelvic	Physical Med
Binder, Breast	Obstetrics/Gynecology

AZTEC MEDICAL PRODUCTS, INC.   800-223-3859
3356 Ironbound Road, Suite 303, Williamsburg, VA 23188
FDA Number: 2243160   Fax: 757-345-3739
E-mail: aztecmed@msn.com
Web site: www.aztecmed.com
Medical Products Sales Volume: $1,000,000
Annual Revenue: $1-$5 Million
Total Employees: 5   *Marketing Staff:* 1   *Sales Staff:* 3
Ownership: Shanghai Zhijiang Biotechnology Co.,Ltd
Produces/Sells CE-marked Devices: N
Federal Procurement Eligibility: Small Business
Distribution: Manufacturer Through Distributor
General Admin.: Richard Newman/President
Endoscope	Gastroenterology/Urology
Loupe, Binocular, Low Power	Ophthalmology
Nasoscope	Ear/Nose/Throat
Surgical Instrument, Non-Powered, Neurosurgical	Cns/Neurology

AZTEC ORTHODONTIC LABORATORY, INC.   888-744-1588
7750 N. Redwing Circle, Tucson, AZ 85741   **520-744-1588**
FDA Number: 3005887326   Fax: 520-572-6985
E-mail: jjhickey@aztecortholab.com
Web site: www.aztecortholab.com
Ownership: Private
Produces/Sells CE-marked Devices: N
Device, Anti-Snoring	Ear/Nose/Throat

AZUR ENVIRONMENTAL
See Strategic Diagnostics Inc.

AZUSA OPTRONICS AND MANUFACTURING INC.   909-659-3011
2409 S. Vineyard Avenue, Suite B& C, Ontario, CA 91761
FDA Number: n/a   Fax: 626-608-9799
Ownership: Private
Produces/Sells CE-marked Devices: N
Microscope And Microscope Accessories, Reproduction, Assisted	Obstetrics/Gynecology

B & B LINGERIE CO., INC.   1-800-262-2789
2417 Bank Dr., Suite 201, P.o. Box 5731,   **208-343-9696**
Boise, ID 83705
FDA Number: 3027754
E-mail: custserv@bosombuddy.com
Web site: www.bosombuddy.com/
Ownership: Private
Produces/Sells CE-marked Devices: N
Prosthesis, Breast, External, No Adhesive	Surgery

B & B LINGERIE COMPANY, INC.   800-262-2789
2417 Bank Dr., Ste. 201, Boise, ID 83705   **208-343-9696**
FDA Number: n/a   Fax: 208-343-9266
E-mail: custserv@bosombuddy.com
Web site: www.bosombuddy.com
Annual Revenue: $0-$1 Million
Year Founded: 1976
Total Employees: 16   *Marketing Staff:* 1   *Sales Staff:* 3
Ownership: Private
Produces/Sells CE-marked Devices: N
Federal Procurement Eligibility: Small Business
Distribution: Manufacturer Direct, Manufacturer Through Distributor, Exporter
General Admin.: Stacie Neely/President, Chief Executive Officer
Prosthesis, Breast, External	Surgery

B & C BIOTECH   951-894-6650
24910 Washington Ave, Suite 204, Murrieta, CA 92562
FDA Number: 3005816806
Ownership: Private
Produces/Sells CE-marked Devices: N
Computer, Chemistry Analyzer	Chemistry

B & H MEDICAL PRODUCTS, INC.   520-296-5544
8925 East Golf Links Rd, Tucson, AZ 85730-1318
FDA Number: 2028806   Fax: 520-885-6787
E-mail: bhmedicalproductsinc@cox.net
Year Founded: 1979
Ownership: Private
Produces/Sells CE-marked Devices: N
Distribution: Manufacturer Direct
Clamp, Surgical, General & Plastic Surgery	Surgery

B & H ORTHOPEDIC LAB., INC.   314-647-1617
2510 Hampton Ave., St. Louis, MO 63139
FDA Number: 1923461
Web site: www.bandhorthopediclab.com

B & H ORTHOPEDIC LAB., INC.   314-647-1617 *(cont'd)*
Ownership: Private
Produces/Sells CE-marked Devices: N
Orthosis, Limb Brace	Physical Med
Orthosis, Lumbar	Physical Med

B & L ENGINEERING   714-505-9492
1901 Carnegie Ave., Suite Q, Santa Ana, CA 92705
FDA Number: 2029197   Fax: 714-505-9493
E-mail: info@bleng.com
Web site: www.bleng.com
Ownership: Private
Produces/Sells CE-marked Devices: N
Electromyograph, Diagnostic	Physical Med

B & M INSTRUMENTS, INC.   574-269-5313
542 East 200 North, Warsaw, IN 46580
FDA Number: n/a   Fax: 574-269-6133
E-mail: info@bminstruments.com
Web site: www.bminstruments.com
Medical Products Sales Volume: $800,000
Annual Revenue: $1-$5 Million
Year Founded: 1986
Ownership: Private
Quality System Registration Information: ISO9001
Produces/Sells CE-marked Devices: N
Federal Procurement Eligibility: Small Business
Distribution: Manufacturer Direct
General Admin.: Peggy Bause/Office Manager
           Mark Workman/President
Contract Manufacturing	General
Service, Maintenance/Repair	General

B & T DAVIS ELECTRIC INC.   812-644-7615
Rr4 Box 150a, Washington, IN 47501
FDA Number: 87877
Ownership: Private
Produces/Sells CE-marked Devices: N
Bed, Manual	General

B&E MEDICAL SYSTEMS   503-233-4872
1006 N.E. Second Ave., Portland, OR 97232
FDA Number: 3026647
Annual Revenue: $0-$1 Million
Year Founded: 1990
Ownership: Private
Produces/Sells CE-marked Devices: N
Federal Procurement Eligibility: Small Business
Distribution: Exclusive Distributor
General Admin.: Harold J. Byrne/Chief Executive Officer
Needle, Dental	Dental And Oral

B-J SCIENTIFIC PRODUCTS, INC.
See Metal Techology, Inc.

B-TEC SOLUTIONS INC.   215-785-2400
913 Cedar Ave., Croydon, PA 19021
FDA Number: n/a   Fax: 215-785-5847
E-mail: info@btecsolutions.com
Web site: www.btecsolutions.com
Medical Products Sales Volume: $1,000,000
Annual Revenue: $25-$50 Million
Total Employees: 80
Ownership: Private
Quality System Registration Information: ISO9001
Produces/Sells CE-marked Devices: N
Federal Procurement Eligibility: Small Business
Distribution: Manufacturer Direct, Manufacturer Through Manufacturer Reps
Component, Electronic	General
Contract Manufacturing	General
Contract R&D, Equipment	General

B. BRAUN MEDICAL   800-854-6851
1940 Olney Ave., Cherry Hill, NJ 08003
FDA Number: 2243801
Web site: www.bbraunusa.com
Annual Revenue: $0-$1 Million
Year Founded: 1839
Ownership: Braun Gmbh & Co.
Quality System Registration Information: ISO9001
Produces/Sells CE-marked Devices: Y
Distribution: Manufacturer Through Distributor, Exporter
General Admin.: Ron Zelzen/President
Mktg./Adv.: Eric Melanson/Director Marketing
Cardiac Output Unit, Indicator Dilution (Thermal)	Cardiovascular
Catheter, Angiographic	Cns/Neurology
Catheter, Cardiac Thermodilution	Cardiovascular
Catheter, Flow Directed	Cardiovascular
Catheter, Other	Gastroenterology/Urology

B. BRAUN MEDICAL
800-854-6851 *(cont'd)*

Catheter, Thermal Dilution	Cardiovascular

B. BRAUN MEDICAL INC., RENAL THERAPIES DIV.
800-854-6851

824 Twelfth Avenue, Bethlehem, PA 18018 610-691-5400
FDA Number: n/a *Fax:* 610-691-1547
E-mail: safetyexpert@bbraun.com
Web site: www.bbraunusa.com
Medical Products Sales Volume: $345,200,000
Annual Revenue: $10-$25 Million
Year Founded: 1979
Total Employees: 600 *Marketing Staff:* 3 *Sales Staff:* 12
Ownership: Private
Quality System Registration Information: ISO9000
Produces/Sells CE-marked Devices: Y
Federal Procurement Eligibility: GSA Contract, VA Contract
Distribution: Manufacturer Direct, Manufacturer Through Distributor, Manufacturer Through Manufacturer Reps, Importer
General Admin.: Caroll Neubauer/Chief Executive Officer
Mktg./Adv.: Samuel Amory/Director Marketing & Sales
 Pete Wells/Manager National Sales
 Lynne Snyder/Marketing Associate
IS: Duane Martz/Manager Tech. Services

Catheter, Intravascular, Therapeutic, Short-term Less Than 30 Days	General
Dialysate Delivery System, Single Patient	Gastroenterology/Urology
Hemodialysis Unit (Kidney Machine)	Gastroenterology/Urology
Kit, Hemodialysis Tubing	Gastroenterology/Urology
Kit, Tubing, Blood, Anti-Regurgitation	Gastroenterology/Urology
Needle, Fistula	Gastroenterology/Urology
Syringe, Piston	General

B. BRAUN MEDICAL INC.,B. BRAUN OEM/INDUSTRIAL DIVISION
See B. Braun Oem Division, B. Braun Medical Inc.

B. BRAUN MEDICAL, INC.
610-596-2536
1601 Wallace Dr., Suite 150, Carrollton, TX 75006
FDA Number: 1641965
Ownership: B. Braun Oem Division, B. Braun Medical Inc.
Produces/Sells CE-marked Devices: N

Pump, Infusion	General
Transfer Unit, IV Fluid	General

B. BRAUN MEDICAL, INC.
610-596-2536
901 Marcon Blvd., Allentown, PA 18109
FDA Number: 2523676
Web site: http://www.bbraunusa.com
Ownership: B. Braun Oem Division, B. Braun Medical Inc.
Produces/Sells CE-marked Devices: N
General Admin.: Carroll Neubauer/Chief Executive Officer, Chairman
 Tim Richards/Senior Vice President
Mktg./Adv.: Carla Carpenter/Director Marketing

Dispenser, Medication, Liquid	General
Filter, Infusion Line	General
Guidewire, Catheter	Cardiovascular
Infusion Stand	General
Injector And Syringe, Angiographic, Balloon Inflation, Reprocessed	Cardiovascular
Introducer, Catheter	Cardiovascular
Irrigator, Ocular Surgery	Ophthalmology
Needle, Aspiration And Injection, Disposable	Surgery
Needle, Hypodermic, Single Lumen With Syringe	General
Needle, Other	General
Set, Administration, Intravenous, Needle-Free	General
Stopcock	General
Syringe, Irrigating	General
Syringe, Piston	General
Tray, Surgical	Surgery

B. BRAUN OEM DIVISION, B. BRAUN MEDICAL INC.
866-8-BBRAUN
824 Twelfth Avenue, 610-691-6785
Bethlehem, PA 18018
FDA Number: 2521402 *Fax:* 610-691-1785
E-mail: contact-usa@bbraunoem.com
Web site: www.bbraunoem.com
Medical Products Sales Volume: $345,200,000
Year Founded: 1979
Total Employees: 600 *Marketing Staff:* 2 *Sales Staff:* 8
Ownership: Private
Produces/Sells CE-marked Devices: Y
Distribution: Manufacturer Through Distributor, OEM
General Admin.: Caroll Neubauer/Chief Executive Officer
 Willem deGoede/Chief Operating Officer
Mktg./Adv.: Dave Williams/Director International Marketing & Sales
 Tom Black/Vice President Marketing & Sales
Research: Dr. Marcus Schabacker/Vice President Research & Engineering

Cannula, Epidural	Obstetrics/Gynecology

B. BRAUN OEM DIVISION, B. BRAUN
866-8-BBRAUN *(cont'd)*

Catheter, Central Venous	General
Catheter, Epidural	Obstetrics/Gynecology
Catheter, Multiple Lumen	Surgery
Catheter, Subcutaneous Intravascular, Implanted	General
Catheter, Subcutaneous Peritoneal, Implanted	General
Check Valve, Retrograde Flow (In-Line)	General
Component, Electronic	General
Container, IV	General
Contract Assembly	General
Contract Laboratory	General
Contract Manufacturing	General
Contract Packaging	General
Controller, Infusion, Intravenous	Cardiovascular
Dispenser, Fluid	General
Filter, Intravenous Tubing	General
Fitting, Luer	General
Fitting, Other	General
General Medical Device	General
Introducer, Catheter	Cardiovascular
Kit, Administration, Blood	General
Kit, Administration, Intra-Arterial	General
Kit, Administration, Intravenous	General
Kit, Anesthesia, Epidural	Anesthesiology
Kit, Catheter Care	General
Kit, First Aid	Surgery
Kit, Intravenous Extension Tubing	General
Molding, Custom	General
Molding, Injection	General
Monitor, Blood Pressure, Venous, Cardiopulmonary Bypass	Cardiovascular
Needle, Blunt	General
Needle, Intravenous	General
Needle, Spinal, Short-Term	General
Packaging, Sterilization	General
Port, Vascular Access	Cardiovascular
Pump, Drug Administration, Closed Loop	General
Pump, Infusion	General
Set, Administration, Intravenous, Needle-Free	General
Solution, Intravenous	General
Stopcock	General
Syringe, Other	General
Transducer, Blood Pressure	General
Transfer Unit, IV Fluid	General
Tubing, Fluid Delivery	General
Tubing, Multi-Lumen	General
Valve, Other	Chemistry
Vascular Access Graft	Gastroenterology/Urology

Medical Product Subsidiaries (Listed Separately)
 B. Braun Medical, Inc.

B. BRAUN OF PUERTO RICO, INC.
610-691-5400
215.7 Insular Rd., Sabana Grande, PR 00637
FDA Number: n/a
Ownership: Private
Produces/Sells CE-marked Devices: N

Accessories, Catheter, G-U	Gastroenterology/Urology
Catheter, Peritoneal Dialysis, Single-Use	Gastroenterology/Urology
Container, IV	General
Dispenser, Medication, Liquid	General
Filter, Infusion Line	General
Kit, Administration, Intravenous	General
Kit, Administration, Peritoneal Dialysis, Disposable	Gastroenterology/Urology
Kit, Blood, Transfusion	Hematology
Kit, Irrigation, Sterile	Gastroenterology/Urology
Monitor, Blood Pressure, Venous, Cardiopulmonary Bypass	Cardiovascular
Stopcock	General
Transfer Unit, Blood	Hematology
Transfer Unit, IV Fluid	General
Tube, Gastrointestinal	Gastroenterology/Urology
Urological Irrigation System	Gastroenterology/Urology
Warmer, Blood, Non-Electromagnetic Radiation	Anesthesiology

B. F. WEHMER CORP.
See Wehmer Corporation

B. GRACZYK, INC.
269-782-2100
27826 Burmax Court, Dowagiac, MI 49047
FDA Number: n/a
Ownership: Private
Produces/Sells CE-marked Devices: N

Caliper, Ophthalmic	Ophthalmology
Cannula, Ophthalmic	Ophthalmology
Clamp, Eyelid, Ophthalmic	Ophthalmology
Clamp, Muscle, Ophthalmic	Ophthalmology
Cleaner, Ultrasonic, Medical Instrument	General
Conformer, Ophthalmic	Ophthalmology
Curette, Ophthalmic	Ophthalmology
Forceps, Ophthalmic	Ophthalmology
Gauge, Lens, Ophthalmic	Ophthalmology
Holder, Needle	Gastroenterology/Urology
Hook, Ophthalmic	Ophthalmology
Knife, Ophthalmic	Ophthalmology

B. GRACZYK, INC.
269-782-2100 *(cont'd)*

Light Source, Photographic, Fiberoptic	Gastroenterology/Urology
Magnet, Permanent	Ophthalmology
Retractor, Ophthalmic	Ophthalmology
Ring, Ophthalmic (Flieringa)	Ophthalmology
Scissors, Ophthalmic	Ophthalmology
Shield, Eye, Ophthalmic	Ophthalmology
Spatula, Ophthalmic	Ophthalmology
Spectacle, Operating (Loupe), Ophthalmic	Ophthalmology
Speculum, Ophthalmic	Ophthalmology
Sponge, Ophthalmic	Ophthalmology
Spoon, Ophthalmic	Ophthalmology
Spud, Ophthalmic	Ophthalmology
Tray, Surgical Instrument	Surgery

B.B.G. ORTHOPEDIC APPLIANCES INC.
1-866-484-4715
514-484-4715
5930 Sherbrooke St. West,
Montreal, QUE H4A-1 Canada
FDA Number: n/a   *Fax:* 514-484-5027
E-mail: info@bbgortho.com
Web site: www.bbgortho.com
Year Founded: 1975
Ownership: Private
Produces/Sells CE-marked Devices: N
Distribution: Manufacturer Direct, Exclusive Distributor

B.E. MEYERS & CO., INC.
800-327-5648
425-881-6648
14540 N.E. 91st Street,
Redmond, WA 98052
FDA Number: n/a   *Fax:* 425-867-1759
E-mail: sales@bemeyers.com
Web site: www.bemeyers.com
Annual Revenue: $25-$50 Million
Year Founded: 1974
Total Employees: 130   *Marketing Staff:* 16   *Sales Staff:* 16
Ownership: Private
Quality System Registration Information: ISO9001
Produces/Sells CE-marked Devices: N
Federal Procurement Eligibility: Small Business
Distribution: Manufacturer Direct, Manufacturer Through Manufacturer Reps, Service Direct
General Admin.: Brad E. Meyers/President
Mktg./Adv.: Bruce Westcoat/Vice President New Business
Production: Tim Franey/Manager Operations

Vision Aid, Electronic, Battery-Powered	Ophthalmology

B.F. LORENZETTI & ASSOCIATES INC.
800-668-5901
416-599-5530
181 University Ave, Suite 1605,
Toronto, ONT M5H 3 Canada
FDA Number: n/a   *Fax:* 416-599-5458
E-mail: Dbarr@bf-lorenzetti.ca
Web site: www.bf-lorenzetti.ca
Year Founded: 1987
Total Employees: 250
Ownership: Private
Produces/Sells CE-marked Devices: N

B.G. INDUSTRIES, INC.
800-822-8288
818-894-0744
8550 Balboa Blvd., Suite 214,
Northridge, CA 91325
FDA Number: n/a   *Fax:* 818-894-7972
E-mail: maxifloat@bgind.com
Web site: www.bgind.com
Medical Products Sales Volume: $8,000,000
Annual Revenue: $5-$10 Million
Year Founded: 1967
Total Employees: 34   *Marketing Staff:* 3   *Sales Staff:* 30
Ownership: Private
Produces/Sells CE-marked Devices: N
Federal Procurement Eligibility: Small Business, GSA Contract
Distribution: Manufacturer Direct, Manufacturer Through Manufacturer Reps
General Admin.: Arnie Balonick/Chief Executive Officer
Larry Lankard/President
Mktg./Adv.: David Buchicchio/Vice President Marketing
Mark Owens/Vice President National Accounts
Richard Bowen/Vice President National Accounts

Mattress, Bed	General
Mattress, Reduction, Pressure	General

B.I.B. COMPANY
See Pace Tech, Inc.

B/R INSTRUMENT CORP.
800-922-9206
410-820-8800
9119 Centreville Road, Easton, MD 21601
FDA Number: 1125771   *Fax:* 410-820-8141
E-mail: brsales@brinstrument.com
Web site: www.brinstrument.com
Annual Revenue: $1-$5 Million

B/R INSTRUMENT CORP.
800-922-9206 *(cont'd)*
Year Founded: 1966
Total Employees: 20
Ownership: Private
Produces/Sells CE-marked Devices: Y
Federal Procurement Eligibility: Small Business, GSA Contract
Distribution: Manufacturer Direct, Manufacturer Through Manufacturer Reps, Exporter
General Admin.: Paul Van Trieste/Executive Vice President
Roger Roark/President
Mktg./Adv.: Richard Roark/Director Marketing
Anne Sanders/Manager Clinical Sales
Richard Roark/Manager International & National Sales
Anne Sanders/Manager National Sales

Formaldehyde (Formalin, Formol)	Pathology
Still, Solvent Recovery	Chemistry

B2 IMPORTS, LLC
918-557-5729
12807 East 90th Street North, Owasso, OK 74055
FDA Number: 3006414075
Ownership: Private
Produces/Sells CE-marked Devices: N

Exerciser, Powered	Anesthesiology
Massager, Therapeutic	Physical Med

BABYKINS PRODUCTS LTD.
800-665-2229
604-275-2255
150 - 12830 Clarke Place,
Richmond, BC V6V 2 Canada
FDA Number: n/a   *Fax:* 604-275-2255
E-mail: taurus@telus.net
Web site: www.babykins.com
Year Founded: 1992
Total Employees: 10
Ownership: Private
Produces/Sells CE-marked Devices: N
Distribution: Manufacturer Direct, Exclusive Distributor, Exporter

BABYTOOTH TECHNOLOGIES, LLC.
802-226-7300
2468 Route 103, Proctorsville, VT 05153
FDA Number: 3006015082

Container, Specimen Mailer And Storage, Temperature Control	Pathology

BACCHUS VASCULAR, INC.
877-622-5082
408-980-8300
3110 Coronado Dr., Santa Clara, CA 95054
FDA Number: 2953724   *Fax:* 408-980-8383
Web site: www.bacchus-vascular.com
Ownership: Private
Produces/Sells CE-marked Devices: N
General Admin.: Mr. Scott Cramer/President, Chief Executive Officer
Finance: Mr. Mike Gandy/Chief Financial Officer, Vice President Finance

Catheter, Continuous Flush	Cardiovascular
Catheter, Peripheral, Atherectomy	Cardiovascular

BACHEM BIOSCIENCE, INC.
800-634-3183
610-239-0300
3700 Horizon Drive, King of Prussia, PA 19406
FDA Number: n/a   *Fax:* 610-239-0800
E-mail: sales@usbachem.com
Web site: www.bachem.com
Medical Products Sales Volume: $300,000
Year Founded: 1971
Total Employees: 35   *Marketing Staff:* 3   *Sales Staff:* 3
Ownership: BACHEM HOLDING AG
Produces/Sells CE-marked Devices: N
Federal Procurement Eligibility: Small Business
Distribution: Manufacturer Direct
General Admin.: Rolf Nyfeler/Chief Executive Officer
Mr. Mike Pennington/Chief Operating Officer
Mktg./Adv.: Lora Gibson/Director Marketing
Jackie Britto/Marketing Coordinator

Antibody, Monoclonal	Microbiology
Antibody, Polyclonal	Microbiology
Contract Laboratory	General
Contract Manufacturing, Pharmaceuticals/Chemicals	General
Peptides	Chemistry
Resin, Ion-Exchange	Pathology

BACK BUBBLE
858-481-8715
621 Seabright Ln., Solana Beach, CA 92075
FDA Number: 2031048

Traction Unit, Non-Powered	Orthopedics

BACK PAIN RELIEF CLINIC, P.C.
574-271-9444
5507 Singer Ct., Granger, IN 46530
FDA Number: 3005344540
Ownership: Private
Produces/Sells CE-marked Devices: N

Orthosis, Limb Brace	Physical Med

BACK PAIN RELIEF CLINIC, P.C.   **574-271-9444** *(cont'd)*
Orthosis, Lumbosacral   Physical Med

BACK SOLUTION, THE   **800-326-2724**
6281 South Park Avenue, Tucson, AZ 85706   **520-889-3997**
FDA Number: n/a   Fax: 520-294-4748
Web site: www.bodybridge.com
Annual Revenue: $0-$1 Million
Ownership: Private
Produces/Sells CE-marked Devices: N
Federal Procurement Eligibility: Small Business
Distribution: Manufacturer Direct
    Table, Other   General

BACK SUPPORT SYSTEMS   **800-669-2225**
67684 San Andreas,   **760-329-1472**
Desert Hot Springs, CA 92240
FDA Number: n/a   Fax: 760-329-1955
E-mail: info@backsupportsystems.com
Web site: www.backsupportsystems.com
Medical Products Sales Volume: $1,500,000
Annual Revenue: $1-$5 Million
Year Founded: 1989
Ownership: Private
Produces/Sells CE-marked Devices: N
Federal Procurement Eligibility: Small Business, Minority Owned
Distribution: Manufacturer Through Distributor, Exporter
    Accessories, Fixation, Orthopedic   Orthopedics
    Chair, Other   General
    Mattress, Bed   General
    Pack, Hot Or Cold, Reusable   Physical Med
    Pillow, Cervical   Orthopedics
    Support, Arm   Physical Med
    Support, Back   Orthopedics
    Support, Hot/Cold Pack   Physical Med
    Traction Unit, Non-Powered   Orthopedics

BACK-MUELLER, INC.   **314-531-6640**
2700 Clark Ave., Saint Louis, MO 63103
FDA Number: 1923491
Ownership: Private
Produces/Sells CE-marked Devices: N
    Forceps, Ophthalmic   Ophthalmology
    Handle, Scalpel   Surgery
    Holder, Needle   Gastroenterology/Urology
    Keratome, AC-Powered   Ophthalmology
    Knife, Ophthalmic   Ophthalmology
    Retractor, Ophthalmic   Ophthalmology
    Spatula, Ophthalmic   Ophthalmology
    Trephine, Manual, Ophthalmic (Corneal)   Ophthalmology

BACKPROJECT CORPORATION   **1-888-470-8100**
170 N Wolfe Rd, Sunnyvale, CA 94086   **1-408-730-1111**
FDA Number: 3006378776   Fax: 1-408-404-8100
E-mail: Info@BackProject.com
Web site: www.backproject.com
Ownership: Private
Produces/Sells CE-marked Devices: N
    Exerciser, Non-Measuring   Physical Med

BACKSAVER   **310-661-3044**
3000 East Imperial Highway, Lynwood, CA 90262
FDA Number: n/a
E-mail: info@backsaver.com
Web site: www.backsaver.com
Annual Revenue: $10-$25 Million
Year Founded: 1958
Ownership: Private
Produces/Sells CE-marked Devices: N
Federal Procurement Eligibility: Small Business
Distribution: Manufacturer Through Distributor, Manufacturer Through Manufacturer Reps, Importer, Exporter
General Admin.: Neil Kimball/Vice President Human Resources
Mktg./Adv.: Phil Angileri/Director Product Development
    Steven Kusmin/Vice President Sales
Production: William Zechello/Manager Materials
    Rob Ayles/Vice President Manufacturing
Research: Phil Angileri/Vice President Research & Development
    Back Rest   General
    Chair, Adjustable, Mechanical   Physical Med
    Cushion, Other   General
    Pillow, Cervical   Orthopedics

BACKSTRONG INTERNATIONAL LLC.   **714-671-1150**
710 N. Brea Blvd., Suite G, Brea, CA 92821
FDA Number: 2438257
Ownership: Private
Produces/Sells CE-marked Devices: N

BACKSTRONG INTERNATIONAL LLC.   **714-671-1150** *(cont'd)*
Exerciser, Non-Measuring   Physical Med

BACON FELT COMPANY, INC.   **508-823-0791**
395 W. Water St., Taunton, MA 02780-4847
FDA Number: n/a   Fax: 508-823-2855
E-mail: baconfelt@aol.com
Total Employees: 15
Ownership: Private
Produces/Sells CE-marked Devices: N
Federal Procurement Eligibility: Small Business
Distribution: Exclusive Distributor, Exporter
Mktg./Adv.: William Founds/Vice President Marketing & Sales
Production: Matthew Landoch/Vice President Manufacturing
    Felt   Surgery

BACOU-DALLOZ
    See Sperian Protection

BACTERIN INTERNATIONAL INC.   **406-388-0480**
664 Cruiser Ln., Belgrade, MT 59714
FDA Number: 3005168462   Fax: 406-388-1354
Web site: http://www.bacterin.com
Ownership: Public
Stock Symbol: BONE
Traded On: AMEX
Produces/Sells CE-marked Devices: N
General Admin.: Mr. Guy Cook/Chief Executive Officer
    Mr. Darrel Holmes/Vice President
    Mr. Jesus Hernandez/Vice President
Finance: Mr. John Gandolfo/Chief Financial Officer
    Accessories, Catheter   Surgery
    Filler, Bone Void, Medicated   Orthopedics
    Filler, Bone Void, Osteoinduction   Physical Med

BACTON ASSAY SYSTEMS, INC.   **760-471-4538**
772-a Twin Oaks Valley Rd., San Marcos, CA 92069
FDA Number: 2026171
Ownership: Private
Produces/Sells CE-marked Devices: N
    Turbidimetric Method, Lipoproteins   Chemistry

BADGE MACHINE PRODUCTS, INC.   **585-394-0330**
2491 Brickyard Rd., Canandaigua, NY 14424
FDA Number: 3005855044   Fax: 585-394-0446
E-mail: sales@badgemachine.com
Web site: www.badgemachine.com
Ownership: Private
Produces/Sells CE-marked Devices: N
    Grid, Radiographic   Radiology

BADGER PHARMACAL CO.
    See Female Health Company, The

BAGBLOCKER, INC   **317-538-6732**
2159 Dockside Drive, Greenwood, IN 46143
FDA Number: 3004976261
Ownership: Private
Produces/Sells CE-marked Devices: N
    Pack, Hot Or Cold, Reusable   Physical Med

BAGCO   **800-533-1931**
1650 Airport Road Suite 104,   **770-422-4187**
Kennesaw, GA 30144
FDA Number: 3002518548   Fax: 770-422-3879
E-mail: sales@bagco.com
Web site: www.bagco.com
Medical Products Sales Volume: $6,000,000
Annual Revenue: $5-$10 Million
Total Employees: 26   *Marketing Staff:* 4   *Sales Staff:* 9
Ownership: TBC GROUP
Quality System Registration Information: ISO9000; ISO9002
Produces/Sells CE-marked Devices: N
Federal Procurement Eligibility: Small Business, Minority Owned, Female Owned
Distribution: Manufacturer Direct, Manufacturer Through Distributor, Importer, Exporter
General Admin.: Nossi Taheri/President
    Katherine Remick/Vice President, General Manager
Mktg./Adv.: Mr. Thammachon/Director Product Development
    Katherine Remick/Manager Contract Sales
    Diana Rollins/Manager International Marketing & Sales
    Craig Griffiths/Manager National Sales
    Katherine Remick/Vice President Marketing
    Craig Griffiths/Vice President Sales
Production: Ms. Janchai/Director Quality Assurance
    Diana Rollins/Manager Materials
    Pehr Lund/Manager Materials
    Bag, Ice   General
    Bag, Plastic   General

BAGCO   800-533-1931 *(cont'd)*
Collector, Specimen   Microbiology

BAGRAD   904-272-6369
84 Sleepy Hollow Rd., Middleburg, FL 32068
FDA Number: 1052422
Ownership: Private
Produces/Sells CE-marked Devices: N
Traction Unit, Non-Powered   Orthopedics

BAGSHAW COMPANY, INC., W.H.   800-343-7467
1 Pine St., Extension, PO Box 766,   603-883-7758
Nashua, NH 03060
FDA Number: n/a   Fax: 603-882-2651
Web site: www.whbagshaw.com
Year Founded: 1970
Ownership: Private
Quality System Registration Information: ISO9001
Produces/Sells CE-marked Devices: N
Federal Procurement Eligibility: Small Business
Distribution: OEM, Exporter
Needle, Other   General
Probe, Other   General

BAILEY INSTRUMENTS
See Physitemp Instruments, Inc.

BAILEY MANUFACTURING CO.   800-321-8372
PO BOX 130, Lodi, OH 44254-0130
FDA Number: n/a   Fax: 800-224-5390
E-mail: baileymfg@baileymfg.com
Web site: www.baileymfg.com
Annual Revenue: $1-$5 Million
Year Founded: 1956
Ownership: Private
Produces/Sells CE-marked Devices: N
Federal Procurement Eligibility: Small Business
Distribution: Manufacturer Through Distributor
Accessories, Traction   Physical Med
Bars, Parallel, Exercise   Physical Med
Bars, Parallel, Walking   Physical Med
Board, Quadriceps (Exerciser)   Physical Med
Cabinet, Other   General
Cart, Multipurpose   General
Cart, Other   General
Chair, Bath   General
Chair, Other   General
Chair, Pediatric   General
Chair, Rehabilitation   General
Component, Exercise   Physical Med
Exercise Stair   Physical Med
Exerciser, Arm   Physical Med
Exerciser, Hand   Physical Med
Exerciser, Leg And Ankle   Physical Med
Exerciser, Other   Physical Med
Exerciser, Shoulder   Physical Med
Exerciser, Wrist   Physical Med
Mirror, Posture   Physical Med
Stool, Bedside   General
Stool, Exercise   Physical Med
Table, Examination/Treatment   General
Table, Other   General
Table, Physical Therapy   Physical Med

BAILEY MEDICAL ENGINEERING   800-413-3216
2216 Sunset Dr., Los Osos, CA 93402   805-528-5781
FDA Number: 2028723   Fax: 805-528-1461
E-mail: folks@baileymed.com
Web site: www.baileymed.com
Ownership: Private
Produces/Sells CE-marked Devices: N
Pump, Breast, Powered   Obstetrics/Gynecology

BAIRD ANALYTICAL, DIV. OF IMO INDUSTRIES
See Thermo - Industrial Hygiene Division

BAIWA, INC.   775-588-8494
630 Alma Way, Zephyr Cove, NV 89448
FDA Number: 74176
E-mail: RickB@baiwa.com
Web site: www.baiwa.com
Ownership: Private
Produces/Sells CE-marked Devices: N
General Admin.: Mr. Richard Baiocchi/President, Chief Executive Officer
Joint, Knee, External Brace   Physical Med

BAK ELECTRONICS, INC.   800-894-6000
PO Box 623, Mount Airy, MD 21771   301-607-8300
FDA Number: 9200096   Fax: 301-607-9018
E-mail: info@bakelectronicsinc.com
Web site: www.bakelectronicsinc.com

BAK ELECTRONICS, INC.   800-894-6000 *(cont'd)*
Medical Products Sales Volume: $200,000
Annual Revenue: $0-$1 Million
Year Founded: 1976
Total Employees: 4
Ownership: Private
Produces/Sells CE-marked Devices: N
Federal Procurement Eligibility: Small Business
Distribution: Manufacturer Direct, Importer, Exporter
General Admin.: Ron Bak/President
Amplifier, Microelectrode   General
Component, Other   General
Electrode, Other   General
Microelectrode   General
Stimulator, Neurological   Surgery

BAKA MANUFACTURING CO.
See Dale Medical Products, Inc.

BAKER COMPANY, THE   800-992-2537
161 Gatehouse Rd., P.O. Drawer E,   207-324-8773
Sanford, ME 04073
FDA Number: n/a   Fax: 207-324-3869
E-mail: bakerco@bakerco.com
Web site: www.bakerco.com
Medical Products Sales Volume: $3,000,000
Year Founded: 1949
Ownership: Private
Quality System Registration Information: ISO9001
Produces/Sells CE-marked Devices: Y
Federal Procurement Eligibility: Small Business
Distribution: Manufacturer Through Manufacturer Reps, Exporter
Box, Glove   Microbiology
Enclosure, Bacteriological Safety   Chemistry
Hood, Fume   Toxicology
Hood, Isolation, Laminar Air Flow   General
Hood, Microbiological   Microbiology
Laminar Air Flow Unit   General
Laminar Air Flow Unit, Fixed (Air Curtain)   Chemistry
Safety Equipment, Laboratory   Chemistry

BALANCE SYSTEMS, INC.   1-888-274-5444
1644 Plaza Way, Suite 317,   541-938-7163
Walla Walla, WA 99362
FDA Number: 3032216   Fax: 541-938-7165
E-mail: customerservice@flextend.com
Web site: www.repetitive-strain.com
Year Founded: 1996
Total Employees: 2   *Marketing Staff:* 4   *Sales Staff:* 20
Ownership: Private
Quality System Registration Information: ISO9002
Produces/Sells CE-marked Devices: Y
Distribution: Manufacturer Through Manufacturer Reps, OEM, Importer, Exporter
Component, Exercise   Physical Med
Compress, Cold   General
Dressing, Wound and Burn, Hydrogel   Surgery
Equipment, Therapy, Handicapped/Physical   Physical Med
Exerciser, Wrist   Physical Med

BALCHEM CORP.
See Arc Specialty Products, Balchem Corporation

BALDOR ELECTRIC
See Wells Dental, Inc.

BALDUR SYSTEMS CORPORATION
See Baldur Systems Corporation/ HTI TRADING

BALDUR SYSTEMS CORPORATION/ HTI TRADING   800-736-4716
33235 Transit Ave., Union City, CA 94587   510-477-9194
FDA Number: 2939291   Fax: 510-477-9634
E-mail: baldur@baldurco.com
Web site: www.baldurco.com
Annual Revenue: $25-$50 Million
Total Employees: 10   *Marketing Staff:* 3   *Sales Staff:* 5
Ownership: Private
Quality System Registration Information: ISO9000; ISO9001; ISO9002
Produces/Sells CE-marked Devices: N
Federal Procurement Eligibility: Small Business, Minority Owned, Female Owned
Distribution: Manufacturer Through Distributor, Importer, Exporter
General Admin.: Dr. David Hu/President
Glove, Other   General
Glove, Patient Examination   General
Glove, Patient Examination, Latex   General
Glove, Patient Examination, Vinyl   General
Gown, Isolation, Surgical   Surgery
Sponge, Gauze   Dental And Oral

BALL DYNAMICS INTERNATIONAL, LLC   800-752-2255
14215 Mead St., Longmont, CO 80504   **970-535-9090**
FDA Number: 1722763   *Fax:* 877-223-2962
E-mail: orders@fitball.com
Web site: www.fitball.com
Medical Products Sales Volume: $1,900,000
Year Founded: 1991
Total Employees: 12
Ownership: Private
Produces/Sells CE-marked Devices: Y
Federal Procurement Eligibility: Small Business, GSA Contract
Distribution: Service Direct

Exerciser, Hand	Physical Med
Exerciser, Non-Measuring	Physical Med
Massager, Therapeutic, Manual	Physical Med
Support, Back	Orthopedics

BALLARD MEDICAL PRODUCTS   770-587-7835
12050 Lone Peak Pkwy., Draper, UT 84020
FDA Number: 1719891

Accessories, Cleaning, Endoscopic	Gastroenterology/Urology
Biopsy Instrument, Mechanical, Gastrointestinal	Gastroenterology/Urology
Brush, Scrub, Operating Room	Surgery
Cable, Electrode	Physical Med
Calibrator Source, Nuclear Sealed	Radiology
Campylobacter Pylori	Microbiology
Catheter, Aspiration	Surgery
Catheter, Biliary	Gastroenterology/Urology
Catheter, Biliary, General & Plastic Surgery	Surgery
Catheter, Irrigation	Surgery
Catheter, Suction (Tracheal Aspirating Tube)	Anesthesiology
Catheter, Suction, With Tip	General
Condenser, Heat And Moisture (Artificial Nose)	Anesthesiology
Connector, Airway (Extension)	Anesthesiology
Defibrillator, Battery-Powered, Low Energy	Cardiovascular
Detector, Beta/Gamma	Chemistry
Dislodger, Store, Biliary	Gastroenterology/Urology
Drain, Tee (Water Trap)	Anesthesiology
ENT Drug Applicator	Ear/Nose/Throat
Electrode, Electrocardiograph	Cardiovascular
Electrode, Electrocardiograph, Multi-Function	Cardiovascular
Electrosurgical Unit, Cutting & Coagulation Device	Surgery
Electrosurgical, Unit, Gastroenterology	Gastroenterology/Urology
Endoscope	Gastroenterology/Urology
Filter, Bacterial, Breathing Circuit	Anesthesiology
Forceps, Biopsy, Bronchoscope (Non-Rigid)	Anesthesiology
Forceps, Biopsy, Electric	Gastroenterology/Urology
Forceps, Biopsy, Non-Electric	Gastroenterology/Urology
Generator, Radiofrequency Lesion	Cns/Neurology
Humidifier, Respiratory Gas, (Direct Patient Interface)	Anesthesiology
Irrigating Solution, Non-Injectable	Surgery
Kit, Anesthesia, Conduction	Anesthesiology
Kit, Biopsy Needle	Gastroenterology/Urology
Kit, Surgical (General)	Surgery
Laparoscope, General & Plastic Surgery	Surgery
Needle, Conduction, Anesthesia (W/Wo Introducer)	Anesthesiology
Needle, Endoscopic	Gastroenterology/Urology
Pacemaker, Cardiac, External Transcutaneous (Non-Invasive)	Cardiovascular
Percussor	Cns/Neurology
Spirometer, Therapeutic (Incentive)	Anesthesiology
Syringe, Irrigating	General
Toothbrush, Manual	Dental And Oral
Tube, Aspirating, Flexible, Connecting	Anesthesiology
Tube, Aspirating, Rigid Bronchoscope Aspirating	Ear/Nose/Throat
Tube, Gastro-Enterostomy	Gastroenterology/Urology
Tube, Gastrointestinal	Gastroenterology/Urology
Tube, Tracheal (Endotracheal)	Anesthesiology

BALLY CASE & COOLER INC.
See Bally Refrigerated Boxes, Inc.

BALLY ENGINEERED STRUCTURES, INC.
See Bally Refrigerated Boxes, Inc.

BALLY REFRIGERATED BOXES, INC.   800-24-BALLY
135 Little Nine Drive, Morehead City, NC 28557   **252-240-2829**
FDA Number: n/a   *Fax:* 252-240-0384
E-mail: ballysales@ballyrefboxes.com
Web site: www.ballyrefboxes.com
Medical Products Sales Volume: $19,200,000
Annual Revenue: $25-$50 Million
Year Founded: 1995
Total Employees: 192
Ownership: Private
Produces/Sells CE-marked Devices: N
Federal Procurement Eligibility: Small Business, GSA Contract
Distribution: Manufacturer Through Manufacturer Reps, Exporter
General Admin.: John Reilly/Chief Executive Officer
      Michael Coyle/President
Mktg./Adv.: William Stompf/Director Marketing

Freezer, Blood Storage	Hematology

BALLY REFRIGERATED BOXES, INC.   800-24-BALLY *(cont'd)*

Freezer, Laboratory, General Purpose	Chemistry
Refrigerator, Biological	Microbiology
Refrigerator, Blood Bank	Hematology
Refrigerator, Morgue, Walk-In	Pathology

BALTIMORE LABORATORIES, INC.   203-445-8423
887 Main St., Monroe, CT 06468
FDA Number: 3002894094
Ownership: Private
Produces/Sells CE-marked Devices: N

Electrode, Ion Selective (Non-Specified)	Chemistry

BAMS MANUFACTURING CO., INC.   847-647-6990
6273 Howard St. West, Niles, IL 60714
FDA Number: 3006055788

Transfer Device, Patient, Manual	General

BANCO HEARING CENTERS   941-753-3131
1133 44th Ave W, Bradenton, FL 34207-1439
FDA Number: 1035388
Total Employees: 2
Ownership: Private
Produces/Sells CE-marked Devices: N
Federal Procurement Eligibility: Small Business

Hearing-Aid	Ear/Nose/Throat

BANGS LABORATORIES, INC.   800-387-0672
9025 Technology Drive, Fishers, IN 46038-2886   **317-570-7020**
FDA Number: n/a   *Fax:* 317-570-7034
E-mail: info@bangslabs.com
Web site: www.bangslabs.com
Medical Products Sales Volume: $2,500,000
Year Founded: 1988
Total Employees: 16   *Marketing Staff:* 1   *Sales Staff:* 1
Ownership: Polysciences, Inc.
Quality System Registration Information: ISO9001
Produces/Sells CE-marked Devices: N
Federal Procurement Eligibility: Small Business
Distribution: Manufacturer Direct, Manufacturer Through Distributor, OEM, Service Direct, Exclusive Distributor, Importer, Exporter
General Admin.: Michael Ott/Chairman, Chief Executive Officer
      Chad Owen/General Manager
      Terry Taylor/Vice President Human Resources
Mktg./Adv.: Robin Bryant/Coord. Marketing
Production: Denise Beemster/Manager Materials
Research: Mary Meza/Vice President Research & Development

Immunoassay, Other	Toxicology
Polymer, Synthetic, Other	General
Reagent, Inoculator Calibration (Laboratory)	Microbiology
Separation Media	Microbiology

BANKIER COMPANIES, INC.   847-647-6565
6151 Gross Point Rd., Niles, IL 60714
FDA Number: 1421062
Ownership: Private
Produces/Sells CE-marked Devices: N

Glove, Patient Examination, Latex	General

BANTA HEALTHCARE PRODUCTS
See Tidi Products, Llc

BANYAN INTERNATIONAL CORP.   800-351-4530
2118 E. Interstate 20, PO Box 1779,   **325-677-1874**
Abilene, TX 79601
FDA Number: 1619634   *Fax:* 325-677-1372
E-mail: customerservice@statkit.com
Web site: www.statkit.com
Medical Products Sales Volume: $5,500,000
Annual Revenue: $5-$10 Million
Year Founded: 1972
Total Employees: 25   *Marketing Staff:* 3   *Sales Staff:* 5
Ownership: Stat Kit, Inc.
Stock Symbol: BNYN
Traded On: OTC Bulletin
Produces/Sells CE-marked Devices: N
Federal Procurement Eligibility: Small Business
Distribution: Manufacturer Direct, Manufacturer Through Distributor
General Admin.: Jim Breckenridge/President, Chief Executive Officer
Mktg./Adv.: Sherri McAuliffe/Director Marketing
      Mike Breckeridge/Manager Contract Sales
      Mike Breckenridge/Vice President Marketing & Sales
Production: Mr. Doug Phariss/Manager Quality Systems
Finance: Mr. Scott Michener/Vice President Finance
Purchasing: Mrs. Toni McDonald/Manager Purchasing

Defibrillator, External, Automatic	Cardiovascular
Kit, Emergency, Anaphylactic	General
Kit, Emergency, Cardiopulmonary Resuscitation	General
Resuscitator, Cardiac, Mechanical, Compressor	Anesthesiology

BANYAN INTERNATIONAL CORP. 800-351-4530 *(cont'd)*
Resuscitator, Emergency Oxygen   Dental And Oral

BAR-RAY PRODUCTS, INC. 800-359-6115
95 Monarch St., Littlestown, PA 17340   **717.359.9100**
FDA Number: 2431606   *Fax:* 717-359-9109
E-mail: bar.ray95@gmail.com
Web site: www.bar-ray.com
Medical Products Sales Volume: $7,500,000
Annual Revenue: $10-$25 Million
Year Founded: 1930
Total Employees: 62   *Marketing Staff:* 2   *Sales Staff:* 2
Ownership: Private
Produces/Sells CE-marked Devices: N
Federal Procurement Eligibility: Small Business
Distribution: Manufacturer Direct, Manufacturer Through Distributor, Exporter
General Admin.: Jeff Stein/President, Chief Executive Officer
Mktg./Adv.: M. Stein/Manager Customer Services & Sales
       R. Buckley Thompson/Vice President Marketing & Sales

Apron, Lead, Radiographic	Radiology
Cabinet, X-Ray Transfer	Radiology
Curtain, Protective, Radiographic	Radiology
Glove, Protective, Radiographic	Radiology
Safelight, X-Ray	Radiology
Shield, Breast	Obstetrics/Gynecology
Shield, Gonadal	Radiology
Shield, Ophthalmic, Radiological	Radiology
Shield, Protective, Personnel	Radiology
Shield, X-Ray	Radiology
Shield, X-Ray, Lead-Plastic	Radiology
Shield, X-Ray, Portable	Radiology
Shield, X-Ray, Throat	Radiology
Shield, X-Ray, Transparent	Radiology
Storage Unit, X-Ray Film	Radiology

Medical Product Subsidiaries (Listed Separately)
   Hearing Technologies

BARCO OF CALIFORNIA 800-421-1932
350 West Rosecrans Ave.,   **310-323-7315**
Gardena, CA 90247
FDA Number: n/a   *Fax:* 310-767-4700
E-mail: CustomerService@BarcoUniforms.com
Web site: www.barcouniforms.com
Medical Products Sales Volume: $25,000,000
Year Founded: 1929
Ownership: Private
Produces/Sells CE-marked Devices: N

Apron, Laboratory	Chemistry
Gown, Operating Room, Reusable	Surgery
Gown, Other	General
Gown, Patient, Reusable	General
Suit, Scrub, Reusable	Surgery

BARCO, INC 678-475-8137
3059 Premiere Parkway, Duluth, GA 30097
FDA Number: 3004578804
Ownership: Private
Produces/Sells CE-marked Devices: N

Image Processing System	Radiology
System, Communication, Image, Digital	Radiology

BARCODES WEST, INC.
   See Barcodes West, Llc

BARCODES WEST, LLC 206-323-8100
1560 First Avenue, S., Seattle, WA 98134
FDA Number: n/a   *Fax:* 206-323-2650
E-mail: info@barcodeswest.com
Web site: www.bcw.com
Annual Revenue: $10-$25 Million
Total Employees: 15   *Marketing Staff:* 4   *Sales Staff:* 11
Ownership: Private
Produces/Sells CE-marked Devices: Y
Federal Procurement Eligibility: Small Business, GSA Contract
Distribution: Manufacturer Direct, Manufacturer Through Distributor, Manufacturer Through Manufacturer Reps
General Admin.: Gary Falconbridge/President
Mktg./Adv.: Dana Milkie/Manager Marketing & Sales
Production: Anna Marietilt/Manager Materials

Label, Bar Code	General

Medical Product Subsidiaries (Listed Separately)
   Brady Corporation

BARD ACCESS SYSTEMS, INC. 800-545-0890
605 N. 5600 West, Salt Lake City, UT 84116   **801-522-5000**
FDA Number: 3006260740   *Fax:* 801-522-49485
E-mail: slc.cs@crbard.com
Web site: www.bardaccess.com
Medical Products Sales Volume: $43,500,000

BARD ACCESS SYSTEMS, INC. 800-545-0890 *(cont'd)*
Annual Revenue: $25-$50 Million
Total Employees: 300   *Marketing Staff:* 3
Ownership: C. R. Bard, Inc.
Stock Symbol: BCR
Traded On: NYSE
Quality System Registration Information: ISO9001
Produces/Sells CE-marked Devices: Y
Federal Procurement Eligibility: Small Business
Distribution: Manufacturer Direct, Exclusive Distributor, Exporter
General Admin.: Len DeCant/Chief Executive Officer, General Manager
Mktg./Adv.: Steve Hagaman/Director Product Development
Production: Ronn C. Gerra/Director Quality Assurance
       William Drugman/Manager Materials
       Ronald Sucky/Manager Regulatory Affairs
Finance: Steve Taylor/Controller

Accessories, AV Shunt	Gastroenterology/Urology
Biopsy Instrument	Gastroenterology/Urology
Brush, Scrub, Operating Room	Surgery
Catheter, Biliary	Gastroenterology/Urology
Catheter, Hemodialysis	Gastroenterology/Urology
Catheter, Intravascular, Therapeutic, Long-term Greater Than 30 Days	General
Catheter, Intravascular, Therapeutic, Short-term Less Than 30 Days	General
Catheter, Irrigation	Surgery
Catheter, Percutaneous	Cardiovascular
Catheter, Peritoneal	Surgery
Catheter, Subclavian	Cardiovascular
Dilator, Vessel	Gastroenterology/Urology
Electrode, Pacemaker, Temporary	Cardiovascular
Equipment, Management, Pain, Radiofrequency, Non-Invasive	General
Guidewire, Catheter	Cardiovascular
Image Processing System	Radiology
Instrument, Manual, General Surgical	Surgery
Introducer, Catheter	Cardiovascular
Needle, Aspiration And Injection, Disposable	Surgery
Needle, Hypodermic, Single Lumen With Syringe	General
Port & Catheter, Infusion, Implanted, Subcut., Intraperit.	General
Port & Catheter, Infusion, Implanted, Subcutaneous, Intraspinal	General
Probe, Ultrasonic	Radiology
Scanner, Ultrasonic (Pulsed Echo)	Radiology
Scanner, Ultrasonic, Other	Radiology
Scanner, Ultrasonic, Vascular	Radiology
Set, Administration, Intravenous, Needle-Free	General
Suction Apparatus, Single Patient, Portable, Non-Powered	Surgery
Transducer, Ultrasonic, Diagnostic	Radiology
Tube, Gastro-Enterostomy	Gastroenterology/Urology
Tube, Gastrointestinal	Gastroenterology/Urology

BARD BRACHYTHERAPY, INC 908-277-8000
295 E. Lies Rd., Carol Stream, IL 60188
FDA Number: 1424526
Ownership: C. R. Bard, Inc.
Stock Symbol: BCR
Traded On: NYSE
Produces/Sells CE-marked Devices: N

Shield, X-Ray, Leaded	Dental And Oral
Source, Brachytherapy, Radionuclide	Radiology

BARD CANADA, INC. 800-632-2109
2345 Stanfield Rd,   **905-275-8000**
Mississauga, ONT L4Y 3 Canada
FDA Number: 8010006   *Fax:* 905-275-5370
E-mail: peter.curry@crbard.com
Web site: www.crbard.com
Year Founded: 1964
Total Employees: 150
Ownership: Private
Quality System Registration Information: ISO9000
Produces/Sells CE-marked Devices: N
Distribution: Manufacturer Direct, Exclusive Distributor, Importer

BARD CARDIOLOGY
   See Bard Electro Physiology

BARD ELECTRO MEDICAL SYSTEM, INC.
   See Conmed Corporation

BARD ELECTRO PHYSIOLOGY 800-824-8724
55 Technology Dr., Lowell, MA 01851   **978-441-6202**
FDA Number: 1222791   *Fax:* 978-323-2222
Web site: www.bardep.com
Total Employees: 1000   *Marketing Staff:* 19   *Sales Staff:* 100
Ownership: C. R. Bard, Inc.
Stock Symbol: BCR
Traded On: NYSE
Quality System Registration Information: ISO9001
Produces/Sells CE-marked Devices: Y
Distribution: Manufacturer Direct, Manufacturer Through Distributor
Mktg./Adv.: Dana Groves/Manager Contract Sales

Adapter, Stopcock, Manifold, Cardiopulmonary Bypass	Cardiovascular

BARD ELECTRO PHYSIOLOGY
800-824-8724 *(cont'd)*

Cable, Electrode	Physical Med
Catheter, Other	Gastroenterology/Urology

BARD PERIPHERAL VASCULAR, INC.
800-321-4254
1625 West Third Street, Tempe, AZ 85281
480-894-9515

FDA Number: 2020394
Fax: 480-303-2767
E-mail: bpv.products@crbard.com
Web site: www.bardpv.com
Medical Products Sales Volume: $50,000,000
Annual Revenue: $50-$100 Million
Total Employees: 300   *Marketing Staff:* 6   *Sales Staff:* 50
Ownership: C. R. Bard, Inc.
Stock Symbol: BCR
Traded On: NYSE
Quality System Registration Information: ISO9000
Produces/Sells CE-marked Devices: Y
Federal Procurement Eligibility: Small Business
Distribution: Manufacturer Direct
General Admin.: John McDermott/President
    Mike Warren/Vice President Human Resources
Mktg./Adv.: Perry Borch/Director Sales
    Regina Thomas/Manager Sales Training
    Peter Fox/Market Manager
    Mark Taylor/Sales Associate
    David Renzi/Vice President Marketing
Production: Bill Bratt/Engineer
    Scott Kreider/Manager Materials
    Bob Calcote/Vice President Manufacturing

Bag, Polymeric Mesh, Pacemaker	Cardiovascular
Catheter, Percutaneous	Cardiovascular
Filter, Intravascular, Cardiovascular	Cardiovascular
Graft, Vascular, Biological	Cardiovascular
Patch, Myocardial	Cardiovascular
Pledget And Intracardiac Patch, PETP, PTFE, Polypropylene	Cardiovascular
Prosthesis, Arterial Graft, Synthetic, Greater Than 6mm	Surgery
Prosthesis, Arterial Graft, Synthetic, Less Than 6mm	Surgery
Prosthesis, Vascular Graft, Less Than 6mm Diameter	Cardiovascular
Prosthesis, Vascular Graft, Of 6mm And Greater Diameter	Cardiovascular
Surgical Instrument, Cardiovascular	Cardiovascular
Tunneler, Surgical	Surgery
Vascular Access Graft	Gastroenterology/Urology

BARD REYNOSA S.A. DE C.V.
908-277-8000
Blvd. Montebello #1, Parque Industrial Colonial,
Reynosa, Tamaulipas Mexico
FDA Number: 9617592

Applicator, Radionuclide, Manual	Radiology
Catheter, Intravascular, Therapeutic, Long-term Greater Than 30 Days	General
Catheter, Intravascular, Therapeutic, Short-term Less Than 30 Days	General
Catheter, Peritoneal, Indwelling, Long-Term	Gastroenterology/Urology
Catheter, Subcutaneous Intravascular, Implanted	General
Guidewire, Catheter	Cardiovascular
Instrument, Manual, General Surgical	Surgery
Introducer, Catheter	Cardiovascular
Kit, Administration, Intravenous	General
Kit, Biopsy Needle	Gastroenterology/Urology
Needle, Hypodermic, Single Lumen With Syringe	General

BARD SHANNON LIMITED
908-277-8000
San Geronimo Industrial Park, Lot # 1, Road # 3, Km 79.7,
Humacao, PR 00791
FDA Number: 3005636544
Ownership: C. R. Bard, Inc.
Stock Symbol: BCR
Traded On: NYSE
Produces/Sells CE-marked Devices: N

Bag, Polymeric Mesh, Pacemaker	Cardiovascular
Biopsy Instrument	Gastroenterology/Urology
Catheter, Intravascular, Therapeutic, Long-term Greater Than 30 Days	General
Catheter, Percutaneous	Cardiovascular
Catheter, Vascular, Cardiopulmonary Bypass	Cardiovascular
Drape, Surgical	Surgery
Endoscope	Gastroenterology/Urology
Laparoscope, General & Plastic Surgery	Surgery
Mesh, Surgical, Polymeric	Surgery
Pledget And Intracardiac Patch, PETP, PTFE, Polypropylene	Cardiovascular
Prosthesis, Vascular Graft, Less Than 6mm Diameter	Cardiovascular
Prosthesis, Vascular Graft, Of 6mm And Greater Diameter	Cardiovascular
Staple, Implantable	Surgery
Tube, Gastro-Enterostomy	Gastroenterology/Urology
Tube, Gastrointestinal	Gastroenterology/Urology
Tube, Tracheostomy (W/Wo Connector)	Anesthesiology

BARD USCI DIV.
See Bard Electro Physiology

BARDEN CORP.
See Lacey Manufacturing Co., LLC

BAREFOOT MEDICAL
760-967-8225
1902 Calle Buena Ventura, Oceanside, CA 92056
FDA Number: n/a
Fax: 760-967-8225
E-mail: bareftent@aol.com
Annual Revenue: $0-$1 Million
Year Founded: 1981
Total Employees: 2   *Marketing Staff:* 1   *Sales Staff:* 2
Ownership: BAREFOOT ENTERPRISES
Produces/Sells CE-marked Devices: N
Federal Procurement Eligibility: Small Business, Female Owned
Distribution: Manufacturer Direct, Manufacturer Through Distributor, Manufacturer Through Manufacturer Reps, Exporter
General Admin.: Gloria L. Flick/President
Mktg./Adv.: Mike Flick/Vice President Marketing & Sales
Production: Mike Flick/Vice President Manufacturing
Research: Mike Flick/Vice President Research & Development

Device, Measurement, Potential, Skin	Cns/Neurology

BARIK MEDICAL INC.
(800) 265-6061
239 Cree Crescent,
204-888-2330
Winnipeg, MAN R3J 3 Canada
FDA Number: n/a
Fax: 204-888-2262
E-mail: sales@barikmedical.com
Web site: www.barikmedical.com
Year Founded: 1992
Total Employees: 25
Ownership: Private
Produces/Sells CE-marked Devices: N
Distribution: Exclusive Distributor

BARJAN MFG., LTD.
800-611-6950
28 Baiting Pl Rd., Farmingdale, NY 11735
631-420-5588
FDA Number: 2434631
Fax: 631-420-5599
E-mail: sales@barjan-mfg.com
Web site: www.barjan-mfg.com
Ownership: Private
Produces/Sells CE-marked Devices: N

Band, Support, Pelvic	Physical Med
Cover, Mattress	General
Gown, Examination	General
Restraint, Protective (Body)	General
Sling, Arm	Physical Med
Transfer Aid	Physical Med

BARLOW MANUFACTURING
See Conmed Linvatec

BARNES, JOHN S.
See Concentric

BARNETT & RAMEL OPTICAL CO.
800-228-9732
7154 N. 16th St., Omaha, NE 68112-0488
FDA Number: n/a
Fax: 800-545-2693
E-mail: info@broptical.com
Web site: secure.broptical.com
Annual Revenue: $0-$1 Million
Ownership: Private
Produces/Sells CE-marked Devices: N
Federal Procurement Eligibility: Small Business
Distribution: Manufacturer Direct, Importer

Eyeglasses	Ophthalmology
Frame, Spectacle (Eyeglasses)	Ophthalmology
Lens, Spectacle/Eyeglasses, Custom (Prescription)	Ophthalmology

BARNETT INTL. CORP.
704-587-0390
610 Greenway Industrial Drive, Charlotte, NC 28273
FDA Number: 1010604
Fax: 704-587-0394
E-mail: sales@barnettinternational.net
Web site: www.barnettinternational.net
Medical Products Sales Volume: $3,500,000
Annual Revenue: $1-$5 Million
Year Founded: 1948
Total Employees: 25   *Marketing Staff:* 2   *Sales Staff:* 2
Ownership: Private
Produces/Sells CE-marked Devices: Y
Federal Procurement Eligibility: Small Business
Distribution: Manufacturer Direct
General Admin.: Jerry M. Barnett/President

Prophylactic (Condom)	General

BARNHARDT MFG. CO.
704-376-0380
1100 Hawthorne Ln., Charlotte, NC 28205
FDA Number: 1010842
Ownership: Private
Produces/Sells CE-marked Devices: N

Cotton, Roll	Dental And Oral
Fiber, Absorbent	General
Mask, Surgical	Surgery

BARNHARDT MFG. CO. 704-376-0380 (cont'd)
Sponge, Gauze   Dental And Oral

BARNHART INDUSTRIES, INC. 800-325-9973
3690 Hwy M, Imperial, MO 63052   636-942-3133
FDA Number: 1925204   *Fax:* 636-948-3152
E-mail: anna@barnhartindustries.com
Web site: www.barnhartindustries.com
Year Founded: 1928
Ownership: Private
Produces/Sells CE-marked Devices: N
General Admin.: Anna Boehm/Owner
    Band, Elastic, Orthodontic   Dental And Oral
    Headgear, Extraoral, Orthodontic   Dental And Oral
    Spring, Orthodontic   Dental And Oral

BARNSTEAD INTERNATIONAL 800-553-0039
2555 Kerper Blvd., Dubuque, IA 52001
FDA Number: 1950043   *Fax:* 563-589-0516
Ownership: Private
Produces/Sells CE-marked Devices: N
    Block, Heating   Chemistry
    Cleaner, Ultrasonic, Medical Instrument   General
    Colorimeter, General Use   Chemistry
    Dispenser, Paraffin   Pathology
    Fluorometer, Chemistry   Chemistry
    Freezer, Blood Storage   Hematology
    Freezer, Laboratory, General Purpose   Chemistry
    Incubator/Water Bath, Microbiology   Microbiology
    Lamp, Slide Warming   Pathology
    Purifier, Water   Chemistry
    Shaker/Stirrer   Chemistry
    Stainer, Slide, Immersion Type   Pathology
    Sterilant, Medical Device   General
    Sterilization Process Indicator, Biological   General
    Sterilization Process Indicator, Physical/Chemical   General
    Sterilizer, Chemical   General
    Sterilizer, Steam (Autoclave)   General

BARNSTEAD/THERMOLYNE CORP.
See Thermo Fisher Scientific Inc.

BARON HOSPITAL MEDICAL SUPPLY, INC.
See Baron Medical Supply

BARON MEDICAL SUPPLY 888-702-2766
709 Grand Street, Brooklyn, NY 11211   718-486-6164
FDA Number: n/a   *Fax:* 718-963-2673
E-mail: baronmedical@verizon.net
Web site: www.baronmedical.com/
Annual Revenue: $0-$1 Million
Ownership: Private
Produces/Sells CE-marked Devices: N
Federal Procurement Eligibility: Small Business
Distribution: Manufacturer Direct
    Binder, Abdominal   General
    Corset   Orthopedics
    Immobilizer, Shoulder   Orthopedics
    Support, Arch   Physical Med

BARR ASSOCIATES, INC. 978-692-7513
2 Lyberty Way, Westford, MA 01886-3616
FDA Number: n/a   *Fax:* 978-692-7443
E-mail: barr@barrassociates.com
Web site: www.barrassociates.com
Medical Products Sales Volume: $61,970,000
Annual Revenue: $50-$100 Million
Year Founded: 1971
Total Employees: 270   *Marketing Staff:* 1
Ownership: Private
Produces/Sells CE-marked Devices: N
Federal Procurement Eligibility: Small Business
Distribution: Manufacturer Direct, Manufacturer Through Distributor, Manufacturer Through Manufacturer Reps, OEM, Exclusive Distributor, Importer
General Admin.: Michael Chung/Chief Operating Officer
    Ali Smajkiewicz/President
Mktg./Adv.: Serena Currie/Marketing Coordinator
Finance: Jeff Maclaren/Chief Financial Officer
    Filter, Lens   Ophthalmology

BARRETT ENGINEERING 714-246-4388
606 L Street, Fortuna, CA 95540
FDA Number: 3005437803
    Amplifier, Physiological Signal   Cns/Neurology

BARRIER EYEWEAR 561-317-5324
840 13th St. #31, Lake Park, FL 33403
FDA Number: n/a   *Fax:* 561-845-0034
Medical Products Sales Volume: $200,000
Total Employees: 3   *Marketing Staff:* 1   *Sales Staff:* 2
Ownership: Private

BARRIER EYEWEAR 561-317-5324 (cont'd)
Produces/Sells CE-marked Devices: N
Distribution: Manufacturer Through Distributor
General Admin.: James Shepard/President
    Bob Nelson/Vice President
Production: Paul Winterlink/Laboratories Product Manager
    Frame, Spectacle (Eyeglasses)   Ophthalmology
    Shield, Ophthalmic, Radiological   Radiology

BARRIER FREE LIFT SYSTEMS, INC.
See Access, Lifts & Mobility Systems, Inc.

BARRON PRECISION INSTRUMENTS, L.L.C. 810-695-2080
8170 Embury Rd., PO Box 973, Grand Blanc, MI 48480
FDA Number: 1835993
Ownership: Private
Produces/Sells CE-marked Devices: N
    Punch, Corneo-Scleral   Ophthalmology
    Trephine, Manual, Ophthalmic (Corneal)   Ophthalmology

BARROWS COMPANY 707-987-0460
18701 Glenwood Road, Hidden Valley Lake, CA 95467
FDA Number: n/a   *Fax:* 707-987-0436
E-mail: wfbarrows@mchsi.com
Web site: www.barrowsco.com
Medical Products Sales Volume: $5,000
Annual Revenue: $0-$1 Million
Year Founded: 1966
Total Employees: 2   *Marketing Staff:* 1   *Sales Staff:* 1
Ownership: Private
Produces/Sells CE-marked Devices: N
Federal Procurement Eligibility: Small Business
Distribution: Manufacturer Direct
General Admin.: Mr. William F. Barrows/President, Chief Executive Officer
Production: Mr. Thomas Hamon/Vice President Manufacturing
    Telemetry Unit, Physiological, Temperature   General
    Transmitter/Receiver System, Physiological, Radiofrequency   Cardiovascular

BARRX MEDICAL, INCORPORATED 888-662-2779
540 Oakmead Parkway, Sunnyvale, CA 94085   408-328-7300
FDA Number: 3004904811   *Fax:* 408-738-1741
Web site: www.barrx.com
Ownership: Private
Produces/Sells CE-marked Devices: N
General Admin.: Mr. Randy Sullivan/Chief Operating Officer
    Mr. Greg Barrett/President, Chief Executive Officer
Medical Admin.: Dr. David Utley/Chief Medical Officer
Mktg./Adv.: Mr. Darin Wilson/Vice President International Marketing & Sales
    Mr. David Thompson/Vice President Marketing
    Mr. Robert Haggerty/Vice President Sales
Finance: Mr. Richard Short/Vice President Finance
    Electrosurgical Unit, Cutting & Coagulation Device   Surgery

BARTON MATTHEW, INC. 734-420-2326
11251 Ridge Road, Plymouth, MI 48170-3067
FDA Number: n/a   *Fax:* 734-453-0506
E-mail: hallgary@comcast.net
Medical Products Sales Volume: $350,000
Annual Revenue: $0-$1 Million
Year Founded: 1981
Total Employees: 10
Ownership: Private
Produces/Sells CE-marked Devices: N
Federal Procurement Eligibility: Small Business
Distribution: Manufacturer Direct
General Admin.: Gary E. Hall/Chief Executive Officer
    Cephalometer   Dental And Oral

BARTON-CAREY MEDICAL PRODUCTS, INC. 423-784-0444
460 Fifth St., Jellico, TN 37762
FDA Number: n/a
Ownership: Private
Produces/Sells CE-marked Devices: N
    Stocking, Support (Anti-Embolic)   General

BARTRONIX
See Nurse Assist ,Inc.

BASELINE - MOCON, INC. 800-321-4665
19661 Highway 36, P.O. Box 649,   303-823-6661
Lyons, CO 80540
FDA Number: n/a   *Fax:* 303-823-5151
E-mail: info@baselineindustries.com
Web site: www.baseline-mocon.com
Annual Revenue: $0-$1 Million
Year Founded: 1969
Ownership: Private
Produces/Sells CE-marked Devices: N
Federal Procurement Eligibility: Small Business

BASELINE - MOCON, INC.   800-321-4665 *(cont'd)*
Distribution: Manufacturer Direct, Exporter
Chromatography Equipment, Gas   Chemistry

BASELINE INDUSTRIES, INC.
See Baseline - Mocon, Inc.

BASHAW MEDICAL, INC.   800-499-3857
4909-B Mobile Hwy., Pensacola, FL 32506-3229   **850-455-7017**
FDA Number: 1048597   *Fax:* 850-456-3076
E-mail: jackie@bashawmedical.com
Medical Products Sales Volume: $200,000
Annual Revenue: $0-$1 Million
Total Employees: 5   *Marketing Staff:* 1   *Sales Staff:* 2
Ownership: Private
Produces/Sells CE-marked Devices: N
Federal Procurement Eligibility: Small Business
Distribution: Manufacturer Through Distributor
General Admin.: Jaqueline Bashaw/President
Immobilizer, Cervical   Orthopedics
Rescue Equipment   General
Restraint   Physical Med
Restraint, Protective (Body)   General
Splint, Other   Orthopedics

BASI (BIOANALYTICAL SYSTEMS, INC.)   800-845-4246
2701 Kent Avenue,   **765-463-4527**
West Lafayette, IN 47906
FDA Number: 9016139   *Fax:* 765-497-1102
E-mail: basi@bioanalytical.com
Web site: www.bioanalytical.com
Medical Products Sales Volume: $43,040,000
Annual Revenue: $25-$50 Million
Year Founded: 1974
Total Employees: 380
Ownership: Public
Stock Symbol: BASI
Traded On: NASDAQ
Produces/Sells CE-marked Devices: Y
Federal Procurement Eligibility: Small Business, GSA Contract
Distribution: Manufacturer Direct
General Admin.: Peter T. Kissinger/President, Chief Executive Officer
    Lina Kerner/Vice President Human Resources
Mktg./Adv.: Alice Schwind/Director Corporate Communications
    Michael Silvon/Vice President Business Development
    Craig S. Bruntlett/Vice President Sales
Production: Cindy Grimes/Manager Materials
    Laurel Branstrator/Manager Regulatory Affairs
Research: Ronald E. Shoup/President Research
    Candice Kissinger/Senior Vice President Research
    Craig S. Bruntlett/Vice President Product Development
Analyzer, Amino Acid   Microbiology
Analyzer, Chemistry, Electrolyte   Chemistry
Chromatographic/Fluorometric Method, Catecholamines   Chemistry
Chromatography Equipment, Liquid   Chemistry
Contract Laboratory   General
Detector, Electrochemical, Chromatography, Liquid   Toxicology
Equipment, In Vitro Fertilization/Embryo Transfer   Obstetrics/Gynecology
Kit, Sampling, Blood   General
Labeling Equipment   General
Mass Spectrometer, Clinical Use   Toxicology
Microelectrode   General
Probe, Other   General
Pump, Infusion   General
Pump, Infusion, Syringe   General
System, Infusion, Administration, Drug, Implantable   General

BASIC AMERICAN MEDICAL PRODUCTS   800-849-6664
2935-A Northeast Pkwy, Atlanta, GA 30360   **770-368-4700**
FDA Number: n/a   *Fax:* 770-368-4701
E-mail: info@basicamerican.com
Web site: www.basicamerican.com
Medical Products Sales Volume: $600,000
Annual Revenue: $25-$50 Million
Year Founded: 1994
Total Employees: 10   *Marketing Staff:* 10   *Sales Staff:* 40
Ownership: Basic American Medical, Inc.
Federal Procurement Eligibility: Small Business, GSA Contract
Distribution: Manufacturer Direct
General Admin.: Wayne Coleman/Executive Vice President
    Gene Minotto/President
Mktg./Adv.: Marc Minotto/Vice President Marketing & Sales
Bed, Electric   General
Bed, Electric, Home-Use   General
Bed, Pediatric (Crib)   General
Bedrail   General
Chair, Geriatric   General
Chair, Seat Lifting (Standing Aid)   General
Commode (Toilet)   General

BASIC AMERICAN MEDICAL PRODUCTS   800-849-6664 *(cont'd)*
Cover, Mattress   General
Furniture, Patient Room   General
Mattress, Bed   General
Table, Overbed   General
Wheelchair, Manual   Physical Med

BASIC AMERICAN METAL PRODUCTS   800-365-2338
336 Trowbridge Drive, PO Box 907,   **920-929-8200**
Fond du Lac, WI 54937
FDA Number: 2183191   *Fax:* 920-929-8210
E-mail: info@bampwi.com
Web site: www.bampwi.com
Medical Products Sales Volume: $10,000,000
Annual Revenue: $10-$25 Million
Year Founded: 1959
Total Employees: 140   *Marketing Staff:* 2   *Sales Staff:* 5
Ownership: GRAHAM-FIELD HEALTH PRODUCTS, INC.
Produces/Sells CE-marked Devices: N
Federal Procurement Eligibility: Small Business, GSA Contract
Distribution: Manufacturer Direct, Manufacturer Through Distributor, Manufacturer Through Manufacturer Reps, Service Direct
General Admin.: Gene Minatto/President
Production: Kurt Hellman/Vice President Manufacturing
Purchasing: Mr. Keith Cramer/Director Contracts
Bed, Manual   General
Bedrail   General
Furniture, Patient Room   General
Monitor, Bed Patient   General
Table, Overbed   General

BASIC BIO SYSTEMS
See Nurture Inc.

BASIC DENTAL IMPLANT SYSTEMS, INC.   505-884-1922
3321 Columbia, N.E., Albuquerque, NM 87107-2001
FDA Number: 1723412   *Fax:* 505-884-1923
E-mail: basicdental@qwest.net
Web site: www.basicdentalimplants.com
Ownership: Private
Produces/Sells CE-marked Devices: N
Burr, Dental   Dental And Oral
Crown, Preformed   Dental And Oral
Gauge, Depth, Instrument, Dental   Dental And Oral
Handle, Instrument, Dental   Dental And Oral
Implant, Endosseous   Dental And Oral
Punch, Biopsy, Surgical   Dental And Oral

BASS MEDICAL, INC   800-214-9084
2539 John Hawkins Parkway, Suite 101,
Birmingham, AL 35244
FDA Number: 2027633   *Fax:* 800-214-9085
E-mail: info@bassmed.com
Web site: www.bassmed.com
Ownership: Private
Produces/Sells CE-marked Devices: N
Federal Procurement Eligibility: Minority Owned, Female Owned
Distribution: Manufacturer Direct, Manufacturer Through Distributor
Suction Apparatus, Operating Room, Wall Vacuum-Powered   Surgery

BATH-TEC WHIRLPOOL BATH   800-526-3301
5142 Hwy 34 W., Ennis, TX 75119-7260   **972-646-5279**
FDA Number: n/a   *Fax:* 972-646-5688
E-mail: sales@bathtec.com
Web site: www.bathtec.com
Medical Products Sales Volume: $1,300,000
Annual Revenue: $1-$5 Million
Year Founded: 1985
Total Employees: 20
Ownership: Private
Quality System Registration Information: ISO9002
Federal Procurement Eligibility: Small Business
Distribution: Manufacturer Direct
General Admin.: Elaine Griffin/Chief Executive Officer
    Chris Griffin/President
Bath, Hydro-Massage (Whirlpool)   Physical Med

BATHEASE INC.   888-747-7845
3815 Darston St., Palm Harbor, FL 34685-3119   **727-786-2604**
FDA Number: 1052206   *Fax:* 727-786-2604
E-mail: bathease@aol.com
Web site: www.bathease.com
Medical Products Sales Volume: $490,000
Annual Revenue: $0-$1 Million
Year Founded: 1988
Total Employees: 4   *Marketing Staff:* 1   *Sales Staff:* 1
Ownership: Private
Produces/Sells CE-marked Devices: N
Federal Procurement Eligibility: Small Business

BATHEASE INC.
888-747-7845 *(cont'd)*
Distribution: Manufacturer Direct, Service Direct, Exclusive Distributor, Exporter
General Admin.: Thomas J. FitzGerald/Chief Executive Officer
Mktg./Adv.: Joseph Magilligan/Manager Advertising
Alison FitzGerald/Manager International & National Sales
Production: Ron D'Amico/Manager Production
Research: Terry Stickler/Manager Research

Bath, Hydro-Massage (Whirlpool)	Physical Med
Bathtub	General

BATTERY SPECIALTIES
800-854-5759
3530 Cadillac Ave., Costa Mesa, CA 92626
714-755-0888
FDA Number: n/a
Fax: 714-755-0889
E-mail: sales@batteryspecialties.com
Web site: www.batteryspecialties.com
Medical Products Sales Volume: $15,000,000
Annual Revenue: $10-$25 Million
Year Founded: 1969
Ownership: Cadex Electronics Inc.
Quality System Registration Information: ISO9002
Produces/Sells CE-marked Devices: N
Federal Procurement Eligibility: Small Business
Distribution: Manufacturer Direct, OEM

Battery	General
Contract Manufacturing, Product, Disposable	General

BATTLE CREEK EQUIPMENT CO.
800-253-0854
307 W. Jackson St., Battle Creek, MI 49017-2306
269-962-6181
FDA Number: 1811605
Fax: 269-962-8058
E-mail: bcec@prodigy.net
Medical Products Sales Volume: $10,000,000
Annual Revenue: $5-$10 Million
Year Founded: 1931
Total Employees: 60   *Marketing Staff:* 2   *Sales Staff:* 2
Ownership: Private
Produces/Sells CE-marked Devices: N
Federal Procurement Eligibility: Small Business
Distribution: Manufacturer Direct, Manufacturer Through Distributor, Manufacturer Through Manufacturer Reps, Service Direct, Exporter
General Admin.: Steven C. Martin/President, Chief Executive Officer
Mary Brown/Vice President
Mktg./Adv.: Gordon Bart/Director Product Development
John W. Doty/Vice President Marketing & Sales
Production: Tom Lewis/Director Quality Assurance

Equipment, Cleaning, Air	General
Exerciser, Bicycle	Physical Med
Exerciser, Non-Measuring	Physical Med
Humidifier, Non-Direct Patient Interface (Home-Use)	Anesthesiology
Moist Therapy Pack	Physical Med
Pack, Cold	General
Pillow, Cervical	Orthopedics
Table, Physical Therapy	Physical Med
Treadmill, Mechanical	Physical Med
Treadmill, Powered	Physical Med

BAUERFEIND USA, INC.
800-423-3405
55 Chastain Road, Suite 112,
770-429-8330
Kennesaw, GA 30144
FDA Number: n/a
Fax: 770-429-8477
E-mail: info@bauerfeindUSA.com
Web site: www.bauerfeindusa.com
Medical Products Sales Volume: $8,700,000
Annual Revenue: $5-$10 Million
Year Founded: 1985
Total Employees: 26
Ownership: Trimas Corporation
Produces/Sells CE-marked Devices: Y
Federal Procurement Eligibility: Small Business
Distribution: Manufacturer Direct, Manufacturer Through Manufacturer Reps, Exclusive Distributor
Mktg./Adv.: Erin Gibson/Director Marketing
Allison Stefanov/Director National Accounts & Sales

Brace, Joint, Ankle (External)	Physical Med
Cushion, Foot	Orthopedics
Holder, Shoulder, Arthroscopy	Surgery
Joint, Knee, External Brace	Physical Med
Orthosis, Lumbar	Physical Med
Pad, Pressure, Foam (Elbow, Heel)	General
Stocking, Support (Anti-Embolic)	General
Support, Ankle	Orthopedics
Support, Back	Orthopedics
Support, Elbow	Orthopedics
Support, Knee	Physical Med
Support, Wrist	Physical Med

BAUMAN & HARNISH
See Griffith Rubber Mills

BAUSCH & LOMB
585-338-6000
1 Bausch & Lomb Place, Rochester, NY 14604-2701
FDA Number: 1313525
Fax: 585-338-6007
Web site: www.bausch.com
Medical Products Sales Volume: $2,292,400,000
Annual Revenue: More than $1 Billion
Year Founded: 1853
Total Employees: 13000
Ownership: Private
Produces/Sells CE-marked Devices: N
Distribution: Manufacturer Direct, Manufacturer Through Distributor
General Admin.: Mr. Brent Saunders/Chief Executive Officer
Mr. Robert Grant/Chief Executive Officer
Mr. Alan Farnsworth/Chief Information Officer
Mr. John Sheets, Jr./Chief Technology Officer
Ms. Susan Roberts/Compliance Officer
Mr. Michael Gowen/Vice President International Operations
Finance: Mr. Brian Harris/Chief Financial Officer

Accessories, Solution, Lens, Contact	Ophthalmology
Case, Contact Lens	Ophthalmology
Lens, Intraocular	Ophthalmology
Lens, Other	Ophthalmology
Lenses, Soft Contact, Daily Wear	Ophthalmology

Medical Product Subsidiaries (Listed Separately)
Bausch & Lomb Inc., Greenville Solutions Plant
Bausch & Lomb Pharmaceutical, Inc.
Bausch & Lomb Surgical
Bausch & Lomb, Inc.
Bausch & Lomb, Vision Care
Eyeonics, Inc.

BAUSCH & LOMB HEARING SYSTEMS DIV.
See Miracle-Ear

BAUSCH & LOMB INC., GREENVILLE SOLUTIONS PLANT
585-338-6000
8507 Pelham Rd., Greenville, SC 29615-9598
FDA Number: 1032500
Ownership: Bausch & Lomb
Stock Symbol: BOL
Traded On: NYSE
Produces/Sells CE-marked Devices: N

Cleaner, Lens, Contact	Ophthalmology
Lens, Contact, Gas-Permeable	Ophthalmology

BAUSCH & LOMB INC., OPTICAL SYSTEMS DIV.
See Leica Microsystems, Inc., Educational & Analytical Division

BAUSCH & LOMB PHARMACEUTICAL, INC.
800-227-1427
8500 Hidden River Pkwy, Tampa, FL 33637
585-338-6000
FDA Number: 1052807
Web site: www.bausch.com
Ownership: Bausch & Lomb
Stock Symbol: BOL
Traded On: NYSE
Produces/Sells CE-marked Devices: N

Cleaner, Lens, Contact	Ophthalmology
Viscoelastic Surgical Aid	Ophthalmology

BAUSCH & LOMB SURGICAL
See Bausch & Lomb, Inc.

BAUSCH & LOMB SURGICAL
636-255-5051
3365 Tree Ct. Indust. Blvd., St. Louis, MO 63122-6615
FDA Number: 1920664
Fax: 909-399-1422
Web site: www.bausch.com
Medical Products Sales Volume: $250,000,000
Total Employees: 1000
Ownership: Bausch & Lomb
Stock Symbol: BOL
Traded On: NYSE
Quality System Registration Information: ISO9000; ISO9001; ISO9002
Produces/Sells CE-marked Devices: Y
Distribution: Manufacturer Direct
Production: Michael Nicoletta/Vice President Manufacturing

Adapter, Tube, Tracheal	Anesthesiology
Adenotome	Ear/Nose/Throat
Applicator, ENT	Ear/Nose/Throat
Aspirator, Ophthalmic	Ophthalmology
Balloon, Epistaxis (Nasal)	Ear/Nose/Throat
Blade, Surgical, Saw, General & Plastic Surgery	Surgery
Block, Cutting, ENT	Ear/Nose/Throat
Burr, Corneal, Manual	Ophthalmology
Burr, Surgical, General & Plastic Surgery	Surgery
Caliper, Ophthalmic	Ophthalmology
Cannula, Bronchial	Ear/Nose/Throat
Cannula, Cyclodialysis (Eye)	Ophthalmology
Cannula, Ear	Ear/Nose/Throat
Cannula, Lacrimal (Eye)	Ophthalmology
Cannula, Nasal	General

BAUSCH & LOMB SURGICAL   636-255-5051 *(cont'd)*

Cannula, Ophthalmic	Ophthalmology
Cannula, Sinus	Ear/Nose/Throat
Cannula, Surgical, General & Plastic Surgery	Surgery
Cannula, Tracheostomy	Ear/Nose/Throat
Catheter, Suction, With Tip	General
Cautery, Radiofrequency, AC-Powered	Ophthalmology
Cautery, Thermal, Battery-Powered	Ophthalmology
Chisel, Bone, Surgical	Dental And Oral
Chisel, Mastoid	Ear/Nose/Throat
Chisel, Middle Ear	Ear/Nose/Throat
Chisel, Nasal	Ear/Nose/Throat
Chisel, Surgical, Manual	Surgery
Clamp, Cannula	Gastroenterology/Urology
Clamp, Eyelid, Ophthalmic	Ophthalmology
Clamp, Muscle, Ophthalmic	Ophthalmology
Clamp, Ossicle Holding	Ear/Nose/Throat
Clamp, Surgical, General & Plastic Surgery	Surgery
Clip, Iris Retractor	Ophthalmology
Container, Sterilization (Tray)	General
Crimper, Wire, ENT	Ear/Nose/Throat
Cuff, Tracheal Tube, Inflatable	Anesthesiology
Cuff, Tracheostomy Tube	Ear/Nose/Throat
Curette, Adenoid	Ear/Nose/Throat
Curette, Ear	Ear/Nose/Throat
Curette, Nasal	Ear/Nose/Throat
Curette, Ophthalmic	Ophthalmology
Curette, Surgical	Surgery
Cutter, Vitreous Aspiration, AC-Powered	Ophthalmology
Cutter, Vitreous Infusion Suction	Ophthalmology
Depressor, Orbital	Ophthalmology
Die, Wire Bending, ENT	Ear/Nose/Throat
Dilator, Lacrimal	Ophthalmology
Dissector, Surgical, General & Plastic Surgery	Surgery
Drill, Manual (With Burr, Trephine & Accessories)	Cns/Neurology
Drill, Powered Compound (With Burr, Trephine & Accessories)	Cns/Neurology
Drum, Eye Knife Test	Ophthalmology
Electrode, Electrosurgical, Active, Foot Controlled	Surgery
Elevator, ENT	Ear/Nose/Throat
Elevator, Surgical, General & Plastic Surgery	Surgery
Erisophake	Ophthalmology
Extractor, Cataract	Ophthalmology
File, Surgical, General & Plastic Surgery	Surgery
Forceps, Dressing	Surgery
Forceps, ENT	Ear/Nose/Throat
Forceps, General & Plastic Surgery	Surgery
Forceps, Hemostatic	Surgery
Forceps, Ophthalmic	Ophthalmology
Forceps, Tissue	Surgery
Forceps, Wire Closure, ENT	Ear/Nose/Throat
Gag, Mouth	Ear/Nose/Throat
Gauge, Mastoid	Ear/Nose/Throat
Gouge, Surgical, General & Plastic Surgery	Surgery
Handle, Scalpel	Surgery
Headlight, ENT	Ear/Nose/Throat
Holder, Needle	Gastroenterology/Urology
Holder, Needle, Other	Surgery
Hook, Incus	Ear/Nose/Throat
Hook, Microsurgical Ear	Ear/Nose/Throat
Hook, Ophthalmic	Ophthalmology
Hook, Rhinoplastic	Surgery
Hook, Scleral Fixation	Ophthalmology
Hook, Skin	Surgery
Hook, Strabismus	Ophthalmology
Hook, Surgical, General & Plastic Surgery	Surgery
Hook, Tonsil Suturing	Ear/Nose/Throat
Hook, Tracheal	Ear/Nose/Throat
Hook, Tracheal, ENT	Ear/Nose/Throat
Instrument, Microsurgical	Cns/Neurology
Introducer, Sphere	Ophthalmology
Irrigator, Sinus	Ear/Nose/Throat
Jig, Piston Cutting, ENT	Ear/Nose/Throat
Keratome, AC-Powered	Ophthalmology
Kit, Irrigation, Eye	Ophthalmology
Kit, Laryngeal Injection	Ear/Nose/Throat
Kit, Tracheotomy	Anesthesiology
Knife, Cataract	Ophthalmology
Knife, Dermatome	Surgery
Knife, Ear	Ear/Nose/Throat
Knife, Keratome	Ophthalmology
Knife, Laryngeal	Ear/Nose/Throat
Knife, Myringotomy	Ear/Nose/Throat
Knife, Nasal	Ear/Nose/Throat
Knife, Ophthalmic	Ophthalmology
Knife, Skin Grafting	Surgery
Knife, Tonsil	Ear/Nose/Throat
Lens, Intraocular	Ophthalmology
Light, Surgical Headlight	Dental And Oral
Magnet, AC-Powered	Ophthalmology
Mallet, Surgical, General & Plastic Surgery	Surgery
Marker, Sclera (Ocular)	Ophthalmology
Microscope, Operating, AC-Powered, Ophthalmic	Ophthalmology

BAUSCH & LOMB SURGICAL   636-255-5051 *(cont'd)*

Mirror, ENT	Ear/Nose/Throat
Mirror, General & Plastic Surgery	Surgery
Mirror, Headband, Ophthalmic	Ophthalmology
Mirror, Laryngeal	Ear/Nose/Throat
Mirror, Middle Ear	Ear/Nose/Throat
Mold, Middle Ear	Ear/Nose/Throat
Monitor, Eye Movement	Ophthalmology
Needle, Aspiration And Injection, Reusable	Surgery
Nipper, Malleus	Ear/Nose/Throat
Obturator, Cleft Palate	Ear/Nose/Throat
Osteotome, Manual (Plastic Surgery)	Surgery
Pachometer	Surgery
Phacoemulsification System	Ophthalmology
Phacofragmentation Unit	Ophthalmology
Pick, Microsurgical Ear	Ear/Nose/Throat
Probe, Lacrimal	Ophthalmology
Probe, Radiofrequency Lesion	Cns/Neurology
Probe, Sinus	Ear/Nose/Throat
Probe, Trabeculotomy	Ophthalmology
Prosthesis, Ear, Internal	Surgery
Prosthesis, Larynx	Ear/Nose/Throat
Punch, Adenoid	Ear/Nose/Throat
Punch, Antrum	Ear/Nose/Throat
Punch, Corneo-Scleral	Ophthalmology
Punch, Ethmoid	Ear/Nose/Throat
Punch, Nasal	Ear/Nose/Throat
Punch, Tonsil	Ear/Nose/Throat
Rasp, Ear	Ear/Nose/Throat
Rasp, Frontal-Sinus	Ear/Nose/Throat
Rasp, Nasal	Ear/Nose/Throat
Rasp, Surgical, General & Plastic Surgery	Surgery
Retractor, Fiberoptic	Gastroenterology/Urology
Retractor, Ophthalmic	Ophthalmology
Retractor, Orbital	Surgery
Retractor, Surgical	Surgery
Ring, Ophthalmic (Flieringa)	Ophthalmology
Rongeur, Lacrimal Sac	Ophthalmology
Rongeur, Mastoid	Ear/Nose/Throat
Saw, Nasal	Ear/Nose/Throat
Scissors, Disposable	General
Scissors, Ear	Ear/Nose/Throat
Scissors, Nasal	Ear/Nose/Throat
Scissors, Ophthalmic	Ophthalmology
Scissors, Plastic Surgery (Dissecting)	Surgery
Scissors, Wire Cutting, ENT	Ear/Nose/Throat
Shield, Eye, Ophthalmic	Ophthalmology
Snare, Ear	Ear/Nose/Throat
Snare, Enucleating	Ophthalmology
Snare, Nasal	Ear/Nose/Throat
Snare, Tonsil	Ear/Nose/Throat
Spatula, Middle Ear	Ear/Nose/Throat
Spatula, Ophthalmic	Ophthalmology
Spatula, Surgical, General & Plastic Surgery	Surgery
Speculum, Ear	Ear/Nose/Throat
Speculum, Nasal	Ear/Nose/Throat
Speculum, Ophthalmic	Ophthalmology
Splint, Nasal	Ear/Nose/Throat
Sponge, Gauze	Dental And Oral
Sponge, Ophthalmic	Ophthalmology
Spoon, Ear	Ear/Nose/Throat
Spoon, Ophthalmic	Ophthalmology
Spud, Ophthalmic	Ophthalmology
Stimulator, Neuromuscular, External Functional	Cns/Neurology
Stripper, Vein, Reusable	Surgery
Stylet, Surgical	Surgery
Syringe, Ear	Ear/Nose/Throat
Syringe, Ophthalmic	Ophthalmology
Tape, Measuring, Ruler And Caliper	Surgery
Tonometer, AC-Powered	Ophthalmology
Tonsillectome	Ear/Nose/Throat
Tray, Surgical Instrument	Surgery
Trephine, Manual, Ophthalmic (Corneal)	Ophthalmology
Trocar, Laryngeal	Ear/Nose/Throat
Tubal Occlusive Device	Obstetrics/Gynecology
Tube, Ear Suction	Ear/Nose/Throat
Tube, Laryngectomy	Ear/Nose/Throat
Tube, Tonsil Suction	Ear/Nose/Throat
Tube, Tracheostomy (Breathing Tube), ENT	Ear/Nose/Throat
Tube, Tympanostomy	Ear/Nose/Throat

BAUSCH & LOMB, INC.   585-338-8731
100 Research Drive, Wlmington, MA 01887
FDA Number: 1281950
Ownership: Bausch & Lomb
Stock Symbol: BOL
Traded On: NYSE
Produces/Sells CE-marked Devices: N

Lens, Contact (Other Material)	Ophthalmology
Lens, Contact (orthokeratology)	Ophthalmology

BAUSCH & LOMB, INC. — 585-338-8731
130 Commerce Dr., Greenville, SC 29615
FDA Number: 1051854
Web site: www.bausch.com
Ownership: Bausch & Lomb
Stock Symbol: BOL
Traded On: NYSE
Produces/Sells CE-marked Devices: N

Accessories, Solution, Lens, Contact	Ophthalmology

BAUSCH & LOMB, INC. — 585-338-8731
1501 Graves Mill Rd., Lynchburg, VA 24502
FDA Number: 1123818
Web site: www.bausch.com
Ownership: Bausch & Lomb
Stock Symbol: BOL
Traded On: NYSE
Produces/Sells CE-marked Devices: N

Burr, Corneal, Manual	Ophthalmology
Cannula, Ophthalmic	Ophthalmology
Forceps, Ophthalmic	Ophthalmology
Handle, Scalpel	Surgery
Needle, Aspiration And Injection, Reusable	Surgery
Punch, Corneo-Scleral	Ophthalmology
Ring, Ophthalmic (Flieringa)	Ophthalmology
Tube, Aspirating, Flexible, Connecting	Anesthesiology
Tubing, Non-Invasive	Surgery

BAUSCH & LOMB, INC. — 813-724-6600
21 Park Place Blvd. N., Clearwater, FL 33759
FDA Number: 1119279   Fax: 813-724-6693
Web site: www.bausch.com
Total Employees: 190
Ownership: Bausch & Lomb
Stock Symbol: BOL
Traded On: NYSE
Quality System Registration Information: ISO9001
Produces/Sells CE-marked Devices: Y
Distribution: Manufacturer Direct, Exporter
General Admin.: Bob Blankemeyer/President
Mktg./Adv.: Jim Tiffany/Vice President Marketing & Sales
Production: Shelly Valdez/Coord. Regulatory Affairs

Contract Manufacturing	General
Folders and Injectors, Intraocular Lens (IOL)	Ophthalmology
Guide, Intraocular Lens	Ophthalmology
Lens, Intraocular	Ophthalmology

BAUSCH & LOMB, INC. — 585-338-8731
499 Sovereign Ct., Manchester, MO 63011
FDA Number: 1932180
Web site: www.bausch.com
Ownership: Bausch & Lomb
Stock Symbol: BOL
Traded On: NYSE
Produces/Sells CE-marked Devices: N

Burr	Ear/Nose/Throat
Cannula, Nasal, Oxygen	Anesthesiology
Forceps, Tube Introduction	Anesthesiology
Holder, Speculum, ENT	Ear/Nose/Throat
Knife, Surgical	Dental And Oral
Nasopharyngoscope (Flexible Or Rigid)	Ear/Nose/Throat
Splint, Nasal	Ear/Nose/Throat
Tube, Aspirating, Flexible, Connecting	Anesthesiology

BAUSCH & LOMB, PERSONAL PRODUCTS DIV.
See Bausch & Lomb, Vision Care

BAUSCH & LOMB, VISION CARE — 800-553-5340 / 585-338-6000
1400 N. Goodman St., Rochester, NY 14609-3547
FDA Number: 1313525   Fax: 585-338-6896
Web site: www.bausch.com
Medical Products Sales Volume: $347,000,000
Total Employees: 4000
Ownership: Bausch & Lomb
Stock Symbol: BOL
Traded On: NYSE
Produces/Sells CE-marked Devices: N
Distribution: Manufacturer Direct
Production: Michael Santalucia/Vice President Regulatory Affairs

Accessories, Solution, Lens, Contact	Ophthalmology
Cleaner, Lens, Contact	Ophthalmology
Keratome, AC-Powered	Ophthalmology
Lens, Contact (Other Material)	Ophthalmology
Sterilizer, Soft Lens, Thermal, AC-Powered	Ophthalmology

BAUSCH & STROEBEL MACHINE COMPANY, INC. — 866-512-2637
112 Nod Road, Unit 17, Clinton, CT 06413
FDA Number: n/a   Fax: 877-512-2637

BAUSCH & STROEBEL MACHINE — 866-512-2637 (cont'd)
E-mail: info@bausch-stroebel.com
Web site: www.bausch-stroebel.com
Medical Products Sales Volume: $800,000,000
Year Founded: 1967
Total Employees: 22
Ownership: Private
Federal Procurement Eligibility: Small Business, GSA Contract, VA Contract
General Admin.: Oliver Bausch/President

Closure, Other	General
Conveyor, Tray	General
Labeling Equipment	General
Washer, Laundry	General

BAXA CORPORATION — 800-567-2292 / 303-690-4204
9540 S Maroon Circle, Suite 400, Englewood, CO 80112
FDA Number: 1419106   Fax: 303-690-4804
E-mail: baxamail@baxa.com
Web site: www.baxa.com
Annual Revenue: $50-$100 Million
Year Founded: 1975
Total Employees: 50   Marketing Staff: 16   Sales Staff: 38
Ownership: Private
Quality System Registration Information: ISO9001
Produces/Sells CE-marked Devices: Y
Federal Procurement Eligibility: Small Business
Distribution: Manufacturer Direct, Manufacturer Through Distributor, Manufacturer Through Manufacturer Reps, OEM, Exclusive Distributor, Importer, Exporter
General Admin.: Greg Baldwin/Chairman, Chief Executive Officer
    Jeffrey Baldwin/President, Chief Operating Officer
    Mr. Jim Morphew/Vice President Information Technology
Mktg./Adv.: Mr. Brendan Parker/Director Sales
    Mr. Dennis Schneider/Senior Vice President Marketing & Business Development
    Marian Robinson/Vice President Marketing
    Pam Price/Vice President Sales
Production: Mr. Joe Tsiakals/Senior Vice President Quality Assurance
    Mr. A. Wahid Khan/Vice President Manufacturing
    Steve VanEngen/Vice President Operations
    Mr. Tim Gordon/Vice President Process Development
    Pat Hynes/Vice President Quality Systems
Finance: Mr. David Runck/Chief Financial Officer

Cap, Tip, Syringe	General
Computer Software	General
Container, Medication, Graduated Liquid	General
Dispenser, Fluid	General
Dispenser, Liquid, Unit-Dose	General
Dispenser, Narcotic	General
Dispenser, Other	General
Filter, Infusion Line	General
Filter, Syringe	General
Injector, Syringe	General
Mixer, Clinical Laboratory	Chemistry
Needle, Intravenous	General
Needle, Other	General
Pin, Transfer, Solution	General
Pump, Industrial	General
Pump, Infusion	General
Pump, Laboratory	Chemistry
Set, Administration, Intravenous, Needle-Free	General
Syringe, Piston	General
System, Delivery, Drug, Unit-Dose	General
Transfer Unit, IV Fluid	General
Tubing, Fluid Delivery	General

BAXANO, INC. — 408-514-2200
655 River Oaks Parkway, San Jose, CA 95134
FDA Number: 3006324586   Fax: 408-514-2201
E-mail: 1-877-6BAXANO
Web site: http://www.baxano.com
Year Founded: 2005
Ownership: Private
Produces/Sells CE-marked Devices: N
General Admin.: Mr. Tony Recupero/President, Chief Executive Officer
Mktg./Adv.: Mr. Amie Borgstrom/Director Marketing
Production: Mr. Greg Weslh/Director Operations
    Mr. Ed Sinclair/Vice President Quality Control & Regulatory Affairs
Research: Mr. Mike Wallace/Senior Vice President Research & Development
Finance: Mr. George Harter, Jr./Chief Financial Officer

Rongeur, Manual, Neurosurgical	Cns/Neurology
Stimulator, Nerve, ENT	Ear/Nose/Throat

BAXTER HEALTHCARE CORP., BAXTER BIOSCIENCE
See Baxter International Inc

BAXTER HEALTHCARE CORP., BIOSCIENCE
See Baxter International Inc

BAXTER HEALTHCARE CORP., FENWAL
See Fenwal Inc.

BAXTER HEALTHCARE CORP., HYLAND
See Baxter International Inc

BAXTER HEALTHCARE CORP., IV SYS. & MEDICAL PRODUCTS
See Baxter Healthcare Corporation, Medication Delivery

BAXTER HEALTHCARE CORP., IV SYSTEMS
See Baxter Healthcare Corporation, Medication Delivery

BAXTER HEALTHCARE CORP., IV SYSTEMS/ALTERNATE CARE TEAM
See Baxter Healthcare Corporporation, Alternate Care And Channel Team

BAXTER HEALTHCARE CORP., IV SYSTEMS/ANESTHESIA
See Baxter Healthcare Corporation, Baxter Pharmaceuticals And Technologies

BAXTER HEALTHCARE CORP., IV SYSTEMS/CLINTEC NUTRITION
See Baxter Healthcare Corporation Nutrition

BAXTER HEALTHCARE CORP., IV SYSTEMS/IV THERAPY
See Baxter Healthcare Corporation, Global Drug Delivery

BAXTER HEALTHCARE CORP., RENAL DIVISION 847-948-2000
7511 114th Avenue North, Largo, FL 33777
FDA Number: 1036337   Fax: 800-756-4952
E-mail: onebaxter@baxter.com
Ownership: Baxter International Inc
Stock Symbol: BAX
Traded On: NYSE
Produces/Sells CE-marked Devices: N

Bag, Blood, Collection	Hematology
Dialysate Delivery System, Peritoneal, Semi-Automatic	Gastroenterology/Urology
Dialysate Delivery System, Single Patient	Gastroenterology/Urology
Dialyzer, High Permeability	Gastroenterology/Urology
Equipment, Laboratory, Gen. Purpose (Specific Medical Use)	Chemistry
Hematocrit, Manual	Hematology
Kit, Administration, Intravenous	General
Kit, Administration, Peritoneal Dialysis, Disposable	Gastroenterology/Urology
Mixer/Scale, Blood	Hematology
Pressure Infusor, IV Container	General
Separator, Blood Cell, Automated	Hematology
Supplies, Blood Bank	Hematology
System, Hemodialysis, Access Recirculation Monitoring	Gastroenterology/Urology
System, Peritoneal Dialysis, Automatic	Gastroenterology/Urology
System/device, Pharmacy Compounding	General

BAXTER HEALTHCARE CORPORATION 847-473-6141
1606 E. University Dr., Phoenix, AZ 85034
FDA Number: 2090142
Ownership: Baxter International Inc
Stock Symbol: BAX
Traded On: NYSE
Produces/Sells CE-marked Devices: N

BAXTER HEALTHCARE CORPORATION 847-473-6141
1900 N. Hwy. 201, Mountain Home, AR 72653
FDA Number: 2314912
Ownership: Baxter International Inc
Stock Symbol: BAX
Traded On: NYSE
Produces/Sells CE-marked Devices: N

Kit, Administration, Peritoneal Dialysis, Disposable	Gastroenterology/Urology
System, Peritoneal Dialysis, Automatic	Gastroenterology/Urology

BAXTER HEALTHCARE CORPORATION 847-473-6141
21026 Alexander Court, Hayward, CA 94545
FDA Number: 2937398
Ownership: Baxter International Inc
Stock Symbol: BAX
Traded On: NYSE
Produces/Sells CE-marked Devices: N

Agent, Hemostatic, Absorbable, Collagen-Based	Surgery
Laparoscope, General & Plastic Surgery	Surgery
Regulator, Pressure, Gas Cylinder	Anesthesiology
Syringe, Irrigating	General

BAXTER HEALTHCARE CORPORATION 847-473-6141
3925 Gateway Blvd, Pinellas Park, FL 33782
FDA Number: 3004096418
Ownership: Baxter International Inc
Stock Symbol: BAX
Traded On: NYSE
Produces/Sells CE-marked Devices: N

BAXTER HEALTHCARE CORPORATION 847-473-6141
4501 Colorado Blvd., Los Angeles, CA 90039
FDA Number: 2011021
Ownership: Baxter International Inc

BAXTER HEALTHCARE CORPORATION 847-473-6141 *(cont'd)*
Stock Symbol: BAX
Traded On: NYSE
Produces/Sells CE-marked Devices: N

BAXTER HEALTHCARE CORPORATION 847-473-6141
4835 S. Mendenhall Rd., Memphis, TN 38141
FDA Number: 1041673
Ownership: Baxter International Inc
Stock Symbol: BAX
Traded On: NYSE
Produces/Sells CE-marked Devices: N

BAXTER HEALTHCARE CORPORATION 847-473-6141
65 Pitts Station Road, Marion, NC 28752
FDA Number: 1025114
Ownership: Baxter International Inc
Stock Symbol: BAX
Traded On: NYSE
Produces/Sells CE-marked Devices: N

Culture Media, Non-Selective And Non-Differential	Microbiology
Humidifier, Respiratory Gas, (Direct Patient Interface)	Anesthesiology

BAXTER HEALTHCARE CORPORATION 847-473-6141
911 North Davis, Cleveland, MS 38732
FDA Number: 1019003
Ownership: Baxter International Inc
Stock Symbol: JNJ
Traded On: NYSE
Produces/Sells CE-marked Devices: N

Kit, Blood, Transfusion	General
Syringe, Piston	General
System, Peritoneal Dialysis, Automatic	Gastroenterology/Urology

BAXTER HEALTHCARE CORPORATION 800-422-9837
One Baxter Parkway, Deerfield, IL 60015
FDA Number: 3005185784   Fax: 800-568-5020
Ownership: BAXTER INTERNATIONAL INC
Produces/Sells CE-marked Devices: N

Pump, Infusion	General

BAXTER HEALTHCARE CORPORATION NUTRITION 888-229-0001

One Baxter Pkwy., Deerfield, IL 60015 847-948-2000
FDA Number: 2032282   Fax: 888-229-0020
E-mail: onebaxter@baxter.com
Web site: www.baxter.com
Year Founded: 1931
Total Employees: 50000
Ownership: BAXTER INTERNATIONAL INC
Stock Symbol: BAX
Traded On: NYSE
Produces/Sells CE-marked Devices: N
Distribution: Manufacturer Direct, Manufacturer Through Distributor
General Admin.: Robert L. Parkinson/Chief Executive Officer
Jane Kiernan/General Manager

Container, IV	General
Sealer, Packaging	General
Solution, Intravenous	General
Solution, Nutrition, Parenteral	Gastroenterology/Urology
Standard, Amino Acid	Chemistry
Transfer Unit, IV Fluid	General

BAXTER HEALTHCARE CORPORATION, BAXTER BIOPHARMA SOLUTIONS 800-353-0887

927 S. Curry Pike Drive, Bloomington, IN 47402 812-333-0887
FDA Number: 1417572   Fax: 812-332-3079
E-mail: onebaxter@baxter.com
Web site: www.baxter.com
Year Founded: 1931
Ownership: Public
Stock Symbol: BAX
Traded On: NASDAQ
Produces/Sells CE-marked Devices: N
Distribution: Manufacturer Direct
General Admin.: Robert Parkinson Jr./Chief Executive Officer

Syringe, Other	General

BAXTER HEALTHCARE CORPORATION, BAXTER PHARMACEUTICALS AND TECHNOLOGIES 800-667-0959

95 Spring St., New Providence, NJ 07974 908-286-7000
FDA Number: n/a   Fax: 908-286-7044
E-mail: onebaxter@baxter.com
Web site: www.baxter.com
Annual Revenue: $100-$500 Million
Year Founded: 1931
Total Employees: 50000

MANUFACTURER PROFILES

BAXTER HEALTHCARE CORPORATION,   **800-667-0959** *(cont'd)*
Ownership: Private
Stock Symbol: BAX
Traded On: NYSE
Produces/Sells CE-marked Devices: N
Distribution: Manufacturer Direct, Manufacturer Through Distributor, Manufacturer Through Manufacturer Reps, Service Direct
General Admin.: Robert L. Parkinson/Chief Executive Officer

Analyzer, Gas, Enflurane, Gaseous Phase (Anesthetic Conc.)	Anesthesiology

BAXTER HEALTHCARE CORPORATION,   **888-229-0001**
GLOBAL DRUG DELIVERY

One Baxter Parkway, Deerfield, IL 60015-4625   **800-422-9837**
FDA Number: n/a   *Fax:* 800-568-5020
E-mail: onebaxter@baxter.com
Web site: www.baxter.com
Annual Revenue: $100-$500 Million
Year Founded: 1931
Total Employees: 50000
Ownership: Public
Stock Symbol: BAX
Traded On: NYSE
Produces/Sells CE-marked Devices: N
Distribution: Manufacturer Direct, Manufacturer Through Distributor
General Admin.: Robert L Parkinson/Chief Executive Officer

Bottle, Evacuated	General
Bottle, Sterile Solution	General
Cap, Tip, Syringe	General
Container, Evacuated	General
Container, IV	General
Hanger, Intravenous	General
Heparin	Pathology
Irrigating Solution, Non-Injectable	Surgery
Liquid Anti-Infectives	General
Premixed Medications	General
Solution, Intravenous	General
Water, Distilled (Irrigation)	Gastroenterology/Urology

BAXTER HEALTHCARE CORPORATION,   **949-851-9066**
MEDICATION DELIVERY

17511 Armstrong Ave, Irvine, CA 92614
FDA Number: 2025695   *Fax:* 800-756-4952
E-mail: onebaxter@baxter.com
Web site: www.baxter.com
Year Founded: 1931
Ownership: Private
Stock Symbol: BAX
Traded On: NYSE
Produces/Sells CE-marked Devices: N
General Admin.: Robert L. Parkinson, Jr./Chief Executive Officer

Agent, Hemostatic, Absorbable, Collagen-Based	Surgery
Infusion Pump, Enteral	General
Laparoscope, General & Plastic Surgery	Surgery
Pump, Infusion, Elastomeric	General
Pump, Infusion, Patient Controlled Analgesia (PCA)	General
Syringe, Piston	General

BAXTER HEALTHCARE CORPORATION,   **888-229-0001**
MEDICATION DELIVERY

25212 W. Illinois Route 120,   **847-948-4770**
Round Lake, IL 60073
FDA Number: n/a   *Fax:* 888-229-0020
E-mail: onebaxter@baxter.com
Web site: www.baxter.com
Year Founded: 1931
Total Employees: 50000
Ownership: Public
Stock Symbol: BAX
Traded On: NYSE
Produces/Sells CE-marked Devices: N
Distribution: Manufacturer Direct, Manufacturer Through Distributor
General Admin.: Robert L Parkinson/Chief Executive Officer
     David Bonderud/President

Accessories, Catheter	Surgery
Arthroscope	Orthopedics
Catheter, Suction, With Tip	General
Container, IV	General
Equipment, Laboratory, Gen. Purpose (Specific Medical Use)	Chemistry
Filter, Infusion Line	General
Kit, Administration, Peritoneal Dialysis, Disposable	Gastroenterology/Urology
Processor, Frozen Blood	Hematology
Set, Administration, Intravenous, Needle-Free	General
Solution, Intravenous	General
Stopcock	General
Syringe, Piston	General
Transfer Unit, IV Fluid	General

BAXTER HEALTHCARE CORPORATION, RENAL   **888-229-0001**
1620 Waukegan Road, McGaw Park, IL 60085   **847-473-6030**
FDA Number: 1423500   *Fax:* 847-574-5829
E-mail: onebaxter@baxter.com
Web site: www.baxter.com
Annual Revenue: $100-$500 Million
Year Founded: 1931
Total Employees: 50000
Ownership: Baxter International Inc
Stock Symbol: BAX
Traded On: NYSE
Produces/Sells CE-marked Devices: N
Distribution: Manufacturer Direct
General Admin.: Robert L Parkinson/Chief Executive Officer
     Bruce McGillivray/Vice President

Accessories, Blood Circuit, Hemodialysis	Gastroenterology/Urology
Accessories, Catheter	Surgery
Adapter, Catheter	Surgery
Dialyzer, Capillary, Hollow Fiber (Hemodialysis)	Gastroenterology/Urology
Dialyzer, High Permeability	Gastroenterology/Urology
Hemodialyzer, Re-use, High Flux	Gastroenterology/Urology
Hemodialyzer, Re-use, Low Flux	Gastroenterology/Urology
Kit, Administration, Peritoneal Dialysis, Disposable	Gastroenterology/Urology
Needle, Fistula	Gastroenterology/Urology
Peritoneal Dialysis Unit (CAPD)	Gastroenterology/Urology
Pump, Blood, Hemodialysis Unit	Gastroenterology/Urology
Solution, Dialysis	Gastroenterology/Urology
System, Peritoneal Dialysis, Automatic	Gastroenterology/Urology

BAXTER HEALTHCARE CORPORPORATION,   **888-229-0001**
ALTERNATE CARE AND CHANNEL TEAM

One Baxter Parkway, Deerfield, IL 60015-4625   **847-948-2000**
FDA Number: 1417572   *Fax:* 800-568-5020
E-mail: onebaxter@baxter.com
Web site: www.baxter.com
Annual Revenue: $100-$500 Million
Year Founded: 1931
Total Employees: 50000
Ownership: Public
Stock Symbol: BAX
Traded On: NYSE
Produces/Sells CE-marked Devices: N
Distribution: Manufacturer Direct, Manufacturer Through Distributor
General Admin.: Robert L. Parkinson/Chief Executive Officer

Kit, Administration, Blood	General
Kit, Administration, Intravenous	General
Kit, Intravenous Extension Tubing	General
Kit, Intravenous, Administration, Buret	General
Needle, Intravenous	General
Pump, Infusion	General
Pump, Infusion, Ambulatory	General
Pump, Infusion, Syringe	General
Set, Administration, Intravenous, Needle-Free	General
Stopcock	General
Transfer Unit, IV Fluid	General
Tubing, Fluid Delivery	General

BAXTER HEALTHCARE OF PUERTO RICO   **847-948-4054**
530 Road #5, Building #1, Bo Juana Matos, PR 00962
FDA Number: 3004483508
Ownership: Baxter International Inc
Stock Symbol: BAX
Traded On: NYSE
Produces/Sells CE-marked Devices: N

BAXTER HEALTHCARE S.A.   **847-948-2000**
Rd. 721, Km. 0.3, Aibonito, PR 00609
FDA Number: 2649614   *Fax:* 800-756-4952
E-mail: onebaxter@baxter.com
Ownership: Baxter International Inc
Stock Symbol: BAX
Traded On: NYSE
Produces/Sells CE-marked Devices: N

Collector, Blood, Vacuum-Assisted	Hematology
Container, IV	General
Kit, Administration, Intravenous	General
Kit, Blood, Transfusion	General
Separator, Blood Cell, Automated	Hematology
Stopcock	General
System, Peritoneal Dialysis, Automatic	Gastroenterology/Urology
Transfer Unit, Blood	Hematology
Transfer Unit, IV Fluid	General
Urological Irrigation System	Gastroenterology/Urology

BAXTER HEALTHCARE, MEDICATION
DELIVERY/ANESTHESIA & CRITICAL

See Baxter Healthcare Corporation, Baxter Pharmaceuticals And Technologies

BAXTER INTERNATIONAL INC
One Baxter Parkway, Deerfield, IL 60015
800-422-9837
847-948-2000
Fax: 847-948-3642
FDA Number: 1417572
E-mail: onebaxter@baxter.com
Web site: www.baxter.com
Annual Revenue: More than $1 Billion
Year Founded: 1931
Total Employees: 46500
Ownership: Public
Stock Symbol: BAX
Traded On: NYSE
Produces/Sells CE-marked Devices: N
Distribution: Manufacturer Direct, Manufacturer Through Manufacturer Reps, OEM, Service Direct
General Admin.: Mr. Robert L Parkinson, Jr/Chairman
    Ms. Karennan Terrell/Chief Information Officer
    Mr. Norbert Riedel/Chief Scientific Officer, Vice President
Production: Mr. James Michael Gatling/Vice President Manufacturing
Finance: Mr. Robert M Davis/Chief Financial Officer

Plasma, Deficient, Factor, Coagulation	Hematology

Medical Product Subsidiaries (Listed Separately)
Baxter Healthcare Corp., Renal Division
Baxter Healthcare Corporation
Baxter Healthcare Corporation Nutrition
Baxter Healthcare Corporation, Baxter Biopharma Solutions
Baxter Healthcare Corporation, Baxter Pharmaceuticals And Technologies
Baxter Healthcare Corporation, Global Drug Delivery
Baxter Healthcare Corporation, Medication Delivery
Baxter Healthcare Corporation, Renal
Baxter Healthcare Corporoation, Alternate Care And Channel Team
Baxter Healthcare Of Puerto Rico
Baxter Healthcare S.A.
Baxter Productos Medicos, Ltda.
Baxter Sales & Distribution Corp

BAXTER SALES & DISTRIBUTION CORP
Rexco Industrial Park, State Road #24, Buchanan, Guaynabo, PR 00968
847-473-6141
FDA Number: 2647689
Ownership: Baxter International Inc
Stock Symbol: BAX
Traded On: NYSE
Produces/Sells CE-marked Devices: N

BAY CORPORATION
867 Canterbury Road, Westlake, OH 44145-1486
888-835-3800
440-835-2212
Fax: 440-835-1377
FDA Number: n/a
E-mail: sales@baycorp.com
Web site: www.baycorporation.com
Medical Products Sales Volume: $5,000,000
Annual Revenue: $1-$5 Million
Year Founded: 1979
Total Employees: 30   *Marketing Staff:* 5   *Sales Staff:* 5
Ownership: Private
Quality System Registration Information: ISO9001
Produces/Sells CE-marked Devices: Y
Federal Procurement Eligibility: Small Business
Distribution: Manufacturer Through Distributor, OEM, Exporter
General Admin.: Brooks G. Hull/President, Chief Executive Officer
Mktg./Adv.: Mark Altstadt/Manager Marketing & Sales
Production: Bruce Wick/Vice President Engineering & Product Development
    Bruce Wick/Vice President Quality Assurance & Regulatory Affairs

Contract Manufacturing, Product, Durable	General
Fitting, Other	General

BAY OPTICAL INSTRUMENTS
2401 15th St., San Francisco, CA 94114
415-431-8711
FDA Number: n/a
Fax: 415-252-9184
E-mail: ergoadap@bayoptical.com
Web site: www.bayoptical.com
Year Founded: 1983
Ownership: Private

Microscope, Laboratory, Optical	Microbiology

BAY SHORE MEDICAL EQUIPMENT CORP.
235 South Fehr Way, Bay Shore, NY 11706
631-586-1991
FDA Number: 3005810333
Fax: 631-467-5734
Ownership: Private
Produces/Sells CE-marked Devices: N

Generator, Diagnostic X-Ray, High Voltage, Single Phase	Radiology
Holder, Radiographic Cassette, Wall-Mounted	Radiology
Mount, X-Ray Tube, Diagnostic	Radiology
Radiographic Unit, Diagnostic, Mammographic	Radiology
Stretcher, Wheeled (Mobile)	General
Table, Radiographic, Non-Tilting, Powered	Radiology

BAYER CONSUMER CARE
See Bayer Healthcare Llc, Consumer Care

BAYER HEALTHCARE LLC
555 White Plains Rd., 5th Floor, Tarrytown, NY 10591
914-366-1800
FDA Number: 1810909
Ownership: Private
Produces/Sells CE-marked Devices: N
General Admin.: Dr. Jaurg Reinhart/Chief Executive Officer
Mktg./Adv.: Paul Bentz/Sales Representative
Production: Chester McCoy/Director Regulatory Affairs

Analyzer, Chemistry, Urinalysis	Chemistry
Azo-Dyes, Colorimetric, Bilirubin And Conjugates	Chemistry
Bath, Tissue Flotation, Pathology	Pathology
Colorimeter, General Use	Chemistry
Colorimetric Method, Triglycerides	Chemistry
Colorimetric, Occult Blood in Urine	Hematology
Computer, Diagnostic, Pre-Programmed, Single-Function	Cardiovascular
Control, Analyte (Assayed And Unassayed)	Chemistry
Control, Urinalysis (Assayed And Unassayed)	Chemistry
Diazo (Colorimetric), Nitrite (Urinary, Non-Quantitative)	Chemistry
Diazonium Colorimetry, Urobilinogen (Urinary, Non-Quant.)	Chemistry
Disc, Strip And Reagent, Microorganism Differentiation	Microbiology
Drying Unit	Chemistry
Enzymatic Method, Blood, Occult, Urinary	Chemistry
Enzymatic Method, Creatinine	Chemistry
Enzymatic Method, Glucose (Urinary, Non-Quantitative)	Chemistry
Glucose Dehydrogenase, Glucose	Chemistry
Indicator Method, Protein Or Albumin (Urinary, Non-Quant.)	Chemistry
Kit, Identification, Yeast	Microbiology
Kit, Yeast Screening	Microbiology
LDL & VLDL Precipitation, HDL	Chemistry
Leukocyte Alkaline Phosphatase	Hematology
Metallic Reduction Method, Glucose (Urinary, Non-Quant.)	Chemistry
Microtome, Cryostat	Pathology
NADH Oxidation/NAD Reduction, AST/SGOT	Chemistry
Nitroprusside, Ketones (Urinary, Non-Quantitative)	Chemistry
Radioassay, 17-Hydroxycorticosteroids	Chemistry
Radioimmunoassay, Human Chorionic Gonadotropin	Chemistry
Reagent, Creatinine (Test System)	Chemistry
Reagent, Glucose (Test System)	Chemistry
Reagent, Protein, Total	Chemistry
SGPT, Ultraviolet	Chemistry
System, Test, Blood Glucose, Over-The-Counter	Chemistry
Test, Urine Leukocyte	Hematology
Tetrazolium Int Dye-Diaphorase, Lactate Dehydrogenase	Chemistry
Urease, Photometric, Urea Nitrogen	Chemistry

Medical Product Subsidiaries (Listed Separately)
Bayer Healthcare Llc, Consumer Care
Bayer Healthcare, Llc

BAYER HEALTHCARE LLC, CONSUMER CARE
36 Columbia Rd., Morristown, NJ 07962
717-866-2141
FDA Number: 2248903
Fax: 717-866-3713
Web site: www.bayerhealthcare.com
Annual Revenue: $5-$10 Million
Total Employees: 53100
Ownership: Bayer Healthcare Llc
Stock Symbol: BAY
Traded On: Frankfurt
Produces/Sells CE-marked Devices: N
Distribution: Manufacturer Direct, Manufacturer Through Distributor
General Admin.: Gary Balkema/President

Contract Manufacturing, Pharmaceuticals/Chemicals	General
Detector/Remover, Lice	General

BAYER HEALTHCARE, LLC
430 South Beiger St., Mishawaka, IN 46544
574-256-3430
FDA Number: 1826988
Ownership: Bayer Healthcare Llc

Analyzer, Chemistry, Urinalysis	Chemistry
Calibrator, Drug Specific	Toxicology
Calibrator, Surrogate, Clinical Chemistry	Chemistry
Colorimeter, General Use	Chemistry
Colorimetric, Occult Blood in Urine	Hematology
Computer, Diagnostic, Pre-Programmed, Single-Function	Cardiovascular
Control, Analyte (Assayed And Unassayed)	Chemistry
Control, Drug Mixture	Toxicology
Control, Urinalysis (Assayed And Unassayed)	Chemistry
Diazonium Colorimetry, Urobilinogen (Urinary, Non-Quant.)	Chemistry
Disc, Strip And Reagent, Microorganism Differentiation	Microbiology
Enzymatic Method, Blood, Occult, Urinary	Chemistry
Enzymatic Method, Creatinine	Chemistry
Enzymatic Method, Glucose (Urinary, Non-Quantitative)	Chemistry
Enzyme Immunoassay, Ethosuximide	Toxicology
Enzyme Immunoassay, N-Acetylprocainamide	Toxicology
Enzyme Immunoassay, Primidone	Toxicology
Enzyme Immunoassay, Procainamide	Toxicology
Enzyme Immunoassay, Valproic Acid	Toxicology
Fluorescent Immunoassay, Tobramycin	Toxicology
Hexokinase, Glucose	Chemistry
Indicator Method, Protein Or Albumin (Urinary, Non-Quant.)	Chemistry
Kit, Identification, Yeast	Microbiology

BAYER HEALTHCARE, LLC   574-256-3430 *(cont'd)*

Lancet, Blood	General
Leukocyte Alkaline Phosphatase	Hematology
Metallic Reduction Method, Glucose (Urinary, Non-Quant.)	Chemistry
Multi Analyte Mixture, Calibrator	Chemistry
Nitroprusside, Ketones (Urinary, Non-Quantitative)	Chemistry
Radioimmunoassay, Gentamicin (125-I), Second Antibody	Toxicology
Radioimmunoassay, Netilmicin (125-I)	Toxicology
Reagent, Glucose (Test System)	Chemistry
Reagent, Occult Blood	Hematology
Stain, Wright's	Pathology
Stainer, Slide, Automated	Pathology
Test, Glycosylated Hemoglobin Assay	Hematology
Test, Urine Leukocyte	Hematology
Urease, Photometric, Urea Nitrogen	Chemistry

BAYER HEALTHCARE, LLC   574-256-3430
510 Oakmead Pkwy., Sunnyvale, CA 94085
FDA Number: 2954361
Ownership: Bayer Healthcare Llc
Produces/Sells CE-marked Devices: N

Test, Glycosylated Hemoglobin Assay	Hematology

BAYLIS MEDICAL COMPANY   800-850-9801   514-488-9801
5959 Trans-Canada Highway,
Montreal, QC H4t 1 Canada
FDA Number: 9710452   *Fax:* 514-488-7209
Web site: www.baylismedical.com
Ownership: Private
Produces/Sells CE-marked Devices: N

BAYLOR BIOMEDICAL SERVICES
See SYSMED

BAYZ SUNWEAR   410-939-2200
920 Revolution St., Havre De Grace, MD 21078
FDA Number: 3003425384   *Fax:* 410-939-5980
E-mail: info@bayz.com
Web site: www.bayz.com
Ownership: Private
Produces/Sells CE-marked Devices: N

Sunglasses (Including Photosensitive)	Ophthalmology

BBA FIBERWEB WASHOUGAL, INC.   800-772-7771   360-835-8787
3720 Grant St., Washougal, WA 98671-2807
FDA Number: n/a   *Fax:* 360-835-2546
E-mail: rkramer@bbafiberweb.com
Web site: www.bbafiberweb.com
Annual Revenue: $25-$50 Million
Total Employees: 100
Ownership: Prudential Overall Supply
Quality System Registration Information: ISO9002
Produces/Sells CE-marked Devices: N
Distribution: Manufacturer Direct
General Admin.: Rick Lundgren/President
Production: Gary Drews/Plant Manager

Linen	General

BBG, INC.   757-366-9211
1708 South Park Ct, Chesapeake, VA 23320
FDA Number: 1123074   *Fax:* 757-366-9170
E-mail: sales@bbginc.com
Web site: www.bbginc.com
Ownership: Private
Produces/Sells CE-marked Devices: N

Stimulator, Nerve, Transcutaneous (Pain Relief, TENS)	Cns/Neurology

BBI DIAGNOSTICS, A DIVISION OF SERACARE LIFE SCIEN   508-244-6428
375 West St., West Bridgewater, MA 02379
FDA Number: 1220394
Ownership: Private
Produces/Sells CE-marked Devices: N

Antibody Igm, If, Cytomegalovirus Virus	Microbiology
Antisera, IF, Toxoplasma Gondii	Microbiology
Control, Analyte (Assayed And Unassayed)	Chemistry
Control, Multi Analyte, All Kinds (Assayed And Unassayed)	Chemistry
Kit, Quality Control, Blood Banking	Hematology
Kit, Serological, Positive Control	Microbiology
Kit, Test(donors), For Bloodborne Pathogen	Immunology
Reagent, Borrelia, Serological	Microbiology

BCI INTERNATIONAL
See Smiths Medical Pm, Inc.

BCL X-RAY CANADA INC.   1-800-561-1214   905-624-0394
1575 Sismet Rd., Unit 5,
Mississauga, ONT L4W-1 Canada
FDA Number: n/a   *Fax:* 905-624-0401
E-mail: bclxray@sympatico.ca

BCL X-RAY CANADA INC.   1-800-561-1214 *(cont'd)*
Year Founded: 1976
Total Employees: 25
Ownership: Private
Produces/Sells CE-marked Devices: N
Distribution: Exclusive Distributor

BCT MIDWEST, INC.   785-856-1414
1220 Wagon Wheel Road, Lawrence, KS 66049
FDA Number: 3006084760

Bandage, Cast	Physical Med
Splint, Extremity, Non-Inflatable, External	Surgery

BD ACCU-GLASS
See Accu-Glass Llc

BD BECTON DICKINSON VACUTAINER SYSTEMS PREANALYTIC
See Becton, Dickinson & Co.

BD BIOSCIENCES   408-954-6307
2350 Qume Dr., San Jose, CA 95131
FDA Number: 2916837   *Fax:* 408-954-2007
Ownership: Becton Dickinson And Company
Produces/Sells CE-marked Devices: N

Counter, Cell Or Particle, Automated	Hematology
Counter, Cell, Differential Classifier, Automated	Hematology
Diluter, Blood Cell, Automated	Hematology
Equipment, Laboratory, Gen. Purpose (Specific Medical Use)	Chemistry
Fluid, Red Cell Lysing	Hematology
Pipetting And Diluting System, Automated	Chemistry
Reagents, Specific, Analyte	Hematology
Stain, Reticulocyte	Hematology

BD BIOSCIENCES DISCOVERY LABWARE   978-901-7431
One Becton Circle, Durham, NC 27712
FDA Number: 1054657

Bottle, Tissue Culture, Roller	Pathology
Dish, Tissue Culture	Pathology
General Purpose Microbiology Diagnostic Device	Microbiology
Labware, Assisted Reproduction	Obstetrics/Gynecology
Pipette, Diluting	Hematology
Pipette, Quantitative, Hematology	Hematology
Pipetting And Diluting System, Automated	Chemistry

BD CARIBE, LTD.
See Aspen Surgical Puerto Rico Corp.

BD DIAGNOSTIC SYSTEMS   800-675-0908
7 Loveton Circle, Sparks, MD 21152
FDA Number: 1119779
E-mail: customer_support@bd.com
Web site: www.bd.com
Year Founded: 1897
Ownership: Becton Dickinson And Company
Quality System Registration Information: ISO9000
Produces/Sells CE-marked Devices: Y
Distribution: Manufacturer Through Distributor, Manufacturer Through Manufacturer Reps
General Admin.: Ed Ludwig/Chief Executive Officer

Animal, Laboratory	Microbiology
Antibody, Treponema Pallidum	Microbiology
Antigen, (Febrile), Agglutination, Brucella SPP.	Microbiology
Antigen, B. Parapertussis	Microbiology
Antigen, B. Pertussis	Microbiology
Antigen, Febrile	Microbiology
Antigen, Febrile, Slide And Tube, Salmonella	Microbiology
Antigen, Non-Treponemal, All	Microbiology
Antigen, Salmonella SPP.	Microbiology
Antigen, Slide And Tube, Francisella Tularensis	Microbiology
Antigen, Slide And Tube, Listeria Monocytogenes	Microbiology
Antigen, Streptococcus SPP.	Microbiology
Antigen, Treponema Pallidum For FTA-ABS Test	Microbiology
Antiserum, Agglutinating, B. Parapertussis	Microbiology
Antiserum, Agglutinating, B. Pertussis, All	Microbiology
Antiserum, Control For Non-Treponemal Test	Microbiology
Antiserum, Escherichia Coli	Microbiology
Antiserum, Fluorescent Antibody For FTA-ABS Test	Microbiology
Antiserum, Fluorescent, B. Parapertussis	Microbiology
Antiserum, Fluorescent, B. Pertussis	Microbiology
Antiserum, Fluorescent, Groups, Streptococcus SPP.	Microbiology
Antiserum, Francisella Tularensis	Microbiology
Antiserum, H. Influenzae	Microbiology
Antiserum, Listeria Monocytogenes	Microbiology
Antiserum, N. Meningitidis	Microbiology
Antiserum, Positive And Negative Febrile Antigen Control	Microbiology
Antiserum, Salmonella SPP.	Microbiology
Antiserum, Shigella SPP.	Microbiology
Antiserum, Streptococcus Pneumoniae	Microbiology
Antiserum, Streptococcus SPP.	Microbiology
Antiserum, Vibrio Cholerae	Microbiology
Centrifuge, Hematocrit	Hematology

BD DIAGNOSTIC SYSTEMS   800-675-0908 *(cont'd)*

Computer, Patient Data Management	General
Corynebacterium Diphtheriae, Virulence Strip	Microbiology
Crystal Violet	Hematology
Culture Media, Amino Acid Assay	Microbiology
Culture Media, Antibiotic Assay	Microbiology
Culture Media, Antimicrobial Susceptibility Test	Microbiology
Culture Media, Enriched	Microbiology
Culture Media, For Isolation Of Pathogenic Neisseria	Microbiology
Culture Media, General Nutrient Broth	Microbiology
Culture Media, Mueller Hinton Agar Broth	Microbiology
Culture Media, Multiple Biochemical Test	Microbiology
Culture Media, Non-Propagating Transport	Microbiology
Culture Media, Non-Selective And Differential	Microbiology
Culture Media, Non-Selective And Non-Differential	Microbiology
Culture Media, Propagating Transport	Microbiology
Culture Media, Selective And Differential	Microbiology
Culture Media, Selective And Non-Differential	Microbiology
Culture Media, Selective Broth	Microbiology
Culture Media, Single Biochemical Test	Microbiology
Culture Media, Supplements	Microbiology
Culture Media, Vitamin Assay	Microbiology
DNA-Probe, Nucleic Acid Amplification, Chlamydia	Microbiology
Disc, Strip And Reagent, Microorganism Differentiation	Microbiology
Disc, Susceptibility, Antimicrobial	Microbiology
Dish, Petri	Chemistry
Dispenser, Disc, Sensitivity, Antibiotic	Microbiology
Enzyme Linked Immunoabsorbent Assay, Cytomegalovirus	Microbiology
Fibrometer	Hematology
Gelatin	Pathology
Generator, Gas, Microbiology	Microbiology
Kit, Identification, Glucose (Non-Ferment)	Microbiology
Kit, Meningitis Detection	Microbiology
Kit, Mycobacteria Identification	Microbiology
Kit, Screening, Staphylococcus Aureus	Microbiology
Loop, Inoculating	Microbiology
Media, Mycoplasma Detection	Pathology
Microplate	General
Monitor, Microbial Growth	Microbiology
Papain	Pathology
Pipette Tip	Chemistry
Pipette, Micro	Chemistry
Pipetter	Hematology
Plasma, Coagulase, Human/Horse/Rabbit	Microbiology
Plate, Culture	Microbiology
Reagent, Clostridium Difficile Toxin	Microbiology
Reagent, Streptolysin O/Antistreptolysin-Titer	Microbiology
Respiratory Syncytial Virus, Antigen, Antibody, IFA	Microbiology
Serum, Biological, General	Toxicology
Serum, Reactive And Non-Specific Control, FTA-ABS Test	Microbiology
Sorbent, FTA-ABS Test	Microbiology
Stain, Acid Fuchsin	Pathology
Stain, Acridine Orange	Pathology
Stain, Auramine O	Pathology
Stain, Biological, General	Pathology
Stain, Brilliant Green	Pathology
Stain, Carbol Fuchsin	Pathology
Stain, Crystal Violet, Histology	Pathology
Stain, Grams Iodine	Pathology
Stain, Malachite Green	Pathology
Stain, Methylene Blue	Pathology
Stain, Microbiological	Microbiology
Stain, Other	Pathology
Stain, Safranin	Pathology
Streptolysin O	Pathology
Swabs, Specimen Collection	General
System, Blood Culturing	Microbiology
Test, Agar Plate	Microbiology
Test, Agar Tube	Microbiology
Test, Antimicrobial Susceptibility	Microbiology
Test, Bacteria Characterization	General
Test, Bacterial Diagnostic	Microbiology
Test, DNA-Probe, Other	Microbiology
Test, Rheumatoid Factor	Immunology
Test, Syphilis (RPR or VDRL)	Microbiology
Transport System, Aerobic	Microbiology
Transport System, Anaerobic	Microbiology
Tube, Transfer	General

BD DIAGNOSTICS (GENEOHM SCIENCES, INC.)   (888) 436-3646
11085 North Torrey Pines Road, Suite 210,   **(858) 334-6300**
La Jolla, CA 92037
FDA Number: 3004788834   *Fax:* (858) 334-6301
E-mail: geneohm_customer_service@bd.com
Ownership: Becton Dickinson And Company
Produces/Sells CE-marked Devices: N

Concentrator, Clinical Sample	Chemistry
Nucleic Acid Amplification Assay System, Group B Streptococcus, Direct Specimen Test	Microbiology
Reagent, Clostridium Difficile Toxin	Microbiology
Reagent, General Purpose	Pathology

BD DIAGNOSTICS (GENEOHM SCIENCES, INC.)   (888) 436-3646
(cont'd)

System, Nucleic Acid Amplification Test, Dna, Methicillin Resistant Staphylococcus Aureus, Direct Specimen	Microbiology

BD LEE LABORATORIES   800-732-9150
1475 Athens Hwy., Grayson, GA 30017   **770-972-4450**
FDA Number: 1025402   *Fax:* 770-979-9570
E-mail: steve_palance@bd.com
Web site: www.leelabs.com
Medical Products Sales Volume: $5,800,000
Annual Revenue: $10-$25 Million
Total Employees: 42   *Marketing Staff:* 1   *Sales Staff:* 2
Ownership: Becton Dickinson And Company
Quality System Registration Information: ISO9001
Produces/Sells CE-marked Devices: N
Federal Procurement Eligibility: Small Business
Distribution: Manufacturer Direct, Manufacturer Through Distributor, Exporter
Mktg./Adv.: Anthony D. Porcelli/Manager National Marketing & Sales
     John W. Deutsch/Manager Product Development
Production: J. Douglas Guthrie/Director Operations
     Thomas Domke/Manager Materials
     Cindi Kisiel-Smith/Manager Quality Assurance & Regulatory Affairs

Antibody, Polyclonal	Microbiology
Antigen, (Febrile), Agglutination, Brucella SPP.	Microbiology
Antigen, Febrile	Microbiology
Antigen, Febrile, Slide And Tube, Salmonella	Microbiology
Antigen, Non-Treponemal, All	Microbiology
Antigen, Slide And Tube, Francisella Tularensis	Microbiology
Antigen, Streptococcus SPP.	Microbiology
Antigen, Treponema Pallidum For FTA-ABS Test	Microbiology
Antiserum, Control For Non-Treponemal Test	Microbiology
Antiserum, Escherichia Coli	Microbiology
Antiserum, Salmonella SPP.	Microbiology
Antiserum, Shigella SPP.	Microbiology
Antiserum, Streptococcus SPP.	Microbiology
Contract Laboratory	General
Culture Media, Supplements	Microbiology
Reagent, Clostridium Difficile Toxin	Microbiology
Reagent, Streptolysin O/Antistreptolysin-Titer	Microbiology

BD MEDICAL   760-631-6520
4665 North Ave., Oceanside, CA 92056
FDA Number: 2029238
Ownership: Private
Produces/Sells CE-marked Devices: N
General Admin.: Ann Gosier/Vice President Government Affairs
     Anthony Lakavage/Vice President Government Affairs
Mktg./Adv.: Robert Hallenbeck/Vice President Business Development

Container, Sharpes	General
Labware, Blood Collection	Chemistry
Needle, Hypodermic, Single Lumen With Syringe	General

BD MEDICAL - DIABETES CARE   201-847-4298
1329 West Hwy 6, Holdrege, NE 68949
FDA Number: 1920898
Ownership: Private
Produces/Sells CE-marked Devices: N

Needle, Aspiration And Injection, Disposable	Surgery
Needle, Hypodermic, Single Lumen With Syringe	General
Pad, Alcohol	General
Syringe, Piston	General

BD MEDICAL - MEDICAL SURGICAL SYSTEMS
See Becton Dickinson Infusion Therapy Systems, Inc.

BD MEDICAL - OPHTHALMIC SYSTEMS
See Becton Dickinson And Co.

BDC LABORATORIES   (303) 456-4665
4060 Youngfield Street, Wheat Ridge, CO 80033-3862
FDA Number: n/a   *Fax:* 303-940-2740
E-mail: craig@bdclabs.com
Web site: www.bdclabs.com
Ownership: Private
Produces/Sells CE-marked Devices: N

BDH, INC.   800-268-0310
350 Evans Ave., Toronto, ONT M8Z 1K5 Canada   **416-255-8521**
FDA Number: n/a   *Fax:* 416-626-1850
E-mail: klewis@bdhinc.com
Web site: www.bdhinc.com
Total Employees: 130   *Marketing Staff:* 10   *Sales Staff:* 10
Ownership: MERCK KGAA
Quality System Registration Information: ISO9002
Produces/Sells CE-marked Devices: Y
Distribution: Manufacturer Direct

BE WELL USA, INC.   229-890-1627
3195 7th St Se, Moultrie, GA 31788
FDA Number: 3004497290   *Fax:* 229-890-1637

BE WELL USA, INC.   229-890-1627 *(cont'd)*
E-mail: bewell@bewell-usa.com
Ownership: Private
Produces/Sells CE-marked Devices: N

Pack, Hot Or Cold, Disposable	Physical Med
Pack, Hot Or Cold, Reusable	Physical Med
Pack, Moist Heat	Physical Med

BEACON BIOLOGICALS, INC.   561-395-1862
5139 pointe alexis Drive, Boca Raton, FL 33433
FDA Number: 1064638   *Fax:* 561-394-7825
E-mail: DrDaya@BeaconBiologicals.com
Medical Products Sales Volume: $900,000
Annual Revenue: $1-$5 Million
Year Founded: 1996
Total Employees: 10
Ownership: Private
Quality System Registration Information: ISO9002
Produces/Sells CE-marked Devices: N
Federal Procurement Eligibility: Small Business, Minority Owned
Distribution: Manufacturer Direct

Antigen, Non-Treponemal, All	Microbiology

BEACON CONVERTERS, INC.   201-797-2600
Bldg. P-1 Andrea Blvd., Saddle Brook, NJ 07663-8208
FDA Number: 2242794   *Fax:* 201-797-3015
E-mail: info@beaconconverters.com
Web site: www.beaconconverters.com
Medical Products Sales Volume: $14,300,000
Annual Revenue: $5-$10 Million
Year Founded: 1947
Total Employees: 260   *Sales Staff:* 4
Ownership: Private
Quality System Registration Information: ISO9000
Produces/Sells CE-marked Devices: N
Federal Procurement Eligibility: Small Business, Female Owned
Distribution: Manufacturer Direct, Manufacturer Through Manufacturer Reps
General Admin.: Mr. William Daly/Chairman
         Ms. Jackie Daly Johnson/President, Chief Executive Officer, Director
Mktg./Adv.: Ms. Kathleen Daly Mascolo/Vice President Marketing & Sales

Pack, Sterilization Wrapper (Bag And Accessories)	Surgery
Packaging Material	General
Packaging, Sterilization	General

BEACON LABORATORIES, INC.
See Conmed Corporation

BEACON PROMOTIONS, INC.   507-354-3900
2121 Bridge St., New Ulm, MN 56073
FDA Number: 3004420206
Ownership: Private
Produces/Sells CE-marked Devices: N

Bandage, Adhesive	Surgery
Gauze/sponge, Nonresorbable For External Use	Surgery
Kit, First Aid	Surgery
Pad, Alcohol	General

BEAM CO.
See Omnimed, Inc. (Beam Products)

BEAN PRODUCTS   800-726-8365
**1500 S. Western Avenue, Suite 4BN,   312-666-3600
Chicago, IL 60608**
FDA Number: n/a   *Fax:* 312-666-3629
E-mail: info@beanproducts.com
Web site: www.beanproducts.com
Medical Products Sales Volume: $1,100,000
Annual Revenue: $0-$1 Million
Year Founded: 1987
Total Employees: 21   *Marketing Staff:* 2   *Sales Staff:* 2
Ownership: Private
Produces/Sells CE-marked Devices: N
Federal Procurement Eligibility: Small Business
Distribution: Manufacturer Direct
General Admin.: Vicky Watts/Office Manager
         Chuck Blumenthal/President
         Juliet Cella/Vice President, General Manager
Mktg./Adv.: Chuck Blumenthal/Manager National Sales
         Ms. Isabella Samovsky/Manager Sales

Fluorophotometer	Chemistry
Pillow	General
Support, Hot/Cold Pack	Physical Med

BEATTY MARKETING & SALES, LLC   425-895-1656
17371 Ne 67th Ct., #a-12, Redmond, WA 98052
FDA Number: 3005670453

Snare, Surgical	Surgery

BEAUMONT PRODUCTS, INC.   800-451-7096
1560 Big Shanty Dr., Kennesaw, GA 30144-3606   770-514-9000
FDA Number: n/a   *Fax:* 770-514-7400
E-mail: citrusII@beaumontproducts.com
Web site: www.citrus2.com
Medical Products Sales Volume: $3,800,000
Annual Revenue: $10-$25 Million
Year Founded: 1984
Total Employees: 45   *Marketing Staff:* 4   *Sales Staff:* 50
Ownership: Private
Produces/Sells CE-marked Devices: N
Federal Procurement Eligibility: Small Business
Distribution: Manufacturer Direct, Manufacturer Through Distributor, Manufacturer Through Manufacturer Reps, Service Direct, Exclusive Distributor, Exporter
General Admin.: Hank Picken/President
Mktg./Adv.: Mr. Mark Woods/Executive Vice President Marketing & Sales

Disinfector, Liquid	General
Sanitizer	General
Solution, Ostomy, Odor Control	Gastroenterology/Urology

BEAVER INC., RUDOLPH
See Becton Dickinson And Co.

BEAVERSTATE DENTAL, INC.   800-237-2303
115 S. Elliott Rd., Newberg, OR 97132   503-538-8756
FDA Number: 3019103   *Fax:* 503-538-2845
E-mail: sales@beaverstatedental.com
Web site: www.beaverstatedental.com
Medical Products Sales Volume: $5,000,000
Annual Revenue: $1-$5 Million
Year Founded: 1970
Total Employees: 22   *Marketing Staff:* 3   *Sales Staff:* 18
Ownership: Private
Produces/Sells CE-marked Devices: N
Federal Procurement Eligibility: Small Business
Distribution: Manufacturer Through Distributor, Manufacturer Through Manufacturer Reps, OEM, Exporter
General Admin.: Aaron Britton/General Manager
         Rick Whitman/President, Chief Executive Officer
         Chuck Whisman/Vice President
Mktg./Adv.: Chuck Whisman/Director National Accounts
         Rick Whitman/Director Product Development
         Chuck Whisman/Vice President Marketing & Sales
Production: Pam Lawrence/Customer Service Representative
         Adam Schieble/Director Quality Assurance

Chair, Dental	Dental And Oral
Cuspidor	Dental And Oral
Light, Dental	Dental And Oral
Operative Dental Treatment Unit	Dental And Oral
Syringe Unit, Air And/Or Water	Dental And Oral

BECK-LEE   800-235-2852
P.O. Box 528, Stratford, CT 06615-0528
FDA Number: n/a   *Fax:* 800-525-4568
E-mail: info@becklee.com
Web site: www.becklee.com
Medical Products Sales Volume: $4,500,000
Annual Revenue: $1-$5 Million
Year Founded: 1950
Ownership: Private
Produces/Sells CE-marked Devices: N
Federal Procurement Eligibility: Small Business
Distribution: Exclusive Distributor

Electrode, Electrocardiograph	Cardiovascular
Electrode, Holter	Cardiovascular
Electrode, Other	General
Gel, Electrode, Electrocardiograph	Cardiovascular
Gel, Ultrasonic Coupling	Physical Med
Glove, Patient Examination	General
Strap, Electrode	General

Medical Product Subsidiaries (Listed Separately)
In Disposables Inc.

BECKER INDUSTRIES, INC.   (281)-590-4900
2712 Frank Road, Houston, TX 77032
FDA Number: n/a   *Fax:* (281)-590-4903
E-mail: sales@beckerind.com
Web site: www.becker-industries.com
Total Employees: 3   *Marketing Staff:* 1   *Sales Staff:* 1
Ownership: Private
Produces/Sells CE-marked Devices: N
Federal Procurement Eligibility: Small Business, Female Owned
Distribution: Manufacturer Direct
General Admin.: Laura Becker/Chief Executive Officer
         Danny Becker/President
Mktg./Adv.: Aaron Becker/Director Marketing

Amputation Protection Unit	General
Board, Scooter, Prone	Physical Med

BECKER INDUSTRIES, INC.
(281)-590-4900 *(cont'd)*
Tray, Foodservice
General

BECKER ORTHOPEDIC APPLIANCE CO.
248-588-7480
635 Executive Dr., Troy, MI 48083
FDA Number: 1824252
Ownership: Private
Produces/Sells CE-marked Devices: N

Brace, Joint, Ankle (External)	Physical Med
Helmet, Cranial, For Protective Use	Physical Med
Joint, Elbow, External Limb Component, Mechanical	Physical Med
Joint, Hip, External Brace	Physical Med
Joint, Knee, External Brace	Physical Med
Orthosis, Cervical	Physical Med
Orthosis, Cervical-Thoracic, Rigid	Physical Med
Orthosis, Cranial	Cns/Neurology
Orthosis, Limb Brace	Physical Med
Orthosis, Lumbar	Physical Med
Orthosis, Lumbosacral	Physical Med
Orthosis, Thoracic	Physical Med
Orthosis, Truncal/Limb	Physical Med
Splint, Hand, And Component	Physical Med
Stirrup, External Brace Component	Physical Med
Twister, Brace Setting	Physical Med

BECKMAN COULTER CORP.
See Beckman Coulter, Inc.

BECKMAN COULTER INC.
800-231-7970
445 Medical Center Blvd., Webster, TX 77598
281-332-9678
FDA Number: 1628193
Fax: 281-338-1895
E-mail: info@dslabs.com
Web site: www.dslabs.com
Medical Products Sales Volume: $9,200,000
Annual Revenue: $10-$25 Million
Year Founded: 1981
Total Employees: 108   *Marketing Staff:* 3   *Sales Staff:* 10
Ownership: Private
Quality System Registration Information: ISO9001
Produces/Sells CE-marked Devices: Y
Federal Procurement Eligibility: Small Business, Minority Owned
Distribution: Manufacturer Direct, Manufacturer Through Distributor, Manufacturer Through Manufacturer Reps, Exporter
General Admin.: SHUBHA SINGH/Director Human Resources
  Gopal Savjani/President
  Scott Garrett/President, Chief Executive Officer
  Rajen Savjani/Vice President
  Michael Schiffer/Vice President, General Counsel
Mktg./Adv.: Preston Reynolds/Director International Sales
  Anthony Morrison/Manager National Sales
  Thomas Verghese/Vice President Business Development
Production: Umesh Bodani/Director Manufacturing
  Dr. Michael Nicar/Director Regulatory Affairs
  John Lindsey/Manager Operations
  Carroll Potts/Manager Regulatory Affairs
Research: Dr. Radha Krishna/Director Research & Development
Finance: Shaila Gupta/Controller

Analyzer, Chemistry, Enzyme Immunoassay	Chemistry
Kit, Test, Alpha-fetoprotein For Testicular Cancer	Immunology
Radioimmunoassay, 17-Hydroxyprogesterone	Chemistry
Radioimmunoassay, ACTH	Chemistry
Radioimmunoassay, Aldosterone	Chemistry
Radioimmunoassay, Androstenedione	Chemistry
Radioimmunoassay, Angiotensin I And Renin	Chemistry
Radioimmunoassay, C Peptides Of Proinsulin	Chemistry
Radioimmunoassay, Calcitonin	Chemistry
Radioimmunoassay, Cortisol	Chemistry
Radioimmunoassay, Dehydroepiandrosterone (Free And Sulfate)	Chemistry
Radioimmunoassay, Estradiol	Chemistry
Radioimmunoassay, Estriol	Chemistry
Radioimmunoassay, Estrone	Chemistry
Radioimmunoassay, Ferritin	Microbiology
Radioimmunoassay, Follicle Stimulating Hormone	Chemistry
Radioimmunoassay, Human Growth Hormone	Chemistry
Radioimmunoassay, Immunoreactive Insulin	Chemistry
Radioimmunoassay, Luteinizing Hormone	Chemistry
Radioimmunoassay, Parathyroid Hormone	Chemistry
Radioimmunoassay, Progesterone	Chemistry
Radioimmunoassay, Prolactin (Lactogen)	Chemistry
Radioimmunoassay, Prostate-Specific Antigen (PSA)	Immunology
Radioimmunoassay, Testosterones And Dihydrotestosterone	Chemistry
Radioimmunoassay, Thyroid Stimulating Hormone	Chemistry
Radioimmunoassay, Total Thyroxine	Chemistry
Radioimmunoassay, Total Triiodothyronine	Chemistry
System, Gonadotropin, Chorionic, Human (Non-RIA)	Chemistry
Test, Erythropoietin	Hematology

BECKMAN COULTER INC. (SAGIAN OPERATION)
800-742-2345
5350 Lakeview Parkway South DR,
317-808-4200
Indianapolis, IN 46268
FDA Number: 3004198394
Fax: 800-643-4366
Web site: www.beckmancoulter.com
Total Employees: 10548
Ownership: Private
Stock Symbol: BEC
Traded On: NYSE
Produces/Sells CE-marked Devices: Y
Distribution: Manufacturer Direct
General Admin.: Charlie Slacik/Chief Financial Officer, Senior Vice President
  Bob Kleinert/Executive Vice President
  Scott Garrett/President, Chief Executive Officer, Chairman
  Pam Miller/Senior Vice President
  Paul Glyer/Senior Vice President
  Russ Bell/Senior Vice President
  Bob Hurley/Senior Vice President Human Resources
  Arnie Pinkston/Senior Vice President, General Counsel
  Cynthia Collins/Vice President
  Mike Whelan/Vice President
  Richard Creager/Vice President
  Scott Atkin/Vice President
Medical Admin.: Peter Heseltine/Vice President, Medical Director
Production: Melina Cimler/Senior Vice President Quality Assurance

Pipetting And Diluting System, Automated	Chemistry
System, Robot	General
Training Manikin, Intravenous Arm	General

BECKMAN COULTER PRIMARY CARE DIAGNOSTICS
714-961-3712
1050 Page Mill Rd., Bldg. 2-B, Palo Alto, CA 94303-0803
FDA Number: 2912312
Web site: www.beckmancoulter.com
Ownership: Beckman Coulter, Inc.
Stock Symbol: BEC
Traded On: NYSE
Produces/Sells CE-marked Devices: N

Reagent, Occult Blood	Hematology

BECKMAN COULTER, INC.
952-368-7629
1000 Lake Hazeltine Dr., Chaska, MN 55318
FDA Number: 2122870
Web site: www.beckmancoulter.com
Ownership: Beckman Coulter, Inc.
Stock Symbol: BEC
Traded On: NYSE
Produces/Sells CE-marked Devices: N

Antigen, Antiserum, Control, Albumin	Immunology
Antigen, Antiserum, Control, Beta Globulin	Immunology
Antigen, Antiserum, Control, Carcinoembryonic Antigen	Immunology
Antigen, Antiserum, Control, FAB, FITC	Immunology
Antigen, Antiserum, Control, Haptoglobin	Immunology
Antigen, Antiserum, Control, IGE	Immunology
Antigen, Antiserum, Control, Myoglobin	Immunology
Antigen, Antiserum, Control, Plasminogen	Immunology
Antigen, Antiserum, Control, Protein, Complement	Immunology
Antigen, Antiserum, Control, Transferrin	Immunology
Antigen, Antiserum, Control, Whole Human Serum	Immunology
Calibrator, Primary, Clinical Chemistry	Chemistry
Calibrator, Secondary, Clinical Chemistry	Chemistry
Electrophoretic Separation, Alkaline Phosphatase Isoenzymes	Chemistry
Fluorometric Method, CPK Or Isoenzymes	Chemistry
Radioimmunoassay, Cortisol	Chemistry
Radioimmunoassay, Estradiol	Chemistry
Radioimmunoassay, Estriol	Chemistry
Radioimmunoassay, Folic Acid	Chemistry
Radioimmunoassay, Follicle Stimulating Hormone	Chemistry
Radioimmunoassay, Free Thyroxine	Chemistry
Radioimmunoassay, Human Chorionic Gonadotropin	Chemistry
Radioimmunoassay, Immunoreactive Insulin	Chemistry
Radioimmunoassay, Luteinizing Hormone	Chemistry
Radioimmunoassay, Parathyroid Hormone	Chemistry
Radioimmunoassay, Prolactin (Lactogen)	Chemistry
Radioimmunoassay, Testosterones And Dihydrotestosterone	Chemistry
Radioimmunoassay, Total Triiodothyronine	Chemistry
Radioimmunoassay, Vitamin B12	Chemistry
Test, Erythropoietin	Hematology
Whole Human Plasma, Antigen, Antiserum, Control	Immunology

BECKMAN COULTER, INC.
800-526-3821
11800 Sw 147th Ave., Kendall, FL 33196
305-380-2730
FDA Number: 1061932
Fax: 800-232-3828
Web site: www.beckmancoulter.com
Ownership: Beckman Coulter, Inc.
Stock Symbol: BEC
Traded On: NYSE
Produces/Sells CE-marked Devices: N

MANUFACTURER PROFILES

BECKMAN COULTER, INC.
800-526-3821 *(cont'd)*

Analyzer, Sedimentation Rate, Automated	Hematology
Counter, Cell Or Particle, Automated	Hematology
Counter, Cell, Differential Classifier, Automated	Hematology
Counter, Platelet, Manual	Hematology
Diluter, Blood Cell, Automated	Hematology
Equipment, Laboratory, Gen. Purpose (Specific Medical Use)	Chemistry
Pipetting And Diluting System, Automated	Chemistry
Spinner, Slide, Automated	Hematology
Stainer, Slide, Automated	Pathology
Timer, General Laboratory	Hematology

BECKMAN COULTER, INC.
714-871-4848

22900 W. Eight Mile Rd., Southfield, MI 48033-4302
FDA Number: 3005864509
Ownership: Beckman Coulter, Inc.
Produces/Sells CE-marked Devices: N

Reagent, General Purpose	Pathology

BECKMAN COULTER, INC.
714-993-8767

2470 Faraday Ave., Carlsbad, CA 92008
FDA Number: 2050010
Web site: www.beckmancoulter.com
Ownership: Beckman Coulter, Inc.
Stock Symbol: BEC
Traded On: NYSE
Produces/Sells CE-marked Devices: N

Electrode, Ion Specific, Chloride	Chemistry
Electrode, Ion Specific, Urea Nitrogen	Chemistry
Electrophoretic, Protein Fractionation	Chemistry
Lipase Hydrolysis/Glycerol Kinase Enzyme, Triglycerides	Chemistry
Urease And Glutamic Dehydrogenase, Urea Nitrogen	Chemistry

BECKMAN COULTER, INC.
800-742-2345
714-871-4848

250 S. Kraemer Boulevard, PO Box 8000,
Brea, CA 92822
FDA Number: 2050012 *Fax:* 714-773-8283
E-mail: info@beckmancoulter.com
Web site: www.beckmancoulter.com
Medical Products Sales Volume: $2,017,000,000
Annual Revenue: More than $1 Billion
Year Founded: 1934
Total Employees: 10100
Ownership: Public
Stock Symbol: BEC
Traded On: NYSE
Quality System Registration Information: ISO9000; ISO9001; ISO9002
Produces/Sells CE-marked Devices: Y
Distribution: Manufacturer Direct, Exporter
General Admin.: Mr. Bob Hurley/Chief Executive Officer
　　　　Mr. Charlie Slacik/Chief Financial Officer, Senior Vice President
　　　　Mr. Bob Kleinert/Executive Vice President
　　　　Mr. Scott Atkin/Executive Vice President
　　　　Arnie Pinkston/Senior Vice President, General Counsel
Medical Admin.: Mr. Peter Haselton/Medical Director

2, 4-dinitrophenylhydrazine, Lactate Dehydrogenase	Chemistry
Accessories, Chromatography (Gas, Gel, Liquid, Thin Layer)	Chemistry
Alpha-1-Acid-Glycoprotein, Antigen, Antiserum, Control	Immunology
Analyzer, Amino Acid	Microbiology
Analyzer, BUN (Blood Urea Nitrogen)	Chemistry
Analyzer, Chemistry, Centrifuge	Chemistry
Analyzer, Chemistry, Desk-Top	Chemistry
Analyzer, Chemistry, ELISA	Chemistry
Analyzer, Chemistry, Electrolyte	Chemistry
Analyzer, Chemistry, Enzyme	Chemistry
Analyzer, Chemistry, Enzyme Immunoassay	Chemistry
Analyzer, Chemistry, Micro	Chemistry
Analyzer, Chemistry, Multi-Channel, Fixed	Chemistry
Analyzer, Chemistry, Multi-Channel, Programmable	Chemistry
Analyzer, Chemistry, Nephelometric Immunoassay	Chemistry
Analyzer, Chemistry, Radioimmunoassay, Automated	Chemistry
Analyzer, Chemistry, Single Channel, Programmable	Chemistry
Analyzer, Combination Chemistry/Hematology/Electrolyte	Chemistry
Analyzer, Glucose	Chemistry
Analyzer, Protein	Chemistry
Antibody, Monoclonal	Microbiology
Antibody, Other	General
Antibody, Polyclonal	Microbiology
Buffer, pH	Hematology
Calibrator, Primary, Clinical Chemistry	Chemistry
Cell, Spectrophotometer	Chemistry
Centrifuge, Blood Bank, Diagnostic	Hematology
Centrifuge, Continuous Flow	Chemistry
Centrifuge, Floor	Pathology
Centrifuge, General (Over 5,000 rpm)	Toxicology
Centrifuge, General (Up to 5,000 rpm)	Pathology
Centrifuge, Hematocrit	Hematology
Centrifuge, Microhematocrit	Hematology
Centrifuge, Refrigerated	Pathology
Centrifuge, Tabletop	Pathology

BECKMAN COULTER, INC.
800-742-2345 *(cont'd)*

Chromatography Equipment, Ion Exchange	Toxicology
Chromatography Equipment, Liquid	Chemistry
Chromatography Equipment, Paper	Chemistry
Chromatography, Liquid, Performance, High	Toxicology
Colorimeter, General Use	Chemistry
Column, Chromatography	Chemistry
Column, Liquid Chromatography	Toxicology
Computer Software	General
Computer, Chemistry Analyzer	Chemistry
Computer, Clinical Laboratory	Chemistry
Contract Manufacturing	General
Control, Electrolyte (Assayed And Unassayed)	Chemistry
Control, Multi Analyte, All Kinds (Assayed And Unassayed)	Chemistry
Counter, Scintillation	Chemistry
Counter, Scintillation, Liquid, Toxicology	Toxicology
Cuvette, Spectrophotometer	Chemistry
Densitometer	Cardiovascular
Densitometer, Laboratory	Chemistry
Diluter	Chemistry
Dispenser, Fluid	General
Dispenser, Liquid, Laboratory	Chemistry
Dispenser, Microbiology Media	Microbiology
Electrode, Laboratory pH	Chemistry
Electrode, Specific Ion	Chemistry
Electrode, pH	Gastroenterology/Urology
Electrophoresis Equipment, Gel	Chemistry
Electrophoresis Equipment, Liquid	Chemistry
Electrophoresis Instrumentation	Immunology
Electrophoretic Separation, Lipoproteins	Chemistry
Enzymatic Esterase-Oxidase, Cholesterol	Chemistry
Enzyme Immunoassay, Carbamazepine	Toxicology
Enzyme Immunoassay, Other	Chemistry
Glucose-6-Phosphate Dehydrogenase (Erythrocytic), Spot	Hematology
Hexokinase, Glucose	Chemistry
High Pressure Liquid Chromatography, Barbiturate	Toxicology
High Pressure Liquid Chromatography, Benzodiazepine	Toxicology
High Pressure Liquid Chromatography, Cocaine & Metabolites	Toxicology
High Pressure Liquid Chromatography, Codeine	Toxicology
High Pressure Liquid Chromatography, Methamphetamine	Toxicology
High Pressure Liquid Chromatography, Opiates	Toxicology
High Pressure Liquid Chromatography, Propoxyphene	Toxicology
High Pressure Liquid Chromatography, Quinine	Toxicology
High Pressure Liquid Chromatography, Tricyclic Drug	Toxicology
Immunoassay, Other	Toxicology
Immunoelectrophoretic, Immunoglobulins, (G, A, M)	Chemistry
Labware, Basic, Reusable	Chemistry
Lactic Dehydrogenase, Antigen, Antiserum, Control	Immunology
Meter, pH, General Use	Toxicology
Meter, pH, Portable	Chemistry
Microdensitometry Method, Lipoproteins	Chemistry
Microelectrode	General
Monitor, Fetal	Obstetrics/Gynecology
Nephelometer	Chemistry
Nephelometer, Immunology	Immunology
Ninhydrin, Nitrogen (Amino-Nitrogen)	Chemistry
Paper, Chart, Record, Medical	General
Phosphatase, Alkaline	Hematology
Photometer	Chemistry
Pipette	Chemistry
Pipette Tip	Chemistry
Pipette, Micro	Chemistry
Pipetter	Hematology
Pipetting And Diluting System, Automated	Chemistry
Pump, Laboratory	Chemistry
Rack, Test Tube	Chemistry
Reagent, Albumin, Colorimetric	Chemistry
Reagent, Amylase, Colorimetric	Chemistry
Reagent, Analyzer, Amino Acid	Microbiology
Reagent, Bilirubin (Total Or Direct Test System)	Chemistry
Reagent, Blood Urea Nitrogen (BUN)	Chemistry
Reagent, Calcium (Test System)	Chemistry
Reagent, Calibration	General
Reagent, Cholesterol (Total Test System)	Chemistry
Reagent, Creatinine (Test System)	Chemistry
Reagent, Glucose (Test System)	Chemistry
Reagent, Protein, Total	Chemistry
Reagent, Quality Control	General
Recorder, Chart, Laboratory	Chemistry
Recorder, Paper Chart	Cardiovascular
SGOT, Ultraviolet	Chemistry
SGPT, Ultraviolet	Chemistry
Solution, pH Buffer	Chemistry
Solvent, Spectrophotometer	Chemistry
Spectrophotometer, U.V./Visible	Chemistry
Spectrophotometer, Ultraviolet	Chemistry
Spectrophotometer, Visible	Chemistry
Standard, Amino Acid	Chemistry
Standard, Ultraviolet Reference	Chemistry
Standard/Control, All Types	Chemistry
Stirrer	Chemistry
Synthesizer, DNA	Chemistry

BECKMAN COULTER, INC.   800-742-2345 *(cont'd)*

Synthesizer, Polynucleotide	Chemistry
System, Robot	General
Test, Bacillus Subtilis Microbiology, Tobramycin	Toxicology
Test, Rheumatoid Factor	Immunology
Tube, Centrifuge	Chemistry
Ultracentrifuge	Chemistry
Uricase (Coulometric), Uric Acid	Chemistry

Medical Product Subsidiaries (Listed Separately)
Beckman Coulter Primary Care Diagnostics
Beckman Coulter, Inc.
Beckman Coulter, Inc. Primary Care Diagnostics

BECKMAN COULTER, INC.   800-635-3497
250 South Kraemer Boulevard,   **(800) 742-2345**
Brea, CA 92821
FDA Number: 1017835   *Fax:* (800) 232-3828
E-mail: iot@immunotech.com
Web site: www.beckmancoulter.com
Total Employees: 13   *Marketing Staff:* 8   *Sales Staff:* 10
Ownership: Beckman Coulter, Inc.
Stock Symbol: BEC
Traded On: NYSE
Quality System Registration Information: ISO9000; ISO9003
Produces/Sells CE-marked Devices: Y
Distribution: Manufacturer Direct, Manufacturer Through Distributor

Analyzer, Chemistry, Centrifuge	Chemistry
Analyzer, Chemistry, Electrolyte	Chemistry
Analyzer, Chemistry, Enzyme	Chemistry
Analyzer, Chemistry, Micro	Chemistry
Analyzer, Chemistry, Multi-Channel, Programmable	Chemistry
Analyzer, Chemistry, Photometric, Discrete	Chemistry
Analyzer, Chemistry, Therapeutic Drug Monitor (TDM)	Chemistry
Analyzer, Particle	Chemistry
Antibody, Monoclonal	Microbiology
Antigen, Antiserum, Control, IGG	Immunology
Antigen, Antiserum, Control, IGG, FITC	Immunology
Antigen, Antiserum, Control, IGM	Immunology
Antigen, Antiserum, Control, IGM (Mu Chain Specific)	Immunology
Antigen, Antiserum, Control, IGM, FITC	Immunology
Calibrator, Cell Indices	Hematology
Calibrator, Platelet Counting	Hematology
Centrifuge, Floor	Pathology
Centrifuge, General (Over 5,000 rpm)	Toxicology
Centrifuge, Tabletop	Pathology
Colorimetric Method, Gamma-Glutamyl Transpeptidase	Chemistry
Colorimetric Method, Triglycerides	Chemistry
Complexone, Cresolphthalein, Calcium	Chemistry
Computer, Chemistry Analyzer	Chemistry
Computer, Hematology Analyzer	Hematology
Control, Cell Counter, Normal And Abnormal	Hematology
Control, Enzyme (Assayed And Unassayed)	Chemistry
Control, Multi Analyte, All Kinds (Assayed And Unassayed)	Chemistry
Control, White Cell	Hematology
Counter, Cell	Microbiology
Counter, Cell Or Particle, Automated	Hematology
Counter, Platelet, Automated	Hematology
Detergent	Hematology
Diluent, Blood Cell	Hematology
Diluter	Chemistry
Diluter, Blood Cell, Automated	Hematology
Dye-Binding, Albumin, Bromcresol, Green	Chemistry
Enzymatic Esterase-Oxidase, Cholesterol	Chemistry
Fluid, Red Cell Lysing	Hematology
Hematology Quality Control Mixture	Hematology
Hemoglobinometer	Hematology
Hexokinase, Glucose	Chemistry
Kit, Quality Control, Blood Banking	Hematology
Mixer, Blood Tube	Hematology
Multi Analyte Mixture, Calibrator	Chemistry
NAD Reduction/NADH Oxidation, Lactate Dehydrogenase	Chemistry
NADH Oxidation/NAD Reduction, AST/SGOT	Chemistry
Nephelometric Inhibition Immunoassay, Phenobarbital	Toxicology
Nephelometric Method, Immunoglobulins (G, A, M)	Immunology
Phosphatase, Acid	Hematology
Phosphatase, Alkaline	Hematology
Phosphorus Reagent (Test System)	Chemistry
Reagent, Albumin, Colorimetric	Chemistry
Reagent, Amylase, Colorimetric	Chemistry
Reagent, Bilirubin (Total Or Direct Test System)	Chemistry
Reagent, Blood Urea Nitrogen (BUN)	Chemistry
Reagent, Calcium (Test System)	Chemistry
Reagent, Calibration	General
Reagent, Chloride (Test System)	Chemistry
Reagent, Cholesterol (Total Test System)	Chemistry
Reagent, Creatinine (Test System)	Chemistry
Reagent, Cyanomethemoglobin, With Standard	Hematology
Reagent, General Purpose	Pathology
Reagent, Glucose (Test System)	Chemistry
Reagent, Kinase, Phosphate, Creatine	Chemistry
Reagent, Protein, Total	Chemistry

BECKMAN COULTER, INC.   800-635-3497 *(cont'd)*

SGOT, Ultraviolet	Chemistry
SGPT, Ultraviolet	Chemistry
Sorter, Cell (Separator)	Pathology
Stain, Hematology	Pathology
Stain, Wright's, Hematology	Hematology
Standard/Control, All Types	Chemistry
Standard/Control, Hemoglobin, Normal/Abnormal	Hematology
Tartrate Inhibited, Acid Phosphatase (Prostatic)	Chemistry
Timer, General Laboratory	Hematology
U.V. Method, CPK Isoenzymes	Chemistry
Urease, Photometric, Urea Nitrogen	Chemistry
Uricase (Coulometric), Uric Acid	Chemistry

BECKMAN COULTER, INC.   (317) 808-4200
5350 Lakeview Parkway S Drive, Indianapolis, IN 46268
FDA Number: n/a   *Fax:* (800) 742-2345
Web site: www.beckmancoulter.com
Ownership: Beckman Coulter, Inc.
Stock Symbol: BEC
Traded On: NYSE
Produces/Sells CE-marked Devices: N

Station Pipetting	Chemistry

BECKMAN COULTER, INC.   305-380-4079
7381 Empire Dr., Florence, KY 41042
FDA Number: 1034886
Web site: www.beckmancoulter.com
Ownership: BECKMAN COULTER, INC.
Stock Symbol: BEC
Traded On: NYSE
Produces/Sells CE-marked Devices: N

Detergent	Hematology
Diluent, Blood Cell	Hematology
Reagent, General Purpose	Pathology

BECKMAN COULTER, INC. PRIMARY CARE DIAGNOSTICS   714-961-3712
606 Elmwood Ave., Elmwood Court Three,
Sharon Hill, PA 19079
FDA Number: 2518658
Web site: www.beckmancoulter.com
Ownership: Beckman Coulter, Inc.
Stock Symbol: BEC
Traded On: NYSE
Produces/Sells CE-marked Devices: N

Antigen, Streptococcus SPP.	Microbiology
Campylobacter Pylori	Microbiology
Radioimmunoassay, Human Chorionic Gonadotropin	Chemistry
Reagent, Guaiac	Hematology
Reagent, Occult Blood	Hematology
Test, Infectious Mononucleosis	Immunology

BECKMAN INSTRUMENTS, INC.
See Beckman Coulter, Inc.

BECKMAN INSTRUMENTS, PHYSIOLOGICAL MEASU
See CAREFUSION 211, INC..

BECTON DICKINSON AND CO.   201-847-6800
1 Becton Drive, Franklin Lakes, NJ 07417
FDA Number: 2243072
Ownership: Becton Dickinson And Company
Produces/Sells CE-marked Devices: N

Blade, Scalpel	Surgery
Bottle, Collection, Vacuum (Aspirator)	General
Cannula, Injection	Gastroenterology/Urology
Catheter, Conduction, Anesthesia	Anesthesiology
Catheter, Intravascular, Therapeutic, Short-term Less Than 30 Days	General
Container, Medication, Graduated Liquid	General
Container, Specimen Mailer And Storage	Pathology
Container, Specimen, All Types	General
Culture Media, Enriched	Microbiology
Culture Media, Non-Selective And Differential	Microbiology
Culture Media, Non-Selective And Non-Differential	Microbiology
Culture Media, Selective And Differential	Microbiology
Culture Media, Selective And Non-Differential	Microbiology
Culture Media, Supplements	Microbiology
Diluent, Blood Cell	Hematology
Dispenser, Medication, Liquid	General
Handle, Scalpel	Surgery
Hematocrit Tube, Rack, Sealer, Holder	Hematology
Kit, Anesthesia, Conduction	Anesthesiology
Lancet, Blood	General
Magnifier, Hand-Held, Low-Vision	Ophthalmology
Needle, Aspiration And Injection, Reusable	Surgery
Needle, Conduction, Anesthesia (W/Wo Introducer)	Anesthesiology
Needle, Hypodermic, Single Lumen With Syringe	General
Scalpel, One-Piece (Knife)	Surgery
Shunt, Peritoneal	Gastroenterology/Urology
Stain, Reticulocyte	Hematology

BECTON DICKINSON AND CO. 201-847-6800 *(cont'd)*

Syringe, Antistick	General
Syringe, Piston	General
Tube, Blood Collection	Chemistry
Tube, Sedimentation Rate	Hematology

BECTON DICKINSON AND CO. 866-906-8080
411 Waverley Oaks Rd., Waltham, MA 02452-8405

FDA Number: 1211998 *Fax:* 781-893-7957
E-mail: special_projects@bd.com
Web site: www.bd.com/ophthalmology
Medical Products Sales Volume: $20,000,000
Total Employees: 200
Ownership: Becton Dickinson And Company
Stock Symbol: BDX
Traded On: NYSE
Produces/Sells CE-marked Devices: N
General Admin.: David Pulsifer/President
Mr. Doug Lawrence/Vice President, General Manager
Production: David Routhier/Director Manufacturing
George Kozlowski/Vice President Operations
Research: Anthony Martino/Director Research & Development

Blade, Bone Cutting	Orthopedics
Blade, Scalpel	Surgery
Blade, Surgical, Saw, General & Plastic Surgery	Surgery
Cannula, Lacrimal (Eye)	Ophthalmology
Cannula, Ophthalmic	Ophthalmology
Cutter, Ring	General
Cystotome, Ophthalmic	Ophthalmology
Electrosurgical Unit, Cutting & Coagulation Device	Surgery
Handle, Knife Blade	Surgery
Handle, Scalpel	Surgery
Holder, Knife	Surgery
Instrument, Dental, Manual	Dental And Oral
Knife, Cataract	Ophthalmology
Knife, ENT	Ear/Nose/Throat
Knife, Ear	Ear/Nose/Throat
Knife, Keratome	Ophthalmology
Knife, Meniscus	Surgery
Knife, Microtome	Pathology
Knife, Myringotomy	Ear/Nose/Throat
Knife, Ophthalmic	Ophthalmology
Knife, Other	Surgery
Knife, Tonsil	Ear/Nose/Throat
Mallet, Surgical, General & Plastic Surgery	Surgery
Marker, Ocular	Ophthalmology
Needle, Knife	Surgery
Nonabsorbable Gauze, Surgical Sponge, & Wound Dressing for External Use (with a Drug)	General
Spoon, Ophthalmic	Ophthalmology
Spud, Ophthalmic	Ophthalmology
Surgical Instrument, Non-Powered, Neurosurgical	Cns/Neurology
Syringe, Irrigating	General
Syringe, Piston	General
Tape, Measuring, Ruler And Caliper	Surgery
Tray, Surgical Instrument	Surgery

BECTON DICKINSON AND COMPANY 800-284-6845
1 Becton Dr., Franklin Lakes, NJ 07417 201-847-6800

FDA Number: 2243072 *Fax:* 201-847-6475
E-mail: customer_support@bd.com
Web site: www.bd.com
Medical Products Sales Volume: $3,940,000,000
Annual Revenue: More than $1 Billion
Year Founded: 1897
Total Employees: 28000
Ownership: Public
Stock Symbol: BDX
Traded On: NYSE
Quality System Registration Information: ISO9000
Produces/Sells CE-marked Devices: Y
Distribution: Manufacturer Direct, Manufacturer Through Distributor
General Admin.: Mr. Vincent Forlenza/Chief Operating Officer
Mr. Scott Bruder/Chief Technology Officer
Mr. Edward J. Ludwig/President, Chief Executive Officer
Mr. Donna M. Boles/Senior Vice President Human Resources
Production: Ms. Patricia Shrader/Vice President Regulatory Affairs
Finance: Mr. David Elkins/Chief Financial Officer

Blade, Scalpel	Surgery
Cannula, Injection	Gastroenterology/Urology
Catheter, Conduction, Anesthesia	Anesthesiology
Catheter, Intravascular, Therapeutic, Long-term Greater Than 30 Days	General
Catheter, Intravascular, Therapeutic, Short-term Less Than 30 Days	General
Container, Specimen Mailer And Storage, Temperature Control	Pathology
Hematocrit Tube, Rack, Sealer, Holder	Hematology
Kit, Anesthesia, Conduction	Anesthesiology
Lancet, Blood	General
Magnifier, Hand-Held, Low-Vision	Ophthalmology
Needle, Conduction, Anesthesia (W/Wo Introducer)	Anesthesiology
Needle, Hypodermic, Single Lumen With Syringe	General

BECTON DICKINSON AND COMPANY 800-284-6845 *(cont'd)*

Stain, Reticulocyte	Hematology
Syringe, Piston	General
Tourniquet, Non-Pneumatic, Surgical	Surgery
Tube, Blood Collection	Chemistry
Tube, Capillary Blood Collection	Hematology
Tube, Sedimentation Rate	Hematology

Medical Product Subsidiaries (Listed Separately)
Bd Biosciences
Bd Diagnostic Systems
Bd Diagnostics (Geneohm Sciences, Inc.)
Bd Lee Laboratories
Becton Dickinson And Co.
Becton Dickinson And Company
Becton Dickinson Caribe Ltd
Becton Dickinson Infusion Therapy Systems, Inc.
Becton Dickinson Medical Systems
Becton, Dickinson & Co
Becton, Dickinson & Co.

BECTON DICKINSON AND COMPANY 201-847-4570
2153 12th Ave., Columbus, NE 68601

FDA Number: 1911916
Ownership: Becton Dickinson And Company
Stock Symbol: BDX
Traded On: NYSE
Produces/Sells CE-marked Devices: N

Cannula, Injection	Gastroenterology/Urology
Catheter, Intravascular, Therapeutic, Short-term Less Than 30 Days	General
Needle, Hypodermic, Single Lumen With Syringe	General
Syringe, Piston	General

BECTON DICKINSON CARIBE LTD 410-316-4000
Vicks Dr, Lot #6, Cayey, PR 00634

FDA Number: 2647876
Ownership: Becton Dickinson And Company
Stock Symbol: BDX
Traded On: NYSE
Produces/Sells CE-marked Devices: N

Disc, Susceptibility, Antimicrobial	Microbiology

BECTON DICKINSON CRITICAL CARE MONIT.
See Becton Dickinson Infusion Therapy Systems, Inc.

BECTON DICKINSON INFUSION THERAPY SYSTEMS, INC. 888-237-2762
9450 S. State St., Sandy, UT 84070

FDA Number: 1710034 *Fax:* 800-847-2220
E-mail: infusion_marketing@bd.com
Web site: www.bd.com/infusion
Annual Revenue: $5-$10 Million
Total Employees: 900 *Marketing Staff:* 11 *Sales Staff:* 60
Ownership: Becton Dickinson And Company
Stock Symbol: BDX
Traded On: NYSE
Produces/Sells CE-marked Devices: N
Distribution: Manufacturer Direct, Exporter
General Admin.: Glen Nash/Director Human Resources
Robert Adrion/President
Derek Wendelken/Vice President Human Resources
Mktg./Adv.: David Dowsett/Director Business Development
Richard Borncamp/Director Development & Sales
Bijan Farhangui/Director Marketing
Kathy Sullivan/Director Marketing
Ernest Mantes/Manager Business Development
Ms. Alicia Mares/Manager Marketing
Bill Marshall/Vice President Business Development
Bill Marshall/Vice President Marketing
Production: Mike Van Couwenberghe/Coord. Distribution
Mr. Curtis Bloch/Senior Product Manager
Cal Alexander/Vice President Operations
Rick Beck/Vice President Regulatory Affairs
Research: Noel Harmon/Director Research & Development

Accessories, Catheter	Surgery
Brush, Scrub, Operating Room	Surgery
Cap, Surgical	Surgery
Catheter, Arterial	Cardiovascular
Catheter, Central Venous	General
Catheter, Intravascular, Therapeutic, Short-term Less Than 30 Days	General
Catheter, Intravenous	Cardiovascular
Catheter, Multiple Lumen	Surgery
Connector, Catheter	Surgery
Dilator, Vascular	Cardiovascular
Dilator, Vessel, Percutaneous Catheterization	Cardiovascular
Dressing, Other	General
Guidewire, Catheter	Cardiovascular
IV Start Kit	Surgery
Introducer, Catheter	Cardiovascular
Kit, Administration, Intravenous	General

BECTON DICKINSON INFUSION THERAPY 888-237-2762 (cont'd)

Kit, Catheterization, Intravenous, Winged	Cardiovascular
Needle, Catheter	Surgery
Needle, Hypodermic, Single Lumen With Syringe	General
Needle, Intravenous	General
Set, Administration, Intravenous, Needle-Free	General
Shield, Syringe	General
Syringe, Piston	General
Valve, Catheter Flush, Continuous	Cardiovascular
Wrap, Sterilization	General

BECTON DICKINSON MEDICAL SYSTEMS   201-847-6800
9630 South 54th St., Franklin, WI 53132
FDA Number: 2134319
Ownership: Becton Dickinson And Company
Produces/Sells CE-marked Devices: N

Catheter, Intravascular, Therapeutic, Short-term Less Than 30 Days	General

BECTON DICKINSON MEDICAL SYSTEMS   201-847-4570
Grace Way, Canaan, CT 06018
FDA Number: 1213809
Ownership: Becton Dickinson And Company
Stock Symbol: BDX
Traded On: NYSE
Produces/Sells CE-marked Devices: N

Cannula, Injection	Gastroenterology/Urology
Filter, Infusion Line	General
Needle, Aspiration And Injection, Disposable	Surgery
Needle, Hypodermic, Single Lumen With Syringe	General
Syringe, Antistick	General
Syringe, Piston	General

BECTON DICKINSON MICROBIOLOGY SYSTEMS
See Bd Diagnostic Systems

BECTON, DICKINSON & CO   410-316-4000
250 Schilling Circle, Cockeysville, MD 21030
FDA Number: 1111096
Ownership: Becton Dickinson And Company
Stock Symbol: BDX
Traded On: NYSE
Produces/Sells CE-marked Devices: N

Antigen, CF, (Including CF Control), Varicella-Zoster	Microbiology
Antigen, HA (Including HA Control), Influenza Virus	Microbiology

BECTON, DICKINSON & CO.   308-872-6811
150 South First St., Broken Bow, NE 68822
FDA Number: 1917413   *Fax:* 308-872-5553
Web site: www.bd.com
Year Founded: 1947
Total Employees: 400
Ownership: Becton Dickinson And Company
Produces/Sells CE-marked Devices: N
Federal Procurement Eligibility: Small Business

Cannula, Injection	Gastroenterology/Urology
Collector, Specimen	Microbiology
Labware, Blood Collection	Chemistry
Needle, Aspiration And Injection, Disposable	Surgery
Syringe, Piston	General
Transport System, Anaerobic	Microbiology

BECTON, DICKINSON & CO., (BD)   201-847-6280
PREANALYTICAL SYSTEM
1575 Airport Rd., Sumter, SC 29153
FDA Number: 1024879

Collector, Specimen	Microbiology
Kit, Administration, Intravenous	General
Labware, Blood Collection	Chemistry
Needle, Aspiration And Injection, Disposable	Surgery

BED-CHECK CORPORATION   800-523-7956
307 E. Brady, Tulsa, OK 74120   **918-592-3338**
FDA Number: 1640702   *Fax:* 918-582-9828
E-mail: info@bedcheck.com
Web site: www.bedcheck.com
Medical Products Sales Volume: $3,800,000
Annual Revenue: $5-$10 Million
Year Founded: 1978
Total Employees: 25   *Marketing Staff:* 2   *Sales Staff:* 4
Ownership: Private
Produces/Sells CE-marked Devices: N
Federal Procurement Eligibility: Small Business, Female Owned
Distribution: Manufacturer Through Distributor, Exclusive Distributor, Exporter
General Admin.: Cheryl Barrett/Manager Human Resources
        Margaret S. Blaker/President, Chief Executive Officer
        David Auten/Vice President, General Manager
Mktg./Adv.: Mr. Kit Sprague/Manager Advertising
        Debbie Jones/Manager Contract Sales
        Jim Stewart/Manager International & National Sales
        Greg Poling/Manager National Sales

BED-CHECK CORPORATION   800-523-7956 (cont'd)
        Jim Stewart/Manager Sales Training
Production: Toby Smith/Director Engineering
        Andy Cobb/Director Quality Assurance
        Sanford Fitzgerald/Director Regulatory Affairs
        Dale Wells/Manager Materials

Chair, Other	General
Monitor, Bed Occupancy	General

BEDCOLAB LTD.   800-461-6414
2305 Francis Hughes,   **514-384-2820**
Laval, QUE H7S 1 Canada
FDA Number: n/a   *Fax:* 514-384-4270
E-mail: information@bedcolab.com
Web site: www.bedcolab.com
Medical Products Sales Volume: $4,000,000
Year Founded: 1976
Total Employees: 25   *Marketing Staff:* 1   *Sales Staff:* 6
Ownership: GERODON CANADA INC.
Quality System Registration Information: ISO9002
Produces/Sells CE-marked Devices: Y
Distribution: Manufacturer Direct, Exclusive Distributor, Exporter

BEDSCAPES INTERNATIONAL
See Healing Environments International, Inc.

BEECH MEDICAL PRODUCTS, INC.   603-355-4843
2 South Winchester St., West Swanzey, NH 03469
FDA Number: 94286
Ownership: Private
Produces/Sells CE-marked Devices: N

Kit, Administration, Intravenous	General

BEECHAM PRODUCTS
See Gsk Consumer Healthcare

BEEKLEY CORP.   860-583-4700
One Prestige Lane, Bristol, CT 06010
FDA Number: 9021987   *Fax:* 860-584-2739
E-mail: info@beekley.com
Ownership: Private
Produces/Sells CE-marked Devices: N

Bandage, Adhesive	Surgery
Container, Specimen, All Types	General
Device, Biopsy, Percutaneous	Surgery
Grid, Radiographic	Radiology
Marker, Skin	Surgery
Pack, Hot Or Cold, Disposable	Physical Med
Radiographic Unit, Diagnostic, Mammographic	Radiology
System, Marking, Film, Radiographic	Radiology
System, Orientation, Identification, Specimen/Tissue	Pathology

BEERE PRECISION MEDICAL INSTRUMENTS,   919-544-8000
KMEDIC, TELEF
5307 95th Ave., Kenosha, WI 53144
FDA Number: 2132732
Ownership: Private
Produces/Sells CE-marked Devices: N

Applier, Hemostatic Clip	Cns/Neurology
Applier, Surgical, Clip	Surgery
Awl	Orthopedics
Bender	Orthopedics
Bit, Drill	Orthopedics
Chisel, Surgical, Manual	Surgery
Clip, Instrument	Surgery
Cutter, Surgical	Surgery
Guide, Surgical, Instrument	Surgery
Mallet, Surgical, General & Plastic Surgery	Surgery
Orthopedic Manual Surgical Instrument	Orthopedics
Osteotome, Manual (Plastic Surgery)	Surgery
Pliers, Surgical	Orthopedics
Probe	Orthopedics
Screwdriver	Orthopedics
Tamp	Orthopedics
Tap, Bone	Orthopedics
Wrench	Orthopedics

BEEVERS MANUFACTURING, INC.   800-818-4025
14670 Baker Creek Road,   **503-472-9055**
Mcminnville, OR 97128
FDA Number: 3023468   *Fax:* 503-434-6303
E-mail: info@beevers.net
Web site: www.beevers.net
Medical Products Sales Volume: $230,000
Annual Revenue: $0-$1 Million
Year Founded: 1987
Total Employees: 2
Ownership: Private
Produces/Sells CE-marked Devices: N
Federal Procurement Eligibility: Small Business

MANUFACTURER PROFILES

BEEVERS MANUFACTURING, INC. 800-818-4025 *(cont'd)*
Distribution: Manufacturer Direct, Manufacturer Through Distributor, Exporter
General Admin.: Mrs. Leslie Harrison/Office Manager
      Mrs. Kate Beevers/President
      Mr. Tim Beevers/Vice President
Connector, Airway (Extension)   Anesthesiology
Continuous Positive Airway Pressure Unit (CPAP, CPPB)   Anesthesiology

BEFOUR, INC. 800-367-7109
102 Progress Drive, Saukville, WI 53080 262-284-5150
FDA Number: 2183494   *Fax:* 262-284-5966
E-mail: mail@befour.com
Web site: www.befour.com
Medical Products Sales Volume: $1,000,000
Year Founded: 1979
Total Employees: 14   *Marketing Staff:* 1   *Sales Staff:* 1
Ownership: Private
Produces/Sells CE-marked Devices: N
Federal Procurement Eligibility: Small Business
Distribution: Manufacturer Direct, Manufacturer Through Distributor, Manufacturer Through Manufacturer Reps, OEM, Service Direct
Scale, Infant   General
Scale, Platform, Wheelchair   Physical Med
Scale, Stand-On   General

BEHAVIORAL TECHNOLOGY, INC. 888-363-9017
24 M St.,, Salt Lake City, UT 84103 801-363-9017
FDA Number: 1722764   *Fax:* 801-363-9022
E-mail: sales@btimonarch.com
Web site: www.btimonarch.com
Medical Products Sales Volume: $500,000
Annual Revenue: $0-$1 Million
Year Founded: 1994
Total Employees: 4   *Marketing Staff:* 1   *Sales Staff:* 1
Ownership: Private
Produces/Sells CE-marked Devices: N
Federal Procurement Eligibility: Small Business
Distribution: Manufacturer Direct, Service Direct
General Admin.: Ms. Mickey Adams Grames/Chief Operating Officer
      Peter M. Byrne/President, Chief Executive Officer
Monitor, Penile Tumescence   Gastroenterology/Urology
Plethysmograph, Impedance   Cardiovascular
Plethysmograph, Photo-Electric, Pneumatic Or Hydraulic   Cardiovascular

BEI SENSORS & MOTION SYSTEMS CO.
See Bei Technologies, Inc.

BEI TECHNOLOGIES, INC. 949-341-9500
170 Technology Drive, Irvine, CA 92618
FDA Number: n/a   *Fax:* 949-453-2700
E-mail: sales@beiduncan.com
Web site: www.beiduncan.com
Medical Products Sales Volume: $1,900,000
Annual Revenue: $25-$50 Million
Year Founded: 2004
Total Employees: 12   *Sales Staff:* 12
Ownership: BEI TECHNOLOGIES, INC.
Quality System Registration Information: ISO9000; ISO9001
Produces/Sells CE-marked Devices: N
Federal Procurement Eligibility: Small Business
Distribution: Manufacturer Through Manufacturer Reps
General Admin.: Roger Wells/General Manager
Mktg./Adv.: Paul C. Cain/Director Marketing
      Paul C. Cain/Manager International & National Sales
Pump, Vacuum, Central   Anesthesiology
Valve, Other   Chemistry

BEI TECHNOLOGIES, INC. DUNCAN ELECTRONICS DIVISION
See Bei Technologies, Inc.

BEIERSDORF, INC.
See 3M Company

BEIERSDORF, INC. 800-233-2340
Wilton Corporate Center, 187 Danbury Rd., 203-563-5800
Wilton, CT 06897
FDA Number: 1250043   *Fax:* 203-563-5895
E-mail: contact-bdfinc@bdfusa.com
Web site: www.beiersdorf.com
Total Employees: 675   *Marketing Staff:* 50   *Sales Staff:* 75
Ownership: Private
Traded On: NYSE
Produces/Sells CE-marked Devices: N
Distribution: Manufacturer Through Distributor
General Admin.: Ian Holding/President
Mktg./Adv.: Susan Lewis/Director Marketing
      Nicolas Maurer/Vice President Marketing
Production: Catherine Lair/Director Manufacturing
Lotion, Skin Care   General
Medical Product Subsidiaries (Listed Separately)

BEIERSDORF, INC. 800-233-2340 *(cont'd)*
3M Company

BEKS INCORPORATED 630-480-0476
401 14th Avenue N.e., Unit 2, Jasper, AL 35501
FDA Number: 3006079103
Source, Heat, Bleaching, Teeth, Dental   Dental And Oral

BELCHER PHARMACEUTICALS, INC. 727-544-8866
12393 Belcher Rd., Ste. 420, Largo, FL 33773
FDA Number: 1000526113
Dressing, Other   General

BELCO ENGINEERING, INC.
See Belco Packaging Systems, Inc.

BELCO PACKAGING SYSTEMS, INC. 800-833-1833
910 S. Mountain Avenue, Monrovia, CA 91016 626-357-9566
FDA Number: n/a   *Fax:* 626-359-3440
E-mail: info@belcopackaging.com
Web site: www.belcomedical.com
Medical Products Sales Volume: $4,700,000
Annual Revenue: $5-$10 Million
Year Founded: 1956
Total Employees: 56   *Marketing Staff:* 3   *Sales Staff:* 10
Ownership: Private
Produces/Sells CE-marked Devices: Y
Federal Procurement Eligibility: Small Business, Female Owned
Distribution: Manufacturer Direct, Manufacturer Through Distributor, Manufacturer Through Manufacturer Reps, OEM, Exporter
General Admin.: Mrs. Helen Misik/Chief Executive Officer
      Mr. Michael Misik/President
Mktg./Adv.: Mr. Thomas Misik/Vice President Business Development
Packaging Equipment   General
Sealer, Packaging   General

BELCON ALLIANCE, INC.
See Brady Corporation

BELIMED 800-457-4117
2284 Clements Ferry Road, 305-252-3338
Charleston, SC 29492
FDA Number: 1054953   *Fax:* 305-234-1115
E-mail: info@belimed.us
Web site: www.belimed.com
Medical Products Sales Volume: $15,000,000
Annual Revenue: $10-$25 Million
Year Founded: 1990
Total Employees: 70   *Sales Staff:* 6
Ownership: Belimed Ag
Quality System Registration Information: ISO9001
Produces/Sells CE-marked Devices: N
Distribution: Manufacturer Through Manufacturer Reps
General Admin.: Joseph McDonald/President, Chief Executive Officer
Mktg./Adv.: Mrs. Denise Thompson/Manager Sales Admin.
Research: Chris Bible/Manager Research & Development
Rack, Instrument, Laparoscopy   Surgery
Sterilizer, Steam, Bulk   General
Washer, Cart   General
Washer/Disinfector   General

BELL DENTAL PRODUCTS, LLC. 800.920.4478
3301 W. Hampden Ave. Unit N, 303-292-2137
Englewood, CO 80205
FDA Number: 3003241008   *Fax:* 303.292.4411
Ownership: Private
Produces/Sells CE-marked Devices: N
Operative Dental Treatment Unit   Dental And Oral

BELL HEARING INSTRUMENTS, INC. 800-535-0516
700 Stevens Avenue, Oldsmar, FL 34677 813-814-2355
FDA Number: 1052259
E-mail: bill.bell@knology.net
Web site: www.bellhearingaids.com
Annual Revenue: $1-$5 Million
Ownership: Private
Produces/Sells CE-marked Devices: N
Distribution: Manufacturer Direct
Hearing-Aid   Ear/Nose/Throat

BELL HELICOPTER TEXTRON, INC. 817-280-2011
600 E. Hurst Blvd., State Highway 10, Hurst, TX 76053
FDA Number: n/a   *Fax:* 817-280-2321
Web site: www.bellhelicopter.com
Annual Revenue: More than $1 Billion
Year Founded: 1935
Ownership: TEXTRON, INC.
Quality System Registration Information: ISO9001
Produces/Sells CE-marked Devices: N

BELL HELICOPTER TEXTRON, INC. 817-280-2011 *(cont'd)*
Distribution: Manufacturer Direct, Exclusive Distributor
General Admin.: Lewis B. Campbell/Chief Executive Officer, Chairman

Ambulance, Air	General

BELL-HORN, INC. 317-228-1144
4511 W. 99th Street, Carmel, IN 46032
FDA Number: n/a *Fax:* 317-228-1155
E-mail: bell-horn@bell-horn.com
Web site: www.bell-horn.com
Annual Revenue: $1-$5 Million
Ownership: Private
Produces/Sells CE-marked Devices: N
Federal Procurement Eligibility: Small Business
Distribution: Manufacturer Direct, Exclusive Distributor

Anklet	Physical Med
Back Rest	General
Belt, Abdominal	Gastroenterology/Urology
Belt, Lumbosacral	Orthopedics
Belt, Rib (Support)	Orthopedics
Binder, Abdominal	General
Collar, Cervical Neck	Orthopedics
Collar, Gingival	Dental And Oral
Corset	Orthopedics
Immobilizer, Knee	Orthopedics
Orthosis, Lumbosacral	Physical Med
Orthosis, Other	Physical Med
Ostomy Appliance (Ileostomy, Colostomy)	Gastroenterology/Urology
Pant, Incontinence	General
Pillow, Cervical	Orthopedics
Shoe, Cast	Physical Med
Sock, Stump Cover	General
Splint, Molded, Plastic	Orthopedics
Splint, Other	Orthopedics
Stocking, Elastic, Physical Medicine	Physical Med
Stocking, Support (Anti-Embolic)	General
Support, Abdominal	Physical Med
Support, Ankle	Orthopedics
Support, Arm	Physical Med
Support, Back	Orthopedics
Support, Hand	Orthopedics
Support, Hernia	Gastroenterology/Urology
Support, Knee	Physical Med
Support, Leg	Physical Med
Support, Thigh	Physical Med
Support, Wrist	Physical Med
Truss, Hernia (Belt)	Gastroenterology/Urology

BELL-MORE LABS, INC. 410-239-7554
4030 Gill Ave., Hampstead, MD 21074
FDA Number: n/a
E-mail: apassmore@bell-more.com
Web site: www.bell-more.com
Medical Products Sales Volume: $1,500,000
Annual Revenue: $1-$5 Million
Year Founded: 1973
Ownership: Private
Produces/Sells CE-marked Devices: N
Federal Procurement Eligibility: Small Business
Distribution: Service Direct

Contract Manufacturing, Pharmaceuticals/Chemicals	General
Contract Manufacturing, Reagent	General

BELLA PRODUCTS, INC. 877-550-5655
27136 Burbank, Foothill Ranch, CA 92610
FDA Number: 2032133
Ownership: Private
Produces/Sells CE-marked Devices: N

Brush, Dermabrasion	Surgery

BELLACURE, INC. 800-795-2070
6327 W. Marginal Wy Sw, Bldg.2, 206-762-2070
Seattle, WA 98106
FDA Number: 3005168844
E-mail: hello@bellacure.com *Fax:* 206-762-2080
Web site: www.bellacure.com
Ownership: Private
Produces/Sells CE-marked Devices: N

Orthosis, Limb Brace	Physical Med

BELLCO BIOTECHNOLOGY INC.
See Bellco Glass, Inc.

BELLCO GLASS, INC. 800-257-7043
340 Edrudo Rd., Vineland, NJ 08360 856-691-1075
FDA Number: n/a *Fax:* 856-691-3247
E-mail: cservice@bellcoglass.com
Web site: www.bellcoglass.com
Medical Products Sales Volume: $12,000,000
Annual Revenue: $10-$25 Million

BELLCO GLASS, INC. 800-257-7043 *(cont'd)*
Ownership: Private
Quality System Registration Information: ISO9001
Produces/Sells CE-marked Devices: Y
Federal Procurement Eligibility: Small Business
Distribution: Manufacturer Direct
General Admin.: Steven J. Harker/President, Chief Executive Officer

Burner	Chemistry
Coverslip, Microscope Slide	Pathology
Dialyzer, Laboratory	Chemistry
Flask, Spinner	Pathology
Freeze Drying Equipment	Chemistry
Homogenizer, Tissue	Microbiology
Hood, Isolation, Laminar Air Flow	General
Hood, Microbiological	Microbiology
Incubator/Water Bath, Microbiology	Microbiology
Labware, Basic, Disposable	Chemistry
Labware, Basic, Reusable	Chemistry
Oven	Chemistry
Pipette, Micro	Chemistry
Pipetter	Hematology
Rack, Test Tube	Chemistry
Roller Apparatus	Pathology
Shaker/Stirrer	Chemistry
Sterilizer, Laboratory	Microbiology
Still, Water	Chemistry
Stirrer	Chemistry
Stopper	General
Tissue Culture Apparatus	Microbiology
Tissue Embedding Equipment/Reagent	Pathology
Tray, Medicine	General
Tray, Micro (Mic Plate)	Microbiology
Tube, Culture	Microbiology

BELMED, INC. 888-723-5893
887 Delta Rd., Red Lion, PA 17356 717-246-5500
FDA Number: 1119231 *Fax:* 717-246-7586
E-mail: bmi@belmedinc.com
Web site: www.belmedinc.com
Medical Products Sales Volume: $2,000,000
Annual Revenue: $1-$5 Million
Year Founded: 1976
Total Employees: 14 *Marketing Staff:* 15 *Sales Staff:* 15
Ownership: Private
Produces/Sells CE-marked Devices: N
Federal Procurement Eligibility: Small Business
Distribution: Manufacturer Through Distributor
General Admin.: Gerald Belcher/President

Dental Laboratory Equipment	Dental And Oral
Yoke, Medical Gas	Anesthesiology

BELMONT EQUIPMENT CORP.
See Takara Belmont Usa, Inc.

BELMONT INSTRUMENT CORP. 866-663-0212
780 Boston Road, Billerica, MA 01821-5925 978-663-0212
FDA Number: 1219702 *Fax:* 978-663-0214
E-mail: sales@belmontinstrument.com
Web site: www.belmontinstrument.com
Medical Products Sales Volume: $3,700,000
Annual Revenue: $5-$10 Million
Year Founded: 1980
Total Employees: 35 *Sales Staff:* 6
Ownership: Private
Quality System Registration Information: ISO9001
Produces/Sells CE-marked Devices: Y
Federal Procurement Eligibility: Small Business, GSA Contract, VA Contract
Distribution: Manufacturer Direct, Manufacturer Through Distributor
General Admin.: George Herzlinger/President, Chief Executive Officer
Mktg./Adv.: Lisa Fornicoia/Director Marketing & Sales
Production: Janet Cichocki/Manager Manufacturing
Uraiwan Labadini/Manager Quality Assurance & Regulatory Affairs
Research: John Landy/Manager Research & Development
Michael Gildersleeve/Manager Research & Development

Pump, Infusion	General
Warmer, Blood, Non-Electromagnetic Radiation	Anesthesiology

BELOIT PRECISION INCORPORATED 800-865-1592
1525 Office Parkway, Beloit, WI 53511 608-362-9085
FDA Number: 3002195840 *Fax:* 608-362-6207
Web site: www.beloitprecision.com
Ownership: Private
Produces/Sells CE-marked Devices: N

Retainer, Screw Expansion, Orthodontic	Dental And Oral

BELPORT CO. INC., GINGI-PAK DIV. 800-437-1514
4825 Calle Alto, Camarillo, CA 93011-0240 805-484-1051
FDA Number: n/a *Fax:* 805-484-5076
E-mail: info@gingi-pak.com

BELPORT CO. INC., GINGI-PAK DIV. 800-437-1514 *(cont'd)*

Web site: www.gingi-pak.com
Annual Revenue: $1-$5 Million
Year Founded: 1954
Ownership: Private
Quality System Registration Information: ISO9001; ISO9002
Produces/Sells CE-marked Devices: Y
Federal Procurement Eligibility: Small Business
Distribution: Manufacturer Through Distributor, Manufacturer Through
Manufacturer Reps

Applicator (Laryngo-Tracheal), Topical Anesthesia	Anesthesiology
Block, Heating	Chemistry
Control, Coagulation, Plasma	Hematology
Hemostat	Orthopedics
Kit, Gingival Retraction	Dental And Oral
Material, Impression	Dental And Oral
Solution, Antibacterial Cleaner	General

BELTONE ELECTRONICS CORP. 800-235-8663
2601 Patriot Blvd., Glenview, IL 60026 **847-832-3300**

FDA Number: 1416900
Web site: www.beltone.com
Medical Products Sales Volume: $95,000,000
Year Founded: 1940
Ownership: Private
Produces/Sells CE-marked Devices: N
Federal Procurement Eligibility: Small Business
Distribution: Manufacturer Through Distributor

Audiometer	Ear/Nose/Throat
Hearing-Aid	Ear/Nose/Throat
Hearing-Aid, Plate, Face	Ear/Nose/Throat
Masker, Tinnitus	Ear/Nose/Throat
Tester, Auditory Impedance	Ear/Nose/Throat

BEMCO, INC. 805-583-4970
2255 Union Pl., Simi Valley, CA 93065

FDA Number: n/a *Fax:* 805-583-5033
E-mail: bemco@bemcoinc.com
Web site: www.bemcoinc.com
Annual Revenue: $1-$5 Million
Year Founded: 1951
Total Employees: 33 *Marketing Staff:* 1 *Sales Staff:* 3
Ownership: Private
Produces/Sells CE-marked Devices: N
Federal Procurement Eligibility: Small Business
Distribution: Manufacturer Direct, OEM, Service Direct, Exporter
General Admin.: Barry Bruskrud/President
Mktg./Adv.: Mr. Bill Pennock/Sales Engineer

Equipment, Control, Pollution	General

BEMIS MFG. CO. 800-558-7651
300 Mill St., Sheboygan Falls, WI 53085-0901 **920-467-4621**

FDA Number: 2133713 *Fax:* 920-467-8573
E-mail: hcg@bemismfg.com
Web site: www.bemishealthcare.com
Year Founded: 1971
Total Employees: 2000 *Marketing Staff:* 2 *Sales Staff:* 3
Ownership: Bemis Manufacturing Company
Produces/Sells CE-marked Devices: Y
Distribution: Manufacturer Through Distributor
General Admin.: Peter Bemis/Chief Executive Officer
    Norman Giertz/President
Mktg./Adv.: Joe Hand/Director Product Development
    Margaret Hand/Manager Market Development
Production: Nancy Steinpreis/Associate Product Manager
    Andy Raml/Director Operations
    John Cutting/Manager Regulatory Affairs
Finance: Frank Poja/Vice President Finance

Bottle, Collection, Vacuum (Aspirator)	General
Canister, Suction	Cardiovascular
Container, Sharpes	General
Container, Specimen, All Types	General
Drain, Suction, Closed	Surgery
Suction Apparatus, Operating Room, Wall Vacuum-Powered	Surgery
Waste Disposal Unit, Sharps	General
Waste Disposal Unit, Surgical Instrument (Sharps)	Surgery
Waste Disposal Unit, Syringe	General

BEMIS MFG. CO. 920-467-4621
300 Mill Street, P.O. Box 901, Sheboygan Falls, WI 53085

FDA Number: 2133713 *Fax:* 920-467-8573
E-mail: corp@BemisMfg.com
Web site: www.bemismfg.com
Ownership: Private
Produces/Sells CE-marked Devices: N

Accessories, Operating Room, Table	Surgery
Bottle, Collection, Vacuum (Aspirator)	General
Container, Sharpes	General
Monitor, Infusion, Gravity Flow	General

BEMIS MFG. CO. 920-467-4621 *(cont'd)*
Needle, Aspiration And Injection, Disposable	Surgery

BENCHER, INC. 847-838-3195
241 Depot St., Antioch, IL 60002

FDA Number: n/a *Fax:* 847-838-3479
Web site: www.bencher.com
Annual Revenue: $1-$5 Million
Year Founded: 1974
Ownership: Private
Produces/Sells CE-marked Devices: N
Federal Procurement Eligibility: Small Business
Distribution: Manufacturer Direct

Copier, Image, Radiographic	Radiology
Stand/Holder, Equipment, Laboratory	Chemistry

BENCHMARK ELECTRONICS, INC. (979) 849-6550
3000 Technology Dr., Angleton, TX 77515

FDA Number: 1641405 *Fax:* 409-848-5271
Web site: www.bench.com
Medical Products Sales Volume: $350,000,000
Total Employees: 6000 *Marketing Staff:* 3 *Sales Staff:* 8
Ownership: Public
Stock Symbol: BHE
Traded On: NYSE
Quality System Registration Information: ISO9003
Produces/Sells CE-marked Devices: N
Distribution: OEM
General Admin.: Donald Nigbor/Chief Executive Officer
    Steve Barton/Executive Vice President
    Cary Fu/President
Mktg./Adv.: Christopher Narwocki/Vice President Sales

Contract Manufacturing	General

Medical Product Subsidiaries (Listed Separately)
Benchmark Electronics, Inc.

BENCHMARK ELECTRONICS, INC. 507-453-4912
3535 Technology Dr., N.w., Rochester, MN 55901

FDA Number: 2133786
Ownership: Private
Produces/Sells CE-marked Devices: N

Glucose Dehydrogenase, Glucose	Chemistry
Stimulator, Auditory, Evoked Response	Cns/Neurology

BENCHMARK ELECTRONICS, INC. 507-452-8932
4065 Theurer Blvd., Winona, MN 55987

FDA Number: 2133641 *Fax:* 507-453-4608
E-mail: doug.darbo@bench.com
Web site: www.bench.com
Annual Revenue: More than $1 Billion
Year Founded: 1986
Total Employees: 800 *Sales Staff:* 2
Ownership: Benchmark Electronics, Inc.
Stock Symbol: BHE
Traded On: NYSE
Quality System Registration Information: ISO9001
Produces/Sells CE-marked Devices: Y
Distribution: Manufacturer Direct, Service Direct
General Admin.: Don Nigbor/Chief Executive Officer, Chairman
    Cary Fu/Chief Operating Officer
    Paul Rice/General Manager
Mktg./Adv.: Doug Darbo/Director Sales
    Chuck Thistle/Vice President Marketing & Sales
Production: Jon Eckhoff/Director Engineering
    Peter Randklev/Director Quality Assurance

Contract Manufacturing	General
Service, Engineering/Design	General

BENCHMARK WINONA 507-452-8932
6301 Bandel Rd. Nw, Rochester, MN 55901

FDA Number: 3005600432
Ownership: Private
Quality System Registration Information: ISO9001
Produces/Sells CE-marked Devices: N

Reagent, Glucose (Test System)	Chemistry
System, Test, Blood Glucose, Over-The-Counter	Chemistry

BENDER, INC. 800-356-4266
700 Fox Chase, Highlands Corp. Center, **610-383-9200**
Coatesville, PA 19320

FDA Number: n/a *Fax:* 610-383-7100
E-mail: info@bender.org
Web site: www.bender.org
Medical Products Sales Volume: $40,000,000
Annual Revenue: $1-$5 Million
Year Founded: 1979
Total Employees: 16 *Sales Staff:* 4
Ownership: Private

BENDER, INC.   800-356-4266 *(cont'd)*
Quality System Registration Information: ISO9002
Produces/Sells CE-marked Devices: Y
Federal Procurement Eligibility: Small Business
Distribution: Manufacturer Direct, Manufacturer Through Manufacturer Reps
General Admin.: Christian Bender/Chief Executive Officer
Mktg./Adv.: Dave Bradley/Manager Regional Sales
    Hans D. Steinke/Vice President Marketing & Sales
Production: Marcel Tremblay/Executive Vice President Production

Analyzer, Electrical Safety	General
Clock, Elapsed Time	General
Monitor, Line Isolation	Cardiovascular
Power System, Isolated	General
Tester, Isolated Power System	General

BENDISTAL PLIERS   636-230-9933
175 Lamp & Lantern Village, Chesterfield, MO 63017-8208
FDA Number: 1954181   *Fax:* 636-230-8467
E-mail: suhailkhouri@sbcglobal.net
Web site: www.bendistalpliers.com
Annual Revenue: $0-$1 Million
Year Founded: 1999
Total Employees: 3   *Marketing Staff:* 3   *Sales Staff:* 3
Ownership: Bendistal Pliers
Quality System Registration Information: ISO9002
Produces/Sells CE-marked Devices: Y
Federal Procurement Eligibility: Small Business
Distribution: Exclusive Distributor
General Admin.: Dr. Suhail Khouri/President, General Director

Pliers, Operative	Dental And Oral

Medical Product Subsidiaries (Listed Separately)
  Bendistal Pliers

BENECHILL INC.   -
10060 Carroll Canyon Rd., Suite 100, San Diego, CA 92131
FDA Number: n/a   *Fax:* -
E-mail: -
Web site: http://www.benechill.com
Year Founded: 2004
Ownership: Private
Produces/Sells CE-marked Devices: N
General Admin.: Mr. Alan Raffensperger/Chief Executive Officer
    Dr. Allen Rozenburg/Chief Operating Officer
Medical Admin.: Ms. Becky Inderbitzen/Vice President Clinical Affairs
Production: Mr. Charles Anderson/Director Manufacturing
    Ms. Nevine Erian/Vice President Quality Assurance
Research: Mr. John Hoffman/Vice President Research & Development

BENEKE
See Sani-Med, A Division Of Sanderson Plumbing Products, Inc.

BENIK CORP.   800-442-8910
11871 Silverdale Way N.w., #107,   360-692-5601
Olympic View, WA 98383
FDA Number: 3023878   *Fax:* 360-692-5600
E-mail: info@benik.com
Web site: www.benik.com
Ownership: Private
Produces/Sells CE-marked Devices: N

Brace, Joint, Ankle (External)	Physical Med
Joint, Knee, External Brace	Physical Med
Joint, Shoulder, External Limb Component	Physical Med
Orthosis, Truncal/Limb	Physical Med
Splint, Hand, And Component	Physical Med

BENJAMIN BIOMEDICAL, INC.   727-343-5503
539 Pasadena Avenue South, St. Petersburg, FL 33710
FDA Number: 1064537   *Fax:* 727-343-4637
E-mail: GPapit@benjaminbiomedical.com
Web site: www.benjaminbiomedical.com
Ownership: Private
Produces/Sells CE-marked Devices: N

Phacofragmentation Unit	Ophthalmology
Table, Ophthalmic, Instrument, Manual	Ophthalmology
Table, Ophthalmic, Instrument, Powered	Ophthalmology

BENLAN INC.   905-829-5004
2760 Brighton Rd., Oakville, ONT L6H 5T4 Canada
FDA Number: 8022210   *Fax:* 905-829-5006
E-mail: sales@benlan.com
Web site: www.benlan.com
Medical Products Sales Volume: $5,000,000
Year Founded: 1980
Total Employees: 100   *Marketing Staff:* 2   *Sales Staff:* 2
Ownership: Private
Quality System Registration Information: ISO9000
Produces/Sells CE-marked Devices: N
Federal Procurement Eligibility: Small Business

BENLAN INC.   905-829-5004 *(cont'd)*
Distribution: Manufacturer Direct, Exporter

BENNETT INDUSTRIES, INC.   931-432-4011
1805 Burgess Falls Rd., Cookeville, TN 38506
FDA Number: 1045031
Ownership: Private
Produces/Sells CE-marked Devices: N

Bed, Pediatric (Crib)	General
Restraint, Protective (Body)	General

BENNETT MANUFACTURING CO., INC.   800-345-2142
13315 Railroad St., Alden, NY 14004-1330   716-937-9161
FDA Number: n/a   *Fax:* 716-937-3137
E-mail: amathis@bennettmfg.com
Web site: www.bennettmfg.com
Medical Products Sales Volume: $16,100,000
Annual Revenue: $0-$1 Million
Year Founded: 1906
Total Employees: 150
Ownership: Private
Produces/Sells CE-marked Devices: N
Federal Procurement Eligibility: Small Business
Distribution: Manufacturer Direct, Manufacturer Through Distributor
General Admin.: Steven Yellen/President
Production: Michael Wacht/Director Quality Assurance
    Danielle Witke/Manager Customer Services

Cart, Housekeeping	General
Waste Receptacle, General Purpose	General

BENSON MEDICAL INDUSTRIES INC.   800-563-3859
151 Esna Park Dr.,   905-475-0401
Markham, ONT L3R-3 Canada
FDA Number: n/a   *Fax:* 905-475-3656
E-mail: hr@bensonmedical.ca
Web site: www.bensonmedical.ca
Year Founded: 1974
Ownership: Private
Produces/Sells CE-marked Devices: N
Distribution: Exclusive Distributor, Importer

BENSON MEDICAL INSTRUMENTS CO.   612-827-2222
310 4th Avenue South, Suite 5000, Minneapolis, MN 55415
FDA Number: 2132504   *Fax:* 612-827-2277
E-mail: sales@bensonmedical.com
Web site: www.bensonmedical.com
Medical Products Sales Volume: $700,000
Year Founded: 1993
Total Employees: 8
Ownership: Private
Produces/Sells CE-marked Devices: N
Federal Procurement Eligibility: Small Business, VA Contract
Distribution: Manufacturer Through Distributor
General Admin.: Mr. Stephen Benson/President
Mktg./Adv.: Mr. David Mayou/Vice President Sales

Audiometer	Ear/Nose/Throat

BENTEC MEDICAL, INC.   757-224-0177
1380 East Beamer St., Woodland, CA 95776
FDA Number: 2939142

Catheter, Biliary	Gastroenterology/Urology
Catheter, Intravascular, Therapeutic, Short-term Less Than 30 Days	General
Catheter, Irrigation	Surgery
Catheter, Nephrostomy	Gastroenterology/Urology
Elastomer, Silicone Block	Surgery
Lens, Contact (Other Material)	Ophthalmology
Mesh, Surgical, Polymeric	Surgery
Tube, Drainage	Gastroenterology/Urology
Tube, Laryngectomy	Ear/Nose/Throat

BENVENUE MEDICAL, INC.   888 717-9333
3052 Bunker Hill Lane, Suite 120,   408-454-9300
Santa Clara, CA 95054
FDA Number: 3007033608   *Fax:* 408-982-9023
E-mail: info@benvenuemedical.com
Web site: http://www.benvenuemedical.com
Year Founded: 2004
Ownership: Private
Produces/Sells CE-marked Devices: N
General Admin.: Mr. Robert Weigle/Chief Executive Officer
    Mr. Laurent Schaller/Chief Technology Officer
Mktg./Adv.: Ben Murdock/Senior Mktg Manager
    Mr. Paul Byerley/Vice President Sales
Production: Mr. Victor Barajas/Vice President Operations
    Mr. Lloyd Griese/Vice President Quality Assurance

Cement, Bone, Pre-formed, Modular, Polymeric, Vertebroplasty	Orthopedics
Intervertebral Fusion Device With Bone Graft, Cervical	Orthopedics

BENVENUE MEDICAL, INC.
888 717-9333 *(cont'd)*
Spinal Channeling Instrument, Vertebroplasty | Orthopedics

BENZ RESEARCH AND DEVELOPMENT CORP.
941-758-8256
6447 Parkland Dr., Sarasota, FL 34243
FDA Number: 1052446 | *Fax:* 941-758-1191
E-mail: lpomroy@benzrd.com
Ownership: Private
Produces/Sells CE-marked Devices: N

Lens, Contact (Other Material)	Ophthalmology
Lens, Intraocular	Ophthalmology
Lenses, Soft Contact, Daily Wear	Ophthalmology

BEOCARE INC., HUDSON
353-643-9400
1905, International Blvd., Hudson, NC 28638
FDA Number: 3006010416

Stocking, Elastic	General

BERAL ENTERPRISES, INC.
See Samco Scientific Corporation

BERAL ENTERPRISES, INC.
See Garren Scientific, Inc.

BERCHTOLD CORP.
800-243-5135
843-569-6100
1950 Hanahan Rd., Charleston, SC 29406
FDA Number: 1220685 | *Fax:* 843-569-6133
E-mail: BERCHTOLDusa@BERCHTOLDusa.com
Web site: www.berchtoldusa.com
Medical Products Sales Volume: $26,000,000
Annual Revenue: $25-$50 Million
Ownership: Berchtold Gmbh & Co.
Quality System Registration Information: ISO9001
Produces/Sells CE-marked Devices: Y
Distribution: Manufacturer Direct

Column, Life Support (Electrical/Gas)	General
Component, Electrical	General
Evacuator, Fume	Chemistry
Lamp, Examination (Light)	General
Lamp, Examination, Ceiling Mounted (Light)	General
Lamp, Operating Room	General
Lamp, Surgical	Surgery
Light, Surgical, Ceiling Mounted	Surgery
Light, Surgical, Floor Standing	Surgery
Table, Surgical, Hydraulic	Surgery
Television Monitor, Operating Room	General

BERG, W. M., INC.
800-232-BERG
499 Ocean Ave., East Rockaway, NY 11518
FDA Number: n/a | *Fax:* (800) 455-BERG
Web site: www.wmberg.com
Ownership: Private
Produces/Sells CE-marked Devices: N
General Admin.: Rich Halen/President
Mktg./Adv.: Joe Amendolara/Director Product Development
  Mary Ann Mandrachia/Manager Advertising
  Maureen Day/Manager Contract Sales
  Jim Ferdenzi/Manager International & National Sales
Production: Alex Klyachko/Director Quality Assurance

Production Equipment	General

BERGAD MATTRESS
888-476-8664
724-763-2883
747 Eljer Way, Ford City, PA 16226
FDA Number: 2531809
E-mail: paulb@bergad.com
Web site: www.bergad.com
Medical Products Sales Volume: $1,100,000
Annual Revenue: $1-$5 Million
Year Founded: 1987
Total Employees: 38 | *Marketing Staff:* 2 | *Sales Staff:* 3
Ownership: Private
Produces/Sells CE-marked Devices: N
Federal Procurement Eligibility: Small Business
Distribution: Manufacturer Direct, Manufacturer Through Distributor, Manufacturer Through Manufacturer Reps
General Admin.: Paul Bergad/Chief Executive Officer

Mattress, Air Flotation	General

BERGERON HEALTH CARE
800-371-2778
585-919-3750
15 South Second St., Dolgeville, NY 13329
FDA Number: 84532 | *Fax:* 315-429-8862
E-mail: jamie@bergeronhealthcare.com
Ownership: Private
Produces/Sells CE-marked Devices: Y
Federal Procurement Eligibility: Small Business
Distribution: Manufacturer Through Distributor

Chair, With Casters	Physical Med
Equipment, Therapy, Handicapped/Physical	Physical Med

BERGHOF/AMERICA
800-544-5004
954-344-2554
3773 NW 126th Avenue, Building 1,
Coral Springs, FL 33065
FDA Number: n/a | *Fax:* 954-344-2008
E-mail: berghof@berfhofusa.com
Web site: www.berghofusa.com
Medical Products Sales Volume: $3,000,000
Annual Revenue: $1-$5 Million
Year Founded: 1992
Total Employees: 14 | *Marketing Staff:* 2 | *Sales Staff:* 3
Ownership: Private
Produces/Sells CE-marked Devices: N
Federal Procurement Eligibility: Small Business
Distribution: Manufacturer Direct, Manufacturer Through Distributor, OEM, Exclusive Distributor
General Admin.: Steve Little/Chief Executive Officer
  Steve Little/President
Mktg./Adv.: Nancy Gregorio/Manager Sales

Bag, Plastic	General
Beaker (Laboratory)	Chemistry
Column, Chromatography	Chemistry
Component, Ceramic	General
Container, Specimen, All Types	General
Contract Manufacturing, Product, Durable	General
Dish, Petri	Chemistry
Dispenser, Liquid, Laboratory	Chemistry
Filter, Membrane	Chemistry
Flask, Spinner	Pathology
Glove, Other	General
Labware, Basic, Reusable	Chemistry
Probe, Temperature	General
Rack, Test Tube	Chemistry
Reaction Apparatus	Microbiology
Stirrer	Chemistry
Stopcock	General
Stopper	General
Tube, Centrifuge	Chemistry
Tube, Test	Chemistry
Tubing, Polytetrafluoroethylene	General
Vial, Other	General

BERGMAN ORAL CARE
877-356-7727
13745 Seminole Dr., Chino, CA 91710
FDA Number: 2032821 | *Fax:* 909-902-9544
Ownership: Private
Produces/Sells CE-marked Devices: N

Floss, Dental	Dental And Oral

BERGQUIST TORRINGTON COMPANY
860-489-0489
89 Commercial Blvd., Torrington, CT 06790
FDA Number: 3000144549

Humidifier, Respiratory Gas, (Direct Patient Interface)	Anesthesiology
Ventilator, Non-Continuous (Respirator)	Anesthesiology

BERKELEY ADVANCED BIOMATERIALS, INC.
510-883-0500
901 Grayson Street, Suite 101, Berkeley, CA 94710
FDA Number: 3003586733 | *Fax:* 510-883-0511
E-mail: info@ostetic.com
Web site: www.ostetic.com
Annual Revenue: $1-$5 Million
Year Founded: 1996
Total Employees: 3
Ownership: Private
Quality System Registration Information: ISO9001
Produces/Sells CE-marked Devices: Y
Federal Procurement Eligibility: Small Business, Female Owned
Distribution: Manufacturer Direct, Manufacturer Through Distributor, OEM
General Admin.: Francois Genin/Chief Executive Officer

Filler, Bone Void, Osteoinduction	Physical Med

BERKELEY HEARTLAB, INC.
510-747-1740
960 Atlantic Avenue, Suite 100, Alameda, CA 94501
FDA Number: 3004180570
Ownership: Private
Produces/Sells CE-marked Devices: N

Electrophoretic Separation, Lipoproteins	Chemistry

BERKELEY MEDEVICES, INC.
800-227-2388
510-231-2474
1330 S. 51st St., Richmond, CA 94804-4628
FDA Number: 2917182 | *Fax:* 510-231-9880
E-mail: contactmedevices@aol.com
Web site: www.berkeleymedevices.com
Medical Products Sales Volume: $7,200,000
Annual Revenue: $1-$5 Million
Year Founded: 1981
Total Employees: 40 | *Marketing Staff:* 1 | *Sales Staff:* 2
Ownership: Private
Produces/Sells CE-marked Devices: Y
Federal Procurement Eligibility: Small Business, GSA Contract

BERKELEY MEDEVICES, INC. 800-227-2388 *(cont'd)*
Distribution: Manufacturer Direct, Manufacturer Through Distributor, Exporter
General Admin.: Dieter Kubny/President
            Donna Kubny/Secretary, Treasurer

Brush, Endometrial	Obstetrics/Gynecology
Cannula, Suction, Uterine	Obstetrics/Gynecology
Catheter, Bartholin Gland	Gastroenterology/Urology
Dilator, Cervical, Fixed Size	Obstetrics/Gynecology
Dilator, Cervical, Hygroscopic-Laminaria	Obstetrics/Gynecology
Forceps, Biopsy, Gynecological	Obstetrics/Gynecology
Kit, Sampling, Endometrial	Obstetrics/Gynecology
Loop, Vascular	Cardiovascular
Pump, Vacuum, Central	Anesthesiology

BERKELEY NUCLEONICS CORP. 800-234-7858
2955 Kerner Blvd., San Rafael, CA 94901   **415-453-9955**
FDA Number: n/a   Fax: 415-453-9956
E-mail: info@berkelevnucleonics.com
Web site: www.berkeleynucleonics.com
Annual Revenue: $1-$5 Million
Year Founded: 1960
Total Employees: 25
Ownership: Private
Produces/Sells CE-marked Devices: N
Federal Procurement Eligibility: Small Business, GSA Contract
Distribution: Manufacturer Direct, Manufacturer Through Manufacturer Reps, OEM
Mktg./Adv.: Mr. Robert Corsetti/Director Marketing & Sales
            John Yee/Manager Product Development
Production: Ms. Kristin Geertsema/Director Operations
Finance: Mr. Mel Brown/Chief Financial Officer
            David Brown/President

Analyzer, Chemistry, Multi-Channel, Fixed	Chemistry
Computer Software	General
Detector, Radioisotope	Radiology
Electrophoretic Separation, Lipoproteins	Chemistry
Tester, Radiology Quality Assurance	Radiology

BERKLEY MEDICAL INDUSTRIES
See Packaging Plus Llc

BERKLEY MEDICAL RESOURCES, INC. 412-438-3000
49 Virginia Ave., Uniontown, PA 15401
FDA Number: 2518423

Dress, Surgical	Surgery
Mask, Surgical	Surgery

BERKLINE/BENCHCRAFT LLC 423-585-1517
One Berkline Dr., Morristown, TN 37813
FDA Number: n/a
Ownership: Private
Produces/Sells CE-marked Devices: N

Chair, Position, Electric	Physical Med

BERLEX CANADA INC. 800-361-0240
334 Avro Avenue,   **514-631-7400**
Pointe-Claire, PQ H9R 5 Canada
FDA Number: n/a   Fax: 514-636-9177
E-mail: webmaster.bci@berlex.ca
Web site: www.berlex.ca
Year Founded: 1960
Total Employees: 100
Ownership: SCHERING, AG
Produces/Sells CE-marked Devices: N
Distribution: Exclusive Distributor

BERNELL CORP.
See Vision Training Products, Inc.

BERNER INTERNATIONAL CORP. 800-245-4455
Shenango Commerce Park   **724-658-3551**
111 Progress Ave.
New Castle, PA 16101
FDA Number: n/a   Fax: 724-652-0682
E-mail: sales@berner.com
Web site: www.berner.com
Medical Products Sales Volume: $6,000,000
Annual Revenue: $5-$10 Million
Year Founded: 1953
Total Employees: 30   *Marketing Staff:* 2   *Sales Staff:* 3
Ownership: Private
Produces/Sells CE-marked Devices: Y
Federal Procurement Eligibility: Small Business, Female Owned
Distribution: Manufacturer Through Manufacturer Reps
General Admin.: Georgia Berner/President, Chief Executive Officer
Mktg./Adv.: Alison Clingensmith/Director Marketing
           Michael Coscarelli/Director National Accounts
           David Johnson/Director Product Development
Production: Jane Ward/Manager Materials

Laminar Air Flow Unit, Fixed (Air Curtain)	Chemistry

BERNER INTERNATIONAL CORP. 800-245-4455 *(cont'd)*
Laminar Air Flow Unit, Mobile   Chemistry

BERRING PRECISION BLADES LLC 352-383-8333
9236 Wildwood Lane, Robertsville, MO 63072
FDA Number: 3005409400

General Use Surgical Scissors	Surgery
Scissors, Ophthalmic	Ophthalmology

BERSA GROUP, INC. 954-920-9991
3430 N. 29th Ave., Hollywood, FL 33020
FDA Number: 3006238785
Ownership: Private
Produces/Sells CE-marked Devices: N

Medical Disinfectants/Cleaners for Instruments	General

BERTEC CORPORATION 877-237-8320
6171 Huntley Rd., Suite J, Columbus, OH 43229   **614-430-5421**
FDA Number: 1530895   Fax: 614-430-5425
E-mail: sales@bertec.com
Web site: www.bertec.com
Year Founded: 1987
Ownership: Private
Produces/Sells CE-marked Devices: Y
General Admin.: Dr. N. Berme/President

Equipment, Therapy, Handicapped/Physical	Physical Med
Platform, Force-Measuring	Physical Med
Treadmill, Mechanical	Physical Med
Treadmill, Powered	Physical Med

BERTEC MEDICAL 800-428-5025
70 5th Ave., P.O. Box 128,   **418-247-3986**
L'Isletville, QUE G0R-2 Canada
FDA Number: n/a   Fax: 418-247-7925
E-mail: bertec@bertecmedical.com
Web site: www.bertecmedical.com
Year Founded: 1920
Total Employees: 100
Ownership: STRYKER CORPORATION
Produces/Sells CE-marked Devices: N
Distribution: Manufacturer Direct, Exporter

BERTEK PHARMACEUTICALS
See Mylan Pharmaceuticals Inc

BERTEK, INC.
See Mylan Technologies, Inc.

BEST GLOVE MANUFACTURING LTD. 800-565-2378
253 Michaud St.,   **819-849-6381**
Coaticook, QUE J1A-1 Canada
FDA Number: n/a   Fax: 819-849-6120
E-mail: info@bestglove.ca
Web site: www.bestglove.com
Year Founded: 1978
Ownership: Tillotson Healthcare Corp.
Produces/Sells CE-marked Devices: N
Distribution: Manufacturer Direct, Exporter

BEST GLOVE, INC. 800-241-0323
579 Edison Street, Cloudland, GA 30731   **706-862-6712**
FDA Number: 3003452481   Fax: 888-393-2666
E-mail: USA@showabestglove.com
Web site: www.showabestglove.com
Ownership: Private
Produces/Sells CE-marked Devices: N

Glove, Protective, Radiographic	Radiology

BEST HOSPITAL SUPPLY
See Best Manufacturing Group Llc

BEST INVESTMENT CO., INC.
See Bestway Products Co.

BEST MANUFACTURING CO. 800-241-0323
579 Edison St., PO Box 8, Menlo, GA 30731   **706-862-2302**
FDA Number: 1066746   Fax: 888-393-2666
E-mail: usa@bestglove.com
Web site: www.bestglove.com
Year Founded: 1951
Total Employees: 1200   *Marketing Staff:* 4   *Sales Staff:* 35
Ownership: Private
Quality System Registration Information: ISO9002
Produces/Sells CE-marked Devices: Y
Federal Procurement Eligibility: Small Business
Distribution: Manufacturer Through Distributor
General Admin.: Mr. Bill Alico/President, Chief Executive Officer
           Jeffrey Richardson/Vice President Personnel
Mktg./Adv.: Mr. Mark Wheeler/Director Marketing
           Mr. Tom Eggleston/Director Marketing & Sales
           Mrs. Vicki Bunn/Marketing Coordinator

BEST MANUFACTURING CO.   800-241-0323 *(cont'd)*
     Mr. Don Groce/Project Manager Marketing
Production: Mrs. Mary Ann Raines/Customer Service Representative
   Glove, Other   General

BEST MANUFACTURING CO.(FAYETTE DIVISION) 706-862-6712
931 Second Ave., S.e., Fayette, AL 35555
FDA Number: 1043622
Ownership: Private
Produces/Sells CE-marked Devices: N
   Glove, Patient Examination   General
   Glove, Patient Examination, Latex   General
   Glove, Protective, Radiographic   Radiology
   Glove, Surgical, Plastic Surgery   Surgery

BEST MANUFACTURING GROUP LLC   800-843-3233
1633 Broadway, 18th Fl.,   **212-974-1100**
New York, NY 10019
FDA Number: 9200115   Fax: 212-245-0385
E-mail: bclickstein@bestmfg.com
Web site: www.bestmfg.com
Medical Products Sales Volume: $20,000,000
Annual Revenue: More than $100 Million
Year Founded: 1914
Total Employees: 850   Sales Staff: 20
Ownership: Private
Federal Procurement Eligibility: VA Contract
Distribution: Manufacturer Direct
General Admin.: Lester Maslow/Chief Executive Officer
       Glenn Palmee/President
       Barry Clickstein/Vice President, General Manager
       Hugh Rovit/Vice President, General Manager
Medical Admin.: Debbie Rodrigues/Manager Health Care
Mktg./Adv.: Barry Clickstein/Director Marketing & Sales
Purchasing: John Hogan/Director Purchasing
   Bag, Laundry, Operating Room   General
   Bib   General
   Blanket, Infant   General
   Cart, Other   General
   Cover, Mattress   General
   Cover, Mattress, Waterproof   General
   Curtain, Cubicle   General
   Diaper, Adult   General
   Diaper, Pediatric   General
   Drape, Surgical, Reusable   Surgery
   Dress, Scrub, Reusable   Surgery
   Gown, Operating Room, Reusable   Surgery
   Gown, Patient, Reusable   General
   Pad, Incontinence (Underpad)   General
   Sheet, Operating Room   Surgery
   Suit, Scrub, Reusable   Surgery
   Towel, Surgical   Surgery
   Wrapper, Surgical Instrument (Sterile)   General

BEST MEDICAL CANADA   877-668-6636
413 March Road, Ottawa, ONT K2K 0E4 Canada   **613-591-2100**
FDA Number: 8043666   Fax: 613-596-5243
E-mail: bmcinfo@TeamBest.com
Web site: www.bestmedicalcanada.com
Year Founded: 1984
Total Employees: 15
Ownership: Best Medical International, Inc.
Produces/Sells CE-marked Devices: N
Distribution: Manufacturer Direct, Exporter

BEST MEDICAL INTERNATIONAL, INC.   800-336-4970
7639 & 7643 Fullerton Road,   **703-451-2378**
Springfield, VA 22153
FDA Number: 1120804   Fax: 703-451-5228
E-mail: nfo@bestmedical.com
Web site: www.bestmedical.com
Medical Products Sales Volume: $3,900,000
Annual Revenue: $1-$5 Million
Year Founded: 1977
Total Employees: 42   Marketing Staff: 3   Sales Staff: 6
Ownership: Private
Quality System Registration Information: ISO9002
Produces/Sells CE-marked Devices: N
Federal Procurement Eligibility: Small Business, Minority Owned
Distribution: Manufacturer Direct
General Admin.: Krishnan Suthanthiran/President
       Ruth Bergen/Senior Vice President
       Bob Wittmer/Vice President
Mktg./Adv.: Shawn Weingast/Manager Business Development
       Sankara I. Ramaswamy/Manager International & National Sales
Production: Sankara Ramaswamy/Director Operations
       David Meade/Director Quality Assurance
       Sankara I. Ramaswamy/Manager Regulatory Affairs

BEST MEDICAL INTERNATIONAL, INC.   800-336-4970 *(cont'd)*
Research: Dr. Manny Subramanian/Director Research & Development
   Applicator, Other   General
   Applicator, Radionuclide, Manual   Radiology
   Applicator, Radionuclide, Remote-Controlled   Radiology
   Source, Brachytherapy, Radionuclide   Radiology
   Source, Isotope, Sealed, Gold, Titanium, Platinum   Radiology
   Source, Teletherapy, Radionuclide   Radiology
   Template   Orthopedics
   Thermometer, Electronic   General
Medical Product Subsidiaries (Listed Separately)
   Best Medical Canada
   Best Nomos Corp.

BEST NOMOS CORP.   800-70-NOMOS
One Best Dr., Pittsburgh, PA 15202   **412-312-6700**
FDA Number: 2434141   Fax: 412-312-6701
E-mail: info@nomos.com
Web site: www.nomos.com
Medical Products Sales Volume: $3,000,000
Annual Revenue: $25-$50 Million
Total Employees: 104   Marketing Staff: 1   Sales Staff: 15
Ownership: Best Medical International, Inc.
Quality System Registration Information: ISO9001
Produces/Sells CE-marked Devices: Y
Federal Procurement Eligibility: Small Business, VA Contract
Distribution: Manufacturer Direct, Exporter
General Admin.: John A. Friede/Chairman
       John Manzetti/President, Chief Executive Officer
Mktg./Adv.: William Wells/Executive Vice President Marketing & Sales
       Judith Hale/Manager Corporate Communications
       Patricia Anders/Manager Marketing & Sales
       Jim Karas/Manager National Sales
Production: Joseph Argyros/Vice President Operations
       Fran Dobscha/Vice President Quality Assurance & Regulatory Affairs
Research: Fred Marroni/Vice President Engineering
   Block, Beam Shaping, Radionuclide   Radiology
   Couch, Radiation Therapy, Powered   Radiology
   Holder, Head, Radiographic   Radiology
   Simulator, Radiotherapy, Special Purpose   Radiology
   Stereotaxy Equipment   Cns/Neurology
   System, Delivery, Drug, Unit-Dose   General
   Ultrasound, Hyperthermia, Cancer Treatment   Radiology

BEST ORTHOPEDIC AND MEDICAL SERVICES, INC.   800-344-5279
2356-B Springs Road NE, Hickory, NC 28601   **828-256-1933**
FDA Number: 1058626   Fax: 828-256-3924
E-mail: customerservices@best-ortho.com
Web site: www.best-ortho.com
Medical Products Sales Volume: $200,000
Annual Revenue: $0-$1 Million
Year Founded: 1987
Total Employees: 10
Ownership: Private
Produces/Sells CE-marked Devices: N
Federal Procurement Eligibility: Small Business
Distribution: Manufacturer Through Distributor, Manufacturer Through Manufacturer Reps, Exporter
General Admin.: Pauline Eckard/President
       G.R. Renchard/President, Chief Executive Officer
   Binder, Abdominal   General
   Joint, Knee, External Brace   Physical Med
   Orthosis, Cervical   Physical Med
   Sling, Arm   Physical Med
   Support, Ankle   Orthopedics
   Support, Wrist   Physical Med

BEST ORTHOPEDIC PRODUCTS, INC.
   See Best Orthopedic And Medical Services, Inc.

BEST VALUE CERAMICS   607-723-2803
19 Chenango St., Binghamton, NY 13901
FDA Number: n/a
Medical Products Sales Volume: $600,000
Annual Revenue: $0-$1 Million
Ownership: Private
Produces/Sells CE-marked Devices: N
Federal Procurement Eligibility: Small Business
Distribution: Importer
   Crown, Preformed   Dental And Oral

BEST VASCULAR, INC.   770-717-0904
4350 International Blvd., Norcross, GA 30093
FDA Number: 1062385
   Intravascular Radiation Delivery System   Cardiovascular

BESTWAY PRODUCTS CO.
310-329-0600
16602 S. Broadway St., Gardena, CA 90248
FDA Number: 2020401   *Fax:* 310-329-0602
E-mail: stuart_gordon@bestwayproductscompany.com
Web site: http://www.bestwayproductscompany.com
Ownership: Private
Produces/Sells CE-marked Devices: N
Federal Procurement Eligibility: Small Business, GSA Contract
Distribution: Manufacturer Direct, Manufacturer Through Distributor, Exporter
General Admin.: Stuart Gordon/President
Saw, Bone Cutting   Orthopedics
Saw, Manual, And Accessories   Surgery
Saw, Manual, Neurological (With Accessories)   Cns/Neurology

BETA BIOMED SERVICES, INC.
800-315-7551
2804 Singleton St., Rowlett, TX 75088
FDA Number: 1650347   *Fax:* 972-475-9814
E-mail: info@betabiomed.com
Web site: www.betabiomed.com
Ownership: Private
Produces/Sells CE-marked Devices: Y
Distribution: Manufacturer Direct, Manufacturer Through Distributor, Manufacturer Through Manufacturer Reps, Exporter
Oximeter, Intracardiac   Cardiovascular

BETA MEDICAL PRODUCTS, INC.
See Surgical Table Services Co.

BETA TECHNOLOGY, INC.
800-858-2382
831-426-0882
2841 Mission St., Santa Cruz, CA 95060
FDA Number: n/a   *Fax:* 831-423-4573
E-mail: lisa.swanson@beta-technology.com
Web site: www.beta-technology.com
Medical Products Sales Volume: $900,000
Annual Revenue: $0-$1 Million
Year Founded: 1976
Ownership: UNILEVER
Quality System Registration Information: ISO9001
Produces/Sells CE-marked Devices: Y
Distribution: Manufacturer Direct
General Admin.: Dermott Corr/General Manager
Mktg./Adv.: Stewart Peterson/Director Marketing
Production: David Collette/Product Manager
Caliper, Skinfold   General

BETCO CORP.
800-462-3826
419-241-2156
P.O. Box 3127, Toledo, OH 43607
FDA Number: n/a   *Fax:* 419-321-1954
E-mail: email@betco.com
Web site: www.betco.com
Annual Revenue: $50-$100 Million
Year Founded: 1950
Total Employees: 200   *Marketing Staff:* 7   *Sales Staff:* 45
Ownership: Private
Produces/Sells CE-marked Devices: N
Distribution: Manufacturer Through Distributor
General Admin.: Paul Betz/Chief Executive Officer
     Greg Chesnutt/President
Mktg./Adv.: Griff Crammond/Director Marketing
     Par Ricketts/Director National Accounts
     Joanna Hunter/Manager Marketing & Communications
     John Reed/Manager Sales Training
     Dan Carr/Vice President Sales
Production: Dorothy Clarke/Manager Materials
     Candice Rushton/Manager Regulatory Affairs
     Jim Betz/Vice President Manufacturing
Disinfector, Liquid   General
Solution, Antibacterial Cleaner   General

BETHESDA RESEARCH LABORATORIES INC.
See Life Technologies Corporation

BETHLEHEM APPARATUS CO., INC.
610-838-7034
890 Front St., Hellertown, PA 18055
FDA Number: n/a   *Fax:* 610-838-6333
E-mail: info@bethlehemapparatus.com
Web site: www.bethapp.com
Medical Products Sales Volume: $9,500,000
Year Founded: 1950
Total Employees: 15   *Marketing Staff:* 1   *Sales Staff:* 4
Ownership: Private
Produces/Sells CE-marked Devices: N
Federal Procurement Eligibility: Small Business
Distribution: Manufacturer Direct, Manufacturer Through Distributor, Manufacturer Through Manufacturer Reps, Service Direct
General Admin.: Bruce Lawrence/President
Burner   Chemistry
Mercury   Dental And Oral

BETTER CONTAINERS MFG. CO., INC.
800-831-6049
530 Hyde Park, Hillside, IL 60162
FDA Number: n/a   *Fax:* 708-547-7106
E-mail: team@bettercontainers.com
Web site: www.bettercontainers.com
Year Founded: 1945
Ownership: Private
Produces/Sells CE-marked Devices: N
General Admin.: Randy Christie/President
Sterilizer, Steam (Autoclave)   General

BETTER DENTAL PRODUCTS
402-934-4996
8540 I St., Omaha, NE 68127
FDA Number: 3006278472
Mouthpiece, Saliva Ejector   Dental And Oral

BETTER HANDS GLOVE PRODUCTS
800-242-2850
925-825-2349
P.O. Box 21641, Concord, CA 94521
FDA Number: 2954278   *Fax:* 209-755-5746
E-mail: brucek@betterhands.com
Web site: http://www.betterhands.com
Annual Revenue: $0-$1 Million
Year Founded: 1992
Total Employees: 1
Ownership: Private
Produces/Sells CE-marked Devices: N
Federal Procurement Eligibility: Small Business
Distribution: Manufacturer Direct, Manufacturer Through Manufacturer Reps
General Admin.: Mr. Bruce Klimoski/Chief Executive Officer
Splint, Other   Orthopedics

BETTER HEALTH, INC.
866-BED-BLOX
865-922-8712
4117 E Emory Road Suite 601, Knoxville, TN 37938
FDA Number: 1054189   *Fax:* 865-922-6362
E-mail: fdjhurst@aol.com
Web site: www.bedblox.com
Medical Products Sales Volume: $100,000
Year Founded: 1991
Total Employees: 3
Ownership: Private
Produces/Sells CE-marked Devices: N
Federal Procurement Eligibility: Small Business
Distribution: Manufacturer Direct
General Admin.: Dr. Fred A. Hurst/President, Chief Executive Officer
Mktg./Adv.: James W. Hurst/Director Marketing
     Regina S. Hurst/Director National Accounts
     Regina S. Hurst/Director Product Development
     Gregory D. Sharpe/Manager Contract Sales
     Gregory D. Sharpe/Manager International & National Sales
     James W. Hurst/Manager Market Research
     Greg Sharpe/Manager National Sales
Production: Robin A. Hurst/Director Quality Assurance
     Andrew Pfeiffer/Manager Materials
Bed, Manual   General

BETTER PARTS CO.
952-881-0234
219 West 90th St., Minneapolis, MN 55420
FDA Number: 2183532
Ownership: Private
Produces/Sells CE-marked Devices: N
Accessories, Catheter   Surgery

BETTER WATER, INC.
615-355-6063
698 Swan Dr., Smyrna, TN 37167
FDA Number: 1055109   *Fax:* 615-355-6065
E-mail: customerservice@betterwater.com
Web site: www.betterwater.com
Annual Revenue: $5-$10 Million
Year Founded: 1971
Total Employees: 30
Ownership: Private
Produces/Sells CE-marked Devices: N
Purification System, Water   Gastroenterology/Urology
Tank, Holding, Dialysis   Gastroenterology/Urology

BEUTLICH LP, PHARMACEUTICALS
800-238-8542
847-473-1100
1541 Shields Drive, Waukegan, IL 60085-8304
FDA Number: 1413399   *Fax:* 847-473-1122
E-mail: beutlich@beutlich.com
Web site: www.beutlich.com
Medical Products Sales Volume: $1,700,000
Year Founded: 1954
Total Employees: 20   *Marketing Staff:* 2   *Sales Staff:* 16
Ownership: Private
Produces/Sells CE-marked Devices: Y
Federal Procurement Eligibility: Small Business, VA Contract

BEUTLICH LP, PHARMACEUTICALS   800-238-8542 *(cont'd)*

Distribution: Manufacturer Direct, Manufacturer Through Distributor, Manufacturer Through Manufacturer Reps, Exporter
General Admin.: F. J. Beutlich/President
Mktg./Adv.: Catherine Gordon/Manager Advertising & Communications
     Erin Loeher/Manager International & National Sales
     Ron Rosenberg/Manager Market Research
     T. Al Harmon/Manager National Sales
Production: Ann Marie Pahlman/Manager Regulatory Affairs

Handle, Instrument, Dental	Dental And Oral
Indicator, pH, Dye (Urinary, Non-Quantitative)	Chemistry
Tooth Bonding Agent, Resin Restoration	Dental And Oral

BEVCO ERGONOMIC SEATING   800-864-2991
2246A Bluemound Road, Waukesha, WI 53186   **262-798-9200**
FDA Number: n/a   *Fax:* 262-798-9201
E-mail: sales@bevco.com
Web site: www.bevco.com
Medical Products Sales Volume: $5,800,000
Annual Revenue: $1-$5 Million
Year Founded: 1950
Total Employees: 16   *Marketing Staff:* 3   *Sales Staff:* 2
Ownership: Private
Produces/Sells CE-marked Devices: N
Federal Procurement Eligibility: Small Business
Distribution: Manufacturer Through Distributor
General Admin.: John R. Bevington/President, Chief Executive Officer
Mktg./Adv.: Ron Buettner/Vice President Marketing & Sales

Chair, Other	General
Furniture, General	General
Office Equipment	General

BEVCO PRECISION MANUFACTURING CO.
See Bevco Ergonomic Seating

BEYOND 21ST CENTURY INC.   888-484-2587
13706 W. 75th Pl., Lenexa, KS 66216-4229   **913-631-4790**
FDA Number: 1933955   *Fax:* 913-725-9324
E-mail: megamind_2000@yahoo.com
Web site: www.badbadbreath.com
Medical Products Sales Volume: $1,500
Annual Revenue: $0-$1 Million
Year Founded: 1997
Ownership: Private
Produces/Sells CE-marked Devices: N
Federal Procurement Eligibility: Small Business
Distribution: Manufacturer Direct
General Admin.: Hemant Thakur/President, Chief Executive Officer
Mktg./Adv.: Margarita Thakur/Director Marketing

Scraper, Tongue	Dental And Oral

BF TECHNOLOGIES
See Agion Technologies Inc.

BG MEDICINE INC.   781-890-1199
610N Lincoln Street, Waltham, MA 02451
FDA Number: 3006424683   *Fax:* 781-895-1119
E-mail: communications@bg-medicine.com
Web site: www.bg-medicine.com
Ownership: Private
Produces/Sells CE-marked Devices: N
General Admin.: Mr. Michael Rogers/Chief Financial Officer, Executive Vice President
     Dr. Pieter Muntendam/President, Chief Executive Officer
Medical Admin.: Dr. Peter Gardiner/Chief Medical Officer
Mktg./Adv.: Mr. Wayne Sheperd/Vice President Marketing & Sales
Production: Ms. Carol Adiletto/Vice President Regulatory & Clinical Affairs

Test, Natriuretic Peptide	Chemistry

BHK, INC.   909-983-2973
1480 N. Claremont Blvd., Claremont, CA 91711-3538
FDA Number: n/a   *Fax:* 909-399-3637
E-mail: info@bhkinc.com
Web site: www.bhkinc.com
Annual Revenue: $5-$10 Million
Year Founded: 1975
Total Employees: 50   *Sales Staff:* 5
Ownership: Private
Quality System Registration Information: ISO9001
Produces/Sells CE-marked Devices: N
Federal Procurement Eligibility: Small Business
Distribution: Manufacturer Direct, Manufacturer Through Distributor, Manufacturer Through Manufacturer Reps, OEM, Exporter
General Admin.: Mr. Steven H. Boland/President, Chief Executive Officer
     Mr. Steven G. Boland/Vice President, General Manager
Mktg./Adv.: Ms. Suzie Garcia/Sales Associate

Component, Electrical	General
Generator, Ozone	Anesthesiology
Lamp, Infrared	Physical Med

BHK, INC.   909-983-2973 *(cont'd)*

Lamp, Other	General
Lamp, Ultraviolet (Spectrum A)	General
Lamp, Ultraviolet, Germicidal	General
Lamp, Ultraviolet, Physical Medicine	Physical Med
Sterilizer, Ultraviolet	General

BHM MEDICAL, INC.   800-868-0441
2001 Tanguay, Magog, QC J1X 5Y5 Canada   **819-868-0441**
FDA Number: 9681684   *Fax:* 819-868-2249
E-mail: bhm@bhm-medical.com
Web site: www.bhm-medical.com
Year Founded: 1991
Total Employees: 50
Ownership: ArjoHuntleigh
Quality System Registration Information: ISO9001
Produces/Sells CE-marked Devices: Y
Federal Procurement Eligibility: Small Business
Distribution: Manufacturer Direct, Manufacturer Through Distributor, Manufacturer Through Manufacturer Reps, Exporter

BHP INC.
See Biomerieux Inc.

BHS INTERNATIONAL, INC.   410-721-5055
2431 Crofton Lane, Ste.9, Crofton, MD 21114
FDA Number: 1122226   *Fax:* 410-721-2942
E-mail: info@bhsinternational.com
Web site: www.bhsinternational.com
Medical Products Sales Volume: $2,900,000
Annual Revenue: $5-$10 Million
Year Founded: 1982
Total Employees: 7   *Marketing Staff:* 2   *Sales Staff:* 2
Ownership: Private
Produces/Sells CE-marked Devices: N
Federal Procurement Eligibility: Small Business, Minority Owned
Distribution: Manufacturer Direct
Mktg./Adv.: Julie Kanoff/Manager National Sales
     Boman Najmi/President, Chief Executive Officer, Marketing Manager

Stethoscope, Manual	Cardiovascular

BI-OPTICAL, INC.
See Newport Glass Works, Ltd.

BIACARE CORPORATION   616-931-1267
140 West Washington, Suite 100, Zeeland, MI 49464
FDA Number: 3005550595

Bandage, Compression	General
Bandage, Elastic	General
Binder, Elastic	General
Binder, Medical, Therapeutic	General
Stocking, Elastic, Physical Medicine	Physical Med

BIBBERO SYSTEMS, INC.   800-242-2376
1300 N. McDowell Blvd., Petaluma, CA 94954   **707-778-3131**
FDA Number: n/a   *Fax:* 800-242-9330
E-mail: info@bibbero.com
Web site: www.bibbero.com
Annual Revenue: $10-$25 Million
Year Founded: 1953
Total Employees: 130   *Marketing Staff:* 4   *Sales Staff:* 20
Ownership: Private
Produces/Sells CE-marked Devices: N
Federal Procurement Eligibility: Small Business
Distribution: Manufacturer Direct
General Admin.: Michael J. Buckley/President
Mktg./Adv.: Carolyn Talesfore/Director Marketing & Sales
     Don Buckley/Manager Market Research
Production: Steve Hackett/Manager Materials
Research: Don Buckley/Vice President Research & Development

Furniture, General	General
Glove, Patient Examination	General
Gown, Patient, Disposable	General
Paper, Chart, Record, Medical	General
Service, Printing	General
Sheet, Examination Table, Disposable	General

BICON, LLC   800-882-4266
501 Arborway, Second Floor, Boston, MA 02130   **617-524-4443**
FDA Number: 1223843   *Fax:* 617-524-0096
E-mail: support@bicon.com
Web site: www.bicon.com
Medical Products Sales Volume: $6,800,000
Annual Revenue: $10-$25 Million
Year Founded: 1985
Total Employees: 80
Ownership: Private
Quality System Registration Information: ISO9001
Produces/Sells CE-marked Devices: Y
Federal Procurement Eligibility: Small Business

BICON, LLC
800-882-4266 (cont'd)
Distribution: Manufacturer Direct
General Admin.: Mr. V.J. Morgan/Chief Operating Officer
Implant, Endosseous — Dental And Oral

BICRON ELECTRONICS
800-624-2766
50 Barlow St., Canaan, CT 06018 — 860-824-5125
FDA Number: n/a — *Fax:* 860-824-1137
Web site: www.bicronusa.com
Year Founded: 1964
Total Employees: 100
Ownership: Private
Quality System Registration Information: ISO9001
Produces/Sells CE-marked Devices: N
Distribution: Manufacturer Through Manufacturer Reps, OEM
General Admin.: Peter Kent/President, Chief Executive Officer
Mktg./Adv.: Jason McHugh/Director Marketing
　　　　Linda Walella/Vice President Sales
Adapter, Cable, Equipment — General
Valve, Other — Chemistry

BIDDLE INSTRUMENTS
See Megger Inc. (Formerly Avo International)

BIDWELL INDUSTRIAL GROUP, INC., BLU-RAY DIVISION
860-343-5353
2055 S. Main St., Middletown, CT 06457
FDA Number: 9200143 — *Fax:* 860-347-8775
E-mail: blu-ray@bidwellinc.com
Web site: www.bidwellinc.com
Medical Products Sales Volume: $4,800,000
Year Founded: 1957
Total Employees: 30
Ownership: Private
Produces/Sells CE-marked Devices: N
Federal Procurement Eligibility: Small Business
Distribution: Manufacturer Through Distributor
General Admin.: Donald Bidwell
Mktg./Adv.: Donald Bidwell/Manager Advertising
　　　　Michael Bidwell/Vice President Marketing & Sales
Duplicator, X-Ray Film — Radiology
Printer, Radiographic Duplicator — Radiology

BIEN AIR USA, INC.
800-433-2636
17880 Sky Park Circle, Ste 140, Irvine, CA 92614 — 949-477-6050
FDA Number: 9034059 — *Fax:* 949-477-6051
E-mail: ba-usa@bienair.com
Web site: www.bienair.com
Year Founded: 1959
Total Employees: 350 — *Marketing Staff:* 5 — *Sales Staff:* 27
Ownership: Private
Quality System Registration Information: ISO9000; ISO9001; ISO9002
Produces/Sells CE-marked Devices: N
Federal Procurement Eligibility: Small Business
Distribution: Manufacturer Through Distributor, OEM, Service Direct, Exporter
General Admin.: Vincent Mosimann/Chief Executive Officer
　　　　Jean Claude Meier/President
　　　　Arthur Mateen/Vice President
Mktg./Adv.: Daniel Kern/Director National Accounts
　　　　Jose Forchelet/Manager Advertising
　　　　Denis Cuendet/Manager Contract Sales
　　　　Arthur Mateen/Manager National Sales
Production: Alain Leoniti/Director Quality Assurance & Regulatory Affairs
　　　　Maxwell Bowman/Manager Materials
Handpiece, Air-Powered, Dental — Dental And Oral
Instrument, Dental, Manual — Dental And Oral

BIG BOYZ INDUSTRIES, INC.
877-574-3233
128 Railroad Dr., Ivyland, PA 18974 — 215-942-9971
FDA Number: 2531688 — *Fax:* 215-942-8803
Web site: www.bariatricbeds.com
Ownership: Private
Produces/Sells CE-marked Devices: N
Bed, Electric — General

BIG D INDUSTRIES, INC.
405-682-2541
5620 S.W. 29th St., Oklahoma City, OK 73179
FDA Number: n/a
Web site: www.bigdind.com
Annual Revenue: $1-$5 Million
Ownership: Private
Produces/Sells CE-marked Devices: N
Federal Procurement Eligibility: Small Business
Distribution: Manufacturer Through Distributor
Housekeeping Equipment — General

BIG THREE INDUSTRIES, INC.
See Air Liquide America Corporation

BILL FRANK PRODUCTIONS BF BIO-SUPPORTS INC.
614-840-0091
665 Old Pond Lane, Powell, OH 43065
FDA Number: n/a
Ownership: Private
Produces/Sells CE-marked Devices: N
Orthosis, Truncal/Limb — Physical Med

BILLEDEAUX HEARING CENTER, LLC
337-989-4327
4414 Johnson St. Ste. D, Lafayette, LA 70503
FDA Number: 3003529241
Ownership: Private
Produces/Sells CE-marked Devices: N
Hearing-Aid — Ear/Nose/Throat

BILLUPS-ROTHENBERG, INC.
877-755-3309
PO Box 977, Del Mar, CA 92014-0977 — 858-535-0545
FDA Number: n/a — *Fax:* 858-535-0546
E-mail: bri@brincubator.com
Web site: www.brincubator.com
Annual Revenue: $0-$1 Million
Year Founded: 1973
Ownership: Private
Produces/Sells CE-marked Devices: N
Federal Procurement Eligibility: Small Business
Distribution: Manufacturer Direct, Manufacturer Through Distributor
Box, Transportation, Container, Specimen — General
Incubator, Anaerobic — Microbiology

BINARY SYSTEMS
See Mediware Information Systems, Inc.

BINDER BIOMEDICAL INC.
561-981-2682
2385 NW Executive Center Drive, Boca Raton, FL 33431
FDA Number: 3007594625 — *Fax:* 561-962-2710
E-mail: info@bindermed.com
Ownership: Private
Produces/Sells CE-marked Devices: N
Intervertebral Fusion Device With Bone Graft, Cervical — Orthopedics

BINDING SITE, INC., THE
800-633-4484
5889 Oberlin Dr., Ste. 101, — 858-453-9177
San Diego, CA 92121
FDA Number: 2083566 — *Fax:* 858-453-9189
E-mail: info@thebindingsite.com
Web site: www.bindingsite.co.uk
Year Founded: 1988
Total Employees: 64 — *Marketing Staff:* 6 — *Sales Staff:* 2082
Ownership: Private
Quality System Registration Information: ISO9001; ISO9002
Produces/Sells CE-marked Devices: Y
Federal Procurement Eligibility: Small Business
Distribution: Exclusive Distributor
Mktg./Adv.: Anne Grainger/Manager National Sales
　　　　Dr. Dick Rowland/Vice President Marketing
2nd Antibody (Species Specific Anti-Animal Gamma Globulin) — Immunology
Alpha-1 Microglobulin, Antigen, Antiserum, Control — Immunology
Alpha-1-Acid-Glycoprotein, Antigen, Antiserum, Control — Immunology
Alpha-1-T-Glycoprotein, Antigen, Antiserum, Control — Immunology
Alpha-2-AP-Glycoprotein, Antigen, Antiserum, Control — Immunology
Anti-DNA Antibody (Enzyme-Labeled), Antigen, Control — Immunology
Anti-DNA Antibody, Antigen and Control — Immunology
Anti-DNA Indirect Immunofluorescent Solid Phase — Immunology
Anti-RNP-Antibody, Antigen And Control — Immunology
Anti-SM-Antibody, Antigen And Control — Immunology
Antibodies, Anti-Ribosomal P — Immunology
Antibodies, Gliadin — Immunology
Antibody, Anti-Smooth Muscle, Indirect Immunofluorescent — Immunology
Antibody, Anti-Thyroid, Indirect Immunofluorescent — Immunology
Antibody, Antimitochondrial, Indirect Immunofluorescent — Immunology
Antibody, Antinuclear, Indirect Immunofluorescent, Antigen — Immunology
Antibody, Other — General
Antigen, Antiserum, Alpha-2-Macroglobulin, Rhodamine — Immunology
Antigen, Antiserum, Complement C1 Inhibitor (Inactivator) — Immunology
Antigen, Antiserum, Control, Albumin — Immunology
Antigen, Antiserum, Control, Albumin, FITC — Immunology
Antigen, Antiserum, Control, Alpha-1-Antichymotrypsin — Immunology
Antigen, Antiserum, Control, Alpha-2-Glycoproteins — Immunology
Antigen, Antiserum, Control, Alpha-2-HS-Glycoprotein — Immunology
Antigen, Antiserum, Control, Alpha-2-Macroglobulin — Immunology
Antigen, Antiserum, Control, Antithrombin III — Immunology
Antigen, Antiserum, Control, Bence-Jones Protein — Immunology
Antigen, Antiserum, Control, Ceruloplasmin — Immunology
Antigen, Antiserum, Control, Complement C1q — Immunology
Antigen, Antiserum, Control, Complement C1r — Immunology
Antigen, Antiserum, Control, Complement C1s — Immunology
Antigen, Antiserum, Control, Complement C3 — Immunology
Antigen, Antiserum, Control, Complement C4 — Immunology
Antigen, Antiserum, Control, Complement C5 — Immunology
Antigen, Antiserum, Control, Complement C8 — Immunology

BINDING SITE, INC., THE   800-633-4484 *(cont'd)*

Antigen, Antiserum, Control, Complement C9	Immunology
Antigen, Antiserum, Control, Factor B	Immunology
Antigen, Antiserum, Control, Free Secretory Component	Immunology
Antigen, Antiserum, Control, Gamma Globulin	Immunology
Antigen, Antiserum, Control, Gamma Globulin, FITC	Immunology
Antigen, Antiserum, Control, Haptoglobin	Immunology
Antigen, Antiserum, Control, IGA	Immunology
Antigen, Antiserum, Control, IGA, FITC	Immunology
Antigen, Antiserum, Control, IGA, Peroxidase	Immunology
Antigen, Antiserum, Control, IGD	Immunology
Antigen, Antiserum, Control, IGE	Immunology
Antigen, Antiserum, Control, IGE, Peroxidase	Immunology
Antigen, Antiserum, Control, IGG	Immunology
Antigen, Antiserum, Control, IGG (Gamma Chain Specific)	Immunology
Immunoassay, Other	Toxicology
Plate, Radial Immunodiffusion	Immunology
Radial Immunodiffusion, Albumin	Chemistry
Radial Immunodiffusion, Lipoproteins	Chemistry
Reader, Radial Immunodiffusion	Microbiology
Test, B Lymphocyte Marker	Hematology
Test, Beta 2 - Microglobulin	Immunology
Test, Qualitative And Quantitative Factor Deficiency	Hematology

BINER ELLISON   800-741-2341
2685 South Melrose Drive, Vista, CA 92081   **760-598-6500**
FDA Number: n/a   *Fax:* 760-598-7600
E-mail: Sales@Binerellison.com
Web site: www.Binerellison.com
Medical Products Sales Volume: $10,000,000
Annual Revenue: $1-$5 Million
Year Founded: 1936
Total Employees: 55   *Marketing Staff:* 2   *Sales Staff:* 10
Ownership: Accutek Pacakging Equipment
Produces/Sells CE-marked Devices: N
Federal Procurement Eligibility: Small Business

Labeling Equipment	General

BIO AIR SYSTEMS DIV.   336-299-2885
PO Box 18547, Greensboro, NC 27419-8547
FDA Number: n/a   *Fax:* 336-294-2472
Web site: www.bioair.com
Annual Revenue: $10-$25 Million
Year Founded: 1960
Ownership: CUSTOM INDUSTRIES, INC.
Produces/Sells CE-marked Devices: N
Federal Procurement Eligibility: Small Business
Distribution: OEM

Hood, Isolation, Laminar Air Flow	General
Laminar Air Flow Unit, Fixed (Air Curtain)	Chemistry

BIO BREEDERS, INC.   617-926-5278
116 Temperton Parkway, Watertown, MA 02472
FDA Number: n/a   *Fax:* 617-926-6789
E-mail: info@biobreeders.com
Medical Products Sales Volume: $1,100,000
Annual Revenue: $0-$1 Million
Year Founded: 1984
Total Employees: 10
Ownership: Private
Produces/Sells CE-marked Devices: N
Federal Procurement Eligibility: Small Business
Distribution: Manufacturer Direct
General Admin.: Dr. VanDongen/President
         Mark Laraway/Supervisor

Animal, Laboratory	Microbiology
Contract Manufacturing	General
Valve, Heart, Tissue	Cardiovascular

BIO COMPRESSION SYSTEMS, INC.   800-888-0908
120 W. Commercial Avenue,   **201-939-0716**
Moonachie, NJ 07074
FDA Number: 2424387   *Fax:* 201-939-4503
E-mail: biosystems@biocompression.com
Web site: www.biocompression.com
Medical Products Sales Volume: $2,100,000
Annual Revenue: $5-$10 Million
Year Founded: 1983
Total Employees: 24   *Marketing Staff:* 3   *Sales Staff:* 6
Ownership: Private
Produces/Sells CE-marked Devices: Y
Federal Procurement Eligibility: Small Business, GSA Contract, VA Contract
Distribution: Manufacturer Through Distributor, OEM
General Admin.: Robert Freidenrich/Chief Executive Officer
         Ronald Motherwell/Vice President, General Manager
Mktg./Adv.: Dolores Freidenrich/Director Marketing

Compression Instrument	Orthopedics
Mattress, Alternating Pressure (Or Pads)	Physical Med

BIO COMPRESSION SYSTEMS, INC.   800-888-0908 *(cont'd)*

Sleeve, Compressible Limb	Cardiovascular

BIO CYBERNETICS INTL.   800-220-4224
1815 Wright Avenue, La Verne, CA 91750   **909-447-7050**
FDA Number: 2029084   *Fax:* 909-363-7311
E-mail: customerservice@cybertechmedical.com
Web site: www.cybertechmedical.com
Medical Products Sales Volume: $1,300,000
Year Founded: 1991
Total Employees: 15   *Sales Staff:* 1
Ownership: Private
Produces/Sells CE-marked Devices: Y
Federal Procurement Eligibility: Small Business, GSA Contract
Distribution: Manufacturer Through Manufacturer Reps

Orthosis, Lumbosacral	Physical Med

BIO DIAGNOSTIC INTL.   562-691-7850
1300-c- Pioneer Street, Brea, CA 92821
FDA Number: 2023751
Ownership: Private
Produces/Sells CE-marked Devices: N

Control, Drug Mixture	Toxicology

BIO MED SCIENCES, INC.   800-257-4566
7584 Morris Court, Suite 218,   **610-530-3193**
Allentown, PA 18106
FDA Number: 2529394   *Fax:* 610-530-3194
E-mail: biomed@silon.com
Web site: www.silon.com
Medical Products Sales Volume: $1,600,000
Annual Revenue: $1-$5 Million
Year Founded: 1987
Total Employees: 20   *Marketing Staff:* 2   *Sales Staff:* 2
Ownership: Private
Quality System Registration Information: ISO9001
Produces/Sells CE-marked Devices: Y
Federal Procurement Eligibility: Small Business
Distribution: Manufacturer Direct, Manufacturer Through Distributor, Manufacturer Through Manufacturer Reps, OEM, Exporter
General Admin.: Mark E. Dillon/President, Chief Executive Officer
Mktg./Adv.: Jay Mundy/Manager Marketing & Sales

Contract Manufacturing	General
Contract Manufacturing, Product, Disposable	General
Dressing, Wound and Burn, Occlusive	Surgery
Elastomer, Silicone (Scar Management)	Surgery

BIO NUCLEAR DIAGNOSTICS INC.   800-668-4033
1791 Albion Road,   **416-674-1545**
Toront, ONT M9W-5 Canada
FDA Number: n/a   *Fax:* 416-674-7280
E-mail: customerservice@bndinc.com
Web site: www.bndinc.com
Year Founded: 1979
Total Employees: 25
Ownership: Private
Produces/Sells CE-marked Devices: N
Distribution: Manufacturer Direct, Exclusive Distributor, Importer

BIO PLAS, INC.   415-472-3777
4340 Redwood Highway, Suite A15, San Rafael, CA 94903
FDA Number: 2916716   *Fax:* 415-472-3758
E-mail: info@bioplas.com
Web site: www.bioplas.com
Medical Products Sales Volume: $2,500,000
Annual Revenue: $1-$5 Million
Year Founded: 1976
Total Employees: 10   *Marketing Staff:* 2   *Sales Staff:* 2
Ownership: Private
Produces/Sells CE-marked Devices: N
Federal Procurement Eligibility: Small Business
Distribution: Manufacturer Through Distributor
General Admin.: Donald H. DeVaughn/Chief Executive Officer, Chairman
         Jeannie McGrath/Chief Financial Officer, Controller
Mktg./Adv.: Jim Slattery/Director National Accounts
Production: Jeannie McGrath/Manager Regulatory Affairs
         Gino Escalante/Supervisor Warehouse Operations

Closure, Other	General
Cuvette, Spectrophotometer	Chemistry
Delivery System, Allergen And Vaccine	General
Equipment, Bank, Blood, Cryogenic (Liquid Nitrogen)	Hematology
Labware, Blood Collection	Chemistry
Pipette Tip	Chemistry
Support, Tube, Test	Chemistry
Tissue Embedding Equipment/Reagent	Pathology
Tube, Centrifuge	Chemistry

BIO-ANALYSIS, INC.   310-828-7423
1701 Berkeley St., Santa Monica, CA 90404
FDA Number: 2018685

Diazo, P-Nitroaniline/Vanillin, Vanilmandelic Acid	Chemistry
Radioimmunoassay, 17-Hydroxyprogesterone	Chemistry
Radioimmunoassay, Estradiol	Chemistry
Radioimmunoassay, Progesterone	Chemistry

BIO-BRITE, INC.   800-621-5483
4330 East-West Hwy., Suite 310,   **301-961-5940**
Bethesda, MD 20814
FDA Number: n/a   *Fax:* 301-961-5943
E-mail: biobrite@aol.com
Web site: www.biobrite.com
Medical Products Sales Volume: $1,000,000
Annual Revenue: $1-$5 Million
Year Founded: 1989
Total Employees: 6
Ownership: Private
Produces/Sells CE-marked Devices: N
Federal Procurement Eligibility: Small Business
Distribution: Manufacturer Direct, Manufacturer Through Distributor
General Admin.: Kirk Renaud/Chief Executive Officer

Light, Therapy, Seasonal Affective Disorder (SAD)	General

BIO-CLIN, INC.   314-647-3244
5977 S.W. Avenue, St. Louis, MO 63139
FDA Number: 1937537   *Fax:* 314-647-2151
Medical Products Sales Volume: $270,000
Annual Revenue: $0-$1 Million
Year Founded: 1982
Total Employees: 5   *Marketing Staff:* 5   *Sales Staff:* 5
Ownership: Private
Produces/Sells CE-marked Devices: N
Federal Procurement Eligibility: Small Business
Distribution: Manufacturer Through Distributor
General Admin.: Bruce Watkins/Chief Executive Officer

Contract R&D, Diagnostics	General

BIO-CONCEPTS, INC.   202-772-5333
2424 East University Dr., Phoenix, AZ 85034
FDA Number: 2022548

Stocking, Elastic	General

BIO-DETEK, INC.   800-225-1310
525 Narragansett Park Drive,   **401-729-1400**
Pawtucket, RI 02861
FDA Number: 1218058   *Fax:* 401-729-1408
E-mail: info@bio-detek.com
Web site: www.bio-detek.com
Medical Products Sales Volume: $9,200,000
Annual Revenue: $5-$10 Million
Total Employees: 100
Ownership: Zoll Medical Corp.
Produces/Sells CE-marked Devices: Y
Federal Procurement Eligibility: Small Business
Distribution: Manufacturer Through Distributor
General Admin.: Mark Totman/President
       Patricia Lyons/Vice President Human Resources
Production: Robert Morse/Director Quality Assurance
       Paula Trabucco/Manager Customer Services
       Bruce Carlson/Manager Materials
Research: Deborah Jones/Vice President Research & Development

Electrode, Electrocardiograph	Cardiovascular

BIO-DYNAMICS INC.
See Roche Diagnostics Operations

BIO-FEEDBACK SYSTEMS, INC.   303-444-1411
2736 47th St., Boulder, CO 80301-2317
FDA Number: n/a   *Fax:* 303-444-1412
E-mail: pitchj@qwest.net
Web site: www.users.qwest.net/~pitchj
Medical Products Sales Volume: $70,000
Annual Revenue: $0-$1 Million
Year Founded: 1969
Ownership: Private
Produces/Sells CE-marked Devices: N
Federal Procurement Eligibility: Small Business
Distribution: Manufacturer Direct, Manufacturer Through Distributor, Manufacturer Through Manufacturer Reps, OEM, Exporter
General Admin.: John Picchiottino/President
       Paul Picchiottino/Secretary, Treasurer

Amplifier, Microelectrode	General
Amplifier, Physiological Signal	Cns/Neurology
Analyzer, Signal Isolation	Cardiovascular
Biofeedback Device	Cns/Neurology
Biofeedback Equipment, Myoelectric, Battery-Powered	Physical Med

BIO-FEEDBACK SYSTEMS, INC.   303-444-1411 *(cont'd)*

Biofeedback Equipment, Myoelectric, Powered	Physical Med
Computer, Patient Monitor	Anesthesiology
Conditioner, Signal, Physiological	Cns/Neurology
Device, Dysfunction, Erectile	Gastroenterology/Urology
Electroencephalograph	Cns/Neurology
Impotence Device, Mechanical/Hydraulic	Gastroenterology/Urology
Material, Training, Audiovisual	General
Meter, Conductivity	Chemistry
Meter, Skin Resistance, Battery-Powered	Physical Med
Monitor, EEG	Cns/Neurology
Monitor, Temperature (With Probe)	Anesthesiology
Monitor, Uterine Contraction, External	Obstetrics/Gynecology
Plethysmograph, Photo-Electric, Pneumatic Or Hydraulic	Cardiovascular
Thermometer, Electronic, Continuous	General

BIO-FLEX INTERNATIONAL, INC.   800-755-4588
1250 E. Hallandale Beach Blvd., Suite 1,   **954-457-2655**
Hallandale Beach, FL 33009
FDA Number: 2084040   *Fax:* 954-457-2688
E-mail: gloves@bio-flex.com
Web site: www.bio-flex.com
Medical Products Sales Volume: $2,800,000
Annual Revenue: $5-$10 Million
Year Founded: 1988
Total Employees: 15   *Marketing Staff:* 4   *Sales Staff:* 8
Ownership: Private
Quality System Registration Information: ISO9002
Produces/Sells CE-marked Devices: N
Federal Procurement Eligibility: Small Business, Female Owned, GSA Contract
Distribution: Exclusive Distributor
General Admin.: Fernando De Paz/Chief Operating Officer
       Steven Ezekiel/President, Chief Executive Officer
Finance: Michael Ezekiel/Chief Financial Officer

Glove, Patient Examination	General
Glove, Patient Examination, Latex	General

BIO-GATE USA, INC.   714-670-2771
6800 Orangethorpe Ave., Unit E, Buena Park, CA 90620
FDA Number: 2032596
Ownership: Private
Produces/Sells CE-marked Devices: N

Exerciser, Powered	Anesthesiology
Otoscope	Ear/Nose/Throat

BIO-HEME   801-277-9392
3710 Ceres Drive, Salt Lake City, UT 84124
FDA Number: 1722359   *Fax:* 801-278-4516
E-mail: randolpotter@networld.com
Medical Products Sales Volume: $40,000
Annual Revenue: $0-$1 Million
Year Founded: 1982
Ownership: Private
Produces/Sells CE-marked Devices: N
Federal Procurement Eligibility: Small Business
Distribution: Manufacturer Direct, Manufacturer Through Distributor, OEM, Exporter
General Admin.: Rand Potter/Director

Whole Human Plasma, Antigen, Antiserum, Control	Immunology

BIO-IMAGING TECHNOLOGIES, INC.
See Bioclinica, Inc.

BIO-LIFE, L.L.C.   800-851-8745
2000 Spring Rd., Suite 600, Hinsdale, IL 60523
FDA Number: 3005841037
Ownership: Private
Produces/Sells CE-marked Devices: N

Implant, Endosseous	Dental And Oral

BIO-LOGICS PRODUCTS, INC.   800-426-7577
PO Box 505, West Jordan, UT 84084   **801-561-9208**
FDA Number: n/a   *Fax:* 801-561-9208
E-mail: sales@biologicsinc.com
Web site: www.biologicsinc.com
Medical Products Sales Volume: $4,000,000
Annual Revenue: $1-$5 Million
Year Founded: 1972
Total Employees: 30   *Marketing Staff:* 4   *Sales Staff:* 5
Ownership: Private
Produces/Sells CE-marked Devices: N
Federal Procurement Eligibility: Small Business
Distribution: Manufacturer Direct, Exporter
General Admin.: C. Eugene McDermott/Chief Executive Officer
Mktg./Adv.: Steven E. McDermott/Director Marketing
       Robert McDermott/Director Product Development
       Jack Van Ry/Manager National Sales
Production: Scott McDermott/Director Quality Assurance
       James Chase/Plant Manager

MANUFACTURER PROFILES

BIO-LOGICS PRODUCTS, INC.
800-426-7577 *(cont'd)*

Bracelet, Identification	General
Cart, Waste	General
Identification, Alert, Medical	General
Kit, Labor and Delivery	Obstetrics/Gynecology
Label, Bar Code	General
Patient Transfer Unit	General
Tag, Device Status	General

BIO-MED DEVICES, INC.
61 Soundview Road, Guilford, CT 06437
800-224-6633
203-458-0202

FDA Number: 1218704   Fax: 203-458-0440
E-mail: custserv@biomeddevices.com
Web site: www.biomeddevices.com
Year Founded: 1985
Ownership: Private
Produces/Sells CE-marked Devices: Y
Federal Procurement Eligibility: Small Business
Distribution: Manufacturer Direct, Manufacturer Through Distributor, Manufacturer Through Manufacturer Reps, OEM, Exporter
General Admin.: Dean J. Bennett/President, Chief Executive Officer

Circuit, Breathing, Ventilator	Anesthesiology
Controller, Oxygen (Blender)	Anesthesiology
Lung, Membrane (For Long-Term Respiratory Support)	Anesthesiology
Monitor, Neonatal	Obstetrics/Gynecology
Monitor, Oxygen (Ventilatory) W/Wo Alarm	Anesthesiology
Monitor, Ventilatory Frequency	Anesthesiology
Ventilator, Emergency, Powered (Resuscitator)	Anesthesiology
Ventilator, Neonatal Respirator	General
Ventilator, Volume (Critical Care)	Anesthesiology

BIO-MED U.S.A. INC.
111 Ellison Street, Paterson, NJ 07505
973-278-5222

FDA Number: 2246683   Fax: 973-278-7152
E-mail: admin@biomedus.com
Web site: www.biomedus.com
Year Founded: 1987
Ownership: Private
Quality System Registration Information: ISO9001; ISO9002
Produces/Sells CE-marked Devices: Y
Federal Procurement Eligibility: Small Business
Distribution: Manufacturer Through Distributor, OEM, Exclusive Distributor, Importer, Exporter

Antigen, Rubella, Other	Microbiology
Grid, Radiographic	Radiology
Holder, X-Ray Film Cassette, Vertical	Radiology
Kit, Pregnancy Test, Over The Counter, HCG	Chemistry

BIO-MEDIA UNLIMITED LTD.
200 Vinyl Court, Unit A,
Woodbridge, ONT L4L-4 Canada
888-476-4276
416-410-2950

FDA Number: n/a   Fax: 905-850-0985
E-mail: drjlabs@istar.ca
Web site: www.bio-media.ca
Year Founded: 1985
Total Employees: 25
Ownership: Private
Produces/Sells CE-marked Devices: N
Distribution: Manufacturer Direct, Exclusive Distributor, Importer

BIO-MEDIC HEALTH SERVICES, INC.
5041B Benois Road, Building B,
Roanoke, VA 24018
800-525-0072
540-772-0072

FDA Number: n/a   Fax: 540-772-1188
E-mail: custservice@bmhsi.com
Web site: www.bmhsi.com
Medical Products Sales Volume: $600,000
Annual Revenue: $0-$1 Million
Year Founded: 1991
Total Employees: 5   Marketing Staff: 2   Sales Staff: 3
Ownership: Private
Produces/Sells CE-marked Devices: N
Federal Procurement Eligibility: Small Business
Distribution: Manufacturer Direct, Importer
General Admin.: Philip Willmott/General Manager

Cane, Safety Walk	Physical Med
Commode (Toilet)	General
Crutch	Physical Med
Diaper, Adult	General
Pad, Incontinence (Underpad)	General
Walker, Mechanical	Physical Med
Wheelchair, Manual	Physical Med

BIO-MEDICAL ASSOCIATES, INC.
See Bio-Medical Products Corp.

BIO-MEDICAL DEVICES
17171 Daimler Ave, Irvine, CA 92614
800-443-3842

FDA Number: 2083467   Fax: 949-752-9658

BIO-MEDICAL DEVICES
800-443-3842 *(cont'd)*

E-mail: info@bmdi.com
Web site: www.bmdi.com
Ownership: Private
Produces/Sells CE-marked Devices: N
Distribution: Manufacturer Direct, Importer
General Admin.: Susan Hurd/Manager
    Ben Trainer/Partner
    Bradford Hack/Partner
    Nick Herbert/President, Chief Executive Officer
Production: Jermayne Calhoun/Customer Service Representative
    Michelle Chu/Customer Service Representative

Accessories, Apparel, Surgical	Surgery
Gown, Surgical	Surgery
Hood, Surgical	Surgery

BIO-MEDICAL INSTRUMENT CO.
15764 Munn Rd., Newbury, OH 44065
440-564-5450

FDA Number: 1520016   Fax: 440-564-5170
E-mail: biothesiometer@aol.com
Web site: www.biothesiometer.com
Ownership: Private
Produces/Sells CE-marked Devices: N

Stimulator, Auditory, Evoked Response	Cns/Neurology
Vibration Threshold Measurement Device	Cns/Neurology

BIO-MEDICAL INSTRUMENTS, INC.
2387 E. 8 Mile Road, Warren, MI 48091-2486
800-521-4640
586-756-5070

FDA Number: 1833896   Fax: 586-756-9891
E-mail: sales@bio-medical.com
Web site: www.bio-medical.com
Medical Products Sales Volume: $300,000
Annual Revenue: $0-$1 Million
Year Founded: 1975
Total Employees: 6   Sales Staff: 2
Ownership: Private
Produces/Sells CE-marked Devices: N
Federal Procurement Eligibility: Small Business
Mktg./Adv.: T. F. Thierbach/Manager Marketing
    Brian Milstead/Manager National Sales

Biofeedback Device	Cns/Neurology
Biofeedback Equipment, Myoelectric, Battery-Powered	Physical Med
Biofeedback Equipment, Myoelectric, Powered	Physical Med
Computer, Patient Data Management	General
Electrode, Electromyographic	Cns/Neurology
Monitor, EEG	Cns/Neurology
Monitor, EMG	Anesthesiology
Monitor, Physiological, Stress Exercise	Cardiovascular
Monitor, Pulse Rate	Anesthesiology
Monitor, Response, Skin, Galvanic	Cns/Neurology
Monitor, Temperature (With Probe)	Anesthesiology
Myograph	Physical Med
Sphygmomanometer, Electronic, Automatic	General

BIO-MEDICAL PRODUCTS CORP.
10 Halstead Rd., Mendham, NJ 07945
800-543-7427
973-543-7434

FDA Number: 2246827   Fax: 973-543-7497
E-mail: biomedicalproductscorp@msn.com
Web site: www.biomedicalproductscorp.com
Annual Revenue: $0-$1 Million
Total Employees: 5   Marketing Staff: 1   Sales Staff: 4
Ownership: Private
Produces/Sells CE-marked Devices: N
Federal Procurement Eligibility: Small Business
Distribution: Manufacturer Direct, Importer, Exporter
General Admin.: John G. Geppert/President
    Chris L. Geppert/Vice President

Analyzer, Chemistry, Fluorescence Immunoassay	Chemistry
Antigen, Prostate-Specific (PSA), Management, Cancer	Immunology
Antiserum, Fluorescent, Mycobacterium Tuberculosis	Microbiology
Campylobacter Pylori	Microbiology
Chlamydia, DNA Reagents	Microbiology
Collector, Urine	Gastroenterology/Urology
Container, Specimen Mailer And Storage	Pathology
Container, Urine Specimen	General
Enzymatic Method, Troponin Subunit	Chemistry
Kit, Pregnancy Test	Obstetrics/Gynecology
Radioimmunoassay, Follicle Stimulating Hormone	Chemistry
Radioimmunoassay, Prolactin (Lactogen)	Chemistry
Radioimmunoassay, Thyroid Stimulating Hormone	Chemistry
Reagent, Cholesterol (Total Test System)	Chemistry
Reagent, Occult Blood	Hematology
Solution, Antibacterial Cleaner	General
Strip, Test	Chemistry
System, Identification, Hepatitis B Antigen	Hematology
System, Test, Drugs of Abuse	Chemistry
Test, Alpha-Fetoprotein	Pathology
Test, Antibody, Acquired Immune Deficiency Syndrome (AIDS)	Hematology
Test, C-Reactive Protein	Immunology

BIO-MEDICAL PRODUCTS CORP.   800-543-7427 *(cont'd)*

Test, Direct Agglutination, Toxoplasma Gondii	Microbiology
Test, Fertility Monitoring	Obstetrics/Gynecology
Test, Hiv Detection	Immunology
Test, Human Chorionic Gonadotropin	Immunology
Test, Infectious Mononucleosis	Immunology
Test, Rheumatoid Factor	Immunology
Test, Systemic Lupus Erythematosus	Immunology
Tube, Culture	Microbiology
Tube, Transfer	General

BIO-MEDICAL SERVICE ASSOC.
See American Bio-Medical Service Corporation (Abmsc)

BIO-METRIC SYSTEMS, INC.
See Surmodics, Inc.

BIO-MOLECULAR DYNAMICS
See Spectrum Laboratories, Inc.

BIO-OPTICS, INC.   503-493-8000
1525 NE 41st Avenue, Portland, OR 97232
FDA Number: 1219413
Fax: 503-493-9000
E-mail: biooptics@aol.com
Web site: www.bio-optics.com
Medical Products Sales Volume: $800,000
Year Founded: 1976
Total Employees: 10   *Marketing Staff:* 3   *Sales Staff:* 4
Ownership: Private
Produces/Sells CE-marked Devices: Y
Federal Procurement Eligibility: Small Business
Distribution: Manufacturer Direct, Manufacturer Through Distributor, Importer, Exporter
General Admin.: Ronald A. Laing/Chief Executive Officer
     Robert Leslie/General Manager
     Dr. Ronald A. Laing/President
Mktg./Adv.: Robert Leslie/Manager Contract Sales

Computer Software	General
Spectacle Microscope, Low-Vision	Ophthalmology

BIO-PLEXUS, INC.   800-223-0010
129 Reservoir Road, Vernon, CT 06066   860-870-6112
FDA Number: 1221924
Fax: 860-870-6118
E-mail: cservice@bio-plexus.com
Web site: www.bio-plexus.com
Medical Products Sales Volume: $2,900,000
Annual Revenue: $5-$10 Million
Year Founded: 1987
Total Employees: 31   *Marketing Staff:* 5   *Sales Staff:* 8
Ownership: Private
Stock Symbol: BPXS
Traded On: NASDAQ
Quality System Registration Information: ISO9001; ISO9002
Produces/Sells CE-marked Devices: Y
Federal Procurement Eligibility: Small Business, GSA Contract, VA Contract
Distribution: Manufacturer Direct, Manufacturer Through Distributor, Manufacturer Through Manufacturer Reps, Exporter
General Admin.: Deborah Mancini/Director Human Resources
     John S. Metz/President, Chief Executive Officer
Mktg./Adv.: Jill Phillips/Director Marketing
     Christopher Zorn/Director National Accounts
     Christopher Zorn/Vice President Sales
Production: Craig Churchill/Director Engineering
     Timothy Rourke/Director Operations
     Dennis Masse/Manager Materials

Collector, Blood, Vacuum-Assisted	Hematology
Kit, Blood Collection, Phlebotomy	Cardiovascular
Needle, Blood Collection	General
Protector, Puncture, Needle	General
Waste Disposal Unit, Syringe	General

BIO-RAD LABORATORIES   800-866-0305
1000 Alfred Nobel Drive, Hercules, CA 94547   510-724-7000
FDA Number: 2919376
Fax: 510-741-5815
E-mail: Tina_Cuccia@bio-rad.com
Web site: www.bio-rad.com
Year Founded: 1952
Ownership: Bio-Rad Laboratories, Inc.
Stock Symbol: BIO
Traded On: AMEX
Produces/Sells CE-marked Devices: Y
Distribution: Manufacturer Direct
General Admin.: Carole Polito/President, Chief Executive Officer
Mktg./Adv.: James Blatt/Vice President Marketing & Sales

Analyzer, Sedimentation Rate, Erythrocyte	Hematology
Control, Cell Counter, Normal And Abnormal	Hematology
Control, Multi Analyte, All Kinds (Assayed And Unassayed)	Chemistry
Control, Urinalysis (Assayed And Unassayed)	Chemistry
Hematology Quality Control Mixture	Hematology

BIO-RAD LABORATORIES INC   425-881-8300
1000 Thomas St., Seattle, WA 98109
FDA Number: 3032700
Ownership: Bio-Rad Laboratories, Inc.
Stock Symbol: BIO
Traded On: AMEX
Produces/Sells CE-marked Devices: Y

BIO-RAD LABORATORIES INC., CLINICAL DIAGNOSTICS GROUP
See Bio-Rad Laboratories Inc., Clinical Systems Div.

BIO-RAD LABORATORIES INC., CLINICAL SYSTEMS DIV.   800-224-6723
4000 Alfred Nobel Dr., Hercules, CA 94547   510-724-7000
FDA Number: 2915274
Fax: 510-741-6373
E-mail: diagcs@bio-rad.com
Ownership: Bio-Rad Laboratories, Inc.
Stock Symbol: BIO
Traded On: AMEX
Produces/Sells CE-marked Devices: Y

Analyzer, Chemistry, Enzyme	Chemistry
Anti-DNA Antibody (Enzyme-Labeled), Antigen, Control	Immunology
Anti-RNP-Antibody, Antigen And Control	Immunology
Anti-SM-Antibody, Antigen And Control	Immunology
Antibodies, Anti-Ribosomal P	Immunology
Antinuclear Antibody (Enzyme-Labeled), Antigen, Controls	Immunology
Antinuclear Antibody, Antigen, Control	Immunology
Calibrator, Hemoglobin And Hematocrit Measurement	Hematology
Chromatographic/Fluorometric Method, Catecholamines	Chemistry
Column, Ion Exchange With Colorimetry, Delta-Aminolevulinic	Chemistry
Diazo, P-Nitroaniline/Vanillin, Vanilmandelic Acid	Chemistry
Extractable Antinuclear Antibody (Rnp/Sm), Antigen/Control	Immunology
Fluorescent Proc. (Qual.), Galactose-1-Phosphate Uridyl	Chemistry
Hemoglobin A2 Quantitation	Hematology
High Pressure Liquid Chromatography, Benzodiazepine	Toxicology
Instrumentation For Clinical Multiplex Test Systems	Chemistry
Instrumentation, High Pressure Liquid Chromatography	Toxicology
Ion Exchange Resin, Ehrlich's Reagent, Porphobilinogen	Chemistry
Liquid Chromatography, Amphetamine	Toxicology
Nitrous Acid & Nitrosonaphthol, 5-Hydroxyindole Acetic Acid	Chemistry
Quantitation, Hemoglobin, Abnormal	Hematology
Radioimmunoassay, Folic Acid	Chemistry
Spectrophotometric, Uroporphyrin	Chemistry
Test, Glycosylated Hemoglobin Assay	Hematology
Test, Hemoglobin Bart's	Hematology
Urinary Homocystine (Non-Quantitative) Test System	Chemistry

BIO-RAD LABORATORIES INC., CLINICAL SYSTEMS DIVISI
See Bio-Rad Laboratories Inc., Clinical Systems Div.

BIO-RAD LABORATORIES, DIAGNOSTIC GROUP   800-224-6723
524 Stone Rd, Suite A, Benicia, CA 94510   510-724-7000
FDA Number: 2919376
Fax: 510-741-6373
E-mail: diagcs@bio-rad.com
Ownership: Bio-Rad Laboratories, Inc.
Stock Symbol: BIO
Traded On: AMEX
Produces/Sells CE-marked Devices: Y

Analyzer, Sedimentation Rate, Erythrocyte	Hematology
Control, Cell Counter, Normal And Abnormal	Hematology
Control, Multi Analyte, All Kinds (Assayed And Unassayed)	Chemistry
Control, Platelet	Hematology
Control, Urinalysis (Assayed And Unassayed)	Chemistry
Detergent	Hematology
Diluent, Blood Cell	Hematology
Fluid, Red Cell Lysing	Hematology
Hematology Quality Control Mixture	Hematology
Reagent, General Purpose	Pathology
Standard/Control, Hemoglobin, Normal/Abnormal	Hematology
Tube, Capillary Blood Collection	Hematology

BIO-RAD LABORATORIES, INC   510-741-6263
5500 East 2nd St, Benicia, CA 94510
FDA Number: 2950880
Web site: www.bio-rad.com
Ownership: Bio-Rad Laboratories, Inc.
Stock Symbol: BIO
Traded On: AMEX
Produces/Sells CE-marked Devices: N

Assay, Enzyme Linked Immunosorbent, Parvovirus B19 Igm	Microbiology
Control, Multi Analyte, All Kinds (Assayed And Unassayed)	Chemistry
Enzyme Linked Immunoabsorbent Assay, Chlamydia Group	Microbiology
Enzyme Linked Immunoabsorbent Assay, Herpes Simplex Virus	Microbiology
Epstein-Barr Virus, Other	Microbiology
Multi Analyte Mixture, Calibrator	Chemistry
Test, Infectious Mononucleosis	Immunology

BIO-RAD LABORATORIES, INC.   800-866-0305
1000 Alfred Nobel Drive,   **510-724-7000**
Hercules, CA 94547
FDA Number: 2950880   Fax: 510-724-5815
Web site: http://www.bio-rad.com
Medical Products Sales Volume: $1,270,000,000
Annual Revenue: More than $1 Billion
Year Founded: 1952
Total Employees: 6300
Ownership: Private
Stock Symbol: BIO
Traded On: NYSE
Produces/Sells CE-marked Devices: N
General Admin.: David Schwartz/Chairman
      Norman Schwartz/President, Chief Executive Officer
Mktg./Adv.: Mr. Giovanni Magni/Vice President International Sales
Finance: Christine Tsingos/Chief Financial Officer
      Ronald Hutton/Treasurer

Anti-DNA Antibody (Enzyme-Labeled), Antigen, Control	Immunology
Anti-RNP-Antibody, Antigen And Control	Immunology
Antibodies, Anti-Ribosomal P	Immunology
Antinuclear Antibody (Enzyme-Labeled), Antigen, Controls	Immunology
Antinuclear Antibody, Antigen, Control	Immunology
Computer Software	General
Extractable Antinuclear Antibody (Rnp/Sm), Antigen/Control	Immunology
Multi Analyte Mixture, Calibrator	Chemistry

Medical Product Subsidiaries (Listed Separately)
Bio-Rad Laboratories
Bio-Rad Laboratories Inc., Clinical Systems Div.
Bio-Rad Laboratories, Diagnostic Group
Bio-Rad Laboratories, Inc
Bio-Rad Laboratories, Inc.
Bio-Rad Laboratories, Life Science Group
Bio-Rad, Diagnostics Group

BIO-RAD LABORATORIES, INC.   425-881-8300
14620 N.E. North Woodinville, Way, Suite 200,
Woodinville, WA 98072
FDA Number: 3032705
Ownership: Bio-Rad Laboratories, Inc.
Produces/Sells CE-marked Devices: Y

Antibody, Antimitochondrial, Indirect Immunofluorescent	Immunology
Antibody, Antinuclear, Indirect Immunofluorescent, Antigen	Immunology
Antibody, Multiple Auto, Indirect Immunofluorescent	Immunology
Antinuclear Antibody (Enzyme-Labeled), Antigen, Controls	Immunology
Antinuclear Antibody, Antigen, Control	Immunology
Antisera, Fluorescent, Herpesvirus Hominis 1, 2	Microbiology
Antiserum, Fluorescent, Chlamydia Trachomatis	Microbiology
Collector, Specimen	Microbiology
Culture Media, Non-Propagating Transport	Microbiology
Enzyme Linked Immunoabsorbent Assay, Chlamydia Group	Microbiology
Enzyme Linked Immunoabsorbent Assay, Cytomegalovirus	Microbiology
Enzyme Linked Immunoabsorbent Assay, Treponema Pallidum	Microbiology
Epstein-Barr Virus, Other	Microbiology
Legionella Direct & Indirect Fluorescent Antibody Regents	Microbiology
Multi Analyte Mixture, Calibrator	Chemistry
Pneumocystis Carinii	Microbiology
Test, Hiv Detection	Immunology
Test, Infectious Mononucleosis	Immunology

BIO-RAD LABORATORIES, INC.   1-800-224-6723
6565 185th Ave., N.E., Redmond, WA 98052   **425-881-8300**
FDA Number: 3022521
Web site: www.bio-rad.com
Ownership: Bio-Rad Laboratories, Inc.
Produces/Sells CE-marked Devices: Y

Antiserum, Neutralization, Respiratory Syncytial Virus	Microbiology
Colorimeter, General Use	Chemistry
Control, Multi Analyte, All Kinds (Assayed And Unassayed)	Chemistry
Enzyme Linked Immunoabsorbent Assay, Herpes Simplex Virus	Microbiology
Enzyme-Linked Immunosorbent Assay, Herpes Simplex Virus, HSV-1	Microbiology
Enzyme-Linked Immunosorbent Assay, Herpes Simplex Virus, HSV-2	Microbiology
Equipment, Cleaning, Air	General
Hepatitis B Test (B Core, BE Antigen & Antibody, B Core IGM)	Microbiology
Legionella Direct & Indirect Fluorescent Antibody Regents	Microbiology
Microtiter Diluting/Dispensing Device	Microbiology
Multi Analyte Mixture, Calibrator	Chemistry
Pipetting And Diluting System, Automated	Chemistry
Pneumocystis Carinii	Microbiology
SGPT, Colorimetric	Chemistry

Medical Product Subsidiaries (Listed Separately)
Bio-Rad Laboratories Inc
Bio-Rad Laboratories, Inc.

BIO-RAD LABORATORIES, LIFE   800-424-6723
SCIENCE GROUP
2000 Alfred Nobel Dr., Hercules, CA 94547   **510-741-1000**
FDA Number: 2939715   Fax: 510-741-1060

BIO-RAD LABORATORIES, LIFE   800-424-6723 *(cont'd)*
Web site: www.bio-rad.com
Medical Products Sales Volume: $844,000,000
Annual Revenue: $500 Million-$1 Billion
Total Employees: 4300
Ownership: Bio-Rad Laboratories, Inc.
Stock Symbol: BIO
Traded On: AMEX
Quality System Registration Information: ISO9000; ISO9001
Produces/Sells CE-marked Devices: Y
General Admin.: David Schwartz/President
      Burton Zabin/Vice President

Accessories, Chromatography (Gas, Gel, Liquid, Thin Layer)	Chemistry
Analyzer, Amino Acid	Microbiology
Analyzer, Protein	Chemistry
Chromatographic/Fluorometric Method, Catecholamines	Chemistry
Chromatography Equipment, Ion Exchange	Toxicology
Chromatography Equipment, Liquid	Chemistry
Chromatography, Liquid, Performance, High	Toxicology
Column, Chromatography	Chemistry
Densitometer, Laboratory	Chemistry
Electrofocusing Equipment	Chemistry
Electrophoresis Equipment, Gel	Chemistry
Electrophoresis Instrumentation	Immunology
Equipment, Immunoelectrophoresis, Rocket	Immunology
Filter, Membrane	Chemistry
Fluorometric Measurement, Porphyrins	Chemistry
Gel, Filter	Chemistry
Immunodiffusion Equipment (Agar Cutter)	Chemistry
Immunofluorescence Equipment	Immunology
Injector, Sample	Chemistry
Isotachophoresis Equipment	Chemistry
Media, Supporting	Chemistry
Monitor, Biological (Contamination Testing)	General
Pipette Tip	Chemistry
Pipette, Micro	Chemistry
Radioimmunoassay, Cortisol	Chemistry
Radioimmunoassay, Digoxin (125-I), Rabbit, Charcoal	Toxicology
Radioimmunoassay, Estriol	Chemistry
Radioimmunoassay, Ferritin	Microbiology
Radioimmunoassay, Folic Acid	Chemistry
Radioimmunoassay, Follicle Stimulating Hormone	Chemistry
Radioimmunoassay, T3 Uptake	Chemistry
Radioimmunoassay, T4	Chemistry
Radioimmunoassay, Thyroid Stimulating Hormone	Chemistry
Radioimmunoassay, Total Thyroxine	Chemistry
Radioimmunoassay, Total Triiodothyronine	Chemistry
Radioimmunoassay, Vitamin B12	Chemistry
Reagent, Analyzer, Amino Acid	Microbiology
Reagent, Protein, Total	Chemistry
Recorder, Chart, Laboratory	Chemistry
Resins, Ion Exchange, Liquid Chromatography	Toxicology
Standard, Amino Acid	Chemistry
Stick, Urinalysis Test	Chemistry
Test, Thyroid Autoantibody	Immunology
Tube, Test	Chemistry

BIO-RAD, DIAGNOSTICS GROUP   800-854-6737
9500 Jeronimo Rd., Irvine, CA 92618-2017   **949-598-1200**
FDA Number: 2016706   Fax: 949-598-1552
Web site: www.bio-rad.com
Total Employees: 200   *Marketing Staff:* 10   *Sales Staff:* 70
Ownership: Bio-Rad Laboratories, Inc.
Stock Symbol: BIO.A
Traded On: AMEX
Quality System Registration Information: ISO9002
Produces/Sells CE-marked Devices: N
Distribution: Service Direct
Mktg./Adv.: Robyn Hawkins/Division Manager

Control, Cell Counter, Normal And Abnormal	Hematology
Control, Heavy Metals	Toxicology
Control, Hemoglobin	Hematology
Control, Multi Analyte, All Kinds (Assayed And Unassayed)	Chemistry
Control, Urinalysis (Assayed And Unassayed)	Chemistry
Multi-analyte Controls Unassayed	Chemistry
Packaging Equipment	General
Standard/Control, All Types	Chemistry

BIO-RAD, ECS DIVISION
See Bio-Rad, Diagnostics Group

BIO-REG ASSOCIATES, INC.   301-623-2500
11800 Baltimore Avenue, Suite 105, Beltsville, MD 20705-1561
FDA Number: n/a   Fax: 301-623-2600
E-mail: marketing@bioreg.com
Web site: www.bioreg.com
Medical Products Sales Volume: $700,000
Year Founded: 1987
Total Employees: 9
Ownership: Private
Produces/Sells CE-marked Devices: N

BIO-REG ASSOCIATES, INC.   301-623-2500 *(cont'd)*
Federal Procurement Eligibility: Small Business
Distribution: Service Direct
General Admin.: James Howard/President, Chief Executive Officer
Mktg./Adv.: Schuyler Ritter/Vice President Marketing & Sales
Service, Consulting	General
Service, Licensing, Device, Medical	General

BIO-RESEARCH ASSOCIATES, INC.   414-357-7525
9275 North 49th Street, Suite 150, Brown Deer, WI 53223
FDA Number: 2183552
Device, Jaw Tracking, For Monitoring Jaw Positions	Dental And Oral
Electrode, Cutaneous	Cns/Neurology
Electromyograph, Diagnostic	Physical Med
Monitor, Muscle, Dental	Dental And Oral
Optical Position/Movement Recording System	Physical Med
Stethoscope, Electronic (Auscultoscope)	Cardiovascular
Stimulator, Nerve, Transcutaneous (Pain Relief, TENS)	Cns/Neurology

BIO-SCIENTIFIC SPECIALTY PRODUCTS, INC.   516-868-2553
197-99 North Main St., P.o. Box 521, Freeport, NY 11520
FDA Number: 2431198
Ownership: Private
Produces/Sells CE-marked Devices: N
Buffer, pH	Hematology
Stain, Orange G	Pathology
Stain, Papanicolau	Pathology
Stain, Wright's	Pathology

BIO-SYNTHESIS, INC   800-227-0627
612 East Main St, Lewisville, TX 75057   972-420-8505
FDA Number: 3005577752   *Fax:* 972-420-0442
E-mail: biosyn@biosyn.com
Web site: www.biosyn.com
Ownership: SYNTHES GMBH
Produces/Sells CE-marked Devices: N
Reagent, General Purpose	Pathology

BIO-TECHNOLOGY USA, INC.   305-512-3522
6175 NW 167th St., Suite # G-8, Miami, FL 33015-4334
FDA Number: 1064494   *Fax:* 305-512-3521
E-mail: biotechusa@yahoo.com
Web site: www.biotechusa.net
Ownership: Private
Produces/Sells CE-marked Devices: N
Hip, Hemi-, Femoral, Metal Ball	Orthopedics
Plate, Fixation, Bone	Orthopedics
Prosthesis, Hip, Acetabular Mesh	Orthopedics
Prosthesis, Hip, Cement Restrictor	Orthopedics
Prosthesis, Hip, Femoral Component, Cemented, Metal	Orthopedics
Prosthesis, Hip, Hemi-, Femoral, Metal/Polymer	Orthopedics
Prosthesis, Hip, Semi-Const., Metal/Ceramic/Ceramic, Cem.	Orthopedics
Prosthesis, Hip, Semi-Constrained Acetabular	Orthopedics
Prosthesis, Knee, Hemi-, Tibial Resurfacing, Uncemented	Orthopedics
Prosthesis, Knee, P/F, Unconst., Uncem., Por., Ctd., P/M/P	Orthopedics
Screw, Fixation, Bone	Orthopedics
System, Appliance, Fixation, Spinal Pedicle Screw	Orthopedics

BIO-TEST MEDICAL, INC.   412-444-0933
1017 Executive Dr., Gibsonia, PA 15044
FDA Number: 2518630
Kit, Quality Control	Microbiology

BIO-TISSUE, INC.   888-296-8858
7000 S.w. 97th Ave., Ste. 211, Miami, FL 33173   305-412-0098
FDA Number: 3003415347   *Fax:* 305-412-4429
E-mail: info@biotissue.com
Web site: www.biotissue.com
Ownership: Private
Produces/Sells CE-marked Devices: N
Conformer, Ophthalmic, Biological Tissue	Ophthalmology

BIO. WORKS CORP.   208-772-5509
12611 N.Chicken Pt. Rd., Hayden, ID 83835-1388
FDA Number: n/a
Ownership: Private
Produces/Sells CE-marked Devices: N
Biofeedback Device	Cns/Neurology

BIO/CAN SCIENTIFIC INC.   800-387-8125
2170 Dunwin Dr., Unit 5,   905-828-2455
Mississauga, ONT L5L-1 Canada
FDA Number: n/a   *Fax:* 905-828-9422
E-mail: orders@biocan.com
Web site: www.biocan.com
Year Founded: 1983
Total Employees: 25
Ownership: Private
Produces/Sells CE-marked Devices: N

BIO/CAN SCIENTIFIC INC.   800-387-8125 *(cont'd)*
Distribution: Exclusive Distributor

BIO/DATA CORP.   215-441-4000
155 Gibraltar Rd., Horsham, PA 19044
FDA Number: 2517686
Aggregometer, Platelet, Thrombokinetogram	Hematology
Analyzer, Coagulation	Hematology
Analyzer, Coagulation, Multipurpose	Hematology
Control, Coagulation, Plasma	Hematology
Partial Thromboplastin Time	Hematology
Plasma, Control, Fibrinogen	Hematology
Plasma, Control, Normal	Hematology
Plasma, Deficient, Factor, Coagulation	Hematology
Prothrombin Time	Hematology
Reagent, Platelet Aggregation	Hematology
Test, Fibrinogen	Hematology
Test, Qualitative And Quantitative Factor Deficiency	Hematology
Test, Thrombin Time	Hematology
Thromboplastin, Activated Partial	Hematology
Timer, Coagulation	Hematology

BIOANALOGICS   503-626-8000
7909 SW Cirrus Drive 27, Beaverton, OR 97008
FDA Number: 3024036   *Fax:* 503-641-4031
E-mail: sales@bioanalogics.com
Web site: www.bioanalogics.com
Medical Products Sales Volume: $400,000
Annual Revenue: $1-$5 Million
Year Founded: 1990
Total Employees: 5   *Marketing Staff:* 1   *Sales Staff:* 5
Ownership: Private
Produces/Sells CE-marked Devices: N
Federal Procurement Eligibility: Small Business
Distribution: Manufacturer Direct, Manufacturer Through Distributor, Manufacturer Through Manufacturer Reps, OEM, Service Direct, Exporter
General Admin.: Mr. Richard Wooten/President
Analyzer, Composition, Weight, Patient	General

BIOBEHAVIORAL DIAGNOSTICS COMPANY   877-246-2397
239 Littleton Road, Suite 6A,   617-213-3013
Westford, MA 01886
FDA Number: 3006224965
E-mail: quotientAõÉ,™É_oadhd@biobdx.com
Web site: www.biobdx.com
Ownership: Private
Produces/Sells CE-marked Devices: N
Recorder, Attention Task Performance	Cns/Neurology

BIOCARDIA, INC.   800-624-1179
125 Shoreway Road, SuiteB,   650-226-0120
San Carlos, CA 94070
FDA Number: 3003610571   *Fax:* 650-631-3731
E-mail: info@biocardia.com
Web site: www.biocardia.com
Ownership: Private
Produces/Sells CE-marked Devices: N
Catheter, Intravascular, Diagnostic	Cardiovascular
Introducer, Catheter	Cardiovascular

BIOCARE MEDICAL, LLC   925-603-8003
4040 Pike Lane, Concord, CA 94520
FDA Number: 3004140393
Ownership: Private
Produces/Sells CE-marked Devices: N
Equipment, Laboratory, Gen. Purpose (Specific Medical Use)	Chemistry
Immunohistochemistry Reagents And Kits	Pathology
Reagent, General Purpose	Pathology
Reagents, Specific, Analyte	Hematology
Stain, Hematoxylin	Pathology
Stainer, Slide, Automated	Pathology

BIOCELL LABORATORIES, INC.   800-222-8382
2001 E. University Dr.,   310-537-3300
Rancho Dominguez, CA 90220
FDA Number: 2077563   *Fax:* 310-637-3927
E-mail: info@biocell.com
Web site: www.biocell.com
Medical Products Sales Volume: $5,000,000
Annual Revenue: $5-$10 Million
Total Employees: 40   *Marketing Staff:* 4   *Sales Staff:* 6
Ownership: Private
Quality System Registration Information: ISO9001
Produces/Sells CE-marked Devices: N
Federal Procurement Eligibility: Small Business
Distribution: Manufacturer Direct
General Admin.: Marc McKonic/President
2nd Antibody (Species Specific Anti-Animal Gamma Globulin)	Immunology
Alpha-1-Acid-Glycoprotein, Antigen, Antiserum, Control	Immunology

BIOCELL LABORATORIES, INC.
800-222-8382 *(cont'd)*

Antigen, Antiserum, Control, Albumin	Immunology
Antigen, Antiserum, Control, Albumin, Fraction V	Immunology
Antigen, Antiserum, Control, Alpha-2-Macroglobulin	Immunology
Antigen, Antiserum, Control, Complement C3	Immunology
Antigen, Antiserum, Control, Complement C4	Immunology
Antigen, Antiserum, Control, Haptoglobin	Immunology
Antigen, Antiserum, Control, IGA	Immunology
Antigen, Antiserum, Control, IGG	Immunology
Antigen, Antiserum, Control, IGM	Immunology
Antigen, Antiserum, Control, Transferrin	Immunology
Antigen, Antiserum, Control, Whole Human Serum	Immunology
Control, Analyte (Assayed And Unassayed)	Chemistry
Control, Electrolyte (Assayed And Unassayed)	Chemistry
Control, Enzyme (Assayed And Unassayed)	Chemistry
Control, Multi Analyte, All Kinds (Assayed And Unassayed)	Chemistry
Control, Urinalysis (Assayed And Unassayed)	Chemistry
Culture Media, Enriched	Microbiology
Culture Media, General Nutrient Broth	Microbiology
Culture Media, Supplements	Microbiology
Multi Analyte Mixture, Calibrator	Chemistry
Reagent, Calibration	General
Reservoir, Spinal Fluid	Cns/Neurology
Serum, Animal	Pathology
Serum, Biological, General	Toxicology
Serum, Control, Digitoxin, RIA	Toxicology
Serum, Human	Pathology
Sponge, Hemostatic, Absorbable Collagen	Surgery
Standard, Lipid	Chemistry
Whole Human Plasma, Antigen, Antiserum, Control	Immunology

BIOCHECK, INC.
650-573-1968

323 Vintage Park Drive, Foster City, CA 94404
FDA Number: 2953756 *Fax:* 650-573-1969
E-mail: info@biocheckinc.com
Web site: www.biocheckinc.com
Medical Products Sales Volume: $2,100,000
Year Founded: 1997
Total Employees: 22
Ownership: Private
Produces/Sells CE-marked Devices: Y
Federal Procurement Eligibility: Small Business
Distribution: OEM
General Admin.: Dr. John Chen/Chief Executive Officer

Antigen, Antiserum, Control, Carcinoembryonic Antigen	Immunology
Antigen, Cancer 549	Immunology
Antigen, Prostate-Specific (PSA), Management, Cancer	Immunology
Campylobacter Pylori	Microbiology
Enzymatic Method, Troponin Subunit	Chemistry
Enzyme Immunoassay, Non-Radiolabeled, Total Thyroxine	Chemistry
Enzyme Linked Immunoabsorbent Assay, Cytomegalovirus	Microbiology
Enzyme Linked Immunoabsorbent Assay, Herpes Simplex Virus	Microbiology
Enzyme Linked Immunoabsorbent Assay, Rubella	Microbiology
Enzyme Linked Immunoabsorbent Assay, Toxoplasma Gondii	Microbiology
Kit, Test, Alpha-fetoprotein For Testicular Cancer	Immunology
Radioimmunoassay, Estradiol	Chemistry
Radioimmunoassay, Ferritin	Microbiology
Radioimmunoassay, Follicle Stimulating Hormone	Chemistry
Radioimmunoassay, Human Chorionic Gonadotropin	Chemistry
Radioimmunoassay, Human Growth Hormone	Chemistry
Radioimmunoassay, Immunoglobulins (D, E)	Immunology
Radioimmunoassay, Luteinizing Hormone	Chemistry
Radioimmunoassay, Progesterone	Chemistry
Radioimmunoassay, Prolactin (Lactogen)	Chemistry
Radioimmunoassay, Testosterones And Dihydrotestosterone	Chemistry
Radioimmunoassay, Thyroid Stimulating Hormone	Chemistry
Radioimmunoassay, Total Triiodothyronine	Chemistry
Test, Antigen (CA125), Tumor-Associated, Ovarian, Epithelial	Immunology
Test, Beta 2 - Microglobulin	Immunology
Test, C-Reactive Protein	Immunology

BIOCHEM INTERNATIONAL
See Smiths Medical Pm, Inc.

BIOCHEMICAL DIAGNOSTICS, INC.
800-223-4835
631-595-9200

180 Heartland Blvd., Edgewood, NY 11717-8314
FDA Number: 2432495
E-mail: support@biochemicaldiagnostics.com *Fax:* 631-595-9204
Web site: www.biochemicaldiagnostics.com
Medical Products Sales Volume: $2,200,000
Year Founded: 1981
Total Employees: 25 *Marketing Staff:* 3 *Sales Staff:* 3
Ownership: Private
Produces/Sells CE-marked Devices: Y
Federal Procurement Eligibility: Small Business
Distribution: Manufacturer Direct, Importer, Exporter
General Admin.: Allen Panetz/President, Chief Executive Officer
Mktg./Adv.: Allen Panetz/Manager Advertising
 Ms. Colleen Gang/Project Manager
Production: Amir Faroogi/Vice President Manufacturing
Research: Amir Faroogi/Vice President Research & Development

BIOCHEMICAL DIAGNOSTICS, INC.
800-223-4835 *(cont'd)*

Calibrator, Drug Specific	Toxicology
Column, Chromatography	Chemistry
Diazo, P-Nitroaniline/Vanillin, Vanilmandelic Acid	Chemistry
Reagent, Quality Control	General
Standard/Control, All Types	Chemistry
System, Test, Drugs of Abuse	Chemistry
Test, Tetrahydrocannabinol	Toxicology

BIOCHEMICAL LABORATORIES INC.
See Spectrum Laboratory Products, Inc.

BIOCISION LLC
888-478-2221

12 East Sir Francis Drake Blvd., Suite B, Lakespur, CA 94939
FDA Number: n/a *Fax:* 415-634-2350
E-mail: info@biocision.com
Ownership: Private
Produces/Sells CE-marked Devices: N

BIOCIUS LIFE SCIENCES INC.
781-928-2700

11 Audubon Road, Wakefield, MA 01880
FDA Number: n/a *Fax:* 781-998-0054
E-mail: info@BIOCIUS.com
Web site: http://www.biocius.com
Ownership: Private
Produces/Sells CE-marked Devices: N
General Admin.: Mr. Jeffrey Leathe/Chairman, Chief Executive Officer
 Dr. Can Ozbal/Chief Operating Officer
Mktg./Adv.: Ms. Jennifer Rossi/Director Marketing & Communications
 Dr. Selena Larkin/Vice President International Sales
Research: Mr. Arrin Katz/Vice President Engineering
 Mr. Donald Green/Vice President Product Development
Finance: Mr. Gary St. Pierre/Chief Financial Officer

BIOCLINICA, INC.
800-748-9032
267-757-3000

826 Newtown-Yardley Rd., Ste. 101, Newtown, PA 18940
FDA Number: n/a *Fax:* 267-757-3010
E-mail: general@bioclininca.com
Web site: www.bioclinica.com
Annual Revenue: $500 Million-$1 Billion
Ownership: Public
Stock Symbol: BIOC
Traded On: NASDAQ
Produces/Sells CE-marked Devices: N
Federal Procurement Eligibility: Small Business
Distribution: Service Direct
General Admin.: Mr. Ted Kaminer/Chief Financial Officer, Senior Vice President
 Mark L. Weinstein/President, Chief Executive Officer
Mktg./Adv.: Colin Miller/Senior Vice President Business Development
Production: David Pitler/Senior Vice President Operations

Computer Software	General

BIOCLINICAL GROUP
See Advanced Magnetics, Inc.

BIOCOAT, INC.
215-734-0888

211 Witmer Road, Horsham, PA 19044
FDA Number: 3004462529 *Fax:* 215-734-0889
E-mail: info@biocoat.com
Web site: www.biocoat.com
Medical Products Sales Volume: $800,000
Annual Revenue: $1-$5 Million
Year Founded: 1991
Total Employees: 7
Ownership: Private
Produces/Sells CE-marked Devices: N
Federal Procurement Eligibility: Small Business
Distribution: Manufacturer Direct, Manufacturer Through Distributor, OEM
General Admin.: Ellington M. Beavers/Chairman
 Djoerd Hoekstra/President, Chief Executive Officer

Device, Semen Analysis	Obstetrics/Gynecology
Labware, Assisted Reproduction	Obstetrics/Gynecology
Media, Reproductive	Obstetrics/Gynecology

BIOCOLD ENVIRONMENTAL
636-349-0300

239 Seebold Spur, Fenton, MO 63026
FDA Number: n/a *Fax:* 636-349-0419
E-mail: biocold@aol.com
Web site: www.biocoldenvironmental.com
Annual Revenue: $1-$5 Million
Total Employees: 12 *Marketing Staff:* 2 *Sales Staff:* 2
Ownership: Private
Produces/Sells CE-marked Devices: N
Federal Procurement Eligibility: Small Business
Distribution: Manufacturer Direct, Manufacturer Through Distributor, OEM
General Admin.: John Herdlein/President

Chamber, Constant Temperature (Environmental)	Microbiology

BIOCOLD ENVIRONMENTAL   **636-349-0300** *(cont'd)*
Refrigerator, Biological   Microbiology

BIOCOM INC.
See U.F.I.

BIOCOMP RESEARCH INSTITUTE
See The Biofeedback Institute Of Los Angeles

BIOCOMP RESEARCH INSTITUTE   **800-246-3526**
    6542 Hayes Dr., Los Angeles, CA 90048   **323-930-8500**
FDA Number: 9200126   *Fax:* 323-930-8505
E-mail: info@biocomp.mpowermail.com
Web site: www.biocompresearch.org
Medical Products Sales Volume: $500,000
Annual Revenue: $0-$1 Million
Year Founded: 1972
Total Employees: 5   *Marketing Staff:* 1   *Sales Staff:* 2
Ownership: Private
Produces/Sells CE-marked Devices: N
Federal Procurement Eligibility: Small Business, Female Owned
Distribution: Manufacturer Direct
General Admin.: Hershel Toomim/President, Chief Executive Officer
Mktg./Adv.: Robert Marsh/Director Marketing
       Hershel Toomim/Director Product Development
   Biofeedback Device   Cns/Neurology
   Biofeedback Equipment, Myoelectric, Powered   Physical Med
   Computer Equipment   General
   Computer Software   General

BIOCOMPATIBLES INC.   **877-783-5463**
    115 Hurley Road, Bldg. 3, Oxford, CT 06478   **203-262-4190**
FDA Number: 1225114   *Fax:* 800-789-0897
E-mail: marketing@biocompatibles.com
Web site: www.biocompatibles.com
Medical Products Sales Volume: $6,000,000
Year Founded: 1996
Total Employees: 30
Ownership: Private
Quality System Registration Information: ISO9001
Produces/Sells CE-marked Devices: Y
Federal Procurement Eligibility: Small Business
General Admin.: Gary Lamoureux/Chief Executive Officer
Mktg./Adv.: Mr. Charlie Jacobs/Manager Business Development
       Dave Hart/Manager National Sales
   Chamber, Decompression, Abdominal   Obstetrics/Gynecology
   Kit, Anesthesia, Conduction   Anesthesiology
   Kit, Biopsy Needle   Gastroenterology/Urology
   Kit, Collection/Transfusion, Marrow, Bone   General
   Ligator, Hemorrhoidal   Gastroenterology/Urology
   Needle, Aspiration And Injection, Disposable   Surgery
   Needle, Gastro-Urology   Gastroenterology/Urology
   Needle, Spinal, Short-Term   General
   Radiographic Unit, Diagnostic, Mammographic   Radiology
   Syringe, Piston   General
   Trocar, Cardiovascular   Cardiovascular

BIOCOMPOSITES INC.   **910-350-8015**
    PO Box 2692, Wilmington, NC 28402
FDA Number: 1065982   *Fax:* 910-350-8072
Web site: www.biocomposites.com
Ownership: Private
Produces/Sells CE-marked Devices: N

BIOCONTROL MEDICAL   **877-494-8770**
    9220 Bass Lake Road, Suite 255,
    New Hope, MN 55427   -
FDA Number: n/a   *Fax:* 763-450-6803
E-mail: info@biocontrol-medical.com
Web site: www.biocontrol-medical.com
Ownership: Private
Produces/Sells CE-marked Devices: N
General Admin.: Mr. Ehud Cohen/Chief Executive Officer
       Mr. Shai Ayal/Chief Technology Officer
Medical Admin.: Mr. Paul Hauptmann/Medical Director
Research: Ms. Susan Peterson-Stejskal/Vice President Clinical Research
Finance: Mr. Offer Erlichmann/Vice President Finance

BIOCORE MEDICAL TECHNOLOGIES, INC.   **301-740-1893**
    13851 90th Street, Oskaloosa, KS 66066
FDA Number: 3003545239
   Bandage, Liquid   Surgery

BIOCRYST PHARMACEUTICALS, INC.   **205-444-4600**
    2190 Parkway Lake Dr., Birmingham, AL 35244
FDA Number: n/a   *Fax:* 205-444-4640
E-mail: info@biocryst.com
Web site: www.biocryst.com
Annual Revenue: $50-$100 Million
Total Employees: 80

BIOCRYST PHARMACEUTICALS, INC.   **205-444-4600** *(cont'd)*
Ownership: Public
Stock Symbol: BCRX
Traded On: NASDAQ
Produces/Sells CE-marked Devices: N
General Admin.: Stuart Grant/Chief Financial Officer, Senior Vice President
       Jon P. Stonehouse/President, Chief Executive Officer
   Contract R&D, Diagnostics   General

BIOCURE, INC.   **800-246-2873**
    2975 Gateway Drive, Suite 100,   **678-966-3400**
    Norcross, GA 30071
FDA Number: 1067143   *Fax:* 770-416-4331
E-mail: information@biocure.com
Web site: www.biocure.com
Ownership: Private
Produces/Sells CE-marked Devices: N
Production: Sameer Shums/Project Director
   Device, Embolization, Artificial   Cns/Neurology
   Embolization Device   Cardiovascular

BIOCURV MEDICAL INSTRUMENTS, INC.   **1-800-589-3043**
    245 Dryden CT SW, Canton, OH 44706   **330-451-1628**
FDA Number: 3003496855   *Fax:* 330-451-1628
E-mail: info@tonguesweeper.com
Web site: www.tonguesweeper.com
Ownership: Private
Produces/Sells CE-marked Devices: N
Federal Procurement Eligibility: Small Business
Distribution: Manufacturer Direct, Manufacturer Through Distributor
   Scraper, Tongue   Dental And Oral

BIODECISION LABORATORIES
See Novum Inc.

BIODECISION, INC.
See Novum Inc.

BIODERM, INC.   **800-373-7006**
    12320 73rd Court North, Largo, FL 33773   **727-507-7655**
FDA Number: 1063299   *Fax:* 727-507-7645
E-mail: customerservice@bioderm-inc.com
Web site: www.bioderm-inc.com
Medical Products Sales Volume: $670,000
Year Founded: 1990
Total Employees: 8
Ownership: Private
Produces/Sells CE-marked Devices: N
Federal Procurement Eligibility: Small Business, GSA Contract
   Accessories, Catheter   Surgery
   Appliance, Incontinence, Urosheath Type   Gastroenterology/Urology
   Device, Incontinence, Paste-On   Gastroenterology/Urology
   Drainage System, Urine, Closed   Gastroenterology/Urology

BIODERMIS CORP.   **800-322-3729**
    1820 Whitney Mesa Dr., Henderson, NV 89014   **702-260-4466**
FDA Number: 2950792
Ownership: Private
Produces/Sells CE-marked Devices: N
   Elastomer, Silicone (Scar Management)   Surgery

BIODERMIS CORP.   **800-322-3729**
    6000 South Eastern, Suite 9-D,   **702-260-4466**
    Las Vegas, NV 89119
FDA Number: 2950792
E-mail: biodermis@biodermis.com
Web site: www.biodermis.com
Annual Revenue: $1-$5 Million
Year Founded: 1985
Ownership: Private
Quality System Registration Information: ISO9001
Produces/Sells CE-marked Devices: Y
Federal Procurement Eligibility: Small Business
Distribution: Manufacturer Direct, Manufacturer Through Distributor, Manufacturer
   Through Manufacturer Reps, OEM, Exclusive Distributor, Exporter
   Compression Instrument   Orthopedics
   Elastomer, Silicone (Scar Management)   Surgery

BIODESIGN INTERNATIONAL
See Meridian Life Science, Inc.

BIODESIX INC   **303-417-0500**
    520 Zang Street, Suite 213, Broomfield, CO 80021
FDA Number: n/a   *Fax:* 303-417-9700
Web site: www.Biodesix.com
Ownership: Private
Produces/Sells CE-marked Devices: N
General Admin.: Mr. David Brunel/Chief Executive Officer
       Mr. Heinrich Roder/Chief Technology Officer
Mktg./Adv.: Mr. Paul Beresford/Vice President Business Development

MANUFACTURER PROFILES

BIODESIX INC 303-417-0500 *(cont'd)*
Mr. Doug Swan/Vice President Commercial Operations
Production: Mr. Jeffery Bojar/Vice President Regulatory Affairs
Finance: Mr. Frank Ronchetti/Chief Financial Officer

BIODEX CORP.
See Biodex Medical Systems, Inc.

BIODEX MEDICAL SYSTEMS, INC. 800-224-6339
20 Ramsay Road, Shirley, NY 11967-4704 631-924-9000
FDA Number: 2431314 *Fax:* 631-924-8355
E-mail: info@biodex.com
Web site: www.biodex.com
Medical Products Sales Volume: $18,300,000
Annual Revenue: $25-$50 Million
Year Founded: 1949
Total Employees: 200
Ownership: Private
Quality System Registration Information: ISO9001
Produces/Sells CE-marked Devices: Y
Federal Procurement Eligibility: Small Business, GSA Contract
Distribution: Manufacturer Direct, Manufacturer Through Manufacturer Reps, OEM, Service Direct
General Admin.: James Reiss/Chief Executive Officer
Mktg./Adv.: Lila Corwin/Director Corporate Marketing
 Adel Holl/Director International Sales
 Robert Ranieri/Vice President Sales
Production: Clyde Schlein/Manager Regulatory Affairs

Analyzer, Motion	General
Calibrator Source, Nuclear Sealed	Radiology
Calibrator, Dose, Radionuclide	Radiology
Chair, Blood Drawing	General
Counter, Gamma, General Use	Toxicology
Detector, Beta/Gamma	Chemistry
Dosimeter, Radiation	Radiology
Exerciser, Measuring	Physical Med
Holder, Syringe, Leaded	Radiology
Hood, Fume	Toxicology
Isokinetic Testing And Evaluation System	Physical Med
Monitor, Radiation	Radiology
Nebulizer, Direct Patient Interface	Anesthesiology
Phantom, Anthropomorphic, Nuclear	Radiology
Phantom, Flood Source, Nuclear	Radiology
Platform, Force-Measuring	Physical Med
Probe, Uptake, Nuclear	Radiology
Rebreathing System, Radionuclide	Radiology
Safe, Radionuclide	Radiology
Shield, Protective, Personnel	Radiology
Shield, Vial	Radiology
Shield, X-Ray	Radiology
Sign, Hospital	General
Station Pipetting	Chemistry
Stretcher, Wheeled (Mobile)	General
Table, Other	General
Table, Radiographic, Tilting	Radiology
Table, Urological, Non-Electrical	Gastroenterology/Urology
Treadmill, Powered	Physical Med

BIODRAIN MEDICAL, INC. 651-389-4800
2060 Centre Pointe Blvd, Suite 7, Mendota Heights, MN 55120
FDA Number: 3006369524 *Fax:* 651-379-5024
E-mail: info@biodrainmedical.com
Web site: http://www.biodrainmedical.com/
Ownership: Private
Produces/Sells CE-marked Devices: N
General Admin.: Mr. Kevin Davidson/Chief Executive Officer, Chief Financial Officer
 Mr. Chad Ruwe/Chief Operating Officer
Mktg./Adv.: Mr. David Dauwalter/Director Product Management
 Ms. Kristen Doerfert/Vice President Marketing & Sales

Suction Apparatus, Operating Room, Wall Vacuum-Powered	Surgery

BIODX
See Scimedx Corporation

BIODX
See Mardx Diagnostics, Inc.

BIODYNAMICS CORP. 206-526-0205
4554 9th Avenue Ne, #100, Seattle, WA 98105
FDA Number: 3023856

Meter, Conductivity, Non-Remote	Gastroenterology/Urology

BIOFEEDBACK INSTRUMENT CORP. 212-222-5665
255 W. 98th St., Suite 3D, New York, NY 10025-5575
FDA Number: n/a *Fax:* 212-222-5667
E-mail: brotmanp@verizon.net
Web site: www.biof.com
Medical Products Sales Volume: $1,000,000
Annual Revenue: $0-$1 Million
Year Founded: 1972

BIOFEEDBACK INSTRUMENT CORP. 212-222-5665 *(cont'd)*
Total Employees: 10 *Marketing Staff:* 5 *Sales Staff:* 5
Ownership: Private
Produces/Sells CE-marked Devices: Y
Federal Procurement Eligibility: Small Business
Distribution: Manufacturer Through Distributor
General Admin.: Dr. Philip Brotman/President

Biofeedback Device	Cns/Neurology
Biofeedback Equipment, Myoelectric, Battery-Powered	Physical Med
Computer Equipment	General
Computer, Brain Mapping	Cns/Neurology
Computer, Patient Data Management	General
Myograph	Physical Med
Stimulator, Nerve, Transcutaneous (Pain Relief, TENS)	Cns/Neurology

BIOFEEDBACK RESEARCH INSTITUTE
See Biocomp Research Institute

BIOFILM, INC. 800-848-5900
3225 Executive Ridge, Vista, CA 92081
FDA Number: 2025771
E-mail: customer.service@biofilm.com
Web site: www.astroglide.com
Annual Revenue: $5-$10 Million
Year Founded: 1991
Ownership: Private
Quality System Registration Information: ISO9000
Produces/Sells CE-marked Devices: Y
Distribution: Manufacturer Direct, Manufacturer Through Manufacturer Reps, Exporter

Condom	Obstetrics/Gynecology
Lubricant, Patient	General
Lubricant, Vaginal, Patient	General

BIOFIT ENGINEERED PRODUCTS 800-597-0246
PO Box 109, Waterville, OH 43566-0109 419-823-1089
FDA Number: 9200033 *Fax:* 419-823-1342
E-mail: biofit@biofit.com
Web site: www.biofit.com
Annual Revenue: $10-$25 Million
Year Founded: 1993
Total Employees: 105 *Marketing Staff:* 2 *Sales Staff:* 25
Ownership: Private
Produces/Sells CE-marked Devices: N
Federal Procurement Eligibility: Small Business, GSA Contract, VA Contract
Distribution: Manufacturer Through Distributor, Manufacturer Through Manufacturer Reps, Exporter
General Admin.: Dale E. Barnard/President
Mktg./Adv.: Max Church/Manager National Sales
 Edward A. Metzger/Vice President Sales
Production: Randy Baldwin/Manager Production

Chair, Adjustable, Mechanical	Physical Med
Chair, Surgical, Non-Electrical	Surgery
Stool, Anesthetist's	Anesthesiology
Stool, Operating Room, Adjustable	Surgery

BIOFLEX MEDICAL MAGNETICS, INC. 800-619-2717
3370 N.E. Fifth Ave., Oakland Park, FL 33334 954-565-8500
FDA Number: 1063920 *Fax:* 954-568-6117
E-mail: info@bioflexmagnets.com
Web site: www.bioflexmagnets.com
Year Founded: 1986
Ownership: Private
Quality System Registration Information: ISO9000; ISO9001; ISO9002; ISO9003
Produces/Sells CE-marked Devices: Y
Federal Procurement Eligibility: Small Business
Distribution: Manufacturer Direct, Manufacturer Through Distributor, Manufacturer Through Manufacturer Reps, OEM, Importer, Exporter

Accessories, Wheelchair	Physical Med
Brace, Joint, Ankle (External)	Physical Med
Component, Exercise	Physical Med
Mattress, Non-Powered Flotation Therapy	Physical Med
Orthosis, Cervical	Physical Med
Orthosis, Corrective Shoe	Physical Med
Orthosis, Limb Brace	Physical Med
Orthosis, Lumbar	Physical Med

BIOFLEX, INC. 614-236-8079
3055 Templeton Rd., Columbus, OH 43209
FDA Number: 1529049
Ownership: Private
Produces/Sells CE-marked Devices: N

Electrode, Cutaneous	Cns/Neurology

BIOFOCUS INCORPORATED 877-864-2329
P.O. Box 25182, Halifax, NS B3M-4H4 Canada 902-864-2329
FDA Number: n/a *Fax:* 902-864-7679
E-mail: chalker@istar.ca
Year Founded: 1997

BIOFOCUS INCORPORATED 877-864-2329 (cont'd)
Ownership: Private
Produces/Sells CE-marked Devices: N
Distribution: Exclusive Distributor

BIOFORM MEDICAL, INC. 262-835-3323
4133 Courtney Road, #10, Franksville, WI 53126
FDA Number: 2135225
Ownership: Public
Stock Symbol: BFRM
Traded On: NASDAQ
Produces/Sells CE-marked Devices: N

Agent, Bulking, Injectable (Gastro-Urology)	Gastroenterology/Urology
Implant, Endosseous (Bone Filling and/or Augmentation)	Dental And Oral
Marker, Radiographic, Implantable	Surgery
Needle, Aspiration And Injection, Disposable	Surgery
Needle, Catheter	Surgery
Prosthesis, Laryngeal (Taub)	Ear/Nose/Throat
System, Vocal Cord Medialization	Ear/Nose/Throat

BIOFREEZE PERFORMANCE HEALTH, INC. 800-246-3733
1245 Home Ave, Akron, OH 44310 330-633-8460
FDA Number: n/a Fax: 330-634-2193
E-mail: web@biofreeze.com
Web site: www.biofreeze.com
Annual Revenue: $10-$25 Million
Year Founded: 1991
Total Employees: 70 Marketing Staff: 6 Sales Staff: 11
Ownership: Private
Produces/Sells CE-marked Devices: Y
Federal Procurement Eligibility: Small Business
Distribution: Manufacturer Through Distributor, Manufacturer Through
Manufacturer Reps, Exclusive Distributor, Exporter
Mktg./Adv.: Mr. Michael Park/Manager International Sales
　　　Mr. Craig M. Cox/Vice President Business Development
　　　Mr. Craig M. Cox/Vice President International Sales
　　　Mr. Perry A. Isenberg/Vice President Marketing
　　　Mr. Bob Poirier/Vice President Sales

Equipment, Management, Pain, Radiofrequency, Non-Invasive	General
Gel, Ultrasonic Coupling	Physical Med
Stimulator, Electro-Analgesic	Cns/Neurology

BIOGENEX LABORATORIES 800-421-4149
4600 Norris Canyon Road, 925-275-0550
San Ramon, CA 94583
FDA Number: 2936532 Fax: 925-275-0580
E-mail: info@biogenex.com
Web site: www.biogenex.com
Medical Products Sales Volume: $15,500,000
Annual Revenue: $10-$25 Million
Year Founded: 1981
Total Employees: 120 Marketing Staff: 6 Sales Staff: 25
Ownership: Private
Quality System Registration Information: ISO9001
Produces/Sells CE-marked Devices: Y
Federal Procurement Eligibility: Small Business, Minority Owned, Female Owned,
GSA Contract
Distribution: Manufacturer Direct, Manufacturer Through Distributor, Exporter
General Admin.: Dr. Krishan Kalra/President, Chief Executive Officer

Antibody, Monoclonal	Microbiology
Antibody, Polyclonal	Microbiology
Antigen, Antiserum, Control, IGG	Immunology
Equipment, Laboratory, Gen. Purpose (Specific Medical Use)	Chemistry
Stain, Chemical Solution	Pathology
Test, Cancer Detection, Monoclonal Antibody	Immunology
Test, DNA-Probe, Other	Microbiology

BIOGENIC DENTAL CORP. 800-367-3322
282-284 Genesee St., P.O. Box 4119, Utica, NY 13504-4119
FDA Number: n/a
Web site: www.biogenicdental.com
Annual Revenue: $0-$1 Million
Year Founded: 1906
Ownership: Private
Produces/Sells CE-marked Devices: N
Distribution: Manufacturer Direct
General Admin.: Paul Giovannone/President, Chief Executive Officer

Prosthesis, Dental	Dental And Oral

BIOGRIP, INC. 888-590-4747
P.O. Box 1375, Rancho Cordova, CA 95741 916-483-2686
FDA Number: 2954956 Fax: 916-483-1654
E-mail: support2009@biogrip.com
Web site: www.biogrip.com
Ownership: Private
Produces/Sells CE-marked Devices: N

Transfer Aid	Physical Med

BIOHIT INC. 800-922-0784
3535 Rte. 66, Bldg. 4, PO Box 308,, 732-922-4900
Neptune, NJ 07754
FDA Number: 9201117 Fax: 732-922-0557
E-mail: pipet@biohit.com
Web site: www.biohit.com
Annual Revenue: $1-$5 Million
Year Founded: 1988
Total Employees: 50 Marketing Staff: 2 Sales Staff: 5
Ownership: Biohit Oyj
Traded On: Helsinki
Quality System Registration Information: ISO9001
Produces/Sells CE-marked Devices: Y
Federal Procurement Eligibility: Small Business, GSA Contract
Distribution: Manufacturer Through Distributor, Manufacturer Through
Manufacturer Reps, Exclusive Distributor, Importer
General Admin.: Robert Gearty/Director
　　　Mr. Jussi HeiniA/President, Chief Executive Officer
Finance: Ms. Tiina Hankonen/Vice President Finance

Equipment, Bank, Blood, Cryogenic (Liquid Nitrogen)	Hematology
Labware, Basic, Disposable	Chemistry
Loop, Inoculating	Microbiology
Pipette, Diluting	Hematology
Pipetter	Hematology
Vial, Other	General

BIOHORIZONS IMPLANT SYSTEMS, INC. 888.246.8338
2300 Riverchase Center, Birmingham, AL 35244 205-967-7880
FDA Number: 1060818 Fax: 205-870-0304
E-mail: customercare@biohorizons.com
Web site: www.biohorizons.com
Annual Revenue: $100-$500 Million
Year Founded: 1994
Total Employees: 1000 Sales Staff: 60
Ownership: Private
Produces/Sells CE-marked Devices: N
General Admin.: R. Steven Boggan/President, Chief Executive Officer

Abutment, Implant, Dental, Endosseous	Dental And Oral
Crown, Preformed	Dental And Oral
Drill, Dental, Intraoral	Dental And Oral
Implant, Endosseous	Dental And Oral
Screw, Fixation, Intraosseous	Dental And Oral

BIOIMPLANT - CANADA
See St. Jude Medical, Inc.

BIOJECT MEDICAL TECHNOLOGIES, INC. 800-683-7221
20245 SW 95th Avenue, Tualatin, OR 97062 503-692-8001
FDA Number: 3023012 Fax: 503-692-6698
E-mail: cfarrell@bioject.com
Web site: www.bioject.com
Medical Products Sales Volume: $12,000,000
Annual Revenue: $10-$25 Million
Year Founded: 1985
Total Employees: 50 Sales Staff: 3
Ownership: Bioject Medical Technologies, Inc.
Stock Symbol: BJCT
Traded On: NASDAQ
Produces/Sells CE-marked Devices: Y
Distribution: Manufacturer Direct
General Admin.: Dr. Richard Stout/Chief Medical Officer, Vice President
　　　Mr. Mark Logomasini/President, Chief Executive Officer
Finance: Chris Farrell/Vice President Admin., Finance

Injector, Fluid, Non-Electric	General
Injector, Insulin	Gastroenterology/Urology
Injector, Jet, Gas-Powered	Dental And Oral
Injector, Jet, Mechanical-Powered	Dental And Oral

Medical Product Subsidiaries (Listed Separately)
Bioject Medical Technologies, Inc.

BIOKINETIC PROSTHETICS INC. 506-455-5462
45 Bromley Ave., Hanwell, NB E3C-1M8 Canada
FDA Number: n/a Fax: 506-455-5462
E-mail: jbush@nbnet.nb.ca
Year Founded: 1997
Total Employees: 10
Ownership: Private
Produces/Sells CE-marked Devices: N
Distribution: Manufacturer Direct, Exclusive Distributor

BIOKINETIX CORP. 203-327-7893
33 Parker Ave., Stamford, CT 06906
FDA Number: 1250016 Fax: 203-975-0949
Ownership: Private
Produces/Sells CE-marked Devices: N

Analyzer, Chemistry, Micro	Chemistry

MANUFACTURER PROFILES

BIOKIT USA, INC.   **800-926-3353**
180 Hartwell Ave., Bedford, MA 02421   **781-861-0710**
FDA Number: 9006551   *Fax:* 781-861-1908
E-mail: biokitusa@biokitusa.com
Web site: www.ilus.com
Medical Products Sales Volume: $5,000,000
Annual Revenue: $1-$5 Million
Year Founded: 1975
Total Employees: 10   *Marketing Staff:* 2   *Sales Staff:* 5
Ownership: Biokit, S.A.
Quality System Registration Information: ISO9001
Produces/Sells CE-marked Devices: N
Federal Procurement Eligibility: Small Business
Distribution: Manufacturer Through Distributor
General Admin.: Fred Russo/General Manager
   Assay, Agglutination, Latex, Rubella   Microbiology
   Reagent, Other   General

BIOLAB EQUIPMENT CANADA LIMITED   **800-268-5035**
505 Iroquois Shore Rd., Unit 14,   **(905) 639-7025**
Oakville, ONT L6H-2 Canada
FDA Number: n/a   *Fax:* 905-639-0425
E-mail: water@biolab.ca
Web site: www.biolab.ca
Year Founded: 1969
Total Employees: 50
Ownership: Private
Produces/Sells CE-marked Devices: N
Distribution: Manufacturer Direct, Service Direct

BIOLASE TECHNOLOGY, INC.   **888-424-6527**
4 Cromwell, Irvine, CA 92618   **949-361-1200**
FDA Number: 2027755   *Fax:* 949-366-3325
Web site: www.biolase.com
Annual Revenue: $50-$100 Million
Year Founded: 1986
Total Employees: 216
Ownership: Public
Stock Symbol: BLTI
Traded On: NASDAQ
Produces/Sells CE-marked Devices: Y
Federal Procurement Eligibility: Small Business
Distribution: Manufacturer Direct, Manufacturer Through Distributor
General Admin.: Jake St. Philip/Chief Executive Officer
     Federico Pignatelli/President
Mktg./Adv.: Keith G. Bateman/Vice President International Marketing & Sales
Research: Dmitri Boutoussov/Vice President Engineering
     Ioana Rizoiu/Vice President Research & Development
Finance: David Mulder/Chief Financial Officer
   Broach, Endodontic   Dental And Oral
   Curette, Endodontic   Dental And Oral
   Drill, Bone, Powered   Dental And Oral
   Endodontic Instrument   Dental And Oral
   Kit, Endodontic   Dental And Oral
   Lamp, Infrared   Physical Med
   Laser, Dental   Dental And Oral
   Laser, Surgical   Surgery
   Syringe, Periodontic, Endodontic   Dental And Oral

BIOLECTRON, INC.   **800-524-0677**
25 Commerce Drive, Allendale, NJ 07401   **201-760-6400**
FDA Number: n/a   *Fax:* 201-760-6441
Web site: www.biolectron.com
Medical Products Sales Volume: $400,000,000
Annual Revenue: $10-$25 Million
Year Founded: 1988
Total Employees: 35
Ownership: Private
Produces/Sells CE-marked Devices: N
Federal Procurement Eligibility: Small Business, Minority Owned, VA Contract
Distribution: Manufacturer Direct, Manufacturer Through Distributor, Manufacturer Through Manufacturer Reps
General Admin.: Jay Penchina/Chief Financial Officer, Controller
     Gary Grenter/President, Chief Executive Officer
Mktg./Adv.: Cindy Schawe/Vice President Marketing
     J. Chris McAuliffe/Vice President Sales
Production: Steven Powell/Director Operations
     Thomas Denaro/Director Quality Assurance
Research: Stephen Zlock/Director Research & Development
   Drill, Bone   Orthopedics
   Stimulator, Osteogenesis, Electric, Non-Invasive   Orthopedics

BIOLIFE SOLUTIONS, INC.   **607-687-4487**
171 Front Street, Owego, NY 13827-1520
FDA Number: n/a   *Fax:* 607-687-6683
E-mail: info@BioLifeSolutions.com
Web site: www.BiolifeSolutions.com

BIOLIFE SOLUTIONS, INC.   **607-687-4487** *(cont'd)*
Ownership: Public
Stock Symbol: BLFS
Traded On: OTC Bulletin
Produces/Sells CE-marked Devices: N
Federal Procurement Eligibility: Small Business
Distribution: Manufacturer Direct
   Media, Culture, Ex Vivo, Tissue And Cell   Gastroenterology/Urology

BIOLIFE, LLC   **800-722-7559**
8163 25th Court East, Sarasota, FL 34243-3271   **941-360-1300**
FDA Number: 1066421   *Fax:* 800-204-1115
E-mail: customer.care@biolife.com
Web site: www.biolife.com
Ownership: Private
Produces/Sells CE-marked Devices: N
General Admin.: Mr. Douglas R. Goodman/President, Chief Executive Officer
   Dressing, Wound, Hydrophilic   Surgery

BIOLITEC, INC.   **800-934-2377**
515 Shaker Road, East Longmeadow, MA 01028   **413-525-0600**
FDA Number: 1222625   *Fax:* 413-525-0611
E-mail: info@biolitec.com
Web site: www.biolitec.com
Medical Products Sales Volume: $3,500,000
Annual Revenue: $10-$25 Million
Year Founded: 1986
Total Employees: 50   *Marketing Staff:* 5   *Sales Staff:* 15
Ownership: Private
Stock Symbol: BIB
Traded On: Frankfurt
Quality System Registration Information: ISO9001
Produces/Sells CE-marked Devices: Y
Federal Procurement Eligibility: Small Business
Distribution: Manufacturer Direct, Manufacturer Through Distributor, Manufacturer Through Manufacturer Reps, OEM
General Admin.: Dr. Wolfgang Neuberger/President, Chief Executive Officer
Production: Brian Foley/Vice President Operations
   Accessories, Laser   General
   Cable, Fiberoptic   General
   Cable, Laser, Fiberoptic   Surgery
   Contract Manufacturing   General
   Contract Manufacturing, Product, Disposable   General
   Laser, Combination   General
   Laser, Ophthalmic   Ophthalmology
   Laser, Surgical   Surgery

BIOLOG, INC.   **800-284-4949**
21124 Cabot Blvd., Hayward, CA 94545-1130   **510-785-2564**
FDA Number: 2919175   *Fax:* 510-782-4639
E-mail: info@biolog.com
Web site: www.biolog.com
Medical Products Sales Volume: $3,600,000
Year Founded: 1984
Total Employees: 40   *Marketing Staff:* 3   *Sales Staff:* 9
Ownership: Private
Produces/Sells CE-marked Devices: Y
Federal Procurement Eligibility: Small Business
Distribution: Manufacturer Direct, Manufacturer Through Manufacturer Reps
General Admin.: Barry Bochner/Chief Scientific Officer
     Timothy P. Mullane/President, Chief Executive Officer
Production: Barbara So/Manager Quality Assurance
     Douglas Rife/Vice President Manufacturing
   Chromatographic Bacterial Identification   Microbiology
   Kit, Identification, Yeast   Microbiology
   Meter, Bacterial Culture Growth   Microbiology
   Microplate   General
   Reader, Microplate   General
   Reagent, Other   General
   Test, Bacteria Characterization   General
   Test, Bacterial Diagnostic   Microbiology

BIOLOGICAL CONTROLS INC.   **800-224-9768**
749 Hope Road, Suite A,   **732-389-8922**
Eatontown, NJ 07724
FDA Number: 2247700   *Fax:* 732-389-8821
E-mail: sales@biologicalcontrols.com
Web site: www.biologicalcontrols.com
Annual Revenue: $1-$5 Million
Year Founded: 1973
Total Employees: 8   *Sales Staff:* 1
Ownership: Private
Produces/Sells CE-marked Devices: N
Federal Procurement Eligibility: Small Business, GSA Contract
Distribution: Manufacturer Direct, Manufacturer Through Manufacturer Reps
   Equipment, Cleaning, Air   General

BIOLOGICAL CORP. OF AMERICA
See Biomerieux Inc.

BIOLOGICAL SIGNAL PROCESSING INC.
See BSP Ltd.

BIOLOGOS, INC.   800-246-4088
2235 Cornell Avenue, Montgomery, IL 60538   **630-801-4740**
FDA Number: 1422674   Fax: 630-801-4766
E-mail: info@biologos.com
Web site: www.biologos.com
Medical Products Sales Volume: $500,000
Annual Revenue: $1-$5 Million
Year Founded: 1976
Total Employees: 9   Marketing Staff: 4   Sales Staff: 4
Ownership: Private
Quality System Registration Information: ISO9002
Produces/Sells CE-marked Devices: N
Federal Procurement Eligibility: Small Business
Distribution: Manufacturer Direct
General Admin.: Dennis Raine/President
   Serum, Animal   Pathology
   Tissue Culture Apparatus   Microbiology

BIOMAGNETICS DIAGNOSTICS CORP.   916-987-7078
8864 Greenback Lane, Suite E, Orangevale, CA 95662
FDA Number: n/a   Fax: 916-987-7922
E-mail: info@biomagneticsbmgp.com
Web site: www.BiomagneticsBMGP.com
Ownership: Biospectrum Technologies
Stock Symbol: BMGP
Traded On: OTC Bulletin
Produces/Sells CE-marked Devices: N
General Admin.: Clayton M. Hardman/President, Chief Executive Officer

BIOMAT SCIENCES, INC.   866-4-BIOMAT
7210A Corporate Court, Frederick, MD 21703   **301-529-7081**
FDA Number: 1125730   Fax: 301-652-3327
E-mail: info@biomatsciences.com
Web site: www.biomatsciences.com
Medical Products Sales Volume: $160,000
Year Founded: 1999
Total Employees: 3
Ownership: Private
Produces/Sells CE-marked Devices: N
Federal Procurement Eligibility: Small Business
Distribution: Manufacturer Direct, OEM
General Admin.: Dr. Ivan Stangel/Chief Executive Officer
   Material, Tooth Shade, Resin   Dental And Oral
   Tooth Bonding Agent, Resin Restoration   Dental And Oral

BIOMATION   888-667-2324
335 Perth St., P.O. Box 156,   **613-256-2821**
Almonte, ON K0A 1 Canada
FDA Number: n/a   Fax: 613-256-5872
E-mail: info@biomation.com
Web site: www.biomation.com
Medical Products Sales Volume: $500,000
Year Founded: 1989
Total Employees: 4   Marketing Staff: 1   Sales Staff: 2
Ownership: Private
Quality System Registration Information: ISO9001
Produces/Sells CE-marked Devices: N
Federal Procurement Eligibility: Small Business
Distribution: Exclusive Distributor, Importer

BIOMECH DESIGNS LTD.   780-446-5303
9627 83 St., Edmonton, ALB T6C-3A3 Canada
FDA Number: n/a   Fax: 780-465-1396
E-mail: info@biomech.com
Web site: www.biomech.net
Year Founded: 1982
Ownership: Private
Produces/Sells CE-marked Devices: N
Distribution: Manufacturer Direct, Exporter

BIOMECHANIC
See Signal Medical Corporation

BIOMED DEVICES CORP.   540-636-7976
1325 Progress Dr., Front Royal, VA 22630
FDA Number: 1123070
Ownership: Private
Produces/Sells CE-marked Devices: N
   Lenses, Soft Contact, Daily Wear   Ophthalmology

BIOMED DIAGNOSTICS, INC.   541-830-3000
1388 Antelope Road, White City, OR 97503
FDA Number: 2951280   Fax: 541-830-3001
E-mail: info@biomeddiagnostics.com

BIOMED DIAGNOSTICS, INC.   541-830-3000 (cont'd)
Web site: www.biomeddiagnostics.com
Medical Products Sales Volume: $400,000
Year Founded: 1989
Total Employees: 7   Marketing Staff: 2   Sales Staff: 2
Ownership: Private
Produces/Sells CE-marked Devices: Y
Federal Procurement Eligibility: Small Business
Distribution: Manufacturer Direct, Manufacturer Through Distributor, Exclusive Distributor
   Culture Media, Enriched   Microbiology
   Culture Media, Selective And Differential   Microbiology

BIOMED INK   720-493-5199
3411 Westhaven Place, Littleton, CO 80126-8036
FDA Number: n/a   Fax: 720-493-5199
E-mail: solutions@biomedink.com
Web site: www.biomedink.com
Medical Products Sales Volume: $100,000
Year Founded: 1992
Ownership: Private
Produces/Sells CE-marked Devices: N
Federal Procurement Eligibility: Small Business, Minority Owned, Female Owned
Distribution: Service Direct
General Admin.: Joy Kocar/President
   Manual, Policies   General
   Service, Consulting   General
   Service, Licensing, Device, Medical   General

BIOMED INSTRUMENTS, INC.
See Advanced American Biotechnology (Aab)

BIOMED LABORATORIES, INC.   972-282-8008
11910 Shiloh Rd., Ste. 142, Dallas, TX 75228
FDA Number: 3006784948   Fax: 419-844-2025
E-mail: nfo@biomedlabs.net
Web site: www.biomedlabs.net
Ownership: Private
Produces/Sells CE-marked Devices: N
   Cement, Stomal Appliance, Ostomy   Gastroenterology/Urology

BIOMED PRODUCTS LLC.   877-424-6633
11300 Sanders Drive, Suite 26,   **916-852-8620**
Rancho Cordova, CA 95742
FDA Number: 2954309   Fax: 916-852-8647
E-mail: Erik@BiomedElectrodes.com
Web site: www.biomedelectrodes.com
Ownership: Private
Produces/Sells CE-marked Devices: N
   Electrode, Cutaneous   Cns/Neurology

BIOMED RESOURCE, INC.   310-323-3888
6646 Doolittle Ave., Riverside, CA 92503
FDA Number: 2087535   Fax: 951-343-8888
Ownership: Private
Produces/Sells CE-marked Devices: N
   Accessories, Apparel, Surgical   Surgery
   Dress, Surgical   Surgery
   Garment, Protective, For Incontinence   Gastroenterology/Urology
   Gown, Examination   General
   Linen, Bed   General

BIOMEDICAL COMPOSITES, LTD.   805-644-4892
4526 Telephone Rd., Suite 204, Ventura, CA 93003
FDA Number: 2183692
Ownership: Private
Produces/Sells CE-marked Devices: N
   Base, Denture, Relining, Repairing, Rebasing, Resin   Dental And Oral
   Bone Mill   Orthopedics

BIOMEDICAL ENTERPRISES, INC.   800-880-6528
14785 Omicron Drive, Suite 205,   **210-677-0354**
San Antonio, TX 78245
FDA Number: 1649263   Fax: 210-677-0355
E-mail: bme@bme-tx.com
Web site: www.bme-tx.com
Medical Products Sales Volume: $7,100,000
Year Founded: 1991
Total Employees: 45
Ownership: Private
Quality System Registration Information: ISO9001
Produces/Sells CE-marked Devices: Y
Federal Procurement Eligibility: Small Business
Distribution: Manufacturer Direct, Manufacturer Through Distributor, Importer, Exporter
General Admin.: Dr. W. Casey Fox/Chief Executive Officer
Mktg./Adv.: Mr. Ken Palmer/Director Sales
Finance: Mr. Bobby Rios/Chief Financial Officer
   Bit, Drill   Orthopedics

BIOMEDICAL ENTERPRISES, INC. 800-880-6528 *(cont'd)*
Kit, Collection/Transfusion, Marrow, Bone — General
Staple, Fixation, Bone — Orthopedics

BIOMEDICAL IMPLANT TECHNOLOGY INC. 800-268-6684
206 King St., 905-685-9822
St. Catharines, ONT L3R-3 Canada
FDA Number: n/a Fax: 905-682-8495
E-mail: Implant@bit123.com
Web site: www.dental-implant.com
Year Founded: 1990
Total Employees: 25
Ownership: Private
Produces/Sells CE-marked Devices: N
Distribution: Manufacturer Direct, Exclusive Distributor, Exporter

BIOMEDICAL INDUSTRY GROUP INC. 613-745-4139
532 Montreal Rd., Ste. 362, Ottawa, ONT K1K-4R4 Canada
FDA Number: n/a Fax: 613-746-2590
E-mail: info@BioMedGroup.com
Web site: www.biomedgroup.com
Year Founded: 1996
Ownership: Private
Produces/Sells CE-marked Devices: N

BIOMEDICAL LIFE SYSTEMS, INC. 800-726-8367
2448 Cades Way, Vista, CA 92085 760-727-5600
FDA Number: 2024292 Fax: 760-727-4220
E-mail: information@bmls.com
Web site: www.bmls.com
Medical Products Sales Volume: $5,000,000
Annual Revenue: $5-$10 Million
Year Founded: 1986
Total Employees: 20 Marketing Staff: 3 Sales Staff: 5
Ownership: Private
Quality System Registration Information: ISO9000; ISO9001; ISO9002; ISO9003
Produces/Sells CE-marked Devices: Y
Federal Procurement Eligibility: Small Business, GSA Contract, VA Contract
Distribution: Manufacturer Through Distributor, Manufacturer Through Manufacturer Reps, OEM, Exporter
General Admin.: Richard Saxon/Chief Executive Officer
　　　　　　Hans Reiss/Vice President
Mktg./Adv.: Hans Reiss/Manager Marketing
Production: Sheri Cole/Manager Regulatory Affairs

Electrode, TENS	Cns/Neurology
Stimulator, Acupuncture	Anesthesiology
Stimulator, Cranial Electrotherapy	Cns/Neurology
Stimulator, Electro-Analgesic	Cns/Neurology
Stimulator, Electro/Acupuncture	Anesthesiology
Stimulator, External, Neuromuscular, Functional	Physical Med
Stimulator, Muscle, Electrical-Powered (EMS)	Physical Med
Stimulator, Nerve, Anesthesia	Anesthesiology
Stimulator, Nerve, Battery-Powered	Anesthesiology
Stimulator, Nerve, Transcutaneous (Pain Relief, TENS)	Cns/Neurology
Stimulator, Neurological	Surgery
Stimulator, Neuromuscular, External Functional	Cns/Neurology
Unit, Therapy, Current, Interferential	Cns/Neurology

BIOMEDICAL MODELS LLC 800-635-4801
327 S. 7th Street, Hudson, WI 54016 715-386-1293
FDA Number: n/a Fax: 715-386-7573
E-mail: info@biomedicalmodels.com
Web site: www.biomedicalmodels.com
Annual Revenue: $0-$1 Million
Ownership: Private
Produces/Sells CE-marked Devices: N
Federal Procurement Eligibility: Small Business
Distribution: Importer
General Admin.: Milton A. Cornwall/President

Anatomical Training Model	General

BIOMEDICAL POLYMERS, INC. 800-253-3684
42 Linus Allain Avenue, Gardner, MA 01440 978-632-2555
FDA Number: 1220502 Fax: 978-632-2524
E-mail: mfaulkner@biomedicalpolymers.com
Web site: www.biomedicalpolymers.com
Medical Products Sales Volume: $9,000,000
Year Founded: 1978
Total Employees: 41 Marketing Staff: 3 Sales Staff: 1
Ownership: Private
Produces/Sells CE-marked Devices: N
Federal Procurement Eligibility: Small Business, GSA Contract
Distribution: Manufacturer Direct
General Admin.: John E. Fay/Chief Executive Officer
　　　　　　Michael T. Faulkner/President
Mktg./Adv.: Christopher Stamas/Vice President Sales
Production: Kevin Duffey/Quality Control, Product Engineer
　　　　　　John Bellorado/Vice President Manufacturing

BIOMEDICAL POLYMERS, INC. 800-253-3684 *(cont'd)*
Contract Manufacturing, Product, Disposable — General

BIOMEDICAL RESEARCH & DEVELOPMENT LABS, INC.
See Brandel

BIOMEDICAL SYSTEMS 800-877-6334
77 Progress Parkway, Building One, 314-576-6800
St. Louis, MO 63043
FDA Number: 1954552 Fax: 314-576-1664
E-mail: info@biomedsys.com
Web site: www.biomedsys.com
Year Founded: 1975
Total Employees: 250
Ownership: Private
Produces/Sells CE-marked Devices: N
Federal Procurement Eligibility: Small Business
Distribution: Exclusive Distributor
Production: K. Michael Kroehnke/Director Quality Assurance & Regulatory Affairs

Protector, Skin Pressure	General

BIOMEDICAL SYSTEMS CORP. 800-877-6334
77 Progress Parkway, Building One, 314-576-6800
St. Louis, MO 63043
FDA Number: 1931795 Fax: 314-576-1664
E-mail: info@biomedsys.com
Web site: www.biomedsys.com
Medical Products Sales Volume: $200,000
Year Founded: 1975
Total Employees: 5 Marketing Staff: 2 Sales Staff: 20
Ownership: Private
Quality System Registration Information: ISO9000; ISO9001
Produces/Sells CE-marked Devices: Y
Federal Procurement Eligibility: Small Business
Distribution: Manufacturer Direct, Manufacturer Through Distributor, Manufacturer Through Manufacturer Reps, OEM
General Admin.: W. Raymond Barrett/Chairman
　　　　Mr. Dan Barrett/Chief Operating Officer
　　　　Dr. Timothy Callahan/Chief Scientific Officer
　　　　Jim Ott/President
　　　　Timothy Barrett/President
　　　　Mr. Tim Barrett/President, Chief Executive Officer
Medical Admin.: Dr. Pierre Maison-Blanche/Chief Medical Officer
Mktg./Adv.: Craig Pennington/Director Marketing
Production: Michael Kroenke/Director Quality Assurance
Finance: Mr. Tom Modglin/Chief Financial Officer

Monitor, ECG	Cardiovascular
Recorder, Long-Term, ECG	Cardiovascular
Recorder, Long-Term, ECG, Portable (Holter Monitor)	Cardiovascular
Scanner, Ultrasonic, Other	Radiology

BIOMEDICAL TECHNOLOGIES, INC. 781-344-9942
378 Page St., Stoughton, MA 02072-1141
FDA Number: n/a Fax: 781-341-1451
E-mail: info@btiinc.com
Web site: www.btiinc.com
Medical Products Sales Volume: $5,000,000
Annual Revenue: $1-$5 Million
Year Founded: 1981
Total Employees: 10 Marketing Staff: 2 Sales Staff: 1
Ownership: Private
Produces/Sells CE-marked Devices: N
Federal Procurement Eligibility: Small Business
Distribution: Manufacturer Direct, Exporter
General Admin.: Maurice Lamarque/President

Antibody, Anti-Smooth Muscle, Indirect Immunofluorescent	Immunology
Antigen, Antiserum, Control, Lipoprotein, Low Density	Immunology
Antigen, Antiserum, Control, Lysozyme	Immunology
Contract R&D, Diagnostics	General
Enzyme Immunoassay, Other	Chemistry
Immunoassay, Other	Toxicology
Immunochemical, Lysozyme (Muramidase)	Chemistry
Pipette Tip	Chemistry
Radioimmunoassay, Cyclic AMP	Chemistry
Radioimmunoassay, Cyclic GMP	Chemistry
Radioimmunoassay, Other	Chemistry
Test, Radioreceptor	Chemistry
Test, Radioreceptor, Neuroleptic Drugs	Toxicology

BIOMEDICAL TECHNOLOGY SOLUTIONS, INC. 303-653-0100
9800 Mt. Pyramid Court, Ste 350, Centennial, CO 80112
FDA Number: 2435368 Fax: 303.653.0120
E-mail: sales@bmtscorp.com
Web site: www.bmtscorp.com
Ownership: Private
Produces/Sells CE-marked Devices: N

Container, Sharpes	General

BIOMEDICS CORPORATION
See Wheelchair Sales And Service Co., Inc.

BIOMEDICS, INC.   949-458-1998
23322 Peralta Drive, Ste. 11, Laguna Hills, CA 92653
FDA Number: n/a   *Fax:* 949-458-1708
E-mail: thebiomedics@yahoo.com
Web site: www.thebiomedics.com
Annual Revenue: $0-$1 Million
Year Founded: 2000
Total Employees: 4   *Marketing Staff:* 1   *Sales Staff:* 2
Ownership: Private
Produces/Sells CE-marked Devices: N
Federal Procurement Eligibility: Small Business
Distribution: Service Direct
General Admin.: Mr. Douglas Green/President, Chief Executive Officer
      Mrs. Lisa Green/Vice President, Corporate Secretary

Aspirator, Surgical	Surgery
Defibrillator/Monitor, Battery-Powered	Cardiovascular
Defibrillator/Monitor, Line-Powered	Cardiovascular
Electrocautery Unit, Line-Powered	Surgery
Electrosurgical Unit, General Purpose (ESU)	Surgery
Extractor, Cataract	Ophthalmology
Fluidic, Phacoemulsification/fragmentation	Ophthalmology
Lamp, Slit	Ophthalmology
Lamp, Surgical, Xenon	Surgery
Laser, Argon, Surgical	Surgery
Laser, Carbon-Dioxide, Microsurgical, ENT	Ear/Nose/Throat
Laser, Carbon-Dioxide, Surgical	Surgery
Laser, Combination	General
Laser, Gastroenterology/Urology	Gastroenterology/Urology
Laser, Nd:YAG, Laparoscopy	Surgery
Laser, Nd:YAG, Surgical	Surgery
Laser, Ophthalmic	Ophthalmology
Laser, Surgical	Surgery
Laser, Surgical, Holmium	Surgery
Microscope, Operating, AC-Powered, Ophthalmic	Ophthalmology
Microscope, Surgical	Ear/Nose/Throat
Microscope, Surgical, General & Plastic Surgery	Surgery
Mount, Surgical Microscope	Surgery
Phacoemulsification System	Ophthalmology
Phacofragmentation Unit	Ophthalmology
System, Cooling, Laser	Surgery
System, Evacuation, Smoke, Laser	Surgery
Table, Surgical, Electrical	Surgery

BIOMEDIX INC.   877-854-0012
178 East Ninth Street, St Paul, MN 55101   651-762-4010
FDA Number: 2134492   *Fax:* 651-762-4014
E-mail: biomedix@biomedix.com
Web site: www.biomedix.com
Medical Products Sales Volume: $10,000,000
Year Founded: 1977
Total Employees: 39
Ownership: Private
Quality System Registration Information: ISO9001
Produces/Sells CE-marked Devices: Y
Federal Procurement Eligibility: Small Business
Distribution: Manufacturer Direct, Manufacturer Through Distributor, Manufacturer Through Manufacturer Reps, Exporter
General Admin.: Will Rogers/Chief Technology Officer
      John Romans/President, Chief Executive Officer
Mktg./Adv.: Todd Aldrich/Vice President Marketing Services
      Mike Lobinsky/Vice President Sales
Production: Rick Grave/Senior Product Manager

Computer and Software, Medical	General
Detector, Blood Flow, Ultrasonic (Doppler)	Cardiovascular
Monitor, Blood Pressure, Indirect (Arterial)	Cardiovascular
Monitor, Ultrasonic, Non-Fetal	Radiology
Plethysmograph, Photo-Electric, Pneumatic Or Hydraulic	Cardiovascular
Probe, Ultrasonic	Radiology
Transducer, Ultrasonic	Cardiovascular

BIOMEDIX, INC.   800-627-2765
3895 W. Vernal Pike, Bloomington, IN 47404   812-355-7000
FDA Number: 1833470   *Fax:* 812-355-7001
E-mail: biomedix@biomedix-inc.com
Web site: www.biomedix-inc.com
Annual Revenue: $1-$5 Million
Year Founded: 1992
Total Employees: 32   *Marketing Staff:* 1   *Sales Staff:* 1
Ownership: Private
Produces/Sells CE-marked Devices: N
Federal Procurement Eligibility: Small Business
Distribution: Manufacturer Direct, Manufacturer Through Distributor
General Admin.: Richard Sweet/President
Mktg./Adv.: Myra Bender/Vice President Marketing & Sales

Fixation Device, Tracheal Tube	Anesthesiology

BIOMEDIX, INC.   800-627-2765 *(cont'd)*
Kit, Administration, Intravenous   General

BIOMEGA CORP.
See Physio-Control, Inc.

BIOMERICA, INC.   800-854-3002
17571 Von Karman Ave, Irvine, CA 92614   949-645-2111
FDA Number: n/a   *Fax:* 949-722-6674
E-mail: bmra@biomerica.com
Web site: www.biomerica.com
Medical Products Sales Volume: $7,200,000
Annual Revenue: $5-$10 Million
Year Founded: 1971
Total Employees: 27   *Marketing Staff:* 4   *Sales Staff:* 20
Ownership: Public
Stock Symbol: BMRA
Traded On: OTC Bulletin
Produces/Sells CE-marked Devices: Y
Federal Procurement Eligibility: Small Business
Distribution: Manufacturer Direct, Manufacturer Through Distributor, Manufacturer Through Manufacturer Reps, OEM, Exclusive Distributor, Exporter
General Admin.: Zack Irani/Chief Executive Officer
      Fran Capitanio/President
Mktg./Adv.: Mr. Patrick Garcia/Director Marketing
Production: Dr. W. Kevin Liddle/Director Manufacturing
      Perry Rucker/Manager Regulatory Affairs
Research: Dr. S. Rao/Vice President Research & Development

Antibody, Anti-Thyroid, Indirect Immunofluorescent	Immunology
Antigen, Antiserum, Control, Luteinizing Hormone	Immunology
Antigen, ID, Candida Albicans	Microbiology
Antigen, Prostate-Specific (PSA), Management, Cancer	Immunology
Campylobacter Pylori	Microbiology
Enzymatic Method, Blood, Occcult, Fecal	Chemistry
Enzyme Immunoassay, Other	Chemistry
Immunoassay, Other	Toxicology
Immunochemical, Thyroglobulin Autoantibody	Immunology
Kit, Pregnancy Test	Obstetrics/Gynecology
Test, Allergy	Immunology
Test, Cancer Detection, Other	Hematology

BIOMERIDIAN, INT   888-224-2337
2440 south 1070 west suite a,   801-5017517
salt lake city, UT 84119
FDA Number: 1723429   *Fax:* 801-501-7518
E-mail: mail@biomeridian.com
Web site: www.biomeridian.com
Year Founded: 1997
Ownership: Private
Stock Symbol: LWAY
Traded On: NYSE
Produces/Sells CE-marked Devices: N
General Admin.: Dennis W Remington/Managing Director

BIOMERIEUX INC.   800-682-2666
100 Rodolphe Ave., Durham, NC 27712   919-620-2000
FDA Number: n/a   *Fax:* 919-620-2615
E-mail: bob.bokerman@na.biomerieux.com
Web site: www.biomerieux-usa.com
Medical Products Sales Volume: $240,000,000
Total Employees: 600   *Marketing Staff:* 25   *Sales Staff:* 150
Ownership: Organon Teknika Bv
Quality System Registration Information: ISO9001
Produces/Sells CE-marked Devices: Y
Distribution: Manufacturer Direct, Manufacturer Through Distributor, Manufacturer Through Manufacturer Reps
General Admin.: Philippe Sans/Chief Executive Officer
Mktg./Adv.: George Goedesky/Director Marketing
      Mark Gnagy/Director National Accounts
      Gail English/Manager Contract Sales
      Allison Williams/Manager Sales Training
Production: Herb Steward/Senior Vice President Operations
Finance: Lloyd Moores/Vice President Finance & Operations

Acetone	Chemistry
Agglutination Method, Human Chorionic Gonadotropin	Chemistry
Alpha-Ketobutyric Acid And NADH (U.V.), Hydroxybutyric	Chemistry
Analyzer, Blood Grouping/Antibody, Automated	Hematology
Analyzer, Chemistry, Electrolyte	Chemistry
Analyzer, Chemistry, Enzyme	Chemistry
Analyzer, Coagulation	Hematology
Analyzer, Coagulation, Automated	Hematology
Analyzer, Coagulation, Manual	Hematology
Analyzer, Coagulation, Whole Blood	Hematology
Antigen, Antiserum, Control, Haptoglobin	Immunology
Antigen, Antiserum, Control, Prothrombin	Immunology
Antigen, Antiserum, Fibrinogen And Fibrin Split Products	Immunology
Antigen, Salmonella SPP.	Microbiology
Antiserum, Fluorescent, Groups, Streptococcus SPP.	Microbiology
Antiserum, Fluorescent, Hemophilus SPP.	Microbiology

BIOMERIEUX INC.
800-682-2666 *(cont'd)*

Bleeding Time Device	Hematology
Chromatographic Separation, CPK Isoenzymes	Chemistry
Colorimetric Method, Triglycerides	Chemistry
Complexone, Cresolphthalein, Calcium	Chemistry
Control, Analyte (Assayed And Unassayed)	Chemistry
Control, Coagulation, Plasma	Hematology
Control, Coombs	Hematology
Control, Multi Analyte, All Kinds (Assayed And Unassayed)	Chemistry
Cuvette, Spectrophotometer	Chemistry
Detector, Air Bubble	Gastroenterology/Urology
Dye-Binding, Albumin, Bromcresol, Green	Chemistry
Electrophoretic, Lactate Dehydrogenase Isoenzymes	Chemistry
Enzymatic Esterase-Oxidase, Cholesterol	Chemistry
Equipment, Apheresis	Hematology
Exoenzyme, Multiple, Streptococcal	Microbiology
Extractor, Plasma	Hematology
Fibrin Monomer Paracoagulation	Hematology
Hematology Quality Control Mixture	Hematology
Immunoassay, Other	Toxicology
Immunodiffusion Method, Immunoglobulins (G, A, M)	Chemistry
Kit, Disc Agar Gel Diffusion, Serum Level	Microbiology
Kit, Identification, Enterobacteriaceae	Microbiology
Kit, Mycobacteria Identification	Microbiology
Kit, Quality Control	Microbiology
Labware, Blood Collection	Chemistry
Lectins/Protectins	Hematology
Leukocyte Alkaline Phosphatase	Hematology
M. Lysodeikticus Cells (Spectrophotometric), Lysozyme	Chemistry
NAD Reduction/NADH Oxidation, Lactate Dehydrogenase	Chemistry
NADH Oxidation/NAD Reduction, AST/SGOT	Chemistry
Nitrophenylphosphate, Alkaline Phosphatase Or Isoenzymes	Chemistry
Partial Thromboplastin Time	Hematology
Partial Thromboplastin Time, Reagent, Control	Hematology
Phenylphosphate, Alkaline Phosphatase Or Isoenzymes	Chemistry
Phosphatase, Acid	Hematology
Phosphatase, Alkaline	Hematology
Phosphorus Reagent (Test System)	Chemistry
Phosphotungstate Reduction, Uric Acid	Chemistry
Photometer	Chemistry
Pipette Tip	Chemistry
Plasma, Deficient, Factor, Coagulation	Hematology
Reagent, Albumin, Colorimetric	Chemistry
Reagent, Amylase, Colorimetric	Chemistry
Reagent, Bilirubin (Total Or Direct Test System)	Chemistry
Reagent, Blood Urea Nitrogen (BUN)	Chemistry
Reagent, Calcium (Test System)	Chemistry
Reagent, Chloride (Test System)	Chemistry
Reagent, Creatinine (Test System)	Chemistry
Reagent, Glucose (Test System)	Chemistry
Reagent, Iron (Test System)	Chemistry
Reagent, Kinase, Phosphate, Creatine	Chemistry
Reagent, NAD-NADH, Alcohol Enzyme Method	Toxicology
Reagent, Protein, Total	Chemistry
SGOT, Colorimetric	Chemistry
SGOT, Ultraviolet	Chemistry
SGPT, Colorimetric	Chemistry
SGPT, Ultraviolet	Chemistry
Seminal Fluid, Antigen, Antiserum, Control	Immunology
Separator, Blood Cell, Automated	Hematology
Serum Separation System	Hematology
Stain, Acid Fuchsin	Pathology
Standard/Control, All Types	Chemistry
Standard/Control, Fibrinogen Determination	Hematology
Streptolysin O	Pathology
System, Blood Culturing	Microbiology
Test, Antibody, Acquired Immune Deficiency Syndrome (AIDS)	Hematology
Test, Bacterial Diagnostic	Microbiology
Test, C-Reactive Protein	Immunology
Test, C-Reactive Protein, FITC	Immunology
Test, Fibrinogen	Hematology
Test, Rheumatoid Factor	Immunology
Test, Sickle Cell	Hematology
Test, Syphilis (RPR or VDRL)	Microbiology
Test, Thrombin Time	Hematology
Test, Thromboplastin Generation	Hematology
Tetrabromo-M-Cresolsulfonphthalein, Albumin	Chemistry

Medical Product Subsidiaries (Listed Separately)
Advanced Bioscience Laboratories, Inc.

BIOMERIEUX INDUSTRY
800-634-7656
595 Anglum Road, Hazelwood, MO 63042-2320
314-731-8500
FDA Number: n/a
Fax: 314-731-8678
E-mail: IndustryCS@na.biomerieux.com
Web site: www.industry.biomerieux-usa.com
Medical Products Sales Volume: $4,300,000
Total Employees: 39
Ownership: Public
Produces/Sells CE-marked Devices: Y
Federal Procurement Eligibility: Small Business

BIOMERIEUX INDUSTRY
800-634-7656 *(cont'd)*
Distribution: Manufacturer Direct, Manufacturer Through Distributor, Importer, Exporter
General Admin.: Douglas Maxwell/President
Mktg./Adv.: Emil Ulstrup/Director Marketing & Sales
Production: Frank Cammarata/Director Quality Assurance

Culture Media, Antimicrobial Susceptibility Test	Microbiology
Culture Media, For Isolation Of Pathogenic Neisseria	Microbiology
Culture Media, General Nutrient Broth	Microbiology
Culture Media, Multiple Biochemical Test	Microbiology
Culture Media, Non-Selective And Non-Differential	Microbiology
Culture Media, Selective Broth	Microbiology
Culture Media, Single Biochemical Test	Microbiology
Disc, Strip And Reagent, Microorganism Differentiation	Microbiology
Reagent, Other	General
Safety Equipment, Laboratory	Chemistry
Serum, Animal	Pathology
Stain, Microbiological	Microbiology
Stain, Other	Pathology
Test, Antibiotic Susceptibility	Microbiology

BIOMET 3I
800-342-5454
4555 Riverside Dr.,
561-776-6700
Palm Beach Gardens, FL 33410
FDA Number: n/a
Fax: 561-776-1272
E-mail: mprescott@3implant.com
Web site: www.biomet3i.com
Ownership: Biomet, Inc.
Produces/Sells CE-marked Devices: Y
Distribution: Manufacturer Through Distributor, Manufacturer Through Manufacturer Reps
Mktg./Adv.: Marilyn Prescott/Public Relations Specialist

Attachment, Precision	Dental And Oral
Bar, Preformed	Dental And Oral
Bone Mill	Orthopedics
Burr, Surgical, General & Plastic Surgery	Surgery
Drill, Dental, Intraoral	Dental And Oral
Graft, Bone	Orthopedics
Handle, Instrument, Dental	Dental And Oral
Handpiece, Contra- And Right-Angle Attachment, Dental	Dental And Oral
Implant, Endosseous	Dental And Oral
Implant, Endosseous (Bone Filling and/or Augmentation)	Dental And Oral
Kit, Surgical (General)	Surgery

BIOMET CANADA INC.
800-263-9447
2891 Portland Drive,
905.825.8066
Oakville, ONT L6H 5 Canada
FDA Number: n/a
Fax: 905-825-8075
E-mail: bmetcan@globalserve.net
Web site: www.biomet.com
Year Founded: 1978
Total Employees: 10
Ownership: Biomet, Inc.
Produces/Sells CE-marked Devices: N
Distribution: Exclusive Distributor

BIOMET MICROFIXATION INC.
800-874-7711
1520 Tradeport Dr., Jacksonville, FL 32218
904-741-4400
FDA Number: 1032347
Fax: 904-741-4470
Web site: www.biometmicrofixation.com
Year Founded: 1965
Ownership: Biomet, Inc.
Produces/Sells CE-marked Devices: N

Accessories, Powered Drill	Cns/Neurology
Accessories, Retractor, Dental	Dental And Oral
Adapter, Holder, Syringe	Physical Med
Adenotome	Ear/Nose/Throat
Applicator, ENT	Ear/Nose/Throat
Applier, Hemostatic Clip	Cns/Neurology
Applier, Surgical, Clip	Surgery
Articulators	Dental And Oral
Awl	Orthopedics
Band, Material, Orthodontic	Dental And Oral
Basin, Emesis	General
Biopsy Instrument	Gastroenterology/Urology
Bit, Drill	Orthopedics
Blade, Scalpel	Surgery
Blade, Surgical, Saw, General & Plastic Surgery	Surgery
Block, Bite	Cns/Neurology
Bone Mill	Orthopedics
Broach, Endodontic	Dental And Oral
Burr	Ear/Nose/Throat
Burr, Orthopedic	Orthopedics
Cannula, Suction, Uterine	Obstetrics/Gynecology
Cannula, Surgical, General & Plastic Surgery	Surgery
Carrier, Amalgam, Operative	Dental And Oral
Carrier, Ligature	Surgery
Catheter, Suction, With Tip	General
Cement, Ear, Nose And Throat	Ear/Nose/Throat
Chisel (Osteotome)	Surgery

BIOMET MICROFIXATION INC.   800-874-7711 *(cont'd)*

Chisel, Bone, Surgical	Dental And Oral
Chisel, Nasal	Ear/Nose/Throat
Chisel, Osteotome, Surgical	Dental And Oral
Chisel, Surgical, Manual	Surgery
Clamp, Bone	Orthopedics
Clamp, Carotid Artery	Cns/Neurology
Clamp, Surgical, General & Plastic Surgery	Surgery
Clamp, Tubing, Blood, Automatic	Gastroenterology/Urology
Clamp, Uterine	Obstetrics/Gynecology
Clamp, Vascular	Cardiovascular
Clamp, Wire, Orthodontic	Dental And Oral
Clip, Tubal Occlusion	Obstetrics/Gynecology
Clip, Vascular	Cardiovascular
Coagulator/Cutter, Endoscopic, Bipolar	Obstetrics/Gynecology
Curette	Orthopedics
Curette, Adenoid	Ear/Nose/Throat
Curette, Biopsy, Bronchoscope (Rigid)	Anesthesiology
Curette, Ear	Ear/Nose/Throat
Curette, Endodontic	Dental And Oral
Curette, Nasal	Ear/Nose/Throat
Curette, Periodontic	Dental And Oral
Curette, Surgical, Dental	Dental And Oral
Curette, Uterine	Obstetrics/Gynecology
Cutter, Surgical	Surgery
Cutter, Wire And Pin	Orthopedics
Depressor, Tongue	General
Dilator, Lacrimal	Ophthalmology
Dilator, Nasal	Ear/Nose/Throat
Dilator, Urethral	Gastroenterology/Urology
Dilator, Vaginal	Obstetrics/Gynecology
Dilator, Vessel, Surgical	Cardiovascular
Dissector, Surgical, General & Plastic Surgery	Surgery
Dissector, Tonsil	Ear/Nose/Throat
Drill, Bone	Orthopedics
Drill, Bone, Powered	Dental And Oral
Drill, Dental, Intraoral	Dental And Oral
Drill, Manual (With Burr, Trephine & Accessories)	Cns/Neurology
Driver, Wire, And Bone Drill, Manual	Dental And Oral
Elevator, ENT	Ear/Nose/Throat
Elevator, Surgical, Dental	Dental And Oral
Elevator, Surgical, General & Plastic Surgery	Surgery
Excavator, Dental, Operative	Dental And Oral
Exerciser, Non-Measuring	Physical Med
Expander, Surgical, Skin Graft	Surgery
Explorer, Operative	Dental And Oral
External Mandibular Fixator And/or Distractor	Dental And Oral
Facial Fracture Appliance, External	Surgery
Fiberoptic Light Source & Carrier	Ear/Nose/Throat
File	Orthopedics
File, Bone, Surgical	Dental And Oral
File, Periodontic	Dental And Oral
File, Surgical, General & Plastic Surgery	Surgery
Fixation Device, Tracheal Tube	Anesthesiology
Forceps	Orthopedics
Forceps, Biopsy, Bronchoscope (Rigid)	Anesthesiology
Forceps, Biopsy, Gynecological	Obstetrics/Gynecology
Forceps, Dressing, Dental	Dental And Oral
Forceps, ENT	Ear/Nose/Throat
Forceps, General & Plastic Surgery	Surgery
Forceps, Obstetrical	Obstetrics/Gynecology
Forceps, Rongeur, Surgical	Dental And Oral
Forceps, Surgical, Gynecological	Obstetrics/Gynecology
Forceps, Tooth Extractor, Surgical	Dental And Oral
Forceps, Wire Closure, ENT	Ear/Nose/Throat
Fork, Tuning	Cns/Neurology
Gag, Mouth	Ear/Nose/Throat
Gauge, Depth, Instrument, Dental	Dental And Oral
General Use Surgical Scissors	Surgery
Goniometer, Non-Powered	Orthopedics
Gouge, Nasal	Ear/Nose/Throat
Gouge, Surgical, General & Plastic Surgery	Surgery
Guide, Surgical, Instrument	Surgery
Guide, Surgical, Needle	Surgery
Hammer, Reflex, Powered	Physical Med
Hammer, Surgical	Surgery
Handle, Instrument, Dental	Dental And Oral
Handle, Scalpel	Surgery
Handpiece (Brace), Drill	Cns/Neurology
Handpiece, Air-Powered, Dental	Dental And Oral
Handpiece, Contra- And Right-Angle Attachment, Dental	Dental And Oral
Headlight, Fiberoptic Focusing	Gastroenterology/Urology
Hemostat, Surgical	Dental And Oral
High Pressure Liquid Chromatography, Quinine	Toxicology
Holder, Needle	Gastroenterology/Urology
Holder, Needle, Orthopedic	Orthopedics
Holder, Speculum, ENT	Ear/Nose/Throat
Hook, Fibroid, Gynecological	Obstetrics/Gynecology
Hook, Gastro-Urology	Gastroenterology/Urology
Hook, Microsurgical Ear	Ear/Nose/Throat
Hook, Surgical, General & Plastic Surgery	Surgery
Implant, Endosseous	Dental And Oral

BIOMET MICROFIXATION INC.   800-874-7711 *(cont'd)*

Implant, Endosseous (Bone Filling and/or Augmentation)	Dental And Oral
Implant, Fixation Device, Condylar Plate	Orthopedics
Implant, Joint, Temporomandibular	Dental And Oral
Kit, Catheterization, Sterile Urethral	Gastroenterology/Urology
Knife, ENT	Ear/Nose/Throat
Knife, Ear	Ear/Nose/Throat
Knife, Nasal	Ear/Nose/Throat
Knife, Orthopedic	Orthopedics
Knife, Periodontic	Dental And Oral
Knife, Surgical	Dental And Oral
Knife, Tonsil	Ear/Nose/Throat
Lock, Wire, And Ligature, Intraoral	Dental And Oral
Loop, Wire	Ear/Nose/Throat
Mallet, Surgical, General & Plastic Surgery	Surgery
Marker, Radiographic, Implantable	Surgery
Mesh, Metal	Gastroenterology/Urology
Metacrylate, Methyl, Cranioplasty	Cns/Neurology
Mirror, Mouth	Dental And Oral
Motor, Surgical Instrument, AC-Powered	Surgery
Needle, Aspiration And Injection, Reusable	Surgery
Needle, Gastro-Urology	Gastroenterology/Urology
Needle, Suture, Disposable	Surgery
Nipper, Malleus	Ear/Nose/Throat
Orthopedic Manual Surgical Instrument	Orthopedics
Osteotome (Orthopedic)	Surgery
Otoscope	Ear/Nose/Throat
Passer, Wire, Orthopedic	Orthopedics
Pelvimeter, External	Obstetrics/Gynecology
Perforator, Antrum	Ear/Nose/Throat
Pick, Microsurgical Ear	Ear/Nose/Throat
Plate, Bone, Orthodontic	Dental And Oral
Plate, Bone, Skull, Preformed, Non-Alterable	Cns/Neurology
Plate, Fixation, Bone	Orthopedics
Pliers, Crimp	Gastroenterology/Urology
Pliers, Surgical	Orthopedics
Plugger, Root Canal, Endodontic	Dental And Oral
Probe, Gastrointestinal	Gastroenterology/Urology
Probe, Lacrimal	Ophthalmology
Prosthesis, Condyle, Mandibular, Temporary	Dental And Oral
Prosthesis, Facial, Mandibular Implant	Ear/Nose/Throat
Prosthesis, Laryngeal (Taub)	Ear/Nose/Throat
Prosthesis, Mandibular Condyle	Dental And Oral
Protector, Wound, Plastic	Gastroenterology/Urology
Punch, Adenoid	Ear/Nose/Throat
Punch, Antrum	Ear/Nose/Throat
Punch, ENT	Ear/Nose/Throat
Punch, Skull	Cns/Neurology
Punch, Surgical	Surgery
Punch, Tonsil	Ear/Nose/Throat
Pusher, Band, Orthodontic	Dental And Oral
Rasp, Bone	Orthopedics
Rasp, Nasal	Ear/Nose/Throat
Rasp, Surgical, General & Plastic Surgery	Surgery
Restraint, Protective (Body)	General
Retractor, All Types	Dental And Oral
Retractor, Fiberoptic	Gastroenterology/Urology
Retractor, Surgical	Surgery
Retractor, Vaginal	Obstetrics/Gynecology
Rod, Fixation, Intramedullary	Orthopedics
Rongeur, Manual, Neurosurgical	Cns/Neurology
Rongeur, Nasal	Ear/Nose/Throat
Saw, Manual, And Accessories	Surgery
Saw, Nasal	Ear/Nose/Throat
Scaler, Periodontic	Dental And Oral
Scissors, Disposable	General
Scissors, Ear	Ear/Nose/Throat
Scissors, Episiotomy	Obstetrics/Gynecology
Scissors, Nasal	Ear/Nose/Throat
Scissors, Orthopedic	Orthopedics
Scissors, Surgical Tissue, Dental (Oral)	Dental And Oral
Scissors, Wire Cutting, ENT	Ear/Nose/Throat
Scoop, Gallstone	Gastroenterology/Urology
Screw, Fixation, Bone	Orthopedics
Screw, Fixation, Intraosseous	Dental And Oral
Screw, Oral	Ear/Nose/Throat
Screwdriver	Orthopedics
Snare, Ear	Ear/Nose/Throat
Snare, Nasal	Ear/Nose/Throat
Snare, Tonsil	Ear/Nose/Throat
Sound, Urethral, Metal Or Plastic	Gastroenterology/Urology
Sound, Uterine	Obstetrics/Gynecology
Spatula, Surgical, General & Plastic Surgery	Surgery
Speculum, Ear	Ear/Nose/Throat
Speculum, Non-Illuminated	Surgery
Speculum, Rectal	Gastroenterology/Urology
Speculum, Vaginal, Metal	Obstetrics/Gynecology
Splint, Hand, And Component	Physical Med
Stethoscope, Electronic (Auscultoscope)	Cardiovascular
Stripper, Surgical	Orthopedics
Stripper, Vein, Reusable	Surgery
Stylet, Surgical	Surgery

MANUFACTURER PROFILES

BIOMET MICROFIXATION INC.   800-874-7711 *(cont'd)*

Surgical Bench Vise	Surgery
Surgical Instrument, Non-Powered, Neurosurgical	Cns/Neurology
Suture, Absorbable, Synthetic	Surgery
Suture, Dental	Dental And Oral
Syringe, Ear	Ear/Nose/Throat
Syringe, Periodontic, Endodontic	Dental And Oral
System, Retroperfusion, Artery, Coronary	Cardiovascular
Tap, Bone	Orthopedics
Tape, Measuring, Ruler And Caliper	Surgery
Tourniquet, Non-Pneumatic, Surgical	Surgery
Tourniquet, Pneumatic	Surgery
Tray, Surgical	Surgery
Tray, Surgical Instrument	Surgery
Trocar, ENT	Ear/Nose/Throat
Trocar, Gastro-Urology	Gastroenterology/Urology
Tube, Ear Suction	Ear/Nose/Throat
Tube, Tonsil Suction	Ear/Nose/Throat
Tube, Tracheostomy (W/Wo Connector)	Anesthesiology
Tucker, Ligature, Orthodontic	Dental And Oral
Twister, Wire	Orthopedics
Valvulotome	Cardiovascular
Wire, Fixation, Intraosseous	Dental And Oral
Wire, Orthodontic	Dental And Oral
Wrench	Orthopedics

BIOMET SPORTS MEDICINE   530-226-5800
6704 Lockheed Dr., Redding, CA 96002
FDA Number: 2950285
Ownership: Biomet, Inc.

Arthroscope	Orthopedics
Camera, Television, Endoscopic (With Audio)	Surgery
Laparoscope, General & Plastic Surgery	Surgery
Light Source, Endoscope, Xenon Arc	Surgery
Motor, Surgical Instrument, AC-Powered	Surgery
Pump, Withdrawal/Infusion	Cardiovascular
Surgical Instrument, Orthopedic, AC-Powered Motor	Orthopedics
Surgical Instrument, Sonic	Orthopedics

BIOMET SPORTS MEDICINE, INC   800-348-9500
56 East Bell Drive, Warsaw, IN 46581-0587   **574-267-6639**
FDA Number: 2027970   *Fax:* 574-267-8137
E-mail: Arthrotek@arthrotek.com
Web site: www.arthrotek.com
Medical Products Sales Volume: $1,800,000
Annual Revenue: $25-$50 Million
Year Founded: 1977
Total Employees: 25
Ownership: Biomet, Inc.
Stock Symbol: BMET
Traded On: NASDAQ
Quality System Registration Information: ISO9001
Produces/Sells CE-marked Devices: Y
Federal Procurement Eligibility: Small Business
Distribution: Manufacturer Direct, Manufacturer Through Distributor, Manufacturer Through Manufacturer Reps, Exclusive Distributor, Importer, Exporter
General Admin.: Tom Prichard/President, Chief Executive Officer
Mktg./Adv.: Brandon Miller/Director Marketing
         Dave Nolan/Vice President Sales
Production: Susan Ladua/Manager Manufacturing
         Fred Edwards/Manager Regulatory Affairs
         Bill Coy/Plant Manager

Forceps	Orthopedics
Orthopedic Implant Material	Orthopedics
Orthopedic Manual Surgical Instrument	Orthopedics

BIOMET, INC.   574-267-6639
56 E. Bell Dr., PO Box 587, Warsaw, IN 46581
FDA Number: 1825034   *Fax:* 574-267-8137
E-mail: biomet@biomet.com
Web site: www.biomet.com
Medical Products Sales Volume: $238,300,000
Annual Revenue: More than $1 Billion
Year Founded: 1977
Ownership: Public
Stock Symbol: BMET
Traded On: NASDAQ
Produces/Sells CE-marked Devices: N
General Admin.: Jeffrey R. Binder/President, Chief Executive Officer
         Glen Kashuba/Senior Vice President
         Gregory W. Sasso/Senior Vice President
         Jon C. Serbousek/Senior Vice President
         Steven S. Schiess/Senior Vice President
Production: Robert Durgin/Vice President Quality Assurance & Regulatory Affairs
Finance: Daniel P. Florin/Chief Financial Officer

Accessories, Traction	Physical Med
Acid, Hyaluoronic	Dental And Oral
Appliance, Fix., Nail/Blade/Plate Comb., Multiple Component	Orthopedics
Applier, Cast	Orthopedics

BIOMET, INC.   574-267-6639 *(cont'd)*

Applier, Cerclage	Orthopedics
Applier, Surgical, Clip	Surgery
Arthroscope	Orthopedics
Assembly, Shoulder/Elbow/Forearm/Wrist/Hand, Mechanical	Physical Med
Awl	Orthopedics
Band, Support, Pelvic	Physical Med
Bandage, Elastic	General
Bars, Parallel, Exercise	Physical Med
Bed, Patient Rotation, Manual	Physical Med
Belt, Traction, Pelvic, Orthopedic	Orthopedics
Bender	Orthopedics
Binder, Abdominal	General
Bit, Drill	Orthopedics
Bit, Surgical	Surgery
Board, Bed	General
Bolt, Nut, Washer	Orthopedics
Bone Cement	Orthopedics
Bone Cement, Antibiotic	Orthopedics
Brace, Drill	Orthopedics
Brace, Joint, Ankle (External)	Physical Med
Broach	Orthopedics
Burr, Orthopedic	Orthopedics
Burr, Surgical, General & Plastic Surgery	Surgery
Caliper	Orthopedics
Cane	Physical Med
Catheter, Irrigation	Surgery
Centrifuge, Cell Washing	Hematology
Cerclage, Fixation	Orthopedics
Chisel (Osteotome)	Surgery
Chisel, Surgical, Manual	Surgery
Clamp, Bone	Orthopedics
Clamp, Surgical, General & Plastic Surgery	Surgery
Clip, Implantable	Surgery
Component, Traction, Invasive	Orthopedics
Compression Instrument	Orthopedics
Contractor, Surgical	Surgery
Corkscrew	Orthopedics
Countersink	Orthopedics
Crimper, Pin	Orthopedics
Crutch	Physical Med
Cuff, Blood Pressure	Cardiovascular
Cuff, Nerve	Cns/Neurology
Curette	Orthopedics
Cutter, Operative	Dental And Oral
Cutter, Orthopedic	Orthopedics
Cutter, Ring	General
Cutter, Wire And Pin	Orthopedics
Dermatome	Surgery
Drape, Surgical	Surgery
Drape, Surgical, Disposable	Surgery
Driver, Prosthesis	Orthopedics
Driver, Surgical, Pin	Surgery
Electrolysis Unit, Ophthalmic	Ophthalmology
Electrosurgical Unit, Cutting & Coagulation Device	Surgery
Elevator, Surgical, General & Plastic Surgery	Surgery
Endoscope, Fiberoptic	Surgery
Evacuator, Vapor, Cement Monomer	Orthopedics
Exhaust System, Surgical	Surgery
Extractor, Nail	Orthopedics
Fastener, Cranioplasty Plate	Cns/Neurology
Fastener, Fixation, Biodegradable, Soft Tissue	Orthopedics
Fastener, Fixation, Non-Biodegradable, Soft Tissue	Orthopedics
File	Orthopedics
Filler, Calcium Sulfate Preformed Pellets	Orthopedics
Fixation Appliance, Multiple Component	Orthopedics
Forceps	Orthopedics
Forceps, General & Plastic Surgery	Surgery
Forceps, Wire Holding	Orthopedics
Gauge, Depth	Orthopedics
Glove, Surgical, Plastic Surgery	Surgery
Goniometer, Non-Powered	Orthopedics
Gown, Surgical	Surgery
Guide, Surgical, Instrument	Surgery
Halter, Head, Traction, Orthopedic	Orthopedics
Hammer, Surgical	Surgery
Hip, Hemi-, Femoral, Metal Ball	Orthopedics
Holder, Needle, Orthopedic	Orthopedics
Hollow Mill Set	Orthopedics
Hook, Surgical, General & Plastic Surgery	Surgery
Impactor	Orthopedics
Implant, Endosseous (Bone Filling and/or Augmentation)	Dental And Oral
Implant, Fixation Device, Condylar Plate	Orthopedics
Implant, Fixation Device, Proximal Femoral	Orthopedics
Implant, Fixation Device, Spinal	Orthopedics
Instrument, Bending (Contouring)	Orthopedics
Instrument, Surgical, Powered, Pneumatic	Orthopedics
Joint, Hip, External Brace	Physical Med
Joint, Knee, External Brace	Physical Med
Knife, Amputation	Surgery
Laparoscope, General & Plastic Surgery	Surgery
Linen, Bed	General

BIOMET, INC.   574-267-6639 (cont'd)

Mallet, Bone	Orthopedics
Marker, Radiographic, Implantable	Surgery
Metacrylate, Methyl, Cranioplasty	Cns/Neurology
Orthopedic Manual Surgical Instrument	Orthopedics
Orthosis, Abdominal	Physical Med
Orthosis, Cervical	Physical Med
Orthosis, Cervical-Thoracic, Rigid	Physical Med
Orthosis, Limb Brace	Physical Med
Orthosis, Lumbosacral	Physical Med
Orthosis, Rib Fracture, Soft	Physical Med
Orthosis, Sacroiliac, Soft	Physical Med
Orthosis, Thoracic	Physical Med
Osteotome (Orthopedic)	Surgery
Pack, Hot Or Cold, Disposable	Physical Med
Passer, Wire, Orthopedic	Orthopedics
Pen, Marking, Surgical	Ophthalmology
Pin, Fixation, Smooth	Orthopedics
Pin, Fixation, Threaded	Orthopedics
Plate, Bone, Orthodontic	Dental And Oral
Plate, Bone, Skull, Preformed, Alterable	Cns/Neurology
Plate, Bone, Skull, Preformed, Non-Alterable	Cns/Neurology
Plate, Fixation, Bone	Orthopedics
Pliers, Surgical	Orthopedics
Pliers, Tube	Gastroenterology/Urology
Probe	Physical Med
Prosthesis Alignment Device	Physical Med
Prosthesis, Elbow, Constrained	Orthopedics
Prosthesis, Elbow, Hemi-, Radial, Polymer	Orthopedics
Prosthesis, Elbow, Semi-Constrained	Orthopedics
Prosthesis, Facial, Mandibular Implant	Ear/Nose/Throat
Prosthesis, Hip, Cement Restrictor	Orthopedics
Prosthesis, Hip, Constrained, Metal/Polymer	Orthopedics
Prosthesis, Hip, Femoral Component, Cemented, Metal	Orthopedics
Prosthesis, Hip, Femoral, Resurfacing	Orthopedics
Prosthesis, Hip, Hemi-, Femoral, Metal/Polymer	Orthopedics
Prosthesis, Hip, Semi-, Uncemented, Osteophilic Finish	Orthopedics
Prosthesis, Hip, Semi-Const., Metal/Ceramic/Ceramic, Cem.	Orthopedics
Prosthesis, Hip, Semi-Const., Metal/Poly., Porous Uncemented	Orthopedics
Prosthesis, Hip, Semi-Const., Uncem., Non-P., M/P, Ca./Phos.	Orthopedics
Prosthesis, Hip, Semi-Constr., Metal/Ceramic, Cemented/NC	Orthopedics
Prosthesis, Hip, Semi-Constrained (Cemented Acetabular)	Orthopedics
Prosthesis, Hip, Semi-Constrained Acetabular	Orthopedics
Prosthesis, Hip, Semi-Constrained, Metal/Polymer	Orthopedics
Prosthesis, Hip, Semi-Constrained, Metal/Polymer, Uncemented	Orthopedics
Prosthesis, Hip, Semi-constrained, Metal/Ceramic/Ceramic/Metal, Cemented Or Uncemented	Orthopedics
Prosthesis, Hip, Semi-constrained, Metal/ceramic/polymer, Cemented Or Non-porous Cemented, Osteophilic Finish	Orthopedics
Prosthesis, Knee, Femorotibial, Constrained, Metal/Polymer	Orthopedics
Prosthesis, Knee, Femorotibial, Non-Constrained	Orthopedics
Prosthesis, Knee, Femorotibial, Semi-Constrained	Orthopedics
Prosthesis, Knee, Patellofemoral, Semi-Constrained	Orthopedics
Prosthesis, Knee, Patellofemorotibial, Semi-Constrained	Orthopedics
Prosthesis, Knee, Patellofemorotibial, Semi-constrained, Metal/polymer, Mobile Bearing	Orthopedics
Prosthesis, Knee, Patfem., S-C., UHMWPE, Pegged, Unc., P/M/P	Orthopedics
Prosthesis, Knee, Patfem., S-C., Unc., Por., Ctd., P/M/P	Orthopedics
Prosthesis, Shoulder, Constr., Metal/Metal or Polymer/Cem.	Orthopedics
Prosthesis, Shoulder, Hemi-, Humeral	Orthopedics
Prosthesis, Shoulder, Humeral, Bipol., Hemi-, Constr., M/P	Orthopedics
Prosthesis, Shoulder, Metal/Polymer, Uncemented	Orthopedics
Prosthesis, Shoulder, Non-Constrained, Metal/Polymer Cem.	Orthopedics
Prosthesis, Shoulder, Semi-Constrained, Metal/Polymer Cem.	Orthopedics
Prosthesis, Toe (Metaphal.), Joint, Met./Poly., Semi-Const.	Orthopedics
Prosthesis, Upper Femoral	Orthopedics
Prosthesis, Wrist, 2 Part Metal-Plastic Articulation	Orthopedics
Prosthesis, Wrist, 3 Part Metal-Plastic-Metal Articulation	Orthopedics
Protector, Skin Pressure	General
Protractor	Orthopedics
Pump, Infusion, Elastomeric	General
Punch, Femoral Neck	Orthopedics
Pusher, Socket	Orthopedics
Rasp, Bone	Orthopedics
Rasp, Surgical, General & Plastic Surgery	Surgery
Reamer	Orthopedics
Restraint, Protective (Body)	General
Retention Device, Suture	Surgery
Retractor, Self-Retaining, Neurology	Cns/Neurology
Retractor, Surgical	Surgery
Rod, Fixation, Intramedullary	Orthopedics
Rongeur, Manual, Neurosurgical	Cns/Neurology
Rongeur, Rib	Orthopedics
Saw, Bone Cutting	Orthopedics
Saw, Manual, And Accessories	Surgery
Scissors, Orthopedic	Orthopedics
Screw, Fixation, Bone	Orthopedics
Screw, Fixation, Intraosseous	Dental And Oral
Screwdriver	Orthopedics
Shoe, Cast	Physical Med
Skid, Bone	Orthopedics
Sling, Arm	Physical Med

BIOMET, INC.   574-267-6639 (cont'd)

Sling, Arm, Overhead Supported	Physical Med
Spatula, Surgical, General & Plastic Surgery	Surgery
Splint, Abduction, Congenital Hip Dislocation	Physical Med
Splint, Clavicle	Physical Med
Splint, Denis Brown	Physical Med
Splint, Extremity, Non-Inflatable, External	Surgery
Splint, Hand, And Component	Physical Med
Splint, Nasal	Ear/Nose/Throat
Splint, Temporary Training	Physical Med
Splint, Traction	Orthopedics
Staple, Fixation, Bone	Orthopedics
Staple, Implantable	Surgery
Stereotaxy Equipment	Cns/Neurology
Stocking, Elastic	General
Stripper, Surgical	Orthopedics
Suction Apparatus, Single Patient, Portable, Non-Powered	Surgery
Supplies, Blood Bank	Hematology
Support, Arm	Physical Med
Support, Patient Position	Anesthesiology
Surgical Instrument, Orthopedic, AC-Powered Motor	Orthopedics
Surgical Instrument, Sonic	Orthopedics
Suture, Absorbable, Synthetic	Surgery
Suture, Non-Absorbable, Steel, Monofilament & Multifilament	Surgery
Suture, Non-Absorbable, Synthetic, Polyester	Surgery
Suture, Non-Absorbable, Synthetic, Polyethylene	Surgery
Syringe, Irrigating	General
Syringe, Piston	General
System, Extraction, Cement Removal	Orthopedics
Tamp	Orthopedics
Tap, Bone	Orthopedics
Tape, Measuring, Ruler And Caliper	Surgery
Template	Orthopedics
Tips And Pads, Cane, Crutch And Walker	Physical Med
Tongs, Skull, Traction	Cns/Neurology
Traction Unit, Hip, Non-Powered, Non-Penetrating	Orthopedics
Traction Unit, Non-Powered	Orthopedics
Tray, Surgical Instrument	Surgery
Trephine, Bone	Orthopedics
Tube, Cement Ventilation	Orthopedics
Twister, Wire	Orthopedics
Walker, Mechanical	Physical Med
Wrench	Orthopedics

Medical Product Subsidiaries (Listed Separately)
Biomet 3i
Biomet Canada Inc.
Biomet Microfixation Inc.
Biomet Sports Medicine
Biomet Sports Medicine, Inc
Ebi, Llc

BIOMIMETIC THERAPEUTICS, INC.   615-844-1280

389 Nichol Mill Lane, Franklin, TN 37067
FDA Number: n/a   *Fax:* 615-844-1281
E-mail: info@biomimetics.com
Web site: www.biomimetics.com
Year Founded: 2001
Total Employees: 85
Ownership: Public
Stock Symbol: BMTI
Traded On: NASDAQ
Produces/Sells CE-marked Devices: N
General Admin.: Earl Douglas/General Counsel
     Dr. Samuel E. Lynch/President, Chief Executive Officer, Director
Production: James Monsor/Vice President Operations
     John McKay/Vice President Quality Systems
     Russ Pagano/Vice President Regulatory & Clinical Affairs
Research: Leo Snel/Vice President Research & Development
Finance: Larry Bullock/Chief Financial Officer

BIOMIRA USA

See Oncothyreon Inc.

BIOMIRA, INC.

See Oncothyreon Inc.

BIOMODA INC.   505-821-0875

609 Broadway NE, Albuquerque, NM 87102
FDA Number: n/a   *Fax:* 866-519-6156
E-mail: askbiomoda@biomoda.com
Web site: www.biomoda.com
Ownership: Public
Stock Symbol: BMOD
Traded On: OTC Bulletin
Produces/Sells CE-marked Devices: N
General Admin.: Ms. Maria Zannes/Chief Executive Officer
     Mr. John Cousins/President, Chief Financial Officer
Production: Ms. Constance Dorian/Vice President Tech. Operations

BIOMOL RESEARCH LABS   800-942-0430
  5120 Butler Pike, Plymouth Meeting, PA 19462   610-941-0430
FDA Number: n/a   Fax: 610-941-9252
E-mail: info@biomol.com
Web site: www.biomol.com
Medical Products Sales Volume: $3,000,000
Total Employees: 38   *Marketing Staff:* 5   *Sales Staff:* 5
Ownership: Private
Produces/Sells CE-marked Devices: N
Federal Procurement Eligibility: Small Business
Distribution: Manufacturer Direct
General Admin.: Robert Zipkin/Chief Executive Officer
Mktg./Adv.: Ira Taffer/Vice President Sales
  Enzyme Linked Immunoabsorbent Assay, Rotavirus   Microbiology
  Enzyme, Cell (Erythrocytic And Leukocytic)   Hematology

BIONESS INC.   800-211-9136
  25103 Rye Canyon Loop, Valencia, CA 91355
FDA Number: 3004553866
Ownership: Private
Produces/Sells CE-marked Devices: N
  Stimulator, Muscle, Electrical-Powered (EMS)   Physical Med
  Stimulator, Neuromuscular, External Functional   Cns/Neurology

BIONETICS CORP.
  See Vmed Technology, Inc. (Formerly Ems Products, Inc.)

BIONETICS LTD.   800-665-9930
  1580 Beaulac St.,   514-331-9930
  St-Laurent, QUE H4R-1 Canada
FDA Number: n/a   Fax: 514-331-1498
E-mail: creitelman@aol.com
Year Founded: 1965
Total Employees: 10
Ownership: Private
Produces/Sells CE-marked Devices: N
Distribution: Exclusive Distributor

BIONEXUS INC.
  See Closure Medical

BIONICA, INC.   916-643-2222
  5112 Bailey Loop, Mcclellan, CA 95652
FDA Number: 3004435660
Ownership: Private   Fax: 916-643-2280
Produces/Sells CE-marked Devices: N
  Pump, Infusion   General

BIONIX DEVELOPMENT CORP.   800-551-7096
  5154 Enterprise Blvd., Toledo, OH 43612   419-727-8421
FDA Number: 1526854   Fax: 800-455-5678
E-mail: bionix@bionix.com
Web site: www.bionixusa.com
Medical Products Sales Volume: $4,300,000
Year Founded: 1984
Total Employees: 35
Federal Procurement Eligibility: Small Business
  Applier, Pressure, Physical Medicine   Physical Med
  Component, Cast   Orthopedics
  Curette, Ear   Ear/Nose/Throat
  ENT Drug Applicator   Ear/Nose/Throat
  Forceps, General & Plastic Surgery   Surgery
  Holder, Head, Radiographic   Radiology
  Housing, X-Ray Tube, Therapeutic   Radiology
  Joint, Knee, External Limb Component   Physical Med
  Light, Examination, Battery-Powered   General
  Locator, Bleeding, Gastrointestinal, String And Tube   Gastroenterology/Urology
  Pack, Hot Or Cold, Reusable   Physical Med
  Radiotherapy Unit, Charged-Particle   Radiology
  Speculum, Ear   Ear/Nose/Throat
  Syringe, Ear   Ear/Nose/Throat
  Syringe, Irrigating   General
  Tester, Radiology   Radiology
  Therapeutic X-Ray System   Radiology
  Transfer Device, Patient, Manual   General

BIONOSTICS, INC.   978-772-7070
  7 Jackson Rd., Devens, MA 01434
FDA Number: 1220649
Ownership: Private
Produces/Sells CE-marked Devices: N
  Buffer, pH   Hematology
  Control, Analyte (Assayed And Unassayed)   Chemistry
  Control, Blood Gas   Chemistry
  Control, Electrolyte (Assayed And Unassayed)   Chemistry
  Control, Multi Analyte, All Kinds (Assayed And Unassayed)   Chemistry
  Electrode, Ion Specific, Potassium   Chemistry
  Hematocrit Control   Hematology
  Hematology Quality Control Mixture   Hematology
  Labware, Blood Collection   Chemistry

BIONOSTICS, INC.   978-772-7070 *(cont'd)*
  Standard/Control, Hemoglobin, Normal/Abnormal   Hematology
  Tonometer (Calibration And Q.C. Of Blood Gas Instruments)   Chemistry
  Tube, Capillary Blood Collection   Hematology

BIOO SCIENTIFIC CORPORATION   512-707-8993
  3913 Todd Lane, Suite 312, Austin, TX 78744
FDA Number: n/a   Fax: 512-707-2051
E-mail: info@biooscientific.com
Ownership: Private
Produces/Sells CE-marked Devices: N

BIOPACIFIC DIAGNOSTIC INC.   800-267-5800
  114 - 828 Harbourside Drive,   604-985-7000
  North Vancouver, BC V7P 3 Canada
FDA Number: n/a   Fax: 604-985-3366
E-mail: biopacific@telus.net
Web site: www.biopacific.ne
Year Founded: 1982
Ownership: Private
Produces/Sells CE-marked Devices: N

BIOPHASE DIAGNOSTIC LABORATORIES   905-567-9165
  6625 Kitimat Rd., Unit 51, Mississauga, ONT L5N-6J1 Canada
FDA Number: n/a   Fax: 905-567-9021
Year Founded: 1989
Total Employees: 10
Ownership: SUM PHASE TRADING INC.
Produces/Sells CE-marked Devices: N
Distribution: Manufacturer Direct, Exclusive Distributor

BIOPHYSIC MEDICAL INC.
  See Alcon Research, Ltd.

BIOPHYSICA INC.   416-766-9333
  67 Constance St., Toront, ONT M6R-1S5 Canada
FDA Number: n/a   Fax: 416-766-0676
E-mail: info@biophysica.com
Web site: www.biophysica.com
Year Founded: 1989
Total Employees: 10
Ownership: Private
Produces/Sells CE-marked Devices: N
Distribution: Manufacturer Direct, Exclusive Distributor

BIOPLASTICS CO.   800-487-2358
  34655 Mills Rd., N. Ridgeville, OH 44039
FDA Number: 1531145
  Restraint, Protective (Body)   General

BIOPLATE, INC.   310-815-2100
  3643 Lenawee Ave., Los Angeles, CA 90016-4310
FDA Number: 2029447   Fax: 310-815-2126
Web site: www.bioplate.com
Ownership: Private
Produces/Sells CE-marked Devices: N
Federal Procurement Eligibility: Female Owned
  Battery, Replacement, Rechargeable   Surgery
  Cover, Burr Hole (Cranial)   Cns/Neurology
  Motor, Surgical Instrument, AC-Powered   Surgery
  Plate, Bone, Orthodontic   Dental And Oral
  Plate, Bone, Skull, Preformed, Non-Alterable   Cns/Neurology
  Plate, Fixation, Bone   Orthopedics
  Screw, Fixation, Intraosseous   Dental And Oral
  Shunt, Central Nerve, With Component   Cns/Neurology
  Surgical Instrument, Non-Powered, Neurosurgical   Cns/Neurology
  Tap, Bone   Orthopedics

BIOPRO, INC.   800-252-7707
  2929 Lapeer Rd., Port Huron, MI 48060-4101   810-982-7777
FDA Number: 1833506   Fax: 810-982-7794
E-mail: info@bioproimplants.com
Web site: www.bioproimplants.com
Medical Products Sales Volume: $4,800,000
Year Founded: 1987
Total Employees: 20   *Marketing Staff:* 2   *Sales Staff:* 100
Ownership: Private
Quality System Registration Information: ISO9001
Produces/Sells CE-marked Devices: Y
Federal Procurement Eligibility: Small Business
Distribution: Manufacturer Direct, Manufacturer Through Distributor, Manufacturer Through Manufacturer Reps, OEM, Exporter
General Admin.: Patrick Pringle/Chief Executive Officer
Mktg./Adv.: Stephen Erdner/Director National Marketing & Sales
         David Mrak/Director New Product Development
  Appliance, Fix., Nail/Blade/Plate Comb., Multiple Component   Orthopedics
  Guide   Orthopedics
  Prosthesis, Elbow, Total   Orthopedics
  Prosthesis, Hip, Femoral, Resurfacing   Orthopedics

BIOPRO, INC.   800-252-7707 *(cont'd)*

Prosthesis, Hip, Semi-constrained, Metal/ceramic/polymer, Cemented Or Non-porous Cemented, Osteophilic Finish	Orthopedics
Prosthesis, Knee, Total	Orthopedics
Prosthesis, Shoulder	Orthopedics
Prosthesis, Toe, Hemi-, Phalangeal	Orthopedics
Rod, Fixation, Intramedullary	Orthopedics
Support, Patient Position, Radiographic	Radiology

BIOPROCESSING, INC.   207-615-0571
1045 Riverside St, Portland, ME 04103
FDA Number: n/a
E-mail: info@bioprocessinginc.com   *Fax:* 202-553-2523
Web site: www.bioprocessinginc.com
Annual Revenue: $1-$5 Million
Year Founded: 1991
Total Employees: 50   *Marketing Staff:* 1   *Sales Staff:* 2
Ownership: Private
Quality System Registration Information: ISO9001
Produces/Sells CE-marked Devices: N
Federal Procurement Eligibility: Small Business
Distribution: Manufacturer Direct, Manufacturer Through Distributor, OEM, Exporter
General Admin.: Mrs. Kathi Daigle/Director, General Manager
Mktg./Adv.: Mrs. Karen Bracy/Director Product Development

Control, Multi Analyte, All Kinds (Assayed And Unassayed)	Chemistry

BIOPTICS, INC.   800.477.8985 / 520-3998180
3440 e. britannia dr. suite 150,
Tucson, AZ 85714
FDA Number: 3004855195
E-mail: sales@bioptic-inc.com   *Fax:* 520.399.8182
Web site: www.bioptics-inc.com
Year Founded: 2001
Ownership: Private
Produces/Sells CE-marked Devices: N
General Admin.: Hugh Cormican/Chief Executive Officer

Cabinet, X-ray System	Radiology

BIOQUEST PROSTHETICS   661-325-3338
412 18th St., Bakersfield, CA 93304
FDA Number: 3005238868
E-mail: bioquest@bioquestpros.com   *Fax:* 661-325-3338
Web site: www.bioquestpros.com
Ownership: Private
Produces/Sells CE-marked Devices: N

Ankle/Foot, External Limb Component	Physical Med

BIOQUIP, INC.
See Bioscience Contract Production Corp.

BIORAD LABORATORIES   800-2BI-ORAD / 510-724-7000
1000 Alfred Nobel Drive, Hercules, CA 94547
FDA Number: 2939715   *Fax:* 510-741-5815
Web site: http://www.bio-rad.com
Total Employees: 2500   *Marketing Staff:* 25   *Sales Staff:* 75
Ownership: Biorad Laboratories
Traded On: AMEX
Quality System Registration Information: ISO9001
Produces/Sells CE-marked Devices: N
Federal Procurement Eligibility: GSA Contract, VA Contract
Distribution: Manufacturer Direct
General Admin.: Mr. David Schwartz/Chairman
    Ms. Christina Tsingos/Chief Financial Officer, Vice President
    Mr. Norman Schwartz/President, Chief Executive Officer
    Mr. Brad Crutchfield/Vice President
Mktg./Adv.: Mr. Giovanni Magni/Vice President International Sales

Test, Antibody, Acquired Immune Deficiency Syndrome (AIDS)	Hematology
Test, Glycosylated Hemoglobin Assay	Hematology

Medical Product Subsidiaries (Listed Separately)
Biorad Laboratories

BIORELIANCE   800-553-5372 / 301-738-1000
14920 Broschart Road, Rockville, MD 20850
FDA Number: n/a   *Fax:* 301-738-1036
E-mail: info@bioreliance.com
Web site: www.bioreliance.com
Medical Products Sales Volume: $36,500,000
Annual Revenue: $50-$100 Million
Year Founded: 1947
Total Employees: 700   *Marketing Staff:* 6   *Sales Staff:* 13
Ownership: Private
Produces/Sells CE-marked Devices: N
Distribution: Manufacturer Direct, Service Direct
General Admin.: Capers McDonald/Chief Executive Officer
    Michael Wiebe/Chief Scientific Officer
    Ralph Adams/Director Human Resources
    John McEntire/President

BIORELIANCE   800-553-5372 *(cont'd)*
Mktg./Adv.: N. Bakowski/Director Sales
    Anne Derrick/Manager Market Research
Production: Claire Courtemanche/Director Quality Assurance
    Gail Sofer/Director Regulatory Affairs
    John Gilly/Vice President Manufacturing
Finance: Patrick Spratt/Chief Financial Officer, Senior Vice President Finance

Equipment/Service, Quality Control	General
Test, DNA-Probe, Other	Microbiology

BIORESOURCE TECHNOLOGY, INC.   954-792-5222
11924 Miramar Pkwy., Flamingo Park Of Commerce,
Miramar, FL 33025
FDA Number: 1058931

Control, Multi Analyte, All Kinds (Assayed And Unassayed)	Chemistry
Standard/Control, Hemoglobin, Normal/Abnormal	Hematology

BIOSCALE INC.   781-430-6800
4 Maguire Street, Lexington, MA 02421
FDA Number: n/a   *Fax:* 781-430-6801
E-mail: info@bioscale.com
Web site: http://www.bioscale.com
Ownership: Private
Produces/Sells CE-marked Devices: N
General Admin.: Mr. Mark Lundstrum/Chief Executive Officer
    Mr. Chip Leveille/Chief Operating Officer
    Mr. Brett Masters/Chief Technology Officer
Research: Dr. Michael Miller/Vice President Product Development

BIOSCAN CONTINENTAL INC.   450-974-0151
350 Industriel Blvd., 2nd Floor,
St-Eustache, QUE J7R-5 Canada
FDA Number: n/a   *Fax:* 450-491-3069
E-mail: bioscan@dsuper.net
Web site: www.bioscancontinental.com
Year Founded: 1981
Total Employees: 10
Ownership: Private
Produces/Sells CE-marked Devices: N
Distribution: Manufacturer Direct, Exclusive Distributor, Exporter

BIOSCAN, INC.   800-255-7226 / 202-338-0974
4590 MacArthur Blvd., Washington, DC 20007
FDA Number: n/a   *Fax:* 202-333-8514
E-mail: sales@bioscan.com
Web site: www.bioscan.com
Medical Products Sales Volume: $2,200,000
Annual Revenue: $1-$5 Million
Year Founded: 1980
Total Employees: 22   *Marketing Staff:* 1   *Sales Staff:* 5
Ownership: Private
Produces/Sells CE-marked Devices: Y
Federal Procurement Eligibility: Small Business, GSA Contract
Distribution: Manufacturer Direct
General Admin.: Seth D. Shulman/President
    Ted Kleinman/President, Chief Operating Officer
Mktg./Adv.: Victor Cao/Director Marketing
    Shell B. Shetti/Vice President Marketing & Sales

Counter, Gamma, General Use	Toxicology

BIOSCIENCE CONTRACT PRODUCTION CORP.   410-563-9200
5901 E. Lombard Street, Baltimore, MD 21224
FDA Number: n/a   *Fax:* 410-563-9206
E-mail: info@bscp.com
Web site: www.bscp.com
Year Founded: 1990
Total Employees: 115   *Marketing Staff:* 1   *Sales Staff:* 2
Ownership: Private
Quality System Registration Information: ISO9002
Distribution: Service Direct
General Admin.: Jaques Rubin/Chief Executive Officer
    Steven Rubin/President
Mktg./Adv.: Stan Zeichner/Director National Accounts

Fermentation Equipment	Microbiology

BIOSCREEN MEDICAL INC.   570-928-7636
Rr I Box 1045a, Mildred, PA 18632
FDA Number: 3005416220
Ownership: Private
Produces/Sells CE-marked Devices: N

Kit, Pregnancy Test, Over The Counter, HCG	Chemistry

BIOSCULPTURE TECHNOLOGY, INC.   212-977-5400
40 Central Park South, New York, NY 10019
FDA Number: 3004199046   *Fax:* 561-651-7808
E-mail: info@biosculpturetechnology.com
Web site: www.biosculpturetechnology.com
Ownership: Private

BIOSCULPTURE TECHNOLOGY, INC. 212-977-5400 *(cont'd)*
Produces/Sells CE-marked Devices: N
System, Suction, Lipoplasty — Surgery

BIOSEAL 800-441-7325
167 W. Orangethorpe Avenue, 714-528-4695
Placentia, CA 92870
FDA Number: 2027062 *Fax:* 714-528-8434
E-mail: Sales@biosealnet.com
Web site: www.biosealnet.com
Medical Products Sales Volume: $3,700,000
Annual Revenue: $1-$5 Million
Year Founded: 1988
Total Employees: 40 *Sales Staff:* 8
Ownership: Private
Produces/Sells CE-marked Devices: N
Federal Procurement Eligibility: Small Business
Distribution: Manufacturer Direct, Manufacturer Through Distributor, Manufacturer Through Manufacturer Reps, OEM
General Admin.: Mr. William L. Runion/President, Chief Executive Officer
Mktg./Adv.: Mr. Kevin Cannan/Vice President Sales
Production: Ms. Martha Reyes/Manager Operations
Mr. Mark McAnallen/Manager Quality Assurance & Regulatory Affairs

Applicator, Tipped, Absorbent	General
Ball, Cotton	General
Band, Elastic, Orthodontic	Dental And Oral
Bandage, Elastic	General
Contract Packaging	General
Dressing, Other	General
Fiber, Absorbent	General
Fixation Device, Tracheal Tube	Anesthesiology
Gauze, Non-Absorbable, Non-Medicated (Internal Sponge)	Surgery
Gauze, Non-Absorbable, X-Ray Detectable (Internal Sponge)	Surgery
Kit, Instruments and Accessories, Surgical	Surgery
Kit, Surgical Instrument, Disposable	Surgery
Padding, Cast/Splint	General
Stockinette	Orthopedics

BIOSEARCH MEDICAL PRODUCTS, INC. 908-722-5000
35 Industrial Pkwy., Branchburg, NJ 08876
FDA Number: 2242547 *Fax:* 908-722-5024
E-mail: jnewmcdyck@hydromer.com
Web site: www.biosearch.com
Year Founded: 1975
Ownership: Private
Produces/Sells CE-marked Devices: N

Analyzer, Coagulation, Semi-Automated	Hematology
Biofeedback Device	Cns/Neurology
Catheter, Biliary	Gastroenterology/Urology
Catheter, Upper Urinary Tract	Gastroenterology/Urology
Catheter, Urological	Gastroenterology/Urology
Electrosurgical Unit, Cutting & Coagulation Device	Surgery
Tube, Feeding	General
Tube, Gastrointestinal	Gastroenterology/Urology
Tube, Nasogastric	Anesthesiology

BIOSENSE CORPORATION 215-348-2977
450 East Street, Doylestown, PA 18901
FDA Number: 3006264427
Ownership: Private
Produces/Sells CE-marked Devices: N

Fertility Diagnostic Device	Obstetrics/Gynecology
Viscometer, Mucus, Cervical	Obstetrics/Gynecology

BIOSENSE WEBSTER 800-729-9010
15715 Arrow Hwy, Irwindale, CA 91706 909-839-8500
FDA Number: 2029046 *Fax:* 909-468-2905
E-mail: CustServ@bwius.jnj.com
Web site: www.biosensewebster.com
Medical Products Sales Volume: $200,000,000
Year Founded: 1978
Total Employees: 150
Ownership: Johnson & Johnson
Produces/Sells CE-marked Devices: N
Federal Procurement Eligibility: Small Business

Catheter, Electrode Recording, Or Probe	Cardiovascular
Catheter, Flow Directed	Cardiovascular
Catheter, Percutaneous	Cardiovascular
Introducer, Catheter	Cardiovascular

BIOSENSE WEBSTER, INC 800-729-9010
3333 Diamond Canyon Road, 909-839-8500
Diamond Bar, CA 91765
FDA Number: 2020638 *Fax:* 909-468-2905
Ownership: Johnson & Johnson
Quality System Registration Information: ISO9001
Produces/Sells CE-marked Devices: Y
Distribution: Manufacturer Direct, Exporter
General Admin.: Dan Simpson/Chief Financial Officer, Vice President

BIOSENSE WEBSTER, INC 800-729-9010 *(cont'd)*
Roy Tanaka/President, Chief Executive Officer
Heather Hand/Vice President Human Resources
Mktg./Adv.: Rob Pike/Director Product Development
Betty Russell/Vice President Marketing

Catheter, Electrode Recording, Or Probe	Cardiovascular
Catheter, Other	Gastroenterology/Urology

BIOSENSORS INTERNATIONAL - USA 949-553-8300
20280 Acacia St., Suite 300, Newport Beach, CA 92660
FDA Number: 2084493 *Fax:* 949-553-9129
E-mail: sales@biosensors-usa.com
Web site: www.biosensors.com
Medical Products Sales Volume: $3,300,000
Annual Revenue: $25-$50 Million
Year Founded: 1990
Total Employees: 44 *Marketing Staff:* 25 *Sales Staff:* 15
Ownership: Private
Quality System Registration Information: ISO9001
Produces/Sells CE-marked Devices: Y
Federal Procurement Eligibility: Small Business, Minority Owned, GSA Contract, VA Contract
Distribution: Manufacturer Direct, Manufacturer Through Distributor, Manufacturer Through Manufacturer Reps, OEM, Service Direct, Exclusive Distributor, Importer, Exporter
General Admin.: Yoh Chie Lu/President, Chief Executive Officer
Mktg./Adv.: Chee Mun Loh/Director New Business Development
Dennis Bassett/Manager Sales
Keith Garmon/Manager Sales
Production: Doug Savage/Director Engineering
Jorge Haider/Director Regulatory Affairs
Thuy Tran/Manager Materials
Scott Olson/Vice President Operations
Research: John Shulze/Vice President, Director Research & Development
Finance: Joe Blow/Accountant
Ron Lung/Controller

Balloon, Angioplasty, Coronary, Heated	Cardiovascular
Catheter, Cardiac Thermodilution	Cardiovascular
Catheter, Embolectomy (Fogarty Type)	Cardiovascular
Catheter, Flow Directed	Cardiovascular
Catheter, Thermal Dilution	Cardiovascular
Kit, Sampling, Blood	General
Stent, Cardiovascular	Cardiovascular
Transducer, Blood Pressure	General

BIOSENTIENT CORPORATION -
700 Gemini St. Suite 210, Houston, TX 77058
FDA Number: 3004483567
Ownership: Private
Produces/Sells CE-marked Devices: N

Biofeedback Device	Cns/Neurology

BIOSERV CORPORATION 858-450-3123
5340 Eastgate Mall, San Diego, CA 92121-2804
FDA Number: 2027352 *Fax:* 858-450-0785
E-mail: info@bioservcorp.com
Web site: www.bioservcorp.com
Medical Products Sales Volume: $5,100,000
Annual Revenue: $25-$50 Million
Year Founded: 1988
Total Employees: 45 *Marketing Staff:* 3 *Sales Staff:* 2
Ownership: Private
Quality System Registration Information: ISO9002
Produces/Sells CE-marked Devices: Y
Federal Procurement Eligibility: Small Business
Distribution: OEM
General Admin.: Jeanne M. Dunham/President, Chief Executive Officer
Sheanett Lett/Supervisor
Mktg./Adv.: Lee Starr/Director Business Development
Production: Dan Juntunen/Director Manufacturing
Mary Richardson/Director Quality Assurance
Janes Walter/Manager Materials
Finance: H. Glenn Dunham/Chief Financial Officer
Purchasing: John Manahan/Purchasing Agent

Contract Manufacturing	General
Contract Packaging	General

BIOSIG INSTRUMENTS INC. 800-463-5470
440 19th Ave., Ste. 100, 514-637-0016
Lachine, QUE H8S-3 Canada
FDA Number: n/a *Fax:* 514-637-1353
E-mail: biosig@biosig.net
Web site: http://www.biosiginstruments.com
Year Founded: 1977
Total Employees: 25
Ownership: Private
Produces/Sells CE-marked Devices: N

BIOSIG INSTRUMENTS INC. 800-463-5470 (cont'd)
Distribution: Manufacturer Direct, Exporter

BIOSIG INSTRUMENTS, INC. 800-463-5470
P.O. Box 860, Champlain, NY 12919 **514-637-0016**
FDA Number: n/a *Fax:* 514-637-1353
E-mail: biosig@biosig.net
Web site: www.biosiginstruments.com
Total Employees: 8
Ownership: Private
Produces/Sells CE-marked Devices: N
Federal Procurement Eligibility: Small Business
Distribution: Manufacturer Direct, Manufacturer Through Manufacturer Reps, OEM
General Admin.: Gregory Lekhtman/President, Chief Executive Officer

Biofeedback Device	Cns/Neurology
Contract Manufacturing	General
Monitor, Heart Rate, R-Wave (ECG)	Cardiovascular

BIOSIGNETICS CORPORATION 603-858-3844
29 Downing Ct., Exeter, NH 03833
FDA Number: 3004512425 *Fax:* 603 772-8706
Ownership: Private
Produces/Sells CE-marked Devices: N

Phonocardiograph	Cardiovascular

BIOSITE INCORPORATED 888-246-7483
9975 Summers Ridge Rd, San Diego, CA 92121 **858-805-3423**
FDA Number: 2027969
E-mail: custservice@biosite.com
Web site: www.biosite.com
Ownership: Alere, Inc.
Produces/Sells CE-marked Devices: N
General Admin.: Kim Blickenstaff/Chief Executive Officer, Chairman
　　　　　Gary King/Vice President International Operations
Medical Admin.: Norman Paradis/Vice President Medical Affairs
Mktg./Adv.: Sarah Gunhouse/Vice President U.S. Sales
Finance: John Cajigas/Vice President Finance

Antigen, Antiserum, Control, Myoglobin	Immunology
Antigen, Antiserum, Fibrinogen And Fibrin Split Products	Immunology
Antigen, Latex Agglutination, Entamoeba Histolytica & Rel.	Microbiology
Calibrator, Secondary, Clinical Chemistry	Chemistry
Chromatography, Thin Layer, Tricyclic Antidepressant Drugs	Toxicology
Colorimeter, General Use	Chemistry
Colorimetric Method, CPK Or Isoenzymes	Chemistry
Colorimetry, Acetaminophen	Toxicology
Control, Analyte (Assayed And Unassayed)	Chemistry
Control, Coagulation, Plasma	Hematology
Control, Drug Mixture	Toxicology
Control, Multi Analyte, All Kinds (Assayed And Unassayed)	Chemistry
Cryptosporidium Spp.	Microbiology
Enzymatic Esterase-Oxidase, Cholesterol	Chemistry
Enzyme Immunoassay, Amphetamine	Toxicology
Enzyme Immunoassay, Barbiturate	Toxicology
Enzyme Immunoassay, Benzodiazepine	Toxicology
Enzyme Immunoassay, Cannabinoids	Toxicology
Enzyme Immunoassay, Cocaine	Toxicology
Enzyme Immunoassay, Cocaine And Cocaine Metabolites	Toxicology
Enzyme Immunoassay, Methadone	Toxicology
Enzyme Immunoassay, Opiates	Toxicology
Enzyme Immunoassay, Phencyclidine	Toxicology
Enzyme Immunoassay, Propoxyphene	Toxicology
Fibrin Split Products	Hematology
Fluorometer, Chemistry	Chemistry
Fluorometric Method, CPK Or Isoenzymes	Chemistry
Gas Chromatography, Methamphetamine	Toxicology
Giardia Spp.	Microbiology
Hydrazone Colorimetry, Aldolase	Chemistry
Liquid Chromatography, Morphine	Toxicology
Radioimmunoassay, Luteinizing Hormone	Chemistry
Reagent, Clostridium Difficile Toxin	Microbiology
System, Test, Drugs of Abuse	Chemistry
Test, C-Reactive Protein	Immunology
Test, Natriuretic Peptide	Chemistry
Test, Qualitative And Quantitative Factor Deficiency	Hematology
Thin Layer Chromatography, Metamphetamine	Toxicology

BIOSOFT INTERNATIONAL CORP. 215-295-0088
102 West Bridge St., Morrisville, PA 19067
FDA Number: n/a *Fax:* 215-295-0899
E-mail: info@biosoft.com
Web site: www.biosoft.com
Ownership: Private
Produces/Sells CE-marked Devices: N

Base, Denture, Relining, Repairing, Rebasing, Resin	Dental And Oral

BIOSONICS, INC. 215-646-7100
260 New York Drive, Fort Washington, PA 19034-2491
FDA Number: 2245553 *Fax:* 215-646-3364
E-mail: biosonics@biosonics.com
Web site: http://www.biosonics.com

BIOSONICS, INC. 215-646-7100 (cont'd)
Medical Products Sales Volume: $20,000,000
Annual Revenue: $10-$25 Million
Total Employees: 7 *Marketing Staff:* 1 *Sales Staff:* 2
Ownership: IMRC
Stock Symbol: BISN
Traded On: OTC Bulletin
Quality System Registration Information: ISO9001
Produces/Sells CE-marked Devices: N
Federal Procurement Eligibility: Small Business
Distribution: Manufacturer Direct
General Admin.: Jack Paller/President, Chief Executive Officer
　　　　　Sandra Pileggi/Vice President, General Manager
Mktg./Adv.: Alice Cavallaro/Director Product Development

Device, Incontinence, Fecal	Gastroenterology/Urology
Ejector, Saliva	Ear/Nose/Throat

BIOSOUND ESAOTE, INC. 800-428-4374
8000 Castleway Drive, **317-813-6000**
Indianapolis, IN 46250
FDA Number: 1826555 *Fax:* 317-813-6600
E-mail: info@biosound.com
Web site: www.biosound.com
Medical Products Sales Volume: $7,100,000
Annual Revenue: $25-$50 Million
Year Founded: 1979
Total Employees: 75 *Marketing Staff:* 8 *Sales Staff:* 18
Ownership: Esaote Spa
Quality System Registration Information: ISO9001
Produces/Sells CE-marked Devices: Y
Federal Procurement Eligibility: Small Business
Distribution: Manufacturer Through Distributor, Manufacturer Through Manufacturer Reps
General Admin.: Fabrizio Landi/Chairman
　　　　　Tom Feick/Chief Financial Officer, Executive Vice President
　　　　　Claudio Bertolini/President
Mktg./Adv.: Jim Chapman/Director Product Marketing
Production: Alan Voils/Director Quality Assurance
　　　　　Adam Koneski/Director Services

Echocardiograph (Ultrasonic Scanner)	Cardiovascular
Scanner, Ultrasonic (Pulsed Echo)	Radiology
Scanner, Ultrasonic, Abdominal	Radiology
Scanner, Ultrasonic, Obstetrical/Gynecological, Mobile	Obstetrics/Gynecology
Scanner, Ultrasonic, Small Parts	Radiology
Scanner, Ultrasonic, Vascular	Radiology

BIOSOURCE INTERNATIONAL INCORPORATED, 800-242-0607
ROCKVILLE DI
1106 Taft Street, Rockville, MD 20850
FDA Number: 3004976189
Ownership: Private
Produces/Sells CE-marked Devices: N

Culture Media, Non-Selective And Non-Differential	Microbiology

BIOSOURCE INTERNATIONAL, INC.
See Invitrogen Corporation

BIOSPACE MED 866-933-5301
120 Interstate N. Pkwy, Ste 116, **678-564-5400**
Atlanta, GA 30339
FDA Number: n/a *Fax:* 678-564-5399
E-mail: info-USA@biospacemed.com
Year Founded: 1989
Ownership: Private
Produces/Sells CE-marked Devices: N
General Admin.: Dr. Marie Meynadier/Chief Executive Officer

BIOSPAN TECHNOLOGIES, INC. 800-730-8980
6540 Meyer Dr., Washington, MO 63090 **636-583-7974**
FDA Number: 1954588 *Fax:* 636-583-1773
E-mail: info@biospantech.com
Web site: www.biospantech.com
Ownership: Private
Produces/Sells CE-marked Devices: N

Medical Disinfectants/Cleaners for Instruments	General

BIOSPHERE MEDICAL, INC.
See BIOSPHERE MEDICAL, INC.

BIOSTAR MEDICAL PRODUCTS INC.
See Thermo Biostar, Inc.

BIOSTRUCTURES, LLC 949-553-1743
3700 Campus Dr. Suite 204, Newport Beach, CA 92660
FDA Number: 3005449756 *Fax:* 949-553-0407
E-mail: mail@biostructures.net
Ownership: Private
Produces/Sells CE-marked Devices: N

BIOSTRUCTURES, LLC 949-553-1743 *(cont'd)*
Filler, Calcium Sulfate Preformed Pellets — Orthopedics

BIOSURE, INC. 800-345-2267
12301 Loma Rica Drive, Suite G, 530-273-5095
Grass Valley, CA 95945
FDA Number: 2938656 *Fax:* 530-273-5097
E-mail: comments@biosure.com
Web site: www.biosure.com
Medical Products Sales Volume: $500,000
Annual Revenue: $0-$1 Million
Year Founded: 1986
Total Employees: 5 *Marketing Staff:* 1 *Sales Staff:* 1
Ownership: Private
Produces/Sells CE-marked Devices: N
Federal Procurement Eligibility: Small Business
Distribution: Manufacturer Direct, Manufacturer Through Manufacturer Reps
General Admin.: Richard Riese/President, Chief Executive Officer
Mktg./Adv.: Marian Hirsch/Director Marketing
Calibrator, Cell Indices — Hematology
Contract Packaging — General
Diluent, Blood Cell — Hematology
Service, Consulting — General
Stain, Dye Solution — Pathology
Sterilization Process Indicator, Physical/Chemical — General

BIOSURFACE TECHNOLOGY, INC.
See Genzyme Corp.

BIOSURPLUS INC. 858-550-0800
10805 Vista Sorrento Pkwy, #200, San Diego, CA 92121
FDA Number: n/a *Fax:* 858-550-0255
E-mail: info@biosurplus.com
Web site: http://www.biosurplus.com
Year Founded: 2003
Ownership: Private
Produces/Sells CE-marked Devices: N
General Admin.: Mr. Arlen Greer/Chief Technology Officer
Mr. Preston Plumb/President, Chief Executive Officer
Mktg./Adv.: Mr. Fred Hill/Vice President Marketing
Production: Ms. Anggie Becorest/Vice President Operations
Finance: Ms. Kathy Scott/Chief Financial Officer

BIOSYNERGY, INC. 800-255-5274
1940 E. Devon Ave., Elk Grove Village, IL 60007 847-956-0471
FDA Number: 1419300 *Fax:* 847-956-6050
E-mail: bsi@icsp.net
Web site: www.biosynergyinc.com
Annual Revenue: $0-$1 Million
Total Employees: 5 *Marketing Staff:* 2 *Sales Staff:* 2
Ownership: Public
Produces/Sells CE-marked Devices: N
Federal Procurement Eligibility: Small Business
Distribution: Manufacturer Direct, Manufacturer Through Distributor, OEM, Exporter
General Admin.: Fred K. Suzuki/President, Chief Executive Officer
Mktg./Adv.: Mary K. Friske/Vice President Marketing Admin.
Production: Larry Mead/Vice President Manufacturing
Monitor, Temperature (Self-Contained) — General
Temperature Strip, Forehead, Liquid Crystal — General
Thermometer, Electronic — General
Thermometer, Liquid Crystals — Surgery

BIOTEC, INC. 616-772-2133
652 East Main Street, Zeeland, MI 49464
FDA Number: 1824362 *Fax:* 616-772-4320
Web site: www.royaldentalgroup.com
Annual Revenue: $1-$5 Million
Ownership: Royal Dental Manufacturing, Inc.
Produces/Sells CE-marked Devices: N
Federal Procurement Eligibility: Small Business
Distribution: Manufacturer Direct
Cabinet, Dental — Dental And Oral
Cuspidor — Dental And Oral
Operative Dental Treatment Unit — Dental And Oral

BIOTECH
See Consolidated Technologies, Inc.

BIOTECH ATLANTIC, INC. 732-389-4789
Bay F, 6 Industrial Way West, Eatontown, NJ 07724
FDA Number: 2248024 *Fax:* 732-389-3837
E-mail: biotechatlantic@verizon.net
Web site: www.lidelabs.com
Ownership: Private
Produces/Sells CE-marked Devices: N
Kit, Pregnancy Test, Over The Counter, HCG — Chemistry
Radioimmunoassay, Human Chorionic Gonadotropin — Chemistry

BIOTECH ATLANTIC, INC. 732-389-4789 *(cont'd)*
Radioimmunoassay, Luteinizing Hormone — Chemistry

BIOTECHNOLOGY DEVELOPMENT CORP.
See Microfluidics International Corporation

BIOTECX LABORATORIES, INC. 800-535-6286
15225 Gulf Hwy, #F106, Houston, TX 77034 713-643-0606
FDA Number: n/a *Fax:* 713-643-3143
E-mail: biotecx@aol.com
Web site: www.biotecx.com
Annual Revenue: $1-$5 Million
Year Founded: 1985
Total Employees: 10
Ownership: Private
Produces/Sells CE-marked Devices: N
Federal Procurement Eligibility: Small Business, Minority Owned
Distribution: Manufacturer Direct, Manufacturer Through Distributor, OEM, Exporter
General Admin.: Mohan Mehra/President
Buffer, pH — Hematology
Enzyme Immunoassay, Non-Radiolabeled, Total Thyroxine — Chemistry
Enzyme Immunoassay, Other — Chemistry
Radioimmunoassay, Other — Chemistry
Test, DNA-Probe, Other — Microbiology

BIOTEK INSTRUMENTS, INC. 888-451-5171
100 Tigan Street, P.O. Box 998, Highland Park, 802-655-4040
Winooski, VT 05404
FDA Number: 1217454 *Fax:* 802-655-7941
E-mail: customercare@biotek.com
Web site: www.biotek.com
Ownership: Private
Produces/Sells CE-marked Devices: N
Alarm, Leakage Current, Portable — Cardiovascular
Analyzer, Pacemaker Generator Function — Cardiovascular
Colorimeter, General Use — Chemistry
Electrocardiograph, Single Channel — Cardiovascular
Fluorometer, Chemistry — Chemistry
Monitor, Blood Pressure, Indirect, Semi-Automatic — Cardiovascular
Monitor, Cardiac (Cardiotachometer & Rate Alarm) — Cardiovascular
Oximeter, Intracardiac — Cardiovascular
Pipetting And Diluting System, Automated — Chemistry
Tester, Defibrillator — Cardiovascular
Transducer, Blood Pressure, Extravascular — Cardiovascular

BIOTEK, INC. 800-269-2918
PO Box 2216, West Lafayette, IN 47996-2216 765-497-9415
FDA Number: n/a *Fax:* 765-497-0092
E-mail: sales@biotekcases.com
Web site: www.biotekcases.com
Medical Products Sales Volume: $100,000
Annual Revenue: $0-$1 Million
Year Founded: 1980
Total Employees: 6 *Marketing Staff:* 1 *Sales Staff:* 1
Ownership: Private
Produces/Sells CE-marked Devices: N
Federal Procurement Eligibility: Small Business, GSA Contract
Distribution: Manufacturer Direct, Manufacturer Through Manufacturer Reps
General Admin.: Andrew Thomas/Chief Executive Officer
Mktg./Adv.: Andrew Thomas/Manager Advertising
Andrew Thomas/Vice President Marketing & Sales
Production: Andrew Thomas/Vice President Manufacturing
Bag, Medical, Physician — General

BIOTELEMETRICS, INC. 561-394-0315
6520 Contempo Ln., Boca Raton, FL 33433-6635
FDA Number: n/a *Fax:* 561-394-0315
E-mail: biotran@ix.netcom.com
Web site: www.biotelemetrics.com
Medical Products Sales Volume: $100,000
Annual Revenue: $0-$1 Million
Year Founded: 1981
Ownership: Private
Produces/Sells CE-marked Devices: N
Federal Procurement Eligibility: Small Business, VA Contract
Distribution: Manufacturer Direct
General Admin.: Carl C. Enger/President
Mktg./Adv.: William J. Enger/Vice President Business Development
Telemetry Unit, Physiological, ECG — Cardiovascular

BIOTEMPS DENTAL LABORATORY 949-440-2683
2181 Dupont Dr., Irvine, CA 92612
FDA Number: 2031503
Device, Anti-Snoring — Ear/Nose/Throat

BIOTEST DIAGNOSTIC CORP. 800-522-0090
400 Commons Way, Rockaway, NJ 07866
FDA Number: 2246961 *Fax:* 973-625-9454

BIOTEST DIAGNOSTIC CORP.   800-522-0090 (cont'd)
E-mail: customerservice@biotestusa.com
Web site: www.biotestusa.com
Year Founded: 1980
Ownership: BIOTEST AG
Quality System Registration Information: ISO9001
Produces/Sells CE-marked Devices: Y
Distribution: Manufacturer Direct, Importer, Exporter
General Admin.: Bill Weiss/President
      Candance Williams/Vice President
Mktg./Adv.: Ken Troia/Director Marketing
Production: Shari States/Product Manager
Antibody, Monoclonal	Microbiology
Sampler, Air	General
Serum, Screening, Blood	Hematology
Tray, Custom/Special Procedure	General

BIOTEX, INC.   713-741-0111
8058 El Rio St., Houston, TX 77054
FDA Number: 3005726841
Laser, Surgical	Surgery

BIOTRAC, INC.   301-496-8290
1 Cloister Court, building 60 Room 237, Bethesda, MD 20833
FDA Number: n/a
E-mail: nardonem@mail.nih.gov
Annual Revenue: $0-$1 Million
Total Employees: 4
Ownership: Private
Produces/Sells CE-marked Devices: N
Federal Procurement Eligibility: Small Business
Distribution: Manufacturer Through Distributor, Exporter
General Admin.: L. C. Hansen/President, Chief Executive Officer
Monitor, Blood Pressure, Venous	Cardiovascular

BIOTROL USA
See Sekisui Diagnostics, LLC

BIOTRONICS INC.
See Dedicated Distribution

BIOTRONICS RESEARCH CORPORATION   604-298-1832
#610-4160 Albert St., Burnaby, BC V5C 6K2 Canada
FDA Number: n/a   Fax: 604-291-8443
E-mail: inquiries@biotronicsresearch.com
Web site: www.biotronicsresearch.com
Year Founded: 1988
Total Employees: 10
Ownership: Private
Produces/Sells CE-marked Devices: N
Distribution: Manufacturer Direct

BIOTRONIK, INC.   503-635-3594
6024 Jean Road, Lake Oswego, OR 97035
FDA Number: 1028232   Fax: 503-635-9936
E-mail: marketing@biotronik.com
Web site: http://www.biotronik.com
Year Founded: 1963
Total Employees: 4800
Ownership: Private
Produces/Sells CE-marked Devices: N
General Admin.: Mr. Jake Langer/President
Mktg./Adv.: Mr. Rex Richmond/Vice President Marketing & Communications
      Mr. Patrick Horan/Vice President Sales
Defibrillator, Implantable, Automatic	Cardiovascular
Electrode, Pacemaker, External	Cardiovascular
Guidewire, Catheter	Cardiovascular

BIOVENTRIX   925-830-1000
12647 Alcosta Blvd., Suite 400, San Ramon, CA 94583
FDA Number: n/a   Fax: 925-830-1002
E-mail: info@bioventrix.com
Web site: www.bioventrix.com
Ownership: Private
Produces/Sells CE-marked Devices: N
General Admin.: Mr. Kenneth Miller/President, Chief Executive Officer
    Medical Admin.: Dr. Lon Annest/Chief Medical Officer
Mktg./Adv.: Mr. David Schickling/Vice President Marketing & Sales
Production: Ms. Tessa Yamut/Director Regulatory Affairs
Research: Mr. Kevin Van Bladel/Vice President Research & Development
Device, Stabilizer, Heart	Cardiovascular

BIOVENTRIX, A CHF TECHNOLOGIES COMPANY
See Bioventrix

BIOVERIS CORPORATION   800-336-4436
16020 Industrial Dr., Gaithersburg, MD 20877   301-869-9800
FDA Number: 1125079   Fax: 301-230-0158
E-mail: bvcorp@bioveris.com
Web site: www.bioveris.com

BIOVERIS CORPORATION   800-336-4436 (cont'd)
Ownership: Private
Produces/Sells CE-marked Devices: N
Colorimeter, General Use	Chemistry

BIOVEST INTERNATIONAL, INC.   866-3BIOVEST
8500 Evergreen Blvd. NW,   763-786-0302
Minneapolis, MN 55433
FDA Number: 2183664   Fax: 763-786-0915
E-mail: Info@Biovest.com
Web site: www.biovest.com
Medical Products Sales Volume: $7,290,000
Annual Revenue: $10-$25 Million
Year Founded: 1981
Total Employees: 10
Ownership: Public
Stock Symbol: BVTI
Traded On: OTC Bulletin
Produces/Sells CE-marked Devices: Y
Federal Procurement Eligibility: Small Business
Distribution: Manufacturer Direct, Exclusive Distributor, Exporter
General Admin.: Frank O'Donnell/Chairman
      Julian Casciano/Chief Medical Officer, Vice President
      Richard Sakowicz/Chief Operating Officer
      Mark Hirschel/Chief Scientific Officer
      Sharon Aleck/Director Human Resources
      Stephane Allard/President, Chief Executive Officer
Finance: James McNulty/Chief Financial Officer
Perfusion Apparatus	Pathology
Suspension System, Cell Culture	Pathology

BIOVIR LABORATORIES, INC.   800-442-7342
685 Stone Rd., Unit 6, Benicia, CA 94510   707-747-5906
FDA Number: 2939599   Fax: 707-747-1751
E-mail: csj@biovir.com
Web site: www.biovir.com
Ownership: Private
Produces/Sells CE-marked Devices: N
Antigen, ID, HA, CEP, Entamoeba Histolytica	Microbiology

BIOVISION TECHNOLOGIES, LLC   303-237-9608
221 Corporate Circle Unit H, Golden, CO 80401
FDA Number: 3004452289
Laparoscope, General & Plastic Surgery	Surgery

BIOWAVE CORPORATION   203-855-8610
16 Knight Street, Norwalk, CT 06851
FDA Number: 3004558433
Nerve, Stimulator, Electrical, Percutaneous (pens) For Pain Relief	Cns/Neurology
Stimulator, Nerve, Transcutaneous (Pain Relief, TENS)	Cns/Neurology

BIOZYME LABORATORIES   800-423-8199
INTERNATIONAL LTD.
9939 Hibert St., Suite 101,   858-549-4484
San Diego, CA 92131
FDA Number: n/a   Fax: 858-549-0138
E-mail: bioinfo@biozyme.com
Web site: www.biozyme.com
Annual Revenue: $1-$5 Million
Year Founded: 1971
Total Employees: 4   Marketing Staff: 4   Sales Staff: 4
Ownership: BIOZYME LABORATORIES LTD.
Quality System Registration Information: ISO9002
Federal Procurement Eligibility: Small Business
Distribution: Manufacturer Direct
General Admin.: John Chesham/Managing Director
Production: Ellen Williams/Vice President Operations
Analyzer, Chemistry, Enzyme	Chemistry
Contract R&D, Diagnostics	General
Phosphatase, Alkaline	Hematology
Urease And Glutamic Dehydrogenase, Urea Nitrogen	Chemistry

BIPORE, INC.
See Bipore, Inc.

BIRCHWOOD LABORATORIES, INC.   800-328-6156
7900 Fuller Road, Eden Prairie, MN 55344-2195   952-937-7943
FDA Number: 2182825   Fax: 952-937-7979
E-mail: medical@birchlabs.com
Web site: www.birchlabs.com
Medical Products Sales Volume: $9,600,000
Annual Revenue: $10-$25 Million
Year Founded: 1979
Total Employees: 80   Marketing Staff: 3   Sales Staff: 35
Ownership: Private
Produces/Sells CE-marked Devices: N
Federal Procurement Eligibility: Small Business

BIRCHWOOD LABORATORIES, INC.   800-328-6156 *(cont'd)*

Distribution: Manufacturer Direct, Manufacturer Through Distributor, Manufacturer Through Manufacturer Reps, OEM
General Admin.: Mr. Dan Brooks/President, Chief Financial Officer
Mktg./Adv.: Mr. Tim Brown/Manager Marketing & Advertising
    Stephen M. Souder/Vice President Marketing & Sales
Production: Mr. Dale Borgeson/Customer Service Representative
    Mike Shelton/Director Quality Assurance & Regulatory Affairs
    Mike Shelton/Manager Regulatory Affairs
    Mike Shelton/President Manufacturing
Research: Stephen M. Souder/Vice President Research & Development

Applicator, Tipped, Absorbent	General
Applicator, Vaginal	Obstetrics/Gynecology
Binder, Perineal	General
Brush, Cytology	General
Dressing, Other	General
Pad, Medicated	General
Swabs, Cotton	General
Swabs, Specimen Collection	General

BIRD & CRONIN, INC.   651-683-1111
1200 Trapp Rd., Saint Paul, MN 55121
FDA Number: 2182345   *Fax:* 800-279-7934
E-mail: sales@birdcronin.com
Web site: www.birdcronin.com
Ownership: Private
Produces/Sells CE-marked Devices: N

Accessories, Traction	Physical Med
Bandage, Elastic	General
Belt, Traction, Pelvic, Orthopedic	Orthopedics
Belt, Wheelchair	Physical Med
Binder, Abdominal	General
Board, Bed	General
Brace, Joint, Ankle (External)	Physical Med
Cage, Knee	Physical Med
Cane	Physical Med
Component, Exercise	Physical Med
Halter, Head, Traction	Physical Med
Orthosis, Cervical	Physical Med
Orthosis, Corrective Shoe	Physical Med
Orthosis, Limb Brace	Physical Med
Orthosis, Lumbosacral	Physical Med
Orthosis, Rib Fracture, Soft	Physical Med
Protector, Skin Pressure	General
Restraint, Protective (Body)	General
Shoe, Cast	Physical Med
Sling, Arm	Physical Med
Splint, Abduction, Congenital Hip Dislocation	Physical Med
Splint, Clavicle	Physical Med
Splint, Traction	Orthopedics
Traction Unit, Non-Powered	Orthopedics
Transfer Device, Patient, Manual	General

BIRD MOYER CO.
See Moyco Technologies, Inc.

BIRD SPACE TECHNOLOGY
See Percussionaire Corporation

BIRKOVA PRODUCTS   888-567-4502   308-537-7300
809 4th Street, Gothenburg, NE 69138
FDA Number: 2247209   *Fax:* 308-537-7363
E-mail: info@birkovaproducts.com
Web site: www.birkovaproducts.com
Medical Products Sales Volume: $140,000
Year Founded: 2003
Total Employees: 4
Ownership: Private
Produces/Sells CE-marked Devices: N
Federal Procurement Eligibility: Small Business
Distribution: Manufacturer Direct, Manufacturer Through Distributor
Mktg./Adv.: Kevin Sitorius/Admin. Sales

Accessories, Operating Room, Table	Surgery
Clamp, Other	Surgery
Stretcher, Transfer	Surgery

BIRTCHER CORP.
See Conmed Corporation

BIRTCHER MEDICAL SYSTEMS, INC.
See Conmed Corporation

BISCO, INC.   630-523-7400
520 Windy Point Drive, Glendale Heights, IL 60193
FDA Number: 1420052   *Fax:* 630-523-7485
E-mail: mkt@biscoind.com
Web site: www.biscoind.com
Ownership: Private
Produces/Sells CE-marked Devices: N

Activator, Ultraviolet, Polymerization	Dental And Oral
Adhesive, Bracket And Conditioner, Resin	Dental And Oral
Airbrush	Dental And Oral

BISCO, INC.   630-523-7400 *(cont'd)*

Base, Denture, Relining, Repairing, Rebasing, Resin	Dental And Oral
Burr, Dental	Dental And Oral
Cement, Dental	Dental And Oral
Coating, Filling Material, Resin	Dental And Oral
Crown And Bridge, Temporary, Resin	Dental And Oral
Drill, Dental, Intraoral	Dental And Oral
Instrument, Dental, Manual	Dental And Oral
Liner, Cavity, Calcium Hydroxide	Dental And Oral
Material, Tooth Shade, Resin	Dental And Oral
Post, Root Canal	Dental And Oral
Powder, Porcelain	Dental And Oral
Resin, Root Canal Filling	Dental And Oral
Sealant, Pit And Fissure, And Conditioner, Resin	Dental And Oral
Syringe, Restorative And Impression Material	Dental And Oral
Tooth Bonding Agent, Resin Restoration	Dental And Oral

BL HEALTHCARE, INC.   508-543-4150
33 Commercial St., Suite #3, Foxboro, MA 02035
FDA Number: 3006782137   *Fax:* 508-543-6150
E-mail: info@blhealthcare.com
Web site: hwww.blhealthcare.com
Ownership: Private
Produces/Sells CE-marked Devices: N

Dialyzer, High Permeability	Gastroenterology/Urology
Transmitter/Receiver System, Physiological, Radiofrequency	Cardiovascular

BLACK DIAMOND VIDEO, INC.   215-348-3896
1151 Harbor Bay Parkway, Suite 208, Alameda, CA 94502
FDA Number: 3005907379

Device, Storage, Image, Digital	Radiology
System, Communication, Image, Digital	Radiology

BLACKHAGEN DESIGN   727-736-0582
811-C Douglas Avenue, Dunedin, FL 34698-5071
FDA Number: n/a   *Fax:* 727-738-0523
E-mail: Jeff@blackhagendesign.com
Web site: www.blackhagendesign.com
Medical Products Sales Volume: $400,000
Annual Revenue: $1-$5 Million
Year Founded: 1995
Total Employees: 7   *Marketing Staff:* 1
Ownership: Private
Produces/Sells CE-marked Devices: N
Federal Procurement Eligibility: Small Business
Distribution: Service Direct
General Admin.: Sean Hagen/President, Owner
Mktg./Adv.: Jeff Herbert/Director Business Development
Research: Philip Remedios/Vice President Research & Development

Monitor, Bed Patient	General

BLACKHAWK BIOSYSTEMS
See Bio-Rad Laboratories

BLACKSTONE INDUSTRIES
See Foredom Electric Co.

BLACKSTONE MEDICAL, INC.   888-298-5400   413-731-8711
90 Brookdale Dr., Springfield, MA 01104
FDA Number: 1225457   *Fax:* 413-731-8750
Web site: www.blackstonemedical.com
Annual Revenue: $10-$25 Million
Total Employees: 25
Ownership: Private
Produces/Sells CE-marked Devices: Y
Distribution: Manufacturer Through Distributor

Accessories, Operating Room, Table	Surgery
Appliance, Fixation, Spinal Intervertebral Body	Orthopedics
Awl	Orthopedics
Bender	Orthopedics
Bit, Drill	Orthopedics
Cannula, Surgical, General & Plastic Surgery	Surgery
Catheter, Suction, With Tip	General
Curette, Surgical	Surgery
Dissector, Surgical, General & Plastic Surgery	Surgery
Driver, Prosthesis	Orthopedics
Elevator, Surgical, General & Plastic Surgery	Surgery
Equipment, Shaving, Disc, Spinal	Orthopedics
Guide, Surgical, Instrument	Surgery
Handle, Scalpel	Surgery
Hook, Surgical, General & Plastic Surgery	Surgery
Impactor	Orthopedics
Instrument, Manual, General Surgical	Surgery
Orthopedic Manual Surgical Instrument	Orthopedics
Orthosis, Cervical	Physical Med
Probe	Orthopedics
Pusher, Socket	Orthopedics
Retractor	Orthopedics
Rongeur, Other	Surgery
Screwdriver	Orthopedics
Spatula, Orthopedic	Orthopedics

BLACKSTONE MEDICAL, INC.　888-298-5400 *(cont'd)*

Stylet, Surgical	Surgery
Tap, Bone	Orthopedics
Tape, Measuring, Ruler And Caliper	Surgery
Template	Orthopedics
Tray, Surgical Instrument	Surgery
Wrench	Orthopedics

BLAINE LABS, INC.　800-307-8818
11037 Lockport Place,　562-906-4477
Santa Fe Springs, CA 90670
FDA Number: 3001744192
Fax: 562-906-4467
Web site: www.blainelabs.com
Ownership: Private
Produces/Sells CE-marked Devices: N

Elastomer, Silicone (Scar Management)	Surgery
Shield, Nipple	Obstetrics/Gynecology
Vibrator, Therapeutic	Physical Med

BLAIREX LABORATORIES, INC.　800-252-4739
PO Box 2127, 1600 Brian Drive,　812-378-1864
Columbus, IN 47202
FDA Number: 1825549
Fax: 812-378-1033
E-mail: info@blairex.com
Web site: www.blairex.com
Medical Products Sales Volume: $400,000
Annual Revenue: $50-$100 Million
Year Founded: 1994
Total Employees: 25　*Marketing Staff:* 4　*Sales Staff:* 10
Ownership: Private
Federal Procurement Eligibility: Small Business
Distribution: Manufacturer Direct, Manufacturer Through Distributor, Manufacturer Through Manufacturer Reps
General Admin.: Anthony Moravec/President
Mktg./Adv.: Ryan Moravec/Vice President Marketing
　　　　Craig Skelton/Vice President Sales

Bottle, Sterile Solution	General

BLAKE INDUSTRIES, INC.　908-233-7240
660 Jerusalem Road, Scotch Plains, NJ 07076-2028
FDA Number: n/a
Fax: 908-233-1354
E-mail: blake4xray@worldnet.att.net
Medical Products Sales Volume: $1,400,000
Annual Revenue: $1-$5 Million
Year Founded: 1968
Total Employees: 6　*Marketing Staff:* 2　*Sales Staff:* 3
Ownership: Private
Produces/Sells CE-marked Devices: N
Federal Procurement Eligibility: Small Business
Distribution: Manufacturer Direct
General Admin.: David Rognlie/President

Densitometer, Laboratory	Chemistry
Diffractometer, X-Ray	Chemistry

BLAKE MANUFACTURING, INC.　813-935-1841
9241 Lazy Ln., Tampa, FL 33614
FDA Number: 1064732
Ownership: Private
Produces/Sells CE-marked Devices: N

Orthosis, Limb Brace	Physical Med
Splint, Hand, And Component	Physical Med

BLANCHARD CONTACT LENS, INC.　603-625-1664
8025 South Willow Street, Bldg #2 Unit 211-212,
Manchester, NH 03103
FDA Number: 1223801
Web site: www.blanchardlab.com
Ownership: Private
Produces/Sells CE-marked Devices: N

Lens, Contact (Other Material)	Ophthalmology
Lens, Contact(rigid Gas Permeable)-extended Wear	Ophthalmology
Lens, Contact, Orthokeratology, Overnight	Ophthalmology
Lens, Contact, Polymethylmethacrylate	Ophthalmology

BLANCHARD OSTOMY PRODUCTS　818-242-6789
1510 Raymond Avenue, Glendale, CA 91201
FDA Number: 2030471
Fax: 818-242-6789
E-mail: familiacerveza@msn.com
Medical Products Sales Volume: $50,000
Annual Revenue: $0-$1 Million
Year Founded: 1984
Total Employees: 1
Ownership: Private
Produces/Sells CE-marked Devices: N
Federal Procurement Eligibility: Small Business
Distribution: Manufacturer Through Distributor, Service Direct

Bag, Drainage, Ostomy (With Adhesive)	General

BLATEK, INC.　814-231-2085
2820 E. College Avenue, Suite F, State College, PA 16801-7548
FDA Number: n/a
Fax: 814-231-2087
E-mail: sales@blatek.com
Web site: www.blatek.com
Medical Products Sales Volume: $4,600,000
Annual Revenue: $1-$5 Million
Year Founded: 1978
Total Employees: 55　*Marketing Staff:* 1　*Sales Staff:* 2
Ownership: Private
Produces/Sells CE-marked Devices: N
Federal Procurement Eligibility: Small Business
Distribution: Manufacturer Direct, Manufacturer Through Manufacturer Reps, OEM
General Admin.: Stuart Blacker/President
Production: Mr. Kevin Knarr/Manager Operations
　　　Mr. Chris Rishel/Manager Quality Assurance
Research: Dr. Xuecang Geng/Chief Scientist

Detector, Blood Flow, Ultrasonic (Doppler)	Cardiovascular
Monitor, Blood Flow, Ultrasonic	Obstetrics/Gynecology
Scanner, Ultrasonic (Pulsed Doppler)	Radiology
Scanner, Ultrasonic (Pulsed Echo)	Radiology
Scanner, Ultrasonic, Abdominal	Radiology
Scanner, Ultrasonic, Ophthalmic	Radiology
Transducer, Ultrasonic	Cardiovascular
Transducer, Ultrasonic, Diagnostic	Radiology
Transducer, Ultrasonic, Intravaginal	Obstetrics/Gynecology
Transducer, Ultrasonic, Obstetrical	Obstetrics/Gynecology

BLEDSOE BRACE SYSTEMS　888-253-3763
2601 Pinewood Drive,　972-647-0884
Grand Prairie, TX 75051
FDA Number: 1640542
Fax: 972-660-5495
E-mail: mhenderson@bledsoebrace.com
Web site: www.bledsoebrace.com
Medical Products Sales Volume: $10,900,000
Annual Revenue: $10-$25 Million
Year Founded: 1982
Total Employees: 160　*Marketing Staff:* 3　*Sales Staff:* 3
Ownership: Private
Produces/Sells CE-marked Devices: Y
Federal Procurement Eligibility: Small Business, GSA Contract, VA Contract
Distribution: Manufacturer Direct, Manufacturer Through Distributor, Manufacturer Through Manufacturer Reps, OEM, Importer, Exporter
General Admin.: Gary R. Bledsoe/President, Chief Executive Officer
Mktg./Adv.: Pete Berney/Director Marketing
　　　Eric Bledsoe/Director Sales
Research: Brett Bledsoe/Vice President Research & Development

Joint, Knee, External Brace	Physical Med
Orthosis, Limb Brace	Physical Med

BLEVINS MEDICAL INC　866-783-3056
207 Broad Street, Marion, VA 24354　276-783-3056
FDA Number: n/a
Fax: 866-783-3056
E-mail: versatran@msn.com
Web site: www.patientlift.net
Medical Products Sales Volume: $230,000
Year Founded: 2002
Total Employees: 2
Ownership: Private
Produces/Sells CE-marked Devices: N
Federal Procurement Eligibility: Small Business, VA Contract
Distribution: Manufacturer Direct
Mktg./Adv.: Mr. Jerry Blevins/Admin. Marketing & Sales

Bath, Portable	General
Bed, Electric	General
Lift, Patient	General

BLICKMAN　800-247-5070
39 Robinson Road, Lodi, NJ 07644　201-909-0807
FDA Number: 2244019
Fax: 201-909-0832
E-mail: info@blickman.com
Web site: www.blickman.com
Year Founded: 1975
Total Employees: 100
Ownership: Private
Produces/Sells CE-marked Devices: N
Federal Procurement Eligibility: Small Business, GSA Contract, VA Contract
Distribution: Manufacturer Through Distributor, Manufacturer Through Manufacturer Reps
General Admin.: Paul Freedman/Chief Financial Officer, Chairman
　　　Rob Freedman/President, Chief Operating Officer
Mktg./Adv.: Seth Flexo/Vice President Marketing & Sales
Production: Dayne Smith/Vice President Manufacturing

Bassinet (Infant Bed)	General
Cabinet Casework, Laboratory	Chemistry
Cabinet, Instrument	General
Cabinet, Narcotic Control	General
Cabinet, Warming	General

MANUFACTURER PROFILES

BLICKMAN   800-247-5070 *(cont'd)*

Cart, Anesthetist's	Anesthesiology
Cart, Instrument	Surgery
Cart, Multipurpose	General
Footstool, Operating Room	Surgery
Infusion Stand	General
Sink, Hospital	General
Stand, Basin	General
Stand, Laundry Hamper	General
Stand, Operating Room Instrument (Mayo)	Surgery
Stool, Anesthetist's	Anesthesiology
Stool, Operating Room, Adjustable	Surgery
Table, Anesthetist's	Anesthesiology
Table, Instrument, Surgical	Surgery
Warmer, Blanket	General
Waste Receptacle, Kick Bucket	General

BLIND & VISION REHABILITATION SERVICES OF PITTSBUR   412-325-7504
1204 Western Ave., Bldg. 4, Pittsburgh, PA 15233
FDA Number: 2522338

Tourniquet, Non-Pneumatic, Surgical	Surgery

BLOCK DRUG CO., INC.   973-889-2578
2149 Harbor Ave., Memphis, TN 38113
FDA Number: 1020379

Carboxymethylcellulose Sodium/Ethylene-Oxide Homopolymer	Dental And Oral
Cleaner, Denture	Dental And Oral
Detector/Remover, Lice	General
Polyvinyl Methylether Maleic Acid-Calcium-Sodium Dbl. Salt	Dental And Oral
Polyvinyl Methylether Maleic Acid/Carboxymethylcellulose	Dental And Oral
Sealant, Pit And Fissure, And Conditioner, Resin	Dental And Oral
Toothbrush, Manual	Dental And Oral

BLOCK MEDICAL DE MEXICO S.A. DE C.V.   949-206-2700
La Mesa Parque Industrial, Paseo Reforma S/n, Fracc., Tijuana, Bc Mexico
FDA Number: 9680425

Kit, Administration, Intravenous	General
Pump, Infusion	General
Pump, Infusion, Elastomeric	General

BLOOD BANK COMPUTER SYSTEMS, INC.   253-333-0046
1002 15th St. Sw, Suite 120, Auburn, WA 98001
FDA Number: 3028885

Software, Blood Bank (Stand-Alone Products)	Hematology

BLOOD TRAC SYSTEMS, INC.   416-364-8441
300-49 Front St E, Toronto M5E 1B3 Canada
FDA Number: 9680679

Software, Blood Bank (Stand-Alone Products)	Hematology

BLOODNETUSA, INC.   863-687-8925
3200 Lakeland Hills Blvd., Lakeland, FL 33805
FDA Number: 1073584

Software, Blood Bank (Stand-Alone Products)	Hematology

BLOOMEX INTERNATIONAL, INC.   201-703-9799
295 Molnar Dr., Elmwood Park, NJ 07407-3211
FDA Number: 2431678   *Fax:* 201-703-9626
E-mail: bloomex@aol.com
Web site: www.bloomex.com
Annual Revenue: $0-$1 Million
Total Employees: 5   *Marketing Staff:* 1   *Sales Staff:* 1
Ownership: Private
Produces/Sells CE-marked Devices: N
Federal Procurement Eligibility: Small Business
Distribution: Manufacturer Direct, Manufacturer Through Distributor, Service Direct, Importer, Exporter
General Admin.: Benjamin Laroux/President
Mktg./Adv.: Juliette Laroux/Admin. Marketing & Sales

Electrode, Neuromuscular Stimulator	Cns/Neurology
Electrode, Other	General
Equipment, Therapy, Handicapped/Physical	Physical Med
Stimulator, External, Neuromuscular, Functional	Physical Med
Stimulator, Muscle, Electrical-Powered (EMS)	Physical Med
Stimulator, Nerve, Transcutaneous (Pain Relief, TENS)	Cns/Neurology

BLS SYSTEMS, LTD.   905-339-1069
1055 Industry St, Oakville L6J 2X3 Canada
FDA Number: 9681848

Mask, Oxygen, Non-Rebreathing	Anesthesiology

BLU-RAY INC.
See Bidwell Industrial Group, Inc., Blu-Ray Division

BLUE BELL BIO-MEDICAL   800-258-3235
1260 Industrial Drive, Van Wert, OH 45891   419-238-4442
FDA Number: 2528968   *Fax:* 419-238-0226
E-mail: info@bluebellcarts.com
Web site: www.bluebellcarts.com

BLUE BELL BIO-MEDICAL   800-258-3235 *(cont'd)*
Medical Products Sales Volume: $2,000,000
Annual Revenue: $1-$5 Million
Year Founded: 1982
Total Employees: 3
Ownership: Private
Produces/Sells CE-marked Devices: N
Federal Procurement Eligibility: Small Business, GSA Contract, VA Contract
Distribution: Manufacturer Direct, Manufacturer Through Distributor, Manufacturer Through Manufacturer Reps, Exclusive Distributor, Exporter
General Admin.: Larry Dineen/President
Mktg./Adv.: Larry Dineen/Director Marketing

Accessories, Cart, Multipurpose	General
Cart, Anesthetist's	Anesthesiology
Cart, Dressing	General
Cart, Emergency, Cardiopulmonary Resuscitation (Crash)	Anesthesiology
Cart, Equipment, Video	General
Cart, Instrument	Surgery
Cart, Monitor	General
Cart, Multipurpose	General
Cart, Other	General
Cart, Supply	General
Cart, Supply, Operating Room	Surgery

BLUE BELL CARTS
See Blue Bell Bio-Medical

BLUE CHIP MEDICAL PRODUCTS, INC.   800-795-6115
7-11 Suffern Place, #2, Suffern, NY 10901   845-369-7535
FDA Number: 2438690   *Fax:* 845-369-7633
E-mail: sales@bluechipmedical.com
Web site: www.bluechipmedical.com
Medical Products Sales Volume: $1,400,000
Year Founded: 1996
Total Employees: 8   *Marketing Staff:* 5   *Sales Staff:* 32
Ownership: Private
Produces/Sells CE-marked Devices: Y
Federal Procurement Eligibility: Small Business, VA Contract
Distribution: Manufacturer Through Distributor, Manufacturer Through Manufacturer Reps, OEM
General Admin.: Mr. Ron Resnick/President
Mktg./Adv.: Mr. Trip Handy/National Sales Representative
    Mr. Jim Acker/Vice President Sales
Production: D. Milchman/Director Quality Assurance

Accessories, Wheelchair	Physical Med
Mattress, Water, Temperature Regulated	General

BLUE EARTH, INC.   518-237-5585
31 Ontario St., 2nd Floor - Front, Cohoes, NY 12047-3745
FDA Number: 3004828796
Ownership: Private
Produces/Sells CE-marked Devices: N

Accessories, Wheelchair	Physical Med
Belt, Wheelchair	Physical Med
Cushion, Wheelchair (Pad)	Physical Med
Support, Head And Trunk, Wheelchair	Physical Med

BLUE HORIZON MEDICAL   321-217-2717
3129 Ginger Cir., Orlando, FL 32826
FDA Number: 3005750748
E-mail: sales@bluehorizonmedical.com
Web site: www.bluehorizonmedical.com
Ownership: Private
Produces/Sells CE-marked Devices: N

Chair, Surgical, AC-Powered	Surgery

BLUE SKY BIO, LLC   888-446-6724
888 E Belvidere Rd., Suite 212,   718-376-0422
Grayslake, IL 60030
FDA Number: 3003402534   *Fax:* 888-234-3685
E-mail: info@blueskybio.com
Web site: www.blueskybio.com
Ownership: Private
Produces/Sells CE-marked Devices: N

Abutment, Implant, Dental, Endosseous	Dental And Oral
Burr, Dental	Dental And Oral
Implant, Endosseous	Dental And Oral
Instrument, Dental, Manual	Dental And Oral
Tray, Impression	Dental And Oral

BLUE SKY MEDICAL GROUP INCORPORATED   727-392-1261
5924 Balfour Ct., Suite 102, Carlsbad, CA 92008
FDA Number: 2032666
Ownership: Private
Produces/Sells CE-marked Devices: N

Accessories, Catheter	Surgery
Drain, Tee (Water Trap)	Anesthesiology
Dressing, Wound, Occlusive	Surgery

BLUE SKY MEDICAL GROUP INCORPORATED   727-392-1261
(cont'd)

Pump, Aspiration, Portable	Anesthesiology

BLUE SPRING CORP.   361-552-8898
45 Blue Spring Rd., Port Lavaca, TX 77979
FDA Number: 2023262   *Fax:* 1-512-287-4039
E-mail: sales@bluspr.com
Web site: www.bluspr.com
Year Founded: 1980
Ownership: Private
Produces/Sells CE-marked Devices: N
Federal Procurement Eligibility: Small Business
Distribution: Manufacturer Direct, Manufacturer Through Manufacturer Reps
Mktg./Adv.: Satish Desal/Representative Tech. Sales

Purification System, Water, Reverse Osmosis	Chemistry
Purifier, Water	Chemistry

BLUE TORCH MEDICAL TECHNOLOGIES   508-231-1080
9700 Great Seneca Highway, Suite 303, Rockville, MD 20850
FDA Number: 3004115203   *Fax:* 443-583-2476
E-mail: sales@bluetorch.com
Web site: www.bluetorchmed.com
Ownership: Private
Produces/Sells CE-marked Devices: N

Stimulator, Nerve, ENT	Ear/Nose/Throat

BLUE WAVE ULTRASONICS   800-373-0144
960 S. Rolff St., Davenport, IA 52802   563-322-0144
FDA Number: n/a   *Fax:* 563-322-7180
E-mail: info@bluewaveinc.com
Web site: www.bluewaveinc.com
Medical Products Sales Volume: $3,300,000
Annual Revenue: $5-$10 Million
Year Founded: 1962
Total Employees: 20   *Marketing Staff:* 3   *Sales Staff:* 3
Ownership: Private
Produces/Sells CE-marked Devices: N
Federal Procurement Eligibility: Small Business, GSA Contract
Distribution: Manufacturer Direct, Manufacturer Through Manufacturer Reps, OEM
General Admin.: Roger Stoneking/President
Mktg./Adv.: Jeff Hancock/Vice President Marketing & Sales

Cleaner, Ultrasonic, Medical Instrument	General
Solution, Instrument Cleaner	General

BLUE WHITE INDUSTRIES, INC.   714-893-8529
5300 Business Drive, Huntington Beach, CA 92649
FDA Number: n/a   *Fax:* 714-894-9492
E-mail: sales@blue-white.com
Web site: http://www.bluwhite.com
Medical Products Sales Volume: $9,000,000
Annual Revenue: $10-$25 Million
Total Employees: 70   *Marketing Staff:* 2   *Sales Staff:* 2
Ownership: Private
Produces/Sells CE-marked Devices: Y
Federal Procurement Eligibility: Small Business
Distribution: Manufacturer Through Distributor, Manufacturer Through Manufacturer Reps
General Admin.: Robin Gladhill/President
Mktg./Adv.: David Cook/Director Marketing
     Jeanie Norman/Manager Advertising
Production: R. King/Vice President Manufacturing
Research: Bill McDowell/Vice President Research & Development

Flowmeter, Back-Pressure Compensated, Thorpe Tube	Anesthesiology
Flowmeter, Gas (Oxygen), Calibrated	Anesthesiology
Pump, Laboratory	Chemistry

BLUEGRASS VASCULAR TECHNOLOGIES
163 E. Main Street, Suite 300, Lexington, KY 40507
FDA Number: n/a
E-mail: info@bluegrassvascular.com
Web site: www.bluegrassvascular.com
Ownership: Private
Produces/Sells CE-marked Devices: N

BLUFF CREEK SYSTEMS
See Omnisys, Inc.

BMC INDUSTRIES
See Vision-Ease Lens

BMW PRECISION MACHINING, INC.   619-439-6813
2379 Industry St., Oceanside, CA 92054
FDA Number: n/a
E-mail: bmw@bmwprecision.com
Web site: www.bmwprecision.com
Total Employees: 48   *Marketing Staff:* 2   *Sales Staff:* 2
Ownership: Private
Quality System Registration Information: ISO9002
Produces/Sells CE-marked Devices: N

BMW PRECISION MACHINING, INC.   619-439-6813 *(cont'd)*
Federal Procurement Eligibility: Small Business
Distribution: Manufacturer Direct
General Admin.: Louie Poloni/Chief Executive Officer
     Richard Blakley/President

Contract Manufacturing	General

BOB J. JOHNSON & ASSOCIATES   218-873-5555
16420 W. Hardy Rd., Ste. 100, Houston, TX 77060
FDA Number: 3003371652

Purification System, Water	Gastroenterology/Urology

BOBBITT LABORATORIES, INC.
See Carolina Biological Supply Co.

BOBRICK WASHROOM EQUIPMENT, INC.   818-764-1000
11611 Hart St., North Hollywood, CA 91605-5882
FDA Number: 7000444   *Fax:* 818-765-2700
E-mail: info@bobrick.com
Web site: www.bobrick.com
Year Founded: 1906
Ownership: Private
Produces/Sells CE-marked Devices: Y
Distribution: Manufacturer Through Distributor
General Admin.: Mark Louchheim/President
Mktg./Adv.: Alan Gettelman/Director Marketing
     Dennis Redman/Manager Marketing
     Chet Webb/Vice President Sales
Production: A. Mark Lawrence/Vice President Manufacturing

Dispenser, Soap	General
Rail, Bath	General
Waste Receptacle, General Purpose	General

BOC GASES   800-262-4273
575 Mountain Ave., Murray Hill, NJ 07974-2002   908-464-8100
FDA Number: n/a   *Fax:* 410-749-4073
E-mail: USweb-inquiries@boc.com
Web site: http://www.lindeus.com
Medical Products Sales Volume: $60,000,000
Ownership: Private
Quality System Registration Information: ISO9002
Produces/Sells CE-marked Devices: N
Distribution: Manufacturer Direct, Manufacturer Through Distributor, Exclusive Distributor, Exporter

Gas Mixtures, Medical	General
Valve, Other	Chemistry

BOCK ORTHOPEDIC INDUSTRY INC., USA, OTTO
See Otto Bock Heathcare

BODE TECHNOLOGY GROUP, INC.   866-263-3443
0430 Furnace Road, Suite 107, Lorton, VA 22079   703-646-9740
FDA Number: n/a   *Fax:* 703-646-9741
E-mail: bode.service@bodetech.com
Web site: http://www.bodetech.com
Ownership: Private
Produces/Sells CE-marked Devices: N
General Admin.: Mr. Barry Watson/President, Chief Executive Officer
Mktg./Adv.: Mr. Randolph Nagy/Vice President Marketing & Sales
Research: Mr. Jangbir Sangha/Vice President Product Development

BODINE ELECTRIC CO.   800-786-3463
201 Northfield Road, Northfield, IL 60093   773-478-3515
FDA Number: n/a   *Fax:* 773-478-3232
Web site: www.bodine-electric.com
Annual Revenue: $50-$100 Million
Total Employees: 600
Ownership: Private
Produces/Sells CE-marked Devices: Y
Distribution: Manufacturer Through Distributor, Manufacturer Through Manufacturer Reps, OEM
General Admin.: John Bodine/President
     Rich Meserve/Vice President Human Resources
Mktg./Adv.: Susan Rexford/Director Marketing
     James Starmont/Vice President Sales
Production: John Horvath/Director Quality Assurance
     Dave Alspaugh/Vice President Manufacturing

Component, Electronic	General

BODY GLOVE   310-374-3441
201 Herondo Street, Redondo Beach, CA 90277
FDA Number: n/a   *Fax:* 310-372-7457
E-mail: pr@bodyglove.com
Web site: www.bodyglove.com
Medical Products Sales Volume: $4,000,000
Annual Revenue: $1-$5 Million
Ownership: Private
Produces/Sells CE-marked Devices: N
Federal Procurement Eligibility: Small Business

BODY GLOVE
310-374-3441 *(cont'd)*

Distribution: Exclusive Distributor

Collar, Ice	General
Equipment, Therapy, Handicapped/Physical	Physical Med
Support, Ankle	Orthopedics
Support, Back	Orthopedics
Support, Elbow	Orthopedics
Support, Wrist	Physical Med

BODY TECH 1 NW
866-315-0640
10727 47th Pl. W, Mukilteo, WA 98275   **425-315-0640**
FDA Number: n/a   *Fax:* 425-315-0879
E-mail: sales@bodytechnw.com
Web site: www.bodytechnw.com
Ownership: Private
Produces/Sells CE-marked Devices: N
Federal Procurement Eligibility: Small Business, Female Owned
Distribution: Manufacturer Direct, Manufacturer Through Distributor, Manufacturer Through Manufacturer Reps, OEM, Exporter
Mktg./Adv.: Ms. LuWane Driskill/Market Manager

Accessories, Wheelchair	Physical Med
Component, Wheelchair	Physical Med
Restraint	Physical Med
Support, Head And Trunk, Wheelchair	Physical Med

BODY THERAPEUTICS, DIV. OF I-REP, INC.
800-530-3722
508 Chaney Street, Suite 13,   **909-674-5722**
Lake Elsinore, CA 92530
FDA Number: n/a   *Fax:* 909-674-8126
E-mail: btwilhelm@juno.com
Web site: www.bodytherapeutics.net
Year Founded: 1982
Total Employees: 12   *Marketing Staff:* 1   *Sales Staff:* 2
Ownership: I-Rep, Inc.
Produces/Sells CE-marked Devices: N
Distribution: Manufacturer Through Distributor

Binder, Abdominal, OB/GYN	Obstetrics/Gynecology
Pillow	General
Pillow, Cervical	Orthopedics
Support, Back	Orthopedics

BODY THERAPEUTICS, INC.
See N-K Products Company, Div. Of I-Rep,Inc.

BODY WELL DESIGN,LLC
866-293-8444
6206 E. Trent Ave., Suite 1a, Spokane Valley, WA 99212
FDA Number: 3034546
Ownership: Private
Produces/Sells CE-marked Devices: N

Massager, Therapeutic	Physical Med

BODYLINE COMFORT SYSTEMS
800-874-7715
3730 Kori Rd., Jacksonville, FL 32257   **904-262-4068**
FDA Number: 1047473   *Fax:* 800-323-2225
E-mail: info@bodyline.com
Web site: www.bodyline.com
Annual Revenue: $1-$5 Million
Year Founded: 1968
Ownership: Private
Produces/Sells CE-marked Devices: N
Distribution: Manufacturer Direct, Importer, Exporter

Collar, Cervical Neck	Orthopedics
Cushion, Flotation, Therapeutic	Physical Med
Orthosis, Limb Brace	Physical Med
Support, Back	Orthopedics

BODYPOINT, INC.
800-547-5716
558 First Avenue So., Suite 300,   **206-405-4555**
Seattle, WA 98104
FDA Number: 3032497   *Fax:* 206-405-4556
E-mail: sales@bodypoint.com
Web site: www.bodypoint.com
Medical Products Sales Volume: $1,700,000
Year Founded: 1991
Total Employees: 30
Ownership: Private
Produces/Sells CE-marked Devices: Y
Federal Procurement Eligibility: Small Business
Distribution: Manufacturer Through Distributor, Manufacturer Through Manufacturer Reps, OEM, Exclusive Distributor, Importer
Mktg./Adv.: Mr. Ryan Malane/Managing Director Marketing
       Mr. David Jones/Managing Director Marketing & Sales
       Mr. Leif Flynn/Marketing Coordinator
       Mr. Thomas Sams/Sales Specialist

Accessories, Wheelchair	Physical Med
Belt, Wheelchair	Physical Med
Chair, With Casters	Physical Med
Mattress, Alternating Pressure (Or Pads)	Physical Med

BOECKELER INSTRUMENTS, INC.
800-552-2262
4650 S. Butterfield Drive, Tucson, AZ 85714   **520-745-0001**
FDA Number: n/a   *Fax:* 520-745-0004
E-mail: info@boeckeler.com
Web site: www.boeckeler.com
Medical Products Sales Volume: $2,600,000
Year Founded: 1942
Total Employees: 30
Ownership: Private
Produces/Sells CE-marked Devices: Y
Federal Procurement Eligibility: Small Business
Distribution: Manufacturer Through Distributor, OEM
General Admin.: Len Ness/Chief Executive Officer
       Len Ness/President
Mktg./Adv.: Richard Earl/Manager Marketing Communications
       Pat Brey/Vice President Marketing & Sales
Production: Greg Becker/Applications Specialist
       Dave Roberts/Senior Product Manager
       Len Ness/Vice President Manufacturing

Accessories, Microtome	Pathology
Knife, Microtome	Pathology
Microtome, Freezing Attachment	Pathology
Microtome, Rotary	Pathology
Microtome, Ultra	Pathology
Tissue Processor, Automated	Pathology
Unit, Imaging, Thermal	Radiology

BOEHM SURGICAL INSTRUMENT CORP.
585-436-6584
966 Chili Ave., Rochester, NY 14611
FDA Number: 1317164   *Fax:* 585-436-6428
E-mail: sales@boehmsurgical.com
Web site: www.boehmsurgical.com
Ownership: Private
Produces/Sells CE-marked Devices: N

Bronchoscope, Rigid	Ear/Nose/Throat
Cord, Electric, Endoscope	Gastroenterology/Urology
Cystoscope	Gastroenterology/Urology
Esophagoscope (Flexible Or Rigid)	Ear/Nose/Throat
Lamp, Surgical, Incandescent	Surgery
Laryngoscope, Surgical	Surgery
Otoscope	Ear/Nose/Throat
Proctoscope	Surgery
Resectoscope	Gastroenterology/Urology
Sigmoidoscope, Rigid, Electrical	Gastroenterology/Urology
Tube, Bronchial (W/Wo Connector)	Anesthesiology

BOEHRINGER INGELHEIM ROXANE INC.
614-241-4135
1809 Wilson Rd., P.o. Box 16532, Columbus, OH 43228
FDA Number: 1510690
Ownership: Private
Produces/Sells CE-marked Devices: N

Saliva, Artificial	Dental And Oral

BOEHRINGER LABORATORIES, INC.
800-642-4945
500 E. Washington St.,   **610-278-0900**
Norristown, PA 19404
FDA Number: 2518417   *Fax:* 610-278-0907
E-mail: info@boehringerlabs.com
Web site: www.boehringerlabs.com
Medical Products Sales Volume: $2,300,000
Year Founded: 1972
Total Employees: 30
Ownership: Private
Quality System Registration Information: ISO9001
Produces/Sells CE-marked Devices: N
Federal Procurement Eligibility: Small Business
Distribution: Manufacturer Direct, Manufacturer Through Manufacturer Reps, Exporter
General Admin.: John Boehringer/President
Mktg./Adv.: Roseann Stadler/Marketing & Advertising Assistant
Production: Pat Paul/Manager Customer Services
       John Karpowicz/Manager Regulatory Affairs

Autotransfusion Unit (Blood)	Anesthesiology
Meter, Peak Flow, Spirometry	Anesthesiology
Monitor, Airway Pressure (Inspiratory Force)	Anesthesiology
Regulator, Suction, Surgical	General
Restraint, Wrist/Hand	General
Spirometer, Diagnostic (Respirometer)	Anesthesiology
Valve, Positive End Expiratory Pressure (PEEP)	Anesthesiology

BOEHRINGER LABS, INC
888-390-4325
500 East Washington St., Suite 2a, Black Horse, PA 19401
FDA Number: 3005925254

Suction Apparatus, Ward Use, Portable, AC-Powered	Surgery
System, Skin Closure	Surgery

BOEHRINGER MANNHEIM CORP.
See Roche Diagnostics Operations

BOEHRINGER MANNHEIM DIAGNOSTICS MICROGENICS
See Microgenics Corporation

BOEKEL INDUSTRIES
See Boekel Scientific

BOEKEL SCIENTIFIC
855 Pennsylvania Blvd., Feasterville, PA 19053
800-336-6929
215-396-8200
FDA Number: n/a   *Fax:* 215-396-8264
E-mail: boekel-info@boekelsci.com
Web site: www.boekelsci.com
Medical Products Sales Volume: $21,800,000
Year Founded: 1868
Total Employees: 200
Ownership: Private
Produces/Sells CE-marked Devices: N
Federal Procurement Eligibility: Small Business
Distribution: Manufacturer Through Distributor, OEM
General Admin.: Leo Synnestvedt/Chief Executive Officer
Mktg./Adv.: Joseph Lessard/Director Product Development
     Chuck Carney/Vice President Marketing & Sales
Production: L. Lanzi/Manager Customer Services
     Joe Lessard/Manager Regulatory Affairs

Bath, Tissue Flotation	Microbiology
Cabinet, Storage, Slide	General
Desiccator	Chemistry
Incubator, Test Tube, Stationary	Microbiology
Incubator/Water Bath, Microbiology	Microbiology
Lamp, Other	General
Oven	Chemistry
Shaker/Stirrer	Chemistry
Washer, Pipette	Chemistry

BOGEN COMMUNICATIONS INTERNATIONAL, INC.
800-999-2809

50 Spring St., Ramsey, NJ 07446-2810
201-934-8500
FDA Number: n/a   *Fax:* 800-999-9016
E-mail: info@bogen.com
Web site: www.bogen.com
Medical Products Sales Volume: $24,000,000
Annual Revenue: $50-$100 Million
Total Employees: 195
Ownership: Public
Stock Symbol: BOGN
Traded On: OTC Bulletin
Produces/Sells CE-marked Devices: N
Distribution: Manufacturer Through Distributor
General Admin.: Jonathan Guss/Chief Executive Officer
     Jeffrey E. Schwarz/Co-Chairman
     Yoav Stern/Co-Chairman
     Michael P. Fleischer/President
Finance: Maureen A. Flotard/Chief Financial Officer, Vice President Finance

Communication Equipment	General
Public Address System	General

BOGEN COMMUNICATIONS, INC.
See Bogen Communications International, Inc.

BOGEN DIV./LEAR SIEGLER COMPANY
See Bogen Communications International, Inc.

BOLT BETHEL, LLC
763-434-5900
23530 University Avenue N.W., PO Box 135, Bethel, MN 55005
FDA Number: 2183910   *Fax:* 763-434-8002
E-mail: sales.bethel@boltindustries.com
Web site: www.boltindustries.com
Medical Products Sales Volume: $9,400,000
Annual Revenue: $25-$50 Million
Year Founded: 2001
Total Employees: 130   *Marketing Staff:* 2   *Sales Staff:* 10
Ownership: Private
Quality System Registration Information: ISO9001
Produces/Sells CE-marked Devices: N
Federal Procurement Eligibility: Small Business
Distribution: Manufacturer Direct, Manufacturer Through Manufacturer Reps
General Admin.: Cindy Holm/General Manager
     Jeff Bell/President, Chief Executive Officer
Mktg./Adv.: Ron Rygiel/Director Marketing & Sales
     Mr. Dave Ohmann/Manager Sales
     Kim Johnson/Sales Representative
Production: Jim Lind/Director Quality Assurance
     John Carter/Manager Manufacturing

Accessories, Fixation, Orthopedic	Orthopedics
Clip, Instrument	Surgery
Component, Ceramic	General
Component, Metal, Other	General
Contract Manufacturing	General
Fixation Appliance, Multiple Component	Orthopedics
Handle, Instrument, Laparoscopic (Electrocautery)	Surgery
Implant, Fixation Device, Spinal	Orthopedics

BOLT BETHEL, LLC
763-434-5900 *(cont'd)*

Instrument, Electrosurgery, Laparoscopic	Surgery
Instrument, Manual, General Surgical	Surgery
Orthopedic Manual Surgical Instrument	Orthopedics
Port & Catheter, Infusion, Implanted, Subcutaneous, Intraspinal	General
Prosthesis, Knee, Hinged (Metal-Metal)	Orthopedics
Surgical Instrument, Cardiovascular	Cardiovascular
Surgical Instrument, Disposable	Surgery

BOLTON MEDICAL, INC.
954-838-9699
799 International Parkway, Sunrise, FL 33325
FDA Number: 2247858   *Fax:* 954-838-8224
E-mail: dbean@boltonmedical.com
Web site: www.boltonmedical.com
Ownership: Private
Produces/Sells CE-marked Devices: N

Catheter, Angioplasty, Coronary, Transluminal, Percut. Oper.	Cardiovascular
Catheter, Angioplasty, Transluminal, Peripheral	Cardiovascular
Stent, Cardiovascular	Cardiovascular
System, Treatment, Aortic Aneurysm, Endovascular Graft	Cardiovascular

BOMED MEDICAL MANUFACTURING, LTD.
See Cardiodynamics International Corp.

BOND CASTER AND WHEEL CORPORATION
800-233-2663
230 South Penn Street, PO Box 339,
717-665-2275
Manheim, PA 17545
FDA Number: n/a   *Fax:* 717-665-3336
E-mail: sales@bondcaster.com
Web site: www.bondcaster.com
Medical Products Sales Volume: $1,400,000
Annual Revenue: $1-$5 Million
Year Founded: 1905
Total Employees: 23   *Marketing Staff:* 2   *Sales Staff:* 4
Ownership: Private
Produces/Sells CE-marked Devices: N
Federal Procurement Eligibility: Small Business
Distribution: Manufacturer Direct, Manufacturer Through Distributor, OEM, Service Direct, Importer, Exporter
General Admin.: Mr. Louis J. Bond/President
Mktg./Adv.: Mrs. Karen C. von Clef/Manager Marketing & Sales

Cart, Instrument	Surgery
Casters, Hospital Equipment	General
Facility, Equipment, Medical, Mobile	General

BONDED LOGISTICS, INC.
704-597-9638
PO Box 480203, 5709 North Graham Street,
Charlotte, NC 28269
FDA Number: 1063309   *Fax:* 704-509-5301
E-mail: m.andrews@bondedlogistics.com
Web site: www.bondedlogistics.com
Medical Products Sales Volume: $10,000,000
Annual Revenue: $1-$5 Million
Year Founded: 1972
Total Employees: 70
Ownership: Private
Quality System Registration Information: ISO9002
Produces/Sells CE-marked Devices: N
Federal Procurement Eligibility: Small Business
Distribution: Service Direct
General Admin.: Mr. Scott Carr/President

Glove, Surgical, Plastic Surgery	Surgery

BONE DENSITY MEASUREMENT INTERNATIONAL, LLC
301-631-0008
550 Highland St., Suite 303, Frederick, MD 21701
FDA Number: 1122857

Densitometer, Bone, Single Photon	Radiology

BONE FOAM
612-338-1400
700 South 10th Ave., Minneapolis, MN 55415
FDA Number: 2321033

Support, Patient Position	Anesthesiology

BONE SOLUTIONS, INC.
214-234-0661
10,000 North Central Expwy, Suite 900, Dallas, TX 75231
FDA Number: n/a   *Fax:* 800-417-8196
E-mail: copp@bonesolutionsinc.com
Web site: http://www.bonesolutionsinc.com
Ownership: Private
Produces/Sells CE-marked Devices: N
General Admin.: Mr. Tony Copp/Chief Operating Officer
     Mr. Tom Lally/Chief Technology Officer

BONITA DENTAL LAB
239-495-3368
10915 Bonita Beach Rd., #1152, Bonita Springs, FL 34135
FDA Number: 1063973
Ownership: Private
Produces/Sells CE-marked Devices: N

BONITA DENTAL LAB   239-495-3368 *(cont'd)*
Crown, Preformed   Dental And Oral
Toothbrush, Manual   Dental And Oral

BONOVO ORTHOPEDICS INC.   480-902.3094
7702 East Doubletree Ranch Road, Suite 300,
Scottsdale, AZ 85258
FDA Number: n/a   *Fax:* 480-902.3093
E-mail: info@bonovo-ortho.com
Web site: http://www.bonovo-ortho.com
Ownership: Private
Produces/Sells CE-marked Devices: N
General Admin.: Mr. Peter Slate/Chief Executive Officer
       Dr. Hansen Yuan/Chief Technology Officer
Production: Dr. Yong Song/Vice President Regulatory & Clinical Affairs
Finance: Mr. Sunny Yen/Vice President Admin., Finance

BONUTTI RESEARCH, INC.   217-342-3412
2600 South Raney, Effingham, IL 62401
FDA Number: 1422428
Bit, Drill   Orthopedics
Fastener, Fixation, Non-Biodegradable, Soft Tissue   Orthopedics
Orthopedic Manual Surgical Instrument   Orthopedics
Orthosis, Limb Brace   Physical Med

BOONE'S INC.
See Mission X-Ray

BOOST TECHNOLOGY, LLC   415-334-8246
1601 Ocean Ave., San Francisco, CA 94112-1717
FDA Number: 3003515980
Ownership: Private
Produces/Sells CE-marked Devices: N
Communication System, Powered   Physical Med

BORDER OPPORTUNITY SAVER SYSTEMS, INC.   830-775-0992
10 Finegan Drive, Del Rio, TX 78841
FDA Number: 1640425   *Fax:* 830-774-3337
E-mail: lmtz@borderopp.com
Web site: www.borderopp.com
Medical Products Sales Volume: $1,500,000
Annual Revenue: $5-$10 Million
Year Founded: 1979
Total Employees: 425   *Marketing Staff:* 1   *Sales Staff:* 1
Ownership: Private
Produces/Sells CE-marked Devices: N
Federal Procurement Eligibility: Small Business, Minority Owned, Female Owned
Distribution: Manufacturer Direct, OEM, Importer
General Admin.: Don P. Newton/Chief Executive Officer
       Leo Martinez/President
       Oralia Newton/Vice President
       Arnulfo E. Ozuna/Vice President, General Manager
Mktg./Adv.: Roy Musquiz/Vice President Marketing & Sales
Adhesive Strip, Waterproof   General
Ball, Cotton   General
Coat, Laboratory   General
Halter, Head, Traction, Orthopedic   Orthopedics
Kit, Prep   General
Kit, Suture Removal   Surgery
Splint, Abduction, Shoulder   Orthopedics
Splint, Padded Stays   Orthopedics
Support, Ankle   Orthopedics
Support, Back   Orthopedics

BOREL ENTERPRISES LLC   337-583-3448
3664 A. Miller Rd., Lake Charles, LA 70605
FDA Number: 3005550422
Ownership: Private
Produces/Sells CE-marked Devices: N
Accessories, Wheelchair   Physical Med

BORNING CORP., THE
See Hill-Rom Holdings, Inc.

BOSE CORPORATION - ELECTROFORCE SYSTEMS GROUP   800-273-0437
    952-278-3070
10250 Valley View Road, Suite 113,
Eden Prairie, MN 55344
FDA Number: n/a   *Fax:* 952-278-3071
E-mail: electroforce@bose.com
Web site: www.bose-electroforce.com
Year Founded: 1964
Ownership: Bose Corporation
Quality System Registration Information: ISO9001
Produces/Sells CE-marked Devices: Y
Distribution: Manufacturer Direct, Manufacturer Through Manufacturer Reps, OEM, Service Direct
General Admin.: Mr. Ed Moriarty/Director, General Manager
Mktg./Adv.: Dave Santo/Manager International & National Sales
Computer Software   General

BOSE CORPORATION - ELECTROFORCE   800-273-0437 *(cont'd)*
Equipment, Laboratory, Gen. Purpose (Specific Medical Use)   Chemistry

BOSOM BUDDY BREAST FORMS
See B & B Lingerie Company, Inc.

BOSS INSTRUMENTS, LTD.   800-210-2677
395 Reas Ford Road, Suite 120,   434-951-0007
Earlysville, VA 22936
FDA Number: 1056350   *Fax:* 800-210-2677
E-mail: boss@bossinst.com
Web site: www.bossinst.com
Medical Products Sales Volume: $800,000
Year Founded: 1990
Total Employees: 10   *Marketing Staff:* 2   *Sales Staff:* 3
Ownership: Private
Quality System Registration Information: ISO9000; ISO9002
Produces/Sells CE-marked Devices: Y
Federal Procurement Eligibility: Small Business
Distribution: Manufacturer Direct, Manufacturer Through Distributor, Manufacturer Through Manufacturer Reps, OEM, Exclusive Distributor, Exporter
General Admin.: Burns Phillips/President, Chief Executive Officer
       Dale Mutryn/Regional Manager
Mktg./Adv.: Larry Griffith/Executive Director Marketing & Sales
       Ashley Robertson/Manager Business Development
Cannula, Extraction, Appendix   Surgery
Clamp, Fixation, Cholangiography   Surgery
Clamp, Laparoscopy   Surgery
Dilator, Blunt   Surgery
ENT Manual Surgical Instrument   Ear/Nose/Throat
Electrode, Electrosurgery, Laparoscopic   Surgery
Endoscope, Electronic (Videoendoscope)   Surgery
Forceps   Orthopedics
Forceps, Grasping, Atraumatic   Surgery
Holder, Needle   Gastroenterology/Urology
Holder, Needle, Laparoscopic   Surgery
Instrument, Dissecting, Laparoscopic   Surgery
Instrument, Knot Tying, Suture, Laparoscopic   Surgery
Instrument, Microsurgical   Cns/Neurology
Instrument, Needle Holder/Knot Tying   Surgery
Needle, Insufflation, Laparoscopic   Surgery
Probe, Suction, Irrigator/Aspirator, Laparoscopic   Surgery
Retractor   Orthopedics
Retractor, ENT (Thoracic)   Ear/Nose/Throat
Scissors, Ophthalmic   Ophthalmology
Scissors, Thoracic   Cardiovascular
Surgical Instrument, Cardiovascular   Cardiovascular
Surgical Instrument, Non-Powered, Neurosurgical   Cns/Neurology
Surgical Instrument, Radial Keratotomy   Ophthalmology

BOSTON BILLOWS, INC.   603-598-1200
114 Perimeter Road, Unit E., Nashua, NH 03063
FDA Number: 3005042377
E-mail: Contact@bostonbillows.com
Ownership: Private
Produces/Sells CE-marked Devices: N
Orthosis, Limb Brace   Physical Med

BOSTON BRACE INTERNATIONAL, INC.   800-262-2235
20 Ledin Dr., Avon, MA 02322
FDA Number: 3001967835   *Fax:* 800-634-5048
E-mail: info@bostonbrace.com
Web site: www.bostonbrace.com
Annual Revenue: $0-$1 Million
Year Founded: 1970
Ownership: Private
Produces/Sells CE-marked Devices: N
Federal Procurement Eligibility: Small Business
Distribution: Manufacturer Direct, Manufacturer Through Distributor
General Admin.: Tom Morrissey/President, Chief Executive Officer
       Robin Meek/Vice President Human Resources
Medical Admin.: James Miller/Vice President Clinical Affairs
Mktg./Adv.: Jonathan Taylor/Vice President Business Development
Production: Derek Ghostlaw/Vice President Manufacturing
Research: James H. Wynne/Vice President Education & Training
Brace, Joint, Ankle (External)   Physical Med
Joint, Knee, External Brace   Physical Med
Orthosis, Corrective Shoe   Physical Med
Orthosis, Lumbar   Physical Med
Orthosis, Lumbosacral   Physical Med
Orthosis, Other   Physical Med
Orthosis, Thoracic   Physical Med
Stimulator, Scoliosis (Orthosis)   Physical Med

BOSTON ENDO-SURGICAL TECHNOLOGIES, INC.   603-929-0066
8 Merrill Drive, Hampton, NH 03842
FDA Number: 1226255   *Fax:* 603-929-0088
E-mail: info@be-st.com

BOSTON ENDO-SURGICAL 603-929-0066 (cont'd)
Web site: www.be-st.com
Ownership: Private
Quality System Registration Information: ISO9001
Produces/Sells CE-marked Devices: N

Drill, Dental, Intraoral	Dental And Oral
Electrosurgical Unit, Cutting & Coagulation Device	Surgery
Knife, Orthopedic	Orthopedics

BOSTON MEDICAL PRODUCTS, INC. 800-433-2674
117 Flanders Road, **508-898-9300**
Westborough, MA 01581
FDA Number: 1219795   *Fax:* 508-898-2373
E-mail: info@bosmed.com
Web site: www.bosmed.com
Medical Products Sales Volume: $2,500,000
Year Founded: 1980
Total Employees: 16
Ownership: Private
Quality System Registration Information: ISO9001
Produces/Sells CE-marked Devices: Y
Federal Procurement Eligibility: Small Business, GSA Contract, VA Contract
Distribution: Manufacturer Direct, Manufacturer Through Manufacturer Reps
General Admin.: Stuart K. Montgomery/President, Chief Executive Officer
Mktg./Adv.: Stuart Montgomery/Director Sales
          C. Robert Woerner/Vice President Business Development
Production: Michael Warren/Manager Regulatory Affairs

Button, Nasal Septal	Ear/Nose/Throat
Cannula, Tracheostomy	Ear/Nose/Throat
Cutter, Surgical	Surgery
Prosthesis, Esophageal	Ear/Nose/Throat
Prosthesis, Laryngeal (Taub)	Ear/Nose/Throat
Prosthesis, Trachea	Surgery
Tube, Nasogastric	Anesthesiology
Tube, Tracheostomy (Breathing Tube), ENT	Ear/Nose/Throat
Valve, Speaking, Tracheal	Ear/Nose/Throat

BOSTON PACICIC MEDICAL,INC.
See Mentor Corp.

BOSTON RHEOLOGY, L.L.C. 617-912-1020
20 Whitney Drive, Chestnut Hill Medical Center,
Sherborn, MA 01770
FDA Number: 1223928   *Fax:* 617-566-6159
E-mail: info@bostonrheology.com
Web site: www.bostonrheology.com
Year Founded: 1992
Total Employees: 6   *Marketing Staff:* 1
Ownership: Private
Quality System Registration Information: ISO9000
Produces/Sells CE-marked Devices: N
Federal Procurement Eligibility: Small Business
Distribution: Manufacturer Through Distributor
General Admin.: Harold J. Kosasky/President, Chief Executive Officer
          Shirley A. Johnston/Vice President, General Manager

Viscometer, Mucus, Cervical	Obstetrics/Gynecology

BOSTON SCIENTIFIC - MAPLE GROVE 800-553-5878
One Scimed Place, **763-494-1700**
Maple Grove, MN 55311
FDA Number: 2134265
Web site: www.bostonscientific.com
Medical Products Sales Volume: $2,400,000,000
Annual Revenue: More than $1 Billion
Total Employees: 14400
Ownership: Boston Scientific Corporation
Stock Symbol: BSX
Traded On: NYSE
Produces/Sells CE-marked Devices: N
Distribution: Manufacturer Direct
General Admin.: Mr. Paul A. LaViolette/Chief Operating Officer
          Paul LaViolette/President
          Mr. William H. (Hank) Kucheman/Senior Vice President
Mktg./Adv.: Nan Upin/Communications Director

Accessories, Catheter	Surgery
Adapter, Stopcock, Manifold, Cardiopulmonary Bypass	Cardiovascular
Adapter, Y	Gastroenterology/Urology
Catheter, Angiographic	Cns/Neurology
Catheter, Angioplasty, Coronary, Transluminal, Percut. Oper.	Cardiovascular
Catheter, Balloon (Foley Type)	Surgery
Catheter, Biliary	Gastroenterology/Urology
Catheter, Cardiovascular, Balloon Type	Cardiovascular
Catheter, Continuous Flush	Cardiovascular
Catheter, Imaging, Ultrasonic	Radiology
Catheter, Intravascular, Diagnostic	Cardiovascular
Catheter, Nephrostomy, General & Plastic Surgery	Surgery
Catheter, Percutaneous	Cardiovascular
Catheter, Percutaneous (Valvuloplasty)	Cardiovascular
Catheter, Peritoneal	Surgery

BOSTON SCIENTIFIC - MAPLE GROVE 800-553-5878 (cont'd)

Filter, Intravascular, Cardiovascular	Cardiovascular
Forceps, Biopsy	Surgery
Guidewire	Cardiovascular
Guidewire, Catheter	Cardiovascular
Injector, Syringe	General
Introducer, Catheter	Cardiovascular
Kit, Biopsy Needle	Gastroenterology/Urology
Stent, Ureteral	Gastroenterology/Urology
Tube, Drainage	Gastroenterology/Urology

BOSTON SCIENTIFIC - MARINA BAY CUSTOMER 617-689-6000
FULFILLMENT CENTER
500 Commander Shea Blvd, Quincy, MA 02171
FDA Number: 1225687
Web site: www.bostonscientific.com
Ownership: BOSTON SCIENTIFIC CORPORATION
Stock Symbol: BSX
Traded On: NYSE
Produces/Sells CE-marked Devices: N

Cannula, Surgical, General & Plastic Surgery	Surgery
Catheter, Angioplasty, Coronary, Transluminal, Percut. Oper.	Cardiovascular
Catheter, Biliary	Gastroenterology/Urology
Catheter, Coronary, Atherectomy	Cardiovascular
Catheter, Percutaneous	Cardiovascular
Dissector, Surgical, General & Plastic Surgery	Surgery
Endoscope	Gastroenterology/Urology
Fastener, Fixation, Non-Biodegradable, Soft Tissue	Orthopedics
Guide, Surgical, Instrument	Surgery
Guide, Surgical, Needle	Surgery
Laparoscope, General & Plastic Surgery	Surgery
Mesh, Surgical, Polymeric	Surgery
Needle, Suture, Disposable	Surgery
Splint, Ureteral	Gastroenterology/Urology
Stent, Cardiovascular	Cardiovascular

BOSTON SCIENTIFIC CORP. 408-517-2800
10231 Bubb Rd., Cupertino, CA 95014-4167
FDA Number: 3005231525
Web site: www.bostonscientific.com
Ownership: Public
Stock Symbol: BSX
Traded On: NYSE
Produces/Sells CE-marked Devices: N

BOSTON SCIENTIFIC CORP. 408-935-3400
150 Baytech Dr., San Jose, CA 95134
FDA Number: 3001236349
Ownership: Boston Scientific Corporation
Produces/Sells CE-marked Devices: N

Catheter, Intravascular Occluding, Temporary	Cardiovascular
Clamp, Vascular	Cardiovascular
Device, Stabilizer, Heart	Cardiovascular
Electrosurgical Unit, Cutting & Coagulation Device	Surgery
Guide, Surgical, Needle	Surgery
Laparoscope, General & Plastic Surgery	Surgery
Lavage Unit, Water Jet	General
Surgical Instrument, Cardiovascular	Cardiovascular
Suture, Non-Absorbable, Synthetic, Polyamide	Surgery
Suture, Non-Absorbable, Synthetic, Polyester	Surgery
System, Albation, Microwave And Accessories	Surgery

BOSTON SCIENTIFIC CORP. 800-323-6472
5905 Nathan Lane, Plymouth, MN 55442-1656 **763-694-5500**
FDA Number: 2183541   *Fax:* 612-550-5880
Medical Products Sales Volume: $60,000,000
Total Employees: 650   *Marketing Staff:* 12   *Sales Staff:* 67
Ownership: Boston Scientific Corporation
Produces/Sells CE-marked Devices: N
Distribution: Manufacturer Direct, Manufacturer Through Manufacturer Reps
General Admin.: Jan Dick/Director Personnel
          David Booth/President
Mktg./Adv.: Diane Davies/Manager Business
          William Gearhart/Vice President Marketing & Sales
Production: John Adams/Vice President Manufacturing
Research: Mike Mikulich/Vice President Research & Development

Catheter, Angiographic	Cns/Neurology
Catheter, Angioplasty, Coronary, Transluminal, Percut. Oper.	Cardiovascular
Catheter, Biliary	Gastroenterology/Urology
Catheter, Cardiovascular	Surgery
Catheter, Percutaneous	Cardiovascular
Guide, Catheter	Cardiovascular
Guide, Wire, Angiographic (And Accessories)	Cns/Neurology
Guidewire, Catheter	Cardiovascular
Introducer, Catheter	Cardiovascular
Kit, Angiographic, Special Procedure	Radiology
Prosthesis, Esophageal	Ear/Nose/Throat
Prosthesis, Trachea	Surgery
Stent, Cardiovascular	Cardiovascular

MANUFACTURER PROFILES

BOSTON SCIENTIFIC CORP.   612-582-7448
6645 185th Ave. N.E., Redmond, WA 98052
FDA Number: n/a
Web site: www.bostonscientific.com
Ownership: BOSTON SCIENTIFIC CORPORATION
Stock Symbol: BSX
Traded On: NYSE
Produces/Sells CE-marked Devices: N

Dual Chamber, Implantable Pulse Generator	Cardiovascular
Pacemaker, Heart, Implantable, Programmable	Cardiovascular
Single Chamber, Sensor Driven, Implantable Pulse Generator	Cardiovascular

BOSTON SCIENTIFIC CORPORATION   508-652-5578
2011 Stierlin Court, Mountain View, CA 94043
FDA Number: 2954755
Ownership: Boston Scientific Corporation
Produces/Sells CE-marked Devices: N

BOSTON SCIENTIFIC CORPORATION   508-652-5578
780 Brookside Drive, Spencer, IN 47460
FDA Number: 1828132
Ownership: Boston Scientific Corporation
Produces/Sells CE-marked Devices: N

Accessories, Catheter	Surgery
Adapter, Bulb, Endoscope, Miscellaneous	Gastroenterology/Urology
Adapter, Catheter, Ureteral	Gastroenterology/Urology
Catheter, Nephrostomy, General & Plastic Surgery	Surgery
Connector, Catheter	Surgery
Connector, Ureteral Catheter	Gastroenterology/Urology
Dilator, Catheter	Surgery
Dislodger, Stone, Basket, Ureteral, Metal	Gastroenterology/Urology
Dislodger, Stone, Flexible	Gastroenterology/Urology
Driver, Prosthesis	Orthopedics
Esterase	Pathology
Evacuator, Bladder, Manually Operated	Gastroenterology/Urology
Evacuator, Fluid	Gastroenterology/Urology
Evacuator, Gastro-Urology	Gastroenterology/Urology
Glove, Protective, Radiographic	Radiology
Guide, Surgical, Instrument	Surgery
Instrument, Passing, Ligature, Knot Tying	Cns/Neurology
Ligator, Esophageal	Gastroenterology/Urology
Ligator, Hemorrhoidal	Gastroenterology/Urology
Mesh, Surgical, Polymeric	Surgery
Needle, Gastro-Urology	Gastroenterology/Urology
Needle, Suture, Disposable	Surgery
Retention Device, Suture	Surgery
Retractor, Vaginal	Obstetrics/Gynecology
Stylet, Catheter, Gastro-Urology	Gastroenterology/Urology
Surgical Instrument, G-U, Manual	Gastroenterology/Urology
Tube, Gastro-Enterostomy	Gastroenterology/Urology
Tube, Gastrointestinal	Gastroenterology/Urology

BOSTON SCIENTIFIC CORPORATION   508-652-5578
8600 N.w. 41st Street, Miami, FL 33166
FDA Number: 1051710
Ownership: Private
Produces/Sells CE-marked Devices: N

Endoscope	Gastroenterology/Urology
Forceps, Biopsy, Non-Electric	Gastroenterology/Urology
Guide, Surgical, Needle	Surgery
Guidewire, Catheter	Cardiovascular
Holder, Needle	Gastroenterology/Urology
Instrument, Manual, General Surgical	Surgery
Needle, Aspiration And Injection, Disposable	Surgery
Needle, Suture, Disposable	Surgery
Stylet, Catheter, Gastro-Urology	Gastroenterology/Urology
Surgical Instrument, G-U, Manual	Gastroenterology/Urology

BOSTON SCIENTIFIC CORPORATION   800-225-2732
One Boston Scientific Place,   **508-650-8000**
Natick, MA 01760
FDA Number: 1225687   Fax: 508-650-8951
Web site: www.bostonscientific.com
Medical Products Sales Volume: $8,357,000,000
Annual Revenue: More than $1 Billion
Year Founded: 1979
Total Employees: 24500   *Marketing Staff:* 3500   *Sales Staff:* 3500
Ownership: Public
Stock Symbol: BSX
Traded On: NYSE
Produces/Sells CE-marked Devices: N
General Admin.: Jeff Capello/Chief Financial Officer, Executive Vice President
     Mr. Samuel Leno/Chief Operating Officer
     Raymond Elliott/President, Chief Executive Officer
Production: Mr. Kenneth Pucel/Executive Vice President Operations
     Mr. Brian Burns/Senior Vice President Quality Assurance

Accessories, Catheter, G-U	Gastroenterology/Urology
Balloon, Intra-Aortic (With Control System)	Cardiovascular
Basket, Biliary Stone Retrieval	Gastroenterology/Urology
Catheter, Angiographic	Cns/Neurology

BOSTON SCIENTIFIC CORPORATION   800-225-2732 *(cont'd)*

Catheter, Angioplasty, Coronary, Transluminal, Percut. Oper.	Cardiovascular
Catheter, Biliary	Gastroenterology/Urology
Catheter, Electrode Recording, Or Probe	Cardiovascular
Catheter, Imaging, Ultrasonic	Radiology
Catheter, Nephrostomy, General & Plastic Surgery	Surgery
Catheter, Occlusion	Cardiovascular
Catheter, Other	Gastroenterology/Urology
Catheter, Pericardium Drainage	Cardiovascular
Catheter, Steerable	Cardiovascular
Dilator, Catheter	Surgery
Dilator, Catheter, Ureteral	Gastroenterology/Urology
Dilator, Esophageal	Gastroenterology/Urology
Dislodger, Stone, Flexible	Gastroenterology/Urology
Dislodger, Store, Biliary	Gastroenterology/Urology
Electrosurgical, Unit, Gastroenterology	Gastroenterology/Urology
Embolization Device	Cardiovascular
Endoscope	Gastroenterology/Urology
Filter, Vena Cava	Cardiovascular
Guidewire, Catheter	Cardiovascular
Guidewire, Coronary, Total Occlusion	Cardiovascular
Kit, Angiographic, Digital	Radiology
Kit, Catheterization, Urinary	Gastroenterology/Urology
Kit, Laparoscopy	Gastroenterology/Urology
Laparoscope, General & Plastic Surgery	Surgery
Lithotriptor, Electro-Hydraulic, Extracorporeal	Gastroenterology/Urology
Lithotriptor, Mechanical, Biliary	Gastroenterology/Urology
Needle, Cardiac	Cardiovascular
Prosthesis, Esophageal	Ear/Nose/Throat
Snare, Flexible	Gastroenterology/Urology
Stent, Cardiovascular	Cardiovascular
Stent, Ureteral	Gastroenterology/Urology
System, Delivery, Drug, Non-invasive	General
Transducer, Ultrasonic, Diagnostic	Radiology
Tube, Drainage	Gastroenterology/Urology
Tube, Gastrointestinal	Gastroenterology/Urology

Medical Product Subsidiaries (Listed Separately)
   Asthmatx, Inc.
   Boston Scientific - Maple Grove
   Boston Scientific Corp.
   Boston Scientific Corporation
   Boston Scientific Neuromodulation Corporation
   Boston Scientific-Neurovascular
   Ep Technologies, Inc.
   Guidant Corporation
   Interventional Technologies, Inc.

BOSTON SCIENTIFIC INTERVENTIONAL   858-268-4488
TECHNOLOGIES
3574 Ruffin Rd., San Diego, CA 92123-2502
FDA Number: n/a   Fax: 858-292-8381
Web site: www.bostonscientific.com
Medical Products Sales Volume: $150,000,000
Year Founded: 1984
Total Employees: 480   *Marketing Staff:* 6
Ownership: BOSTON SCIENTIFIC CORPORATION
Stock Symbol: BSX
Traded On: NYSE
Quality System Registration Information: ISO9001; ISO9003
Produces/Sells CE-marked Devices: Y
Distribution: Manufacturer Direct, Exporter
General Admin.: Tom O'Connell/Director Human Resources
     Matthew Jenusaites/General Manager
Production: Bob Salvucci/Director Quality Assurance
     Paul Mason/Director Regulatory Affairs
     Doug Rimer/Vice President Operations
Research: Herb Radisch/Vice President Research & Development
Finance: Chase Morrison/Controller

Catheter, Balloon, Dilatation, Vessel	Gastroenterology/Urology
Stent, Other	Obstetrics/Gynecology

BOSTON SCIENTIFIC NEUROMODULATION   508-652-5578
CORPORATION
25155 Rye Canyon Loop, Valencia, CA 91355
FDA Number: 3006630150
Web site: www.bostonscientific.com
Annual Revenue: $100-$500 Million
Ownership: Boston Scientific Corporation
Stock Symbol: BSX
Traded On: NYSE
Produces/Sells CE-marked Devices: N
General Admin.: Mr. Paul A. LaViolette/Chief Operating Officer
     Mr. Michael Onuscheck/President

Stimulator, Cerebellar, Full Implant (Pain Relief)	Cns/Neurology

BOSTON SCIENTIFIC VASCULAR
   See Maquet Cardiovascular LLC

BOSTON SCIENTIFIC-NEUROVASCULAR   510-440-7700
47900 Bayside Pkwy., Fremont, CA 94538-6515
FDA Number: 2939204
Web site: www.bostonscientific.com
Annual Revenue: $100-$500 Million
Ownership: Stryker Corp.
Stock Symbol: BSX
Traded On: NYSE
Produces/Sells CE-marked Devices: N
General Admin.: Mr. Paul A. LaViolette/Chief Operating Officer
     Mr. Joseph M. Fitzgerald/President

Catheter, Balloon (Foley Type)	Surgery
Catheter, Continuous Flush	Cardiovascular
Catheter, Coronary, Atherectomy	Cardiovascular
Catheter, Infusion	Surgery
Catheter, Intravascular, Diagnostic	Cardiovascular
Computer, Diagnostic, Programmable	Cardiovascular
Device, Embolization, Artificial	Cns/Neurology
Electrode, Ablation, Tissue, Conduction, Percutaneous	Cardiovascular
Scanner, Ultrasonic (Pulsed Doppler)	Radiology
Scanner, Ultrasonic (Pulsed Echo)	Radiology
Transducer, Ultrasonic, Diagnostic	Radiology

BOUND TREE ALS MEDICAL PRODUCTS
See Bound Tree Medical

BOUND TREE CORP.
See Bound Tree Medical

BOUND TREE MEDICAL   800-533-0523
PO Box 8023, Dublin, OH 43016-2023   614-760-5000
FDA Number: n/a   *Fax:* 800-257-5713
E-mail: info@boundtree.com
Web site: www.boundtree.com
Total Employees: 270   *Marketing Staff:* 5   *Sales Staff:* 60
Ownership: Private
Produces/Sells CE-marked Devices: N
Distribution: Manufacturer Through Distributor, Exclusive Distributor
General Admin.: Matthew Walter/Chief Executive Officer
     Linden Joseph/President

Board, Spine	Orthopedics

BOUND TREE MEDICAL, LLC   800-533-0523
5200 Rings Road, Suite A, Dublin, OH 43017   614-878-8581
FDA Number: 3004986234   *Fax:* 800-257-5713
E-mail: info@boundtree.com
Web site: www.boundtree.com
Medical Products Sales Volume: $39,300,000
Year Founded: 1978
Total Employees: 80
Ownership: Private
Produces/Sells CE-marked Devices: N
Federal Procurement Eligibility: Small Business
Distribution: Manufacturer Direct
General Admin.: Lendy Joseph/Chief Executive Officer
     Matt Walter/President
Mktg./Adv.: Ross Baum/Market Manager

Board, Spine	Orthopedics
Tray, Custom/Special Procedure	General

BOVIE MEDICAL CORP.   800-537-2790
5115 Ulmerton Road, Clearwater, FL 33760   727-384-2323
FDA Number: 3007593903
Web site: www.boviemedical.com
Total Employees: 163   *Sales Staff:* 11
Ownership: Public
Stock Symbol: BVX
Traded On: AMEX
Quality System Registration Information: ISO9001
Produces/Sells CE-marked Devices: Y
Federal Procurement Eligibility: Small Business
Distribution: Manufacturer Through Distributor, OEM, Exporter
General Admin.: Moshe Citronowicz/Chief Operating Officer, Vice President
     Mr. J. Robert Saron/President
     Andrew Makrides/President, Chief Executive Officer
Mktg./Adv.: Genard McCauley/Product & Sales Manager
     Mr. Jeff Rencher/Vice President Marketing & Sales
Finance: Gary Pickett/Chief Financial Officer

Arthroscope	Orthopedics
Bandage, Other	General
Burr, Corneal, Battery-Powered	Ophthalmology
Burr, Corneal, Manual	Ophthalmology
Cautery, Thermal, Battery-Powered	Ophthalmology
Depressor, Tongue	General
Electrocautery Unit, Battery-Powered	Surgery
Electrocautery Unit, Gynecologic	Obstetrics/Gynecology
Electrode, Electrosurgical, Return (Ground, Dispersive)	Surgery
Electrode, Other	General
Electrosurgical Unit, Cutting & Coagulation Device	Surgery
Electrosurgical, Unit, Gastroenterology	Gastroenterology/Urology

BOVIE MEDICAL CORP.   800-537-2790 *(cont'd)*

Illuminator, Non-Remote	Surgery
Light, Other	General
Penlight, Battery-Powered	Ophthalmology
Power Supply, Endoscopic, Battery-Operated	General
Shield, Eye, Ophthalmic	Ophthalmology
Stimulator, Nerve Locating	Cns/Neurology
Stimulator, Nerve Locating, Facial	Cns/Neurology
Stylet, Tracheal Tube	Anesthesiology

BOVIE MEDICAL CORPORATION
See Bovie Medical Corp.

BOWEN MEDICAL SERVICES, INC.   800-726-8377
709 Industrial Ave., Live Oak, FL 32064   386-362-1345
FDA Number: 1055584   *Fax:* 386-362-1345
E-mail: info@bowenmed.com
Web site: www.bowenmed.com
Ownership: Private
Produces/Sells CE-marked Devices: N

Cuff, Blood Pressure	Cardiovascular

BOWER, INC.   205-884-7918
830 Pine Harbor Rd., Pell City, AL 35128-6763
FDA Number: 3003722308
Ownership: Private
Produces/Sells CE-marked Devices: N

Accessories, Wheelchair	Physical Med
Tips And Pads, Cane, Crutch And Walker	Physical Med

BOWERS MEDICAL SUPPLY CO.   800-663-0047
3691 Viking Way, Unit 9,   604-278-7566
Richmond, BC V6V 2 Canada
FDA Number: 9680511   *Fax:* 604-278-7525
E-mail: bowersmed@bowersmedical.com
Web site: www.bowersmedical.com
Year Founded: 1972
Total Employees: 100
Ownership: NORTHWEST MEDICAL GROUP
Produces/Sells CE-marked Devices: N
Distribution: Manufacturer Direct, Exclusive Distributor, Importer

BOWMAN
See Bowman Manufacturing Company, Inc.

BOWMAN MANUFACTURING COMPANY, INC.   360-435-5005
17301 51st Ave NE, Arlington, WA 98223
FDA Number: n/a   *Fax:* 360-435-5277
E-mail: info@bowmanmfg.com
Web site: www.bowmanmfg.com
Medical Products Sales Volume: $6,500,000
Annual Revenue: $5-$10 Million
Year Founded: 1971
Total Employees: 80   *Marketing Staff:* 2   *Sales Staff:* 3
Ownership: BOWMAN MANUFACTURING COMPANY, INC.
Quality System Registration Information: ISO9001
Produces/Sells CE-marked Devices: N
Federal Procurement Eligibility: Small Business, GSA Contract, VA Contract
Distribution: Manufacturer Through Distributor
General Admin.: Randy L. Bellon/President
Mktg./Adv.: Greg Hill/Vice President Marketing
     Gene A. Bellon/Vice President National Sales

Dispenser, Other	General

BOY BOY APPLE NON WOVENS WASHOUGAL, INC.
See Bba Fiberweb Washougal, Inc.

BOYD ASSOCIATES INC.   330-854-5433
465 Trelake Dr., Canal Fulton, OH 44614
FDA Number: 3004537832
Ownership: Private
Produces/Sells CE-marked Devices: N

Dilator, Nasal	Ear/Nose/Throat

BOYD CONVERTING CO., INC.   800-262-2242
PO BOX 287, South Lee, MA 01260   413-243-2200
FDA Number: 1287317   *Fax:* 413-243-4460
E-mail: schase@boydconverting.com
Web site: www.boydconverting.com
Medical Products Sales Volume: $3,000,000
Annual Revenue: $25-$50 Million
Year Founded: 1979
Total Employees: 130   *Marketing Staff:* 3   *Sales Staff:* 8
Ownership: Boyd Technologies LLC
Quality System Registration Information: ISO9001
Produces/Sells CE-marked Devices: N
Federal Procurement Eligibility: Small Business
Distribution: Manufacturer Direct, Service Direct, Exclusive Distributor
General Admin.: Stephen Boyd/President
Mktg./Adv.: Andrew Diamond/Vice President Business Development

BOYD CONVERTING CO., INC.   800-262-2242 *(cont'd)*
Matthew Boyd/Vice President Sales

Drape, Surgical	Surgery
Sheet, Burn	General
Wrap, Sterilization	General

BOYD INDUSTRIES, INC.   800-255-2693
12900 44th St. North, Clearwater, FL 33762   **727-561-9292**
FDA Number: 1062917   Fax: 727-561-9393
Web site: www.boydindustries.com
Ownership: Private
Produces/Sells CE-marked Devices: N

Chair, Dental (With Unit)	Dental And Oral
Light, Surgical Operating, Dental	Dental And Oral
Operative Dental Treatment Unit	Dental And Oral

BP MEDICAL SYSTEMS, INC.
See Allied Healthcare Products, Inc.

BPSP CO. (MEDICAL Z CORP.)   800-368-7478
6800 Alamo Downs Pkwy,   **210-521-7074**
San Antonio, TX 78238
FDA Number: 1644436   Fax: 210-521-6874
E-mail: info.us@medicalz.com
Web site: www.medicalz.com
Medical Products Sales Volume: $800,000
Annual Revenue: $0-$1 Million
Total Employees: 15   *Marketing Staff:* 1   *Sales Staff:* 3
Ownership: Private
Produces/Sells CE-marked Devices: N
Federal Procurement Eligibility: Small Business
Distribution: Exclusive Distributor, Importer, Exporter
General Admin.: Andre Zagame/President

Bandage, Elastic	General
Contract Manufacturing	General
Electrode, Gel	Cardiovascular

BRADEN SHIELDING SYSTEMS   918-624-2888
9260 Broken Arrow Expressway, Tulsa, OK 74145-1229
FDA Number: n/a   Fax: 918-624-2886
E-mail: info@bradenshielding.com
Web site: www.bradenshielding.com
Medical Products Sales Volume: $2,300,000
Annual Revenue: $10-$25 Million
Year Founded: 1986
Total Employees: 40   *Marketing Staff:* 2   *Sales Staff:* 6
Ownership: Private
Produces/Sells CE-marked Devices: N
Federal Procurement Eligibility: Small Business
Distribution: Manufacturer Direct, OEM, Exporter
General Admin.: Mr. Steve Pittman/Chief Financial Officer, Vice President
    Mr. Tom Foyil/President, Chief Executive Officer
Mktg./Adv.: Mr. Stefan Hipskind/Manager Sales
    Mr. Gil Raymond/Sales Associate
    Mr. John Dattilio/Sales Associate
    Mr. Tony Steffens/Sales Associate
Production: Mr. Dave Moss/Manager Operations
    Mr. Harold Jimison/Manager Operations
    Mr. Q.L. Bell/Manager Quality Control
Finance: Ms. Joy Pittman/Controller

Shield, Magnetic Field	Radiology

BRADFORD MEDICAL, LLC   816-584-8100
8350 N. St. Clair Ave., #230, Kansas City, MO 64151
FDA Number: 3004477123
Ownership: Private
Produces/Sells CE-marked Devices: N

Linen, Bed	General

BRADLEY ALARM SYSTEMS   402-791-2388
28801 S. 96th Street, Firth, NE 68358
FDA Number: 3006278572
Ownership: Private
Produces/Sells CE-marked Devices: N

Regulator, Pressure, Gas Cylinder	Anesthesiology

BRADLEY CO.
See Bradley Company, A Sub. Of Xerox Corporation

BRADLEY COMPANY, A SUB. OF XEROX CORPORATION   216-292-7220
4829 Galaxy Parkway, Cleveland, OH 44128
FDA Number: n/a   Fax: 216-292-9101
E-mail: info@bradleycompany.com
Web site: www.bradleycompany.com
Medical Products Sales Volume: $2,500,000
Annual Revenue: $1-$5 Million
Year Founded: 1983
Total Employees: 40   *Marketing Staff:* 2   *Sales Staff:* 8

BRADLEY COMPANY, A SUB. OF XEROX   216-292-7220 *(cont'd)*
Ownership: Xerox Corp.
Produces/Sells CE-marked Devices: N
Federal Procurement Eligibility: Small Business
Distribution: Service Direct
General Admin.: John S. Zitzner/President, Chief Executive Officer
Mktg./Adv.: Mary Martin/Manager Marketing Communications
    Eric Baumgartner/Vice President Marketing
Production: Terry Light/Vice President Manufacturing

Computer Software	General

BRADROCK INDUSTRIES, INC.   847-299-8151
75 E. Bradrock Drive, Des Plaines, IL 60018   **757-224-0177**
FDA Number: 3000151870   Fax: 847-299-8157
E-mail: information@bradrock.com
Web site: www.bradrock.com
Ownership: Private
Produces/Sells CE-marked Devices: N

Cup, Prophylaxis	Dental And Oral

BRADY CORPORATION   800-541-1686
6555 West Good Hope Road, PO Box 571, Milwaukee, WI 53223
FDA Number: n/a   Fax: 800-292-2289
Web site: www.bradycorp.com
Annual Revenue: More than $1 Billion
Year Founded: 1914
Total Employees: 45
Ownership: Public
Stock Symbol: BRC
Traded On: NYSE
Quality System Registration Information: ISO9002
Produces/Sells CE-marked Devices: Y
Distribution: Manufacturer Direct, OEM
General Admin.: Thomas J. Felmer/Chief Financial Officer, Senior Vice President
    Mr. Bentley Curran/Chief Information Officer
    Dr. Robert Tatterson/Chief Technology Officer, Vice President
    Frank M. Jaehnert/President, Chief Executive Officer
Finance: Mr. Aaron Pearce/Vice President, Treasurer

Adhesive Strip, Hypoallergenic	General
Adhesive Strip, Waterproof	General
Bandage, Butterfly	General
Contract Assembly	General
Contract Manufacturing	General
Contract Manufacturing, Product, Disposable	General
Dressing, Gel	General
Electrode, Other	General
Pad, Dressing	General
Patch, Transdermal	General
Service, Printing	General

BRADY MEDICAL SOLUTIONS
See Brady Corporation

BRADY PRECISION CONVERTING, LLC   214-275-9595
1801 Big Town Blvd., Suite 100, Mesquite, TX 75149
FDA Number: 1648579   Fax: 214-275-6748
E-mail: bdavies@pcitechnology.com
Web site: www.pcitechnology.com
Medical Products Sales Volume: $100,000
Annual Revenue: $10-$25 Million
Year Founded: 1995
Ownership: Private
Quality System Registration Information: ISO9001
Produces/Sells CE-marked Devices: N
Federal Procurement Eligibility: Small Business
Distribution: OEM
General Admin.: Mr. Roger A. Liebelt/President, Chief Executive Officer
    Mr. Brian Davies/Vice President
Production: Mr. Hank Meza/Manager Production
    Mr. Greg White/Vice President Quality Assurance & Quality Control

Adhesive, Wound Closure	Surgery
Bandage, Adhesive	Surgery
Contract Manufacturing	General
Contract Manufacturing, Product, Disposable	General
Contract Packaging	General
Dressing, Gel	General
Dressing, Permeable, Moisture	General
Dressing, Wound, Hydrophilic	Surgery
Dressing, Wound, Occlusive	Surgery
Patch, Transdermal	General
Shield, Eye, Ophthalmic	Ophthalmology
Tape, Adhesive	General
Tape, Adhesive, Hypoallergenic	General

BRAEMAR, INC   803-407-3044
400 Arbor Lake Dr., Suite B450, Columbia, SC 29223-4571
FDA Number: 1319022
E-mail: info@braemarinc.com
Web site: www.braemarinc.com

BRAEMAR, INC
803-407-3044 *(cont'd)*

Ownership: Private
Produces/Sells CE-marked Devices: N
Computer, Diagnostic, Programmable — Cardiovascular
Electrocardiograph, Ambulatory(without Analysis) — Cardiovascular
Monitor, Blood Pressure, Indirect, Semi-Automatic — Cardiovascular
Scanner, Ultrasonic (Pulsed Doppler) — Radiology

BRAEMAR, INC.
800-328-2719
651-286-8620
1285 Corporate Center Dr., Suite 150,
Eagan, MN 55121

FDA Number: 2133409 — *Fax:* 651-286-8630
E-mail: info@braemarinc.com
Web site: www.braemarinc.com
Medical Products Sales Volume: $11,200,000
Year Founded: 1998
Total Employees: 41 — *Marketing Staff:* 1 — *Sales Staff:* 1
Ownership: BIOTEL, INC.
Quality System Registration Information: ISO9001
Produces/Sells CE-marked Devices: Y
Distribution: OEM
General Admin.: Harry Strandquist/President
Mktg./Adv.: Andy McLaughlin/Manager Sales
Production: Darren Dershem/Director Engineering
Betty Matschiner/Director Operations
Finance: Judy Naus/Vice President Admin., Chief Financial Officer
Electrocardiograph, Ambulatory(without Analysis) — Cardiovascular
Pump, Infusion — General
Recorder, Long-Term, ECG — Cardiovascular
Recorder, Long-Term, ECG, Portable (Holter Monitor) — Cardiovascular
Recorder, Magnetic Tape/Disc — Cardiovascular
Scanner, Long-Term, ECG, Recording — Cardiovascular
Transmitter/Receiver System, ECG, Telephone Single-Channel — Cardiovascular

BRAILSFORD & CO., INC.
603-588-2880
15 Elm Avenue, Antrim, NH 03440

FDA Number: n/a — *Fax:* 603-588-7172
E-mail: askus@brailsfordco.com
Web site: www.brailsfordco.com
Medical Products Sales Volume: $1,500,000
Annual Revenue: $1-$5 Million
Year Founded: 1944
Total Employees: 25
Ownership: Private
Produces/Sells CE-marked Devices: N
Federal Procurement Eligibility: Small Business
Distribution: Manufacturer Direct, OEM
General Admin.: R. E. Drummond/President, Chief Executive Officer
R. Drummond/Vice President, General Manager
Mktg./Adv.: John Halper/Manager Market Research
Elizabeth Drummond/Vice President Marketing & Advertising
Blower, Powder, ENT — Ear/Nose/Throat
Motor, Surgical Instrument, DC-Powered — Surgery
Pump, Aspiration, Portable — Anesthesiology
Pump, Inflator — General
Pump, Vacuum, Central — Anesthesiology

BRAIN POWER, INC.
800-327-2250
305-264-4465
4470 S.W. 74th Ave., Miami, FL 33155

FDA Number: n/a — *Fax:* 305-264-1467
E-mail: bpi@callbpi.com
Web site: www.callbpi.com
Year Founded: 1971
Total Employees: 45
Ownership: Private
Produces/Sells CE-marked Devices: Y
Federal Procurement Eligibility: Small Business
Distribution: Manufacturer Direct, OEM, Exporter
General Admin.: Herbert Wertheim/President
Mktg./Adv.: Jean Brill/Manager International & National Sales
J. R. Blackwood/Manager Marketing & Sales
Research: William Moore/Manager Research & Development
Apron, Laboratory — Chemistry
Cleaner, Ultrasonic, Medical Instrument — General
Glove, Other — General
Photometer — Chemistry
Wipe, Instrument — General

BRAIN TUNNELGENIX TECHNOLOGIES CORP.
203-922-0105
375 mather street, Hamden, CT 06514

FDA Number: n/a
Web site: http://www.braintunnelgenix.com
Ownership: Private
Produces/Sells CE-marked Devices: N
General Admin.: Dr. M. Marc Abreu/Chief Scientific Officer
Mr. Rick Foreman/President
Research: Ms. Maria Altieri/Vice President Research
Mr. J. Roger Titone/Vice President Research & Development

BRAIN TUNNELGENIX TECHNOLOGIES CORP.
203-922-0105
(cont'd)

Finance: Mr. Paul Caiafa/Chief Financial Officer
Pack, Hot Or Cold, Disposable — Physical Med
Thermometer, Electronic — General

BRAINMASTER TECHNOLOGIES
440-232-6000
195 Willis Street, Bedford, OH 44146

FDA Number: 1531052 — *Fax:* 440-232-7171
Web site: www.brainmaster.com
Ownership: Private
Produces/Sells CE-marked Devices: N
Biofeedback Device — Cns/Neurology
Electroencephalograph — Cns/Neurology

BRAINSCOPE COMPANY INC.
240-752-7680
8120 Woodmont Avenue, Suite 250, Bethesda, MD 20814

FDA Number: n/a
E-mail: info@brainscope.com
Ownership: Private
Produces/Sells CE-marked Devices: N
General Admin.: Mr. Michael Singer/Chief Executive Officer
Mr. Douglas Oberly/Director Clinical Affairs
Mktg./Adv.: Dr. Neil Rothman/Executive Director Product Development & Marketing

BRAMSTEDT INSTRUMENT SERVICE CO., INC.
See Minnesota Bramstedt Surgical, Inc.

BRANAN MEDICAL CORP.
866-468-3287
949-598-7166
140 Technology, Suite 400, Irvine, CA 92618

FDA Number: 2032137 — *Fax:* 949-598-7167
E-mail: info@brananmedical.com
Web site: www.brananmedical.com
Ownership: Private
Produces/Sells CE-marked Devices: N
Chromatography, Thin Layer, Tricyclic Antidepressant Drugs — Toxicology
Enzyme Immunoassay, Amphetamine — Toxicology
Enzyme Immunoassay, Barbiturate — Toxicology
Enzyme Immunoassay, Benzodiazepine — Toxicology
Enzyme Immunoassay, Cannabinoids — Toxicology
Enzyme Immunoassay, Cocaine And Cocaine Metabolites — Toxicology
Enzyme Immunoassay, Methadone — Toxicology
Enzyme Immunoassay, Opiates — Toxicology
Enzyme Immunoassay, Phencyclidine — Toxicology
Fixative, Alcohol Containing — Pathology
Fluorometry, Morphine — Toxicology
Gas Chromatography, Methamphetamine — Toxicology
Radioimmunoassay, Morphine (125-I), Goat Antibody — Toxicology
Radioimmunoassay, Tricyclic Antidepressant Drugs — Toxicology
Thin Layer Chromatography, Metamphetamine — Toxicology
U.V. Spectrometry, Tricyclic Antidepressant Drugs — Toxicology

BRAND X-RAY CO., INC.
630-543-5331
910 Westwood Ave., Addison, IL 60101-4917

FDA Number: 1450560 — *Fax:* 630-543-8551
E-mail: e-mail@brandx-ray.com.
Web site: www.brandx-ray.com
Ownership: Private
Produces/Sells CE-marked Devices: N
Radiographic/Fluoroscopic Unit, Image-Intensified — Radiology

BRANDEL
800-948-6506
301-948-6506
8561 Atlas Dr., Gaithersburg, MD 20877-4135

FDA Number: n/a — *Fax:* 301-869-5570
E-mail: sales@brandel.com
Web site: www.brandel.com
Annual Revenue: $0-$1 Million
Ownership: Bmr Teo.
Produces/Sells CE-marked Devices: Y
Federal Procurement Eligibility: Small Business
Distribution: Manufacturer Direct, Manufacturer Through Manufacturer Reps, Exporter
Contract R&D, Diagnostics — General
Harvester, Cell — Microbiology
Pump, Infusion — General
System, Robot — General

BRANDRUD FURNITURE, INC.
253-838-6500
1502 20th St. NW, Auburn, WA 98001-3428

FDA Number: n/a — *Fax:* 253-735-2576
E-mail: info@brandrud.com
Web site: www.brandrud.com
Medical Products Sales Volume: $3,700,000
Annual Revenue: $10-$25 Million
Year Founded: 1955
Total Employees: 50 — *Marketing Staff:* 3 — *Sales Staff:* 35
Ownership: Private
Produces/Sells CE-marked Devices: N
Federal Procurement Eligibility: Small Business, GSA Contract

MANUFACTURER PROFILES

BRANDRUD FURNITURE, INC.   **253-838-6500** *(cont'd)*
Distribution: Manufacturer Direct, Manufacturer Through Distributor, Manufacturer Through Manufacturer Reps
General Admin.: Bobby Holt/President
Mktg./Adv.: Lee Falck/President, Director Sales
Production: Jeanette Barrett/Manager Customer Services
  Chair, Other   General
  Furniture, General   General

BRANDT INDUSTRIES, INC.   **800-221-8031**
  4461 Bronx Blvd., Bronx, NY 10470-1496   **718-994-0800**
FDA Number: 2410630   Fax: 718-325-7995
E-mail: info@brandtind.com
Web site: www.brandtind.com
Medical Products Sales Volume: $1,800,000
Annual Revenue: $1-$5 Million
Year Founded: 1930
Total Employees: 9   Marketing Staff: 1   Sales Staff: 2
Ownership: Private
Produces/Sells CE-marked Devices: N
Federal Procurement Eligibility: Small Business
Distribution: Manufacturer Through Distributor, OEM
General Admin.: Neil Brandt/President, Chief Executive Officer
           Susan Brandt/Vice President
Production: Angenol Santiago/Foreman
           Kathy Rice/Manager Production
  Cart, Multipurpose   General
  Chair, Blood Donor   General
  Chair, Examination And Treatment   General
  Chair, Other   General
  Cushion, Stool   General
  Dispenser, Narcotic   General
  Footstool   General
  Footstool, Non-Conductive   General
  Hanger, Intravenous   General
  Illuminator, Radiographic Film   Radiology
  Infusion Stand   General
  Lamp, Examination (Light)   General
  Lamp, Infrared   Physical Med
  Lamp, Other   General
  Lamp, Surgical, Incandescent   Surgery
  Lamp, Ultraviolet, Physical Medicine   Physical Med
  Stand, Operating Room Instrument (Mayo)   Surgery
  Stool, Exercise   Physical Med
  Stool, Operating Room, Adjustable   Surgery
  Table, Examination/Treatment   General
  Table, Other   General
  Table, Overbed   General
  Table, Surgical, Hydraulic   Surgery
  Tray, Surgical Instrument   Surgery
  Waste Receptacle, Kick Bucket   General

BRANFORD LABORATORIES   **843-832-8004**
  PO Box 51000, Summerville, SC 29485-1000
FDA Number: 1221899   Fax: 843-832-0803
E-mail: customerservice@branfordlabs.com
Web site: www.branfordlabs.com
Annual Revenue: $1-$5 Million
Total Employees: 7
Ownership: Private
Produces/Sells CE-marked Devices: Y
Federal Procurement Eligibility: Small Business
Distribution: Manufacturer Through Manufacturer Reps, Exporter
General Admin.: Kenneth W. Kubofcik/President, Chief Executive Officer
Production: Christopher Kubofcik/Vice President Operations
  Eyeglasses, Safety   Ophthalmology
  Glove, Surgical   General

BRANSON ULTRASONICS CORP.   **203-796-2235**
  41 Eagle Rd., P.o. Box 1961, Danbury, CT 06813
FDA Number: 1219133
Ownership: Private
Produces/Sells CE-marked Devices: N
  Cleaner, Ultrasonic, Medical Instrument   General

BRANT-WALD SURGICALS, INC.   **865-483-5230**
  368 E. Tennessee Ave., Oak Ridge, TN 37830-4962
FDA Number: n/a   Fax: 865-482-4186
E-mail: info@brantwald.com
Web site: www.brantwald.com
Medical Products Sales Volume: $250,000
Year Founded: 1974
Total Employees: 5   Marketing Staff: 1   Sales Staff: 2
Ownership: Private
Produces/Sells CE-marked Devices: Y
Federal Procurement Eligibility: Small Business
Distribution: Manufacturer Direct, Manufacturer Through Distributor, Exclusive Distributor, Exporter
General Admin.: Mr. Rayburn C. Waldrop/President, Owner

BRANT-WALD SURGICALS, INC.   **865-483-5230** *(cont'd)*
  Apron, Surgical   Surgery

BRANTLIN   **954-691-6476**
  1511 N.e. 40th St., Pompano Beach, FL 33064
FDA Number: 3005761470
  Insoles, Medical   General

BRASEL PRODUCTS, INC.   **630-879-3759**
  715 Hunter Dr., Batavia, IL 60510-1425
FDA Number: n/a   Fax: 630-879-6912
E-mail: mark@brasel.com
Web site: www.brasel.com
Medical Products Sales Volume: $1,500,000
Annual Revenue: $1-$5 Million
Total Employees: 12
Ownership: Private
Produces/Sells CE-marked Devices: Y
Federal Procurement Eligibility: Small Business, Female Owned
Distribution: Manufacturer Through Distributor
General Admin.: Melody B. Davoust/President
           Mark J. Davoust/Vice President, General Manager
Mktg./Adv.: Mark J. Davoust/Vice President Marketing
Production: Brian Davoust/Director Distribution
  Bandage, Gauze   General
  Bandage, Other   General

BRASSELER CANADA INC.   **800-363-3838**
  5757 Decelles Ave., Ste. 234,   **514-737-8857**
  Montreal, QUE H3S-2 Canada
FDA Number: n/a   Fax: 514-737-7427
E-mail: larrychapdelaine@brasseler.attcanada.net
Web site: www.brasseler.de
Year Founded: 1987
Total Employees: 25
Ownership: Private
Produces/Sells CE-marked Devices: N
Distribution: Exclusive Distributor

BRASSELER USA - KOMET MEDICAL   **800-535-6638**
  One Brassler Blvd., Savannah, GA 31419-9565   **912-925-8525**
FDA Number: 1032227   Fax: 912-921-7578
E-mail: komet@kometmedical.com
Web site: www.kometmedical.com
Total Employees: 150   Marketing Staff: 4   Sales Staff: 125
Ownership: Private
Quality System Registration Information: ISO9001
Produces/Sells CE-marked Devices: Y
Federal Procurement Eligibility: GSA Contract, VA Contract
Distribution: Manufacturer Direct, Manufacturer Through Manufacturer Reps, OEM, Importer, Exporter
General Admin.: Mr. Ken Kitzarow/Managing Director
Mktg./Adv.: Mr. Jens Haverkamp/Director Marketing & Sales
Production: Ms. Sandra Mueller/Product Manager
  Accessories, Powered Drill   Cns/Neurology
  Battery   General
  Blade, Bone Cutting   Orthopedics
  Blade, Saw, Cast Cutting   Orthopedics
  Blade, Surgical, Saw, General & Plastic Surgery   Surgery
  Burr, Cranial   Cns/Neurology
  Burr, Dental   Dental And Oral
  Burr, Dental Excavating   Dental And Oral
  Burr, Orthopedic   Orthopedics
  Burr, Other   Surgery
  Burr, Podiatric   Orthopedics
  Burr, Surgical, General & Plastic Surgery   Surgery
  Forceps, Tooth Extractor, Surgical   Dental And Oral
  Handle, Scalpel   Surgery
  Orthopedic Manual Surgical Instrument   Orthopedics
  Pin, Fixation, Smooth   Orthopedics
  Pin, Fixation, Threaded   Orthopedics
  Saw, Other   Surgery

BRASSELER USA - MEDICAL   **805-650-5209**
  4837 McGrath Street, Suite J, Ventura, CA 93003
FDA Number: 2025102   Fax: 805-650-5260
E-mail: customerservice@brasselerusamedical.com
Web site: www.brasselerusamedical.com
Year Founded: 1987
Ownership: Private
Produces/Sells CE-marked Devices: Y
Production: Mr. Christopher Feitel/Director Regulatory Affairs
  Accessories, Powered Drill   Cns/Neurology
  Blade, Surgical, Saw, General & Plastic Surgery   Surgery
  Burr   Ear/Nose/Throat
  Burr, Dental   Dental And Oral
  Burr, Surgical, General & Plastic Surgery   Surgery
  Instrument, Surgical, Powered, Pneumatic   Orthopedics
  Lavage Unit, Water Jet   General

BRASSELER USA - MEDICAL   805-650-5209 *(cont'd)*
Motor, Drill, Pneumatic	Cns/Neurology
Pin, Fixation, Smooth	Orthopedics
Pin, Fixation, Threaded	Orthopedics
Saw, Powered, And Accessories	Cns/Neurology
Suction Apparatus, Operating Room, Wall Vacuum-Powered	Surgery
Surgical Instrument, Orthopedic, AC-Powered Motor	Orthopedics
Wrap, Sterilization	General

BRATON BIOTECH, INC.   301-762-5301
1 Taft Ct., Suite 101, Rockville, MD 20850
FDA Number: n/a   *Fax:* 301-294-9467
E-mail: labs@bratonbiotech.com
Web site: http://www.bratonbiotech.com/
Medical Products Sales Volume: $2,500,000
Annual Revenue: $0-$1 Million
Year Founded: 1984
Total Employees: 15   *Marketing Staff:* 2   *Sales Staff:* 5
Ownership: Private
Produces/Sells CE-marked Devices: N
Federal Procurement Eligibility: Small Business, Minority Owned
Distribution: Service Direct
General Admin.: Sharma Vedbrat/Chief Executive Officer
Antibody, Monoclonal	Microbiology
Antibody, Polyclonal	Microbiology

BRAUN BIOTECH, B.
See Sartorius Stedim Sus Inc.

BRAUN INDUSTRIES, INC.   800-222-7286
1170 Production Drive, Van Wert, OH 45891   419-232-7020
FDA Number: 9200158   *Fax:* 419-232-7070
E-mail: contactus@braunambulances.com
Web site: www.braunambulances.com
Medical Products Sales Volume: $19,200,000
Annual Revenue: $10-$25 Million
Year Founded: 1972
Total Employees: 190   *Marketing Staff:* 1   *Sales Staff:* 5
Ownership: Private
Produces/Sells CE-marked Devices: N
Federal Procurement Eligibility: Small Business, Female Owned
Distribution: Manufacturer Through Distributor, Exporter
General Admin.: Phillip C. Braun/Chairman, Chief Executive Officer
    Philip Braun/President
Mktg./Adv.: Charma Braun/Vice President Business Development
    Jim Biedenharn/Vice President Marketing & Sales
Production: Gary Kohls/Vice President Manufacturing
Ambulance	General

BRAUN INSTRUMENTS, B.
See Sartorius Stedim Sus Inc.

BRAUN MEDICAL EQUIPMENT, B.
See B. Braun Medical Inc., Renal Therapies Div.

BRAUN MEDICAL, INC., B.
See B. Braun Oem Division, B. Braun Medical Inc.

BRAUN NORTHWEST, INC.   800-245-6303
PO BOX 1204, Chehalis, WA 98532
FDA Number: n/a   *Fax:* 360-748-0256
E-mail: sales@braunnorthwest.com
Web site: www.braunnorthwest.com
Medical Products Sales Volume: $7,500,000
Annual Revenue: $5-$10 Million
Year Founded: 1986
Ownership: Private
Produces/Sells CE-marked Devices: N
Distribution: Manufacturer Direct
Ambulance	General

BRAUN, B.
See B. Braun Medical

BRAVA, LLC   305-856-4242
14221 SW 142nd Street, Miami, FL 33186
FDA Number: 3005643748   *Fax:* 305-856-4494
E-mail: info@brava.com
Web site: www.brava.com
Ownership: Private
Produces/Sells CE-marked Devices: N
Expander, Skin, Inflatable	Surgery

BRAY CORPORATION   760-345-6689
14149 Calle Contesa, Victorville, CA 92392
FDA Number: 2031356
Ownership: Private
Produces/Sells CE-marked Devices: N
Component, Traction, Non-Invasive	Orthopedics
Equipment, Traction, Powered	Physical Med

BREATHE E-Z SYSTEMS, INC.   800-490-5052
P.O. Box 7813, Shawnee Mission, KS 66207
FDA Number: 3004141536   *Fax:* 913-338-2826
E-mail: info@testbreath.com
Web site: www.testbreath.com
Ownership: Private
Produces/Sells CE-marked Devices: N
Analyzer, Gas, Carbon-Monoxide, Gaseous Phase	Anesthesiology
Analyzer, Gas, Hydrogen	Anesthesiology

BREATHE TECHNOLOGIES INC.   925-359-1500
4000 Executive Parkway, Suite 190, San Ramon, CA 94583
FDA Number: 3008778542
E-mail: info@breathetechnologies.com
Web site: http://www.breathetechnologies.com
Year Founded: 2005
Ownership: Private
Produces/Sells CE-marked Devices: N
General Admin.: Mr. Lawrence Mastrovich/President, Chief Executive Officer
    Medical Admin.: Mr. Anthony Gerber/Chief Medical Officer
Mktg./Adv.: Ms. Rebecca Mabry/Vice President Marketing & Sales
Production: Mr. Mohan Sancheti/Vice President Operations
Research: Mr. Joseph Cipollone/Vice President Research & Development
IS: Mr. Tony Wondka/Vice President Technology
Ventilator, Other	Anesthesiology

BREATHE WITH EEZ CORP.   800-826-7077
PO Box 37, Albertson, NY 11507   516-625-4331
FDA Number: 2435077   *Fax:* 516-295-2605
E-mail: dds4kids@aol.com
Web site: www.breathewitheez.com
Ownership: Private
Produces/Sells CE-marked Devices: N
Dilator, Nasal	Ear/Nose/Throat

BREATHING AIDS, INC.
See Allied Medco, Inc.

BREAZEALE & ASSOCIATES, INC.   770-447-4418
2909 Langford Road, Suite 500B, Norcross, GA 30071
FDA Number: n/a   *Fax:* 770-446-5229
E-mail: corp@baiusa.com
Ownership: Private
Produces/Sells CE-marked Devices: N
Distribution: Service Direct
General Admin.: L. Derryl Breazeale/Chief Executive Officer
Mktg./Adv.: L. Nolan Breazeale/Vice President Marketing
Production: L. Adam Breazeale/Vice President Operations
Service, Consulting	General

BRECON KNITTING MILLS, INC.   800-841-2821
PO BOX 478, Talladega, AL 35161
FDA Number: n/a   *Fax:* 256-362-6143
Web site: www.breconknittingmill.com
Annual Revenue: $1-$5 Million
Year Founded: 1948
Ownership: Private
Produces/Sells CE-marked Devices: N
Federal Procurement Eligibility: Small Business
Distribution: Manufacturer Direct, Manufacturer Through Distributor, Manufacturer Through Manufacturer Reps, Service Direct, Importer, Exporter
Bandage, Tubular	General
Dressing, Other	General
Dressing, Wound and Burn, Occlusive	Surgery
Stockinette	Orthopedics
Stockinette, Cast	Orthopedics

BRECONRIDGE MANUFACTURING SOLUTIONS   315-393-8000
120 Chimney Point Dr., Ogdensburg, NY 13669
FDA Number: 3005569144
Ownership: Private
Produces/Sells CE-marked Devices: N
Monitor, Blood Pressure, Indirect, Semi-Automatic	Cardiovascular

BREEN HEALTHCARE INC.
See Sunrise Medical, Inc.

BREG, INC., AN ORTHOFIX COMPANY   800-897-2734
2611 Commerce Way, Vista, CA 92081   760-599-3000
FDA Number: 2028253   *Fax:* 800-329-2734
E-mail: info@breg.com
Web site: www.breg.com
Year Founded: 1989
Ownership: ORTHOFIX
Stock Symbol: OFIX
Traded On: NASDAQ
Produces/Sells CE-marked Devices: N
General Admin.: Brad Lee/President
    Dave Brengle/Vice President

BREG, INC., AN ORTHOFIX COMPANY   800-897-2734 *(cont'd)*
Kathy Barber/Vice President
Finance: Bill Hopson/Financial Executive

Bag, Ice	General
Bandage, Adhesive	Surgery
Brace, Joint, Ankle (External)	Physical Med
Component, Exercise	Physical Med
Cover, Limb	Physical Med
Exerciser, Measuring	Physical Med
Exerciser, Non-Measuring	Physical Med
Exerciser, Powered	Anesthesiology
Insoles, Medical	General
Joint, Knee, External Brace	Physical Med
Kit, Wound Dressing	Surgery
Labware, Blood Collection	Chemistry
Orthosis, Corrective Shoe	Physical Med
Orthosis, Limb Brace	Physical Med
Orthosis, Lumbar	Physical Med
Orthosis, Lumbosacral	Physical Med
Pack, Hot Or Cold, Reusable	Physical Med
Pack, Hot Or Cold, Water Circulating	Physical Med
Pump, Infusion	General
Pump, Infusion, Elastomeric	General
Shoe, Cast	Physical Med
Sling, Arm	Physical Med
Splint, Hand, And Component	Physical Med
Splint, Temporary Training	Physical Med
Traction Unit, Non-Powered	Orthopedics
Tube, Aspirating, Flexible, Connecting	Anesthesiology

BREMER MEDICAL, INC.
See Depuy Mitek, Inc.

BRENDAN SCIENTIFIC
See Brendan Technologies Inc.

BRENDAN TECHNOLOGIES INC.   760-929-7500
Research Center Plaza, 2236 Rutherford Rd., Ste. 107,
Carlsbad, CA 92008
FDA Number: n/a
E-mail: sales@brendan.com
Web site: www.brendan.com
Ownership: Public
Produces/Sells CE-marked Devices: N
Distribution: Manufacturer Direct

Computer Software	General
Enzyme Immunoassay, Other	Chemistry
Radioimmunoassay, Other	Chemistry

BRENNEN MEDICAL, LLC   800-328-9105
1290 Hammond Rd., St. Paul, MN 55110   651-429-7413
FDA Number: 2132242   *Fax:* 651-429-8020
E-mail: customerservice@brennenmed.com
Web site: www.brennenmed.com
Ownership: Private
Produces/Sells CE-marked Devices: N

Accessories, Apparel, Surgical	Surgery
Apron, Lead, Radiographic	Radiology
Bandage, Adhesive	Surgery
Bandage, Elastic	General
Dressing, Burn, Porcine	Surgery
Dressing, Other	General
Dressing, Wound and Burn, Hydrogel	Surgery
Elastomer, Silicone (Scar Management)	Surgery
Expander, Surgical, Skin Graft	Surgery
Fiber, Absorbent	General
Mesh, Surgical (Steel Gauze)	Surgery
Orthosis, Limb Brace	Physical Med
Protector, Skin Pressure	General

BRENNER METAL PRODUCTS   (973) 778-0084.
16 Main Ave., Wallington, NJ 07057
FDA Number: n/a   *Fax:* 973-778-2466
Annual Revenue: $0-$1 Million
Ownership: Private
Produces/Sells CE-marked Devices: N
Federal Procurement Eligibility: Small Business
Distribution: Manufacturer Direct

Infusion Stand	General
Traction Unit, Non-Powered	Orthopedics

BRENTWOOD DIV.
See Alcon Research, Ltd.

BRENTWOOD INDUSTRIES, INC.   610-374-5109
610 Morgantown Rd., Reading, PA 19611
FDA Number: n/a   *Fax:* 610-376-6022
Web site: www.brentwoodindustries.com
Medical Products Sales Volume: $4,500,000
Annual Revenue: $50-$100 Million
Year Founded: 1965
Ownership: Private

BRENTWOOD INDUSTRIES, INC.   610-374-5109 *(cont'd)*
Quality System Registration Information: ISO9001
Produces/Sells CE-marked Devices: Y
Federal Procurement Eligibility: Female Owned
Distribution: Manufacturer Direct

Accessories, Catheter	Surgery
Packaging Material	General

BRENTWOOD INSTRUMENTS, INC.
See Midmark Diagnostics Group

BRETTON SQUARE INDUSTRIES   800-360-6126
812 E. Jolly Rd., Ste. 216, Lansing, MI 48910   517-346-9607
FDA Number: 1827789   *Fax:* 517-394-2150
E-mail: brettonsquare@ceicmh.org
Web site: www.brettonsquare.com
Medical Products Sales Volume: $1,000,000
Annual Revenue: $1-$5 Million
Total Employees: 100   *Marketing Staff:* 1   *Sales Staff:* 3
Ownership: Private
Produces/Sells CE-marked Devices: N
Distribution: Manufacturer Through Distributor
General Admin.: Thomas O. Knudtson/Chief Executive Officer
Production: Sherry Kletke/Customer Service Representative
    Steve Frese/Customer Service Representative

Toothbrush, Manual	Dental And Oral

BREUER ELECTRIC MANUFACTURING CO.
See Tornado Industries

BREVET, INC.   949-474-7000
16661 Jamboree Blvd., Irvine, CA 92606
FDA Number: 2025870   *Fax:* 949-553-1498
E-mail: wtomblin@brevet.com
Web site: www.brevet.com
Medical Products Sales Volume: $13,000,000
Annual Revenue: $10-$25 Million
Year Founded: 1978
Total Employees: 60   *Marketing Staff:* 1   *Sales Staff:* 1
Ownership: Private
Produces/Sells CE-marked Devices: N
Federal Procurement Eligibility: Small Business
Distribution: OEM
General Admin.: C. Brewer/President
Production: Wayne Tomblin/General Manager Operations

Catheter, Percutaneous	Cardiovascular
Connector, Tubing, Blood	Cardiovascular

BREVIS CORP.   800-383-3377
225 West 2855 South, Salt Lake City, UT 84115   801-466-6677
FDA Number: n/a   *Fax:* 801-485-2844
E-mail: info@brevis.com
Web site: www.brevis.com
Total Employees: 10
Ownership: Private
Produces/Sells CE-marked Devices: N
Federal Procurement Eligibility: Small Business
Distribution: Manufacturer Direct
General Admin.: J. Gordon Short/Chief Executive Officer
    Barry Short/President
Mktg./Adv.: Lovina Short/Manager Marketing
Production: Barry Short/General Manager Production

Dispenser, Other	General
Lamp, Ultraviolet (Spectrum A)	General
Sign, Hospital	General

BREWER CO., E. F.
See Brewer Company, The

BREWER COMPANY, THE   888-873-9371
N88 W13901 Main St.,   262-251-9530
Menomonee Falls, WI 53051
FDA Number: 2182536   *Fax:* 262-251-2332
E-mail: sales@brewercompany.com
Web site: www.brewercompany.com
Medical Products Sales Volume: $1,000,000
Annual Revenue: $10-$25 Million
Year Founded: 1947
Total Employees: 115   *Marketing Staff:* 6   *Sales Staff:* 38
Ownership: MAIN STREET INDUSTRIES
Produces/Sells CE-marked Devices: N
Federal Procurement Eligibility: Small Business
Distribution: Manufacturer Through Distributor, OEM
General Admin.: Paul Siepmann/President
Mktg./Adv.: Jody Dobson/Director Corporate Accounts
    Erica Mitchell/Marketing Manager, Design and OEM
    Melinda Bohlmann/Marketing Manager, Medical
    Mark Stecker/Senior Director Business Development
    Cheryl Miller/Vice President Medical Sales and Marketing

BREWER COMPANY, THE   888-873-9371 (cont'd)
Production: Ken Bettin/Product Manager
Finance: Tom Tellefson/Chief Financial Officer
    Deb Byington/Director Sales, Specialty Seating

Cart, Supply	General
Chair, Other	General
Footstool	General
Footstool, Non-Conductive	General
Infusion Stand	General
Laundry Hamper	General
Light, Other	General
Liner, Laundry Hamper	General
Powered Medical Examination Table	General
Stand, Operating Room Instrument (Mayo)	Surgery
Stool, Bedside	General
Table, Examination/Treatment	General
Table, Overbed	General
Waste Receptacle, General Purpose	General

BRIDGEPOINT MEDICAL   763-225-8500
2800 Campus Drive, #50, Plymouth, MN 55441
FDA Number: 3007210311   Fax: 763-225-8718
Web site: http://www.bridgepointmedical.com
Year Founded: 2006
Ownership: Private
Produces/Sells CE-marked Devices: N
General Admin.: Mr. Chad Kugler/President, General Manager
Medical Admin.: Mr. John Shultz/Vice President Clinical Affairs
Production: Mr. Peter Jacobs/Manager Operations
    Mr. Craig Schlawin/Vice President Quality Assurance
Research: Mr. Matt Olson/Vice President Research & Development

Catheter, Percutaneous	Cardiovascular
Guidewire, Catheter	Cardiovascular

BRIDGER BIOMED, INC.   908-277-8000
2430 North 7th Ave., Bozeman, MT 59715
FDA Number: 3031159
Ownership: C. R. Bard, Inc.
Produces/Sells CE-marked Devices: N

Balloon, Epistaxis (Nasal)	Ear/Nose/Throat
Dura-Substitute	Cns/Neurology
Mesh, Surgical, Polymeric	Surgery
Pledget And Intracardiac Patch, PETP, PTFE, Polypropylene	Cardiovascular

BRIGGS CORPORATION   800-247-2343
7300 Westown Pkwy., PO Box 1698,   515-327-6400
Des Moines, IA 50306
FDA Number: 1650560   Fax: 800-222-1996
E-mail: kbecker@briggscorp.com
Web site: www.briggscorp.com
Year Founded: 1947
Total Employees: 350   Marketing Staff: 100   Sales Staff: 100
Ownership: Private
Produces/Sells CE-marked Devices: N
Federal Procurement Eligibility: Small Business
Distribution: Manufacturer Direct, Exclusive Distributor
General Admin.: Merwyn Dan/Chief Executive Officer
    Dennis Billings/President
Mktg./Adv.: Kelly Becker/Communication Specialist
    Dave Davis/Manager Corporate Communications
    Michael Ness/Vice President Marketing & Sales

Bag, Urinary Collection	General
Bandage, Adhesive	Surgery
Bandage, Elastic	General
Bandage, Gauze	General
Camera, Other	General
Eyeglasses	Ophthalmology
Label, Device	General

BRIGGS HEALTH CARE PRODUCTS
See Briggs Corporation

BRIGHT IDEAS 4 THERAPY, LLC   805-390-0330
1630 Sophia Dr., PO BOX 7396, Oxnard, CA 93031
FDA Number: 2032630
E-mail: info@brightideas4therapy.com
Web site: www.brightideas4therapy.com
Ownership: Private
Produces/Sells CE-marked Devices: N

Component, Exercise	Physical Med

BRIGHTON COLLECTIBLES INC.   800-628-7687
14022 Nelson Ave., City of Industry, CA 91746
FDA Number: 2086573   Fax: 626-961-9380
Web site: www.brighton.com
Year Founded: 1991
Ownership: Private
Produces/Sells CE-marked Devices: N

Lens, Spectacle/Eyeglasses, Non-Custom	Ophthalmology

BRIGHTON COLLECTIBLES INC.   800-628-7687 (cont'd)

Sunglasses (Including Photosensitive)	Ophthalmology

BRIMMS, INC.
See Combe, Inc.

BRISSMAN-KENNEDY INC.
See AmSan

BRISTOL C&D, INC.   877-255-1181
14317 S.W. 142 Avenue, Miami, FL 33186   305-255-1181
FDA Number: 1035939   Fax: 305-235-9734
E-mail: info@bcdlens.com
Web site: www.bcdlens.com
Annual Revenue: $0-$1 Million
Year Founded: 1958
Ownership: Private
Produces/Sells CE-marked Devices: N
Federal Procurement Eligibility: Small Business
Distribution: Manufacturer Direct
General Admin.: Alexander C. Bristol/President, Chief Executive Officer
Production: Alexander N. Bristol/Manager Production

Lens, Other	Ophthalmology

BRISTOL CONSULTING & DEVELOPMENT, INC.
See Bristol C&D, Inc.

BRISTOL-MYERS GROUP COMPANY   800-332-2056
P.O. Box 4500, Princeton, NJ 08543   609-252-4000
FDA Number: n/a
Web site: www.bms.com
Medical Products Sales Volume: $1,430,000,000
Ownership: Bristol-Myers Squibb Company
Produces/Sells CE-marked Devices: Y
Distribution: Manufacturer Direct, Manufacturer Through Distributor, Manufacturer Through Manufacturer Reps, Service Direct, Exclusive Distributor

Contract Manufacturing, Pharmaceuticals/Chemicals	General

BRISTOL-MYERS SQUIBB   732-227-7564
2400 West Lloyd Expressway, Evansville, IN 47721
FDA Number: 1819504

Indicator, pH, Dye (Urinary, Non-Quantitative)	Chemistry
Protector, Ostomy	Gastroenterology/Urology

BRISTOL-MYERS SQUIBB MEDICAL IMAGING
See Lantheus Medical Imaging

BRIT SYSTEMS INC.   800-230-7227
1909 Hi-Line Drive, Suite A, Dallas, TX 75207   214-630-0636
FDA Number: 1647172   Fax: 214-630-1638
E-mail: sales@brit.com
Web site: www.brit.com
Medical Products Sales Volume: $5,700,000
Year Founded: 1993
Total Employees: 22   Marketing Staff: 2   Sales Staff: 5
Ownership: Private
Produces/Sells CE-marked Devices: N
Federal Procurement Eligibility: Small Business, Female Owned, GSA Contract
Distribution: Manufacturer Direct, Manufacturer Through Distributor, Manufacturer Through Manufacturer Reps
General Admin.: R. Garvey/Chairman
    Robert Murry/Chief Executive Officer
    Michele Fisher/President
    Kim Herman/Vice President Human Resources
Mktg./Adv.: Tom D'Apice/Director Marketing & Advertising
    Michele Fisher/Vice President Sales
Production: Chris Ciardo/Director Customer Services
    Bob Murry/Vice President Engineering & Product Development
IS: Robbie Barton/Vice President Software

Image Digitizer	Radiology
Radiographic Picture Archiving/Communication System (PACS)	Radiology

BRITESMILE, INC.
See Bsml, Inc.

BRITISH-AMERICAN MEDICAL, INC.
See Arkray Usa

BROADWEST CORP.   800-232-2948
304 Elati St, Denver,, CO 80223
FDA Number: 2434071   Fax: 800-625-1381
E-mail: info@broadwest.com
Web site: www.broadwest.com
Medical Products Sales Volume: $200,000
Annual Revenue: $1-$5 Million
Year Founded: 1984
Total Employees: 4   Marketing Staff: 1   Sales Staff: 2
Ownership: Private
Produces/Sells CE-marked Devices: N
Federal Procurement Eligibility: Small Business
Distribution: Manufacturer Through Distributor, Exclusive Distributor, Importer, Exporter

BROADWEST CORP. 800-232-2948 (cont'd)
General Admin.: Jack F. Donovan/President

Illuminator, Radiographic Film	Radiology
Magnifier, Hand-Held, Low-Vision	Ophthalmology
Viewer, Radiographic Film, Motorized	Radiology

BROCK TECHNICAL SERVICES 888-287-2433
20 Spencer Street,, **705-646-2225**
Bracebridge, ONT P1L 1 Canada
FDA Number: n/a Fax: 705-646-2264
E-mail: brocktec@muskoka.com
Year Founded: 1989
Ownership: Private
Produces/Sells CE-marked Devices: N
Distribution: Service Direct

BRODA ENTERPRISES INC. 800-668-0637
385 Phillip St., Waterloo, ONT N2L 5R8 Canada **519-746-8080**
FDA Number: 8043392 Fax: 519-746-8616
E-mail: sales@brodaseating.com
Web site: www.brodaseating.com
Medical Products Sales Volume: $3,000,000
Annual Revenue: $5-$10 Million
Year Founded: 1981
Total Employees: 50
Ownership: MITY-LITE, INC.
Produces/Sells CE-marked Devices: Y
Federal Procurement Eligibility: Small Business
Distribution: Manufacturer Through Distributor, Manufacturer Through
Manufacturer Reps, Exporter
General Admin.: David Heap/President
Mktg./Adv.: Shane Green/Manager International & National Sales
Production: Rob Deans/Manager Production
Research: Ian Brotherston/Manager Research & Development

Chair, Geriatric	General
Chair, Geriatric, Wheeled	General
Chair, Other	General
Cushion, Wheelchair (Pad)	Physical Med
Tray, Wheelchair	Physical Med
Wheelchair, Manual	Physical Med

BRODA SEATING 800-668-0637
385 Phillip St., Waterloo, ONT N2L-5R8 Canada **519-746-8080**
FDA Number: n/a Fax: 519-746-8616
E-mail: Sales@brodaseating.com
Web site: www.brodaseating.com
Ownership: Private
Produces/Sells CE-marked Devices: N

BRONTES TECHNOLOGIES 781-541-5200
10 Maguire Road, Suite 310, Lexington, MA 02421
FDA Number: 3006095883

System, Optical Impression, Computer Assisted Design And Manufacturing (cad/cam) Of Dental Restorations	Dental And Oral

BROOKDALE MEDICAL SPECIALTIES LTD. 800-655-1155
418 Hanlan Rd., Unit 27, **905-856-5006**
Woodbridge, ONT L4L-3 Canada
FDA Number: n/a Fax: 905-856-5019
E-mail: info@brookdalemedical.com
Web site: www.Brookdalemedical.com
Year Founded: 1984
Ownership: Private
Produces/Sells CE-marked Devices: N
Distribution: Manufacturer Direct, Exclusive Distributor, Importer

BROOKFIELD OPTICAL SYSTEMS 508-867-6675
218 Wigwam Rd., West Brookfield, MA 01585
FDA Number: 1226076
Ownership: Private
Produces/Sells CE-marked Devices: N

Refractometer, Ophthalmic	Ophthalmology

BROOKLYN THERMOMETER CO., INC. 800-241-6316
90 Verdi Street, Farmingdale, NY 11735-6318 **631-694-7610**
FDA Number: 7000067 Fax: 631-694-6329
E-mail: custserv@brooklynthermometer.com
Web site: www.brooklynthermometer.com
Medical Products Sales Volume: $24,000,000
Annual Revenue: $10-$25 Million
Year Founded: 1903
Ownership: Private
Produces/Sells CE-marked Devices: N
Federal Procurement Eligibility: Small Business
Distribution: Manufacturer Direct, OEM, Importer, Exporter
General Admin.: Todd Teichert/President

Thermistor	General

BROOKLYN THERMOMETER CO., INC. 800-241-6316 (cont'd)

Thermometer, Laboratory	Chemistry

BROTHERSTON HOMECARE INC., PXI DIV. 800-695-9729
1388 Bridgewater Rd., Bensalem, PA 19020 **215-633-7300**
FDA Number: n/a Fax: 215-633-7304
E-mail: jim@brotherstonhomecare.com
Web site: www.brotherstonhomecare.com
Annual Revenue: $0-$1 Million
Ownership: Private
Produces/Sells CE-marked Devices: N
Federal Procurement Eligibility: Small Business, Female Owned
Distribution: Manufacturer Direct
General Admin.: James P. Feeney/President

Compression Unit, Intermittent (Anti-Embolism Pump)	Cardiovascular
Holder, Radiographic Cassette, Wall-Mounted	Radiology
Immobilizer, Infant (Circumcision Board)	Orthopedics

BROWN & SHARPE INC. 800-343-7933
250 Circuit Drive, N. Kingstown, RI 02852 **401-886-2000**
FDA Number: n/a Fax: 401-886-2727
E-mail: bwnshp@us.bnsmc.com
Web site: www.brownandsharpe.com
Medical Products Sales Volume: $95,100,000
Year Founded: 1968
Total Employees: 700
Ownership: Hexagon AB
Quality System Registration Information: ISO9000; ISO9001
Produces/Sells CE-marked Devices: Y
Distribution: Manufacturer Direct, Manufacturer Through Distributor, Manufacturer
Through Manufacturer Reps, OEM, Service Direct, Exporter
General Admin.: Mr. William Gruber/President, Chief Executive Officer
Mktg./Adv.: Mr. Jack Rosignal/Vice President Sales

Equipment/Service, Quality Control	General

BROWN ENGINEERING CORP. 800-726-4233
289 Chesterfield Road, **413-527-3510**
Westhampton, MA 01027
FDA Number: n/a Fax: 413-303-1774
E-mail: info@bedbar.com
Web site: www.bedbar.com
Medical Products Sales Volume: $500,000
Year Founded: 1993
Total Employees: 6
Ownership: Private
Produces/Sells CE-marked Devices: N
Federal Procurement Eligibility: Small Business

Bedrail	General

BROWN MANUFACTURING OF HARTLEY INC.
See Brown Medical Industries

BROWN MEDICAL INDUSTRIES 800-843-4395
1300 Lundberg Dr. W., Spirit Lake, IA 51360 **712-336-4395**
FDA Number: 1926174 Fax: 712-336-2874
E-mail: info@brownmed.com
Web site: www.brownmed.com
Annual Revenue: $5-$10 Million
Year Founded: 1965
Total Employees: 30 Marketing Staff: 1 Sales Staff: 2
Ownership: Private
Quality System Registration Information: ISO9001
Produces/Sells CE-marked Devices: Y
Federal Procurement Eligibility: Small Business
Distribution: Manufacturer Through Distributor, OEM, Exporter
General Admin.: Janet Brown/Manager Human Resources
Ivan E. Brown/President, Chief Executive Officer
Mktg./Adv.: Paul Katzfey/Director International Marketing & Sales
Kylia Brown/Manager Marketing Services
Matt Henry/Manager Sales
Production: Terry Kounkel/Vice President Operations
Finance: Tony Poncelet/Director Finance
IS: Brian Miller/Vice President Information Systems

Ankle/Foot, External Limb Component	Physical Med
Brace, Joint, Ankle (External)	Physical Med
Cover, Limb	Physical Med
Hand, External Limb Component, Mechanical	Physical Med
Orthosis, Limb Brace	Physical Med
Pack, Hot Or Cold, Reusable	Physical Med
Pad, Pressure, Foam (Elbow, Heel)	General
Splint, Extremity, Non-Inflatable, External	Surgery
Splint, Hand, And Component	Physical Med
Stirrup, External Brace Component	Physical Med

BROWNE MEDICAL, A DIVISION OF TIMM RESEARCH CO.
See Timm Medical Technologies, Inc.

BROWNING ENTERPRISES, INC.
616-849-2420
1234 Zoschke Rd., Benton Harbor, MI 49022
FDA Number: 3003891457
Ownership: Private
Produces/Sells CE-marked Devices: N

Bag, Leg   Gastroenterology/Urology

BRUCE COOK, PROSTHETICS
314-567-7585
2821 North Ballas, #215, Crystal Lake Park, MO 63131
FDA Number: 1933145

Eye, Artificial, Non-Custom   Ophthalmology

BRUDER HEALTHCARE COMPANY
888-827-8337
770-569-5994
3150 Engineering Parkway,
Alpharetta, GA 30004
FDA Number: 1039131   *Fax:* 770-521-5557
E-mail: info@bruder.com
Web site: www.bruder.com
Medical Products Sales Volume: $700,000
Annual Revenue: $1-$5 Million
Year Founded: 1986
Total Employees: 10   *Marketing Staff:* 1   *Sales Staff:* 2
Ownership: Private
Produces/Sells CE-marked Devices: N
Federal Procurement Eligibility: Small Business
Distribution: Manufacturer Through Distributor, Manufacturer Through
Manufacturer Reps
General Admin.: Mark H. Bruder/Chief Executive Officer
       Aaron Ingram/Vice President, General Manager

Bag, Ice   General
Bottle, Hot/Cold Water   General
Compress, Cold   General
Moist Therapy Pack   Physical Med
Pack, Cold   General
Pack, Hot Or Cold, Reusable   Physical Med
Pack, Moist Heat   Physical Med
Pad, Heating, Electrical   Physical Med
Support, Hot/Cold Pack   Physical Med

BRUDER SAFEGUARD
See Bruder Healthcare Company

BRUIN PLASTICS CO.
800-556-7764
401-568-3081
61 Joslin Rd., Glendale, RI 02826-0700
FDA Number: n/a   *Fax:* 401-568-0019
E-mail: sales@bruinplastics.com
Web site: www.bruinplastics.com
Year Founded: 1964
Total Employees: 55
Ownership: Private
Produces/Sells CE-marked Devices: N
Federal Procurement Eligibility: Small Business
Distribution: OEM
General Admin.: Dennis Angelone/President
       Steve Angelone/Vice President
Mktg./Adv.: Mr. Walter Conine/Vice President Marketing & Sales

Component, Plastic   General
Cover, Laundry Hamper   General
Cover, Mattress   General
Cover, Mattress, Conductive   General
Cover, Mattress, Waterproof   General
Curtain, Cubicle   General
Curtain, Shower   General
Mattress, Bed   General
Screen, Bedside   General
Stretcher, Hand-Carried   General

BRUKER CORPORATION
978-663-3660
40 Manning Road, Billerica, MA 01821
FDA Number: n/a   *Fax:* 978-663-5585
E-mail: ms-sales@bdal.com
Web site: www.bruker.com
Ownership: Private
Stock Symbol: BRKR
Traded On: NASDAQ
Produces/Sells CE-marked Devices: N
General Admin.: Mr. William Knight/Chief Operating Officer
       Dr. Frank Laukian/President, Chief Executive Officer
Finance: Mr. Brian Monohan/Chief Financial Officer

BRULIN & CO. INC.
800-776-7149
317-923-3211
2920 Drive A.J. Brown Avenue,
Indianapolis, IN 46205
FDA Number: n/a   *Fax:* 317-925-4596
E-mail: mfalkowski@brulin.com
Web site: www.brulin.com
Medical Products Sales Volume: $12,900,000
Annual Revenue: $25-$50 Million
Year Founded: 1935

BRULIN & CO. INC.
800-776-7149 *(cont'd)*
Total Employees: 50   *Marketing Staff:* 6   *Sales Staff:* 50
Ownership: Private
Quality System Registration Information: ISO9002
Produces/Sells CE-marked Devices: N
Federal Procurement Eligibility: Small Business
Distribution: Manufacturer Direct, Manufacturer Through Distributor, Exporter
General Admin.: Charles Pollnow/President, Chief Executive Officer
       Jolee Chaartrand/Vice President Personnel
Mktg./Adv.: Louis Amici/Director Marketing
       Michael Beeks/Director Product Development
       Janet Salisbury/Manager Advertising
       Chris Jones/Manager International Marketing & Sales
       George Brodnicki/Manager National Sales
       Michael Falkowski/Vice President Marketing & Sales
Production: Brad Arnold/Director Operations
       Berma Zootman/Manager Regulatory Affairs

Disinfector, Liquid   General
Solution, Antibacterial Cleaner   General
Washer/Sterilizer   General

BRUNO INDEPENDENT LIVING AIDS, INC.
800-882-8183
262-567-4990
1780 Executive Drive,
Oconomowoc, WI 53066
FDA Number: 2131358   *Fax:* 262-953-5501
E-mail: webmaster@bruno.com
Web site: www.bruno.com
Medical Products Sales Volume: $10,000,000
Annual Revenue: $50-$100 Million
Year Founded: 1987
Total Employees: 225   *Marketing Staff:* 2   *Sales Staff:* 15
Ownership: Private
Quality System Registration Information: ISO9001
Produces/Sells CE-marked Devices: N
Federal Procurement Eligibility: Small Business, GSA Contract, VA Contract
General Admin.: Michael R. Bruno/Chief Executive Officer
       Beverly A. Bruno/Corporate Secretary
       Michael Bruno/President
Mktg./Adv.: Jack Sheehan/Director Marketing
       Dick Keller/Director Product Development
       Anne Tyler/Manager Advertising
       Pat Foy/Manager National Sales
Production: William W. Belson/Director Engineering
       Tom Habeck/Director Quality Assurance
       Joseph Popelka/Manager Materials
       Terry Andrus/Manager Regulatory Affairs
       Jerry Gnabasik/Plant Manager

Conveyor, Guided Vehicle   General
Lift, Stair Climbing   General
Lift, Wheelchair   General
Scooter (Motorized 3-Wheeled Vehicle)   Physical Med

BRUNSWICK BIOMEDICAL TECHNOLOGIES, INC.
See Brunswick Laboratories

BRUNSWICK LABORATORIES
800-362-3482
508-285-2006
50 Commerce Way, Norton, MA 02766
FDA Number: 1216827   *Fax:* 508-285-8002
E-mail: info@brunswicklabs.com
Web site: www.brunswicklabs.com
Medical Products Sales Volume: $900,000
Annual Revenue: $1-$5 Million
Total Employees: 10   *Marketing Staff:* 1   *Sales Staff:* 1
Ownership: Private
Produces/Sells CE-marked Devices: N
Federal Procurement Eligibility: Small Business
Distribution: Manufacturer Direct, Manufacturer Through Distributor, Exporter
General Admin.: James G. Nichols/President, Chief Executive Officer

Airway, Esophageal (Obturator)   Anesthesiology
Compressor, External, Cardiac, Powered   General
Resuscitator, Cardiac, Mechanical, Compressor   Anesthesiology
Tube, Esophageal, Blakemore   Gastroenterology/Urology

BRUNSWICK MANUFACTURING COMPANY, INC.
See Brunswick Laboratories

BRY-AIR, INC.
877-379-2479
740-965-2974
10793 State Rt. 37 W., Sunbury, OH 43074
FDA Number: n/a   *Fax:* 740-965-5470
E-mail: info@bry-air.com
Web site: www.bry-air.com
Medical Products Sales Volume: $5,000,000
Annual Revenue: $10-$25 Million
Year Founded: 1964
Total Employees: 43   *Marketing Staff:* 1   *Sales Staff:* 5
Ownership: Private
Produces/Sells CE-marked Devices: N
Federal Procurement Eligibility: Small Business
Distribution: Manufacturer Through Manufacturer Reps

MANUFACTURER PROFILES

BRY-AIR, INC.
877-379-2479 *(cont'd)*
General Admin.: Mr. Melvyn Meyers/President
Mktg./Adv.: Mr. Kenneth Baker/Vice President Corporate Affairs

Dehumidifier	General
Dryer, Labware	Chemistry

BRYAN CORP.
800-343-7711
4 Plympton St., Woburn, MA 01801-2908 **781-935-0004**
FDA Number: 1221129 Fax: 781-935-7602
E-mail: info@bryancorp.com
Web site: www.bryancorp.com
Medical Products Sales Volume: $10,000,000
Annual Revenue: $5-$10 Million
Year Founded: 1979
Total Employees: 20 *Marketing Staff:* 3 *Sales Staff:* 2
Ownership: Private
Produces/Sells CE-marked Devices: Y
Federal Procurement Eligibility: Small Business, GSA Contract
Distribution: Manufacturer Direct, Manufacturer Through Distributor
General Admin.: Bridget Rodrigue/Manager Human Resources
Frank Abrano/President, Chief Executive Officer
Mktg./Adv.: Paivi Mikkola/Director Marketing
Bryan Abrano/Manager Market Research

Bronchoscope, Rigid	Ear/Nose/Throat
Bronchoscope, Rigid, Non-Ventilating	Anesthesiology
Bronchoscope, Rigid, Ventilating	Anesthesiology
Camera, Video, Endoscopic	General
Cord, Electric, Endoscope	Gastroenterology/Urology
Endoscope, Direct Vision	Surgery
Endoscope, Rigid	Surgery
Equipment, Suction/Irrigation, Laparoscopic	Surgery
Forceps, Endoscopic	Gastroenterology/Urology
Forceps, Grasping, Atraumatic	Surgery
Forceps, Grasping, Traumatic	Surgery
Instrument, Dissecting, Laparoscopic	Surgery
Media, Gastroenterographic Contrast (Barium Sulfate)	Radiology
Nebulizer, Medicinal	Ear/Nose/Throat
Needle, Endoscopic	Gastroenterology/Urology
Scissors, Wire Cutting, ENT	Ear/Nose/Throat
Service, Maintenance/Repair	General
Stent, Other	Obstetrics/Gynecology

BRYMILL CORPORATION
800-777-2796
105 Windermere Ave, Ellington, CT 06029 **860-875-2460**
FDA Number: 1216795 Fax: 860-872-2371
E-mail: brymill@brymill.com
Web site: www.brymill.com
Year Founded: 1966
Ownership: Private
Quality System Registration Information: ISO9003
Produces/Sells CE-marked Devices: Y
Federal Procurement Eligibility: Small Business
Distribution: Manufacturer Direct, Manufacturer Through Distributor, Manufacturer Through Manufacturer Reps, Importer, Exporter

Container, Liquid Nitrogen	Anesthesiology
Controller, Temperature, Other	General
Cryosurgical Unit	Surgery
Equipment, Cryotherapy	Physical Med
Flask, Dewar	Chemistry
Monitor, Lesion Temperature	Cns/Neurology
Needle, Other	General

BRYTECH INC.
613-731-5800
2301 St. Laurent Blvd., Suite 400, Ottawa ON K1G 4J7 Canada
FDA Number: 8022111 Fax: 613-731-5812
E-mail: inquiries@brytech.com
Web site: www.brytech.com
Year Founded: 1982
Total Employees: 25 *Marketing Staff:* 2 *Sales Staff:* 5
Ownership: Private
Produces/Sells CE-marked Devices: N
Federal Procurement Eligibility: Small Business
Distribution: Manufacturer Through Distributor

BRYTON CORP.
800-567-9500
4310 Guion Rd., Indianapolis, IN 46254-3111 **317-334-8700**
FDA Number: 1834026 Fax: 317-334-8787
E-mail: info@brytoncorp.com
Web site: www.brytoncorp.com
Year Founded: 1981
Ownership: Private
Produces/Sells CE-marked Devices: N
Federal Procurement Eligibility: Small Business

Accessories, Operating Room, Table	Surgery
Arm Rest	Physical Med
Bed, Birthing	General
Board, Arm	Anesthesiology
Chair, Birthing	Obstetrics/Gynecology
Clamp, Other	Surgery

BRYTON CORP.
800-567-9500 *(cont'd)*

Clamp, Surgical, General & Plastic Surgery	Surgery
Cover, Arm Board	General
Cover, Mattress, Conductive	General
Cover, Stool	General
Cushion, Other	General
Cushion, Stool	General
Cushion, Table, Surgical	Surgery
Equipment/Service, Quality Control	General
Holder, Leg	Surgery
Holder, Leg, Arthroscopy	Orthopedics
Leg Rest	General
Mattress, Operating Table	General
Pad, Pressure, Gel, Operating Table	General
Restraint, Ankle/Foot	General
Restraint, Arm	General
Restraint, Patient, Conductive	Anesthesiology
Restraint, Protective (Body)	General
Screen, Anesthesia	Anesthesiology
Service, Equipment Leasing	General
Service, Maintenance/Repair	General
Service, Parts, Repair	General
Service, Used Equipment	General
Stirrup	Gastroenterology/Urology
Strap, Restraining	General
Support, Arm	Physical Med
Support, Knee	Physical Med
Support, Leg	Physical Med
Support, Patient Position	Anesthesiology
Table, Cystometric, Non-Electrical	Gastroenterology/Urology
Table, Examination/Treatment	General
Table, Instrument, Surgical	Surgery
Table, Obstetrical	Obstetrics/Gynecology
Table, Obstetrical, AC-Powered	Obstetrics/Gynecology
Table, Obstetrical, Manual	Obstetrics/Gynecology
Table, Operating Room, AC-Powered	Surgery
Table, Operating Room, Mechanical	Surgery
Table, Radiographic, Stationary Top	Radiology
Table, Surgical With Orthopedic Accessories, AC-Powered	Surgery
Table, Surgical, Electrical	Surgery
Table, Surgical, Hydraulic	Surgery
Table, Surgical, Manual	General
Table, Surgical, Orthopedic	Orthopedics
Table, Urological (Cystological)	Gastroenterology/Urology
Table, Urological, Non-Electrical	Gastroenterology/Urology
Table, Urological, Radiographic	Gastroenterology/Urology

BSD MEDICAL CORPORATION
801-972-5555- 2
2188 W. 2200 S., Salt Lake City, UT 84119
FDA Number: 1719106 Fax: 801-972-5930
E-mail: info@bsdmc.com
Web site: www.bsdmc.com
Medical Products Sales Volume: $3,000,000
Annual Revenue: $1-$5 Million
Year Founded: 1978
Total Employees: 45 *Marketing Staff:* 2 *Sales Staff:* 8
Ownership: Public
Stock Symbol: BSDM
Traded On: NASDAQ
Quality System Registration Information: ISO9000; ISO9001; ISO9002; ISO9003
Produces/Sells CE-marked Devices: Y
Federal Procurement Eligibility: Small Business
Distribution: Manufacturer Direct, Manufacturer Through Distributor, Manufacturer Through Manufacturer Reps, OEM, Service Direct, Exclusive Distributor, Exporter
General Admin.: Dr. Damian Dupuy/Chairman
Paul F. Turner/Chief Technology Officer, Senior Vice President
Mktg./Adv.: Richard A. White/Vice President Business Development
Mr. Steven Smith/Vice President Marketing & Business Development
Brian Ferrand/Vice President Sales
Production: Dixie Toolson Sells/Vice President Regulatory Affairs
Research: Mr. Todd Turnlund/Vice President Engineering
Finance: Mr. Dennis Gauger/Chief Financial Officer

Hyperthermia Unit, Microwave	Radiology
Probe, Temperature	General
System, Cancer Treatment, Hyperthermia, RF/Microwave	Radiology
Thermometer, Electronic	General

BSI CORPORATION
See Surmodics, Inc.

BSML, INC.
561-988-4098
7777 Glades Road, Suite 100, Boca Raton, FL 33434
FDA Number: 3005960071
E-mail: info@britesmile.com
Web site: www.britesmile.com
Annual Revenue: $50-$100 Million
Year Founded: 1983
Total Employees: 7 *Marketing Staff:* 5 *Sales Staff:* 2
Ownership: Public
Stock Symbol: BSML

BSML, INC.   561-988-4098 *(cont'd)*
Traded On: NASDAQ
Produces/Sells CE-marked Devices: N
Federal Procurement Eligibility: Small Business
Distribution: Manufacturer Direct
  Source, Heat, Bleaching, Teeth, Dental   Dental And Oral

BSN MEDICAL, INC   800-552-1157
5825 Carnegie Boulevard, Charlotte, NC 28209   **704-554-9933**
FDA Number: 7000609   *Fax:* 704-331-8785
E-mail: BSNorthopaedics@bsnmedical.com
Web site: www.bsnmedical.com
Medical Products Sales Volume: $11,400,000
Annual Revenue: $10-$25 Million
Year Founded: 2001
Total Employees: 110   *Marketing Staff:* 1   *Sales Staff:* 6
Ownership: Private
Quality System Registration Information: ISO9001
Produces/Sells CE-marked Devices: Y
Federal Procurement Eligibility: Small Business, GSA Contract
Distribution: Manufacturer Direct, Manufacturer Through Distributor, OEM, Exporter
General Admin.: Barry Price/Chief Operating Officer
    James Martin/President, Chief Executive Officer
    Lana Ellingsworth/Vice President Human Resources
Mktg./Adv.: Milt Moravek/Director National Accounts
    Barry Price/Manager International Marketing & Sales
    Lisa Phlegar/Manager Marketing Services
Production: Larry DeCamp/Director Manufacturing
    Holly Hayes/Manager Customer Services
    George Schulz/Manager Regulatory Affairs
Finance: John Pointer/Chief Financial Officer, Vice President Finance

Bandage, Cast	Physical Med
Bandage, Elastic	General
Blade, Saw, Cast Cutting	Orthopedics
Cart, Orthopedic Supply (Cast)	Orthopedics
Cast	Orthopedics
Cast Walking Heel	Orthopedics
Cutter, Cast	Orthopedics
Immobilizer, Cervical	Orthopedics
Immobilizer, Knee	Orthopedics
Immobilizer, Wrist/Hand	Orthopedics
Padding, Cast/Splint	General
Protector, Finger	Orthopedics
Saw, Autopsy	Pathology
Shoe, Orthopedic	Orthopedics
Splint, Temporary Training	Physical Med
Spreader, Plaster (Cast)	Orthopedics
Stockinette, Cast	Orthopedics
Vacuum, Cast Cutter	Orthopedics

BSN MEDICAL, INC.   800-552-1157
5825 Carnegie Boulevard, Charlotte, NC 28209   **704-554-9933**
FDA Number: 1928508   *Fax:* 704-331-8785
E-mail: BSNorthopaedics@bsnmedical.com
Web site: www.bsnmedical.com
Ownership: Private
Produces/Sells CE-marked Devices: N

Cutter, Cast, AC-Powered	Orthopedics
Splint, Extremity, Non-Inflatable, External	Surgery

BSN-JOBST   704-554-9933
5825 Carnagie Blvd., Charlotte, NC 28209
FDA Number: 1043537   *Fax:* 704-551-8582
E-mail: andrea.smith@bsnmedical.com
Web site: www.jobst-usa.com
Medical Products Sales Volume: $90,500,000
Year Founded: 1950
Total Employees: 200
Ownership: Private
Produces/Sells CE-marked Devices: Y
Federal Procurement Eligibility: Small Business

Adaptor, Dressing	Physical Med
Bandage, Adhesive	Surgery
Bandage, Elastic	General
Binder, Breast	Obstetrics/Gynecology
Dressing, Other	General
Kit, Wound Dressing	Surgery
Stocking, Elastic	General
Stocking, Support (Anti-Embolic)	General

BSP LTD.   +972 3 6474840
22a Wallenberg Street, Tel-Aviv 69719
FDA Number: 3006223083   *Fax:* +972 3 6471498
Web site: http://www.bsp.co.il/
Ownership: Public
Stock Symbol: BSP
Produces/Sells CE-marked Devices: N
General Admin.: Dr. Amir Beker/Chief Executive Officer

BSP LTD.   +972 3 6474840 *(cont'd)*
    Mr. Nissim Greisas/Chief Executive Officer
Research: Dr. Linda Davrath/Director Clinical Research
    Dr. Eran Toledo/Vice President Research & Development
Finance: Ms. Meirav Dudek/Chief Financial Officer
IS: Dr. Guy Amit/Chief Technologist

Monitor, Physiological, Patient(without Arrhythmia Detection Or Alarms)	Cardiovascular

BTE TECHNOLOGIES, INC.   800-331-8845
7455-L New Ridge Rd., Hanover, MD 21076   **410-850-0333**
FDA Number: n/a   *Fax:* 410-850-5244
E-mail: info@btetech.com
Web site: www.btetech.com
Year Founded: 1979
Total Employees: 75
Ownership: Private
Quality System Registration Information: ISO9001
Produces/Sells CE-marked Devices: Y
Federal Procurement Eligibility: Small Business, GSA Contract, VA Contract
Distribution: Manufacturer Direct, Manufacturer Through Manufacturer Reps, OEM, Service Direct, Exclusive Distributor, Exporter
General Admin.: Tom Rogan/Chief Executive Officer
    Chuck Wetherington/President
Mktg./Adv.: Tim Collins/Manager National Sales
Production: Ken Johnson/Product Specialist
    Joe Perret/Vice President Operations

Dynamometer, Physical Medicine, Electronic	Physical Med
Equipment, Therapy, Handicapped/Physical	Physical Med
Exerciser, Hand	Physical Med
Exerciser, Measuring	Physical Med
Exerciser, Shoulder	Physical Med
Isokinetic Testing And Evaluation System	Physical Med

BTI FILTRATION   405-842-2517
7317 N. Classen Blvd., Oklahoma City, OK 73116
FDA Number: 1651723   *Fax:* 405-842-3626
E-mail: BTIFiltration@birch.net
Medical Products Sales Volume: $300,000
Total Employees: 4
Ownership: Bio Medical Technologies Co., Ltd.
Produces/Sells CE-marked Devices: N
Federal Procurement Eligibility: Small Business, Minority Owned
Distribution: Manufacturer Direct, Manufacturer Through Distributor

Purification System, Water	Gastroenterology/Urology

BTL INDUSTRIES, INC.   866-285-1656
47 Loring Drive, Framingham, MA 01702
FDA Number: n/a   *Fax:* 888-499-2502
E-mail: sales@btlnet.com
Web site: www.btlaesthetics.com
Ownership: Private
Produces/Sells CE-marked Devices: N

BTU INTERNATIONAL, INC.   978-667-4111
23 Esquire Rd., North Billerica, MA 01862
FDA Number: n/a   *Fax:* 978-667-9068
E-mail: sales@btu.com
Web site: www.btu.com
Medical Products Sales Volume: $60,000,000
Annual Revenue: $50-$100 Million
Total Employees: 381   *Sales Staff:* 77
Ownership: Public
Stock Symbol: BTUI
Traded On: NASDAQ
Quality System Registration Information: ISO9001
Produces/Sells CE-marked Devices: N
Distribution: Manufacturer Direct, Manufacturer Through Manufacturer Reps
General Admin.: Paul J. van der Wansem/Chief Executive Officer, Chairman
Mktg./Adv.: James M. Griffin/Vice President Sales
Production: John J. McCaffrey/Vice President Operations
Finance: Thomas P. Kealy/Vice President, Chief Administrative Officer

Oven	Chemistry

BTX TECH   800-666-0996
5 Skyline Drive, Hawthorne, NY 10532   **914-592-1800**
FDA Number: n/a   *Fax:* 800-569-4244
E-mail: info@btx.com
Web site: http://www.btx.com
Medical Products Sales Volume: $4,900,000
Annual Revenue: $5-$10 Million
Year Founded: 1967
Total Employees: 35   *Marketing Staff:* 2   *Sales Staff:* 10
Ownership: Private
Produces/Sells CE-marked Devices: N
Federal Procurement Eligibility: Small Business
Distribution: Manufacturer Direct, Manufacturer Through Distributor, Manufacturer Through Manufacturer Reps, OEM, Exclusive Distributor, Importer, Exporter
General Admin.: Greg Schwartz/President

BTX TECH

800-666-0996 *(cont'd)*

Adapter, Cable, Equipment	General
Regulator, Line Voltage	General

BUBBLE TECHNOLOGY INDUSTRIES INC.

613-589-2456

P.O. Box 100, Highway 17, Chalk River, ONT K0J-1J0 Canada

FDA Number: n/a *Fax:* 613-589-2763
E-mail: inquiries@bubbletech.ca
Web site: www.magma.ca/~bubble/
Year Founded: 1988
Total Employees: 25
Ownership: Private
Produces/Sells CE-marked Devices: N
Distribution: Manufacturer Direct, Service Direct, Exclusive Distributor, Exporter

BUCHMANN OPTICAL, INC.

See Abb Concise Optical Group Llc

BUCK SCIENTIFIC, INC.

800-562-5566
203-853-9444

58 Fort Point St., East Norwalk, CT 06855

FDA Number: n/a *Fax:* 203-853-0569
E-mail: sales@bucksci.com
Web site: www.bucksci.com
Medical Products Sales Volume: $4,000,000
Annual Revenue: $1-$5 Million
Year Founded: 1970
Ownership: Private
Produces/Sells CE-marked Devices: Y
Federal Procurement Eligibility: Small Business
Distribution: Manufacturer Direct, Manufacturer Through Manufacturer Reps, OEM, Exclusive Distributor, Importer, Exporter

Adsorbents, Liquid Chromatography	Toxicology
Analyzer, Chemistry, Electrolyte	Chemistry
Analyzer, Mercury	Chemistry
Chromatography Equipment, Gas	Chemistry
Cuvette, Spectrophotometer	Chemistry
Photometer, Flame, General Use	Toxicology
Recorder, Chart, Laboratory	Chemistry
Solvent, Spectrophotometer	Chemistry
Spectrophotometer, Atomic Absorption, General Use	Toxicology
Spectrophotometer, Infrared	Chemistry
Spectrophotometer, U.V./Visible	Chemistry

BUCKBEE-MEARS CO.

See Vision-Ease Lens

BUCKSTAFF CO.

800-755-5890
920-235-5890

1127 S. Main St., Oshkosh, WI 54902

FDA Number: n/a *Fax:* 920-235-2018
E-mail: tmugerauer@buckstaff.com
Web site: www.buckstaff.com
Medical Products Sales Volume: $450,000
Annual Revenue: $10-$25 Million
Year Founded: 1850
Total Employees: 200 *Marketing Staff:* 5 *Sales Staff:* 30
Ownership: Private
Quality System Registration Information: ISO9000
Produces/Sells CE-marked Devices: N
Federal Procurement Eligibility: Small Business, GSA Contract
Distribution: Manufacturer Direct, Manufacturer Through Distributor, Manufacturer Through Manufacturer Reps
General Admin.: John D. Buckstaff/President
Mktg./Adv.: Thom Madden/Director Marketing
 Thomas Mugerauer/Manager Sales
Production: Terry Young/Plant Manager

Furniture, General	General
Furniture, Patient Room	General

BUDENHEIM USA, INC

800-645-3044
516-683-6900

245 Newtown Road, Suite 305,
Plainview, NY 11803

FDA Number: 2410981 *Fax:* 516-683-6990
E-mail: lguerin@gallard.com
Web site: www.gallard.com
Medical Products Sales Volume: $55,000,000
Annual Revenue: $25-$50 Million
Year Founded: 2001
Total Employees: 27 *Sales Staff:* 12
Ownership: CHEMISCHE FABRIK BUDENHEIM
Produces/Sells CE-marked Devices: N
Federal Procurement Eligibility: Small Business
Distribution: Importer
Mktg./Adv.: Sandra Riquelme/Manager Advertising
Production: Henry Medollo/Product Manager

Electrophoretic, Protein Fractionation	Chemistry
Medium, Lymphocyte Separation	Hematology
Reagent, Other	General
Stain, Alizarin Red	Pathology

BUDENHEIM USA, INC

800-645-3044 *(cont'd)*

Stain, Biological, General	Pathology

BUDGET BUDDY COMPANY, INC.

800-208-3375
816-322-2290

P.O. Box 590, Belton, MO 64012-0590

FDA Number: n/a *Fax:* 816-322-6332
E-mail: office@budgetbuddy.com
Web site: www.budgetbuddy.com
Medical Products Sales Volume: $250,000
Annual Revenue: $0-$1 Million
Year Founded: 1953
Total Employees: 3 *Marketing Staff:* 2
Ownership: Private
Produces/Sells CE-marked Devices: N
Federal Procurement Eligibility: Small Business
Distribution: Manufacturer Through Distributor
General Admin.: Kenneth D. Tompkins/President
Mktg./Adv.: Barbara J. Tompkins/Vice President Sales

Furniture, General	General
Furniture, Patient Room	General
Holder, Medical Chart	General
Office Equipment	General
Storage Unit, X-Ray Film	Radiology

BUFFALO DENTAL MANUFACTURING CO., INC.

800-828-0203
516-496-7200

159 Lafayette Dr., PO BOX 678,
Syosset, NY 11791

FDA Number: 2411056 *Fax:* 516-496-7751
E-mail: jeannieb@bdm1.com
Web site: www.buffalodental.com
Annual Revenue: $0-$1 Million
Ownership: Private
Produces/Sells CE-marked Devices: N
Federal Procurement Eligibility: Small Business
Distribution: Manufacturer Through Distributor, Importer, Exporter

Adhesive, Liquid	General
Airbrush	Dental And Oral
Apron, Lead, Radiographic	Radiology
Articulators	Dental And Oral
Base, Denture, Relining, Repairing, Rebasing, Resin	Dental And Oral
Brush, Burr Cleaning	Dental And Oral
Burnisher, Operative, Dental	Dental And Oral
Burr, Dental	Dental And Oral
Carrier, Amalgam, Operative	Dental And Oral
Carver, Wax, Dental	Dental And Oral
Casting Unit, Dental	Dental And Oral
Condenser, Amalgam And Foil, Operative	Dental And Oral
Cup, Prophylaxis	Dental And Oral
Dental Laboratory Equipment	Dental And Oral
Engine, Dental	Dental And Oral
Floss, Dental	Dental And Oral
Foil, Dental	Dental And Oral
Forceps, Articulation Paper	Dental And Oral
Handpiece, Belt and/or Gear Driven, Dental	Dental And Oral
Hemostat, Surgical	Dental And Oral
Instrument, Dental, Manual	Dental And Oral
Kit, Dental Prophylaxis	Dental And Oral
Knife, Margin Finishing, Operative	Dental And Oral
Knife, Plaster	Orthopedics
Mallet, Dental	Dental And Oral
Mandrel	Dental And Oral
Material, Impression Tray, Resin	Dental And Oral
Point, Abrasive	Dental And Oral
Regulator, Vacuum	General
Ring, Dental (Casting)	Dental And Oral
Scissors, Collar And Crown	Dental And Oral
Spatula, Cement	Dental And Oral
Spatula, Other	Surgery
Syringe, Dental	Dental And Oral
Toothbrush, Manual	Dental And Oral
Wax, Dental	Dental And Oral
Wheel, Polishing Agent	Dental And Oral

BUFFALO DENTAL MFG. CO., INC.

516-496-7200

159 Lafayette Dr., Syosset, NY 11791

FDA Number: 2411056

Airbrush	Dental And Oral
Articulators	Dental And Oral
Base, Denture, Relining, Repairing, Rebasing, Resin	Dental And Oral
Burr, Dental	Dental And Oral
Carrier, Amalgam, Operative	Dental And Oral
Carver, Wax, Dental	Dental And Oral
Condenser, Amalgam And Foil, Operative	Dental And Oral
Cup, Prophylaxis	Dental And Oral
Disk, Abrasive	Dental And Oral
Forceps, Articulation Paper	Dental And Oral
Handpiece, Direct Drive, AC-Powered	Dental And Oral
Hemostat, Surgical	Dental And Oral
Material, Impression Tray, Resin	Dental And Oral
Point, Abrasive	Dental And Oral

BUFFALO DENTAL MFG. CO., INC. 516-496-7200 (cont'd)
Scissors, Collar And Crown	Dental And Oral
Toothbrush, Manual	Dental And Oral

BUFFALO FILTER, A DIVISION OF MEDTEK 800-343-2324
DEVICES INC.

595 Commerce Drive, Buffalo, NY 14228 716-835-7000
FDA Number: 1319774 *Fax:* 716-835-3414
E-mail: info@buffalofilter.com
Web site: www.buffalofilter.com
Medical Products Sales Volume: $7,000,000
Annual Revenue: $5-$10 Million
Year Founded: 1991
Total Employees: 50   *Marketing Staff:* 2   *Sales Staff:* 6
Ownership: Private
Quality System Registration Information: ISO9000
Produces/Sells CE-marked Devices: Y
Federal Procurement Eligibility: Small Business
Distribution: Manufacturer Direct, Manufacturer Through Distributor, Manufacturer Through Manufacturer Reps, OEM, Exporter
General Admin.: Christopher A. Palmerton/President, Chief Executive Officer
Mktg./Adv.: Mr. Joseph Lynch/Director Marketing
    Mr. Greg Pepe/Vice President Business Development
    Daniel Palmerton/Vice President Sales
Production: Karen A. Loretto/Director Quality Assurance & Quality Control
    Ms. Carrie Termin/Director Quality Assurance & Regulatory Affairs
    Robert O. Dean/Vice President Operations, General Manager
Finance: Mr. David McKay/Director Finance
    Ms. Nicole Piciulo/Director Finance
Accessories, Laser	General
Adapter, Unit, Electrosurgical, Hand-Controlled	Surgery
Bottle, Collection, Vacuum (Aspirator)	General
Electrosurgical Equipment, General Purpose	Surgery
Equipment/Accessories, Laser, Laparoscopy	Surgery
Exhaust System, Surgical	Surgery
System, Evacuation, Smoke, Laser	Surgery
Tubing, Non-Invasive	Surgery

BUFFALO NOVOCOL
See Buffalo Dental Manufacturing Co., Inc.

BUGLAB LLC 925-208-1952
310 Freitas Court, Danville, CA 94526
FDA Number: n/a *Fax:* 925-208-1917
E-mail: info@buglab.com
Web site: http://www.buglab.com
Ownership: Private
Produces/Sells CE-marked Devices: N

BULBMAN, INC. 800-648-1163
630 Sunshine Lane, Reno, NV 89502 775-788-5661
FDA Number: n/a *Fax:* 800-548-6216
E-mail: service@bulbman.com
Web site: www.bulbman.com
Medical Products Sales Volume: $12,600,000
Annual Revenue: $10-$25 Million
Year Founded: 1975
Total Employees: 38
Ownership: Private
Produces/Sells CE-marked Devices: N
Federal Procurement Eligibility: Small Business
Distribution: Exclusive Distributor
Lamp, Operating Room	General

BULBTRONICS, INC. 800-624-2852
45 Banfi Plaza N, Farmingdale, NY 11735-1539 631-249-2272
FDA Number: n/a *Fax:* 631-249-6066
E-mail: bulbs@bulbtronics.com
Web site: www.bulbtronics.com
Medical Products Sales Volume: $19,300,000
Year Founded: 2000
Total Employees: 45   *Marketing Staff:* 2   *Sales Staff:* 40
Ownership: Private
Produces/Sells CE-marked Devices: Y
Federal Procurement Eligibility: Small Business
Distribution: Exclusive Distributor
General Admin.: Howard Smith/Chief Operating Officer
    Bruce Thaw/President, Chief Executive Officer
Mktg./Adv.: Barbara Kaplan/Manager Marketing
    Lee Vestrich/Vice President Sales
Headlamp, Operating, AC-Powered	Ophthalmology
Lamp, Endoscopic, Incandescent	Surgery
Lamp, Examination (Light)	General
Lamp, Fluorescein, AC-Powered	Surgery
Lamp, Heat	General
Lamp, Infrared	Physical Med
Lamp, Microscope	Pathology
Lamp, Operating Room	General

BULBTRONICS, INC. 800-624-2852 (cont'd)
Lamp, Other	General
Lamp, Slit	Ophthalmology
Lamp, Slit, Biomicroscope, AC-Powered	Ophthalmology
Lamp, Sun, Incandescent	General
Lamp, Surgical	Surgery
Lamp, Surgical, Xenon	Surgery
Lamp, Ultraviolet (Spectrum A)	General
Lamp, Ultraviolet, Germicidal	General
Lamp, Ultraviolet, Physical Medicine	Physical Med
Light Source, Endoscope, Xenon Arc	Surgery
Light Source, Endoscopic	Obstetrics/Gynecology
Light Source, Fiberoptic, Routine	Gastroenterology/Urology
Light Source, Flash	Chemistry
Light Source, Incandescent, Diagnostic	Gastroenterology/Urology
Light Source, Photographic, Fiberoptic	Gastroenterology/Urology
Light, Dental	Dental And Oral
Light, Other	General
Light, Surgical, Fiberoptic	Surgery
Safelight, X-Ray	Radiology

BULBWORKS, INC. 800-334-2852
Unit 5, 80 North Dell Avenue, Kenvil, NJ 07847 973-584-7171
FDA Number: n/a *Fax:* 973-584-0300
E-mail: bulbwork@bulbworks.com
Web site: www.bulbworks.com
Medical Products Sales Volume: $1,200,000
Annual Revenue: $1-$5 Million
Year Founded: 1993
Total Employees: 8   *Marketing Staff:* 1   *Sales Staff:* 3
Ownership: Private
Produces/Sells CE-marked Devices: N
Federal Procurement Eligibility: Small Business
Distribution: Manufacturer Direct, Manufacturer Through Distributor
General Admin.: Mr. Dennis Barker/President
Accessories, Light, Surgical	Surgery
Camera, Video, Headlight, Surgical	Surgery
Fiberoptic Light Source & Carrier	Ear/Nose/Throat
Lamp, Endoscopic, Incandescent	Surgery
Lamp, Examination (Light)	General
Lamp, Heat	General
Lamp, Infrared	Physical Med
Lamp, Laryngoscope	Ear/Nose/Throat
Lamp, Microscope	Pathology
Lamp, Operating Room	General
Lamp, Other	General
Lamp, Ultraviolet, Germicidal	General
Light, Other	General
Phototherapy Unit (Bilirubin Lamp)	General
Safelight, X-Ray	Radiology

BUNNELL INCORPORATED 800-800-4358
436 Lawndale Dr., Salt Lake City, UT 84115-2917 801-467-0800
FDA Number: 1719232 *Fax:* 801-467-0867
E-mail: info@bunl.com
Web site: www.bunl.com
Annual Revenue: $1-$5 Million
Year Founded: 1980
Total Employees: 30   *Marketing Staff:* 2   *Sales Staff:* 7
Ownership: Private
Produces/Sells CE-marked Devices: N
Federal Procurement Eligibility: Small Business
Distribution: Manufacturer Direct, Service Direct, Exclusive Distributor
General Admin.: J. Bert Bunnell/Chief Executive Officer
    J. Bert Bunnell/President
Mktg./Adv.: David R. Platt/Director Marketing
    Ken Hekking/Manager National Sales
Production: Greg Jex/Manager Operations
    Diane Goodman/Manager Regulatory Affairs
Research: Jeff Orth/Vice President Research & Development
Adapter, Tube, Tracheal	Anesthesiology
Cart, Other	General
Circuit, Breathing, Ventilator	Anesthesiology
Ventilator, High-Frequency	Anesthesiology

BUNTING DIV.
See Pdi Communication Systems

BURCH MANUFACTURING CO., INC. 515-573-4136
618 1st Avenue North, Fort Dodge, IA 50501-0876
FDA Number: n/a *Fax:* 515-573-4138
E-mail: info@burchmfg.com
Web site: www.burchmfg.com
Medical Products Sales Volume: $260,000
Year Founded: 1882
Total Employees: 7
Ownership: Private
Produces/Sells CE-marked Devices: N
Federal Procurement Eligibility: Small Business, Female Owned

BURCH MANUFACTURING CO., INC. 515-573-4136 *(cont'd)*
Distribution: Manufacturer Through Distributor, Manufacturer Through Manufacturer Reps, OEM
General Admin.: Karla Skaggs/President, Chief Executive Officer
Production: Kathleen Ramthun/Manager Materials

Decontamination Kit	Surgery
Tank, Full Body (Bath)	General

BURDICK & JACKSON
See Honeywell Burdick & Jackson

BURDICK, INC.
See Cardiac Science Corp.

BURKE L. MAYS AND ASSOCIATES, INC. 615-791-6247
315 Springhouse Circle, Franklin, TN 37067
FDA Number: 3005550372

Electroencephalograph	Cns/Neurology

BURKE MEDICAL, LLC 727-532-8333
2310 Tall Pines Dr., Suite 210, Largo, FL 33771
FDA Number: 1059264
Ownership: Private
Produces/Sells CE-marked Devices: N

Epilator, High-Frequency, Tweezer Type	Surgery
Joint, Knee, External Brace	Physical Med
Pack, Hot Or Cold, Water Circulating	Physical Med
Twister, Brace Setting	Physical Med

BURKE MOBILITY PRODUCTS, INC.
See Leisure-Lift, Inc.

BURKE, INC.
See Leisure-Lift, Inc.

BURKHART ROENTGEN INTL. INC. 800-USA-XRAY
5201 8th Ave. S., St. Petersburg, FL 33707 727-327-6950
FDA Number: 1219074 *Fax:* 727-327-3255
E-mail: survice@usaxray.com
Web site: www.usaxray.com
Annual Revenue: $1-$5 Million
Total Employees: 25
Ownership: Private
Quality System Registration Information: ISO9001
Produces/Sells CE-marked Devices: Y
Federal Procurement Eligibility: Small Business
Distribution: Manufacturer Through Distributor, Manufacturer Through Manufacturer Reps, OEM, Importer, Exporter
General Admin.: George D. Burkhart/President
Mktg./Adv.: Richard Burkhart/International Sales Representative
　　　Angel Hernandez/Manager International & National Sales
　　　Julia Karcher/Manager Marketing & Advertising

Accessories, Laser	General
Accessories, Radiotherapy	Radiology
Apron, Lead, Radiographic	Radiology
Battery, Mobile Radiographic Unit	Radiology
Cassette, Radiographic Film	Radiology
Eyeglasses, Safety	Ophthalmology
Film, X-Ray	Radiology
Grid, Radiographic	Radiology
Illuminator, Radiographic Film	Radiology
Light, High Intensity	Radiology
Light, Surgical, Ceiling Mounted	Surgery
Processor, Radiographic Film, Automatic	Radiology
Radiographic Unit, Diagnostic	Radiology
Recovery Equipment, Waste Heat	General
Recovery Equipment, Water	General
Scale, Laboratory	Chemistry
Screen, Intensifying, Radiographic	Radiology
Shield, Ophthalmic, Radiological	Radiology
Shield, Protective, Personnel	Radiology
Shield, X-Ray	Radiology
Shield, X-Ray, Portable	Radiology
Shield, X-Ray, Throat	Radiology
Support, Patient Position	Anesthesiology
System, Marking, Film, Radiographic	Radiology
Training Aid	Orthopedics

BURLING INSTRUMENTS, INC. 973-635-9481
16 River Rd., Chatham, NJ 07928-0298
FDA Number: n/a *Fax:* 973-635-9530
E-mail: burlinginstruments@yahoo.com
Web site: www.burlinginstruments.com
Ownership: Private
Produces/Sells CE-marked Devices: Y
Federal Procurement Eligibility: Small Business
Distribution: Manufacturer Through Distributor, Manufacturer Through Manufacturer Reps, OEM

Controller, Temperature, Other	General
Probe, Temperature	General
Regulator, Temperature	Chemistry

BURLINGTON MEDICAL SUPPLIES, INC. 800-221-3466
3 Elmhurst Str., PO Box 3194, 757-888-8994
Newport News, VA 23603
FDA Number: 1222742 *Fax:* 757-887-5894
E-mail: info@burmed.com
Web site: www.burmed.com
Medical Products Sales Volume: $7,000,000
Annual Revenue: $1-$5 Million
Year Founded: 1969
Total Employees: 40　　*Marketing Staff:* 2　　*Sales Staff:* 12
Ownership: Private
Quality System Registration Information: ISO9001
Produces/Sells CE-marked Devices: N
Federal Procurement Eligibility: Small Business, GSA Contract, VA Contract
Distribution: Manufacturer Direct, Manufacturer Through Manufacturer Reps, Exporter
General Admin.: Dennis F. Swartz/President
Mktg./Adv.: Elaine R. Swartz/Manager Contract Sales
　　　Elaine Swartz/Vice President Marketing

Apron, Lead, Dental	Dental And Oral
Apron, Lead, Radiographic	Radiology
Cushion, Table, Surgical	Surgery
Eyeglasses	Ophthalmology
Glove, Protective, Radiographic	Radiology
Grid, Radiographic	Radiology
Shield, X-Ray, Leaded	Dental And Oral
Support, Patient Position, Radiographic	Radiology

BURNFREE PRODUCTS DIVISION 888-909-2876
9382 S. 670 W., Sandy, UT 84070 801-569-9090
FDA Number: 9011104 *Fax:* 801-569-3733
E-mail: info@burnfree.com
Web site: www.burnfree.com
Medical Products Sales Volume: $660,000
Annual Revenue: $1-$5 Million
Year Founded: 1994
Total Employees: 5　　*Marketing Staff:* 2　　*Sales Staff:* 3
Ownership: Private
Quality System Registration Information: ISO9001
Produces/Sells CE-marked Devices: Y
Federal Procurement Eligibility: Small Business
Distribution: Manufacturer Through Distributor, OEM, Exporter
General Admin.: Bob Daniels/President
　　　Karen Horton/Vice President, General Manager
Mktg./Adv.: Daniel Mulvany/Director National Accounts

Blanket, Fire	General
Dressing, Wound and Burn, Hydrogel	Surgery

BURNISHINE PRODUCTS
See Weiman Healthcare Solutions

BURRELL CORPORATION
See Burrell Scientific, Inc

BURRELL SCIENTIFIC, INC 800-637-6074
2223 Fifth Avenue, Pittsburgh, PA 15219-5597 412-471-2527
FDA Number: 9320051 *Fax:* 412-391-4231
E-mail: burrellsci@sprintmail.com
Web site: www.burrellsci.com
Medical Products Sales Volume: $3,200,000
Annual Revenue: $1-$5 Million
Year Founded: 1917
Total Employees: 14　　*Sales Staff:* 3
Ownership: Private
Produces/Sells CE-marked Devices: Y
Federal Procurement Eligibility: Small Business
Distribution: Manufacturer Direct, Manufacturer Through Distributor
General Admin.: Loren Holmes/President
Mktg./Adv.: Joesph Mattis/Vice President, Manager Sales

Labware, Basic, Disposable	Chemistry
Labware, Basic, Reusable	Chemistry
Mixer, Clinical Laboratory	Chemistry

BURRON MEDICAL, INC., HOSPITAL DIV.
See B. Braun Oem Division, B. Braun Medical Inc.

BURRON OEM DIV., B. BRAUN MEDICAL INC.
See B. Braun Oem Division, B. Braun Medical Inc.

BURTON CO., R.H. 800-848-0410
3965 Brookham Drive, 614-875-9600
Grove City, OH 43123
FDA Number: 1525679 *Fax:* 614-875-8839
E-mail: sales@rhburton.com
Web site: www.rhburton.com
Medical Products Sales Volume: $200,000
Annual Revenue: $10-$25 Million
Year Founded: 1947
Total Employees: 3　　*Marketing Staff:* 2　　*Sales Staff:* 4
Ownership: Private

BURTON CO., R.H. 800-848-0410 (cont'd)

Quality System Registration Information: ISO9001; ISO9002
Produces/Sells CE-marked Devices: N
Federal Procurement Eligibility: Small Business
Distribution: OEM, Service Direct, Exclusive Distributor, Importer, Exporter
General Admin.: Kevin W. Intrieri/President
Mktg./Adv.: Kevin W. Intrieri/Manager Marketing
　　　　Brent B. Ludington/Manager National Sales
Production: David Wood/Manager Production Services

Chair, Ophthalmic, AC-Powered	Ophthalmology
Keratometer	Ophthalmology
Lamp, Slit	Ophthalmology
Measurer, Lens Radius, Ophthalmic	Ophthalmology
Measurer, Lens, AC-Powered	Ophthalmology
Projector, Ophthalmic	Ophthalmology
Pupillometer	Ophthalmology
Refractor, Ophthalmic	Ophthalmology
Tonometer, Manual	Ophthalmology

BURTON MEDICAL PRODUCTS, INC. 800-444-9909
21100 Lassen St., Chatsworth, CA 91311 818-701-8700
FDA Number: 2018492 *Fax:* 818-701-8725
E-mail: jthomas@burtonmedical.com
Web site: www.burtonmedical.com
Annual Revenue: $5-$10 Million
Total Employees: 45 *Marketing Staff:* 2 *Sales Staff:* 4
Ownership: Private
Quality System Registration Information: ISO9001
Produces/Sells CE-marked Devices: Y
Federal Procurement Eligibility: VA Contract
Distribution: Manufacturer Through Distributor, Manufacturer Through Manufacturer Reps, OEM
General Admin.: Mr. George Preston/President, Chief Executive Officer
Production: Mr. Scot Kinghorn/Manager Quality Assurance & Regulatory Affairs

Accessories, Light, Surgical	Surgery
Contract Manufacturing	General
Examination Device, AC-Powered	General
Illuminator, Radiographic Film	Radiology
Lamp, Examination (Light)	General
Lamp, Examination, Ceiling Mounted (Light)	General
Lamp, Operating Room	General
Lamp, Surgical	Surgery
Lamp, Ultraviolet, Germicidal	General
Lamp, Ultraviolet, Physical Medicine	Physical Med
Light Source, Fiberoptic, Routine	Gastroenterology/Urology
Light, Bilirubin (Phototherapy)	General
Light, Overbed	General
Light, Surgical Headlight	Dental And Oral
Light, Surgical Operating, Dental	Dental And Oral
Light, Surgical, Ceiling Mounted	Surgery
Light, Surgical, Floor Standing	Surgery
Nebulizer, Medicinal	Ear/Nose/Throat
Phototherapy Unit (Bilirubin Lamp)	General
Television Monitor, Operating Room	General

BURTON PARSONS & CO. INC.
See Alcon Research, Ltd.

BUSAK+SHAMBAN, TRELLEBORG AMERICAN VARISEAL
See Trelleborg Sealing Solutions

BUSCH, INC 800-872-7867
516 Viking Drive, Virginia Beach, VA 23452-7316 757-463-7800
FDA Number: n/a *Fax:* 757-463-7407
E-mail: marketing@buschinc.com
Web site: www.buschpump.com
Medical Products Sales Volume: $50,000,000
Annual Revenue: $50-$100 Million
Year Founded: 1975
Total Employees: 155 *Marketing Staff:* 4 *Sales Staff:* 16
Ownership: Private
Quality System Registration Information: ISO9001
Produces/Sells CE-marked Devices: Y
Federal Procurement Eligibility: Small Business
Distribution: Manufacturer Direct
General Admin.: Charles Kane/President
Mktg./Adv.: Amie Banis/Manager Advertising

Pump, Vacuum, Central	Anesthesiology

BUSHNELL
See Bausch & Lomb

BUSINESS AVIATION SERVICES 800-888-1646
3501 Aviation Avenue, 605-336-7791
Sioux Falls, SD 57104
FDA Number: n/a *Fax:* 605-336-8009
E-mail: busav@busav.com
Web site: www.busav.com
Medical Products Sales Volume: $6,000,000
Annual Revenue: $0-$1 Million
Year Founded: 1992

BUSINESS AVIATION SERVICES 800-888-1646 (cont'd)
Total Employees: 35 *Marketing Staff:* 3 *Sales Staff:* 2
Ownership: BUSINESS AVIATION
Federal Procurement Eligibility: Small Business, Female Owned
Distribution: Manufacturer Direct
General Admin.: Dale Froehlich/Chief Executive Officer
　　　　Dale Froehlich/President
　　　　Richard Smith/Vice President, General Manager
Mktg./Adv.: Koni Schiller/Director Marketing
　　　　Koni Schiller/Manager National Sales
　　　　Linda Barker/Vice President Business Development
　　　　Linda Barker/Vice President Marketing
Production: Scott Barber/Manager Materials

Ambulance	General
Ambulance, Air	General

BUSINESS SYSTEMS SPECIALTIES, INC.
See Pacifiq Systems Llc

BUSSARD & SON INC., R.D. 800-252-2692
415 S.W. 25th AVE., Albany, OR 97322 541-926-7747
FDA Number: n/a *Fax:* 541-926-4361
E-mail: sales@rdbussard.com
Web site: www.rdbussard.com
Medical Products Sales Volume: $1,000,000
Annual Revenue: $1-$5 Million
Total Employees: 18 *Marketing Staff:* 2 *Sales Staff:* 2
Ownership: Private
Produces/Sells CE-marked Devices: N
Federal Procurement Eligibility: Small Business
Distribution: Manufacturer Through Distributor, OEM
General Admin.: William Harris/President

Bag, Laundry, Infection Control	General
Cover, Cart	General
Liner, Laundry Hamper	General

BUSSE HOSPITAL DISPOSABLES, INC. 800-645-6526
75 Arkay Dr., Hauppauge, NY 11788 631-435-4711
FDA Number: 2433012 *Fax:* 631-435-4721
E-mail: mail@busseinc.com
Web site: www.busseinc.com
Ownership: Private
Produces/Sells CE-marked Devices: N

Accessories, Apparel, Surgical	Surgery
Amniotome	Obstetrics/Gynecology
Apron, Lead, Radiographic	Radiology
Bag, Ice	General
Biopsy Instrument	Gastroenterology/Urology
Cannula, Suction, Uterine	Obstetrics/Gynecology
Cap, Surgical	Surgery
Catheter, Straight	Gastroenterology/Urology
Catheter, Urethral	Gastroenterology/Urology
Clamp And Cutter, Umbilical	Obstetrics/Gynecology
Clamp, Circumcision	Obstetrics/Gynecology
Clip, Instrument, Forming/Cutting	Cns/Neurology
Collector, Specimen	Microbiology
Cover, Shoe, Operating Room	Surgery
Curette, Uterine	Obstetrics/Gynecology
Drape, Surgical	Surgery
Dressing, Other	General
Forceps	Orthopedics
Gown, Isolation, Surgical	Surgery
Instrument, Manual, General Surgical	Surgery
Kit, Anesthesia, Conduction	Anesthesiology
Kit, Biopsy, Gastro-Urology	Gastroenterology/Urology
Kit, Suture Removal	Surgery
Kit, Wound Dressing	Surgery
Label/Tag, Sterile	Surgery
Linen, Bed	General
Manometer, Spinal Fluid	General
Mask, Surgical	Surgery
Needle, Aspiration And Injection, Disposable	Surgery
Needle, Conduction, Anesthesia (W/Wo Introducer)	Anesthesiology
Needle, Hypodermic, Single Lumen With Syringe	General
Pad, Menstrual, Unscented	Obstetrics/Gynecology
Pump, Suction Operatory	Dental And Oral
Qualitative Chemical Reactions, Urinary Calculi (Stone)	Chemistry
Sampler, Amniotic Fluid (Amniocentesis Tray)	Obstetrics/Gynecology
Scissors, Disposable	General
Surgical Instrument, Disposable	Surgery
Syringe Unit, Air And/Or Water	Dental And Oral
Syringe, Irrigating	General
Syringe, Piston	General
Trap, Sterile Specimen	Anesthesiology
Tray, Surgical Instrument	Surgery
Tube, Aspirating, Flexible, Connecting	Anesthesiology
Tube, Tracheostomy (W/Wo Connector)	Anesthesiology
Tubing, Flexible, Medical Gas, Low-Pressure	Anesthesiology
Wrap, Sterilization	General

BUTLER STAIRLIFT
See Flinchbaugh-Kurtz Company

BUXCO RESEARCH SYSTEMS   910-794-6980
219 Station Road, Suite 202, Wilmington, NC 28405
FDA Number: 9200177   *Fax:* 910-794-6981
E-mail: sales@buxco.com
Web site: www.buxco.com
Medical Products Sales Volume: $2,800,000
Year Founded: 1968
Total Employees: 30
Ownership: Private
Produces/Sells CE-marked Devices: Y
Federal Procurement Eligibility: Small Business, GSA Contract
Distribution: Manufacturer Direct, Manufacturer Through Manufacturer Reps,
    Service Direct, Exclusive Distributor, Exporter
General Admin.: Joseph M. Lomask/President, Chief Executive Officer
Mktg./Adv.: Mr. Richard Shafer/Manager Marketing & Sales
Research: Morton R Lomask/Director Development

Computer Equipment	General
Computer Software	General
Meter, Volume, Blood	Hematology
Monitor, Blood Pressure, Indirect (Arterial)	Cardiovascular
Monitor, Hemodynamic	Anesthesiology

BUXTON MEDICAL EQUIPMENT CORP.   631-957-4500
1178 Route 109, Lindenhurst, NY 11757
FDA Number: 2433867   *Fax:* 631-957-3884
E-mail: cnewman@buxtonmed.com
Web site: www.buxtonmed.com
Medical Products Sales Volume: $4,000,000
Annual Revenue: $1-$5 Million
Year Founded: 1980
Total Employees: 30   *Marketing Staff:* 3   *Sales Staff:* 14
Ownership: Private
Produces/Sells CE-marked Devices: N
Federal Procurement Eligibility: Small Business, GSA Contract
Distribution: Manufacturer Direct, Service Direct
General Admin.: Carl B. Newman/President
Mktg./Adv.: Philip McCann/Manager International & National Sales
       Philip McCann/Vice President, Director Marketing

Cleaner, Ultrasonic, Medical Instrument	General
Sterilizer, Laboratory	Microbiology
Sterilizer, Steam (Autoclave)	General
Sterilizer, Steam (Autoclave), Surgical	Surgery
Sterilizer, Steam, Bulk	General
Washer, Cart	General
Washer, Labware	Chemistry
Washer, Pipette	Chemistry
Washer, Utensil	General
Washer/Sterilizer	General

BVR AERO PRECISION CORPORATION   815-874-2471
3358-60 Publishers Dr., Rockford, IL 61109
FDA Number: n/a   *Fax:* 815-874-4415
Web site: www.bvraero.com
Total Employees: 60   *Marketing Staff:* 6   *Sales Staff:* 6
Ownership: Private
Stock Symbol: ESL
Quality System Registration Information: ISO9001
Produces/Sells CE-marked Devices: N
Federal Procurement Eligibility: Small Business
General Admin.: Mr. Jerry Leitman/Chairman
       Mr. R. Brad Lawrence/President, Chief Executive Officer
Mktg./Adv.: Craig Legault/Vice President Sales
Research: Mr. James Morris/Vice President Engineering

Drill, Oral Surgery	Dental And Oral

BVS, INC.   877-877-4821
949 Poplar Road, Honey Brook, PA 19344-0250   610-273-2841
FDA Number: n/a   *Fax:* 610-273-2843
E-mail: info@bvssamplers.com
Web site: www.bvssamplers.com
Medical Products Sales Volume: $800,000
Year Founded: 1971
Total Employees: 3
Ownership: Private
Produces/Sells CE-marked Devices: N
Federal Procurement Eligibility: Small Business
Distribution: Manufacturer Direct, Manufacturer Through Distributor, Manufacturer
    Through Manufacturer Reps
General Admin.: Robert M. Blechman/President
       Ursita S. Aparre/Vice President
Finance: Joseph J. Meehan/Treasurer

Compressor, Air, Portable	Anesthesiology
Equipment, Control, Pollution	General

BWELL INC.   865-982-2184
1723 St. Ives Blvd., Alcoa, TN 37701
FDA Number: 3005080523
Ownership: Private
Produces/Sells CE-marked Devices: N

Dilator, Nasal	Ear/Nose/Throat

BYK GULDEN INC.
See Altana, Inc.

BYRNE MEDICAL, INC.   800-490-9869
2021 Airport Road, Conroe, TX 77304
FDA Number: 1651395   *Fax:* 936-539-0392
E-mail: rusty@byrnemedical.com
Web site: www.byrnemedical.com
Medical Products Sales Volume: $6,400,000
Year Founded: 1997
Total Employees: 60
Ownership: Private
Produces/Sells CE-marked Devices: N
Federal Procurement Eligibility: Small Business
Production: Mr. Rusty Smith/Manager Production & RA
       Mr. David B. Moore/Manager Quality Systems

Endoscope	Gastroenterology/Urology

BYRON MEDICAL   800-777-3434
602 W. Rillito, Tucson, AZ 85705   520-573-0857
FDA Number: 2025576   *Fax:* 520-746-1757
E-mail: bleavenworth@byronmedical.com
Web site: www.byronmedical.com
Medical Products Sales Volume: $8,900,000
Annual Revenue: $10-$25 Million
Year Founded: 2002
Total Employees: 55   *Marketing Staff:* 2   *Sales Staff:* 14
Ownership: Mentor Corp.
Quality System Registration Information: ISO9001
Produces/Sells CE-marked Devices: Y
Federal Procurement Eligibility: Small Business
Distribution: Manufacturer Direct, OEM, Service Direct, Exclusive Distributor
Mktg./Adv.: Todd Lane/Director Sales
       Brett Leavenworth/National Sales Representative

Aspirator, Liposuction	Surgery
Binder, Elastic	General
Cannula, Surgical, General & Plastic Surgery	Surgery
Pump, Aspiration, Portable	Anesthesiology
Pump, Infusion	General
Suction Apparatus, Single Patient, Portable, Non-Powered	Surgery
Syringe, Irrigating	General
Tubing, Non-Invasive	Surgery
Unit, Filter, Membrane	Chemistry

C & A SCIENTIFIC CO. INC.   703-330-1413
7241 Gabe Court, Manassas, VA 20109
FDA Number: 1122839   *Fax:* 703-330-7510
E-mail: sales@cnascientific.com
Web site: www.cnascientific.com
Medical Products Sales Volume: $1,100,000
Annual Revenue: $1-$5 Million
Year Founded: 1990
Total Employees: 9   *Marketing Staff:* 2   *Sales Staff:* 5
Ownership: Private
Quality System Registration Information: ISO9001; ISO9002
Produces/Sells CE-marked Devices: N
Federal Procurement Eligibility: Small Business, Minority Owned
Distribution: Manufacturer Through Distributor, Importer
General Admin.: Ming Xiang/Chief Executive Officer
Mktg./Adv.: Karla Carias/Manager Market Research
       Trenton Middleton/Manager National Sales

Blade, Scalpel	Surgery
Container, Slide Mailer	Microbiology
Container, Specimen Mailer And Storage	Pathology
Container, Specimen, All Types	General
Coverslip, Microscope Slide	Pathology
Depressor, Tongue, ENT, Wood	Ear/Nose/Throat
Floss, Dental	Dental And Oral
Handle, Scalpel	Surgery
Lamp, Microscope	Pathology
Lancet, Blood	General
Microscope	Hematology
Pipette, Quantitative, Hematology	Hematology
Scalpel, One-Piece (Knife)	Surgery
Slide, Microscope	Pathology
Spatula, Cervical, Cytology	Obstetrics/Gynecology
Thermometer, Mercury	General

C & C OXYGEN CO.   423-867-2369
3615 Rossville Blvd., Chattanooga, TN 37407
FDA Number: n/a
Annual Revenue: $0-$1 Million

C & C OXYGEN CO. 423-867-2369 *(cont'd)*
Ownership: Private
Produces/Sells CE-marked Devices: N
Federal Procurement Eligibility: Small Business, Female Owned
Distribution: Manufacturer Through Manufacturer Reps
Oxygen — Anesthesiology

C & D INDUSTRIES, INC. 413-493-1200
28 Appleton St., Holyoke, MA 01040
FDA Number: 1225804 *Fax:* 413-493-1212
Ownership: Private
Produces/Sells CE-marked Devices: N
Tampon, Menstrual, Unscented — Obstetrics/Gynecology

C & D TECHNOLOGIES INC., DYNASTY DIV. 414-967-6500
900 East Keefe Ave., Milwaukee, WI 53212
FDA Number: 2132466 *Fax:* 414-964-2419
Ownership: Private
Produces/Sells CE-marked Devices: N
Component, Wheelchair — Physical Med

C & J PRECISION PLASTICS
See C&J Industries, Inc.

C & K MANUFACTURING & SALES 800-821-7795
28825 Ranney Pkwy., Westlake, OH 44145 440-871-4078
FDA Number: 1527697 *Fax:* 440-871-4070
E-mail: ckmfg1@ckmfg.com
Web site: www.ckmfg.com
Year Founded: 1964
Total Employees: 100 *Marketing Staff:* 6 *Sales Staff:* 20
Ownership: MAIN STREET CAPITAL
Produces/Sells CE-marked Devices: N
Federal Procurement Eligibility: Small Business
Distribution: Manufacturer Through Distributor
Mktg./Adv.: Mary Stieger/Director Marketing
Glove, Patient Examination, Latex — General
Glove, Patient Examination, Vinyl — General
Medical Product Subsidiaries (Listed Separately)
Changzhou Jiuhong Medical Instruments Co., Ltd

C & S ELECTRONICS, INC. 402-563-3596
2565 16th Ave., Columbus, NE 68601
FDA Number: 1933113 *Fax:* 402-564-5800
E-mail: info@cselectronicsinc.com
Web site: www.cselectronicsinc.com
Ownership: Private
Produces/Sells CE-marked Devices: N
General Admin.: Mr. Carl Seckel/President
Mktg./Adv.: Mr. Rod Behlen/Sales Manager
Purchasing: Mr. jeri Rosno/Purchasing Agent
Iontophoresis Device, Dental — Dental And Oral

C CHANGE SURGICAL LLC 877.989.3737
101 North Chestnut Street, Suite 301, 336-723-0200
Winston-salem, NC 27101
FDA Number: 3005853119
E-mail: service@cchangesurgical.com
Web site: www.cchangesurgical.com
Ownership: Private
Produces/Sells CE-marked Devices: N

C&E GP SPECIALISTS 800-346-2626
1015 Calle Amanecer, San Clemente, CA 92673
FDA Number: 2032336 *Fax:* 888-418-2626
E-mail: chrisa@cevision.com
Web site: www.cevision.com
Medical Products Sales Volume: $1,300,000
Annual Revenue: $0-$1 Million
Year Founded: 1987
Total Employees: 15 *Marketing Staff:* 3 *Sales Staff:* 4
Ownership: C&E VISION SERVICES, INC.
Produces/Sells CE-marked Devices: N
Federal Procurement Eligibility: Small Business, Minority Owned
Distribution: Manufacturer Direct, Manufacturer Through Distributor, Exporter
General Admin.: Dr. HARVEY YAMAMOTO/President
Lens, Contact, Gas-Permeable — Ophthalmology

C&H CONTACT LENS, INC. 800-527-5060
2836 Walnut Hill Lane, P.O. Box 29081, 214-358-4433
Dallas, TX 75229
FDA Number: n/a *Fax:* 214-358-2599
Web site: www.chcontacts.com
Medical Products Sales Volume: $2,500,000
Annual Revenue: $1-$5 Million
Ownership: Private
Produces/Sells CE-marked Devices: N
Distribution: Manufacturer Direct

C&H CONTACT LENS, INC. 800-527-5060 *(cont'd)*
Lens, Contact, Extended-Wear — Ophthalmology

C&H GAUGE CO. INC.
See Accellent Inc.

C&J INDUSTRIES, INC. 814-724-4950
760 Water St., Meadville, PA 16335-3338
FDA Number: 2522206 *Fax:* 814-724-4959
E-mail: stephaniegoss@cjindustries.com
Web site: www.cjindustries.com
Medical Products Sales Volume: $6,000,000
Annual Revenue: $10-$25 Million
Year Founded: 1962
Total Employees: 250 *Marketing Staff:* 2 *Sales Staff:* 8
Ownership: Private
Quality System Registration Information: ISO9001
Produces/Sells CE-marked Devices: N
Federal Procurement Eligibility: Small Business
Distribution: Manufacturer Direct
General Admin.: C. Richard Johnston/Chief Executive Officer
Sandra Hurban/Director Human Resources
Dennis R. Frampton/President
Mktg./Adv.: Mark Fuhrman/Market Manager
Production: Maria Porter/Director Quality Assurance
David W. Lennox/Vice President Operations
Component, Plastic — General
Contract Manufacturing — General
Contract Packaging — General
Insufflator, Laparoscopic — Obstetrics/Gynecology
Molding, Custom — General
Retractor, Self-Retaining, Neurology — Cns/Neurology
System, Suction, Lipoplasty — Surgery

C&S RESEARCH CORPORATION 800-545-8460
625 Clark Avenue, Suite 21B, King of Prussia, PA 19406
FDA Number: n/a *Fax:* 610-265-0786
E-mail: support@csrc.com
Web site: www.csrc.com
Annual Revenue: $0-$1 Million
Year Founded: 1978
Ownership: Private
Produces/Sells CE-marked Devices: N
Distribution: Manufacturer Direct, Manufacturer Through Manufacturer Reps,
Service Direct
Computer, Patient Data Management — General

C-AXIS P.R., INC. 787-286-0590
Parque Industrial Valle Polima, Edif Multifabril 14-a-2,
Caguas, PR 00727
FDA Number: 3005029036 *Fax:* 787-286-1601
Ownership: Private
Produces/Sells CE-marked Devices: N
Anchor, Suture, Bone Fixation, Metallic — Orthopedics

C. L. STURKEY, INC. 800-274-3446
824 Cumberland Street, Avon, PA 17042 717-274-9441
FDA Number: 2531348 *Fax:* 717-274-9442
Web site: www.sturkey.com
Ownership: Private
Produces/Sells CE-marked Devices: N
Accessories, Microtome — Pathology

C. R. BARD, INC. 908-277-8481
289 Bay Rd., Queensbury, NY 12804
FDA Number: 1313046
Ownership: C. R. Bard, Inc.
Stock Symbol: BCR
Traded On: NYSE
Produces/Sells CE-marked Devices: N
Cable/Lead, ECG, With Transducer And Electrode — Cardiovascular
Catheter, Electrode Recording, Or Probe — Cardiovascular
Catheter, Percutaneous — Cardiovascular
Filter, Intravascular, Cardiovascular — Cardiovascular
Guidewire, Catheter — Cardiovascular

C. R. BARD, INC. 908-277-8481
428 Powerhouse Rd., Moncks Corner, SC 29461
FDA Number: 1030583
Web site: www.crbard.com
Ownership: C. R. Bard, Inc.
Stock Symbol: BCR
Traded On: NYSE
Produces/Sells CE-marked Devices: N
Catheter, Coude — Gastroenterology/Urology
Catheter, Retention Type, Balloon — Gastroenterology/Urology
Catheter, Urological — Gastroenterology/Urology
Tube, Tracheostomy (W/Wo Connector) — Anesthesiology

C. R. BARD, INC.
730 Central Ave., Murray Hill, NJ 07974
800-367-2273
908-277-8000
FDA Number: n/a
Fax: 908-277-8412
E-mail: bard.helpline@crbard.com
Web site: www.crbard.com
Medical Products Sales Volume: $1,980,000,000
Annual Revenue: More than $1 Billion
Year Founded: 1907
Total Employees: 210
Ownership: Public
Stock Symbol: BCR
Traded On: NYSE
Quality System Registration Information: ISO9001
Produces/Sells CE-marked Devices: N
Federal Procurement Eligibility: Small Business
Distribution: Manufacturer Direct, Manufacturer Through Distributor, OEM
General Admin.: Timothy M. Ring/Chief Executive Officer, Chairman
John H. Weiland/President, Chief Operating Officer
Finance: Todd Schermerhorn/Chief Financial Officer
Mr. Todd Garner/Vice President Investor Relations

Guidewire	Cardiovascular

Medical Product Subsidiaries (Listed Separately)
Bard Access Systems, Inc.
Bard Brachytherapy, Inc
Bard Electro Physiology
Bard Peripheral Vascular, Inc.
Bard Shannon Limited
Bridger Biomed, Inc.
C. R. Bard, Inc.
C. R. Bard, Inc., Bard Medical Div.
C. R. Bard, Inc., Bard Urological Div.
Davol Inc., Sub. C.R. Bard, Inc.
Dymax Corp.
Medchem Products, Inc.
Senorx, Inc.
Venetec International., Inc.

C. R. BARD, INC., BARD MEDICAL DIV.
8195 Industrial Blvd., Covington, GA 30209
800-526-4455
770-784-6100
FDA Number: 3006082230
Fax: 770-784-6731
E-mail: bard.medical@crbard.com
Web site: www.bardmedical.com
Ownership: C. R. Bard, Inc.
Stock Symbol: BCR
Traded On: NYSE
Quality System Registration Information: ISO9001
Produces/Sells CE-marked Devices: N
Distribution: Manufacturer Direct, Manufacturer Through Distributor
General Admin.: Bill Midgette/President
Keith Collins/Vice President Human Resources
Mktg./Adv.: Bob Anderson/Director National Accounts
Ben Trammell/Manager National Sales
Brett Giffin/Vice President Marketing
Dan LaFever/Vice President Sales
Production: Andre Mailliez/Vice President Manufacturing
Mary Mayo/Vice President Quality Assurance
Research: Vern Liebman/Vice President Research & Development

Accessories, Catheter	Surgery

C. R. BARD, INC., BARD UROLOGICAL DIV.
8195 Industrial Boulevard, Covington, GA 30014
800-526-4455
770-784-6100
FDA Number: 1018233
Fax: 770-784-6731
E-mail: bard.medical@crbard.com
Web site: www.bardurological.com
Year Founded: 1904
Total Employees: 109 *Marketing Staff:* 17 *Sales Staff:* 60
Ownership: C.R. BARD, INC.
Stock Symbol: BCR
Traded On: NYSE
Quality System Registration Information: ISO9001
Produces/Sells CE-marked Devices: N
Distribution: Manufacturer Direct, Manufacturer Through Distributor
General Admin.: Tim Ring/Chief Executive Officer
Burt Mirsky/President
Paul Murphy/Vice President Human Resources
Mktg./Adv.: Gary Teague/Director Marketing
Bob Anderson/Director National Accounts
George Cavagnaro/Vice President Business Development
Tom Woods/Vice President Sales
Production: Wayne Williamson/Director Quality Assurance
Research: Scott Britton/Vice President Research & Development

Accessories, Catheter	Surgery
Adapter, Stopcock, Manifold, Cardiopulmonary Bypass	Cardiovascular
Amplifier, Transducer Signal (W Signal Conditioner)	Cardiovascular
Antigen, Tumor Marker, Bladder (Basement Membrane Complexes)	Immunology
Basket, Biliary Stone Retrieval	Gastroenterology/Urology
Biopsy Instrument	Gastroenterology/Urology

C. R. BARD, INC., BARD UROLOGICAL DIV. 800-526-4455 *(cont'd)*

Catheter and Accessories, Urological	Gastroenterology/Urology
Catheter, Biliary	Gastroenterology/Urology
Catheter, Cardiovascular, Balloon Type	Cardiovascular
Catheter, Nephrostomy	Gastroenterology/Urology
Catheter, Suprapubic	Gastroenterology/Urology
Catheter, Urological	Gastroenterology/Urology
Clamp, Penile	Gastroenterology/Urology
Collector, Urine	Gastroenterology/Urology
Connector, Catheter	Surgery
Container, Specimen, All Types	General
Device, Cystometric, Hydraulic	Gastroenterology/Urology
Dilator, Catheter, Ureteral	Gastroenterology/Urology
Dilator, Urethral	Gastroenterology/Urology
Dislodger, Stone, Basket, Ureteral, Metal	Gastroenterology/Urology
Endoscope	Gastroenterology/Urology
Evacuator, Bladder, Manually Operated	Gastroenterology/Urology
Evacuator, Gastro-Urology	Gastroenterology/Urology
Flowmeter, Urine, Disposable	Gastroenterology/Urology
Glove, Surgical	General
Guidewire, Catheter	Cardiovascular
Implant, Collagen (Non-Aesthetic Use)	Surgery
Implant, Collagen, Dermal (Aesthetic Use)	Surgery
Injector, Angiographic (Cardiac Catheterization)	Cardiovascular
Kit, Biopsy Needle	Gastroenterology/Urology
Kit, Catheterization, Sterile Urethral	Gastroenterology/Urology
Laser, Surgical	Surgery
Splint, Ureteral	Gastroenterology/Urology
Stent, Ureteral	Gastroenterology/Urology
Surgical Instrument, G-U, Manual	Gastroenterology/Urology
Syringe, Irrigating, Sterile	General
Syringe, Piston	General
Uroflowmeter	Gastroenterology/Urology

C. R. NEWTON CO. LTD.
1575 S. Beretania St., Honolulu, HI 96826
800-545-2078
808-949-8389
FDA Number: n/a
Fax: 808-955-4721
Web site: www.crnewton.com
Annual Revenue: $1-$5 Million
Ownership: Private
Produces/Sells CE-marked Devices: N
Federal Procurement Eligibility: Small Business
Distribution: Manufacturer Direct, Service Direct

Bed, Electric	General
Bed, Manual	General
Collar, Cervical Neck	Orthopedics
Cushion, Other	General
Joint, Knee, External Brace	Physical Med
Support, Back	Orthopedics
Wheelchair, Manual	Physical Med

C.A.M. GRAPHICS CO., INC.
166 New Highway, Amityville, NY 11701
516-842-3400
FDA Number: n/a
Fax: 516-842-1005
E-mail: info@camgraphics.com
Web site: www.camgraphics.com
Medical Products Sales Volume: $3,500,000
Annual Revenue: $1-$5 Million
Total Employees: 50 *Marketing Staff:* 1 *Sales Staff:* 3
Ownership: Private
Produces/Sells CE-marked Devices: N
Federal Procurement Eligibility: Small Business
Distribution: Manufacturer Direct
General Admin.: Emanuel Cardinale/President
Mktg./Adv.: Emanuel Cardinale/Director Marketing
Brian Heiser/Director Product Development
Production: Pat Oltayem/Director Quality Assurance
Elizabeth Cardinale/Manager Materials
Brian Heiser/Vice President Operations
Research: Mike DeMartino/Manager Design
Finance: Peg Pawlowski/Manager Acctg.

Component, Electronic	General

C.A.M. SUPPLY, INC.
490 East Menlo Ave., Hemet, CA 92543
909-851-7114
FDA Number: 2085835
Ownership: Private
Produces/Sells CE-marked Devices: N

Needle, Acupuncture, Single Use	General

C.B. FLEET COMPANY INC.
PO Box 11349, 4615 Murray Place, Lynchburg, VA 24506-1349
804-528-4000
FDA Number: 1111503
Fax: 434-847-6110
E-mail: dimterh@cbfleet.com
Web site: www.cbfleet.com
Medical Products Sales Volume: $213,700,000
Year Founded: 1869
Total Employees: 400 *Marketing Staff:* 8 *Sales Staff:* 30
Ownership: Private

C.B. FLEET COMPANY INC.   804-528-4000 *(cont'd)*
Federal Procurement Eligibility: Small Business, Female Owned, GSA Contract, VA Contract
Distribution: Manufacturer Direct
General Admin.: William Chambers/Chief Executive Officer
     Crystal Sax/Director Human Resources
     Douglas Ballaire/President
     Sarah Post/Vice President Admin.
Mktg./Adv.: Robert Reznek/Director National Accounts
     Timothy Whalen/Manager Contract Sales
     Jeff Rowan/Vice President Business Development
     William Parsanko/Vice President Marketing
     Howard Dimter/Vice President Sales
Production: David Vaughan/Director Quality Assurance
     Joseph Kanapka/Manager Regulatory Affairs
     George Hricz/Vice President Operations

Applicator, Other	General
Bag, Enema	General
Kit, Bowel	Gastroenterology/Urology
Kit, Enema	General
Pad, Medicated	General

C.B. MEDICAL L.L.C.   860-693-2103
26 Center Street, Canton, CT 06019
FDA Number: 3004189022
Ownership: Private
Produces/Sells CE-marked Devices: N

Bandage, Adhesive	Surgery

C.C.I.
See Custom Comfort

C.D. DENISON ORTHOPAEDIC APPLIANCE CORP.   410-235-9645
220 W. 28th St., Baltimore, MD 21211-3089
FDA Number: 1119197   *Fax:* 410-243-7043
E-mail: denison@erols.com
Web site: www.cddenison.com
Medical Products Sales Volume: $2,500,000
Annual Revenue: $1-$5 Million
Year Founded: 1922
Total Employees: 18   *Marketing Staff:* 1
Ownership: Private
Produces/Sells CE-marked Devices: N
Federal Procurement Eligibility: Small Business
Distribution: Manufacturer Direct, Manufacturer Through Distributor
General Admin.: Harold E. Thompson/President

Orthosis, Cervical	Physical Med
Orthosis, Limb Brace	Physical Med
Splint, Temporary Training	Physical Med

C.E. TECH   800-333-7477
800 Prudential Dr., Jacksonville, FL 32207   904-202-5294
FDA Number: n/a   *Fax:* 904-399-3455
E-mail: scott.long@ce-tech.net
Web site: www.ce-tech.net
Medical Products Sales Volume: $4,500,000
Annual Revenue: $1-$5 Million
Year Founded: 1981
Total Employees: 28
Ownership: Private
Produces/Sells CE-marked Devices: N
Federal Procurement Eligibility: Small Business
Distribution: Service Direct
General Admin.: Scott Long/Vice President

Service, Maintenance/Repair	General

C.E.J. DENTAL PRODUCTS INC.   949-493-2449
32332 Camino Capistrano #101, San Juan Capistrano, CA 92675
FDA Number: 1000540886   *Fax:* 949-493-2492
E-mail: Steve@cejdental.com
Web site: www.cejdental.com
Ownership: Private
Produces/Sells CE-marked Devices: N

Contouring, Instrument, Matrix, Operative	Dental And Oral
Gel, Electrode, Pulp Tester	Dental And Oral
Matrix, Dental	Dental And Oral
Retainer, Matrix	Dental And Oral

C.F. ELECTRONICS, INC.   307-742-5200
2052 North Third Street, Laramie, WY 82072
FDA Number: 2435731   *Fax:* 307-742-8510
E-mail: ecyluick@aol.com
Medical Products Sales Volume: $500,000
Year Founded: 1974
Total Employees: 24
Ownership: Private

C.F. ELECTRONICS, INC.   307-742-5200 *(cont'd)*
Produces/Sells CE-marked Devices: N
Federal Procurement Eligibility: Small Business
Distribution: Manufacturer Direct, Manufacturer Through Distributor

Heater, Breathing System W/Wo Controller	Anesthesiology
Warmer, Infusion Fluid, Thermal	General

C.G. LABORATORIES, INC.   817-279-1945
1410 Southtown Dr., Granbury, TX 76048
FDA Number: 1649664
Ownership: Private
Produces/Sells CE-marked Devices: N

Bandage, Elastic	General
Dressing, Wound and Burn, Hydrogel	Surgery
Support, Arm	Physical Med

C.J.T. ENTERPRISES, INC.   714-751-6295
PO Box 10028, Costa Mesa, CA 92627
FDA Number: n/a   *Fax:* 714-751-5775
E-mail: yescjt@prodigy.net
Web site: www.cjt-yes.com
Medical Products Sales Volume: $300,000
Annual Revenue: $0-$1 Million
Year Founded: 1991
Total Employees: 5   *Sales Staff:* 3
Ownership: Private
Produces/Sells CE-marked Devices: Y
Federal Procurement Eligibility: Small Business, Female Owned
Distribution: Manufacturer Direct, Manufacturer Through Distributor

Accessories, Walker	General
Accessories, Wheelchair	Physical Med
Cart, Other	General
Mount, Equipment	General

C.M.S. INDUSTRIES LTD.   800-668-8821
1320 Alberta Ave., Saskatoon, SK S7K 1 Canada   306-955-8821
FDA Number: 9615398   *Fax:* 306-955-3090
E-mail: sales@redimedic.com
Web site: www.redimedic.com
Year Founded: 1986
Total Employees: 12
Ownership: Private
Produces/Sells CE-marked Devices: N
Distribution: Manufacturer Through Distributor

C.O.R.E. TECH, INC.   574-267-5744
542 E. 200 N., Warsaw, IN 46582
FDA Number: 1833679   *Fax:* 574-267-5856
E-mail: rreynolds@coretech-inc.com
Web site: www.coretech-inc.com
Year Founded: 1985
Total Employees: 26   *Sales Staff:* 1
Ownership: Private
Produces/Sells CE-marked Devices: N
Federal Procurement Eligibility: Small Business, Female Owned
Distribution: Manufacturer Direct
General Admin.: Maria Peacock/Chief Executive Officer

Implant, Fixation Device, Condylar Plate	Orthopedics
Orthopedic Implant Material	Orthopedics

C/S GROUP
See Construction Specialties Inc.

C3 INTERNATIONAL
See Cartwright Consulting Co.

CA PLUS ADHESIVES, INC.   803-772-4138
701 Kingsbridge Road, Columbia, SC 29210
FDA Number: n/a   *Fax:* 803-753-0024
E-mail: CustomerService@CA-PLUS.com
Web site: www.CA-PLUS.com
Medical Products Sales Volume: $1,400,000
Annual Revenue: $0-$1 Million
Year Founded: 1972
Total Employees: 4   *Marketing Staff:* 1   *Sales Staff:* 2
Ownership: Private
Produces/Sells CE-marked Devices: N
Federal Procurement Eligibility: Small Business
Distribution: Manufacturer Direct, Manufacturer Through Distributor, Manufacturer Through Manufacturer Reps, Importer, Exporter
General Admin.: Mr. William Burgi/Chief Executive Officer
     Mr. David Bushman/General Manager

Adhesive, Liquid	General

CABLESTRAND CORP.   562-595-4527
2660 Signal Pkwy., Signal Hill, CA 90755
FDA Number: 2083936

Wire, Orthodontic	Dental And Oral

MANUFACTURER PROFILES

CABOT SAFETY CORP., AO SAFETY PRODUCTS
See Aearo Company

CADCO DENTAL PRODUCTS
800-833-8267
600 E. Hueneme Rd., Oxnard, CA 93033-8634 **805-488-1122**
FDA Number: n/a *Fax:* 805-488-2266
E-mail: tkarst@duxdental.com
Web site: www.cadcodental.com
Annual Revenue: $5-$10 Million
Ownership: Van R Dental Products, Inc.
Produces/Sells CE-marked Devices: Y
Federal Procurement Eligibility: Small Business
Distribution: Manufacturer Through Distributor, Manufacturer Through
Manufacturer Reps, Service Direct, Exclusive Distributor, Importer
General Admin.: Paul Porteas/President
Frank Rovelli/Vice President, General Manager
Mktg./Adv.: Bob Zettler/Vice President Sales
Production: Frank Rovelli/Vice President Operations
Research: Paul Wittrock/Vice President Research & Development

Agent, Polishing, Abrasive, Oral Cavity	Dental And Oral
Apron, Lead, Dental	Dental And Oral
Component, Plastic	General
Illuminator, Radiographic Film	Radiology
Instrument, Diamond, Dental	Dental And Oral
Liner, Cavity, Calcium Hydroxide	Dental And Oral
Material, Impression	Dental And Oral
Mirror, Mouth	Dental And Oral
Mixer, Alginate	Dental And Oral
Mixing Slab	Dental And Oral
Needle, Dental	Dental And Oral
Occluder, Umbilical	General
Packaging, Sterilization	General
Primer, Cavity, Resin	Dental And Oral
Sealant, Pit And Fissure, And Conditioner, Resin	Dental And Oral
Service, Engineering/Design	General
Syringe, Restorative And Impression Material	Dental And Oral
Test, Equipment, Sterilization	General
Tray, Custom/Special Procedure	General
Tray, Impression	Dental And Oral
Tray, Surgical Instrument	Surgery
Varnish	Dental And Oral
Washer/Sterilizer	General
Zinc Oxide Eugenol	Dental And Oral

CADDY CORPORATION
856-467-4222
509 Sharptown Road, Bridgeport, NJ 08014-0345
FDA Number: n/a *Fax:* 856-467-5511
E-mail: tcarter@caddycorp.com
Web site: www.caddycorp.com
Medical Products Sales Volume: $7,500,000
Annual Revenue: $5-$10 Million
Year Founded: 1945
Total Employees: 52 *Marketing Staff:* 1 *Sales Staff:* 78
Ownership: Private
Federal Procurement Eligibility: Small Business, GSA Contract
Distribution: Manufacturer Through Distributor, Manufacturer Through
Manufacturer Reps, Exporter
Mktg./Adv.: James T. Krier/Vice President Marketing & Sales

Compactor, Fixed	General
Conveyor, Tray	General
Foodservice Product/Equipment	General
Ventilator, Other	Anesthesiology

CADENCE SCIENCE INC.
888-717-7677
516-248-0300
1979 Marcus Ave, Suite 215,
Lake Success, NY 11042
FDA Number: 1213649 *Fax:* 516-747-1188
E-mail: sales@cadencescience.com
Web site: http://www.cadencescience.com
Medical Products Sales Volume: $10,800,000
Year Founded: 1922
Total Employees: 27
Ownership: Private
Quality System Registration Information: ISO9001
Produces/Sells CE-marked Devices: Y
Federal Procurement Eligibility: Small Business
Distribution: Manufacturer Direct, Manufacturer Through Manufacturer Reps, OEM,
Exporter
General Admin.: Joseph A. Popper/President
Mktg./Adv.: Zev Asch/Vice President Marketing & Sales
Production: Vin Altruda/Vice President Manufacturing & Development
Ira L. Zuckerman/Vice President Operations

Accessories, Chromatography (Gas, Gel, Liquid, Thin Layer)	Chemistry
Adapter, Anesthesia	Anesthesiology
Adapter, Catheter	Surgery
Adapter, Stopcock, Manifold, Cardiopulmonary Bypass	Cardiovascular
Adapter, Syringe	General
Cannula, Arterial	Cardiovascular
Cannula, Aspirating	Cardiovascular

CADENCE SCIENCE INC.
888-717-7677 *(cont'd)*

Cannula, Brain	Cns/Neurology
Cannula, Catheter	Cardiovascular
Cannula, Epidural	Obstetrics/Gynecology
Cannula, Injection	Gastroenterology/Urology
Cannula, Lacrimal (Eye)	Ophthalmology
Cannula, Other	General
Cannula, Surgical, General & Plastic Surgery	Surgery
Cap, Tip, Syringe	General
Component, Metal, Other	General
Connector, Catheter	Surgery
Contract Manufacturing	General
Coverslip, Microscope Slide	Pathology
Dispenser, Fluid	General
Euthyscope, AC-Powered	Ophthalmology
Fitting, Luer	General
Immunodiffusion Equipment (Agar Cutter)	Chemistry
Injector, Syringe	General
Introducer, Syringe Needle	General
Manifold, Liquid	Chemistry
Microtiter Diluting/Dispensing Device	Microbiology
Needle, Angiographic	Cns/Neurology
Needle, Biopsy, Cardiovascular	Cardiovascular
Needle, Blood Collection	General
Needle, Blunt	General
Needle, Bone Marrow	Surgery
Needle, Cardiac	Cardiovascular
Needle, Catheter	Surgery
Needle, Cholangiography	Cardiovascular
Needle, Conduction, Anesthesia (W/Wo Introducer)	Anesthesiology
Needle, Fistula	Gastroenterology/Urology
Needle, Hypodermic	General
Needle, Intra-Arterial	Cardiovascular
Needle, Intravenous	General
Needle, Ophthalmic	Ophthalmology
Needle, Radiographic	Radiology
Needle, Spinal, Short-Term	General
Pipetter	Hematology
Stopcock	General
Stylet, Needle	General
Syringe, Anesthesia	Anesthesiology
Syringe, Angiographic	Cns/Neurology
Syringe, Bulb	General
Syringe, Catheter	General
Syringe, Drug, Luer-Lock	Dental And Oral
Syringe, Ear	Ear/Nose/Throat
Syringe, Hypodermic	General
Syringe, Insulin	General
Syringe, Irrigating, Dental	Dental And Oral
Syringe, Laboratory	Chemistry
Syringe, Tuberculin	General
Tissue Culture Apparatus	Microbiology
Trocar, Laryngeal	Ear/Nose/Throat
Trocar, Other	General

CADENT, INC.
201-842-0800
640 Gotham Pkwy., Carlstadt, NJ 07072-2405
FDA Number: 3003664745 *Fax:* 201-842-0850
E-mail: info@cadent.biz
Ownership: Private
Produces/Sells CE-marked Devices: N

Bracket, Metal, Orthodontic	Dental And Oral
Bracket, Plastic, Orthodontic	Dental And Oral
Operative Dental Treatment Unit	Dental And Oral

CADEX ELECTRONICS INC.
800-565-5228
604-231-7777
22000 Fraserwood Way,
Richmond, BC V6W-1 Canada
FDA Number: 3003800159 *Fax:* 604-231-7755
E-mail: info@cadex.com
Web site: www.cadex.com
Medical Products Sales Volume: $4,000,000
Total Employees: 50 *Marketing Staff:* 6 *Sales Staff:* 6
Ownership: Private
Quality System Registration Information: ISO9001
Produces/Sells CE-marked Devices: Y
Distribution: Manufacturer Through Distributor, Manufacturer Through
Manufacturer Reps, OEM, Exporter

CADMET, INC.
800-543-7282
610- 640-1234
155 Planebrook Road, P.O. Box 24,
Malvern, PA 19355
FDA Number: n/a *Fax:* 610-695-0290
Web site: www.cadmet.com
Annual Revenue: $0-$1 Million
Year Founded: 1987
Ownership: Private
Produces/Sells CE-marked Devices: N
Federal Procurement Eligibility: Small Business
Distribution: Exclusive Distributor

CADMET, INC. 800-543-7282 (cont'd)

General Admin.: James M. Cadmus/President

Component, Optical	General
Electrode, Other	General
Monitor, Video, Endoscope	General
Printer, Image, Video	General

CADWELL LABORATORIES 800-245-3001
909 N. Kellogg Street, 509-735-6481
Kennewick, WA 99336
FDA Number: 3020018 *Fax:* 509-783-6503
E-mail: info@cadwell.com
Web site: www.cadwell.com
Medical Products Sales Volume: $8,800,000
Annual Revenue: $10-$25 Million
Year Founded: 1979
Total Employees: 40 *Marketing Staff:* 3 *Sales Staff:* 16
Ownership: Private
Produces/Sells CE-marked Devices: Y
Federal Procurement Eligibility: Small Business
Distribution: Manufacturer Direct, Manufacturer Through Distributor, Manufacturer Through Manufacturer Reps, OEM, Service Direct, Exclusive Distributor, Exporter
General Admin.: C. M. Cadwell/President, Chief Executive Officer
Cathy Alton/Vice President Human Resources
Mktg./Adv.: Lori Kaufman/Director Marketing
John Cadwell/Director Product Development
Virginia Kellogg/Manager Contract Sales
Carlton Cadwell/Manager International & National Sales
Production: John Cadwell/Director Quality Assurance
Chris Bolken/Manager Regulatory Affairs
Richard Webber/Vice President Manufacturing & Materials
Research: John Cadwell/Vice President Research & Development

Device, Measurement, Velocity, Conduction, Nerve	Cns/Neurology
Electrode, Cutaneous	Cns/Neurology
Electrode, Needle	Cns/Neurology
Electroencephalograph	Cns/Neurology
Electromyograph, Diagnostic	Physical Med
Evoked Response Unit	Cns/Neurology
Gel, Electrode, Stimulator	Cns/Neurology
Monitor, ECG, Ambulatory, Real-Time	Cardiovascular
Monitor, EEG	Cns/Neurology
Monitor, EMG	Anesthesiology
Photostimulator, AC-Powered	Ophthalmology
Recorder, Long-Term, EEG	Cns/Neurology
Sleep Assessment Equipment	Cns/Neurology
Stimulator, Auditory, Evoked Response	Cns/Neurology
Stimulator, Electrical, Evoked Response	Cns/Neurology
Stimulator, Nerve, AC-Powered	Anesthesiology
Stimulator, Photic, Evoked Response	Cns/Neurology
Tester, Electrode/Lead, Electroencephalograph	Cns/Neurology

CAE ELECTRONICS, INC.
See Medsim-Eagle Simulation Inc.

CAE SERVICES CORP. 630-761-9898
280 Belleview Lane, Batavia, IL 60510
FDA Number: n/a *Fax:* 630-761-9391
E-mail: mark@caeservices.com
Web site: www.caeservices.com
Ownership: Private
Produces/Sells CE-marked Devices: N
General Admin.: Keith Schauer/Chief Executive Officer
Mktg./Adv.: Mark Solberg/Director Marketing

Contract R&D, Diagnostics	General

CAE-LINK CORPORATION
See Medsim-Eagle Simulation Inc.

CAFRAMO LTD. 800-567-3556
RR#2 Airport Rd., 519-534-1080
Wiarton, ONT N0H 2 Canada
FDA Number: 7000782 *Fax:* 519-534-1088
E-mail: caframo@caframo.com
Web site: www.caframo.com
Annual Revenue: $1-$5 Million
Total Employees: 30 *Marketing Staff:* 2 *Sales Staff:* 4
Ownership: Private
Produces/Sells CE-marked Devices: Y
Federal Procurement Eligibility: Small Business
Distribution: Manufacturer Through Distributor
General Admin.: Tony Solecki/President, Chief Executive Officer
Mktg./Adv.: Marta LaForest/Manager Marketing & Sales
Production: Scott Cruickshank/Manager Production

Equipment, Cleaning, Air	General
Humidifier, Heat/Moisture Exchange	Anesthesiology
Stirrer	Chemistry

CAGUAS ORTHOPEDIC CENTER, INC. 787-744-2325
Ff4, Calle 11, 4th Secc., Villa Del Rey, Caguas, PR 00625
FDA Number: 2649884

CAGUAS ORTHOPEDIC CENTER, INC. 787-744-2325 (cont'd)

Ownership: Private
Produces/Sells CE-marked Devices: N

Assembly, Shoulder/Elbow/Forearm/Wrist/Hand, Mechanical	Physical Med
Cage, Knee	Physical Med
Orthosis, Cervical	Physical Med
Orthosis, Limb Brace	Physical Med
Orthosis, Lumbosacral	Physical Med
Orthosis, Thoracic	Physical Med
Prosthesis, Thigh Socket, External Component	Physical Med

CAIG LABORATORIES, INC. 800-224-4123
12200 Thatcher Court, Poway, CA 92064-6876 858-486-8388
FDA Number: 9330020 *Fax:* 858-486-8398
E-mail: jhopp@caig.com
Web site: www.caig.com
Annual Revenue: $1-$5 Million
Year Founded: 1956
Total Employees: 14 *Marketing Staff:* 2 *Sales Staff:* 2
Ownership: Private
Stock Symbol: N/A
Produces/Sells CE-marked Devices: N
Federal Procurement Eligibility: Small Business
Distribution: Manufacturer Direct, Manufacturer Through Distributor, Manufacturer Through Manufacturer Reps, Exporter
General Admin.: Mark Lohkemper/President, Chief Executive Officer

Cleaner, Ultrasonic, Medical Instrument	General
Wipe, Instrument	General

CAIRE, INC. 800-482-2473
1800 Sandy Plains Industrial Parkway 770-425-4470
Suite 316
Marietta, GA 30066
FDA Number: 3004972304 *Fax:* 770-425-4740
E-mail: anita.conrade@chart-ind.com
Web site: www.cairemedical.com
Medical Products Sales Volume: $15,500,000
Annual Revenue: $25-$50 Million
Year Founded: 1993
Total Employees: 200 *Marketing Staff:* 1
Ownership: Chart Industries, Inc.
Quality System Registration Information: ISO9001
Produces/Sells CE-marked Devices: Y
Federal Procurement Eligibility: Small Business
Distribution: Manufacturer Through Manufacturer Reps, Service Direct
General Admin.: Steve Shaw/President
Production: Pat Burke/Product Manager

Canister, Liquid Oxygen, Portable	Anesthesiology
Container, Liquid Oxygen	Anesthesiology

CAIRE, INC. 770-479-6531
2000 Airport Industrial Dr., Ball Ground, GA 30107
FDA Number: 3004822415
Ownership: Private
Produces/Sells CE-marked Devices: N

CAL BIONICS, INC. 415-892-1892
1777 Indian Valley Rd., Novato, CA 94947-4223
FDA Number: n/a *Fax:* 415-892-1740
E-mail: thjcbi@worldnet.att.net
Annual Revenue: $0-$1 Million
Total Employees: 5 *Marketing Staff:* 2 *Sales Staff:* 2
Ownership: Private
Produces/Sells CE-marked Devices: Y
Federal Procurement Eligibility: Small Business
Distribution: Manufacturer Direct, Exporter
General Admin.: Harbo P. Jensen/President
Tyna D. Jensen/Vice President

Component, Plastic	General
Lens, Contact, Tinted	Ophthalmology

CAL HUSH LLC 505-763-0770
108 Calle De Oro, Clovis, NM 88101
FDA Number: 1066000
Ownership: Private
Produces/Sells CE-marked Devices: N

Toothbrush, Manual	Dental And Oral

CAL-U MEDICAL MANUFACTURING, INC.
See Galaxy Medical Manufacturing Co.

CALA DIAGNOSTICS
See More Diagnostics, Inc.

CALBIOTECH, INC. 866-calbiotech
10461 Austin Dr., #g, Spring Valley, CA 91978 619-660-6162
FDA Number: 2090110 *Fax:* 619-660-6970
E-mail: info@calbiotech.com
Web site: www.calbiotech.com

CALBIOTECH, INC.
866-calbiotech *(cont'd)*

Ownership: Private
Produces/Sells CE-marked Devices: N

Antigen, Enzyme Linked Immunoabsorbent Assay, Cryptococcus	Microbiology
Antigen, Salmonella SPP.	Microbiology
Enzymatic (U.V.), Pyruvic Acid	Chemistry
Enzyme Linked Immunoabsorbent Assay, Mumps Virus	Microbiology
Enzyme Linked Immunoabsorbent Assay, Mycoplasma SPP.	Microbiology
Enzyme Linked Immunoabsorbent Assay, Rubeola	Microbiology
Radioassay, Triiodothyronine Uptake	Chemistry
Radioimmunoassay, Dehydroepiandrosterone (Free And Sulfate)	Chemistry
Radioimmunoassay, Estradiol	Chemistry
Radioimmunoassay, Estriol	Chemistry
Radioimmunoassay, Estrone	Chemistry
Radioimmunoassay, Follicle Stimulating Hormone	Chemistry
Radioimmunoassay, Human Growth Hormone	Chemistry
Radioimmunoassay, Luteinizing Hormone	Chemistry
Radioimmunoassay, Progesterone	Chemistry
Radioimmunoassay, Prolactin (Lactogen)	Chemistry
Radioimmunoassay, Total Triiodothyronine	Chemistry
Reagent, General Purpose	Pathology
Reagents, Specific, Analyte	Hematology
Strip, HAMA IGG, ELISA, In Vitro Test System	Immunology

CALCITEK, INC.
See Zimmer Dental, Inc.

CALDERA MEDICAL INC.
866-422-5337
5171 Clareton Drive, Agoura Hills, CA 91301 818-879-6555

FDA Number: 3003990090 *Fax:* 818.879.6556
Web site: http://www.calderamedical.com
Year Founded: 2002
Ownership: Private
Produces/Sells CE-marked Devices: N
Mktg./Adv.: Mr. Perry Needham/Senior Vice President International Sales
Ms. Dov Tamler/Vice President Business Development

Mesh, Surgical, Polymeric	Surgery

CALDON BIOSCIENCE, INC.
877-CALDON1
2100 South Reservoir St., Pomona, CA 91766 909-628-9944

FDA Number: 3004169036 *Fax:* 909-465-1616
E-mail: info@caldonbioscience.com
Web site: www.caldonbioscience.com
Ownership: Private
Produces/Sells CE-marked Devices: N

Colorimetric Method, Triglycerides	Chemistry
Complexone, Cresolphthalein, Calcium	Chemistry
Dye-Binding, Albumin, Bromcresol, Green	Chemistry
Enzymatic Esterase-Oxidase, Cholesterol	Chemistry
Hexokinase, Glucose	Chemistry
Kinetic Method, Gamma-Glutamyl Transpeptidase	Chemistry
LDL & VLDL Precipitation, Cholesterol Via Esterase-Oxidase	Chemistry
NAD Reduction/NADH Oxidation, CPK Or Isoenzymes	Chemistry
NAD Reduction/NADH Oxidation, Lactate Dehydrogenase	Chemistry
NADH Oxidation/NAD Reduction, AST/SGOT	Chemistry
Nitrophenylphosphate, Alkaline Phosphatase Or Isoenzymes	Chemistry
Phosphorus Reagent (Test System)	Chemistry
Photometric Method, Iron (Non-Heme)	Chemistry
Photometric Method, Magnesium	Chemistry
Reagent, Bilirubin (Total Or Direct Test System)	Chemistry
Reagent, Creatinine (Test System)	Chemistry
Reagent, Protein, Total	Chemistry
SGPT, Ultraviolet	Chemistry
Saccharogenic, Amylase	Chemistry
Urease And Glutamic Dehydrogenase, Urea Nitrogen	Chemistry
Uricase (Colorimetric), Uric Acid	Chemistry

CALDWELL, JUSTISS & CO., INC.
800-643-4343
622 W. Sycamore, Fayetteville, AR 72702 479-442-7553

FDA Number: n/a *Fax:* 479-442-9102
Annual Revenue: $0-$1 Million
Total Employees: 4
Ownership: Private
Produces/Sells CE-marked Devices: N
Federal Procurement Eligibility: Small Business
Distribution: Manufacturer Direct, Manufacturer Through Distributor
General Admin.: Charles W. Caldwell/President

Device, Measurement, Potential, Skin	Cns/Neurology

CALDYNE, INC.
215-830-3076
2425 Maryland Road, Willow Grove, PA 19090

FDA Number: 3005351302 *Fax:* 215.830.8761
E-mail: mjh@caldyne-inc.com
Web site: www.caldyne-inc.com
Ownership: Private
Produces/Sells CE-marked Devices: N

Calibrator, Gas, Volume	Anesthesiology

CALEDON LABORATORIES LTD.
877-225-3366
40 Armstrong Ave., 905-877-0101
Georgetown, ONT L7G 4 Canada

FDA Number: n/a *Fax:* 905-877-6666
E-mail: service@caledonlabs.com
Web site: www.caledonlabs.com
Total Employees: 30 *Marketing Staff:* 2 *Sales Staff:* 10
Ownership: Private
Quality System Registration Information: ISO9002
Produces/Sells CE-marked Devices: N
Distribution: Manufacturer Direct

CALIBRA MEDICAL INC.
650-298-4710
220 saginaw drive, Redwood City, CA 94063

FDA Number: 3008272700
E-mail: abasu@calibra.com
Web site: http://www.myfinesse.com/
Ownership: Private
Produces/Sells CE-marked Devices: N
Mktg./Adv.: Mr. Abu Basu/Vice President Marketing
Finance: Mr. William Albright/Chief Financial Officer

Pump, Infusion	General

CALIBUR DENTAL TECHNOLOGIES, INC.
905-833-5122
2189 King Rd, Po Box 520, King City L7B 1A7 Canada

FDA Number: 9615333

Burr, Dental	Dental And Oral

CALIFORNIA LATEX, INC.
See California Medical Innovations

CALIFORNIA MEDICAL ELECTRONICS
707-456-0990
2325 Perch Drive, Willits, CA 95490

FDA Number: 2938172 *Fax:* 707-456-0660
E-mail: Calmedical@saber.net
Annual Revenue: $0-$1 Million
Year Founded: 1972
Ownership: Private
Produces/Sells CE-marked Devices: N
Distribution: Service Direct

Service, Maintenance/Repair	General
Shield, X-Ray, Lead-Plastic	Radiology

CALIFORNIA MEDICAL INNOVATIONS
800-229-5871
873 E. Arrow Highway, Pomona, CA 91767 909-621-5871

FDA Number: n/a *Fax:* 909-621-3911
E-mail: pcoye@cal-med-innovations.com
Web site: www.cal-med-innovations.com
Medical Products Sales Volume: $1,300,000
Annual Revenue: $5-$10 Million
Year Founded: 1986
Total Employees: 17 *Marketing Staff:* 1 *Sales Staff:* 2
Ownership: Private
Produces/Sells CE-marked Devices: N
Federal Procurement Eligibility: Small Business, VA Contract
Distribution: Manufacturer Direct, OEM
General Admin.: Peter L. Coye/President, Chief Executive Officer
Amabel Francisco/Vice President Human Resources
Mktg./Adv.: Yousof Nathie/Director Product Development
Production: Lizbeth Santana/Director Quality Assurance
Carlos Granados/Vice President Manufacturing

Bag, Leg	Gastroenterology/Urology
Catheter, Balloon (Foley Type)	Surgery
Component, Rubber	General
Contract Manufacturing, Product, Disposable	General
Device, Incontinence, Fecal	Gastroenterology/Urology

CALIFORNIA MEDICAL LABORATORIES, INC.
714-556-7365
1570 Sunland Lane, Costa Mesa, CA 92646

FDA Number: 2028837 *Fax:* 714-556-7997
E-mail: cml@calmedlab.com
Web site: www.calmedlab.com
Medical Products Sales Volume: $2,100,000
Annual Revenue: $1-$5 Million
Year Founded: 1993
Total Employees: 22 *Marketing Staff:* 1 *Sales Staff:* 2
Ownership: Private
Quality System Registration Information: ISO9001
Produces/Sells CE-marked Devices: Y
Federal Procurement Eligibility: Small Business, Minority Owned
Distribution: Manufacturer Direct, Manufacturer Through Distributor, Manufacturer Through Manufacturer Reps, Exclusive Distributor, Exporter
General Admin.: Mr. Mehmet Bicakci/President
Production: Mr. Michael Webb/General Manager Operations

Catheter, Vascular, Cardiopulmonary Bypass	Cardiovascular
Drain, Thoracic (Chest)	Anesthesiology
Sucker, Cardiotomy Return, Cardiopulmonary Bypass	Cardiovascular

Medical Product Subsidiaries (Listed Separately)

2013 MEDICAL DEVICE REGISTER

CALIFORNIA MEDICAL LABORATORIES, INC.   714-556-7365
(cont'd)
   Burak Healthcare

CALIFORNIA MOUNTAIN CO. LTD.
   See Cmc Rescue, Inc.

CALIFORNIA SCIENTIFIC   800-284-8112
   4005 Seaport, West Sacramento, CA 95691   916-372-6800
   FDA Number: n/a   *Fax:* 530-478-9041
   E-mail: sales@calsci.com
   Web site: www.calsci.com
   Medical Products Sales Volume: $1,000,000
   Year Founded: 1985
   Total Employees: 3   *Marketing Staff:* 1   *Sales Staff:* 2
   Ownership: Private
   Produces/Sells CE-marked Devices: N
   Federal Procurement Eligibility: Small Business
   Distribution: Manufacturer Direct
   General Admin.: Alison Augustson/General Manager
     Mark Lawrence/President, Chief Executive Officer
   Mktg./Adv.: Alison Augustson/Director Marketing & Sales
   Computer Software   General

CALIFORNIA TECHNICS LTD.
   See Engler Engineering Corp.

CALIGOR   800-472-4346
   846 Pelham Pkwy., Pelham Manor, NY 10803
   FDA Number: n/a
   E-mail: custserv@henryschein.com
   Web site: www.henryschein.com
   Medical Products Sales Volume: $900,000,000
   Year Founded: 2000
   Total Employees: 36   *Marketing Staff:* 10   *Sales Staff:* 300
   Ownership: American Greetings
   Quality System Registration Information: ISO9003
   Produces/Sells CE-marked Devices: Y
   Federal Procurement Eligibility: Small Business
   Distribution: Exclusive Distributor
   General Admin.: Stan Bergman/Chief Executive Officer
     Michael Racioppi/President
     Art Moran/Vice President
     Brad Connett/Vice President
   Mktg./Adv.: Mary-Anne Disimile/Director Marketing
   Finance: Gary Butler/Treasurer
   Equipment, Laboratory, Gen. Purpose (Specific Medical Use)   Chemistry
   Kit, Emergency Drug   General
   Kit, First Aid   Surgery
   Ventilator, Emergency, Manual (Resuscitator)   Anesthesiology

CALIPER LIFE SCIENCES, INC.   508-435-9500
   68 Elm Street, Hopkinton, MA 01748
   FDA Number: n/a   *Fax:* 508-435-3439
   Web site: www.caliperls.com
   Total Employees: 550
   Ownership: Public
   Stock Symbol: CALP
   Traded On: NASDAQ
   Produces/Sells CE-marked Devices: N
   General Admin.: David M. Manyak/Executive Vice President
     Kevin Hrusovsky/President, Chief Executive Officer
     Peter F. McAree/Senior Vice President
     Paula J. Cassidy/Vice President, Vice President Human
   Resources
   Production: Bruce J. Bal/Senior Vice President Operations
   System, Imaging, Fluorescence   Ear/Nose/Throat

CALIPER SYSTEMS, INC.   781-687-9222
   23 Crosby Drive, Bedford, MA 01730
   FDA Number: 3003827268   *Fax:* 781-687-8881
   E-mail: bmillett@calipersystems.com
   Web site: www.calipersystems.com
   Annual Revenue: $0-$1 Million
   Year Founded: 2002
   Total Employees: 6
   Ownership: Private
   Stock Symbol: CALP
   Traded On: NASDAQ
   Produces/Sells CE-marked Devices: N
   Federal Procurement Eligibility: Small Business
   Distribution: OEM
   General Admin.: Mr. Bryan Millett/President
   LDL & VLDL Precipitation, HDL   Chemistry

CALL LIGHT COMMUNICATIONS
   See Pioneer Medical Systems

CALLCARE   800-345-9414
   1370 Arcadia Road, Lancaster, PA 17601   717-393-9653
   FDA Number: n/a   *Fax:* 717-393-0646
   E-mail: callcare@callcareonline.com
   Web site: www.callcareonline.com
   Medical Products Sales Volume: $6,800,000
   Year Founded: 1989
   Total Employees: 45   *Marketing Staff:* 3   *Sales Staff:* 4
   Federal Procurement Eligibility: Small Business
   General Admin.: Carol J. Hammond/Manager
     John D. Hessen/President
   Mktg./Adv.: Lloyd D. Miller/Director National Accounts
     Edward J. Hockenberry/Vice President Marketing
   Production: Caroline Eshelman/Manager Materials
   Cable   Physical Med
   Communication System, Room Status   General
   Light, Other   General
   Nurse Call System   General
   Security Equipment/Supplies   General

CALMAQUIP ENGINEERING CORP.   305-592-4510
   7240 N.W. 12th St., Miami, FL 33126-1909
   FDA Number: n/a   *Fax:* 305-593-9618
   E-mail: mhidalgo@calmaquip.com
   Web site: www.calmaquip.com
   Year Founded: 1959
   Ownership: Calmaquip Engineering Corp
   Produces/Sells CE-marked Devices: N
   Federal Procurement Eligibility: Small Business, Minority Owned
   Distribution: Exporter
   General Admin.: Raul J Gutierrez/President, Chief Executive Officer
     Sara Davalos/Director Medical Div.
   Mktg./Adv.: Patricia Cabarcos/Director Marketing
     Manuel J. Hidalgo/Medical Equipment Specialist
   Finance: Angel Rodriguez/Vice President Finance
   Ambulance   General
   Bed, Birthing   General
   Bed, Electric   General
   Bed, Manual   General
   Endoscope, Electronic (Videoendoscope)   Surgery
   Equipment, Laboratory, Gen. Purpose (Specific Medical Use)   Chemistry
   Facility, Equipment, Medical, Mobile   General
   Furniture, Patient Room   General
   Gas-Machine, Anesthesia   Anesthesiology
   General Medical Device   General
   Monitor, Cardiac (Cardiotachometer & Rate Alarm)   Cardiovascular
   Radiographic Unit, Diagnostic   Radiology
   Scanner, Computed Tomography, X-Ray, Full Body   Radiology
   Service, Architectural   General
   Service, Consulting   General
   Service, Import/Export   General
   Stretcher, Transfer   Surgery
   Table, Surgical, Electrical   Surgery

CALMAR ORTHOPAEDICS   1.888.879.9330
   760 Birchmount Rd., Unit 33,   416-757-6296
   Scarborough, ONT M1K-5 Canada
   FDA Number: n/a   *Fax:* 416-757-3771
   E-mail: info@calmarorthopaedics.com
   Web site: www.calmarcare.com
   Year Founded: 1988
   Total Employees: 10
   Ownership: Private
   Produces/Sells CE-marked Devices: N
   Distribution: Manufacturer Direct, Exclusive Distributor

CALMIA MEDICAL, INC.   416-441-9009
   7-15 Lesmill Rd, Toronto M3B 2T3 Canada
   FDA Number: 9615297
   Pessary, Vaginal   Obstetrics/Gynecology

CALMOSEPTINE, INC.   800-800-3405
   16602 Burke Lane,   714-840-3405
   Huntington Beach, CA 92647
   FDA Number: n/a   *Fax:* 714-840-9810
   E-mail: info@calmoseptineointment.com
   Web site: www.calmoseptineointment.com
   Ownership: Private
   Produces/Sells CE-marked Devices: N
   Federal Procurement Eligibility: Small Business
   Distribution: Manufacturer Through Distributor, Manufacturer Through
   Manufacturer Reps
   General Admin.: Gregory Dixon/Chief Executive Officer
   Lotion, Skin Care   General
   Pad, Incontinence (Underpad)   General

CALPAC
   See Regency Product International

CALTECH INDUSTRIES, INC.
800-234-7700
2420 Schuette Drive, Midland, MI 48642-5974
989-496-3110
FDA Number: n/a
Fax: 989-496-0811
E-mail: info@caltechind.com
Web site: www.caltechind.com
Medical Products Sales Volume: $5,000,000
Annual Revenue: $1-$5 Million
Total Employees: 20   *Marketing Staff:* 2   *Sales Staff:* 16
Ownership: Private
Produces/Sells CE-marked Devices: N
Federal Procurement Eligibility: Small Business, Female Owned
Distribution: Manufacturer Through Distributor
General Admin.: C. G. Anders/Chief Executive Officer
     Sue Hohlbein/Vice President Human Resources
Mktg./Adv.: Curt Goeders/Director National Accounts
     Phil Donatelli/Director Product Development
     Curt Goeders/Director Sales
     Jessica Dub/Manager Marketing & Communications
Production: Phil Donatelli/Director Quality Assurance
     Cathy Anders/Manager Regulatory Affairs

Decontamination Kit	Surgery
Disinfector, Liquid	General
Towel/Towelette, Paper	General

CALUMET COACH COMPANY
See Oshkosh Specialty Vehicles

CALUTECH CORPORATION
6615 W. 111th St., Worth, IL 60482
FDA Number: 3004464240
Ownership: Private
Produces/Sells CE-marked Devices: N

Purifier, Air, Ultraviolet	General

CALYPSO MEDICAL TECHNOLOGIES INC
206-254-0600
2101 Fourth Ave, Suite 500, Seattle, WA 98121
FDA Number: 3004837948
Fax: 206-254-0606
Web site: http://calypsomedical.com
Year Founded: 2000
Ownership: Private
Produces/Sells CE-marked Devices: N
General Admin.: Mr. Alfred Merriweather/Chief Financial Officer, Executive Vice President
     Mr. J. Nelson Wright/Chief Technology Officer
     Dr. Ed Vertatschitsch/President, Chief Executive Officer
Mktg./Adv.: Ms. Lorraine Wright/Director Marketing
     Mr. Mark Querry/Vice President Commercial Operations
Production: Ms. Marcia Page/Vice President Quality Assurance & Regulatory Affairs

Accelerator, Linear, Medical	Radiology

CALYPTE BIOMEDICAL CORPORATION
877-CALYPTE
16290 SW Upper Boones Ferry Road,
503-726-2227
Portland, OR 97224
FDA Number: 2955343
Fax: 503-601-6299
E-mail: customerservice@calypte.com
Web site: www.calypte.com
Annual Revenue: $1-$5 Million
Year Founded: 1988
Ownership: Public
Stock Symbol: CALY
Traded On: OTC Bulletin
Quality System Registration Information: ISO9001
Produces/Sells CE-marked Devices: N
Distribution: Manufacturer Through Distributor
General Admin.: Adel Karas/President, Chief Executive Officer, Chief Financial Officer

Equipment, Test, Western Blot	Microbiology
Test, Antibody, Acquired Immune Deficiency Syndrome (AIDS)	Hematology

CALZYME LABORATORIES, INC.
800-523-9127
3443 Miguelito Court,
805-541-5754
San Luis Obispo, CA 93401
FDA Number: n/a
Fax: 805-541-8310
Web site: www.calzyme.com
Medical Products Sales Volume: $1,750,000
Ownership: Private
Produces/Sells CE-marked Devices: N
Federal Procurement Eligibility: Minority Owned, Female Owned
Distribution: Manufacturer Direct, Service Direct, Exporter

Enzyme Immunoassay, Other	Chemistry

CAMAG SCIENTIFIC, INC.
800-334-3909
515 Cornelius Harnett Dr.,
910-343-1833
Wilmington, NC 28401
FDA Number: n/a
Fax: 910-343-1834
E-mail: tlc@camagusa.com
Web site: www.camag.com/usa

CAMAG SCIENTIFIC, INC.
800-334-3909 *(cont'd)*
Annual Revenue: $0-$1 Million
Year Founded: 1980
Total Employees: 6   *Marketing Staff:* 1   *Sales Staff:* 1
Ownership: Private
Quality System Registration Information: ISO9001
Produces/Sells CE-marked Devices: N
Federal Procurement Eligibility: Small Business
Distribution: Exclusive Distributor
General Admin.: Roger James/General Manager
     Dieter Jaenchen/President

Accessories, Chromatography (Gas, Gel, Liquid, Thin Layer)	Chemistry
Cabinet, Chromatography (U.V.) Viewing	Chemistry
Chromatography Equipment, Thin Layer	Toxicology
Densitometer, Laboratory	Chemistry
Electrophoresis Equipment, Cellulose Acetate Membrane	Chemistry
Scanner, Ultraviolet	Chemistry
Sprayer, Thin Layer Chromatography	Chemistry
Transilluminator, Laboratory	Chemistry

CAMBRIDGE CHEMICAL PRODUCTS
See Cambridge Diagnostic Products, Inc.

CAMBRIDGE DIAGNOSTIC PRODUCTS, INC.
800-525-6262
6880 N.W. 17th Avenue,
954-971-4040
Fort Lauderdale, FL 33309
FDA Number: 1029182
Fax: 954-975-5609
E-mail: techinfo@ecamco.com
Web site: www.ecamco.com
Medical Products Sales Volume: $1,100,000
Year Founded: 1953
Total Employees: 11   *Marketing Staff:* 4   *Sales Staff:* 3
Ownership: Private
Produces/Sells CE-marked Devices: N
Federal Procurement Eligibility: Small Business, GSA Contract
Distribution: Manufacturer Direct, Manufacturer Through Distributor, OEM, Exporter
General Admin.: Ms. Jane Walk/Administrator
     Roy & Gary Gold/Chief Executive Officer
     Roy & Gary Gold/President
Mktg./Adv.: Mr. Roy Gold/Director Marketing
     Tom Mauthner/Director Product Development
Production: Mr. Gary Gold/Director Operations
     Roy Gold/Director Quality Assurance
     Roy Gold/Manager Regulatory Affairs
Research: Tom Mauthner/Vice President Research & Development

Counter, Platelet, Manual	Hematology
Enzymatic Method, Blood, Occcult, Fecal	Chemistry
Enzymatic Method, Blood, Occult, Urinary	Chemistry
Fixative, Alcohol Containing	Pathology
Reagent, Guaiac	Hematology
Reagent, Occult Blood	Hematology
Soap	General
Solution, Instrument Cleaner	General
Stain, Giemsa, Hematology	Hematology
Stain, Wright's	Pathology
Stain, Wright's, Hematology	Hematology

CAMBRIDGE FILTER CORP
See Camfil Farr

CAMBRIDGE HEART INC.
888-CAM-WAVE
100 Ames Pond Dr, Suite 100,
978-654-7600
Tewksbury, MA 01876
FDA Number: 1225215
Fax: 978-654-4501
E-mail: Info@CambridgeHeart.com
Web site: www.cambridgeheart.com
Ownership: Private
Produces/Sells CE-marked Devices: N
General Admin.: Mr. Roderick de Greef/Chairman
     Mr. Ali Haghighi-Mood/Chief Executive Officer
Finance: Mr. Vincenzo LiCausi/Vice President Finance

Computer, Diagnostic, Programmable	Cardiovascular
Electrode, Electrocardiograph	Cardiovascular

CAMBRIDGE HEART, INC.
888-226-9283
100 Ames Pond Drive, Suite 100,
978-654-7600
Tewksbury, MA 01876
FDA Number: 1225215
Fax: 978-654-4501
Web site: www.cambridgeheart.com
Ownership: Public
Stock Symbol: CAMH
Traded On: OTC Bulletin
Produces/Sells CE-marked Devices: N
General Admin.: Mr. Ali Haghighi-Mood/Chief Executive Officer
Finance: Mr. Vincenzo LiCausi/Chief Financial Officer, Vice President Finance

Computer, Diagnostic, Programmable	Cardiovascular
Electrocardiograph, Single Channel	Cardiovascular

CAMBRIDGE HEART, INC.   888-226-9283 (cont'd)
Electrode, Electrocardiograph   Cardiovascular

CAMBRIDGE INSTRUMENTS
See Leica Microsystems, Inc., Educational & Analytical Division

CAMBRIDGE RESEARCH &   800-383-7924
INSTRUMENTATION (CRI)

35-B Cabot Road, Woburn, MA 01801   781-935-9099
FDA Number: n/a   Fax: 781-935-3388
E-mail: sales@cri-inc.com
Web site: www.cri-inc.com
Ownership: Private
Quality System Registration Information: ISO9001
Produces/Sells CE-marked Devices: N
Distribution: Manufacturer Direct
General Admin.: Theodare Les/Chief Financial Officer, Vice President
               Peter J. Miller/Chief Scientific Officer, Vice President
               Clifford Hoyt/Chief Technology Officer, Vice President
               George A. Abe/President, Chief Executive Officer
Instrumentation For Clinical Multiplex Test Systems   Chemistry
Microscope, Fluorescence/U.V.   Pathology
System, Image Management, Ophthalmic   Ophthalmology
System, Imaging, Fluorescence   Ear/Nose/Throat

CAMBRIDGE RESEARCH LABORATORY
See Covance Research Products Inc.

CAMBRIDGE SCIENTIFIC INDUSTRIES
See Beta Technology, Inc.

CAMBRO MANUFACTURING   800-833-3003
5801 Skylab Rd., Huntington Beach, CA 92647   714-848-1555
FDA Number: n/a   Fax: 714-842-3430
E-mail: gfischer@cambro.com
Web site: www.cambro.com
Ownership: Private
Produces/Sells CE-marked Devices: N
Distribution: Manufacturer Through Manufacturer Reps
Cart, Foodservice   General
Tray, Foodservice   General

CAMDA CORP.   213-381-0888
3435 Wilshire Blvd.,#990, Los Angeles, CA 90010
FDA Number: 2031516
Ownership: Private
Produces/Sells CE-marked Devices: N
Epilator, High-Frequency, Tweezer Type   Surgery

CAMELOT SYSTEMS, INC.
See Speedline Technologies, Inc.

CAMERON HEALTH INC   877-742-3411
905 Calle Amanecer, Suite 300, San Clemente, CA 92673
FDA Number: n/a   Fax: 949-498-5932
Web site: 949-498-5932
Ownership: Private
Produces/Sells CE-marked Devices: N
General Admin.: Mr. Mitch Hill/Chief Financial Officer, Vice President
               Mr. Kevin Hykes/President, Chief Executive Officer
Mktg./Adv.: Mr. Ward Dykstra/Vice President Commercial Operations
Production: Mr. David Hackbarth/Vice President Operations
           Mr. Ryan Majkrzak/Vice President Quality Systems
           Dr. Jon Hunt/Vice President Regulatory & Clinical Affairs
Research: Mr. Todd Kerkow/Vice President Product Development

CAMERON-MILLER, INC.   800-621-0142
5410 West Roosevelt, Road #241,   773-379-2624
Chicago, IL 60644
FDA Number: 1415191   Fax: 773-379-2686
E-mail: info@cameron-miller.com
Web site: http://cameron-miller.com/
Medical Products Sales Volume: $1,700,000
Annual Revenue: $25-$50 Million
Year Founded: 1915
Total Employees: 25
Ownership: Private
Quality System Registration Information: ISO9000
Produces/Sells CE-marked Devices: N
Federal Procurement Eligibility: Small Business
Distribution: Manufacturer Through Manufacturer Reps, OEM, Exporter
Mktg./Adv.: John W. Martin/President, Director Marketing
Adapter, Electrosurgical Unit, Cable   Surgery
Adapter, Unit, Electrosurgical, Hand-Controlled Surgery
Anoscope, Non-Powered   Gastroenterology/Urology
Assay, Enzyme Linked Immunosorbent, Parvovirus B19 Igg   Microbiology
Cabinet, Table And Tray, Anesthesia   Anesthesiology
Cable, Electrosurgical Unit   Surgery
Cart, Instrument   Surgery
Coagulator, Laparoscopic, Unipolar   Obstetrics/Gynecology
Coagulator/Cutter, Endoscopic, Unipolar   Obstetrics/Gynecology

CAMERON-MILLER, INC.   800-621-0142 (cont'd)
Electrode, Electrosurgery, Laparoscopic   Surgery
Electrode, Electrosurgical, Active (Blade)   Surgery
Electrode, Electrosurgical, Active, Foot Controlled Surgery
Electrode, Electrosurgical, Return (Ground, Dispersive) Surgery
Electrode, Flexible Suction Coagulator   Gastroenterology/Urology
Electrosurgical Equipment, General Purpose   Surgery
Electrosurgical Equipment, Special Purpose   Surgery
Electrosurgical Unit, Cardiovascular   Cardiovascular
Electrosurgical Unit, Cutting & Coagulation Device Surgery
Electrosurgical Unit, Gastroenterology   Gastroenterology/Urology
Electrosurgical Unit, General Purpose (ESU)   Surgery
Endoscope, Rigid   Surgery
Examination Device, AC-Powered   General
Excavator, Dental, Operative   Dental And Oral
Forceps, Biopsy, Non-Electric   Gastroenterology/Urology
Forceps, Electrosurgical   Surgery
Headlight, ENT   Ear/Nose/Throat
Headlight, Fiberoptic Focusing   Gastroenterology/Urology
Holder, Ear Speculum   Ear/Nose/Throat
Holder, Needle, Other   Surgery
Infusion Stand   General
Instrument, Microsurgical   Cns/Neurology
Lamp, Endoscopic, Incandescent   Surgery
Lamp, Examination (Light)   General
Lift, Bath, Non-AC-Powered   General
Light Source, Endoscopic   Obstetrics/Gynecology
Light Source, Fiberoptic, Routine   Gastroenterology/Urology
Light, Headband, Surgical   Surgery
Light, Surgical Headlight   Dental And Oral
Microelectrode   General
Nasoscope   Ear/Nose/Throat
Otoscope   Ear/Nose/Throat
Papillotome   Surgery
Plate, Patient   Gastroenterology/Urology
Power Supply, Endoscopic, Line-Operated   General
Proctoscope   Surgery
Proctosigmoidoscope   Gastroenterology/Urology
Punch, Biopsy   Gastroenterology/Urology
Sigmoidoscope, Rigid, Non-Electrical   Gastroenterology/Urology
Snare, Endoscopic   Surgery
Snare, Flexible   Gastroenterology/Urology
Snare, Nasal   Ear/Nose/Throat
Snare, Other   Surgery
Snare, Polyp   Surgery
Snare, Rigid Self-Opening   Gastroenterology/Urology
Snare, Surgical   Surgery
Snare, Tonsil   Ear/Nose/Throat
Speculum, Ear   Ear/Nose/Throat
Speculum, Illuminated   Surgery
Speculum, Vaginal, Metal   Obstetrics/Gynecology
Speculum, Vaginal, Non-Metal   Obstetrics/Gynecology
Stand, Operating Room Instrument (Mayo)   Surgery
Stool, Anesthetist's   Anesthesiology
Stretcher, Wheeled (Mobile)   General
Surgical Instrument, Obstetric/Gynecologic, General Obstetrics/Gynecology
System, Evacuation, Smoke, Laser   Surgery
Tip, Suction   Anesthesiology
Tip, Suction Tube (Yankauer, Poole, Etc.)   Surgery
Tip, Suction, Electrosurgical   Surgery
Tip, Suction, Fiberoptic Illuminated   Anesthesiology
Transfer Device, Patient, Manual   General
Wristlet, Patient Return   Gastroenterology/Urology

CAMFIL FARR   800-300-3277
2121 E Paulhan Street,   310-668-6355
Rancho Dominguez, CA 90220
FDA Number: n/a   Fax: 310-609-2164
Web site: www.camfilfarr.com
Ownership: Private
Quality System Registration Information: ISO9001
Produces/Sells CE-marked Devices: Y
Federal Procurement Eligibility: Small Business
Distribution: Manufacturer Direct, Manufacturer Through Distributor, Manufacturer
Through Manufacturer Reps, OEM, Exporter
Cleanroom Equipment   General
Filter, Air   General
Filter, Bacterial, Breathing Circuit   Anesthesiology
Filter, Bacteriological, Laboratory   Chemistry
Laminar Air Flow Unit, Fixed (Air Curtain)   Chemistry

CAMP CANADA LTD.   800-267-2812
39 Davis St., P.O. Box 495,   613-392-6528
Trenton, ONT K8V-5 Canada
FDA Number: n/a   Fax: 613-392-4139
E-mail: camphealthcare@symaptico.ca
Web site: http://www.camphealthcare.com
Year Founded: 1957
Total Employees: 25
Ownership: Private

CAMP CANADA LTD.   800-267-2812 *(cont'd)*
Produces/Sells CE-marked Devices: N
Distribution: Manufacturer Direct, Exclusive Distributor

CAMSIGHT CO., INC.   323-259-1900
3380 N. San Fernando Road, Glassell, CA 90065
FDA Number: 2032365

Microscope, Surgical	Ear/Nose/Throat
System, X-ray, Extraoral Source, Digital	Radiology

CAMTEC   410-228-1156
1959 Church Creek Rd., Cambridge, MD 21613
FDA Number: 1121219

Accessories, Operating Room, Table	Surgery
Bed, Electric	General
Chair, Posture, For Cardiac And Pulmonary Treatment	Anesthesiology
Infusion Stand	General
Stool, Anesthetist's	Anesthesiology
Stretcher, Wheeled (Mobile)	General
Transfer Device, Patient, Manual	General
Wheelchair, Manual	Physical Med

CAN-DAN REHATEC LTD.   905-648-7522
3-1378 Sandhill Dr., Ancaster, ONT L9G-4V5 Canada
FDA Number: n/a   *Fax:* 905-648-7799
E-mail: info@can-dan.com
Web site: www.can-dan.com
Year Founded: 1986
Ownership: Private
Produces/Sells CE-marked Devices: N
Distribution: Manufacturer Through Distributor

CAN-MED SURGICAL SUPPLIES LIMITED   800-565-7553
7037 Mumford Rd., P.O. Box 518,   902-455-4649
Halifax, NS B3J-2 Canada
FDA Number: n/a   *Fax:* 902-455-1028
E-mail: canmed@canmedsurgical.com
Web site: www.canmedhealthcare.com
Year Founded: 1974
Total Employees: 50
Ownership: Imp Group Ltd.
Produces/Sells CE-marked Devices: N
Distribution: Service Direct

CANADA CARE MEDICAL INC.   800-267-8855
1644 Bank St., Ottawa, ONT K1V-7Y6 Canada   613-234-1222
FDA Number: n/a   *Fax:* 613-731-4135
E-mail: ottawa@canadacaremedical.com
Web site: www.canadacaremedical.com
Year Founded: 1969
Total Employees: 25
Ownership: Private
Produces/Sells CE-marked Devices: N
Distribution: Service Direct

CANADA ENDOSCOPE CORP.   800-563-2907
4-160 Konrad Cres., Unit,   905-479-2277
Markham, ONT L3R 9 Canada
FDA Number: n/a   *Fax:* 905-479-6495
E-mail: info@canadaendoscope.ca
Web site: http://www.canadaendoscope.ca/
Year Founded: 1991
Ownership: Private
Produces/Sells CE-marked Devices: N
Distribution: Manufacturer Direct, Service Direct, Exclusive Distributor

CANADA MICROSURGICAL LTD.   1-800-263-6693
311 Enterprise Drive, Plainsboro, NJ 08536   905-632-7888
FDA Number: n/a   *Fax:* 1-905-632-7938
E-mail: custsvcnj@integralife.com
Web site: www.canadamicrosurgical.ca
Year Founded: 1982
Ownership: Private
Produces/Sells CE-marked Devices: N
Distribution: Exclusive Distributor
General Admin.: Bill MacDonald/President

CANADA OPTIX, INC.   905-238-3332
5181 Bradco Blvd, Mississauga L4W 2A6 Canada
FDA Number: 9615073

Lens, Spectacle/Eyeglasses, Non-Custom	Ophthalmology

CANADAWIDE SCIENTIFIC LTD.   800-267-2362
2300 Walkley Rd., Ottawa, ONT K1G-6B1 Canada   613-736-8178
FDA Number: n/a   *Fax:* 613-736-8133
E-mail: cwsales@canadawide.ca
Web site: canadawide.ca
Ownership: Private

CANADAWIDE SCIENTIFIC LTD.   800-267-2362 *(cont'd)*
Quality System Registration Information: ISO9001
Produces/Sells CE-marked Devices: N
Distribution: Exclusive Distributor

CANADIAN HOSPITAL SPECIALTIES LTD.   800-461-1423
2810 Coventry Road,   905-825-9300
Oakville, ONT L6H 6 Canada
FDA Number: n/a   *Fax:* 905-825-9600
E-mail: chs@chsltd.com
Web site: www.chsltd.com
Ownership: Private
Produces/Sells CE-marked Devices: N
Distribution: Exclusive Distributor, Importer

CANADIAN MEDICAL BRUSH INC.   905-405-1075
7065 Fir Tree Drive, Mississauga, ONT L55 1J7 Canada
FDA Number: 9615339
Ownership: Private
Produces/Sells CE-marked Devices: N
Distribution: Manufacturer Direct, Exporter

CANADIAN MEDICAL BRUSH, INC.   905-405-1075
11-7686 Kimbel St, Mississauga L5S 1E9 Canada
FDA Number: 9615339

Kit, Smear, Cervical	Obstetrics/Gynecology
Spatula, Cervical, Cytology	Obstetrics/Gynecology

CANADIAN MEDICAL PRODUCTS, LTD.   800-267-0572
850 Tapscott Rd., Unit 21,   416-298-0572
Scarborough, ONT M1X-1 Canada
FDA Number: 8022189   *Fax:* 416-298-8990
E-mail: ccrawford@canmedprod.com
Web site: www.canmedprod.com
Year Founded: 1978
Total Employees: 10
Ownership: Private
Produces/Sells CE-marked Devices: N
Distribution: Manufacturer Direct, Exclusive Distributor, Importer

CANADIAN ORTHOTICS LABORATORY LTD.   1(877)265-2248
40 Bradwick Drive Units 12-15,   905-669-5655
Concord, ON L4K 1 Canada
FDA Number: 8020406   *Fax:* 905-669-8772
E-mail: canadianorthoticslabtry@bellnet.ca
Web site: www.canadianorthotics.com
Total Employees: 15
Ownership: Private
Produces/Sells CE-marked Devices: N
Distribution: Manufacturer Direct, Exporter

CANADIAN SCIENTIFIC PRODUCTS LTD.   800-265-3460
1055 Sarnia Rd., Unit B2,   519-473-2277
London, ONT N6H-5 Canada
FDA Number: n/a   *Fax:* 519-473-2585
E-mail: sales@cspmedical.com
Web site: www.cspmedicalstore.com
Year Founded: 1971
Ownership: Private
Produces/Sells CE-marked Devices: N
Distribution: Exclusive Distributor

CANADIAN TECHNICAL TAPE LTD.   800-334-1567
455 Cote Vertu Rd.,   514-334-1510
Montreal, QUE H4N-1 Canada
FDA Number: n/a   *Fax:* 514-745-0764
E-mail: info@cttgroup.com
Web site: www.cttgroup.com
Year Founded: 1950
Total Employees: 250
Ownership: Private
Produces/Sells CE-marked Devices: N
Distribution: Manufacturer Direct, Exporter

CANBERRA   800-255-6370
800 Research Parkway, Meriden, CT 06450   203-238-235
FDA Number: n/a   *Fax:* 203-639-2067
E-mail: techsupport@canberra.com
Web site: www.canberra.com
Annual Revenue: $1-$5 Million
Ownership: Private
Produces/Sells CE-marked Devices: N
Federal Procurement Eligibility: Small Business
Distribution: Manufacturer Direct

Counter, Radiation	Radiology
Dosimeter, Radiation	Radiology

CANBERRA   800-255-6370 (cont'd)
Monitor, Radiation   Radiology

CANBERRA CORP.   419-841-6616
3610 Holland-Sylvania Road, Toledo, OH 43615
FDA Number: n/a
E-mail: info@canberracorp.com
Web site: www.canberracorp.com
Annual Revenue: $1-$5 Million
Year Founded: 1965
Ownership: Private
Produces/Sells CE-marked Devices: N
Distribution: Manufacturer Through Distributor, OEM
  Disinfector, Liquid   General
  Solution, Antibacterial Cleaner   General

CANBERRA INDUSTRIES   800-243-3955
800 Research Pkwy., Meriden, CT 06450-3215   **203-238-2351**
FDA Number: 7000783   Fax: 203-235-1347
E-mail: customersupport@canberra.com
Web site: www.canberra.com
Medical Products Sales Volume: $43,900,000
Annual Revenue: $100-$500 Million
Year Founded: 2005
Total Employees: 365   Marketing Staff: 60   Sales Staff: 55
Ownership: AREVA Group
Quality System Registration Information: ISO9001
Produces/Sells CE-marked Devices: Y
Federal Procurement Eligibility: Small Business, GSA Contract
Distribution: Manufacturer Direct
General Admin.: Christian Petit/President, Chief Executive Officer
    Mike Charland/Vice President, General Manager
Mktg./Adv.: Hank Palasek/Director Marketing Communications
    Markku Koskelo/Vice President Marketing
    Mike Catalano/Vice President Sales
  Counter, Radiation   Radiology
  Counter, Scintillation   Chemistry
  Spectrometer, Nuclear   Chemistry

CANBERRA-PACKARD CANADA   800-387-9559
6300 Northwest Dr., Bldg. 312,   **905-673-8028**
Mississauga, ONT L4V-1 Canada
FDA Number: n/a   Fax: 905-673-8129
E-mail: sales@cpcan.ca
Web site: www.pharmindex.com
Year Founded: 1985
Total Employees: 50
Ownership: Private
Produces/Sells CE-marked Devices: N
Distribution: Service Direct, Exclusive Distributor

CANBERRA/R M C
See Rmc Medical

CANDELA CORP.   800-733-8550
530 Boston Post Rd., Wayland, MA 01778-1833   **508-358-7637**
FDA Number: 1218402   Fax: 508-358-5602
Web site: www.candelalaser.com
Medical Products Sales Volume: $30,413,000
Annual Revenue: $25-$50 Million
Year Founded: 1970
Total Employees: 195   Sales Staff: 50
Ownership: Public
Stock Symbol: CLZR
Traded On: NASDAQ
Produces/Sells CE-marked Devices: Y
Federal Procurement Eligibility: Small Business
Distribution: Manufacturer Direct, Manufacturer Through Distributor
General Admin.: Gerard Puorro/Chief Executive Officer
    F. Paul Broyer/Chief Financial Officer, Vice President
    Bunny Montgomery/Manager Human Resources
    Richard J. Olsen/Senior Vice President
    Kenji Shimizu/Vice President
Production: Jay Caplan/Vice President Operations
Research: James Hsia/Senior Vice President Research & Development
  Catheter, Percutaneous   Cardiovascular
  Endoscope   Gastroenterology/Urology
  Laser, Dye   General
  Laser, Surgical   Surgery
  Lithotriptor, Laser   Gastroenterology/Urology
  Sound, Urethral, Metal Or Plastic   Gastroenterology/Urology

CANDELA LASER CORP.
See Candela Corp.

CANDELIS, INC.   800 800 8600
18821 Bardeen Ave., Irvine, CA 92612   **1 949 852 1000**
FDA Number: 3005919188   Fax: 1 949 752-7317
E-mail: info@candelis.com

CANDELIS, INC.   800 800 8600 (cont'd)
Web site: www.candelis.com
Ownership: Private
Produces/Sells CE-marked Devices: N
  Device, Storage, Image, Digital   Radiology
  Image Processing System   Radiology

CANDENT   888-243-6065
21 2601 Matheson Blvd. East,   **905-629-7688**
Mississauga, ONT L4W-5 Canada
FDA Number: n/a   Fax: 905-629-0825
E-mail: info@candent.net
Web site: www.candent.net
Year Founded: 1971
Total Employees: 10
Ownership: Private
Produces/Sells CE-marked Devices: N
Distribution: Manufacturer Direct, Exclusive Distributor, Importer

CANDO, INC.
See Budget Buddy Company, Inc.

CANICA DESIGN INC.   800-705-8312
36 Mill Street, Almonte, ON K0A 1A0 Canada   **613-256-0350**
FDA Number: 9616525   Fax: 613-256-0360
E-mail: sales@canica.com
Web site: www.canica.com
Year Founded: 1998
Ownership: Private
Quality System Registration Information: ISO9001
Produces/Sells CE-marked Devices: N

CANIX STERILIZER INC.   905-670-8299
7085 Tomken Rd., Mississauga, ONT L5S-1R7 Canada
FDA Number: n/a   Fax: 905-670-0195
E-mail: stardish@phoenix-biomed.com
Web site: www.phoenix-biomed.com
Year Founded: 1981
Total Employees: 10
Ownership: Phoenix Biomedical Products, Inc.
Produces/Sells CE-marked Devices: N

CANNON AVENT
See Philips Avent

CANNON INSTRUMENT CO.   800-676-6232
2139 High Tech Road, State College, PA 16803   **814-353-8000**
FDA Number: 7000082   Fax: 814-353-8007
E-mail: cannon@cannon-ins.com
Web site: www.cannoninstrument.com
Annual Revenue: $5-$10 Million
Year Founded: 1938
Total Employees: 75   Marketing Staff: 2   Sales Staff: 3
Ownership: Private
Quality System Registration Information: ISO9001; ISO9002
Produces/Sells CE-marked Devices: N
Federal Procurement Eligibility: Small Business
Distribution: Manufacturer Direct
General Admin.: Patrick Maggi/President
Mktg./Adv.: Frank Saylor/Vice President Marketing
Production: Edgar S. Titlar/Customer Service Representative
Research: Kenneth Henderson/Vice President Research & Development
  Bath, Kinematic Viscosity   Chemistry
  Incubator/Water Bath, Microbiology   Microbiology
  Viscometer   Chemistry

CANNON RUBBER LTD.
See Philips Avent

CANON
See UBM Canon

CANON COMMUNICATIONS LLC
See UBM Canon

CANON DEVELOPMENT AMERICAS, INC   949-932-3100
15955 Alton Parkway, Irvine, CA 92618-3731
FDA Number: 8030410   Fax: 949-932-3510
E-mail: staffing@cda.canon.com
Web site: www.cda.canon.com/
Medical Products Sales Volume: $20,600,000
Annual Revenue: $25-$50 Million
Total Employees: 125   Marketing Staff: 4   Sales Staff: 10
Ownership: Canon, Inc.
Quality System Registration Information: ISO9000; ISO9001
Produces/Sells CE-marked Devices: N
Federal Procurement Eligibility: Small Business, GSA Contract, VA Contract
Distribution: Manufacturer Direct, Manufacturer Through Distributor
  Medical Admin.: Neo Imai/Medical Director
Mktg./Adv.: Toru Yoneyama/Manager International & National Sales
    Toru Yoneyama/Manager Market Research

CANON DEVELOPMENT AMERICAS, INC 949-932-3100 *(cont'd)*

Toru Yoneyama/Manager Marketing

Camera, Ophthalmic, AC-Powered (Fundus)	Ophthalmology
Image Digitizer	Radiology
Imager, X-Ray, Solid State (Flat Panel/Digital)	Radiology
Keratometer	Ophthalmology
Refractometer, Ophthalmic	Ophthalmology
Tonometer, AC-Powered	Ophthalmology

CANON U.S.A., INC. 516-328-5000

One Canon Plaza, Lake Success, NY 92618-3731

FDA Number: 2029102
E-mail: pr@cusa.canon.com
Web site: www.canon.com
Ownership: Private
Produces/Sells CE-marked Devices: N
General Admin.: Mr. Seymour Liebman/Chief Administrative Officer
　Mr. Kunihiko Tedo/Chief Executive Officer, Chief Financial Officer
　Mr. Shunichi Izawa/Chief Technology Officer
　Mr. Shunichi Uzawa/Chief Technology Officer, Executive Vice President
　Mr. Joe Adachi/President, Chief Executive Officer
Finance: Mr. Kunihiko Tedo/Chief Financial Officer

Camera, Ophthalmic, AC-Powered (Fundus)	Ophthalmology
Device, Communications, Images, Ophthalmic	Ophthalmology
Device, Storage, Image, Digital	Radiology
Device, Storage, Images, Ophthalmic	Ophthalmology
Grid, Radiographic	Radiology
System, Image Management, Ophthalmic	Ophthalmology

CANRAD INC., HANOVIA DIV

See Hanovia Specialty Lighting Llc

CANREG INC. 905-689-3980

7 Innovation Dr., Unit 118, Flamborough, ONT L9H-7H9 Canada

FDA Number: n/a　　　　　　　*Fax:* 905-689-1465
E-mail: atomalin@canreg.on.ca
Web site: www.canreg.on.ca
Year Founded: 1996
Total Employees: 50
Ownership: Private
Produces/Sells CE-marked Devices: N
Distribution: Service Direct

CANTEL MEDICAL CORP. 973-890-7220

150 Clove Road, 9th Floor, Little Falls, NJ 07424

FDA Number: n/a　　　　　　　*Fax:* 973-890-7270
Web site: www.cantelmedical.com
Annual Revenue: $100-$500 Million
Total Employees: 838
Ownership: Public
Stock Symbol: CMN
Traded On: NYSE
Produces/Sells CE-marked Devices: N
General Admin.: Charles M. Diker/Chairman
　Andrew A. Krakauer/President
　Seth R. Segel/Senior Vice President
　Eric W. Nodiff/Senior Vice President, General Counsel
Finance: Craig A. Sheldon/Chief Financial Officer, Senior Vice President Finance
　Steven C. Anaya/Vice President, Controller
Medical Product Subsidiaries (Listed Separately)
　Confirm Monitoring Systems, Inc.

CANTYLIGHT 716-625-4227

6100 Donner, Buffalo, NY 14094

FDA Number: n/a　　　　　　　*Fax:* 716-625-4228
E-mail: sales@jmcanty.com
Web site: www.cantylight.com
Annual Revenue: $10-$25 Million
Total Employees: 40　　　*Sales Staff:* 5
Ownership: Private
Quality System Registration Information: ISO9000
Produces/Sells CE-marked Devices: Y
Federal Procurement Eligibility: Small Business
Distribution: Manufacturer Direct, Manufacturer Through Manufacturer Reps, OEM, Service Direct, Exclusive Distributor, Importer
General Admin.: Mr. Thomas M. Canty/President
Mktg./Adv.: Mr. Paul O'Brien/Manager Advertising
　Mr. THOMAS CANTY/Manager Sales
Production: Mr. Mike Rizzo/Vice President Manufacturing
Research: Mr. Jack Doescher/Vice President Research & Development

Chamber, Hyperbaric	Anesthesiology
Chamber, Hypobaric	General
Lamp, Examination (Light)	General
Lamp, Examination, Ceiling Mounted (Light)	General
Light Source, Fiberoptic, Routine	Gastroenterology/Urology
Light, Surgical, Fiberoptic	Surgery
Sterilizer, Steam (Autoclave)	General

CANVAS SPECIALTIES, INC. 210-662-6412

5923 Distribution, San Antonio, TX 78218-5532

FDA Number: 3004057055　　　*Fax:* 210-662-6925
E-mail: canvasspecialties@satx.rr.com
Web site: www.canvasspecialties.com
Medical Products Sales Volume: $380,000
Year Founded: 1987
Total Employees: 8
Ownership: Private
Produces/Sells CE-marked Devices: N
Federal Procurement Eligibility: Small Business

Tourniquet, Non-Pneumatic, Surgical	Surgery

CAO GROUP, INC. 801-256-9282

4628 West Skyhawk Drive, West Jordan, UT 84084

FDA Number: 1725006
Ownership: Private
Produces/Sells CE-marked Devices: N

Activator, Ultraviolet, Polymerization	Dental And Oral
Dam, Rubber	Dental And Oral
Lamp, Infrared	Physical Med
Laser, Surgical	Surgery
Sealant, Pit And Fissure, And Conditioner, Resin	Dental And Oral
Source, Heat, Bleaching, Teeth, Dental	Dental And Oral
Tooth Bonding Agent, Resin Restoration	Dental And Oral
Varnish, Cavity	Dental And Oral

CAPINTEC, INC. 800-631-3826

6 Arrow Road, Ramsey, NJ 07446-1205　　201-825-9500

FDA Number: n/a　　　　　　　*Fax:* 201-825-4859
E-mail: getinfo@capintec.com
Web site: www.capintec.com
Medical Products Sales Volume: $7,700,000
Annual Revenue: $10-$25 Million
Year Founded: 1964
Total Employees: 80　　*Marketing Staff:* 5　　*Sales Staff:* 10
Ownership: Private
Quality System Registration Information: ISO9001
Produces/Sells CE-marked Devices: Y
Federal Procurement Eligibility: Small Business
Distribution: Manufacturer Direct, Manufacturer Through Distributor, Manufacturer Through Manufacturer Reps, OEM, Service Direct, Exclusive Distributor, Exporter
General Admin.: Mr. Arthur Weis/Chairman
　Mr. Ralph Monaco/Chief Financial Officer, Vice President
　Ms. Jessica Bede/President, Chief Executive Officer
Mktg./Adv.: Mr. Roy Eve/Vice President International Sales
Production: Mary Anne Dell/Vice President Manufacturing
Research: Mr. Bill Tyberg/Vice President Engineering

Accelerator, Linear, Medical	Radiology
Accessories, Radiotherapy	Radiology
Analyzer, Chemistry, Radioimmunoassay, Automated	Chemistry
Analyzer, ECG	Cardiovascular
Cabinet, Other	General
Calibrator Source, Nuclear Sealed	Radiology
Calibrator, Beam	Radiology
Calibrator, Dose, Radionuclide	Radiology
Calibrator, Radioisotope	Radiology
Cardiac Output Unit, Other	Cardiovascular
Cardiac Output Unit, Radioisotope Probe	Cardiovascular
Computer, Nuclear Medicine	Radiology
Computer, Radiographic Data	Radiology
Contract Manufacturing	General
Counter, Gamma, General Use	Toxicology
Counter, Gamma, Radioimmunoassay (Manual)	Toxicology
Counter, Radiation	Radiology
Counter, Scintillation	Chemistry
Detector, Beta/Gamma	Chemistry
Dosimeter, Radiation	Radiology
Hood, Fume	Toxicology
Monitor, Physiological, Stress Exercise	Cardiovascular
Monitor, Radiation	Radiology
Monitor, X-Ray Tube	Radiology
Phantom, Anthropomorphic, Nuclear	Radiology
Phantom, Anthropomorphic, Radiographic	Radiology
Phantom, Computed Axial Tomography (CAT, CT)	Radiology
Phantom, Flood Source, Nuclear	Radiology
Phantom, Radiotherapy	Radiology
Probe, Uptake, Nuclear	Radiology
Pyrometer	General
Recorder, Long-Term, ECG, Portable (Holter Monitor)	Cardiovascular
Safe, Radionuclide	Radiology
Shield, Syringe	General
Shield, Vial	General
Source, Radioisotope Reference	Chemistry
Test Pattern/Phantom, Radionuclide	Radiology
Tester, Radiology Quality Assurance	Radiology
Thermometer, Laboratory	Chemistry
Thyroid Uptake System	Radiology

CAPISTRANO LABS, INC.   949-492-0390
150 Calle Iglesia, Unit B, San Clemente, CA 92672
FDA Number: n/a   Fax: 949-492-3041
E-mail: clisales@capolabs.com
Web site: www.capolabs.com
Medical Products Sales Volume: $4,700,000
Annual Revenue: $1-$5 Million
Year Founded: 1984
Total Employees: 20   Marketing Staff: 1   Sales Staff: 1
Ownership: Private
Produces/Sells CE-marked Devices: Y
Federal Procurement Eligibility: Small Business
Distribution: Manufacturer Direct, OEM
General Admin.: Paul Meyers/President, Chief Executive Officer
Mktg./Adv.: Jeff Johnson/Vice President Marketing
Production: Doug Petersen/Manager Production
Finance: Matt Stabley/Chief Financial Officer
     Paul Meyers/Treasurer
   Probe, Ultrasonic   Radiology

CAPITAL BEDDING, INCORPORATED   757-224-0177
5262 South Raymond Street, Verona, MS 38879
FDA Number: 3006365764
   Mattress, Non-Powered Flotation Therapy   Physical Med

CAPITAL CONTROLS CO., INC.
See Capital Controls, MicroChem

CAPITAL CONTROLS, MICROCHEM   215-997-4000
3000 Advance Lane, Colmar, PA 18915
FDA Number: n/a   Fax: 215-997-4062
E-mail: jblundi@severntrentservices.com
Web site: www.severntrentservices.com
Annual Revenue: $25-$50 Million
Ownership: SOUVERN TRENT
Produces/Sells CE-marked Devices: N
Distribution: Manufacturer Through Distributor
   Meter, pH, General Use   Toxicology
   Washer/Disinfector   General

CAPITAL INSTRUMENTS, LTD.   425-271-3756
6210 Lake Washington Blvd., Se, Bellevue, WA 98006
FDA Number: 3026633
Ownership: Private
Produces/Sells CE-marked Devices: N
   Forceps, Ophthalmic   Ophthalmology
   Measurer, Lens Radius, Ophthalmic   Ophthalmology

CAPITOL MANAGEMENT CONSULTING, INC.   609-737-9963
30 Pleasant Valley Harbourton, Titusville, NJ 08560-2101
FDA Number: n/a   Fax: 609-737-9964
E-mail: jk@capitolmgmt.com
Web site: www.capitolmgmt.com
Annual Revenue: $0-$1 Million
Year Founded: 1984
Total Employees: 6
Ownership: Private
Federal Procurement Eligibility: Small Business
Distribution: Service Direct, Exporter
General Admin.: Joseph J. Kowalski/President
   Service, Consulting   General

CAPITOL VIAL   334-887-8311
2039 Mcmillan Street, Auburn, AL 36832
FDA Number: 1062700   Fax: 334-887-9102
Ownership: Private
Produces/Sells CE-marked Devices: N
   Container, Specimen Mailer And Storage, Temperature Controlled, Non-sterile
     Pathology
   Container, Specimen, Non-sterile   General
   Pipetting And Diluting System, Automated   Chemistry

CAPLUGS WEST   310-537-2300
18704 S. Ferris Place, Rancho Dominguez, CA 90220
FDA Number: 2032895
Ownership: Private
Produces/Sells CE-marked Devices: N
   Cannula, Nasal, Oxygen   Anesthesiology

CAPPEL LABORATORIES
See Biomerieux Inc.

CAPRI OPTICS, INC.   800-221-3544
1421 38th St., Brooklyn, NY 11218-3678   718-633-2300
FDA Number: n/a
E-mail: capri@caprioptics.com
Web site: www.caprioptics.com
Annual Revenue: $0-$1 Million
Ownership: Private
Produces/Sells CE-marked Devices: N

CAPRI OPTICS, INC.   800-221-3544 (cont'd)
Federal Procurement Eligibility: Small Business
Distribution: Manufacturer Direct, Importer, Exporter
   Frame, Spectacle (Eyeglasses)   Ophthalmology

CAPRIUS INC.   201-342-0900
One University Plaza, Suite 400, Hackensack, NJ 07601
FDA Number: n/a   Fax: 201-342-0991
E-mail: ir@caprius.com
Web site: www.caprius.com
Ownership: Public
Stock Symbol: CAPI
Traded On: OTC Bulletin
Produces/Sells CE-marked Devices: N
General Admin.: Jonathan Joels/Chief Financial Officer, Treasurer
     Dwight Morgan/President, Chief Executive Officer, Chairman
     George Aaron/Vice President International Affairs

CAPRO SOLUTIONS, LLC   518-456-1145
8 Corporate Cir., Karner Park, Albany, NY 12203
FDA Number: 1317498
Ownership: Private
Produces/Sells CE-marked Devices: N
   Prosthesis Alignment Device   Physical Med

CAPROCK DEVELOPMENTS INC.   800-222-0325
475 Speedwell Avenue, PO Box 95,   973-267-9292
Morris Plains, NJ 07950
FDA Number: n/a   Fax: 973-292-0614
E-mail: info@caprockdev.com
Web site: www.caprockdev.com
Year Founded: 1953
Ownership: Private
Produces/Sells CE-marked Devices: Y
Federal Procurement Eligibility: Small Business
Distribution: Manufacturer Direct, Manufacturer Through Distributor, Exclusive
     Distributor, Importer, Exporter
General Admin.: Alan Schwartz/President
   Densitometer   Cardiovascular
   Lamp, Endoscopic, Incandescent   Surgery
   Lamp, Infrared   Physical Med
   Lamp, Microscope   Pathology
   Lamp, Other   General
   Lamp, Slit   Ophthalmology
   Lamp, Surgical, Xenon   Surgery
   Lamp, Ultraviolet (Spectrum A)   General
   Lamp, Ultraviolet, Germicidal   General
   Light, High Intensity   Radiology
   Magnifier, Hand-Held, Low-Vision   Ophthalmology
   Meter, Conductivity   Chemistry
   Meter, pH, General Use   Toxicology
   Meter, pH, Portable   Chemistry
   Viewer/Magnifier   Hematology

CAPSTONE THERAPEUTICS   800-937-5520
1275 W. Washington St., Tempe, AZ 85281   602-286-5520
FDA Number: n/a
E-mail: investorinquiries@capstonethx.com
Web site: www.capstonehx.com
Medical Products Sales Volume: $77,049,000
Annual Revenue: $50-$100 Million
Ownership: Public
Stock Symbol: CAPS
Traded On: NASDAQ
Produces/Sells CE-marked Devices: N
Federal Procurement Eligibility: Small Business
Distribution: Manufacturer Direct
General Admin.: Terry Meier/Chief Financial Officer, Vice President
     Tom Trotter/President, Chief Executive Officer
     MaryAnn Miller/Vice President Human Resources
Mktg./Adv.: Bill Rieger/Vice President Marketing
Production: Jon Brockman/Director Quality Assurance
     Reggie Ponder/Manager Regulatory Affairs
Research: Frank Magee/Executive Vice President Research & Development
     James Koeneman/Vice President Engineering
   Brace, Joint, Ankle (External)   Physical Med
   Exerciser, Passive, Non-Measuring (CPM Machine)   Physical Med
   Fixation Device, Spinal (External)   Orthopedics
   Stimulator, Growth, Bone, Non-Invasive   Orthopedics
   Stimulator, Wound Healing   Physical Med
Medical Product Subsidiaries (Listed Separately)
   Orthomotion Inc.

CAPTIVA SOFTWARE CORPORATION   800-783-3378
601 Oakmont Lane, Suite 200,   630-654-8800
Westmont, IL 60559
FDA Number: n/a   Fax: 630-654-1607
E-mail: info@captivasoftware.com

MANUFACTURER PROFILES

CAPTIVA SOFTWARE CORPORATION   800-783-3378 *(cont'd)*
Web site: www.captivasoftware.com
Year Founded: 1988
Total Employees: 375
Ownership: Private
Stock Symbol: ADP
Traded On: NYSE
Produces/Sells CE-marked Devices: N
Federal Procurement Eligibility: Small Business
Distribution: Manufacturer Direct, Exclusive Distributor
Production: Mark Earles/Vice President Operations
Computer Software	General
Computer, Patient Data Management	General

CAR-MAY   970-532-2816
308 Mountain View Rd, Unit D, Berthoud, CO 80513
FDA Number: n/a   Fax: 970-532-2817
E-mail: info@car-may.com
Web site: www.encynova.com
Year Founded: 1994
Total Employees: 50   *Marketing Staff:* 1   *Sales Staff:* 4
Ownership: Private
Produces/Sells CE-marked Devices: Y
Federal Procurement Eligibility: Small Business
Distribution: Manufacturer Direct, Manufacturer Through Distributor, OEM
General Admin.: Robert Mulverhill/President
Mktg./Adv.: David Miller/Director Product Development
         Heather Botarelli/Manager Marketing & Business Development
Dispenser, Fluid	General
Pump, Laboratory	Chemistry
System, Infusion, Administration, Drug, Implantable	General

CARBO-FUNG LABS INC./TRUETT LABS
See Truett Labs

CARBON MEDICAL TECHNOLOGIES, INC.   877-277-1788
1290 Hammond Road, Saint Paul, MN 55110   **651-653-8512**
FDA Number: 2134494   Fax: 651-407-1975
E-mail: info@carbonmed.com
Web site: www.carbonmed.com
Medical Products Sales Volume: $5,200,000
Year Founded: 1994
Total Employees: 14
Ownership: Private
Quality System Registration Information: ISO9001
Produces/Sells CE-marked Devices: Y
Federal Procurement Eligibility: Small Business
Distribution: Manufacturer Through Distributor
General Admin.: Dean Klein/President, Chief Executive Officer
Production: Robert Johnson/Vice President Quality Assurance & Regulatory Affairs
Agent, Injectable, Embolic	Surgery
Endoscope	Gastroenterology/Urology
Mesh, Surgical (Steel Gauze)	Surgery

CARBYLAN BIOSURGERY, INC.   650-855-6777
3181 Porter Drive, Palo Alto, CA 94304
FDA Number: 3006287117
Splint, Septal, Intranasal	Ear/Nose/Throat

CARCLO TECHNICAL PLASTICS - EXPORT   724-539-1833
6009 Enterprise Drive, Export, PA 15632
FDA Number: n/a
Ownership: Private
Produces/Sells CE-marked Devices: N
Equipment, Laboratory, Gen. Purpose (Specific Medical Use)	Chemistry

CARCLO TECHNICAL PLASTICS - TUCSON   724-539-1833
1141 W. Grant Road, Kino, AZ 85705
FDA Number: 3005203111
Ownership: Private
Produces/Sells CE-marked Devices: N
Antigen, Antiserum, Control, IGE	Immunology
Radioimmunoassay, Total Triiodothyronine	Chemistry
Ventilator, Continuous (Respirator)	Anesthesiology

CARD TECHNOLOGY CORPORATION
See Nbs Technologies Inc.

CARDEA TECHNOLOGY INC.   877-392-7763
359 Green Street, Cambridge, MA 02139
FDA Number: 3004512404
Ownership: Private
Produces/Sells CE-marked Devices: N
System, Communication, Image, Digital	Radiology

CARDENT INTERNATIONAL, INC.   866-764-6832
1568 NW 89th Ct., Miami, FL 33172   **305-994-8000**
FDA Number: 1062152   Fax: 305-994-7800
E-mail: dei@cardent.com
Web site: www.cardent.com

CARDENT INTERNATIONAL, INC.   866-764-6832 *(cont'd)*
Medical Products Sales Volume: $8,500,000
Annual Revenue: $5-10 Million
Year Founded: 1981
Total Employees: 10   *Marketing Staff:* 1   *Sales Staff:* 4
Ownership: Private
Produces/Sells CE-marked Devices: N
Federal Procurement Eligibility: Small Business
Distribution: Exclusive Distributor, Exporter
General Admin.: Mr. Carlos Grande/President
Dam, Dental	Dental And Oral
Teeth, Porcelain	Dental And Oral

CARDEON CORP.   408-253-3319
10600 North Tantau Ave., Cupertino, CA 95014
FDA Number: 2954753
Ownership: Private
Produces/Sells CE-marked Devices: N
Catheter, Vascular, Cardiopulmonary Bypass	Cardiovascular

CARDIA INC.   651-691-4100
2900 Lone Oak Parkway, Suite 130, Eagan, MN 55121
FDA Number: 3003215458
Ownership: Private
Produces/Sells CE-marked Devices: N
Device, Occlusion, Cardiac, Transcatheter	Cardiovascular

CARDIAC ASSIST, INC.   412-963-7770
240 Alpha Dr., Pittsburgh, PA 15238
FDA Number: 2531527
Web site: www.cardiacassist.com
Year Founded: 1996
Ownership: Private
Produces/Sells CE-marked Devices: N
General Admin.: Michael Garippa/President, Chief Executive Officer
   Medical Admin.: Mr. Cory Cortese/Director Clinical Affairs
Production: Robert Svitek/Director Engineering
         Jeffrey Stuckley/Director Manufacturing
         Mr. Robert Bollinger/Director Quality Assurance & Regulatory Affairs
Finance: Mr. Robert Dickson/Chief Financial Officer
Cannula, Catheter	Cardiovascular
Circulatory Assist Unit, Left Ventricular	Cardiovascular
Pump, Blood, Cardiopulmonary Bypass, Non-Roller Type	Cardiovascular

CARDIAC CARE UNITS, INC.   818-592-6004
7745 Alabama Avenue, Canoga Park, CA 91304
FDA Number: 2082647   Fax: 818-592-6004
E-mail: hklee4@hotmail.com
Web site: www.ubsca.tripod.com
Medical Products Sales Volume: $1,000,000
Annual Revenue: $0-$1 Million
Total Employees: 3
Ownership: Private
Produces/Sells CE-marked Devices: Y
Federal Procurement Eligibility: Small Business
Distribution: Manufacturer Direct, Manufacturer Through Distributor, Exporter
General Admin.: Thomas M. Curran/President, Chief Executive Officer
         Dale Curran/Vice President, General Manager
Mktg./Adv.: Dale Curran/Director Marketing
Production: Gerald McVicker/Director Engineering
Monitor, ECG, Ambulatory, Real-Time	Cardiovascular

CARDIAC CONCEPTS INC.   952-540-4470
12400 Whitewater Dr., Suite 500, Minnetonka, MN 55343
FDA Number: n/a
E-mail: info@cardiacconcepts.com
Web site: http://www.cardiacconcepts.com
Year Founded: 2006
Ownership: Private
Produces/Sells CE-marked Devices: N
General Admin.: Ms. Bonnie Labosky/President, Chief Executive Officer

CARDIAC DATACORP
See Philips Remote Cardiac Services

CARDIAC DIMENSIONS, INC.   425- 605-5900
5540 Lake Washington Blvd. NE, Kirkland, WA 98033
FDA Number: n/a   Fax: 425-605-5901
E-mail: info@cardiacdimensions.com
Web site: www.cardiacdimensions.com
Ownership: Private
Produces/Sells CE-marked Devices: N
General Admin.: Mr. Rick Stewart/President, Chief Executive Officer
   Medical Admin.: Dr. David Reuter/Chief Medical Officer
         Dr. Nawzer Mehta/Vice President Clinical Affairs
Production: Mr. Gary Swinford/Vice President Operations
         Mr. Paul Cornelison/Vice President Regulatory Affairs
Research: Mr. Bob Conta/Vice President Research & Development

CARDIAC DIMENSIONS, INC.   425- 605-5900 (cont'd)
Finance: Mr. Rich Wypych/Chief Financial Officer

CARDIAC RESUSCITATOR CORP.
See Laerdal Medical Corporation

CARDIAC SCIENCE CORP.   800-777-1777
500 Burdick Pkwy., Deerfield, WI 53531-9692   **608-764-1919**
FDA Number: 2112020   Fax: 608-764-7194
E-mail: info@burdick.com
Web site: www.burdick.com
Medical Products Sales Volume: $50,000,000
Annual Revenue: $50-$100 Million
Year Founded: 1926
Total Employees: 550   Marketing Staff: 5   Sales Staff: 30
Ownership: Cardiac Science Corporation
Stock Symbol: CSCX
Traded On: NYSE
Quality System Registration Information: ISO9001
Produces/Sells CE-marked Devices: Y
Distribution: Manufacturer Direct, Manufacturer Through Distributor, Manufacturer Through Manufacturer Reps, Importer, Exporter
Mktg./Adv.: Nancy Sandy/Director Marketing
    Darryl Lustig/Vice President Marketing & Sales
Production: Feroze Motafram/Vice President Manufacturing

Analyzer, ECG	Cardiovascular
Analyzer, Pulmonary Function	Anesthesiology
Cable, Electrode	Physical Med
Computer, Patient Data Management	General
Computer, Stress Exercise	Cardiovascular
Defibrillator, External, Automatic	Cardiovascular
Defibrillator, Line-Powered	Cardiovascular
Detector, Arrhythmia Alarm	Cardiovascular
Electrocardiograph, Multi-Channel	Cardiovascular
Electrocardiograph, Single Channel	Cardiovascular
Electrode, Electrocardiograph	Cardiovascular
Gel, Electrode, Electrocardiograph	Cardiovascular
Gel, Ultrasonic Coupling	Physical Med
Oximeter, Pulse	General
Recorder, Long-Term, Trend	General
Spirometer, Diagnostic (Respirometer)	Anesthesiology
Syringe, Calibration Testing, Spirometer	Anesthesiology
Treadmill, Powered	Physical Med

CARDIAC SCIENCE CORPORATION (CA)   1.800.426.0337
3303 Monte Villa Parkway, Bothell, WA 98021   **1.425.402.2000**
FDA Number: 3004495806   Fax: 1.425.402.2001
E-mail: care@cardiacscience.com
Web site: www.cardiacscience.com
Medical Products Sales Volume: $66,000,000
Annual Revenue: $50-$100 Million
Year Founded: 1991
Total Employees: 250   Marketing Staff: 6   Sales Staff: 58
Ownership: Cardiac Science Corporation
Stock Symbol: CSCX
Traded On: NASDAQ
Quality System Registration Information: ISO9001
Produces/Sells CE-marked Devices: Y
Federal Procurement Eligibility: Small Business
Distribution: Manufacturer Direct, Manufacturer Through Distributor, Manufacturer Through Manufacturer Reps, Exporter
General Admin.: Raymond W. Cohen/Chief Executive Officer
    Michael Gioffredi/Chief Medical Officer, Vice President
    Howard Evers/Chief Operating Officer
    Kenneth F. Olson/Chief Technology Officer
    Sandra Thomson/Vice President Human Resources
Mktg./Adv.: Stephanie Jones/Manager Marketing
    Kurt Lemvigh/Vice President International Sales
    Peter Foster/Vice President Sales
Production: Prabodh Mathur/Chief Engineer
Research: Dr. Don Lin/Chief Scientist
    Mark Altmann/Vice President Education & Training
Finance: Roderick De Greef/Chief Financial Officer

Defibrillator, External, Automatic	Cardiovascular

CARDIAC SERVICES, INC.   800-722-5742
618 Grassmere Park Dr., Ste. 17,   **615-333-6341**
Nashville, TN 37211
FDA Number: n/a   Fax: 615-833-1619
E-mail: info@CardiacServicesInc.com
Web site: www.cardiacservicesinc.com
Annual Revenue: $5-$10 Million
Total Employees: 10
Ownership: Private
Produces/Sells CE-marked Devices: N
Federal Procurement Eligibility: Small Business
Distribution: Service Direct
General Admin.: Kent Simpkins/President

CARDIAC SERVICES, INC.   800-722-5742 (cont'd)
Computer, Cardiac Catheterization Laboratory   Cardiovascular

CARDIAC TELECOM CORPORATION   800-355-2594
212 Outlet Way, Suite 1, Greensburg, PA 15601
FDA Number: 2529601   Fax: 800-403-7682
E-mail: sales@cardiactelecom.com
Web site: www.cardiactelecom.com
Medical Products Sales Volume: $1,600,000
Annual Revenue: $0-$1 Million
Year Founded: 1988
Total Employees: 17   Marketing Staff: 1   Sales Staff: 4
Ownership: TELEMED TECHNOLOOGIES INTERNATIONAL CORP.
Produces/Sells CE-marked Devices: N
Federal Procurement Eligibility: Small Business
Distribution: Manufacturer Direct, Service Direct, Exporter
General Admin.: Alois Langer/Chief Technology Officer
    Mr. Lee B. Ehrlichman/President
Production: Mr. Lee Deneault/Director Operations
Finance: Mary Margaret Galdes/Manager Finance

Detector, Arrhythmia Alarm	Cardiovascular
Monitor, ECG	Cardiovascular

CARDIAQ VALVE TECHNOLOGIES   617-957-8945
1 Orient Street, Winchester, MA 01890
FDA Number: n/a
E-mail: info@cardiaq.com
Web site: http://www.cardiaq.com
Ownership: Private
Produces/Sells CE-marked Devices: N
General Admin.: Mr. Rob Michiels/Chief Executive Officer
    Mr. Brent Ratz/Chief Operating Officer
Medical Admin.: Dr. Arshad Quadri/Chief Medical Officer

CARDICA, INC.   888-544-7194
900 Saginaw Dr., Redwood City, CA 94063   **650-364-9975**
FDA Number: 3004114958   Fax: 650-364-3134
Web site: www.cardica.com
Year Founded: 1997
Total Employees: 68   Sales Staff: 10
Ownership: Public
Stock Symbol: CRDC
Traded On: NASDAQ
Produces/Sells CE-marked Devices: Y
General Admin.: Bernard Hausen/President, Chief Executive Officer
    Medical Admin.: Dr. Lee Swanstrom/Medical Director
Mktg./Adv.: Christopher Littel/Vice President Marketing & Sales
Production: Mr. Frederick Bauer/Vice President Operations
Research: Bryan Knodel/Vice President Research & Development
Finance: Robert Newell/Chief Financial Officer, Vice President Finance

Clip, Implantable	Surgery
Device, Suturing, Stapling, Graft, Aortic	Surgery
Surgical Instrument, Cardiovascular	Cardiovascular

CARDIMA, INC.   888-354-0300
47266 Benicia St., Fremont, CA 94538-1372   **510-354-0166**
FDA Number: 2951009   Fax: 510-657-4476
Web site: www.cardima.com
Ownership: Public
Stock Symbol: CADM
Traded On: OTC Bulletin
Produces/Sells CE-marked Devices: Y
General Admin.: Mr. Robert Cheney/Chief Executive Officer
    Dr. Richard Gaston/Director
Medical Admin.: Dr. Sung Chun/Chief Medical Officer

Cable, Electrode	Physical Med
Cable/Lead, ECG, With Transducer And Electrode	Cardiovascular
Catheter, Electrode Recording, Or Probe	Cardiovascular
Catheter, Percutaneous	Cardiovascular
Electrode, Ablation, Tissue, Conduction, Percutaneous	Cardiovascular

CARDINAL HEALTH   888-571-5950
7000 Cardinal Place, Dublin, OH 43017   **614.757.5000**
FDA Number: n/a   Fax: 416-213-5152
E-mail: lafortg@allegiance.net
Web site: www.cardinal.com
Annual Revenue: $50-$100 Million
Year Founded: 1996
Total Employees: 50
Ownership: CARDINAL HEALTH, INC.
Produces/Sells CE-marked Devices: N
Distribution: Manufacturer Direct
General Admin.: Gordon LaFortune/General Manager
Mktg./Adv.: Carol Bentley/Manager Marketing
    Lianne MacMillan/Manager Marketing
    Rita Forman/Manager Marketing
    Vafa Jamali/Manager Marketing & Sales

MANUFACTURER PROFILES

CARDINAL HEALTH
See Cardinal Health Inc.

CARDINAL HEALTH   847-785-3323
State Rd. 402, Km 0.9, Anasco, PR 00610
FDA Number: 2640138
Web site: www.cardinal.com
Ownership: Cardinal Health Inc.
Stock Symbol: CAH
Traded On: NYSE
Produces/Sells CE-marked Devices: N

Catheter, Irrigation	Surgery
Container, Specimen Mailer And Storage	Pathology
Dislodger, Stone, Basket, Ureteral, Metal	Gastroenterology/Urology
Forceps, Biopsy, Non-Electric	Gastroenterology/Urology
Knife, Ear	Ear/Nose/Throat
Suction Apparatus, Operating Room, Wall Vacuum-Powered	Surgery
Suction Apparatus, Single Patient, Portable, Non-Powered	Surgery

CARDINAL HEALTH 200, INC   847-578-4515
1240 Waukegan Rd, Park City, IL 60085
FDA Number: 1419729
Web site: www.cardinal.com
Ownership: Cardinal Health Inc.
Stock Symbol: CAH
Traded On: NYSE
Produces/Sells CE-marked Devices: N

Analyzer, Gas, Carbon-Dioxide, Gaseous Phase (Capnograph)	Anesthesiology
Dilator, Vessel	Gastroenterology/Urology

CARDINAL HEALTH 200, INC   800-964-5227
1430 Waukegan Rd, McGaw Park, IL 60085   847-689-8410
FDA Number: 1423537
Web site: www.cardinal.com
Ownership: Cardinal Health Inc.
Stock Symbol: CAH
Traded On: NYSE
Produces/Sells CE-marked Devices: N

Catheter, Irrigation	Surgery
Glove, Patient Examination, Poly	General
Glove, Surgical	General
Lavage Unit, Water Jet	General
Mask, Surgical	Surgery
Tubing, Non-Invasive	Surgery

CARDINAL HEALTH 200, INC   847-473-1500
1430 Waukegan Rd. KB-3B, McGaw Park, IL 60085
FDA Number: 1423339
Web site: www.cardinal.com
Ownership: Cardinal Health Inc.
Stock Symbol: CAH
Traded On: NYSE
Produces/Sells CE-marked Devices: N

Analyzer, Gas, Carbon-Dioxide, Gaseous Phase (Capnograph)	Anesthesiology
Bandage, Elastic	General
Basin, Emesis	General
Catheter, Suction (Tracheal Aspirating Tube)	Anesthesiology
Container, Specimen, All Types	General
Cotton, Roll	Dental And Oral
Cover, Shoe, Operating Room	Surgery
Depressor, Tongue	General
Dilator, Vessel	Gastroenterology/Urology
Drainage System, Urine, Closed	Gastroenterology/Urology
Fiber, Absorbent	General
Gown, Surgical	Surgery
Guidewire, Catheter	Cardiovascular
Kit, Laparoscopy	Gastroenterology/Urology
Needle, Hypodermic	General
Oxygenator, Cardiopulmonary Bypass	Cardiovascular
Set, Administration, Intravenous, Needle-Free	General
Sponge, Gauze	Dental And Oral
Syringe, Piston	General
Tape, Measuring, Ruler And Caliper	Surgery
Tray, Surgical Instrument	Surgery
Truss, Umbilical	Gastroenterology/Urology
Wrap, Sterilization	General

CARDINAL HEALTH 200, INC   847-578-6610
1660 Iowa Ave.,, Suite 100/200, Box Springs, CA 92507
FDA Number: 2020472
Web site: www.cardinal.com
Ownership: Cardinal Health Inc.
Stock Symbol: CAH
Traded On: NYSE
Produces/Sells CE-marked Devices: N

CARDINAL HEALTH 200, INC
See Cardinal Health 2200, Inc

CARDINAL HEALTH 200, INC   847-785-3323
200 Mcknight St, Jacksonville, TX 75766
FDA Number: 1623486
Web site: www.cardinal.com
Ownership: Cardinal Health Inc.
Stock Symbol: CAH
Traded On: NYSE
Produces/Sells CE-marked Devices: N

Basin, Emesis	General
Container, Medication, Graduated Liquid	General
Container, Specimen Mailer And Storage	Pathology
Forceps	Orthopedics
Infusion Stand	General
Tube, Aspirating, Flexible, Connecting	Anesthesiology

CARDINAL HEALTH 200, INC
See Cardinal Health 2200, Inc

CARDINAL HEALTH 200, INC   847-785-3323
4551 East Philadelphia St, Ontario, CA 91761
FDA Number: 2020289
Web site: www.cardinal.com
Ownership: Cardinal Health Inc.
Stock Symbol: CAH
Traded On: NYSE
Produces/Sells CE-marked Devices: N

CARDINAL HEALTH 200, INC
See Cardinal Health 2200, Inc

CARDINAL HEALTH 200, INC
See Cardinal Health 2200, Inc

CARDINAL HEALTH 200, INC   847-785-3323
785 Fort Mill Hwy, Fort Mill, SC 29715
FDA Number: 1065831
Web site: www.cardinal.com
Ownership: Cardinal Health Inc.
Stock Symbol: CAH
Traded On: NYSE
Produces/Sells CE-marked Devices: N

Analyzer, Gas, Carbon-Dioxide, Gaseous Phase (Capnograph)	Anesthesiology
Catheter, Intravascular, Diagnostic	Cardiovascular
Catheter, Retention Type, Balloon	Gastroenterology/Urology
Catheter, Suction (Tracheal Aspirating Tube)	Anesthesiology
Cotton, Roll	Dental And Oral
Depressor, Tongue	General
Dilator, Vessel	Gastroenterology/Urology
Drainage System, Urine, Closed	Gastroenterology/Urology
Guidewire, Catheter	Cardiovascular
Holder, Needle, Other	Surgery
Kit, Laparoscopy	Gastroenterology/Urology
Kit, Urinary Drainage Collection	Gastroenterology/Urology
Oxygenator, Cardiopulmonary Bypass	Cardiovascular
Sponge, Gauze	Dental And Oral
Truss, Umbilical	Gastroenterology/Urology

CARDINAL HEALTH 200, INC   847-785-3323
808 Hwy. 24 West, Moberly, MO 65270
FDA Number: 1940373
Web site: www.cardinal.com
Ownership: Cardinal Health Inc.
Stock Symbol: CAH
Traded On: NYSE
Produces/Sells CE-marked Devices: N

Bag, Ice	General
Pack, Hot Or Cold, Disposable	Physical Med
Pack, Hot Or Cold, Reusable	Physical Med
Warmer, Heel, Infant	Physical Med

CARDINAL HEALTH 200, INC   847-785-3323
One Butterfield Trail, El Paso, TX 79906
FDA Number: 1623223
Web site: www.cardinal.com
Ownership: Cardinal Health Inc.
Stock Symbol: CAH
Traded On: NYSE
Produces/Sells CE-marked Devices: N

Bandage, Elastic	General
Drape, Pure Latex Sheet, With Self-Retaining Finger Cot	Gastroenterology/Urology
Gown, Examination	General
Gown, Surgical	Surgery
Kit, Administration, Intravenous	General
Kit, Biopsy Needle	Gastroenterology/Urology
Kit, Blood, Transfusion	General
Mask, Surgical	Surgery
Nebulizer, Direct Patient Interface	Anesthesiology
Needle, Hypodermic, Single Lumen With Syringe	General
Wrap, Sterilization	General

CARDINAL HEALTH 200, INC.   847-785-3323
1300 Waukegan Rd., Waukegan, IL 60085
FDA Number: 1419729
Web site: www.cardinal.com
Ownership: Cardinal Health Inc.
Stock Symbol: CAH
Traded On: NYSE
Produces/Sells CE-marked Devices: N

CARDINAL HEALTH 200, INC.   800-964-5227
1500 Waukegan Road, McGaw Park, IL 60085   847-578-2325
FDA Number: 1423507
Web site: www.cardinal.com
Ownership: Cardinal Health Inc.
Stock Symbol: CAH
Traded On: NYSE
Produces/Sells CE-marked Devices: N

CARDINAL HEALTH 200, INC.   913-451-0880
1550 Northwestern Dr., El Paso, TX 79912
FDA Number: 3004932373
Web site: www.cardinal.com
Ownership: Cardinal Health Inc.
Stock Symbol: CAH
Traded On: NYSE
Produces/Sells CE-marked Devices: N
Bandage, Liquid   Surgery

CARDINAL HEALTH 200, LLC   847-785-3323
500 Neelytown Rd, Montgomery, NY 12549
FDA Number: 1319736
Web site: www.cardinal.com
Ownership: Cardinal Health Inc.
Stock Symbol: CAH
Traded On: NYSE
Produces/Sells CE-marked Devices: N
Catheter, Suction (Tracheal Aspirating Tube)   Anesthesiology

CARDINAL HEALTH 203, INC   763-398-8305
17400 Medina Road, Suite 100, Minneapolis, MN 55447
FDA Number: 2031702
Web site: www.cardinal.com
Ownership: Cardinal Health Inc.
Stock Symbol: CAH
Traded On: NYSE
Produces/Sells CE-marked Devices: N
Ventilator, Continuous (Respirator)   Anesthesiology

CARDINAL HEALTH 203, INC   763-398-8305
3555 Holly Lane, Suite 65, Minneapolis, MN 55447
FDA Number: n/a
Web site: www.cardinal.com
Ownership: Cardinal Health Inc.
Stock Symbol: CAH
Traded On: NYSE
Produces/Sells CE-marked Devices: N

CARDINAL HEALTH 203, INC.   763-398-8305
1016 East Cooley Dr, Suite N, Colton, CA 92324
FDA Number: 3005016214
Web site: www.cardinal.com
Ownership: Cardinal Health Inc.
Stock Symbol: CAH
Traded On: NYSE
Produces/Sells CE-marked Devices: N

CARDINAL HEALTH 207, INC   760-778-7255
8822 Flower Road, Suite 140, Rancho Cucamonga, CA 91730
FDA Number: 3006346857
Web site: www.cardinal.com
Ownership: Cardinal Health Inc.
Stock Symbol: CAH
Traded On: NYSE
Produces/Sells CE-marked Devices: N

CARDINAL HEALTH 207, INC.   610-862-0800
1100 Bird Center Dr., Palm Springs, CA 92262
FDA Number: 2021710
Web site: www.cardinal.com
Ownership: Cardinal Health Inc.
Stock Symbol: CAH
Produces/Sells CE-marked Devices: N
Circuit, Breathing (W Connector, Adapter, Y Piece)   Anesthesiology
Compressor, Air, Portable   Anesthesiology
Computer, Pulmonary Function Data   Anesthesiology
Computer, Pulmonary Function, Predicted Values   Anesthesiology
Hood, Oxygen, Infant   General
Humidifier, Respiratory Gas, (Direct Patient Interface)   Anesthesiology
Mask, Oxygen, Non-Rebreathing   Anesthesiology

CARDINAL HEALTH 207, INC.   610-862-0800 *(cont'd)*
Mixer, Breathing Gases, Anesthesia Inhalation   Anesthesiology
Monitor, Ventilatory Frequency   Anesthesiology
Plethysmograph, Volume   Anesthesiology
Recorder, Ventilatory Effort   Anesthesiology
Regulator, Pressure, Gas Cylinder   Anesthesiology
Spirometer, Monitoring (Volumeter)   Anesthesiology
Valve, Non-Rebreathing   Anesthesiology
Ventilator, Continuous (Respirator)   Anesthesiology
Ventilator, Non-Continuous (Respirator)   Anesthesiology

CARDINAL HEALTH 207, INC.
See CAREFUSION 211, INC..

CARDINAL HEALTH 208, INC.
See Corpak Medsystems, Inc.

CARDINAL HEALTH 2200, INC   847-578-6442
17820 Englewood Dr, Cleveland, OH 44130
FDA Number: 1526531
Web site: www.cardinal.com
Ownership: Cardinal Health Inc.
Stock Symbol: CAH
Traded On: NYSE
Produces/Sells CE-marked Devices: N
Tray, Surgical Instrument   Surgery
Wrap, Sterilization   General

CARDINAL HEALTH 2200, INC   847-578-6610
400 East Foster Rd, Mannford, OK 74044
FDA Number: 1625685
Web site: www.cardinal.com
Ownership: Cardinal Health Inc.
Stock Symbol: CAH
Traded On: NYSE
Produces/Sells CE-marked Devices: N
Biopsy Instrument   Gastroenterology/Urology
Catheter, Peritoneal Dialysis, Single-Use   Gastroenterology/Urology
Kit, Biopsy Needle   Gastroenterology/Urology
Needle, Hypodermic, Single Lumen With Syringe   General
Suction Apparatus, Single Patient, Portable, Non-Powered   Surgery
Tray, Surgical   Surgery

CARDINAL HEALTH 2200, INC   847-578-6442
5 Sunnen Dr, Maplewood, MO 63143
FDA Number: 1923569
Web site: www.cardinal.com
Ownership: Cardinal Health Inc.
Stock Symbol: CAH
Traded On: NYSE
Produces/Sells CE-marked Devices: N
Cannula, Catheter   Cardiovascular
Clamp, Vascular   Cardiovascular
Trocar, Other   General

CARDINAL HEALTH 2200, INC   847-578-6442
6215 Ferris Square, Suite 100, San Diego, CA 92121
FDA Number: 3006186449
Web site: www.cardinal.com
Ownership: Cardinal Health Inc.
Stock Symbol: CAH
Traded On: NYSE
Produces/Sells CE-marked Devices: N
Endoscope   Gastroenterology/Urology
Laparoscope, General & Plastic Surgery   Surgery

CARDINAL HEALTH 303, INC   800-854-7128
10020 Pacific Mesa Blvd, San Diego, CA 92121   858-458-7000
FDA Number: 2016493   *Fax:* 858-458-7760
Web site: www.cardinal.com
Ownership: Cardinal Health Inc.
Stock Symbol: CAH
Traded On: NYSE
Produces/Sells CE-marked Devices: N
Analyzer, Gas, Carbon-Dioxide, Gaseous Phase (Capnograph)   Anesthesiology
Cabinet, Table And Tray, Anesthesia   Anesthesiology
Kit, Blood, Transfusion   General
Thermometer, Electronic   General

CARDINAL HEALTH 303, INC
See CareFusion MANUFACTURING LLC

CARDINAL HEALTH 303, INC.   571-521-8907
12120 Sunset Hills Road, 3rd Floor, Reston, VA 20190
FDA Number: 3003560006
Web site: www.cardinal.com
Ownership: Cardinal Health Inc.
Stock Symbol: CAH
Traded On: NYSE
Produces/Sells CE-marked Devices: N
Computer, Chemistry Analyzer   Chemistry

CARDINAL HEALTH 303, INC.
Software, Blood Bank (Stand-Alone Products) — 571-521-8907 *(cont'd)*
Hematology

CARDINAL HEALTH 303,INC.
1515 Ivac Way, Creedmoor, NC 27522 — 858-458-7830
FDA Number: 1034172
Web site: www.cardinal.com
Ownership: Cardinal Health Inc.
Stock Symbol: CAH
Traded On: NYSE
Produces/Sells CE-marked Devices: N
General Admin.: Mr. George Barrett/Chairman, Chief Executive Officer
    Ms. Carole Watkins/Chief Human Resources
    Ms. PAtricia Morrison/Chief Information Officer
    Mr. Craig Morford/Chief Legal Officer
    Mr. Mark Blake/Executive Vice President
    Ms. Shelley Bird/Executive Vice President
    Ms. Lisa Ashby/President
    Mr. Jeffery Scott/Senior Vice President & General Manager,
Central Lab
Mktg./Adv.: Mr. Tony Caprio/Executive Vice President Sales
Finance: Mr. Jeff Henderson/Chief Financial Officer

Accessories, Pump, Infusion	General
Kit, Administration, Intravenous	General
Monitor, Blood Pressure, Indirect, Semi-Automatic	Cardiovascular
Set, Administration, Intravenous, Needle-Free	General
Stopcock	General
Syringe, Piston	General
Thermometer, Electronic	General
Thermometer, Electronic, Continuous	General
Transfer Unit, IV Fluid	General

CARDINAL HEALTH INC.
7000 Cardinal Place, q&r department, Dublin, OH 43017 — 614-757-5000
FDA Number: 3004008697
Web site: www.cardinal.com
Annual Revenue: More than $1 Billion
Year Founded: 1971
Total Employees: 41300
Ownership: Public
Stock Symbol: CAH
Traded On: NYSE
Produces/Sells CE-marked Devices: N
General Admin.: Mr. George Barrett/Chief Executive Officer, Chairman
Mktg./Adv.: Ms. Shelley Bird/Vice President Public Affairs
Production: Mr. Mike Duffy/Executive Vice President Operations
Finance: Mr. Jeff Henderson/Chief Financial Officer
Medical Product Subsidiaries (Listed Separately)
CARDINAL HEALTH 200, LLC
Cardinal Health
Cardinal Health 200, Inc
Cardinal Health 200, Inc.
Cardinal Health 203, Inc
Cardinal Health 203, Inc.
Cardinal Health 207, Inc
Cardinal Health 207, Inc.
Cardinal Health 2200, Inc
Cardinal Health 303, Inc
Cardinal Health 303, Inc.
Cardinal Health 303,Inc.
Cardinal Health Manufacturing Llc
Cardinal Healthcare 209, Inc.
CareFusion 2200, Inc.,
CareFusion MANUFACTURING LLC
Corpak Medsystems, Inc.
Nitric Bio, Inc.

CARDINAL HEALTH MANUFACTURING LLC
3750 Torrey View Court, San Diego, CA 92130 — 858-617-5889
FDA Number: n/a
Web site: www.cardinal.com
Ownership: Cardinal Health Inc.
Stock Symbol: CAH
Traded On: NYSE
Produces/Sells CE-marked Devices: N

CARDINAL HEALTH MANUFACTURING LLC
See CARDINAL HEALTH 200, LLC

CARDINAL HEALTH, SNOWDEN PENCER PRODUCTS
See CareFusion 2200, Inc.,

CARDINAL HEALTH-MEDICAL PRODUCTS AND SERVICES
See CARDINAL HEALTH 200, LLC

CARDINAL HEALTHCARE 209, INC.
5225 Verona Rd., Madison, WI 53711-4495 — 610-862-0800
FDA Number: 2126317
Ownership: Cardinal Health Inc.
Stock Symbol: CAH

CARDINAL HEALTHCARE 209, INC.
610-862-0800 *(cont'd)*
Traded On: NYSE
Produces/Sells CE-marked Devices: N

Amplifier, Physiological Signal	Cns/Neurology
Analyzer, Spectrum, EEG Signal	Cns/Neurology
Audiometer	Ear/Nose/Throat
Biofeedback Device	Cns/Neurology
Calibrator, Hearing-Aid/Earphone And Analysis Systems	Ear/Nose/Throat
Cannula, Suction, Uterine	Obstetrics/Gynecology
Computer, Blood Pressure	Cardiovascular
Electrocardiograph, Single Channel	Cardiovascular
Electrode, Corneal	Ophthalmology
Electrode, Cortical	Cns/Neurology
Electrode, Cutaneous	Cns/Neurology
Electrode, Depth	Cns/Neurology
Electrode, Nasopharyngeal	Cns/Neurology
Electrode, Needle	Cns/Neurology
Electrode, Needle, Diagnostic Electromyograph	Physical Med
Electroencephalograph	Cns/Neurology
Electromyograph, Diagnostic	Physical Med
Flowmeter, Blood, Intravenous	Cardiovascular
Image Processing System	Radiology
Monitor, Blood Flow, Ultrasonic	Obstetrics/Gynecology
Monitor, Fetal, Ultrasonic	Obstetrics/Gynecology
Monitor, Fetal, Ultrasonic, Heart Rate	Obstetrics/Gynecology
Monitor, Fetal, Ultrasonic, Heart Sound	Obstetrics/Gynecology
Monitor, Perinatal	Obstetrics/Gynecology
Monitor, Ultrasonic, Non-Fetal	Radiology
Photostimulator, AC-Powered	Ophthalmology
Plethysmograph, Photo-Electric, Pneumatic Or Hydraulic	Cardiovascular
Scanner, Ultrasonic (Pulsed Doppler)	Radiology
Scanner, Ultrasonic (Pulsed Echo)	Radiology
Sleep Assessment Equipment	Cns/Neurology
Stethoscope, Electronic (Auscultoscope)	Cardiovascular
Stimulator, Auditory, Evoked Response	Cns/Neurology
Stimulator, Electrical, Evoked Response	Cns/Neurology
Stimulator, Nerve, ENT	Ear/Nose/Throat
Stimulator, Photic, Evoked Response	Cns/Neurology
Telemetry Unit, Physiological, Neurological	Cns/Neurology
Tester, Auditory Impedance	Ear/Nose/Throat
Transducer, Ultrasonic	Cardiovascular
Transducer, Ultrasonic, Diagnostic	Radiology

CARDINAL MEDICAL SPECIALTIES, INC.
4708 Pinewood Rd., Louisville, KY 40218 — 502-969-9652
FDA Number: 3002864976
Ownership: Private
Produces/Sells CE-marked Devices: N

Absorber, Carbon-Dioxide	Anesthesiology
Gas-Machine, Anesthesia	Anesthesiology

CARDINAL SCALE MANUFACTURING CO.
See Detecto Scale Co.

CARDINAL SCALE MFG. CO.
203 East Daugherty, Box 151,
Webb City, MO 64870 — 800-641-2008 / 417-673-4631
FDA Number: 1929045
Fax: 417-673-5001
E-mail: detecto@cardet.com
Web site: www.detectoscale.com
Year Founded: 1950
Ownership: CARDINAL HEALTH
Quality System Registration Information: ISO9002
Produces/Sells CE-marked Devices: N
Distribution: Manufacturer Through Manufacturer Reps

Scale, Infant	General
Scale, Platform, Wheelchair	Physical Med
Scale, Stand-On	General

Medical Product Subsidiaries (Listed Separately)
Detecto Scale Co.

CARDIO CATH INC.
See Origen Biomedical, Inc.

CARDIO COMMAND, INC.
4920 W. Cypress St., Suite 110,
Tampa, FL 33607 — 800-231-6370 / 813-289-5555
FDA Number: n/a
Fax: 813-289-5454
E-mail: jmaass@cardiocommand.com
Web site: www.cardiocommand.com
Medical Products Sales Volume: $2,800,000
Annual Revenue: $0-$1 Million
Year Founded: 1988
Total Employees: 17   *Marketing Staff:* 1
Ownership: Private
Produces/Sells CE-marked Devices: N
Federal Procurement Eligibility: Small Business
Distribution: Manufacturer Through Distributor, Manufacturer Through Manufacturer Reps
General Admin.: Al Williams/Chief Operating Officer, Vice President
    Maynard Ramsey/President, Chief Executive Officer

CARDIO COMMAND, INC.   800-231-6370 *(cont'd)*

Production: Jack Samorajczyk/Manager Regulatory Affairs
Research: Maynard Ramsey/Chief Scientist
   Darryl Parmet/Director Research & Development

Electrode, Electrocardiograph	Cardiovascular
Electrode, Esophageal	Gastroenterology/Urology
Electrode, Pacemaker, External	Cardiovascular
Pacemaker, Heart, External	Cardiovascular
Stethoscope, Esophageal, With Electrical Conductors	Anesthesiology

CARDIO SYSTEMS, INC.
See Asi Medical Equipment, Ltd.

CARDIO-DYNAMICS INC.
See Clinical Data Inc

CARDIO-NEF, S.A. DE C.V.   800-024-0240
Rio Grijalva 186, Col. Mitras Norte,   **52 81 8371 2340**
Monterrey, N.L. 64320 Mexico
FDA Number: n/a   *Fax:* 52 81 8373 4009
E-mail: v.gonzalez@prodigy.net.mx
Web site: www.cardionef.com
Medical Products Sales Volume: $1,500,000
Year Founded: 1991
Total Employees: 17   *Marketing Staff:* 2   *Sales Staff:* 10
Ownership: Private
Quality System Registration Information: ISO9002
Produces/Sells CE-marked Devices: Y
Federal Procurement Eligibility: Small Business
Distribution: Service Direct, Exclusive Distributor, Importer

CARDIO-PULMONARY INST. CO.
See CAREFUSION 211, INC..

CARDIO-VASCULAR SALES   888-287-8700
27111 Aliso Creek Rd., Ste. 130,   **949-448-0609**
Aliso Viejo, CA 92656
FDA Number: n/a   *Fax:* 949-448-0626
E-mail: chrisW@cvsales.net
Web site: www.cvsales.com
Medical Products Sales Volume: $10,000,000
Annual Revenue: $5-$10 Million
Year Founded: 1992
Total Employees: 20   *Marketing Staff:* 2   *Sales Staff:* 7
Ownership: Private
Quality System Registration Information: ISO9001
Produces/Sells CE-marked Devices: N
Federal Procurement Eligibility: Small Business
Distribution: Manufacturer Direct, Importer, Exporter
General Admin.: Mr. Chase Thompson/Chief Operating Officer
   Mr. Kirk Foate/General Manager
   Mr. Bill Ward/Manager
   Chris Walker/President, CTO
Mktg./Adv.: Chris Walker/Director Marketing
   Mr. Jonathan Ames/Director Marketing
   Nal Aronson/Manager International & National Sales
   Ms. Arlana Franklin/Manager Training
Production: Tom Smith/Director Materials
   Eryn Thompson/Director Quality Assurance
   Bill Ward/Director Services
   Bob Thomas/Director Services
Finance: Ms. Jennifer Thompson/Controller

Service, Used Equipment	General

CARDIOANALYSIS SYSTEMS
See Lifeclinic International, Inc.

CARDIOBEAT.COM   480-419-3957
Suite 118, Box 210, 29834 North Cave Creek Road,
Cave Creek,, AZ 85331
FDA Number: 3005503665
E-mail: gmcbride@CardiolertSystems.com
Web site: www.cardiolertsystems.com
Ownership: Private
Produces/Sells CE-marked Devices: N

Plethysmograph, Impedance	Cardiovascular

CARDIOCOM LLC   888-243-8881
7980 Century Blvd., Chanhassen, MN 55317   **952-361-6467**
FDA Number: 3004954267   *Fax:* 888-320-8881
E-mail: info@cardiocom.com
Web site: www.cardiocom.com
Year Founded: 1997
Ownership: Private
Produces/Sells CE-marked Devices: N

Computer, Chemistry Analyzer	Chemistry
Monitor, Blood Pressure, Indirect, Semi-Automatic	Cardiovascular
Scale, Stand-On	General
System, Test, Blood Glucose, Over-The-Counter	Chemistry

CARDIOCONTROL, INC.   973-340-8000
101425 Overseas Hwy, P.O. Box 615, Key Largo, FL 33037
FDA Number: n/a   *Fax:* 973-340-5522
E-mail: sales@ekgcharts.com
Web site: www.ekgcharts.com
Medical Products Sales Volume: $3,000,000
Annual Revenue: $1-$5 Million
Ownership: Private
Produces/Sells CE-marked Devices: N
Federal Procurement Eligibility: Small Business
Distribution: Manufacturer Through Distributor

Paper, Recording, ECG/EEG	General

CARDIODATA
See Mortara Instrument, Inc.

CARDIODX   650-475-2788
2500 Faber Place, Palo Alto, CA 94303
FDA Number: n/a   *Fax:* 650-475-2799
E-mail: info@cardiodx.com
Web site: www.cardiodx.com
Ownership: Private
Produces/Sells CE-marked Devices: N
General Admin.: Dr. Steven Rosenberg/Chief Scientific Officer
   Mr. David Levison/President, Chief Executive Officer
Medical Admin.: Dr. Mark Monane/Chief Medical Officer
Mktg./Adv.: Mr. Eric Sandberg/Vice President Sales
Finance: Mr. Andrew Guggenhime/Chief Financial Officer

CARDIODYNAMICS INTERNATIONAL CORP.   888-482-9449
21919 30th Drive SE, Bothell, WA 98021   **425-951-1200**
FDA Number: 2022575
E-mail: customer-service@cardiodynamics.com
Web site: www.cardiodynamics.com
Medical Products Sales Volume: $30,300,000
Annual Revenue: $25-$50 Million
Year Founded: 1980
Total Employees: 151   *Marketing Staff:* 6   *Sales Staff:* 50
Ownership: Sonosite, Inc.
Stock Symbol: CDIC
Traded On: NASDAQ
Quality System Registration Information: ISO9001
Produces/Sells CE-marked Devices: Y
Federal Procurement Eligibility: Small Business, GSA Contract, VA Contract
Distribution: Manufacturer Direct, Manufacturer Through Distributor, OEM, Exporter
General Admin.: Michael Perry/Chief Executive Officer
   Richard Trayler/Chief Operating Officer
   Rhonda Rhyne/President
Mktg./Adv.: Paul Jansen/Director Marketing
   Ashlee Gora/Manager Advertising
   Matt Borer/Manager Market Research
   Matt Barer/Manager Sales Training
   Pat Bradley/Vice President Business Development
Production: Norma Karbasi/Manager Materials
   Brian Park/Manager Regulatory Affairs
   Russ Berger/Vice President Manufacturing
Research: Dennis Hepp/Vice President Research & Development

Monitor, Hemodynamic	Anesthesiology

CARDIOFOCUS INC.   (508) 658-7200
500 Nickerson Road, Suite 500-200, Marlborough, MA 01752
FDA Number: 1225698   *Fax:* (508) 480-0600
E-mail: information@cardiofocus.com
Web site: www.cardiofocus.com
Ownership: Private
Produces/Sells CE-marked Devices: N

Laser, Surgical	Surgery
Lens, Surgical, Laser	Ophthalmology

CARDIOFOCUS, INC.   508-658-7200
500 Nickerson Road, Suite 500-200, Marlborough, MA 01752
FDA Number: n/a   *Fax:* 508-480-0600
E-mail: information@cardiofocus.com
Web site: www.cardiofocus.com
Annual Revenue: $0-$1 Million
Total Employees: 26
Ownership: Private
Quality System Registration Information: ISO9001
Produces/Sells CE-marked Devices: N
Federal Procurement Eligibility: Small Business
Distribution: Manufacturer Direct, Exporter
General Admin.: Jeff Arnold/President, Chief Executive Officer
Production: Mark Olsen/Vice President Operations
   Burke Barrett/Vice President Regulatory & Clinical Affairs
IS: Edward L. Sinofsky/Chief Tech. Manager

Accessories, Laser	General

CARDIOFOCUS, INC. 508-658-7200 *(cont'd)*
Probe, Other General

CARDIOGENICS INC. 905-673-8501
6295 Northam Drive, Unit 8, Mississauga, ON L4V 1W8
FDA Number: n/a
E-mail: info@cardiogenics.com
Web site: www.cardiogenics.com
Year Founded: 1997
Ownership: Private
Produces/Sells CE-marked Devices: N
General Admin.: Dr. Yahia Gawad/Chief Executive Officer
　　　　　Ms. Linda Sterling/Corporate Counsel
Finance: Mr. James Essex/Chief Financial Officer

CARDIOGRAPHICS
See Precision Charts, Inc.

CARDIOINSIGHT TECHNOLOGIES INC. 216-453-5950
11000 Cedar Avenue, Suite 210, Cleveland, OH 44106
FDA Number: n/a
E-mail: info@CardioInsight.com
Web site: www.ecgimaging.com
Year Founded: 2006
Ownership: Private
Produces/Sells CE-marked Devices: N
General Admin.: Mr. Steve Arless/Chairman, Chief Executive Officer
Production: Ms. Christina Vacca/Vice President Quality Control & Regulatory Affairs
Research: Dr. Charu Ramanathan/Vice President Clinical Development
　　　　　Dr. Harold Wodlinger/Vice President Product Development
Finance: Mr. Kevin Mendelsohn/Vice President Finance

CARDIOINTEGRAPH, INC.
See Ocg Technology, Inc.

CARDIOMAG IMAGING, INC. 518-381-1000
450 Duane Ave., Schenectady, NY 12304
FDA Number: 3004786036
E-mail: contact@cardiomag.com *Fax:* 518-381-4400
Web site: www.cardiomag.com
Year Founded: 1999
Ownership: Private
Produces/Sells CE-marked Devices: N
General Admin.: Mr. Carl Rosner/Chairman, Chief Executive Officer
Electrocardiograph, Single Channel Cardiovascular

CARDIOMED SUPPLIES INC. 800-387-9757
199 Saint David Street, 705-328-2518
Lindsay, ONT K9V5K Canada
FDA Number: 8020347
E-mail: mail@cardiomed.com
Web site: www.cardiomed.com
Medical Products Sales Volume: $7,000,000
Year Founded: 1979
Total Employees: 25 *Marketing Staff:* 2 *Sales Staff:* 8
Ownership: Cardiomed Supplies Inc.
Quality System Registration Information: ISO9001
Produces/Sells CE-marked Devices: Y
Federal Procurement Eligibility: Small Business
Distribution: Manufacturer Through Distributor, Exclusive Distributor

CARDIOMEDICS, INC. 888-849-0200
7 Whatney, Suite B, Irvine, CA 92618-2849 (949) 598-2900
FDA Number: 2025845 *Fax:* (949) 598-2999
E-mail: info@cardiomedics.com
Web site: www.cardiomedics.com
Ownership: Private
Produces/Sells CE-marked Devices: N
Monitor, Cardiopulmonary Level Sensing Cardiovascular
Monitor, ECG Cardiovascular
Pump, Counterpulsating, External Cardiovascular

CARDIOMEMS, INC. 866-240-3335
387 Technology Circle NW, Suite 500, 678-651-2300
Atlanta, GA 30313
FDA Number: 3004936110
E-mail: info@cardiomems.com
Web site: www.cardiomems.com
Ownership: Private
Produces/Sells CE-marked Devices: N
General Admin.: Dr. Jay S. Yadav/Chairman, Chief Executive Officer
　　　　　Sandeep S. Yadav/Chief Operating Officer
　　　　　Dr. Mark G. Allen/Chief Technology Officer
Mktg./Adv.: Mr. Kevin Corcoran/Vice President Marketing
Finance: Daniel H. Bauer, CPA/Chief Financial Officer
Sensor, Pressure, Aneurysm, Implantable Cardiovascular

CARDIONET 888-312-BEAT
227 Washington Street, #300, Conshohocken, PA 19428
FDA Number: n/a *Fax:* 610-828-8048
E-mail: info@cardionet.com
Web site: www.cardionet.com
Ownership: Private
Produces/Sells CE-marked Devices: N
General Admin.: Mr. Joseph Capper/President, Chief Executive Officer
Mktg./Adv.: Mr. Dan Wisniewski/Senior Vice President Business Development
　　　　　Mr. Matthew Margolies/Senior Vice President Marketing
　　　　　Mr. Andy Broadyway/Vice President Marketing
Research: Mr. Charles Gropper/Senior Vice President Research & Development
Finance: Ms. Heather Getz/Chief Financial Officer
Detector, Arrhythmia Alarm Cardiovascular
Electrocardiograph, Ambulatory (With Analysis Algorithm) Cardiovascular

CARDIONICS, INC. 800-364-5901
910 Bay Star Blvd., Webster, TX 77598 281-488-5901
FDA Number: 1629623 *Fax:* 281-488-3195
E-mail: info@cardionics.com
Web site: www.cardionics.com
Medical Products Sales Volume: $1,750,000
Annual Revenue: $1-$5 Million
Year Founded: 1980
Ownership: Private
Produces/Sells CE-marked Devices: Y
Federal Procurement Eligibility: Small Business, Female Owned
Distribution: Manufacturer Direct, Manufacturer Through Distributor
Material, Training, Audiovisual General
Monitor, EEG Cns/Neurology
Simulator, ECG Cardiovascular
Simulator, Heart Sound Cardiovascular
Simulator, Lung Anesthesiology
Stethoscope, Amplified General
Stethoscope, Electronic-Amplified Surgery
Training Manikin, Other General
Transmitter/Receiver, Physiological Signal, Infrared Cardiovascular

CARDIOPULMONARY CORP. 203-877-1999
200 Cascade Blvd., Milford, CT 06460
FDA Number: 1225489
Ventilator, Continuous (Respirator) Anesthesiology

CARDIOPULMONARY INSTRUMENTATION, INC. 305-592-8196
3002 N.w. 79th Avenue, Miami, FL 33122
FDA Number: 1034275 *Fax:* 305-593-5056
E-mail: cardio@cpiinst.com
Web site: www.cpiinst.com
Medical Products Sales Volume: $1,600,000
Year Founded: 1976
Total Employees: 12
Ownership: Private
Produces/Sells CE-marked Devices: N
Federal Procurement Eligibility: Small Business

CARDIOSOFT, L.P. 713-623-4009
1776 Yorktown, Suite LI-30, Houston, TX 77056
FDA Number: 3003786840
Ownership: Private
Produces/Sells CE-marked Devices: N
Electrocardiograph, Single Channel Cardiovascular

CARDIOSOLUTIONS INC. 781-344-0801
75 Mill St., Stoughton, MA 02072
FDA Number: n/a *Fax:* 781-344-0803
E-mail: info@cardiosolutionsinc.com
Web site: www.cardiosolutionsinc.com
Year Founded: 2006
Ownership: Private
Produces/Sells CE-marked Devices: N
General Admin.: Ross Garofalo/Chief Financial Officer, Vice President
　　　　　Jon Wilson/Chief Operating Officer
　　　　　Steven Tallarida/President
Medical Admin.: Dr. Thomas Piemonte/Medical Director
Production: Chris Maurer/Director Engineering
Finance: Ron Murphy/Vice President Public Communications & Investor Relations

CARDIOSTREAM, LLC 770-457-5337
12600 Deerfield Parkway, Ste. 100, Alpharetta, GA 30004
FDA Number: 3005393814 *Fax:* 678-623-0439
E-mail: info@cardiostream.com
Web site: www.cardiostream.com
Ownership: Private
Produces/Sells CE-marked Devices: N

CARDIOTECH INTERNATIONAL, INC.
See Advansource Biomaterials Corp.

CARDIOTRONICS INC.   1-866-932-1702
5025 Sherbrooke St. W.,, Suite 660,   514-932-1702
Westmount, QUE H4A 1 Canada
FDA Number: n/a   Fax: 514-486-3866
E-mail: info@cardiotronics.ca
Web site: www.meditech.net
Year Founded: 1995
Total Employees: 10
Ownership: MEDITECH LTD., BUDAPEST, HUNGARY
Produces/Sells CE-marked Devices: N
Distribution: Service Direct, Exclusive Distributor

CARDIOVASCULAR DYNAMICS
See Endologix, Inc.

CARDIOVASCULAR IMAGING   816-531-2842
TECHNOLOGIES, LLC
4320 Wornall Rd., Suite 55, Kansas City, MO 64111
FDA Number: 3004504920   Fax: 816-531-0643
E-mail: scourter@cvit.com
Web site: www.cvit.com
Ownership: Private
Produces/Sells CE-marked Devices: N
Scanner, Emission Computed Tomography   Radiology

CARDIOVASCULAR RESEARCH, INC.   813-832-6222
4810 W. Gandy Blvd., Tampa, FL 33611
FDA Number: n/a   Fax: 813-832-6506
E-mail: cardiovascularrs@aol.com
Web site: www.cardiovascuaarresearch.com
Annual Revenue: $0-$1 Million
Total Employees: 5   *Marketing Staff:* 3   *Sales Staff:* 3
Ownership: Private
Quality System Registration Information: ISO9002
Produces/Sells CE-marked Devices: N
Federal Procurement Eligibility: Small Business
Distribution: Manufacturer Direct, Service Direct, Exporter
General Admin.: Dean M. Razi/President, Chief Executive Officer
  Cameron Dean/Vice President, General Manager
Mktg./Adv.: Neal Jason/Vice President Business Development
Balloon, Angioplasty, Coronary, Heated   Cardiovascular
Camera, Video   General
Cannula, Other   General
Kit, Instruments and Accessories, Surgical   Surgery
Tenaculum, Other (Forceps)   Surgery

CARDIOVASCULAR SYSTEMS INC.
See Sorin Group Usa

CARDIOVASCULAR SYSTEMS, INC.   877-CSI-0360
651 Campus Drive, St. Paul, MN 55112   651-259-1600
FDA Number: 3004742232   Fax: 612-677-3355
E-mail: generalinquiries@csi360.com
Web site: www.csi360.com
Ownership: Private
Produces/Sells CE-marked Devices: N
General Admin.: James E. Flaherty/Chief Administrative Officer
  Robert J. Thatcher/Executive Vice President
  David L. Martin/President, Chief Executive Officer
Mktg./Adv.: Paul Tyska/Vice President Business Development
  Scott Kraus/Vice President Sales
Production: Mr. Paul Koehn/Vice President Manufacturing
  Brian Doughty/Vice President Operations
Finance: Laurence L. Betterley/Chief Financial Officer
Catheter, Peripheral, Atherectomy   Cardiovascular
Introducer, Catheter   Cardiovascular
Tape, Measuring, Ruler And Caliper   Surgery

CARDIOVENTION, INC.   408-873-3400
19200 Stevens Creek Blvd., #200, Cupertino, CA 95014
FDA Number: 3003598413
Ownership: Private
Produces/Sells CE-marked Devices: N
Console, Heart-Lung Machine, Cardiopulmonary Bypass   Cardiovascular
Defoamer, Cardiopulmonary Bypass   Cardiovascular
Heat Exchanger, Heart-Lung Bypass   Cardiovascular
Oxygenator, Cardiopulmonary Bypass   Cardiovascular
Pump, Blood, Cardiopulmonary Bypass, Non-Roller Type   Cardiovascular

CARDIUM THERAPEUTICS INC.   858-436-1000
12255 El Camino Rea, Suite 250, San Diego, CA 92130
FDA Number: n/a   Fax: 858-436-1001
E-mail: investorrelations@cardiumthx.com
Web site: www.cardiumthx.com
Year Founded: 2005
Total Employees: 61
Ownership: Public
Stock Symbol: CXM
Traded On: AMEX

CARDIUM THERAPEUTICS INC.   858-436-1000 *(cont'd)*
Produces/Sells CE-marked Devices: Y
General Admin.: Christopher Reinhard/Chief Executive Officer, Treasurer
  Gabor Rubanyi/Chief Scientific Officer
  Tyler Dylan-Hyde/Executive Vice President
Medical Admin.: Dr. Robert Engler/Chief Medical Officer
Mktg./Adv.: Mark McCutchen/Vice President Business Development
  Ted Williams/Vice President Marketing & Operations
Finance: Dennis Mulroy/Chief Financial Officer
  Ms. Bonnie Ortega/Director Investment & Public Relations
Agent, Hemostatic, Absorbable, Collagen-Based   Surgery
Device, Closure, Puncture, Hemostatic   Cardiovascular

CARDIVA MEDICAL, INC.   650-964-8900
888 W. Maude Avenue, Sunnyvale, CA 94085
FDA Number: 3004182619   Fax: 650-964-8911
E-mail: customerservice@cardivamedical.com
Web site: www.cardivamedical.com
Ownership: Private
Produces/Sells CE-marked Devices: N
General Admin.: Mr. Charles Maroney/President, Chief Executive Officer
  Medical Admin.: Ms. Marlys Chellew/Vice President Clinical Affairs
Mktg./Adv.: Mr. John McCurdy/Vice President Sales
Production: Mr. Justin Ballotta/Vice President Operations
  Mr. Michael Daniel/Vice President Regulatory Affairs
Research: Mr. Zia Yassinzadeh/Vice President Research & Development
Finance: Mr. Macolm Farnsworth/Chief Financial Officer, Vice President Finance
Clamp, Vascular   Cardiovascular

CARDON REHABILITATION PRODUCTS   905-761-7868
8001 Jane St., Unit 1, Concord, ONT L4K-2M7 Canada
FDA Number: n/a   Fax: 905-761-7877
E-mail: sales@cardonrehab.com
Web site: sales@cardonrehab.com
Year Founded: 1977
Ownership: Private
Produces/Sells CE-marked Devices: N
Distribution: Manufacturer Direct, Exclusive Distributor

CARDON REHABILITATION PRODUCTS INC   800-944-7868 x
Wurlitzer Industrial Park   800-944-7868 x2
908 Niagara Falls Blvd.
N.Tonawanda, NY 14120
FDA Number: 8020417   Fax: 716-297-0411
E-mail: sales@cardonrehab.com
Web site: www.cardonrehab.com
Year Founded: 1978
Total Employees: 25   *Marketing Staff:* 5   *Sales Staff:* 5
Ownership: Private
Produces/Sells CE-marked Devices: N
Federal Procurement Eligibility: Small Business
Distribution: Manufacturer Direct, Manufacturer Through Distributor, Exclusive Distributor
General Admin.: Holly J. Cardon/General Manager
  Charles Cardon/President, Chief Executive Officer
Mktg./Adv.: Charles Cardon/Director Marketing
  Charles Cardon/Manager International & National Sales
Production: Chester Lake/Vice President Manufacturing
Equipment, Therapy, Handicapped/Physical   Physical Med
Table, Examination/Treatment   General
Table, Other   General
Table, Physical Therapy   Physical Med
Table, Traction   Orthopedics

CARE APPAREL INDUSTRIES   800-326-6262
127-09 91st Ave., Richmond Hill, NY 11418   718-577-0888
FDA Number: n/a
Web site: www.careapparel.com
Annual Revenue: $5-$10 Million
Ownership: Private
Produces/Sells CE-marked Devices: N
Distribution: Manufacturer Direct, Manufacturer Through Manufacturer Reps
General Admin.: David C. Welner/Chief Executive Officer
Assembly, Thigh/Knee/Shank/Ankle/Foot, External   Physical Med
Cushion, Foot   Orthopedics
Garment, Protective, For Incontinence   Gastroenterology/Urology
Gown, Patient   Surgery

CARE CATALOG SERVICES
See Care Medical Equipment, Inc.

CARE ELECTRONICS, INC.   303-444-2273
4700 Sterling Drive, Suite D, Boulder, CO 80301-2305
FDA Number: 1722392   Fax: 303-447-3502
E-mail: tom@medicalshoponline.com
Web site: www.careelectronics.com
Medical Products Sales Volume: $520,000
Annual Revenue: $1-$5 Million

MANUFACTURER PROFILES

CARE ELECTRONICS, INC. 303-444-2273 *(cont'd)*
Year Founded: 1988
Total Employees: 6   Marketing Staff: 1   Sales Staff: 4
Ownership: Private
Produces/Sells CE-marked Devices: N
Federal Procurement Eligibility: Small Business
Distribution: Manufacturer Direct, Manufacturer Through Distributor, Exporter
General Admin.: Thomas O. Moody/President, Chief Executive Officer
        Bonnie Moody/Vice President, General Manager
Mktg./Adv.: Tom Moody/Manager Contract Sales
        Donna Lewis/Manager International & National Sales
        Merle Gleiforst/Manager Marketing & Sales
        Donna Lewis/Manager Sales Training
Production: Tim Zessin/Director Quality Assurance
        Bonnie Moody/Vice President Operations

Accessories, Wheelchair	Physical Med
Bracelet, Identification	General
Device, Incontinence, Paste-On	Gastroenterology/Urology
Monitor, Bed Occupancy	General
Monitor, Bed Patient	General
Security Equipment/Supplies	General

CARE FUSION 205, INC. 610-862-0800
4153 W. 166th St., Oak Forest, IL 60452
FDA Number: 1424490
Ownership: Private
Produces/Sells CE-marked Devices: N

Tubing, Ventilator	Anesthesiology
Ventilator, Non-Continuous (Respirator)	Anesthesiology

CARE LINE, INC. 800-251-1157
2210 Lake Road, Greenbrier, TN 37073   615-643-4797
FDA Number: 1034116   Fax: 615-643-5728
E-mail: sales@carelineinc.com
Web site: www.carelineinc.com
Medical Products Sales Volume: $24,100,000
Annual Revenue: $25-$50 Million
Year Founded: 1986
Total Employees: 80   Marketing Staff: 5   Sales Staff: 32
Ownership: Private
Produces/Sells CE-marked Devices: N
Federal Procurement Eligibility: Small Business
Distribution: Manufacturer Through Distributor
General Admin.: Mr. David C. Love/Chief Executive Officer
        Mr. John D. Love/President, Chief Operating Officer
Mktg./Adv.: Mr. Don Kusterer/Vice President Sales
        Mr. Tyler Crouch/Vice President Sales
Production: Ms. Becky Hitchens/Manager Customer Services
        Mr. James Love/Vice President Operations, General Manager

Contract Packaging	General
Pillow	General

CARE MEDICAL
See Care Medical Equipment, Inc.

CARE MEDICAL EQUIPMENT, INC. 800-952-9566
1877 NE 7th Avenue, Portland, OR 97212   503-288-8174
FDA Number: 1000127199   Fax: 503-288-8817
E-mail: portland@caremedical.com
Web site: www.caremedical.com
Annual Revenue: $5-$10 Million
Ownership: Private
Produces/Sells CE-marked Devices: N
Federal Procurement Eligibility: Small Business
Distribution: Manufacturer Through Distributor, Importer, Exporter

Garment, Protective, For Incontinence	Gastroenterology/Urology
Lift, Wheelchair	General
Wheelchair, Manual	Physical Med

CARE PRODUCTS INC. 800-445-7345
10701 N. Ware Rd., PO Box 720193,   757-224-0177
Mc Allen, TX 78504
FDA Number: 3004839392   Fax: 800-580-1044
E-mail: info@careproductsinc.com
Web site: www.careproductsinc.com
Ownership: Private
Produces/Sells CE-marked Devices: N

Basin, Emesis	General
Cart, Emergency, Cardiopulmonary Resuscitation (Crash)	Anesthesiology
Chair, Adjustable, Mechanical	Physical Med
Chair, Geriatric	General
Chair, With Casters	Physical Med
Device, Anti-Tip, Wheelchair	Physical Med
Stretcher, Wheeled (Mobile)	General
Walker, Mechanical	Physical Med

CARE REHAB AND ORTHOPAEDIC 703-448-9644
PRODUCTS, INC.
3930 Horseshoe Bend Road, Keysville, VA 23947
FDA Number: 1124681
Ownership: Private
Produces/Sells CE-marked Devices: N

Biofeedback Device	Cns/Neurology
Component, Traction, Non-Invasive	Orthopedics
Exerciser, Powered	Anesthesiology
Stimulator, Muscle, Electrical-Powered (EMS)	Physical Med
Stimulator, Nerve, Transcutaneous (Pain Relief, TENS)	Cns/Neurology
Stimulator, Transcutaneous Electrical, For Cosmetic Use	Cns/Neurology
Unit, Therapy, Current, Interferential	Cns/Neurology

CARE WARE DESIGNS FOR ACTIVE LIVING 800-261-5552
P.O. Box 48111, RPO Lakewood,   204-254-8296
Winnipeg, MAN R2J-4 Canada
FDA Number: n/a   Fax: 204-253-3495
E-mail: mcelhoes@mts.net
Web site: http://www.mts.net/~mcelhoes/cw8.htm
Year Founded: 1994
Total Employees: 10
Ownership: Private
Produces/Sells CE-marked Devices: N
Distribution: Manufacturer Direct, Exclusive Distributor

CARE WISE MEDICAL PRODUCTS CORP. 888-462-8725
P.O. Box 1655, Morgan Hill, CA 95037   408-779-5531
FDA Number: 2939478   Fax: 408-779-3185
E-mail: marketing@carewise.com
Web site: www.carewise.com
Ownership: Private
Produces/Sells CE-marked Devices: Y
Federal Procurement Eligibility: Small Business
Distribution: Manufacturer Direct, Manufacturer Through Distributor, Manufacturer Through Manufacturer Reps, Exporter
General Admin.: Ms. Ann Wise/General Counsel
        Robin Wise/President, Chief Executive Officer
Mktg./Adv.: Mrs. Rhonda Butler/Vice President Sales
Production: Mr. Tom Frazier/Director Operations

Instrument, Manual, General Surgical	Surgery
Kit, Instruments and Accessories, Surgical	Surgery
Probe, Other	General
Probe, Uptake, Nuclear	Radiology

CARE-TEK 888-879-3746
5012 Lakeshore Rd.,   905-634-6975
Burllington, ONT L7L-4 Canada
FDA Number: n/a   Fax: 905-634-1262
E-mail: info@caretek.on.ca
Web site: www.caretek.com
Year Founded: 1993
Total Employees: 10
Ownership: Private
Produces/Sells CE-marked Devices: N
Distribution: Exclusive Distributor

CARECENTRIC, INC. 800-441-2331
2839 Paces Ferry Road, Suite 900,   678-264-4400
Atlanta, GA 33039
FDA Number: n/a   Fax: 770-384-1650
E-mail: info@carecentric.com
Web site: www.carecentric.com
Year Founded: 1996
Total Employees: 158   Marketing Staff: 3   Sales Staff: 17
Ownership: Private
Produces/Sells CE-marked Devices: N
Federal Procurement Eligibility: Small Business
Distribution: Manufacturer Direct
General Admin.: H. Darrell Young/Chief Executive Officer
        David Dasinger/Senior Vice President Software Development
        Gene Weiland/Vice President Information Technology
Mktg./Adv.: Richk Sackett/Sales Representative
        Terry McGuire/Sales Representative
        Ralph Capasso/Senior Vice President Sales
Finance: Stephen Shea/Chief Financial Officer

Computer, Patient Data Management	General

CAREFUSION 211, INC.. 800-231-2466
22745 Savi Ranch Pkwy.,   714-283-2228
Yorba Linda, CA 92887
FDA Number: 2050001   Fax: 714-283-8493
E-mail: productinfo.eur@sensormedics.com
Web site: www.viasyshealthcare.com
Medical Products Sales Volume: $23,000,000
Annual Revenue: $50-$100 Million
Year Founded: 2001

CAREFUSION 211, INC.. 800-231-2466 *(cont'd)*

Total Employees: 230   *Marketing Staff:* 10   *Sales Staff:* 30
Ownership: CARDINAL HEALTH, INC.
Stock Symbol: CAH
Traded On: NYSE
Quality System Registration Information: ISO9001
Produces/Sells CE-marked Devices: Y
Distribution: Manufacturer Through Distributor, Manufacturer Through Manufacturer Reps
General Admin.: Randy Thurman/Chief Executive Officer
        Arie Cohen/President
        Michelle Santamuero/Vice President Human Resources
Mktg./Adv.: Kevin Siana/Coord. Marketing
        Gregory C. Gunderson/Director National Accounts
        William Preuit/Vice President International Sales
        Chris Kondo/Vice President Marketing & Product Development
        Arthur B. Gillespie/Vice President Sales
Production: Yvette Lloyd/Manager Regulatory Affairs
        Gary Fulbright/Vice President Manufacturing
Research: Edmund Chu/Vice President Research & Development

Analyzer, Metabolism	Anesthesiology
Analyzer, Pulmonary Function	Anesthesiology
Attachment, Breathing, Positive End Expiratory Pressure	Anesthesiology
Bag, Reservoir (Blood)	Anesthesiology
Catheter, Suction (Tracheal Aspirating Tube)	Anesthesiology
Computer, Pulmonary Function Data	Anesthesiology
Computer, Stress Exercise	Cardiovascular
Condenser, Heat And Moisture (Artificial Nose)	Anesthesiology
Continuous Positive Airway Pressure Unit (CPAP, CPPB)	Anesthesiology
Filter, Bacterial, Breathing Circuit	Anesthesiology
Humidifier, Respiratory Gas, (Direct Patient Interface)	Anesthesiology
Mask, Oxygen, Low Concentration, Venturi	Anesthesiology
Mask, Oxygen, Other	General
Monitor, Airway Pressure, Continuous	Anesthesiology
Nebulizer, Direct Patient Interface	Anesthesiology
Plethysmograph, Pressure (Body)	Anesthesiology
Sensor, Oxygen	Anesthesiology
Sleep Assessment Equipment	Cns/Neurology
Spirometer, Therapeutic (Incentive)	Anesthesiology
Strap, Head, Gas Mask	Anesthesiology
Suction Apparatus, Single Patient, Portable, Non-Powered	Surgery
Treadmill, Powered	Physical Med
Tube, Tracheostomy (W/Wo Connector)	Anesthesiology
Ventilator, Emergency, Manual (Resuscitator)	Anesthesiology
Ventilator, Non-Continuous (Respirator)	Anesthesiology

CAREFUSION 2200, INC., 847-689-8410

5175 South Royal Atlanta Dr., Tucker, GA 30084-3053
FDA Number: 1038548
Web site: www.cardinal.com
Ownership: Cardinal Health Inc.
Stock Symbol: CAH
Traded On: NYSE
Produces/Sells CE-marked Devices: N

Brush, Dermabrasion, Manual	Surgery
Cannula, Suprapubic, With Trocar	Gastroenterology/Urology
Clamp, Bone	Orthopedics
Clip, Aneurysm (Intracranial)	Cns/Neurology
Curette, Surgical	Surgery
Diathermy, Ultrasonic (Physical Therapy)	Physical Med
Dissector, Surgical, General & Plastic Surgery	Surgery
ENT Manual Surgical Instrument	Ear/Nose/Throat
Electrode, Electrosurgical, Return (Ground, Dispersive)	Surgery
Electrosurgical Unit, Cutting & Coagulation Device	Surgery
Elevator, Surgical, General & Plastic Surgery	Surgery
Endoscope	Gastroenterology/Urology
Forceps, General & Plastic Surgery	Surgery
General Use Surgical Scissors	Surgery
Hemostat	Orthopedics
Holder, Needle	Gastroenterology/Urology
Hook, Surgical, General & Plastic Surgery	Surgery
Instrument, Manual, General Surgical	Surgery
Insufflator, Laparoscopic	Obstetrics/Gynecology
Knife, Surgical	Dental And Oral
Laparoscope, General & Plastic Surgery	Surgery
Laparoscope, Gynecologic	Obstetrics/Gynecology
Light Source, Endoscope, Xenon Arc	Surgery
Osteotome, Manual (Plastic Surgery)	Surgery
Rasp, Surgical, General & Plastic Surgery	Surgery
Retractor, Fiberoptic	Gastroenterology/Urology
Retractor, Surgical	Surgery
Screwdriver, Surgical	Surgery
Speculum, Non-Illuminated	Surgery
Tape, Measuring, Ruler And Caliper	Surgery
Tape, Television & Video, Endoscopic	Gastroenterology/Urology

CAREFUSION CORPORATION 888-876-4287

3750 Torrey View Court, San Diego, CA 92130   **858-617-2000**
FDA Number: n/a   *Fax:* 858-617-2900
Web site: http://www.carefusion.com

CAREFUSION CORPORATION 888-876-4287 *(cont'd)*

Ownership: Public
Stock Symbol: CFN
Traded On: NYSE
Produces/Sells CE-marked Devices: N
General Admin.: Mr. Kieran T. Gallahue/Chairman, Chief Executive Officer
        Mr. Dwight Winstead/Chief Operating Officer
Medical Admin.: Dr. Steve Lewis/Chief Medical Officer
Production: Mr. Don Abbey/Senior Vice President Regulatory Affairs
Finance: Mr. Edward Borkowski/Chief Financial Officer

CAREFUSION MANUFACTURING LLC 800-367-9947

3750 Torrey View Court, San Diego, CA 92130   **858-480-6000**
FDA Number: 3003879246   *Fax:* 858-480-6329
Web site: www.cardinal.com
Ownership: Cardinal Health Inc.
Stock Symbol: CAH
Traded On: NYSE
Produces/Sells CE-marked Devices: N

CAREMARK LTD. 888 9096199a__

2785 Skymark Ave., Unit 2,   **905 624 1234a__**
Mississauga, ONT L4W-4 Canada
FDA Number: n/a   *Fax:* 905-629-0123
E-mail: mesterhammer@caremark.ca
Year Founded: 1992
Total Employees: 100
Ownership: Fresenius Ag
Produces/Sells CE-marked Devices: N
Distribution: Manufacturer Direct

CAREMATIX INC. 312-371-3050

120 S. Riverside Plaza, Suite 2100, Chicago, IL 60606
FDA Number: 3003982635

Monitor, Blood Pressure, Indirect, Semi-Automatic	Cardiovascular

CARESTREAM DENTAL LLC 800-944-6365

1765 The Exchange, Atlanta, GA 30339
FDA Number: 1226003
E-mail: practiceworkssupport@kodakdental.com
Web site: www.kodakdental.com
Ownership: Carestream Health, Inc.
Stock Symbol: OCX
Traded On: TSX Venture Exchange
Produces/Sells CE-marked Devices: N
General Admin.: Dr. David Gane/Vice President

Device, Storage, Image, Digital	Radiology
Radiographic Unit, Diagnostic, Dental, Extraoral	Dental And Oral
System, X-ray, Extraoral Source, Digital	Radiology

CARESTREAM HEALTH, INC. 888-777-2072

1 Imation Way, Oakdale, MN 55128
FDA Number: 2133929
E-mail: info@carestreamhealth.com
Web site: www.carestreamhealth.com
Ownership: Carestream Health, Inc.
Stock Symbol: OCX
Traded On: TSX Venture Exchange
Produces/Sells CE-marked Devices: N

Camera, Multi Format	Radiology

CARESTREAM HEALTH, INC. 585-722-4565

1049 West Ridge Road, Rochester, NY 14615
FDA Number: 1317307   *Fax:* 585-722-0160
E-mail: info@carestreamhealth.com
Web site: www.carestreamhealth.com
Ownership: Carestream Health, Inc.
Stock Symbol: OCX
Traded On: TSX Venture Exchange
Produces/Sells CE-marked Devices: N

Accelerator, Linear, Medical	Radiology
Camera, Multi Format	Radiology
Cassette, Radiographic Film	Radiology
Grid, Radiographic	Radiology
Image Digitizer	Radiology
Imager, X-Ray, Solid State (Flat Panel/Digital)	Radiology
Screen, Intensifying, Radiographic	Radiology
Table, Radiographic	Radiology

CARESTREAM HEALTH, INC. 888-777-2072

150 Verona Street, Rochester, NY 14608   **585-627-1800**
FDA Number: 1315356
E-mail: info@carestreamhealth.com
Web site: www.carestreamhealth.com
Annual Revenue: More than $1 Billion
Total Employees: 8000
Ownership: Public
Stock Symbol: OCX

CARESTREAM HEALTH, INC.   888-777-2072 *(cont'd)*
Traded On: TSX Venture Exchange
Produces/Sells CE-marked Devices: N
General Admin.: Mr. Robert M. LeBlanc/Chairman
         Mr. Kevin J. Hobert/Chief Executive Officer
         Mr. Michael C. Pomeroy/Chief Financial Officer, Vice President
         Mr. Bruce D. Leidal/Chief Information Officer
         Ms. Holly M. Hillberg/Chief Technology Officer
         Mr. James M. Quinn/Secretary, General Counsel

Camera, Multi Format	Radiology
Film, X-Ray, Special Purpose	Radiology
System, Communication, Image, Digital	Radiology

Medical Product Subsidiaries (Listed Separately)
Carestream Dental LLC
Carestream Health, Inc.

CARESTREAM HEALTH, INC.   888-777-2072
1669 Lake Ave., Rochester, NY 14652
FDA Number: 1317267
E-mail: info@carestreamhealth.com
Web site: www.carestreamhealth.com
Ownership: Carestream Health, Inc.
Stock Symbol: OCX
Traded On: TSX Venture Exchange
Produces/Sells CE-marked Devices: N

Screen, Intensifying, Radiographic	Radiology

CARESTREAM HEALTH, INC.   888-777-2072
2000 Howard Smith Avenue West, Windsor, CO 80550
FDA Number: 1718432
E-mail: info@carestreamhealth.com
Web site: www.carestreamhealth.com
Ownership: Carestream Health, Inc.
Stock Symbol: OCX
Traded On: TSX Venture Exchange
Produces/Sells CE-marked Devices: N

CARESTREAM HEALTH, INC.   541-831-7222
8124 Pacific Ave., White City, OR 97503
FDA Number: 3029911
E-mail: info@carestreamhealth.com
Web site: www.carestreamhealth.com
Ownership: Carestream Health, Inc.
Stock Symbol: OCX
Traded On: TSX Venture Exchange
Produces/Sells CE-marked Devices: N

CARESTREAM MEDICAL LTD.   888-310-2186
                                       604-552-5486
8800 Dufferin Street,, Suite 201,
Vaughan, ONTAR L4K 0 Canada
FDA Number: n/a   *Fax:* 604-552-5487
E-mail: info@carestream.com
Web site: www.carestream.com
Year Founded: 1998
Total Employees: 10
Ownership: Private
Produces/Sells CE-marked Devices: N
Distribution: Manufacturer Direct, Exclusive Distributor, Importer

CAREX HEALTH BRANDS   800-526-8051
                                       800-526-8051
921 East Amidon St, PO Box 2526,
Sioux Falls, SD 57101
FDA Number: 2182780   *Fax:* 888-616-4297
E-mail: customerservice@carex.com
Web site: http://www.carex.com
Medical Products Sales Volume: $100,000
Annual Revenue: $25-$50 Million
Ownership: Private
Produces/Sells CE-marked Devices: Y
Federal Procurement Eligibility: Small Business
Distribution: Manufacturer Through Distributor, Manufacturer Through Manufacturer Reps, OEM, Importer, Exporter

Care Kit, Baby	General
Container, Medication, Home-Use	General
Dispenser, Medication, Liquid	General
Dropper, Medicine	General
Identification, Alert, Medical	General
Protector, Finger	Orthopedics
Spoon, Medicine	General
Temperature Strip, Forehead, Liquid Crystal	General

CARGILLE LABORATORIES   973-239-6633
55 Commerce Rd., Cedar Grove, NJ 07009-1289
FDA Number: 2210661   *Fax:* 973-239-6096
E-mail: cargillelabs@aol.com
Web site: www.cargille.com
Annual Revenue: $1-$5 Million
Year Founded: 1924

CARGILLE LABORATORIES   973-239-6633 *(cont'd)*
Total Employees: 25   *Marketing Staff:* 2
Ownership: Private
Quality System Registration Information: ISO9001
Produces/Sells CE-marked Devices: N
Federal Procurement Eligibility: Small Business
Distribution: Manufacturer Direct, Manufacturer Through Distributor
Mktg./Adv.: Dorothy Schneider/Manager Advertising
IS: William J. Sacher/Vice President, Tech. Director

Beaker (Laboratory)	Chemistry
Bin, Storage	General
Container, Urine Specimen	General
Indicator Method, Protein Or Albumin (Urinary, Non-Quant.)	Chemistry
Labware, Basic, Disposable	Chemistry
Media, Mounting	Pathology
Oil, Immersion	Hematology
Turbidimetric Method, Protein Or Albumin (Urinary)	Chemistry
Viscometer	Chemistry

CARGOCAIRE ENGINEERING CORP.
See Munters Corp. - Cargocaire Division

CARI-ALL CO.
See Gillis Associated Industries

CARI-ALL INC.   1.888.640.1414
                         514-640-1414
12 425, boul. Industriel,
Montreal, QUE H1B 5 Canada
FDA Number: n/a   *Fax:* 514-645-2661
E-mail: cariall@cari-all.com
Web site: www.cari-all.com
Year Founded: 1969
Total Employees: 100
Ownership: Private
Produces/Sells CE-marked Devices: N
Distribution: Manufacturer Direct, Exporter

CARIDIANBCT INC.   800-525-2623
                         303-232-6800
10810 W. Collins Ave., Lakewood, CO 80215
FDA Number: 1722028   *Fax:* 303-231-4949
E-mail: bob.sullivan@gambrobct.com
Medical Products Sales Volume: $300,000,000
Year Founded: 1964
Total Employees: 2000   *Marketing Staff:* 22   *Sales Staff:* 60
Ownership: Private
Quality System Registration Information: ISO9001
Produces/Sells CE-marked Devices: Y
Distribution: Manufacturer Direct
General Admin.: Teresa Ayers/Chief Operating Officer, Vice President
         David Perez/President
         David Perez/President, Chief Executive Officer
         Bill Mercer/Vice President
         Stacey Klein/Vice President Human Resources
Mktg./Adv.: Bob Sullivan/Director National Sales
         Steve Urdahl/Vice President Business Development
         Bob Cole/Vice President Marketing
         Tom Jordan/Vice President Sales
Production: Craig Rinehardt/Vice President Manufacturing
         Mark Holmes/Vice President Regulatory Affairs
Research: Tim Gordon/Vice President Research & Development
Finance: Taras Skibicky/Chief Financial Officer, Vice President Finance

Autotransfusion Unit (Blood)	Anesthesiology
Bag, Blood, Collection	Hematology
Equipment, Apheresis	Hematology
Separator, Blood Cell, Automated	Hematology
Separator, Blood Cell/Plasma, Therapeutic	Gastroenterology/Urology
Separator, Semi-automated, Blood Component	Hematology
Software, Blood Bank (Stand-Alone Products)	Hematology
Washer, Cell (Frozen Blood Processor)	Hematology

CARING HANDS, INC.   208-691-9524
4347 N Alderbrook Dr, CDA, ID 83815
FDA Number: n/a   *Fax:* 208-691-1020
Web site: http://www.whenyagottago.com
Annual Revenue: $0-$1 Million
Year Founded: 1997
Total Employees: 4   *Sales Staff:* 2
Ownership: Private
Produces/Sells CE-marked Devices: N
Federal Procurement Eligibility: Small Business
Distribution: Manufacturer Direct, Manufacturer Through Distributor, Exporter
General Admin.: Charles W. Robertson/Chief Executive Officer

Collector, Urine	Gastroenterology/Urology

CARL HEYER, INC.   800-284-5550
                         516-783-7800
1872 Bellmore Avenue,
North Bellmore, NY 11710
FDA Number: n/a
E-mail: CarlHeyer@aol.com

CARL HEYER, INC.　800-284-5550 (cont'd)
Web site: www.dexiter.com
Year Founded: 1976
Ownership: Private
Quality System Registration Information: ISO9000
Produces/Sells CE-marked Devices: N
Federal Procurement Eligibility: Small Business
Distribution: Manufacturer Through Distributor

Blade, Scalpel	Surgery
Curette	Orthopedics
Cutter, Operative	Dental And Oral
Dilator, Other	Surgery
Forceps	Orthopedics
General Use Surgical Scissors	Surgery
Glove, Patient Examination	General
Handle, Scalpel	Surgery
Hook, Other	Surgery
Retractor	Orthopedics
Scissors, Bandage/Gauze/Plaster	General
Tweezers	General

CARL ZEISS MEDITEC INC.　877-486-7473
5160 Hacienda Drive, Dublin, CA 94568　**925-557-4100**
FDA Number: 2918630　*Fax:* 925-557-4298
E-mail: info@meditec.zeiss.com
Web site: www.meditec.zeiss.com
Medical Products Sales Volume: $1,000,000
Annual Revenue: $0-$1 Million
Year Founded: 2000
Total Employees: 2100　*Marketing Staff:* 14　*Sales Staff:* 50
Ownership: Carl Zeiss Surgical, Inc.
Stock Symbol: AFX
Traded On: Frankfurt
Quality System Registration Information: ISO9000; ISO9001
Produces/Sells CE-marked Devices: Y
Federal Procurement Eligibility: Minority Owned
Distribution: Manufacturer Direct, Manufacturer Through Distributor, Manufacturer Through Manufacturer Reps, Service Direct, Importer, Exporter
General Admin.: John Moore/President, Chief Executive Officer
　　　　Mimi Hui/Vice President Human Resources
Mktg./Adv.: James Laux/Director Marketing
　　　　Gina Crabb/Manager Advertising
　　　　James Carter/Manager International Marketing & Sales
　　　　Joe Donahoe/Vice President Marketing & Sales
Production: Steve Williams/Vice President Manufacturing
Research: Charlie Campbell/Vice President Research & Development

Camera, Video	General
Computer and Software, Medical, Ophthalmic Use	Ophthalmology
Computer, Radiographic Data	Radiology
Keratometer	Ophthalmology
Lamp, Slit	Ophthalmology
Lamp, Slit, Biomicroscope, AC-Powered	Ophthalmology
Lensometer	Ophthalmology
Measurer, Corneal Radius	Ophthalmology
Microscope, Surgical	Ear/Nose/Throat
Pachometer	Ophthalmology
Perimeter, Automatic, AC-Powered	Ophthalmology
Probe, Other	General
Refractor, Ophthalmic	Ophthalmology
Scanner, Computed Tomography, X-Ray, Head	Radiology

CARL ZEISS MEDITEC, INC.　800-722-6393
10805 Rancho Benardo Road, Suite 210,　**858-673-7900**
San Diego, CA 92127
FDA Number: 2028397　*Fax:* 858-673-7909
E-mail: i.info@meditec.zeiss.com
Web site: www.meditec.zeiss.com
Medical Products Sales Volume: $2,200,000
Annual Revenue: $10-$25 Million
Total Employees: 28　*Marketing Staff:* 7　*Sales Staff:* 20
Ownership: Public
Stock Symbol: AFXG
Quality System Registration Information: ISO9001
Produces/Sells CE-marked Devices: N
Federal Procurement Eligibility: Small Business
Distribution: Manufacturer Direct, Manufacturer Through Distributor
General Admin.: Kris Vinluan/Manager Human Resources
　　　　John Moore/President, Chief Executive Officer
Mktg./Adv.: Jeff Keeling/Director Sales
　　　　Rob Foster/Manager Advertising
　　　　Rob Foster/Vice President Marketing
　　　　James Gardner/Vice President Sales
Production: Kitty Legerton/Director Quality Assurance
　　　　Kitty Legerton/Director Regulatory Affairs
　　　　Steve Bailey/Manager Materials
　　　　Patrick Scott/Manager Quality Assurance & Regulatory Affairs
Research: Maurice Blais/Vice President Engineering

CARL ZEISS MEDITEC, INC.　800-722-6393 (cont'd)
Ophthalmoscope, AC-Powered　Ophthalmology

CARL ZEISS MICROIMAGING AIS, INC　949-425-5700
31 Columbia, Aliso Viejo, CA 92656
FDA Number: 2031113

Locator, Cell, Automated	Hematology

CARL ZEISS SURGICAL, INC.　1 800 233 2343
One Zeiss Dr., Thornwood, NY 10594-1939　**914-747-1800**
FDA Number: 2431026　*Fax:* 1 914 681 7446
Web site: www.zeiss.com/micro
Total Employees: 240　*Marketing Staff:* 100　*Sales Staff:* 100
Ownership: Private
Produces/Sells CE-marked Devices: N
Distribution: Manufacturer Direct, Manufacturer Through Manufacturer Reps, Importer, Exporter
General Admin.: Eric Timko/President
　　　　Jim Kelly/President, Chief Executive Officer
　　　　Meg Donohue/Vice President Human Resources
Mktg./Adv.: Jeff Rospert/Director National Accounts
　　　　Carl O'Connell/Vice President Marketing

Camera, Microscope	Microbiology
Camera, Ophthalmic, AC-Powered (Fundus)	Ophthalmology
Colposcope	Obstetrics/Gynecology
Computer, Imaging, Presurgery	Surgery
Drape, Surgical, Disposable	Surgery
Drape, Surgical, Reusable	Surgery
Endoscope	Gastroenterology/Urology
Gown, Patient, Reusable	General
Image Processing System	Radiology
Lamp, Microscope	Pathology
Lamp, Slit	Ophthalmology
Laser, Carbon-Dioxide, Surgical	Surgery
Laser, Nd:YAG, Surgical	Surgery
Laser, Ophthalmic	Ophthalmology
Light Source, Fiberoptic, Routine	Gastroenterology/Urology
Loupe, Diagnostic/Surgical	Surgery
Micromanipulator	General
Microscope	Hematology
Microscope, Ear	Ear/Nose/Throat
Microscope, Fluorescence/U.V.	Pathology
Microscope, Inverted Stage, Tissue Culture	Pathology
Microscope, Laboratory, Optical	Microbiology
Microscope, Operating, AC-Powered, Ophthalmic	Ophthalmology
Microscope, Phase Contrast	Pathology
Microscope, Surgical	Ear/Nose/Throat
Microscope, Surgical, General & Plastic Surgery	Surgery
Microscope, Surgical, Neurosurgical	Cns/Neurology
Ophthalmoscope, Direct	Ophthalmology
Ophthalmoscope, Indirect	Ophthalmology

Medical Product Subsidiaries (Listed Separately)
　Carl Zeiss Meditec Inc.
　Zeiss Jena Gmbh, Carl

CARL ZEISS VISION INC.　707-763-9911
1030 Worldwide Blvd., Hebron, KY 41048
FDA Number: 3004022413
Ownership: Private
Produces/Sells CE-marked Devices: N

Lens, Spectacle/Eyeglasses, Non-Custom	Ophthalmology

CARL ZEISS VISION-KENTUCKY　866-289-7652
1050 World Wide Blvd., Hebron, KY 41048
FDA Number: 3003473777　*Fax:* 866-329-7652
E-mail: customercare@sola.com
Web site: www.solatechnologies.com
Ownership: Private
Produces/Sells CE-marked Devices: N

Lens, Spectacle/Eyeglasses, Non-Custom	Ophthalmology

CARL ZEISS, INC.
　See Carl Zeiss Surgical, Inc.

CARLETON LIFE SUPPORT SYSTEMS INC.　563-383-6204
2734 Hickory Grove Rd., Davenport, IA 52804
FDA Number: 3002840531　*Fax:* 563-383-6430
Web site: www.cobham.com
Ownership: Private
Produces/Sells CE-marked Devices: N

Generator, Oxygen, Portable	Anesthesiology

CARLEY LAMPS　310-325-8474
1502 W. 228th St., Torrance, CA 90501
FDA Number: n/a　*Fax:* 310-534-2912
E-mail: sales@carleylamps.com
Web site: www.carleylamps.com
Medical Products Sales Volume: $20,100,000
Year Founded: 1960
Total Employees: 300　*Marketing Staff:* 2　*Sales Staff:* 5

CARLEY LAMPS
310-325-8474 *(cont'd)*

Ownership: Private
Produces/Sells CE-marked Devices: N
Federal Procurement Eligibility: Small Business, GSA Contract, VA Contract
Distribution: Manufacturer Direct, OEM, Exporter
General Admin.: James A. Carley/President
    Curt Carley/Vice President, General Manager
Mktg./Adv.: Craig Carley/Director Marketing
    Todd Cecil/Director Product Development
    Craig Carley/Manager International & National Sales
    Sobeida De La Mora-Mares/Manager Sales Training
Production: Julie Giannette/Director Quality Assurance
    Claudia Gomez/Manager Materials
    Margarette Tsang/Manager Regulatory Affairs

Contract Manufacturing	General
Lamp, Endoscopic, Incandescent	Surgery
Lamp, Infrared	Physical Med
Lamp, Laryngoscope	Ear/Nose/Throat
Lamp, Other	General
Lamp, Surgical	Surgery
Lamp, Surgical, Xenon	Surgery
Laryngoscope	Ear/Nose/Throat
Laryngoscope, Rigid	Anesthesiology
Laryngoscope, Surgical	Surgery
Ophthalmoscope, Battery-Powered	Ophthalmology

CARLISLE STREET LLC
610-821-4222

321 South Carlisle St., Allentown, PA 18109
FDA Number: 100113
Ownership: Private
Produces/Sells CE-marked Devices: N

Cart, Emergency, Cardiopulmonary Resuscitation (Crash)	Anesthesiology

CARLSBAD INTERNATIONAL EXPORT, INC.
760-438-5323

1954 Kellogg Ave., Carlsbad, CA 92008
FDA Number: 2023169

Humidifier, Respiratory Gas, (Direct Patient Interface)	Anesthesiology
Pneumotachometer	Anesthesiology

CAROCHEM, INC.
919-682-5121

744 E. Markham Avenue, Box 15699, Durham, NC 27701
FDA Number: 1038132   Fax: 919-682-3174
E-mail: carochemInc@aol.com
Medical Products Sales Volume: $850,000
Annual Revenue: $1-$5 Million
Year Founded: 1977
Total Employees: 8   Marketing Staff: 1   Sales Staff: 2
Ownership: Private
Produces/Sells CE-marked Devices: N
Federal Procurement Eligibility: Small Business
Distribution: Manufacturer Through Distributor
General Admin.: S. Thomas Amore/President, Chief Executive Officer
    Thomas J. Carr/Vice President, General Manager
Mktg./Adv.: Sherry Earp/Vice President Sales
Production: John Durrett/General Manager Production
    Thomas J Carr III/Vice President Manufacturing

Detergent	Hematology
Disinfector, Liquid	General
Lubricant, Instrument	General
Soap	General
Solution, Instrument Cleaner	General

CAROL COLE COMPANY
888-360-9171
760-734-4545

3146 Tiger Run Court, Suite 109, Carlsbad, CA 92010
FDA Number: 3006459199   Fax: 760-734-4565
Web site: www.mynuface.com
Ownership: Private
Produces/Sells CE-marked Devices: N

Stimulator, Nerve, Transcutaneous (Pain Relief, TENS)	Cns/Neurology

CAROLE LEWIS STOLPE' B.C.O.
310-271-8801

435 N. Bedford Drive, Suite 411, Beverly Hills, CA 90210
FDA Number: 2029328
Ownership: Private
Produces/Sells CE-marked Devices: N

Eye, Artificial, Non-Custom	Ophthalmology

CAROLINA ABSORBENT COTTON
775 856 2444, e

4969 Energy Way, Reno, NV 89502
FDA Number: 3006180768
Fax: 775 856 1223
Ownership: Private
Produces/Sells CE-marked Devices: N

Fiber, Absorbent	General

CAROLINA ABSORBENT COTTON CO.
800-277-0377
704-376-0380

1100 Hawthorne Lane, Charlotte, NC 28205
FDA Number: 3006180768   Fax: 704-342-1892
E-mail: custserv@barnhardt.net

CAROLINA ABSORBENT COTTON CO.
800-277-0377 *(cont'd)*

Web site: www.barnhardt.net
Annual Revenue: $5-$10 Million
Year Founded: 1900
Total Employees: 25
Ownership: BARNHARDT MANUFACTURING CO.
Produces/Sells CE-marked Devices: Y
Federal Procurement Eligibility: Small Business
Distribution: Manufacturer Direct, Manufacturer Through Distributor
General Admin.: T. M. Barnhardt/Chairman
    Tom L. Barnhardt/Chief Executive Officer
    Lewis Barnhardt/President
    Randy Godfrey/Vice President Human Resources
Mktg./Adv.: George Hargrove/Director Marketing & Advertising
    Ashley Chilton/Sales Representative
    Donna Harris/Sales Representative
    George M. Hargrove/Vice President Marketing & Sales
Production: MaryAnn Bujak/Customer Service Representative
Research: David Spinks/Director Tech. Affairs

Ball, Cotton	General
Cotton, Roll	Dental And Oral
Fiber, Absorbent	General

CAROLINA BIOLOGICAL SUPPLY CO.
800-334-5551

2700 York Rd., Burlington, NC 27215-3398
FDA Number: 1048439   Fax: 336.538.6330
E-mail: customer_service@carolina.com
Web site: www.carolina.com
Annual Revenue: $0-$1 Million
Year Founded: 1927
Total Employees: 450
Ownership: Private
Produces/Sells CE-marked Devices: N
Federal Procurement Eligibility: Small Business
Distribution: Manufacturer Through Distributor

Anatomical Training Model	General
Lamp, Ultraviolet (Spectrum A)	General
Microscope	Hematology
Power System, Isolated	General

CAROLINA BIOLOGICAL SUPPLY CO.
800-334-5551
336-584-0381

2700 York Road, Burlington, NC 27215-3398
FDA Number: 3003783142   Fax: 800-222-7112
E-mail: carolina@carolina.com
Web site: www.carolina.com
Medical Products Sales Volume: $25,400,000
Year Founded: 1927
Total Employees: 100   Sales Staff: 3
Ownership: Private
Produces/Sells CE-marked Devices: N
Federal Procurement Eligibility: Small Business
Distribution: Manufacturer Direct, Exclusive Distributor, Importer, Exporter
General Admin.: Thomas E. Powell/Chairman
    Richard Cooper/Chief Financial Officer, Vice President
    Jim Parrish/President
    Ray Gladden/Vice President
    Leon Joyce/Vice President Admin., Personnel
Mktg./Adv.: Mike Webb/Director Advertising
    Dan Woodlief/Manager Market Research
    Daniel James/Vice President Business Development
    George Ross/Vice President Marketing
Production: Roger Phillips/Vice President Production

Blanket, Fire	General
Blender/Mixer	Chemistry
Board, Dissecting	Pathology
Bulb, Inflation	General
Buret	Chemistry
Cabinet Casework, Laboratory	Chemistry
Cabinet, Laboratory	Chemistry
Cabinet, Storage, Slide	General
Cage, Animal	Microbiology
Camera, Microscope	Microbiology
Camera, Video	General
Cart, Equipment, Video	General
Clamp, Tubing	General
Coat, Laboratory	General
Coverslip, Microscope Slide	Pathology
Culture Media, General Nutrient Broth	Microbiology
Culture Media, Mueller Hinton Agar Broth	Microbiology
Desiccator	Chemistry
Dish, Petri	Chemistry
Electrocardiograph, Multi-Channel	Cardiovascular
Glove, Utility	General
Incubator, Aerobic	Microbiology
Labware, Basic, Disposable	Chemistry
Labware, Basic, Reusable	Chemistry
Microscope, Laboratory, Optical	Microbiology
Microscope, Light	Pathology
Otoscope	Ear/Nose/Throat

CAROLINA BIOLOGICAL SUPPLY CO.   800-334-5551 (cont'd)

Pipette, Micro	Chemistry
Rack, Test Tube	Chemistry
Spatula, Other	Surgery
Sphygmomanometer, Aneroid (Arterial Pressure)	General
Sphygmomanometer, Electronic, Automatic	General
Sphygmomanometer, Electronic, Manual	General
Stain, Biological, General	Pathology
Stethoscope, Manual	Cardiovascular
Stirrer	Chemistry
Table, Other	General
Tube, Culture	Microbiology
Tube, Test	Chemistry
Tubing, Connecting	General
Tubing, Latex	General
Tubing, Other	General
Tubing, Plastic	General

CAROLINA EYE PROSTHETICS, INC.   336-228-7877
420 Maple Ave., Burlington, NC 27215
FDA Number: 1062253

Eye, Artificial, Non-Custom	Ophthalmology

CAROLINA LIQUID CHEMISTRIES CORP.   800-471-7272
510 W. Central Ave., Suite C, Brea, CA 92821
FDA Number: 2030861

Absorption, Atomic, Lithium	Toxicology
Alcohol Dehydrogenase, Spec. Reagent - Ethanol Enzyme	Toxicology
Alpha-1-Lipoprotein, Antigen, Antiserum, Control	Immunology
Antigen, Antiserum, Control, Complement C3	Immunology
Antigen, Antiserum, Control, Complement C4	Immunology
Antigen, Antiserum, Control, Haptoglobin	Immunology
Antigen, Antiserum, Control, Lipoprotein, Low Density	Immunology
Antigen, Antiserum, Control, Prealbumin, FITC	Immunology
Antigen, Antiserum, Control, Transferrin	Immunology
Calibrator, Primary, Clinical Chemistry	Chemistry
Catalytic Method, Amylase	Chemistry
Colorimetry, Acetaminophen	Toxicology
Complexone, Cresolphthalein, Calcium	Chemistry
Control, Analyte (Assayed And Unassayed)	Chemistry
Control, Multi Analyte, All Kinds (Assayed And Unassayed)	Chemistry
Dye-Binding, Albumin, Bromcresol, Green	Chemistry
Dye-Binding, Albumin, Bromcresol, Purple	Chemistry
Electrode, Ion Specific, Sodium	Chemistry
Enzymatic Esterase-Oxidase, Cholesterol	Chemistry
Enzymatic Method, Ammonia	Chemistry
Enzyme Immunoassay, Amphetamine	Toxicology
Enzyme Immunoassay, Barbiturate	Toxicology
Enzyme Immunoassay, Benzodiazepine	Toxicology
Enzyme Immunoassay, Cannabinoids	Toxicology
Enzyme Immunoassay, Cocaine And Cocaine Metabolites	Toxicology
Enzyme Immunoassay, Methadone	Toxicology
Enzyme Immunoassay, Opiates	Toxicology
Enzyme Immunoassay, Phencyclidine	Toxicology
Enzyme Immunoassay, Propoxyphene	Toxicology
Ferrozine (Colorimetric) Iron Binding Capacity	Chemistry
Hemoglobinometer, Electrophoretic Analysis System	Hematology
Hexokinase, Glucose	Chemistry
Immunoelectrophoretic, Immunoglobulins, (G, A, M)	Chemistry
Kinetic Method, Gamma-Glutamyl Transpeptidase	Chemistry
LDL & VLDL Precipitation, HDL	Chemistry
Lipase Hydrolysis/Glycerol Kinase Enzyme, Triglycerides	Chemistry
Lipase-Esterase, Enzymatic, Photometric, Lipase	Chemistry
Multi Analyte Mixture, Calibrator	Chemistry
NAD Reduction/NADH Oxidation, CPK Or Isoenzymes	Chemistry
NAD Reduction/NADH Oxidation, Lactate Dehydrogenase	Chemistry
NADH Oxidation/NAD Reduction, AST/SGOT	Chemistry
Nitrophenylphosphate, Alkaline Phosphatase Or Isoenzymes	Chemistry
Phosphorus Reagent (Test System)	Chemistry
Photometric Method, Magnesium	Chemistry
Pipetting And Diluting System, Automated	Chemistry
Reagent, Bilirubin (Total Or Direct Test System)	Chemistry
Reagent, Creatinine (Test System)	Chemistry
Reagent, Glucose (Test System)	Chemistry
Reagent, Iron (Test System)	Chemistry
Reagent, Protein, Total	Chemistry
SGPT, Ultraviolet	Chemistry
Test, C-Reactive Protein, FITC	Immunology
Test, Glycosylated Hemoglobin Assay	Hematology
Test, Rheumatoid Factor	Immunology
Urease And Glutamic Dehydrogenase, Urea Nitrogen	Chemistry
Uricase (Colorimetric), Uric Acid	Chemistry
Urinary Homocystine (Non-Quantitative) Test System	Chemistry
pH Rate Measurement, Carbon-Dioxide	Chemistry

CAROLINA MEDICAL PRODUCTS CO.   800-227-6637
8026 Us 264 Alternate, P.o. Box 147,   252-753-7111
Farmville, NC 27828
FDA Number: 1050589
E-mail: cmp@carolinamedical.com   *Fax:* 252-753-3882
Web site: www.carolinamedical.com

CAROLINA MEDICAL PRODUCTS CO.   800-227-6637 (cont'd)
Ownership: Private
Produces/Sells CE-marked Devices: N

Kit, Enema (For Cleaning Purposes)	Gastroenterology/Urology

CAROLINA MEDICAL, INC.   800-334-4531
157 Industrial Dr., King, NC 27021-0307   336-983-5132
FDA Number: 1017913   *Fax:* 336-983-8992
E-mail: info@caromed.com
Web site: www.caromed.com
Annual Revenue: $5-$10 Million
Total Employees: 25
Ownership: Private
Quality System Registration Information: ISO9001; ISO9002
Produces/Sells CE-marked Devices: Y
Federal Procurement Eligibility: Small Business
Distribution: Manufacturer Direct, Manufacturer Through Distributor, Manufacturer Through Manufacturer Reps, OEM
General Admin.: Dr. Carroll L. Turner/President, Chief Executive Officer
Mktg./Adv.: B. Leon Wilson/Director Product Development
    Renea Bennett/Manager Exports
Production: Daniel Edwards/Director Quality Assurance
    Samuel D. Brown/Plant Manager

Cuff, Blood Pressure	Cardiovascular
Flowmeter, Blood, Intravenous	Cardiovascular
Monitor, Penile Tumescence	Gastroenterology/Urology
Probe, Blood Flow, Extravascular	Cardiovascular

CAROLINA NARROW FABRIC CO.   336-631-3000
1100 Patterson Ave., Winston-salem, NC 27101
FDA Number: 1064808

Bandage, Cast	Physical Med
Cover, Cast	General
Protector, Skin Pressure	General
Splint, Extremity, Non-Inflatable, External	Surgery

CAROLON COMPANY   800-334-0414
601 Forum Pkwy., Rural Hall, NC 27045   336-969-6001
FDA Number: 1043551   *Fax:* 336.969.6999
E-mail: carolon@carolon.com
Web site: www.carolon.com
Ownership: Private
Produces/Sells CE-marked Devices: Y
Federal Procurement Eligibility: Small Business
Distribution: Manufacturer Through Distributor

Bag, Ice	General
Bandage, Elastic	General
Gown, Examination	General
Legging, Compression, Non-Inflatable	General
Pack, Hot Or Cold, Disposable	Physical Med
Pack, Hot Or Cold, Reusable	Physical Med
Pack, Moist Heat	Physical Med
Slippers	General
Stocking, Support (Anti-Embolic)	General

CARON PRODUCTS AND SERVICES, INC.   800-648-3042
PO Box 715, Marietta, OH 45750   740-373-6809
FDA Number: n/a   *Fax:* 740-374-3760
E-mail: sales@caronproducts.com
Web site: www.caronproducts.com
Annual Revenue: $1-$5 Million
Year Founded: 1985
Total Employees: 20   *Marketing Staff:* 1   *Sales Staff:* 4
Ownership: Private
Produces/Sells CE-marked Devices: Y
Federal Procurement Eligibility: Small Business
Distribution: Manufacturer Direct, Manufacturer Through Distributor, Service Direct, Exporter
General Admin.: Terry St. Peter/General Manager

Chamber, Environmental, Platelet Storage	Hematology
Circulator, Water Bath	Chemistry

CARPAL DOCTORS LLC   866-401-1213
701 Brickell Avenue, Suite 1550, Miami, FL 33131
FDA Number: 3006084857
E-mail: info@carpaldoctors.com
Web site: www.carpaldoctors.com
Ownership: Private
Produces/Sells CE-marked Devices: N

Traction Unit, Non-Powered	Orthopedics

CARPAL THERAPY, INC.   317-313-0680
1201 Main St., Suite 200, Speedway, IN 46224
FDA Number: n/a
E-mail: David@sastm.com
Web site: www.sastm.com
Annual Revenue: $1-$5 Million
Ownership: Private
Produces/Sells CE-marked Devices: N

CARPAL THERAPY, INC.   317-313-0680 *(cont'd)*

Distribution: Manufacturer Direct, Manufacturer Through Distributor
General Admin.: David Graston/President

Massager, Therapeutic, Manual	Physical Med

CARR CORPORATION   800-952-2398
1547 11th St., Santa Monica, CA 90401   **310-587-1113**

FDA Number: n/a   Fax: 310-395-9751
E-mail: carrcorp@aol.com
Web site: www.carrcorporation.com
Medical Products Sales Volume: $5,000,000
Annual Revenue: $1-$5 Million
Year Founded: 1946
Ownership: Private
Produces/Sells CE-marked Devices: N
Federal Procurement Eligibility: Small Business
Distribution: Manufacturer Direct, OEM

Apron, Lead, Radiographic	Radiology
Cabinet Casework, Laboratory	Chemistry
Cabinet, X-Ray Transfer	Radiology
Dryer, Film, Radiographic	Dental And Oral
File	Orthopedics
Glove, Protective, Radiographic	Radiology
Illuminator, Radiographic Film	Radiology
Safelight, X-Ray	Radiology
Shield, X-Ray	Radiology
Storage Unit, X-Ray Film	Radiology
Tank, Developing, TLC	Toxicology

CARR METAL PRODUCTS, INC.
See Greatbatch Medical

CARROLL CO.   800-527-5722
2900 W. Kingsley Rd., Garland, TX 75041

FDA Number: n/a
E-mail: customerservice@carrollco.com
Web site: www.carrollco.com
Year Founded: 1921
Total Employees: 13
Ownership: Private
Produces/Sells CE-marked Devices: N
Federal Procurement Eligibility: Small Business
Distribution: Manufacturer Through Distributor, Exporter

Disinfector, Liquid	General
Soap	General
Solution, Antibacterial Cleaner	General

CARSAN ENGINEERING, INC.   303-237-9608
221 Corporate Circle, Suite H, Golden, CO 80401

FDA Number: n/a   Fax: 303-237-0757
Web site: www.carsaneng.com
Medical Products Sales Volume: $5,000,000
Annual Revenue: $1-$5 Million
Ownership: Private
Produces/Sells CE-marked Devices: N
Federal Procurement Eligibility: Small Business
Distribution: Manufacturer Direct, Manufacturer Through Manufacturer Reps
General Admin.: John K. Small/Vice President
Mktg./Adv.: Cora Schmidt/Admin. Sales

Light Source, Fiberoptic, Routine	Gastroenterology/Urology

CARSEN GROUP INC.   800-837-0437
151 Telson Rd., Markham, ONT L3R-1E7 Canada   **905-479-4100**

FDA Number: n/a   Fax: 905-479-1610
E-mail: info@carsengroup.com
Web site: www.carsengroup.com
Year Founded: 1947
Total Employees: 100
Ownership: CANTEL INDUSTRIES INC.
Produces/Sells CE-marked Devices: N
Distribution: Service Direct, Exclusive Distributor

CARTER DENTAL LAB, LLC   870-673-1568
301 S. Grand St., Stuttgart, AR 72160

FDA Number: 3004766121
Ownership: Private
Produces/Sells CE-marked Devices: N

Teeth, Porcelain	Dental And Oral

CARTER-HOFFMANN   800-323-9793
1551 McCormick Ave.,   **847-362-5500**
Mundelein, IL 60060

FDA Number: n/a   Fax: 847-367-8981
E-mail: sales@carterhoffmann.com
Web site: www.carter-hoffmann.com
Annual Revenue: $10-$25 Million
Total Employees: 130   Marketing Staff: 1   Sales Staff: 7
Ownership: TOKIBO Co., LTD.
Produces/Sells CE-marked Devices: Y

CARTER-HOFFMANN   800-323-9793 *(cont'd)*

Distribution: Manufacturer Through Distributor, Manufacturer Through Manufacturer Reps, Exporter
Mktg./Adv.: Kim Aaron/Manager Marketing
       Mark Anderson/Manager Regional Sales
       Roger Laskowski/Manager Regional Sales
       Rick Steffen/Vice President Natl Accounts & Sales
Research: Jerry Henke/Manager Development

Cart, Foodservice	General
Foodservice Product/Equipment	General

CARTICEPT MEDICAL, INC   (770) 754-3800
6120 Windward Parkway, Suite 220, Alpharetta, GA 30005

FDA Number: 3006693771   Fax: (770) 754-3808
Ownership: Public
Produces/Sells CE-marked Devices: N
General Admin.: Mr. Timothy Patrick/President, Chief Executive Officer
Mktg./Adv.: Mr. Barry Hassett/Vice President Marketing
       Mr. Robert Singer/Vice President Sales
Production: Mr. Richard Knostman/Vice President Operations
       Ms. Deborah Moore/Vice President Regulatory & Clinical Affairs
Research: Mr. Steven Walsh/Vice President Research & Development
Finance: Mr. Peter Pizzo/Chief Financial Officer, Senior Vice President Finance

Bit, Drill	Orthopedics
Orthopedic Manual Surgical Instrument	Orthopedics
Prosthesis, Toe, Hemi-, Phalangeal	Orthopedics
Pump, Infusion	General
Tray, Surgical	Surgery

CARTIER CHEMICALS LTD.   800-361-9432
445 21st Ave., Lachine, QUE H8S-3T8 Canada   **514-637-4631**

FDA Number: n/a   Fax: 514-637-8804
E-mail: info@vytac.com
Web site: www.vytac.com
Year Founded: 1939
Total Employees: 50
Ownership: Private
Produces/Sells CE-marked Devices: N
Distribution: Manufacturer Direct, Exporter

CARTWRIGHT CONSULTING CO.   952-854-4911
8324 16th Avenue S., Minneapolis, MN 55425-1742

FDA Number: n/a   Fax: 952-854-6964
E-mail: pscartwright@msn.com
Web site: http://cartwright-consulting.com/
Medical Products Sales Volume: $100,000
Annual Revenue: $0-$1 Million
Year Founded: 1974
Total Employees: 2   Marketing Staff: 1   Sales Staff: 2
Ownership: Private
Produces/Sells CE-marked Devices: N
Federal Procurement Eligibility: Small Business
General Admin.: P. S. Cartwright/President

Purification Filter, Water, Charcoal	Chemistry
Ultrafiltration Equipment	Chemistry

CARVER INC.   260-563-7577
1569 Morris St., Wabash, IN 46992-0544

FDA Number: 7000084   Fax: 260-563-7625
E-mail: carverpress@corpemail.com
Web site: www.carverpress.com
Medical Products Sales Volume: $430,000
Annual Revenue: $10-$25 Million
Year Founded: 1977
Total Employees: 7   Marketing Staff: 3   Sales Staff: 12
Ownership: Aec, Inc.
Produces/Sells CE-marked Devices: Y
Federal Procurement Eligibility: Small Business
Distribution: Manufacturer Direct, Manufacturer Through Distributor, Manufacturer Through Manufacturer Reps, Exporter
General Admin.: Mr. Joel Kline/Regional Manager
Mktg./Adv.: Mr. David Singer/Manager Marketing & Sales

Contract Manufacturing	General
Disintegrator, Biological Cell	Microbiology
Equipment, Laboratory, Gen. Purpose (Specific Medical Use)	Chemistry
Equipment, Molding	General
Plate, Hot	Chemistry

CARWILD CORP.   860-442-4914
3 State Pier Road, New London, CT 06320

FDA Number: 1219313   Fax: 860-442-5895
E-mail: trudy@carwild.net
Web site: www.carwild.net
Medical Products Sales Volume: $6,000,000
Annual Revenue: $5-$10 Million
Total Employees: 250   Marketing Staff: 3   Sales Staff: 3
Ownership: Private
Quality System Registration Information: ISO9002

CARWILD CORP.   860-442-4914 (cont'd)
Produces/Sells CE-marked Devices: N
Federal Procurement Eligibility: Small Business, GSA Contract
Distribution: OEM
General Admin.: Joel S. Wildstein/President
Mktg./Adv.: Trudy Richard/Director Marketing & Sales
Production: Mr. David Wildstein/Director Operations
    Beth Casler/Manager Regulatory Affairs
Purchasing: Ms. Melissa Lowry/Manager Purchasing

Dissector, Surgical, General & Plastic Surgery	Surgery
Gauze, Absorbable	Surgery
Gauze, Non-Absorbable, Non-Medicated (Internal Sponge)	Surgery
Gauze, Non-Absorbable, X-Ray Detectable (Internal Sponge)	Surgery
Sponge, Internal	Cns/Neurology
Sponge, Neuro	Cns/Neurology

CAS MEDICAL SYSTEMS, INC.   800-227-4414
44 E. Industrial Rd., Branford, CT 06405   203-488-6056
FDA Number: 2244861   Fax: 203-488-9438
E-mail: custsrv@casmed.com
Web site: www.casmed.com
Annual Revenue: $25-$50 Million
Year Founded: 1984
Total Employees: 150
Ownership: Public
Stock Symbol: CASM
Traded On: NASDAQ
Quality System Registration Information: ISO9001
Produces/Sells CE-marked Devices: Y
Federal Procurement Eligibility: GSA Contract, VA Contract
Distribution: Manufacturer Direct, Manufacturer Through Distributor, Manufacturer Through Manufacturer Reps, OEM, Exporter
General Admin.: Louis Scheps/Chairman
    Andrew Kersey/President, Chief Executive Officer
Mktg./Adv.: Steve Otis/Director Sales
Finance: Jeffery Baird/Chief Financial Officer

Board, Arm	Anesthesiology
Cuff, Blood Pressure	Cardiovascular
Electrode, ECG, Radiolucent	Cardiovascular
Electrode, Electrocardiograph	Cardiovascular
Electrode, Gel	Cardiovascular
Monitor, Blood Pressure, Indirect, Anesthesiology	Anesthesiology
Monitor, Blood Pressure, Indirect, Automatic	Cardiovascular
Monitor, Fetal, Ultrasonic	Obstetrics/Gynecology
Monitor, Physiological, Patient	Cardiovascular
Oximeter, Tissue Saturation	Cardiovascular
Probe, Temperature	General
Shield, Heat, Infant	General
Sphygmomanometer, Electronic, Automatic	General

CASA FUTURA TECHNOLOGIES   303-417-9752
720 31st St, Boulder, CO 80303-2402
FDA Number: n/a   Fax: 303-413-0853
E-mail: sales@casafuturatech.com
Web site: www.casafuturatech.com
Medical Products Sales Volume: $250,000
Annual Revenue: $0-$1 Million
Year Founded: 1992
Ownership: Private
Produces/Sells CE-marked Devices: N
Federal Procurement Eligibility: Small Business
Distribution: Manufacturer Direct, Manufacturer Through Distributor

Biofeedback Device	Cns/Neurology

CASA PLARRE, S.A. DE C.V.   +51 34 02 70
Av. Cuahtemoc 220-201, Mexico D.F. 06720 Mexico
FDA Number: n/a   Fax: +51 34 02 82
E-mail: ventas@casaplarre.com
Medical Products Sales Volume: $11,000,000
Total Employees: 90   Marketing Staff: 4   Sales Staff: 26
Ownership: Private
Produces/Sells CE-marked Devices: N
Federal Procurement Eligibility: Small Business
Distribution: Manufacturer Direct, Manufacturer Through Distributor, OEM, Service Direct, Importer, Exporter

CASCADE DAFO, INC.   800-848-7332
1360 Sunset Avenue, Ferndale, WA 98248
FDA Number: 3003475336   Fax: 877-856-2160
E-mail: bizdev@dafo.com
Web site: www.dafo.com
Ownership: Private
Produces/Sells CE-marked Devices: N

Orthosis, Limb Brace	Physical Med

CASCADE DENTAL PRODUCTS CO.   800-939-9926
3960 Grandview Drive, Hood River, OR 97031   541-386-2012
FDA Number: 3029778

CASCADE DENTAL PRODUCTS CO.   800-939-9926 (cont'd)
E-mail: info@cascadedentalproducts.com
Web site: www.cascadedentalproducts.com
Ownership: Private
Produces/Sells CE-marked Devices: N

Cleaner, Denture	Dental And Oral

CASCADE DESIGNS, INC.   206-505-9500
4000 1st Avenue South, Seattle, WA 98134
FDA Number: 3024102   Fax: 206-343-5795
E-mail: consumer@cascadedesigns.com
Web site: www.cascadedesigns.com
Annual Revenue: $1-$5 Million
Year Founded: 1972
Ownership: Private
Produces/Sells CE-marked Devices: Y
Federal Procurement Eligibility: Small Business
Distribution: Manufacturer Through Manufacturer Reps, OEM, Exporter

Accessories, Wheelchair	Physical Med
Cushion, Flotation	Physical Med
Cushion, Wheelchair (Pad)	Physical Med

CASCADE LIFE SOLUTIONS, LLC   616-977-2505
3710 Sysco Court Se, Grand Rapids, MI 49512
FDA Number: 3005728568
Ownership: Private
Produces/Sells CE-marked Devices: N

Catheter, Vascular, Cardiopulmonary Bypass	Cardiovascular
Clamp, Surgical, General & Plastic Surgery	Surgery
Suction Apparatus, Operating Room, Wall Vacuum-Powered	Surgery
Surgical Instrument, Cardiovascular	Cardiovascular

CASCADE MEDICAL, INC.
See Quest Star Medical, Inc.

CASCADE ORTHOTICS LTD.   403-283-7872
2636 Parkdale Blvd. NW, Calgary, ALB T2N-3S6 Canada
FDA Number: n/a   Fax: 403-283-7853
E-mail: cascadeinfo@cascadeorthotics.com
Web site: www.cascadeorthotics.com
Year Founded: 1993
Total Employees: 10
Ownership: Private
Produces/Sells CE-marked Devices: N
Distribution: Manufacturer Direct

CASCO MANUFACTURING SOLUTIONS, INC.   800-843-1339
3107 Spring Grove Avenue,   513-681-0003
Cincinnati, OH 45225
FDA Number: 1528695   Fax: 513-853-3605
E-mail: inquiries@cascosolutions.com
Web site: www.cascosolutions.com
Medical Products Sales Volume: $12,100,000
Annual Revenue: $10-$25 Million
Year Founded: 1959
Total Employees: 151   Marketing Staff: 2   Sales Staff: 7
Ownership: Private
Quality System Registration Information: ISO9001
Produces/Sells CE-marked Devices: N
Federal Procurement Eligibility: Small Business, Female Owned, GSA Contract
Distribution: Manufacturer Direct, Manufacturer Through Distributor, Manufacturer Through Manufacturer Reps, OEM, Exclusive Distributor, Exporter
General Admin.: Melissa Mangold/President
Mktg./Adv.: Mr. KERRY FLICKNER/Director Marketing & Sales

Contract Manufacturing	General
Contract R&D, Diagnostics	General
Cover, Mattress	General
Cover, Mattress, Conductive	General
Cover, Mattress, Waterproof	General
Mattress, Alternating Pressure (Or Pads)	Physical Med
Mattress, Bed	General
Mattress, Reduction, Pressure	General
Sheeting, Stretcher	General

CASCO PRODUCTS, INC.
See Casco Manufacturing Solutions, Inc.

CASE DESIGN CORP.   800-847-4176
333 School Lane, Telford, PA 18969   215-703-0130
FDA Number: n/a   Fax: 215-703-0139
E-mail: sales@casedesigncorp.com
Web site: www.casedesigncorp.com
Medical Products Sales Volume: $5,300,000
Annual Revenue: $1-$5 Million
Year Founded: 1921
Total Employees: 83   Marketing Staff: 2   Sales Staff: 5
Ownership: Private
Produces/Sells CE-marked Devices: N
Federal Procurement Eligibility: Small Business
Distribution: Manufacturer Direct

CASE DESIGN CORP.   800-847-4176 *(cont'd)*
General Admin.: Roger Ernst/President
Mktg./Adv.: Paul Lowman/Manager Marketing
     Blair Wagner/Sales Engineer
Production: Jody Licker/Manager Production

Case, Protection, Equipment	General
Container, Surgical Instrument	Surgery

CASE IN POINT   801-647-5437
3917 E Viewcrest Drive, Salt Lake City, UT 84124
FDA Number: 3003526496

Freezer, Blood Storage	Hematology

CASE MEDICAL, INC.   888-227-2273
65 Railroad Avenue, Ridgefield, NJ 07657   **201-313-1999**
FDA Number: 2248608   Fax: 201-313-9090
E-mail: casemed@casemed.com
Web site: www.casemed.com
Medical Products Sales Volume: $10,000,000
Annual Revenue: $5-$10 Million
Year Founded: 1992
Total Employees: 40   *Marketing Staff:* 3   *Sales Staff:* 57
Ownership: Private
Quality System Registration Information: ISO9001
Produces/Sells CE-marked Devices: Y
Federal Procurement Eligibility: Small Business, Female Owned, GSA Contract, VA Contract
Distribution: Manufacturer Direct, Manufacturer Through Distributor, Manufacturer Through Manufacturer Reps, OEM, Service Direct
General Admin.: Marcia Frieze/Chief Executive Officer
     Allan S. Frieze/President
Mktg./Adv.: Ron Amster/Director Product Development
Production: Tania Lupu/Manager Regulatory Affairs
     Marcia A. Frieze/Vice President Manufacturing

Brush, Other	General
Cart, Other	General
Case, Protection, Equipment	General
Cleaner, Medical Device	General
Container, Sterilization (Tray)	General
Container, Surgical Instrument	Surgery
Lubricant, Instrument	General
Reamer	Orthopedics
Solution, Instrument Cleaner	General
Sterilization Process Indicator, Chemical	General
Wrap, Sterilization	General

CASPIAN DESIGNS, INC.   310-396-5258
2632 Lincoln Blvd., Santa Monica, CA 90405
FDA Number: 3005823000

Component, Wheelchair	Physical Med

CASTLE CO.
See Getinge Usa, Inc.

CASTLE PINES MEDICAL, INC.   303-442-4514
14883 E Hinsdale Ave, Suite 2, Centennial, CO 80112
FDA Number: 3005907133

Blood System, Extracorporeal (With Accessories)	Gastroenterology/Urology
Connector, Tubing, Dialysate	Gastroenterology/Urology
Dialyzer, Capillary, Hollow Fiber (Hemodialysis)	Gastroenterology/Urology

CATACHEM INC.   203-262-0330
353 Christian Street, Suite 2, Oxford, CT 06478
FDA Number: 2434178   Fax: 203-262-9836
E-mail: catachem@catacheminc.com
Web site: www.catacheminc.com
Annual Revenue: $0-$1 Million
Year Founded: 1984
Ownership: Private
Produces/Sells CE-marked Devices: N
Federal Procurement Eligibility: Minority Owned
Distribution: Manufacturer Direct, Manufacturer Through Distributor
General Admin.: Louis Leon/President, Chief Executive Officer

5-AMP-Phosphate Release (Colorimetric), 5'-Nucleotidase	Chemistry
Calibrator, Primary, Clinical Chemistry	Chemistry
Colorimetric Method, Gamma-Glutamyl Transpeptidase	Chemistry
Colorimetric Method, Triglycerides	Chemistry
Enzymatic Esterase-Oxidase, Cholesterol	Chemistry
Kinetic Method, Gamma-Glutamyl Transpeptidase	Chemistry
Lipase Hydrolysis/Glycerol Kinase Enzyme, Triglycerides	Chemistry
NAD Reduction/NADH Oxidation, Lactate Dehydrogenase	Chemistry
NADH Oxidation/NAD Reduction, AST/SGOT	Chemistry
Radioimmunoassay, Cholyglycine, Bile Acids	Chemistry
Reagent, Other	General

CATALENT PHARMA SOLUTIONS   866-720-3148
2200 Lake Shore Dr., Woodstock, IL 60098   **815-338-9500**
FDA Number: 1419377   Fax: 815-206-1335
E-mail: patricia.mcgee@catalent.com
Web site: www.catalent.com

CATALENT PHARMA SOLUTIONS   866-720-3148 *(cont'd)*
Ownership: Private
Produces/Sells CE-marked Devices: N
General Admin.: Mr. Matthew Walsh/Chief Financial Officer, Senior Vice President
     Mr. Roy Satchell/Chief Information Officer
     Mr. John Chiminski/President, Chief Executive Officer
Mktg./Adv.: Mr. Will Downie/Senior Vice President Marketing & Sales
Production: Mr. Steve Leonard/Senior Vice President Operations
     Ms. Sharon Johnson/Senior Vice President Regulatory Affairs

Catheter, Intravascular, Therapeutic, Short-term Less Than 30 Days	General
Catheter, Suction, With Tip	General
Humidifier, Respiratory Gas, (Direct Patient Interface)	Anesthesiology
Lubricant, Vaginal, Patient	General
Nebulizer, Direct Patient Interface	Anesthesiology
Saliva, Artificial	Dental And Oral
Tube, Tracheostomy (Breathing Tube), ENT	Ear/Nose/Throat

CATALINA CYLINDERS   714-890-0999
7300 Anaconda Avenue, Garden Grove, CA 92841
FDA Number: n/a   Fax: 714-890-1744
E-mail: sales@catalinacylinders.com
Web site: www.catalinacylinders.com
Year Founded: 1992
Total Employees: 80   *Marketing Staff:* 2   *Sales Staff:* 4
Ownership: ALUMINUM PRECISION PRODUCTS INC.
Produces/Sells CE-marked Devices: N
Federal Procurement Eligibility: Small Business
Distribution: Manufacturer Through Distributor, Manufacturer Through Manufacturer Reps
General Admin.: Thomas R. Newell/Vice President, General Manager
Mktg./Adv.: Michael T. Krupsky/Manager International & National Sales

Cylinder, Compressed Gas, With Valve	Anesthesiology
Cylinder, Gas (Empty)	Anesthesiology
Cylinder, Oxygen	Anesthesiology

CATCH INCORPORATED   425-402-8960
11822 North Creek Parkway N., Suite 107, Bothell, WA 98011
FDA Number: 3005002431

Urinary Homocystine (Non-Quantitative) Test System	Chemistry

CATH-LABS CORP.   201-883-0008
282 Hudson St., Hackensack, NJ 07601
FDA Number: 3004378578
Ownership: Private
Produces/Sells CE-marked Devices: N

Catheter, Occluding, Cardiovascular, Implantable	Cardiovascular

CATHEFFECTS, LLC.   916-677-1790
1100 Melody Ln., Roseville, CA 95678
FDA Number: 3003571830
Ownership: Private
Produces/Sells CE-marked Devices: N

Catheter, Electrode Recording, Or Probe	Cardiovascular
Computer, Diagnostic, Programmable	Cardiovascular

CATHETER CONNECTIONS INC.   1-888-706-8883
615 Arapeen Dr, Suite 302a, Salt Lake City, UT 84108
FDA Number: n/a
E-mail: info@cathconn.com
Web site: http://www.catheterconnections.com
Ownership: Private
Produces/Sells CE-marked Devices: N
General Admin.: Ms. Vicki Farrar/Chief Executive Officer
     Dr. Donald Soloman/Chief Operating Officer
Mktg./Adv.: Ms. Charity Williams/Director Business
     Mr. Bryan Gerzsenyi/Vice President Sales
Research: Dr. Robert Hitchcock/Vice President Product Development

Accessories, Catheter	Surgery

CATHETER INNOVATIONS, INC.   800-418-2828
3598 West 1820 South,   **801-954-8444**
Salt Lake City, UT 84104
FDA Number: n/a   Fax: 801-954-8484
Web site: www.bostonscientific.com
Ownership: BOSTON SCIENTIFIC CORPORATION
Produces/Sells CE-marked Devices: N

Catheter, Intravascular, Therapeutic, Long-term Greater Than 30 Days	General
Catheter, Subcutaneous Intravascular, Implanted	General
Kit, Administration, Intravenous	General

CATHETER RESEARCH, INC. (CRI)   317-872-0074
5610 W. 82nd St., Indianapolis, IN 46278
FDA Number: 1833117   Fax: 317-872-0169
E-mail: info@catheterresearch.com
Web site: www.catheterresearch.com
Medical Products Sales Volume: $8,100,000
Year Founded: 1987
Total Employees: 100
Ownership: Private

CATHETER RESEARCH, INC. (CRI)　317-872-0074 (cont'd)

Quality System Registration Information: ISO9002
Produces/Sells CE-marked Devices: N
Federal Procurement Eligibility: Small Business, GSA Contract
Distribution: Manufacturer Direct, Manufacturer Through Distributor, OEM
General Admin.: John A. Steen, Ph.D./President, Chief Executive Officer

Catheter, Cardiovascular	Surgery
Catheter, Intravascular, Therapeutic, Short-term Less Than 30 Days	General
Catheter, Occlusion	Cardiovascular
Catheter, Other	Gastroenterology/Urology
Catheter, Steerable	Cardiovascular
Contract Assembly	General
Contract Manufacturing	General
Contract Manufacturing, Product, Disposable	General
Contract Packaging	General

CATON CONNECTOR CORP.　877-522-2866
26 Wapping Road, Kingston, MA 02364-1302　781-585-4315
FDA Number: n/a　　　　　　　　　　　Fax: 781-585-2973
E-mail: info@caton.com
Web site: www.caton.com
Medical Products Sales Volume: $5,700,000
Annual Revenue: $5-$10 Million
Year Founded: 1973
Total Employees: 42　　Marketing Staff: 1　　Sales Staff: 3
Ownership: Private
Produces/Sells CE-marked Devices: N
Federal Procurement Eligibility: Small Business
Distribution: Manufacturer Direct, Manufacturer Through Distributor
General Admin.: Daniel Galambos/President, Chief Executive Officer
　　　　　　　Pat Ottino/Vice President Human Resources
Mktg./Adv.: James Tantillo/Director National Accounts
　　　　　Kevin Magwood/Director Product Development
　　　　　Daniel Galambos/Manager Advertising
Production: Warren Slyvester/Director Quality Assurance
　　　　　Guy Detrani/Manager Materials
　　　　　Paul Tantillo/Vice President Manufacturing

Component, Electronic	General
Packaging Material	General

CAVITAT MEDICAL TECHNOLOGIES, INC.　903-473-1710
118 South Texas St, PO Box 879, Emory, TX 75440
FDA Number: 3003672013　　　　　　Fax: 903-473-1717
E-mail: bjones@cavitat.com
Web site: www.cavitatmedtech.homestead.com
Medical Products Sales Volume: $920,000
Total Employees: 2
Ownership: Private
Produces/Sells CE-marked Devices: Y
Federal Procurement Eligibility: Small Business

Radiographic Unit, Diagnostic, Dental, Extraoral	Dental And Oral

CAVITRON CORP., BURTON DIV.
See Burton Medical Products, Inc.

CAVITRON DENTAL SYSTEMS
See Dentsply Professional

CAVITRON SURGICAL SYSTEMS INC.
See Valleylab

CAVRO SCIENTIFIC INSTRUMENTS, INC.
See Tecan Systems

CB SCIENCES, INC.
See iWorx Systems, Inc.

CBS MEDICAL TECHNOLOGIES INC.　514-582-9098
225 Chemin des Grands Ducs,
Piedmont, QUEBE J0R 1 Canada
FDA Number: n/a　　　　　　　　　　Fax: 450-240-0627
E-mail: info@cbs-medical.com
Web site: www.cbs-medical.com
Year Founded: 1997
Total Employees: 3
Ownership: Private
Produces/Sells CE-marked Devices: N
Distribution: Manufacturer Direct, Exclusive Distributor

CBS SCIENTIFIC CO., INC.　800-243-4959
po Box 856, Del Mar, CA 92014　858-755-4959
FDA Number: 7000074　　　　　　　Fax: 858-755-0733
E-mail: sales@cbssci.com
Web site: www.cbsscientific.com
Annual Revenue: $0-$1 Million
Total Employees: 50　　Marketing Staff: 1　　Sales Staff: 5
Ownership: Private
Produces/Sells CE-marked Devices: Y
Federal Procurement Eligibility: Small Business, Female Owned
Distribution: Manufacturer Direct
General Admin.: Charles B. Scott/Chief Executive Officer

CBS SCIENTIFIC CO., INC.　800-243-4959 (cont'd)
Mktg./Adv.: Jocelyn B. Scott/Vice President Marketing & Sales

Electrophoresis Equipment, Gel	Chemistry
Shield, X-Ray	Radiology
Tissue Culture Apparatus	Microbiology

CC MEDICAL DEVICES, INC.　913-269-8400
14131 S. Mur Len Rd., Olathe, KS 66062
FDA Number: 1954571
Ownership: Private
Produces/Sells CE-marked Devices: N

Orthosis, Limb Brace	Physical Med

CCL CONTAINERS　724-981-4420
One Llodio Drive, Hermitage, PA 16148
FDA Number: n/a　　　　　　　　　　Fax: 724-342-1116
Web site: www.cclcontainer.com
Annual Revenue: $0-$1 Million
Ownership: Private
Produces/Sells CE-marked Devices: N
Federal Procurement Eligibility: Small Business
Distribution: Manufacturer Direct, Service Direct

Bottle, Sterile Solution	General
Container, Medication, Graduated Liquid	General
Contract Packaging	General

CCL CUSTOM MANUFACTURING INC.
See KIK Custom Products

CCR MEDICAL, INC.　888-883-7331
967 43 Avenue NE,　　　　　　　727-822-1420
St. Petersburg, FL 33703
FDA Number: 1064565　　　　　　　Fax: 727-894-6650
E-mail: info@ccrmed.com
Web site: www.ccrmed.com
Year Founded: 1998
Ownership: Private
Produces/Sells CE-marked Devices: N
Federal Procurement Eligibility: Small Business, Female Owned
Distribution: Manufacturer Direct
Production: Mr. Charles Harstad/Product Manager

Connector, Airway (Extension)	Anesthesiology
Laryngoscope, Rigid	Anesthesiology
Stylet, Tracheal Tube	Anesthesiology
Transducer, Stethoscope	Anesthesiology

CCT LASER SERVICES　800-808-5273
25421 South Schulte Road, Tracy, CA 95377　209-833-1110
FDA Number: n/a　　　　　　　　　　Fax: 209-833-1116
E-mail: glove@cctlaser.com
Web site: www.cctlaser.com
Annual Revenue: $1-$5 Million
Year Founded: 1984
Total Employees: 10　　Marketing Staff: 1　　Sales Staff: 1
Ownership: Private
Produces/Sells CE-marked Devices: N
Federal Procurement Eligibility: Small Business
Distribution: Service Direct
General Admin.: Roger Underwood/Chief Executive Officer
Production: Michael Acosta/Manager Operations

Service, Printing	General

CD NELSON MANUFACTURING CO.　847-487-4870
26920 N Grace St, Wauconda, IL 60084
FDA Number: n/a　　　　　　　　　　Fax: 847-487-4873
E-mail: CN999@aol.com
Web site: www.cdnelson.com
Medical Products Sales Volume: $30,000
Annual Revenue: $0-$1 Million
Year Founded: 1978
Ownership: Private
Produces/Sells CE-marked Devices: Y
Federal Procurement Eligibility: Small Business
Distribution: Manufacturer Direct, Service Direct, Exporter
General Admin.: Agnes Nelson/Office Manager
　　　　　　　Clinton Nelson/President, Chief Executive Officer

Sterilizer, Steam (Autoclave)	General

CDB CORPORATION　910-383-6464
9201 Industrial Blvd. NE, Leland, NC 28451
FDA Number: 1054415
E-mail: info@cdbcorp.net
Web site: http://www.cdbcorp.net
Annual Revenue: $1-$5 Million
Ownership: Private
Quality System Registration Information: ISO9000
Produces/Sells CE-marked Devices: Y
Federal Procurement Eligibility: Small Business
Distribution: Manufacturer Direct, Manufacturer Through Distributor, OEM

MANUFACTURER PROFILES

CDB CORPORATION   910-383-6464 *(cont'd)*
Band, Material, Orthodontic   Dental And Oral
Bracket, Plastic, Orthodontic   Dental And Oral

CDC PRODUCTS CORP.   800-636-7363
1801 Falmouth Avenue,   516-437-3570
New Hyde Park, NY 11040
FDA Number: 2435053   Fax: 516-437-4126
E-mail: info@cdcproductscorp.com
Web site: www.cdcproductscorp.com
Annual Revenue: $5-$10 Million
Year Founded: 1970
Total Employees: 35   Marketing Staff: 2   Sales Staff: 5
Ownership: Mettis Group
Stock Symbol: ACET
Traded On: NASDAQ
Produces/Sells CE-marked Devices: N
Federal Procurement Eligibility: Small Business
Distribution: Manufacturer Through Distributor
General Admin.: Barbara Newman/Office Manager
     Hal Yerys/Regional Manager
     Michelle DeVito/Senior Vice President
Mktg./Adv.: Uday Gosalia/Division Manager
     Cindy Tomich/Manager International Marketing & Sales
     Les Brodie/Vice President, Manager Sales
IS: Bruce Victor/Technical Director
Encapsulator, Fluid   General
Housekeeping Equipment   General

CDI MEDICAL SERVICES
See Philips Remote Cardiac Services

CDL TECHNOLOGIES INC.   619-702-1806
645 Front St., Suite 2007, San Diego, CA 92101
FDA Number: 3004840176
Ownership: Private
Produces/Sells CE-marked Devices: N
Powder, Porcelain   Dental And Oral

CDM DENTAL   541-928-4444
812 Water St NE, Albany, OR 97321
FDA Number: 3034600   Fax: 541-928-2444
E-mail: info@cdmdental.com
Web site: www.duracetal.com
Medical Products Sales Volume: $500,000
Total Employees: 8
Ownership: Private
Produces/Sells CE-marked Devices: N
Clasp, Preformed   Dental And Oral
Crown And Bridge, Temporary, Resin   Dental And Oral
Dam, Rubber   Dental And Oral

CDS ANALYTICAL, INC.   800-541-6593
465 Limestone Road, Oxford, PA 19363-0277   610-932-3636
FDA Number: n/a   Fax: 610-932-4158
E-mail: cds@cdsanalytical.com
Web site: www.cdsanalytical.com
Annual Revenue: $1-$5 Million
Year Founded: 1969
Total Employees: 25   Marketing Staff: 3   Sales Staff: 3
Ownership: Private
Produces/Sells CE-marked Devices: Y
Federal Procurement Eligibility: Small Business
Distribution: Manufacturer Direct
Mktg./Adv.: Mr. Neil Cornelssen/Director Market Research & Planning
Analyzer, Chemistry, Multi-Channel, Fixed   Chemistry
Analyzer, Chemistry, Multi-Channel, Programmable   Chemistry
Analyzer, Chemistry, Single Channel, Programmable   Chemistry
Concentrator, Clinical Sample   Chemistry
Gas Chromatograph, Alcohol (Dedicated Instruments)   Toxicology
Sampler, Air   General

CEA INSTRUMENTS, INC.   888-893-9640
16 Chestnut St., Emerson, NJ 07630   201-967-5660
FDA Number: n/a   Fax: 201-967-8450
E-mail: ceainstr@aol.com
Web site: www.ceainstr.com
Medical Products Sales Volume: $1,000,000
Annual Revenue: $1-$5 Million
Year Founded: 1972
Total Employees: 12   Marketing Staff: 2   Sales Staff: 3
Ownership: Private
Quality System Registration Information: ISO9001
Produces/Sells CE-marked Devices: Y
Federal Procurement Eligibility: Small Business
Distribution: Manufacturer Through Distributor, Exclusive Distributor
General Admin.: Martin Adelman/Vice President, General Manager
Mktg./Adv.: Steven Adelman/Vice President Marketing & Sales
Analyzer, Ethylene-Oxide   General

CEA INSTRUMENTS, INC.   888-893-9640 *(cont'd)*
Analyzer, Gas, Nitrous-Oxide, Gaseous Phase   Anesthesiology

CEDARLANE LABORATORIES LTD.   800-268-5058
5516 8th Line R.R. 2,   905-878-8891
Hornby, ONT L0P 1 Canada
FDA Number: n/a   Fax: 905-878-7800
E-mail: info@cedarlanelabs.com
Web site: www.cedarlanelabs.com
Medical Products Sales Volume: $3,000,000
Year Founded: 1975
Total Employees: 45   Marketing Staff: 4   Sales Staff: 5
Ownership: Private
Quality System Registration Information: ISO9001
Produces/Sells CE-marked Devices: Y
Federal Procurement Eligibility: Female Owned
Distribution: Manufacturer Direct, Exclusive Distributor, Importer, Exporter

CEDARON MEDICAL, INC.   800-424-1007
PO Box 2100, Davis, CA 95617   530-758-7007
FDA Number: n/a   Fax: 530-759-1699
E-mail: cedaron@cedaron.com
Web site: www.cedaron.com
Medical Products Sales Volume: $7,700,000
Annual Revenue: $5-$10 Million
Year Founded: 1990
Total Employees: 40   Marketing Staff: 1   Sales Staff: 25
Ownership: Private
Produces/Sells CE-marked Devices: Y
Federal Procurement Eligibility: Small Business, Female Owned, GSA Contract, VA Contract
Distribution: Manufacturer Direct, Manufacturer Through Distributor, Manufacturer Through Manufacturer Reps, Service Direct, Exclusive Distributor, Exporter
General Admin.: Josh Segal/Administrator
     Karen Bond/President, Chief Executive Officer
Mktg./Adv.: Clay Chase/Director Marketing
     Malcolm L. Bond, Ph.D./Director Product Development
Production: George Van Derven/Director Quality Assurance
Research: Gary Engle/Vice President Research & Development
Computer Software   General

CEJAY ENGINEERING, LLC   888-584-3060
24600 South Tamiami Trail, Suite 212-353,   239-498-8923
Bonita Springs, FL 34134
FDA Number: 3004413478
E-mail: info@cejayeng.com
Ownership: Private
Produces/Sells CE-marked Devices: N
Light, Examination, Battery-Powered   General

CEL U DEX CORP.
See Aigner Index, Inc.

CELL BIOSCIENCES, INC.   888-607-9692
3040 Oakmead Village Drive,   408-510-5500
Santa Clara, CA 95051
FDA Number: n/a   Fax: 408-510-5599
E-mail: info@cellbiosciences.com
Web site: www.cellbiosciences.com
Year Founded: 2004
Ownership: Private
Produces/Sells CE-marked Devices: N
General Admin.: Tim Harkness/President, Chief Executive Officer
Mktg./Adv.: Ms. Jocelyn Dave/Director Marketing
     Dr. Trent Basarsky/Vice President Corporate Development
     Dr. Walter Ausserer/Vice President Marketing
Finance: Jason Novi/Chief Financial Officer

CELL MARQUE CORP.   916-746-8977
6600 Sierra College Blvd., Rocklin, CA 95677
FDA Number: 1649339
Cytokeratins   Immunology
Immunohistochemistry Assay, Antibody, Estrogen Receptor   Pathology
Immunohistochemistry Assay, Antibody, Progesterone Receptor   Pathology

CELL SCIENCE SYSTEMS, LTD. CORP.   954-426-2304
1239 E. Newport Center Dr., Suite 101,
Deerfield Beach, FL 33442
FDA Number: 1051901
Ownership: Private
Produces/Sells CE-marked Devices: N
Counter, Cell Or Particle, Automated   Hematology
Massager, Therapeutic   Physical Med
Whole Human Plasma, Antigen, Antiserum, Control   Immunology

CELL SOURCE
See Tulip Medical Products

CELLERATION, INC.
866-307-6478
6321 Bury Drive, Suite 15,
Eden Prairie, MN 55346
952-224-8700
FDA Number: 3004580659
Fax: 952-224-8750
Web site: http://www.celleration.com
Year Founded: 1999
Ownership: Private
Produces/Sells CE-marked Devices: N
General Admin.: Mr. Mark Wagner/President, Chief Executive Officer
Mktg./Adv.: Mr. Julie Higginson/Vice President Marketing & Sales
Research: Ms. Pamela Unger/Vice President Clinical Research
   Mr. Douglas Duchon/Vice President Research & Development
Finance: Mr. Christopher Geyen/Chief Financial Officer
Wound Cleaner, Ultrasound
Surgery

CELLEX BIOSCIENCES, INC.
See Biovest International, Inc.

CELLTRAK DIAGNOSTIC SYSTEMS, INC.
See Nova Biomedical

CELLUCAP MANUFACTURING CO.
800-523-3814
4626 N. 15th St., Philadelphia, PA 19140-1109
215-324-0213
FDA Number: 2523138
Fax: 215-324-1290
E-mail: sales@cellucap.com
Web site: www.cellucap.com
Medical Products Sales Volume: $14,500,000
Annual Revenue: $10-$25 Million
Year Founded: 1954
Total Employees: 30
Ownership: Private
Produces/Sells CE-marked Devices: N
Federal Procurement Eligibility: Small Business, Female Owned
Distribution: Manufacturer Through Distributor
General Admin.: Jane Harris/President
   Mark Davis/Vice President, General Manager
Mktg./Adv.: Damon Goodwin/Manager National Accounts & Sales
Production: Hank Wagenfeld/Director Quality Assurance
   Frank Schrier/Plant Manager
Accessories, Apparel, Surgical | Surgery
Cap, Surgical | Surgery
Cover, Head, Surgical | Surgery
Cover, Shoe, Conductive | General
Cover, Shoe, Operating Room | Surgery

CELLULAR DYNAMICS INTERNATIONAL
877-310-6688
525 Science Drive, Madison, WI 53711
608-310-5100
FDA Number: n/a
Web site: http://www.cellulardynamics.com
Ownership: Private
Produces/Sells CE-marked Devices: N
General Admin.: Mr. Robert Palay/Chief Executive Officer
   Mr. David Snyder/Chief Financial Officer, Vice President
   Dr. Emile Nuwaysir/Chief Operating Officer, Vice President
   Dr. James Thompson/Chief Scientific Officer
   Mr. Nicholas Seay/Chief Technology Officer
   Dr. Thomas Palay/President

CELLULAR PRODUCTS, INC.
See Zeptometrix Corporation

CELONOVA BIOSCIENCES INC.
1.770.632.2450
401 Westpark Court, Suite 100, Peachtree City, GA 30269
FDA Number: n/a
Fax: 1.770.631.7621
E-mail: info@celonova.com
Web site: www.celonova.com
Ownership: Private
Produces/Sells CE-marked Devices: N
General Admin.: Dr. Harry Jacobson/Chairman
   Thomas Gordy/President, Chief Executive Officer
Embolization Device | Cardiovascular

CELSION CORPORATION
800-262-0394
10220-L Old Columbia Road,
Columbia, MD 21046
410-290-5390
FDA Number: 1122126
Fax: 410-290-5394
E-mail: celsion@celsion.com
Web site: www.celsion.com
Medical Products Sales Volume: $11,200,000
Annual Revenue: $0-$1 Million
Year Founded: 1982
Total Employees: 29
Ownership: Public
Stock Symbol: CLN
Traded On: AMEX
Quality System Registration Information: ISO9002
Produces/Sells CE-marked Devices: Y
Federal Procurement Eligibility: Small Business
Distribution: Exclusive Distributor

CELSION CORPORATION
800-262-0394 *(cont'd)*
General Admin.: Mr. Tony Deasey/Chief Financial Officer, Vice President Operations
   Augustine Cheung/President, Chief Executive Officer
System, Cancer Treatment, Hyperthermia, RF/Microwave | Radiology
System, Hyperthermia, Rf/microwave (benign Prostatic Hyperplasia), Thermotherapy | Gastroenterology/Urology

CELSIS LABORATORY GROUP
800-523-5227
165 Fieldcrest Avenue, Edison, NJ 08837
732-346-5100
FDA Number: 2210008
Fax: 732-346-5115
E-mail: info@celsislabs.com
Web site: www.celsislabs.com
Medical Products Sales Volume: $3,000,000
Annual Revenue: $10-$25 Million
Year Founded: 1997
Total Employees: 50 | *Marketing Staff:* 1 | *Sales Staff:* 3
Ownership: CELSIS INTERNATIONAL PLC
Quality System Registration Information: ISO9001
Produces/Sells CE-marked Devices: N
Federal Procurement Eligibility: Small Business
Distribution: Service Direct
General Admin.: Anthony Grilli/Vice President, General Manager
Mktg./Adv.: Ken Giebe/Vice President Marketing & Sales
Production: Andrea Perewijnyk/Director Quality Assurance
   Dennis Fleming/Vice President Regulatory Affairs
Absorption, Atomic, Antimony | Toxicology
Absorption, Atomic, Arsenic | Toxicology
Absorption, Atomic, Calcium | Chemistry
Absorption, Atomic, Iron (Non-Heme) | Chemistry
Absorption, Atomic, Lead | Toxicology
Absorption, Atomic, Lithium | Toxicology
Absorption, Atomic, Magnesium | Chemistry
Absorption, Atomic, Mercury | Toxicology
Chromatography (Gas), Clinical Use | Toxicology
Chromatography, Liquid, Performance, High | Toxicology
Contract R&D, Diagnostics | General
Equipment/Service, Quality Control | General
Radioimmunoassay, ACTH | Chemistry
Radioimmunoassay, Follicle Stimulating Hormone | Chemistry
Radioimmunoassay, Luteinizing Hormone | Chemistry
Test, Antibiotic Susceptibility | Microbiology
Test, Heparin (Clotting Time) | Hematology
Test, Human Chorionic Gonadotropin | Immunology

CENOGENICS CORP.
800-747-9457
100 Route 520, Drawer 308,
Morganville, NJ 07751
732-536-6457
FDA Number: 2250030
Fax: 732-972-8527
E-mail: info@cenogenics.com
Web site: www.cenogenics.net
Annual Revenue: $1-$5 Million
Ownership: Private
Produces/Sells CE-marked Devices: N
Federal Procurement Eligibility: Small Business
Distribution: Manufacturer Direct, OEM, Service Direct, Exporter
General Admin.: Michael Katz/President
   Nitza Hernandez-Katz/Vice President
Antigen, (Febrile), Agglutination, Brucella SPP. | Microbiology
Antigen, Febrile | Microbiology
Antigen, Febrile, Slide And Tube, Salmonella | Microbiology
Antigen, Non-Treponemal, All | Microbiology
Antigen, Salmonella SPP. | Microbiology
Antiserum, Positive And Negative Febrile Antigen Control | Microbiology
Kit, Pregnancy Test | Obstetrics/Gynecology
Radioimmunoassay, Infectious Mononucleosis | Microbiology
Reagent, Guaiac | Hematology
Reagent, Occult Blood | Hematology
Reagent, Streptolysin O/Antistreptolysin-Titer | Microbiology
Serum, Reactive And Non-Specific Control, FTA-ABS Test | Microbiology
Standard/Control, All Types | Chemistry
Streptolysin O | Pathology
Test, C-Reactive Protein | Immunology
Test, Rheumatoid Factor | Immunology
Test, Syphilis (RPR or VDRL) | Microbiology

CENORIN
800-426-1042
6324 S. 199th Place, Suite 107, Kent, WA 98032
253-395-2400
FDA Number: 3004153171
Fax: 253-395-2650
E-mail: info@cenorin.com
Web site: www.cenorin.com
Medical Products Sales Volume: $1,500,000
Annual Revenue: $1-$5 Million
Year Founded: 2001
Total Employees: 26 | *Marketing Staff:* 1 | *Sales Staff:* 4
Ownership: Private
Produces/Sells CE-marked Devices: N
Federal Procurement Eligibility: Small Business

CENORIN
800-426-1042 (cont'd)

Distribution: Manufacturer Direct, Manufacturer Through Distributor, Manufacturer Through Manufacturer Reps, Exporter
General Admin.: Richard Radford/Chief Executive Officer
　　　Kaye Counts/President
Mktg./Adv.: Ms. Valerie Thomson/Marketing Coordinator
　　　Mr. Todd Medley/Vice President Sales

Disinfector, Pasteurization	General
Dressing, Other	General
Dryer, Respiratory/Anesthesia Equipment	General
Soap	General

CENTENNIAL OPTICAL LTD.
800-561-0681
158 Norfinch Dr.,
416-739-8539
Toronto, ONTAR M3N 1 Canada
FDA Number: 9680743　　　　　*Fax:* 416-739-6504
E-mail: info@centennialoptical.com
Web site: www.centennialoptical.com
Year Founded: 1967
Total Employees: 200　　*Marketing Staff:* 5　　*Sales Staff:* 30
Ownership: Private
Produces/Sells CE-marked Devices: Y
Federal Procurement Eligibility: Small Business
Distribution: Exclusive Distributor

CENTENNIAL PRODUCTS INC.
888-604-1004
6900 Philips Hwyd, Suite 45,
904-332-0404
Jacksonville, FL 32216
FDA Number: n/a　　　　　*Fax:* 904-332-0406
E-mail: sales@centennialproducts.com
Web site: www.centennialproducts.com
Medical Products Sales Volume: $1,170,000
Annual Revenue: $1-$5 Million
Year Founded: 1999
Total Employees: 3　　*Marketing Staff:* 1　　*Sales Staff:* 4
Ownership: Private
Quality System Registration Information: ISO9000
Produces/Sells CE-marked Devices: N
Federal Procurement Eligibility: Small Business, Female Owned
Distribution: Manufacturer Direct, Manufacturer Through Distributor, Manufacturer Through Manufacturer Reps
General Admin.: Ms. Jane M. Everson/President, Chief Executive Officer
Mktg./Adv.: Ms. Lisa Smith/Admin. Marketing & Sales
　　　Ms. Jane M. Everson/Manager National Sales
Finance: Ms. Cindy Maguire/Controller, Credit Manager
IS: Ms. Lisa Smith/Web Master

Bag, Body	General

CENTER FOR OCULAR PROSTHETICS, LLC.
503-229-8490
2525 N.w. Lovejoy, Suite 306, Portland, OR 97210
FDA Number: 3030033

Eye, Artificial, Non-Custom	Ophthalmology

CENTER FOR OCULAR RECONSTRUCTION
(800) 982-EYES
4833 Rugby Ave., 4th Flr., Bethesda, MD 20814
301-652-9282
FDA Number: 3004552445　　　*Fax:* (301) 652-7585
E-mail: contact@frieleyes.com
Web site: www.frieleyes.com
Ownership: Private
Produces/Sells CE-marked Devices: N

Conformer, Ophthalmic	Ophthalmology
Eye, Artificial, Non-Custom	Ophthalmology
Shell, Scleral	Ophthalmology

CENTER FOR ORTHOTIC & PROSTHETIC CARE
812-941-0966
1931 West St., New Albany, IN 47150
FDA Number: 3003144682　　　*Fax:* 812-941-0958
Ownership: Private
Produces/Sells CE-marked Devices: N

Orthosis, Cranial	Cns/Neurology

CENTERPULSE ORTHOPEDICS INC.
877-768-7349
9900 Spectrum Drive, Austin, TX 78717
512-432-9900
FDA Number: 2935620　　　　*Fax:* 512-432-9014
E-mail: kelly.erickson@sous.com
Web site: www.sulzerorthopedics.com
Total Employees: 125　*Marketing Staff:* 50　*Sales Staff:* 275
Ownership: SULZER MEDICA
Stock Symbol: SM
Traded On: NYSE
Quality System Registration Information: ISO9001
Produces/Sells CE-marked Devices: Y
Federal Procurement Eligibility: Small Business, GSA Contract
Distribution: Manufacturer Through Distributor, Manufacturer Through Manufacturer Reps
General Admin.: Stephen Rieticker/Chief Executive Officer
　　　David Floyd/President
　　　Renee Rogers/Vice President Human Resources

CENTERPULSE ORTHOPEDICS INC.
877-768-7349 (cont'd)

　　　Pete Vescolen/Vice President, General Manager
Mktg./Adv.: Kelly Carper Erickson/Director Communications
　　　Frank Jensen/Director National Sales
　　　Janet Stacey/Manager Market Research
　　　Dana Kolflat/Manager Sales Training
　　　Jerry DeVries/Vice President Marketing
Production: Rob McCollough/Director Quality Assurance
　　　Mitchell Dhority/Manager Regulatory Affairs
Research: Steve Whitlock/Vice President Research & Development
　　　Larry Beeman/Vice President Scientific Affairs
Finance: Jeff Frizell/Vice President Finance

Plate, Fixation, Bone	Orthopedics
Prosthesis, Elbow, Constrained	Orthopedics
Prosthesis, Hip, Femoral Component, Cemented, Metal	Orthopedics
Prosthesis, Hip, Femoral, Resurfacing	Orthopedics
Prosthesis, Hip, Hemi-, Femoral, Metal/Polymer	Orthopedics
Prosthesis, Hip, Semi-Const., Metal/Poly., Porous Uncemented	Orthopedics
Prosthesis, Hip, Semi-Const., Uncem., Non-P., M/P, Ca./Phos.	Orthopedics
Prosthesis, Hip, Semi-Constr., Metal/Ceramic, Cemented/NC	Orthopedics
Prosthesis, Hip, Semi-Constrained Acetabular	Orthopedics
Prosthesis, Hip, Semi-Constrained, Metal/Polymer	Orthopedics
Prosthesis, Knee, Femorotibial, Semi-Constrained	Orthopedics
Prosthesis, Knee, Hemi-, Tibial Resurfacing, Uncemented	Orthopedics
Prosthesis, Knee, Patellofemoral, Semi-Constrained	Orthopedics
Prosthesis, Knee, Patellofemorotibial, Semi-Constrained	Orthopedics
Prosthesis, Shoulder, Non-Constrained, Metal/Polymer Cem.	Orthopedics
Prosthesis, Shoulder, Semi-Constrained, Metal/Polymer Cem.	Orthopedics

Medical Product Subsidiaries (Listed Separately)
　Sulzer Orthopedics

CENTERS FOR DISEASE CONTROL
See Centers For Disease Control And Prevention

CENTERS FOR DISEASE CONTROL AND PREVENTION
800-232-4636
1600 Clifton Rd., Atlanta, GA 30333
888-232-6348
FDA Number: 1050190
E-mail: cdcinfo@cdc.gov
Web site: www.cdc.gov
Total Employees: 14000
Ownership: Private
Produces/Sells CE-marked Devices: N
Distribution: Manufacturer Through Distributor
General Admin.: Jim Seligman/Chief Information Officer
　　　Richard E. Besser/Director
Finance: Barbara Harris/Chief Financial Officer

Anti-Human Globulin, FTA-ABS Test (Coombs)	Microbiology
Antigen, (Febrile), Agglutination, Brucella SPP.	Microbiology
Antigen, Blastomyces Dermatitidis, Other	Microbiology
Antigen, CF (Including CF Control), Adenovirus 1-33	Microbiology
Antigen, CF (Including CF Control), Coxsackievirus A 1-24	Microbiology
Antigen, CF (Including CF Control), Echovirus 1-34	Microbiology
Antigen, CF (Including CF Control), Equine Encephalitis	Microbiology
Antigen, CF (Including CF Control), Influenza Virus	Microbiology
Antigen, CF (Including CF Control), Mumps Virus	Microbiology
Antigen, CF (Including CF Control), Parainfluenza Virus	Microbiology
Antigen, CF (Including CF Control), Poliovirus 1-3	Microbiology
Antigen, CF (Including CF Controls), Respiratory Syncytial	Microbiology
Antigen, CF And/Or ID, Coccidioides Immitis	Microbiology
Antigen, CF, (Including CF Control), Rubeola	Microbiology
Antigen, CF, (Including CF Control), Varicella-Zoster	Microbiology
Antigen, CF, B. Dermatitidis	Microbiology
Antigen, CF, Mycoplasma SPP.	Microbiology
Antigen, CF, Psittacosis (Chlamydia Group)	Microbiology
Antigen, CF, Q Fever	Microbiology
Antigen, CF, Spotted Fever Group	Microbiology
Antigen, CF, Typhus Fever Group	Microbiology
Antigen, Cf (including Cf Control), Herpesvirus Hominis 1, 2	Microbiology
Antigen, HA (Including HA Control), Influenza Virus	Microbiology
Antigen, HA (Including HA Control), Mumps Virus	Microbiology
Antigen, HA (Including HA Control), Parainfluenza Virus	Microbiology
Antigen, HA (Including HA Control), Reovirus 1-3	Microbiology
Antigen, HA (Including HA Control), Rubella	Microbiology
Antigen, HA (Including HA Control), Rubeola	Microbiology
Antigen, Histoplasma Capsulatum, All	Microbiology
Antigen, IF, Toxoplasma Gondii	Microbiology
Antigen, Non-Treponemal, All	Microbiology
Antigen, Positive Control, Cryptococcus Neoformans	Microbiology
Antigen, Slide And Tube, Francisella Tularensis	Microbiology
Antigen, Treponema Pallidum For FTA-ABS Test	Microbiology
Antisera, Cf, Herpesvirus Hominis 1, 2	Microbiology
Antisera, Fluorescent, Herpesvirus Hominis 1, 2	Microbiology
Antiserum, Arizona SPP.	Microbiology
Antiserum, Blastomyces Dermatitidis, Other	Microbiology
Antiserum, CF, Adenovirus 1-33	Microbiology
Antiserum, CF, Coxsackievirus A 1-24, B 1-6	Microbiology
Antiserum, CF, Echovirus 1-34	Microbiology
Antiserum, CF, Equine Encephalitis Virus, EEE, WEE	Microbiology
Antiserum, CF, Influenza Virus A, B, C	Microbiology

CENTERS FOR DISEASE CONTROL AND
800-232-4636 (cont'd)

Antiserum, CF, Mumps Virus	Microbiology
Antiserum, CF, Parainfluenza Virus 1-4	Microbiology
Antiserum, CF, Psittacosis (Chlamydia Group)	Microbiology
Antiserum, CF, Q Fever	Microbiology
Antiserum, CF, Rubeola	Microbiology
Antiserum, CF, Varicella-Zoster	Microbiology
Antiserum, Control For Non-Treponemal Test	Microbiology
Antiserum, Escherichia Coli	Microbiology
Antiserum, Fluorescent (Direct Test), N. Gonorrhoeae	Microbiology
Antiserum, Fluorescent, All Globulins, Salmonella SPP.	Microbiology
Antiserum, Fluorescent, B. Pertussis	Microbiology
Antiserum, Fluorescent, Cryptococcus Neoformans	Microbiology
Antiserum, Fluorescent, Escherichia Coli	Microbiology
Antiserum, Fluorescent, Francisella Tularensis	Microbiology
Antiserum, Fluorescent, Groups, Streptococcus SPP.	Microbiology
Antiserum, Fluorescent, Hemophilus SPP.	Microbiology
Antiserum, Fluorescent, Histoplasma Capsulatum	Microbiology
Antiserum, Fluorescent, N. Meningitidis	Microbiology
Antiserum, Fluorescent, Pseudomonas Pseudomallei	Microbiology
Antiserum, Fluorescent, Rabies Virus	Microbiology
Antiserum, Fluorescent, Shigella SPP., All Globulins	Microbiology
Antiserum, Fluorescent, Sporothrix Schenckii	Microbiology
Antiserum, Fluorescent, Streptococcus Pneumoniae	Microbiology
Antiserum, Francisella Tularensis	Microbiology
Antiserum, H. Influenzae	Microbiology
Antiserum, HAI (Including HAI Control), Rubella	Microbiology
Antiserum, HAI, Influenza Virus A, B, C	Microbiology
Antiserum, HAI, Mumps Virus	Microbiology
Antiserum, HAI, Parainfluenza Virus 1-4	Microbiology
Antiserum, HAI, Reovirus 1-3	Microbiology
Antiserum, HAI, Rubeola	Microbiology
Antiserum, Klebsiella SPP.	Microbiology
Antiserum, Latex Agglutination, Cryptococcus Neoformans	Microbiology
Antiserum, Leptospira SPP.	Microbiology
Antiserum, Mycoplasma SPP.	Microbiology
Antiserum, N. Meningitidis	Microbiology
Antiserum, Neutralization, Adenovirus 1-33	Microbiology
Antiserum, Neutralization, Coxsackievirus A 1-24, B 1-6	Microbiology
Antiserum, Neutralization, Echovirus 1-34	Microbiology
Antiserum, Neutralization, Herpes Virus Hominis	Microbiology
Antiserum, Neutralization, Parainfluenza Virus 1-4	Microbiology
Antiserum, Neutralization, Poliovirus 1-3	Microbiology
Antiserum, Neutralization, Respiratory Syncytial Virus	Microbiology
Antiserum, Neutralization, Rubeola	Microbiology
Antiserum, Neutralizing, Reovirus 1-3	Microbiology
Antiserum, Positive And Negative Febrile Antigen Control	Microbiology
Antiserum, Positive Control, Blastomyces Dermatitidis	Microbiology
Antiserum, Positive Control, Coccidioides Immitis	Microbiology
Antiserum, Positive Control, Histoplasma Capsulatum	Microbiology
Antiserum, Salmonella SPP.	Microbiology
Antiserum, Streptococcus Pneumoniae	Microbiology
Antiserum, Streptococcus SPP.	Microbiology
Antiserum, Typhus Fever	Microbiology
Antiserum, Vibrio Cholerae	Microbiology
Kit, Identification, Yeast	Microbiology
Neuramininase (Sialidase)	Pathology
Phages, Staphylococcal Typing, All Types	Microbiology
Serum, Reactive And Non-Specific Control, FTA-ABS Test	Microbiology
Sorbent, FTA-ABS Test	Microbiology

CENTINEL SPINE INC.
952-885-0500
505 Park Ave., 14th Floor, New York, NY 10022
FDA Number: 3007494564 — Fax: 952-885-0200
E-mail: info@centinelspine.com
Web site: http://www.centinelspine.com
Ownership: Private
Produces/Sells CE-marked Devices: N

Appliance, Fixation, Spinal Interlaminal	Orthopedics
Appliance, Fixation, Spinal Intervertebral Body	Orthopedics
Awl	Orthopedics
Driver, Prosthesis	Orthopedics
Impactor	Orthopedics
Intervertebral Fusion Device With Bone Graft, Cervical	Orthopedics
Orthopedic Manual Surgical Instrument	Orthopedics
Rongeur, Other	Surgery
Screwdriver	Orthopedics
Template	Orthopedics
Tray, Surgical Instrument	Surgery

CENTOCOR, INC.
800-457-6399
800/850 Ridgeview Drive, Horsham, PA 19044
610-651-6000
FDA Number: n/a — Fax: 610-651-6100
Web site: www.centocor.com
Medical Products Sales Volume: $32,863,000
Annual Revenue: $25-$50 Million
Ownership: JOHNSON & JOHNSON
Stock Symbol: JNJ
Traded On: NYSE
Quality System Registration Information: ISO9000
Produces/Sells CE-marked Devices: N

CENTOCOR, INC.
800-457-6399 (cont'd)
Distribution: Manufacturer Through Distributor
General Admin.: David P. Holveck/President, Chief Executive Officer
Mktg./Adv.: Aris Petropoulos/Vice President Marketing & Sales
Research: Richard Malklosky/Director Research & Development

Contract Manufacturing, Pharmaceuticals/Chemicals	General
Contract R&D, Diagnostics	General
Cytomegalovirus, DNA Reagents	Microbiology
System, Identification, Hepatitis B Antigen	Hematology
Test, Cancer Detection, Monoclonal Antibody	Immunology
Test, Chemotherapy Sensitivity (Tumor Colony Forming)	Immunology
Test, Syphilis (RPR or VDRL)	Microbiology

CENTORR FURNACES
See Centorr Vacuum Industries

CENTORR VACUUM INDUSTRIES
800-962-8631
55 Northeastern Blvd., Nashua, NH 03062
603-595-7233
FDA Number: n/a — Fax: 603-595-9220
E-mail: sales@centorr.com
Web site: www.centorr.com
Medical Products Sales Volume: $7,500,000
Annual Revenue: $10-$25 Million
Ownership: Private
Produces/Sells CE-marked Devices: Y
Federal Procurement Eligibility: Small Business
Distribution: Manufacturer Direct
General Admin.: William J. Nareski/Chief Executive Officer
Production: Stephen Hewitt/Vice President Operations

Oven	Chemistry

CENTRAL ASSOC. FOR BLIND & VISUALLY IMPAIRED
877-719-9996
507 Kent St., Utica, NY 13501
315-797-2233
FDA Number: 1319302
Web site: www.cabvi.org
Medical Products Sales Volume: $5,000,000
Annual Revenue: $5-$10 Million
Year Founded: 1929
Total Employees: 163
Ownership: Private
Produces/Sells CE-marked Devices: N
Distribution: Manufacturer Direct, Manufacturer Through Distributor, Service Direct

Contract Packaging	General
Glove, Patient Examination	General
Glove, Patient Examination, Latex	General
Glove, Patient Examination, Poly	General
Glove, Patient Examination, Vinyl	General

CENTRAL BIOMEDIA, INC.
800-448-0016
9900 Pflumm Rd., Unit 61-63, Lenexa, KS 66215
913-541-0090
FDA Number: n/a — Fax: 913-541-1712
Web site: www.centralbiomedia.com
Annual Revenue: $0-$1 Million
Year Founded: 1985
Total Employees: 30 — Marketing Staff: 3 — Sales Staff: 3
Ownership: Private
Quality System Registration Information: ISO9000
Produces/Sells CE-marked Devices: N
Federal Procurement Eligibility: Small Business
Distribution: OEM
General Admin.: William G. Skelly/President
Mktg./Adv.: Cathy Wright/Vice President Sales
Production: Donald Myers/Manager Regulatory Affairs

Serum, Animal	Pathology

CENTRAL CANADA CONTACT LENSES INC.
877-223-9807
3075 14th Ave., Markham, ONT L3R 5L2 Canada
905-968-2000
FDA Number: n/a — Fax: 905-968-2400
Web site: www.jnjcanada.com
Year Founded: 1979
Total Employees: 10
Ownership: Private
Produces/Sells CE-marked Devices: N
Distribution: Manufacturer Direct, Exclusive Distributor

CENTRAL NEW YORK MEDICAL PRODUCTS
315-428-9945
749 W. Genesee St, Syracuse, NY 13204
FDA Number: 1319259
E-mail: customerservice@cnymedpro.com
Web site: www.cnymedpro.com
Medical Products Sales Volume: $250,000
Annual Revenue: $0-$1 Million
Year Founded: 1981
Ownership: Private
Produces/Sells CE-marked Devices: N
Distribution: Manufacturer Direct

Bed, Manual	General

CENTRAL NEW YORK MEDICAL PRODUCTS   315-428-9945
(cont'd)

Halter, Head, Traction, Orthopedic	Orthopedics
Wheelchair, Manual	Physical Med

CENTRAL PAPER PRODUCTS COMPANY   800-339-4065
P.O. Box 4480, Manchester, NH 03108-4480   603-624-4064
FDA Number: n/a   *Fax:* 603-624-8795
E-mail: customerservice@centralpaper.com
Web site: www.centralpaper.com
Total Employees: 45   *Marketing Staff:* 1   *Sales Staff:* 15
Ownership: Private
Produces/Sells CE-marked Devices: N
Federal Procurement Eligibility: Small Business
Distribution: Manufacturer Through Distributor
General Admin.: Fred Kfoury/President
Mktg./Adv.: Fred Kfoury/Manager Marketing
     David Martineau/Manager Sales
Production: Robert Dalzell/Manager Warehouse
Purchasing: Christine Kfoury/Manager Purchasing

Foodservice Product/Equipment	General
Garment, Protective, For Incontinence	Gastroenterology/Urology
Glove, Patient Examination	General
Housekeeping Equipment	General
Pad, Incontinence (Underpad)	General
Towel/Towelette, Paper	General

CENTRAL SOLUTIONS, INC.   913-621-6542
401 Funston Road, Kansas City, KS 66115
FDA Number: 1932672

Medical Disinfectants/Cleaners for Instruments	General

CENTRAL WELDER'S SUPPLY, INC.   800-728-2068
127-d Lee Road, Watsonville, CA 95076   831-728-2068
FDA Number: 2938477   *Fax:* 831-728-1364
E-mail: Medmanatcw@aol.com
Web site: www.centralwelderssupply.com
Medical Products Sales Volume: $3,800,000
Year Founded: 1975
Total Employees: 21
Ownership: Private
Produces/Sells CE-marked Devices: N
Federal Procurement Eligibility: Small Business
Distribution: Manufacturer Direct
Production: Mr. Jason Norman/Director Operations

Cryosurgical, Unit, Urology	Surgery
Handpiece, Belt and/or Gear Driven, Dental	Dental And Oral

CENTRICO, INC.
   See Gea Westfalia Separator, Inc.

CENTRIMED
   See Terumo Cardiovascular Systems, Corp

CENTRIX, INC.   800-235-5862
770 River Rd., Shelton, CT 06484-5458   203-929-5582
FDA Number: 1281412   *Fax:* 203-929-6804
Web site: www.centrixdental.com
Annual Revenue: $5-$10 Million
Total Employees: 110   *Marketing Staff:* 7   *Sales Staff:* 25
Ownership: Private
Quality System Registration Information: ISO9000
Produces/Sells CE-marked Devices: Y
Federal Procurement Eligibility: Small Business
Distribution: Manufacturer Direct, Manufacturer Through Manufacturer Reps, OEM, Importer, Exporter
General Admin.: William Dragan/Chairman
     John Discko/Executive Vice President
     William Dragan/President
     Arthur Fattibene/Vice President Legal Services
Mktg./Adv.: Leif Klein/Vice President Marketing & Sales

Brush, Other	General
Coating, Filling Material, Resin	Dental And Oral
Material, Dental Filling	Dental And Oral
Syringe, Cartridge	Dental And Oral
Syringe, Dental	Dental And Oral
Syringe, Periodontic, Endodontic	Dental And Oral
Syringe, Restorative And Impression Material	Dental And Oral

CENTRON TECHNOLOGIES, INC.   215-501-0430
10601 Decatur Road, Suite 100, Philadelphia, PA 19154
FDA Number: 3005824261

Heat-Sealing Device	Hematology
Mixer/Scale, Blood	Hematology

CENTURION MEDICAL PRODUCTS CORP.   517-545-1135
3310 South Main St., Salisbury, NC 28147
FDA Number: 1038445
Web site: www.tristate.com
Ownership: Private

CENTURION MEDICAL PRODUCTS CORP.   517-545-1135 *(cont'd)*
Produces/Sells CE-marked Devices: N

Accessories, Catheter	Surgery
Applicator, Tipped, Absorbent, Sterile	General
Applicator, Vaginal	Obstetrics/Gynecology
Bag, Leg	Gastroenterology/Urology
Bandage, Cast	Physical Med
Bandage, Elastic	General
Basin, Emesis	General
Bath, Sitz, Non-Powered	Physical Med
Bedpan	General
Binder, Abdominal	General
Binder, Breast	Obstetrics/Gynecology
Binder, Elastic	General
Brush, Cleaning, Tracheal Tube	Ear/Nose/Throat
Cannula, Surgical, General & Plastic Surgery	Surgery
Catheter, Intravascular, Therapeutic, Short-term Less Than 30 Days	General
Catheter, Suction (Tracheal Aspirating Tube)	Anesthesiology
Cleaner, Denture	Dental And Oral
Container, Medication, Graduated Liquid	General
Container, Specimen, All Types	General
Cover, Limb	Physical Med
Decontamination Kit	Surgery
Dispenser, Medication, Liquid	General
Drainage System, Urine, Closed	Gastroenterology/Urology
Drape, Surgical	General
Ear Irrigation Kit	General
Fiber, Absorbent	General
Forceps, General & Plastic Surgery	Surgery
Gas, Collecting Vessel	Anesthesiology
Gauze, Non-Absorbable, X-Ray Detectable (Internal Sponge)	Surgery
Gauze/sponge, Nonresorbable For External Use	Surgery
General Use Surgical Scissors	Surgery
Gown, Examination	General
Holder, Intravascular Catheter	General
IV Start Kit	Surgery
Kit, Administration, Intravenous	General
Kit, Irrigation, Sterile	Gastroenterology/Urology
Kit, Labor and Delivery	Obstetrics/Gynecology
Kit, Pelvic Exam	Obstetrics/Gynecology
Kit, Surgical (General)	Surgery
Kit, Surgical Instrument, Disposable	Surgery
Kit, Suture Removal	Surgery
Kit, Urinary Drainage Collection	Gastroenterology/Urology
Kit, Wound Dressing	Surgery
Label/Tag, Sterile	Surgery
Linen, Bed	General
Lubricant, Patient	General
Marker, Skin	Surgery
Nebulizer, Medicinal, Non-Ventilatory (Atomizer)	Anesthesiology
Occluder, Umbilical	General
Pad, Eye	Ophthalmology
Pad, Menstrual, Unscented	Obstetrics/Gynecology
Patient Personal Hygiene Kit	Dental And Oral
Retractor, Vaginal	Obstetrics/Gynecology
Scissors, Disposable	General
Spatula, Cervical, Cytology	Obstetrics/Gynecology
Speculum, Ear	Ear/Nose/Throat
Speculum, Vaginal, Metal	Obstetrics/Gynecology
Stethoscope, Manual	Cardiovascular
Surgical Instrument, Disposable	Surgery
Surgical Instrument, Obstetric/Gynecologic	Obstetrics/Gynecology
Surgical, Razor	Surgery
Syringe, Irrigating	Surgery
Syringe, Irrigating, Dental	Dental And Oral
Toothbrush, Manual	Dental And Oral
Tourniquet, Non-Pneumatic, Surgical	Surgery
Tray, Surgical	Surgery
Tube, Aspirating, Flexible, Connecting	Anesthesiology
Urinal	General
Washer, Receptacle, Waste, Body	General

CENTURION MEDICAL PRODUCTS CORPORATION   866-386-0530
3173 East 43rd St., Yuma, AZ 85365   517-546-5400
FDA Number: 2032758   *Fax:* 517-546-1195
E-mail: info@tshsc.com
Ownership: Private
Produces/Sells CE-marked Devices: N

Accessories, Catheter	Surgery
Applicator, Tipped, Absorbent, Sterile	General
Applicator, Vaginal	Obstetrics/Gynecology
Bag, Leg	Gastroenterology/Urology
Bandage, Cast	Physical Med
Bandage, Elastic	General
Basin, Emesis	General
Bath, Sitz, Non-Powered	Physical Med
Bedpan	General
Binder, Abdominal	General
Binder, Breast	Obstetrics/Gynecology
Binder, Elastic	General

CENTURION MEDICAL PRODUCTS   866-386-0530 (cont'd)

Brush, Cleaning, Tracheal Tube	Ear/Nose/Throat
Cannula, Surgical, General & Plastic Surgery	Surgery
Catheter, Intravascular, Therapeutic, Short-term Less Than 30 Days	General
Catheter, Suction (Tracheal Aspirating Tube)	Anesthesiology
Cleaner, Denture	Dental And Oral
Container, Medication, Graduated Liquid	General
Container, Specimen, All Types	General
Cover, Limb	Physical Med
Decontamination Kit	Surgery
Dispenser, Medication, Liquid	General
Drainage System, Urine, Closed	Gastroenterology/Urology
Drape, Surgical	Surgery
Ear Irrigation Kit	General
Fiber, Absorbent	General
Forceps, General & Plastic Surgery	Surgery
Gas, Collecting Vessel	Anesthesiology
Gauze, Non-Absorbable, X-Ray Detectable (Internal Sponge)	Surgery
Gauze/sponge, Nonresorbable For External Use	Surgery
General Use Surgical Scissors	Surgery
Gown, Examination	General
Holder, Intravascular Catheter	General
IV Start Kit	Surgery
Kit, Administration, Intravenous	General
Kit, Irrigation, Sterile	Gastroenterology/Urology
Kit, Labor and Delivery	Obstetrics/Gynecology
Kit, Pelvic Exam	Obstetrics/Gynecology
Kit, Surgical (General)	Surgery
Kit, Surgical Instrument, Disposable	Surgery
Kit, Suture Removal	Surgery
Kit, Urinary Drainage Collection	Gastroenterology/Urology
Kit, Wound Dressing	Surgery
Label/Tag, Sterile	Surgery
Linen, Bed	General
Lubricant, Patient	General
Marker, Skin	General
Nebulizer, Medicinal, Non-Ventilatory (Atomizer)	Anesthesiology
Occluder, Umbilical	General
Pad, Eye	Ophthalmology
Pad, Menstrual, Unscented	Obstetrics/Gynecology
Patient Personal Hygiene Kit	Dental And Oral
Retractor, Vaginal	Obstetrics/Gynecology
Scissors, Disposable	General
Spatula, Cervical, Cytology	Obstetrics/Gynecology
Speculum, Ear	Ear/Nose/Throat
Speculum, Vaginal, Metal	Obstetrics/Gynecology
Stethoscope, Manual	Cardiovascular
Surgical Instrument, Disposable	Surgery
Surgical Instrument, Obstetric/Gynecologic	Obstetrics/Gynecology
Surgical, Razor	Surgery
Syringe, Irrigating	General
Syringe, Irrigating, Dental	Dental And Oral
Toothbrush, Manual	Dental And Oral
Tourniquet, Non-Pneumatic, Surgical	Surgery
Tray, Surgical	Surgery
Tube, Aspirating, Flexible, Connecting	Anesthesiology
Urinal	General
Washer, Receptacle, Waste, Body	General

CENTURY MANUFACTURING CO.
See ArjoHuntleigh

CENTURY PHARMACEUTICALS, INC.   317-849-4210
10377 Hague Rd., Indianapolis, IN 46256
FDA Number: 1819174

Concentrate, Dialysis, Hemodialysis (Liquid or Powder)	Gastroenterology/Urology
Saliva, Artificial	Dental And Oral

CENTURY WOODWORKING CORP.   330-753-2024
846 Coventry Road, Barberton, OH 44203
FDA Number: n/a   *Fax:* 330-753-3930
Total Employees: 12
Ownership: Private
Produces/Sells CE-marked Devices: N
Federal Procurement Eligibility: Small Business
Distribution: Manufacturer Direct
General Admin.: Russ Snyder/President
        Connie Snyder/Secretary

Furniture, General	General

CEPHEID   408-541-4191
904 Caribbean Drive, Sunnyvale, CA 94089
FDA Number: 3004530256   *Fax:* 408-541-4192
Web site: http://www.cepheid.com
Ownership: Private
Stock Symbol: CPHD
Traded On: NASDAQ
Produces/Sells CE-marked Devices: N
General Admin.: John L. Bishop/Chief Executive Officer
        Andrew D. Miller/Chief Financial Officer, Senior Vice President

CEPHEID   408-541-4191 (cont'd)
Humberto Reyes/Chief Operating Officer, Executive Vice President
  Medical Admin.: Dr. David Persing/Chief Medical Officer
  Production: Nicolaas Arnold/Executive Vice President Operations
  Research: Dr. Peter Dailey/Senior Vice President Research & Development

Assay, Enterovirus Nucleic Acid	Microbiology
Nucleic Acid Amplification Assay System, Group B Streptococcus, Direct Specimen Test	Microbiology
Reagent, General Purpose	Pathology
System, Nucleic Acid Amplification Test, Dna, Methicillin Resistant Staphylococcus Aureus, Direct Specimen	Microbiology
Test, Influenza	Microbiology

CEPHEID   408-541-4191
904 Caribbean Drive, Sunnyvale, CA 94089
FDA Number: 3004530258   *Fax:* 408-541-4192
Web site: www.cepheid.com
Ownership: Private
Produces/Sells CE-marked Devices: N

Assay, Enterovirus Nucleic Acid	Microbiology
Nucleic Acid Amplification Assay System, Group B Streptococcus, Direct Specimen Test	Microbiology
Nucleic Acid Amplification, Novel Influenza A Virus, A/h5 (asian Lineage) Rna	Microbiology
Reagent, Clostridium Difficile Toxin	Microbiology
System, Nucleic Acid Amplification Test, Dna, Methicillin Resistant Staphylococcus Aureus, Direct Specimen	Microbiology
System, Test, Genotypic Detection, Resistant Markers, Enterococcus Species	Microbiology
Test, Factor Ii G20210a Mutations, Genomic Dna Pcr	Hematology
Test, Factor V Leiden Mutations, Genomic Dna Pcr	Hematology

CERAGROUP INDUSTRIES INC.   954-670-0208
6555 N.w. 9th Ave., Suite 211, Ft. Lauderdale, FL 33309
FDA Number: 1064583
Ownership: Private
Produces/Sells CE-marked Devices: N

Metal, Base	Dental And Oral
Powder, Porcelain	Dental And Oral
Tray, Impression	Dental And Oral

CERAPEDICS INC.   303-974-6275
11025 Dover Street, Suite 1600, Westminster, CO 80021
FDA Number: 3007155473   *Fax:* 303-974-6285
E-mail: info@cerapedics.com
Web site: www.cerapedics.com
Ownership: Private
Produces/Sells CE-marked Devices: N
General Admin.: Mr. Paul Mraz/Chief Executive Officer
        Mr. Andy Handwerker/Chief Operating Officer
Production: Mr. Roger White/Vice President Regulatory & Clinical Affairs
Research: Dr. Jim Benedict/Vice President Research & Development

Filler, Bone Void, Non-Osteoinduction	Physical Med
Orthopedic Manual Surgical Instrument	Orthopedics

CEREMED, INC.   310-815-2125
3643 Lenawee Ave., Los Angeles, CA 90016
FDA Number: 3004961344   *Fax:* 800-303-0963
E-mail: information@ceremed.com
Web site: www.ceremed.com
Ownership: Private
Produces/Sells CE-marked Devices: N

Wax, Bone	Surgery

CEREVAST THERAPEUTICS INC   425-821-1939
12277 134th Court NE, Suite 202, Redmond, WA 98052
FDA Number: 3008781398   *Fax:* 425-821-9313
E-mail: cerevast@cerevast.com
Web site: www.cerevast.com
Ownership: Private
Produces/Sells CE-marked Devices: N
General Admin.: Mr. Dilip Worah/Chief Scientific Officer
        Mr. Bradford Zakes/President, Chief Executive Officer
  Medical Admin.: Dr. Gordon Brandt/Chief Medical Officer
  Production: Mr. Anthony Alleman/Vice President Operations
        Mr. Andrew Leo/Vice President Quality Control
  Finance: Mr. Kendall Stever/Chief Financial Officer

CERMOPTEC INC.
See Biolitec, Inc.

CERNER CORP.   866-221-8877   816-221-1024
2800 Rockcreek Parkway, Kansas City, MO 64117
FDA Number: 1931259   *Fax:* 816-474-1742
E-mail: info@cerner.com
Web site: www.cerner.com
Annual Revenue: More than $1 Billion
Year Founded: 1979

CERNER CORP.   866-221-8877 (cont'd)
Total Employees: 7300
Ownership: Public
Stock Symbol: CERN
Traded On: NASDAQ
Quality System Registration Information: ISO9001; ISO9002
Produces/Sells CE-marked Devices: N
Distribution: Manufacturer Direct
General Admin.: Neal Patterson/Chief Executive Officer
     Donald Trigg/Chief Medical Officer, Vice President
     Trace Devanny/President
     Julie Wilson/Vice President Human Resources
Mktg./Adv.: Mike Valentine/Executive Vice President Sales
     John Landis/Manager Contract Sales
     Angela Betts/Manager Marketing
Finance: Scott Siemers/Vice President Finance

Computer Software	General
Software, Blood Bank (Stand-Alone Products)	Hematology

CERNER CORPORATION INNOVATION CAMPUS   816-201-1368
10234 Marion Park Drive, Kansas City, MO 64137
FDA Number: 3006801809
Ownership: Private
Produces/Sells CE-marked Devices: N

Computer, Chemistry Analyzer	Chemistry
Transmitter/Receiver System, Physiological, Radiofrequency	Cardiovascular
Transmitter/Receiver System, Physiological, Telephone	Cardiovascular

CERT HEALTH SCIENCES, LLC   866-990-4444
7036 Golden Ring Rd., Baltimore, MD 21237
FDA Number: 3003905623
Ownership: Private
Produces/Sells CE-marked Devices: N

Equipment, Traction, Powered	Physical Med

CERTIFIED FACILITIES CORP.   206-622-2508
208 Columbia St., Seattle, WA 98104-1508
FDA Number: n/a   *Fax:* 206-622-2807
E-mail: info@certifiedfacilites.com
Web site: www.certifiedfacilities.com
Annual Revenue: $10-$25 Million
Total Employees: 15
Ownership: Private
Produces/Sells CE-marked Devices: N
Federal Procurement Eligibility: Small Business
General Admin.: Gerald A. Miltner/President, Chief Financial Officer
     J. Scott Kemp/Senior Vice President

Service, Engineering/Design	General

CERTIFIED SAFETY MANUFACTURING   800-854-7474
1400 Chestnut, Kansas City, MO 64127   816-483-9090
FDA Number: 1932902   *Fax:* 816-483-9091
E-mail: egerson@certifiedsafety.com
Web site: www.certifiedsafety.com
Medical Products Sales Volume: $10,000,000
Annual Revenue: $10-$25 Million
Year Founded: 1987
Total Employees: 130   *Marketing Staff:* 2   *Sales Staff:* 8
Ownership: Private
Produces/Sells CE-marked Devices: N
Federal Procurement Eligibility: Small Business
Distribution: Manufacturer Through Distributor
General Admin.: Ed Gerson/President, Chief Executive Officer
     Pam Gerson/Vice President, General Manager
Mktg./Adv.: Ed Gerson/Director Marketing & Sales

Bag, Ice	General
Bandage, Adhesive	Surgery
Compress, Cold	General
Compress, Gauze	General
Device, Assist, CPR	Anesthesiology
Dressing, Wound and Burn, Occlusive	Surgery
Kit, First Aid	Surgery
Pack, Hot Or Cold, Disposable	Physical Med
Protector, Mouth Guard	Dental And Oral
Sponge, Gauze	Dental And Oral
Stimulator, Wound Healing	Physical Med

CERTOL INTERNATIONAL, LLC   303-799-9401
6120 E. 58th Ave., Adams City, CO 80022
FDA Number: 1720499

Block, Heating	Chemistry
Glove, Patient Examination, Vinyl	General
Mask, Surgical	Surgery
Medical Disinfectants/Cleaners for Instruments	General
Radiographic Unit, Diagnostic, Intraoral	Dental And Oral
Sterilant, Medical Device	General

CERVICAL BARRIER ADVANCEMENT SOCIETY
P.O. Box 38203, Cambridge, MA 02238-2031
FDA Number: n/a   *Fax:* 617-349-0041
E-mail: info@cervicalbarriers.org
Web site: www.cervicalbarriers.org
Medical Products Sales Volume: $500,000
Annual Revenue: $0-$1 Million
Year Founded: 2004
Ownership: Private
Produces/Sells CE-marked Devices: N
Federal Procurement Eligibility: Female Owned
Distribution: Exclusive Distributor

Cap, Cervical	Obstetrics/Gynecology

CERVICAL CAP LTD.
See Cervical Barrier Advancement Society

CET TECHNOLOGY   603-894-6100
27 Roulston Rd., Windham, NH 03087-1210
FDA Number: n/a   *Fax:* 603-894-6161
E-mail: cet@cettech.com
Web site: www.cettech.com
Annual Revenue: $10-$25 Million
Total Employees: 300   *Sales Staff:* 25
Ownership: Private
Produces/Sells CE-marked Devices: Y
Federal Procurement Eligibility: Small Business
Distribution: Manufacturer Direct, Manufacturer Through Manufacturer Reps, OEM
General Admin.: Bob Mirabella/Vice President, General Manager
Mktg./Adv.: Sue Oliveri/Director Marketing
     Dave Hill/Manager International & National Sales

Component, Electronic	General

CETAC TECHNOLOGIES, INC.   800-369-2822
14306 Industrial Rd., Omaha, NE 68144   402-733-2829
FDA Number: n/a   *Fax:* 402-733-1932
E-mail: custserv@cetac.com
Web site: www.cetac.com
Annual Revenue: $1-$5 Million
Ownership: Private
Produces/Sells CE-marked Devices: Y
Federal Procurement Eligibility: Small Business, Minority Owned
Distribution: Manufacturer Direct

Applicator, Sample	Chemistry
Injector, Sample	Chemistry

CETYLITE INDUSTRIES, INC.   800-257-7740
9051 River Rd., Pennsauken, NJ 08110   856-665-6111
FDA Number: 2242327   *Fax:* 856-665-5408
E-mail: karlm@cetylite.com
Web site: www.cetylite.com
Ownership: Private
Produces/Sells CE-marked Devices: N

Cleaner, Ultrasonic, Medical Instrument	General
Sterilant, Medical Device	General
Varnish, Cavity	Dental And Oral

CFI MEDICAL SOLUTIONS (CONTOUR FABRICATORS, INC.)   810-750-5300
14241 Fenton Road, Fenton, MI 48430
FDA Number: 1825560   *Fax:* 810-750-5310
E-mail: sales@cfimedical.com
Web site: www.cfimedical.com
Medical Products Sales Volume: $2,700,000
Annual Revenue: $10-$25 Million
Year Founded: 1970
Total Employees: 300   *Marketing Staff:* 3   *Sales Staff:* 10
Ownership: RAWCAR GROUP, LLC
Produces/Sells CE-marked Devices: Y
Federal Procurement Eligibility: Small Business, GSA Contract
Distribution: Manufacturer Direct, Manufacturer Through Distributor, Manufacturer Through Manufacturer Reps, OEM
General Admin.: Michael Czop/President
     Richard A. Weaver/President, Chief Executive Officer
     Ms. Kim Weaver/Vice President
Mktg./Adv.: John Lochner/Market Manager
Research: John Schaefer/Research Engineer

Applicator, Tipped, Absorbent, Sterile	General
Apron, Lead, Radiographic	Radiology
Camera, Still, Surgical	Surgery
Cushion, Wheelchair (Pad)	Physical Med
Drape, Surgical, Disposable	Surgery
Exerciser, Hand	Physical Med
Exerciser, Leg And Ankle	Physical Med
Exerciser, Other	Physical Med
Immobilizer, Arm	Orthopedics
Immobilizer, Knee	Orthopedics
Immobilizer, Wrist/Hand	Orthopedics

CFI MEDICAL SOLUTIONS (CONTOUR   810-750-5300 (cont'd)

Mattress, Immobilization	General
Microscope, Surgical	Ear/Nose/Throat
Orthosis, Other	Physical Med
Pad, Pressure, Foam Convoluted	General
Restraint, Wheelchair	General
Sand Bag	Radiology
Splint, Molded, Plastic	Orthopedics
Splint, Padded Stays	Orthopedics
Sponge, Other	General
Support, Patient Position, Radiographic	Radiology

CFT, INC./LIFE MASK   800-331-8844
14602 N. Cave Creek Road, Suite B,   **602-992-1220**
Phoenix, AZ 85022
FDA Number: 2029073   *Fax:* 602-992-5530
E-mail: info@cprlifemask.com
Web site: www.cprlifemask.com
Medical Products Sales Volume: $400,000
Year Founded: 1989
Total Employees: 5   *Marketing Staff:* 1   *Sales Staff:* 4
Ownership: Private
Quality System Registration Information: ISO9000; ISO9002
Produces/Sells CE-marked Devices: N
Federal Procurement Eligibility: Small Business
Distribution: Manufacturer Through Distributor, Manufacturer Through Manufacturer Reps, OEM, Importer, Exporter
General Admin.: Rick L. Stockett/President, Chief Executive Officer
    Diana Stockett/Vice President Personnel
Mktg./Adv.: Shelly Cohen/Manager National Sales

Aid, Resuscitation, Cardiopulmonary	Cardiovascular
Mask, Oxygen, Non-Rebreathing	Anesthesiology
Valve, Non-Rebreathing	Anesthesiology

CH ELLIS COMPANY INC.   800-466-3351
2432 Southeastern Avenue,   **317-636-3351**
Indianapolis, IN 46201
FDA Number: n/a   *Fax:* 317-635-5140
E-mail: tomrich@chellis.com
Web site: www.chellis.com
Medical Products Sales Volume: $6,000,000
Annual Revenue: $5-$10 Million
Year Founded: 1997
Total Employees: 40   *Marketing Staff:* 5   *Sales Staff:* 5
Ownership: Private
Produces/Sells CE-marked Devices: N
Federal Procurement Eligibility: Small Business
Distribution: Manufacturer Direct, Manufacturer Through Distributor, OEM, Importer
Mktg./Adv.: Tom Rich/Manager Sales
    George Celtrick/Sales Specialist

Bag, Medical, Physician	General
Case, Protection, Equipment	General
Service, Consulting	General

CHAD THERAPEUTICS, INC.   800-423-8870
21622 Plummer St., Chatsworth, CA 91311   **818-882-0883**
FDA Number: 2024040   *Fax:* 818-882-1809
E-mail: info@chadtherapeutics.com
Web site: www.chadtherapeutics.com
Medical Products Sales Volume: $19,000,000
Annual Revenue: $10-$25 Million
Year Founded: 1982
Total Employees: 130   *Marketing Staff:* 3   *Sales Staff:* 50
Ownership: Public
Stock Symbol: CTU
Traded On: AMEX
Quality System Registration Information: ISO9000; ISO9001
Produces/Sells CE-marked Devices: Y
Federal Procurement Eligibility: Small Business, GSA Contract, VA Contract
Distribution: Manufacturer Through Distributor, Manufacturer Through Manufacturer Reps
General Admin.: Tom Jones/Chief Executive Officer
    Barb Muskin/Manager Human Resources
    Earl L. Yager/President, Chief Operating Officer
Mktg./Adv.: Erika Laskey/Director Marketing & Sales
    Holly Dysart-Ward/Manager Advertising & Media
    Carla Laureano/Market Manager
    Oscar Sanchez/Vice President Business Development
Production: Shahan Moses/Director Quality Assurance
    Shahan Moses/Manager Regulatory Affairs
    Alfonzo DelToro/Vice President Manufacturing
Research: Kevin McCulloh/Vice President Research & Development & Engineering

Carrier, Container, Oxygen, Portable	General
Cylinder, Oxygen	Anesthesiology
Regulator, Oxygen, Mechanical	General
Tubing, Oxygen Connecting	General

CHAGRIN SAFETY SUPPLY, INC.   800-227-0468
8227 East Washington Ave.,   **440-543-2777**
Chagrin Falls, OH 44023
FDA Number: 1528667   *Fax:* 440-543-7373
E-mail: sales@chagrinsafetysupply.com
Web site: www.chagrinsafetysupply.com
Medical Products Sales Volume: $3,500,000
Annual Revenue: $1-$5 Million
Year Founded: 1988
Total Employees: 7   *Marketing Staff:* 1   *Sales Staff:* 5
Ownership: Private
Quality System Registration Information: ISO9002
Produces/Sells CE-marked Devices: Y
Federal Procurement Eligibility: Small Business
Distribution: OEM, Importer, Exporter
General Admin.: William H. Oler/Chief Executive Officer
    Bill Oler/President
Mktg./Adv.: Rick McEntee/Director National Accounts
    Tom Scully/Manager Sales Training
    Peter Oler/Vice President Sales

Bib	General
Blade, Scalpel	Surgery
Cap, Surgical	Surgery
Container, Urine Specimen	General
Cotton, Roll	Dental And Oral
Depressor, Tongue	General
Ejector, Saliva	Ear/Nose/Throat
Facial Tissue	General
Glove, Other	General
Glove, Patient Examination, Latex	General
Glove, Patient Examination, Vinyl	General
Glove, Protective, Radiographic	Radiology
Glove, Surgical, Powder-Free	Surgery
Gown, Examination	General
Gown, Isolation, Surgical	Surgery
Mask, Face	General
Needle, Hypodermic	General
Pack, Sterilization Wrapper (Bag And Accessories)	Surgery
Pad, Alcohol	General
Shoe And Shoe Cover, Conductive	Anesthesiology
Sponge, Gauze	Dental And Oral
Stick, Urinalysis Test	Chemistry
Strip, Test	Chemistry
Swabs, Antiseptic	General
Swabs, Cotton	General
Syringe, Hypodermic	General
Syringe, Insulin	General
Syringe, Other	General
Syringe, Tuberculin	General
Tape, Gauze, Adhesive	General
Wrapper, Surgical Instrument (Sterile)	General

CHAIR CARE-MOBILE COT, INC.   803-564-3698
6241 Wagener Rd., Wagener, SC 29164
FDA Number: 3006117030

Stretcher, Hand-Carried	General
Stretcher, Wheeled (Mobile)	General

CHAIR CARRIER PRODUCTS INC.
    See Travel Ramp, Inc.

CHALGREN ENTERPRISES, INC.   408-847-3994
380 Tomkins Ct., Gilroy, CA 95020-6315
FDA Number: 2939713   *Fax:* 408-847-3620
E-mail: chalgren@garlic.com
Annual Revenue: $1-$5 Million
Year Founded: 1965
Total Employees: 12   *Marketing Staff:* 3   *Sales Staff:* 3
Ownership: Private
Quality System Registration Information: ISO9002
Produces/Sells CE-marked Devices: N
Federal Procurement Eligibility: Small Business
Distribution: Manufacturer Through Distributor
General Admin.: Richard L. Kaiser/President
Mktg./Adv.: Becky Kaiser/Vice President Business Development
Production: Michael Kaiser/Director Quality Assurance
    Laurie Salaiz/Manager Materials
    Carol Hopf/Manager Production

Electrode, Cutaneous	Cns/Neurology
Electrode, Electromyographic	Cns/Neurology

CHALLENGE PRINTING COMPANY, THE   800-654-1234
2 Bridewell Place, Clifton, NJ 07014   **973-471-4700**
FDA Number: n/a   *Fax:* 973-471-2562
E-mail: info@challengeprintingco.com
Web site: www.challprint.com
Medical Products Sales Volume: $29,200,000
Annual Revenue: $10-$25 Million
Year Founded: 1911

CHALLENGE PRINTING COMPANY, THE   800-654-1234 *(cont'd)*
Total Employees: 203
Ownership: Private
Produces/Sells CE-marked Devices: N
Federal Procurement Eligibility: Small Business
Distribution: Manufacturer Direct
Mktg./Adv.: Tony Kapsaskis/Vice President Marketing & Sales
Production: Tim Gelsinger/Vice President Manufacturing
     Service, Printing   General

CHAMBERLIN RUBBER COMPANY, INC.   585-427-7780
3333 Brighton Henrietta Town Line Road, PO Box 22700,
Rochester, NY 14692
FDA Number: n/a   *Fax:* 585-427-2429
E-mail: sales@crubber.com
Web site: www.chamberlinrubber.com
Medical Products Sales Volume: $6,100,000
Year Founded: 1865
Total Employees: 28   *Marketing Staff:* 1   *Sales Staff:* 5
Ownership: Private
Quality System Registration Information: ISO9001
Produces/Sells CE-marked Devices: N
Federal Procurement Eligibility: Small Business
Distribution: Manufacturer Direct, Manufacturer Through Distributor, Manufacturer Through Manufacturer Reps, Service Direct, Exclusive Distributor
General Admin.: Mr. Bill Lanigan/Chief Executive Officer
Mktg./Adv.: Mr. Andrew Chase/Market Manager
Component, Other	General
Component, Rubber	General
Cushion, Other	General
Cushion, Ring, Foam Rubber	General
Elastomer, Other	General
Elastomer, Silicone Rubber	General
Fitting, Other	General
Floor Mat, Antibacterial	General
Pad, Pressure, Soft Rubber	General
Padding, Cast/Splint	General
Silicone Sheeting	General
Splint, Padded Stays	Orthopedics
Sponge, External, Rubber	Surgery
Strip, Adhesive	Surgery
Tubing, Braided	General
Tubing, Polypropylene	General
Tubing, Silicone	General

CHAMBERMAID PRODUCTS , INC.   800-549-5356
12050 Suellen Circle, Wellington, FL 33414   561-795-9127
FDA Number: 1058823   *Fax:* 561-795-9142
E-mail: payson1@bellsouth.com
Web site: chambermaid.us
Year Founded: 1995
Ownership: Private
Produces/Sells CE-marked Devices: Y
Distribution: Manufacturer Through Distributor
     Sterilizer, Steam (Autoclave)   General

CHAMCO, INC.   888-674-6683
798 Clearlake Rd., Cocoa, FL 32922   321-639-3314
FDA Number: 1063298   *Fax:* 775-201-0151
E-mail: jimcummins@cfl.rr.com
Web site: www.chamcousa.com
Medical Products Sales Volume: $1,000,000
Year Founded: 1989
Total Employees: 9
Ownership: Private
Produces/Sells CE-marked Devices: Y
Federal Procurement Eligibility: Small Business
     Nuclear Magnetic Resonance Imaging System   Radiology

CHAMELEON DENTAL PRODUCTS, INC.   913-281-5552
200 North Sixth St., Kansas City, KS 66101
FDA Number: 1931030
Cement, Dental	Dental And Oral
Powder, Porcelain	Dental And Oral
Tray, Fluoride, Disposable	Dental And Oral

CHAMPION AMERICA   800-521-7000
PO Box 3092, Stony Creek, CT 06405   203-315-1181
FDA Number: n/a   *Fax:* 800-336-3707
E-mail: teamca@champion-america.com
Web site: www.champion-america.com
Year Founded: 1989
Total Employees: 250
Distribution: Manufacturer Direct
Mktg./Adv.: CYNTHIA CZYZ/Marketing Officer
Communication System, Non-Powered	Physical Med
Labeling Equipment	General
Sign, Hospital	General

CHAMPION AMERICA   800-521-7000 *(cont'd)*
   System, Marking, Laser   General

CHAMPION BUS INC.   800-776-4943
331 Graham Rd., Imlay City, MI 48444   800-331-5761 Ex
FDA Number: n/a   *Fax:* 810-724-1844
E-mail: sales@championbus.com
Web site: www.championbus.com
Medical Products Sales Volume: $70,000,000
Annual Revenue: $50-$100 Million
Year Founded: 1972
Total Employees: 350   *Marketing Staff:* 2   *Sales Staff:* 8
Ownership: THOR INDUSTRIES
Quality System Registration Information: ISO9001
Produces/Sells CE-marked Devices: N
Distribution: Manufacturer Through Distributor
General Admin.: Dan Roberts/Chief Executive Officer
Mktg./Adv.: Paul Allmacher/Director Marketing
       Matt Dougherty/Director National Accounts
       Rick Lee/Manager National Sales
Production: David Carter/Director Engineering
       Warren Marsh/Vice President Manufacturing
   Vehicle, Handicapped   Physical Med

CHAMPION MACHINERY CO., INC.
See Champion, A Gardner Denver Co.

CHAMPION MANUFACTURING, LLC.   800-998-5018
2601 Industrial Pwy., Elkhart, IN 46516   219-295-6893
FDA Number: n/a   *Fax:* 219-293-5760
E-mail: info@championchair.com
Medical Products Sales Volume: $2,500,000
Annual Revenue: $1-$5 Million
Total Employees: 23   *Marketing Staff:* 1   *Sales Staff:* 10
Ownership: Private
Produces/Sells CE-marked Devices: N
Federal Procurement Eligibility: Small Business
Distribution: Manufacturer Direct, Manufacturer Through Distributor
General Admin.: Paul Romanetz/President
Mktg./Adv.: Pat Cooper/Manager Market Research
       Paul Romanetz/Manager National Sales
Production: Diane Cameron/Manager Materials
Chair, Other	General
Chair/Table, Medical	General
Exerciser, Bicycle	Physical Med

CHAMPION MFG. INC.   800-998-5018
2601 Industrial Pkwy., Elkhart, IN 46516   574-295-6893
FDA Number: 1834066   *Fax:* 574-293-5760
Web site: www.championchair.com
Ownership: Invacare Corporation
Produces/Sells CE-marked Devices: N
Chair, Surgical, AC-Powered	Surgery
Chair/Table, Medical	General
Scale, Infant	General

CHAMPION MOTOR COACH, INC.
See Champion Bus Inc.

CHAMPION, A GARDNER DENVER CO.   800 232 0865
1800 Gardner Expressway, Quincy, IL 62305
FDA Number: n/a   *Fax:* 815-872-0421
E-mail: customerservice@championpneumatic.com
Web site: www.championpneumatic.com
Annual Revenue: $25-$50 Million
Ownership: GARDNER DENVER
Quality System Registration Information: ISO9001
Produces/Sells CE-marked Devices: N
Federal Procurement Eligibility: Small Business
Distribution: Manufacturer Through Manufacturer Reps
   Compressor, Air, Portable   Anesthesiology

CHANNEL INDUSTRIES, INC.   805-967-0171
839 Ward Drive, Santa Barbara, CA 93111-2920
FDA Number: 9200198   *Fax:* 805-683-3420
E-mail: ciisales@channeltech.com
Web site: www.channelindustries.com
Medical Products Sales Volume: $23,800,000
Year Founded: 1984
Total Employees: 104
Ownership: Private
Produces/Sells CE-marked Devices: N
Federal Procurement Eligibility: Small Business
Distribution: Manufacturer Direct
General Admin.: Robert F. Carlson/Chief Executive Officer
       John Prizler/President
Mktg./Adv.: Marie Puchli/Manager International & National Sales
       Edward Bickel/Manager Tech. Sales

CHANNEL INDUSTRIES, INC.   805-967-0171 (cont'd)
Transducer, Ultrasonic   Cardiovascular

CHARLES B. SCHWED CO., INC.   800-847-4073
124-02 Metropolitan Ave.,   **718-441-0526**
Kew Gardens, NY 11415
FDA Number: 2430119   *Fax:* 718-441-4507
E-mail: info@schwed.com
Web site: www.schwed.com
Medical Products Sales Volume: $1,300,000
Annual Revenue: $1-$5 Million
Ownership: Private
Produces/Sells CE-marked Devices: Y
Federal Procurement Eligibility: Small Business, Female Owned
Distribution: Manufacturer Direct, Manufacturer Through Distributor, Importer

Cotton, Roll	Dental And Oral
Curette, Endodontic	Dental And Oral
Endodontic Instrument	Dental And Oral
Evacuator, Oral Cavity	Dental And Oral
File, Pulp Canal, Endodontic	Dental And Oral
Forceps, Dressing, Dental	Dental And Oral
Lamp, Operating Room	General
Mandrel	Dental And Oral
Plugger, Root Canal, Endodontic	Dental And Oral
Post, Root Canal	Dental And Oral
Spreader, Pulp Canal Filling Material, Endodontic	Dental And Oral

CHARTER MEDICAL LTD.   866-458-3116
3948-A Westpoint Blvd,   **336-768-6447**
Winston Salem, NC 27103
FDA Number: 1066733   *Fax:* 336-714-4241
E-mail: chartercustomerservice@lydall.com
Web site: www.chartermedical.com
Total Employees: 130   *Marketing Staff:* 3   *Sales Staff:* 5
Ownership: LYDALL, INC.
Quality System Registration Information: ISO9001
Produces/Sells CE-marked Devices: N
Distribution: Manufacturer Direct, Manufacturer Through Distributor, OEM

Bag, Blood	Hematology
Catheter, Intravenous	Cardiovascular
Kit, Blood, Transfusion	General
Microfilter, Blood Transfusion	Anesthesiology
Set, Administration, Intravenous, Needle-Free	General

CHARTEX INTERNATIONAL
See The Female Health Co.

CHARTEX RESOURCES, LTD.
See Female Health Company, The

CHARTS-INC.   800-882-9357
12977 Arroyo St., San Fernando, CA 91340   **818-898-3707**
FDA Number: n/a   *Fax:* 818-361-3038
E-mail: sales@recordingcharts.com
Web site: www.recordingcharts.com
Annual Revenue: $0-$1 Million
Total Employees: 30   *Marketing Staff:* 1   *Sales Staff:* 6
Ownership: Private
Produces/Sells CE-marked Devices: N
Federal Procurement Eligibility: Small Business
Distribution: Manufacturer Through Distributor, Exclusive Distributor
General Admin.: Marvin Solomon/President
     Howard Yudell/Vice President
Mktg./Adv.: Judi Minke/Manager Advertising

Recorder, Chart, Laboratory	Chemistry

CHASE ERGONOMICS, INC.   800-621-5436
5921 Midway Park Blvd NE,   **505-345-8488**
Albuquerque, NM 87109
FDA Number: n/a   *Fax:* 505-345-2340
E-mail: marketing@chaseergo.com
Web site: www.chaseergo.com
Annual Revenue: $5-$10 Million
Year Founded: 1991
Total Employees: 50   *Marketing Staff:* 2   *Sales Staff:* 30
Ownership: Private
Produces/Sells CE-marked Devices: Y
Federal Procurement Eligibility: Small Business
Distribution: Manufacturer Through Distributor, Manufacturer Through Manufacturer Reps, OEM, Importer, Exporter
General Admin.: David Chase/Chief Executive Officer
     Gary Shumate/President

Orthosis, Abdominal	Physical Med
Orthosis, Lumbar	Physical Med
Orthosis, Lumbosacral	Physical Med
Splint, Extremity, Non-Inflatable, External	Surgery
Support, Arm	Physical Med

CHASE MEDICAL, LP   800-787-0378
1876 Firman Dr., Richardson, TX 75081   **972-783-0644**
FDA Number: 1649139   *Fax:* 972-235-3446
E-mail: cust_svc@chasemedical.com
Web site: www.chasemedical.com
Ownership: Private
Produces/Sells CE-marked Devices: N

Accessories, Cardiopulmonary Bypass	Cardiovascular
Cannula, Surgical, General & Plastic Surgery	Surgery
Catheter, Intravascular Occluding, Temporary	Cardiovascular
Catheter, Vascular, Cardiopulmonary Bypass	Cardiovascular
Clamp, Surgical, General & Plastic Surgery	Surgery
Image Processing System	Radiology
Lavage Unit, Water Jet	General
Pledget And Intracardiac Patch, PETP, PTFE, Polypropylene	Cardiovascular
Suction Apparatus, Operating Room, Wall Vacuum-Powered	Surgery
Surgical Instrument, Cardiovascular	Cardiovascular
Surgical Instrument, Disposable	Surgery

CHASE SCIENTIFIC GLASS
See Kimble Chase Life Science And Research Products Llc

CHASE SCIENTIFIC GLASS, INC.   412-490-8425
234 Cardiff Valley Rd., Rockwood, TN 37854
FDA Number: 1047986
Ownership: Private
Produces/Sells CE-marked Devices: N

Hematocrit Tube, Rack, Sealer, Holder	Hematology
Labware, Blood Collection	Chemistry
Pipette, Pasteur	Hematology
Tube, Capillary Blood Collection	Hematology
Tube, Sedimentation Rate	Hematology
Tube, Tissue Culture	Pathology

CHATTANOOGA GROUP   800-321-9549
1430 Decision Street, Vista, CA 37343-0489   **760-727-1280**
FDA Number: n/a   *Fax:* 800-242-8329
Web site: www.chattgroup.com
Medical Products Sales Volume: $90,000,000
Annual Revenue: $50-$100 Million
Year Founded: 1947
Total Employees: 300
Ownership: ReAble Therapeutics, Inc.
Quality System Registration Information: ISO9001
Produces/Sells CE-marked Devices: Y
Federal Procurement Eligibility: Small Business, VA Contract
Distribution: Manufacturer Through Distributor, Manufacturer Through Manufacturer Reps, OEM, Exclusive Distributor, Exporter
General Admin.: Chris Ramsay/Director Human Resources
     Scott Klosterman/President
     Paul Chapman/President, Chief Executive Officer
Mktg./Adv.: Debbie Joles/Manager International Marketing
     Keith Hagy/Manager Marketing
     Jeff Gephart/Manager National Sales
     Chuck Thomas/Vice President International Marketing & Sales
     Ed Dunlay/Vice President Marketing
     Dwayne Hofstatter/Vice President Sales
Production: Theresa Danberry/Director Materials
     Bo Whiteside/Director Quality Assurance
     Mike Treas/Director Regulatory Affairs

Accessories, Traction	Physical Med
Belt, Traction, Pelvic, Orthopedic	Orthopedics
Chair, Adjustable, Mechanical	Physical Med
Chilling Unit	Physical Med
Compression Unit, Intermittent (Anti-Embolism Pump)	Cardiovascular
Diathermy, Ultrasonic (Physical Therapy)	Physical Med
Electrotherapeutic Unit	General
Equipment, Traction, Powered	Physical Med
Exerciser, Passive, Non-Measuring (CPM Machine)	Physical Med
Halter, Head, Traction, Orthopedic	Orthopedics
Heating Unit, Powered	Physical Med
Lotion, Skin Care	General
Moist Therapy Pack	Physical Med
Pack, Cold	General
Pack, Hot Or Cold, Reusable	Physical Med
Pack, Moist Heat	Physical Med
Sleeve, Compressible Limb	Cardiovascular
Stimulator, Cranial Electrotherapy	Cns/Neurology
Stimulator, Muscle, Electrical-Powered (EMS)	Physical Med
Stimulator, Neuromuscular, External Functional	Cns/Neurology
Stimulator, Ultrasound, Muscle	Physical Med
Table, Examination/Treatment	General
Table, Traction	Orthopedics
Unit, Therapy, Current, Interferential	Cns/Neurology

CHATTECX CORPORATION
See Chattanooga Group

CHATTEM DRUG & CHEMICAL COMPANY
See Chattem, Inc.

CHATTEM, INC.
800-366-6077
423-821-4571

1715 W. 38th St., Chattanooga, TN 37409-1259
Fax: 423-821-0395
FDA Number: 1022556
E-mail: customer_relations@chattem.com
Web site: www.chattem.com
Medical Products Sales Volume: $300,500,000
Year Founded: 1879
Total Employees: 350
Ownership: Public
Stock Symbol: CHTT
Traded On: NASDAQ
Produces/Sells CE-marked Devices: N
Federal Procurement Eligibility: Small Business
Distribution: Manufacturer Through Distributor
General Admin.: Mr. Zan Guerry/Chairman
 Mr. Alec Taylor/President, Chief Operating Officer
 Mr. Thad Whitfield/Vice President Legal Services
Mktg./Adv.: Mr. Ron Galante/Vice President Business Development
 Mr. Rick Kornhauser/Vice President Marketing
 Ms. Andrea Crouch/Vice President Marketing
Research: Dr. Don Riker/Vice President Research & Development, Chief Scientific Officer
Finance: Mr. Rick Moss/Vice President Finance
 Contract Manufacturing, Pharmaceuticals/Chemicals   General

CHAYES VIRGINIA INC.
See Dentalez Group

CHED MARKAY, INC.
312-566-3307

1065 High St., Mundelein, IL 60060
FDA Number: 1419245
 Paper, Articulation   Dental And Oral

CHEETAH MEDICAL
866-751-9097
360-828-8685

600 SE Maritime Ave Suite 220,
Vancouver, WA 98661
FDA Number: 3007319130
Fax: 360-718-8154
E-mail: cheetah-us@cheetah-medical.com
Ownership: Private
Produces/Sells CE-marked Devices: N
 Oximeter, Ear   Cardiovascular
 Plethysmograph, Impedance   Cardiovascular
 Pressure Measurement, System, Intermittent   Physical Med

CHEK-MED SYSTEMS, INC.
800-451-5797

200 Grandview Ave., Camp Hill, PA 17011
FDA Number: n/a
Web site: www.chekmed.com
Ownership: Private
Produces/Sells CE-marked Devices: N
Federal Procurement Eligibility: Small Business, Female Owned
Distribution: Manufacturer Direct
 Material, Training, Audiovisual   General
Medical Product Subsidiaries (Listed Separately)
 Gi Supply

CHEM-TAINER INDUSTRIES, INC.
800-ASK-CHEM
631-661-8300

361 Neptune Avenue, West Babylon, NY 11704
Fax: 631-661-8209
FDA Number: n/a
E-mail: sales@chemtainer.com
Web site: www.chemtainer.com
Medical Products Sales Volume: $18,900,000
Annual Revenue: $25-$50 Million
Total Employees: 50   *Marketing Staff:* 2   *Sales Staff:* 20
Ownership: Private
Produces/Sells CE-marked Devices: N
Federal Procurement Eligibility: Small Business, GSA Contract
Distribution: Manufacturer Through Distributor, OEM
General Admin.: James B. Glen/Chief Executive Officer
 Anthony Lamb/Vice President, General Manager
Mktg./Adv.: Anthony Lamb/Vice President Sales
 Cart, Supply   General
 Waste Receptacle, General Purpose   General

CHEMATICS, INC.
574-834-4080

Hwy. 13 South, North Webster, IN 46555
FDA Number: 1825396
 Collector, Specimen   Microbiology
 Enzymatic Esterase-Oxidase, Cholesterol   Chemistry
 Lancet, Blood   General
 Reagent, Glucose (Test System)   Chemistry
 Test, Ethyl Alcohol   Toxicology

CHEMBIO DIAGNOSTIC SYSTEMS, INC.
631-924-1135

3661 Horseblock Rd., Medford, NY 11763
FDA Number: 2431980
Fax: 631-924-6033
E-mail: info@chembio.com
Web site: www.chembio.com
Year Founded: 1985

CHEMBIO DIAGNOSTIC SYSTEMS, INC.
631-924-1135 *(cont'd)*

Ownership: Private
Produces/Sells CE-marked Devices: N
Production: Mr. Richard Bruce/Vice President Operations
 Mr. Tom Ippolito/Vice President Regulatory Affairs
Research: Mr. Javan Esfandiari/Senior Vice President Research & Development
Finance: Mr. Richard Larkin/Chief Financial Officer
 Mr. Lawrence Siebert/President
 Antigen, Prostate-Specific (PSA), Management, Cancer   Immunology
 Antigen, Streptococcus SPP.   Microbiology
 Antiserum, CF, Equine Encephalitis Virus, EEE, WEE   Microbiology
 Antiserum, Fluorescent, Mycobacterium Tuberculosis   Microbiology
 Campylobacter Pylori   Microbiology
 Chlamydia Trachomatis   Microbiology
 Control, Analyte (Assayed And Unassayed)   Chemistry
 Control, Hemoglobin   Hematology
 Enzymatic Method, Troponin Subunit   Chemistry
 Enzyme Linked Immunoabsorbent Assay, Resp. Syncytial Virus   Microbiology
 Enzyme Linked Immunoabsorbent Assay, Rotavirus   Microbiology
 Enzyme Linked Immunoabsorbent Assay, T. Cruzi   Microbiology
 Hepatitis B Test (B Core, BE Antigen & Antibody, B Core IGM)   Microbiology
 Kit, Test, Saliva, Hiv-1&2   Hematology
 Radioimmunoassay, Luteinizing Hormone   Chemistry
 Reagent, Borrelia, Serological   Microbiology
 System, Nucleic Acid Amplification, Mycobacterium Tuberculosis Complex   Microbiology
 Test, Hiv Detection   Immunology
 Test, Human Chorionic Gonadotropin, Serum   Immunology
 Test, Sickle Cell   Hematology

CHEMDEV INSTRUMENTS, INC.
408-541-8535

1289 Reamwood Ave., #b, Sunnyvale, CA 94089
FDA Number: 2954748
Ownership: Private
Produces/Sells CE-marked Devices: N
 Analyzer, Chemistry, Photometric, Discrete   Chemistry

CHEMENCE MEDICAL PRODUCTS INC.
770-664-6624

185 Bluegrass Valley Parkway, Suite 100,
Alpharetta, GA 30005
FDA Number: 1067168
Ownership: Private
Produces/Sells CE-marked Devices: N
 Bandage, Liquid   Surgery
 Protectant, Skin   Surgery

CHEMETRICS INC.
See Biomerieux Inc.

CHEMETRON MEDICAL PRODUCTS
See Allied Healthcare Products, Inc.

CHEMICAL SERVICE LABS, LLC
214-691-3484

5543 Dyer St., Dallas, TX 75206
FDA Number: 1613616
Fax: 214-691-8555
E-mail: cslab@sbcglobal.net
Medical Products Sales Volume: $100,000
Year Founded: 1970
Total Employees: 3
Ownership: Private
Produces/Sells CE-marked Devices: N
Federal Procurement Eligibility: Small Business
Distribution: Manufacturer Direct
 Stain, Giemsa, Hematology   Hematology
 Stain, Wright's, Hematology   Hematology

CHEMISPHERE CORP.
314-644-1300

2101 Clifton Ave., Saint Louis, MO 63139
FDA Number: 100158477
Ownership: Private
Produces/Sells CE-marked Devices: N
 Sterilizer, Chemical   General

CHEMLAND INC.
See Preserve International

CHEMLINK LABORATORIES, LLC.
770-499-8008

1590 N. Roberts Rd. Nw, Suite 111, Kennesaw, GA 30144
FDA Number: 1058458
Fax: 770-421-1984
E-mail: smeske@chemlinklabs.com
Web site: smeske@chemlinklabs.com
Ownership: Private
Produces/Sells CE-marked Devices: N
 Medical Disinfectants/Cleaners for Instruments   General

CHEMPLAST INC.
See Saint-Gobain Performance Plastics--Akron

CHEMPLEX INDUSTRIES, INC.
800-424-3675
772-283-2700

2820 SW 42nd Avenue, Palm City, FL 34990
Fax: 772-283-2774
FDA Number: 9200202
E-mail: sales@chemplex.com
Web site: www.chemplex.com

CHEMPLEX INDUSTRIES, INC.   800-424-3675 *(cont'd)*
Medical Products Sales Volume: $2,000,000
Annual Revenue: $1-$5 Million
Year Founded: 1971
Total Employees: 12   *Marketing Staff:* 5   *Sales Staff:* 5
Ownership: Private
Quality System Registration Information: ISO9000
Produces/Sells CE-marked Devices: N
Federal Procurement Eligibility: Small Business
Distribution: Manufacturer Direct
General Admin.: Monte J. Solazzi/President
   Film, X-Ray   Radiology

CHEMSW, INC.   800-536-0404
4771 Mangels Blvd, Fairfield, CA 94534   **707-864-0845**
FDA Number: n/a   *Fax:* 707-864-2815
E-mail: info@chemsw.com
Web site: www.chemsw.com
Medical Products Sales Volume: $1,800,000
Annual Revenue: $1-$5 Million
Year Founded: 1991
Total Employees: 12   *Marketing Staff:* 2   *Sales Staff:* 3
Ownership: Private
Produces/Sells CE-marked Devices: N
Federal Procurement Eligibility: Small Business
Distribution: Manufacturer Direct
General Admin.: Brian Stafford/President
Mktg./Adv.: Dave Hessler/Director Product Development
Research: Patrick Spink/Vice President Research & Development
IS: Rick Musselman/Tech. Specialist
   Computer Software   General

CHEMUX BIOSCIENCE, INC.   650-872-1800
50 South Linden Ave. #7, South San Francisco, CA 94080
FDA Number: 3004189868
Ownership: Private
Produces/Sells CE-marked Devices: N
   Enzyme Immunoassay, Non-Radiolabeled, Total Thyroxine   Chemistry
   Radioimmunoassay, C Peptides Of Proinsulin   Chemistry
   Radioimmunoassay, Free Thyroxine   Chemistry
   Radioimmunoassay, Thyroid Stimulating Hormone   Chemistry
   Radioimmunoassay, Total Triiodothyronine   Chemistry

CHENEY COMPANY OF LOUISIANA, THE
See Thyssenkrupp Access Corp.

CHENEY DIVISION OF ACCESS INDUSTRIES
See Thyssenkrupp Access Corp.

CHERRY BLOSSOM ENTERPRISES INC.   864-972-2920
305 South Union Rd., S-37-85, Westminster, SC 29693
FDA Number: 1061111
Ownership: Private
Produces/Sells CE-marked Devices: N
   Pack, Hot Or Cold, Reusable   Physical Med

CHESEBROUGH-POND'S INC.
See Covidien Lp

CHESSON LABORATORY ASSOCIATES, INC.   919-636-5773
603 Ellis Road, Durham, NC 27703
FDA Number: 3006317783
Ownership: Private
Produces/Sells CE-marked Devices: N
   Insoles, Medical   General
   Protectant, Skin   Surgery

CHESTECH CORP.
See CAREFUSION 211, INC..

CHESTER LABS, INC.   800-354-9709
1900 Section Road, Cincinnati, OH 45237   **513-458-3840**
FDA Number: 1022110   *Fax:* 800-235-3995
E-mail: jack.armstrong@chester-labs.com
Web site: www.chester-labs.com
Medical Products Sales Volume: $20,000,000
Annual Revenue: $10-$25 Million
Year Founded: 1939
Total Employees: 125   *Marketing Staff:* 1   *Sales Staff:* 20
Ownership: Private
Quality System Registration Information: ISO9001
Produces/Sells CE-marked Devices: N
Federal Procurement Eligibility: Small Business, GSA Contract
Distribution: Manufacturer Through Distributor
General Admin.: Kay Erdman/Manager Human Resources
     John Armstrong/President, Chief Executive Officer
Mktg./Adv.: Stuart Hyde/Vice President Marketing
     Jack Armstrong/Vice President Sales
Production: Ken Miller/Director Quality Assurance
     Mike Griggs/Manager Materials
     Mark Kramer/Plant Manager

CHESTER LABS, INC.   800-354-9709 *(cont'd)*
     Dodd Rheinfrank/Vice President Manufacturing
Research: Chuck Ficker/Chemist
Finance: Tom Twilling/Chief Financial Officer
     Steve Tharp/Controller
   Detergent   Hematology
   Dispenser, Soap   General
   Gel, Ultrasonic Coupling   Physical Med
   Irrigator, Perineal   Gastroenterology/Urology
   Jelly, Lubricating   General
   Kit, Enema   General
   Lotion, Skin Care   General
   Soap   General
   Solution, Antibacterial Cleaner   General
   Towel/Towelette, Paper   General

CHESTNUT RIDGE FOAM, INC.   800-234-2734
P.O. Box 781, Latrobe, PA 15650-0781   **724-537-9000**
FDA Number: n/a   *Fax:* 724-537-9003
E-mail: crfoamsales@verizon.net
Web site: www.chestnutridgefoam.com
Medical Products Sales Volume: $2,000,000
Annual Revenue: $10-$25 Million
Year Founded: 1986
Total Employees: 150   *Marketing Staff:* 2   *Sales Staff:* 8
Ownership: Private
Stock Symbol: N/A
Produces/Sells CE-marked Devices: N
Federal Procurement Eligibility: Small Business
Distribution: Manufacturer Direct, Manufacturer Through Distributor, Manufacturer Through Manufacturer Reps, Exporter
General Admin.: Mr. Larry Garrity/Chairman
     Mr. Carl Ogburn/Executive Vice President
Mktg./Adv.: Linda Patterson/Marketing Representative
Production: Laura Young/Director Quality Assurance
     Mr. George Romanish/Vice President Manufacturing
   Cushion, Other   General
   Cushion, Wheelchair (Pad)   Physical Med
   Mattress, Bed   General
   Mattress, Reduction, Pressure   General

CHEWRITE CO., A SUBSIDIARY OF MAGNESIA   513-746-5509
PRODUCTS, I
265 Pioneer Blvd., Springboro, OH 45066
FDA Number: 1510414
Ownership: Private
Produces/Sells CE-marked Devices: N
   Acacia And Karaya With Sodium Borate   Dental And Oral

CHF SOLUTIONS, INC.   763-463-4600
7601 Northland Dr. Ste. 170, Brooklyn Center, MN 55428
FDA Number: 3003504604   *Fax:* 763-463-4606
E-mail: info@chfsolutions.com
Ownership: Private
Produces/Sells CE-marked Devices: N
   Dialysate Delivery System, Single Patient   Gastroenterology/Urology
   Dialyzer, High Permeability   Gastroenterology/Urology

CHI INSTITUTE   949-361-3976
27130a Paseo Espada, Ste 1407,
San Juan Capistrano, CA 92675
FDA Number: 2027987
Ownership: Private
Produces/Sells CE-marked Devices: N
   Massager, Therapeutic   Physical Med

CHI'AM INTERNATIONAL   727-647-3940
4155 Grandchamp Circle, Palm Harbor, FL 34685
FDA Number: 2131836   *Fax:* 727-786-0847
E-mail: chiam@usinternet.com
Medical Products Sales Volume: $1,000,000
Annual Revenue: $1-$5 Million
Total Employees: 2
Ownership: Private
Produces/Sells CE-marked Devices: Y
Federal Procurement Eligibility: Small Business
Distribution: Exporter
General Admin.: Andrew W. Wolf/Chief Executive Officer
Mktg./Adv.: Susan G. Wolf/Vice President Advertising
   Accessories, Traction   Physical Med

CHICK SURGICAL SYSTEMS
See Midmark Corporation

CHIEF POWER CHAIR, LLC   520-722-5265
8051 E. Lakeside Pkwy, #113, Tucson, AZ 85730
FDA Number: 3004620958
Ownership: Private
Produces/Sells CE-marked Devices: N

CHIEF POWER CHAIR, LLC 520-722-5265 (cont'd)
Wheelchair, Powered
Physical Med

CHILDREN'S HOSPITAL 800-437-0272
8200 Dodge St., Omaha, NE 68114 402-955-3857
FDA Number: 3000930743
Ownership: Private
Produces/Sells CE-marked Devices: N
Orthosis, Cranial
Cns/Neurology

CHILDREN'S MEDICAL VENTURES, INC. 800-345-6443
191 Wyngate Drive, Monroeville, PA 15146
FDA Number: n/a
E-mail: info@childmed.com
Web site: www.childmed.com
Medical Products Sales Volume: $10,000,000
Annual Revenue: $10-$25 Million
Ownership: Philips Healthcare
Quality System Registration Information: ISO9001
Produces/Sells CE-marked Devices: N
Distribution: Manufacturer Direct, Manufacturer Through Distributor, Manufacturer Through Manufacturer Reps, Service Direct, Exclusive Distributor
Bumper Guard, Corner General
Diaper, Pediatric General
Holder, Infant Position General
Kit, Feeding, Pediatric (Enteral) General
Mattress, Water, Temperature Regulated General
Pacifier General

CHINDEX INTERNATIONAL, INC. 301-215-7777
4340 East West Highway, Suite 1100, Bethesda, MD 20814
FDA Number: n/a Fax: 301-215-7719
Web site: http://www.chindex.com
Year Founded: 1981
Total Employees: 1328
Ownership: Public
Stock Symbol: CHDX
Traded On: NASDAQ
Produces/Sells CE-marked Devices: N
General Admin.: Ms. Elyse Beth Silverberg/Executive Vice President
   Ms. Roberta Lipson/President, Chief Executive Officer
Production: Ms. Judy Sakreski/Vice President Operations
Finance: Mr. Lawrence Pemble/Chief Financial Officer

CHIRAL TECHNOLOGIES, INC. 800-6-Chiral
800 North Five Points Road, 610-594-2100
West Chester, PA 19380
FDA Number: n/a Fax: 610-594-2325
E-mail: chiral@chiraltech.com
Web site: www.chiraltech.com
Medical Products Sales Volume: $11,200,000
Annual Revenue: $10-$25 Million
Year Founded: 1990
Total Employees: 22 Marketing Staff: 2 Sales Staff: 5
Ownership: Private
Produces/Sells CE-marked Devices: N
Federal Procurement Eligibility: Small Business
Distribution: Manufacturer Direct
General Admin.: Thomas B. Lewis/President
Chromatography, Liquid, Performance, High Toxicology
Column, Chromatography Chemistry

CHIROTRON, INC. 206-364-1262
20126 Ballinger Way Ne, #295, Seattle, WA 98155
FDA Number: 3018985
Ownership: Private
Produces/Sells CE-marked Devices: N
Scale, Stand-On General

CHISOLM BIOLOGICAL LAB. 803-663-9618
542 Legion Rd, Warrenville, SC 29851-3403
FDA Number: 1047739 Fax: 803-663-6019
E-mail: cbiolab@mindspring.com
Annual Revenue: $0-$1 Million
Total Employees: 10 Marketing Staff: 2 Sales Staff: 2
Ownership: Private
Produces/Sells CE-marked Devices: N
Federal Procurement Eligibility: Small Business, Minority Owned, Female Owned
Distribution: Manufacturer Direct
General Admin.: Minter H. Dopson/Chief Executive Officer
   Michelle DiMaria Dopson/Vice President
Serum, Animal Pathology
Serum, Biological, General Toxicology

CHIU TECHNICAL CORP. 631-544-0606
252 Indian Head Road, Kings Park, NY 11754-4814
FDA Number: n/a Fax: 631-544-0809
Web site: www.chiutech.com

CHIU TECHNICAL CORP. 631-544-0606 (cont'd)
Medical Products Sales Volume: $1,800,000
Annual Revenue: $1-$5 Million
Year Founded: 1972
Total Employees: 18 Marketing Staff: 1 Sales Staff: 2
Ownership: Private
Produces/Sells CE-marked Devices: Y
Federal Procurement Eligibility: Small Business, Minority Owned
Distribution: OEM, Exporter
General Admin.: Eva Chiu/President
Fiberoptic Light Source & Carrier Ear/Nose/Throat
Illuminator, Fiberoptic (For Endoscope) Gastroenterology/Urology
Illuminator, Fiberoptic, Surgical Field Cns/Neurology
Lamp, Microscope Pathology
Lamp, Surgical, Xenon Surgery
Light Source, Endoscope, Xenon Arc Surgery
Light Source, Fiberoptic, Routine Gastroenterology/Urology
Light, Surgical, Fiberoptic Surgery
Power Supply, Endoscopic, Battery-Operated General
Transilluminator, AC-Powered, Other Ophthalmology

CHO-PAT 800-221-1601
Lippincott Lane, Unit 6 609-261-1336
Mt. Holly Industrial Commons
Mt. Holly, NJ 08060
FDA Number: 2243659 Fax: 609-261-7593
E-mail: sales@cho-pat.com
Web site: www.cho-pat.com
Medical Products Sales Volume: $1,600,000
Annual Revenue: $1-$5 Million
Year Founded: 1980
Total Employees: 16 Marketing Staff: 1 Sales Staff: 3
Ownership: Private
Produces/Sells CE-marked Devices: N
Federal Procurement Eligibility: Small Business
Distribution: Manufacturer Direct, Manufacturer Through Distributor
General Admin.: David Daily/President, Chief Executive Officer
Brace, Joint, Ankle (External) Physical Med
Joint, Knee, External Brace Physical Med
Protector, Skin Pressure General
Restraint, Wheelchair General
Splint, Extremity, Non-Inflatable, External Surgery
Support, Ankle Orthopedics
Support, Arm Physical Med
Support, Elbow Orthopedics
Support, Knee Physical Med
Support, Leg Physical Med
Support, Wrist Physical Med

CHOICE MEDICAL SYSTEMS, INC. 727-347-8833
1426 Pasadena Avenue, S., St. Petersburg, FL 33707
FDA Number: 1063114 Fax: 727-347-7140
E-mail: choice@choicemedical.com
Web site: www.choicemedical.com
Medical Products Sales Volume: $1,000,000
Year Founded: 1991
Total Employees: 7
Ownership: Private
Produces/Sells CE-marked Devices: N
Federal Procurement Eligibility: Small Business
General Admin.: Derrell McCrary/Owner
Facility, Equipment, Medical, Mobile General

CHOICES TECHNOLOGIES 425-765-9400
21730-176th Ave. South East, Kent, WA 98042-7210
FDA Number: 3006017650
Ownership: Private
Produces/Sells CE-marked Devices: N
Denture, Plastic, Teeth Dental And Oral

CHOLERAPREP 800-523-0502
11400 Tomahawk Creek Pkwy, Suite 310, 913-451-0880
Leawood, KS 66211
FDA Number: n/a Fax: 913-451-8509
E-mail: sales@medi-flex.com
Web site: www.medi-flex.com
Annual Revenue: $100-$500 Million
Year Founded: 1985
Total Employees: 650 Marketing Staff: 14 Sales Staff: 100
Ownership: Private
Quality System Registration Information: ISO9002
Produces/Sells CE-marked Devices: N
Federal Procurement Eligibility: Small Business, GSA Contract, VA Contract
Distribution: Manufacturer Through Distributor, Exporter
General Admin.: Jim Mitchum/President, Chief Executive Officer
   Brian Jackson/Vice President Human Resources
Medical Admin.: Cindi Crosby/Vice President Medical Affairs
Mktg./Adv.: Sonya Butler/Director Corporate Communications

CHOLERAPREP
800-523-0502 *(cont'd)*
Juan Bournas/Director International Business Development
Bill Brandmeyer/Director Product Development
Mark Brandmeyer/Senior Vice President Sales
Diarmuid Boran/Vice President Business Development
Jan Creidenberg/Vice President Marketing
Production: Mary Wilson/Director Customer Services
Ray Cramer/Senior Vice President Operations
Orlando Cordova/Senior Vice President Quality Assurance
Research: Dr. Mike Baltezor/Chief Scientist
Finance: Steve Braun/Chief Financial Officer
Applicator, Antiseptic — General
Material, Preparation, Skin — Hematology

CHOLESTECH CORP.
800-733-0404
3347 Investment Blvd., Hayward, CA 94545-3808
510-732-7200
FDA Number: 2950138
Fax: 510-732-7227
E-mail: ctec_pr@cholestech.com
Web site: www.cholestech.com
Medical Products Sales Volume: $69,500,000
Annual Revenue: $50-$100 Million
Year Founded: 1998
Total Employees: 220   *Marketing Staff:* 5   *Sales Staff:* 25
Ownership: Alere, Inc.
Quality System Registration Information: ISO9001
Produces/Sells CE-marked Devices: Y
Federal Procurement Eligibility: Small Business
Distribution: Manufacturer Direct, Manufacturer Through Distributor, Manufacturer Through Manufacturer Reps
General Admin.: Warren E. Pinckert/President, Chief Executive Officer
Mktg./Adv.: Steve Wray/Director Tech. Sales
Colleen Wagener/Manager National Sales
Kenneth F. Miller/Vice President Marketing & Sales
Production: Steve Gottlieb/Director Quality Assurance
Barry McCormally/Manager Materials
Dr. Tom Worthy/Manager Regulatory Affairs
Don Wood/Vice President Manufacturing
Donald P. Wood/Vice President Operations
Research: Gregory L. Bennett/Vice President Research & Development
Finance: John F. Glenn/Vice President Finance
Reagent, Other — General

CHOOSE MANUFACTURING, CO. LLC
714-327-1698
3310 W. Macarthur Blvd, Santa Ana, CA 92704
FDA Number: 3004524266
Fax: 714-327-1699
E-mail: help@choosemfg.com
Web site: www.choosemfg.com
Ownership: Private
Produces/Sells CE-marked Devices: N

CHRISTENSEN ORTHOPEDIC INC.
See Cosco

CHRISTIE GROUP LTD.
800-361-8750
516 rue de Parc,
450-472-9120
St-Eustache, QUE J7R-5 Canada
FDA Number: n/a
Fax: 450-472-9410
E-mail: info@christieinnomed.com
Web site: www.christiegrp.com
Year Founded: 1954
Total Employees: 100
Ownership: VAC INC.
Produces/Sells CE-marked Devices: N
Distribution: Manufacturer Direct, Service Direct, Exclusive Distributor, Importer

CHRISTIE MEDICAL HOLDINGS
901-252-3700
1256 Union Ave., 3 Floor, Memphis, TN 38104
FDA Number: 3008161930
Fax: 901-252-3701
Web site: http://www.christiedigital.com
Ownership: Private
Produces/Sells CE-marked Devices: N
Locator, Vein, Liquid Crystal — General

CHRISTY MANUFACTURING CORP.
925-462-7982
1228-f Quarry Ln., Pleasanton, CA 94566
FDA Number: 2939854
Ownership: Private
Produces/Sells CE-marked Devices: N
Dynamometer, Non-Powered — Orthopedics
Elastomer, Silicone (Scar Management) — Surgery
Esthesiometer — Cns/Neurology
Exerciser, Non-Measuring — Physical Med

CHROMABEC INC.
888-624-7662
5475 Industriel, Waterloo, QUE J0E 2N0 Canada
514-335-6288
FDA Number: n/a
Fax: 1.450.539.6489
E-mail: info@chromabec.ca
Web site: www.chromabec.ca

CHROMABEC INC.
888-624-7662 *(cont'd)*
Year Founded: 1991
Ownership: Private
Produces/Sells CE-marked Devices: N
Distribution: Exclusive Distributor

CHROMATOGRAPHY SCIENCES CO. (CSC)
800-668-4752
5750 Vanden Abeele,
514-334-1892
St-Laurent, QUE H4S 1 Canada
FDA Number: n/a
Fax: 514-334-1898
E-mail: csc.inc@sympztico.ca
Web site: www.chromataographysciences.com
Medical Products Sales Volume: $1,000,000
Year Founded: 1980
Total Employees: 6   *Sales Staff:* 3
Ownership: Private
Quality System Registration Information: ISO9003
Produces/Sells CE-marked Devices: N
Federal Procurement Eligibility: Small Business
Distribution: Manufacturer Direct, Exclusive Distributor

CHROMODYNAMICS
732-730-1877
1195 Airport Road, # !, Lakewood, NJ 08701
FDA Number: n/a
Fax: 732-730-3547
E-mail: info@chromodynamics.net
Web site: www.chromodynamics.net
Ownership: GOOCH & HOUSEGO
Produces/Sells CE-marked Devices: N
Federal Procurement Eligibility: Small Business
Distribution: Manufacturer Direct
Research: Mr. Elliot Wachman/Chief Scientist
Radiographic/Fluoroscopic Unit, Angiographic — Radiology

CHRONIMED, INC.
See Arkray Usa

CHRONO-LOG CORP.
800-247-6665
2 W. Park Rd., Havertown, PA 19083-4691
610-853-1130
FDA Number: 2518152
Fax: 610-853-3972
E-mail: chronolog@chronolog.com
Web site: www.chronolog.com
Medical Products Sales Volume: $2,500,000
Annual Revenue: $1-$5 Million
Total Employees: 20   *Sales Staff:* 4
Ownership: Private
Produces/Sells CE-marked Devices: Y
Federal Procurement Eligibility: Small Business
Distribution: Manufacturer Direct
General Admin.: Nicholas Veriabo/Executive Director
Mktg./Adv.: Kathy Jacobs/Manager National Sales
Production: Al Roy/Manager Production
Aggregometer, Platelet — Hematology
Aggregometer, Platelet, Photo-Optical Scanning — Hematology
Analyzer, Platelet Aggregation — Hematology
Analyzer, Platelet Aggregation, Automated — Hematology
Clock, Elapsed Time — General
Reagent, Platelet Aggregation — Hematology
Test, Qualitative And Quantitative Factor Deficiency — Hematology

CHRONTROL CORPORATION
800-854-1999
PO Box 19537, San Diego, CA 92159
619-282-8686
FDA Number: 9200650
Fax: 619-563-6563
E-mail: info@chrontrol.com
Web site: www.chrontrol.com
Medical Products Sales Volume: $1,000,000
Annual Revenue: $0-$1 Million
Year Founded: 1977
Total Employees: 10   *Marketing Staff:* 2   *Sales Staff:* 2
Ownership: Private
Produces/Sells CE-marked Devices: N
Federal Procurement Eligibility: Small Business
Distribution: Manufacturer Direct, Manufacturer Through Distributor, Manufacturer Through Manufacturer Reps, Importer, Exporter
Research: James Durham/Vice President Research & Development
Timer, General Laboratory — Hematology
Timer, Radiographic — Radiology

CHURCH & DWIGHT CO., INC.
609-279-7715
1851 Touchstone Rd., Colonial Heights, VA 23834
FDA Number: 1122329
Ownership: Private
Produces/Sells CE-marked Devices: N
Condom — Obstetrics/Gynecology
Condom With Nonoxynol-9 — Obstetrics/Gynecology
Condom, Non-Latex — Obstetrics/Gynecology

CHURCHILL MEDICAL SYSTEMS, INC.
800-468-0585
103a Park Drive, Montgomeryville, PA 19044
215-956-0585
FDA Number: n/a
Fax: 215-672-6740

CHURCHILL MEDICAL SYSTEMS, INC.   800-468-0585 *(cont'd)*
E-mail: CMS935@aol.com
Web site: www.ChurchillMedicalSystems.com
Medical Products Sales Volume: $9,800,000
Annual Revenue: $10-$25 Million
Year Founded: 1987
Total Employees: 4
Ownership: Vygon Corp.
Quality System Registration Information: ISO9002
Produces/Sells CE-marked Devices: N
Federal Procurement Eligibility: Small Business, GSA Contract, VA Contract
Distribution: Manufacturer Direct, Manufacturer Through Distributor, OEM
General Admin.: Mr. Bob Combs/President, Chief Executive Officer
Mktg./Adv.: Mr. Ron Metro/Vice President Marketing & Sales

Filter, Intravenous Tubing	General
Fitting, Luer	General
Kit, Intravenous Extension Tubing	General
Needle, Aspiration And Injection, Disposable	Surgery
Needle, Other	General
Stopcock	General
Transfer Unit, IV Fluid	General

CHX TECHNOLOGIES, INC.   416-233-3737
105-4800 Dundas St W, Toronto M9A 1B1 Canada
FDA Number: 9680945

Varnish, Cavity	Dental And Oral

CIANNA MEDICAL, INC.   866-920-9444
6 Journey, Suite 125, Aliso Viejo, CA 92656   949-360-0059
FDA Number: 2032338   *Fax:* 949-297-4527
E-mail: info@ciannamedical.com
Web site: http://www.ciannamedical.com
Ownership: Private
Produces/Sells CE-marked Devices: N
General Admin.: Mr. Christopher Serocke/Chief Operating Officer
         Dr. James Stubbs/Chief Scientific Officer
         Ms. Jill Anderson/President, Chief Executive Officer
Mktg./Adv.: Mr. Brian Driscoll/Vice President Marketing
Production: Mr. Gary Mocnik/Vice President Quality Assurance & Regulatory Affairs
Research: Mr. Eduardo Chi Sing/Vice President Research & Development
Finance: Mr. Hugh Neuharth/Chief Financial Officer

Applicator, Radionuclide, Remote-Controlled	Radiology
Catheter, Balloon (Foley Type)	Surgery

CIBA CORNING DIAGNOSTIC CORP.
    See Siemens Healthcare Diagnostics Inc

CIBA VISION   800-875-3001
11460 Johns Creek Parkway, Duluth, GA 30097   678-415-3937
FDA Number: 1065835   *Fax:* 847-321-7894
E-mail: sales@cibavision.com
Web site: www.cibavision.com/
Medical Products Sales Volume: $412,900,000
Year Founded: 1980
Total Employees: 6500   *Marketing Staff:* 30   *Sales Staff:* 200
Ownership: WESLEY JESSEN VISIONCARE, INC.
Quality System Registration Information: ISO9001; ISO9002
Produces/Sells CE-marked Devices: Y
Distribution: Manufacturer Direct, Manufacturer Through Distributor, Manufacturer Through Manufacturer Reps, OEM, Exporter
General Admin.: Ms. Andrea Saia/President
Mktg./Adv.: Mr. Ed Vlacic/Director Marketing
Research: Mr. Frank Leveiller/Director Research & Development
Finance: Mr. John Mckenna/Chief Financial Officer

Lens, Contact (Other Material)	Ophthalmology
Lens, Contact, Extended-Wear	Ophthalmology
Lens, Contact, Gas-Permeable	Ophthalmology
Lens, Contact, Hydrophilic	Ophthalmology
Lens, Contact, Polymethylmethacrylate	Ophthalmology
Lens, Contact, Tinted	Ophthalmology

CIBA VISION CORPORATION   800-875-3001
11460 Johns Creek Pkwy., Duluth, GA 30097   678-415-3646
FDA Number: 1053053   *Fax:* 678-415-3592
E-mail: kristie.madara@cibavision.com
Web site: www.cibavision.com
Medical Products Sales Volume: $412,900,000
Annual Revenue: More than $1 Billion
Year Founded: 1985
Total Employees: 1900
Ownership: NOVARTIS
Produces/Sells CE-marked Devices: Y
Distribution: Manufacturer Direct, Manufacturer Through Distributor
General Admin.: Joe Mallof/Chief Executive Officer

Accessories, Solution, Lens, Contact	Ophthalmology
Cleaner, Lens, Contact	Ophthalmology
Lens, Contact (Other Material)	Ophthalmology
Lens, Contact, Bifocal	Ophthalmology

CIBA VISION CORPORATION   800-875-3001 *(cont'd)*

Lens, Contact, Hydrophilic	Ophthalmology
Lens, Contact, Polymethylmethacrylate	Ophthalmology

CIBA VISION CORPORATION   678-415-3638
2930 Amwiler Court, Atl, GA 30360
FDA Number: 1030321
Ownership: CIBA VISION CORPORATION
Produces/Sells CE-marked Devices: N

CIBA VISION CORPORATION   1 847-321-7002
333 East Howard Avenue, Des Plaines, IL 60018
FDA Number: 1422160
Ownership: CIBA VISION CORPORATION
Produces/Sells CE-marked Devices: N

Lens, Contact, Extended-Wear	Ophthalmology

CIBA VISION PUERTO RICO, INC.   678-415-3638
El Jibaro Industrial Park, PO Box 1360, Cidra, PR 00739
FDA Number: 2648694
Ownership: Private
Produces/Sells CE-marked Devices: N

Lens, Intraocular	Ophthalmology
Lenses, Soft Contact, Daily Wear	Ophthalmology

CIF FURNITURE LTD.   905-738-5821
56 Edilcan Dr., Concord, ONT L4K-3S6 Canada
FDA Number: n/a   *Fax:* 905-738-6537
E-mail: dross@ciffurniture.com
Web site: www.ciffurniture.com
Year Founded: 1969
Total Employees: 50   *Marketing Staff:* 1   *Sales Staff:* 3
Ownership: Private
Produces/Sells CE-marked Devices: Y
Distribution: Manufacturer Direct, Exclusive Distributor, Exporter

CILCO INC.
    See Alcon Research, Ltd.

CIMA SCIENTIFIC   972-293-1605
P.O. Box 1237, De Soto, TX 75123
FDA Number: n/a   *Fax:* 972-293-1615
Web site: www.cimascientific.com
Annual Revenue: $0-$1 Million
Ownership: Private
Produces/Sells CE-marked Devices: N
Federal Procurement Eligibility: Small Business
Distribution: Manufacturer Through Distributor

Agglutination Method, Human Chorionic Gonadotropin	Chemistry
Chromatographic, Cystine	Chemistry
Enzymatic Esterase-Oxidase, Cholesterol	Chemistry
Hexokinase, Glucose	Chemistry
LDL & VLDL Precipitation, Cholesterol Via Esterase-Oxidase	Chemistry
NAD Reduction/NADH Oxidation, CPK Or Isoenzymes	Chemistry
NAD Reduction/NADH Oxidation, Lactate Dehydrogenase	Chemistry
NADH Oxidation/NAD Reduction, AST/SGOT	Chemistry
Nitrophenylphosphate, Alkaline Phosphatase Or Isoenzymes	Chemistry
Phosphorus Reagent (Test System)	Chemistry
Reagent, Bilirubin (Total Or Direct Test System)	Chemistry
Reagent, Cholesterol (Total Test System)	Chemistry
Reagent, Iron (Test System)	Chemistry
SGPT, Colorimetric	Chemistry
Test, Glycosylated Hemoglobin Assay	Hematology
Thymolphthalein Monophosphate, Acid Phosphatase	Chemistry
Thymolphthalein Monophosphate, Alkaline Phosphatase	Chemistry
Urease And Glutamic Dehydrogenase, Urea Nitrogen	Chemistry
Urease, Photometric, Urea Nitrogen	Chemistry
Uricase (Oxygen Rate), Uric Acid	Chemistry

CIMA TECHNOLOGY, INC.   724-733-2627
3253-C Old Frankstown Road, Pittsburgh, PA 15239
FDA Number: 2529709
Ownership: Private
Produces/Sells CE-marked Devices: N

Fluid, Intraocular	Ophthalmology
Lens, Intraocular	Ophthalmology

CIMEX MEDICAL INNOVATIONS, LLC   985-871-0802
72385 Industry Park, Covington, LA 70435
FDA Number: 2320472

Component, Traction, Non-Invasive	Orthopedics
Protector, Skin Pressure	General

CINCINNATI ASSOCIATION FOR THE BLIND   888-687-3935
2045 Gilbert Ave., Cincinnati, OH 45202-1403   513-221-8558
FDA Number: 1527107   *Fax:* 513-221-2995
Medical Products Sales Volume: $800,000
Annual Revenue: $5-$10 Million
Total Employees: 100   *Marketing Staff:* 1   *Sales Staff:* 1
Ownership: Private
Produces/Sells CE-marked Devices: N

CINCINNATI ASSOCIATION FOR THE BLIND   888-687-3935
(cont'd)
Distribution: Manufacturer Through Distributor
General Admin.: Hank Baud/Executive Director
Mktg./Adv.: Jane McGraw/Commercial Admin.
Production: Rick Wellman/Industrial Engineer
Finance: Stephen A. Wesseler/Chief Financial Officer
  Sheeting, Examination Table   General

CINCINNATI SUB-ZERO PRODUCTS, INC.,   800-989-7373
MEDICAL DIVISION

12011 Mosteller Road,   **513-772-8810**
Cincinnati, OH 45241
FDA Number: 1516825   Fax: 513-772-9119
E-mail: medsales@cszinc.com
Web site: www.cszmedical.com
Annual Revenue: $10-$25 Million
Year Founded: 1940
Total Employees: 240   *Marketing Staff:* 2   *Sales Staff:* 55
Ownership: Private
Quality System Registration Information: ISO9001
Produces/Sells CE-marked Devices: Y
Federal Procurement Eligibility: Small Business, Female Owned, VA Contract
Distribution: Manufacturer Direct, Manufacturer Through Distributor, Manufacturer Through Manufacturer Reps, Exporter
General Admin.: Steven J. Berke/President, Chief Executive Officer
    Eileen Berke/Vice President Human Resources
    Jerry Silvertooth/Vice President, General Manager
Mktg./Adv.: Dennis Daar/Director National Accounts
    Dan Koewler/Director Product Development
    Dave Frederick/Director Sales
    Kristal Yelton/Manager Advertising
    Dave Frederick/Manager Contract Sales
    Dave Frederick/Manager Market Research
    Julie C Fogt/Manager Sales Admin.
    Jerry Silvertooth/Vice President Business Development
Production: Crystal Morrison/Director Quality Assurance
    Victoria Meyer/Manager Materials
    Jerry Silvertooth/Manager Regulatory Affairs
    Aron Jarret/Vice President Manufacturing

Chamber, Constant Temperature (Environmental)	Microbiology
Compress, Cold	General
Controller, Temperature, Cardiopulmonary Bypass	Cardiovascular
Hypo/Hyperthermia Blanket	General
Hypo/Hyperthermia Unit, Mobile	General
Hypothermia Unit	General
Hypothermic Equipment	Microbiology
Probe, Temperature	General
Warmer, Blanket	General

CINCINNATI SURGICAL COMPANY   800-544-3100
11256 Cornell Park Dr.,   **513-489-6640**
Cincinnati, OH 45242
FDA Number: 1517254   Fax: 513-489-6683
E-mail: info@cincinnatisurgical.com
Web site: www.cincinnatisurgical.com
Annual Revenue: $1-$5 Million
Year Founded: 1938
Total Employees: 7
Ownership: Private
Quality System Registration Information: ISO9001
Produces/Sells CE-marked Devices: Y
Federal Procurement Eligibility: Small Business
Distribution: Manufacturer Through Distributor, Manufacturer Through Manufacturer Reps, OEM, Exclusive Distributor
General Admin.: Jason Greiner/President, Chief Executive Officer
    Richard F. Gregory/Vice President, General Manager
Mktg./Adv.: Richard F. Gregory/Vice President Marketing & Sales

Blade, Scalpel	Surgery
Blade, Surgical Saw, General & Plastic Surgery	Surgery
Cutter, Surgical	Surgery
Cutter, Suture	Surgery
Handle, Scalpel	Surgery
Knife, Scalpel	Surgery
Needle, Suture, Disposable	Surgery
Needle, Suture, Reusable	Surgery
Remover, Blade, Scalpel	General
Scalpel, One-Piece (Knife)	Surgery
Suture, Other	Surgery

CINEREX IMAGING SYSTEMS
  See Agfa Corp.

CINTAS CORP.
6800 Cintas Blvd, P. O. Box 625737,   **800-246-8271**
Cincinnati, OH 45262   **513-459-1200.**
FDA Number: 1121142
Web site: www.cintas.com

CINTAS CORP.   800-246-8271 *(cont'd)*
Medical Products Sales Volume: $3,700,000,000
Annual Revenue: More than $1 Billion
Total Employees: 31000
Ownership: Public
Stock Symbol: CTAS
Traded On: NASDAQ
Quality System Registration Information: ISO9001
Produces/Sells CE-marked Devices: N
Distribution: Manufacturer Direct, Service Direct, Exclusive Distributor
General Admin.: Richard T. Farmer/Chairman
    Scott D. Farmer/Chief Executive Officer
    William C. Gale/Chief Financial Officer, Senior Vice President
    J. Phillip Holloman/President, Chief Operating Officer
    Robert J. Kohlhepp/Vice Chairman
    Thomas Frooman/Vice President, Secretary
Finance: Michael L. Thompson/Vice President, Treasurer

Dress, Surgical	Surgery
Gown, Isolation, Surgical	Surgery
Gown, Operating Room, Reusable	Surgery
Gown, Surgical	Surgery
Housekeeping Equipment	General
Suit, Scrub, Reusable	Surgery
Suit, Surgical	Surgery

CIR SYSTEMS INC   914-734-8178
8 John Walsh Blvd., Suite 429, Peekskill, NY 10566
FDA Number: 3006462771
Ownership: Private
Produces/Sells CE-marked Devices: N
  Pressure Measurement, System, Intermittent   Physical Med

CIRCADIAN SYSTEMS   800-669-7001
8099 Savage Way, Valley Springs, CA 95252   **209-786-6000**
FDA Number: 2918203   Fax: 209-786-4864
Medical Products Sales Volume: $500,000
Annual Revenue: $1-$5 Million
Total Employees: 4
Ownership: Private
Produces/Sells CE-marked Devices: N
Federal Procurement Eligibility: Small Business, GSA Contract
Distribution: Manufacturer Direct
General Admin.: James L. Bothwell/Owner
    Daun M. Krahn/Vice President, General Manager
Mktg./Adv.: Jo Ann Varady/Manager Contract Sales

Analyzer, Pulmonary Function	Anesthesiology
Computer, Ultrasound	Radiology
Electrocardiograph, Multi-Channel	Cardiovascular
Monitor, Blood Pressure, Indirect, Automatic	Cardiovascular
Recorder, Long-Term, ECG, Portable (Holter Monitor)	Cardiovascular

CIRCADIANCE LLC   1-888-825-9640
1060 Corporate Lane, Export, PA 15632   **724-858-2837**
FDA Number: 3006182632   Fax: 412-202-4583
E-mail: info@circadiance.com
Ownership: Private
Produces/Sells CE-marked Devices: N

Mask, Oxygen, Venturi	Anesthesiology
Ventilator, Non-Continuous (Respirator)	Anesthesiology

CIRCAID MEDICAL PRODUCTS, INC.   800-247-2243
9323 Chesapeake Dr., Suite B2,   **858-576-3550**
San Diego, CA 92123
FDA Number: 2243150   Fax: 858-576-3555
E-mail: info@circaid.com
Web site: www.circaid.com
Annual Revenue: $0-$1 Million
Ownership: Private
Produces/Sells CE-marked Devices: N
Federal Procurement Eligibility: Small Business
Distribution: Manufacturer Direct, Manufacturer Through Distributor, Manufacturer Through Manufacturer Reps
Mktg./Adv.: Ingrid Adams/Director Sales

Ankle/Foot, External Limb Component	Physical Med
Binder, Medical, Therapeutic	General
Brace, Joint, Ankle (External)	Physical Med

CIRCLE MEDICAL DEVICES   408-395-0443
101 Cooper Court, Los Gatos, CA 95032
FDA Number: 3004737415   Fax: 408.395.0465
E-mail: info@cirtecmed.com
Ownership: Private
Produces/Sells CE-marked Devices: N
  Electrosurgical Unit, Cutting & Coagulation Device   Surgery

CIRCLE SEAL CORP., AERODYNE CONTROLS DIVISION
  See Aerodyne Controls, Inc., A Circor International Company

CIRCUIT EQUIPMENT CO.
  See Air Techniques International

CIRCUIT TREE MEDICAL, INC. 626-303-7902
  1911 Walker Avenue, Monrovia, CA 91016
  FDA Number: 2030501
  Ownership: Staar Surgical Co.
    Phacofragmentation Unit Ophthalmology

CIRCULAR TRACTION SUPPLY, INC. 800-247-6535
  7602 Talbert Avenue, Unit 9, 714-847-8334
  Huntington Beach, CA 92648
  FDA Number: 3005083774
  E-mail: info@circular Traction.com Fax: 714-847-8666
  Web site: www.circulartraction.com
  Year Founded: 1986
  Ownership: Private
  Produces/Sells CE-marked Devices: N
    Accessories, Traction Physical Med
    Component, Exercise Physical Med
    Orthosis, Cervical Physical Med
    Orthosis, Thoracic Physical Med

CIRCULATOR BOOT CORP. 610-240-9980
  72 Pennsylvania Avenue, Malvern, PA 19355
  FDA Number: 2518635
  E-mail: circboot@op.net Fax: 610-240-9982
  Web site: www.circulatorboot.com
  Medical Products Sales Volume: $500,000
  Annual Revenue: $0-$1 Million
  Total Employees: 4 *Marketing Staff:* 2
  Ownership: Private
  Produces/Sells CE-marked Devices: N
  Federal Procurement Eligibility: Small Business, GSA Contract, VA Contract
  Distribution: Manufacturer Direct
  General Admin.: Richard S. Dillon/President, Chief Executive Officer
      Susan Holt Dillon/Vice President
  Mktg./Adv.: Joseph Makowski/Vice President Marketing & Sales
    Compression Instrument Orthopedics
    Cover, Limb Physical Med
    Sleeve, Compressible Limb Cardiovascular

CIRCULATORY TECHNOLOGY, INC. 516-624-2424
  21 Singworth St., Oyster Bay, NY 11771
  FDA Number: 2436790
    Catheter, Vascular, Cardiopulmonary Bypass Cardiovascular
    Pressure Infusor, IV Container General
    Reservoir, Blood, Cardiopulmonary Bypass Cardiovascular
    Valve, Pressure Relief, Cardiopulmonary Bypass Cardiovascular

CIRCULITE 201-543-2430
  250 Pehle Avenue, Park 80 West, Suite 403,
  Saddle Brook, NJ 07663
  FDA Number: n/a
  Web site: www.circulite.net.
  Ownership: Private
  Produces/Sells CE-marked Devices: N
  General Admin.: Mr. John Budris/Chief Technology Officer
      Mr. Pauk Southworth/President, Chief Executive Officer
  Medical Admin.: Dr. Daniel Burkhoff/Chief Medical Officer
  Mktg./Adv.: Ms. Gail Farnan/Vice President Marketing
  Finance: Mr. Peter Pfreundschuh/Chief Financial Officer

CIRIUS GROUP INC. 925-685-9300
  140 Gregory Lane, Suite 240, Pleasant Hill, CA 94523
  FDA Number: n/a Fax: 925-685-6526
  E-mail: admin@ciriusgroup.com
  Web site: www.ciriusgroup.com
  Annual Revenue: $0-$1 Million
  Ownership: Private
  Produces/Sells CE-marked Devices: N
  Federal Procurement Eligibility: Small Business
  Distribution: Manufacturer Direct
  General Admin.: Paul Bartlett/President
    Computer Software, Hospital/Nursing Management General

CIRRUS DIAGNOSTICS, INC.
  See Siemens Healthcare Diagnostics Inc

CISSELL MANUFACTURING COMPANY 888-223-2980
  PO Box 990, Shepard Street, Ripon, WI 54971
  FDA Number: n/a Fax: 502-585-2333
  E-mail: cissell@thepoint.net
  Web site: www.cissellmfg.com
  Medical Products Sales Volume: $30,000,000
  Annual Revenue: $0-$1 Million
  Total Employees: 150
  Ownership: IPSO CORPORATION
  Produces/Sells CE-marked Devices: N

CISSELL MANUFACTURING COMPANY 888-223-2980 *(cont'd)*
  Federal Procurement Eligibility: Small Business
  Distribution: Manufacturer Through Distributor
  Mktg./Adv.: Mr. Fred Quarles/Vice President Sales
  Production: Ms. Phyllis Decker/General Manager Manufacturing
    Laundry Equipment General

CITATION COMPUTER SYSTEM
  See Cerner Corp.

CITIZENS DEVELOPMENT CENTER 214-637-2911
  8800 Ambassador Row, Dallas, TX 75247-4621
  FDA Number: 1626364
  E-mail: info@cdcdallas.org Fax: 214-637-2929
  Web site: www.cdcdallas.org
  Medical Products Sales Volume: $2,200,000
  Annual Revenue: $1-$5 Million
  Year Founded: 1951
  Total Employees: 40
  Ownership: Private
  Produces/Sells CE-marked Devices: N
  Federal Procurement Eligibility: Small Business
  General Admin.: Rita De Young/Executive Managing Director
  Mktg./Adv.: Tim DeGrendele/Managing Director Marketing & Sales
    Bag, Blood, Collection Hematology
    Drill, Dental, Intraoral Dental And Oral
    Tray, Impression Dental And Oral

CITMED 800-224-8633
  18601 South Main St., Citronelle, AL 36522 251-866-5519
  FDA Number: 1043545 Fax: 251-866-7541
  E-mail: info@citmedcorp.com
  Web site: www.citmedcorp.com
  Ownership: Private
  Produces/Sells CE-marked Devices: N
    Applicator, Tipped, Absorbent, Non-Sterile General
    Applicator, Tipped, Absorbent, Sterile General
    Depressor, Tongue General
    Scraper, Specimen, Skin Surgery

CITOW CERVICAL VISUALIZER COMPANY 877-272-4869
  712 South Milwaukee Avenue, 646-460-2984
  Libertyville, IL 60048
  FDA Number: 3006785224
  E-mail: customerservice@citowcv.com
  Ownership: Private
  Produces/Sells CE-marked Devices: N
    Glove, Protective, Radiographic Radiology
    Table, Surgical, Orthopedic Orthopedics

CITRA ANTICOAGULANTS, INC. 800-299-3411
  55 Messina Drive, Braintree, MA 02184 781-848-2174
  FDA Number: n/a Fax: 781-848-6781
  E-mail: TeamCustomer@t3cc.com
  Web site: www.citraanticoagulants.com
  Annual Revenue: $1-$5 Million
  Year Founded: 1997
  Ownership: Cytosol Laboratories, Inc.
  Quality System Registration Information: ISO9002
  Produces/Sells CE-marked Devices: N
  Federal Procurement Eligibility: Small Business
  Distribution: Manufacturer Direct, Manufacturer Through Distributor
  General Admin.: Ron Lewis/President, Chief Executive Officer
    Contract Manufacturing, Pharmaceuticals/Chemicals General

CIVCO MEDICAL INSTRUMENTS CO., INC. 800.445.6741
  102 First St. South, Kalona, IA 52247 319-656-4447
  FDA Number: 1937223 Fax: 319.656.4451
  E-mail: info@civco.com
  Web site: www.civco.com
  Ownership: Private
  Produces/Sells CE-marked Devices: N
    Clamp, Surgical, General & Plastic Surgery Surgery
    Communication System, Non-Powered Physical Med
    Cover, Mattress General
    Cover, Shoe, Operating Room Surgery
    Densitometer Cardiovascular
    Evacuator, Gastro-Urology Gastroenterology/Urology
    Holder, Radiographic Cassette, Wall-Mounted Radiology
    Needle, Biopsy, Cardiovascular Cardiovascular
    Probe Orthopedics
    Scanner, Ultrasonic (Pulsed Echo) Radiology
    System, Marking, Film, Radiographic Radiology
    Table, Anesthetist's Anesthesiology
    Tank, Holding, Dialysis Gastroenterology/Urology
    Transducer, Ultrasonic, Diagnostic Radiology

CJPS MEDICAL SYSTEMS
2333 E. Walton Blvd., Auburn Hills, MI 48326
248-593-5926
FDA Number: 3008629890
Fax: 248-593-1265
E-mail: Inquiries@CJPS-MedicalSystems.com
Web site: http://www.cjps.com
Ownership: Private
Produces/Sells CE-marked Devices: N

CJV MFG., INC.
See Vancare, Inc.

CLAREBLEND, INC.
3555 Airway Dr., Suite 307, Reno, NV 89511
800-334-7126
775-332-3850
FDA Number: 2020958
Fax: 775-332-3852
E-mail: staff@clareblend.com
Web site: www.clareblend.com
Medical Products Sales Volume: $150,000
Annual Revenue: $0-$1 Million
Year Founded: 1927
Total Employees: 5   *Marketing Staff:* 2   *Sales Staff:* 10
Ownership: Private
Produces/Sells CE-marked Devices: N
Federal Procurement Eligibility: Small Business, Female Owned
Distribution: Manufacturer Direct, Manufacturer Through Distributor, Manufacturer Through Manufacturer Reps, OEM, Exporter
General Admin.: Mr. Richard Klukovich/President, Owner
    Mrs. Nadia Klukovich/Secretary, Treasurer

Epilator, High-Frequency, Needle-Type	Surgery
Lamp, Infrared	Physical Med
Laser, Surgical	Surgery
Massager, Therapeutic	Physical Med

CLARIANT
4000 Monroe Road, Charlotte, NC 28205
704-331-7000
FDA Number: n/a
E-mail: info@clariant.com
Web site: www.clariant.us
Annual Revenue: $1-$5 Million
Ownership: Private
Quality System Registration Information: ISO9001
Produces/Sells CE-marked Devices: N
Distribution: Manufacturer Direct, Manufacturer Through Distributor

Concentrate, Dialysis, Hemodialysis (Liquid or Powder)	Gastroenterology/Urology

CLARIANT CORPORATION
4000 Monroe Road, Charlotte, NC 28205
1 704 331 7000
FDA Number: 2531100
Web site: www.clariant.us
Ownership: Private
Produces/Sells CE-marked Devices: N

Disinfector, Medical Device	General

CLARIENT, INC.
31 Columbia, Aliso Viejo, CA 92656
888-443-3310
949-425-5700
FDA Number: n/a
Fax: 949-425-5701
E-mail: info@clarientinc.com
Web site: http://www.clarientinc.com
Year Founded: 1993
Ownership: Public
Stock Symbol: CLRT
Traded On: NASDAQ
Produces/Sells CE-marked Devices: N
General Admin.: Ron A. Andrews/Chief Executive Officer, Vice Chairman
    Mr. Michael Rodriguez/Chief Financial Officer, Senior Vice President
    Mr. Ronald Collette/Chief Information Officer
    Dr. Douglas Ross/Chief Scientific Officer
    Michael J. Pellini/President, Chief Operating Officer
Medical Admin.: Dr. Kenneth Bloom/Chief Medical Officer

CLARIO MEDICAL IMAGING, INC.
520 Pike Street, Suite 1005, Seattle, WA 98101
866 941-6412
206 315-5410
FDA Number: 3005847781
Fax: 206 315 5409
E-mail: info@clariomedical.com
Web site: www.clariomedical.com
Ownership: Private
Produces/Sells CE-marked Devices: N

Image Processing System	Radiology

CLARITY MEDICAL SYSTEMS
5775 West Las Positas Blvd., Suite 200, Pleasanton, CA 94588
925-463-7984
FDA Number: 2952489

Camera, Ophthalmic, AC-Powered (Fundus)	Ophthalmology
Device, Analysis, Anterior Segment	Ophthalmology
Device, Communications, Images, Ophthalmic	Ophthalmology
Device, Storage, Images, Ophthalmic	Ophthalmology

CLARK COMPANY INC., DAVID
360 Franklin St., Worcester, MA 01615-0054
800-900-3434
508-756-6216
FDA Number: 9200210
Fax: 508-753-5827
E-mail: sales@davidclark.com
Web site: www.davidclark.com
Medical Products Sales Volume: $1,000,000
Annual Revenue: $25-$50 Million
Total Employees: 298   *Marketing Staff:* 3   *Sales Staff:* 17
Ownership: Private
Produces/Sells CE-marked Devices: Y
Federal Procurement Eligibility: Small Business
Distribution: Manufacturer Through Distributor
General Admin.: Robert Vincent/President
Mktg./Adv.: Richard M. Urella/Vice President Marketing & Sales
Production: D. Hansen */Product Manager

Pressure Infusor, IV Container	General
Protector, Hearing (Circumaural)	Ear/Nose/Throat
Suit, Pneumatic Counterpressure (Anti-Shock)	Cardiovascular

CLARK LABORATORIES, INC.
See Trinity Biotech, Inc.

CLARK MANUFACTURING (SUNDANCE SPAS)
See Sundance Spas, Inc.

CLARK MEDICAL PRODUCTS, INC.
10-5510 Ambler Drive,
Mississauga, ONT L4W- Canada
800-889-5295
905-238-6163
FDA Number: n/a
Fax: 905-624-3161
E-mail: info@clarkmedical.com
Web site: www.clarkmedical.com
Year Founded: 1987
Total Employees: 10   *Marketing Staff:* 1   *Sales Staff:* 1
Ownership: Private
Produces/Sells CE-marked Devices: N
Federal Procurement Eligibility: Small Business
Distribution: Manufacturer Through Distributor, Exclusive Distributor

CLARKE HEALTH CARE PRODUCTS, INC.
1003 International Dr., Oakdale, PA 15071-9226
888-347-4537
724-695-2122
FDA Number: 2523870
Fax: 724-695-2922
E-mail: info@clarkehealthcare.com
Web site: www.clarkehealthcare.com
Medical Products Sales Volume: $1,000,000
Annual Revenue: $1-$5 Million
Year Founded: 1994
Total Employees: 17   *Marketing Staff:* 4   *Sales Staff:* 6
Ownership: Private
Produces/Sells CE-marked Devices: N
Federal Procurement Eligibility: Small Business
Distribution: Service Direct, Exclusive Distributor
General Admin.: Gerard C. Clarke/President, General Manager
Mktg./Adv.: Susan Grabel/Manager Advertising
    Mr. Jay Everett/Manager National Sales

Bag, Urinary Collection	General
Chair, Pediatric	General
Chair, Shower	General
Commode (Toilet)	General
Lift, Bath, Non-AC-Powered	General
Lift, Patient	General
Rail, Bath	General
Training Aid	Orthopedics
Walker, Mechanical	Physical Med

CLARKE MANUFACTURING, INC.
3000 W. Clarke St., Milwaukee, WI 53210
414-444-7003
FDA Number: 2184047
Fax: 414-444-9365
E-mail: mktg@clarkemanufacturing.com
Web site: www.clarkemanufacturing.com
Medical Products Sales Volume: $900,000
Year Founded: 1960
Total Employees: 17
Ownership: Private
Quality System Registration Information: ISO9001
Produces/Sells CE-marked Devices: N
Federal Procurement Eligibility: Small Business, Female Owned
Distribution: Service Direct
General Admin.: Eileen Nelson/President, Chief Executive Officer
    Tom Nelson/Vice President
Production: Steve Detrie/Plant Manager

Contract Manufacturing	General

CLAROS DIAGNOSTICS INC.
4 Constitution Way, Suite E, Woburn, MA 01801
781-933-8012
FDA Number: n/a
Fax: 781-933-8011
Web site: http://www.clarosdx.com
Ownership: Private
Produces/Sells CE-marked Devices: N
General Admin.: Dr. David Steinmiller/Chief Operating Officer

CLAROS DIAGNOSTICS INC.
781-933-8012 *(cont'd)*
Dr. Vincent Linder/Chief Technology Officer
Dr. Michael Magliochetti/President, Chief Executive Officer

CLARUS MEDICAL, LLC.
800-359-2372
1000 Boone Ave. North, Suite 300,
763-525-8400
Minneapolis, MN 55427
FDA Number: 2183911
Fax: 763-525-8656
Web site: www.clarus-medical.com
Ownership: Private
Produces/Sells CE-marked Devices: N

Accessories, Photographic, Endoscopic	Gastroenterology/Urology
Accessories, Pump, Infusion	General
Arthroscope	Orthopedics
Camera, Television, Endoscopic (Without Audio)	Surgery
Endoscope	Gastroenterology/Urology
Endoscope, Fiberoptic	Surgery
Endoscope, Flexible	Gastroenterology/Urology
Endoscope, Neurological	Cns/Neurology
Instrument, Surgical, Powered, Pneumatic	Orthopedics
Laparoscope, Gynecologic	Obstetrics/Gynecology
Laryngoscope, Flexible	Anesthesiology
Laser, Surgical	Surgery
Light Source, Endoscope, Xenon Arc	Surgery
Motor, Surgical Instrument, Pneumatic-Powered	Surgery
Sheath, Endoscopic	Gastroenterology/Urology

CLASSIC HEALTH SUPPLIES LTD.
888-421-0488
8317 Argyll Road,
780-421-4372
Edmonton, AB T5H-3 Canada
FDA Number: n/a
Fax: 780-421-4507
E-mail: email@classichealth.com
Web site: www.classichealth.com
Year Founded: 1991
Total Employees: 10
Ownership: Private
Produces/Sells CE-marked Devices: N
Distribution: Exclusive Distributor

CLASSIC MEDICAL PRODUCTS, INC.
See Covidien Lp, Formerly Registered As Uni-Patch

CLASSONE ORTHODONTICS, INC.
806-799-0608
5064 50th St., Lubbock, TX 79414
FDA Number: 1643189
Ownership: Private
Produces/Sells CE-marked Devices: N

Adhesive, Bracket And Conditioner, Resin	Dental And Oral
Adhesive, Wound Closure	Surgery
Band, Elastic, Orthodontic	Dental And Oral
Band, Material, Orthodontic	Dental And Oral
Band, Preformed, Orthodontic	Dental And Oral
Bracket, Ceramic, Orthodontic	Dental And Oral
Bracket, Metal, Orthodontic	Dental And Oral
Face Bow	Dental And Oral
Handle, Instrument, Dental	Dental And Oral
Headgear, Extraoral, Orthodontic	Dental And Oral
Maintainer, Space Preformed, Orthodontic	Dental And Oral
Material, Impression Tray, Resin	Dental And Oral
Mirror, Mouth	Dental And Oral
Pack, Sterilization Wrapper (Bag And Accessories)	Surgery
Retainer, Screw Expansion, Orthodontic	Dental And Oral
Retractor, All Types	Dental And Oral
Spring, Orthodontic	Dental And Oral
Toothbrush, Manual	Dental And Oral
Tube, Orthodontic	Dental And Oral
Wax, Dental	Dental And Oral
Wire, Orthodontic	Dental And Oral

CLAUSS TOOLS
800-225-2877
1931 Black Rock Turnpike, Fairfield, CT 06825
419-898-3870
FDA Number: 1523524
Fax: 419-898-3871
E-mail: info@claussco.com
Web site: www.claussco.com
Annual Revenue: $10-$25 Million
Year Founded: 1877
Total Employees: 55   *Marketing Staff:* 2   *Sales Staff:* 180
Ownership: Private
Produces/Sells CE-marked Devices: N
Federal Procurement Eligibility: GSA Contract
Distribution: Manufacturer Through Manufacturer Reps
General Admin.: Scott F. Sprouse/President
Mktg./Adv.: William Miller/Manager Marketing
       E. Ted Mills/Manager Sales

General Use Surgical Scissors	Surgery

CLEAN AIR ENGINEERING
800-627-0033
500 W. Wood St., Palatine, IL 60067
847-991-3300
FDA Number: n/a
Fax: 847-991-3385
E-mail: contact@cleanair.com

CLEAN AIR ENGINEERING
800-627-0033 *(cont'd)*
Web site: www.cleanair.com
Annual Revenue: $10-$25 Million
Year Founded: 1972
Total Employees: 100
Ownership: Private
Produces/Sells CE-marked Devices: N
Federal Procurement Eligibility: Small Business
Distribution: Manufacturer Direct
General Admin.: William J. Walker/President
Mktg./Adv.: Allen Kephart/Vice President Business Development
       Steve Rees/Vice President Marketing & Sales
Production: Dan Rybarski/Vice President Manufacturing
Research: John Chapman/Vice President Research & Development

Balance, Analytical	Chemistry
Equipment, Cleaning, Air	General

CLEAN AIR RESEARCH & ENVIRONMENTAL, INC.
972-233-2777
13628 Beta Rd., Suite B, Dallas, TX 75244
FDA Number: 1648585

Purifier, Air, Ultraviolet	General

CLEAN AIR TECHNOLOGY, INC.
800 459 6320
41105 Capital, Canton, MI 48187
734-459-6320
FDA Number: n/a
Fax: 734-459-9437
E-mail: rkos@cleanairtechnology.com
Web site: www.cleanairtechnology.com
Medical Products Sales Volume: $1,000,000
Annual Revenue: $5-$10 Million
Year Founded: 1980
Total Employees: 55   *Marketing Staff:* 5   *Sales Staff:* 5
Ownership: Private
Quality System Registration Information: ISO9001
Produces/Sells CE-marked Devices: Y
Federal Procurement Eligibility: Small Business, VA Contract
Distribution: Manufacturer Direct, Manufacturer Through Manufacturer Reps, OEM, Service Direct, Exporter
General Admin.: Ms. Beverly Favor/Manager Admin. & Finance
       Frank X. Austin/President, Chief Executive Officer, General Manager
Mktg./Adv.: Ron Kosmalski/Director Marketing
       Ron Kosmalski/Manager International & National Sales
Production: Mr. Casey Bell/Manager Production

Building Material	General
Cabinet, Pass Through	General
Chamber, Isolation, Patient Care	General
Chamber, Isolation, Patient Transport	General
Cleanroom Equipment	General
Controller, Temperature, Humidifier	General
Equipment, Cleaning, Air	General
Filter, Air	General
Light, Other	General
Service, Consulting	General
Service, Engineering/Design	General

CLEAN ESD PRODUCTS, INC.
510-257-5080
48340 Milmont Drive, Fremont, CA 94538
FDA Number: 2939593
Fax: 510-257-5079
E-mail: cleanesd@cleanesd.com
Web site: www.cleanesd.com
Medical Products Sales Volume: $1,800,000
Annual Revenue: $1-$5 Million
Year Founded: 1987
Total Employees: 12   *Marketing Staff:* 2   *Sales Staff:* 6
Ownership: Private
Quality System Registration Information: ISO9001
Produces/Sells CE-marked Devices: N
Federal Procurement Eligibility: Small Business, Minority Owned, Female Owned
Distribution: Manufacturer Through Distributor, Manufacturer Through Manufacturer Reps, Importer
General Admin.: Elsie Katin/Chief Executive Officer
       Steve Katin/President
Mktg./Adv.: Elsie Katin/Manager Contract Sales
       Steve Katin/Manager Marketing
       Elsie Katin/Manager National Sales
       Elsie Katin/Manager Sales

Cap, Surgical	Surgery
Coat, Laboratory	General
Cover, Shoe, Operating Room	Surgery
Glove, Other	General
Glove, Patient Examination	General
Mask, Face	General
Swabs, Cotton	General

CLEAN ROOM TECHNOLOGY INC.
See Cleanroom Systems

CLEANROOM SYSTEMS
7000 Performance Dr., Syracuse, NY 13212
800-825-3268
315-452-7400
FDA Number: n/a
Fax: 315-452-7420
E-mail: info@airinnovations.com
Web site: www.cleanroomsystems.com
Annual Revenue: $1-$5 Million
Year Founded: 1983
Total Employees: 40   *Marketing Staff:* 3   *Sales Staff:* 10
Ownership: AIR INNOVATIONS, INC.
Produces/Sells CE-marked Devices:
Federal Procurement Eligibility: Small Business
Distribution: Manufacturer Through Distributor, Manufacturer Through Manufacturer Reps
General Admin.: Larry Wetzel/Chief Executive Officer
     Mike Wetzel/President
     Anne Tindall/Vice President Human Resources
Mktg./Adv.: Mike Militi/Manager International & National Sales
     Debbie Pelow/Manager Marketing Communications
Production: Mike Wetzel/Director Engineering
     Rich Goziqian/Vice President Manufacturing
   Cleanroom Equipment   General
   Controller, Temperature, Humidifier   General
Medical Product Subsidiaries (Listed Separately)
   Cleanroom Systems

CLEANWEAR PRODUCTS LTD.
54 Crockford Rd., Toronto, ON M1R-3C3 Canada
(416) 751-7307
FDA Number: n/a
Fax: (416) 751-8771
E-mail: jmharris@cleanwear.com
Web site: www.cleanwear.com
Year Founded: 1978
Total Employees: 50   *Marketing Staff:* 2   *Sales Staff:* 2
Ownership: Private
Quality System Registration Information: ISO9002
Produces/Sells CE-marked Devices: N
Distribution: Manufacturer Direct, Exclusive Distributor

CLEAR CATHETER SYSTEMS
20380 Halfway Road Ste. 4, Bend, OR 97701
541-382-8346
FDA Number: 3008782989
E-mail: info@clearcatheter.com
Web site: www.clearcatheter.com
Ownership: Private
Produces/Sells CE-marked Devices: N
General Admin.: Dr. Edward Boyle/Chief Executive Officer
   Catheter, Irrigation   Surgery

CLEAR STREAM MEDIA
4440 PGA Blvd-Suite 403, Palm Beach Gardens, FL 33410
561) 622-5995
FDA Number: n/a
E-mail: supply@medsite.com
Web site: www.clearstreammedia.com
Annual Revenue: $0-$1 Million
Total Employees: 10
Ownership: Private
Produces/Sells CE-marked Devices: N
Federal Procurement Eligibility: Small Business
Distribution: Exclusive Distributor
Mktg./Adv.: Donna Rothman/Vice President Marketing & Sales
Production: Jo Ellen Luedke/Manager Operations
   Training Aid   Orthopedics

CLEARCOUNT MEDICAL SOLUTIONS, INC.
101 Bellevue Road,, Suite 203, Pittsburgh, PA 15229
412-931-7233
FDA Number: 3005841380
Web site: www.clearcount.com
Ownership: Private
Produces/Sells CE-marked Devices: N
General Admin.: Mr. Steven Fleck/Chief Technology Officer
     Mr. David Palmer/President, Chief Executive Officer
Mktg./Adv.: Mr. Jim Sweeney/Vice President Marketing
     Mr. Curtis Groppe/Vice President Marketing & Sales
Production: Mr. Jim Sroc/Vice President Engineering & Operations
Finance: Mr. David Haffner/Chief Financial Officer
   Counter, Sponge, Surgical   Surgery
   Gauze, Non-Absorbable, X-Ray Detectable (Internal Sponge)   Surgery

CLEARFIELD/FOG CITY ENTERPRISES
See Primesource Healthcare, Inc.

CLEARMEDICAL, INC.
See Cenorin

CLEARMEDICAL, INC.
PMB - 357, 14150 NE 20th F-1, Bellevue, WA 98007
425-883-1522
FDA Number: 9031041
Fax: 425-883-1599
E-mail: orders@clearmedical.com
Web site: www.clearmedical.com
Annual Revenue: $5-$10 Million

CLEARMEDICAL, INC.
425-883-1522 *(cont'd)*
Year Founded: 1997
Total Employees: 50
Ownership: Private
Quality System Registration Information: ISO9001
Produces/Sells CE-marked Devices: N
Federal Procurement Eligibility: Small Business
Distribution: Manufacturer Direct
General Admin.: Mr. Gregg Bennett/Chief Executive Officer
     Mr. Vic Breed/Executive Vice President
Production: Mr. Mike Kovacs/Vice President Production
     Ms. Leslie Honda/Vice President Quality Assurance & Regulatory Affairs
   Circuit, Breathing, Ventilator   Anesthesiology

CLEARWATER COLON HYDROTHERAPY, INC.
3145 S.w. 74th Terrace, Ocala, FL 34474
888-869-6191
352-401-0303
FDA Number: 1062839
Fax: 352-401-9197
E-mail: sales@colonhydrotherapy.com
Web site: www.colonhydrotherapy.com
Medical Products Sales Volume: $500,000
Year Founded: 1992
Total Employees: 4
Ownership: Clearwater Colon Hydrotherapy, Inc.
Produces/Sells CE-marked Devices: N
Federal Procurement Eligibility: Small Business, Female Owned
Distribution: Manufacturer Direct, Manufacturer Through Distributor, Service Direct, Exporter
   Irrigator, Colonic   Gastroenterology/Urology
   Speculum, Rectal   Gastroenterology/Urology

CLESTRA CLEAN ROOM TECHNOLOGY, INC.
See Cleanroom Systems

CLESTRA CLEANROOM, INC.
See Cleanroom Systems

CLEVELAND MEDICAL DEVICES, INC.
4415 Euclid Avenue, Suite 400, Cleveland, OH 44103
877-253-8363
216-791-6720
FDA Number: 1530224
Fax: 216-791-6744
E-mail: sales@clevemed.com
Web site: www.clevemed.com
Medical Products Sales Volume: $4,000,000
Annual Revenue: $1-$5 Million
Year Founded: 1991
Total Employees: 40   *Marketing Staff:* 1   *Sales Staff:* 3
Ownership: Private
Produces/Sells CE-marked Devices: N
Federal Procurement Eligibility: Small Business
Distribution: Manufacturer Direct, Manufacturer Through Distributor, Manufacturer Through Manufacturer Reps, OEM, Exporter
General Admin.: Robert N. Schmidt/President, Chief Executive Officer
Mktg./Adv.: Kevin J. Farrell/Director Marketing & Sales
Production: Mary Varghai/Director Manufacturing
     Christy Robey/Manager Regulatory Affairs
Research: Mohammad Modarreszadeh/Director Research & Development
   Collector, Urine   Gastroenterology/Urology
   Electroencephalograph   Cns/Neurology
   Protector, Skin Pressure   General
   Transducer, Miniature Pressure   Physical Med

CLEVER SOLUTIONS, INC.
10163 Faetano Lane, Milan, MI 48160
800-743-6165
FDA Number: 1836002
Fax: 734-439-0213
E-mail: infor@cleversolutions.net
Web site: www.cleversolutions.net
Medical Products Sales Volume: $200,000
Year Founded: 1997
Total Employees: 3
Ownership: Private
Produces/Sells CE-marked Devices: N
Federal Procurement Eligibility: Small Business
   Transfer Device, Patient, Manual   General

CLIFF KEYES MANUFACTURING & SUPPLY CO., INC.
See Keyes Manufacturing & Supply Llc.

CLIMATRONICS CORP.
140 Wilbur Place, Bohemia, NY 11716
631-567-7300
FDA Number: n/a
Fax: 631-567-7585
E-mail: support@climatronics.com
Web site: www.climatronics.com
Annual Revenue: $0-$1 Million
Ownership: Private
Quality System Registration Information: ISO9001
Produces/Sells CE-marked Devices: Y
Federal Procurement Eligibility: Small Business
Distribution: Manufacturer Direct, Manufacturer Through Distributor, Manufacturer Through Manufacturer Reps, Importer, Exporter

CLIMATRONICS CORP. — 631-567-7300 *(cont'd)*
Recorder, Chart, Laboratory — Chemistry

CLIMET INSTRUMENTS CO. — 909-793-2788
1320 W. Colton Ave., Redlands, CA 92374
FDA Number: n/a — *Fax:* 909-793-1738
E-mail: sales@climet.com
Web site: www.climet.com
Total Employees: 50 — *Marketing Staff:* 3 — *Sales Staff:* 20
Ownership: VENTUREDYNE LTD
Produces/Sells CE-marked Devices: Y
Distribution: Manufacturer Direct, Manufacturer Through Distributor, Exporter
General Admin.: Raymond Felbinger/General Manager
    Brian Nahigh/President
Mktg./Adv.: David Chandler/Director Product Development
    Bart Groninger/Manager Marketing
Production: Bill Ferguson/Manager Manufacturing
    Randy Grater/Manager Quality Assurance
Cleanroom Equipment — General
Counter, Cell — Microbiology
Monitor, Biological (Contamination Testing) — General
Monitor, Gas, Atmospheric, Environmental — General

CLINDAR INC.
See Novum Inc.

CLINE PRODUCTS INC. — 941-776-0230
11446 Savannah Lakes Dr., Parrish, FL 34219
FDA Number: 3005619676
Ownership: Private
Produces/Sells CE-marked Devices: N
Table, Ophthalmic, Instrument, Powered — Ophthalmology

CLINETICS — 518-477-6886
25 Hy Drive, East Schodack, NY 12063
FDA Number: 1321174
Ownership: Private
Produces/Sells CE-marked Devices: N
Accessories, Apparel, Surgical — Surgery

CLINICAL COMPUTER SYSTEMS, INC. — 847-622-0847
715 Tollgate Rd., Elgin, IL 60123
FDA Number: 3004423584
Ownership: Private
Produces/Sells CE-marked Devices: N

CLINICAL CONTROLS INTERNATIONAL — 805-528-4039
2131 10th Street, Los Osos, CA 93402
FDA Number: n/a
Ownership: Private
Produces/Sells CE-marked Devices: N
Antigen, Antiserum, Fibrinogen And Fibrin Split Products — Immunology
Control, Alcohol — Toxicology
Control, Analyte (Assayed And Unassayed) — Chemistry
Control, Drug Mixture — Toxicology
Control, Drug Specific — Toxicology
Control, Enzyme (Assayed And Unassayed) — Chemistry
Control, Multi Analyte, All Kinds (Assayed And Unassayed) — Chemistry
IGG, Ferritin, Antigen, Antiserum, Control — Immunology
Plasma, Control, Fibrinogen — Hematology

CLINICAL DATA INC — 800-937-5449 / 617 527-9933
One Gateway Center, Suite 702,
Newton, MA 02458
FDA Number: n/a — *Fax:* 401-233-6480
E-mail: info@CLDA.com
Web site: www.clda.com
Medical Products Sales Volume: $9,700,000
Annual Revenue: $10-$25 Million
Year Founded: 1972
Total Employees: 300
Ownership: Public
Stock Symbol: CLDA
Traded On: NASDAQ
Quality System Registration Information: ISO9000
Produces/Sells CE-marked Devices: Y
Federal Procurement Eligibility: Small Business
Distribution: Manufacturer Through Distributor
General Admin.: Mr. C. Evan Ballantyne/Chief Financial Officer, Senior Vice President
    Dr. Carol Reed/Executive Vice President
    Mr. Caesar J Belbel/Executive Vice President
    Mr. Drew Fromkin/President, Chief Executive Officer
    Ms. Lynn Ferrucci/Vice President Human Resources
Analyzer, Chemistry, Enzyme — Chemistry
Colorimeter, General Use — Chemistry
Prothrombin Time — Hematology

CLINICAL DATA INSTRUMENTS, INC.
See Clinical Data Inc

CLINICAL DIAGNOSTIC SOLUTIONS, INC. — 800-453-3328 / 954-791-1773
1800 N.w. 65th Ave., Plantation, FL 33313
FDA Number: 1064130 — *Fax:* 954-791-7118
E-mail: sales@cdsolinc.com
Web site: www.cdsolinc.com
Ownership: Private
Produces/Sells CE-marked Devices: N
Analyzer, Coagulation, Semi-Automated — Hematology
Calibrator, Cell Indices — Hematology
Calibrator, Red Cell And White Cell Counting — Hematology
Cleaner, Medical Device — General
Fluid, Red Cell Lysing — Hematology
Hematology Quality Control Mixture — Hematology
Solution, Balanced Salt — Pathology
Stain, Reticulocyte — Hematology

CLINICAL DYNAMICS CORP. — 800-247-6427 / 203-269-0090
10 Capital Dr., Wallingford, CT 06492
FDA Number: n/a — *Fax:* 203-269-3402
E-mail: sales@clinicaldynamics.com
Web site: www.clinicaldynamics.com
Annual Revenue: $1-$5 Million
Total Employees: 10 — *Marketing Staff:* 3 — *Sales Staff:* 5
Ownership: Private
Produces/Sells CE-marked Devices: Y
Federal Procurement Eligibility: Small Business
Distribution: Manufacturer Direct, Manufacturer Through Distributor, Manufacturer Through Manufacturer Reps, OEM, Service Direct, Exclusive Distributor
General Admin.: Leo Costello/President
Mktg./Adv.: Joseph R. Rebot/Vice President Sales
Oximeter, Pulse — General
Simulator, Blood Pressure — Cardiovascular

CLINICAL IMMUNOLOGICAL LABORATORIES INC.
See Specialty Laboratories, Inc.

CLINICAL INNOVATIONS, INC. — 888-268-6222 / 801-268-8200
747 West 4170 South, Murray, UT 84123
FDA Number: 1722684 — *Fax:* 801-266-7373
E-mail: mail@clinicalinnovations.com
Web site: www.clinicalinnovations.com
Annual Revenue: $10-$25 Million
Year Founded: 1993
Total Employees: 100 — *Marketing Staff:* 7 — *Sales Staff:* 7
Ownership: Argon Medical Devices Inc.
Produces/Sells CE-marked Devices: Y
Federal Procurement Eligibility: Small Business
Distribution: Manufacturer Direct, Exclusive Distributor, Exporter
General Admin.: Paul Mooney/President, Chief Executive Officer
    Christopher A. Cutler/Vice President
Mktg./Adv.: Paul Huish/Director Marketing
    Mark Landon/Senior Vice President Sales
Production: Steven R. Smith/Director Engineering
    Gerry D. Adair/Manager Operations
Research: William Dean Wallace/Senior Vice President Research & Development
Catheter, Intrauterine, With Introducer — Obstetrics/Gynecology
Elevator, Uterine — Obstetrics/Gynecology
Extractor, Vacuum, Fetal — Obstetrics/Gynecology
Injector & Accessories, Manipulator, Uterine — Obstetrics/Gynecology
Probe, Electrosurgery, Endoscopy — Surgery
Sound, Uterine — Obstetrics/Gynecology
Transducer, Pressure, Intrauterine — Obstetrics/Gynecology

CLINICAL INSTRUMENTS INTL., INC. — 508-764-2200
278 Worcester St., Southbridge, MA 01550
FDA Number: 1219038 — *Fax:* 508-764-2244
E-mail: ec@clinicalinstrument.com
Web site: www.clinicalinstrument.com
Ownership: Private
Produces/Sells CE-marked Devices: N
Catheter, Balloon (Foley Type) — Surgery
Catheter, Continuous Flush — Cardiovascular
Catheter, Continuous Irrigation — Surgery
Catheter, Embolectomy (Fogarty Type) — Cardiovascular
Catheter, Femoral — Gastroenterology/Urology
Catheter, Flow Directed — Cardiovascular
Catheter, Infusion — Surgery
Catheter, Intravascular Occluding — Cns/Neurology
Catheter, Intravascular, Diagnostic — Cardiovascular
Catheter, Irrigation — Surgery
Catheter, Multiple Lumen — Surgery
Catheter, Straight — Gastroenterology/Urology
Catheter, Vascular, Cardiopulmonary Bypass — Cardiovascular
Introducer, Catheter — Cardiovascular
Mirror, Endoscopic — Surgery

CLINICAL MICROSYSTEMS INTL. — 703-920-4345
620 22nd St. South, Arlington, VA 22202
FDA Number: 1181143

CLINICAL MICROSYSTEMS INTL.   703-920-4345 *(cont'd)*
Ownership: Private
Produces/Sells CE-marked Devices: N
  Tester, Radiology   Radiology

CLINICAL PHARMACIES, INC.   800-669-6973
21622 Surveyor Circle, #8-C,   **714-969-6818**
Huntington Beach, CA 92646
FDA Number: n/a   Fax: 714-969-2320
E-mail: carl@cpmednet.com
Web site: www.cpmednet.com
Medical Products Sales Volume: $1,500,000
Annual Revenue: $1-$5 Million
Year Founded: 1981
Total Employees: 8   Marketing Staff: 1   Sales Staff: 1
Ownership: Private
Produces/Sells CE-marked Devices: N
Federal Procurement Eligibility: Small Business
Distribution: Manufacturer Direct
Production: Desserie Cuttery/Director Quality Assurance
  Concentrate, Dialysis, Hemodialysis (Liquid or Powder)   Gastroenterology/Urology
  Kit, Administration, Intravenous   General
  Kit, Surgical Instrument, Disposable   Surgery
  Protector, Transducer, Dialysis   Gastroenterology/Urology
  Surgical Instrument, Disposable   Surgery

CLINICAL REFERENCE SYSTEMS   800-237-8401
335 Interlocken Pkway, Broomfield, CO 80021   **303-664-6485**
FDA Number: n/a   Fax: 303-460-6282
E-mail: crs-info@cliniref.com
Web site: www.patienteducation.com
Ownership: MCKESSON HBOC INC.
Produces/Sells CE-marked Devices: N
Mktg./Adv.: Mark Dwyer/Director Marketing
  Computer Software   General

CLINICAL RESOLUTION LABORATORY   213-384-0500
14401 Chambers Road, #200, Tustin, CA 92780
FDA Number: 3005727243
  Instrument, Manual, General Surgical   Surgery

CLINICAL SCIENCES, INC.
See Diasorin Inc

CLINICAL SYSTEMS, INC.
See Mediq/Prn

CLINICOMP INTL.   800-350-8202
9655 Towne Centre Drive, San Diego, CA 92121   **858-546-8202**
FDA Number: 2028916   Fax: 858-546-1801
E-mail: sales_info@clinicomp.com
Web site: www.clinicomp.com
Medical Products Sales Volume: $8,700,000
Year Founded: 1983
Total Employees: 80
Ownership: Private
Produces/Sells CE-marked Devices: N
Federal Procurement Eligibility: Small Business, GSA Contract
Distribution: Service Direct
  Computer and Software, Medical   General

CLINICON CORP.   1-800-CLINICON
3025 Industry St., Suite A,   **760-439-1700**
Oceanside, CA 92054
FDA Number: 2086015   Fax: 760-439-1798
E-mail: purebeam@clinicon.com
Web site: www.clinicon.com
Ownership: Private
Produces/Sells CE-marked Devices: N
  Laser, Surgical   Surgery

CLINIMED, INCORPORATED   877-CLINIMED
303 Markus Court, Sandy Brae Industrial Park,   **302-454-8400**
Newark, DE 19713
FDA Number: 2431788   Fax: 302-737-8900
E-mail: info@clinimed.us
Web site: www.clinimed.us
Medical Products Sales Volume: $1,200,000
Annual Revenue: $1-$5 Million
Year Founded: 1978
Total Employees: 16   Marketing Staff: 2   Sales Staff: 3
Ownership: Private
Produces/Sells CE-marked Devices: Y
Federal Procurement Eligibility: Small Business, Minority Owned
Distribution: Manufacturer Through Distributor, OEM, Exporter
General Admin.: Mr. Aasim Saber/Managing Director
       Mr. M. Saber/President, Chief Executive Officer
Mktg./Adv.: Mr. Alan Azpurua/Director International Sales
       Mr. Fayyaz Memon/Director Marketing & Sales

CLINIMED, INCORPORATED   877-CLINIMED *(cont'd)*
Adenotome   Ear/Nose/Throat
Applicator, ENT   Ear/Nose/Throat
Base, Roller, Tank, Oxygen   General
Basin, Sponge   General
Bed Cradle   General
Bed, Manual   General
Blade, Saw, Surgical, Cardiovascular   Cardiovascular
Bowl, Solution   General
Cabinet, Bedside   General
Cabinet, Other   General
Cable, Fiberoptic   General
Camera, Video, Endoscopic   General
Cannula, Ear   Ear/Nose/Throat
Cart, Equipment, Video   General
Chisel, Mastoid   Ear/Nose/Throat
Chisel, Middle Ear   Ear/Nose/Throat
Chisel, Nasal   Ear/Nose/Throat
Clamp, Aorta   Cardiovascular
Clamp, Bronchus   Ear/Nose/Throat
Clamp, Peripheral Vascular   Cardiovascular
Clamp, Tubing   General
Clamp, Vascular   Cardiovascular
Contract Manufacturing   General
Contract Manufacturing, Product, Durable   General
Crimper, Wire, ENT   Ear/Nose/Throat
Cuff, Inflation   General
Curette, Adenoid   Ear/Nose/Throat
Curette, Ear   Ear/Nose/Throat
Curette, Ethmoid   Ear/Nose/Throat
Cutter, Ring   General
Depressor, Tongue   Ear/Nose/Throat
Depressor, Tongue, ENT, Metal   Ear/Nose/Throat
Die, Wire Bending, ENT   Ear/Nose/Throat
Dilator, Tracheal   Ear/Nose/Throat
Dilator, Vessel, Surgical   Cardiovascular
Dissector, Tonsil   Ear/Nose/Throat
Drill, Surgical, ENT (Electric Or Pneumatic)   Ear/Nose/Throat
Elevator, ENT   Ear/Nose/Throat
Esophagoscope (Flexible Or Rigid)   Ear/Nose/Throat
Fiberoptic Light Source & Carrier   Ear/Nose/Throat
Footstool   General
Forceps, ENT   Ear/Nose/Throat
Forceps, Sterilizer Transfer   General
Forceps, Tonsil   Ear/Nose/Throat
Forceps, Wire Closure, ENT   Ear/Nose/Throat
Fork, Tuning, ENT   Ear/Nose/Throat
Furniture, Patient Room   General
Gag, Mouth   Ear/Nose/Throat
Gauge, Mastoid   Ear/Nose/Throat
Gouge, Nasal   Ear/Nose/Throat
Headlight, ENT   Ear/Nose/Throat
Hook, Microsurgical Ear   Ear/Nose/Throat
Infusion Stand   General
Irrigator, Suction   General
Lamp, Examination (Light)   General
Laryngoscope, Rigid   Anesthesiology
Mirror, ENT   Ear/Nose/Throat
Nasopharyngoscope (Flexible Or Rigid)   Ear/Nose/Throat
Otoscope   Ear/Nose/Throat
Pharyngoscope   Ear/Nose/Throat
Rasp, Ear   Ear/Nose/Throat
Rasp, Nasal   Ear/Nose/Throat
Rhinoscope   Ear/Nose/Throat
Rongeur, Mastoid   Ear/Nose/Throat
Rongeur, Nasal   Ear/Nose/Throat
Saw, Laryngeal   Ear/Nose/Throat
Saw, Nasal   Ear/Nose/Throat
Saw, Surgical, ENT (Electric Or Pneumatic)   Ear/Nose/Throat
Scissors, Bandage/Gauze/Plaster   General
Scissors, Ear   Ear/Nose/Throat
Scissors, General Dissecting   General
Scissors, Nasal   Ear/Nose/Throat
Scissors, Wire Cutting, ENT   Ear/Nose/Throat
Snare, Ear   Ear/Nose/Throat
Solution, Instrument Cleaner   General
Thermometer, Electronic   General
Tourniquet   General

CLINIQA CORPORATION   800-728-9558
774 North Twin Oaks Valley Road, Suite C,   **760-744-1900**
San Marcos, CA 92069
FDA Number: 2085064   Fax: 760-736-3773
E-mail: info@cliniqa.com
Web site: www.cliniqa.com
Medical Products Sales Volume: $2,800,000
Annual Revenue: $10-$25 Million
Year Founded: 1975
Total Employees: 12   Marketing Staff: 6   Sales Staff: 6
Ownership: Private
Quality System Registration Information: ISO9001

CLINIQA CORPORATION 800-728-9558 *(cont'd)*

Produces/Sells CE-marked Devices: Y
Federal Procurement Eligibility: Small Business, GSA Contract, VA Contract
Distribution: Manufacturer Direct, Manufacturer Through Distributor, Exporter
General Admin.: Dean Harriman/Chief Operating Officer, Chief Financial Officer
    Lisa Rodrigues/Manager Human Resources
    Granger Haugh/President, Chief Executive Officer
Mktg./Adv.: Mike Hoskins/Director Special Projects
    Yu Xin/Manager Marketing
    Kimberly Dimpel/Manager Marketing Admin.
    Barry Rhodes/Vice President International Sales
    John Fewster/Vice President Marketing & Sales
Production: Lisa Burgess/Manager Facilities
    Jonie Bales/Manager Materials
    Carol Ruggiero/Manager Quality Assurance & Regulatory Affairs
    Bob Elms/Vice President Operations
Research: Larry Beaty/Vice President Research & Development
Purchasing: Doris Kent/Buyer
IS: Linda McLaren/Manager Tech. Support

Antibody, Monoclonal	Microbiology
Antibody, Polyclonal	Microbiology
Control, Multi Analyte, All Kinds (Assayed And Unassayed)	Chemistry
Reagent, Calibration	General
Standard, Lipid	Chemistry

CLINITRON

    See Hill-Rom Manufacturing, Inc.

CLINTON INDUSTRIES, INC 717-848-3519
1140 Edison St., Botts, PA 17403
FDA Number: 3001452523

Chair/Table, Medical	General
Table, Physical Medicine, Powered	Physical Med

CLIVE CRAIG CO. 800-833-8267
600 East Hueneme Rd., Oxnard, CA 93033 805-488-1122
FDA Number: n/a Fax: 805-422-2266
Ownership: Private
Produces/Sells CE-marked Devices: N

Apron, Lead, Dental	Dental And Oral
Mirror, Mouth	Dental And Oral
Needle, Dental	Dental And Oral
Wrap, Sterilization	General

CLOPAY CORP., PLASTIC PROD. DIV.

    See Clopay Plastic Products Company

CLOPAY PLASTIC PRODUCTS COMPANY 800-282-2260
8585 Duke Blvd, Mason, OH 45040-3101 513-770-4800
FDA Number: n/a Fax: 513-770-3965
Web site: www.clopayplastics.com
Medical Products Sales Volume: $21,800,000
Year Founded: 1859
Total Employees: 1080 *Marketing Staff:* 2 *Sales Staff:* 10
Ownership: GRIFFON CORPORATION
Quality System Registration Information: ISO9001
Produces/Sells CE-marked Devices: N
Federal Procurement Eligibility: Small Business
Distribution: Manufacturer Through Distributor
General Admin.: Gary A. Abyad/President
Mktg./Adv.: Ronald E. Zinco/Vice President Marketing & Sales
Production: Michael C. Carlson/Vice President Operations
Research: Rick Jezzi/Vice President Research & Development

Clothing, Protective	General
Drape, Surgical	Surgery
Dress, Surgical	Surgery
Linen	General

CLOSE CALL CORP. 630-663-0189
4617 Cumnor Rd., Downers Grove, IL 60515
FDA Number: 1424246
Ownership: Private
Produces/Sells CE-marked Devices: N

Monitor, Bed Patient	General

CLOSURE MEDICAL 888-257-7633
5250 Greens Dairy Rd., Raleigh, NC 27616 919-876-7800
FDA Number: 1034548 Fax: 919-790-1041
E-mail: info@closuremed.com
Web site: http://www.closuremed.com/
Medical Products Sales Volume: $7,500,000
Annual Revenue: $10-$25 Million
Total Employees: 75 *Marketing Staff:* 3
Ownership: Johnson & Johnson
Quality System Registration Information: ISO9001
Produces/Sells CE-marked Devices: Y
Federal Procurement Eligibility: Small Business
Distribution: OEM, Exclusive Distributor
General Admin.: Daniel A. Pelak/President, Chief Executive Officer
    Robert Toni/President, Chief Executive Officer

CLOSURE MEDICAL 888-257-7633 *(cont'd)*

    Gabe Szabo/Vice President
    Mike Hoban/Vice President Human Resources
    Dennis Burns/Vice President, General Manager
Mktg./Adv.: Anthony Sherbondy/Vice President Business Development
Production: Mark Spain/Director Quality Assurance
    Cherie Kennedy/Manager Materials
    Tony Voiers/Manager Production
    Tom Stephens/Manager Regulatory Affairs
    Bill Cotter/Vice President Manufacturing
    Joe B. Barefoot/Vice President Quality Assurance & Regulatory Affairs
Research: Jeff Clark/Vice President Research & Development
Finance: Benny Ward/Chief Financial Officer

Adhesive Strip, Waterproof	General
Adhesive, Tissue, Ophthalmology	Ophthalmology
Adhesive, Wound Closure	Surgery
Embolization Device	Cardiovascular

CLOUD 9 630-595-5000
777 Edgewood Avenue, Wood Dale, IL 60191-1254
FDA Number: n/a Fax: 630-595-5902
E-mail: we@4cloud9.com
Web site: www.4cloud9.com
Medical Products Sales Volume: $3,200,000
Year Founded: 1971
Total Employees: 45
Ownership: Private
Federal Procurement Eligibility: Small Business, GSA Contract
Distribution: Manufacturer Direct, Manufacturer Through Manufacturer Reps, Exporter
General Admin.: Jon E. Spranger/President
Mktg./Adv.: Jerry Ladin/Vice President Business Development
    Fred Green/Vice President Marketing
    Jerry Ladin/Vice President Sales
Production: Fred Green/Vice President Manufacturing
Research: Fred Green/Vice President Research & Development

Filter, Air	General
Purifier, Air, Ultraviolet	General

CLOVER MEDICAL EQUIPMENT SERVICES, INC. 800-550-4111
117 Albert Drive, Lancaster, NY 14086 716-686-0515
FDA Number: 1131919 Fax: 716-686-9694
E-mail: clomedequip@aol.com
Web site: www.clovermedical.com
Medical Products Sales Volume: $390,000
Year Founded: 1988
Total Employees: 3
Ownership: Private
Produces/Sells CE-marked Devices: N
Federal Procurement Eligibility: Small Business
General Admin.: Robert Thomson/Vice President, General Manager

Vaporizer	General
Vaporizer, Anesthesia, Non-Heated	Anesthesiology

CLOWARD INSTRUMENT CORPORATION 808-734-3511
3787 Diamond Head Road, Honolulu, HI 96816
FDA Number: 2950729 Fax: 808-734-3511
E-mail: cloward@aol.com
Web site: www.cloward.com
Medical Products Sales Volume: $180,000
Annual Revenue: $1-$5 Million
Year Founded: 1991
Total Employees: 2 *Sales Staff:* 3
Ownership: Private
Quality System Registration Information: ISO9000; ISO9001
Produces/Sells CE-marked Devices: Y
Federal Procurement Eligibility: Small Business
Distribution: Manufacturer Direct
General Admin.: Ms. Cindy Chung/Office Manager
    Mr. Kerry Cloward/President

Arm Rest	Physical Med
Kit, Instruments and Accessories, Surgical	Surgery
Retractor	Orthopedics
Support, Patient Position	Anesthesiology
Surgical Instrument, Orthopedic, AC-Powered Motor	Orthopedics

CLYNCH TECHNOLOGIES INC. 403-247-2755
#3 Montgomery Plaza, 4703 Bowness Rd. NW, Calgary, ALB T3B-0 Canada
FDA Number: n/a Fax: 403-286-0157
E-mail: info@clynch-tech.com
Web site: http://www.clynch-tech.com/
Year Founded: 1992
Total Employees: 10
Ownership: Private
Produces/Sells CE-marked Devices: N
Distribution: Manufacturer Direct

CMC RESCUE, INC.
800-235-5741
P.O. Box 6870, Santa Barbara, CA 93160   **805-562-9120**
FDA Number: n/a   *Fax:* 805-562-9870
E-mail: info@cmcrescue.com
Web site: www.cmcrescue.com
Medical Products Sales Volume: $6,000,000
Annual Revenue: $5-$10 Million
Year Founded: 1978
Ownership: Private
Quality System Registration Information: ISO9001
Federal Procurement Eligibility: Small Business
Distribution: Manufacturer Direct, Manufacturer Through Distributor, Importer, Exporter
Blanket, Rescue	General
Rescue Equipment	General

CME MEDICAL EQUIPMENT CORP.
908-561-0906
1130 Donamy Glen, Scotch Plains, NJ 07076-2403
FDA Number: n/a   *Fax:* 908-561-0906
E-mail: akreit@aol.com
Annual Revenue: $0-$1 Million
Ownership: Private
Produces/Sells CE-marked Devices: N
Federal Procurement Eligibility: Small Business, Female Owned
Distribution: Exclusive Distributor
General Admin.: Anita Kreitman/President
       Edward Kreitman/Vice President
Reacher (Handicapped)	General
Utensil, Handicapped Aid	Physical Med

CMI, INC.
270-685-6200
316 East Ninth St., Owensboro, KY 42303
FDA Number: 1530303
Ownership: Private
Produces/Sells CE-marked Devices: N
Alcohol Breath Trapping Device	Toxicology

CMP INDUSTRIES LLC
800-888-5868
413 N. Pearl St., Albany, NY 12201   **518-434-3147**
FDA Number: 1315551   *Fax:* 518-434-1288
E-mail: info@cmpindustries.com
Web site: http://cmpindustry.com/
Medical Products Sales Volume: $8,000,000
Annual Revenue: $5-$10 Million
Year Founded: 1889
Total Employees: 65   *Marketing Staff:* 3   *Sales Staff:* 6
Ownership: Private
Quality System Registration Information: ISO9002
Produces/Sells CE-marked Devices: Y
Federal Procurement Eligibility: Small Business, VA Contract
Distribution: Manufacturer Direct, Exporter
General Admin.: Bob Briggs/Director Admin.
       William Regan/President
       Bob Briggs/Vice President Human Resources
Mktg./Adv.: Dean Quackenbush/Manager Advertising
Research: Abdul Kahn/Vice President Research & Development
Base, Denture, Relining, Repairing, Rebasing, Resin	Dental And Oral
Crown And Bridge, Temporary, Resin	Dental And Oral
Material, Impression Tray, Resin	Dental And Oral

CMS GILBRETH
800.630.2413
3001 State Rd., Croydon, PA 19021   **215-185-3350**
FDA Number: n/a   *Fax:* 215-244-8362
E-mail: info@gilbreth.com
Web site: www.gilbrethusa.com
Ownership: Private
Produces/Sells CE-marked Devices: N
Federal Procurement Eligibility: Small Business
Distribution: Manufacturer Direct
General Admin.: Richard Majewski/Chief Executive Officer
Mktg./Adv.: Rotanda Thompson/Vice President Marketing
       George Landes/Vice President Sales
Labeling Equipment	General
Packaging Equipment	General

CMT, INC.
800-659-9140
Post Office Box 297, Hamilton, MA 01936-0297   **978-768-2555**
FDA Number: n/a   *Fax:* 978-768-2555
E-mail: info@habitatmonitor.com
Web site: www.habitatmonitor.com
Medical Products Sales Volume: $100,000
Annual Revenue: $0-$1 Million
Year Founded: 1984
Ownership: Private
Produces/Sells CE-marked Devices: N
Federal Procurement Eligibility: Small Business

CMT, INC.
800-659-9140 *(cont'd)*
Distribution: Manufacturer Direct, Manufacturer Through Distributor, OEM, Service Direct, Exporter
General Admin.: David C. de Sieyes/President
Alarm, Refrigerator	Hematology
Chamber, Constant Temperature (Environmental)	Microbiology
Contract R&D, Diagnostics	General
Contract R&D, Equipment	General
Controller, Temperature, Humidifier	General
Controller, Temperature, Other	General
Controller, Temperature, Programmable	Chemistry
Hygrometer (Humidity Indicator)	Anesthesiology
Insufflator, Carbon-Dioxide, Automatic (For Endoscope)	Gastroenterology/Urology
Insufflator, Laparoscopic	Obstetrics/Gynecology
Monitor, Temperature (Self-Contained)	General
Pump, Infusion	General
Pump, Infusion, Syringe	General
Regulator, Temperature	Chemistry
Security Equipment/Supplies	General
Sensor, Moisture	General
Service, Consulting	General
Service, Engineering/Design	General

CN GOEDERS
See Caltech Industries, Inc.

CNS, INC.
800-441-0417
7615 Smetana Lane, Eden Prairie, MN 55344   **952-229-1500**
FDA Number: 2183550   *Fax:* 952-229-1700
E-mail: cns@breathright.com
Web site: www.cns.com
Medical Products Sales Volume: $8,300,000
Annual Revenue: $100-$500 Million
Total Employees: 1000
Ownership: Private
Stock Symbol: CNXS
Traded On: NASDAQ
Quality System Registration Information: ISO9001
Produces/Sells CE-marked Devices: Y
Distribution: Manufacturer Through Distributor
Production: Ms. Elaine Grotbeck/Manager Regulatory Affairs
Dilator, Nasal	Ear/Nose/Throat

CO-ORAL-ITE DENTAL MFG. CO.
530-621-4913
6635 Merchandise Way, Diamond Springs, CA 95619
FDA Number: 2950685
Base, Denture, Relining, Repairing, Rebasing, Resin	Dental And Oral

CO/OP OPTICAL VISION DESIGNS
866-733-2667
2424 E. Eight Mile Road, E. of Dequindre,   **313-366-5100**
Detroit, MI 48234
FDA Number: n/a   *Fax:* 313-366-7314
E-mail: bedwards@coopoptical.com
Web site: www.coopoptical.com
Medical Products Sales Volume: $3,000,000
Annual Revenue: $1-$5 Million
Year Founded: 1960
Total Employees: 200   *Marketing Staff:* 5
Ownership: Private
Produces/Sells CE-marked Devices: N
Federal Procurement Eligibility: Small Business
Distribution: Manufacturer Direct
General Admin.: Dr. Ken Feinauer/Executive Director
       Mrs. Jackee Smith/President, Chief Executive Officer
Mktg./Adv.: Mrs. Nicole Weldon/Director Marketing & Advertising
Production: Mr. Charles A. Benson/Director Manufacturing
       Mr. Benjamin L. Edwards Jr./Director Operations
       Mr. Melvin Evans/Director Tech. Operations
Finance: Ms. Debora Matthews/Chief Financial Officer
Eyeglasses, Safety	Ophthalmology
Frame, Spectacle (Eyeglasses)	Ophthalmology
Laboratory Equipment, Ophthalmic	Ophthalmology
Lens, Contact, Bifocal	Ophthalmology
Lens, Contact, Disposable	Ophthalmology
Lens, Contact, Extended-Wear	Ophthalmology
Lens, Spectacle/Eyeglasses, Custom (Prescription)	Ophthalmology
Lens, Spectacle/Eyeglasses, Non-Custom	Ophthalmology

COACTIV MEDICAL BUSINESS SOLUTIONS
877-262-2848
900 Ethan Allen Highway, Ridgefield, CT 06877   **203-894-1651**
FDA Number: 3004957385   *Fax:* 203-438-5004
E-mail: info@coactiv.com
Web site: www.coactiv.com
Ownership: Private
Produces/Sells CE-marked Devices: N
Image Processing System	Radiology

MANUFACTURER PROFILES

COAPT SYSTEMS, INC. 650-461-7600
1820 Embarcadero Rd., Palo Alto, CA 94303
FDA Number: 3003644133
Ownership: Private
Produces/Sells CE-marked Devices: N
Dissector, Surgical, General & Plastic Surgery — Surgery
Fastener, Fixation, Biodegradable, Soft Tissue — Orthopedics
Screw, Fixation, Bone — Orthopedics
Suture, Absorbable, Synthetic, Polyglycolic Acid — Surgery

COAST HEARING AID LAB, LLC 228-539-5400
12100 Highway 49 North, Suite 314, Gpt, MS 39503
FDA Number: 2319195
Hearing-Aid — Ear/Nose/Throat

COAST HEARING SERVICES 541-265-6273
1217 N. Coast Hwy Suite D, Newport, OR 97365
FDA Number: 3029033
E-mail: info@caosthearingservice.com
Web site: www.coasthearingservices.com
Ownership: Private
Produces/Sells CE-marked Devices: N
Hearing-Aid — Ear/Nose/Throat

COAST SCIENTIFIC 800-445-1544
1445 Engineer St., Vista, CA 92081 760-598-9494
FDA Number: 2085469 *Fax:* 760-598-2147
E-mail: information@coastscientific.com
Web site: www.coastscientific.com
Medical Products Sales Volume: $3,200,000
Year Founded: 1999
Total Employees: 30
Ownership: Private
Produces/Sells CE-marked Devices: N
Federal Procurement Eligibility: Small Business
Distribution: Manufacturer Direct, Importer, Exporter
Mktg./Adv.: Stacy Camp/Director Marketing
    Alex Sardarian/Manager Sales Training
Accessories, Apparel, Surgical — Surgery
Glove, Patient Examination — General
Glove, Patient Examination, Latex — General
Glove, Patient Examination, Vinyl — General

COASTAL BIOCARE 714-751-0121
2737 South Croddy Way, Unit D, Santa Ana, CA 92704
FDA Number: 3005888740
Ownership: Private
Produces/Sells CE-marked Devices: N
Abutment, Implant, Dental, Endosseous — Dental And Oral
Accessories, Implant, Dental, Endosseous — Dental And Oral
Implant, Endosseous — Dental And Oral

COASTAL LIFE SYSTEMS, INC. 800-727-6814
1803 Grandstand Drive, Suite 101, 210-684-7553
San Antonio, TX 78238
FDA Number: 3003643846 *Fax:* 210-684-7587
E-mail: clssales@clsssp.com
Web site: www.coastallifesystems.com
Year Founded: 1989
Ownership: Private
Produces/Sells CE-marked Devices: N
Distribution: Service Direct
Catheter, Cholangiography — Surgery
Fiberoptic Light Source & Carrier — Ear/Nose/Throat
Laser, Surgical — Surgery

COASTAL LIFE TECHNOLOGIES, INC.
See Coastal Life Systems, Inc.

COASTVISION, INC.
See Coopervision, Inc.

COATS AMERICAN, INC. 704-329-5800
Rt. 64 West, Hendersonville, NC 27739
FDA Number: 1035752
Ownership: Private
Produces/Sells CE-marked Devices: N
Floss, Dental — Dental And Oral

COAXIA, INC. 763-315-1809
10900 73rd Ave. N., Suite 102, Maple Grove, MN 55369
FDA Number: 3004020311 *Fax:* 763-315-3660
Web site: www.coaxia.com
Ownership: Private
Produces/Sells CE-marked Devices: N
Catheter, Intravascular Occluding, Temporary — Cardiovascular
Catheter, Neuro-vasculature, Occluding Ballon — Cns/Neurology

COBE BCT, INC.
See Caridianbct Inc.

COBE CARDIOVASCULAR, A SORIN GROUP COMPANY
See Sorin Group Usa

COBE CHEMICAL CO. 562-942-2426
8616 Slauson Ave., Pico Rivera, CA 90660
FDA Number: n/a *Fax:* 562-942-9985
Web site: www.cobechem.com
Ownership: Private
Produces/Sells CE-marked Devices: N
Dressing, Wound and Burn, Hydrogel — Surgery

COBER ELECTRONICS, INC. 203-855-8755
151 Woodward Avenue, Norwalk, CT 06854-4730
FDA Number: n/a *Fax:* 203-855-7511
E-mail: sales@cober.com
Web site: www.cober.com
Medical Products Sales Volume: $270,000
Annual Revenue: $5-$10 Million
Year Founded: 1999
Total Employees: 2
Ownership: Private
Produces/Sells CE-marked Devices: Y
Federal Procurement Eligibility: Small Business
Distribution: Manufacturer Direct, Manufacturer Through Manufacturer Reps, Exporter
General Admin.: Bernard Krieger/President
Production: Vern Magnuson/Vice President Manufacturing
Research: Martin Yonnone/Vice President Engineering
Detector, Microwave Leakage — General
Oven — Chemistry

COBERT ASSOCIATES, INC. 800-972-4766
2302 Weldon Parkway, St. Louis, MO 63146 314-993-2390
FDA Number: 7000096 *Fax:* 314-993-2491
E-mail: cobert@cobertassoc.com
Web site: www.cobertassoc.com
Medical Products Sales Volume: $3,000,000
Annual Revenue: $1-$5 Million
Year Founded: 1973
Total Employees: 14 *Marketing Staff:* 2 *Sales Staff:* 4
Ownership: Private
Produces/Sells CE-marked Devices: N
Federal Procurement Eligibility: Small Business
Distribution: Manufacturer Direct, Exclusive Distributor
General Admin.: P. J. Cobert/President
    Carolyn Harkins/Vice President
    Cheryl Cobert/Vice President
Accessories, Chromatography (Gas, Gel, Liquid, Thin Layer) — Chemistry
Chromatography Equipment, Gas — Chemistry
Chromatography Equipment, Liquid — Chemistry
Chromatography Equipment, Thin Layer — Toxicology
Chromatography, Liquid, Performance, High — Toxicology

COBURN OPTICAL INDUSTRIES INC.
See Bausch & Lomb, Inc.

COBURN OPTICAL INDUSTRIES INC. LENS DIV.
See Bausch & Lomb, Inc.

COBURN OPTICAL INDUSTRIES, INC.
See Gerber Coburn Optical Inc.

COBURN OPTICAL INDUSTRIES, PROF. PROD. D
See Bausch & Lomb, Inc.

COCHLEAR AMERICAS 303-790-9010
400 Inverness Parkway, Suite 400, Englewood, CO 80112-5128
FDA Number: n/a *Fax:* 303-792-9025
E-mail: info@cochlear.com
Web site: www.cochlearamericas.com
Medical Products Sales Volume: $452,260,000
Year Founded: 1985
Total Employees: 135 *Marketing Staff:* 12 *Sales Staff:* 11
Ownership: Cochlear Ltd.
Stock Symbol: COH
Traded On: Sydney
Quality System Registration Information: ISO9000
Produces/Sells CE-marked Devices: Y
Federal Procurement Eligibility: Small Business
Distribution: Manufacturer Direct, Exclusive Distributor, Importer, Exporter
General Admin.: Steve Ray/Director Human Resources
    Chris Smith/President
Mktg./Adv.: Christopher Bertrand/Senior Vice President Sales
    Peter Billing/Vice President International Sales
    Rick Giancola/Vice President International Sales
    Susan Van Horne/Vice President Marketing
Research: Chris Van Der Honert/Vice President Research
Finance: David Williams/Vice President Finance
Implant, Cochlear — Ear/Nose/Throat

COCHRAN, STEPHENSON & DONKERVOET, INC. ARCHITECTS
410-539-2080

323 W. Camden St., Ste. 700
The Warehouse at Camden Yards
Baltimore, MD 21201
FDA Number: n/a   Fax: 410-752-5263
Web site: www.csdarch.com
Medical Products Sales Volume: $7,000,000
Annual Revenue: $5-$10 Million
Year Founded: 1947
Total Employees: 84
Ownership: Private
Produces/Sells CE-marked Devices: N
Federal Procurement Eligibility: Small Business
Distribution: Service Direct
General Admin.: Jose Galvez/Chief Operating Officer
    David Dillard/President
Finance: Mark Debinski/Chief Financial Officer
  Service, Architectural   General

CODAN MEDLON, INC.
See Codan Us Corporation

CODAN US CORPORATION
800-332-6326
714-545-2111

3511 W. Sunflower Avenue,
Santa Ana, CA 92704
FDA Number: 2016945   Fax: 714-545-9111
E-mail: info@codanus.com
Web site: www.codanus.com
Annual Revenue: $10-$25 Million
Total Employees: 160   *Marketing Staff:* 2   *Sales Staff:* 3
Ownership: Private
Produces/Sells CE-marked Devices: N
Federal Procurement Eligibility: Small Business
Distribution: OEM, Exclusive Distributor
General Admin.: Bernd Larsen/President
Mktg./Adv.: Janice Tarwater/Manager Contract Sales
    Janice Tarwater/Vice President National Marketing & Sales
Production: Marilyn Pourazar/Director Quality Assurance
Finance: Mr. Lance Gordan/Chief Financial Officer
  Kit, Administration, Blood   General
  Kit, Administration, Intravenous   General
  Kit, Intravenous Extension Tubing   General
  Kit, Intravenous, Administration, Buret   General
  Tubing, Fluid Delivery   General

CODE ALERT
See Rf Technologies

CODMAN & SHURTLEFF, INC
800-382-4682
877-744-5617

325 Paramount Dr., Raynham, MA 02767
FDA Number: 1226348   Fax: 508-880-8122
E-mail: wworderdesk@dpyus.jnj.com
Web site: www.depuy.com
Medical Products Sales Volume: $230,000
Annual Revenue: $0-$1 Million
Year Founded: 1857
Total Employees: 1200
Ownership: Johnson & Johnson
Quality System Registration Information: ISO9000
Produces/Sells CE-marked Devices: N
Distribution: Manufacturer Direct, OEM
General Admin.: David M. Hable/President
Mktg./Adv.: Debbie Williams/Market Manager
    Dan Wildman/Vice President Marketing & Sales
Production: Rich Manginelli/Vice President Operations
Finance: Greg Collins/Vice President Finance
  Adapter, Shunt   Gastroenterology/Urology
  Anoscope, Non-Powered   Gastroenterology/Urology
  Applicator, Clip (Forceps)   General
  Bougie, Urological   Gastroenterology/Urology
  Burr, Cranial   Cns/Neurology
  Button, Surgical   Surgery
  Cable, Fiberoptic   General
  Cannula, Brain   Cns/Neurology
  Carrier, Ligature   Surgery
  Catheter, Intravascular, Diagnostic   Cardiovascular
  Catheter, Percutaneous   Cardiovascular
  Catheter, Ventricular   Cns/Neurology
  Clamp, Aorta   Cardiovascular
  Clamp, Hemorrhoidal   Gastroenterology/Urology
  Clamp, Intestinal   Gastroenterology/Urology
  Clamp, Patent Ductus   Surgery
  Clamp, Peripheral Vascular   Cardiovascular
  Clamp, Vascular   Cardiovascular
  Clip, Aneurysm (Intracranial)   Cns/Neurology
  Clip, Removable (Skin)   Surgery
  Clip, Scalp   Cns/Neurology
  Clip, Towel   Surgery

CODMAN & SHURTLEFF, INC
800-382-4682 *(cont'd)*

  Clip, Wound   Surgery
  Colposcope   Obstetrics/Gynecology
  Container, Sterilization (Tray)   General
  Cover, Burr Hole (Cranial)   Cns/Neurology
  Curette, Surgical   Surgery
  Depressor, Tongue   General
  Dilator, Common Duct   Gastroenterology/Urology
  Dilator, Tracheal   Ear/Nose/Throat
  Dilator, Uterine   Obstetrics/Gynecology
  Dispenser, Cement   Orthopedics
  Dissector, Surgical, General & Plastic Surgery   Surgery
  Drill, Cranial   Cns/Neurology
  Drill, Perforator   Cns/Neurology
  Drill, Powered Compound (With Burr, Trephine & Accessories)   Cns/Neurology
  Elevator, Adson   Surgery
  Elevator, Neurosurgical   Cns/Neurology
  Elevator, Orthopedic   Orthopedic
  Elevator, Surgical, General & Plastic Surgery   Surgery
  Endoscope And Accessories, AC-Powered   Surgery
  Endoscope, Neurological   Cns/Neurology
  Fiberoptic Light Source & Carrier   Ear/Nose/Throat
  Forceps, Biopsy, Gynecological   Obstetrics/Gynecology
  Forceps, Dressing   Surgery
  Forceps, Electrosurgical   Surgery
  Forceps, Gallbladder (Biliary Duct)   Gastroenterology/Urology
  Forceps, General & Plastic Surgery   Surgery
  Forceps, Hemostatic   Surgery
  Forceps, Intestinal (Clamps)   Gastroenterology/Urology
  Forceps, Obstetrical   Obstetrics/Gynecology
  Forceps, Sponge   Surgery
  Forceps, Stone Manipulation   Gastroenterology/Urology
  Forceps, Suction   Surgery
  Forceps, Tissue   Surgery
  Forceps, Utility   Surgery
  Gag, Mouth   Ear/Nose/Throat
  Guidewire, Catheter   Cardiovascular
  Hammer, Neurological   Cns/Neurology
  Hammer, Percussion   Cns/Neurology
  Handle, Knife Blade   Surgery
  Headlight, ENT   Ear/Nose/Throat
  Headlight, Fiberoptic Focusing   Gastroenterology/Urology
  Holder, Head, Neurosurgical (Skull Clamp)   Cns/Neurology
  Holder, Needle, Other   Surgery
  Hook, Cordotomy   Ear/Nose/Throat
  Hook, Skin   Surgery
  Hook, Tracheal   Ear/Nose/Throat
  Illuminator, Fiberoptic (For Endoscope)   Gastroenterology/Urology
  Instrument, Forming, Material, Cranioplasty   Cns/Neurology
  Instrument, Implantation, Shunt   Cns/Neurology
  Instrument, Manual, General Surgical   Surgery
  Instrument, Microsurgical   Cns/Neurology
  Knife, Dura Hook   Cns/Neurology
  Knife, Plaster   Orthopedic
  Knife, Sternum   Surgery
  Light Source, Fiberoptic, Routine   Gastroenterology/Urology
  Loop, Endarterectomy   Cardiovascular
  Loupe, Diagnostic/Surgical   Surgery
  Mallet, Bone   Orthopedics
  Marker, Skin   Surgery
  Material, Casting   Dental And Oral
  Metacrylate, Methyl, Cranioplasty   Cns/Neurology
  Methyl Metacrylate   Cns/Neurology
  Microscope, Surgical, General & Plastic Surgery   Surgery
  Mirror, General & Plastic Surgery   Surgery
  Obturator, Cement   Orthopedics
  Osteotome (Orthopedic)   Surgery
  Paddie, Cottonoid   Cns/Neurology
  Pelvimeter   Obstetrics/Gynecology
  Percussor   Cns/Neurology
  Perforator, Antrum   Ear/Nose/Throat
  Proctoscope   Surgery
  Punch, Aortic   Cardiovascular
  Punch, Biopsy   Gastroenterology/Urology
  Punch, Bone   Orthopedics
  Rack, Surgical Instrument   Surgery
  Rasp, Nasal   Ear/Nose/Throat
  Raspatory   Surgery
  Resinous Compound, Cranial   Cns/Neurology
  Retractor, Abdominal   Surgery
  Retractor, Bladder   Gastroenterology/Urology
  Retractor, Brain   Cns/Neurology
  Retractor, Brain Decompression   Cns/Neurology
  Retractor, ENT (Thoracic)   Ear/Nose/Throat
  Retractor, Fiberoptic   Gastroenterology/Urology
  Retractor, Laminectomy   Surgery
  Retractor, Rectal   Gastroenterology/Urology
  Retractor, Rib   Orthopedics
  Retractor, Self-Retaining   Gastroenterology/Urology
  Retractor, Self-Retaining, Neurology   Cns/Neurology
  Retractor, Vaginal   Obstetrics/Gynecology
  Retractor, Vessel   Cardiovascular

CODMAN & SHURTLEFF, INC   800-382-4682 *(cont'd)*

Rongeur, Manual, Neurosurgical	Cns/Neurology
Rongeur, Rib	Orthopedics
Scissors, Bandage/Gauze/Plaster	General
Scissors, Cardiovascular	Cardiovascular
Scissors, Corneal	Ophthalmology
Scissors, General Dissecting	General
Scissors, Gynecological	Obstetrics/Gynecology
Scissors, Nasal	Ear/Nose/Throat
Scissors, Neurosurgical (Dura)	Cns/Neurology
Scissors, Ophthalmic	Ophthalmology
Scissors, Suture	Surgery
Scissors, Tenotomy	Ophthalmology
Scissors, Thoracic	Cardiovascular
Scoop, Gallstone	Gastroenterology/Urology
Separator, Dural	Cns/Neurology
Shunt, Central Nerve, With Component	Cns/Neurology
Shunt, Hydrocephalic	Cns/Neurology
Sound, Urethral, Metal Or Plastic	Gastroenterology/Urology
Sound, Uterine	Obstetrics/Gynecology
Spatula, Brain	Cns/Neurology
Speculum, Ear	Ear/Nose/Throat
Speculum, Nasal	Ear/Nose/Throat
Speculum, Rectal	Gastroenterology/Urology
Speculum, Vaginal, Metal	Obstetrics/Gynecology
Speculum, Vaginal, Metal, Fiberoptic	Obstetrics/Gynecology
Sponge, X-Ray Detectable	Surgery
Spreader, Plaster (Cast)	Orthopedics
Spreader, Vein	Cardiovascular
Stand, Operating Room Instrument (Mayo)	Surgery
Stripper, Tendon	Surgery
Stripper, Vein, Disposable	Surgery
Stripper, Vein, Reusable	Surgery
Surgical Instrument, Cardiovascular	Cardiovascular
Surgical Instrument, Manual (General Use)	Surgery
Tip, Suction Tube (Yankauer, Poole, Etc.)	Surgery
Tip, Suction, Fiberoptic Illuminated	Anesthesiology
Tongs, Skull	Cns/Neurology
Tongs, Skull, Traction	Cns/Neurology
Tourniquet, Non-Pneumatic, Surgical	Surgery
Tray, Surgical Instrument	Surgery
Trephine, Skull	Cns/Neurology
Trocar, Amniotic	Obstetrics/Gynecology
Trocar, Gallbladder	Gastroenterology/Urology
Tube, Tracheal (Endotracheal)	Anesthesiology
U.V. Method, CPK Isoenzymes	Chemistry

CODMAN & SHURTLEFF, INC.
See Codman & Shurtleff, Inc

CODMAN AND SHURTLEFF, INC   508-880-8100
325 Paramount Drive, Raynham, MA 02767
FDA Number: 3003921133   *Fax:* 508-880-8122
Web site: www.codman.com
Year Founded: 1857
Ownership: Johnson & Johnson
Stock Symbol: JNJ
Traded On: NYSE
Produces/Sells CE-marked Devices: N

Battery, Replacement, Rechargeable	Surgery
Gag, Mouth	Ear/Nose/Throat
Saw, Pneumatically Powered	Surgery

CODONICS   800-444-1198
17991 Englewood Drive,   440-243-1198
Middleburg Heights, OH 44130
FDA Number: 1530958   *Fax:* 440-243-1334
E-mail: info@codonics.com
Web site: www.codonics.com
Medical Products Sales Volume: $26,200,000
Annual Revenue: $50-$100 Million
Year Founded: 1982
Total Employees: 210
Ownership: Private
Quality System Registration Information: ISO9001
Produces/Sells CE-marked Devices: Y
Federal Procurement Eligibility: Small Business
Distribution: Manufacturer Direct, Manufacturer Through Distributor, Manufacturer Through Manufacturer Reps, Exporter
Mktg./Adv.: Cristy Granger/Director Communications

Camera, Multi Format	Radiology
Camera, Other	General
Film, X-Ray, Special Purpose	Radiology

COE LABORATORIES, INC.
See G-C America Inc.

COEUR INC., SHEBOYGAN   800-874-4240
3411 Behrens Pkwy., Sheboygan, WI 53081   920-458-4664
FDA Number: 1220497   *Fax:* 920-458-1368
Web site: www.vpicorp.com

COEUR INC., SHEBOYGAN   800-874-4240 *(cont'd)*
Year Founded: 1951
Ownership: Coeur, Inc
Quality System Registration Information: ISO9002
Produces/Sells CE-marked Devices: N
Federal Procurement Eligibility: Small Business
Distribution: Manufacturer Direct

Component, Plastic	General
Contract Assembly	General
Contract Manufacturing	General
Kit, Administration, Enteral	Gastroenterology/Urology
Kit, Administration, Intravenous	General
Tube, Connecting	General
Tubing, Conductive	General
Tubing, Flexible, Medical Gas, Low-Pressure	Anesthesiology
Tubing, Non-Conductive	General
Tubing, Oxygen Connecting	General
Tubing, Polyethylene	General
Tubing, Polyvinyl Chloride	General
Tubing, Urethane	General

COEUR LABORATORIES, INC.
See Coeur, Inc

COEUR, INC   800-296-5893
100 Physicians Way, Lebanon, TN 37087   615-547-7923
FDA Number: 1038185   *Fax:* 615-547-7937
E-mail: customer.service@coeurinc.com
Web site: www.coeurinc.com
Medical Products Sales Volume: $8,200,000
Annual Revenue: $10-$25 Million
Year Founded: 1999
Total Employees: 9
Ownership: Private
Quality System Registration Information: ISO9002
Produces/Sells CE-marked Devices: Y
Federal Procurement Eligibility: Small Business
Distribution: Manufacturer Direct, Manufacturer Through Distributor, Manufacturer Through Manufacturer Reps, OEM, Exporter
General Admin.: William J. Cude/President, Chief Executive Officer
Mktg./Adv.: Don F. McClintock/Vice President Marketing & Sales
Production: Debra F. Manning/Vice President Quality Assurance & Regulatory Affairs
Research: J. Michael Cude/Vice President Engineering
Finance: Ms. Jacqueline Wheeler/Chief Financial Officer

Injector, Contrast Medium, Automatic	Radiology
Syringe, Angiographic	Cns/Neurology
Syringe, Angioplasty	Cardiovascular
Syringe, Piston	General
Tubing, Polyethylene	General
Tubing, Polyvinyl Chloride	General
Tubing, Urethane	General

Medical Product Subsidiaries (Listed Separately)
Coeur Inc., Sheboygan

COEYE, INC.   321-543-2219
2025 West New Haven Ave., West Melbourne, FL 32904
FDA Number: n/a
Ownership: Private
Produces/Sells CE-marked Devices: N

Lens, Spectacle/Eyeglasses, Non-Custom	Ophthalmology

COHERENT, INC.   800-527-3786
5100 Patrick Henry Drive, Santa Clara, CA 95054   408-764-4000
FDA Number: n/a   *Fax:* 408-764-4800
E-mail: tech.sales@coherent.com
Web site: www.Coherent.com
Annual Revenue: $500 Million-$1 Billion
Year Founded: 1966
Total Employees: 2189
Ownership: Public
Stock Symbol: COHR
Traded On: NASDAQ
Quality System Registration Information: ISO9000; ISO9001; ISO9002
Produces/Sells CE-marked Devices: Y
Distribution: Manufacturer Direct, Manufacturer Through Distributor, Manufacturer Through Manufacturer Reps, OEM
General Admin.: Mr. Helene Simonet/Chief Financial Officer, Executive Vice President
    Mr. Luis Spinelli/Chief Technology Officer, Executive Vice President
    Mr. Bret DiMarco/Executive Vice President
    Mr. Ronald A. Victor/Executive Vice President Human Resources
    Dr. John R. Ambroseo/President, Chief Executive Officer
Mktg./Adv.: Rosemarie Smith-Wood/Manager Advertising & Communications
    Savina Angel/Marketing Coordinator
    Thomas Hutches/Vice President Marketing & Sales

Accessories, Laser	General
Laser, Laboratory	Chemistry

COHERENT, INC.   800-527-3786 *(cont'd)*
Microscope, Laser, Scanning, Acoustic	Microbiology
Photocoagulator	Ophthalmology
Radiometer, Laser	General
System, Marking, Film, Radiographic	Radiology
System, Marking, Laser	General
Tester, Alignment, Laser Beam	General

COHEREX MEDICAL INC.   800-390-9107
3598 West 1820 South, Salt Lake City, UT 84104   **801-433-9900**
FDA Number: 3006186509   Fax: 801-433-9901
E-mail: info@coherex.com
Web site: http://www.coherex.com
Year Founded: 2003
Ownership: Private
Produces/Sells CE-marked Devices: N
General Admin.: Mr. Ronald Watkins/Chief Operating Officer
      Mr. Richard Linder/President, Chief Executive Officer
Medical Admin.: Dr. Randall Jones/Chief Medical Officer
Mktg./Adv.: Mr. Rudy Davis/Marketing Officer
Production: Mr. Abraham Mathews/Vice President Quality Assurance & Regulatory Affairs
      Mr. Gary Snow/Vice President Quality Control
Research: Mr. Phillip Carter/Vice President Product Development
      Mr. Daryl Edminston/Vice President Research & Development

COHR INC./MEDIQUIP DIVISION
See Medical Technologies Co.

COLD ICE, INC.   800-525-4435
9999 San Leandro St., Oakland, CA 94603   **510-568-8129**
FDA Number: n/a   Fax: 510-568-2355
E-mail: info@coldice.com
Web site: www.coldice.com
Annual Revenue: $5-$10 Million
Year Founded: 1982
Ownership: Private
Produces/Sells CE-marked Devices: N
Federal Procurement Eligibility: Small Business
Distribution: Manufacturer Direct, Manufacturer Through Distributor, Manufacturer Through Manufacturer Reps
Pack, Hot Or Cold, Reusable	Physical Med

COLD RIVER UNLIMITED, INC.   662-286-3558
2070a South Tate St., Corinth, MS 38834
FDA Number: n/a
Ownership: Private
Produces/Sells CE-marked Devices: N
Sunglasses (Including Photosensitive)	Ophthalmology

COLDSTAR INTERNATIONAL, INC.   423-538-5551
677 Mountain View Dr., Piney Flats, TN 37686
FDA Number: 1060934
Pack, Hot Or Cold, Reusable	Physical Med

COLDSTREAM PRODUCTS CORP.   204-669-1201
1001 Regent Ave W, Winnipeg, MB R2C 4M2 Canada
FDA Number: n/a   Fax: 204-222-0655
Total Employees: 150   *Marketing Staff:* 10   *Sales Staff:* 10
Ownership: Private
Produces/Sells CE-marked Devices: N
Distribution: Manufacturer Direct, Exporter

COLE VISION COROPRATION   770-305-7352
2465 Joe Field Rd., Dallas, TX 75229
FDA Number: 1627826
Ownership: Private
Produces/Sells CE-marked Devices: N
Lens, Spectacle/Eyeglasses, Non-Custom	Ophthalmology

COLE VISION CORP.   770-305-7352
2150 Bixby Road, Lockbourne, OH 43137
FDA Number: n/a
Ownership: Private
Produces/Sells CE-marked Devices: N
Lens, Spectacle/Eyeglasses, Non-Custom	Ophthalmology

COLE VISION CORPORATION   770-305-7352
1887 S. 3230 West, Salt Lake City, UT 84104
FDA Number: 3005694511
Lens, Spectacle/Eyeglasses, Non-Custom	Ophthalmology

COLE VISION CORPORATION   770-305-7352
4435 Anderson Rd., Knoxville, TN 37918
FDA Number: 3005740134
Lens, Spectacle/Eyeglasses, Non-Custom	Ophthalmology

COLE VISION CORPORATION   770-305-7352
5780 E. Shelby Dr., Memphis, TN 38141
FDA Number: 3002902099

COLE VISION CORPORATION   770-305-7352 *(cont'd)*
Lens, Spectacle/Eyeglasses, Non-Custom	Ophthalmology

COLE VISION CORPORATION   513-765-6300
820 Southlake Blvd., Richmond, VA 23236
FDA Number: 3003991833
Ownership: Private
Produces/Sells CE-marked Devices: N
Lens, Spectacle/Eyeglasses, Non-Custom	Ophthalmology

COLE VISION CORPORATION   770-305-7352
9926 International Blvd., Cincinnati, OH 45246
FDA Number: 3005713451
Lens, Spectacle/Eyeglasses, Non-Custom	Ophthalmology

COLE-PARMER INSTRUMENT INC.   800-323-4340
625 E. Bunker Ct., Vernon Hills, IL 60061-1844   **847-549-7600**
FDA Number: n/a   Fax: 847-247-2929
E-mail: info@coleparmer.com
Web site: www.coleparmer.com
Ownership: Ismatec Sa Labortechnik/Analytik
Produces/Sells CE-marked Devices: N
Federal Procurement Eligibility: Small Business
Distribution: Exclusive Distributor, Importer, Exporter
Apron, Laboratory	Chemistry
Balance, Macro (0.1 mg Accuracy)	Chemistry
Balance, Semimicro (0.01 mg Accuracy)	Chemistry
Bath, Water (Constant Temperature)	Chemistry
Cart, Multipurpose	General
Circulator, Water Bath	Chemistry
Cleaner, Ultrasonic, Medical Instrument	General
Cleanroom Equipment	General
Controller, pH	Chemistry
Desiccator	Chemistry
Electrode, Laboratory pH	Chemistry
Electrode, pH	Gastroenterology/Urology
Evaporator	Chemistry
Flask, Dewar	Chemistry
Flowmeter, Gas (Oxygen), Calibrated	Anesthesiology
Gauge, Measuring	Ear/Nose/Throat
Heater, Immersion	Microbiology
Homogenizer, Tissue	Microbiology
Hood, Fume	Toxicology
Incubator/Water Bath, Microbiology	Microbiology
Labware, Basic, Disposable	Chemistry
Labware, Basic, Reusable	Chemistry
Lamp, Other	General
Manometer, Laboratory	Chemistry
Meter, pH, Portable	Chemistry
Mixer, Clinical Laboratory	Chemistry
Monitor, Contamination, Environmental, Personal	General
Oven	Chemistry
Pipette Tip	Chemistry
Pipette, Diluting	Hematology
Plate, Hot	Chemistry
Pump, Food (Enteral Feeding)	General
Pump, Infusion, Laboratory	Chemistry
Pump, Laboratory	Chemistry
Pyrometer	General
Recorder, Chart, Laboratory	Chemistry
Recorder, Paper Chart	Cardiovascular
Scale, Laboratory	Chemistry
Solution, pH Buffer	Chemistry
Stirrer	Chemistry
Tachometer	General
Thermistor	General
Thermometer, Laboratory	Chemistry
Tubing, Polyethylene	General
Tubing, Silicone	General
Tubing, Vinyl	General

COLGATE JUNCOS, INC.   212-310-2000
Rd #31 No 100, Juncos, PR 00777
FDA Number: 2648973
Ownership: Private
Produces/Sells CE-marked Devices: N
Toothbrush, Manual	Dental And Oral

COLGATE ORAL PHARMACEUTICALS, INC.   212-310-2000
300 Park Avenue, New York, NY 10022
FDA Number: 1644728
E-mail: directors@colpal.com
Web site: www.colgate.com
Ownership: Private
Produces/Sells CE-marked Devices: N
General Admin.: Mr. Ian Cook/Chairman, Chief Executive Officer
Agent, Polishing, Abrasive, Oral Cavity	Dental And Oral
Dental Cement w/out Zinc-Oxide Eugenol as an Ulcer Covering for Pain Relief	Dental And Oral
Floss, Dental	Dental And Oral
Sterilant, Medical Device	General

COLGATE ORAL PHARMACEUTICALS, INC. 212-310-2000
(cont'd)

Toothbrush, Manual	Dental And Oral
Varnish, Cavity	Dental And Oral

COLGON VESTAL
See Steris Corporation

COLIBRI HEART VALVE, LLC 303-460-8667
2150 West 6th Avenue, Suite M, Broomfield, CO 80020
FDA Number: n/a *Fax:* 303-460-1527
E-mail: info@ColibriHV.com
Web site: http://www.colibrihv.com
Ownership: Private
Produces/Sells CE-marked Devices: N
General Admin.: Mr. Joseph Horn/President, Chief Executive Officer
Mktg./Adv.: Mr. Eric Schauble/Vice President Corporate Development

COLIGHT
See Hanovia Specialty Lighting Llc

COLIN MEDICAL INSTRUMENTS CORP.
See Mediana Technologies Corp

COLLA-TEC, INC.
See Integra Lifesciences Holdings Corp.

COLLAGEN MATRIX, INC. 888-405-1001
  201-405-1477
15 Thornton Road, Oakland, NJ 07436
FDA Number: 2249852 *Fax:* 201-405-1355
E-mail: mlane@collagenmatrix.com
Web site: www.collagenmatrix.com
Ownership: Private
Produces/Sells CE-marked Devices: N

Bone Grafting Material, Animal Source	Dental And Oral
Cuff, Nerve	Cns/Neurology
Dressing, Burn, Porcine	Surgery
Dura-Substitute	Cns/Neurology
Filler, Calcium Sulfate Preformed Pellets	Orthopedics
Implant, Endosseous (Bone Filling and/or Augmentation)	Dental And Oral
Needle, Aspiration And Injection, Disposable	Surgery

COLLARD-ROSE OPTICAL LAB 562-698-2286
12402 Philadelphia St., Whittier, CA 90601
FDA Number: 2082813
Ownership: Private
Produces/Sells CE-marked Devices: N

Lens, Spectacle/Eyeglasses, Non-Custom	Ophthalmology

COLLEGE PARK INDUSTRIES, INC. 800-728-7950
  586-294-7950
17505 Helro Drive, Fraser, MI 48026
FDA Number: 1834241 *Fax:* 586-294-0067
E-mail: info@college-park.com
Web site: www.college-park.com
Medical Products Sales Volume: $3,300,000
Year Founded: 1988
Total Employees: 45 *Sales Staff:* 5
Ownership: Private
Produces/Sells CE-marked Devices: Y
Federal Procurement Eligibility: Small Business
Distribution: Manufacturer Direct
General Admin.: Eric L. Robinson/President
Mktg./Adv.: Eric L. Robinson/Vice President Marketing & Sales
Production: Mike Wilson/Vice President Manufacturing
IS: Michael Link/Technical Director

Prosthesis, Foot	Orthopedics

COLLINS BUS CORPORATION 800-354-9802
  620-662-9000
**415 W. 6th St., P.O. Box 2946,
South Hutchinson, KS 67504**
FDA Number: n/a *Fax:* 800-513-2501
Web site: www.collinsbus.com
Year Founded: 1967
Total Employees: 150 *Sales Staff:* 5
Ownership: Public
Produces/Sells CE-marked Devices: N
Federal Procurement Eligibility: Small Business
Distribution: Manufacturer Through Distributor, Exporter

Vehicle, Handicapped	Physical Med

COLLIS CURVE, INC. 800-298-4818
  956-546-4818
6110 California Rd., Brownsville, TX 78521
FDA Number: 2183594 *Fax:* 956-546-1426
E-mail: brushteeth@aol.com
Web site: www.colliscurve.com
Ownership: Private
Produces/Sells CE-marked Devices: N
Federal Procurement Eligibility: Small Business
Distribution: Manufacturer Direct
General Admin.: George Collis/President

COLLIS CURVE, INC. 800-298-4818 *(cont'd)*

Toothbrush, Manual	Dental And Oral

COLMAN PROSTHETICS & ORTHOTICS INC. 403-270-2941
2340 1st Ave. NW, Calgary, ALB T2N-0B8 Canada
FDA Number: n/a *Fax:* 403-270-7884
E-mail: info@cpoi.com
Web site: www.cpoi.com
Year Founded: 1983
Total Employees: 25
Ownership: Private
Produces/Sells CE-marked Devices: N
Distribution: Manufacturer Direct, Service Direct, Exclusive Distributor

COLON-EZ LLC 936-756-1970
12126 Kimberly Trace, Conroe, TX 77304
FDA Number: 3006137648

Kit, Enema (For Cleaning Purposes)	Gastroenterology/Urology

COLONIAL CARTON CO.
See 3c Packaging

COLONIAL MEDICAL SUPPLY 800-634-9334
  800-634-9334
**1350 E. Flamingo Rd. # 343,
Las Vegas, NV 89119**
FDA Number: 2031999 *Fax:* 949-481-3704
E-mail: colonialmedicalsupply@cox.net
Web site: www.kegelme.com
Year Founded: 1994
Total Employees: 2 *Marketing Staff:* 2 *Sales Staff:* 2
Ownership: Private
Produces/Sells CE-marked Devices: N
Federal Procurement Eligibility: Small Business, Female Owned
Distribution: Manufacturer Through Manufacturer Reps

Perineometer	Obstetrics/Gynecology

COLONIAL METALS, INC. 410-398-7200
505 Blue Ball Rd., Bldg. 20, Elkton, MD 21921
FDA Number: 1118598

Osmium Tetroxide	Pathology

COLONIAL SCIENTIFIC LTD. 902-468-1811
201 Brownlow Ave., Unit 52, Dartmouth, NS B3B-1W2 Canada
FDA Number: n/a *Fax:* 902-468-4363
E-mail: cslhfx@istar.ca
Medical Products Sales Volume: $3,500,000
Year Founded: 1971
Total Employees: 8 *Marketing Staff:* 1 *Sales Staff:* 5
Ownership: Private
Produces/Sells CE-marked Devices: N
Federal Procurement Eligibility: Small Business
Distribution: Exclusive Distributor

COLONIAL SPRING
See Colonial/Han-Dee Spring, Llc

COLONIAL/HAN-DEE SPRING, LLC 860-589-3231
95 Valley St., PO Box 1079, Bristol, CT 06011
FDA Number: n/a *Fax:* 860-582-9875
E-mail: sales@colonialspringco.com
Web site: www.colonialspringco.com
Medical Products Sales Volume: $5,000,000
Annual Revenue: $1-$5 Million
Year Founded: 1946
Total Employees: 40 *Marketing Staff:* 1 *Sales Staff:* 2
Ownership: Private
Quality System Registration Information: ISO9002
Produces/Sells CE-marked Devices: N
Federal Procurement Eligibility: Small Business
Distribution: Manufacturer Direct
General Admin.: Bill Lathrop/President
Mktg./Adv.: Loren Godrey/Director Product Development
  Bill Lathrop/Vice President Sales
Production: Howard Herman/Director Quality Assurance
Research: Loren Godfrey/Vice President Research & Development

Service, Engineering/Design	General

COLONICS DIVERSFIED, INC.
See Dotolo Research Corp.

COLOPLAST CORP., NORTH AMERICAN SALES DIVISION
See Coloplast Manufacturing Us, Llc

COLOPLAST MANUFACTURING US, LLC 800-533-0464
  507-345-6200
**1601 West River Road North,
Minneapolis, MN 55411**
FDA Number: 1046831 *Fax:* 507-345-8960
E-mail: usmedweb@coloplast.com
Web site: www.us.coloplast.com
Medical Products Sales Volume: $5,600,000
Year Founded: 1957

2013 MEDICAL DEVICE REGISTER

COLOPLAST MANUFACTURING US, LLC 800-533-0464 *(cont'd)*
Total Employees: 650   Marketing Staff: 37   Sales Staff: 125
Ownership: Public
Stock Symbol: COLOB
Traded On: Copenhagen
Quality System Registration Information: ISO9001
Produces/Sells CE-marked Devices: Y
Distribution: Manufacturer Direct, Manufacturer Through Distributor, OEM
Mktg./Adv.: Peter Romanot/Director National Accounts
　　　　　Keith Johnson/Director Sales
　　　　　Ralph Ferguson/Manager Corporate Sales
　　　　　Dave Hotchkiss/Vice President Marketing & Sales
Production: Tom Ryan/President Manufacturing Services
Research: Jesper Jul/Vice President Consumer Health Care

Bag, Drainage (Incontinence)	Gastroenterology/Urology
Bag, Leg	Gastroenterology/Urology
Bag, Stomal	Surgery
Bag, Urinary Collection	General
Bag, Urinary, Ileostomy	Gastroenterology/Urology
Bandage, Compression	General
Catheter, Coude	Gastroenterology/Urology
Catheter, Olive Tip	Gastroenterology/Urology
Catheter, Retention Type, Balloon	Gastroenterology/Urology
Catheter, Straight	Gastroenterology/Urology
Catheter, Urethral	Gastroenterology/Urology
Catheter, Urinary	Gastroenterology/Urology
Catheter, Urinary, Condom	Gastroenterology/Urology
Catheter, Urological	Gastroenterology/Urology
Collector, Ostomy	Gastroenterology/Urology
Collector, Urine, Disposable	Gastroenterology/Urology
Colostomy Appliance, Disposable	Gastroenterology/Urology
Dressing, Foam	General
Dressing, Gel	General
Dressing, Other	General
Dressing, Skin Graft, Donor Site	General
Dressing, Universal	General
Dressing, Wound and Burn, Occlusive	Surgery
Irrigator, Ostomy	Gastroenterology/Urology
Legging, Compression, Non-Inflatable	General
Lotion, Skin Care	General
Ostomy Appliance (Ileostomy, Colostomy)	Gastroenterology/Urology
Pant, Incontinence	General
Plug, Ostomy	Gastroenterology/Urology
Pouch, Colostomy	Gastroenterology/Urology
Prosthesis, Breast, External	Surgery
Soap	General
Solution, Ostomy, Odor Control	Gastroenterology/Urology
Tubal Occlusive Device	Obstetrics/Gynecology

Medical Product Subsidiaries (Listed Separately)
Amoena

COLOPLAST, INC.
See Coloplast Manufacturing Us, Llc

COLOR CHANGE CORP. 630-289-0900
1545 Burgundy Pkwy., Streamwood, IL 60107
FDA Number: 1424366   Fax: 630-289-0909
E-mail: info@colorchange.com
Web site: www.ColorChange.com
Ownership: Private
Produces/Sells CE-marked Devices: N
Federal Procurement Eligibility: Small Business
General Admin.: Margo Musial/Office Manager
　　　　　Mr. Timothy Homola/President
Temperature Strip, Forehead, Liquid Crystal	General

COLORADO SERUM COMPANY 303-295-7527
4950 York St., PO Box 16428, Denver, CO 80216-2266
FDA Number: 7000097   Fax: 303-295-1923
E-mail: colorado-serum@colorado-serum.com
Web site: www.colorado-serum.com
Medical Products Sales Volume: $5,800,000
Year Founded: 1923
Total Employees: 99
Ownership: Private
Produces/Sells CE-marked Devices: N
Federal Procurement Eligibility: Small Business
Distribution: Manufacturer Direct, Manufacturer Through Distributor
General Admin.: J. N. Huff/President
Needle, Other	General
Serum, Biological, General	Toxicology
Syringe, Bulb	General

COLORCODE MEDICAL PRODUCTS, INC.
See R&Da Co.

COLORED PLASTICS, LLC 888-807-9554
3902 Grant Street South, Bondurant, IA 50035 515-957-9367
FDA Number: n/a
E-mail: info@coloredplastics.com
Web site: www.coloredplastics.com

COLORED PLASTICS, LLC 888-807-9554 *(cont'd)*
Ownership: Private
Produces/Sells CE-marked Devices: N
Cane	Physical Med

COLORS IN OPTICS LTD. 866-465-2656
366 5th Ave., #1003, New York, NY 10001-2211 212-465-1200
FDA Number: 2432297   Fax: 212-465-0939
E-mail: info@colorsinopticsusa.com
Web site: www.colorsinoptics.com
Total Employees: 100   Sales Staff: 30
Ownership: Private
Produces/Sells CE-marked Devices: N
Federal Procurement Eligibility: Small Business
Distribution: Manufacturer Direct, Exclusive Distributor, Importer
General Admin.: Sanford Hutton/President, Chief Executive Officer
Frame, Spectacle (Eyeglasses)	Ophthalmology

COLOURS 'N MOTION, INC.
See Colours Wheelchair

COLOURS WHEELCHAIR 800-892-8998
860 E. Parkridge Avenue, Corona, CA 92879 951-808-9131
FDA Number: 2029329   Fax: 951-808-9949
E-mail: kristachamberlain@colourswheelchair.com
Web site: www.colourswheelchair.com
Medical Products Sales Volume: $100,000
Annual Revenue: $1-$5 Million
Year Founded: 1992
Total Employees: 1   Marketing Staff: 1   Sales Staff: 25
Ownership: Private
Quality System Registration Information: ISO9003
Produces/Sells CE-marked Devices: Y
Federal Procurement Eligibility: Small Business, Minority Owned, VA Contract
Distribution: Manufacturer Through Distributor, OEM
General Admin.: Mr. Toshi Tamba/Chief Executive Officer
Mktg./Adv.: Mr. Rick Hayden/Vice President Sales
Wheelchair, Special Grade	Physical Med

COLSON CASTER CORPORATION 800-643-5515
3700 Airport Road, Jonesboro, AR 72401 870-932-4501
FDA Number: n/a   Fax: 800-356-6708
E-mail: info1@colsoncaster.com
Web site: www.colsoncaster.com
Year Founded: 1885
Total Employees: 300
Ownership: Private
Produces/Sells CE-marked Devices: N
Federal Procurement Eligibility: Small Business
Distribution: Exclusive Distributor
Mktg./Adv.: Russell Candell/Vice President Marketing & Sales
Production: Chad Kaderabek/Product Manager
Casters, Hospital Equipment	General

COLTENE/WHALEDENT INC. 330-916-8858
235 Ascot Parkway, Cuyahoga Falls, OH 44223
FDA Number: 2416455   Fax: 330-916-7077
E-mail: info@coltenewhaledent.com
Web site: www.coltene.com
Ownership: Private
Produces/Sells CE-marked Devices: N

Absorber, Saliva, Paper	Dental And Oral
Activator, Ultraviolet, Polymerization	Dental And Oral
Aligner, Bracket, Orthodontic	Dental And Oral
Attachment, Precision	Dental And Oral
Base, Denture, Relining, Repairing, Rebasing, Resin	Dental And Oral
Burr, Dental	Dental And Oral
Chisel, Bone, Surgical	Dental And Oral
Clamp, Rubber Dam	Dental And Oral
Cleaner, Ultrasonic, Medical Instrument	General
Crown And Bridge, Temporary, Resin	Dental And Oral
Dam, Rubber	Dental And Oral
Drill, Dental, Intraoral	Dental And Oral
Electrosurgical Unit, Dental	Dental And Oral
Evacuator, Oral Cavity	Dental And Oral
Forceps, Rubber Dam Clamp	Dental And Oral
Frame, Rubber Dam	Dental And Oral
Gauge, Depth, Instrument, Dental	Dental And Oral
Gutta Percha	Dental And Oral
Handle, Instrument, Dental	Dental And Oral
Handpiece, Contra- And Right-Angle Attachment, Dental	Dental And Oral
Hemostat, Surgical	Dental And Oral
Liner, Cavity, Calcium Hydroxide	Dental And Oral
Material, Impression Tray, Resin	Dental And Oral
Material, Tooth Shade, Resin	Dental And Oral
Pack, Sterilization Wrapper (Bag And Accessories)	Surgery
Pin, Retentive And Splinting	Dental And Oral
Pliers, Orthodontic	Dental And Oral
Plugger, Root Canal, Endodontic	Dental And Oral
Point, Paper, Endodontic	Dental And Oral

COLTENE/WHALEDENT INC.   330-916-8858 *(cont'd)*

Post, Root Canal	Dental And Oral
Probe, Periodontic	Dental And Oral
Pusher, Band, Orthodontic	Dental And Oral
Resin, Root Canal Filling	Dental And Oral
Scaler, Ultrasonic	Dental And Oral
Scissors, Collar And Crown	Dental And Oral
Spreader, Pulp Canal Filling Material, Endodontic	Dental And Oral
Sterilizer, Dry Heat	General
Tester, Pulp	Dental And Oral
Tooth Bonding Agent, Resin Restoration	Dental And Oral
Tray, Impression	Dental And Oral
Tucker, Ligature, Orthodontic	Dental And Oral
Wax, Dental	Dental And Oral
Wrap, Sterilization	General

COLUMBIA DENTOFORM CORP.
See Dentalez Group

COLUMBIA MEDICAL MANUFACTURING LLC   800-454-6612
13577 Larwin Circle,   **310-454-6612**
Santa Fe Springs, CA 90670
FDA Number: 3005328749   *Fax:* 310-305-1718
E-mail: info@columbiamedical.com
Web site: www.columbiamedical.com
Year Founded: 1978
Total Employees: 50
Ownership: Private
Produces/Sells CE-marked Devices: N
Federal Procurement Eligibility: Small Business
Distribution: Manufacturer Through Distributor
General Admin.: Gary Werschmidt/President
Mktg./Adv.: Mr. Alan Rushing/Director Business Development
    Ms. Kristine Storle/Marketing Consultant
Production: Mrs. Brandi Mayclin/Customer Service Representative

Chair, Bath	General
Chair, Other	General
Commode (Toilet)	General
Cover, Seat, Toilet, Sanitary	General
Exerciser, Other	Physical Med

COLUMBIA-INLAND CORPORATION   503-657-6676
415 17th St., Suite #2, Oregon City, OR 97045
FDA Number: 3005675206
Ownership: Private
Produces/Sells CE-marked Devices: N

Exerciser, Non-Measuring	Physical Med

COLUMBUS MCKINNON CORP., MOBILITY PRODUCTS DIV.   800-888-0985
140 John James Audubon Pkwy, Amherst,   **716-689-5400**
Amherst, NY 14228
FDA Number: 1319258   *Fax:* 716-689-5598
E-mail: rob.beightol@cmworks.com
Web site: http://cmworks.com/
Medical Products Sales Volume: $589,800,000
Year Founded: 1875
Ownership: Public
Stock Symbol: CMCO
Traded On: NASDAQ
Produces/Sells CE-marked Devices: N
General Admin.: Timothy T Tevens/Chief Executive Officer
Mktg./Adv.: Craig P. Johnston/Manager International Marketing & Sales

Lift, Patient	General

COMAR APPLICATOR
See Comar, Inc.

COMAR PUERTO RICO
See Marcoop Molding

COMAR, INC.   800-962-6627
1 Comar Place, Buena, NJ 08310-9901
FDA Number: 2220100
E-mail: information@comar.com
Web site: www.comar.com
Medical Products Sales Volume: $55,000,000
Annual Revenue: $50-$100 Million
Year Founded: 1949
Total Employees: 260
Ownership: Private
Quality System Registration Information: ISO9002
Produces/Sells CE-marked Devices: Y
Federal Procurement Eligibility: Small Business
Distribution: Manufacturer Direct

Closure, Other	General
Container, Medication, Graduated Liquid	General
Dispenser, Medication, Liquid	General
Dropper, Medicine	General
Molding, Injection	General

COMAR, INC.   800-962-6627 *(cont'd)*

Service, Engineering/Design	General
Vial, Other	General

COMBE INCORPORATED   800-873-7400
1101 Westchester Ave., White Plains, NY 10604
FDA Number: n/a
Web site: www.combe.com
Year Founded: 1949
Ownership: Private
Produces/Sells CE-marked Devices: N
Distribution: Manufacturer Direct

Cushion, Denture, OTC	Dental And Oral

COMBE LABORATORIES, INC.   800-873-7400
200 Shelhouse Dr., Rantoul, IL 61866   **217-893-4490**
FDA Number: 1450238
Web site: www.combe.com
Year Founded: 1949
Ownership: Private
Produces/Sells CE-marked Devices: N

Adhesive, Denture, Acacia & Karaya with Sodium Borate	Dental And Oral
Detector/Remover, Lice	General
Homopolymer, Karaya and Ethylene-Oxide	Dental And Oral
pH Paper, Obstetric	Obstetrics/Gynecology

COMBE, INC.   (800) 873-7400
1101 Westchester Avenue,   **716-694-7100**
White Plains, NY 10604
FDA Number: n/a
Medical Products Sales Volume: $10,000,000
Annual Revenue: $10-$25 Million
Year Founded: 1945
Ownership: Private
Produces/Sells CE-marked Devices: N
Federal Procurement Eligibility: Small Business
Distribution: Manufacturer Through Manufacturer Reps

Adhesive, Denture, OTC	Dental And Oral
Brush, Dental Plate (Denture)	Dental And Oral
Cleaner, Denture	Dental And Oral
Cushion, Denture, OTC	Dental And Oral
Kit, Denture Repair, OTC	Dental And Oral
Lotion, Skin Care	General
Protector, Mouth Guard	Dental And Oral

COMBINED OPTICAL INDUSTRIES LTD.
See Ctp Coil Inc.

COMCO, INC.   800-796-6626
2151 N. Lincoln St., Burbank, CA 91504   **818-841-5500**
FDA Number: n/a   *Fax:* 818-955-8365
E-mail: sales@COMCOinc.com
Web site: www.COMCOinc.com
Medical Products Sales Volume: $3,500,000
Annual Revenue: $1-$5 Million
Year Founded: 1968
Total Employees: 33
Ownership: Private
Produces/Sells CE-marked Devices: Y
Federal Procurement Eligibility: Small Business
Distribution: Manufacturer Direct, Manufacturer Through Manufacturer Reps
General Admin.: Neil Weightman/President
Mktg./Adv.: Ms. Jill Bassett/Coord. Marketing Communications
    Mr. Neil Weightman/Manager National Sales

Brush, Burr Cleaning	Dental And Oral
Burr, Other	Surgery
Production Equipment	General
Screw, Fixation, Bone	Orthopedics
Stent, Cardiovascular	Cardiovascular

COMERCIALIZADORA MEDICA ALVASAN S.A. 01 800-71026-33 DE C.V.
Eulalio Gutierrez #303, Col. Francisco Villa,   **(01-81) 8383-24**
San Nicolas De Los Garza, NL 66430 Mexico
FDA Number: n/a   *Fax:* (01-81) 8350-17
Total Employees: 4   *Marketing Staff:* 1   *Sales Staff:* 4
Ownership: Private
Produces/Sells CE-marked Devices: N
Federal Procurement Eligibility: Female Owned
Distribution: Manufacturer Through Distributor, Service Direct

COMFORT ACRYLICS, INC.   360-834-9218
2103 N.e. 272nd Ave., Camas, WA 98607
FDA Number: 3025124
Web site: www.comfortacrylics.com
Ownership: Private
Produces/Sells CE-marked Devices: N

COMFORT ACRYLICS, INC.   360-834-9218 *(cont'd)*

Base, Denture, Relining, Repairing, Rebasing, Resin   Dental And Oral

COMFORT CARE PRODUCTS

See Smith & Nephew Inc.- Orthopaedics Division

COMFORT PRODUCTS, INC.   800-822-7500

931 River Road, Croydon, PA 19021-6850   **215-781-0300**
FDA Number: n/a   Fax: 215-785-5737
E-mail: frebern@aol.com
Web site: www.comfortoandp.com
Annual Revenue: $1-$5 Million
Total Employees: 20
Ownership: Private
Produces/Sells CE-marked Devices: Y
Federal Procurement Eligibility: Small Business, Female Owned
Distribution: Manufacturer Direct, Manufacturer Through Distributor, Manufacturer Through Manufacturer Reps, Exporter
General Admin.: Harold Bernhardt/President
     Fred Bernhardt/Vice President, General Manager
Mktg./Adv.: Frederick Bernhardt/Vice President Sales

Sheath, Endoscopic	Gastroenterology/Urology
Sock, Fracture	Orthopedics
Sock, Stump Cover	General
Stockinette	Orthopedics
Stockinette, Cast	Orthopedics

COMFORT STRAP CO.   605-997-3810

212 Second Ave East, Egan, SD 57024-9701
FDA Number: 2183811
Ownership: Private
Produces/Sells CE-marked Devices: N

Cannula, Nasal, Oxygen	Anesthesiology

COMFORT TECHNOLOGIES, INC.   800-321-7846

381 Mountain Blvd., Watchung, NJ 07069   **908-757-3200**
FDA Number: 2246474   Fax: 908-757-7200
E-mail: sytech@optonline.net
Web site: www.comforttechnologies.com
Annual Revenue: $1-$5 Million
Year Founded: 1986
Total Employees: 12   *Marketing Staff:* 4   *Sales Staff:* 18
Ownership: Private
Quality System Registration Information: ISO9000; ISO9001
Produces/Sells CE-marked Devices: Y
Federal Procurement Eligibility: Small Business
Distribution: Manufacturer Direct, Manufacturer Through Distributor, Exclusive Distributor, Importer, Exporter
General Admin.: Sy Gelbard/President, Chief Executive Officer

Electrode, Other	General
Stimulator, Muscle, Electrical-Powered (EMS)	Physical Med
Stimulator, Muscle, Low Intensity	Physical Med
Stimulator, Nerve, Transcutaneous (Pain Relief, TENS)	Cns/Neurology
Stimulator, Neuromuscular, External Functional	Cns/Neurology

COMFORT TOUCH   888-8BR-IEFS

P.O Box 630104, Miami, FL 33163   **305-770-1336**
FDA Number: n/a   Fax: 305-770-4636
E-mail: sales@comfort-touch.com
Web site: www.comfort-touch.com/
Medical Products Sales Volume: $300,000
Annual Revenue: $1-$5 Million
Year Founded: 1992
Total Employees: 2
Ownership: Private
Produces/Sells CE-marked Devices: N
Federal Procurement Eligibility: Small Business
Distribution: Exclusive Distributor, Importer
General Admin.: Susan Shalev/President
     Lior Shalev/Vice President, General Manager

Diaper, Adult	General

COMFORTEX, INC.   800-445-4007

1680 Wilkie Dr., P.O. Box 850, Winona, MN 55987   **507-454-6579**
FDA Number: 2183571   Fax: 507-454-6581
E-mail: info@comfortexinc.com
Web site: prevent-injuries.com
Annual Revenue: $5-$10 Million
Ownership: Private
Produces/Sells CE-marked Devices: N
Federal Procurement Eligibility: Small Business
Distribution: Manufacturer Direct, Manufacturer Through Manufacturer Reps, Exporter

Cover, Mattress	General
Cushion, Flotation	Physical Med
Cushion, Other	General
Mattress, Air Flotation	General
Mattress, Bed	General
Mattress, Reduction, Pressure	General

COMFORTEX, INC.   800-445-4007 *(cont'd)*

Splint, Extremity, Non-Inflatable, External	Surgery
Traction Unit, Non-Powered	Orthopedics

COMMAND MEDICAL PRODUCTS, INC.   386-672-8116

15 Signal Avenue, Ormond Beach, FL 32174-2984
FDA Number: 1526611   Fax: 386-677-7781
E-mail: sales@commandmedical.com
Web site: www.commandmedical.com
Medical Products Sales Volume: $7,200,000
Year Founded: 1987
Total Employees: 90   *Marketing Staff:* 2   *Sales Staff:* 3
Ownership: Private
Produces/Sells CE-marked Devices: N
Federal Procurement Eligibility: Small Business
Distribution: Manufacturer Through Distributor, OEM
General Admin.: David Slick/President, Chief Executive Officer
Mktg./Adv.: Stephanie McGee/Director Marketing & Sales
Production: Jim Skelly/Manager Operations
     Mr. Michael Clayton/Manager Quality Assurance & Regulatory Affairs

Bag, Blood	Hematology
Bag, Drainage (Incontinence)	Gastroenterology/Urology
Bag, Drainage, Nasogastric	General
Bag, Drainage, Ostomy (With Adhesive)	General
Contract Assembly	General
Contract Manufacturing	General
Contract Manufacturing, Product, Disposable	General
Contract Packaging	General
Molding, Custom	General
System, Delivery, Drug, Ocular	Ophthalmology
Thermoforming, Extrusion, Custom	General
Tubing, Polyvinyl Chloride	General

COMMERCE ATLANTIC CORP.   626-448-8905

2239 Tyler Ave., Suite B, South El Monte, CA 91733
FDA Number: n/a
Ownership: Private
Produces/Sells CE-marked Devices: N

Orthosis, Corrective Shoe	Physical Med

COMMERCE FACILITATORS   703-352-3569

3924 Tedrich Blvd., Fairfax, VA 22031
FDA Number: 1125870
Ownership: Private
Produces/Sells CE-marked Devices: N

Linen, Bed	General

COMMERCIAL/MEDICAL ELECTRONICS, INC.   800-324-4844

1519 S. Lewis Avenue, Tulsa, OK 74104-4919   **918-749-6151**
FDA Number: 1628548   Fax: 918-749-3023
E-mail: hugh@cme-usa.com
Web site: www.cme-usa.com
Medical Products Sales Volume: $1,500,000
Annual Revenue: $1-$5 Million
Year Founded: 1976
Total Employees: 13   *Marketing Staff:* 2   *Sales Staff:* 3
Ownership: Private
Produces/Sells CE-marked Devices: N
Federal Procurement Eligibility: Small Business, Minority Owned
Distribution: Manufacturer Direct, Service Direct, Exclusive Distributor, Exporter
General Admin.: Hugh Holly/President
     Perry Youngblood/Vice President Human Resources
Mktg./Adv.: William C. Ninke/Manager Contract Sales
     Hugh Holly/Manager International & National Sales
     Clint Wilkins/Manager National Sales
     Charles Youngblood/Manager Sales
     Hugh Holly/Manager Sales Training
     C. Clint Wilkins/Vice President Marketing & Sales
Production: Anna M. Vaughn/Director Quality Assurance
     Elizabeth Brooks/Manager Materials
     Anna Vaughn/Manager Regulatory Affairs
Research: Jonathan Black/Biomedical Engineer
     William C. Ninke/Vice President Research & Development

Defibrillator, Battery-Powered	Cardiovascular
Equipment, Therapy, Handicapped/Physical	Physical Med
Monitor, Cardiac (Cardiotachometer & Rate Alarm)	Cardiovascular
Monitor, ECG	Cardiovascular
Monitor, Respiratory	Surgery
Oximeter, Pulse	General
Spirometer, Diagnostic (Respirometer)	Anesthesiology
Transmitter/Receiver System, ECG, Telephone Multi-Channel	Cardiovascular
Transmitter/Receiver System, ECG, Telephone Single-Channel	Cardiovascular
Transmitter/Receiver System, Fetal Monitor, Telephone	General
Transmitter/Receiver System, Physiological, Telephone	Cardiovascular
Transmitter/Receiver System, Pulmonary Monitor, Telephone	General
Ventilator, Non-Continuous (Respirator)	Anesthesiology

COMMON SENSE DENTAL INC.   888-853-5773
14998 Cleveland St., Suite A,   616-935-0704
Spring Lake, MI 49456
FDA Number: n/a
Annual Revenue: $1-$5 Million   *Fax:* 616-935-0711
Total Employees: 7   *Marketing Staff:* 7   *Sales Staff:* 7
Ownership: Private
Produces/Sells CE-marked Devices: N
Federal Procurement Eligibility: Small Business
Distribution: Manufacturer Direct
General Admin.: John Garrison/President
     Amy Garrison/Vice President

Block, Bite	Cns/Neurology
Handle, Instrument, Dental	Dental And Oral

COMMON SENSE DENTAL PRODUCTS,
See Common Sense Dental Inc.

COMMONWEALTH H2O SERVICES, INC.   434-975-4426
325 Greenbrier Drive, Charlottesville, VA 22901-1618
FDA Number: 1124834   *Fax:* 434-978-1999
E-mail: jdavis@h-two-o.com
Web site: www.h-two-o.com
Year Founded: 1994
Ownership: Private
Produces/Sells CE-marked Devices: N
Federal Procurement Eligibility: Small Business, Female Owned
Distribution: Manufacturer Direct
General Admin.: Mrs. Linda Schroeder/President, Owner
     Mr. Jon Davis/Vice President

Purifier, Water	Chemistry

COMMUNITY BLOOD CENTER OF GREATER K.C.   888-647-4040
4040 Main St., Kansas City, MO 64111   816-753-4040
FDA Number: 1972933   *Fax:* 816-968-4047
Ownership: Private
Produces/Sells CE-marked Devices: N
General Admin.: Mr. Jay Menitove/President, Chief Executive Officer
     Mr. David Graham/Vice President
     Ms. Lori Wolfe/Vice President Human Resources
Production: Ms. Kim Peck/Vice President Quality Assurance

Software, Blood Bank (Stand-Alone Products)	Hematology

COMMUNITY PRODUCTS, LLC   845-658-7723
2032 Route 213, Rifton, NY 12471
FDA Number: 1319061

Board, Scooter, Prone	Physical Med
Chair, Adjustable, Mechanical	Physical Med
Exerciser, Non-Measuring	Physical Med
Lift, Bath, Non-AC-Powered	General
Table, Mechanical	Physical Med
Walker, Mechanical	Physical Med

COMMUNITY PRODUCTS, LLC   845-658-7723
Platte Clove Rd., Elka Park, NY 12427
FDA Number: 1319558
Ownership: Private
Produces/Sells CE-marked Devices: N

Chair, Adjustable, Mechanical	Physical Med
Restraint	Physical Med

COMP EQUIPMENT CORP.
See Ergodyne

COMPANION WALKER LTD.   403-250-1888
4 1420 40th Ave. NE, Calgary, ALB T2E-6L1 Canada
FDA Number: n/a   *Fax:* 403-275-5678
E-mail: info@companionwalker.com
Web site: www.companionwalker.com
Year Founded: 1990
Total Employees: 10
Ownership: Private
Produces/Sells CE-marked Devices: N
Distribution: Manufacturer Direct, Exclusive Distributor, Exporter

COMPASS BIOSCIENCE   626-359-9645
1850 Evergreen St., Duarte, CA 91010-2906
FDA Number: 2032652   *Fax:* 626-359-7697
E-mail: info@seraplex.com
Web site: www.seraplex.com
Medical Products Sales Volume: $1,000,000
Annual Revenue: $5-$10 Million
Year Founded: 1974
Total Employees: 15   *Marketing Staff:* 1   *Sales Staff:* 1
Ownership: Seraplex Biologicals Inc.
Produces/Sells CE-marked Devices: N
Federal Procurement Eligibility: Small Business
Distribution: Manufacturer Direct, OEM, Exporter
General Admin.: Ms. Evy Johnson/Chief Operating Officer

COMPASS BIOSCIENCE   626-359-9645 *(cont'd)*
     Mr. Philip Rossi/President, Chief Executive Officer
Production: Ms. Mary Anne St. John/Director Quality Assurance & Regulatory Affairs

Control, Multi Analyte, All Kinds (Assayed And Unassayed)	Chemistry
Control, Urinalysis (Assayed And Unassayed)	Chemistry

COMPASS INTERNATIONAL, INC.   800-933-2143
1815 14th Street NW, Rochester, MN 55901   507-281-2143
FDA Number: 2183671   *Fax:* 507-281-1736
E-mail: info@compass.com
Web site: www.compass.com
Annual Revenue: $1-$5 Million
Year Founded: 1986
Total Employees: 8   *Marketing Staff:* 2   *Sales Staff:* 18
Ownership: Private
Produces/Sells CE-marked Devices: N
Federal Procurement Eligibility: Small Business
Distribution: Manufacturer Direct, Manufacturer Through Distributor, Manufacturer Through Manufacturer Reps, Service Direct, Importer, Exporter
General Admin.: Jon S. Rousu/General Manager
     Bruce Kall/President
Production: Jon S. Rousu/Director Engineering
     Scott Brue/Engineer
     William Jackson/Manager Regulatory Affairs
IS: Mike Goodman/Tech. Specialist

Accessories, Wheelchair	Physical Med
Electrosurgical Unit, Neurological	Cns/Neurology
Image Processing System	Radiology
Needle, Aspiration And Injection, Disposable	Surgery
Retractor, Self-Retaining, Neurology	Cns/Neurology
Stereotaxy Equipment	Cns/Neurology

COMPENSATION ECONOMICS INFORMATION SYS.
See Rehabilitation Services, Inc.

COMPETITIVE ENGINEERING INC.   520-746-0270
3371 E. Hemisphere Loop, Tucson, AZ 85706
FDA Number: 3002619448

Knife, Surgical	Dental And Oral

COMPEX TECHNOLOGIES, INC.   866-676-6489
1811 Old Hwy. 8, New Brighton, MN 55112   651-631-0590
FDA Number: 2126518   *Fax:* 651-638-0476
E-mail: info@rehabilicare.com
Web site: www.compextechnologies.com
Medical Products Sales Volume: $96,100,000
Annual Revenue: $50-$100 Million
Year Founded: 1972
Total Employees: 481
Ownership: Private
Stock Symbol: CMPX
Traded On: NASDAQ
Produces/Sells CE-marked Devices: Y
Federal Procurement Eligibility: Small Business, VA Contract
General Admin.: John Maley/Chairman
     Sonja Grunlan/Director Human Resources
     Dan Gladney/President, Chief Executive Officer
Mktg./Adv.: Mike Goodpaster/Vice President Sales
Production: Gary Moore/Director Engineering
     Brian Edwards/Director Quality Assurance & Regulatory Affairs
     Paul Taft/Manager Materials
     Wayne Chrystal/Vice President Manufacturing
Finance: Scott Youngstrom/Vice President Finance

Catheter, Olive Tip	Gastroenterology/Urology
Electrode, Neurological	Cns/Neurology
Electrode, Neuromuscular Stimulator	Cns/Neurology
Electrode, Other	General
Stimulator, Muscle, Electrical-Powered (EMS)	Physical Med
Stimulator, Nerve, Transcutaneous (Pain Relief, TENS)	Cns/Neurology
Stimulator, Neuromuscular, External Functional	Cns/Neurology

COMPIX INCORPORATED   503-639-8496
15824 Sw Upper Boones Ferry Rd,
Lake Oswego, OR 97035
FDA Number: 3004125952
Ownership: Private
Produces/Sells CE-marked Devices: N

Telethermographic System (Adjunctive Use)	Radiology

COMPLETE MEDICAL SUPPLIES, INC.   800-242-2674
10 Ford Products Rd., Valley Cottage, NY 10989   845-353-0434
FDA Number: n/a   *Fax:* 845-353-1379
E-mail: sales@completemedical.com
Web site: www.completemedical.com
Annual Revenue: $10-$25 Million
Year Founded: 1988
Total Employees: 58   *Marketing Staff:* 4   *Sales Staff:* 24
Ownership: Private

COMPLETE MEDICAL SUPPLIES, INC. 800-242-2674 *(cont'd)*
Produces/Sells CE-marked Devices: N
Distribution: Manufacturer Through Distributor, Manufacturer Through
Manufacturer Reps, Importer, Exporter
General Admin.: Seth Klein/President, Chief Executive Officer
Mktg./Adv.: Tony Jackson/Vice President Business Development
    Manny Levy/Vice President Sales
Purchasing: Manny Levy/Director Exports
    Jerry Raiani/Director Purchasing
  Aid, Living, Handicapped   General

COMPLETE MOBILITY SYSTEMS INC.
See IMED Mobility Inc.

COMPLETE SYSTEM DIAGNOSTICS, INC. 800-722-4273
1170 North Lincoln, Suite 108, Dixon, CA 95620 707-678-1909
FDA Number: 2950359   *Fax:* 707-678-1328
E-mail: cmorse@csd-ultrasound.com
Web site: www.csd-ultrasound.com
Medical Products Sales Volume: $1,700,000
Annual Revenue: $0-$1 Million
Year Founded: 1984
Total Employees: 11   *Marketing Staff:* 1   *Sales Staff:* 3
Ownership: Private
Produces/Sells CE-marked Devices: N
Federal Procurement Eligibility: Small Business
Distribution: Manufacturer Through Distributor
General Admin.: Ken Bushey/President
  Computer, Ultrasound   Radiology

COMPLEWARE CORP. 800-369-8888
2865 Stoner Court, North Liberty, IA 52317 319-626-8888
FDA Number: 3003619818   *Fax:* 319-626-8725
E-mail: info@compleware.com
Web site: www.compleware.com
Ownership: Private
Produces/Sells CE-marked Devices: N
  Spirometer, Diagnostic (Respirometer)   Anesthesiology

COMPLEX MEDICAL PRODUCTS, INC.
See Coeur Inc., Sheboygan

COMPOSIFLEX, INC. 800-673-2544
8100 Hawthorne Circle, Erie, PA 16509 814-866-8616
FDA Number: n/a   *Fax:* 814-866-0563
E-mail: info@composiflex.com
Web site: www.composiflex.com
Medical Products Sales Volume: $7,000,000
Annual Revenue: $5-$10 Million
Year Founded: 1985
Total Employees: 75   *Marketing Staff:* 2   *Sales Staff:* 2
Ownership: Private
Quality System Registration Information: ISO9001
Produces/Sells CE-marked Devices: N
Federal Procurement Eligibility: Small Business
Distribution: Manufacturer Direct, OEM
General Admin.: Alan J. Hannibal/President
Mktg./Adv.: Nancy B. Potter/Director Marketing & Sales

Accessories, Operating Room, Table	Surgery
Accessories, Radiotherapy	Radiology
Bed, Scanning, Nuclear/Fluoroscopic	Radiology
Board, Spine	Orthopedics
Cassette, Radiographic Film	Radiology
Couch, Radiation Therapy, Powered	Radiology
Cradle, Patient, Radiographic	Radiology
Grid, Radiographic	Radiology
Holder, Head, Radiographic	Radiology
Resin, Plastic	General
Stretcher, Radiographic	Radiology
Support, Patient Position, Radiographic	Radiology
Table, Nuclear Medicine	Radiology
Table, Radiographic	Radiology
Table, Radiographic, Non-Tilting, Powered	Radiology
Table, Radiographic, Stationary Top	Radiology
Table, Radiographic, Tilting	Radiology
Table, Surgical With Orthopedic Accessories, AC-Powered	Surgery
Table, Surgical, Electrical	Surgery
Table, Surgical, Manual	General
Table, Surgical, Orthopedic	Orthopedics
Table, Urological, Radiographic	Gastroenterology/Urology

COMPOSITE MANUFACTURING, INC. 949-361-7580
970 B Calle Amanecer, San Clemente, CA 92673
FDA Number: 2030380
  Holder, Head, Neurosurgical (Skull Clamp)   Cns/Neurology
  Regulator, Vacuum   General

COMPOSITES HORIZONS, INC. 626-331-0861
1471 Industrial Park St., Covina, CA 91722
FDA Number: 2026030   *Fax:* 626-339-3220

COMPOSITES HORIZONS, INC. 626-331-0861 *(cont'd)*
E-mail: chi@chi-covina.com
Web site: www.chi-covina.com
Medical Products Sales Volume: $5,000,000
Annual Revenue: $10-$25 Million
Year Founded: 1981
Total Employees: 95   *Marketing Staff:* 2   *Sales Staff:* 2
Ownership: Public
Stock Symbol: HAMP
Traded On: London
Quality System Registration Information: ISO9001
Produces/Sells CE-marked Devices: N
Distribution: Manufacturer Direct
General Admin.: Jeff Hynes/President, Chief Executive Officer
Production: Steve Peery/Vice President Quality Assurance
Research: Kevin Synder/Vice President Engineering
  Board, Spine   Orthopedics
  Head Rest, Neurosurgical   Cns/Neurology
  Table, Radiographic, Stationary Top   Radiology

COMPREHENSIVE SAFETY COMPLIANCE, INC. 412-826-5480
295 William Pitt Way, Pittsburgh, PA 15238-1328
FDA Number: n/a   *Fax:* 412-826-5486
Web site: www.csc-inc.cc
Medical Products Sales Volume: $1,800,000
Annual Revenue: $1-$5 Million
Ownership: Private
Produces/Sells CE-marked Devices: N
Federal Procurement Eligibility: Small Business
Distribution: Service Direct
General Admin.: Amy Lecocq/Assistant Manager
    John Frye/President, Chief Executive Officer
  Service, Consulting   General
  Service, Maintenance/Repair   General
  Training Aid   Orthopedics

COMPRESSION DESIGN 866-421-1267
140 W. Washington Ave., Suite 200, 616-931-1267
Zeeland, MI 49464
FDA Number: 3005694039   *Fax:* 616-582-5911
E-mail: info@compressiondesign.com
Web site: www.compressiondesign.com
Ownership: Private
Produces/Sells CE-marked Devices: N
  Binder, Elastic   General
  Stocking, Elastic, Physical Medicine   Physical Med

COMPRESSOR TECHNOLOGIES
See Dntlworks Equipment Corporation

COMPRESSUS INC. 202-742-4307
101 Constitution Ave. N.w., Suite 800, Washington, DC 20001
FDA Number: 3004849214   *Fax:* 202-742-4286
E-mail: info@compressus.com
Web site: www.compressus.com
Ownership: Private
Produces/Sells CE-marked Devices: N
  System, Communication, Image, Digital   Radiology

COMPSEE OPTICAL DATA COLLECTION SYSTEMS
See Compsee, Inc.

COMPSEE, INC. 800-628-3888
400 N. Main St., PO Box 1209, 321-724-4321
Mount Gilead, NC 27306
FDA Number: n/a   *Fax:* 321-723-2895
E-mail: sales@compsee.com
Web site: www.compsee.com
Medical Products Sales Volume: $17,000,000
Annual Revenue: $10-$25 Million
Year Founded: 1985
Total Employees: 100   *Marketing Staff:* 4   *Sales Staff:* 17
Ownership: MCRAE INDUSTRIES
Produces/Sells CE-marked Devices: Y
Federal Procurement Eligibility: Small Business
Distribution: Manufacturer Direct, Manufacturer Through Distributor, Exporter
General Admin.: Gary McRae/Chief Executive Officer
    Gary McRae/President
Mktg./Adv.: Billy Graham/Director Marketing
    Sally Morgan/Manager Advertising
    Billy Graham/Manager International & National Sales
    Billy Graham/Vice President Sales
  Computer Software   General

COMPU TECH INC 407-788-6353
407 Wekiva Springs Road, Suite 347, Longwood, FL 32779
FDA Number: 1064588   *Fax:* 407-788-2476
E-mail: info@tims.com
Web site: www.tims.com

COMPU TECH INC   407-788-6353 *(cont'd)*
- *Ownership:* Private
- *Produces/Sells CE-marked Devices:* N
  - Device, Storage, Image, Digital   Radiology

COMPUCHEM
- *See Lab Corp Of America*

COMPUMED MEDICATION DISPENSER, INC.
- *See Compumed, Inc.*

COMPUMED, INC.   800-421-3395
5777 West Century Blvd.,, Suite 360,   310-258-5000
Los Angeles, CA 90045
- *FDA Number:* 2020657   *Fax:* 310-645-5880
- *E-mail:* sales@compumed.net
- *Web site:* http://www.compumed.net
- *Total Employees:* 18
- *Ownership:* Public
- *Stock Symbol:* CMPD
- *Traded On:* OTC Bulletin
- *Produces/Sells CE-marked Devices:* N
- *General Admin.:* Mr. Xiaoli Bi/Chief Technology Officer
  - Mr. Maurizio Vecchione/President, Chief Executive Officer
- *Research:* Dr. Louai Al-Dayeh/Director Scientific Affairs
  - Analyzer, ECG   Cardiovascular
  - Densitometer, Bone, Single Photon   Radiology
  - Electrocardiograph, Single Channel   Cardiovascular
  - Spirometer, Diagnostic (Respirometer)   Anesthesiology
  - Transmitter/Receiver System, Physiological, Telephone   Cardiovascular

COMPUMED, INC.   800-722-4417
P.O. Box 126, 574 Lane 40, Burlington, WY 82433   307-868-2555
- *FDA Number:* n/a   *Fax:* 307-868-2550
- *E-mail:* info@compumed.com
- *Web site:* www.compumed.com
- *Annual Revenue:* $0-$1 Million
- *Year Founded:* 1988
- *Total Employees:* 3   *Marketing Staff:* 1   *Sales Staff:* 1
- *Ownership:* COMPUMED, INC.
- *Produces/Sells CE-marked Devices:* N
- *Federal Procurement Eligibility:* Small Business
- *Distribution:* Manufacturer Direct, Manufacturer Through Distributor
- *General Admin.:* Steve Christiansen/President, Chief Executive Officer
  - Dispenser, Other   General

COMPUMEDICS USA, LTD.   877-717-3975
6605 West WT Harris Blvd, Suite F,   704-749-3200
Charlotte, NC 28269
- *FDA Number:* 1650946   *Fax:* 704-749-3299
- *Ownership:* Private
- *Produces/Sells CE-marked Devices:* N
  - Electrode, Cutaneous   Cns/Neurology
  - Electroencephalograph   Cns/Neurology
  - Electromyograph, Diagnostic   Physical Med
  - Stimulator, Auditory, Evoked Response   Cns/Neurology
  - Stimulator, Electrical, Evoked Response   Cns/Neurology
  - Stimulator, Photic, Evoked Response   Cns/Neurology

COMPUTATIONAL DIAGNOSTICS, INC.   412-681-9990
5001 Baum Blvd., Suite 530, Pittsburgh, PA 15213
- *FDA Number:* 2530126   *Fax:* 412-681-9994
- *E-mail:* enos@cdi.com
- *Web site:* cdi.com
- *Annual Revenue:* $1-$5 Million
- *Year Founded:* 1988
- *Total Employees:* 20   *Marketing Staff:* 6   *Sales Staff:* 4
- *Ownership:* Private
- *Produces/Sells CE-marked Devices:* N
- *Federal Procurement Eligibility:* Small Business
- *Distribution:* Manufacturer Direct
- *General Admin.:* Dr. Robert Sclabassi/Chief Executive Officer
  - Dr. Sheri Enos Ph.D./President
  - Electroencephalograph   Cns/Neurology
  - Stimulator, Electrical, Evoked Response   Cns/Neurology

COMPUTER INSTRUMENTS CORP.
- *See Polar Electro Inc.*

COMPUTER MARKETPLACE
- *See Medical Marketplace*

COMPUTER OPTICS INC.   603-889-2116
120 Derry Road, Hudson, NH 03051
- *FDA Number:* n/a   *Fax:* 603-889-2393
- *E-mail:* contact@computeroptics.com
- *Web site:* www.computeroptics.com
- *Medical Products Sales Volume:* $1,800,000
- *Annual Revenue:* $1-$5 Million
- *Year Founded:* 1985
- *Total Employees:* 19   *Marketing Staff:* 1   *Sales Staff:* 4

COMPUTER OPTICS INC.   603-889-2116 *(cont'd)*
- *Ownership:* Private
- *Produces/Sells CE-marked Devices:* N
- *Federal Procurement Eligibility:* Small Business, VA Contract
- *Distribution:* Manufacturer Direct, OEM, Importer, Exporter
  - Light, Surgical, Ceiling Mounted   Surgery

COMPUTER PROGRAMS AND SYSTEMS, INC.   251-639-8100
6600 Wall Street, Mobile, AL 36695
- *FDA Number:* n/a   *Fax:* 251-639-8214
- *Ownership:* Private
- *Produces/Sells CE-marked Devices:* N
  - System, Communication, Image, Digital   Radiology

COMPUTER SPORTS MEDICINE, INC.   781-297-2034
101 Tosca Dr., Stoughton, MA 02072
- *FDA Number:* 1224631
  - Isokinetic Testing And Evaluation System   Physical Med

COMPUTERIZED IMAGING REFERENCE   800-617-1177
SYSTEMS, INC.
2428 Almeda Ave. Suite 212, Norfolk, VA 23513   757-855-2765
- *FDA Number:* 1121267   *Fax:* 757-857-0523
- *E-mail:* admin@cirsinc.com
- *Web site:* www.cirsinc.com
- *Ownership:* Private
- *Produces/Sells CE-marked Devices:* N
  - Phantom, Anthropomorphic, Radiographic   Radiology

COMPUTERIZED MEDICAL SYSTEMS, INC.   468-587-2550
1145 Corporate Lake Dr., Olivette, MO 63132
- *FDA Number:* 1937649
- *Ownership:* Private
- *Produces/Sells CE-marked Devices:* N
  - Accelerator, Linear, Medical   Radiology
  - Applicator, Radionuclide, Manual   Radiology
  - Block, Beam Shaping, Radionuclide   Radiology
  - Radiotherapy Unit, Charged-Particle   Radiology
  - Simulator, Radiotherapy, Special Purpose   Radiology
  - System, Communication, Image, Digital   Radiology
  - System, Planning, Radiation Therapy Treatment   Radiology
  - Tester, Radiology   Radiology

COMPUTERIZED RADIATION SCANNERS, INC.   (800) 848-3852
140 Sopwith Dr., Vero Beach, FL 32968   772-562-0405
- *FDA Number:* 1054745   *Fax:* (772) 562-7472
- *E-mail:* crs7@bellsouth.net
- *Annual Revenue:* $0-$1 Million
- *Year Founded:* 1979
- *Ownership:* Private
- *Produces/Sells CE-marked Devices:* N
- *Federal Procurement Eligibility:* Small Business
- *Distribution:* Manufacturer Direct, Manufacturer Through Distributor
  - Accessory - Film Dosimetry System   Radiology
  - Block, Therapy, Radiation   Radiology
  - Collimator, Therapeutic X-Ray, Orthovoltage   Radiology
  - Device, Limiting, Beam, Diagnostic, X-Ray   Radiology

COMPUTERIZED SCREENING, INC. (CSI)   800-533-9230
9550 Gateway Drive, Reno, NV 89521-8924   775-359-1191
- *FDA Number:* 2022315   *Fax:* 775-359-7879
- *E-mail:* sales@computerized-screening.com
- *Web site:* www.computerized-screening.com
- *Medical Products Sales Volume:* $2,000,000
- *Annual Revenue:* $1-$5 Million
- *Year Founded:* 1978
- *Total Employees:* 50   *Marketing Staff:* 2   *Sales Staff:* 3
- *Ownership:* Private
- *Produces/Sells CE-marked Devices:* Y
- *Federal Procurement Eligibility:* Small Business, GSA Contract
- *Distribution:* Manufacturer Direct, Manufacturer Through Distributor
- *General Admin.:* Charles P. Bluth/President, Chief Executive Officer
- *Mktg./Adv.:* Mr. Charles R. Sullivan/Executive Vice President Marketing & Sales
  - Mrs. Tracy Sullivan/Vice President Sales
- *Production:* Mr. Mike Estelle/Vice President Manufacturing & Operations
- *Research:* Mr. Chris Munz/Director Technology
  - Computer, Blood Pressure   Cardiovascular
  - Monitor, Blood Pressure, Indirect, Automatic   Cardiovascular

COMPUTERIZED THERMAL IMAGING CO.   801-776-4700
1719 West 2800 South, Ogden, UT 84401
- *FDA Number:* 3002222542
- *Ownership:* Private
- *Produces/Sells CE-marked Devices:* N
  - Lamp, Infrared   Physical Med

COMPUTERS UNLIMITED   406-255-9500
2407 Montana Avenue, Billings, MT 59101-2336
- *FDA Number:* n/a   *Fax:* 406-255-9595

COMPUTERS UNLIMITED 406-255-9500 (cont'd)
E-mail: sales@cu.net
Web site: www.cu.net
Medical Products Sales Volume: $15,000,000
Annual Revenue: $10-$25 Million
Year Founded: 1978
Total Employees: 165   Marketing Staff: 3   Sales Staff: 7
Ownership: Private
Produces/Sells CE-marked Devices: N
Federal Procurement Eligibility: Small Business
Distribution: Manufacturer Direct, Exporter
General Admin.: Dr. Michael Schaer/President
Mktg./Adv.: Heidi Thometz/Director Marketing & Sales
   Deanna Carpenter/Manager Market Research
   Computer Software   General

COMPUTRITION, INC. 800-222-4488
19808 Nordhoff Place, 800-222-4458
Chatsworth, CA 91311
FDA Number: n/a   Fax: 818-701-1702
E-mail: info@computrition.com
Web site: www.computrition.com
Medical Products Sales Volume: $6,400,000
Annual Revenue: $10-$25 Million
Year Founded: 1980
Total Employees: 60   Marketing Staff: 6   Sales Staff: 8
Ownership: Private
Produces/Sells CE-marked Devices: N
Federal Procurement Eligibility: Small Business, Female Owned, GSA Contract
Distribution: Manufacturer Direct
General Admin.: Brian Andrews/Chief Information Officer
   Scott Saklad/Chief Operating Officer
   Ellyn Luros-Elson/President, Chief Executive Officer
Mktg./Adv.: Marty Yadrick/Managing Director Marketing
Production: Kim Goldberg/Vice President Operations
   Bridget Harvey-Elliott/Vice President Services
Research: Joseph Bibbo/Executive Vice President Research & Development
   Computer Software   General

COMPUTRON MEDICAL CORP. 847-952-8800
1697 W. Imperial Court, Mount Prospect, IL 60056
FDA Number: 3003982553
Ownership: Private
Produces/Sells CE-marked Devices: N
   Table, Radiographic   Radiology

COMPVIEW MEDICAL LLC 503-641-8439
10035 Sw Arctic Drive, Beaverton, OR 97005
FDA Number: 3006293618
   System, Communication, Image, Digital   Radiology

COMTECH EFDATA 480-333-2200
2114 West 7th Street, Tempe, AZ 85281
FDA Number: 3005124123   Fax: 480-333-2540
E-mail: sales@comtechefdata.com
Web site: www.comtechefdata.com
Ownership: Private
Produces/Sells CE-marked Devices: N
General Admin.: Larry Dumouchel/Chief Financial Officer, Vice President
   Robert McCollum/Senior Vice President
   Diathermy, Shortwave   Physical Med

CON MED
See Conmed Corporation

CON-CISE CONTACT LENS CO. 800-772-3911
14450 Doolittle Drive, PO Box 2198, 510-483-9400
San Leandro, CA 94577
FDA Number: n/a   Fax: 510-483-0292
E-mail: support@con-cise.com
Web site: www.con-cise.com
Medical Products Sales Volume: $8,300,000
Annual Revenue: $25-$50 Million
Year Founded: 1959
Total Employees: 100   Marketing Staff: 4   Sales Staff: 8
Ownership: Private
Produces/Sells CE-marked Devices: N
Federal Procurement Eligibility: Small Business
Distribution: Manufacturer Direct
General Admin.: Carl Moore/President, Chief Executive Officer
   Roxanne Goggin/Vice President Human Resources
   Lynda Baker/Vice President, General Manager
Mktg./Adv.: Lynda Baker/Vice President Marketing
   Dan Davis/Vice President Sales
Production: Greg Goodhart/Vice President Manufacturing
Research: Robert Mandell, O.D./Research & Development Associate
   Lens, Contact(rigid Gas Permeable)-extended Wear   Ophthalmology
   Lens, Contact, Bifocal   Ophthalmology

CON-CISE CONTACT LENS CO. 800-772-3911 (cont'd)
   Lens, Contact, Extended-Wear   Ophthalmology
   Lens, Contact, Gas-Permeable   Ophthalmology

CONAIR CORP. 203-351-9000
150 Milford Rd., East Windsor, NJ 08520
FDA Number: 2242745   Fax: 203-351-9180
Ownership: Private
Produces/Sells CE-marked Devices: N
   Massager, Therapeutic   Physical Med
   Toothbrush, Powered   Dental And Oral

CONCENTRIC 800-572-7867
2222 15th St., Rockford, IL 61104 815-398-4400
FDA Number: n/a   Fax: 815-398-5977
E-mail: info.usro@concentricAB.com
Web site: www.concentricab.com
Annual Revenue: $50-$100 Million
Total Employees: 490
Ownership: Private
Quality System Registration Information: ISO9001
Produces/Sells CE-marked Devices: N
Distribution: Manufacturer Through Distributor, Importer, Exporter
General Admin.: John Pepe/President
   Corbett Howard/Vice President Human Resources
Mktg./Adv.: Steve Zarembski/Director Marketing
   John Larson/Vice President Sales
Production: Mike Moris/Vice President Manufacturing
Research: Mark Kemmer/Vice President Research & Development
   Pump, Laboratory   Chemistry
   Valve, Other   Chemistry

CONCENTRIC MEDICAL, INC. 650-938-2100
301 East Evelyn Ave., Mountain View, CA 94041
FDA Number: 2954917   Fax: 650-938-2700
Web site: http://concentric-medical.com
Ownership: Private
Produces/Sells CE-marked Devices: N
General Admin.: Ms. Maria Sainz/Chief Executive Officer
Mktg./Adv.: Ms. Kimberly Bridges/Vice President Sales
Production: Mr. Robert Nichols/Vice President Operations
   Ms. Kirsten Valley/Vice President Regulatory Affairs
Finance: Mr. Brett Hale/Chief Financial Officer
   Catheter, Intravascular, Diagnostic   Cardiovascular
   Catheter, Percutaneous   Cardiovascular
   Catheter, Thrombus Retriever   Cardiovascular
   Embolization Device   Cardiovascular
   Guidewire, Catheter   Cardiovascular

CONCEPT HEALTH, LLC 215-364-3600
3600 Boundbrook Ave., Trevose, PA 19053
FDA Number: 2530957   Fax: 215-364-7290
E-mail: info@gentell.com
Web site: www.gentell.com
Annual Revenue: $1-$5 Million
Year Founded: 1999
Total Employees: 36   Marketing Staff: 1   Sales Staff: 12
Ownership: Private
Produces/Sells CE-marked Devices: N
Federal Procurement Eligibility: Small Business
Distribution: Manufacturer Through Distributor, Exporter
General Admin.: David A. Navazio/Executive Vice President
   Bandage, Adhesive   Surgery
   Dressing, Wound and Burn, Hydrogel   Surgery

CONCEPT II, INC. 800-245-5676
105 Industrial Park Drive, 802-888-7971
Morrisville, VT 05661
FDA Number: n/a   Fax: 802-888-4791
E-mail: rowing@concept2.com
Web site: http://rowing.concept2.com
Medical Products Sales Volume: $4,300,000
Year Founded: 1976
Total Employees: 55   Marketing Staff: 5   Sales Staff: 10
Ownership: Private
Produces/Sells CE-marked Devices: N
Federal Procurement Eligibility: Small Business, GSA Contract
Distribution: Manufacturer Direct
General Admin.: Richard A. Dreissigacker/President
Mktg./Adv.: Peter D. Dreissigacker/Vice President Marketing
   Robert Brody/Vice President Marketing
   Ergometer, Other   Anesthesiology

CONCEPT INTERNATIONAL
See Conmed Linvatec

CONCEPT MARKETING, INC. 800-926-3277
1000 Arendell St., Morehead City, NC 28557
FDA Number: 1039016   Fax: 800-247-7290

CONCEPT MARKETING, INC.   800-926-3277 *(cont'd)*
E-mail: info@Conceptsjewelry.com
Web site: www.concept-marketing-inc.com
Ownership: Private
Produces/Sells CE-marked Devices: N
  Perforator, Ear-Lobe   Ear/Nose/Throat

CONCEPT PLASTICS, INC.   336-889-2001
1210 Hickory Chapel, High Point, NC 27260
FDA Number: 1062244
Ownership: Private
Produces/Sells CE-marked Devices: N
  Bed, Manual   General

CONCEPTION TECHNOLOGIES   800-995-8081
6835 Flanders Dr. Suite 500,   858-824-0888
San Diego, CA 92121
FDA Number: 2031824   *Fax:* 858-824-0891
Ownership: Private
Produces/Sells CE-marked Devices: N
  Media, Reproductive   Obstetrics/Gynecology
  Microtools, Assisted Reproduction   Obstetrics/Gynecology
  System, Water, Reproduction, Assisted, And Purification   Obstetrics/Gynecology

CONCEPTS INTERNATIONAL, INC.   800-627-9729
224 East Main Street, Summerton, SC 29148   866-467-6352
FDA Number: n/a   *Fax:* 864-508-8022
E-mail: info@conceptsintl.com
Web site: www.conceptsintl.com
Annual Revenue: $0-$1 Million
Year Founded: 1975
Total Employees: 5
Ownership: Private
Produces/Sells CE-marked Devices: N
Federal Procurement Eligibility: Small Business
Distribution: Manufacturer Through Distributor
General Admin.: Donna J. Price/Chief Financial Officer, Vice President
           Allen L. Price/President, Chief Executive Officer
  Curing Unit, Acrylic   Dental And Oral
  Dispenser, Soap   General
  Eyeglasses, Safety   Ophthalmology
  Fountain, Eye Wash   Chemistry
  Goggles, Protective, Eye   Ophthalmology
  Lamp, Other   General
  Loupe, Diagnostic/Surgical   Surgery
  Magnifier, Hand-Held, Low-Vision   Ophthalmology
  Marker, X-Ray   Radiology
  Mask, Face   General
  Mount, Equipment   General
  Sink, Hospital   General
  Viewer/Magnifier   Hematology

CONCEPTUS, INC.   650-962-4000
331 East Evelyn Ave., Mountain View, CA 94041
FDA Number: 2951250   *Fax:* 650-962-5200
E-mail: publicrelations@conceptus.com
Web site: www.conceptus.com
Year Founded: 1992
Ownership: Public
Stock Symbol: CPTS
Traded On: NASDAQ
Produces/Sells CE-marked Devices: N
Distribution: Manufacturer Direct, Manufacturer Through Distributor, Manufacturer Through Manufacturer Reps, Importer, Exporter
General Admin.: Gregory Lichtwardt/Chief Financial Officer, Treasurer
           Ms. Julie Brooks/Executive Vice President
           Mark Sieczkarek/President, Chief Executive Officer
Mktg./Adv.: Ulric Cote/Executive Vice President Sales
           Mr. Todd Sloan/Vice President Marketing
Research: Mr. Edward Yu/Vice President Clinical Research
  Catheter, Assisted Reproduction   Obstetrics/Gynecology
  Catheter, Intrauterine, With Introducer   Obstetrics/Gynecology
  Catheter, Transcervical, Balloon Tuboplasty   Obstetrics/Gynecology
  Guidewire, Catheter   Cardiovascular
  Hysteroscope   Obstetrics/Gynecology
  Insert, Tubal Occlusion   Obstetrics/Gynecology
  Resectoscope   Gastroenterology/Urology

CONCISE CONTACT LENS CO.
See Con-Cise Contact Lens Co.

CONCO MEDICAL COMPANY
See Hartmann-Conco Inc.

CONCOA   800-225-0473
1501 Harpers Road,   757-422-8330
Virginia Beach, VA 23454
FDA Number: 1121335
E-mail: e-mail@concoa.com   *Fax:* 757-422-3125
Web site: www.concoa.com

CONCOA   800-225-0473 *(cont'd)*
Medical Products Sales Volume: $12,900,000
Annual Revenue: $10-$25 Million
Year Founded: 1987
Total Employees: 130   *Marketing Staff:* 15   *Sales Staff:* 10
Ownership: Private
Quality System Registration Information: ISO9001
Produces/Sells CE-marked Devices: Y
Federal Procurement Eligibility: Small Business
Distribution: Manufacturer Through Distributor, OEM
General Admin.: Sande Dukas/President
Mktg./Adv.: Pat Carlucci/Vice President Marketing & Sales
Production: Ernest Filomarino/Director Quality Assurance
  Flowmeter, Back-Pressure Compensated, Thorpe Tube   Anesthesiology
  Regulator, Pressure, Gas Cylinder   Anesthesiology

CONCORD CONSULTING GROUP, INC.   978-369-8744
30 Monument Square, Suite 215, Concord, MA 01742-1895
FDA Number: n/a   *Fax:* 978-369-7823
E-mail: corp@concordcg.com
Web site: www.concordcg.com
Medical Products Sales Volume: $2,500,000
Annual Revenue: $1-$5 Million
Year Founded: 1976
Total Employees: 14
Ownership: Private
Produces/Sells CE-marked Devices: N
Federal Procurement Eligibility: Small Business
Distribution: Manufacturer Direct
General Admin.: Lawrence D. Lorah/President
           Michael J. Lydon/Principal
           Philip G. Drew/Principal
Mktg./Adv.: Paul E. Mawn/Vice President Business Development
  Service, Consulting   General
  Service, Engineering/Design   General

CONCORD MEDICAL PRODUCTS   978-857-5884
72 Bristers Hill Rd., Concord, MA 01742-3502
FDA Number: n/a
Ownership: Private
Produces/Sells CE-marked Devices: N
  Defibrillator, Automatic, External, For Out-of-hospital Use   Cardiovascular

CONCORDE BATTERY   626-813-1234
2009 San Bernardino Rd., West Covina, CA 91790-1006
FDA Number: n/a   *Fax:* 626-813-1235
E-mail: customer-service@concordebattery.com
Web site: www.concordebattery.com
Medical Products Sales Volume: $55,000
Annual Revenue: $1-$5 Million
Year Founded: 1977
Total Employees: 150   *Marketing Staff:* 3   *Sales Staff:* 7
Ownership: Private
Quality System Registration Information: ISO9001
Produces/Sells CE-marked Devices: N
Federal Procurement Eligibility: Small Business
Distribution: Manufacturer Through Distributor, Manufacturer Through Manufacturer Reps
Mktg./Adv.: Mr. Skip Koss/Vice President Marketing
Production: Ms. Shelley Johnson/Director Customer Services
  Battery   General

CONDEX INTERNATIONAL, INC.   310-618-8444
2441 W. 205th St. Suite C200e, Torrance, CA 90501
FDA Number: 2032899
Ownership: Private
Produces/Sells CE-marked Devices: N
  Protector, Skin Pressure   General

CONE BIOPRODUCTS   830-379-0197
1012 N. Austin St., Seguin, TX 78155
FDA Number: 3004152597   *Fax:* 830-379-0471
E-mail: wkcone@conebio.com
Web site: www.conebio.com
Ownership: Private
Produces/Sells CE-marked Devices: N
  Control, Hemoglobin   Hematology

CONE BIOTECH, INC.
See Consolidated Technologies, Inc.

CONE INSTRUMENTS, INC.   800-321-6964
5201 Naiman Pkwy., Solon, OH 44139-1005   440-248-1035
FDA Number: 1525771   *Fax:* 440-248-9477
E-mail: info@coneinstruments.com
Web site: www.coneinstruments.com
Medical Products Sales Volume: $12,000,000
Annual Revenue: $5-$10 Million
Year Founded: 2000

CONE INSTRUMENTS, INC.　800-321-6964 *(cont'd)*

Total Employees: 23　　Marketing Staff: 2　　Sales Staff: 8
Ownership: Private
Produces/Sells CE-marked Devices: Y
Federal Procurement Eligibility: Small Business, VA Contract
Distribution: Manufacturer Through Distributor, Service Direct, Exclusive
Distributor, Importer, Exporter
General Admin.: Mary Ann Griffith/Administrator
　　　　　　Patrick C. Beck/President
Mktg./Adv.: Bill Kahle/Manager Marketing

Apron, Lead, Radiographic	Radiology
Cable/Lead, ECG	Cardiovascular
Detector, Blood Flow, Ultrasonic (Doppler)	Cardiovascular
Gel, Ultrasonic Transmission	General
Illuminator, Radiographic Film	Radiology
Marker, X-Ray	Radiology
Monitor, Fetal, Ultrasonic	Obstetrics/Gynecology
Monitor, X-Ray Film Processor Quality Control	Radiology
Phantom, Dental, Radiographic	Dental And Oral
Phantom, Ultrasound	Radiology
Printer, Image, Video	General
Scanner, Ultrasonic, General Purpose	Radiology
Scanner, Ultrasonic, Obstetrical/Gynecological	Obstetrics/Gynecology
Scanner, Ultrasonic, Obstetrical/Gynecological, Mobile	Obstetrics/Gynecology
Scanner, Ultrasonic, Other	Radiology
Scanner, Ultrasonic, Small Parts	Radiology
Screen, Intensifying, Radiographic, Dental	Dental And Oral
Shield, X-Ray	Radiology
Storage Unit, X-Ray Film	Radiology
System, Marking, Film, Radiographic	Radiology
Table, Ultrasound	General
Towel/Towelette, Paper	General
Transducer, Ultrasonic	Cardiovascular

CONFECTION MEDICALE D.R. INC.　514-252-5553

200-4220 Rue De Rouen, Montreal H1V 3T2 Canada
FDA Number: 9616605

Fiber, Absorbent	General

CONFI DENTAL LAB, INC.　201-385-8777

50 Park Ave. Suite # 200-201, Dumont, NJ 07628
FDA Number: 3005396474
Ownership: Private
Produces/Sells CE-marked Devices: N

CONFIDANT INTERNATIONAL, LLC　919-806-4323

2530 Meridian Parkway, Suite 300, Durham, NC 27713
FDA Number: 3005175625

Transmitter/Receiver System, Physiological, Radiofrequency	Cardiovascular

CONFIRM MONITORING SYSTEMS, INC.　303-699-3356

109 inverness Drive East, Unit F, Englewood, CO 80112-5105
FDA Number: 1725050　　　　　　　　Fax: 303-699-8255
E-mail: sales@confirmmonitoring.com
Web site: www.confirmmonitoring.com
Medical Products Sales Volume: $2,600,000
Year Founded: 2001
Total Employees: 16
Ownership: Cantel Medical Corp.
Produces/Sells CE-marked Devices: Y
Federal Procurement Eligibility: Female Owned

Sterilization Process Indicator, Biological	General

CONFIRMA, INC.　877-811-2356
　　　　　　　　　　　　　　　425-691-1400

11040 Main Street, Suite 100,
Bellevue, WA 98004
FDA Number: 3003982333　　　　　　Fax: 425-691-1599
E-mail: support@confirma.com
Web site: www.confirma.com
Medical Products Sales Volume: $10,800,000
Year Founded: 1998
Total Employees: 79
Ownership: Private
Stock Symbol: 11
Traded On: Tokyo
Quality System Registration Information: ISO9001
Produces/Sells CE-marked Devices: Y
Federal Procurement Eligibility: Small Business
General Admin.: Daniel Bickford/Executive Vice President
　　　　　　Wayne Wager/President, Chief Executive Officer
Mktg./Adv.: Ward Sparacio/Vice President International Sales
　　　　　　Mary Gatewood/Vice President Marketing
Research: Paul Budak/Vice President Research & Development & Operations
Finance: Nick Dykstra/Chief Financial Officer

Coil, Magnetic Resonance, Specialty	Radiology
Image Processing System	Radiology

CONFLEX　800-225-4296
　　　　　　262-512-2665

W130 N10751 Washington Drive,
Germantown, WI 53022
FDA Number: n/a　　　　　　　　Fax: 262-512-1665
E-mail: conflex@execpc.com
Web site: www.conflex.com
Annual Revenue: $5-$10 Million
Total Employees: 25
Ownership: Private
Produces/Sells CE-marked Devices: N
Distribution: Manufacturer Through Distributor, Manufacturer Through
Manufacturer Reps
General Admin.: Kevin Laird/Chief Executive Officer
　　　　　　Kevin Laird/President
　　　　　　Bill Morrissey/Vice President, General Manager
Mktg./Adv.: Joe Morrissey/Director Marketing
　　　　　　Mark Kubisiak/Director Product Development
　　　　　　Joe Morrissey/Manager International & National Sales
Production: Wayne Fredricks/Vice President Manufacturing

Wrap, Sterilization	General

CONFLUENT SURGICAL,INC　888-734-2583
　　　　　　781-693-2300

101A First Ave., Waltham, MA 02451
FDA Number: 3003157248　　　　　　Fax: 781-693-2331
E-mail: info@confluentsurgical.com
Web site: www.confluentsurgical.com
Ownership: Covidien Ltd.
Produces/Sells CE-marked Devices: N

Applicator, Vaginal	Obstetrics/Gynecology
Barrier, Adhesion, Absorbable	Obstetrics/Gynecology
Laparoscope, General & Plastic Surgery	Surgery
Regulator, Pressure, Gas Cylinder	Anesthesiology
Sealant, Polymerizing	General
Surgical Instrument, Obstetric/Gynecologic	Obstetrics/Gynecology
Syringe, Piston	General

CONFORMA LABORATORIES, INC.　800-426-1700
　　　　　　757-321-0200

4705 Colley Ave., Norfolk, VA 23508
FDA Number: n/a　　　　　　　　Fax: 757-321-0201
E-mail: info@conforma.com
Web site: www.conforma.com
Annual Revenue: $1-$5 Million
Ownership: Private
Produces/Sells CE-marked Devices: N
Federal Procurement Eligibility: Small Business
Distribution: Manufacturer Direct
General Admin.: Kevin Sanford/President

Lens, Other	Ophthalmology

CONFORMIS INC.　(781) 345-9001

11 North Ave., Burlington, MA 01803
FDA Number: 3004153240　　　　　Fax: (781) 345-0147
E-mail: conformis@racepointgroup.com
Web site: www.conformis.com
Ownership: Private
Produces/Sells CE-marked Devices: N
General Admin.: Mr. Philipp Lang/President, Chairman, Chief Executive Officer
　　　　　　Mr. David Cerveny/Senior Vice President
Mktg./Adv.: Mr. Jong Lee/Senior Vice President Marketing
　　　　　　Mr. Robert Phelps/Senior Vice President Sales
Finance: Ms. Judith Huber/Chief Financial Officer

Forceps	Orthopedics
Prosthesis, Knee, Femorotibial, Non-Constrained	Orthopedics
Prosthesis, Knee, Hemi-, Tibial Resurfacing	Orthopedics
Prosthesis, Knee, Hemi-, Tibial Resurfacing, Uncemented	Orthopedics
Prosthesis, Knee, Patellofemoral, Semi-Constrained	Orthopedics

CONFORMIS, INC.　781-345-9001

11 North Ave., Burlington, MA 01803
FDA Number: 3004153240　　　　　Fax: 781-345-0147
Web site: www.conformis.com
Year Founded: 2004
Ownership: Private
Produces/Sells CE-marked Devices: N
General Admin.: Mr. Klaus Rademacher/Chairman
　　　　　　Dr. Philipp Lang/President, Chief Executive Officer
Mktg./Adv.: Mr. Jong Lee/Senior Vice President Marketing
　　　　　　Mr. Robert Phelps/Senior Vice President Sales
Production: Mr. Robert Calcote/Senior Vice President Operations
　　　　　　Mr. Amit Shah/Vice President Quality Assurance & Regulatory Affairs
Research: Dr. Dan Steines/Senior Vice President Research & Development
Finance: Ms. Judith Huber/Chief Financial Officer

Forceps	Orthopedics
Orthopedic Manual Surgical Instrument	Orthopedics
Prosthesis, Knee Patellofemorotibial, Partial, Semi-constrained, Cemented, Polymer/metal/polymer	Orthopedics
Prosthesis, Knee, Femorotibial, Non-Constrained	Orthopedics
Prosthesis, Knee, Hemi-, Tibial Resurfacing, Uncemented	Orthopedics

CONFORMIS, INC. — 781-345-9001 *(cont'd)*
Prosthesis, Knee, Patellofemorotibial, Semi-Constrained — Orthopedics

CONFORTAIRE INC — 662-842-2966
2133 South Veterans Blvd., Tupelo, MS 38804
FDA Number: 3004723313
Fax: 662-842-2912
Ownership: Private
Produces/Sells CE-marked Devices: N
General Admin.: Mr. Mike Hurst/General Manager
   Ms. Gayle Dillard/Human Resources Representative
   Ms. Laura Plyler/Owner
   Mr. Mike Plyler/Owner, Chief Executive Officer
   Mr. Drew Lawson/Shipping Manager
Production: Ms. Tanya Edwards/Customer Service Representative
   Mr. James Parker/Production Supervisor
Research: Mr. Ken Steele/Product Development Specialist
Finance: Ms. Tammy Pettit/Controller

Cushion, Wheelchair (Pad)	Physical Med
Head Rest, Neurosurgical	Cns/Neurology
Mattress, Non-Powered Flotation Therapy	Physical Med
Orthosis, Cervical-Thoracic, Rigid	Physical Med
Protector, Skin Pressure	General
Splint, Abduction, Congenital Hip Dislocation	Physical Med
Support, Patient Position	Anesthesiology

CONFROM MEDICAL PRODUCTS DIV
See Ansell Healthcare, Inc.

CONGER DENTAL SUPPLY, INC. — 800-255-3983
302 Rosedale Lane, Bristol, TN 37620
FDA Number: n/a
Fax: 866-526-6437
E-mail: info@congerdental.net
Web site: www.congerdental.net
Annual Revenue: $0-$1 Million
Year Founded: 1916
Ownership: Private
Produces/Sells CE-marked Devices: N
Federal Procurement Eligibility: Small Business
Distribution: Manufacturer Direct, Manufacturer Through Distributor, Manufacturer Through Manufacturer Reps, Service Direct, Exclusive Distributor, Importer

Dental Laboratory Equipment	Dental And Oral

CONGLOM — 514-333-6666
2600, Marie-Curie Ave., St-Laurent, QUE H4S 2C3 Canada
FDA Number: n/a
Fax: 514-333-4070
E-mail: mail@conglom.com
Year Founded: 1922
Ownership: Private
Produces/Sells CE-marked Devices: N
Distribution: Exclusive Distributor, Importer

CONKIN SURGICAL INSTRUMENTS LTD. — 416-922-9496
30 Lesmill Road, Unit 4, Toronto, ON M3B 2T6 Canada
FDA Number: 8022078
Fax: 416-922-3501
E-mail: info@conkinsurgical.com
Web site: http://www.conkinsurgical.com
Year Founded: 1974
Total Employees: 10
Ownership: Private
Produces/Sells CE-marked Devices: N
Distribution: Manufacturer Direct, OEM, Exclusive Distributor, Exporter

CONMED CORPORATION — 800-448-6506
310 Broad Street, Utica, NY 13501
FDA Number: 1317214
Fax: 800-438-3051
E-mail: customer_service@mail.conmed.com
Web site: www.conmed.com
Year Founded: 1970
Total Employees: 3100
Ownership: Conmed Corporation
Stock Symbol: CNMD
Traded On: NASDAQ
Produces/Sells CE-marked Devices: N
Distribution: Manufacturer Direct, OEM
General Admin.: Joe Corasanti/President, Chief Executive Officer

Adapter, Electrosurgical Unit, Cable	Surgery
Adapter, Unit, Electrosurgical, Hand-Controlled	Surgery
Autotransfusion Unit (Blood)	Anesthesiology
Blade, Electrosurgery, Laparoscopic	Surgery
Bottle, Collection, Vacuum (Aspirator)	General
Cable, Electrode	Physical Med
Cable, Electrosurgical Unit	Surgery
Cable/Lead, TENS	Cns/Neurology
Camera, Video, Multi-Image	General
Cannula, Suction/Irrigation, Laparoscopic	Surgery
Coagulator, Laparoscopic, Unipolar	Obstetrics/Gynecology
Coagulator/Cutter, Endoscopic, Bipolar	Obstetrics/Gynecology
Coagulator/Cutter, Endoscopic, Unipolar	Obstetrics/Gynecology
Controller, Foot, Handpiece And Cord	Dental And Oral
Electrocautery Unit, Endoscopic	Obstetrics/Gynecology

CONMED CORPORATION — 800-448-6506 *(cont'd)*

Electrocautery Unit, Line-Powered	Surgery
Electrode, Defibrillator	Cardiovascular
Electrode, Electrocardiograph	Cardiovascular
Electrode, Electrosurgery, Laparoscopic	Surgery
Electrode, Electrosurgical, Active (Blade)	Surgery
Electrode, Electrosurgical, Active, Foot Controlled	Surgery
Electrode, Electrosurgical, Return (Ground, Dispersive)	Surgery
Electrode, Esophageal	Gastroenterology/Urology
Electrode, Holter	Cardiovascular
Electrode, Metallic With Soft Pad Covering	Physical Med
Electrode, Needle	Cns/Neurology
Electrode, Neuromuscular Stimulator	Cns/Neurology
Electrode, Other	General
Electrosurgical Equipment, General Purpose	Surgery
Electrosurgical Equipment, Special Purpose	Surgery
Electrosurgical Unit, Anesthesiology Accessories	Surgery
Electrosurgical Unit, Cardiovascular	Cardiovascular
Electrosurgical Unit, Cutting & Coagulation Device	Surgery
Electrosurgical Unit, Gastroenterology	Gastroenterology/Urology
Electrosurgical Unit, General Purpose (ESU)	Surgery
Equipment, Suction/Irrigation, Laparoscopic	Surgery
Forceps, Electrosurgical	Surgery
Forceps, Endoscopic	Gastroenterology/Urology
Forceps, Grasping, Atraumatic	Surgery
Forceps, Grasping, Traumatic	Surgery
Gel, Ultrasonic Coupling	Physical Med
Gel, Ultrasonic Transmission	General
Generator, Power, Electrosurgical	Surgery
Holder, Intravascular Catheter	General
Instrument, Dissecting, Laparoscopic	Surgery
Instrument, Electrosurgery, Laparoscopic	Surgery
Irrigator, Suction	General
Kit, Administration, Intravenous	General
Kit, Cholecystectomy	Gastroenterology/Urology
Light Source, Endoscope, Xenon Arc	Surgery
Light, Surgical, Endoscopic	Surgery
Module, Control, Electrosurgery	Surgery
Needle, Insufflation, Laparoscopic	Surgery
Probe, Electrocauterization, Multi-Use	Surgery
Probe, Electrocauterization, Single-Use	Surgery
Probe, Electrosurgery, Endoscopy	Surgery
Probe, Other	General
Probe, Suction, Irrigator/Aspirator, Laparoscopic	Surgery
Scissors, Disposable	General
Scissors, Laparoscopy	Surgery
System, Evacuation, Smoke, Laser	Surgery
Tip, Suction, Electrosurgical	Surgery
Trocar, Abdominal	Gastroenterology/Urology
Trocar, Gallbladder	Gastroenterology/Urology
Trocar, Laparoscopic	Surgery
Trocar, Other	General

CONMED CORPORATION
See Conmed Corporation

CONMED CORPORATION — 800-448-6506
5836 Success Drive, Rome, NY 13440
FDA Number: n/a
Fax: 800-438-3051
E-mail: customer_service@mail.conmed.com
Web site: www.conmed.com
Total Employees: 3100
Ownership: Conmed Corporation
Stock Symbol: CNMD
Traded On: NASDAQ
Produces/Sells CE-marked Devices: N
General Admin.: Joe Corasanti/President, Chief Executive Officer

Electrode, Cutaneous	Cns/Neurology
Electrode, Electrocardiograph	Cardiovascular
Electrode, Electrosurgical, Active (Blade)	Surgery
Electrosurgical Unit, Cutting & Coagulation Device	Surgery

CONMED CORPORATION (HQ)
See Conmed Corporation

CONMED ELECTROSURGERY — 800-448-6506
14603 E. Fremont Avenue, Centennial, CO 80112
FDA Number: 1720159
Fax: 800-438-3051
E-mail: customer_service@mail.conmed.com
Web site: www.conmed.com
Total Employees: 3100
Ownership: Conmed Corporation
Stock Symbol: CNMD
Traded On: NASDAQ
Produces/Sells CE-marked Devices: N
General Admin.: Joe Corasanti/President, Chief Executive Officer

Electrosurgical Unit, Cutting & Coagulation Device	Surgery
Exhaust System, Surgical	Surgery
Unit, Electrosurgical, Endoscopic (with Or Without Accessories), Reprocessed	Gastroenterology/Urology

CONMED ENDOSCOPIC TECHNOLOGIES 315-797-8375
525 French Road, Utica, NY 13502
FDA Number: 1223688
Fax: 315-797-0321
E-mail: customer_service@mail.conmed.com
Web site: www.conmed.com
Total Employees: 3100
Ownership: Conmed Corporation
Stock Symbol: CNMD
Traded On: NASDAQ
Produces/Sells CE-marked Devices: N
General Admin.: Joe Corasanti/President, Chief Executive Officer

Accessories, Bite Blocks (For Endoscope)	Gastroenterology/Urology
Accessories, Bronchoscope	Ear/Nose/Throat
Accessories, Cleaning Brushes (For Endoscope)	Gastroenterology/Urology
Bronchoscope, Rigid	Ear/Nose/Throat
Brush, Biopsy, Bronchoscope (Non-Rigid)	Anesthesiology
Brush, Biopsy, General & Plastic Surgery	Surgery
Brush, Cytology, Endoscopic	Gastroenterology/Urology
Catheter, Biliary	Gastroenterology/Urology
Dilator, Esophageal	Gastroenterology/Urology
Electrosurgical Unit, Gastroenterology	Gastroenterology/Urology
Electrosurgical, Unit, Gastroenterology	Gastroenterology/Urology
Endoscope	Gastroenterology/Urology
Forceps, Biopsy, Electric	Gastroenterology/Urology
Forceps, Biopsy, Non-Electric	Gastroenterology/Urology
Ligator, Esophageal	Gastroenterology/Urology
Needle, Aspiration And Injection, Disposable	Surgery
Needle, Endoscopic	Gastroenterology/Urology
Snare, Flexible	Gastroenterology/Urology
Snare, Non-Electrical	Gastroenterology/Urology
Tube, Gastrointestinal	Gastroenterology/Urology

CONMED LINVATEC 800-448-6506
11311 Concept Blvd, Largo, FL 33773-4908
FDA Number: 1017294
Fax: 800-438-3051
E-mail: customer_service@mail.conmed.com
Web site: www.conmed.com
Year Founded: 1963
Total Employees: 3100
Ownership: Conmed Corporation
Stock Symbol: CNMD
Traded On: NASDAQ
Quality System Registration Information: ISO9001
Produces/Sells CE-marked Devices: Y
Distribution: Manufacturer Direct, Manufacturer Through Distributor, Manufacturer Through Manufacturer Reps, Exporter
General Admin.: Joe Corasanti/President, Chief Executive Officer

Arthroscope	Orthopedics
Bit, Drill	Orthopedics
Blade, Surgical, Saw, General & Plastic Surgery	Surgery
Burr	Ear/Nose/Throat
Burr, Dental	Dental And Oral
Burr, Surgical, General & Plastic Surgery	Surgery
Camera, Cine, Endoscopic (Without Audio)	Surgery
Camera, Television, Surgical (Without Audio)	Surgery
Curette, Adenoid	Ear/Nose/Throat
Drill, Surgical, ENT (Electric Or Pneumatic)	Ear/Nose/Throat
Driver, Surgical, Pin	Surgery
Electrode, Electrosurgical, Return (Ground, Dispersive)	Surgery
Electrosurgical Unit, Cutting & Coagulation Device	Surgery
Endoscope	Gastroenterology/Urology
Fastener, Fixation, Biodegradable, Soft Tissue	Orthopedics
Guide	Orthopedics
Instrument, Surgical, Powered, Pneumatic	Orthopedics
Knife, Orthopedic	Orthopedics
Laparoscope, Gynecologic	Obstetrics/Gynecology
Motor, Drill, Pneumatic	Cns/Neurology
Motor, Surgical Instrument, AC-Powered	Surgery
Motor, Surgical Instrument, Pneumatic-Powered	Surgery
Needle, Suture, Disposable	Surgery
Orthopedic Manual Surgical Instrument	Orthopedics
Pump, Infusion	General
Rasp, Bone	Orthopedics
Rasp, Surgical, General & Plastic Surgery	Surgery
Reamer	Orthopedics
Retractor, Surgical	Surgery
Saw, Pneumatically Powered	Surgery
Screw, Fixation, Bone	Orthopedics
Staple, Absorbable	Orthopedics
Staple, Implantable	Surgery
Surgical Instrument, Orthopedic, AC-Powered Motor	Orthopedics
System, Extraction, Cement Removal	Orthopedics
Tape, Television & Video, Endoscopic	Gastroenterology/Urology

CONMED LINVATEC ENDOSCOPY 800-448-6506
7416 Hollister Avenue, Goleta, CA 93117
FDA Number: 2028292
Fax: 800-438-3051
E-mail: customer_service@mail.conmed.com
Web site: www.conmed.com
Total Employees: 3100

CONMED LINVATEC ENDOSCOPY 800-448-6506 (cont'd)
Ownership: Conmed Corporation
Stock Symbol: CNMD
Traded On: NASDAQ
Produces/Sells CE-marked Devices: N
General Admin.: Joe Corasanti/President, Chief Executive Officer

Accessories, Arthroscope	Orthopedics
Accessories, Arthroscopic	Orthopedics
Accessories, Surgical Camera	Surgery
Arthroscope	Orthopedics
Camera, Television, Endoscopic (Without Audio)	Surgery
Camera, Television, Surgical (Without Audio)	Surgery
Device, Storage, Image, Digital	Radiology
Endoscope	Gastroenterology/Urology
Fiberoptic Light Source & Carrier	Ear/Nose/Throat
Hysteroscope	Obstetrics/Gynecology
Image Processing System	Radiology
Insufflator, Laparoscopic	Obstetrics/Gynecology
Laparoscope, General & Plastic Surgery	Surgery
Light Source, Endoscope, Xenon Arc	Surgery
Nasopharyngoscope (Flexible Or Rigid)	Ear/Nose/Throat
Tray, Surgical Instrument	Surgery

CONNECT IMAGING, INC. 866-949-7227
850 West Hind Dr., Suite 116, Honolulu, HI 96821 808-373-7048
FDA Number: 3004061281
Fax: 808-373-7017
E-mail: info@connectimaging.com
Web site: www.connectimaging.com
Ownership: Private
Produces/Sells CE-marked Devices: N

Image Processing System	Radiology

CONNECTED MEDICAL SYSTEMS LLC 662-455-4523
2005 Highway 82 West, Greenwood, MS 38930
FDA Number: 3004582444
Ownership: Private
Produces/Sells CE-marked Devices: N

Device, Storage, Images, Ophthalmic	Ophthalmology

CONNECTICUT HYPODERMICS, INC. 203-265-4881
519 Main St., Yalesville, CT 06492-1723
FDA Number: n/a
Fax: 203-284-1520
E-mail: sales@connhypo.com
Web site: www.connhypo.com
Medical Products Sales Volume: $10,000,000
Annual Revenue: $10-$25 Million
Year Founded: 1979
Total Employees: 90   Marketing Staff: 1   Sales Staff: 5
Ownership: Private
Produces/Sells CE-marked Devices: N
Federal Procurement Eligibility: Small Business
Distribution: Manufacturer Direct, Service Direct
General Admin.: Leonard Tutolo/Chief Executive Officer
    Steven Tutolo/President
    Mr. Mark Tutolo/Vice President
Mktg./Adv.: Chris Tutolo/Vice President Sales

Cannula, Injection	Gastroenterology/Urology
Cannula, Venous	Cardiovascular

CONNECTOR CONTACTS 877-463-9029
714 East Edna Place, Covina, CA 91723
FDA Number: n/a
Fax: 877-263-9029
E-mail: sales@connectorcontacts.com
Web site: www.connectorcontacts.com
Annual Revenue: $0-$1 Million
Ownership: Private
Produces/Sells CE-marked Devices: N
Federal Procurement Eligibility: Small Business
Distribution: Manufacturer Direct

Light, Surgical, Connector	Surgery

CONNEXMD 206-356-4568
800 W Park Avenue, Suite 3, Leland, WA 98368
FDA Number: 3004111564
Web site: www.connexmd.com
Ownership: Private
Produces/Sells CE-marked Devices: N

Image Processing System	Radiology

CONNOR-WINFIELD CORP. 630-851-4722
2111 Comprehensive Dr., Aurora, IL 60505-1345
FDA Number: n/a
Fax: 630-851-5040
E-mail: sales@conwin.com
Web site: www.conwin.com
Annual Revenue: $50-$100 Million
Total Employees: 500   Marketing Staff: 2   Sales Staff: 16
Ownership: Private
Quality System Registration Information: ISO9001; ISO9002
Produces/Sells CE-marked Devices: N

CONNOR-WINFIELD CORP. 630-851-4722 *(cont'd)*
Federal Procurement Eligibility: Small Business
Distribution: Manufacturer Direct, Manufacturer Through Manufacturer Reps
General Admin.: Robert Olp/President, Chief Executive Officer
    Cindy Garbe/Vice President Human Resources
    Dan Olp/Vice President, General Manager
Mktg./Adv.: Bob Dranter/Director Marketing
    Ken Hartman/Director Product Development
    Mary Antich/Manager International Sales
    Ray Kepka/Manager National Sales
Production: Joe Bloch/Director Quality Assurance
    Dave Jahr/Manager Materials
  Component, Electronic   General

CONOPTICS, INC. 800-748-3349
19 Eagle Rd., Danbury, CT 06810-4127   **203-743-3349**
FDA Number: n/a   Fax: 203-790-6145
E-mail: sales@conoptics.com
Web site: www.conoptics.com
Annual Revenue: $1-$5 Million
Year Founded: 1981
Total Employees: 11   *Marketing Staff:* 2   *Sales Staff:* 2
Ownership: Private
Produces/Sells CE-marked Devices: Y
Federal Procurement Eligibility: Small Business
Distribution: Manufacturer Direct, Service Direct, Exporter
General Admin.: Ronald Pizzo/President
Mktg./Adv.: Richard Kocka/Vice President Marketing
Research: Robert Enscoe/Vice President Engineering
  Accessories, Laser   General
  Production Equipment   General

CONQUEST CONDOMS LLC 305-279-0089
9020 S.w. 83rd. St., Miami, FL 33173
FDA Number: 3006312204
  Condom   Obstetrics/Gynecology

CONRAC CORP., DISPLAY PRODUCTS GROUP
See Conrac, Inc.

CONRAC, INC. 626-480-0095
5124 Commerce Drive, Baldwin Park, CA 91706
FDA Number: n/a   Fax: 626-480-0077
E-mail: monitors@conrac.com
Web site: www.conrac.com
Medical Products Sales Volume: $2,200,000
Annual Revenue: $5-$10 Million
Year Founded: 2001
Total Employees: 15   *Marketing Staff:* 1   *Sales Staff:* 2
Ownership: Private
Produces/Sells CE-marked Devices: Y
Federal Procurement Eligibility: Small Business
Distribution: Manufacturer Direct, Service Direct
General Admin.: Ray Allen/Chief Financial Officer, Vice President
    William Moeller/President
  Monitor, Video, Endoscope   General

CONRAY, INC. 623-465-7881
1950 East Watkins Rd.,, Suite 110, Phoenix, AZ 85034
FDA Number: 2028808
  Exerciser, Powered   Anesthesiology

CONSOLIDATED INSTRUMENTS CORP. 410-391-9116
8825 Kelso Dr., Essex, MD 21221
FDA Number: n/a
Annual Revenue: $0-$1 Million
Ownership: Private
Produces/Sells CE-marked Devices: N
Distribution: Manufacturer Through Distributor, Manufacturer Through
Manufacturer Reps, OEM, Service Direct, Exporter
  Equipment/Service, Quality Control   General

CONSOLIDATED MACHINE CORP.
See Consolidated Stills & Sterilizers

CONSOLIDATED MACHINE CORP. 617-782-6072
76 Ashford Street, Boston, MA 02134-0003
FDA Number: 1219189   Fax: 617-787-5865
E-mail: info@consteril.com
Web site: www.consteril.com
Medical Products Sales Volume: $100,000
Annual Revenue: $5-$10 Million
Year Founded: 1946
Total Employees: 2   *Marketing Staff:* 1   *Sales Staff:* 4
Ownership: Private
Produces/Sells CE-marked Devices: N
Federal Procurement Eligibility: Small Business
Distribution: Manufacturer Direct, Manufacturer Through Distributor, Manufacturer Through Manufacturer Reps

CONSOLIDATED MACHINE CORP. 617-782-6072 *(cont'd)*
  Sterilizer, Steam (Autoclave)   General

CONSOLIDATED MEDICAL EQUIPMENT INC.
See Conmed Corporation

CONSOLIDATED MEDICAL TECHNOLOGIES
See Habley Medical Technology Corp.

CONSOLIDATED POLYMER TECHNOLOGIES
See Saint-Gobain Performance Plastics/Clearwater

CONSOLIDATED STILLS & STERILIZERS 617-782-6072
76 Ashford Street, Boston, MA 02134-0003
FDA Number: n/a   Fax: 617-787-5865
E-mail: info@consteril.com
Web site: www.consteril.com
Medical Products Sales Volume: $100,000
Annual Revenue: $1-$5 Million
Year Founded: 1946
Total Employees: 2   *Marketing Staff:* 2   *Sales Staff:* 4
Ownership: Private
Produces/Sells CE-marked Devices: N
Federal Procurement Eligibility: Small Business
Distribution: Manufacturer Direct, Manufacturer Through Manufacturer Reps,
Exporter
General Admin.: William A. Barnstead/President, Chief Executive Officer
Mktg./Adv.: George H. Lowe/Vice President Marketing & Sales
Production: W. A. Barnstead/Production Engineer
  Distilling Unit   Chemistry
  Purifier, Water   Chemistry
  Sterilizer, Laboratory   Microbiology
  Sterilizer, Steam (Autoclave)   General
  Sterilizer, Steam, Bulk   General
  Sterilizer, Vapor   General
  Washer/Sterilizer   General

CONSOLIDATED TECHNOLOGIES, INC. 512-445-5100
4401 Sedrich Lane, Building 1, Suite 107,
Austin, TX 78744
FDA Number: 1650189
Medical Products Sales Volume: $4,000,000
Annual Revenue: $1-$5 Million
Ownership: Private
Produces/Sells CE-marked Devices: N
Federal Procurement Eligibility: Small Business
Distribution: Manufacturer Direct, OEM
  Antibody, Polyclonal   Microbiology
  Contract Laboratory   General
  Reagent, Other   General
  Serum, Animal   Pathology
  Standard/Control, All Types   Chemistry

CONSTRUCTION SPECIALTIES INC. 800-233-8493
6696 Route. 405, Muncy, PA 17756   **570-546-2255**
FDA Number: n/a
Web site: www.c-sgroup.com
Medical Products Sales Volume: $10,000,000
Ownership: Private
Produces/Sells CE-marked Devices: N
Federal Procurement Eligibility: Female Owned
Distribution: Manufacturer Through Manufacturer Reps
  Bumper Guard, Corner   General
  Cover, Other   General
  Floor Mat   General
  Rail, Wall Side   General
  Security Equipment/Supplies   General
  Wallpaper, Antibacterial   General

CONSULTANTS FOR MEDICAL TECHNOLOGY, INC.
See Cmt, Inc.

CONSUMAQUIP CORPORATION 305-592-4510
7240 NW 12th Street, Miami, FL 33126-1909
FDA Number: n/a   Fax: 305-593-9618
E-mail: pcbarcos@calmaquip.com
Annual Revenue: $10-$25 Million
Total Employees: 49   *Marketing Staff:* 3   *Sales Staff:* 16
Ownership: Private
Produces/Sells CE-marked Devices: N
Federal Procurement Eligibility: Small Business, Minority Owned
Distribution: Exclusive Distributor, Importer, Exporter
General Admin.: Mr. Raul J Gutierrez III/President, Chief Executive Officer
Mktg./Adv.: Ms. Patricia Cabarcos/Director Marketing & Sales
Production: Mr. Bo Hollsten/Consumables Product Manager
  Balloon, Angioplasty, Peripheral, Heated   Cardiovascular
  Catheter, Biliary, General & Plastic Surgery   Surgery
  Scanner, Computed Tomography, X-Ray (CAT, CT)   Cns/Neurology
  Scanner, Magnetic Resonance (NMR/MRI)   Radiology
  Transducer, Ultrasonic, Diagnostic   Radiology
  Transducer, Ultrasonic, Intravaginal   Obstetrics/Gynecology

CONSUMAQUIP CORPORATION
305-592-4510 *(cont'd)*
Washer, Laundry .... General

CONTAINER RESEARCH CORP.
610-459-2160
Hollow Hill Road, PO Box 0159, Glen Riddle, PA 19037-0159
FDA Number: 2529959   Fax: 610-558-4578
E-mail: wconner@crc-flex.com
Web site: www.crc-flex.com/
Medical Products Sales Volume: $24,700,000
Year Founded: 1955
Total Employees: 120   *Marketing Staff:* 3   *Sales Staff:* 3
Ownership: Private
Produces/Sells CE-marked Devices: N
Federal Procurement Eligibility: Small Business
Distribution: Manufacturer Direct
Sterilizer, Laboratory .... Microbiology

CONTAMINATION CONTROL PRODUCTS
877-553-2676
1 Third Avenue, Box 578, Neptune, NJ 07753   732-869-3400
FDA Number: n/a   Fax: 732-869-2999
E-mail: info@ccpcleanroom.com
Web site: www.ccpcleanroom.com
Medical Products Sales Volume: $2,000,000
Annual Revenue: $5-$10 Million
Year Founded: 1988
Total Employees: 1500   *Marketing Staff:* 2   *Sales Staff:* 10
Ownership: Supply King, Inc.
Produces/Sells CE-marked Devices: N
Distribution: Manufacturer Direct
General Admin.: Sheldon Kawut/President, Chief Executive Officer
     Adrienne Levine/Vice President, General Manager
Mktg./Adv.: Henry Levenstein/Director Marketing
     Henry Levenstein/Vice President Marketing
Purchasing: Ann-Marie Nichols/Manager Materials, Director Purchasing
Cleanroom Equipment .... General
Equipment, Control, Pollution .... General
Laminar Air Flow Unit .... General
Table, Other .... General

CONTEC, INC.
800-289-5762
525 Locust Grove, Spartanburg, SC 29303   864-503-8333
FDA Number: n/a   Fax: 864-503-8444
E-mail: wipers@contecinc.com
Web site: www.contecinc.com
Year Founded: 1988
Total Employees: 157   *Marketing Staff:* 2
Ownership: Private
Produces/Sells CE-marked Devices: N
Distribution: Manufacturer Direct, Exclusive Distributor
General Admin.: Jack McBride/President
Mktg./Adv.: Fernando Costanzo/Manager International Sales
     Melissa Sullivan/Manager Marketing
     Cara Ritchie/Manager National Sales
     Rick Harward/Manager National Sales
Cleaner, Medical Device .... General
Sponge, Other .... General

CONTECH MEDICAL, INC.
401-351-4890
99 Hartford Ave., Providence, RI 02909-3326
FDA Number: 1221541   Fax: 401-421-5072
E-mail: info@contechmedical.com
Web site: www.contechmedical.com
Medical Products Sales Volume: $7,500,000
Annual Revenue: $5-$10 Million
Year Founded: 1987
Total Employees: 75   *Marketing Staff:* 2   *Sales Staff:* 3
Ownership: Private
Quality System Registration Information: ISO9002
Produces/Sells CE-marked Devices: Y
Federal Procurement Eligibility: Small Business
Distribution: OEM
General Admin.: Raymond A. Byrnes/President, Chief Executive Officer
Mktg./Adv.: Frank Barrett/Vice President Sales
Production: Chris Byrnes/Vice President Operations
Contract Manufacturing .... General
Contract Packaging .... General
Fitting, Luer .... General
Guidewire .... Cardiovascular
Molding, Injection .... General
System, Infusion, Administration, Drug, Implantable .... General
Tubing, Non-Invasive .... Surgery

CONTECH PACKAGING, INC.
See Contech Medical, Inc.

CONTEMPORARY PRODUCTS, INC.
800-424-2444
2055 South Main St.,   868-343-1100
Middletown, CT 04103
FDA Number: n/a   Fax: 868-343-1118

CONTEMPORARY PRODUCTS, INC.
800-424-2444 *(cont'd)*
E-mail: cpi@contemporaryproducts.com
Web site: www.contemporaryproducts.com
Medical Products Sales Volume: $400,000
Annual Revenue: $5-$10 Million
Year Founded: 1988
Total Employees: 7
Ownership: Private
Produces/Sells CE-marked Devices: N
Federal Procurement Eligibility: Small Business
Distribution: Manufacturer Direct, Manufacturer Through Manufacturer Reps, OEM
General Admin.: Bill Smith/Chief Executive Officer
     Barry Schwartz/President
Mktg./Adv.: Barry Schwartz/Manager Contracts
     Barry Schwartz/Manager International Accounts
     Barry Schwartz/Manager National Sales
Production: Joe Newman/Director Operations
     Kevin Fijak/Director Quality Assurance
     Joe Newman/Vice President Manufacturing
Cart, Gas Cylinder (Carrier) .... Anesthesiology
Cart, Multipurpose .... General
Cart, Supply .... General
Cylinder, Oxygen .... Anesthesiology
Nebulizer, Direct Patient Interface .... Anesthesiology
Pump, Aspiration, Portable .... Anesthesiology
Regulator, Oxygen, Mechanical .... General
Suction Apparatus, Ward Use, Portable, AC-Powered .... Surgery
Tank, Full Body (Bath) .... General

CONTEX, INC.
800-626-6839
4505 Van Nuys Blvd., Sherman Oaks, CA 91403   818-788-5836
FDA Number: 2031102   Fax: 818-788-5078
E-mail: info@contexusa.com
Web site: www.oklens.com
Medical Products Sales Volume: $810,000
Year Founded: 1962
Total Employees: 15
Ownership: Private
Produces/Sells CE-marked Devices: N
Federal Procurement Eligibility: Small Business
Lens, Contact (Other Material) .... Ophthalmology

CONTEXT SOFTWARE SYSTEMS, INC.
See Captiva Software Corporation

CONTINENTAL ACRYLICS
See Plaskolite West Inc.

CONTINENTAL FELT CO. INC.
See Aetna Foot Products/Div. Of Aetna Felt Corporation

CONTINENTAL FUELS, INC.
713-231-0330
600 Travis, Suite 6910, Houston, TX 77002
FDA Number: n/a
Year Founded: 1989
Ownership: Public
Stock Symbol: CNFU
Traded On: OTC Bulletin
Produces/Sells CE-marked Devices: N

CONTINENTAL HYDRODYNE SYSTEMS, INC.
See Continental Hydrodyne Systems, Inc.

CONTINENTAL MANUFACTURING CO.
800-325-1051
13330 Lake Front Drive, Earth City, MO 63045   314-770-9949
FDA Number: n/a   Fax: 314-770-9938
E-mail: contmfg@contico.com
Web site: www.continental-mfg.com
Annual Revenue: $50-$100 Million
Total Employees: 500   *Sales Staff:* 50
Ownership: Private
Distribution: Manufacturer Through Distributor
General Admin.: Michael D. Boland/President
Mktg./Adv.: Rex Thompson/Manager National Sales
Housekeeping Equipment .... General
Waste Receptacle, General Purpose .... General

CONTINENTAL MEDICAL LABORATORIES, INC.
262-534-2787
813 Ela Avenue, Waterford, WI 53185
FDA Number: 2128604   Fax: 262-534-7611
E-mail: cmlinc@tds.net
Web site: www.cmlmedicalkits.com
Medical Products Sales Volume: $2,200,000
Year Founded: 1988
Total Employees: 14
Ownership: Private
Produces/Sells CE-marked Devices: N
Federal Procurement Eligibility: Small Business
Kit, Catheterization, Sterile Urethral .... Gastroenterology/Urology
Kit, Suctioning, Tracheostomy and Nasal .... Surgery

CONTINENTAL MEDICAL LABORATORIES, INC. 262-534-2787
(cont'd)

    Kit, Wound Dressing   Surgery

CONTINENTAL METAL PRODUCTS CO., INC. 800-221-4439
35 Olympia Avenue, Woburn, MA 01801   781-935-4400
FDA Number: n/a   Fax: 781-935-4404
E-mail: sales@continentalmetal.com
Web site: www.continentalmetal.com
Medical Products Sales Volume: $5,000,000
Year Founded: 1948
Total Employees: 45
Ownership: Private
Produces/Sells CE-marked Devices: N
Federal Procurement Eligibility: Small Business, VA Contract
Distribution: Manufacturer Direct, Manufacturer Through Distributor, OEM, Service Direct, Exclusive Distributor, Importer
General Admin.: Paul Siegal/President, Chief Executive Officer
Mktg./Adv.: Paul Siegal/Manager Advertising
           Stephen Siegal/Vice President Marketing
Research: Paul Malenchini/Vice President Research & Development
Finance: S. Streiff/Controller
  Cabinet Casework, General Purpose   General
  Cabinet Casework, Modular   General
  Cabinet, Warming   General
  Sink, Hospital   General
  Station, Nourishment   General

CONTINENTAL SCIENTIFIC   800-523-7138
539 Dunksferry Rd., Bensalem, PA 19020-5908   215-244-1400
FDA Number: n/a   Fax: 215-244-9579
E-mail: jjh@continental-refrig.com
Web site: www.continentalscientific.com
Annual Revenue: $1-$5 Million
Ownership: Private
Produces/Sells CE-marked Devices: Y
Federal Procurement Eligibility: Small Business
Distribution: Manufacturer Direct, Manufacturer Through Distributor, Manufacturer Through Manufacturer Reps, OEM, Exporter
  Refrigerator, Foodservice   General

CONTINENTAL SOFT LENS, INC.   303-795-2130
9350 Yale Lane, Hghlnds Ranch, CO 80130
FDA Number: 1721765
Ownership: Private
Produces/Sells CE-marked Devices: N
  Lenses, Soft Contact, Daily Wear   Ophthalmology

CONTINENTAL WATER CONDITIONING
  See Millipore Corporation

CONTINUUM, INC.   888-532-1064
3150 Central Expressway,   408-727-3240
Santa Clara, CA 95051
FDA Number: 2918486   Fax: 408-727-3550
E-mail: info@continuumlasers.com
Web site: www.continuumlasers.com
Medical Products Sales Volume: $6,100,000
Year Founded: 1975
Total Employees: 55
Ownership: Private
Stock Symbol: XLTC
Traded On: NASDAQ
Quality System Registration Information: ISO9001
Produces/Sells CE-marked Devices: Y
Federal Procurement Eligibility: Small Business
Distribution: Manufacturer Direct, Manufacturer Through Distributor, OEM
General Admin.: Dr. Laurence Cramer/Executive Vice President, General Manager
Mktg./Adv.: Mr. Mark Ortiz/Director Medical Marketing
Finance: Mr. Timothy Gehlmann/Vice President Finance
  Laser, Dental   Dental And Oral
  Laser, Surgical   Surgery
Medical Product Subsidiaries (Listed Separately)
  Continuum

CONTOUR FORM PRODUCTS   800-223-8808
38 Stewart Avenue, PO Box 328,   724-588-4452
Greenville, PA 16125
FDA Number: 2523708   Fax: 724-588-8641
E-mail: info@contourform.com
Web site: www.warmandform.com
Annual Revenue: $0-$1 Million
Year Founded: 1978
Total Employees: 20   Sales Staff: 1
Ownership: Private
Produces/Sells CE-marked Devices: N
Federal Procurement Eligibility: Small Business
Distribution: Manufacturer Direct

CONTOUR FORM PRODUCTS   800-223-8808 *(cont'd)*
General Admin.: Robert Kroner/Chief Executive Officer
  Orthosis, Other   Physical Med
  Support, Back   Orthopedics
  Support, Wrist   Physical Med

CONTOUR MEDICAL, INC.
  See Cfi Medical Solutions (Contour Fabricators, Inc.)

CONTOUR PAK, INC.   800-926-2228
346 Rheem Blvd., Suite 104, Moraga, CA 94556 925-631-9601
FDA Number: n/a   Fax: 925-631-9607
E-mail: info@contourpak.com
Web site: www.contourpak.com
Medical Products Sales Volume: $2,100,000
Year Founded: 1990
Total Employees: 25
Ownership: Private
Produces/Sells CE-marked Devices: N
Federal Procurement Eligibility: Small Business, Female Owned
Distribution: Manufacturer Direct, Manufacturer Through Distributor, Manufacturer Through Manufacturer Reps
General Admin.: Mr. David Bayliss/Chief Executive Officer, Chief Operating Officer
          Ms. Alice M. Mayn/President, Chief Executive Officer
  Pack, Cold   General

CONTRA ANGLE; PROPHY ANGLE   513-682-2520
9790 Inter-Ocean Dr., Cincinnati, OH 45246
FDA Number: n/a   Fax: 513-682-2525
Web site: www.professionalcase.com
Annual Revenue: $0-$1 Million
Total Employees: 15   *Marketing Staff:* 1   *Sales Staff:* 2
Ownership: Private
Produces/Sells CE-marked Devices: N
Federal Procurement Eligibility: Small Business, Minority Owned, Female Owned
Distribution: Manufacturer Direct, Manufacturer Through Distributor
General Admin.: Dianne Brown/Chief Executive Officer
          Paul Biel/General Manager
          Thomas Brown/President
Mktg./Adv.: Erin R. Biel/Vice President Sales
Production: Paul Biel/Vice President Production
  Bag, Medical, Physician   General

CONTROL BIONICS   202-257-7090
333 North Broad St., Fairborn, OH 45324
FDA Number: 3006789226
Ownership: Private
Produces/Sells CE-marked Devices: N
  Communication System, Powered   Physical Med
  Environmental Control System, Powered   Physical Med

CONTROL PRODUCTS INC.   952-448-2217
1724 Lake Dr. W., Chanhassen, MN 55317
FDA Number: n/a   Fax: 952-448-1606
E-mail: sales@controlproductsinc.com
Web site: www.controlproductsinc.com
Annual Revenue: $10-$25 Million
Year Founded: 1985
Ownership: Private
Produces/Sells CE-marked Devices: N
Federal Procurement Eligibility: Small Business
Distribution: Manufacturer Through Distributor, OEM
General Admin.: Chris Berghoff/Chief Executive Officer
  Monitor, Temperature (Self-Contained)   General

CONTROL RESEARCH, INC.   847-392-4770
1775 Winnetka Circle, Rolling Meadows, IL 60008
FDA Number: 3004188986
Ownership: Private
Produces/Sells CE-marked Devices: N
  Illuminator, Radiographic Film   Radiology

CONTROL SOLUTIONS, INC.   630-806-7062
2520 Diehl Road, Aurora, IL 60502
FDA Number: 1424661   Fax: 630-802-7065
E-mail: sales@controls.com
Web site: www.controls.com
Annual Revenue: $25-$50 Million
Year Founded: 1989
Total Employees: 50   *Marketing Staff:* 2   *Sales Staff:* 2
Ownership: Private
Quality System Registration Information: ISO9001
Produces/Sells CE-marked Devices: Y
Federal Procurement Eligibility: Small Business
Distribution: Manufacturer Direct, Manufacturer Through Distributor, OEM, Exclusive Distributor
  Stimulator, Muscle, Electrical-Powered (EMS)   Physical Med
  Unit, Therapy, Current, Interferential   Cns/Neurology

CONTROL-X MEDICAL, INC.
800-777-9729
1755 Atlas Street, Columbus, OH 43228-9648
614-777-9729
FDA Number: 1528327
Fax: 614-777-0395
E-mail: sales@cxmed.com
Web site: www.cxmed.com
Medical Products Sales Volume: $4,200,000
Annual Revenue: $1-$5 Million
Total Employees: 15
Ownership: Private
Quality System Registration Information: ISO9002
Produces/Sells CE-marked Devices: Y
Federal Procurement Eligibility: Small Business
Distribution: Manufacturer Direct, Manufacturer Through Distributor, OEM, Exclusive Distributor, Importer, Exporter
General Admin.: Zsigmond Kovacs/President
Mktg./Adv.: Larry M. Hurd/Vice President Marketing & Sales
Production: Laszlo Adrovitz/Vice President Operations

Collimator, Radiographic, Automatic	Radiology
Collimator, Radiographic, Manual	Radiology
Generator, Diagnostic X-Ray, High Voltage, 3-Phase	Radiology
Generator, Diagnostic X-Ray, High Voltage, Single Phase	Radiology
Holder, Radiographic Cassette, Wall-Mounted	Radiology
Radiographic Unit, Diagnostic, Chest	Radiology
Radiographic Unit, Diagnostic, Fixed (X-Ray)	Radiology
Table, Radiographic, Non-Tilting, Powered	Radiology
Table, Radiographic, Stationary Top	Radiology
Table, Radiographic, Tilting	Radiology

CONTROLAIR, INC.
800-216-3636
8 Columbia Drive, Amherst, NH 03031
603-886-9400
FDA Number: n/a
Fax: 603-889-1844
E-mail: sales@controlair.com
Web site: www.controlair.com
Annual Revenue: $5-$10 Million
Year Founded: 1987
Ownership: Private
Quality System Registration Information: ISO9001
Produces/Sells CE-marked Devices: Y
Federal Procurement Eligibility: Small Business
Distribution: Manufacturer Direct, Manufacturer Through Distributor
General Admin.: Scott Comstock/President
Mktg./Adv.: Mark Levine/Director Marketing & Sales
James Doyle/Director Product Development

Ventilator, Other	Anesthesiology

CONTROLLED CHEMICALS, INC.
734-769-5940
317 South Division, Suite 9, Ann Arbor, MI 48104
FDA Number: 1835319

Supplies, Blood Bank	Hematology

CONTROLLED ENVIRONMENT EQUIPMENT CORP.
800-569-5444
59 Sanford Drive, Suite 32, Gorham, ME 04038
207-854-9126
FDA Number: n/a
Fax: 207-854-4357
E-mail: ceec@ceecusa.com
Web site: www.ceecusa.com
Medical Products Sales Volume: $1,100,000
Annual Revenue: $1-$5 Million
Year Founded: 1960
Total Employees: 10
Ownership: Private
Produces/Sells CE-marked Devices: N
Federal Procurement Eligibility: Small Business
Distribution: Manufacturer Direct, Manufacturer Through Distributor, Exporter
General Admin.: Robert Crichton/President, Chief Executive Officer

Equipment, Cleaning, Air	General
Floor Mat, Antibacterial	General

CONTROLLED MOLDING, INC.
724-253-3550
3043 Perry Highway, Hadley, PA 16130
FDA Number: 2531824
Fax: 724-253-3555
E-mail: sales@controlledmolding.com
Web site: www.controlledmolding.com
Ownership: Private
Produces/Sells CE-marked Devices: N

Scalpel, One-Piece (Knife)	Surgery

CONTROLS CORP. OF AMERICA
See Concoa

CONTROLTEK, INC.
360-896-9375
3905 NE 112th Avenue, Vancouver, WA 98682
FDA Number: 3029922
Fax: 360-896-9913
E-mail: info@controltek.com
Web site: www.controltek.com
Year Founded: 1971
Total Employees: 105

CONTROLTEK, INC.
360-896-9375 *(cont'd)*
Ownership: Private
Quality System Registration Information: ISO9000
Produces/Sells CE-marked Devices: Y
Federal Procurement Eligibility: Small Business, VA Contract
Distribution: Manufacturer Direct, Manufacturer Through Manufacturer Reps, Service Direct

Contract Assembly	General
Contract Manufacturing	General
Contract Manufacturing, Product, Durable	General
Service, Engineering/Design	General

CONVAID INC.
888-266-8243
PO Box 4209, Palos Verdes, CA 90274-9579
310-618-0111
FDA Number: 2022883
Fax: 310-618-8811
E-mail: custservice@convaid.com
Web site: www.convaid.com
Medical Products Sales Volume: $9,400,000
Annual Revenue: $5-$10 Million
Year Founded: 1976
Total Employees: 89   *Marketing Staff:* 2   *Sales Staff:* 8
Ownership: Private
Produces/Sells CE-marked Devices: Y
Federal Procurement Eligibility: Small Business
Distribution: Manufacturer Through Distributor, Manufacturer Through Manufacturer Reps, Exporter
General Admin.: Martha Kozik/Executive Assistant
Mervyn M. Watkins/President, Chief Executive Officer
Mktg./Adv.: Sue Johnson/Director Marketing & Sales
Mervyn M. Watkins/Director Product Development
Gina Reed/Supervisor Marketing & Sales
Production: Nathan A. Watkins/Director Production
Donald Griggs/Manager Quality Assurance & Regulatory Affairs
Finance: Rodolfo Restelli/Controller
Purchasing: Rodolfo Restelli/Director Exports

Stroller, Adaptive	Physical Med
Wheelchair, Manual	Physical Med

CONVAQUIP INDUSTRIES, INC.
800-637-8436
4834 Derrick Drive, PO Box 3417, Abilene, TX 79604
325-677-4177
FDA Number: 1629847
Fax: 325-677-7217
E-mail: info@convaquip.com
Web site: www.convaquip.com
Medical Products Sales Volume: $2,000,000
Annual Revenue: $1-$5 Million
Year Founded: 1974
Total Employees: 8   *Marketing Staff:* 1   *Sales Staff:* 2
Ownership: Private
Produces/Sells CE-marked Devices: Y
Federal Procurement Eligibility: Small Business
Distribution: Manufacturer Direct
General Admin.: Terry Goodman/President
Brad Goodman/Vice President, General Manager
Mktg./Adv.: Brad Goodman/Manager Advertising
Brad Goodman/Vice President Marketing & Sales
Production: Brad Goodman/Director Quality Assurance
Larry Holt/Vice President Manufacturing
Research: Brad Goodman/Vice President Research & Development

Accessories, Wheelchair	Physical Med
Bed, Electric, Home-Use	General
Cane	Physical Med
Chair, Bath	General
Chair, Shower	General
Commode (Toilet)	General
Crutch	Physical Med
Footstool	General
Lift, Patient	General
Rail, Commode	General
Scale, Bed	General
Walker, Mechanical	Physical Med

CONVATEC
800-422-8811
211 American Ave., Greensboro, NC 27409
FDA Number: 1049092
Web site: www.convatec.com
Total Employees: 3400
Ownership: Private
Produces/Sells CE-marked Devices: N
General Admin.: Dave Johnson/Chief Executive Officer

Bag, Collection, Urine, Newborn	General
Bag, Drainage, Ostomy (With Adhesive)	General
Bag, Urinary, Ileostomy	Gastroenterology/Urology
Collector, Ostomy	Gastroenterology/Urology
Colostomy Appliance, Disposable	Gastroenterology/Urology
Dressing, Wound, Hydrogel W/out Drug And/or Biologic	Surgery
Dressing, Wound, Hydrophilic	Surgery
Dressing, Wound, Occlusive	Surgery

CONVATEC   800-422-8811 *(cont'd)*

Irrigator, Ostomy	Gastroenterology/Urology
Orthosis, Abdominal	Physical Med
Pouch, Colostomy	Gastroenterology/Urology
Protector, Ostomy	Gastroenterology/Urology
Rod, Colostomy	Gastroenterology/Urology

CONVATEC CANADA   800-465-6302

555 Dr. Frederick Phillips, Ste. 110,   **514-747-8000**
St-Laurent, QUE H4M-2 Canada
FDA Number: n/a   *Fax:* 514-744-8124
E-mail: ccanada@usccmail.bms.com
Web site: www.convatec.com
Year Founded: 1978
Total Employees: 50
Ownership: Bristol Myers Squibb
Distribution: Exclusive Distributor

CONVATEC PROFESSIONAL SERVICES   800-422-8811

100 Headquarters Park Dr., Skillman, NJ 08558
FDA Number: 2243969
E-mail: CIC@convatec.com
Web site: www.convatec.com
Annual Revenue: $0-$1 Million
Total Employees: 3400
Ownership: Private
Produces/Sells CE-marked Devices: Y
Distribution: Manufacturer Direct
General Admin.: Dave Johnson/Chief Executive Officer
Finance: Mr. George Kegler/Chief Financial Officer

Bag, Drainage, Ostomy (With Adhesive)	General
Bag, Urinary Collection	General
Bandage, Cast	Physical Med
Bandage, Elastic	General
Catheter, Urinary, Condom	Gastroenterology/Urology
Collector, Ostomy	Gastroenterology/Urology
Collector, Urine	Gastroenterology/Urology
Colostomy Appliance, Disposable	Gastroenterology/Urology
Compression Unit, Intermittent (Anti-Embolism Pump)	Cardiovascular
Dressing, Gel	General
Dressing, Universal	General
Dressing, Wound and Burn, Occlusive	Surgery
Fiber, Absorbent	General
Irrigator, Ostomy	Gastroenterology/Urology
Nonabsorbable Gauze, Surgical Sponge, & Wound Dressing for External Use (with a Drug)	General
Orthosis, Abdominal	Physical Med
Ostomy Appliance (Ileostomy, Colostomy)	Gastroenterology/Urology
Pouch, Colostomy	Gastroenterology/Urology
Protector, Ostomy	Gastroenterology/Urology
Rod, Colostomy	Gastroenterology/Urology
Sleeve, Compressible Limb	Cardiovascular
Sponge, Other	General
Tubing, Other	General

CONVATEC, A DIVISION OF E.R. SQUIBB
See Convatec

CONVATECH
See Steris Corporation

CONVERGENCE MEDICAL DEVICES   888-362-8824

400 TradeCenter, Suite 5900, Woburn, MA 01801
FDA Number: n/a
E-mail: info@cmdevices.com
Web site: http://cmdevices.com
Ownership: Private
Produces/Sells CE-marked Devices: N
General Admin.: Dr. Seward Rutkove/Chairman
     Dr. Jose Bohorquez/President, Chief Executive Officer
Mktg./Adv.: Mr. David Freeman/Vice President Marketing & Business Development
Research: Dr. E.C. Lupton/Vice President Research & Development

CONVERGENT LASER TECHNOLOGIES   800-848-8200

1660 S. Loop Road, Alameda, CA 94502   **510-832-2130**
FDA Number: n/a   *Fax:* 510-832-1600
E-mail: sales@convergentlaser.com
Web site: www.convergentlaser.com
Medical Products Sales Volume: $2,900,000
Year Founded: 1984
Total Employees: 25
Ownership: XINTEC CORPORATION
Quality System Registration Information: ISO9003
Produces/Sells CE-marked Devices: N
Federal Procurement Eligibility: Small Business, Minority Owned, Female Owned, VA Contract
Distribution: Manufacturer Direct, Manufacturer Through Distributor, Manufacturer Through Manufacturer Reps, OEM, Exclusive Distributor, Exporter
General Admin.: Marilyn M. Chou, PhD/Executive Vice President

CONVERGENT LASER TECHNOLOGIES   800-848-8200 *(cont'd)*
     Mark H. K. Chim/President

Accessories, Laser	General
Endoscope, Flexible	Gastroenterology/Urology
Laser, Nd:YAG, Surgical	Surgery
Laser, Surgical	Surgery
Laser, Surgical, Holmium	Surgery

CONWAY MILL
See KIMBERLY-CLARK CORP. CONWAY MILL

COOK (CANADA) INC,   800-668-0300

111 Sandiford Dr.,   **905-640-7110**
Stouffville, ONT L4A-7 Canada
FDA Number: n/a   *Fax:* 905-640-7408
E-mail: inquiries@cookcanada.com
Web site: www.cookgroup.com
Year Founded: 1973
Total Employees: 100
Ownership: COOK GROUP
Produces/Sells CE-marked Devices: N
Distribution: Manufacturer Direct, Exclusive Distributor

COOK BIOTECH, INCORPORATED   888-299-4224

1425 Innovation Place, West Lafayette, IN 47906   **765-497-3355**
FDA Number: 1835959   *Fax:* 765-497-2361
E-mail: info@cookbiotech.com
Web site: www.cookbiotech.com
Year Founded: 1995
Total Employees: 50
Ownership: COOK GROUP
Quality System Registration Information: ISO9001
Produces/Sells CE-marked Devices: Y
Federal Procurement Eligibility: Small Business
Distribution: Manufacturer Direct, Manufacturer Through Distributor
General Admin.: Mr. Mark Bleyer/President, Chief Executive Officer
Mktg./Adv.: Mrs. Madia Milks/Coord. Communications
Production: Mr. Joe Ely/Director Operations
Research: Mr. Mike Hiles/Vice President Research

Device, Incontinence, Occlusion, Urethral	Gastroenterology/Urology
Dressing, Other	General
Dura-Substitute	Cns/Neurology
Mesh, Surgical, Polymeric	Surgery

COOK ENDOSCOPY   336-744-0157

4900 Bethania Station Rd. &, 5951 Grassy Creek Blvd.,
Winston Salem, NC 27105
FDA Number: 1037905
E-mail: Sales.Ops@cookmedical.com
Web site: www.cookmedical.com
Ownership: Private
Produces/Sells CE-marked Devices: N

Accessories, Cleaning Brushes (For Endoscope)	Gastroenterology/Urology
Adapter, Bulb, Endoscope, Miscellaneous	Gastroenterology/Urology
Adapter, Holder, Syringe	Physical Med
Analyzer, Motility, Gastrointestinal, Electrical	Gastroenterology/Urology
Bag, Leg	Gastroenterology/Urology
Brush, Biopsy, Bronchoscope (Non-Rigid)	Anesthesiology
Brush, Cytology, Endoscopic	Gastroenterology/Urology
Cannula, Injection	Gastroenterology/Urology
Catheter, Balloon (Foley Type)	Surgery
Catheter, Biliary	Gastroenterology/Urology
Catheter, Biliary, General & Plastic Surgery	Surgery
Catheter, Cholangiography	Surgery
Catheter, Continuous Irrigation	Surgery
Clip, Hemostatic	Surgery
Dilator, Catheter	Surgery
Dilator, Esophageal	Gastroenterology/Urology
Dilator, Esophageal, ENT	Ear/Nose/Throat
Dislodger, Stone, Basket, Ureteral, Metal	Gastroenterology/Urology
Electrosurgical Unit, Cutting & Coagulation Device	Surgery
Electrosurgical, Unit, Gastroenterology	Gastroenterology/Urology
Endoscope	Gastroenterology/Urology
Forceps	Orthopedics
Forceps, Biopsy, Bronchoscope (Non-Rigid)	Anesthesiology
Forceps, Biopsy, Electric	Gastroenterology/Urology
Forceps, Biopsy, Non-Electric	Gastroenterology/Urology
General Use Surgical Scissors	Surgery
Kit, Biopsy Needle	Gastroenterology/Urology
Laparoscope, General & Plastic Surgery	Surgery
Ligator, Esophageal	Gastroenterology/Urology
Ligator, Hemorrhoidal	Gastroenterology/Urology
Lithotriptor, Mechanical, Biliary	Gastroenterology/Urology
Mesh, Surgical (Steel Gauze)	Surgery
Needle, Aspiration And Injection, Disposable	Gastroenterology/Urology
Pressure Measurement, System, Intermittent	Physical Med
Prosthesis, Esophageal	Ear/Nose/Throat
Prosthesis, Trachea	Surgery
Snare, Flexible	Gastroenterology/Urology
Snare, Non-Electrical	Gastroenterology/Urology

COOK ENDOSCOPY
336-744-0157 (cont'd)

Stent, Colonic, Metalic, Expandable	Gastroenterology/Urology
Syringe, Balloon Inflation	Cardiovascular
System, Laser, Fiber Optic, Photodynamic Therapy	Surgery
Tube, Double Lumen For Intestinal Decompression	Gastroenterology/Urology
Tube, Gastro-Enterostomy	Gastroenterology/Urology
Tube, Gastrointestinal	Gastroenterology/Urology

COOK INC.
800-457-4500
PO Box 489, Bloomington, IN 47402-0489   **812-339-2235**

FDA Number: 1820334   *Fax:* 812-339-5369
E-mail: info@cook-inc.com
Web site: www.cookgroup.com
Medical Products Sales Volume: $1,500,000,000
Year Founded: 1963
Total Employees: 9000
Ownership: Private
Quality System Registration Information: ISO9001
Produces/Sells CE-marked Devices: Y
Distribution: Manufacturer Direct
General Admin.: Kem Hawkins/President, Chief Executive Officer
Mktg./Adv.: Rick Mellinger/Advisor Tech. Marketing
    John Brumleve/Director Marketing
    Michael Hughes/Director National Accounts
    J. Heckman/Manager Advertising
    Mr. Rob Doracle/Vice President Communications
    R. Mellinger/Vice President Marketing
    D. Reed/Vice President Sales
Production: A. Lavender/Manager Regulatory Affairs
    S. Eells/Vice President Manufacturing
Research: T. Osborne/Vice President Research & Development

Airway, Obstruction Removal (Choke Saver)	General
Bag, Bile Collection	Gastroenterology/Urology
Basket, Biliary Stone Retrieval	Gastroenterology/Urology
Catheter, Angiographic	Cns/Neurology
Catheter, Angioplasty, Coronary, Transluminal, Percut. Oper.	Cardiovascular
Catheter, Angioplasty, Transluminal, Peripheral	Cardiovascular
Catheter, Balloon, Dilatation, Vessel	Gastroenterology/Urology
Catheter, Biliary	Gastroenterology/Urology
Catheter, Cardiovascular, Balloon Type	Cardiovascular
Catheter, Cholangiography	Surgery
Catheter, Infusion	Surgery
Catheter, Intravascular, Therapeutic, Short-term Less Than 30 Days	General
Catheter, Jejunostomy	Gastroenterology/Urology
Catheter, Malecot (Gastrostomy Tube)	Gastroenterology/Urology
Catheter, Nephrostomy	Gastroenterology/Urology
Catheter, Pericardium Drainage	Cardiovascular
Catheter, Septostomy	Cardiovascular
Catheter, Vascular, Cardiopulmonary Bypass	Cardiovascular
Clamp, Fixation, Cholangiography	Surgery
Dilator, Vessel, Percutaneous Catheterization	Cardiovascular
Filter, Vena Cava	Cardiovascular
Forceps, Biopsy	Surgery
Guide, Catheter	Cardiovascular
Guidewire	Cardiovascular
Guidewire, Catheter	Cardiovascular
Guidewire, Catheter, Radiological	Radiology
Injector, Contrast Medium, Automatic	Radiology
Injector, Lymphangiographic	Cns/Neurology
Introducer, Catheter	Cardiovascular
Kit, Biopsy Needle	Gastroenterology/Urology
Kit, Cricothyrotomy	Anesthesiology
Kit, First Aid	Surgery
Kit, Lymphangiographic	Cns/Neurology
Marker, Ostia, Aorto-Saphenous Vein	Surgery
Needle, Angiographic	Cns/Neurology
Occluder, Catheter Tip	Cardiovascular
Stent, Cardiovascular	Cardiovascular
Stopcock	General
Syringe, Angiographic	Cns/Neurology
System, Infusion, Enzyme, Thrombolytic	Cardiovascular
Tube, Decompression	General
Tube, Double Lumen For Intestinal Decompression	Gastroenterology/Urology
Tube, Gastrointestinal	Gastroenterology/Urology
Vascular Access Graft	Gastroenterology/Urology

Medical Product Subsidiaries (Listed Separately)
    Cook Medical Inc.
    Cook Urological, Inc.
    Wilson-Cook Medical, Inc.

COOK MEDICAL INC.
800-457-4500
400 daniels way, Bloomington, IN 47404   **812-339-2235**

FDA Number: 3005580113   *Fax:* 800-554-8335
E-mail: Sales.Ops@cookmedical.com
Web site: www.cookmedical.com
Year Founded: 2003
Ownership: Cook Inc.
Produces/Sells CE-marked Devices: N

COOK OB/GYN
800-457-4500
812-339-2235
P.O. Box 4195, Bloomington, IN 47402-4195

FDA Number: n/a   *Fax:* 800-554-8335
E-mail: Sales.Ops@cookmedical.com
Web site: www.cookgroup.com
Total Employees: 345
Ownership: Cook Urological, Inc.
Quality System Registration Information: ISO9000
Produces/Sells CE-marked Devices: Y
Federal Procurement Eligibility: Small Business
Distribution: Manufacturer Direct
General Admin.: Tammie Lawrence/Human Resources Representative
    Charles W. Franz/President
    Fred Roemer/Vice President
    Jerry French/Vice President
Production: Chris Kilander/Manager Quality Assurance
    Debbie Schmitt/Manager Regulatory Affairs
    Frank Fischer/Vice President Manufacturing & Operations
Research: Frank Fischer/Manager Research & Development
    Jessica Miller/Manager Research & Development

Accessory, Assisted Reproduction	Obstetrics/Gynecology
Cannula, Intrauterine Insemination	Obstetrics/Gynecology
Cap, Cervical	Obstetrics/Gynecology
Catheter, Assisted Reproduction	Obstetrics/Gynecology
Catheter, Other	Gastroenterology/Urology
Forceps, Obstetrical	Obstetrics/Gynecology
Laparoscope, Gynecologic	Obstetrics/Gynecology
Microtools, Assisted Reproduction	Obstetrics/Gynecology
Needle, Assisted Reproduction	Obstetrics/Gynecology
Sampler, Amniotic Fluid (Amniocentesis Tray)	Obstetrics/Gynecology
Sound, Uterine	Obstetrics/Gynecology

COOK PACEMAKER CORP.
See Cook Vascular, Incorporated

COOK SURGICAL INC.
See Cook Inc.

COOK UROLOGICAL, INC.
800-457-4500
812-829-4891
1100 West Morgan St., P.O. Box 227, Spencer, IN 47460

FDA Number: 1825146   *Fax:* 800-554-8335
E-mail: Sales.Ops@cookmedical.com
Web site: www.cookmedical.com
Medical Products Sales Volume: $40,000,000
Year Founded: 1977
Ownership: Cook Inc.
Produces/Sells CE-marked Devices: Y
Federal Procurement Eligibility: Small Business
Distribution: Manufacturer Direct

Adapter, Catheter, Ureteral	Gastroenterology/Urology
Bag, Bile Collection	Gastroenterology/Urology
Bag, Urinary Collection, Ureterostomy	Gastroenterology/Urology
Bag, Urinary, Ileostomy	Gastroenterology/Urology
Biopsy Instrument	Gastroenterology/Urology
Brush, Cytology, Endoscopic	Gastroenterology/Urology
Catheter, Balloon, Dilatation, Vessel	Gastroenterology/Urology
Catheter, Malecot (Gastrostomy Tube)	Gastroenterology/Urology
Catheter, Nephrostomy	Gastroenterology/Urology
Catheter, Retention Type	Gastroenterology/Urology
Catheter, Retention Type, Balloon	Gastroenterology/Urology
Catheter, Straight	Gastroenterology/Urology
Catheter, Suprapubic	Gastroenterology/Urology
Catheter, Suprapubic, With Tube	Gastroenterology/Urology
Catheter, Upper Urinary Tract	Gastroenterology/Urology
Catheter, Ureteral Disposable (X-Ray)	Gastroenterology/Urology
Catheter, Ureteral, Gastro-Urology	Gastroenterology/Urology
Catheter, Urinary, Irrigation	Gastroenterology/Urology
Catheter, Urological	Gastroenterology/Urology
Collector, Urine, Disposable	Gastroenterology/Urology
Colostomy Appliance, Disposable	Gastroenterology/Urology
Dilator, Catheter, Ureteral	Gastroenterology/Urology
Dilator, Urethral	Gastroenterology/Urology
Dislodger, Stone, Basket, Ureteral, Metal	Gastroenterology/Urology
Dislodger, Stone, Flexible	Gastroenterology/Urology
Dressing, Wound and Burn, Occlusive	Surgery
Filiform, With Filiform Follower	Gastroenterology/Urology
Forceps, Grasping, Flexible Endoscopic	Gastroenterology/Urology
Forceps, Obstetrical	Obstetrics/Gynecology
Forceps, Stone Manipulation	Gastroenterology/Urology
Guidewire	Cardiovascular
Guidewire, Catheter	Cardiovascular
Holder, Needle	Gastroenterology/Urology
Kit, Biopsy Needle	Gastroenterology/Urology
Mesh, Surgical (Steel Gauze)	Surgery
Needle, Endoscopic	Gastroenterology/Urology
Ostomy Appliance (Ileostomy, Colostomy)	Gastroenterology/Urology
Punch, Catheter	Gastroenterology/Urology
Stent, Ureteral	Gastroenterology/Urology
Tube, Drainage	Gastroenterology/Urology
Tube, Nephrostomy	Gastroenterology/Urology

COOK UROLOGICAL, INC.   800-457-4500 (cont'd)
Medical Product Subsidiaries (Listed Separately)
Cook Ob/Gyn

COOK VASCULAR, INCORPORATED   800-457-4500
1186 Montgomery Lane, Vandergrift, PA 15690   724-845-8621
FDA Number: 2522007   *Fax:* 724-845-0914
E-mail: info@cookmedical.com
Web site: www.cookmedical.com
Medical Products Sales Volume: $16,000,000
Year Founded: 1981
Total Employees: 150   *Marketing Staff:* 3   *Sales Staff:* 10
Ownership: Private
Quality System Registration Information: ISO9001
Produces/Sells CE-marked Devices: Y
Federal Procurement Eligibility: Small Business
Distribution: Manufacturer Direct, Manufacturer Through Manufacturer Reps, OEM, Importer, Exporter
General Admin.: Louis Goode/President
    Vic Sheaffer/Vice President, General Manager
Mktg./Adv.: Barry Norlander/Manager Marketing
    Kris Domenick/Manager National Sales
Production: Kathy Emmert/Manager Production
    Tom Kardos/Manager Regulatory Affairs

Catheter, Subcutaneous Intravascular, Implanted	General
Device, Removal, Pacemaker Electrode, Percutaneous	Cardiovascular
Dilator, Vessel, Percutaneous Catheterization	Cardiovascular
Electrosurgical Unit, Cutting & Coagulation Device	Surgery
Guidewire, Catheter	Cardiovascular
Surgical Instrument, Manual (General Use)	Surgery
Transducer, Ultrasonic, Diagnostic	Radiology

COOKGAS LLC   314-781-5700
1167 Hillside Dr., St. Louis, MO 63117
FDA Number: 3004594307
Web site: www.cookgas.com
Ownership: Private
Produces/Sells CE-marked Devices: N

Airway, Oropharyngeal, Anesthesia	Anesthesiology
Stylet, Tracheal Tube	Anesthesiology

COOL VIEW, LLC   865-982-5552
9530 Gladiolus Blossom Ct., Fort Myers, FL 33908
FDA Number: 3006095511

Headlamp, Operating, Battery-Operated	Ophthalmology

COOLEY & COOLEY, LTD.   800-215-4487
8550 Westland W. Blvd., Houston, TX 77041   281-897-0009
FDA Number: 1620228   *Fax:* 281-897-8040
E-mail: admin@copalite.com
Web site: www.copalite.com
Annual Revenue: $0-$1 Million
Total Employees: 8   *Marketing Staff:* 1   *Sales Staff:* 3
Ownership: Private
Quality System Registration Information: ISO9001
Produces/Sells CE-marked Devices: Y
Federal Procurement Eligibility: Small Business, Female Owned
Distribution: Manufacturer Through Distributor, Exporter
General Admin.: Talbot Cooley/Chief Operating Officer
    Marianna Cooley/President, Chief Executive Officer
Mktg./Adv.: Dan Hendricks/Director Marketing
    Dr Timothy Fraser/Director Product Development
    Pamela Wade/Manager Sales Training

Adhesive, Dental	Dental And Oral
Cement, Dental	Dental And Oral
Dam, Rubber	Dental And Oral
Instrument, Dental, Manual	Dental And Oral
Mouthguard	Dental And Oral
Resin, Root Canal Filling	Dental And Oral
Tray, Impression	Dental And Oral
Unit, Sanitation/Sterilization, Toothbrush, Ultraviolet	Dental And Oral
Varnish	Dental And Oral

COOLSYSTEMS, INC.   510-868-5378
1201 Marina Village Parkway, Suite 200, Alameda, CA 94501
FDA Number: 2954777
Ownership: Private
Produces/Sells CE-marked Devices: N

Massager, Powered Inflatable Tube	Physical Med
Pack, Hot Or Cold, Water Circulating	Physical Med

COOPER BIOMEDICAL
See Biomerieux Inc.

COOPER DEVELOPMENT CO.
See Biomerieux Inc.

COOPER DIAGNOSTICS
See Biomerieux Inc.

COOPER LASERSONICS INC./SURG. LASER DIV.
See Ams Innovative Center-San Jose

COOPER MEDICAL CORP.
See Valleylab

COOPER VISION CARRIBBEAN   925-460-3600
500 Road 584 Lot 7, Amuelas Industrial Park,
Juana Diaz, PR 00795
FDA Number: 2640128
Web site: www.coopercos.com
Ownership: Public
Stock Symbol: COO
Traded On: NYSE
Produces/Sells CE-marked Devices: N

Lens, Contact (Other Material)	Ophthalmology
Lens, Contact, (disposable)	Ophthalmology
Lenses, Soft Contact, Daily Wear	Ophthalmology
Lenses, Soft Contact, Extended Wear	Ophthalmology

COOPER VISION, INC.   510-460-3600
1215 Boissevain Ave., Norfolk, VA 23507
FDA Number: 1118577
Web site: www.coopervision.com
Ownership: Public
Stock Symbol: COO
Traded On: NYSE
Produces/Sells CE-marked Devices: N
General Admin.: Jeff McLean/President

Lenses, Soft Contact, Daily Wear	Ophthalmology

COOPER-HEWITT CORP.
See Kbd, Inc.

COOPERATIVE WORKSHOPS, INC.   888-615-6332
1500 Ewing Drive, Sedalia, MO 65301   660-826-4400 ex
FDA Number: 1932233   *Fax:* 866-495-6424
E-mail: agraff@chs-mo.org
Web site: www.chs-mo.org
Medical Products Sales Volume: $2,100,000
Annual Revenue: $1-$5 Million
Year Founded: 1965
Total Employees: 295   *Marketing Staff:* 1   *Sales Staff:* 1
Ownership: Private
Produces/Sells CE-marked Devices: N
Federal Procurement Eligibility: Small Business
Distribution: Manufacturer Direct, Manufacturer Through Distributor, Manufacturer Through Manufacturer Reps
General Admin.: James Canter/President
    Debbie Milligan/Secretary
    Jean Jensen/Vice President
Mktg./Adv.: Mrs. Angela Eckstrom/Coord. Sales
Finance: Ann Tettlebaum/Treasurer

Kit, First Aid	Surgery

COOPERCARE INC.
See Oral-B Laboratories, Inc.

COOPERCARE LASTRAP INC   416-741-9675
Highway H, Koopman Ln., Elkhorn, WI 53121
FDA Number: 1319118   *Fax:* 416-741-2873
E-mail: sales@coopercare.com
Web site: www.coopercare.com
Annual Revenue: $1-$5 Million
Year Founded: 1989
Total Employees: 7
Ownership: Monarch-Mclaren, Inc.
Produces/Sells CE-marked Devices: Y
Federal Procurement Eligibility: Small Business
Distribution: Manufacturer Direct

Band, Support, Pelvic	Physical Med
Splint, Molded, Aluminum	Orthopedics
Support, Back	Orthopedics
Support, Elbow	Orthopedics
Support, Hand	Orthopedics

COOPERCARE-LASTRAP INC.   416-741-9675
329 Deerhide Crescent, Toronto, ONT M9M-2Z2 Canada
FDA Number: n/a   *Fax:* 416-741-2873
E-mail: mail@coopercare.ca
Web site: www.coopercare.ca
Year Founded: 1988
Total Employees: 10
Ownership: Monarch-Mclaren, Inc.
Produces/Sells CE-marked Devices: N
Distribution: Manufacturer Direct

COOPERSURGICAL, INC.   800-243-2974
95 Corporate Drive, Trumbull, CT 06611   203-601-5200
FDA Number: 1216677   *Fax:* 800-262-0105
E-mail: e-mail@coopersurgical.com

COOPERSURGICAL, INC.   800-243-2974 (cont'd)
Web site: www.coopersurgical.com
Medical Products Sales Volume: $125,000,000
Annual Revenue: $100-$500 Million
Year Founded: 1990
Total Employees: 426   *Marketing Staff:* 10   *Sales Staff:* 50
Ownership: The Cooper Companies
Stock Symbol: COO
Traded On: NYSE
Quality System Registration Information: ISO9001
Produces/Sells CE-marked Devices: Y
Federal Procurement Eligibility: Small Business
Distribution: Manufacturer Direct, Manufacturer Through Manufacturer Reps, Service Direct
General Admin.: Nicholas Pichotta/Chief Executive Officer
     Paul Remmell/President, Chief Operating Officer
Mktg./Adv.: Mark Curtis/Vice President Sales
Production: Frank Schepp/Director Operations
     Kerry Blair/Vice President Engineering & Operations
Finance: Alan Tucker/Controller

Accessories, Cleaning, Endoscopic	Gastroenterology/Urology
Accessories, Laser	General
Accessories, Photographic, Endoscopic	Gastroenterology/Urology
Applicator, Other	General
Applier, Clip, Laparoscopic	Surgery
Applier, Clip, Repair, Hernia, Laparoscopic	Gastroenterology/Urology
Bougie, Urological	Gastroenterology/Urology
Cable, Fiberoptic	General
Camera, Still, Endoscopic	Surgery
Camera, Still, Surgical	Surgery
Camera, Television, Microsurgical (Without Audio)	Surgery
Camera, Television, Surgical (Without Audio)	Surgery
Camera, Video, Endoscopic	General
Catheter, Suction (Tracheal Aspirating Tube)	Anesthesiology
Colposcope	Obstetrics/Gynecology
Computer, Pulmonary Function Data	Anesthesiology
Cryosurgical Unit	Surgery
Cryosurgical Unit, Gynecologic	Obstetrics/Gynecology
Curette, Uterine	Obstetrics/Gynecology
Densitometer, Bone, Dual Photon	Radiology
Device, Cystometric, Hydraulic	Gastroenterology/Urology
Dilator, Blunt	Surgery
Dilator, Cervical, Expandable	Obstetrics/Gynecology
Dilator, Rectal	Gastroenterology/Urology
Electrode, Other	General
Electrosurgical Equipment, General Purpose	Surgery
Electrosurgical Unit, Cutting & Coagulation Device	Surgery
Fixation Device, Tracheal Tube	Anesthesiology
Gel, Ultrasonic Transmission	General
Generator, Power, Electrosurgical	Surgery
Holder, Instrument, Laparoscopic	Surgery
Holder, Needle	Gastroenterology/Urology
Hysteroscope	Obstetrics/Gynecology
Instrument, Knot Tying, Suture, Laparoscopic	Surgery
Instrument, Needle Holder/Knot Tying	Surgery
Laparoscope, General & Plastic Surgery	Surgery
Monitor, Fetal Doppler Ultrasound	Obstetrics/Gynecology
Punch, Biopsy, Surgical	Dental And Oral
Retractor, Vaginal	Obstetrics/Gynecology
Speculum, Vaginal, Metal	Obstetrics/Gynecology
Stretcher, Hand-Carried	General
System, Evacuation, Smoke, Laser	Surgery
Tenaculum, Uterine	Obstetrics/Gynecology
Thermometer, Electronic	General
Tube, Aspirating, Flexible, Connecting	Anesthesiology
Tube, Smoke Removal, Endoscopic	Gastroenterology/Urology
Ventilator, Non-Continuous (Respirator)	Anesthesiology
Warmer, Gel	General

COOPERVISION   (585) 421-0100
370 Woodcliff Drive, Suite 200, Fairport, NY 14450
FDA Number: 9929062
E-mail: info@coopervision.com
Web site: www.coopervision.com
Ownership: Private
Produces/Sells CE-marked Devices: N

Lenses, Soft Contact, Daily Wear	Ophthalmology
Lenses, Soft Contact, Extended Wear	Ophthalmology

COOPERVISION INC.   800-341-2020
370 Woodcliff Drive, Suite 200,   **949-597-8130**
Fairport, NY 14450
FDA Number: 3005724763   *Fax:* 949-597-0665
E-mail: dfancher@coopervision.com
Web site: www.coopervision.com
Annual Revenue: $25-$50 Million
Year Founded: 1911
Total Employees: 700   *Marketing Staff:* 12   *Sales Staff:* 50
Ownership: THE COOPER COMPANIES, INC.
Stock Symbol: COO

COOPERVISION INC.   800-341-2020 (cont'd)
Traded On: NYSE
Quality System Registration Information: ISO9000
Produces/Sells CE-marked Devices: N
Distribution: Manufacturer Direct
General Admin.: Janice Jones/Director Human Resources
     Jeff McLean/President
     Tom Bender/President, Chief Executive Officer
Mktg./Adv.: Dave Fancher/Senior Vice President Marketing & Sales
     Greg Fryling/Vice President Business Development
     Thom Freytag/Vice President International Sales
     Tom Shone/Vice President Marketing
     Tom Stone/Vice President Marketing
     Mike Stulak/Vice President Sales
Production: Amy Blazak/Director Regulatory Affairs
     Peter Brierley/Vice President Manufacturing
     Dennis Snyder/Vice President Manufacturing, General Manager

Lens, Contact, Disposable	Ophthalmology
Lens, Contact, Extended-Wear	Ophthalmology
Lenses, Soft Contact, Daily Wear	Ophthalmology

COOPERVISION INC.   925- 251-6600
5870 Stoneridge Drive # 1, Pleasanton, CA 94588-2733
FDA Number: 3005124956   *Fax:* 716-889-5688
Web site: www.coopervision.com
Annual Revenue: $0-$1 Million
Total Employees: 750
Ownership: THE COOPER COMPANIES, INC.
Stock Symbol: COO
Traded On: NYSE
Quality System Registration Information: ISO9001
Produces/Sells CE-marked Devices: Y
Distribution: Manufacturer Direct, Importer, Exporter
General Admin.: A. Thomas Bender/Chief Executive Officer
     Greg Fryling/President
Mktg./Adv.: Rick Mark/Director National Accounts
     Thom Freytag/Vice President International Sales
     Dave Fancher/Vice President Marketing
     Thomas Ghone/Vice President Marketing
Production: Bernard F. Hallatt/Director Quality Assurance
     Bonnie Tsymbal/Manager Regulatory Affairs
     Dennis Snyder/Vice President Manufacturing

Lens, Contact, Disposable	Ophthalmology
Lens, Contact, Extended-Wear	Ophthalmology
Lenses, Soft Contact, Daily Wear	Ophthalmology

COOPERVISION/COASTVISION, INC.
See Coopervision Inc.

COPAN DIAGNOSTICS, INC.   800-216-4016
26055 Jefferson Avenue, Murrieta, CA 92562   **951-696-6957**
FDA Number: 2436875   *Fax:* 951-600-1832
E-mail: info@copanusa.com
Web site: http://www.copanusa.com
Year Founded: 1994
Ownership: Private
Produces/Sells CE-marked Devices: N
General Admin.: Mr. Norman Sharples/Executive Vice President

Container, Specimen Mailer And Storage	Pathology
Equipment, Laboratory, Gen. Purpose (Specific Medical Use)	Chemistry
Kit, Quality Control	Microbiology
Pipette, Micro	Chemistry

CORA DISPOSABLES INC.
See New York Hospital Disposables, Inc.

CORAL BIOTECHNOLOGY   760-727-8224
110 Bosstick Blvd., San Marcos, CA 92069
FDA Number: n/a
Ownership: Private
Produces/Sells CE-marked Devices: N

Colorimeter, General Use	Chemistry
Kit, Screening, Urine	Microbiology

CORALITE DENTAL PRODUCTS
See Harry J. Bosworth Company

CORDIS CORPORATION   800-447-7585
430 Route 22 East, Bridgewater, NJ 08807   **908-541-4100**
FDA Number: 2249557   *Fax:* 800-997-1122
Web site: www.cordis.com
Year Founded: 1959
Total Employees: 7000
Ownership: Johnson & Johnson
Produces/Sells CE-marked Devices: N
General Admin.: Rick Anderson/President
     Todd Pope/President
     Dennis Donohoe/Vice President
     Liesl Cooper/Vice President
Production: Nancy Coulson/Director Regulatory Affairs

MANUFACTURER PROFILES

CORDIS CORPORATION   800-447-7585 *(cont'd)*
Catheter, Biliary   Gastroenterology/Urology
Stent, Cardiovascular   Cardiovascular
Stent, Other   Obstetrics/Gynecology

CORDIS ENDOVASCULAR   877-338-4235
7 Powder Horn Drive, Warren, NJ 07059   **908-755-8300**
FDA Number: 2249557   *Fax:* 908-927-5786
E-mail: cordis_endo@crdus.jnj.com
Web site: www.cordis.com
Year Founded: 1959
Total Employees: 7000
Ownership: Johnson & Johnson
Produces/Sells CE-marked Devices: N
Distribution: Manufacturer Direct
General Admin.: Carol Zilm/President
     Rick Anderson/President
     Todd Pope/President
     Dennis Donohoe/Vice President
     Liesl Cooper/Vice President
     Ken Koharki/Vice President Human Resources
Mktg./Adv.: Shawn McCarthy/Director Marketing
     Lisa Ippoliti/Manager Advertising
     Mark Valentine/Manager National Sales
     Michael Madden/Manager Sales Training
     Chris Frederick/Vice President Marketing
     Jack Springer/Vice President Marketing & Sales
Production: Dennis Genito/Vice President Regulatory Affairs
Research: David Wilson/Vice President Research & Development
Catheter, Biliary   Gastroenterology/Urology
Shunt, Carotid   Cardiovascular
Stent, Cardiovascular   Cardiovascular
Stent, Metallic, Expandable   Anesthesiology
Stent, Vascular   Cardiovascular

CORDIS LABORATORIES, INC.
See Diamedix Corp.

CORDIS LLC   877-338-4235
Road 362 Km 0.5, San German, PR 00683   **786-313-2000**
FDA Number: 3003742446
Web site: www.cordis.com
Year Founded: 1959
Total Employees: 7000
Ownership: Johnson & Johnson
Produces/Sells CE-marked Devices: N
General Admin.: Rick Anderson/President
     Dennis Donohoe/Vice President
     Liesl Cooper/Vice President
Stent, Cardiovascular   Cardiovascular
Stent, Coronary, Drug-eluting   Cardiovascular

CORDIS NEUROVASCULAR, INC.   800-327-7714
14201 NW 60 Avenue, Miami Lakes, FL 33014   **786-313-6550**
FDA Number: 1058196
Web site: www.cordis.com
Year Founded: 1959
Total Employees: 7000
Ownership: Johnson & Johnson
Produces/Sells CE-marked Devices: N
General Admin.: Guy j. Lebeau/Chairman
     Rick Anderson/President
     Staffan Ternstrom/President
     Brian Firth/Vice President
     Dennis Donohoe/Vice President
     Liesl Cooper/Vice President
     Sidney Cohen/Vice President
Agent, Injectable, Embolic   Surgery
Catheter, Continuous Flush   Cardiovascular
Catheter, Intravascular, Diagnostic   Cardiovascular
Catheter, Percutaneous   Cardiovascular
Device, Embolization, Artificial   Cns/Neurology
Embolization Device   Cardiovascular
Guidewire, Catheter   Cardiovascular
Stent, Intracranial Neurovascular   Cns/Neurology

CORDIS WEBSTER, INC.
See Biosense Webster, Inc

CORDIS, A JOHNSON & JOHNSON CO.
See Cordis Endovascular

CORE ESSENCE ORTHOPAEDICS INC.   215-310-9534
575A Virginia Drive, Fort Washington, PA 19034
FDA Number: 3006283823   *Fax:* 215-660-5014
E-mail: Info@ceortho.com
Web site: www.ceortho.com
Ownership: Private
Produces/Sells CE-marked Devices: N
General Admin.: Shawn Huxel/President, Chief Executive Officer

CORE ESSENCE ORTHOPAEDICS INC.   215-310-9534 *(cont'd)*
Mktg./Adv.: Alan Miller/Executive Vice President International Marketing & Sales
Production: Jeff Miller/Vice President Operations
Fastener, Fixation, Non-Biodegradable, Soft Tissue   Orthopedics
Orthopedic Manual Surgical Instrument   Orthopedics
Screw, Fixation, Bone   Orthopedics
Staple, Fixation, Bone   Orthopedics
Suture, Non-Absorbable, Steel, Monofilament & Multifilament   Surgery
Suture, Non-Absorbable, Synthetic, Polyamide   Surgery

CORE PRODUCTS INTERNATIONAL, INC.   800-365-3047
808 Prospect Avenue, Osceola, WI 54020   **715-294-2050**
FDA Number: 2020254   *Fax:* 715-294-2622
E-mail: info@coreproducts.com
Web site: www.coreproducts.com
Medical Products Sales Volume: $12,100,000
Annual Revenue: $5-$10 Million
Year Founded: 1988
Total Employees: 110   *Marketing Staff:* 3   *Sales Staff:* 5
Ownership: Private
Produces/Sells CE-marked Devices: Y
Federal Procurement Eligibility: Small Business
Distribution: Manufacturer Through Distributor
General Admin.: Philip Mattison/President, Chief Executive Officer
     Tammy Frank/Vice President
Mktg./Adv.: Kevin McArdle/Vice President Marketing & Sales
Production: Deb Larson/Vice President Manufacturing
Research: Paul Norstrem/Research & Development Associate
Accessories, Traction   Physical Med
Bandage, Elastic   General
Belt, Traction, Pelvic, Orthopedic   Orthopedics
Cushion, Other   General
Joint, Knee, External Brace   Physical Med
Orthosis, Cervical   Physical Med
Orthosis, Lumbosacral   Physical Med
Pack, Hot Or Cold, Reusable   Physical Med
Pillow, Cervical   Orthopedics
Sling, Arm   Physical Med
Splint, Clavicle   Physical Med
Support, Ankle   Orthopedics
Support, Knee   Physical Med
Traction Unit, Non-Powered   Orthopedics

COREN   877-267-3677
15 Fruean Ave, South Yarmouth, MA 02664
FDA Number: n/a   *Fax:* 508-760-1872
E-mail: Sales@CorenPS.com
Web site: www.corenps.com
Annual Revenue: $0-$1 Million
Ownership: Private
Produces/Sells CE-marked Devices: Y
Federal Procurement Eligibility: Small Business
Distribution: Manufacturer Through Distributor
Perforator, Ear-Lobe   Ear/Nose/Throat

COREVALVE, INC.   949-679-2707
2 Jenner, Suite 100, Irvine, CA 92618
FDA Number: 3005140434
Ownership: Private
Produces/Sells CE-marked Devices: N
General Admin.: Jacques SÇguin/Chief Executive Officer, Chairman

CORFLEX, INC.   800-426-7353
669 E. Industrial Park Dr.,   **603-623-3344**
Manchester, NH 03109
FDA Number: 1218997   *Fax:* 603-623-4111
E-mail: sales@corflex.com
Web site: www.corflex.com
Annual Revenue: $5-$10 Million
Total Employees: 50
Ownership: Private
Produces/Sells CE-marked Devices: Y
Federal Procurement Eligibility: Small Business
Distribution: Manufacturer Through Distributor, Manufacturer Through Manufacturer Reps
General Admin.: Paul Lorenzetti/Chief Executive Officer
Mktg./Adv.: Ted Lorenzetti/Vice President Sales
Belt, Rib (Support)   Orthopedics
Binder, Abdominal   General
Collar, Cervical Neck   Orthopedics
Equipment, Cryotherapy   Physical Med
Finger Cot   General
Immobilizer, Knee   Orthopedics
Immobilizer, Shoulder   Orthopedics
Immobilizer, Wrist/Hand   Orthopedics
Joint, Knee, External Brace   Physical Med
Orthosis, Lumbosacral   Physical Med
Orthosis, Other   Physical Med
Pack, Hot Or Cold, Reusable   Physical Med

CORFLEX, INC.   800-426-7353 (cont'd)

Pillow	General
Shoe, Cast	Physical Med
Sling, Arm	Physical Med
Splint, Abduction, Shoulder	Orthopedics
Splint, Molded, Aluminum	Orthopedics
Splint, Other	Orthopedics
Strap, Clavicle	Orthopedics
Support, Back	Orthopedics

CORGENIX MEDICAL CORPORATION   800-729-5661
11575 Main Street, Broomfield, CO 80020   303-457-4345
FDA Number: 1721937
E-mail: info@corgenix.com
Web site: www.corgenix.com
Year Founded: 1990
Ownership: Public
Stock Symbol: CONX
Traded On: OTC Bulletin
Produces/Sells CE-marked Devices: N
General Admin.: Luis R. Lopez/Chairman
       William H. Critchfield/Chief Financial Officer, Senior Vice President
       Douglass T. Simpson/President, Chief Executive Officer
Production: Ms. Ann Steinbarger/Senior Vice President Operations
IS: Ms. Taryn Reynolds/Vice President Technology

11-dehydro Thromboxane B2 Kit, Urinary	Hematology
Anti-RNP-Antibody, Antigen And Control	Immunology
Anti-SM-Antibody, Antigen And Control	Immunology
Antinuclear Antibody (Enzyme-Labeled), Antigen, Controls	Immunology
Control, Plasma, Abnormal	Hematology
Extractable Antinuclear Antibody (Rnp/Sm), Antigen/Control	Immunology
System, Test, Antibodies, B2 - Glycoprotein I (b2 - Gpi)	Immunology
System, Test, Anticardiolipin, Immunological	Immunology
Test, Systemic Lupus Erythematosus	Immunology

CORINDUS INC.   508-653-3335
11 Erie Dr., Natick, MA 01760
FDA Number: n/a   Fax: 508-653-3355
E-mail: info@corindus.com
Web site: http://www.corindus.com
Ownership: Private
Produces/Sells CE-marked Devices: N
General Admin.: Mr. David Handler/President, Chief Executive Officer
Mktg./Adv.: Mr. Tal Wenderow/Executive Vice President Marketing
Production: Mr. Paul Pelletier/Director Quality Assurance
       Mr. Erik Bates/Vice President Operations
       Dr. Michail Pankratov/Vice President Regulatory & Clinical Affairs
Research: Mr. Jerry Jennings/Vice President Research & Development
Finance: Mr. Eamonn Fahy/Director Finance

CORION CORP.
See Newport Franklin, Inc.

CORIUM INTERNATIONAL, INC.   616-656-4563
235 Constitution Drive, Menlo Park, CA 94025
FDA Number: 3003693105   Fax: 616-698-5070
Ownership: Private
Produces/Sells CE-marked Devices: N
General Admin.: Mr. Steve Klemm/Chief Operating Officer
       Mr. Peter Staple/President, Chief Executive Officer
Mktg./Adv.: Ms. Christina Dickerson/Vice President Corporate Development
Research: Dr. Bobby Singh/Vice President Research & Development
Finance: Mr. Tim Sweemer/Chief Financial Officer

Dressing, Wound and Burn, Hydrogel	Surgery
Dressing, Wound, Hydrogel W/out Drug And/or Biologic	Surgery
Dressing, Wound, Occlusive	Surgery
Holder, Intravascular Catheter	General

CORMATRIX CARDIOVASCULAR INC.   877-651-2628
155-a Moffett Park Drive, Suite 240,   408-734-2628
Sunnyvale, CA 94089
FDA Number: 3005619880   Fax: 408-734-2629
E-mail: ecm@cormatrix.com
Web site: www.cormatrix.com
Year Founded: 2001
Ownership: Private
Produces/Sells CE-marked Devices: N
General Admin.: Mr. David Camp/Chairman, Chief Executive Officer
       Dr. Robert Matheny/Chief Scientific Officer
       Mr. Beecher Lewis/President, Chief Operating Officer
Production: Mr. Michael Billig/Vice President Quality Control & Regulatory Affairs
Finance: Mr. John Thomas, Jr./Chief Financial Officer

Pledget And Intracardiac Patch, PETP, PTFE, Polypropylene	Cardiovascular

CORNEAL LENS LAB, INC.   816-455-0500
621-f Moorefield Park Dr., Richmond, VA 23236
FDA Number: 1119146
Ownership: Private

CORNEAL LENS LAB, INC.   816-455-0500 (cont'd)
Produces/Sells CE-marked Devices: N

Lens, Contact (Other Material)	Ophthalmology

CORNERSTONE SENSORS, INC.   800-955-1470
2128 ARNOLD WAY, Suite 4, Alpine, CA 91901   619-445-1172
FDA Number: n/a   Fax: 619-445-9859
E-mail: Info@CornerstoneSensors.com
Web site: WWW.CORNERSTONESENSORS.COM
Annual Revenue: $1-$5 Million
Year Founded: 1992
Ownership: Private
Produces/Sells CE-marked Devices: N
Federal Procurement Eligibility: Small Business
Distribution: Manufacturer Direct
General Admin.: Gregg Lavenuta/President
Mktg./Adv.: Dan McGillicuddy/Director Marketing
       Dan McGillicuddy/Manager National Sales
Production: Timothy McGehee/Vice President Manufacturing
Finance: Mr. David Botting/Vice President Finance, Controller

Probe, Temperature	General
Thermistor	General

CORNERSTONE SURGICAL, LLC   503-680-7281
10175 Sw Barbur Blvd., Suite # 214-b, Portland, OR 97219-5955
FDA Number: 3005762030
Ownership: Private
Produces/Sells CE-marked Devices: N

Surgical Instrument, Disposable	Surgery

CORNING CLINICAL LABORATORIES
See Quest Diagnostics, Inc.

CORNING FREQUENCY CONTROL
See Vectron International

CORNING GLASS WORKS
See Corning Inc., Science Products Division

CORNING HAZLETON
See Covance Laboratories ,Inc

CORNING INC.
See Corning Inc., Science Products Division

CORNING INC., LIFE SCIENCES   207-985-5310
2 Alfred Rd., Kennebunk, ME 04043
FDA Number: 1218905

Flask, Tissue Culture	Pathology

CORNING INC., SCIENCE PRODUCTS DIVISION   800-492-1110
45 Nagog Park, Acton, MA 01720   978-635-2200
FDA Number: 1350014   Fax: 978-635-2476
E-mail: clswebmail@corning.com
Web site: www.scienceproducts.corning.com
Total Employees: 20000
Ownership: Private
Quality System Registration Information: ISO9000; ISO9001; ISO9002
Produces/Sells CE-marked Devices: Y
Distribution: Manufacturer Direct, Manufacturer Through Distributor, Manufacturer Through Manufacturer Reps
General Admin.: Roger Ackerman/Chief Executive Officer
       R. Pierce Baker/President, Chief Executive Officer
       Kathy Schrock/Vice President Human Resources
Mktg./Adv.: Andrew Niemann/Director Marketing
       Christopher Cunanan/Director Marketing
       John Lubniewski/Director Marketing
       Mike Cupo/Manager Business Development
       Susan Britton/Manager Contract Sales
       Rick Darcangelo/Manager Marketing
       Pamela D'Arcangelo/Manager Marketing Communications
       Dave Whitehouse/Manager National Sales
       Lydia Kenton/Manager National Sales
Production: John Ryan/Manager Regulatory Affairs
       Stan Zelek/Vice President Manufacturing
Research: David Root/Vice President Research & Development

Buret	Chemistry
Coverslip, Microscope Slide	Pathology
Electrode, pH	Gastroenterology/Urology
Filter, Bacteriological, Laboratory	Chemistry
Filter, Cell Collection, Tissue Processing	Pathology
Filter, Membrane	Chemistry
Heater, Immersion	Microbiology
Homogenizer, Tissue	Microbiology
Labware, Basic, Disposable	Chemistry
Labware, Basic, Reusable	Chemistry
Manometer, Laboratory	Chemistry
Meter, pH, General Use	Toxicology
Meter, pH, Portable	Chemistry
Microfilter, Blood Transfusion	Anesthesiology
Microplate	General
Pipette	Chemistry

CORNING INC., SCIENCE PRODUCTS DIVISION   800-492-1110
(cont'd)

Pipette Tip	Chemistry
Pipette, Diluting	Hematology
Pipette, Micro	Chemistry
Pipette, Quantitative, Hematology	Hematology
Plate, Hot	Chemistry
Purifier, Water	Chemistry
Tissue Culture Apparatus	Microbiology
Unit, Filter, Membrane	Chemistry

Medical Product Subsidiaries (Listed Separately)
Samco Scientific Corporation

CORNING SAMCO CORPORATION
See Samco Scientific Corporation

CORNING WAX   631-738-0041
1744 Julia Goldbach Avenue, Ronkonkoma, NY 11779
FDA Number: 3004375181   *Fax:* 631-738-0045
Ownership: Private
Produces/Sells CE-marked Devices: N

Wax, Dental	Dental And Oral

CORNING, INC.   607-433-3100
275 River St., Oneonta, NY 13820
FDA Number: 1316282   *Fax:* 607-433-3161
E-mail: Inquiries@corning.com
Web site: http://www.corning.com
Ownership: Private
Produces/Sells CE-marked Devices: N
General Admin.: Mr. Wendell Weeks/Chief Executive Officer
     Mr. Peter Volanikis/Chief Operating Officer
     Dr. Joseph Miller/Chief Technology Officer, Executive Vice
President
Mktg./Adv.: Mr. Lawrence McRae/Senior Vice President Corporate Development
Production: Ms. Pamela Schneider/Senior Vice President Operations
Finance: Mr. James Flaws/Chief Financial Officer

Filter, Cell Collection, Tissue Processing	Pathology

CORNUCOPIA TOOL & PLASTICS, INC.   800-235-4144
448 Sherwood Road, P.O. Box 1915,   805-369-0030
Paso Robles, CA 93447
FDA Number: n/a   *Fax:* 805-369-0033
E-mail: info@cornucopiaplastics.com
Web site: www.cornucopiaplastics.com
Annual Revenue: $0-$1 Million
Total Employees: 15   *Marketing Staff:* 2   *Sales Staff:* 2
Ownership: Private
Quality System Registration Information: ISO9000
Produces/Sells CE-marked Devices: N
Federal Procurement Eligibility: Small Business
Distribution: Manufacturer Direct
General Admin.: Larry Horn/President
     Art Horn/Vice President

Contract Manufacturing	General

CORPAK MEDSYSTEMS, INC.   800-323-6305
100 Chaddick Dr., Wheeling, IL 60090   847-403-3400
FDA Number: 1419949   *Fax:* 847-541-9526
E-mail: questions@corpakmedsystems.com
Web site: www.corpakmedsystems.com
Year Founded: 1979
Total Employees: 150
Ownership: Cardinal Health Inc.
Produces/Sells CE-marked Devices: N

Attachment, Breathing, Positive End Expiratory Pressure	Anesthesiology
Catheter, Intravascular, Therapeutic, Long-term Greater Than 30 Days	General
Catheter, Peritoneal Dialysis, Single-Use	Gastroenterology/Urology
Catheter, Suction (Tracheal Aspirating Tube)	Anesthesiology
Endoscope	Gastroenterology/Urology
Exhaust System, Surgical	Surgery
Helmet, Surgical	Surgery
Humidifier, Respiratory Gas, (Direct Patient Interface)	Anesthesiology
Infusion Pump, Enteral	General
Mask, Gas, Anesthesia	Anesthesiology
Mask, Oxygen, Aerosol Administration	Anesthesiology
Mask, Oxygen, Non-Rebreathing	Anesthesiology
Pump, Infusion	General
Strap, Head, Gas Mask	Anesthesiology
Tube, Feeding	General
Tube, Gastrointestinal	Gastroenterology/Urology
Tubing, Flexible, Medical Gas, Low-Pressure	Anesthesiology
Valve, Non-Rebreathing	Anesthesiology
Ventilator, Emergency, Manual (Resuscitator)	Anesthesiology

CORRIDOR GROUP, INC., THE   800-343-4163
6405 Metcalf, Ste. 108, Overland Park, KS 66202   913-362-0600
FDA Number: n/a   *Fax:* 913-362-5378
E-mail: tcg@corridorgroup.com
Web site: www.corridorgroup.com

CORRIDOR GROUP, INC., THE   800-343-4163 *(cont'd)*
Annual Revenue: $1-$5 Million
Ownership: Private
Produces/Sells CE-marked Devices: N
Federal Procurement Eligibility: Small Business, Female Owned
Distribution: Manufacturer Direct
General Admin.: Katheen Dodd/Chief Executive Officer
     Jeannee Parker Martin/President
Mktg./Adv.: Ann Ruder/Coord. Public Relations
     Randy Weast/Vice President Sales
Finance: terri Kirley/Chief Financial Officer

Manual, Policies	General
Service, Consulting	General

CORTECHS LABS, INC.   858-459-9702
1020 Prospect St., Suite 304, La Jolla, CA 92037
FDA Number: 1226773   *Fax:* 858-459-9705
E-mail: info@cortechslabs.com
Web site: www.cortechs.net
Ownership: Private
Produces/Sells CE-marked Devices: N

Image Processing System	Radiology
Test Pattern, Radiographic	Radiology

CORTEK ENDOSCOPY, INC.   847-526-2266
260 Jamie Lane, Unit D, Wauconda, IL 60084
FDA Number: 3003816595   *Fax:* 847-526-2251
E-mail: ct@cortek-endoscopy.com
Web site: www.cortek-endoscopy.com
Ownership: Private
Produces/Sells CE-marked Devices: N

Arthroscope	Orthopedics
Cystoscope	Gastroenterology/Urology
Hysteroscope	Obstetrics/Gynecology
Laparoscope, General & Plastic Surgery	Surgery
Laparoscope, Gynecologic	Obstetrics/Gynecology
Ureteroscope	Gastroenterology/Urology

CORTEK ENDOSCOPY, INC.   847-526-2266
260 Jamie Lane, Unit D, Lake Barrington, IL 60084
FDA Number: 3003816595   *Fax:* 847) 526-2251 f
E-mail: ct@cortek-endoscopy.com
Web site: /www.cortek-endoscopy.com
Ownership: Private
Produces/Sells CE-marked Devices: N

Arthroscope	Orthopedics
Ureteroscope	Gastroenterology/Urology

CORTICAL SYSTEMATICS LLC.   520-444-0666
5324 E. 18th Street, Tucson, AZ 85711
FDA Number: 3006268778
E-mail: info@corticalsystematics.net
Web site: www.corticalsystematics.net
Ownership: Private
Produces/Sells CE-marked Devices: N

Component, Wheelchair	Physical Med

COSA CORP.
See Hansco Technologies, Inc.

COSCO   800-582-6853
1602 Lakeside Drive, Redding, CA 96001
FDA Number: 9320061   *Fax:* 530-244-2644
E-mail: gailpc@digitalpath.net
Web site: www.cosco.net
Medical Products Sales Volume: $100,000
Annual Revenue: $0-$1 Million
Year Founded: 1952
Total Employees: 2   *Sales Staff:* 2
Ownership: Private
Quality System Registration Information: ISO9000
Produces/Sells CE-marked Devices: N
Federal Procurement Eligibility: Small Business, Female Owned
Distribution: Manufacturer Direct, Manufacturer Through Distributor, Exclusive
Distributor
General Admin.: Gail Christensen/President, Chief Executive Officer
     James A. Bumsted/Vice President, General Manager

Orthosis, Limb Brace	Physical Med
Orthosis, Other	Physical Med
Splint, Hand, And Component	Physical Med
Splint, Other	Orthopedics

COSEM NEUROSTIM LTD.   418-849-9047
P.O. Box 4199 , Terminus, Quebec, QUE G1K 7R9 Canada
FDA Number: n/a   *Fax:* 418-849-9160
E-mail: jgauthier@quebectel.com
Year Founded: 1987
Total Employees: 10
Ownership: Private

COSEM NEUROSTIM LTD.   418-849-9047 *(cont'd)*
Produces/Sells CE-marked Devices: N
Distribution: Manufacturer Direct

COSMAN COMPANY, INC.   888-886-7686
76 Cambridge St., Burlington, MA 01803-4140   **781-272-6561**
FDA Number: 3004867882   Fax: 781-272-6563
E-mail: info@cosmanmedical.com
Web site: www.cosmanmedical.com
Ownership: Private
Produces/Sells CE-marked Devices: N
General Admin.: Dr. Eric Cosman Sr./Chairman
         Dr. Michael Arnold/President
Research: Dr. Eric Cosman Jr./Director Scientific Affairs
   Electrosurgical Unit, Cutting & Coagulation Device   Surgery
   Generator, Radiofrequency Lesion   Cns/Neurology
   Probe, Radiofrequency Lesion   Cns/Neurology

COSMEDENT, INC.   800-621-6729
401 N. Michigan Ste. 2500, Chicago, IL 60611
FDA Number: 1450653   Fax: 312-644-9752
Annual Revenue: $0-$1 Million
Year Founded: 1982
Ownership: Private
Produces/Sells CE-marked Devices: N
Federal Procurement Eligibility: Small Business
Distribution: Manufacturer Direct
   Adhesive, Bracket And Conditioner, Resin   Dental And Oral
   Agent, Polishing, Abrasive, Oral Cavity   Dental And Oral
   Cement, Dental   Dental And Oral
   Coating, Filling Material, Resin   Dental And Oral
   Crown And Bridge, Temporary, Resin   Dental And Oral
   Cup, Prophylaxis   Dental And Oral
   Disk, Abrasive   Dental And Oral
   Handle, Instrument, Dental   Dental And Oral
   Material, Impression   Dental And Oral
   Material, Tooth Shade, Resin   Dental And Oral
   Point, Abrasive   Dental And Oral
   Sealant, Pit And Fissure, And Conditioner, Resin   Dental And Oral
   Strip, Polishing Agent   Dental And Oral
   Tooth Bonding Agent, Resin Restoration   Dental And Oral
   Varnish, Cavity   Dental And Oral
   Wheel, Polishing Agent   Dental And Oral

COSMETECH   951-677-5472
26435 John Adams St., Murrieta, CA 92563
FDA Number: 2026028
Ownership: Private
Produces/Sells CE-marked Devices: N

COSMETIC LABORATORIES OF AMERICA   818-717-1301
20245 Sunburst Street, Chatsworth, CA 91311-6219
FDA Number: 2018526   Fax: 818-717-6156
E-mail: akoenig@cla-cosmeticlabs.com
Web site: www.cla-cosmeticlabs.com
Ownership: Private
Produces/Sells CE-marked Devices: N
   Lubricant, Patient, Vaginal, Latex Compatible   Obstetrics/Gynecology

COSMO HEALTH, INC.   626-248-7917
15310 Elliot Avenue, Suite 4112, La Puente, CA 91747
FDA Number: 2249807   Fax: 626-839-9995
E-mail: contact@cosmohealthinc.com
Web site: www.cosmohealthinc.com
Medical Products Sales Volume: $1,000,000
Annual Revenue: $0-$1 Million
Year Founded: 1994
Total Employees: 5   *Marketing Staff:* 5   *Sales Staff:* 5
Ownership: Private
Produces/Sells CE-marked Devices: Y
Federal Procurement Eligibility: Small Business
Distribution: Manufacturer Through Distributor, Manufacturer Through
Manufacturer Reps, Exclusive Distributor
   Massager, Therapeutic   Physical Med

COSTA DEL MAR SUNGLASSES, INC.   800-447-3700
2361 Mason Avenue, Suite 100,   **386-274-4000**
Daytona Beach, FL 32117
FDA Number: 1052217   Fax: 386-274-4001
Web site: www.costadelmar.com
Annual Revenue: $5-$10 Million
Ownership: Private
Produces/Sells CE-marked Devices: Y
Federal Procurement Eligibility: Small Business
Distribution: Manufacturer Direct, Manufacturer Through Distributor, Manufacturer
Through Manufacturer Reps, Exporter
   Sunglasses (Including Photosensitive)   Ophthalmology

COSTONDE PRODUCTS LLC   810-743-1167
419 Tennyson Ave, P.O. Box 7179Flint, Flint, MI 48507
FDA Number: 3006224479   Fax: 810-743-1167
Web site: www.costondeproducts.com
Ownership: Private
Produces/Sells CE-marked Devices: N
   Transfer Aid   Physical Med

COTRAN CORP.   800-345-4449
574 Park Avenue, PO Box 130,   **401-682-1555**
Portsmouth, RI 02871
FDA Number: 1220401   Fax: 401-682-1775
E-mail: info@cotrancorp.com
Web site: www.cotrancorp.com
Medical Products Sales Volume: $670,000
Annual Revenue: $0-$1 Million
Year Founded: 1986
Total Employees: 5   *Marketing Staff:* 1   *Sales Staff:* 6
Ownership: Private
Produces/Sells CE-marked Devices: N
Federal Procurement Eligibility: Small Business
Distribution: Manufacturer Through Distributor, Importer, Exporter
General Admin.: Bertrand Dumont/President, Chief Executive Officer
Mktg./Adv.: Paul Botvin/Director Marketing
   IV Start Kit   Surgery
   Needle, Hypodermic   General
   Syringe, Hypodermic   General

COULOMETRICS
See Uic, Inc.

COULTER CORPORATION
See Beckman Coulter, Inc.

COULTER ELECTRONICS
See Beckman Coulter, Inc.

COUNTRY MEDICAL EQUIPMENT   302-845-2462
3758 Williamsville Rd., Houston, DE 19954
FDA Number: 2531615
Ownership: Private
Produces/Sells CE-marked Devices: N
   Table, Physical Medicine, Powered   Physical Med

COURION   800-533-5760
3044 Lambdin Ave., St. Louis, MO 63115-2899   **314-533-5700**
FDA Number: n/a   Fax: 314-533-5720
E-mail: sales@couriondoors.com
Web site: www.couriondoors.com
Annual Revenue: $0-$1 Million
Total Employees: 25
Ownership: Private
Produces/Sells CE-marked Devices: N
Distribution: Manufacturer Direct
General Admin.: Mike Gamer/President
Mktg./Adv.: Joe Desimone/Manager Sales
   Cart, Other   General
   Component, Metal, Other   General

COURTAULDS AEROSPACE
See Vermont Composites, Inc.

COURTAULDS STRUCTURAL COMPOSITES
See Vermont Composites, Inc.

COVALON TECHNOLOGIES LTD.   905-568-8400
405 Britannia Rd. East, Suite 106,
Mississauga, ON L4Z 3 Canada
FDA Number: 3005004019   Fax: 905-568-5200
E-mail: office@covalon.com
Web site: www.covalon.com
Ownership: Public
Stock Symbol: COV
Traded On: TSX Venture Exchange
Produces/Sells CE-marked Devices: N

COVANCE CARDIAC SAFETY SERVICES, INC.   215-282-5588
9390 Gateway Drive, Reno, NV 89521
FDA Number: 2916493
Ownership: COVANCE INC.
   Transmitter/Receiver System, Physiological, Telephone   Cardiovascular

COVANCE INC.   888-268-2623
210 Carnegie Center, Princeton, NJ 08540   **609-419-2240**
FDA Number: n/a
Web site: www.covance.com
Ownership: Private
Stock Symbol: CVD
Traded On: NYSE
Produces/Sells CE-marked Devices: N
General Admin.: Mr. Joseph Herring/Chairman, Chief Executive Officer

COVANCE INC. 888-268-2623 (cont'd)
Mr. John Replo/Chief Information Officer
Mktg./Adv.: Mr. Nigel Brown/Vice President Business Development
Finance: Mr. William Klitgaard/Chief Financial Officer

COVANCE LABORATORIES ,INC 800-742-8378
3301 Kinsman Blvd., Madison, WI 53704 608-241-4471
FDA Number: n/a
E-mail: info@covance.com Fax: 703-759-6947
Web site: www.covance.com
Medical Products Sales Volume: $135,700,000
Annual Revenue: $500 Million-$1 Billion
Year Founded: 1997
Total Employees: 1250 *Marketing Staff:* 6 *Sales Staff:* 15
Ownership: COVANCE INC.
Produces/Sells CE-marked Devices: N
Distribution: Service Direct
General Admin.: Christopher A. Kuebler/Chief Executive Officer
Ed Murray/Director Human Resources
Wendel Barr/President
Mktg./Adv.: Roger Greathead/Director Marketing
Production: Lydia Dickerell/Director Quality Assurance
Anthony Clemento/Manager Regulatory Affairs

Contract R&D, Diagnostics	General
Serum, Animal	Pathology

COVANCE RESEARCH PRODUCTS INC. 800-223-0796
180 Rustcraft Road, Suite 140, 781-329-7919
Dedham, MA 02026
FDA Number: 1225972
E-mail: pfluckiger@signetlabs.com Fax: 781-461-2456
Web site: www.covance.com
Medical Products Sales Volume: $1,300,000
Annual Revenue: $1-$5 Million
Year Founded: 1989
Total Employees: 17 *Marketing Staff:* 2 *Sales Staff:* 4
Ownership: COVANCE INC.
Produces/Sells CE-marked Devices: N
Federal Procurement Eligibility: Small Business
Distribution: Manufacturer Direct, Manufacturer Through Distributor, OEM,
Exclusive Distributor
General Admin.: Ronald J. Casciato/Executive Chairman
Richard D. Gill/President, Chief Executive Officer
Mktg./Adv.: Terri Daly/Corporate Communications Specialist
Paul Fluckiger/Vice President Marketing & Sales
Finance: John Hallinan/Chief Financial Officer

Antibody, Monoclonal	Microbiology
Antibody, Other	General
Stain, Chemical Solution	Pathology
Test, Cancer Detection, Monoclonal Antibody	Immunology

COVARIS INC. 781-932-3959
14 Gill Street, Unit H, Woburn, MA 01801
FDA Number: n/a Fax: 781-932-8705
E-mail: info@covarisinc.com
Web site: http://www.covarisinc.com
Year Founded: 1999
Ownership: Private
Produces/Sells CE-marked Devices: N

COVENTINA HEALTHCARE ENTERPRISES, INC. 412-915-6442
1297 Royal Park Blvd., South Park, PA 15129
FDA Number: n/a
Ownership: Private
Produces/Sells CE-marked Devices: N

Diathermy, Shortwave	Physical Med

COVIDIEN 303-305-2382
5870 Stoneridge Drive, Suite 6, Pleasanton, CA 94588
FDA Number: 3006400630
Web site: www.covidien.com
Ownership: Public
Stock Symbol: COV
Traded On: NYSE
Produces/Sells CE-marked Devices: N
General Admin.: Tracy Berns/General Counsel
Mktg./Adv.: Matt Bastardi/Vice President Business Development
Dennis Crowley/Vice President Corporate Development
Scott Miller/Vice President Corporate Development
Production: Amy Hinton/Product Manager

Accessories, Cardiopulmonary Bypass	Cardiovascular
Analyzer, Gas, Carbon-Dioxide, Gaseous Phase (Capnograph)	Anesthesiology
Attachment, Breathing, Positive End Expiratory Pressure	Anesthesiology
Catheter, Suction, With Tip	General
Humidifier, Respiratory Gas, (Direct Patient Interface)	Anesthesiology
Injector, Angiographic (Cardiac Catheterization)	Cardiovascular
Mask, Oxygen, Other	General
Oximeter, Ear	Cardiovascular

COVIDIEN 303-305-2382 (cont'd)

Pressure Infusor, IV Container	General
Spirometer, Diagnostic (Respirometer)	Anesthesiology
Stopcock	General
System, Network And Communication, Physiological Monitors	Cardiovascular
Thermometer, Electronic	General
Tracheobronchial Suction Catheter Kit	Anesthesiology
Ventilator, Continuous (Respirator), Accessory	Anesthesiology
Ventilator, Emergency, Manual (Resuscitator)	Anesthesiology

COVIDIEN (FORMERLY NELLCOR PURITAN 800-962-9888
BENNETT / TYCO HEALTHCARE)
6135 Gunbarrel Ave, Boulder, CO 80301 303-530-2300
FDA Number: 2936999
E-mail: customersupport@covidien.com
Web site: www.covidien.com
Annual Revenue: More than $1 Billion
Total Employees: 41700
Ownership: COVIDIEN LTD.
Stock Symbol: COV
Traded On: NYSE
Quality System Registration Information: ISO9000; ISO9001
Produces/Sells CE-marked Devices: Y
Distribution: Manufacturer Direct, Manufacturer Through Distributor, Manufacturer
Through Manufacturer Reps
General Admin.: Charles J. Dockendorff/Chief Financial Officer, Executive Vice
President
Richard J. Meelia/President, Chief Executive Officer
Finance: Richard G. Brown/Vice President Accounting

Analyzer, Gas, Carbon-Dioxide, Gaseous Phase (Capnograph)	Anesthesiology
Canister, Liquid Oxygen, Portable	Anesthesiology
Canister, Oxygen	Anesthesiology
Cannula, Nasal, Oxygen	Anesthesiology
Computer, Patient Monitor	Anesthesiology
Computer, Pulmonary Function Data	Anesthesiology
Container, Liquid Oxygen	Anesthesiology
Continuous Positive Airway Pressure Unit (CPAP, CPPB)	Anesthesiology
Cuff, Tracheostomy Tube	Ear/Nose/Throat
Filter, Bacterial, Breathing Circuit	Anesthesiology
Filter, Ventilator	Anesthesiology
Holder, Tracheostomy Tube	Anesthesiology
Humidifier, Heat/Moisture Exchange	Anesthesiology
Monitor, Carbon-Dioxide, Cutaneous	Anesthesiology
Monitor, Temperature (With Probe)	Anesthesiology
Oximeter, Pulse	General
Probe, Temperature	General
Sensor, Oxygen	Anesthesiology
Spirometer, Diagnostic (Respirometer)	Anesthesiology
Tube, Tracheal (Endotracheal)	Anesthesiology
Tube, Tracheostomy (W/Wo Connector)	Anesthesiology
Tubing, Ventilator	Anesthesiology
Ventilator, Continuous (Respirator)	Anesthesiology
Ventilator, Continuous (Respirator), Accessory	Anesthesiology
Ventilator, Emergency, Manual (Resuscitator)	Anesthesiology
Ventilator, Neonatal Respirator	General
Ventilator, Volume (Critical Care)	Anesthesiology
Warmer, Blanket	General
Warmer, Infusion Fluid, Thermal	General

COVIDIEN LP 508-261-8000
15 Hampshire St., Mansfield, MA 02048
FDA Number: 1282497
E-mail: todd.carpenter@covidien.com
Web site: www.covidien.com
Medical Products Sales Volume: $1,100,000,000
Annual Revenue: More than $1 Billion
Total Employees: 41000
Ownership: TYCO INTERNATIONAL LTD.
Stock Symbol: COV
Traded On: NYSE
Quality System Registration Information: ISO9001; ISO9002
Produces/Sells CE-marked Devices: Y
Distribution: Manufacturer Direct, OEM
General Admin.: Mr. Richard Meelia/Chairman, Chief Executive Officer
Mr. Charles Dockendorff/Chief Financial Officer, Executive Vice
President
Mr. Steve McManama/Chief Information Officer
Mr. Jose Almeida/President
Ms. Amy Wendell/Senior Vice President Planning and
Development
Mktg./Adv.: Mr. Eric Kraus/Vice President Corporate Communications

Airway, Bi-Nasopharyngeal (With Connector)	Anesthesiology
Airway, Esophageal (Obturator)	Anesthesiology
Airway, Nasopharyngeal (Breathing Tube)	Anesthesiology
Analyzer, Pulmonary Function	Anesthesiology
Applicator, Tipped, Absorbent	General
Applicator, Tipped, Absorbent, Sterile	General
Applier, Clip, Repair, Hernia, Laparoscopic	Gastroenterology/Urology
Aspirator, Wound Suction Pump	General

COVIDIEN LP   508-261-8000 *(cont'd)*

Autotransfusion Unit (Blood)	Anesthesiology
Bag, Drainage (Incontinence)	Gastroenterology/Urology
Bag, Urinary Collection	General
Bandage, Elastic	General
Bolster, Suture (Bumper)	Surgery
Bottle, Blow (Exerciser)	Anesthesiology
Brush, Scrub, Operating Room	Surgery
Cable	Physical Med
Cannula, Nasal, Oxygen	Anesthesiology
Cap, Tip, Syringe	General
Catheter, Aspiration	Surgery
Catheter, Balloon (Foley Type)	Surgery
Catheter, Biliary	Gastroenterology/Urology
Catheter, Embolectomy (Fogarty Type)	Cardiovascular
Catheter, Epidural	Obstetrics/Gynecology
Catheter, Infusion	Surgery
Catheter, Intravascular, Therapeutic, Short-term Less Than 30 Days	General
Catheter, Intravenous	Cardiovascular
Catheter, Intravenous, Central	Cardiovascular
Catheter, Nasal, Oxygen (Tube)	Anesthesiology
Catheter, Occlusion	Cardiovascular
Catheter, Other	Gastroenterology/Urology
Catheter, Oxygen, Tracheal	Anesthesiology
Catheter, Perfusion	Cardiovascular
Catheter, Retention Type, Balloon	Gastroenterology/Urology
Catheter, Straight	Gastroenterology/Urology
Catheter, Suprapubic	Gastroenterology/Urology
Catheter, Suprapubic, With Tube	Gastroenterology/Urology
Catheter, Ureteral Disposable (X-Ray)	Gastroenterology/Urology
Catheter, Urethral	Gastroenterology/Urology
Catheter, Urinary	Gastroenterology/Urology
Catheter, Urinary, Irrigation	Gastroenterology/Urology
Catheter, Vascular, Cardiopulmonary Bypass	Cardiovascular
Chair, Blood Drawing	General
Clip, Vascular	Cardiovascular
Closure, Other	General
Collector, Sputum	Anesthesiology
Collector, Urine	Gastroenterology/Urology
Collector, Urine, Disposable	Gastroenterology/Urology
Connector, Airway (Extension)	Anesthesiology
Connector, Catheter	Surgery
Connector, Suction/Irrigation	Surgery
Container, Specimen Mailer And Storage, Temperature Control	Pathology
Container, Specimen, All Types	General
Container, Urine Specimen	General
Device, Anastomosis, Biofragmentable	Surgery
Device, Embolization, Artificial	Cns/Neurology
Diluter	Chemistry
Dispenser, Medication, Liquid	General
Dispenser, Other	General
Drain, Penrose	Gastroenterology/Urology
Drain, Sump	Gastroenterology/Urology
Drain, Thoracic (Chest)	Anesthesiology
Drain, Thoracic, Water Seal	Anesthesiology
Drainage System, Urine, Closed	Gastroenterology/Urology
Drainage Unit, Urinary	General
Dressing, Gel	General
Dressing, Non-Adherent	General
Dressing, Other	General
Dressing, Roller Gauze	General
Dressing, Universal	General
Dressing, Wound and Burn, Occlusive	Surgery
Ejector, Saliva	Ear/Nose/Throat
Electrode, Pacemaker, External	Cardiovascular
Exerciser, Respiratory	Anesthesiology
Gauze Roll	Surgery
Gauze, Absorbable	Surgery
Hematocrit Tube, Rack, Sealer, Holder	Hematology
Holder, Needle, Other	Surgery
Introducer, Catheter	Cardiovascular
Introducer, Spinal Needle	Anesthesiology
Introducer, Syringe Needle	General
Jelly, Lubricating	General
Kit, Administration, Enteral	Gastroenterology/Urology
Kit, Administration, Parenteral	Gastroenterology/Urology
Kit, Anesthesia, Caudal	Anesthesiology
Kit, Anesthesia, Epidural	Anesthesiology
Kit, Anesthesia, Other	Anesthesiology
Kit, Anesthesia, Paracervical	Obstetrics/Gynecology
Kit, Anesthesia, Pudendal	Obstetrics/Gynecology
Kit, Anesthesia, Spinal	Anesthesiology
Kit, Biopsy	General
Kit, Burn	General
Kit, Catheter Care	General
Kit, Catheterization, Intravenous, Winged	Cardiovascular
Kit, Catheterization, Sterile Urethral	Gastroenterology/Urology
Kit, Catheterization, Urinary	Gastroenterology/Urology
Kit, Chest Drainage (Thoracentesis Tray)	General
Kit, Feeding, Adult (Enteral)	General
Kit, Feeding, Pediatric (Enteral)	General
Kit, Irrigation, Bladder	Gastroenterology/Urology

COVIDIEN LP   508-261-8000 *(cont'd)*

Kit, Irrigation, Sterile	Gastroenterology/Urology
Kit, Irrigation, Wound	General
Kit, Lumbar Puncture	Cns/Neurology
Kit, Sampling, Arterial Blood	Anesthesiology
Kit, Sampling, Blood	General
Kit, Sampling, Blood Gas	General
Kit, Suction, Airway (Tracheal)	Anesthesiology
Kit, Tracheostomy Care	Anesthesiology
Kit, Urinary Drainage Collection	Gastroenterology/Urology
Kit, Wound Dressing	Surgery
Labware, Basic, Disposable	Chemistry
Labware, Blood Collection	Chemistry
Lancet, Blood	General
Ligature, Laparoscopic	Surgery
Loop, Inoculating	Microbiology
Lotion, Skin Care	General
Mesh, Surgical, Polymeric	Surgery
Monitor, Ventilation	Anesthesiology
Needle, Aspiration And Injection, Disposable	Surgery
Needle, Biopsy, Cardiovascular	Cardiovascular
Needle, Blood Collection	General
Needle, Blunt	General
Needle, Cardiac	Cardiovascular
Needle, Conduction, Anesthesia (W/Wo Introducer)	Anesthesiology
Needle, Dental	Dental And Oral
Needle, Gastro-Urology	Gastroenterology/Urology
Needle, Hypodermic	General
Needle, Intravenous	General
Needle, Other	General
Needle, Spinal, Short-Term	General
Pad, Dressing	General
Pad, Medicated	General
Pad, Pressure, Gel, Operating Table	General
Paraffin, All Formulations	Pathology
Pipette Tip	Chemistry
Pipette, Diluting	Hematology
Pipette, Micro	Chemistry
Pipetting And Diluting System, Automated	Chemistry
Pledget, Dacron, Teflon, Polypropylene	Cardiovascular
Pump, Aspiration, Portable	Anesthesiology
Pump, Food (Enteral Feeding)	General
Punch, Aortic	Cardiovascular
Remover, Staple, Surgical	Surgery
Retention Device, Suture	Surgery
Serum Separation System	Hematology
Shunt, Arteriovenous	Gastroenterology/Urology
Shunt, Carotid	Cardiovascular
Sizer, Device, Anastomosis	Surgery
Solution, Surgical Scrub	General
Spirometer, Therapeutic (Incentive)	Anesthesiology
Standard/Control, All Types	Chemistry
Stapler, Surgical	Surgery
Sterilizer, Laboratory	Microbiology
Stethoscope, Esophageal	Anesthesiology
Stick, Urinalysis Test	Chemistry
Stimulator, Wound Healing	Physical Med
Stopcock	General
Suction Apparatus, Single Patient, Portable, Non-Powered	Surgery
Support, Patient Position	Anesthesiology
Suture, Absorbable	Surgery
Suture, Absorbable, Ophthalmic	Ophthalmology
Suture, Absorbable, Synthetic, Polyglycolic Acid	Surgery
Suture, Cardiovascular	Cardiovascular
Suture, Catgut	Surgery
Suture, Cotton	Surgery
Suture, Laparoscopy	Surgery
Suture, Multifilament Steel	Surgery
Suture, Non-Absorbable	Surgery
Suture, Non-Absorbable, Ophthalmic	Ophthalmology
Suture, Non-Absorbable, Silk	Surgery
Suture, Non-Absorbable, Steel, Monofilament & Multifilament	Surgery
Suture, Non-Absorbable, Synthetic, Polyamide	Surgery
Suture, Non-Absorbable, Synthetic, Polyester	Surgery
Suture, Non-Absorbable, Synthetic, Polyethylene	Surgery
Suture, Other	Surgery
Suture, Polypropylene Monofilament	Surgery
Suture, Silk	Surgery
Suture, Stainless Steel	Surgery
Syringe, Anesthesia	Anesthesiology
Syringe, Antistick	General
Syringe, Bulb	General
Syringe, Bulb, Air Or Water	Dental And Oral
Syringe, Catheter	General
Syringe, Dental	Dental And Oral
Syringe, Hypodermic	General
Syringe, Insulin	General
Syringe, Irrigating, Dental	Dental And Oral
Syringe, Periodontic, Endodontic	Dental And Oral
Syringe, Piston	General
Syringe, Tuberculin	General
Tape, Adhesive	General

COVIDIEN LP
508-261-8000 *(cont'd)*

Tape, Gauze, Adhesive	General
Tape, Umbilical	General
Thermometer, Electronic	General
Thermometer, Electronic, Continuous	General
Thermometer, Tympanic	Ear/Nose/Throat
Timer, Clot, Automated	Hematology
Timer, Coagulation	Hematology
Tip, Suction	Anesthesiology
Tip, Suction Tube (Yankauer, Poole, Etc.)	Surgery
Trap, Mucus	Anesthesiology
Trap, Sterile Specimen	Anesthesiology
Tray, Medicine	General
Tube, Blood Collection	Chemistry
Tube, Blood Microcollection	Chemistry
Tube, Bronchoscope, Aspirating	Anesthesiology
Tube, Capillary	Chemistry
Tube, Capillary Blood Collection	Hematology
Tube, Centrifuge	Chemistry
Tube, Connecting	General
Tube, Culture	Microbiology
Tube, Double Lumen For Intestinal Decompression	Gastroenterology/Urology
Tube, Drainage	Gastroenterology/Urology
Tube, Esophageal, Replogle	Gastroenterology/Urology
Tube, Feeding	General
Tube, Levine	General
Tube, Nasogastric	Anesthesiology
Tube, Single Lumen, W Mercury Wt Balloon	Gastroenterology/Urology
Tube, Tracheal (Endotracheal)	Anesthesiology
Tube, Tracheostomy (Breathing Tube), ENT	Ear/Nose/Throat
Tube, Vacuum Sample, With Anticoagulant	Hematology
Tubing, Conductive	General
Tubing, Flexible, Medical Gas, Low-Pressure	Anesthesiology
Tubing, Irrigation	Surgery
Tubing, Non-Conductive	General
Tubing, Non-Invasive	Surgery
Tubing, Oxygen Connecting	General
Tubing, Polyethylene	General
Tubing, Polyvinyl Chloride	General
Tubing, Silicone	General
Waste Disposal Unit, Sharps	General
Waste Disposal Unit, Surgical Instrument (Sharps)	Surgery
Waste Disposal Unit, Syringe	General

Medical Product Subsidiaries (Listed Separately)
Nippon Sherwood Medical Ind. Ltd.
Somanetics Corp.
U.S. Clinical Products, Div. Sherwood Medical Co.

COVIDIEN LP, FORMERLY REGISTERED AS KENDALL
800-962-9888

130 South Main St., Oriskany Falls, NY 13425 **315-821-7233**
FDA Number: 1314412
E-mail: customersupport@covidien.com
Web site: www.covidien.com
Total Employees: 41700
Ownership: Covidien Ltd.
Stock Symbol: COV
Traded On: NYSE
Produces/Sells CE-marked Devices: N
General Admin.: Charles J. Dockendorff/Chief Financial Officer, Executive Vice President

Richard J. Meelia/President, Chief Executive Officer
Finance: Richard G. Brown/Vice President Accounting

Applicator, Tipped, Absorbent, Non-Sterile	General
Applicator, Tipped, Absorbent, Sterile	General
Bandage, Elastic	General
Catheter, Percutaneous	Cardiovascular
Catheter, Umbilical Artery	General
Catheter, Vascular, Cardiopulmonary Bypass	Cardiovascular
Dressing, Other	General
Dressing, Wound and Burn, Hydrogel	Surgery
Syringe, Piston	General
Tube, Gastrointestinal	Gastroenterology/Urology

COVIDIEN LP, FORMERLY REGISTERED AS KENDALL
800-962-9888

1430 Marvin Griffin Rd, Augusta, GA 30906 **706-793-3030**
FDA Number: 1018120
E-mail: customersupport@covidien.com
Web site: www.covidien.com
Annual Revenue: More than $1 Billion
Total Employees: 41700
Ownership: Covidien Ltd.
Stock Symbol: COV
Traded On: NYSE
Produces/Sells CE-marked Devices: N
General Admin.: Charles J. Dockendorff/Chief Financial Officer, Executive Vice President

Richard J. Meelia/President, Chief Executive Officer

COVIDIEN LP, FORMERLY REGISTERED AS
800-962-9888
(cont'd)
Finance: Richard G. Brown/Vice President Accounting

Bandage, Cast	Physical Med
Bandage, Liquid	Surgery
Bandage, Other	General
Dressing, Wound and Burn, Hydrogel	Surgery
Dressing, Wound, Occlusive	Surgery
Fiber, Absorbent	General
Gauze, Non-Absorbable, X-Ray Detectable (Internal Sponge)	Surgery
Gauze/sponge, Nonresorbable For External Use	Surgery
Pad, Alcohol	General
Pad, Eye	Ophthalmology
Solvent, Adhesive Tape	Surgery
Tape, Adhesive	General

COVIDIEN LP, FORMERLY REGISTERED AS KENDALL
800-962-9888

1448 Blue Ridge Blvd, Seneca, SC 29672 **864-882-7203**
FDA Number: 1017072
E-mail: customersupport@covidien.com
Web site: www.covidien.com
Annual Revenue: More than $1 Billion
Total Employees: 41700
Ownership: Covidien Ltd.
Stock Symbol: COV
Traded On: NYSE
Produces/Sells CE-marked Devices: N
General Admin.: Charles J. Dockendorff/Chief Financial Officer, Executive Vice President

Richard J. Meelia/President, Chief Executive Officer
Finance: Richard G. Brown/Vice President Accounting

Bandage, Cast	Physical Med
Bandage, Elastic	General
Collector, Urine	Gastroenterology/Urology
Dressing, Wound, Occlusive	Surgery
Sleeve, Compressible Limb	Cardiovascular
Sponge, Internal	Cns/Neurology
Stocking, Support (Anti-Embolic)	General

COVIDIEN LP, FORMERLY REGISTERED AS KENDALL
See Covidien Lp, Formerly Registered As Tyco Healthcare

COVIDIEN LP, FORMERLY REGISTERED AS KENDALL
800-962-9888

2010 East International, Speedway Boulevard, Deland, FL 32724 **386-738-8212**
FDA Number: 1017768
E-mail: customersupport@covidien.com
Web site: www.covidien.com
Annual Revenue: More than $1 Billion
Total Employees: 41700
Ownership: Covidien Ltd.
Stock Symbol: COV
Traded On: NYSE
Produces/Sells CE-marked Devices: N
General Admin.: Charles J. Dockendorff/Chief Financial Officer, Executive Vice President

Richard J. Meelia/President, Chief Executive Officer
Finance: Richard G. Brown/Vice President Accounting

Instrument, Manual, General Surgical	Surgery
Lancet, Blood	General
Needle, Aspiration And Injection, Disposable	Surgery
Needle, Conduction, Anesthesia (W/Wo Introducer)	Anesthesiology
Needle, Dental	Dental And Oral
Needle, Hypodermic, Single Lumen With Syringe	General
Syringe, Cartridge	Dental And Oral
Syringe, Periodontic, Endodontic	Dental And Oral
Syringe, Piston	General

COVIDIEN LP, FORMERLY REGISTERED AS KENDALL
800-962-9888

400 Maple St, Commerce, TX 75428 **903-886-3153**
FDA Number: 1650158
E-mail: customersupport@covidien.com
Web site: www.covidien.com
Annual Revenue: More than $1 Billion
Total Employees: 41700
Ownership: Covidien Ltd.
Stock Symbol: COV
Traded On: NYSE
Produces/Sells CE-marked Devices: N
General Admin.: Charles J. Dockendorff/Chief Financial Officer, Executive Vice President

Richard J. Meelia/President, Chief Executive Officer
Finance: Richard G. Brown/Vice President Accounting

Connector, Catheter	Surgery
Container, Medication, Graduated Liquid	General

COVIDIEN LP, FORMERLY REGISTERED AS   800-962-9888
(cont'd)

Container, Specimen Mailer And Storage	Pathology
Equipment, Laboratory, Gen. Purpose (Specific Medical Use)	Chemistry
Kit, Surgical Instrument, Disposable	Surgery
Needle, Hypodermic, Single Lumen With Syringe	General
Syringe, Piston	General
Tube, Connecting	General
Tubing, Other	General

COVIDIEN LP, FORMERLY REGISTERED AS   800-962-9888
KENDALL

444 Mcdonnell Blvd., Hazelwood, MO 63042
FDA Number: 1921846
E-mail: customersupport@covidien.com
Web site: www.covidien.com
Total Employees: 41700
Ownership: Covidien Ltd.
Stock Symbol: COV
Traded On: NYSE
Produces/Sells CE-marked Devices: N
General Admin.: Charles J. Dockendorff/Chief Financial Officer, Executive Vice President
     Richard J. Meelia/President, Chief Executive Officer
Finance: Richard G. Brown/Vice President Accounting

Needle, Hypodermic, Single Lumen With Syringe	General
Pump, Infusion	General
Set, Administration, Intravenous, Needle-Free	General
Syringe, Piston	General
Thermometer, Electronic	General

COVIDIEN LP, FORMERLY REGISTERED AS   800-962-9888
KENDALL

525 North Emerald Rd, Greenwood, SC 29646   **864-223-4281**
FDA Number: 1033903
E-mail: customersupport@covidien.com
Web site: www.covidien.com
Total Employees: 41700
Ownership: Covidien Ltd.
Stock Symbol: COV
Traded On: NYSE
Produces/Sells CE-marked Devices: N
General Admin.: Charles J. Dockendorff/Chief Financial Officer, Executive Vice President
     Richard J. Meelia/President, Chief Executive Officer
Finance: Richard G. Brown/Vice President Accounting

Fiber, Absorbent	General
Garment, Protective, For Incontinence	Gastroenterology/Urology
Sheet, Examination Table, Disposable	General

COVIDIEN LP, FORMERLY REGISTERED AS   800-962-9888
KENDALL

5439 State Rte. 40, Argyle, NY 12809   **518-638-6101**
FDA Number: 1317749   *Fax:* 518-638-8493
E-mail: customersupport@covidien.com
Web site: www.covidien.com
Annual Revenue: More than $1 Billion
Total Employees: 41700
Ownership: COVIDIEN LTD.
Stock Symbol: COV
Traded On: NYSE
Quality System Registration Information: ISO9000
Produces/Sells CE-marked Devices: Y
Federal Procurement Eligibility: Small Business
Distribution: Manufacturer Through Distributor
General Admin.: Charles J. Dockendorff/Chief Financial Officer, Executive Vice President
     Richard J. Meelia/President, Chief Executive Officer
Finance: Richard G. Brown/Vice President Accounting

Catheter, Balloon (Foley Type)	Surgery
Catheter, Other	Gastroenterology/Urology
Probe, Temperature	General
Stethoscope, Esophageal	Anesthesiology
Stylet, Tracheal Tube	Anesthesiology
Tube, Tracheal (Endotracheal)	Anesthesiology

COVIDIEN LP, FORMERLY REGISTERED AS   800-962-9888
KENDALL

815 Tek Dr., Crystal Lake, IL 60039   **815-444-2500**
FDA Number: 1424643
E-mail: customersupport@covidien.com
Web site: www.covidien.com
Annual Revenue: More than $1 Billion
Total Employees: 41700
Ownership: Covidien Ltd.
Stock Symbol: COV
Traded On: NYSE

COVIDIEN LP, FORMERLY REGISTERED AS   800-962-9888
(cont'd)

Produces/Sells CE-marked Devices: N
General Admin.: Charles J. Dockendorff/Chief Financial Officer, Executive Vice President
     Richard J. Meelia/President, Chief Executive Officer
Finance: Richard G. Brown/Vice President Accounting

Container, Sharpes	General
Infusion Stand	General
Needle, Hypodermic, Single Lumen With Syringe	General
Waste Disposal Unit, Surgical Instrument (Sharps)	Surgery

COVIDIEN LP, FORMERLY REGISTERED AS LUDLOW
   See Covidien Lp, Formerly Registered As Tyco Healthcare

COVIDIEN LP, FORMERLY REGISTERED   800-962-9888
AS LUDLOW

Two Ludlow Park Dr., Chicopee, MA 01022   **413-593-6400**
FDA Number: 1219103
E-mail: customersupport@covidien.com
Web site: www.covidien.com
Annual Revenue: More than $1 Billion
Total Employees: 41700
Ownership: Covidien Ltd.
Stock Symbol: COV
Traded On: NYSE
Produces/Sells CE-marked Devices: N
General Admin.: Charles J. Dockendorff/Chief Financial Officer, Executive Vice President
     Richard J. Meelia/President, Chief Executive Officer
Finance: Richard G. Brown/Vice President Accounting

Accessories, Operating Room, Table	Surgery
Applicator, Tipped, Absorbent, Non-Sterile	General
Clamp, Surgical, General & Plastic Surgery	Surgery
Container, IV	General
Container, Specimen Mailer And Storage	Pathology
Counter, Sponge, Surgical	Surgery
Cutter, Surgical	Surgery
Drape, Surgical	Surgery
Dressing, Wound and Burn, Hydrogel	Surgery
Dressing, Wound, Hydrogel W/out Drug And/or Biologic	Surgery
Electrode, Electrocardiograph	Cardiovascular
Electrode, Electrocardiograph, Multi-Function	Cardiovascular
Electrosurgical Unit, Cutting & Coagulation Device	Surgery
Equipment, Laboratory, Gen. Purpose (Specific Medical Use)	Chemistry
Glove, Patient Examination, Specialty	General
Gown, Examination	General
Holder, Needle	Gastroenterology/Urology
Lamp, Operating Room	General
Laparoscope, General & Plastic Surgery	Surgery
Marker, Skin	Surgery
Pack, Hot Or Cold, Disposable	Physical Med
Pack, Hot Or Cold, Reusable	Physical Med
Pack, Sterilization Wrapper (Bag And Accessories)	Surgery
Pad, Menstrual, Unscented	Obstetrics/Gynecology
Recorder, Paper Chart	Cardiovascular
Restraint, Patient, Conductive	Anesthesiology
Stapler, Surgical	Surgery
Surgical Instrument, Obstetric/Gynecologic	Obstetrics/Gynecology
Syringe, Piston	General
Toothbrush, Manual	Dental And Oral
Transfer Unit, IV Fluid	General
Warmer, Heel, Infant	Physical Med

COVIDIEN LP, FORMERLY REGISTERED AS TYCO HEALTHCAR
   See First Quality Retail Services, Llc.

COVIDIEN LP, FORMERLY REGISTERED AS   800-962-9888
TYCO HEALTHCARE

110 Kendall Park Lane, Atlanta, GA 30336   **404-344-7400**
FDA Number: 1067165
E-mail: customersupport@covidien.com
Web site: www.covidien.com
Annual Revenue: More than $1 Billion
Total Employees: 41700
Ownership: Covidien Ltd.
Stock Symbol: COV
Traded On: NYSE
Produces/Sells CE-marked Devices: N
General Admin.: Charles J. Dockendorff/Chief Financial Officer, Executive Vice President
     Richard J. Meelia/President, Chief Executive Officer
Finance: Richard G. Brown/Vice President Accounting

COVIDIEN LP, FORMERLY REGISTERED AS   800-962-9888
TYCO HEALTHCARE

15 Hampshire Street, Mansfield, MA 02048   **508-261-8000**
FDA Number: 1282497

COVIDIEN LP, FORMERLY REGISTERED AS   800-962-9888
(cont'd)

E-mail: customersupport@covidien.com
Web site: www.covidien.com
Annual Revenue: More than $1 Billion
Total Employees: 41700
Ownership: Covidien Ltd.
Stock Symbol: COV
Traded On: NYSE
Produces/Sells CE-marked Devices: N
General Admin.: Charles J. Dockendorff/Chief Financial Officer, Executive Vice President

Mr. Jose Almedia/President, Chief Executive Officer
Mr. Michael Dunford/Senior Vice President Human Resources
Mr. John Masterson/Senior Vice President, General Counsel
Medical Admin.: Mr. Michael Tarnoff/Chief Medical Officer
Production: Mr. Mike Sgrignari/Senior Vice President Quality Assurance
Finance: Richard G. Brown/Vice President Accounting
Mr. Coleman Lannum/Vice President Investor Relations

Applicator, Tipped, Absorbent, Non-Sterile	General
Cable/Lead, ECG, With Transducer And Electrode	Cardiovascular
Connector, Airway (Extension)	Anesthesiology
Container, IV	General
Counter, Sponge, Surgical	Surgery
Dressing, Wound, Hydrogel W/out Drug And/or Biologic	Surgery
Electrode, Circular (Spiral), Scalp And Applicator	Obstetrics/Gynecology
Electrode, Electrocardiograph	Cardiovascular
Electrode, Electrocardiograph, Multi-Function	Cardiovascular
Electrosurgical Unit, Cutting & Coagulation Device	Surgery
Equipment, Laboratory, Gen. Purpose (Specific Medical Use)	Chemistry
Fixation Device, Tracheal Tube	Anesthesiology
Garment, Protective, For Incontinence	Gastroenterology/Urology
Glove, Patient Examination, Specialty	General
Handpiece, Air-Powered, Dental	Dental And Oral
Kit, Trocar	Surgery
Pacemaker, Cardiac, External Transcutaneous (Non-Invasive)	Cardiovascular
Pack, Hot Or Cold, Disposable	Physical Med
Pack, Hot Or Cold, Reusable	Physical Med
Pad, Menstrual, Unscented	Obstetrics/Gynecology
Recorder, Paper Chart	Cardiovascular
Support, Patient Position	Anesthesiology
Surgical Instrument, Obstetric/Gynecologic	Obstetrics/Gynecology
Syringe, Piston	General
Warmer, Heel, Infant	Physical Med

COVIDIEN LP, FORMERLY REGISTERED AS   800-962-9888
TYCO HEALTHCARE

4651 E. Francis Street, Ontario, CA 91761   **508-261-8587**
FDA Number: 3005120631
E-mail: customersupport@covidien.com
Web site: www.covidien.com
Annual Revenue: More than $1 Billion
Total Employees: 41700
Ownership: Covidien Ltd.
Stock Symbol: COV
Traded On: NYSE
Produces/Sells CE-marked Devices: N
General Admin.: Charles J. Dockendorff/Chief Financial Officer, Executive Vice President

Richard J. Meelia/President, Chief Executive Officer
Finance: Richard G. Brown/Vice President Accounting

COVIDIEN LP, FORMERLY REGISTERED AS   800-962-9888
UNI-PATCH

1313 Grant Blvd, Wabasha, MN 55981   **651-565-2601**
FDA Number: 2183164
E-mail: customersupport@covidien.com
Web site: www.covidien.com
Annual Revenue: More than $1 Billion
Total Employees: 41700
Ownership: Covidien Ltd.
Stock Symbol: COV
Traded On: NYSE
Quality System Registration Information: ISO9000; ISO9001; ISO9002; ISO9003
Produces/Sells CE-marked Devices: Y
Distribution: Manufacturer Through Distributor, Exporter
General Admin.: Charles J. Dockendorff/Chief Financial Officer, Executive Vice President

Richard J. Meelia/President, Chief Executive Officer
Finance: Richard G. Brown/Vice President Accounting

Bandage, Elastic	General
Electrode, Neuromuscular Stimulator	Cns/Neurology
Electrode, TENS	Cns/Neurology
Lotion, Skin Care	General
Pack, Hot Or Cold, Reusable	Physical Med
Solution, Patient Preparation	General
Solvent, Adhesive Tape	Surgery

COVIDIEN LP, FORMERLY REGISTERED AS   800-962-9888
(cont'd)
Support, Hot/Cold Pack   Physical Med

COVIDIEN LP, FORMERLY REGISTERED AS   800-962-9888
UNITED STATES SURGICAL

150 Glover Ave., Norwalk, CT 06856-5080   **203-845-1000**
FDA Number: 1219161
E-mail: customersupport@covidien.com
Web site: www.ussurg.com
Annual Revenue: More than $1 Billion
Total Employees: 41700
Ownership: Covidien Ltd.
Stock Symbol: COV
Traded On: NYSE
Quality System Registration Information: ISO9001; ISO9002
Produces/Sells CE-marked Devices: Y
Distribution: Manufacturer Direct, Manufacturer Through Distributor, Manufacturer Through Manufacturer Reps, Exporter
General Admin.: Charles J. Dockendorff/Chief Financial Officer, Executive Vice President

Richard J. Meelia/President, Chief Executive Officer
Finance: Richard G. Brown/Vice President Accounting

Adhesive, Wound Closure	Surgery
Applier, Clip, Laparoscopic	Surgery
Applier, Clip, Repair, Hernia, Laparoscopic	Gastroenterology/Urology
Applier, Surgical Staple	Surgery
Applier, Surgical, Clip	Surgery
Bag, Specimen, Laparoscopic	Surgery
Cannula With Inflatable Balloon (Distal Tip)	Surgery
Cannula, Suprapubic, With Trocar	Gastroenterology/Urology
Carrier, Ligature	Surgery
Clip, Hemostatic	Surgery
Clip, Implantable	Surgery
Clip, Instrument	Surgery
Device, Suturing, Endoscopic	Surgery
Equipment, Suction/Irrigation, Laparoscopic	Surgery
Forceps, Endoscopic	Gastroenterology/Urology
Forceps, Grasping, Atraumatic	Surgery
Forceps, Grasping, Flexible Endoscopic	Gastroenterology/Urology
Forceps, Grasping, Traumatic	Surgery
Gauge, Thickness, Tissue	Surgery
Indirect Fluorescent Antibody Test, Entamoeba Histolytica	Microbiology
Instrument, Dissecting, Laparoscopic	Surgery
Instrument, Manual, General Surgical	Surgery
Instrument, Passing, Ligature, Knot Tying	Cns/Neurology
Instrument, Surgical, Powered, Pneumatic	Orthopedics
Irrigator, Suction	General
Kit, Laparoscopy	Gastroenterology/Urology
Kit, Suture Removal	Surgery
Laparoscope, General & Plastic Surgery	Surgery
Mesh, Surgical, Polymeric	Surgery
Needle, Endoscopic	Gastroenterology/Urology
Needle, Insufflation, Laparoscopic	Surgery
Needle, Pneumoperitoneum, Simple	Gastroenterology/Urology
Needle, Suture, Reusable	Surgery
Obturator, Endoscopic	Gastroenterology/Urology
Peritoneoscope	Gastroenterology/Urology
Retractor, Fan-Type, Laparoscopy	Surgery
Retractor, Laparoscopy, Other	Surgery
Retractor, Other	Surgery
Scissors, Disposable	General
Scissors, Suture	Surgery
Staple, Absorbable	Orthopedics
Staple, Implantable	Surgery
Staple, Removable (Skin)	Surgery
Stapler, Laparoscopic	Surgery
Stapler, Surgical	Surgery
Surgical Instrument, Disposable	Surgery
Suture, Absorbable	Surgery
Suture, Absorbable, Synthetic	Surgery
Suture, Laparoscopy	Surgery
Suture, Non-Absorbable, Silk	Surgery
Suture, Non-Absorbable, Steel, Monofilament & Multifilament	Surgery
Suture, Non-Absorbable, Synthetic, Polyamide	Surgery
Suture, Non-Absorbable, Synthetic, Polyester	Surgery
Suture, Non-Absorbable, Synthetic, Polypropylene	Surgery
Suture, Other	Surgery
Trainer, Laparoscopy	Surgery
Tray, Surgical	Surgery
Trocar, Abdominal	Gastroenterology/Urology
Trocar, Gallbladder	Gastroenterology/Urology
Trocar, Laparoscopic	Surgery
Trocar, Other	General
Trocar, Short	Surgery
Trocar, Thoracic	Cardiovascular

Medical Product Subsidiaries (Listed Separately)
Medolas, Gesellschaft Fur Medizintechnik

COVIDIEN LP, FORMERLY REGISTERED AS UNITED STATES SURGICAL
800-962-9888

195 Mcdermott Road, North Haven, CT 06473   **203-492-5000**

FDA Number: 1219930
Web site: www.covidien.com
Annual Revenue: More than $1 Billion
Total Employees: 41700
Ownership: Covidien Ltd.
Stock Symbol: COV
Traded On: NYSE
Produces/Sells CE-marked Devices: N
General Admin.: Charles J. Dockendorff/Chief Financial Officer, Executive Vice President

    Richard J. Meelia/President, Chief Executive Officer

Finance: Richard G. Brown/Vice President Accounting

Accessories, Cleaning, Endoscopic	Gastroenterology/Urology
Appliance, Fixation, Spinal Intervertebral Body	Orthopedics
Applier, Surgical, Clip	Surgery
Arthroscope	Orthopedics
Biopsy Instrument	Gastroenterology/Urology
Catheter, Intravascular, Therapeutic, Long-term Greater Than 30 Days	General
Catheter, Subcutaneous Intravascular, Implanted	General
Catheter, Suction, With Tip	General
Catheter, Vascular, Cardiopulmonary Bypass	Cardiovascular
Cerclage, Fixation	Orthopedics
Clamp, Vascular	Cardiovascular
Clip, Implantable	Surgery
Container, Specimen Mailer And Storage, Temperature Control	Pathology
Curette	Orthopedics
Cutter, Surgical	Surgery
Dissector, Surgical, General & Plastic Surgery	Surgery
Electrosurgical Unit, Cutting & Coagulation Device	Surgery
Elevator, Surgical, General & Plastic Surgery	Surgery
Endoscope	Gastroenterology/Urology
Fastener, Fixation, Biodegradable, Soft Tissue	Orthopedics
Forceps, Obstetrical	Obstetrics/Gynecology
Gauge, Depth	Orthopedics
Gouge, Surgical, General & Plastic Surgery	Surgery
Illuminator, Fiberoptic, Surgical Field	Cns/Neurology
Impactor	Orthopedics
Instrument, Manual, General Surgical	Surgery
Instrument, Passing, Ligature, Knot Tying	Cns/Neurology
Insufflator, Laparoscopic	Obstetrics/Gynecology
Laparoscope, General & Plastic Surgery	Surgery
Laparoscope, Gynecologic	Obstetrics/Gynecology
Mesh, Surgical (Steel Gauze)	Surgery
Mesh, Surgical, Polymeric	Surgery
Motor, Surgical Instrument, Pneumatic-Powered	Surgery
Needle, Pneumoperitoneum, Spring Loaded	Gastroenterology/Urology
Orthopedic Manual Surgical Instrument	Orthopedics
Orthosis, Fusion, Intervertebral, Spinal	Orthopedics
Plate, Fixation, Bone	Orthopedics
Pledget And Intracardiac Patch, PETP, PTFE, Polypropylene	Cardiovascular
Pump, Aspiration, Portable	Anesthesiology
Retractor, Fiberoptic	Gastroenterology/Urology
Retractor, Surgical	Surgery
Rongeur, Rib	Orthopedics
Screw, Fixation, Bone	Orthopedics
Staple, Fixation, Bone	Orthopedics
Staple, Implantable	Surgery
Staple, Removable (Skin)	Surgery
Stapler, Surgical	Surgery
Surgical Instrument, Cardiovascular	Cardiovascular
Surgical Instrument, Orthopedic, AC-Powered Motor	Orthopedics
Surgical Instrument, Ultrasonic	Surgery
Suture Apparatus, Stomach And Intestinal	Gastroenterology/Urology
Suture, Absorbable	Surgery
Suture, Absorbable, Natural	Surgery
Suture, Absorbable, Synthetic	Surgery
Suture, Non-Absorbable, Silk	Surgery
Suture, Non-Absorbable, Steel, Monofilament & Multifilament	Surgery
Suture, Non-Absorbable, Synthetic, Polyamide	Surgery
Suture, Non-Absorbable, Synthetic, Polyethylene	Surgery
Suture, Non-Absorbable, Synthetic, Polypropylene	Surgery
Trocar, Gastro-Urology	Gastroenterology/Urology
Tube, Aspirating, Flexible, Connecting	Anesthesiology

COVIDIEN, FORMERLY PURITAN BENNETT CORP
800-962-9888

2101 Faraday Avenue, Carlsbad, CA 92008   **303-305-2382**

FDA Number: 2024500
E-mail: customersupport@covidien.com
Web site: www.covidien.com
Annual Revenue: More than $1 Billion
Total Employees: 41700
Ownership: Covidien Ltd.
Stock Symbol: COV
Traded On: NYSE
Produces/Sells CE-marked Devices: N

COVIDIEN, FORMERLY PURITAN
800-962-9888 *(cont'd)*

General Admin.: Charles J. Dockendorff/Chief Financial Officer, Executive Vice President

    Richard J. Meelia/President, Chief Executive Officer

Finance: Richard G. Brown/Vice President Accounting

Tubing, Ventilator	Anesthesiology
Ventilator, Continuous (Respirator)	Anesthesiology

COVIDIEN, FORMERLY TYCO HEALTHCARE MALLINCKRODT
See Mallinckrodt, Inc.

COVOC CORP.
800-725-3266

1194 E. Valencia Drive, Fullerton, CA 92831   **714-879-0341**

FDA Number: n/a   Fax: 714-879-9365
E-mail: info@covoc.com
Web site: www.covoc.com
Annual Revenue: $0-$1 Million
Year Founded: 1970
Total Employees: 8
Ownership: Private
Produces/Sells CE-marked Devices: N
Federal Procurement Eligibility: Small Business, GSA Contract
Distribution: Manufacturer Direct
General Admin.: Bradley J. Condon/President
Mktg./Adv.: Sam Raneri/Vice President Marketing

Accessories, Decorative	General
Curtain, Cubicle	General
Curtain, Shower	General
Track And Carrier, Cubicle Curtain	General
Track And Carrier, Intravenous	General

COWAN PLASTICS, LLC
401-351-1400

610 Manton Avenue, Providence, RI 02909

FDA Number: 1223835   Fax: 401-751-3481
E-mail: kpetti@cowanplastics.com
Web site: www.cowanplastics.com
Medical Products Sales Volume: $4,000,000
Annual Revenue: $1-$5 Million
Year Founded: 1950
Total Employees: 50   Marketing Staff: 1   Sales Staff: 2
Ownership: Private
Quality System Registration Information: ISO9000; ISO9001; ISO9002
Produces/Sells CE-marked Devices: N
Federal Procurement Eligibility: Small Business
General Admin.: Mr. William Dessel/President, Chief Executive Officer
Production: Mr. Nelson Rego/Manager Quality Assurance & Regulatory Affairs

Floss, Dental	Dental And Oral
General Medical Device	General

COY LABORATORY PRODUCTS, INC.
734-475-2200

14500 Coy Drive, Grass Lake, MI 49240

FDA Number: 1824208   Fax: 734-475-1846
E-mail: sales@coylab.com
Web site: www.coylab.com
Medical Products Sales Volume: $3,500,000
Annual Revenue: $1-$5 Million
Year Founded: 1969
Total Employees: 16   Marketing Staff: 1
Ownership: Private
Quality System Registration Information: ISO9000
Produces/Sells CE-marked Devices: N
Federal Procurement Eligibility: Small Business
Distribution: Manufacturer Direct
General Admin.: Richard Coy/Chief Executive Officer
Mktg./Adv.: Brian Coy/Director Marketing

Box, Glove	Microbiology
Chamber, Anaerobic	Microbiology
Incubator/Water Bath, Microbiology	Microbiology
Planchet	Chemistry
Sterilizer, Loop, Inoculating	Microbiology

CP MEDICAL CORPORATION
800-950-2763

803 NE 25th Avenue, Portland, OR 97232   **503-232-1555**

FDA Number: 3032563   Fax: 503-230-9993
E-mail: cpmedical@aol.com
Web site: www.cpmedical.com
Annual Revenue: $10-$25 Million
Year Founded: 1989
Total Employees: 75   Marketing Staff: 3   Sales Staff: 5
Ownership: Theragenics Corp.
Quality System Registration Information: ISO9001
Produces/Sells CE-marked Devices: Y
Federal Procurement Eligibility: Small Business
Distribution: Manufacturer Direct, Manufacturer Through Distributor, OEM
General Admin.: Patrick Ferguson/President
Mktg./Adv.: Wayne Black/Director Sales
Production: Madalyn Duncan/Director Quality Assurance & Regulatory Affairs
Research: Tom Brammer/Director Research & Development

Accessories, Cardiopulmonary Bypass	Cardiovascular

CP MEDICAL CORPORATION 800-950-2763 (cont'd)

Cable/Lead, ECG	Cardiovascular
Source, Brachytherapy, Radionuclide	Radiology
Suture, Absorbable	Surgery
Suture, Absorbable, Natural	Surgery
Suture, Non-Absorbable	Surgery
Suture, Non-Absorbable, Synthetic, Polyethylene	Surgery

CPAC EQUIPMENT, INC. 800-333-9729
2364 Leicester Road, Leicester, NY 14481-0175 585-382-3223
FDA Number: 2431273 Fax: 585-382-9481
E-mail: imaginginfo@cpac.com
Web site: www.cpacequipment.com
Medical Products Sales Volume: $93,000,000
Year Founded: 1972
Total Employees: 473 Marketing Staff: 1 Sales Staff: 4
Ownership: New World Medical, Inc.
Produces/Sells CE-marked Devices: N
Federal Procurement Eligibility: Small Business
Distribution: Manufacturer Through Distributor, Manufacturer Through
Manufacturer Reps, Exclusive Distributor, Exporter
Mktg./Adv.: Frank Manfre/Manager Marketing & Sales
Production: Bryan Murphy/Product Manager

Evacuator, Oral Cavity	Dental And Oral
Sterilizer, Dry Heat, Dental	Dental And Oral
Tip, Suction Tube (Yankauer, Poole, Etc.)	Surgery

Medical Product Subsidiaries (Listed Separately)
Allied Diagnostic Imaging Resources, Inc.

CPC HEALTHCARE INC. 800-661-4250
958 Heathorne St., Unit 1, 905-686-2723
London, ONT N5Z-3 Canada
FDA Number: n/a Fax: 905-686-0171
E-mail: cpc@on.aibn.com
Web site: www.cpchealthcare.on.ca
Year Founded: 1982
Total Employees: 10
Ownership: Private
Produces/Sells CE-marked Devices: N
Distribution: Service Direct, Exclusive Distributor, Importer

CPI
See CAREFUSION 211, INC..

CPR MEDICAL DEVICES INC. 416-691-2669
161 Don Park Rd., Markham, ONT L3R-1C2 Canada
FDA Number: n/a Fax: 416-691-7951
E-mail: haro@cprmedic.com
Web site: www.cprmedic.com
Year Founded: 1992
Total Employees: 10
Ownership: Private
Produces/Sells CE-marked Devices: N
Distribution: Manufacturer Direct, Exporter

CPT MED, INC. 770-242-1165
195 A Commerce Center, Gville, SC 29615
FDA Number: 3006098247

Tray, Surgical	Surgery

CRAFTMASTER CONTOUR EQUIPMENT, INC. 817-396-0900
6900 South Freeway, #9-b, P.O. Box 278, Cresson, TX 76035
FDA Number: 1644863
E-mail: info@ccei.net
Web site: www.ccei.net
Ownership: Private
Produces/Sells CE-marked Devices: N

Chair, Dental (With Unit)	Dental And Oral

CRAFTSMEN/ACCESS UNLIMITED 800-849-2143
570 Hance Rd., Binghamton, NY 13903
FDA Number: n/a Fax: 607-669-4595
Web site: www.accessunlimited.com
Ownership: Private
Produces/Sells CE-marked Devices: N

Lift, Bath, Non-AC-Powered	General

CRAMER PRODUCTS, INC. 1-800-345-2231
153 W. Warren, Gardner, KS 66030-1151 913-856-7511
FDA Number: 1910082 Fax: 913-884-5626
E-mail: info@cramersportsmed.com
Web site: www.cramersportsmed.com
Annual Revenue: $0-$1 Million
Total Employees: 75 Marketing Staff: 4 Sales Staff: 4
Ownership: Private
Produces/Sells CE-marked Devices: N
Distribution: Manufacturer Through Distributor, Importer, Exporter
General Admin.: Thomas Rogge/President
Mktg./Adv.: Ed Christman/Vice President Marketing

CRAMER PRODUCTS, INC. 1-800-345-2231 (cont'd)
Jack Patterson/Vice President Sales
Production: Bob Yoksh/Vice President Operations

Applicator, Tipped, Absorbent	General
Bag, Ice	General
Bandage, Adhesive	Surgery
Bandage, Elastic	General
Binder, Medical, Therapeutic	General
Brace, Joint, Ankle (External)	Physical Med
Depressor, Tongue	General
Dressing, Wound and Burn, Hydrogel	Surgery
Gauze/sponge, Nonresorbable For External Use	Surgery
Joint, Knee, External Brace	Physical Med
Kit, First Aid	Surgery
Orthosis, Limb Brace	Physical Med
Pack, Cold, Chemical	General
Pack, Hot Or Cold, Reusable	Physical Med
Refrigerant, Topical (Vapocoolant)	Physical Med
Sling, Arm	Physical Med
Solvent, Adhesive Tape	Surgery
Splint, Extremity, Non-Inflatable, External	Surgery
Splint, Vacuum	Orthopedics

CRANDALL MEDICAL DEVICES 949-369-9954
2209 Via Gavilan, San Clemente, CA 92673-5643
FDA Number: 2028824 Fax: 949-369-9961
E-mail: nvcrandall@earthlink.net
Medical Products Sales Volume: $100,000
Annual Revenue: $0-$1 Million
Year Founded: 1996
Total Employees: 1
Ownership: Private
Produces/Sells CE-marked Devices: N
Federal Procurement Eligibility: Small Business
General Admin.: Norman Crandall/President

Tube, Tracheostomy (W/Wo Connector)	Anesthesiology

CRANFORD X-RAY CO. 800-285-8329
8106 Berwyn Dr., Houston, TX 77037 281-999-2990
FDA Number: n/a Fax: 281-999-7339
E-mail: service@cranfordx-ray.com
Web site: www.cranfordx-ray.com
Annual Revenue: $1-$5 Million
Year Founded: 1946
Ownership: Private
Produces/Sells CE-marked Devices: N
Distribution: Exclusive Distributor

Service, Used Equipment	General

CRANIAL SOLUTIONS 973-835-7929
602 Lincoln Ave., Pompton Lakes, NJ 07442
FDA Number: 3003524425
Ownership: Private
Produces/Sells CE-marked Devices: N

Orthosis, Cranial	Cns/Neurology

CRANIAL TECHNOLOGIES, INC. 866-362-2263
1395 West Auto Dr., Tempe, AZ 85284 480-505-1840
FDA Number: 2030829 Fax: 480-505-1842
Web site: www.cranialtech.com
Ownership: Private
Produces/Sells CE-marked Devices: N

Orthosis, Cervical-Thoracic, Rigid	Physical Med
Orthosis, Cranial	Cns/Neurology

CREATIONS MAGIQUES C.M. INC. 514-753-3892
3001 Rue Visitation, Saint-Charles-Borromee J6E 7Y8 Canada
FDA Number: 9681198

Pack, Hot Or Cold, Reusable	Physical Med
Pack, Moist Heat	Physical Med

CREATIVE BEDDING TECHNOLOGIES, INC. 815-444-9088
300 Exchange Dr., Unit A, Crystal Lake, IL 60014
FDA Number: 1424528
Ownership: Private
Produces/Sells CE-marked Devices: N

Mattress, Non-Powered Flotation Therapy	Physical Med

CREATIVE BIOMEDICS, INC.
See Creative Biotech Inc.

CREATIVE BIOTECH INC. 949-481-5500
814 Calle Negocio, San Clemente, CA 92673
FDA Number: 2029330 Fax: 949-481-5559
E-mail: cbi@creative-biotech.com
Web site: http://creative-biotech.com
Annual Revenue: $1-$5 Million
Year Founded: 1999
Ownership: Private
Quality System Registration Information: ISO9001

CREATIVE BIOTECH INC.   949-481-5500 *(cont'd)*
Produces/Sells CE-marked Devices: Y
Federal Procurement Eligibility: Female Owned
Distribution: Manufacturer Direct, Manufacturer Through Distributor, Manufacturer Through Manufacturer Reps, OEM, Service Direct

Analyzer, Gas, Carbon-Dioxide, Gaseous Phase (Capnograph)	Anesthesiology
Clip, Nose	Anesthesiology
Filter, Bacterial, Breathing Circuit	Anesthesiology
Meter, Peak Flow, Spirometry	Anesthesiology
Spirometer, Diagnostic (Respirometer)	Anesthesiology

CREATIVE ENGINEERING, INC.
See Creative Health Products, Inc.

CREATIVE FOAM MEDICAL SYSTEMS   800-446-4644
405 N Industrial Drive, Bremen, IN 46506   **574-546-4238**
FDA Number: 1835830   *Fax:* 574-546-5093
E-mail: info@creativefoammedicalsystems.com
Web site: www.bremencorp.com
Year Founded: 1990
Total Employees: 40
Ownership: Private
Quality System Registration Information: ISO9000
Produces/Sells CE-marked Devices: Y
Federal Procurement Eligibility: Small Business
Distribution: Manufacturer Direct

Attachment, Commode, Wheelchair	Physical Med
Cushion, Wheelchair (Pad)	Physical Med
Holder, Head, Radiographic	Radiology
Mattress, Non-Powered Flotation Therapy	Physical Med
Support, Patient Position	Anesthesiology

CREATIVE HEALTH PRODUCTS, INC.   800-742-4478
5148 Saddle Ridge Road,   **734-996-5900**
Plymouth, MI 48170
FDA Number: 1831289   *Fax:* 734-996-4650
E-mail: websales@chponline.com
Web site: www.chponline.com
Medical Products Sales Volume: $1,500,000
Annual Revenue: $1-$5 Million
Year Founded: 1976
Total Employees: 12   *Marketing Staff:* 1   *Sales Staff:* 4
Ownership: Private
Produces/Sells CE-marked Devices: N
Federal Procurement Eligibility: Small Business, Female Owned, GSA Contract
Distribution: Manufacturer Direct, Manufacturer Through Distributor, OEM, Service Direct, Importer, Exporter
General Admin.: Marlene Donoghue/President
Mktg./Adv.: Robin Larsen-Mack/Manager National Sales
         Wallace C. Donoghue/Vice President Marketing

Analyzer, Composition, Weight, Patient	General
Caliper, Skinfold	General
Cuff, Blood Pressure	Cardiovascular
Dynamometer, Grip-Strength (Squeeze)	Anesthesiology
Exerciser, Arm	Physical Med
Exerciser, Bicycle	Physical Med
Exerciser, Hand	Physical Med
Exerciser, Measuring	Physical Med
Exerciser, Respiratory	Anesthesiology
Goniometer, Orthopedic	Orthopedics
Monitor, Blood Pressure, Indirect, Automatic	Cardiovascular
Mouthpiece, Breathing	Anesthesiology
Ophthalmoscope, Battery-Powered	Ophthalmology
Otoscope	Ear/Nose/Throat
Scale, Stand-On	General
Spirometer, Diagnostic (Respirometer)	Anesthesiology
Spirometer, Monitoring (Volumeter)	Anesthesiology
Stethoscope, Manual	Cardiovascular
Tape, Measuring, Ruler And Caliper	Surgery
Unit, Pad, Heating, Portable	Physical Med

CREATIVE LABORATORY PRODUCTS, INC.   317-293-2991
6420 N. Guion Rd., Indianapolis, IN 46268
FDA Number: 1832818   *Fax:* 317-293-7991
E-mail: sales@clplipids.com
Web site: www.clplipids.com
Annual Revenue: $0-$1 Million
Year Founded: 1987
Total Employees: 3
Ownership: Private
Produces/Sells CE-marked Devices: N
Federal Procurement Eligibility: Small Business
Distribution: OEM
General Admin.: Gary J. Proksch/President, Chief Executive Officer

Antigen, Antiserum, Control, Lipoprotein, Low Density	Immunology
Cholinesterase, Antigen, Antiserum, Control	Toxicology
Electrophoretic, Lactate Dehydrogenase Isoenzymes	Chemistry
Standard, Lipid	Chemistry

CREATIVE LABORATORY PRODUCTS, INC.   317-293-2991
(cont'd)

Test, Sickle Cell	Hematology

CREATIVE MARKETING CONCEPTS, INC.   978-532-7517
96 Audubon Road, Wakefield, MA 01880
FDA Number: 1287334

Booth, Sun Tan	Physical Med

CREATIVE MEDICAL DESIGNS, INC.   813-875-9999
13914 Shady Shores Dr., Tampa, FL 33613
FDA Number: 1055920

Plate, Bone, Orthodontic	Dental And Oral
Plate, Fixation, Bone	Orthopedics

CREATIVE MEDICAL TECHNOLOGIES   (888) 535-8180
6060 Phyllis Drive, Cypress, CA 90630   -
FDA Number: n/a   *Fax:* (714) 891-3140
E-mail: customerservice@medcominc.com
Web site: www.medcom.com
Annual Revenue: $0-$1 Million
Total Employees: 3
Ownership: Private
Produces/Sells CE-marked Devices: N
Federal Procurement Eligibility: Small Business
Distribution: Service Direct, Exclusive Distributor
General Admin.: Dave Palmer/General Manager

Service, Maintenance/Repair	General

CREATIVE OPTICS INC.
See Marcolin Usa

CREATIVE SCIENTIFIC TECHNOLOGY, INC.
See Cst Technologies, Inc.

CREGANNA-TACTX MEDICAL   408-364-7100
1353 Dell Ave., Campbell, CA 95008
FDA Number: 3004036480
Ownership: Private
Produces/Sells CE-marked Devices: N

Catheter, Balloon (Foley Type)	Surgery

CREIDY, INC.
See Primus Diagnostics

CRELLIN, INC.
See Sonoco Crellin, Inc.

CRES COR   877-273-7267
5925 Heisley Rd., Mentor, OH 44060-1833   **440-350-1100**
FDA Number: 9330030   *Fax:* 800-822-0393
E-mail: crescor@crescor.com
Web site: www.crescor.com
Year Founded: 1936
Total Employees: 200
Ownership: Private
Produces/Sells CE-marked Devices: N
Distribution: Manufacturer Through Distributor
General Admin.: Clifford D. Baggott/President, Chief Executive Officer
         Rio DeGennaro/Vice President
Mktg./Adv.: Michael Capretta/Director National Marketing & Sales
         Stacey Shriver/Marketing Assistant
Production: Mary Nemanic/Manager Customer Services

Foodservice Product/Equipment	General

CRESC-COR CROWN-X, CRESCENT METAL PROD.
See Cres Cor

CRESCENT CHEMICAL CO., INC.   800-877-3225
2 Oval Drive, Islandia, NY 11749   **631-348-0333**
FDA Number: n/a   *Fax:* 631-348-0913
E-mail: crescent@creschem.com
Web site: www.crescentchemical.com
Medical Products Sales Volume: $1,900,000
Year Founded: 1947
Total Employees: 11
Ownership: Private
Produces/Sells CE-marked Devices: N
Federal Procurement Eligibility: Small Business, Female Owned
Distribution: Manufacturer Direct, Manufacturer Through Manufacturer Reps, OEM, Exclusive Distributor
General Admin.: Ilene S. Cohen/Chief Executive Officer

Electrophoresis Equipment, Gel	Chemistry
Reagent, Other	General
Solution, pH Buffer	Chemistry

CRESCENT DESIGN, INC.   858-452-3240
9932 Mesa Rim Rd., Suite B, San Diego, CA 92121
FDA Number: n/a   *Fax:* 858-452-3241
E-mail: sroyce@crescentdesign.com
Web site: www.crescentdesign.com
Year Founded: 1994

CRESCENT DESIGN, INC. 858-452-3240 (cont'd)
Ownership: Private
Produces/Sells CE-marked Devices: Y
Federal Procurement Eligibility: Small Business
Distribution: Manufacturer Direct
General Admin.: Steven D. Royce/President
  Production Equipment .... General

CRESCENT MANUFACTURING COMPANY 419-332-6484
4615 Progress Drive, Columbus, IN 47201
FDA Number: 3004973335
Ownership: Private
Produces/Sells CE-marked Devices: N
  Accessories, Microtome .... Pathology

CRESCENT METAL PRODUCTS
See Cres Cor

CRESCENT MFG. CO. 800-537-1330
1310 Majestic Dr., Fremont, OH 43420   419-332-6484
FDA Number: 1520597   Fax: 419-332-6564
Web site: www.crescentblades.com
Medical Products Sales Volume: $3,000,000
Annual Revenue: $10-$25 Million
Year Founded: 1898
Total Employees: 120   Marketing Staff: 1   Sales Staff: 5
Ownership: Private
Quality System Registration Information: ISO9001
Produces/Sells CE-marked Devices: N
Federal Procurement Eligibility: Small Business
Distribution: Manufacturer Direct, OEM, Importer, Exporter
General Admin.: Mike Walyerszak/President, Chief Executive Officer
Mktg./Adv.: Frank Wojcik/Director Product Development
    Chuck Bayer/Vice President Marketing & Sales
Production: Linda Smith/Director Quality Assurance
    Kara Bork/Manager Materials
  Accessories, Microtome .... Pathology
  Blade, Knife, Laparoscopic .... Surgery
  Blade, Surgical, Saw, General & Plastic Surgery .... Surgery
  Knife, Keratome .... Ophthalmology
Medical Product Subsidiaries (Listed Separately)
  Crescent Medical

CRESPAC INC. 770-938-1900
5032 N. Royal Atlanta Dr., Tucker, GA 30084
FDA Number: n/a   Fax: 770-939-4900
E-mail: sales@crespac.com
Web site: www.atp-plastic.com
Annual Revenue: $0-$1 Million
Ownership: Private
Produces/Sells CE-marked Devices: N
Federal Procurement Eligibility: Small Business, Minority Owned
Distribution: Manufacturer Direct
  Adaptor, Grooming .... Physical Med
  Bathtub, Portable .... General
  Packaging Material .... General
  Thermoforming, Extrusion, Custom .... General
  Tray, Custom/Special Procedure .... General
  Tray, Medicine .... General
  Tray, Surgical .... Surgery
  Tray, Surgical Instrument .... Surgery

CREST ELECTRONICS
See Crest Healthcare Supply

CREST FOAM INDUSTRIES 201-807-0809
100 Carol Place, Moonachie, NJ 07074-1304
FDA Number: 7000475   Fax: 201-807-1113
E-mail: info@crestfoam.com
Web site: www.crestfoam.com
Medical Products Sales Volume: $23,000,000
Annual Revenue: $25-$50 Million
Year Founded: 1997
Total Employees: 94   Marketing Staff: 3   Sales Staff: 8
Ownership: BRITISH VITA
Quality System Registration Information: ISO9002
Produces/Sells CE-marked Devices: N
Federal Procurement Eligibility: Small Business
Distribution: Manufacturer Through Distributor
General Admin.: Mr. Raj Mehta/President
Mktg./Adv.: Thomas Myers/Director Marketing
    Thomas Myers/Manager Advertising
Production: Mr. Tom Walker/Director Manufacturing
  Foam, Plastic .... General

CREST HEALTHCARE SUPPLY 800-328-8908
195 Third Street South, Dassel, MN 55325   320-275-3382
FDA Number: n/a   Fax: 320-275-2306
E-mail: customerservice@cresthealthcare.com
Web site: www.cresthealthcare.com

CREST HEALTHCARE SUPPLY 800-328-8908 (cont'd)
Year Founded: 1968
Ownership: Private
Quality System Registration Information: ISO9001
Produces/Sells CE-marked Devices: N
Distribution: Manufacturer Direct
General Admin.: Corey Tisthammer/General Manager
    Larry Lautt/President, Chief Executive Officer
Mktg./Adv.: Jean Dockendorf/Director Marketing
Production: Mark Sowada/Director Engineering
Finance: Diane Hedlund/Controller
  Bedrail .... General
  Cable, Electric .... General
  Cable/Lead, ECG .... Cardiovascular
  Cart, Emergency, Cardiopulmonary Resuscitation (Crash) ... Anesthesiology
  Cart, Housekeeping .... General
  Cart, Medicine .... General
  Casters, Hospital Equipment .... General
  Clock, Elapsed Time .... General
  Communication Equipment .... General
  Communication System, Emergency Alert, Personal ... General
  Communication System, Room Status .... General
  Component, Electrical .... General
  Component, Electronic .... General
  Component, Wheelchair .... Physical Med
  Cover, Cart .... General
  Cover, Mattress .... General
  Curtain, Cubicle .... General
  Cushion, Other .... General
  Equipment, Extruding/Molding .... General
  Housekeeping Equipment .... General
  IV Start Kit .... Surgery
  Infusion Stand .... General
  Lamp, Examination (Light) .... General
  Lift, Patient .... General
  Light, Other .... General
  Light, Overbed .... General
  Mattress, Bed .... General
  Mirror, Corridor Safety .... General
  Mount, Television Set .... General
  Nurse Call System .... General
  Pager, Visual .... General
  Physician Registry .... General
  Pillow .... General
  Receptacle, Electrical .... General
  Security Equipment/Supplies .... General
  Service, Parts, Repair .... General
  Sign, Hospital .... General
  Sphygmomanometer, Electronic, Manual ...... General
  Stethoscope, Mechanical .... General
  Table, Other .... General
  Telephone Equipment .... General
  Timeclock .... General
  Track And Carrier, Cubicle Curtain .... General
  Unit, Control, Bed, Patient, Powered .... General

CREST ULTRASONICS CORP. 800-992-7378
P.O. Box 7266, Scotch Road, Trenton, NJ 08628   609-883-4000
FDA Number: 3001547782   Fax: 609-883-6452
E-mail: info@crest-ultrasonics.com
Annual Revenue: $0-$1 Million
Year Founded: 1961
Total Employees: 960
Ownership: Private
Produces/Sells CE-marked Devices: N
Federal Procurement Eligibility: Small Business
Distribution: Manufacturer Direct, Manufacturer Through Distributor, Manufacturer Through Manufacturer Reps, Service Direct, Exclusive Distributor
  Cleaner, Ultrasonic, Dental Laboratory ...... Dental And Oral
  Cleaner, Ultrasonic, Medical Instrument ..... General
  Lubricant, Instrument .... General
  Sink, Sonic .... General
  Solution, Instrument Cleaner .... General
  Washer, Pipette, Ultrasonic .... Chemistry
Medical Product Subsidiaries (Listed Separately)
  Forward Technology

CREST-FOAM CORPORATION
See Crest Foam Industries

CRESTLINE COACH LTD. 888-887-6886
802 57th St. East,   306-934-8844
Saskatoon, SK S7K-5 Canada
FDA Number: n/a   Fax: 306-242-5838
E-mail: padsten@cclnet.ca
Web site: www.crestlinecoach.com
Ownership: Private
Produces/Sells CE-marked Devices: N
Distribution: Manufacturer Direct, Exclusive Distributor

CRESTLINE PRODUCTS INC.   407-859-6428
PO Box 2108, Orlando, FL 32802-2108
FDA Number: 1054957   Fax: 407-859-6409
E-mail: easyup@msn.com
Medical Products Sales Volume: $300,000
Year Founded: 1990
Total Employees: 4
Ownership: Private
Produces/Sells CE-marked Devices: N
Federal Procurement Eligibility: Small Business, Female Owned
Distribution: Manufacturer Direct, Exporter
General Admin.: Penny H. Cunningham/Chief Executive Officer
              Thomas W. Cunningham/President
   Accessories, Walker   General

CRF HEALTH   1 267 498 2300
4000 Chemical Road, Suite 400, Plymouth Meeting, PA 19462
FDA Number: 3009129501   Fax: 1 215 565 0001
E-mail: info-us@crfhealth.com
Web site: www.crfhealth.com
Ownership: Private
Produces/Sells CE-marked Devices: N
General Admin.: Ms. Rachael King/Chief Executive Officer
              Mr. John Larson/Chief Operating Officer
              Mr. Pekka Keskiivari/Chief Technology Officer
Mktg./Adv.: Ms. Mary Briggs/Vice President Global Marketing
Finance: Mr. Jeffery Payne/Chief Financial Officer

CRI
See Catheter Research, Inc. (Cri)

CRISS OPTICAL MANUFACTURING CO., INC.   800-835-2023
3628 S.West St., Wichita, KS 67217   316-529-0414
FDA Number: 1922662   Fax: 316-529-3006
E-mail: sales@crissoptical.com
Medical Products Sales Volume: $1,300,000
Annual Revenue: $1-$5 Million
Year Founded: 2002
Total Employees: 8   Sales Staff: 1
Ownership: Private
Quality System Registration Information: ISO9001
Produces/Sells CE-marked Devices: N
Federal Procurement Eligibility: Small Business, Female Owned, GSA Contract
Distribution: Manufacturer Through Distributor, Service Direct, Exporter
General Admin.: Diane Loveall/President
   Frame, Spectacle (Eyeglasses)   Ophthalmology

CRIST INSTRUMENT CO., INC.   301-393-8615
111 W. First St., Hagerstown, MD 21740
FDA Number: n/a   Fax: 301-393-8618
E-mail: neurotoys@msn.com
Web site: www.cristinstrument.com
Medical Products Sales Volume: $1,900,000
Annual Revenue: $0-$1 Million
Year Founded: 1990
Total Employees: 15   Marketing Staff: 1   Sales Staff: 1
Ownership: Private
Produces/Sells CE-marked Devices: N
Federal Procurement Eligibility: Small Business, Female Owned
Distribution: Manufacturer Direct
General Admin.: J. Burkholder/President, Chief Executive Officer
Mktg./Adv.: Pat Crist/Vice President Marketing
Research: K. Crist/Vice President Engineering
         C. F. Crist/Vice President Research & Development
   Chair, Neurosurgical   Cns/Neurology
   Chamber, Isolation, Patient Care   General
   Component, Electronic   General
   Contract R&D, Equipment   General
   Fixation Device, Extra-Cranial (Head Frame)   Orthopedics
   Recorder, Attention Task Performance   Cns/Neurology
   Stimulator, Audio   Cns/Neurology

CRITICAL CARE SYSTEMS, INC.   954-989-4400
5000 Hollywood Blvd., Hollywood, FL 33021
FDA Number: 1036218
Ownership: Private
Produces/Sells CE-marked Devices: N
   Computer, Diagnostic, Programmable   Cardiovascular

CRITICAL DIAGNOSTICS   877-700-1250
3030 Bunker Hill St., Suite 115A,   858-270-2400
San Diego, CA 92109
FDA Number: n/a   Fax: 858) 270-2400
E-mail: info@criticaldiagnostics.com
Web site: http://criticaldiagnostics.com
Ownership: Private
Produces/Sells CE-marked Devices: N
General Admin.: Mr. Patrick Arensdorf/Chief Executive Officer

CRITICAL DIAGNOSTICS   877-700-1250 (cont'd)
Dr. James Snider/President

CRITICARE SYSTEMS, INC.   262-798-8282
N7W22025 Johnson Drive, Waukesha, WI 53186
FDA Number: 2183600   Fax: 262-798-8290
Ownership: Private
Produces/Sells CE-marked Devices: N
   Analyzer, Gas, Halothane, Gaseous Phase (Anesthetic Conc.)   Anesthesiology
   Detector, Arrhythmia Alarm   Cardiovascular
   Monitor, Cardiac (Cardiotachometer & Rate Alarm) Cardiovascular
   Monitor, Physiological, Patient   Cardiovascular
   Monitor, Physiological, Patient(without Arrhythmia Detection Or Alarms)   Cardiovascular
   Oximeter, Intracardiac   Cardiovascular
   Telemetry Unit, Physiological, Neurological   Cns/Neurology
   Transmitter/Receiver System, Physiological, Radiofrequency   Cardiovascular

CRITIKON COMPANY L.L.C.
See Ge Medical Systems Information Technologies

CRITIKON, INC.
See Ge Medical Systems Information Technologies

CROCS, INC.   801-455-8558
6328 Monarch Park Place, Niwot, CO 80503
FDA Number: 3005087292
Ownership: Private
Produces/Sells CE-marked Devices: N
   Orthosis, Corrective Shoe   Physical Med
   Stocking, Elastic   General

CROLL REYNOLDS COMPANY, INC.   908-232-4200
Six Campus Drive, Parsippany, NJ 07054
FDA Number: n/a   Fax: 908-232-2146
E-mail: info@croll.com
Web site: www.croll.com
Medical Products Sales Volume: $2,500,000
Annual Revenue: $10-$25 Million
Year Founded: 1917
Total Employees: 20   Marketing Staff: 1   Sales Staff: 9
Ownership: Private
Produces/Sells CE-marked Devices: N
Federal Procurement Eligibility: Small Business
Distribution: Manufacturer Direct, Manufacturer Through Manufacturer Reps, OEM, Exporter
General Admin.: Samuel W. Croll/Chief Executive Officer
Mktg./Adv.: Mr. Henry Hage/Sales Manager
   Column, Adsorption, Lipid   Cardiovascular
   Environmental Control System, Powered   Physical Med
   Precipitator, Radioimmunoassay Multiple Sampling Chemistry

CROMWELL ARCHITECT FIRM
See Cromwell Architects Engineers

CROMWELL ARCHITECTS ENGINEERS   501-372-2900
101 S. Spring St., Little Rock, AR 72201-2490
FDA Number: n/a   Fax: 501-372-0482
E-mail: cromwell@cromwell.com
Web site: www.cromwell.com
Medical Products Sales Volume: $13,000,000
Year Founded: 1885
Total Employees: 108
Ownership: Private
Produces/Sells CE-marked Devices: N
Federal Procurement Eligibility: Small Business
Distribution: Service Direct
General Admin.: Mr. Brent Thompson, AIA/Chief Executive Officer
              Mr. Charley Penix, AIA/President
Mktg./Adv.: Mr. Joe Johnson, AIA/Vice President Marketing & Sales
   Service, Architectural   General

CROPPER MEDICAL, INC./BIO SKIN   800-541-2455
240 East Hersey Street, Suite 2,   541-488-0600
Ashland, OR 97520
FDA Number: 2024235   Fax: 541-482-2119
E-mail: custserv@bioskin.com
Web site: www.Bioskin.com
Medical Products Sales Volume: $4,000,000
Year Founded: 1981
Total Employees: 47
Ownership: Private
Produces/Sells CE-marked Devices: Y
Federal Procurement Eligibility: Small Business, VA Contract
Distribution: Manufacturer Direct, Manufacturer Through Manufacturer Reps, OEM, Exclusive Distributor
General Admin.: Michelle Hallett/Executive Assistant
   Bandage, Elastic   General
   Immobilizer, Ankle   Orthopedics
   Support, Ankle   Orthopedics
   Support, Back   Orthopedics
   Support, Elbow   Orthopedics

CROPPER MEDICAL, INC./BIO SKIN　　　800-541-2455 *(cont'd)*
　　Support, Foot　　　　　　　　　　　　　　　　　Orthopedics
　　Support, Hand　　　　　　　　　　　　　　　　Orthopedics

CROSS COUNTRY PAPER PRODUCTS CORP/CROSSTEX
　　See Crosstex International, Inc.

CROSSLINK-D, INC　　　　　　　　　　　203-318-8270
3480 Industrial Blvd #105, West Sacramento, CA 95691
　　FDA Number: 3005905522
　　Dressing, Other　　　　　　　　　　　　　　　General

CROSSTEX INTERNATIONAL　　　　　　800-223-2497
10 Ranick Road, Hauppauge, NY 11788　　631-582-6777
　　FDA Number: 2433773　　　　　　　*Fax:* 631-582-1726
　　E-mail: crosstex@mindspring.com
　　Web site: www.crosstex.com
　　Annual Revenue: $100-$500 Million
　　Year Founded: 1953
　　Total Employees: 100　　*Marketing Staff:* 4　　*Sales Staff:* 4
　　Ownership: Crosstex International, Inc.
　　Quality System Registration Information: ISO9002
　　Produces/Sells CE-marked Devices: Y
　　Federal Procurement Eligibility: Small Business
　　Distribution: Manufacturer Through Distributor, Exporter
　　General Admin.: Mitchell Steinberg/Vice President, General Manager
　　Mktg./Adv.: Gary Steinberg/Vice President Business Development
　　　　　　Mr. Andrew Whitehead/Vice President Marketing
　　　　　　Ron Psimas/Vice President Sales
　　　　　　Mr. Les Gershon/Vice President Sales
　　　　　　Mr. Sheldon Fisher/Vice President Sales
　　Absorber, Saliva, Paper　　　　　　　　　Dental And Oral
　　Apron, Lead, Radiographic　　　　　　　　　　Radiology
　　Bandage, Gauze　　　　　　　　　　　　　　　General
　　Bib　　　　　　　　　　　　　　　　　　　　General
　　Cotton, Roll　　　　　　　　　　　　　　Dental And Oral
　　Cup, Medicine　　　　　　　　　　　　　　　General
　　Disinfector, Liquid　　　　　　　　　　　　　General
　　Dress, Surgical　　　　　　　　　　　　　　　Surgery
　　Ejector, Saliva　　　　　　　　　　　　Ear/Nose/Throat
　　Gauze/sponge, Nonresorbable For External Use　　Surgery
　　Glove, Patient Examination　　　　　　　　　　General
　　Handpiece, Belt and/or Gear Driven, Dental　　Dental And Oral
　　Kit, Disposable Procedure　　　　　　　　　Cardiovascular
　　Mask, Face　　　　　　　　　　　　　　　　General
　　Mask, Surgical　　　　　　　　　　　　　　　Surgery
　　Packaging, Sterilization　　　　　　　　　　　General
　　Sanitizer　　　　　　　　　　　　　　　　　General
　　Solution, Antibacterial Cleaner　　　　　　　　General
　　Towel/Towelette, Paper　　　　　　　　　　　General
　　Vial, Other　　　　　　　　　　　　　　　　General
　　Wrap, Sterilization　　　　　　　　　　　　　General

CROSSTEX INTERNATIONAL LTD., W. REGION　　800-707-2737
14059 Stage Rd., Santa Fe Springs, CA 90670　　562-921-3343
　　FDA Number: n/a　　　　　　　　*Fax:* 562-921-8070
　　E-mail: Crosstexca@crosstex.com
　　Annual Revenue: $25-$50 Million
　　Total Employees: 10　　*Marketing Staff:* 1　　*Sales Staff:* 3
　　Ownership: Private
　　Quality System Registration Information: ISO9000
　　Produces/Sells CE-marked Devices: N
　　Distribution: Manufacturer Through Distributor
　　General Admin.: Mitchell Steinberg/Chief Executive Officer
　　　　　　Norman Steinberg/President
　　　　　　Sheldon M. Fisher/Vice President
　　Mktg./Adv.: Andy Whitehead/Director National Accounts
　　　　　　Paul Orofino/Manager Advertising
　　　　　　Richard Allen/Vice President Marketing
　　　　　　Ron Psmis/Vice President Sales
　　　　　　Sheldon M. Fisher/Vice President Sales
　　Bandage, Gauze　　　　　　　　　　　　　　General
　　Bib　　　　　　　　　　　　　　　　　　　　General
　　Cup, Medicine　　　　　　　　　　　　　　　General
　　Ejector, Saliva　　　　　　　　　　　　Ear/Nose/Throat
　　Facial Tissue　　　　　　　　　　　　　　　General
　　Glove, Patient Examination　　　　　　　　　　General
　　Glove, Patient Examination, Latex　　　　　　　General
　　Kit, Disposable Procedure　　　　　　　　　Cardiovascular
　　Lotion, Skin Care　　　　　　　　　　　　　General
　　Mask, Face　　　　　　　　　　　　　　　　General
　　Packaging, Sterilization　　　　　　　　　　　General
　　Solution, Antibacterial Cleaner　　　　　　　　General
　　Towel/Towelette, Paper　　　　　　　　　　　General
　　Vial, Other　　　　　　　　　　　　　　　　General

CROSSTEX INTERNATIONAL, INC.　　　516-482-9001
534 Vine Street, Sharon, PA 16146
　　FDA Number: 3006008984
　　Ownership: Private

CROSSTEX INTERNATIONAL, INC.　　　516-482-9001 *(cont'd)*
　　Produces/Sells CE-marked Devices: N
　　Mouthpiece, Saliva Ejector　　　　　　　　Dental And Oral

CROSSTEX INTERNATIONAL, INC.　　　800 743 3490
621 Hurricane Shoals Rd. Nw, Suite G,　　770 682 3369
Lawrenceville, GA 30045
　　FDA Number: 3003675658　　　　*Fax:* 770 682 3174
　　E-mail: Crosstexga@crosstex.com
　　Web site: www.crosstex.com
　　Ownership: Private
　　Produces/Sells CE-marked Devices: N
　　Absorber, Saliva, Paper　　　　　　　　　Dental And Oral
　　Gauze/sponge, Nonresorbable For External Use　　Surgery

CROSSTEX INTERNATIONAL, INC.　　　888-276-7783
10 Ranick Rd., Hauppauge, NY 11788-4209　　631-582-6777
　　FDA Number: 2433773　　　　　　*Fax:* 631-582-1726
　　E-mail: crosstex@crosstex.com
　　Web site: www.crosstex.com
　　Medical Products Sales Volume: $4,000,000
　　Annual Revenue: $50-$100 Million
　　Year Founded: 1953
　　Total Employees: 125　　*Marketing Staff:* 5　　*Sales Staff:* 12
　　Ownership: Cantel Medical Corporation
　　Produces/Sells CE-marked Devices: Y
　　Federal Procurement Eligibility: Small Business
　　Distribution: Manufacturer Through Distributor, OEM, Importer, Exporter
　　General Admin.: Richard Allen Orofino/Chief Executive Officer
　　　　　　Gary Steinberg/Executive Vice President
　　　　　　Mitchell Steinberg/Executive Vice President
　　Mktg./Adv.: Andrew Whitehead/Vice President Marketing & Sales
　　　　　　Les Gershon/Vice President Regional Sales
　　　　　　Ronald Psimas/Vice President Regional Sales
　　　　　　Sheldon Fisher/Vice President Regional Sales
　　Production: Richard Orofino Jr./Manager Regulatory Affairs
　　Bandage, Gauze　　　　　　　　　　　　　　General
　　Bib　　　　　　　　　　　　　　　　　　　　General
　　Cup, Medicine　　　　　　　　　　　　　　　General
　　Ejector, Saliva　　　　　　　　　　　　Ear/Nose/Throat
　　Eyeglasses, Safety　　　　　　　　　　　　Ophthalmology
　　Facial Tissue　　　　　　　　　　　　　　　General
　　Glove, Patient Examination　　　　　　　　　　General
　　Kit, Disposable Procedure　　　　　　　　　Cardiovascular
　　Mask, Face　　　　　　　　　　　　　　　　General
　　Packaging, Sterilization　　　　　　　　　　　General
　　Solution, Antibacterial Cleaner　　　　　　　　General
　　Solution, Antimicrobial　　　　　　　　　　Microbiology
　　Solution, Patient Preparation　　　　　　　　　General
　　Sterilizer, Steam (Autoclave)　　　　　　　　　General
　　Towel/Towelette, Paper　　　　　　　　　　　General
　　Vial, Other　　　　　　　　　　　　　　　　General
　　Medical Product Subsidiaries (Listed Separately)
　　Crosstex International

CROSSTEX/CROSS COUNTY PAPER PRODUCTS
　　See Crosstex International

CROSSTREES MEDICAL, INC.　　　　　866-442-2328
4735 Walnut St. Suite E, Boulder, CO 80301
　　FDA Number: 3005255976　　　　*Fax:* 303-442-2369
　　E-mail: info@crosstreesmedical.com
　　Web site: www.crosstreesmedical.com
　　Ownership: Private
　　Produces/Sells CE-marked Devices: N
　　Bit, Drill　　　　　　　　　　　　　　　　Orthopedics
　　Cannula, Surgical, General & Plastic Surgery　　Surgery
　　Device, Biopsy, Percutaneous　　　　　　　　Surgery
　　Guide, Surgical, Needle　　　　　　　　　　Surgery
　　Impactor　　　　　　　　　　　　　　　　Orthopedics
　　Kit, Surgical Instrument, Disposable　　　　　　Surgery
　　Orthopedic Manual Surgical Instrument　　　　Orthopedics
　　Positioner, Socket　　　　　　　　　　　　Orthopedics
　　Reamer　　　　　　　　　　　　　　　　Orthopedics

CROSSWELL INTERNATIONAL
　　See Hospital Specialty Company

CROSSWELL INTERNATIONAL CORPORATION　　305-648-0777
101 Madeira Avenue, Coral Gables, FL 33134
　　FDA Number: 1066225　　　　　　*Fax:* 305-648-1613
　　E-mail: hl@crosswell.com
　　Web site: www.crosswell.com
　　Medical Products Sales Volume: $9,900,000
　　Annual Revenue: $5-$10 Million
　　Year Founded: 1992
　　Total Employees: 10　　　　　　*Sales Staff:* 65
　　Ownership: Crosswell International Corporation
　　Federal Procurement Eligibility: Small Business, Minority Owned
　　Distribution: Exporter

CROSSWELL INTERNATIONAL CORPORATION   305-648-0777
(cont'd)
  General Admin.: Hector Lans/Chief Executive Officer
    Hector Lans/President
  Mktg./Adv.: Charles Haylock/Director Marketing
    Antonio Visiola/Director Product Development
  Bandage, Other   General
  Diaper, Pediatric   General
  Kit, Enema   General
  Swabs, Cotton   General
  Test, Antibody, Acquired Immune Deficiency Syndrome (AIDS)   Hematology
  Test, Fertility Monitoring   Obstetrics/Gynecology
  Medical Product Subsidiaries (Listed Separately)
  Crosswell International Corporation

CROTHALL   800-447-4476
13111 E. Briarwood Ave. #225, Englewood, CO 80112-3926
  FDA Number: n/a
  E-mail: bradley.giles@crothall.com
  Web site: http://www.crothall.com
  Annual Revenue: $10-$25 Million
  Year Founded: 1979
  Total Employees: 185   *Sales Staff:* 3
  Ownership: Private
  Produces/Sells CE-marked Devices: N
  Federal Procurement Eligibility: Small Business
  Distribution: Service Direct
  General Admin.: Randy Scott/Executive Vice President
    Scott C. Brown/President
    Nancy J. Lake/Vice President Admin.
  Mktg./Adv.: Scott Brown/Manager Marketing
  Service, Consulting   General

CROWN DELTA CORP.   914-245-8910
1550 Front St., Yorktown Heights, NY 10598
  FDA Number: 2431069   *Fax:* 914-245-8912
  E-mail: sales@crowndelta.com
  Web site: www.crowndelta.com
  Medical Products Sales Volume: $3,000,000
  Annual Revenue: $1-$5 Million
  Year Founded: 1975
  Ownership: Private
  Quality System Registration Information: ISO9001
  Produces/Sells CE-marked Devices: N
  Federal Procurement Eligibility: Small Business
  Distribution: Manufacturer Direct, OEM
  Elastomer, Silicone Rubber   General
  Hearing Aid, Air Conduction, Transcutaneous System   Ear/Nose/Throat
  Material, Impression   Dental And Oral

CROWN HEALTH CARE LAUNDRY SERVICES, INC.   850-438-7578
3805 Highway 41 North, Selma, AL 36701
  FDA Number: 3006197597
  Drape, Surgical   Surgery

CROWN MATS   800-628-5463
2100 Commerce Drive, Fremont, OH 43420-1014   419-332-5531
  FDA Number: 9330071   *Fax:* 419-332-4180
  E-mail: sales@crown-mats.com
  Web site: www.crown-mats.com
  Medical Products Sales Volume: $14,000,000
  Annual Revenue: $25-$50 Million
  Year Founded: 1943
  Total Employees: 180   *Marketing Staff:* 1   *Sales Staff:* 4
  Ownership: Private
  Produces/Sells CE-marked Devices: N
  Federal Procurement Eligibility: Small Business
  Distribution: Manufacturer Through Distributor, Manufacturer Through Manufacturer Reps, Importer, Exporter
  General Admin.: R. J. Moran/President, Chief Executive Officer
  Mktg./Adv.: Phyllis Lark/Admin. Marketing
    Phyllis Lark/Manager Advertising
    Thomas M. McLaughlin/Vice President Sales
  Production: Ann Bolyard/Manager Customer Services
  Finance: Randy Dobbs/Vice President Admin., Finance
  Floor Mat   General
  Foam, Plastic   General
  Insoles, Medical   General
  Tubing, Vinyl   General

CROWN MFG. CO.   905-545-2546
53 Gibson Ave, Hamilton L8L 6J7 Canada
  FDA Number: 9617859
  Cushion, Flotation   Physical Med

CROWN THERAPEUTICS INC.
  See Roho Group, The

CROWN ZELLERBACH CORP.
  See Bba Fiberweb Washougal, Inc.

CRS MEDICAL DIAGNOSTICS INC.   262-432-5900
PO Box 510137, New Berlin, WI 53151
  FDA Number: 3005517198   *Fax:* 262-355-4478
  Ownership: Private
  Produces/Sells CE-marked Devices: N
  Catheter, Intravascular, Therapeutic, Long-term Greater Than 30 Days   General

CRUX BIOMEDICAL INC.   650-321-9903
1455 Adams Drive, #1170, Menlo Park, CA 94025
  FDA Number: n/a
  E-mail: info@cruxbiomedical.com
  Web site: http://cruxbiomedical.com/
  Year Founded: 2004
  Ownership: Private
  Produces/Sells CE-marked Devices: N
  General Admin.: Mr. Mel Schatz/President, Chief Executive Officer
  Production: Mr. Murli Srinivasan/Director Operations
    Ms. Elisa Hebb/Vice President Regulatory & Clinical Affairs
  Research: Mr. Eric Johnson/Vice President Research & Development
  Finance: Mr. Chris Schaffer/Chief Financial Officer

CRX MEDICAL INC.
  See Closure Medical

CRYO-CELL INTERNATIONAL, INC.   800-786-7235
700 Brooker Creek Blvd., Suite 1800,   813-749-2100
Oldsmar, FL 34677
  FDA Number: n/a   *Fax:* 813-855-4745
  E-mail: ajohnson@cryo-cell.com
  Web site: www.cryo-cell.com
  Medical Products Sales Volume: $17,200,000
  Year Founded: 1989
  Total Employees: 34   *Marketing Staff:* 3
  Ownership: Public
  Stock Symbol: CCEL
  Traded On: OTC Bulletin
  Produces/Sells CE-marked Devices: Y
  Federal Procurement Eligibility: Small Business
  Distribution: Service Direct
  General Admin.: Mrs. Mercedes Walton/Chief Executive Officer, Chairman
    Medical Admin.: Dr. Buff Mair/Medical Director
  Research: Dr. Julie Allickson/Vice President Research & Development
  Finance: Mrs. Jill Taymans/Chief Financial Officer, Vice President Finance
  Bin, Storage   General

CRYOCATH TECHNOLOGIES INC.   877-694-1212
16771 Chemin Ste-Marie, Montreal, QUE H9H-5H3 Canada
  FDA Number: 3002648230   *Fax:* 514 694 6279
  E-mail: rs.cscryocathorders@medtronic.com
  Web site: www.cryocath.com
  Year Founded: 1995
  Total Employees: 210
  Ownership: Medtronic, Inc.
  Produces/Sells CE-marked Devices: N
  Distribution: Manufacturer Direct

CRYOCOR, INC.   858-909-2213
9717 Pacific Heights Blvd., San Diego, CA 92121
  FDA Number: n/a
  Ownership: Private
  Produces/Sells CE-marked Devices: N
  Electrode, Ablation, Tissue, Conduction, Percutaneous   Cardiovascular
  Introducer, Catheter   Cardiovascular

CRYOFAB, INC.   800-426-2186
540 N. Michigan Ave., Kenilworth, NJ 07033-1023   908-686-3636
  FDA Number: 2246710   *Fax:* 908-686-9538
  E-mail: sales@cryofab.com
  Web site: www.cryofab.com
  Annual Revenue: $5-$10 Million
  Total Employees: 48   *Marketing Staff:* 4   *Sales Staff:* 3
  Ownership: Private
  Produces/Sells CE-marked Devices: Y
  Federal Procurement Eligibility: Small Business
  Distribution: Manufacturer Direct, Manufacturer Through Manufacturer Reps, OEM, Service Direct, Exporter
  General Admin.: Vincent J. Grillo/Executive Vice President
  Production: Frank Durantino/Manager Operations & Services
  Carrier, Container, Oxygen, Portable   General
  Container, Liquid Oxygen   Anesthesiology
  Equipment, Bank, Blood, Cryogenic (Liquid Nitrogen)   Hematology
  Service, Maintenance/Repair   General

CRYOGENIC ASSOCIATION
  See Caire, Inc.

CRYOLIFE, INC.
800-438-8285
1655 Roberts Blvd. NW., Kennesaw, GA 30144
770-419-3355
FDA Number: 1063481
Fax: 770-426-0031
E-mail: info@cryolife.com
Web site: http://www.cryolife.com
Medical Products Sales Volume: $44,712,000
Annual Revenue: $50-$100 Million
Year Founded: 1984
Total Employees: 405
Ownership: Public
Stock Symbol: CRY
Traded On: NYSE
Quality System Registration Information: ISO9001
Produces/Sells CE-marked Devices: Y
Federal Procurement Eligibility: Small Business
Distribution: Manufacturer Direct, Manufacturer Through Distributor, Manufacturer Through Manufacturer Reps, Importer, Exporter
General Admin.: Steven G. Anderson/President, Chief Executive Officer
  Medical Admin.: Dr. William F. Northrup/Vice President Medical & Consumer Affairs
Mktg./Adv.: Mr. Gerald B. Seery/Senior Vice President Marketing & Sales
      Mr. Richard C. Gridley/Vice President International Marketing & Sales
      Mr. David Lang/Vice President Market Development
      Mr. Bruce G. Anderson/Vice President U.S. Sales
Production: Mr. David M. Fronk/Vice President Quality Assurance & Regulatory Affairs
Research: Dr. Albert E. Heacox/Senior Vice President Research & Development
      Mr. Scott B. Capps/Vice President Clinical Research
      Mr. Timothy M. Neja/Vice President Lab. Operations
Finance: Amy D. Horton/Chief Accountant
      Ms. Ashley Lee/Chief Financial Officer

Agent, Hemostatic, Absorbable, Collagen-Based	Surgery
Allograft, Heart Valve	Cardiovascular
Glue, Surgical Tissue	Surgery
Graft, Arterial, Biological	Cardiovascular
Mesh, Surgical (Steel Gauze)	Surgery
Pledget And Intracardiac Patch, PETP, PTFE, Polypropylene	Cardiovascular
Prosthesis, Cardiac Valve	Cardiovascular
Prosthesis, Cardiac Valve, Biological	Cardiovascular
Prosthesis, Ligament	Orthopedics
Prosthesis, Tendon	Surgery
Prosthesis, Vascular Graft, Less Than 6mm Diameter	Cardiovascular
Prosthesis, Vascular Graft, Of 6mm And Greater Diameter	Cardiovascular
Tissue Graft of 6mm and Greater	Cardiovascular
Valve, Heart, Mechanical	Cardiovascular
Valve, Heart, Tissue	Cardiovascular

CRYOPAK INDUSTRIES, INC.
732-346-9200
55 Raritan Center Parkway, Edison, NJ 08837 Canada
FDA Number: 9680689
Fax: 732-346-0295
E-mail: sales@cryopak.com
Web site: www.cryopak.com
Year Founded: 1981
Total Employees: 70   *Marketing Staff:* 1   *Sales Staff:* 7
Ownership: Private
Produces/Sells CE-marked Devices: N
Distribution: Manufacturer Direct, Manufacturer Through Distributor, OEM, Service Direct

CRYOPEN INC.
888-246-3928
800 North Shoreline, Suite 900, Corpus Christi, TX 78401
FDA Number: 3005607001
Fax: 985-871-0804
E-mail: sales@cryopen.com
Web site: http://cryopen.com
Ownership: Private
Produces/Sells CE-marked Devices: N

Cryosurgical Unit	Surgery

CRYOSURGERY, INC.
800-729-1624
5829 Old Harding Road, Nashville, TN 37205
615-354-0414
FDA Number: 1056356
Fax: 615-354-0466
E-mail: info@cryosurgeryinc.com
Web site: www.cryosurgeryinc.com
Ownership: Private
Produces/Sells CE-marked Devices: N
Federal Procurement Eligibility: Small Business
Distribution: Manufacturer Through Distributor, Exporter
General Admin.: Ronald A. McDow/President
Mktg./Adv.: Laura Reline/Vice President Marketing

Cryosurgical Unit	Surgery

CRYOTHERAPY PAIN RELIEF PRODUCTS, INC.
954-893-9059
3460 Laurel Oaks Lane, Hollywood, FL 33021-8448
FDA Number: 1063212
Ownership: Private
Produces/Sells CE-marked Devices: N

Pack, Hot Or Cold, Water Circulating	Physical Med

CRYSCHEM
  See Qed Bioscience, Inc.

CRYSTAL COMPUTER LENSES
214-773-3457
104 E. Us Hwy 80, Suite 100, Forney, TX 75126
FDA Number: 3006432230

Lens, Spectacle (prescription), For Reading Discomfort	Ophthalmology

CRYSTAL MEDICAL TECHNOLOGY
205-733-0901
153 Cahaba Valley Pkwy., Pelham, AL 35124
FDA Number: 1065595
Fax: 205-733-8509
E-mail: Acfolsomjr2@cs.com
Web site: www.crystalmedicaltech.com
Medical Products Sales Volume: $900,000
Year Founded: 1994
Total Employees: 7
Ownership: Private
Produces/Sells CE-marked Devices: N
Federal Procurement Eligibility: Small Business

Accessories, Fixation, Orthopedic	Orthopedics
Implant, Endosseous	Dental And Oral

CRYSTAL TONE HEARING INSTRUMENTS
515-255-4144
4217 University Ave., Des Moines, IA 50311
FDA Number: n/a
Ownership: Private
Produces/Sells CE-marked Devices: N

Hearing-Aid	Ear/Nose/Throat
Hearing-Aid, Plate, Face	Ear/Nose/Throat

CRYSTALMARK DENTAL SYSTEMS, INC.
818-240-7596
621 Ruberta Ave., Glendale, CA 91201
FDA Number: 2029314

Airbrush	Dental And Oral
Mirror, Mouth	Dental And Oral

CS&D ARCHITECTS
  See Cochran, Stephenson & Donkervoet, Inc. Architects

CSA MEDICAL, INC.
866.481.7786
1101 E 33rd Street, Third Floor, Ste. E305,
443-921-8053
Baltimore, MD 21218
FDA Number: 3004534508
Fax: 866.300.5183
Web site: http://www.csamedical.com
Ownership: Private
Produces/Sells CE-marked Devices: N
General Admin.: Mr. William Floyd/Chief Executive Officer
      Dr. Rob Burr/Chief Technology Officer
Mktg./Adv.: Mr. Richard Hughen/Vice President Marketing & Business Development
      Ms. Kimberly Strusky/Vice President Sales
Finance: Mr. Steven Schaefer/Chief Financial Officer

Cryosurgical Unit	Surgery
System, Cryosurgical, Liquid Nitrogen, For Gastroenterology	Gastroenterology/Urology

CSAM, INC.
563-359-7917
1890 14th St., Bettendorf, IA 52722
FDA Number: 1954126
Fax: 563-359-7917
E-mail: skim@PyMath.com
Web site: http://pygame.com/
Medical Products Sales Volume: $340,000
Year Founded: 1995
Total Employees: 6   *Marketing Staff:* 2   *Sales Staff:* 2
Ownership: Csam, Inc.
Produces/Sells CE-marked Devices: N
Federal Procurement Eligibility: Small Business, Minority Owned
Distribution: Manufacturer Direct
General Admin.: Sun Kim/Vice President

Computer and Software, Medical	General

Medical Product Subsidiaries (Listed Separately)
  Csam, Inc.

CSC SCIENTIFIC CO.
800-621-4778
2810 Old Lee Hwy., Fairfax, VA 22031-4304
703-876-4030
FDA Number: n/a
Fax: 703-280-5142
E-mail: info@cscscientific.com
Web site: www.cscscientific.com
Annual Revenue: $1-$5 Million
Total Employees: 19   *Sales Staff:* 6
Ownership: Private
Produces/Sells CE-marked Devices: N
Federal Procurement Eligibility: Small Business
Distribution: Manufacturer Direct, Manufacturer Through Distributor, Exclusive Distributor
General Admin.: Art Gatenby/President
      Ellie Gatenby/Vice President Human Resources
Mktg./Adv.: Wendy Liu/Coord. Marketing

Balance, Electronic	Chemistry

CSC SCIENTIFIC CO.
800-621-4778 *(cont'd)*
Shaker/Stirrer — Chemistry

CSI HOLDINGS
615-452-9633
170 Commerce Way, Gallatin, TN 37066
FDA Number: 2320386
Fax: 615-452-9451
E-mail: fknox@csiholdings.com
Web site: www.csimed.com
Medical Products Sales Volume: $2,400,000
Annual Revenue: $5-$10 Million
Total Employees: 30 — Marketing Staff: 2 — Sales Staff: 4
Ownership: Csi Holdings
Quality System Registration Information: ISO9001
Produces/Sells CE-marked Devices: N
Federal Procurement Eligibility: Small Business
Distribution: Manufacturer Direct, OEM, Importer, Exporter
General Admin.: Mr. Fred Knox/Principal

Bandage, Gauze	General
Contract Assembly	General
Contract Manufacturing	General
Contract Manufacturing, Product, Disposable	General
Dressing, Non-Adherent	General
Retractor	Orthopedics
Strip, Adhesive	Surgery
Tape, Adhesive	General
Tape, Adhesive, Hypoallergenic	General
Tubing, Polyvinyl Chloride	General

Medical Product Subsidiaries (Listed Separately)
  Csi Holdings

CSI INTERNATIONAL, INC.
303-795-8273
4301 S. Federal Blvd., Suite 116, Englewood, CO 80110-5310
FDA Number: 1720903
Fax: 303-795-9982
Total Employees: 6
Ownership: Private
Quality System Registration Information: ISO9000
Produces/Sells CE-marked Devices: N
Federal Procurement Eligibility: Small Business
Distribution: Service Direct, Importer
General Admin.: Lance Ferrin/President

Bag, Breathing	Anesthesiology
Bag, Urinary Collection	General
Cable	Physical Med
Cap, Tip, Syringe	General
Component, Rubber	General
Component, Silicone	General
Molding, Custom	General
Service, Import/Export	General
Stopper	General

CSI RUBBER PRODUCTS, INC.
See Csi International, Inc.

CSL BEHRING
610-878-4000
1020 First Ave., P.O. Box 61501, King of Prussia, PA 19406-0901
FDA Number: 7000427
Fax: 610-878-4009
Web site: www.cslbehring.com
Medical Products Sales Volume: $500,000,000
Annual Revenue: More than $1 Billion
Total Employees: 8400
Ownership: Private
Produces/Sells CE-marked Devices: Y
Distribution: Manufacturer Direct, Manufacturer Through Distributor, Importer
General Admin.: Gordon Naylor/Executive Vice President
        Peter Turner/President
Production: Paul Perreault/Executive Vice President Operations
Research: Val Romberg/Senior Vice President Research & Development

Controller, Infusion, Intravascular	General
Kit, Administration, Intravenous	General
Test, Thyroid Autoantibody	Immunology

CSP INC.
See Delval Glass, Inc.

CST TECHNOLOGIES, INC.
800-448-4407
55 Northern Blvd., Suite 200,
516-482-9001
Great Neck, NY 11021
FDA Number: n/a
Fax: 516-482-0186
E-mail: info@cstti.com
Web site: www.cstti.com
Medical Products Sales Volume: $900,000
Annual Revenue: $1-$5 Million
Year Founded: 1986
Total Employees: 10 — Marketing Staff: 2 — Sales Staff: 7
Ownership: Private
Produces/Sells CE-marked Devices: N
Federal Procurement Eligibility: Small Business, Minority Owned
Distribution: Manufacturer Direct
General Admin.: Anand Akerkar/President, Chief Executive Officer
        Alan P. Schwartz/Vice President

CST TECHNOLOGIES, INC.
800-448-4407 *(cont'd)*
Production: Linda O'Brien/Manager Materials

Analyzer, Chemistry, Micro	Chemistry
Antibody, Other	General
Antigen, Antiserum, Control, Whole Human Serum	Immunology
Control, Urinalysis (Assayed And Unassayed)	Chemistry
Diluent, Blood Cell	Hematology

CTBR (INVERESK RESEARCH GROUP MEMBER) 514-630-8200
87 Senneville Rd., Senneville, QUE H9X-3R3 Canada
FDA Number: n/a
Fax: 514-630-8230
E-mail: marketing@ctbr.com
Web site: www.ctbr.com
Year Founded: 1965
Total Employees: 250
Ownership: Private
Produces/Sells CE-marked Devices: N

CTE CHEM TEC EQUIPMENT CO.
800-222-2177
234 S.W. 12th Avenue,
954-428-8259
Deerfield Beach, FL 33442
FDA Number: n/a
Fax: 954-428-8745
E-mail: info@chemtec.com
Web site: www.chemtec.com
Medical Products Sales Volume: $4,000,000
Annual Revenue: $1-$5 Million
Year Founded: 1968
Total Employees: 30 — Marketing Staff: 2 — Sales Staff: 4
Ownership: Private
Produces/Sells CE-marked Devices: Y
Federal Procurement Eligibility: Small Business
Distribution: Manufacturer Direct, Manufacturer Through Distributor, Manufacturer Through Manufacturer Reps, OEM
General Admin.: William A. Nolan/President, Chief Executive Officer
Mktg./Adv.: Christian Nolan/Manager International & National Sales
        Shannon Kantor/Vice President Marketing
        Christian Nolan/Vice President Sales
Production: Rajen Jairam/Director Quality Assurance
        Darlene Panella/Manager Regulatory Affairs

Component, Other	General
Flowmeter, Dialysate	Gastroenterology/Urology
Valve, Other	Chemistry

CTI MEDICAL EQUIPMENT, INC.
856-424-0503
1910 Route 70 (e), Ste.10, Cherry Hill, NJ 08003
FDA Number: 2249862
Ownership: Private
Produces/Sells CE-marked Devices: N

Epilator, High-Frequency, Needle-Type	Surgery

CTP COIL INC.
800-933-2645
1801-D Howard Street,
847-228-8818
Elk Grove Village, IL 60007
FDA Number: 8010133
Fax: 847-593-3930
E-mail: jpope@iwic.net
Web site: www.ctpcoil.co.uk
Medical Products Sales Volume: $200,000
Year Founded: 1994
Total Employees: 2 — Marketing Staff: 1 — Sales Staff: 5
Ownership: CARLCO ENGINEERING GROUP PLC
Quality System Registration Information: ISO9000; ISO9001
Produces/Sells CE-marked Devices: Y
Federal Procurement Eligibility: Small Business
Distribution: Manufacturer Through Distributor, Importer, Exporter
General Admin.: Ian Williamsom/President
Mktg./Adv.: John Newth/Director International Business Development
        Janice Pope/Director National Accounts
        John Newth/Director Product Development
        John Newth/Manager International & National Sales
        John Newth/Manager National Sales
        John Newth/Manager Sales Training
Production: Patrick Ward/Director Manufacturing

Lens, Spectacle/Eyeglasses, Non-Custom	Ophthalmology
Loupe, Binocular, Low Power	Ophthalmology
Magnifier, Hand-Held, Low-Vision	Ophthalmology
Reader, Bar, Ophthalmic	Ophthalmology
Shield, Eye, Ophthalmic	Ophthalmology
Spectacle, Magnifier	Ophthalmology
Sunglasses (Including Photosensitive)	Ophthalmology
Telescope, Spectacle, Low-Vision	Ophthalmology
Vision Aid, Image Intensification, Battery-Powered	Ophthalmology
Vision Aid, Optical, AC-Powered	Ophthalmology
Vision Aid, Optical, Battery-Powered	Ophthalmology

CTRONICS
800-472-9909
6333 Pacific Avenue, PMB 294,
209-467-3800
Stockton, CA 95207
FDA Number: n/a
Fax: 209-982-0243

CTRONICS 800-472-9909 *(cont'd)*
E-mail: info@CTronics.com
Web site: www.CTronics.com
Annual Revenue: $1-$5 Million
Year Founded: 1980
Total Employees: 50   *Marketing Staff:* 3   *Sales Staff:* 3
Ownership: Private
Produces/Sells CE-marked Devices: N
Federal Procurement Eligibility: Small Business
Distribution: Service Direct, Importer, Exporter
General Admin.: John Taylor/President
     Aimee St. Georges/Vice President Personnel
Mktg./Adv.: William Blackford/Manager International Sales
     Aimee St. Georges/Vice President Advertising
     Paul Ackerman/Vice President Marketing & Sales
Production: William Blackford/Manager Materials

Service, Parts, Repair	General
Service, Used Equipment	General

CUDA FIBEROPTICS
See Sunoptic Technologies

CUDA PRODUCTS CORPORATION
See Sunoptic Technologies

CUFF TOUGHENER 601-853-3966
103 Weldon Dr., Madison, MS 39110
FDA Number: 3003604812
Ownership: Private
Produces/Sells CE-marked Devices: N

Component, Exercise	Physical Med

CULLIGAN INTERNATIONAL CO. 866-775-0260
9399 West Higgins Road, Rosemont, IL 60018 847-430-2800
FDA Number: 2135346
Web site: www.culligan.com
Medical Products Sales Volume: $304,500,000
Year Founded: 1936
Ownership: Private
Quality System Registration Information: ISO9000
Produces/Sells CE-marked Devices: Y
Distribution: Manufacturer Through Distributor

Purification Filter, Water, Charcoal	Chemistry
Purification Filter, Water, Particulate	Chemistry
Purification System, Water	Gastroenterology/Urology
Purification System, Water, Deionization	Chemistry
Purification System, Water, Reverse Osmosis	Chemistry
Purification System, Water, Reverse Osmosis, Reagent Grade	Chemistry
Purification System, Water, Ultraviolet	Chemistry
Reverse Osmosis Membrane Equipment	Chemistry

CULLIGAN SOFT WATER SERVICE CO. 952-933-7200
6030 Culligan Way, Minnetonka, MN 55345
FDA Number: 2135346
Web site: www.culligan.com
Year Founded: 1936
Ownership: Private
Produces/Sells CE-marked Devices: N

Purification System, Water	Gastroenterology/Urology

CULTURE KITS, INC. 888-680-6853
**14 Prentice St., PO Box 748, 607-336-1422
Norwich, NY 13815**
FDA Number: 1318700   *Fax:* 607-336-8573
E-mail: info@culturekits.com
Web site: www.culturekits.com
Medical Products Sales Volume: $920,000
Annual Revenue: $0-$1 Million
Year Founded: 1983
Total Employees: 11   *Marketing Staff:* 2   *Sales Staff:* 2
Ownership: Private
Produces/Sells CE-marked Devices: N
Federal Procurement Eligibility: Small Business
Distribution: Manufacturer Direct
General Admin.: Anne D. Lauenstein/Secretary, Treasurer
Mktg./Adv.: Lisa Smith/Director Marketing
     Lynne Fleming/Director National Accounts
     Holly Sweet/Director Product Development
     Raymond Lauenstein/Manager Advertising
     Lynne Fleming/Manager Contract Sales
     Raymond J. Lauenstein/Manager National Sales
     Ursula Yearton/Manager Product Development
     Raymond J. Lauenstein/President Marketing
Production: Ursula Yearton/Director Quality Assurance
     Holly Sweet/Manager Regulatory Affairs
Research: Holly Sweet/Manager Laboratories

Antigen, Streptococcus SPP.	Microbiology
Container, Specimen, All Types	General
Culture Media, Antimicrobial Susceptibility Test	Microbiology

CULTURE KITS, INC. 888-680-6853 *(cont'd)*

Culture Media, Enriched	Microbiology
Culture Media, For Isolation Of Pathogenic Neisseria	Microbiology
Culture Media, Mueller Hinton Agar Broth	Microbiology
Culture Media, Non-Selective And Differential	Microbiology
Culture Media, Selective And Differential	Microbiology
Culture Media, Selective And Non-Differential	Microbiology
Dispenser, Disc, Sensitivity, Antibiotic	Microbiology
Jelly, Lubricating, Transurethral Surgical Instrument	Gastroenterology/Urology
Kit, Identification, Neisseria Gonorrhoeae	Microbiology
Kit, Screening, Urine	Microbiology
Kit, Yeast Screening	Microbiology
Oxidase Test Device for Gonorrhea	Microbiology
Test, Bacterial Diagnostic	Microbiology

CUMBERLAND PHARMACEUTICALS INC. 877-484-2700
**2525 West End Ave, Suite 500, 615-255-0068
Nashville, TN 37203**
FDA Number: n/a   *Fax:* 615-255-0094
E-mail: info@cumberlandpharma.com
Web site: http://www.cumberlandpharma.com
Ownership: Public
Stock Symbol: CPIX
Traded On: NASDAQ
Produces/Sells CE-marked Devices: N
General Admin.: Mr. A.J. Kazimi/Chairman, Chief Executive Officer
     Mr. David Lowrance/Chief Financial Officer, Senior Vice President
     Mr. Martin Cearnal/Senior Vice President
Medical Admin.: Dr. Gordon Bernard/Medical Director
Production: Mr. Leo Pavliv/Senior Vice President Operations

CUNO FILTER SYSTEMS 800-243-6894
400 Research Pkwy., Meriden, CT 06450 203-237-5541
FDA Number: n/a   *Fax:* 203-238-8977
Web site: www.cuno.com
Annual Revenue: $25-$50 Million
Year Founded: 1912
Total Employees: 350   *Sales Staff:* 25
Ownership: 3M COMPANY
Quality System Registration Information: ISO9001
Produces/Sells CE-marked Devices: N
Distribution: OEM

Service, Consulting	General
Service, Modification, Product	General

CURAE'LASE INC. 843-455-7020
2315 Hwy 701 South, Loris, SC 29569
FDA Number: 3005535133
Ownership: Private
Produces/Sells CE-marked Devices: N

Lamp, Infrared	Physical Med

CURAPHARM, INC. 619-449-7388
10054 Prospect Ave., Suite F, Santee, CA 92071
FDA Number: 2032469

Dressing, Wound and Burn, Hydrogel	Surgery

CURBELL ELECTRONICS INC. 716-667-3377
20 Centre Dr., Orchard Park, NY 14127
FDA Number: 1320360

Bed, Electric	General
Cable/Lead, ECG, With Transducer And Electrode	Cardiovascular
Communication System, Powered	Physical Med
Monitor, Bed Patient	General

CURBELL, INC. ELECTRONICS 800-235-7500
7 Cobham Dr., Orchard Park, NY 14127 716-667-3377
FDA Number: n/a   *Fax:* 716-667-7775
E-mail: info@curbellelectronics.com
Web site: www.curbellelectronics.com
Ownership: CURBELL, INC.
Quality System Registration Information: ISO9001
Produces/Sells CE-marked Devices: N
Distribution: Manufacturer Direct
General Admin.: Thomas Leone/President, Chief Executive Officer
     Art Ghost/Vice President, General Manager
Mktg./Adv.: Douglas Rockwood/Manager International & National Sales
     Jeni Becker/Market Manager
     Katie Zoratti/Marketing Associate
Production: Abdul Sarac/Director Quality Assurance

Casters, Hospital Equipment	General
Monitor, Bed Patient	General
Nurse Call System	General

CURETIS AG +49 0 7031 4919
Max-Eyth-Str. 42, Holzgerlingen 71088
FDA Number: n/a
E-mail: contact@curetis.com
Web site: www.curetis.com

CURETIS AG   +49 0 7031 4919 *(cont'd)*
Ownership: Private
Produces/Sells CE-marked Devices: N
General Admin.: Mr. Oliver Schacht/Chief Executive Officer
     Mr. Johannes Bacher/Chief Operating Officer
     Mr. Andreas Boos/Chief Technology Officer
Mktg./Adv.: Dr. Anne Thews/Director Medical Marketing
     Dr. Klaus Brinkmann/Director Sales
Finance: Ms. Anne Burger/Chief Financial Officer

CURMED, INC.
See Currie Medical Specialties, Inc.

CURRENT CONTROLS, INC.   585-593-1544
353 S. Brooklyn Avenue, Wellsville, NY 14895
FDA Number: n/a   Fax: 585-593-1713
E-mail: SALES@CURRENTCONTROLS.COM
Web site: www.currentcontrols.com
Medical Products Sales Volume: $8,400,000
Annual Revenue: $5-$10 Million
Year Founded: 1982
Total Employees: 150
Ownership: Private
Quality System Registration Information: ISO9001
Produces/Sells CE-marked Devices: N
Federal Procurement Eligibility: Small Business
Distribution: Manufacturer Direct, OEM
Mktg./Adv.: Sylvia A. Landon/Director Marketing
     Sylvia A. Landon/Director National Accounts
     Component, Electronic   General

CURRENT MEDICINE GROUP LLC   800-427-1796
400 Market St., Suite 700,   **215-574-2266**
Philadelphia, PA 19106
FDA Number: n/a   Fax: 215-574-2225
E-mail: info@phl.cursci.com
Web site: www.current-medicine.com
Medical Products Sales Volume: $4,800,000
Annual Revenue: $0-$1 Million
Year Founded: 1990
Total Employees: 45   Marketing Staff: 2
Ownership: Private
Produces/Sells CE-marked Devices: N
Federal Procurement Eligibility: Small Business
Distribution: Manufacturer Direct
General Admin.: Abe Krieger/President
Mktg./Adv.: Linda Lee/Director Marketing
     Computer Software   General
     Material, Training, Audiovisual   General
     Printer, Image, Video   General

CURRENT SCIENCE
See Current Medicine Group Llc

CURRENT TECHNOLOGIES INC   800-456-4022
PO Box 21, Crawfordsville, IN 47933-0021   **765-364-0490**
FDA Number: n/a   Fax: 765-364-1607
Medical Products Sales Volume: $670,000
Year Founded: 1968
Total Employees: 12
Ownership: Private
Produces/Sells CE-marked Devices: Y
Federal Procurement Eligibility: Small Business, Female Owned, GSA Contract
Distribution: Manufacturer Direct, Manufacturer Through Distributor
General Admin.: Susan Hapak/President
     Strip, Test   Chemistry

CURRENT TECHNOLOGY CORPORATION   800-661-4247
530 800 West Pender St.,   **604-684-2727**
Vancouver, BC V6C-2 Canada
FDA Number: n/a   Fax: 604-684-0526
E-mail: ctc@axionet.com
Web site: www.currentech.com
Year Founded: 1987
Total Employees: 10
Ownership: Public
Stock Symbol: CRTCF
Traded On: OTC Bulletin
Produces/Sells CE-marked Devices: N
Distribution: Manufacturer Direct, Exclusive Distributor, Exporter

CURRIE MEDICAL SPECIALTIES, INC.   800-669-3521
730 E. Los Angeles Avenue,   **626-303-3521**
Monrovia, CA 91016
FDA Number: 2023637   Fax: 626-303-2947
E-mail: cmsweb@curriemedical.com
Web site: www.curriemedical.com
Medical Products Sales Volume: $6,000,000

CURRIE MEDICAL SPECIALTIES, INC.   800-669-3521 *(cont'd)*
Annual Revenue: $5-$10 Million
Total Employees: 100   Marketing Staff: 10   Sales Staff: 6
Ownership: Private
Quality System Registration Information: ISO9000
Produces/Sells CE-marked Devices: N
Federal Procurement Eligibility: Small Business
Distribution: Manufacturer Direct, Manufacturer Through Distributor, Manufacturer Through Manufacturer Reps
General Admin.: Rick Roeder/President, Chief Executive Officer
Production: Natalia Cueto/Director Quality Assurance
     Judy McAllister/Vice President Customer Service
     Sean Souney/Vice President Operations
     Connie Wong/Vice President Regulatory Affairs
Purchasing: Eric Warfield/Vice President Purchasing
     Contract Laboratory   General
     Contract Manufacturing   General

CUSTOM BOTTLE/LERMAN CONTAINER   800-315-6681
10 Great Hill Road, Naugatuck, CT 06770-0979   **203-723-6681**
FDA Number: 1220480   Fax: 203-723-6687
E-mail: sales@bottles.com
Web site: www.bottles.com
Medical Products Sales Volume: $29,300,000
Annual Revenue: $25-$50 Million
Year Founded: 1979
Total Employees: 200   Marketing Staff: 2   Sales Staff: 5
Ownership: Private
Produces/Sells CE-marked Devices: N
Federal Procurement Eligibility: Small Business
Distribution: Exclusive Distributor
General Admin.: Robert Lerman/Chief Executive Officer
     Barry Lerman/President
     Lynn S. Quinn/Vice President Human Resources
     Neil Bloomberg/Vice President, General Manager
Mktg./Adv.: Lisa Calabrese/Manager Advertising
     Kate Harrington/Manager Marketing
     Barry Lerman/Manager National Sales
     Joseph Fragala/Vice President Business Development
Production: Paul Jessell/Vice President Manufacturing
     Collector, Specimen   Microbiology
     Packaging Material   General

CUSTOM COMFORT
See Custom Comfort Medtek

CUSTOM COMFORT   800-749-0933
PO Box 4779, Winter Park, FL 32793-4779   **407-366-1626**
FDA Number: n/a   Fax: 407-366-8246
E-mail: sales@customcomfort.com
Web site: www.customcomfort.com
Annual Revenue: $1-$5 Million
Year Founded: 1987
Total Employees: 17   Marketing Staff: 4   Sales Staff: 4
Ownership: Private
Produces/Sells CE-marked Devices: N
Federal Procurement Eligibility: Small Business
Distribution: Manufacturer Direct
General Admin.: Mr. Peter Gaughn/President, Owner
Mktg./Adv.: Mr. Doug Patton/Vice President Sales
Production: Mr. Gary Newton/General Manager Manufacturing
     Cabinet, Other   General
     Cart, Supply   General
     Chair, Infant Treatment   General
     Chair, Other   General
     Chair/Table, Medical   General

CUSTOM COMFORT MEDTEK   800-749-0933
3939 Forsyth Road, Suite A,   **407-332-0062**
Winter Park, FL 32792
FDA Number: n/a   Fax: 407-332-0025
E-mail: sales@customcomfort.com
Web site: www.customcomfort.com
Medical Products Sales Volume: $4,700,000
Annual Revenue: $5-$10 Million
Year Founded: 1985
Total Employees: 22   Marketing Staff: 4   Sales Staff: 6
Ownership: Private
Produces/Sells CE-marked Devices: N
Federal Procurement Eligibility: Small Business
Distribution: Manufacturer Direct
Mktg./Adv.: Mr. Doug Patton/General Manager, Manager International Marketing and Sales
     Accessories, Cart, Multipurpose   General
     Cabinet, Other   General
     Cart, Equipment, Video   General
     Cart, Supply   General
     Chair, Blood Donor   General

MANUFACTURER PROFILES

CUSTOM COMFORT MEDTEK　800-749-0933 *(cont'd)*
Chair, Blood Drawing　General
Footstool　General
Furniture, Patient Room　General
Table, Examination/Treatment　General

CUSTOM CONTACT LENSES　866-273-4125
3075 14th Ave., Unit 15,　905-477-5038
Markham, ONT L3R-0 Canada
FDA Number: n/a　*Fax:* 905-477-4902
Web site: www.customcontactlenses.com
Year Founded: 2000
Total Employees: 10
Ownership: Private
Produces/Sells CE-marked Devices: N
Distribution: Manufacturer Direct

CUSTOM DURABLE PRODUCTS, INC　800 478-2363
21279 Protecta Drive, Elkhart, IN 46516　574 522-7201
FDA Number: n/a　*Fax:* 574 293-0202
E-mail: info@pvcdme.com
Web site: www.pvcdme.com
Medical Products Sales Volume: $1,000,000
Annual Revenue: $1-$5 Million
Total Employees: 15
Ownership: Private
Produces/Sells CE-marked Devices: Y
Federal Procurement Eligibility: Small Business, Female Owned
Distribution: Manufacturer Direct, Manufacturer Through Distributor, OEM, Exporter
General Admin.: Tom Roberts/Chief Executive Officer
　　　　　Dawn Slabach/President
Cart, Laundry　General
Cart, Multipurpose　General
Chair, Other　General
Commode (Toilet)　General

CUSTOM DURABLE PRODUCTS, PUC DURABLE MEDICAL EQUIP
See Custom Durable Products, Inc

CUSTOM HEALTHCARE SYSTEMS, INC.　804-421-5959
4205 Eubank Rd., Richmond, VA 23231
FDA Number: 1121091
Annual Revenue: $1-$5 Million
Total Employees: 15　*Marketing Staff:* 3　*Sales Staff:* 3
Ownership: Private
Produces/Sells CE-marked Devices: N
Federal Procurement Eligibility: Small Business
Distribution: Manufacturer Through Distributor
General Admin.: Larry Heath/President
　　　　　Carol Heath/Vice President
Applicator, Tipped, Absorbent, Sterile　General
Ball, Cotton　General
Bandage, Cast　Physical Med
Bandage, Elastic　General
Kit, Administration, Intravenous　General
Kit, Skin Scrub　General
Kit, Surgical Instrument, Disposable　Surgery
Kit, Tracheostomy Care　Anesthesiology
Kit, Wound Dressing　Surgery
Sponge, Other　General
Stockinette　Orthopedics
Tray, Surgical　Surgery

CUSTOM INDUSTRIES INC., BIO AIR SYSTEMS
See Bio Air Systems Div.

CUSTOM MEDICAL PRODUCTS　407-865-7211
3909 East Semoran Blvd., Bldg. 599, Apopka, FL 32703
FDA Number: 1066315
Ownership: Private
Produces/Sells CE-marked Devices: N
Kit, Collection/Transfusion, Marrow, Bone　General
Kit, Cord Blood Collection　Hematology
Kit, Instruments and Accessories, Surgical　Surgery
Kit, Surgical (Lacrimal)　Surgery

CUSTOM OCULAR PROSTHETICS　206-522-4222
10212 5th Avenue NE, Suite 210, Seattle, WA 98125-7471
FDA Number: 3030005　*Fax:* 206-525-1496
E-mail: cop@artificialeye.com
Web site: www.artificialeye.com
Medical Products Sales Volume: $300,000
Total Employees: 3
Ownership: Private
Produces/Sells CE-marked Devices: N
Federal Procurement Eligibility: Small Business
Prosthesis, Eye, Internal (Sphere)　Surgery

CUSTOM ORTHOTIC DESIGN GROUP LTD.　(866) 829-2969
4120 Ridgeway Dr., Unit 24,　905-828-2969
Mississauga, ONT L5L-5 Canada
FDA Number: n/a　*Fax:* 905-828-1091
E-mail: lindalaakso@customorthotic.ca
Web site: www.customorthotic.ca
Year Founded: 1996
Total Employees: 25
Ownership: Private
Produces/Sells CE-marked Devices: N
Distribution: Manufacturer Direct

CUSTOM ORTHOTICS OF LONDON　519-850-4721
1 Adelaide St. North, London, ONT N6B-3P8 Canada
FDA Number: n/a　*Fax:* 519-850-1816
E-mail: orthotic@execulink.com
Year Founded: 1987
Total Employees: 10
Ownership: Private
Produces/Sells CE-marked Devices: N
Distribution: Manufacturer Direct, Service Direct

CUSTOM PAPER TUBES INC.　800-864-1793
15900 Industrial Parkway, Cleveland, OH 44135　216-362-2964
FDA Number: 3005017508　*Fax:* 216-362-2980
Ownership: Private
Produces/Sells CE-marked Devices: N
Mouthpiece, Breathing　Anesthesiology

CUSTOM PROSTHETIC DESIGN, INC.　703-723-4668
20608 Gordon Park Square, Suite 150, Ashburn, VA 20147
FDA Number: n/a　*Fax:* 703-723-7130
E-mail: cpdrbarron@prosthesis.com
Web site: www.prosthesis.com
Ownership: Private
Produces/Sells CE-marked Devices: N
Custom Prosthesis　Orthopedics
Eye, Artificial, Custom　Ophthalmology
Prosthesis, Ear, Internal　Surgery
Prosthesis, Finger　Orthopedics

CUSTOM SCIENTIFIC PRODUCTS
See Delval Glass, Inc.

CUSTOM SPINE INC　973-808-0019
1140 Parsippany Boulevard, Suite #201, Parsippany, NJ 07054
FDA Number: 3005129649　*Fax:* 973-808-0707
E-mail: info@customspine.com
Web site: www.customspine.com
Ownership: Private
Produces/Sells CE-marked Devices: N
Mktg./Adv.: Mr. Frank Herrington/Senior Vice President Marketing & Sales
Appliance, Fixation, Spinal Interlaminal　Orthopedics
Appliance, Fixation, Spinal Intervertebral Body　Orthopedics
Awl　Orthopedics
Bender　Orthopedics
Cannula, Surgical, General & Plastic Surgery　Surgery
Compression Instrument　Orthopedics
Driver, Bone Staple　Orthopedics
Forceps　Orthopedics
Gauge, Depth　Orthopedics
Guide, Surgical, Instrument　Surgery
Instrument, Bending (Contouring)　Orthopedics
Intervertebral Fusion Device With Bone Graft, Cervical　Orthopedics
Orthodontic Instrument　Dental And Oral
Orthopedic Manual Surgical Instrument　Orthopedics
Orthosis, Fixation, Spinal, Spondylolisthesis　Orthopedics
Orthosis, Spinal Pedicle Fixation, For Degenerative Disc Disease　Orthopedics
Probe　Orthopedics
Rasp, Other　Surgery
Rongeur, Other　Surgery
Screwdriver　Orthopedics
Tap, Bone　Orthopedics
Template　Orthopedics
Tray, Surgical Instrument　Surgery
Wrench　Orthopedics

CUSTOM TAPE COMPANY　888-259-3521
6288 Claude Way, Inver Grove Heights, MN 55077
FDA Number: 3004181163
Web site: www.customtapecompany.com
Ownership: Private
Produces/Sells CE-marked Devices: N
Container, IV　General

CUSTOM ULTRASONICS, INC.　215-364-1477
144 Railroad Dr., Hartsville, PA 18974
FDA Number: n/a　*Fax:* 215-364-7674
E-mail: q-net@msn.com
Web site: www.customultrasonics.com

CUSTOM ULTRASONICS, INC.   215-364-1477 *(cont'd)*
Total Employees: 23
Ownership: Private
Produces/Sells CE-marked Devices: Y
Federal Procurement Eligibility: Small Business
Distribution: Manufacturer Through Manufacturer Reps
General Admin.: Frank Weber/President, Chief Executive Officer
Mktg./Adv.: Bob Blanchard/Director Marketing
       George Raudenbush/Manager Product Marketing
Production: Craig Weber/Vice President Manufacturing

Cabinet, Storage, Endoscope	Gastroenterology/Urology
Cleaner, Ultrasonic, Medical Instrument	General
Monitor, Contamination, Environmental, Personal	General
Sterilizer/Washer, Endoscope	General
Washer, Respiratory/Anesthesia Equipment	General

CUSTOM X-RAY SERVICE, INC.   (800) 230 - XRA
2120 West Encanto, Phoenix, AZ 85009   **602-439-3100**
FDA Number: 2022141   *Fax:* (602) 252 - 595
E-mail: cathy@customxray.com
Web site: www.customxray.com
Ownership: Private
Produces/Sells CE-marked Devices: N

Generator, Diagnostic X-Ray, High Voltage, Single Phase	Radiology

CUSTOMED, INC.   787-801-0101
Calle Igualdad #7, Fajardo, PR 00738
FDA Number: 2648727

Accessories, Apparel, Surgical	Surgery
Circuit, Breathing (W Connector, Adapter, Y Piece)	Anesthesiology
Drape, Surgical	Surgery
ENT Drug Applicator	Ear/Nose/Throat
Gown, Surgical	Surgery
IV Start Kit	Surgery
Kit, Catheterization, Sterile Urethral	Gastroenterology/Urology
Kit, Irrigation, Sterile	Gastroenterology/Urology
Kit, Sampling, Arterial Blood	Anesthesiology
Kit, Suctioning, Tracheostomy and Nasal	Surgery
Kit, Surgical (General)	Surgery
Kit, Suture Removal	Surgery
Kit, Wound Dressing	Surgery
Phacofragmentation Unit	Ophthalmology

CUSTOMS HOSPITAL PRODUCTS, INC   800-426-2780
12452 SE Capps Rd., Clackamas, OR 97015
FDA Number: 3019260   *Fax:* 800-427-6929
Web site: www.customhospital.com
Ownership: Private
Produces/Sells CE-marked Devices: N

Applicator, Tipped, Absorbent, Non-Sterile	General
Bandage, Cast	Physical Med
Container, Specimen, All Types	General
Cotton, Roll	Dental And Oral
Fiber, Absorbent	General
Gauze/sponge, Nonresorbable For External Use	Surgery
Strip, Adhesive	Surgery

CUTERA, INC.   888-4-CUTERA
3240 Bayshore Blvd, Brisbane, CA 94005   **415-657-5500**
FDA Number: 2954354   *Fax:* 415-330-2444
Web site: www.cutera.com
Year Founded: 1998
Total Employees: 221
Ownership: Public
Stock Symbol: CUTR
Traded On: NASDAQ
Produces/Sells CE-marked Devices: N
General Admin.: Annette J. Campbell-White/Director
       David B. Apfelberg/Director
       Jerry P. Widman/Director
       Mark Lortz/Director
       Kevin P. Connors/President, Chief Executive Officer

Lamp, Infrared	Physical Med
Laser, Surgical	Surgery
System, Vocal Cord Medialization	Ear/Nose/Throat

CUTTING EDGE INSTRUMENTS INC.   330-916-8858
312 River Rd., Bridgewater Corners, VT 05035
FDA Number: 1223868
Ownership: Private
Produces/Sells CE-marked Devices: N

Burr, Dental	Dental And Oral
Instrument, Diamond, Dental	Dental And Oral

CVRX INC.   763-416-2840
9201 W. Broadway Ave., Suite 650, Minneapolis, MN 55445
FDA Number: n/a   *Fax:* 763-416-2841
Web site: www.cvrx.com
Ownership: Private

CVRX INC.   763-416-2840 *(cont'd)*
Produces/Sells CE-marked Devices: N
General Admin.: Nadim Yared/President, Chief Executive Officer

CW MEDICAL, INC.   909-591-5220
5595 Daniels St, Suite E, Chino, CA 91710
FDA Number: 2087524   *Fax:* 909-591-5769
E-mail: customerservice@cwmedical.us
Web site: www.cwmedical.us
Medical Products Sales Volume: $550,000
Annual Revenue: $1-$5 Million
Year Founded: 1994
Total Employees: 6   *Marketing Staff:* 1   *Sales Staff:* 3
Ownership: Private
Produces/Sells CE-marked Devices: Y
Federal Procurement Eligibility: Small Business
Distribution: Manufacturer Direct, OEM, Importer, Exporter
General Admin.: Mr. Joseph Tsao/Chief Executive Officer

Airway, Nasopharyngeal (Breathing Tube)	Anesthesiology
Bed, Manual	General
Catheter, Intravascular, Therapeutic, Short-term Less Than 30 Days	General
Catheter, Suction (Tracheal Aspirating Tube)	Anesthesiology
Drain, Tee (Water Trap)	Anesthesiology
Drape, Surgical	Surgery
Electrode, ECG, Hand-Held	Cardiovascular
Gown, Surgical	Surgery
Kit, Administration, Intravenous	General
Laryngoscope, Rigid	Anesthesiology
Mask, Oxygen, Low Concentration, Venturi	Anesthesiology
Mouthpiece, Breathing	Anesthesiology
Needle, Fistula	Gastroenterology/Urology
Pressure Infusor, IV Container	General
Resuscitator, Cardiopulmonary	Cardiovascular
Syringe, Irrigating	General

CWECO, INC.   800-292-9326
1156 W. 135th St., P.O. Box 2456,   **310-538-9440**
Gardena, CA 90247
FDA Number: n/a   *Fax:* 310-715-9188
Web site: www.cwecoinc.com
Medical Products Sales Volume: $3,000,000
Annual Revenue: $1-$5 Million
Year Founded: 1966
Ownership: Private
Produces/Sells CE-marked Devices: N
Federal Procurement Eligibility: Small Business
Distribution: Manufacturer Through Manufacturer Reps

Chair, Shower	General
Rail, Bath	General
Rail, Commode	General
Rail, Wall Side	General

CYALUME TECHNOLOGIES, INC.   (888) 858-7881
96 Windsor St., West Springfield, MA 01089   **413-858-2500**
FDA Number: 1223443
E-mail: info@cyalume.com
Web site: http://www.cyalume.com
Ownership: Private
Produces/Sells CE-marked Devices: N

CYBER MEDICAL IMAGING, INC.   310-859-3802
3054 Franklin Canyon Dr., Beverly Hills, CA 90210
FDA Number: n/a
Ownership: Private
Produces/Sells CE-marked Devices: N

System, X-ray, Extraoral Source, Digital	Radiology

CYBERBIOMED, LLC   561-582-1955
3605 S. Ocean Blvd. #a-335, Palm Beach, FL 33480
FDA Number: 3004181153
Ownership: Private
Produces/Sells CE-marked Devices: N

Larynx, Artificial Battery-Powered	Ear/Nose/Throat

CYBERKINETICS NEUROTECHNOLOGY SYSTEMS, INC.   508-549-9981
100 Foxborough Blvd., Suite 240, Foxborough, MA 02035
FDA Number: n/a
E-mail: info@braingate.com
Web site: www.cyberkineticsinc.com
Ownership: Public
Stock Symbol: CYKN
Traded On: OTC Bulletin
Produces/Sells CE-marked Devices: N
General Admin.: Timothy R. Surgenor/President, Chief Executive Officer
Finance: David A. Keene/Vice President Finance

Amplifier, Physiological Signal	Cns/Neurology
Electrode, Depth	Cns/Neurology

CYBERKINETICS NEUROTECHNOLOGY   **508-549-9981** *(cont'd)*
Electroencephalograph   Cns/Neurology

CYBERMDX, INC.   **401-228-3772**
850 Waterman Ave, East Providence, RI 02914
FDA Number: 3005660963
Ownership: Private
Produces/Sells CE-marked Devices: N
Image Processing System   Radiology

CYBERNET SYSTEMS CORP.   **734-668-2567**
3885 Research Park Drive, Ann Arbor, MI 48108
FDA Number: 3004198411   *Fax:* 734-668-8780
E-mail: info@cybernet.com
Web site: www.cybernet.com
Ownership: Private
Produces/Sells CE-marked Devices: N
Transmitter/Receiver System, Physiological, Telephone   Cardiovascular

CYBERNETIC RESEARCH LABORATORIES, INC.   **520-571-8065**
3562 E. 42nd Stravenue, Tucson, AZ 85713
FDA Number: 3006250175
Ownership: Private
Produces/Sells CE-marked Devices: N
Discriminator, Two-point   Cns/Neurology
Dynamometer, AC-Powered   Orthopedics

CYBERONICS BELTWAY 8 DISTRIBUTION   **800-332-1375**
FACILITY
100 Cyberonics Boulevard W,   **800-332-1375**
Houston, TX 77058
FDA Number: 3006705088   *Fax:* 281-218-9332
E-mail: ir@cyberonics.com
Web site: www.cyberonics.com
Year Founded: 1987
Ownership: CYBERONICS, INC.
Produces/Sells CE-marked Devices: N
Magnet, Test, Pacemaker   Cardiovascular
Stimulator, Nerve, Autonomic, Implantable (Epilepsy)   Cns/Neurology
Surgical Instrument, Non-Powered, Neurosurgical   Cns/Neurology

CYBERONICS, INC.   **800-332-1375**
The Cyberonics Building   **281-228-7262**
100 Cyberonics Boulevard
Houston, TX 77058
FDA Number: 1644487   *Fax:* 281-218-9332
E-mail: ir@cyberonics.com
Web site: www.cyberonics.com
Annual Revenue: $50-$100 Million
Year Founded: 1987
Total Employees: 438   *Marketing Staff:* 20   *Sales Staff:* 235
Ownership: Public
Stock Symbol: CYBX
Traded On: NASDAQ
Quality System Registration Information: ISO9001; ISO9002
Produces/Sells CE-marked Devices: Y
Federal Procurement Eligibility: Small Business
Distribution: Manufacturer Direct
General Admin.: Daniel J. Moore/President, Chief Executive Officer
Medical Admin.: Dr. Brian Olin/Vice President Clinical Affairs
Mktg./Adv.: James A. Reinstein/Vice President Sales
Production: Randal L. Simpson/Vice President Operations
Research: Dr. Milton Morris/Vice President Research & Development
Finance: Gregory H. Browne/Chief Financial Officer, Vice President Finance
Instrument, Manual, General Surgical   Surgery
Magnet, Test, Pacemaker   Cardiovascular
Stimulator, Nerve, Autonomic, Implantable (Epilepsy)   Cns/Neurology
Stimulator, Nerve, Cranial, Implanted (Pain Relief)   Cns/Neurology
Stimulator, Vagus Nerve, Implanted (Coma And Vegetative State)   Cns/Neurology

CYBERSONICS, INC.   **814-899-4220**
5325 Kuhl Rd., Erie, PA 16510
FDA Number: 3004216443   *Fax:* 814-898-4737
E-mail: info@cybersonics-inc.com
Web site: www.cybersonics-inc.com
Ownership: Private
Produces/Sells CE-marked Devices: N
Lithotriptor   Gastroenterology/Urology

CYBEX / TECTRIX
See CYBEX INTERNATIONAL, INC.

CYBEX INTERNATIONAL, INC.   **800-667-6544**
10 Trotter Dr., Medway, MA 02053   **508-533-4300**
FDA Number: 2027766   *Fax:* 508-533-5500
Medical Products Sales Volume: $138,466,000
Ownership: Public
Stock Symbol: CYBI

CYBEX INTERNATIONAL, INC.   **800-667-6544** *(cont'd)*
Traded On: NASDAQ
Produces/Sells CE-marked Devices: N
Distribution: Manufacturer Direct, Manufacturer Through Distributor, Manufacturer Through Manufacturer Reps, Importer, Exporter
General Admin.: Elise Dierlam/Director Human Resources
Production: Tom Oliver/Plant Manager
Computer, Stress Exercise   Cardiovascular
Dynamometer, Physical Medicine, Electronic   Physical Med
Ergometer, Bicycle   Cardiovascular
Ergometer, Other   Anesthesiology
Ergometer, Treadmill   Cardiovascular
Exerciser, Chest   Physical Med
Exerciser, Leg And Ankle   Physical Med
Exerciser, Measuring   Physical Med
Exerciser, Other   Physical Med
Isokinetic Testing And Evaluation System   Physical Med
Stimulator, Electrical, Evoked Response   Cns/Neurology

CYBEX INTERNATIONAL, INC.   **508-533-4300**
10 Trotter Drive, Medway, MA 02053
FDA Number: 2027766   *Fax:* 508-533-5500
E-mail: info@cybexintl.com
Web site: www.cybexintl.com
Annual Revenue: $25-$50 Million
Total Employees: 600
Ownership: Public
Stock Symbol: CYBI
Traded On: NASDAQ
Produces/Sells CE-marked Devices: N
Distribution: Manufacturer Through Distributor, Manufacturer Through Manufacturer Reps
General Admin.: John Aglialoro/Chairman, Chief Executive Officer
     Arthur W. Hicks Jr./President, Chief Operating Officer
Mktg./Adv.: Mr. John Young/Senior Vice President International Sales
Production: Mr. Edward Kurzontkowski/Senior Vice President Manufacturing
Research: Mr. Raymond Gianelli/Senior Vice President Research & Development
Component, Exercise   Physical Med
Exercise Stair   Physical Med
Exerciser, Bicycle   Physical Med
Monitor, Physiological, Stress Exercise   Cardiovascular

CYGNUS IMAGING
See Progeny Dental

CYGNUS INC.   **973-523-0668**
510 E. 41st. St., Paterson, NJ 07504
FDA Number: 2247717   *Fax:* 973-523-0375
E-mail: don@cygnusnj.com
Annual Revenue: $5-$10 Million
Total Employees: 55   *Marketing Staff:* 1   *Sales Staff:* 1
Ownership: Private
Produces/Sells CE-marked Devices: N
Federal Procurement Eligibility: Small Business
Distribution: Manufacturer Direct, OEM, Exporter
General Admin.: Gabor Lederer/President, Chief Executive Officer
Mktg./Adv.: Donald Wilcox/Vice President Marketing & Sales
Production: James Kearney/Director Quality Assurance
     Kathleen Nicholas/Manager Materials
Centrifuge, General (Up to 5,000 rpm)   Pathology

CYGNUS INSTRUMENTS, INC.
See Progeny Dental

CYLEX, INC.   **888-33-CYEX**
8980-i Old Annapolis Rd., Columbia, MD 21045   **410-964-0236**
FDA Number: 3003920771   *Fax:* 410-964-0367
Web site: www.cylex.net
Ownership: Private
Produces/Sells CE-marked Devices: N
Assay, Proliferation, In Vitro, T Lymphocyte   Hematology

CYMED OSTOMY CO.   **800-582-0707**
1440 4th St # C, Berkeley, CA 94710   **510-558-1926**
FDA Number: n/a
Web site: cymedostomy.com
Medical Products Sales Volume: $1,000,000
Annual Revenue: $1-$5 Million
Year Founded: 1985
Ownership: Private
Produces/Sells CE-marked Devices: N
Federal Procurement Eligibility: Small Business, Female Owned
Distribution: Manufacturer Through Distributor
General Admin.: Dianne Eastman/President, Chief Executive Officer
Collector, Ostomy   Gastroenterology/Urology

CYNERGY, INC.
See Plexus Corp

CYNOSURE, INC.   800-886-2966
5 Carlisle Road, Westford, MA 01886   978-256-4200
FDA Number: 1222993
Web site: www.cynosurelaser.com
Annual Revenue: $25-$50 Million
Ownership: Public
Stock Symbol: CYNO
Traded On: NASDAQ
Quality System Registration Information: ISO9001
Produces/Sells CE-marked Devices: Y
Federal Procurement Eligibility: Small Business, Minority Owned
Distribution: Manufacturer Direct, Manufacturer Through Distributor, Manufacturer Through Manufacturer Reps, Service Direct, Exporter
General Admin.: Timothy W. Baker/Chief Financial Officer, Executive Vice President
   Mr. Rafael Sierra/Chief Technology Officer
   Michael R. Davin/President, Chief Executive Officer, Chairman
Mktg./Adv.: Mr. William Kelley/Senior Vice President International Sales
   Mr. Douglas Delaney/Vice President Sales
Production: Mr. David Mackle/Executive Vice President Operations

Accessories, Laser	General
Laser, Surgical	Surgery
Massager, Therapeutic	Physical Med
Massager, Vacuum, Light Induced Heating	Surgery

CYPRANE
See Datex-Ohmeda, Inc. (Madison)

CYPRESS MEDICAL PRODUCTS   800-334-3646
1202 S. Rte. 31, McHenry, IL 60050
FDA Number: n/a   Fax: 815-385-0114
E-mail: info@cypressmed.com
Web site: www.cypressmed.com
Medical Products Sales Volume: $18,800,000
Annual Revenue: $50-$100 Million
Year Founded: 1988
Total Employees: 125   Marketing Staff: 5   Sales Staff: 30
Ownership: Private
Produces/Sells CE-marked Devices: N
Federal Procurement Eligibility: Small Business
Distribution: Manufacturer Through Distributor
General Admin.: Alan Bagliore/Chief Executive Officer
   Tim Sabatka/Chief Operating Officer, Chief Financial Officer
   Varun Soni/Vice President
Mktg./Adv.: Jennifer Yormark/Director Marketing
   Greg Meagher/Vice President Business Development
Production: Anthony Giacco/Director Quality Assurance
   John Carr/Manager Materials

Bag, Leg	Gastroenterology/Urology
Bag, Urinary Collection	General
Bandage, Elastic	General
Bandage, Other	General
Cap, Surgical	Surgery
Cover, Shoe, Operating Room	Surgery
Crutch	Physical Med
Cup, Medicine	General
Glove, Patient Examination, Latex	General
Glove, Patient Examination, Specialty	General
Glove, Patient Examination, Vinyl	General
Gown, Isolation, Surgical	Surgery
IV Start Kit	Surgery
Kit, Suture Removal	Surgery
Remover, Staple, Surgical	Surgery
Sphygmomanometer, Aneroid (Arterial Pressure)	General
Sponge, Gauze	Dental And Oral
Sponge, Other	General
Stethoscope, Manual	Cardiovascular
Tape, Gauze, Adhesive	General
Tray, Custom/Special Procedure	General

CYPRUS PERSONAL CARE PRODUCTS, INC.   415-771-0333
2269 Chestnut Ave., #237, San Francisco, CA 94123
FDA Number: 2939000
Ownership: Private
Produces/Sells CE-marked Devices: N

Condom	Obstetrics/Gynecology
Condom With Nonoxynol-9	Obstetrics/Gynecology

CYR DESIGNS, LLC   207-723-6766
112 New York St, Millinocket, ME 04462
FDA Number: 3006015254

Bed, Manual	General

CYTEK DEVELOPMENT, INC.   510-657-0102
4059 Clipper Court, Fremont, CA 94538
FDA Number: 1000292377

Counter, Cell, Differential Classifier, Automated	Hematology

CYTO DIOGNOSTICS
See Dianon Systems - Labcorp

CYTOCOLOR, INC.   800-776-6455
P.O. Box 401, Hinckley, OH 44233-9747   330-273-6455
FDA Number: 1527216   Fax: 330-225-3865
E-mail: sales@cytocolor.com
Web site: http://www.cytocolor.com
Total Employees: 10   Marketing Staff: 2   Sales Staff: 2
Ownership: Private
Produces/Sells CE-marked Devices: N
Federal Procurement Eligibility: Small Business, Female Owned
Distribution: Manufacturer Direct
General Admin.: S. F. Kass/President, Chief Executive Officer

Reagent, Calibration	General
Stain, Hematology	Pathology
Stain, Other	Pathology

CYTOCORE, INC.   312-379-4790
414 North Orlean, Suite 510, Chicago, IL 60654
FDA Number: 3003592854   Fax: 312-222-9580
E-mail: info@cytocoreinc.com
Web site: www.cytocoreinc.com
Ownership: Public
Stock Symbol: CYOE
Traded On: OTC Bulletin
Produces/Sells CE-marked Devices: N

Reagent, General Purpose	Pathology
Reagents, Specific, Analyte	Hematology

CYTOGEN CORP.   800-833-3533
600 College Road E., Suite 3100,   609-750-8200
Princeton, NJ 08540
FDA Number: 2246903   Fax: 609-452-2476
E-mail: cytoinfo@corpcomm.cytogen.com
Web site: www.cytogen.com
Medical Products Sales Volume: $17,300,000
Annual Revenue: $10-$25 Million
Year Founded: 1980
Total Employees: 32   Marketing Staff: 5   Sales Staff: 15
Ownership: Public
Stock Symbol: CYTO
Traded On: NASDAQ
Produces/Sells CE-marked Devices: N
Federal Procurement Eligibility: Small Business
Distribution: Manufacturer Through Distributor
General Admin.: H. Joseph Reiser/President, Chief Executive Officer
   Medical Admin.: Nick Borys/Vice President Medical Affairs
Mktg./Adv.: June Jobern/Director Marketing
   Charmie Pitchford/Director National Accounts

Antibody, Monoclonal	Microbiology
Brush, Other	General
Unit, Imaging, Thermal	Radiology

CYTORI THERAPEUTICS, INC.   877-470-8000
3020 Callan Road, San Diego, CA 92121-4148   858-458-0900
FDA Number: 3002642958   Fax: 858-458-0994
E-mail: info@cytoritx.com
Web site: www.cytori.com
Ownership: Private
Produces/Sells CE-marked Devices: N

Appliance, Fixation, Spinal Intervertebral Body	Orthopedics
Centrifuge, Refrigerated	Pathology
Fastener, Fixation, Biodegradable, Soft Tissue	Orthopedics
Mesh, Metal	Gastroenterology/Urology
Mesh, Surgical, Polymeric	Surgery
Prosthesis, Hip, Semi-Constrained, Metal/Polymer	Orthopedics
System, Suction, Lipoplasty	Surgery
Trypsin	Pathology
Warmer, Infusion Fluid, Thermal	General

CYTORI THERAPEUTICS, INC.   877-470-8000
3020 Callan Road, San Diego, CA 92121   858-458-0900
FDA Number: 3002642958   Fax: 858-458-0994
E-mail: info@cytoritx.com
Web site: http://www.cytori.com
Ownership: Public
Stock Symbol: CYTX
Traded On: NASDAQ
Produces/Sells CE-marked Devices: N
General Admin.: Mr. Christopher Calhoun/Chief Executive Officer
   Mr. Marc Hedrick/President
Mktg./Adv.: Mr. Bruce Reuter/Senior Vice President International Sales
   Mr. David Oxley/Vice President Marketing
Production: Dr. Douglas Arm/Senior Vice President Operations
   Mr. Kenneth Kleinhenz/Vice President Quality Assurance & Regulatory Affairs
Research: Mr. Alexander Milstein/Vice President Clinical Development
Finance: Mr. Mark Saad/Chief Financial Officer

Autotransfusion Unit (Blood)	Anesthesiology
Separator, Blood Cell/Plasma, Therapeutic	Gastroenterology/Urology

CYTORI THERAPEUTICS, INC. 877-470-8000 *(cont'd)*
Syringe, Irrigating General
System, Suction, Lipoplasty Surgery

CYTOTECH, INC.
See Quidel Corporation

CYTOTHERM 800-747-9699
110 Sewell Ave., Trenton, NJ 08610-6059 609-396-1456
FDA Number: 2248707 *Fax:* 609-396-9395
E-mail: serve@cytotherm.com
Web site: www.cytotherm.com
Medical Products Sales Volume: $500,000
Annual Revenue: $0-$1 Million
Total Employees: 6 *Marketing Staff:* 3 *Sales Staff:* 3
Ownership: Private
Quality System Registration Information: ISO9001
Produces/Sells CE-marked Devices: Y
Federal Procurement Eligibility: Small Business
Distribution: Manufacturer Direct
General Admin.: Natalie Kuzyk/President
  Roman Kuzyk/President
Warmer, Blood and Plasma Hematology

CYTYC CORPORATION
See Hologic, Inc.

CYTYC CORPORATION
See HOLOGIC, INC.

CYTYC CORPORATION
See Hologic, Inc.

CYTYC SURGICAL PRODUCTS
See HOLOGIC, INC.

D & D VIDEO SPECIALISTS, LLC 405-720-3180
6444 Nw Expressway Street, Suite 225E, Okc, OK 73132
FDA Number: 3003194165 *Fax:* 405-720-3951
Ownership: Private
Produces/Sells CE-marked Devices: N
Camera, Television, Endoscopic (Without Audio) Surgery

D & N MICRO PRODUCTS, INC. 260-484-6414
2721 Corrinado Court, Fort Wayne, IN 46808
FDA Number: n/a
Web site: www.dnmicroproducts.com
Annual Revenue: $0-$1 Million
Year Founded: 1999
Ownership: Private
Produces/Sells CE-marked Devices: N
Federal Procurement Eligibility: Small Business
Distribution: Manufacturer Through Distributor
Radiographic Unit, Diagnostic, Dental (X-Ray) Dental And Oral

D&D TECHNOLOGIES INC. 780-918-6616
7535 94 Avenue, Edmonton, AB T6C 1V9 Canada
FDA Number: n/a *Fax:* 780-450-2617
E-mail: info@danddtech.net
Web site: www.danddtech.net
Ownership: Private
Produces/Sells CE-marked Devices: N
Federal Procurement Eligibility: Small Business
Distribution: Manufacturer Direct, Manufacturer Through Manufacturer Reps,
Exporter

D&M SOOMEKH INTERNATIONAL, INC. 323-266-2500
1260 South Boyle Ave., Los Angeles, CA 90023
FDA Number: 2028005
Ownership: Private
Produces/Sells CE-marked Devices: N
Pack, Hot Or Cold, Disposable Physical Med

D&S DENTAL, LLC 423-928-1299
3111 Hanover Road, Jc, TN 37604
FDA Number: 3006365702
Broach, Endodontic Dental And Oral
Drill, Dental, Intraoral Dental And Oral
File, Pulp Canal, Endodontic Dental And Oral

D-TEK LLC 267 306 3430
3580 Progress Dr., Suite J3, Bensalem, PA 19020
FDA Number: 3005981046 *Fax:* 215 245 5270
E-mail: dtekllc@comcast.net
Web site: www.dtekllc.net
Ownership: Private
Produces/Sells CE-marked Devices: N
Kit, Pregnancy Test, Over The Counter, HCG Chemistry
Nitroprusside, Ketones (Urinary, Non-Quantitative) Chemistry
Reagent, Antistreptolysin-Titer/Streptolysin O Microbiology

D. SIGN DENTAL LAB, INC. 757-224-0177
690 W. Fremont Avenue, Suite 9c, Sunnyvale, CA 94087
FDA Number: 3005940438
Alloy, Gold Based, For Clinical Use Dental And Oral
Denture, Plastic, Teeth Dental And Oral
Metal, Base Dental And Oral
Powder, Porcelain Dental And Oral

D. Y. INSTRUMENT, INC. 516-482-9001
59 Westervelt Avenue, Tenafly, NJ 07670
FDA Number: 3005376704
Ownership: Private
Produces/Sells CE-marked Devices: N

D.B.I. AMERICA CORP. 813-909-9005
254 Crystal Grove Blvd., Lutz, FL 33548
FDA Number: 1056087
Electrosurgical Unit, Neurological Cns/Neurology
Scaler, Ultrasonic Dental And Oral

D.C.A. (DENTAL CORPORATION OF AMERICA) 800-638-6684
889 South Matlack, West Chester, PA 19382 610-344-7488
FDA Number: 1119195 *Fax:* 610-431-6500
E-mail: ortho@dentalcorp.com
Web site: www.dentalcorp.com
Annual Revenue: $0-$1 Million
Total Employees: 10 *Marketing Staff:* 3 *Sales Staff:* 3
Ownership: Private
Produces/Sells CE-marked Devices: N
Federal Procurement Eligibility: Small Business
Distribution: Manufacturer Direct
General Admin.: Don Taylor/Chief Executive Officer
Mktg./Adv.: Barbara Hamilton/Manager National Marketing & Sales
Band, Elastic, Orthodontic Dental And Oral
Cement, Dental Dental And Oral
Film, X-Ray, Dental, Extraoral Dental And Oral
Material, Impression Dental And Oral
Orthodontic Instrument Dental And Oral
Protector, Mouth Guard Dental And Oral
Tray, Impression Dental And Oral
Wire, Orthodontic Dental And Oral

D.G.H. TECHNOLOGY, INC. 800-722-3883
110 Summit Drive, Suite B, Exton, PA 19341 610-594-9100
FDA Number: 2522950 *Fax:* 610-594-0390
E-mail: info@dghkoi.com
Web site: www.dghkoi.com
Medical Products Sales Volume: $720,000
Year Founded: 1982
Total Employees: 10 *Marketing Staff:* 2 *Sales Staff:* 2
Ownership: Private
Produces/Sells CE-marked Devices: N
Federal Procurement Eligibility: Small Business
Distribution: Manufacturer Direct, Manufacturer Through Manufacturer Reps, OEM,
Exporter
General Admin.: Earl Henderson/President
Production: Luther Detweiler/Vice President Production
Pachometer Ophthalmology
Scanner, Ultrasonic, Ophthalmic Radiology

D.J. ORTHO
See DJO Inc.

D.M. DAVIS INC. 201-833-0513
460 Warwick Ave., PO Box 536, Teaneck, NJ 07666
FDA Number: n/a *Fax:* 101-100-1000
E-mail: davinc@juno.com
Web site: www.dmdavis.com
Ownership: Private
Produces/Sells CE-marked Devices: N
Federal Procurement Eligibility: Small Business
Distribution: Manufacturer Direct
General Admin.: David Davis/President
Monitor, Penile Tumescence Gastroenterology/Urology
Simulator, Respiration Anesthesiology

D.O. INDUSTRIES, INC.
See Navitar, Inc.

D.R.E., INC. 800-462-8195
1800 Williamson Ct., Louisville, KY 40223 502-244-4444
FDA Number: 1528118 *Fax:* 502-244-0369
E-mail: info@dremed.com
Web site: www.dremed.com
Medical Products Sales Volume: $7,000,000
Annual Revenue: $5-$10 Million
Year Founded: 1984
Total Employees: 30 *Marketing Staff:* 2 *Sales Staff:* 10
Ownership: Private
Produces/Sells CE-marked Devices: N

D.R.E., INC.　800-462-8195 (cont'd)
Federal Procurement Eligibility: Small Business, GSA Contract
Distribution: Manufacturer Direct, Exclusive Distributor
General Admin.: Michael J. Dirr/President
　　　　Charles Vitittow/Secretary
Mktg./Adv.: Charles Vitittow/Manager Advertising
Finance: Michael Spencer/Treasurer

Electrosurgical Unit, General Purpose (ESU)	Surgery
Gas-Machine, Anesthesia	Anesthesiology
Monitor, Bed Patient	General
Monitor, Blood Pressure, Indirect, Surgery, Powered	Surgery
Service, Used Equipment	General

D4D TECHNOLOGIES, LLC　972-234-3880
650 International Pkwy., Richardson, TX 75081
FDA Number: 3004998675　　　*Fax:* 972-479-1128
Web site: www.d4dtech.com
Ownership: Private
Produces/Sells CE-marked Devices: N

System, Optical Impression, Computer Assisted Design And Manufacturing (cad/cam) Of Dental Restorations	Dental And Oral

DA-LITE SCREEN CO., INC.　800-622-3737
3100 N. Detroit St., PO Box 137,　**574-267-8101**
Warsaw, IN 46581
FDA Number: n/a　　　*Fax:* 574-267-7804
E-mail: info@da-lite.com
Web site: www.da-lite.com
Medical Products Sales Volume: $169,800,000
Annual Revenue: $100-$500 Million
Year Founded: 1909
Total Employees: 300
Ownership: Private
Produces/Sells CE-marked Devices: N
Federal Procurement Eligibility: Small Business, Female Owned, GSA Contract
Distribution: Manufacturer Through Distributor, Manufacturer Through Manufacturer Reps, Exporter
General Admin.: Rich Lundin/President, Chief Executive Officer
Mktg./Adv.: Matt Teevan/Market Manager
　　　　Judy Loughran/Vice President Marketing & Sales

Cart, Other	General
Mount, Monitor (Support)	General
Mount, Television Set	General
Table, Other	General

DAC INC./DIAGNOSTIC AUDIOLOGY CORP.　800-551-3277
351 Bank St. Suite 105, Southlake, TX 76092-9126
FDA Number: 2320465
Ownership: Private
Produces/Sells CE-marked Devices: N

Audiometer	Ear/Nose/Throat

DAC INTERNATIONAL, INC.　888-373-3027
6390 Rose Lane, Carpinteria, CA 93013　**805-684-8307**
FDA Number: n/a　　　*Fax:* 805-566-2196
E-mail: info@dac-intl.com
Web site: www.dac-intl.com
Medical Products Sales Volume: $4,700,000
Annual Revenue: $5-$10 Million
Year Founded: 1964
Total Employees: 53　　*Marketing Staff:* 1　　*Sales Staff:* 7
Ownership: Private
Produces/Sells CE-marked Devices: Y
Federal Procurement Eligibility: Small Business
Distribution: Manufacturer Direct
General Admin.: Jim Drain/President, Chief Executive Officer
Mktg./Adv.: Keith Swanson/Vice President Marketing & Sales
Research: Rod Keller/Vice President Research & Development

Laboratory Equipment, Ophthalmic	Ophthalmology

DACOR MANUFACTURING CO., INC.　618-939-8700
8718 Hanover Industrial Dr., Columbia, IL 62236
FDA Number: n/a　　　*Fax:* 618-939-8898
E-mail: dacor400@worldnet.att.net
Web site: www.dacormfg.com
Annual Revenue: $0-$1 Million
Ownership: Private
Produces/Sells CE-marked Devices: Y
Distribution: Manufacturer Direct, OEM, Exporter
General Admin.: Dan Sweet/President

Chair, Blood Donor	General
Contract Manufacturing	General

DADSON MFG. CORP.　816-847-2388
1109 Valley Ridge Drive, Blue Springs, MO 64029
FDA Number: 1925538

Dermatome	Surgery

DAGE-MTI, INC.
See Dage-MTI, Inc.

DAHER MFG., INC.　204-663-3299
Mazenod Rd, Winnipeg R2J 4H2 Canada
FDA Number: 9615404

Armboard, Wheelchair	Physical Med
Belt, Wheelchair	Physical Med
Support, Head And Trunk, Wheelchair	Physical Med

DAHLIN LABORATORY　952-541-9622
393 South Harlan, Suite 210, Lakewood, CO 80226
FDA Number: 3004147962
Ownership: Private
Produces/Sells CE-marked Devices: N

Mouthguard	Dental And Oral

DAI SHIN TECHNOLOGIES, INC.　262-347-0500
W238 N1690 N Rockwood Dr, Suite 400, Waukesha, WI 53188
FDA Number: 2135336　　　*Fax:* 262-347-0600
E-mail: sales@daishintech.com
Web site: www.daishintech.com
Year Founded: 1997
Ownership: Private
Quality System Registration Information: ISO9001
Produces/Sells CE-marked Devices: Y

Oximeter, Intracardiac	Cardiovascular

DAILY MEDICAL PRODUCTS, INC.　800-550-1553
4620 Goldenrod Lane, Plymouth, MN 55442
FDA Number: 2083299
Ownership: Private
Produces/Sells CE-marked Devices: N

Controller, Temperature, Cardiopulmonary Bypass	Cardiovascular
Surgical Instrument, Cardiovascular	Cardiovascular

DAISY PRODUCTS
See Griffith Rubber Mills

DAISY PRODUCTS COMPANY
See Iron Duck, A Div. Of Fleming Industries, Inc.

DAKO COLORADO, INC.　454-485-9500
4850 Innovation Dr., Fort Collins, CO 80525-5776
FDA Number: 3004485389
Ownership: Private
Produces/Sells CE-marked Devices: N
General Admin.: Mr. Lars Holmkvist/Chief Executive Officer
Mktg./Adv.: Ms. Lisa Miller/Vice President Global Marketing
Production: Mr. Henrik Archer-Jensen/Vice President Operations
　　　　Mr. henrik Jensen/Vice President Operations
　　　　Ms. Annika Berg/Vice President Regulatory Affairs
Research: Mr. Jacob Thaysen/Vice President Research & Development
Finance: Mr. Egil Madsen/Chief Financial Officer

Locator, Cell, Automated	Hematology
Stainer, Slide, Automated	Pathology

DAKO CORP.
See Dako North America, Inc

DAKO DIAGNOSTICS CANADA INC.　800-668-4630
12 Falconer Dr., Unit 4,　**905-858-8510**
Mississauga, ONT L5N-3 Canada
FDA Number: n/a　　　*Fax:* 905-858-8801
E-mail: techservice@dako.ca
Web site: www.dako.ca
Year Founded: 1985
Total Employees: 25
Ownership: Private
Produces/Sells CE-marked Devices: N
Distribution: Exclusive Distributor, Exporter

DAKO NORTH AMERICA, INC　805-566-6655
6392 Via Real, Carpinteria, CA 93013
FDA Number: 2022180　　　*Fax:* 805-566-6688
E-mail: general@dako.com
Web site: www.dakousa.com
Medical Products Sales Volume: $45,000,000
Annual Revenue: $25-$50 Million
Year Founded: 1966
Total Employees: 1000
Ownership: Private
Quality System Registration Information: ISO9001
Produces/Sells CE-marked Devices: N
Federal Procurement Eligibility: Small Business
Distribution: Manufacturer Direct, Manufacturer Through Manufacturer Reps, OEM, Exclusive Distributor
General Admin.: Lars Holmkvist/President, Chief Executive Officer
Production: Mr. Henrich Anker-Jensen/Executive Vice President Operations
　　　　Ms. Annika Berg/Executive Vice President Quality Assurance & Regulatory Affairs

DAKO NORTH AMERICA, INC   805-566-6655 *(cont'd)*
  Research: Mr. Rudolph Seibl/Executive Vice President Research & Development
  Finance: Per Toelstang/Chief Financial Officer

2nd Antibody (Species Specific Anti-Animal Gamma Globulin)	Immunology
Alpha-1-Acid-Glycoprotein, Antigen, Antiserum, Control	Immunology
Antibody, Antinuclear, Indirect Immunofluorescent, Antigen	Immunology
Antibody, Monoclonal	Microbiology
Antigen, Antiserum, Control, Albumin	Immunology
Antigen, Antiserum, Control, Albumin, FITC	Immunology
Antigen, Antiserum, Control, Alpha-1-Antichymotrypsin	Immunology
Antigen, Antiserum, Control, Alpha-1-Antitrypsin	Immunology
Antigen, Antiserum, Control, Antithrombin III	Immunology
Antigen, Antiserum, Control, Carcinoembryonic Antigen	Immunology
Antigen, Antiserum, Control, Ceruloplasmin	Immunology
Antigen, Antiserum, Control, Complement C1q	Immunology
Antigen, Antiserum, Control, Complement C3	Immunology
Antigen, Antiserum, Control, Complement C4	Immunology
Antigen, Antiserum, Control, Complement C5	Immunology
Antigen, Antiserum, Control, Factor B	Immunology
Antigen, Antiserum, Control, Ferritin	Immunology
Antigen, Antiserum, Control, Fibrinogen And Split Products	Immunology
Antigen, Antiserum, Control, Free Secretory Component	Immunology
Antigen, Antiserum, Control, Gamma Globulin	Immunology
Antigen, Antiserum, Control, Gamma Globulin, FITC	Immunology
Antigen, Antiserum, Control, Haptoglobin	Immunology
Antigen, Antiserum, Control, Hemopexin	Immunology
Antigen, Antiserum, Control, IGA	Immunology
Antigen, Antiserum, Control, IGA, FITC	Immunology
Antigen, Antiserum, Control, IGA, Peroxidase	Immunology
Antigen, Antiserum, Control, IGA, Rhodamine	Immunology
Antigen, Antiserum, Control, IGD	Immunology
Antigen, Antiserum, Control, IGD, FITC	Immunology
Antigen, Antiserum, Control, IGD, Peroxidase	Immunology
Antigen, Antiserum, Control, IGD, Rhodamine	Immunology
Antigen, Antiserum, Control, IGE	Immunology
Antigen, Antiserum, Control, IGE, FITC	Immunology
Antigen, Antiserum, Control, IGE, Peroxidase	Immunology
Antigen, Antiserum, Control, IGG	Immunology
Antigen, Antiserum, Control, IGG (Fc Fragment Specific)	Immunology
Antigen, Antiserum, Control, IGG (Gamma Chain Specific)	Immunology
Antigen, Antiserum, Control, IGG, FITC	Immunology
Antigen, Antiserum, Control, IGG, Peroxidase	Immunology
Antigen, Antiserum, Control, IGG, Rhodamine	Immunology
Antigen, Antiserum, Control, IGM	Immunology
Antigen, Antiserum, Control, IGM (Mu Chain Specific)	Immunology
Antigen, Antiserum, Control, IGM, FITC	Immunology
Antigen, Antiserum, Control, IGM, Peroxidase	Immunology
Antigen, Antiserum, Control, IGM, Rhodamine	Immunology
Antigen, Antiserum, Control, Inter-Alpha Trypsin Inhibitor	Immunology
Antigen, Antiserum, Control, Kappa	Immunology
Antigen, Antiserum, Control, Kappa, FITC	Immunology
Antigen, Antiserum, Control, Kappa, Rhodamine	Immunology
Antigen, Antiserum, Control, Lactoferrin	Immunology
Antigen, Antiserum, Control, Lambda	Immunology
Antigen, Antiserum, Control, Lambda, FITC	Immunology
Antigen, Antiserum, Control, Lambda, Rhodamine	Immunology
Antigen, Antiserum, Control, Luteinizing Hormone	Immunology
Antigen, Antiserum, Control, Lymphocyte Typing	Immunology
Antigen, Antiserum, Control, Lysozyme	Immunology
Antigen, Antiserum, Control, Myoglobin	Immunology
Antigen, Antiserum, Control, Plasminogen	Immunology
Antigen, Antiserum, Control, Prealbumin	Immunology
Antigen, Antiserum, Control, Protein, Complement	Immunology
Antigen, Antiserum, Control, Prothrombin	Immunology
Antigen, Antiserum, Control, Transferrin	Immunology
Antigen, Antiserum, Control, Whole Human Serum	Immunology
Antigen, Antiserum, Fibrinogen And Fibrin Split Products	Immunology
Antigen, Antiserum, Fibrinogen And Split Products, FITC	Immunology
Antinuclear Antibody (Enzyme-Labeled), Antigen, Controls	Immunology
Antisera, Fluorescent, Herpesvirus Hominis 1, 2	Microbiology
Antiserum, Escherichia Coli	Microbiology
Estrogen Receptor Assay Kit	Chemistry
FC, Antigen, Antiserum, Control	Immunology
FC, FITC, Antigen, Antiserum, Control	Immunology
IGA, Ferritin, Antigen, Antiserum, Control	Immunology
IGE, Ferritin, Antigen, Antiserum, Control	Immunology
IGG, Ferritin, Antigen, Antiserum, Control	Immunology
IGM, Ferritin, Antigen, Antiserum, Control	Immunology
Immunochemical, Lysozyme (Muramidase)	Chemistry
Immunoelectrophoretic, Immunoglobulins, (G, A, M)	Chemistry
Kit, Assay, Receptor, Progesterone	Chemistry
Kit, RIA, Basic Protein, Myelin	Immunology
Lectins/Protectins	Hematology
Reagent, Virus, General	Pathology
Respiratory Syncytial Virus, Antigen, Antibody, IFA	Microbiology
Retinol-Binding Protein, Antigen, Antiserum, Control	Immunology
Serum, Animal	Pathology
System, Identification, Hepatitis B Antigen	Hematology
Test, Alpha-Fetoprotein	Pathology
Test, Cancer Detection, Monoclonal Antibody	Immunology
Test, Cancer Detection, Other	Hematology
Test, Human Chorionic Gonadotropin	Immunology

DAKO NORTH AMERICA, INC   805-566-6655 *(cont'd)*

Test, Human Placental Lactogen	Immunology
Whole Human Plasma, Antigen, Antiserum, Control	Immunology

DAKOTA HEARING INSTRUMENTS, INC.   888-373-1283
370 W Anchor Dr, Dakota Dunes, SD 57049   605-487-7661
FDA Number: 2184053
Ownership: Private
Produces/Sells CE-marked Devices: N

Hearing-Aid	Ear/Nose/Throat

DALCO INTERNATIONAL, INC.   888-354-5515
8433 Glazebrook Ave., Richmond, VA 23228   804-266-7702
  Fax: 804-266-7740
E-mail: mail@dalcointernational.com
Web site: www.dalcointernational.com
Annual Revenue: $1-$5 Million
Ownership: Private
Quality System Registration Information: ISO9001
Produces/Sells CE-marked Devices: Y
Federal Procurement Eligibility: Small Business
Distribution: Manufacturer Through Distributor, Manufacturer Through Manufacturer Reps, Importer, Exporter
General Admin.: Mr. Leif Daleng/President
Production: Mr. Craig Organ/Manager Operations

Brace, Joint, Ankle (External)	Physical Med
Collar, Cervical Neck	Orthopedics
Immobilizer, Knee	Orthopedics
Joint, Knee, External Brace	Physical Med
Splint, Hand, And Component	Physical Med
Splint, Other	Orthopedics

DALE MEDICAL PRODUCTS, INC.   800-343-3980
7 Cross St., Plainville, MA 02762-0556   508-695-9316
  Fax: 508-695-6587
FDA Number: 1214422
E-mail: info@dalemed.net
Web site: www.dalemed.net
Medical Products Sales Volume: $20,500,000
Annual Revenue: $10-$25 Million
Year Founded: 1961
Total Employees: 151   *Marketing Staff:* 6   *Sales Staff:* 3
Ownership: Private
Produces/Sells CE-marked Devices: N
Federal Procurement Eligibility: Small Business
Distribution: Manufacturer Through Distributor
General Admin.: John Vandegrift/Executive Vice President
      Donna Bibeault/Human Resources Representative
      John C. Brezack/President, Chairman
Mktg./Adv.: Allison Frazer/Director Marketing & Sales
      Sharon Steeves/Director Product Development
      Lionel Rush/Manager International Sales
Production: Marge Enders/Manager Materials
      Joseph Kovacs/Vice President Manufacturing
Finance: Irving Forman/Vice President Finance

Accessories, Apparel, Surgical	Surgery
Airway, Nasopharyngeal (Breathing Tube)	Anesthesiology
Belt, Abdominal	Gastroenterology/Urology
Belt, Rib (Support)	Orthopedics
Binder, Abdominal	General
Binder, Abdominal, OB/GYN	Obstetrics/Gynecology
Binder, Chest	General
Board, Arm	Anesthesiology
Cuff, Tracheostomy Tube	Ear/Nose/Throat
Dressing, Other	General
Holder, Catheter	Gastroenterology/Urology
Holder, Tracheostomy Tube	Anesthesiology
Orthosis, Rib Fracture, Soft	Physical Med
Support, Abdominal	Physical Med

DALLAS EYE PROSTHETICS   214-739-5355
8226 Douglas Ave., #415, Dallas, TX 75225
FDA Number: 1646980

Eye, Artificial, Non-Custom	Ophthalmology

DALLAS TRIM INDUSTRIES CORP.   972-278-3598
2511 National Dr., Garland, TX 75041
FDA Number: 1649943
Ownership: Private
Produces/Sells CE-marked Devices: N

Accessories, Wheelchair	Physical Med
Cushion, Flotation, Therapeutic	Physical Med
Cushion, Wheelchair (Pad)	Physical Med

DALORE, INC.
  See Angiosystems, Inc.

DALSA CORP.   519-886-6000
605 McMurray Road, Waterloo, ONT N2V 2E9 Canada
FDA Number: n/a   *Fax:* 519-886-8023
Web site: www.dalsa.com

DALSA CORP.
519-886-6000 *(cont'd)*
Year Founded: 1980
Ownership: Public
Stock Symbol: DSA
Traded On: Toronto
Quality System Registration Information: ISO9001; ISO9002
Produces/Sells CE-marked Devices: Y
Distribution: Manufacturer Direct, Manufacturer Through Distributor, Manufacturer Through Manufacturer Reps, OEM, Service Direct, Exclusive Distributor

DALTON CHEMICAL LABORATORIES INC.
800-567-5060
349 Wildcat Rd., Toronto, ON M3J 2S3 Canada
416-736-5394
FDA Number: n/a
Fax: 416-736-5846
E-mail: chemist@dalton.com
Web site: www.dalton.com
Year Founded: 1987
Total Employees: 50
Ownership: Private
Produces/Sells CE-marked Devices: N
Distribution: Manufacturer Direct, Exporter

DALTON MEDICAL CORP.
972-418-5129
1103 Venture, Carrollton, TX 75006
FDA Number: 1649595
Fax: 972-418-5706
E-mail: service@daltonmedical.com
Web site: www.daltonmedical.com
Medical Products Sales Volume: $6,000,000
Annual Revenue: $5-$10 Million
Year Founded: 1984
Ownership: Private
Produces/Sells CE-marked Devices: N
Federal Procurement Eligibility: Small Business
Distribution: Importer

Attachment, Commode, Wheelchair	Physical Med
Cover, Mattress	General
Cushion, Wheelchair (Pad)	Physical Med
Lift, Bath, Non-AC-Powered	General
Mattress, Alternating Pressure (Or Pads)	Physical Med
Orthosis, Corrective Shoe	Physical Med
Regulator, Pressure, Gas Cylinder	Anesthesiology
Table, Mechanical	Physical Med
Walker, Mechanical	Physical Med
Wheelchair, Manual	Physical Med
Wheelchair, Powered	Physical Med

DALYNN BIOLOGICALS INC.
888-404-4045
3253 - 34 Avenue N.E.,
403-291-0067
Calgary, ALB T1Y 6 Canada
FDA Number: n/a
Fax: 403-250-9010
E-mail: info@dalynn.com
Web site: www.dalynn.com
Year Founded: 1985
Total Employees: 10
Ownership: Private
Produces/Sells CE-marked Devices: N
Distribution: Manufacturer Direct, Exclusive Distributor

DALZELL USA MEDICAL SYSTEMS
540-253-7715
PO Box 162, Marshall, VA 20116-0162
FDA Number: 1062170
Fax: 540-253-7734
E-mail: DalzellUSA@aol.com
Ownership: Private
Produces/Sells CE-marked Devices: N
Federal Procurement Eligibility: Female Owned

Caliper	Orthopedics

DAN KAR CORPORATION
800-942-5542
192 New Boston St C, Woburn, MA 01801
781-935-9221
FDA Number: n/a
Fax: 781-935-4343
E-mail: quality@dan-kar.com
Web site: www.dan-kar.com
Medical Products Sales Volume: $800,000
Year Founded: 1976
Total Employees: 10
Ownership: Private
Produces/Sells CE-marked Devices: N
Federal Procurement Eligibility: Small Business
Distribution: Manufacturer Direct, Manufacturer Through Manufacturer Reps, OEM
General Admin.: Terrance Hahn/President

Component, Electrical	General
Labware, Basic, Reusable	Chemistry
Rack, Test Tube	Chemistry
Shield, X-Ray	Radiology
Waste Receptacle, Radioactive	Radiology

DANA DOUGLAS MEDICAL INC.
800-267-3552
155 Colonnade Rd., Unit 10,
613-723-6734
Nepean, ONT K2E-7 Canada
FDA Number: n/a
Fax: 613-723-1058
E-mail: info@danadouglas.com
Web site: www.danadouglas.com
Year Founded: 1987
Total Employees: 10
Ownership: Private
Produces/Sells CE-marked Devices: N
Distribution: Manufacturer Direct, Exclusive Distributor

DANA MOLDED PRODUCTS, INC.
847-255-2000
6 N. Hickory Avenue, Arlington Heights, IL 60004
FDA Number: n/a
Fax: 847-255-1298
E-mail: info@danamolded.com
Web site: www.danamolded.com
Medical Products Sales Volume: $500,000
Annual Revenue: $5-$10 Million
Year Founded: 1965
Total Employees: 65
Sales Staff: 3
Ownership: Private
Produces/Sells CE-marked Devices: N
Federal Procurement Eligibility: Small Business
Distribution: Manufacturer Direct, Exporter
General Admin.: Daniel Hidding/Chief Executive Officer, Chairman
David Hidding/President
Mktg./Adv.: David Hidding/Director National Accounts

Molding, Custom	General

DANA PRODUCTS, INC.
847-455-2881
11457 Melrose St., Franklin Park, IL 60131
FDA Number: 3007412809
Fax: 847-455-2886
E-mail: info@danaproducts.com
Web site: www.danaproducts.com
Ownership: Private
Produces/Sells CE-marked Devices: N

Sterilization Process Indicator, Physical/Chemical	General

DANAHER
See Danaher Corporation

DANAHER CORPORATION
202-828-0850
2000 Pennsylvania Avenue, NW, Suite 800 West,
Washington, DC 20006
FDA Number: n/a
Fax: 202-828-0860
Web site: www.danaher.com
Medical Products Sales Volume: $2,997,986,000
Annual Revenue: More than $1 Billion
Total Employees: 50000
Ownership: Public
Stock Symbol: DHR
Traded On: NYSE
Produces/Sells CE-marked Devices: N
General Admin.: Steven M Rales/Chairman
Daniel L Comas/Chief Financial Officer, Executive Vice President
Thomas P Joyce/Executive Vice President
Mr. J. Lawrence Kulp Jr./President, Chief Executive Officer
Jonathan P Graham/Senior Vice President, General Counsel
Finance: James H Ditkoff/Senior Vice President Finance
Medical Product Subsidiaries (Listed Separately)
Imaging Sciences International, Llc
Kaltenbach & Voigt Gmbh & Co.
Kavo Dental Corp.
Kavo Dental Manufacturing Inc
Leica Biosystems - St. Louis, Llc
Leica Microsystems Inc.
Pelton & Crane

DANAM ELECTRONICS, INC.
See Drew Scientific, Inc.

DANARA INTL. LTD.
800-526-7048
8101 Tonnelle Ave., North Bergen, NJ 07047
201-295-1448
FDA Number: 2242795
Fax: 201-295-1573
E-mail: info@danaraint.com
Web site: www.danaraint.com
Ownership: Private
Produces/Sells CE-marked Devices: N

Ring, Teething, Fluid-Filled	Dental And Oral

DANBI, INC.
310-398-0013
12099 West Washington Blvd., Suite 304,
Los Angeles, CA 90066
FDA Number: 2025109

Regulator, Thermal, Cardiopulmonary Bypass	Cardiovascular
Thermometer, Electronic, Continuous	General

DANE TECHNOLOGIES
7105 Northland Terrace,
Brooklyn Park, MN 55428
1-888-544-7779
763-746-4423
FDA Number: 3003857817
E-mail: info@danetechnologies.com
Web site: www.danetechnologies.com
Ownership: Private
Produces/Sells CE-marked Devices: N
Fax: 763-544-4234

Wheelchair, Powered	Physical Med
Wheelchair, Standup	Physical Med

DANEK MANUFACTURING, INC.
See Medtronic Sofamor Danek Usa, Inc

DANIEL T ACOSTA
635 C Street, Suite 502, San Diego, CA 92101
619-235-8950
FDA Number: 2029242

Eye, Artificial, Non-Custom	Ophthalmology

DANIEL WOODHEAD CO.
See Woodhead L.P.

DANIELS SHARPSMART, INC.
4144 E. Therese Avenue, Fresno, CA 93727
559-351-9593
FDA Number: 3006185230
Ownership: Private
Produces/Sells CE-marked Devices: N

Needle, Hypodermic, Single Lumen With Syringe	General

DANLEE MEDICAL PRODUCTS, INC.
6075 Molloy Rd. E., Bldg. 5, Syracuse, NY 13211
800-433-7797
315-431-0143
FDA Number: 3004531359
E-mail: info@danleemedical.com
Web site: www.danleemedical.com
Medical Products Sales Volume: $2,300,000
Annual Revenue: $1-$5 Million
Year Founded: 1994
Total Employees: 11   *Marketing Staff:* 2   *Sales Staff:* 4
Ownership: Private
Produces/Sells CE-marked Devices: N
Federal Procurement Eligibility: Female Owned
Distribution: Manufacturer Direct, Manufacturer Through Distributor, Exclusive Distributor
General Admin.: Joni L. Walton/Chief Executive Officer
Production: Amy Sommer/Manager Customer Services
Fax: 315-431-0149

Electrode, Electrocardiograph	Cardiovascular
Electrode, Other	General
Kit, Disposable Procedure	Cardiovascular

DANLIN PRODUCTS, INC.
3321 Columbia, N.E., Albuquerque, NM 87107-2001
505-884-1922
FDA Number: 1723551
E-mail: danlinproducts@qwest.net
Medical Products Sales Volume: $600,000
Year Founded: 1986
Total Employees: 6
Ownership: Private
Produces/Sells CE-marked Devices: N
Federal Procurement Eligibility: Small Business
Fax: 505-884-1923

Implant, Endosseous	Dental And Oral

DANMAR PRODUCTS, INC.
221 Jackson Industrial Dr., Ann Arbor, MI 48103
734-761-1990
FDA Number: 1831680

Orthosis, Cranial	Cns/Neurology
Support, Head And Trunk, Wheelchair	Physical Med

DANSEREAU HEALTH PRODUCTS, INC.
210 & 250 E. Harrison Street, Corona, CA 92879
800-423-5657
951-549-1400
FDA Number: 2027216
E-mail: harry@dhpdental.com
Web site: www.dhpdental.com
Medical Products Sales Volume: $5,200,000
Annual Revenue: $5-$10 Million
Year Founded: 1961
Total Employees: 43   *Marketing Staff:* 5   *Sales Staff:* 5
Ownership: Private
Produces/Sells CE-marked Devices: Y
Federal Procurement Eligibility: Small Business
Distribution: Manufacturer Direct, Manufacturer Through Distributor, Manufacturer Through Manufacturer Reps, OEM
General Admin.: Harry P. Nelson/President, Chief Executive Officer
    Harry C. Nelson/Vice President
    Tamera Davis/Vice President, General Manager
Mktg./Adv.: Harry C. Nelson/Director Marketing & Advertising
    Harry C. Nelson/Director Product Development
Production: Leo Alvarado/Manager Production
Fax: 951-549-1411

Chair, Dental	Dental And Oral
Chair, Dental (With Unit)	Dental And Oral

DANSEREAU HEALTH PRODUCTS, INC.
800-423-5657 *(cont'd)*

Chair, Examination And Treatment	General
Chair, Other	General
Compressor, Air, Portable	Anesthesiology
Pump, Vacuum, Central	Anesthesiology
Stool, Dental	Dental And Oral

DANVILLE MATERIALS
3420 Fostoria Way, Suite A200,
San Ramon, CA 94583
800-827-7940
925-973-0710
FDA Number: 2954330
E-mail: dsimpson2@daneng.com
Web site: www.danvillematerials.com
Medical Products Sales Volume: $2,500,000
Year Founded: 1970
Total Employees: 35   *Marketing Staff:* 2   *Sales Staff:* 4
Ownership: Private
Quality System Registration Information: ISO9003
Produces/Sells CE-marked Devices: Y
Federal Procurement Eligibility: Small Business
Distribution: Manufacturer Through Distributor, Service Direct, Exclusive Distributor
General Admin.: Craig Bruns/President, Chief Executive Officer, Chief Financial Officer
    Mark Fernwood/Vice President
Production: Debbie Simpson/Director Customer Services
Finance: Elane Atterbury/Controller
Fax: 925-973-0764

Adhesive, Dental	Dental And Oral
Airbrush	Dental And Oral
Cabinet, Dental	Dental And Oral
Compound, Resinous, Composite	Dental And Oral
Crown And Bridge, Temporary, Resin	Dental And Oral
Dental Laboratory Equipment	Dental And Oral
Detector, Caries	Dental And Oral
Instrument, Dental, Manual	Dental And Oral
Prophylaxis Unit, Ultrasonic, Dental	Dental And Oral

DAPCO INDUSTRIES
241 Ethan Allen Hwy., Ridgefield, CT 06877-6208
800-597-2726
203-438-9696
FDA Number: n/a
E-mail: generalinfo@DapcoNDT.com
Web site: www.dapcondt.com
Medical Products Sales Volume: $2,800,000
Annual Revenue: $1-$5 Million
Year Founded: 1970
Total Employees: 20   *Marketing Staff:* 1   *Sales Staff:* 2
Ownership: Private
Produces/Sells CE-marked Devices: N
Federal Procurement Eligibility: Small Business
Distribution: Manufacturer Direct, OEM
General Admin.: Dominick Pagano/President, Chief Executive Officer
Mktg./Adv.: Joe Zaccone/Manager Marketing & Sales
    David Giragosian/Vice President Business Development
Production: Mike Pagano/Manager Regulatory Affairs
Fax: 203-438-1794

Needle, Other	General
Transducer, Ultrasonic	Cardiovascular

DARBY DENTAL SUPPLY CO.
300 Jericho Quadrangle, Jericho, NY 11753
800-645-2310
FDA Number: 3003459843
Web site: www.darbydental.com
Year Founded: 1948
Ownership: Private
Produces/Sells CE-marked Devices: N

Cement, Dental	Dental And Oral

DARBY DENTAL SUPPLY CO.
4460 Holmes Rd., Memphis, TN 38118
800-645-2310
FDA Number: 2320982
Web site: www.darbydental.com
Year Founded: 1948
Ownership: DARBY DENTAL SUPPLY CO.
Produces/Sells CE-marked Devices: N
Federal Procurement Eligibility: Small Business
Distribution: Manufacturer Direct, Exclusive Distributor

Cement, Dental	Dental And Oral
Disk, Abrasive	Dental And Oral
Explorer, Operative	Dental And Oral
Liner, Cavity, Calcium Hydroxide	Dental And Oral
Material, Impression	Dental And Oral
Material, Impression Tray, Resin	Dental And Oral
Mercury	Dental And Oral
Retainer, Screw Expansion, Orthodontic	Dental And Oral

DARCO INTERNATIONAL, INC.
810 Memorial Blvd, Huntington, WV 25701
800-999-8866
304-522-4883
FDA Number: 1122845
E-mail: info@darcointernational.com
Web site: www.darcointernational.com
Fax: 304-522-0037

DARCO INTERNATIONAL, INC.　800-999-8866 (cont'd)
Medical Products Sales Volume: $2,400,000
Year Founded: 1985
Total Employees: 15
Ownership: Private
Produces/Sells CE-marked Devices: Y
Federal Procurement Eligibility: Small Business
Distribution: Manufacturer Through Distributor, OEM, Importer, Exporter
General Admin.: Mr. Darrel Darby/President, Chief Executive Officer
Mktg./Adv.: Mr. George Borak/Vice President Marketing & Sales
Finance: Brent Fulks/Director Finance

Brace, Joint, Ankle (External)	Physical Med
Cast Walking Heel	Orthopedics
Cover, Shoe, Operating Room	Surgery
Immobilizer, Knee	Orthopedics
Immobilizer, Shoulder	Orthopedics
Immobilizer, Wrist/Hand	Orthopedics
Padding, Cast/Splint	General
Shoe, Cast	Physical Med
Sock, Cast Toe	Orthopedics
Splint, Temporary Training	Physical Med
Support, Back	Orthopedics

DAREN INDUSTRIES, INC　574-534-3418
2452 Lincolnway East, Goshen, IN 46526
FDA Number: 3004033067　　　*Fax:* 574-975-0408
Ownership: Private
Produces/Sells CE-marked Devices: N

Splint, Hand, And Component	Physical Med

DAREX CONTAINER PRODUCTS　617-498-4357
6050 West 51st St., Chicago, IL 60638
FDA Number: n/a
Ownership: Private
Produces/Sells CE-marked Devices: N

Absorbent, Carbon-Dioxide	Anesthesiology

DARNELL-ROSE CASTERS　800-327-6355
**17915 Railroad St.,　　　　　　626-912-1688
City of Industry, CA 91748**
FDA Number: n/a　　　　　*Fax:* 626-912-3765
E-mail: joe@casters.com
Web site: www.casters.com
Annual Revenue: $10-$25 Million
Year Founded: 1921
Total Employees: 120
Ownership: Private
Quality System Registration Information: ISO9001
Produces/Sells CE-marked Devices: N
Federal Procurement Eligibility: Small Business
Distribution: Manufacturer Direct, Manufacturer Through Distributor, OEM, Service Direct, Exclusive Distributor, Exporter
General Admin.: Salvatore Aliotta/Chief Executive Officer
Mktg./Adv.: Rick Chichester/Manager National Sales
Production: John Posen/Vice President Manufacturing

Casters, Hospital Equipment	General

DARTNELL CORPORATION　800-223-8720
222 Sedwick Dr., Durham, NC 27713
FDA Number: n/a　　　　*Fax:* 800-508-2592
E-mail: customerservice@dartnellcorp.com
Web site: www.dartnellcorp.com
Annual Revenue: $10-$25 Million
Total Employees: 95　　　*Marketing Staff:* 6
Ownership: Private
Produces/Sells CE-marked Devices: N
Federal Procurement Eligibility: Small Business, Female Owned
Distribution: Manufacturer Direct, Exclusive Distributor
General Admin.: Clark Fetridge/Chairman, Chief Executive Officer
　　　　　Ken Khn/President, Chief Executive Officer
Mktg./Adv.: Dayna Eynom/Marketing & Sales Representative

Cart, Equipment, Video	General
Office Product	General

DASH MEDICAL GLOVES, INC.　800-523-2055
10180 S. 54th St., Franklin, WI 53132
FDA Number: 2183812　　　*Fax:* 800-523-7795
E-mail: info@dashmedical.com
Web site: www.dashmedical.com
Medical Products Sales Volume: $10,000,000
Annual Revenue: $10-$25 Million
Year Founded: 1988
Ownership: Private
Produces/Sells CE-marked Devices: N
Federal Procurement Eligibility: Small Business
Distribution: Manufacturer Through Distributor, Importer

Glove, Patient Examination	General
Glove, Patient Examination, Latex	General

DASH MEDICAL GLOVES, INC.　800-523-2055 (cont'd)

Glove, Patient Examination, Vinyl	General
Glove, Surgical, Powder-Free	Surgery

DATA HUNTER LLC　714-892-5461
5412 Balsa Ave, Unit G, Huntington Beach, CA 92649
FDA Number: n/a　　　　*Fax:* 714-892-9768
E-mail: info@datahunter.com
Web site: www.datahunter.com
Annual Revenue: $0-$1 Million
Year Founded: 1983
Ownership: Private
Quality System Registration Information: ISO9002
Produces/Sells CE-marked Devices: Y
Federal Procurement Eligibility: Small Business, Female Owned
Distribution: Manufacturer Direct, Manufacturer Through Distributor, Importer, Exporter

Reader, Bar Code	General
Shield Radio Frequency	Radiology

DATA INNOVATIONS, INC.　802-658-2850
120 Kimball Ave., Suite 100, Btv, VT 05403
FDA Number: 1225673

Computer, Chemistry Analyzer	Chemistry

DATABASE, INC.　919-493-6969
3100 Tower Blvd., Suite 304, Durham, NC 27707-7105
FDA Number: n/a　　　　*Fax:* 919-493-3691
E-mail: kay@dbvax.mc.duke.edu
Web site: www.dbtmr.com
Medical Products Sales Volume: $750,000
Annual Revenue: $0-$1 Million
Total Employees: 10　　*Marketing Staff:* 2　　*Sales Staff:* 2
Ownership: Private
Federal Procurement Eligibility: Small Business
Distribution: Exclusive Distributor
General Admin.: W. Edward Hammond/Chairman
　　　　　Lois C. Funderburk/Chief Executive Officer
Mktg./Adv.: Wayland Johnosn/Manager Product Development
　　　　　Lois C. Funderburk/Manager Training
　　　　　Kay F. Hammond/Vice President Marketing & Sales

Computer Software	General
Computer, Patient Data Management	General

DATACARD GROUP　800-621-6972
**11111 Bren Road W.,　　　　952-933-1223
Minnetonka, MN 55343**
FDA Number: 9310022　　　*Fax:* 952-931-0418
E-mail: info@datacard.com
Web site: www.datacard.com
Medical Products Sales Volume: $130,100,000
Year Founded: 1987
Total Employees: 800
Ownership: Private
Quality System Registration Information: ISO9000
Produces/Sells CE-marked Devices: N
Distribution: Manufacturer Direct, Manufacturer Through Distributor
Mktg./Adv.: Kevin Gillick/Director Marketing Communications
　　　　　Mike Schnaus/Vice President Business Development

Card, Identification	General
Computer, Patient Data Management	General
Printer, Bar Code	General

DATACUBE INC.　978-777-4200
300 Rosewood Drive, Danvers, MA 01923-4505
FDA Number: n/a　　　　*Fax:* 978-777-3117
E-mail: info@datacube.com
Web site: www.datacube.com
Annual Revenue: $10-$25 Million
Year Founded: 1978
Total Employees: 50　　*Marketing Staff:* 2　　*Sales Staff:* 10
Ownership: Private
Quality System Registration Information: ISO9001
Produces/Sells CE-marked Devices: Y
Federal Procurement Eligibility: Small Business
Distribution: Manufacturer Direct, Manufacturer Through Distributor, Manufacturer Through Manufacturer Reps, Service Direct, Exclusive Distributor
General Admin.: Stanley Karandanis/Chairman
　　　　　Barry Egan/Chief Operating Officer
Mktg./Adv.: Tom Hospod/Vice President Marketing & Sales

Image Processing System	Radiology

DATAFIRST CORP.　800-634-8504
5124 Departure Drive, Raleigh, NC 27616　919-876-6650
FDA Number: 1065566　　　*Fax:* 919-876-6651
E-mail: sales@datafirst.com
Web site: www.datafirst.com
Medical Products Sales Volume: $1,700,000

DATAFIRST CORP. 800-634-8504 *(cont'd)*
Year Founded: 1990
Total Employees: 10
Ownership: Private
Produces/Sells CE-marked Devices: N
Federal Procurement Eligibility: Small Business
  Device, Storage, Image, Digital — Radiology

DATASCOPE CARDIAC ASSIST DIV. 800-777-4222
15 Law Drive, Fairfield, NJ 07004 973-244-6100
FDA Number: 2248146 *Fax:* 973-244-6279
Web site: www.datascope.com
Annual Revenue: $5-$10 Million
Total Employees: 290 *Marketing Staff:* 6 *Sales Staff:* 40
Ownership: DATASCOPE CORP.
Stock Symbol: DSCP
Traded On: NASDAQ
Quality System Registration Information: ISO9000
Produces/Sells CE-marked Devices: Y
Distribution: Manufacturer Direct, Manufacturer Through Distributor, Exporter
General Admin.: Susan Peterson/Assistant President
      Lawrence Saper/Chief Executive Officer
      Paul Fein/Director Human Resources
      Paul Southworth/President
Mktg./Adv.: Bill Friedberg/Vice President Marketing
      Ken Waters/Vice President Sales
Production: Kevin Crossen/Director Quality Assurance
Research: Tom Lindstrand/Vice President Research & Development & Operations
  Balloon, Intra-Aortic (With Control System) — Cardiovascular
  Bandage, Adhesive — Surgery
  Catheter, Balloon (Foley Type) — Surgery
  Catheter, Intra-Aortic Balloon — Cardiovascular
  Circulatory Assist Unit, Intra-Aortic Balloon — Cardiovascular
  Clamp, Vascular — Cardiovascular
  Guidewire, Catheter — Cardiovascular
  Introducer, Catheter — Cardiovascular
  Tube, Pump, Cardiopulmonary Bypass — Cardiovascular

DATASCOPE CORP.
See MAQUET

DATASCOPE CORP., CARDIAC ASSIST DIVISION 1 800 777 4222
1300 Macarthur Blvd., Mahwah, NJ 07430 1-201-307-5400
FDA Number: 2249723 *Fax:* 1 201 995 8910
Ownership: DATASCOPE CORP.
Stock Symbol: DSCP
Traded On: NASDAQ
Produces/Sells CE-marked Devices: N
  Balloon, Intra-Aortic (With Control System) — Cardiovascular
  Dilator, Vessel, Percutaneous Catheterization — Cardiovascular
  Guidewire, Catheter — Cardiovascular
  Introducer, Catheter — Cardiovascular
  Tubing, Flexible, Medical Gas, Low-Pressure — Anesthesiology

DATCARD SYSTEMS INC 877-543-3898
7 Goodyear, Irvine, CA 92618 949-932-1300
FDA Number: 3003341080 *Fax:* 949-932-1373
E-mail: Sales@datcard.com
Web site: www.datcard.com
Ownership: Private
Produces/Sells CE-marked Devices: N
  Device, Storage, Image, Digital — Radiology
  System, Communication, Image, Digital — Radiology

DATEL MEDICAL STORAGE SYSTEMS INC.
See Windquest

DATEX-OHMEDA (CANADA) 800-268-1472
1093 Meyerside Dr., Unit 2, Mississauga, ONT L5T-1 Canada 905-565-8572
FDA Number: 9200717 *Fax:* 905-565-8592
Web site: www.datex-ohmeda.com
Year Founded: 1918
Total Employees: 100 *Marketing Staff:* 2 *Sales Staff:* 13
Ownership: Instrumentarium Corp.
Produces/Sells CE-marked Devices: Y
Distribution: Service Direct, Exclusive Distributor

DATEX-OHMEDA INC. 608-221-1551
3030 Ohmeda Drive, Madison, WI 53718
FDA Number: 2112667
Web site: www.gehealthcare.com
Ownership: Ge Healthcare
Produces/Sells CE-marked Devices: N
  Absorber, Carbon-Dioxide — Anesthesiology
  Analyzer, Gas, Carbon-Dioxide, Gaseous Phase (Capnograph) — Anesthesiology
  Analyzer, Gas, Nitrous-Oxide, Gaseous Phase — Anesthesiology
  Apparatus, Nitric Oxide Delivery — Anesthesiology

DATEX-OHMEDA INC. 608-221-1551 *(cont'd)*
  Bottle, Collection, Breathing System (Uncalibrated) — Anesthesiology
  Flowmeter, Gas (Oxygen), Calibrated — Anesthesiology
  Gas-Machine, Anesthesia — Anesthesiology
  Monitor, Airway Pressure (Gauge/Alarm) — Anesthesiology
  Tube, Gastrointestinal — Gastroenterology/Urology
  Tubing, Flexible, Medical Gas, Low-Pressure — Anesthesiology
  Vaporizer, Anesthesia, Non-Heated — Anesthesiology
  Ventilator, Continuous (Respirator) — Anesthesiology

DATEX-OHMEDA INC., A DIVISION OF INSTRUMENTARIUM C
See Datex-Ohmeda Inc.

DATEX-OHMEDA, INC. (MADISON) 800-345-2700
3030 Ohmeda Dr., Madison, WI 53707-7550 6082211551
FDA Number: 2112667 *Fax:* 608-222-9147
E-mail: don.spence@ohmeda.boc.com
Web site: www.ohmedamedical.com
Total Employees: 200 *Marketing Staff:* 15 *Sales Staff:* 120
Ownership: Datex-Ohmeda
Traded On: Helsinki
Produces/Sells CE-marked Devices: Y
Distribution: Manufacturer Direct, Exporter
General Admin.: Richard Atkin/President
  Analyzer, Gas, Carbon-Dioxide, Gaseous Phase (Capnograph) — Anesthesiology
  Analyzer, Gas, Nitrous-Oxide, Gaseous Phase — Anesthesiology
  Gas Machine, Analgesia — Anesthesiology
  Monitor, Airway Pressure (Gauge/Alarm) — Anesthesiology
  Tube, Gastrointestinal — Gastroenterology/Urology
  Vaporizer, Anesthesia, Non-Heated — Anesthesiology
  Ventilator, Continuous (Respirator) — Anesthesiology

DATREND SYSTEMS INC. 800-667-6557
5355 Parkwood Place, Richmond, BC V6V 2 Canada 604-291-7747
FDA Number: 9515335 *Fax:* 604-294-2355
E-mail: customerservice@datrend.com
Web site: www.datrend.com
Year Founded: 1993
Total Employees: 17
Ownership: Private
Produces/Sells CE-marked Devices: N
Distribution: Manufacturer Direct, Manufacturer Through Distributor, Service Direct, Exporter

DATRIX 760-480-8874
340 State Place, Escondido, CA 92029
FDA Number: 2028530
Ownership: Private
Produces/Sells CE-marked Devices: N
  Electrocardiograph, Ambulatory(without Analysis) — Cardiovascular
  Recorder, Magnetic Tape/Disc — Cardiovascular

DAVID CLARK COMPANY, INC. 800-900-3434
360 Franklin St., Worcester, MA 01604 508-751-5800
FDA Number: 1217478 *Fax:* 508-753-5827
E-mail: sales@davidclark.com
Web site: www.davidclark.com
Medical Products Sales Volume: $1,000,000
Annual Revenue: $25-$50 Million
Year Founded: 1935
Total Employees: 302 *Marketing Staff:* 2 *Sales Staff:* 15
Ownership: Private
Quality System Registration Information: ISO9000
Produces/Sells CE-marked Devices: Y
Federal Procurement Eligibility: Small Business
Distribution: Manufacturer Through Distributor
  Communication Equipment — General
  Infuser, Pressure (Blood Pump) — General
  Pressure Infusor, IV Container — General
  Suit, Pneumatic Counterpressure (Anti-Shock) — Cardiovascular
  Trousers, Anti-Shock — Anesthesiology

DAVID SCOTT COMPANY 800-804-0333
59 Fountain St., Framingham, MA 01702 508-875-3333
FDA Number: 1219214 *Fax:* 508-875-3375
E-mail: sales@davidscottco.com
Web site: www.davidscottco.com
Medical Products Sales Volume: $3,500,000
Year Founded: 1972
Total Employees: 35 *Marketing Staff:* 3 *Sales Staff:* 54
Ownership: ROBERT H. KAPLAN ASSOCIATES, INC.
Produces/Sells CE-marked Devices: Y
Federal Procurement Eligibility: Small Business, GSA Contract, VA Contract
Distribution: Manufacturer Direct, Manufacturer Through Distributor, Manufacturer Through Manufacturer Reps, OEM, Exporter
General Admin.: David M. Kaplan/President
Mktg./Adv.: David M. Kaplan/Director Marketing & Sales
      David M. Kaplan/Director Product Development

DAVID SCOTT COMPANY
800-804-0333 *(cont'd)*

Production: Joseph Baum/Manager Regulatory Affairs

Catheter, Other	Gastroenterology/Urology
Cuff, Blood Pressure	Cardiovascular
Cushion, Wheelchair (Pad)	Physical Med
Infuser, Pressure (Blood Pump)	General
Kit, Biopsy	General
Kit, Disposable Procedure	Cardiovascular
Kit, Wound Drainage, Closed	Cns/Neurology
Monitor, Blood Pressure, Indirect (Arterial)	Cardiovascular
Monitor, Blood Pressure, Invasive (Arterial), Anesthesia	Anesthesiology
Pad, Pressure, Gel	General
Stopcock	General
Stretcher, Transfer	Surgery
Surgical Instrument, Disposable	Surgery
Thermometer, Liquid Crystals	Surgery
Transducer, Blood Pressure	General
Transfer Aid	Physical Med
Tray, Custom/Special Procedure	General
Trocar, Laparoscopic	Surgery

DAVID ZELLER'S WHEELCHAIR BRAKE & ATTACHMENT BRKT.
610-759-5134

182 Bath Pike, Nazareth, PA 18064
FDA Number: 3006226273
Ownership: Private
Produces/Sells CE-marked Devices: N

Accessories, Wheelchair	Physical Med

DAVIS & GECK DIV., AMERICAN HOME PRO.
See Covidien Lp

DAVIS INSTRUMENT COMPANY, INC.
(800) 522-7442
920-478-3579

5850 Cherry Lane, Marshall, WI 53559-0100
FDA Number: n/a   *Fax:* 920-478-2760
E-mail: info@davisinstrument.com
Web site: www.davisinstrument.com
Ownership: Private
Produces/Sells CE-marked Devices: N
General Admin.: Lisa Kruesel/President

Centrifuge, General (Over 5,000 rpm)	Toxicology
Centrifuge, General (Up to 5,000 rpm)	Pathology
Microscope	Hematology

DAVIS LEAD APRON, INC.
800-483-3979
713-681-6561

4560 West 34th St., PO Box 924585, Houston, TX 77092
FDA Number: 1645308   *Fax:* 713-680-8185
E-mail: davisleadapron@swbell.net
Web site: www.apronco.com
Medical Products Sales Volume: $200,000
Annual Revenue: $0-$1 Million
Year Founded: 1997
Total Employees: 5   *Marketing Staff:* 1   *Sales Staff:* 6
Ownership: Private
Produces/Sells CE-marked Devices: N
Federal Procurement Eligibility: Small Business
Distribution: Manufacturer Direct, Manufacturer Through Manufacturer Reps
General Admin.: Jeffrey P. Burkett/President

Apron, Lead, Dental	Dental And Oral
Apron, Lead, Radiographic	Radiology
Eyeglasses	Ophthalmology
Glove, Patient Examination	General

DAVIS MEDICAL ELECTRONICS, INC.
800-422-3547
760-477-2000

2441 Cades Way, Suite 200, Vista, CA 92081
FDA Number: n/a   *Fax:* 760-727-7518
E-mail: info@davismedical.com
Web site: www.davismedical.com
Medical Products Sales Volume: $1,500,000
Annual Revenue: $1-$5 Million
Ownership: Private
Produces/Sells CE-marked Devices: N
Federal Procurement Eligibility: Small Business
Distribution: Service Direct, Exporter
General Admin.: Randy Davis/President
Mktg./Adv.: Marion Davis/Vice President Marketing & Sales

Computer, Ultrasound	Radiology
Service, Used Equipment	General

DAVISMADE, INC.
866-742-0581
810-233-9706

2511 Davison Road, Flint, MI 48506-3649
FDA Number: 1833039   *Fax:* 810-715-0946
E-mail: info@standingdani.com
Web site: www.standingdani.com
Medical Products Sales Volume: $700,000
Annual Revenue: $0-$1 Million
Year Founded: 1985
Total Employees: 10   *Marketing Staff:* 1   *Sales Staff:* 4

DAVISMADE, INC.
866-742-0581 *(cont'd)*

Ownership: Private
Quality System Registration Information: ISO9000
Produces/Sells CE-marked Devices: N
Federal Procurement Eligibility: Small Business
Distribution: Manufacturer Direct, Manufacturer Through Manufacturer Reps
General Admin.: Dan Davis/President

Wheelchair, Standup	Physical Med

DAVOL INC., SUB. C.R. BARD, INC.
800-556-6275
401-463-7000

100 Crossings Blvd., Warwick, RI 02886
FDA Number: 1213643   *Fax:* 401-464-9446
Web site: www.davol.com
Year Founded: 1874
Ownership: C. R. Bard, Inc.
Produces/Sells CE-marked Devices: N

Agent, Hemostatic, Absorbable, Collagen-Based	Surgery
Arthroscope	Orthopedics
Autotransfusion Unit (Blood)	Anesthesiology
Drape, Surgical	Surgery
Electrosurgical Unit, Cutting & Coagulation Device	Surgery
Endoscope	Gastroenterology/Urology
Holder, Needle	Gastroenterology/Urology
Insufflator, Hysteroscopic	Obstetrics/Gynecology
Laparoscope, General & Plastic Surgery	Surgery
Lavage Unit, Water Jet	General
Mesh, Surgical, Polymeric	Surgery
Microfilter, Blood Transfusion	Anesthesiology
Staple, Implantable	Surgery
Suture, Non-Absorbable, Steel, Monofilament & Multifilament	Surgery
Tray, Surgical Instrument	Surgery

DAVOL/EMS
See Conmed Corporation

DAVRON
See King Pharmaceuticals, Inc.

DAVTAIR INDUSTRIES INC.
613-831-1266

P.O. Box 11448, Station H, Ottawa, ONT K2H-7V1 Canada
FDA Number: n/a   *Fax:* 613-831-1971
E-mail: sales@davtair.com
Web site: www.davtair.com
Year Founded: 1987
Total Employees: 25
Ownership: Private
Produces/Sells CE-marked Devices: N
Distribution: Service Direct, Exclusive Distributor

DAW INDUSTRIES
800-252-2828
858-550-6848

5737 Pacific Center Blvd., San Diego, CA 92121
FDA Number: n/a
E-mail: info@daw-usa.com
Web site: www.daw-usa.com
Ownership: Private
Produces/Sells CE-marked Devices: N
Distribution: Exclusive Distributor
General Admin.: Hugo Belzidsky/President, Chief Executive Officer

Adhesive, Prosthesis, External	Surgery

DAWNING TECHNOLOGIES, INC.
800-332-0499
239-931-6004

8140 College Parkway, Suite 202, Fort Myers, FL 33919
FDA Number: 300728920   *Fax:* 239-931-0085
E-mail: sales@dawning.com
Web site: www.dawning.com
Medical Products Sales Volume: $2,000,000
Annual Revenue: $1-$5 Million
Total Employees: 20   *Marketing Staff:* 2   *Sales Staff:* 3
Ownership: Private
Produces/Sells CE-marked Devices: Y
Federal Procurement Eligibility: Small Business
Distribution: Manufacturer Direct, Manufacturer Through Distributor, OEM, Service Direct, Exclusive Distributor, Exporter
General Admin.: John Selmyer/President

Computer, Clinical Laboratory	Chemistry
General Purpose Microbiology Diagnostic Device	Microbiology

DAXOR CORPORATION
865-425-0555

107 Meco Lane, Oak Ridge, TN 37830
FDA Number: 3003529145
Ownership: Private
Produces/Sells CE-marked Devices: N

Collector, Blood, Vacuum-Assisted	Hematology
Detector, Beta/Gamma	Chemistry
Equipment, Laboratory, Gen. Purpose (Specific Medical Use)	Chemistry
Meter, Volume, Blood	Hematology
Syringe, Piston	General
Tray, Blood Collection	Hematology

DAXOR CORPORATION
212-244-0805
350 5th Ave., Ste. 7120, New York, NY 10118
FDA Number: n/a
Fax: 212-244-0806
E-mail: info@daxor.com
Web site: www.daxor.com
Medical Products Sales Volume: $1,000,000
Annual Revenue: $1-$5 Million
Year Founded: 1971
Total Employees: 30
Sales Staff: 6
Ownership: Public
Stock Symbol: DXR
Traded On: AMEX
Produces/Sells CE-marked Devices: Y
Federal Procurement Eligibility: Small Business
Distribution: Manufacturer Direct, Manufacturer Through Manufacturer Reps
General Admin.: Stephen Feldschuh/Chief Financial Officer, Vice President
Dr. Joseph Feldschuh/President, Chief Executive Officer
Stephen Feldschuh/Vice President Human Resources
Stephen Feldschuh/Vice President, General Manager
Mktg./Adv.: John Reyes-Guerra/Director Marketing
Ron Baldry/Director Product Development
John Reyes-Guerra/Manager International & National Sales
Dr. Gary Fischman/Manager Market Research
John Reyes-Garcia/Manager Sales Training
John Reyes-Guerra/Vice President Sales
Production: Dr. Gary J. Fischman/Director Quality Assurance
Deanna O'Brien/Manager Materials
Ron Baldry/Manager Regulatory Affairs
Ron Baldry/Vice President Manufacturing
Research: Dr. Gary J. Fischman/Vice President Research & Development
Analyzer, Blood Grouping — Hematology
Medical Product Subsidiaries (Listed Separately)
Scientific Medical Systems Ltd.

DAY & ZIMMERMANN VALIDATION SERVICES
215-299-8000
1818 Market St., Philadelphia, PA 19103
FDA Number: n/a
Fax: 215-299-2273
E-mail: ValidationServices@dayzim.com
Web site: www.dayzim.com
Medical Products Sales Volume: $1,900,000,000
Annual Revenue: $10-$25 Million
Year Founded: 1901
Total Employees: 23000
Marketing Staff: 2
Sales Staff: 4
Ownership: DAY & ZIMMERMANN INTERNATIONAL, INC.
Produces/Sells CE-marked Devices: N
Distribution: Service Direct
General Admin.: Joseph Ucciferro/Chief Executive Officer
Mr. Hal Baseman/President
Mktg./Adv.: Ms. Alveretta Pressley/Manager Marketing
Mr. Marc Waldman/Vice President Sales
Service, Consulting — General
Service, Engineering/Design — General

DAY CO., J.H.
See Littleford Day, Inc.

DAYSTAR MANUFACTURING, INCORPORATED
620-342-4440
3701 W. 6th Avenue, Emporia, KS 66801
FDA Number: 3006001889
Ownership: Private
Produces/Sells CE-marked Devices: N
Chair, Adjustable, Mechanical — Physical Med

DAZIAN FABRICS,LLC.
877-232-9426
201-549-1000
124 Enterprise Ave South, PO Box 2121,
Secaucus, NJ 07094
FDA Number: 622630
Fax: 201-549-1055
E-mail: info@dazian.com
Web site: www.dazian.com
Medical Products Sales Volume: $7,000,000
Annual Revenue: $0-$1 Million
Year Founded: 1998
Total Employees: 30
Ownership: Private
Produces/Sells CE-marked Devices: N
Federal Procurement Eligibility: Small Business
Distribution: Manufacturer Direct
General Admin.: Jon Weingarten/President
Mktg./Adv.: Karen Loftus/Director Marketing
Cover, Other — General
Curtain, Cubicle — General
Linen — General

DAZOR MANUFACTURING CORP.
800-345-9103
314-652-2400
2079 Congressional St., St. Louis, MO 63146
FDA Number: n/a
Fax: 314-652-2069
E-mail: info@dazor.com
Web site: www.dazor.com

DAZOR MANUFACTURING CORP.
800-345-9103 *(cont'd)*
Medical Products Sales Volume: $4,300,000
Annual Revenue: $5-$10 Million
Year Founded: 1940
Total Employees: 50
Marketing Staff: 2
Sales Staff: 3
Ownership: Private
Produces/Sells CE-marked Devices: Y
Federal Procurement Eligibility: Small Business, GSA Contract
Distribution: Manufacturer Direct, Manufacturer Through Distributor, Manufacturer Through Manufacturer Reps, OEM, Exporter
General Admin.: David Morley/Chairman
Stan Hogrebe/President
Mktg./Adv.: Kirk Cressey/Director Marketing
Donna Cronin/Director National Sales
Production: Stan Hogrebe/Manager Materials
Lamp, Examination (Light) — General
Lamp, Other — General

DAZTECH, INC.
215-669-3102
424 Broad Street, Perkasie, PA 18944
FDA Number: 3004355508
Ownership: Private
Produces/Sells CE-marked Devices: N
Cleaner, Ultrasonic, Medical Instrument — General

DB CONSULTANTS, INC
See Db Consultants, Inc

DB SQUARE, LLC
402-292-2383
101 Hickory Grove Church Rd., Sumrall, MS 39482
FDA Number: 3005842955
Medical Disinfectants/Cleaners for Instruments — General

DBA SYSTEMS, INC.
See Titan Corporation/Systems & Imagery Division

DCCT,INC
See Quest Star Medical, Inc.

DCI INCORPORATED
See Elecsys Corporation

DCI, INC.
913.647.0158
846 N Mart-Way Court, Olathe, KS 66061
FDA Number: n/a
Fax: 913-647-0132
E-mail: dcisales@dciincorporated.com
Web site: www.dciincorporated.com
Medical Products Sales Volume: $2,000,000
Annual Revenue: $5-$10 Million
Total Employees: 100
Marketing Staff: 1
Sales Staff: 5
Ownership: Public
Traded On: AMEX
Produces/Sells CE-marked Devices: N
Distribution: Manufacturer Through Manufacturer Reps, OEM
General Admin.: Keith Cowan/Chief Executive Officer
Karl Gemperli/President
Chris Hammond/Vice President, General Manager
Mktg./Adv.: Tyson Hoffman/Manager Advertising
Larry Shelton/Manager International & National Sales
Bill Cook/Vice President Marketing
Production: Ron Peck/Director Quality Assurance
Mary Owens/Manager Materials
Mike Morgan/Vice President Manufacturing
Contract Manufacturing — General

DDC TECHNOLOGIES, INC.
866-346-3527
516-594-1533
311 Woods Ave, Oceanside, NY 11572
FDA Number: 2438558
Fax: 516-764-4412
E-mail: sales@ddctech.com
Web site: www.ddctech.com
Medical Products Sales Volume: $600,000
Annual Revenue: $1-$5 Million
Year Founded: 1999
Total Employees: 6
Marketing Staff: 1
Sales Staff: 1
Ownership: Private
Produces/Sells CE-marked Devices: N
Federal Procurement Eligibility: Small Business
Distribution: Manufacturer Direct, Manufacturer Through Distributor, Service Direct
General Admin.: Mr. Dmitry Donskoy/Chief Executive Officer, Chief Financial Officer
Mktg./Adv.: Mr. Alex Chernovets/Admin. Marketing & Sales
Laser, Nd:YAG, Surgical — Surgery
Laser, Surgical — Surgery

DDS SERVICES, INC.
720-435-9052
15000 W. 6th Ave., Ste. 150, Golden, CO 80401
FDA Number: 3004738905
Ownership: Private
Produces/Sells CE-marked Devices: N
Powder, Porcelain — Dental And Oral

DE GOOD DIMENSIONAL CONCEPTS, INC. 574-834-5437
7815 Sr 13 N, North Webster, IN 46555
FDA Number: 3003866219   *Fax:* 574-834-5736
E-mail: mary@degooddc.com
Web site: www.degooddc.com
Ownership: Private
Produces/Sells CE-marked Devices: N
  Orthopedic Manual Surgical Instrument   Orthopedics

DE MEDCO 865-457-4077
851 Old Emory Rd., Clinton, TN 37716
FDA Number: n/a
E-mail: customerservice@deroyal.com
Web site: www.deroyal.com
Ownership: DEROYAL INDUSTRIES, INC.
Produces/Sells CE-marked Devices: N

DE NOVO SOFTWARE 213-384-7000
3250 Wilshire Blvd., Suite 803, Los Angeles, CA 90010
FDA Number: 3005798890
Web site: http://www.denovosoftware.com/
Year Founded: 1998
Ownership: Private
Produces/Sells CE-marked Devices: N
General Admin.: Mr. David Novo/President
Mktg./Adv.: Mr. Tanya Tolmachoff/Director Marketing & Sales
  Computer, Chemistry Analyzer   Chemistry

DEAN B. SCOTT, OCULARIST 847-965-4455
1319 Butterfield Rd.,, Suite 524, Downers Grove, IL 60515
FDA Number: 1423757
Ownership: Private
Produces/Sells CE-marked Devices: N
  Eye, Artificial, Non-Custom   Ophthalmology

DEAN B. SCOTT, OCULARIST 847-965-4455
1901 S. Osprey Ave., Sarasota, FL 34239
FDA Number: 1057997
Ownership: Private
Produces/Sells CE-marked Devices: N
  Eye, Artificial, Non-Custom   Ophthalmology

DEAN B. SCOTT, OCULARIST 847-965-4455
4101 Evans Ave., Ft. Myers, FL 33901
FDA Number: 1058005
Ownership: Private
Produces/Sells CE-marked Devices: N
  Eye, Artificial, Non-Custom   Ophthalmology

DEAN B. SCOTT, OCULARIST 847-965-4455
5225 Old Orchard Rd.,, Suite 27-b, Skokie, IL 60077
FDA Number: 1423758
Ownership: Private
Produces/Sells CE-marked Devices: N
  Eye, Artificial, Non-Custom   Ophthalmology

DEAN MEDICAL INSTRUMENTS, INC. 714-893-2772
15502 Commerce Lane, Huntington Beach, CA 92649
FDA Number: 2024452   *Fax:* 562-493-4852
Medical Products Sales Volume: $170,000
Annual Revenue: $0-$1 Million
Year Founded: 1984
Total Employees: 2
Ownership: Private
Federal Procurement Eligibility: Small Business
Distribution: Manufacturer Direct, Importer, Exporter
General Admin.: Anton Magnet/President
  Aspirator, Surgical   Surgery

DEB SBS, INC. 704-263-4240
1100 Highway 27, Stanley, NC 28164
FDA Number: n/a   *Fax:* 704-263-9601
E-mail: cser@debsbs.com
Web site: www.debsbs.com
Medical Products Sales Volume: $500,000
Year Founded: 1941
Ownership: Private
Produces/Sells CE-marked Devices: N
Federal Procurement Eligibility: Small Business
Distribution: Manufacturer Through Distributor, Manufacturer Through
Manufacturer Reps
  Lotion, Skin Care   General
  Soap   General

DEBMAR DISTRIBUTING INC. 800-265-3354
17 Wexford Rd.,   905-846-4528
Brampton, ONT L6Z-2 Canada
FDA Number: n/a   *Fax:* 905-846-5689
E-mail: customerservice@debmar.com

DEBMAR DISTRIBUTING INC. 800-265-3354 *(cont'd)*
Web site: www.debmar.com
Year Founded: 1989
Total Employees: 10
Ownership: Private
Produces/Sells CE-marked Devices: N
Distribution: Exclusive Distributor, Importer, Exporter

DEBUS, INC.
  See Deb Sbs, Inc.

DEBUS/SBS PRODUCTS, INC.
  See Deb Sbs, Inc.

DEBUSK ORTHOPEDIC CASTING (DOC) 865-362-2334
420 Straight Creek Road,, Suite 1, New Tazewell, TN 37825
FDA Number: 1624487
Ownership: Private
Produces/Sells CE-marked Devices: N
  Bandage, Cast   Physical Med
  Bandage, Elastic   General
  Component, Cast   Orthopedics
  Cover, Limb   Physical Med
  Cutter, Cast, AC-Powered   Orthopedics
  Orthosis, Limb Brace   Physical Med
  Pack, Hot Or Cold, Water Circulating   Physical Med
  Tape, Orthopedic   Orthopedics

DECIMAL 1.800.255.1613
121 Central Park Place, Sanford, FL 32771   407-330-3300
FDA Number: 3003586672   *Fax:* 407.322.7546
E-mail: rsweat@dotdecimal.com
Web site: http://www.dotdecimal.com/
Ownership: Private
Produces/Sells CE-marked Devices: N
  Accelerator, Linear, Medical   Radiology
  Block, Beam Shaping, Radionuclide   Radiology
  System, Planning, Radiation Therapy Treatment   Radiology

DECOMPRESSION TECHNOLOGY 903-667-3802
INTERNATIONAL
1235 Cr 4244, Dekalb, TX 75559-9739
FDA Number: 3004140821
Ownership: Private
Produces/Sells CE-marked Devices: N
  Massager, Therapeutic   Physical Med

DECON LABORATORIES LTD. (800) 332-6647
460 Glennie Circle, King of Prussia, PA 19406   (610) 755-0800
FDA Number: n/a   *Fax:* (610) 270-8905
Total Employees: 12   *Sales Staff:* 3
Ownership: Private
Produces/Sells CE-marked Devices: N
Distribution: Manufacturer Direct, Importer, Exporter
General Admin.: Robert N. Taylor/Chief Executive Officer
Mktg./Adv.: Keith Sullivan/Manager Sales
Production: Peter Hood/Manager Manufacturing
  Cleaner, Ultrasonic, Medical Instrument   General
  Washer/Disinfector   General

DECTRO INTERNATIONAL 800-463-5566
1000 Parc-Technologique Blvd.,   418-650-0303
Quebec, QUE G1P-4 Canada
FDA Number: n/a   *Fax:* 418-650-0707
E-mail: info@dectro.com
Web site: www.dectro.com
Year Founded: 1984
Total Employees: 50
Ownership: Private
Produces/Sells CE-marked Devices: N
Distribution: Manufacturer Direct, Exporter

DEDECO INTERNATIONAL, INC. 888-433-3326
Route 97, Long Eddy, NY 12760   845-887-4840
FDA Number: 3003149349   *Fax:* 845-887-5281
E-mail: service@dedeco.com
Web site: www.dedeco.com
Medical Products Sales Volume: $4,500,000
Annual Revenue: $25-$50 Million
Year Founded: 1937
Total Employees: 55
Ownership: Private
Produces/Sells CE-marked Devices: N
Federal Procurement Eligibility: Small Business
Distribution: Manufacturer Direct, Manufacturer Through Distributor
General Admin.: Steven Antler/President, Chief Executive Officer
Mktg./Adv.: Joseph Lancellotti/Director Marketing
    Steven Antler/Vice President Marketing & Sales

DEDECO INTERNATIONAL, INC. 888-433-3326 (cont'd)
Agent, Polishing, Abrasive, Oral Cavity Dental And Oral

DEDECO INTL., INC. 845-887-4840
11617 Route 97, Long Eddy, NY 12760
FDA Number: 1316367
E-mail: service@dedeco.com Fax: 845-887-5281
Web site: www.dedeco.com
Ownership: Private
Produces/Sells CE-marked Devices: N
Agent, Polishing, Abrasive, Oral Cavity Dental And Oral
Burr, Dental Dental And Oral
Disk, Abrasive Dental And Oral
Instrument, Diamond, Dental Dental And Oral
Point, Abrasive Dental And Oral

DEDICATED DISTRIBUTION 800-325-8367
640 Miami Avenue, Kansas City, KS 66105-2140 913-371-2200
FDA Number: n/a Fax: 877-371-2252
E-mail: ddinfo@dedicateddistribution.com
Web site: www.dedicateddistribution.com
Medical Products Sales Volume: $4,100,000
Annual Revenue: $10-$25 Million
Year Founded: 1989
Total Employees: 25 Marketing Staff: 2 Sales Staff: 10
Ownership: Dedicated Distribution
Produces/Sells CE-marked Devices: N
Federal Procurement Eligibility: Small Business
Distribution: Exclusive Distributor
General Admin.: Steven E. Cole/President, Chief Executive Officer
Mktg./Adv.: Jennifer Cisneros/Admin. Marketing Communications
Production: Gary Strub/Vice President Operations
Analyzer, Ultrasonic Unit General
Cannula, Other General
Exerciser, Bicycle Physical Med
Exerciser, Passive, Non-Measuring (CPM Machine) Physical Med
Inhaler, Nasal Ear/Nose/Throat
Monitor, Blood Gas, Oxygen Anesthesiology
Monitor, Blood Glucose (Test) Gastroenterology/Urology
Monitor, Blood Pressure, Venous Cardiovascular
Nebulizer, Non-Heated Anesthesiology
Pack, Moist Heat Physical Med
Regulator, Oxygen, Mechanical General
Stimulator, Electrical, For Incontinence Gastroenterology/Urology
Stimulator, Muscle, Low Intensity Physical Med
Stocking, Support (Anti-Embolic) General
Treadmill, Powered Physical Med
Tubing, Oxygen Connecting General
Medical Product Subsidiaries (Listed Separately)
Dedicated Distribution

DEEM PRECISION PRODUCTS 562-692-5416
4203 Durfee Avenue, Pico Rivera, CA 90660-0182
FDA Number: 2087019 Fax: 562-692-8484
E-mail: res04dp1@verizon.com
Ownership: Private
Produces/Sells CE-marked Devices: N
Holder, Needle Gastroenterology/Urology

DEEPAK PRODUCTS, INC. 305-482-9669
5220 N.w. 72nd Ave., Bay 15, Miami, FL 33166
FDA Number: 3004185272
Ownership: Private
Produces/Sells CE-marked Devices: N
Activator, Ultraviolet, Polymerization Dental And Oral
Agent, Polishing, Abrasive, Oral Cavity Dental And Oral
Amalgamator, Dental, AC-Powered Dental And Oral
Cotton, Roll Dental And Oral
Cover, Shoe, Conductive General
Eraser, Dental Stain Dental And Oral
Handpiece, Air-Powered, Dental Dental And Oral
Handpiece, Contra- And Right-Angle Attachment, Dental Dental And Oral
Instrument, Dental, Manual Dental And Oral
Material, Tooth Shade, Resin Dental And Oral
Mirror, Mouth Dental And Oral
Mouthpiece, Saliva Ejector Dental And Oral
Needle, Dental Dental And Oral
Paper, Articulation Dental And Oral
Syringe Unit, Air And/Or Water Dental And Oral
Tooth Bonding Agent, Resin Restoration Dental And Oral
Tray, Fluoride, Disposable Dental And Oral

DEFENSE BLOOD STANDARD SYSTEM (DBSS) 703-681-3901
5205 Leesburg Pike, Suite 1000, Falls Church, VA 22041
FDA Number: 1119523
Software, Blood Bank (Stand-Alone Products) Hematology

DEFIANCE METAL PROD CO. 419-784-5332
21 Seneca St., Defiance, OH 43512
FDA Number: 1526185

DEFIANCE METAL PROD CO. 419-784-5332 (cont'd)
Ownership: Private
Produces/Sells CE-marked Devices: N
Lamp, Ultraviolet, Physical Medicine Physical Med

DEFIBTECH LLC 866-333-4248
741Boston Post Rd., Suite 201, 203-453-4507
Guilford, CT 06437
FDA Number: n/a Fax: 203-453-6657
E-mail: sales@defibtech.com.
Web site: www.defibtech.com
Ownership: Private
Produces/Sells CE-marked Devices: N
Defibrillator, External, Automatic Cardiovascular

DEFLECTO CORP. 800-428-4328
7035 E. 86th St., Indianapolis, IN 46250 317-849-9555
FDA Number: n/a Fax: 877-333-5351
E-mail: tomb@deflecto.com
Web site: www.deflecto.com
Medical Products Sales Volume: $54,500,000
Annual Revenue: $10-$25 Million
Total Employees: 726
Ownership: JORDAN INDUSTRIES
Produces/Sells CE-marked Devices: N
Federal Procurement Eligibility: GSA Contract
Distribution: Manufacturer Through Distributor, Manufacturer Through Manufacturer Reps, Exporter
General Admin.: Henry Janzen/President, Chief Executive Officer
Mktg./Adv.: Tammy McKnight/Manager Advertising
John Wood/Manager National Sales
Tom Bratton/Vice President Sales
Cabinet, Other General
Hook, Other Surgery
Office Product General
Paper, Chart, Record, Medical General

DEGANIA SILICONE, INC. 401-349-5373
14 Thurber Boulevard, Suite A, Smithfield, RI 02917
FDA Number: 8030107 Fax: 401-349-5374
E-mail: info@deganiasilicone.com
Web site: www.deganiasilicone.com
Year Founded: 1984
Total Employees: 220
Ownership: Degania Silicone, Ltd.
Quality System Registration Information: ISO9001
Produces/Sells CE-marked Devices: Y
Distribution: Manufacturer Direct, Manufacturer Through Distributor, OEM
General Admin.: Nancy Jones/Office Manager
Steve Bellin/President
Catheter, Balloon (Foley Type) Surgery
Catheter, Retention Type, Balloon Gastroenterology/Urology
Catheter, Ureteral, General & Plastic Surgery Surgery
Component, Silicone General
Contract Manufacturing General
Drain, Suction, Closed Surgery
Drain, Thoracic (Chest) Anesthesiology
Tubing, Silicone General

DEGASA, S.A. DE C.V. 525-5-483 31
Prolongacion Canal De, Miramontes #3775 Col. Ex-,
Hacienda San Juan Del. Tlalpan Mexico
FDA Number: 8030654
Bandage, Cast Physical Med
Bandage, Elastic General
Cotton, Roll Dental And Oral
Gauze, Absorbable Surgery
Gauze, Non-Absorbable, Non-Medicated (Internal Sponge) Surgery
Paddie, Cottonoid Cns/Neurology

DEGUSSA - NEY DENTAL INC. 800-221-0168
65 W. Dudley Town Rd., Bloomfield, CT 06002 -
FDA Number: n/a Fax: 877-630-2894
Web site: www.neydental.com
Annual Revenue: $50-$100 Million
Total Employees: 155 Marketing Staff: 4 Sales Staff: 45
Ownership: Public
Traded On: NYSE
Produces/Sells CE-marked Devices: N
Distribution: Manufacturer Through Distributor
Dental Laboratory Equipment Dental And Oral
Metal, Medical General
Powder, Porcelain Dental And Oral

DEJARNETTE RESEARCH SYSTEMS 410-583-0680
401 Washington Avenue, Suite 1010, Towson, MD 21204
FDA Number: 1123714 Fax: 410-583-0696
E-mail: info@dejarnette.com

DEJARNETTE RESEARCH SYSTEMS — 410-583-0680 (cont'd)
Web site: www.dejarnette.com
Medical Products Volume: $3,500,000
Year Founded: 1985
Total Employees: 60
Ownership: Private
Quality System Registration Information: ISO9001
Produces/Sells CE-marked Devices: N
Federal Procurement Eligibility: Small Business, GSA Contract, VA Contract
Distribution: OEM

Camera, Multi Format	Radiology
Device, Storage, Image, Digital	Radiology
System, Communication, Image, Digital	Radiology

DEKA MEDICAL — 662-327-9950
665 3rd st ste 20, san francisco, CA 94107
FDA Number: 3007771416   Fax: 662-329-2349
E-mail: contactdeka@dekaresearch.com
Total Employees: 600
Ownership: Private
Quality System Registration Information: ISO9000
Produces/Sells CE-marked Devices: N
Distribution: OEM
General Admin.: Kim Vought/President
          Joni Withers/Vice President
Mktg./Adv.: Kathy Zachry/Vice President Marketing & Sales
Production: Gerald Nelson/Vice President Operations

Contract Manufacturing	General
Cover, Mattress	General
Equipment, Extruding/Molding	General

DEKA RESEARCH & DEVELOPMENT CORP. — 603-669-5139
340 Commercial St., Manchester, NH 03101-1121
FDA Number: 1220973   Fax: 603-624-0573
E-mail: contactdeka@dekaresearch.com
Web site: www.dekaresearch.com
Total Employees: 175
Ownership: Private
Quality System Registration Information: ISO9001
Produces/Sells CE-marked Devices: Y
Federal Procurement Eligibility: Small Business
Distribution: Service Direct
General Admin.: Dean Kamen/President
Mktg./Adv.: Charlie Grinell/Director Product Development
Production: Roger Leroux/Director Quality Assurance
          Roger Leroux/Manager Regulatory Affairs
          Robert Manning/Vice President Manufacturing

Contract R&D, Equipment	General
Controller, Infusion, Intravascular	General
Extracorporeal Photopheresis System	Gastroenterology/Urology
Infusion Pump, Enteral	General
Monitor, Infusion, Gravity Flow	General
Peritoneal Dialysis Unit (CAPD)	Gastroenterology/Urology
Service, Engineering/Design	General
Wheelchair, Stair Climbing	Physical Med

DEL DENT DENTAL SUPPLIED LTD. — 800-268-6657 / 416-222-8469
127 Willowdale Ave.,
Willowdale, ONT M2N-4 Canada
FDA Number: n/a   Fax: 416-223-2526
E-mail: DDS@DelDent.ca
Web site: www.deldent.ca
Year Founded: 1983
Total Employees: 10
Ownership: Private
Produces/Sells CE-marked Devices: N
Distribution: Service Direct, Exclusive Distributor

DEL ELECTRONICS CORP.
See Del Global Technologies Corp.

DEL GLOBAL TECHNOLOGIES CORP. — 914-686-3600
1 Commerce Pk., Valhalla, NY 10595-1455
FDA Number: n/a   Fax: 914-686-5425
Annual Revenue: $1-$5 Million
Total Employees: 290   Marketing Staff: 4   Sales Staff: 6
Ownership: Public
Stock Symbol: DGTC
Traded On: OTC Bulletin
Quality System Registration Information: ISO9000
Produces/Sells CE-marked Devices: Y
Federal Procurement Eligibility: Small Business
Distribution: Manufacturer Direct, Manufacturer Through Manufacturer Reps, Exporter
General Admin.: Lenard A. Trugman/Chief Executive Officer
          George Solomon/President
          Louis Farin/Vice President, General Manager
Mktg./Adv.: Jeremy Simon/Director Marketing & Sales
          Karl Weybig/Vice President Sales

DEL GLOBAL TECHNOLOGIES CORP. — 914-686-3600 (cont'd)
Finance: Michael Taber/Chief Financial Officer

Power System, Isolated	General

DEL MEDICAL SYSTEMS — 800-800-6006 / 847-288-7000
50 B. N. Gary Avenue, Roselle, IL 60172
FDA Number: 1418964   Fax: 847-288-7011
E-mail: usa_sales@delmedical.com
Web site: www.delmedical.com
Medical Products Sales Volume: $83,010,000
Annual Revenue: $50-$100 Million
Year Founded: 1929
Total Employees: 230   Marketing Staff: 3   Sales Staff: 8
Ownership: DEL GLOBAL TECHNOLOGIES CORPORATION
Quality System Registration Information: ISO9000; ISO9001
Produces/Sells CE-marked Devices: Y
Federal Procurement Eligibility: Small Business, Minority Owned
Distribution: Manufacturer Through Distributor, OEM, Exporter
General Admin.: Walt Schneider/President, Chief Executive Officer
Mktg./Adv.: Jennifer Fisher/Coord. Marketing & Sales
          Scott Loehrke/Director Marketing & Advertising
          Tony Bavuso/Director Product Development
          Joe Bavuso/Manager International Sales
          Steve Dahlquist/Vice President International Marketing & Sales
          Scott Loehrke/Vice President Marketing & Sales
Production: Steve Schiera/Director Quality Assurance & Regulatory Affairs
          Steve Schiera/Plant Manager
          Scott Loehrke/Product Manager

Generator, Diagnostic X-Ray, High Voltage, Single Phase	Radiology
Holder, Radiographic Cassette, Wall-Mounted	Radiology
Holder, X-Ray Film	Dental And Oral
Mount, X-Ray Tube, Diagnostic	Radiology
Radiographic Unit, Diagnostic, Chest	Radiology
Radiographic Unit, Diagnostic, Dental (X-Ray)	Dental And Oral
Radiographic Unit, Diagnostic, Fixed (X-Ray)	Radiology
Radiographic Unit, Diagnostic, Head	Radiology
Radiographic Unit, Diagnostic, Intraoral	Dental And Oral
Radiographic Unit, Diagnostic, Mammographic	Radiology
Radiographic Unit, Diagnostic, Tomographic	Radiology
System, X-Ray, Mobile	Radiology
Table, Radiographic	Radiology
Table, Radiographic, Stationary Top	Radiology

DEL PHARMACEUTICALS, INC.(SUBSIDIARY OF DEL LABORA — 516-844-2020
1830 Carver Drive, Rocky Point, NC 28457
FDA Number: 3001238190
Ownership: Private
Produces/Sells CE-marked Devices: N

Bandage, Liquid	Surgery
Detector/Remover, Lice	General
Toothbrush, Manual	Dental And Oral
Toothbrush, Powered	Dental And Oral

DELAWARE DIAMOND KNIVES — 800-222-5143 / 302-999-7476
3825 Lancaster Pike, Wilmington, DE 19805
FDA Number: n/a   Fax: 302-999-8320
Web site: www.ddk.com
Ownership: Private
Produces/Sells CE-marked Devices: N
Federal Procurement Eligibility: Small Business
Distribution: Manufacturer Direct, Manufacturer Through Distributor
General Admin.: Joe Tabeling/Chief Executive Officer
Mktg./Adv.: Pete Montr/Director Marketing

Instrument, Diamond, Dental	Dental And Oral
Knife, Other	Surgery
Scalpel, One-Piece (Knife)	Surgery

DELCATH SYSTEMS INC. — 212-489-2100
810 Seventh Avenue, Suite 3505, New York City, NY 10019
FDA Number: 3008822486   Fax: 212-489-2102
E-mail: info@delcath.com
Web site: www.delcath.com
Ownership: Public
Stock Symbol: DCTH
Traded On: NASDAQ
Produces/Sells CE-marked Devices: N
General Admin.: Mr. Graham Miao/Chief Financial Officer, Executive Vice President
          Dr. Krishna Kandarpa/Chief Medical Officer, Vice President
          Mr. Harold Mapes/Executive Vice President
          Mr. Eamonn Hobbs/President, Chief Executive Officer
Medical Admin.: Mr. Jason Rifkin/Senior Vice President Clinical Affairs
Mktg./Adv.: Mr. Agustin Gago/Executive Vice President Marketing & Sales
Production: Mr. John Pupura/Executive Vice President Quality Assurance & Regulatory Affairs
          Mr. Chuck Frigon/Vice President Operations

DELCATH SYSTEMS INC. 212-489-2100 *(cont'd)*
Finance: Mr. David Mcdonald/Chief Financial Officer
Hemoperfusion System, Sorbent — Gastroenterology/Urology

DELCO WIRE WINDING COMPANY 610-296-0350
59 Street Rd., Newtown Square, PA 19073
FDA Number: 2521541 — Fax: 610-296-7809
E-mail: dwwcollc@verizon.net
Web site: www.delcowirewinding.com
Annual Revenue: $0-$1 Million
Year Founded: 1958
Ownership: Private
Produces/Sells CE-marked Devices: N
Federal Procurement Eligibility: Small Business, Female Owned
Distribution: Exclusive Distributor
General Admin.: Gloria Pyle/President
Suture, Laparoscopy	Surgery
Suture, Non-Absorbable, Steel, Monofilament & Multifilament	Surgery
Suture, Stainless Steel	Surgery
Wire, Ligature	Surgery

DELFI MEDICAL INNOVATIONS INC. 800-933-3022
Suite 106, 1099 West 8th Avenue, 604-742-0600
Vancouver, BC V6H 1 Canada
FDA Number: 9681444 — Fax: 604-742-3800
E-mail: info@delfimedical.com
Web site: www.delfimedical.com
Year Founded: 1994
Total Employees: 10
Ownership: Private
Produces/Sells CE-marked Devices: Y
Distribution: Manufacturer Direct, Exclusive Distributor, Exporter

DELMARK COMPANY, THE
See Novartis Nutrition

DELPHI CORPORATION 888-526-1426
5725 Delphi Dr., Troy, MI 48098 248-813-2000
FDA Number: 3004973301 — Fax: 248-813-5008
E-mail: medical@delphi.com
Web site: delphimedical.com
Ownership: Public
Stock Symbol: DPHIQ
Traded On: OTC Bulletin
Quality System Registration Information: ISO9000
Produces/Sells CE-marked Devices: Y
General Admin.: Jim Brown/Business Manager
Nasser Lukmani/Business Manager
Production: John Mann/Manager Quality Assurance & Regulatory Affairs

DELPHI MEDICAL SYSTEMS
See Delphi Corporation

DELSTAR TECHNOLOGIES, INC. 800-521-6713
601 Industrial Dr., Middletown, DE 19709 302-378-8888
FDA Number: n/a — Fax: 302-378-4482
E-mail: info@delstarinc.com
Web site: www.delstarinc.com
Annual Revenue: $25-$50 Million
Year Founded: 2001
Total Employees: 250 — *Marketing Staff:* 2 — *Sales Staff:* 7
Ownership: APPLIED EXTRUSION TECHNOLOGIES, INC.
Stock Symbol: AETC
Traded On: NASDAQ
Produces/Sells CE-marked Devices: N
Distribution: Manufacturer Direct, Manufacturer Through Manufacturer Reps, OEM, Exporter
General Admin.: Mark Abrahams/Chief Executive Officer
Mktg./Adv.: Marjorie Wilcox/Director Marketing
D. Timothy Cullen/Vice President Sales
Dressing, Non-Adherent	General
Dressing, Other	General
Pad, Dressing	General
Retainer, Bandage (Elastic Net)	General
Tape, Adhesive	General

DELSYS, INC. 617-236-0599
650 Beacon St., 6th Flr., Boston, MA 02215
FDA Number: 1226013 — Fax: 617-236-0549
E-mail: delsys@delsys.com
Web site: www.delsys.com
Ownership: Private
Produces/Sells CE-marked Devices: N
Biofeedback Device	Cns/Neurology
Electromyograph, Diagnostic	Physical Med

DELTA GLOVES 800-220-1262
6865 Shiloh Rd. E., Ste. 400, 770-886-1400
Alpharetta, GA 30005
FDA Number: n/a — Fax: 770-886-1500
E-mail: tbdelta@bellsouth.net
Web site: www.deltagloves.com
Annual Revenue: $5-$10 Million
Year Founded: 1987
Total Employees: 16 — *Marketing Staff:* 4 — *Sales Staff:* 8
Ownership: Private
Quality System Registration Information: ISO9002
Produces/Sells CE-marked Devices: N
Federal Procurement Eligibility: Small Business
Distribution: Manufacturer Direct, Manufacturer Through Distributor, Exclusive Distributor
Glove, Patient Examination	General
Glove, Patient Examination, Latex	General
Glove, Patient Examination, Vinyl	General

DELTA HEALTH TECHNOLOGIES, LLC 800-444-1651
400 Lakemont Park Blvd., Altoona, PA 16603 814-944-1651
FDA Number: n/a — Fax: 814-942-0125
E-mail: Sales@DeltaHealthTech.com
Web site: www.deltahealth.com
Medical Products Sales Volume: $20,000,000
Annual Revenue: $25-$50 Million
Year Founded: 1974
Ownership: Private
Produces/Sells CE-marked Devices: N
Computer Software, Home Healthcare	General

DELTA INDUSTRIAL SERVICES, INC. 800-279-3358
11501 Eagle St. N.W., 763-755-7744
Minneapolis, MN 55448
FDA Number: n/a — Fax: 763-755-7799
E-mail: delta@deltaind.com
Web site: www.deltaind.com
Medical Products Sales Volume: $3,600,000
Annual Revenue: $10-$25 Million
Year Founded: 1977
Total Employees: 45 — *Marketing Staff:* 1 — *Sales Staff:* 7
Ownership: Private
Quality System Registration Information: ISO9001
Produces/Sells CE-marked Devices: N
Federal Procurement Eligibility: Small Business
Distribution: Manufacturer Direct
General Admin.: Vic Schiebout/General Manager
David Schiebout/President, Chief Executive Officer
Toby Fuerst/Vice President, Vice President Human Resources
Mktg./Adv.: Joel Oakes/Manager International Marketing & Sales
Packaging Equipment	General
Production Equipment	General

DELTA MEDICAL
See Delta Gloves

DELTA PRODUCTS CORP. 510-668-5100
4405 Cushing Parkway, Fremont, CA 94538
FDA Number: n/a — Fax: 510-668-0680
Web site: www.delta.com
Year Founded: 1971
Ownership: DELTA ELECTRONICS INC.
Quality System Registration Information: ISO9000
Produces/Sells CE-marked Devices: N
Distribution: Manufacturer Direct, Manufacturer Through Distributor, Manufacturer Through Manufacturer Reps, OEM
Computer Equipment	General
Filter, Radiographic	Radiology

DELTA SCIENTIFIC LABORATORY PRODUCTS LTD. 800-387-3256
1287 Matheson Blvd. East, 905-629-4545
Mississauga, ONT L4W-1 Canada
FDA Number: n/a — Fax: 905-629-7249
E-mail: info@delta-sci.com
Web site: http://www.delta-sci.com
Year Founded: 1985
Total Employees: 10
Ownership: Private
Produces/Sells CE-marked Devices: N
Distribution: Exclusive Distributor

DELTA SURGICAL SPECIALTIES LTD. 800-838-8585
8726 Barnard St., P.O. Box 95008, 604-325-8333
Vancouver, BC V6P-6 Canada
FDA Number: n/a — Fax: 604-325-0517
Year Founded: 1982

DELTA SURGICAL SPECIALTIES LTD. 800-838-8585 *(cont'd)*
Ownership: Private
Produces/Sells CE-marked Devices: N
Distribution: Exclusive Distributor

DELTA SYSTEMS DE MEXICO 702-331-1890
Prolongacion Las Lomas No. 16, Tijuana, B.c. Mexico
FDA Number: 9616077
Cannula, Nasal, Oxygen   Anesthesiology

DELTAGEN INC. 650-345-7600
1900 S. Norfolk St., Suite 105, San Mateo, CA 94403
FDA Number: n/a
Web site: http://www.deltagen.com
Ownership: Public
Stock Symbol: DGEN
Traded On: OTC Bulletin
Produces/Sells CE-marked Devices: N
General Admin.: Dr. Winston Thomas/Chief Operating Officer
    Dr. Robert Driscoll/President, Chief Executive Officer
Finance: Mr. Daniel Ratto/Chief Financial Officer

DELTATRAK, INC. 800-962-6776
PO Box 398, Pleasanton, CA 94566 925-249-2250
FDA Number: n/a   *Fax:* 925-249-2251
E-mail: FWU@deltatrak.com
Web site: www.deltatrak.com
Medical Products Sales Volume: $8,600,000
Annual Revenue: $5-$10 Million
Year Founded: 1989
Total Employees: 75   *Marketing Staff:* 3   *Sales Staff:* 20
Ownership: Private
Produces/Sells CE-marked Devices: Y
Federal Procurement Eligibility: Small Business, Minority Owned
Distribution: Manufacturer Direct, Manufacturer Through Manufacturer Reps
General Admin.: Fred Wu/President, Chief Executive Officer
Mktg./Adv.: Fred Wu/Manager International & National Sales
Production: Alan Hui/Vice President Operations
Cleanroom Equipment   General
Regulator, Temperature   Chemistry
Thermometer, Electronic   General
Thermometer, Infrared   General

DELTEC SYSTEMS
See Smiths Medical Asd, Inc.

DELTRONIC CORP. 800-451-6922
3900 West Segerstrom Avenue, 714-545-0401
Santa Ana, CA 92704
FDA Number: n/a   *Fax:* 800-969-3358
E-mail: sales@deltronic.com
Web site: www.deltronic.com
Annual Revenue: $0-1 Million
Year Founded: 1955
Ownership: Private
Produces/Sells CE-marked Devices: Y
Federal Procurement Eligibility: Small Business
Distribution: Manufacturer Through Distributor
Component, Optical   General

DELVAL GLASS, INC. 302-656-6606
1135 E. 7th St., Wilmington, DE 19801-4501
FDA Number: n/a
Medical Products Sales Volume: $150,000
Annual Revenue: $0-1 Million
Ownership: Private
Produces/Sells CE-marked Devices: N
Federal Procurement Eligibility: Small Business
Distribution: Manufacturer Direct, Service Direct
Service, Parts, Repair   General

DEMETECH CORP. 888-324-2447
3530 N.w. 115th Ave., Miami, FL 33178 305-597-5277
FDA Number: n/a   *Fax:* 305-437-7607
E-mail: info@demetech.us
Web site: www.demetech.us
Ownership: Private
Produces/Sells CE-marked Devices: N
Applicator, Tipped, Absorbent, Sterile   General
Bandage, Elastic   General
Blade, Scalpel   Surgery
Caliper, Ophthalmic   Ophthalmology
Cannula, Ophthalmic   Ophthalmology
Cuff, Blood Pressure   Cardiovascular
Curette, Ophthalmic   Ophthalmology
Forceps, Ophthalmic   Ophthalmology
Glove, Patient Examination, Latex   General
Glove, Surgical, Plastic Surgery   Surgery
Holder, Needle   Gastroenterology/Urology

DEMETECH CORP. 888-324-2447 *(cont'd)*
Hook, Ophthalmic   Ophthalmology
Monitor, Blood Pressure, Indirect, Semi-Automatic Cardiovascular
Needle, Conduction, Anesthesia (W/Wo Introducer) Anesthesiology
Percussor   Cns/Neurology
Scale, Stand-On   General
Scissors, Ophthalmic   Ophthalmology
Spatula, Ophthalmic   Ophthalmology
Spud, Ophthalmic   Ophthalmology
Stapler, Surgical   Surgery
Stethoscope, Manual   Cardiovascular
Suture, Absorbable, Natural   Surgery
Suture, Absorbable, Synthetic, Polyglycolic Acid Surgery
Suture, Dental   Dental And Oral
Suture, Non-Absorbable, Silk   Surgery
Suture, Non-Absorbable, Synthetic, Polyamide   Surgery
Suture, Non-Absorbable, Synthetic, Polyethylene Surgery
Suture, Non-Absorbable, Synthetic, Polypropylene Surgery
Template   Orthopedics
Tray, Surgical Instrument   Surgery
Walker, Mechanical   Physical Med
Wheelchair, Manual   Physical Med

DEMLAR MONITOR
See Monitor Instruments Inc.

DEN-MAT HOLDINGS, LLC 800-433-6628
2727 Skyway Dr., Santa Maria, CA 93455 805-922-8491
FDA Number: 2018957
E-mail: info@denmat.com
Web site: www.denmat.com
Ownership: Private
Produces/Sells CE-marked Devices: N
General Admin.: Mr. Todd Tiberi/Chief Administrative Officer
    Mr. Steven Semmelmayer/Chief Executive Officer
    Mr. Robert Cartagena/Chief Operating Officer
Adhesive, Bracket And Conditioner, Resin   Dental And Oral
Agent, Polishing, Abrasive, Oral Cavity   Dental And Oral
Alloy, Amalgam   Dental And Oral
Alloy, Precious Metal, For Clinical Use   Dental And Oral
Carver, Dental Amalgam, Operative   Dental And Oral
Cement, Dental   Dental And Oral
Cleaner, Denture, Mechanical   Dental And Oral
Cleanser, Root Canal   Dental And Oral
Coating, Filling Material, Resin   Dental And Oral
Crown And Bridge, Temporary, Resin   Dental And Oral
Crown, Preformed   Dental And Oral
Dam, Rubber   Dental And Oral
Disk, Abrasive   Dental And Oral
Floss, Dental   Dental And Oral
Instrument, Diamond, Dental   Dental And Oral
Light, Fiberoptic, Dental   Dental And Oral
Material, Impression   Dental And Oral
Material, Tooth Shade, Resin   Dental And Oral
Matrix, Dental   Dental And Oral
Point, Abrasive   Dental And Oral
Post, Root Canal   Dental And Oral
Powder, Porcelain   Dental And Oral
Sealant, Pit And Fissure, And Conditioner, Resin Dental And Oral
Solution, Cement Dissolving   Dental And Oral
Tooth Bonding Agent, Resin Restoration   Dental And Oral

DENALI R&D CORPORATION 781-826-9190
134 Old Washington Street, Hanover, MA 02339
FDA Number: 3006367836
Material, Tooth Shade, Resin   Dental And Oral
Sealant, Pit And Fissure, And Conditioner, Resin Dental And Oral

DENART AESTHETIC DESIGN, S.F. 415-392-2233
450 Sutter St., Suite 1215, San Francisco, CA 94108
FDA Number: n/a
Ownership: Private
Produces/Sells CE-marked Devices: N
Crown, Preformed   Dental And Oral

DENBUR, INC. 630-969-6865
433 Plaza Drive, Unit 4, Westmont, IL 60559
FDA Number: 3006264569
Ownership: Private
Produces/Sells CE-marked Devices: N
Applicator, Resin   Dental And Oral
Filling, Instrument Plastic, Dental   Dental And Oral
Light, Fiberoptic, Dental   Dental And Oral
Syringe, Periodontic, Endodontic   Dental And Oral

DENCRAFT 800-328-9729
PO Box 57, Moorestown, NJ 08057-0057 856-784-0154
FDA Number: n/a   *Fax:* 856-784-5428
E-mail: sales@dencraftonline.com
Web site: www.dencraftonline.com
Annual Revenue: $1-$5 Million

DENCRAFT · 800-328-9729 (cont'd)

Total Employees: 18
Ownership: Private
Produces/Sells CE-marked Devices: N
Federal Procurement Eligibility: Small Business
Distribution: Manufacturer Through Distributor, OEM, Importer, Exporter
Mktg./Adv.: David Duer/Director Marketing

Cabinet, Table And Tray, Anesthesia	Anesthesiology
Casting Unit, Dental	Dental And Oral
Cleaner, Ultrasonic, Medical Instrument	General
Compressor, External, Cardiac, Powered	General
Electrosurgical Unit, Dental	Dental And Oral
Handpiece, Air-Powered, Dental	Dental And Oral
Jar, Operating Room	Surgery
Light, Dental	Dental And Oral
Pump, Suction Operatory	Dental And Oral
Radiographic Unit, Diagnostic, Dental (X-Ray)	Dental And Oral
Retainer, Matrix	Dental And Oral
Sterilizer, Dry Heat	General
Sterilizer, Steam (Autoclave), Dental	Dental And Oral
Tray, Surgical Instrument	Surgery

DENDREON CORP. · 866-477-6782
3005 First Avenue, Seattle, WA 98121 · **206-256-4545**

FDA Number: 2953124 — *Fax:* 206-256-0571
E-mail: ir@dendreon.com
Web site: www.dendreon.com
Medical Products Sales Volume: $300,000
Year Founded: 1992
Total Employees: 208
Ownership: Public
Stock Symbol: DNDN
Traded On: NASDAQ
Produces/Sells CE-marked Devices: N
Federal Procurement Eligibility: Small Business

Medium, Lymphocyte Separation	Hematology
System, Concentration, Hematopoietic Stem Cell	Hematology

DENISON ORTHOPAEDIC APPLIANCE CORP.
See C.D. Denison Orthopaedic Appliance Corp.

DENLOK, INC.
See Denovo Dental, Inc.

DENMED TECHNOLOGIES, INC. · 866-433-6633
1531 West Orangewood Avenue, · **714-532-1107**
Orange, CA 92868

FDA Number: 2032547 — *Fax:* 714-532-2063
E-mail: Sales@denmedtech.com
Web site: www.denmedtech.com
Medical Products Sales Volume: $1,000,000
Annual Revenue: $0-$1 Million
Year Founded: 2000
Total Employees: 4 — *Marketing Staff:* 2 — *Sales Staff:* 4
Ownership: Private
Produces/Sells CE-marked Devices: Y
Federal Procurement Eligibility: Small Business, Minority Owned
Distribution: Manufacturer Direct, Manufacturer Through Distributor, OEM, Service Direct, Exclusive Distributor, Importer, Exporter

Material, Tooth Shade, Resin	Dental And Oral
Operative Dental Treatment Unit	Dental And Oral

DENNISON MANUFACTURING CO.
See Avery Dennison Corporation

DENOVO DENTAL, INC. · 800-854-7949
5130 Commerce Drive, Baldwin Park, CA 91706 · **626-939-5000**

FDA Number: 2032006 — *Fax:* 626-939-5020
E-mail: info@denovodental.com
Web site: www.denovodental.com
Medical Products Sales Volume: $3,000,000
Annual Revenue: $1-$5 Million
Year Founded: 1988
Total Employees: 16 — *Marketing Staff:* 1 — *Sales Staff:* 2
Ownership: Private
Produces/Sells CE-marked Devices: Y
Federal Procurement Eligibility: Small Business
Distribution: Manufacturer Direct, Service Direct, Exclusive Distributor, Exporter
General Admin.: Richard Parker/President, Chief Executive Officer
Joe Parker/Vice President, General Manager
Kim Altomare/Vice President, General Manager

Band, Matrix	Dental And Oral
Forceps	Orthopedics
Maintainer, Space Preformed, Orthodontic	Dental And Oral

DENPLUS INC. · 888-344-4424
2186 de la Province, · **450-646-1330**
Longueuil, QUE J4G 1 Canada

FDA Number: 9613743 — *Fax:* 450-646-1350
E-mail: info@denplus.com

DENPLUS INC. · 888-344-4424 (cont'd)

Web site: www.denplus.com
Year Founded: 1997
Total Employees: 10
Ownership: Private
Quality System Registration Information: ISO9001
Produces/Sells CE-marked Devices: N
Federal Procurement Eligibility: Small Business
Distribution: Manufacturer Direct, Manufacturer Through Distributor, Manufacturer Through Manufacturer Reps, Exclusive Distributor, Importer, Exporter

DENT ZAR, INC. · 800-444-1241
6362 Hollywood Blvd., #214, · **323-465-3621**
Los Angeles, CA 90028

FDA Number: 2027375 — *Fax:* 323-465-2994
E-mail: dentzar@yahoo.com
Web site: www.dentzar.com
Annual Revenue: $0-$1 Million
Year Founded: 1988
Total Employees: 30 — *Sales Staff:* 15
Ownership: Private
Produces/Sells CE-marked Devices: N

Adhesive, Bracket And Conditioner, Resin	Dental And Oral
Agent, Polishing, Abrasive, Oral Cavity	Dental And Oral
Cement, Dental	Dental And Oral
Coating, Filling Material, Resin	Dental And Oral
Crown And Bridge, Temporary, Resin	Dental And Oral
Instrument, Diamond, Dental	Dental And Oral
Light, Fiberoptic, Dental	Dental And Oral
Material, Tooth Shade, Resin	Dental And Oral
Sealant, Pit And Fissure, And Conditioner, Resin	Dental And Oral
Tooth Bonding Agent, Resin Restoration	Dental And Oral
Varnish, Cavity	Dental And Oral

DENTAL COMPONENTS, INC. · 800-624-2793
305 N. Springbrook Road, Newberg, OR 97132 · **503-538-8343**

FDA Number: n/a — *Fax:* 503-538-9302
E-mail: orderdesk@dcionline.com
Web site: www.dcionline.com
Medical Products Sales Volume: $10,000,000
Annual Revenue: $50-$100 Million
Total Employees: 140 — *Marketing Staff:* 8 — *Sales Staff:* 8
Ownership: Private
Produces/Sells CE-marked Devices: N
Federal Procurement Eligibility: Small Business
Distribution: Manufacturer Through Distributor, Manufacturer Through Manufacturer Reps, OEM, Exporter
General Admin.: Regina Arrigo/Director Human Resources
John Spencer/President, Chief Executive Officer
Mktg./Adv.: Peggy Fisher/Director Marketing
Lee Shook/Director National Accounts
Mike Welstad/Director Product Development
Production: Steve Freeman/Manager Customer Services
Sid Brown/Manager Materials
Finance: Nancy Hanson/Controller

Evacuator, Oral Cavity	Dental And Oral
Syringe, Dental	Dental And Oral
Unit, Operative Dental, Accessories	Dental And Oral

DENTAL CONCEPTS LLC · 800-592-6661
90 north broadway, irvington, NYÿ 10533 · **914-524-6894**

FDA Number: 2433180 — *Fax:* 201-576-9780
E-mail: medtech@sourceoneglobal.com
Web site: www.dentalconcepts.com
Year Founded: 1981
Ownership: Private
Produces/Sells CE-marked Devices: N

Hand Instrument, Calculus Removal	Dental And Oral
Pick, Massaging	Dental And Oral

DENTAL CONTROL PRODUCTS
See Ranir, Llc

DENTAL HEALTH PRODUCTS, INC. · 800-828-6868
4011 Creek Rd., Youngstown, NY 14174-0355 · **716-754-2696**

FDA Number: n/a — *Fax:* 716-754-4352
E-mail: 71603.1103@compuserve.com
Web site: http://dhpinc.com/
Annual Revenue: $0-$1 Million
Total Employees: 6 — *Sales Staff:* 2
Ownership: Private
Produces/Sells CE-marked Devices: N
Federal Procurement Eligibility: Small Business
Distribution: Manufacturer Direct, Manufacturer Through Distributor
General Admin.: Peter Owen/President
John Owen/Vice President, General Manager
Mktg./Adv.: Denise Wood/Manager International & National Sales
Production: Janice Mariani/Manager Materials

DENTAL HEALTH PRODUCTS, INC. 800-828-6868 (cont'd)
Dental Laboratory Equipment — Dental And Oral
Office Equipment — General

DENTAL HEALTH PRODUCTS, INC. 716-754-2696
4011 Creek Rd., Youngstown, NY 14174
FDA Number: 3004927689
Ownership: Private
Produces/Sells CE-marked Devices: N
Absorber, Saliva, Paper — Dental And Oral

DENTAL INNOVATORS, INC. 877-921-3919
3016 grandoaks drive, 714-921-3919
Westlake Village, CA 91361
FDA Number: 2020685 Fax: 714-283-8603
E-mail: BahiaJo@aol.com
Annual Revenue: $0-$1 Million
Year Founded: 1975
Total Employees: 4
Ownership: Private
Produces/Sells CE-marked Devices: N
Federal Procurement Eligibility: Small Business, Female Owned
Distribution: OEM, Exclusive Distributor
General Admin.: W. Grant Johnson/President
Mktg./Adv.: Joanne Johnson/Vice President Marketing & Sales
Evacuator, Oral Cavity — Dental And Oral
Mouthpiece, Saliva Ejector — Dental And Oral

DENTAL PROCEDURES, INC. L.L.C. 973-267-6195
9 Baer Court, Morristown, NJ 07960
FDA Number: 3004837179
Ownership: Private
Produces/Sells CE-marked Devices: N
Denture, Preformed — Dental And Oral

DENTAL PROSTHETIC SERVICES, INC. 319-393-1990
1150 Old Marion Road Ne, Cedar Rapids, IA 52402
FDA Number: 3000171384
Ownership: Private
Produces/Sells CE-marked Devices: N
Device, Anti-Snoring — Ear/Nose/Throat

DENTAL RESOURCES 717-866-7571
52 West King St., Myerstwn, PA 17067
FDA Number: 2182674
Ownership: Private
Produces/Sells CE-marked Devices: N
Agent, Polishing, Abrasive, Oral Cavity — Dental And Oral
Articulators — Dental And Oral
Base, Denture, Relining, Repairing, Rebasing, Resin — Dental And Oral
Cup, Prophylaxis — Dental And Oral
Material, Impression Tray, Resin — Dental And Oral
Scraper, Tongue — Dental And Oral
Sealant, Pit And Fissure, And Conditioner, Resin — Dental And Oral
Tray, Fluoride, Disposable — Dental And Oral
Varnish, Cavity — Dental And Oral

DENTAL SERVICES GROUP OF PITTSBURGH 80-322-7080
101 South 10th Street, Pittsburgh, PA 15203 421-431-3353
FDA Number: 3004142463 Fax: 412-431-6208
E-mail: gturnbull@dentalservices.net
Web site: www.dentalservices.net
Ownership: Private
Produces/Sells CE-marked Devices: N
Crown, Preformed — Dental And Oral
Device, Anti-Snoring — Ear/Nose/Throat
Device, Repositioning, Jaw — Dental And Oral
Mouthguard — Dental And Oral
Reliner, Denture, OTC — Dental And Oral

DENTAL SYSTEMS GROUP 800- 332-3151
601 State Street, Utica, NY 13502 315-732-3151
FDA Number: 3003624475 Fax: 315-797-4836
E-mail: fred@dentalsystemsgroup.com
Web site: www.dentalsystemsgroup.com
Ownership: Private
Produces/Sells CE-marked Devices: N
Device, Anti-Snoring — Ear/Nose/Throat

DENTAL TECHNOLOGIES, INC. 800-229-0936
5601 Arnold Rd, Dublin, CA 94568 925-829-3611
FDA Number: 1413475 Fax: 925-828-0153
Ownership: Private
Produces/Sells CE-marked Devices: N
General Admin.: Mr. Bob Starr/Chief Administrative Officer
Mr. Lee Culp/Chief Technology Officer
Ms. Kimberly Bradshaw-Sickinger/President, Chief Executive Officer
Mktg./Adv.: Mr. Len Liptak/Vice President Marketing

DENTAL TECHNOLOGIES, INC. 800-229-0936 (cont'd)
Finance: Mr. Jeff Zellmer/Chief Financial Officer
Adhesive, Bracket And Conditioner, Resin — Dental And Oral
Agent, Polishing, Abrasive, Oral Cavity — Dental And Oral
Cement, Dental — Dental And Oral
Coating, Filling Material, Resin — Dental And Oral
Crown And Bridge, Temporary, Resin — Dental And Oral
Dam, Rubber — Dental And Oral
Material, Impression — Dental And Oral
Material, Impression Tray, Resin — Dental And Oral
Material, Tooth Shade, Resin — Dental And Oral
Sealant, Pit And Fissure, And Conditioner, Resin — Dental And Oral
Tray, Impression — Dental And Oral

DENTAL USA, INC. 866-439-3400
5005 Mccullom Lake Rd., Mchenry, IL 60050 815-363-8003
FDA Number: 3003969055 Fax: 15-363-3545
E-mail: info@mydentalusa.com
Web site: www.mydentalusa.com
Ownership: Private
Produces/Sells CE-marked Devices: N
Burnisher, Operative, Dental — Dental And Oral
Caliper — Orthopedics
Carrier, Amalgam, Operative — Dental And Oral
Carver, Dental Amalgam, Operative — Dental And Oral
Carver, Wax, Dental — Dental And Oral
Chisel, Bone, Surgical — Dental And Oral
Chisel, Surgical, Manual — Surgery
Curette — Orthopedics
Curette, Endodontic — Dental And Oral
Curette, Operative — Dental And Oral
Curette, Periodontic — Dental And Oral
Curette, Surgical, Dental — Dental And Oral
Cutter, Operative — Dental And Oral
Elevator, Surgical, Dental — Dental And Oral
Excavator, Dental, Operative — Dental And Oral
Explorer, Operative — Dental And Oral
File, Bone, Surgical — Dental And Oral
File, Margin Finishing, Operative — Dental And Oral
File, Periodontic — Dental And Oral
File, Pulp Canal, Endodontic — Dental And Oral
Filling, Instrument Plastic, Dental — Dental And Oral
Forceps — Orthopedics
Forceps, Articulation Paper — Dental And Oral
Forceps, Dressing, Dental — Dental And Oral
Forceps, Rongeur, Surgical — Dental And Oral
Forceps, Rubber Dam Clamp — Dental And Oral
Forceps, Tooth Extractor, Surgical — Dental And Oral
Gauge, Depth, Instrument, Dental — Dental And Oral
Handle, Instrument, Dental — Dental And Oral
Handle, Scalpel — Surgery
Hoe, Periodontic — Dental And Oral
Knife, Margin Finishing, Operative — Dental And Oral
Knife, Periodontic — Dental And Oral
Knife, Surgical — Dental And Oral
Matrix, Dental — Dental And Oral
Mirror, Mouth — Dental And Oral
Pliers, Operative — Dental And Oral
Pliers, Orthodontic — Dental And Oral
Pliers, Surgical — Orthopedics
Plugger, Root Canal, Endodontic — Dental And Oral
Preparer, Root Canal, Endodontic — Dental And Oral
Probe — Orthopedics
Probe, Periodontic — Dental And Oral
Remover, Crown — Dental And Oral
Retainer, Matrix — Dental And Oral
Retractor, All Types — Dental And Oral
Rongeur, Rib — Orthopedics
Scaler, Periodontic — Dental And Oral
Scissors, Orthopedic — Orthopedics
Spatula, Surgical, General & Plastic Surgery — Surgery
Speculum, Vaginal, Metal — Obstetrics/Gynecology
Spreader, Pulp Canal Filling Material, Endodontic — Dental And Oral
Syringe, Ear — Ear/Nose/Throat
Tray, Impression — Dental And Oral
Tray, Surgical Instrument — Surgery

DENTAL/MEDICAL OPTICS MFG., INC. 516-889-5857
4217 Austin Blvd., Island Park, NY 11558
FDA Number: 2435774
Ownership: Private
Produces/Sells CE-marked Devices: N
Accessories, Apparel, Surgical — Surgery

DENTALAIRE PRODUCTS 800-866-6881
17150 Newhope #407, Fountain Valley, CA 92708 714-540-9969
FDA Number: 2087127 Fax: 714-540-9947
E-mail: klieber@dentalaireproducts.com
Web site: www.dentalaireproducts.com
Medical Products Sales Volume: $1,600,000
Annual Revenue: $1-$5 Million

DENTALAIRE PRODUCTS   800-866-6881 *(cont'd)*

Year Founded: 1988
Total Employees: 9   Sales Staff: 5
Ownership: Private
Quality System Registration Information: ISO9002
Produces/Sells CE-marked Devices: N
Federal Procurement Eligibility: Small Business
Distribution: Manufacturer Direct, Manufacturer Through Distributor
General Admin.: Kurt Leiber/Chief Executive Officer
                Kurt Leiber/President
                Ron Anderson/Vice President, General Manager
Production: John Voskuhl/Manager Materials

Dental Laboratory Equipment	Dental And Oral

DENTALAIRE PRODUCTS INTERNATIONAL INC.

See Dentalaire Products

DENTALEZ GROUP   866-DTE-INFO

2 West Liberty Boulevard, Ste. 160,   (610) 725-8004
Malvern, PA 19355
FDA Number: 2520265
E-mail: efficiency@dentalez.com   Fax: 610-725-9898
Web site: www.dentalez.com
Annual Revenue: $5-$10 Million
Total Employees: 135   Marketing Staff: 7   Sales Staff: 45
Ownership: Private
Quality System Registration Information: ISO9001
Produces/Sells CE-marked Devices: N
Federal Procurement Eligibility: Small Business
Distribution: Manufacturer Through Distributor
General Admin.: Carl Bretko/Chief Executive Officer
                Carl Bretko/President
Mktg./Adv.: Ed Schmitt/Manager Contract Sales
            Paco Rodriguez/Manager International & National Sales
            Aggie Pennington/Manager Product Development
            Ms. Randy Arner/Vice President Marketing
Production: John Morris/Director Quality Assurance
            Ed Holland/Vice President Manufacturing
Finance: Marc Rose/Chief Financial Officer

Base, Denture, Relining, Repairing, Rebasing, Resin	Dental And Oral
Burr, Dental	Dental And Oral
Burr, Dental Excavating	Dental And Oral
Cabinet, Dental	Dental And Oral
Capsule, Dental, Amalgam	Dental And Oral
Carver, Dental Amalgam, Operative	Dental And Oral
Cement, Dental	Dental And Oral
Chair, Dental	Dental And Oral
Chair, Operative	Dental And Oral
Coating, Filling Material, Resin	Dental And Oral
Condenser, Amalgam And Foil, Operative	Dental And Oral
Controller, Foot, Handpiece And Cord	Dental And Oral
Curette, Periodontic	Dental And Oral
Dam, Dental	Dental And Oral
Dispenser, Mercury And/Or Alloy	Dental And Oral
Drill, Dental, Intraoral	Dental And Oral
Electrosurgical Unit, Dental	Dental And Oral
Endodontic Instrument	Dental And Oral
Evacuator, Oral Cavity	Dental And Oral
Excavator, Dental, Operative	Dental And Oral
Explorer, Operative	Dental And Oral
File, Pulp Canal, Endodontic	Dental And Oral
Filling, Instrument Plastic, Dental	Dental And Oral
Forceps, Dressing, Dental	Dental And Oral
Frame, Rubber Dam	Dental And Oral
Gas-Machine, Analgesia	Anesthesiology
Gauge, Depth, Instrument, Dental	Dental And Oral
Gutta Percha	Dental And Oral
Hand Instrument, Calculus Removal	Dental And Oral
Handle, Instrument, Dental	Dental And Oral
Handpiece, Air-Powered, Dental	Dental And Oral
Handpiece, Belt and/or Gear Driven, Dental	Dental And Oral
Handpiece, Contra- And Right-Angle Attachment, Dental	Dental And Oral
Illuminator, Radiographic Film	Radiology
Instrument, Dental, Manual	Dental And Oral
Instrument, Diamond, Dental	Dental And Oral
Knife, Periodontic	Dental And Oral
Light, Dental	Dental And Oral
Light, Fiberoptic, Dental	Dental And Oral
Light, Surgical Operating, Dental	Dental And Oral
Material, Dental Filling	Dental And Oral
Material, Impression	Dental And Oral
Material, Tooth Shade, Resin	Dental And Oral
Matrix, Dental	Dental And Oral
Mercury	Dental And Oral
Microscope, Surgical	Ear/Nose/Throat
Mirror, Mouth	Dental And Oral
Operative Dental Treatment Unit	Dental And Oral
Periodontal Instrument	Dental And Oral
Pliers, Operative	Dental And Oral
Plugger, Root Canal, Endodontic	Dental And Oral

DENTALEZ GROUP   866-DTE-INFO *(cont'd)*

Point, Paper, Endodontic	Dental And Oral
Point, Silver, Endodontic	Dental And Oral
Post, Root Canal	Dental And Oral
Probe, Periodontic	Dental And Oral
Pump, Suction Operatory	Dental And Oral
Radiographic Unit, Diagnostic, Dental, Extraoral	Dental And Oral
Reamer, Pulp Canal, Endodontic	Dental And Oral
Remover, Crown	Dental And Oral
Scaler, Periodontic	Dental And Oral
Scaler, Rotary	Dental And Oral
Scaler, Ultrasonic	Dental And Oral
Splint, Endodontic Stabilizer	Dental And Oral
Spreader, Pulp Canal Filling Material, Endodontic	Dental And Oral
Sterilizer, Dry Heat, Dental	Dental And Oral
Sterilizer, Glass Bead	Dental And Oral
Stool, Dental	Dental And Oral
Syringe Unit, Air And/Or Water	Dental And Oral
Syringe, Dental	Dental And Oral
Syringe, Irrigating, Dental	Dental And Oral

Medical Product Subsidiaries (Listed Separately)
Ramvac Dental Products Inc

DENTALEZ GROUP, STARDENTAL DIVISION   717-291-1161

1816 Colonial Village Ln., Lancaster, PA 17601
FDA Number: 2520265

Burr, Dental	Dental And Oral
Carver, Dental Amalgam, Operative	Dental And Oral
Cement, Dental	Dental And Oral
Controller, Foot, Handpiece And Cord	Dental And Oral
Curette, Periodontic	Dental And Oral
Device, Limiting, Beam, Diagnostic, X-Ray	Radiology
Drill, Dental, Intraoral	Dental And Oral
Excavator, Dental, Operative	Dental And Oral
Explorer, Operative	Dental And Oral
Frame, Rubber Dam	Dental And Oral
Hand Instrument, Calculus Removal	Dental And Oral
Handle, Instrument, Dental	Dental And Oral
Handpiece, Air-Powered, Dental	Dental And Oral
Handpiece, Contra- And Right-Angle Attachment, Dental	Dental And Oral
Instrument, Diamond, Dental	Dental And Oral
Knife, Periodontic	Dental And Oral
Material, Impression	Dental And Oral
Matrix, Dental	Dental And Oral
Mirror, Mouth	Dental And Oral
Operative Dental Treatment Unit	Dental And Oral
Pliers, Operative	Dental And Oral
Plugger, Root Canal, Endodontic	Dental And Oral
Point, Silver, Endodontic	Dental And Oral
Preparer, Root Canal, Endodontic	Dental And Oral
Probe, Periodontic	Dental And Oral
Radiographic Unit, Diagnostic, Dental, Extraoral	Dental And Oral
Radiographic Unit, Diagnostic, Intraoral	Dental And Oral
Scaler, Periodontic	Dental And Oral
Scaler, Ultrasonic	Dental And Oral
Scissors, Surgical Tissue, Dental (Oral)	Dental And Oral
Spreader, Pulp Canal Filling Material, Endodontic	Dental And Oral
Syringe Unit, Air And/Or Water	Dental And Oral

DENTALEZ MANUFACTURING CO.

See Dentalez Group

DENTALEZ OF ALABAMA   251-937-6781

2500 U.s. Highway 31 South, Bay Minette, AL 36507
FDA Number: 1049061

Chair, Dental (With Unit)	Dental And Oral
Evacuator, Oral Cavity	Dental And Oral
Light, Surgical Operating, Dental	Dental And Oral
Operative Dental Treatment Unit	Dental And Oral

DENTALIUM DENTAL CERAMICS, INC.   949-440-2600

4141 Macarthur Blvd., Newport Beach, CA 92660
FDA Number: 1058855
Ownership: Private
Produces/Sells CE-marked Devices: N

Alloy, Precious Metal, For Clinical Use	Dental And Oral
Metal, Base	Dental And Oral

DENTAMERICA INC.   626-912-1388

18688 E. San Jise Ave., City of Industry, CA 91748
FDA Number: n/a   Fax: 626-913-0510
E-mail: info@dentamerica.com
Web site: www.dentamerica.com
Annual Revenue: $0-$1 Million
Year Founded: 1986
Ownership: Private
Quality System Registration Information: ISO9002
Produces/Sells CE-marked Devices: N
Federal Procurement Eligibility: Small Business
Distribution: Manufacturer Direct, Importer, Exporter

DENTAMERICA INC.   626-912-1388 *(cont'd)*
Light, Surgical Operating, Dental   Dental And Oral

DENTECH EQUIPMENT   800-826-5004
901 West Front Street, Sumas, WA 98295   **360-988-7080**
FDA Number: 3024061   *Fax:* 360-988-4050
E-mail: sales@dentechcorp.com
Web site: www.alliancehinc.com
Ownership: Private
Produces/Sells CE-marked Devices: N
Chair, Dental (With Unit)   Dental And Oral
Light, Surgical Operating, Dental   Dental And Oral
Unit, Operative Dental, Accessories   Dental And Oral

DENTECH PRODUCTS LIMITED   800-826-5004
31 Scarsdale Road, Unit #2,   **416-447-9500**
Toronto, ONTAR M3B 2 Canada
FDA Number: n/a   *Fax:* 416-447-3500
E-mail: canplant@dentechcorp.com
Web site: www.alliancehinc.com
Year Founded: 1972
Total Employees: 100
Ownership: Private
Produces/Sells CE-marked Devices: N
Distribution: Manufacturer Direct, Exporter

DENTECON, INC.   800-423-6088
1249 S. La Cienega Blvd.,   **310-854-3854**
Los Angeles, CA 90035
FDA Number: 2028264   *Fax:* 310-854-3852
E-mail: dentecon@pacbell.net
Annual Revenue: $0-$1 Million
Total Employees: 11   *Marketing Staff:* 2   *Sales Staff:* 6
Ownership: Private
Produces/Sells CE-marked Devices: N
Federal Procurement Eligibility: Small Business, Minority Owned
Distribution: Manufacturer Direct, Manufacturer Through Distributor, Manufacturer Through Manufacturer Reps, Service Direct, Importer
General Admin.: John Yavrouian/President
Mktg./Adv.: Vicky Yavrouian/Manager Marketing
Production: Raffi Bezjian/Manager Production & Engineering
Material, Casting   Dental And Oral

DENTEK ORAL CARE, INC.   865-983-1300
307 Excellence Way, Maryville, TN 37801
FDA Number: 2938386   *Fax:* 865-983-2444
E-mail: info@usdentek.com
Medical Products Sales Volume: $24,000,000
Year Founded: 1983
Total Employees: 65
Ownership: Private
Quality System Registration Information: ISO9001
Produces/Sells CE-marked Devices: Y
Federal Procurement Eligibility: Small Business
Distribution: Manufacturer Direct, Manufacturer Through Manufacturer Reps, Exclusive Distributor
Floss, Dental   Dental And Oral
Hand Instrument, Calculus Removal   Dental And Oral
Handle, Instrument, Dental   Dental And Oral
Mirror, Mouth   Dental And Oral
Pick, Massaging   Dental And Oral
Polyvinyl Methylether Maleic Acid-Calcium-Sodium Dbl. Salt   Dental And Oral
Scraper, Tongue   Dental And Oral
Toothbrush, Manual   Dental And Oral
Toothbrush, Powered   Dental And Oral
Wax, Dental   Dental And Oral
Zinc Oxide Eugenol   Dental And Oral

DENTICATOR CO., INC.
See Denticator International, Inc.

DENTICATOR INTERNATIONAL, INC.   866-469-6864
13705 Shoreline Court East,   **800-325-1881**
Earth City, MO 63045
FDA Number: 2939420   *Fax:* 314-344-0021
E-mail: info@denticator.com
Web site: http://www.denticator.com
Total Employees: 120   *Marketing Staff:* 3   *Sales Staff:* 3
Ownership: Young Innovations, Inc.
Stock Symbol: YDNT
Traded On: NASDAQ
Quality System Registration Information: ISO9001
Produces/Sells CE-marked Devices: Y
Federal Procurement Eligibility: Minority Owned
Distribution: Manufacturer Through Distributor, OEM, Importer, Exporter
General Admin.: Rick Richmand/President
Mktg./Adv.: John Rappe/Director Marketing
Agent, Polishing, Abrasive, Oral Cavity   Dental And Oral

DENTICATOR INTERNATIONAL, INC.   866-469-6864 *(cont'd)*
Cup, Prophylaxis   Dental And Oral
Handpiece, Air-Powered, Dental   Dental And Oral
Handpiece, Contra- And Right-Angle Attachment, Dental   Dental And Oral
Mirror, Mouth   Dental And Oral
Pick, Massaging   Dental And Oral
Tip, Rubber, Oral-Hygiene   Dental And Oral
Varnish, Cavity   Dental And Oral

DENTICATOR, DIV. OF SYNDEX LAB.
See Denticator International, Inc.

DENTICON INTERNATIONAL INC.   952-541-9622
840 North Grand Ave., Suite#13, Nogales, AZ 85621
FDA Number: 2032808
Ownership: Private
Produces/Sells CE-marked Devices: N
Mouthguard   Dental And Oral

DENTLIGHT INC.   972-889-8857
1411 E. Campbell Rd., Suite 500, Richardson, TX 75081
FDA Number: 3005515469
Activator, Ultraviolet, Polymerization   Dental And Oral
Bracket, Metal, Orthodontic   Dental And Oral
Explorer, Operative   Dental And Oral
Instrument, Manual, General Surgical   Surgery

DENTO-PROFILE SCALE CO.   800-936-8610
1010 Eighth Street, Suite A,   **619-435-4444**
Coronado, CA 92118
FDA Number: 2122521   *Fax:* 619-435-5379
E-mail: info@drpopp.com
Web site: www.drpopp.com
Medical Products Sales Volume: $300,000
Annual Revenue: $0-$1 Million
Total Employees: 2
Ownership: Private
Produces/Sells CE-marked Devices: N
Federal Procurement Eligibility: Small Business, Female Owned
Distribution: Manufacturer Direct, Service Direct, Exporter
General Admin.: Dr. Suzanne M. M. Popp/President, Chief Executive Officer
Instrument, Dental, Manual   Dental And Oral

DENTON VACUUM, INC.   856-439-9100
1259 North Church St., Moorestown, NJ 08057
FDA Number: n/a   *Fax:* 856-439-9111
E-mail: info@dentonvacuum.com
Web site: www.dentonvacuum.com
Annual Revenue: $0-$1 Million
Ownership: Private
Produces/Sells CE-marked Devices: N
Federal Procurement Eligibility: Small Business
Distribution: Manufacturer Direct, Manufacturer Through Manufacturer Reps, Service Direct
General Admin.: Rod Moore/President
Finance: Ellen Carson/Director Finance
Drying Unit   Chemistry
Evaporator   Chemistry

DENTRONIX, INC.   800-523-5944
235 Ascot Parkway, Cuyahoga Falls, OH 44223   **330-916-7300**
FDA Number: 2518439   *Fax:* 330-916-7333
E-mail: info@dentronix.com
Web site: www.dentronix.com
Medical Products Sales Volume: $5,500,000
Year Founded: 1977
Total Employees: 50   *Marketing Staff:* 1   *Sales Staff:* 11
Ownership: Coltene-Whaledent, Inc.
Quality System Registration Information: ISO9003
Produces/Sells CE-marked Devices: Y
Federal Procurement Eligibility: Small Business, VA Contract
Distribution: Manufacturer Direct, Manufacturer Through Distributor, Exporter
General Admin.: Jerry Sullivan/Chief Executive Officer
     Gerri Cevetillo/General Manager
Cleaner, Ultrasonic, Medical Instrument   General
Disinfector, Liquid   General
Pliers, Orthodontic   Dental And Oral
Pusher, Band, Orthodontic   Dental And Oral
Scaler, Ultrasonic   Dental And Oral
Scissors, Collar And Crown   Dental And Oral
Sterilizer, Dry Heat   General
Sterilizer, Dry Heat, Dental   Dental And Oral
Washer/Disinfector   General

DENTSPLY CANADA, LTD.   800-263-1437
161 Vinyl Ct., Woodbridge, ONT L4L 4A3 Canada   **905-851-6060**
FDA Number: n/a   *Fax:* 905-851-2453
E-mail: info@dentsply.ca
Web site: www.dentsply.ca

DENTSPLY CANADA, LTD.   800-263-1437 *(cont'd)*
Year Founded: 1899
Total Employees: 75   *Marketing Staff:* 6   *Sales Staff:* 30
Ownership: Dentsply International, Inc.
Stock Symbol: XRAY
Traded On: NASDAQ
Produces/Sells CE-marked Devices: N
Distribution: Manufacturer Direct, Service Direct, Exclusive Distributor

DENTSPLY CAULK   800-532-2855
38 West Clarke Avenue, Milford, DE 19963
FDA Number: 2515379   Fax: 800-788-4110
Web site: www.caulk.com
Medical Products Sales Volume: $80,000,000
Year Founded: 1877
Total Employees: 9400
Ownership: Dentsply International, Inc.
Stock Symbol: XRAY
Traded On: NASDAQ
Quality System Registration Information: ISO9000; ISO9001
Produces/Sells CE-marked Devices: Y
Federal Procurement Eligibility: Small Business
Distribution: Manufacturer Through Distributor
General Admin.: Bret W. Wise/Chief Executive Officer, Chairman
     William R. Jellison/Chief Financial Officer, Senior Vice President
     Tom Leonardi/Vice President, General Manager

Activator, Ultraviolet, Polymerization	Dental And Oral
Adhesive, Bracket And Conditioner, Resin	Dental And Oral
Agent, Polishing, Abrasive, Oral Cavity	Dental And Oral
Alloy, Amalgam	Dental And Oral
Amalgamator, Dental, AC-Powered	Dental And Oral
Cement, Dental	Dental And Oral
Crown, Preformed	Dental And Oral
Gutta Percha	Dental And Oral
Liner, Cavity, Calcium Hydroxide	Dental And Oral
Material, Impression	Dental And Oral
Material, Tooth Shade, Resin	Dental And Oral
Matrix, Dental	Dental And Oral
Point, Paper, Endodontic	Dental And Oral
Primer, Cavity, Resin	Dental And Oral
Retractor, Abdominal, Padded, Flexible	Surgery
Syringe, Restorative And Impression Material	Dental And Oral
Tray, Impression	Dental And Oral

DENTSPLY CERAMCO
See Dentsply Prosthetics

DENTSPLY FRIADENT CERAMED   717-849-4229
12860 West Cedar Dr.,suite 110, Lakewood, CO 80228
FDA Number: 1721411
Ownership: Private
Produces/Sells CE-marked Devices: N

Bone Grafting Material, Dental, With Biologic Component	Dental And Oral
Implant, Endosseous (Bone Filling and/or Augmentation)	Dental And Oral

DENTSPLY GAC INTERNATIONAL
See Dentsply Gac International

DENTSPLY GENDEX
See Dentsply Professional

DENTSPLY INTERNATIONAL, INC.   800-877-0020
Susquehanna Commerce Center   **717-845-7511**
221 W. Philadelphia Street
York, PA 17405
FDA Number: n/a
E-mail: webmaster@dentsply.com
Web site: www.dentsply.com
Medical Products Sales Volume: $1,810,000,000
Annual Revenue: More than $1 Billion
Year Founded: 1899
Total Employees: 9400
Ownership: Public
Stock Symbol: XRAY
Traded On: NASDAQ
Quality System Registration Information: ISO9001
Produces/Sells CE-marked Devices: Y
Distribution: Manufacturer Direct, Manufacturer Through Distributor
General Admin.: Bret W. Wise/Chief Executive Officer, Chairman
     William R. Jellison/Chief Financial Officer, Senior Vice President

Activator, Ultraviolet, Polymerization	Dental And Oral
Alloy, Precious Metal, For Clinical Use	Dental And Oral
Amalgamator, Dental, AC-Powered	Dental And Oral
Anchor, Preformed	Dental And Oral
Articulators	Dental And Oral
Base, Denture, Relining, Repairing, Rebasing, Resin	Dental And Oral
Bone Cement	Orthopedics
Capsule, Dental, Amalgam	Dental And Oral
Cement, Dental	Dental And Oral
Cement, Orthopedic (Bone)	Orthopedics
Chair, Dental	Dental And Oral

DENTSPLY INTERNATIONAL, INC.   800-877-0020 *(cont'd)*

Cleaner, Ultrasonic, Medical Instrument	General
Contract Manufacturing, Product, Durable	General
Crown, Preformed	Dental And Oral
Dental Laboratory Equipment	Dental And Oral
Denture, Plastic, Teeth	Dental And Oral
Dispenser, Mercury And/Or Alloy	Dental And Oral
Electrosurgical Unit, Dental	Dental And Oral
Evacuator, Oral Cavity	Dental And Oral
Filling, Instrument Plastic, Dental	Dental And Oral
Handle, Instrument, Dental	Dental And Oral
Instrument, Dental, Manual	Dental And Oral
Instrument, Diamond, Dental	Dental And Oral
Kit, Denture Repair, OTC	Dental And Oral
Material, Dental Filling	Dental And Oral
Material, Impression	Dental And Oral
Material, Investment	Dental And Oral
Material, Tooth Shade, Resin	Dental And Oral
Matrix, Dental	Dental And Oral
Plate, Base, Shellac	Dental And Oral
Powder, Porcelain	Dental And Oral
Prophylaxis Unit, Ultrasonic, Dental	Dental And Oral
Prosthesis, Dental	Dental And Oral
Pump, Vacuum, Central	Anesthesiology
Resin, Root Canal Filling	Dental And Oral
Retractor, All Types	Dental And Oral
Stool, Dental	Dental And Oral
Syringe Unit, Air And/Or Water	Dental And Oral
Syringe, Dental	Dental And Oral
Teeth, Artificial, Backing And Facing	Dental And Oral
Teeth, Artificial, Posterior With Metal Insert	Dental And Oral
Teeth, Porcelain	Dental And Oral
Varnish, Cavity	Dental And Oral
Wax, Dental	Dental And Oral
Wheel, Polishing Agent	Dental And Oral

Medical Product Subsidiaries (Listed Separately)
Dentsply Canada, Ltd.
Dentsply Caulk
Dentsply Gac International
Dentsply North America (Dna)
Dentsply Professional
Dentsply Prosthetics
Dentsply Rinn
Dentsply Specialty Materials
Dentsply Tulsa Dental Products
Dentsply Tulsa Dental Specialties
Dshealthcare Inc.
Glenroe Technologies
Orthodental Intl., Inc
Prident International Inc.
Roydent Dental Products
United Dental Mfg., Inc.

DENTSPLY NORTH AMERICA (DNA)   800-877-0020
400 1st St., Suite 250, Middletown, PA 17057
FDA Number: 3006186796
E-mail: webmaster@dentsply.com
Web site: www.dentsply.com
Annual Revenue: More than $1 Billion
Year Founded: 1899
Total Employees: 9400
Ownership: Dentsply International, Inc.
Stock Symbol: XRAY
Traded On: NASDAQ
Produces/Sells CE-marked Devices: N
General Admin.: Bret W. Wise/Chief Executive Officer, Chairman
     William R. Jellison/Chief Financial Officer, Senior Vice President

DENTSPLY PREVENTIVE CARE
See Dentsply Professional

DENTSPLY PROFESSIONAL   800-989-8825
1301 Smile Way, York, PA 17404   **717-767-8250**
FDA Number: 2424472
Web site: www.prevent.dentsply.com
Medical Products Sales Volume: $160,000,000
Annual Revenue: More than $1 Billion
Year Founded: 1899
Total Employees: 9400
Ownership: Dentsply International, Inc.
Stock Symbol: XRAY
Traded On: NASDAQ
Quality System Registration Information: ISO9001
Produces/Sells CE-marked Devices: Y
Distribution: Manufacturer Through Distributor, OEM, Exporter
General Admin.: Bret W. Wise/Chief Executive Officer, Chairman
     William R. Jellison/Chief Financial Officer, Senior Vice President

Airbrush	Dental And Oral
Bone Grafting Material, Dental, With Biologic Component	Dental And Oral
Dispenser, Medication, Liquid	General

DENTSPLY PROFESSIONAL   800-989-8825 (cont'd)

Handpiece, Air-Powered, Dental	Dental And Oral
Prophylaxis Unit, Ultrasonic, Dental	Dental And Oral
Scaler, Ultrasonic	Dental And Oral
Sealant, Pit And Fissure, And Conditioner, Resin	Dental And Oral
Syringe Unit, Air And/Or Water	Dental And Oral
Varnish, Cavity	Dental And Oral

DENTSPLY PROFESSIONAL   800-800-2888
901 West Oakton St., Des Plaines, IL 60018
FDA Number: 1419322   Fax: 847-640-6165
Web site: www.prevent.dentsply.com
Year Founded: 1899
Total Employees: 9400
Ownership: Dentsply International, Inc.
Stock Symbol: XRAY
Traded On: NASDAQ
Produces/Sells CE-marked Devices: N
General Admin.: Bret W. Wise/Chief Executive Officer, Chairman
    William R. Jellison/Chief Financial Officer, Senior Vice President

Burr, Dental	Dental And Oral
Camera, Television, Surgical (Without Audio)	Surgery
Collimator, X-Ray	Dental And Oral
Cup, Prophylaxis	Dental And Oral
Handpiece, Air-Powered, Dental	Dental And Oral
Handpiece, Contra- And Right-Angle Attachment, Dental	Dental And Oral
Handpiece, Direct Drive, AC-Powered	Dental And Oral
Holder, Radiographic Cassette, Wall-Mounted	Radiology
Instrument, Diamond, Dental	Dental And Oral
Light, Fiberoptic, Dental	Dental And Oral
Operative Dental Treatment Unit	Dental And Oral
Processor, Radiographic Film, Automatic, Dental	Dental And Oral
Radiographic Unit, Diagnostic, Dental, Extraoral	Dental And Oral
Radiographic Unit, Diagnostic, Intraoral	Dental And Oral
Radiographic/Fluoroscopic Unit, Image-Intensified	Radiology
Scaler, Ultrasonic	Dental And Oral
Sterilizer, Steam (Autoclave)	General
Syringe, Cartridge	Dental And Oral
System, X-Ray, Mobile	Radiology
Table, Radiographic, Stationary Top	Radiology

DENTSPLY PROSTHETICS   800-877-0020
183 State Road, K.M. 19.6, Las Piedras, PR 00771   787-733-8303
FDA Number: 2647456
E-mail: webmaster@dentsply.com
Web site: www.dentsply.com
Annual Revenue: More than $1 Billion
Year Founded: 1899
Total Employees: 9400
Ownership: Dentsply International, Inc.
Stock Symbol: XRAY
Traded On: NASDAQ
Produces/Sells CE-marked Devices: N
General Admin.: Bret W. Wise/Chief Executive Officer, Chairman
    Mr. William R. Jellison/Chief Financial Officer, Senior Vice President

Alloy, Precious Metal, For Clinical Use	Dental And Oral
Articulators	Dental And Oral
Material, Tooth Shade, Resin	Dental And Oral
Powder, Porcelain	Dental And Oral

DENTSPLY PROSTHETICS   800-621-0381
570 West College Avenue, York, PA 17404
FDA Number: 2585114   Fax: 1-877-630-2894
Web site: austenal.dentsply.com
Medical Products Sales Volume: $30,000,000
Annual Revenue: $25-$50 Million
Year Founded: 1928
Total Employees: 9400
Ownership: Private
Stock Symbol: XRAY
Traded On: NASDAQ
Quality System Registration Information: ISO9001; ISO9002
Produces/Sells CE-marked Devices: Y
Distribution: Manufacturer Direct, Manufacturer Through Distributor
General Admin.: Bret W. Wise/Chief Executive Officer, Chairman
    William R. Jellison/Chief Financial Officer, Senior Vice President

Alloy, Gold Based, For Clinical Use	Dental And Oral
Alloy, Precious Metal, For Clinical Use	Dental And Oral
Attachment, Precision	Dental And Oral
Base, Denture, Relining, Repairing, Rebasing, Resin	Dental And Oral
Crown And Bridge, Temporary, Resin	Dental And Oral
Denture, Plastic, Teeth	Dental And Oral
Implant, Subperiosteal	Dental And Oral
Material, Investment	Dental And Oral
Material, Tooth Shade, Resin	Dental And Oral
Metal, Base	Dental And Oral
Powder, Porcelain	Dental And Oral
Teeth, Artificial, Posterior With Metal Insert	Dental And Oral

DENTSPLY PROSTHETICS   800-621-0381 (cont'd)

Teeth, Porcelain	Dental And Oral

Medical Product Subsidiaries (Listed Separately)
Myerson Company Ltd.

DENTSPLY PROSTHETICS   800-877-0020
Six Terri Lane, Burlington, NJ 08016   609-386-8900
FDA Number: 2248025
E-mail: webmaster@dentsply.com
Web site: www.dentsply.com
Year Founded: 1899
Total Employees: 9400
Ownership: Dentsply International, Inc.
Stock Symbol: XRAY
Traded On: NASDAQ
Produces/Sells CE-marked Devices: N
General Admin.: Bret W. Wise/Chief Executive Officer, Chairman
    William R. Jellison/Chief Financial Officer, Senior Vice President

Alloy, Amalgam	Dental And Oral
Alloy, Gold Based, For Clinical Use	Dental And Oral
Articulators	Dental And Oral
Cement, Dental	Dental And Oral
Implant, Endosseous	Dental And Oral
Material, Tooth Shade, Resin	Dental And Oral
Powder, Porcelain	Dental And Oral
Teeth, Porcelain	Dental And Oral

DENTSPLY RINN   800-323-0970
1212 Abbot Drive, Elgin, IL 60123
FDA Number: 1418963   Fax: 800-544-0787
E-mail: service@rinncorp.com
Web site: www.rinncorp.com
Annual Revenue: More than $1 Billion
Year Founded: 1923
Total Employees: 9400
Ownership: Dentsply International, Inc.
Stock Symbol: XRAY
Traded On: NASDAQ
Produces/Sells CE-marked Devices: Y
Distribution: Manufacturer Through Distributor
General Admin.: Bret W. Wise/Chief Executive Officer, Chairman
    William R. Jellison/Chief Financial Officer, Senior Vice President

Aligner, Beam, X-Ray (Collimator)	Dental And Oral
Amalgamator, Dental, AC-Powered	Dental And Oral
Apron, Lead, Dental	Dental And Oral
Articulators	Dental And Oral
Capsule, Dental, Amalgam	Dental And Oral
Collimator, X-Ray	Dental And Oral
Cup, Prophylaxis	Dental And Oral
Forceps, Articulation Paper	Dental And Oral
Gutta Percha	Dental And Oral
Holder, X-Ray Film	Dental And Oral
Illuminator, Radiographic Film	Radiology
Injector, Jet, Mechanical-Powered	Dental And Oral
Irrigator, Oral	Dental And Oral
Needle, Dental	Dental And Oral
Needle, Hypodermic, Single Lumen With Syringe	General
Phantom, Anthropomorphic, Radiographic	Radiology
Probe, Periodontic	Dental And Oral
Protector, Dental	Anesthesiology
Resin, Root Canal Filling	Dental And Oral
Syringe, Cartridge	Dental And Oral
Syringe, Periodontic, Endodontic	Dental And Oral

DENTSPLY SPECIALTY MATERIALS   800-877-0020
1301 Smile Way, York, PA 17404   717-849-4229
FDA Number: 2424472   Fax: 717-767-8250
E-mail: webmaster@dentsply.com
Web site: www.dentsply.com
Annual Revenue: More than $1 Billion
Year Founded: 1899
Total Employees: 9400
Ownership: Dentsply International, Inc.
Stock Symbol: XRAY
Traded On: NASDAQ
Produces/Sells CE-marked Devices: N
General Admin.: Bret W. Wise/Chief Executive Officer, Chairman
    William R. Jellison/Chief Financial Officer, Senior Vice President

Agent, Polishing, Abrasive, Oral Cavity	Dental And Oral
Bone Grafting Material, Dental, With Biologic Component	Dental And Oral
Handpiece, Air-Powered, Dental	Dental And Oral
Handpiece, Direct Drive, AC-Powered	Dental And Oral
Implant, Endosseous (Bone Filling and/or Augmentation)	Dental And Oral
Instrument, Diamond, Dental	Dental And Oral
Material, Tooth Shade, Resin	Dental And Oral
Needle, Dental	Dental And Oral
Sealant, Pit And Fissure, And Conditioner, Resin	Dental And Oral
Syringe, Bulb, Air Or Water	Dental And Oral

DENTSPLY TULSA DENTAL PRODUCTS
800-662-1202

608 Rolling Hills Dr., Johnson City, TN 37604
FDA Number: 2320721
Fax: 800-597-2779
Web site: www.tulsadental.com
Annual Revenue: More than $1 Billion
Year Founded: 1988
Total Employees: 9400
Ownership: Dentsply International, Inc.
Stock Symbol: XRAY
Traded On: NASDAQ
Produces/Sells CE-marked Devices: N
General Admin.: Bret W. Wise/Chief Executive Officer, Chairman
Finance: William R. Jellison/Chief Financial Officer

Bone Grafting Material, Dental, With Biologic Component	Dental And Oral
Broach, Endodontic	Dental And Oral
Burr, Dental	Dental And Oral
Cleanser, Root Canal	Dental And Oral
Dam, Rubber	Dental And Oral
Drill, Dental, Intraoral	Dental And Oral
File, Periodontic	Dental And Oral
File, Pulp Canal, Endodontic	Dental And Oral
Gutta Percha	Dental And Oral
Hand Instrument, Calculus Removal	Dental And Oral
Handle, Instrument, Dental	Dental And Oral
Handpiece, Air-Powered, Dental	Dental And Oral
Handpiece, Contra- And Right-Angle Attachment, Dental	Dental And Oral
Instrument, Diamond, Dental	Dental And Oral
Locator, Apex, Root	Dental And Oral
Motor, Surgical Instrument, AC-Powered	Surgery
Needle, Dental	Dental And Oral
Plugger, Root Canal, Endodontic	Dental And Oral
Point, Paper, Endodontic	Dental And Oral
Post, Root Canal	Dental And Oral
Preparer, Root Canal, Endodontic	Dental And Oral
Reamer, Pulp Canal, Endodontic	Dental And Oral
Resin, Root Canal Filling	Dental And Oral
Scaler, Ultrasonic	Dental And Oral
Spreader, Pulp Canal Filling Material, Endodontic	Dental And Oral
Syringe, Periodontic, Endodontic	Dental And Oral

DENTSPLY TULSA DENTAL SPECIALTIES
800-662-1202

5100 East Skelly Drive, Suite 300, Tulsa, OK 74136
FDA Number: 1643003
Fax: 800-597-2779
Web site: www.tulsadental.com
Annual Revenue: More than $1 Billion
Year Founded: 1988
Total Employees: 9400
Ownership: Dentsply International, Inc.
Stock Symbol: XRAY
Traded On: NASDAQ
Produces/Sells CE-marked Devices: N
General Admin.: Bret W. Wise/Chief Executive Officer, Chairman
William R. Jellison/Chief Financial Officer, Senior Vice President

Bone Grafting Material, Dental, With Biologic Component	Dental And Oral
Broach, Endodontic	Dental And Oral
Burr, Dental	Dental And Oral
Condenser, Amalgam And Foil, Operative	Dental And Oral
File, Periodontic	Dental And Oral
File, Pulp Canal, Endodontic	Dental And Oral
Graft, Bone	Orthopedics
Instrument, Diamond, Dental	Dental And Oral
Preparer, Root Canal, Endodontic	Dental And Oral
Sterilizer, Endodontic Dry Heat	Dental And Oral

DENTSPLY TULSA DENTAL SPECIALTIES
See Dentsply Tulsa Dental Products

DENTSPLY-CAVITRON
See Dentsply Professional

DENVER INSTRUMENT COMPANY
800-321-1135
303-431-7255

5 Orville Dr., Bohemia, NY 11716
FDA Number: n/a
Fax: 303-423-4831
Web site: www.denverinstrumentusa.com
Annual Revenue: $0-$1 Million
Year Founded: 1880
Ownership: Private
Quality System Registration Information: ISO9001
Produces/Sells CE-marked Devices: Y
Distribution: Manufacturer Through Distributor

Balance, Analytical	Chemistry
Balance, Electronic	Chemistry
Calibrator, Primary, Clinical Chemistry	Chemistry
Hood, Fume	Toxicology
Meter, pH, General Use	Toxicology
Meter, pH, Portable	Chemistry
Molecular Weight Equipment	Chemistry
Titrator	Chemistry

DENVER OPTIC COMPANY
303-649-9494

14 Inverness Dr. East, Building D, Suite 146, Englewood, CO 80112
FDA Number: n/a
Fax: 303-790-4055
E-mail: Eyeguyz@aol.com
Web site: www.eyeprosthetics.com
Annual Revenue: $0-$1 Million
Year Founded: 1906
Ownership: Private
Produces/Sells CE-marked Devices: N
Federal Procurement Eligibility: Small Business
Distribution: Manufacturer Direct
Mktg./Adv.: Albert E. Johnson/General Manager Marketing

Eye, Artificial, Custom	Ophthalmology

DENVER SPLINT CO., INC.
See Shippert Medical Technologies Corp.

DEPARTMENT OF VETERANS AFFAIRS MEDICAL CENTER
503-220-8262

3710 S.w. U.s. Veterans, Hospital Rd., Portland, OR 97207-1034
FDA Number: 3073275
Ownership: Private
Produces/Sells CE-marked Devices: N

Eye, Artificial, Non-Custom	Ophthalmology

DEPUY ACE MEDICAL COMPANY
See Depuy Ace, A Johnson & Johnson Company

DEPUY ACE, A JOHNSON & JOHNSON COMPANY
800-473-3789

700 Orthopedic Drive, Warsaw, IN 46581
574-267-8143
FDA Number: 2020231
Fax: 574-267-7196
E-mail: info@dpyus.jnj.com
Web site: www.depuyace.com
Medical Products Sales Volume: $392,800,000
Year Founded: 2002
Total Employees: 800
Ownership: Depuy Orthopaedics, Inc.
Produces/Sells CE-marked Devices: Y
Distribution: Manufacturer Through Distributor, Manufacturer Through Manufacturer Reps, Service Direct, Exporter
General Admin.: Andrew Balaity/Executive Vice President

Accessories, Fixation, Orthopedic	Orthopedics
Nail, Fixation, Bone	Orthopedics
Orthosis, Cervical-Thoracic, Rigid	Physical Med
Pin, Fixation, Threaded	Orthopedics
Plate, Fixation, Bone	Orthopedics
Screw, Fixation, Bone	Orthopedics
Splint, Abduction, Congenital Hip Dislocation	Physical Med
Traction Unit, Hip, Non-Powered, Non-Penetrating	Orthopedics

DEPUY ACROMED
See Depuy Mitek, Inc.

DEPUY BRIDGEWATER
800-473-3789

50 Scotland Park Dr., Bridgewater, MA 02324
574-371-4865
FDA Number: 3004464325
Fax: 574-267-8143
Web site: www.depuy.com
Year Founded: 1895
Ownership: Johnson & Johnson
Produces/Sells CE-marked Devices: N
General Admin.: Michael Mahoney/Chairman
Kevin Dwyer/Vice President
Mktg./Adv.: Sarah Colamarino/Vice President Communications
Production: Sarah Deegan/Vice President Quality Systems
Finance: Peter Batesko III/Vice President Finance

Pin, Fixation, Smooth	Orthopedics
Prosthesis, Elbow, Semi-Constrained	Orthopedics
Prosthesis, Hip, Semi-Const., M/P, Por. Uncem., Calc./Phos.	Orthopedics
Prosthesis, Knee, Femorotibial, Semi-Constrained, Trunnion	Orthopedics
Screw, Fixation, Bone	Orthopedics

DEPUY CODMAN
See Codman & Shurtleff, Inc

DEPUY MITEK, A JOHNSON & JOHNSON COMPANY
800-451-2006

50 Scotland Blvd., Bridgewater, MA 02324
508-880-8100
FDA Number: 3004065025
Fax: 508-880-8122
E-mail: wworderdesk@ethus.jnj.com
Web site: www.depuy.com
Year Founded: 1895
Ownership: Johnson & Johnson
Stock Symbol: DPU
Traded On: NYSE
Produces/Sells CE-marked Devices: N
General Admin.: Michael Mahoney/Chairman
Earl R. Fender/President

DEPUY MITEK, A JOHNSON & JOHNSON 800-451-2006 *(cont'd)*

Kevin Dwyer/Vice President
Mktg./Adv.: Sarah Colamarino/Vice President Communications
Production: Sarah Deegan/Vice President Quality Systems
Finance: Peter Batesko III/Vice President Finance

Applier, Surgical Staple	Surgery
Arthroscope	Orthopedics
Awl	Orthopedics
Bit, Drill	Orthopedics
Bit, Surgical	Surgery
Bolt, Nut, Washer	Orthopedics
Cannula, Surgical, General & Plastic Surgery	Surgery
Cutter, Surgical	Surgery
Electrosurgical Unit, Cutting & Coagulation Device	Surgery
Elevator, Surgical, General & Plastic Surgery	Surgery
Extractor, Nail	Orthopedics
Fastener, Fixation, Biodegradable, Soft Tissue	Orthopedics
Fastener, Fixation, Non-Biodegradable, Soft Tissue	Orthopedics
Gauge, Depth	Orthopedics
Guide, Surgical, Instrument	Surgery
Instrument, Passing, Ligature, Knot Tying	Cns/Neurology
Knife, Orthopedic	Orthopedics
Needle, Suture, Disposable	Surgery
Orthopedic Manual Surgical Instrument	Orthopedics
Passer	Orthopedics
Pin, Fixation, Smooth	Orthopedics
Pin, Fixation, Threaded	Orthopedics
Probe	Orthopedics
Reamer	Orthopedics
Scalpel, One-Piece (Knife)	Surgery
Screw, Fixation, Bone	Orthopedics
Screwdriver	Orthopedics
Staple, Fixation, Bone	Orthopedics
Suture, Absorbable, Synthetic, Polyglycolic Acid	Surgery
Suture, Non-Absorbable, Synthetic, Polyester	Surgery
Tap, Bone	Orthopedics
Tray, Surgical Instrument	Surgery

DEPUY MITEK, INC. 800-451-2006
325 Paramount Dr., Raynham, MA 02767 508-880-8100

FDA Number: 1221934 Fax: 508-880-8122
E-mail: DePuySpine@dpyus.jnj.com
Web site: www.depuyspine.com
Annual Revenue: $1-$5 Million
Year Founded: 1895
Total Employees: 24
Ownership: Johnson & Johnson
Stock Symbol: DPU
Traded On: NYSE
Produces/Sells CE-marked Devices: Y
Federal Procurement Eligibility: Small Business
Distribution: Manufacturer Through Manufacturer Reps
General Admin.: Michael Mahoney/Chairman
Kevin Dwyer/Vice President
Mktg./Adv.: Sarah Colamarino/Vice President Communications
Production: John Knapik/Director Operations
Sarah Deegan/Vice President Quality Systems
Finance: Peter Batesko III/Vice President Finance

Accessories, Traction	Physical Med
Cutter, Surgical	Surgery
Fixation Appliance, Multiple Component	Orthopedics
Guide, Surgical, Instrument	Surgery
Head Rest, Neurosurgical	Cns/Neurology
Immobilizer, Cervical	Orthopedics
Immobilizer, Upper Body	Orthopedics
Infusion Stand	General
Needle, Suture, Disposable	Surgery
Resectoscope Working Element	Gastroenterology/Urology
Splint, Abduction, Shoulder	Orthopedics
Suture, Non-Absorbable, Synthetic, Polyamide	Surgery
Suture, Non-Absorbable, Synthetic, Polyester	Surgery
Traction Unit, Non-Powered	Orthopedics
Tray, Surgical Instrument	Surgery

DEPUY ORTHOPAEDICS, INC. 800-473-3789
700 Orthopaedic Dr., Warsaw, IN 46581 574-267-8143

FDA Number: 1818910 Fax: 574-371-4865
E-mail: info@dpyus.jnj.com
Web site: www.depuyorthopedics.com
Year Founded: 1895
Ownership: Johnson & Johnson
Stock Symbol: DPU
Traded On: NYSE
Produces/Sells CE-marked Devices: N
General Admin.: Harry Kotlarz/Director
Tom Till/Manager
David Floyd/President
George Grobe/Vice President
Randy Kilburn/Vice President

DEPUY ORTHOPAEDICS, INC. 800-473-3789 *(cont'd)*

Mktg./Adv.: Alicia Whitaker/Sales Representative

Accessories, Apparel, Surgical	Surgery
Accessories, Fixation, Orthopedic	Orthopedics
Appliance, Fix., Nail/Blade/Plate Comb., Multiple Component	Orthopedics
Bandage, Cast	Physical Med
Bandage, Elastic	General
Bit, Surgical	Surgery
Bolt, Nut, Washer	Orthopedics
Bone Cement	Orthopedics
Bone Cement, Antibiotic	Orthopedics
Bone Mill	Orthopedics
Component, Traction, Invasive	Orthopedics
Cover, Shoe, Operating Room	Surgery
Dispenser, Cement	Orthopedics
Drape, Surgical	Surgery
Dress, Surgical	Surgery
Evacuator, Vapor, Cement Monomer	Surgery
Exerciser, Non-Measuring	Physical Med
Exhaust System, Surgical	Surgery
Fastener, Fixation, Biodegradable, Hard Tissue	Orthopedics
Fastener, Fixation, Non-Biodegradable, Soft Tissue	Orthopedics
Fixation Appliance, Multiple Component	Orthopedics
Fixation Appliance, Single Component	Orthopedics
Gauge, Depth	Orthopedics
Glove, Surgical, Plastic Surgery	Surgery
Gown, Surgical	Surgery
Guide, Surgical, Instrument	Surgery
Helmet, Surgical	Surgery
Hip, Hemi-, Femoral, Metal Ball	Orthopedics
Hood, Surgical	Surgery
Instrument, Manual, General Surgical	Surgery
Instrument, Surgical, Powered, Pneumatic	Orthopedics
Kit, Surgical (General)	Surgery
Mask, Surgical	Surgery
Mesh, Surgical (Steel Gauze)	Surgery
Mixing Equipment, Cement	Orthopedics
Motor, Surgical Instrument, AC-Powered	Surgery
Nail, Fixation, Bone	Orthopedics
Obturator, Cement	Orthopedics
Orthopedic Manual Surgical Instrument	Orthopedics
Pin, Fixation, Smooth	Orthopedics
Pin, Fixation, Threaded	Orthopedics
Plate, Fixation, Bone	Orthopedics
Prosthesis, Ankle, Semi-Constrained, Metal/Polymer	Orthopedics
Prosthesis, Elbow, Constrained	Orthopedics
Prosthesis, Elbow, Hemi-, Radial, Polymer	Orthopedics
Prosthesis, Elbow, Semi-Constrained	Orthopedics
Prosthesis, Finger, Constrained, Polymer	Orthopedics
Prosthesis, Hip, Acetabular Mesh	Orthopedics
Prosthesis, Hip, Cement Restrictor	Orthopedics
Prosthesis, Hip, Constrained, Metal/Polymer	Orthopedics
Prosthesis, Hip, Femoral Component, Cemented, Metal	Orthopedics
Prosthesis, Hip, Hemi-, Femoral, Metal	Orthopedics
Prosthesis, Hip, Hemi-, Femoral, Metal/Polymer	Orthopedics
Prosthesis, Hip, Semi-Const., M/P, Por. Uncem., Calc./Phos.	Orthopedics
Prosthesis, Hip, Semi-Const., Metal/Poly., Porous Uncemented	Orthopedics
Prosthesis, Hip, Semi-Const., Uncem., Non-P., M/P, Ca./Phos.	Orthopedics
Prosthesis, Hip, Semi-Constr., Metal/Ceramic, Cemented/NC	Orthopedics
Prosthesis, Hip, Semi-Constrained (Cemented Acetabular)	Orthopedics
Prosthesis, Hip, Semi-Constrained Acetabular	Orthopedics
Prosthesis, Hip, Semi-Constrained, Metal/Polymer	Orthopedics
Prosthesis, Hip, Semi-Constrained, Metal/Polymer, Uncemented	Orthopedics
Prosthesis, Hip, Semi-constrained, Metal/Ceramic/Ceramic/Metal, Cemented Or Uncemented	Orthopedics
Prosthesis, Knee, Femorotibial, Constrained, Metal/Polymer	Orthopedics
Prosthesis, Knee, Femorotibial, Non-Constrained	Orthopedics
Prosthesis, Knee, Femorotibial, Semi-Constrained	Orthopedics
Prosthesis, Knee, Patellofemoral, Semi-Constrained	Orthopedics
Prosthesis, Knee, Patellofemorotibial, Semi-Constrained	Orthopedics
Prosthesis, Knee, Patellofemorotibial, Semi-constrained, Metal/polymer, Mobile Bearing	Orthopedics
Prosthesis, Knee, Patfem., S-C., Unc., Por., Ctd., P/M/P	Orthopedics
Prosthesis, Shoulder, Hemi-, Humeral	Orthopedics
Prosthesis, Shoulder, Metal/Polymer, Uncemented	Orthopedics
Prosthesis, Shoulder, Non-Constrained, Metal/Polymer Cem.	Orthopedics
Prosthesis, Shoulder, Semi-Constrained, Metal/Polymer Cem.	Orthopedics
Prosthesis, Wrist, 3 Part Metal-Plastic-Metal Articulation	Orthopedics
Punch, Surgical	Surgery
Regulator, Pressure, Gas Cylinder	Anesthesiology
Rod, Fixation, Intramedullary	Orthopedics
Saw, Pneumatically Powered	Surgery
Saw, Powered, And Accessories	Cns/Neurology
Screw, Fixation, Bone	Orthopedics
Spacer, Cement	Orthopedics
Staple, Fixation, Bone	Orthopedics
Stereotaxy Equipment	Cns/Neurology
Suction Apparatus, Single Patient, Portable, Non-Powered	Surgery
Suction Apparatus, Ward Use, Portable, AC-Powered	Surgery
Surgical Instrument, Orthopedic, AC-Powered Motor	Surgery
Table, Anesthetist's	Anesthesiology
Tourniquet, Pneumatic	Surgery

DEPUY ORTHOPAEDICS, INC.   800-473-3789 *(cont'd)*

Traction Unit, Non-Powered	Orthopedics
Trocar, Cardiovascular	Cardiovascular

DEPUY ORTHOTECH

See DJO Inc.

DEPUY SPINE, INC.   800-227-6633

325 Paramount Dr., Raynham, MA 02767   508-880-8100
FDA Number: 1526439   *Fax:* 800-446-0234
E-mail: DePuySpine@dpyus.jnj.com
Web site: www.depuyspine.com
Year Founded: 1895
Ownership: Johnson & Johnson
Stock Symbol: DPU
Traded On: NYSE
Produces/Sells CE-marked Devices: N
General Admin.: Mike Dormer/Chairman
Mike Mahoney/Chairman
Kevin Sidow/President
Ian Burgess/Vice President
Richard Toselli/Vice President

Accessories, Operating Room, Table	Surgery
Appliance, Fixation, Spinal Interlaminal	Orthopedics
Appliance, Fixation, Spinal Intervertebral Body	Orthopedics
Arthroscope	Orthopedics
Awl	Orthopedics
Bit, Drill	Orthopedics
Bolt, Nut, Washer	Orthopedics
Broach	Orthopedics
Caliper	Orthopedics
Cannula, Surgical, General & Plastic Surgery	Surgery
Centrifuge, Cell Washing	Hematology
Curette	Orthopedics
Cutter, Orthopedic	Orthopedics
Cutter, Wire And Pin	Orthopedics
Device, Spinal Vertebral Body Replacement	Orthopedics
Driver, Surgical, Pin	Surgery
Elevator, Orthopedic	Orthopedics
Equipment, Laboratory, Gen. Purpose (Specific Medical Use)	Chemistry
Filler, Calcium Sulfate Preformed Pellets	Orthopedics
Forceps	Orthopedics
Gauge, Depth	Orthopedics
Goniometer, Non-Powered	Orthopedics
Guide, Surgical, Instrument	Surgery
Implant, Fixation Device, Spinal	Orthopedics
Instrument, Bending (Contouring)	Orthopedics
Knife, Orthopedic	Orthopedics
Mesh, Surgical (Steel Gauze)	Surgery
Nail, Fixation, Bone	Orthopedics
Needle, Aspiration And Injection, Disposable	Surgery
Orthopedic Manual Surgical Instrument	Orthopedics
Orthosis, Fixation, Cervical Intervertebral Body, Spinal	Orthopedics
Orthosis, Fixation, Pedicle, Spinal	Orthopedics
Orthosis, Fixation, Spinal, Spondylolisthesis	Orthopedics
Orthosis, Fusion, Intervertebral, Spinal	Orthopedics
Osteotome, Manual (Plastic Surgery)	Surgery
Plate, Fixation, Bone	Orthopedics
Pliers, Surgical	Orthopedics
Probe	Orthopedics
Prosthesis, Spine, Intervertebral Disc	Orthopedics
Punch, Femoral Neck	Orthopedics
Reamer	Orthopedics
Retainer, Surgical	Surgery
Retractor, Self-Retaining, Neurology	Cns/Neurology
Retractor, Surgical	Surgery
Rongeur, Rib	Orthopedics
Screw, Fixation, Bone	Orthopedics
Screwdriver	Orthopedics
Surgical Instrument, Non-Powered, Neurosurgical	Cns/Neurology
Syringe, Piston	General
Tamp	Orthopedics
Tap, Bone	Orthopedics
Template	Orthopedics
Tray, Surgical Instrument	Surgery
Trephine, Bone	Orthopedics
Wrench	Orthopedics

DEPUY SPINE, INC.   800-227-6633

365 Ravendale Dr., Mountain View, CA 94043   508-880-8100
FDA Number: 1000453488   *Fax:* 800-446-0234
E-mail: DePuySpine@dpyus.jnj.com
Web site: www.depuyspine.com
Year Founded: 1895
Ownership: Johnson & Johnson
Stock Symbol: DPU
Traded On: NYSE
Produces/Sells CE-marked Devices: N
General Admin.: Mike Mahoney/Chairman
Gary Fischetti/President
Mktg./Adv.: Sarah Colamarino/Vice President Communications

DEPUY SPINE, INC.   800-227-6633 *(cont'd)*

Production: Sarah Deegan/Vice President Quality Systems
Finance: Peter Batesko/Vice President Finance

Filler, Bone Void, Osteoinduction	Physical Med
Filler, Calcium Sulfate Preformed Pellets	Orthopedics
Graft, Bone	Orthopedics
Syringe, Piston	General

DEPUY-RAYNHAM, A DIV. OF DEPUY ORTHOPAEDICS   800-451-2006

325 Paramount Dr., Raynham, MA 02767-0350   574-267-8143
FDA Number: 1219655   *Fax:* 508-880-8122
E-mail: wworderdesk@ethus.jnj.com
Web site: www.depuy.com
Year Founded: 1895
Ownership: Johnson & Johnson
Stock Symbol: DPU
Traded On: NYSE
Produces/Sells CE-marked Devices: N
General Admin.: Michael Mahoney/Chairman
Earl R. Fender/President
Kevin Dwyer/Vice President
Mktg./Adv.: Sarah Colamarino/Vice President Communications
Production: Sarah Deegan/Vice President Quality Systems
Finance: Peter Batesko III/Vice President Finance

Appliance, Fixation, Spinal Intervertebral Body	Orthopedics
Bandage, Cast	Physical Med
Bit, Surgical	Surgery
Bolt, Nut, Washer	Orthopedics
Clamp, Carotid Artery	Cns/Neurology
Clip, Implantable, Malleable	Cns/Neurology
Clip, Removable (Skin)	Surgery
Cutter, Wire And Pin	Orthopedics
Dilator, Vessel, Surgical	Cardiovascular
Dispenser, Cement	Orthopedics
Electrosurgical Unit, Cutting & Coagulation Device	Surgery
Fastener, Fixation, Biodegradable, Hard Tissue	Orthopedics
Fastener, Fixation, Non-Biodegradable, Soft Tissue	Orthopedics
Fixation Appliance, Multiple Component	Orthopedics
Forceps, General & Plastic Surgery	Surgery
Gauge, Depth	Orthopedics
Implant, Fixation Device, Spinal	Orthopedics
Instrument, Manual, General Surgical	Surgery
Instrument, Surgical, Powered, Pneumatic	Orthopedics
Marker, Skin	Surgery
Motor, Surgical Instrument, AC-Powered	Surgery
Nail, Fixation, Bone	Orthopedics
Orthopedic Manual Surgical Instrument	Orthopedics
Percussor	Cns/Neurology
Pin, Fixation, Smooth	Orthopedics
Pin, Fixation, Threaded	Orthopedics
Prosthesis, Elbow, Semi-Constrained	Orthopedics
Prosthesis, Hip, Cement Restrictor	Orthopedics
Prosthesis, Hip, Constrained, Metal/Polymer	Orthopedics
Prosthesis, Hip, Femoral Component, Cemented, Metal	Orthopedics
Prosthesis, Hip, Hemi-, Femoral, Metal/Polymer	Orthopedics
Prosthesis, Hip, Semi-Const., Metal/Poly., Porous Uncemented	Orthopedics
Prosthesis, Hip, Semi-Const., Uncem., Non-P., M/P, Ca./Phos.	Orthopedics
Prosthesis, Hip, Semi-Constr., Metal/Ceramic, Cemented/NC	Orthopedics
Prosthesis, Hip, Semi-Constrained (Cemented Acetabular)	Orthopedics
Prosthesis, Hip, Semi-Constrained Acetabular	Orthopedics
Prosthesis, Hip, Semi-Constrained, Metal/Polymer	Orthopedics
Prosthesis, Hip, Semi-Constrained, Metal/Polymer, Uncemented	Orthopedics
Prosthesis, Knee, Femorotibial, Constrained, Metal/Polymer	Orthopedics
Prosthesis, Knee, Femorotibial, Non-Constrained	Orthopedics
Prosthesis, Knee, Femorotibial, Semi-Constrained	Orthopedics
Prosthesis, Knee, Patellofemoral, Semi-Constrained	Orthopedics
Prosthesis, Knee, Patellofemorotibial, Semi-Constrained	Orthopedics
Prosthesis, Knee, Patellofemorotibial, Semi-constrained, Metal/polymer, Mobile Bearing	Orthopedics
Prosthesis, Knee, Patfem., S-C., Unc., Por., Ctd., P/M/P	Orthopedics
Pusher, Socket	Orthopedics
Saw, Pneumatically Powered	Surgery
Saw, Powered, And Accessories	Cns/Neurology
Screw, Fixation, Bone	Orthopedics
Spacer, Cement	Orthopedics
Splint, Extremity, Non-Inflatable, External	Surgery
Staple, Fixation, Bone	Orthopedics
Stereotaxy Equipment	Cns/Neurology
Stripper, Surgical	Orthopedics
Stripper, Vein, Disposable	Surgery
Surgical Instrument, Non-Powered, Neurosurgical	Cns/Neurology
Tray, Surgical Instrument	Surgery
Trocar, Cardiovascular	Cardiovascular
Vision Aid, Optical, Battery-Powered	Ophthalmology

DERATA CORP.

See Antares Pharma, Inc.

DERBY INDUSTRIES
757-224-0177
24350 Sr 23 South, South Bend, IN 46614
FDA Number: 3005864972
Cover, Mattress — General

DERBY, INC.
219-233-4500
24350 State Rd. 23 S., South Bend, IN 46614
FDA Number: n/a — *Fax:* 219-288-4550
E-mail: derbyinc@earthlink.net
Web site: www.derbycase.com
Annual Revenue: $1-$5 Million
Total Employees: 128 — *Marketing Staff:* 8 — *Sales Staff:* 8
Ownership: Private
Produces/Sells CE-marked Devices: N
Federal Procurement Eligibility: Small Business
Distribution: Manufacturer Direct
General Admin.: Andrew Karafa/President
David Karafa/Vice President
Andrew Karafa/Vice President, General Manager
Mktg./Adv.: Timothy Shelby/Manager International & National Sales
Production: Bev Norton/Design Engineer
Bag, Medical, Physician — General
Case, Protection, Equipment — General
Mattress, Alternating Pressure (Or Pads) — Physical Med

DERINGER-NEY, INC.
860-242-2281
Ney Industrial Park, 2 Douglas Street, Bloomfield, CT 06002
FDA Number: 1218814 — *Fax:* 860-242-5688
E-mail: info@deringerney.com
Web site: www.deringerney.com
Ownership: Private
Quality System Registration Information: ISO9000; ISO9001
Produces/Sells CE-marked Devices: N
Distribution: Manufacturer Direct
Component, Metal, Other — General
Component, Other — General
Component, Plastic — General
Contract Assembly — General
Implant, Endosseous — Dental And Oral
Metal, Medical — General

DERMA SAFE COMPANY
See Derma-Safe Company

DERMA SCIENCES
609-514-4744
214 Carnegie Center, Suite 300, Princeton, NJ 08540
FDA Number: 9680091
E-mail: jroseman@dermasciences.com
Web site: www.dermasciences.com
Annual Revenue: $0-$1 Million
Total Employees: 20 — *Marketing Staff:* 3 — *Sales Staff:* 20
Ownership: Public
Stock Symbol: DSCI
Traded On: NASDAQ
Produces/Sells CE-marked Devices: N
Distribution: Manufacturer Through Distributor
General Admin.: Edward Quilty/Chief Executive Officer
Mr. John Yetter/Chief Financial Officer, Vice President
Mktg./Adv.: Mr. Barry Wolfenson/Executive Vice President Business Development
Mr. Robert Cole/Executive Vice President Sales
Production: Mr. Frederic Eigner/Executive Vice President Operations
Anoscope, Non-Powered — Gastroenterology/Urology
Bandage, Cast — Physical Med
Bandage, Elastic — General
Bandage, Liquid — Surgery
Bottle, Hot/Cold Water — General
Dressing, Non-Adherent — General
Dressing, Other — General
Sanitizer — General
Sponge, Gauze — Dental And Oral
Strip, Adhesive — Surgery

DERMA-SAFE COMPANY
973-839-6383
32 Juniper Road, Wayne, NJ 07470-6156
FDA Number: 2246445 — *Fax:* 973-839-6383
E-mail: razors@derma-safe.com
Web site: www.derma-safe.com
Medical Products Sales Volume: $400,000
Annual Revenue: $0-$1 Million
Year Founded: 1982
Total Employees: 2
Ownership: Private
Produces/Sells CE-marked Devices: Y
Federal Procurement Eligibility: Small Business, VA Contract
Distribution: Manufacturer Through Distributor
General Admin.: Warren Grosjean/President
Mktg./Adv.: Paul Grosjean/Vice President Marketing
Surgical, Razor — Surgery

DERMAMED INTL, INC.
610-358-4447
394 Parkmount Rd., Lenni, PA 19052
FDA Number: 2531692
Dermatome — Surgery

DERMAPAC, INC.
203-924-7148
33 Hull St., Shelton, CT 06484
FDA Number: 1221362 — *Fax:* 203-924-4932
E-mail: dermapac@sbcglobal.net
Web site: http://www.dermapac.net
Year Founded: 1986
Ownership: Private
Produces/Sells CE-marked Devices: N
Federal Procurement Eligibility: Small Business, Female Owned
Distribution: Manufacturer Direct, Manufacturer Through Distributor, OEM
General Admin.: Steven Tuchband/General Manager
Arlene Tuchband/President, Chief Executive Officer
Bandage, Cast — Physical Med
Bandage, Compression — General
Bandage, Elastic — General
Bandage, Gauze — General
Gauze Roll — Surgery
Sponge, Gauze — Dental And Oral
Stockinette — Orthopedics
Tray, Surgical Instrument — Surgery

DERMASWEEP, INC.
916) 632-9134
3715 Atherton Drive,, Suite 2, Rocklin, CA 95765
FDA Number: 3007035827 — *Fax:* 916) 630-9125
Ownership: Private
Produces/Sells CE-marked Devices: N
Brush, Dermabrasion — Surgery

DERMATEC INDUSTRIES, LLC
765-427-0092
970 Cape Marco Dr., #405, Marco Island, FL 34145
FDA Number: n/a
Ownership: Private
Produces/Sells CE-marked Devices: N
Brush, Dermabrasion — Surgery

DERMATOLOGIC LAB & SUPPLY, INC.
800-831-6273
608 13th Ave., Council Bluffs, IA 51501
712-323-3269
FDA Number: 1930126 — *Fax:* 800-320-9612
E-mail: questions@delasco.com
Web site: www.delasco.com
Year Founded: 1980
Ownership: Private
Produces/Sells CE-marked Devices: Y
Federal Procurement Eligibility: Small Business, Female Owned
Cautery, Thermal, AC-Powered — Ophthalmology
Cryosurgical Unit — Surgery
Curette — Orthopedics
Cutter, Ring — General
Electrode, Electrosurgical, Active (Blade) — Surgery
Electrosurgical Unit, General Purpose (ESU) — Surgery
Elevator, Surgical, General & Plastic Surgery — Surgery
Exhaust System, Surgical — Surgery
Forceps — Orthopedics
Forceps, Electrosurgical — Surgery
General Use Surgical Scissors — Surgery
Hemostat — Orthopedics
Holder, Needle — Gastroenterology/Urology
Instrument, Manual, General Surgical — Surgery
Needle, Aspiration And Injection, Reusable — Surgery
Punch, Surgical — Surgery
Medical Product Subsidiaries (Listed Separately)
Sleep Sauna, Inc.

DERMAWAVE, LLC
561-784-0599
15693 83rd Lane North, Loxahatchee, FL 33470
FDA Number: 3003921083
Ownership: Private
Produces/Sells CE-marked Devices: N
Electrode, Cutaneous — Cns/Neurology
Stimulator, Nerve, Transcutaneous (Pain Relief, TENS) — Cns/Neurology
Stimulator, Ultrasound, Muscle — Physical Med
Unit, Therapy, Current, Interferential — Cns/Neurology

DERMED DIAGNOSTICS, INC.
630-668-4644
2-S 558 White Birch Ln., Wheaton, IL 60187
FDA Number: 1423755
Web site: www.dermeddirect.com
Year Founded: 1988
Ownership: Private
Produces/Sells CE-marked Devices: N
Plethysmograph, Impedance — Cardiovascular

DEROYAL INDUSTRIES, INC.
800-251-9864
200 DeBusk Lane, Powell, TN 37849
865-362-6022
FDA Number: 1048770 — *Fax:* 800-543-2182

DEROYAL INDUSTRIES, INC. 800-251-9864 *(cont'd)*

E-mail: customerservice@deroyal.com
Web site: www.deroyal.com
Medical Products Sales Volume: $168,300,000
Year Founded: 1973
Ownership: Private
Quality System Registration Information: ISO9000
Produces/Sells CE-marked Devices: Y
Federal Procurement Eligibility: Small Business
Distribution: Manufacturer Direct, Manufacturer Through Manufacturer Reps, OEM, Exclusive Distributor, Importer, Exporter
General Admin.: Mr. Pete DeBusk/Chairman
  Mr. Brian DeBusk/Chief Executive Officer
  Mr. David Metz/Chief Financial Officer, Executive Vice President
  Ms. Tracy Edmunson/Chief Legal Officer
  Mr. Bill Pittman/President, Chief Operating Officer
Medical Admin.: Dr. Bob Haralson/Medical Director
Production: Mr. Gary Burchett/Executive Vice President Manufacturing

Accessories, Light, Surgical	Surgery
Accessories, Operating Room, Table	Surgery
Ankle/Foot, External Limb Component	Physical Med
Applicator, Cotton	Dental And Oral
Bandage, Cast	Physical Med
Bandage, Elastic	General
Belt, Traction, Pelvic, Orthopedic	Orthopedics
Binder, Abdominal	General
Blade, Tongue	Surgery
Brush, Cleaning, Tracheal Tube	Ear/Nose/Throat
Clasp, Preformed	Dental And Oral
Component, Exercise	Physical Med
Cotton, Roll	Dental And Oral
Counter, Needle	Surgery
Counter, Sponge, Surgical	Surgery
Cover, Limb	Physical Med
Dissector, Surgical, General & Plastic Surgery	Surgery
Drape, Incision, Surgical	Surgery
Drape, Surgical Instrument, Magnetic	Surgery
Drape, Surgical, Disposable	Surgery
Dressing, Other	General
Elevator, Orthopedic	Orthopedics
Fiber, Absorbent	General
Gauze, Absorbable	Surgery
Gauze, Non-Absorbable, Non-Medicated (Internal Sponge)	Surgery
Holder, Needle	Gastroenterology/Urology
Instrument, Manual, General Surgical	Surgery
Insufflator, Laparoscopic	Obstetrics/Gynecology
Jar, Operating Room	Surgery
Kit, Burn	General
Marker, Skin	Surgery
Orthosis, Limb Brace	Physical Med
Restraint, Protective (Body)	General
Sheet, Burn	General
Splint, Clavicle	Physical Med
Splint, Traction	Orthopedics
Sponge, Gauze	Dental And Oral
Sponge, Internal	Cns/Neurology
Sponge, Laparotomy	Surgery
Sponge, Ophthalmic	Ophthalmology
Staple, Removable (Skin)	Surgery
Stapler, Surgical	Surgery
Stockinette	Orthopedics
Support, Patient Position	Anesthesiology
Tray, Surgical	Surgery
Wick, Ear	Ear/Nose/Throat
Wrap, Sterilization	General

DEROYAL SURGICAL - ROSE HILL 800-251-9864

100 Rose Hill Industrial Park, 865-362-6022
Rose Hill, VA 24281
FDA Number: 1046367
E-mail: customerservice@deroyal.com
Web site: www.deroyal.com
Year Founded: 1973
Ownership: DEROYAL INDUSTRIES, INC.
Produces/Sells CE-marked Devices: N

Accessories, Apparel, Surgical	Surgery
Accessories, Cardiopulmonary Bypass	Cardiovascular
Accessories, Catheter	Gastroenterology/Urology
Accessories, Cleaning, Endoscopic	Gastroenterology/Urology
Accessories, Light, Surgical	Surgery
Accessories, Surgical Camera	Surgery
Adapter, Stopcock, Manifold, Cardiopulmonary Bypass	Cardiovascular
Amniotome	Obstetrics/Gynecology
Applicator, Tipped, Absorbent, Non-Sterile	General
Applicator, Tipped, Absorbent, Sterile	General
Bag, Blood, Collection	Hematology
Bandage, Adhesive	Surgery
Bandage, Cast	Physical Med
Bandage, Compression	General
Bandage, Elastic	General

DEROYAL SURGICAL - ROSE HILL 800-251-9864 *(cont'd)*

Bandage, Liquid	Surgery
Basin, Emesis	General
Blade, Scalpel	Surgery
Blade, Surgical, Saw, General & Plastic Surgery	Surgery
Brush, Cytology, Endoscopic	Gastroenterology/Urology
Brush, Scrub, Operating Room	Surgery
Catheter, Intravascular, Diagnostic	Cardiovascular
Catheter, Irrigation	Surgery
Catheter, Peritoneal	Surgery
Catheter, Suction (Tracheal Aspirating Tube)	Anesthesiology
Catheter, Upper Urinary Tract	Gastroenterology/Urology
Circuit, Breathing (W Connector, Adapter, Y Piece)	Anesthesiology
Clamp, Bone	Orthopedics
Clamp, Circumcision	Obstetrics/Gynecology
Clamp, Vascular	Cardiovascular
Clasp, Preformed	Dental And Oral
Component, Traction, Non-Invasive	Orthopedics
Container, Medication, Graduated Liquid	General
Container, Sharpes	General
Container, Specimen, All Types	General
Container, Specimen, Non-sterile	General
Cotton, Roll	Dental And Oral
Counter, Sponge, Surgical	General
Cover, Limb	Physical Med
Cuff, Blood Pressure	Cardiovascular
Depressor, Tongue	General
Depressor, Tongue, ENT, Metal	Ear/Nose/Throat
Dilator, Vessel, Percutaneous Catheterization	Cardiovascular
Dissector, Surgical, General & Plastic Surgery	Surgery
Drape, Surgical	Surgery
Dressing, Other	General
Dressing, Wound And Burn, Occlusive, Heated	Surgery
Dressing, Wound and Burn, Hydrogel	Surgery
Dressing, Wound and Burn, Occlusive	Surgery
Dressing, Wound, Hydrophilic	Surgery
Dressing, Wound, Occlusive	Surgery
Electrocautery Unit, Gynecologic	Obstetrics/Gynecology
Electrosurgical Unit, Cutting & Coagulation Device	Surgery
Endoscope	Gastroenterology/Urology
Fiber, Absorbent	General
Filter, Bacterial, Breathing Circuit	Anesthesiology
Forceps	Orthopedics
Forceps, General & Plastic Surgery	Surgery
Gauze, Non-Absorbable, X-Ray Detectable (Internal Sponge)	Surgery
Gauze/sponge, Nonresorbable For External Use	Surgery
General Use Surgical Scissors	Surgery
Hemostat	Orthopedics
Injector, Angiographic (Cardiac Catheterization)	Cardiovascular
Instrument, Manual, General Surgical	Surgery
Instrument, Passing, Ligature, Knot Tying	Cns/Neurology
Insufflator, Laparoscopic	Obstetrics/Gynecology
Kit, Administration, Intravenous	General
Kit, Surgical Instrument, Disposable	Surgery
Label/Tag, Sterile	Surgery
Laparoscope, General & Plastic Surgery	Surgery
Light, Surgical, Floor Standing	Surgery
Linen, Bed	General
Lubricant, Patient	General
Marker, Skin	General
Mask, Gas, Anesthesia	Anesthesiology
Needle, Aspiration And Injection, Disposable	Surgery
Needle, Hypodermic, Single Lumen With Syringe	General
Needle, Suture, Disposable	Surgery
Occluder, Umbilical	General
Pad, Neonatal Eye	General
Pledget And Intracardiac Patch, PETP, PTFE, Polypropylene	Cardiovascular
Retractor, Surgical	Surgery
Scalpel, One-Piece (Knife)	Surgery
Scissors, Disposable	General
Sheet, Burn	General
Slide, Microscope	Pathology
Snare, Surgical	Surgery
Sponge, External	Surgery
Sponge, Gauze	Dental And Oral
Sponge, Ophthalmic	Ophthalmology
Staple, Removable (Skin)	Surgery
Stapler, Surgical	Surgery
Stethoscope, Esophageal	Anesthesiology
Stethoscope, Esophageal, With Electrical Conductors	Anesthesiology
Stethoscope, Manual	Cardiovascular
Suction Apparatus, Operating Room, Wall Vacuum-Powered	Surgery
Suction Apparatus, Single Patient, Portable, Non-Powered	Surgery
Surgical Instrument, Disposable	Surgery
Surgical Instrument, Non-Powered, Neurosurgical	Cns/Neurology
Syringe, Irrigating	General
Tape, Measuring, Ruler And Caliper	Surgery
Temperature Strip, Forehead, Liquid Crystal	General
Thermometer, Electronic, Continuous	General
Toothbrush, Manual	Dental And Oral
Tourniquet, Non-Pneumatic, Surgical	Surgery
Transfer Unit, IV Fluid	General

DEROYAL SURGICAL - ROSE HILL 800-251-9864 *(cont'd)*

Tray, Surgical	Surgery
Tray, Surgical Instrument	Surgery
Tube, Aspirating, Flexible, Connecting	Anesthesiology
Tubing, Flexible, Medical Gas, Low-Pressure	Anesthesiology
Tubing, Non-Invasive	Surgery
Warmer, Radiant, Infant	General
Wick, Ear	Ear/Nose/Throat
Wrap, Sterilization	General

DEROYAL SURGICAL TRAY DIVISION 800-251-9864
1595 Highway 33 South, 865-362-6022
New Tazewell, TN 37825
FDA Number: 2320762
E-mail: customerservice@deroyal.com
Web site: www.deroyal.com
Year Founded: 1973
Ownership: DEROYAL INDUSTRIES, INC.
Produces/Sells CE-marked Devices: N

Drape, Surgical	Surgery
Gown, Surgical	Surgery
Kit, Surgical (General)	Surgery
Kit, Surgical Instrument, Disposable	Surgery

DEROYAL TECHNOLOGIES, INC. 800-251-9864
1595 Highway 33 South, 865-362-6022
New Tazewell, TN 37825
FDA Number: 3004616094
E-mail: customerservice@deroyal.com
Web site: www.deroyal.com
Year Founded: 1973
Ownership: Private
Produces/Sells CE-marked Devices: N

Bandage, Liquid	Surgery
Dressing, Other	General
Dressing, Wound and Burn, Hydrogel	Surgery
Pack, Hot Or Cold, Water Circulating	Physical Med

DEROYAL TEXTILES, INC. 800-251-9864
125 East York, Camden, SC 29020 865-362-6022
FDA Number: 1061092
E-mail: customerservice@deroyal.com
Web site: www.deroyal.com
Year Founded: 1973
Ownership: DEROYAL INDUSTRIES, INC.
Produces/Sells CE-marked Devices: N

Dressing, Other	General
Fiber, Absorbent	General
Gauze/sponge, Nonresorbable For External Use	Surgery
Sponge, Gauze	Dental And Oral

DEROYAL WOUND CARE 800-251-9864
164 giles hollow road, P.O. Box 309, 865-362-6022
Rose Hill, VA 24281
FDA Number: 1123071
E-mail: customerservice@deroyal.com
Web site: www.deroyal.com
Year Founded: 1973
Ownership: DEROYAL INDUSTRIES, INC.
Produces/Sells CE-marked Devices: N

Adapter, Stopcock, Manifold, Cardiopulmonary Bypass	Cardiovascular
Catheter, Intravascular, Diagnostic	Cardiovascular
Dressing, Other	General
Dressing, Wound and Burn, Hydrogel	Surgery
Injector, Angiographic (Cardiac Catheterization)	Cardiovascular
Orthosis, Lumbosacral	Physical Med
Sheet, Burn	General
Sponge, External, Synthetic	Surgery
Strip, Adhesive	Surgery
Tape, Gauze, Adhesive	General
Transfer Unit, IV Fluid	General
Tray, Surgical	Surgery

DEROYAL/LMB, INC. 800-251-9864
712 Fiero Lane, No. 37, 865-362-6022
San Luis Obispo, CA 93401
FDA Number: 2021791
E-mail: customerservice@deroyal.com
Web site: www.deroyal.com
Year Founded: 1973
Ownership: DEROYAL INDUSTRIES, INC.
Produces/Sells CE-marked Devices: N

Component, Exercise	Physical Med
Exerciser, Non-Measuring	Physical Med
Orthosis, Limb Brace	Physical Med
Protector, Skin Pressure	General
Splint, Hand, And Component	Physical Med

DERRON SURGICAL INSTRUMENTS, INC. 888-374-3622
1055 Scherer Way, Osprey, FL 34229 941-918-8852
FDA Number: 1424471 *Fax:* 941-918-8862
E-mail: gkderron@cs.com
Annual Revenue: $0-$1 Million
Year Founded: 1999
Total Employees: 2
Ownership: Private
Produces/Sells CE-marked Devices: N
Federal Procurement Eligibility: Small Business, Minority Owned, Female Owned
Distribution: Manufacturer Through Distributor

Orthopedic Manual Surgical Instrument	Orthopedics
Surgical Instrument, Manual (General Use)	Surgery
Surgical Instrument, Obstetric/Gynecologic, General	Obstetrics/Gynecology

DESACC, INC. 866-638-0936
0844 Sw Curry St., Portland, OR 97239
FDA Number: 3003230585
Ownership: Private
Produces/Sells CE-marked Devices: N

System, Communication, Image, Digital	Radiology

DESCENT CONTROL SYSTEMS, INC. 801-304-9299
8100 South 1300 West, #d, West Jordan, UT 84088
FDA Number: 3004828791

Lift, Bath, Non-AC-Powered	General
Stretcher, Hand-Carried	General
Stretcher, Wheeled (Mobile)	General

DESCHUTES MEDICAL PRODUCTS, INC. 800-383-2588
1011 S.w. Emkay Drive, Suite 104, 541-385-0350
Bend, OR 97702
FDA Number: 3021763 *Fax:* 541-382-2079
E-mail: info@DependOnMyself.com
Web site: www.deschutesmed.com
Year Founded: 1992
Total Employees: 9 *Marketing Staff:* 3 *Sales Staff:* 2
Ownership: Private
Quality System Registration Information: ISO9001
Produces/Sells CE-marked Devices: Y
Federal Procurement Eligibility: Small Business
Distribution: Manufacturer Direct
General Admin.: Michael Wax/President, Chief Executive Officer
Mktg./Adv.: Lisa Hammermann/Director Marketing
    Matt Hoskins/Director Product Development
    Chris Bridges/Vice President Natl Accounts & Sales

Perineometer	Obstetrics/Gynecology

DESERET LABORATORIES INC. 435-628-8786
1414 East 3850 South, St. George, UT 84790
FDA Number: 1000160324 *Fax:* 435-673-1202
E-mail: sales@deseretlabs.com
Web site: www.deseretlabs.com
Ownership: Private
Produces/Sells CE-marked Devices: N

Cleaner, Denture	Dental And Oral

DESERET MEDICAL, INC.
See Becton Dickinson Infusion Therapy Systems, Inc.

DESIGN & EVALUATION, INC. 856-228-3800
1451-B Chews Landing Road, Laurel Springs, NJ 08021
FDA Number: n/a *Fax:* 856-228-9687
E-mail: walt.smith@designandevaluation.com
Web site: www.designandevaluation.com
Medical Products Sales Volume: $900,000
Year Founded: 1976
Total Employees: 9
Ownership: Private
Produces/Sells CE-marked Devices: N
Federal Procurement Eligibility: Small Business

Service, Consulting	General
Service, Engineering/Design	General

DESIGN PRINCIPLES, INC.
See Allied Healthcare Products, Inc.

DESIGN STANDARDS CORP. 603-826-7744
Box 1620, 957 Claremont Road, Charlestown, NH 03603
FDA Number: 1222274 *Fax:* 603-826-4406
E-mail: hr@designstandards.com
Web site: www.designstandards.com
Ownership: Private
Produces/Sells CE-marked Devices: N

Extractor, Nail	Orthopedics
Staple, Removable (Skin)	Surgery

DESIGN TECHNOLOGY CORP. 978-663-7000
5 Suburban Park Dr., Billerica, MA 01821-3904
FDA Number: n/a *Fax:* 978-663-6841

MANUFACTURER PROFILES

DESIGN TECHNOLOGY CORP.   978-663-7000 *(cont'd)*
- *E-mail:* sales@design-technology.com
- *Web site:* www.design-technology.com
- *Annual Revenue:* $5-$10 Million
- *Total Employees:* 40
- *Ownership:* Private
- *Produces/Sells CE-marked Devices:* Y
- *Federal Procurement Eligibility:* Small Business
- *Distribution:* Manufacturer Direct
- *General Admin.:* Marvin Menzin/Chief Executive Officer

Contract R&D, Equipment	General
Foodservice Product/Equipment	General
Packaging Equipment	General
Production Equipment	General
Service, Engineering/Design	General
System, Robot	General

DESIGNER CARE CO., LTD.   800-848-6335
474 Main Avenue, Neche, ND 58265   701-886-7778
- *FDA Number:* 2183845   *Fax:* 701-866-7797
- *E-mail:* wecare@polarcomm.com
- *Web site:* www.designercare.com
- *Year Founded:* 0
- *Ownership:* Private
- *Produces/Sells CE-marked Devices:* N

Glove, Patient Examination, Latex	General
Glove, Patient Examination, Poly	General
Glove, Patient Examination, Vinyl	General

DESIGNS FOR COMFORT, INC.   800-443-9226
P.O. Box 671044, Marietta, GA 30066   770-565-8246
- *FDA Number:* n/a   *Fax:* 770-565-8425
- *Web site:* www.headlinerhats.com
- *Annual Revenue:* $0-$1 Million
- *Ownership:* Private
- *Produces/Sells CE-marked Devices:* N
- *Federal Procurement Eligibility:* Small Business
- *Distribution:* Manufacturer Direct

Adaptor, Grooming	Physical Med
Clothing, Protective	General

DESTAL INDUSTRIES, INC.   973-227-1830
201 Washington St., Columbus, IN 47201
- *FDA Number:* 2031865

Nebulizer, Direct Patient Interface	Anesthesiology

DETECTO SCALE CO.   800-641-2008
203 E. Daugherty, PO Box 151,   417-673-4631
Webb City, MO 64870
- *FDA Number:* n/a   *Fax:* 417-673-5001
- *E-mail:* detecto@cardet.com
- *Web site:* www.detectoscale.com
- *Medical Products Sales Volume:* $40,000,000
- *Year Founded:* 1950
- *Total Employees:* 450   *Marketing Staff:* 5   *Sales Staff:* 10
- *Ownership:* Cardinal Scale Mfg. Co.
- *Quality System Registration Information:* ISO9001; ISO9002
- *Produces/Sells CE-marked Devices:* N
- *Federal Procurement Eligibility:* Small Business
- *Distribution:* Manufacturer Direct, Manufacturer Through Distributor, Manufacturer Through Manufacturer Reps, Service Direct, Exporter
- *General Admin.:* W. H. Perry/Chief Executive Officer
  - David Perry/President
- *Mktg./Adv.:* Ron Vocelka/Manager Advertising
  - Fred Cox/Vice President Sales

Analyzer, Composition, Weight, Patient	General

DETERLINE CORP.
- *See* Titan Corporation/Systems & Imagery Division

DEUTERONOMY MANAGEMENT SERVICES,INC.   850-897-3321
1439 Live Oak St., Suite A, Niceville, FL 32578-8829
- *FDA Number:* 1064327
- *Ownership:* Private
- *Produces/Sells CE-marked Devices:* N

Container, IV	General
Cover, Barrier, Protective	General
Kit, Administration, Intravenous	General
Wrap, Sterilization	General

DEVAR INC.   800-566-6822
706 Bostwick Avenue,   203-368-6751
Bridgeport, CT 06605
- *FDA Number:* 7000113
- *E-mail:* info@devarinc.com
- *Web site:* www.devarinc.com
- *Medical Products Sales Volume:* $2,300,000
- *Annual Revenue:* $1-$5 Million
- *Year Founded:* 1961

DEVAR INC.   800-566-6822 *(cont'd)*
- *Total Employees:* 30   *Marketing Staff:* 3   *Sales Staff:* 2
- *Ownership:* Private
- *Quality System Registration Information:* ISO9001
- *Produces/Sells CE-marked Devices:* Y
- *Federal Procurement Eligibility:* Small Business
- *Distribution:* Manufacturer Direct, Manufacturer Through Manufacturer Reps
- *General Admin.:* A. J. Ruscito/President, Chief Executive Officer
  - Diane Billings/Vice President Human Resources
- *Mktg./Adv.:* T. W. Tomasko/Vice President Marketing & Sales
- *Production:* J. C. Head/General Manager Production
- *Research:* Andy Gura/Vice President Research & Development

Meter, pH, General Use	Toxicology
Recorder, Chart, Laboratory	Chemistry
Regulator, Temperature	Chemistry

DEVAX, INC.   949-334-2333
20996 Bake Parkway, Suite 106, Lake Forest, CA 92630
- *FDA Number:* n/a   *Fax:* 949-334-2330
- *E-mail:* info@devax.net
- *Web site:* www.devax.net
- *Total Employees:* 32
- *Ownership:* Private
- *Produces/Sells CE-marked Devices:* N
- *Federal Procurement Eligibility:* Small Business
- *General Admin.:* Mr. Jeff Thiel/President, Chief Executive Officer

Stent, Cardiovascular	Cardiovascular

DEVICES AND SERVICES CO.
- *See* Images-On-Call

DEVICOR MEDICAL PRODUCTS INC.   513.864.9000
300 E-Business Way, Fifth Floor, Cincinnati, OH 45241
- *FDA Number:* 300849246   *Fax:* 513.864.9011
- *E-mail:* customersupport@mammotome.com
- *Web site:* http://www.devicormedical.com
- *Year Founded:* 2008
- *Ownership:* Private
- *Produces/Sells CE-marked Devices:* N
- *General Admin.:* Mr. Tom Daulton/Chief Executive Officer
  - Mr. Kent Rex/Chief Operating Officer
- *Mktg./Adv.:* Mr. Jonathan Salkin/Senior Vice President Corporate Development
- *Production:* Mr. Bruce Bruce Marchioni/Vice President Quality Assurance & Regulatory Affairs
- *Research:* Mr. Mike Ehlert/Senior Vice President Scientific Affairs
- *Finance:* Mr. Joe Trentacosta/Chief Financial Officer
  - Mr. Sean Burke/Vice President Finance

Biopsy Instrument	Gastroenterology/Urology
Clip, Implantable	Surgery
Forceps, General & Plastic Surgery	Surgery
Marker, Radiographic, Implantable	Surgery
Scanner, Ultrasonic (Pulsed Doppler)	Radiology
Staple, Implantable	Surgery

DEVON MEDICAL PRODUCTS   800-571-3135
1100 First Ave., Ste 202, King of Prussia, PA 19406
- *FDA Number:* 3006516543   *Fax:* 484-636-3380
- *E-mail:* info@devonmedicalsupplies.com
- *Web site:* www.devonmedicalinc.com
- *Year Founded:* 5
- *Total Employees:* 15   *Marketing Staff:* 2   *Sales Staff:* 5
- *Ownership:* Devon International Group
- *Produces/Sells CE-marked Devices:* N
- *Federal Procurement Eligibility:* Small Business
- *Distribution:* Manufacturer Direct, Manufacturer Through Distributor, Manufacturer Through Manufacturer Reps, Importer
- *Mktg./Adv.:* Ms. Nicole Rivera/Marketing Product Specialist
  - Ms. Keyscha Schofield/Sales Representative
- *Production:* Ms. Ruth Wu/Manager Medical Products

Biofeedback Device	Cns/Neurology
Chromatography (Thin Layer), Clinical Use	Toxicology
Defibrillator, External, Automatic	Cardiovascular
Enzyme Immunoassay, Amphetamine	Toxicology
Enzyme Immunoassay, Barbiturate	Toxicology
Enzyme Immunoassay, Benzodiazepine	Toxicology
Enzyme Immunoassay, Cannabinoids	Toxicology
Enzyme Immunoassay, Cocaine And Cocaine Metabolites	Toxicology
Enzyme Immunoassay, Methadone	Toxicology
Enzyme Immunoassay, Opiates	Toxicology
Enzyme Immunoassay, Phencyclidine	Toxicology
Monitor, Blood Pressure, Indirect, Automatic	Cardiovascular
Oximeter, Pulse	General
Pump, Blood, Extra-Luminal	Gastroenterology/Urology
Sleeve, Compressible Limb	Cardiovascular
Syringe, Ear	Ear/Nose/Throat
U.V. Spectrometry, Tricyclic Antidepressant Drugs	Toxicology

DEXALL BIOMEDICAL LABS, INC.   301-840-1884
18904 Bonanza Way, Gaithersburg, MD 20879
- *FDA Number:* 1121520   *Fax:* 301-330-0883

DEXALL BIOMEDICAL LABS, INC.　301-840-1884 (cont'd)
E-mail: info@dexall.com
Web site: www.dexall.com
Annual Revenue: $1-$5 Million
Year Founded: 1978
Ownership: Private
Produces/Sells CE-marked Devices: Y
Federal Procurement Eligibility: Small Business
Distribution: Manufacturer Through Distributor
General Admin.: Dr. Thomas T. Hubscher/President
Mktg./Adv.: Glen M. Ford/Director Product Development
Production: Eric I. Thompson/Manager Production
　　　　　C. R. Ruth Lee/Manager Regulatory Affairs
Research: Dr. Thomas T. Hubscher/Director Research & Development

Test, Allergy	Immunology
Test, C-Reactive Protein	Immunology
Urease, Photometric, Urea Nitrogen	Chemistry

DEXCOM, INC.　858-200-0200
6340 Sequence Drive, San Diego, CA 92121
FDA Number: 3004753838　　　　Fax: 858-200-0201
E-mail: info@dexcom.com
Web site: www.dexcom.com
Year Founded: 1999
Ownership: Public
Stock Symbol: DXCM
Traded On: NASDAQ
Produces/Sells CE-marked Devices: N
General Admin.: Mr. Jess Roper/Chief Financial Officer, Vice President
　　　　Mr. Steven Pacelli/Chief Operating Officer
　　　　Mr. Terrance H. Gregg/President, Chief Executive Officer
Mktg./Adv.: Mr. Peter Gerhardsson/Vice President Business Development
　　　　Ms. Claudia Graham/Vice President Marketing
　　　　Mr. Richard Doubleday/Vice President Sales
Production: Mr. Jorge A. Valdes/Senior Vice President Operations
　　　　Mr. Andrew K. Balo/Senior Vice President Regulatory Affairs

Bandage, Adhesive	Surgery
Sensor, Glucose, Invasive	General

DEXON MANUFACTURING
See La Calhene

DEXTA CORPORATION　800-733-3982
962 Kaiser Rd., Napa, CA 94558　707-255-2454
FDA Number: 2916273　　　　Fax: 707-255-8520
Web site: www.dexta.com
Medical Products Sales Volume: $2,000,000
Annual Revenue: $25-$50 Million
Ownership: Private
Produces/Sells CE-marked Devices: Y
Federal Procurement Eligibility: Small Business
Distribution: Manufacturer Direct, Manufacturer Through Distributor

Band, Elastic, Orthodontic	Dental And Oral
Chair, Dental	Dental And Oral
Chair, Examination And Treatment	General
Chair, Ophthalmic, AC-Powered	Ophthalmology
Chair, Surgical, AC-Powered	Surgery
Stool, Operating Room, Adjustable	Surgery
Table, Surgical, Electrical	Surgery

DEXTER APACHE HOLDINGS, INC.　800-524-2954
2211 W. Grimes, Fairfield, IA 52556　641-472-5131
FDA Number: n/a　　　　Fax: 641-472-6336
E-mail: akretz@dxtrco.com
Web site: www.dexter.com
Annual Revenue: $50-$100 Million
Year Founded: 1972
Total Employees: 540　Marketing Staff: 6　Sales Staff: 6
Ownership: Private
Produces/Sells CE-marked Devices: Y
Distribution: Manufacturer Through Distributor
Mktg./Adv.: Mr. Andrew Kretz/Director Marketing & Sales

Laundry Equipment	General
Washer, Laundry	General

DEXTER CORP.
See Ahlstrom Windsor Locks Llc

DEY, L.P.　800-755-5560
2751 Napa Valley Corporate Drive,　707-224-3200
Napa, CA 94558
FDA Number: n/a　　　　Fax: 707-224-0495
E-mail: deyhr@dey.com
Web site: www.dey.com
Medical Products Sales Volume: $127,400,000
Year Founded: 1978
Total Employees: 1000　Marketing Staff: 16　Sales Staff: 220
Ownership: An Affiliate of EMD, Inc.
Produces/Sells CE-marked Devices: N

DEY, L.P.　800-755-5560 (cont'd)
Distribution: Manufacturer Direct, Manufacturer Through Distributor
General Admin.: J. Melville Engle/Chief Executive Officer
　Medical Admin.: Michelle Carpenter/Executive Vice President Clinical Affairs
Mktg./Adv.: Colin Chan/Director Business Development
　　　　Ray Joske/Executive Vice President Marketing
　　　　Christy Taylor/Executive Vice President Sales
　　　　Jan Prazak/Manager Sales Training
Production: Don Hume/Director Materials
　　　　Mary Lou Freathy/Director Quality Assurance
　　　　Larry Lavi/Director Quality Control
　　　　Gary Michaud/Executive Vice President Operations
　　　　Susan Schnars/Product Manager

Flowmeter, Gas (Oxygen), Calibrated	Anesthesiology
Inhaler, Nasal	Ear/Nose/Throat
Valve, Breathing	Anesthesiology
Water, Therapy, Respiratory	Microbiology

DFINE INC.　866-963-3463
3047 Orchard Parkway, San Jose, CA 95134　408-321-9401
FDA Number: 3006396387　　　　Fax: 408-321-9401
E-mail: info@dfineinc.com
Web site: www.dfineinc.com
Year Founded: 2004
Ownership: Private
Produces/Sells CE-marked Devices: N
General Admin.: Mr. Kevin Mosher/Chief Executive Officer
Mktg./Adv.: Mr. James Mazzerella/Vice President Sales
Production: Mr. Gabor Gran/Vice President Operations
　　　　Mr. Sandeep Saboo/Vice President Quality Assurance & Regulatory
Affairs
Research: Mr. Robert Poser/Vice President Scientific Affairs
Finance: Mr. Lewis Yee/Chief Financial Officer

Cement, Bone, Vertebroplasty, Pre-formed, Modular	Orthopedics
Dispenser, Cement	Orthopedics
Mixing Equipment, Cement	Orthopedics
Orthopedic Manual Surgical Instrument	Orthopedics

DGH TECHNOLOGY, INC.　800-722-3883
110 Summit Dr., Ste.B, Exton, PA 19341　610-594-9100
FDA Number: 2522950　　　　Fax: 610-594-0390
Web site: www.dghkoi.com
Annual Revenue: $5-$10 Million
Total Employees: 20　Marketing Staff: 4　Sales Staff: 16
Ownership: Private
Produces/Sells CE-marked Devices: N
Federal Procurement Eligibility: Small Business, Minority Owned
Distribution: Manufacturer Direct, Manufacturer Through Distributor, Manufacturer
Through Manufacturer Reps, OEM, Service Direct, Exporter
General Admin.: Earl Henderson/President, Chief Executive Officer
Mktg./Adv.: Thomas H. McSunas/Director Marketing & Sales
　　　　Lou Detweiler/Director Product Development
Production: Lou Detweiler/Director Quality Assurance
Research: William Grenoble/Vice President Research & Development

Blade, Scalpel	Surgery
Cleaner, Ultrasonic, Medical Instrument	General
Handle, Knife Blade	Surgery
Knife, Cataract	Ophthalmology
Knife, Keratome	Ophthalmology
Knife, Ophthalmic	Ophthalmology
Knife, Scalpel	Surgery
Knife, Surgical	Dental And Oral

DGH-KOI, INC.
See Dgh Technology, Inc.

DGIMED ORTHO INC.　952-582-6700
12400 Whitewater Dr, Suite 2010, Minnetonka, MN 55343
FDA Number: 3007710313　　　　Fax: 952-582-6701
E-mail: info@dgimedortho.com
Web site: http://dgimedortho.com
Ownership: Private
Produces/Sells CE-marked Devices: N
General Admin.: Mr. Scott Youngstrom/Chief Operating Officer, Vice President
　　　　Mr. Mark McMahan/President, Chief Executive Officer
Mktg./Adv.: Mr. Erik Martz/Director Product Development
Production: Mr. Gary Graham/Director Operations

Rod, Fixation, Intramedullary	Orthopedics

DGR, INC.
See Eyekon Medical, Inc

DH BIOMEDICAL, INC.　800-600-8791
1712 9th St. W., Bradenton, FL 34205
FDA Number: n/a　　　　Fax: 941-714-0210
E-mail: sales@dhbiomedical.com
Web site: www.dhbiomedical.com
Ownership: Private
Produces/Sells CE-marked Devices: N

MANUFACTURER PROFILES

DH BIOMEDICAL, INC.   **800-600-8791** *(cont'd)*
Electrocardiograph, Multi-Channel   Cardiovascular

DHS SYSTEMS LLC   **845-359-6066**
33 Kings Hwy., Orangeburg, NY 10962-1802
FDA Number: n/a   *Fax:* 845-365-2114
E-mail: drash@drash.com
Web site: www.drash.com
Annual Revenue: $25-$50 Million
Ownership: Private
Quality System Registration Information: ISO9000; ISO9001
Produces/Sells CE-marked Devices: N
Federal Procurement Eligibility: Small Business
Distribution: Manufacturer Direct
  Facility, Equipment, Medical, Mobile   General

DI-CHEM CONCENTRATE, INC.   **763-422-8311**
509 Fishing Creek Rd., Lewisberry, PA 17339
FDA Number: 1528807
  Concentrate, Dialysis, Hemodialysis (Liquid or Powder)   Gastroenterology/Urology

DI-CHEM, INC.   **800-847-2598**
12297 Ensign Ave. North, Champlin, MN 55316   **763-422-8311**
FDA Number: 2183415   *Fax:* 763-422-8472
E-mail: info@dichem-us.com
Web site: www.dichem-us.com
Ownership: Private
Produces/Sells CE-marked Devices: N
  Concentrate, Dialysis, Hemodialysis (Liquid or Powder)   Gastroenterology/Urology

DIABETES SENTRY PRODUCTS   **360-738-1200**
1200 Dupont St, Suite 1-D, Bellingham, WA 98225
FDA Number: 3003636198
E-mail: Info@DiabetesSentry.com   *Fax:* 360-671-1996
Web site: www.diabetessentry.com/index.html
Medical Products Sales Volume: $400,000
Annual Revenue: More than $1 Billion
Total Employees: 4   *Marketing Staff:* 4   *Sales Staff:* 2
Ownership: Private
Produces/Sells CE-marked Devices: N
Federal Procurement Eligibility: Small Business
Distribution: Manufacturer Direct
General Admin.: Marvin Meier/President, Chief Executive Officer
Production: Marlene Riviere/General Manager Operations
  Alarm, Hypoglycemia   Gastroenterology/Urology

DIABETES SUPPLIES
See Diabetes Sentry Products

DIABETES TECHNOLOGIES, INC.   **888-872-2443**
184 Big Star Drive, Thomasville, GA 31757   **229-227-1245**
FDA Number: 1065559
Web site: www.diabetestechnologies.com
Ownership: Private
Produces/Sells CE-marked Devices: N
  Test, Glycosylated Hemoglobin Assay   Hematology

DIABETICA SOLUTIONS, INC.   **210-692-1114**
12665 Silicon Dr., San Antonio, TX 78249
FDA Number: 3004982763
  Thermometer, Electronic, Continuous   General
  Vibration Threshold Measurement Device   Cns/Neurology

DIABLO SALES & MARKETING, INC.   **925-648-1611**
PO Box 408, Diablo, CA 94526
FDA Number: n/a   *Fax:* 925-648-1711
E-mail: info@diablosales.com
Web site: www.diablosales.com
Year Founded: 1987
Ownership: Private
Produces/Sells CE-marked Devices: N
Federal Procurement Eligibility: Small Business
  Cannula, Aortic   Cardiovascular
  Cannula, Brain   Cns/Neurology
  Cannula, Catheter   Cardiovascular
  Cannula, Ventricular   Cns/Neurology
  Catheter, Arterial   Cardiovascular
  Catheter, Central Venous   General
  Catheter, Imaging, Ultrasonic   Radiology
  Catheter, Intraspinal, Percutaneous, Short-Term   General
  Catheter, Intravascular Occluding   Cns/Neurology
  Catheter, Intravascular, Therapeutic, Short-term Less Than 30 Days   General
  Catheter, Intravenous   Cardiovascular
  Catheter, Perfusion   Cardiovascular
  Catheter, Steerable   Cardiovascular
  Guide, Wire, Angiographic (And Accessories)   Cns/Neurology
  Guidewire, Catheter, Radiological   Radiology
  Introducer, Catheter   Cardiovascular
  Stylet, Catheter   Cardiovascular
  Trocar, Cardiovascular   Cardiovascular

DIABLO SALES & MARKETING, INC.   **925-648-1611** *(cont'd)*
  Trocar, Other   General
  Trocar, Thoracic   Cardiovascular
  Tubing, Braided   General
  Tubing, Multi-Lumen   General
  Tubing, Polyethylene   General
  Tubing, Radiopaque   General
  Tubing, Silicone   General
  Tubing, Urethane   General

DIACK
See Thorn Smith Laboratories

DIACOR, INC.   **800-342-2679**
2550 Decker Lane, Suite 26,   **801-467-0050**
West Valley City, UT 84119
FDA Number: 1721113   *Fax:* 801-487-3258
E-mail: info@diacorinc.com
Web site: www.diacorinc.com
Medical Products Sales Volume: $500,000
Year Founded: 1983
Total Employees: 5
Ownership: Private
Quality System Registration Information: ISO9001
Produces/Sells CE-marked Devices: Y
Federal Procurement Eligibility: Small Business, GSA Contract
Distribution: Manufacturer Direct, Manufacturer Through Distributor, Manufacturer Through Manufacturer Reps, OEM, Importer, Exporter
General Admin.: Glenn N. Waterman/President, Chief Executive Officer
Mktg./Adv.: Kevin Anderson/Director Marketing
  Accelerator, Linear, Medical   Radiology
  Block, Therapy, Radiation   Radiology
  Cabinet, Other   General
  Cart, Other   General
  Immobilizer, Therapy, Radiation   Radiology
  Monitor, Patient Position, Light Beam   Radiology
  Table, Radiographic   Radiology
  Therapeutic X-Ray System   Radiology

DIADEXUS, INC.   **650-246-6400**
343 Oyster Point Blvd., South San Francisco, CA 94080
FDA Number: 3003643666   *Fax:* 650-246-6499
Ownership: Private
Produces/Sells CE-marked Devices: N
General Admin.: Mr. David Foster/Chief Financial Officer, Executive Vice President
                Dr. Robert Wolfert/Chief Scientific Officer & Executive Vice President
                Mr. Bernard Alfano/Executive Vice President
                Mr. Patrick Plewman/President, Chief Executive Officer
  Antigen, Antiserum, Control, Lipoprotein, Low Density   Immunology
  Calibrator, Secondary, Clinical Chemistry   Chemistry
  Control, Analyte (Assayed And Unassayed)   Chemistry
  Reagents, Specific, Analyte   Hematology
  Test, System, Immunoassay, Lipoprotein-associated Phospholipase A2   Immunology

DIAGNOCURE, INC.   **418-527-6100**
4535 Wilfrid-Hamel Blvd, Suite 250,
QUEBEC CITY, QUE G1P 2 Canada
FDA Number: n/a   *Fax:* 418-527-0240
E-mail: communications@diagnocure.com
Web site: www.diagnocure.com
Year Founded: 1994
Ownership: Public
Stock Symbol: CUR
Traded On: Toronto
Quality System Registration Information: ISO9001
Produces/Sells CE-marked Devices: N
Distribution: Manufacturer Direct, Exclusive Distributor, Exporter

DIAGNOSIS, LLC   **978.458.1600**
Suite 500, 175 Cabot Street, Lowell,, MA 01854
FDA Number: n/a   *Fax:* 978.458.1755
E-mail: mail@diagnosysllc.com
Web site: www.diagnosysllc.com
Annual Revenue: $0-$1 Million
Total Employees: 5
Ownership: Private
Produces/Sells CE-marked Devices: N
Federal Procurement Eligibility: Small Business
Distribution: Manufacturer Through Manufacturer Reps
General Admin.: Bruce Doran/President
Mktg./Adv.: Anne Doran/Vice President Marketing & Sales
Production: Alan Crist/Design Engineer
  Electrode, Corneal   Ophthalmology
  Electroretinograph (ERG)   Ophthalmology
  Stimulator, Photic, Evoked Response   Cns/Neurology
  Telemetry Unit, Physiological, EOG   Cns/Neurology

DIAGNOSOFT, INC.   650-320-9397
3461 Kenneth Drive, Palo Alto, CA 94303
FDA Number: 3006015847
Nuclear Magnetic Resonance Imaging System   Radiology

DIAGNOSTIC AUTOMATION/ CORTEZ DIAGNOSTICS INC,.   818-591-3030
23961 Craftsman Rd, Suite E/F, Calabasas, CA 91302
FDA Number: 2029372   *Fax:* 818-591-8383
E-mail: onestep@rapidtest.com.
Web site: www.diagnosticautomation.com
Ownership: Private
Produces/Sells CE-marked Devices:
Diazonium Colorimetry, Urobilinogen (Urinary, Non-Quant.)	Chemistry
Enzyme Linked Immunoabsorbent Assay, Chlamydia Group	Microbiology
Radioimmunoassay, Estriol	Chemistry
Radioimmunoassay, Estrone	Chemistry
Radioimmunoassay, Free Thyroxine	Chemistry
Radioimmunoassay, Human Growth Hormone	Chemistry
Radioimmunoassay, Luteinizing Hormone	Chemistry
Radioimmunoassay, Prolactin (Lactogen)	Chemistry
Radioimmunoassay, Testosterones And Dihydrotestosterone	Chemistry
Radioimmunoassay, Total Thyroxine	Chemistry
Radioimmunoassay, Total Triiodothyronine	Chemistry
Spirometer, Diagnostic (Respirometer)	Anesthesiology
Urease, Photometric, Urea Nitrogen	Chemistry

DIAGNOSTIC BIOSYSTEMS   888-896-3350
1020 Serpentine Lane, Suite # 114,   925-484-3350
Pleasanton, CA 94566
FDA Number: 3007035884
E-mail: customersupport@dbiosys.com
Web site: http://dbiosys.com
Ownership: Private
Produces/Sells CE-marked Devices: N
Buffer, pH	Hematology
Immunohistochemistry Reagents And Kits	Pathology
Reagent, General Purpose	Pathology
Reagents, Specific, Analyte	Hematology

DIAGNOSTIC DEVICES INC.   704-285-6400
9300 Harris Corners Parkway, Suite 450, Charlotte, NC 28269
FDA Number: 3004622211
Ownership: Private
Produces/Sells CE-marked Devices: N
Control, Analyte (Assayed And Unassayed)	Chemistry
Reagent, Glucose (Test System)	Chemistry
System, Test, Blood Glucose, Over-The-Counter	Chemistry

DIAGNOSTIC GROUP LLC   952-278-4457
7625 Golden Triangle Drive, Suite F, Eden Prairie, MN 55344
FDA Number: 2113281
Ownership: Private
Produces/Sells CE-marked Devices: N
Audiometer	Ear/Nose/Throat
Hearing-Aid	Ear/Nose/Throat
Stimulator, Auditory, Evoked Response	Cns/Neurology
Tester, Auditory Impedance	Ear/Nose/Throat

DIAGNOSTIC HEALTH GROUP   800-669-3442
PO Box 747, Frederick, MD 21703
FDA Number: n/a   *Fax:* 301-695-7940
E-mail: info@dhgsonomed
Medical Products Sales Volume: $1,000,000
Annual Revenue: $1-$5 Million
Total Employees: 1   *Marketing Staff:* 2   *Sales Staff:* 4
Ownership: Private
Produces/Sells CE-marked Devices: N
Federal Procurement Eligibility: Small Business
Distribution: Exclusive Distributor
General Admin.: Dennis H. Grizzle/President
Mktg./Adv.: Rich Waxham/Vice President Sales
Monitor, Fetal, Cardiac	Obstetrics/Gynecology
Scanner, Ultrasonic, Other	Radiology
Service, Maintenance/Repair	General

DIAGNOSTIC HYBRIDS, INC.   800-344-5847
1055 East State St., Suite 100, Athens, OH 45701   740-589-3300
FDA Number: 1528450   *Fax:* 740-592-9820
E-mail: customer_service@dhiusa.com
Web site: www.dhiusa.com
Ownership: Private
Produces/Sells CE-marked Devices: N
Antigen, Cf (including Cf Control), Herpesvirus Hominis 1, 2	Microbiology
Antisera, Fluorescent, Coxsackievirus A 1-24, B 1-6	Microbiology
Antisera, Fluorescent, Echovirus 1-34	Microbiology
Antisera, Fluorescent, Poliovirus 1-3	Microbiology
Antiserum, CF, Influenza Virus A, B, C	Microbiology
Applicator, Tipped, Absorbent, Sterile	General

DIAGNOSTIC HYBRIDS, INC.   800-344-5847 *(cont'd)*
Block, Heating	Chemistry
Control, Analyte (Assayed And Unassayed)	Chemistry
Control, Multi Analyte, All Kinds (Assayed And Unassayed)	Chemistry
Culture Media, Synthetic Cell And Tissue	Pathology
Cultured Animal And Human Cells	Pathology
Media, Mounting	Pathology
Reagents, Specific, Analyte	Hematology
Slide, Control, Quality	Microbiology
Solution, Balanced Salt	Pathology
Test, Thyroid Autoantibody	Immunology

DIAGNOSTIC INCORPORATED
See Lifecore Biomedical, Inc.

DIAGNOSTIC INSTRUMENTS INC.   586-731-6000
6540 Burroughs St., Sterling Heights, MI 48314-2133
FDA Number: n/a   *Fax:* 586-731-6469
E-mail: info@diaginc.com
Web site: www.diaginc.com
Medical Products Sales Volume: $1,800,000
Year Founded: 1985
Total Employees: 26
Ownership: Private
Produces/Sells CE-marked Devices: Y
Federal Procurement Eligibility: Small Business
Distribution: Manufacturer Through Distributor
General Admin.: Patrick Merlo/President
     Philip Merlo/Vice President
Mktg./Adv.: Dan Dayley/Manager National Sales
Camera, Microscope	Microbiology
Stand/Holder, Equipment, Laboratory	Chemistry

DIAGNOSTIC MEDICAL INSTRUMENTS, INC.
See Cardiac Science Corp.

DIAGNOSTIC MONITORING SOFTWARE   775-589-6049
292 Kingsbury Grade, #32, P.o. Box 3109, Stateline, NV 89449
FDA Number: 2028190
Ownership: Private
Produces/Sells CE-marked Devices: N
Electrocardiograph, Single Channel	Cardiovascular

DIAGNOSTIC SPECIALTIES   732-549-4011
4 Leonard St., Metuchen, NJ 08840-1220
FDA Number: 2242674   *Fax:* 732-549-4711
E-mail: dsmetuchen@aol.com
Web site: http://diagnosticspecialties.com
Medical Products Sales Volume: $1,000,000
Annual Revenue: $0-$1 Million
Total Employees: 12
Ownership: Private
Produces/Sells CE-marked Devices: N
Federal Procurement Eligibility: Small Business, Minority Owned
Distribution: Manufacturer Direct, OEM
General Admin.: Praful K. Raja/President
Mktg./Adv.: Rinaldo Pagnucco/Vice President Marketing
Analyzer, Chemistry, ELISA	Chemistry
Colorimetric Method, Triglycerides	Chemistry
Complexone, Cresolphthalein, Calcium	Chemistry
Diacetyl-Monoxime, Urea Nitrogen	Chemistry
Enzymatic Esterase-Oxidase, Cholesterol	Chemistry
Kit, Pregnancy Test	Obstetrics/Gynecology
LDL & VLDL Precipitation, HDL	Chemistry
Phosphorus Reagent (Test System)	Chemistry
Phosphotungstate Reduction, Uric Acid	Chemistry
Reagent, Bilirubin (Total Or Direct Test System)	Chemistry
Reagent, Creatinine (Test System)	Chemistry
Reagent, Cyanomethemoglobin, With Standard	Hematology
SGOT, Colorimetric	Chemistry
SGPT, Colorimetric	Chemistry
Tetraphenyl Borate, Colorimetry, Potassium	Chemistry
Tetrazolium Int Dye-Diaphorase, Lactate Dehydrogenase	Chemistry
Thymolphthalein Monophosphate, Alkaline Phosphatase	Chemistry

DIAGNOSTIC SUPPORT USA INC.   305-532-1586
1900 Sunset Harbour Dr., Suite 1902, Miami Beach, FL 33139
FDA Number: 3004732018
Ownership: Private
Produces/Sells CE-marked Devices: N
Transducer, Miniature Pressure	Physical Med

DIAGNOSTIC TECHNOLOGY, INC.   631-582-4949
175 Commerce Dr., Unit L, Hauppauge, NY 11788
FDA Number: 2424478
Antibody, Antinuclear, Indirect Immunofluorescent, Antigen	Immunology
Antiserum, Fluorescent, Epstein-Barr Virus	Microbiology
Control, Hemoglobin, Abnormal	Hematology
Control, Platelet	Hematology
Counter, Cell Or Particle, Automated	Hematology
Detergent	Hematology

DIAGNOSTIC TECHNOLOGY, INC.   631-582-4949 *(cont'd)*

Diluent, Blood Cell	Hematology
Fluid, Red Cell Lysing	Hematology
Formalin, Neutral Buffered	Pathology
Hematology Quality Control Mixture	Hematology
Reagent, Antistreptolysin-Titer/Streptolysin O	Microbiology
Reagent, Cyanomethemoglobin, With Standard	Hematology
Standard/Control, Hemoglobin, Normal/Abnormal	Hematology
Test, C-Reactive Protein	Immunology
Test, Human Chorionic Gonadotropin, Serum	Immunology
Test, Infectious Mononucleosis	Immunology
Test, Rheumatoid Factor	Immunology

DIAGNOSTICA STAGO, INC.   800-222-COAG
5 Century Drive, Parsippany, NJ 07054   973-631-1200
FDA Number: 2245451   *Fax:* 973-631-1618
E-mail: general.info@stago-us.com
Web site: www.stago-us.com
Medical Products Sales Volume: $32,700,000
Annual Revenue: $50-$100 Million
Year Founded: 1985
Total Employees: 200   *Marketing Staff:* 6   *Sales Staff:* 35
Ownership: Private
Quality System Registration Information: ISO9001
Produces/Sells CE-marked Devices: Y
Federal Procurement Eligibility: Small Business, GSA Contract
Distribution: Exclusive Distributor
General Admin.: Gerard Perrot/General Manager
Mktg./Adv.: Pascal Boulanger/Director Marketing
Steve Hintze/Director National Accounts
Frank Toffoloni/Director Sales
Laura Worfolk/Manager Marketing Research
Production: James Barrow/Director Quality Assurance
Karen Wrona/Product Manager

Analyzer, Coagulation	Hematology
Control, Coagulation, Plasma	Hematology
Enzyme Immunoassay, Other	Chemistry
Fibrin Monomer Paracoagulation	Hematology
Partial Thromboplastin Time	Hematology
Partial Thromboplastin Time, Reagent, Control	Hematology
Quantitation, Antithrombin III	Hematology
Radioimmunoassay, Platelet Factor 4	Hematology
Reagent, Thromboplastin, With Control	Hematology
Standard/Control, All Types	Chemistry
Test, Heparin (Clotting Time)	Hematology
Test, Qualitative And Quantitative Factor Deficiency	Hematology
Thromboplastin, Activated Partial	Hematology

DIAGNOSTICS BIOCHEM CANADA INC.   519-681-8731
1020 Hargrieve Rd., London, ONT N6E 1P5 Canada
FDA Number: 8010132   *Fax:* 519-681-8731
E-mail: dbc@dbc-labs.com
Web site: www.dbc-labs.com
Year Founded: 1973
Total Employees: 10   *Marketing Staff:* 2   *Sales Staff:* 2
Ownership: Private
Produces/Sells CE-marked Devices: N
Federal Procurement Eligibility: Small Business
Distribution: Manufacturer Direct, Exporter

DIAGNOSTICS FOR THE REAL WORLD, LTD.   408-773-1511
840 Del Rey Avenue, Sunnyvale, CA 94085
FDA Number: 3006247421   *Fax:* 408-773-1553
E-mail: sales.drw@drw-ltd.com
Ownership: Private
Produces/Sells CE-marked Devices: N

Container, Specimen, All Types	General
Enzyme Linked Immunoabsorbent Assay, Chlamydia Group	Microbiology

DIAGNOSTIX LTD.   800-282-4075
400 Matheson Blvd. East, Units 14 & 15,   905-890-6023
Mississauga, ONT L4Z-2 Canada
FDA Number: n/a   *Fax:* 905-890-6024
E-mail: sales.diagnostics.ca@thermofisher.com
Web site: www.diagnostix.ca
Year Founded: 1989
Total Employees: 10
Ownership: Private
Produces/Sells CE-marked Devices: N
Distribution: Manufacturer Direct, Exclusive Distributor

DIAGNOSTIX PLUS, INC.   516-536-2670
100 North Village Ave., Suite # 33, Rockville Centre, NY 11570
FDA Number: n/a   *Fax:* 516-536-2095
E-mail: info@diagplus.com
Web site: www.diagplus.com
Medical Products Sales Volume: $1,500,000
Annual Revenue: $1-$5 Million
Year Founded: 1983

DIAGNOSTIX PLUS, INC.   516-536-2670 *(cont'd)*
Total Employees: 6
Ownership: Private
Produces/Sells CE-marked Devices: N
Federal Procurement Eligibility: Small Business
Distribution: Manufacturer Direct, Manufacturer Through Manufacturer Reps, Exporter
General Admin.: Barbara Zinno/Administrator
Wayne Webster/Managing Director
Donald P. Bogutski/President, Chief Executive Officer
Production: Michael Molnar/Manager Production Services

Calibrator Source, Nuclear Sealed	Radiology
Calibrator, Dose, Radionuclide	Radiology
Camera, Gamma (Nuclear/Scintillation)	Radiology
Camera, Multi-Image	Radiology
Camera, Positron	Radiology
Computer, Nuclear Medicine	Radiology
Scanner, Nuclear Emission Computed Tomography (ECT)	Radiology
Scanner, Positron Emission Tomography (PET)	Radiology
Synchronizer, Nuclear Camera	Radiology

DIAL CORPORATION., THE
See The Dial Corporation, A Henkel Company

DIALYSIS DIMENSIONS, INC.   615-292-0333
2003 Blair Blvd., Nashville, TN 37212
FDA Number: n/a
Ownership: Private
Produces/Sells CE-marked Devices: N

Purification System, Water	Gastroenterology/Urology
Tank, Holding, Dialysis	Gastroenterology/Urology

DIALYSIS SERVICES, INC.   615-384-4810
130 Elder Dr., Springfield, TN 37172
FDA Number: 3004486997
Ownership: Private
Produces/Sells CE-marked Devices: N

Purification System, Water	Gastroenterology/Urology

DIALYSIS SOLUTIONS INC.   905-669-3832
380 Elgin Mills Rd E, Richmond Hill L4C 5H2 Canada
FDA Number: 9616842

Concentrate, Dialysis, Hemodialysis (Liquid or Powder)	Gastroenterology/Urology

DIAMED LAB SUPPLIES INC.   800-434-2633
3069 Universal Dr.,   905-625-6021
Mississauga, ONT L4X-2 Canada
FDA Number: n/a   *Fax:* 905-625-6280
E-mail: sales@diamedlab.com
Web site: www.diamedlab.com
Year Founded: 1978
Ownership: Private
Produces/Sells CE-marked Devices: N
Distribution: Manufacturer Direct, Manufacturer Through Distributor, Importer

DIAMEDIX CORP.   800-327-4565
2140 N. Miami Avenue, Miami, FL 33127-4933   305-324-2300
FDA Number: 1044713   *Fax:* 800-578-3377
E-mail: info@diamedix.com
Web site: www.diamedix.com
Medical Products Sales Volume: $5,800,000
Annual Revenue: $5-$10 Million
Year Founded: 1985
Total Employees: 50   *Marketing Staff:* 3   *Sales Staff:* 11
Ownership: Avid Medical Inc.
Produces/Sells CE-marked Devices: Y
Federal Procurement Eligibility: Small Business
Distribution: Manufacturer Direct, Manufacturer Through Distributor
General Admin.: Duane Steele/Chief Operating Officer
Giorgio D'Urso/President, Chief Executive Officer
Mark Deutsch/Vice President Human Resources
Mktg./Adv.: Maria Perez/Manager Contract Sales
Raul Alvarez/Manager International & National Sales
Jean-Nate Fonte/Manager Marketing Communications
Nevin Breedlove/Manager National Accounts & Sales
Linda Schwartz/Market Manager
Duane Steele/Vice President Business Development
Ray Earl/Vice President National Sales
Production: Lynne Stirling/Director Product Development & Regulatory Affairs
Vivian Roman/Director Quality Assurance
Liliana Sanz/Manager Materials
Stefanie Ellis/Product Manager
Pat Ahmad/Senior Product Manager
Jim Rugg/Vice President Manufacturing
Finance: Mark Deutsch/Chief Financial Officer
Marc Segal/Controller
IS: Lynne Stirling/Technical Manager

Anti-DNA Antibody, Antigen and Control	Immunology
Anti-RNP-Antibody, Antigen And Control	Immunology

DIAMEDIX CORP.   800-327-4565 *(cont'd)*

Anti-SM-Antibody, Antigen And Control	Immunology
Enzyme Linked Immunoabsorbent Assay, Cytomegalovirus	Microbiology
Enzyme Linked Immunoabsorbent Assay, Herpes Simplex Virus	Microbiology
Enzyme Linked Immunoabsorbent Assay, Mumps Virus	Microbiology
Enzyme Linked Immunoabsorbent Assay, Rubella	Microbiology
Enzyme Linked Immunoabsorbent Assay, Rubeola	Microbiology
Enzyme Linked Immunoabsorbent Assay, Toxoplasma Gondii	Microbiology
Enzyme Linked Immunoabsorbent Assay, Treponema Pallidum	Microbiology
Enzyme Linked Immunoabsorbent Assay, Varicella-Zoster	Microbiology
Immunoassay, Other	Toxicology
Test, Disease, Lyme	Immunology
Test, Rheumatoid Factor	Immunology

DIAMICS, INC.   415-883-0414
Six Hamilton Landing Suite 200, Novato, CA 94949
FDA Number: 3006180907   *Fax:* 415-883-0415
Ownership: Alere, Inc.
Produces/Sells CE-marked Devices: N

Spatula, Cervical, Cytology	Obstetrics/Gynecology

DIAMODENT   888-281-8850   714-701-0171
1577 North Harmony Circle, Anaheim, CA 92806
FDA Number: 2031884   *Fax:* 714-237-0087
E-mail: jrassoli@diamodent.com
Web site: www.diamodent.com
Ownership: Private
Produces/Sells CE-marked Devices: N

Implant, Endosseous	Dental And Oral

DIAMOND DENTAL, INC.   770-381-3799
3545 Cruse Rd., Suite 203, Lawrenceville, GA 30044
FDA Number: 3005901698
Ownership: Private
Produces/Sells CE-marked Devices: N

Matrix, Dental	Dental And Oral

DIAMOND DIAGNOSTICS, INC.   508-429-0450
333 Fiske St., Holliston, MA 01746
FDA Number: 3003030793
Ownership: Private
Produces/Sells CE-marked Devices: N

Analyzer, Chemistry, Photometric, Discrete	Chemistry
Analyzer, Chemistry, Sequential Multiple, Continuous Flow	Chemistry
Electrode, Ion Specific, Calcium	Chemistry
Electrode, Ion Specific, Chloride	Chemistry
Electrode, Ion Specific, Potassium	Chemistry
Electrode, Ion Specific, Sodium	Chemistry
Fluorometer, Chemistry	Chemistry

DIAMOND EDGE CO.   727-586-2927
801 West Bay Drive, Suite 700, Largo, FL 33770
FDA Number: 1063239
Ownership: Private
Produces/Sells CE-marked Devices: N

Caliper, Ophthalmic	Ophthalmology
Cannula, Ophthalmic	Ophthalmology
Counter, Sponge, Surgical	Surgery
Forceps, Ophthalmic	Ophthalmology
Knife, Ophthalmic	Ophthalmology
Retractor, Ophthalmic	Ophthalmology
Scissors, Ophthalmic	Ophthalmology
Spatula, Ophthalmic	Ophthalmology
Speculum, Ophthalmic	Ophthalmology
Tape, Measuring, Ruler And Caliper	Surgery
Tray, Surgical Instrument	Surgery

DIAMOND OPHIR OPTICS INC.
See Ophir Optronics, Inc.

DIAMOND POLYMERS, INC.   888-437-4674   330-773-2700
1353 Exeter Rd., Akron, OH 44306
FDA Number: n/a   *Fax:* 330-773-2799
E-mail: custservice@diamondpolymers.com
Web site: www.diamondpolymers.com
Medical Products Sales Volume: $500,000
Annual Revenue: $50-$100 Million
Year Founded: 1989
Total Employees: 85   *Marketing Staff:* 1   *Sales Staff:* 12
Ownership: Private
Produces/Sells CE-marked Devices: N
Federal Procurement Eligibility: Small Business
Distribution: Manufacturer Direct, Importer, Exporter
General Admin.: Alan Woll/Chief Executive Officer
       Alan Woll/President
Mktg./Adv.: Denny Sanzone/Director Sales
       Jeff Stachler/Sales Representative
Production: Steve Blazey/Vice President Manufacturing
Research: Steve Blazey/Vice President Research & Development

Elastomer, Other	General

DIAMOND POLYMERS, INC.   888-437-4674 *(cont'd)*

Polymer, Synthetic, Other	General

DIANON SYSTEMS - LABCORP   800-328-2666   203-926-7100
1 Forest Parkway, Shelton, CT 06484
FDA Number: n/a   *Fax:* 203-381-4079
Web site: www.dianon.com
Annual Revenue: $25-$50 Million
Ownership: Private
Produces/Sells CE-marked Devices: N
Federal Procurement Eligibility: Small Business
Distribution: Manufacturer Through Distributor, Manufacturer Through Manufacturer Reps, Service Direct

Contract Laboratory	General

DIAPEDIA, LLC   814-234-0700
200 Innovation Blvd., Ste. 241, State College, PA 16803
FDA Number: 3005085138

Insoles, Medical	General

DIASOL, INC.   800-366-0546   818-255-1800
1110 Arroyo, North Hollywood, CA 91340
FDA Number: 2031664   *Fax:* 818-982-8539
E-mail: DISCOUNT.MEDICAL@att.net
Web site: www.dialysissupply.com
Medical Products Sales Volume: $5,500,000
Annual Revenue: $5-$10 Million
Year Founded: 2001
Total Employees: 7   *Marketing Staff:* 1   *Sales Staff:* 5
Ownership: Private
Produces/Sells CE-marked Devices: N
Federal Procurement Eligibility: Small Business, Female Owned
Distribution: Manufacturer Direct, Manufacturer Through Distributor, OEM, Importer, Exporter
General Admin.: Monica Abeles/President, Chief Executive Officer
Mktg./Adv.: Monica Abeles/Director Marketing & Sales
       Mary Castillo/Manager Contract Sales
       Marisol Castillo/Vice President Sales

Bag, Blood, Collection	Hematology
Chair, Dialysis, Unpowered (Without Scale)	Gastroenterology/Urology
Concentrate, Dialysis, Hemodialysis (Liquid or Powder)	Gastroenterology/Urology
Needle, Fistula	Gastroenterology/Urology

DIASONICS INC.
See Ge Oec Medical Systems Inc.

DIASONICS INC., MRI DIV.
See Toshiba America Medical Systems

DIASORIN INC   800-328-1482   651-439-9710
1951 Northwestern Avenue, PO Box 285, Stillwater, MN 55082
FDA Number: 2182595   *Fax:* 651-351-5669
E-mail: info@diasorin.com
Web site: www.diasorin.com
Medical Products Sales Volume: $100,000
Annual Revenue: $50-$100 Million
Total Employees: 2   *Marketing Staff:* 10   *Sales Staff:* 25
Ownership: Private
Quality System Registration Information: ISO9001
Produces/Sells CE-marked Devices: Y
Federal Procurement Eligibility: Small Business, GSA Contract, VA Contract
Distribution: Manufacturer Direct, Manufacturer Through Distributor, Manufacturer Through Manufacturer Reps
General Admin.: Kay Williams/Director General Affairs
       Stephen P. Gouze/General Manager
Mktg./Adv.: Carroll Streetman/Director Business Development
       Gordon MacFarlane/Director Product Development
       Keith Bevers/Director Sales
       Chen Even/General Manager, Manager International Marketing and Sales
Production: John Walter/Director Operations
Finance: Elaine Jacklin/Director Accounting

Analyzer, Chemistry, Radioimmunoassay	Chemistry
Antigen, Antiserum, Control, Complement C3	Immunology
Antigen, Antiserum, Control, Complement C4	Immunology
Antigen, Antiserum, Control, IGA	Immunology
Antigen, Antiserum, Control, IGA, FITC	Immunology
Antigen, Antiserum, Control, IGA, Peroxidase	Immunology
Antigen, Antiserum, Control, IGG	Immunology
Antigen, Antiserum, Control, IGG (FAB Fragment Specific)	Immunology
Antigen, Antiserum, Control, IGM	Immunology
Antigen, Antiserum, Control, Prealbumin	Immunology
Antisera, Conjugated Fluorescent, Cytomegalovirus	Microbiology
Control, Analyte (Assayed And Unassayed)	Chemistry
Epstein-Barr Virus, Other	Microbiology
Hepatitis B Test (B Core, BE Antigen & Antibody, B Core IGM)	Microbiology
Nephelometer, Immunology	Immunology
Phosphatase, Alkaline	Hematology
Radioimmunoassay, C Peptides Of Proinsulin	Chemistry

MANUFACTURER PROFILES

DIASORIN INC — 800-328-1482 (cont'd)

Radioimmunoassay, Cyclic AMP	Chemistry
Radioimmunoassay, Estradiol	Chemistry
Radioimmunoassay, Other	Chemistry
Radioimmunoassay, Parathyroid Hormone	Chemistry
Radioimmunoassay, Testosterones And Dihydrotestosterone	Chemistry
Radioimmunoassay, Total Thyroxine	Chemistry
System, Determination, Fibrinogen	Hematology
System, Identification, Hepatitis B Antigen	Hematology
Test, C-Reactive Protein	Immunology
Test, Erythropoietin	Hematology
Test, Fibrinogen	Hematology
Test, Hepatitis A (Antibody and IGM Antibody)	Microbiology

DIASYS CORPORATION — 800-360-2003 / 203-755-5083
**21, West Main Street,
Waterbury, CT 06702**
FDA Number: 1223854
Fax: 203-755-5105
E-mail: sales@diasys.com
Web site: www.diasys.com
Medical Products Sales Volume: $1,690,000
Year Founded: 1992
Total Employees: 12   Marketing Staff: 3   Sales Staff: 6
Ownership: Public
Stock Symbol: DYXC
Traded On: OTC Bulletin
Quality System Registration Information: ISO9000
Produces/Sells CE-marked Devices: Y
Federal Procurement Eligibility: Small Business, GSA Contract, VA Contract
Distribution: Manufacturer Direct, Manufacturer Through Distributor, Manufacturer Through Manufacturer Reps, Service Direct, Exporter
General Admin.: Greg Witchel/President
Mktg./Adv.: Richard Sledziona/Director Product Development
Production: Werner Sigrist/Manager Manufacturing
    Mark Wissing/Vice President Operations
Finance: Mr. Jeff Aaronson/Chief Financial Officer

Microscope, Light	Pathology

DIAZYME LABORATORIES — 858-455-4761
12889 Gregg Court, Poway, CA 92064
FDA Number: 2032900
Fax: 858-455-3701
E-mail: sales@diazyme.com
Web site: www.diazyme.com
Ownership: Private
Produces/Sells CE-marked Devices: N

5-AMP-Phosphate Release (Colorimetric), 5'-Nucleotidase	Chemistry
Absorption, Atomic, Lithium	Toxicology
Calibrator, Primary, Clinical Chemistry	Chemistry
Control, Analyte (Assayed And Unassayed)	Chemistry
Radioimmunoassay, Cholyglycine, Bile Acids	Chemistry
System, Test, Sodium, Enzymatic Method	Chemistry
Test, Glycosylated Hemoglobin Assay	Hematology
Test, System, Potassium, Enzymatic Method	Chemistry
Urinary Homocystine (Non-Quantitative) Test System	Chemistry

DICK MEDICAL SUPPLY, LLC — 614-444-2300
630 Marion Rd., Columbus, OH 43207
FDA Number: 3005831263

Joint, Wrist, External Limb Component, Mechanical	Physical Med
Transfer Device, Patient, Manual	General

DICKSON CO — 800-757-3747 / 630-543-3747
930 S. Westwood Avenue, Addison, IL 60101
FDA Number: n/a
Fax: 800-676-0498
E-mail: dicksoncsr@dicksondata.com
Web site: www.dicksonweb.com
Year Founded: 1923
Total Employees: 15   Marketing Staff: 6   Sales Staff: 6
Ownership: Private
Produces/Sells CE-marked Devices: Y
Federal Procurement Eligibility: Small Business
Distribution: Manufacturer Direct, Manufacturer Through Distributor, OEM, Importer, Exporter
General Admin.: Mike Unger/President
Mktg./Adv.: Kelly Giardino/Coord. Marketing
    Chris Sorensen/Director Marketing & Sales
    Kelly Giardino/Manager Advertising
    Kelly Temple/Manager International Marketing & Sales
    Tommie Spears/Manager Sales
Production: Dana Hyland/Manager Materials

Gauge, Pressure	General
Hygrometer (Humidity Indicator)	Anesthesiology
Monitor, Temperature (Self-Contained)	General
Monitor, Temperature (With Probe)	Anesthesiology
Monitor, Temperature, Surgery	Surgery
Probe, Temperature	General
Recorder, Chart, Laboratory	Chemistry

DICOMIT DICOM INFORMATION TECHNOLOGIES CORP. — 905-477-3354
12-250 Cochrane Dr, Markham L3R 8E5 Canada
FDA Number: 9681780

Scanner, Ultrasonic (Pulsed Echo)	Radiology

DICTATOR U.S., INC. — 877-366-7439 / 770-427-9555
**3939 Royal Drive NW Suite 214,
Kennesaw, GA 30144**
FDA Number: n/a
Fax: 770-427-0600
E-mail: info@dictator.com
Web site: www.dictator.com
Medical Products Sales Volume: $100,000
Annual Revenue: $25-$50 Million
Total Employees: 75   Marketing Staff: 30   Sales Staff: 15
Ownership: Private
Quality System Registration Information: ISO9001
Produces/Sells CE-marked Devices: N
Federal Procurement Eligibility: Small Business
Distribution: Manufacturer Direct, Exclusive Distributor, Importer, Exporter
General Admin.: Joachim Stech/President
Mktg./Adv.: Greg Rowell/Manager National Sales

Equipment, Building Security	General

DICTATOR-TECHNIK GMBH
See Dictator U.S., Inc.

DIELECTRICS, INC. — 800-472-7286 / 413-594-8111
300 Burnett Road, Chicopee, MA 01020
FDA Number: 1220351
Fax: 413-594-2343
E-mail: sales@dielectrics.com
Web site: www.dielectrics.com
Medical Products Sales Volume: $34,900,000
Annual Revenue: $25-$50 Million
Year Founded: 1954
Total Employees: 250
Ownership: Private
Quality System Registration Information: ISO9001
Produces/Sells CE-marked Devices: N
Federal Procurement Eligibility: Small Business
Distribution: Manufacturer Through Distributor, Manufacturer Through Manufacturer Reps
General Admin.: John Kusler/Chief Operating Officer
Mktg./Adv.: Joanne Lyons/Sales Associate
    Shanna Sutton/Sales Associate
    Sherri Duffy-Denaut/Sales Associate
    Bart Rietkerk/Vice President Business Development
    Adam Epstein/Vice President Sales
Finance: Martha Benoit/Controller, Credit Manager
Purchasing: Robert Merrill/Purchasing Agent

Drain, Suction, Closed	Surgery

DIESTCO MANUFACTURING CORP. — 800-795-2392 / 530-893-3136
PO Box 6504, Chico, CA 95927
FDA Number: n/a
Fax: 530-893-2635
E-mail: info@diestco.com
Web site: www.diestco.com
Medical Products Sales Volume: $740,000
Total Employees: 9
Ownership: Private
Produces/Sells CE-marked Devices: N
Federal Procurement Eligibility: Small Business
Distribution: Manufacturer Through Distributor, OEM
General Admin.: Daniel G. Diestel/Partner
Mktg./Adv.: Chris Cawthon/Director Marketing

Accessories, Wheelchair	Physical Med
Attachment, Bag (Crutch, Walker, Wheelchair)	Physical Med
Cover, Other	General
Service, Parts, Repair	General
Tray, Wheelchair	Physical Med

DIETZ LABORATORIES, INC. — 800-792-8934 / 817-926-6611
3124 Stuart Drive, Fort Worth, TX 76110-4318
FDA Number: n/a
Fax: 817-923-6681
E-mail: dietzlab@aol.com
Medical Products Sales Volume: $1,000,000
Annual Revenue: $1-$5 Million
Total Employees: 25   Marketing Staff: 1   Sales Staff: 3
Ownership: Private
Produces/Sells CE-marked Devices: N
Federal Procurement Eligibility: Small Business, Female Owned
Distribution: Manufacturer Direct
General Admin.: Angie Brown/Office Manager
    Ed Dietz/President
    Barbara Dietz/Vice President

Lens, Spectacle/Eyeglasses, Non-Custom	Ophthalmology

DIGENE CORP.
See Qiagen Gaithersburg, Inc.

DIGI-COM ELECTRONICS   805-522-6223
5327 Jacuzzi Street, Richmond, CA 94804
FDA Number: 3006367638
  Stimulator, Nerve, Transcutaneous (Pain Relief, TENS)   Cns/Neurology

DIGI-TRAX CORP.   847-613-2100
650 Heathrow Drive, Lincolnshire, IL 60069
FDA Number: 1424004   *Fax:* 847-465-9055
E-mail: info@digi-trax.com
Web site: www.digi-trax.com
Medical Products Sales Volume: $1,600,000
Annual Revenue: $1-$5 Million
Year Founded: 1986
Total Employees: 16   *Marketing Staff:* 1   *Sales Staff:* 3
Ownership: Private
Produces/Sells CE-marked Devices: N
Federal Procurement Eligibility: Small Business
Distribution: Manufacturer Direct, Manufacturer Through Distributor, Service Direct
Mktg./Adv.: Richard Kriozere/Vice President Marketing
    Jeff Kriozere/Vice President Sales
Research: Larry Cullen/Vice President Research & Development
  Software, Blood Bank (Stand-Alone Products)   Hematology

DIGIRAD CORP.   800-947-6134
13950 Stowe Drive, Poway, CA 92064-8803   858-726-1600
FDA Number: 2031050   *Fax:* 858-726-1700
Web site: www.digirad.com
Year Founded: 1985
Ownership: Public
Stock Symbol: DRAD
Traded On: NASDAQ
Produces/Sells CE-marked Devices: N
General Admin.: Mr. Todd Clyde/President, Chief Executive Officer
Mktg./Adv.: Mr. Randy L Weatherhead/Senior Vice President Business Development
Finance: Mr. Richard Slanksy/Chief Financial Officer
  Camera, Gamma (Nuclear/Scintillation)   Radiology
  Probe, Uptake, Nuclear   Radiology
  Scanner, Emission Computed Tomography   Radiology

DIGIRAY INCORPORATED   800-268-9917
44 Fasken Dr., Unit 3,   416-674-9955
Toronto, ONT M9W-5 Canada
FDA Number: n/a   *Fax:* 416-674-2692
E-mail: turow@globalserve.net
Web site: http://www.digiray.com
Year Founded: 1982
Ownership: Private
Produces/Sells CE-marked Devices: N
Distribution: Service Direct, Exclusive Distributor

DIGISONICS, INC.   713-529-7979
3701 Kirby Drive, Suite 930, Houston, TX 77098-3903
FDA Number: 1626313   *Fax:* 713-529-7999
E-mail: info@digison.net
Web site: www.digisonicsinc.com
Medical Products Sales Volume: $2,100,000
Year Founded: 1974
Total Employees: 15   *Sales Staff:* 4
Ownership: Private
Produces/Sells CE-marked Devices: N
Federal Procurement Eligibility: Small Business, Female Owned
Distribution: Manufacturer Direct
General Admin.: Diana McSherry/President, Chairman
    Diana McSherry/President, Chairman, Chief Executive Officer
    Ernest Jackson/Vice President
  Computer Software   General

DIGISPLINT CANADA   888-377-5468
489 Main St. South,   519-235-2981
Exeter, ONT N0M-1 Canada
FDA Number: n/a   *Fax:* 519-235-2984
E-mail: splintinfo@digisplint.ca
Web site: http://www.digisplint.ca
Year Founded: 1996
Total Employees: 10
Ownership: Private
Produces/Sells CE-marked Devices: N
Distribution: Manufacturer Direct, Exclusive Distributor, Importer

DIGITAL ANGEL CORP.   651-554-1574
490 Villuame Avenue, South Saint Paul, MN 55075
FDA Number: 3003309171
  Implantable Radio Frequency Transponder System   General

DIGITAL DYNAMICS, INC.   800-765-1288
5 Victor Square, Scotts Valley, CA 95066   831-438-4444
FDA Number: n/a   *Fax:* 831-438-6825
E-mail: sales@digitaldynamics.com
Web site: www.digitaldynamics.com
Medical Products Sales Volume: $7,300,000
Year Founded: 1974
Total Employees: 40
Ownership: Private
Quality System Registration Information: ISO9001
Produces/Sells CE-marked Devices: Y
Federal Procurement Eligibility: Small Business, GSA Contract
Distribution: Manufacturer Direct, OEM
General Admin.: James B. Jerde/President
  Computer Equipment   General
  Service, Computer   General

DIGITAL HEARING AID CENTER   530-877-3808
6032 Clark Rd.,suite C, Paradise, CA 95969
FDA Number: 2954768
Ownership: Private
Produces/Sells CE-marked Devices: N
  Hearing-Aid   Ear/Nose/Throat

DIGITAL HEARING SYSTEMS CORP.   479-925-7700
9679 East High Meadows, Rogers, AR 72756
FDA Number: 1832533
E-mail: sales@dhsc.com
Web site: www.dhsc.com
Medical Products Sales Volume: $70,000
Year Founded: 1975
Ownership: Private
Produces/Sells CE-marked Devices: N
Federal Procurement Eligibility: Small Business
Distribution: Manufacturer Direct, Manufacturer Through Manufacturer Reps
General Admin.: Anthony Miltich II/President
  Audiometer   Ear/Nose/Throat

DIGITAL VISION, INC   678-222-5200
301 Perimeter Center North, Suite 600, Atlanta, GA 30346
FDA Number: 1066656
  Aberrometer, Ophthalmic   Ophthalmology

DIGITCARE CORPORATION   888-287-2990
2999 Overland Ave., Ste. 209,   310-287-2990
Los Angeles, CA 90064
FDA Number: 2083593   *Fax:* 310-287-2991
E-mail: info@digitcare.net
Web site: www.digitcare.com
Annual Revenue: $5-$10 Million
Total Employees: 7
Ownership: Private
Quality System Registration Information: ISO9002
Produces/Sells CE-marked Devices: N
Distribution: Manufacturer Through Distributor
General Admin.: William Jordan/President
  Glove, Patient Examination   General
  Glove, Patient Examination, Latex   General
  Glove, Patient Examination, Specialty   General
  Glove, Surgical, Hypoallergenic   General
  Glove, Surgical, Powder-Free   Surgery
  Gown, Examination   General
  Gown, Operating Room, Disposable   Surgery
  Gown, Patient   Surgery

DIGITONE TECHNOLOGY, INC.   847-413-1688
890 E. Higgins Rd., Suite 158, Schaumburg, IL 60173
FDA Number: 3004998724
Ownership: Private
Produces/Sells CE-marked Devices: N
  Hearing-Aid   Ear/Nose/Throat

DIGITRACE CARE SERVICES
See Sleepmed Incorporated

DIGIVISION, INC.
See Enhanced Video Devices, Inc.

DIGNIFIED PRODUCTS CORP.
See Electric Mobility Corporation

DILLON OPTICS   480-948-8009
8009 E. Dillon's Way, Scottsdale, AZ 85260
FDA Number: 3004875810
E-mail: info@dillonoptics.com
Web site: www.dillonoptics.com
Ownership: Private
Produces/Sells CE-marked Devices: N
  Sunglasses (Including Photosensitive)   Ophthalmology

DILON DIAGNOSTICS LLC
877-GO-DILON
12050 Jefferson Avenue, Suite 340,
Newport News, VA 23606
757-269-4910
FDA Number: 1125612
Fax: 757-269-4912
E-mail: sales@dilon.com
Web site: www.dilon.com
Medical Products Sales Volume: $2,100,000
Year Founded: 1997
Total Employees: 18
Ownership: Private
Produces/Sells CE-marked Devices: N
Federal Procurement Eligibility: Small Business
Distribution: Manufacturer Direct, Manufacturer Through Distributor
General Admin.: Mr. Robert Moussa/President, Chief Executive Officer
Mktg./Adv.: Nancy Morter/Director Marketing & Business Development
    Scott Yarde/Vice President Sales
    Mr. John Reyes/Vice President Sales
Production: Mr. Vijay Singh/Director Operations
Research: Lee Fairchild/Vice President Engineering
    Mr. Douglas Kieper/Vice President Science & Technology
  Camera, Gamma (Nuclear/Scintillation)   Radiology

DILON TECHNOLOGIES LLC
See Dilon Diagnostics Llc

DIMCO GRAY CO.
800-876-8353
900 Dimco Way, Centerville, OH 45458-2709
937-433-7600
FDA Number: 9200288
Fax: 937-433-0520
E-mail: dgsales@dimcogray.com
Web site: www.dimco-gray.com
Medical Products Sales Volume: $6,800,000
Annual Revenue: $10-$25 Million
Year Founded: 1924
Total Employees: 90   *Marketing Staff:* 1   *Sales Staff:* 5
Ownership: Private
Quality System Registration Information: ISO9001
Produces/Sells CE-marked Devices: Y
Federal Procurement Eligibility: Small Business
Distribution: Manufacturer Direct, Manufacturer Through Distributor, Exporter
General Admin.: Dollie Mabe/Manager Human Resources
    David Scott/President, Chief Executive Officer
Mktg./Adv.: Donald Eadie/Manager Marketing
    Phyllis Snell/Manager Sales
Production: Jim Daulton/Manager Manufacturing & Engineering
    Vince Ferraro/Manager Materials
    Michael Cassidy/Manager Quality Assurance
  Timer, Radiographic   Radiology

DIMENSIONAL DOSING SYSTEMS, INC.
724-933-7874
2465 Dogwood Dr., Wexford, PA 15090
FDA Number: 1066338
  Plethysmograph, Impedance   Cardiovascular

DIO USA
213-300-7979
3435 Wilshire Blvd, Suite 2210, Los Angeles, CA 90010
FDA Number: 3006400105
Ownership: Private
Produces/Sells CE-marked Devices: N
  Implant, Endosseous   Dental And Oral

DIOMEDICS, INC.
888-972-4699
342 S.E. 35th St., Keystone Heights, FL 32656
352-478-2370
FDA Number: 1058095
Fax: 352-478-2371
E-mail: info@diomedics.com
Web site: www.diomedics.com
Medical Products Sales Volume: $200,000
Annual Revenue: $5-$10 Million
Year Founded: 1993
Total Employees: 3   *Marketing Staff:* 4   *Sales Staff:* 30
Ownership: Private
Produces/Sells CE-marked Devices: N
Federal Procurement Eligibility: Small Business
Distribution: Manufacturer Direct, Manufacturer Through Distributor, Manufacturer Through Manufacturer Reps, Exclusive Distributor, Exporter
General Admin.: Randall Everett/Chief Executive Officer
  Lamp, Infrared   Physical Med

DIONEX CORP.
408-737-0700
1228 Titan Way, P.O. Box 3603, Sunnyvale, CA 94088-3603
FDA Number: n/a
Fax: 408-730-9403
Web site: www.dionex.com
Annual Revenue: $0-$1 Million
Ownership: Thermo Fisher Scientific Inc.
Produces/Sells CE-marked Devices: N
Federal Procurement Eligibility: Small Business
Distribution: Manufacturer Direct
  Column, Liquid Chromatography   Toxicology

DIOPSYS INC.
973-244-0622
16 Chapin Road, Suite 912, Pine Brook, NJ 07058
FDA Number: 3004174467
Fax: 973-244-0670
E-mail: info@diopsys.com
Web site: http://www.diopsys.com
Ownership: Private
Produces/Sells CE-marked Devices: N
General Admin.: Mr. Joseph Fontanetta/Chief Executive Officer

DIOPTICS MEDICAL PRODUCTS, INC.
800-959-9040
125 Venture Drive, San Luis Obispo, CA 93401
805-781-3300
FDA Number: 2024748
Fax: 805-781-3322
E-mail: info@dioptics.com
Web site: www.dioptics.com
Medical Products Sales Volume: $7,100,000
Total Employees: 99
Ownership: Private
Produces/Sells CE-marked Devices: Y
Federal Procurement Eligibility: Small Business
Distribution: Manufacturer Through Distributor
General Admin.: Henry Lane/President
Mktg./Adv.: Stephanie Schmidt/Director Sales
    Melissa Malephansakul/Manager Marketing
    Robin Leonino/Manager National Sales
Production: Valerie Reiss/Product Manager
Finance: Janice Langley/Director Finance
  Sunglasses (Including Photosensitive)   Ophthalmology

DIRECT CROWN, LLC
888-910-4490
895 Country Club Rd., Ste. B-100,
Eugene, OR 97401
541-344-5876
FDA Number: 3032791
Fax: 541-431-1187
Web site: www.directcrown.com
Year Founded: 1998
Ownership: Private
Produces/Sells CE-marked Devices: N
General Admin.: David Correale/Chief Executive Officer
  Crown And Bridge, Temporary, Resin   Dental And Oral
  Crown, Preformed   Dental And Oral

DIRECT RADIOGRAPHY
302-631-2700
600 Technology Drive, Newark, DE 19702
FDA Number: 2531544
Fax: 302-731-7438
E-mail: sales@hologic.com
Web site: www.hologic.com
Medical Products Sales Volume: $9,700,000
Total Employees: 85
Ownership: Hologic, Inc.
Stock Symbol: HOLX
Traded On: NASDAQ
Produces/Sells CE-marked Devices: N
Federal Procurement Eligibility: Small Business
  Image Processing System   Radiology
  Imager, X-Ray, Solid State (Flat Panel/Digital)   Radiology

DIRECTIONAL HEARING AID SERVICE
208-376-9431
6876 Fairview, Boise, ID 83704
FDA Number: 3032332
Medical Products Sales Volume: $280,000
Year Founded: 1971
Total Employees: 5
Federal Procurement Eligibility: Small Business
  Hearing-Aid   Ear/Nose/Throat

DIRECTMED, INC.
516-656-3377
150 Pratt Oval, Glen Cove, NY 11542
FDA Number: n/a
Fax: 516-656-5574
E-mail: cs@directmed.com
Web site: www.directmed.com
Medical Products Sales Volume: $1,500,000
Annual Revenue: $1-$5 Million
Year Founded: 1997
Total Employees: 5   *Marketing Staff:* 2   *Sales Staff:* 2
Ownership: Private
Quality System Registration Information: ISO9002
Produces/Sells CE-marked Devices: Y
Federal Procurement Eligibility: Small Business, Female Owned
Distribution: Manufacturer Direct, OEM, Exclusive Distributor, Importer, Exporter
General Admin.: Louis Pagliara/President
Mktg./Adv.: Dana H. Pagliara/Vice President Marketing
  Adapter, Y   Gastroenterology/Urology
  Bag, Breathing   Anesthesiology
  Brush, Cytology   General
  Cannula, Nasal, Oxygen   Anesthesiology
  Clamp, Line   Gastroenterology/Urology
  Clamp, Tubing   General
  Clamp, Umbilical   Obstetrics/Gynecology
  Clip, Nose   Anesthesiology

DIRECTMED, INC.
516-656-3377 *(cont'd)*

Clip, Other	Surgery
Component, Other	General
Component, Plastic	General
Connector, Tubing, Dialysate	Gastroenterology/Urology
Contract Manufacturing, Product, Disposable	General
Controller, Infusion	Cardiovascular
Depressor, Tongue	General
Drain, Tee (Water Trap)	Anesthesiology
Filter, Bacterial, Breathing Circuit	Anesthesiology
Filter, Intravenous Tubing	General
Fitting, Luer	General
Forceps, Dressing	Surgery
Forceps, Sponge	Surgery
Kit, Administration, Intravenous	General
Kit, Intravenous Extension Tubing	General
Speculum, Vaginal, Non-Metal	Obstetrics/Gynecology
Stopcock	General
Transfer Unit, IV Fluid	General
Valve, Other	Chemistry

DIREX SYSTEMS CORP.
339-502-6013

437 Turnpike St., Canton, MA 02021
FDA Number: 1224828
Ownership: Private
Produces/Sells CE-marked Devices: N

Accelerator, Linear, Medical	Radiology
Image Processing System	Radiology
Lithotriptor, Extracorporeal Shock-wave, Urological	Gastroenterology/Urology
Radiographic/Fluoroscopic Unit, Image-Intensified	Radiology
Table, Cystometric, Electric	Gastroenterology/Urology

DIROS TECHNOLOGY, INC.
905-415-3440

232 Hood Road, Markham, ON L3R 3K8 Canada
FDA Number: 8043398   Fax: 905-415-0667
E-mail: info@dirostech.com
Web site: www.dirostech.com
Year Founded: 1983
Total Employees: 15   Marketing Staff: 1   Sales Staff: 1
Ownership: Private
Quality System Registration Information: ISO9001
Produces/Sells CE-marked Devices: Y
Distribution: Manufacturer Direct, Service Direct, Exclusive Distributor, Exporter

DISCOUNT DME
714-630-9590

1265 N. Grove St, Suite A, Anaheim, CA 92806
FDA Number: 3005034350
Ownership: Private
Produces/Sells CE-marked Devices: N

Component, Exercise	Physical Med
Exerciser, Powered	Anesthesiology
Pack, Hot Or Cold, Water Circulating	Physical Med
Stimulator, Muscle, Electrical-Powered (EMS)	Physical Med

DISCOUNT MEDICAL SUPPLY, INC.
See Diasol, Inc.

DISCOVERY DIAGNOSTICS
888-883-9101
905-465-2252

P.O. Box 5186, Claremont, ONT L1Y-1A4 Canada
FDA Number: n/a   Fax: 905-649-5559
E-mail: info@discovery-diagnostics.com
Web site: www.discovery-diagnostics.com
Year Founded: 1998
Total Employees: 10
Ownership: Private
Produces/Sells CE-marked Devices: N
Distribution: Exclusive Distributor, Importer

DISCOVERY ENGINEERING INTL., INC.
785-272-3781

3115 S.w. Westwood Dr., Topeka, KS 66614
FDA Number: 1933084
Biofeedback Device   Cns/Neurology

DISCOVERY HEARING AID CO-OP, INC.
800-736-9903
251-342-1144

4318 Downtowner Loop North,, #k,
Mobile, AL 36609
FDA Number: 2320981
Ownership: Private
Produces/Sells CE-marked Devices: N
Hearing-Aid   Ear/Nose/Throat

DISENOS TERMOELECTRICOS LUYFEL
16-17-0425

7424 Juarez Porvenir, Cd. Juarez Mexico
FDA Number: 9614029
Pad, Heating, Powered   Physical Med

DISETRONIC MEDICAL SYSTEMS
See Roche Insulin Delivery Systems Inc.

DISETRONIC STERILE PRODUCTS
800-280-7801
603-427-5511

124 Heritage Avenue,
Portsmouth, NH 03801
FDA Number: 1220894   Fax: 603-431-1612
E-mail: Jay.Riley@DSPUSA.tv
Web site: www.dspusa.tv
Annual Revenue: $10-$25 Million
Year Founded: 1985
Total Employees: 125
Ownership: DISETRONIC AG
Quality System Registration Information: ISO9002
Produces/Sells CE-marked Devices: Y
Federal Procurement Eligibility: Small Business
Distribution: Manufacturer Direct, OEM
General Admin.: John J. Riley/President, Chief Executive Officer
Production: Jack McCaughey/Director Manufacturing
          John Mitzel/Director Quality Assurance
Finance: Darryl Brown/Controller

Contract Manufacturing	General
Contract Packaging	General

DISMED INC.
800-361-3581
514-355-4711

9950 Parkway Blvd., Anjou, QUE H1J-1P5 Canada
FDA Number: n/a   Fax: 514-354-6051
E-mail: infocontact@dismed.com
Web site: www.dismed.com
Year Founded: 1979
Total Employees: 100
Ownership: Private
Produces/Sells CE-marked Devices: N

DISPENSERS OPTICAL SERVICE CORP.
800-626-4545
502-491-3440

1815 Plantside Dr., Louisville, KY 40299
FDA Number: 1034043   Fax: (502) 499-8445
E-mail: mdr@dosc.com
Web site: www.dosc.com
Medical Products Sales Volume: $7,000,000
Annual Revenue: $5-$10 Million
Year Founded: 1954
Total Employees: 10
Ownership: Private
Produces/Sells CE-marked Devices: N
Federal Procurement Eligibility: Small Business
Distribution: Manufacturer Direct, Importer, Exporter
General Admin.: Charles S. Arensberg/President, Chief Executive Officer
          Richard T. Schneider/Vice President Government Affairs
Mktg./Adv.: Cathy L. Carter/Manager Sales Admin.
Production: Gary W. Grove/Senior Vice President Operations
IS: Mark Woodcock./Director Information Systems

Eyeglasses	Ophthalmology
Frame, Spectacle (Eyeglasses)	Ophthalmology
Laboratory Equipment, Ophthalmic	Ophthalmology
Lens, Spectacle/Eyeglasses, Custom (Prescription)	Ophthalmology

DISPOMED, INC.
See Adex Medical, Inc.

DISPOS-ALLS CORP.
See Nurses Choice Specialty Textiles

DISPOSABLE SURGICAL INNOVATIONS
516-377-1497

958 Church Street, Baldwin, NY 11510
FDA Number: 3004370651
Ownership: Private
Produces/Sells CE-marked Devices: N
Scaler, Periodontic   Dental And Oral

DISTRIBUIDORA CAISA,S.A.DE C.V.
5-534-3044

Adolfo Prieto 1759-b, Del Valle,
Ciudad De Mexico, DF 03100 Mexico
FDA Number: n/a   Fax: 5-534-3043
E-mail: info@distribuidorcaisa.com
Web site: www.distribuidoracaisa.com
Total Employees: 6   Marketing Staff: 2   Sales Staff: 3
Ownership: Private
Produces/Sells CE-marked Devices: N
Federal Procurement Eligibility: Female Owned
Distribution: Manufacturer Direct, Exclusive Distributor, Importer, Exporter

DITEC MFG.
800-332-7083
805-566-7800

1019 Mark Avenue, Carpinteria, CA 93013
FDA Number: 2025796   Fax: 805-566-7802
E-mail: contact@ditecmfg.com
Web site: www.ditecmfg.com
Medical Products Sales Volume: $1,200,000
Annual Revenue: $1-$5 Million
Year Founded: 1985
Total Employees: 13   Marketing Staff: 1   Sales Staff: 1

DITEC MFG. 800-332-7083 (cont'd)
Ownership: Private
Quality System Registration Information: ISO9002
Produces/Sells CE-marked Devices: N
Federal Procurement Eligibility: Small Business
Distribution: Manufacturer Direct, OEM
General Admin.: Mr. Don L. Cooper/President

Burr, Dental	Dental And Oral
Burr, Surgical, General & Plastic Surgery	Surgery
Instrument, Diamond, Dental	Dental And Oral

DIV. OF FLEXBAR MACHINE CORP.
See Mediflex Surgical Products

DIVERSIFIED DIAGNOSTIC PRODUCTS, INC. 281-955-5323
11603 Windfern Road, Houston, TX 77064-4801
FDA Number: 1628192
E-mail: bkrueger@ddpixray.com *Fax:* 281-955-8522
Web site: www.ddpixray.com
Medical Products Sales Volume: $1,100,000
Annual Revenue: $1-$5 Million
Year Founded: 1982
Total Employees: 15 *Marketing Staff:* 2 *Sales Staff:* 1
Ownership: Private
Quality System Registration Information: ISO9001
Produces/Sells CE-marked Devices: N
Federal Procurement Eligibility: Small Business, VA Contract
Distribution: Manufacturer Direct, Manufacturer Through Manufacturer Reps
General Admin.: Gerald M. Timpe/President
Mktg./Adv.: Ms. Brenda Krueger/Director Marketing & Sales
Production: Walter Barnett/Manager Regulatory Affairs
Research: Terry Deville/Vice President Research & Development

Flowmeter, Meter, Cerebral Blood, Xenon Clearance	Cns/Neurology
Illuminator, Radiographic Film	Radiology
Rebreathing System, Radionuclide	Radiology

DIVERSIFIED OPHTHALMICS, INC. 800-626-2281
250 McCullough St., Cincinnati, OH 45226-2145 513-321-7988
FDA Number: n/a
E-mail: do-infor@divopt.com *Fax:* 513-321-6355
Web site: www.divopt.com
Annual Revenue: $0-$1 Million
Total Employees: 200 *Marketing Staff:* 2 *Sales Staff:* 12
Ownership: Private
Produces/Sells CE-marked Devices: N
Distribution: Exclusive Distributor
General Admin.: Ronald Cooke/President, Chief Executive Officer
  Deborah Youngblood/Vice President Human Resources
Mktg./Adv.: Harry Fagedes/Manager Business Development
  Dan Woebkenberg/Vice President Marketing & Sales
Research: Harry Fadges/Vice President Research & Development

Frame, Spectacle (Eyeglasses)	Ophthalmology
Lens, Contact, Hydrophilic	Ophthalmology
Lens, Other	Ophthalmology

DIVERSITY EQUIPMENT TECHNOLOGY
See Beta Technology, Inc.

DIVINE SKIN SOLUTIONS, INC. 888-404-7770
119-51 Metropolitan Ave., Suite G4, 207-993-8254
Kew Gardens, NY 11415
FDA Number: 2438817
E-mail: CONTACT@DSLABORATORIES.COM *Fax:* 646-219-2572
Web site: www.dslaboratories.com
Ownership: Private
Produces/Sells CE-marked Devices: N

Epilator, High-Frequency, Tweezer Type	Surgery

DIVISION COLORCODE UNLIMITED CORP.
See R&Da Co.

DIXIE EMS SUPPLY 800-347-3494
10101 Foster Ave, Brooklyn, NY 11211 718-257-6400
FDA Number: 9200290
E-mail: customerservice@dixieems.com *Fax:* 718-257-6401
Web site: www.dixieems.com
Annual Revenue: $1-$5 Million
Year Founded: 1965
Total Employees: 26 *Marketing Staff:* 26 *Sales Staff:* 26
Ownership: Private
Produces/Sells CE-marked Devices: N
Federal Procurement Eligibility: Small Business, Female Owned
Distribution: Manufacturer Direct, Manufacturer Through Distributor
General Admin.: Eva Silverstein/President, Chief Executive Officer
Mktg./Adv.: Leah Jacobs/Director Marketing
  Israel Greenwald/Manager Contract Sales

Airway, Esophageal (Obturator)	Anesthesiology
Anatomical Training Model	General
Aspirator, Emergency Suction	General
Bag, Breathing	Anesthesiology

DIXIE EMS SUPPLY 800-347-3494 (cont'd)

Bandage, Adhesive	Surgery
Bandage, Gauze	General
Board, Bed	General
Board, Cardiopulmonary Resuscitation	General
Board, Spine	Orthopedics
Cannula, Nasal	General
Cart, Emergency, Cardiopulmonary Resuscitation (Crash)	Anesthesiology
Cart, Gas Cylinder (Carrier)	Anesthesiology
Collar, Cervical Neck	Orthopedics
Cutter, Ring	General
Dressing, Universal	General
Extrication Equipment	General
Flowmeter, Gas (Oxygen), Calibrated	Anesthesiology
Forceps, Hemostatic	Surgery
Glove, Patient Examination	General
Humidifier, Non-Heated	Anesthesiology
Kit, First Aid	Surgery
Kit, Snake Bite	General
Kit, Tracheotomy	Anesthesiology
Laryngoscope	Ear/Nose/Throat
Mask, Oxygen, Aerosol Administration	Anesthesiology
Regulator, Oxygen, Mechanical	General
Rescue Equipment	General
Restraint, Ankle/Foot	General
Restraint, Wrist/Hand	General
Resuscitator, Cardiopulmonary	Cardiovascular
Resuscitator, Emergency Oxygen	Dental And Oral
Scissors, Bandage/Gauze/Plaster	General
Sheet, Burn	General
Simulator, Lung	Anesthesiology
Sphygmomanometer, Aneroid (Arterial Pressure)	General
Splint, Extremity, Inflatable, External	Surgery
Stethoscope, Amplified	General
Stethoscope, Mechanical	General
Stretcher, Hand-Carried	General
Stretcher, Wheeled (Mobile)	General
Training Manikin, CPR (Resuscitation)	General
Training Manikin, Wound Moulage	General
Transfer Device, Patient, Manual	General
Tube, Tracheal (Endotracheal)	Anesthesiology
Tube, Tracheostomy (Breathing Tube), ENT	Ear/Nose/Throat

DIXON MEDICAL INC 770-457-0602
3710 Long View Drive, Atlanta, GA 30341
FDA Number: 1054087
E-mail: dixon@dixonmed.com *Fax:* 770-454-7548
Web site: www.dixonmed.com
Annual Revenue: $0-$1 Million
Total Employees: 2
Ownership: DIXON MEDICAL, INC.
Federal Procurement Eligibility: Small Business
Distribution: Importer
General Admin.: William Dixon/President

Arthroscope	Orthopedics
Endoscope	Gastroenterology/Urology

DJ ORTHOPEDICS DE MEXICO, S.A. DE C.V. 690-727-1280
Ave. Venustiano Carranza 6802, Castillo,
Tijuana 22100 Mexico
FDA Number: 9616087

Accessories, Catheter	Surgery
Accessories, Traction	Physical Med
Accessories, Wheelchair	Physical Med
Belt, Traction, Pelvic, Orthopedic	Orthopedics
Binder, Abdominal	General
Binder, Elastic	General
Brace, Joint, Ankle (External)	Physical Med
Cage, Knee	Physical Med
Component, Cast	Orthopedics
Component, Exercise	Physical Med
Cover, Limb	Physical Med
Drainage System, Urine, Closed	Gastroenterology/Urology
Exerciser, Non-Measuring	Physical Med
Joint, Hip, External Brace	Physical Med
Joint, Knee, External Brace	Physical Med
Joint, Knee, External Limb Component	Physical Med
Orthosis, Abdominal	Physical Med
Orthosis, Cervical	Physical Med
Orthosis, Limb Brace	Physical Med
Orthosis, Lumbar	Physical Med
Orthosis, Lumbosacral	Physical Med
Orthosis, Rib Fracture, Soft	Physical Med
Protector, Skin Pressure	General
Sling, Arm	Physical Med
Sling, Arm, Overhead Supported	Physical Med
Splint, Abduction, Congenital Hip Dislocation	Physical Med
Splint, Extremity, Non-Inflatable, External	Surgery
Splint, Hand, And Component	Physical Med
Stirrup, External Brace Component	Physical Med
Support, Arm	Physical Med

DJ ORTHOPEDICS DE MEXICO, S.A. DE C.V.   690-727-1280
(cont'd)

Traction Unit, Non-Powered	Orthopedics

DJ ORTHOPEDICS DE MEXICO, S.A. DE C.V.   690-727-1280
Blvd., Delagacion La Presa, Tijuana 22397 Mexico
FDA Number: 9616086

Accessories, Catheter	Surgery
Accessories, Traction	Physical Med
Accessories, Wheelchair	Physical Med
Belt, Traction, Pelvic, Orthopedic	Orthopedics
Binder, Abdominal	General
Binder, Elastic	General
Brace, Joint, Ankle (External)	Physical Med
Cage, Knee	Physical Med
Component, Cast	Orthopedics
Component, Exercise	Physical Med
Cover, Limb	Physical Med
Drainage System, Urine, Closed	Gastroenterology/Urology
Exerciser, Non-Measuring	Physical Med
Joint, Hip, External Brace	Physical Med
Joint, Knee, External Brace	Physical Med
Joint, Knee, External Limb Component	Physical Med
Orthosis, Abdominal	Physical Med
Orthosis, Cervical	Physical Med
Orthosis, Limb Brace	Physical Med
Orthosis, Lumbar	Physical Med
Orthosis, Lumbosacral	Physical Med
Orthosis, Rib Fracture, Soft	Physical Med
Protector, Skin Pressure	General
Sling, Arm	Physical Med
Sling, Arm, Overhead Supported	Physical Med
Splint, Abduction, Congenital Hip Dislocation	Physical Med
Splint, Extremity, Non-Inflatable, External	Surgery
Splint, Hand, And Component	Physical Med
Stirrup, External Brace Component	Physical Med
Support, Arm	Physical Med
Traction Unit, Non-Powered	Orthopedics

DJO INC.   800-336-6569
1430 Decision Street, Vista, CA 92081   760-727-1280
FDA Number: 2020737   *Fax:* 800-936-6569
Web site: http://www.djoglobal.com
Annual Revenue: $100-$500 Million
Total Employees: 4690
Ownership: Private
Produces/Sells CE-marked Devices: Y
Federal Procurement Eligibility: Small Business
Distribution: Manufacturer Direct
General Admin.: Mr. Leslie Cross/Chief Executive Officer
     Mr. Luke Faulstick/Chief Operating Officer
Mktg./Adv.: Mr. Stephen Murphy/Executive Vice President Marketing & Sales
Finance: Ms. Vickie Capps/Chief Financial Officer

Accessories, Fixation, Orthopedic	Orthopedics
Accessories, Traction	Physical Med
Awl	Orthopedics
Bandage, Cast	Physical Med
Bandage, Elastic	General
Belt, Traction, Pelvic	Physical Med
Belt, Traction, Pelvic, Orthopedic	Orthopedics
Binder, Abdominal	General
Bit, Drill	Orthopedics
Bolt, Nut, Washer	Orthopedics
Brace, Joint, Ankle (External)	Physical Med
Burr, Orthopedic	Orthopedics
Compression Instrument	Orthopedics
Crutch	Physical Med
Curette	Orthopedics
Driver, Prosthesis	Orthopedics
Exerciser, Non-Measuring	Physical Med
Forceps	Orthopedics
Glove, Surgical, Plastic Surgery	Surgery
Gouge, Surgical, General & Plastic Surgery	Surgery
Guide	Orthopedics
Halter, Head, Traction	Physical Med
Helmet, Surgical	Surgery
Insoles, Medical	General
Joint, Knee, External Brace	Physical Med
Joint, Shoulder, External Limb Component	Physical Med
Mallet, Bone	Orthopedics
Orthopedic Manual Surgical Instrument	Orthopedics
Orthosis, Cervical	Physical Med
Orthosis, Limb Brace	Physical Med
Orthosis, Lumbar	Physical Med
Orthosis, Lumbosacral	Physical Med
Orthosis, Rib Fracture, Soft	Physical Med
Orthosis, Sacroiliac, Soft	Physical Med
Osteotome (Orthopedic)	Surgery
Pack, Hot Or Cold, Reusable	Physical Med
Pack, Hot Or Cold, Water Circulating	Physical Med
Pad, Medicated, Adhesive, Non-Electric	General

DJO INC.   800-336-6569 *(cont'd)*

Pin, Fixation, Threaded	Orthopedics
Protector, Skin Pressure	General
Punch, Surgical	Surgery
Rasp, Bone	Orthopedics
Reamer	Orthopedics
Restraint, Protective (Body)	General
Retractor, Surgical	Surgery
Scissors, Orthopedic	Orthopedics
Screw, Fixation, Bone	Orthopedics
Screwdriver	Orthopedics
Shoe, Cast	Physical Med
Sling, Arm	Physical Med
Sling, Arm, Overhead Supported	Physical Med
Splint, Clavicle	Physical Med
Splint, Extremity, Non-Inflatable, External	Surgery
Splint, Hand, And Component	Physical Med
Splint, Traction	Orthopedics
Stocking, Support (Anti-Embolic)	General
Support, Arm	Physical Med
Support, Hernia	Gastroenterology/Urology
Tap, Bone	Orthopedics
Tips And Pads, Cane, Crutch And Walker	Physical Med
Tray, Surgical Instrument	Surgery
Trephine, Bone	Orthopedics
Wire, Fixation, Intraosseous	Dental And Oral
Wrench	Orthopedics

DJO SURGICAL   800-456-8696
9800 Metric Blvd., Austin, TX 78758   512-832-9500
FDA Number: n/a   *Fax:* 512-834-6300
Web site: http://www.djosurgical.com
Medical Products Sales Volume: $46,000,000
Annual Revenue: $100-$500 Million
Year Founded: 1992
Total Employees: 150
Ownership: DJO Surgical
Stock Symbol: ENMC
Traded On: NASDAQ
Quality System Registration Information: ISO9001
Produces/Sells CE-marked Devices: Y
Federal Procurement Eligibility: Small Business, GSA Contract, VA Contract
Distribution: Manufacturer Through Distributor, Manufacturer Through Manufacturer Reps, OEM, Exclusive Distributor, Importer, Exporter
General Admin.: Kenneth W. Davidson/Chief Executive Officer, Chairman
     William Burke/Chief Financial Officer, Executive Vice President
     Harry Zimmerman/Executive Vice President
     Jack Cahill/President
     Paul Chapman/President, Chief Operating Officer
     Kathy Wiederkehr/Vice President Human Resources
Mktg./Adv.: William Fain/Director Sales
     Davis Henley/Vice President Business Development
     Bryan Monroe/Vice President Marketing
Production: Perry Barrs/Vice President Manufacturing & Operations
     Al Alonso/Vice President Quality Assurance & Quality Control
Research: Craig Smith, PhD/Chief Scientist

Fixation Device, Spinal (External)	Orthopedics
Prosthesis, Femoral	Orthopedics
Prosthesis, Knee, Patellar	Orthopedics
Prosthesis, Shoulder, Hemi-, Glenoid, Metal	Orthopedics
Prosthesis, Tibial	Orthopedics
Stimulator, Scoliosis, Neuromuscular, Functional	Orthopedics

Medical Product Subsidiaries (Listed Separately)
   Chattanooga Group
   DJO Surgical

DJO, LLC
   See DJO Inc.

DKL CONSTRUCTION MANAGEMENT, INC.   231-947-6450
323 East Welch Court, Suite B, Traverse City, MI 49686
FDA Number: 1836366   *Fax:* 231-947-9894
E-mail: kentgray@dklconstruction.com
Web site: www.dklconstruction.com
Ownership: Private
Produces/Sells CE-marked Devices: N

Irradiator, Blood, Extracorporeal	Gastroenterology/Urology

DLC LABORATORIES, INC.
7008 Marcelle Street, Paramount, CA 90723
FDA Number: 2020223

Lubricant, Patient, Vaginal, Latex Compatible	Obstetrics/Gynecology

DM SYSTEMS, INC.   800-254-5438
1316 Sherman Avenue, Evanston, IL 60201   847-328-9541
FDA Number: 1424774   *Fax:* 847-328-9561
E-mail: info@dmsystems.com
Web site: www.dmsystems.com
Medical Products Sales Volume: $1,100,000
Year Founded: 1979

DM SYSTEMS, INC.   800-254-5438 (cont'd)

Total Employees: 8   *Marketing Staff:* 3
Ownership: Private
Produces/Sells CE-marked Devices: Y
Federal Procurement Eligibility: Small Business, GSA Contract, VA Contract
Distribution: Manufacturer Direct, Manufacturer Through Distributor, Manufacturer Through Manufacturer Reps
General Admin.: Denis Drennan/President, Chief Executive Officer
Mktg./Adv.: Larry Clayman/Director Marketing
    Denis Drennan/Director National Accounts
    Denis Drennan/Director Product Development
    Denis Drennan/Manager International Sales
    Daniela Robinson/Manager Marketing
Production: Donna Schwartz/Manager Operations

Cast Walking Heel	Orthopedics
Component, Cast	Orthopedics
Component, Traction, Non-Invasive	Orthopedics
Exerciser, Leg And Ankle	Physical Med
Exerciser, Other	Physical Med
Orthosis, Other	Physical Med
Pad, Pressure, Foam (Elbow, Heel)	General
Protector, Heel	General
Shoe, Cast	Physical Med

DMA MED-CHEM CORPORATION   800-362-1833
49 Water Mill Lane, Great Neck, NY 11021-4234   **516-829-1200**

FDA Number: 2432416   *Fax:* 516-487-1239
E-mail: info@dmamed.com
Web site: www.dmamed.com
Medical Products Sales Volume: $2,900,000
Annual Revenue: $10-$25 Million
Year Founded: 1982
Total Employees: 15   *Marketing Staff:* 4   *Sales Staff:* 12
Ownership: Private
Quality System Registration Information: ISO9000; ISO9001; ISO9002; ISO9003
Produces/Sells CE-marked Devices: Y
Federal Procurement Eligibility: Small Business, GSA Contract, VA Contract
Distribution: Exclusive Distributor, Importer, Exporter
General Admin.: Leo R. Mindick/Chief Executive Officer, Chairman
    Daniel Plante/Manager Human Resources
    Russell Mindick/President, Chief Operating Officer
Mktg./Adv.: Joseph Parisi/Manager Business Development
    Ruby Singh/Manager Contract Sales
    Joseph Parisi/Manager Sales Training
    Angad Jhingan/Vice President Market Research
    Angad Jhingan/Vice President Marketing & International Sales
Production: Robert Deschak/Director Quality Assurance & Regulatory Affairs
Finance: Alvin Smilow/Chief Financial Officer
Purchasing: Susan Mindick/Vice President Contract Admin.

Accessories, Catheter	Surgery
Accessories, Surgical Camera	Surgery
Agent, Hemostatic, Absorbable, Collagen-Based	Surgery
Bag, Urinary Collection	General
Barrier, Adhesion, Absorbable	Obstetrics/Gynecology
Cart, Instrument/Equipment, Laparoscopy	Surgery
Catheter, Cholangiography	Surgery
Catheter, Epidural	Obstetrics/Gynecology
Catheter, Suction, With Tip	General
Catheter, Thermal Dilution	Cardiovascular
Clamp, Other	Surgery
Colonoscope, General & Plastic Surgery	Surgery
Cryosurgical Unit	Surgery
Cryosurgical Unit, Gynecologic	Obstetrics/Gynecology
Diaper, Pediatric	General
Dilator, Port, Laparoscopic	Surgery
Electrode, Electrocardiograph	Cardiovascular
Electrode, Other	General
Glove, Patient Examination	General
Glove, Surgical	General
Glove, Surgical, Hypoallergenic	General
Glove, Surgical, Powder-Free	Surgery
Guidewire	Cardiovascular
Holder, Instrument, Laparoscopic	Surgery
Infuser, Pressure (Blood Pump)	General
Introducer, Catheter	Cardiovascular
Kit, Anesthesia, Epidural	Anesthesiology
Kit, Anesthesia, Other	Anesthesiology
Laryngoscope, Rigid	Anesthesiology
Light, Surgical, Fiberoptic	Surgery
Needle, Blood Collection	General
Needle, Hypodermic	General
Needle, Other	General
Oximeter, Pulse	General
Pacifier	General
Port, Vascular Access	Cardiovascular
Probe, Temperature	General
Pump, Infusion	General
Pump, Infusion, Implantable, General	General
Service, Consulting	General

DMA MED-CHEM CORPORATION   800-362-1833 (cont'd)

Stimulator, Nerve Locating	Cns/Neurology
Syringe, Other	General
Trocar, Laparoscopic	Surgery
Tube, Tracheal (Endotracheal)	Anesthesiology

DMEDICUS, LLC.   469-698-9939
842 Canterbury Dr., Rockwall, TX 75032

FDA Number: 3003763347
Ownership: Private
Produces/Sells CE-marked Devices: N

Stimulator, Muscle, Powered, Invasive	Physical Med
Stimulator, Neuromuscular, External Functional	Cns/Neurology

DMS   410-757-8400
530 College Pkwy., Suite D, Annapolis, MD 21409

FDA Number: 1123652   *Fax:* 410-757-3878
E-mail: FDEJACMA@POWERPEEL.IT
Web site: WWW.POWERPEEL.COM
Medical Products Sales Volume: $750,000
Annual Revenue: $0-$1 Million
Year Founded: 1996
Total Employees: 3   *Marketing Staff:* 1
Ownership: Private
Quality System Registration Information: ISO9002
Produces/Sells CE-marked Devices: Y
Federal Procurement Eligibility: Small Business
Distribution: Manufacturer Through Distributor, Importer
General Admin.: Fred DeJacma/Chief Executive Officer
Mktg./Adv.: FRED DE JACMA/Director Product Development

Brush, Dermabrasion	Surgery

DMS LABORATORIES, INC.   800-567-4367
2 Darts Mill Road, Flemington, NJ 08822   **908-782-3353**

FDA Number: n/a   *Fax:* 908-782-0832
E-mail: dmslabs@aol.com
Web site: www.rapidvet.com
Medical Products Sales Volume: $1,000,000
Year Founded: 1982
Total Employees: 6
Ownership: Private
Quality System Registration Information: ISO9002
Produces/Sells CE-marked Devices: N
Federal Procurement Eligibility: Small Business, GSA Contract, VA Contract
Distribution: Manufacturer Direct, Manufacturer Through Distributor
General Admin.: Nicholas A. Gallo/President, Chief Executive Officer
Mktg./Adv.: Denise G. Darmanian/Vice President Business Development

Analyzer, Blood Grouping	Hematology
Kit, Identification, Dermatophyte	Microbiology
Kit, Platelet Associated IGG	Hematology
Test, Allergy	Immunology

DMV CORPORATION   800-522-9465
1024 Military Rd., Zanesville, OH 43702-0878   **740-452-4787**

FDA Number: 1523955   *Fax:* 740-452-4501
E-mail: info@dmvcorp.com
Web site: www.dmvcorp.com
Medical Products Sales Volume: $350,000
Annual Revenue: $0-$1 Million
Year Founded: 1968
Total Employees: 8
Ownership: Private
Produces/Sells CE-marked Devices: Y
Federal Procurement Eligibility: Small Business
Distribution: Manufacturer Through Distributor
General Admin.: Robert C. England/President
Production: Patricia A. Burkhart/Director Operations

Inserter/Remover, Lens, Contact	Ophthalmology
Laboratory Equipment, Ophthalmic	Ophthalmology

DMX-WORKS, INC.   800-839-6757
4159-b Corporate Court, Palm Harbor, FL 34683   **727-942-8324**

FDA Number: 1058051
Web site: www.dmxworks.com
Ownership: Private
Produces/Sells CE-marked Devices: N

Radiographic/Fluoroscopic Unit, Image-Intensified	Radiology

DMZ/TIMCO MACHINE COMPANY   440-942-4001
35530 Lakeland Blvd., Eastlake, OH 44095-5305

FDA Number: n/a
E-mail: sales@dmztimco.com
Web site: dmztimco.com
Annual Revenue: $0-$1 Million
Ownership: Private
Produces/Sells CE-marked Devices: N
Federal Procurement Eligibility: Small Business
Distribution: OEM

DMZ/TIMCO MACHINE COMPANY 440-942-4001 (cont'd)
Contract Manufacturing General
Medical Product Subsidiaries (Listed Separately)
Timco Machine

DNA
See Noshok, Inc.

DNA PRODUCTS, LLC 800-535-3189
P.O. Box 306, New York, NY 10032-0306 800-535-3189
FDA Number: n/a *Fax:* 800-535-3189
E-mail: support@dnaproductsonline.com
Web site: www.dnaproductsonline.com
Medical Products Sales Volume: $300,000
Annual Revenue: $0-$1 Million
Year Founded: 2001
Total Employees: 4
Ownership: Private
Produces/Sells CE-marked Devices: N
Federal Procurement Eligibility: Small Business, Minority Owned, Female Owned
Distribution: Exclusive Distributor
General Admin.: Danita Harris/President
Mktg./Adv.: Danita Harris/Director Marketing
    David Harris/Vice President Sales
Gown, Patient, Disposable General
Linen, Bed General
Suit, Scrub, Disposable Surgery

DNI NEVADA
See Fluke Biomedical

DNMS INSTITUTE, LLC 210-561-7881
6421 Mondean St., San Antonio, TX 78240-2533
FDA Number: 1649881 *Fax:* 210-561-7806
Ownership: Private
Produces/Sells CE-marked Devices: N
Vibrator, Therapeutic Physical Med

DNTLWORKS EQUIPMENT CORPORATION 800-847-0694
7300 South Tucson Way, Centennial, CO 80112 303-693-1410
FDA Number: n/a *Fax:* 303-693-6189
E-mail: info@DNTLworks.com
Web site: www.DNTLworks.com
Medical Products Sales Volume: $2,000,000
Annual Revenue: $1-$5 Million
Year Founded: 1986
Total Employees: 6 *Marketing Staff:* 2 *Sales Staff:* 2
Ownership: Private
Produces/Sells CE-marked Devices: N
Federal Procurement Eligibility: Small Business
Distribution: Manufacturer Through Distributor, OEM, Exporter
General Admin.: Steven R. Knight/President, Chief Executive Officer
Mktg./Adv.: Thomas L. Meighan/Director Sales
Production: Robert J. Kennedy/Director Quality Assurance
    Paul W. Miskimon/Manager Materials
Cabinet, Dental Dental And Oral
Cart, Instrument Surgery
Chair, Dental Dental And Oral
Compressor, Air, Portable Anesthesiology
Evacuator, Oral Cavity Dental And Oral
Light, Dental Dental And Oral
Light, Dental, Intraoral Dental And Oral
Operative Dental Treatment Unit Dental And Oral
Radiographic Unit, Diagnostic, Dental (X-Ray) Dental And Oral
Suction Apparatus, Ward Use, Portable, AC-Powered Surgery

DO NOT DISTURB, INC. 770-750-0065
5665 Highway 9 N 10, Alpharetta, GA 30004-3959
FDA Number: 1066057 *Fax:* 770-346-0035
E-mail: mary@dodisturb.com
Web site: www.dodisturb.com
Medical Products Sales Volume: $90,000
Year Founded: 2000
Total Employees: 3
Ownership: Private
Produces/Sells CE-marked Devices: N
Federal Procurement Eligibility: Small Business
General Admin.: Mrs. Mary Geoghagan/Owner
Hexokinase, Glucose Chemistry

DOBI MEDICAL INTERNATIONAL, INC. 201-760-6464
1200 Macarthur Boulevard, Mahwah, NJ 07430
FDA Number: 3003601351
Ownership: Private
Produces/Sells CE-marked Devices: N

DOBI-SYMPLEX
See Seattle Systems

DOC'S PROPLUGS, INC. 800-521-2982
719 Swift st, Suite 100, Santa Cruz, CA 95060 831-425-5920
FDA Number: 2937200 *Fax:* 831-425-0178
E-mail: info@proplugs.com
Web site: www.proplugs.com
Medical Products Sales Volume: $1,500,000
Annual Revenue: $0-$1 Million
Year Founded: 1977
Total Employees: 9 *Marketing Staff:* 3 *Sales Staff:* 7
Ownership: Private
Produces/Sells CE-marked Devices: N
Federal Procurement Eligibility: Small Business
Distribution: Manufacturer Direct, Manufacturer Through Distributor, Manufacturer Through Manufacturer Reps, Exporter
General Admin.: Mrs. Janice Scott/Vice President
Mktg./Adv.: Mr. Rawley Bushman/Admin. Marketing & Sales
Production: Mrs. Brenda Rogers/Director Distribution
Finance: Mr. Les Hill/Accountant
    Mrs. Lisa Larsen/Accountant
Amplifier, Voice Ear/Nose/Throat
Device, Assistive Listening Ear/Nose/Throat
Hearing-Aid Ear/Nose/Throat
Plug, Ear Ear/Nose/Throat
Protector, Hearing (Insert) Ear/Nose/Throat
Unit, Therapy, Tinnitus Ear/Nose/Throat

DOCKUM RESEARCH LAB 626-794-1821
844 East Mariposa St., Altadena, CA 91001
FDA Number: 2017608
Retainer, Matrix Dental And Oral

DOCTOR DOWN, INC. 888-883-3696
802 1st Street East, P.O. Box 1, 406-883-3052
Polson, MT 59860
FDA Number: 3029057
E-mail: info@doctordown.com
Web site: www.doctordown.com
Ownership: Private
Produces/Sells CE-marked Devices: N
Linen, Bed General

DOCTORS ORDERS 866-356-0771
731 B Construction Ct., Zeeland, MI 49464 616-931-9939
FDA Number: n/a *Fax:* 616-582-6200
E-mail: info@do-engineering.com
Web site: www.do-engineering.com
Year Founded: 2001
Ownership: Private
Produces/Sells CE-marked Devices: N
Component, Exercise Physical Med

DOCXS BIOMEDICAL PRODUCTS AND 707-462-2351
ACCESSORIES
564 South Dora, Suite A-1, Ukiah, CA 95482
FDA Number: 3003693585 *Fax:* 707-462-2751
E-mail: info@docxs.net
Web site: www.docxs.net
Medical Products Sales Volume: $100,000
Annual Revenue: $0-$1 Million
Year Founded: 2001
Total Employees: 2 *Marketing Staff:* 2 *Sales Staff:* 1
Ownership: Private
Produces/Sells CE-marked Devices: Y
Federal Procurement Eligibility: Small Business, Female Owned
Distribution: Manufacturer Direct, Manufacturer Through Distributor, OEM
Cable/Lead, ECG, With Transducer And Electrode Cardiovascular
Electrode, Cutaneous Cns/Neurology
Gel, Electrode, Stimulator Cns/Neurology
Vena Cava Balloon Occluder Cardiovascular

DODGE
See Regupol America

DOH,DDSD,CSB 505-841-5287
1000 Main St., Nw, P.o. Box 1269, Los Lunas, NM 87031
FDA Number: 3004980950
Ownership: Private
Produces/Sells CE-marked Devices: N
Cushion, Wheelchair (Pad) Physical Med

DOLPHIN IMAGING SYSTEMS 800-548-7241
9200 Eton Avenue, Chatsworth, CA 91311-5807 818-435-1368
FDA Number: n/a *Fax:* 818-435-1369
E-mail: info@dolphinimaging.com
Web site: www.dolphinimaging.com
Ownership: Private
Produces/Sells CE-marked Devices: N
Distribution: Manufacturer Direct, Exporter

DOLPHIN IMAGING SYSTEMS   800-548-7241 *(cont'd)*
Computer, Radiographic Data   Radiology
System, Communication, Image, Digital   Radiology

DOLPHIN MEDICAL INC.   310-978-0516
12525 Chadron Ave., Hawthorne, CA 90250
FDA Number: 2021846
Ownership: Private
Produces/Sells CE-marked Devices: N
Oximeter, Intracardiac   Cardiovascular

DOME PUBLISHING COMPANY, INC.   401-738-7900
10 New England Way, Warwick, RI 02887
FDA Number: 3003437498
Ownership: Private
Produces/Sells CE-marked Devices: N
Bandage, Elastic   General

DOMINATOR RADIOLOGY SYSTEMS, INC.
See Dr Systems, Inc.

DOMINION BIOLOGICALS LTD.   800-565-0653
5 Isnor Dr., Dartmouth, NS B3B 1M1 Canada   902-468-3992
FDA Number: n/a   *Fax:* 902-468-3599
E-mail: general@dominionbio.ns.ca
Web site: http://www.immucor.com/site/home_orig.jsp?lang=en-ca
Medical Products Sales Volume: $4,000,000
Year Founded: 1972
Total Employees: 50   *Marketing Staff:* 1   *Sales Staff:* 4
Ownership: IMMUCORGAMMA Corp.
Quality System Registration Information: ISO9001
Produces/Sells CE-marked Devices: Y
Distribution: Manufacturer Direct, Manufacturer Through Distributor, OEM,
Exclusive Distributor, Exporter

DOMINION MEDICAL SUPPLY INC.   800-660-3674
7563 Regional Rd. #63, RR#1,   905-701-5083
Dunnville, ONT N1A-2 Canada
FDA Number: n/a   *Fax:* 905-701-5084
E-mail: kjshaw@niagara.com
Web site: www.dominionmedical.com
Year Founded: 1996
Total Employees: 10
Ownership: Private
Produces/Sells CE-marked Devices: N
Distribution: Service Direct, Exclusive Distributor

DON JOHNSTON INCORPORATED   800-999-4660
26799 Commerce Dr., Volo, IL 60073   847-740-0749
FDA Number: n/a   *Fax:* 847-740-7326
E-mail: info@donjohnston.com
Web site: www.donjohnston.com
Ownership: Private
Produces/Sells CE-marked Devices: N
Federal Procurement Eligibility: Small Business
Distribution: Manufacturer Direct
General Admin.: Don Johnston/Chief Executive Officer
    Ruth Ziolkowski/President
    Cheryll Johnston/Vice President Human Resources
Mktg./Adv.: Mary Mourousias/Manager Advertising
    Roxanne Butterfield/Manager Marketing
Communication System, Non-Powered   Physical Med
Computer Software   General

DON TAY INDUSTRIES   262-789-9102
2383 South 162nd St., New Berlin, WI 53151
FDA Number: 2134215
Ownership: Private
Produces/Sells CE-marked Devices: N
Electrode, Electrocardiograph   Cardiovascular

DONALDSON COMPANY, INC.   952-887-3131
1400 W. 94th St., Bloomington, MN 55431
FDA Number: n/a
Web site: www.donaldson.com
Medical Products Sales Volume: $3,000,000
Annual Revenue: More than $1 Billion
Ownership: Lifeline Systems, Inc.
Stock Symbol: DCI
Traded On: NYSE
Quality System Registration Information: ISO9000
Produces/Sells CE-marked Devices: Y
Distribution: Manufacturer Direct, Manufacturer Through Distributor, OEM,
Exporter
General Admin.: William M. Cook/President, Chief Executive Officer, Chairman
    Charles J. McMurray/Senior Vice President
    Jay L. Ward/Senior Vice President
Production: Lowell F. Schwab/Senior Vice President Operations
Equipment, Cleaning, Air   General

DONALDSON COMPANY, INC.   952-887-3131 *(cont'd)*
Equipment, Control, Pollution   General
Equipment, Filtering, Air, ETO   General
Media, Filter   General
Medical Product Subsidiaries (Listed Separately)
Donaldson Europe N.V.
Nippon Donaldson, Ltd.

DONATELLE   651-746-2900
501 County Rd. E-2 Extension, New Brighton, MN 55112
FDA Number: 3004961578
Ownership: Private
Produces/Sells CE-marked Devices: N
Mixing Equipment, Cement   Orthopedics

DONELL   800-324-7455
1801 Taylor Avenue, Louisville, KY 40213   502-452-6079
FDA Number: 9020600   *Fax:* 502-452-6059
E-mail: info@donellskin.com
Web site: www.donellskin.com
Medical Products Sales Volume: $600,000
Annual Revenue: $0-$1 Million
Year Founded: 1989
Total Employees: 5
Ownership: Private
Produces/Sells CE-marked Devices: N
Federal Procurement Eligibility: Small Business, Minority Owned
Distribution: Manufacturer Through Distributor, Exclusive Distributor
General Admin.: Stacey Johnson/President, Chief Executive Officer
Dressing, Gel   General
Elastomer, Silicone (Scar Management)   Surgery
Lotion, Skin Care   General
Silicone Sheeting   General
Stabilizer, Vein   General

DONOVAN INDUSTRIES   800-334-4404
13401 McCormick Drive, Tampa, FL 33626   813-854-1547
FDA Number: 1051193   *Fax:* 813-855-6569
E-mail: marketing@dawnmist.com
Web site: www.donovanindustries.com
Medical Products Sales Volume: $4,800,000
Annual Revenue: $10-$25 Million
Year Founded: 1979
Total Employees: 22   *Marketing Staff:* 3
Ownership: Private
Quality System Registration Information: ISO9002
Produces/Sells CE-marked Devices: N
Federal Procurement Eligibility: Small Business, GSA Contract
Distribution: Manufacturer Through Distributor
General Admin.: Jim Donovan/President
Mktg./Adv.: Brian Cupari/Manager Market Planning
    Samuel J. Whyel/Vice President Marketing & Sales
Production: Laura Dawson/Customer Service Representative
    Jodi Hutchins/Manager Quality Assurance & Regulatory Affairs
Bag, Plastic   General
Dentifrice   Dental And Oral
Lotion, Skin Care   General
Toothbrush, Manual   Dental And Oral
Tourniquet, Non-Pneumatic, Surgical   Surgery

DORAN INSTRUMENTS, INC.
See Diagnosis, Llc

DOREL DESIGN & DEVELOPMENT CENTER   800-909-7133
25 Forbes Blvd., Foxboro, MA 02035   781-364-3542
FDA Number: 1223794
E-mail: consumer@djgusa.com
Web site: www.dorel.com
Ownership: Private
Produces/Sells CE-marked Devices: N
Disinfector, Medical Device   General
Dispenser, Medication, Liquid   General
Humidifier, Non-Direct Patient Interface (Home-Use)   Anesthesiology
Nebulizer, Medicinal   Ear/Nose/Throat
Otoscope   Ear/Nose/Throat
Pack, Hot Or Cold, Reusable   Physical Med
Pump, Nebulizer, Manual   Ear/Nose/Throat
Ring, Teething, Fluid-Filled   Dental And Oral
Syringe, Ear   Ear/Nose/Throat
Temperature Strip, Forehead, Liquid Crystal   General
Thermometer, Electronic   General
Toothbrush, Manual   Dental And Oral

DOREX, INC.   714-639-0700
954 N. Lemon St., Orange, CA 92867
FDA Number: 2026347   *Fax:* 714-639-4951
E-mail: mkutas@earthlink.net
Web site: WWW.DOREXIR.COM
Medical Products Sales Volume: $100,000

DOREX, INC.   714-639-0700 (cont'd)
Annual Revenue: $1-$5 Million
Year Founded: 1968
Total Employees: 6   *Marketing Staff:* 2   *Sales Staff:* 11
Ownership: Private
Produces/Sells CE-marked Devices: N
Federal Procurement Eligibility: Small Business, Female Owned
Distribution: Manufacturer Direct, Exporter
General Admin.: Jean Kutas/Chief Executive Officer
     Mel Kutas/President
Mktg./Adv.: Christie Bishop/Vice President Sales
Production: Mark Yoshihara/Vice President Manufacturing
   Thermographic Device, Infrared   Obstetrics/Gynecology
   Unit, Imaging, Thermal   Radiology

DORMER LABORATORIES INC.   416-242-6167
91 Kelfield Rd., Unit 5, Rexdale, ONT M9W-5A3 Canada
FDA Number: n/a   *Fax:* 416-242-9487
Web site: http://www.dormer.ca
Year Founded: 1992
Total Employees: 10
Ownership: Private
Produces/Sells CE-marked Devices: N
Distribution: Manufacturer Direct, Exporter

DORMER LABORATORIES INC.   800-363-5040
91 Kelfield St., Unit 5,   416-242-6167
Toronto, ONT M9W-5 Canada
FDA Number: n/a   *Fax:* 416-242-9487
E-mail: info@dormer.com
Web site: www.dormer.com
Year Founded: 1979
Total Employees: 10
Ownership: Private
Produces/Sells CE-marked Devices: N
Distribution: Exclusive Distributor, Importer

DORNIER MEDICAL SYSTEMS, INC.
   See Dornier Medtech America

DORNIER MEDTECH AMERICA   800-367-6437
1155 Roberts Blvd., Kennesaw, GA 30144   770-426-1315
FDA Number: 1037955   *Fax:* 770-426-6115
E-mail: info@dornier.com
Web site: www.dornier.com
Medical Products Sales Volume: $36,000,000
Year Founded: 1984
Total Employees: 110   *Marketing Staff:* 3   *Sales Staff:* 13
Ownership: Ffm Med Reps, Llc
Quality System Registration Information: ISO9001
Produces/Sells CE-marked Devices: Y
Federal Procurement Eligibility: Small Business, GSA Contract, VA Contract
Distribution: Manufacturer Direct, Manufacturer Through Distributor, OEM, Service Direct, Importer
General Admin.: Brian Walsh/General Manager
     Christy Loewenstern/Manager Human Resources
     Brian Walsh/President
Mktg./Adv.: Martha Yannessa/Vice President Sales
Production: Tim Thomas/Manager Quality Assurance & Regulatory Affairs
   Facility, Equipment, Medical, Mobile   General
   Image Digitizer   Radiology
   Laser, Nd:YAG, Surgical   Surgery
   Lithotriptor, Multipurpose   Gastroenterology/Urology

DORNOCH MEDICAL SYSTEMS, INC.   888-466-6633
200 Northwest Parkway, Riverside, MO 64150   816-505-2226
FDA Number: 1954182   *Fax:* 816-505-1050
Ownership: Private
Produces/Sells CE-marked Devices: N
   Basin, Emesis   General
   Bottle, Collection, Vacuum (Aspirator)   General
   Regulator, Vacuum   General
   Suction Apparatus, Single Patient, Portable, Non-Powered   Surgery
   Urinal   General
   Washer, Receptacle, Waste, Body   General

DOSIMETER CORP. OF AMERICA
   See Dosimeter Division Of Arrow Tech Inc

DOSIMETER DIVISION OF ARROW TECH INC   800-322-8258
5 Eastmans Road, Parsippany, NJ 07054   973-887-7100
FDA Number: 9200291   *Fax:* 973-887-4732
E-mail: bfinnegan@dosimeter.com
Web site: www.dosimeter.com
Medical Products Sales Volume: $5,000,000
Annual Revenue: $5-$10 Million
Total Employees: 55   *Marketing Staff:* 2   *Sales Staff:* 6
Ownership: MORGAN-CRUCIBLE, PLC
Stock Symbol: MGCR

DOSIMETER DIVISION OF ARROW TECH INC   800-322-8258
(cont'd)
Traded On: London
Quality System Registration Information: ISO9001
Produces/Sells CE-marked Devices: N
Distribution: Manufacturer Direct, Manufacturer Through Distributor, Exporter
General Admin.: Mary Crawford/Manager Human Resources
     Paul A. Roba/President, Chief Executive Officer
     Peter Petruzela/Vice President, General Manager
Mktg./Adv.: Paul A. Roba/Director Marketing
     Carolyn Murat/Manager International & National Sales
Production: Paul L. Fierro/Director Quality Assurance
     Robert M. Rich/Manager Regulatory Affairs
     Peter Petruzela/Vice President Manufacturing
   Counter, Gamma, General Use   Toxicology
   Counter, Radiation   Radiology
   Detector, Beta/Gamma   Chemistry
   Dosimeter, Radiation   Radiology
   Safety Equipment, Laboratory   Chemistry

DOSS K. TANNEHILL - OCULARIST   808-738-5300
752 17th Ave., Honolulu, HI 96816
FDA Number: 3004939306   *Fax:* 808-738-5304
E-mail: doss@pacificeyes.net
Web site: www.pacificeyes.net
Ownership: Private
Produces/Sells CE-marked Devices: N
   Eye, Artificial, Non-Custom   Ophthalmology

DOTOLO RESEARCH CORP.   800-237-8458
2875 MCI Drive, Pinellas Park, FL 33782   727-217-9300
FDA Number: 1036507   *Fax:* 727-217-9500
E-mail: rhdotolo@DotoloResearch.com
Web site: www.dotoloresearch.com
Medical Products Sales Volume: $1,100,000
Annual Revenue: $1-$5 Million
Year Founded: 1984
Total Employees: 16   *Marketing Staff:* 2   *Sales Staff:* 2
Ownership: Private
Quality System Registration Information: ISO9001
Produces/Sells CE-marked Devices: Y
Federal Procurement Eligibility: Small Business
Distribution: Manufacturer Direct, Manufacturer Through Distributor, Manufacturer Through Manufacturer Reps
General Admin.: Raymond Dotolo/Chief Executive Officer
Mktg./Adv.: Ms. Kaori Yamauchi Azzi/Manager International Sales
Production: Rose Kennedy/Manager Regulatory Affairs
   Irrigator, Colonic   Gastroenterology/Urology
   Irrigator, Perineal   Gastroenterology/Urology
   Kit, Irrigation, Perineal   Gastroenterology/Urology

DOTOLO RESEARCH WESTERN DIV.   623-936-0500
10199 W. Van Buren, Suite 10, Tolleson, AZ 85353
FDA Number: 3005598712
   Irrigator, Colonic   Gastroenterology/Urology

DOTRONIX, INC.   651-633-1742
160 First St. S.E., New Brighton, MN 55112
FDA Number: n/a   *Fax:* 651-633-2152
E-mail: sales@dotronix.com
Web site: www.dotronix.com
Annual Revenue: $1-$5 Million
Total Employees: 185
Ownership: Public
Stock Symbol: DOTX
Traded On: NASDAQ
Produces/Sells CE-marked Devices: N
Federal Procurement Eligibility: Small Business
Distribution: Manufacturer Direct
General Admin.: William Sadler/President, Chief Executive Officer
Mktg./Adv.: Dick Lemke/Manager National Sales
Production: William R. Sadler/Manager Materials
     Kurt Sadler/Manager Operations
     Robert Andrews/Vice President Operations
   Computer Equipment   General

DOUGLAS & HARPER MFG. CO., INC.   912-367-4149
1126 South Main St., Baxley, GA 31513
FDA Number: 1049813
Ownership: Private
Produces/Sells CE-marked Devices: N
   Garment, Protective, For Incontinence   Gastroenterology/Urology
   Sling, Arm   Physical Med

DOVER UROLOGICAL PRODUCTS
   See Covidien Lp

DOW CHEMICAL INSTRUMENTS
   See Seradyn, Inc.

DOW CORNING WRIGHT
See Wright Medical Group, Inc.

DOW HICKAM PHARMACEUTICALS, INC.
See Mylan Pharmaceuticals Inc

DOWLING TEXTILES   770-957-3981
615 Macon Rd., Mcdonough, GA 30253
FDA Number: 1043644

Binder, Abdominal	General
Cap, Surgical	Surgery
Cover, Mattress	General
Dress, Surgical	Surgery
Gown, Isolation, Surgical	Surgery
Gown, Patient	Surgery
Gown, Surgical	Surgery
Mask, Surgical	Surgery
Suit, Surgical	Surgery
Wrap, Sterilization	General

DOWNEY INDUSTRIES INC.
See Zevex Incorporated

DOXTECH, LLC.   503-641-1865
10025 S.W. Allen Blvd., Beaverton, OR 97005
FDA Number: 2950338   Fax: 503-626-8298
E-mail: sales@doxtech.com
Web site: www.doxtech.com
Annual Revenue: $1-$5 Million
Ownership: Private
Produces/Sells CE-marked Devices: N
Federal Procurement Eligibility: Small Business, GSA Contract
Distribution: Manufacturer Direct, Service Direct
Mktg./Adv.: Susan Russell/Vice President Marketing & Sales

Container, Specimen Mailer And Storage	Pathology
Container, Specimen, All Types	General
Thermometer, Liquid Crystals	Surgery

DP MANUFACTURE CORP.   800-403-1890
1460 N.w. 107th Ave., Ste. H, Miami, FL 33172   305-640-9894
FDA Number: 1063774   Fax: 305-477-3205
E-mail: dpmusaco@msn.com
Web site: www.dpmusacorp.com
Ownership: Private
Produces/Sells CE-marked Devices: N

Activator, Ultraviolet, Polymerization	Dental And Oral
Amalgamator, Dental, AC-Powered	Dental And Oral
Handpiece, Air-Powered, Dental	Dental And Oral
Handpiece, Contra- And Right-Angle Attachment, Dental	Dental And Oral
Handpiece, Direct Drive, AC-Powered	Dental And Oral
Light, Fiberoptic, Dental	Dental And Oral
Radiographic Unit, Diagnostic, Dental, Extraoral	Dental And Oral
Scaler, Periodontic	Dental And Oral
Source, Heat, Bleaching, Teeth, Dental	Dental And Oral
Sterilizer, Boiling Water	Dental And Oral
Syringe Unit, Air And/Or Water	Dental And Oral

DPIX, LLC   650-842-9600
3406 Hillview Ave., Palo Alto, CA 94304
FDA Number: n/a   Fax: 650-842-9793
E-mail: info@dpix.com
Web site: http://www.dpix.com
Total Employees: 100
Ownership: Private
Quality System Registration Information: ISO9001
Produces/Sells CE-marked Devices: N
Distribution: Manufacturer Direct, OEM
General Admin.: Dr. Richard Weisfield/Chief Technology Officer, Vice President
          Mr. Frank Caris/President, Chief Executive Officer
Mktg./Adv.: Mr. Bob Tolan/Vice President Marketing
Production: Mrs. Terri Pederson/Director Quality Assurance
          Mrs. Maria Batey/Vice President Manufacturing
Finance: Mr. Jason Lachance/Chief Financial Officer

Imager, X-Ray, Solid State (Flat Panel/Digital)	Radiology

DPS, INC.   800-654-4689
3685 Priority Way South Drive, Suite 100,   317-574-4300
Indianapolis, IN 46240
FDA Number: n/a   Fax: 317-574-4322
E-mail: sales@dpslink.com
Web site: www.dpslink.com
Medical Products Sales Volume: $15,300,000
Annual Revenue: $5-$10 Million
Year Founded: 1972
Total Employees: 55   Marketing Staff: 15   Sales Staff: 8
Ownership: Private
Federal Procurement Eligibility: Small Business
Distribution: Manufacturer Direct
General Admin.: Dan Barrow/President, Chief Executive Officer
Mktg./Adv.: Kevin Kennedy/Vice President Marketing & Sales

DPS, INC.   800-654-4689 (cont'd)
Research: Michael Henegham/Vice President Research & Development

Computer Software	General
Computer Software, Hospital/Nursing Management	General

DPT LABORATORIES, LTD.   866-225-5378
4040 Broadway, Suite 401,   210-476-8159
San Antonio, TX 78209
FDA Number: 1628114   Fax: 210-829-8733
E-mail: confidence@dptlabs.com
Web site: www.dptlabs.com
Annual Revenue: More than $100 Million
Year Founded: 1990
Total Employees: 1400   Marketing Staff: 2   Sales Staff: 20
Ownership: Private
Produces/Sells CE-marked Devices: N
Mktg./Adv.: Paul Josephs/Vice President Marketing & Sales

Contract Manufacturing, Pharmaceuticals/Chemicals	General
Contract Manufacturing, Reagent	General
Contract Packaging	General
Contract R&D, Diagnostics	General
Equipment/Service, Quality Control	General
Packaging System, Unit-Dose	General

DR SYSTEMS, INC.   800-794-5955
10140 Mesa Rim Rd., San Diego, CA 92121-2914   858-625-3344
FDA Number: 2028802   Fax: 858-625-3335
E-mail: sales@dominator.com
Web site: www.dominator.com
Annual Revenue: $25-$50 Million
Year Founded: 1992
Total Employees: 180   Marketing Staff: 5   Sales Staff: 15
Ownership: Private
Quality System Registration Information: ISO9000
Produces/Sells CE-marked Devices: N
Federal Procurement Eligibility: Small Business
Distribution: Manufacturer Direct, Manufacturer Through Distributor, Manufacturer Through Manufacturer Reps, Service Direct
General Admin.: Murray A. Reicher/Chairman
          Kent Curtis/Chief Operating Officer
          Richard C. Porritt/President, Chief Executive Officer
Mktg./Adv.: Douglas Dill/Director Marketing
          Mark Herndon/Vice President Sales
Finance: Charles Zuckerman/Chief Financial Officer

Radiographic Picture Archiving/Communication System (PACS)	Radiology
Transmitter, Image & Data, Radiographic	Radiology

DR. LEN'S MEDICAL PRODUCTS LLC   678-908-8180
412 Atwood Rd., Erdenheim, PA 19038
FDA Number: 3004153498
Ownership: Private
Produces/Sells CE-marked Devices: N

Bandage, Compression	General
Binder, Medical, Therapeutic	General
Dressing, Other	General
Dressing, Wound, Hydrophilic	Surgery
Dressing, Wound, Occlusive	Surgery
Orthosis, Cervical	Physical Med
Splint, Extremity, Non-inflatable, External, Non-sterile	Surgery
Splint, Extremity, Non-Inflatable, External	Surgery
Stocking, Elastic	General

DR. ROTH'S FOOTCARE PRODUCTS, LLC.   800-486-0325
261 E. Imperial Hwy, Suite #570,   949-646-8413
Costa Mesa, CA 92835
FDA Number: 2031076   Fax: 949-646-8489
E-mail: customerservice@drroths.com
Web site: www.drroths.com
Annual Revenue: $0-$1 Million
Ownership: Private
Produces/Sells CE-marked Devices: N
Distribution: Manufacturer Direct, Manufacturer Through Distributor, Manufacturer Through Manufacturer Reps, Exclusive Distributor, Exporter

Orthosis, Corrective Shoe	Physical Med
Support, Foot	Orthopedics

DR. SCHOLL'S
See Schering-Plough Health Care Products

DR.'S PAGE   888-297-9109
P.O. Box 801764, Santa Clarita, CA 91380-1764   661-294-9509
FDA Number: n/a   Fax: 661-294-9837
E-mail: info@homeaid.com
Web site: www.homeaid.com
Medical Products Sales Volume: $700,000
Annual Revenue: $0-$1 Million
Total Employees: 6   Marketing Staff: 4   Sales Staff: 4
Ownership: Home-Aid-Healthcare, Inc.
Produces/Sells CE-marked Devices: N

DR.'S PAGE   888-297-9109 *(cont'd)*

Federal Procurement Eligibility: Small Business, Minority Owned, Female Owned
Distribution: Manufacturer Direct, Manufacturer Through Distributor, Manufacturer Through Manufacturer Reps
General Admin.: Roland A. Hinds/President
     Robin J. Yamashita/Vice President

Anatomical Training Model	General
Chart, Anatomical Training	General
Material, Training, Audiovisual	General

DRAEGER MEDICAL SYSTEMS, INC   800-437-2437
3135 Quarry Rd, Telford, PA 18969   **215-721-5400**
FDA Number: 2510954   *Fax:* 215-723-5935
Web site: http://www.draeger.com
Ownership: Draeger Medical Ag & Co. Kg
Stock Symbol: DRW3
Traded On: Frankfurt
Produces/Sells CE-marked Devices: N

Bilirubin (Total and Unbound) Neonate Test System	Chemistry
Incubator, Neonatal	General
Incubator, Neonatal Transport	General
Phototherapy Unit, Neonatal	General
Thermometer, Electronic	General
Warmer, Radiant, Infant	General

DRAEGER MEDICAL SYSTEMS, INC   215-660-2626
6 Tech Drive, Andover, MA 01810
FDA Number: 3005783425
Web site: www.draeger-medical.com
Ownership: Draeger Medical Ag & Co. Kg
Stock Symbol: DRW3
Traded On: Frankfurt
Produces/Sells CE-marked Devices: N

Analyzer, Gas, Carbon-Dioxide, Gaseous Phase (Capnograph)	Anesthesiology
Gas Machine, Analgesia	Anesthesiology
Spirometer, Monitoring (Volumeter)	Anesthesiology

DRAEGER MEDICAL SYSTEMS, INC.   215-660-2626
16 Electronics Ave., Danvers, MA 01923
FDA Number: 1220063
Web site: www.draeger-medical.com
Ownership: Draeger Medical Ag & Co. Kg
Stock Symbol: DRW3
Traded On: Frankfurt
Produces/Sells CE-marked Devices: N

Amplifier, Transducer Signal (W Signal Conditioner)	Cardiovascular
Analyzer, Gas, Carbon-Dioxide, Gaseous Phase (Capnograph)	Anesthesiology
Analyzer, Gas, Oxygen, Gaseous Phase	Anesthesiology
Analyzer, Gas, Sevoflurane, Gaseous-phase (anesthetic Concentration)	Anesthesiology
Analyzer, Spectrum, EEG Signal	Cns/Neurology
Computer and Software, Medical	General
Computer, Blood Pressure	Cardiovascular
Computer, Chemistry Analyzer	Chemistry
Computer, Diagnostic, Programmable	Cardiovascular
Detector, Arrhythmia Alarm	Cardiovascular
Display, Cathode-Ray Tube	Cardiovascular
Electroencephalograph	Cns/Neurology
Gas-Machine, Anesthesia	Anesthesiology
Monitor, Apnea	General
Monitor, Blood Pressure, Indirect, Semi-Automatic	Cardiovascular
Monitor, Carbon-Dioxide, Cutaneous	Anesthesiology
Monitor, Cardiac (Cardiotachometer & Rate Alarm)	Cardiovascular
Monitor, Oxygen, Cutaneous	Anesthesiology
Monitor, Physiological, Patient	Cardiovascular
Monitor, ST Segment (With Alarm)	General
Monitor, Ventilatory Frequency	Anesthesiology
Oximeter, Ear	Cardiovascular
Oximeter, Intracardiac	Cardiovascular
Recorder, Paper Chart	Cardiovascular
Spirometer, Monitoring (Volumeter)	Anesthesiology
Stimulator, Nerve, Anesthesia	Anesthesiology
System, Network And Communication, Physiological Monitors	Cardiovascular
Thermometer, Electronic, Continuous	General
Transmitter/Receiver System, Physiological, Radiofrequency	Cardiovascular
Ventilator, Continuous (Respirator)	Anesthesiology

DRAEGER SAFETY, INC.   215-660-2186
3135 Quarry Road, Telford, PA 18969
FDA Number: 2517967
E-mail: prodinfo@draeger.net
Web site: www.draeger.net
Annual Revenue: $0-$1 Million
Total Employees: 200
Ownership: DRAEGERWERK, AG
Quality System Registration Information: ISO9001
Produces/Sells CE-marked Devices: N
Distribution: Manufacturer Through Distributor, Importer, Exporter
General Admin.: Wes Kenneweg/President, Chief Executive Officer

Analyzer, Gas, Carbon-Monoxide, Gaseous Phase	Anesthesiology
Dryer, Respiratory/Anesthesia Equipment	General

DRAEGER SAFETY, INC.   215-660-2186 *(cont'd)*

Sampler, Gas	Chemistry
Test, Ethyl Alcohol	Toxicology
Ventilator, Continuous (Respirator)	Anesthesiology

DRAPER PRODUCTS, INC.
See R. Sabee Company

DRAVON MEDICAL, INC.   800-654-1976
11465 SE Highway 212, PO Box 69,   **503-656-6600**
Clackamas, OR 97015
FDA Number: 3021643   *Fax:* 503-655-5229
E-mail: dravon@mindspring.com
Web site: www.dravon.com
Medical Products Sales Volume: $3,000,000
Annual Revenue: $1-$5 Million
Year Founded: 1974
Total Employees: 30   *Marketing Staff:* 1   *Sales Staff:* 2
Ownership: Private
Produces/Sells CE-marked Devices: Y
Federal Procurement Eligibility: Small Business
Distribution: Manufacturer Direct, OEM
General Admin.: Michael P. Napoli/President, Chief Executive Officer
Mktg./Adv.: Michael Napoli/Director Marketing
     Richard Parker/Manager National Sales
     Alan Crowe/Sales Engineer
Production: Darlene Berg/Director Quality Assurance
     Mary Ann Murray/Manager Materials
     Richard Kluempke/Manager Production
Finance: Richard Parker/Controller

Bag, Plastic	General
Clamp, Hemodialysis Unit Blood Line	Gastroenterology/Urology
Clamp, Other	Surgery
Clamp, Tubing, Blood, Automatic	Gastroenterology/Urology
Contract Assembly	General
Contract Manufacturing	General
Contract Packaging	General
Contract Sterilization	General

DRAXIMAGE INC.   888-633-5343
16751 TransCanada Hwy,   **514-694-8220**
Kirkland, QUE H9H-4 Canada
FDA Number: n/a   *Fax:* 514-694-9295
E-mail: info@draximage.com
Web site: www.draximage.com
Year Founded: 1950
Ownership: Draxis Health Inc.
Produces/Sells CE-marked Devices: N
Distribution: Manufacturer Direct, Exclusive Distributor

DRB TECHNOLOGIES, INC   610-356-4258
3612 Chapel Rd., Suite B, Newtown Square, PA 19073
FDA Number: 97924
Ownership: Private
Produces/Sells CE-marked Devices: N

Larynx, Artificial Battery-Powered	Ear/Nose/Throat

DREAM INVENTORS DESIGN LLC   208-882-3082
4805 Robinson Park Rd., Moscow, ID 83843
FDA Number: 3004945833
Ownership: Private
Produces/Sells CE-marked Devices: N

Chair, Position, Electric	Physical Med

DREAM SYSTEMS, L.L.C.   650-369-9227
6 Malory Ct., Redwood City, CA 94061
FDA Number: 3004769094
Ownership: Private
Produces/Sells CE-marked Devices: N

Device, Anti-Snoring	Ear/Nose/Throat
Dilator, Nasal	Ear/Nose/Throat

DREAMWRX DENTAL LABORATORY   949-448-9985
1911 Colorado Blvd., Los Angeles, CA 90041
FDA Number: 3005034462
Ownership: Private
Produces/Sells CE-marked Devices: N

Device, Repositioning, Jaw	Dental And Oral

DRESCH/TOLSON DENTAL LAB   952-345-6300
4024 North Holland-sylvania Rd, Toledo, OH 43623
FDA Number: 3004363473
Ownership: Private
Produces/Sells CE-marked Devices: N

Device, Anti-Snoring	Ear/Nose/Throat
Device, Repositioning, Jaw	Dental And Oral
Mouthguard	Dental And Oral

DRESSER INC., DRESSER MEASUREMENT DIVISION   203-426-3115

PO Box 5605, Newtown, CT 06470
FDA Number: n/a
E-mail: brucetibbitts@dresser.com   Fax: 203-426-4349
Web site: www.heise.com
Annual Revenue: $10-$25 Million
Total Employees: 100   *Marketing Staff:* 8   *Sales Staff:* 30
Ownership: Private
Traded On: NYSE
Quality System Registration Information: ISO9000; ISO9001
Produces/Sells CE-marked Devices: Y
Distribution: Manufacturer Through Manufacturer Reps
General Admin.: Jim Cummings/General Manager
Mktg./Adv.: Bruce Tibbitts/Manager Marketing & Sales
Production: Bill Steer/Vice President Manufacturing
Research: Ron Deschenes/Manager Research & Development
   Calibrator, Pressure Transducer   Anesthesiology
   Gauge, Gas Pressure, Cylinder/Pipeline   Anesthesiology

DRESSER INDUSTRIES, INC., INSTRUMENT DIV.
See Dresser Inc., Dresser Measurement Division

DREW SCIENTIFIC
See Drew Scientific, Inc.

DREW SCIENTIFIC, INC.   800-433-0945
4230 Shilling Way, Dallas, TX 75237-1023   **214-210-4900**
FDA Number: 1629992
E-mail: pruductsusa@.drew-scientific.com   Fax: 214-210-4949
Web site: www.drew-scientific.com
Annual Revenue: $5-$10 Million
Total Employees: 60
Ownership: Drew Scientific Ltd.
Produces/Sells CE-marked Devices: Y
Federal Procurement Eligibility: Small Business, GSA Contract
Distribution: Manufacturer Direct, Manufacturer Through Distributor, OEM, Exporter
General Admin.: Jerry West/President
Mktg./Adv.: Roger Bourree/Vice President International Marketing & Sales
Production: Susan Tisza/Manager Customer Services
       Philip West/Vice President Manufacturing
Research: Roger Bourree/Vice President Research & Development
   Counter, Cell   Microbiology
   Counter, Cell Or Particle, Automated   Hematology
   Counter, Cell, Differential Classifier, Automated   Hematology
   Detergent   Hematology
   Diluent, Blood Cell   Hematology

DREXLER TECHNOLOGY
See Lasercard Systems Corporation

DRG INTERNATIONAL, INC.   800-321-1167
1167 US Highway 22 E.,   **908-233-2079**
Mountainside, NJ 07092
FDA Number: 2245285
E-mail: corp@drg-international.com   Fax: 908-233-0758
Web site: www.drg-international.com
Medical Products Sales Volume: $20,000,000
Annual Revenue: $10-$25 Million
Year Founded: 1970
Total Employees: 95   *Marketing Staff:* 8   *Sales Staff:* 25
Ownership: Private
Quality System Registration Information: ISO9000; ISO9001
Produces/Sells CE-marked Devices: Y
Federal Procurement Eligibility: Small Business
Distribution: Manufacturer Direct, Manufacturer Through Distributor, Manufacturer Through Manufacturer Reps, OEM, Exclusive Distributor, Importer, Exporter
General Admin.: E. Geacintov/Executive Vice President
       D. Kekalo/General Manager
       Cyril E. Geacintov/President, Chief Executive Officer
Mktg./Adv.: W. Saenger/Director Marketing
       A. Janetzko/Director Product Development
       Vlad V. Kaluzhny/Manager Business Development
Production: B. Roeder/Director Regulatory Affairs
   Analyzer, Chemistry, ELISA   Chemistry
   Analyzer, ECG   Cardiovascular
   Antibody, Monoclonal   Microbiology
   Antibody, Multiple Auto, Indirect Immunofluorescent   Immunology
   Balloon, Intra-Aortic (With Control System)   Cardiovascular
   Catheter, Angioplasty, Coronary, Transluminal, Percut. Oper.   Cardiovascular
   Computer Software   General
   Computer Software, Hospital/Nursing Management   General
   Enzyme Immunoassay, Other   Chemistry
   Kit, Pregnancy Test   Obstetrics/Gynecology
   Radioimmunoassay, Other   Chemistry
   Stent, Cardiovascular   Cardiovascular
   Stent, Vascular   Cardiovascular
   Surgical Instrument, Cardiovascular   Cardiovascular

DRG INTERNATIONAL, INC.   800-321-1167 *(cont'd)*
   System, Test, Drugs of Abuse   Chemistry
   Test, Fertility Monitoring   Obstetrics/Gynecology
Medical Product Subsidiaries (Listed Separately)
   Drg - Cr
   Drg Instruments Gmbh
   Drg Medtek Sp. Z O.O.
   Drg Techsystems

DRG MEDICAL PACKAGING
See Amcor Flexibles, Inc.

DRI MARK PRODUCTS, INC.   516-484-6200
15 Harbor Park Dr., Port Washington, NY 11050
FDA Number: 2436880
E-mail: info@drimark.com   Fax: 800-645-9662
Web site: www.drimark.com
Ownership: Private
Produces/Sells CE-marked Devices: N
   Pen, Marking, Surgical   Ophthalmology

DRI-DEK/KENDALL PRODUCTS   800-348-2398
901 Sarasota Center Blvd., Naples, FL 34104   **239-643-0448**
FDA Number: n/a
E-mail: info@dri-dek.com   Fax: 800-828-4248
Web site: www.dri-dek.com
Ownership: Private
Produces/Sells CE-marked Devices: N
Federal Procurement Eligibility: Small Business
Distribution: Manufacturer Direct, Manufacturer Through Distributor, Exclusive Distributor
General Admin.: Lee Dees/President, Chief Executive Officer
   Floor Mat   General

DRI-LINE PRODUCTS LTD.   780-466-2953
7210- 76 Avenue, Edmonton, ALB T6B 0B2 Canada
FDA Number: n/a
E-mail: info@dri-line.com   Fax: 780-466-7598
Web site: http://www.dri-line.com
Year Founded: 1989
Total Employees: 10
Ownership: Private
Produces/Sells CE-marked Devices: N
Distribution: Manufacturer Direct, Exporter

DRICAST ORTHOPAEDICS, INC.
See Professional's Choice Sports Medicine Products, Inc.

DRIPRIDE
See Sca Personal Care, North America

DRIVE-MASTER CO., INC.   973-808-9709
37 DANIEL ROAD W, Fairfield, NJ 07004
FDA Number: n/a
E-mail: sales@drivemaster.net   Fax: 973-808-9713
Web site: www.drivemaster.net
Medical Products Sales Volume: $1,200,000
Annual Revenue: $1-$5 Million
Year Founded: 1952
Total Employees: 24   *Sales Staff:* 2
Ownership: Private
Federal Procurement Eligibility: Small Business, GSA Contract, VA Contract
Distribution: Manufacturer Direct, Manufacturer Through Manufacturer Reps, Service Direct, Exporter
General Admin.: Peter B. Ruprecht/President
Mktg./Adv.: Adrienne Ruprecht/Manager Advertising
Production: Christina Ruprecht/Manager Manufacturing
   Control, Foot Driving, Automobile, Mechanical   Physical Med
   Control, Hand Driving, Automobile, Mechanical   Physical Med
   Lift, Patient   General

DRIVING AIDS DEVELOPMENT CORPORATION   800-767-6435
9417 Delancey Dr., Vienna, VA 22182   **703-938-6435**
FDA Number: n/a
E-mail: dadc500@drivingaids.com   Fax: 270-574-9952
Web site: www.drivingaids.com
Ownership: Private
Produces/Sells CE-marked Devices: N
Federal Procurement Eligibility: Small Business
Distribution: Manufacturer Through Distributor
   Control, Hand Driving, Automobile, Mechanical   Physical Med

DRM RESEARCH LABORATORIES, INC.   203-488-5555
29 Business Park Dr., Branford, CT 06405
FDA Number: 1225491
   Coating, Filling Material, Resin   Dental And Oral
   Crown And Bridge, Temporary, Resin   Dental And Oral
   Tooth Bonding Agent, Resin Restoration   Dental And Oral

DRUMMOND INDUSTRIES, INC. 260-356-6837
254 W. Mccrum St., Huntington, IN 46750
FDA Number: n/a Fax: 260-356-5091
E-mail: info10@sitz-bath.com
Web site: www.sitz-bath.com
Ownership: Private
Produces/Sells CE-marked Devices: N
  Bath, Sitz, Non-Powered Physical Med

DRUMMOND SCIENTIFIC CO. 800-523-7480
500 Pkwy, Box 700, Broomall, PA 19008 610-353-0200
FDA Number: 2518153 Fax: 610-353-6204
E-mail: info@drummondsci.com
Web site: www.drummondsci.com
Medical Products Sales Volume: $5,700,000
Year Founded: 1948
Total Employees: 69 *Marketing Staff:* 1 *Sales Staff:* 1
Ownership: Private
Produces/Sells CE-marked Devices: Y
Federal Procurement Eligibility: Small Business
Distribution: Manufacturer Direct, OEM, Exporter
General Admin.: Jack Walker/General Manager
  R.J. Drummond/President
Mktg./Adv.: Jim Kenney/Director Product Development
  Chuck Locke/Manager International & National Sales
Production: Bert Moses/Director Quality Assurance
  Larry Piccirilli/Manager Operations
  Component, Plastic General
  Hematocrit Tube, Rack, Sealer, Holder Hematology
  Molding, Injection General
  Pipette, Diluting Hematology
  Pipetter Hematology
  Production Equipment General
  Service, Engineering/Design General
  Tube, Blood Collection Chemistry
  Tube, Blood Microcollection Chemistry
  Tube, Capillary Chemistry
  Tube, Centrifuge Chemistry
  Tubing, Other General

DSHEALTHCARE INC. 201-871-1232
85 West Forest Ave., Englewood, NJ 07631
FDA Number: 2219682
Web site: www.dentsply.com
Ownership: Dentsply International, Inc.
Produces/Sells CE-marked Devices: N
  Agent, Polishing, Abrasive, Oral Cavity Dental And Oral
  Cement, Dental Dental And Oral
  Cleaner, Ultrasonic, Medical Instrument General
  Crown And Bridge, Temporary, Resin Dental And Oral
  Hemostat, Surgical Dental And Oral
  Liner, Cavity, Calcium Hydroxide Dental And Oral
  Material, Impression Dental And Oral
  Needle, Dental Dental And Oral
  Pack, Sterilization Wrapper (Bag And Accessories) Surgery
  Preparer, Root Canal, Endodontic Dental And Oral
  Sterilant, Medical Device General
  Varnish, Cavity Dental And Oral
  Zinc Oxide Eugenol Dental And Oral

DSL (DIAGNOSTIC SYSTEMS LABORATORIES, INC.)
See Beckman Coulter Inc.

DSM DESOTECH INC. (800) 222-7189
1122 St. Charles St., Elgin, IL 60120 847-697-0400
FDA Number: n/a Fax: 847-468-7795
E-mail: info.desotech@dsm.com
Web site: www.dsm.com
Annual Revenue: $0-$1 Million
Total Employees: 110 *Marketing Staff:* 10 *Sales Staff:* 10
Ownership: DSM, NV
Quality System Registration Information: ISO9000
Produces/Sells CE-marked Devices: N
General Admin.: Dan Zacharski/Director Human Resources
  Ken Lawson/President
Mktg./Adv.: Jim Reese/Vice President Marketing & Sales
Production: Les Nack/Vice President Manufacturing
  Service, Device Coating, Protective General

DTEC
See Wheelchairs Of Kansas

DTI DIMARTINO DENTAL LAB 800.562.0300
345 Burnett Ave. North, Renton, WA 98055 425.228.5400
FDA Number: 3004945121 Fax: 425.228.8949
E-mail: dimartino@dtidental.com
Web site: www.dtidental.com
Ownership: Private
Produces/Sells CE-marked Devices: N

DU-AL CORP. 770-784-9062
1912 Hwy. 142 E., Covington, GA 30014-8830
FDA Number: 1047987 Fax: 770-385-7216
Annual Revenue: $0-$1 Million
Total Employees: 5 *Marketing Staff:* 1 *Sales Staff:* 2
Ownership: Public
Traded On: NASDAQ
Produces/Sells CE-marked Devices: N
Federal Procurement Eligibility: Small Business
Distribution: Manufacturer Direct, OEM, Exporter
General Admin.: Robert E. Allen/President, Chief Executive Officer
  Contract R&D, Equipment General
  Extractor, Cataract Ophthalmology

DU-MORE, INC. 425-489-6088
1751 South First St., Rogers, AR 72756
FDA Number: 1628024 Fax: 425-485-1472
E-mail: info@du-ore.com
Web site: www.du-ore.com
Medical Products Sales Volume: $4,500,000
Year Founded: 2002
Total Employees: 15
Ownership: Private
Produces/Sells CE-marked Devices: N
Federal Procurement Eligibility: Small Business
  Floss, Dental Dental And Oral

DUALL PLASTICS, INC.
See Filtrona Extrusion, Inc./PexcoA,Ar Medical Products Div.

DUBIN PAPER CO., INC. 800-653-8246
1910 S. Columbus Blvd., Philadelphia, PA 19148 215-462-7900
FDA Number: n/a Fax: 215-463-0210
Web site: www.dubinpaper.com
Annual Revenue: $0-$1 Million
Year Founded: 1919
Ownership: Private
Produces/Sells CE-marked Devices: N
Federal Procurement Eligibility: Small Business
Distribution: Exclusive Distributor
General Admin.: Joan Weber/Human Resources Associate
Mktg./Adv.: Frank Dubin/Vice President Sales
Production: Celeste Lane/Customer Service Representative
  Frank Hockman/Vice President Operations
Purchasing: Ken Hockman/Vice President Purchasing
  Foodservice Product/Equipment General
  Glove, Patient Examination General
  Liner, Kick Bucket General
  Pad, Incontinence (Underpad) General
  Towel/Towelette, Paper General

DUFFENS OPTICAL 800-432-2475
400 S.E. Quincy Street, Topeka, KS 66603 785-234-3481
FDA Number: n/a Fax: 785-235-0347
Web site: www.duffens-optical.com
Annual Revenue: $1-$5 Million
Year Founded: 1919
Ownership: Omega Group
Quality System Registration Information: ISO9000
Produces/Sells CE-marked Devices: N
Federal Procurement Eligibility: Small Business
  Eyepiece, Lens, Prescription, Endoscopic Gastroenterology/Urology

DUFORT & LAVIGNE LTEE. 800-361-0655
2165 Parthenais Street, 514-527-9381
Montreal, QUE H2K 3 Canada
FDA Number: n/a Fax: 514-527-6883
E-mail: dufort@dufortlavigne.com
Web site: www.dufortlavigne.com
Medical Products Sales Volume: $22,000,000
Year Founded: 1962
Total Employees: 70 *Sales Staff:* 22
Ownership: Private
Produces/Sells CE-marked Devices: N

DUKAL CORPORATION 800-243-0741
5 Plant Avenue, Hauppauge, NY 11788 631-656-3800
FDA Number: 2435946 Fax: 631-656-3810
E-mail: customerservice@dukal.com
Web site: www.hermitageonline.com
Medical Products Sales Volume: $50,000,000
Annual Revenue: $25-$50 Million
Year Founded: 1991
Total Employees: 45 *Marketing Staff:* 3 *Sales Staff:* 6
Ownership: Private
Quality System Registration Information: ISO9002
Produces/Sells CE-marked Devices: N
Federal Procurement Eligibility: Small Business

DUKAL CORPORATION
800-243-0741 *(cont'd)*

Distribution: Manufacturer Through Distributor, Manufacturer Through Manufacturer Reps, OEM
General Admin.: Albert Shen/Chief Executive Officer
    Gerry LoDuca/President
Mktg./Adv.: Stephanie Lee/Director Product Development
    Christopher Brooks/Manager Advertising
    Christopher Brooks/Vice President Marketing & Sales
Production: Bryan Smith/Director Quality Assurance & Regulatory Affairs
    John Grasso/Vice President Operations

Applicator, Tipped, Absorbent, Non-Sterile	General
Applicator, Tipped, Absorbent, Sterile	General
Bandage, Elastic	General
Bandage, Gauze	General
Dressing, Non-Adherent	General
Dressing, Other	General
Dressing, Universal	General
Dressing, Wound and Burn, Occlusive	Surgery
Fiber, Absorbent	General
Gauze Roll	Surgery
Gauze, Non-Absorbable, X-Ray Detectable (Internal Sponge)	Surgery
Service, Import/Export	General
Sponge, Gauze	Dental And Oral
Sponge, Laparotomy	Surgery
Sponge, Other	General
Tape, Adhesive	General
Towel, Surgical	Surgery

DUKE DIAGNOSTIC RESALE
516-496-3503
257 Cold Spring Road, Syosset, NY 11791
FDA Number: n/a
E-mail: info@dukediagnostic.com   *Fax:* 516-496-7872
Web site: http://websites.medmatrix.com/duke
Year Founded: 1993
Total Employees: 5   *Marketing Staff:* 1   *Sales Staff:* 4
Ownership: Private
Produces/Sells CE-marked Devices: N
Federal Procurement Eligibility: Female Owned
General Admin.: Lisa DeVito/President
    Vincent DeVito/Vice President, General Manager
Mktg./Adv.: Rosa Hildebrandt/Manager International Sales
    Carla Benjamin/Manager National Sales

Facility, Equipment, Medical, Mobile	General

DUKE LABS
See Beiersdorf, Inc.

DUMEX MEDICAL SURGICAL PRODUCTS LTD.
800-463-9613
416-299-4003
104 Shorting Rd.,
Scarborough, ONT M1S 3 Canada
FDA Number: 9006771
E-mail: feigner@dermasciences.com   *Fax:* 416-299-4912
Web site: www.dumex.com
Year Founded: 1982
Total Employees: 100   *Marketing Staff:* 3   *Sales Staff:* 9
Ownership: Private
Produces/Sells CE-marked Devices: N
Federal Procurement Eligibility: Small Business
Distribution: Manufacturer Through Distributor, Manufacturer Through Manufacturer Reps, Exclusive Distributor

DUNE MEDICAL DEVICES INC.
646 429-1452
28 West 44th Street, 16th Floor, New York City, NY 10036
FDA Number: n/a   *Fax:* 646 429-1455
E-mail: infousa@dunemedical.com
Web site: www.dunemedical.com
Year Founded: 2002
Ownership: Private
Produces/Sells CE-marked Devices: N
General Admin.: Mr. Daniel Levangie/Chief Executive Officer
    Dr. Dan Hashimshony/Chief Technology Officer, Vice President
Production: Ms. Kristine Burke/Vice President Quality Control & Regulatory Affairs
Research: Mr. Gal Aharonowitz/Vice President Engineering
Finance: Mr. Gil Rosen/Vice President Finance

DUNLEE
800-238-3780
630-585-2100
555 North Commerce St., Aurora, IL 60504
FDA Number: 1483239   *Fax:* 630-585-2125
E-mail: info@dunlee.de
Web site: www.dunlee.com
Medical Products Sales Volume: $90,000,000
Annual Revenue: $50-$100 Million
Year Founded: 1946
Total Employees: 280
Ownership: Public
Stock Symbol: PHG
Traded On: NYSE
Quality System Registration Information: ISO9001
Produces/Sells CE-marked Devices: Y

DUNLEE
800-238-3780 *(cont'd)*

Federal Procurement Eligibility: Small Business
Mktg./Adv.: Mr. Tom Spees/Director National Sales
    Mr. Michael Stiefvater/Director Sales
    Ms. Laura Hafner/Manager Contract Sales
    Mr. Jeff Kendrick/Manager Sales
    Mr. David Kuehn/Vice President Marketing & Sales

Housing, X-Ray Tube, Diagnostic	Radiology

DUNLEE-RICHMOND FACILITY
800-526-0555
8819 Whitepine Road, Richmond, VA 23237
804-714-2501
FDA Number: 1423539   *Fax:* 804-714-2507
E-mail: info@dunlee.de
Web site: www.dunlee.com
Year Founded: 1946
Ownership: Public
Stock Symbol: PHG
Traded On: NYSE
Produces/Sells CE-marked Devices: N
Mktg./Adv.: Mr. Tom Spees/Director National Sales
    Mr. Michael Stiefvater/Director Sales
    Ms. Laura Hafner/Manager Contract Sales
    Mr. Jeff Kendrick/Manager Sales
    Mr. David Kuehn/Vice President Marketing & Sales

DUNLEE-TUBEMASTER FACILITY
800-544-9729
2312 Avenue J, Arlington, TX 76006
817-640-7666
FDA Number: 1646916   *Fax:* 817-640-6644
E-mail: info@dunlee.de
Web site: www.dunlee.com
Year Founded: 1946
Ownership: Private
Produces/Sells CE-marked Devices: N
Mktg./Adv.: Mr. Tom Spees/Director National Sales
    Mr. Michael Stiefvater/Director Sales
    Ms. Laura Hafner/Manager Contract Sales
    Mr. Jeff Kendrick/Manager Sales
    Mr. David Kuehn/Vice President Marketing & Sales

Housing, X-Ray Tube, Diagnostic	Radiology

DUO-DENT DENTAL IMPLANT SYSTEMS LLC.
800-386-3368
340 Butterfield Road, Suite 2A,
Elmhurst, IL 60126
FDA Number: 1422368   *Fax:* 630-941-0310
E-mail: OBDC@aol.com
Web site: www.duodent.com
Annual Revenue: $1-$5 Million
Year Founded: 1995
Total Employees: 6   *Marketing Staff:* 2   *Sales Staff:* 3
Ownership: Private
Quality System Registration Information: ISO9001
Produces/Sells CE-marked Devices: Y
Federal Procurement Eligibility: Small Business
Distribution: Manufacturer Direct
General Admin.: Dr. James D'Alise/Chief Executive Officer, Chairman

Implant, Endosseous	Dental And Oral

DUOJECT MEDICAL SYSTEMS
877-534-3666
50 chemin de GaspAc, Complex B5,
450-534-3666
Bromont, QUE J2L-2 Canada
FDA Number: n/a   *Fax:* 450-534-3700
E-mail: e-novations@duoject.com
Web site: www.duoject.com
Year Founded: 1985
Total Employees: 10
Ownership: Private
Produces/Sells CE-marked Devices: N
Distribution: Service Direct, Exporter

DUOTEK DIVISION, STS DUOTEK
See Sts Duotek, Inc

DUOTEK INC.
See Sts Duotek, Inc

DUPACO, INC.
800-546-4550
4144 Avenida de la Plata,
760-758-4550
Oceanside, CA 92056
FDA Number: 2021969   *Fax:* 760-758-1465
E-mail: customerservice@dupacoinc.com
Web site: www.dupacoinc.com
Medical Products Sales Volume: $5,000,000
Annual Revenue: $1-$5 Million
Year Founded: 1975
Total Employees: 25   *Marketing Staff:* 2   *Sales Staff:* 2
Ownership: Private
Produces/Sells CE-marked Devices: Y
Federal Procurement Eligibility: Small Business

DUPACO, INC.   800-546-4550 (cont'd)
Distribution: Manufacturer Through Distributor
General Admin.: Greg Jordan/President, Chief Executive Officer
Mktg./Adv.: Greg Jordan/Manager International & National Sales
Production: An Vu/Director Quality Assurance & Product Development
Goggles, Protective, Eye	Ophthalmology
Support, Patient Position	Anesthesiology

DUPAGE KINETIC LABS INC.
See Apex Engineering Products Corp.

DUPONT CO.
See Micro Care Corp.

DUR-A-FLEX, INC.   800-253-3539
95 Goodwin St., East Hartford, CT 06108   **860-528-9838**
FDA Number: n/a   *Fax:* 860-528-2802
E-mail: info@dur-a-flex.com
Web site: www.dur-a-flex.com
Medical Products Sales Volume: $21,500,000
Annual Revenue: $10-$25 Million
Year Founded: 1967
Total Employees: 64   *Marketing Staff:* 3   *Sales Staff:* 12
Ownership: Private
Produces/Sells CE-marked Devices: N
Federal Procurement Eligibility: Small Business
Distribution: Manufacturer Direct, Exporter
General Admin.: Robert Smith/President
Mktg./Adv.: Mark Paggioli/Director Marketing
Production: Nick Wallick/Vice President Production
Research: William Greider/Director Tech. Affairs
Flooring	General
Resin, Plastic	General

DURA PHARMACEUTICALS, INC.
See Elan

DURA-KOLD CORP.   800-541-7199
3525 S. Purdue, Oklahoma City, OK 73179   **405-943-8811**
FDA Number: 1640923   *Fax:* 405-943-9339
E-mail: durakold@theshop.net
Web site: www.dura-kold.com
Medical Products Sales Volume: $2,000,000
Annual Revenue: $1-$5 Million
Year Founded: 1986
Total Employees: 19   *Marketing Staff:* 2   *Sales Staff:* 2
Ownership: Private
Produces/Sells CE-marked Devices: Y
Federal Procurement Eligibility: Small Business
Distribution: Manufacturer Direct
General Admin.: Jim Dixon/Chief Executive Officer
    J. T. Dixon/President, Chief Executive Officer
Mktg./Adv.: Dan Gibson/Vice President Marketing & Sales
Production: Keith Brink/Vice President Manufacturing
Compress, Cold	General
Pack, Cold	General

DURABLE CORPORATION   877-938-7225
75 N. Pleasant St., Norwalk, OH 44857-0290   **419-668-8138**
FDA Number: 9330034   *Fax:* 800-537-6287
E-mail: sales@durablecorp.com
Web site: www.durablecorp.com
Medical Products Sales Volume: $3,900,000
Annual Revenue: $5-$10 Million
Year Founded: 1923
Total Employees: 60   *Marketing Staff:* 2   *Sales Staff:* 5
Ownership: Private
Produces/Sells CE-marked Devices: N
Federal Procurement Eligibility: Small Business
Distribution: Manufacturer Through Distributor, Exporter
General Admin.: Tom Secor/Chief Executive Officer
Mktg./Adv.: Kaci Hartlaub/Director Marketing
    Phil Lorcher/Manager National Sales
Floor Mat	General

DURABLE MAT CO.
See Durable Corporation

DURABUILT MEDICAL CORP.   800-321-9729
1901 East 50th St., Texarkana, AR 71854   **908-387-1875**
FDA Number: 3005065295   *Fax:* 858-404-0000
E-mail: sales@c-arm.com
Web site: www.durabuiltmedical.net
Ownership: Private
Produces/Sells CE-marked Devices: N
Powered Medical Examination Table	General

DURACELL USA   800-551-2355
8 Research Dr., Berkshire Corporate Park, Bethel, CT 06801
FDA Number: n/a   *Fax:* 800-796-4565

DURACELL USA   800-551-2355 (cont'd)
Web site: www.duracell.com
Medical Products Sales Volume: $2,079,000,000
Year Founded: 1920
Ownership: PROCTER & GAMBLE
Produces/Sells CE-marked Devices: N
Distribution: Manufacturer Through Distributor
Battery	General
Battery, Hearing-Aid	Ear/Nose/Throat

DURALIFE, INC.   800-443-5433
195 Phillips Park Dr., Williamsport, PA 17702   **570-323-9743**
FDA Number: 2523969   *Fax:* 570-323-9762
E-mail: duralfe@aol.com
Web site: www.duralife-usa.com
Annual Revenue: $0-$1 Million
Year Founded: 1988
Total Employees: 22
Ownership: Private
Produces/Sells CE-marked Devices: N
Federal Procurement Eligibility: Small Business
Distribution: Manufacturer Through Distributor
General Admin.: Daniel E. Day/President
Mktg./Adv.: Timothy J. Ludgate/Manager Advertising
    Timothy J. Ludgate/Vice President Marketing & Sales
Research: Daniel E. Day/Vice President Research & Development
Cart, Laundry	General
Cart, Other	General
Chair, Shower	General
Commode (Toilet)	General
Laundry Hamper	General
Stretcher, Wheeled (Mobile)	General
Transfer Device, Patient, Manual	General
Walker, Mechanical	Physical Med

DURALINE MEDICAL PRODUCTS   800-667-6996
Box 849, 111 3rd Ave. West,   **306-948-2331**
Biggar, SK S0K-0 Canada
FDA Number: n/a   *Fax:* 306-948-2333
E-mail: duraline@sympatico.sk
Year Founded: 1909
Total Employees: 10
Ownership: Private
Produces/Sells CE-marked Devices: N
Distribution: Exclusive Distributor

DURALINE MEDICAL PRODUCTS, INC.   800-654-3376
324 Werner St., P.O. Box 67, Leipsic, OH 45856   **419-943-2044**
FDA Number: n/a   *Fax:* 419-943-3637
E-mail: duraline@fairpoint.net
Web site: www.dmponline.com
Annual Revenue: $1-$5 Million
Year Founded: 1984
Ownership: Private
Produces/Sells CE-marked Devices: N
Federal Procurement Eligibility: Small Business
Distribution: Exclusive Distributor
Production: Kathy Peck/General Manager Operations
Diaper, Adult	General
Diaper, Pediatric	General
Garment, Protective, For Incontinence	Gastroenterology/Urology
Pad, Incontinence (Underpad)	General
Pant, Incontinence	General

DURASOL CORP.   978-388-2020
1 Oakland St., P.o. Box 35, Amesbury, MA 01913
FDA Number: 1211545
Ownership: Private
Produces/Sells CE-marked Devices: N
Pad, Denture, OTC	Dental And Oral

DURDEN ENTERPRISES   800-554-5673
1317 4th Ave., P.O. Box 909, Auburn, GA 30011   **770-963-0637**
FDA Number: 1042100   *Fax:* 770-995-7067
E-mail: steriorders@durdene.com
Web site: www.sterisystems.com
Medical Products Sales Volume: $800,000
Annual Revenue: $0-$1 Million
Year Founded: 1971
Total Employees: 10   *Sales Staff:* 2
Ownership: Durden Enterprises
Quality System Registration Information: ISO9001
Produces/Sells CE-marked Devices: N
Federal Procurement Eligibility: Small Business
Distribution: Manufacturer Direct
General Admin.: Bill Durden/Chief Operating Officer
    John G. Durden/President
    Bill Durden/Vice President, General Manager

DURDEN ENTERPRISES 800-554-5673 *(cont'd)*

Production: Debbie Sharpton/Director Quality Assurance

Bandage, Adhesive	Surgery
Bandage, Butterfly	General
Condom	Obstetrics/Gynecology
Container, IV	General
Dressing, Other	General
Electrode, Electrosurgical, Active, Foot Controlled	Surgery
Electrosurgical Unit, Cutting & Coagulation Device	Surgery
Oral Irrigation Kit	Dental And Oral

Medical Product Subsidiaries (Listed Separately)
Durden Enterprises

DURECT CORP. 408.777.1417

2 Results Way, Cupertino, CA 95014
FDA Number: 1723978
E-mail: mike.arenberg@durect.com *Fax:* 408.777.3577
Web site: www.intraear.com
Ownership: Public
Stock Symbol: DRRX
Traded On: NASDAQ
Produces/Sells CE-marked Devices: N

Catheter, Irrigation	Surgery
ENT Manual Surgical Instrument	Ear/Nose/Throat
Tube, Tympanostomy	Ear/Nose/Throat

DURFOLD CORPORATION 800-345-6849
601-922-4144

102 Upton Drive, Jackson, MS 39209-2525
FDA Number: n/a *Fax:* 601-922-6244
E-mail: durfold@netdoor.com
Web site: www.durfold.com
Medical Products Sales Volume: $1,200,000
Annual Revenue: $1-$5 Million
Year Founded: 1983
Total Employees: 27 *Marketing Staff:* 6 *Sales Staff:* 6
Ownership: Private
Produces/Sells CE-marked Devices: N
Federal Procurement Eligibility: Small Business, Minority Owned, Female Owned
Distribution: Manufacturer Direct, Manufacturer Through Distributor
General Admin.: WENDY COLSON/President

Furniture, Patient Room	General

DURHAM MANUFACTURING COMPANY 800-243-3774

201 Main Street, Durham, CT 06422
FDA Number: n/a *Fax:* 800-782-5499
E-mail: info@durhammfg.com
Web site: www.durhammfg.com
Annual Revenue: $5-$10 Million
Year Founded: 1922
Ownership: Private
Produces/Sells CE-marked Devices: N
Federal Procurement Eligibility: Small Business
Distribution: Manufacturer Through Distributor, Manufacturer Through Manufacturer Reps

Cabinet Casework, General Purpose	General
Cart, Anesthetist's	Anesthesiology
Cart, Emergency, Cardiopulmonary Resuscitation (Crash)	Anesthesiology
Cart, Foodservice	General
Cart, Gas Cylinder (Carrier)	Anesthesiology
Cart, Instrument	Surgery
Cart, Multipurpose	General
Cart, Other	General
Cart, Supply	General
Rack, Drying	Chemistry
Waste Receptacle, General Purpose	General

DURHAM MEDICAL LTD. 1-888-479-4687
905-728-1112

92 Simcoe St. North,
Oshawa, ONT L1H 1 Canada
FDA Number: n/a *Fax:* 905-728-8037
E-mail: sales@durhammedical.ca
Web site: http://www.durhammedical.ca
Year Founded: 1983
Ownership: Private
Produces/Sells CE-marked Devices: N
Distribution: Exclusive Distributor

DURO-MED INDUSTRIES 800-526-4753

1788 W. Cherry St., Jesup, GA 31545
FDA Number: 1219232 *Fax:* 800-479-7968
Web site: www.mabisdmi.com
Medical Products Sales Volume: $2,500,000
Annual Revenue: $1-$5 Million
Ownership: Private
Produces/Sells CE-marked Devices: N
Federal Procurement Eligibility: Small Business
Distribution: Manufacturer Through Manufacturer Reps
General Admin.: Ray Thornton/Supervisor

DURO-MED INDUSTRIES 800-526-4753 *(cont'd)*

Production: Linda Jones/Customer Service Representative

Airway, Esophageal (Obturator)	Anesthesiology
Aspirator, Emergency Suction	General
Bag, Ice	General
Bag, Urinary Collection	General
Bandage, Elastic	General
Bedpan	General
Binder, Abdominal	General
Board, Bed	General
Brace, Joint, Ankle (External)	Physical Med
Chair, With Casters	Physical Med
Clamp, Umbilical	Obstetrics/Gynecology
Collar, Cervical Neck	Orthopedics
Component, Wheelchair	Physical Med
Cushion, Flotation	Physical Med
Dressing, Other	General
Dressing, Wound and Burn, Occlusive	Surgery
Exerciser, Non-Measuring	Physical Med
Garment, Protective, For Incontinence	Gastroenterology/Urology
Gown, Examination	General
Kit, Burn	General
Kit, First Aid	Surgery
Kit, Snake Bite, Suction	General
Mask, Oxygen, Non-Rebreathing	Anesthesiology
Pack, Custom/Special Procedure	General
Pack, Hot Or Cold, Disposable	Physical Med
Pack, Hot Or Cold, Reusable	Physical Med
Pack, Moist Heat	Physical Med
Pad, Heating, Powered	Physical Med
Penlight, Battery-Powered	Ophthalmology
Protector, Skin Pressure	General
Sheet, Burn	General
Shoe, Cast	Physical Med
Sling, Arm	Physical Med
Splint, Extremity, Inflatable, External	Surgery
Splint, Extremity, Non-Inflatable, External	Surgery
Splint, Other	Orthopedics
Splint, Temporary Training	Physical Med
Splint, Traction	Orthopedics
Support, Head, Surgical, ENT	Ear/Nose/Throat
Support, Hernia	Gastroenterology/Urology
Syringe, Irrigating	General
Tips And Pads, Cane, Crutch And Walker	Physical Med
Transfer Aid	Physical Med
Urinal	General

DURO-TEST CANADA INC. 800-268-4749
416-675-1623

419 Attwell Dr.,
Etobicoke, ONT M9W-5 Canada
FDA Number: n/a *Fax:* 416-675-8875
E-mail: info@duro-test.ca
Web site: www.duro-test.ca
Year Founded: 1955
Total Employees: 100
Ownership: Private
Produces/Sells CE-marked Devices: N
Distribution: Exclusive Distributor

DURO-TEST LIGHTING 800-289-3876

12401 McNulty Road, Suite 101, Philidelphia, PA 19154
FDA Number: n/a *Fax:* 888-959-7250
E-mail: info@duro-test.com
Web site: www.duro-test.com
Annual Revenue: $0-$1 Million
Ownership: Private
Produces/Sells CE-marked Devices: N
Distribution: Manufacturer Direct, Importer, Exporter

Lamp, Examination (Light)	General
Light, Dental	Dental And Oral
Light, Other	General

DURR-FILLAUER MEDICAL, ORTHOPEDIC DIV.
See Fillauer Companies, Inc.

DUSA PHARMACEUTICALS, INC. 978-657-7500

25 Upton Dr., Wilmington, MA 01887
FDA Number: 1226354 *Fax:* 978-657-9193
E-mail: customerservice@dusapharma.com
Web site: http://www.dusapharma.com
Total Employees: 86 *Marketing Staff:* 46 *Sales Staff:* 46
Ownership: Public
Stock Symbol: DUSA
Traded On: NASDAQ
Produces/Sells CE-marked Devices: N
General Admin.: Dr. Stuart Marcus/Chief Medical Officer, Vice President
Mr. Mark Carota/Chief Operating Officer
Mr. Robert Doman/President, Chief Executive Officer
Mktg./Adv.: Mr. William O'Dell/Vice President Marketing & Sales
Production: Mr. Scott Lundahl/Vice President Regulatory Affairs

DUSA PHARMACEUTICALS, INC.   978-657-7500 (cont'd)

Finance: Mr. Richard Christopher/Chief Financial Officer, Vice President Finance

Laser, Surgical	Surgery
System, Laser, Photodynamic Therapy	Surgery
System, Non-coherent Light, Photodynamic Therapy	Surgery

DUSOUTH INDUSTRIES   707-745-5117
651 Stone Rd., Benicia, CA 94510
FDA Number: 3005992126
Ownership: Private
Produces/Sells CE-marked Devices: N

Brush, Dermabrasion	Surgery

DUTCH OPHTHALMIC USA, INC.   800-753-8824
10 Continental Drive, Building 1, Exeter, NH 03833
FDA Number: 1222074

Cannula, Ophthalmic	Ophthalmology
Forceps, Ophthalmic	Ophthalmology
Scissors, Ophthalmic	Ophthalmology

DUX DENTAL   800-833-8267
600 E. Hueneme Rd., Oxnard, CA 93033-8600   805-488-1122
FDA Number: 2011107   *Fax:* 800-444-5170
E-mail: duxoffice@duxdental.com
Web site: www.duxdental.com
Annual Revenue: $10-$25 Million
Ownership: Van R Dental Products, Inc.
Quality System Registration Information: ISO9000
Produces/Sells CE-marked Devices: Y
Federal Procurement Eligibility: Small Business
Distribution: Manufacturer Through Distributor, Manufacturer Through Manufacturer Reps, Service Direct, Exclusive Distributor, Importer
General Admin.: Don Porteous/President
    Carl Barlow/Vice President
    Frank Rovelli/Vice President, General Manager
Mktg./Adv.: Carl Barlow/Vice President Marketing
    Bob Zettler/Vice President Sales
Production: Frank Rovelli/Vice President Operations

Agent, Polishing, Abrasive, Oral Cavity	Dental And Oral
Apron, Lead, Dental	Dental And Oral
Component, Plastic	General
Floss, Dental	Dental And Oral
Illuminator, Radiographic Film	Radiology
Instrument, Diamond, Dental	Dental And Oral
Liner, Cavity, Calcium Hydroxide	Dental And Oral
Material, Impression	Dental And Oral
Mirror, Mouth	Dental And Oral
Mixer, Alginate	Dental And Oral
Mixing Slab	Dental And Oral
Needle, Dental	Dental And Oral
Occluder, Umbilical	General
Packaging, Sterilization	General
Sealant, Pit And Fissure, And Conditioner, Resin	Dental And Oral
Service, Engineering/Design	General
Syringe, Restorative And Impression Material	Dental And Oral
Test, Equipment, Sterilization	General
Tray, Custom/Special Procedure	General
Tray, Impression	Dental And Oral
Tray, Surgical Instrument	Surgery
Varnish	Dental And Oral
Washer/Sterilizer	General
Wrap, Sterilization	General
Zinc Oxide Eugenol	Dental And Oral

DUX SALES, INC.
See Dux Dental

DUXBURY SYSTEMS, INC.   978-692-3000
270 Littleton Road, #6, Westford, MA 01886
FDA Number: 3001643234   *Fax:* 978-692-7912
E-mail: info@duxsys.com
Web site: www.duxburysystems.com
Medical Products Sales Volume: $700,000
Year Founded: 1975
Total Employees: 12
Ownership: Private
Produces/Sells CE-marked Devices: N
Federal Procurement Eligibility: Small Business
Distribution: Manufacturer Direct, Manufacturer Through Distributor

Computer Software	General
Vision Aid, Braille	General

DWFRITZ AUTOMATION, INC.   503-598-9393
17750 SW Upper Boones Ferry Road, Portland, OR 97224
FDA Number: n/a   *Fax:* 503-624-2799
E-mail: mfritz@dwfritz.com
Web site: www.dwfritz.com
Medical Products Sales Volume: $2,200,000
Annual Revenue: $5-$10 Million
Year Founded: 1973

DWFRITZ AUTOMATION, INC.   503-598-9393 (cont'd)
Total Employees: 40
Ownership: Private
Produces/Sells CE-marked Devices: Y
Federal Procurement Eligibility: Small Business, Female Owned
Distribution: Manufacturer Direct, Service Direct

Adapter, Cable, Equipment	General

DWYER PRECISION PRODUCTS, INC.   800-422-3894
266 N. 20th St.,   904-249-3545
Jacksonville Beach, FL 32250
FDA Number: 1095802   *Fax:* 904-249-1120
E-mail: dwyerprecision@gmail.com
Web site: www.dwyerprecisionproducts.com
Annual Revenue: $0-$1 Million
Year Founded: 1964
Total Employees: 9   *Marketing Staff:* 1   *Sales Staff:* 1
Ownership: Private
Produces/Sells CE-marked Devices: Y
Federal Procurement Eligibility: Small Business
Distribution: Manufacturer Through Distributor, OEM
Production: Alex King/Plant Manager
    Bert Wechtenhiser/Vice President, General Manager Production

Nurse Call System	General

DYATRON HEALTH SYSTEMS DIV.
See Medical Systems Support, Inc.

DYMAX CORP.   908-277-8481
110 Marshall Dr., Warrendale, PA 15086
FDA Number: 2523003
Web site: http://www.dymax.com
Ownership: C. R. Bard, Inc.
Produces/Sells CE-marked Devices: N
General Admin.: Mr. Greg Bachman/President

Catheter, Intravascular, Therapeutic, Long-term Greater Than 30 Days	General
Image Processing System	Radiology
Transducer, Ultrasonic, Diagnostic	Radiology

DYMEDIX CORPORATION   888-212-1100
5985 Rice Creek Pkwy, Suite 201,   763-789-8280
Shoreview, MN 55126
FDA Number: 2134563   *Fax:* 763-781-4120
E-mail: info@dymedix.com
Web site: www.dymedix.com
Year Founded: 1998
Ownership: Private
Produces/Sells CE-marked Devices: N
Federal Procurement Eligibility: Small Business
Distribution: Manufacturer Direct, Manufacturer Through Distributor
General Admin.: Eric Silvertson/President, Chief Executive Officer

Electrode, Cutaneous	Cns/Neurology
Electrode, Surface	Anesthesiology
Monitor, Ventilatory Frequency	Anesthesiology
Recorder, Ventilatory Effort	Anesthesiology

DYNA MEDICAL CORP.   800-268-1181
843 Wellington St.,   519-642-0424
London, ONT N6A-3 Canada
FDA Number: 9613805   *Fax:* 519-642-0426
E-mail: info@dynamedical.com
Web site: www.dynamedical.com
Year Founded: 1994
Total Employees: 10
Ownership: Private
Produces/Sells CE-marked Devices: N
Distribution: Exclusive Distributor, Importer

DYNA VOX SYSTEMS INC., DIVISION OF SUNRISE MEDICAL
See Dynavox Systems Inc.

DYNA-PLAST, INC.   763-780-8674
13911 Unity St. Nw, Ramsey, MN 55303
FDA Number: 3004028690   *Fax:* 763-780-5348
Ownership: Private
Produces/Sells CE-marked Devices: N

DYNA-TEK, INC.   913-438-6363
8369 Nieman Rd., Lenexa, KS 66214
FDA Number: 1932270
Ownership: Private
Produces/Sells CE-marked Devices: N

Test, Tetrahydrocannabinol	Toxicology

DYNACON ENT. LTD.   905-672-8828
2nd Fl, 3565 Nashua Dr, Mississauga L4V 1R1 Canada
FDA Number: 9612747

Microtiter Diluting/Dispensing Device	Microbiology

DYNACON, INC.   573-594-3813
4924 Pike 451, Curryville, MO 63339
FDA Number: n/a   Fax: 573-594-2306
E-mail: dynaconmedicalproducts@yahoo.com
Medical Products Sales Volume: $2,900,000
Annual Revenue: $1-$5 Million
Year Founded: 1981
Total Employees: 10   *Marketing Staff:* 2   *Sales Staff:* 6
Ownership: Private
Produces/Sells CE-marked Devices: N
Federal Procurement Eligibility: Small Business, Minority Owned
Distribution: Exclusive Distributor, Importer, Exporter
General Admin.: Ms. Elena Criasnova/Admin. Operations
     German Cordoba/Chief Executive Officer
Mktg./Adv.: David J. Cordoba/Manager Advertising

Ambulance	General
Lithotriptor, Laser	Gastroenterology/Urology
System, Pipeline, Gas	General
System, X-Ray, Mobile	Radiology

DYNACOR
See Medline Industries, Inc.

DYNAMET, INC.   800-237-9655   724-229-4187
195 Museum Rd., Washington, PA 15301
FDA Number: n/a   Fax: 724-229-4195
E-mail: twagner@cartech.com
Web site: www.cartech.com
Year Founded: 1972
Ownership: Carpenter Technology Corp.
Quality System Registration Information: ISO9002
Produces/Sells CE-marked Devices: N
Distribution: Manufacturer Direct, Manufacturer Through Distributor, Manufacturer Through Manufacturer Reps, Exporter

DYNAMIC DENTAL CORP.   954-753-4693
10791 Nw. 53rd. St., Ste. 102, Sunrise, FL 33351
FDA Number: 1058957
Ownership: Private
Produces/Sells CE-marked Devices: N

Handpiece, Air-Powered, Dental	Dental And Oral
Handpiece, Contra- And Right-Angle Attachment, Dental	Dental And Oral

DYNAMIC ENERGY SYSTEMS, INC.   800-326-0314   972-548-0444
1500 South Central Expressway, McKinney, TX 75070
FDA Number: n/a   Fax: 972-548-0395
E-mail: dessales@dynamicenergy.com
Web site: www.dynamicenergy.com
Medical Products Sales Volume: $1,000,000
Annual Revenue: $1-$5 Million
Year Founded: 1982
Total Employees: 11   *Marketing Staff:* 3   *Sales Staff:* 6
Ownership: Private
Produces/Sells CE-marked Devices: N
Federal Procurement Eligibility: Small Business, Female Owned
Distribution: Manufacturer Direct
General Admin.: Nancy Matz/Chief Executive Officer
     Nancy Matz/President
     Phil Cody/Vice President, General Manager
Mktg./Adv.: Phil Cody/Director Sales
     Jack Matz/Vice President Business Development
     Paul Miller/Vice President Marketing
     Phil Cody/Vice President Sales

Service, Computer	General
Service, Consulting	General

DYNAMIC SYSTEMS, INC.   828-683-3523
104 Morrow Branch, Leicester, NC 28748
FDA Number: n/a   Fax: 828-683-3511
E-mail: dsi@sunmatecushions.com
Web site: www.sunmatecushions.com
Annual Revenue: $1-$5 Million
Total Employees: 30
Ownership: Private
Produces/Sells CE-marked Devices: N
Distribution: Manufacturer Direct
Mktg./Adv.: Cathy Ramsey/Executive Director Product Development & Marketing
Production: Ellie Brown/Executive Director Production
Finance: Mimi Chang/Chief Financial Officer

Cushion, Wheelchair (Pad)	Physical Med
Mattress, Non-Powered Flotation Therapy	Physical Med
Pad, Pressure, Foam (Elbow, Heel)	General
Support, Patient Position	Anesthesiology

DYNAMICS RESEARCH CORP.   800-522-4321   978-289-1500
Two Tech Drive, Andover, MA 01810-5498
FDA Number: n/a   Fax: 978-289-1887

DYNAMICS RESEARCH CORP.   800-522-4321 *(cont'd)*
Web site: www.drc.com
Year Founded: 1955
Total Employees: 1600   *Marketing Staff:* 1   *Sales Staff:* 3
Ownership: SDI Medical Consultants
Stock Symbol: DRCO
Traded On: NASDAQ
Produces/Sells CE-marked Devices: N
Distribution: Manufacturer Direct, Manufacturer Through Distributor, Manufacturer Through Manufacturer Reps, OEM, Exporter
General Admin.: James Regan/President
     Chet Ju/Vice President, General Manager
Mktg./Adv.: Fred Pitman/Director Marketing
     Peter Stratis/Vice President Marketing

Component, Ceramic	General
Component, Electronic	General
Component, Optical	General
Connector, Catheter	Surgery
Contract Manufacturing	General
Electrode, Catheter Tip	Cardiovascular
Lens, Fresnel, Flexible, Diagnostic	Ophthalmology
Microelectrode	General
Transducer, Flow, Catheter Tip	Cardiovascular

DYNAMIT NOBEL OF AMERICA
See Hpg International, Inc.

DYNAREX CORP.   888-356-2739   845-365-8200
10 Glenshaw St., Orangeburg, NY 10962
FDA Number: 2431014   Fax: 845-365-8201
E-mail: sales@dynarex.com
Web site: www.dynarex.com
Annual Revenue: $25-$50 Million
Total Employees: 30   *Marketing Staff:* 4   *Sales Staff:* 6
Ownership: Private
Produces/Sells CE-marked Devices: Y
Federal Procurement Eligibility: Small Business
Distribution: Manufacturer Through Distributor
General Admin.: George Deutsch/President, Chief Executive Officer
     John Moulden/Vice President, General Manager
Mktg./Adv.: John Moulden/Director Marketing
     John Moulden/Manager Contract Sales
Production: Za;wam Temeubaum/Manager Regulatory Affairs

Airway, Oropharyngeal, Anesthesia	Anesthesiology
Bandage, Cast	Physical Med
Bandage, Elastic	General
Bandage, Gauze	General
Cover, Shoe, Operating Room	Surgery
Dressing, Other	General
Glove, Patient Examination, Latex	General
Glove, Patient Examination, Vinyl	General
Glove, Surgical	General
Gown, Examination	General
Gown, Isolation, Surgical	Surgery
Handle, Scalpel	Surgery
Iodine (Tincture)	Pathology
Pad, Alcohol	General
Pad, Eye	Ophthalmology

DYNASIL CORPORATION OF AMERICA   856-767-4600
385 Cooper Road, West Berlin, NJ 08091
FDA Number: n/a   Fax: 856-767-6813
Web site: http://dynasilcorp.com
Year Founded: 2004
Ownership: Private
Produces/Sells CE-marked Devices: N
General Admin.: Mr. Craig Dunham/President, Chief Executive Officer
Finance: Mr. Richard Johnson/Chief Financial Officer

DYNASPLINT SYSTEMS, INC.   800-638-6771   410-544-9530
770 Ritchie Highway, River Reach, Suite W21, Severna Park, MD 21146
FDA Number: 1121034   Fax: 800-380-3784
E-mail: info@dynasplint.com
Web site: www.dynasplint.com
Medical Products Sales Volume: $9,000,000
Annual Revenue: $5-$10 Million
Year Founded: 1981
Ownership: Private
Produces/Sells CE-marked Devices: Y
Federal Procurement Eligibility: Small Business
Distribution: Manufacturer Through Distributor, Manufacturer Through Manufacturer Reps, Exporter

Immobilizer, Ankle	Orthopedics
Immobilizer, Elbow	Orthopedics
Immobilizer, Knee	Orthopedics
Immobilizer, Wrist/Hand	Orthopedics
Orthosis, Other	Physical Med

DYNASPLINT SYSTEMS, INC.　　800-638-6771 *(cont'd)*
　Splint, Hand, And Component　　　　　　　　　Physical Med

DYNATEC SCIENTIFIC LABS, INC.　　915-849-1322
　11940 Golden Gate, El Paso, TX 79936
　FDA Number: 1645338　　　　　　　　*Fax:* 915-849-0092
　E-mail: dynatec@sbcglobal.net
　Web site: www.dynatec-labs.com
　Medical Products Sales Volume: $900,000
　Annual Revenue: $1-$5 Million
　Year Founded: 1989
　Total Employees: 19　　*Marketing Staff:* 1　　*Sales Staff:* 2
　Ownership: Private
　Quality System Registration Information: ISO9002
　Produces/Sells CE-marked Devices: N
　Federal Procurement Eligibility: Small Business, Minority Owned
　Distribution: Service Direct
　General Admin.: Rudy M. Pina/President, Chief Executive Officer
　　　　　　Julie Pina/Vice President Human Resources
　Mktg./Adv.: Jan Kimball/Director National Accounts
　Production: David Ballard/Director Quality Assurance
　　Contract Laboratory　　　　　　　　　　　　General

DYNATECH ELECTRO-OPTICS
　See Sensors, Inc.

DYNATECH NEVADA, INC.
　See Fluke Biomedical

DYNATRONICS CORP.　　　　　　　800-874-6251
　7030 Park Centre Dr., Salt Lake City, UT 84121　801-568-7000
　FDA Number: 1719362　　　　　　　　*Fax:* 801-568-7711
　E-mail: info@dynatron.com
　Web site: www.dynatronics.com
　Medical Products Sales Volume: $17,000,000
　Annual Revenue: $10-$25 Million
　Total Employees: 100　*Marketing Staff:* 5　　*Sales Staff:* 5
　Ownership: Public
　Stock Symbol: DYNT
　Traded On: NASDAQ
　Quality System Registration Information: ISO9000; ISO9001
　Produces/Sells CE-marked Devices: Y
　Federal Procurement Eligibility: Small Business
　Distribution: Manufacturer Through Distributor, Exclusive Distributor, Exporter
　General Admin.: Kelvyn H. Cullimore/President, Chief Executive Officer
　Mktg./Adv.: Larry K. Beardall/Vice President Marketing & Sales
　Research: Mr. Douglas Sampson/Vice President Research & Development & Production
　Finance: Mr. Terry Atkinson/Chief Financial Officer
　　Analyzer, Motion　　　　　　　　　　　　General
　　Diathermy, Ultrasonic (Physical Therapy)　　　Physical Med
　　Dynamometer, Grip-Strength (Squeeze)　　　Anesthesiology
　　Goniometer, AC-powered　　　　　　　　Orthopedics
　　Isokinetic Testing And Evaluation System　　　Physical Med
　　Lamp, Infrared　　　　　　　　　　　　Physical Med
　　Laser, Therapeutic　　　　　　　　　　　Radiology
　　Stimulator, Nerve, Transcutaneous (Pain Relief, TENS)　Cns/Neurology
　　Stimulator, Ultrasound, Muscle　　　　　　Physical Med
　　Transducer, Miniature Pressure　　　　　　Physical Med
　　Unit, Therapy, Current, Interferential　　　　Cns/Neurology

DYNATRONICS CORP. CHATTANOOGA　　801-568-7000
OPERATIONS
　6607 Mountain View Rd., Ooltewah, TN 37363
　FDA Number: 1000643136
　Ownership: Private
　Produces/Sells CE-marked Devices: N
　　Accessories, Traction　　　　　　　　　Physical Med
　　Accessories, Wheelchair　　　　　　　　Physical Med
　　Adapter, Hygiene　　　　　　　　　　　Physical Med
　　Adaptor, Dressing　　　　　　　　　　Physical Med
　　Adaptor, Grooming　　　　　　　　　　Physical Med
　　Brace, Joint, Ankle (External)　　　　　　Physical Med
　　Cable, Electrode　　　　　　　　　　　Physical Med
　　Cane　　　　　　　　　　　　　　　Physical Med
　　Crutch　　　　　　　　　　　　　　Physical Med
　　Exerciser, Non-Measuring　　　　　　　　Physical Med
　　Halter, Head, Traction　　　　　　　　　Physical Med
　　Heating Unit, Powered　　　　　　　　　Physical Med
　　Joint, Knee, External Brace　　　　　　　Physical Med
　　Orthosis, Abdominal　　　　　　　　　Physical Med
　　Orthosis, Cervical　　　　　　　　　　Physical Med
　　Orthosis, Limb Brace　　　　　　　　　Physical Med
　　Orthosis, Lumbar　　　　　　　　　　Physical Med
　　Orthosis, Lumbosacral　　　　　　　　Physical Med
　　Orthosis, Rib Fracture, Soft　　　　　　　Physical Med
　　Orthosis, Sacroiliac, Soft　　　　　　　　Physical Med
　　Pack, Hot Or Cold, Reusable　　　　　　　Physical Med
　　Pack, Moist Heat　　　　　　　　　　　Physical Med
　　Pad, Heating, Powered　　　　　　　　　Physical Med

DYNATRONICS CORP. CHATTANOOGA　　801-568-7000 *(cont'd)*
　　Plinth　　　　　　　　　　　　　　Physical Med
　　Sling, Arm　　　　　　　　　　　　　Physical Med
　　Support, Arm　　　　　　　　　　　　Physical Med
　　Table, Mechanical　　　　　　　　　　Physical Med
　　Table, Physical Medicine, Powered　　　　　Physical Med
　　Traction Unit, Non-Powered　　　　　　　Orthopedics
　　Utensil, Handicapped Aid　　　　　　　　Physical Med
　　Vibrator, Therapeutic　　　　　　　　　Physical Med
　　Walker, Mechanical　　　　　　　　　　Physical Med

DYNATRONICS LASER CORP.
　See Dynatronics Corp.

DYNAVOX SYSTEMS INC.　　　　　866-396-2869
　2100 Wharton St., Suite 400,　　　　412-381-4883
　Pittsburgh, PA 15203
　FDA Number: n/a　　　　　　　　　*Fax:* 412-381-5241
　E-mail: sales@dynavoxsys.com
　Web site: www.dynavoxsys.com
　Year Founded: 1983
　Ownership: Sunrise Medical
　Produces/Sells CE-marked Devices: Y
　Distribution: Manufacturer Direct
　General Admin.: Ed Donnelly/Chief Executive Officer
　　　　　　Lawrence Stephens/Chief Information Officer
　　　　　　Michelle Heying/Chief Operating Officer
　　　　　　Bob Cunningham/Chief Technology Officer, Senior Vice President
　Mktg./Adv.: Jim Shea/Vice President Marketing
　　Communication Equipment　　　　　　　General

DYNAWAVE RESEARCH INC.　　　800-732-7877
　Broadway W Prof Centre, 412-2150 Broadway W,
　Vancouver V6K 4 Canada
　FDA Number: 9680915
　　Stimulator, Nerve, Transcutaneous (Pain Relief, TENS)　Cns/Neurology

DYNEX TECHNOLOGIES, INC.　　　800-288-2354
　14340 Sullyfield Cir., Chantilly, VA 20151　703-631-7800
　FDA Number: 1117676　　　　　　　*Fax:* 703-803-1441
　E-mail: customerservice@dynextechnologies.com
　Web site: www.dynextechnologies.com
　Medical Products Sales Volume: $74,400,000
　Year Founded: 1952
　Total Employees: 50
　Ownership: Private
　Produces/Sells CE-marked Devices: N
　Federal Procurement Eligibility: Small Business
　Distribution: OEM
　General Admin.: Mr. Adrian Bunce/President
　Mktg./Adv.: Mr. Simon Price/Vice President Marketing & Sales
　Production: Mr. John Enescu/Manager Operations
　Finance: Mr. Doug Kaspar/Vice President Admin., Finance
　IS: Mr. Dean Sequera/Technical Director
　　Colorimeter, General Use　　　　　　　Chemistry
　　Equipment, Laboratory, Gen. Purpose (Specific Medical Use)　Chemistry
　　Fluorometer　　　　　　　　　　　Immunology
　　Microtiter Diluting/Dispensing Device　　　Microbiology
　　Pipetting And Diluting System, Automated　　Chemistry

DYNOMAX INC　　　　　　　　　847-680-8833
　1535 Abbott Drive, Wheeling, IL 60090
　FDA Number: n/a　　　　　　　　　*Fax:* 847-680-8838
　E-mail: pmartucci@dynomaxinc.com
　Web site: www.dynomaxinc.com
　Ownership: Private
　Produces/Sells CE-marked Devices: N
　General Admin.: Dr. Richard Zic/Chief Executive Officer

DYNORTHOTICS LTD.
　See Palumbo Orthopaedics

DYNORTHOTICS, INC.
　See Palumbo Orthopaedics

DYONICS, INC.
　See Smith & Nephew, Inc., Endoscopy Division

E & G SPORTSCHAIRS
　See Eagle Sports Chairs

E G & G WALLAC INC.
　See Perkin Elmer Wallac, Inc.

E K INDUSTRIES, INC.　　　　　　877-EKI-CHEM
　1403 Herklmer St, Joliet, IL 60432-1059　　815-732-4000
　FDA Number: 1419699　　　　　　　*Fax:* 815-723-5502
　E-mail: info@eki-chem.com
　Web site: www.eki-chem.com
　Medical Products Sales Volume: $1,000,000
　Year Founded: 1976
　Total Employees: 25　*Marketing Staff:* 5　　*Sales Staff:* 5

E K INDUSTRIES, INC.   877-EKI-CHEM *(cont'd)*

Ownership: Private
Produces/Sells CE-marked Devices: N
Federal Procurement Eligibility: Small Business, GSA Contract, VA Contract
Distribution: Manufacturer Direct, Manufacturer Through Distributor, OEM, Importer

Adhesive, Albumin Based	Pathology
Clearing Agent	Pathology
Diluent, Blood Cell	Hematology
Fluid, Bouin's	Pathology
Fluid, Red Cell Diluting	Hematology
Fluid, White Cell Diluting	Hematology
Formaldehyde (Formalin, Formol)	Pathology
Formalin, Neutral Buffered	Pathology
Glutaraldehyde (Fixative)	Pathology
Hyaluronidase	Pathology
Indicator Method, Protein Or Albumin (Urinary, Non-Quant.)	Chemistry
Mounting Media, Oil Soluble	Pathology
Reagent, Cyanomethemoglobin, With Standard	Hematology
Reagent, General Purpose	Pathology
Solution, Pathology, Carnoy's	Pathology
Solution, Pathology, Decalcifier, Acid Containing	Pathology
Solution, Pathology, Formalin-Alcohol-Acetic Acid	Pathology
Solution, Pathology, Zenker's	Pathology
Stain, Carbol Fuchsin	Pathology
Stain, Giemsa	Pathology
Stain, Grams Iodine	Pathology
Stain, Hematoxylin, Harris's	Pathology
Stain, Light Green	Pathology
Stain, Methylene Blue	Pathology
Stain, Microbiological	Microbiology
Stain, Mucicarmine	Pathology
Stain, Orange G	Pathology
Stain, Papanicolau	Pathology
Stain, Reagent, Schiff	Pathology
Stain, Safranin	Pathology
Stain, Wright's	Pathology
Sudan III	Pathology
Sudan IV	Pathology
Tube, Gastro-Enterostomy	Gastroenterology/Urology

E&M SCIENCE   513-631-0445

2909 Highland Ave., Cincinnati, OH 45212
FDA Number: n/a
Annual Revenue: $0-$1 Million
Ownership: Private
Quality System Registration Information: ISO9001
Produces/Sells CE-marked Devices: Y
Distribution: Manufacturer Through Distributor, Manufacturer Through Manufacturer Reps

Stainer, Slide, Hematology	Hematology

E-GLOBAL MEDICAL EQUIPMENT, L.L.C.   866-422-1845

2f 500 Lincoln St., Allston, MA 02134
FDA Number: 3005037851
Ownership: Private
Produces/Sells CE-marked Devices: N

Airway, Oropharyngeal, Anesthesia	Anesthesiology
Blade, Surgical, Saw, General & Plastic Surgery	Surgery
Cannula, Suprapubic, With Trocar	Gastroenterology/Urology
Curette, Surgical	Surgery
Cushion, Flotation	Physical Med
Cushion, Table, Surgical	Surgery
Cushion, Wheelchair (Pad)	Physical Med
Dilator, Nasal	Ear/Nose/Throat
Mask, Gas, Anesthesia	Anesthesiology
Mask, Oxygen, Aerosol Administration	Anesthesiology
Motor, Surgical Instrument, AC-Powered	Surgery
Suction Apparatus, Single Patient, Portable, Non-Powered	Surgery

E-MED CORP.   800-974-3633   513-489-3633

8307 Marigold Lane, Maineville, OH 45039-9542
FDA Number: n/a   Fax: 513-683-5633
E-mail: mail@emedcorp.com
Web site: www.emedcorp.com
Medical Products Sales Volume: $270,000
Year Founded: 1972
Total Employees: 5
Ownership: Private
Produces/Sells CE-marked Devices: Y
Federal Procurement Eligibility: Small Business
Distribution: Manufacturer Direct, Manufacturer Through Distributor, Manufacturer Through Manufacturer Reps, Exporter
General Admin.: Don R. Zaleski/Chief Executive Officer
Production: Philip M. Buttaravoli/Manager Production

Adhesive Strip, Hypoallergenic	General

E-ONE   352-237-1122

1601 S.W. 37th Ave., Ocala, FL 34474
FDA Number: n/a   Fax: 352-237-1151
E-mail: info@e-one.com

E-ONE   352-237-1122 *(cont'd)*

Web site: www.e-one.com
Year Founded: 1974
Total Employees: 900
Ownership: Private
Quality System Registration Information: ISO9000
Produces/Sells CE-marked Devices: N
Federal Procurement Eligibility: Small Business
Distribution: Manufacturer Through Distributor

Ambulance	General

E-SCOPE

See Cardionics, Inc.

E-STAT PLASTICS, DIVISION OF FRAM TRAK INDUSTRIES   732-424-1600

205 Hallock Ave., Middlesex, NJ 08846
FDA Number: 3003718026
Ownership: Private
Produces/Sells CE-marked Devices: N

Orthosis, Cervical	Physical Med

E-Y LABORATORIES, INC.   800-821-0044   650-342-3296

107 North Amphlett Blvd.,
San Mateo, CA 94401
FDA Number: 2917572   Fax: 650-342-2648
E-mail: sales@eylabs.com
Web site: www.eylabs.com
Medical Products Sales Volume: $3,000,000
Year Founded: 1978
Total Employees: 10
Ownership: Private
Quality System Registration Information: ISO9001
Produces/Sells CE-marked Devices: Y
Federal Procurement Eligibility: Small Business, Minority Owned, Female Owned
Distribution: Manufacturer Direct, Manufacturer Through Distributor, OEM, Exporter

Exoenzyme, Multiple, Streptococcal	Microbiology
Kit, Identification, Neisseria Gonorrhoeae	Microbiology
Oxidase Test Device for Gonorrhea	Microbiology

E-Z FLOSS   760-325-1888

P.O. BOX 2292, Palm Springs, CA 92263
FDA Number: n/a
Ownership: Private
Produces/Sells CE-marked Devices: N

Handle, Instrument, Dental	Dental And Oral
Toothbrush, Manual	Dental And Oral

E-Z SALES & MANUFACTURING INC.   310-324-5980

1432 West 166th Street, Gardena, CA 90247
FDA Number: 3003730594
Ownership: Private
Produces/Sells CE-marked Devices: N

Stretcher, Hand-Carried	General

E-Z-EM, INC.   516-333-8230

750 Summa Ave, Westbury, NY 11590
FDA Number: 2411512
Web site: www.ezem.com
Year Founded: 1962
Ownership: Private
Produces/Sells CE-marked Devices: N

Catheter, Infusion	Surgery
Catheter, Intravascular, Diagnostic	Cardiovascular
Container, Specimen, All Types	General
Gel, Electrode, Stimulator	Cns/Neurology
Kit, Barium Enema, Disposable	Gastroenterology/Urology
Rongeur, Powered	Cns/Neurology
Spectacle, Magnifier	Ophthalmology
System, Thermographic, Liquid Crystal	Obstetrics/Gynecology
Tray, Surgical	Surgery
Trocar, Cardiovascular	Cardiovascular
Urinal	General

E-Z-ON PRODUCTS INC. OF FLORIDA   800-323-6598   561-747-6920

605 Commerce Way W., Jupiter, FL 33458-8893
FDA Number: n/a   Fax: 561-747-8779
Web site: www.ezonpro.com
Medical Products Sales Volume: $840,000
Annual Revenue: $0-$1 Million
Total Employees: 8   Marketing Staff: 1   Sales Staff: 1
Ownership: Private
Produces/Sells CE-marked Devices: N
Federal Procurement Eligibility: Small Business, Female Owned
Distribution: Manufacturer Direct, Manufacturer Through Distributor, Exporter
General Admin.: Connie Murray/President, Chief Executive Officer
Leanne Huxtable/Vice President, General Manager
Mktg./Adv.: Wendi Fitz-Hancock/Director Marketing

E-Z-ON PRODUCTS INC. OF FLORIDA   800-323-6598 *(cont'd)*
Tonya Ferguson/Director Product Development
Joyce Guthrie/Manager National Sales

Restraint, Vest	General
Restraint, Wheelchair	General
Service, Consulting	General

E. BENSON HOOD LABORATORIES, INC.   800-942-5227
575 Washington St., Pembroke, MA 02359-2318   **781-826-7573**
FDA Number: 1220850   Fax: 781-826-3899
E-mail: customerservice@hoodlabs.com
Web site: www.hoodlabs.com
Medical Products Sales Volume: $1,100,000
Annual Revenue: $1-$5 Million
Year Founded: 1962
Total Employees: 15
Ownership: Private
Quality System Registration Information: ISO9001
Produces/Sells CE-marked Devices: Y
Federal Procurement Eligibility: Small Business
Distribution: Manufacturer Direct, Manufacturer Through Distributor, OEM, Exclusive Distributor, Importer, Exporter
General Admin.: Lewis Marten/President, Chief Executive Officer
    Dennis F. Creedon/Vice President, General Manager
Mktg./Adv.: Dennis F. Creedon/Vice President Business Development
    Dennis F. Creedon/Vice President Marketing & Sales
Production: Lewis Marten/Vice President Manufacturing
Research: Lewis Marten/Vice President Research & Development

Button, Nasal Septal	Ear/Nose/Throat
Button, Tracheostomy Tube	Anesthesiology
Cannula, Sinus	Ear/Nose/Throat
Cannula, Tracheostomy	Ear/Nose/Throat
Device, Anti-Snoring	Ear/Nose/Throat
Device, Ultrasound, Sinus	Ear/Nose/Throat
Equipment, Therapy, Apnea	Anesthesiology
Implant, Eye Valve	Ophthalmology
Larynx, Artificial Battery-Powered	Ear/Nose/Throat
Prosthesis, Esophageal	Ear/Nose/Throat
Prosthesis, Esophagus	Surgery
Prosthesis, Laryngeal (Taub)	Ear/Nose/Throat
Prosthesis, Larynx	Ear/Nose/Throat
Prosthesis, Trachea	Surgery
Rhinoanemometer (Measurement Of Nasal Decongestion)	Anesthesiology
Rhinomanometer	Anesthesiology
Splint, Nasal	Ear/Nose/Throat
Stent, Tracheal	Anesthesiology
Tube, Bronchial (W/Wo Connector)	Anesthesiology
Tube, Esophageal, Sengstaken	Gastroenterology/Urology
Tube, Laryngectomy	Ear/Nose/Throat
Tube, Shunt, Endolymphatic	Ear/Nose/Throat
Tube, Shunt, Endolymphatic, With Valve	Ear/Nose/Throat
Tube, Tracheostomy (Breathing Tube), ENT	Ear/Nose/Throat
Valve, Ear	Ear/Nose/Throat
Valve, Ophthalmic	Ophthalmology
Valve, Prosthesis	Physical Med
Valve, Speaking, Tracheal	Ear/Nose/Throat

E. Q., INC.   215-997-1765
3469 Limekiln Ave., Chalfont, PA 18914
FDA Number: 2528880   Fax: 215-997-1282
E-mail: Customer@GaitMat.Com
Web site: www.GaitMat.Com
Year Founded: 1983
Ownership: Private
Produces/Sells CE-marked Devices: N
Federal Procurement Eligibility: Small Business
Distribution: Manufacturer Direct
General Admin.: Ronald French/General Manager
    Donald Taylor/President

Alarm, Overload, External Limb, Powered	Physical Med
Pressure Measurement, System, Intermittent	Physical Med

E.A. BECK & CO.   949-645-4072
657 West 19th St. Ste. E, P O Box 10857, Costa Mesa, CA 92627
FDA Number: 2080222   Fax: 949-645-4085
E-mail: eabeck@sbcglobal.net
Web site: www.beckinstruments.com
Year Founded: 1954
Total Employees: 9
Ownership: Private
Produces/Sells CE-marked Devices: Y
Federal Procurement Eligibility: Small Business, Female Owned
Distribution: Manufacturer Direct, Service Direct, Importer, Exporter

Blade, Scalpel	Surgery
Carver, Dental Amalgam, Operative	Dental And Oral
Carver, Wax, Dental	Dental And Oral
Catheter, Suction, With Tip	General
Chisel (Osteotome)	Surgery
Chisel, Bone, Surgical	Dental And Oral

E.A. BECK & CO.   949-645-4072 *(cont'd)*

Depressor, Tongue	General
Elevator, Surgical, Dental	Dental And Oral
Excavator, Dental, Operative	Dental And Oral
Explorer, Operative	Dental And Oral
File, Bone, Surgical	Dental And Oral
File, Periodontic	Dental And Oral
Filling, Instrument Plastic, Dental	Dental And Oral
Forceps, Articulation Paper	Dental And Oral
Forceps, Dressing, Dental	Dental And Oral
Forceps, Rongeur, Surgical	Dental And Oral
Forceps, Tooth Extractor, Surgical	Dental And Oral
Gag, Mouth	Ear/Nose/Throat
Handle, Scalpel	Surgery
Hemostat, Surgical	Dental And Oral
Hoe, Periodontic	Dental And Oral
Holder, Needle	Gastroenterology/Urology
Instrument, Passing, Ligature, Knot Tying	Cns/Neurology
Knife, Periodontic	Dental And Oral
Lock, Wire, And Ligature, Intraoral	Dental And Oral
Mallet, Surgical, General & Plastic Surgery	Surgery
Osteotome (Orthopedic)	Surgery
Pliers, Orthodontic	Dental And Oral
Plugger, Root Canal, Endodontic	Dental And Oral
Pusher, Band, Orthodontic	Dental And Oral
Retainer, Matrix	Dental And Oral
Retractor, Surgical	Surgery
Scaler, Periodontic	Dental And Oral
Scissors, Collar And Crown	Dental And Oral
Scissors, Surgical Tissue, Dental (Oral)	Dental And Oral
Screw, Oral	Ear/Nose/Throat
Tube, Tonsil Suction	Ear/Nose/Throat
Wire, Surgical	Orthopedics

E.C. WALKER INC.   416) 744-2011
375 Rexdale Boulevard, Toronto, ONT M9W 1R9 Canada
FDA Number: n/a   Fax: (416) 744-2374
E-mail: rick@ecwalkers.com
Web site: www.ecwalkers.com
Year Founded: 1883
Total Employees: 25
Ownership: Private
Produces/Sells CE-marked Devices: N
Distribution: Manufacturer Direct, Exclusive Distributor

E.CARE SOLUTIONS, INC.   912-897-6480
1345 Wilmington Island Road, Savannah, GA 31410
FDA Number: 3005535119

Monitor, Perinatal	Obstetrics/Gynecology

E.G.& G. ENVIRONMENTAL EQUIPMENT DIV.
See Edgetech

E.M. ADAMS CO.   800-225-4788
7496 Commercial Circle, Fort Pierce, FL 34951
FDA Number: 1054786
E-mail: questions@EMAdamsCo.com
Web site: www.emadamsco.com
Annual Revenue: $5-$10 Million
Year Founded: 1958
Ownership: Private
Produces/Sells CE-marked Devices: N
Federal Procurement Eligibility: Female Owned
Distribution: Manufacturer Direct, Manufacturer Through Distributor, Manufacturer Through Manufacturer Reps, Importer, Exporter

Belt, Traction, Pelvic	Physical Med
Binder, Abdominal	General
Board, Bed	General
Cover, Mattress	General
Joint, Knee, External Brace	Physical Med
Orthosis, Lumbar	Physical Med
Pack, Sterilization Wrapper (Bag And Accessories)	Surgery
Protector, Skin Pressure	General
Restraint, Protective (Body)	General
Shoe, Cast	Physical Med

E.S.W.L. PRODUCTS, INC.   847-419-6844
1542 Barclay Blvd., Buffalo Grove, IL 60089
FDA Number: 1424723
Ownership: Private
Produces/Sells CE-marked Devices: N

Lithotriptor, Extracorporeal Shock-wave, Urological	Gastroenterology/Urology

E.T.D. INC. (ELECTRO-THERAPEUTIC DEVICES)   800-268-3834
70 Esna Park Drive,, Unit 4,   **905-475-8344**
Markham, ONT L3R 6 Canada
FDA Number: n/a   Fax: 905-475-5143
E-mail: info@etdinc.ca
Web site: http://www.etdinc.ca
Year Founded: 1981
Total Employees: 10

E.T.D. INC. (ELECTRO-THERAPEUTIC DEVICES) 800-268-3834
(cont'd)
Ownership: Private
Produces/Sells CE-marked Devices: N
Distribution: Manufacturer Direct

E.V.F. INC.
See Emergency Vehicles, Inc.

E.W. PIKE & COMPANY 908-352-0630
501-517 Pennsylvania Avenue, Elizabeth, NJ 07201-1101
FDA Number: n/a
E-mail: info@ewpike.com   *Fax:* 908-352-4199
Web site: www.ewpike.com
Medical Products Sales Volume: $1,000,000
Annual Revenue: $0-$1 Million
Total Employees: 25   *Marketing Staff:* 1   *Sales Staff:* 3
Ownership: Private
Produces/Sells CE-marked Devices: N
Federal Procurement Eligibility: Small Business, Female Owned, GSA Contract
Distribution: Manufacturer Direct
General Admin.: Susan Wacaster/President
              Thomas Wacaster/Vice President
Mktg./Adv.: Jay Wacaster/Director Marketing
Magnifier, Hand-Held, Low-Vision   Ophthalmology
Vision Aid, Optical, AC-Powered   Ophthalmology

E2 TECHNOLOGY, A MIKRON COMPANY
See Mikron Infrared, Inc.

EAGLE HEALTH CARE, INC.
See Eagle Health Supplies, Inc.

EAGLE HEALTH SUPPLIES, INC. 800-755-8999
535 W. Walnut Ave., Orange, CA 92868 **714-532-1777**
FDA Number: n/a
E-mail: andychao@eaglehealth.com   *Fax:* 714-532-9777
Web site: www.eaglehealth.com
Medical Products Sales Volume: $1,500,000
Annual Revenue: $1-$5 Million
Year Founded: 1984
Total Employees: 10   *Marketing Staff:* 3   *Sales Staff:* 5
Ownership: Private
Produces/Sells CE-marked Devices: N
Federal Procurement Eligibility: Small Business, Minority Owned, Female Owned
Distribution: Manufacturer Through Distributor, Service Direct, Importer
General Admin.: Amy Chao/Chief Executive Officer
              Andy Chao/President
Mktg./Adv.: Brent Yamamoto/Director Marketing
          Andy Chao/Director National Accounts
          Roger Cheng/Director Product Development
          Andy Chao/Manager Contract Sales
Production: Roger Cheng/Manager Materials
          Steven Liu/Manager Operations
Device, Assist, CPR   Anesthesiology
Patient Transfer Unit   General
Walker, Mechanical   Physical Med
Wheelchair, Powered   Physical Med

EAGLE LABORATORIES 800-782-6534
10201-A Trademark Street, **909-481-0011**
Rancho Cucamonga, CA 91730
FDA Number: 2027619   *Fax:* 909-481-4481
E-mail: rdecamp@eaglelabs.com
Web site: www.eaglelabs.com
Medical Products Sales Volume: $5,000,000
Annual Revenue: $1-$5 Million
Year Founded: 1988
Total Employees: 50   *Marketing Staff:* 4   *Sales Staff:* 4
Ownership: Pharma-Sept Ltd.
Quality System Registration Information: ISO9001
Produces/Sells CE-marked Devices: Y
Federal Procurement Eligibility: Small Business, GSA Contract, VA Contract
Distribution: Manufacturer Direct, Manufacturer Through Manufacturer Reps, OEM, Exporter
General Admin.: Dennis M. De Camp/President, Chief Executive Officer
              Richard J. De Camp/Vice President, General Manager
Mktg./Adv.: Michael P. De Camp/Vice President International Marketing & Sales
Production: Terry Moore/Director Quality Assurance
          Donna Green/Manager Customer Services
          Elvia Esmerio/Plant & Production Manager
Finance: Ines Avila/Controller
Blade, Scalpel   Surgery
Blade, Surgical, Saw, General & Plastic Surgery   Surgery
Cannula, Lacrimal (Eye)   Ophthalmology
Cannula, Ophthalmic   Ophthalmology
Cystotome, Ophthalmic   Ophthalmology
Extractor, Cataract   Ophthalmology
Instrument, Microsurgical   Cns/Neurology
Kit, Intravenous Extension Tubing   General

EAGLE LABORATORIES 800-782-6534 *(cont'd)*
Knife, Keratome   Ophthalmology
Knife, Ophthalmic   Ophthalmology
Shield, Eye, Ophthalmic   Ophthalmology
Sponge, Ophthalmic   Ophthalmology
Surgical Instrument, Disposable   Surgery
Wick, Ear   Ear/Nose/Throat
Wipe, Instrument   General

EAGLE MANUFACTURING 304-737-3171
2400 Charles St., Wellsburg, WV 26070
FDA Number: n/a   *Fax:* 304-737-1752
E-mail: sales@eagle-mfg.com
Web site: www.eagle-mfg.com
Year Founded: 1894
Total Employees: 150   *Marketing Staff:* 2   *Sales Staff:* 5
Ownership: Private
Quality System Registration Information: ISO9001
Produces/Sells CE-marked Devices: N
Distribution: Manufacturer Through Distributor
General Admin.: James Paull/President
Mktg./Adv.: Joe Eddy/Director Marketing
          Jerry Gillespie/Director Product Development
          John Mitchell/Manager National Sales
          John Mitchell/Vice President Marketing & Sales
Production: Jack Knox/Vice President Manufacturing
Waste Receptacle, General Purpose   General

EAGLE MHC 800-637-5100
100 Industrial Blvd., Clayton, DE 19938 **302-653-3000**
FDA Number: n/a   *Fax:* 302-653-2065
E-mail: eaglemhc@eaglegrp.com
Web site: www.eaglegrp.com
Annual Revenue: $25-$50 Million
Total Employees: 500
Ownership: Private
Produces/Sells CE-marked Devices: N
Federal Procurement Eligibility: Small Business
Distribution: Manufacturer Through Manufacturer Reps
General Admin.: Larry McAllister/President
Mktg./Adv.: Paul Northam/Manager National Sales
Accessories, Cart, Multipurpose   General
Cart, Dressing   General
Cart, Gas Cylinder (Carrier)   Anesthesiology
Cart, Instrument   Surgery
Cart, Other   General
Cart, Supply   General
Cart, Supply, Operating Room   Surgery
Table, Instrument, Surgical   Surgery

EAGLE PARTS & PRODUCTS, INC. 888-972-9911
1411 Marvin Griffin Rd., Augusta, GA 30906 **706-790-6687**
FDA Number: 1065497   *Fax:* 706-790-6066
E-mail: lstringfield@eagleproducts.us
Web site: www.eagleproducts.us
Ownership: Private
Produces/Sells CE-marked Devices: N
General Admin.: Mr. Robert Hoffman/Executive Vice President
              Mr. Frank Dolan/President
Scooter (Motorized 3-Wheeled Vehicle)   Physical Med
Wheelchair, Powered   Physical Med

EAGLE SIMULATION INC.
See Medsim-Eagle Simulation Inc.

EAGLE SPORTS CHAIRS 800-932-9380
2351 Parkwood Rd., Snellville, GA 30039 **770-972-0763**
FDA Number: n/a   *Fax:* 770-985-4885
E-mail: bewing@bellsouth.net
Web site: www.eaglesportschairs.com
Medical Products Sales Volume: $500,000
Annual Revenue: $0-$1 Million
Year Founded: 1980
Total Employees: 10   *Marketing Staff:* 1   *Sales Staff:* 2
Ownership: Private
Produces/Sells CE-marked Devices: N
Federal Procurement Eligibility: Small Business
Distribution: Manufacturer Direct, Manufacturer Through Distributor, Service Direct, Exporter
General Admin.: Barry M. Ewing/President, Chief Executive Officer
Mktg./Adv.: Beverly Rousseau/Manager Advertising
Treadmill, Mechanical   Physical Med
Wheelchair, Manual   Physical Med
Wheelchair, Special Grade   Physical Med

EAGLE STAINLESS CONTAINER 215-957-9333
816 Nina Way, Warminster, PA 18974-2206
FDA Number: n/a   *Fax:* 215-957-9330
Web site: www.eaglestainless.com

EAGLE STAINLESS CONTAINER   215-957-9333 *(cont'd)*
Medical Products Sales Volume: $2,500,000
Annual Revenue: $1-$5 Million
Year Founded: 1990
Ownership: EAGLE FAR EAST
Quality System Registration Information: ISO9000; ISO9001
Produces/Sells CE-marked Devices: N
Federal Procurement Eligibility: Small Business, Minority Owned, Female Owned
Distribution: Manufacturer Direct, Manufacturer Through Manufacturer Reps, Importer
General Admin.: Hsihu Lin/President

Beaker (Laboratory)	Chemistry
Bin, Storage	General
Container, Specimen Mailer And Storage	Pathology
Container, Specimen, All Types	General
Material, Metallic-Stainless Steel, Tantalum, Platinum	Ear/Nose/Throat
Suspension System, Cell Culture	Pathology
Tray, Custom/Special Procedure	General
Tubing, Hypodermic	General
Tubing, Other	General

EAGLE VISION, INC.   800-222-7584
8500 Wolf Lake Drive, Suite 110,   **901-380-7000**
Memphis, TN 38133
FDA Number: 1034718   Fax: 901-380-7001
E-mail: info@eaglevis.com
Web site: www.eaglevis.com
Year Founded: 1983
Total Employees: 33   *Marketing Staff:* 2   *Sales Staff:* 45
Ownership: Private
Produces/Sells CE-marked Devices: Y
Federal Procurement Eligibility: Small Business
Distribution: Manufacturer Direct, Manufacturer Through Distributor, Manufacturer Through Manufacturer Reps, Exporter
General Admin.: Jerry Dowdy/Chief Operating Officer
    Murray L. Beard/President, Chief Executive Officer
Mktg./Adv.: Robert Brosnahan/Senior Vice President Product Development
    Wade Allen/Vice President Marketing & Sales
Production: Jeff Cobb/Senior Vice President Regulatory Affairs
Finance: Amy James/Chief Financial Officer

Burr, Corneal, Battery-Powered	Ophthalmology
Clip, Iris Retractor	Ophthalmology
Dilator, Lacrimal	Ophthalmology
Exophthalmometer	Ophthalmology
Forceps, Ophthalmic	Ophthalmology
Gauge, Measuring	Ear/Nose/Throat
Head Rest, Neurosurgical	Cns/Neurology
Material, Training, Audiovisual	General
Plug, Punctum	Ophthalmology
Probe, Lacrimal	Ophthalmology
Strip, Schirmer	Ophthalmology
System, Delivery, Drug, Ocular	Ophthalmology
Tray, Surgical Instrument	Surgery

EAGLE WATER SYSTEMS OF THE TRIANGLE   919-688-1111
507-C Cornerstone Court, Hillsborough, NC 27278
FDA Number: 1061126
E-mail: twhicker@eaglewatersystems.com
Web site: www.eaglewatersystems.com
Ownership: Private
Produces/Sells CE-marked Devices: N

Purifier, Water	Chemistry

EAR LAB   301-790-3300
363 South Cleveland Ave., Hagerstown, MD 21740
FDA Number: 1181086
Ownership: Private
Produces/Sells CE-marked Devices: N

Hearing-Aid	Ear/Nose/Throat

EAR TECH, INC.   941-747-8193
3904 9th Ave., West, Bradenton, FL 34205
FDA Number: 1051705
Ownership: Private
Produces/Sells CE-marked Devices: N

Hearing-Aid	Ear/Nose/Throat

EAR TECHNOLOGY CORP.   800-327-8547
207 E. Myrtle Avenue, PO Box 1516,   **423-928-9060**
Johnson City, TN 37605
FDA Number: n/a   Fax: 423-928-0515
E-mail: info@eartech.com
Web site: www.eartech.com
Medical Products Sales Volume: $480,000
Annual Revenue: $0-$1 Million
Year Founded: 1992
Total Employees: 7
Ownership: Private

EAR TECHNOLOGY CORP.   800-327-8547 *(cont'd)*
Quality System Registration Information: ISO9001
Produces/Sells CE-marked Devices: N
Federal Procurement Eligibility: Small Business
Distribution: Manufacturer Direct
General Admin.: Rick Gilbert/General Manager
    Dan Schumaier/President

Component, Other	General
Curette, Ear	Ear/Nose/Throat

EAR-CLEAR, INC.   866-290-4260
1920 Brunns Rd., #29, Sebring, FL 33872
FDA Number: 1062060
Ownership: Private
Produces/Sells CE-marked Devices: N

Syringe, Ear	Ear/Nose/Throat
Syringe, Irrigating	General

EAR-TECH OF PUERTO RICO   787-841-6913
Urb. Mercedita, 1469 Calle Aloa, Ponce, PR 00717-2622
FDA Number: 2640046
Ownership: Private
Produces/Sells CE-marked Devices: N

Hearing-Aid	Ear/Nose/Throat

EAR-TRONICS, INC.   239-275-7655
7181 College Pkwy, Suite 14, Fort Myers, FL 33907
FDA Number: 1051293
Web site: www.eartronics.com
Annual Revenue: $0-$1 Million
Ownership: Private
Produces/Sells CE-marked Devices: N
Federal Procurement Eligibility: Small Business
Distribution: Manufacturer Direct
General Admin.: Robert L. Hooper/President, Chief Executive Officer

Hearing-Aid	Ear/Nose/Throat

EARCRAFTERS, INC.   800-688-3277
5000 Nations Crossing Road #205,   **704-522-1020**
Charlotte, NC 28217
FDA Number: 1065237   Fax: 704-522-1429
E-mail: HAToday2@aol.com
Medical Products Sales Volume: $510,000
Total Employees: 4
Ownership: Private
Produces/Sells CE-marked Devices: N
Federal Procurement Eligibility: Small Business

Hearing-Aid	Ear/Nose/Throat

EARLYSENSE   617-517-0095
990 Washington Street,, Suite 204, Dedham, MA 02026
FDA Number: n/a   Fax: 617-608-0232
Web site: http://www.earlysense.com
Year Founded: 2004
Ownership: Private
Produces/Sells CE-marked Devices: N
General Admin.: Mr. Avner Halperin/Chief Executive Officer
Production: Mr. Amir Cohn/Vice President Operations
    Ms. Dalia Argaman/Vice President Regulatory & Clinical Affairs
Research: Dr. Danny Lange/Chief Scientist
    Mr. Guy Meger/Vice President Research & Development

EARMOLD CONNECTION   507-289-9318
6538 Ranch View Ln. S.e., Eyota, MN 55934
FDA Number: 2134607
Ownership: Private
Produces/Sells CE-marked Devices: N

Hearing-Aid	Ear/Nose/Throat

EASE LABS, INC.   650-872-7788
338 North Canal St., #9, South San Francisco, CA 94080
FDA Number: 3003526437
Ownership: Private
Produces/Sells CE-marked Devices: N

Buffer, pH	Hematology
IGG Immunoassay Reagents	Immunology

EASE OF LIFE PRODUCTS, LLC   914-834-3480
515 Larchmont Acres East, D, Larchmont, NY 10538
FDA Number: 3006258083
Ownership: Private
Produces/Sells CE-marked Devices: N

Accessories, Wheelchair	Physical Med

EASI FILE CORP.   800-800-5563
6 Wrigley St., Irvine, CA 92618   **949-855-4121**
FDA Number: n/a   Fax: 949-380-0561
E-mail: info@easifileusa.com
Web site: www.easifileusa.com

EASI FILE CORP.   800-800-5563 *(cont'd)*
Medical Products Sales Volume: $1,100,000
Annual Revenue: $1-$5 Million
Year Founded: 1971
Total Employees: 10   *Marketing Staff:* 1   *Sales Staff:* 3
Ownership: Private
Produces/Sells CE-marked Devices: N
Federal Procurement Eligibility: Small Business
Distribution: Manufacturer Direct
General Admin.: Dixie Russo/Office Manager
         Brad Barrett/President
Mktg./Adv.: Dixie Russo/Manager Sales
Production: Larry Grable/Vice President Manufacturing
Research: Larry Grable/Vice President Research & Development
   Office Equipment   General

EAST ATLANTIC TRADING/TRIANGLE   800-243-4635
HEALTHCARE INC.
76 National Road, Edison, NJ 08817-2809   **732-287-6100**
FDA Number: 2249432   *Fax:* 732-287-9292
E-mail: eatco@aol.com
Web site: www.trianglegloves.com
Annual Revenue: $1-$5 Million
Total Employees: 6
Ownership: Private
Quality System Registration Information: ISO9001; ISO9002
Produces/Sells CE-marked Devices: N
Federal Procurement Eligibility: Small Business
Distribution: Importer
General Admin.: Peter Kurani/President
         Marge Kurani/Vice President, General Manager
Diaper, Adult	General
Gauze Roll	Surgery
Glove, Patient Examination	General
Glove, Patient Examination, Latex	General
Glove, Patient Examination, Vinyl	General
Glove, Surgical, Powder-Free	Surgery
Pad, Incontinence (Underpad)	General

EAST COAST SURGICAL INC.   717-361-0400
64 Pheasant Ct., Elizabethtown, PA 17022
FDA Number: 3005215838
Coagulator/Cutter, Endoscopic, Unipolar	Obstetrics/Gynecology
Tubing, Flexible, Medical Gas, Low-Pressure	Anesthesiology

EAST PENN MANUFACTURING   610-682-6361
Deka Road, Lyon Station, PA 19536-0147
FDA Number: n/a   *Fax:* 610-682-4781
E-mail: eastpenn@eastpenn-deka.com
Web site: www.eastpenn-deka.com
Year Founded: 1946
Total Employees: 750
Ownership: Private
Quality System Registration Information: ISO9001
Produces/Sells CE-marked Devices: N
Distribution: Manufacturer Through Distributor
General Admin.: DeLight Breidegam/Chief Executive Officer
      Dan Langdon/President
      Robert Harrop/Vice President Human Resources
Mktg./Adv.: Joel Brady/Coord. Advertising
      Donna Snyder/Director Marketing & Sales
      Clyde Elium/Vice President International Sales
      Jim Sikora/Vice President Marketing
      Dan Fetherolf/Vice President Sales
      Harold Eberly/Vice President Sales
Service, Parts, Repair	General

EAST RIVER VENTURES LP   212-644-2322
c/o East River Ventures LP, 590 Madison Avenue,
New York, NY 10022
FDA Number: n/a   *Fax:* 212-644-5498
E-mail: WCarozza@EastRiverVC.com
Web site: www.eastrivervc.com
Medical Products Sales Volume: $17,000,000
Ownership: Private
Produces/Sells CE-marked Devices: N
Monitor, Apnea	General

EAST TEXAS LIGHTHOUSE FOR THE BLIND   903-595-3444
500 North Bois D'arc, Tyler, TX 75702
FDA Number: 1640864   *Fax:* 903-595-3447
E-mail: sales@horizonind.com
Web site: www.horizonind.com
Medical Products Sales Volume: $16,300,000
Annual Revenue: $10-$25 Million
Year Founded: 1976
Total Employees: 90
Ownership: Private

EAST TEXAS LIGHTHOUSE FOR THE BLIND   903-595-3444
(cont'd)
Produces/Sells CE-marked Devices: N
Federal Procurement Eligibility: Small Business
Distribution: Manufacturer Direct, Manufacturer Through Distributor
General Admin.: Mr. J. Gordon Bryson/President
Production: Mr. Nick Vandagriff/Manager Materials
   Wrap, Sterilization   General

EASTER SERVICES, INC.   309-754-8303
3031 North Shore Dr., Moline, IL 61265
FDA Number: 1450766
Ownership: Private
Produces/Sells CE-marked Devices: N
Sterilizer, Steam (Autoclave)	General

EASTERN CRANIAL AFFILIATES   703-807-5899
1600 Wilson Blvd., Ste. 200, Arlington, VA 22209
FDA Number: 3005021665   *Fax:* 703-807-1183
E-mail: contactus@infinitetech.org
Web site: www.infinitetech.org
Ownership: Private
Produces/Sells CE-marked Devices: N
Orthosis, Cranial	Cns/Neurology

EASTERN RAIL SYSTEMS, INC.   800-327-0443
2014 Ford Rd., Unit G, Bristol, PA 19007   -
FDA Number: n/a   *Fax:* 800-476-8276
E-mail: webmaster@easternrail.com
Web site: http://www.easternrail.com/
Annual Revenue: $0-$1 Million
Total Employees: 3
Ownership: Private
Produces/Sells CE-marked Devices: N
Federal Procurement Eligibility: Small Business
Distribution: Manufacturer Direct, Manufacturer Through Manufacturer Reps
General Admin.: James Gunnerson/Chief Executive Officer
         James Gunnerson/President
Mktg./Adv.: Richard Heraty/Manager Advertising
Research: Richard Heraty/Vice President Research & Development
   Rails, Equipment   General

EASTERN STEEL RACK COMPANY
   See Servolift/Eastern Corp.

EASTMAN MEDICAL PRODUCTS INC.   800-373-4410
2000 Powell St., Suite 1540,   **510-652-2961**
Emeryville, CA 94608
FDA Number: 2939832   *Fax:* 510-655-6940
E-mail: deastman@eastmanmedical.com
Medical Products Sales Volume: $200,000
Year Founded: 1988
Total Employees: 5   *Sales Staff:* 1
Ownership: Private
Produces/Sells CE-marked Devices: N
Federal Procurement Eligibility: Small Business, Female Owned
Distribution: Manufacturer Through Distributor
General Admin.: Ms. Dianne Eastman/President, Chief Executive Officer
Finance: Mr. Robert S. Meadowcroft/Chief Financial Officer
Aid, Living, Handicapped	General
Drainage Unit, Urinary	General
Sterilizer, Chemical	General
Sterilizer, Laboratory	Microbiology

EASTMED ENTERPRISES, INC.   856-797-0131
11 Brandywine Drive, Marlton, NJ 08053-1101
FDA Number: 2246453   *Fax:* 856-797-0151
E-mail: Mona_putatunda2003@yahoo.com
Web site: www.eastmedent.com
Medical Products Sales Volume: $180,000
Year Founded: 1987
Total Employees: 2
Ownership: Private
Produces/Sells CE-marked Devices: N
Federal Procurement Eligibility: Small Business
Airway, Nasopharyngeal (Breathing Tube)	Anesthesiology
Airway, Oropharyngeal, Anesthesia	Anesthesiology
Circuit, Breathing (W Connector, Adapter, Y Piece)	Anesthesiology
Forceps, Tube Introduction	Anesthesiology
Laryngoscope, Rigid	Anesthesiology
Mask, Gas, Anesthesia	Anesthesiology
Strap, Head, Gas Mask	Anesthesiology
Stylet, Tracheal Tube	Anesthesiology
Valve, Non-Rebreathing	Anesthesiology
Ventilator, Emergency, Manual (Resuscitator)	Anesthesiology

EASY SEAT LLC
2361 South 1560w Suite 200,
Woods Cross, UT 84087
877-327-9732
801-294-2700
FDA Number: 1724773
E-mail: rford@easy-seat.com
Fax: 801-294-2733
Web site: www.easy-seat.com
Medical Products Sales Volume: $510,000
Annual Revenue: $0-$1 Million
Year Founded: 1998
Total Employees: 6   *Marketing Staff:* 1   *Sales Staff:* 1
Ownership: Private
Produces/Sells CE-marked Devices: N
Federal Procurement Eligibility: Small Business, VA Contract
Distribution: Manufacturer Through Manufacturer Reps
General Admin.: Rodney Ford/Chief Executive Officer
Mktg./Adv.: Rex Haddock/Director Marketing
　　　　Blaine Ford/Director Product Development
Cushion, Wheelchair (Pad)   Physical Med

EATON CARE TELEMETRY, INC.
See Eaton Medical Devices, Inc.

EATON ELECTRONICS LTD.
11811 95th Ave., North Delta, BC V4C-3T7 Canada
604-589-5997
FDA Number: n/a
Fax: 604-589-0190
Year Founded: 1986
Total Employees: 10
Ownership: Private
Produces/Sells CE-marked Devices: N
Distribution: Manufacturer Direct, Exclusive Distributor

EATON MEDICAL DEVICES, INC.
254 S Wagner Rd, P.O. Box 1002, Ann Arbor, MI 48106
734-428-0000
FDA Number: n/a
E-mail: info@eatonmedical.com
Web site: http://www.eatonmedical.com
Medical Products Sales Volume: $18,203,000
Annual Revenue: $10-$25 Million
Ownership: EATON INDUSTRIES, INC.
Quality System Registration Information: ISO9002
Produces/Sells CE-marked Devices: N
Federal Procurement Eligibility: Small Business
Distribution: Manufacturer Direct, Manufacturer Through Distributor, Manufacturer Through Manufacturer Reps, OEM, Service Direct, Importer, Exporter
Monitor, Cardiac (Cardiotachometer & Rate Alarm)   Cardiovascular
Monitor, ECG   Cardiovascular
Telemetry Unit, Physiological, ECG   Cardiovascular

EATON MEDICAL DEVICES, INC.
254 South Wagner Rd., Ann Arbor, MI 48103-1940
734-428-0000
FDA Number: 1827783
E-mail: info@eatonmedical.com
Web site: http://www.eatonmedical.com
Ownership: Private
Produces/Sells CE-marked Devices: N
Electrocardiograph, Single Channel   Cardiovascular

EATON MEDICAL GROUP
See Eaton Medical Devices, Inc.

EBERBACH CORP.
505 S. Maple Rd., Ann Arbor, MI 48106-1024
800-422-2558
734-665-8877
FDA Number: 9330154
E-mail: info@eberbachlabtools.com
Fax: 734-665-9099
Web site: www.eberbachlabtools.com
Annual Revenue: $1-$5 Million
Total Employees: 40
Ownership: Private
Quality System Registration Information: ISO9001
Produces/Sells CE-marked Devices: Y
Federal Procurement Eligibility: Small Business
Distribution: Manufacturer Direct, Manufacturer Through Distributor, Exporter
Mktg./Adv.: Ralph O. Boehnke/President, Director Marketing
Production: Christopher Boehnke/Manager Materials
Blender/Mixer   Chemistry
Homogenizer, Tissue   Microbiology
Manometer, Laboratory   Chemistry
Shaker, Waterbath   Chemistry
Shaker/Stirrer   Chemistry
Stirrer   Chemistry
Tissue Culture Apparatus   Microbiology
Tissue Embedding Equipment/Reagent   Pathology

EBERLINE ANALYTICAL CORP.
See Eberline Services

EBERLINE SERVICES
7021 Pan American Hwy. N.E.,
Albuquerque, NM 87109
877-477-898
505-262-2694
FDA Number: n/a
Fax: 505-262-2698

EBERLINE SERVICES
877-477-898 *(cont'd)*
E-mail: info@eberlineservices.com
Web site: www.becorp.com
Annual Revenue: $0-$1 Million
Ownership: THERMORETEC
Quality System Registration Information: ISO9000
Produces/Sells CE-marked Devices: N
Distribution: Manufacturer Direct, Manufacturer Through Manufacturer Reps
Dosimeter, Radiation   Radiology
Service, Consulting   General
Source, Radioisotope Reference   Chemistry

EBI MEDICAL SYSTEMS, INC.
See Ebi, Llc

EBI PATIENT CARE, INC.
1 Electro-biology Blvd., Guaynabo, PR 00657
973-299-9300
FDA Number: 3003435252
Web site: www.biomet.com
Ownership: Private
Produces/Sells CE-marked Devices: N
Arthroscope   Orthopedics
Bandage, Cast   Physical Med
Catheter, Conduction, Anesthesia   Anesthesiology
Orthosis, Limb Brace   Physical Med
Pack, Hot Or Cold, Water Circulating   Physical Med

EBI, LLC
100 Interpace Pky., Parsippany, NJ 07054
800-526-2579
973-299-9300
FDA Number: 2242816
Fax: 973-299-0906
Web site: www.biomet.com
Total Employees: 550   *Marketing Staff:* 25   *Sales Staff:* 250
Ownership: Biomet, Inc.
Quality System Registration Information: ISO9001; ISO9002
Produces/Sells CE-marked Devices: Y
Distribution: Manufacturer Through Manufacturer Reps, Exporter
General Admin.: James R. Pastena/Chief Executive Officer
　　　　James R. Pastena/President
Mktg./Adv.: Chris Denicola/Admin. Sales
　　　　Grover Braswell/Director International Marketing
　　　　Richard Dickerson/Director Marketing
　　　　Jim Bechtold/Director National Accounts
　　　　Linda Smyth/Director Product Development
　　　　Chris Denicola/Manager Admin. Sales
　　　　Marc Davis/Manager Advertising
　　　　Karen Zawisha/Manager Contract Sales
　　　　Grover Braswell/Manager International Sales
　　　　Ed Graubart/Manager Sales Training
　　　　Jack Ritter/Manager Sales Training
　　　　Marshall Perez/Vice President Marketing
　　　　Sal Bracco/Vice President Sales
Production: Mike Taggart/Director Quality Assurance
　　　　John Capparotta/Manager Regulatory Affairs
　　　　Bart Gamundi/Vice President Manufacturing
Research: Dan Page/Vice President Research & Development
IS: Bill Russo/Director Systems
Appliance, Fixation, Spinal Interlaminal   Orthopedics
Fixation Device, Jaw Fracture   Orthopedics
Fixation Device, Spinal (External)   Orthopedics
Orthosis, Other   Physical Med
Pack, Cold   General
Stimulator, Dorsal Column   Cns/Neurology
Stimulator, Osteogenesis, Electric, Invasive   Orthopedics
Stimulator, Osteogenesis, Electric, Non-Invasive   Orthopedics
Support, Patient Position   Anesthesiology

EBIOSCIENCE
10255 Science Center Drive,
San Diego, CA 92121
888-999-1371
858-642-2058
FDA Number: 3007206953
Fax: 858-642-2046
E-mail: info@eBioscience.com
Ownership: Private
Produces/Sells CE-marked Devices: N
Reagent, General Purpose   Pathology

EBM TECHNOLOGIES USA, LLC
641 Keeaumoku Street Unit 5, Hon, HI 96814
1.866.212.6127
808-945-3100
FDA Number: 3003643634
Fax: 1.808.945.3105
E-mail: info@ebmtech.com
Web site: www.ebmtech.com
Ownership: Private
Produces/Sells CE-marked Devices: N
System, Communication, Image, Digital   Radiology

EBR SYSTEMS, INC.
686 W. Maude Ave. - Suite 102, Sunnyvale, CA 94085
1 408 720 1906
FDA Number: n/a
Fax: 1 408 720 1996
Web site: www.ebrsystemsinc.com
Ownership: Private

EBR SYSTEMS, INC.
1 408 720 1906 *(cont'd)*
Produces/Sells CE-marked Devices: N
General Admin.: Mr. Rick Riley/Chief Executive Officer
　　　　　Mr. Alan Will/President, Chief Executive Officer

EC MOORE COMPANY, INC
800-331-3548
13325 Leonard Street, Dearborn, MI 48126-3633 **313-581-7878**
FDA Number: 1824299
Fax: 313-581-8348
E-mail: customerservice@ecmoore.com
Web site: www.ecmoore.com
Medical Products Sales Volume: $5,200,000
Annual Revenue: $5-$10 Million
Year Founded: 1898
Total Employees: 44
Ownership: Private
Produces/Sells CE-marked Devices: Y
Federal Procurement Eligibility: Small Business
Distribution: Manufacturer Through Distributor
General Admin.: Mr. George Aho/President, Chief Executive Officer
Production: Mrs. Shari Bodinus/Customer Service Representative
　Disk, Abrasive
Dental And Oral

ECARDIO DIAGNOSTICS
888-747-1442
1717 N. Sam Houston Parkway West, **281-465-5200**
Houston, TX 77038
FDA Number: 300533208
Fax: 281-465-5200
E-mail: info@ecardio.com
Web site: www.eCardio.com
Annual Revenue: $10-$25 Million
Year Founded: 2004
Total Employees: 65　　　*Marketing Staff:* 4　　　*Sales Staff:* 60
Ownership: Private
Produces/Sells CE-marked Devices: Y
Federal Procurement Eligibility: Small Business
Distribution: Manufacturer Through Distributor, Manufacturer Through
Manufacturer Reps
General Admin.: Mr. Larry Lawson/President, Chief Executive Officer, Chairman
　　　　　Mr. Thomas Strachan/Vice President
　　　　　Mr. Andrew Arroyo/Vice President Information Technology
Medical Admin.: Mr. Paul Minardi/Vice President Medical Affairs
Mktg./Adv.: Mr. Robert Jordan/Executive Vice President Sales
　　　　　Mr. Jim Tassone/Vice President Business Development
　　　　　Mr. Paul Davis/Vice President Marketing & Sales
Production: Mr. Jim Dilger/Vice President Operations
Finance: Mr. John Untereker/Chief Financial Officer
　Electrocardiograph, Ambulatory (With Analysis Algorithm)
Cardiovascular
　Electrocardiograph, Ambulatory(without Analysis)
Cardiovascular
　Monitor, ECG, Arrhythmia
Cardiovascular
　Transmitter/Receiver System, Physiological, Radiofrequency
Cardiovascular

ECHO THERAPEUTICS, INC.
215-717-4100
8 Penn Center, 1628 JFK Boulevard Suite 300,
Philadelphia, PA 19103
FDA Number: n/a
E-mail: info@echotx.com
Web site: www.echotx.com
Ownership: Public
Stock Symbol: ECTE
Traded On: OTC Bulletin
Produces/Sells CE-marked Devices: N
General Admin.: Ms. Kimberly Burke/General Counsel
　　　　　Dr. Patrick T. Mooney/President, Chief Executive Officer,
Chairman
Production: Mr. Marshall Deweese/Senior Vice President Operations
Research: Mr. Kenneth Gary/Senior Vice President Research & Development
Finance: Mr. Christopher Schnittker/Chief Financial Officer
　Tester, Electrode, Surface, Electrocardiograph
Cardiovascular
　Ultrasound, Skin Permeation
Surgery

ECHO ULTRASOUND INC.
　See Johnson & Johnson

ECI MEDICAL TECHNOLOGIES, INC.
800-668-5289
2 Cook Rd., Bridgewater, NS B4V 3W7 Canada **902-543-6665**
FDA Number: 9680785
Fax: 902-543-6644
E-mail: general@ecimedical.com
Web site: www.elastyfree.com
Year Founded: 1992
Total Employees: 100　　　*Marketing Staff:* 3　　　*Sales Staff:* 23
Ownership: Private
Quality System Registration Information: ISO9000; ISO9001
Produces/Sells CE-marked Devices: Y
Federal Procurement Eligibility: Small Business
Distribution: Manufacturer Through Distributor, OEM, Exporter

ECKEL INDUSTRIES OF CANADA LIMITED
800-563-3574
15 Allison Ave., P.O. Box 776, **613-543-2967**
Morrisburg, ONT K0C 1 Canada
FDA Number: 9310025
Fax: 613-543-4173
E-mail: eckel@eckel.ca
Web site: www.eckel.ca/eckel
Year Founded: 1962
Total Employees: 25
Ownership: Private
Produces/Sells CE-marked Devices: N
Federal Procurement Eligibility: Small Business
Distribution: Manufacturer Through Distributor, Manufacturer Through
Manufacturer Reps, Exporter

ECKERT & ZIEGLER ISOTOPE PRODUCTS
661-309-1034
24937 Avenue Tibbitts, Valencia, CA 91355
FDA Number: 2032766
Ownership: Private
Produces/Sells CE-marked Devices: N
　Calibrator Source, Nuclear Sealed
Radiology
　Source, Brachytherapy, Radionuclide
Radiology
　Test Pattern/Phantom, Radionuclide
Radiology

ECLECTIC GREY MATER DESIGNS
801-296-0741
279 East 650 North, Bountiful, UT 84010
FDA Number: 3005168348
Ownership: Private
Produces/Sells CE-marked Devices: N
　Transfer Device, Patient, Manual
General

ECLIPSE MEDICAL, INC.
877-600-0042
12105 S.w. 129th Ct., #104, Miami, FL 33186
FDA Number: 3006146722
Ownership: Private
Produces/Sells CE-marked Devices: N
　Holder, Catheter
Gastroenterology/Urology

ECLIPSYS CORPORATION
800-869-8300
3 Ravinia Drive, Atlanta, GA 30346-2156 **404-847-5000**
FDA Number: n/a
Fax: 404-847-5700
E-mail: proposals@eclipsys.com
Web site: www.eclipsys.com
Annual Revenue: $100-$500 Million
Ownership: Public
Stock Symbol: ECLP
Traded On: NASDAQ
Produces/Sells CE-marked Devices: N
Distribution: Manufacturer Direct, Service Direct
General Admin.: W. David Morgan/Chief Financial Officer, Treasurer
　　　　　Phillip M. Pead/President, Chief Executive Officer
　Computer Software, Hospital/Nursing Management
General
　Computer, Diagnostic, Pre-Programmed, Single-Function
Cardiovascular
　Computer, Diagnostic, Programmable
Cardiovascular

ECO MEDICAL EQUIPMENT
800-232-9450
18303 107 Ave., **780-483-6232**
Edmonton, ALB T5S-1 Canada
FDA Number: n/a
Fax: 780-484-8238
E-mail: info@ecomedical.ca
Web site: http://www.ecomedical.ca
Year Founded: 1978
Total Employees: 25
Ownership: Private
Produces/Sells CE-marked Devices: N
Distribution: Service Direct

ECODYNE WATER TREATMENT, INC.
800-228-9326
1270 Frontenac Road, Naperville, IL 60563 **630-961-5043**
FDA Number: n/a
Fax: 800-671-8846
E-mail: sales@ecodyneind.com
Web site: www.ecodyneindustrial.com
Medical Products Sales Volume: $1,700,000
Year Founded: 1956
Total Employees: 20
Ownership: Private
Produces/Sells CE-marked Devices: N
Federal Procurement Eligibility: Small Business
Distribution: Manufacturer Through Distributor, Manufacturer Through
Manufacturer Reps, OEM, Exporter
　Purifier, Water
Chemistry

ECOLAB INC.
800-232-6522
370 Wabasha Street N., St. Paul, MN 55102
FDA Number: n/a
Web site: www.ecolab.com
Annual Revenue: More than $1 Billion
Year Founded: 1923
Total Employees: 26500

ECOLAB INC.   800-232-6522 *(cont'd)*
Ownership: Private
Stock Symbol: ECL
Traded On: NYSE
Produces/Sells CE-marked Devices: N
Distribution: Manufacturer Direct, Manufacturer Through Distributor, Manufacturer Through Manufacturer Reps, Importer, Exporter
General Admin.: Douglas M. Baker/President, Chairman, Chief Executive Officer
        Michael L. Meyer/Senior Vice President Human Resources
        Lawrence T. Bell/Senior Vice President, General Counsel
Research: Larry L. Berger/Senior Vice President Research & Development
Finance: Steven L. Fritze/Chief Financial Officer
        John J. Corkrean/Vice President, Corporate Controller

Cleaner, Ultrasonic, Medical Instrument	General
Disinfector, Liquid	General
Dispenser, Brush	Surgery
Dispenser, Fluid	General
Dispenser, Liquid, Unit-Dose	General
Dispenser, Soap	General
Housekeeping Equipment	General
Lotion, Skin Care	General
Sanitizer	General
Solution, Antibacterial Cleaner	General
Solution, Instrument Cleaner	General
Solution, Patient Preparation	General
Solution, Skin Degreaser	General
Solution, Surgical Scrub	General

ECOLAB PROFESSIONAL PRODUCTS DIV.
See Ecolab Inc.

ECONNECTECH LLC.   415-810-9436
2434- 14 Avenue, San Francisco, CA 94116
FDA Number: 3006125661

Massager, Therapeutic	Physical Med

ECONOMICS LABORATORY INC.
See Ecolab Inc.

ECP HEALTH, INC.   817-881-4499
8416 Prairie Rose Lane, Fort Worth, TX 76123
FDA Number: 3005726773
Ownership: Private
Produces/Sells CE-marked Devices: N

Pump, Counterpulsating, External	Cardiovascular

EDCOR SAFETY
See Certified Safety Manufacturing

EDDA TECHNOLOGY, INC.   609-919-9889
5 Independence Way, Suite 210, Princeton, NJ 08540
FDA Number: 3004857110   *Fax:* 609-919-9779
Web site: http://www.edda-tech.com
Ownership: Private
Produces/Sells CE-marked Devices: N

Image Processing System	Radiology

EDER INDUSTRIES, INC.
See Apw Eder Industries, Inc.

EDGE BIOLOGICALS, INC.   800-238-5004
598 North Second St., Memphis, TN 38105   **901-523-0034**
FDA Number: n/a   *Fax:* 901-527-3343
E-mail: lowe@edgebiological.com
Web site: www.edgebiologicals.com
Medical Products Sales Volume: $500,000
Annual Revenue: $0-$1 Million
Ownership: Private
Produces/Sells CE-marked Devices: N
Federal Procurement Eligibility: Small Business, Minority Owned, Female Owned
Distribution: Manufacturer Direct, Manufacturer Through Manufacturer Reps

Culture Media, Amino Acid Assay	Microbiology
Culture Media, Anaerobic Transport	Microbiology
Culture Media, Antibiotic Assay	Microbiology
Culture Media, Antimicrobial Susceptibility Test	Microbiology
Culture Media, For Isolation Of Pathogenic Neisseria	Microbiology
Culture Media, General Nutrient Broth	Microbiology
Culture Media, Mueller Hinton Agar Broth	Microbiology
Culture Media, Multiple Biochemical Test	Microbiology
Culture Media, Non-Propagating Transport	Microbiology
Culture Media, Non-Selective And Differential	Microbiology
Culture Media, Non-Selective And Non-Differential	Microbiology
Culture Media, Propagating Transport	Microbiology
Culture Media, Selective And Differential	Microbiology
Culture Media, Selective And Non-Differential	Microbiology
Culture Media, Selective Broth	Microbiology
Culture Media, Single Biochemical Test	Microbiology
Culture Media, Supplements	Microbiology
Culture Media, Vitamin Assay	Microbiology
Labware, Basic, Disposable	Chemistry
Pipette, Micro	Chemistry
Pipetter	Hematology

EDGE BIOLOGICALS, INC.   800-238-5004 *(cont'd)*

Stain, Microbiological	Microbiology

EDGE DIAGNOSTICS INC.
See Edge Biologicals, Inc.

EDGE I-WEAR CORP.   909-598-7679
1775 Curtiss Ct., La Verne, CA 91750
FDA Number: 2032332
Ownership: Private
Produces/Sells CE-marked Devices: N

Shield, Eye, Ophthalmic	Ophthalmology

EDGE MEDICAL IMAGING, INC.   703-919-4732
6003 Woodlake Lane, Alexandria, VA 22315-2638
FDA Number: 3006422811
Ownership: Private
Produces/Sells CE-marked Devices: N

Diluent, Blood Cell	Hematology
Reagent, General Purpose	Pathology

EDGE SYSTEMS CORPORATION   800-603-4996
2277 REDONDO AVENUE, Signal Hill, CA 90755   **562-597-0102**
FDA Number: 2031227   *Fax:* 562-597-0148
E-mail: sales@edgesystem.net
Web site: www.edgesystem.net
Year Founded: 1997
Total Employees: 25
Ownership: Private
Produces/Sells CE-marked Devices: Y
Federal Procurement Eligibility: Small Business
Distribution: Manufacturer Direct, Manufacturer Through Distributor, Manufacturer Through Manufacturer Reps, OEM

Brush, Dermabrasion	Surgery
Camera, Still, Surgical	Surgery
Dermatome	Surgery
Epilator, High-Frequency, Needle-Type	Surgery
Exhaust System, Surgical	Surgery
Laser, Surgical	Surgery

EDGECO   800-833-4326
P.O. Box 338, Little Ferry, NJ 07643   **201-641-3222**
FDA Number: n/a
E-mail: edgecoamerica@msn.com
Web site: www.edgecoamerica.com
Ownership: Private
Produces/Sells CE-marked Devices: N
Federal Procurement Eligibility: Small Business, Female Owned
Distribution: Manufacturer Direct

Bin, Storage	General
Cabinet, Narcotic Control	General
Cart, Emergency, Cardiopulmonary Resuscitation (Crash)	Anesthesiology
Cart, Housekeeping	General
Cart, Laundry	General
Cart, Medicine	General
Cart, Supply	General
Cover, Laundry Hamper	General
Floor Mat	General

EDGETECH   800-276-3729
19 Brigham St., Unit #8, Marlborough, MA 01752   **508-263-5900**
FDA Number: 7000119   *Fax:* 508-486-9348
E-mail: h20@edgetech.com
Web site: www.edgetech.com
Medical Products Sales Volume: $8,700,000
Year Founded: 1965
Total Employees: 45   *Marketing Staff:* 5
Ownership: EdgeOne L.L.C.
Produces/Sells CE-marked Devices: Y
Federal Procurement Eligibility: Small Business
Distribution: Manufacturer Through Manufacturer Reps
General Admin.: Charles Francisco/Chief Executive Officer
        Richard Jablonski/President
        Ken Murray/Vice President, General Manager

Hygrometer (Humidity Indicator)	Anesthesiology
Sensor, Moisture	General

EDGEWATER MEDICAL SYSTEMS INC.
See Taga Medical Technologies

EDIMS, LLC   800.626.4583
651 West Mount Pleasant Avenue, Livingston, NJ 07039
FDA Number: n/a
E-mail: info@edims.net
Web site: http://edims.net
Ownership: Private
Produces/Sells CE-marked Devices: N
General Admin.: Mr. Shane Hade/Chief Executive Officer
   Medical Admin.: Dr. John Fontanetta/Chief Medical Officer

EDIMS, LLC   800.626.4583 (cont'd)
Finance: Mr. Alan Sugerman/Chief Financial Officer

EDITEK, INC.
See Medtox Diagnostics Inc.

EDLUND CO.   800-772-2126
159 Industrial; Parkway, Burlington, VT 05401   **802-862-9661**
FDA Number: n/a   *Fax:* 802-862-4822
E-mail: customerservice@edlundco.com
Web site: www.edlundco.com
Annual Revenue: $10-$25 Million
Year Founded: 1925
Total Employees: 125   *Marketing Staff:* 2   *Sales Staff:* 5
Ownership: Private
Quality System Registration Information: ISO9001
Produces/Sells CE-marked Devices: Y
Federal Procurement Eligibility: GSA Contract
Distribution: Manufacturer Through Distributor, Manufacturer Through
Manufacturer Reps, Exporter
General Admin.: Willett S. Foster/President, Chief Executive Officer
Mktg./Adv.: Peter G. Nordell/Vice President Marketing & Sales
Production: Steven Foster/Vice President Production
  Foodservice Product/Equipment   General

EDMONDS DENTAL PROSTHETICS, INC.   1.800.462.3569
2065 W. Woodland, Springfield, MO 65807   **417-881-8572**
FDA Number: 3000279043   *Fax:* 417.881.0484
E-mail: jimb@edplabs.com
Web site: www.edmondsdentallabs.com
Ownership: Private
Produces/Sells CE-marked Devices: N
  Restoration, Base Metal
  Restoration, Noble Metal
  Restoration, Porcelain-fused-to-metal

EDMUND INDUSTRIAL OPTICS   800-363-1992
101 E. Gloucester Pike,   **856-573-6250**
Barrington, NJ 08007
FDA Number: n/a   *Fax:* 856-573-6295
E-mail: sales@edmundoptics.com
Web site: www.edmundoptics.com
Medical Products Sales Volume: $76,190,000
Annual Revenue: $50-$100 Million
Year Founded: 1942
Total Employees: 220   *Marketing Staff:* 10   *Sales Staff:* 13
Ownership: EDMUND SCIENTIFIC
Quality System Registration Information: ISO9001
Produces/Sells CE-marked Devices: Y
Federal Procurement Eligibility: Small Business
Distribution: OEM, Exclusive Distributor
General Admin.: Robert Edmund/Chief Executive Officer
    John Stack/President
Mktg./Adv.: Nicole Edmund/Vice President Marketing
    Jeff Barney/Vice President Sales
  Balance, Electronic   Chemistry
  Balance, Mechanical   Chemistry
  Caliper, Ophthalmic   Ophthalmology
  Camera, Microscope   Microbiology
  Cleaner, Lens, Contact   Ophthalmology
  Component, Optical   General
  Contract Manufacturing   General
  Cuff, Blood Pressure   Cardiovascular
  Dish, Petri   Chemistry
  Glove, Other   General
  Goggles, Protective, Eye   Ophthalmology
  Labware, Basic, Reusable   Chemistry
  Lamp, Microscope   Pathology
  Laser, Diode, Laparoscopy   Surgery
  Laser, Ophthalmic   Ophthalmology
  Magnifier, Hand-Held, Low-Vision   Ophthalmology
  Microscope, Laboratory, Optical   Microbiology
  Monitor, Blood Pressure, Invasive (Arterial)   Cardiovascular
  Oil, Immersion   Hematology
  Ophthalmoscope, Battery-Powered   Ophthalmology
  Otoscope   Ear/Nose/Throat
  Plate, Hot   Chemistry
  Printer, Image, Video   General
  Scale, Laboratory   Chemistry
  Slide And Coverslip   Hematology
  Slide, Microscope   Pathology
  Spectacle, Magnifier   Ophthalmology
  Stage, Microscope   Pathology
  Stethoscope, Electronic (Auscultoscope)   Cardiovascular
  Stirrer   Chemistry
  Thermometer, Electronic, Continuous   General
  Timer, General Laboratory   Hematology
  Tube, Test   Chemistry
  Tweezers   General

EDMUND INDUSTRIAL OPTICS   800-363-1992 (cont'd)
pH Paper, Obstetric   Obstetrics/Gynecology

EDMUND SCIENTIFIC CO., INDUSTRIAL OPTICS DIVISION
See Edmund Industrial Optics

EDP BIOTECH CORPORATION   866-883-7389
6701 Baum Dr, Suite 110, Knoxville, TN 37919   **865-246-0514**
FDA Number: n/a   *Fax:* 865-971-1969
Web site: http://www.colomarker.com
Ownership: Private
Produces/Sells CE-marked Devices: N
General Admin.: Ms. Meg Ritinger/Chief Administrative Officer
    Mr. Tom Boyd/Chief Executive Officer
Production: Ms. Deanna O'Brien/Director Quality Control & Regulatory
Affairs
Research: Dr. Lawrence Thompson/Director Research & Development
Finance: Ms. Janet Parkey/Chief Financial Officer

EDROY PRODUCTS CO., INC.   800-233-8803
245 N. Midland Avenue, PO Box 998,   **845-358-6600**
Nyack, NY 10960
FDA Number: 2431025   *Fax:* 845-358-4098
E-mail: info@edroyproducts.com
Web site: www.edroyproducts.com
Medical Products Sales Volume: $600,000
Year Founded: 1937
Total Employees: 7
Ownership: Private
Produces/Sells CE-marked Devices: N
Federal Procurement Eligibility: Small Business
Distribution: Manufacturer Through Distributor
General Admin.: Steve Stoltze/President
Mktg./Adv.: Steve Stoltze/Vice President Sales
  Loupe, Diagnostic/Surgical   Surgery
  Magnifier, Operating   Surgery
  Spectacle, Magnifier   Ophthalmology
  Viewer/Magnifier   Hematology

EDUCATIONAL SOFTWARE CONCEPTS, INC.   800-748-7734
660 S. Fourth St., Edwardsville, KS 66113-0267   **913-441-2881**
FDA Number: 1220134   *Fax:* 913-441-2119
E-mail: escinc@concentric.net
Medical Products Sales Volume: $600,000
Total Employees: 10   *Marketing Staff:* 2
Ownership: Private
Produces/Sells CE-marked Devices: N
Federal Procurement Eligibility: Small Business
Distribution: Manufacturer Direct
General Admin.: David Assmann/President, Chief Executive Officer
  Computer Software   General
  Computer Software, Hospital/Nursing Management General
  Computer and Software, Medical   General

EDUSA CORP.   651-733-4365
11751 Alameda St., El Paso, TX 79927
FDA Number: 1641303
Ownership: Private
Produces/Sells CE-marked Devices: N
  Staple, Implantable   Surgery
  Staple, Removable (Skin)   Surgery

EDWARD HINES VA HOSPITAL   708-786-5905
5th Ave & Roosevelt Rd., Hines, IL 60141
FDA Number: 1649879
  Software, Blood Bank (Stand-Alone Products)   Hematology

EDWARDS COMPANY, INC.
See Edwards Signaling & Security Systems

EDWARDS LIFESCIENCES RESEARCH MEDICAL 949-250-2500
6864 South 300 West, Midvale, UT 84047
FDA Number: 1713910
Ownership: Edwards Lifesciences, Llc.
Stock Symbol: EW
Traded On: NYSE
Produces/Sells CE-marked Devices: Y
  Adapter, Stopcock, Manifold, Cardiopulmonary Bypass   Cardiovascular
  Cannula, Catheter   Cardiovascular
  Catheter, Intravascular, Diagnostic   Cardiovascular
  Catheter, Vascular, Cardiopulmonary Bypass   Cardiovascular
  Clamp, Vascular   Cardiovascular
  Filter, Blood, Cardiopulmonary Bypass, Arterial Line   Cardiovascular
  Gauge, Pressure, Coronary, Cardiopulmonary Bypass   Cardiovascular
  Introducer, Catheter   Cardiovascular
  Kit, Administration, Intravenous   General
  Lavage Unit, Water Jet   General
  Sucker, Cardiotomy Return, Cardiopulmonary Bypass   Cardiovascular
  Surgical Instrument, Cardiovascular   Cardiovascular

EDWARDS LIFESCIENCES TECHNOLOGY SARL 949-250-2500
State Rd. 402 N.km 1.4, Anasco, PR 00610-1577
FDA Number: 2648045
Ownership: Edwards Lifesciences, Llc.
Stock Symbol: EW
Traded On: NYSE
Produces/Sells CE-marked Devices: Y

Catheter, Cholangiography	Surgery
Catheter, Continuous Flush	Cardiovascular
Catheter, Embolectomy (Fogarty Type)	Cardiovascular
Catheter, Flow Directed	Cardiovascular
Catheter, Intravascular Occluding	Cns/Neurology
Catheter, Intravascular Occluding, Temporary	Cardiovascular
Catheter, Intravascular, Diagnostic	Cardiovascular
Catheter, Intravascular, Therapeutic, Short-term Less Than 30 Days	General
Catheter, Irrigation	Surgery
Catheter, Oximeter, Fiberoptic	Cardiovascular
Catheter, Percutaneous	Cardiovascular
Catheter, Peripheral, Atherectomy	Cardiovascular
Catheter, Septostomy	Cardiovascular
Clamp, Surgical, General & Plastic Surgery	Surgery
Clamp, Vascular	Cardiovascular
Dilator, Vessel	Gastroenterology/Urology
Electrode, Pacemaker, Temporary	Cardiovascular
Introducer, Catheter	Cardiovascular
Kit, Administration, Intravenous	General
Kit, Sampling, Arterial Blood	Anesthesiology
Lead, Pacemaker, Implantable Myocardial	Cardiovascular
Monitor, Physiological, Patient	Cardiovascular
Probe, Thermodilution	Cardiovascular
Stopcock	General
Suction Apparatus, Single Patient, Portable, Non-Powered	Surgery
Transducer, Blood Pressure, Extravascular	Cardiovascular
Tubing, Fluid Delivery	General

EDWARDS LIFESCIENCES, LLC. 800-424-3278
One Edwards Way, Irvine, CA 92614 949-250-2500
FDA Number: 2015691 *Fax:* 949-250-2525
Web site: www.edwards.com
Annual Revenue: $1-$5 Million
Year Founded: 1958
Total Employees: 5600
Ownership: Public
Stock Symbol: EW
Traded On: NYSE
Quality System Registration Information: ISO9001
Produces/Sells CE-marked Devices: Y
General Admin.: Michael A. Mussallem/Chief Executive Officer, Chairman
Mr. Thomas M. Abate/Chief Financial Officer, Treasurer
Mr. Bruce P. Garren/Corporate Vice President
Mr. Donald E. Bobo, Jr./Corporate Vice President
Mr. John H. Kehl Jr./Corporate Vice President
Dirksen Lehman/Vice President Government Affairs
Medical Admin.: Jodi Akin/Vice President Clinical Affairs

Angioscope	Cardiovascular
Cannula, Catheter	Cardiovascular
Catheter, Biliary	Gastroenterology/Urology
Catheter, Cholangiography	Surgery
Catheter, Continuous Flush	Cardiovascular
Catheter, Embolectomy (Fogarty Type)	Cardiovascular
Catheter, Flow Directed	Cardiovascular
Catheter, Infusion	Surgery
Catheter, Intravascular Occluding	Cns/Neurology
Catheter, Intravascular, Diagnostic	Cardiovascular
Catheter, Intravascular, Therapeutic, Short-term Less Than 30 Days	General
Catheter, Irrigation	Surgery
Catheter, Oximeter, Fiberoptic	Cardiovascular
Catheter, Percutaneous	Cardiovascular
Catheter, Peripheral, Atherectomy	Cardiovascular
Catheter, Septostomy	Cardiovascular
Catheter, Vascular, Cardiopulmonary Bypass	Cardiovascular
Clamp, Vascular	Cardiovascular
Device, Embolization, Artificial	Cns/Neurology
Dislodger, Stone, Basket, Ureteral, Metal	Gastroenterology/Urology
Electrode, Pacemaker, Temporary	Cardiovascular
Holder, Heart Valve Prosthesis	Cardiovascular
Instrument, Manual, General Surgical	Surgery
Kit, Sampling, Arterial Blood	Anesthesiology
Monitor, Physiological, Patient	Cardiovascular
Probe, Thermodilution	Cardiovascular
Prosthesis, Cardiac Valve, Biological	Cardiovascular
Prosthesis, Vascular Graft, Less Than 6mm Diameter	Cardiovascular
Prosthesis, Vascular Graft, Of 6mm And Greater Diameter	Cardiovascular
Recorder, Paper Chart	Cardiovascular
Ring, Annuloplasty	Cardiovascular
Sizer, Heart Valve Prosthesis	Cardiovascular
Surgical Instrument, Cardiovascular	Cardiovascular
Transducer, Blood Pressure, Catheter Tip	Cardiovascular
Transducer, Blood Pressure, Extravascular	Cardiovascular
Tray, Surgical Instrument	Surgery

EDWARDS LIFESCIENCES, LLC. 800-424-3278 *(cont'd)*

Valve, Heart, Mechanical	Cardiovascular
Valve, Heart, Tissue	Cardiovascular
Valvulotome	Cardiovascular

Medical Product Subsidiaries (Listed Separately)
Edwards Lifesciences Research Medical
Edwards Lifesciences Technology Sarl

EDWARDS SIGNALING & SECURITY SYSTEMS 800-336-4206
41 Woodford Avenue, Plainville, CT 06062 860-793-5301
FDA Number: n/a *Fax:* 203-699-3108
E-mail: customerservice@edwards-signals.com/
Web site: www.edwards-signals.com
Medical Products Sales Volume: $200,000
Year Founded: 1872
Total Employees: 2
Ownership: General Signal Corp.
Stock Symbol: GENSI
Traded On: NYSE
Quality System Registration Information: ISO9000; ISO9001; ISO9002; ISO9003
Produces/Sells CE-marked Devices: N
Federal Procurement Eligibility: Small Business
Distribution: Manufacturer Through Distributor, OEM, Exporter
General Admin.: Paul Suzio/Vice President, General Manager
Mktg./Adv.: Jerry Jenkins/Manager Marketing Services
Bob Hoeppner/Vice President Marketing
Bob Beck/Vice President Sales

Communication System, Emergency Alert, Personal	General

EDWIN CORP. 1-888-323-3941
425 Hill Dr., Ste. H, Glendale, CA 91206 818-507-7854
FDA Number: 1450450 *Fax:* 818-507-7854
E-mail: edwincorp@sbcglobal.net
Web site: www.ecimmobilizer.com
Year Founded: 1975
Total Employees: 7 *Marketing Staff:* 2 *Sales Staff:* 1
Ownership: Private
Produces/Sells CE-marked Devices: N
Federal Procurement Eligibility: Small Business, Minority Owned
Distribution: Manufacturer Direct

Cradle, Patient, Radiographic	Radiology
Holder, Radiographic Cassette, Wall-Mounted	Radiology
Immobilizer, Therapy, Radiation	Radiology

EEL ELECTRONICS MFG. CO. 910-944-4780
160 South May St., Suite #2, Southern Pines, NC 28387
FDA Number: 1053045 *Fax:* 910-692-7226
E-mail: leecole007@aol.com
Web site: www.rejuvenu.com
Annual Revenue: $0-$1 Million
Year Founded: 1995
Total Employees: 30 *Marketing Staff:* 1 *Sales Staff:* 3
Ownership: Private
Produces/Sells CE-marked Devices: N
Federal Procurement Eligibility: Small Business
Distribution: Manufacturer Direct

Electrolysis Equipment, Other	General

EELE LABORATORIES, LLC 631-244-0051
50 Orville Drive, Bohemia, NY 11716
FDA Number: n/a
Ownership: Private
Produces/Sells CE-marked Devices: N

Activator, Ultraviolet, Polymerization	Dental And Oral

EFOTOXPRESS INC. 510-979-9100
46560 Fremont Blvd., Unit 115, Fremont, CA 94538
FDA Number: 3006015800
Ownership: Private
Produces/Sells CE-marked Devices: N

Device, Storage, Image, Digital	Radiology

EG & G AMORPHOUS SILICON 800-528-4225
4250 E. Broadway Rd., Phoenix, AZ 85040 602-437-1315
FDA Number: n/a *Fax:* 602-437-4459
E-mail: ftmarket@ftimeters.com
Web site: www.ftimeters.com
Annual Revenue: $10-$25 Million
Total Employees: 85 *Marketing Staff:* 2 *Sales Staff:* 10
Ownership: Eg & G, Inc.
Stock Symbol: EGG
Traded On: NYSE
Quality System Registration Information: ISO9001
Produces/Sells CE-marked Devices: Y
Distribution: Manufacturer Through Manufacturer Reps
Mktg./Adv.: Ladd Howell/Manager International Sales
Mike McCoy/Manager National Sales
Rey Mann/Manager National Sales

EG & G AMORPHOUS SILICON
800-528-4225 *(cont'd)*
Dave Florian/Vice President Marketing
Flowmeter, Meter, Cerebral Blood, Xenon Clearance — Cns/Neurology
Service, Maintenance/Repair — General

EG & G FLOW TECHNOLOGY, INC.
See Eg & G Amorphous Silicon

EG & G MOISTURE & HUMIDITY
See Edgetech

EG & G OPTOELECTRONICS CANADA LTD. (450) 424-3300
22001 Dumberry Rd, Vaudreuil-Dorion, QC J7V 8P7 Canada
FDA Number: n/a — *Fax:* (450) 424-3413
E-mail: maurice.lacharite@perkinelmer.com
Web site: http://www.perkinelmer.com
Total Employees: 200 — *Marketing Staff:* 10 — *Sales Staff:* 10
Ownership: Eg & G, Inc.
Produces/Sells CE-marked Devices: N
Distribution: Manufacturer Direct, Exclusive Distributor, Exporter

EG & G ORTEC
See Ortec - (Advanced Measurement Technology)

EG & G WALLAC INC.
See Perkinelmer Life And Analytical Sciences

EHOB, INC.
800-899-5553
250 N. Belmont Avenue, Indianapolis, IN 46222 — **317-972-4600**
FDA Number: 1832066 — *Fax:* 317-972-4625
E-mail: corporate@ehob.com
Web site: www.ehob.com
Medical Products Sales Volume: $8,400,000
Year Founded: 1985
Total Employees: 120 — *Marketing Staff:* 3 — *Sales Staff:* 50
Ownership: Private
Quality System Registration Information: ISO9001
Produces/Sells CE-marked Devices: Y
Federal Procurement Eligibility: Small Business
Distribution: Manufacturer Direct, Manufacturer Through Distributor, Manufacturer Through Manufacturer Reps, Exporter
General Admin.: James G. Spahn/Chief Executive Officer
 Scott Rogers/President
 Kelly Walsh/Vice President Human Resources
Mktg./Adv.: Dave Denton/Director National Accounts
 Margaret Prentice/Manager Advertising
 Stephen Langley/Manager Contract Sales
 Jerry Garriott/Manager International Marketing & Sales
 Nancy Pugh/Vice President Marketing
 Brian Conway/Vice President Sales
Production: Ken Turro/Manager Materials
Cushion, Foot — Orthopedics
Mattress, Non-Powered Flotation Therapy — Physical Med
Support, Back — Orthopedics

EHW DESIGN ENGINEERING CO.
See H&W Technology, Llc.

EIE-ANALYTIC
See Sybronendo

EIGEN
888-924-2020
13366 Grass Valley Avenue, — **530-265-2020**
Grass Valley, CA 95945
FDA Number: 2937707 — *Fax:* 530-274-3656
E-mail: sales@eigen.com
Web site: www.eigen.com
Medical Products Sales Volume: $550,000
Year Founded: 1975
Total Employees: 7
Ownership: Private
Quality System Registration Information: ISO9001
Produces/Sells CE-marked Devices: Y
Federal Procurement Eligibility: Small Business
Distribution: Manufacturer Direct, Manufacturer Through Distributor, OEM, Service Direct, Exporter
General Admin.: Michael Castorino/President
Mktg./Adv.: Dan Uranga/Director Sales
Production: Paul Phillips/Manager Regulatory Affairs
Recorder, Videotape/Videodisc — General
Recorder, X-Ray Image — Radiology

EIRSAN CARE INC.
201-880-8615
624 Monroe St., #2a, Hoboken, NJ 07030
FDA Number: n/a
Ownership: Private
Produces/Sells CE-marked Devices: N
Cover, Mattress — General

EISCHCO, INC.
503-492-2232
1232 Se 282nd Ave, Gresham, OR 97080
FDA Number: 3034602

EISCHCO, INC.
503-492-2232 *(cont'd)*
Ownership: Private
Produces/Sells CE-marked Devices: N
Orthosis, Limb Brace — Physical Med

EIT INSTRUMENTATION PRODUCTS
See Eit, Inc.

EIT, INC.
703-478-0700
108 Carpenter Drive, Sterling, VA 20164
FDA Number: n/a — *Fax:* 703-478-0291
E-mail: uv@eitinc.com
Web site: www.eitinc.com
Medical Products Sales Volume: $37,200,000
Annual Revenue: $1-$5 Million
Year Founded: 1977
Total Employees: 230 — *Marketing Staff:* 3 — *Sales Staff:* 3
Ownership: Private
Quality System Registration Information: ISO9001
Produces/Sells CE-marked Devices: N
Federal Procurement Eligibility: Small Business
Distribution: Manufacturer Direct, Manufacturer Through Distributor, Manufacturer Through Manufacturer Reps
General Admin.: Joe T. May/President
Mktg./Adv.: David Snyder/Director Marketing
 Sue Casacia/Manager Advertising
 David Snyder/Manager International Marketing & Sales
 David Snyder/Manager National Sales
Detector, Ultraviolet — Dental And Oral
Production Equipment — General

EKCO PRODUCTS, INC.
See Pactiv Corporation

EKCOMED, LLC
314-303-9757
629 Bemis Heights Pl, St. Charles, MO 63303
FDA Number: 3004715120
Ownership: Private
Produces/Sells CE-marked Devices: N
Bandage, Elastic — General
Gown, Examination — General
Stocking, Support (Anti-Embolic) — General

EKLIN MEDICAL SYSTEMS
408-492-0057
1605 Wyatt Dr., Santa Clara, CA 95054
FDA Number: 85323 — *Fax:* 408-904-5713
E-mail: info@eklin.com
Web site: www.eklin.com
Year Founded: 2002
Ownership: Private
Produces/Sells CE-marked Devices: N
General Admin.: Gary Cantu/Chief Executive Officer, Chairman
 Jim Drury/President
Mktg./Adv.: Christine Stafford/Division Manager
 Dannis Ballance/Division Manager
 Laurie Hallwyler/Vice President Corporate Communications
 Rob Royea/Vice President Worldwide sales and service
Research: Andy Fu/Vice President Engineering
Imager, X-Ray, Electrostatic — Radiology

EKOS CORP.
888-400-3567
11911 N Creek Parkway South, — **425-415-3100**
Bothell, WA 98011
FDA Number: 3001627457 — *Fax:* 425-415-3102
E-mail: Ekosmarketing@ekoscorp.com
Web site: www.ekoscorp.com
Year Founded: 1995
Ownership: Private
Produces/Sells CE-marked Devices: N
General Admin.: Douglas Hansmann/Chief Operating Officer
 Robert Hubert/President, Chief Executive Officer
Production: Jocelyn Kersten/Vice President Quality Assurance & Regulatory Affairs
Finance: Matt Stupfel/Vice President Admin., Finance
Catheter, Continuous Flush — Cardiovascular
Infusion Stand — General
Ultrasound, Infusion, System — Cardiovascular

EL CAJON HEARING AID CENTER
619-442-5634
761 Arnele Ave., El Cajon, CA 92020
FDA Number: 2031695
Hearing-Aid — Ear/Nose/Throat

EL MAR, INC.
860-729-7232
43 Cody St., West Hartford, CT 06110
FDA Number: 1225490 — *Fax:* 860-953-8889
E-mail: elmarubtc@aol.com
Web site: www.slivergripper.com
Medical Products Sales Volume: $700,000
Annual Revenue: $0-$1 Million
Year Founded: 1995

EL MAR, INC. 860-729-7232 (cont'd)
Total Employees: 9 *Marketing Staff:* 1 *Sales Staff:* 1
Ownership: Private
Produces/Sells CE-marked Devices: N
Federal Procurement Eligibility: Small Business
Distribution: Manufacturer Direct
Mktg./Adv.: Mr. Paul Cleveland/Director Marketing Accounts
  Surgical Instrument, Manual (General Use)   Surgery

EL PASO LIGHTHOUSE FOR THE BLIND 915-532-4495
200 Washington St., El Paso, TX 79905
FDA Number: 1648144   *Fax:* 915-532-6338
Ownership: Private
Produces/Sells CE-marked Devices: N
  Pad, Alcohol   General

EL-FAX COMPANY, INC. (LUNG GYM) 610-896-6853
32 Llanfair Road, PO Box 407, Ardmore, PA 19003
FDA Number: 2523535
E-mail: breathe@lunggym.com
Web site: www.lunggym.com
Medical Products Sales Volume: $1,000,000
Annual Revenue: $0-$1 Million
Ownership: Private
Produces/Sells CE-marked Devices: N
Distribution: Manufacturer Direct
General Admin.: Mr. Ted Fitz/Owner
  Mouthpiece, Breathing   Anesthesiology
  Spirometer, Therapeutic (Incentive)   Anesthesiology

ELA MEDICAL, INC. 800-352-6466
2950 Xenium Lane N., Plymouth, MN 55441   763-519-9400
FDA Number: 7000801   *Fax:* 888-352-3299
E-mail: info@ela-usa.com
Web site: www.elamedical.com
Year Founded: 1979
Total Employees: 100   *Marketing Staff:* 3   *Sales Staff:* 50
Ownership: Sorin Group Usa
Quality System Registration Information: ISO9001
Produces/Sells CE-marked Devices: N
Federal Procurement Eligibility: Small Business
Distribution: Manufacturer Direct, Manufacturer Through Manufacturer Reps
General Admin.: David Merrill/President
Mktg./Adv.: Didier Theret/Director Marketing
Research: Peter Jacobson/Vice President Research & Development
  Adapter, Lead, Pacemaker   Cardiovascular
  Analyzer, Pacemaker Generator Function   Cardiovascular
  Defibrillator, Implantable, Automatic   Cardiovascular
  Electrode, Myocardial   Cardiovascular
  Lead, Pacemaker, Implantable Endocardial   Cardiovascular
  Lead, Pacemaker, Implantable Myocardial   Cardiovascular
  Monitor, Blood Pressure, Indirect (Arterial)   Cardiovascular
  Pacemaker, Heart, Implantable, Programmable   Cardiovascular
  Programmer, Pacemaker   Cardiovascular
  Recorder, Long-Term, ECG, Portable (Holter Monitor)   Cardiovascular

ELABSUPPLY 714-446-8740
1001 Starbuck Street, Suite C306, Fullerton, CA 92833
FDA Number: n/a   *Fax:* 714-446-8740
E-mail: info@elabsupply.com
Web site: www.elabsupply.com
Medical Products Sales Volume: $250,000
Year Founded: 2000
Total Employees: 6   *Marketing Staff:* 1   *Sales Staff:* 2
Ownership: Private
Quality System Registration Information: ISO9001; ISO9002
Produces/Sells CE-marked Devices: Y
Federal Procurement Eligibility: Small Business, Minority Owned
Distribution: Manufacturer Direct, Manufacturer Through Distributor, Manufacturer Through Manufacturer Reps, OEM, Service Direct, Exclusive Distributor, Importer, Exporter
Mktg./Adv.: Mr. Terry Lynch/Director Development & Sales
  Analyzer, Chemistry, ELISA   Chemistry
  Analyzer, Chemistry, Urinalysis   Chemistry
  Analyzer, Chemistry, Urine   Chemistry
  Analyzer, Combination Chemistry/Hematology/Electrolyte   Chemistry
  Kit, Pregnancy Test, Over The Counter, HCG   Chemistry
  Reagent, Bilirubin (Total Or Direct Test System)   Chemistry
  Reagent, Calcium (Test System)   Chemistry
  Reagent, Chloride (Test System)   Chemistry
  Reagent, Kinase, Phosphate, Creatine   Chemistry
  Test, Cancer Detection, Other   Hematology
  Test, Infectious Mononucleosis   Immunology
  Tube, Test   Chemistry

ELAMEX S.A. DE C.V. 52-16-164333
Av. Insurgentes 4145 lote., Cd. Jiarex, Chih Mexico
FDA Number: 9616374
  Jelly, Lubricating, Transurethral Surgical Instrument   Gastroenterology/Urology

ELAMEX S.A. DE C.V. 52-16-164333 (cont'd)
  Kit, Surgical (General)   Surgery
  Lubricant, Vaginal, Patient   General
  Nonabsorbable Gauze, Surgical Sponge, & Wound Dressing for External Use (with a Drug)   General
  Tray, Surgical   Surgery
  Tray, Surgical Instrument   Surgery

ELAN 650-877-0900
800 Gateway Boulevard, South San Francisco, CA 94080
FDA Number: n/a   *Fax:* 650-877-7669
Web site: www.elan.com
Annual Revenue: $500 Million-$1 Billion
Total Employees: 1687
Ownership: Private
Stock Symbol: ELN
Traded On: NYSE
Produces/Sells CE-marked Devices: N
Federal Procurement Eligibility: Small Business
Distribution: Manufacturer Direct
General Admin.: Kelly Martin/Chief Executive Officer
          Carlos Paya M.D./President
  Contract Manufacturing, Pharmaceuticals/Chemicals   General
  Inhaler, Nasal   Ear/Nose/Throat

ELAN PHARMACEUTICAL RESEARCH CORP. 800-859-8586
1300 Gould Drive, Gainesville, GA 30504   770-534 8239
FDA Number: n/a   *Fax:* 770-534 8247
Web site: www.elan.com
Annual Revenue: $500 Million-$1 Billion
Total Employees: 1687   *Sales Staff:* 123
Ownership: ELAN CORPORATION PLC.
Stock Symbol: ELN
Traded On: NYSE
Produces/Sells CE-marked Devices: N
Federal Procurement Eligibility: Small Business
Distribution: Service Direct
General Admin.: G. Kelly Martin/Chief Executive Officer
          Shane Cook/Chief Financial Officer, Executive Vice President
          Carlos V. Paya, M.D./President
  System, Delivery, Drug, Unit-Dose   General

ELANTEC MED, INC. 303-278-7672
85 S. Union Blvd., Suite M160, Lakewood, CO 80228-2207
FDA Number: 1721695   *Fax:* 303-278-7672
E-mail: tagoff@tagoff.com
Web site: www.elantecmed.com
Medical Products Sales Volume: $390,000
Annual Revenue: $0-$1 Million
Year Founded: 1989
Total Employees: 5   *Marketing Staff:* 1   *Sales Staff:* 1
Ownership: Private
Produces/Sells CE-marked Devices: N
Federal Procurement Eligibility: Small Business, Female Owned, GSA Contract, VA Contract
Distribution: Manufacturer Direct, Manufacturer Through Manufacturer Reps, Exporter
General Admin.: Rose Mary Allen/Chief Executive Officer
          Larry M. Allen/Vice President, General Manager
  Solvent   Chemistry
  Solvent, Adhesive Tape   Surgery

ELASTIC CORPORATION OF AMERICA 205-669-3101
455 Highway 70 West, Columbiana, AL 35051
FDA Number: 1051834
Ownership: Private
Produces/Sells CE-marked Devices: N
  Bandage, Elastic   General
  Belt, Traction, Pelvic, Orthopedic   Orthopedics
  Gauze/sponge, Nonresorbable For External Use   Surgery
  Sponge, Gauze   Dental And Oral

ELASTIC THERAPY, INC. 800-849-2497
718 Industrial Park Ave., P.O. Box 4068,   336-625-0529
Asheboro, NC 27204
FDA Number: 1057079   *Fax:* 336-626-7732
E-mail: info@elastictherapy.com
Web site: www.elastictherapy.com
Medical Products Sales Volume: $20,000,000
Annual Revenue: $10-$25 Million
Total Employees: 180
Ownership: Private
Quality System Registration Information: ISO9000; ISO9001
Produces/Sells CE-marked Devices: N
Federal Procurement Eligibility: Small Business
Distribution: Manufacturer Through Distributor
General Admin.: J. M. Ramsay/Chief Executive Officer
          D. Neal Hughes/Vice President

ELASTIC THERAPY, INC. 800-849-2497 (cont'd)
Melinda Lambeth/Vice President Human Resources
Mktg./Adv.: P. Amatangelo/Manager International Marketing & Sales
Production: Ginger Dawkins/Manager Materials
Greg Russell/Manager Production
Sherri Hicks/Manager Regulatory Affairs
Joey Coats/Vice President Manufacturing
Research: George Bryant/Vice President Research & Development
Legging, Compression, Non-Inflatable — General
Stocking, Support (Anti-Embolic) — General

ELB & ASSOC., MONITOR INSTRUENTS DIV.
See Monitor Instruments Inc.

ELCAM MEDICAL ASSOCIATES NETWORK
See Medical Associates Network

ELCAM MEDICAL, INC. 800-530-2441
2 University Plaza, suite 620, **201-457-1120**
Hackensack, NJ 07601
FDA Number: 2087368 *Fax:* 201-457-1125
E-mail: info@elcam-medical.com
Web site: www.elcam-medical.com
Medical Products Sales Volume: $470,000
Annual Revenue: $10-$25 Million
Year Founded: 1970
Total Employees: 5
Ownership: Elcam Medical
Quality System Registration Information: ISO9001
Produces/Sells CE-marked Devices: Y
Federal Procurement Eligibility: Small Business
General Admin.: Mr. Bruce Ward/General Manager
Mktg./Adv.: Mr. Ron Reid/Director Sales
Ms. Sandee Queally/Manager Business Development
Lloyd Fishman/Vice President Business Development
Production: Mrs. Heather Boettcher/Manager Operations
Adapter, Stopcock, Manifold, Cardiopulmonary Bypass — Cardiovascular
Stopcock — General

ELCAM PLASTIC MEDICAL PRODUCTS
See Medical Associates Network

ELCOMA METAL FABRICATING CANADA 705-526-9636
878 William St., Midland, ONT L4R-4P4 Canada
FDA Number: n/a *Fax:* 705-526-7555
E-mail: salesca@elcoma.com
Year Founded: 1989
Total Employees: 50 *Marketing Staff:* 2 *Sales Staff:* 3
Ownership: Elcoma Metal Fabricating Canada
Produces/Sells CE-marked Devices: N
Distribution: Manufacturer Direct, Manufacturer Through Manufacturer Reps, OEM, Exclusive Distributor, Exporter

ELDER OXYGEN COMPANY
See Allied Healthcare Products, Inc.

ELDEX LABORATORIES 800-969-3533
30 Executive Ct., Napa, CA 94558-6278 **707-224-8800**
FDA Number: n/a *Fax:* 707-224-0688
E-mail: sales@eldex.com
Web site: www.eldex.com
Ownership: Private
Produces/Sells CE-marked Devices: N
Federal Procurement Eligibility: Small Business
Distribution: Manufacturer Direct
Chromatography Equipment, Liquid — Chemistry
Chromatography, Liquid, Performance, High — Toxicology
Collector, Fraction — Chemistry
Pump, Laboratory — Chemistry

ELEC WESTERN MEDICAL DEVICES LTD. 800-387-8326
1015 Matheson Blvd., Ste. 8, **905-238-4860**
Mississauga, ONT L4W-3 Canada
FDA Number: n/a *Fax:* 905-238-9140
E-mail: info@centurion-systems.com
Web site: www.centurion-systems.com
Year Founded: 1980
Total Employees: 25
Ownership: Private
Produces/Sells CE-marked Devices: N
Distribution: Manufacturer Direct, Exclusive Distributor, Exporter

ELECSYS CORPORATION 913-647-0158
846 N. Mart-way Court, Olathe, KS 66061
FDA Number: 3002744013 *Fax:* 913-647-0132
E-mail: info@elecsyscorp.com
Web site: www.elecsyscorp.com
Ownership: Private
Produces/Sells CE-marked Devices: N

ELECSYS CORPORATION 913-647-0158 (cont'd)
Spirometer, Monitoring (Volumeter) — Anesthesiology

ELECTA CORPORATION
See Elekta Inc.

ELECTONE, A DIVISION OF SIEMENS HEARING 407-831-2555
INSTRUMENTS, INC.
1124 Florida Central Pkwy, Longwood, FL 32750
FDA Number: 1028145 *Fax:* 407-830-4678
E-mail: info@electoneonline.com
Web site: www.electoneonline.com
Ownership: Siemens Ag
Produces/Sells CE-marked Devices: N
Federal Procurement Eligibility: Small Business
Distribution: Manufacturer Direct, Importer, Exporter
Hearing-Aid — Ear/Nose/Throat

ELECTONE, INC.
See Electone, A Division Of Siemens Hearing Instruments, Inc.

ELECTRA-TEC INC. 800-225-3532
P.O. Box 17, 567 West M-89, **269-694-2058**
Otsego, MI 49078
FDA Number: n/a *Fax:* 269-694-5880
E-mail: sales@electratec.com
Web site: www.electratec.com
Annual Revenue: $1-$5 Million
Year Founded: 1977
Total Employees: 18
Ownership: Private
Produces/Sells CE-marked Devices: N
Federal Procurement Eligibility: Small Business
Distribution: Manufacturer Direct, Manufacturer Through Manufacturer Reps
General Admin.: Julie Wilson/Office Manager
Karla Zantello/Office Manager
Robert Pawlowski/President
Cabinet, Laboratory — Chemistry
Sink, Laboratory — Chemistry

ELECTRI-TEC, INC. 219-665-1252
509 Growth Pkwy., Angola, IN 46703
FDA Number: n/a *Fax:* 219-665-1132
E-mail: sales@electritec.com
Web site: www.electritec.com
Medical Products Sales Volume: $1,200,000
Annual Revenue: $1-$5 Million
Total Employees: 50 *Sales Staff:* 3
Ownership: Private
Quality System Registration Information: ISO9002
Produces/Sells CE-marked Devices: N
Federal Procurement Eligibility: Small Business
Distribution: Manufacturer Direct, Manufacturer Through Manufacturer Reps
General Admin.: Neal A. Gaff/President
Troy N. Weimer/Vice President, General Manager
Mktg./Adv.: Dan Stewart/Vice President Marketing & Sales
Production: Rod Frye/Manager Materials
Research: Denny Springer/Vice President Research & Development
Component, Electronic — General
Equipment, Molding — General

ELECTRIC MOBILITY CORPORATION 800-718-2082
591 Mantua Blvd., PO Box 450, Sewell, NJ 08080
FDA Number: 2246719 *Fax:* 877-282-1447
E-mail: emcinsurance@electricmobility.com
Web site: www.rascalinsurance.com
Medical Products Sales Volume: $90,000,000
Annual Revenue: $100-$500 Million
Year Founded: 1947
Total Employees: 500
Ownership: Private
Quality System Registration Information: ISO9001
Produces/Sells CE-marked Devices: N
Federal Procurement Eligibility: VA Contract
Distribution: Manufacturer Direct, Manufacturer Through Distributor, Manufacturer Through Manufacturer Reps, Service Direct, Importer, Exporter
General Admin.: Mr. Michael Johns/Director
Accessories, Wheelchair — Physical Med
Ramp, Wheelchair — General
Scooter (Motorized 3-Wheeled Vehicle) — Physical Med
Wheelchair, Powered — Physical Med

ELECTRICAL GEODESICS, INC. 541-687-7962
2979 Chad Dr., Eugene, OR 97408
FDA Number: 3005657763
Electroencephalograph — Cns/Neurology

ELECTRICAL GEODESICS, INCORPORATED   541-687-7962
1600 Millrace Drive, Suite 307, Eugene, OR 97403
FDA Number: 3001090553   *Fax:* 541-687-7963
E-mail: info@egi.com
Web site: www.egi.com
Medical Products Sales Volume: $7,700,000
Annual Revenue: $5-$10 Million
Year Founded: 1992
Total Employees: 9   *Marketing Staff:* 2   *Sales Staff:* 6
Ownership: Private
Quality System Registration Information: ISO9001
Produces/Sells CE-marked Devices: Y
Federal Procurement Eligibility: Small Business
Distribution: Manufacturer Direct, Manufacturer Through Distributor, Manufacturer Through Manufacturer Reps, Service Direct
Mktg./Adv.: Ono Olivieri/Director International Sales
     Dee Dee Carver/Manager Sales
     Dr. Ann Bunnenberg/President Marketing & Sales
   Electroencephalograph   Cns/Neurology

ELECTRO ASSEMBLIES CORP.   847-498-6520
2909 MacArthur Boulevard, Northbrook, IL 60062-2368
FDA Number: n/a   *Fax:* 847-272-2915
E-mail: easales@electroassemblies.com
Web site: www.electroassemblies.com
Annual Revenue: $1-$5 Million
Ownership: Private
Produces/Sells CE-marked Devices: N
Distribution: Manufacturer Direct, Manufacturer Through Manufacturer Reps
General Admin.: William L. Nettelhorst/President
Production: William S. Nettelhorst/Vice President Manufacturing
   Contract Manufacturing   General

ELECTRO MECHANICAL PRODUCTS INC.   772-286-8848
41 SE Kindred St., Stuart, FL 34994
FDA Number: 3005310849
Ownership: Private
Produces/Sells CE-marked Devices: N
   Platform, Force-Measuring   Physical Med

ELECTRO MEDICAL EQUIPMENT CO., INC.   800-423-2926
12015 Industriplex Blvd.,   225-756-0351
Baton Rouge, LA 70809
FDA Number: n/a   *Fax:* 225-753-0719
E-mail: info@emecompany.com
Web site: www.emecompany.com
Annual Revenue: $5-$10 Million
Year Founded: 1976
Total Employees: 35   *Marketing Staff:* 2   *Sales Staff:* 12
Ownership: Private
Produces/Sells CE-marked Devices: N
Federal Procurement Eligibility: Small Business, Minority Owned, GSA Contract
Distribution: Manufacturer Direct, Manufacturer Through Distributor, Manufacturer Through Manufacturer Reps, OEM, Importer
General Admin.: Mr. leonard carmouche/President, Chief Executive Officer, General Manager
   Bag, Ice   General
   Electrode, Holter   Cardiovascular
   Recorder, Magnetic Tape/Disc   Cardiovascular
   Recorder, Paper Chart   Cardiovascular

ELECTRO MEDICAL INC.   918-663-0297
9736 E. 55th Pl., Tulsa, OK 74146
FDA Number: 1000117937
E-mail: info@electro-medical.com
Web site: www.electro-medical.com
Ownership: Private
Produces/Sells CE-marked Devices: N
   Stimulator, Nerve, Transcutaneous (Pain Relief, TENS)   Cns/Neurology

ELECTRO MEDICAL SYSTEMS
   See Conmed Corporation

ELECTRO SURFACE TECHNOLOGIES, INC.   760-431-8306
2281 Las Palmas Drive, Suite 101, Carlsbad, CA 92011
FDA Number: 2029162   *Fax:* 760-431-8715
E-mail: info@est.com
Web site: www.est.com
Ownership: Private
Produces/Sells CE-marked Devices: N
   Stimulator, Nerve, Transcutaneous (Pain Relief, TENS)   Cns/Neurology

ELECTRO SURGICAL INSTRUMENT CO., INC.   888-464-2784
37 Centennial St., Rochester, NY 14611   716-235-1430
FDA Number: 1315756   *Fax:* 585-235-1438
E-mail: sales@electrosurgicalinstrument.com
Web site: www.electrosurgicalinstrument.com
Annual Revenue: $0-$1 Million

ELECTRO SURGICAL INSTRUMENT CO., INC.   888-464-2784
(cont'd)
Year Founded: 1896
Ownership: Private
Produces/Sells CE-marked Devices: N
Federal Procurement Eligibility: Small Business
Distribution: Manufacturer Direct, OEM, Service Direct, Exporter
General Admin.: Mr. Michael McAndrews/President
   Accessories, Cleaning, Endoscopic   Gastroenterology/Urology
   Accessories, Speculum   Surgery
   Anoscope, Non-Powered   Gastroenterology/Urology
   Block, Bite   Cns/Neurology
   Box, Battery, Pocket (Endoscopic)   Gastroenterology/Urology
   Bronchoscope, Rigid   Ear/Nose/Throat
   Cannula, Bronchial   Ear/Nose/Throat
   Carrier, Sponge, Endoscopic   Gastroenterology/Urology
   Cord, Electric, Endoscope   Gastroenterology/Urology
   Cystoscope   Gastroenterology/Urology
   Depressor, Tongue   General
   Endoscope, Fiberoptic   Surgery
   Esophagoscope (Flexible Or Rigid)   Ear/Nose/Throat
   Fiberoptic Light Source & Carrier   Ear/Nose/Throat
   Forceps, General & Plastic Surgery   Surgery
   Gag, Mouth   Ear/Nose/Throat
   Headlight, Fiberoptic Focusing   Gastroenterology/Urology
   Knife, Tonsil   Ear/Nose/Throat
   Lamp, Endoscopic, Incandescent   Surgery
   Laryngoscope, Surgical   Surgery
   Light, Surgical, Fiberoptic   Surgery
   Mirror, ENT   Ear/Nose/Throat
   Proctoscope   Surgery
   Retractor, Fiberoptic   Gastroenterology/Urology
   Snare, Surgical   Surgery
   Speculum, Illuminated   Surgery
   Speculum, Rectal   Gastroenterology/Urology
   Transformer, Endoscope   Surgery
   Transilluminator, AC-Powered, Ophthalmic   Ophthalmology

ELECTRO THERAPEUTIC DEVICES INC.   877-475-8344
70 Esna Park Drive, Unit 4,   905-475-8344
Markham, ONT L3R 6 Canada
FDA Number: 8022039   *Fax:* 905-475-5143
E-mail: info@etdinc.ca
Web site: www.etdinc.ca
Medical Products Sales Volume: $1,500,000
Year Founded: 1979
Total Employees: 4   *Marketing Staff:* 4   *Sales Staff:* 4
Ownership: Private
Produces/Sells CE-marked Devices: Y
Federal Procurement Eligibility: Small Business
Distribution: Manufacturer Direct, Manufacturer Through Distributor, Exclusive Distributor, Exporter

ELECTRO VAN LIFT, INC.
   See IMED Mobility Inc.

ELECTRO-BIOLOGY INC.
   See Ebi, Llc

ELECTRO-CAP INTERNATIONAL, INC.   800-527-2193
1011 W. Lexington Road, PO Box 87,   937-456-6099
Eaton, OH 45320
FDA Number: 1626185   *Fax:* 937-456-7323
E-mail: eci@infinet.com
Web site: www.electro-cap.com
Medical Products Sales Volume: $1,100,000
Annual Revenue: $1-$5 Million
Year Founded: 1988
Total Employees: 18   *Marketing Staff:* 2   *Sales Staff:* 3
Ownership: Private
Quality System Registration Information: ISO9001
Produces/Sells CE-marked Devices: Y
Federal Procurement Eligibility: Small Business
Distribution: Manufacturer Direct, Manufacturer Through Distributor, OEM, Exclusive Distributor, Exporter
General Admin.: W. Nelson Hardin/President, Chief Executive Officer
Mktg./Adv.: Amy Swallows/Director Marketing
   Cap, Nerve   Cns/Neurology
   Electrode, Biopotential, Surface, Metallic   Physical Med
   Electrode, Electroencephalographic   Cns/Neurology
   Electrode, Neurological   Cns/Neurology
   Electrode, Other   General
   Electroencephalograph   Cns/Neurology
   Gel, Electrode, TENS   Physical Med

ELECTRO-DIAGNOSTIC IMAGING, INC.   650-367-9293
200f Twin Dolphin Drive, Redwood City, CA 94065
FDA Number: 2954355
   Photostimulator, AC-Powered   Ophthalmology

MANUFACTURER PROFILES

ELECTRO-MED HEALTH INDUSTRIES 800-232-3644
PO Box 610484, Miami, FL 33261-0484 305-892-2866
FDA Number: 1028751 *Fax:* 305-892-2980
E-mail: info@egs-emhi.com
Web site: www.egs-emhi.com
Year Founded: 1972
Ownership: S & P ELECTRICAL INDUSTRIES, INC.
Produces/Sells CE-marked Devices: N
Federal Procurement Eligibility: Small Business, Female Owned
Distribution: Manufacturer Direct, Manufacturer Through Distributor, Service Direct
General Admin.: Phyllis Lehman/President
  Electrode, Other   General
  Stimulator, Muscle, Electrical-Powered (EMS)   Physical Med

ELECTRO-MEDICAL INSTRUMENT CO. 905-822-3188
1-2359 Royal Windsor Dr., Mississauga, ONT L5J-4S9 Canada
FDA Number: n/a *Fax:* 905-822-9920
E-mail: emi@honson.com
Web site: www.emi-canada.com
Year Founded: 1993
Total Employees: 10
Ownership: Private
Produces/Sells CE-marked Devices: N
Distribution: Service Direct, Exclusive Distributor

ELECTRO-OPTICAL SCIENCES, INC. 914-591-3783
3 W. Main St., Ste. 201, Irvington, NY 10533
FDA Number: n/a *Fax:* 914-591-3785
Ownership: Private
Produces/Sells CE-marked Devices: N
General Admin.: Mr. Breaux Castleman/Chairman
     Mr. Joseph Gulfo/President, Chief Executive Officer, Director
Finance: Mr. Richard Steinhart/Chief Financial Officer, Vice President Finance
  Caries Detector, Laser Light, Transmission   Dental And Oral
  Operative Dental Treatment Unit   Dental And Oral

ELECTRO-STEAM GENERATOR CORP. 888-783-2624
1000 Bernard Street, Alexandria, VA 22314 703-549-0664
FDA Number: 9200320 *Fax:* 703-836-2581
E-mail: sales@electrosteam.com
Web site: www.electrosteam.com
Year Founded: 1952
Ownership: Private
Produces/Sells CE-marked Devices: Y
Federal Procurement Eligibility: Small Business
Distribution: Manufacturer Direct, Manufacturer Through Distributor, Manufacturer Through Manufacturer Reps, Exporter
Mktg./Adv.: Jack Harlin/Manager International & National Sales
  Bath, Steam   General
  Foodservice Product/Equipment   General
  Laundry Equipment   General
  Sterilizer, Steam, Table Top   General
  Vaporizer   General

ELECTRO-SUPPORT SYSTEMS
See Ims-Ess

ELECTRO-TECH PRODUCTS INC. 909-592-1434
2001 E. Gladstone Street,#a, Glendora, CA 91740
FDA Number: 2023825
  Stimulator, Nerve, Transcutaneous (Pain Relief, TENS)   Cns/Neurology

ELECTRODE ARRAYS (888) 267.6157
612 N. Resler, El Paso, TX 79912 915-273-7600
FDA Number: 3006413966
E-mail: info@electrodearrays.com
Web site: www.electrodearrays.com
Ownership: Private
Produces/Sells CE-marked Devices: N

ELECTRODYNE, INC. 503-654-0711
11200 S.E. 21st Ave., Milwaukie, OR 97222
FDA Number: n/a *Fax:* 503-654-1959
E-mail: leon@electrodyne-nw..com
Web site: www.electrodyne-nw.com
Annual Revenue: $0-$1 Million
Total Employees: 7   *Marketing Staff:* 1   *Sales Staff:* 1
Ownership: Private
Produces/Sells CE-marked Devices: N
Federal Procurement Eligibility: Small Business
Distribution: Manufacturer Direct
General Admin.: Leon Fuller/President, Chief Executive Officer
  Valve, Other   Chemistry

ELECTROLUX HOME PRODUCTS - NORTH AMERICA 877-435-3287
250 Bobby Jones Expressway, PO Box 212378, Augusta, GA 30917 706-651-1751
FDA Number: n/a *Fax:* 706-651-7769
E-mail: info@frigidaire.com
Web site: www.electroluxusa.com
Medical Products Sales Volume: $4,000,000
Annual Revenue: More than $100 Million
Total Employees: 40
Ownership: Private
Stock Symbol: ELUXF
Produces/Sells CE-marked Devices: N
Federal Procurement Eligibility: Small Business, Female Owned
Distribution: Manufacturer Through Distributor, Service Direct
General Admin.: Robert E. Cook/President
     Roger Leon/Vice President
Mktg./Adv.: Carol Rice/Manager Advertising
     Mark Chambers/Manager Marketing & Sales
     Jay Penney/Vice President Sales
  Facility, Equipment, Medical, Mobile   General
  Refrigerator, Foodservice   General
  Washer, Laundry   General

ELECTROMAGNETIC INDUSTRIES INC.
See Square D Company

ELECTROMED IMAGING INC. 450-681-6810
440 Armand Frappier Blvd., Ste. 250, Laval, QUE H7V-4 Canada
FDA Number: n/a *Fax:* 450-681-3925
E-mail: info@electromed.com
Web site: www.electromed.com
Year Founded: 2000
Total Employees: 50
Ownership: Private
Produces/Sells CE-marked Devices: N
Distribution: Manufacturer Direct, Service Direct

ELECTROMED, INC. 800-462-1045
500 Sixth Ave. N.W., New Prague, MN 56071 952-758-9299
FDA Number: 2134852 *Fax:* 952-758-1941
E-mail: info@electromed.com
Web site: www.electromed.com
Year Founded: 1992
Ownership: Public
Stock Symbol: ELMD
Traded On: NASDAQ
Quality System Registration Information: ISO9001
Produces/Sells CE-marked Devices: Y
Federal Procurement Eligibility: Small Business
Distribution: Manufacturer Direct
General Admin.: Mr. Robert Hansen/Chief Executive Officer
Mktg./Adv.: Ms. Pankti Shah/Manager Marketing
     Mr. Martin Davij/National Sales Manager
     Mr. Rick Leonard/Regional Marketing Manager
Finance: Mr. Jeremy Brock/Chief Financial Officer
     Mr. Terry Belford/Chief Financial Officer
  Percussor, Powered   Anesthesiology

ELECTROMEDICAL PRODUCTS INTERNATIONAL, INC. 800-367-7246
2201 Garrett Morris Pkwy., Mineral Wells, TX 76067 940-328-0788
FDA Number: 2020648 *Fax:* 940-328-0888
E-mail: alpha-stim@epii.com
Web site: www.alpha-stim.com
Medical Products Sales Volume: $800,000
Annual Revenue: $1-$5 Million
Year Founded: 1981
Total Employees: 12   *Marketing Staff:* 3   *Sales Staff:* 4
Ownership: Private
Quality System Registration Information: ISO9001
Produces/Sells CE-marked Devices: Y
Federal Procurement Eligibility: Small Business, GSA Contract
Distribution: Manufacturer Through Distributor, Service Direct, Exporter
General Admin.: Dr. Daniel Kirsch/Chairman
     Tracey B. Kirsch/President
Mktg./Adv.: Douglas McCauley/Manager Customer Services & Sales
     Ms. Krissa Brewer/Manager Market Information
  Stimulator, Cranial Electrotherapy   Cns/Neurology
  Stimulator, Cranial Electrotherapy (Situational Anxiety)   Cns/Neurology
  Stimulator, Nerve, Transcutaneous (Pain Relief, TENS)   Cns/Neurology

ELECTRON MICROSCOPY SCIENCES
800-523-5874
215-412-8400
1560 Industry Road, P.O. Box 550,
Hatfield, PA 19440
FDA Number: 7000128   Fax: 215-412-8450
E-mail: sgkcck@aol.com
Web site: www.emsdiasum.com
Medical Products Sales Volume: $1,250,000
Annual Revenue: $1-$5 Million
Year Founded: 1988
Total Employees: 17   *Marketing Staff:* 2   *Sales Staff:* 7
Ownership: Private
Produces/Sells CE-marked Devices: Y
Federal Procurement Eligibility: Small Business, Female Owned
Distribution: Manufacturer Direct
General Admin.: Stacie Kirsch/President, Chief Executive Officer
Mktg./Adv.: Bang Nguyen/Director Product Development
Production: Bojour Burlacu/Director Quality Assurance
     Bang Nguyrn/Manager Production
   Microscope, Laboratory, Electron   Microbiology
   Radioautographic Equipment   Chemistry
   Reagent, Other   General

ELECTRONETICS CORP.
See General Transco Inc.

ELECTRONIC CONTROL CONCEPTS
800-847-9729
845-246-9013
160 Partition St., Saugerties, NY 12477
FDA Number: 1320182   Fax: 845-247-9028
E-mail: eccxray@verizon.net
Web site: www.eccxray.com
Medical Products Sales Volume: $170,000
Annual Revenue: $0-$1 Million
Year Founded: 1994
Total Employees: 2
Ownership: Private
Produces/Sells CE-marked Devices: Y
Federal Procurement Eligibility: Small Business
Distribution: Manufacturer Direct, Manufacturer Through Distributor, Exporter
   Monitor, Radiation   Radiology
   Phototimer, Radiographic Mobile   Radiology
   Radiographic Unit, Diagnostic, Dental, Extraoral   Dental And Oral

ELECTRONIC DESIGN & RESEARCH CO., INC.
502-433-8660
7331 Intermodal Dr., Louisville, KY 40258
FDA Number: 1034860   Fax: 502-933-3422
E-mail: info@vsholding.com
Web site: www.vsholding.com
Medical Products Sales Volume: $120,000
Annual Revenue: $1-$5 Million
Year Founded: 1984
Total Employees: 15   *Marketing Staff:* 1   *Sales Staff:* 1
Ownership: Private
Produces/Sells CE-marked Devices: N
Federal Procurement Eligibility: Small Business
Distribution: Manufacturer Direct
General Admin.: Dr. Vladimir Shvartsman/President, Chief Executive Officer
   Monitor, Cardiac (Cardiotachometer & Rate Alarm)   Cardiovascular

ELECTRONIC DEVELOPMENT LABS, INC.
800-342-5335
434-799-0807
244 Oakland Drive, Danville, VA 24540-9287
FDA Number: 2410808   Fax: 434-799-0847
E-mail: sales@edl-inc.com
Web site: www.edl-inc.com
Medical Products Sales Volume: $1,000,000
Annual Revenue: $1-$5 Million
Year Founded: 1943
Total Employees: 35   *Marketing Staff:* 2   *Sales Staff:* 2
Ownership: Private
Produces/Sells CE-marked Devices: N
Federal Procurement Eligibility: Small Business
Distribution: Manufacturer Direct, Manufacturer Through Distributor, OEM, Exporter
General Admin.: Donald Polsky/President, Chief Executive Officer
     Kenny Sloneker/Vice President
Mktg./Adv.: Jean Moore/Manager International & National Sales
   Pyrometer   General
   Thermometer, Electronic   General

ELECTRONIC INDUSTRIES ALLIANCE
703-907-7500
2500 Wilson Blvd., Arlington, VA 22201-3834
FDA Number: n/a
Web site: www.eia.org
Annual Revenue: $0-$1 Million
Ownership: Private
Produces/Sells CE-marked Devices: N
Distribution: Manufacturer Direct, Service Direct
General Admin.: Matthew Flanigan/President, Chief Executive Officer
   Component, Electronic   General

ELECTRONIC INDUSTRIES ALLIANCE
703-907-7500 *(cont'd)*
   Service, Consulting   General
   Service, Engineering/Design   General

ELECTRONIC INDUSTRIES ASSOCIATION
See Electronic Industries Alliance

ELECTRONIC MFG. CO.
813-855-4068
13440 Wright Circle, Tampa, FL 33626
FDA Number: 1054469   Fax: 813-854-3924
E-mail: normb@electronicmanufacturingco.com
Web site: www.electronicmanufacturingco.com
Ownership: Private
Produces/Sells CE-marked Devices: N
   Bed, Flotation Therapy, Powered   Physical Med
   Electromyograph, Diagnostic   Physical Med

ELECTRONIC SERVICES MART
See Rahd Oncology Products

ELECTRONIC SYSTEMS ENGINEERING COMPANY
800-331-5904
One ESECO Road, Cushing, OK 74023
918-225-1266
FDA Number: 1000257786   Fax: 918-225-1284
Ownership: Private
Produces/Sells CE-marked Devices: N
   Tester, Radiology   Radiology

ELECTRONIC WAVEFORM LABORATORY, INC.
800-874-9283
16168 Beach Blvd., Suite 232,
714-843-0463
Huntington Beach, CA 92647
FDA Number: 2023152   Fax: 714-843-1992
E-mail: painrelief@h-wave.com
Web site: www.h-wave.com
Medical Products Sales Volume: $2,200,000
Annual Revenue: $1-$5 Million
Year Founded: 1981
Total Employees: 25
Ownership: Private
Produces/Sells CE-marked Devices: N
Federal Procurement Eligibility: Small Business
Distribution: Manufacturer Direct
General Admin.: W. J. Heaney/President
Mktg./Adv.: W. J. Heaney/Vice President Sales
Research: W. J. Heaney/Vice President Research & Development
Finance: Francis Nixon/Accountant
   Monitor, Muscle, Dental   Dental And Oral
   Stimulator, Nerve, Transcutaneous (Pain Relief, TENS)   Cns/Neurology

ELECTROSCOPE, INC.
See Encision Inc.

ELECTROSTIM MEDICAL SERVICES, INC.
800-588-8383
3504 Cragmont Dr., Suite #100, Tampa, FL 33619
813-931-2369
FDA Number: 3003573572   Fax: 800-588-9282
E-mail: mgarcia@wecontrolpain.com
Web site: www.wecontrolpain.com
Year Founded: 1995
Total Employees: 85   *Sales Staff:* 40
Ownership: Private
Produces/Sells CE-marked Devices: N
Federal Procurement Eligibility: Small Business, Minority Owned
   Electrode, Cutaneous   Cns/Neurology
   Stimulator, Nerve, AC-Powered   Anesthesiology
   Stimulator, Nerve, Transcutaneous (Pain Relief, TENS)   Cns/Neurology
   Unit, Therapy, Current, Interferential   Cns/Neurology

ELECTROTHERAPY SYSTEMS, INC.
503-779-7039
476 Winding Ct.,se, Salem, OR 97302
FDA Number: 3005056646
Ownership: Private
Produces/Sells CE-marked Devices: N
   Stimulator, Muscle, Electrical-Powered (EMS)   Physical Med

ELEKTA INC.
800-535-7355
4775 Peachtree Industrial Blvd.
770-300-9725
Bldg. 300, Suite 300
Norcross, GA 30092
FDA Number: 1037831   Fax: 770-448-6338
E-mail: info.america@elekta.com
Web site: www.elekta.com
Medical Products Sales Volume: $9,200,000
Year Founded: 1983
Total Employees: 60
Ownership: Private
Stock Symbol: ELEKTA
Traded On: Stockholm
Quality System Registration Information: ISO9000; ISO9002
Produces/Sells CE-marked Devices: Y

ELEKTA INC.   800-535-7355 (cont'd)
Federal Procurement Eligibility: Small Business
Distribution: Manufacturer Direct, Manufacturer Through Distributor, Manufacturer Through Manufacturer Reps, Importer, Exporter
General Admin.: Thomas Puusepp/President, Chief Executive Officer
     PJ Gaccione/Vice President, General Manager
Mktg./Adv.: James Rose/Vice President Marketing
     Ray Rau/Vice President Marketing & Sales

Accelerator, Linear, Medical	Radiology
Fixation Device, Extra-Cranial (Head Frame)	Orthopedics
Retractor, Self-Retaining, Neurology	Cns/Neurology

ELEKTA INSTRUMENTS, INC.
See Elekta, Inc.

ELEKTA, INC.
See Elekta, Inc.

ELEMAC MEDICAL   877-333-5306
     603-816-1920
Heron Cove Office Park
10 Al Paul Lane, Suite 102
Merrimack, NH 03054
FDA Number: n/a   *Fax:* 603-882-4762
E-mail: info@elememedical.com
Web site: www.elememedical.com
Ownership: Private
Produces/Sells CE-marked Devices: N
Distribution: Manufacturer Through Distributor
General Admin.: Nancy M. Briefs/President, Chief Executive Officer
Finance: Christopher Joyce/Vice President Finance

ELEMAC MEDICAL, INCORPORATED   877-333-5306
     603-816-1920
Heron Cove Office Park
10 Al Paul Lane, Suite 102
Merrimack, NH 03054
FDA Number: 3006182507   *Fax:* 603-882-4762
E-mail: mmarkham-burns@elememedical.com
Web site: http://www.elememedical.com
Ownership: Private
Produces/Sells CE-marked Devices: N

ELEMENTIS PERFORMANCE POLYMERS
See Elementis Specialties

ELEMENTIS SPECIALTIES   800-866-6800
     609-443-2000
329 Wyckoffs Mill Road, Hightstown, NJ 08520
FDA Number: n/a   *Fax:* 609-443-2422
E-mail: peter.russo@elementis-na.com
Web site: www.elementis-specialties.com
Medical Products Sales Volume: $86,900,000
Annual Revenue: More than $100 Million
Year Founded: 1957
Total Employees: 572   *Marketing Staff:* 3   *Sales Staff:* 11
Ownership: Private
Stock Symbol: ELM
Traded On: London
Quality System Registration Information: ISO9001
Produces/Sells CE-marked Devices: N
Federal Procurement Eligibility: GSA Contract
Distribution: Manufacturer Direct
General Admin.: Neil Carr/President, Chief Executive Officer
Mktg./Adv.: Peter B. Russo/Director Business
     Frank Lee/Manager Market Development

Strip, Adhesive	Surgery

ELGAR DENTAL PRODUCTS, INC.   702-699-5655
3374 Racquet St., Las Vegas, NV 89121
FDA Number: 2030597
Ownership: Private
Produces/Sells CE-marked Devices: N

Crown, Preformed	Dental And Oral

ELGINEX CORPORATION   800-279-3762
     630-268-1000
270 N. Eisenhower Lane, Unit 4-A,
Lombard, IL 60148
FDA Number: 1419188   *Fax:* 630-268-1007
E-mail: elginsales@sbcglobal.net
Web site: www.elginex.com
Annual Revenue: $1-$5 Million
Total Employees: 8   *Marketing Staff:* 2   *Sales Staff:* 3
Ownership: Private
Produces/Sells CE-marked Devices: N
Federal Procurement Eligibility: Small Business
Distribution: Manufacturer Through Distributor
General Admin.: Robert Boules/President
     Mr. Graham R. Boules/Vice President

Exerciser, Arm	Physical Med
Exerciser, Chest	Physical Med
Exerciser, Leg And Ankle	Physical Med

ELGINEX CORPORATION   800-279-3762 (cont'd)

Exerciser, Non-Measuring	Physical Med
Exerciser, Shoulder	Physical Med
Exerciser, Wrist	Physical Med
Pillow	General
Pillow, Cervical	Orthopedics

ELI LILLY AND CO.   317-276-4000
Lilly Corporate Center, Drop Code 2622, Indianapolis, IN 46285
FDA Number: 3005192253
Ownership: Private
Produces/Sells CE-marked Devices: N
General Admin.: James Collins/Executive Director

Disc, Susceptibility, Antimicrobial	Microbiology
Metallic Reduction Method, Glucose (Urinary, Non-Quant.)	Chemistry
Syringe, Piston	General

ELITE DENTAL SERVICE   954-825-6392
10188 Nw 47th Street, Sunrise, FL 33351
FDA Number: 3007074536
E-mail: support@eds-usa.com
Web site: www.eds-usa.com
Ownership: Private
Produces/Sells CE-marked Devices: N

Metallic Reduction Method, Glucose (Urinary, Non-Quant.)	Chemistry

ELITE MATTRESS MANUFACTURING   800-332-5878
     314-353-0800
4999 Rear Fyler Avenue, St. Louis, MO 63139
FDA Number: n/a   *Fax:* 314-353-6078
E-mail: info@elitemattress.com
Web site: www.elitemattress.com
Medical Products Sales Volume: $720,000
Year Founded: 1991
Total Employees: 9   *Sales Staff:* 1
Ownership: Private
Produces/Sells CE-marked Devices: N
Federal Procurement Eligibility: Small Business, Female Owned
Distribution: Manufacturer Direct
General Admin.: Jeff Massey/President

Bed, Electric	General
Mattress, Bed	General

ELITE MEDICAL EQUIPMENT   719-659-7926
5470 Kates Drive, Co Spgs, CO 80919
FDA Number: 3004889490   *Fax:* 720-941-1227
E-mail: inforequest@elite-med.com
Web site: www.elite-med.com
Ownership: Private
Produces/Sells CE-marked Devices: N

Accessories, Operating Room, Table	Surgery
Cutter, Cast, AC-Powered	Orthopedics
Reamer	Orthopedics
Traction Unit, Non-Powered	Orthopedics

ELITE MEDICAL PRODUCTS, INC.   661-273-6518
38606 Roma Court, Palmdale, CA 93550
FDA Number: 3005727179   *Fax:* 661-273-8963
E-mail: daniel@elitemedicalproductsinc.com
Web site: www.elitemedicalproductsinc.com
Ownership: Private
Produces/Sells CE-marked Devices: N

Suction Apparatus, Operating Room, Wall Vacuum-Powered	Surgery

ELITE ORTHOPAEDICS, INC.   800-284-1688
     626-452-0758
1535 Santa Anita Avenue, S. El Monte, CA 91733
FDA Number: 2028810   *Fax:* 626-452-1806
E-mail: info@elite-ortho.com
Web site: www.elite-ortho.com
Year Founded: 1992
Total Employees: 7
Ownership: Private
Produces/Sells CE-marked Devices: N
Federal Procurement Eligibility: Small Business
Distribution: Manufacturer Direct, Manufacturer Through Distributor
General Admin.: Christine Cespedes/Assistant Manager
     David Chang/Chief Executive Officer

Brace, Joint, Ankle (External)	Physical Med
Joint, Knee, External Brace	Physical Med

ELIXIR MEDICAL CORPORATION   408-636-2000
870 Hermosa Ave., Sunnyvale, CA 94085
FDA Number: 3005092783
E-mail: info@elixirmedical.com
Web site: www.elixirmedical.com
Ownership: Private
Produces/Sells CE-marked Devices: N
General Admin.: Mr. Motasim Sirhan/President, Chief Executive Officer

Stent, Coronary, Drug-eluting	Cardiovascular

ELLIPSE TECHNOLOGIES, INC
949-837-3600
13900 Alton Parkway, Irvine, CA 92618
FDA Number: 3006179046   *Fax:* 949-837-3664
E-mail: cs@ellipse-tech.com
Web site: www.ellipse-tech.com
Ownership: Private
Produces/Sells CE-marked Devices: N

Accessories, Fixation, Spinal Interlaminal	Orthopedics
Appliance, Fixation, Spinal Interlaminal	Orthopedics
Rod, Fixation, Intramedullary	Orthopedics

ELLIQUENCE LLC
(516) 277-9000
2455 Grand Avenue, Baldwin, NY 11510
FDA Number: 3007024186
Ownership: Private
Produces/Sells CE-marked Devices: N

Arthroscope	Orthopedics
Electrosurgical Unit, Cutting & Coagulation Device	Surgery

ELLIS OPHTHALMIC TECHNOLOGIES, INC.
718-656-7390
147-39, 175 St.,, Suite #128, Jamaica, NY 11434
FDA Number: 2438659   *Fax:* 718-656-7394
E-mail: info@eye-ellis.com
Web site: www.eye-ellis.com
Ownership: Private
Produces/Sells CE-marked Devices: N

Lens, Intraocular	Ophthalmology
Scanner, Ultrasonic (Pulsed Echo)	Radiology
Transducer, Ultrasonic	Cardiovascular

ELLKAR CORPORATION
727-442-8231
1137 Sunnydale Dr., Clearwater, FL 33755
FDA Number: 3004552892
Ownership: Private
Produces/Sells CE-marked Devices: N

Utensil, Food	Physical Med

ELLMAN INTERNATIONAL, INC.
800-835-5355
3333 Royal Ave, Oceanside, NY 11572
516-594-3333
FDA Number: 2428235   *Fax:* 516-569-0054
Web site: www.ellman.com
Ownership: Private
Produces/Sells CE-marked Devices: N

Arthroscope	Orthopedics
Burr, Dental	Dental And Oral
Condenser, Amalgam And Foil, Operative	Dental And Oral
Cryosurgical Unit	Surgery
Electrocautery Unit, Gynecologic	Obstetrics/Gynecology
Electrode, Flexible Suction Coagulator	Gastroenterology/Urology
Electrosurgical Unit, Cutting & Coagulation Device	Surgery
Evacuator, Vapor, Cement Monomer	Orthopedics
Exhaust System, Surgical	Surgery
Instrument, Dental, Manual	Dental And Oral
Kit, Anesthesia, Paracervical	Obstetrics/Gynecology
Liner, Cavity, Calcium Hydroxide	Dental And Oral
Pin, Retentive And Splinting	Dental And Oral
Post, Root Canal	Dental And Oral
Retractor, All Types	Dental And Oral
Shield, Eye, Ophthalmic	Ophthalmology
Snare, Surgical	Surgery
Speculum, Rectal	Gastroenterology/Urology

ELLMAN INTERNATIONAL, INC.
800-835-5355
3333 Royal Avenue, Oceanside, NY 11572
516-594-3333
FDA Number: 2428235   *Fax:* 516-569-0054
E-mail: vip@ellman.com
Web site: www.ellman.com
Medical Products Sales Volume: $15,000,000
Annual Revenue: $25-$50 Million
Total Employees: 85   *Sales Staff:* 10
Ownership: Private
Quality System Registration Information: ISO9001
Produces/Sells CE-marked Devices: Y
Federal Procurement Eligibility: Small Business
Distribution: Manufacturer Direct
General Admin.: Rick Epstein/Chief Executive Officer
     Jon Garito/President
Mktg./Adv.: Bill Bernstein/Vice President Sales

Burr, Dental	Dental And Oral
Coagulator/Cutter, Endoscopic, Bipolar	Obstetrics/Gynecology
Condenser, Amalgam And Foil, Operative	Dental And Oral
Crown And Bridge, Temporary, Resin	Dental And Oral
Electrocautery Unit, Gynecologic	Obstetrics/Gynecology
Electrode, Electrosurgery, Laparoscopic	Surgery
Electrosurgical Equipment, General Purpose	Surgery
Electrosurgical Unit, Cutting & Coagulation Device	Surgery
Electrosurgical Unit, Dental	Dental And Oral
Generator, Power, Electrosurgical	Surgery
Instrument, Dental, Manual	Dental And Oral

ELLMAN INTERNATIONAL, INC.
800-835-5355 *(cont'd)*

Instrument, Electrosurgical, Field Focused	Cns/Neurology
Kit, Anesthesia, Paracervical	Obstetrics/Gynecology
Liner, Cavity, Calcium Hydroxide	Dental And Oral
Locator, Apex, Root	Dental And Oral
Matrix, Dental	Dental And Oral
Pin, Retentive And Splinting	Dental And Oral
Post, Root Canal	Dental And Oral
Retractor, All Types	Dental And Oral
Scaler, Rotary	Dental And Oral
Snare, Surgical	Surgery
Speculum, Rectal	Gastroenterology/Urology
System, Evacuation, Smoke, Laser	Surgery
Tester, Pulp	Dental And Oral

ELMA MEDTEC PRODUCTS INC.
204-348-7164
Po Box 160, Elma R0E 0Z0 Canada
FDA Number: 8043837

Depressor, Tongue	General

ELMED, INC.
630-543-2792
60 W. Fay Avenue, Addison, IL 60101-5106
FDA Number: 1412854   *Fax:* 630-543-2102
E-mail: medical@elmed.com
Web site: www.elmed.com
Medical Products Sales Volume: $1,700,000
Annual Revenue: $1-$5 Million
Total Employees: 22
Ownership: Private
Produces/Sells CE-marked Devices: N
Federal Procurement Eligibility: Small Business
Distribution: Manufacturer Direct, Manufacturer Through Distributor, Manufacturer Through Manufacturer Reps, Service Direct, Importer, Exporter
General Admin.: Mr. Werner Hausner/President
Mktg./Adv.: Mr. Othmar Goettel/Manager Product Sales

Adapter, Electrosurgical Unit, Cable	Surgery
Adapter, Unit, Electrosurgical, Hand-Controlled	Surgery
Blade, Knife, Laparoscopic	Surgery
Cabinet, Storage, Endoscope	Gastroenterology/Urology
Cable, Electrosurgical Unit	Surgery
Cable, Fiberoptic	General
Cable/Lead, ECG	Cardiovascular
Caliper, Ophthalmic	Ophthalmology
Caliper, Orthopedic	Orthopedics
Camera, Video, Endoscopic	General
Cannula, Lacrimal (Eye)	Ophthalmology
Cannula, Ophthalmic	Ophthalmology
Cannula, Suction, Pool-Tip	Surgery
Cardiograph, Impedance	Cardiovascular
Cart, Equipment, Video	General
Cart, Instrument/Equipment, Laparoscopy	Surgery
Chair, Surgical, AC-Powered	Surgery
Chisel, Bone, Surgical	Dental And Oral
Clamp, Fixation, Cholangiography	Surgery
Clamp, Laparoscopy	Surgery
Clip, Hemostatic	Surgery
Clip, Towel	Surgery
Coagulator, Hysteroscopic (With Accessories)	Obstetrics/Gynecology
Coagulator, Laparoscopic, Unipolar	Obstetrics/Gynecology
Coagulator/Cutter, Endoscopic, Bipolar	Obstetrics/Gynecology
Coagulator/Cutter, Endoscopic, Unipolar	Obstetrics/Gynecology
Colposcope	Obstetrics/Gynecology
Container, Surgical Instrument	Surgery
Cord, Electric, Endoscope	Gastroenterology/Urology
Cover, Laparoscope	Surgery
Cryosurgical Unit	Surgery
Cuff, Blood Pressure	Cardiovascular
Curette, Surgical	Surgery
Cutter, Ring	General
Cutter, Vitreous Aspiration, AC-Powered	Ophthalmology
Diathermy, Shortwave	Physical Med
Diathermy, Ultrasonic (Physical Therapy)	Physical Med
Dilator, Blunt	Surgery
Dynamometer, Grip-Strength (Squeeze)	Anesthesiology
Electrocardiograph, Multi-Channel	Cardiovascular
Electrocardiograph, Single Channel	Cardiovascular
Electrocautery Unit, Endoscopic	Obstetrics/Gynecology
Electrocautery Unit, Line-Powered	Surgery
Electrode, Electrocardiograph	Cardiovascular
Electrode, Electrosurgical, Active (Blade)	Surgery
Electrode, Electrosurgical, Active, Foot Controlled	Surgery
Electrode, Electrosurgical, Return (Ground, Dispersive)	Surgery
Electrosurgical Equipment, General Purpose	Surgery
Electrosurgical Unit, General Purpose (ESU)	Surgery
Endoscope, Rigid	Surgery
Epilator, High-Frequency, Needle-Type	Surgery
Equipment, Suction/Irrigation, Laparoscopic	Surgery
Ergometer, Bicycle	Cardiovascular
Exerciser, Bicycle	Physical Med
Fiberoptic Light Source & Carrier	Ear/Nose/Throat
File	Orthopedics

MANUFACTURER PROFILES

ELMED, INC. 630-543-2792 *(cont'd)*

File, Bone, Surgical	Dental And Oral
Forceps, Biopsy, Gynecological	Obstetrics/Gynecology
Forceps, Dressing	Surgery
Forceps, Electrosurgical	Surgery
Forceps, Endoscopic	Gastroenterology/Urology
Forceps, Fixation	Surgery
Forceps, Gallbladder (Biliary Duct)	Gastroenterology/Urology
Forceps, Grasping, Atraumatic	Surgery
Forceps, Grasping, Flexible Endoscopic	Gastroenterology/Urology
Forceps, Grasping, Traumatic	Surgery
Forceps, Hemostatic	Surgery
Forceps, Intestinal (Clamps)	Gastroenterology/Urology
Forceps, Obstetrical	Obstetrics/Gynecology
Forceps, Ophthalmic	Ophthalmology
Forceps, Rongeur, Surgical	Dental And Oral
Forceps, Sponge	Surgery
Forceps, Stone Manipulation	Gastroenterology/Urology
Forceps, Surgical, Gynecological	Obstetrics/Gynecology
Forceps, Tissue	Surgery
Forceps, Tonsil	Ear/Nose/Throat
Forceps, Utility	Surgery
Gel, Electrode, TENS	Physical Med
Hammer, Neurological	Cns/Neurology
Hammer, Percussion	Cns/Neurology
Hammer, Surgical	Surgery
Handle, Knife Blade	Surgery
Headlight, ENT	Ear/Nose/Throat
Hemostat, Surgical	Dental And Oral
Holder, Electrosurgical Electrode	Surgery
Holder, Laparoscope	Obstetrics/Gynecology
Holder, Needle	Gastroenterology/Urology
Holder, Needle, Curved, Laparoscopic	Surgery
Holder, Needle, Laparoscopic	Surgery
Holder, Needle, Other	Surgery
Holder/Scissors, Needle, Laparoscopic	Surgery
Hook, Cordotomy	Ear/Nose/Throat
Hook, Rhinoplastic	Surgery
Hook, Strabismus	Ophthalmology
Hook, Surgical, General & Plastic Surgery	Surgery
Hook, Sympathectomy	Cns/Neurology
Hook, Tracheal	Ear/Nose/Throat
Illuminator, Fiberoptic (For Endoscope)	Gastroenterology/Urology
Inflator, Cuff	General
Instrument, Dissecting, Laparoscopic	Surgery
Instrument, Dissecting, Myoma, Laparoscopic	Surgery
Instrument, Knot Tying, Suture, Laparoscopic	Surgery
Instrument, Manual, General Surgical	Surgery
Instrument, Microsurgical	Cns/Neurology
Instrument, Needle Holder/Knot Tying	Surgery
Instrument, Passing, Suture, Laparoscopic	Surgery
Insufflator, Carbon-Dioxide, Automatic (For Endoscope)	Gastroenterology/Urology
Insufflator, Hysteroscopic	Obstetrics/Gynecology
Insufflator, Laparoscopic	Obstetrics/Gynecology
Kit, Cholecystectomy	Gastroenterology/Urology
Kit, Laparoscopy	Gastroenterology/Urology
Knife, Amputation	Surgery
Knife, Cataract	Ophthalmology
Knife, Ear	Ear/Nose/Throat
Knife, Meniscus	Surgery
Knife, Scalpel	Surgery
Knife, Surgical	Dental And Oral
Knife, Tonsil	Ear/Nose/Throat
Lamp, Examination (Light)	General
Lamp, Examination, Ceiling Mounted (Light)	General
Lamp, Surgical	Surgery
Laparoscope, General & Plastic Surgery	Surgery
Laparoscope, Gynecologic	Obstetrics/Gynecology
Light Source, Endoscope, Xenon Arc	Surgery
Light Source, Fiberoptic, Routine	Gastroenterology/Urology
Light, Surgical, Ceiling Mounted	Surgery
Loupe, Diagnostic/Surgical	Surgery
Mallet, Bone	Orthopedics
Microelectrode	General
Microscope, Surgical, General & Plastic Surgery	Surgery
Mirror, Laryngeal	Ear/Nose/Throat
Monitor, Heart Rate, Other	Cardiovascular
Monitor, Heart Rate, R-Wave (ECG)	Cardiovascular
Monitor, Pulse Rate	Anesthesiology
Monitor, Video, Endoscope	General
Needle, Insufflation, Laparoscopic	Surgery
Needle, Pneumoperitoneum, Simple	Gastroenterology/Urology
Osteotome (Orthopedic)	Surgery
Paper, Recording, ECG/EEG	General
Plethysmograph, Impedance	Cardiovascular
Plethysmograph, Photo-Electric, Pneumatic Or Hydraulic	Cardiovascular
Plethysmograph, Pressure (Body)	Anesthesiology
Pliers, Surgical	Orthopedics
Probe, Suction, Irrigator/Aspirator, Laparoscopic	Surgery
Punch, Biopsy	Gastroenterology/Urology
Punch, Biopsy, Surgical	Dental And Oral
Retractor	Orthopedics

ELMED, INC. 630-543-2792 *(cont'd)*

Retractor, Abdominal	Surgery
Retractor, Bladder	Gastroenterology/Urology
Retractor, Brain	Cns/Neurology
Retractor, Cardiac	Cardiovascular
Retractor, ENT (Thoracic)	Ear/Nose/Throat
Retractor, Fan-Type, Laparoscopy	Surgery
Retractor, Fiberoptic	Gastroenterology/Urology
Retractor, Laminectomy	Surgery
Retractor, Manual	Cns/Neurology
Retractor, Mastoid	Ear/Nose/Throat
Retractor, Ophthalmic	Ophthalmology
Retractor, Orbital	Surgery
Retractor, Other	Surgery
Retractor, Rectal	Gastroenterology/Urology
Retractor, Rib	Orthopedics
Retractor, Self-Retaining	Gastroenterology/Urology
Retractor, Self-Retaining, Neurology	Cns/Neurology
Retractor, Surgical	Surgery
Retractor, Vaginal	Obstetrics/Gynecology
Retractor, Vessel	Cardiovascular
Rongeur, Manual, Neurosurgical	Cns/Neurology
Rongeur, Other	Surgery
Rongeur, Rib	Orthopedics
Saw, Bone Cutting	Orthopedics
Saw, Manual, And Accessories	Surgery
Scissors, Bandage/Gauze/Plaster	General
Scissors, Cardiovascular	Cardiovascular
Scissors, Corneal	Ophthalmology
Scissors, Enucleation	Ophthalmology
Scissors, General Dissecting	General
Scissors, Gynecological	Obstetrics/Gynecology
Scissors, Iris	Ophthalmology
Scissors, Nasal	Ear/Nose/Throat
Scissors, Neurosurgical (Dura)	Cns/Neurology
Scissors, Ophthalmic	Ophthalmology
Scissors, Orthopedic	Orthopedics
Scissors, Pediatric	General
Scissors, Plastic Surgery (Dissecting)	Surgery
Scissors, Rectal	Gastroenterology/Urology
Scissors, Suture	Surgery
Scissors, Tenotomy	Ophthalmology
Scissors, Thoracic	Cardiovascular
Scissors, Wire Cutting, ENT	Ear/Nose/Throat
Service, Maintenance/Repair	General
Sleeve, Trocar	Surgery
Snare, Endoscopic	Surgery
Snare, Polyp	Surgery
Snare, Surgical	Surgery
Snare, Tonsil	Ear/Nose/Throat
Speculum, Ear	Ear/Nose/Throat
Speculum, Nasal	Ear/Nose/Throat
Speculum, Ophthalmic	Ophthalmology
Speculum, Other	General
Speculum, Rectal	Gastroenterology/Urology
Speculum, Vaginal, Metal	Obstetrics/Gynecology
Stand, Operating Room Instrument (Mayo)	Surgery
Stimulator, External, Neuromuscular, Functional	Physical Med
Stimulator, Muscle, Diagnostic	Physical Med
Stimulator, Muscle, Electrical-Powered (EMS)	Physical Med
Stimulator, Nerve, Transcutaneous (Pain Relief, TENS)	Cns/Neurology
Stimulator, Neurological	Surgery
Stimulator, Neuromuscular, External Functional	Cns/Neurology
Stimulator, Ultrasound, Muscle	Physical Med
Strap, Electrode	General
Surgical Instrument, Cardiovascular	Cardiovascular
Surgical Instrument, Non-Powered, Neurosurgical	Cns/Neurology
Table, Examination/Treatment	General
Table, Instrument, Surgical	Surgery
Table, Obstetrical, Manual	Obstetrics/Gynecology
Table, Other	General
Table, Surgical, Manual	General
Table, Surgical, Orthopedic	Orthopedics
Table, Urological (Cystological)	Gastroenterology/Urology
Tenaculum, Thyroid	Gastroenterology/Urology
Tenaculum, Uterine	Obstetrics/Gynecology
Tester, Electrode	General
Transducer, Ultrasonic	Cardiovascular
Treadmill, Mechanical	Physical Med
Trocar, Abdominal	Gastroenterology/Urology
Trocar, Gallbladder	Gastroenterology/Urology
Trocar, Laryngeal	Ear/Nose/Throat
Vectorcardiograph	Cardiovascular
Warmer, Endoscope	Surgery

ELRA INDUSTRIES, INC. 800-654-3066 / 513-868-6228
550 South Erie Highway,
Hamilton, OH 45011
FDA Number: n/a
E-mail: elraind@one.net Fax: 513-863-6555
Web site: www.elra.com

ELRA INDUSTRIES, INC. 800-654-3066 *(cont'd)*
Medical Products Sales Volume: $500,000
Annual Revenue: $0-$1 Million
Ownership: Private
Produces/Sells CE-marked Devices: N
Federal Procurement Eligibility: Small Business
Distribution: Manufacturer Direct, Manufacturer Through Manufacturer Reps, Importer
General Admin.: Eldon Smith/President
  Bag, Plastic   General

ELSOHLY LABS, INC. 662-236-2609
5 Industrial Park Dr., Oxford, MS 38655
FDA Number: 2319772   *Fax:* 662-234-0253
E-mail: elimae@watervalley.net
Web site: www.elsohly.com
Year Founded: 1985
Total Employees: 15
Ownership: Private
Produces/Sells CE-marked Devices: N
Distribution: Manufacturer Direct
  Control, Drug Mixture   Toxicology
  Control, Urinalysis (Assayed And Unassayed)   Chemistry

ELVEX CORPORATION 800-888-6582
13 Trowbridge Dr., Bethel, CT 06801 203-743-2488
FDA Number: n/a   *Fax:* 203-791-2278
E-mail: info@elvex.com
Web site: www.elvex.com
Annual Revenue: $5-$10 Million
Total Employees: 13   *Marketing Staff:* 2   *Sales Staff:* 20
Ownership: Private
Produces/Sells CE-marked Devices: Y
Federal Procurement Eligibility: Small Business
Distribution: Manufacturer Through Distributor, Manufacturer Through Manufacturer Reps
General Admin.: Roland Westerdal/President
Mktg./Adv.: Bob Marczak/Director National Accounts
    Bob Maczak/Manager Contract Sales
    Fred Ravetto/Senior Vice President International & National Sales
Finance: Ms. Leslie Hegedus/Financial Executive
  Goggles, Protective, Eye   Ophthalmology
  Safety Equipment, Laboratory   Chemistry

ELWYN INDUSTRIES PRODUCTS. Elwyn Industrie
2047 Bridgewater Rd., Aston, PA 19014 610-364-3551
FDA Number: 2522836
Ownership: Private
Produces/Sells CE-marked Devices: N
  Bandage, Cast   Physical Med

ELYRIA PLASTIC PRODUCTS 440-322-8577
710 Taylor St., Elyria, OH 44035
FDA Number: 3003414634   *Fax:* 440-322-7979
E-mail: jkastler@elyriapp.com
Web site: www.elyriapp.com
Ownership: Private
Produces/Sells CE-marked Devices: N
General Admin.: James Kastler/Owner
    James Reichlin/Owner
  Walker, Mechanical   Physical Med

EM DIAGNOSTIC SYSTEMS INC.
See Emd Chemicals Inc.

EM-PROBE INC. 360-297-6858
4110 Ne Carver Dr., Port Gamble, WA 98364
FDA Number: 3004450978
Ownership: Private
Produces/Sells CE-marked Devices: N
  Lamp, Non-heating, For Adjunctive Use In Pain Therapy   Physical Med

EMAGEON INC. 262-369-3379
1200 Corporate Dr, Suite 200, Birmingham, AL 35242
FDA Number: 2320709
Web site: www.emageon.com
Ownership: Private
Produces/Sells CE-marked Devices: N
  Device, Storage, Image, Digital   Radiology
  Image Processing System   Radiology

EMBASSY CREATIONS, INC. 800-367-3341
122 Manton Avenue, Box L4, 401-273-9389
Providence, RI 02909
FDA Number: 2518603
E-mail: info@embassycreations.com   *Fax:* 800-683-3186
Web site: www.embassycreations.com
Annual Revenue: $0-$1 Million
Total Employees: 47

EMBASSY CREATIONS, INC. 800-367-3341 *(cont'd)*
Ownership: Private
Produces/Sells CE-marked Devices: N
Federal Procurement Eligibility: Small Business
Distribution: Manufacturer Through Distributor
General Admin.: Joe Caruso/President
Mktg./Adv.: Joe Caruso/Vice President Marketing & Sales
Production: Joe Caruso/Vice President Manufacturing
  Frame, Spectacle (Eyeglasses)   Ophthalmology

EMBLA SYSTEMS, INC. 716-691-0718
55 Pineview Dr., Suite 100, Buffalo, NY 14228
FDA Number: 3004361429
Ownership: Private
Produces/Sells CE-marked Devices: N
  Amplifier, Physiological Signal   Cns/Neurology
  Electroencephalograph   Cns/Neurology
  Monitor, Apnea   General

EMBO-OPTICS, LLC. 887-885-6400
100 cumming center 326-B, Beverly, MA 01915
FDA Number: 3004409134   *Fax:* 978-921-6404
E-mail: joel@embo-optics.com
Web site: www.embo-optics.com
Medical Products Sales Volume: $270,000
Year Founded: 1997
Total Employees: 3
Ownership: Private
Produces/Sells CE-marked Devices: N
Federal Procurement Eligibility: Small Business
Distribution: Manufacturer Direct, Manufacturer Through Distributor, Manufacturer Through Manufacturer Reps
Research: Mr. Joel Rodriguez/Managing Partner
  Accessories, Light, Surgical   Surgery
  Ambulance   General
  Ambulance, Air   General
  Balloon, Angioplasty, Coronary, Heated   Cardiovascular
  Catheter, Angioplasty, Coronary, Ultrasonic   Cardiovascular
  Catheter, Conduction, Anesthesia   Anesthesiology
  Catheter, Imaging, Ultrasonic   Radiology
  Catheter, Intravascular, Therapeutic, Long-term Greater Than 30 Days   General
  Drill, Oral Surgery   Dental And Oral

EMBRACE HEALTHCARE LLC (800) 255-3311
100 Factory Street, Suite C3, Nashua, NH 03060 603-578-1320
FDA Number: 3002680644   *Fax:* (603) 578-1322
Ownership: Private
Produces/Sells CE-marked Devices: N
  Accessories, Apparel, Surgical   Surgery

EMBRELLA CARDIOVASCULAR, INC. 610-783-1100
880 E. Swedesford Road, Suite 220, Wayne, PA 19087
FDA Number: n/a   *Fax:* 484-831-5401
Ownership: Private
Produces/Sells CE-marked Devices: N
General Admin.: Mr. Jeffrey O'Donnell/Chairman, Chief Executive Officer
    Mr. Jeffrey Carpenter/Chief Scientific Officer
Research: Ms. Carol Burns/Vice President Product Development
  Catheter, Carotid, Temporary, For Embolization Capture   Cardiovascular

EMBRYOTECH LABORATORIES, INC. 800-673-7500
323 Andover St., Wilmington, MA 01887-1035 978-658-4600
FDA Number: 1225480   *Fax:* 978-658-5777
E-mail: edorman@embryotech.com
Web site: www.embryotech.com
Medical Products Sales Volume: $1,100,000
Annual Revenue: $0-$1 Million
Year Founded: 1994
Total Employees: 10   *Sales Staff:* 1
Ownership: Private
Produces/Sells CE-marked Devices: N
Federal Procurement Eligibility: Small Business
Distribution: Manufacturer Through Distributor
General Admin.: Eric V. Dorman/President
  Device, Semen Analysis   Obstetrics/Gynecology
  Equipment, In Vitro Fertilization/Embryo Transfer   Obstetrics/Gynecology
  Fertility Diagnostic Device   Obstetrics/Gynecology
  Test, Cervical Mucous Penetration   Pathology
  Test, Fertility Monitoring   Obstetrics/Gynecology

EMD ASSOCIATES, INC.
See Benchmark Electronics, Inc.

EMD CHEMICALS INC. 800-222-0342
480 S. Democrat Road, Gibbstown, NJ 08027 856-423-6300
FDA Number: 9610140   *Fax:* 856-423-4389
E-mail: info@emdchemicals.com
Web site: www.emdchemicals.com
Medical Products Sales Volume: $346,870,000

EMD CHEMICALS INC. 800-222-0342 (cont'd)

Annual Revenue: $100-$500 Million
Year Founded: 1970
Total Employees: 700　　Marketing Staff: 21　　Sales Staff: 34
Ownership: Merck KGaA, Darmstadt, Germany
Quality System Registration Information: ISO9001
Produces/Sells CE-marked Devices: N
Distribution: Manufacturer Direct, Manufacturer Through Distributor, OEM, Service Direct, Exclusive Distributor, Exporter
General Admin.: Doug Brown/President
Mktg./Adv.: Gene Desotelle/Director Product Development
　　　Mike Frangiosa/Manager Contract Sales
　　　Ingolf Smrke/Manager Marketing Services
　　　Rebecca Vaiarelli/Marketing Specialist
　　　Bill Molnar/Vice President Marketing
　　　Jim Mazziotta/Vice President Sales
Production: Anna Bentley/Director Regulatory Affairs
　　　Robert Jones/Manager Manufacturing
Research: Norman Jordan/Manager Research & Development
Finance: Kathie Lamb/Chief Financial Officer

Culture Media, Antimicrobial Susceptibility Test	Microbiology
Disc, Strip And Reagent, Microorganism Differentiation	Microbiology
Reagent, Iron (Test System)	Chemistry
Stain, Hematoxylin	Pathology
Stain, Hematoxylin, Harris's	Pathology
Stain, Microbiological	Microbiology
Stain, Papanicolau	Pathology
Stainer, Slide, Hematology	Hematology

EMED TECHNOLOGIES 866-363-3669
76 Blanchard Road, Burlington, MA 01803-5125 781-862-0000

FDA Number: 1224848
E-mail: info03@emed.com　　　　Fax: 781-272-4333
Web site: www.emed.com
Medical Products Sales Volume: $15,000,000
Annual Revenue: $25-$50 Million
Year Founded: 1992
Total Employees: 135　　Marketing Staff: 1　　Sales Staff: 15
Ownership: Private
Federal Procurement Eligibility: Small Business
Distribution: Manufacturer Direct, OEM, Service Direct
General Admin.: Mark Smith/Chief Executive Officer
Mktg./Adv.: Johnathan Bis/Manager International & National Sales
　　　Kristen Kohler/Manager Marketing
　　　Dave Mahoney/Vice President Sales
Production: Barbara Dumery/Senior Product Manager
Research: Johnathan Go/Vice President Engineering & Development

Television System, Slow Scan	Radiology
Transmitter, Image & Data, Radiographic	Radiology

EMEPE INTERNATIONAL, INC. 813-994-9690
18108 Sugar Brooke Drive, Tampa, FL 33647

FDA Number: n/a　　　　Fax: 813-994-9691
E-mail: emepeint@aol.com
Web site: www.emepe.us
Medical Products Sales Volume: $800,000
Annual Revenue: $0-$1 Million
Year Founded: 1992
Total Employees: 3　　Marketing Staff: 1　　Sales Staff: 1
Ownership: Private
Produces/Sells CE-marked Devices: N
Federal Procurement Eligibility: Small Business, Minority Owned
Distribution: Exporter
General Admin.: Jose Moronta/Owner, Chief Executive Officer

Compressor, Air, Portable	Anesthesiology
Cylinder, Compressed Gas, With Valve	Anesthesiology
Flowmeter, Gas (Oxygen), Calibrated	Anesthesiology
Humidifier, Respiratory Gas, (Direct Patient Interface)	Anesthesiology
Mask, Gas, Anesthesia	Anesthesiology
Pump, Vacuum, Central	Anesthesiology
Regulator, Pressure, Gas Cylinder	Anesthesiology
Regulator, Suction, Surgical	General
Regulator, Suction, Thoracic	Anesthesiology
Resuscitator, Emergency Oxygen	Dental And Oral
System, Pipeline, Gas	General

EMERALD MEDICAL PRODUCTS CORP. 206-781-9450
1338 Shark Reef Road, Lopez Island, WA 98107

FDA Number: n/a　　　　Fax: 206-781-4646
E-mail: emerald@alert2.com
Web site: http://emeraldmedicalproducts.com
Year Founded: 1990
Ownership: Private
Produces/Sells CE-marked Devices: N
Federal Procurement Eligibility: Small Business
Distribution: Manufacturer Direct

Cushion, Foot	Orthopedics

EMERALD MEDICAL PRODUCTS CORP. 206-781-9450 (cont'd)

General Medical Device	General

EMERGE MEDICAL INC. 866-553-0376
1530 Blake Street, Suite 204, Denver, CO 80202

FDA Number: 3008500488　　　　Fax: 800-698-1440
E-mail: info@emergemedical.com
Ownership: Private
Produces/Sells CE-marked Devices: N

Bit, Drill	Orthopedics
Instrument, Manual, General Surgical	Surgery
Screw, Fixation, Bone	Orthopedics

EMERGENCIA 2000, INC. 757-224-0177
8578 Nw 23rd St, Miami, FL 33122

FDA Number: 3003291342
Ownership: Private
Produces/Sells CE-marked Devices: N

Armrest, Wheelchair	Physical Med
Stretcher, Wheeled (Mobile)	General

EMERGENCY FILTRATION PRODUCTS, INC.

See Nano Mask Inc.

EMERGENCY FIRST AID PRODUCTS (USA), INC. 518-562-9911
53 Area Development Dr.,, Unit B, Plattsburgh, NY 12901

FDA Number: 1319630
Ownership: Private
Produces/Sells CE-marked Devices: N

Kit, First Aid	Surgery

EMERGENCY MEDICAL INTERNATIONAL 305-362-6050
6065 N.W. 167th St., #B-18, Miami, FL 33015-4315

FDA Number: 9010636　　　　Fax: 305-362-6052
E-mail: emi@emi-medical.com
Web site: www.emi-medical.com
Medical Products Sales Volume: $800,000
Annual Revenue: $1-$5 Million
Year Founded: 1981
Total Employees: 3　　Marketing Staff: 1　　Sales Staff: 2
Ownership: Private
Quality System Registration Information: ISO9000; ISO9001; ISO9002
Produces/Sells CE-marked Devices: Y
Federal Procurement Eligibility: Small Business, Minority Owned
Distribution: Manufacturer Direct, Manufacturer Through Distributor, Service Direct, Importer, Exporter
General Admin.: Mr. Juan A. Manfredi/President
　　　Mrs. Elsa Manfredi/Vice President
　　　Ms. Mercedes Alvarez/Vice President, General Manager

Ambulance	General
Radiographic Unit, Digital Subtraction Angiographic (DSA)	Radiology
Radiographic/Fluoroscopic Unit, Angiographic	Radiology
Ventilator, Continuous (Respirator)	Anesthesiology

EMERGENCY MEDICAL SUPPLY, INC. 502-955-9233
238 Saltwell Rd., P.o.. Box 99, Shepherdsville, KY 40165

FDA Number: 1531016
Ownership: Private
Produces/Sells CE-marked Devices: N

Orthosis, Cervical	Physical Med
Orthosis, Cervical-Thoracic, Rigid	Physical Med

EMERGENCY MEDICAL SYSTEMS 214-704-7077
PO Box 111034, Carrollton, TX 75011

FDA Number: 1649984　　　　Fax: 972-231-9587
E-mail: monty.neel@cityofcarrollton.com
Ownership: Private
Produces/Sells CE-marked Devices: N
Mktg./Adv.: Mr. Monty Neel/Vice President, General Manager Marketing

Nebulizer, Medicinal, Non-Ventilatory (Atomizer)	Anesthesiology

EMERGENCY ONE

See E-One

EMERGENCY POWER ENGINEERING

See Mge Ups Sytems, Inc.

EMERGENCY PRODUCTS AND RESEARCH 305-304-6933
890 West Main Street, Kent, OH 44240

FDA Number: 3002754225　　　　Fax: 330-673-4940
E-mail: info@epandr.com
Ownership: Private
Produces/Sells CE-marked Devices: N

Orthosis, Cervical-Thoracic, Rigid	Physical Med
Restraint, Protective (Body)	General
Splint, Extermity, Non-inflatable, External, Non-sterile	Surgery
Splint, Traction	Orthopedics
Stretcher, Hand-Carried	General

EMERGENCY VEHICLES, INC. 800-848-6652
705 13th street, Lake Park, FL 33403-2303 561-848-6652
FDA Number: n/a *Fax:* 561-848-6658
E-mail: evi@evi-fl.com
Web site: www.evi-fl.com
Annual Revenue: $5-$10 Million
Year Founded: 1971
Total Employees: 28 *Sales Staff:* 3
Ownership: Private
Produces/Sells CE-marked Devices: N
Federal Procurement Eligibility: Small Business, Female Owned
Distribution: Manufacturer Direct, Manufacturer Through Manufacturer Reps
General Admin.: Mr. Ernst R. Temme/President
    Mr. Ernst R. Temme/Vice President, General Manager
Mktg./Adv.: Ms. Jo Anne Antonacci/Manager Advertising
    Mr. Dave M. Taliercio/Vice President Sales
  Rescue Equipment General

EMERGING HEALTHCARE SOLUTIONS, INC. 713-821-1486
5847 San Felipe, Suite 1700, Houston, TX 77057
FDA Number: n/a
E-mail: info@emerginghealthcaresolutionsinc.com
Ownership: Private
Produces/Sells CE-marked Devices: N

EMERGING HEALTHCARE SOLUTIONS, LLC 770-923-7391
1285 Denmark Dr. SW, Lilburn, GA 30047
FDA Number: n/a *Fax:* 770-923-6212
E-mail: sales@emerginghcs.com
Web site: http://emerginghcs.com
Ownership: Public
Stock Symbol: EHSI
Produces/Sells CE-marked Devices: N

EMKINETICS, INC. 650-384-0008
583 Division St., Suite A, Campbell,, CA 95008
FDA Number: n/a *Fax:* 866-596-5087
Web site: www.emkinetics.com
Ownership: Private
Produces/Sells CE-marked Devices: N

EMO
  See Invensys Process Systems

EMPI 800.328.2536
599 Cardigan Road, St. Paul, MN 55126-4099 651-415-9000
FDA Number: 1721293
E-mail: support@empi.com
Web site: http://www.empi.com
Ownership: DJO INCORPORATED
Stock Symbol: DJO
Traded On: NYSE
Produces/Sells CE-marked Devices: N
  Biofeedback Device Cns/Neurology
  Exerciser, Non-Measuring Physical Med
  Iontophoresis Device, Dental Dental And Oral
  Orthosis, Limb Brace Physical Med
  Stimulator, Muscle, Electrical-Powered (EMS) Physical Med
  Stimulator, Nerve, Transcutaneous (Pain Relief, TENS) Cns/Neurology
  Stimulator, Neuromuscular, External Functional Cns/Neurology

EMPI CANADA 800-463-3674
16773 Hymus Blvd., 514-426-4444
Kirkland, QUE H9H-3 Canada
FDA Number: n/a *Fax:* 514-426-4333
E-mail: info@empi.ca
Web site: www.empi.ca
Year Founded: 1980
Total Employees: 250
Ownership: Private
Produces/Sells CE-marked Devices: N
Distribution: Exclusive Distributor

EMPI, INC. 800-328-2536
599 Cardigan Rd., St. Paul, MN 55126-4099 651-415-9000
FDA Number: 2182686 *Fax:* 800-450-3593
E-mail: support@empi.com
Web site: www.empi.com
Medical Products Sales Volume: $61,300,000
Annual Revenue: $50-$100 Million
Total Employees: 514 *Marketing Staff:* 15 *Sales Staff:* 93
Ownership: DJO INCORPORATED
Quality System Registration Information: ISO9000
Produces/Sells CE-marked Devices: Y
Federal Procurement Eligibility: Small Business
Distribution: Manufacturer Direct, Manufacturer Through Manufacturer Reps
General Admin.: Barb Hutto/Director Human Resources
    Phillip Vierling/President, Chief Executive Officer

EMPI, INC. 800-328-2536 *(cont'd)*
Mktg./Adv.: Rick Rides/Director International Marketing & Sales
    Priscilla Gunderson/Manager Marketing
Production: Rob Clapp/Vice President Manufacturing
  Electrode, Neuromuscular Stimulator Cns/Neurology
  Exerciser, Passive, Non-Measuring (CPM Machine) Physical Med
  Stimulator, Electrical, For Incontinence Gastroenterology/Urology
  Stimulator, Incontinence (Non-Implantable), Electrical Gastroenterology/Urology
  Stimulator, Nerve, Transcutaneous (Pain Relief, TENS) Cns/Neurology
  Stimulator, Neuromuscular, External Functional Cns/Neurology

EMPIRIC SYSTEMS, LLC 866-367-4742
3800 Paramount Pkwy, Suite 130, Morrisville, NC 27560
FDA Number: n/a
Web site: www.fujifilmusa.com
Ownership: Fujifilm Medical Systems Usa, Inc.
Produces/Sells CE-marked Devices: N
  Device, Storage, Image, Digital Radiology
  System, Communication, Image, Digital Radiology

EMPLEX SYSTEMS, INC. 800-265-1775
2045 Midland Ave., Toronto, ON MIP 3E2 Canada 416-291-8085
FDA Number: n/a *Fax:* 416-298-4328
E-mail: info@plexpack.com
Web site: www.emplex.com
Year Founded: 1973
Total Employees: 30 *Marketing Staff:* 1 *Sales Staff:* 2
Ownership: Private
Produces/Sells CE-marked Devices: Y
Distribution: OEM

EMPORIUM SPECIALTIES CO., INC. 814-647-8661
10 Foster Avenue, Austin, PA 16720
FDA Number: n/a *Fax:* 814-647-5536
E-mail: info@empspec.com
Web site: www.empspec.com
Medical Products Sales Volume: $1,500,000
Annual Revenue: $5-$10 Million
Year Founded: 1947
Total Employees: 50 *Marketing Staff:* 1 *Sales Staff:* 4
Ownership: Private
Quality System Registration Information: ISO9002
Produces/Sells CE-marked Devices: N
Federal Procurement Eligibility: Small Business, GSA Contract
Distribution: Manufacturer Direct, OEM, Service Direct
General Admin.: Marvin Deupree/President, Chief Executive Officer
Mktg./Adv.: Kris Rees/Director Marketing
    Kris Rees/Manager International & National Sales
Production: B. D. Fowler/Director Quality Assurance
  Pliers, Orthodontic Dental And Oral
  Wrench Orthopedics

EMPOWER, INC.
  See Medimaging Tecnology, Inc.

EMR TOOLS, LLC 602-579-2694
4814 W. Laurel Ln., Glendale, AZ 85304
FDA Number: 3005482741
Ownership: Private
Produces/Sells CE-marked Devices: N
  Accessories, Surgical Camera Surgery

EMS MEDICAL INC.
  See Vmed Technology, Inc. (Formerly Ems Products, Inc.)

EMS PACIFIC, INC. 800-575-5093
4480 Enterprise St., Unit D, Fremont, CA 94538 510-668-0405
FDA Number: n/a *Fax:* 510-668-1012
E-mail: info@emspacific.com
Web site: www.emspacific.com
Annual Revenue: $0-$1 Million
Ownership: Private
Produces/Sells CE-marked Devices: N
Federal Procurement Eligibility: Small Business, Minority Owned, Female Owned
Distribution: Manufacturer Direct, Manufacturer Through Manufacturer Reps, OEM
General Admin.: Ely Soriano/President
Mktg./Adv.: Edward Soriano/Manager Market Research
Production: Oscar Macaranas/Director Quality Assurance
Finance: Mila Soriano/Controller
  Dispenser, Fluid General
  Dispenser, Liquid, Laboratory Chemistry
  Dispenser, Other General
  Pump, Laboratory Chemistry

EMSENSE INC. 866-574-7014
150 Spear St., Suite 200, San Francisco, CA 94105
FDA Number: n/a
E-mail: Info@emsense.com
Web site: http://www.emsense.com
Year Founded: 2004

EMSENSE INC. 866-574-7014 (cont'd)
Ownership: Private
Produces/Sells CE-marked Devices: N
General Admin.: Mr. Michael Lee/Chief Scientific Officer
   Mr. Hans Lee/Chief Technology Officer
   Mr. Keith Winter/President, Chief Executive Officer
Mktg./Adv.: Mr. Mark Mallardi/Senior Vice President Marketing & Sales
Production: Mr. Kirk Henderson/Vice President Operations
Finance: Mr. Jeff Kirkley/Vice President Finance

EMT MEDICAL CO., INC. 800-473-5333
PO Box 294ÿÿÿÿÿÿÿÿÿÿÿÿÿÿÿÿÿÿÿÿÿÿÿÿÿÿÿÿÿÿÿ, 360-394-4600
POULSBO, WA 92691
FDA Number: 2028189   *Fax:* 949-452-0029
E-mail: emtmedicalco@cs.com
Web site: www.emtmedicalco.com
Medical Products Sales Volume: $300,000
Annual Revenue: $0-$1 Million
Year Founded: 1990
Total Employees: 3   *Marketing Staff:* 1
Ownership: Private
Produces/Sells CE-marked Devices: Y
Federal Procurement Eligibility: Small Business
Distribution: Manufacturer Direct
General Admin.: Brian Burns/President, Chief Executive Officer

Cover, Probe, Transducer	Surgery

EMTECH LABORATORIES, INC. 1-800-336-5719
7745 Garland Circle, Roanoke, VA 24019 540-265-9156
FDA Number: n/a   *Fax:* 540-265-9164
E-mail: emtech@emtech-labs.com
Web site: www.emtech-labs.com
Annual Revenue: $10-$25 Million
Total Employees: 50   *Marketing Staff:* 3   *Sales Staff:* 3
Ownership: Private
Produces/Sells CE-marked Devices: N
Federal Procurement Eligibility: Small Business
Distribution: Manufacturer Direct, Manufacturer Through Manufacturer Reps
General Admin.: Moses Nakhley/President, Chief Executive Officer
Production: Kim Hodges/Manager Customer Services

Mold, Middle Ear	Ear/Nose/Throat

ENABLE MEDICAL CORP.
See ATRICURE, INC.

ENABLING TECHNOLOGIES COMPANY 800-7773687
1601 N.E. Braille Pl., Jensen Beach, FL 34957 772-225-3687
FDA Number: n/a   *Fax:* 772-225-3299
E-mail: info@brailler.com
Web site: www.brailler.com
Annual Revenue: $1-$5 Million
Total Employees: 40   *Marketing Staff:* 5   *Sales Staff:* 4
Ownership: Private
Produces/Sells CE-marked Devices: Y
Federal Procurement Eligibility: Small Business
Distribution: Manufacturer Direct, Manufacturer Through Distributor
General Admin.: Tony Schenk/President
Mktg./Adv.: Greg Schenk/Manager International Marketing & Sales

Vision Aid, Braille	General

ENCISION INC. 303-444-2600
6797 Winchester Circle, Boulder, CO 80301
FDA Number: 1722040   *Fax:* 303-444-2693
E-mail: feedback@encision.com
Web site: www.encision.com
Medical Products Sales Volume: $11,000,000
Annual Revenue: $10-$25 Million
Year Founded: 1991
Total Employees: 46   *Marketing Staff:* 2   *Sales Staff:* 9
Ownership: Public
Stock Symbol: ECI
Traded On: AMEX
Produces/Sells CE-marked Devices: Y
Federal Procurement Eligibility: Small Business
Distribution: Manufacturer Direct, Manufacturer Through Distributor, Manufacturer Through Manufacturer Reps, Exporter
General Admin.: Mr. Fred Perner/Chief Executive Officer
Mktg./Adv.: Roger Odell/Vice President Business Development
Production: Judith King/Director Quality Assurance & Regulatory Affairs
   Richard Smoot/Vice President Operations
Finance: Marcia McHaffie/Corporate Controller
IS: David Newton/Vice President Technology

Accessories, Cleaning Brushes (For Endoscope)	Gastroenterology/Urology
Electrode, Electrosurgery, Laparoscopic	Surgery
Electrosurgical Equipment, General Purpose	Surgery
Instrument, Electrosurgical, Field Focused	Cns/Neurology

ENCOLL CORP. 510-795-8581
4576 Enterprise Street, Fremont, CA 94538
FDA Number: 3004117927
Ownership: Private
Produces/Sells CE-marked Devices: N

ENCOMPAS UNLIMITED, INC. 800-825-7701
2219 Whitfield Park Dr,, Sarasota, FL 34243 941-751-3385
FDA Number: 1056035   *Fax:* 941-727-7986
E-mail: encompas2@aol.com
Medical Products Sales Volume: $2,000,000
Annual Revenue: $1-$5 Million
Year Founded: 1979
Total Employees: 6   *Sales Staff:* 1
Ownership: Private
Produces/Sells CE-marked Devices: Y
Federal Procurement Eligibility: Small Business, Female Owned
Distribution: Manufacturer Direct, Exporter
General Admin.: Mary E. Flynn/President, Chief Executive Officer
   Marybeth Flynn/Vice President, General Manager
Mktg./Adv.: Marybeth Flynn/Vice President Marketing & Sales

Accessories, Bite Blocks (For Endoscope)	Gastroenterology/Urology
Accessories, Cleaning, Endoscopic	Gastroenterology/Urology
Cabinet, Storage, Endoscope	Gastroenterology/Urology
Cart, Equipment, Video	General
Cleaner, Ultrasonic, Medical Instrument	General
Container, Specimen, All Types	General
Container, Specimen, Laparoscopic	Surgery
Container, Sterilization (Tray)	General
Dilator, Other	Surgery
Endoscope	Gastroenterology/Urology
Pump, Aspiration, Portable	Anesthesiology
Rack, Surgical Instrument	Surgery
Sponge, Other	General
Sterilizer/Washer, Endoscope	General
Support, Patient Position	Anesthesiology

ENCOMPASS MEDICAL 800-826-4490
16415 Addison Road, Suite 660, 972-732-7694
Addison, TX 75001
FDA Number: n/a   *Fax:* 972-732-7842
E-mail: info@encompassmed.net
Web site: www.encompassgroup.net
Ownership: Private
Quality System Registration Information: ISO9001
Produces/Sells CE-marked Devices: N
Federal Procurement Eligibility: Small Business
Distribution: Manufacturer Direct, Manufacturer Through Distributor

Box, Glove	Microbiology
Gown, Patient	Surgery

ENCOMPASS THERAPEUTIC SUPPORT 818-546-2466
SYSTEMS
100 E. Corson St, Suite 310, Pasadena, CA 91103
FDA Number: 2032648
Ownership: Private
Produces/Sells CE-marked Devices: N

Cover, Mattress	General
Cushion, Flotation	Physical Med
Cushion, Table, Surgical	Surgery
Cushion, Wheelchair (Pad)	Physical Med
Mattress, Air Flotation	General
Protector, Skin Pressure	General

ENCON MANUFACTURING CO.
See Encon Safety Products

ENCON SAFETY PRODUCTS 800-283-6266
6825 West Sam Houston Pkwy. N., 713-466-1449
Houston, TX 77041
FDA Number: n/a   *Fax:* 713-466-1703
E-mail: customerservice@EnconSafety.com
Web site: www.enconsafety.com
Year Founded: 1964
Ownership: HAGEMEYER
Quality System Registration Information: ISO9001
Produces/Sells CE-marked Devices: N
Distribution: Manufacturer Through Distributor

Clothing, Protective	General
Eyeglasses, Safety	Ophthalmology
Fountain, Eye Wash	Chemistry
Goggles, Protective, Eye	Ophthalmology
Protector, Hearing (Insert)	Ear/Nose/Throat
Rescue Equipment	General
Shower, Emergency	Chemistry

ENCORE MEDICAL CORPORATION
See DJO Surgical

ENCORE ORTHOPEDICS
See DJO Surgical

ENCORE PLASTICS CORPORATION   419-626-8000
725 Water Street, Cambridge, OH 43725
FDA Number: 1525927
Surgical, Razor   Surgery

ENCORE, INC.   800-221-6603
7696 15th STREET EAST, SARASOTA, FL 34243   941-359-3599
FDA Number: 1527982   *Fax:* 941-359-3509
E-mail: impoaid@earthlink.net
Medical Products Sales Volume: $1,200,000
Annual Revenue: $1-$5 Million
Year Founded: 1987
Total Employees: 16   *Marketing Staff:* 2   *Sales Staff:* 5
Ownership: Private
Produces/Sells CE-marked Devices: Y
Federal Procurement Eligibility: Small Business
Distribution: Manufacturer Direct, Exclusive Distributor
General Admin.: Margaret Bennett/President, Chief Executive Officer
Mktg./Adv.: Kevin Chitwood/Director Marketing
  Impotence Device, Mechanical/Hydraulic   Gastroenterology/Urology

ENCYNOVA
See Car-May

ENDLESS POOLS, INC.   800-233-0741
200 East Dutton Mill Rd., Aston, PA 19014
FDA Number: 2531355   *Fax:* 610-497-5421
E-mail: swim@endlesspools.com
Web site: www.endlesspools.com
Year Founded: 1987
Total Employees: 70
Ownership: Private
Produces/Sells CE-marked Devices: N
Distribution: Manufacturer Direct
  Exerciser, Powered   Anesthesiology

ENDO OPTIKS, INC.   800-756-3636
39 Sycamore Avenue, Little Silver, NJ 07739   732-530-6762
FDA Number: 2247224   *Fax:* 732-530-5344
E-mail: psonntag@endooptiks.com
Web site: www.endo-optiks.com
Medical Products Sales Volume: $600,000
Year Founded: 1991
Total Employees: 4   *Marketing Staff:* 2
Ownership: Private
Produces/Sells CE-marked Devices: Y
Federal Procurement Eligibility: Small Business
Distribution: Manufacturer Direct, Manufacturer Through Distributor, Manufacturer Through Manufacturer Reps, Exporter
General Admin.: Martin Uram/Chief Executive Officer
           Steve Kohn/President
Mktg./Adv.: Paula Ender/Vice President Marketing & Sales
Production: Keith Hertz/Manager Regulatory Affairs
           Gene Boccia/Vice President Manufacturing
Research: Tim Boyce/Vice President Research & Development
  Endoscope, Ophthalmic   Gastroenterology/Urology

ENDO TECHNIC CORP.
See Biolase Technology, Inc.

ENDO-THERAPEUTICS, INC.   888-294-2377
15251 Roosevelt Blvd, Suite #204,   727-524-4100
Clearwater, FL 33760
FDA Number: 1056129   *Fax:* 727-524-4111
E-mail: info@bioceps.com
Web site: www.bioceps.com
Medical Products Sales Volume: $4,600,000
Annual Revenue: $1-$5 Million
Year Founded: 1992
Total Employees: 55   *Marketing Staff:* 2   *Sales Staff:* 10
Ownership: Private
Quality System Registration Information: ISO9001
Produces/Sells CE-marked Devices: Y
Federal Procurement Eligibility: Small Business, Female Owned
Distribution: Manufacturer Through Distributor, Manufacturer Through Manufacturer Reps, OEM, Exporter
General Admin.: Charles T. Hardy/Chief Executive Officer
           Robert Querido/President
Mktg./Adv.: Brett Loggains/Vice President Marketing & Sales
Production: Cindi Noel/Manager Quality Assurance
           Todd Adkisson/Manager Regulatory Affairs
           Debbie Gray/Product Manager
Finance: Tania Cefaratti/Chief Financial Officer
  Accessories, Bite Blocks (For Endoscope)   Gastroenterology/Urology
  Accessories, Cleaning Brushes (For Endoscope)   Gastroenterology/Urology
  Endoscope And Accessories, AC-Powered   Surgery

ENDO-THERAPEUTICS, INC.   888-294-2377 *(cont'd)*
  Forceps, Biopsy   Surgery
  Needle, Endoscopic   Gastroenterology/Urology

ENDOCARE, INC.   (888) 252-6575
9825 Spectrum Dr. Bldg. 3, Austin, TX 78717   (512) 328-2892
FDA Number: 2030653   *Fax:* (512) 439-8303
E-mail: customerservice@endocare.com
Web site: www.endocare.com
Ownership: Public
Stock Symbol: ENDO
Traded On: NASDAQ
Produces/Sells CE-marked Devices: N
General Admin.: Mary Syiek/Vice President
  Cryosurgical Unit   Surgery

ENDOCHOICE INC.   888-682-3636
11810 Wills Rd, Suite 100, Alpharetta, GA 30009
FDA Number: 300759133   *Fax:* 866-567-8218
E-mail: bizdev@endochoice.com
Ownership: Private
Produces/Sells CE-marked Devices: N
General Admin.: Mr. Lou Malice/Chief Operating Officer
          Mr. Brit Young/General Counsel
          Mr. Mark Gilreath/President, Chairman, Chief Executive Officer
Mktg./Adv.: Mr. Will Parks/Vice President Business Development
          Mr. Scott Fraser/Vice President Marketing
          Mr. Gregg Costantino/Vice President Sales
Finance: Mr. Ed Mithcell/Vice President Finance
  Accessories, Cleaning Brushes (For Endoscope)   Gastroenterology/Urology
  Blood And Urine Collection Kit (excludes Hiv Testing)   Chemistry
  Catheter, Biliary   Gastroenterology/Urology
  Endoscope   Gastroenterology/Urology
  Forceps, Biopsy, Non-Electric   Gastroenterology/Urology
  Prosthesis, Esophagus   Surgery

ENDODENT, INC.   626-359-5715
851 Meridian St., Duarte, CA 91010
FDA Number: 2023852   *Fax:* 626-303-1844
Annual Revenue: $1-$5 Million
Total Employees: 30   *Marketing Staff:* 2
Ownership: Private
Quality System Registration Information: ISO9002
Produces/Sells CE-marked Devices: Y
Federal Procurement Eligibility: Small Business
Distribution: Manufacturer Through Distributor, Exporter
General Admin.: Max Lenz/Chief Executive Officer
Mktg./Adv.: Elisabeth Lenz/Executive Vice President Sales
          Nicolas Lenz/Vice President Marketing
Production: Nicolas Lenz/Vice President Manufacturing
Research: Nicolas Lenz/Vice President Research & Development
  Gutta Percha   Dental And Oral
  Point, Paper, Endodontic   Dental And Oral
  Resin, Root Canal Filling   Dental And Oral

ENDOGASTRIC SOLUTIONS, INC.   425-307-9226
8210 154th Ave. Ne, Redmond, WA 98052
FDA Number: 3005473391   *Fax:* 425-307-9201
Web site: http://www.endogastricsolutions.com
Ownership: Private
Produces/Sells CE-marked Devices: N
General Admin.: Mr. Thierry Thaure/President, Chief Executive Officer
 Medical Admin.: Dr. Alex Porter/Medical Director
Mktg./Adv.: Mr. David Schummers/Vice President Marketing
          Mr. Chris Marrus/Vice President Sales
Research: Mr. Rick Romley/Senior Vice President Research & Development
Finance: Mr. Tom Hoster/Chief Financial Officer
  Device, Suturing, Endoscopic   Surgery
  Endoscope   Gastroenterology/Urology
  Endoscopic Suture/plication System, Gastroesophageal Reflux Disease (gerd) Gastroenterology/Urology
  Endoscopic Tissue Approximation Device   Gastroenterology/Urology

ENDOGEN, INC.
See Pierce Biotechnology

ENDOLITE NORTH AMERICA, LTD.   800-548-3534
1031 Byers Road, Miamisburg, OH 45342   937-291-3636
FDA Number: 1058311   *Fax:* 937-291-0789
E-mail: info@endolite.com
Web site: www.endolite.com
Ownership: Private
Produces/Sells CE-marked Devices: N
General Admin.: Mr. Chris Nolan/Vice President
Mktg./Adv.: Ms. Sue Borondy/Marketing & Communications Officer
Production: Ms. Teresa Stratton/Manager Customer Services
  Ankle/Foot, External Limb Component   Physical Med
  Cover, Limb   Physical Med
  Joint, Hip, External Limb Component   Physical Med

ENDOLITE NORTH AMERICA, LTD.   800-548-3534 (cont'd)
Joint, Knee, External Limb Component   Physical Med

ENDOLOGIX, INC.   800-983-2284
11 Studebaker, Irvine, CA 92618   **949-595-7200**
FDA Number: 2031527   *Fax:* 949-457-9561
E-mail: customerservice@endologix.com
Web site: http://www.endologix.com
Annual Revenue: $1-$5 Million
Year Founded: 1992
Ownership: Public
Stock Symbol: ELGX
Traded On: NASDAQ
Produces/Sells CE-marked Devices: Y
Federal Procurement Eligibility: Small Business
Distribution: Manufacturer Through Distributor, Manufacturer Through Manufacturer Reps
General Admin.: John McDermott/President, Chief Executive Officer
Mktg./Adv.: Mr. Joseph DeJohn/Vice President Sales
Production: Mr. Todd Abraham/Vice President Operations
    Mr. Gary Sorsher/Vice President Quality Assurance
    Ms. Janet Fauls/Vice President Regulatory & Clinical Affairs
Finance: Robert J. Krist/Chief Financial Officer
IS: Dr. Stefan Schreck/Vice President Technology
Catheter, Percutaneous	Cardiovascular
Introducer, Catheter	Cardiovascular
System, Treatment, Aortic Aneurysm, Endovascular Graft	Cardiovascular

ENDOPLUS INC.   800-236-5972
431 Lexington Drive, Suite A,   **847-325-5660**
Buffalo Grove, IL 60089
FDA Number: 1423714   *Fax:* 847-325-5661
Web site: http://www.endoplususa.com
Ownership: Private
Produces/Sells CE-marked Devices: N
Laparoscope, Gynecologic	Obstetrics/Gynecology

ENDOPLUS, INC.   847-325-5660
431 Lexington Drive, Suite A, Buffalo Grove, IL 60089
FDA Number: 1423714   *Fax:* 847-325-5661
E-mail: mgudeman@endoplususa.com
Web site: www.endoplususa.com
Medical Products Sales Volume: $1,100,000
Year Founded: 1992
Total Employees: 16
Ownership: Private
Produces/Sells CE-marked Devices: N
Federal Procurement Eligibility: Small Business
Distribution: Manufacturer Through Distributor, OEM
Coagulator, Culdoscopic	Obstetrics/Gynecology
Laparoscope, Gynecologic	Obstetrics/Gynecology

ENDORPHIN CORPORATION   800-940-9844
6901 90th Avenue North,   **727-545-9848**
Pinellas Park, FL 33782
FDA Number: 1066296   *Fax:* 727-546-0613
E-mail: sales@endorphin.net
Web site: www.endorphin.net
Medical Products Sales Volume: $1,000,000
Annual Revenue: $0-$1 Million
Year Founded: 1985
Total Employees: 15   *Marketing Staff:* 1   *Sales Staff:* 3
Ownership: Private
Produces/Sells CE-marked Devices: N
Federal Procurement Eligibility: Small Business
Distribution: Manufacturer Direct, Manufacturer Through Distributor, Manufacturer Through Manufacturer Reps
Mktg./Adv.: Mr. John Primrose/Vice President Sales
Traction Unit, Non-Powered	Orthopedics

ENDOSCOPY SUPPORT SERVICES, INC.   800-349-3636
3 Fallsview Lane, Brewster, NY 10509   **845-277-1700**
FDA Number: n/a   *Fax:* 845-277-7300
E-mail: ess@endoscopy.com
Web site: www.endoscopy.com
Annual Revenue: $1-$5 Million
Year Founded: 1988
Total Employees: 13   *Marketing Staff:* 2   *Sales Staff:* 6
Ownership: Private
Produces/Sells CE-marked Devices: Y
Federal Procurement Eligibility: Small Business
Distribution: Manufacturer Direct, Service Direct, Exporter
General Admin.: James Burns/General Manager
    Robert Savitt/President
    Chris Siddall/Vice President
Mktg./Adv.: James Stewart/Director Marketing & Sales
Camera, Video, Endoscopic	General

ENDOSCOPY SUPPORT SERVICES, INC.   800-349-3636 (cont'd)
Endoscope	Gastroenterology/Urology
Endoscope, Flexible	Gastroenterology/Urology
Endoscope, Rigid	Surgery
Forceps	Orthopedics
Lamp, Surgical, Xenon	Surgery
Light Source, Flash	Chemistry
Service, Repair, Endoscopic	General

ENDOTEC, INC.   973-762-6100
2546 Hansrob Road, Orlando, FL 32804
FDA Number: 2280596
Hip, Hemi-, Femoral, Metal Ball	Orthopedics
Prosthesis, Ankle, Non-Constrained	Orthopedics
Prosthesis, Hip, Constrained, Metal/Polymer	Orthopedics
Prosthesis, Hip, Femoral Component, Cemented, Metal	Orthopedics
Prosthesis, Hip, Hemi-, Acetabular, Metal	Orthopedics
Prosthesis, Knee, Patellofemorotibial, Semi-Constrained	Orthopedics
Prosthesis, Shoulder, Hemi-, Glenoid, Metal	Orthopedics
Prosthesis, Shoulder, Hemi-, Humeral	Orthopedics
Prosthesis, Shoulder, Non-Constrained, Metal/Polymer Cem.	Orthopedics
Screw, Fixation, Bone	Orthopedics

ENDOTRONICS, INC.
See Biovest International, Inc.

ENDOVASCULAR INSTRUMENTS, INC.   360-750-1150
2501 S.E. Columbia Way, Suite 150, Vancouver, WA 98661-8038
FDA Number: 3032561   *Fax:* 360-750-1101
E-mail: tomwiita@aol.com
Medical Products Sales Volume: $750,000
Annual Revenue: $0-$1 Million
Year Founded: 1990
Total Employees: 8
Ownership: Private
Quality System Registration Information: ISO9001
Produces/Sells CE-marked Devices: N
Federal Procurement Eligibility: Small Business
Distribution: Manufacturer Through Distributor
General Admin.: Thomas A. Wiita/President, Chief Executive Officer
Mktg./Adv.: Thomas L. Kelly/Director Product Development
Dilator, Vascular	Cardiovascular
Loop, Endarterectomy	Cardiovascular
Prosthesis, Vascular Graft, Less Than 6mm Diameter	Cardiovascular
Prosthesis, Vascular Graft, Of 6mm And Greater Diameter	Cardiovascular

ENDOVIA MEDICAL, INC.   781-255-1888
150 Kerry Place, Norwood, MA 02062
FDA Number: n/a   *Fax:* 781-255-5525
E-mail: rwc@brockrogers.com
Web site: www.brockrogers.com
Annual Revenue: $0-$1 Million
Year Founded: 1996
Total Employees: 7
Ownership: Private
Produces/Sells CE-marked Devices: N
Federal Procurement Eligibility: Small Business
Distribution: Manufacturer Direct
General Admin.: Robert W. Cunningham/Chief Executive Officer
Research: David L. Brock/Vice President Research & Development
Computer Software	General
Kit, Laparoscopy	Gastroenterology/Urology

ENDURE MEDICAL, INC.   800-736-3873
1455 Ventura Drive, Cumming, GA 30040   **770-888-3755**
FDA Number: 1062308   *Fax:* 770-888-3991
E-mail: info@enduremed.com
Web site: www.enduremed.com
Ownership: Private
Produces/Sells CE-marked Devices: N
Microscope, Operating, AC-Powered, Ophthalmic	Ophthalmology

ENDURO MEDICAL TECHNOLOGY, INC.   860-289-2299
310 Nutmeg Road South, Unit C-5, South Windsor, CT 06074
FDA Number: 84724   *Fax:* 860-289-2008
E-mail: enduromedical@aol.com
Web site: www.enduromedical.com
Year Founded: 2001
Total Employees: 6   *Sales Staff:* 4
Ownership: Private
Produces/Sells CE-marked Devices: N
Federal Procurement Eligibility: Small Business
Distribution: Manufacturer Direct
General Admin.: Kenneth Messier/President
    Patrick Summers/Vice President
Equipment, Therapy, Handicapped/Physical	Physical Med
Walker, Mechanical	Physical Med

ENERGETICS SCIENCE
See Draeger Safety, Inc.

ENERGEX SYSTEMS INC.   201-995-1919
80 Commerce Dr., Allendale, NJ 07401
FDA Number: 3004414423   Fax: 201-995-0095
E-mail: info@energexsystems.com
Web site: www.energexsystems.com
Year Founded: 1999
Ownership: Private
Produces/Sells CE-marked Devices: N

ENERGIZER PERSONAL CARE DIVISION   888-310-4290
300 Nyala Farms Rd., Westport, CT 06880   203-341-4000
FDA Number: 2515444
Web site: www.playtexproductsinc.com
Year Founded: 1932
Ownership: Public
Stock Symbol: PYX
Traded On: NYSE
Produces/Sells CE-marked Devices: N
Distribution: Manufacturer Direct, Manufacturer Through Manufacturer Reps, Service Direct

Bottle, Nursing	Obstetrics/Gynecology
Glove, Patient Examination	General
Lotion, Skin Care	General
Nipple, Feeding	General
Pump, Breast, Non-Powered	Obstetrics/Gynecology
Pump, Breast, Powered	Obstetrics/Gynecology
Ring, Teething, Non-Fluid-Filled	Dental And Oral
Tampon, Menstrual, Scented	Obstetrics/Gynecology
Tampon, Menstrual, Unscented	Obstetrics/Gynecology
Toothbrush, Manual	Dental And Oral

ENERGIZER POWER SYSTEMS
See Moltech Power Systems Inc

ENERGY BEAM SCIENCES, INC.   800-992-9037
29 B Kripes Road, East Granby, CT 06026-9669   860-653-0411
FDA Number: 1225709   Fax: 860-653-0422
E-mail: ebs@ebsciences.com
Web site: www.ebsciences.com
Medical Products Sales Volume: $2,000,000
Annual Revenue: $1-$5 Million
Year Founded: 2000
Total Employees: 17   Marketing Staff: 2   Sales Staff: 5
Ownership: Private
Produces/Sells CE-marked Devices: Y
Federal Procurement Eligibility: Small Business
Distribution: Manufacturer Direct, Manufacturer Through Distributor, Manufacturer Through Manufacturer Reps, OEM
General Admin.: Michael R. Nesta/Managing Director
Mktg./Adv.: Sandy White/Sales Assistant
Production: Paul Kenney/Director Operations
       Mr. Mike Dufraine/Product Manager
       Mr. Phil McArdle/Product Manager
Research: Mike Whittlesey/Director Technology

Desiccator	Chemistry
Microtome, Rotary	Pathology
Unit, Microwave, Transurethral	Gastroenterology/Urology

ENERGY MEDICINE CENTER   781-545-1277
88 Front Street, Suite 31, Scituate, MA 02066
FDA Number: n/a
E-mail: energymedc@yahoo.com
Ownership: Private
Produces/Sells CE-marked Devices: N

Kit, Enema (For Cleaning Purposes)	Gastroenterology/Urology

ENERGY PROSTHETICS   818-675-5083
20438 Acre Street, Winnetka, CA 91306
FDA Number: 3005823146
Ownership: Private
Produces/Sells CE-marked Devices: N

Ankle/Foot, External Limb Component	Physical Med

ENERSYS   610-208-1991
2366 Bernville Road, Reading, PA 19605
FDA Number: n/a   Fax: 610-372-8457
E-mail: special.batteries@uk.enersysinc.com
Web site: www.enersys.com
Medical Products Sales Volume: $1,280,000,000
Year Founded: 1965
Total Employees: 200
Ownership: Public
Stock Symbol: ENS
Traded On: NYSE
Quality System Registration Information: ISO9001
Produces/Sells CE-marked Devices: N
Federal Procurement Eligibility: Small Business, GSA Contract
Distribution: Manufacturer Direct, Manufacturer Through Distributor, Manufacturer Through Manufacturer Reps, OEM, Importer, Exporter

ENERSYS   610-208-1991 (cont'd)
General Admin.: Mr. Richard Zuidema/Executive Vice President
       Mr. John Craig/President, Chairman, Chief Executive Officer
Mktg./Adv.: Todd Sechrist/Vice President Sales
Finance: Mr. Michael Schmidtlein/Chief Financial Officer

Battery	General

ENGINEERED MEDICAL SOLUTIONS CO. LLC.   908-213-9001
85 Industrial Dr., Building B, Phillipsburg, NJ 08865
FDA Number: 3005977121

Catheter, Suction, With Tip	General
Light, Examination, Battery-Powered	General
Retractor, Surgical	Surgery
Suction Apparatus, Single Patient, Portable, Non-Powered	Surgery

ENGINEERED MEDICAL SYSTEMS   317-246-5500
2055 Executive Dr., Drexel Gardens, IN 46241
FDA Number: 1832562   Fax: 317-246-5501
E-mail: info@EngMedSys.com
Web site: www.engmedsys.com
Ownership: Private
Produces/Sells CE-marked Devices: N

Kit, Suctioning, Tracheostomy and Nasal	Surgery
Mask, Gas, Anesthesia	Anesthesiology
Monitor, Airway Pressure (Gauge/Alarm)	Anesthesiology
Ventilator, Emergency, Manual (Resuscitator)	Anesthesiology

ENGINEERED PRODUCTS
See Haskel International, Inc.

ENGINEERING & RESEARCH ASSOC., INC.   800-225-5242
(D.B.A. SEBRA)
400 Wood Rd, Braintree, MA 02184
FDA Number: n/a   Fax: 800-860-1512
E-mail: info@sebra.com
Web site: www.sebra.com
Medical Products Sales Volume: $12,400,000
Annual Revenue: $10-$25 Million
Year Founded: 1974
Total Employees: 80
Ownership: HAEMONETICS CORP.
Produces/Sells CE-marked Devices: Y
Federal Procurement Eligibility: Small Business
Distribution: Manufacturer Direct, Manufacturer Through Distributor, Manufacturer Through Manufacturer Reps, OEM
General Admin.: Loren C. Acker/Chief Executive Officer
       Alan Smith/President
Research: Bill Thomasson/Vice President Research & Development

Generator, Radiofrequency Lesion	Cns/Neurology
Heat-Sealing Device	Hematology
Kit, Blood Collection, Phlebotomy	Cardiovascular
Mixer, Blood Bank, Donor Blood	Hematology
Mixer/Scale, Blood	Hematology
Molding, Custom	General
Packaging Equipment	General
Production Equipment	General
Scale, Blood	Hematology

ENGINEERING MARKETING ASSOC. DBA   800-964-2362
IMPULSE TRAINING SYSTEMS
339 Millard Farmer Industrial Blvd, PO Box 2312,   770-253-7037
Newnan, GA 30263
FDA Number: 1038925   Fax: 770-251-0808
E-mail: impulse@impulsepower.com
Web site: www.impulsepower.com
Medical Products Sales Volume: $200,000
Year Founded: 1982
Total Employees: 3
Ownership: Private
Produces/Sells CE-marked Devices: N
Federal Procurement Eligibility: Small Business
Distribution: Manufacturer Direct, Manufacturer Through Manufacturer Reps

Exerciser, Non-Measuring	Physical Med
Exerciser, Other	Physical Med

ENGINEERING SERVICES KENNETH C.   888-364-7782
SALTRICK INC.
2200 East Enterprise Parkway,   330-425-9279
Twinsburg, OH 44087
FDA Number: n/a   Fax: 330-425-0919
E-mail: ken@eng-services.com
Web site: www.eng-services.com
Ownership: Private
Produces/Sells CE-marked Devices: N

Nuclear Magnetic Resonance Imaging System	Radiology

ENGINEERS EXPRESS, INC.
See Microgroup

ENGINIVITY LLC
781-862-7008
1 Militia Drive, Lla, Lexington, MA 02421
FDA Number: 3006095475
Web site: www.enginivity.com
Ownership: Vital Signs, Inc.
Produces/Sells CE-marked Devices: N
Warmer, Infusion Fluid, Thermal   General

ENGLE DENTAL SYSTEMS, INC.
503-359-9390
4115 24th Avenue, Suite A, Forest Grove, OR 97116
FDA Number: 3020989   Fax: 503-357-7286
E-mail: info@engledental.com
Web site: www.engledental.com
Medical Products Sales Volume: $2,300,000
Annual Revenue: $1-$5 Million
Year Founded: 1978
Total Employees: 30
Ownership: Private
Produces/Sells CE-marked Devices: N
Federal Procurement Eligibility: Small Business
Distribution: Manufacturer Through Distributor
General Admin.: Marvin Fox/President
Chair, Dental (With Unit)   Dental And Oral
Operative Dental Treatment Unit   Dental And Oral

ENGLER ENGINEERING CORP.
800-445-8581
1099 E. 47 St., Hialeah, FL 33013-2139
305-688-8581
FDA Number: 1036336   Fax: 305-685-7671
E-mail: info@engler-engineering.com
Web site: www.engler-engineering.com
Medical Products Sales Volume: $2,600,000
Annual Revenue: $1-$5 Million
Year Founded: 1964
Total Employees: 26   Marketing Staff: 2   Sales Staff: 2
Ownership: Private
Produces/Sells CE-marked Devices: N
Federal Procurement Eligibility: Small Business, Female Owned
Distribution: Manufacturer Direct, Manufacturer Through Distributor, Manufacturer Through Manufacturer Reps, OEM, Service Direct, Importer, Exporter
General Admin.: Eva K. Engler/President, Chief Executive Officer
Mktg./Adv.: Steven Menaged/Director Marketing
         Joel katz/Director National Accounts
         Mike Engler/Director Product Development
         Steven Menaged/Manager International & National Sales
         Steven Menaged/Manager Market Research
         Steven Menaged/Manager Sales Training
         Steven S. Menaged/Vice President Marketing & Sales
Production: Raya Engler/Director Quality Assurance
         Eva K. Engler/Manager Materials
         Mike Engler/Vice President Manufacturing
Gas-Machine, Anesthesia   Anesthesiology
Handle, Instrument, Dental   Dental And Oral
Monitor, Respiratory   Surgery
Prophylaxis Unit, Ultrasonic, Dental   Dental And Oral
Scaler, Ultrasonic   Dental And Oral

ENHANCED MOBILITY SOLUTIONS
651-451-1637
6910 Dixie Ave. E., Inver Grove Heights, MN 55076
FDA Number: 3004962723
Ownership: Private
Produces/Sells CE-marked Devices: N
Wheelchair, Powered   Physical Med

ENHANCED MOBILITY TECHNOLOGIES
612-310-4408
1615 Aguila Ave. N, Golden Valley, MN 55427
FDA Number: 2135143
Ownership: Private
Produces/Sells CE-marked Devices: N
Biofeedback Device   Cns/Neurology

ENHANCED VIDEO DEVICES, INC.
858-530-0100
9830 Summers Ridge Road, San Diego, CA 92121
FDA Number: n/a   Fax: 858-530-0500
Web site: www.digivision.com
Medical Products Sales Volume: $2,500,000
Annual Revenue: $1-$5 Million
Ownership: Private
Produces/Sells CE-marked Devices: Y
Federal Procurement Eligibility: Small Business
Distribution: Manufacturer Direct, Manufacturer Through Manufacturer Reps, OEM
Computer, Imaging, Presurgery   Surgery

ENMET CORP.
734-761-1270
680 Fairfield Ct., Ann Arbor, MI 48106-0979
FDA Number: n/a   Fax: 734-761-3220
E-mail: info@enmet.com
Web site: www.enmet.com
Annual Revenue: $1-$5 Million

ENMET CORP.
734-761-1270 (cont'd)
Total Employees: 35   Marketing Staff: 3   Sales Staff: 6
Ownership: Private
Produces/Sells CE-marked Devices: N
Federal Procurement Eligibility: GSA Contract
Distribution: Manufacturer Direct, Manufacturer Through Distributor, Manufacturer Through Manufacturer Reps, OEM, Service Direct, Exclusive Distributor, Importer, Exporter
General Admin.: Verne B. Brown/President
Mktg./Adv.: Nancy Aulisa/Manager Marketing Services
         Mr. Ray Kelley/Manager Sales
         Elwood Boomus/Vice President Marketing & Sales
Alarm, Central Gas System   Anesthesiology
Analyzer, Ethylene-Oxide   General
Detector, Leakage, Medical Gas   General
Monitor, Oxygen   General

ENNEKING MEDICAL INC.
888-685-9699
10940 Parallel Parkway, K102, Kansas City, KS 66109
FDA Number: 3004578190   Fax: 815-346-5853
Web site: www.ennekingmedical.com
Ownership: Private
Produces/Sells CE-marked Devices: N
Bath, Hydro-Massage (Whirlpool)   Physical Med
Lift, Bath, Non-AC-Powered   General
Lift, Patient   General

ENOCHS EXAMINING ROOM FURNITURE, INC.
800-428-2305
P.O. Box 50559, Indianapolis, IN 46250
317-580-2940
FDA Number: 1825436   Fax: 317-580-2944
E-mail: enochs@enochsmed.com
Web site: www.enochsmed.com
Medical Products Sales Volume: $3,000,000
Annual Revenue: $1-$5 Million
Year Founded: 1932
Total Employees: 75   Marketing Staff: 2   Sales Staff: 10
Ownership: Private
Quality System Registration Information: ISO9001
Produces/Sells CE-marked Devices: N
Federal Procurement Eligibility: Small Business, Female Owned
Distribution: Manufacturer Through Distributor
General Admin.: Ms. Marla Foster/President, Chief Executive Officer
Mktg./Adv.: Ms. Marla Foster/Vice President Marketing
         Ms. Dena McKenna/Vice President Sales
Production: Ms. Kristy Yount/Manager Customer Services
Cabinet, Instrument   General
Cabinet, Other   General
Chair, Blood Drawing   General
Chair, Examination And Treatment   General
Furniture, General   General
Table, Examination/Treatment   General
Table, Obstetrical   Obstetrics/Gynecology
Table, Obstetrical, AC-Powered   Obstetrics/Gynecology
Table, Physical Medicine, Powered   Physical Med
Waste Receptacle, General Purpose   General

ENOVA MEDICAL TECHNOLOGIES
866-773-0539
1839 Buerkle Road, St. Paul, MN 55110-5246
651-773-3181
FDA Number: 2127132   Fax: 651-773-3190
E-mail: info@enovamedical.com
Web site: www.enovamedical.com
Medical Products Sales Volume: $1,400,000
Annual Revenue: $1-$5 Million
Year Founded: 1965
Total Employees: 20   Marketing Staff: 1   Sales Staff: 3
Ownership: Private
Quality System Registration Information: ISO9001
Produces/Sells CE-marked Devices: N
Federal Procurement Eligibility: Small Business
Distribution: Manufacturer Direct, Manufacturer Through Manufacturer Reps, OEM, Service Direct
General Admin.: Thomas Brust/Chief Executive Officer
         Dawn Mountin/Office Manager
         Randall Seeliger/President
Mktg./Adv.: Joan Will/Director Marketing
         Ms. Nicole Juettner/Manager Sales
         Gary Haugen/Senior Manager Accounts
Production: Mark Schrom/Senior Engineer
         Bruce Church/Vice President Operations
Research: Dr. Michael Hoey/Vice President Research & Development
Bag, Collection, Urine, Newborn   General
Contract Assembly   General
Contract Manufacturing   General
Contract Packaging   General
Contract Sterilization   General
Lamp, Surgical   Surgery
Light, Surgical Headlight   Dental And Oral

ENOVA MEDICAL TECHNOLOGIES   866-773-0539 *(cont'd)*
Service, Consulting   General

ENPAC CORP.   800-936-7229
34355 Vokes Drive, Eastlake, OH 44095-4033   440-975-0070
FDA Number: n/a   *Fax:* 440-975-0047
E-mail: info@enpac.com
Web site: www.enpac.com
Medical Products Sales Volume: $3,300,000
Year Founded: 1998
Total Employees: 50   *Marketing Staff:* 2   *Sales Staff:* 6
Ownership: Private
Federal Procurement Eligibility: Small Business, GSA Contract
Distribution: Manufacturer Through Distributor
General Admin.: Tim Reed/Chief Executive Officer
         Douglas Horner/President
Mktg./Adv.: Chris Hilty/Vice President Marketing & Sales
   Waste Receptacle, Contaminated   General

ENPATH MEDICAL, INC.
See Greatbach Medical

ENSIGN-BICKFORD OPTICS CO.
See Ofs, Specialty Photonics Division

ENSURE MEDICAL, INC.   408-745-7610
762 San Aleso Ave., Sunnyvale, CA 94085
FDA Number: 3004859522
Ownership: Private
Produces/Sells CE-marked Devices: N
   Device, Hemostasis, Vascular   Cardiovascular

ENTECH   800-451-0591
7300 West Detroit Street, Chandler, AZ 85226   602-747-9081
FDA Number: n/a   *Fax:* 602-747-9082
E-mail: e.l.gordon@bannerhealth.com
Medical Products Sales Volume: $5,000,000
Annual Revenue: $1-$5 Million
Total Employees: 72   *Marketing Staff:* 2   *Sales Staff:* 2
Ownership: Private
Produces/Sells CE-marked Devices: N
Distribution: Service Direct
General Admin.: Timothy K. McFarlan/General Manager
         E.L. Gordon/Manager
Mktg./Adv.: James Sullivan/Manager Contract Sales
Production: Shane Gilman/Manager Production
         Terry Allen/Manager Production
   Service, Maintenance/Repair   General

ENTELLUS MEDICAL   866-620-7615
6705 Wedgwood Court North,   763-463-1595
Maple Grove, MN 55311
FDA Number: 3006345872
E-mail: info@entellusmedical.com   *Fax:* 866-620-7616
Web site: www.entellusmedical.com
Year Founded: 2006
Ownership: Private
Produces/Sells CE-marked Devices: N
Distribution: Manufacturer Direct
General Admin.: Peter Keith/Chief Technology Officer
         Mr. Brian Farley/President, Chief Executive Officer
Mktg./Adv.: Thomas Ressemann/Senior Director Business Development
         Mr. James Surek/Vice President Sales
Production: Mr. Stephen Paidosh/Vice President Operations
         Ms. Karen Paterson/Vice President Quality Assurance & Regulatory
Affairs
Finance: Thomas E. Griffin/Chief Financial Officer
   Instrument, Manual, General Surgical   Surgery
   Nasopharyngoscope (Flexible Or Rigid)   Ear/Nose/Throat

ENTERIX INC.   800-531-3681
236 Fernwood Ave., Edison, NJ 08837   732-429-1899
FDA Number: 1226769   *Fax:* 732-429-1898
Ownership: Private
Produces/Sells CE-marked Devices: N
   Reagent, Occult Blood   Hematology

ENTERNET MEDICAL, INC.   888-887-6638
1676 village green, Crofton, MD 21114   888-729-9674
FDA Number: 2953152   *Fax:* 702-943-0117
E-mail: term2@aol.com
Web site: www.enternetmedical.com
Medical Products Sales Volume: $300,000
Annual Revenue: $1-$5 Million
Year Founded: 1994
Total Employees: 5   *Marketing Staff:* 1   *Sales Staff:* 2
Ownership: Private
Produces/Sells CE-marked Devices: N
Federal Procurement Eligibility: Small Business

ENTERNET MEDICAL, INC.   888-887-6638 *(cont'd)*
Distribution: Manufacturer Direct, Manufacturer Through Distributor
   Filter, Bacterial, Breathing Circuit   Anesthesiology
   Humidifier, Heat/Moisture Exchange   Anesthesiology
   Humidifier, Heated   Anesthesiology

ENTEROMEDICS   651-634-3003
2800 Patton Road, St. Paul, MN 55113
FDA Number: n/a
Web site: http://www.enteromedics.com
Year Founded: 2002
Total Employees: 34
Ownership: Public
Stock Symbol: ETRM
Traded On: NASDAQ
Produces/Sells CE-marked Devices: N
General Admin.: Mr. Gregory Lea/Chief Financial Officer, Senior Vice President
         Dr. Mark Knudson/President, Chief Executive Officer
Medical Admin.: Dr. Scott Shikora/Chief Medical Officer
Production: Mr. Adrianus Donders/Senior Vice President Operations
Research: Ms. Katherine Tweden/Vice President Clinical Research

ENTHERMICS MEDICAL SYSTEMS, INC.   800-862-9276
W164 N9221 Water St.,   414-251-8356
Menomonee Falls, WI 53051
FDA Number: n/a   *Fax:* 414-251-7067
E-mail: generalinfo@enthermics.com
Web site: www.enthermics.com
Annual Revenue: $1-$5 Million
Total Employees: 10   *Sales Staff:* 3
Ownership: Private
Produces/Sells CE-marked Devices: Y
Federal Procurement Eligibility: Small Business, Female Owned
Distribution: Manufacturer Direct, Manufacturer Through Distributor, Manufacturer
Through Manufacturer Reps
General Admin.: Karen A. Hansen/Chief Executive Officer
Mktg./Adv.: Mark Suszkowski/Vice President Marketing & Sales
Research: William J. Hansen/Vice President Engineering
   Cabinet, Warming   General

ENTRACARE, LLC   913-451-2234
11315 Strang Line Rd., Lenexa, KS 66215
FDA Number: 1931566
   Container, IV   General
   Filter, Infusion Line   General
   Infusion Pump, Enteral   General
   Kit, Administration, Intravenous   General
   Pneumoperitoneum Apparatus, Automatic   Gastroenterology/Urology
   Thermometer, Electronic, Continuous   General
   Tube, Feeding   General

ENTURIA, INC. (FORMERLY MEDI-FLEX)
See CholeraPrep

ENTYLON LTD.   info@enlyton.ne
7700 Rivers Edge Drive, Columbus, OH 43235   614-888-9220
FDA Number: n/a   *Fax:* 614-436-0057
Web site: http://www.enlyton.net
Year Founded: 2004
Ownership: Private
Produces/Sells CE-marked Devices: N
General Admin.: Mr. Jeffrey Bergen/Chief Executive Officer
         Mr. Edward Martin III/Chief Operating Officer
         Dr. Edward Martin Jr./Chief Scientific Officer
Medical Admin.: Dr. Mark Arnold/Chief Medical Officer

ENURESIS SOLUTIONS, LLC   912-353-7675
51 W. Fairmont Avenue, Suite 2, Savannah, GA 31406
FDA Number: 3004135078
E-mail: service@drybuddy.com
Web site: www.drybuddy.com
Ownership: Private
Produces/Sells CE-marked Devices: N
   Alarm, Enuresis   Gastroenterology/Urology

ENVIRO GUARD, INC.   800-438-1152
201 Shannon Oaks Circle, Suite 115,   866-742-3133
Cary, NC 27511
FDA Number: n/a   *Fax:* 919-355-1041
E-mail: admin@enviroguard.com
Web site: www.enviroguard.com
Medical Products Sales Volume: $3,500,000
Annual Revenue: $1-$5 Million
Year Founded: 2000
Total Employees: 27   *Marketing Staff:* 1   *Sales Staff:* 8
Ownership: Private
Produces/Sells CE-marked Devices: N
Federal Procurement Eligibility: Small Business

ENVIRO GUARD, INC.
800-438-1152 (cont'd)

Distribution: Manufacturer Direct, Manufacturer Through Distributor, Manufacturer Through Manufacturer Reps, Service Direct, Exclusive Distributor
General Admin.: Dustin C. Blackwell/President, Chief Operating Officer
Production: Mrs. Jody Alt/Laboratories Product Manager

Alarm, Central Gas System	Anesthesiology
Compressor, Air, Portable	Anesthesiology
Dosimeter, Ethylene-Oxide	General
Dosimeter, Nitrous-Oxide	Anesthesiology
Monitor, Biological (Contamination Testing)	General
Monitor, Contamination, Environmental, Personal	General
Monitor, Gas, Atmospheric, Environmental	General
Pump, Vacuum, Central	Anesthesiology
Sensor, Moisture	General
System, Pipeline, Gas	General

ENVIRO MED
See Access, Lifts & Mobility Systems, Inc.

ENVIRON CORP.
703-516-2300
4350 North Fairfax Drive, Suite 300, Arlington, VA 22203
FDA Number: n/a
Fax: 703-516-2345
Web site: www.environcorp.com
Annual Revenue: $0-$1 Million
Year Founded: 1982
Ownership: Private
Quality System Registration Information: ISO9003
Produces/Sells CE-marked Devices: Y
Federal Procurement Eligibility: Small Business, Minority Owned
Distribution: Service Direct

Service, Consulting	General

ENVIRONETICS
See Idexx Laboratories, Inc.

ENVIRONMENTAL CHEMICAL SPECIALTIES, INC
See Bio-Rad, Diagnostics Group

ENVIRONMENTAL DIAGNOSTICS, INC.
See Medtox Diagnostics Inc.

ENVIRONMENTAL GROWTH CHAMBERS
800-321-6854
510 E. Washington St., Chagrin Falls, OH 44022
440-247-5100
FDA Number: 9200333
Fax: 440-247-8710
E-mail: Info@egc.com
Web site: www.egc.com
Annual Revenue: $10-$25 Million
Year Founded: 1952
Total Employees: 88   *Marketing Staff:* 2   *Sales Staff:* 8
Ownership: Private
Produces/Sells CE-marked Devices: N
Federal Procurement Eligibility: Small Business
Distribution: Manufacturer Direct
General Admin.: Frank N. Beaven/Director Admin.
Mktg./Adv.: Steven Griggs/Manager Marketing
　　　　Adrian O. Rule/President, Director Sales
　　　　Steven H. Griggs/Vice President Corporate Development
Production: Tom McGrath/Chief Engineering Officer
　　　　Adrian Rule/Vice President Operations, General Manager
Finance: Ray Pletcher/Treasurer

Chamber, Constant Temperature (Environmental)	Microbiology
Chamber, Freezing	Chemistry
Freezer, Blood Storage	Hematology
Freezer, Laboratory, Biological	Chemistry
Freezer, Laboratory, General Purpose	Chemistry
Incubator, Aerobic	Microbiology
Refrigerator, Morgue, Walk-In	Pathology

ENVIRONMENTAL PROTECTION LABORATORIES
See Micro-Bio-Logics.Inc

ENVIRONMENTAL SCIENCES ASSOC., INC
See Esa, Inc.

ENVIRONMENTAL TECTONICS CORP.
215-355-9100
125 James Way, Southampton, PA 18966
FDA Number: 2518447
Fax: 215-357-4000
E-mail: info@etcusa.com
Web site: www.etcusa.com
Medical Products Sales Volume: $17,400,000
Annual Revenue: $25-$50 Million
Year Founded: 1969
Total Employees: 175   *Marketing Staff:* 2   *Sales Staff:* 20
Ownership: Public
Stock Symbol: ETC
Traded On: AMEX
Produces/Sells CE-marked Devices: N
Federal Procurement Eligibility: Small Business, GSA Contract
Distribution: Manufacturer Direct, Manufacturer Through Manufacturer Reps, Service Direct, Exporter
General Admin.: Tom Loughlin/Chief Operating Officer
　　　　William F. Mitchell/President, Chief Executive Officer

ENVIRONMENTAL TECTONICS CORP.
215-355-9100 (cont'd)

Mktg./Adv.: Donna Averell/Director Marketing
　　　　Mr. David Mitchell/Division Manager
　　　　Gene A. Davis/Vice President Marketing & Sales
Production: Tom G. Loughlin/Vice President Manufacturing
Finance: Duane Deaner/Chief Financial Officer

Cabinet, Aerator, Ethylene-Oxide Gas	General
Chamber, Hyperbaric Oxygen	Physical Med
Sterilizer, Bulk, Steam & Ethylene-Oxide	General
Sterilizer, Ethylene-Oxide Gas	General
Sterilizer, Vapor	General
Washer/Sterilizer	General

ENVIROPAK LLC
(800)308-8371
218 claridge curve, Peachtree City, GA 30269
770-632-1991
FDA Number: 1056276
E-mail: info@enviropouch.com
Ownership: Private
Produces/Sells CE-marked Devices: N

Wrap, Sterilization	General

ENVISION DENTAL SOLUTIONS
800-372-3010
2515 Channing Way, Idaho Falls, ID 83404
FDA Number: 3004046445
Fax: 208-529-8609
Web site: www.envisiondental.com
Ownership: Private
Produces/Sells CE-marked Devices: N

Contouring, Instrument, Matrix, Operative	Dental And Oral

ENVISION EYES, LLC
303-880-1031
5368 Wildcat Ct., Morrison, CO 80465
FDA Number: 3005802870

Speculum, Ophthalmic	Ophthalmology

ENVISIONEERING MEDICAL TECHNOLOGIES
314-429-7367
1982 Innerbelt Business Center, Drive, Overland, MO 63114
FDA Number: 3005673110

Applicator, Radionuclide, Manual	Radiology
Kit, Biopsy Needle	Gastroenterology/Urology
Scanner, Ultrasonic (Pulsed Echo)	Radiology

ENVOY MEDICAL CORPORATION
1-866-950-4327
5000 Township Parkway,
651-361-8041
Saint Paul, MN 55110
FDA Number: 3004007782
Ownership: Private
Produces/Sells CE-marked Devices: N

Cement, Ear, Nose And Throat	Ear/Nose/Throat

ENZO BIOCHEM, INC.
212-583-0100
527 Madison Ave., New York, NY 10022
FDA Number: n/a
Fax: 212-679-7999
Web site: http://www.enzo.com
Medical Products Sales Volume: $19,801,300
Annual Revenue: $50-$100 Million
Year Founded: 1976
Total Employees: 200
Ownership: Public
Stock Symbol: ENZ
Traded On: NYSE
Produces/Sells CE-marked Devices: N
Federal Procurement Eligibility: Small Business
Distribution: Manufacturer Direct, Manufacturer Through Distributor
General Admin.: Elazar Rabbani/Chief Executive Officer
　　　　Barry Weiner/President
Mktg./Adv.: David Goldberg/Vice President Corporate Development
Finance: Herbert Bass/Vice President Finance

Antibody, Monoclonal	Microbiology
Filter Paper	Chemistry
Genetic Engineering	Microbiology
Test, DNA-Probe, Other	Microbiology

ENZYME SOLUTIONS, INC.
260-497-0851
7601 Honeywell Dr., Fort Wayne, IN 46825
FDA Number: 3003879366
Ownership: Private
Produces/Sells CE-marked Devices: N

Cleaner, Ultrasonic, Medical Instrument	General

EP MEDICAL, INC.
See Eastman Medical Products Inc.

EP TECHNOLOGIES, INC.
888-272-1001
2710 Orchard Pkwy., San Jose, CA 95134
508-650-8172
FDA Number: 2953184
Web site: www.bostonscientific.com
Annual Revenue: $100-$500 Million
Ownership: BOSTON SCIENTIFIC CORPORATION
Produces/Sells CE-marked Devices: N
General Admin.: Mr. Joseph M. Fitzgerald/President

EP TECHNOLOGIES, INC.   888-272-1001 *(cont'd)*

Catheter, Electrode Recording, Or Probe	Cardiovascular
Catheter, Intracardiac Mapping, High-density Array	Cardiovascular
Electrode, Ablation, Tissue, Conduction, Percutaneous	Cardiovascular
Electrosurgical Unit, Cutting & Coagulation Device	Surgery
Introducer, Catheter	Cardiovascular
Radiographic/Fluoroscopic Unit, Image-Intensified	Radiology

EPCOM INC.
See Vmed Technology, Inc. (Formerly Ems Products, Inc.)

EPCOM MEDICAL SYSTEMS INC.
See Vmed Technology, Inc. (Formerly Ems Products, Inc.)

EPE TECHNOLOGIES, INC.
See Mge Ups Sytems, Inc.

EPIC MEDICAL EQUIPMENT SERVICES, INC.   800-327-3742
1800 10th St., Suite 300, Plano, TX 75074   972-801-9854
FDA Number: n/a   *Fax:* 972-801-9859
E-mail: mail@epicmedical.com
Web site: www.epicmedical.com
Annual Revenue: $5-$10 Million
Total Employees: 41   *Marketing Staff:* 1
Ownership: Private
Quality System Registration Information: ISO9001
Produces/Sells CE-marked Devices: Y
Federal Procurement Eligibility: Small Business
Distribution: Manufacturer Direct, Manufacturer Through Distributor, OEM, Service Direct
General Admin.: Keneth Perdue/Chief Executive Officer
    Nancy Hall/Vice President Human Resources
Mktg./Adv.: Becky Erman/Director Marketing
    Jeffrey Secunda/Director Product Development
    Roberto Conti/Manager International Sales
    Jeffrey Secunda/Manager Market Research
Production: Les Posey/Director Quality Assurance
    Nancy Hall/Manager Materials
    Les Posey/Manager Regulatory Affairs
Research: Jeff Secunda/Vice President Research & Development

Cable	Physical Med
Oximeter, Finger	General
Service, Maintenance/Repair	General
Service, Parts, Repair	General
Transducer, Ultrasonic, Obstetrical	Obstetrics/Gynecology

EPIC SYSTEMS CORP.   608-271-9000
1979 Milky Way, Verona, WI 53593
FDA Number: n/a   *Fax:* 608-271-7237
E-mail: info@epicsystems.com
Web site: www.epicsystems.com
Year Founded: 1979
Total Employees: 2400
Ownership: Private
Produces/Sells CE-marked Devices: N
Distribution: Manufacturer Direct, Service Direct
General Admin.: Carl Dvorak/Executive Vice President
    Judith R. Faulkner/President, Chief Executive Officer

Computer Software	General

EPIC SYSTEMS, INC.   800-338-2812
4488 Thorning Loop, P.O. BOX 908,   406-821-3900
Darby, MT 59829
FDA Number: n/a   *Fax:* 406-821-3918
E-mail: epicsystemsinc.com
Web site: www.epicsystemsinc.com
Medical Products Sales Volume: $650,000
Annual Revenue: $0-$1 Million
Total Employees: 5   *Marketing Staff:* 2   *Sales Staff:* 1
Ownership: Private
Produces/Sells CE-marked Devices: N
Federal Procurement Eligibility: Small Business
Distribution: Manufacturer Direct, Manufacturer Through Distributor, Manufacturer Through Manufacturer Reps, Service Direct, Exclusive Distributor
General Admin.: Jay Estus/President

Transmitter/Receiver System, Physiological, Telephone	Cardiovascular

EPICENTRE TECHNOLOGIES   800-284-8474
726 Post Rd., Madison, WI 53713   608-258-3080
FDA Number: n/a   *Fax:* 608-258-3088
E-mail: customerservice@epibio.com
Web site: www.epicentre.com
Annual Revenue: $0-$1 Million
Year Founded: 1987
Ownership: Illumina, Inc.
Produces/Sells CE-marked Devices: N
Federal Procurement Eligibility: Small Business
Distribution: Manufacturer Direct, Manufacturer Through Distributor, Manufacturer Through Manufacturer Reps, OEM, Exporter

Gel, Support	Immunology

EPICENTRE TECHNOLOGIES   800-284-8474 *(cont'd)*

Kit, DNA Detection, Human Papillomavirus	Microbiology

EPIEN MEDICAL, INC.   651-653-3380
4225 White Bear Parkway, Suite 600, Birchwood, MN 55110
FDA Number: 3003428492

Protectant, Skin	Surgery

EPIKEIA, INC.   210-313-4600
500 Sandau, Suite 200, San Antonio, TX 78216-3636
FDA Number: 1651194
Ownership: Private
Produces/Sells CE-marked Devices: N

Bandage, Liquid	Surgery
Protectant, Skin	Surgery

EPIMED INTERNATIONAL, INC.   800-866-3342
141 Sal Landrio Drive   518-725-0209
Crossroads Business Park
Johnstown, NY 12095
FDA Number: 1316297   *Fax:* 518-725-0207
E-mail: cserve@epimedint.com
Web site: www.epimedint.com
Medical Products Sales Volume: $7,500,000
Year Founded: 1992
Total Employees: 43
Ownership: Private
Quality System Registration Information: ISO9001
Produces/Sells CE-marked Devices: Y
Federal Procurement Eligibility: Small Business
Distribution: Manufacturer Direct, Manufacturer Through Distributor, Manufacturer Through Manufacturer Reps, OEM
General Admin.: Gabor J. Racz/President
    Sandor Racz/Vice President, General Manager
Mktg./Adv.: SteveN Loretz/Director Marketing & Sales
    Gary Bullard/Director Product Development
Production: Chris Lake/Director Quality Assurance
    Donald R. Henderson/Director Regulatory Affairs
    Chris Lake/Manager Regulatory Affairs
    Bruce Whitcavitch/Vice President Manufacturing

Apron, Lead, Radiographic	Radiology
Catheter, Conduction, Anesthesia	Anesthesiology
Catheter, Epidural	Obstetrics/Gynecology
Needle, Conduction, Anesthesia (W/Wo Introducer)	Anesthesiology
Needle, Spinal, Short-Term	General
Set, Administration, Intravenous, Needle-Free	General

EPITOPE DIAGNOSTICS, INC.   858-693-7877
8940 Activity Rd., Suite G, San Diego, CA 92126
FDA Number: 2032839   *Fax:* 1-858-693-7678
E-mail: cs@epitopediagnostics.com
Web site: www.epitopediagnostics.com
Ownership: Private
Produces/Sells CE-marked Devices: N

Alpha 2, 2N-Glycoprotein, Antigen, Antiserum, Control	Immunology
Antibodies, Gliadin	Immunology
Antigen, CF (Including CF Control), Adenovirus 1-33	Microbiology
Calibrator, Secondary, Clinical Chemistry	Chemistry
Immunochemical, Thyroglobulin Autoantibody	Immunology

EPITOPE, INC.
See Orasure Technologies, Inc.

EPIX PHARMACEUTICALS, INC   781-761-7600
4 Maguire Road, Lexington, MA 02421
FDA Number: n/a   *Fax:* 781-761-7641
E-mail: info@EPIXpharma.com
Web site: www.epixmed.com
Medical Products Sales Volume: $6,000,000
Year Founded: 1988
Total Employees: 46
Ownership: Public
Stock Symbol: EPIX
Traded On: NASDAQ
Produces/Sells CE-marked Devices: N
Federal Procurement Eligibility: Small Business
General Admin.: Michael D. Webb/Chief Executive Officer
Mktg./Adv.: Gregg Mayer/Vice President Marketing
Research: Alan Carpenter/Executive Vice President Research & Development

Injector, Contrast Medium, Automatic	Radiology
Media, Radiographic Injectable Contrast	Radiology

EPIX, INC.   847-465-1818
381 Lexington Drive, Buffalo Grove, IL 60089-6934
FDA Number: n/a   *Fax:* 847-465-1919
E-mail: epix@epixinc.com
Web site: www.epixinc.com
Medical Products Sales Volume: $1,700,000
Annual Revenue: $1-$5 Million

EPIX, INC.   847-465-1818 *(cont'd)*
Year Founded: 1983
Total Employees: 9   Marketing Staff: 1   Sales Staff: 3
Ownership: Private
Produces/Sells CE-marked Devices: Y
Federal Procurement Eligibility: Small Business
Distribution: Manufacturer Direct, Manufacturer Through Distributor, Manufacturer Through Manufacturer Reps
Mktg./Adv.: Kirsten Gimm/Director Advertising
    Mr. Charlie Dijak/Sales Engineer
    Computer Equipment   General

EPL INC./MICRO-BIO-LOGICS
See Micro-Bio-Logics.Inc

EPOCRATES INC.   650-227-1700
1100 Park Place, Suite 300, San Mateo, CA 94403
FDA Number: n/a   Fax: 650-227-2770
Web site: http://www.epocrates.com
Year Founded: 1998
Total Employees: 250
Ownership: Public
Stock Symbol: EPOC
Traded On: NASDAQ
Produces/Sells CE-marked Devices: N
General Admin.: Mr. Dave Burlington/Chief Operating Officer
    Mr. Joe Kleine/Executive Vice President
    Ms. Rose Crane/President, Chief Executive Officer
Medical Admin.: Dr. Thomas Giannulli/Chief Medical Officer
Finance: Mr. Burt Podbere/Senior Vice President Finance

EPPENDORF NORTH AMERICA   800-645-3050
102 Motor Parkway, Hauppauge, NY 11788   **516-334-7500**
FDA Number: 8010471   Fax: 516-334-7506
E-mail: info@eppendorf.com
Ownership: Eppendorf Ag
Produces/Sells CE-marked Devices: N
Mktg./Adv.: Ms. Andrea Dickstein/Director Marketing

EPROGEN, INC.   800-556-4272
8205 S. Cass Avenue, Suite 106,   **630-963-1481**
Darien, IL 60561
FDA Number: n/a   Fax: 630-963-6432
E-mail: info@eprogen.com
Web site: www.eprogen.com
Medical Products Sales Volume: $440,000
Year Founded: 2001
Total Employees: 4
Ownership: Private
Produces/Sells CE-marked Devices: N
Federal Procurement Eligibility: Small Business
Distribution: Manufacturer Direct, Manufacturer Through Manufacturer Reps, Service Direct, Exporter
General Admin.: Dr. Tim Barder/Chief Scientific Officer
    Bruce Grotefend/President, Chief Executive Officer
Mktg./Adv.: John Taulien/Director Sales
    Cara Tomasek/Manager Market Development
    Dr. Jim Harvey/Vice President Product Services
    Chromatography, Liquid, Performance, High   Toxicology
    Column, Chromatography   Chemistry

EPRT TECHNOLOGIES, INC.   805-522-6223
2139 Tapo St., Suite 228, Simi Valley, CA 93063
FDA Number: 2032288
    Stimulator, Nerve, Transcutaneous (Pain Relief, TENS)   Cns/Neurology

EQM RESEARCH, INC.   513-661-0560
3638 Glenmore Ave., Cheviot, OH 45211
FDA Number: 3003502294
Ownership: Private
Produces/Sells CE-marked Devices: N
    Colorimetry, Cholinesterase   Toxicology

EQUAL DIAGNOSTICS, INC.
See Sekisui Diagnostics, LLC

EQUILASERS, INC   408-588-1212
3350 Scott Blvd., Bldg. 5, Santa Clara, CA 95054
FDA Number: 3001854602
Ownership: Private
Produces/Sells CE-marked Devices: N
    Laser, Surgical   Surgery

EQUIP FOR INDEPENDENCE, INC.   800-216-4881
333 Mamaroneck Avenue, Suite 383,   **914-328-7230**
White Plains, NY 10605
FDA Number: 2436266
E-mail: LIFTALIMB@aol.com   Fax: 914-428-2261
Web site: www.LIFTALIMB.com

EQUIP FOR INDEPENDENCE, INC.   800-216-4881 *(cont'd)*
Year Founded: 1992
Ownership: Private
Produces/Sells CE-marked Devices: N
Federal Procurement Eligibility: Small Business, Female Owned
Distribution: Manufacturer Direct, Manufacturer Through Distributor
General Admin.: Ms. Walda B. Lipson/President
Mktg./Adv.: Ms. Terri L. Lipson/Manager Marketing & Sales
    Elevator, Orthopedic   Orthopedics
    Holder, Leg, Arthroscopy   Orthopedics
    Orthosis, Limb Brace   Physical Med
    Support, Elbow   Orthopedics
    Support, Foot   Orthopedics
    Support, Hand   Orthopedics

EQUIPMENT SHOP, INC.   800-525-7681
P.O. Box 33, Bedford, MA 01730-2246   **781-275-7681**
FDA Number: n/a   Fax: 781-275-4094
E-mail: info@equipmentshop.com
Web site: www.equipmentshop.com
Medical Products Sales Volume: $500,000
Annual Revenue: $0-$1 Million
Total Employees: 2
Ownership: Private
Produces/Sells CE-marked Devices: N
Federal Procurement Eligibility: Small Business
Distribution: Manufacturer Direct
General Admin.: Ken Larson/President
Mktg./Adv.: Carrie Larson/Director Marketing
Production: Paul Druan/Manager Production
    Exerciser, Other   Physical Med
    Utensil, Food   Physical Med

EQUIPMENT TECHNOLOGY CONVEYANCE   408-483-1894
125 Connemara Way #164, Sunnyvale, CA 94087
FDA Number: n/a   Fax: 408-483-4413
E-mail: info@etcsales.com
Web site: www.etcsales.com
Annual Revenue: $1-$5 Million
Ownership: Private
Produces/Sells CE-marked Devices: N
Distribution: Exclusive Distributor
General Admin.: Bob Kinder/Chief Executive Officer
Mktg./Adv.: Ray Brachelli/Director National Accounts
    Ray Brachelli/Vice President Sales
    Equipment, Device Coating, Protective   General

EQUIPOIS INC.   866-601-2070
6601 Santa Monica Blvd.,   **310-736-4130**
Los Angeles, CA 90038
FDA Number: n/a
E-mail: info@equipoisinc.com
Web site: http://www.equipoisinc.com
Ownership: Private
Produces/Sells CE-marked Devices: N
General Admin.: Mr. Eric Golden/President, Chief Executive Officer
Mktg./Adv.: Mr. Tony Wisniewski/Vice President Business Development
    Mr. Jeff Disbrow/Vice President Sales
Production: Mr. Paul Stahlke/Director Manufacturing
Research: Mr. Tony Stacksteder/Vice President Product Development

EQUIPRO EQUIPMENT DE BEAUTE   514-324-2226
11005 Rue Masse, Montreal-Nord H1G 4G5 Canada
FDA Number: 9615152
    Light, Wood's, Fluorescence   Microbiology

ERAD/IMAGE MEDICAL CORP.   864-234-7430
9 Pilgrim Road, Suite 312, Greenville, SC 29607
FDA Number: 2954766   Fax: 864-234-7412
E-mail: info@eradimagemedical.com
Web site: www.eradimagemedical.com
Medical Products Sales Volume: $2,800,000
Year Founded: 1999
Total Employees: 28
Ownership: Private
Produces/Sells CE-marked Devices: N
Federal Procurement Eligibility: Small Business
Distribution: Manufacturer Direct, OEM, Exclusive Distributor
General Admin.: Mr. Gabor Ligeti/Chief Technology Officer
    Mr. Stephen Friedman/Executive Vice President
Mktg./Adv.: Mr. Seth Koeppel/Senior Vice President Sales
Production: Mike Young/Senior Product Manager
    Mr. Randy Phillips/Vice President Operations
Research: James Connors/Vice President Product Development
    Device, Storage, Image, Digital   Radiology
    Radiographic Picture Archiving/Communication System (PACS)   Radiology
    System, Communication, Image, Digital   Radiology

ERAGEN BIOSCIENCES INC.   608-662-9000
918 Deming Way, Suite 201, Madison, WI 53717
FDA Number: n/a   Fax: 608-662-9003
E-mail: info@eragen.com
Web site: http://www.eragen.com
Ownership: Private
Produces/Sells CE-marked Devices: N
General Admin.: Dr. Irene Hrusovsky/President, Chief Executive Officer
Mktg./Adv.: Ms. Maria Foster/Vice President Commercial Operations
Production: Mr. Brian Loeffler/Vice President Operations
     Mr. Ronald Dunn/Vice President Quality Control & Regulatory Affairs
Research: Dr. Scott Johnson/Vice President Product Development
Finance: Ms. Linda Pauls Flemming/Chief Financial Officer
   Reagents, Specific, Analyte   Hematology

ERASER COMPANY, INC.   800-724-0594
123 Oliva Drive, Mattydale, NY 13211   315-454-3237
FDA Number: n/a   Fax: 315-454-3090
E-mail: info@eraser.com
Web site: www.eraser.com
Medical Products Sales Volume: $4,300,000
Annual Revenue: $5-$10 Million
Year Founded: 1911
Total Employees: 55   *Marketing Staff:* 3   *Sales Staff:* 6
Ownership: Private
Quality System Registration Information: ISO9001
Produces/Sells CE-marked Devices: Y
Federal Procurement Eligibility: Small Business, GSA Contract
Distribution: Manufacturer Direct, Manufacturer Through Distributor
General Admin.: Mr. Marcus BeVard/Chief Executive Officer
Mktg./Adv.: Mrs. Laura Prattico/Assistant Director Marketing
     Ms. Eileen Donovan/Manager Sales
Production: Mr. William Jackson/Manager Factory
Finance: Mr. Richard DePaulis/Vice President Finance, Controller
   Lamp, Infrared   Physical Med
   Sealer, Packaging   General
   Stripper, Other   Surgery
   Tubing, Other   General

ERB INDUSTRIES INC.   800-800-6522
#1 Safety Way, Woodstock, GA 30188   770-926-7944
FDA Number: n/a   Fax: 800-232-9372
E-mail: customerservice@e-erb.com
Web site: www.e-erb.com
Medical Products Sales Volume: $17,100,000
Annual Revenue: $10-$25 Million
Year Founded: 1970
Total Employees: 100   *Marketing Staff:* 4   *Sales Staff:* 16
Ownership: Private
Quality System Registration Information: ISO9002
Produces/Sells CE-marked Devices: N
Federal Procurement Eligibility: GSA Contract
Distribution: Manufacturer Direct
General Admin.: Bill Erb/Chairman
Mktg./Adv.: Jackie Barker/Manager Advertising
     D. Peter Burke/Manager International & National Sales
     Julie Charyna/Manager National Sales
     Cinja Williams/Manager Sales Training
     Shirley Miley/National Accounts Representative
Production: Vicki Scott/Manager Materials
     Jud Crosby/Manager Regulatory Affairs
   Goggles, Protective, Eye   Ophthalmology
   Kit, First Aid   Surgery

ERB SAFETY
See Erb Industries Inc.

ERBE MEDICAL INSTRUMENTS
See Conmed Corporation

ERBE USA, INC.   800-778-3723
2225 Northwest Parkway, Marietta, GA 30067
FDA Number: 1057212   Fax: 770-955-2577
E-mail: info@erbe-usa.com
Web site: www.erbe-usa.com
Medical Products Sales Volume: $9,400,000
Annual Revenue: $10-$25 Million
Year Founded: 1992
Ownership: ERBE ELEKTROMEDIZIN GMBH
Quality System Registration Information: ISO9001
Produces/Sells CE-marked Devices: N
Federal Procurement Eligibility: Small Business
Distribution: Manufacturer Direct, Manufacturer Through Manufacturer Reps, OEM, Service Direct, Exclusive Distributor, Importer
   Cord, Electric, Endoscope   Gastroenterology/Urology
   Electrocautery Unit, Endoscopic   Obstetrics/Gynecology
   Electrosurgical Equipment, General Purpose   Surgery
   Electrosurgical Unit, Cutting & Coagulation Device   Surgery
   Electrosurgical Unit, Gastroenterology   Gastroenterology/Urology

ERBE USA, INC.   800-778-3723 *(cont'd)*
   Electrosurgical Unit, General Purpose (ESU)   Surgery
   Electrosurgical Unit, Neurological   Cns/Neurology
   Electrosurgical, Unit, Gastroenterology   Gastroenterology/Urology
   Generator, Power, Electrosurgical   Surgery
   Instrument, Electrosurgical, Field Focused   Cns/Neurology

ERCHONIA MEDICAL   888-242-0571
2021 Commerce Dr, Mckinney, TX 75069   214-544-2227
FDA Number: 2032513   Fax: 214-544-2228
Ownership: Private
Produces/Sells CE-marked Devices: N
   Iontophoresis Device, Dental   Dental And Oral
   Lamp, Non-heating, For Adjunctive Use In Pain Therapy   Physical Med
   Laser, Surgical   Surgery

ERESEARCHTECHNOLOGY INC.   215-972-0420
1818 Market Street, Suite 1000, Philadelphia, PA 19103-3638
FDA Number: 2916493   Fax: 215-972-0414
Web site: http://www.ert.com
Year Founded: 1977
Ownership: Public
Stock Symbol: ERES
Traded On: NASDAQ
Produces/Sells CE-marked Devices: N
General Admin.: Keith Schneck/Chief Financial Officer, Executive Vice President
     Mr. Eric Schwartz/Chief Legal Officer
     Joel Morganroth/Chief Scientific Officer
     Dr. Jeffery Litwin/President, Chief Executive Officer
Medical Admin.: Dr. Jeffrey Litwin/Chief Medical Officer
Mktg./Adv.: Mr. John Blakely/Executive Vice President Marketing & Sales
Research: Mr. Tom Devine/Director Development
   Electrocardiograph, Interpretive   Cardiovascular
   Oximeter, Pulse   General
   Plethysmograph, Volume   Anesthesiology
   Spirometer, Diagnostic (Respirometer)   Anesthesiology
   Transmitter/Receiver System, ECG, Telephone Multi-Channel   Cardiovascular
   Transmitter/Receiver System, ECG, Telephone Single-Channel   Cardiovascular

ERG INTERNATIONAL   800-446-1186
361 N. Bernoulli Circle, Oxnard, CA 93030
FDA Number: n/a
Web site: www.ergcontract.com
Medical Products Sales Volume: $1,500,000
Annual Revenue: $5-$10 Million
Year Founded: 1981
Ownership: Private
Produces/Sells CE-marked Devices: N
Federal Procurement Eligibility: Small Business
Distribution: Manufacturer Through Manufacturer Reps
   Furniture, General   General

ERGODYNE   800-225-8238
1021 Bandana Boulevard East, Suite 220,   651-642-9889
St. Paul, MN 55108
FDA Number: 2183520   Fax: 651-642-1882
E-mail: azemke@beehivepr.biz
Web site: www.ergodyne.com
Medical Products Sales Volume: $45,500,000
Year Founded: 1983
Total Employees: 250   *Marketing Staff:* 3   *Sales Staff:* 20
Ownership: Private
Produces/Sells CE-marked Devices: Y
Federal Procurement Eligibility: Small Business, GSA Contract
Distribution: Manufacturer Through Distributor, Service Direct
General Admin.: Thomas F. Votel/President, Chief Executive Officer
Mktg./Adv.: Howard Huber/Manager Marketing
Production: Mike Bazal/Vice President Manufacturing
   Board, Foot   Orthopedics
   Chair, Seat Lifting (Standing Aid)   General
   Support, Back   Orthopedics
   Support, Hand   Orthopedics
   Support, Knee   Physical Med
   Support, Wrist   Physical Med
   Transfer Device, Patient, Manual   General

ERGOGENESIS, LLC   800-364-5299
One Bodybilt Pl., Navasota, TX 77868   936-825-1700
FDA Number: 1640211   Fax: 936-825-1725
E-mail: info@ergogenesis.com
Web site: www.ergogenesis.com
Medical Products Sales Volume: $19,500,000
Year Founded: 2002
Total Employees: 122
Ownership: Private
Produces/Sells CE-marked Devices: N
Federal Procurement Eligibility: Small Business, GSA Contract
Distribution: Manufacturer Direct

MANUFACTURER PROFILES

ERGOGENESIS, LLC   800-364-5299 *(cont'd)*
  Chair, Adjustable, Mechanical   Physical Med

ERGOMED, INC.   800-333-3746
  5426 Billington Dr., San Antonio, TX 78230   210-377-2217
  FDA Number: 1647162   *Fax:* 210-366-1075
  Ownership: Private
  Produces/Sells CE-marked Devices: N
  Fixation Device, Tracheal Tube   Anesthesiology

ERGOTRON, INC.   800-888-8458
  1181 Trapp Road, St. Paul, MN 55121   651-681-7600
  FDA Number: n/a   *Fax:* 651-681-7715
  E-mail: sales@ergotron.com
  Web site: www.ergotron.com
  Medical Products Sales Volume: $95,000,000
  Annual Revenue: $50-$100 Million
  Year Founded: 1982
  Total Employees: 275   *Marketing Staff:* 10   *Sales Staff:* 70
  Ownership: Private
  Produces/Sells CE-marked Devices: Y
  Federal Procurement Eligibility: Small Business, GSA Contract
  Distribution: Manufacturer Direct, Manufacturer Through Distributor, Manufacturer Through Manufacturer Reps, OEM, Service Direct, Importer
  General Admin.: Joel Hazzard/Chief Executive Officer, Chief Operating Officer
    Diane Kaufman/Vice President Human Resources
  Mktg./Adv.: Jane Payfer/Director Marketing
    Lynn Spieker/Manager Advertising
    Lee Schalk/Vice President Sales
  Production: Joe Carroll/Director Quality Assurance
  Cart, Other   General
  Cart, Supply   General
  Mount, Equipment   General
  Mount, Monitor (Support)   General

ERGOUNLIMITED, INC.   205-591-9977
  5401 9th Ave. South, Birmingham, AL 35212
  FDA Number: 3005977711
  Adapter, Hygiene   Physical Med
  Kit, Enema (For Cleaning Purposes)   Gastroenterology/Urology

ERIC ARMIN INC.   800-272-0272
  118 Bauer Drive, PO Box 7046,   201-891-9466
  Oakland, NJ 07436
  FDA Number: n/a   *Fax:* 201-891-5689
  E-mail: info@eaiusa.com
  Web site: www.eaiusa.com
  Medical Products Sales Volume: $3,000,000
  Annual Revenue: $5-$10 Million
  Year Founded: 1981
  Total Employees: 30   *Marketing Staff:* 5   *Sales Staff:* 10
  Ownership: Private
  Produces/Sells CE-marked Devices: N
  Federal Procurement Eligibility: Small Business
  Distribution: Manufacturer Through Distributor, Manufacturer Through Manufacturer Reps, OEM, Exclusive Distributor, Importer
  General Admin.: Eric Guglberger/President
  Mktg./Adv.: Eric Guglberger/Manager National Sales
  Timer, General Laboratory   Hematology

ERICKSON LABS NORTHWEST   425-823-1861
  12911 120th Ave. Ne, Suite C10, Kirkland, WA 98034
  FDA Number: 3005290929
  Button, Iris, Eye, Artificial   Ophthalmology
  Eye, Artificial, Non-Custom   Ophthalmology
  Shell, Scleral   Ophthalmology

ERICKSON'S ARTIFICIAL EYES   800-665-0538
  805 W. Broadway, Ste. 703,   604-876-1211
  Vancouver, BC V5Z-1 Canada
  FDA Number: n/a
  E-mail: leif@ericksoneyes.com
  Web site: www.ericksoneyes.com
  Year Founded: 1985
  Total Employees: 10
  Ownership: Private
  Produces/Sells CE-marked Devices: N
  Distribution: OEM

ERICOMP, INC.   800-541-8471
  10211 Pacific Mesa Blvd., Suite 411,   858-457-1888
  San Diego, CA 92121
  FDA Number: n/a   *Fax:* 858-457-2937
  E-mail: webinfo@ericomp.com
  Web site: www.ericomp.com
  Total Employees: 20
  Ownership: Private
  Produces/Sells CE-marked Devices: Y

ERICOMP, INC.   800-541-8471 *(cont'd)*
  Federal Procurement Eligibility: Small Business, GSA Contract
  Distribution: Manufacturer Direct, Manufacturer Through Distributor
  General Admin.: Lonnie Adelman/President, Chief Executive Officer
  Mktg./Adv.: Craig Alvis/Director Marketing & Sales
  Centrifuge, Cell Washing   Hematology
  Computer Software   General
  Incubator/Water Bath, Microbiology   Microbiology

ERICSSON GE MOBILE COMMUNICATIONS, INC.
  See Ericsson, Inc.

ERICSSON, INC.   434-528-7000
  100 Mountain View Drive, Lynchburg, VA 24502-0197
  FDA Number: 9330043   *Fax:* 434-592-3902
  Annual Revenue: $10-$25 Million
  Total Employees: 4200
  Ownership: Private
  Quality System Registration Information: ISO9000
  Federal Procurement Eligibility: GSA Contract, VA Contract
  Distribution: Manufacturer Direct, Exporter
  General Admin.: Tom Sherrier/Vice President Human Resources
    Dennis C. Conners/Vice President International Operations
  Communication Equipment   General

ERIE MEDICAL   800-932-2293
  10225 82nd Avenue, Pleasant Prairie, WI 53158   262-947-9000
  FDA Number: 2127064   *Fax:* 262-947-9020
  E-mail: sales@eriemedical.com
  Web site: www.eriemedical.com
  Medical Products Sales Volume: $12,700,000
  Year Founded: 1977
  Total Employees: 160   *Marketing Staff:* 2   *Sales Staff:* 30
  Ownership: OCENCO INCORPORATED
  Quality System Registration Information: ISO9001
  Produces/Sells CE-marked Devices: N
  Federal Procurement Eligibility: Small Business
  Distribution: Manufacturer Direct, Manufacturer Through Distributor, Manufacturer Through Manufacturer Reps, OEM, Importer, Exporter
  General Admin.: J. P. Droppleman/President, Chief Executive Officer
    Richard A. Van Derveer/Vice President, General Manager
  Mktg./Adv.: Robert Rakers/Vice President Marketing & Sales
  Production: B. P. Sorensen/Director Quality Assurance & Regulatory Affairs
    M. Frost/Manager Materials
    Fred Kohlscheen/Manager Production
    S. C. Berning/Vice President Engineering & Operations
  Research: S. C. Berning/Vice President Product Development
  Finance: Dan Ambrowiak/Manager Finance
  Canister, Oxygen   Anesthesiology
  Cylinder, Compressed Gas, With Valve   Anesthesiology
  Cylinder, Oxygen   Anesthesiology
  Flowmeter, Gas (Oxygen), Calibrated   Anesthesiology
  Regulator, Oxygen, Mechanical   General
  Resuscitator, Emergency Oxygen   Dental And Oral
  Resuscitator, Pulmonary, Gas   General
  Suction Apparatus, Single Patient, Portable, Non-Powered   Surgery
  Suction Apparatus, Ward Use, Portable, AC-Powered   Surgery

ERIE SCIENTIFIC   603-431-8410
  Portsmouth Park, 20 Post Road, Newington, NH 03801
  FDA Number: n/a
  Ownership: Private
  Produces/Sells CE-marked Devices: N
  Chamber, Slide Culture   Pathology
  Coverslip, Microscope Slide   Pathology
  Slide, Microscope   Pathology

ERIEM SURGICAL   800-833-3380
  28438 Ballard Dr., Lake Forest, IL 60045   847-549-1410
  FDA Number: n/a   *Fax:* 847-549-1510
  Web site: www.micrins.com
  Ownership: Private
  Produces/Sells CE-marked Devices: N
  Federal Procurement Eligibility: Small Business
  Distribution: Exclusive Distributor
  Dilator, Vessel, Surgical   Cardiovascular
  Instrument, Microsurgical   Cns/Neurology
  Tray, Surgical Instrument   Surgery

ERIGON   361-387-8276
  1301 Dakota St., Robstown, TX 78380
  FDA Number: 3004196246
  Ownership: Private
  Produces/Sells CE-marked Devices: N
  Component, Exercise   Physical Med

ERIKA DE REYNOSA, S.A. DE C.V.   781-402-9068
Brecha E99 Sur; Parque, Industrial Reynos, Bldg. Ii,
Cd, Reynosa, Tamps Mexico
FDA Number: 8030665

Accessories, Blood Circuit, Hemodialysis	Gastroenterology/Urology
Connector, Tubing, Blood, Infusion, T-Type	Gastroenterology/Urology
Kit, Administration, Intravenous	General
Kit, Administration, Peritoneal Dialysis, Disposable	Gastroenterology/Urology
Kit, Perfusion, Kidney, Disposable	Gastroenterology/Urology
Meter, Conductivity, Induction, Remote Type	Gastroenterology/Urology
Meter, Conductivity, Non-Remote	Gastroenterology/Urology
System, Peritoneal Dialysis, Automatic	Gastroenterology/Urology
Tray, Start/Stop (Including Contents), Dialysis	Gastroenterology/Urology

ERNEST F. FULLAM, INC.
See Ted Pella, Inc.

ERNST FLOW INDUSTRIES   800-992-2843
116 Main St., Farmingdale, NJ 07727-1495   732-938-5641
FDA Number: n/a   *Fax:* 888-992-2843
E-mail: info@ernstflow.com
Web site: www.ernstflow.com
Medical Products Sales Volume: $1,200,000
Annual Revenue: $1-$5 Million
Year Founded: 1962
Total Employees: 14   *Marketing Staff:* 3   *Sales Staff:* 3
Ownership: Private
Produces/Sells CE-marked Devices: N
Federal Procurement Eligibility: Small Business
Distribution: Manufacturer Direct
General Admin.: Eugene Ernst/Chief Executive Officer
Mktg./Adv.: Susan Montgomery/Manager International & National Sales
     Roger Ernst/President, Director Marketing
     John Ernst/Vice President Marketing & Sales

Component, Other	General
Stopcock	General

ERP GROUP PROFESSIONAL PRODUCTS LTD.   800-361-3537
3232 Autoroute Laval W.,   450-687-0780
Laval, QUEBE H7T 2 Canada
FDA Number: n/a   *Fax:* 450-687-8035
E-mail: info@erp.ca
Web site: www.erp.ca
Year Founded: 1978
Total Employees: 25   *Marketing Staff:* 2   *Sales Staff:* 5
Ownership: Private
Produces/Sells CE-marked Devices: N
Distribution: Exclusive Distributor, Importer

ERP GROUP PROFESSIONAL PRODUCTS LTD.   800-361-3537
3232 Autoroute Laval West,   450-687-0780
Laval, QUE H7T-2 Canada
FDA Number: n/a   *Fax:* 450-687-8035
E-mail: info@erp.ca
Web site: www.erp.ca
Year Founded: 1978
Total Employees: 25
Ownership: Private
Produces/Sells CE-marked Devices: N
Distribution: Service Direct, Exclusive Distributor, Importer

ERTELALSOP   800-553-7835
321 Fair St, P.O. Box 3449,   845-331-4552
Kingston, NY 12402
FDA Number: n/a   *Fax:* 845-339-1063
E-mail: sales@ertelalsop.com
Web site: www.ertelalsop.com
Annual Revenue: $1-$5 Million
Year Founded: 1920
Ownership: Private
Produces/Sells CE-marked Devices: N
Federal Procurement Eligibility: Small Business
Distribution: Manufacturer Direct, Manufacturer Through Manufacturer Reps, Exporter

Blender/Mixer	Chemistry
Filter Paper	Chemistry
Filter, Bacteriological, Laboratory	Chemistry
Filter, Membrane	Chemistry

ES INDUSTRIES   800-356-6140
701 South Route 73, West Berlin, NJ 08091   856-753-8400
FDA Number: n/a   *Fax:* 856-753-8484
Web site: www.esind.com
Ownership: Private
Produces/Sells CE-marked Devices: N
Federal Procurement Eligibility: Small Business
Distribution: Manufacturer Direct, OEM

Chromatography, Liquid, Performance, High	Toxicology

ES INDUSTRIES   800-356-6140 *(cont'd)*

Column, Chromatography	Chemistry

ESA, INC.   800-959-5095
22 Alpha Road, Chelmsford, MA 01824-4171   978-250-7000
FDA Number: 1218996   *Fax:* 978-250-7090
E-mail: info@esainc.com
Web site: www.esainc.com
Medical Products Sales Volume: $12,700,000
Annual Revenue: $10-$25 Million
Year Founded: 1968
Total Employees: 84   *Marketing Staff:* 3   *Sales Staff:* 10
Ownership: Private
Quality System Registration Information: ISO9001
Produces/Sells CE-marked Devices: Y
Federal Procurement Eligibility: Small Business, GSA Contract
Distribution: Manufacturer Direct, Manufacturer Through Distributor, Manufacturer Through Manufacturer Reps, OEM, Service Direct, Exclusive Distributor, Importer, Exporter
General Admin.: Walter DiGiusto/President
Mktg./Adv.: K. Oakes/Coord. Marketing
     John Waraska/Director Marketing & Business Development
     K. G. Oakes/Manager Advertising
     Helmer Korb/Manager National Sales
Production: Harold Asp/Manager Regulatory Affairs

Analyzer, Chemistry, Multi-Channel, Programmable	Chemistry
Analyzer, Chemistry, Single Channel, Programmable	Chemistry
Analyzer, Lead	General
Chromatography Equipment, Liquid	Chemistry
Detector, Electrochemical, Chromatography, Liquid	Toxicology
Filter, Air	General
Kit, Sampling, Blood	General
Sampler, Air	General

ESB ENTERPRISES, LLC   847-429-9990
1490 Crispin Dr., Elgin, IL 60123
FDA Number: 1422570

Booth, Sun Tan	Physical Med

ESB MEDCOR INC.
See St. Jude Medical Atrial Fibrillation

ESBE SCIENTIFIC INDUSTRIES INC.   800-268-3477
80 McPherson St.,   905-475-8232
Markham, ONT L3R-3 Canada
FDA Number: n/a   *Fax:* 905-475-5688
E-mail: info@esbe.com
Web site: www.esbe.com
Year Founded: 1968
Total Employees: 100
Ownership: Private
Produces/Sells CE-marked Devices: N
Distribution: Exclusive Distributor

ESCALON MEDICAL CORP.   610-688-6830
435 Devon Park Drive, Building 100, Wayne, PA 19087
FDA Number: n/a   *Fax:* 610-688-3641
E-mail: info@escalonmed.com
Web site: www.escalonmed.com
Medical Products Sales Volume: $7,600,000
Annual Revenue: $5-$10 Million
Year Founded: 1987
Total Employees: 25   *Marketing Staff:* 2   *Sales Staff:* 7
Ownership: Public
Stock Symbol: ESMC
Traded On: NASDAQ
Produces/Sells CE-marked Devices: N
Federal Procurement Eligibility: Small Business
Distribution: Manufacturer Direct, OEM
General Admin.: Richard J. DePiano/Chief Executive Officer
     Ronald Hueneke/President, Chief Operating Officer
Mktg./Adv.: William Anton/Vice President Marketing
Finance: Douglas McGonegal/Vice President Admin., Finance

Endoscope, Ophthalmic	Gastroenterology/Urology
Light Source, Fiberoptic, Routine	Gastroenterology/Urology
Light, Surgical, Fiberoptic	Surgery

Medical Product Subsidiaries (Listed Separately)
Drew Scientific Ltd.
Escalon Trek Medical
Sonomed, Inc.

ESCALON OPHTHALMICS
See Escalon Medical Corp.

ESCALON TREK MEDICAL   800-433-8197
2440 S. 179th St., New Berlin, WI 53146   262-821-9182
FDA Number: 2183477   *Fax:* 262-821-9927
E-mail: sales@escalonmed.com
Web site: www.escalonmed.com

ESCALON TREK MEDICAL   800-433-8197 (cont'd)

Ownership: Escalon Medical Corp.
Produces/Sells CE-marked Devices: N

Camera, Ophthalmic, AC-Powered (Fundus)	Ophthalmology
Cannula, Ophthalmic	Ophthalmology
Endoilluminator	Ophthalmology
Flowmeter, Blood, Intravenous	Cardiovascular
Illuminator, Fiberoptic, Surgical Field	Cns/Neurology
Knife, Ophthalmic	Ophthalmology
Light, Surgical, Fiberoptic	Surgery
Needle, Suture, Ophthalmic	Ophthalmology
Pump, Infusion, Ophthalmic	Ophthalmology
Retractor, Ophthalmic	Ophthalmology
Syringe, Piston	General
Transducer, Blood Pressure, Catheter Tip	Cardiovascular
Transducer, Ultrasonic, Diagnostic	Radiology

ESCHENBACH OPTIK OF AMERICA, INC.   800-487-5389
904 Ethan Allen Hwy., Ridgefield, CT 06877-2826   203-438-7471

FDA Number: 1220848   Fax: 203-438-1670
E-mail: info@eschenbach.com
Web site: www.eschenbach.com
Ownership: Private
Quality System Registration Information: ISO9001
Produces/Sells CE-marked Devices: N
Distribution: Exclusive Distributor, Importer
General Admin.: Kenneth Bradley/President
Mktg./Adv.: Timothy J. Gels/Director Marketing

Loupe, Binocular, Low Power	Ophthalmology
Loupe, Diagnostic/Surgical	Surgery
Magnifier, Hand-Held, Low-Vision	Ophthalmology
Magnifier, Operating	Surgery
Material, Training, Audiovisual	General
Spectacle, Magnifier	Ophthalmology
Spectacle, Operating (Loupe), Ophthalmic	Ophthalmology
Sunglasses (Including Photosensitive)	Ophthalmology
Telescope, Spectacle, Low-Vision	Ophthalmology
Viewer/Magnifier	Hematology
Vision Aid, Electronic, AC-Powered	Ophthalmology
Vision Aid, Image Intensification, Battery-Powered	Ophthalmology
Vision Aid, Optical, AC-Powered	Ophthalmology
Vision Aid, Optical, Battery-Powered	Ophthalmology

ESCO MEDICAL INSTRUMENTS, INC.
See Esco Medical Instruments, Inc.

ESCO PRECISION, INC.
See Esco Medical Instruments, Inc.

ESCREEN, INC.   800-881-0722
7500 W. 110th Street, Suite 500,   913-327-8606
Overland Park, KS 66210

FDA Number: 2032801   Fax: 913-327-8606
Ownership: Private
Produces/Sells CE-marked Devices: N

Enzyme Immunoassay, Cannabinoids	Toxicology
Enzyme Immunoassay, Cocaine And Cocaine Metabolites	Toxicology
Enzyme Immunoassay, Opiates	Toxicology
Enzyme Immunoassay, Phencyclidine	Toxicology
Gas Chromatography, Methamphetamine	Toxicology
Kit, Screening, Urine	Microbiology

ESE ACQUISITION LLC.   609-716-0600
666 Plainsboro Rd. Suite 1271, Plainsboro, NJ 08536

FDA Number: 2183644
Ownership: Private
Produces/Sells CE-marked Devices: N

Surgical Instrument, Disposable	Surgery

ESHA RESEARCH   503-585-6242
4747 skyline Rd S Suite 100, Salem, OR 97306

FDA Number: n/a   Fax: 503-585-5543
E-mail: info@esha.com
Web site: www.esha.com
Medical Products Sales Volume: $2,000,000
Annual Revenue: $1-$5 Million
Year Founded: 1981
Total Employees: 22   Marketing Staff: 3   Sales Staff: 3
Ownership: Private
Produces/Sells CE-marked Devices: N
Federal Procurement Eligibility: Small Business
Distribution: Manufacturer Direct, Exporter
General Admin.: Robert B. Geltz/Chief Executive Officer
    Elizabeth S. Hands/President
Mktg./Adv.: Layne Westover/Vice President Marketing & Sales
Production: Alicia Triplett/Customer Service Representative

Computer Software	General

ESI, INC.   763-473-2533
2915 Everest Ln. N., Plymouth, MN 55447

FDA Number: 3004181533

ESI, INC.   763-473-2533 (cont'd)

Ownership: Private
Produces/Sells CE-marked Devices: N

Shell, Scleral	Ophthalmology

ESMA, INC.   800-276-2466
450 WestTaft Dr., South Holland, IL 60473   708-331-1855

FDA Number: n/a   Fax: 708-331-8919
E-mail: sales@esmainc.com
Web site: www.esmainc.com
Year Founded: 1972
Ownership: Private
Produces/Sells CE-marked Devices: N
Federal Procurement Eligibility: Small Business
Distribution: Manufacturer Direct
General Admin.: Tim Beezhold/President
Mktg./Adv.: Paul Beezhold/Vice President Sales

Cleaner, Ultrasonic, Dental Laboratory	Dental And Oral
Cleaner, Ultrasonic, Medical Instrument	General
Prophylaxis Unit, Ultrasonic, Dental	Dental And Oral

ESSENTIAL DENTAL SYSTEMS, INC.   800-223-5394
89 Leuning St., South Hackensack, NJ 07606   201-487-9090

FDA Number: 2433629   Fax: 201-487-5120
E-mail: info@edsdental.com
Web site: www.edsdental.com
Medical Products Sales Volume: $1,900,000
Year Founded: 1981
Total Employees: 25
Ownership: Private
Quality System Registration Information: ISO9001
Produces/Sells CE-marked Devices: Y
Federal Procurement Eligibility: Small Business
Distribution: Manufacturer Through Distributor
General Admin.: Dr. N/A N/A/Chief Executive Officer
    Allan S. Deutsch/Executive Vice President
    Barry Lee Musikant/President
Mktg./Adv.: Rick Willson/Manager National Sales
Production: Gary Cofrancesco/Manager Operations
Finance: N/A N/A/Controller

Cement, Dental	Dental And Oral
Compound, Resinous, Composite	Dental And Oral
Post, Root Canal	Dental And Oral

ESSENTIAL INDUSTRIES INC.   800-551-9679
28391 Essential Road, P.O. Box 12,   262-538-1122
Merton, WI 53056

FDA Number: n/a   Fax: 262-538-1354
E-mail: service@essind.com
Web site: www.essind.com
Annual Revenue: $1-$5 Million
Year Founded: 1898
Ownership: Private
Produces/Sells CE-marked Devices: N
Federal Procurement Eligibility: Small Business
Distribution: Manufacturer Through Distributor, Manufacturer Through
Manufacturer Reps

Disinfector, Liquid	General
Solution, Antibacterial Cleaner	General

ESSENTIAL MEDICAL SUPPLY, INC.   800-826-8423
6420 Hazeltine National Drive, Orlando, FL 32822   407-770-0710

FDA Number: 1056127   Fax: 407-770-0624
E-mail: essmed@aol.com
Web site: www.essentialmedicalsupply.com
Medical Products Sales Volume: $4,900,000
Annual Revenue: $5-$10 Million
Year Founded: 1985
Total Employees: 30   Marketing Staff: 2   Sales Staff: 7
Ownership: Private
Quality System Registration Information: ISO9002
Produces/Sells CE-marked Devices: N
Federal Procurement Eligibility: Small Business
Distribution: Manufacturer Direct, Manufacturer Through Distributor, Manufacturer
Through Manufacturer Reps
General Admin.: Carol Ann Hoepner/Co-Owner, Vice President
    J. Michael Hoepner/President, Owner

Attachment, Commode, Wheelchair	Physical Med
Cane	Physical Med
Cushion, Wheelchair (Pad)	Physical Med
Equipment, Therapy, Handicapped/Physical	Physical Med
Gown, Patient, Reusable	General
Linen, Bed	General
Mattress, Alternating Pressure (Or Pads)	Physical Med
Pad, Incontinence (Underpad)	General
Pant, Incontinence	General
Pillow	General
Pillow, Cervical	Orthopedics

ESSENTIAL MEDICAL SUPPLY, INC. 800-826-8423 *(cont'd)*

Pump, Inflator	General
Walker, Mechanical	Physical Med
Wheelchair, Manual	Physical Med

ESSEX CRYOGENICS OF MISSOURI, INC. 314-832-8077
8007 Chivvis Dr., St. Louis, MO 63123
FDA Number: 1937980   *Fax:* 314-832-8208
Ownership: Private
Produces/Sells CE-marked Devices: N

Canister, Liquid Oxygen, Portable	Anesthesiology
Conserver, Oxygen	Anesthesiology

ESSILOR INDUSTRIES 011-331-4977422
Sabanetas Industrial Park, Mercedita, PR 00715
FDA Number: 2648462   *Fax:* 787-848-4690
E-mail: jpannone@essilorusa.com
Year Founded: 1980
Total Employees: 250
Ownership: Private
Quality System Registration Information: ISO9002
Produces/Sells CE-marked Devices: N

Lens, Spectacle/Eyeglasses, Non-Custom	Ophthalmology

ESSILOR OF AMERICA, INC. 800-843-3937
4970 Park St. North, St. Petersburg, FL 33709
FDA Number: 1043713
Web site: http://essilorusa.com
Annual Revenue: $0-$1 Million
Ownership: ESSILOR INTL.
Produces/Sells CE-marked Devices: N
Distribution: Manufacturer Through Manufacturer Reps
General Admin.: Kevin A. Rupp/Chief Financial Officer, Senior Vice President
      John Carrier/President
      Leslie Wilemon/Vice President Human Resources
Mktg./Adv.: John Walborn/Vice President Business Development
      Carl Bracy/Vice President Market Development

Lens, Spectacle/Eyeglasses, Non-Custom	Ophthalmology

ESSILOR OF AMERICA, INC., MFG. DIV.
See Essilor Of America, Inc.

ESTECH, INC. 888-378-3240
2603 Camino Ramon, Suite 100,   925-866-7111
San Ramon, CA 94583
FDA Number: 2953686   *Fax:* 925-866-7117
E-mail: customerservice@estech.com
Web site: http://www.estech.com
Ownership: Private
Produces/Sells CE-marked Devices: N

Catheter, Vascular, Cardiopulmonary Bypass	Cardiovascular
Retractor, Manual	Cns/Neurology
Sucker, Cardiotomy Return, Cardiopulmonary Bypass	Cardiovascular
Surgical Device, For Ablation Of Cardiac Tissue	Surgery

ESTILL MEDICAL TECHNOLOGIES, INC. 877-354-0286
4144 North Central Expressway, Ste. 260,   214-561-6001
Dallas, TX 75204
FDA Number: 1650754   *Fax:* 214-561-1930
E-mail: brandonlopez@thermalangel.com
Web site: www.thermalangel.com
Medical Products Sales Volume: $1,200,000
Annual Revenue: $1-$5 Million
Year Founded: 1997
Total Employees: 5   *Marketing Staff:* 1   *Sales Staff:* 1
Ownership: Private
Produces/Sells CE-marked Devices: N
Federal Procurement Eligibility: Small Business
Distribution: Manufacturer Through Manufacturer Reps
General Admin.: Mr. Leo Lopez/Chief Executive Officer
      Mr. Jay Lopez/Chief Operating Officer
Production: Mr. Michael Ben/Director Engineering
      Mr. Michael Ben/Director Quality Assurance & Regulatory Affairs
      Mr. Brandon Lopez/Vice President Operations, General Manager
Finance: Mr. David Newby/Controller

Warmer, Blood, Non-Electromagnetic Radiation	Anesthesiology
Warmer, Infusion Fluid, Thermal	General

ET TRAINING SYSTEMS, LLC 313-864-1317
3494 Cambridge, Detroit, MI 48221
FDA Number: 105343
Ownership: Private
Produces/Sells CE-marked Devices: N

Exerciser, Non-Measuring	Physical Med

ETC
See Environmental Tectonics Corp.

ETCHELLS TECHNOLOGY CORP. 413-587-3922
82 Industrial Dr., Northampton, MA 01060-2327
FDA Number: 1226495
Ownership: Private
Produces/Sells CE-marked Devices: N

Bandage, Adhesive	Surgery

ETEX CORPORATION 617-577-7270
38 Sidney St., Suite 370, The Clark Bldg.,
Cambridge, MA 02139
FDA Number: 1225112   *Fax:* 617-577-7170
E-mail: Info@etexcorp.com
Web site: www.etexcorp.com
Medical Products Sales Volume: $2,800,000
Year Founded: 1989
Total Employees: 65
Ownership: Private
Quality System Registration Information: ISO9001
Produces/Sells CE-marked Devices: Y
Federal Procurement Eligibility: Small Business
Distribution: Exclusive Distributor
General Admin.: Steve Kim/Chief Financial Officer, Vice President
      Pamela Adams/Chief Operating Officer, Senior Vice President
      Brian Ennis/President, Chief Executive Officer
Mktg./Adv.: Mrs. Suneela Frary/Product & Sales Manager
      Jeffrey Wellkamp/Vice President Sales
Production: Charles Capps/Director Manufacturing & Operations
Research: Jerry Chang/Senior Director Research & Development

Bone Grafting Material, Human Source	Dental And Oral
Filler, Bone Void, Osteoinduction	Physical Med
Graft, Bone	Orthopedics
Metacrylate, Methyl, Cranioplasty	Cns/Neurology

ETHICARE 954-742-3599
P.O. Box 5027, Ft. Lauderdale, FL 33310
FDA Number: 1032351
Ownership: Private
Produces/Sells CE-marked Devices: N

Irrigator, Oral	Dental And Oral
Irrigator, Powered Nasal	Ear/Nose/Throat
Irrigator, Sinus	Ear/Nose/Throat
Toothbrush, Manual	Dental And Oral

ETHICARE PRODUCTS 800-253-3599
PO Box 5027, Fort Lauderdale, FL 33310-5027   954-742-3599
FDA Number: 9200343   *Fax:* 954-741-6367
E-mail: mail@ethicare.com
Web site: www.ethicare.com
Annual Revenue: $0-$1 Million
Total Employees: 9
Ownership: Private
Produces/Sells CE-marked Devices: N
Federal Procurement Eligibility: Small Business, Female Owned
Distribution: Manufacturer Direct, Service Direct
General Admin.: Kenneth E. Mullenix/President
      Barbara T. Mullenix/Vice President, General Manager

Kit, Irrigation, Ear	Ear/Nose/Throat
Lavage Unit, ENT	Ear/Nose/Throat

ETHICON ENDO-SURGERY, INC. 877-384-4266
3801 University Blvd., S.E.,   513-337-7000
Albuquerque, NM 87106
FDA Number: 1628808
Web site: www.ethicon.com
Total Employees: 9000
Ownership: Johnson & Johnson
Produces/Sells CE-marked Devices: N
General Admin.: Robert N. Wilson/Chairman
      W. C. Weldon/Chairman
      Lesley Fishman/Director
      Tina Pinto/Director
      Brian Perkins/President

Applier, Hemostatic Clip	Cns/Neurology
Biopsy Instrument	Gastroenterology/Urology
Cannula, Surgical, General & Plastic Surgery	Surgery
Clip, Hemostatic	Surgery
Clip, Implantable	Surgery
Electrocautery Unit, Gynecologic	Obstetrics/Gynecology
Electrosurgical Unit, Cutting & Coagulation Device	Surgery
Endoscope	Gastroenterology/Urology
Instrument, Manual, General Surgical	Surgery
Laparoscope, General & Plastic Surgery	Surgery
Laparoscope, Gynecologic	Obstetrics/Gynecology
Laser, Surgical	Surgery
Ligator, Esophageal	Gastroenterology/Urology
Ligator, Hemorrhoidal	Gastroenterology/Urology
Marker, Radiographic, Implantable	Surgery
Mesh, Surgical, Polymeric	Surgery

ETHICON ENDO-SURGERY, INC.   877-384-4266 *(cont'd)*

Needle, Pneumoperitoneum, Simple	Gastroenterology/Urology
Needle, Pneumoperitoneum, Spring Loaded	Gastroenterology/Urology
Retention Device, Suture	Surgery
Staple, Implantable	Surgery
Staple, Removable (Skin)	Surgery
Surgical Instrument, Ultrasonic	Surgery
Suture, Absorbable	Surgery
Suture, Absorbable, Synthetic	Surgery
Suture, Absorbable, Synthetic, Polyglycolic Acid	Surgery
Suture, Non-Absorbable, Silk	Surgery
Suture, Non-Absorbable, Synthetic, Polyamide	Surgery
Suture, Non-Absorbable, Synthetic, Polyester	Surgery
Suture, Non-Absorbable, Synthetic, Polyethylene	Surgery
Truss, Umbilical	Gastroenterology/Urology

ETHICON ENDO-SURGERY, INC.   800-USE-ENDO
4545 Creek Rd., MI #132, Cincinnati, OH 45242   **513-337-7000**
FDA Number: 1628808   *Fax:* 513-337-7912
E-mail: customersupport@eesus.jnj.com
Web site: www.ethiconendo.com
Annual Revenue: $1-$5 Million
Total Employees: 3000
Ownership: JOHNSON & JOHNSON
Produces/Sells CE-marked Devices: Y
Mktg./Adv.: Christian Williams/Manager PR
         Katen Licitra/Vice President Marketing & Sales

Applier, Clip, Laparoscopic	Surgery
Applier, Surgical, Clip	Surgery
Bag, Specimen, Laparoscopic	Surgery
Biopsy Instrument	Gastroenterology/Urology
Cannula, Surgical, General & Plastic Surgery	Surgery
Catheter, Balloon (Foley Type)	Surgery
Clamp, Laparoscopy	Surgery
Clip, Ligature	Surgery
Cord, Electric, Endoscope	Gastroenterology/Urology
Cutter, Linear, Laparoscopic	Surgery
Cutter, Surgical	Surgery
Electrode, Electrosurgery, Laparoscopic	Surgery
Electrosurgical Equipment, General Purpose	Surgery
Electrosurgical Unit, Cutting & Coagulation Device	Surgery
Endoscope	Gastroenterology/Urology
Equipment, Suction/Irrigation, Laparoscopic	Surgery
Forceps, Endoscopic	Gastroenterology/Urology
Forceps, Grasping, Atraumatic	Surgery
Forceps, Lung	Surgery
Forceps, Tissue	Surgery
Handle, Instrument, Laparoscopic (Electrocautery)	Surgery
Handle, Instrument, Laparoscopic (Irrigation)	Surgery
Holder, Needle, Curved, Laparoscopic	Surgery
Holder, Needle, Laparoscopic	Surgery
Instrument, Dissecting, Laparoscopic	Surgery
Instrument, Electrosurgery, Laparoscopic	Surgery
Instrument, Manual, General Surgical	Surgery
Introducer, Catheter	Cardiovascular
Kit, Bowel	Gastroenterology/Urology
Kit, Cholecystectomy	Gastroenterology/Urology
Kit, Herniorrhaphy	Gastroenterology/Urology
Kit, Hysterectomy	Obstetrics/Gynecology
Laparoscope, Gynecologic	Obstetrics/Gynecology
Mesh, Surgical, Polymeric	Surgery
Needle, Insufflation, Laparoscopic	Surgery
Obturator, Endoscopic	Gastroenterology/Urology
Probe, Electrosurgery, Endoscopy	Surgery
Probe, Suction, Irrigator/Aspirator, Laparoscopic	Surgery
Remover, Staple, Surgical	Surgery
Retention Device, Suture	Surgery
Scissors, Disposable	General
Sleeve, Trocar	Surgery
Staple, Implantable	Surgery
Staple, Removable (Skin)	Surgery
Stapler, Laparoscopic	Surgery
Stapler, Surgical	Surgery
Surgical Instrument, Disposable	Surgery
Surgical Instrument, Ultrasonic	Surgery
Suture, Non-Absorbable, Synthetic, Polyamide	Surgery
Thread, Stability, Trocar	Surgery
Trainer, Laparoscopy	Surgery
Trocar, Laparoscopic	Surgery
Trocar, Short	Surgery
Trocar, Surgical	Surgery
Trocar, Thoracic	Cardiovascular

ETHICON ENDO-SURGERY, LLC   513-337-3134
475 Calle C, Guaynabo, PR 00969
FDA Number: 3005075853
Web site: www.ethicon.com
Total Employees: 9000
Ownership: Johnson & Johnson
Produces/Sells CE-marked Devices: N

Biopsy Instrument, Suction	Gastroenterology/Urology

ETHICON ENDO-SURGERY, LLC   513-337-3134 *(cont'd)*

Clip, Implantable	Surgery
Stapler, Surgical	Surgery
Suture, Non-Absorbable, Synthetic, Polyamide	Surgery
Suture, Non-Absorbable, Synthetic, Polyester	Surgery
Suture, Non-Absorbable, Synthetic, Polyethylene	Surgery

ETHICON, INC   908-218-2996
3348 Pulliam St., San Angelo, TX 76905
FDA Number: 1614993
Web site: www.ethicon.com
Total Employees: 9000
Ownership: Johnson & Johnson
Produces/Sells CE-marked Devices: N
General Admin.: Dan Wildman/President
         Gary Pruden/President
         Renee Selman/President
Production: Robert Nunez/Plant Manager

Bandage, Adhesive	Surgery
Clip, Implantable	Surgery
Kit, Surgical Instrument, Disposable	Surgery
Mesh, Surgical, Polymeric	Surgery
Pledget And Intracardiac Patch, PETP, PTFE, Polypropylene	Cardiovascular
Suture, Absorbable, Synthetic	Surgery
Suture, Non-Absorbable, Synthetic, Polyamide	Surgery

ETHICON, INC.
See Artegraft, Inc.

ETHICON, INC.   908-218-2996
655 Ethicon Cir., Cornelia, GA 30531
FDA Number: 1049223
Web site: www.ethiconinc.com
Total Employees: 9000
Ownership: Johnson & Johnson
Produces/Sells CE-marked Devices: N
General Admin.: Dan Wildman/President
         Gary Pruden/President
         Renee Selman/President
Production: Robert Nunez/Plant Manager

Mesh, Surgical, Polymeric	Surgery

ETHICON, INC.   800-4-ETHICON
Route 22 West, p.o. box 151,   **908-218-0707**
Somerville, NJ 08876
FDA Number: 2210968   *Fax:* 908-218-2471
Web site: www.ethicon.com
Total Employees: 9000
Ownership: Johnson & Johnson
Stock Symbol: JNJ
Traded On: NYSE
Produces/Sells CE-marked Devices: N
Distribution: Manufacturer Direct, Manufacturer Through Distributor, Exclusive Distributor
General Admin.: Dan Wildman/President
         Gary Pruden/President
         Renee Selman/President
Production: Robert Nunez/Plant Manager

Agent, Hemostatic, Absorbable, Collagen-Based	Surgery
Bandage, Adhesive	Surgery
Barrier, Adhesion, Absorbable	Obstetrics/Gynecology
Button, Surgical	Surgery
Cabinet Casework, General Purpose	General
Cannula, Surgical, General & Plastic Surgery	Surgery
Cart, Multipurpose	General
Catheter, Suction, With Tip	General
Catheter, Transcervical, Balloon Tuboplasty	Obstetrics/Gynecology
Electrode, Pacemaker, Temporary	Cardiovascular
Endoscope	Gastroenterology/Urology
Fastener, Fixation, Biodegradable, Soft Tissue	Orthopedics
Fastener, Fixation, Non-Biodegradable, Soft Tissue	Orthopedics
Hysteroscope	Obstetrics/Gynecology
Infusion Stand	General
Laparoscope, General & Plastic Surgery	Surgery
Lead, Pacemaker, Implantable Myocardial	Cardiovascular
Mesh, Surgical (Steel Gauze)	Surgery
Mesh, Surgical, Polymeric	Surgery
Needle, Cardiac	Cardiovascular
Needle, Ophthalmic	Ophthalmology
Needle, Suture, Disposable	Surgery
Pledget And Intracardiac Patch, PETP, PTFE, Polypropylene	Cardiovascular
Pledget, Dacron, Teflon, Polypropylene	Cardiovascular
Polymer, Synthetic, Other	General
Prosthesis, Suture, Cerclage	Obstetrics/Gynecology
Retention Device, Suture	Orthopedics
Retractor	Orthopedics
Staple, Implantable	Surgery
Stent, Vaginal, Special Purpose	Obstetrics/Gynecology
Strip, Adhesive	Surgery
Surgical Instrument, Cardiovascular	Cardiovascular

ETHICON, INC.　800-4-ETHICON *(cont'd)*

Suture, Absorbable, Natural	Surgery
Suture, Absorbable, Synthetic	Surgery
Suture, Catgut	Surgery
Suture, Laparoscopy	Surgery
Suture, Multifilament Steel	Surgery
Suture, Non-Absorbable	Surgery
Suture, Non-Absorbable, Silk	Surgery
Suture, Non-Absorbable, Steel, Monofilament & Multifilament	Surgery
Suture, Non-Absorbable, Synthetic, Polyamide	Surgery
Suture, Non-Absorbable, Synthetic, Polyester	Surgery
Suture, Non-Absorbable, Synthetic, Polypropylene	Surgery
Suture, Other	Surgery
Suture, Polypropylene Monofilament	Surgery
Suture, Silk	Surgery
Suture, Stainless Steel	Surgery
Syringe, Irrigating	General
Tape, Measuring, Ruler And Caliper	Surgery
Tape, Umbilical	General
Truss, Umbilical	Gastroenterology/Urology
Wax, Bone	Surgery

Medical Product Subsidiaries (Listed Separately)
Mitek Products

ETHICON, LLC.　908-218-2887
Rd. 183, Km. 8.3,, Industrial Area Hato, San Lorenzo, PR 00754
FDA Number: 2648650
Web site: www.ethicon.com
Total Employees: 9000
Ownership: Johnson & Johnson
Produces/Sells CE-marked Devices: N

Agent, Hemostatic, Absorbable, Collagen-Based	Surgery
Agent, Hemostatic, Non-Absorbable, Collagen-Based	Surgery
Barrier, Adhesion, Absorbable	Obstetrics/Gynecology
Clip, Implantable	Surgery
Electrode, Pacemaker, Temporary	Cardiovascular
Mesh, Surgical, Polymeric	Surgery
Pledget And Intracardiac Patch, PETP, PTFE, Polypropylene	Cardiovascular
Prosthesis, Suture, Cerclage	Obstetrics/Gynecology
Retention Device, Suture	Surgery
Suture, Absorbable, Natural	Surgery
Suture, Non-Absorbable, Silk	Surgery
Suture, Non-Absorbable, Synthetic, Polyamide	Surgery
Suture, Non-Absorbable, Synthetic, Polyester	Surgery
Suture, Non-Absorbable, Synthetic, Polypropylene	Surgery
Truss, Umbilical	Gastroenterology/Urology
Wax, Bone	Surgery

ETHIX MEDICAL　514-935-5593
3465 Cote-des-Neiges, Ste. 702,
Montreal, QUE H3H-1 Canada
FDA Number: n/a　　*Fax:* 514-935-4305
E-mail: sales@ethixmedical.com
Web site: www.ethixmedical.com
Year Founded: 1994
Total Employees: 10
Ownership: Private
Produces/Sells CE-marked Devices: N
Distribution: Manufacturer Direct, Exclusive Distributor, Exporter

ETHOX INTERNATIONAL　800-521-1022
251 Seneca St., Buffalo, NY 14204　**716-842-4000**
FDA Number: 1314417　　*Fax:* 716-842-4040
E-mail: mpd@ethoxint.com
Web site: www.ethoxint.com
Medical Products Sales Volume: $27,000,000
Year Founded: 1966
Ownership: Moog Inc.
Produces/Sells CE-marked Devices: N
General Admin.: Ms. Matilda Lorenzo/Director Human Resources
　　　Mr. Thomas J. Bienias/President, Chief Executive Officer
　　　Ms. Anne Rowlands/Vice President, General Manager
Mktg./Adv.: Mr. Paul Baer/Marketing & Communications Officer
　　　John E. Creighton/Vice President Marketing & Sales
　　　Mr. John DeLuca/Vice President Sales
　　　Mr. Richard J. Malo/Vice President Sales
Production: Mr. Joe Gugino/Executive Vice President Operations
Finance: Mr. Brian Berkman/Chief Financial Officer

Bag, Blood, Collection	Hematology
Block, Bite	Cns/Neurology
Catheter, Aspiration	Surgery
Cuff, Blood Pressure	Cardiovascular
Decalcifier Device, Electrolytic	Pathology
Flask, Tissue Culture	Pathology
Infuser, Pressure (Blood Pump)	General
Kit, Surgical Instrument, Disposable	Surgery
Pack, Sterilization Wrapper (Bag And Accessories)	Surgery
Pressure Infusor, IV Container	General
Protector, Skin Pressure	General
Pump, Infusion	General

ETHOX INTERNATIONAL　800-521-1022 *(cont'd)*

Syringe, Irrigating	General
Transfer Unit, IV Fluid	General
Tube, Feeding	General
Tube, Gastro-Enterostomy	Gastroenterology/Urology
Tube, Gastrointestinal	Gastroenterology/Urology

Medical Product Subsidiaries (Listed Separately)
Sts Division Of Ethox International

ETKON USA, INC.
See Straumann Manufacturing, Inc.

ETONIC WORLDWIDE LLC　781-419-3060
260 Charles Street, Waltham, MA 02453
FDA Number: 3005241435
Ownership: Private
Produces/Sells CE-marked Devices: N
General Admin.: Mr. Tom Elwell/Chief Executive Officer

Shoe, Cast	Physical Med

ETS, INC.　317-554-3500
7445 Company Dr., Indianapolis, IN 46237
FDA Number: 1422143

Booth, Sun Tan	Physical Med

ETYMONIC DESIGN INC.　800-265-2093
41 Byron Ave.,　　519-268-3313
Dorchester, ONT N0L 1 Canada
FDA Number: 8022229　　*Fax:* 519-268-3256
E-mail: joanne@etymonic.com
Web site: www.audioscan.com
Annual Revenue: $1-$5 Million
Total Employees: 18
Ownership: Private
Produces/Sells CE-marked Devices: N
Distribution: Manufacturer Through Distributor, Exclusive Distributor
General Admin.: William A. Cole/President
　　　J. M. Jonkman/Secretary
Mktg./Adv.: Roger Whittle/Director Sales
　　　J. A. Jonkman/Manager Product Development

Calibrator, Hearing-Aid/Earphone And Analysis Systems	Ear/Nose/Throat

ETYMOTIC RESEARCH, INC.　888-389-6684
61 Martin Lane, Elk Grove Village, IL 60007　**847-228-0006**
FDA Number: 1450042　　*Fax:* 847-228-6836
E-mail: customer-service@etymotic.com
Web site: www.etymotic.com
Medical Products Sales Volume: $10,000,000
Annual Revenue: $10-$25 Million
Year Founded: 1983
Ownership: Private
Produces/Sells CE-marked Devices: N
Federal Procurement Eligibility: Small Business
Distribution: OEM
General Admin.: Mark E. Piepenbrink/Chief Executive Officer
　　　Mead Killion/President
Mktg./Adv.: Michael Shaver/Director International Sales
　　　Gail Gudmundsen/Director Marketing & Sales
Finance: Ms. Fran Wroble/Chief Financial Officer

Audiometer	Ear/Nose/Throat
Calibrator, Hearing-Aid/Earphone And Analysis Systems	Ear/Nose/Throat
Cushion, Earphone (For Audiometric Testing)	Ear/Nose/Throat
Electrode, Cutaneous	Cns/Neurology
Protector, Hearing (Insert)	Ear/Nose/Throat
Tester, Auditory Impedance	Ear/Nose/Throat

EUCARDIO LABORATORY, INC.　760-632-1824
2216 Silver Peak Place, Encinitas, CA 92024
FDA Number: 2027963
Ownership: Private
Produces/Sells CE-marked Devices: N

Kit, Pregnancy Test, Over The Counter, HCG	Chemistry
Turbidimetric Method, Lipoproteins	Chemistry

EUGENE ERNST PROD. CO.
See Ernst Flow Industries

EUMEDIC INCORPORATED
1369 Forest Park Circle, Ste 100, Lafayette, CO 80026
FDA Number: 3004935902
Ownership: Private
Produces/Sells CE-marked Devices: N

Biofeedback Device	Cns/Neurology
Stimulator, Nerve, Transcutaneous (Pain Relief, TENS)	Cns/Neurology

EURO-FRAMES, INC.　800-422-2773
2985 Glendale Blvd.,　　323-662-4225
Los Angeles, CA 90039
FDA Number: 2081262　　*Fax:* 323-662-7971
E-mail: info@euroframes.com

EURO-FRAMES, INC.   800-422-2773 *(cont'd)*

Web site: www.euroframes.com
Medical Products Sales Volume: $900,000
Annual Revenue: $0-$1 Million
Total Employees: 4   *Sales Staff:* 8
Ownership: Private
Produces/Sells CE-marked Devices: Y
Federal Procurement Eligibility: Small Business
Distribution: Service Direct, Exclusive Distributor, Importer, Exporter
General Admin.: Adour Douzjian/President
Mktg./Adv.: Houri Douzjian/Vice President Sales

Frame, Spectacle (Eyeglasses)	Ophthalmology
Sunglasses (Including Photosensitive)	Ophthalmology

EUROGENTEC

See Eurogentec North America, Inc.

EUROGENTEC NORTH AMERICA, INC.   877-387-6436
11111 Flintkote Avenue, San Diego, CA 92121   858-793-2661

FDA Number: 3008004341   *Fax:* 858-793-2666
E-mail: ivd.na@eurogentec.com
Web site: www.eurogentec.com
Ownership: Private
Produces/Sells CE-marked Devices: N
General Admin.: Mr. Jean-Pierre Delwart/Chief Executive Officer
    Mr. Takamune Yasuda/Chief Operating Officer
    Mr. Philippe Cronet/Chief Scientific Officer
Mktg./Adv.: Mr. Pierre Lacaze/Director Marketing & Sales
Finance: Ms. Veronique Distexhe/Chief Financial Officer

Reagents, Specific, Analyte	Hematology

EUROMED, INC.   877-238-76329
25 Corporate Drive, Orangeburg, NY 10962   845-359-4039

FDA Number: 3006358042   *Fax:* 845-359-1315
E-mail: Rlovell@euromedinc.com
Web site: www.euromedinc.com
Year Founded: 1991
Ownership: Private
Stock Symbol: N/A
Quality System Registration Information: ISO9001
Produces/Sells CE-marked Devices: Y
Distribution: Manufacturer Direct, Manufacturer Through Distributor, Manufacturer Through Manufacturer Reps, OEM, Exclusive Distributor
General Admin.: Mr. Thomas Gardner/President, Chief Executive Officer
Production: Mr. Stephen Powell/Vice President Operations
Research: Dr. Ravi Ramjit/Manager Research & Development

EUROPEAN EYEWEAR CORP.   941-322-6771
630 Myakka Rd., Sarasota, FL 34240

FDA Number: 1063916
Ownership: Private
Produces/Sells CE-marked Devices: N

Frame, Spectacle (Eyeglasses)	Ophthalmology
Lens, Spectacle/Eyeglasses, Non-Custom	Ophthalmology
Sunglasses (Including Photosensitive)	Ophthalmology

EUROTECH DENTAL LABORATORY, INC.   307-234-6808
301 N. Mckinley St., Casper, WY 82601

FDA Number: 3004828661
Ownership: Private
Produces/Sells CE-marked Devices: N

Alloy, Precious Metal, For Clinical Use	Dental And Oral
Teeth, Porcelain	Dental And Oral

EUROTHERM INC.   703-443-0000
741-F Miller Drive, Leesburg, VA 20175-8993

FDA Number: n/a   *Fax:* 703-669-1300
E-mail: info@eurotherm.com
Web site: www.eurotherm.com
Medical Products Sales Volume: $40,000,000
Annual Revenue: $50-$100 Million
Year Founded: 1965
Total Employees: 30   *Marketing Staff:* 10   *Sales Staff:* 18
Ownership: INVENSYS PLC
Quality System Registration Information: ISO9001; ISO9002
Produces/Sells CE-marked Devices: Y
Federal Procurement Eligibility: Small Business
Distribution: Manufacturer Direct, Manufacturer Through Distributor, Manufacturer Through Manufacturer Reps, OEM
General Admin.: John Searle/President
    Francine Markbein/Vice President Human Resources
Mktg./Adv.: Monique Watkins/Marketing Communications Specialist
    Al Betz/Vice President Sales

Controller, Temperature, Other	General
Recorder, Long-Term, Trend	General
Recorder, Paper Chart	Cardiovascular
Transmitter/Receiver, Physiological Signal, Infrared	Cardiovascular

EUTECTIC ELECTRONICS, INC.

See Suntech Medical, Inc.

EV3 INC.   800-716-6700
3033 Campus Drive, Plymouth, MN 55441   763-398-7000

FDA Number: 3005544822   *Fax:* 763-398-7200
E-mail: customerservice@ev3.net
Web site: www.ev3.net
Year Founded: 2000
Total Employees: 1600
Ownership: Ev3 Inc.
Produces/Sells CE-marked Devices: N
General Admin.: Mr. Patrick Spangler/Chief Financial Officer, Senior Vice President
    Pascal E.R. Girin/Executive Vice President
    Mr. Robert J. Palmisano/President, Chief Executive Officer
    Ms. Stacy Enxing Seng/Senior Vice President
    Gregory Morrison/Senior Vice President Human Resources

Catheter, Biliary	Gastroenterology/Urology
Catheter, Carotid, Temporary, For Embolization Capture	Cardiovascular
Catheter, Percutaneous	Cardiovascular
Catheter, Peripheral, Atherectomy	Cardiovascular
Device, Coronary Saphenous Vein Bypass Graft, Temporary, For Embolization Protection	Cardiovascular
Device, Retrieval, Percutaneous	Cardiovascular
Guidewire, Catheter	Cardiovascular
Introducer, Catheter	Cardiovascular
Prosthesis, Esophageal	Ear/Nose/Throat
Prosthesis, Trachea	Surgery
Stent, Superficial Femoral Artery	Cardiovascular

EV3 NEUROVASCULAR   800-716-6700
9775 Toledo Way, Irvine, CA 92618   949-837-3700

FDA Number: 2029214   *Fax:* 949-837-2044
E-mail: webmaster@ev3.net
Web site: www.ev3.net
Medical Products Sales Volume: $22,300,000
Year Founded: 2000
Total Employees: 240   *Marketing Staff:* 6   *Sales Staff:* 12
Ownership: Ev3 Inc.
Stock Symbol: EVVV
Traded On: NASDAQ
Produces/Sells CE-marked Devices: N

Agent, Injectable, Embolic	Surgery
Catheter, Continuous Flush	Cardiovascular
Catheter, Intravascular Occluding, Temporary	Cardiovascular
Catheter, Intravascular, Therapeutic, Short-term Less Than 30 Days	General
Catheter, Peripheral, Atherectomy	Cardiovascular
Device, Embolization, Artificial	Cns/Neurology
Dilator, Vessel, Percutaneous Catheterization	Cardiovascular
Guidewire, Catheter	Cardiovascular
Syringe, Piston	General

EVA HEALTH USA, INC.

See Cygnus Inc.

EVACU TECHNOLOGIES INC.   905-372-0322
2-20 Strathy Rd, Cobourg K9A 5J7 Canada

FDA Number: 9680534

Transfer Device, Patient, Manual	General

EVANS MEDICAL INC.   916-939-2451
1529 Terracina Drive, El Dorado Hills, CA 95762

FDA Number: 2523167
Ownership: Private
Produces/Sells CE-marked Devices: N

Kit, Administration, Intravenous	General

EVAPORATED METAL FILMS CORP.   800-456-7070
239 Cherry St., Ithaca, NY 14850

FDA Number: 3004936638   *Fax:* 800-456-3227
E-mail: info@emf-corp.com
Web site: www.emf-corp.com
Ownership: Private
Produces/Sells CE-marked Devices: N

Mirror, Mouth	Dental And Oral

EVELYN CO., INC.   800-221-0518
P.O. Box 35265, Tulsa, OK 74153-0265   918-665-3952

FDA Number: n/a   *Fax:* 19186656027
E-mail: dirk@evelyndental.com
Web site: evelyndental.com
Annual Revenue: $0-$1 Million
Year Founded: 1971
Ownership: Private
Produces/Sells CE-marked Devices: N
Federal Procurement Eligibility: Small Business
Distribution: Manufacturer Direct

Handpiece, Contra- And Right-Angle Attachment, Dental	Dental And Oral

EVENFLO COMPANY, INC.
800-233-5921
1801 Commerce Dr., Piqua, OH 45356 **937-773-3971**
FDA Number: 3001329238
Web site: www.evenflo.com
Annual Revenue: $10-$25 Million
Ownership: Private
Produces/Sells CE-marked Devices: N
Distribution: Manufacturer Direct
General Admin.: Rob Matteucci/Chief Executive Officer

Fiber, Absorbent	General
Pump, Breast, Non-Powered	Obstetrics/Gynecology
Pump, Breast, Powered	Obstetrics/Gynecology
Shield, Nipple	Obstetrics/Gynecology

EVENFLO PRODUCTS CO.
See Evenflo Company, Inc.

EVENVIEW TELEVISION INC.
See Pdi Communication Systems

EVEREADY BATTERY CO.
314-985-1569
Checkerboard Square, St. Louis, MO 63164
FDA Number: n/a
E-mail: evang.nunn@energizer.com Fax: 314-985-2205
Total Employees: 18000   Marketing Staff: 50   Sales Staff: 250
Ownership: Private
Produces/Sells CE-marked Devices: N
Distribution: Manufacturer Through Distributor
General Admin.: J. P. Mulcahy/Chief Executive Officer
Evan G. Nunn/Vice President, General Manager
Mktg./Adv.: Scott Viebranz/Vice President Sales

Battery	General

EVEREST & JENNINGS DE MEXICO S.A. DE C.V.
333-145-1045
Calle 3 No.631, Zona Industrial,
Guadalajara, JALIS 44940 Mexico
FDA Number: 8030605 Fax: 333-145-1060
E-mail: www.everestjennings.com
Medical Products Sales Volume: $3,490,000
Total Employees: 285   Marketing Staff: 2   Sales Staff: 8
Ownership: Everest & Jennings
Produces/Sells CE-marked Devices: N
Distribution: Manufacturer Direct, Exclusive Distributor

EVEREST BIOMEDICAL INSTRUMENTS CO.
636-305-9900
1732 Gilsinn Ln., Fenton, MO 63026
FDA Number: 1954453
Ownership: STRYKER CORPORATION
Produces/Sells CE-marked Devices: N

Audiometer	Ear/Nose/Throat

EVEREST INTERSCIENCE, INC.
800-422-4342
1891 North Oracle Road, Tucson, AZ 85705 **520-792-4545**
FDA Number: 7000802 Fax: 520-792-4546
E-mail: info@everestinterscience.com
Web site: www.everestinterscience.com
Medical Products Sales Volume: $1,000,000
Year Founded: 1980
Total Employees: 6   Marketing Staff: 1   Sales Staff: 2
Ownership: Private
Produces/Sells CE-marked Devices: N
Federal Procurement Eligibility: Small Business, Female Owned
Distribution: Manufacturer Direct
General Admin.: Charles E. Everest/President, Chief Executive Officer
Marilyn M. Everest/Vice President, General Manager
Mktg./Adv.: Marilyn M. Everest/Vice President Marketing & Sales
Research: N/A N/A/Vice President Research & Development

Controller, Temperature, Other	General
Monitor, Temperature (With Probe)	Anesthesiology
Reagent, Calibration	General
Thermographic Device, Infrared	Obstetrics/Gynecology
Thermometer, Electronic	General
Thermometer, Electronic, Continuous	General
Thermometer, Infrared	General
Thermometer, Laboratory, Recording	General

EVEREST MEDICAL CORP.
See Gyrus Medical, Inc.

EVERGREEN HEALTH INC.
877-742-3555
401 Audubon St., Adair, IA 50002 **641-742-3555**
FDA Number: 3003517441 Fax: 641-742-3556
E-mail: harris@visitevergreen.com
Web site: www.visitevergreen.com
Ownership: Private
Produces/Sells CE-marked Devices: N
Federal Procurement Eligibility: Small Business
Distribution: Manufacturer Direct, Manufacturer Through Manufacturer Reps

Utensil, Food	Physical Med

EVERGREEN MEDICAL PRODUCTS INC.
See C. R. Bard, Inc., Bard Urological Div.

EVERGREEN MEDICAL TECHNOLOGIES
See Welch Allyn Protocol Inc.

EVERGREEN RESEARCH, INC.
303-526-7402
433 Park Point Drive, Suite 140, Golden, CO 80401
FDA Number: 1722641 Fax: 303-526-7416
E-mail: HR@evergreenresearch.com
Web site: www.evergreenresearch.com
Medical Products Sales Volume: $1,400,000
Annual Revenue: $1-$5 Million
Year Founded: 1988
Total Employees: 16   Marketing Staff: 1   Sales Staff: 1
Ownership: Private
Quality System Registration Information: ISO9002
Produces/Sells CE-marked Devices: Y
Federal Procurement Eligibility: Small Business
Distribution: OEM
General Admin.: George Eilers/Chief Executive Officer
David Mabe/President
Finance: Linda Steinhoff/Controller

Computer Software	General
Contract Assembly	General
Contract Manufacturing, Product, Disposable	General
Contract Manufacturing, Product, Durable	General
Contract R&D, Diagnostics	General
Contract R&D, Equipment	General
Service, Consulting	General
Service, Engineering/Design	General
Weight, IV Pole	General

EVERGREEN SALES & MARKETING, INC.
651-222-2885
1010 W. University Avenue Suite 211, St. Paul, MN 55104
FDA Number: n/a Fax: 651-222-2960
E-mail: mike@evergreensales.com
Web site: www.evergreensales.com
Medical Products Sales Volume: $4,000,000
Annual Revenue: $1-$5 Million
Year Founded: 1990
Total Employees: 5   Marketing Staff: 1   Sales Staff: 4
Ownership: Private
Produces/Sells CE-marked Devices: N
Federal Procurement Eligibility: Small Business, Female Owned
Distribution: Manufacturer Direct, Manufacturer Through Manufacturer Reps
General Admin.: Mr. Patricia Fowler/Owner
Mr. Michael Fowler/President

Cable, Electrode	Physical Med
Cable, Electrosurgical Unit	Surgery
Cable/Lead, ECG	Cardiovascular
Cable/Lead, ECG, With Transducer And Electrode	Cardiovascular
Cable/Lead, EEG	Cns/Neurology
Cable/Lead, EMG	Cns/Neurology
Cable/Lead, TENS	Cns/Neurology

EVERIST GENOMICS
855-383-7478
709 W. Ellsworth Road, Ann Arbor, MI 48108
FDA Number: n/a Fax: 866-793-9041
E-mail: furban@everistgenomics.com
Web site: www.everistgenomics.com
Ownership: Private
Produces/Sells CE-marked Devices: N
General Admin.: Dr. Prasad Sunkara/Chief Executive Officer
Dr. David Fry/Chief Scientific Officer
Mr. Bill Worzel/Chief Technology Officer
Medical Admin.: Dr. Peter Lenehan/Chief Medical Officer
Mktg./Adv.: Mr. Frank Urban/Director Medical Marketing

EVERMED
See C. R. Bard, Inc., Bard Urological Div.

EVERMED CORP.
714-777-9997
4999 E. La Palma Ave., Anaheim, CA 92807
FDA Number: 2086716
Ownership: Private
Produces/Sells CE-marked Devices: N

Bed, Electric	General
Chair, With Casters	Physical Med
Wheelchair, Manual	Physical Med
Wheelchair, Powered	Physical Med

EVERYBYTE, LLC
805-279-3228
3940 Verde Vista Dr., Thousand Oaks, CA 91360-2650
FDA Number: 3004951213
Ownership: Private
Produces/Sells CE-marked Devices: N

System, Communication, Image, Digital	Radiology

EVOLUTION MEDICAL PRODUCTS, INC.   877-223-3999
74 Eastwood Drive, Deerfield, IL 60015   **847-945-5392**
FDA Number: n/a   Fax: 847-940-0401
E-mail: sales@evolutionmedical.com
Web site: www.cordcaddy.com
Medical Products Sales Volume: $400,000
Annual Revenue: $0-$1 Million
Year Founded: 1998
Total Employees: 3   *Marketing Staff:* 2   *Sales Staff:* 25
Ownership: Private
Produces/Sells CE-marked Devices: N
Federal Procurement Eligibility: Small Business
Distribution: Manufacturer Direct, Manufacturer Through Distributor
General Admin.: Bruce A. Glass/President, Chief Executive Officer
Mktg./Adv.: Randi F. Glass/Vice President Marketing
   Component, Electrical   General

EVOLVE MANUFACTURING TECHNOLOGIES INC. 650-968-9292
960 Linda Vista Avenue, Mountain View, CA 94043
FDA Number: 3006262888
   Scanner, Ultrasonic (Pulsed Doppler)   Radiology

EVS SPORTS PROTECTION   800-229-4EVS
2146 . Gladwick St,   **310-637-5000**
Rancho Dominguez, CA 90220
FDA Number: n/a   Fax: 310-325-5125
E-mail: lanticusa@aol.com
Web site: www.kneebrace.com
Annual Revenue: $1-$5 Million
Total Employees: 14   *Marketing Staff:* 1   *Sales Staff:* 4
Ownership: LANTIC USA
Produces/Sells CE-marked Devices: N
Distribution: Manufacturer Direct, Manufacturer Through Distributor, Exporter
General Admin.: Guido Rietdijk/President
   Kevin Hinyub/Vice President, General Manager
   Brace, Joint, Ankle (External)   Physical Med
   Joint, Knee, External Brace   Physical Med
   Support, Ankle   Orthopedics
   Support, Elbow   Orthopedics
   Support, Knee   Physical Med
   Support, Wrist   Physical Med

EXACT LABORATORIES, INC.
See Exact Sciences, Inc.

EXACT SCIENCES, INC.   866-333-9228
441 Charmany Drive, Madison, WI 53719   **608-284-5700**
FDA Number: n/a   Fax: 5608-284-5701
E-mail: brochelle@exactsciences.com
Web site: www.exactsciences.com
Annual Revenue: $0-$1 Million
Year Founded: 1995
Total Employees: 14
Ownership: Public
Stock Symbol: EXAS
Traded On: NASDAQ
Produces/Sells CE-marked Devices: N
Federal Procurement Eligibility: Small Business
Distribution: Manufacturer Through Distributor, Manufacturer Through Manufacturer Reps
General Admin.: Mr. Maneesh Arora/Chief Financial Officer, Senior Vice President
   Barry Berger/Chief Medical Officer, Vice President
   Mr. Graham Lidgard/Chief Scientific Officer
   Mr. Kevn Conroy/President, Chief Executive Officer
   Test, Cancer Detection, Other   Hematology

EXACTECH, INC.   800-392-2832
2320 N.W. 66 Court, Gainesville, FL 32653   **352-377-1140**
FDA Number: 1038671   Fax: 352-378-2617
E-mail: human.resources@exac.com
Web site: www.exac.com
Annual Revenue: $50-$100 Million
Year Founded: 1985
Total Employees: 215   *Marketing Staff:* 18   *Sales Staff:* 230
Ownership: Public
Stock Symbol: EXAC
Traded On: NASDAQ
Quality System Registration Information: ISO9001
Produces/Sells CE-marked Devices: Y
Federal Procurement Eligibility: Small Business
Distribution: Manufacturer Through Distributor, Manufacturer Through Manufacturer Reps
General Admin.: William Petty/Chief Executive Officer
   David Petty/President, Director
   Betty B. Petty/Vice President Human Resources
Research: Gary J. Miller/Vice President Research & Development
Finance: Joel Phillips/Chief Financial Officer
   Assembly, Knee/Shank/Ankle/Foot, External   Physical Med

EXACTECH, INC.   800-392-2832 *(cont'd)*
   Bit, Drill   Orthopedics
   Brace, Drill   Orthopedics
   Broach   Orthopedics
   Compression Instrument   Orthopedics
   Driver, Prosthesis   Orthopedics
   Gauge, Depth   Orthopedics
   Graft, Bone   Orthopedics
   Guide, Surgical, Instrument   Surgery
   Plate, Fixation, Bone   Orthopedics
   Prosthesis, Hip (Metal Stem/Ceramic Self-Locking Ball)   Orthopedics
   Prosthesis, Hip, Constrained, Metal   Orthopedics
   Prosthesis, Hip, Femoral Component, Cemented, Metal   Orthopedics
   Prosthesis, Hip, Semi-Const., Uncem., Non-P., M/P, Ca./Phos.   Orthopedics
   Prosthesis, Hip, Semi-constrained, Metal/Ceramic/Ceramic/Metal, Cemented Or Uncemented   Orthopedics
   Prosthesis, Knee, Femorotibial, Semi-Constrained   Orthopedics
   Prosthesis, Knee, Patellofemorotibial, Constrained, Metal   Orthopedics
   Prosthesis, Shoulder   Orthopedics
   Prosthesis, Shoulder, Hemi-, Humeral   Orthopedics
   Punch, Femoral Neck   Orthopedics
   Reamer   Orthopedics
   Screwdriver   Orthopedics
   Surgical Instrument, Orthopedic, AC-Powered Motor   Orthopedics
   Tamp   Orthopedics
   Template   Orthopedics
   Tray, Surgical Instrument   Surgery

EXAKT TECHNOLOGIES, INC.   800-866-7172
7002 N. Broadway Ext.,   **405-848-5800**
Oklahoma City, OK 73116
FDA Number: 1643230   Fax: 405-848-7701
E-mail: info@exaktusa.com
Web site: www.exaktusa.com
Annual Revenue: $1-$5 Million
Total Employees: 12
Ownership: Private
Produces/Sells CE-marked Devices: N
Federal Procurement Eligibility: Small Business, Female Owned
Distribution: Manufacturer Direct, Exclusive Distributor, Importer
General Admin.: Linda Durbin/President, Chief Executive Officer
Mktg./Adv.: West Williams/Sales Representative
   Ms. Debbie Walters/Sales Representative
   Janice Porter/Vice President Marketing
   Container, Specimen Mailer And Storage   Pathology
   Container, Specimen Mailer And Storage, Temperature Control   Pathology
   Grinder, Tissue   Pathology
   Tissue Processor (Infiltrator)   Pathology

EXAMI-GOWNS, INC.   800-962-4696
8647 Ridgely's Choice Drive,   **410-248-2825**
Baltimore, MD 21236
FDA Number: n/a   Fax: 410-248-0765
E-mail: egi@exami-gowns.com
Web site: www.exami-gowns.com
Medical Products Sales Volume: $1,300,000
Annual Revenue: $0-$1 Million
Year Founded: 1994
Total Employees: 7   *Marketing Staff:* 2   *Sales Staff:* 3
Ownership: Private
Produces/Sells CE-marked Devices: N
Federal Procurement Eligibility: Small Business, Female Owned, VA Contract
Distribution: Manufacturer Direct, Manufacturer Through Distributor
General Admin.: Patricia Blume/President
Mktg./Adv.: R. Craig Blume/Vice President Sales
   Gown, Examination   General
   Gown, Patient   Surgery
   Gown, Patient, Reusable   General
   Gown, Surgical   Surgery

EXAXOL CHEMICAL CORP.   800-739-2965
14325 60th St. North, Clearwater, FL 33760   **727-524-7732**
FDA Number: 1052985   Fax: 727-532-8221
Ownership: Private
Produces/Sells CE-marked Devices: N
   Reagent, General Purpose   Pathology

EXCEL LABS   763-391-7413
106 Central Ave., Suite B, Osseo, MN 55369
FDA Number: 2131667
Ownership: Private
Produces/Sells CE-marked Devices: N
   Hearing-Aid   Ear/Nose/Throat

EXCEL MEDICAL PRODUCTS, LLC   810-714-4775
3145 Copper Avenue, Fenton, MI 48430
FDA Number: 3004198398   Fax: 810-714-4059
E-mail: Info@excelmedicalproducts.com
Web site: www.angioplast.com

EXCEL MEDICAL PRODUCTS, LLC   810-714-4775 (cont'd)
Medical Products Sales Volume: $900,000
Total Employees: 6   *Marketing Staff:* 2   *Sales Staff:* 2
Ownership: Ffm Med Reps, Llc
Quality System Registration Information: ISO9001
Produces/Sells CE-marked Devices: N
Federal Procurement Eligibility: Small Business
Distribution: Manufacturer Direct, Manufacturer Through Distributor, Manufacturer Through Manufacturer Reps, OEM
General Admin.: Mr. Adam Cole/General Manager
Mktg./Adv.: Mr. Rick Moller/Manager Marketing & Sales

Accessories, Catheter	Surgery
Component, Silicone	General
Connector, Tubing, Blood	Cardiovascular
Contract Manufacturing	General
Contract Packaging	General
Device, Hemostasis, Vascular	Cardiovascular
Kit, Catheterization, Cardiac	Cardiovascular
Kit, Disposable Procedure	Cardiovascular
Syringe, Balloon Inflation	Cardiovascular

EXCEL TECH. LTD.   905-829-5300
2568 Bristol Cir, Oakville L6H 5S1 Canada
FDA Number: 9612330
Ownership: Natus Medical Inc.

Electromyograph, Diagnostic	Physical Med
Stimulator, Muscle, Electrical-Powered (EMS)	Physical Med
Stimulator, Nerve, Transcutaneous (Pain Relief, TENS)	Cns/Neurology
Stimulator, Ultrasound, Muscle	Physical Med
Vibrator, Therapeutic	Physical Med

EXCEL TECHNOLOGY, INC.   631-784-6100
41 Research Way, East Setauket, NY 11733
FDA Number: n/a   *Fax:* 631-246-9742
Web site: www.exceltechinc.com
Medical Products Sales Volume: $32,000,000
Total Employees: 90   *Marketing Staff:* 8   *Sales Staff:* 12
Ownership: Private
Produces/Sells CE-marked Devices: N
Distribution: Manufacturer Direct
General Admin.: ANTOINE DOMINIC/Chief Executive Officer

Laser, Dental	Dental And Oral

Medical Product Subsidiaries (Listed Separately)
Photo Research, Inc.

EXCELLADERM CORP.   877-969-7546
300065 Comercio, Rancho Santa Margarita, CA 92688
FDA Number: n/a   *Fax:* 877-807-7546
E-mail: info@excelladerm.com
Web site: www.excelladerm.com
Medical Products Sales Volume: $5,000,000
Annual Revenue: $1-$5 Million
Year Founded: 1998
Total Employees: 11
Ownership: Private
Produces/Sells CE-marked Devices: N
Distribution: Manufacturer Direct, Manufacturer Through Distributor, Manufacturer Through Manufacturer Reps, OEM, Exporter
General Admin.: Karen Monzo/General Manager
     Diane Carrier/President

Dermabrasion Unit	Surgery

EXCELLANCE, INC.   800-882-9799
453 Lanier Rd., Madison, AL 35758-1896   256-772-9321
FDA Number: n/a   *Fax:* 256-772-8792
Web site: www.excellance.com
Medical Products Sales Volume: $8,500,000
Annual Revenue: $5-$10 Million
Total Employees: 98   *Marketing Staff:* 6   *Sales Staff:* 6
Ownership: Private
Produces/Sells CE-marked Devices: N
Federal Procurement Eligibility: Small Business
Distribution: Manufacturer Direct, Manufacturer Through Distributor, Manufacturer Through Manufacturer Reps
General Admin.: Charlie Epps/President, Chief Executive Officer
Mktg./Adv.: Kevin Harrell/Manager National Sales
     Steve Vaughan/Vice President Sales
Production: Mike Davis/Vice President Manufacturing

Ambulance	General

EXCELSIOR MEDICAL CORP.   800-487-4276
1933 Heck Ave., Neptune, NJ 07753   732-776-7525
FDA Number: 2027791   *Fax:* 732-776-7600
Web site: www.excelsiormedical.com
Ownership: Private
Produces/Sells CE-marked Devices: N

Catheter, Hemodialysis	Gastroenterology/Urology
Catheter, Intravascular, Therapeutic, Short-term Less Than 30 Days	General

EXCELSIOR MEDICAL CORP.   800-487-4276 (cont'd)

Device, Flush, Vascular Access	General
Heparin	Pathology
Kit, Administration, Intravenous	General
Pad, Alcohol	General
Pump, Infusion	General
Transfer Unit, IV Fluid	General

EXCHANGE CART ACCESSORIES   800-823-1490
1 Commerce Drive, Freeburg, IL 62243   618-539-5006
FDA Number: n/a   *Fax:* 618-539-6202
E-mail: denise@peaknet.net
Web site: www.exchangecart.com
Medical Products Sales Volume: $400,000
Annual Revenue: $0-$1 Million
Year Founded: 1983
Total Employees: 4   *Marketing Staff:* 2   *Sales Staff:* 4
Ownership: Private
Produces/Sells CE-marked Devices: N
Federal Procurement Eligibility: Small Business
Distribution: Manufacturer Direct, OEM
General Admin.: Donald Gebhart/President
Mktg./Adv.: Denise Albers/Vice President Marketing & Sales

Accessories, Cart, Multipurpose	General
Cart, Equipment, Video	General
Cart, Instrument/Equipment, Laparoscopy	Surgery
Cart, Isolation	General
Cart, Other	General
Cart, Supply	General
Cart, Supply, Operating Room	Surgery
Cover, Cart	General

EXCITON TECHNOLOGIES INC.   780-248-5868
10230 Jasper Ave, Suite 4000,
Edmonton, AB AB T5 Canada
FDA Number: 3007963765   *Fax:* 780-248-5878
E-mail: info@excitontech.com
Web site: www.excitontech.com
Ownership: Private
Produces/Sells CE-marked Devices: N

EXECUTIVE DENTAL SUPPLY LTD.   800-211-7888
6984 MacPherson Ave.,   604-439-0024
Burnaby, BC V5J-4 Canada
FDA Number: n/a   *Fax:* 604-439-1059
E-mail: info@execdent.com
Web site: www.execdent.com
Year Founded: 1977
Total Employees: 10
Ownership: Private
Produces/Sells CE-marked Devices: N
Distribution: Manufacturer Direct, Importer

EXELINT INTERNATIONAL CO.   800-940-3935
5840 W. Centinela Ave., Los Angeles, CA 90045   727-827-1922
FDA Number: 1035907   *Fax:* 727-827-1635
E-mail: info@exelint.com
Web site: www.exelint.com
Annual Revenue: $5-$10 Million
Total Employees: 35   *Marketing Staff:* 8   *Sales Staff:* 20
Ownership: Private
Quality System Registration Information: ISO9001
Produces/Sells CE-marked Devices: Y
Federal Procurement Eligibility: Small Business
Distribution: Manufacturer Direct, Manufacturer Through Distributor, OEM, Exclusive Distributor, Importer, Exporter
General Admin.: E. Hamid/President, Chief Executive Officer
Mktg./Adv.: Armand Hamid/Director Advertising
     Keith Fredericks/Manager National Sales
     Robert Fredericks/Vice President Marketing & Sales

Accessories, Catheter	Surgery
Bandage, Other	General
Blade, Scalpel	General
Catheter, Intravenous	Cardiovascular
Glove, Other	General
Kit, Administration, Intravenous	General
Kit, Urinary Drainage Collection	Gastroenterology/Urology
Needle, Aspiration And Injection, Disposable	Surgery
Needle, Dental	Dental And Oral
Needle, Fistula	Gastroenterology/Urology
Needle, Hypodermic	General
Needle, Other	General
Needle, Scalp	Cns/Neurology
Needle, Spinal, Short-Term	General
Syringe, Hypodermic	General
Syringe, Insulin	General
Syringe, Other	General
Syringe, Tuberculin	General
System, Infusion, Administration, Drug, Implantable	General

EXELINT INTERNATIONAL CO.   800-940-3935 *(cont'd)*
- Tube, Blood Collection   Chemistry
- Tubing, Connecting   General

EXERCYCLE CORPORATION   800-367-6712 **X**
667 Providence St.,   401-769-7160
Woonsocket, RI 02895
FDA Number: 1218831   *Fax:* 401-762-0797
E-mail: exercycle@exercycle.com
Web site: www.exercycle.com
Annual Revenue: $1-$5 Million
Total Employees: 25   *Marketing Staff:* 3   *Sales Staff:* 3
Ownership: Private
Produces/Sells CE-marked Devices: N
Federal Procurement Eligibility: Small Business
Distribution: Manufacturer Direct, OEM, Service Direct, Exclusive Distributor, Exporter
General Admin.: David St.Germain/President
- Exerciser, Passive, Non-Measuring (CPM Machine)   Physical Med

EXERGEN CORP.   800-422-3006
400 Pleasant Street, Watertown, MA 02472   617-923-9900
FDA Number: 1221195   *Fax:* 617-923-9911
E-mail: marketing@exergen.com
Web site: www.exergen.com
Year Founded: 1980
Ownership: Private
Produces/Sells CE-marked Devices: N
Federal Procurement Eligibility: Small Business
Distribution: Manufacturer Direct, Manufacturer Through Distributor
General Admin.: Francesco Pompei/President, Chief Executive Officer
- Thermographic Device, Liquid Crystal, Adjunctive   Radiology
- Thermometer, Electronic, Continuous   General

EXFO AMERICA INC.   800-663-3936
3701 Plano Parkway, Suite 160, Plano, TX 75075   972-907-1505
FDA Number: 7000072   *Fax:* 716-924-9072
E-mail: Orders.EXFO.America@exfo.com
Web site: www.exfo.com
Medical Products Sales Volume: $9,000,000
Annual Revenue: $10-$25 Million
Year Founded: 1993
Total Employees: 24   *Marketing Staff:* 3   *Sales Staff:* 6
Ownership: Private
Traded On: NASDAQ
Produces/Sells CE-marked Devices: Y
Federal Procurement Eligibility: Small Business
Distribution: Manufacturer Direct, Manufacturer Through Distributor, Manufacturer Through Manufacturer Reps
General Admin.: David Farrell/President, Chief Executive Officer
Mktg./Adv.: Tim Klimasawski/Director Marketing Operations
    Ed Friedrich/Manager International & National Sales
    Don Jarvie/Manager National Sales
    David Henderson/Manager Product Development
Production: Cynthia Payne/Manager Production
Research: David Henderson/Vice President Research & Development
Finance: Peter Battisti/Vice President Finance
IS: William Gornall/Vice President Technology
- Micromanipulators and Microinjectors, Assisted Reproduction   Obstetrics/Gynecology

EXIQON INC.   800-576-6326
15501 Red Hill Avenue, Tustin, CA 92780   714-566-0420
FDA Number: n/a   *Fax:* 714-566-0421
E-mail: info@oncotech.com
Web site: www.exiqon.com
Ownership: Private
Produces/Sells CE-marked Devices: N
Distribution: Service Direct
- Test, Chemotherapy Sensitivity (Tumor Colony Forming)   Immunology

EXOCELL, INC.   800-234-3962
1880 JFK Boulevard, Suite 200,   215-557-8021
Philadelphia, PA 19103
FDA Number: 2528952   *Fax:* 215-557-8053
E-mail: exocellinc@aol.com
Web site: www.exocell.com
Medical Products Sales Volume: $1,000,000
Year Founded: 1988
Total Employees: 20
Ownership: Private
Produces/Sells CE-marked Devices: N
Federal Procurement Eligibility: Small Business, GSA Contract, VA Contract
Distribution: Manufacturer Direct, Manufacturer Through Distributor
Production: Dr. Gregory Lautenslager/Manager Quality Assurance & Quality Control
- Antigen, Antiserum, Control, Albumin   Immunology
- Colorimeter, General Use   Chemistry

EXOCELL, INC.   800-234-3962 *(cont'd)*
- Reagent, Other   General

EXOGEN, INC.   800-836-0849
10 Constitution Ave., Piscataway, NJ 08855   732-981-0990
FDA Number: 2248073   *Fax:* 732-981-0648
E-mail: exogen@worldnet.att.net
Web site: www.exogen.com
Medical Products Sales Volume: $12,000,000
Annual Revenue: $10-$25 Million
Total Employees: 46
Ownership: Private
Stock Symbol: EXGN
Quality System Registration Information: ISO9003
Produces/Sells CE-marked Devices: Y
Federal Procurement Eligibility: Small Business
Distribution: Manufacturer Through Distributor, Manufacturer Through Manufacturer Reps
General Admin.: John P. Ryaby/Chairman
    Richard H. Reisner/Chief Financial Officer, Vice President
    Susan Kelley/Executive Assistant
    Patrick A. McBrayer/President, Chief Executive Officer
Mktg./Adv.: Timothy Fenton/Manager International Marketing & Sales
Production: David Brintzinghoffer/General Manager Operations
    Teri Bolyog/Manager Quality Assurance
    John P. Ryaby/Manager Regulatory Affairs
    Roger J. Talish/Vice President Operations
Research: John P. Ryaby/Vice President Research & Development
- Analyzer, Bone, Sonic, Non-Invasive   Orthopedics
- Stimulator, Osteogenesis, Electric, Non-Invasive   Orthopedics

EXPANDOVER
See Covidien Lp

EXPRESS DIAGNOSTICS INT'L, INC.   507-526-3951
1550 Industrial Dr., Blue Earth, MN 56013
FDA Number: 3005411947
- Chromatography, Thin Layer, Tricyclic Antidepressant Drugs   Toxicology
- Enzyme Immunoassay, Amphetamine   Toxicology
- Enzyme Immunoassay, Barbiturate   Toxicology
- Enzyme Immunoassay, Benzodiazepine   Toxicology
- Enzyme Immunoassay, Cannabinoids   Toxicology
- Enzyme Immunoassay, Cocaine And Cocaine Metabolites   Toxicology
- Enzyme Immunoassay, Methadone   Toxicology
- Enzyme Immunoassay, Opiates   Toxicology
- Enzyme Immunoassay, Phencyclidine   Toxicology
- Enzyme Immunoassay, Propoxyphene   Toxicology
- Gas Chromatography, Methamphetamine   Toxicology
- Thin Layer Chromatography, Metamphetamine   Toxicology

EXPRESS MANUFACTURING, INC.   714-979-2228
3519 West Warner Ave., Santa Ana, CA 92704
FDA Number: 2087572   *Fax:* 714-556-0575
E-mail: info@eminc.com
Web site: www.eminc.com
Ownership: Private
Produces/Sells CE-marked Devices: N
- Scale, Stand-On   General

EXPRESS OPTICS, INC.
See Newport Optical Laboratories, Inc.

EXPRESS SYSTEMS AND PARTS   (888) 550-3776
NETWORK INC
325 Harris Drive, Aurora, OH 44202   330-995-4350
FDA Number: 3001334979   *Fax:* (330) 995-2320
Ownership: Private
Produces/Sells CE-marked Devices: N
- Equipment, Laboratory, Gen. Purpose (Specific Medical Use)   Chemistry

EXTA, INC.
See Smiths Medical Asd

EXTECH INSTRUMENTS CORP.   781-890-7440
285 Bear Hill Rd., Boston, MA 02451
FDA Number: n/a   *Fax:* 781-890-7864
Web site: www.extech.com
Medical Products Sales Volume: $6,000,000
Year Founded: 1970
Total Employees: 100
Ownership: FLIR SYSTEMS
Quality System Registration Information: ISO9001
Produces/Sells CE-marked Devices: Y
Federal Procurement Eligibility: Small Business
Distribution: Manufacturer Direct, Manufacturer Through Distributor
- Electrode, Laboratory pH   Chemistry
- Hygrometer (Humidity Indicator)   Anesthesiology
- Meter, Conductivity   Chemistry
- Meter, pH, General Use   Toxicology
- Meter, pH, Portable   Chemistry

EXTECH INSTRUMENTS CORP.   781-890-7440 *(cont'd)*
Solution, pH Buffer	Chemistry
Tachometer	General
Thermometer, Electronic	General

EXTENDED CARE AIR THERAPY SYSTEMS, INC. 740-697-0845
7165 Payne Rd., Roseville, OH 43777
FDA Number: 1530898
Ownership: Private
Produces/Sells CE-marked Devices: N
Bed, Electric	General
Restraint, Protective (Body)	General

EXTRA PACKAGING, CORP.   800-872-7548
631 Golden Harbour Drive, Boca Raton, FL 33432   **561-416-2060**
FDA Number: n/a   *Fax:* 561-416-9545
E-mail: sales@extrapackaging.com
Web site: www.extrapackaging.com
Medical Products Sales Volume: $7,700,000
Annual Revenue: $10-$25 Million
Year Founded: 1988
Total Employees: 33   *Marketing Staff:* 2   *Sales Staff:* 15
Ownership: Private
Quality System Registration Information: ISO9002
Produces/Sells CE-marked Devices: N
Federal Procurement Eligibility: Small Business, Female Owned, GSA Contract
Distribution: Manufacturer Direct, Manufacturer Through Distributor, Manufacturer Through Manufacturer Reps
General Admin.: Donna Kramer/Chief Executive Officer
    Matt Nesbitt/General Manager
    Gerald S. Kramer/President
Production: Joeseph Bertalome/Vice President Manufacturing
Research: Mr. Deon Rodden/Director Technology
Accessories, Decorative	General
Bag, Body	General
Bag, Plastic	General
Packaging Material	General
Packaging, Sterilization	General

EXTRANUCLEAR LABORATORIES INC.
See Extrel Cms

EXTREL CMS   412-963-7530
575 Epsilon Dr., Pittsburgh, PA 15238-2838
FDA Number: n/a   *Fax:* 412-963-6578
E-mail: info@extrel.com
Web site: www.extrel.com
Annual Revenue: $0-$1 Million
Year Founded: 1964
Total Employees: 48
Ownership: Private
Produces/Sells CE-marked Devices: N
Distribution: Manufacturer Through Distributor, Manufacturer Through Manufacturer Reps, Importer, Exporter
General Admin.: Luke Kephart/Chief Executive Officer
Production: Rick Schaeffer/Vice President Manufacturing
Mass Spectrometer, Clinical Use	Toxicology

EXTREL CORPORATION
See Extrel Cms

EXTREME ADHESIVES, INC.   800-888-4583
63 Epping Road, P.O. Box 1445,   **603-895-4028**
Raymond, NH 03077
FDA Number: n/a   *Fax:* 603-895-6236
E-mail: info@extremeadhesives.com
Web site: www.extremeadhesives.com
Medical Products Sales Volume: $1,000,000
Annual Revenue: $1-$5 Million
Year Founded: 1987
Ownership: Private
Produces/Sells CE-marked Devices: N
Federal Procurement Eligibility: Small Business
Distribution: Manufacturer Direct, Manufacturer Through Distributor, Exclusive Distributor
Adhesive, Liquid	General
Component, Other	General
Conveyor, Tray	General
Dispenser, Other	General
Tape, Adhesive, Hypoallergenic	General

EXTRUMED, INC.
See Vesta

EYE CARE AND CURE   800-486-6169
4646 S Overland Dr, Tucson, AZ 85714
FDA Number: 2085143
Bandage, Adhesive	Surgery
Caliper, Ophthalmic	Ophthalmology
Curette, Ophthalmic	Ophthalmology
Dilator, Lacrimal	Ophthalmology

EYE CARE AND CURE   800-486-6169 *(cont'd)*
Dish, Tissue Culture	Pathology
Forceps, Ophthalmic	Ophthalmology
Frame, Trial, Ophthalmic	Ophthalmology
Instrument, Manual, General Surgical	Surgery
Knife, Ophthalmic	Ophthalmology
Lens, Maddox	Ophthalmology
Lens, Set, Trial, Ophthalmic	Ophthalmology
Magnifier, Hand-Held, Low-Vision	Ophthalmology
Measurer, Lens, AC-Powered	Ophthalmology
Probe, Lacrimal	Ophthalmology
Pupillometer, Manual	Ophthalmology
Scissors, Ophthalmic	Ophthalmology
Simultan (Including Crossed Cylinder)	Ophthalmology
Spectacle, Magnifier	Ophthalmology
Speculum, Ophthalmic	Ophthalmology
Spud, Ophthalmic	Ophthalmology
Sunglasses (Including Photosensitive)	Ophthalmology

EYE EXPERT, LLC.   866-393-3973
2501-B Stantonsburg Rd., Greenville, NC 27834   **252-758-2402**
FDA Number: 1065974   *Fax:* 252-317-0374
E-mail: info@eyeExpert.com
Web site: www.eyeExpert.com
Ownership: Private
Produces/Sells CE-marked Devices: N
Camera, Ophthalmic, AC-Powered (Fundus)	Ophthalmology

EYE PROSTHETICS OF UTAH, INC.   801-942-1600
7400 Union Park Ave., Suite 102, Midvale, UT 84047
FDA Number: 1722804   *Fax:* 801-942-1717
E-mail: epuinc@aol.com
Web site: www.epu-inc.com
Year Founded: 1992
Total Employees: 2
Ownership: Private
Produces/Sells CE-marked Devices: N
Federal Procurement Eligibility: Small Business
General Admin.: Richard T. Caruso/President
Eye, Artificial, Non-Custom	Ophthalmology
Shell, Scleral	Ophthalmology

EYE PROSTHETICS OF WISCONSIN, INC.   262-363-1528
4781 Hayes Rd., Madison, WI 53704
FDA Number: 3004028951
Ownership: Private
Produces/Sells CE-marked Devices: N
Eye, Artificial, Non-Custom	Ophthalmology

EYE RESTORATION CLINIC   866-364-6544
4606 South Garnett, Suite 302,   **918-664-6544**
Tulsa, OK 74146
FDA Number: 1646981   *Fax:* 918-664-0668
E-mail: eyemakers2@easytelmail.com
Web site: elsiejoybco.tripod.com
Year Founded: 1982
Ownership: Private
Produces/Sells CE-marked Devices: N
Eye, Artificial, Non-Custom	Ophthalmology

EYEKON MEDICAL, INC   800-633-9248
2451 Enterprise Road, Clearwater, FL 33763   **727-793-0170**
FDA Number: 1038833   *Fax:* 727-799-2212
E-mail: info@eyekonmedical.com
Web site: www.eyekonmedical.com
Medical Products Sales Volume: $900,000
Annual Revenue: $1-$5 Million
Year Founded: 1987
Total Employees: 12   *Marketing Staff:* 3   *Sales Staff:* 30
Ownership: Private
Produces/Sells CE-marked Devices: Y
Federal Procurement Eligibility: Small Business
Distribution: Manufacturer Through Distributor, Manufacturer Through Manufacturer Reps, OEM, Exporter
General Admin.: Tina D. Baack/General Manager
    Mark D. Robinson/President, Chief Executive Officer
Mktg./Adv.: Chuck Jones/Director National Sales
Folders and Injectors, Intraocular Lens (IOL)	Ophthalmology
Lens, Intraocular	Ophthalmology
Viscoelastic Surgical Aid	Ophthalmology

EYEONICS, INC.   949-916-9352
10574 Acacia St., Suite D-1, Rancho Cucamonga, CA 91730
FDA Number: 2031924
Ownership: Bausch & Lomb
Produces/Sells CE-marked Devices: N
Lens, Intraocular	Ophthalmology

EYEQUIP, DIV OF ALLIANCE MEDICAL MARKETING
800-393-8676

5150 Palm Valley Road, Suite 305,
Ponte Vedra Beach, FL 32082
904-280-1900

FDA Number: 9011651
Fax: 904-280-1888
E-mail: info@eyequip.com
Web site: www.eyequip.com
Medical Products Sales Volume: $400,000
Annual Revenue: $1-$5 Million
Year Founded: 1994
Total Employees: 5   Marketing Staff: 3   Sales Staff: 11
Ownership: Private
Produces/Sells CE-marked Devices: Y
Federal Procurement Eligibility: Small Business
Distribution: Manufacturer Through Manufacturer Reps, Importer, Exporter
General Admin.: Scott E. Lewis/President
Production: Wayne A. Starling/Manager Regulatory Affairs
  Keratoscope, AC-Powered   Ophthalmology

EYESUPPLY USA, INC.
800-521-5257

10770 North 46th St.,, Suite C-700,
Tampa, FL 33617
813-975-2020

FDA Number: 1056058
Fax: 813-975-1000
E-mail: custserv@eyesupplyusa.com
Web site: www.eyesupplyusa.com
Medical Products Sales Volume: $3,500,000
Annual Revenue: $1-$5 Million
Year Founded: 1989
Total Employees: 12   Marketing Staff: 2   Sales Staff: 4
Ownership: Private
Produces/Sells CE-marked Devices: N
Federal Procurement Eligibility: Small Business
General Admin.: Susan Maida/President, Chief Executive Officer
  Catheter, Intravascular, Diagnostic   Cardiovascular

EYESYS VISION, INC.
281-885-3800

225 Pennbright Dr., Suite 100, Houston, TX 77090

FDA Number: 3003846583
Fax: 281-749-8139
E-mail: info@eyesys.com
Web site: www.eyesys.com
Ownership: Private
Produces/Sells CE-marked Devices: N
  Keratoscope, AC-Powered   Ophthalmology

EYETECH LTD.
847-470-1777

9408 Normandy Ave., Morton Grove, IL 60053

FDA Number: 1422635
Fax: 847-470-1778
E-mail: eyetech@usa.com
Web site: www.eyetechusa.com
Year Founded: 1985
Ownership: Private
Produces/Sells CE-marked Devices: N
Federal Procurement Eligibility: Small Business
Distribution: Manufacturer Direct
Production: Mr. Marek Mori/Product Manager
  Applicator, Ocular Pressure   Ophthalmology
  Button, Iris, Eye, Artificial   Ophthalmology
  Reducer, Pressure, Intraocular   Ophthalmology
  Sterilizer, Tonometer   Ophthalmology
  Tonometer, Manual   Ophthalmology

EYETEL IMAGING, INC.
888-222-3875

9130 Guilford Rd., Columbia, MD 21046
781-890-9989

FDA Number: 1126083
Fax: 888-668-7475
Ownership: Private
Produces/Sells CE-marked Devices: N
General Admin.: Mr. Gary Gregory/President, Chief Executive Officer
Research: Mr. Shazhou Zou/Vice President Engineering
  Camera, Ophthalmic, AC-Powered (Fundus)   Ophthalmology

EZ WAY, INC.
800-627-8940

710 E. Main Street, PO Box 89, Clarinda, IA 51632
712-542-5102

FDA Number: 2183887
Fax: 712-542-1899
Web site: www.ezlifts.com
Annual Revenue: $1-$5 Million
Year Founded: 1994
Ownership: Private
Produces/Sells CE-marked Devices: N
Federal Procurement Eligibility: Small Business
Distribution: Manufacturer Through Distributor, Manufacturer Through Manufacturer Reps
  Bath, Sitz, Non-Powered   Physical Med
  Bed, Hydraulic   General
  Lift, Patient   General
  Stretcher, Wheeled, Mechanical   Physical Med
  Transfer Device, Patient, Manual   General

EZY-RAMP CO.
800-835-8513

4502 North Armenia Avenue, Tampa, FL 33603
813-875-6302

FDA Number: 1035822
Fax: 813-876-2621
E-mail: info@healthaidonline.com
Web site: www.healthaidonline.com
Year Founded: 1972
Ownership: Private
Produces/Sells CE-marked Devices: N
  Component, Other   General
Medical Product Subsidiaries (Listed Separately)
  2c Optics, Inc.

F & L MEDICAL PRODUCTS CO.
724-845-7028

1129 Industrial Park Rd., Box 3, Vandergrift, PA 15690

FDA Number: 2529126
Fax: 724-845-5439
E-mail: Info@fandlmedicalproducts.com
Web site: www.fandlmedicalproducts.com
Ownership: Private
Produces/Sells CE-marked Devices: N
  Glove, Patient Examination, Specialty   General
  Shield, Protective, Personnel   Radiology

F & M SCIENTIFIC CORP.
See Agilent Technologies, Inc.

F.A.S.T. FIRST AID & SURVIVAL TECHNOLOGIES LTD.
604-540-8300

1687 Cliveden Ave, Delta V3M 6V5 Canada

FDA Number: 9680765
  Kit, First Aid   Surgery

FABLOK MILLS, INC.
908-464-1950

140 Spring St., Murray Hill, NJ 07974

FDA Number: n/a
Fax: 908-464-6520
E-mail: info@fablokmills.com
Web site: www.fablokmills.com
Annual Revenue: $0-$1 Million
Year Founded: 1952
Total Employees: 50   Sales Staff: 10
Ownership: Private
Quality System Registration Information: ISO9001
Produces/Sells CE-marked Devices: N
Federal Procurement Eligibility: Small Business
Distribution: Manufacturer Direct, Manufacturer Through Manufacturer Reps
General Admin.: Alex Fisher/President
  Curtain, Cubicle   General
  Lift, Patient   General

FABRICATION ENT., INC.
See Fabrication Enterprises Inc.

FABRICATION ENTERPRISES INC.
800-431-2830

Post Office Box 1500, White Plains, NY 10602
914-345-9300

FDA Number: 2432177
Fax: 914-345-9800
E-mail: info@FabricationEnterprises.com
Web site: www.FabricationEnterprises.com
Year Founded: 1974
Ownership: Private
Produces/Sells CE-marked Devices: N
General Admin.: Elliot Goldberg/President
Mktg./Adv.: Andrew Goldberg/Director Marketing
      Linda Goldberg/Director Sales
  Algesimeter, Manual   Anesthesiology
  Board, Scooter, Prone   Physical Med
  Chair, Adjustable, Mechanical   Physical Med
  Chair, With Casters   Physical Med
  Chair/Table, Medical   General
  Component, Exercise   Physical Med
  Discriminator, Two-point   Cns/Neurology
  Dynamometer, Non-Powered   Orthopedics
  Esthesiometer   Cns/Neurology
  Exerciser, Non-Measuring   Physical Med
  Fork, Tuning   Cns/Neurology
  Goniometer, Non-Powered   Orthopedics
  Pack, Hot Or Cold, Reusable   Physical Med
  Pack, Moist Heat   Physical Med
  Percussor   Cns/Neurology
  Pinwheel   Cns/Neurology

FABRITE LAMINATING CORP.
973-777-1406

70 Passaic St., Wood Ridge, NJ 07075-1004

FDA Number: n/a
Fax: 973-777-6707
E-mail: info@fabrite.com
Web site: www.fabrite.com
Annual Revenue: $5-$10 Million
Total Employees: 55   Marketing Staff: 2   Sales Staff: 4
Ownership: Private
Produces/Sells CE-marked Devices: N
Federal Procurement Eligibility: Female Owned
Distribution: Manufacturer Direct

FABRITE LAMINATING CORP. 973-777-1406 *(cont'd)*
General Admin.: Melody Levy/Chief Operating Officer
    Frank Olejarz/General Manager
    Annabelle Levy/President
Mktg./Adv.: Sid Sharma/Director Tech. Sales

Apron, Lead, Dental	Dental And Oral
Bib	General
Clothing, Protective	General
Cushion, Foot	Orthopedics
Cushion, Other	General
Diaper, Adult	General
Gown, Isolation, Surgical	Surgery
Mattress, Alternating Pressure (Or Pads)	Physical Med

FACEMASTER OF BEVERLY HILLS, INC. 818-222-2461
23961 Craftsman Rd.,suite I, Calabasas, CA 92302
FDA Number: 2087073
Ownership: Private
Produces/Sells CE-marked Devices: N

Massager, Therapeutic	Physical Med
Stimulator, Transcutaneous Electrical, For Cosmetic Use	Cns/Neurology

FACET TECHNOLOGIES, LLC 888-526-2387
112 Town Park Drive, Kennesaw, GA 30144 770-767-8800
FDA Number: 2082882
E-mail: busdev@facettechnologies.com
Ownership: Facet Technologies, Llc
Produces/Sells CE-marked Devices: N

Bandage, Adhesive	Surgery
Lancet, Blood	General

FACET TECHNOLOGIES, LLC 800-526-2387
112 Townpark Dr., Ste. 300, 770-590-6400
Kennesaw, GA 30144
FDA Number: 3005408301   *Fax:* 770-767-7320
E-mail: info@facettechnologies.com
Web site: www.facettechnologies.com
Annual Revenue: $50-$100 Million
Year Founded: 1969
Total Employees: 50   *Marketing Staff:* 2   *Sales Staff:* 6
Ownership: Private
Stock Symbol: MATR
Traded On: NASDAQ
Quality System Registration Information: ISO9001
Produces/Sells CE-marked Devices: Y
Federal Procurement Eligibility: Small Business, GSA Contract
Distribution: Manufacturer Direct, Manufacturer Through Distributor, Service Direct, Importer, Exporter
General Admin.: Kevin Selfert/Chief Executive Officer
    Anthony Cruz/General Manager
Mktg./Adv.: Mr. Michael Flater/Director Business Development
Production: Glenn Dill/Vice President Manufacturing
Research: Michael Lipoma/Vice President Development
    Doug Vine/Vice President Engineering
Finance: Don Jackson/Chief Financial Officer

Bandage, Adhesive	Surgery
Bandage, Compression	General
Lancet, Blood	General
Packaging Material	General
Packaging, Sterilization	General

Medical Product Subsidiaries (Listed Separately)
Facet Technologies, Llc

FACTOR II, INC. 928-537-8387
5642 White Mountain Avenue, Lakeside, AZ 85929-1339
FDA Number: 2023623   *Fax:* 928-537-0893
E-mail: factor2@whitemtos.com
Web site: www.factor2.com
Annual Revenue: $1-$5 Million
Total Employees: 6   *Marketing Staff:* 2   *Sales Staff:* 4
Ownership: Private
Produces/Sells CE-marked Devices: N
Federal Procurement Eligibility: Small Business, Minority Owned, Female Owned
Distribution: Manufacturer Through Distributor, Manufacturer Through Manufacturer Reps, Exporter
General Admin.: John McFall/Chief Executive Officer
Mktg./Adv.: Shannon Barton/Manager Advertising
    David Tearner/Manager International & National Sales
    David Tearner/Manager Sales Training
Production: John McFall/Director Quality Assurance
    John McFall/Manager Materials

Cap, Surgical	Surgery
Elastomer, Other	General
Elastomer, Silicone Rubber	General

FACTS AND COMPARISONS 800-223-0554
77 Westport Plaza, Suite 450, 314-216-2176
St. Louis, MO 63146
FDA Number: n/a
E-mail: rbrown@fandc.com   *Fax:* 317-735-5390
Web site: www.drugfacts.com
Ownership: Public
Stock Symbol: WK
Traded On: Amsterdam
Produces/Sells CE-marked Devices: N
General Admin.: Michael Riley/President
Mktg./Adv.: Robert Brown/Director Marketing

Computer Software	General

FAICHNEY MEDICAL CO. 800-548-0817
433 Scenic Drive, Suite # 103, 636-240-9501
St. Peters, MO 63376
FDA Number: 1933255   *Fax:* 636-272-6986
E-mail: fmcsales@msn.com
Web site: www.faichneymedical.com
Year Founded: 1886
Total Employees: 39091   *Marketing Staff:* 1   *Sales Staff:* 2
Ownership: Cantel Medical Corporation
Quality System Registration Information: ISO9001
Produces/Sells CE-marked Devices: Y
Federal Procurement Eligibility: Small Business
Distribution: Manufacturer Direct, Manufacturer Through Distributor, OEM, Importer
Mktg./Adv.: Mr. Jim Davis/General Manager Marketing & Sales

Thermometer, Electronic	General

FAIRBANKS SCALES, INC. 800-451-4107
821 Locust Street, Kansas City, MO 64106 816-471-0231
FDA Number: 1222929   *Fax:* 816-471-5951
E-mail: ingrid.l.adel@fancor.com
Web site: www.Fairbanks.com
Year Founded: 1830
Ownership: Private
Quality System Registration Information: ISO9000
Produces/Sells CE-marked Devices: N
Distribution: Manufacturer Direct, Manufacturer Through Distributor, Manufacturer Through Manufacturer Reps, Service Direct, Importer, Exporter
Mktg./Adv.: Mr. Bob Jozwiak/Vice President Marketing & Sales

Scale, Platform, Wheelchair	Physical Med
Scale, Stand-On	General

FAIRDALE ORTHODONTIC CO., INC. 513-421-2620
312 West 4th St., Cincinnati, OH 45202
FDA Number: 1523527
Ownership: Private
Produces/Sells CE-marked Devices: N

Band, Elastic, Orthodontic	Dental And Oral
Headgear, Extraoral, Orthodontic	Dental And Oral

FALCK MEDICAL CORPORATION 860-536-5162
35 Washington St., Suite 200, Mystic, CT 06355
FDA Number: 1226586
Ownership: Private
Produces/Sells CE-marked Devices: N

Tonometer, AC-Powered	Ophthalmology

FALCON PRODUCTS, INC. 800-873-3252
10650 Gateway Blvd., St. Louis, MO 63132-2214 314-991-9200
FDA Number: 9200348   *Fax:* 314-991-9227
E-mail: info@falconproducts.com
Web site: www.falconproducts.com
Annual Revenue: $50-$100 Million
Year Founded: 1959
Total Employees: 500
Ownership: Private
Produces/Sells CE-marked Devices: N
Distribution: Manufacturer Through Distributor, Manufacturer Through Manufacturer Reps
General Admin.: Frank Jacobs/Chief Executive Officer
    Rick Powers/Vice President
Mktg./Adv.: Lynda Garrison/Vice President Marketing
    Robert Rohlman/Vice President National Accounts
    Richard Hatek/Vice President Sales
Production: Darryl Rosser/Vice President Operations
Finance: Mike Dreller/Chief Financial Officer

Chair, Geriatric	General
Table, Other	General
Tray, Wheelchair	Physical Med

Medical Product Subsidiaries (Listed Separately)
Shelby-Williams Industries

FALCON REHABILITATION PRODUCTS, INC.
See Phoenix Group, The

FALICK/KLEIN PARTNERSHIP INC., THE
See Fkp Architects,Inc

FALL PREVENTION TECHNOLOGIES, LLC 937-434-5455
4601 Gateway Circle, Kettering, OH 45440
FDA Number: 3005049286
Ownership: Private
Produces/Sells CE-marked Devices: N

Nystagmograph	Cns/Neurology
Platform, Force-Measuring	Physical Med

FALLGARD LLC 800-828-0702
631 Alexandria Dr., Naperville, IL 60565
FDA Number: 1424460   Fax: 630-369-5219
E-mail: ellsta@aol.com
Web site: www.fallgard.com
Year Founded: 1999
Total Employees: 10   Marketing Staff: 5
Ownership: Private
Produces/Sells CE-marked Devices: N
Distribution: Manufacturer Direct, Manufacturer Through Manufacturer Reps, Importer, Exporter
General Admin.: Stanley Wiener/President, Chief Executive Officer

Orthosis, Limb Brace	Physical Med
Orthosis, Truncal/Limb	Physical Med

FARABLOC DEVELOPMENT CORP. 604-941-8201
211-3030 Lincoln Ave, Coquitlam V3B 6B4 Canada
FDA Number: 9615149

Cover, Limb	Physical Med

FARALLON MEDICAL, INC. 510-785-0800
3521 Investment Blvd., Suite 1, Hayward, CA 94545
FDA Number: 3005438989
Ownership: Private
Produces/Sells CE-marked Devices: N

Analyzer, Coagulation, Multipurpose	Hematology

FARETEC, INC. 440-350-9510
1610 W. Jackson St. #6, Concord Twp, OH 44077
FDA Number: 1528440

Sling, Arm	Physical Med
Splint, Clavicle	Physical Med
Splint, Hand, And Component	Physical Med
Splint, Traction	Orthopedics
Traction Unit, Non-Powered	Orthopedics

FARLEY INC., W.T. 800-327-5397
931 Via Alondra, Camarillo, CA 93012   805-437-7090
FDA Number: 2080309   Fax: 805-437-7098
E-mail: heather@wtfarley.com
Web site: www.wtfarley.com
Medical Products Sales Volume: $1,800,000
Year Founded: 1968
Total Employees: 12
Ownership: Private
Produces/Sells CE-marked Devices: N
Federal Procurement Eligibility: Small Business
Distribution: Manufacturer Direct, Manufacturer Through Manufacturer Reps
General Admin.: W. T. Farley/Chief Executive Officer
Mktg./Adv.: Sean Farley/Director Marketing & Product Development
     Karolina Zajac/Manager International & National Sales
Finance: Heather Farley/Chief Financial Officer

Aspirator, Emergency Suction	General
Attachment, Oxygen Canister/IV Pole, Wheelchair	General
Canister, Oxygen	Anesthesiology
Carrier, Container, Oxygen, Portable	General
Cart, Gas Cylinder (Carrier)	Anesthesiology
Cart, Other	General
Flowmeter, Gas (Oxygen), Calibrated	Anesthesiology
Holder, Gas Cylinder	Anesthesiology
Infusion Stand	General
Manifold, Gas	Chemistry
Regulator, Anesthesia	Anesthesiology
Regulator, Oxygen, Mechanical	General
Stand, Gas Cylinder	Anesthesiology
Stretcher, Hand-Carried	General
Ventilator, Other	Anesthesiology
Walker, Mechanical	Physical Med

FARMACEUTICOS ALTAMIRANO DE MEXICO, S.A. 52 (55) 52-71-4
BLVD. Adolfo Lopez Mateos NO .- 957,, COL. AUGUST 8, DEL., ALVARO OBREGON, DF CP 01 Mexico
FDA Number: n/a   Fax: 52 (55) 52-72-4
Medical Products Sales Volume: $1,000,000
Total Employees: 20   Marketing Staff: 1   Sales Staff: 3
Ownership: Private
Produces/Sells CE-marked Devices: N

FARMACEUTICOS ALTAMIRANO DE 52 (55) 52-71-4 (cont'd)
Federal Procurement Eligibility: Small Business
Distribution: Manufacturer Through Distributor

FARMATAP S.A. DE C.V.
117 Alfonso Esparza Oteo, Mexico Df 01020 Mexico
FDA Number: 8030618

Bag, Leg	Gastroenterology/Urology
Collector, Urine, Disposable	Gastroenterology/Urology
Drainage System, Urine, Closed	Gastroenterology/Urology
Stopcock	General
Tube, Feeding	General

FARNAM CUSTOM PRODUCTS 828-684-3766
90 Bradley Branch Rd., Arden, NC 28704
FDA Number: n/a   Fax: 828-684-3768
E-mail: info@farnam-custom.com
Web site: www.farnam-custom.com
Ownership: Private
Produces/Sells CE-marked Devices: N
Distribution: Manufacturer Direct, Manufacturer Through Distributor, Manufacturer Through Manufacturer Reps, OEM

Component, Electronic	General

FARPIN, INC. 801-262-8406
333 East 4500 South, #13, Murray, UT 84107-3965
FDA Number: n/a
Ownership: Private
Produces/Sells CE-marked Devices: N

Post, Root Canal	Dental And Oral

FARR COMPANY
See Camfil Farr

FARRAND OPTICAL COMPONENTS & 914-287-4035
INSTRUMENTS, DIV. OF RUHLE CO.
99 Wall St., Valhalla, NY 10595
FDA Number: n/a   Fax: 914-287-4025
E-mail: sales@farrandoptical.com
Web site: farrandoptical.com
Year Founded: 1949
Total Employees: 60   Sales Staff: 3
Ownership: Private
Produces/Sells CE-marked Devices: N
Federal Procurement Eligibility: Small Business
Distribution: Manufacturer Direct, Manufacturer Through Manufacturer Reps, OEM, Service Direct

Chromatography Equipment, Thin Layer	Toxicology
Fluorometer	Immunology

FARROW MEDICAL INNOVATIONS, INC. 877-417-5187
801 North Bryan, Bryan, TX 77803   979-822-9120
FDA Number: 3004537780   Fax: 979-775-5205
Web site: www.farrowmedical.com
Ownership: Private
Produces/Sells CE-marked Devices: N

Binder, Elastic	General
Binder, Medical, Therapeutic	General
Stocking, Support (Anti-Embolic)	General

FASER MEDICAL PACKAGING GROUP
See Beacon Converters, Inc.

FASSON
See Avery Dennison Corporation

FASSTECH 978-663-2800
76 Treble Cove Rd., Building 3, North Billerica, MA 01862
FDA Number: 1223851   Fax: 978-663-0999
E-mail: info@Fasstech.com
Web site: www.fasstech.com
Medical Products Sales Volume: $3,000,000
Annual Revenue: $1-$5 Million
Year Founded: 1993
Ownership: Private
Quality System Registration Information: ISO9001
Produces/Sells CE-marked Devices: N
Federal Procurement Eligibility: Small Business
Distribution: Manufacturer Direct, Manufacturer Through Manufacturer Reps, OEM, Exporter

Biofeedback Device	Cns/Neurology
Goniometer, AC-powered	Orthopedics

FASTEC MEDICAL SYSTEMS 866-463-3633
802 Whitewater Drive, Fullerton, CA 92833
FDA Number: 3004588200
E-mail: info@fastecmedical.com.
Web site: www.fastecmedical.com
Ownership: Private
Produces/Sells CE-marked Devices: N

FASTEC MEDICAL SYSTEMS   866-463-3633 (cont'd)
Device, Storage, Image, Digital   Radiology

FAULTLESS RUBBER CO.
See Hospira

FAUSTEL   262-253-3333
W194 N11301 McCormick Drive, Germantown, WI 53022
FDA Number: n/a   Fax: 262-253-3334
E-mail: sales@faustel.com
Web site: www.faustel.com
Medical Products Sales Volume: $4,200,000
Annual Revenue: $10-$25 Million
Year Founded: 1956
Total Employees: 60   Marketing Staff: 2   Sales Staff: 8
Ownership: Private
Produces/Sells CE-marked Devices: N
Federal Procurement Eligibility: Small Business
Distribution: Manufacturer Direct
General Admin.: Milton Kuyers/Chief Executive Officer
     John Hartley/President
Mktg./Adv.: Richard Greer/Vice President Sales
Production Equipment   General

FAWN VENDORS, INC.   800-548-1982
8040 University Blvd., Des Moines, IA 50325   866-657-7549
FDA Number: n/a   Fax: 515-271-8530
E-mail: contact@vending.com
Web site: www.fawnvendors.com
Medical Products Sales Volume: $1,000,000
Annual Revenue: $5-$10 Million
Year Founded: 1931
Total Employees: 50   Marketing Staff: 12   Sales Staff: 12
Ownership: Private
Produces/Sells CE-marked Devices: N
Distribution: Manufacturer Direct, Manufacturer Through Distributor, Manufacturer Through Manufacturer Reps, Service Direct
Foodservice Product/Equipment   General

FAXITRON X-RAY, LLC   888-465-9729
575 Bond Street, Lincolnshire, IL 60069   1 847 276 3427
FDA Number: n/a   Fax: 847.276.3437
E-mail: sales@faxitron.com
Web site: www.faxitron.com
Year Founded: 1994
Ownership: Private
Produces/Sells CE-marked Devices: N
Federal Procurement Eligibility: Small Business
Distribution: Manufacturer Direct, Manufacturer Through Manufacturer Reps, Exclusive Distributor
General Admin.: Mr. Allan Little/Chief Executive Officer
Mktg./Adv.: Mr. Brad Jackson/Vice President Marketing
     Mr. Don C. Whitehead/Vice President Sales
Research: Mr. Doug Wiegman/Vice President Engineering
Computer, Radiographic Image Analysis   Radiology
Radiographic Unit, Diagnostic   Radiology

FC INDUSTRIES INC.   937-275-8700
4900 Webster Street, Dayton, OH 45414
FDA Number: n/a   Fax: 937-275-9510
E-mail: afc@afctool.com
Web site: www.afctool.com
Annual Revenue: $50-$100 Million
Year Founded: 1989
Total Employees: 25
Ownership: Private
Quality System Registration Information: ISO9001
Produces/Sells CE-marked Devices: N
Federal Procurement Eligibility: Small Business
Distribution: Manufacturer Direct, Manufacturer Through Distributor
Drill, Oral Surgery   Dental And Oral

FCI OPHTHALMICS   800-932-4202
64 Schoosett Street, Pembroke, MA 02359   781-826-9060
FDA Number: 1225124   Fax: 781-826-9062
E-mail: info@fci-ophthalmics.com
Web site: www.fci-ophthalmics.com
Annual Revenue: $1-$5 Million
Year Founded: 1996
Total Employees: 5
Ownership: Scivex
Quality System Registration Information: ISO9002
Produces/Sells CE-marked Devices: Y
Federal Procurement Eligibility: Small Business
Distribution: Manufacturer Through Distributor, Manufacturer Through Manufacturer Reps, Exclusive Distributor
General Admin.: Bruno Chermette/President
Mktg./Adv.: Anne Bohsack/Vice President Sales

FCI OPHTHALMICS   800-932-4202 (cont'd)
Crutch, Ptosis   Ophthalmology
Dilator, Expansive Iris (Accessory)   Ophthalmology
Implant, Orbital, Extra-Ocular   Ophthalmology
Implant, Retinal   Ophthalmology
Ocular Peg   Ophthalmology
Plug, Punctum   Ophthalmology
Probe, Lacrimal   Ophthalmology
Retractor, Ophthalmic   Ophthalmology
Ring, Endocapsular   Ophthalmology
Ring, Symblepharon   Ophthalmology

FCI OPTOMETRICS
See Fci Ophthalmics

FECOM CORPORATION   800-292-3362
12 Stults Road, Suite 103, Dayton, NJ 08810   609-409-1720
FDA Number: n/a   Fax: 609-409-1721
E-mail: sales@fecomcorp.com
Web site: www.fecomcorp.com
Medical Products Sales Volume: $10,300,000
Year Founded: 1985
Total Employees: 30
Ownership: Private
Quality System Registration Information: ISO9000; ISO9001; ISO9002
Produces/Sells CE-marked Devices: Y
Federal Procurement Eligibility: Small Business, Minority Owned
Distribution: Manufacturer Direct, Manufacturer Through Distributor, Manufacturer Through Manufacturer Reps, Service Direct
Mktg./Adv.: Mr. Cliff Cheng/Sales Associate
     Ms. Monica Tartsanyi/Sales Associate
Analyzer, Battery   General
Battery, Hearing-Aid   Ear/Nose/Throat
Component, Metal, Other   General
System, Analysis, Hearing-Aid   Ear/Nose/Throat
Tester, Auditory Impedance   Ear/Nose/Throat
Unit, Measuring, Potential, Evoked, Auditory   Ear/Nose/Throat

FEDERAL ELEVATOR SYSTEMS INC.   888-785-5438
1090 Lorimar Drive,   905-458-4015
Mississauga, ONT L5S 2 Canada
FDA Number: n/a   Fax: 905-458-0680
E-mail: sales@federalelevator.com
Web site: www.federalelevator.com
Year Founded: 1988
Total Employees: 50
Ownership: Private
Produces/Sells CE-marked Devices: N
Distribution: Manufacturer Direct, Exporter

FEDERAL FOAM TECHNOLOGIES, INC.   800-457-3626
312 Industrial Rd., Ellsworth, WI 54011-5065   715-273-6700
FDA Number: 3003616072   Fax: 715-273-6717
E-mail: sales@federalfoam.com
Web site: www.federalfoam.com
Ownership: Private
Produces/Sells CE-marked Devices: N
Cushion, Flotation   Physical Med
Mattress, Non-Powered Flotation Therapy   Physical Med

FEELS GOOD FOOTWEAR, INC   203-740-8504
1 Whispering Way, Brookfld Ctr, CT 06804
FDA Number: 3005453670
Monitor, Orthotic/prosthetic   Physical Med

FEHLING SURGICAL INSTRUMENTS   800-FEHLING
509 Broadstone Lane, Acworth, GA 30101   770-794-0111
FDA Number: 1055706   Fax: 770-794-0122
E-mail: info@fehlingsurgical.com
Web site: www.fehlingsurgical.com
Annual Revenue: $1-$5 Million
Ownership: Private
Produces/Sells CE-marked Devices: Y
Federal Procurement Eligibility: Small Business
Distribution: Manufacturer Direct, Manufacturer Through Manufacturer Reps
General Admin.: Peter Skott/President, Chief Executive Officer
Mktg./Adv.: Peter Skott/Vice President Marketing & Sales
Production: Peter Skott/Vice President Manufacturing & Development
Biopsy Device, Endomyocardial   Cardiovascular
Chisel, Orthopedic   Orthopedics
Clamp, Aorta   Cardiovascular
Clamp, Peripheral Vascular   Cardiovascular
Clamp, Vascular   Cardiovascular
Clip, Vascular   Cardiovascular
Clip, Vena Cava   Cardiovascular
Curette   Orthopedics
Dilator, Blunt   Surgery
Dilator, Vascular   Cardiovascular
Dilator, Vessel, Surgical   Cardiovascular

FEHLING SURGICAL INSTRUMENTS 800-FEHLING *(cont'd)*

Elevator, Adson	Surgery
Forceps	Orthopedics
Forceps, Grasping, Atraumatic	Surgery
Forceps, Hemostatic	Surgery
Holder, Needle, Orthopedic	Orthopedics
Instrument, Manual, General Surgical	Surgery
Instrument, Microsurgical	Cns/Neurology
Instrument, Needle Holder/Knot Tying	Surgery
Punch, Bone	Orthopedics
Punch, Femoral Neck	Orthopedics
Punch, Surgical	Surgery
Retractor, Brain	Cns/Neurology
Retractor, Laminectomy	Surgery
Retractor, Surgical	Surgery
Retractor, Vessel	Cardiovascular
Rongeur, Manual, Neurosurgical	Cns/Neurology
Scissors, Cardiovascular	Cardiovascular
Scissors, Neurosurgical (Dura)	Cns/Neurology
Scissors, Plastic Surgery (Dissecting)	Surgery
Spreader, Rib	Orthopedics
Surgical Instrument, Cardiovascular	Cardiovascular
Surgical Instrument, Manual (General Use)	Surgery

FEITER'S INC 414-355-7575
8700 West Port Ave., Milwaukee, WI 53224
FDA Number: 2184103
Ownership: Private
Produces/Sells CE-marked Devices: N

Accessories, Wheelchair	Physical Med
Armrest, Wheelchair	Physical Med
Bedpan	General
Holder, Crutch and Cane, Wheelchair	Physical Med
Wrench	Orthopedics

FELTON INTERNATIONAL, INC. 913-599-1590
8210 Marshall Dr., Lenexa, KS 66214
FDA Number: 1000407601
Ownership: Private
Produces/Sells CE-marked Devices: N

Injector, Fluid, Non-Electric	General

FEMALE HEALTH COMPANY, THE 800-884-1601
515 N. State, Suite 2250, Suite 2225, 312-595-9123
Chicago, IL 60655
FDA Number: 1422723   *Fax:* 312-595-9122
E-mail: info@femalehealth.com
Web site: www.femalehealth.com
Medical Products Sales Volume: $14,800,000
Year Founded: 1996
Total Employees: 87   *Marketing Staff:* 1   *Sales Staff:* 1
Ownership: Public
Stock Symbol: FHC
Traded On: AMEX
Produces/Sells CE-marked Devices: Y
Federal Procurement Eligibility: Small Business
Distribution: Manufacturer Direct, Exporter
General Admin.: O. B. Parrish/Chairman, Chief Executive Officer
    Robert Zic/Director Admin. & Finance
    Mary Ann Leeper/President, Chief Operating Officer
    Mitchell Warren/Vice President International Affairs
    Michael Pope/Vice President, General Manager
Mktg./Adv.: Jack Weissman/Vice President Sales

Condom	Obstetrics/Gynecology

FEMASYS INC. 770-500-3910
5000 Research Court, Suite 100, Suwanee, GA 30024
FDA Number: 3007800906   *Fax:* 770-500-3980
E-mail: info@femasys.com
Web site: www.femasys.com
Ownership: Private
Produces/Sells CE-marked Devices: N

Cannula, Manipulator/Injector, Uterine	Obstetrics/Gynecology

FEMCAP INCORPORATED 858-792-2624
14058 Mira Montana Drive, Del Mar, CA 92014
FDA Number: 3002764647
Ownership: Private
Produces/Sells CE-marked Devices: N

Contraceptive Cervical Cap	Obstetrics/Gynecology

FEMINICA INC. 514-875-4422
3216 Rue Monsabre, Montreal H1N 2L5 Canada
FDA Number: 9616524

Speculum, Vaginal, Non-Metal	Obstetrics/Gynecology

FEMSUITE, LLC 415-561-2565
16A Funston Ave., San Francisco, CA 94129
FDA Number: 3004769119
Ownership: Private

FEMSUITE, LLC 415-561-2565 *(cont'd)*
Produces/Sells CE-marked Devices: N

Accessories, Surgical Camera	Surgery
Curette, Suction, Endometrial	Obstetrics/Gynecology
Curette, Uterine	Obstetrics/Gynecology
Speculum, Vaginal, Non-Metal	Obstetrics/Gynecology

FEN DENTAL MFG., INC. 305-556-5259
2665 West 81st St., Hialeah, FL 33016
FDA Number: 1058077
E-mail: sales@fendental.com   *Fax:* 305-826-0106
Web site: www.fendental.com
Ownership: Private
Produces/Sells CE-marked Devices: N

Activator, Ultraviolet, Polymerization	Dental And Oral
Alloy, Amalgam	Dental And Oral
Blade, Scalpel	Surgery
Burnisher, Operative, Dental	Dental And Oral
Material, Impression	Dental And Oral
Needle, Dental	Dental And Oral
Suture, Non-Absorbable, Synthetic, Polyamide	Surgery
Syringe, Cartridge	Dental And Oral
Wrap, Sterilization	General

FENWAL INC. 800-766-1077
Three Corporate Drive, Lake Zurich, IL 60073 847-550-2300
FDA Number: 3004548776
E-mail: info@fenwalinc.com   *Fax:* 847-550-5788
Web site: www.fenwalinc.com
Medical Products Sales Volume: $500,000,000
Annual Revenue: $100-$500 Million
Year Founded: 1949
Total Employees: 3500
Ownership: Private
Produces/Sells CE-marked Devices: N
Distribution: Manufacturer Direct
General Admin.: Ron K. Labrum/Chief Executive Officer
    Jo Anne Fasetti/Chief Human Resources
    Mr. William Cork/Chief Technology Officer, Senior Vice President
    Tony Orsini/Senior Vice President
    Angela Goodwin/Senior Vice President, Chief Information Officer
Mktg./Adv.: Mr. Geoffrey Fenton/Vice President Communications
Production: Mr. Dean Gregory/Senior Vice President Operations
Finance: Michael Johnson/Chief Financial Officer

Bag, Blood	Hematology
Bag, Blood, Collection	Hematology
Bracelet, Identification	General
Equipment, Apheresis	Hematology
Flask, Tissue Culture	Pathology
Kit, Blood Collection, Phlebotomy	Cardiovascular
Kit, Sampling, Blood	General
Microfilter, Blood Transfusion	Anesthesiology
Needle, Blood Collection	General
Needle, Other	General
Pressure Infusor, IV Container	General
Separator, Blood Cell, Automated	Hematology
Stripper, Donor Tube	Hematology
Supplies, Blood Bank	Hematology
Transfer Unit, Blood	Hematology
Tubing, Other	General

Medical Product Subsidiaries (Listed Separately)
Fenwal International, Inc.

FENWAL INTERNATIONAL, INC. 847-550-7908
Camino Real Industrial Park,, Road #122,
Ext Mans San German, PR 00683
FDA Number: 2648979
Ownership: Fenwal Inc.

Separator, Blood Cell, Automated	Hematology

FENWAL INTERNATIONAL, INC. 847-550-7908
Road 357, Km. 0.8, Maricao, PR 00606
FDA Number: 2627511
Ownership: Fenwal Inc.

Bag, Blood, Collection	Hematology
Separator, Blood Cell, Automated	Hematology

FENWICK HEARING INSTRUMENTS 503-464-9441
2888 NW Westover Rd., Portland, OR 97210
FDA Number: 3026267
Ownership: Private
Produces/Sells CE-marked Devices: N

Hearing-Aid	Ear/Nose/Throat

FERENCE WEICKER & COMPANY 1-866-680-3926
475 W. Georgia St., Ste. 550, 604-688-2424
Vancouver, BC V6B-4 Canada
FDA Number: n/a   *Fax:* 604-688-2369
E-mail: tweicker@direct.ca

FERENCE WEICKER & COMPANY 1-866-680-3926 (cont'd)
Web site: www.fwco.com
Year Founded: 1979
Total Employees: 10
Ownership: Private
Produces/Sells CE-marked Devices: N
Distribution: Exporter

FERGUSON PRODUCTION, INC. (620) 241-2400
2130 Industrial Drive, Conway, KS 67460
FDA Number: 300209807   Fax: (620) 241-2084
E-mail: nfo@fergusonproduction.com
Web site: www.fergusonproduction.com
Ownership: Private
Produces/Sells CE-marked Devices: N
  Shield, Eye, Ophthalmic   Ophthalmology

FERNANDEZ INDUSTRIES, INC. 978-371-8431
43 Oak Knoll Rd., Carlisle, MA 01741
FDA Number: 1226421
E-mail: sales@fernandez.com
Web site: www.fernandez.com
Ownership: Private
Produces/Sells CE-marked Devices: N
  Image Processing System   Radiology

FERNDALE LABORATORIES, INC. 888-548-0900
780 West Eight Mile Rd., Ferndale, MI 48220 248-548-0900
FDA Number: 1811212
E-mail: contactus@ferndalelabs.com
Ownership: Private
Produces/Sells CE-marked Devices: N
  Bandage, Adhesive   Surgery
  Drape, Adhesive, Aerosol   Surgery
  Dressing, Other   General
  Solvent, Adhesive Tape   Surgery

FERNO-FORGE
  See Getinge Usa, Inc.

FERNO-WASHINGTON, INC. 800-733-3766
70 Weil Way, Wilmington, OH 45177-9371 973-382-1451
FDA Number: 1523574   Fax: 937-382-1191
E-mail: info@ferno.com
Web site: www.ferno.com
Medical Products Sales Volume: $360,000
Annual Revenue: $25-$50 Million
Year Founded: 1956
Total Employees: 440
Ownership: Private
Produces/Sells CE-marked Devices: Y
Federal Procurement Eligibility: Small Business, VA Contract
Distribution: Manufacturer Through Distributor, Manufacturer Through
  Manufacturer Reps, Importer, Exporter
General Admin.: Elroy E. Bourgraf/Chairman
    Joe Bourgraf/Chief Executive Officer
    Paul Riordan/Chief Financial Officer, Senior Vice President
    Ron Beymer/Executive Vice President
    Joe Bourgraf/President
    Robert Ginter/Vice President Human Resources
Mktg./Adv.: John Meehan/Director Corporate Communications
    Ron Beymer/Director Marketing
    Chris Boise/Director Product Development
    Gary Hiles/Manager International & National Sales
    Gary Hiles/Vice President International Sales
  Bath, Hydro-Massage (Whirlpool)   Physical Med
  Board, Spine   Orthopedics
  Collar, Cervical Neck   Orthopedics
  Disinfector, Liquid   General
  Lift, Stair Climbing   General
  Orthosis, Cervical   Physical Med
  Orthosis, Limb Brace   Physical Med
  Orthosis, Pneumatic Structure, Rigid   Physical Med
  Rescue Equipment   General
  Splint, Pneumatic   Orthopedics
  Stretcher, Basket, Portable   General
  Stretcher, Emergency, Other   General
  Stretcher, Hand-Carried   General
  Stretcher, Orthopedic   Orthopedics
  Stretcher, Wheeled (Mobile)   General
  Stretcher, Wheeled, Mechanical   Physical Med
  Tank, Full Body (Bath)   General

FERNWOOD GUN SUPPLY INC.
  See Danville Materials

FERRIS MFG CORP. 800-765-9636
16 W300 83rd St., Burr Ridge, IL 60527-5848 630-887-9797
FDA Number: 1419520   Fax: 630-887-1008
E-mail: info@ferrispolymem.com

FERRIS MFG CORP. 800-765-9636 (cont'd)
Web site: http://www.polymem.com
Annual Revenue: $10-$25 Million
Year Founded: 1977
Total Employees: 40
Ownership: Private
Quality System Registration Information: ISO9001
Produces/Sells CE-marked Devices: Y
Federal Procurement Eligibility: Small Business
Distribution: Manufacturer Direct, Manufacturer Through Distributor, Exporter
General Admin.: Roger C. Sessions/Chief Executive Officer
    Clayton Kain/Chief Financial Officer, Treasurer
    Jim Arnold/President
Mktg./Adv.: John Newton/Director Marketing & Product Development
    Myron Troschuk/Vice President Sales
Production: Paul Kay/Director Quality Assurance & Regulatory Affairs
    Paul Zimmerman/Manager Materials
  Bandage, Liquid   Surgery
  Bandage, Other   General
  Dressing, Foam   General
  Dressing, Wound and Burn, Hydrogel   Surgery
  Nursing Pad, Polyurethane Pad With Starch Copolymer, Glycerin, And Surfactant (f-68)
  General
  Orthosis, Limb Brace   Physical Med
  Orthosis, Lumbosacral   Physical Med
  Pad, Dressing   General

FERTILITY SOLUTIONS, INC. 800-959-7656
13000 Shaker Blvd., Cleveland, OH 44120 216-491-0030
FDA Number: 3003750510   Fax: 216-491-0032
E-mail: areese@fertilitysolutions.com
Web site: www.fertilitysolutions.com
Medical Products Sales Volume: $310,000
Year Founded: 1992
Total Employees: 9
Ownership: Private
Produces/Sells CE-marked Devices: N
Federal Procurement Eligibility: Small Business, Female Owned
Distribution: Manufacturer Direct
General Admin.: Dr. Susan Rothmann/President
Mktg./Adv.: Ms. Angela Reese/Manager Customer Services & Sales
  Control, Cell Counter, Normal And Abnormal   Hematology
  Reagent, General Purpose   Pathology
  Slide, Control, Quality   Microbiology
  Stain, Chemical Solution   Pathology
  Whole Human Plasma, Antigen, Antiserum, Control   Immunology

FERTILITY TECH. INC 702-233-2601
9405 Darwell Drive, Las Vegas, NV 89117
FDA Number: 3004422844
E-mail: info@fertilitytechinc.com
Web site: www.fertilitytechinc.com
Ownership: Private
Produces/Sells CE-marked Devices: N
  Test, Luteinizing Hormone (lh), Over The Counter   Chemistry

FFM MED REPS, LLC
  See Excel Medical Products, Llc

FHC, INC 800-326-2905
1201 Main Street, Bowdoin, ME 04287 207-666-8190
FDA Number: 3005677147   Fax: 207-666-8292
E-mail: fhcinc@fh-co.com
Web site: www.fh-co.com
Medical Products Sales Volume: $5,000,000
Annual Revenue: $1-$5 Million
Year Founded: 1987
Total Employees: 50   *Marketing Staff:* 4   *Sales Staff:* 4
Ownership: Private
Quality System Registration Information: ISO9001
Produces/Sells CE-marked Devices: Y
Federal Procurement Eligibility: Small Business
Distribution: Manufacturer Direct
General Admin.: Frederick Haer/President
  Electrode, Depth   Cns/Neurology
  Stereotaxy Equipment   Cns/Neurology

FIBER PROCESS
  See Lydall, Inc.

FIBERBILT CASES, INC.
  See Case Design Corp.

FIBERGUIDE INDUSTRIES, INC. 908-647-6601
3409 East Linden St., Caldwell, ID 83605
FDA Number: 3024758   Fax: 908-647-8464
E-mail: info@fiberguide.com
Web site: www.fiberguide.com
Year Founded: 1977
Ownership: Private

FIBERGUIDE INDUSTRIES, INC.   908-647-6601 *(cont'd)*
Produces/Sells CE-marked Devices: N
Federal Procurement Eligibility: Small Business
Distribution: Manufacturer Direct
Cable, Fiberoptic	General
Contract Manufacturing	General
Endoscope, Accessories, Narrow Band Spectrum	Gastroenterology/Urology
Eyepiece, Lens, Prescription, Endoscopic	Gastroenterology/Urology

FIBERLITE CENTRIFUGE INC.   408-988-1103
422 Aldo Avenue, Santa Clara, CA 95054
FDA Number: 3005459215
Ownership: Private
Produces/Sells CE-marked Devices: N
Analyzer, Chemistry, Centrifuge	Chemistry

FIBEROPTIC COMPONENTS, LLC   978-422-0422
2 Spratt Tech. Way, Sterling, MA 01564
FDA Number: 3003683459   Fax: 978-422-0050
E-mail: sales@lightguides.com
Web site: www.lightguides.com
Medical Products Sales Volume: $3,000,000
Annual Revenue: $1-$5 Million
Year Founded: 1989
Total Employees: 12   *Marketing Staff:* 1   *Sales Staff:* 2
Ownership: Private
Produces/Sells CE-marked Devices: N
Federal Procurement Eligibility: Small Business
Distribution: OEM
Mktg./Adv.: Mr. Jack Castonguay/Manager Marketing
Production: Mr. Bob Palo/Manager Engineering
Fiberoptic Light Source & Carrier	Ear/Nose/Throat
Headlight, Fiberoptic Focusing	Gastroenterology/Urology
Light, Fiberoptic, Dental	Dental And Oral

FIBEROPTICS TECHNOLOGY, INC.   800-433-5248
1 Fiber Rd., Pomfret, CT 06258   860-928-0443
FDA Number: 1222275   Fax: 860-928-7664
E-mail: tbeeman@fiberoptix.com
Web site: www.fiberoptix.com
Annual Revenue: $10-$25 Million
Total Employees: 170
Ownership: Private
Produces/Sells CE-marked Devices: Y
Federal Procurement Eligibility: Small Business, Minority Owned, Female Owned
Distribution: OEM
General Admin.: Robert F. Dowling/President
Mktg./Adv.: Tim Beeman/Manager Sales
Light, Surgical, Fiberoptic	Surgery

FIBERWEB
See Bba Fiberweb Washougal, Inc.

FIBRA-SONICS, A DIVISION OF MISONIX, INC.   631-694-9555
1938 New Highway, E Farmingdale, NY 11735
FDA Number: 1419218
Caliper, Ophthalmic	Ophthalmology
Diathermy, Ultrasonic (Physical Therapy)	Physical Med
Lithotriptor, Ultrasonic	Gastroenterology/Urology
Phacofragmentation Unit	Ophthalmology
Pump, Aspiration, Portable	Anesthesiology
Surgical Instrument, Ultrasonic	Surgery

FIBREWORKS CORPORATION   800-843-0063
2417 Data Drive, Louisville, KY 40299   502-499-9944
FDA Number: n/a   Fax: 502-499-9880
E-mail: natural@fibreworks.com
Web site: www.fibreworks.com
Annual Revenue: $5-$10 Million
Ownership: Private
Produces/Sells CE-marked Devices: N
Federal Procurement Eligibility: Small Business
Distribution: Manufacturer Direct
General Admin.: Steve Stooksberry/President
Mktg./Adv.: Kim Lewis/Vice President Marketing
Carpeting	General
Floor Mat	General

FIELDING MANUFACTURING   800-230-8690
780 Wellington Ave., Cranscon, RI 02910-2938   401-461-0400
FDA Number: 1222305   Fax: 401-941-2222
E-mail: info@fieldingmfg.com
Web site: www.fieldingmfg.com
Annual Revenue: $5-$10 Million
Total Employees: 150   *Marketing Staff:* 3   *Sales Staff:* 6
Ownership: Private
Quality System Registration Information: ISO9001; ISO9002
Produces/Sells CE-marked Devices: N
Federal Procurement Eligibility: Small Business

FIELDING MANUFACTURING   800-230-8690 *(cont'd)*
Distribution: Manufacturer Direct
General Admin.: Steven Fielding/President, Chief Executive Officer
    Nancy Roderick/Vice President Human Resources
    Skip Cook/Vice President, General Manager
Mktg./Adv.: Skip Cook/Director Product Development
    Janet Carroll/Manager Contract Sales
    Brian Fielding/Manager Sales Training
    Skip Cook/Vice President Business Development
    Skip Cook/Vice President Marketing & Sales
Production: Denise Mullins/Director Quality Assurance
    Pezer Burke/Manager Materials
    Skip Cook/Vice President Manufacturing
Contract Manufacturing	General
Periodontal Instrument	Dental And Oral

FIELDTEX PRODUCTS, INC.   800-772-4816
3055 Brighton-Henrietta TL Road,   585-427-2940
Rochester, NY 14623
FDA Number: 1320537   Fax: 585-427-8666
E-mail: sales@fieldtex.com
Web site: www.fieldtex.com
Medical Products Sales Volume: $7,500,000
Annual Revenue: $1-$5 Million
Year Founded: 1972
Total Employees: 50   *Marketing Staff:* 2   *Sales Staff:* 4
Ownership: Private
Produces/Sells CE-marked Devices: N
Federal Procurement Eligibility: Small Business
Distribution: Manufacturer Direct
General Admin.: Sanford Abbey/President, Chief Executive Officer
Mktg./Adv.: Pattie Draper/Director Marketing & Advertising
Production: Fred Kwan/Manager Materials
Case, Protection, Equipment	General
Kit, First Aid	Surgery

FIL-CHEM, INC.   919-788-0909
PO Box 90833, Raleigh, NC 27675
FDA Number: n/a   Fax: 919-788-0908
E-mail: fil-chem@juno.com
Web site: www.Fil-Chem.com
Total Employees: 10   *Marketing Staff:* 1   *Sales Staff:* 2
Ownership: Private
Produces/Sells CE-marked Devices: N
Federal Procurement Eligibility: Small Business, Female Owned
Distribution: Manufacturer Direct, Importer, Exporter
General Admin.: Jerome Bogus/Chief Executive Officer
Mktg./Adv.: Felice Bogus/Vice President Marketing & Sales
Strip, Test	Chemistry
pH Paper, Obstetric	Obstetrics/Gynecology

FILLAUER COMPANIES, INC.   800-251-6398
2710 Amnicola Hwy.,   423-624-0946
Chattanooga, TN 37406
FDA Number: 1022826   Fax: 423-622-7836
E-mail: fillauer@fillauer.com
Web site: www.fillauer.com
Medical Products Sales Volume: $12,500,000
Year Founded: 1914
Total Employees: 106   *Marketing Staff:* 4   *Sales Staff:* 6
Ownership: Private
Quality System Registration Information: ISO9001
Produces/Sells CE-marked Devices: Y
Distribution: Manufacturer Direct, Importer, Exporter
General Admin.: Karl Fillauer, CPO/Chief Executive Officer, Chairman
    B. Kenneth Driver/President, Chief Operating Officer
Mktg./Adv.: Gerald Stark, CP/Director Education
    Fran Jenkins/Vice President Marketing
    Dennis Williams/Vice President Marketing
Production: Todd Smith/Vice President Manufacturing & Operations
Finance: Ed Connelly/Chief Financial Officer
Band, Support, Pelvic	Physical Med
Cover, Limb	Physical Med
Joint, Hip, External Brace	Physical Med
Joint, Knee, External Brace	Physical Med
Joint, Knee, External Limb Component	Physical Med
Orthosis, Cervical	Physical Med
Orthosis, Limb Brace	Physical Med
Orthosis, Lumbar	Physical Med
Orthosis, Thoracic	Physical Med
Prosthesis Alignment Device	Physical Med
Prosthesis, Arm	Orthopedics
Prosthesis, Leg	Orthopedics
Splint, Abduction, Congenital Hip Dislocation	Physical Med
Splint, Denis Brown	Physical Med
Stirrup, External Brace Component	Physical Med
Valve, Prosthesis	Physical Med
Medical Product Subsidiaries (Listed Separately)

FILLAUER COMPANIES, INC.   800-251-6398 *(cont'd)*
Hosmer-Dorrance Corp.
Motion Control, Inc.

FILLAUER ORTHOPEDIC
See Fillauer Companies, Inc.

FILTERSPUN   800-432-0108
624 N Fairfield St, Amarillo, TX 79107   **806-383-3840**
FDA Number: n/a   *Fax:* 806-383-3842
E-mail: sales@filterspun.com
Web site: www.filterspun.com
Annual Revenue: $10-$25 Million
Total Employees: 25
Ownership: Private
Produces/Sells CE-marked Devices: N
Federal Procurement Eligibility: Small Business
Distribution: Manufacturer Direct, Manufacturer Through Manufacturer Reps, OEM, Exclusive Distributor, Exporter
General Admin.: Jack H. Berg/President
    Philip Wittlinger/Vice President, General Manager
Production: Julie Stiles/Manager Customer Services
    M. Stiles/Manager Production

Electrode, pH	Gastroenterology/Urology
Filter, Air	General

FILTERTEK INC.   800-248-2461
11411 Price Rd., Hebron, IL 60034   **815-648-2416**
FDA Number: 1419411   *Fax:* 815-648-2929
E-mail: sales@filtertek.com
Web site: www.filtertek.com
Medical Products Sales Volume: $93,000,000
Annual Revenue: $50-$100 Million
Year Founded: 1965
Total Employees: 290
Ownership: Private
Quality System Registration Information: ISO9001; ISO9002
Produces/Sells CE-marked Devices: N
Federal Procurement Eligibility: Small Business
Distribution: OEM
Mktg./Adv.: Mr. M. Scott Farese/Director Business
Production: Tom Weier/Plant Manager

Filter, Air	General
Filter, Gas	Anesthesiology
Filter, Membrane	Chemistry
Filter, Syringe	General
Molding, Injection	General
Recovery Equipment, Water	General
Unit, Filter, Membrane	Chemistry
Valve, Other	Chemistry

FILTRONA EXTRUSION, INC.
See Filtrona Extrusion, Inc./PexcoA,Ar Medical Products Div.

FILTRONA EXTRUSION, INC./PEXCOA,AR   800-755-7528
MEDICAL PRODUCTS DIV.
764 south athol road, Athol, MA 01331   **404-564-8560**
FDA Number: 1220945   *Fax:* 404-584-8579
Web site: www.filtronaextrusion.com
Medical Products Sales Volume: $17,000,000
Annual Revenue: $25-$50 Million
Year Founded: 1949
Total Employees: 170   *Marketing Staff:* 1   *Sales Staff:* 5
Ownership: Public
Stock Symbol: FLTR
Traded On: London
Quality System Registration Information: ISO9001
Produces/Sells CE-marked Devices: N
Distribution: Manufacturer Direct, Manufacturer Through Distributor, Manufacturer Through Manufacturer Reps, Exporter
General Admin.: Ray Hackney/Vice President, General Manager
Mktg./Adv.: Richard Brooks/Vice President Marketing & Sales
Production: Ivan Green/Manager Quality Systems

Accessories, Catheter	Surgery
Cannula, Nasal	General
Catheter, Oxygen, Tracheal	Anesthesiology
Catheter, Suction (Tracheal Aspirating Tube)	Anesthesiology
Connector, Tubing, Dialysate	Gastroenterology/Urology
Contract Manufacturing	General
Contract R&D, Equipment	General
Delivery System, Pneumatic Tube	General
Drain, Thoracic (Chest)	Anesthesiology
Kit, Administration, Enteral	Gastroenterology/Urology
Kit, Administration, Intravenous	General
Kit, Feeding, Adult (Enteral)	General
Kit, Feeding, Pediatric (Enteral)	General
Kit, Intravenous Extension Tubing	General
Polymer, Synthetic, Other	General
Tube, Blood Collection	Chemistry

FILTRONA EXTRUSION, INC./PEXCOA,AR   800-755-7528 *(cont'd)*

Tube, Connecting	General
Tube, Double Lumen For Intestinal Decompression	Gastroenterology/Urology
Tube, Drainage	Gastroenterology/Urology
Tube, Enema	Gastroenterology/Urology
Tube, Feeding	General
Tube, Suction	General
Tube, Tracheal (Endotracheal)	Anesthesiology
Tube, Transfer	General
Tubing, Braided	General
Tubing, Conductive	General
Tubing, Connecting	General
Tubing, Flexible, Medical Gas, Low-Pressure	Anesthesiology
Tubing, Fluid Delivery	General
Tubing, Irrigation	Surgery
Tubing, Multi-Lumen	General
Tubing, Non-Conductive	General
Tubing, Non-Invasive	Surgery
Tubing, Nylon	General
Tubing, Other	General
Tubing, Oxygen Connecting	General
Tubing, Plastic	General
Tubing, Polyethylene	General
Tubing, Polypropylene	General
Tubing, Polyvinyl Chloride	General
Tubing, Radiopaque	General
Tubing, Urethane	General
Tubing, Vinyl	General
Warmer, Blood, Coil	Hematology

FILTRONA POROUS TECHNOLOGIES   804-524-4983
1625 Ashton Park Drive, Colonial Heights, VA 23834
FDA Number: n/a   *Fax:* 804-518-0105
E-mail: FPT-USA@filtrona.com
Web site: http://www.filtronaporoustechnologies.com
Ownership: Private
Produces/Sells CE-marked Devices: N
Mktg./Adv.: Mr. Russell Rogers/Division Manager
Production: Thomas Beaudet/Vice President Operations
Research: Dr. Chandrasiri Jayakody/Director Research & Development
    Dr. Bennett Ward/Vice President Research & Development

FINE & PARTICULAR EY   (914) 834-9227
1723 nw 82nd ave, doral, FL 33126
FDA Number: 2438249
Ownership: Private
Produces/Sells CE-marked Devices: N

Frame, Spectacle (Eyeglasses)	Ophthalmology
Sunglasses (Including Photosensitive)	Ophthalmology

FINE PITCH TECHNOLOGIES, INC., A   408-957-8500
SOLECTRON SUBSIDI
1077 Gibraltar Drive, Milpitas, CA 95035
FDA Number: 86294
Ownership: Private
Produces/Sells CE-marked Devices: N

Laser, Ophthalmic	Ophthalmology

FINE SURGICAL INSTRUMENT, INC.   800-851-5155
741 Peninsula Blvd., Hempstead, NY 11550   **516-292-7400**
FDA Number: 2433092   *Fax:* 516-292-7484
E-mail: sales@finesurgical.com
Web site: www.finesurgical.com
Year Founded: 1975
Total Employees: 20   *Marketing Staff:* 3   *Sales Staff:* 3
Ownership: Private
Quality System Registration Information: ISO9002
Produces/Sells CE-marked Devices: N
Federal Procurement Eligibility: Small Business, Minority Owned
Distribution: Manufacturer Through Distributor, Exclusive Distributor, Importer, Exporter
General Admin.: M. Mirza/President
Mktg./Adv.: Ron Wertheimer/Manager National Sales

Forceps, Dressing	Surgery
Forceps, Hemostatic	Surgery
Forceps, Intestinal (Clamps)	Gastroenterology/Urology
Holder, Needle	Gastroenterology/Urology
Retractor	Orthopedics
Scissors, Bandage/Gauze/Plaster	General
Speculum, Vaginal, Metal	Obstetrics/Gynecology

FINE-CUT DIAMOND TOOL CO.   440-563-5505
2811 Rome-Rock Creek Rd., Rock Creek, OH 44084-0457
FDA Number: n/a   *Fax:* 440-563-5503
E-mail: finecutdia@ncweb.com
Medical Products Sales Volume: $200,000
Annual Revenue: $0-$1 Million
Total Employees: 10   *Marketing Staff:* 3   *Sales Staff:* 2
Ownership: Private

FINE-CUT DIAMOND TOOL CO. 440-563-5505 (cont'd)
Produces/Sells CE-marked Devices: N
Federal Procurement Eligibility: Small Business, Minority Owned, Female Owned
Distribution: Manufacturer Direct, Service Direct
General Admin.: Bowen D. Morris/General Manager
    Michelle White/Office Manager
    Marilyn E. Morris/President
Mktg./Adv.: Marilyn E. Morris/Director Marketing
    Bowen E. Morris/Director Product Development
    Michelle Morris/Manager Contract Sales
Production: Ken Schley/Director Quality Assurance
    Thomas Camp/Production Engineer
Research: Bowen D. Morris/Vice President Engineering

Knife, Cataract	Ophthalmology
Knife, Keratome	Ophthalmology
Knife, Microtome	Pathology
Knife, Other	Surgery
Lens, Intraocular	Ophthalmology
Needle, Other	General

FINEBRAND CO. 323-588-3228
3720 S. Santa Fe Ave., Los Angeles, CA 90058
FDA Number: n/a
E-mail: info@finebrand.net
Web site: www.finebrand.net
Medical Products Sales Volume: $1,000,000
Annual Revenue: $0-$1 Million
Ownership: Private
Produces/Sells CE-marked Devices: N
Federal Procurement Eligibility: Small Business
Distribution: Manufacturer Direct

Pad, Breast	Obstetrics/Gynecology
Prosthesis, Breast, External	Surgery

FINETONE HEARING INSTRUMENTS 207-893-2920
885 Roosevelt Trail, Windham, ME 04062
FDA Number: 1220631

Hearing-Aid	Ear/Nose/Throat

FIREHOUSE MEDICAL, INC. 714-688-1575
1045 Armando St. # D, Anaheim, CA 92806
FDA Number: 2085508
Fax: 714-688-1577
E-mail: brentp@fhmed.com
Web site: www.firehousemedical.com
Ownership: Private
Produces/Sells CE-marked Devices: N

Bag, Intestine	Surgery
Reagent, Glucose (Test System)	Chemistry
Regulator, Pressure, Gas Cylinder	Anesthesiology
Stretcher, Hand-Carried	General

FIRESTONE OPTICS, INC. 816-455-0500
3901 E N.e., 33rd. Terr., Kansas City, MO 64117
FDA Number: 1929429

Lens, Contact (Other Material)	Ophthalmology
Lens, Contact, Polymethylmethacrylate	Ophthalmology

FIRST AID BANDAGE CO., INC. 888-813-8214
3 State Pier Road, New London, CT 06320 860-443-8499
FDA Number: 1211226
Fax: 860-442-8699
E-mail: customerservice@fabco.net
Web site: www.fabco.net
Medical Products Sales Volume: $3,000,000
Annual Revenue: $1-$5 Million
Total Employees: 24   Marketing Staff: 1   Sales Staff: 3
Ownership: Private
Produces/Sells CE-marked Devices: Y
Federal Procurement Eligibility: Small Business
Distribution: Manufacturer Direct, Manufacturer Through Distributor
General Admin.: Joel S. Wildstein/President, Chief Executive Officer
Mktg./Adv.: Trudy Richard/Director National Accounts & Sales
Production: Beth Casler/Manager Regulatory Affairs
    Mr. David Wildstein/Vice President, Director Operations

Applicator, Tipped, Absorbent, Sterile	General
Bandage, Elastic	General
Depressor, Tongue	General
Dissector, Surgical, General & Plastic Surgery	Surgery
Gauze, Non-Absorbable, Non-Medicated (Internal Sponge)	Surgery
Gauze, Non-Absorbable, X-Ray Detectable (Internal Sponge)	Surgery
Kit, Forensic Evidence, Sexual Assault	Obstetrics/Gynecology
Marker, Skin	Surgery
Sponge, External	Surgery
Wick, Ear	Ear/Nose/Throat

FIRST CALL, INC. 317-596-3280
660 E. 200 N, Warsaw, IN 46582
FDA Number: 3005693976
E-mail: Indianapolis@fcqs.com
Ownership: Private

FIRST CALL, INC. 317-596-3280 (cont'd)
Produces/Sells CE-marked Devices: N

Marker, Cardiopulmonary Bypass (Vein Marker)	Cardiovascular

FIRST GULF INTERNATIONAL 713-961-7793
3055 Sage Road #210, Suite 1690, Houston, TX 77056
FDA Number: n/a
Fax: 713-961-7722
E-mail: fgirfq@aol.com
Web site: www.fgico.com
Medical Products Sales Volume: $5,000,000
Annual Revenue: $1-$5 Million
Total Employees: 9   Marketing Staff: 3   Sales Staff: 3
Ownership: Private
Produces/Sells CE-marked Devices: N
General Admin.: Dr. Osama Hamonie/President
    Sam Hamonie/Vice President, General Manager
Mktg./Adv.: Max Hamonie/Director Marketing
    Lukas Katona/Director National Sales
    Albert Pinnelli/Manager International & National Sales
    Martin Hamonie/Manager National Sales
    Ken Huegel/Manager Sales Training
Production: Basel Harb/Manager Materials

Equipment/Accessories, Laser, Laparoscopy	Surgery
Facility, Equipment, Medical, Mobile	General
Surgical Instrument, Disposable	Surgery

FIRST HEALTHCARE PRODUCTS 800-854-8304
6125 Lendell Drive, Sanborn, NY 14132 716-731-6608
FDA Number: n/a
Fax: 800-542-7225
E-mail: info@firstproducts.com
Web site: www.firstproducts.com
Medical Products Sales Volume: $6,500,000
Annual Revenue: $5-$10 Million
Year Founded: 1945
Total Employees: 40   Marketing Staff: 1   Sales Staff: 20
Ownership: FIRST HOSPITAL PRODUCTS, INC.
Produces/Sells CE-marked Devices: N
Distribution: Manufacturer Direct, Manufacturer Through Distributor, Manufacturer Through Manufacturer Reps, Service Direct, Exclusive Distributor, Exporter
General Admin.: Tom Maloney/Chief Financial Officer, Vice President Operations
    Paul Smith/President, Chief Executive Officer
Mktg./Adv.: Nancy Pigoni/Director Marketing
    Carl Decarlo/Director National Accounts
    Paul Smith/Manager International & National Sales
    Nancy Pigoni/Manager Market Research
    Carl Decarlo/Manager Sales
Production: Mike Caillier/Director Quality Assurance
    Jim Klein/Manager Materials
    Tom Maloney/Manager Regulatory Affairs

Holder, Medical Chart	General
Rack, Medical Chart	General

FIRST HOSPITAL PRODUCTS, INC.
See First Healthcare Products

FIRST LEVEL INC 717-266-2450
3109 Espresso Way, York, PA 17406
FDA Number: n/a
Fax: 717-266-7410
E-mail: info@firstlevelinc.com
Web site: www.firstlevelinc.com
Medical Products Sales Volume: $200,000
Annual Revenue: $1-$5 Million
Year Founded: 2001
Total Employees: 15   Marketing Staff: 1   Sales Staff: 1
Ownership: Private
Quality System Registration Information: ISO9001
Produces/Sells CE-marked Devices: N
Federal Procurement Eligibility: Small Business
Distribution: Manufacturer Through Manufacturer Reps, Service Direct

Service, Engineering/Design	General

FIRST QUALITY ENTERPRISE, INC. 516-829-3030
80 Cuttermill Road, Suite 500, Great Neck, NY 11021
FDA Number: n/a
Fax: 516-829-4949
E-mail: fqe@firstquality.com
Web site: www.firstquality.com
Medical Products Sales Volume: $50,500,000
Total Employees: 3000
Ownership: Private
Quality System Registration Information: ISO9000
Produces/Sells CE-marked Devices: Y
Federal Procurement Eligibility: Small Business, Minority Owned
Distribution: Manufacturer Through Distributor
General Admin.: Nader Damaghi/President, Chief Executive Officer
    Kambiz Damagh/Vice President

Diaper, Adult	General
Diaper, Pediatric	General
Pad, Incontinence (Underpad)	General

FIRST QUALITY ENTERPRISE, INC. 516-829-3030 (cont'd)

Pant, Incontinence	General
Tampon, Menstrual, Unscented	Obstetrics/Gynecology

Medical Product Subsidiaries (Listed Separately)
First Quality Hygienic, Inc.
First Quality Products, Inc.

FIRST QUALITY HYGIENIC, INC. 800-488-3130 Ex

North Rd., Clinton County Industrial Park,
Mcelhattan, PA 17748
FDA Number: 2529605
E-mail: fqhsales@firstquality.com
Web site: www.firstquality.com
Ownership: First Quality Enterprise, Inc.
Quality System Registration Information: ISO9001
Produces/Sells CE-marked Devices: N
Distribution: Manufacturer Through Manufacturer Reps

Tampon, Menstrual, Scented	Obstetrics/Gynecology
Tampon, Menstrual, Unscented	Obstetrics/Gynecology

FIRST QUALITY PRODUCTS, INC. 800-227-3551 Ex

North Rd., Clinton County Industrial Park,
Mcelhattan, PA 17748
FDA Number: 2529604
E-mail: fqpsales@firstquality.com
Web site: www.firstquality.com
Ownership: First Quality Enterprise, Inc.
Produces/Sells CE-marked Devices: N
Distribution: Manufacturer Through Manufacturer Reps

Garment, Protective, For Incontinence	Gastroenterology/Urology

FIRST QUALITY RETAIL SERVICES, LLC. 516-829-3030

601 Allendale Rd., King Of Prussia, PA 19406
FDA Number: 2522297
Ownership: Private
Produces/Sells CE-marked Devices: N

Garment, Protective, For Incontinence	Gastroenterology/Urology
Pad, Menstrual, Scented	Obstetrics/Gynecology
Pad, Menstrual, Unscented	Obstetrics/Gynecology
Pads, Menstrual, Scented-deodorized	Obstetrics/Gynecology

FIRST RESPONSE SOLUTIONS 310-537-3300

2015 University Dr., Rancho Dominguez, CA 90220
FDA Number: 2032812
Ownership: Private
Produces/Sells CE-marked Devices: N

Bandage, Adhesive	Surgery

FIRST UNITED LEASING CORP.
See Ge Capital

FIRST YEARS, THE
See Learning Curve Brands Inc. THE FIRST YEARS

FISCHER IMAGING CORPORATION
See Fischer Medical Technologies Inc.

FISCHER INDUSTRIES, INC. 630-232-2803

2630 Kaneville Court, Geneva, IL 60134
FDA Number: 1417466
Ownership: Private
Produces/Sells CE-marked Devices: N

Processor, Radiographic Film, Automatic	Radiology

FISCHER MEDICAL TECHNOLOGIES INC. 800-777-5345
303-280-2311

325 Interlocken Parkway, Building C,
Broomfield, CO 80021
FDA Number: 3006188092
Web site: www.fischerimaging.com
Annual Revenue: $0-$1 Million
Ownership: Private
Produces/Sells CE-marked Devices: N
Federal Procurement Eligibility: Small Business
Distribution: Manufacturer Direct, Exporter
Fax: 303-920-0836

Generator, Diagnostic X-Ray, High Voltage, 3-Phase	Radiology
Generator, Diagnostic X-Ray, High Voltage, Single Phase	Radiology
Holder, Radiographic Cassette, Wall-Mounted	Radiology
Image Processing System	Radiology
Mount, X-Ray Tube, Diagnostic	Radiology
Pacemaker, Heart, External, Programmable	Cardiovascular
Pulse Generator, Pacemaker, Implantable, With Cardiac Resynchronization Cardiovascular	
Radiographic Unit, Diagnostic	Radiology
Radiographic Unit, Diagnostic, Chest	Radiology
Radiographic Unit, Diagnostic, Fixed (X-Ray)	Radiology
Radiographic Unit, Diagnostic, Mammographic	Radiology
Radiographic Unit, Diagnostic, Portable (X-Ray)	Radiology
Radiographic Unit, Diagnostic, Tomographic	Radiology
Radiographic Unit, Digital Subtraction Angiographic (DSA)	Radiology
Radiographic/Fluoroscopic Unit, Fixed	Radiology
Radiographic/Fluoroscopic Unit, Mobile C-Arm	Radiology

FISCHER MEDICAL TECHNOLOGIES INC. 800-777-5345 (cont'd)

System, X-Ray, Mobile	Radiology
Table, Radiographic, Tilting	Radiology
Table, Surgical, Manual	General
Tube, X-Ray	Radiology

Medical Product Subsidiaries (Listed Separately)
Robot Research, Inc., Sensomatics Div.

FISCHER SURGICAL INC. 866-622-2221
314-303-7753

1343 Pine Drive, Arnold, MO 63010
FDA Number: 3004571672
E-mail: info@firstsurgical.com
Web site: www.fischersurgical.com
Ownership: Private
Produces/Sells CE-marked Devices: N
Fax: 636-464-8192

Forceps, Ophthalmic	Ophthalmology
Hook, Ophthalmic	Ophthalmology
Instrument, Microsurgical	Cns/Neurology
Needle, Suture, Ophthalmic	Ophthalmology
Probe, Lacrimal	Ophthalmology
Scissors, Ophthalmic	Ophthalmology
Spatula, Ophthalmic	Ophthalmology
Speculum, Ophthalmic	Ophthalmology
Spud, Ophthalmic	Ophthalmology
Surgical Instrument, Non-Powered, Neurosurgical	Cns/Neurology

FISHER DIAGNOSTICS 877-722-4366
704-875-0494

11515 Vanstory Drive, Suite 125,
Huntersville, NC 28078
FDA Number: 1055411
E-mail: Paul-Gee@fishersci.com
Medical Products Sales Volume: $3,790,000,000
Total Employees: 30500   *Marketing Staff:* 2   *Sales Staff:* 6
Ownership: FISHER SCIENTIFIC COMPANY L.L.C.
Stock Symbol: TMO
Traded On: NYSE
Produces/Sells CE-marked Devices: N
Federal Procurement Eligibility: Small Business
Distribution: Manufacturer Through Distributor, Exclusive Distributor, Exporter
General Admin.: Paul Montrone/Chief Executive Officer
   David Hanlon/Vice President, General Manager
Mktg./Adv.: Paul Gee/Director Marketing
   Bruno Borganti/Manager International & National Sales
   Paul Gee/Manager National Sales
Production: Kathy Napier/Director Quality Assurance
   Bill Ellithorpe/Manager Materials
   Larry Kopyta/Manager Regulatory Affairs
Research: Gerald Steiner/Manager Research & Development
Fax: 704-875-9862

Control, Coagulation, Plasma	Hematology
Fibrin Split Products	Hematology
Heparin	Pathology
Multi Analyte Mixture, Calibrator	Chemistry
Plasma, Control, Fibrinogen	Hematology
Plasma, Deficient, Factor, Coagulation	Hematology
Prothrombin Time	Hematology
Quantitation, Antithrombin III	Hematology
Standard, Fibrinogen	Hematology
System, Determination, Fibrinogen	Hematology
Test, Fibrinogen	Hematology
Test, Heparin (Clotting Time)	Hematology
Test, Sickle Cell	Hematology
Thromboplastin, Activated Partial	Hematology

FISHER HAMILTON SCIENTIFIC INC.
See Thermo Scientific Hamilton

FISHER HEALTHCARE 800-766-7000
800-766-7000

9999 Veterans Memorial Dr.,
Houston, TX 77038
FDA Number: n/a
E-mail: robert.kovar@fishersci.com
Web site: www.fishersci.com
Total Employees: 2300
Ownership: FISHER SCIENTIFIC CO.
Stock Symbol: FSH
Traded On: NYSE
Produces/Sells CE-marked Devices: N
Distribution: Exclusive Distributor
Mktg./Adv.: Robert Kovar/Director Marketing
   Cory Stevenson/Senior Vice President Marketing
Fax: 800-926-1166

Analyzer, Blood Gas pH	Anesthesiology
Bath, Water (Constant Temperature)	Chemistry
Blender/Mixer	Chemistry
Counter, Cell	Microbiology
Diluter, Blood Cell, Automated	Hematology
Equipment, Test, Western Blot	Microbiology
Labware, Basic, Disposable	Chemistry
Labware, Basic, Reusable	Chemistry
Stain, Crystal Violet, Histology	Pathology

FISHER HEALTHCARE

800-766-7000 *(cont'd)*

Sterilizer, Loop, Inoculating	Microbiology

Medical Product Subsidiaries (Listed Separately)
Biochemical Sciences, Inc.

FISHER HEARING AID SERVICE

330-627-2002

25 Public Square, Carrollton, OH 44615
FDA Number: 3004082437
Ownership: Private
Produces/Sells CE-marked Devices: N

Hearing-Aid	Ear/Nose/Throat

FISHER MEDICAL DIVISION

See Instrumentation Laboratory Company

FISHER SCIENTIFIC CO., LLC.

800-766-7000
412-490-8816

2000 Park Lane, Pittsburgh, PA 15275
FDA Number: 2517925
Fax: 800-926-1166
Web site: www.fishersci.com
Annual Revenue: $50-$100 Million
Ownership: Private
Produces/Sells CE-marked Devices: N
Distribution: Manufacturer Through Distributor

5-AMP-Phosphate Release (Colorimetric), 5'-Nucleotidase	Chemistry
Absorbent, Carbon-Dioxide	Anesthesiology
Acetone	Chemistry
Adapter, Centrifuge Tube	Chemistry
Alarm, Central Gas System	Anesthesiology
Alarm, Voltage	General
Ampule	Gastroenterology/Urology
Analyzer, Chemistry, Electrolyte	Chemistry
Analyzer, Glucose	Chemistry
Anatomical Training Model	General
Antigen, CF (Including CF Control), Rubella	Microbiology
Antigen, Febrile	Microbiology
Antigen, Febrile, Slide And Tube, Salmonella	Microbiology
Antigen, Non-Treponemal, All	Microbiology
Antiserum, Control For Non-Treponemal Test	Microbiology
Antiserum, Positive And Negative Febrile Antigen Control	Microbiology
Antiserum, Salmonella SPP.	Microbiology
Antiserum, Shigella SPP.	Microbiology
Apron, Laboratory	Chemistry
Azo-Dye, Calcium	Chemistry
Azo-Dyes, Colorimetric, Bilirubin And Conjugates	Chemistry
Balance, Electronic	Chemistry
Balance, Mechanical	Chemistry
Ball, Cotton	General
Bandage, Adhesive	Surgery
Bath, Dry (Constant Temperature)	Chemistry
Bath, Freezing	Chemistry
Bath, Ice	Microbiology
Bath, Portable	General
Bath, Tissue Flotation	Microbiology
Bath, Tissue Flotation, Pathology	Pathology
Bath, Viscosity	Chemistry
Bath, Water (Constant Temperature)	Chemistry
Beaker (Laboratory)	Chemistry
Blender/Mixer	Chemistry
Brilliant Cresyl Blue	Hematology
Buret	Chemistry
Burner	Chemistry
Cabinet Casework, Laboratory	Chemistry
Cabinet, Laboratory	Chemistry
Cabinet, Microbiological	Microbiology
Cabinet, Other	General
Cage, Animal	Microbiology
Calibrator, Primary, Clinical Chemistry	Chemistry
Cart, Gas Cylinder (Carrier)	Anesthesiology
Cart, Multipurpose	General
Catalytic Method, Amylase	Chemistry
Catalytic Method, Creatine Phosphokinase	Chemistry
Centrifuge, Blood Bank, Diagnostic	Hematology
Centrifuge, General (Up to 5,000 rpm)	Pathology
Centrifuge, Hematocrit	Hematology
Centrifuge, Microhematocrit	Hematology
Centrifuge, Microsedimentation	Hematology
Chair, Blood Drawing	General
Chair, Other	General
Chloridimeter	Gastroenterology/Urology
Chromatographic/Fluorometric Method, Catecholamines	Chemistry
Chromatography Equipment, Gas	Chemistry
Chromatography Equipment, Liquid	Chemistry
Chromatography Equipment, Paper	Chemistry
Chromatography, Liquid, Performance, High	Toxicology
Circulator, Water Bath	Chemistry
Citrulline, Arsenate, Nessler (Colorimetry), Ornithine CT	Chemistry
Clamp, Other	Surgery
Clamp, Tubing, Blood, Automatic	Gastroenterology/Urology
Clearing Oil	Pathology
Collector, Fraction	Chemistry
Collector, Sputum	Anesthesiology
Collector, Urine, Disposable	Gastroenterology/Urology

FISHER SCIENTIFIC CO., LLC.

800-766-7000 *(cont'd)*

Colorimeter, General Use	Chemistry
Colorimetric Method, CPK Or Isoenzymes	Chemistry
Colorimetric Method, Lipoproteins	Chemistry
Column, Chromatography	Chemistry
Compressor, Air, Portable	Anesthesiology
Computer, Clinical Laboratory	Chemistry
Concentrator, Clinical Sample	Chemistry
Container, Slide Mailer	Microbiology
Container, Specimen Mailer And Storage	Pathology
Container, Specimen Mailer And Storage, Temperature Control	Pathology
Container, Specimen, All Types	General
Control, Cell Counter, Normal And Abnormal	Hematology
Control, Multi Analyte, All Kinds (Assayed And Unassayed)	Chemistry
Control, Platelet	Hematology
Control, Red Cell	Hematology
Control, Urinalysis (Assayed And Unassayed)	Chemistry
Control, White Cell	Hematology
Copper Reduction, Glucose	Chemistry
Counter, Bacteria	Microbiology
Counter, Cell	Microbiology
Counter, Colony	Microbiology
Coverslip, Microscope Slide	Pathology
Culture Media, General Nutrient Broth	Microbiology
Demineralizer	Chemistry
Densitometer	Cardiovascular
Densitometer/Scanner (Integrating, Reflectance, TLC, Radio)	Chemistry
Depressor, Tongue	General
Desiccator	Chemistry
Diluent, Blood Cell	Hematology
Diluter	Chemistry
Dish, Petri	Chemistry
Dispenser, Disc, Sensitivity, Antibiotic	Microbiology
Dispenser, Paraffin	Pathology
Dispenser, Pipette	Chemistry
Dispenser, Slide	Chemistry
Distilling Unit	Chemistry
Drying Unit	Chemistry
Dye-Binding, Albumin, Bromcresol, Green	Chemistry
Electrode, Ion Selective (Non-Specified)	Chemistry
Electrode, Laboratory pH	Chemistry
Electrode, pH	Gastroenterology/Urology
Electrophoresis Equipment, Liquid	Chemistry
Electrophoresis Instrumentation	Immunology
Electrophoretic Separation, Alkaline Phosphatase Isoenzymes	Chemistry
Electrophoretic, Protein Fractionation	Chemistry
Evaporator	Chemistry
Filter Paper	Chemistry
Finger Cot	General
Flask, Dewar	Chemistry
Fluid, Red Cell Diluting	Hematology
Fluid, Red Cell Lysing	Hematology
Forceps, Hemostatic	Surgery
Formaldehyde (Formalin, Formol)	Pathology
Formalin, Neutral Buffered	Pathology
Freezer, Blood Storage	Hematology
Freezer, Laboratory, General Purpose	Chemistry
Glove, Other	General
Glove, Surgical	General
Glutaraldehyde (Fixative)	Pathology
Heater, Immersion	Microbiology
Hematology Quality Control Mixture	Hematology
Hemoglobinometer, Automated	Hematology
Holder, Needle	Gastroenterology/Urology
Homogenizer, Tissue	Microbiology
Hood, Isolation, Laminar Air Flow	General
Hood, Microbiological	Microbiology
Hygrometer (Humidity Indicator)	Anesthesiology
Immunodiffusion Equipment (Agar Cutter)	Chemistry
Incubator, Aerobic	Microbiology
Incubator, Anaerobic	Microbiology
Incubator, Test Tube, Portable	Microbiology
Incubator, Test Tube, Stationary	Microbiology
Incubator/Water Bath	Chemistry
Incubator/Water Bath, Microbiology	Microbiology
Indicator, pH, Dye (Urinary, Non-Quantitative)	Chemistry
Kit, First Aid	Surgery
Kit, Pregnancy Test	Obstetrics/Gynecology
Knife, Other	Surgery
Labware, Basic, Disposable	Chemistry
Labware, Basic, Reusable	Chemistry
Lamp, Other	General
Lamp, Ultraviolet (Spectrum A)	General
Lipase Hydrolysis/Glycerol Kinase Enzyme, Triglycerides	Chemistry
Loop, Inoculating	Microbiology
Metallic Reduction Method, Glucose (Urinary, Non-Quant.)	Chemistry
Meter, Conductivity	Chemistry
Meter, Conductivity, Non-Remote	Gastroenterology/Urology
Meter, Resistivity	Chemistry
Meter, pH, Blood	Chemistry
Meter, pH, Portable	Chemistry
Microscope	Hematology

FISHER SCIENTIFIC CO., LLC.   800-766-7000 *(cont'd)*

Microscope, Laboratory, Optical	Microbiology
Microscope, Light	Pathology
Microscope, Phase Contrast	Pathology
Microtiter Diluting/Dispensing Device	Microbiology
Microtome, Cryostat	Pathology
Microtome, Rotary	Pathology
Mixer, Blood Bank, Donor Blood	Hematology
Mixer, Clinical Laboratory	Chemistry
Multi Analyte Mixture, Calibrator	Chemistry
Needle, Blood Collection	General
Needle, Hypodermic	General
Needle, Other	General
Opener, Ampule	Gastroenterology/Urology
Osmometer	Chemistry
Oven	Chemistry
Oven, Paraffin	Pathology
Paper, Chart, Record, Medical	General
Phosphatase, Acid	Hematology
Phosphorus Reagent (Test System)	Chemistry
Photometer	Chemistry
Photometric Method, Iron (Non-Heme)	Chemistry
Pipette Tip	Chemistry
Pipette, Diluting	Hematology
Pipette, Micro	Chemistry
Pipette, Pasteur	Hematology
Pipette, Quantitative, Hematology	Hematology
Pipette, Sahli	Hematology
Pipetter	Hematology
Pipetting And Diluting System, Automated	Chemistry
Plate, Hot	Chemistry
Probe, Other	General
Pump, Laboratory	Chemistry
Purification System, Water, Deionization	Chemistry
Purifier, Water	Chemistry
Pyrometer	General
Rack, Test Tube	Chemistry
Radioimmunoassay, Cortisol	Chemistry
Radioimmunoassay, Follicle Stimulating Hormone	Chemistry
Radioimmunoassay, Luteinizing Hormone	Chemistry
Radioimmunoassay, Prolactin (Lactogen)	Chemistry
Radioimmunoassay, T3 Uptake	Chemistry
Radioimmunoassay, Testosterones And Dihydrotestosterone	Chemistry
Radiometer, Phototherapy	General
Reagent, Albumin, Colorimetric	Chemistry
Reagent, Bilirubin (Total Or Direct Test System)	Chemistry
Reagent, Calcium (Test System)	Chemistry
Reagent, Calibration	General
Reagent, Cholesterol (Total Test System)	Chemistry
Reagent, Cyanomethemoglobin, With Standard	Hematology
Reagent, Glucose (Test System)	Chemistry
Reagent, Iron (Test System)	Chemistry
Reagent, Kinase, Phosphate, Creatine	Chemistry
Reagent, Protein, Total	Chemistry
Reagent, Streptolysin O/Antistreptolysin-Titer	Microbiology
Refractometer, Ophthalmic	Ophthalmology
Refrigerator, Biological	Microbiology
Refrigerator, Blood Bank	Hematology
Refrigerator, Explosion-Proof	Chemistry
Regulator, Oxygen, Mechanical	General
Regulator, Pressure, Gas Cylinder	Anesthesiology
Regulator, Temperature	Chemistry
SGOT, Ultraviolet	Chemistry
SGPT, Ultraviolet	Chemistry
Safety Equipment, Laboratory	Chemistry
Scanner, Long-Term Recording, Respiration	Anesthesiology
Scissors, Bandage/Gauze/Plaster	General
Scissors, Iris	Ophthalmology
Scissors, Plastic Surgery (Dissecting)	Surgery
Serum Separation System	Hematology
Shaker/Stirrer	Chemistry
Sink, Laboratory	Chemistry
Solution, Antibacterial Cleaner	General
Solution, Pathology, Decalcifier, Acid Containing	Pathology
Solution, Pathology, Zenker's	Pathology
Solution, pH Buffer	Chemistry
Solvent	Chemistry
Spatula, Cervical, Cytology	Obstetrics/Gynecology
Spatula, Other	Surgery
Spectrophotometer, Infrared	Chemistry
Stain, Acid Fuchsin	Pathology
Stain, Acridine Orange	Pathology
Stain, Alcian Blue	Pathology
Stain, Alizarin Red	Pathology
Stain, Azure A	Pathology
Stain, Biebrich Scarlet	Pathology
Stain, Carbol Fuchsin	Pathology
Stain, Eosin Y	Pathology
Stain, Grams Iodine	Pathology
Stain, Hematoxylin, Mayer's	Pathology
Stain, Mallory's Trichrome	Pathology
Stain, Microbiological	Microbiology

FISHER SCIENTIFIC CO., LLC.   800-766-7000 *(cont'd)*

Stain, Papanicolau	Pathology
Stain, Reagent, Schiff	Pathology
Stain, Wright's	Pathology
Stain, Wright's, Hematology	Hematology
Stainer, Slide, Cytology	Microbiology
Stainer, Slide, Hematology	Hematology
Stainer, Slide, Histology	Microbiology
Stand, Gas Cylinder	Anesthesiology
Standard/Control, All Types	Chemistry
Standard/Control, Hemoglobin, Normal/Abnormal	Hematology
Station Pipetting	Chemistry
Sterilizer, Steam (Autoclave)	General
Stirrer	Chemistry
Streptolysin O	Pathology
Swabs, Specimen Collection	General
Syringe, Hypodermic	General
Syringe, Insulin	General
Syringe, Tuberculin	General
System, Blood Culturing	Microbiology
Table, Blood Donor	Hematology
Table, Ophthalmic, Instrument, Manual	Ophthalmology
Table, Other	General
Table, Slide Warming	Pathology
Test, Systemic Lupus Erythematosus	Immunology
Tester, Conductivity, Floor And Equipment	General
Thermometer, Electronic, Continuous	General
Thermometer, Mercury	General
Timer, Coagulation	Hematology
Timer, General Laboratory	Hematology
Tissue Culture Apparatus	Microbiology
Tissue Processor, Automated	Pathology
Titrator	Chemistry
Titrator, Calcium	Chemistry
Training Manikin, Other	General
Transilluminator, AC-Powered, Ophthalmic	Ophthalmology
Tube, Blood Collection	Chemistry
Tube, Capillary	Chemistry
Tube, Centrifuge	Chemistry
Tube, Culture	Microbiology
Tube, Sedimentation Rate	Hematology
Tube, Test	Chemistry
Tubing, Braided	General
Tubing, Polyethylene	General
Unit, Filter, Membrane	Chemistry
Urease And Glutamic Dehydrogenase, Urea Nitrogen	Chemistry
Urease, Photometric, Urea Nitrogen	Chemistry
Urinometer, Non-Electrical	Gastroenterology/Urology
View Box, Rh Typing	Hematology
Viewer/Magnifier	Hematology
Voltmeter	Chemistry
Washer, Labware	Chemistry
Washer, Pipette	Chemistry

Medical Product Subsidiaries (Listed Separately)
Fisher Scientific U.K.
Fisher Scientific Worldwide
Nalge Nunc International
Remel
Thermo Fisher Scientific

FISHER SCIENTIFIC CO., LLC.   201-703-3131
One Reagent Ln., Fair Lawn, NJ 07410
FDA Number: 2214740

Electrode, Cutaneous	Cns/Neurology
Formaldehyde (Formalin, Formol)	Pathology
Formalin, Neutral Buffered	Pathology
Paraffin, All Formulations	Pathology
Reagent, General Purpose	Pathology
Solution, Pathology, Decalcifier, Acid Containing	Pathology
Stain, Dye Powder	Pathology
Stain, Eosin Y	Pathology
Stain, Hematoxylin, Harris's	Pathology
Stain, Papanicolau	Pathology

FISHER SCIENTIFIC INTERNATIONAL, INC.
See Fisher Scientific Co., Llc.

FISHER SCIENTIFIC LIMITED   800-237-7437
112 Colonnade Rd.,   **613-226-8874**
Ottawa, ONT K2E-7 Canada
FDA Number: n/a   *Fax:* 613-226-7658
E-mail: help@fishersci.ca
Web site: www.fishersci.ca
Year Founded: 1926
Total Employees: 250
Ownership: Private
Produces/Sells CE-marked Devices: N
Distribution: Service Direct, Exclusive Distributor, Importer

FITNESS MOTIVATION INSTITUTE OF AMERICA, INC.
800-538-7790

26685 Sussex Highway Suite A,   **302-628-3488**
Seaford, DE 19973
FDA Number: 2921545
E-mail: isoghq@aol.com   *Fax:* 302-629-4646
Web site: www.fmia.com
Medical Products Sales Volume: $800,000
Annual Revenue: $1-$5 Million
Year Founded: 2002
Total Employees: 4   *Marketing Staff:* 3   *Sales Staff:* 10
Ownership: Private
Produces/Sells CE-marked Devices: N
Federal Procurement Eligibility: Small Business, Female Owned
Distribution: Manufacturer Direct, Manufacturer Through Distributor, Service Direct, Exclusive Distributor, Importer, Exporter
General Admin.: Mary Ellen Watkins/Chief Executive Officer
     C. Travis Watkins/President
     Kevin Useldinger/Vice President
Mktg./Adv.: Susan Crampton/Director Marketing
     Kevin Useldinger/Manager National Sales
Production: Michael Duerr/Manager Materials

Caliper, Skinfold	General
Exerciser, Isorobic	Physical Med
Exerciser, Measuring	Physical Med
Monitor, Pulse Rate	Anesthesiology

FITNESS PLUS, INC.
888-778-4019

PO Box 516, Suite 280, Valley City, ND 58072   **701-845-4774**
FDA Number: 9021954   *Fax:* 701-845-5883
E-mail: info@fitnessplusinc.com
Web site: www.fitnessplusinc.com
Year Founded: 1990
Total Employees: 2   *Marketing Staff:* 2   *Sales Staff:* 2
Ownership: Private
Produces/Sells CE-marked Devices: N
Federal Procurement Eligibility: Small Business
Distribution: Manufacturer Direct, Manufacturer Through Distributor, Exporter
General Admin.: George Gaukler/Chief Executive Officer
     Duane Fast/Vice President
Mktg./Adv.: Skip Frappier/Manager International & National Sales

Exerciser, Chest	Physical Med
Exerciser, Leg And Ankle	Physical Med
Exerciser, Non-Measuring	Physical Med
Exerciser, Other	Physical Med
Exerciser, Shoulder	Physical Med

FITTER INTERNATIONAL INC.
800-348-8371

3050, 2600 Portland Street SE,   **403-243-6830**
Calgary, ALB T2G 4 Canada
FDA Number: n/a   *Fax:* 403-229-1230
E-mail: orders@fitter1.com
Web site: www.fitter1.com
Year Founded: 1985
Total Employees: 25
Ownership: Private
Produces/Sells CE-marked Devices: N
Distribution: Manufacturer Direct, Exporter

FITZCO, INC.
800-367-8760

4300 Shoreline Drive, Spring Park, MN 55384   **952-471-1185**
FDA Number: 2183989   *Fax:* 952-471-0787
E-mail: Fitzco@FitzcoInc.com
Web site: www.fitzcoinc.com
Ownership: Private
Produces/Sells CE-marked Devices: N

Container, Specimen, Urine, Drugs Of Abuse, Over The Counter	Chemistry
Transport System, Anaerobic	Microbiology

FITZGERALD INDUSTRIES INTERNATIONAL, INC. 800-370-2222

30 Sudbury Road, Suite 1A North,   **978-371-6446**
Action, MA 01720
FDA Number: n/a   *Fax:* 978-371-2266
E-mail: antibodies@fitzgerald-fii.com
Web site: www.fitzgerald-fii.com
Medical Products Sales Volume: $2,400,000
Annual Revenue: $5-$10 Million
Year Founded: 2004
Total Employees: 14
Ownership: Private
Quality System Registration Information: ISO9000; ISO9002; ISO9003
Produces/Sells CE-marked Devices: N
Federal Procurement Eligibility: Small Business
Distribution: OEM, Exclusive Distributor
General Admin.: Edward Fitzgerald/Chief Executive Officer
     Kevin Fitzgerald/President

FITZGERALD INDUSTRIES INTERNATIONAL, INC. 800-370-2222
(cont'd)
Mktg./Adv.: Kevin Fitzgerald/Manager International & National Sales
     Bernie Hodson/Vice President Business Development
     Pamela Williams/Vice President Sales
Production: Judy Amelotte/Director Quality Assurance
     Karl Leeman/Manager Materials

Whole Human Plasma, Antigen, Antiserum, Control	Immunology

FITZPATRICK MANAGEMENT RESOURCES
800-357-0509

9116 Fishers Pond Drive,   **704-542-2685**
Charlotte, NC 28277
FDA Number: n/a   *Fax:* 704-542-6279
E-mail: fitzpatrickmgmt@aol.com
Medical Products Sales Volume: $500,000
Annual Revenue: $0-$1 Million
Year Founded: 1994
Total Employees: 2
Ownership: Private
Produces/Sells CE-marked Devices: N
Federal Procurement Eligibility: Small Business
Distribution: Service Direct
General Admin.: William Fitzpatrick/President, Owner
Mktg./Adv.: Colleen Schute/Vice President Marketing & Sales

Service, Consulting	General

FIWAY MANUFACTURING CORP.
See U.S. Orthotics, Inc.

FIXANO
See Small Bone Innovations, Inc.

FKP ARCHITECTS,INC
713-621-2100

8 Greenway Plaza, Suite 300, Houston, TX 77046-0899
FDA Number: n/a   *Fax:* 713-621-2178
E-mail: fkp@fkp.com
Web site: www.fkp.com
Medical Products Sales Volume: $10,700,000
Annual Revenue: $10-$25 Million
Year Founded: 1971
Total Employees: 158   *Marketing Staff:* 3
Ownership: Private
Produces/Sells CE-marked Devices: N
Federal Procurement Eligibility: Small Business
General Admin.: John S. Crane/President, Chief Executive Officer, Chief Operating Officer
     Paul G. Pedersen/Senior Vice President
Mktg./Adv.: Judith McClain/Director Marketing

Service, Architectural	General

FL INDUSTRIES, PNEUMOTIVE DIV.
See Thomas Products Division

FLA ORTHOPEDICS, INC.
800-327-4110

2881 Corporate Way, Miramar, FL 33025   **954-704-4484**
FDA Number: 1044691   *Fax:* 954-431-8781
E-mail: BSNMarketing@bsnmedical.com
Web site: www.flaorthopedics.com
Year Founded: 1975
Total Employees: 200   *Marketing Staff:* 6   *Sales Staff:* 69
Ownership: Private
Produces/Sells CE-marked Devices: N
Federal Procurement Eligibility: Small Business
Distribution: Manufacturer Direct, Manufacturer Through Distributor, Manufacturer Through Manufacturer Reps
General Admin.: Rex Niles/President, Chief Executive Officer
Mktg./Adv.: Rhonda Newman/Vice President Marketing
     John Slautterback/Vice President Sales
Production: Isabel Rosende/Manager Materials

Belt, Rib (Support)	Orthopedics
Binder, Abdominal	General
Collar, Cervical Neck	Orthopedics
Immobilizer, Knee	Orthopedics
Immobilizer, Wrist/Hand	Orthopedics
Joint, Knee, External Brace	Physical Med
Orthosis, Lumbosacral	Physical Med
Orthosis, Rib Fracture, Soft	Physical Med
Orthosis, Sacroiliac, Soft	Physical Med
Support, Ankle	Orthopedics
Support, Arm	Physical Med
Support, Back	Orthopedics
Support, Knee	Physical Med
Support, Wrist	Physical Med

FLAGHOUSE, INC.
800-793-7900

601 Flaghouse Dr.,   **201-288-7600**
Hasbrouck Heights, NJ 07604
FDA Number: n/a   *Fax:* 201-288-7887
Web site: www.flaghouse.com
Annual Revenue: $25-$50 Million

FLAGHOUSE, INC. 800-793-7900 (cont'd)
Year Founded: 1954
Ownership: Private
Produces/Sells CE-marked Devices: N
Distribution: Exclusive Distributor

Cane	Physical Med
Chair, Bath	General
Equipment, Therapy, Handicapped/Physical	Physical Med
Tray, Wheelchair	Physical Med
Walker, Mechanical	Physical Med

FLAMANCO INTERNATIONAL
See Florida Manufacturing Corp.

FLAT-D INNOVATIONS, INC. 866-354-0056
7531 Berkshire Dr. N.e., PO Box 10342, 319-447-4840
Cedar Rapids, IA 52402
FDA Number: 3004129939
E-mail: info@flat-d.com
Web site: www.flat-d.com
Ownership: Private
Produces/Sells CE-marked Devices: N

Insoles, Medical	General

FLEETWOOD GROUP, INCORPORATED 800-257-6390
11832 James Street, Holland, MI 49422-1259 616-396-1142
FDA Number: n/a Fax: 616-396-8022
E-mail: info@fleetwoodgroup.com
Web site: www.fleetwoodgroup.com
Medical Products Sales Volume: $14,000,000
Annual Revenue: $10-$25 Million
Year Founded: 1955
Total Employees: 110   Marketing Staff: 1   Sales Staff: 10
Ownership: Private
Produces/Sells CE-marked Devices: Y
Federal Procurement Eligibility: Small Business, Minority Owned
Distribution: Manufacturer Through Distributor, OEM
General Admin.: Doug Ruch/President, Chief Executive Officer
Mktg./Adv.: Al Dogger/Manager Contract Sales
          Matthew Rothert/Vice President Marketing & Sales

Cabinet Casework, General Purpose	General
Chair, Other	General
Computer Equipment	General
Furniture, General	General
Table, Examination/Treatment	General
Table, Other	General

FLEMING INDUSTRIES INC.
See Iron Duck, A Div. Of Fleming Industries, Inc.

FLETCHER & CO.
See Fletcher Spaght Ventures

FLETCHER SPAGHT VENTURES 617-247-6700
222 Berkeley St., 20th Floor, Boston, MA 02116-3761
FDA Number: n/a Fax: 617-247-7757
E-mail: jf@fletcherspaght.com
Web site: www.fletcherspaght.com
Annual Revenue: $0-$1 Million
Year Founded: 1983
Ownership: Private
Produces/Sells CE-marked Devices: N
Distribution: Service Direct
General Admin.: R. John Fletcher/Chief Executive Officer
          Pearson Spaght/President

Service, Consulting	General

FLEX-A-BED, INC. 800-421-2277
1825 Hillsdale Rd., Lafayette, GA 30728 310-543-3030
FDA Number: n/a Fax: 310-543-3011
E-mail: info@flexabed.com
Web site: www.flexabeddealers.com
Total Employees: 30
Ownership: Private
Produces/Sells CE-marked Devices: N
Federal Procurement Eligibility: Small Business
Distribution: Manufacturer Direct
General Admin.: Max Morrison/President
Mktg./Adv.: Sandy Thomas/Manager Advertising
          Sandy Thomas/Marketing & Sales Specialist
Production: Max Morrison/Vice President Manufacturing

Bed, Electric	General

FLEXI-WALL SYSTEMS 800-843-5394
208 Carolina Dr., P.O. Box 89, 864-843-3104
Liberty, SC 29657
FDA Number: n/a Fax: 864-843-9318
E-mail: flexiwall@bellsouth.net
Web site: www.flexiwall.com
Annual Revenue: $1-$5 Million

FLEXI-WALL SYSTEMS 800-843-5394 (cont'd)
Ownership: Private
Produces/Sells CE-marked Devices: N
Federal Procurement Eligibility: Small Business
Distribution: Manufacturer Direct, Manufacturer Through Manufacturer Reps

Wallpaper, Antibacterial	General

FLEXIBLE DIMENSIONS LLC
See Direct Crown, Llc

FLEXIBLE STENTING SOLUTIONS INC. 732-578-0060
23 Christopher Way, Eatontown, NJ 07724
FDA Number: 3006982370 Fax: 732-578-0068
E-mail: info@flexiblestent.com
Web site: www.flexiblestent.com
Ownership: Private
Produces/Sells CE-marked Devices: N
General Admin.: Janet Burpee/Chief Executive Officer
Research: Bradley Beach/Vice President Research & Development

Catheter, Biliary	Gastroenterology/Urology
Stent, Other	Obstetrics/Gynecology

FLEXITE COMPANY 1-866-FLEXITE
40 Roselle Street, Mineola, NY 11501 516-746-2622
FDA Number: 2432071 Fax: 516-741-8147
E-mail: Flexite@aol.com
Web site: www.flexitecompany.com
Ownership: Private
Produces/Sells CE-marked Devices: N

Mouthguard	Dental And Oral

FLEXLENS INC.
See Optikem International, Inc.

FLEXPOINT SENSOR SYSTEMS INC 801-568-5111
106 West 12200 South, Draper, UT 84020
FDA Number: n/a Fax: 801-568-2405
Web site: www.flexpoint.com
Ownership: Private
Produces/Sells CE-marked Devices: N
General Admin.: Mr. John Sindt/Chairman
          Mr. Ruland Gill/Director
          Mr. Clark Mower/President, Chief Executive Officer

FLEXSEAL INTERNATIONAL PACKAGING CORP.
See Extra Packaging, Corp.

FLEXSITE DIAGNOSTICS, INC. 772-221-8893
3543 S.W. Corporate Pkwy., Palm City, FL 34990
FDA Number: 1063260
Web site: www.flexsite.com
Annual Revenue: $0-$1 Million
Year Founded: 1997
Total Employees: 8   Marketing Staff: 2   Sales Staff: 2
Ownership: Private
Produces/Sells CE-marked Devices: N
Federal Procurement Eligibility: Small Business
Distribution: Manufacturer Direct, Manufacturer Through Distributor, Manufacturer Through Manufacturer Reps, OEM

Reagent, Creatinine (Test System)	Chemistry
Test, Glycosylated Hemoglobin Assay	Hematology

FLEXTRONICS INTERNATIONAL LTD. 408-576-7000
Flextronics International, 2090 Fortune Dr.,
San Jose, CA 95131
FDA Number: n/a Fax: 408-576-7454
E-mail: Medical@flextronics.com
Web site: www.flextronics.com
Year Founded: 1990
Ownership: Private
Stock Symbol: FLEX
Traded On: NASDAQ
Produces/Sells CE-marked Devices: N
General Admin.: Dan Croteau/President
Mktg./Adv.: Renee Brotherton/Senior Director Corporate Marketing Communications
Finance: Thomas J. Smach/Chief Financial Officer
Medical Product Subsidiaries (Listed Separately)
Flextronics International

FLEXUSPINE 412-539-1520
381 Mansfield Ave, Ste. 205, Pittsburgh, PA 15220
FDA Number: n/a Fax: 412-539-1524
E-mail: info@flexuspine.com
Web site: http://www.flexuspine.com
Year Founded: 2004
Ownership: Private
Produces/Sells CE-marked Devices: N
General Admin.: Erik Wagner/Chief Technology Officer
          Mr. Vin Jannetty/President, Chief Executive Officer

FLEXUSPINE 412-539-1520 *(cont'd)*
Mktg./Adv.: Mike Dapper/Vice President Sales

FLINCHBAUGH CO., INC.
See Flinchbaugh-Kurtz Company

FLINCHBAUGH-KURTZ COMPANY 717-266-2202
245 Beshore School Rd., Manchester, PA 17345
FDA Number: n/a
Fax: 717-266-7055
Web site: www.flinchbaugh.com
Medical Products Sales Volume: $750,000
Annual Revenue: $1-$5 Million
Year Founded: 1936
Ownership: Private
Quality System Registration Information: ISO9001
Produces/Sells CE-marked Devices: N
Federal Procurement Eligibility: Small Business
Distribution: Manufacturer Direct

Lift, Stair Climbing	General
Lift, Wheelchair	General
Power System, Isolated	General

FLIR SYSTEMS
See Sea Horse Bio Science

FLO HEALTHCARE 877-356-4040
5801 Goshen Springs Road NW, Suite A, 678-990-6360
Norcross, GA 30071
FDA Number: n/a
Fax: 678-990-6370
E-mail: info@flohealthcare.com
Web site: http://www.flohealthcare.com
Ownership: Emerson Storage Solutions
Produces/Sells CE-marked Devices: N
Mktg./Adv.: Mr. Dan Fitzpatrick/Vice President Sales

Cart, Medicine	General
Cart, Monitor	General
Computer Equipment	General

FLOCAST LLC. 315-429-8407
15 South Second St., Dolgeville, NY 13329
FDA Number: 3004462857
Ownership: Private
Produces/Sells CE-marked Devices: N

Chair, With Casters	Physical Med

FLORIDA BRACE CORPORATION 800-327-0870
601 W Webster Ave., Winter Park, FL 32789 407-644-2650
FDA Number: 1044130
Fax: 407-644-4698
E-mail: flabrace@earthlink.net
Web site: www.flabrace.com
Annual Revenue: $0-$1 Million
Total Employees: 10
Ownership: Private
Produces/Sells CE-marked Devices: N
Federal Procurement Eligibility: Small Business
Distribution: Manufacturer Direct
General Admin.: Ben Moss/Chief Executive Officer

Orthosis, Cervical	Physical Med
Orthosis, Cervical-Thoracic, Rigid	Physical Med

FLORIDA LIFE SYSTEMS 727-321-9554
2632 NW 43rd Street Suite #E-9, Gainesville, FL 32606
FDA Number: 1044336
Fax: 727-327-4943
E-mail: classic@flalife.com
Web site: www.flalife.com
Annual Revenue: $0-$1 Million
Total Employees: 3
Ownership: Private
Produces/Sells CE-marked Devices: N
Federal Procurement Eligibility: Small Business
Distribution: Manufacturer Through Distributor, Manufacturer Through
Manufacturer Reps, Service Direct
General Admin.: E. Schadow/President, Chief Executive Officer
Mktg./Adv.: E. Schadow/Vice President Marketing & Sales
Production: E. Schadow/Vice President Manufacturing
Research: E. Schadow/Vice President Research & Development

Cabinet, Instrument	General
Electrosurgical Equipment, General Purpose	Surgery
Electrosurgical Equipment, Special Purpose	Surgery
Instrument, Manual, General Surgical	Surgery
Lamp, Examination (Light)	General
Lamp, Examination, Ceiling Mounted (Light)	General
Light, Surgical, Fiberoptic	Surgery
Monitor, Heart Rate, Other	Cardiovascular
Service, Engineering/Design	General
Stretcher, Emergency, Other	General
Table, Examination/Treatment	General
Table, Surgical, Electrical	Surgery

FLORIDA MANUFACTURING CORP. 800-447-2372
501 Beville Road, Daytona Beach, FL 32119 386-767-2372
FDA Number: 1014214
Fax: 800-447-6167
E-mail: info@flamanco.com
Web site: www.flamanco.com
Medical Products Sales Volume: $400,000
Annual Revenue: $0-$1 Million
Year Founded: 1947
Total Employees: 8 Sales Staff: 2
Ownership: Private
Produces/Sells CE-marked Devices: Y
Federal Procurement Eligibility: Small Business
Distribution: Manufacturer Through Distributor, OEM, Exporter
General Admin.: Tom Moore/Chief Executive Officer
            Ann Moore/Vice President

Accessories, Traction	Physical Med
Accessories, Traction (Cart, Frame, Cord, Weight)	Orthopedics
Collar, Cervical Neck	Orthopedics
Frame, Traction	Orthopedics
Halter, Head, Traction	Physical Med
Halter, Head, Traction, Orthopedic	Orthopedics
Orthosis, Cervical	Physical Med
Traction Unit, Static, Bed	Orthopedics
Traction Unit, Static, Other	Orthopedics

FLORIDA PILLOW COMPANY 800-560-1631
1012 Sligh Blvd., Orlando, FL 32806 407-648-3121
FDA Number: 3003520239
Fax: 407-648-4700
E-mail: Sales@FloridaPillow.com
Web site: www.floridapillow.com
Ownership: Private
Produces/Sells CE-marked Devices: N

Pillow, Cervical(for Mild Sleep Apnea)	Ear/Nose/Throat

FLORIDA PROBE CORP. 352-372-1142
3700 N.w. 91st St., Suite C100, Gainesville, FL 32606
FDA Number: 1039382

Probe, Periodontic	Dental And Oral

FLOSS & GO, INC. 310-394-6700
1112 Montana Ave.; Suite D, Santa Monica, CA 90403
FDA Number: 2032877

Cup, Prophylaxis	Dental And Oral
Toothbrush, Manual	Dental And Oral

FLOSSAID CORPORATION 800-528-3384
3045 Copper Road, Santa Clara, CA 95051-0701 408-730-0500
FDA Number: n/a
Fax: 408-730-3350
E-mail: info@flossaid.com
Web site: www.flossaid.com
Medical Products Sales Volume: $1,000,000
Annual Revenue: $0-$1 Million
Year Founded: 1966
Ownership: Private
Produces/Sells CE-marked Devices: N
Federal Procurement Eligibility: Small Business
Distribution: Exclusive Distributor

Floss, Dental	Dental And Oral

FLOTEC, INC. 800-401-1723
7625 W. New York St., 317-273-6960
Indianapolis, IN 46214
FDA Number: 1832475
Fax: 317-273-6979
E-mail: flotec@floteco2.com
Web site: www.floteco2.com
Medical Products Sales Volume: $3,000,000
Year Founded: 1983
Total Employees: 75 Marketing Staff: 1 Sales Staff: 38
Ownership: Private
Quality System Registration Information: ISO9001
Produces/Sells CE-marked Devices: Y
Federal Procurement Eligibility: Small Business
Distribution: Manufacturer Direct, Manufacturer Through Distributor, Manufacturer
Through Manufacturer Reps, OEM, Service Direct, Exclusive Distributor, Exporter
General Admin.: Brian Davidson/President
Mktg./Adv.: David T. Pucillo/Executive Vice President Marketing & Sales

Cylinder, Compressed Gas, With Valve	Anesthesiology
Flowmeter, Gas (Oxygen), Calibrated	Anesthesiology
Regulator, Oxygen, Mechanical	General
Regulator, Pressure, Gas Cylinder	Anesthesiology
Regulator, Vacuum	General

FLOW CYTOMETRY STANDARDS CORP.
See Bangs Laboratories, Inc.

FLOW TECHNOLOGY INC.
See Eg & G Amorphous Silicon

FLOW X-RAY CORP.
See Wolf X-Ray Corporation

FLOW X-RAY CORPORATION
800-356-9729
631-242-9729
100 West Industry Ct., Deer Park, NY 11729
FDA Number: 242700
Fax: 631-242-1001
E-mail: info@flowxray.com
Web site: www.flowxray.com
Medical Products Sales Volume: $2,000,000
Annual Revenue: $10-$25 Million
Year Founded: 1931
Total Employees: 114 *Marketing Staff:* 2 *Sales Staff:* 20
Ownership: Private
Quality System Registration Information: ISO9001; ISO9002
Produces/Sells CE-marked Devices: Y
Distribution: Manufacturer Through Distributor
General Admin.: Martin Wolf/Chief Executive Officer
    Howard Wolf/President
Mktg./Adv.: John Ambrose/Manager National Sales
    William Winters/Vice President Marketing
Production: John Nedelka/Vice President Manufacturing

Cover, Film, X-Ray	Radiology
Film, X-Ray	Radiology
Holder, X-Ray Film	Dental And Oral
Illuminator, Radiographic Film	Radiology
Image Processing System	Radiology
Light, Other	General
Marker, X-Ray	Radiology
Mount, X-Ray Tube, Diagnostic	Radiology
Sand Bag, X-Ray	Radiology
Screen, Intensifying, Radiographic	Radiology
Shield, Ophthalmic, Radiological	Radiology
Shield, X-Ray	Radiology
Storage Unit, X-Ray Film	Radiology
Support, Patient Position, Radiographic	Radiology
System, Marking, Film, Radiographic	Radiology
Timer, Radiographic	Radiology
Tube, Image Amplifier, X-Ray	Radiology

Medical Product Subsidiaries (Listed Separately)
  Wolf X-Ray Corporation

FLOWCARDIA, INC.
408-617-0352
745 N. Pastoria Ave., Sunnyvale, CA 94085
FDA Number: 3005007189
Ownership: Private
Produces/Sells CE-marked Devices: N

Catheter, Percutaneous	Cardiovascular
Catheter, Peripheral, Atherectomy	Cardiovascular
Guidewire, Catheter	Cardiovascular
Injector, Syringe	General

FLOWTRONICS, INC.
602-997-1364
10250 N. 19th Ave. Suite B, Phoenix, AZ 85021-1945
FDA Number: 2023773
Fax: 602-997-1378
E-mail: sales@flowtronics.net
Web site: www.flowtronics.net
Annual Revenue: $0-$1 Million
Year Founded: 1978
Total Employees: 5
Ownership: Private
Produces/Sells CE-marked Devices: Y
Federal Procurement Eligibility: Small Business, Female Owned
Distribution: Manufacturer Direct, Manufacturer Through Distributor, Manufacturer Through Manufacturer Reps, Exclusive Distributor
General Admin.: Margaret Sullivan/President, Chief Executive Officer
    Richard Reinig/Vice President, General Manager

Monitor, Cerebral Blood Flow, Thermal Diffusion	Cns/Neurology
Monitor, Cerebral Function	Cns/Neurology
Monitor, Intracranial Pressure, Continuous	Cns/Neurology
Monitor, Temperature, Neurosurgery, Direct Contact, Powered	Cns/Neurology
Transducer, Blood Flow, Invasive	Anesthesiology

FLUIDIGM CORPORATION
1-866-358-4354
650-266-6000
7000 Shoreline Court, Suite 100,
South San Francisco, CA 94080
FDA Number: n/a
Fax: 650-871-7152
Web site: http://www.fluidigm.com
Ownership: Private
Produces/Sells CE-marked Devices: N
General Admin.: Mr. Gajus Worthington/Chief Executive Officer
Production: Ms. Grace Yow/President Manufacturing
Research: Mr. Robert Jones/Executive Vice President Research & Development
Finance: Mr. Vikram Jog/Chief Financial Officer

FLUITRON, INC.
215-355-9970
30 Industrial Drive, Ivyland, PA 18974
FDA Number: n/a
Fax: 215-355-9074
E-mail: info@fluitron.com
Web site: www.fluitron.com
Medical Products Sales Volume: $5,000,000
Annual Revenue: $1-$5 Million

FLUITRON, INC.
215-355-9970 *(cont'd)*
Year Founded: 1976
Total Employees: 35 *Marketing Staff:* 1 *Sales Staff:* 3
Ownership: Private
Produces/Sells CE-marked Devices: N
Federal Procurement Eligibility: Small Business
Distribution: Manufacturer Direct, OEM
General Admin.: Anthony Chiccarine/President, Chief Executive Officer
Mktg./Adv.: Michael Bennis/Sales Engineer
    Raymond Wozniak/Sales Engineer
Production: James Leaming/Director Quality Assurance

Sterilizer, Steam (Autoclave)	General

FLUKE BIOMEDICAL
800-648-7952
425-347-6100
6920 Seaway Blvd, Everett, WA 98203
FDA Number: 2921581
Fax: 425-446-5116
E-mail: sales@flukebiomedical.com
Web site: www.flukebiomedical.com
Ownership: DANAHER CORPORATION
Quality System Registration Information: ISO9001
Produces/Sells CE-marked Devices: Y
Distribution: Manufacturer Direct, Manufacturer Through Distributor, Manufacturer Through Manufacturer Reps, Service Direct, Exporter
Mktg./Adv.: Heidi Stuelpnagel/Manager Advertising Communications

Alarm, Leakage Current, Portable	Cardiovascular
Analyzer, Electrical Safety	General
Analyzer, Electrosurgical Unit	Surgery
Analyzer, Infusion Pump	General
Analyzer, Pacemaker Generator Function	Cardiovascular
Computer Software	General
Cuff, Inflation	General
Electrosurgical Unit, Cutting & Coagulation Device	Surgery
Flowmeter, Gas (Oxygen), Calibrated	Anesthesiology
Monitor, Blood Pressure, Indirect, Surgery	Surgery
Monitor, Cardiac (Cardiotachometer & Rate Alarm)	Cardiovascular
Monitor, Line Isolation	Cardiovascular
Oximeter, Intracardiac	Cardiovascular
Oximeter, Pulse	General
Printer, Bar Code	General
Reader, Bar Code	General
Simulator, Arrhythmia	Cardiovascular
Simulator, Blood Pressure	Cardiovascular
Simulator, ECG	Cardiovascular
Simulator, Respiration	Anesthesiology
Tester, Defibrillator	Cardiovascular
Tester, Ground Fault Circuit Interrupter	General
Tester, Infusion Pump	General
Tester, Isolated Power System	General
Transducer, Gas Flow	Anesthesiology

FLUOROMED, L.P.
512-255-6877
2350 Double Creek Dr., Round Rock, TX 78664-3801
FDA Number: 1649547
Fax: 512-255-8298
E-mail: information@fluoromed.com
Web site: www.fluoromed.com
Ownership: Private
Produces/Sells CE-marked Devices: N

Fluid, Intraocular	Ophthalmology

FLUXION BIOSCIENCES INC.
866-266-8380
650-241-4777
384 Oyster Point Blvd. #6,
South San Francisco, CA 94080
FDA Number: n/a
Fax: 650-873-3665
E-mail: info@fluxionbio.com
Web site: http://www.fluxionbio.com
Year Founded: 2005
Ownership: Private
Produces/Sells CE-marked Devices: N
General Admin.: Mr. Jeff Jensen/Chief Executive Officer
    Dr. Christian Ionescu-Zanetti/Chief Technology Officer
Mktg./Adv.: Mr. Mark Atlas/Director Sales
Production: Mr. Steve Kushman/Manager Manufacturing
Research: Mr. Scott Lockard/Vice President Research & Development

FMD, LLC
703-880-4642
7200-e Telegraph Square Dr., P.O. Box 1500, Lorton, VA 22079
FDA Number: 3003483103
E-mail: info@fmdco.com
Web site: www.fmdco.com
Ownership: Private
Produces/Sells CE-marked Devices: N

Arthroscope	Orthopedics
Camera, Television, Endoscopic (Without Audio)	Surgery
Cystoscope	Gastroenterology/Urology
Forceps, Biopsy, Non-Electric	Gastroenterology/Urology
Forceps, ENT	Ear/Nose/Throat
Laparoscope, Gynecologic	Obstetrics/Gynecology
Light Source, Fiberoptic, Routine	Gastroenterology/Urology
Lithotriptor, Extracorporeal Shock-wave, Urological	Gastroenterology/Urology

FMD, LLC   703-880-4642 *(cont'd)*
Surgical Instrument, G-U, Manual   Gastroenterology/Urology

FOAM CRAFT   714-459-9971
2441 Cypress Way, Fullerton, CA 92831
FDA Number: 3007008421
Ownership: Private
Produces/Sells CE-marked Devices: N
Cover, Mattress   General
Mattress, Non-Powered Flotation Therapy   Physical Med

FOAM CUTTING ENGINEERS, INC.
See Ufp Technologies, Inc.

FOAMEX INNOVATIONS   800-355-3626
1400 Providence Road, Suite 2000,   610-744-2300
Media, PA 19063
FDA Number: 3007536941
Web site: www.fxi.com
Total Employees: 791
Ownership: Private
Stock Symbol: FMXL
Traded On: NASDAQ
Quality System Registration Information: ISO9001
Produces/Sells CE-marked Devices: N
Distribution: Manufacturer Through Distributor, OEM
General Admin.: Harold J. Earley/Chief Financial Officer, Executive Vice President
    David J. Prilutski/Chief Operating Officer, Executive Vice President
    John G. Johnson/President, Chief Executive Officer
Mktg./Adv.: Mr. Frederick Rullo/Senior Vice President Sales
Research: Mr. Chiu Chan/Vice President Research & Development
Cushion, Ring, Foam Rubber   General
Dressing, Foam   General
Mattress, Air Flotation   General

FOAMEX L.P.   800-355-3626
2211 S. Wayne St., Auburn, IN 46706   757-224-0177
FDA Number: 3004728444
Web site: www.fxi.com
Annual Revenue: More than $1 Billion
Total Employees: 791
Ownership: FOAMEX INNOVATIONS
Quality System Registration Information: ISO9001
Produces/Sells CE-marked Devices: N
General Admin.: Harold J. Earley/Chief Financial Officer, Executive Vice President
    David J. Prilutski/Chief Operating Officer, Executive Vice President
    John G. Johnson/President, Chief Executive Officer
Mattress, Air Flotation   General

FOCAL POINT OPTICIANS   510-923-0568
2638 Ashby Avenue, Berkeley, CA 94705
FDA Number: 2939471
Ownership: Private
Produces/Sells CE-marked Devices: N
Frame, Spectacle (Eyeglasses)   Ophthalmology

FOCUS DIAGNOSTICS, INC.   800-838-4548
11331 Valley View Street, Cypress, CA 90630   562-240-6500
FDA Number: 2023365   Fax: 562-240-6510
Web site: www.focusdx.com
Ownership: Private
Produces/Sells CE-marked Devices: N
General Admin.: Dr. John Hurrell/Vice President
Medical Admin.: Dr. Jay Lieberman/Medical Director
Mktg./Adv.: Mr. Carl Stubbings/Vice President Marketing & Sales
Production: Ms. Ronda Elliott/Vice President Quality Assurance & Regulatory Affairs
Research: Mr. Mark Wobken/Vice President Diagnostics
    Dr. Maurice Exner/Vice President Research & Development
Antisera, Fluorescent, Chlamydia SPP.   Microbiology
Antiserum, CF, Equine Encephalitis Virus, EEE, WEE   Microbiology
Enzyme Linked Immunoabsorbent Assay, Coccidioides Immitis   Microbiology
Enzyme Linked Immunoabsorbent Assay, Herpes Simplex Virus   Microbiology
Enzyme Linked Immunoabsorbent Assay, Histoplasma Capsulatum   Microbiology
General Purpose Microbiology Diagnostic Device   Microbiology
Legionella Direct & Indirect Fluorescent Antibody Regents   Microbiology
Rickettsia Serological Reagents, Other   Microbiology
Test, Nuclear Antigen, Epstein-Barr Virus   Microbiology

FOCUS MEDICAL PRODUCTS
See Medi-Hut Co., Inc.

FOCUS MEDICAL, LLC.   866-633-5273
23 Francis J. Clarke Circle, Bethel, CT 06801   203-730-8885
FDA Number: 1226486   Fax: 203-730-8851
E-mail: info@FocusMedical.com
Web site: www.focusmedical.com
Year Founded: 2000

FOCUS MEDICAL, LLC.   866-633-5273 *(cont'd)*
Ownership: Private
Produces/Sells CE-marked Devices: Y
Distribution: Manufacturer Direct, Manufacturer Through Distributor, Manufacturer Through Manufacturer Reps, Service Direct, Exclusive Distributor, Exporter
Forceps, General & Plastic Surgery   Surgery
Laser, Nd:YAG, Surgical   Surgery
Laser, Surgical   Surgery
Motor, Surgical Instrument, AC-Powered   Surgery

FOCUS SURGERY, INC.   317-541-1580
3940 Pendleton Way, Indianapolis, IN 46226
FDA Number: 2951226   Fax: 317-541-1581
E-mail: mmarcum@focus-surgery.com
Web site: www.focus-surgery.com
Medical Products Sales Volume: $4,500,000
Annual Revenue: $1-$5 Million
Year Founded: 1996
Total Employees: 13   Marketing Staff: 1   Sales Staff: 1
Ownership: Private
Quality System Registration Information: ISO9001
Produces/Sells CE-marked Devices: Y
Federal Procurement Eligibility: Small Business
Distribution: Manufacturer Direct, Manufacturer Through Distributor
General Admin.: Narendra T. Sanghvi/Chief Executive Officer
Device, Ablation, Thermal, Ultrasonic   Gastroenterology/Urology
System, Hyperthermia, Rf/microwave (benign Prostatic Hyperplasia), Thermotherapy   Gastroenterology/Urology

FOCUS TECHNOLOGIES   800-445-0185
5785 Corporate Avenue,   714-220-1900
Cypress, CA 90630
FDA Number: n/a   Fax: 714-220-1683
E-mail: jvargas@mrlinfo.com
Web site: www.focustechnologies.com
Total Employees: 400
Ownership: FOCUS/MRL, INC.
Produces/Sells CE-marked Devices: N
Distribution: Manufacturer Direct, Manufacturer Through Distributor, Manufacturer Through Manufacturer Reps
General Admin.: Laurence R. McCarthy/President
Mktg./Adv.: Lilly Kong, DVM./Director Product Development
    Jane Markley/Manager International Marketing & Sales
    Mary Kay Mosch/Vice President Marketing & Sales
Production: Christine Yang/Director Quality Assurance
    Christina Yang/General Manager Production
    Michael Wagner/Manager Regulatory Affairs
    Josie Vargas-Cunningham/Product Manager
Research: Lilly Kong/Vice President Research & Development
Antigen, Antiserum, Control, IGM   Immunology
Antigen, Leptospira SPP.   Microbiology
Antisera, Fluorescent, Chlamydia SPP.   Microbiology
Antiserum, Fluorescent, Epstein-Barr Virus   Microbiology
Antiserum, Fluorescent, Q Fever   Microbiology
Antiserum, Typhus Fever   Microbiology
Contract Manufacturing, Reagent   General
IGG Immunoassay Reagents   Immunology
Reagent, Borrelia, Serological   Microbiology
Reagent, Legionella Detection   Microbiology
Rickettsia Serological Reagents, Other   Microbiology
Test, Disease, Lyme   Immunology
Test, Nuclear Antigen, Epstein-Barr Virus   Microbiology

FOLLETT CORP.   800-523-9361
801 Church Lane, Easton, PA 18044   610-252-7301
FDA Number: 3005883510   Fax: 610-250-0696
E-mail: marketing@follettice.com
Web site: www.follettice.com
Medical Products Sales Volume: $15,100,000
Year Founded: 1948
Total Employees: 175
Ownership: Private
Produces/Sells CE-marked Devices: Y
Federal Procurement Eligibility: Small Business
Distribution: Manufacturer Direct, Manufacturer Through Distributor, Manufacturer Through Manufacturer Reps
General Admin.: Steve Follett/President, Chief Executive Officer
Mktg./Adv.: Lois Schneck/Director Marketing
    Jim Frantz/Director Product Development
    Dan Chilson/Manager International Marketing & Sales
    Jack Miller/Manager National Operations
    Gary Gutman/Manager National Sales
    Ed Barr/Vice President Sales
Production: Matt Hood/Manager Manufacturing
    Chris Zirkle/Manager Materials
    Robert Bryson/Vice President Manufacturing
Dispenser, Ice   General

FOLLETT CORP.   800-523-9361 *(cont'd)*
Refrigerator, Laboratory   General

FONAR CORP.   888-NEEDMRI
110 Marcus Drive, Melville, NY 11747   **631-694-2929**
FDA Number: 2432211   *Fax:* 631-753-5150
E-mail: sales@fonar.com
Web site: www.fonar.com
Annual Revenue: $1-$5 Million
Year Founded: 1978
Total Employees: 168
Ownership: Public
Stock Symbol: FONR
Traded On: NASDAQ
Quality System Registration Information: ISO9001
Produces/Sells CE-marked Devices: N
Federal Procurement Eligibility: Small Business
Distribution: Manufacturer Direct, Importer
General Admin.: Raymond V. Damadian/President, Chief Executive Officer
     David Terry/Secretary, Treasurer
     Luciano B. Bonanni/Vice President
Mktg./Adv.: Kurt W. Reimann/Vice President Marketing
     Timothy Damadian/Vice President Sales
Production: Timothy Damadian/Vice President Operations
Research: Jay Butterman/Vice President Research & Development

Nuclear Magnetic Resonance Imaging System	Radiology
Scanner, Magnetic Resonance (NMR/MRI)	Radiology

FOOT LEVELERS, INC.   540-345-0008
P.o. Box 12611, Roanoke, VA 24027
FDA Number: 1911617
E-mail: service@footlevelers.com
Ownership: Private
Produces/Sells CE-marked Devices: N

Cover, Limb	Physical Med
Exerciser, Non-Measuring	Physical Med
Orthosis, Limb Brace	Physical Med
Orthosis, Lumbosacral	Physical Med

FOOTENT, LLC   757-224-0177
3392 W. 8600 South, W Jordan, UT 84088
FDA Number: 3006024432

Bed, Manual	General

FOOTHILLS INDUSTRIES, INC.   828-652-4088
300 Rockwell Drive, Marion, NC 28752
FDA Number: 1054069   *Fax:* 828-652-7527
E-mail: awebb@foothillsindustries.com
Web site: www.foothillsindustries.com
Medical Products Sales Volume: $500,000
Annual Revenue: $1-$5 Million
Year Founded: 1972
Total Employees: 115   *Marketing Staff:* 1   *Sales Staff:* 1
Ownership: Private
Produces/Sells CE-marked Devices: N
Distribution: Manufacturer Direct, Manufacturer Through Distributor, Manufacturer Through Manufacturer Reps, Exporter
General Admin.: Ms. Joy Shuford/Chief Executive Officer
Mktg./Adv.: Mr. Andy Webb/Director Marketing & Sales
     Mr. Steve Early/Director Special Projects
Production: Ms. Janet Owens/Director Operations

Contract Manufacturing	General
Drape, Incision, Surgical	Surgery
Drape, Microscope, Ophthalmic	Ophthalmology
Drape, Patient, Ophthalmic	Ophthalmology
Drape, Surgical	Surgery
Drape, Surgical, Disposable	Surgery
Drape, Urological, Disposable	Gastroenterology/Urology
Light, Fiberoptic, Dental	Dental And Oral
Pack, Surgical (Drape)	Surgery
Sheet, Drape	Surgery
Sheet, Drape, Disposable	Surgery
Sudan IV	Pathology

FOOTMAXX HOLDINGS INC.   800-779-3668
468 Queen St. E, Ste. 400,   **416-366-3668**
Toronto, ONT M5A-1 Canada
FDA Number: 1225983   *Fax:* 416-366-8087
E-mail: webmaster@footmaxx.com
Web site: www.footmaxx.com
Year Founded: 1994
Total Employees: 100
Ownership: Private
Produces/Sells CE-marked Devices: N
Distribution: Manufacturer Direct, Exporter

FOOTSPLY INC.
See Pedifix, Inc.

FOREDOM ELECTRIC CO.   203-7304548 EXT
16 Stony Hill Rd., Bethel, CT 06801
FDA Number: 1217202   *Fax:* 203-796-7861
E-mail: company16@aol.com
Web site: www.foredom.net
Annual Revenue: $10-$25 Million
Total Employees: 90
Ownership: Private
Produces/Sells CE-marked Devices: N
Distribution: Manufacturer Through Distributor
General Admin.: Willard P. Nelson/President
Mktg./Adv.: Barbara Heilweil/Manager Advertising
     Tom Degnan/Manager Sales
Production: Robert Horton/Vice President Manufacturing
Research: Ralph Costa/Vice President Research & Development
Finance: Willard P. Nelson/Chief Financial Officer

Drill, Dental, Intraoral	Dental And Oral
Engine, Dental	Dental And Oral
Handpiece, Belt and/or Gear Driven, Dental	Dental And Oral
Handpiece, Contra- And Right-Angle Attachment, Dental	Dental And Oral
Handpiece, Direct Drive, AC-Powered	Dental And Oral
Pad, Percussion	Cns/Neurology
Percussor	Cns/Neurology

FOREMOST DENTAL LLC.   201-894-5500
242 South Dean St., Englewood, NJ 07631
FDA Number: 2244812

Agent, Polishing, Abrasive, Oral Cavity	Dental And Oral
Alloy, Amalgam	Dental And Oral
Applicator, Resin	Dental And Oral
Capsule, Dental, Amalgam	Dental And Oral
Coating, Filling Material, Resin	Dental And Oral
Post, Root Canal	Dental And Oral
Sealant, Pit And Fissure, And Conditioner, Resin	Dental And Oral

FOREST DENTAL PRODUCTS INC   800-423-3535
6200 N.E. Campus Court, Hillsboro, OR 97124   **503-640-3012**
FDA Number: 3022226   *Fax:* 503-640-4008
E-mail: sales@forestmed.com
Web site: www.forestmed.com
Medical Products Sales Volume: $10,000,000
Annual Revenue: $10-$25 Million
Year Founded: 1977
Total Employees: 85   *Marketing Staff:* 5   *Sales Staff:* 17
Ownership: Private
Quality System Registration Information: ISO9002
Produces/Sells CE-marked Devices: Y
Federal Procurement Eligibility: Small Business, Minority Owned
Distribution: Manufacturer Through Distributor, Manufacturer Through Manufacturer Reps, OEM, Importer, Exporter
General Admin.: Franklin Mascarenhas/Chief Executive Officer, Treasurer
     Hank Barton/President
Mktg./Adv.: Jeff Bunker/Vice President Sales
Production: Chuck Lewis/Manager Engineering
     Leah Rosenoff/Supervisor Customer Service

Chair, Dental	Dental And Oral
Chair, Dental (With Unit)	Dental And Oral
Contract Manufacturing	General
Cuspidor	Dental And Oral
Dental Laboratory Equipment	Dental And Oral
Instrument, Dental, Manual	Dental And Oral
Light, Dental	Dental And Oral
Stool, Dental	Dental And Oral
Syringe Unit, Air And/Or Water	Dental And Oral
System, Delivery, Drug, Unit-Dose	General

FOREST IMAGING, INC   619-218-6460
5288 Eastgate Mall, San Diego, CA 92121
FDA Number: 3005278403

Cradle, Patient, Radiographic	Radiology

FOREST PHARMACEUTICAL, INC.   314-493-7000
13600 Shoreline Drive, St. Louis, MO 63045
FDA Number: 1921065
Web site: www.forestpharm.com
Ownership: Private
Produces/Sells CE-marked Devices: N

Nebulizer, Direct Patient Interface	Anesthesiology

FORESTADENT USA   800-721-4940
2315 Weldon Parkway, St. Louis, MO 63146   **314-878-5985**
FDA Number: 3005014825   *Fax:* 314-878-7604
E-mail: info@forestadentusa.com
Web site: www.forestadent.com
Ownership: Private
Produces/Sells CE-marked Devices: N

Activator, Ultraviolet, Polymerization	Dental And Oral
Adhesive, Bracket And Conditioner, Resin	Dental And Oral
Band, Elastic, Orthodontic	Dental And Oral

FORESTADENT USA   800-721-4940 (cont'd)

Band, Preformed, Orthodontic	Dental And Oral
Bracket, Metal, Orthodontic	Dental And Oral
Clamp, Wire, Orthodontic	Dental And Oral
Clasp, Preformed	Dental And Oral
Headgear, Extraoral, Orthodontic	Dental And Oral
Pliers, Orthodontic	Dental And Oral
Retainer, Screw Expansion, Orthodontic	Dental And Oral
Spring, Orthodontic	Dental And Oral
Tube, Orthodontic	Dental And Oral
Wire, Orthodontic	Dental And Oral

FORMED PLASTICS, INC.   516-334-2300

207 Stonehinge Lane, Carle Place, NY 11514
FDA Number: 3005562032

Stretcher, Hand-Carried	General

FORMEDICA LTD.   800-361-9671

7109, Trans, Montreal, (QUEB H4T 1A2 Canada   **514-336-4821**
FDA Number: 9200363   *Fax:* 514-336-2418
E-mail: rfortin@formedica.com
Web site: www.formedica.com
Medical Products Sales Volume: $4,500,000
Year Founded: 1972
Total Employees: 60   *Marketing Staff:* 2   *Sales Staff:* 10
Ownership: Private
Produces/Sells CE-marked Devices: Y
Distribution: Manufacturer Direct, Manufacturer Through Distributor, Manufacturer Through Manufacturer Reps, Importer, Exporter

FORSAN MANUFACTURING
See Hamilton Bell Company

FORSAN MFG.   201-391-4100

30 Craig Rd., Montvale, NJ 07645
FDA Number: 2246613
Ownership: Private
Produces/Sells CE-marked Devices: N

Centrifuge, Cell Washing	Hematology

FORT WAYNE METALS RESEARCH PROD. CORP.   260-747-4154

9609 Indianapolis Road, Fort Wayne, IN 46809
FDA Number: 1824313   *Fax:* 260-747-0398
E-mail: info@fwmetals.com
Web site: www.fwmetals.com
Medical Products Sales Volume: $42,700,000
Annual Revenue: $25-$50 Million
Year Founded: 1970
Total Employees: 30   *Marketing Staff:* 4   *Sales Staff:* 21
Ownership: Fort Wayne Metals Research Products
Quality System Registration Information: ISO9000; ISO9002
Produces/Sells CE-marked Devices: N
Federal Procurement Eligibility: Small Business
Distribution: Manufacturer Direct, Exporter
General Admin.: Scott Glaze/Chief Executive Officer
     Mark Michael/President
Mktg./Adv.: Robert Myers/Vice President, Director Marketing
Production: David Bradley/Director Quality Assurance
     Jerry Litchfield/Manager Customer Services
Purchasing: Ken Hendrickson/Manager Purchasing

Endoscope	Gastroenterology/Urology
Guide, Wire, Angiographic (And Accessories)	Cns/Neurology
Guidewire	Cardiovascular
Guidewire, Catheter	Cardiovascular
Guidewire, Catheter, Radiological	Radiology
Lead, Pacemaker, Implantable Myocardial	Cardiovascular
Stylet, Catheter	Cardiovascular
Suture, Laparoscopy	Surgery
Suture, Multifilament Steel	Surgery
Suture, Non-Absorbable, Steel, Monofilament & Multifilament	Surgery
Suture, Stainless Steel	Surgery
Wire, Bone	Orthopedics
Wire, Ligature	Surgery
Wire, Orthodontic	Dental And Oral

FORT WORTH EYE PROSTHETICS, INC.   817-429-8086

1350 South Main, #2450, Fort Worth, TX 76104
FDA Number: 1649382

Eye, Artificial, Non-Custom	Ophthalmology

FORTRAD EYE INSTRUMENTS CORP.   973-543-2371

8 Franklin Road, Mendham, NJ 07945
FDA Number: 2243869   *Fax:* 973-543-5446
Medical Products Sales Volume: $300,000
Annual Revenue: $0-$1 Million
Year Founded: 1979
Total Employees: 2   *Marketing Staff:* 2   *Sales Staff:* 2
Ownership: Private
Produces/Sells CE-marked Devices: N

FORTRAD EYE INSTRUMENTS CORP.   973-543-2371 (cont'd)

Federal Procurement Eligibility: Small Business
Distribution: Manufacturer Direct, Importer, Exporter
General Admin.: Karl H. Grohn/President, Chief Executive Officer
Mktg./Adv.: Inge A. Grohn/Manager Marketing

Blade, Scalpel	Surgery
Burr, Corneal, Battery-Powered	Ophthalmology
Burr, Corneal, Manual	Ophthalmology
Caliper, Ophthalmic	Ophthalmology
Cannula, Lacrimal (Eye)	Ophthalmology
Cannula, Ophthalmic	Ophthalmology
Clamp, Eyelid, Ophthalmic	Ophthalmology
Clip, Suture	Surgery
Container, Surgical Instrument	Surgery
Curette	Orthopedics
Curette, Ophthalmic	Ophthalmology
Depressor, Orbital	Ophthalmology
Dilator, Lacrimal	Ophthalmology
Expressor	Ophthalmology
Expressor, Lens Loop	Ophthalmology
Forceps	Orthopedics
Forceps, Dressing	Surgery
Forceps, Hemostatic	Surgery
Forceps, Ophthalmic	Ophthalmology
Forceps, Tissue	Surgery
Guide, Intraocular Lens	Ophthalmology
Handle, Knife Blade	Surgery
Hook, Ophthalmic	Ophthalmology
Hook, Other	Surgery
Hook, Scleral Fixation	Ophthalmology
Hook, Strabismus	Ophthalmology
Keratome, AC-Powered	Ophthalmology
Knife, Ophthalmic	Ophthalmology
Lens, Other	Ophthalmology
Loop, Lens	Ophthalmology
Measurer, Corneal Radius	Ophthalmology
Needle, Knife	Surgery
Needle, Suture, Ophthalmic	Ophthalmology
Probe, Lacrimal	Ophthalmology
Protector, Surgical Instrument	Surgery
Retractor, Manual	Cns/Neurology
Retractor, Ophthalmic	Ophthalmology
Retractor, Other	Surgery
Ruler, Nearpoint (Punctometer)	Ophthalmology
Scissors, Corneal	Ophthalmology
Scissors, Enucleation	Ophthalmology
Scissors, Iris	Ophthalmology
Scissors, Ophthalmic	Ophthalmology
Scissors, Tenotomy	Ophthalmology
Spatula, Ophthalmic	Ophthalmology
Spatula, Other	Surgery
Speculum, Ophthalmic	Ophthalmology
Speculum, Other	General
Spud, Ophthalmic	Ophthalmology
Tenaculum, Other (Forceps)	Surgery
Tonometer, Manual	Ophthalmology

FORTRESS SCIENTIFIQUE DU QUEBEC LTEE.   418-847-5225

2160 Rue De Celles, Quebec G2C 1X8 Canada
FDA Number: 8022036

Accessories, Wheelchair	Physical Med
Component, Wheelchair	Physical Med
Wheelchair, Manual	Physical Med
Wheelchair, Powered	Physical Med

FORUM INDUSTRIES INC.   210-225-9600

1903 Hormel Dr., Kirby, TX 78219
FDA Number: 3005381858
Ownership: Private
Produces/Sells CE-marked Devices: N

Mattress, Non-Powered Flotation Therapy	Physical Med

FORWARD MOTIONS, INC.   877-364-8267

214 Valley St., Dayton, OH 45404-1839   **937-222-5001**
FDA Number: n/a   *Fax:* 937-222-4001
E-mail: fmotions@aol.com
Web site: www.forwardmotions.com
Medical Products Sales Volume: $800,000
Annual Revenue: $0-$1 Million
Year Founded: 1977
Total Employees: 8   *Sales Staff:* 2
Ownership: Private
Produces/Sells CE-marked Devices: N
Federal Procurement Eligibility: Small Business
Distribution: Manufacturer Direct, Manufacturer Through Distributor, Service Direct, Exclusive Distributor
General Admin.: Roger E. Flint/Chief Executive Officer
     Laura Sims/Office Manager
     Roger E. Flint/President
Mktg./Adv.: Clark Shockley/Director Marketing

FORWARD MOTIONS, INC.　877-364-8267 (cont'd)
Clark Shockley/Manager National Accounts & Sales
Production: Gilbert Smith/Manager Production

Control, Foot Driving, Automobile, Mechanical	Physical Med
Control, Hand Driving, Automobile, Mechanical	Physical Med
Lift, Wheelchair	General
Ramp, Wheelchair	General
Utensil, Handicapped Aid	Physical Med
Vehicle, Handicapped	Physical Med

FORWARD TECHNOLOGY　320-286-2578
260 Jenks Avenue, Cokato, MN 55321
FDA Number: n/a　　*Fax:* 320-286-2467
E-mail: info@forwardtech.com
Web site: www.forwardtech.com
Medical Products Sales Volume: $6,100,000
Annual Revenue: $10-$25 Million
Year Founded: 2001
Total Employees: 73　　*Marketing Staff:* 1　　*Sales Staff:* 10
Ownership: Crest Ultrasonics Corp.
Produces/Sells CE-marked Devices: Y
Federal Procurement Eligibility: Small Business
Distribution: Manufacturer Through Manufacturer Reps, Exporter
General Admin.: Michael Goodson/Chief Executive Officer
Mktg./Adv.: David Kralovetz/Marketing Coordinator
　　　　　David Kralovetz/Vice President Sales
　　　　　Wayne Mouser/Vice President Sales
Production: Brian Kivisto/Plant Manager
Finance: Brad Henke/Chief Financial Officer

Cleaner, Ultrasonic, Medical Instrument	General
Contract Manufacturing	General
Detector, Leakage, Medical Gas	General
Heat-Sealing Device	Hematology

FOSTEC, INC.
See Schott North America, Inc.

FOSTER HARD FURNITURE
See Hard Manufacturing Co.

FOSTER MANUFACTURING CORP.　262-633-7073
1652 Phillips Avenue, Racine, WI 53403
FDA Number: 7000808　　*Fax:* 262-633-4458
E-mail: info@fostermfgcorp.com
Web site: www.fostermfgcorp.com
Medical Products Sales Volume: $600,000
Annual Revenue: $1-$5 Million
Total Employees: 11
Federal Procurement Eligibility: Small Business
Distribution: Manufacturer Through Distributor
General Admin.: Tim Seils/Office Manager
　　　　　Douglas Foster/President
　　　　　Steve Sharkozy/Vice President

Prosthesis, Hip, Femoral Component, Cemented, Metal	Orthopedics
Prosthesis, Knee, Hinged (Metal-Metal)	Orthopedics

FOSTER REFRIGERATOR L.L.C.　888-828-3311
97 7th St., P.O.Box 718, Kinderhook, NY 12106　518-828-3311
FDA Number: n/a　　*Fax:* 518-828-3315
E-mail: fosterusa@yahoo.com
Web site: www.foster-us.com
Medical Products Sales Volume: $3,000,000
Annual Revenue: $1-$5 Million
Total Employees: 15　　*Marketing Staff:* 2　　*Sales Staff:* 2
Ownership: Private
Quality System Registration Information: ISO9000
Produces/Sells CE-marked Devices: Y
Federal Procurement Eligibility: Small Business
Distribution: Manufacturer Through Distributor, Service Direct
General Admin.: Jim M. Danardi/Owner
Mktg./Adv.: Larry Foster/Vice President Marketing & Sales
Production: Gene O'Reilley/Vice President Manufacturing
Research: Gene O'Reilley/Vice President Research & Development

Freezer, Blood Storage	Hematology
Freezer, Laboratory, Biological	Chemistry
Freezer, Laboratory, General Purpose	Chemistry
Refrigerator, Biological	Microbiology
Refrigerator, Blood Bank	Hematology
Refrigerator, Bone	Orthopedics
Refrigerator, Explosion-Proof	Chemistry
Refrigerator, Eye Bank	Ophthalmology
Refrigerator, Foodservice	General
Refrigerator, Laboratory	General
Refrigerator, Pharmacy	General

FOTHERGILL COMPOSITES INC.
See Vermont Composites, Inc.

FOTODYNE, INC.　800-362-3686
950 Walnut Ridge Dr., Hartland, WI 53029　262-369-7000
FDA Number: n/a　　*Fax:* 262-309-7017

FOTODYNE, INC.　800-362-3686 (cont'd)
E-mail: info@fotodyne.com
Web site: www.fotodyne.com
Annual Revenue: $1-$5 Million
Year Founded: 1980
Ownership: Private
Produces/Sells CE-marked Devices: Y
Federal Procurement Eligibility: Small Business
Distribution: Manufacturer Through Manufacturer Reps

Computer Software	General
Computer, Radiographic Image Analysis	Radiology
Controller, Temperature, Other	General
Electrophoresis Equipment, Gel	Chemistry
Genetic Engineering	Microbiology
Image Processing System	Radiology
Lamp, Ultraviolet, Physical Medicine	Physical Med
Power System, Isolated	General
Shield Radio Frequency	Radiology
Training Aid	Orthopedics
Transilluminator, Laboratory	Chemistry

FOTOFINDER SYSTEMS, INC.　443-283-3865
9693 Gerwig Lane, Suite S, Columbia, MD 21046
FDA Number: 3004575032
Ownership: Private
Produces/Sells CE-marked Devices: N

Device, Storage, Image, Digital	Radiology

FOUGERA　800-645-9833
60 Baylis Road, PO Box 2006, Melville, NY 11747　631-454-6996
FDA Number: n/a　　*Fax:* 631-454-1572
E-mail: info@fougera.com
Web site: www.fougera.com
Year Founded: 1849
Total Employees: 625　　*Marketing Staff:* 5　　*Sales Staff:* 20
Ownership: Altana, Inc.
Stock Symbol: AAA
Traded On: NYSE
Produces/Sells CE-marked Devices: N
Federal Procurement Eligibility: Small Business
Distribution: Manufacturer Through Distributor
General Admin.: George Cole/President
　　　　　Mindy Kirsch/Vice President Human Resources
Mktg./Adv.: Joyce M. Schlener/Manager Marketing
　　　　　David Klaum/Vice President Marketing & Sales
Production: Helen Corso/Vice President Manufacturing

Jelly, Lubricating	General

FOUNDATION MEDICINE INC.　617-418-2200
One Kendall Square, Suite B3501, Cambridge, MA 02139
FDA Number: n/a　　*Fax:* 617-418-2201
E-mail: info@foundationmedicine.com
Web site: www.foundationmedicine.com
Ownership: Private
Produces/Sells CE-marked Devices: N
General Admin.: Dr. Kevin Krenitsky/Chief Operating Officer
　　　　　Dr. Michael Pellini/President, Chief Executive Officer
　　　　　Mr. Gary Cohen/Vice President
Medical Admin.: Dr. Jeffery Rocc/Medical Director
　　　　　Dr. Gary Palmer/Senior Vice President Medical Affairs
Research: Dr. Maureen Cronin/Senior Vice President Research & Development

FOUNDATION MILLING CENTRE　716-579-3724
235 Aero Dr., Suite 2, Buffalo, NY 14225
FDA Number: 3005910901

Powder, Porcelain	Dental And Oral

FOUR PROCESS, LTD.　636-677-5650
1480 West Lark Industrial Park, Fenton, MO 63026
FDA Number: 1954550　　*Fax:* 636-677-4751
E-mail: mhf4process@aol.com
Medical Products Sales Volume: $600,000
Annual Revenue: $1-$5 Million
Year Founded: 1974
Total Employees: 15
Ownership: Private
Produces/Sells CE-marked Devices: N
Federal Procurement Eligibility: Small Business
Distribution: Manufacturer Through Distributor
General Admin.: Mr. Mark Fox/President

Holder, Intravascular Catheter	General

FOX MANUFACTURING, INC.　479-646-1656
5305 Towson Ave., Fort Smith, AR 72901
FDA Number: n/a　　*Fax:* 479-646-1757
Annual Revenue: $0-$1 Million
Total Employees: 2
Ownership: Private

FOX MANUFACTURING, INC.
479-646-1656 *(cont'd)*
Produces/Sells CE-marked Devices: N
Federal Procurement Eligibility: Small Business
Distribution: Manufacturer Direct
General Admin.: Cynthia Fox/President
  Evacuator, Fume — Chemistry

FOXBORO CO./ENVIRONMENTAL MONITORING OPERATIONS
See Invensys Process Systems

FOXBORO ENVIRONMENTAL
See Invensys Process Systems

FOXBORO/ICT
See Sensym Ict

FPP, INC.
352-622-4595
6800 S.W. 66th St., Ocala, FL 34476-5526
FDA Number: n/a   Fax: 352-237-4855
E-mail: bpetti5570@aol.com
Total Employees: 18172   *Marketing Staff:* 2   *Sales Staff:* 2
Ownership: Private
Produces/Sells CE-marked Devices: N
Federal Procurement Eligibility: Small Business, Female Owned
Distribution: Manufacturer Direct
General Admin.: Barbara Petti/President
Production: Beverly J. Fuller/Manager Production
  Board, Arm — Anesthesiology
  Strap, Restraining — General

FR CHEMICAL
603-648-2194
524 South Columbus Ave., Mount Vernon, NY 10550
FDA Number: 3003908491
Ownership: Private
Produces/Sells CE-marked Devices: N
  Film, X-Ray, Special Purpose — Radiology

FR MEDICAL X-RAY SUPPLIES
See Medlink Imaging, Inc.

FRAIN INDUSTRIES, INC.
630-629-9900
9377 Grand Ave., Franklin Park, IL 60131
FDA Number: n/a   Fax: 630-629-6575
Web site: www.fraingroup.com
Annual Revenue: $10-$25 Million
Ownership: FRAIN GROUP, INC.
Produces/Sells CE-marked Devices: N
Federal Procurement Eligibility: Small Business
Distribution: Manufacturer Direct, Exclusive Distributor
  Service, Used Equipment — General

FRANCIS L. FREAS GLASS WORKS, INC.
610-828-0430
148 East Ninth Avenue, Conshohocken, PA 19428
FDA Number: 2522598   Fax: 610-834-0430
E-mail: sales@freasglass.com
Web site: www.freasglass.com
Medical Products Sales Volume: $2,600,000
Annual Revenue: $0-$1 Million
Year Founded: 1905
Total Employees: 36
Ownership: Private
Produces/Sells CE-marked Devices: N
Federal Procurement Eligibility: Small Business, Minority Owned, Female Owned, GSA Contract
Distribution: Manufacturer Direct
General Admin.: Douglas Marzella/Vice President
Mktg./Adv.: Norma Ramey/Director Marketing
  Labware, Basic, Reusable — Chemistry
  Thermometer, Fluid Column — Surgery
  Urinometer, Non-Electrical — Gastroenterology/Urology

FRANK J. MAY, INC.
215-923-3165
256 South 11th St., Philadelphia, PA 19107
FDA Number: 2520656
Ownership: Private
Produces/Sells CE-marked Devices: N
  Excavator, Dental, Operative — Dental And Oral

FRANK SCHOLZ X-RAY CORP.
508-586-8308
244 Liberty St., Brockton, MA 02401-5522
FDA Number: 1217398   Fax: 508-588-6784
Annual Revenue: $0-$1 Million
Year Founded: 1936
Total Employees: 50
Ownership: Private
Produces/Sells CE-marked Devices: N
Federal Procurement Eligibility: Small Business, Female Owned
Distribution: Manufacturer Direct
General Admin.: Thomas E. Richter/President, General Manager
  Apron, Lead, Radiographic — Radiology
  Bin, Storage — General

FRANK SCHOLZ X-RAY CORP.
508-586-8308 *(cont'd)*
  Compressor, Air, Portable — Anesthesiology
  Holder, Head, Neurosurgical (Skull Clamp) — Cns/Neurology
  Holder, Head, Radiographic — Radiology
  Holder, Radiographic Cassette, Wall-Mounted — Radiology
  Patient Transfer Unit — General
  Radiographic Unit, Diagnostic, Mammographic — Radiology
  Support, Patient Position — Anesthesiology
  Support, Patient Position, Radiographic — Radiology
  Table, Surgical With Orthopedic Accessories, AC-Powered — Surgery
  Table, Surgical, Orthopedic — Orthopedics

FRANK STUBBS CO., INC
800-223-1713
1830 Eastman Avenue, Oxnard, CA 93030
805-278-4300
FDA Number: 2014871   Fax: 805-278-6609
E-mail: dpearson@fstubbs.com
Web site: www.fstubbs.com
Medical Products Sales Volume: $8,800,000
Year Founded: 1968
Total Employees: 120   *Marketing Staff:* 3   *Sales Staff:* 5
Ownership: Private
Produces/Sells CE-marked Devices: N
Federal Procurement Eligibility: Small Business, GSA Contract, VA Contract
Distribution: Manufacturer Through Distributor, OEM, Exporter
General Admin.: Patricia Farber/Manager Human Resources
      David Pearson/President, Chief Executive Officer
Mktg./Adv.: Mary Hagerty-Goldberg/Manager Customer Services & Sales
      Allison Lowman/Manager Sales
Finance: Iliana Chan/Admin. Finance
      Jeff Miyasaka/Admin. Finance
      Glenn Slensker/Chief Financial Officer
Purchasing: Dan Berthoodu/Purchasing Agent
  Belt, Rib (Support) — Orthopedics
  Binder, Abdominal — General
  Brace, Joint, Ankle (External) — Physical Med
  Collar, Cervical Neck — Orthopedics
  Joint, Knee, External Brace — Physical Med
  Orthosis, Lumbar — Physical Med
  Orthosis, Sacroiliac, Soft — Physical Med
  Protector, Skin Pressure — General
  Restraint, Arm — General
  Shoe, Cast — Physical Med
  Sling, Arm — Physical Med
  Sling, Arm, Overhead Supported — Physical Med
  Splint, Clavicle — Physical Med
  Splint, Hand, And Component — Physical Med
  Stocking, Elastic — General
  Support, Ankle — Orthopedics
  Support, Back — Orthopedics
  Support, Knee — Physical Med
  Support, Wrist — Physical Med

FRANK TANAKA, OCULARIST, INC.
813-978-1142
3000 East Fletcher Ave.,, Suite 310, Tampa, FL 33613
FDA Number: 1058233
Ownership: Private
Produces/Sells CE-marked Devices: N
  Eye, Artificial, Non-Custom — Ophthalmology
  Shell, Scleral — Ophthalmology

FRANKLIN (MOI) OPHTHALMIC INSTRUMENTS INC.
See Lombart Instruments

FRANKLIN CORP.
662-456-4286
600 Franklin Dr., P.o. Box 569, Houston, MS 38851
FDA Number: 1037199
Ownership: Private
Produces/Sells CE-marked Devices: N
  Chair, Position, Electric — Physical Med

FRANKLIN MILLER INC
800-932-0599
60 Okner Pkwy., Livingston, NJ 07039-1604
973-535-9200
FDA Number: n/a   Fax: 973-535-6269
E-mail: info@franklinmiller.com
Web site: www.franklinmiller.com
Medical Products Sales Volume: $3,500,000
Year Founded: 1953
Total Employees: 40
Ownership: Franklin Miller Inc.
Produces/Sells CE-marked Devices: N
Federal Procurement Eligibility: Small Business
Distribution: Manufacturer Direct
General Admin.: William Galanty/President
Mktg./Adv.: David Schuppe/Manager National Sales
  Crusher, Syringe — General
  Cutter, Syringe And Needle — General
  Office Equipment — General

FRANKLIN PROSTHETIC COVERS   610-666-6645
98 Highland Ave., P.O. Box 313, Oaks, PA 19456-0313
FDA Number: 2532141   Fax: 610-666-0173
Ownership: Private
Produces/Sells CE-marked Devices: N
   Hand, External Limb Component, Mechanical   Physical Med

FRANTZ DESIGN, INC.   512-451-3311
3202 Oakmont Blvd., Austin, TX 78703
FDA Number: 1649919
Ownership: Private
Produces/Sells CE-marked Devices: N
   Device, Anti-Snoring   Ear/Nose/Throat

FRANTZ MEDICAL DEVELOPMENT LTD.   440-255-1155
7740 Metric Drive, Mentor, OH 44060-4862
FDA Number: 1526605   Fax: 440-255-6975
E-mail: info@frantzgroup.com
Web site: www.frantzgroup.com
Medical Products Sales Volume: $16,300,000
Annual Revenue: $10-$25 Million
Year Founded: 1979
Total Employees: 75
Ownership: Private
Quality System Registration Information: ISO9001
Produces/Sells CE-marked Devices: Y
Federal Procurement Eligibility: Small Business, GSA Contract
Distribution: Manufacturer Through Distributor, OEM
General Admin.: Mark G. Frantz/President, Chief Executive Officer
Production: Tom Livingston/Director Quality Assurance
        Marianna Friend/Manager Materials
        Paul Hanson/Vice President Operations, General Manager
Finance: John McGann/Vice President Finance
   Accessories, Traction, Invasive   Orthopedics
   Contract Manufacturing, Product, Disposable   General
   Contract R&D, Equipment   General
   Forceps, Endoscopic   Gastroenterology/Urology
   Keratome, AC-Powered   Ophthalmology
   Kit, Feeding, Adult (Enteral)   General
   Molding, Injection   General
   Obturator, Endoscopic   Gastroenterology/Urology
   Pump, Air, Non-Manual, Endoscopic   Gastroenterology/Urology
   Pump, Food (Enteral Feeding)   General
   Trocar, Laparoscopic   Surgery

FRASER HARLAKE INC.
See Matrx By Midmark

FRASER SWEATMAN INC.
See Matrx By Midmark

FRAY PRODUCTS CORP.
See HealthLink

FRAZER, INC.   888-372-9371
7227 A Rampart, Houston, TX 77081   713-772-5511
FDA Number: n/a   Fax: 713-995-0541
E-mail: webmaster@frazerbilt.com
Web site: www.frazerbilt.com
Ownership: Private
Produces/Sells CE-marked Devices: N
Federal Procurement Eligibility: Small Business, Female Owned
Distribution: Manufacturer Direct
   Ambulance   General

FREAS GLASS WORKS, INC.
See Francis L. Freas Glass Works, Inc.

FREDERICK LEE INC   787-834-4880
Balboa St. #191, PO Box 3287, Mayaguez, PR 00680
FDA Number: 2649612   Fax: 787-833-9320
E-mail: fred@fredericklee.com
Web site: www.fredericklee.com
Medical Products Sales Volume: $1,800,000
Annual Revenue: $1-$5 Million
Year Founded: 1949
Total Employees: 80   Marketing Staff: 1   Sales Staff: 1
Ownership: Private
Produces/Sells CE-marked Devices: N
Federal Procurement Eligibility: Small Business
Distribution: Manufacturer Direct
General Admin.: Richard L. Freeman/Chief Executive Officer
        Norman J. Ramirez/President
Mktg./Adv.: Vivian Caballer/Manager Market Research
Production: Elizabeth Martinez/Manager Materials
        Maritza Rivera/Manager Production
   Binder, Abdominal   General
   Orthosis, Lumbar   Physical Med
   Orthosis, Lumbosacral   Physical Med
   Orthosis, Rib Fracture, Soft   Physical Med
   Orthosis, Sacroiliac, Soft   Physical Med

FREDERICK LEE INC   787-834-4880 (cont'd)
   Support, Hernia   Gastroenterology/Urology

FREDERICK TOOL CORP.   800-443-9618
24615 C.R. 45 Ste.4, Elkhart, IN 46516   -
FDA Number: n/a   Fax: 574-970-1598
E-mail: fredtool@aol.com
Web site: www.Fredericktool.com
Medical Products Sales Volume: $1,000,000
Total Employees: 25   Sales Staff: 2
Ownership: Private
Produces/Sells CE-marked Devices: N
Federal Procurement Eligibility: Small Business
Distribution: Manufacturer Through Distributor, Manufacturer Through
Manufacturer Reps
General Admin.: Jack E. Wait/President
   Cart, Gas Cylinder (Carrier)   Anesthesiology

FREEDOM CONCEPTS, INC.   800-661-9915
2087 Plessis Road,   204-654-1074
Winnipeg, MB R3W 1 Canada
FDA Number: 9615313   Fax: 204-654-1149
E-mail: mobility@freedomconcepts.com
Web site: www.freedomconcepts.com
Year Founded: 1991
Total Employees: 25
Ownership: Private
Produces/Sells CE-marked Devices: N
Distribution: Manufacturer Direct, Exporter

FREEDOM DATA SYSTEMS, INC.   800-932-9000
228 Maple St Fl 1, Manchester, NH 03103   603-668-8095
FDA Number: n/a   Fax: 603-668-8097
E-mail: lczerw@freedomdata.com
Web site: www.freedomdata.com
Medical Products Sales Volume: $1,400,000
Annual Revenue: $0-$1 Million
Total Employees: 15   Marketing Staff: 1   Sales Staff: 3
Ownership: Private
Produces/Sells CE-marked Devices: N
Federal Procurement Eligibility: Small Business
Distribution: Exclusive Distributor
General Admin.: Kerry Rook/General Manager
Mktg./Adv.: Laura Czerw/Coord. Sales
   Computer Software   General

FREEDOM DESIGNS, INC.   800-331-8551
2241N. Madera Rd., Simi Valley, CA 93065   805-582-0077
FDA Number: 2081283   Fax: 805-582-1509
E-mail: customerservice@freedomdesigns.com
Web site: www.freedomdesigns.com
Total Employees: 85   Marketing Staff: 3   Sales Staff: 23
Ownership: INVACARE CORPORATION
Produces/Sells CE-marked Devices: Y
Federal Procurement Eligibility: Small Business, Female Owned
Distribution: Manufacturer Through Distributor, Manufacturer Through
Manufacturer Reps
General Admin.: Ginny Maloco/President, Chief Executive Officer
Mktg./Adv.: Tyler Robuck/Director Marketing & Advertising
        Michael Maloco/Vice President Marketing & Sales
Production: Terry Robuck/Vice President Manufacturing
   Accessories, Wheelchair   Physical Med
   Cushion, Wheelchair (Pad)   Physical Med
   Shield, Heat, Infant   General
   Support, Patient Position   Anesthesiology
   Tray, Wheelchair   Physical Med
   Wheelchair, Manual   Physical Med
   Wheelchair, Powered   Physical Med

FREEDOM FABRICATION   800-304-FREE
815 N. Main St., Suite B, Havana, FL 32333   850-539-4194
FDA Number: n/a   Fax: 850-539-4195
Web site: www.freedomfabrication.com
Ownership: Private
Produces/Sells CE-marked Devices: N
General Admin.: Tony Wickman/President
   Assembly, Knee/Shank/Ankle/Foot, External   Physical Med
   Orthosis, Corrective Shoe   Physical Med
   Prosthesis, Tibial   Orthopedics

FREEDOM INNOVATIONS, INC.   888-818-6777
30 Fairbanks, Suite 114, Irvine, CA 92618   949-672-0032
FDA Number: 2032649   Fax: 949-672-0084
E-mail: info@freedom-innovations.com
Web site: www.freedom-innovations.com
Medical Products Sales Volume: $2,000,000
Total Employees: 24
Ownership: Private

FREEDOM INNOVATIONS, INC.   888-818-6777 *(cont'd)*
Quality System Registration Information: ISO9000
Produces/Sells CE-marked Devices: N
Federal Procurement Eligibility: Small Business
Distribution: OEM
General Admin.: Maynard Carkhuff/President, Chief Operating Officer
Mktg./Adv.: Meghan Eilbeck/Marketing Specialist

Ankle/Foot, External Limb Component	Physical Med

FREEDOM INNOVATIONS, LLC   435-528-7199
425 East 400 North, P.O Box 9, Gunnison, UT 84634
FDA Number: 3004737223
Ownership: Private
Produces/Sells CE-marked Devices: N
General Admin.: Mr. Roland Christensen/Chief Technology Officer
     Mr. Maynard Carkhuff/President, Chief Executive Officer
Mktg./Adv.: Mr. Gary Wertz/Executive Vice President Sales
     Mr. Mark Testerman/Vice President Sales
Research: Mr. Steven Reinecke/Executive Vice President Research & Development
Finance: Mr. Lee Kim/Chief Financial Officer

Ankle/Foot, External Limb Component	Physical Med
Joint, Knee, External Limb Component	Physical Med
Prosthesis, Thigh Socket, External Component	Physical Med

FREEDOM MEDITECH, INC.   619-683-3937
10455 Pacific Center Court, San Diego, CA 92121
FDA Number: n/a
E-mail: info@freedom-meditech.com
Web site: http://www.freedom-meditech.com.
Ownership: Private
Produces/Sells CE-marked Devices: N

Enzyme Immunoassay, Amphetamine	Toxicology
Enzyme Immunoassay, Cannabinoids	Toxicology
Enzyme Immunoassay, Cocaine And Cocaine Metabolites	Toxicology
Enzyme Immunoassay, Opiates	Toxicology
Enzyme Immunoassay, Phencyclidine	Toxicology
Gas Chromatography, Methamphetamine	Toxicology

FREEDOM SCIENTIFIC BLV GROUP, LLC.   727-803-8000
11800 31st Court North, St. Petersburg, FL 33716
FDA Number: 1123650

Magnifier, Hand-Held, Low-Vision	Ophthalmology
Vision Aid, Optical, Battery-Powered	Ophthalmology

FREEMAN MANUFACTURING COMPANY   800-253-2091
900 W. Chicago Road, PO Box J,   269-651-2371
Sturgis, MI 49091
FDA Number: 1811757   Fax: 269-651-8248
E-mail: freeman@freemanmfg.com
Web site: www.freemanmfg.com
Annual Revenue: $5-$10 Million
Total Employees: 45
Ownership: Private
Produces/Sells CE-marked Devices: N
Federal Procurement Eligibility: Small Business, VA Contract
Distribution: Manufacturer Direct, Exporter
General Admin.: Richard L. Freeman/Chief Executive Officer
     Thomas P. Rock/President, Chief Operating Officer
Mktg./Adv.: Frederick J. Wine/Vice President Sales
Finance: Jodi Pant/Controller

Accessories, Traction (Cart, Frame, Cord, Weight)	Orthopedics
Back Rest	General
Bars, Spreader	Orthopedics
Belt, Abdominal	Gastroenterology/Urology
Belt, Lumbosacral	Orthopedics
Belt, Rib (Support)	Orthopedics
Belt, Traction, Pelvic, Orthopedic	Orthopedics
Binder, Abdominal	General
Binder, Elastic	General
Brace, Joint, Ankle (External)	Physical Med
Brassiere, Surgical	Surgery
Cane	Physical Med
Collar, Cervical Neck	Orthopedics
Compression Unit, Intermittent (Anti-Embolism Pump)	Cardiovascular
Corset	Orthopedics
Custom Prosthesis	Orthopedics
Frame, Traction	Orthopedics
Halter, Head, Traction	Physical Med
Halter, Head, Traction, Orthopedic	Orthopedics
Immobilizer, Knee	Orthopedics
Joint, Knee, External Brace	Physical Med
Orthosis, Cervical	Physical Med
Orthosis, Cervical-Thoracic, Rigid	Physical Med
Orthosis, Limb Brace	Physical Med
Orthosis, Lumbar	Physical Med
Orthosis, Lumbosacral	Physical Med
Orthosis, Other	Physical Med
Orthosis, Rib Fracture, Soft	Physical Med

FREEMAN MANUFACTURING COMPANY   800-253-2091 *(cont'd)*

Orthosis, Sacroiliac, Soft	Physical Med
Orthosis, Thoracic	Physical Med
Prosthesis, Breast, External	Surgery
Shoe, Cast	Physical Med
Sling, Arm	Physical Med
Sock, Stump Cover	General
Splint, Clavicle	Physical Med
Splint, Denis Brown	Physical Med
Splint, Extremity, Non-Inflatable, External	Surgery
Splint, Hand, And Component	Physical Med
Stockinette, Cast	Orthopedics
Stocking, Elastic, Physical Medicine	Physical Med
Stocking, Support (Anti-Embolic)	General
Support, Abdominal	Physical Med
Support, Ankle	Orthopedics
Support, Arm	Physical Med
Support, Back	Orthopedics
Support, Clavicle	Orthopedics
Support, Elbow	Orthopedics
Support, Foot	Orthopedics
Support, Hand	Orthopedics
Support, Hernia	Gastroenterology/Urology
Support, Knee	Physical Med
Support, Leg	Physical Med
Support, Wrist	Physical Med
Traction Unit, Static, Bed	Orthopedics
Traction Unit, Static, Chair	Orthopedics
Tray, Impression, Foot	Orthopedics
Truss, Hernia (Belt)	Gastroenterology/Urology

FREQUENCY AND TIME SYSTEMS, INC.
See Symmetricom Timing, Test & Measurement

FRESENIUS KABI, LLC   425-242-2000
14715 NE 95th St, Suite 100, Redmond, WA 98052
FDA Number: 3004152132
E-mail: GHR@fresenius-kabi.com
Web site: www.fresenius-kabi.com
Annual Revenue: More than $1 Billion
Total Employees: 64666
Ownership: FRESENIUS KABI AG
Produces/Sells CE-marked Devices: N

FRESENIUS MEDICAL CARE NORTH AMERICA   781-699-9068
28157 Cedar Park Blvd, Perrysburg, OH 43551
FDA Number: 1527681
Web site: www.fmc-ag.com
Ownership: FRESENIUS MEDICAL CARE AG & CO. KGAA
Produces/Sells CE-marked Devices: N

FRESENIUS MEDICAL CARE NORTH AMERICA   781-699-9068
420 Industrial Dr, Livingston, CA 95334
FDA Number: 2937116
Web site: www.fmcna.com
Annual Revenue: More than $1 Billion
Total Employees: 64666
Ownership: FRESENIUS MEDICAL CARE AG & CO. KGAA
Produces/Sells CE-marked Devices: N

Catheter, Vascular, Cardiopulmonary Bypass	Cardiovascular
Dialysate Delivery System, Central Multiple Patient	Gastroenterology/Urology

FRESENIUS MEDICAL CARE NORTH AMERICA   781-699-9068
475 West 13th St, Ogden, UT 84404
FDA Number: 1713747
Web site: www.fmcna.com
Annual Revenue: More than $1 Billion
Total Employees: 64666
Ownership: FRESENIUS MEDICAL CARE AG & CO. KGAA
Produces/Sells CE-marked Devices: N

Catheter, Vascular, Cardiopulmonary Bypass	Cardiovascular
Dialysate Delivery System, Central Multiple Patient	Gastroenterology/Urology

FRESENIUS MEDICAL CARE NORTH AMERICA   781-699-9068
5201 Regent Blvd, Irving, TX 75063
FDA Number: 1651896
Web site: www.fmcna.com
Annual Revenue: More than $1 Billion
Total Employees: 64666
Ownership: FRESENIUS MEDICAL CARE AG & CO. KGAA
Produces/Sells CE-marked Devices: N

Dialysate Delivery System, Central Multiple Patient	Gastroenterology/Urology

FRESENIUS MEDICAL CARE NORTH AMERICA   781-699-9068
750 North Lallendorf Rd, Oregon, OH 43616
FDA Number: 3005162618
Web site: www.fmcna.com
Annual Revenue: More than $1 Billion
Total Employees: 64666
Ownership: FRESENIUS MEDICAL CARE AG & CO. KGAA
Stock Symbol: FMS

FRESENIUS MEDICAL CARE NORTH AMERICA 781-699-9068
(cont'd)

Produces/Sells CE-marked Devices: N

Dialysate Delivery System, Central Multiple Patient	Gastroenterology/Urology

FRESENIUS MEDICAL CARE NORTH AMERICA 800-662-1237
920 Winter Street, Waltham, MA 02451   **781-699-9000**

FDA Number: 1225714
Web site: www.fmcna.com
Annual Revenue: More than $1 Billion
Total Employees: 64666
Ownership: FRESENIUS MEDICAL CARE AG & CO. KGAA
Produces/Sells CE-marked Devices: N

Accessories, Blood Circuit, Hemodialysis	Gastroenterology/Urology
Clamp, Other	Surgery
Connector, Catheter	Surgery
Dialysate Delivery System, Central Multiple Patient	Gastroenterology/Urology
Dialyzer Reprocessing System	Gastroenterology/Urology
Dialyzer, Capillary, Hollow Fiber (Hemodialysis)	Gastroenterology/Urology
Dialyzer, High Permeability	Gastroenterology/Urology
Hemodialyzer, Re-use, High Flux	Gastroenterology/Urology
Hemodialyzer, Re-use, Low Flux	Gastroenterology/Urology
Peritoneal Dialysis Unit (CAPD)	Gastroenterology/Urology
Protector, Transducer, Dialysis	Gastroenterology/Urology
Set, Administration, Intravenous, Needle-Free	General
System, Peritoneal Dialysis, Automatic	Gastroenterology/Urology
Tray, Start/Stop (Including Contents), Dialysis	Gastroenterology/Urology

FRESENIUS USA, INC. 800-662-1237
920 Winter Street, Waltham, MA 02451-1457   **781-699-900**

FDA Number: 2937457
Web site: www.fmc-ag.com
Medical Products Sales Volume: $4,900,000,000
Annual Revenue: More than $1 Billion
Total Employees: 64666
Ownership: Fresenius Ag
Stock Symbol: FMS
Traded On: NYSE
Produces/Sells CE-marked Devices: N
Distribution: Manufacturer Direct, Manufacturer Through Distributor, Service Direct, Exclusive Distributor, Importer

Accessories, Blood Circuit, Hemodialysis	Gastroenterology/Urology
Computer, Patient Monitor	Anesthesiology
Dialysate Delivery System, Peritoneal, Semi-Automatic	Gastroenterology/Urology
Dialysate Delivery System, Sealed	Gastroenterology/Urology
Dialysate Delivery System, Single Pass	Gastroenterology/Urology
Dialysate Delivery System, Single Patient	Gastroenterology/Urology
Dialysis Unit Test Equipment	Gastroenterology/Urology
Dialyzer Reprocessing System	Gastroenterology/Urology
Dialyzer, Capillary, Hollow Fiber (Hemodialysis)	Gastroenterology/Urology
Dialyzer, High Permeability	Gastroenterology/Urology
Hemodialysis Unit (Kidney Machine)	Gastroenterology/Urology
Kit, Hemodialysis Tubing	Gastroenterology/Urology
Pump, Blood, Hemodialysis Unit	Gastroenterology/Urology
Set, Administration, Intravenous, Needle-Free	General
System, Peritoneal Dialysis, Automatic	Gastroenterology/Urology
Tank, Holding, Dialysis	Gastroenterology/Urology

FRESNEL PRISM & LENS CO. 800-544-4760
6824 Washington Avenue,   **952-496-0432**
Eden Prairie, MN 55344

FDA Number: 2086350   *Fax:* 952-403-7900
E-mail: INFO@FRESNELPRISM.COM
Web site: www.fresnel-prism.com
Ownership: Private
Produces/Sells CE-marked Devices: N

Lens, Set, Trial, Ophthalmic	Ophthalmology
Prism, Fresnel, Ophthalmic	Ophthalmology
Shield, Eye, Ophthalmic	Ophthalmology

FREUND CAN COMPANY
See Freund Container

FREUND CONTAINER 800-363-9822
Corporate Center II   **708-272-7099**
4200 Commerce Court Suite 206
Lisle, IL 60532

FDA Number: n/a   *Fax:* 800-423-7545
E-mail: customerservice@freundcontainer.com
Web site: www.freundcontainer.com
Annual Revenue: $10-$25 Million
Total Employees: 45   *Marketing Staff:* 8   *Sales Staff:* 8
Ownership: Berlin Packaging
Produces/Sells CE-marked Devices: N
Federal Procurement Eligibility: GSA Contract
Distribution: Exclusive Distributor
Production: MIKE WEST/Manager Customer Services

Bin, Storage	General
Container, Specimen, All Types	General

FREUND CONTAINER 800-363-9822 (cont'd)

Contract Manufacturing	General
Jar, Dressing	Surgery
Waste Receptacle, General Purpose	General

FRICKE DENTAL MANUFACTURING CO. 800-537-4253
165 Roma Jean Pkwy, Streamwood, IL 60107   **630-540-1900**

FDA Number: 1417846   *Fax:* 630-833-3148
E-mail: customerservice@frickedental.com
Web site: www.frickedental.com
Annual Revenue: $1-$5 Million
Total Employees: 15   *Marketing Staff:* 4   *Sales Staff:* 5
Ownership: Private
Produces/Sells CE-marked Devices: N
Federal Procurement Eligibility: Small Business
Distribution: Manufacturer Direct, Manufacturer Through Manufacturer Reps, Importer, Exporter
General Admin.: L. R. Fricke/President
Mktg./Adv.: Ron Schumann/Vice President Sales

Base, Denture, Relining, Repairing, Rebasing, Resin	Dental And Oral

FRIDDLE'S ORTHOPEDIC APPLIANCES, INC. 800-528-9339
12306 Belton Honea-Path Hwy.,   **864-369-2328**
Honea Path, SC 29654

FDA Number: n/a   *Fax:* 864-369-1149
E-mail: info@friddles.com
Web site: www.friddles.com
Annual Revenue: $1-$5 Million
Total Employees: 12   *Marketing Staff:* 2   *Sales Staff:* 2
Ownership: Private
Quality System Registration Information: ISO9001
Produces/Sells CE-marked Devices: Y
Federal Procurement Eligibility: Small Business
Distribution: Manufacturer Direct
General Admin.: Frank Friddle/President

Orthosis, Cervical-Thoracic, Rigid	Physical Med
Shoe, Orthopedic	Orthopedics

FRIEDHEIM TOOL COMPANY 619-474-3600
1433 Roosevelt Ave., National City, CA 91950

FDA Number: 3005033500   *Fax:* 619-474-1300
E-mail: info@ftcsteamers.com
Web site: www.ftcsteamers.com
Ownership: Private
Produces/Sells CE-marked Devices: N

Cleaner, Medical Device	General

FRIEDRICH & DIMMOCK, INC. 800-524-1131
2127 Wheaton Avenue, PO Box 230,   **856-825-0305**
Millville, NJ 08332

FDA Number: n/a   *Fax:* 856-327-4299
E-mail: sales@fdglass.com
Web site: www.fdglass.com
Medical Products Sales Volume: $6,000,000
Annual Revenue: $5-$10 Million
Year Founded: 1919
Total Employees: 48   *Marketing Staff:* 1   *Sales Staff:* 6
Ownership: Private
Quality System Registration Information: ISO9001
Produces/Sells CE-marked Devices: N
Federal Procurement Eligibility: Small Business
Distribution: Manufacturer Direct, Manufacturer Through Distributor, OEM, Importer, Exporter
General Admin.: John T. Plumbo/Chief Executive Officer
     Robert Goffredi/President

Pipette	Chemistry
Reagent, Platelet Aggregation	Hematology

FRIO TECHNOLOGIES, INC. 210-308-5635
500 Sandau Rd., Suite 200, San Antonio, TX 78216

FDA Number: 1651422
Ownership: Private
Produces/Sells CE-marked Devices: N

Medical Disinfectants/Cleaners for Instruments	General

FROG LEGS, INC. 319-472-4972
500 East 6th St., Vinton, IA 52349

FDA Number: 1934422
Ownership: Private
Produces/Sells CE-marked Devices: N

Accessories, Wheelchair	Physical Med

FROHOCK-STEWART, INC.
See Invecare

FRONTIER COMPUTING
2221 Yonge St., Ste. 406,
Toronto, ONT M4S-2 Canada
888-480-0000
416-489-6690
FDA Number: n/a
E-mail: sales@frontiercomputing.on.ca
Web site: www.frontiercomputing.on.ca
Fax: 416-489-6693
Year Founded: 1986
Ownership: Private
Produces/Sells CE-marked Devices: N

FRONTIER CONTACT LENSES INC.
See Vistakon, Inc.

FRONTIER DENTAL LABORATORY
7916 Alta Sunrise Dr., Ste. 205, Citrus Heights, CA 95610
916-965-4471
FDA Number: n/a
Web site: www.frontierdentallab.com
Fax: 916-965-3738
Ownership: Private
Produces/Sells CE-marked Devices: N
Crown And Bridge, Temporary, Resin — Dental And Oral
Crown, Preformed — Dental And Oral

FRONTIER DEVICES
153-a Cahaba Valley Parkway, Pelham, AL 35124
205-733-0901
FDA Number: 3006803588
E-mail: cbarney@frontierdevices.com
Fax: 205.733.8445
Web site: www.frontierdevices.com
Ownership: Private
Produces/Sells CE-marked Devices: N
Retainer, Surgical — Surgery

FRONTIER MEDICAL PRODUCTS, INC.
140 S. Park St., Port Washington, WI 53074
800-367-6828
262-284-1055
FDA Number: n/a
E-mail: customercare@frontiermedicalproducts.com
Fax: 262-284-1056
Web site: www.frontiermedicalproducts.com
Annual Revenue: $1-$5 Million
Total Employees: 10
Ownership: Private
Produces/Sells CE-marked Devices: N
Distribution: Manufacturer Through Distributor
General Admin.: Robert Griesmeyer/Chief Executive Officer
Mktg./Adv.: Robert Griesmeyer/Manager Advertising
　　　　Robert Griesmeyer/Vice President Marketing & Sales
Production: Robert Griesmeyer/Vice President Manufacturing
Research: Robert Griesmeyer/Vice President Research & Development
Bag, Ice — General
Cuff, Blood Pressure — Cardiovascular
Sphygmomanometer, Electronic, Manual — General

FRONTIER SCIENTIFIC, INC.,
PO Box 31, Logan, UT 84323-0031
453-753-1901
FDA Number: n/a
E-mail: info@frontiersci.com
Fax: 453-753-6731
Web site: www.frontiersci.com/
Annual Revenue: $1-$5 Million
Year Founded: 1974
Total Employees: 50
Ownership: FRONTIER SCIENTIFIC INC.
Federal Procurement Eligibility: Small Business
Distribution: Manufacturer Direct
General Admin.: Jerry C. Bommer/President
Mktg./Adv.: Bert V. Israelsen/Vice President Marketing & Sales
Accessories, Chromatography (Gas, Gel, Liquid, Thin Layer) — Chemistry
Fluorometric Measurement, Porphyrins — Chemistry
Standard/Control, All Types — Chemistry

FRONTLINE MEDICAL SUPPLIES
See E-One

FRY CONSTRUCTION COMPANY
3212 Commander Drive, Carrollton, TX 75006
972-248-9696
FDA Number: n/a
E-mail: info@fryco.com
Fax: 972-248-1627
Web site: http://www.fryco.com
Year Founded: 1983
Ownership: Private
Produces/Sells CE-marked Devices: N
General Admin.: Ms. Cynthia Fry/Chief Executive Officer, Vice President
　　　　Mr. Benton Fry/President
Mktg./Adv.: Mr. Bruce Fry/Vice President Marketing

FRYE ELECTRONICS, INC.
9826 S.W. Tigard Street, Tigard, OR 97223-5243
800-547-8209
503-620-2722
FDA Number: 3018639
E-mail: sales@frye.com
Fax: 503-639-0128
Web site: www.frye.com
Medical Products Sales Volume: $4,000,000
Annual Revenue: $5-$10 Million

FRYE ELECTRONICS, INC.
800-547-8209 *(cont'd)*
Year Founded: 1973
Total Employees: 34　　Marketing Staff: 7　　Sales Staff: 1
Ownership: Private
Produces/Sells CE-marked Devices: Y
Federal Procurement Eligibility: Small Business, Female Owned, VA Contract
Distribution: Manufacturer Direct, Manufacturer Through Distributor, Manufacturer Through Manufacturer Reps
General Admin.: George J. Frye/President
Mktg./Adv.: Sallie A. Frye/Manager Marketing
Production: Kristina Frye/Director Quality Assurance
　　　　John Burwell/Manager Manufacturing
Audiometer — Ear/Nose/Throat
System, Analysis, Hearing-Aid — Ear/Nose/Throat

FTS SYSTEMS
3538 Main Street, PO Box 158,
Stone Ridge, NY 12484
800-824-0400
845-687-0071
FDA Number: 1318828
E-mail: fts@SPindustries.com
Fax: 845-687-7481
Web site: www.ftssystems.com
Medical Products Sales Volume: $12,900,000
Annual Revenue: $10-$25 Million
Total Employees: 85　　Marketing Staff: 6　　Sales Staff: 6
Ownership: Private
Quality System Registration Information: ISO9000
Produces/Sells CE-marked Devices: N
Federal Procurement Eligibility: Small Business
Distribution: Manufacturer Direct, Manufacturer Through Manufacturer Reps
General Admin.: Gary Schlegel/General Manager
Production: Allen Kolb/Product Manager
Bath, Tissue Flotation — Microbiology
Chamber, Constant Temperature (Environmental) — Microbiology
Filter, Air — General
Freeze Drying Equipment — Chemistry
Stirrer — Chemistry

FTS SYSTEMS, INC.
See Fts Systems

FUJIFILM MANUFACTURING USA, INC.
850 Central Ave, Hanover Park, IL 60133
203-602-3664
FDA Number: 3004532636
Ownership: Private
Produces/Sells CE-marked Devices: N
Film, X-Ray, Special Purpose — Radiology
Screen, Intensifying, Radiographic — Radiology

FUJIFILM MEDICAL SYSTEMS USA, INC.
419 West Avenue, Stamford, CT 06902
800-431-1850
203-324-2000
FDA Number: 2443168
E-mail: info@fujimed.com
Fax: 203-353-0926
Web site: www.fujimed.com
Medical Products Sales Volume: $63,800,000
Year Founded: 1965
Total Employees: 425
Ownership: FujiFilm Holdings Corporation
Produces/Sells CE-marked Devices: N
Federal Procurement Eligibility: Small Business
Distribution: Manufacturer Direct, OEM, Importer
General Admin.: Takushi Nasu/President
Mktg./Adv.: Steven Marchese/Coord. Marketing Communications
　　　　Randy Nagel/Director Corporate Communications
　　　　Paul Genovese/Vice President Business Development
　　　　Clay Larsen/Vice President Marketing
　　　　Tony Gales/Vice President Sales
Production: Rob Berry/Director Regulatory Affairs
　　　　John Weber/Vice President Operations
Camera, Multi Format — Radiology
Cassette, Radiographic Film — Radiology
Changer, Cassette, Radiographic — Radiology
Computer, Radiographic Image Analysis — Radiology
Imager, X-Ray, Electrostatic — Radiology
Laser, Therapeutic — Radiology
Printer, Radiographic Duplicator — Radiology
Processor, Cine Film — Radiology
Processor, Radiographic Film, Automatic — Radiology
Medical Product Subsidiaries (Listed Separately)
Empiric Systems, Llc

FUJINON, INC.
10 High Point Dr., Wayne, NJ 07470-7434
800-385-4666
973-686-2417
FDA Number: 2431293
E-mail: edwin.lee@fujinon.com
Fax: 973-686-2465
Web site: www.fujinon.com
Ownership: Fujinon Corporation
Quality System Registration Information: ISO9000
Produces/Sells CE-marked Devices: N
Distribution: Manufacturer Direct, Manufacturer Through Manufacturer Reps

FUJINON, INC.   800-385-4666 *(cont'd)*

General Admin.: Martin Morici/Manager
Tami Amico/Service Coordinator
Eddie Lee/Service Manager

Accessories, Electrical Power (Electrocautery)	Surgery
Adapter, Cable, Equipment	General
Basket, Biliary Stone Retrieval	Gastroenterology/Urology
Bottle, Endoscopic Wash	Gastroenterology/Urology
Bronchoscope, Non-Rigid	Ear/Nose/Throat
Brush, Cleaning, Tracheal Tube	Ear/Nose/Throat
Brush, Cytology, Endoscopic	Gastroenterology/Urology
Camera, Still, Endoscopic	Surgery
Cannula, Other	General
Cart, Equipment, Video	General
Cart, Other	General
Choledochoscope, Flexible Or Rigid	Gastroenterology/Urology
Colonoscope, Gastro-Urology	Gastroenterology/Urology
Colonoscope, General & Plastic Surgery	Surgery
Computer, Clinical Laboratory	Chemistry
Computer, Radiographic Image Analysis	Radiology
Duodenoscope, Esophago/Gastro	Gastroenterology/Urology
Electrocautery Unit, Line-Powered	Surgery
Electrode, Flexible Suction Coagulator	Gastroenterology/Urology
Electrode, Other	General
Endoscope	Gastroenterology/Urology
Endoscope, Electronic (Videoendoscope)	Surgery
Film, X-Ray	Radiology
Forceps, Biopsy	Surgery
Forceps, Biopsy, Electric	Gastroenterology/Urology
Forceps, Biopsy, Non-Electric	Gastroenterology/Urology
Forceps, Grasping, Flexible Endoscopic	Gastroenterology/Urology
Gastroscope, Flexible	Gastroenterology/Urology
Gastroscope, Gastro-Urology	Gastroenterology/Urology
Gastroscope, General & Plastic Surgery	Gastroenterology/Urology
Hysteroscope	Obstetrics/Gynecology
Image Processing System	Radiology
Kit, Laparoscopy	Gastroenterology/Urology
Lamp, Other	General
Laparoscope, Flexible	Surgery
Laparoscope, General & Plastic Surgery	Surgery
Laryngoscope	Ear/Nose/Throat
Light Source, Fiberoptic, Routine	Gastroenterology/Urology
Light Source, Incandescent, Diagnostic	Gastroenterology/Urology
Light Source, Photographic, Fiberoptic	Gastroenterology/Urology
Module, Control, Electrosurgery	Surgery
Monitor, Video, Endoscope	General
Mount, Monitor (Support)	General
Nasopharyngoscope (Flexible Or Rigid)	Ear/Nose/Throat
Nasoscope	Ear/Nose/Throat
Panendoscope (Gastroduodenoscope)	Gastroenterology/Urology
Papillotome	Surgery
Radiographic Picture Archiving/Communication System (PACS)	Radiology
Recorder, Videotape/Videodisc	General
Retriever, Endomagnetic	Gastroenterology/Urology
Sigmoidoscope, Flexible	Gastroenterology/Urology
Snare, Polyp	Surgery
Thoracoscope	Cardiovascular

FUJIREBIO AMERICA, INC.

See Fujirebio Diagnostics, Inc. (Fdi)

FUJIREBIO DIAGNOSTICS, INC. (FDI)   877-861-7246
201 Great Valley Pkwy., Malvern, PA 19355-3809   **610-240-3800**
FDA Number: 2521625   *Fax:* 610-240-3803
E-mail: customerservice@fdi.com
Web site: www.fdi.com
Medical Products Sales Volume: $17,900,000
Annual Revenue: $25-$50 Million
Year Founded: 1998
Total Employees: 100   *Marketing Staff:* 3   *Sales Staff:* 3
Ownership: Fujirebio, Inc.
Quality System Registration Information: ISO9001
Produces/Sells CE-marked Devices: Y
Federal Procurement Eligibility: Small Business
Distribution: Manufacturer Direct, Manufacturer Through Distributor, OEM, Service Direct, Importer, Exporter
General Admin.: Takeo Hayashi/Chief Executive Officer

Antigen, Carbohydrate (CA19-9)	Immunology
Antiserum, Fluorescent, Rabies Virus	Microbiology
Calibrator, Drug Specific	Toxicology
Calibrator, Secondary, Clinical Chemistry	Chemistry
Control, Analyte (Assayed And Unassayed)	Chemistry
Cyclosporine	Toxicology
Enzymatic Method, Blood, Occcult, Fecal	Chemistry
Fluorometric, Cortisol	Chemistry
Immunoassay, Other	Toxicology
Radioassay, Angiotensin Converting Enzyme	Chemistry
Test, Antigen (CA125), Tumor-Associated, Ovarian, Epithelial	Immunology
Test, Discrimination, Temperature	Cns/Neurology
Test, Syphilis (RPR or VDRL)	Microbiology

FUKUDA DENSHI USA, INC.   800-365-6668
17725 N.E. 65th St., Bldg. C,   **425-588-1661**
Redmond, WA 98052
FDA Number: 3031158
E-mail: lvannoy@fukuda.com   *Fax:* 425-869-2018
Web site: www.fukuda.com
Annual Revenue: $10-$25 Million
Year Founded: 1939
Ownership: Private
Quality System Registration Information: ISO9002
Produces/Sells CE-marked Devices: Y
Federal Procurement Eligibility: Small Business
Distribution: Manufacturer Through Distributor, Manufacturer Through Manufacturer Reps
General Admin.: Mr. Loran Van noy/General Manager
Mktg./Adv.: Mr. Harvey Hauschildt/Director Product Marketing

Analyzer, ECG	Cardiovascular
Analyzer, Gas, Carbon-Dioxide, Gaseous Phase (Capnograph)	Anesthesiology
Detector, Arrhythmia Alarm	Cardiovascular
Display, Cathode-Ray Tube	Cardiovascular
Electrocardiograph, Single Channel	Cardiovascular
Monitor, Blood Pressure, Indirect, Semi-Automatic	Cardiovascular
Monitor, Cardiac (Cardiotachometer & Rate Alarm)	Cardiovascular
Oximeter, Intracardiac	Cardiovascular
Scanner, Ultrasonic (Pulsed Echo)	Radiology
Transducer, Ultrasonic, Diagnostic	Radiology
Transmitter/Receiver System, Physiological, Radiofrequency	Cardiovascular

FULFLEX OF VERMONT, INC.   800-283-2500
32 Justin Holden Dr., Brattleboro, VT 05304
FDA Number: 3003684315
Ownership: Private
Produces/Sells CE-marked Devices: N

Bandage, Elastic	General
Tourniquet, Non-Pneumatic, Surgical	Surgery

FULL VISION, INC.   316-283-3344
3017 Full Vision Dr., Newton, KS 67114
FDA Number: 3001040337   *Fax:* 316-283-3350
E-mail: Sales@Full-Vision.com
Web site: www.full-vision.com
Ownership: Private
Produces/Sells CE-marked Devices: N

Treadmill, Powered	Physical Med

FULLER LABORATORIES   888-826-7660
1135 E. Truslow Avenue, Fullerton, CA 92831   **714-525-7660**
FDA Number: 3004036192   *Fax:* 714-525-7614
E-mail: Chris_Shapiro@FullerLabs.com
Web site: www.fullerlabs.com
Ownership: Private
Produces/Sells CE-marked Devices: N

Epstein-Barr Virus, Other	Microbiology
Rickettsia Serological Reagents, Other	Microbiology

FULLER MEDICAL CO.   256-547-4991
1019 South 4th Street, Gadsden, AL 35901
FDA Number: n/a   *Fax:* 256-547-6258
E-mail: tony@fullermedical.com
Web site: www.fullermedical.com
Medical Products Sales Volume: $300,000
Annual Revenue: $0-$1 Million
Year Founded: 1974
Ownership: Private
Produces/Sells CE-marked Devices: N
Federal Procurement Eligibility: Small Business
Distribution: Exclusive Distributor

Bed, Manual	General
Canister, Liquid Oxygen, Portable	Anesthesiology
Concentrator, Oxygen	Anesthesiology
Lift, Wheelchair	General
Monitor, Apnea	General
Regulator, Pressure, Gas Cylinder	Anesthesiology
Ventilator, Volume (Critical Care)	Anesthesiology
Wheelchair, Manual	Physical Med

FULLER ULTRAVIOLET CORP.   815-469-3301
9416 Gulfstream Road, Frankfort, IL 60423-2521
FDA Number: 9200371   *Fax:* 815-469-1438
E-mail: fulleruvcorp@mindspring.com
Web site: www.fulleruv.com
Medical Products Sales Volume: $500,000
Annual Revenue: $0-$1 Million
Year Founded: 1951
Total Employees: 10   *Sales Staff:* 1
Ownership: Private
Produces/Sells CE-marked Devices: N
Federal Procurement Eligibility: GSA Contract, VA Contract

MANUFACTURER PROFILES

FULLER ULTRAVIOLET CORP.   815-469-3301 (cont'd)
Distribution: Manufacturer Direct
General Admin.: M. K. Eckstrom/General Manager
     William R. Eckstrom/President
Mktg./Adv.: R.A. Schultz/Manager International & National Sales
Production: D. Hommes/Manager Materials
     C. Foresta/Supervisor Production
Finance: E. A. Kelly/Vice President Finance

Generator, Ozone	Anesthesiology
Lamp, Ultraviolet, Germicidal	General
Lamp, Ultraviolet, Physical Medicine	Physical Med
Purification System, Water, Ultraviolet	Chemistry
Sterilizer, Ultraviolet	General

FUMEX INC.   800-432-7550
1150 Cobb International Place, Suite D,   **770-514-7907**
Kennesaw, GA 30152
FDA Number: n/a   *Fax:* 770-514-1547
E-mail: info@fumexinc.com
Web site: www.fumexinc.com
Medical Products Sales Volume: $21,500,000
Year Founded: 1985
Total Employees: 100
Ownership: Private
Produces/Sells CE-marked Devices: Y
Federal Procurement Eligibility: Small Business
Distribution: Manufacturer Direct, Manufacturer Through Distributor, Manufacturer Through Manufacturer Reps, OEM, Importer, Exporter
Mktg./Adv.: Mr. Kevin East/Vice President Sales

Equipment, Filtering, Air, ETO	General
Equipment/Service, Quality Control	General
Evacuator, Fume	Chemistry
Hood, Fume, Chemical	Chemistry
System, Evacuation, Smoke, Laser	Surgery

FUNCTION TECHNOLOGIES, INC.   866-324-1771
8002 Upton Road, Laingsburg, MI 48848   **517-702-0912**
FDA Number: 2133690   *Fax:* 517-833-9154
E-mail: CustomerService@FunctionTechnologies.com
Web site: www.functiontechnologies.com
Ownership: Private
Produces/Sells CE-marked Devices: N

Exerciser, Non-Measuring	Physical Med

FUSED FIBEROPTICS L.L.C.   508-765-1652
79 Golf St., Southbridge, MA 01550-2809
FDA Number: n/a   *Fax:* 508-765-1704
E-mail: info@fusedfiberoptics.com
Web site: www.fusedfiberoptics.com
Medical Products Sales Volume: $1,400,000
Annual Revenue: $1-$5 Million
Year Founded: 1997
Total Employees: 13   *Sales Staff:* 1
Ownership: Private
Produces/Sells CE-marked Devices: N
Federal Procurement Eligibility: Small Business
Distribution: OEM
General Admin.: Robert Dowling/Chief Executive Officer
     Thomas Dowling/President

Light, Fiberoptic, Dental	Dental And Oral

FUSED KONTACTS, INC.   816-455-0500
3901 N.E. 33rd Terrace, Suite E, Kansas City, MO 64117
FDA Number: n/a
E-mail: info@bifocalcontacts.biz
Web site: www.tangentstreak.com
Medical Products Sales Volume: $1,500,000
Annual Revenue: $1-$5 Million
Ownership: Private
Produces/Sells CE-marked Devices: N
Distribution: Manufacturer Direct, Manufacturer Through Distributor
General Admin.: David T. Rusch/President

Lens, Contact (Other Material)	Ophthalmology
Lens, Contact, Bifocal	Ophthalmology
Lens, Contact, Extended-Wear	Ophthalmology
Lens, Contact, Trifocal	Ophthalmology

FUTURE DENTAL TECHNOLOGIES, INC.   909-894-4203
26398 Deere Ct., Suite 105, Murrieta, CA 92562
FDA Number: 2032346
Ownership: Private
Produces/Sells CE-marked Devices: N

Gutta Percha	Dental And Oral

FUTURE HEALTH CONCEPT'S, INC.   888-282-8644
1211 30th St., Sanford, FL 32773   **407-322-3672**
FDA Number: 1033902   *Fax:* 407-322-3871
Web site: www.futurehealthconcepts.com

FUTURE HEALTH CONCEPT'S, INC.   888-282-8644 (cont'd)
Ownership: Private
Produces/Sells CE-marked Devices: N
General Admin.: Mr. Greg Karleskint/President, Chief Executive Officer

Electrocautery Unit, Gynecologic	Obstetrics/Gynecology
Electrosurgical Unit, Cutting & Coagulation Device	Surgery
Hot Water Pasteurization Device	General
Light, Surgical, Ceiling Mounted	Surgery
Microscope, Surgical, General & Plastic Surgery	Surgery
Oximeter, Pulse	General
Sterilizer, Steam (Autoclave)	General
Stretcher, Wheeled (Mobile)	General
Table, Operating Room, AC-Powered	Surgery
Warmer, Irrigation Solution	General

FUTURE IMPEX
See Futuremed America, Inc.

FUTURE MEDICAL PRODUCTS, INC.
See Vasomedical Inc.

FUTURE MEDICAL SYSTEMS, INC.   800-367-6021
504 McCormick Drive Suite T,   **410-761-9411**
Glen Burnie, MD 21061
FDA Number: n/a   *Fax:* 410-761-9422
E-mail: fmsgroup@fmsgroup.com
Web site: www.fmsusa.com
Medical Products Sales Volume: $3,500,000
Annual Revenue: $10-$25 Million
Year Founded: 1986
Total Employees: 15
Ownership: Crest Ultrasonics
Quality System Registration Information: ISO9001
Produces/Sells CE-marked Devices: Y
Federal Procurement Eligibility: Small Business, GSA Contract, VA Contract
Distribution: Manufacturer Through Distributor, Manufacturer Through Manufacturer Reps, Importer, Exporter
General Admin.: Patrick Janin/General Manager

Accessories, Arthroscope	Orthopedics
Cannula, Other	General

FUTUREMED AMERICA, INC.   800-222-6780
15700 Devonshire St.,   **818-830-2500**
Granada Hills, CA 91344
FDA Number: 2433214   *Fax:* 818-891-4755
E-mail: Mail@futuremedamerica.com
Web site: www.futuremedamerica.com
Medical Products Sales Volume: $3,300,000
Annual Revenue: $1-$5 Million
Year Founded: 1979
Total Employees: 9   *Marketing Staff:* 7   *Sales Staff:* 5
Ownership: Private
Quality System Registration Information: ISO9002
Produces/Sells CE-marked Devices: Y
Federal Procurement Eligibility: Small Business, Female Owned, GSA Contract, VA Contract
Distribution: Manufacturer Through Distributor, OEM, Exclusive Distributor, Exporter
General Admin.: Susan Lukenbill/President
     P. Davidson/Vice President, General Manager
Mktg./Adv.: Ed Hakim/Director Clinical Support & Sales
     Fay Hakim/Director National Accounts
     Mike Davidson/Director Product Development
     Fay Hakim/Manager Advertising
     Albert De La Cruz/Manager Sales Training
     Michael Davidson/Vice President International Marketing & Sales
     P. Davidson/Vice President Sales
Production: Susan Watkins/Customer Service Representative

Analyzer, ECG	Cardiovascular
Meter, Peak Flow, Spirometry	Anesthesiology
Monitor, Apnea	General
Monitor, ECG	Cardiovascular
Nebulizer, Direct Patient Interface	Anesthesiology
Spirometer, Diagnostic (Respirometer)	Anesthesiology
Spirometer, Therapeutic (Incentive)	Anesthesiology
Warmer, Infusion Fluid, Thermal	General

FUTUREMED HEALTH CARE PRODUCTS INC.   800-381-7025
280 Basaltic Rd., Concord, ONT L4K-1G6 Canada   **905-761-0068**
FDA Number: n/a   *Fax:* 905-761-9929
E-mail: lillian@fmed.com
Web site: www.futmed.com
Year Founded: 1985
Total Employees: 50
Ownership: Private
Produces/Sells CE-marked Devices: N
Distribution: Exclusive Distributor, Exporter

FZIOMED, INC.   805-546-0610
231 Bonetti Drive, San Luis Obispo, CA 93401
FDA Number: 2031637   Fax: 805-546-0571
E-mail: sales@fziomed.com
Web site: www.fziomed.com
Medical Products Sales Volume: $3,700,000
Year Founded: 1996
Total Employees: 40   Marketing Staff: 3
Ownership: Private
Quality System Registration Information: ISO9001
Produces/Sells CE-marked Devices: Y
Federal Procurement Eligibility: Small Business
Distribution: Manufacturer Through Distributor, OEM

Barrier, Control Panel, X-Ray, Moveable	Radiology
Implant, Collagen, Dermal (Aesthetic Use)	Surgery
Inhibitor, Peridural Fibrosis (Adhesion Barrier)	Physical Med

G & F INDUSTRIES, INC.   508-347-9132
Rt. 20 Box 515, Sturbridge, MA 01566
FDA Number: 1225699

Orthosis, Truncal/Limb	Physical Med

G & G MEDICAL PRODUCTS, INC.   518-542-0395
6 White Fir Dr., Loudonville, NY 12211
FDA Number: 1318662
Ownership: Private
Produces/Sells CE-marked Devices: N

Otoscope	Ear/Nose/Throat

G & H WIRE CO.   800-526-1026   317-346-6655
2165 Earlywood Drive, Franklin, IN 46131
FDA Number: 1833132   Fax: 317-346-6663
E-mail: ghmail@ghwire.com
Web site: www.ghwire.com
Medical Products Sales Volume: $2,200,000
Year Founded: 1981
Total Employees: 33   Marketing Staff: 3   Sales Staff: 8
Ownership: Private
Produces/Sells CE-marked Devices: Y
Federal Procurement Eligibility: Small Business
Distribution: Manufacturer Direct, Manufacturer Through Distributor, Exclusive Distributor, Importer, Exporter

Adhesive, Bracket And Conditioner, Resin	Dental And Oral
Agent, Polishing, Abrasive, Oral Cavity	Dental And Oral
Aligner, Bracket, Orthodontic	Dental And Oral
Band, Elastic, Orthodontic	Dental And Oral
Band, Preformed, Orthodontic	Dental And Oral
Bracket, Metal, Orthodontic	Dental And Oral
Bracket, Plastic, Orthodontic	Dental And Oral
Burr, Dental	Dental And Oral
Clamp, Wire, Orthodontic	Dental And Oral
Clasp, Preformed	Dental And Oral
Clasp, Wire	Dental And Oral
Disk, Abrasive	Dental And Oral
Driver, Band, Orthodontic	Dental And Oral
Film, X-Ray, Dental, Extraoral	Dental And Oral
Guard, Disk	Dental And Oral
Headgear, Extraoral, Orthodontic	Dental And Oral
Material, Impression	Dental And Oral
Mirror, Mouth	Dental And Oral
Orthodontic Instrument	Dental And Oral
Pliers, Orthodontic	Dental And Oral
Positioner, Tooth, Preformed	Dental And Oral
Pusher, Band, Orthodontic	Dental And Oral
Retainer, Screw Expansion, Orthodontic	Dental And Oral
Retractor, All Types	Dental And Oral
Setter, Band, Orthodontic	Dental And Oral
Spring, Orthodontic	Dental And Oral
Strip, Polishing Agent	Dental And Oral
Tray, Impression	Dental And Oral
Tube, Orthodontic	Dental And Oral
Tucker, Ligature, Orthodontic	Dental And Oral
Wax, Dental	Dental And Oral
Wire, Orthodontic	Dental And Oral

Medical Product Subsidiaries (Listed Separately)
Flexmedics

G & K SERVICES   510) 293-5840
3444 Depot Rd., Hayward,, CA 94545
FDA Number: n/a
E-mail: gkweb@gkservices.com
Web site: www.gkservices.com
Annual Revenue: $0-$1 Million
Total Employees: 60   Sales Staff: 10
Ownership: Private
Produces/Sells CE-marked Devices: N
Distribution: Service Direct, Exclusive Distributor
Mktg./Adv.: Jim Hancock/Director Marketing

G & K SERVICES   510) 293-5840 (cont'd)

Cleanroom Equipment	General

G & S INSTRUMENT CO.   972-723-0856
6851 Montgomery Rd., Midlothian, TX 76065
FDA Number: 1644254
Ownership: Private
Produces/Sells CE-marked Devices: N

Stimulator, Collection, Sperm, Electrical	Gastroenterology/Urology

G H MEDICAL INC., DIVISION OF TSJ INC.   612-331-6299
2010 East Hennepin Ave., Minneapolis, MN 55413
FDA Number: 2183792
Ownership: Private
Produces/Sells CE-marked Devices: N

Monitor, Blood Pressure, Indirect, Semi-Automatic	Cardiovascular

G&F MANUFACTURING CO.
See Microcision Llc

G&M RESEARCH COMPANY, INC.   603-645-6655
31 Hale Ave., Hooksett, NH 03106
FDA Number: 3004579046
Ownership: Private
Produces/Sells CE-marked Devices: N
General Admin.: Mr. Louis Mariano Jr./President

Pack, Hot Or Cold, Disposable	Physical Med

G-C AMERICA INC.   800-323-7063   708-597-0900
3737 W. 127th St., Aslip, IL 60803
FDA Number: 2080962   Fax: 800-423-2963
E-mail: gca_sales@gcamerica.com
Web site: www.gcamerica.com
Annual Revenue: $1-$5 Million
Total Employees: 150   Marketing Staff: 8   Sales Staff: 30
Ownership: GCC INTERNATIONAL
Quality System Registration Information: ISO9001
Produces/Sells CE-marked Devices: N
Federal Procurement Eligibility: Small Business
Distribution: Manufacturer Through Distributor
General Admin.: Dean Porter/President, Chief Operating Officer
Mktg./Adv.: George Geffe/Director Marketing
    John O'Neill/Vice President Marketing & Sales
Production: Tom Bartnett/Director Manufacturing & Operations
    Terry Jeritz/Director Regulatory Affairs
Research: Richard Demke/Vice President Research & Development

Cement, Dental	Dental And Oral
Material, Impression	Dental And Oral
Material, Investment	Dental And Oral
Material, Tooth Shade, Resin	Dental And Oral
Powder, Porcelain	Dental And Oral

G. BRUNATTI & SONS LIMITED   705-746-5622
85 River Street, Parry Sound, ONT P2A 2T8 Canada
FDA Number: n/a   Fax: 705-746-8688
E-mail: gbrunatti@cogeco.net
Web site: www.brunattiandsons.com
Year Founded: 1939
Total Employees: 10
Ownership: Private
Produces/Sells CE-marked Devices: N
Distribution: Manufacturer Direct

G. DUNDAS CO.,INC.   253-631-8008
24301 Roberts Dr., Black Diamond, WA 98010
FDA Number: 3019855

Gas-Machine, Anesthesia	Anesthesiology

G. HIRSCH & CO.   650-692-6435
1815 Rollins Rd., Burlingame, CA 94010
FDA Number: n/a
Annual Revenue: $10-$25 Million
Ownership: Private
Produces/Sells CE-marked Devices: N
Distribution: Manufacturer Direct, Manufacturer Through Distributor, Manufacturer Through Manufacturer Reps

Device, Incontinence, Fecal	Gastroenterology/Urology
Diaper, Adult	General
Pad, Incontinence (Underpad)	General

G. HIRSCH AND CO., INC.   650-692-8770
870 Mahler Road, Burlingame, CA 94010
FDA Number: 2938074
Ownership: Private
Produces/Sells CE-marked Devices: N

Cane	Physical Med
Cover, Mattress	General
Crutch	Physical Med
Garment, Protective, For Incontinence	Gastroenterology/Urology
Lift, Bath, Non-AC-Powered	General

G. HIRSCH AND CO., INC.
650-692-8770 *(cont'd)*
Walker, Mechanical — Physical Med
Wheelchair, Manual — Physical Med

G.A.I.
See Gillis Associated Industries

G.E.M. WATER SYSTEMS, INT'L., LLC
800-755-1707
714-736-9990
6351 Orangethorpe Avenue,
Buena Park, CA 90620
FDA Number: 2025607
Fax: 714-736-9402
E-mail: jack@gemwater.com
Web site: www.gemwater.com
Medical Products Sales Volume: $1,700,000
Annual Revenue: $1-$5 Million
Year Founded: 1981
Total Employees: 15   Marketing Staff: 2   Sales Staff: 3
Ownership: Private
Produces/Sells CE-marked Devices: N
Federal Procurement Eligibility: Small Business
Distribution: Manufacturer Direct, Manufacturer Through Manufacturer Reps, Exporter
General Admin.: Mr. Jack Enkowitz/President, Chief Executive Officer
Production: Deo Siron/Vice President Manufacturing
Chair, Dialysis, Powered (Without Scale) — Gastroenterology/Urology
Chair, Dialysis, Unpowered (Without Scale) — Gastroenterology/Urology
Dialysate Delivery System, Single Patient — Gastroenterology/Urology
Dialyzer Reprocessing System — Gastroenterology/Urology
Purification Filter, Water, Particulate — Chemistry
Purification System, Water, Reverse Osmosis — Chemistry
Purification System, Water, Reverse Osmosis, Reagent Grade — Chemistry
Tank, Holding, Dialysis — Gastroenterology/Urology

G.L. INSTRUMENTS, LTD.
See Biosig Instruments, Inc.

G.T. LABORATORIES, INC.
847-998-4776
Central Park Of Lisle Center, 3333 Warrenville Rd.,suite 200,
Lisle, IL 60532
FDA Number: 1419801
Lens, Contact (Other Material) — Ophthalmology

GAC INTERNATIONAL LLC
See Dentsply Gac International

GAERTNER SCIENTIFIC CORP.
847-673-5006
3650 Jarvis Avenue, Skokie, IL 60076
FDA Number: n/a
Fax: 847-673-5009
E-mail: email@gaertnerscientific.com
Web site: www.gaertnerscientific.com
Medical Products Sales Volume: $4,500,000
Annual Revenue: $1-$5 Million
Year Founded: 1896
Ownership: Private
Produces/Sells CE-marked Devices: Y
Federal Procurement Eligibility: Small Business
Distribution: Manufacturer Through Manufacturer Reps
Lamp, Microscope — Pathology

GAGNE, INC.
800-800-5954
607-729-3366
41 Commercial Drive, Johnson City, NY 13790
FDA Number: n/a
Fax: 607-729-7644
E-mail: sales@gagneinc.com
Web site: http://gagneinc.com/
Year Founded: 1953
Total Employees: 25   Marketing Staff: 2
Ownership: Private
Produces/Sells CE-marked Devices: N
Federal Procurement Eligibility: Small Business
Distribution: Manufacturer Through Distributor, Manufacturer Through Manufacturer Reps
General Admin.: Thom Holland/President
Mktg./Adv.: Cary B. Dunlay/Vice President Sales
Production: Kim Pentice/Customer Service Representative
Illuminator, Radiographic Film — Radiology
Light, Other — General

GAIA HOLISTIC,INC
212-799-9711
20 West 64th St. Suite 24e, New York, NY 10023
FDA Number: 3004057530
Fax: 212-799-1661
E-mail: info@gaiahh.com
Web site: www.gaiahh.com
Medical Products Sales Volume: $200,000
Total Employees: 2
Federal Procurement Eligibility: Small Business, Female Owned
Massager, Therapeutic — Physical Med

GAINOR MEDICAL USA, INC.
See Facet Technologies, Llc

GAIT-AID INC.
800-677-1796
416-234-6805
5468 Dundas St. W., Ste. 1000,
Toronto, ONT M9B 6 Canada
FDA Number: n/a
Fax: 416-234-1564
E-mail: sales@gait-aid.com
Web site: www.gait-aid.com
Year Founded: 1986
Total Employees: 10
Ownership: Private
Produces/Sells CE-marked Devices: N
Distribution: Manufacturer Direct, Exporter

GALAXY AQUATICS, INC.
713-464-0303
1075 W. Sam Houston Pkwy. N., Ste. 210,
Houston, TX 77043
FDA Number: n/a
Fax: 713-464-0399
E-mail: galaxy@galaxy-aquatics.com
Web site: www.galaxy-aquatics.com
Annual Revenue: $0-$1 Million
Year Founded: 1982
Total Employees: 10   Marketing Staff: 1   Sales Staff: 3
Ownership: Private
Produces/Sells CE-marked Devices: N
Federal Procurement Eligibility: Small Business
Distribution: Manufacturer Through Distributor, Manufacturer Through Manufacturer Reps, Exporter
General Admin.: Klaus P. Klosterman/President, Chief Executive Officer
Marianne Klosterman/Vice President, General Manager
Mktg./Adv.: Marianne Klosterman/Director National Accounts
Herbert E. Kellner/Manager International & National Sales
Marianne Klosterman/Vice President Marketing
Bath, Portable — General
Tank, Full Body (Bath) — General

GALAXY MEDICAL MANUFACTURING CO.
800-876-4599
323-728-3980
5411 Sheila Street, Commerce, CA 90040-2103
FDA Number: 9320014
Fax: 323-728-5971
E-mail: sales@galaxymfg.com
Web site: www.galaxymfg.com
Medical Products Sales Volume: $2,000,000
Annual Revenue: $1-$5 Million
Year Founded: 1949
Total Employees: 50   Marketing Staff: 6   Sales Staff: 5
Ownership: Private
Produces/Sells CE-marked Devices: N
Federal Procurement Eligibility: Small Business, Minority Owned
Distribution: Manufacturer Through Distributor
General Admin.: John Talei/President
Mktg./Adv.: Henry Talei/Director Marketing
Production: Henry Talei/Vice President Production
Research: Ben Yamini/Manager Research
Chair, Dental — Dental And Oral
Infusion Stand — General
Lamp, Examination (Light) — General
Pillow — General
Stand, Operating Room Instrument (Mayo) — Surgery
Stool, Anesthetist's — Anesthesiology
Stool, Bedside — General
Stool, Dental — Dental And Oral
Stool, Operating Room, Adjustable — Surgery
Table, Examination/Treatment — General
Table, Mechanical — Physical Med
Table, Obstetrical — Obstetrics/Gynecology
Table, Other — General
Table, Physical Therapy — Physical Med

GALEN MEDICAL LTD.
800-980-3003
604-980-9006
408 Kent Ave South E, Suite 126,
Vancouver, BC V5X2X Canada
FDA Number: n/a
Fax: 604-980-3433
E-mail: custserv@galenmed.bc.ca
Web site: www.galenmed.com
Year Founded: 1988
Total Employees: 10
Ownership: Private
Produces/Sells CE-marked Devices: N
Distribution: Exclusive Distributor

GALENICARE
877-309-0560
(403) 342-1900
4621 63 St. #4, Red Deer, ALB T4N-7A6 Canada
FDA Number: n/a
Fax: 403-340-1995
E-mail: peridot@telusplanet.net
Year Founded: 1995
Total Employees: 10
Ownership: Private
Produces/Sells CE-marked Devices: N

GALENICARE
877-309-0560 (cont'd)
Distribution: Manufacturer Direct, Exporter

GALIA TEXTIL S.A. DE C.V.
246-1-6-066
Lote 3 Manzana 4, Parque Industrial, Tlaxcala Mexico
FDA Number: 9680708

Drape, Surgical	Surgery
Sponge, Gauze	Dental And Oral

GALIX BIOMEDICAL INSTRUMENTATION, INC.
305-534-5905
2555 Collins Avenue, Suite C-5, Miami Beach, FL 33140
FDA Number: 1063225   *Fax:* 305-534-8222
E-mail: galix@the-beach.net
Web site: www.galix-gbi.com
Medical Products Sales Volume: $1,300,000
Annual Revenue: $1-$5 Million
Year Founded: 1993
Total Employees: 15   *Marketing Staff:* 1   *Sales Staff:* 3
Ownership: Private
Quality System Registration Information: ISO9001
Produces/Sells CE-marked Devices: Y
Federal Procurement Eligibility: Small Business
Distribution: Manufacturer Direct, Manufacturer Through Distributor, Manufacturer Through Manufacturer Reps, OEM, Exporter
General Admin.: Mr. Jordan Gavrielides/President, Chief Executive Officer
Mktg./Adv.: Mr. Eduardo Rey/Director Product Development
Mr. Greg Velez/Manager Marketing & Sales
Mr. Norberto Lerendegui/Vice President Business Development
Production: Mr. Guillermo Di Primio/Vice President Manufacturing
Research: Mr. Ricardo Tomsic/Director Development
Mr. Agustin Reibel/Vice President Research & Development

Analyzer, ECG	Cardiovascular
Electrocardiograph, Multi-Channel	Cardiovascular
Ergometer, Treadmill	Cardiovascular
Pacemaker, Heart, External	Cardiovascular
Pacemaker, Heart, External, Programmable	Cardiovascular
Polygraph	General
Recorder, Long-Term, ECG, Portable (Holter Monitor)	Cardiovascular

GALIX INSTRUMENTACION BIOMEDICA
See Galix Biomedical Instrumentation, Inc.

GALLOWAY PLASTICS, INC.
847-615-8900
940 North Shore Dr., Lake Bluff, IL 60044
FDA Number: n/a   *Fax:* 847-615-8920
E-mail: sales@gpianatomicals.com
Web site: www.gpianatomicals.com
Annual Revenue: $5-$10 Million
Total Employees: 20   *Marketing Staff:* 2   *Sales Staff:* 6
Ownership: Private
Produces/Sells CE-marked Devices: N
Federal Procurement Eligibility: Small Business
Distribution: Manufacturer Direct, Manufacturer Through Manufacturer Reps
General Admin.: Scott Galloway/Chief Executive Officer
Mktg./Adv.: Adam Galloway/Manager International & National Sales
Scott Galloway/Manager National Sales

Anatomical Training Model	General
Chart, Anatomical Training	General
Contract Manufacturing	General

GALLOWAY TECHNOLOGIES, LLC
801-766-1636
3736 Panarama Dr., Saratoga Springs, UT 84043
FDA Number: 3003843036
Annual Revenue: $1-$5 Million
Ownership: Private
Produces/Sells CE-marked Devices: N
General Admin.: Joe Galloway/Chief Executive Officer
Mark Galloway/President

Monitor, Response, Skin, Galvanic	Cns/Neurology

GALT MEDICAL CORP.
800-639-2800
2220 Merritt Dr., Garland, TX 75041   972-271-5177
FDA Number: 1649395   *Fax:* 972-271-4706
Web site: www.galtmedical.com
Year Founded: 1991
Ownership: Theragenics Corp.
Produces/Sells CE-marked Devices: N

Dilator, Vessel, Percutaneous Catheterization	Cardiovascular
Guide, Catheter	Cardiovascular
Guidewire, Catheter	Cardiovascular
Introducer, Catheter	Cardiovascular

GALVESTON MANUFACTURING CO., INC.
(800) 634-3309
7810 FM 646 S., Santa Fe, TX 77510-9535   409-925-1891
FDA Number: 1621255   *Fax:* (800) 634-3369
E-mail: info@galvestonmed.com
Web site: www.galvestonmedicalmfg.com
Year Founded: 1987
Ownership: Private

GALVESTON MANUFACTURING CO., INC.
(800) 634-3309 (cont'd)
Produces/Sells CE-marked Devices: N
Federal Procurement Eligibility: Small Business, Female Owned
General Admin.: Carol Owens/President, Chief Operating Officer
Susan Feltner/Vice President

Sling, Arm	Physical Med
Splint, Extremity, Non-Inflatable, External	Surgery
Splint, Hand, And Component	Physical Med

GAM INDUSTRIES, INC.
See Duro-Med Industries

GAM LASER INC
407-851-8999
6901 TPC Drive, Suite 300, Orlando, FL 32822
FDA Number: n/a   *Fax:* 407-850-0700
E-mail: sales@gamlaser.com
Web site: www.gamlaser.com
Year Founded: 1984
Total Employees: 20
Ownership: Private
Produces/Sells CE-marked Devices: Y
Federal Procurement Eligibility: Small Business
Distribution: Manufacturer Direct, OEM
General Admin.: Dr. Gordan A, Murray/Chief Executive Officer
Mktg./Adv.: Mr. Joseph Batcho/Director Marketing
Production: Ms. Aruna Bala/Applications Engineer

Accessories, Laser	General

GAM LASER INC.
See Gam Laser Inc

GAM RAD, INC.
540-646-5466
Star Rt. 608 (river Rd.), Chilhowie, VA 24319
FDA Number: 1824336
Ownership: Private
Produces/Sells CE-marked Devices: N

Stain, Giemsa	Pathology
Stain, Wright's	Pathology

GAMBRO BCT, INC.
See Caridianbct Inc.

GAMBRO INC.
514-327-1635
9157, du Champ DA,A'eau Street,
St. Leonard, MONTR H1P 3 Canada
FDA Number: n/a   *Fax:* 514-327-0822
Web site: www.gambro.com
Ownership: Private
Produces/Sells CE-marked Devices: N
Distribution: Manufacturer Direct, Importer

GAMBRO RENAL PRODUCTS
800-525-2623
14143 Denver West Parkway, Lakewood, CO 80401
FDA Number: 1051129   *Fax:* (303) 222-6810
E-mail: americas.webmaster@us.gambro.com
Web site: www.gambroamericas.com
Ownership: Private
Produces/Sells CE-marked Devices: N

Accessories, Blood Circuit, Hemodialysis	Gastroenterology/Urology
Container, Sharpes	General

GAMBRO RENAL PRODUCTS, INC.
800-525-2623
14143 Denver West Parkway, Lakewood, CO 80401
FDA Number: 2087532   *Fax:* 303-231-4310
E-mail: americas.webmaster@us.gambro.com
Web site: www.gambroamericas.com
Ownership: Private
Produces/Sells CE-marked Devices: N

Accessories, Blood Circuit, Hemodialysis	Gastroenterology/Urology
Concentrate, Dialysis, Hemodialysis (Liquid or Powder)	Gastroenterology/Urology
Dialyzer, Capillary, Hollow Fiber (Hemodialysis)	Gastroenterology/Urology
Dialyzer, High Permeability	Gastroenterology/Urology
Hemodialyzer, Re-use, High Flux	Gastroenterology/Urology
Hemoperfusion System, Sorbent	Gastroenterology/Urology
Kit, Tubing, Blood, Anti-Regurgitation	Gastroenterology/Urology
Purification System, Water	Gastroenterology/Urology
Separator, Blood Cell/Plasma, Therapeutic	Gastroenterology/Urology

GAMETRICS LTD.
307-878-4494
426 Lonesome Country Rd, Alzada, MT 59311
FDA Number: n/a   *Fax:* 307-878-4499
E-mail: gametrics@childselect.com
Web site: www.childselect.com
Medical Products Sales Volume: $300,000
Total Employees: 10
Ownership: Private
Produces/Sells CE-marked Devices: N
Federal Procurement Eligibility: Small Business
Distribution: Manufacturer Through Manufacturer Reps, Exclusive Distributor, Exporter
General Admin.: Ronald Ericsson, PhD/Chief Executive Officer

GAMETRICS LTD.
307-878-4494 *(cont'd)*
Kit, Sex Selection — Obstetrics/Gynecology

GAMMA MEDICA-IDEAS, INC
877-426-2633
19355 Business Center Dr., Ste. 8,
Northridge, CA 91324
818-709-2468
FDA Number: 2032285
Fax: 818-709-2464
E-mail: info@gm-ideas.com
Web site: www.gm-ideas.com
Ownership: Private
Produces/Sells CE-marked Devices: N
Mktg./Adv.: David Wilk/Senior Vice President Sales
Patrick Moody/Vice President Marketing
Camera, Gamma (Nuclear/Scintillation) — Radiology

GAMMADIRECT MEDICAL DIVISION
847-267-5929
PO Box 383, Lake Forest, IL 60045
FDA Number: n/a
Fax: 847-267-9078
E-mail: info@gammahealth.com
Web site: www.gammahealth.com
Year Founded: 1984
Total Employees: 419   Marketing Staff: 23   Sales Staff: 18
Ownership: Private
Quality System Registration Information: ISO9001
Produces/Sells CE-marked Devices: Y
Distribution: Manufacturer Through Distributor, OEM, Exclusive Distributor, Exporter

Apron, Lead, Dental	Dental And Oral
Apron, Lead, Radiographic	Radiology
Condom, Non-Latex	Obstetrics/Gynecology
Dam, Dental	Dental And Oral
Device, Biopsy, Percutaneous	Surgery
Film, X-Ray	Radiology
Glove, Other	General
Glove, Patient Examination, Poly	General
Glove, Protective, Radiographic	Radiology
Lens, Other	Ophthalmology
Mask, Surgical	Surgery
Probe, Other	General
Resuscitator, Pulmonary, Manual (Demand Valve)	General
Scissors, Umbilical	Obstetrics/Gynecology
Ventilator, Emergency, Powered (Resuscitator)	Anesthesiology

GAMMASONICS
800-253-0145
170 Dutcher St., Hopedale, MA 01747-1028
508-878-4730
FDA Number: n/a
Fax: 508-478-2911
E-mail: skip@kersur.net
Annual Revenue: $0-$1 Million
Total Employees: 3   Sales Staff: 2
Ownership: Private
Produces/Sells CE-marked Devices: N
Federal Procurement Eligibility: Small Business
Distribution: Manufacturer Direct, Service Direct
General Admin.: Ian Macdonald/President
Mktg./Adv.: Frank Ley/Manager Sales
Production: Alister Shaw/Vice President Production
Transmitter, Image & Data, Radiographic — Radiology

GAMMEX LASERS CORP.
See Gammex Rmi

GAMMEX RMI
800-426-6391
7600 Discovery Drive, Middleton, WI 53562-0327
608-828-7000
FDA Number: 2939370
Fax: 608-828-7500
E-mail: sales@gammex.com
Web site: www.gammex.com
Annual Revenue: $10-$25 Million
Year Founded: 1969
Total Employees: 75   Marketing Staff: 3   Sales Staff: 8
Ownership: Private
Quality System Registration Information: ISO9001
Produces/Sells CE-marked Devices: Y
Federal Procurement Eligibility: Small Business, Minority Owned
Distribution: Manufacturer Direct, Manufacturer Through Distributor, OEM, Exporter
General Admin.: Dr. Charles Lescrenier/Chief Executive Officer
Mr. Ken Windisch/General Manager
Dr. Charles Lescrenier/President
Mktg./Adv.: Mrs. Petra Kilian-Gehring/Coord. Marketing & Trade Show
Mr. Lyle Ruble/Director Sales
Mrs. Petra Kilian-Gehring/Manager Advertising
Mrs. Nikki Zorman/Supervisor Sales
Production: Mr. Ken Windisch/Director Quality Assurance
Mr. Don Engelhart/Manager Materials
Mr. Ken Windisch/Manager Regulatory Affairs
Mr. Robert Steinhauser/Product Specialist
Finance: Mrs. Amanda Robinson/Admin. Finance

Monitor, Patient Position, Light Beam	Radiology
Phantom, Anthropomorphic, Radiographic	Radiology

GAMMEX RMI
800-426-6391 *(cont'd)*

Phantom, Computed Axial Tomography (CAT, CT)	Radiology
Phantom, Mammographic	Radiology
Phantom, Ultrasound	Radiology
Radiotherapy Treatment Planning Unit	Radiology
Support, Patient Position, Radiographic	Radiology

GAMMEX, INC.
See Gammex Rmi

GAPER PRODUCTS LTD.
800-667-5858
4060 Ridgeway Dr. #18,
Mississauga, ONT L5L-5 Canada
905-820-0004
FDA Number: n/a
Fax: 905-820-8002
E-mail: fgagne@gaperproducts.com
Web site: www.gaperproducts.com
Year Founded: 1995
Total Employees: 10
Ownership: Private
Produces/Sells CE-marked Devices: N
Distribution: Exclusive Distributor, Importer

GARAVENTA (CANADA) LTD.
800-663-6556
7505 - 134A St., Surrey, BC V3W-7B3 Canada
604-594-0422
FDA Number: n/a
Fax: 604-594-9915
E-mail: productinfo@garaventa.ca
Web site: www.garaventa.ca
Year Founded: 1974
Total Employees: 170   Marketing Staff: 2   Sales Staff: 8
Ownership: Private
Quality System Registration Information: ISO9001
Produces/Sells CE-marked Devices: Y
Federal Procurement Eligibility: Small Business
Distribution: Manufacturer Through Distributor, Manufacturer Through Manufacturer Reps, Importer, Exporter

GARDEN CITY MEDICAL, INC.
732-683-1900
512 Union Grove Rd., Calhoun, GA 30701
FDA Number: 1125779
Ownership: Invacare Corporation
Produces/Sells CE-marked Devices: N

GARDNER DENVER THOMAS INC.
920-457-4891
1419 Illinois Ave, Sheboygan, WI 53082
FDA Number: 2182215
Fax: 920-451-4237
E-mail: td.usa@gardnerdenver.com
Web site: www.gd-thomas.com
Year Founded: 1948
Total Employees: 1200
Ownership: Gardner Denver, Inc.
Produces/Sells CE-marked Devices: N
Distribution: OEM

Compressor, Air, Portable	Anesthesiology
Nebulizer, Direct Patient Interface	Anesthesiology
Pump, Aspiration, Portable	Anesthesiology
Pump, Breast, Powered	Obstetrics/Gynecology
Pump, Nebulizer, Electric	Ear/Nose/Throat
Suction Apparatus, Ward Use, Portable, AC-Powered	Surgery

GARDNER DENVER, INC.
217-222-5400
1800 Gardner Expressway, Quincy, IL 62305
FDA Number: n/a
Fax: 217-228-8243
Web site: www.gardnerdenver.com
Ownership: Public
Stock Symbol: GDI
Traded On: NYSE
Produces/Sells CE-marked Devices: N
General Admin.: Donald G. Barger/Chairman
Helen W. Cornell/Chief Financial Officer, Executive Vice President
Barry L. Pennypacker/President, Chief Executive Officer

GARGOYLES EYEWEAR
800-426-6396
500 George Washington Hwy, Smithfield, RI 02917
FDA Number: n/a
Web site: http://gargoyleseyewear.com
Annual Revenue: $25-$50 Million
Ownership: TRILLIUM CORP.
Stock Symbol: GOYL
Traded On: NASDAQ
Produces/Sells CE-marked Devices: N
Distribution: Manufacturer Direct, Manufacturer Through Distributor, Manufacturer Through Manufacturer Reps

Goggles, Protective, Eye	Ophthalmology
Shield, Eye, Ophthalmic	Ophthalmology
Sunglasses (Including Photosensitive)	Ophthalmology

GARGOYLES, INC.
See Gargoyles Eyewear

GARREN SCIENTIFIC, INC.

15916 Blythe St., Unit A, Van Nuys, CA 91406   **800-342-3725**
818-989-6340
FDA Number: 2020546   *Fax:* 818-908-9189
E-mail: info@garren-scientific.com
Web site: www.garren-scientific.com
Medical Products Sales Volume: $200,000
Annual Revenue: $1-$5 Million
Year Founded: 1982
Total Employees: 2   *Marketing Staff:* 1   *Sales Staff:* 1
Ownership: Private
Federal Procurement Eligibility: Small Business
Distribution: Manufacturer Direct, Manufacturer Through Distributor, Manufacturer Through Manufacturer Reps, Service Direct, Exclusive Distributor, Exporter
General Admin.: Elsa Ramirez/Office Manager
         Steven Garren/President, Chief Executive Officer
Finance: Karen Garren/Chief Financial Officer

Analyzer, Chemistry, Urinalysis	Chemistry
Container, Specimen, All Types	General
Dispenser, Fluid	General
Kit, Forensic Evidence	Pathology
Needle, Blood Collection	General
Pipette	Chemistry
Pipette, Diluting	Hematology
Pipette, Pasteur	Hematology
Slide, Microscope	Pathology
Tube, Centrifuge	Chemistry
Tube, Culture	Microbiology

GARRETT OPTICAL, INC.
See Abb Concise Optical Group Llc

GARRISON DENTAL SOLUTIONS

150 Dewitt Ln., Spring Lake, MI 49456   **888-437-0032**
616-842-2244
FDA Number: 1836088   *Fax:* 616-842-2430
E-mail: gds@garrisondental.com
Web site: www.garrisondental.com
Ownership: Private
Produces/Sells CE-marked Devices: N
Mktg./Adv.: Mr. Tom Garrison/Vice President Marketing & Sales
Production: Mr. Robert Anderson/Vice President Manufacturing
Finance: Dr. John Garrison/President

Absorber, Saliva, Paper	Dental And Oral
Filling, Instrument Plastic, Dental	Dental And Oral
Handle, Instrument, Dental	Dental And Oral
Instrument, Diamond, Dental	Dental And Oral
Medical Disinfectants/Cleaners for Instruments	General
Operative Dental Treatment Unit	Dental And Oral
Retainer, Matrix	Dental And Oral

GARY E. HALL
See Barton Matthew, Inc.

GAS MONITORING, INC.
See Enviro Guard, Inc.

GAST MANUFACTURING

P.O. Box 97, Benton Harbor, MI 49023-0097   **269.926.6171**
FDA Number: n/a   *Fax:* 269.925.8288
E-mail: marketing@gastmfg.com
Web site: www.gastmfg.com
Total Employees: 650   *Marketing Staff:* 7   *Sales Staff:* 20
Ownership: IDEX CORPORATION
Quality System Registration Information: ISO9001
Produces/Sells CE-marked Devices: Y
Distribution: Manufacturer Through Distributor
General Admin.: Don Rimes/President
Mktg./Adv.: Roger Csepregi/Manager Advertising
         Jim Folk/Manager International & National Sales
         Dennis Kugle/Manager National Sales

Compressor, Air, Portable	Anesthesiology
Pump, Vacuum, Central	Anesthesiology

GASTROTECH INC.
See Applied Medical Technology, Inc.

GATES ENERGY PRODUCTS, INC.
See Moltech Power Systems Inc

GATOR CUSTOM MOBILITY, INC.

501 NE 23rd Ave., Gainesville, FL 32609   **352-373-9673**
FDA Number: 95193   *Fax:* 352-271-9070
E-mail: info@gatorcustom.com
Web site: www.gatorcustom.com
Ownership: Private
Produces/Sells CE-marked Devices: N

Stretcher, Wheeled, Powered	Physical Med

GAUTHIER BIOMEDICAL, INC.

1235 North Dakota Drive, Suite G,   **866-546-0010**
262-546-0010
Grafton, WI 53024
FDA Number: 2134947   *Fax:* 262-546-0011
E-mail: Dean.Poulos@gauthierbiomedical.com

GAUTHIER BIOMEDICAL, INC.   **866-546-0010** *(cont'd)*
Web site: www.gauthierbiomedical.com
Ownership: Private
Produces/Sells CE-marked Devices: N
General Admin.: Mr. Mike Gauthier/President
         Ms. Stacy Gauthier/Vice President

Orthopedic Manual Surgical Instrument	Orthopedics
Screwdriver	Orthopedics
Template	Orthopedics

GAUTHIER INDUSTRIES INC.
See Medical Innovations International Inc.

GAUTHIER MEDICAL, INC.
See Medical Innovations International Inc.

GAYMAR INDUSTRIES, INC.

10 Centre Drive, Orchard Park, NY 14127-2280   **800-828-7341**
716-662-2551
FDA Number: 1313850   *Fax:* 716-662-0748
E-mail: websalescontact@gaymar.com
Web site: www.gaymar.com
Medical Products Sales Volume: $84,000,000
Year Founded: 1956
Total Employees: 180
Ownership: Stryker Corp.
Quality System Registration Information: ISO9001
Produces/Sells CE-marked Devices: Y
Federal Procurement Eligibility: Small Business, GSA Contract
Distribution: Manufacturer Direct, Manufacturer Through Distributor, Manufacturer Through Manufacturer Reps, OEM, Importer, Exporter
General Admin.: Dr. Thomas Stewart/President
Mktg./Adv.: Mr. Donald Woodworth/Director New Business Development
         Mr. John Holder III/President Sales
Production: Mr. Dan Murphy/Vice President Operations

Bed, Adjustable Hospital	General
Bed, Flotation Therapy, Powered	Physical Med
Bed, Patient Rotation, Powered	Physical Med
Hypo/Hyperthermia Blanket	General
Hypo/Hyperthermia Unit, Mobile	General
Hypothermia Unit	General
Mattress, Air Flotation	General
Mattress, Alternating Pressure (Or Pads)	Physical Med
Mattress, Bed	General
Mattress, Non-Powered Flotation Therapy	Physical Med
Pad, Heating, Circulating Fluid	General
Pad, Pressure, Gel, Operating Table	General
Pressure Pad, Alternating, Disposable	General
Pressure Pad, Alternating, Reusable	General
Protector, Heel	General
Pump, Alternating Pressure Pad	General
Warmer, Infusion Fluid, Thermal	General

GBC, INC.

190 South Union Blvd., Lakewood, CO 80228   **(303) 988-6450**
FDA Number: n/a   *Fax:* 303) 989-5923
E-mail: info@gbcinc.com
Web site: www.gbcinc.com
Total Employees: 4   *Marketing Staff:* 2   *Sales Staff:* 2
Ownership: Private
Produces/Sells CE-marked Devices: N
Federal Procurement Eligibility: Small Business
Distribution: Manufacturer Direct, OEM, Importer, Exporter
General Admin.: C. Applegate/President

Lamp, Surgical, Incandescent	Surgery

GBF GRAPHICS, INC.

7300 Niles Center Road, Skokie, IL 60077-3286   **800-GBF-TEAM**
847-677-1700
FDA Number: n/a   *Fax:* 847-677-2598
E-mail: info@gbfgraphics.com
Web site: www.gbfgraphics.com
Annual Revenue: $5-$10 Million
Year Founded: 1951
Total Employees: 350   *Marketing Staff:* 6   *Sales Staff:* 6
Produces/Sells CE-marked Devices: N
General Admin.: Tony Sorrentino/Manager Human Resources
         Richard S. Kuntz/President
Mktg./Adv.: Janice Long/Coord. Marketing
         Jill Snodgrass/Manager Marketing
         Ron Marak/Manager Marketing & Sales
         Greg Herzog/Supervisor Sales
Production: Randal K. Hopson/Senior Vice President Manufacturing
         Fred Raumann/Vice President Quality Assurance

Labware, Blood Collection	Chemistry

GC AMERICA, INC.

3737 W. 127th St., Aslip, IL 60803   **800-323-3386**
708-597-0900
FDA Number: 1410097   *Fax:* 708-371-5148
E-mail: gca_sales@gcamerica.com
Web site: www.gcamerica.com
Annual Revenue: $25-$50 Million

GC AMERICA, INC.
800-323-3386 *(cont'd)*

Total Employees: 150   *Marketing Staff:* 32   *Sales Staff:* 32
Ownership: Private
Quality System Registration Information: ISO9001
Produces/Sells CE-marked Devices: N
Distribution: Manufacturer Through Distributor
Mktg./Adv.: John O'Neil/Director Marketing & Sales

Activator, Ultraviolet, Polymerization	Dental And Oral
Adhesive, Bracket And Conditioner, Resin	Dental And Oral
Agent, Polishing, Abrasive, Oral Cavity	Dental And Oral
Base, Denture, Relining, Repairing, Rebasing, Resin	Dental And Oral
Cement, Dental	Dental And Oral
Crown And Bridge, Temporary, Resin	Dental And Oral
Dam, Rubber	Dental And Oral
Handle, Instrument, Dental	Dental And Oral
Implant, Endosseous	Dental And Oral
Material, Impression	Dental And Oral
Material, Tooth Shade, Resin	Dental And Oral
Post, Root Canal	Dental And Oral
Powder, Porcelain	Dental And Oral
Sterilant, Medical Device	General
Tooth Bonding Agent, Resin Restoration	Dental And Oral
Varnish, Cavity	Dental And Oral

GC AMERICA, INC.
800-323-7063
3737 West 127th St., Alsip, IL 60803   **708-597-0900**
FDA Number: 1410097   *Fax:* 800-GCF-AXME
E-mail: gca_sales@gcamerica.com
Web site: www.gcamerica.com
Ownership: Private
Produces/Sells CE-marked Devices: N

Cement, Dental	Dental And Oral
Crown And Bridge, Temporary, Resin	Dental And Oral
Material, Impression	Dental And Oral
Material, Tooth Shade, Resin	Dental And Oral
Powder, Porcelain	Dental And Oral
Remover, Crown	Dental And Oral
Strip, Polishing Agent	Dental And Oral
Tooth Bonding Agent, Resin Restoration	Dental And Oral
Varnish, Cavity	Dental And Oral

GCX CORP.
800-228-2555
3875 Cypress Drive, Petaluma, CA 94954-5635   **707-773-1100**
FDA Number: n/a   *Fax:* 707-773-1180
E-mail: sales@gcx.com
Web site: www.gcx.com
Annual Revenue: $50-$100 Million
Year Founded: 1971
Total Employees: 155   *Marketing Staff:* 2   *Sales Staff:* 12
Ownership: Private
Quality System Registration Information: ISO9001
Produces/Sells CE-marked Devices: Y
Federal Procurement Eligibility: Small Business
Distribution: Manufacturer Direct, Manufacturer Through Distributor, Manufacturer Through Manufacturer Reps, OEM, Exporter
General Admin.: Mark Ross/General Manager
       John M. Kruger/President
Mktg./Adv.: Bradley Cohen/Division Manager
       Mr. Clint Thompson/Manager Sales
Production: Mark Ross/Director Quality Assurance
       Mr. Cris Daugbjerg/Manager Engineering

Cart, Monitor	General
Cart, Other	General
Headwall System (Patient Room)	General
Mount, Equipment	General
Mount, Monitor (Support)	General
Mount, Television Set	General

GDM ELECTRONIC AND MEDICAL
408-945-4100
2070 Ringwood Ave., San Jose, CA 95131
FDA Number: 2950196   *Fax:* 408-945-4070
E-mail: sales@gdm1.com
Web site: www.gdm1.com
Medical Products Sales Volume: $9,600,000
Annual Revenue: $5-$10 Million
Year Founded: 1983
Total Employees: 100   *Marketing Staff:* 5   *Sales Staff:* 5
Ownership: Private
Quality System Registration Information: ISO9001
Produces/Sells CE-marked Devices: Y
Federal Procurement Eligibility: Small Business
Distribution: Manufacturer Direct
General Admin.: Grant Murphy/Chief Executive Officer
       Shawn Gorham/Vice President
Mktg./Adv.: Susie Perches/Manager Business
Production: Abdulaziz Karimi/Director Quality Assurance

Computer, Bar Code	General
Contract Assembly	General
Contract Manufacturing	General

GDM ELECTRONIC AND MEDICAL
408-945-4100 *(cont'd)*

Contract Manufacturing, Pharmaceuticals/Chemicals	General
Contract Manufacturing, Product, Disposable	General
Contract Manufacturing, Product, Durable	General
Contract Packaging	General
Kit, Identification, Glucose (Non-Ferment)	Microbiology
Pack, Custom/Special Procedure	General
Packaging Material	General
Sealer, Packaging	General
Service, Printing	General

GDM ELECTRONIC ASSEMBLY
See Gdm Electronic And Medical

GE CAPITAL
800-323-6217
3000 Lakeside Drive, Suite 200N,
Bannockburn, IL 60015
FDA Number: n/a   *Fax:* 800-443-3432
E-mail: robert.herb@gecapital.com
Web site: www.gecapital.com
Annual Revenue: More than $100 Million
Total Employees: 130   *Marketing Staff:* 4   *Sales Staff:* 35
Ownership: General Electric Company
Stock Symbol: GE
Traded On: NYSE
Produces/Sells CE-marked Devices: N
Distribution: Manufacturer Direct, Manufacturer Through Distributor, Manufacturer Through Manufacturer Reps
Mktg./Adv.: Rob Herb/Manager Sales
       Roger Dalgleish/National Sales Representative
       Stacey Kuhfuss/National Sales Representative

Service, Equipment Leasing	General

GE CLINICAL SERVICES
888-367-2773
2300 Meadowvale Blvd.,   **905-858-5100**
Mississauga, ONT L5N-5 Canada
FDA Number: n/a   *Fax:* 905-567-3778
E-mail: david.baxter@med.ge.com
Web site: www.ge.com
Year Founded: 1998
Total Employees: 50
Ownership: Private
Produces/Sells CE-marked Devices: N
Distribution: Service Direct

GE HEALTHCARE
877-446-3743
200 E. Randolph Street, Suite 2435,   **312-565-6868**
Chicago, IL 60601
FDA Number: 2183926   *Fax:* 312-565-6870
E-mail: marketing@merge.com
Web site: www.merge.com
Medical Products Sales Volume: $37,000,000
Annual Revenue: $25-$50 Million
Year Founded: 1987
Total Employees: 50   *Marketing Staff:* 6   *Sales Staff:* 19
Ownership: Public
Stock Symbol: MRGE
Traded On: NASDAQ
Quality System Registration Information: ISO9001
Produces/Sells CE-marked Devices: Y
Federal Procurement Eligibility: Small Business
Distribution: Manufacturer Direct, Manufacturer Through Distributor, OEM, Service Direct, Exclusive Distributor
General Admin.: Mr. Jeff Surges/Chief Executive Officer
       Mr. Justin Dearborn/President
Research: Mr. Antonia Wells/Executive Vice President Research & Development
Finance: Mr. Steve Oreskovich/Chief Financial Officer

Computer, Diagnostic, Programmable	Cardiovascular
Computer, Imaging, Presurgery	Surgery
Gas Machine, Analgesia	Anesthesiology
Guide, Surgical, Needle	Surgery
Image Processing System	Radiology
Radiographic Picture Archiving/Communication System (PACS)	Radiology

GE HEALTHCARE
See Ge Medical Systems Information Technologies

GE HEALTHCARE IITS LLC
201-934-8644
40 Boroline Rd., Allendale, NJ 07401
FDA Number: 3003966370
Web site: www.gehealthcare.com
Ownership: Private
Stock Symbol: GE
Traded On: NYSE
Produces/Sells CE-marked Devices: N

Image Processing System	Radiology

GE HEALTHCARE INTEGRATED IT SOLUTIONS
877-519-4471
40 Idx Drive, P.O. Box 1070, Burlington, VT 05402   **802-862-1022**
FDA Number: 1225057
Web site: www2.gehealthcare.com
Year Founded: 1969
Total Employees: 2400
Ownership: Ge Healthcare
Stock Symbol: IDXC
Traded On: NASDAQ
Produces/Sells CE-marked Devices: N
General Admin.: Vishal Wanchoo/President, Chief Executive Officer
  Image Processing System   Radiology

GE HEALTHCARE INTEGRATED IT SOLUTIONS
  See Ge Healthcare It

GE HEALTHCARE IT
847-277-5000
540 W Northwest Highway, Barrington, IL 60010
FDA Number: 3004526608   Fax: 847-277-5240
Web site: www.gehealthcare.com
Ownership: Ge Healthcare
Stock Symbol: GE
Traded On: NYSE
Produces/Sells CE-marked Devices: N
  Device, Storage, Image, Digital   Radiology
  Image Processing System   Radiology
  Monitor, Perinatal   Obstetrics/Gynecology
  System, Communication, Image, Digital   Radiology

GE HEALTHCARE TECHNOLOGIES SURGERY NAVIGATION
800-708-3856
439 South Union Street, Lawrence, MA 01843   **978-552-5200**
FDA Number: 9025003   Fax: 978-552-5193
Web site: www.gehealthcare.com
Total Employees: 73   Marketing Staff: 6   Sales Staff: 13
Ownership: Ge Healthcare Technologies Surgery Navigation
Quality System Registration Information: ISO9001
Produces/Sells CE-marked Devices: Y
Distribution: Manufacturer Direct
General Admin.: Linda Brown/Director Human Resources
    Maurice R. Ferre`/President, Chief Executive Officer
Mktg./Adv.: Jonathan Lauer/Director Marketing
    Lewis Levine/Director Product Development
    Rich Grant/Manager National Sales
    Rich Grant/Vice President Marketing & Sales
Production: Patricia A. Carpenter/Vice President Manufacturing
    Peter Ohanian/Vice President Quality Assurance & Regulatory Affairs
Research: Allan G. Dennison/Vice President Product Development
    Allan G. Dennison/Vice President Research & Development
Finance: Reed Malleck/Vice President Admin., Finance
Purchasing: Kevin Rembis/Manager Purchasing
  Computer, Image, Endoscopic   General
Medical Product Subsidiaries (Listed Separately)
Ge Healthcare Technologies Surgery Navigation

GE INDUSTRIAL, SENSING
800-833-9438
1100 Technology Park Drive,   **978-437-1000**
Billerica, MA 01821
FDA Number: 1218944   Fax: 215-953-2569
E-mail: sensing@ge.com
Web site: www.gesensing.com
Medical Products Sales Volume: $68,900,000
Year Founded: 1892
Total Employees: 600
Ownership: General Electric Company
Stock Symbol: GE
Traded On: NYSE
Quality System Registration Information: ISO9001
Produces/Sells CE-marked Devices: Y
Distribution: Manufacturer Direct, Manufacturer Through Distributor, Manufacturer Through Manufacturer Reps
General Admin.: Caroline Reda/President, Chief Executive Officer
Mktg./Adv.: Kermit Hoffman/Manager Sales
Finance: Andrew Cring/Chief Financial Officer
  Catheter, Cardiac Thermodilution   Cardiovascular
  Electrode, Myocardial   Cardiovascular
  Incubator, Neonatal   General
  Monitor, Respiratory   Surgery
  Stethoscope, Esophageal   Anesthesiology
  Thermistor   General
  Thermometer, Electronic   General
  Thermometer, Electronic, Continuous   General

GE INFRASTRUCTURE WATER & PROCESS TECHNOLOGIES
877-522-7867
5951 Clearwater Drive,   **952-988-6665**
Minnetonka, MN 55343
FDA Number: n/a
E-mail: lab.store@ge.com   Fax: 952-988-6662
Web site: www.gewater.com
Total Employees: 3900   Marketing Staff: 4   Sales Staff: 3
Ownership: GE Infrastructure
Stock Symbol: GE
Traded On: NYSE
Quality System Registration Information: ISO9001
Produces/Sells CE-marked Devices: N
Distribution: Manufacturer Through Distributor, OEM
Mktg./Adv.: Julia M. Kravchenko/Manager Marketing & Advertising Communications
  Filter, Bacteriological, Laboratory   Chemistry
  Filter, Intravenous Tubing   General
  Filter, Membrane   Chemistry
  Filter, Syringe   General
  Unit, Filter, Membrane   Chemistry

GE INSPECTION TECHNOLOGIES, LP
717-447-1278
50 Industrial Park Rd., Lewistown, PA 17044
FDA Number: 2519904   Fax: 717) 242-2606
Ownership: Private
Produces/Sells CE-marked Devices: N
  Transducer, Ultrasonic   Cardiovascular
  Transducer, Ultrasonic, Diagnostic   Radiology

GE IONICS, INC.
214-339-2135
4740 Bronze Way, Dallas, TX 75236-1999
FDA Number: 1651791
Ownership: Private
Produces/Sells CE-marked Devices: N
  Purification System, Water   Gastroenterology/Urology

GE MAGNETS
847-277-5002
3001 West Radio Dr., Florence, SC 29501
FDA Number: 3005326970
Web site: www.gehealthcare.com
Ownership: Ge Healthcare
Stock Symbol: GE
Traded On: NYSE
Produces/Sells CE-marked Devices: N
  Nuclear Magnetic Resonance Imaging System   Radiology

GE MEDICAL SYSTEMS INFORMATION TECHNOLOGIES
800-558-5544
4502 Woodland Corp. Blvd, Tampa, FL 33614   **877-274-8456**
FDA Number: 1030184   Fax: 813-887-2413
Web site: www.gehealthcare.com
Ownership: Ge Healthcare
Stock Symbol: GE
Traded On: NYSE
Quality System Registration Information: ISO9001
Produces/Sells CE-marked Devices: N
Distribution: Manufacturer Direct
General Admin.: Carol Brooks/Executive Assistant
    Heath T. Menshouse/General Manager
Mktg./Adv.: Amy Lee/Manager Business
Production: George Charles/Product Manager
  Cuff, Blood Pressure   Cardiovascular
  Facility, Equipment, Medical, Mobile   General
  Monitor, Blood Pressure, Indirect, Anesthesiology   Anesthesiology
  Monitor, Blood Pressure, Indirect, Automatic   Cardiovascular
  Monitor, Pulse Rate   Anesthesiology

GE MEDICAL SYSTEMS INFORMATION TECHNOLOGIES
414-721-2584
465 Pan American Dr, Suite 11, El paso, TX 79907
FDA Number: 1651104
Web site: www.gehealthcare.com
Ownership: Ge Healthcare
Stock Symbol: GE
Traded On: NYSE
Produces/Sells CE-marked Devices: N

GE MEDICAL SYSTEMS INFORMATION TECHNOLOGIES
800-643-6439
8200 West Tower Avenue,   **414-355-5000**
Milwaukee, WI 53223
FDA Number: 2124823   Fax: 414-355-3790
E-mail: Annette.Busateri@med.ge.com
Web site: www.gehealthcare.com
Medical Products Sales Volume: $16,600,000,000

GE MEDICAL SYSTEMS INFORMATION   800-643-6439 *(cont'd)*
Year Founded: 2000
Total Employees: 46000
Ownership: Ge Healthcare
Stock Symbol: GE
Traded On: NYSE
Quality System Registration Information: ISO9000
Produces/Sells CE-marked Devices: Y
Distribution: Manufacturer Direct, Manufacturer Through Distributor, Manufacturer Through Manufacturer Reps
General Admin.: Dow Wilson/Chief Executive Officer
        Pam Krop/Vice President, General Counsel
Mktg./Adv.: Ellen van Oostenbrugge/Director Marketing & Communications
        Mike Minogue/Vice President Marketing & Sales
Production: Bill Berezowitz/Vice President Manufacturing
        Gary Bobb/Vice President Services
Finance: Scott Schenkel/Chief Financial Officer

Analyzer, ECG	Cardiovascular
Analyzer, Gas, Argon, Gaseous Phase	Anesthesiology
Analyzer, Gas, Carbon-Dioxide, Blood Phase, Indwelling	Anesthesiology
Analyzer, Gas, Carbon-Dioxide, Gaseous Phase (Capnograph)	Anesthesiology
Analyzer, Gas, Carbon-Dioxide, Partial Pressure, Blood	Anesthesiology
Analyzer, Gas, Carbon-Monoxide, Gaseous Phase	Anesthesiology
Analyzer, Gas, Halothane, Gaseous Phase (Anesthetic Conc.)	Anesthesiology
Analyzer, Gas, Helium, Gaseous Phase	Anesthesiology
Analyzer, Gas, Neon, Gaseous Phase	Anesthesiology
Analyzer, Gas, Nitrogen, Gaseous Phase	Anesthesiology
Analyzer, Gas, Oxygen, Partial Pressure, Blood Phase	Anesthesiology
Analyzer, Gas, Water Vapor, Gaseous Phase	Anesthesiology
Cable/Lead, ECG	Cardiovascular
Cardiac Output Unit, Indicator Dilution (Thermal)	Cardiovascular
Communication Equipment	General
Computer Software	General
Computer Software, Hospital/Nursing Management	General
Computer, Blood Pressure	Cardiovascular
Computer, Diagnostic, Pre-Programmed, Single-Function	Cardiovascular
Computer, Diagnostic, Programmable	Cardiovascular
Computer, Patient Monitor	Anesthesiology
Computer, Stress Exercise	Cardiovascular
Defibrillator, Battery-Powered, High Energy	Cardiovascular
Drain, Tee (Water Trap)	Anesthesiology
Electrocardiograph, Interpretive	Cardiovascular
Electrocardiograph, Multi-Channel	Cardiovascular
Electrocardiograph, Single Channel	Cardiovascular
Electrode, Electrocardiograph	Cardiovascular
Gas, Calibrated (Specified Concentration)	Anesthesiology
Heater, Perineal, Radiant, Non-Contact	Obstetrics/Gynecology
Mass Spectrometer, Clinical Use	Toxicology
Monitor, Apnea	General
Monitor, Blood Pressure, Indirect, Anesthesiology	Anesthesiology
Monitor, Blood Pressure, Indirect, Automatic	Cardiovascular
Monitor, Blood Pressure, Invasive (Arterial)	Cardiovascular
Monitor, Cardiac (Cardiotachometer & Rate Alarm)	Cardiovascular
Monitor, Cardiac Output, Thermal (Balloon Type Catheter)	Surgery
Monitor, Cardiac Output, Trend (Arterial Pressure Pulse)	Surgery
Monitor, ECG	Cardiovascular
Monitor, ECG, Ambulatory, Real-Time	Cardiovascular
Monitor, ECG, Arrhythmia	Cardiovascular
Monitor, Fetal	Obstetrics/Gynecology
Monitor, Heart Rate, R-Wave (ECG)	Cardiovascular
Monitor, Neonatal, Heart Rate	General
Monitor, Physiological, Stress Exercise	Cardiovascular
Monitor, Pulse Rate	Anesthesiology
Monitor, Respiratory	Surgery
Monitor, Temperature (With Probe)	Anesthesiology
Monitor, Temperature, Surgery	Surgery
Monitor, Ventilatory Frequency	Anesthesiology
Oximeter, Intracardiac	Cardiovascular
Paper, Recording, ECG/EEG	General
Recorder, Long-Term, ECG	Cardiovascular
Recorder, Long-Term, ECG, Portable (Holter Monitor)	Cardiovascular
Recorder, Paper Chart	Cardiovascular
Scanner, Long-Term, ECG, Recording	Cardiovascular
Telemetry Unit, Physiological, ECG	Cardiovascular
Telemetry Unit, Physiological, Multiple Channel	General
Telemetry Unit, Physiological, Neurological	Cns/Neurology
Transmitter/Receiver System, ECG, Telephone Multi-Channel	Cardiovascular
Transmitter/Receiver System, ECG, Telephone Single-Channel	Cardiovascular
Transmitter/Receiver System, Physiological, Radiofrequency	Cardiovascular
Transmitter/Receiver System, Pulmonary Monitor, Telephone	General
Treadmill, Powered	Physical Med
Ventilator, Anesthesia Unit	Anesthesiology

Medical Product Subsidiaries (Listed Separately)
Data Critical Corp.
Instrumentarium Imaging, Inc.
Marquette Medical Systems, Inc.
Vitalcom, Inc.

GE MEDICAL SYSTEMS INFORMATION TECHNOLOGIES   888-202-5528
9900 Innovation Dr., Wauwatosa, WI 53226   414-721-2584
FDA Number: 3005860720
Web site: www.gehealthcare.com
Ownership: Ge Healthcare
Stock Symbol: GE
Traded On: NYSE
Produces/Sells CE-marked Devices: N

GE MEDICAL SYSTEMS INFORMATION TECHNOLOGIES, INC.   414-721-2584
100 Marquette Drive, Jupiter, FL 33468
FDA Number: 1051778
Web site: www.gehealthcare.com
Ownership: Ge Healthcare
Stock Symbol: GE
Traded On: NYSE
Produces/Sells CE-marked Devices: N

GE MEDICAL SYSTEMS ULTRASOUND AND PRIMARY CARE DIA   608-826-7050
3030 ohmeda dr, Madison, WI 53718
FDA Number: 2183066
Web site: www.gehealthcare.com   *Fax: 608-826-7106*
Ownership: Ge Healthcare
Stock Symbol: GE
Traded On: NYSE
Produces/Sells CE-marked Devices: N

Densitometer, Bone, Single Photon	Radiology
Scanner, Ultrasonic (Pulsed Doppler)	Radiology
Scanner, Ultrasonic (Pulsed Echo)	Radiology
Sonometer, Bone	Radiology
System, X-Ray, Mobile	Radiology

GE MEDICAL SYSTEMS, LLC   262-548-2355
3000 N Grandview Blvd., W-417, Waukesha, WI 53188
FDA Number: 2126677
E-mail: gehealthcare.community@ge.com
Web site: www.gehealthcare.com
Ownership: Ge Healthcare
Stock Symbol: GE
Traded On: NYSE
Produces/Sells CE-marked Devices: N

Changer, Radiographic Film/Cassette	Radiology
Collimator, Radiographic, Automatic	Radiology
Defibrillator, Battery-Powered, High Energy	Cardiovascular
Dryer, Film, Radiographic	Dental And Oral
Generator, Diagnostic X-Ray, High Voltage, Single Phase	Radiology
Holder, Radiographic Cassette, Wall-Mounted	Radiology
Holder, X-Ray Film	Dental And Oral
Illuminator, Radiographic Film	Radiology
Illuminator, Radiographic Film, Explosion-Proof	Radiology
Image Processing System	Radiology
Imager, X-Ray, Solid State (Flat Panel/Digital)	Radiology
Media, Contrast, Radiologic	Radiology
Mount, X-Ray Tube, Diagnostic	Radiology
Phantom, Anthropomorphic, Radiographic	Radiology
Processor, Radiographic Film, Automatic	Radiology
Radiographic Unit, Diagnostic	Radiology
Radiographic Unit, Diagnostic, Intraoral	Dental And Oral
Radiographic Unit, Diagnostic, Mammographic	Radiology
Radiographic Unit, Diagnostic, Tomographic	Radiology
Radiographic/Fluoroscopic Unit, Image-Intensified	Radiology
Restraint, Protective (Body)	General
Scanner, Computed Tomography, X-Ray, Special Procedure	Radiology
Scanner, Emission Computed Tomography	Radiology
Screen, Intensifying, Radiographic, Dental	Dental And Oral
Shield, Gonadal	Radiology
Shield, Protective, Personnel	Radiology
Spot Film Device	Radiology
System, Marking, Film, Radiographic	Radiology
System, X-Ray, Mobile	Radiology
Table, Radiographic, Tilting	Radiology
Tape, Measuring, Ruler And Caliper	Surgery
Test Pattern, Radiographic	Radiology

GE MEDICAL SYSTEMS, LLC   262-312-7117
3200 N. Grandview Blvd., Waukesha, WI 53188
FDA Number: 2183553
Web site: www.gehealthcare.com
Ownership: Ge Healthcare
Stock Symbol: GE
Traded On: NYSE
Produces/Sells CE-marked Devices: N

Coil, Magnetic Resonance, Specialty	Radiology
Nuclear Magnetic Resonance Imaging System	Radiology

GE MEDICAL SYSTEMS, LLC — 262-312-7117 (cont'd)
Nuclear Magnetic Resonance Spectroscopic System — Radiology

GE MEDICAL SYSTEMS, LLC — 847-277-5002
4855 West Electric Ave., West Milwaukee, WI 53219
FDA Number: 2122726
Web site: www.gehealthcare.com
Ownership: Ge Healthcare
Stock Symbol: GE
Traded On: NYSE
Produces/Sells CE-marked Devices: N
Housing, X-Ray Tube, Diagnostic — Radiology
Scanner, Ultrasonic (Pulsed Doppler) — Radiology
Scanner, Ultrasonic (Pulsed Echo) — Radiology
Transducer, Ultrasonic, Diagnostic — Radiology

GE MEDICAL SYSTEMS, ULTRASOUND & PRIMARY CARE DIAGNOSTICS
See Ambassador Medical

GE OEC MEDICAL SYSTEMS — 978-552-5200
439 South Union St., Lawrence, MA 01843
FDA Number: 1225258
Web site: www.gehealthcare.com
Ownership: Ge Healthcare
Stock Symbol: GE
Traded On: NYSE
Produces/Sells CE-marked Devices: N
Image Processing System — Radiology
Radiographic/Fluoroscopic Unit, Image-Intensified — Radiology

GE OEC MEDICAL SYSTEMS INC. — 800-874-7378
384 Wright Brothers Drive, — 801-328-9300
Salt Lake City, UT 84116
FDA Number: 1720753 — *Fax:* 801-328-4300
Web site: www.gehealthcare.com
Medical Products Sales Volume: $2,700,000
Year Founded: 2002
Total Employees: 34 — *Marketing Staff:* 8
Ownership: Ge Healthcare
Stock Symbol: GE
Traded On: NYSE
Quality System Registration Information: ISO9000
Produces/Sells CE-marked Devices: Y
Federal Procurement Eligibility: Small Business
Distribution: Manufacturer Direct, Manufacturer Through Distributor, Manufacturer Through Manufacturer Reps
General Admin.: Pete McCabe/President, Chief Executive Officer
　Marsha Fish/Vice President Human Resources
Mktg./Adv.: Hurley Raynor/Director National Accounts
　Heinz Gloor/Manager International Marketing & Sales
　Steve Hauenstein/Manager Marketing & Communications
　Larry Harrawood/Vice President Business Development
　Larry E. Harrawood/Vice President Marketing
　Dan Edwards/Vice President Sales
Production: Dick Peterson/Manager Materials
　John Sawyer/Manager Regulatory Affairs
　Gary Glowe/Vice President Manufacturing
　Ted Parrot/Vice President Regulatory Affairs
Research: Barry Hanover/Vice President Engineering
Finance: Clarence Verhoef/Controller
Guide, Surgical, Instrument — Surgery
Image Intensification System — Radiology
Image Processing System — Radiology
Monitor, Patient Position, Light Beam — Radiology
Radiographic Unit, Digital Subtraction Angiographic (DSA) — Radiology
Radiographic/Fluoroscopic Unit, Image-Intensified — Radiology
Radiographic/Fluoroscopic Unit, Mobile C-Arm — Radiology
System, X-Ray, Mobile — Radiology
Table, Cystometric, Non-Electrical — Gastroenterology/Urology
Table, Operating Room, Mechanical — Surgery

GE PARALLEL DESIGN, INC. — 480-222-7000
4313 E Cotton Center Blvd, Suite 100, Phoenix, AZ 85040
FDA Number: 2032350 — *Fax:* 208-474-3374
Ownership: Private
Produces/Sells CE-marked Devices: N
Scanner, Ultrasonic (Pulsed Doppler) — Radiology
Scanner, Ultrasonic (Pulsed Echo) — Radiology
Transducer, Ultrasonic, Diagnostic — Radiology

GE PARALLEL DESIGN, INC. — 414-721-2584
4313 East Cotton Center Blvd., Suite 100, Phoenix, AZ 85040
FDA Number: n/a
Web site: www.gehealthcare.com
Ownership: Ge Healthcare
Stock Symbol: GE
Traded On: NYSE
Produces/Sells CE-marked Devices: N

GE PARALLEL DESIGN, INC. — 414-721-2584 (cont'd)
Scanner, Ultrasonic (Pulsed Doppler) — Radiology
Scanner, Ultrasonic (Pulsed Echo) — Radiology
Transducer, Ultrasonic, Diagnostic — Radiology

GEA WESTFALIA SEPARATOR, INC. — 201-767-3900
100 Fairway Court, Northvale, NJ 07647
FDA Number: n/a — *Fax:* 201-767-3416
E-mail: salesinfo@wsus.com
Web site: www.wsus.com
Annual Revenue: $5-$10 Million
Ownership: WEST FALIA SEPARATOR, INC.
Quality System Registration Information: ISO9001
Produces/Sells CE-marked Devices: Y
Distribution: Service Direct, Exclusive Distributor, Importer
Mktg./Adv.: Kim Trager/Director Marketing & Sales
Finance: Greg Robinson/Chief Financial Officer
Service, Maintenance/Repair — General

GEBAUER COMPANY — 800-321-9348
4444 East 153rd Street, Cleveland, OH 44128 — 216-581-3030
FDA Number: 1519179 — *Fax:* 216-581-4970
E-mail: information@gebauerco.com
Web site: www.gebauerco.com
Medical Products Sales Volume: $2,600,000
Year Founded: 1898
Total Employees: 34 — *Marketing Staff:* 1 — *Sales Staff:* 3
Ownership: Private
Produces/Sells CE-marked Devices: N
Federal Procurement Eligibility: Small Business
Distribution: Manufacturer Direct, Manufacturer Through Distributor
General Admin.: John A. Giltinan/President, Chief Executive Officer
　Ted Kulak/Vice President Human Resources
　Bill Evans/Vice President, General Manager
Mktg./Adv.: Libby Tamas/Director International Sales
　Ralph Stilphen/Director National Accounts
　Heather Poltorek/Manager Advertising
　Ralph Stilphen/Vice President Marketing & Sales
Production: Suzanne Wojcik/Director Quality Assurance & Regulatory Affairs
　Ron Coleman/Manager Materials
Refrigerant, Topical (Vapocoolant) — Physical Med
Saliva, Artificial — Dental And Oral

GEEN HEALTHCARE INC. — 800-565-4336
931 Progress Ave. Ste.13, — 416-439-2237
Scarborough, ONT M1G 3 Canada
FDA Number: n/a — *Fax:* 416-439-6934
E-mail: geenhealth@earthlink.net
Year Founded: 1994
Total Employees: 10
Ownership: Private
Produces/Sells CE-marked Devices: Y
Federal Procurement Eligibility: Small Business
Distribution: Manufacturer Through Distributor, Exclusive Distributor, Importer

GEERPRES — 800-253-0373
1780 Harvey St., Muskegon, MI 49443-0658 — 231-773-3211
FDA Number: n/a — *Fax:* 231-773-8263
E-mail: sales@geerpres.com
Web site: www.geerpres.com
Year Founded: 1935
Total Employees: 30 — *Marketing Staff:* 4 — *Sales Staff:* 2
Ownership: Private
Produces/Sells CE-marked Devices: N
Federal Procurement Eligibility: Small Business
Distribution: Manufacturer Through Distributor, Manufacturer Through Manufacturer Reps
General Admin.: Michael D. Gluhanich/President
Mktg./Adv.: Gail Baldwin/Director National Accounts
　Joe Fodrocy/Director Product Development
　Dave Maurer/Vice President Marketing & Sales
Production: Rudy Fierros/Manager Materials
Cart, Housekeeping — General
Housekeeping Equipment — General

GEIGER INSTRUMENT CO., INC
See Geiger Medical Technologies

GEIGER MEDICAL TECHNOLOGIES — 800-320-9612
608 13th Avenue, Council Bluffs, IA 15101-6401 — 712-323-3432
FDA Number: n/a — *Fax:* 712-323-1156
E-mail: info@geigermedical.com
Web site: www.geigermedical.com
Year Founded: 1913
Ownership: Private
Produces/Sells CE-marked Devices: N
Federal Procurement Eligibility: Small Business, Female Owned
Distribution: Manufacturer Direct, Manufacturer Through Distributor

GEIGER MEDICAL TECHNOLOGIES
800-320-9612 *(cont'd)*
Production: Diana Grothe/Manager Operations
  Cautery, Thermal, AC-Powered — Ophthalmology
  System, Evacuation, Smoke, Laser — Surgery

GEL CONCEPTS LLC.
973-884-8995
30 Leslie Court, Whippany, NJ 07981
FDA Number: 3003712571 — *Fax:* 972-884-1331
E-mail: info@gelconcepts.com
Web site: www.gelconcepts.com
Ownership: Private
Produces/Sells CE-marked Devices: N
  Protectant, Skin — Surgery

GELSMART LLC
973-884-8995
30 Leslie Ct., Suite B-202, Whippany, NJ 07981
FDA Number: 3005846541
  Bandage, Elastic — General
  Dressing, Wound, Occlusive — Surgery
  Orthosis, Limb Brace — Physical Med
  Protector, Skin Pressure — General
  Splint, Temporary Training — Physical Med

GEM MEDICAL INDUSTRIES, INC.
See Gem Medical Supplies Llc

GEM MEDICAL SUPPLIES LLC
877-436-6334
2165 Shermer Road, Unit B,
847-562-9890
Northbrook, IL 60062
FDA Number: n/a — *Fax:* 847-562-9894
E-mail: sales@gemmedicalsupplies.com
Web site: www.gemmedicalsupplies.com
Annual Revenue: $0-$1 Million
Ownership: Private
Produces/Sells CE-marked Devices: N
Federal Procurement Eligibility: Small Business
Distribution: Manufacturer Through Distributor, Manufacturer Through Manufacturer Reps
  Bag, Plastic — General
  Container, Sterilization (Tray) — General
  Isolation Unit, Surgical — General
  Liner, Laundry Hamper — General
  Waste Receptacle, Contaminated — General
  Wrap, Sterilization — General

GEM REFRIGERATOR CO.
877-436-7374
7340 Milnor Street, Philadelphia, PA 19136
215-568-0514
FDA Number: n/a — *Fax:* 215-568-3295
E-mail: info@gemref.com
Web site: www.gemref.com
Medical Products Sales Volume: $1,500,000
Annual Revenue: $1-$5 Million
Year Founded: 1925
Ownership: Private
Produces/Sells CE-marked Devices: N
Federal Procurement Eligibility: Small Business
Distribution: OEM
  Alarm, Refrigerator — Hematology
  Freezer, Blood Storage — Hematology
  Refrigerator, Biological — Microbiology
  Refrigerator, Blood Bank — Hematology

GEMA, INC.
773-878-2445
2434 W. Peterson Ave., Chicago, IL 60659
FDA Number: 1424555
Ownership: Private
Produces/Sells CE-marked Devices: N
  Orthosis, Cranial — Cns/Neurology

GEMINI BIO-PRODUCTS, INC.
916-273-5215
930 Riverside Parkway, West Sacramento, CA 95605
FDA Number: 3006236690
  Serum, Animal — Pathology

GEMINI, INC.
800-533-3631
103 Mensing Way, Cannon Falls, MN 55009-1143
507-263-3957
FDA Number: n/a — *Fax:* 507-263-4887
E-mail: sales@geminiplaques.com
Web site: www.geminiplaques.com
Annual Revenue: $0-$1 Million
Ownership: Private
Produces/Sells CE-marked Devices: N
Federal Procurement Eligibility: Small Business
Distribution: Manufacturer Direct
General Admin.: Jim Weinel/President
Mktg./Adv.: Patty Zimmerman/Manager Advertising
    Mark Hedin/Manager Contract Sales
    Jim Seeley/Manager National Sales

GEMINI, INC.
800-533-3631 *(cont'd)*
  Case, Protection, Equipment — General

GEMSPRO, S.A. DE C.V.
262-544-3894
Calle B #504 Parque Industrial, Almacetro, Apodaca, N.I. Mexico
FDA Number: 9616047
  Housing, X-Ray Tube, Diagnostic — Radiology

GEMTECH PRODUCTS, INC.
866-436-8321
10623 Tower Oaks Blvd., Houston, TX 77070
281-469-4042
FDA Number: n/a — *Fax:* 281-469-4409
E-mail: sales@gemtechmedical.com
Web site: www.gemtechmedical.com
Ownership: Private
Produces/Sells CE-marked Devices: N
  Binder, Medical, Therapeutic — General

GEN TRAK, INC.
800-221-7407
121 W. Swannanoa Ave., P.O. Box 1290,
336-622-5266
Liberty, NC 27298
FDA Number: 2523746 — *Fax:* 336-622-1750
E-mail: steve@gentrakinc.com
Web site: www.gentrakinc.com
Ownership: Private
Produces/Sells CE-marked Devices: N
  Reagents, Specific, Analyte — Hematology
  Test, B Lymphocyte Marker — Hematology
  Test, Quantitative, For Hla, Non-diagnostic — Hematology

GEN-PROBE, INC.
800-523-5001
10210 Genetic Center Drive,
858-410-8000
San Diego, CA 92121
FDA Number: 2024800 — *Fax:* 800-288-3141
E-mail: customerservice@gen-probe.com
Web site: www.gen-probe.com
Medical Products Sales Volume: $13,990,000
Annual Revenue: $100-$500 Million
Year Founded: 1983
Total Employees: 74 — *Marketing Staff:* 28 — *Sales Staff:* 39
Ownership: Public
Stock Symbol: GPRO
Traded On: NASDAQ
Quality System Registration Information: ISO9001
Produces/Sells CE-marked Devices: Y
Federal Procurement Eligibility: Small Business
Distribution: Manufacturer Direct, Manufacturer Through Distributor, Manufacturer Through Manufacturer Reps
General Admin.: Mr. Brad Phillips/Chief Information Officer
    Daniel L. Kacian/Chief Scientific Officer & Executive Vice President
    Mr. Carl Hull/President, Chief Executive Officer
    R. William Bowen/Vice President, General Counsel
Mktg./Adv.: Paul Gargan/Vice President Business Development
    Mr. Stephen Kondor/Vice President Marketing & Sales
Production: Mr. Jorgine Ellerbrock/Senior Vice President Operations
Research: Dr. Cristina Giachetti,/Vice President Product Development
Finance: Herm Rosenman/Chief Financial Officer, Vice President Finance
  Campylobacter SPP. — Microbiology
  Chlamydia Trachomatis — Microbiology
  DNA-Probe, Nucleic Acid Amplification, Chlamydia — Microbiology
  DNA-Probe, Reagent — Microbiology
  Disc, Strip And Reagent, Microorganism Differentiation — Microbiology
  EIA, Blastomyces Dermatitidis — Microbiology
  Kit, Identification, Neisseria Gonorrhoeae — Microbiology
  Kit, Mycobacteria Identification — Microbiology
  Kit, Screening, Urine — Microbiology
  Luminometer — Chemistry
  Mycoplasma SPP. DNA Reagents — Microbiology
  Photometer — Chemistry
  Reagent, DNA-Probe, Streptococcal — Microbiology
  Reagents, Specific, Analyte — Hematology
  Software, Blood Bank (Stand-Alone Products) — Hematology
  System, Automated, Microbiological — Microbiology
  Test, Bacterial Diagnostic — Microbiology
  Test, Reagent, Biochemical, Neisseria Gonorrhoeae — Microbiology
  Transport System, Aerobic — Microbiology
  Tube, Culture — Microbiology

GENADYNE BIOTECHNOLOGIES, INC.
800-208-2025
65 Watermill Lane, Great Neck, NY 11021
516-487-8787
FDA Number: 2435947 — *Fax:* 877-487-7878
E-mail: info@genadyne.com
Web site: www.genadyne.com
Ownership: Private
Produces/Sells CE-marked Devices: N
  Accessories, Wheelchair — Physical Med
  Armrest, Wheelchair — Physical Med

GENADYNE BIOTECHNOLOGIES, INC.   800-208-2025 *(cont'd)*
Mattress, Air Flotation   General
Mattress, Non-Powered Flotation Therapy   Physical Med
Pump, Nebulizer, Electric   Ear/Nose/Throat
Stimulator, Nerve, Transcutaneous (Pain Relief, TENS)   Cns/Neurology

GENBIO
See Innominata dba GENBIO

GENCHEM, INC.   714-529-1616
510 W. Central Avenue, Suite D, Brea, CA 92821
FDA Number: 3005432203
Complexone, Cresolphthalein, Calcium   Chemistry
Dye-Binding, Albumin, Bromcresol, Green   Chemistry
Electrode, Ion Specific, Sodium   Chemistry
Electrode, Ion Specific, Urea Nitrogen   Chemistry
Enzymatic Esterase-Oxidase, Cholesterol   Chemistry
Hexokinase, Glucose   Chemistry
Kinetic Method, Gamma-Glutamyl Transpeptidase   Chemistry
LDL & VLDL Precipitation, Cholesterol Via Esterase-Oxidase Chemistry
NAD Reduction/NADH Oxidation, Lactate Dehydrogenase   Chemistry
NADH Oxidation/NAD Reduction, AST/SGOT   Chemistry
Nitrophenylphosphate, Alkaline Phosphatase Or Isoenzymes   Chemistry
Phosphorus Reagent (Test System)   Chemistry
Photometric Method, Iron (Non-Heme)   Chemistry
Photometric Method, Magnesium   Chemistry
Reagent, Bilirubin (Total Or Direct Test System)   Chemistry
Reagent, Creatinine (Test System)   Chemistry
Reagent, Glucose (Test System)   Chemistry
Reagent, Protein, Total   Chemistry
SGPT, Ultraviolet   Chemistry
Saccharogenic, Amylase   Chemistry
Syringe, Piston   General
Urease And Glutamic Dehydrogenase, Urea Nitrogen   Chemistry
Uricase (Colorimetric), Uric Acid   Chemistry
pH Rate Measurement, Carbon-Dioxide   Chemistry

GENCOSOFT LLC.   714-625-8972
17042 Pinehurst Lane, Suite B, Huntington Beach, CA 92647
FDA Number: 3005971388
System, Communication, Image, Digital   Radiology

GENDEX CORP.
See Del Medical Systems

GENDEX, A DIVISION OF DENTSPLY
See Del Medical Systems

GENDEX-DEL MEDICAL IMAGING
See Del Medical Systems

GENDEX-DEL MEDICAL SYSTEMS GROUP
See Del Medical Systems

GENDRON, INC.   800-537-2521
400 E Lugbill Road, Archbold, OH 43502   419-445-6060
FDA Number: 1523528   *Fax:* 419-446-2631
E-mail: sales@gendronic.com
Web site: www.gendroninc.com
Year Founded: 1871
Total Employees: 60   *Marketing Staff:* 5   *Sales Staff:* 40
Ownership: Private
Produces/Sells CE-marked Devices: N
Federal Procurement Eligibility: Small Business, VA Contract
Distribution: Manufacturer Through Distributor, Manufacturer Through
Manufacturer Reps, Exporter
General Admin.: Fred Strobel/Chief Executive Officer
              Steven Cotter/President
Mktg./Adv.: Steven Cotter/Director Marketing
Finance: Linda Rossworm/Controller
Accessories, Wheelchair   Physical Med
Bed, Obese   General
Cart, Patient (Stretcher)   Anesthesiology
Chair, Other   General
Commode (Toilet)   General
Crutch   Physical Med
Footrest, Wheelchair   Physical Med
Patient Transfer Unit   General
Rail, Bath   General
Stretcher, Transfer   Surgery
Stretcher, Wheeled (Mobile)   General
Stretcher, Wheeled, Mechanical   Physical Med
Tips And Pads, Cane, Crutch And Walker   Physical Med
Transfer Device, Patient, Manual   General
Walker, Mechanical   Physical Med
Wheelchair, Manual   Physical Med
Wheelchair, Special Grade   Physical Med

GENE LOGIC   800-436-3564
**50 West Watkins Mill Road,   301-987-1700
Gaithersburg, MD 20878**
FDA Number: n/a   *Fax:* 301-987-1701
E-mail: info@genelogic.com

GENE LOGIC   800-436-3564 *(cont'd)*
Web site: www.genelogic.com
Medical Products Sales Volume: $24,340,000
Year Founded: 1994
Total Employees: 151
Ownership: Private
Produces/Sells CE-marked Devices: N
Federal Procurement Eligibility: Small Business
Distribution: Manufacturer Direct
General Admin.: Mark Gessler/President, Chief Executive Officer
              Tracey Espada/Vice President Human Resources
Mktg./Adv.: David Murray/Vice President Sales
Production: David Murray/Vice President Manufacturing
Research: Douglas Dolgivow/Vice President Research & Development
Computer Software   General

GENEGO INC.   269-983-7629
500 Renaissance Drive, #106, St. Joseph, MI 49085
FDA Number: n/a   *Fax:* 269-983-7654
Web site: http://www.genego.com
Ownership: Private
Produces/Sells CE-marked Devices: N
General Admin.: Dr. Yuri Nikolsky/Chief Executive Officer
              Dr. Andrej Bugrim/Chief Scientific Officer
              Dr. Tatiana Nikolskaya/Chief Scientific Officer
Mktg./Adv.: Ms. Julie Bryant/Vice President Business Development

GENENEWS LIMITED   866-375-0442
**2 East Beaver Creek Road, Building 2,   905-739-2030
Richmond Hill, ONTAR L4B 2 Canada**
FDA Number: n/a   *Fax:* 905-739-2031
E-mail: contact@genenews.com
Web site: www.genenews.com
Ownership: Private
Produces/Sells CE-marked Devices: N

GENENTECH, INC.   888-835-2555
1 DNA Way, South San Francisco, CA 94080-4990   650-225-1000
FDA Number: 2917293   *Fax:* 650-225-6000
Web site: www.gene.com
Annual Revenue: More than $1 Billion
Total Employees: 11186
Ownership: Public
Stock Symbol: GNE
Traded On: NYSE
Produces/Sells CE-marked Devices: N
Distribution: Manufacturer Direct
General Admin.: Pascal Soriot/Chief Executive Officer
              Steve Krognes/Chief Financial Officer, Senior Vice President
Antibody, Monoclonal   Microbiology
Genetic Engineering   Microbiology
Test, Antibody, Acquired Immune Deficiency Syndrome (AIDS) Hematology
Thromboplastin, Activated Partial   Hematology

GENEQ INC.   800-463-4363
8047 Jerry St. E, Montreal, QUE H1J-1H6 Canada   514-354-2511
FDA Number: n/a   *Fax:* 514-354-6948
E-mail: info@geneq.com
Web site: www.geneq.com
Year Founded: 1972
Total Employees: 25
Ownership: Private
Produces/Sells CE-marked Devices: N
Distribution: Service Direct, Exclusive Distributor

GENERAL AIR SERVICE AND SUPPLY   303-892-7003
6330 Colorado Blvd, Adams City, CO 80022
FDA Number: 1717152
Electrode, Blood pH   Chemistry
Gas, Calibrated (Specified Concentration)   Anesthesiology
Laser, Surgical   Surgery

GENERAL ASSEMBLY CORPORATION   877-GACNC4U
**140 Industrial Park Way,   336-246-5143
West Jefferson, NC 28694**
FDA Number: 1058500   *Fax:* 336-846-1676
E-mail: info@gacnc.com
Web site: www.gacnc.com
Medical Products Sales Volume: $7,700,000
Annual Revenue: $1-$5 Million
Year Founded: 2005
Total Employees: 55   *Marketing Staff:* 2   *Sales Staff:* 3
Ownership: Private
Produces/Sells CE-marked Devices: Y
Federal Procurement Eligibility: Small Business
Distribution: Manufacturer Direct, Importer
Production: Mr. Terry Van Natta/Manager Quality Assurance

GENERAL ASSEMBLY CORPORATION   877-GACNC4U *(cont'd)*
Device, Measurement, Potential, Skin   Cns/Neurology

GENERAL BIOMEDICAL SERVICE, INC.   800-558-9449
1900 25th St., Kenner, LA 70062   504-468-8597
FDA Number: n/a   *Fax:* 504-469-3723
E-mail: info@generalbiomedical.com
Web site: www.generalbiomedical.com
Medical Products Sales Volume: $2,000,000
Annual Revenue: $1-$5 Million
Year Founded: 1982
Total Employees: 9   *Marketing Staff:* 2   *Sales Staff:* 3
Ownership: Private
Produces/Sells CE-marked Devices: N
Federal Procurement Eligibility: Small Business
Distribution: Manufacturer Direct, Exporter
General Admin.: Steve Saladino/President
Mktg./Adv.: Ana M. Ortega/Manager Marketing & Sales

Oximeter, Pulse	General
Service, Import/Export	General
Service, Maintenance/Repair	General
Service, Parts, Repair	General
Service, Used Equipment	General
Ventilator, Continuous (Respirator)	Anesthesiology
Ventilator, Neonatal Respirator	General
Ventilator, Other	Anesthesiology
Ventilator, Pressure Cycled (IPPB Machine)	Anesthesiology
Ventilator, Volume (Critical Care)	Anesthesiology

GENERAL BUSINESS FORMS, INC.
See Gbf Graphics, Inc.

GENERAL CARDIAC TECHNOLOGY, INC.   831-471-2940
15814 Winchester Blvd #105, Los Gatos, CA 95030
FDA Number: 2938604
Ownership: Private
Produces/Sells CE-marked Devices: N

Binder, Breast	Obstetrics/Gynecology

GENERAL CHEMICAL CORP.
See Genlabs.

GENERAL CUBICLE CO.   800-869-4606
49 Meeker Avenue, Cranford, NJ 07016
FDA Number: n/a   *Fax:* 830-774-0357
E-mail: customerservice@generalcubicle.com
Web site: www.generalcubicle.com
Medical Products Sales Volume: $2,500,000
Annual Revenue: $1-$5 Million
Year Founded: 1962
Total Employees: 20
Ownership: C/S Group
Produces/Sells CE-marked Devices: N
Federal Procurement Eligibility: Small Business
Distribution: Manufacturer Direct, Manufacturer Through Manufacturer Reps
Mktg./Adv.: Dave Bronovicki/General Manager Sales
     Stacey Gaskill/Manager Marketing
Production: Mike Bradley/Vice President Manufacturing

Track And Carrier, Cubicle Curtain	General

GENERAL DENTAL PRODUCTS, INC.   888-367-6212
201 Ogden Avenue, Ely, NV 89301-1888   775-289-4461
FDA Number: 1450398   *Fax:* 775-289-6152
E-mail: gendentl@mwpower.net
Medical Products Sales Volume: $500,000
Annual Revenue: $0-$1 Million
Year Founded: 1982
Total Employees: 3   *Marketing Staff:* 1   *Sales Staff:* 1
Ownership: Bath Lumber/Ace Hardware
Produces/Sells CE-marked Devices: N
Federal Procurement Eligibility: Small Business
Distribution: Manufacturer Direct, Manufacturer Through Distributor, Manufacturer Through Manufacturer Reps, Exporter
General Admin.: Jed A. Peeler/President
Production: Jed A. Peeler/Manager Regulatory Affairs
Finance: Mr. Thomas Bath/Chief Financial Officer

Base, Denture, Relining, Repairing, Rebasing, Resin	Dental And Oral
Material, Investment	Dental And Oral
Mouthguard	Dental And Oral
Tray, Custom/Special Procedure	General
Wax, Dental	Dental And Oral

GENERAL DEVICES   201-313-7075
1000 River St., Ridgefield, NJ 07657
FDA Number: 2244646   *Fax:* 201-313-5671
E-mail: info@general-devices.com
Web site: www.general-devices.com
Annual Revenue: $1-$5 Million
Year Founded: 1979
Ownership: Private

GENERAL DEVICES   201-313-7075 *(cont'd)*
Quality System Registration Information: ISO9002
Produces/Sells CE-marked Devices: N
Federal Procurement Eligibility: Small Business
Distribution: Manufacturer Direct, Manufacturer Through Manufacturer Reps, OEM, Service Direct
General Admin.: Michael Smith/President, Chief Executive Officer
     Curtis M. Bashford/Vice President, General Manager
Mktg./Adv.: Rhea Lazarus-Smith/Director Sales
Production: Gregory Lowe/Director Engineering

Communication Equipment	General
Device, Measurement, Potential, Skin	Cns/Neurology
Recorder, Magnetic Tape/Disc	Cardiovascular
Service, Engineering/Design	General
Tester, Electrocardiograph Cable	Cardiovascular
Tester, Electrode, Surface, Electrocardiograph	Cardiovascular
Transmitter/Receiver, Physiological Signal, Infrared	Cardiovascular

GENERAL DEVICES CO., INC.   800-626-9484
1410 S. Post Road, Indianapolis, IN 46239   317-897-7000
FDA Number: n/a   *Fax:* 317-898-2917
E-mail: sales@generaldevices.com
Web site: www.generaldevices.com
Medical Products Sales Volume: $16,100,000
Annual Revenue: $25-$50 Million
Year Founded: 1953
Total Employees: 225   *Marketing Staff:* 3   *Sales Staff:* 17
Ownership: Private
Produces/Sells CE-marked Devices: N
Federal Procurement Eligibility: Small Business
Distribution: Manufacturer Direct, Manufacturer Through Distributor, Manufacturer Through Manufacturer Reps, OEM
General Admin.: Gladys Fall/Chairman
     Diane Thompson/Director Personnel
     Martin Fall/Executive Vice President
     Maxwell Fall/President, Chief Executive Officer
Mktg./Adv.: Kimberly O'Neil/Director Marketing
     Ron Stalzle/Vice President Marketing & Sales
Production: David Willis/Field Director
     Ed Hansen/Vice President Manufacturing
Research: Phillip Cutler/Vice President Engineering
Finance: Curt Vander Meer/Vice President Finance

Cabinet Casework, General Purpose	General
Cabinet, Instrument	General
Cabinet, Other	General

GENERAL DIAGNOSTICS
See Biomerieux Inc.

GENERAL ECONOPAK, INC.   888-871-8568
1725 N. 6th St., Philadelphia, PA 19122   215-763-8200
FDA Number: 2515314   *Fax:* 215-763-8118
E-mail: info@generaleconopak.com
Web site: www.generaleconopak.com
Medical Products Sales Volume: $5,500,000
Year Founded: 1966
Total Employees: 75   *Marketing Staff:* 3   *Sales Staff:* 6
Ownership: Private
Produces/Sells CE-marked Devices: N
Federal Procurement Eligibility: Small Business
Distribution: Manufacturer Direct
General Admin.: James G. Baxter/President, Chief Executive Officer
Mktg./Adv.: John Sincavage/Director Marketing & Product Development
     James Hallman/Manager International & National Sales
Production: James Hallman/Director Quality Assurance
     Steve Libros/Vice President Manufacturing & Materials
Finance: Jeffrey Markowitz/Treasurer

Apron, Surgical	Surgery
Bag, Body	General
Band, Sweat	General
Blanket, Infant	General
Blanket, Rescue	General
Care Kit, Baby	General
Coat, Laboratory	General
Cover, Arm Board	General
Cover, Cart	General
Cover, Laundry Hamper	General
Cover, Mattress, Waterproof	General
Cover, Other	General
Cover, Shoe, Conductive	General
Cover, Shoe, Non-Conductive	General
Cover, Shoe, Operating Room	Surgery
Curtain, Cubicle	General
Drape, Surgical, Disposable	Surgery
Dress, Scrub, Disposable	Surgery
Dressing, Other	General
Gown, Isolation, Surgical	Surgery
Gown, Other	General
Gown, Patient	Surgery

GENERAL ECONOPAK, INC.   888-871-8568 *(cont'd)*

Gown, Patient, Disposable	General
Gown, Surgical	Surgery
Hood, Surgical	Surgery
Kit, Shroud	Pathology
Linen	General
Linen, Bed	General
Mask, Face	General
Mitt/Washcloth, Patient	General
Pack, Custom/Special Procedure	General
Packaging, Sterilization	General
Pouch, Telemetry	General
Sheeting, Examination Table	General
Sheeting, Stretcher	General
Shoe, Operating Room	Surgery
Sponge, Gauze	Dental And Oral
Suit, Scrub, Disposable	Surgery
Suit, Surgical	Surgery
Towel/Towelette, Paper	General
Wrapper, Surgical Instrument (Sterile)	General

GENERAL ELECTRIC CO.   800-417-0575

3135 Easton Turnpike, Fairfield, CT 06828   **203-373-2211**

FDA Number: n/a
Web site: www.ge.com
Annual Revenue: More than $1 Billion
Year Founded: 1900
Total Employees: 323000
Ownership: Public
Stock Symbol: GE
Traded On: NYSE
Produces/Sells CE-marked Devices: N
Distribution: Manufacturer Through Distributor
General Admin.: Jeffrey R. Immelt/Chief Executive Officer, Chairman
         John Krenicki/Vice Chairman
         John G. Rice/Vice Chairman
         Michael A. Neal/Vice Chairman
         Keith S. Sherin/Vice Chairman, Chief Financial Officer

Lamp, Infrared	Physical Med
Lamp, Sun, Incandescent	General
Lamp, Ultraviolet (Spectrum A)	General
Lamp, Ultraviolet, Germicidal	General
Lamp, Ultraviolet, Physical Medicine	Physical Med
Light, Bilirubin (Phototherapy)	General
Receptacle, Electrical	General

GENERAL ELECTRIC LIGHTING

See General Electric Co.

GENERAL GASES & SUPPLIES CORP.

See Aga Linde Healthcare P.R. Inc.

GENERAL HEARING INSTRUMENTS, INC.   800-824-3021

175 Brookhollow Espl., Harahan, LA 70123   **504-733-3767**

FDA Number: 2317393
Web site: www.generalhearing.comÉ_Z
Ownership: Private
Produces/Sells CE-marked Devices: N

Hearing-Aid	Ear/Nose/Throat

GENERAL HEATH SYSTEMS INC.

See Healthcare Labels, Inc.

GENERAL HOSPITAL SUPPLY CORP.   704-225-9500

2844 Gray Fox Rd., Monroe, NC 28110

FDA Number: 1223662
Ownership: Private
Produces/Sells CE-marked Devices: N

Accessories, Operating Room, Table	Surgery
Table, Surgical, Orthopedic	Orthopedics
Tray, Surgical	Surgery
Tray, Surgical Instrument	Surgery
Wrap, Sterilization	General

GENERAL MEDICAL CO.   800-432-5362

1935 Armacost Ave.,   **310-820-5881**
Los Angeles, CA 90025

FDA Number: 2012353
E-mail: drionic@generalmedical.com   *Fax:* 310-826-5778
Web site: www.generalmedical.com
Year Founded: 1962
Ownership: Private
Produces/Sells CE-marked Devices: N
Federal Procurement Eligibility: Small Business
Distribution: Manufacturer Direct, Manufacturer Through Distributor
General Admin.: Robert Tapper/President

Epilator, High-Frequency, Needle-Type	Surgery
Iontophoresis Unit, Physical Medicine	Physical Med
System, Delivery, Drug, Non-invasive	General

GENERAL MEDICAL MANUFACTURING CO.

See Mckesson General Medical

GENERAL PYSIOTHERAPY, INC.   800-237-1832

13222 Lakefront Drive,   **314-291-1442**
Earth City, MO 63045

FDA Number: 1937060
E-mail: info@g5.com   *Fax:* 314-291-1485
Web site: www.g5.com
Year Founded: 1972
Total Employees: 75   *Marketing Staff:* 3   *Sales Staff:* 1
Ownership: GENERAL MEDVENTURES INT'L., LLC
Produces/Sells CE-marked Devices: N
Federal Procurement Eligibility: Small Business
Distribution: Manufacturer Direct, Manufacturer Through Distributor, Manufacturer Through Manufacturer Reps, Service Direct, Exporter
General Admin.: Thomas Muchisky/Chief Executive Officer
         Jeff W. Robertson/President

Massager, Therapeutic	Physical Med
Percussor	Cns/Neurology

GENERAL REFINERIES

See Harry J. Bosworth Company

GENERAL SCIENTIFIC CORP.   800-959-0153

77 Enterprise Drive, Ann Arbor, MI 48103   **734-996-9200**

FDA Number: 1834177
E-mail: info@surgitel.com   *Fax:* 734-662-0520
Web site: www.surgitel.com
Medical Products Sales Volume: $3,500,000
Annual Revenue: $5-$10 Million
Year Founded: 1990
Total Employees: 45
Ownership: Private
Produces/Sells CE-marked Devices: Y
Federal Procurement Eligibility: Small Business, Minority Owned, VA Contract
Distribution: Manufacturer Direct, Manufacturer Through Manufacturer Reps, Exporter
General Admin.: B. J. Chang/President, Chief Executive Officer
         Hank Gretzinger/Vice President
Mktg./Adv.: David Nowak/Director Marketing
         Sharon Chang/Vice President Marketing & Sales
Research: Charles Willoughby/Vice President Research & Development

Accessories, Light, Surgical	Surgery
Headlight, ENT	Ear/Nose/Throat
Lens, Other	Ophthalmology
Light Source, Endoscopic	Obstetrics/Gynecology
Light, Examination, Battery-Powered	General
Light, Surgical Headlight	Dental And Oral
Light, Surgical, Endoscopic	Surgery
Loupe, Diagnostic/Surgical	Surgery

GENERAL SCIENTIFIC INSTRUMENT SERVICES INC.   519-659-2275

1764 Oxford St. E, Ste. 1160, London, ONT N5V-3R6 Canada

FDA Number: n/a   *Fax:* 519-659-8893
E-mail: gsis@cscn.com
Web site: www.cscn.com/gsis.html
Year Founded: 1993
Total Employees: 10
Ownership: Private
Produces/Sells CE-marked Devices: N
Distribution: Service Direct

GENERAL SCIENTIFIC SAFETY EQUIPMENT CO.   800-523-0166

2553 E Somerset St. 1st Floor,   **215-739-7559**
Philadelphia, PA 19134

FDA Number: 9200386   *Fax:* 215-739-7441
Medical Products Sales Volume: $500,000
Year Founded: 1988
Total Employees: 2   *Sales Staff:* 2
Ownership: MEDICAL & SAFETY GROUP, INC.
Produces/Sells CE-marked Devices: N
Federal Procurement Eligibility: Small Business
Distribution: Manufacturer Through Distributor
General Admin.: Leon D'Amico/President
Mktg./Adv.: Angela D'Amico/Manager Contract Sales

Apron, Conductive	Surgery
Apron, Laboratory	Chemistry
Blanket, Rescue	General
Cutter, Ring	General
Eyeglasses	Ophthalmology
Finger Cot	General
Glove, Other	General
Kit, Burn	General
Kit, First Aid	Surgery
Shield, Eye, Ophthalmic	Ophthalmology
Stretcher, Hand-Carried	General
Stretcher, Wheeled (Mobile)	General

GENERAL SCIENTIFIC SAFETY EQUIPMENT CO. 800-523-0166
(cont'd)

Thermometer, Chemical Color Change	General

GENERAL TRANSCO INC.   **727-535-2534**
13265 Park Blvd, Seminole, FL 33776
FDA Number: n/a   *Fax:* 727-397-9374
E-mail: pgordy@worldnet.att.net
Web site: www.generaltransco.com
Medical Products Sales Volume: $500,000
Annual Revenue: $0-$1 Million
Ownership: Private
Produces/Sells CE-marked Devices: Y
Federal Procurement Eligibility: Small Business
Distribution: Manufacturer Direct

Surfactometer	Anesthesiology

GENERATIONS, INC.   **360-840-6550**
22895 Apple Ln, Sedro Woolley, WA 98284
FDA Number: 3004945415
Ownership: Private
Produces/Sells CE-marked Devices: N

Adaptor, Recreational	Physical Med

GENERIC MEDICAL DEVICE, INC.   **253-853-3594**
5727 Baker Way Nw, Suite 201, Gig Harbor, WA 98332
FDA Number: 3006142121

Clamp, Circumcision	Obstetrics/Gynecology
Mesh, Surgical, Polymeric	Surgery

GENERIC MEDICAL, INC.   **678-879-1000**
4064 D Nine Mcfarland Dr., Alpharetta, GA 30004
FDA Number: 1063314
Ownership: Private
Produces/Sells CE-marked Devices: N

Cuff, Blood Pressure	Cardiovascular

GENESEE BIOMEDICAL, INC.   **800-786-4890**
1308 S. Jason St., Denver, CO 80223   **303-777-3000**
FDA Number: 1723241   *Fax:* 303-777-8866
E-mail: support@geneseebiomedical.com
Web site: www.geneseebiomedical.com
Medical Products Sales Volume: $7,100,000
Year Founded: 1994
Total Employees: 43   *Marketing Staff:* 2
Ownership: Private
Quality System Registration Information: ISO9001
Produces/Sells CE-marked Devices: Y
Federal Procurement Eligibility: Small Business
Distribution: Manufacturer Direct, Manufacturer Through Distributor, Manufacturer Through Manufacturer Reps, OEM
General Admin.: John T. Wright/Chief Executive Officer
      Woody Mathison/President
Mktg./Adv.: Ms. Denise Frahler/Director Marketing & Sales
Production: Jon Potter/Manager Quality Assurance

Clip, Iris Retractor	Ophthalmology
Device, Stabilizer, Heart	Cardiovascular
Glove, Surgical	General
Marker, Cardiopulmonary Bypass (Vein Marker)	Cardiovascular
Monitor, Heart Rate, Other	Cardiovascular
Occluder, Cardiovascular	Cardiovascular
Pad, Insulation, Cardiac	General
Probe, Blood Flow, Extravascular	Cardiovascular
Punch, Aortic	Cardiovascular
Retractor	Orthopedics
Retractor, Cardiac	Cardiovascular

GENESEN PAN AMERICA, INC.   **714-799-1735**
7245 Garden Grove Blvd., #d, Garden Grove, CA 92841
FDA Number: 2087134
Ownership: Private
Produces/Sells CE-marked Devices: N

Massager, Therapeutic, Manual	Physical Med
Percussor	Cns/Neurology

GENESIS BIOSYSTEMS, INC.   **888-577-7335**
1500 Eagle Court, Lewisville, TX 75057   **972-315-7888**
FDA Number: 1652111   *Fax:* 972-315-7818
E-mail: info@genesisbiosystems.com
Web site: www.genesisbiosystems.com
Medical Products Sales Volume: $4,500,000
Annual Revenue: $1-$5 Million
Year Founded: 2001
Total Employees: 30   *Marketing Staff:* 4   *Sales Staff:* 4
Ownership: Private
Produces/Sells CE-marked Devices: Y
Federal Procurement Eligibility: Small Business
Distribution: Manufacturer Through Manufacturer Reps, Exporter
General Admin.: Jim Lafferty/President

GENESIS BIOSYSTEMS, INC.   **888-577-7335** *(cont'd)*

Dermatome	Surgery
Electrosurgical Unit, Cutting & Coagulation Device	Surgery
Light, Surgical Headlight	Dental And Oral
Shield, Eye, Ophthalmic	Ophthalmology
Syringe, Irrigating	General

GENESIS BUSINESS SYSTEMS INC.
See Achieve Healthcare Technologies

GENESIS DENTAL TECHNOLOGIES, LLC   **715-778-5816**
200 Main Street, Elmwood, WI 54740
FDA Number: 3004961419
Ownership: Private
Produces/Sells CE-marked Devices: N

Operative Dental Treatment Unit	Dental And Oral

GENESIS DIGITAL IMAGING, INC.   **(888) 436-3444**
12921 W. Washington Blvd,   **(310) 305-7358**
Los Angeles, CA 90066
FDA Number: 3005872153   *Fax:* (323) 784-8585
Web site: www.genesisdi.com
Ownership: Private
Produces/Sells CE-marked Devices: N

Device, Storage, Image, Digital	Radiology
Imager, X-Ray, Solid State (Flat Panel/Digital)	Radiology
System, Communication, Image, Digital	Radiology

GENESIS INDUSTRIES/MATERNAL CONCEPTS   **800-310-5817**
130 S Public St, Elmwood, WI 54740   **715-639-4050**
FDA Number: 2183741   *Fax:* 715-639-2739
E-mail: sales@maternalconcepts.com
Web site: www.maternalconcepts.com
Medical Products Sales Volume: $5,600,000
Annual Revenue: $0-$1 Million
Year Founded: 1985
Total Employees: 35   *Marketing Staff:* 2   *Sales Staff:* 2
Ownership: GENESIS INDUSTRIES
Produces/Sells CE-marked Devices: N
Federal Procurement Eligibility: Small Business
Distribution: Manufacturer Through Distributor
General Admin.: Mark Anderson/President

Kit, Feeding, Pediatric (Enteral)	General
Pump, Breast, Non-Powered	Obstetrics/Gynecology

GENESIS INSTRUMENTS, INC.   **(800) 826-3301**
601 Pro-Ject Drive, Elmwood, WI 54740   **715-639-9209**
FDA Number: 3003697955   *Fax:* 715-639-2335
E-mail: sales@genesisinstruments.com
Ownership: Private
Produces/Sells CE-marked Devices: N

Applicator, Vaginal	Obstetrics/Gynecology
Labware, Assisted Reproduction	Obstetrics/Gynecology
Pump, Breast, Non-Powered	Obstetrics/Gynecology

GENESIS MANUFACTURING, INC.   **317-485-7887**
720 E. Broadway, Fortville, IN 46040
FDA Number: 9066714   *Fax:* 317-485-7888
E-mail: TRYDER@genesisrf.com
Web site: www.genesisrf.com
Medical Products Sales Volume: $1,000,000
Annual Revenue: $1-$5 Million
Total Employees: 50   *Marketing Staff:* 1   *Sales Staff:* 2
Ownership: Private
Produces/Sells CE-marked Devices: Y
Federal Procurement Eligibility: Small Business
Distribution: Manufacturer Direct, Manufacturer Through Distributor, OEM
General Admin.: Thomas R. Ryder/President, Chief Executive Officer
Mktg./Adv.: Mr. Mark Vermillion/Manager Sales
Production: Dale Wagner/Manager Operations
      Mr. Scott Hartman/Manager Quality Assurance & Engineering

Component, Plastic	General
Contract Manufacturing	General
Contract Manufacturing, Product, Disposable	General
Cover, Bedrail	General
Cover, Mattress, Waterproof	General
Cuff, Blood Pressure	Cardiovascular
Cuff, Inflation	General
Cushion, Other	General
Cushion, Wheelchair (Pad)	Physical Med
Mattress, Alternating Pressure (Or Pads)	Physical Med
Mattress, Water	General
Pack, Hot Or Cold, Water Circulating	Physical Med
Pad, Heating, Circulating Fluid	General
Pad, Incontinence (Underpad)	General
Pad, Pressure, Air	General
Pad, Pressure, Gel	General
Pad, Pressure, Water Cushion	General
Pressure Pad, Alternating, Disposable	General
Protector, Wound, Plastic	Gastroenterology/Urology

GENESIS MANUFACTURING, INC.
317-485-7887 *(cont'd)*

Service, Modification, Product	General
Warmer, Blanket	General
Warmer, Gel	General

GENESIS MEDICAL INTERVENTIONAL, INC.
650-367-7667
652 Bair Island Road, Suite 103, Redwood City, CA 94063
FDA Number: 3005310846

Catheter, Embolectomy (Fogarty Type)	Cardiovascular

GENESIS MEDICAL PRODUCTS, INC.
508-876-1063
40 Farmhill Rd., Wrentham, MA 02093
FDA Number: 1225419
Ownership: Private
Produces/Sells CE-marked Devices: N

Holder, Intravascular Catheter	General
Pad, Neonatal Eye	General
Support, Head, Surgical, ENT	Ear/Nose/Throat

GENETIC LABORATORIES - CARDIOVASCULAR IM
See Synovis Surgical Innovations

GENETIC TESTING INSTITUTE
800-233-1843
262-754-1000
20925 Crossroads Circle, Suite 200,
Waukesha, WI 53186
FDA Number: 2183608   *Fax:* 262-754-9831
E-mail: customerservice@gen-probe.com
Web site: www.gtidiagnostics.com
Ownership: Private
Produces/Sells CE-marked Devices: N

DNA-Probe, Chromosome, Human	Hematology
Kit, Platelet Associated IGG	Hematology
Media, Potentiating	Hematology
Radioimmunoassay, Platelet Factor 4	Hematology
Reagents, Specific, Analyte	Hematology
Substance, Grouping, Blood (Non-Human Origin)	Hematology
Test, Leukocyte Typing	Hematology
Test, Platelet Antibody	Hematology
Test, Qualitative And Quantitative Factor Deficiency	Hematology
Test, Qualitative, For Hla, Non-diagnostic	Hematology

GENEVA MEDICAL INC.
630-232-2507
2571 Kaneville Court, Geneva, IL 60134
FDA Number: 1419305
Ownership: Private
Produces/Sells CE-marked Devices: N

Catheter, Biliary, General & Plastic Surgery	Surgery
Catheter, Cholangiography	Surgery
Catheter, Peritoneal	Surgery
Insufflator, Laparoscopic	Obstetrics/Gynecology
Laparoscope, General & Plastic Surgery	Surgery
Tube, Drainage	Gastroenterology/Urology

GENICON
800-936-1020
407-657-4851
6869 Stapoint Court, Suite 114,
Winter Park, FL 32792
FDA Number: 1064003   *Fax:* 407-677-9773
E-mail: contact@geniconendo.com
Web site: www.geniconendo.com
Medical Products Sales Volume: $1,700,000
Annual Revenue: $1-$5 Million
Year Founded: 1998
Total Employees: 22   *Marketing Staff:* 2   *Sales Staff:* 8
Ownership: Private
Traded On: NYSE
Produces/Sells CE-marked Devices: Y
Federal Procurement Eligibility: Small Business
Distribution: Manufacturer Direct, Manufacturer Through Distributor, Manufacturer Through Manufacturer Reps, OEM, Exporter
General Admin.: Mr. Gary Haberland/Chief Executive Officer, Vice President Marketing
    Mr. Michael Athey/Chief Operating Officer
Mktg./Adv.: Mr. Gary Haberland/Director International Sales
    Mr. Clinton Hollowell/Director National Sales
    Mr. Matthew Athey/Manager Marketing
Production: Ms. Helaina Jeannot/Customer Service Representative
Finance: Mr. Thomas Calcaterra/Chief Financial Officer
    Mrs. Teri Rhinehart/Controller, Credit Manager

Accessories, Surgical Camera	Surgery
Applier, Surgical, Clip	Surgery
Cannula, Suction/Irrigation, Laparoscopic	Surgery
Equipment, Suction/Irrigation, Laparoscopic	Surgery
Forceps, Laparoscopy, Bipolar, Electrosurgical	Surgery
Instrument, Dissecting, Laparoscopic	Surgery
Insufflator, Laparoscopic	Obstetrics/Gynecology
Irrigator/Coagulator/Cutter, Suction, Laparoscopic	Surgery
Laparoscope, General & Plastic Surgery	Surgery
Laparoscope, Microlaparoscopy	Surgery
Lens, Camera, Surgical	Surgery
Light, Surgical, Endoscopic	Surgery

GENICON
800-936-1020 *(cont'd)*

Needle, Insufflation, Laparoscopic	Surgery
Scissors, Laparoscopy	Surgery
Scissors, Laparoscopy, Bipolar, Electrosurgical	Surgery
Scissors, Laparoscopy, Unipolar, Electrosurgical	Surgery
Surgical Instrument, Disposable	Surgery
Trocar, Laparoscopic	Surgery

GENIE AUDIO INC.
800-363-0793
514-856-9212
125 Gagnon St., Ste. 102,
St-Laurent, QUE H4N-1 Canada
FDA Number: n/a   *Fax:* 514-856-9002
E-mail: info@genieaudio.com
Web site: www.genieaudio.com
Year Founded: 1965
Ownership: Private
Produces/Sells CE-marked Devices: N

GENIE CORP.
See Genie Scientific, Inc.

GENIE SCIENTIFIC, INC.
800-545-8816
714-545-1838
17442 Mt. Cliffwood Circle,
Fountain Valley, CA 92708
FDA Number: n/a   *Fax:* 714-641-0496
E-mail: holliday@geniescientific.com
Web site: www.geniescientific.com
Medical Products Sales Volume: $1,000,000
Annual Revenue: $1-$5 Million
Year Founded: 1974
Total Employees: 12
Ownership: Private
Produces/Sells CE-marked Devices: N
Federal Procurement Eligibility: Small Business
Distribution: Manufacturer Direct, Service Direct
General Admin.: Kim Holliday/Manager
    Mel Levan/President
    Moya O'Neill/Vice President, General Manager

Cabinet, Laboratory	Chemistry
Furniture, General	General
Hood, Fume, Chemical	Chemistry

GENLABS
800-882-5227
909-591-8451
5568 Schaefer Ave., Chino, CA 91710
FDA Number: 2027941   *Fax:* 909-627-7072
E-mail: generalinfo@genlabscorp.com
Web site: www.genlabscorp.com
Annual Revenue: $0-$1 Million
Year Founded: 1973
Ownership: Private
Produces/Sells CE-marked Devices: N
Distribution: Manufacturer Direct

Disinfector, Liquid	General

GENLEE
650-697-5831
769 Morningside Drive, Millbrae, CA 94030
FDA Number: 2083941   *Fax:* 650-697-5832
E-mail: gloves@genlee.com
Web site: www.genlee.com
Medical Products Sales Volume: $100,000
Year Founded: 1989
Total Employees: 1   *Sales Staff:* 2
Ownership: Private
Quality System Registration Information: ISO9000
Produces/Sells CE-marked Devices: N
Federal Procurement Eligibility: Small Business
Distribution: Manufacturer Direct, Manufacturer Through Distributor, Manufacturer Through Manufacturer Reps, Importer, Exporter
Mktg./Adv.: C. Breder/Vice President Marketing & Sales

Glove, Patient Examination, Latex	General

GENMARK DIAGNOSTICS INC.
1-800-373-6767
760-448-4300
5964 La Place Court, Carlsbad, CA 92008
FDA Number: 3008632402   *Fax:* 760-448-4301
E-mail: info@genmarkdx.com
Web site: www.genmarkdx.com
Ownership: Private
Produces/Sells CE-marked Devices: N
General Admin.: Dr. John Faiz Kayyem/Chief Scientific Officer
    Mr. Hany Massarany/President, Chief Executive Officer
Mktg./Adv.: Dr. Pankaj Singhal/Senior Vice President Product Development
    Mr. John Bellano/Vice President Commercial Operations
Research: Ms. Sue Pierce/Vice President Product Development
Finance: Mr. Paul Ross/Chief Financial Officer

Cytochrome P450 2c9 (cyp450 2c9) Drug Metabolizing Enzyme Genotyping System	Toxicology
Instrumentation For Clinical Multiplex Test Systems	Chemistry

GENMARK DIAGNOSTICS INC.   1-800-373-6767 *(cont'd)*

System, Cystic Fibrosis Transmembrane Conductance Regulator, Gene Mutation
Detection   Immunology
Test, Factor Ii G20210a Mutations, Genomic Dna Pcr   Hematology
Test, Factor V Leiden Mutations, Genomic Dna Pcr   Hematology
Vitamin K Epoxide Reductase Complex Subunit One (vkorc1) Genotyping System
Hematology

GENNUM CORPORATION   905-632-2996
P.O. Box 489, Station A, Burlington, ONT L7R-3Y3 Canada
FDA Number: n/a   *Fax:* 905-632-2055
E-mail: corporate@gennum.com
Web site: www.gennum.com
Year Founded: 1973
Ownership: Private
Produces/Sells CE-marked Devices: N
Distribution: Manufacturer Direct, Exporter

GENO LLC.   321-785-2645
2941 Oxbow Circle, Cocoa, FL 32926
FDA Number: n/a
E-mail: contactus@genollc.com
Web site: http://www.genollc.com
Year Founded: 2006
Ownership: Private
Produces/Sells CE-marked Devices: N
General Admin.: Mr. David Fine/Chairman, Chief Executive Officer
    Dr. Robert Roscigno/Vice President
Production: Mr. Nick Samiotes/Vice President Manufacturing

GENOMIC HEALTH INC.   866-662-6897
101 Galveston Drive, Redwood City, CA 94063   650-556-9300
FDA Number: n/a   *Fax:* 650-556-1132
E-mail: customerservice@genomichealth.com
Web site: www.genomichealth.com
Year Founded: 2000
Ownership: Public
Stock Symbol: GHDX
Traded On: NASDAQ
Produces/Sells CE-marked Devices: N
General Admin.: Brad Cole/Chief Operating Officer, Chief Financial Officer
    Joffre Baker/Chief Scientific Officer
    Randy Scott/Executive Chairman
    Kim Popovits/President, Chief Executive Officer
Medical Admin.: Steve Shak/Chief Medical Officer

GENOVA DIAGNOSTICS   828-253-0621
63 Zillicoa St., Asheville, NC 28801
FDA Number: 1055886
Colorimetric, Xylose   Chemistry

GENPORE, A DIVISION OF GENERAL POLYMERIC CORP.   800-654-4391
1136 Morgantown Road, Reading, PA 19607   610-374-5171
FDA Number: n/a   *Fax:* 610-374-4990
E-mail: sales@genpore.com
Web site: www.genpore.com
Medical Products Sales Volume: $9,500,000
Annual Revenue: $5-$10 Million
Year Founded: 1968
Total Employees: 62   *Marketing Staff:* 3   *Sales Staff:* 9
Ownership: Private
Produces/Sells CE-marked Devices: N
Federal Procurement Eligibility: Small Business
Distribution: Manufacturer Direct, Manufacturer Through Manufacturer Reps, OEM,
Exporter
General Admin.: Ken Kreska/Manager Plant
    Joseph Ferri/President
Mktg./Adv.: Mr. Jack Willey/Sales Representative
    Mr. Kevin Katerndahl/Sales Representative
IS: Matthew Kreska/Manager Systems
Accessories, Catheter   Surgery
Component, Plastic   General
Media, Filter   General

GENTEC ELECTRO-OPTICS INC.   888-543-6832
445 St-Jean-Baptiste, Ste. 160,   418-651-8003
Quebec, QUE G2E-5 Canada
FDA Number: n/a   *Fax:* 418-651-1174
E-mail: nbecotte@gentec-eo.com
Web site: www.gentec-eo.com
Medical Products Sales Volume: $300,000
Year Founded: 1973
Total Employees: 50
Ownership: Private
Quality System Registration Information: ISO9001
Produces/Sells CE-marked Devices: Y

GENTEC ELECTRO-OPTICS INC.   888-543-6832 *(cont'd)*
Distribution: Manufacturer Direct, Manufacturer Through Distributor, Exporter

GENTELL   800-840-9041
3600 Bound Brook Rd., Trevose, PA 19053   215-364-3600
FDA Number: 9020543   *Fax:* 215-364-7290
E-mail: info@gentell.com
Web site: www.gentell.com
Medical Products Sales Volume: $2,800,000
Annual Revenue: $1-$5 Million
Year Founded: 1995
Total Employees: 30   *Marketing Staff:* 5   *Sales Staff:* 5
Ownership: Private
Produces/Sells CE-marked Devices: N
Federal Procurement Eligibility: Small Business
Distribution: Manufacturer Direct, Manufacturer Through Distributor, Manufacturer
Through Manufacturer Reps, Importer, Exporter
General Admin.: David Navazio/Executive Vice President, General Manager
    Fredric Brotz/President
Mktg./Adv.: Mathew Brotz/Director National Accounts
    Paul Moore/Director Product Development
    John Sadri/Manager Contract Sales
    Brian Sehorn/Manager International & National Sales
    David Navazio/Manager International Marketing & Sales
Production: Paul Moore/Manager Materials
    Joseph Milestone/Manager Regulatory Affairs
Bandage, Gauze   General
Bandage, Other   General
Beads, Hydrophilic, Wound Exudate Absorption   Surgery
Dressing, Foam   General
Dressing, Gel   General
Dressing, Non-Adherent   General
Dressing, Other   General
Sanitizer   General
Solution, Antibacterial Cleaner   General
Solution, Ostomy, Odor Control   Gastroenterology/Urology
Washer, Receptacle, Waste, Body   General

GENTEX CORPORATION   570-282-8350
324 Main St., P.o. Box 315, Simpson, PA 18407
FDA Number: 3002742064
Ownership: Private
Produces/Sells CE-marked Devices: N
Mask, Oxygen, Low Concentration, Venturi   Anesthesiology
Patient Isolation Chamber   General

GENTEX CORPORATION OPTICS   570-282-3550
P.O. Box 336, Carbondale, PA 18407-0315
FDA Number: 2518613   *Fax:* 570-282-8555
E-mail: filtron@gentexcorp.com
Web site: www.gentexcorp.com
Annual Revenue: $50-$100 Million
Total Employees: 500
Ownership: Private
Quality System Registration Information: ISO9001
Produces/Sells CE-marked Devices: N
Distribution: Manufacturer Direct
General Admin.: Peter Frieder/President
Mktg./Adv.: Charles Rudolf/Director Marketing
    Thomas Blaine/Manager Advertising
Lens, Spectacle/Eyeglasses, Non-Custom   Ophthalmology
Sunglasses (Including Photosensitive)   Ophthalmology

GENTEX OPTICS, INC.   508-943-3860
183 W. Main St., Dudley, MA 01571
FDA Number: 1215866   *Fax:* 508-949-0261
Web site: www.gentexoptics.com
Annual Revenue: $25-$50 Million
Ownership: Private
Quality System Registration Information: ISO9001
Produces/Sells CE-marked Devices: Y
Distribution: Manufacturer Through Distributor
Lens, Spectacle/Eyeglasses, Non-Custom   Ophthalmology
Sunglasses (Including Photosensitive)   Ophthalmology

GENTRA SYSTEMS, INC.   763-543-0678
13355 10th Ave. N., Suite 120, Minneapolis, MN 55441
FDA Number: 2132481
Ownership: Private
Produces/Sells CE-marked Devices: N
Equipment, Laboratory, Gen. Purpose (Specific Medical Use)   Chemistry
Reagent, General Purpose   Pathology

GENTRAN, INC.   510-226-9343
42025 Osgood Rd, Fremont, CA 94539
FDA Number: 9200388   *Fax:* 510-226-1112
E-mail: info@gentran-corp.com
Web site: www.gentran-corp.com
Annual Revenue: $0-$1 Million

GENTRAN, INC.   510-226-9343 (cont'd)

Total Employees: 30   *Marketing Staff:* 1   *Sales Staff:* 3
Ownership: INVIVO CORPORATION
Stock Symbol: SAFE
Traded On: NASDAQ
Produces/Sells CE-marked Devices: N
Federal Procurement Eligibility: Small Business
Distribution: Manufacturer Direct, Manufacturer Through Distributor, Manufacturer Through Manufacturer Reps, Importer, Exporter
General Admin.: James Hawkins/President
Mktg./Adv.: Teresa Sutton/Director Marketing
    Teresa Sutton/Director National Accounts
    Michelle Lewis/Manager Advertising
    Teresa Sutton/Manager International & National Sales
    Michelle Lewis/Vice President Marketing
    Teresa Sutton/Vice President Marketing & Sales
    Teresa Sutton/Vice President Sales
Research: Teresa Sutton/Vice President Research & Development
    Transducer, Blood Pressure   General

GENTRONICS   800-950-3265

8721 Santa Monica Blvd., Suite 210,   **310-358-1997**
Los Angeles, CA 90069
FDA Number: 2025590   *Fax:* 310-358-1974
E-mail: Gentronics@hotmail.com
Web site: www.GentronicsEpilators.com
Medical Products Sales Volume: $200,000
Year Founded: 1976
Ownership: Private
Produces/Sells CE-marked Devices: N
Federal Procurement Eligibility: Small Business
Distribution: Manufacturer Direct, OEM, Exporter
    Epilator, High-Frequency, Needle-Type   Surgery

GENTURADX   510-725-4767

24590 Clawiter Road, Hayward, CA 94545
FDA Number: n/a
Ownership: Private
Produces/Sells CE-marked Devices: N
General Admin.: Mr. Jesus Ching/Chief Scientific Officer
    Mr. Mark Bagnall/President, Chief Executive Officer
Mktg./Adv.: Mr. Dylan Bird/Senior Director Business Development
Production: Ms. Juliet Carrara/Vice President Regulatory & Clinical Affairs
Research: Dr. Geoffrey McKinley/Senior Vice President Research & Development

GENUINE CARE REHAB. SVC., INC.   405-604-5907

2401 N.w. 23rd St. Ste. 17, Oklahoma City, OK 73107
FDA Number: 1651699
Ownership: Private
Produces/Sells CE-marked Devices: N
    Garment, Protective, For Incontinence   Gastroenterology/Urology
    Prosthesis, Thigh Socket, External Component   Physical Med

GENX INTERNATIONAL   888-GEN-XNOW

393 Soundview Road, Guilford, CT 06437   **203-453-1700**
FDA Number: 9003605   *Fax:* 203-453-1769
E-mail: sales@genxintl.com
Medical Products Sales Volume: $4,000,000
Annual Revenue: $1-$5 Million
Year Founded: 1996
Total Employees: 16   *Sales Staff:* 4
Ownership: Private
Quality System Registration Information: ISO9001
Produces/Sells CE-marked Devices: Y
Federal Procurement Eligibility: Small Business
Distribution: Manufacturer Direct, Importer, Exporter
General Admin.: Michael Cecchi/President
    Accessory, Assisted Reproduction   Obstetrics/Gynecology
    Aspirator, Endocervical   Obstetrics/Gynecology
    Catheter, Assisted Reproduction   Obstetrics/Gynecology
    Equipment, In Vitro Fertilization/Embryo Transfer   Obstetrics/Gynecology
    Filter, Air   General
    Media, Reproductive   Obstetrics/Gynecology
    Needle, Assisted Reproduction   Obstetrics/Gynecology

GENZYME   800-332-1042

500 Kendall Street, Cambridge, MA 02139   **617-252-7500**
FDA Number: 1226230   *Fax:* 617-252-7600
Web site: www.genzyme.com
Total Employees: 10000
Ownership: Public
Stock Symbol: GENZ
Traded On: NASDAQ
Produces/Sells CE-marked Devices: Y
Distribution: Manufacturer Direct
General Admin.: Henri Termeer/President, Chief Executive Officer, Chairman
    Peter Wirth/Senior Vice President, General Counsel
Research: Alan Smith/Senior Vice President Research & Development

GENZYME   800-332-1042 (cont'd)

    Acid, Hyaluronic   Dental And Oral
    Antibody, Monoclonal   Microbiology
    Antibody, Polyclonal   Microbiology
    Antigen, Antiserum, Control, Lymphocyte Typing   Immunology
    Container, Specimen Mailer And Storage   Pathology
    Enzyme Immunoassay, Other   Chemistry
    Kit, Surgical Instrument, Disposable   Surgery
    LDL & VLDL Precipitation, HDL   Chemistry
Medical Product Subsidiaries (Listed Separately)
    Genzyme Corp.
    Genzyme Corporation
    Genzyme Diagnostics
    Genzyme Diagnostics P.E.I. Inc.
    Sekisui Diagnostics, LLC

GENZYME BIOSURGERY

    See Genzyme Corp.

GENZYME CORP.   617-252-7500

500 Kendall Street, Cambridge, MA 02142
FDA Number: 1220423   *Fax:* 617 252 7600
Ownership: Genzyme
Produces/Sells CE-marked Devices: N
    Barrier, Adhesion, Absorbable   Obstetrics/Gynecology
    Calibrator, Primary, Clinical Chemistry   Chemistry
    Calibrator, Secondary, Clinical Chemistry   Chemistry
    Splint, Septal, Intranasal   Ear/Nose/Throat

GENZYME CORP.   800-284-2876

64 Sidney St., Cambridge, MA 02139-4136   **617-252-7999**
FDA Number: 1226230   *Fax:* 617-252-0877
Web site: www.genzyme.com
Ownership: Genzyme
Stock Symbol: GENZT
Traded On: NASDAQ
Quality System Registration Information: ISO9002
Produces/Sells CE-marked Devices: Y
Federal Procurement Eligibility: Small Business
Distribution: Manufacturer Direct
General Admin.: Russell Herndon/Senior Vice President
    Container, Specimen Mailer And Storage   Pathology
    Dressing, Wound and Burn, Occlusive   Surgery
    Graft, Skin   Surgery
    Kit, Surgical Instrument, Disposable   Surgery
    Stimulator, Wound Healing   Physical Med

GENZYME CORPORATION   617-252-7500

1125 Pleasantview Terrace, Ridgefield, NJ 07657-2397
FDA Number: 2246315
Ownership: Genzyme
Produces/Sells CE-marked Devices: N
    Acid, Hyaluronic, Intraarticular   Physical Med
    Implant, Collagen, Dermal (Aesthetic Use)   Surgery
    Lens, Contact, Gas-Permeable   Ophthalmology
    Polymer, ENT Synthetic Polyamide (Mesh Or Foil Material)   Ear/Nose/Throat
    Splint, Septal, Intranasal   Ear/Nose/Throat

GENZYME DIAGNOSTICS

    See Sekisui Diagnostics, LLC

GENZYME DIAGNOSTICS   617-252-7500

6659 Top Gun St., San Diego, CA 92121
FDA Number: 2030538
Ownership: Genzyme
Produces/Sells CE-marked Devices: N
    Antigen, CF (Including CF Control), Influenza Virus   Microbiology
    Antigen, Streptococcus SPP.   Microbiology
    Antiserum, Streptococcus SPP.   Microbiology
    Control, Analyte (Assayed And Unassayed)   Chemistry
    Giardia Spp.   Microbiology
    Kit, Pregnancy Test, Over The Counter, HCG   Chemistry
    Kit, Quality Control   Microbiology
    Kit, Trichomonas Screening   Microbiology
    Microdensitometry Method, Lipoproteins   Chemistry
    Radioimmunoassay, Human Chorionic Gonadotropin   Chemistry
    Test, Infectious Mononucleosis   Immunology

GENZYME DIAGNOSTICS P.E.I. INC.   800-565-0265

70 Watts Ave.,   **902-566-1396**
Charlottetown, PEI C1E-2 Canada
FDA Number: 8020316   *Fax:* 902-566-2498
E-mail: sales@dclchem.com
Web site: www.dclchem.com
Year Founded: 1970
Total Employees: 160
Ownership: Genzyme
Quality System Registration Information: ISO9001
Produces/Sells CE-marked Devices: N
Federal Procurement Eligibility: Small Business

GENZYME DIAGNOSTICS P.E.I. INC. 800-565-0265 *(cont'd)*
Distribution: Manufacturer Direct, Manufacturer Through Distributor, Manufacturer Through Manufacturer Reps, Exporter

GENZYME TISSUE REPAIR
See Genzyme Corp.

GEON/SYNERGISTICS
See Polyone

GEORGE C. BISHOP COMPANY 800-476-7374
PO Box 684, Horsham, PA 19044-0684 215-672-1202
FDA Number: 1043613
Annual Revenue: $0-$1 Million
Total Employees: 2
Ownership: Private
Produces/Sells CE-marked Devices: N
Federal Procurement Eligibility: Small Business
Distribution: Manufacturer Direct, Exporter
General Admin.: George C. Bishop/President
  Exerciser, Hand   Physical Med

GEORGE COUREY INC. 800-361-1087
5550 Ferrier St., 514-342-6315
Mont-Royal, QUE H4P-1 Canada
FDA Number: n/a   Fax: 514-342-8027
E-mail: info@georgecourey.com
Web site: www.georgecourey.com
Year Founded: 1934
Total Employees: 100
Ownership: Private
Produces/Sells CE-marked Devices: N
Distribution: Manufacturer Direct, Importer

GEORGE GLOVE COMPANY, INC. 800-631-4292
301 Greenwood Avenue, 201-251-1200
Midland Park, NJ 07432
FDA Number: 2242350   Fax: 201-251-8431
E-mail: roy@georgeglove.com
Web site: www.georgeglove.com
Medical Products Sales Volume: $1,800,000
Annual Revenue: $1-$5 Million
Year Founded: 1932
Total Employees: 8   *Marketing Staff:* 2   *Sales Staff:* 2
Ownership: Private
Produces/Sells CE-marked Devices: N
Federal Procurement Eligibility: Small Business, Female Owned
Distribution: Importer, Exporter
General Admin.: Clark Bullock/Chairman
Mktg./Adv.: Roy Miller/Vice President Sales
  Glove, Other   General

GEORGE J. KAMILAR 516-665-7167
240 Windsor Ave., Brightwaters, NY 11718
FDA Number: 2434068
Ownership: Private
Produces/Sells CE-marked Devices: N
  Transfer Aid   Physical Med

GEORGE KING BIO-MEDICAL, INC. 800-255-5108
11771 W. 112th St., 913-469-5464
Overland Park, KS 66210
FDA Number: 1928890   Fax: 913-469-0871
E-mail: plasma@kingbiomed.com
Web site: www.kingbiomed.com
Year Founded: 1973
Total Employees: 15
Ownership: Private
Stock Symbol: SRLSE
Traded On: Toronto
Produces/Sells CE-marked Devices: N
Federal Procurement Eligibility: Small Business, Female Owned
Distribution: Manufacturer Direct
  Control, Coagulation, Plasma   Hematology
  Control, Plasma, Abnormal   Hematology
  Plasma, Control, Normal   Hematology
  Plasma, Deficient, Factor, Coagulation   Hematology
  Reagent, Other   General

GEORGE MEDICAL
See Xero Products

GEORGE TAUB PRODUCTS & FUSION CO., INC. 800-828-2634
277 New York Ave., Jersey City, NJ 07307-1501 201-798-5353
FDA Number: 2241860   Fax: 201-659-7186
E-mail: sales@taubdental.com
Web site: www.taubdental.com
Medical Products Sales Volume: $970,000
Annual Revenue: $0-$1 Million

GEORGE TAUB PRODUCTS & FUSION CO., INC. 800-828-2634
(cont'd)
Year Founded: 1952
Total Employees: 7   *Marketing Staff:* 1   *Sales Staff:* 3
Ownership: Taub Products, Inc., Laurence
Produces/Sells CE-marked Devices: N
Federal Procurement Eligibility: Small Business
Distribution: Manufacturer Direct, Manufacturer Through Distributor, Importer, Exporter
General Admin.: Lawrence Taub/President, Chief Executive Officer
Mktg./Adv.: Lawrence Taub/Manager International Marketing & Sales
        Mr. Jordan Taub/Market Manager
Production: Lawrence Taub/Manager Production
        Lawrence Taub/Manager Regulatory Affairs

Absorber, Saliva, Paper	Dental And Oral
Agent, Polishing, Abrasive, Oral Cavity	Dental And Oral
Burnisher, Operative, Dental	Dental And Oral
Carver, Wax, Dental	Dental And Oral
Cleaner, Denture	Dental And Oral
Coating, Filling Material, Resin	Dental And Oral
Compound, Resinous, Composite	Dental And Oral
Dental Laboratory Equipment	Dental And Oral
Forceps, Dressing, Dental	Dental And Oral
Kit, Denture Repair, OTC	Dental And Oral
Liner, Cavity, Calcium Hydroxide	Dental And Oral
Material, Tooth Shade, Resin	Dental And Oral
Microscope, Laboratory, Optical	Microbiology
Paper, Articulation	Dental And Oral
Primer, Cavity, Resin	Dental And Oral
Remover, Crown	Dental And Oral
Scissors, Surgical Tissue, Dental (Oral)	Dental And Oral

GEORGE TIEMANN & CO. 800-843-6266
25 Plant Ave., Hauppauge, NY 11788-3804 631-273-6199
FDA Number: 2424531   Fax: 631-273-6199
E-mail: richard@georgetiemann.com
Web site: www.georgetiemann.com
Medical Products Sales Volume: $3,500,000
Annual Revenue: $1-$5 Million
Total Employees: 20
Ownership: Private
Produces/Sells CE-marked Devices: N
Federal Procurement Eligibility: Small Business
Distribution: Manufacturer Direct, OEM, Importer
General Admin.: Richard Moriarty/President
Mktg./Adv.: Kenneth Moriarty/Vice President Marketing

Awl	Orthopedics
Blade, Scalpel	Surgery
Chart, Visual Acuity	Ophthalmology
Chisel, Bone, Surgical	Dental And Oral
Clamp, Eyelid, Ophthalmic	Ophthalmology
Clamp, Non-Electrical	Gastroenterology/Urology
Curette	Orthopedics
Curette, Ear	Ear/Nose/Throat
Curette, Surgical	Surgery
Dilator, Lacrimal	Ophthalmology
Dissector, Surgical, General & Plastic Surgery	Surgery
Dissector, Tonsil	Ear/Nose/Throat
Drill, Manual (With Burr, Trephine & Accessories)	Cns/Neurology
Electrocautery Unit, Endoscopic	Obstetrics/Gynecology
Elevator, ENT	Ear/Nose/Throat
Elevator, Orthopedic	Orthopedics
Elevator, Surgical, General & Plastic Surgery	Surgery
Expressor	Ophthalmology
Fixation Device, Extra-Cranial (Head Frame)	Orthopedics
Fixation Device, Jaw Fracture	Orthopedics
Forceps	Orthopedics
Forceps, Fixation	Surgery
Forceps, General & Plastic Surgery	Surgery
Forceps, Obstetrical	Obstetrics/Gynecology
Forceps, Utility	Surgery
Gouge, Surgical, General & Plastic Surgery	Surgery
Hemostat, Surgical	Dental And Oral
Holder, Needle	Gastroenterology/Urology
Hook, Microsurgical Ear	Ear/Nose/Throat
Hook, Ophthalmic	Ophthalmology
Hook, Surgical, General & Plastic Surgery	Surgery
Impactor	Orthopedics
Infiltrator	Pathology
Knife, Ear	Ear/Nose/Throat
Loop, Wire	Ear/Nose/Throat
Mallet, Bone	Orthopedics
Orthodontic Instrument	Dental And Oral
Osteotome, Manual (Plastic Surgery)	Surgery
Pick, Microsurgical Ear	Ear/Nose/Throat
Pump, Aspiration, Portable	Anesthesiology
Punch, Biopsy, Surgical	Dental And Oral
Retractor	Orthopedics
Retractor, All Types	Dental And Oral
Retractor, Ophthalmic	Ophthalmology

GEORGE TIEMANN & CO. 800-843-6266 (cont'd)

Retractor, Vaginal	Obstetrics/Gynecology
Scissors, Ophthalmic	Ophthalmology
Scissors, Orthopedic	Orthopedics
Scissors, Suture	Surgery
Shield, Eye, Ophthalmic	Ophthalmology
Skid, Bone	Orthopedics
Sound, Uterine	Obstetrics/Gynecology
Spatula, Ophthalmic	Ophthalmology
Suture, Silk	Surgery
Tenaculum, Uterine	Obstetrics/Gynecology
Tube, Tonsil Suction	Ear/Nose/Throat

GEORGIA STEEL & CHEMICAL COMPANY, INC. 800-296-0351
**10810 Guilford Rd., Suite 104, 301-317-5502
Annapolis Junction, MD 20701**
FDA Number: n/a *Fax:* 301-470-6313
E-mail: info@georgiasteelco.com
Web site: www.georgiasteelco.com
Annual Revenue: $0-$1 Million
Ownership: Private
Produces/Sells CE-marked Devices: N
Federal Procurement Eligibility: Small Business
Distribution: Manufacturer Direct, Importer, Exporter

Bin, Storage	General
Cleaner, Medical Device	General
Disinfector, Liquid	General
Drying Unit	Chemistry
Encapsulator, Fluid	General
Glove, Other	General
Housekeeping Equipment	General
Solution, Antibacterial Cleaner	General
Towel/Towelette, Paper	General

GEORGIA-PACIFIC LLC 404-652-4000
133 Peachtree Street, N.E., Atlanta, GA 30303
FDA Number: n/a
Web site: www.gp.com
Year Founded: 1927
Ownership: Private
Quality System Registration Information: ISO9002
Produces/Sells CE-marked Devices: N
Distribution: Manufacturer Through Distributor
General Admin.: David L. Robertson/Chairman
　　　Tyler Woolson/Chief Financial Officer, Senior Vice President
　　　James Hannan/President, Chief Executive Officer

Dispenser, Soap	General
Tissue, Toilet	General
Towel, Surgical	Surgery

GERBER CHAIR MATES, INC. 814-269-9531
1171 Ringling Ave., Johnstown, PA 15902
FDA Number: 2529004 *Fax:* 814-269-3814
E-mail: jgerber@gerberchairmates.com
Web site: www.gerberchairmates.com
Medical Products Sales Volume: $330,000
Annual Revenue: $0-$1 Million
Year Founded: 1988
Total Employees: 5
Ownership: Private
Produces/Sells CE-marked Devices: N
Federal Procurement Eligibility: Small Business, Female Owned
Distribution: Manufacturer Direct
General Admin.: Dorothy A. Gerber/President, Treasurer, General Manager
Production: James Gerber II/Manager Manufacturing

Accessories, Wheelchair	Physical Med
Component, Wheelchair	Physical Med

GERBER COBURN OPTICAL INC. 800-262-8761
55 Gerber Rd., South Windsor, CT 06074 800-843-1479
FDA Number: n/a *Fax:* 800-648-6601
Web site: www.gerbercoburn.com
Annual Revenue: $500 Million-$1 Billion
Year Founded: 1990
Total Employees: 2200
Ownership: Private
Produces/Sells CE-marked Devices: N
Distribution: Manufacturer Direct, Manufacturer Through Distributor, Manufacturer Through Manufacturer Reps, OEM
General Admin.: Alex Incera/President
　　　Mike Dolen/Vice President Human Resources
Mktg./Adv.: Randy Baldwin/Director Marketing
　　　Clement Patry/Executive Director Sales
　　　Wayne Labrecque/Vice President National Sales
Production: Steve Bedford/Director Engineering

Production Equipment	General

Medical Product Subsidiaries (Listed Separately)

GERBER COBURN OPTICAL INC. 800-262-8761 (cont'd)
Stereo Optical Co., Inc.

GERBER FAMILY HEALTH CARE
See Sca Personal Care, North America

GERBER PRODUCTS CO. 800-430-0150
120 N.commercial,4th floor, Neenah, WI 54956 231-928-2000
FDA Number: 2024305 *Fax:* 920-751-5888
E-mail: stesei@altaresources.com
Web site: www.gerber.com
Medical Products Sales Volume: $60,000,000
Annual Revenue: More than $100 Million
Year Founded: 1927
Total Employees: 30
Ownership: Private
Traded On: NYSE
Produces/Sells CE-marked Devices: N
Federal Procurement Eligibility: Small Business
Distribution: Manufacturer Through Distributor
General Admin.: Al Piergallini/President, Chief Executive Officer
Mktg./Adv.: Lee Van Syckle/Manager National Sales
　　　Steve Seidl/Sales Associate
　　　Lee Van Syckle/Senior Vice President Sales

Bottle, Nursing	Obstetrics/Gynecology
Pacifier	
Pump, Breast, Powered	Obstetrics/Gynecology

GEREONICS, INC. 949-929-9319
25501 Aria Drive, Mission Viejo, CA 92692
FDA Number: 2025694

Electrode, Electrocardiograph	Cardiovascular
Monitor, Ventilatory Frequency	Anesthesiology

GERI-CARE PRODUCTS 201-440-0409
250 Moonachie Avenue, Moonachie, NJ 07074
FDA Number: 2242944 *Fax:* 201-440-2899
E-mail: sales@geri-careproducts.com
Web site: www.geri-careproducts.com
Medical Products Sales Volume: $6,600,000
Annual Revenue: $10-$25 Million
Total Employees: 100 *Marketing Staff:* 2 *Sales Staff:* 4
Ownership: Private
Produces/Sells CE-marked Devices: N
Federal Procurement Eligibility: Small Business
Distribution: Manufacturer Through Distributor
General Admin.: Frank Hedges/President
Mktg./Adv.: Jeffrey Knowles/Manager Marketing
　　　Gary Geiger/Vice President Sales
　　　Leslie Farkas/Vice President Sales
　　　Lloyd Sheffer/Vice President Sales
　　　Sharle Camp/Vice President Sales

Bib	General
Diaper, Adult	General
Garment, Protective, For Incontinence	Gastroenterology/Urology
Linen	General
Pad, Incontinence (Underpad)	General
Pant, Incontinence	General

GERIATRIC PRODUCTS, INC. 718-384-5700
72 Division Place, Brooklyn, NY 11222
FDA Number: 2431955
Ownership: Private
Produces/Sells CE-marked Devices: N

Restraint, Protective (Body)	General

GERITREX CORP. 800-736-3437
**144 Kingbridge Road East, 914-668-4003
Mount Vernon, NY 10550**
FDA Number: 54612 *Fax:* 914-668-4047
E-mail: geritrex@aol.com
Web site: www.geritrex.com
Medical Products Sales Volume: $3,800,000
Annual Revenue: $1-$5 Million
Year Founded: 1978
Total Employees: 35 *Marketing Staff:* 2 *Sales Staff:* 5
Ownership: Private
Produces/Sells CE-marked Devices: N
Federal Procurement Eligibility: Small Business, Female Owned, GSA Contract, VA Contract
Distribution: Manufacturer Direct, Manufacturer Through Manufacturer Reps, Exclusive Distributor
General Admin.: Anthony Madaio/President
Mktg./Adv.: Mr. Maxie Rivers/National Accounts Representative
　　　John Gwynne/Vice President Marketing & Sales
Production: Jennifer Nuccitelli/Director Quality Assurance & Product Development

Crusher, Pill	General
Dressing, Wound and Burn, Occlusive	Surgery
Lotion, Skin Care	General

GERITREX CORP.   800-736-3437 *(cont'd)*
Solution, Antibacterial Cleaner   General

GERMAINE LABORATORIES, INC.   210-692-4192
11030 Wye Drive, San Antonio, TX 78217
FDA Number: 1649661   Fax: 210-692-4198
E-mail: sales@germainelabs.com
Web site: www.germainelabs.com
Ownership: Private
Produces/Sells CE-marked Devices: N

Antigen, (Febrile), Agglutination, Brucella SPP.	Microbiology
Antigen, Febrile, Slide And Tube, Salmonella	Microbiology
Antigen, Salmonella SPP.	Microbiology
Antigen, Slide And Tube, Francisella Tularensis	Microbiology
Antigen, Streptococcus SPP.	Microbiology
Antisera, Fluorescent, All Globulins, Proteus SPP.	Microbiology
Antiserum, Fluorescent, Brucella SPP.	Microbiology
Antiserum, Francisella Tularensis	Microbiology
Antiserum, Positive And Negative Febrile Antigen Control	Microbiology
Antiserum, Salmonella SPP.	Microbiology
Campylobacter Pylori	Microbiology
Enzyme Immunoassay, Amphetamine	Toxicology
Enzyme Immunoassay, Barbiturate	Toxicology
Enzyme Immunoassay, Benzodiazepine	Toxicology
Enzyme Immunoassay, Cannabinoids	Toxicology
Enzyme Immunoassay, Cocaine And Cocaine Metabolites	Toxicology
Enzyme Immunoassay, Methadone	Toxicology
Enzyme Immunoassay, Opiates	Toxicology
Enzyme Immunoassay, Phencyclidine	Toxicology
Enzyme Immunoassay, Propoxyphene	Toxicology
Gas Chromatography, Methamphetamine	Toxicology
Kit, Pregnancy Test, Over The Counter, HCG	Chemistry
Radioimmunoassay, Luteinizing Hormone	Chemistry
Radioimmunoassay, Tricyclic Antidepressant Drugs	Toxicology
Strip, Test, Reagent, Residuals For Dialysate, Disinfectant	Gastroenterology/Urology
Test, Human Chorionic Gonadotropin, Serum	Immunology
Test, Infectious Mononucleosis	Immunology
Test, Tetrahydrocannabinol	Toxicology

GERMGARD LIGHTING   (973) 607-1538
3328 Belt Road # 2, dover, NJ 07801-5769
FDA Number: n/a   Fax: 973-607-1543
E-mail: pgordon@germgardlighting.com
Web site: www.germgardlighting.com
Ownership: Private
Produces/Sells CE-marked Devices: N
General Admin.: Dr. Eugene Gordon/Chief Executive Officer
Mktg./Adv.: Dr. Edward David Jr./Advisor Tech. Marketing
    Mr. Peter Gordon/Vice President Marketing

GERMIPHENE CORP.   519-759-7100
1379 Colborne St. E, Brantford, ONT N3T-5M1 Canada
FDA Number: 9615418   Fax: 519-759-1625
E-mail: leslie@germiphene.com
Web site: www.germiphene.com
Year Founded: 1958
Total Employees: 100
Ownership: Private
Produces/Sells CE-marked Devices: N
Distribution: Manufacturer Direct, Exclusive Distributor

GERSON CO. INC., LOUIS M.   800-225-8623
15 Sproat St., Middleboro, MA 02346-2268   508-947-4000
FDA Number: 1219752   Fax: 508-947-5442
E-mail: custserv@gersonco.com
Web site: www.gersonco.com
Annual Revenue: $25-$50 Million
Total Employees: 175   Marketing Staff: 2   Sales Staff: 6
Ownership: Private
Produces/Sells CE-marked Devices: Y
Federal Procurement Eligibility: Small Business, GSA Contract, VA Contract
Distribution: Manufacturer Through Distributor, OEM, Importer, Exporter
General Admin.: R. L. Gerson/President, Chairman
Medical Admin.: Ms. Marsha Emond/Senior Vice President Health Care
Mktg./Adv.: R. L. Gerson/Vice President Marketing & Sales
Production: Bob Brunell/Manager Regulatory Affairs

Filter, Kidney Stone	Gastroenterology/Urology
Mask, Face	General
Mask, Other	General
Mask, Surgical	Surgery

GERSTNER & SONS INC.   937-228-1662
20 Gerstner Way, Dayton, OH 45402-3408
FDA Number: 7000525   Fax: 937-228-8557
E-mail: info@gerstnerusa.com
Web site: www.gerstnerusa.com
Medical Products Sales Volume: $200,000
Annual Revenue: $1-$5 Million
Year Founded: 1906

GERSTNER & SONS INC.   937-228-1662 *(cont'd)*
Total Employees: 20   Marketing Staff: 1   Sales Staff: 1
Ownership: Private
Produces/Sells CE-marked Devices: N
Federal Procurement Eligibility: Small Business, VA Contract
Distribution: Manufacturer Direct, Manufacturer Through Distributor
General Admin.: John H. Campbell/President, Chief Executive Officer
Mktg./Adv.: Kim Campbell/Director Marketing
    Scott Campbell/Director Product Development

Cabinet, Instrument	General
Contract Manufacturing	General

GESTURETEK HEALTH-GESTURETEK INC   408-216-8087
530 Lakeside Drive,, Suite 280, Sunnyvale, CA 94085
FDA Number: n/a   Fax: 408-732-3977
Web site: http://www.gesturetek.com/
Year Founded: 1986
Ownership: Private
Produces/Sells CE-marked Devices: N
General Admin.: Mr. Ralph Linsalata/Chief Executive Officer
    Mr. Francis MacDougall/Chief Technology Officer
Finance: Mr. Gary Nobrega/Vice President Finance & Operations

Exerciser, Non-Measuring	Physical Med

GETINGE SOURCING LLC   800-475-9040
1777 East Henrietta Rd., Rochester, NY 14623
FDA Number: 1314329   Fax: 585-272-5033
E-mail: info@getingeusa.com
Web site: www.getinge.com
Year Founded: 1904
Total Employees: 11500
Ownership: GETINGE AB
Produces/Sells CE-marked Devices: N

Disinfector, Medical Device	General
Hot Water Pasteurization Device	General
Sterilization Process Indicator, Biological	General
Sterilizer, Steam (Autoclave)	General

GETINGE USA, INC
See Maquet, Inc.

GETINGE USA, INC.   800-475-9040
1777 E. Henrietta Rd., Rochester, NY 14623-3133   585-475-1400
FDA Number: 3004147784   Fax: 585-272-5033
E-mail: info@getingeusa.com
Web site: www.getingeusa.com
Medical Products Sales Volume: $220,000,000
Annual Revenue: $100-$500 Million
Year Founded: 1883
Total Employees: 550   Marketing Staff: 15   Sales Staff: 125
Ownership: GETINGE AB
Quality System Registration Information: ISO9001
Produces/Sells CE-marked Devices: N
Distribution: Manufacturer Direct, Importer
Mktg./Adv.: Ms. Julie Shanahan/Manager Marketing & Communications

Accessories, Light, Surgical	Surgery
Cabinet Casework, General Purpose	General
Cabinet Casework, Modular	General
Cabinet, Warming	General
Cleaner, Bedpan (Sterilizer)	General
Cleaner, Ultrasonic, Medical Instrument	General
Culture Media, Non-Selective And Non-Differential	Microbiology
Indicator, Physical/chemical, Storage Temperature	General
Sink, Hospital	General
Sterilization Process Indicator, Biological	General
Sterilization Process Indicator, Chemical	General
Sterilizer, Laboratory	Microbiology
Sterilizer, Steam (Autoclave)	General
Sterilizer, Steam, Bulk	General
Table, Operating Room, AC-Powered	Surgery
Table, Other	General
Table, Surgical With Orthopedic Accessories, AC-Powered	Surgery
Table, Surgical, Electrical	Surgery
Timer, Scrub Station	Surgery
Washer, Cart	General
Washer, Labware	Chemistry
Washer, Pipette	Chemistry
Washer, Utensil	General
Washer/Disinfector	General

GETTIG PHARMACEUTICAL INSTRUMENT CO.,   814-422-8892
DIV OF GETTIG TECHNOLOGIES INC.
1 Streamside Pl. W., Spring Mills, PA 16875-0085
FDA Number: n/a   Fax: 814-422-8011
E-mail: tech1@gettig.com
Web site: www.gettig.com
Annual Revenue: $25-$50 Million
Year Founded: 1952
Total Employees: 7   Marketing Staff: 1   Sales Staff: 2

GETTIG PHARMACEUTICAL INSTRUMENT CO., 814-422-8892
(cont'd)
Ownership: GETTIG TECHNOLOGIES, INC.
Quality System Registration Information: ISO9000
Produces/Sells CE-marked Devices: Y
Federal Procurement Eligibility: Small Business
Distribution: Manufacturer Direct, Manufacturer Through Distributor, Manufacturer Through Manufacturer Reps, OEM, Service Direct, Exclusive Distributor, Exporter
General Admin.: Larry Obreiter/General Manager
　　　　　William Gettig/President, Chief Executive Officer
Production: James Benz/Manager Regulatory Affairs
IS: Jay Shah/Director Tech. Services

Contract Manufacturing	General
Needle, Hypodermic, Single Lumen With Syringe	General
Syringe, Hypodermic	General

Medical Product Subsidiaries (Listed Separately)
Stelrema Corp.

GF HEALTH PRODUCTS, INC 800-347-5678
2935 Northeast Pkwy, Atlanta, GA 30360
FDA Number: 2428983　　　*Fax:* 800-726-0601
E-mail: cs@grahamfield.com
Web site: www.grahamfield.com
Medical Products Sales Volume: $25,100,000
Annual Revenue: $25-$50 Million
Year Founded: 1946
Ownership: Basic American Medical, Inc.
Quality System Registration Information: ISO9000
Produces/Sells CE-marked Devices: N
Federal Procurement Eligibility: Small Business
Distribution: Manufacturer Through Distributor, Manufacturer Through Manufacturer Reps, Exclusive Distributor, Importer, Exporter
General Admin.: Kenneth Spett/Executive Vice President
　　　　　Beatrice Scherer/President, Chief Executive Officer
　　　　　Cherie Antoniazzi/Senior Vice President Human Resources

Bed, Electric	General
Bed, Electric, Home-Use	General
Bed, Manual	General
Bed, Pediatric (Crib)	General
Chair, Geriatric	General
Furniture, Patient Room	General
Mattress, Bed	General
Stretcher, Wheeled, Mechanical	Physical Med
Table, Mechanical	Physical Med
Table, Overbed	General

GF HEALTH PRODUCTS, INC. 770-368-4700
2935 Northeast Parkway, Atlanta, GA 30360
FDA Number: 3004539406　　*Fax:* 770-368-3234
E-mail: cs@grahamfield.com
Ownership: Private
Produces/Sells CE-marked Devices: N

Cuff, Blood Pressure	Cardiovascular
Thermometer, Electronic	General

GF HEALTH PRODUCTS, INC. 800-365-2338
336 Trowbridge Rd., North Fond Du Lac, WI 54937
FDA Number: 2183191　　*Fax:* 920-929-8210
E-mail: cs@grahamfield.com
Web site: www.grahamfield.com
Year Founded: 1946
Ownership: GF HEALTH PRODUCTS, INC
Produces/Sells CE-marked Devices: N
General Admin.: Kenneth Spett/Executive Vice President
　　　　　Beatrice Scherer/President, Chief Executive Officer
　　　　　Cherie Antoniazzi/Senior Vice President Human Resources

Bed, Electric	General
Bed, Electric, Home-Use	General
Bed, Manual	General
Bed, Pediatric (Crib)	General
Chair/Table, Medical	General
Stretcher, Wheeled (Mobile)	General

GFS CHEMICALS, INC. 800-858-9682
867 Mckinley Avenue, 614-224-5345
Columbus, OH 43222
FDA Number: 3002983930　　*Fax:* 614-225-1175
E-mail: sales@gfschemicals.com
Web site: www.gfschemicals.com
Year Founded: 1928
Total Employees: 60
Ownership: Private
Quality System Registration Information: ISO9000
Produces/Sells CE-marked Devices: N
Federal Procurement Eligibility: Small Business
Distribution: Manufacturer Through Distributor

Tricalcium Phosphate Granules for Dental Bone Repair	Dental And Oral

GH GUNTHER HUETTLIN MANUFACTURING, INC. 613-961-8860
101 Petrie Pl, Belleville K8N 4Z6 Canada
FDA Number: 9613808

Pad, Menstrual, Scented	Obstetrics/Gynecology
Pad, Menstrual, Unscented	Obstetrics/Gynecology

GI DYNAMICS, INC. 781-357-3300
1 Maguire Road, Lexington, MA 02421
FDA Number: n/a　　*Fax:* 781-357-3301
E-mail: info@gidynamics.com
Web site: http://www.gidynamics.com
Ownership: Private
Produces/Sells CE-marked Devices: N
General Admin.: Mr. Andy Levine/Chief Technology Officer
　　　　　Mr. Stuart Randle/President, Chief Executive Officer
Mktg./Adv.: Mr. Wade Fox/Vice President Marketing
Production: Ms. Sherrie Coval-Goldsmith/Vice President Regulatory & Clinical Affairs
Finance: Mr. Robert Crane/Chief Financial Officer

GI SUPPLY 800-451-5797
200 Grandview Ave., Camp Hill, PA 17011-1706 717-761-1170
FDA Number: 2529592　　*Fax:* 717-761-0216
E-mail: info@gi-supply.com
Ownership: Chek-Med Systems, Inc.
Produces/Sells CE-marked Devices: Y
Federal Procurement Eligibility: Small Business, Female Owned
Distribution: Manufacturer Direct, Manufacturer Through Manufacturer Reps
General Admin.: Frank C. Carter/Chief Executive Officer
Mktg./Adv.: Wade Schoenecker/Director Marketing & Sales

Accessories, Cart, Multipurpose	General
Bag, Plastic	General
Bib	General
Biopsy Instrument	Gastroenterology/Urology
Block, Bite	Cns/Neurology
Campylobacter Pylori	Microbiology
Cannula, Nasal, Oxygen	Anesthesiology
Cart, Multipurpose	General
Cart, Tissue	General
Cart, Waste	General
Catheter, Biliary	Gastroenterology/Urology
Cryosurgical Unit	Surgery
Endoscope	Gastroenterology/Urology
Gown, Examination	General
Gown, Other	General
Gown, Patient, Disposable	General
Gown, Surgical	Surgery
Kit, Surgical Instrument, Disposable	Surgery
Marker, Colon	Gastroenterology/Urology
Pump, Aspiration, Portable	Anesthesiology

GIBCO LABORATORIES
See Life Technologies Corporation

GIBCO/LIFE TECHNOLOGIES
See Life Technologies Corporation

GIBSON LABORATORIES 800-477-4763
1040 Manchester St., Lexington, KY 40508-2422 859-254-9500
FDA Number: 1050138　　*Fax:* 859-253-1476
E-mail: customerservice@gibsonlabs.com
Web site: www.gibsonlabs.com
Annual Revenue: $0-$1 Million
Total Employees: 14
Ownership: Private
Produces/Sells CE-marked Devices: N
Federal Procurement Eligibility: Small Business
Distribution: Manufacturer Direct, Manufacturer Through Distributor, OEM
General Admin.: Jeff Gibson/General Manager
　　　　　Cecil Gibson/President

Culture Media, For Isolation Of Pathogenic Neisseria	Microbiology
Culture Media, General Nutrient Broth	Microbiology
Culture Media, Mueller Hinton Agar Broth	Microbiology
Culture Media, Multiple Biochemical Test	Microbiology
Culture Media, Non-Propagating Transport	Microbiology
Culture Media, Non-Selective And Differential	Microbiology
Culture Media, Non-Selective And Non-Differential	Microbiology
Culture Media, Selective And Differential	Microbiology
Culture Media, Selective And Non-Differential	Microbiology
Culture Media, Selective Broth	Microbiology
Culture Media, Single Biochemical Test	Microbiology
Kit, Quality Control	Microbiology
Stain, Microbiological	Microbiology
Test, Agar Plate	Microbiology
Test, Agar Tube	Microbiology

GIBSON LABORATORIES, INC. 800-477-4763
1040 Manchester St., Lexington, KY 40508 859-254-9500
FDA Number: 1050138　　*Fax:* 859-253-1476
E-mail: customerservice@gibsonlabs.com

GIBSON LABORATORIES, INC.   800-477-4763 *(cont'd)*
Web site: www.gibsonlabs.com
Ownership: Private
Produces/Sells CE-marked Devices: N

Culture Media, For Isolation Of Pathogenic Neisseria	Microbiology
Culture Media, Mueller Hinton Agar Broth	Microbiology
Culture Media, Non-Selective And Differential	Microbiology
Culture Media, Non-Selective And Non-Differential	Microbiology
Culture Media, Selective And Differential	Microbiology
Culture Media, Selective And Non-Differential	Microbiology
Culture Media, Selective Broth	Microbiology
Culture Media, Single Biochemical Test	Microbiology
Kit, Quality Control	Microbiology

GIFT SALES CO.   800-992-0181
517 South St. Francis, Wichita, KS 67217   **316-267-0671**
FDA Number: 1929420   *Fax:* 316-267-2930
Ownership: Private
Produces/Sells CE-marked Devices: N

Brush, Scrub, Operating Room	Surgery

GILEAD SCIENCES   650-574-3000
333 Lakeside Dr., Foster City, CA 94404
FDA Number: n/a   *Fax:* 650-578-9264
E-mail: corporate_communications@gilead.com
Web site: www.gilead.com
Annual Revenue: $1-$5 Million
Ownership: Public
Stock Symbol: GILD
Traded On: NASDAQ
Produces/Sells CE-marked Devices: N
Federal Procurement Eligibility: Small Business
Distribution: Manufacturer Direct, Exporter
General Admin.: Pat Mahaffy/President

Contract R&D, Diagnostics	General
Standard, Lipid	Chemistry

GILES SCIENTIFIC, INC.   800-603-9290
PO Box 4306, Santa Barbara, CA 93140-4306   **805-963-3876**
FDA Number: 2433947   *Fax:* 805-963-7768
E-mail: giles@biomic.com
Web site: www.biomic.com
Medical Products Sales Volume: $600,000
Annual Revenue: $1-$5 Million
Year Founded: 1984
Total Employees: 5
Ownership: Private
Quality System Registration Information: ISO9001
Produces/Sells CE-marked Devices: Y
Federal Procurement Eligibility: Small Business, GSA Contract, VA Contract
Distribution: Manufacturer Direct, Manufacturer Through Distributor, Manufacturer Through Manufacturer Reps, OEM, Service Direct, Exporter
General Admin.: Dr. David Gibbs/Chief Executive Officer

Reader, Zone, Automated	Microbiology
Test, Antibiotic Susceptibility	Microbiology

GILIAN INSTRUMENT CORP.
See Sensidyne, Inc.

GILLEN INDUSTRIES   877-444-5536
1576 Bella Vista Cruz Drive, Suite 320,   **352-430-0841**
the villages, FL 32159
FDA Number: 1223403   *Fax:* 401-274-2148
E-mail: gillenindustries@cs.com
Web site: www.gillenindustries.com
Annual Revenue: $0-$1 Million
Year Founded: 1992
Total Employees: 1
Ownership: Private
Produces/Sells CE-marked Devices: N
Distribution: Manufacturer Direct
General Admin.: John F. Fillen/President

Restraint, Protective (Body)	General

GILLETTE CHILDREN'S SPECIALTY HEALTHCARE   612-229-3805
200 East University Ave., St. Paul, MN 55101
FDA Number: 2133507

Brace, Joint, Ankle (External)	Physical Med
Chair, Adjustable, Mechanical	Physical Med

GILLIAM ENTERPRISES, LLC   866-655-0517
5830 Briercliff Rd., Knoxville, TN 37918
FDA Number: n/a
Ownership: Private
Produces/Sells CE-marked Devices: N

Traction Unit, Non-Powered	Orthopedics

GILLIS ASSOCIATED INDUSTRIES   800-397-1675
750 Pinecrest Drive, Prospect Heights, IL 60070   **847-541-0858**
FDA Number: n/a   *Fax:* 847-541-0858
E-mail: info@gillisindustries.com
Web site: www.gillisindustries.com
Medical Products Sales Volume: $100,000
Annual Revenue: $50-$100 Million
Year Founded: 1950
Total Employees: 23   *Marketing Staff:* 5   *Sales Staff:* 25
Ownership: LEGGETT AND PLATT
Produces/Sells CE-marked Devices: N
Federal Procurement Eligibility: Small Business
Distribution: Manufacturer Direct, Manufacturer Through Distributor, Manufacturer Through Manufacturer Reps, Importer
General Admin.: Jim Anderson/President, General Manager
Mktg./Adv.: Nancy Novak/Manager Marketing
    Ed Granger/Vice President Sales

Cabinet Casework, General Purpose	General
Cart, Multipurpose	General
Cart, Other	General
Cart, Supply	General

GILMORE LIQUID AIR CO., INC.   626-443-1361
9503 E. Rush St., South El Monte, CA 91733
FDA Number: n/a   *Fax:* 626-443-1917
E-mail: lorraine.kaiban@gilmoreliquidair.com
Web site: www.gilmoreliquidair.com
Medical Products Sales Volume: $15,000
Annual Revenue: $1-$5 Million
Year Founded: 1955
Ownership: Private
Produces/Sells CE-marked Devices: N
Federal Procurement Eligibility: Small Business, Minority Owned, Female Owned
Distribution: Manufacturer Through Distributor
General Admin.: Virginia Mailander/Chief Executive Officer
    Jim Gilmore/President

Cryosurgical Unit	Surgery
Refrigerator, Bone	Orthopedics
Refrigerator, Eye Bank	Ophthalmology

GILSON COMPANY, INC.   800-444-1508
PO Box 200, Lewis Center, OH 43035-0200   **740-548-7298**
FDA Number: n/a   *Fax:* 740-548-5314
E-mail: sales@gilsonco.com
Web site: www.globalgilson.com
Medical Products Sales Volume: $190,000
Annual Revenue: $10-$25 Million
Year Founded: 1939
Total Employees: 2   *Marketing Staff:* 1   *Sales Staff:* 5
Ownership: Private
Produces/Sells CE-marked Devices: N
Federal Procurement Eligibility: Small Business, GSA Contract
Distribution: Manufacturer Direct, Manufacturer Through Distributor, Manufacturer Through Manufacturer Reps, Exclusive Distributor, Importer, Exporter
General Admin.: Robert H. Smith/Chief Executive Officer
    Trent Smith/President
Mktg./Adv.: Patricia Butler/Director Marketing
    Ray Miller/Manager International Marketing & Sales

Balance, Analytical	Chemistry
Burner	Chemistry
Calorimeter	Chemistry
Desiccator	Chemistry
Mixer, Clinical Laboratory	Chemistry
Sieve, Hematology	Hematology
Sieve, Tissue	Pathology

GIVEN IMAGING INC.   770-662-0870
3950 Shackleford Rd., Suite 500, Duluth, GA 30096-1852
FDA Number: 3005708125   *Fax:* 770-662-0510
E-mail: infousa@givenimaging.com
Web site: www.givenimaging.com
Ownership: Given Imaging Ltd.
Stock Symbol: GIVN
Traded On: NASDAQ
Produces/Sells CE-marked Devices: N
General Admin.: Mr. Israel Makov/Chairman
    Mr. James M. Cornelius/Director
    Mr. Michael Grobstein/Director
    Mr. Nachum (Homi) Shamir/President, Chief Executive Officer
Medical Admin.: Anat Loewenstein/Director Medical Div.

System, Imaging, Esophageal, Wireless, Capsule	Gastroenterology/Urology
System, Imaging, Gastrointestinal, Wireless, Capsule	Gastroenterology/Urology

GKR INDUSTRIES, INC.   800-526-7879
13653 Kenton Ave., Crestwood, IL 60445   **708-389-2003**
FDA Number: n/a   *Fax:* 708-389-3267
E-mail: rich@gkrindustries.com
Web site: www.gkrindustries.com

GKR INDUSTRIES, INC. 800-526-7879 *(cont'd)*
Medical Products Sales Volume: $1,600,000
Annual Revenue: $1-$5 Million
Year Founded: 1987
Total Employees: 14   *Marketing Staff:* 1
Ownership: Private
Produces/Sells CE-marked Devices: N
Federal Procurement Eligibility: Small Business
Distribution: Manufacturer Direct, Manufacturer Through Distributor, Manufacturer Through Manufacturer Reps, Exporter
General Admin.: Richard Fleury/President, Chief Executive Officer
Mktg./Adv.: Kris Fleury/Manager National Sales
  Bag, Urinary Collection   General
  Basin, Emesis   General

GLACIER CROSS, INC. 800-388-4828
1694 Whalebone Dr., Kalispell, MT 59901 406-257-8822
FDA Number: 9000761   *Fax:* 406-257-8880
E-mail: info@glaciercross.com
Web site: www.glaciercross.com
Year Founded: 1992
Total Employees: 7   *Marketing Staff:* 2   *Sales Staff:* 2
Ownership: Private
Produces/Sells CE-marked Devices: Y
Federal Procurement Eligibility: Small Business, Female Owned
Distribution: Manufacturer Through Distributor, Exporter
General Admin.: Susan Nickell/President
  Traction Unit, Non-Powered   Orthopedics

GLADES PHARMACEUTICALS, INC.
See Stiefel

GLADIATOR SPORTS 703-878-9434
3499 Cowes Mews, Woodbridge, VA 22193
FDA Number: ÿ1123830   *Fax:* 703-878-4570
E-mail: usgladiators@aol.com
Web site: www.gladiator-sports.com
Medical Products Sales Volume: $1,700,000
Annual Revenue: $0-$1 Million
Year Founded: 1987
Total Employees: 10   *Marketing Staff:* 5   *Sales Staff:* 2
Ownership: Private
Produces/Sells CE-marked Devices: N
Federal Procurement Eligibility: Small Business
Distribution: Importer
General Admin.: Amgad Rafi/Chief Executive Officer
  Sunglasses (Including Photosensitive)   Ophthalmology

GLAS-COL , LLC 800-452-7265
711 Hulman St., PO Box 2128, 812-235-6167
Terre Haute, IN 47802
FDA Number: 9200394   *Fax:* 812-234-6975
E-mail: pinnacle@glascol.com
Web site: www.glascol.com
Medical Products Sales Volume: $1,000,000
Year Founded: 1939
Total Employees: 90   *Marketing Staff:* 3   *Sales Staff:* 6
Ownership: Private
Quality System Registration Information: ISO9002
Produces/Sells CE-marked Devices: Y
Federal Procurement Eligibility: Small Business
Distribution: Manufacturer Through Distributor
General Admin.: Steve Sterrett/President
Mktg./Adv.: Karen Elliott/Manager International Accounts
    Jim Jacso/Manager National Sales
Finance: Paul Adams/Controller
  Evaporator   Chemistry
  Grinder, Tissue   Pathology
  Heating Mantle   Microbiology
  Polarimeter   Chemistry
  Shaker/Stirrer   Chemistry
  Stirrer   Chemistry

GLASROCK PLASTICS
See Porex Corporation

GLASROCK PRODUCTS INC.
See Porex Corporation

GLASS FAB, INC. 585-262-4000
257 Ormond St., PO Box 31880, Rochester, NY 14605
FDA Number: n/a   *Fax:* 585-454-4305
E-mail: info@glassfab.com
Web site: www.glassfab.com
Medical Products Sales Volume: $2,800,000
Annual Revenue: $5-$10 Million
Year Founded: 1974
Total Employees: 38   *Sales Staff:* 4
Ownership: Private
Produces/Sells CE-marked Devices: N

GLASS FAB, INC. 585-262-4000 *(cont'd)*
Federal Procurement Eligibility: Small Business
Distribution: Manufacturer Direct
General Admin.: Robert Saltzman/Chief Executive Officer
    Dan Saltzman/President
Mktg./Adv.: Wayne Leon/Manager National Sales
Production: Tom Kirk/Director Quality Assurance
Purchasing: George Dean/Purchasing Agent
  Filter, Lens   Ophthalmology

GLASS INSTRUMENTS, INC. 323-681-0011
2285 E. Foothill Blvd., Pasadena, CA 91107-3687
FDA Number: n/a   *Fax:* 626-792-7959
E-mail: glassins@earthlink.net
Web site: www.glassinstruments.com
Medical Products Sales Volume: $600,000
Annual Revenue: $0-$1 Million
Year Founded: 1946
Total Employees: 10   *Marketing Staff:* 1   *Sales Staff:* 1
Ownership: Private
Produces/Sells CE-marked Devices: N
Federal Procurement Eligibility: Small Business
Distribution: Manufacturer Direct, OEM, Exporter
General Admin.: Thurston C. LeVay/President, Chief Executive Officer
Production: Royce L. Worley/Manager Materials
    Anthony Mills/Manager Production
  Labware, Basic, Reusable   Chemistry
  Lamp, Ultraviolet, Germicidal   General
  Lamp, Ultraviolet, Physical Medicine   Physical Med

GLASSPAN, INC. 610-363-2300
The Commons at Lincoln Center, 101 J.R. Thomas Drive, Exton, PA 19341
FDA Number: 2530151
E-mail: drjscharf@aol.com
Web site: www.glasspan.com
Ownership: Private
Produces/Sells CE-marked Devices: N
  Cement, Dental   Dental And Oral
  Splint, Endodontic Stabilizer   Dental And Oral

GLAUKOS CORP. 949-367-9600
26051 Merit Cr #103, Laguna Hills, CA 92653
FDA Number: 2032546   *Fax:* 949-367-9984
E-mail: contact@glaukos.com
Web site: www.glaukos.com
Ownership: Private
Produces/Sells CE-marked Devices: N
  Forceps, Ophthalmic   Ophthalmology
  Gonioscope (Prism)   Ophthalmology
  Implant, Eye Valve   Ophthalmology
  Trephine, Manual, Ophthalmic (Corneal)   Ophthalmology

GLAXOSMITHKLINE CONSUMER HEALTHCARE, L.P. 215-751-4000
65 Industrial South, Clifton, NJ 07012
FDA Number: 2210777
Ownership: Private
Produces/Sells CE-marked Devices: N
  Cleaner, Denture   Dental And Oral

GLENN MEDICAL SYSTEMS, INC. 800-394-0173
511 12th Street, N.e., Canton, OH 44704 330-453-1177
FDA Number: 84399   *Fax:* 330-452-5163
E-mail: INFO@GLENNMEDICAL.COM
Web site: www.glennmedical.com
Ownership: Private
Produces/Sells CE-marked Devices: N
  Generator, Oxygen, Portable   Anesthesiology

GLENN REAMS, OCULARIST 800-426-8995
1020 West Buena Vista, Evansville, IN 47710
FDA Number: 1835046
Ownership: Private
Produces/Sells CE-marked Devices: N
  Eye, Artificial, Non-Custom   Ophthalmology

GLENN REAMS, OCULARIST 800-426-8995
221 N.w. Mcnary Court, Lee's Summit, MO 64086
FDA Number: 1933220
Ownership: Private
Produces/Sells CE-marked Devices: N
  Eye, Artificial, Non-Custom   Ophthalmology

GLENN REAMS, OCULARIST 800-426-8995
2845 Farrell Crescent, Owensboro, KY 42303
FDA Number: 1529973
Ownership: Private

GLENN REAMS, OCULARIST 800-426-8995 (cont'd)
Produces/Sells CE-marked Devices: N
  Eye, Artificial, Non-Custom   Ophthalmology

GLENN REAMS, OCULARIST 800-426-8995
610 South Floyd, Louisville, KY 40202
FDA Number: 1529972
  Eye, Artificial, Non-Custom   Ophthalmology

GLENROE TECHNOLOGIES 800-237-4060
1912 44th Ave., East, Bradenton, FL 34203 941-748-0857
FDA Number: 1036212   *Fax:* 941-748-1350
E-mail: glenroe@glenroe.com
Web site: www.glenroe.com
Year Founded: 1984
Ownership: Dentsply International, Inc.
Stock Symbol: XRAY
Traded On: NASDAQ
Produces/Sells CE-marked Devices: N
General Admin.: John Bozman/President
  Accessories, Retractor, Dental   Dental And Oral
  Adhesive, Bracket And Conditioner, Resin   Dental And Oral
  Aligner, Bracket, Orthodontic   Dental And Oral
  Band, Elastic, Orthodontic   Dental And Oral
  Bracket, Metal, Orthodontic   Dental And Oral
  Bracket, Plastic, Orthodontic   Dental And Oral
  Cement, Dental   Dental And Oral
  Depressor, Tongue   General
  Dispenser, Paraffin   Pathology
  Driver, Band, Orthodontic   Dental And Oral
  Filling, Instrument Plastic, Dental   Dental And Oral
  Lock, Wire, And Ligature, Intraoral   Dental And Oral
  Material, Impression Tray, Resin   Dental And Oral
  Mouthpiece, Breathing   Anesthesiology
  Mouthpiece, Saliva Ejector   Dental And Oral
  Pliers, Orthodontic   Dental And Oral
  Positioner, Tooth, Preformed   Dental And Oral
  Pusher, Band, Orthodontic   Dental And Oral
  Retractor, All Types   Dental And Oral
  Screw, Fixation, Intraosseous   Dental And Oral
  Splint, Temporary Training   Physical Med
  Tucker, Ligature, Orthodontic   Dental And Oral
  Wax, Dental   Dental And Oral
  Wire, Orthodontic   Dental And Oral

GLENROE TECHNOLOGIES 800-237-4060
210 Industrial Park Road, Baldwin, GA 30511 717-849-4229
FDA Number: n/a   *Fax:* 941-748-1350
Web site: www.glenroe.com
Year Founded: 1984
Ownership: Dentsply International, Inc.
Stock Symbol: XRAY
Traded On: NASDAQ
Produces/Sells CE-marked Devices: N
General Admin.: John Bozman/President

GLENVEIGH MEDICAL 423-933-3939
401 Chestnut St, Suite 230, Chattanooga, TN 37402
FDA Number: 3007532103
Web site: http://www.glenveigh.com
Year Founded: 2004
Ownership: Private
Produces/Sells CE-marked Devices: N
General Admin.: Mr. C. David Adair/Chief Scientific Officer
       Mr. Rick Proctor/President, Chief Executive Officer
Medical Admin.: Dr. Andy Johnson/Director Clinical Affairs
  Surgical Instrument, Obstetric/Gynecologic   Obstetrics/Gynecology

GLENWOOD LABORATORIES 800-361-9506
2392 Speers Rd., Oakville, ONT L6L-5M2 Canada 905-825-8244
FDA Number: n/a   *Fax:* 905-825-9543
E-mail: CService.glenwood@bellnet.ca
Web site: http://glenwoodmed-cpr.com
Year Founded: 1985
Total Employees: 10
Ownership: Private
Produces/Sells CE-marked Devices: N
Distribution: Exclusive Distributor, Importer

GLENWOOD LLC
See Western Medical, Ltd.

GLIATECH MEDICAL, INC. 216-831-3200
27070 Miles Rd., Solon, OH 44139
FDA Number: n/a
Ownership: Private
Produces/Sells CE-marked Devices: N
  Inhibitor, Peridural Fibrosis (Adhesion Barrier)   Physical Med

GLINES AND RHODES, INC. 800-343-1196
189 East St., P.O. Box 2285, Attleboro, MA 02703 508-226-2000
FDA Number: n/a   *Fax:* 508-226-7136
E-mail: sales@glinesandrhodes.com
Web site: www.glinesandrhodes.com
Year Founded: 1915
Ownership: Private
Produces/Sells CE-marked Devices: N
Mktg./Adv.: Mike Powers/Vice President Sales
  Metal, Medical   General

GLOBAL BIOMEDICS CORPORATION 800-473-1122
11005 Indian Trail #102, Dallas, TX 75229-3515
FDA Number: 3003681036
Ownership: Private
Produces/Sells CE-marked Devices: N
  Dressing, Wound, Hydrogel W/out Drug And/or Biologic   Surgery

GLOBAL CARE QUEST 949-330-7450
65 Enterprise, Suite 350, Aliso Viejo, CA 92656
FDA Number: 3005916650
  Computer, Chemistry Analyzer   Chemistry

GLOBAL DENTAL PRODUCTS 516-221-8844
PO Box 537, Bellmore, NY 11710
FDA Number: 8030898
E-mail: globaldent@aol.com   *Fax:* 516-785-7885
Web site: www.GDPDENTAL.com
Medical Products Sales Volume: $1,500,000
Annual Revenue: $1-$5 Million
Total Employees: 7   *Marketing Staff:* 3   *Sales Staff:* 4
Ownership: Private
Quality System Registration Information: ISO9000; ISO9002
Produces/Sells CE-marked Devices: Y
Federal Procurement Eligibility: Small Business
Distribution: OEM, Importer, Exporter
General Admin.: Jerry L. Bartick/President, Chief Executive Officer
Mktg./Adv.: Jerry Bartick/Director Product Development
       Berndt Lagerstedt/Manager International Marketing & Sales
       Renee Vivenzio/Manager Market Research
       Barry Stolzenberg/Manager National Sales
       Robin Stone/Vice President Marketing
Production: Kenneth Larsson/Director Quality Assurance
       Grethe Gartner/Manager Materials
  Coating, Denture Hydrophilic, Resin   Dental And Oral
  Irrigator, Oral   Dental And Oral
  Liner, Cavity, Calcium Hydroxide   Dental And Oral
  Material, Acrylic, Dental   Dental And Oral
  Soap   General
  Solution, Antibacterial Cleaner   General
  Varnish, Cavity   Dental And Oral

GLOBAL DENTECH INC. 215-654-1237
1116 Horsham Rd., North Wales, PA 19454
FDA Number: 3006115130
  Alloy, Precious Metal, For Clinical Use   Dental And Oral
  Denture, Plastic, Teeth   Dental And Oral
  Material, Impression   Dental And Oral
  Teeth, Porcelain   Dental And Oral

GLOBAL DOSIMETRY SOLUTIONS, INC.
See Mirion Technologies

GLOBAL ENDOSCOPY, INC. 888-434-3398
1507 Industrial Drive, Itasca, IL 60193-4426 630-773-3660
FDA Number: n/a   *Fax:* 630-773-3640
E-mail: info@globalendo.com
Web site: www.globalendo.com
Medical Products Sales Volume: $600,000
Year Founded: 1997
Total Employees: 5
Ownership: Private
Produces/Sells CE-marked Devices: N
Federal Procurement Eligibility: Small Business
Distribution: Manufacturer Direct, OEM
  Arthroscope   Orthopedics
  Cystoscope   Gastroenterology/Urology
  Hysteroscope   Obstetrics/Gynecology
  Laparoscope, General & Plastic Surgery   Surgery
  Laparoscope, Gynecologic   Obstetrics/Gynecology
  Otoscope   Ear/Nose/Throat
  Ureteroscope   Gastroenterology/Urology

GLOBAL FOCUS (G.F.M.D. LTD.) 800-527-2320
2280 Spring Lake Rd., Ste. 106, Dallas, TX 75234 972-919-1780
FDA Number: n/a   *Fax:* 972-247-3690
E-mail: info@gfmd.com
Web site: www.gfmd.com
Ownership: Private

GLOBAL FOCUS (G.F.M.D. LTD.)   800-527-2320 (cont'd)
Quality System Registration Information: ISO9000
Produces/Sells CE-marked Devices: Y
Federal Procurement Eligibility: Small Business
Distribution: Manufacturer Direct, Manufacturer Through Distributor, Exclusive Distributor, Importer, Exporter
General Admin.: Bert R. Williams/Chief Executive Officer
    Jack Horner/President
Production: Eric S. Hoy/Manager Regulatory Affairs

Analyzer, Chemistry, Enzyme Immunoassay	Chemistry
Anti-DNA Antibody (Enzyme-Labeled), Antigen, Control	Immunology
Anti-DNA Indirect Immunofluorescent Solid Phase	Immunology
Anti-RNP-Antibody, Antigen And Control	Immunology
Anti-SM-Antibody, Antigen And Control	Immunology
Antibody, Antimitochondrial, Indirect Immunofluorescent	Immunology
Antibody, Antinuclear, Indirect Immunofluorescent, Antigen	Immunology
Antibody, Multiple Auto, Indirect Immunofluorescent	Immunology
Centrifuge, Floor	Pathology
Centrifuge, Refrigerated	Pathology
Centrifuge, Tabletop	Pathology
Test System, Antineutrophil Cytoplasmic Antibodies (ANCA)	Immunology

GLOBAL FRANCHISE CONSULTANTS, INC.   330-848-1956
3656 Durham Road, Norton, OH 44203-6353
FDA Number: 1531226   *Fax:* 330-848-1956
E-mail: donaldabrown@hotmail.com
Medical Products Sales Volume: $100,000
Ownership: Private
Produces/Sells CE-marked Devices: N

Tips And Pads, Cane, Crutch And Walker	Physical Med

GLOBAL HEALTH PRODUCTS, INC   585-235-8815
1099 Jay St., Suite E, Rochester, NY 14611
FDA Number: 3003617794
E-mail: info1@globalhp.com
Web site: www.globalhp.com
Ownership: Private
Produces/Sells CE-marked Devices: N

Dressing, Wound, Hydrogel W/out Drug And/or Biologic	Surgery
Dressing, Wound, Occlusive	Surgery

GLOBAL HEALTHCARE   800-601-3880
1495 Hembree Rd., Ste. 700, Roswell, GA 30076   770-522-7520
FDA Number: 1057199   *Fax:* 770-522-7518
E-mail: info@globalhealthcare.net
Web site: www.globalhealthcare.net
Medical Products Sales Volume: $6,000,000
Annual Revenue: $5-$10 Million
Year Founded: 1993
Total Employees: 25   *Marketing Staff:* 5   *Sales Staff:* 5
Ownership: Private
Quality System Registration Information: ISO9000; ISO9001
Produces/Sells CE-marked Devices: Y
Federal Procurement Eligibility: Small Business, Minority Owned
Distribution: Manufacturer Through Distributor, Importer
General Admin.: Alam Ahmed/President
Mktg./Adv.: Inaki Chopeitia/Manager National Sales
    Mauricio Restrepo/Sales Associate
    Fabian Restrepo/Vice President Marketing

Bag, Body	General
Bag, Ice	General
Bandage, Elastic	General
Blade, Scalpel	Surgery
Blanket, Infant	General
Bracelet, Identification	General
Cap, Surgical	Surgery
Catheter, Balloon (Foley Type)	Surgery
Catheter, Suction (Tracheal Aspirating Tube)	Anesthesiology
Coat, Laboratory	General
Collector, Urine	Gastroenterology/Urology
Cover, Shoe, Operating Room	Surgery
Drape, Surgical	Surgery
Dress, Scrub, Disposable	Surgery
Gauze/sponge, Nonresorbable For External Use	Surgery
Gown, Examination	General
Gown, Isolation, Surgical	Surgery
Gown, Other	General
Gown, Surgical	Surgery
Kit, Administration, Intravenous	General
Kit, Prep	General
Lancet, Blood	General
Linen	General
Mask, Surgical	Surgery
Shield, Protective, Personnel	Radiology
Shoe And Shoe Cover, Conductive	Anesthesiology
Speculum, Vaginal, Non-Metal	Obstetrics/Gynecology
Sphygmomanometer, Aneroid (Arterial Pressure)	General
Sponge, Rayon Cellulose	General
Stethoscope, Manual	Cardiovascular
Syringe, Bulb	General

GLOBAL HEALTHCARE   800-601-3880 (cont'd)

Tape, Adhesive, Hypoallergenic	General
Thermometer, Mercury	General
Tip, Suction Tube (Yankauer, Poole, Etc.)	Surgery
Wrap, Sterilization	General

GLOBAL HEALTHCARE EXCHANGE INC. CANADA   416-798-1029
10 Carlson Ct., Ste. 610, Etobicoke, ONT M9W-6L2 Canada
FDA Number: n/a   *Fax:* 416-798-8287
Web site: www.ghx.com
Year Founded: 2000
Total Employees: 25
Ownership: Private
Produces/Sells CE-marked Devices: N
Distribution: Service Direct

GLOBAL HEALTHCHECK, INC.   949-757-0639
2417 34th Street, Suite 17, Santa Monica, CA 90405
FDA Number: 3004127564
Ownership: Private
Produces/Sells CE-marked Devices: N

Nitroprusside, Ketones (Urinary, Non-Quantitative)	Chemistry

GLOBAL IMAGING
See Narragansett Imaging

GLOBAL INSTRUMENTATION, LLC   315-682-0272
8104 Cazenovia Rd., Manlius, NY 13104
FDA Number: 3005737664   *Fax:* 1-315-682-0278
E-mail: info@gi-med.com
Web site: www.globalinstrumentation.com
Ownership: Private
Produces/Sells CE-marked Devices: N

Electrocardiograph, Ambulatory (With Analysis Algorithm)	Cardiovascular

GLOBAL MEDICAID PRODUCTS INC.   905-339-0666
3-1100 Invicta Dr, Oakville L6H 2K9 Canada
FDA Number: 9615915

Bandage, Adhesive	Surgery

GLOBAL MEDICAL COMPANY   801-746-0208
3450 S. Highland Dr., #303, Salt Lake City, UT 84106
FDA Number: 3005423322
Ownership: Private
Produces/Sells CE-marked Devices: N

Prosthesis, Hip, Semi-Const., Metal/Poly., Porous Uncemented	Orthopedics

GLOBAL MEDICAL FOAM, INC.   419-529-9354
124 Plymouth Street, Suite A, Lexington, OH 44904
FDA Number: 1530883   *Fax:* 419-884-9344
E-mail: GlobalFoam@aol.com
Web site: www.GlobalmedFoam.com
Medical Products Sales Volume: $100,000
Year Founded: 1992
Total Employees: 2   *Sales Staff:* 7
Ownership: Private
Produces/Sells CE-marked Devices: N
Federal Procurement Eligibility: Small Business, Minority Owned, Female Owned
Distribution: Manufacturer Direct, Manufacturer Through Distributor, Manufacturer Through Manufacturer Reps

Support, Patient Position	Anesthesiology

GLOBAL MEDICAL IMAGING   800-958-9986
222 Rampart Street, CHARLOTTE, NC 28203   704-940-7755
FDA Number: 3007103202
E-mail: rdienst@gmi3.com
Web site: www.gmi3.com
Ownership: Private
Produces/Sells CE-marked Devices: N

Scanner, Ultrasonic (Pulsed Doppler)	Radiology
Scanner, Ultrasonic (Pulsed Echo)	Radiology
Transducer, Ultrasonic, Diagnostic	Radiology

GLOBAL MEDICAL PRODUCTS INC.   800-387-6095
5230 S. Service Rd.,   905-634-7799
Burlington, ONT L7L-5 Canada
FDA Number: n/a   *Fax:* 905-634-2868
E-mail: glomed@on.aibn.com
Year Founded: 1980
Total Employees: 25
Ownership: Private
Produces/Sells CE-marked Devices: N
Distribution: Exclusive Distributor, Importer

GLOBAL ONE MEDICAL, INC.   561-842-7727
3707 Interstate Park Rd. S., Riviera Beach, FL 33404
FDA Number: n/a
Ownership: Private

GLOBAL ONE MEDICAL, INC. 561-842-7727 *(cont'd)*

Produces/Sells CE-marked Devices: N

Cushion, Wheelchair (Pad)	Physical Med
Thermometer, Electronic, Continuous	General
Thermometer, Mercury	General

GLOBAL PHARMAEUTICALS: A DIVISION OF IMPAX LABS INC. 800-296-9227

**3735 Castor Avenue, 215-289-2220
Philadelphia, PA 19124**
FDA Number: n/a *Fax:* 215-289-2223
E-mail: cs@globalphar.com
Web site: www.globalphar.com
Medical Products Sales Volume: $555,500,000
Annual Revenue: $50-$100 Million
Total Employees: 500 *Marketing Staff:* 2 *Sales Staff:* 9
Ownership: IMPAX LABORATORIES, INC.
Stock Symbol: IPXL
Traded On: NASDAQ
Produces/Sells CE-marked Devices: N
Federal Procurement Eligibility: Small Business
Distribution: Manufacturer Through Distributor, Manufacturer Through Manufacturer Reps, Exclusive Distributor
General Admin.: Barry Edwards/Chief Executive Officer
Larry Hsu/President
Mktg./Adv.: Laura Williams/Director Marketing
Gary Skalski/National Accounts Representative
Howard Marcus/National Accounts Representative
Rich Matchett/National Accounts Representative
Production: Gerard Cravello/Director Quality Assurance
Mark Shaw/Vice President Regulatory Affairs

Contract Manufacturing, Pharmaceuticals/Chemicals	General

GLOBAL SERVICES GROUP 757-220-8282

350 Mclaws Circle, Suite:2, Williamsburg, VA 23185
FDA Number: 3005847026
Ownership: Private
Produces/Sells CE-marked Devices: N

Goniometer, AC-powered	Orthopedics
Transducer, Miniature Pressure	Physical Med

GLOBAL SPORT TECHNOLOGY, INC 719-574-0584

4745 Signal Rock Rd., Colorado Springs, CO 80922
FDA Number: 3005147474
E-mail: info@globsport.org
Web site: www.globsport.org
Ownership: Private
Produces/Sells CE-marked Devices: N

Vibrator, Therapeutic	Physical Med

GLOBAL SURGICAL CORP. 800-861-3585
  636-861-3388
**3610 Tree Ct. Industrial Blvd.,
St. Louis, MO 63122**
FDA Number: 1937051 *Fax:* 636-861-2969
E-mail: info@globalsurgical.com
Web site: www.globalsurgical.com
Annual Revenue: $10-$25 Million
Year Founded: 1994
Total Employees: 60
Ownership: Private
Produces/Sells CE-marked Devices: N
Distribution: Manufacturer Through Manufacturer Reps
General Admin.: Mr. Jerry Oarbutt/President
Mktg./Adv.: Ms. Erin Boyd/Vice President Sales

Chair, Adjustable, Mechanical	Physical Med
Chair, Examination And Treatment	General
Chair, With Casters	Physical Med
Examination Device, AC-Powered	General
Light, Surgical Operating, Dental	Dental And Oral
Microscope, Surgical	Ear/Nose/Throat
Stand, Instrument, AC-Powered, Ophthalmic	Ophthalmology
Unit, Examining/Treatment, ENT	Ear/Nose/Throat

GLOBALMED INC. 613-394-9844

155 N. Murray St., Trenton, ONT K8V-5R5 Canada
FDA Number: n/a *Fax:* 613-394-9845
E-mail: info@globalmedinc.com
Web site: www.globalmedinc.com
Year Founded: 1999
Total Employees: 100
Ownership: Private
Quality System Registration Information: ISO9002
Produces/Sells CE-marked Devices: N
Distribution: Manufacturer Direct, Exporter

GLOBE ENTERPRISES INC.

See Globe Medical Tech, Inc.

GLOBE MEDICAL TECH, INC. 713-365-9595

1766 W. Sam Houston Pkwy N., Houston, TX 77043
FDA Number: n/a *Fax:* 713-365-9935
E-mail: sales@globemedtech.com
Web site: www.globemedtech.com
Medical Products Sales Volume: $7,000,000
Annual Revenue: $5-$10 Million
Total Employees: 265 *Marketing Staff:* 2 *Sales Staff:* 4
Ownership: Private
Quality System Registration Information: ISO9000; ISO9001; ISO9002
Produces/Sells CE-marked Devices: Y
Federal Procurement Eligibility: Small Business, Minority Owned
Distribution: Manufacturer Direct, Manufacturer Through Distributor, OEM, Importer, Exporter
General Admin.: Andy S. Hu/President, Chief Executive Officer
Mktg./Adv.: Mr. Joshua Rodriguez/Vice President Business Development
Production: Mr. John Liu/Senior Engineer
Finance: Ms. Tina Chang/Vice President Finance

Catheter, Intravenous	Cardiovascular
Component, Plastic	General
Contract Assembly	General
Contract Manufacturing	General
Equipment, Molding	General
General Medical Device	General
Glove, Surgical, Plastic Surgery	Surgery
Kit, Administration, Intravenous	General
Kit, Intravenous, Administration, Buret	General
Scalpel, One-Piece (Knife)	Surgery
Service, Engineering/Design	General
Service, Import/Export	General
Set, Administration, Intravenous, Needle-Free	General
Syringe, Hypodermic	General
Syringe, Other	General

GLOBE MOTORS 937-228-3171

2275 Stanley Ave., Dayton, OH 45404
FDA Number: n/a *Fax:* 937-229-8531
E-mail: info@globe-motors.com
Web site: www.globe-motors.com
Total Employees: 800
Ownership: Public
Traded On: Paris
Quality System Registration Information: ISO9001
Produces/Sells CE-marked Devices: N
Distribution: Manufacturer Through Manufacturer Reps
General Admin.: Steven A. McHenry/Vice President, General Manager
Mktg./Adv.: Derek J. Keegan/Director Marketing & Sales

Motor, Drill, Electric	Cns/Neurology

GLOBE SCIENTIFIC, INC. 800-394-4562
  201-599-1400
610 Winters Ave., Paramus, NJ 07653-1625
FDA Number: 2244900 *Fax:* 201-599-1406
E-mail: mail@globescientific.com
Web site: www.globescientific.com
Annual Revenue: $5-$10 Million
Year Founded: 1982
Total Employees: 24 *Marketing Staff:* 3 *Sales Staff:* 5
Ownership: Private
Produces/Sells CE-marked Devices: N
Federal Procurement Eligibility: Small Business, Female Owned
Distribution: Manufacturer Through Distributor
General Admin.: Milton Diamond/President
Mktg./Adv.: David Ackley/Manager International & National Sales
Dara Diamond/Vice President Marketing & Sales
Finance: Lisa Diamond Berger, CPA/Vice President Finance & Operations

Analyzer, Chemistry, Urine	Chemistry
Analyzer, Sedimentation Rate, Erythrocyte	Hematology
Brush, Cytology	General
Container, Embedding	Pathology
Container, Specimen, All Types	General
Cuvette, Spectrophotometer	Chemistry
Equipment, Laboratory, Gen. Purpose (Specific Medical Use)	Chemistry
General Purpose Hematology Device	Hematology
Loop, Inoculating	Microbiology
Microplate	General
Pipette	Chemistry
Pipette Tip	Chemistry
Pipette, Micro	Chemistry
Pipette, Pasteur	Hematology
Pipette, Quantitative, Hematology	Hematology
Rack, Test Tube	Chemistry
Transport System, Aerobic	Microbiology
Tube, Centrifuge	Chemistry
Tube, Culture	Microbiology
Tube, Sedimentation Rate	Hematology
Tube, Test	Chemistry
Tube, Transfer	General
Vial, Hematology	General

GLOBE SCIENTIFIC, INC.
800-394-4562 *(cont'd)*
Vial, Liquid Scintillation Counting — Chemistry

GLOBUS MEDICAL INC.
610-930-1800
Valley Forge Business Center, 2560 General Armistead Ave.,
Audobon, PA 19403
FDA Number: 3004142400
Fax: 610-930-2042
E-mail: info@globusmedical.com
Web site: www.globusmedical.com
Year Founded: 2003
Ownership: Private
Produces/Sells CE-marked Devices: N
General Admin.: Mr. Daniel Lemaitre/Chairman
David Paul/Chief Executive Officer
Dave Demski/President, Chief Operating Officer
Mktg./Adv.: Rick Kienzle/Executive Vice President Marketing & Sales
Mr. Kevin Carouge/Senior Vice President Corporate Development
Production: David Davidar/Vice President Operations
Finance: Mr. Al Thorp/Chief Financial Officer

Appliance, Fixation, Spinal Interlaminal	Orthopedics
Appliance, Fixation, Spinal Intervertebral Body	Orthopedics
Calcium Salt Bone Void Filler, Drillable, Non-screw Augmentation	Orthopedics
Device, Spinal Vertebral Body Replacement	Orthopedics
Filler, Bone Void, Osteoinduction	Physical Med
Orthosis, Fixation, Pedicle, Spinal	Orthopedics
Orthosis, Fixation, Spinal, Spondylolisthesis	Orthopedics
Prosthesis, Elbow, Hemi-, Radial, Polymer	Orthopedics
System, Facet Screw Spinal Device	Orthopedics

GLUCOTEC, INC.
864-370-3297
665 north academy street, Greenville, SC 29601
FDA Number: 3005853093
Ownership: Private
Produces/Sells CE-marked Devices: N
Research: Robert Booth/Senior Vice President Research & Development

Accessories, Pump, Infusion	General
Calculator, Drug Dose	Surgery

GML, INC.
651-486-3691
500 Oak Grove Pkwy., St. Paul, MN 55127
FDA Number: 2135339
Ownership: Private
Produces/Sells CE-marked Devices: N

Catheter, Biliary, General & Plastic Surgery	Surgery
Reagent, Glucose (Test System)	Chemistry

GMZ ASSOCIATES, LTD.
800-581-5088
86 Cain Drive, Brentwood, NY 11717
631-273-5088
FDA Number: 2436933
Fax: 631-273-0617
E-mail: wetnbrush@aol.com
Web site: www.wetnbrush.com
Medical Products Sales Volume: $200,000
Year Founded: 1994
Total Employees: 4
Ownership: Private
Produces/Sells CE-marked Devices: N
Federal Procurement Eligibility: Small Business
Distribution: Manufacturer Through Distributor, Manufacturer Through
Manufacturer Reps, Importer

Toothbrush, Manual	Dental And Oral

GN OTOMETRICS
800-289-2150
50 Commerce Drive, Ste 180,
847-534-2150
Schaumburg, IL 60173
FDA Number: 1450453
Fax: 847-534-2151
E-mail: sales@icsmedical.com
Web site: www.icsmedical.com
Medical Products Sales Volume: $7,000,000
Annual Revenue: $5-$10 Million
Total Employees: 30
Ownership: Gn Resound Corp.
Quality System Registration Information: ISO9000
Produces/Sells CE-marked Devices: Y
Federal Procurement Eligibility: Small Business
Distribution: Manufacturer Through Distributor
Production: Peta Gates/Product Manager

Drum, Opticokinetic	Ophthalmology
Electrode, Electronystagmographic	Ophthalmology
Electronystagmograph (ENG)	Ophthalmology
Gel, Electrode, TENS	Physical Med
Irrigator, Caloric	Ear/Nose/Throat
Lens, Fresnel, Flexible, Diagnostic	Ophthalmology
Stimulator, Caloric Water	Ear/Nose/Throat
Unit, Examining/Treatment, ENT	Ear/Nose/Throat
Unit, Measuring, Potential, Evoked, Auditory	Ear/Nose/Throat

GN OTOMETRICS NORTH AMERICA
800-289-2150
125 Commerce Dr., Hoffman Est, IL 60173
FDA Number: n/a

GN OTOMETRICS NORTH AMERICA
800-289-2150 *(cont'd)*
Ownership: Private
Produces/Sells CE-marked Devices: N

Analyzer, Apparatus, Vestibular	Ear/Nose/Throat
Drum, Opticokinetic	Ophthalmology
Lens, Fresnel, Flexible, Diagnostic	Ophthalmology
Nystagmograph	Cns/Neurology
Stimulator, Auditory, Evoked Response	Cns/Neurology
Stimulator, Caloric Air	Ear/Nose/Throat
Stimulator, Caloric Water	Ear/Nose/Throat
Unit, Examining/Treatment, ENT	Ear/Nose/Throat

GN RESOUND
800-248-4327
8001 Bloomington Freeway,
952-769-8000
Bloomington, MN 55420
FDA Number: 2182204
Fax: 952-769-8001
E-mail: gnresound@gnresound.com
Web site: http://www.gnresound.com
Ownership: Private
Produces/Sells CE-marked Devices: N

Hearing Aid, Air Conduction, Transcutaneous System	Ear/Nose/Throat
Hearing-Aid	Ear/Nose/Throat
Hearing-Aid, Plate, Face	Ear/Nose/Throat
Masker, Tinnitus	Ear/Nose/Throat

GN RESOUND CORPORATION
800-582-4327
Seaport Center, 220 Saginaw Drive,
650-780-7800
Redwood City, CA 94063
FDA Number: n/a
Fax: 650-367-0675
E-mail: info@gnresound.com
Web site: www.gnresound.com
Annual Revenue: More than $100 Million
Year Founded: 1984
Total Employees: 500
Ownership: Gn Resound Corporation
Stock Symbol: RSND
Traded On: NASDAQ
Quality System Registration Information: ISO9001
Federal Procurement Eligibility: Small Business
Distribution: Manufacturer Through Distributor, Importer, Exporter
General Admin.: Jesper Mailand/Chief Executive Officer
Carsten Trads/President
Mktg./Adv.: Nikolai Bisgaard/Vice President Business Development
Research: Chaslav Pavlovic/Vice President Research & Development
Finance: Jeris Daugbjerg/Chief Financial Officer

Communication System, Powered	Physical Med

Medical Product Subsidiaries (Listed Separately)
Gn Resound Corporation

GNATHODONTICS LTD.
800-234-9515
10488 West 6th Place, Lakewood, CO 80215
303-424-9515
FDA Number: n/a
Web site: www.gnatho.com
Annual Revenue: $0-$1 Million
Year Founded: 1975
Ownership: Private
Produces/Sells CE-marked Devices: N
Distribution: Manufacturer Direct
General Admin.: Kevin Kelly/Manager
Myron Wilson/Manager
Steve Kelly/Manager
Mktg./Adv.: John Bozis/Sales Associate

Crown, Preformed	Dental And Oral
Prosthesis, Dental	Dental And Oral

GO-MI, INC.
415-453-3409
740 Fawn Dr., San Anselmo, CA 94960
FDA Number: 2939479
Ownership: Private
Produces/Sells CE-marked Devices: N

Computer, Pulmonary Function Data	Anesthesiology

GODARD INSTRUMENTS
See CAREFUSION 211, INC..

GOETZE DENTAL
800-692-0804
3939 N.E. 33rd Terrace, Kansas City, MO 64117
816-413-1200
FDA Number: n/a
Fax: 816-413-0475
Web site: www.goetzedental.com
Year Founded: 1884
Ownership: Private
Produces/Sells CE-marked Devices: N
Federal Procurement Eligibility: Small Business, Female Owned

Film, X-Ray, Dental, Extraoral	Dental And Oral
Film, X-Ray, Dental, Intraoral	Dental And Oral

GOJO INDUSTRIES, INC
800-321-9647
One GOJO Plaza, Suite 500, Akron, OH 44311
330-255-6000
FDA Number: n/a
Fax: 330-255-6119

GOJO INDUSTRIES, INC   800-321-9647 *(cont'd)*
Web site: www.gojo.com
Year Founded: 1946
Ownership: Private
Produces/Sells CE-marked Devices: N
Federal Procurement Eligibility: Small Business
Distribution: Manufacturer Through Distributor

Dispenser, Soap	General
Soap	General
Solution, Antibacterial Cleaner	General

GOLD CARE MEDICAL GROUP   800-282-3909
91 Ave. #4619, Edmonton, ALB T6B-2M7 Canada   **780-468-4002**
FDA Number: n/a   Fax: 780-465-3879
E-mail: sales@goldcare.com
Web site: www.goldcare.com
Year Founded: 1978
Ownership: Private
Produces/Sells CE-marked Devices: N
Distribution: Service Direct

GOLD STANDARD DIAGNOSTICS   530-759-8000
2851 Spafford St., Suite A, Davis, CA 95618
FDA Number: 3007208259   Fax: 530-759-8012
E-mail: info@GoldStandardDiagnostics.com
Web site: www.goldstanddiagnostics.com
Ownership: Private
Produces/Sells CE-marked Devices: N
General Admin.: Mr. Jim Thompson/Chief Executive Officer
     Mr. John Griffiths/President
Mktg./Adv.: Mr. Robert Hatch/Vice President Business Development
Research: Ms. Jennifer Roth/Director Tech. Affairs

GOLD'N BRACES, INC.   800-785-1970
2595 Tampa Road, Suite 1,   **727-785-5491**
Palm Harbor, FL 34684
FDA Number: 1054747   Fax: 727-787-5000
E-mail: nanrs@aol.com
Web site: www.goldnbraces.com
Medical Products Sales Volume: $300,000
Year Founded: 1991
Ownership: Private
Produces/Sells CE-marked Devices: N
Federal Procurement Eligibility: Small Business
Distribution: Manufacturer Direct, OEM, Service Direct, Exporter

Bracket, Metal, Orthodontic	Dental And Oral
Wire, Orthodontic	Dental And Oral

GOLDA, INC.   800-321-4804
24050 Commerce Park,   **216-464-5490**
Cleveland, OH 44122
FDA Number: 1525724   Fax: 216-464-9365
E-mail: sales@surgi-solutions.com
Web site: www.goldainc.com
Annual Revenue: $1-$5 Million
Year Founded: 1976
Total Employees: 5
Ownership: Private
Produces/Sells CE-marked Devices: N
Federal Procurement Eligibility: Small Business
Distribution: Manufacturer Direct, Manufacturer Through Distributor
General Admin.: Alfred Corrado/President
Mktg./Adv.: Catherine Foley/Manager Advertising
     Donald Burck/Vice President Marketing
     Mark Corrado/Vice President Sales

Binder, Abdominal	General
Binder, Breast	Obstetrics/Gynecology
Binder, Medical, Therapeutic	General

GOLDEN EMPIRE DENTAL LAB CORP.   661-327-1888
929 21st Street, Bakersfield, CA 93301
FDA Number: 3004714238
Ownership: Private
Produces/Sells CE-marked Devices: N

Teeth, Porcelain	Dental And Oral

GOLDEN GATE PUMP CO.
See Ems Pacific, Inc.

GOLDEN METAL PRODUCTS CO.   800-978-9058
50 BUSHES LANE, Elmwood Park, NJ 07407-3296   **201-797-8855**
FDA Number: n/a   Fax: 201-398-9326
E-mail: cwclaudia@goldmetal.com
Web site: www.goldmetal.com
Medical Products Sales Volume: $2,000,000
Annual Revenue: $5-$10 Million
Total Employees: 60   *Marketing Staff:* 2   *Sales Staff:* 2
Ownership: Private

GOLDEN METAL PRODUCTS CO.   800-978-9058 *(cont'd)*
Federal Procurement Eligibility: Small Business, Minority Owned, GSA Contract, VA Contract
Distribution: Exporter
General Admin.: Neila Pomar/Assistant Manager
     Thomas Abella/President
Mktg./Adv.: Claudette Wilson/Vice President Sales

Mount, Equipment	General

GOLDEN TECHNOLOGIES, INC.   800-624-6374
401 Bridge St., Old Forge, PA 18518   **570-451-7477**
FDA Number: 2523955   Fax: 800-628-5165
E-mail: info@goldentech.com
Web site: www.goldentech.com
Medical Products Sales Volume: $9,900,000
Year Founded: 1985
Total Employees: 150   *Marketing Staff:* 5   *Sales Staff:* 47
Ownership: Private
Produces/Sells CE-marked Devices: N
Federal Procurement Eligibility: Small Business, VA Contract
Distribution: Manufacturer Direct, Manufacturer Through Manufacturer Reps
General Admin.: Richard Golden/Chief Executive Officer
     Bob Golden/President
     Frederick J. Kiwak/Vice President
Mktg./Adv.: Donna Payer/Director National Accounts
     C.J. Copley/Vice President Marketing
     Randy Walsh/Vice President Marketing & Sales
Production: Ed Pollard/Manager Production
Research: Fred Kiwak/Vice President Research & Development

Bed, Electric	General
Chair, Seat Lifting (Standing Aid)	General
Scooter (Motorized 3-Wheeled Vehicle)	Physical Med
Wheelchair, Powered	Physical Med

GOLDEN TRIANGLE DENTAL LABORATORY INC.   972-910-9912
7475 Las Colinas Blvd., Suite A, Irving, TX 75063
FDA Number: 3006230769
Ownership: Private
Produces/Sells CE-marked Devices: N

Alloy, Gold Based, For Clinical Use	Dental And Oral
Alloy, Precious Metal, For Clinical Use	Dental And Oral
Metal, Base	Dental And Oral
Powder, Porcelain	Dental And Oral

GOLDENTONE HEARING AIDS   800-826-6789
10597 Kansas Ave., Hayward, WI 54843-0751   **715-634-8435**
FDA Number: n/a   Fax: 715-634-8435
Annual Revenue: $0-$1 Million
Ownership: Private
Produces/Sells CE-marked Devices: N
Federal Procurement Eligibility: Small Business
Distribution: Manufacturer Direct, Manufacturer Through Distributor, Manufacturer Through Manufacturer Reps, Exclusive Distributor
General Admin.: Karen Mullally/President
Mktg./Adv.: Thomas Ruby/Vice President Sales

Hearing-Aid	Ear/Nose/Throat

GOLDLINE MOBILITY AND CONVERSIONS   800-561-9621
1759 Trafalgar St.,   **519-453-0480**
London, ONT N5W-1 Canada
FDA Number: n/a   Fax: 519-455-5915
Year Founded: 1970
Total Employees: 10
Ownership: Private
Produces/Sells CE-marked Devices: N
Distribution: Manufacturer Direct

GOLDMAN PRODUCTS, INC.   847-526-1166
379 Hollow Hill Dr., Wauconda, IL 60084
FDA Number: 1419982   Fax: 847-526-1363
E-mail: sales@dentalmaker.com
Web site: www.goldmandental.com
Medical Products Sales Volume: $2,900,000
Annual Revenue: $1-$5 Million
Ownership: Private
Produces/Sells CE-marked Devices: N
Federal Procurement Eligibility: Small Business, Minority Owned
Distribution: Manufacturer Direct, Manufacturer Through Manufacturer Reps, Service Direct

Burnisher, Operative, Dental	Dental And Oral
Carver, Dental Amalgam, Operative	Dental And Oral
Condenser, Amalgam And Foil, Operative	Dental And Oral
Curette, Endodontic	Dental And Oral
Curette, Periodontic	Dental And Oral
Curette, Surgical, Dental	Dental And Oral
Elevator, Surgical, Dental	Dental And Oral
Excavator, Dental, Operative	Dental And Oral
Explorer, Operative	Dental And Oral

GOLDMAN PRODUCTS, INC.   847-526-1166 (cont'd)

File, Margin Finishing, Operative	Dental And Oral
Filling, Instrument Plastic, Dental	Dental And Oral
Handle, Instrument, Dental	Dental And Oral
Knife, Periodontic	Dental And Oral
Knife, Surgical	Dental And Oral
Pliers, Operative	Dental And Oral
Plugger, Root Canal, Endodontic	Dental And Oral
Probe, Periodontic	Dental And Oral
Scaler, Periodontic	Dental And Oral
Scissors, Surgical Tissue, Dental (Oral)	Dental And Oral
Surgical Instrument, Manual (General Use)	Surgery

GOLDSMITH & REVERE, INC.   201-894-5500
242 S. Dean St., Englewood, NJ 07631-4139
FDA Number: 2243988   Fax: 201-894-0213
Annual Revenue: $1-$5 Million
Ownership: Private
Produces/Sells CE-marked Devices: N
Federal Procurement Eligibility: Small Business
Distribution: Manufacturer Through Distributor, Exclusive Distributor

Alloy, Amalgam	Dental And Oral
Amalgamator, Dental, AC-Powered	Dental And Oral
Capsule, Dental, Amalgam	Dental And Oral

GOMCO
See Allied Healthcare Products, Inc.

GOMEZ PACKAGING CORP.   973-569-9500
75 Wood St., Paterson, NJ 07524
FDA Number: 3003829558   Fax: 973-569-0208
E-mail: info@gomezpack.com
Web site: www.gomezpack.com
Ownership: Private
Produces/Sells CE-marked Devices: N

Bandage, Compression	General
Garment, Protective, For Incontinence	Gastroenterology/Urology
Pads, Menstrual, Scented-deodorized	Obstetrics/Gynecology
Tampon, Menstrual, Scented	Obstetrics/Gynecology

GOOD SPORTS   412-731-3032
1701 Monongahela Avenue, Pittsburgh, PA 15218
FDA Number: n/a   Fax: 412-731-3052
E-mail: staff@sportmasterinc.com
Web site: www.sportmasterinc.com
Medical Products Sales Volume: $50,000
Annual Revenue: $0-$1 Million
Year Founded: 1967
Total Employees: 10   Sales Staff: 3
Ownership: Private
Federal Procurement Eligibility: Small Business
Distribution: Manufacturer Direct
General Admin.: Lou Brom/President
Mktg./Adv.: Mary Fullen/Manager Contract Sales
            Jean McCue/Sales Associate

Chair, Rehabilitation	General
Table, Examination/Treatment	General
Wheelchair, Manual	Physical Med

GOOD-LITE CO.   800-362-3860
1155 Jansen Farm Drive, Elgin, IL 60123   847-841-1145
FDA Number: 9200396   Fax: 888-362-2576
E-mail: info@good-lite.com
Web site: www.good-lite.com
Medical Products Sales Volume: $900,000
Annual Revenue: $0-$1 Million
Total Employees: 5
Ownership: Private
Produces/Sells CE-marked Devices: N
Federal Procurement Eligibility: Small Business
Distribution: Manufacturer Through Distributor
General Admin.: Rob Rogers/President

Analyzer, Visual Function	Ophthalmology
Chart, Visual Acuity	Ophthalmology
Tester, Color Vision	Ophthalmology

GOODWILL INDUSTRIES OF CENTRAL INDIANA, INC.   317-524-4313
1635 West Michigan St., Indianapolis, IN 46222
FDA Number: 1832711   Fax: 317-524-4336
E-mail: goodwill@goodwillindy.org
Web site: www.goodwillindy.org
Ownership: Private
Produces/Sells CE-marked Devices: N

Orthosis, Cervical-Thoracic, Rigid	Physical Med

GOODWIN MANUFACTURING, INC.   800-282-5267
6980 Pike View Drive, PO Box 5981,   336-476-4147
Thomasville, NC 27370
FDA Number: n/a   Fax: 336-476-4026
E-mail: info@giraffelamps.com
Web site: www.giraffelamps.com
Medical Products Sales Volume: $1,000,000
Year Founded: 1979
Total Employees: 8   Marketing Staff: 3   Sales Staff: 12
Ownership: Private
Produces/Sells CE-marked Devices: N
Federal Procurement Eligibility: Small Business
Distribution: Manufacturer Direct, Manufacturer Through Distributor, Manufacturer Through Manufacturer Reps, Service Direct
General Admin.: Bill Gurney/President, Chief Executive Officer
            Marty Cagle/Vice President, General Manager
Production: Dwan Richardson/Manager Production

Lamp, Examination (Light)	General
Lamp, Other	General

GOSHEN AMERICANA, INC.
See Bio-Med U.S.A. Inc.

GOSHEN COACH DIV. WARRICK INDUSTRIES, INC.   800-326-2062
25161 LEER DRIVE, Elkhart, IN 46514   219-264-7511
FDA Number: n/a   Fax: 219-266-5866
E-mail: bus@goshencoach.com
Web site: www.goshencoach.com
Medical Products Sales Volume: $36,000,000
Total Employees: 230   Sales Staff: 5
Ownership: Private
Federal Procurement Eligibility: Small Business, GSA Contract
Distribution: Manufacturer Through Distributor
Mktg./Adv.: Randy Nemitz/Director Marketing

Vehicle, Handicapped	Physical Med

GOSPRO, INC.   808-842-2282
2305 Kamehameha Hwy., Honolulu, HI 96819
FDA Number: n/a
Ownership: Private
Produces/Sells CE-marked Devices: N

Gas, Calibrated (Specified Concentration)	Anesthesiology
Laser, Surgical	Surgery

GOTTFRIED MEDICAL, INC.   419-474-2973
4105 W. Alexis Rd., Toledo, OH 43623
FDA Number: 1526072

Stocking, Elastic	General

GOTTFRIED MEDICAL, INC.   (800) 537-1968
P.O. Box 350457, Toledo, OH 43617-0457   419-474-2973
FDA Number: 1526072   Fax: (866) 474-8822
Web site: www.gottfriedmedical.com
Annual Revenue: $0-$1 Million
Total Employees: 12   Sales Staff: 1
Ownership: Private
Produces/Sells CE-marked Devices: N
Federal Procurement Eligibility: Small Business
Distribution: Manufacturer Direct, Manufacturer Through Distributor, Manufacturer Through Manufacturer Reps, Exporter
General Admin.: Brent Gottfried/President
Production: Lisa King/Manager Production

Dressing, Wound and Burn, Occlusive	Surgery
Elastomer, Silicone (Scar Management)	Surgery
Stocking, Elastic	General

GOULD BATTERY
See Duracell Usa

GOULD DISCOUNT MEDICAL   800-876-6846
3901 Dutchmans LN #100, Louisville, KY 40207   502-491-1943
FDA Number: n/a   Fax: 502-491-2000
Web site: www.bruno.gouldsdiscountmedical.com
Medical Products Sales Volume: $3,000,000
Annual Revenue: $1-$5 Million
Total Employees: 75   Marketing Staff: 2   Sales Staff: 3
Ownership: Private
Produces/Sells CE-marked Devices: N
Federal Procurement Eligibility: Small Business
Distribution: Service Direct
General Admin.: Ed Gould/President, Chief Executive Officer
            Kens Gould/Vice President, General Manager
Mktg./Adv.: David Gould/Vice President Business Development

Service, Parts, Repair	General
Wheelchair, Powered	Physical Med

GOULD ELECTRONICS
See Lds Life Science (Formerly Gould Instrument Systems Inc.)

MANUFACTURER PROFILES

GOULD INC., CARDIOPULMONARY DIV.
See CAREFUSION 211, INC..

GOULD INC., DAYTON DIV.
See CAREFUSION 211, INC..

GOULD INC., RECORDING SYSTEMS DIV.
See Lds Life Science (Formerly Gould Instrument Systems Inc.)

GOULD INC., TEST & MSMT. REC. SYST. DIV.
See Lds Life Science (Formerly Gould Instrument Systems Inc.)

GOW TRAINER LTD.   **705-721-9994**
310 Georgian Dr., R.R#1, Barrie, ONT L4M 7B7 Canada
FDA Number: n/a   Fax: 705-721-8485
E-mail: info@shoulderstrength.com
Web site: http://gow-trainer.com
Year Founded: 1974
Ownership: Private
Produces/Sells CE-marked Devices: N
Distribution: Manufacturer Direct, Manufacturer Through Distributor

GOW-MAC INSTRUMENT CO.   **610-954-9000**
277 Brodhead Rd., Bethlehem, PA 18017
FDA Number: 7000158
    Fax: 610-954-0599
E-mail: sales@gow-mac.com
Web site: www.gow-mac.com
Medical Products Sales Volume: $100,000
Annual Revenue: $5-$10 Million
Year Founded: 1935
Total Employees: 36   Marketing Staff: 2   Sales Staff: 4
Ownership: Private
Produces/Sells CE-marked Devices: N
Federal Procurement Eligibility: Small Business
Distribution: Manufacturer Direct, Manufacturer Through Manufacturer Reps, OEM, Exporter
General Admin.: J. Lawson/President, Chairman
Mktg./Adv.: M. Pardovich/Director National Sales
       Gail S. Johnson/Manager Advertising
       K. Fincke/Vice President Marketing & Sales
Research: W. Robertson/Director Research & Development

Chromatography Equipment, Gas	Chemistry

GP INSTRUMENTS   **888-215-6855**
11130 Kingston Pike, Suite 1200, Knoxville, TN 37934
FDA Number: n/a
Web site: www.alcottchromatography.com
Medical Products Sales Volume: $1,500,000
Annual Revenue: $1-$5 Million
Year Founded: 1985
Total Employees: 9   Marketing Staff: 1   Sales Staff: 2
Ownership: Private
Quality System Registration Information: ISO9001
Produces/Sells CE-marked Devices: N
Federal Procurement Eligibility: Small Business
Distribution: Manufacturer Through Distributor, Manufacturer Through Manufacturer Reps, OEM, Service Direct, Exclusive Distributor, Importer, Exporter
General Admin.: Mr. Robert Fincher/President
Mktg./Adv.: Mr. Joe Stoner/Manager Sales

Chromatography, Liquid, Performance, High	Toxicology
Injector, Sample	Chemistry

GRACE BIO-LABS, INC.   **541-318-1208**
Po Box 238, 325 SW Cyber Drive, Bend, OR 97709
FDA Number: 1834178   Fax: 541-318-0242
Web site: www.gracebio.com
Ownership: Private
Produces/Sells CE-marked Devices: N

Slide, Microscope	Pathology

GRACE ENGINEERING CORP.   **810-392-2181**
34775 Potter St., Memphis, MI 48041-0202
FDA Number: 3005403279   Fax: 810-392-2993
E-mail: sales@graceeng.com
Web site: www.graceeng.com
Ownership: Private
Produces/Sells CE-marked Devices: N
General Admin.: Mr. Louis Grace/President
       Mr. Matthew Grace/Vice President
Mktg./Adv.: Mr. Jeff Olley/Sales Manager
Production: Mr. Paul Sulkowski/Customer Service Representative

Burr, Orthopedic	Orthopedics
Burr, Surgical, General & Plastic Surgery	Surgery
Rasp, Surgical, General & Plastic Surgery	Surgery
Tap, Bone	Orthopedics

GRACE MANUFACTURING, INC.   **479-968-5455**
614 SR 247, Russellville, AR 72802
FDA Number: n/a   Fax: 479-968-5460
E-mail: Information@GraceMFG.com
Web site: www.gracemfg.com

GRACE MANUFACTURING, INC.   **479-968-5455** (cont'd)
Medical Products Sales Volume: $12,000,000
Annual Revenue: $10-$25 Million
Year Founded: 1966
Total Employees: 80   Marketing Staff: 1   Sales Staff: 3
Ownership: Private
Quality System Registration Information: ISO9001
Produces/Sells CE-marked Devices: Y
Federal Procurement Eligibility: Small Business
Distribution: Manufacturer Direct, OEM
General Admin.: Mr. Chris Grace/Chief Executive Officer
       Mr. Chris Grace/General Manager
       Richard Grace/President, Owner
Mktg./Adv.: Mr. Jim Bergemann/Manager Sales
Production: Mr. Donnie Elliott/Manager Materials

Blade, Surgical, Saw, General & Plastic Surgery	Surgery
Component, Metal, Other	General
Rasp, Bone	Orthopedics
Rasp, Surgical, General & Plastic Surgery	Surgery
Reamer	Orthopedics

GRACE MEDICAL, INC.   **866-472-2363**
8500 Wolf Lake Dr., Ste. 110,   **901-386-0990**
Memphis, TN 38133
FDA Number: 1057421
    Fax: 901-386-0950
Web site: www.gracemedical.com
Year Founded: 1996
Ownership: Private
Produces/Sells CE-marked Devices: N
General Admin.: Amy James/Chief Financial Officer, Senior Vice President
       Jerry Dowdy/Chief Operating Officer
       Murray Beard/President, Chief Executive Officer
Mktg./Adv.: Mike Crook/Senior Vice President Marketing & Sales
Production: Tony Prescott/Vice President Manufacturing
       Alfred Chung/Vice President Operations

ENT Manual Surgical Instrument	Ear/Nose/Throat
Gauge, Measuring	Ear/Nose/Throat
Prosthesis, Ossicular	Ear/Nose/Throat
Prosthesis, Ossicular, Total	Ear/Nose/Throat
Tray, Surgical, ENT	Ear/Nose/Throat
Tube, Tympanostomy	Ear/Nose/Throat

GRADY RESEARCH, INC.   **978-772-3303**
323 West Main St., Ayer, MA 01432
FDA Number: 3005144617
Ownership: Private
Produces/Sells CE-marked Devices: N

Table, Radiographic	Radiology

GRAHAM BAYCARE
See Graham Medical Products/Div. Of Little Rapids Corp

GRAHAM MEDICAL PRODUCTS/DIV. OF LITTLE   **866-429-1408**
RAPIDS CORP
2273 Larsen Road, Green Bay, WI 54303   **920-494-8701**
FDA Number: 2182303   Fax: 800-494-7877
E-mail: info@grahammedical.com
Web site: www.grahammedical.com
Total Employees: 550   Marketing Staff: 3   Sales Staff: 6
Ownership: Private
Quality System Registration Information: ISO9001
Produces/Sells CE-marked Devices: Y
Federal Procurement Eligibility: Small Business
Distribution: Manufacturer Through Distributor, OEM
General Admin.: Kent Tippy/Chief Executive Officer
       Kirk Ryan/Vice President, General Manager
Mktg./Adv.: Stephanie Bohrer/Director Marketing
       Jeff Anderson/Manager Business
       Amy Foor-Noland/Manager National Sales

Bib	General
Drape, Surgical, Reusable	Surgery
Gown, Examination	General
Gown, Isolation, Surgical	Surgery
Gown, Patient, Disposable	General
Gown, Patient, Reusable	General
Linen	General
Linen, Bed	General
Material, Raw, Production	General
Mitt/Washcloth, Patient	General
Sheet, Drape, Disposable	Surgery
Sheet, Examination Table, Disposable	General
Sheeting, Examination Table	General

GRAIN PROCESSING CORPORATION   **800-448-4472**
1600 Oregon Street, Muscatine, IA 52761-1404   **563-264-4265**
FDA Number: 1910695   Fax: 563-264-4289
E-mail: sales@grainprocessing.com
Web site: www.grainprocessing.com
Ownership: Private

GRAIN PROCESSING CORPORATION   800-448-4472 (cont'd)
Produces/Sells CE-marked Devices: N
Distribution: Manufacturer Direct, Manufacturer Through Distributor, Manufacturer Through Manufacturer Reps
Mktg./Adv.: Diane Rieke/Manager Marketing & Advertising Communications
     Brian Tompoles/Vice President Marketing & Sales
Production: Richard Antrim/Manager Regulatory Affairs

Dusting Powder, Surgical	Surgery

GRAMS MEDICAL INC   949-548-7337
2443 Norse Avenue, Costa Mesa, CA 92627-1369
FDA Number: 2021743   Fax: 949-548-1056
E-mail: service@gramsmedical.com
Web site: www.gramsmedical.com
Medical Products Sales Volume: $700,000
Year Founded: 1975
Total Employees: 5
Ownership: Private
Produces/Sells CE-marked Devices: N
Federal Procurement Eligibility: Small Business
Distribution: Manufacturer Direct
General Admin.: Byron Grams/Owner
     Guenter Grams/Owner

Aspirator, Surgical	Surgery
Headlight, ENT	Ear/Nose/Throat

GRAND MEDICAL PRODUCTS   800-521-2055
7222 Ertel Road, Houston, TX 77040   **713-849-6886**
FDA Number: 1642894   Fax: 713-849-5066
E-mail: allanm@grandmedical.net
Web site: www.grandmedical.net
Medical Products Sales Volume: $800,000
Annual Revenue: $5-$10 Million
Year Founded: 1978
Total Employees: 6   Marketing Staff: 2   Sales Staff: 2
Ownership: Private
Quality System Registration Information: ISO9000; ISO9002
Produces/Sells CE-marked Devices: N
Federal Procurement Eligibility: Small Business, Minority Owned
Distribution: Manufacturer Direct, Manufacturer Through Manufacturer Reps, OEM, Service Direct
General Admin.: Derick Li/President
Mktg./Adv.: Allan Mayhall/Marketing Associate
Purchasing: Jackie Wong/Purchasing Agent

Cap, Surgical	Surgery
Gown, Isolation, Surgical	Surgery
Shoe And Shoe Cover, Conductive	Anesthesiology
Sponge, Gauze	Dental And Oral
Sponge, Laparotomy	Surgery
Sponge, Other	General
Towel, Surgical	Surgery

GRAND RAPIDS FOAM TECHNOLOGIES   877-GET-GRFT
2788 Remico St SW, Wyoming, MI 49519   **616-726-1677**
FDA Number: 1834244   Fax: 616-726-1676
E-mail: jleech@grfoamtech.com
Web site: www.grfoamtech.com
Year Founded: 1948
Total Employees: 250   Marketing Staff: 4   Sales Staff: 4
Ownership: Private
Quality System Registration Information: ISO9001
Produces/Sells CE-marked Devices: N
Distribution: Manufacturer Direct, Manufacturer Through Distributor, Manufacturer Through Manufacturer Reps, OEM, Service Direct, Exclusive Distributor, Importer, Exporter

Contract Manufacturing, Product, Disposable	General
Cushion, Foot	Orthopedics
Cushion, Other	General
Cushion, Ring, Foam Rubber	General
Cushion, Stool	General
Cushion, Table, Surgical	Surgery
Cushion, Wheelchair (Pad)	Physical Med
Foam, Plastic	General
Hemorrhoid Cushion	Gastroenterology/Urology
Mattress, Non-Powered Flotation Therapy	Physical Med
Mattress, Silicone, And Chair Cushion	General
Padding, Cast/Splint	General

GRAND TECHNOLOGY, INC.   562-316-7869
12145 Mora Drive, Unit 1, PO Box 4746, CERRITOS, CA 90703
FDA Number: 90703   Fax: 562-921-3124
E-mail: sales@grandtechinc.com
Web site: www.grandtechinc.com
Medical Products Sales Volume: $420,000
Year Founded: 1997
Total Employees: 3
Ownership: Private
Produces/Sells CE-marked Devices: N

GRAND TECHNOLOGY, INC.   562-316-7869 (cont'd)
Federal Procurement Eligibility: Small Business

Stimulator, Nerve, Transcutaneous (Pain Relief, TENS)	Cns/Neurology

GRANITE DIAGNOSTICS INC.
See Medtox Diagnostics Inc.

GRANT AIRMASS CORPORATION   800-243-5237
126 Chestnut Hill Road., PO Box 3456,   **203-321-3460**
Stamford, CT 06905
FDA Number: 1825709   Fax: 203-321-3465
E-mail: grant@grantairmass.com
Web site: www.grantairmassage.com
Medical Products Sales Volume: $1,300,000
Annual Revenue: $1-$5 Million
Year Founded: 1961
Total Employees: 5
Ownership: Private
Produces/Sells CE-marked Devices: Y
Federal Procurement Eligibility: Small Business, VA Contract
Distribution: Manufacturer Direct, Exporter
General Admin.: Irene H. Grant/President
Mktg./Adv.: Irene H. Grant/Vice President Marketing & Sales

Cover, Mattress	General
Cushion, Flotation	Physical Med
Cushion, Wheelchair (Pad)	Physical Med
Lift, Patient	General
Mattress, Alternating Pressure (Or Pads)	Physical Med
Pressure Pad, Alternating, Disposable	General
Pressure Pad, Alternating, Reusable	General

GRANT CHIROPRACTIC, LLC   770-719-1917
155 Bradford Square, Suite C, Fayetteville, GA 30215
FDA Number: 3004063538
Ownership: Private
Produces/Sells CE-marked Devices: N

Table, Mechanical	Physical Med

GRANT HOSPITAL HARDWARE
See Salsbury Industries

GRANT MEMORIAL   304-257-1026
HOSPITAL/PETERSBURG, WV
Grant Memorial Drive, Petersburg, WV 26847
FDA Number: n/a   Fax: 304-257-2537
E-mail: mhuffman@grantmemorial.com
Web site: www.grantmemorial.com
Medical Products Sales Volume: $28,000,000
Year Founded: 1958
Total Employees: 300
Ownership: Private
Produces/Sells CE-marked Devices: N
Federal Procurement Eligibility: Small Business
Distribution: Service Direct
General Admin.: Myra Huffman/Executive Assistant
     Robert Harman/President, Chief Executive Officer
     Ronnie Arbaugh/Vice President Human Resources
Mktg./Adv.: Frances Welton/Director Marketing
     Joyce Dayton/Vice President Marketing & Sales
Production: Gayann Veach/Director Quality Assurance
     Joyce Dayton/Manager Materials

Service, Consulting	General

GRAPHCO COMPANY
See Tyco Healthcare Group Lp

GRAPHIC CONTROLS CORP.   800-669-1535
400 Exchange St., Buffalo, NY 14204
FDA Number: 1317188   Fax: 800-347-2420
Web site: www.graphiccontrols.com
Medical Products Sales Volume: $20,000,000
Annual Revenue: $10-$25 Million
Total Employees: 90
Ownership: Private
Quality System Registration Information: ISO9001
Produces/Sells CE-marked Devices: Y
Distribution: Manufacturer Through Distributor, OEM

Accessories, Light, Surgical	Surgery
Belt, Abdominal	Gastroenterology/Urology
Cable	Physical Med
Cable, Electrode	Physical Med
Cable/Lead, ECG	Cardiovascular
Cable/Lead, ECG, With Transducer And Electrode	Cardiovascular
Cap, Tip, Syringe	General
Clamp, Surgical, General & Plastic Surgery	Surgery
Clamp, Tubing, Blood, Automatic	Gastroenterology/Urology
Cleaner, Electrosurgical Tip	Surgery
Clip, Drape, Lithotomy	Obstetrics/Gynecology
Clip, Towel	Surgery
Container, Sterilization (Tray)	General

GRAPHIC CONTROLS CORP.   800-669-1535 (cont'd)

Counter, Needle	Surgery
Counter, Sponge, Surgical	Surgery
Drape, Surgical	Surgery
Drape, Surgical Instrument, Magnetic	Surgery
Electrode, Circular (Spiral), Scalp And Applicator	Obstetrics/Gynecology
Electrode, Electrocardiograph	Cardiovascular
Electrode, Electroencephalographic	Cns/Neurology
Electrode, Fetal Scalp	Obstetrics/Gynecology
Endoscope And Accessories, AC-Powered	Surgery
Gel, Electrode, Electrocardiograph	Cardiovascular
Gel, Ultrasonic Transmission	General
Holder, Leg	Surgery
Kit, Quality Control	Microbiology
Kit, Surgical Instrument, Disposable	Surgery
Loop, Lens	Ophthalmology
Marker, Skin	Surgery
Monitor, Pressure, Intrauterine	Obstetrics/Gynecology
Packaging, Sterilization	General
Paper, Chart, Record, Medical	General
Paper, Recording, ECG/EEG	General
Restraint, Patient, Conductive	Anesthesiology
Restraint, Protective (Body)	General
Support, Patient Position	Anesthesiology
Tray, Surgical	Surgery
Waste Disposal Unit, Sharps	General
Waste Disposal Unit, Surgical Instrument (Sharps)	Surgery

GRASEBY ALLEN
See Thermo Fisher Scientific - Checkweighing, Metal And X-Ray Detection

GRASEBY ANDERSEN, SPIROTECH DIV.
See Thermo Fisher Scientific

GRASEBY MEDICAL
See Marcal Medical, Inc.

GRASON & ASSOCIATES, LLC   603-899-3089
71 Conifer Rd, P.o. Box 289, Rindge, NH 03461
FDA Number: 1225529

Cushion, Earphone (For Audiometric Testing)	Ear/Nose/Throat

GRASON-STADLER
See Cardinal Healthcare 209, Inc.

GRASS TECHNOLOGIES, AN ASTRO-MED, INC.   401-828-4002
PRODUCT GRO
53 Airport Park Drive, Rockland, MA 02370
FDA Number: n/a
Ownership: Astro-Med, Inc.
Produces/Sells CE-marked Devices: N

Amplifier, Biopotential (W Signal Conditioner)	Cardiovascular
Amplifier, Physiological Signal	Cns/Neurology
Amplifier, Transducer Signal (W Signal Conditioner)	Cardiovascular
Analyzer, Signal Isolation	Cardiovascular
Cable/Lead, ECG, With Transducer And Electrode	Cardiovascular
Conditioner, Signal, Physiological	Cns/Neurology
Display, Cathode-Ray Tube	Cardiovascular
Electrode, Cortical	Cns/Neurology
Electrode, Cutaneous	Cns/Neurology
Electrode, Nasopharyngeal	Cns/Neurology
Electrode, Needle	Cns/Neurology
Electroencephalograph	Cns/Neurology
Gel, Electrode, Stimulator	Cns/Neurology
Monitor, Apnea	General
Monitor, Ventilatory Frequency	Anesthesiology
Oximeter, Intracardiac	Cardiovascular
Plethysmograph, Photo-Electric, Pneumatic Or Hydraulic	Cardiovascular
Recorder, Paper Chart	Cardiovascular
Stimulator, Auditory, Evoked Response	Cns/Neurology
Stimulator, Nerve, AC-Powered	Anesthesiology
Stimulator, Nerve, ENT	Ear/Nose/Throat
Stimulator, Photic, Evoked Response	Cns/Neurology
Tester, Electrode/Lead, Electroencephalograph	Cns/Neurology
Transducer, Blood Pressure, Extravascular	Cardiovascular
Transducer, Gas Pressure, Differential	Anesthesiology
Transducer, Heart Sound	Cardiovascular
Transducer, Tremor	Cns/Neurology

GRAV-TRAC   813-932-8710
6040 Country Club Rd., Wesley Chapel, FL 33544
FDA Number: n/a
Ownership: Private
Produces/Sells CE-marked Devices: N

Component, Exercise	Physical Med

GRAYMILLS CORP.   800-478-8673
3705 N. Lincoln Avenue, Chicago, IL 60613-3517   **773-477-4100**
FDA Number: n/a   *Fax:* 773-477-4133
E-mail: info@graymills.com
Web site: www.graymills.com
Medical Products Sales Volume: $16,000,000
Annual Revenue: $10-$25 Million

GRAYMILLS CORP.   800-478-8673 (cont'd)
Year Founded: 1939
Total Employees: 78   *Marketing Staff:* 5   *Sales Staff:* 25
Ownership: Private
Stock Symbol: NC
Traded On: NYSE
Produces/Sells CE-marked Devices: N
Federal Procurement Eligibility: Small Business, GSA Contract
Distribution: Manufacturer Through Distributor, OEM, Importer
General Admin.: Jerry Shields/President
　　　　Elliot Fowler/Vice President Human Resources
Mktg./Adv.: John Bosselli/Director Marketing
　　　　Dawn Roberts/Manager Advertising
　　　　Kristen DeNoble/Vice President Marketing
　　　　Steve Cotra/Vice President Marketing

Pump, Infusion	General
Solution, Antibacterial Cleaner	General

GRAYSON O COMPANY   800-435-1508
6509 Newell Ave., Kannapolis, NC 28081
FDA Number: 1041429
Ownership: Private
Produces/Sells CE-marked Devices: N

Laser, Surgical	Surgery

GREAT AGE CONTAINER   800.631.7392
220 Frontage Rd., New Haven, CT 06516   **718-378-4100**
FDA Number: 2433168   *Fax:* 203-934-7172
E-mail: info@oberk.com
Web site: oberk.com
Medical Products Sales Volume: $8,000,000
Annual Revenue: $10-$25 Million
Total Employees: 11   *Marketing Staff:* 2   *Sales Staff:* 3
Ownership: Private
Produces/Sells CE-marked Devices: N
Federal Procurement Eligibility: Small Business
Distribution: Manufacturer Through Distributor
General Admin.: Larry Stein/President, Chief Executive Officer

Diaper, Adult	General
Diaper, Pediatric	General
Glove, Other	General
Glove, Patient Examination	General
Glove, Surgical	General

GREAT BASIN CORPORATION   801-990-1055
2441 South 3850 West, Salt Lake City, UT 84120
FDA Number: n/a   *Fax:* 801-990-1051
E-mail: aolson@gbscience.com
Web site: www.gbscience.com
Ownership: Private
Produces/Sells CE-marked Devices: N
General Admin.: Mr. Robert Jenison/Chief Technology Officer
　　　　Mr. Ryan Ashton/President, Chief Executive Officer
Mktg./Adv.: Dr. Wesley Lindsey/Director Product Development
　　　　Ms. Sandra Nielsen/Vice President Marketing
　　　　Mr. Andrew Olson/Vice President Sales
Production: Mr. Charles Owen/Director Engineering
　　　　Mr. Laurence Rea/Senior Vice President Operations
Research: Dr. Brian Hicke/Director Research

GREAT LAKES EARMOLD LAB   800-842-8184
12740 York Delta Drive, PO Box 338004,   **440-877-9090**
North Royalton, OH 44133
FDA Number: 1523525   *Fax:* 440-877-9190
E-mail: greatlakesearmold@sbcglobal.net
Web site: www.greatlakesearmold.com
Ownership: Private
Produces/Sells CE-marked Devices: N

Hearing-Aid	Ear/Nose/Throat

GREAT LAKES FILTERS/FILPACO INDUSTRIES   517-639-8470
301 Arch Avenue, hillsdale, MI 49242
FDA Number: 7000805   *Fax:* 517-437-2635
E-mail: johnh@acmemill.com
Web site: www.greatlakesfilters.com
Medical Products Sales Volume: $250,000
Annual Revenue: $5-$10 Million
Total Employees: 20   *Sales Staff:* 5
Ownership: The Acme Group
Produces/Sells CE-marked Devices: N
Federal Procurement Eligibility: Small Business
Distribution: Manufacturer Direct, Service Direct
General Admin.: Brian Balliet/President
Mktg./Adv.: Mr. Anthony Vissman/Sales Associate
　　　　Mr. Doug Vissman/Sales Associate
　　　　Mr. John Hughes/Sales Associate
　　　　Mrs. Bev Callahan/Sales Associate

Filter Paper	Chemistry

GREAT LAKES FILTERS/FILPACO INDUSTRIES   517-639-8470
(cont'd)
Filter, Air	General

GREAT LAKES INNOVATION INC   248-680-8671
1103 Winthrop Drive, Troy, MI 48083
FDA Number: 9056288
Medical Products Sales Volume: $100,000
Year Founded: 2003
Adapter, Hygiene	Physical Med
Bandage, Cast	Physical Med
Wheelchair, Manual	Physical Med

GREAT LAKES MEDICAL   800-337-8243
18683 Sheldon Rd., Cleveland, OH 44130   216-898-5002
FDA Number: n/a   *Fax:* 800-897-2192
E-mail: greatlakesmed@aol.com
Web site: www.viatro.com
Medical Products Sales Volume: $2,000,000
Annual Revenue: $1-$5 Million
Total Employees: 12   *Marketing Staff:* 1
Ownership: Private
Quality System Registration Information: ISO9001
Produces/Sells CE-marked Devices: Y
Federal Procurement Eligibility: Small Business, Female Owned
Distribution: Manufacturer Through Distributor, Manufacturer Through Manufacturer Reps, Exclusive Distributor
General Admin.: Patrick Beck/Chief Executive Officer
Mktg./Adv.: Tricia A. Waltz/Director Corporate Accounts
       Tricia Waltz/Manager Marketing
Production: Joan M. Bennett/Product Manager
Research: Jan J. Lewandowski/Vice President Research & Development
Encapsulator, Fluid	General
Medical Disinfectants/Cleaners for Instruments	General

GREAT LAKES ORTHODONTICS, LTD.   800-828-7626
200 Cooper Ave.Dr., Tonawanda, NY 14150   716-871-1161
FDA Number: 1316408   *Fax:* 716-871-0550
E-mail: info@greatlakesortho.com
Web site: www.greatlakesortho.com
Year Founded: 1965
Total Employees: 180
Ownership: Private
Produces/Sells CE-marked Devices: N
Distribution: Importer
Accessories, Retractor, Dental	Dental And Oral
Articulators	Dental And Oral
Base, Denture, Relining, Repairing, Rebasing, Resin	Dental And Oral
Clasp, Preformed	Dental And Oral
Crown And Bridge, Temporary, Resin	Dental And Oral
Device, Anti-Snoring	Ear/Nose/Throat
Exerciser, Measuring	Physical Med
Face Bow	Dental And Oral
Gauge, Measuring	Ear/Nose/Throat
Headgear, Extraoral, Orthodontic	Dental And Oral
Material, Impression	Dental And Oral
Occluder, Umbilical	General
Retainer, Screw Expansion, Orthodontic	Dental And Oral
Tray, Fluoride, Disposable	Dental And Oral
Tray, Impression	Dental And Oral
Tube, Orthodontic	Dental And Oral
Wire, Orthodontic	Dental And Oral

GREAT MIDWEST PACKAGING, LLC   800-788-9873
712 Anita Ave., Antioch, IL 60002-1857   847-395-4500
FDA Number: n/a   *Fax:* 847-395-4814
E-mail: gmp@gmpllc.net
Web site: www.gmpllc.net
Medical Products Sales Volume: $3,000,000
Annual Revenue: $1-$5 Million
Year Founded: 1975
Ownership: Private
Quality System Registration Information: ISO9001
Produces/Sells CE-marked Devices: N
Federal Procurement Eligibility: Small Business
Distribution: Manufacturer Through Distributor, Manufacturer Through Manufacturer Reps, OEM
Contract Packaging	General
Kit, Prep	General
Swabs, Cotton	General

GREAT VALLEY TECHNOLOGIES   610-647-2210
95 Great Valley Pkwy., Malvern, PA 19355
FDA Number: n/a
E-mail: gvti@practice-alt.com
Web site: www.practice-alt.com
Annual Revenue: $1-$5 Million
Ownership: Private
Produces/Sells CE-marked Devices: N

GREAT VALLEY TECHNOLOGIES   610-647-2210 *(cont'd)*
Federal Procurement Eligibility: Small Business
Distribution: Service Direct
Computer Software	General
System, Communication, Image, Digital	Radiology

GREATBACH MEDICAL   800-559-2613
2300 Berkshire Lane N, Minneapolis, MN 55441   763-951-8181
FDA Number: 2183787   *Fax:* 763-559-0148
E-mail: info@enpathmed.com
Web site: www.enpathmedical.com
Medical Products Sales Volume: $36,800,000
Annual Revenue: $25-$50 Million
Year Founded: 1985
Total Employees: 221
Ownership: Greatbatch Inc
Quality System Registration Information: ISO9001
Produces/Sells CE-marked Devices: Y
Federal Procurement Eligibility: Small Business
Distribution: OEM
Mktg./Adv.: Jim Mellor/Vice President Marketing & Sales
Production: Tami Presler/Manager Customer Services
       Tim Bredahi/Manager Quality Assurance
Adapter, Lead, Pacemaker	Cardiovascular
Catheter, Steerable	Cardiovascular
Contract Assembly	General
Contract Manufacturing	General
Contract Manufacturing, Product, Disposable	General
Dilator, Vessel, Percutaneous Catheterization	Cardiovascular
Introducer, Catheter	Cardiovascular
Lead, Pacemaker, Implantable Endocardial	Cardiovascular
Lead, Pacemaker, Implantable Myocardial	Cardiovascular
Service, Engineering/Design	General

GREATBATCH INC   1 216-937-2800
1771 East 30th St., Cleveland, OH 44114
FDA Number: n/a   *Fax:* 1 216-937-2812
Web site: www.greatbatchmedical.com
Ownership: Greatbatch Inc
Stock Symbol: GB
Traded On: NYSE
Produces/Sells CE-marked Devices: N
Instrument, Manual, General Surgical	Surgery
Recorder, Ventilatory Effort	Anesthesiology
Retractor, Vaginal	Obstetrics/Gynecology

GREATBATCH INC   716-759-5600
x, Clarence, NY 14031
FDA Number: n/a   *Fax:* 716-759-5560
Web site: www.greatbatch.com
Year Founded: 1970
Ownership: Public
Stock Symbol: GB
Traded On: NYSE
Quality System Registration Information: ISO9002
Produces/Sells CE-marked Devices: N
Federal Procurement Eligibility: Small Business
Distribution: Manufacturer Through Distributor
General Admin.: Thomas J. Mazza/Chief Financial Officer, Senior Vice President
       Thomas J. Hook/President, Chief Executive Officer
       Mr. Maurice Arellano/Senior Vice President
       Barbara M. Davis/Vice President Human Resources
Battery	General
Component, Metal, Other	General
Medical Product Subsidiaries (Listed Separately)
Greatbach Medical
Greatbatch Inc

GREATBATCH MEDICAL   716-759-5600
10000 Wehrle Drive, Clarence, NY 14031
FDA Number: 1832228   *Fax:* 716-759-5560
Web site: www.greatbatch.com
Medical Products Sales Volume: $15,000,000
Annual Revenue: $10-$25 Million
Ownership: Private
Quality System Registration Information: ISO9001; ISO9002
Produces/Sells CE-marked Devices: N
Federal Procurement Eligibility: Small Business
Distribution: Manufacturer Direct, OEM
General Admin.: Thomas J. Hook/President, Chief Executive Officer
Container, Sterilization (Tray)	General
Container, Surgical Instrument	Surgery
Molding, Custom	General
Packaging, Sterilization	General
Tray, Custom/Special Procedure	General
Medical Product Subsidiaries (Listed Separately)
C/T Med-Systems Ltd., Inc.

GREATBATCH MEDICAL
260-244-6300
4532 Park 30 Drive, Columbia City, IN 46725
FDA Number: 3004976965
Fax: 260-244-6308
E-mail: orthopaedicsna@greatbatchmedical.com
Ownership: Private
Produces/Sells CE-marked Devices: N

Appliance, Fix., Nail/Blade/Plate Comb., Multiple Component	Orthopedics
Orthopedic Manual Surgical Instrument	Orthopedics
Screw, Fixation, Bone	Orthopedics

GREATTEC VISION S.A. DE C.V.
Circuito De La Amistad #2700, Mexicali B.c. Mexico
FDA Number: 8044009

Shield, Eye, Ophthalmic	Ophthalmology
Spectacle, Magnifier	Ophthalmology
Sunglasses (Including Photosensitive)	Ophthalmology

GREEN FIELD MEDICAL SOURCING, INC.
512-894-3002
14141 Highway 290 West, Suite 410, Austin, TX 78737
FDA Number: n/a
Ownership: Private
Produces/Sells CE-marked Devices: N

Airway, Oropharyngeal, Anesthesia	Anesthesiology
Dressing, Wound and Burn, Occlusive	Surgery
Stylet, Tracheal Tube	Anesthesiology

GREENCO INDUSTRIES, INC.
608-328-8311
1601 4th Ave. West, Monroe, WI 53566
FDA Number: n/a
Fax: 608-328-1993
E-mail: jzweifel@greencoind.com
Web site: www.greencoind.com
Ownership: Private
Produces/Sells CE-marked Devices: N

Accessories, Wheelchair	Physical Med
Drape, Surgical	Surgery
Holder, Infant Position	General
Protector, Skin Pressure	General
Restraint	Physical Med

GREENWALD SURGICAL CO., INC.
888-962-1829
2688 Dekalb St., Lake Station, IN 46405
219-962-1604
FDA Number: 1818662
Fax: 219-962-4009
E-mail: sales@greenwaldsurgical.com
Web site: www.greenwaldsurgical.com
Ownership: Private
Produces/Sells CE-marked Devices: N

Bougie, Urological	Gastroenterology/Urology
Cannula, Suprapubic, With Trocar	Gastroenterology/Urology
Clamp, Penile	Gastroenterology/Urology
Coagulator/Cutter, Endoscopic, Bipolar	Obstetrics/Gynecology
Cord, Electric, Instrument, Surgical, Transurethral	Gastroenterology/Urology
Dislodger, Stone, Basket, Ureteral, Metal	Gastroenterology/Urology
Electrocautery Unit, Gynecologic	Obstetrics/Gynecology
Electrode, Electrosurgical, Active (Blade)	Surgery
Electrosurgical Unit, Cutting & Coagulation Device	Surgery
Needle, Endoscopic	Gastroenterology/Urology
Retractor, Non-Self-Retaining	Gastroenterology/Urology
Sound, Urethral, Metal Or Plastic	Gastroenterology/Urology
Stylet, Catheter, Gastro-Urology	Gastroenterology/Urology
Surgical Instrument, G-U, Manual	Gastroenterology/Urology
Urethrotome	Gastroenterology/Urology

GREER LABORATORIES, INC.
800-419-7302
639 NuWay Circle, PO Box 800,
828-754-5327
Lenoir, NC 28645
FDA Number: 1011574
Fax: 828-754-5320
E-mail: sales@greerlabs.com
Web site: www.greerlabs.com
Medical Products Sales Volume: $13,000,000
Annual Revenue: $10-$25 Million
Year Founded: 1904
Total Employees: 214   *Marketing Staff:* 7   *Sales Staff:* 12
Ownership: Private
Produces/Sells CE-marked Devices: N
Federal Procurement Eligibility: Small Business, Female Owned
Distribution: Manufacturer Direct, Exclusive Distributor, Exporter
General Admin.: Craig Kennedy/Chief Operating Officer
     Anita Ruka/Director Human Resources
     Jenni Witherspoon/Manager
     John Roby/President, Chief Executive Officer
Mktg./Adv.: William Mahoney/Director International Marketing & Sales
     Mark Kleinke/Director Sales
     Catherine Lankewicz/Manager Market Development
     Tracy Woody/Vice President Sales
Research: Robert E. Esch/Vice President Research & Development
Finance: Tony Palombo/Chief Financial Officer

Syringe, Other	General
Test, Allergy	Immunology

GREER MEDICAL, INC.
(800) 424-2155
314 East Carrillo St., Suite 1,
805-962-5883
Santa Barbara, CA 93101
FDA Number: 2028175
Fax: (805) 962-4615
E-mail: nfo@greer-medical.com
Ownership: Private
Produces/Sells CE-marked Devices: N

Retainer, Surgical	Surgery
Suction Apparatus, Single Patient, Portable, Non-Powered	Surgery

GREGSTROM CORP.
781-935-6600
64 Holton St., P.O. Box 609, Woburn, MA 01801
FDA Number: 1223955
Fax: 781-935-4905
E-mail: info@gregstrom.com
Web site: www.gregstrom.com
Ownership: Private
Produces/Sells CE-marked Devices: N

Tray, Surgical Instrument	Surgery

GREIF BROS. CORP.
See Greif, Inc.

GREIF, INC.
502-245-6599
425 Winter Road, Delaware, OH 43015
FDA Number: n/a
Fax: 502-245-4492
E-mail: al.clark@greif.com
Web site: www.greif.com
Year Founded: 1877
Total Employees: 9600
Ownership: Public
Stock Symbol: GEF
Traded On: NYSE
Quality System Registration Information: ISO9002
Produces/Sells CE-marked Devices: N
Distribution: Manufacturer Direct
General Admin.: Michael J. Gasser/Chairman, Chief Executive Officer
     Donald S. Huml/Chief Financial Officer, Executive Vice President
     David B. Fischer/President, Chief Operating Officer

Packaging Material	General
Waste Receptacle, Contaminated	General

GREINER BIO-ONE NORTH AMERICA, INC.
410-592-2060
4238 Capital Dr., Monroe, NC 28110
FDA Number: 1125230
Ownership: Private
Produces/Sells CE-marked Devices: N

Labware, Blood Collection	Chemistry
Tube, Vacuum Sample, With Anticoagulant	Hematology

GRESCO PRODUCTS, INC.
800-527-3250
13391 Murphy Rd., P.o. Box 865,
281-261-1811
Stafford, TX 77477
FDA Number: 1642632
Fax: 281-499-6515
Ownership: Private
Produces/Sells CE-marked Devices: N

Adhesive, Bracket And Conditioner, Resin	Dental And Oral
Agent, Polishing, Abrasive, Oral Cavity	Dental And Oral
Detector, Caries	Dental And Oral
Powder, Porcelain	Dental And Oral
Sealant, Pit And Fissure, And Conditioner, Resin	Dental And Oral

GRESHAM DRIVING AIDS, INC.
800-521-8930
30800 Wixom Rd., Wixom, MI 48393
248-624-1533
FDA Number: n/a
Fax: 248-624-6358
E-mail: gpersons@greshamdrivingaids.com
Web site: www.greshamdrivingaids.com
Annual Revenue: $1-$5 Million
Year Founded: 1958
Ownership: Private
Quality System Registration Information: ISO9000
Produces/Sells CE-marked Devices: N
Federal Procurement Eligibility: Small Business
Distribution: Manufacturer Direct, Service Direct, Exporter

Accessories, Wheelchair	Physical Med
Control, Hand Driving, Automobile, Mechanical	Physical Med
Lift, Wheelchair	General

GREYLOR CO.
(239) 574-2011
2340 Andalusia Blvd., Cape Coral, FL 33909
FDA Number: n/a
Fax: (239) 574-2036
E-mail: sales@greylor.com
Web site: www.greylor.com
Annual Revenue: $1-$5 Million
Total Employees: 8   *Marketing Staff:* 2   *Sales Staff:* 2
Ownership: Private
Produces/Sells CE-marked Devices: N
Distribution: Manufacturer Direct, Manufacturer Through Distributor, OEM, Exporter

GREYLOR CO.   (239) 574-2011 *(cont'd)*
Pump, Infusion   General

GREYSTONE OF LINCOLN, INC.   800-446-7161
7 Wellington Rd., Lincoln, RI 02865   401-333-0444
FDA Number: 1222776   *Fax:* 401-334-5745
E-mail: davesaur@greyst.com
Web site: www.greyst.com
Ownership: Private
Produces/Sells CE-marked Devices: N
  Bit, Drill   Orthopedics
  Surgical Instrument, Obstetric/Gynecologic, General   Obstetrics/Gynecology
  Transducer, Stethoscope   Anesthesiology

GRI MEDICAL PRODUCTS, INC.   800-291-9425
4937 E Red Range Way, Cave Creek, AZ 85331
FDA Number: 1222612   *Fax:* 480-595-9933
E-mail: info@grimedical.com
Web site: www.grimedical.com
Year Founded: 1990
Total Employees: 1   *Marketing Staff:* 1   *Sales Staff:* 1
Ownership: Private
Produces/Sells CE-marked Devices: N
Federal Procurement Eligibility: Small Business
Distribution: Manufacturer Direct, Manufacturer Through Distributor
  Evacuator, Gastro-Urology   Gastroenterology/Urology
  Labeler, X-Ray Film   Radiology
  Recorder, Paper Chart   Cardiovascular

GRIFF INDUSTRIES, INC.   800-709-4743
19761 Bahama St., Northridge, CA 91324   818-709-4743
FDA Number: 2031528   *Fax:* 818-709-4768
E-mail: sales@griffindustries.com
Web site: www.griffindustries.com
Medical Products Sales Volume: $2,300,000
Annual Revenue: $1-$5 Million
Year Founded: 1999
Total Employees: 19   *Marketing Staff:* 1   *Sales Staff:* 1
Ownership: Private
Quality System Registration Information: ISO9001
Produces/Sells CE-marked Devices: N
Federal Procurement Eligibility: Small Business
Distribution: Manufacturer Direct, Manufacturer Through Distributor, Manufacturer Through Manufacturer Reps, OEM
General Admin.: Michael Griffin/President
Mktg./Adv.: Rudy Gaba/Director Product Development
Production: George Austria/Director Quality Assurance & Regulatory Affairs
           Carlos Anania/Vice President Manufacturing
Research: Rudy Gaba/Vice President Research & Development
  Accessories, Operating Room, Table   Surgery
  Holder, Needle   Gastroenterology/Urology
  Marker, Skin   Surgery
  Needle, Hypodermic, Single Lumen With Syringe   General
  Pack, Sterilization Wrapper (Bag And Accessories)   Surgery
  Restraint, Patient, Conductive   Anesthesiology
  Scalpel, One-Piece (Knife)   Surgery

GRIFFIN LABORATORIES   800-330-5969
43391 Business Park Dr., #c5, Rancho California, CA 92590
FDA Number: 2030504
  Anti-Stammering Device   Ear/Nose/Throat
  Larynx, Artificial Battery-Powered   Ear/Nose/Throat

GRIFFIN MEDICAL PRODUCTS, INC.   800-366-6870
80 Manheim Avenue, PO Box 457,   856-455-6870
Bridgeton, NJ 08302
FDA Number: 2247743   *Fax:* 856-455-6849
E-mail: Griffbab@aol.com
Web site: www.BuddiesbyGriffin.com
Medical Products Sales Volume: $4,700,000
Annual Revenue: $10-$25 Million
Year Founded: 1984
Total Employees: 80   *Marketing Staff:* 2   *Sales Staff:* 4
Ownership: Private
Produces/Sells CE-marked Devices: N
Federal Procurement Eligibility: Small Business
Distribution: Manufacturer Through Distributor
Mktg./Adv.: Mr. James V. Bennett/National Director Marketing
  Bed, Hydraulic   General

GRIFFITH MICRO SCIENCE
See Sterigenics International, Inc.

GRIFFITH RUBBER MILLS   260-357-3125
400 N. Taylor, Garrett, IN 46738
FDA Number: 7000842   *Fax:* 260-357-3130
E-mail: info@griffithrubber.com
Web site: www.griffithrubber.com
Annual Revenue: $0-$1 Million

GRIFFITH RUBBER MILLS   260-357-3125 *(cont'd)*
Total Employees: 150   *Sales Staff:* 2
Ownership: Private
Quality System Registration Information: ISO9000
Produces/Sells CE-marked Devices: N
Distribution: Manufacturer Direct
General Admin.: Hulem Branscum/General Manager
           Scott Laney/President
  Tips And Pads, Cane, Crutch And Walker   Physical Med

GRIMM SCIENTIFIC IND., INC.   800-223-5395
1403 Pike St., PO Box 2143,   740-374-3412
Marietta, OH 45750
FDA Number: 1526475   *Fax:* 740-374-5745
E-mail: grimm@ee.net
Web site: www.grimmscientific.com
Medical Products Sales Volume: $800,000
Annual Revenue: $0-$1 Million
Year Founded: 1983
Total Employees: 10   *Sales Staff:* 1
Ownership: Private
Produces/Sells CE-marked Devices: N
Federal Procurement Eligibility: Small Business
Distribution: Manufacturer Direct
General Admin.: Mr. Joseph E. Grimm/Chief Executive Officer
  Bath, Hydro-Massage (Whirlpool)   Physical Med
  Bath, Paraffin   Physical Med
  Massager, Powered Inflatable Tube   Physical Med
  Paraffin, All Formulations   Pathology

GRISWOLD TOOL AND DIE, INC.   517-741-7433
8500 M-60 East, P.o. Box 86, Union City, MI 49094
FDA Number: 1831089
Ownership: Private
Produces/Sells CE-marked Devices: N
  Lavage Unit, Water Jet   General
  Shoe, Cast   Physical Med

GROBET FILE CO.   800-847-4188
750 Washington Avenue, Carlstadt, NJ 07072   201-939-6700
FDA Number: 1220428   *Fax:* 201-939-5067
E-mail: email@grobetusa.com
Web site: www.grobetusa.com
Ownership: Private
Produces/Sells CE-marked Devices: N
Federal Procurement Eligibility: Small Business
  Burr, Dental   Dental And Oral
  Forceps, Dressing, Dental   Dental And Oral
  Forceps, General & Plastic Surgery   Surgery
  Wheel, Polishing Agent   Dental And Oral

GROMAN INC.   954-649-8008
4900 Nw 15th St., Ste 4494, Margate, FL 33063
FDA Number: 3004361444
Ownership: Private
Produces/Sells CE-marked Devices: N
  Airbrush   Dental And Oral

GROSFILLEX, INC.   800-233-3186
230 Old West Penn Avenue,   610-693-5835
Robesonia, PA 19551
FDA Number: n/a   *Fax:* 610-693-5414
E-mail: info@grosfillexfurniture.com
Web site: www.grosfillexfurniture.com
Total Employees: 200   *Marketing Staff:* 2   *Sales Staff:* 5
Ownership: Private
Produces/Sells CE-marked Devices: N
Federal Procurement Eligibility: Small Business
Distribution: Manufacturer Through Manufacturer Reps
General Admin.: Guy David/President, Chief Executive Officer
Mktg./Adv.: Ms. Lesley Widergren/Admin. Marketing & Sales
           Susan Castillo/Manager Advertising
           Bruce South/Manager Regional Sales
Production: Dan Yearick/Vice President Manufacturing
Research: John Flemm/Vice President Research & Development
Purchasing: Andre Bourrie/Vice President Contracts
  Furniture, General   General

GROUPE MEDICUS INC.   877-678-8872
5135 10th Ave., Montreal, QUE H1Y-2G5 Canada   514-525-3757
FDA Number: n/a   *Fax:* 514-525-9915
E-mail: medicus@qc.aira.com
Web site: www.medicus.ca
Year Founded: 1957
Total Employees: 100
Ownership: Private
Produces/Sells CE-marked Devices: N

GROUPE MEDICUS INC. 877-678-8872 *(cont'd)*
Distribution: Manufacturer Direct, Service Direct, Exclusive Distributor, Importer

GROUPE NOVALAB INC. 819-474-2580
2350 Rue Power, Drummondville J2C 7Z4 Canada
FDA Number: 9616852
  Cleaner, Denture   Dental And Oral

GROVE INSTRUMENTS INC 508-799-8800
100 Grove Street, Suite 315, Worcester, MA 01605
FDA Number: n/a
E-mail: É_
Web site: info@groveinstruments.com
Ownership: Private
Stock Symbol: N
General Admin.: Mr. Arthur Combs/Chairman, Chief Executive Officer
        Dr. Craig Mello/Director

GRUPO INDUSTRIAL C&A, S.A. DE C.V. 525-562-0660
Circuito Misioneros #26, Cd. Satelite,anucal-Pan,edo Mexico
FDA Number: 9617323
  Linen, Bed   General

GRUPO INDUSTRIAL LATEX, S.A. DE C.V. 011-523-7653
Riveras Del Pilar, Ave. San Jorge 250-A, Chapala 45900 Mexico
FDA Number: 9614027
  Glove, Surgical, Plastic Surgery   Surgery

GRUPO MANUFACTURERO RIO GRANDE, S.A. 878-237-70
DE C.V.
Privada Aldama #113, Piedras Negras, Coah. Mexico
FDA Number: 9680955
  Suture, Absorbable, Natural   Surgery

GRUPO SERVISAN 5-396-3620
Mar Baltico 26, Col.Popotla,
Ciudad De Mexico, DF 11400 Mexico
FDA Number: n/a   *Fax:* 5-396-7094
E-mail: ventas@servisan.com
Web site: www.servisan.com
Medical Products Sales Volume: $4,000,000
Total Employees: 350   *Marketing Staff:* 1   *Sales Staff:* 3
Ownership: Private
Produces/Sells CE-marked Devices: N
Federal Procurement Eligibility: Small Business
Distribution: Manufacturer Direct, Exclusive Distributor, Importer, Exporter

GRYPHUS DIAGNOSTICS, L.L.C. 800-924-4195
2200 Sutherland Ave., Knoxville, TN 37919 865-251-0101
FDA Number: 3006546675   *Fax:* 865-251-0108
E-mail: customerservice@gryphus.com
Web site: www.gryphus.com
Ownership: Private
Produces/Sells CE-marked Devices: N
  Test, Vaginal, Bacterial Sialidase   Chemistry

GS MEDICAL PACKAGING INC. 800-489-7125
501 Lakeshore Road East, Suite 201, 905-271-1532
Mississauga, ONT L5G 1 Canada
FDA Number: 3003067378   *Fax:* 905-271-1526
E-mail: info@gsmedicalpackaging.com
Web site: www.gsmedicalpackaging.com
Year Founded: 1986
Total Employees: 30
Ownership: Private
Produces/Sells CE-marked Devices: Y
Distribution: Manufacturer Direct, OEM, Exclusive Distributor, Exporter

GSI GROUP 800-342-3757
125 Middlesex Tpke, Bedford, MA 01730 781-266-5700
FDA Number: n/a   *Fax:* 781-266-5112
Web site: http://www.gsig.com
Ownership: Private
Produces/Sells CE-marked Devices: N
General Admin.: Mr. John Roush/Chief Executive Officer
Finance: Mr. Robert Buckley/Chief Financial Officer
  Recorder, Paper Chart   Cardiovascular

GSI LUMONICS
  See Gsi Group

GSK CONSUMER HEALTHCARE 888-825-5249
65 Industrial South, Clifton, NJ 07012
FDA Number: 2210777
Web site: www.gsk.com
Ownership: Smithkline Beecham
Stock Symbol: GSK
Traded On: NYSE
Produces/Sells CE-marked Devices: N

GSK CONSUMER HEALTHCARE 888-825-5249 *(cont'd)*
Distribution: Manufacturer Direct, Manufacturer Through Distributor
General Admin.: Andrew Witty/Chief Executive Officer
        Bill Louv/Chief Information Officer
        John Clarke/President
        Simon Bicknell/Senior Vice President
Finance: Julian Heslop/Chief Financial Officer
  Adhesive, Denture, OTC   Dental And Oral
  Dentifrice   Dental And Oral
  Douche, Vaginal   Obstetrics/Gynecology

GT UROLOGICAL, LLC 612-379-3578
1313 5th St. S.e., Minneapolis, MN 55414
FDA Number: 3004961297
  Clamp, Penile   Gastroenterology/Urology

GTE HEALTH SYSTEMS
  See Siemens Medical Solutions Health Services Corp.

GTE PRODUCTS CORP.
  See Osram Sylvania Inc.

GTE SYLVANIA, INC.
  See Osram Sylvania Inc.

GTR LABS, INC. 888-871-9232
510 Elk St., Gassaway, WV 26624 304-364-2211
FDA Number: 1124974   *Fax:* 304-364-2212
E-mail: gtr@gtrllc.com
Web site: www.gtrllc.com
Medical Products Sales Volume: $2,500,000
Annual Revenue: $1-$5 Million
Year Founded: 1996
Total Employees: 8   *Marketing Staff:* 1   *Sales Staff:* 2
Ownership: Private
Quality System Registration Information: ISO9000
Produces/Sells CE-marked Devices: Y
Federal Procurement Eligibility: Small Business
Distribution: Manufacturer Through Distributor, Manufacturer Through
Manufacturer Reps, OEM, Exporter
General Admin.: Ewell Ferguson/Chief Operating Officer
        Peter Silitch/President
        Ewell Ferguson/Vice President, General Manager
Mktg./Adv.: Ewell Ferguson/Director Marketing
Production: Denise Mowery/Director Quality Assurance
        Ewell Ferguson/Manager Regulatory Affairs
  Generator, Diagnostic X-Ray, High Voltage, 3-Phase   Radiology
  Generator, Diagnostic X-Ray, High Voltage, Single Phase   Radiology

GTR X-RAY GENERATOR MANUFACTURING
  See Gtr Labs, Inc.

GUANTES QUIRURGICOS, S.A. DE C.V. 525-760-5122
366 Henry Ford Ave.,, Deleg. Gustavo A. Madero,
Mexico City, D.f. Mexico
FDA Number: 8043918
  Glove, Surgical, Plastic Surgery   Surgery

GUAVA TECHNOLOGIES, INC. 866-448-2827
25801 Industrial Blvd., Hayward, CA 94545 510-576-1400
FDA Number: 3004422899   *Fax:* 510-576-1500
E-mail: communications@guavatechnologies.com
Web site: www.guavatechnologies.com
Year Founded: 1998
Ownership: Private
Produces/Sells CE-marked Devices: N
General Admin.: John Walker/Chairman
        Lawrence Bruder/President, Chief Executive Officer
Mktg./Adv.: Paul Wheeler/Vice President Sales
Research: David King/Vice President Research & Development
Finance: Donald Huffman/Chief Financial Officer
  Counter, Cell, Differential Classifier, Automated   Hematology

GUERILLA TECHNOLOGIES INC. 772-283-0500
4203 SW High Meadows Ave., Palm City, FL 34990
FDA Number: 3005699848   *Fax:* 772-287-0960
E-mail: info@guerillatechnologies.com
Web site: www.guerillatechnologies.com
Ownership: Private
Produces/Sells CE-marked Devices: N
  Vision Aid, Electronic, AC-Powered   Ophthalmology

GUIDANT - REDMOND
  See Boston Scientific Corp.

GUIDANT CANADA CORPORATION 800-268-4487
505 Apple Creek Blvd., Unit 4, 905-947-5800
Markham, ONT L3R-5 Canada
FDA Number: n/a   *Fax:* 905-947-5830
Web site: www.bostonscientific.com
Year Founded: 1992

GUIDANT CANADA CORPORATION 800-268-4487 *(cont'd)*
Total Employees: 50
Ownership: BOSTON SCIENTIFIC CORPORATION
Produces/Sells CE-marked Devices: N
Distribution: Exclusive Distributor

GUIDANT CORPORATION 408-845-3995
8934 Kirby Drive, Houston, TX 77054
FDA Number: n/a
Web site: www.bostonscientific.com
Ownership: BOSTON SCIENTIFIC CORPORATION
Produces/Sells CE-marked Devices: N
  Intravascular Radiation Delivery System Cardiovascular

GUIDANT CORPORATION, CARDIAC SURGERY
See Boston Scientific Corp.

GUIDANT PUERTO RICO B.V.
See Maquet Puerto Rico Inc.

GUIDED THERAPEUTICS INC. 770-242-8723
5835 Peachtree Corners East, Suite D, Norcross, GA 30092
FDA Number: n/a *Fax:* 770-242-8639
E-mail: info@guidedinc.com
Web site: www.guidedinc.com
Ownership: Public
Stock Symbol: GTHP
Traded On: OTC Bulletin
Produces/Sells CE-marked Devices: N
General Admin.: Mr. Ronald Allen/Chairman
  Dr. Mark Faupel/President, Chief Executive Officer
Research: Richard Fowler/Vice President Engineering
  Dr. Shabbir Bambot/Vice President Research & Development

GUIDED WAVE INC. 916-939-4300
5190 Golden Foothill Pkwy., El Dorado Hills, CA 95762-9608
FDA Number: n/a *Fax:* 916-939-4307
E-mail: GWInfo@guided-wave.com
Web site: www.guided-wave.com
Medical Products Sales Volume: $1,200,000
Annual Revenue: $5-$10 Million
Year Founded: 1983
Total Employees: 20
Ownership: Private
Quality System Registration Information: ISO9001
Produces/Sells CE-marked Devices: Y
Federal Procurement Eligibility: Small Business
Distribution: Manufacturer Direct
Mktg./Adv.: Mr. Michael Broussard/Manager Sales
  Analyzer, Ethylene-Oxide General
  Spectrometer, Infrared Chemistry

GUIDED WAVE, INC.
See Guided Wave Inc.

GUIDEWIRE TECHNOLOGIES, INC. 800-894-4399
26 Keewaydin Dr., Salem, NH 03079-2839 **603-894-4399**
FDA Number: 1221806 *Fax:* 603-894-4473
E-mail: prez1@ix.netcom.com
Web site: www.guidewiretech.com
Medical Products Sales Volume: $2,500,000
Annual Revenue: $1-$5 Million
Year Founded: 1988
Total Employees: 29 *Marketing Staff:* 1 *Sales Staff:* 3
Ownership: Private
Produces/Sells CE-marked Devices: N
Federal Procurement Eligibility: Small Business
Distribution: Manufacturer Through Distributor, OEM, Exporter
General Admin.: Douglas J. Curtis/Chief Executive Officer
Mktg./Adv.: Richard Wisneski/Director Sales
  Linda Curtis/Manager Advertising
  Beth Newell/Manager Contract Sales
Production: Selina Par/Director Quality Assurance
  Debbie Shea/Manager Production
Research: Cong Hua/Director Research & Development
  Guide, Wire, Angiographic (And Accessories) Cns/Neurology
  Guidewire Cardiovascular
  Guidewire, Catheter Cardiovascular
  Guidewire, Catheter, Radiological Radiology

GUILD OPTICAL ASSOCIATES, INC. 603-889-6247
11 Columbia Drive, Amherst, NH 03031
FDA Number: n/a *Fax:* 603-889-8361
E-mail: info@guildoptics.com
Web site: www.guildoptics.com
Medical Products Sales Volume: $750,000
Year Founded: 1990
Total Employees: 10
Ownership: Private
Produces/Sells CE-marked Devices: N

GUILD OPTICAL ASSOCIATES, INC. 603-889-6247 *(cont'd)*
Federal Procurement Eligibility: Small Business
Distribution: Manufacturer Direct
General Admin.: Mark Breda/President, Chief Executive Officer
  Frank A. Reed/Vice President
Mktg./Adv.: Anthony M. DeFeo/Senior Sales Manager
  Contract Manufacturing General

GUITAR SUSPENSION SOLUTIONS 207-324-5717
183A Jagger Mill Road, Sanford, ME 04073-2467
FDA Number: 3004824627
E-mail: info@guitarsuspensionsolutions.com
Ownership: Private
Produces/Sells CE-marked Devices: N
  Sling, Arm, Overhead Supported Physical Med

GULDEN & CO. INC., R.O.
See Gulden Ophthalmics

GULDEN OPHTHALMICS 800-659-2250
225 Cadwalader Avenue, **215-884-8105**
Elkins Park, PA 19027
FDA Number: 2518410 *Fax:* 215-884-0418
E-mail: info@guldenindustries.com
Web site: www.guldenindustries.com
Medical Products Sales Volume: $700,000
Annual Revenue: $0-$1 Million
Year Founded: 1938
Total Employees: 7 *Marketing Staff:* 1 *Sales Staff:* 2
Ownership: Private
Quality System Registration Information: ISO9002
Produces/Sells CE-marked Devices: Y
Federal Procurement Eligibility: Small Business
Distribution: Manufacturer Through Distributor
General Admin.: Thomas D. Cockley/President
Mktg./Adv.: Richard Wehr/Director Marketing
  Richard Wehr/Manager Market Research
  Bar, Prism, Ophthalmic Ophthalmology
  Button, Tracheostomy Tube Anesthesiology
  Calibrator, Tonometer Ophthalmology
  Clip, Lens, Trial, Ophthalmic Ophthalmology
  Conformer, Ophthalmic Ophthalmology
  Disk, Pinhole, Ophthalmic Ophthalmology
  Exophthalmometer Ophthalmology
  Frame, Trial, Ophthalmic Ophthalmology
  Lens, Maddox Ophthalmology
  Occluder, Ophthalmic Ophthalmology
  Retractor, Ophthalmic Ophthalmology
  Ruler, Nearpoint (Punctometer) Ophthalmology
  Screen, Tangent, Target Ophthalmology
  Shield, Eye, Ophthalmic Ophthalmology
  Sphere, Ophthalmic (Implant) Ophthalmology
  Sterilizer, Tonometer Ophthalmology
  Test, Spectacle Dissociation, Battery-Powered (Lancaster) Ophthalmology
  Tester, Color Vision Ophthalmology
  Tonometer, Manual Ophthalmology

GULF COAST HYPERBARICS, INC. 850-271-1441
1100 West 26th St., Lynn Haven, FL 32444
FDA Number: 1058256 *Fax:* 850-271-1449
E-mail: mail@gulfcoasthyperbarics.com
Web site: www.gulfcoasthyperbarics.com
Year Founded: 1984
Ownership: Private
Quality System Registration Information: ISO9001
Produces/Sells CE-marked Devices: N
Federal Procurement Eligibility: Small Business
General Admin.: Jim McCarthy/President
  Chamber, Hyperbaric Anesthesiology

GULF INDUSTRIES
See Bound Tree Medical

GULF MEDICAL FIBEROPTICS 813-891-1993
448 commerce blvd, Oldsmar, FL 34677
FDA Number: 3003768921 *Fax:* 813-855-6627
E-mail: contact@gulffiberoptics.com
Web site: www.gulffiberoptics.com
Ownership: Private
Produces/Sells CE-marked Devices: N
  Illuminator, Fiberoptic, Surgical Field Cns/Neurology
  Light, Surgical, Fiberoptic Surgery

GULF STREAM MEDICAL, INC.
See Gulf Stream Medical, Inc. / Alden Scientific

GULF STREAM MEDICAL, INC. / ALDEN 561-478-5688
SCIENTIFIC
1810 Okeechobee Rd, West Palm Beach, FL 33409
FDA Number: n/a
Ownership: Private

GULF STREAM MEDICAL, INC. / ALDEN — 561-478-5688 (cont'd)
Produces/Sells CE-marked Devices: N
Federal Procurement Eligibility: Small Business
Distribution: Manufacturer Direct, Exclusive Distributor

Disinfector, Liquid	General
Medical Disinfectants/Cleaners for Instruments	General

GULL WORKS MFG. LLC — 801-423-2812
685 East 600 South, Salem, UT 84653
FDA Number: 3005597867
Ownership: Private
Produces/Sells CE-marked Devices: N

Exerciser, Non-Measuring	Physical Med

GUNNELL, INC. — 800-551-0055
8440 State Rd., Millington, MI 48746-9401 — 989-871-4529
FDA Number: 1831114 — Fax: 989-871-4563
E-mail: info@gunnell-inc.com
Web site: www.gunnell-inc.com
Medical Products Sales Volume: $2,500,000
Annual Revenue: $1-$5 Million
Year Founded: 1957
Total Employees: 10 — *Marketing Staff:* 1 — *Sales Staff:* 2
Ownership: Private
Produces/Sells CE-marked Devices: N
Federal Procurement Eligibility: Small Business
Distribution: Manufacturer Direct, Manufacturer Through Distributor, Manufacturer Through Manufacturer Reps
Mktg./Adv.: Mr. Dwight Gay/Manager International & National Sales
　　　　Mr. Dwight Gay/President, Director Marketing
Production: Mrs. Denise Surdu/Customer Service Representative
　　　　Mrs. Jaime Higgins/Customer Service Representative
　　　　Mr. Chris Clothier/Engineer
Purchasing: Mrs. Jaime Higgins/Purchasing Agent

Accessories, Wheelchair	Physical Med
Arm Rest	Physical Med
Attachment, Commode, Wheelchair	Physical Med
Chair, Other	General
Chair, Pediatric	General
Walker, Mechanical	Physical Med
Wheelchair, Special Grade	Physical Med

GUNTHER WEISS SCIENTIFIC GLASSBLOWING CO., INC. — 503-621-3463
14640 Nw Rock Creek Rd., Burlington, OR 97231
FDA Number: 3005489143

Probe, Lacrimal	Ophthalmology

GUPPIE ENT., INC. — 541-548-0748
9251 S.w. Geneva View Rd., Crooked River Ranch, OR 97760
FDA Number: 3025261
Ownership: Private
Produces/Sells CE-marked Devices: N

Device, Assist, CPR	Anesthesiology

GUY GRIFFITHS ORTHODONTIC LAB (1984) INC. — 514-482-1267
4927 Rue Sherbrooke O, Westmount H3Z 1H2 Canada
FDA Number: 8021986

Retainer, Matrix	Dental And Oral

GVI TECHNOLOGY PARTNERS — 330-963-4083
1470 Enterprise Pkwy., Twinsburg, OH 44087
FDA Number: 3003917438
Ownership: Private
Produces/Sells CE-marked Devices: N

Camera, Gamma (Nuclear/Scintillation)	Radiology
Image Processing System	Radiology

GVS - NEW YORK — 631-753-2100
46 Central Avenue, Farmingdale, NY 11735
FDA Number: n/a — Fax: 631-753-2134
E-mail: Sales@GVS-NY.com
Web site: www.gvs-ny.com
Annual Revenue: $0-$1 Million
Year Founded: 1987
Total Employees: 9 — *Marketing Staff:* 4 — *Sales Staff:* 4
Ownership: Private
Produces/Sells CE-marked Devices: N
Federal Procurement Eligibility: Small Business
General Admin.: Anthony Palermo/President
Mktg./Adv.: Ruben Gonzalez/Vice President Sales

Service, Used Equipment	General

GVS FILTER TECHNOLOGY INC. — 317-471-3700
5353 W. 79th St., Indianapolis, IN 46268
FDA Number: 3004360546 — Fax: 317-471-8370
E-mail: gvsusa@gvs.com
Web site: http://www.gvs.com
Annual Revenue: $25-$50 Million

GVS FILTER TECHNOLOGY INC. — 317-471-3700 (cont'd)
Year Founded: 1979
Total Employees: 350 — *Marketing Staff:* 3 — *Sales Staff:* 10
Ownership: Private
Quality System Registration Information: ISO9000; ISO9001
Produces/Sells CE-marked Devices: Y
Federal Procurement Eligibility: Small Business, Female Owned
Distribution: OEM
General Admin.: Mr. Hugh Chilton/President
Mktg./Adv.: Mr. Dan Stratton/Manager Health Care Marketing
Research: Mr. Jose Miguel Burgos/Director Laboratories

Cannula, Epidural	Obstetrics/Gynecology
Component, Plastic	General
Filter, Air	General
Filter, Blood, Dialysis	Gastroenterology/Urology
Filter, Infusion Line	General
Filter, Intravenous Tubing	General
Microfilter, Blood Transfusion	Anesthesiology

GW PLASTICS, INC. — 802-234-9941
239 Pleasant St., Bethel, VT 05032
FDA Number: 1219536 — Fax: 802-234-9940
E-mail: tim.reis@gwplastics.com
Web site: www.gwplastics.com
Medical Products Sales Volume: $25,000,000
Annual Revenue: $50-$100 Million
Year Founded: 1955
Total Employees: 450 — *Marketing Staff:* 2 — *Sales Staff:* 10
Ownership: Private
Quality System Registration Information: ISO9002
Produces/Sells CE-marked Devices: N
Distribution: Manufacturer Direct, Manufacturer Through Manufacturer Reps, Exporter
General Admin.: Mr. Frederic Riehl/Chairman
　　　　Mr. Thomas Johansen/Chief Financial Officer, Vice President
　　　　Brenan Riehl/President, Chief Executive Officer
　　　　Art Bennert/Vice President, General Manager
Medical Admin.: Tim Reis/Vice President Health Care
　　　　Timothy P. Reis/Vice President Health Care
Production: Robert Carpenter/Director Quality Assurance
　　　　Mr. John Silvia/Vice President Manufacturing & Engineering
Research: Tim Holmes/Vice President Engineering
　　　　Craig Hadden/Vice President Research & Development

Component, Plastic	General
Contract Assembly	General
Molding, Custom	General
Molding, Injection	General
Pump, Nebulizer, Manual	Ear/Nose/Throat
Service, Engineering/Design	General
Stapler, Surgical	Surgery
Syringe, Hypodermic	General
System, Delivery, Drug, Unit-Dose	General

GWB INTERNATIONAL, LTD. — 888-436-4826
PO Box 370, 76 Prospect Street, — 781-837-2993
Marshfield Hills, MA 02051
FDA Number: 1221818 — Fax: 781-837-2998
E-mail: GWBIntl@comcast.net
Web site: http://gwbinternational.com/
Medical Products Sales Volume: $200,000
Annual Revenue: $0-$1 Million
Year Founded: 1988
Total Employees: 2
Ownership: Private
Quality System Registration Information: ISO9001
Produces/Sells CE-marked Devices: Y
Federal Procurement Eligibility: Small Business, Female Owned
Distribution: Exclusive Distributor, Importer, Exporter
General Admin.: Georg W. Bohsack/President, Chief Executive Officer

Anatomical Training Model	General
Computer, Ultrasound	Radiology
Knife, Cataract	Ophthalmology

GYMSTANDY LLC — 503-684-4990
9055 Sw Mountain View Ln., Tigard, OR 97224
FDA Number: 3005673518
Ownership: Private
Produces/Sells CE-marked Devices: N

Transfer Device, Patient, Manual	General

GYNECARE — 888-496-3227
235 Constitution Dr., Menlo Park, CA 94025
FDA Number: n/a
Annual Revenue: $0-$1 Million
Total Employees: 40 — *Marketing Staff:* 5 — *Sales Staff:* 1
Ownership: Public
Stock Symbol: GYNE
Traded On: NASDAQ

GYNECARE · 888-496-3227 (cont'd)

Quality System Registration Information: ISO9001
Produces/Sells CE-marked Devices: Y
Federal Procurement Eligibility: Small Business
Distribution: Manufacturer Direct
General Admin.: Lan Burgin/Chief Executive Officer
Production: Augie Lien/Vice President Manufacturing

Catheter, Balloon (Foley Type)	Surgery

GYNESONICS INC. · 650-216-3860

604 Fifth Avenue, Redwood City, CA 94063

FDA Number: n/a   Fax: 650-299-1566
E-mail: info@gynesonics.com
Web site: http://www.gynesonics.com
Year Founded: 2005
Ownership: Private
Produces/Sells CE-marked Devices: N
General Admin.: Mr. Jordan Bajor/Chief Operating Officer
  Mr. Darren Ueker/President, Chief Executive Officer
Medical Admin.: Mr. David Toub/Medical Director
Production: Ms. Diane King/Vice President Regulatory Affairs
Research: Mr. David Danitz/Vice President Research & Development
IS: Mr. Michael Munrow/Vice President Systems

GYRUS ACMI, INC. · 508-804-2739

300 Stillwater P.o.box 1971, Stamford, CT 06902

FDA Number: 1218764
Ownership: Private
Produces/Sells CE-marked Devices: N

Accessories, Surgical Camera	Surgery
Brush, Cytology, Endoscopic	Gastroenterology/Urology
Choledochoscope, Flexible Or Rigid	Gastroenterology/Urology
Culdoscope	Obstetrics/Gynecology
Cystoscope	Gastroenterology/Urology
Cystourethroscope	Gastroenterology/Urology
Electrode, Electrosurgical, Active (Blade)	Surgery
Electrosurgical Unit, Cutting & Coagulation Device	Surgery
Endoscope	Gastroenterology/Urology
Hysteroscope	Obstetrics/Gynecology
Laparoscope, General & Plastic Surgery	Surgery
Laryngoscope, Rigid	Anesthesiology
Needle, Pneumoperitoneum, Spring Loaded	Gastroenterology/Urology
Obturator, Endoscopic	Gastroenterology/Urology
Resectoscope Working Element	Gastroenterology/Urology
Scissors, Cystoscopic	Gastroenterology/Urology
Sheath, Endoscopic	Gastroenterology/Urology
Stylet, Tracheal Tube	Anesthesiology
Telescope, Rigid, Endoscopic	Gastroenterology/Urology
Tube, Tracheal (Endotracheal)	Anesthesiology
Tubing, Non-Invasive	Surgery
Ureteroscope	Gastroenterology/Urology
Urethroscope	Gastroenterology/Urology
Urethrotome	Gastroenterology/Urology

GYRUS ACMI, INC. · 508-804-2739

93 North Pleasant St., Norwalk, OH 44857

FDA Number: 1519132
Ownership: Private
Produces/Sells CE-marked Devices: N

Accessories, Cleaning Brushes (For Endoscope)	Gastroenterology/Urology
Accessories, Surgical Camera	Surgery
Adapter, Bulb, Endoscope, Miscellaneous	Gastroenterology/Urology
Brush, Cleaning, Tracheal Tube	Ear/Nose/Throat
Brush, Cytology, Endoscopic	Gastroenterology/Urology
Catheter, Suprapubic	Gastroenterology/Urology
Colposcope	Obstetrics/Gynecology
Culdoscope	Obstetrics/Gynecology
Curette, Uterine	Obstetrics/Gynecology
Cystoscope	Gastroenterology/Urology
Cystourethroscope	Gastroenterology/Urology
Dislodger, Stone, Flexible	Gastroenterology/Urology
Electrode, Electrosurgical, Active (Blade)	Surgery
Electrosurgical Unit, Cutting & Coagulation Device	Surgery
Electrosurgical, Unit, Gastroenterology	Gastroenterology/Urology
Endoscope	Gastroenterology/Urology
Evacuator, Gastro-Urology	Gastroenterology/Urology
Forceps, Biopsy, Non-Electric	Gastroenterology/Urology
Forceps, General & Plastic Surgery	Surgery
General Use Surgical Scissors	Surgery
Hysteroscope	Obstetrics/Gynecology
Illuminator, Fiberoptic (For Endoscope)	Gastroenterology/Urology
Laparoscope, General & Plastic Surgery	Surgery
Laparoscope, Gynecologic	Obstetrics/Gynecology
Laryngoscope, Rigid	Anesthesiology
Lithotriptor, Electro-Hydraulic, Percutaneous	Gastroenterology/Urology
Needle, Endoscopic	Gastroenterology/Urology
Needle, Pneumoperitoneum, Spring Loaded	Gastroenterology/Urology
Obturator, Endoscopic	Gastroenterology/Urology
Pack, Sterilization Wrapper (Bag And Accessories)	Surgery
Resectoscope	Gastroenterology/Urology

GYRUS ACMI, INC. · 508-804-2739 (cont'd)

Resectoscope Working Element	Gastroenterology/Urology
Retractor, Surgical	Surgery
Scissors, Cystoscopic	Gastroenterology/Urology
Sheath, Endoscopic	Gastroenterology/Urology
Stylet, Tracheal Tube	Anesthesiology
Suction Apparatus, Operating Room, Wall Vacuum-Powered	Surgery
Surgical Instrument, G-U, Manual	Gastroenterology/Urology
Telescope, Rigid, Endoscopic	Gastroenterology/Urology
Tube, Tracheal (Endotracheal)	Anesthesiology
Tubing, Non-Invasive	Surgery
Ureteroscope	Gastroenterology/Urology
Urethroscope	Gastroenterology/Urology
Urethrotome	Gastroenterology/Urology

GYRUS ENT L.L.C., SUB. OF GYRUS ACMI, INC. · 800-773-4301 · 901-373-0200

2925 Appling Rd., Bartlett, TN 38133

FDA Number: 1037007   Fax: 901-373-0220
E-mail: CustomerServiceENT@gyrusacmi.com
Web site: www.gyrusacmi.com
Ownership: Private
Produces/Sells CE-marked Devices: N

Accessories, Surgical Camera	Surgery
Applicator, ENT	Ear/Nose/Throat
Balloon, Epistaxis (Nasal)	Ear/Nose/Throat
Block, Cutting, ENT	Ear/Nose/Throat
Bronchoscope, Rigid	Ear/Nose/Throat
Burr	Ear/Nose/Throat
Caliper, Ophthalmic	Ophthalmology
Cannula, Sinus	Ear/Nose/Throat
Ceramics, Triphos./Hydroxyapatite, Ca. (Non-Load Bearing)	Orthopedics
Chisel, Nasal	Ear/Nose/Throat
Die, Wire Bending, ENT	Ear/Nose/Throat
Drape, Microscope, Ophthalmic	Ophthalmology
Drape, Patient, Ophthalmic	Ophthalmology
Drape, Surgical	Surgery
Drape, Surgical, ENT	Ear/Nose/Throat
Drill, Surgical, ENT (Electric Or Pneumatic)	Ear/Nose/Throat
ENT Manual Surgical Instrument	Ear/Nose/Throat
Electrosurgical Unit, Cutting & Coagulation Device	Surgery
Endoscope	Gastroenterology/Urology
Endoscope, Rigid	Surgery
Fiberoptic Light Source & Carrier	Ear/Nose/Throat
Forceps, Ophthalmic	Ophthalmology
Forceps, Wire Closure, ENT	Ear/Nose/Throat
Gauze/sponge, Nonresorbable For External Use	Surgery
Hearing Aid, Air Conduction, Transcutaneous System	Ear/Nose/Throat
Holder, Ear Speculum	Ear/Nose/Throat
Implant, Endosseous (Bone Filling and/or Augmentation)	Dental And Oral
Jig, Piston Cutting, ENT	Ear/Nose/Throat
Knife, Ophthalmic	Ophthalmology
Knife, Surgical	Dental And Oral
Laparoscope, General & Plastic Surgery	Surgery
Lens, Fundus, Hruby, Diagnostic	Ophthalmology
Light, Surgical Headlight	Dental And Oral
Mold, Middle Ear	Ear/Nose/Throat
Nasopharyngoscope (Flexible Or Rigid)	Ear/Nose/Throat
Otoscope	Ear/Nose/Throat
Plate, Fixation, Bone	Orthopedics
Polymer, ENT Synthetic Polyamide (Mesh Or Foil Material)	Ear/Nose/Throat
Probe, Lacrimal	Ophthalmology
Prosthesis, Nose, Internal	Surgery
Prosthesis, Ossicular	Ear/Nose/Throat
Prosthesis, Ossicular, Total	Ear/Nose/Throat
Protector, Hearing (Circumaural)	Ear/Nose/Throat
Rasp, Ear	Ear/Nose/Throat
Retractor, Ophthalmic	Ophthalmology
Scissors, Ophthalmic	Ophthalmology
Scissors, Wire Cutting, ENT	Ear/Nose/Throat
Screw, Fixation, Bone	Orthopedics
Speculum, Ear	Ear/Nose/Throat
Splint, Nasal	Ear/Nose/Throat
Splint, Septal, Intranasal	Ear/Nose/Throat
Staple, Implantable	Surgery
Stimulator, Nerve, ENT	Ear/Nose/Throat
Support, Head, Surgical, ENT	Ear/Nose/Throat
System, Vocal Cord Medialization	Ear/Nose/Throat
Tack, Sacculotomy (Cody)	Ear/Nose/Throat
Tray, Surgical Instrument	Surgery
Tube, Ear Suction	Ear/Nose/Throat
Tube, Tympanostomy	Ear/Nose/Throat
Tubing, Non-Invasive	Surgery
Vise, Ossicular Finger	Ear/Nose/Throat
Wick, Ear	Ear/Nose/Throat

GYRUS MEDICAL, INC. · 800-852-9361 · 763-416-3000

6655 Wedgwood Road, Suite #105, Maple Grove, MN 55311

FDA Number: 2183680   Fax: 763-416-3001
E-mail: info@gyrusmed.com
Web site: www.gyrusmed.com

GYRUS MEDICAL, INC.   800-852-9361 (cont'd)

Medical Products Sales Volume: $23,800,000
Annual Revenue: $50-$100 Million
Year Founded: 2000
Total Employees: 240   *Marketing Staff:* 9   *Sales Staff:* 100
Ownership: OLYMPUS CORPORATION
Stock Symbol: GYG
Traded On: London
Quality System Registration Information: ISO9001
Produces/Sells CE-marked Devices: Y
Federal Procurement Eligibility: Small Business
Distribution: Manufacturer Through Manufacturer Reps, OEM
General Admin.: Mr. Brian Steer/Chairman
        Tom Murphy/President, Chief Executive Officer
Mktg./Adv.: Scott Sanders/Director Business Development
        Michael Geraghty/Vice President, Manager Sales
Production: Craig Swandall/Vice President Manufacturing
Finance: Shelly Olsen/Chief Financial Officer

Adapter, Electrosurgical Unit, Cable	Surgery
Cannula, Other	General
Coagulator/Cutter, Endoscopic, Bipolar	Obstetrics/Gynecology
Dissector, Surgical, General & Plastic Surgery	Surgery
Electrode, Needle	Cns/Neurology
Electrosurgical Equipment, General Purpose	Surgery
Electrosurgical Equipment, Special Purpose	Surgery
Electrosurgical Unit, Cutting & Coagulation Device	Surgery
Electrosurgical Unit, Gastroenterology	Gastroenterology/Urology
Electrosurgical Unit, General Purpose (ESU)	Surgery
Forceps, Electrosurgical	Surgery
Forceps, Endoscopic	Gastroenterology/Urology
Forceps, General & Plastic Surgery	Surgery
Forceps, Laparoscopy, Bipolar, Electrosurgical	Surgery
Forceps, Laparoscopy, Electrosurgical	Surgery
General Use Surgical Scissors	Surgery
Generator, Power, Electrosurgical	Surgery
Needle, Cutting, Bipolar, Electrocauterization	Surgery
Needle, Other	General
Probe	Orthopedics
Probe, Electrocauterization, Multi-Use	Surgery
Probe, Gastrointestinal	Gastroenterology/Urology
Scissors, Laparoscopy, Bipolar, Electrosurgical	Surgery
Scissors, Laparoscopy, Electrosurgical	Surgery
Snare, Polyp	Surgery

GYRX, LLC   904-641-2599
10302 Deerwood Park Blvd., Ste. 209, Jacksonville, FL 32256

FDA Number: 3004588227
Ownership: Private
Produces/Sells CE-marked Devices: N
General Admin.: Mr. Bill Dennis/Chief Executive Officer

Clamp, Penile	Gastroenterology/Urology
Clip, Implantable	Surgery
Clip, Vas Deferens	Surgery
Garment, Protective, For Incontinence	Gastroenterology/Urology

H & H ASSOCIATES, INC.   800-326-5708
4173 George Washington Memorial Highway,   **757-224-0177**
Ordinary, VA 23131

FDA Number: 1126195
E-mail: info@gohandh.com
Web site: www.gohandh.com
Ownership: Private
Produces/Sells CE-marked Devices: N

Bandage, Elastic	General
Dressing, Wound and Burn, Occlusive	Surgery
Kit, Cricothyrotomy	Anesthesiology
Sheet, Burn	General
Shield, Eye, Ophthalmic	Ophthalmology
Tourniquet, Non-Pneumatic, Surgical	Surgery

H & H CO.   909-390-0373
4435 East Airport Dr., #108, Ontario, CA 91761

FDA Number: 1126195
Ownership: Private
Produces/Sells CE-marked Devices: N

Accessories, Implant, Dental, Endosseous	Dental And Oral
Accessories, Retractor, Dental	Dental And Oral
Bone Mill	Orthopedics
Bone Particle Collector	Ear/Nose/Throat
Burr, Dental	Dental And Oral
Chisel, Bone, Surgical	Dental And Oral
Chisel, Osteotome, Surgical	Dental And Oral
Clamp, Wire, Orthodontic	Dental And Oral
Condenser, Amalgam And Foil, Operative	Dental And Oral
Curette, Operative	Dental And Oral
Curette, Periodontic	Dental And Oral
Dressing, Other	General
Drill, Dental, Intraoral	Dental And Oral
Elevator, Surgical, Dental	Dental And Oral
Explorer, Operative	Dental And Oral

H & H CO.   909-390-0373 (cont'd)

File, Bone, Surgical	Dental And Oral
File, Periodontic	Dental And Oral
Forceps	Orthopedics
Forceps, Dressing, Dental	Dental And Oral
Forceps, Rongeur, Surgical	Dental And Oral
Forceps, Tooth Extractor, Surgical	Dental And Oral
Handle, Scalpel	Surgery
Hemostat, Surgical	Dental And Oral
Hoe, Periodontic	Dental And Oral
Irrigator, Sinus	Ear/Nose/Throat
Knife, Periodontic	Dental And Oral
Light, Fiberoptic, Dental	Dental And Oral
Light, Surgical Operating, Dental	Dental And Oral
Mallet, Bone	Orthopedics
Matrix, Dental	Dental And Oral
Mirror, Mouth	Dental And Oral
Mouthpiece, Saliva Ejector	Dental And Oral
Osteotome, Manual (Plastic Surgery)	Surgery
Pliers, Surgical	Orthopedics
Probe, Periodontic	Dental And Oral
Punch, Biopsy, Surgical	Dental And Oral
Remover, Crown	Dental And Oral
Retractor, All Types	Dental And Oral
Scaler, Periodontic	Dental And Oral
Scissors, Surgical Tissue, Dental (Oral)	Dental And Oral
Speculum, Ear	Ear/Nose/Throat
Trephine, Sinus	Ear/Nose/Throat

H & S MANUFACTURING, INC.   800-827-3091
727 E. Broadway, Williston, ND 58801-6105   **701-572-5400**

FDA Number: 2183885   *Fax:* 701-774-3091
E-mail: hsmfg@nemontel.net
Web site: www.h-and-smfg.com
Medical Products Sales Volume: $360,000
Annual Revenue: $0-$1 Million
Total Employees: 8   *Sales Staff:* 2
Ownership: Private
Produces/Sells CE-marked Devices: N
Federal Procurement Eligibility: Small Business, Female Owned
Distribution: Manufacturer Through Distributor, Manufacturer Through Manufacturer Reps
General Admin.: Kathy Zent/President
Mktg./Adv.: Kathy Zent/Manager National Sales

Dispenser, Fluid	General
Encapsulator, Fluid	General

H & S TECHNICAL SERVICES, INC.   800-923-2486
1833 W. Main St., Suite 119, Mesa, AZ 85201   **480-517-4918**

FDA Number: 3003145976   *Fax:* 480-517-4924
E-mail: Info@hstechsvc.com
Ownership: Private
Produces/Sells CE-marked Devices: N

Solution-Test, Standard-Conductivity, Dialysis	Gastroenterology/Urology

H&H INSTRUMENTS   904-797-1502
4950 Crescent Technical Ct, St Augustine, FL 32086

FDA Number: 1052908
Ownership: Private
Produces/Sells CE-marked Devices: N

Drill, Surgical, ENT (Electric Or Pneumatic)	Ear/Nose/Throat
Handpiece, Direct Drive, AC-Powered	Dental And Oral
Saw, Electric	Cardiovascular

H&M RUBBER COMPANY, INC.   330-678-3323
4200 Mogadore Rd., Kent, OH 44240-7258

FDA Number: n/a   *Fax:* 330-678-8460
Web site: www.kingsystems.com
Medical Products Sales Volume: $6
Annual Revenue: $5-$10 Million
Ownership: KING SYSTEMS CORP.
Produces/Sells CE-marked Devices: N
Federal Procurement Eligibility: Small Business

Bag, Breathing	Anesthesiology
Component, Other	General
Component, Plastic	General
Component, Rubber	General

H&W TECHNOLOGY, LLC.   585-218-0385
PO Box 20281, Rochester, NY 14602-0281

FDA Number: n/a   *Fax:* 585-218-4271
E-mail: info@stericert.com
Web site: www.stericert.com
Medical Products Sales Volume: $300,000
Annual Revenue: $0-$1 Million
Year Founded: 1998
Total Employees: 6   *Marketing Staff:* 1   *Sales Staff:* 1
Ownership: Private
Produces/Sells CE-marked Devices: N

H&W TECHNOLOGY, LLC.   585-218-0385 *(cont'd)*
Federal Procurement Eligibility: Small Business
Distribution: Manufacturer Direct, Service Direct, Exporter
General Admin.: Jonathan A. Wilder/Chief Executive Officer
Mktg./Adv.: Jonathan A. Wilder/Director Marketing
    Jonathan A. Wilder/Director Product Development
    Jonathan A. Wilder/Manager Advertising
Production: Charles Hancock/Director Quality Assurance
    Charles Hancock/Manager Regulatory Affairs

Contract R&D, Diagnostics	General
Sterilizer, Ethylene-Oxide Gas	General
Sterilizer, Steam (Autoclave)	General

H. A. STILES CO.   800-447-8537
170 Forest St., Westbrook, ME 04092   **207-854-2339**
FDA Number: 1218881   *Fax:* 207-854-3863
E-mail: info@hastiles.com
Web site: www.hastiles.com
Medical Products Sales Volume: $1,900,000
Year Founded: 1911
Total Employees: 10
Ownership: Private
Produces/Sells CE-marked Devices: N
Federal Procurement Eligibility: Small Business, Female Owned
Distribution: Manufacturer Direct, Importer, Exporter

Depressor, Tongue	General

H.B. FULLER COMPANY   800-328-9673
1200 Willow Lake Blvd., PO Box 64683,   **651-236-5900**
St. Paul, MN 55110
FDA Number: n/a   *Fax:* 651-236-5215
E-mail: nathan.weaver@hbfuller.com
Web site: www.hbfuller.com
Medical Products Sales Volume: $1,460,000,000
Year Founded: 1887
Total Employees: 100
Ownership: Public
Stock Symbol: FUL
Traded On: NYSE
Quality System Registration Information: ISO9000; ISO9001; ISO9002
Produces/Sells CE-marked Devices: N
Distribution: OEM
General Admin.: Carlos Mendivil/Program Manager
Mktg./Adv.: Nathan Weaver/Manager Regional Sales

Tape, Adhesive, Hypoallergenic	General

H.B. GORDON MFG. CO., INC.   310-327-5240
751 East Artesia Blvd., Carson, CA 90746
FDA Number: 2012546
Ownership: Private
Produces/Sells CE-marked Devices: N

Gel, Electrode, Stimulator	Cns/Neurology

H.B. LABORATORIES INC.
See Bio-Med Devices, Inc.

H.E. INC. (HAROD ENTERPRISES)   706-228-5165
4052 Indian Creek Rd, Augusta, GA 30907
FDA Number: n/a
E-mail: rush@hesales.com
Web site: www.hesales.com
Medical Products Sales Volume: $600,000
Annual Revenue: $0-$1 Million
Ownership: Private
Produces/Sells CE-marked Devices: N
Federal Procurement Eligibility: Small Business
Distribution: Manufacturer Direct, Manufacturer Through Distributor, Manufacturer Through Manufacturer Reps, Importer, Exporter

Dressing, Foam	General
Kit, Wound Dressing	Surgery

H.G. FISCHER, INC.
See Fischer Medical Technologies Inc.

H.K. EYECAN LTD.   800-356-3362
2849 Ahearn Ave, Ottawa, ONT K2B-6J8 Canada   **613-860-0333**
FDA Number: n/a   *Fax:* 613-596-4300
E-mail: info@eyecan.ca
Web site: www.eyecan.ca
Year Founded: 1990
Total Employees: 10
Ownership: Private
Produces/Sells CE-marked Devices: N
Distribution: Manufacturer Direct

H.L. BOUTON CO., INC.   800-426-1881
PO Box 840, Buzzards Bay, MA 02532   **508-295-3300**
FDA Number: 1293515   *Fax:* 508-295-3521
E-mail: eyewear@hlbouton.com

H.L. BOUTON CO., INC.   800-426-1881 *(cont'd)*
Web site: www.hlbouton.com
Annual Revenue: $10-$25 Million
Year Founded: 1940
Total Employees: 50   *Marketing Staff:* 8   *Sales Staff:* 35
Ownership: BOUTON CORP.
Produces/Sells CE-marked Devices: N
Federal Procurement Eligibility: Small Business
Distribution: Manufacturer Through Distributor, Manufacturer Through Manufacturer Reps
General Admin.: David F. Miller/President, Chief Executive Officer
Mktg./Adv.: David Roll/Vice President Marketing & Sales
Production: Gary Sullivan/Vice President Manufacturing

Eyeglasses	Ophthalmology
Eyeglasses, Safety	Ophthalmology
Goggles, Protective, Eye	Ophthalmology
Lavage Unit, Water Jet	General
Lens, Other	Ophthalmology

H.L. BOUTON COMPANY, INC.   800-426-1881
P.O. Box 840, Buzzards Bay, MA 02532   **508-295-3300**
FDA Number: n/a   *Fax:* 508-295-3521
E-mail: eyewear@hlbouton.com
Web site: hlbouton.com
Annual Revenue: $10-$25 Million
Total Employees: 120   *Marketing Staff:* 2   *Sales Staff:* 8
Ownership: Private
Produces/Sells CE-marked Devices: N
Federal Procurement Eligibility: Small Business
Distribution: Manufacturer Through Distributor, Manufacturer Through Manufacturer Reps
General Admin.: David F. Miller/President, Chief Executive Officer
Mktg./Adv.: Neil Harold/Manager International & National Sales
    Timothy Flaherty/Manager National Sales
    David Roll/Vice President Marketing & Sales
Production: Gary Sullivan/Vice President Manufacturing

Cup, Eye	Ophthalmology

H.M.B. SURGICAL REPAIR SERVICE
See Hmb Endoscopy Products

H.S. CROCKER   847-669-3600
12100 Smith Dr., Huntley, IL 60142
FDA Number: n/a   *Fax:* 847-669-1170
E-mail: lmsulma@hscrocker.com
Web site: www.hscrocker.com
Annual Revenue: $0-$1 Million
Ownership: Private
Produces/Sells CE-marked Devices: N
Federal Procurement Eligibility: Small Business
Distribution: Manufacturer Direct, Service Direct
General Admin.: Ron Giordano/Chief Executive Officer

Contract Packaging	General
Service, Printing	General

H.S. INTERNATIONAL CO., INC.   800-811-0072
5040 Commercial Circle,, Unit A,   **925-674-1515**
Concord, CA 94520
FDA Number: n/a   *Fax:* 925-674-1509
E-mail: sales@hsisurgical.com
Web site: www.hsisurgical.com
Medical Products Sales Volume: $1,000,000
Year Founded: 1980
Total Employees: 25   *Marketing Staff:* 3   *Sales Staff:* 3
Ownership: Private
Quality System Registration Information: ISO9000; ISO9001; ISO9002; ISO9003
Produces/Sells CE-marked Devices: N
Federal Procurement Eligibility: Small Business
Distribution: Manufacturer Direct, OEM, Service Direct, Exporter
General Admin.: Henry Shapiro/President, Chief Executive Officer

Cutter, Vitreous Aspiration, AC-Powered	Ophthalmology
Scissors, Laparoscopy, Electrosurgical	Surgery
Scissors, Ophthalmic	Ophthalmology
Surgical Instrument, Radial Keratotomy	Ophthalmology

H2OONLY CO.   800-338-4905
1101 Columbus Ave., Bay City, MI 48708
FDA Number: 67874
Ownership: Private
Produces/Sells CE-marked Devices: N

Purification System, Water	Gastroenterology/Urology

H2O RAMPS AND LIFTS, LLC   501-825-8838
7010 Greers Ferry Rd., Greers Ferry, AR 72067
FDA Number: 3005619574
Ownership: Private
Produces/Sells CE-marked Devices: N

Lift, Bath, Non-AC-Powered	General

H2OR, INC.   918-744-4267
1638 South Main, Tulsa, OK 74119
FDA Number: 3004858958
Ownership: Private
Produces/Sells CE-marked Devices: N
Bottle, Collection, Vacuum (Aspirator)	General
Tube, Aspirating, Flexible, Connecting	Anesthesiology

HAAG-STREIT GROUP   800-787-5426
3535 Kings Mills Road, Mason, OH 45040-2303
FDA Number: 1223498
Web site: www.haag-streit-usa.com
Annual Revenue: $10-$25 Million
Ownership: Interzeag Ag
Quality System Registration Information: ISO9000
Produces/Sells CE-marked Devices: N
Federal Procurement Eligibility: Small Business
Distribution: Manufacturer Direct, Manufacturer Through Distributor, Importer
Accessories, Laser	General
Adaptometer (Biophotometer)	Ophthalmology
Computer Software	General
Distometer	Ophthalmology
Keratometer	Ophthalmology
Lamp, Slit	Ophthalmology
Lens, Contact, Polymethylmethacrylate, Diagnostic	Ophthalmology
Lens, Other	Ophthalmology
Pachometer	Ophthalmology
Perimeter, AC-Powered	Ophthalmology
Perimeter, Automatic, AC-Powered	Ophthalmology
Tape, Television & Video, Endoscopic	Gastroenterology/Urology
Tonometer, Manual	Ophthalmology
Visometer	Ophthalmology
Medical Product Subsidiaries (Listed Separately)
  Clement Clarke Internat'L Ltd.
  John Weiss & Son Ltd.

HAAG-STREIT USA, INC.   800-787-5426
3535 Kings Mills Rd., Mason, OH 45040-2303
FDA Number: 1223498
Web site: www.haag-streit-usa.com
Annual Revenue: $10-$25 Million
Year Founded: 1898
Ownership: HAAG STREIT A/G
Quality System Registration Information: ISO9000
Produces/Sells CE-marked Devices: Y
Federal Procurement Eligibility: Small Business
Distribution: Manufacturer Through Distributor
Cabinet, ENT Treatment	Ear/Nose/Throat
Chair, Examination And Treatment	General
Chair, Ophthalmic, AC-Powered	Ophthalmology
Chair, Ophthalmic, Manual	Ophthalmology
Chair, Other	General
Stand, Instrument, Ophthalmic	Ophthalmology
Stool, Bedside	General
Stool, Operating Room, Adjustable	Surgery
Stretcher, Wheeled (Mobile)	General
Table, Ophthalmic, Instrument, Manual	Ophthalmology
Table, Ophthalmic, Instrument, Powered	Ophthalmology
Unit, Examining/Treatment, ENT	Ear/Nose/Throat

HABILIS, INC.   203-377-8835
155 Hill St., Milford, CT 06460
FDA Number: n/a
Ownership: Private
Produces/Sells CE-marked Devices: N
Lens, Spectacle/Eyeglasses, Non-Custom	Ophthalmology

HABLEY MEDICAL TECHNOLOGY CORP.   800-729-1994
15721 Bernardo Heights Parkway, Suite B-30,   760-751-9756
San Diego, CA 92128
FDA Number: n/a   *Fax:* 916-404-5199
E-mail: info@hableymedical.com
Web site: www.hableymedical.com
Medical Products Sales Volume: $48,000,000
Annual Revenue: $1-$5 Million
Year Founded: 1982
Total Employees: 41   *Marketing Staff:* 2
Ownership: Private
Produces/Sells CE-marked Devices: N
Federal Procurement Eligibility: Small Business, Minority Owned
Distribution: Manufacturer Direct, Manufacturer Through Distributor, Manufacturer Through Manufacturer Reps, Service Direct, Exporter
General Admin.: Matthew Kashani/President, Chief Executive Officer
Research: Clark Foster/Vice President Research & Development
Collector, Blood, Vacuum-Assisted	Hematology
Contract R&D, Diagnostics	General
Controller, Infusion, Intravenous	Cardiovascular
Glove, Surgical	General
Nebulizer, Ultrasonic	Anesthesiology

HABLEY MEDICAL TECHNOLOGY CORP.   800-729-1994 *(cont'd)*
Needle, Blood Collection	General
Scalpel, One-Piece (Knife)	Surgery
Service, Engineering/Design	General
Syringe, Other	General

HABONA INC.
  See Pedifix, Inc.

HACH COMPANY / ENVIRONMENTAL TEST SYSTEMS   800-548-4381
23575 County Road 106, PO Box 4659,   574-262-2060
Elkhart, IN 46514
FDA Number: 1833407   *Fax:* 574-262-2495
E-mail: etscustomerservice@hach.com
Web site: www.sterichek.com
Annual Revenue: $100-$500 Million
Ownership: DANAHER CORP.
Quality System Registration Information: ISO9001
Produces/Sells CE-marked Devices: Y
Distribution: Manufacturer Through Distributor
Mktg./Adv.: Jon Brew/Director Marketing
           Ron Merwin/Director Sales
           Drew Chuppe/Market Manager
           John Simon/Vice President Marketing & Sales
Research: Dan Morris/Director Technology
Test, Equipment, Sterilization	General

HACKER INDUSTRIES, INC.   803-712-6100
1132 Kincaid Bridge Rd., Winnsboro, SC 29180
FDA Number: 2248970   *Fax:* 803-712-6116
E-mail: HACKERLAB@AOL.COM
Web site: www.hackerinstruments.com
Ownership: Private
Produces/Sells CE-marked Devices: N
Absorber, Carbon-Dioxide	Anesthesiology
Microtome, Freezing Attachment	Pathology
Microtome, Rotary	Pathology
Microtome, Sliding	Pathology
Stainer, Slide, Automated	Pathology
Tissue Processor, Automated	Pathology

HACKER INSTRUMENTS AND INDUSTRIES INC.   800-442-2537
1132 Kincaid Bridge Road, PO Box 1176,   803-712-6100
Winnsboro,, SC 29180
FDA Number: 9200408   *Fax:* 803-712-6116
E-mail: hackerlab@aol.com
Web site: www.hackerinstruments.com
Medical Products Sales Volume: $1,500,000
Annual Revenue: $1-$5 Million
Year Founded: 1942
Total Employees: 8   *Marketing Staff:* 2   *Sales Staff:* 8
Ownership: Private
Produces/Sells CE-marked Devices: Y
Federal Procurement Eligibility: Small Business, Female Owned
Distribution: Manufacturer Direct, Exclusive Distributor
General Admin.: Elfi L. Hacker/President, Chief Executive Officer
           James Mullen/Vice President, General Manager
Mktg./Adv.: James Mullen/Manager International Marketing & Sales
           Dorothy Murphy/Manager National Sales
Production: Lewis Merikas/Director Quality Assurance
Coverslip, Microscope Slide	Pathology
Dispenser, Paraffin	Pathology
Hood, Fume	Toxicology
Microtome, Cryostat	Pathology
Microtome, Rotary	Pathology
Sharpener, Microtome Blade	Pathology
Stainer, Slide, Automated	Pathology
Stainer, Slide, Hematology	Hematology
Stainer, Slide, Histology	Microbiology
Tissue Processor, Automated	Pathology

HAEMACHEM, INC.   314-644-3277
2335 South Hanley Rd., St. Louis, MO 63144
FDA Number: 1927803
Ownership: Private
Produces/Sells CE-marked Devices: N
Test, Heparin (Clotting Time)	Hematology
Test, Qualitative And Quantitative Factor Deficiency	Hematology
Test, Thrombin Time	Hematology

HAEMACURE CORP.   888-721-8076
2001 University St., Ste. 430,   514-282-3350
Montreal, QUE 34236 Canada
FDA Number: 1064637   *Fax:* 514-282-3358
E-mail: khammes@haemacurecorp.com
Web site: www.haemacurecorp.com
Year Founded: 1991
Total Employees: 50

HAEMACURE CORP.
888-721-8076 *(cont'd)*
Ownership: Private
Produces/Sells CE-marked Devices: N
Distribution: Manufacturer Direct, Exclusive Distributor

HAEMO-SOL, INC.
800-821-5676
7301 York Rd., Baltimore, MD 21204-7631
410-821-5676
FDA Number: n/a
Fax: 410-828-8461
E-mail: haemosol@haemo-sol.com
Web site: www.haemo-sol.com
Annual Revenue: $0-$1 Million
Total Employees: 10
Ownership: Private
Produces/Sells CE-marked Devices: N
Federal Procurement Eligibility: Small Business
Distribution: Manufacturer Through Distributor, Exporter
Mktg./Adv.: William Hermann/General Manager Marketing
Production: Sierra Silkman/Customer Service Representative

Detergent	Hematology
Solution, Instrument Cleaner	General

HAEMONETICS CORP.
781-356-9488
179 Campanelli Parkway, Stoughton, MA 02072
FDA Number: 1225648
Ownership: Haemonetics Corp.
Stock Symbol: HAE
Traded On: NYSE
Produces/Sells CE-marked Devices: N

HAEMONETICS CORP.
800-225-5242
400 Wood Road, Braintree, MA 02184
781-848-7100
FDA Number: 1219343
Web site: www.haemonetics.com
Ownership: Private
Produces/Sells CE-marked Devices: Y
Finance: Mr. Gerry Gould/Vice President Investor Relations

Accessories, Catheter	Surgery
Autotransfusion Unit (Blood)	Anesthesiology
Catheter, Intravascular, Therapeutic, Short-term Less Than 30 Days	General
Centrifuge, Continuous Flow	Chemistry
Freezer, Blood Storage	Hematology
Kit, Blood, Transfusion	General
Microfilter, Blood Transfusion	Anesthesiology
Pump, Aspiration, Portable	Anesthesiology
Separator, Blood Cell, Automated	Hematology
Shaker/Stirrer	Chemistry
Software, Blood Bank (Stand-Alone Products)	Hematology

HAEMONETICS CORP.
781-356-9488
Buncher Industrial Park, Avenue C, Building 18, Leetsdale, PA 15056
FDA Number: 2529337
Ownership: Haemonetics Corp.
Stock Symbol: HAE
Traded On: NYSE
Produces/Sells CE-marked Devices: N

Accessories, Catheter	Surgery
Centrifuge, Refrigerated	Pathology
Separator, Blood Cell, Automated	Hematology
Shaker/Stirrer	Chemistry

HAEMOSCOPE CORP.
800-438-2834
6231 West Howard Street, Niles, IL 60714-3403
847-588-0453
FDA Number: 2429444
Fax: 847-588-0455
E-mail: info@haemoscope.com
Web site: www.haemoscope.com
Medical Products Sales Volume: $5,300,000
Year Founded: 1976
Total Employees: 34
Ownership: Private
Produces/Sells CE-marked Devices: N
Federal Procurement Eligibility: Small Business
Distribution: Manufacturer Direct, Manufacturer Through Distributor, Service Direct, Exclusive Distributor, Exporter
General Admin.: Margalit Tocher/Chief Operating Officer
　　　　　Millie Aponte/Office Manager
　　　　　Dr. Eli Cohen/President, Chief Executive Officer
Production: Gabriel Raviv/Vice President Manufacturing
Finance: Carole S. Cohen/Manager Finance

Analyzer, Coagulation	Hematology
Analyzer, Coagulation, Whole Blood	Hematology

HAEMOTRONIC INC.
See Lucomed Inc.

HAER AND COMPANY, FREDERICK
See Fhc, Inc

HAGER WORLDWIDE, INC.
800-328-2335
13322 Byrd Drive, Odessa, FL 33556-5312
813-926-7474
FDA Number: 1044031
Fax: 800-573-9392
E-mail: contact@hagerworldwide.com
Web site: www.hagerworldwide.com
Medical Products Sales Volume: $1,300,000
Annual Revenue: $1-$5 Million
Year Founded: 1976
Total Employees: 8　　*Marketing Staff:* 3　　*Sales Staff:* 18
Ownership: Hager & Werken Gmbh & Co. Kg
Quality System Registration Information: ISO9002
Produces/Sells CE-marked Devices: Y
Federal Procurement Eligibility: Small Business
Distribution: Manufacturer Through Distributor, Manufacturer Through Manufacturer Reps, OEM, Exclusive Distributor, Importer, Exporter
General Admin.: Mark Schneider/Chief Operating Officer, Vice President
　　　　　Michael Hager/President, Chief Executive Officer
Production: Les Gederos/Manager Operations & Services
Finance: Nancy Schneider/Controller
Purchasing: Sandra Hillard/Manager Merchandise

Accessories, Retractor, Dental	Dental And Oral
Anatomical Training Model	General
Articulators	Dental And Oral
Band, Matrix	Dental And Oral
Bib	General
Burr, Dental	Dental And Oral
Carrier, Amalgam, Operative	Dental And Oral
Carver, Wax, Dental	Dental And Oral
Chart, Anatomical Training	General
Clamp, Rubber Dam	Dental And Oral
Cup, Denture	Dental And Oral
Dental Laboratory Equipment	Dental And Oral
Evacuator, Oral Cavity	Dental And Oral
Eyeglasses, Safety	Ophthalmology
Filling, Instrument Plastic, Dental	Dental And Oral
Floss, Dental	Dental And Oral
Forceps, Rubber Dam Clamp	Dental And Oral
Frame, Rubber Dam	Dental And Oral
Holder, Needle	Gastroenterology/Urology
Holder, X-Ray Film	Dental And Oral
Mask, Surgical	Surgery
Mirror, Mouth	Dental And Oral
Mouthpiece, Saliva Ejector	Dental And Oral
Punch, Dental, Rubber Dam	Dental And Oral
Remover, Crown	Dental And Oral
Retainer, Matrix	Dental And Oral
Retractor, All Types	Dental And Oral
Scissors, Suture	Surgery
Toothbrush, Manual	Dental And Oral
Tray, Impression	Dental And Oral
Tray, Surgical Instrument	Surgery
Tube, Suction	General
Well, Amalgam	Dental And Oral

HAI LABORATORIES, INC.
781-862-9884
320 Massachusetts Ave., Lexington, MA 02420
FDA Number: 1226587
Fax: 781-860-7722
Ownership: Private
Produces/Sells CE-marked Devices: N

Caliper, Ophthalmic	Ophthalmology
Cannula, Ophthalmic	Ophthalmology
Cannula, Ophthalmic, Posterior Capsular Polishing, Polyvinyl Acetal	Ophthalmology
Forceps, Ophthalmic	Ophthalmology
Hook, Ophthalmic	Ophthalmology
Knife, Ophthalmic	Ophthalmology
Lamp, Slit, Biomicroscope, AC-Powered	Ophthalmology
Needle, Suture, Ophthalmic	Ophthalmology
Ophthalmoscope, AC-Powered	Ophthalmology
Scanner, Ultrasonic (Pulsed Echo)	Radiology
Scissors, Ophthalmic	Ophthalmology
Spatula, Ophthalmic	Ophthalmology
Speculum, Ophthalmic	Ophthalmology
Spoon, Ophthalmic	Ophthalmology
Transducer, Ultrasonic, Diagnostic	Radiology
Trephine, Manual, Ophthalmic (Corneal)	Ophthalmology

HAKO-MED USA, INC.
888-913-7900
905-C Makahiki Way, Honolulu, HI 96826
808-848-6111
FDA Number: 3004050897
Fax: 808-845-1013
E-mail: info@electromedicine.com
Web site: www.electromedicine.com/
Medical Products Sales Volume: $1,800,000
Annual Revenue: $10-$25 Million
Year Founded: 1991
Total Employees: 10
Ownership: Private
Quality System Registration Information: ISO9002
Produces/Sells CE-marked Devices: N
Federal Procurement Eligibility: Small Business

MANUFACTURER PROFILES

HAKO-MED USA, INC.
888-913-7900 *(cont'd)*

Distribution: Manufacturer Direct, Manufacturer Through Distributor, Manufacturer Through Manufacturer Reps, OEM, Importer, Exporter
General Admin.: Kai Hans Jurgens/President
John Mihok/Vice President
Stimulator, Nerve, Transcutaneous (Pain Relief, TENS) — Cns/Neurology

HAL-HEN COMPANY, INC.
800-242-5436
516-294-3200

180 Atlantic Avenue,
Garden City Park, NY 11040

FDA Number: 2428157 — Fax: 516-739-5248
E-mail: sales@halhen.com
Web site: www.halhenpro.com
Medical Products Sales Volume: $3,600,000
Annual Revenue: $5-$10 Million
Year Founded: 1946
Total Employees: 50   *Marketing Staff:* 2   *Sales Staff:* 4
Ownership: Private
Produces/Sells CE-marked Devices: Y
Federal Procurement Eligibility: Small Business, GSA Contract
Distribution: Manufacturer Direct, Manufacturer Through Distributor, Exporter
General Admin.: Eric Spar/President
Mktg./Adv.: Lee Frankel/Manager Marketing
Production: Mr. Joe Vespe/Director Operations
Mr. George Schiffner/Manager Materials
Finance: Harold Spar/Treasurer

Battery	General
Fork, Tuning, ENT	Ear/Nose/Throat
Masker, Tinnitus	Ear/Nose/Throat
Otoscope	Ear/Nose/Throat
Plug, Ear	Ear/Nose/Throat
Stethoscope, Electronic (Auscultoscope)	Cardiovascular
Unit, Therapy, Tinnitus	Ear/Nose/Throat

HALBAR NORTH, INC.
650-349-4700

#3 West 37th Avenue, San Mateo, CA 94403-4457

FDA Number: n/a — Fax: 650-349-0134
E-mail: halbar@halbarnorth.com
Web site: www.halbarnorth.com
Medical Products Sales Volume: $920,000
Year Founded: 1989
Total Employees: 4
Ownership: Private
Produces/Sells CE-marked Devices: N
Federal Procurement Eligibility: Small Business
Component, Electronic — General

HALDEX BARNES
See Concentric

HALE FIRE PUMP CO.
See Hale Products Inc.

HALE IMAGING SYSTEMS, INC.
800-321-4253
614-877-4357

5314 Mill St., P.O. Box 184, Orient, OH 43146-0184

FDA Number: n/a — Fax: 614-877-3293
E-mail: halemed@aol.com
Web site: www.halseimaging.com
Year Founded: 1961
Total Employees: 22
Ownership: Private
Quality System Registration Information: ISO9000
Produces/Sells CE-marked Devices: N
Federal Procurement Eligibility: Small Business, Female Owned
Distribution: Manufacturer Direct, Manufacturer Through Distributor
General Admin.: Bernice Hale Walsh/Chief Executive Officer
Mktg./Adv.: Daniel Walsh/Vice President Sales

Processor, Radiographic Film, Automatic	Radiology
Radiographic Unit, Diagnostic	Radiology
Storage Unit, X-Ray Film	Radiology

HALE MANUFACTURING CO., F.E.
800-USE-HALE
315-894-5490

120 Benson Place, PO Box 186,
Frankfort, NY 13340

FDA Number: n/a — Fax: 315-894-5046
E-mail: sales@halebookcases.com
Web site: www.halebookcases.com
Medical Products Sales Volume: $4,300,000
Annual Revenue: $5-$10 Million
Year Founded: 1907
Total Employees: 65   *Marketing Staff:* 1   *Sales Staff:* 20
Ownership: Private
Produces/Sells CE-marked Devices: N
Federal Procurement Eligibility: Small Business, GSA Contract
Distribution: Manufacturer Through Distributor
General Admin.: James Benson/President
Mktg./Adv.: Russell Blanchard/Vice President Marketing & Sales
Production: Jon Benson/Vice President Manufacturing

HALE MANUFACTURING CO., F.E.
800-USE-HALE *(cont'd)*

Furniture, General — General

HALE PRODUCTS INC.
800-220-4253
610-825-6300

700 Spring Mill Ave., Conshohocken, PA 19428

FDA Number: n/a — Fax: 610-825-6440
E-mail: TechnicalServices@idexcorp.com
Web site: www.haleproducts.com
Annual Revenue: $0-$1 Million
Year Founded: 1914
Ownership: IDEX CORPORATION
Produces/Sells CE-marked Devices: N
Distribution: Manufacturer Direct
Extrication Equipment — General

HALKEY MEDICAL
See Halkey-Roberts Corp.

HALKEY-ROBERTS CORP.
1.800.303.4384
1.727.471.4200

2700 Halkey-Roberts Place North,
St. Petersburg, FL 33716

FDA Number: 1000324175 — Fax: 1.727.578.0450
E-mail: sales@halkeyroberts.com
Web site: www.halkeyroberts.com
Year Founded: 1941
Total Employees: 200
Ownership: Atrion Medical Products, Inc.
Quality System Registration Information: ISO9001
Produces/Sells CE-marked Devices: N
Federal Procurement Eligibility: Small Business
Distribution: Manufacturer Direct
General Admin.: David Battat/President
Mktg./Adv.: Lewis Lecceardone/Vice President Marketing & Sales
Production: Gordon Hicks/Director Quality Assurance
Karen Prescott/Manager Materials
Jim Bowling/Vice President Operations
Research: John Lucius/Vice President Product Development
Finance: Jeff Strickland/Chief Financial Officer

Accessories, Catheter	Surgery
Check Valve, Retrograde Flow (In-Line)	General
Clamp, Tubing	General
Closure, Other	General
Fitting, Luer	General
Needle, Other	General
Pump, Inflator	General
Stopcock	General
Valve, Other	Chemistry

HALLMARK INSURANCE BROKERS LTD.
800-492-4070
416-492-4070

4 Lansing Square,, Suite 100,
Toronto, ONT M2J 5 Canada

FDA Number: n/a — Fax: 416-492-4321
E-mail: hib@hallmarkins.com
Web site: www.hallmarkins.com
Year Founded: 1948
Total Employees: 50
Ownership: Private
Produces/Sells CE-marked Devices: N

HALLMARK REFINING CORP. INC.
360-428-5880

1016 Dale Lane, Mount Vernon, WA 98273

FDA Number: n/a — Fax: 360-424-8118
E-mail: mark@hallmarkrefining.com
Web site: www.hallmarkrefining.com
Medical Products Sales Volume: $8,800,000
Annual Revenue: $5-$10 Million
Year Founded: 1972
Total Employees: 57   *Marketing Staff:* 6   *Sales Staff:* 4
Ownership: Private
Produces/Sells CE-marked Devices: N
Federal Procurement Eligibility: Small Business
Distribution: Manufacturer Direct
General Admin.: Anthony N. Senff/Chief Executive Officer
Mktg./Adv.: Mark Osborn/Director Sales
Silver Recovery Equipment — Radiology

HALO OPTICAL PRODUCTS, INC.
518-773-4256

9 Phair St., Gloversville, NY 12078

FDA Number: n/a
Annual Revenue: $0-$1 Million
Ownership: Private
Quality System Registration Information: ISO9000
Produces/Sells CE-marked Devices: Y
Federal Procurement Eligibility: Small Business
Distribution: Manufacturer Direct
Frame, Spectacle (Eyeglasses) — Ophthalmology

HALOSOURCE, INC.   425-881-6464
1631 220th Street SE, Bothell, WA 98021
FDA Number: n/a   *Fax:* 425-882-2476
E-mail: info@halosource.com
Web site: www.halosource.com
Year Founded: 2002
Ownership: Private
Produces/Sells CE-marked Devices: N

HALT MEDICAL INC.   925-634-7943
131 Sand Creek Road, Suite B, Brentwood, CA 94513
FDA Number: 3006443171
E-mail: info@haltmedical.com
Web site: http://www.haltmedical.com
Year Founded: 2004
Ownership: Private
Produces/Sells CE-marked Devices: N
General Admin.: Dr. Gordon Epstein/Chief Technology Officer
　　　　　　　Mr. Jeffrey Cohen/President, Chief Executive Officer
　　　　　　　Mr. Russell DeLonzor/President, Chief Operating Officer
Medical Admin.: Dr. Bruce Lee/Chief Medical Officer
　　　　　　　Ms. Laura Kemp/Vice President Clinical Affairs
Production: Mr. Robert Skidmore/Vice President Manufacturing & Operations
Research: Ms. Rick Spero/Vice President Research & Development
　Electrosurgical Unit, Cutting & Coagulation Device   Surgery

HALTONE ELECTRONICS LIMITED   800-263-4864
1221 Barton St.,   905-643-0000
Stoney Creek, ONT L8E 5 Canada
FDA Number: n/a   *Fax:* 450-643-0001
E-mail: tph@cogeco.net
Web site: http://www.haltone.ca
Year Founded: 1969
Total Employees: 10
Ownership: Private
Produces/Sells CE-marked Devices: N
Distribution: Manufacturer Direct, Exclusive Distributor, Importer

HAMAMATSU CORP.   800-524-0504
360 Foothill Road, Bridgewater, NJ 08807-2920   908-231-0960
FDA Number: n/a   *Fax:* 908-231-1218
E-mail: usa@hamamatsu.com
Web site: sales.hamamatsu.com
Medical Products Sales Volume: $740,000
Annual Revenue: $50-$100 Million
Year Founded: 1969
Total Employees: 200
Ownership: HAMAMATSU PHOTONICS K.K. - JAPAN
Quality System Registration Information: ISO9000
Produces/Sells CE-marked Devices: Y
Federal Procurement Eligibility: Small Business
Distribution: Manufacturer Direct, Exclusive Distributor, Importer
General Admin.: David Leinwand/General Manager
　　　　　　　Ralph Eno/President
　　　　　　　Carol Simola/Vice President Human Resources & Personnel
Mktg./Adv.: George Marshall/Assistant Vice President Marketing & Sales
　　　　　　　Craig Walling/Director Market Research
　　　　　　　Robert Wisner/Vice President Marketing & Sales
Production: Brenda Battista/Customer Service Representative
　　　　　　　Yuji Shinoda/Vice President Quality Assurance
　Component, Electronic   General
　Sorter, Cell (Separator)   Pathology

HAMAMATSU PHOTONIC SYSTEMS   800-524-0504
360 Foothill Road, Bridgewater, NJ 08807-0910   908-231-1116
FDA Number: n/a   *Fax:* 908-231-0852
E-mail: usa@hamamatsu.com
Web site: www.hps-systems.com
Annual Revenue: $10-$25 Million
Year Founded: 1969
Total Employees: 28   *Marketing Staff:* 3   *Sales Staff:* 8
Ownership: HAMAMATSU PHOTONICS K.K. - JAPAN
Quality System Registration Information: ISO9001
Produces/Sells CE-marked Devices: N
Distribution: Manufacturer Through Manufacturer Reps, Service Direct
General Admin.: Ralph Eno/President
　　　　　　　Akira Hiruma/Vice President, General Manager
　Monitor, Oxygen   General

HAMILTON ASSOCIATES
See Air Techniques International

HAMILTON BELL COMPANY   800-526-0864
30 Craig Rd., Montvale, NJ 07645-1709   201-391-4100
FDA Number: n/a   *Fax:* 201-391-5994
E-mail: hamiltonbell@mindspring.com
Web site: www.hamiltonbell.com
Medical Products Sales Volume: $3,500,000

HAMILTON BELL COMPANY   800-526-0864 *(cont'd)*
Annual Revenue: $1-$5 Million
Total Employees: 15
Ownership: Private
Produces/Sells CE-marked Devices: N
Federal Procurement Eligibility: Small Business
Distribution: Manufacturer Through Distributor
General Admin.: James SanVito/President, Chief Executive Officer
　Centrifuge, Tabletop   Pathology

HAMILTON CASTER & MFG. CO.   888-699-7164
1637 Dixie Hwy., Hamilton, OH 45011-4087   513-863-3300
FDA Number: 7000817   *Fax:* 513-863-5508
E-mail: info@hamiltoncaster.com
Web site: www.hamiltoncaster.com
Annual Revenue: $10-$25 Million
Year Founded: 1907
Total Employees: 80   *Marketing Staff:* 4
Ownership: Private
Produces/Sells CE-marked Devices: N
Federal Procurement Eligibility: Small Business, GSA Contract
Distribution: Manufacturer Direct, Manufacturer Through Distributor
General Admin.: Steven J. Lippert/Executive Vice President
　　　　　　　David R. Lippert/President
Mktg./Adv.: Mark Lippert/Manager Advertising
　Bumper Guard, Corner   General
　Cart, Multipurpose   General
　Casters, Hospital Equipment   General

HAMILTON COMPANY   800-648-5950
4970 Energy Way, Reno, NV 89520-0012   775-858-3000
FDA Number: 2915796   *Fax:* 775-856-7259
E-mail: sales@hamiltoncompany.com
Web site: www.hamiltoncompany.com
Year Founded: 1953
Total Employees: 250   *Marketing Staff:* 18   *Sales Staff:* 15
Ownership: Private
Quality System Registration Information: ISO9001
Produces/Sells CE-marked Devices: Y
Federal Procurement Eligibility: Small Business, GSA Contract
Distribution: Manufacturer Direct, Manufacturer Through Distributor, OEM
General Admin.: Will Frazzi/Director Personnel
　　　　　　　Steven Hamilton/President
Mktg./Adv.: Ron Lewis/Director Marketing
　　　　　　　Gary Englehart/Manager National Sales
Production: Bob West/Director Manufacturing
　　　　　　　Wayne McAuliffe/Manager Quality Assurance
Research: Tom Peterson/Director Research & Development
Finance: Leonard Smith/Director Finance
　Cleaner, Needle   General
　Cleaner, Syringe   General
　Column, Chromatography   Chemistry
　Diluter   Chemistry
　Dispenser, Fluid   General
　Fitting, Luer   General
　Injector, Syringe   General
　Needle, Blunt   General
　Pipette, Diluting   Hematology
　Pipette, Micro   Chemistry
　Pipetter   Hematology
　Pipetting And Diluting System, Automated   Chemistry
　Sampler, Air   General
　Sampler, Gas   Chemistry
　Syringe, Laboratory   Chemistry
　Syringe, Other   General
　System, Robot   General

HAMILTON INDUSTRIES INC.
See Thermo Scientific Hamilton

HAMILTON MEDICAL, INC.   800-426-6331
4990 Energy Way, Reno, NV 89502   775-858-3200
FDA Number: 2937708   *Fax:* 775-856-5621
E-mail: info@hamiltonmedical.net
Web site: www.hamilton-medical.com
Annual Revenue: $5-$10 Million
Year Founded: 1983
Ownership: Private
Quality System Registration Information: ISO9001
Produces/Sells CE-marked Devices: Y
Federal Procurement Eligibility: Small Business
Distribution: Service Direct, Exclusive Distributor, Importer, Exporter
General Admin.: Bob Hamilton/President
　Compressor, Air, Portable   Anesthesiology
　Continuous Positive Airway Pressure Unit (CPAP, CPPB)   Anesthesiology
　Ventilator, Continuous (Respirator)   Anesthesiology
　Ventilator, Other   Anesthesiology
　Ventilator, Volume (Critical Care)   Anesthesiology

HAMILTON MFG. CO.
888-871-5600
128 Berkeley Cir., Summerville, SC 29483-7302   **843-871-5600**
FDA Number: 1063488   *Fax:* 843-871-2007
E-mail: hammed@hotmail.com
Medical Products Sales Volume: $1,900,000
Year Founded: 1996
Total Employees: 30
Ownership: Private
Produces/Sells CE-marked Devices: N
Federal Procurement Eligibility: Small Business, GSA Contract, VA Contract
Distribution: Manufacturer Through Manufacturer Reps
Table, Mechanical   Physical Med
Table, Physical Medicine, Powered   Physical Med

HAMILTON THORNE BIOSCIENCES
800-323-0503
100 Cummings Center-suite 465e,   **978-921-2050**
Beverly, MA 01915
FDA Number: 1221433   *Fax:* 978-921-0250
E-mail: info@hamiltonthorne.com
Web site: www.hamiltonthorne.com
Ownership: Private
Produces/Sells CE-marked Devices: N
General Admin.: Mr. David Wolf/President, Chief Executive Officer
Mktg./Adv.: Mr. Anthony McCook/Vice President Sales
Research: Mr. Diarmaid Douglas-Hamilton/Senior Vice President Research & Development
        Mr. Thomas Kenny/Vice President Engineering
Finance: Mr. Michael Burns/Chief Financial Officer, Vice President Finance
Counter, Cell Or Particle, Automated   Hematology
System, Laser Assisted Hatching   Obstetrics/Gynecology

HAMMER-PLANE INC.
800-398-3017
2245 Homewood Avenue, Simi Valley, CA 93063   **805-583-1268**
FDA Number: 2028338
E-mail: info@hammerplane.com
Ownership: Private
Produces/Sells CE-marked Devices: N
Fixation Device, Tracheal Tube   Anesthesiology
Support, Breathing Tube   Anesthesiology

HAMMILL INTERNATIONAL
800-228-2129
PO Box 4968, Orange, CA 92613   **714-637-0344**
FDA Number: n/a   *Fax:* 714-777-0907
E-mail: plogs@juno.com
Web site: www.plogs.com
Year Founded: 1985
Ownership: Private
Produces/Sells CE-marked Devices: N
Federal Procurement Eligibility: Small Business, Female Owned
Distribution: Exclusive Distributor
Shoe, Operating Room   Surgery

HAMPTON MEDICAL DEVICES
636-225-3100
3550 Crowndun Dr., St. Louis, MO 63129
FDA Number: n/a   *Fax:* 636-225-3103
E-mail: HamptonMed@aol.com
Web site: www.hamptondevices.com
Ownership: Private
Produces/Sells CE-marked Devices: N
Trephine, Manual, Ophthalmic (Corneal)   Ophthalmology
Tube, Tympanostomy   Ear/Nose/Throat

HAMPTON RESEARCH
800-452-3899
34 Journey, Aliso Viejo, CA 92656-3317   **949-425-1321**
FDA Number: n/a   *Fax:* 949-425-1611
E-mail: info@hrmail.com
Web site: http://hamptonresearch.com
Annual Revenue: $0-$1 Million
Ownership: Private
Produces/Sells CE-marked Devices: Y
Federal Procurement Eligibility: Small Business
Distribution: Manufacturer Direct
Coverslip, Microscope Slide   Pathology
Equipment, Laboratory, Gen. Purpose (Specific Medical Use)   Chemistry

HAMPTON RESEARCH & ENGINEERING, INC.
800-800-6369
2726 N. Oklahoma, Oklahoma City, OK 73105   **405-232-5103**
FDA Number: n/a   *Fax:* 405-232-5104
E-mail: hamptondental.com@gmail.com
Web site: www.hamptondental.com
Year Founded: 1966
Ownership: Private
Produces/Sells CE-marked Devices: N
Federal Procurement Eligibility: Small Business
Distribution: Manufacturer Direct
General Admin.: William Harris/President
Electrosurgical Unit, Dental   Dental And Oral

HAMPTON RESEARCH & ENGINEERING, INC.
800-800-6369
(cont'd)
Operative Dental Treatment Unit   Dental And Oral

HANCOCK/JAFFE LABORATORIES
949-261-2900
2807 Mcgaw Ave., Irvine, CA 92614
FDA Number: 2031002
Graft, Vascular, Biological   Cardiovascular

HAND BIOMECHANICS LAB, INC.
800-522-5778
77 Scripps Drive, Suite 104,   **916-923-5073**
Sacramento, CA 95825
FDA Number: 2919128   *Fax:* 916-920-2215
E-mail: wristjack@handbiolab.com
Web site: www.handbiolab.com
Medical Products Sales Volume: $1,300,000
Year Founded: 1979
Total Employees: 16
Ownership: Private
Federal Procurement Eligibility: Small Business
Distribution: Manufacturer Direct, Manufacturer Through Manufacturer Reps
General Admin.: John Agee/President
Mktg./Adv.: Cindy Kerfoot/Director Marketing
Production: Timothy Stallings/Director Manufacturing
Finance: Kimberly Sutton/Accountant
Bit, Drill   Orthopedics
Immobilizer, Wrist/Hand   Orthopedics

HAND INNOVATIONS, LLC.
800-800-8188
6303 Blue Lagoon Drive, Suite 100,   **305-412-8010**
Miami, FL 33126
FDA Number: 3003506715
E-mail: raisingexpectations@dpyus.jnj.com
Web site: www.handinnovations.com
Year Founded: 2001
Ownership: Johnson & Johnson
Stock Symbol: JNJ
Traded On: NYSE
Produces/Sells CE-marked Devices: N
Mktg./Adv.: Claudia Arenas/Marketing Coordinator
Appliance, Fix., Nail/Blade/Plate Comb., Multiple Component   Orthopedics
Bolt, Nut, Washer   Orthopedics
Pin, Fixation, Smooth   Orthopedics
Plate, Fixation, Bone   Orthopedics
Rod, Fixation, Intramedullary   Orthopedics
Screw, Fixation, Bone   Orthopedics
Surgical Instrument, Manual (General Use)   Surgery

HANDI-CAP AIDS COMPANY
800-689-0511
730 West Hefner Road,   **405-842-0511**
Oklahoma City, OK 73114
FDA Number: n/a   *Fax:* 405-840-9170
E-mail: Pat@HandicapAids.net
Web site: www.handicapaids.net
Medical Products Sales Volume: $1,240,000
Year Founded: 1978
Total Employees: 9   *Marketing Staff:* 1   *Sales Staff:* 3
Ownership: Private
Produces/Sells CE-marked Devices: N
Federal Procurement Eligibility: Small Business
General Admin.: Mike Bradshaw/President
Mktg./Adv.: Pat Bradshaw/Sales Representative
Lift, Wheelchair   General
Utensil, Handicapped Aid   Physical Med

HANDI-MOVE/T.F.HERCEG
See Surehands Lift & Care Systems

HANDI-RAMP
800-876-7267
510 North Avenue, Libertyville, IL 60048   **847-680-7700**
FDA Number: 7000534   *Fax:* 847-816-8866
E-mail: info@handiramp.com
Web site: www.handiramp.com
Annual Revenue: $1-$5 Million
Year Founded: 1958
Total Employees: 20   *Marketing Staff:* 2   *Sales Staff:* 5
Ownership: Private
Produces/Sells CE-marked Devices: N
Federal Procurement Eligibility: Small Business
Distribution: Manufacturer Direct, Manufacturer Through Manufacturer Reps
General Admin.: Thomas R. Disch/Chief Executive Officer
Mktg./Adv.: Scott Longueil/Manager Sales
Lift, Stair Climbing   General
Lift, Wheelchair   General
Rail, Wall Side   General
Ramp, Wheelchair   General
Restraint, Wheelchair   General

HANDICAP UNLIMITED, INC.
5640 Summer Avenue, Suite 3,
Memphis, TN 38134
888-371-0095
901-373-0095
FDA Number: n/a
E-mail: monte@handicapunlimited.com
Web site: www.handicapunlimited.com
Fax: 901-388-0901
Medical Products Sales Volume: $810,000
Year Founded: 1983
Total Employees: 12   *Marketing Staff:* 1   *Sales Staff:* 3
Ownership: Private
Stock Symbol: 1500000
Produces/Sells CE-marked Devices: N
Federal Procurement Eligibility: Small Business

Lift, Wheelchair	General
Ramp, Wheelchair	General
Scooter (Motorized 3-Wheeled Vehicle)	Physical Med
Walker, Mechanical	Physical Med
Wheelchair, Manual	Physical Med
Wheelchair, Powered	Physical Med

HANDICAPS, INC.
4335 S. Santa Fe Drive, Englewood, CO 80110
800-782-4335
303-781-2062
FDA Number: n/a
E-mail: forest77@earthlink.net
Web site: www.handicapsinc.com
Fax: 303-761-6811
Annual Revenue: $0-$1 Million
Year Founded: 1959
Total Employees: 8   *Marketing Staff:* 1
Ownership: Private
Produces/Sells CE-marked Devices: N
Federal Procurement Eligibility: Small Business, Female Owned
Distribution: Manufacturer Direct, Manufacturer Through Manufacturer Reps, OEM, Exporter
General Admin.: Geraldine O'Dell/Owner
     Geraldine O'Dell/President
     Ernestine Kittle/Vice President
Mktg./Adv.: Jeanenne Phillips/Manager Marketing & Sales

Control, Foot Driving, Automobile, Mechanical	Physical Med
Control, Hand Driving, Automobile, Mechanical	Physical Med
Lift, Wheelchair	General
Ramp, Wheelchair	General

HANDLER MANUFACTURING CO.
612 N. Avenue E., Westfield, NJ 07090-0520
800-274-2635
908-233-7796
FDA Number: n/a
E-mail: info@handlermfg.com
Web site: www.handlermfg.com
Fax: 908-233-7340
Medical Products Sales Volume: $3,000,000
Annual Revenue: $1-$5 Million
Year Founded: 1920
Total Employees: 42   *Marketing Staff:* 1   *Sales Staff:* 4
Ownership: Private
Quality System Registration Information: ISO9001
Produces/Sells CE-marked Devices: Y
Federal Procurement Eligibility: Small Business
Distribution: Manufacturer Through Distributor
General Admin.: William A. Lehman/Chairman, Chief Executive Officer
     Lorraine Lehman/Secretary Treasurer
Mktg./Adv.: Rick LaDuca/Manager International & National Sales
     Rick LaDuca/Vice President Marketing & Sales
Production: Al Valero/Manager Materials
     Alberto Valero/Vice President Production

Cabinet, Dental	Dental And Oral
Dental Laboratory Equipment	Dental And Oral
Grinder, Tissue	Pathology
Regulator, Vacuum	General
Wheel, Polishing Agent	Dental And Oral

HANDPIECE PARTS & PRODUCTS, INC.
707 West Angus Ave., Orange, CA 92868
800-368-3684
714-997-4331
FDA Number: 2031715
E-mail: michelle@handpieceparts.com
Web site: www.handpieceparts.com
Fax: 714-997-5440
Ownership: Private
Produces/Sells CE-marked Devices: N

Handpiece, Air-Powered, Dental	Dental And Oral

HANDYLAB
5230 South State Rd., Ann Arbor, MI 48108
734-663-4719
FDA Number: n/a
E-mail: info@handylab.com
Web site: www.handylab.com
Fax: 734-663-7437
Ownership: Private
Produces/Sells CE-marked Devices: N
General Admin.: Kalyan Handique/Chief Technology Officer
     Jeffrey Williams/President, Chief Executive Officer
Mktg./Adv.: Kerry Wilson/Director Product Management

HANDYLAB
734-663-4719 *(cont'd)*
   Mark Powelson/Vice President Marketing & Sales
Production: Ted Springer/Vice President Manufacturing
Research: Sundaresh Brahmasandra/Vice President Product Development
Finance: Kimberlee Kochan/Controller

Assay, Nucleic Acid Amplification, Growth Identification, Mycobacterium Tuberculosis	Microbiology
Concentrator, Clinical Sample	Chemistry
Reagent, General Purpose	Pathology

HANGER NATIONAL FABRICATION FACILITY
1119 West Geneva Dr., Tempe, AZ 85282
912-691-2030
FDA Number: 2032381
Ownership: HANGER ORTHOPEDIC GROUP, INC.
Produces/Sells CE-marked Devices: N

Orthosis, Cranial	Cns/Neurology

HANGER ORTHOPEDIC GROUP, INC.
10910 Domain Drive, Suite 300, Austin, TX 78758
877-442-6437
301-986-0701
FDA Number: n/a
E-mail: info@hanger.com
Web site: www.hanger.com
Fax: 301-986-0702
Annual Revenue: $500 Million-$1 Billion
Year Founded: 1861
Total Employees: 3364
Ownership: Public
Stock Symbol: HGR
Traded On: NYSE
Quality System Registration Information: ISO9001
Produces/Sells CE-marked Devices: N
Distribution: Manufacturer Direct
General Admin.: George E. McHenry/Chief Financial Officer, Executive Vice President
     Mr. Walt Meffert/Chief Information Officer
     Thomas F. Kirk/President, Chief Executive Officer
     Richmond L. Taylor/President, Chief Operating Officer

Custom Prosthesis	Orthopedics
Prosthesis, Elbow, Total	Orthopedics
Prosthesis, Knee, Total	Orthopedics
Support, Foot	Orthopedics

HANGER SABOLICH
See Hanger Orthopedic Group, Inc.

HANKISON INTERNATIONAL
1000 Philadelphia St., Canonsburg, PA 15317
724-745-1555
FDA Number: n/a
Web site: www.hankisonintl.com
Fax: 724-745-6040
Annual Revenue: $25-$50 Million
Year Founded: 1948
Ownership: Private
Quality System Registration Information: ISO9001
Produces/Sells CE-marked Devices: N
Federal Procurement Eligibility: Small Business
Distribution: Manufacturer Through Distributor

Filter, Air	General

HANNA INSTRUMENTS CANADA INC.
3156 Industriel Blvd.,
Laval, QUE H7L-4 Canada
800-842-6629
450-629-1444
FDA Number: n/a
E-mail: info@hannacan.com
Web site: www.hannacan.com
Fax: 450-629-3335
Year Founded: 1978
Total Employees: 25
Ownership: Private
Produces/Sells CE-marked Devices: N
Distribution: Manufacturer Direct, Exclusive Distributor

HANNAH'S MIRACLE SHOE, INC.
11237 S. Aubrey Meadow Cir., South Jordan, UT 84095-2231
801-329-9802
FDA Number: 3003604718
Ownership: Private
Produces/Sells CE-marked Devices: N

Wheelchair, Manual	Physical Med

HANOVIA SPECIALTY LIGHTING LLC
6 Evans Street, Fairfield, NJ 07004
800-229-3666
973-651-5510
FDA Number: n/a
E-mail: sales@hanovia-uv.com
Web site: www.hanovia-uv.com/
Fax: 973-651-5550
Medical Products Sales Volume: $3,300,000
Annual Revenue: $10-$25 Million
Year Founded: 1905
Total Employees: 50   *Marketing Staff:* 3   *Sales Staff:* 10
Ownership: Private
Produces/Sells CE-marked Devices: N
Federal Procurement Eligibility: Small Business
Distribution: Manufacturer Direct, OEM, Exporter

HANOVIA SPECIALTY LIGHTING LLC   800-229-3666 (cont'd)

General Admin.: Len Perre/Chief Executive Officer
Mktg./Adv.: Robert Majka/Manager Product Development
Production: Tom Gaven/Vice President Manufacturing

Lamp, Other	General
Lamp, Ultraviolet, Germicidal	General
Lamp, Ultraviolet, Physical Medicine	Physical Med
Sterilizer, Ultraviolet	General
Sterilizer/Compactor	General

HANS RUDOLPH, INC.   913-422-7788

8325 Cole Parkway, Shawnee, KS 66227
FDA Number: 1922553   *Fax:* 913-422-3337
E-mail: hri@rudolphkc.com
Web site: www.rudolphkc.com
Ownership: Private
Produces/Sells CE-marked Devices: N

Bag, Reservoir (Blood)	Anesthesiology
Calibrator, Gas, Volume	Anesthesiology
Clip, Nose	Anesthesiology
Computer, Pulmonary Function Data	Anesthesiology
Mask, Gas, Anesthesia	Anesthesiology
Mask, Oxygen, Aerosol Administration	Anesthesiology
Mask, Oxygen, Non-Rebreathing	Anesthesiology
Mouthpiece, Breathing	Anesthesiology
Plethysmograph, Pressure (Body)	Anesthesiology
Pneumotachometer	Anesthesiology
Support, Breathing Tube	Anesthesiology
Tubing, Flexible, Medical Gas, Low-Pressure	Anesthesiology
Valve, Non-Rebreathing	Anesthesiology
Ventilator, Non-Continuous (Respirator)	Anesthesiology

HANSCO TECHNOLOGIES, INC.   201-391-0700

17 Philips Pkwy., Montvale, NJ 07645-1810
FDA Number: 7000100   *Fax:* 201-391-4261
E-mail: sales@hanscotech.com
Web site: www.hanscotech.com
Annual Revenue: $1-$5 Million
Total Employees: 15
Ownership: Private
Produces/Sells CE-marked Devices: N
Federal Procurement Eligibility: Small Business
Distribution: Exclusive Distributor, Importer
General Admin.: Hans U. Berlinger/President
Mktg./Adv.: Guy Metz/Vice President Sales

Production Equipment	General

HANSEN DENTAL LAB   952-541-9622

6700 Squibb Road, Suite 208, Mission, KS 66202
FDA Number: 3001160287
Ownership: Private
Produces/Sells CE-marked Devices: N

Mouthguard	Dental And Oral

HANSEN MEDICAL, INC.   888-404-5801

800 East Middlefield Road,   650-404-5800
Mountain View, CA 94043
FDA Number: 3006026430   *Fax:* 650-404-5901
E-mail: info@hansenmedical.com
Web site: www.hansenmedical.com
Year Founded: 2002
Total Employees: 96
Ownership: Public
Stock Symbol: HNSN
Traded On: NASDAQ
Produces/Sells CE-marked Devices: N

Catheter, Steerable	Cardiovascular
Control System, Catheter, Steerable	Cardiovascular
Dilator, Vessel	Gastroenterology/Urology
Trocar, Cardiovascular	Cardiovascular

HANSEN OPHTHALMIC DEVELOPMENT LAB   319-338-1285

745 Avalon Pl., Coralville, IA 52241
FDA Number: 1935505

Electrode, Corneal	Ophthalmology
Fixation Device, AC-Powered, Ophthalmic	Ophthalmology
Probe, Gastrointestinal	Gastroenterology/Urology
Shell, Scleral	Ophthalmology
Tape, Measuring, Ruler And Caliper	Surgery

HANSEN OPHTHALMIC DEVELOPMENT LAB., INC.   319-338-1285

2590 Auburn Hills Ln. N.E., Solon, IA 52333
FDA Number: 1935505   *Fax:* 319-338-7970
E-mail: hansenlb@inav.net
Web site: www.hansenlab.com
Annual Revenue: $0-$1 Million
Total Employees: 2   *Marketing Staff:* 2   *Sales Staff:* 2
Ownership: Private

HANSEN OPHTHALMIC DEVELOPMENT   319-338-1285 (cont'd)

Produces/Sells CE-marked Devices: N
Federal Procurement Eligibility: Small Business
Distribution: Manufacturer Direct, Exclusive Distributor, Exporter
General Admin.: Jeff Hansen/Office Manager
       Gary Hansen/President
Mktg./Adv.: Gary Hansen/Vice President Marketing & Sales
Production: Gary Hansen/Vice President Manufacturing
Research: Gary Hansen/Vice President Research & Development

Electrode, Corneal	Ophthalmology
Fixation Device, AC-Powered, Ophthalmic	Ophthalmology
Probe	Orthopedics
Prosthesis, Evisceration	Ophthalmology
Shell, Scleral	Ophthalmology
Tape, Measuring, Ruler And Caliper	Surgery

HANSON MEDICAL, INC.   800-771-2215

825 Riverside Avenue, Building #2,   360-297-1997
Paso Robles, CA 93446
FDA Number: 2031444   *Fax:* 360-297-1998
E-mail: info@hansonmedical.com
Web site: www.hansonmedical.com
Medical Products Sales Volume: $2,500,000
Annual Revenue: $1-$5 Million
Year Founded: 1997
Total Employees: 9   *Marketing Staff:* 3   *Sales Staff:* 3
Ownership: Private
Quality System Registration Information: ISO9001
Produces/Sells CE-marked Devices: N
Federal Procurement Eligibility: Small Business
Distribution: Manufacturer Direct, Importer, Exporter

Bandage, Liquid	Surgery
Binder, Abdominal	General
Drain, Suction, Closed	Surgery
Elastomer, Silicone (Scar Management)	Surgery
Elastomer, Silicone Block	Surgery
General Use Surgical Scissors	Surgery
Implant, Muscle, Pectoralis	Surgery
Instrument, Manual, General Surgical	Surgery
Malar Implant	Surgery
Prosthesis, Chin, Internal	Surgery
Prosthesis, Nose, Internal	Surgery

HANTEL TECHNOLOGIES   510-487-1561

721 Sandoval Way, Hayward, CA 94544
FDA Number: 2954912   *Fax:* 510-487-1569
E-mail: info@hanteltech.com
Web site: www.hanteltech.com
Ownership: Private
Produces/Sells CE-marked Devices: N
General Admin.: Ms. Mary Pascual-Gallup/Chief Executive Officer
Production: Ms. Marina Weinstock/Vice President Operations
Research: Mr. David Gallup/Vice President Engineering
Finance: Mr. Sunil Mehra/Controller

Catheter, Flow Directed	Cardiovascular
Electrode, Electrosurgical, Return (Ground, Dispersive)	Surgery

HAPAD, INC.   800-544-2723

5301 Enterprise Blvd.,   412-835-2220
Bethel Park, PA 15102
FDA Number: 600087   *Fax:* 412-835-6460
E-mail: hapadinc@aol.com
Web site: www.hapad.com
Medical Products Sales Volume: $1,625,350
Annual Revenue: $1-$5 Million
Year Founded: 1963
Total Employees: 14   *Marketing Staff:* 1   *Sales Staff:* 1
Ownership: Private
Produces/Sells CE-marked Devices: N
Federal Procurement Eligibility: Small Business
Distribution: Manufacturer Direct, Manufacturer Through Distributor, Exporter
General Admin.: John P. Hauser/President, Chief Executive Officer
Mktg./Adv.: Sandra J. Kardos/Director Marketing
Production: Robert Diesing/Manager Materials

Cushion, Foot	Orthopedics

HARBOR METALCRAFTERS, INC./MEDPRO   631-242-2428

208 Fehr Way, Bay Shore, NY 11706
FDA Number: 2437738
Ownership: Private
Produces/Sells CE-marked Devices: N

Stretcher, Wheeled (Mobile)	General

HARC MERCANTILE LTD.   800-445-9968

1111 West Centre Avenue, Portage, MI 49024   269-324-1615
FDA Number: n/a   *Fax:* 269-324-2387
E-mail: info@harc.com
Web site: www.harcmercantile.com

HARC MERCANTILE LTD.   800-445-9968 (cont'd)
Annual Revenue: $1-$5 Million
Year Founded: 1960
Total Employees: 15   *Marketing Staff:* 1   *Sales Staff:* 3
Ownership: HAC OF AMERICA, INC.
Produces/Sells CE-marked Devices: N
Federal Procurement Eligibility: Small Business
Distribution: Service Direct
General Admin.: Ronald Slager/President, Chief Executive Officer
    Joann Newsted/Vice President
Mktg./Adv.: Roberta Taylor/Director National Accounts
    Joyce L. Thorson/Manager International & National Sales
    Roberta Taylor/Manager National Sales

Battery, Hearing-Aid	Ear/Nose/Throat
Hearing-Aid	Ear/Nose/Throat
Plug, Ear	Ear/Nose/Throat
Telephone, Handicapped Use	Physical Med

HARCO CO., LTD.   905-890-1220
5915 Coopers Avenue, Mississauga, ONT L4Z 1R9 Canada
FDA Number: n/a   *Fax:* 905-890-7039
Web site: www.harcoco.com
Total Employees: 25   *Marketing Staff:* 3   *Sales Staff:* 4
Ownership: Private
Produces/Sells CE-marked Devices: N
Distribution: Exclusive Distributor

HARD MANUFACTURING CO.   800-873-4273
230 Grider St., Buffalo, NY 14215-3797   **716-893-1800**
FDA Number: 1317178   *Fax:* 716-896-2579
Web site: www.hardmfg.com
Annual Revenue: $5-$10 Million
Total Employees: 75
Ownership: Private
Quality System Registration Information: ISO9000
Produces/Sells CE-marked Devices: Y
Federal Procurement Eligibility: Small Business
Distribution: Manufacturer Through Manufacturer Reps
General Admin.: William Godin/President
Mktg./Adv.: Mary Bias/Manager Sales

Bed, Electric	General
Bed, Manual	General
Bed, Pediatric (Crib)	General
Bedrail	General
Cabinet, Bedside	General
Chair, Other	General
Furniture, Patient Room	General
Mattress, Bed	General
Table, Overbed	General

HARDING MEDICAL SUPPLIES LTD.   1-877-457-8600
1158 Grand Lake Road,   **902-567-1144**
Sydney, NS B1M 1 Canada
FDA Number: n/a   *Fax:* 902-567-1150
E-mail: harding.cb@hardingmedical.com
Web site: http://www.hardingmedical.com
Year Founded: 1987
Total Employees: 14
Ownership: Private
Produces/Sells CE-marked Devices: N
Distribution: Service Direct

HARDMAN
See Elementis Specialties

HARDWOOD PRODUCTS COMPANY LLC
See Puritan Medical Products Company Llc

HARDY DIAGNOSTICS   800-226-2222
1430 West McCoy Lane, Santa Maria, CA 93455   **805-346-2766**
FDA Number: 2022807   *Fax:* 805-346-2760
E-mail: sales@hardydiagnostics.com
Web site: www.hardydiagnostics.com
Medical Products Sales Volume: $18,000,000
Annual Revenue: $10-$25 Million
Year Founded: 1980
Total Employees: 100   *Marketing Staff:* 2   *Sales Staff:* 10
Ownership: Private
Produces/Sells CE-marked Devices: N
Federal Procurement Eligibility: Small Business, GSA Contract, VA Contract
Distribution: Manufacturer Direct
General Admin.: Joe Altavilla/Chief Operating Officer, Chief Financial Officer
    Jay Hardy/President
Mktg./Adv.: Christopher Catani/Director Marketing
    Joe Plummer/Market Manager
Production: Melissa Traylor/Director Quality Assurance
    Melissa Traylor/Director Regulatory Affairs
    Rick Treinen/Manager Materials
    Len Kovalski/Product Manager

HARDY DIAGNOSTICS   800-226-2222 (cont'd)
Purchasing: Eric Hardy/Purchasing Agent

Analyzer, Parasite Concentration	Microbiology
Culture Media, Antimicrobial Susceptibility Test	Microbiology
Culture Media, For Isolation Of Pathogenic Neisseria	Microbiology
Culture Media, General Nutrient Broth	Microbiology
Culture Media, Multiple Biochemical Test	Microbiology
Culture Media, Non-Propagating Transport	Microbiology
Culture Media, Selective And Differential	Microbiology
Culture Media, Supplements	Microbiology
Disc, Strip And Reagent, Microorganism Differentiation	Microbiology

HARDY MEDIA
See Hardy Diagnostics

HARLECO
See Emd Chemicals Inc.

HARLOFF COMPANY, INC.   800-433-4064
650 Ford Street,   **719-637-0300**
Colorado Springs, CO 80915
FDA Number: 3001109397   *Fax:* 719-597-8273
E-mail: customerservice@harloff.com
Web site: www.harloff.com
Year Founded: 1951
Total Employees: 75   *Marketing Staff:* 1   *Sales Staff:* 46
Ownership: Winsford Corporation
Produces/Sells CE-marked Devices: N
Federal Procurement Eligibility: Small Business, GSA Contract
Distribution: Manufacturer Through Distributor, OEM, Exporter
General Admin.: John Sweetland/President
Mktg./Adv.: Joel Charles/Manager International & National Sales

Cart, Anesthetist's	Anesthesiology
Cart, Emergency, Cardiopulmonary Resuscitation (Crash)	Anesthesiology
Cart, Instrument	Surgery
Cart, Medicine	General
Cart, Monitor	General
Cart, Multipurpose	General
Cart, Orthopedic Supply (Cast)	Orthopedics
Cart, Supply, Operating Room	Surgery

HARMAC INDUSTRIES INC.
See Harmac Medical Products, Inc.

HARMAC MEDICAL PRODUCTS, INC.   716-897-4500
2201 Bailey Avenue, Buffalo, NY 14211-1797
FDA Number: 1317547   *Fax:* 716-897-0016
E-mail: info@harmac.com
Web site: www.harmac.com
Medical Products Sales Volume: $25,900,000
Total Employees: 70   *Marketing Staff:* 2   *Sales Staff:* 5
Ownership: Private
Quality System Registration Information: ISO9001
Produces/Sells CE-marked Devices: Y
Federal Procurement Eligibility: Small Business
Distribution: Manufacturer Direct, OEM, Service Direct, Exporter
Production: James Wagner/Manager Engineering

Bag, Blood	Hematology
Bag, Drainage, Nasogastric	General
Bag, Enteral Feeding	General
Bag, Plastic	General
Contract Assembly	General
Contract Manufacturing	General
Contract Manufacturing, Product, Disposable	General
Contract Packaging	General
Kit, Administration, Intravenous	General
Kit, Intravenous Extension Tubing	General
Molding, Custom	General
Molding, Injection	General
Needle, Other	General
Pump, Infusion	General
Pump, Infusion, Ambulatory	General
Service, Engineering/Design	General
Set, Administration, Intravenous, Needle-Free	General

HARMON
See Brandrud Furniture, Inc.

HARMONIZER   330-677-0771
448 Silver Oaks Drive Unit 5, Kent, OH 44240
FDA Number: 1059123
Ownership: Private
Produces/Sells CE-marked Devices: N

Exerciser, Non-Measuring	Physical Med

HAROD ENTERPRISES
See H.E. Inc. (Harod Enterprises)

HARRICK SCIENTIFIC PRODUCTS, INC.

FDA Number: n/a
Annual Revenue: $1-$5 Million
General Admin.: Milan Milosevic/President, CTO

HARRICK SCIENTIFIC PRODUCTS, INC. *(cont'd)*

Mktg./Adv.: Laurie Miller/Senior Vice President Marketing & Business Development

Cell, Spectrophotometer	Chemistry
Spectrophotometer, Infrared	Chemistry
Spectrophotometer, Ultraviolet	Chemistry
Washer/Sterilizer	General

HARRIS CALORIFIC DIVISION

See Harris Products Group

HARRIS ENVIRONMENTAL SYSTEMS, INC.   888-771-4200

11 Connector Rd., Andover, MA 01810-5993   **978-470-8600**
FDA Number: 7000168   *Fax:* 978-475-7903
E-mail: smith@harris-env.com
Web site: www.harris-env.com
Medical Products Sales Volume: $9,000,000
Annual Revenue: $10-$25 Million
Total Employees: 75   *Sales Staff:* 4
Ownership: Private
Produces/Sells CE-marked Devices: N
Federal Procurement Eligibility: Small Business
Distribution: Manufacturer Direct
General Admin.: P. W. Hunt/President
Mktg./Adv.: Robert Smith/Manager National Sales
Production: Alex Murray/Vice President Manufacturing

Chamber, Constant Temperature (Environmental)	Microbiology
Cleanroom Equipment	General
Dehumidifier	General
Freezer, Blood Storage	Hematology
Refrigerator, Laboratory	General

HARRIS LAKE, INC.

See Matrx By Midmark

HARRIS MANUFACTURING

See Kendro Laboratory Products

HARRIS PRODUCTS GROUP   800-241-0804

2345 Murphy Blvd., Gainesville, GA 30504-6001   **770-536-8801**
FDA Number: 7000167   *Fax:* 770-535-0544
Medical Products Sales Volume: $50,000,000
Annual Revenue: $25-$50 Million
Total Employees: 220   *Marketing Staff:* 2   *Sales Staff:* 20
Ownership: Lincoln Electric Co.
Quality System Registration Information: ISO9002
Produces/Sells CE-marked Devices: N
Distribution: Manufacturer Through Distributor
General Admin.: David Nangle/Chief Executive Officer
Mktg./Adv.: Eugene Moon/Manager Advertising
Production: Dave Mueller/Vice President Operations

Calorimeter	Chemistry
Flowmeter, Back-Pressure Compensated, Thorpe Tube	Anesthesiology
Regulator, Pressure, Gas Cylinder	Anesthesiology

HARRIS RESEARCH & DEVELOPMENT, LLC.   800-802-2228

528 East 800 North, Orem, UT 84097-4146
FDA Number: 3004452319
Ownership: Private
Produces/Sells CE-marked Devices: N

Hearing Aid, Air Conduction, Transcutaneous System	Ear/Nose/Throat

HARRISON & CARDILLO DENTAL LAB   800-525-5913

725 Powell Street, Renton, WA 98057   **425-271-4421**
FDA Number: 3004160976   *Fax:* 425-917-5715
E-mail: vthomas@dentalservices.net
Web site: www.dentalservicesgroup.com
Ownership: Private
Produces/Sells CE-marked Devices: N

Base, Denture, Relining, Repairing, Rebasing, Resin	Dental And Oral
Crown, Preformed	Dental And Oral
Device, Anti-Snoring	Ear/Nose/Throat
Device, Repositioning, Jaw	Dental And Oral
Mouthguard	Dental And Oral

HARROP INDUSTRIES LABORATORY INSTRUMENTS GROUP

See Harrop Industries, Inc.

HARROP INDUSTRIES, INC.   614-231-3621

3470 E. Fifth Ave., Columbus, OH 43219-1797
FDA Number: n/a   *Fax:* 614-235-3699
E-mail: info@harropusa.com
Web site: www.harropusa.com
Annual Revenue: $0-$1 Million
Year Founded: 1919
Ownership: Private
Produces/Sells CE-marked Devices: N
Federal Procurement Eligibility: Small Business
Distribution: Manufacturer Direct, Exporter

Thermogravimetric Analysis Equipment	Chemistry

HARRY J. BOSWORTH COMPANY   800-323-4352

7227 N. Hamlin Avenue, Skokie, IL 60076-3999   **847-679-3400**
FDA Number: 1410638   *Fax:* 847-679-2080
E-mail: hjbinfo@bosworth.com
Web site: www.bosworth.com
Medical Products Sales Volume: $4,100,000
Annual Revenue: $1-$5 Million
Year Founded: 1912
Total Employees: 40   *Marketing Staff:* 3   *Sales Staff:* 11
Ownership: Private
Quality System Registration Information: ISO9000; ISO9001; ISO9002
Produces/Sells CE-marked Devices: N
Federal Procurement Eligibility: Small Business, Female Owned
Distribution: Manufacturer Through Distributor
General Admin.: Martin C. Herbst/General Manager
        Mildred M. Goldstein/President
        Herbert L. Pozen/Vice President

Adhesive, Dental	Dental And Oral
Adhesive, Denture, OTC	Dental And Oral
Adhesive, Prosthesis, External	Surgery
Agent, Polishing, Abrasive, Oral Cavity	Dental And Oral
Base, Denture, Relining, Repairing, Rebasing, Resin	Dental And Oral
Cement, Dental	Dental And Oral
Cleaner, Denture	Dental And Oral
Cleaner, Ultrasonic, Medical Instrument	General
Crown And Bridge, Temporary, Resin	Dental And Oral
Crown, Preformed	Dental And Oral
Dental Laboratory Equipment	Dental And Oral
Dispenser, Mercury And/Or Alloy	Dental And Oral
Handle, Instrument, Dental	Dental And Oral
Kit, Gingival Retraction	Dental And Oral
Kit, Plaque Disclosing	Dental And Oral
Lamp, Ultraviolet (Spectrum A)	General
Material, Acrylic, Dental	Dental And Oral
Material, Dental Filling	Dental And Oral
Material, Impression	Dental And Oral
Material, Impression Tray, Resin	Dental And Oral
Material, Investment	Dental And Oral
Material, Tooth Shade, Resin	Dental And Oral
Mercury	Dental And Oral
Mouthpiece, Saliva Ejector	Dental And Oral
Paper, Articulation	Dental And Oral
Protector, Silicate	Dental And Oral
Syringe, Restorative And Impression Material	Dental And Oral
Tray, Fluoride	Dental And Oral
Tray, Impression	Dental And Oral
Varnish	Dental And Oral
Wax, Dental	Dental And Oral

HART ENTERPRISES, INC.   616-887-0400

400 Applejack Ct., Sparta, MI 49345
FDA Number: 1828424   *Fax:* 616-887-5400
E-mail: sales@hartneedles.com
Web site: www.hartneedles.com
Medical Products Sales Volume: $5,300,000
Year Founded: 1976
Total Employees: 78   *Marketing Staff:* 1   *Sales Staff:* 6
Ownership: Private
Produces/Sells CE-marked Devices: N
Federal Procurement Eligibility: Small Business
Distribution: OEM
General Admin.: Robert Striebel/Executive Vice President
        Alan Taylor/President
Mktg./Adv.: Larry Swan/Director Marketing & Sales
Production: Robert Striebel/Director Quality Assurance
Research: Ken Chettleburgh/Vice President Engineering

Component, Metal, Other	General
Component, Plastic	General
Contract Manufacturing	General
General Medical Device	General
Introducer, Catheter	Cardiovascular
Molding, Custom	General
Needle, Aspiration And Injection, Disposable	Surgery
Needle, Biopsy, Cardiovascular	Cardiovascular
Needle, Conduction, Anesthesia (W/Wo Introducer)	Anesthesiology
Needle, Other	General
Needle, Spinal, Short-Term	General

HART SPECIALTIES, INC.   800-221-6966

5000 New Horizons Blvd., Amityville, NY 11701   **631-226-5600**
FDA Number: n/a   *Fax:* 631-226-5884
Web site: www.newyorkeye.net
Year Founded: 1978
Ownership: Private
Produces/Sells CE-marked Devices: N
Federal Procurement Eligibility: Small Business
Distribution: Manufacturer Direct
General Admin.: Arthur Jankolovits/President
Mktg./Adv.: Shannon Johnson/Vice President Product Services

HART SPECIALTIES, INC. 800-221-6966 *(cont'd)*
Eyeglasses	Ophthalmology
Sunglasses (Including Photosensitive)	Ophthalmology

HARTFORD WALKING SYSTEMS INC. 315-735-1659
22 Pearl St., New Hartford, NY 13413
FDA Number: 3006152534
Ankle/Foot, External Limb Component	Physical Med
Walker, Mechanical	Physical Med

HARTMANN USA, INC. 812-332-3703
4265 West Vernal Pike, Bloomington, IN 47404
FDA Number: 3004360577 *Fax:* 812-333-3270
E-mail: customerservice@whitestonecorp.com
Web site: www.whitestonecorp.com
Medical Products Sales Volume: $90,000,000
Year Founded: 1949
Ownership: Private
Produces/Sells CE-marked Devices: N
Distribution: Manufacturer Through Distributor
Device, Incontinence, Fecal	Gastroenterology/Urology
Diaper, Adult	General
Diaper, Pediatric	General
Garment, Protective, For Incontinence	Gastroenterology/Urology
Mitt/Washcloth, Patient	General
Pad, Incontinence (Underpad)	General
Pant, Incontinence	General

HARTMANN-CONCO INC. 800-243-2294
481 Lakeshore Pkwy., Rock Hill, SC 29730-4205 803-325-7600
FDA Number: 1218946 *Fax:* 803-325-7606
E-mail: info@hartmann-conco.com
Web site: www.hartmann-conco.com
Medical Products Sales Volume: $34,000,000
Year Founded: 2001
Total Employees: 87 *Marketing Staff:* 4 *Sales Staff:* 9
Ownership: Private
Produces/Sells CE-marked Devices: Y
Federal Procurement Eligibility: Small Business, GSA Contract, VA Contract
Distribution: Manufacturer Through Distributor
General Admin.: Jacques Lemmetti/President, Chief Executive Officer
Mktg./Adv.: Ernie Goulet/Director Marketing
Mike Weiner/Director Sales
Production: Bob Trahan/Director Quality Assurance
Kevin Colangelo/Supervisor Customer Service
Bandage, Adhesive	Surgery
Bandage, Cast	Physical Med
Bandage, Compression	General
Bandage, Elastic	General
Bandage, Gauze	General
Bandage, Other	General
Bandage, Tubular	General
Dressing, Other	General
Dressing, Wound and Burn, Hydrogel	Surgery
Splint, Hand, And Component	Physical Med
Splint, Molded, Aluminum	Orthopedics
Splint, Nasal	Ear/Nose/Throat
Tape, Adhesive	General
Tape, Cotton	General

HARTWELL MEDICAL CORP. 800-633-5900
6352 Corte del Abeto, Suite J, 760-438-5500
Carlsbad, CA 92011
FDA Number: 2028459 *Fax:* 760-438-2783
E-mail: info@hartwellmedical.com
Web site: www.HartwellMedical.com
Medical Products Sales Volume: $950,000
Annual Revenue: $1-$5 Million
Year Founded: 1989
Total Employees: 6
Ownership: Private
Produces/Sells CE-marked Devices: Y
Federal Procurement Eligibility: Small Business, Female Owned, GSA Contract
Distribution: Manufacturer Through Distributor, Exclusive Distributor, Exporter
General Admin.: Gary R. Williams/President, Chief Executive Officer
Bag, Medical, Physician	General
Laryngoscope, Rigid	Anesthesiology
Mattress, Immobilization	General
Splint, Vacuum	Orthopedics
Stretcher, Orthopedic	Orthopedics
Ventilator, Emergency, Powered (Resuscitator)	Anesthesiology

HARTZELL & SON, G. 800-950-2206
2372 Stanwell Circle, Concord, CA 94520-4807 925-798-2206
FDA Number: 2910921 *Fax:* 925-798-2053
E-mail: sales@ghartzellandson.com
Web site: www.ghartzellandson.com
Medical Products Sales Volume: $2,100,000
Year Founded: 1935

HARTZELL & SON, G. 800-950-2206 *(cont'd)*
Total Employees: 30
Ownership: Private
Produces/Sells CE-marked Devices: Y
Federal Procurement Eligibility: Small Business
Distribution: Manufacturer Through Distributor
General Admin.: Andrew McIver/Chief Executive Officer
Kerry McIver/Vice President, General Manager
Mktg./Adv.: Rich Schmitt/Manager International & National Sales
Explorer, Operative	Dental And Oral
Filling, Instrument Plastic, Dental	Dental And Oral
Hemostat	Orthopedics
Holder, Needle	Gastroenterology/Urology
Scaler, Periodontic	Dental And Oral
Scissors, Surgical Tissue, Dental (Oral)	Dental And Oral

HARVARD APPARATUS CANADA 514-335-0792
6010 Vanden Abeele St., St. Laurent, QUE H4S 1R9 Canada
FDA Number: n/a *Fax:* 514-335-3482
E-mail: sales@harvardapparatus.ca
Medical Products Sales Volume: $1,500,000
Total Employees: 5 *Marketing Staff:* 1 *Sales Staff:* 5
Ownership: Private
Produces/Sells CE-marked Devices: Y
Federal Procurement Eligibility: Small Business
Distribution: Exclusive Distributor

HARVARD APPARATUS, INC. 800-272-2775
84 October Hill Road, Holliston, MA 01746 508-893-8999
FDA Number: 7000171 *Fax:* 508-429-5732
E-mail: bioscience@harvardapparatus.com
Web site: www.harvardapparatus.com
Medical Products Sales Volume: $67,430,000
Year Founded: 1901
Total Employees: 50 *Marketing Staff:* 4 *Sales Staff:* 8
Ownership: Ismatec Sa Labortechnik/Analytik
Stock Symbol: HBIO
Traded On: NASDAQ
Produces/Sells CE-marked Devices: Y
Federal Procurement Eligibility: Small Business, GSA Contract
Distribution: Manufacturer Direct, Manufacturer Through Distributor, Manufacturer Through Manufacturer Reps, Service Direct, Exporter
Mktg./Adv.: Ms. Mara Potter/Manager Marketing Communications
Mr. Ron Sostek/Vice President Sales
Column, Liquid Chromatography	Toxicology
Dialyzer	Chemistry
Electrode, Other	General
Forceps	Orthopedics
Pipette Tip	Chemistry
Pump, Infusion	General
Pump, Infusion, Laboratory	Chemistry
Pump, Infusion, Syringe	General
Pump, Withdrawal/Infusion	Cardiovascular
Syringe, Laboratory	Chemistry
Transducer, Blood Pressure, Extravascular	Cardiovascular

HARVARD BIOSCIENCE INC. 800-272-2775
84 October Hill Road, Holliston, MA 01746 508-893-8999
FDA Number: n/a *Fax:* 508-429-5732
E-mail: info@harvardbioscience.com
Web site: http://www.harvardbioscience.com
Ownership: Public
Stock Symbol: HBIO
Traded On: NASDAQ
Produces/Sells CE-marked Devices: N
General Admin.: Mr. Chane Graziano/Chief Executive Officer
Ms. Susan Luscinski/Chief Operating Officer
Mr. David Green/President
Finance: Mr. Thomas McNaughton/Chief Financial Officer
Analyzer, Chemistry, Micro	Chemistry

HARVEST TECHNOLOGIES, CORP. 508-732-7500
40 Grissom Rd, Suite 100, Plymouth, MA 02360
FDA Number: 1225520 *Fax:* 508-732-0400
E-mail: info@harvesttech.com
Web site: www.harvesttech.com
Ownership: Private
Produces/Sells CE-marked Devices: N
Autotransfusion Unit (Blood)	Anesthesiology
Bone Grafting Material, Dental, With Biologic Component	Dental And Oral
Centrifuge, Cell Washing	Hematology
Supplies, Blood Bank	Hematology
Syringe, Piston	General

HARVEY PRECISION INSTRUMENTS 707-793-2600
217 Fairway Road, Cape Haze, FL 33947
FDA Number: 3004632098
Ownership: Private
Produces/Sells CE-marked Devices: N

HARVEY PRECISION INSTRUMENTS

707-793-2600 *(cont'd)*

Cannula, Ophthalmic	Ophthalmology
Forceps, Ophthalmic	Ophthalmology
Hook, Ophthalmic	Ophthalmology
Needle, Suture, Ophthalmic	Ophthalmology
Scissors, Ophthalmic	Ophthalmology
Speculum, Ophthalmic	Ophthalmology

HARVEY, R.J. INSTRUMENT CORP.

201-664-1380

123 Patterson St., Hillsdale, NJ 07642
FDA Number: 2250031 — Fax: 201-664-5578
E-mail: rjhinst@aol.com
Web site: www.rjharveyinst.com
Annual Revenue: $0-$1 Million
Total Employees: 10
Ownership: Private
Produces/Sells CE-marked Devices: Y
Federal Procurement Eligibility: Small Business
Distribution: Manufacturer Direct
General Admin.: Robert Maines/President
Angelo D'Imperio/Vice President

Analyzer, Combination Chemistry/Hematology/Electrolyte	Chemistry
Colorimetric Method, Triglycerides	Chemistry
Electrode, Ion Specific, Sodium	Chemistry
Enzymatic Esterase-Oxidase, Cholesterol	Chemistry
Fluid, Red Cell Diluting	Hematology
Reagent, Glucose (Test System)	Chemistry

HASBRO, INC.

401-431-8697

1027 Newport Ave., Pawtucket, RI 02862-1059
FDA Number: 1211011
Web site: www.hasbro.com
Ownership: Private
Produces/Sells CE-marked Devices: N

Sunglasses (Including Photosensitive)	Ophthalmology
Syringe, Irrigating	General
Toothbrush, Manual	Dental And Oral
Vibrator, Therapeutic	Physical Med

HASKEL INTERNATIONAL, INC.

818-843-4000

100 E. Graham Place, Burbank, CA 91502-2027
FDA Number: n/a — Fax: 818-841-4291
E-mail: sales@haskel.com
Web site: www.haskel.com
Medical Products Sales Volume: $36,600,000
Annual Revenue: $50-$100 Million
Year Founded: 1946
Total Employees: 335 — Marketing Staff: 3 — Sales Staff: 15
Ownership: Private
Quality System Registration Information: ISO9001
Produces/Sells CE-marked Devices: N
Federal Procurement Eligibility: Small Business
Distribution: Manufacturer Direct, Manufacturer Through Distributor, Manufacturer Through Manufacturer Reps, OEM, Exporter
General Admin.: R. Needham/Chief Executive Officer
Mark Petty/President
Pam Karno/Vice President Human Resources
Mktg./Adv.: G. Volk/Director National Accounts
Cindy Zawaski/Manager Advertising
P. Duffy/Manager International & National Sales
Peter Duffy/Vice President Marketing & Sales
Production: Lavon McVay/Director Quality Assurance

Regulator, Oxygen, Mechanical	General

HASKEL MFG, INC.

See Haskel International, Inc.

HATCH CORPORATION

800-347-1200
909-923-7300

42374 Avenida Alvarado, Suite A,
Temecula, CA 92590
FDA Number: 3005471875 — Fax: 909-923-7400
E-mail: info@hatch-corp.com
Web site: www.hatch-corp.com
Medical Products Sales Volume: $1,000,000
Annual Revenue: $5-$10 Million
Year Founded: 1967
Total Employees: 15 — Marketing Staff: 4 — Sales Staff: 4
Ownership: Private
Produces/Sells CE-marked Devices: Y
Federal Procurement Eligibility: Small Business
Distribution: Manufacturer Through Distributor
General Admin.: Bob Hatch/President
Mktg./Adv.: Rich Wilde/Director National Sales
Everett Smith/Vice President Sales
Research: Bill Hatch/Vice President Research & Development

Accessories, Wheelchair	Physical Med
Glove, Other	General

HATCH GLOVES & ACCESSORIES

See Hatch Corporation

HAUN SPECIALTY GASES, INC.

315-463-5241

5921 Court Street Road, Syracuse, NY 13206
FDA Number: 1314971 — Fax: 315-463-5784
E-mail: lnash@thehaunedge.com
Web site: www.thehaunedge.com
Ownership: Private
Produces/Sells CE-marked Devices: N

Gas, Calibrated (Specified Concentration)	Anesthesiology

HAUSMANN INDUSTRIES, INC.

888-428-7626
201-767-0255

130 Union St., Northvale, NJ 07647-2207
FDA Number: 2242467 — Fax: 201-767-1369
E-mail: info@hausmann.com
Web site: www.hausmann.com
Annual Revenue: $10-$25 Million
Total Employees: 75 — Marketing Staff: 1 — Sales Staff: 6
Ownership: Private
Produces/Sells CE-marked Devices: N
Federal Procurement Eligibility: Small Business
Distribution: Manufacturer Through Distributor
General Admin.: David Hausmann/Chief Executive Officer
Werner R. Hausmann/General Manager
Mktg./Adv.: George Batchelor/Director Marketing & Sales

Bars, Parallel, Exercise	Physical Med
Bars, Parallel, Walking	Physical Med
Board, Arm	Anesthesiology
Board, Quadriceps (Exerciser)	Physical Med
Cabinet, Bedside	General
Cabinet, Instrument	General
Cart, Multipurpose	General
Chair/Table, Medical	General
Exercise Stair	Physical Med
Exerciser, Arm	Physical Med
Exerciser, Chest	Physical Med
Exerciser, Leg And Ankle	Physical Med
Exerciser, Non-Measuring	Physical Med
Exerciser, Shoulder	Physical Med
Footstool, Non-Conductive	General
Furniture, General	General
Furniture, Patient Room	General
Mirror, Posture	Physical Med
Plinth	Physical Med
Stirrup	Gastroenterology/Urology
Stool, Exercise	Physical Med
Table, Examination/Treatment	General
Table, Other	General
Table, Physical Medicine, Powered	Physical Med
Table, Physical Therapy	Physical Med

HAUSSER SCIENTIFIC

215-675-7769

935 Horsham Rd., Suite C, Horsham, PA 19044
FDA Number: 2518612 — Fax: 215-672-9602
E-mail: admin@hausserscientific.com
Web site: www.hausserscientific.com
Annual Revenue: $0-$1 Million
Ownership: Private
Produces/Sells CE-marked Devices: N
Federal Procurement Eligibility: Small Business
Distribution: Manufacturer Direct, Exporter

Coverslip, Microscope Slide	Pathology
Hemocytometer	Hematology

HAVEL'S INC.

800-638-4770
513-271-2117

3726 Lonsdale, Cincinnati, OH 45227-3637
FDA Number: 1526069 — Fax: 800-628-3458
E-mail: customercare@havels.com
Web site: www.havels.com
Annual Revenue: $5-$10 Million
Year Founded: 1981
Total Employees: 16
Ownership: Private
Produces/Sells CE-marked Devices: Y
Federal Procurement Eligibility: Small Business
Distribution: Manufacturer Direct, Manufacturer Through Distributor, Exclusive Distributor, Importer, Exporter
General Admin.: Barbara Rauen/Chief Executive Officer
Mktg./Adv.: Patrick Carrothers/Vice President Marketing

Biopsy Instrument	Gastroenterology/Urology
Blade, Scalpel	Surgery
Blade, Surgical, Saw, General & Plastic Surgery	Surgery
Burr, Dental	Dental And Oral
Dermatome	Surgery
Device, Biopsy, Percutaneous	Surgery
Guide, Surgical, Needle	Surgery
Kit, Anesthesia, Conduction	Anesthesiology
Kit, Anesthesia, Epidural	Anesthesiology
Kit, Lumbar Puncture	Cns/Neurology

HAVEL'S INC.   800-638-4770 *(cont'd)*

Knife, Cataract	Ophthalmology
Knife, ENT	Ear/Nose/Throat
Knife, Keratome	Ophthalmology
Knife, Meniscus	Surgery
Knife, Microtome	Pathology
Knife, Myringotomy	Ear/Nose/Throat
Knife, Ophthalmic	Ophthalmology
Knife, Orthopedic	Orthopedics
Needle, Aspiration And Injection, Disposable	Surgery
Needle, Aspiration And Injection, Reusable	Surgery
Needle, Biopsy, Mammary	Obstetrics/Gynecology
Needle, Bone Marrow	Surgery
Needle, Conduction, Anesthesia (W/Wo Introducer)	Anesthesiology
Needle, Radiographic	Radiology
Needle, Suture, Reusable	Surgery
Scalpel, One-Piece (Knife)	Surgery
Scissors, Suture	Surgery
Suture, Absorbable	Surgery
Suture, Absorbable, Synthetic	Surgery
Suture, Non-Absorbable, Silk	Surgery

HAWKEN INDUSTRIES   216-831-6782
26650 Renaissance Pkwy.,, Bedford Heights, OH 44128
FDA Number: 3003542113
Ownership: Private
Produces/Sells CE-marked Devices: N

HAWORTH, INC.   800-426-8562
One Haworth Center, Holland, MI 49423-9570   **616-393-3000**
FDA Number: n/a   *Fax:* 616-393-1570
E-mail: al.lanning@haworth.com
Web site: www.haworth-furn.com
Medical Products Sales Volume: $1,390,000,000
Annual Revenue: More than $100 Million
Year Founded: 1948
Total Employees: 3000   *Marketing Staff:* 2   *Sales Staff:* 2
Ownership: Private
Quality System Registration Information: ISO9001
Produces/Sells CE-marked Devices: N
Federal Procurement Eligibility: Small Business, GSA Contract
Distribution: Manufacturer Through Manufacturer Reps
General Admin.: Richard G. Haworth/Chairman
    Gerald B. Johanneson/President, Chief Operating Officer
Mktg./Adv.: Al Lanning/Vice President Sales
Production: Craig Speck/Vice President Manufacturing

Furniture, General	General

HAWS CORPORATION   775-359-4712
1455 Kleppe Ln., Sparks, NV 89431
FDA Number: n/a   *Fax:* 775-359-7424
E-mail: info@hawsco.com
Web site: www.hawsco.com
Medical Products Sales Volume: $27,000,000
Annual Revenue: $25-$50 Million
Total Employees: 120   *Marketing Staff:* 3   *Sales Staff:* 8
Ownership: Private
Quality System Registration Information: ISO9001
Produces/Sells CE-marked Devices: N
Federal Procurement Eligibility: Small Business, GSA Contract
Distribution: Manufacturer Through Distributor, Exporter
General Admin.: Michael H. Traynor/Chief Executive Officer
    Sallie Haws/President
Mktg./Adv.: John Guhin/Manager International Sales
    Ray Doane/Vice President Marketing & Sales
Production: Tom White/Vice President Manufacturing

Fountain, Eye Wash	Chemistry

HAYDAY IRRIT-EASERS   416-434-1400
883 Derry Crt, Oshawa L1J 6X8 Canada
FDA Number: 8020441

Table, Physical Therapy	Physical Med

HAYES MANUFACTURING SERVICES, INC.   1AŽ408AŽ730AŽ50
1178 Sonora Court, Sunnyvale, CA 94086
FDA Number: 3006785390   *Fax:* 1AŽ408AŽ730AŽ58
E-mail: mail@hayesms.com
Ownership: Private
Produces/Sells CE-marked Devices: N

Film, X-Ray, Special Purpose	Radiology

HAYES MEDICAL, INC.   800-240-0500
1115 Windfield Way, Suite 100,   **916-355-7100**
El Dorado Hills, CA 95762
FDA Number: 2952369   *Fax:* 916-355-7190
E-mail: info@hayesmed.com
Web site: www.hayesmed.com
Medical Products Sales Volume: $4,000,000
Annual Revenue: $5-$10 Million

HAYES MEDICAL, INC.   800-240-0500 *(cont'd)*
Year Founded: 1992
Total Employees: 48   *Marketing Staff:* 3   *Sales Staff:* 3
Ownership: Private
Quality System Registration Information: ISO9001
Produces/Sells CE-marked Devices: Y
Federal Procurement Eligibility: Small Business
Distribution: Manufacturer Through Distributor, Manufacturer Through Manufacturer Reps
General Admin.: Colleen Gray/Chief Executive Officer
Mktg./Adv.: Curt Wiedenhoefer/Vice President Marketing

Contract R&D, Equipment	General
Equipment/Service, Quality Control	General
Prosthesis, Hip, Semi-Constrained Acetabular	Orthopedics
Prosthesis, Hip, Semi-Constrained, Metal/Polymer	Orthopedics
Prosthesis, Knee, Total	Orthopedics
Service, Engineering/Design	General

HAYWOOD VOCATIONAL OPPORTUNITIES
See HVO

HAZELTON LABORATORIES CORP.
See Covance Laboratories ,Inc

HAZELTON SYSTEMS INC.
See Covance Laboratories ,Inc

HAZLETON WASHINGTON
See Covance Laboratories ,Inc

HBR HEALTHCARE COMPANY, INC.   765-966-1400
2211 Williamsburg Pike, Chester, IN 47374
FDA Number: 3002350580
Ownership: Private
Produces/Sells CE-marked Devices: N

Bed, Electric	General

HCI   800-783-8105
113 Commerce Blvd, Cincinnati, OH 45140   **513-271-8100**
FDA Number: n/a   *Fax:* 513-271-8108
E-mail: sales@hci-tv.com
Web site: www.hcic.com
Medical Products Sales Volume: $15,000,000
Annual Revenue: $10-$25 Million
Ownership: Private
Produces/Sells CE-marked Devices: N
Federal Procurement Eligibility: Small Business
Distribution: Manufacturer Direct, Service Direct

Television, Patient Room	General

HCMI, INC.   773-588-2444
2146 East Pythian St., Springfield, MO 65802
FDA Number: 1450503
Ownership: Private
Produces/Sells CE-marked Devices: N

Curette, Biopsy, Bronchoscope (Non-Rigid)	Anesthesiology
Generator, Diagnostic X-Ray, High Voltage, Single Phase	Radiology
Table, Physical Medicine, Powered	Physical Med
Table, Physical Therapy	Physical Med

HCS
See Health Care Software, Inc. (Hcs)

HDR POWER SYSTEMS INC.
See Ametek Solidstate Controls

HDS SPECIALTY VEHICLES
See Hds Specialty Vehicles

HEADWALL PHOTONICS, INC.   978-353-4100
601 River St., Fitchburg, MA 01420
FDA Number: n/a   *Fax:* 978-348-1864
E-mail: information@headwallphotonics.com
Web site: www.HeadwallPhotonics.com
Medical Products Sales Volume: $3,200,000
Annual Revenue: $10-$25 Million
Year Founded: 2003
Total Employees: 32
Ownership: Private
Traded On: NYSE
Quality System Registration Information: ISO9001
Produces/Sells CE-marked Devices: N
Federal Procurement Eligibility: Small Business, GSA Contract
Distribution: Manufacturer Direct, OEM
General Admin.: David Bannon/Chief Executive Officer
    Larry Barstow/President, Chief Operating Officer
Mktg./Adv.: Mr. Jay Zakrzewski/Director Business Development
Production: Mr. Richard Driver/Director Engineering

Mass Spectrometer, Clinical Use	Toxicology
Spectrograph, Mass	Chemistry
Spectrophotometer, U.V./Visible	Chemistry

Medical Product Subsidiaries (Listed Separately)

HEADWALL PHOTONICS, INC.   978-353-4100 *(cont'd)*
Invitrogen Dynal

HEALER PRODUCTS, LLC   914-663-6300
427 Commerce Lane, Unit 1, West Berlin, NJ 08091
FDA Number: 3000209486
Ownership: Private
Produces/Sells CE-marked Devices: N

Applicator, Tipped, Absorbent, Non-Sterile	General
Bandage, Adhesive	Surgery
Bandage, Compression	General
Bandage, Elastic	General
Container, Sharpes	General
Cup, Eye	Ophthalmology
Depressor, Tongue	General
Dressing, Other	General
Dressing, Wound and Burn, Hydrogel	Surgery
Dressing, Wound and Burn, Occlusive	Surgery
Finger Cot	General
Forceps	Orthopedics
Gauze/sponge, Nonresorbable For External Use	Surgery
Glove, Patient Examination	General
Glove, Patient Examination, Latex	General
Kit, First Aid	Surgery
Kit, Snake Bite, Suction	General
Mask, Oxygen, Aerosol Administration	Anesthesiology
Monitor, Blood Pressure, Indirect, Semi-Automatic	Cardiovascular
Pack, Hot Or Cold, Disposable	Physical Med
Pad, Eye	Ophthalmology
Protector, Hearing (Insert)	Ear/Nose/Throat
Scalpel, One-Piece (Knife)	Surgery
Scissors, Disposable	General
Sheet, Burn	General
Splint, Extermity, Non-inflatable, External, Non-sterile	Surgery
Stethoscope, Manual	Cardiovascular
Strip, Adhesive	Surgery
Temperature Strip, Forehead, Liquid Crystal	General
Thermometer, Mercury	General
Tourniquet, Non-Pneumatic, Surgical	Surgery

HEALING ENVIRONMENTS   800-233-7433
INTERNATIONAL, INC.
4623 NE 110th Street, Seattle, WA 98125
FDA Number: n/a
E-mail: info@bedscapes.com
Web site: www.bedscapes.com
Ownership: Private
Produces/Sells CE-marked Devices: N
Federal Procurement Eligibility: Small Business
General Admin.: Yosaif August/President, Chief Executive Officer

Screen, Bedside	General

HEALING SOLUTIONS, LLC.   636-376-8100
2112 Penta Dr, High Ridge, MO 63049
FDA Number: 3005632311

Bed, Flotation Therapy, Powered	Physical Med

HEALTH & EDUCATION SERVICES CORP.
See Novel Products, Inc.

HEALTH & HYGIENE, INC.   239-403-9919
4406 Exchange Ave., #127, Naples, FL 34104
FDA Number: 3005787322
Ownership: Private
Produces/Sells CE-marked Devices: N

Irrigator, Oral	Dental And Oral

HEALTH & RADIOLOGICAL SEMINARS, INC.   800-969-4774
550 Highland St., Suite 100, Frederick, MD 21701
FDA Number: n/a   *Fax:* 724-871-5568
E-mail: info@hrsiseminars.com
Web site: www.hrsiseminars.com
Annual Revenue: $0-$1 Million
Ownership: Private
Produces/Sells CE-marked Devices: N
Federal Procurement Eligibility: Small Business, Female Owned
Distribution: Service Direct

Training Aid, Arrhythmia Recognition	Cardiovascular

HEALTH CARE EXPORTS, INC.   800-847-0173
5701 N.W. 74 Ave., Miami, FL 33166   305-594-0026
FDA Number: n/a   *Fax:* 305-594-0768
E-mail: info@ahce.com
Web site: www.ahce.com
Medical Products Sales Volume: $2,000,000
Annual Revenue: $1-$5 Million
Year Founded: 1979
Total Employees: 12   *Marketing Staff:* 3   *Sales Staff:* 7
Ownership: Private
Produces/Sells CE-marked Devices: N

HEALTH CARE EXPORTS, INC.   800-847-0173 *(cont'd)*
Federal Procurement Eligibility: Small Business, Minority Owned
Distribution: Manufacturer Through Distributor, Exporter
General Admin.: Mr. Peter Ehrlich/President, Chief Executive Officer
     Angela Ehrlich/Vice President Human Resources
Mktg./Adv.: Mr. Alan Ehrlich/Vice President Marketing & Sales

Camera, Gamma (Nuclear/Scintillation)	Radiology
Densitometer, Radiographic	Radiology
Radiographic Unit, Diagnostic, Mammographic	Radiology
Radiographic Unit, Diagnostic, Mobile, Explosion-Safe	Radiology
Radiographic/Fluoroscopic Unit, Mobile C-Arm	Radiology
Recorder, Long-Term, ECG, Portable (Holter Monitor)	Cardiovascular
Scanner, Ultrasonic, Abdominal	Radiology
Scanner, Ultrasonic, General Purpose	Radiology
Scanner, Ultrasonic, Obstetrical/Gynecological	Obstetrics/Gynecology
Scanner, Ultrasonic, Small Parts	Radiology
Scanner, Ultrasonic, Vascular	Radiology
Service, Used Equipment	General

HEALTH CARE FURNISHINGS, INC.   800-648-5744
63 Pebble Beach Drive, Little Rock, AR 72212   501-221-2033
FDA Number: n/a   *Fax:* 501-221-2783
E-mail: design@healthcarefurnishings.com
Web site: www.heathcarefurnishings.com
Medical Products Sales Volume: $330,000
Annual Revenue: $0-$1 Million
Year Founded: 1988
Total Employees: 3
Ownership: Private
Produces/Sells CE-marked Devices: N
Federal Procurement Eligibility: Small Business, Female Owned
Distribution: Service Direct
General Admin.: Delena Morrison/Chief Executive Officer
     Miki Butler/Office Manager

Furniture, General	General

HEALTH CARE INFORMATION CORPORATION
See HCI

HEALTH CARE LOGISTICS, INC.   800-848-1633
450 East Town St., PO Box 25,   740-477-1686
Circleville, OH 43113
FDA Number: 1530671   *Fax:* 800-447-2923
E-mail: hcl@healthcarelogistics.com
Web site: www.healthcarelogistics.com
Year Founded: 1978
Total Employees: 125   *Marketing Staff:* 5   *Sales Staff:* 30
Ownership: Private
Produces/Sells CE-marked Devices: N
Federal Procurement Eligibility: Small Business, GSA Contract
Distribution: Service Direct, Importer, Exporter

Accessories, Catheter, G-U	Gastroenterology/Urology
Adapter, Hygiene	Physical Med
Airway, Oropharyngeal, Anesthesia	Anesthesiology
Applicator, Vaginal	Obstetrics/Gynecology
Bandage, Elastic	General
Basin, Emesis	General
Blade, Scalpel	Surgery
Board, Cardiopulmonary Resuscitation	General
Cart, Emergency, Cardiopulmonary Resuscitation (Crash)	Anesthesiology
Catheter, Umbilical Artery	General
Catheter, Urological	Gastroenterology/Urology
Cleaner, Medical Device	General
Container, IV	General
Container, Specimen, All Types	General
Cuff, Blood Pressure	Cardiovascular
Curette, Ear	Ear/Nose/Throat
Dispenser, Medication, Liquid	General
Fiberoptic Light Source & Carrier	Ear/Nose/Throat
Fixation Device, Tracheal Tube	Anesthesiology
Forceps	Orthopedics
Forceps, General & Plastic Surgery	Surgery
General Use Surgical Scissors	Surgery
Glove, Patient Examination, Latex	General
Guide, Surgical, Needle	Surgery
Holder, Intravascular Catheter	General
Infusion Stand	General
Mask, Oxygen, Aerosol Administration	Anesthesiology
Medical Disinfectants/Cleaners for Instruments	General
Needle, Hypodermic, Single Lumen With Syringe	General
Orthotoluidine, Glucose	Chemistry
Pad, Neonatal Eye	General
Pressure Infusor, IV Container	General
Pump, Aspiration, Portable	Anesthesiology
Restraint, Protective (Body)	General
Scalpel, One-Piece (Knife)	Surgery
Scissors, Disposable	General
Solution, Isotonic	Hematology
Solution, Saline(wound Dressing)	Surgery
Speculum, Vaginal, Metal	Obstetrics/Gynecology

HEALTH CARE LOGISTICS, INC.   800-848-1633 *(cont'd)*

Stylet, Tracheal Tube	Anesthesiology
Support, Arm	Physical Med
Support, Breathing Tube	Anesthesiology
Support, Patient Position	Anesthesiology
Surgical Instrument, Obstetric/Gynecologic	Obstetrics/Gynecology
Syringe, Irrigating	General
Syringe, Piston	General
Tourniquet, Non-Pneumatic, Surgical	Surgery
Tourniquet, Pneumatic	Surgery
Transfer Unit, IV Fluid	General
Tube, Capillary Blood Collection	Hematology
Tube, Feeding	General
Tubing, Fluid Delivery	General
Vaporizer, Anesthesia, Non-Heated	Anesthesiology
Ventilator, Emergency, Manual (Resuscitator)	Anesthesiology

HEALTH CARE PRODUCTS, INC.   419-678-9620
410 Nisco St., Coldwater, OH 45828
FDA Number: 3006073016

Pad, Menstrual, Unscented	Obstetrics/Gynecology
Tampon, Menstrual, Unscented	Obstetrics/Gynecology

HEALTH CARE SOFTWARE, INC. (HCS)   800-524-1038
PO Box 2430, Farmingdale, NJ 07727-2430   **732-938-5600**
FDA Number: n/a   *Fax:* 732-938-5380
E-mail: marketing@hcsinteractant.com
Web site: www.hcsinteractant.com
Medical Products Sales Volume: $5,500,000
Annual Revenue: $10-$25 Million
Year Founded: 1969
Total Employees: 80   *Marketing Staff:* 3   *Sales Staff:* 5
Ownership: Private
Produces/Sells CE-marked Devices: N
Federal Procurement Eligibility: Small Business
Distribution: Manufacturer Direct
General Admin.: Joseph Manzi/Executive Vice President
    Joseph Fahey/President
Mktg./Adv.: Tom Fahey/Vice President Sales

Computer Software	General
Computer Software, Hospital/Nursing Management	General

HEALTH CAREER LEARNING SYSTEMS, INC.
See Medical Safety Systems Inc.

HEALTH CHEM DIAGNOSTICS LLC   954-979-3845
3341 S.w. 15th St., Pompano Beach, FL 33069
FDA Number: 1048532

Alpha-Ketobutyric Acid And NADH (U.V.), Hydroxybutyric	Chemistry
Alpha-Naphthyl Phosphate, Alkaline Phosphatase Or Isoenzyme	Chemistry
Antigen, Antiserum, Control, Albumin	Immunology
Antigen, Antiserum, Control, Alpha-1-Antitrypsin	Immunology
Antigen, Antiserum, Control, IGA	Immunology
Antigen, Antiserum, Control, IGD	Immunology
Antigen, Antiserum, Control, IGE	Immunology
Antigen, Antiserum, Control, IGE, Peroxidase	Immunology
Antigen, Antiserum, Control, IGG	Immunology
Antigen, Antiserum, Control, IGM	Immunology
Antigen, Antiserum, Control, Kappa	Immunology
Antigen, Antiserum, Control, Lambda	Immunology
Antigen, Antiserum, Control, Spinal Fluid, Total	Immunology
Antigen, Antiserum, Control, Whole Human Serum	Immunology
Antiserum, Digitoxin	Toxicology
Antiserum, Positive And Negative Febrile Antigen Control	Microbiology
Calibrator, Primary, Clinical Chemistry	Chemistry
Chromatographic Separation, CPK Isoenzymes	Chemistry
Chromatographic, Phospholipids	Chemistry
Colorimetric Method, CPK Or Isoenzymes	Chemistry
Colorimetry, Cresol Red, Carbon-Dioxide	Chemistry
Complexone, Cresolphthalein, Calcium	Chemistry
Control, Analyte (Assayed And Unassayed)	Chemistry
Control, Blood Gas	Chemistry
Control, Coagulation, Plasma	Hematology
Control, Drug Mixture	Toxicology
Control, Electrolyte (Assayed And Unassayed)	Chemistry
Control, Enzyme (Assayed And Unassayed)	Chemistry
Control, Multi Analyte, All Kinds (Assayed And Unassayed)	Chemistry
Control, Plasma, Abnormal	Hematology
Control, Urinalysis (Assayed And Unassayed)	Chemistry
Diacetyl-Monoxime, Urea Nitrogen	Chemistry
Differential Rate Kinetic Method, CPK Or Isoenzymes	Chemistry
Diluent, Blood Cell	Hematology
Disc, Strip And Reagent, Microorganism Differentiation	Microbiology
Dye-Binding, Albumin, Bromcresol, Green	Chemistry
Electrode, Ion Specific, Potassium	Chemistry
Electrode, Ion Specific, Sodium	Chemistry
Electrophoretic Separation, Alkaline Phosphatase Isoenzymes	Chemistry
Electrophoretic, Lactate Dehydrogenase Isoenzymes	Chemistry
Enzymatic Esterase-Oxidase, Cholesterol	Chemistry
Ferrozine (Colorimetric) Iron Binding Capacity	Chemistry
Fluid, Red Cell Lysing	Hematology

HEALTH CHEM DIAGNOSTICS LLC   954-979-3845 *(cont'd)*

Glucose-6-Phosphate Dehydrogenase (Erythrocytic), Screening	Hematology
Hexokinase, Glucose	Chemistry
Lipase Hydrolysis/Glycerol Kinase Enzyme, Triglycerides	Chemistry
Multi Analyte Mixture, Calibrator	Chemistry
NAD Reduction/NADH Oxidation, Lactate Dehydrogenase	Chemistry
NADH Oxidation/NAD Reduction, AST/SGOT	Chemistry
Nitrophenylphosphate, Alkaline Phosphatase Or Isoenzymes	Chemistry
Orthotoluidine, Glucose	Chemistry
Partial Thromboplastin Time, Reagent, Control	Hematology
Phosphorus Reagent (Test System)	Chemistry
Phosphotungstate Reduction, Uric Acid	Chemistry
Plasma, Coagulase, Human/Horse/Rabbit	Microbiology
Plasma, Control, Normal	Hematology
Plasma, Deficient, Factor, Coagulation	Hematology
Radioassay, Triiodothyronine Uptake	Chemistry
Radioimmunoassay, Aldosterone	Chemistry
Radioimmunoassay, Angiotensin I And Renin	Chemistry
Radioimmunoassay, Cortisol	Chemistry
Radioimmunoassay, Cyclic GMP	Chemistry
Radioimmunoassay, Desoxycorticosterone	Chemistry
Radioimmunoassay, Digitoxin (3-H), Rabbit Antibody, Char.	Toxicology
Radioimmunoassay, Digoxin (3-H), Rabbit, Charcoal	Toxicology
Radioimmunoassay, Folic Acid	Chemistry
Radioimmunoassay, Follicle Stimulating Hormone	Chemistry
Radioimmunoassay, Immunoreactive Insulin	Chemistry
Radioimmunoassay, Progesterone	Chemistry
Radioimmunoassay, Testosterones And Dihydrotestosterone	Chemistry
Radioimmunoassay, Thyroid Stimulating Hormone	Chemistry
Radioimmunoassay, Total Triiodothyronine	Chemistry
Radioimmunoassay, Vitamin B12	Chemistry
Reagent, Albumin, Colorimetric	Chemistry
Reagent, Bilirubin (Total Or Direct Test System)	Chemistry
Reagent, Chloride (Test System)	Chemistry
Reagent, Cholesterol (Total Test System)	Chemistry
Reagent, Creatinine (Test System)	Chemistry
Reagent, Cyanomethemoglobin, With Standard	Hematology
Reagent, Glucose (Test System)	Chemistry
Reagent, Protein, Total	Chemistry
Reagent, Thromboplastin, With Control	Hematology
SGOT, Ultraviolet	Chemistry
SGPT, Colorimetric	Chemistry
SGPT, Ultraviolet	Chemistry
Serum, Control, Digoxin, RIA	Toxicology
Standard/Control, Hemoglobin, Normal/Abnormal	Hematology
Test, Antithrombin III, Two Stage Clotting Time	Hematology
Test, Human Chorionic Gonadotropin, Serum	Immunology
Tetrabromophenolphthalein, Albumin	Chemistry
Tetrazolium Int Dye-Diaphorase, Lactate Dehydrogenase	Chemistry
Thromboplastin, Activated Partial	Hematology
Thymolphthalein Monophosphate, Acid Phosphatase	Chemistry
Thymolphthalein Monophosphate, Alkaline Phosphatase	Chemistry
Tray, Blood Collection	Hematology
Tryptophan Measurement (Colorimetric), Globulin	Chemistry
U.V. Method, CPK Isoenzymes	Chemistry
Urease, Photometric, Urea Nitrogen	Chemistry
Uricase (Oxygen Rate), Uric Acid	Chemistry
Uricase (U.V.), Uric Acid	Chemistry
Ventilator, Continuous (Respirator)	Anesthesiology
Whole Human Plasma, Antigen, Antiserum, Control	Immunology

HEALTH ED. CO., INC.
See Wrs Group, Ltd.

HEALTH EDCO   800-299-3366
PO Box 21207, Waco, TX 76702   **254-776-6461**
FDA Number: n/a   *Fax:* 254-751-0221
E-mail: sales@wrsgroup.com
Web site: www.healthedco.com
Annual Revenue: $10-$25 Million
Total Employees: 125   *Marketing Staff:* 4
Ownership: Wrs Group, Ltd.
Produces/Sells CE-marked Devices: N
Federal Procurement Eligibility: Small Business
Distribution: Manufacturer Through Distributor, Manufacturer Through Manufacturer Reps

Anatomical Training Model	General

HEALTH ENT., INC.   800-633-4243
90 George Leven Dr.,   **508-695-0727**
North Attleboro, MA 02760
FDA Number: 1224962   *Fax:* 508-695-3061
Web site: www.healthenterprises.com
Ownership: Private
Produces/Sells CE-marked Devices: N

Brace, Joint, Ankle (External)	Physical Med
Cushion, Flotation	Physical Med
Detector/Remover, Lice	General
Dressing, Wound, Occlusive	Surgery
Gauze/sponge, Nonresorbable For External Use	Surgery
Joint, Knee, External Brace	Physical Med

MANUFACTURER PROFILES

HEALTH ENT., INC.   **800-633-4243** (cont'd)
  Otoscope   Ear/Nose/Throat
  Splint, Hand, And Component   Physical Med
  Syringe, Irrigating   General
  Unit, Sanitation/Sterilization, Toothbrush, Ultraviolet   Dental And Oral

HEALTH ENTERPRISES   **800-633-4243**
90 George Leven Dr.,   **508-695-0727**
North Attleboro, MA 02760
  FDA Number: 1224962   *Fax:* 508-695-3061
  E-mail: Sales-HE@healthenterprises.com
  Web site: www.healthenterprises.com
  Medical Products Sales Volume: $8,000,000
  Annual Revenue: $5-$10 Million
  Year Founded: 1973
  Ownership: Private
  Produces/Sells CE-marked Devices: N
  Federal Procurement Eligibility: Small Business
  Distribution: Manufacturer Direct, Manufacturer Through Manufacturer Reps,
  Importer, Exporter
  Bracelet, Identification   General
  Card, Identification   General
  Container, Medication, Home-Use   General
  Cutter, Pill   General
  Detector/Remover, Lice   General
  Dropper, Medicine   General
  Kit, Emergency, Insect Sting   General
  Lotion, Skin Care   General
  Splint, Other   Orthopedics
  Spoon, Medicine   General

HEALTH EQUIPMENT MANUFACTURERS, INC.   **269-962-6181**
702 S. Reed Street, Fremont, IN 46737
  FDA Number: 1832415
  Exerciser, Non-Measuring   Physical Med
  Pad, Heating, Powered   Physical Med

HEALTH HERO NETWORK, INC.   **888-947-8957**
2400 Geng Road, Ste. 200, Palo Alto, CA 94303   **650-690-9100**
  FDA Number: 3004142783   *Fax:* 650-798-3770
  Ownership: Private
  Produces/Sells CE-marked Devices: N
  Reagent, Glucose (Test System)   Chemistry
  Scale, Stand-On   General
  Transmitter/Receiver System, Physiological, Radiofrequency Cardiovascular

HEALTH IMAGING CORP.   **800-468-7874**
1011 Campus Drive, Mundelein, IL 60060   **847-680-7040**
  FDA Number: n/a   *Fax:* 847-680-7160
  E-mail: ed@crgq.com
  Annual Revenue: $1-$5 Million
  Total Employees: 25   *Marketing Staff:* 3   *Sales Staff:* 3
  Ownership: Private
  Produces/Sells CE-marked Devices: N
  Federal Procurement Eligibility: Small Business, Female Owned
  Distribution: Manufacturer Direct
  General Admin.: Edward Halpern/Chairman
                   Gregory Halpern/President
  Material, Training, Audiovisual   General

HEALTH IMPRESSIONS
  See Health Edco

HEALTH INFORMATION DESIGNS, INC.   **334-502-3262**
391 Industry Drive, Auburn, AL 36832
  FDA Number: n/a   *Fax:* 334-466-6947
  E-mail: bill.mixon@hidinc.com
  Web site: www.hidinc.com
  Annual Revenue: $0-$1 Million
  Year Founded: 1976
  Total Employees: 250
  Ownership: Private
  Produces/Sells CE-marked Devices: N
  Distribution: Manufacturer Direct
  General Admin.: Guy Robert DiBenedetto/Chief Operating Officer
                   William R. Mixon/President, Chief Executive Officer
  Computer, Patient Data Management   General

HEALTH KEEPER 9000 USA INC.   **213-385-3933**
680 S. Wilshire Pl., #405, Los Angeles, CA 90005
  FDA Number: 2032498
  Ownership: Private
  Produces/Sells CE-marked Devices: N
  Massager, Therapeutic   Physical Med

HEALTH LEARNING SYSTEMS, INC.   **800-388-1000**
402 Interpace Parkway   **973-785-8500**
Wayne Interchange Plaza II
Parsippany, NJ 07454
  FDA Number: n/a   *Fax:* 973-785-4457
  E-mail: ssinger@commonhealth.com
  Web site: www.commonhealth.com
  Medical Products Sales Volume: $17,500,000
  Annual Revenue: $25-$50 Million
  Total Employees: 545
  Ownership: WPP GROUP
  Traded On: NASDAQ
  Federal Procurement Eligibility: Small Business
  Distribution: Service Direct
  General Admin.: Joseph A. Mastracchio/Chief Executive Officer
    Material, Training, Audiovisual   General

HEALTH LIGHT INC.   **800-265-6020**
P.O. Box 3899, LCD 4,   **905-545-4997**
Hamilton, ONT L8H-7 Canada
  FDA Number: n/a   *Fax:* 905-545-8963
  E-mail: dworthington@healthlight.net
  Web site: www.healthlight.net
  Year Founded: 1988
  Total Employees: 10
  Ownership: Private
  Produces/Sells CE-marked Devices: N
  Federal Procurement Eligibility: Small Business
  Distribution: Manufacturer Direct

HEALTH PHYSICS SERVICES, INC.
  See Health & Radiological Seminars, Inc.

HEALTH SCIENCE PRODUCTS, INC.   **800-237-5794**
1489 Hueytown Road,   **800-237-5794**
Birmingham, AL 35023
  FDA Number: 7000820   *Fax:* 205-251-0419
  E-mail: hspinc@wwisp.com
  Web site: www.hspinc.com
  Medical Products Sales Volume: $1,500,000
  Annual Revenue: $1-$5 Million
  Year Founded: 1969
  Total Employees: 6   *Marketing Staff:* 1   *Sales Staff:* 2
  Ownership: Private
  Produces/Sells CE-marked Devices: N
  Federal Procurement Eligibility: Small Business, Female Owned
  Distribution: Manufacturer Direct, Manufacturer Through Distributor, Importer,
  Exporter
  General Admin.: Ms. Anita Bedford/President, Chief Executive Officer
  Mktg./Adv.: Mr. Michael Muscari/Senior Vice President International & National
  Sales
            Mr. Michael Muscari/Senior Vice President Marketing & Business
  Development
  Production: Mr. Earl Wells/Plant General Manager
  Finance: Mr. Jimmy Glenn/Director Accounting
  Cabinet, Dental   Dental And Oral
  Chair, Dental   Dental And Oral
  Light, Dental   Dental And Oral
  Light, Surgical Operating, Dental   Dental And Oral
  Operative Dental Treatment Unit   Dental And Oral
  Scaler, Ultrasonic   Dental And Oral
  Sink, Hospital   General
  Stool, Dental   Dental And Oral

HEALTH SCIENCE PRODUCTS, LLC   **757-224-0177**
1010 S. Beeline Hwy, Payson, AZ 85541
  FDA Number: 2032679
  Ownership: Private
  Produces/Sells CE-marked Devices: N
  Electrode, Ion Selective (Non-Specified)   Chemistry

HEALTH SOLUTIONS MEDICAL   **310-837-9594**
PRODUCTS, CORP.
9027 Monte Mar Dr., Los Angeles, CA 90035
  FDA Number: 2032685
  Ownership: Private
  Produces/Sells CE-marked Devices: N
  Irrigator, Oral   Dental And Oral

HEALTH WATCH PERSONAL RESPONSE   **561-994-6699**
SYSTEMS
6400 Park Of Commerce Blvd., Suite 1a, Boca Raton, FL 33487
  FDA Number: 1054748
  Ownership: Private
  Produces/Sells CE-marked Devices: N
  Environmental Control System, Powered   Physical Med

HEALTH-DENT INTERNATIONAL, INC.
See Healthdent'L L.L.C.

HEALTH-PAK, INC.   315-724-8370
2005 Beechgrove Pl., Utica, NY 13501-1703
FDA Number: 1318989   Fax: 315-724-7895
E-mail: info@health-pak.com
Web site: www.health-pak.com
Medical Products Sales Volume: $2,000,000
Annual Revenue: $1-$5 Million
Total Employees: 30   *Marketing Staff:* 2   *Sales Staff:* 4
Ownership: LIFE ENERGY & TECHNOLOGY HOLDINGS INC.
Stock Symbol: LETH
Traded On: OTC Bulletin
Produces/Sells CE-marked Devices: Y
Federal Procurement Eligibility: Small Business
Distribution: Manufacturer Through Distributor, Manufacturer Through
Manufacturer Reps
General Admin.: Anthony Liberatore/President
         Michael Liberatore/Vice President

Bib	General
Cap, Surgical	Surgery
Clothing, Protective	General
Coat, Laboratory	General
Cover, Shoe, Operating Room	Surgery
Dress, Scrub, Disposable	Surgery
Gown, Examination	General
Gown, Isolation, Surgical	Surgery
Gown, Surgical	Surgery
Linen	General
Mitt/Washcloth, Patient	General
Pack, Sterilization Wrapper (Bag And Accessories)	Surgery
Sheet, Drape	Surgery
Sheeting, Examination Table	General
Suit, Scrub, Disposable	Surgery
Wrap, Sterilization	General

HEALTHCARE & REHAB SPECIALTIES   800-232-9408   780-424-6094
10611 Kingsway Ave., Unit 114,
Edmonton, ALB T5G-3 Canada
FDA Number: n/a   Fax: 780-426-1734
E-mail: health@mail.worldgate.com
Web site: www.healthcareandrehab.com
Year Founded: 1984
Total Employees: 100
Ownership: Private
Produces/Sells CE-marked Devices: N
Distribution: Exclusive Distributor

HEALTHCARE AFFILIATED SVCS. LAB SYSTEMS
See Labfusions

HEALTHCARE COMPUTER CORP.   888-727-5422   817-531-8992
2601 Scott Ave., Suite 600,
Fort Worth, TX 76103
FDA Number: n/a   Fax: 817-536-6615
E-mail: sales1@hcc-care.com
Web site: www.hcc-care.com
Ownership: Private
Produces/Sells CE-marked Devices: N
Federal Procurement Eligibility: Small Business
Distribution: Manufacturer Direct
General Admin.: Rex Akers/Chief Executive Officer

Computer and Software, Medical	General

HEALTHCARE INFORMATION, L.L.C.
See HCI

HEALTHCARE LABELS, INC.   800-323-8323   847-382-3993
245 Honey Lake Ct., N. Barrington, IL 60010
FDA Number: 1419465   Fax: 847-382-1648
E-mail: healthcarelabels@aol.com
Web site: www.healthcarelabels.com
Medical Products Sales Volume: $1,700,000
Annual Revenue: $1-$5 Million
Year Founded: 1983
Total Employees: 19
Ownership: Private
Produces/Sells CE-marked Devices: N
Federal Procurement Eligibility: Small Business, GSA Contract
Distribution: Manufacturer Through Distributor
General Admin.: Ronald F. Gagnier/President
Mktg./Adv.: Terry Gagnier/Vice President Marketing

Label, Device	General
Labeling Equipment	General

HEALTHCARE MANAGEMENT SYSTEMS, INC.   800-383-3317   615-383-7300
3102 West End Ave., Suite 400,
Nashville, TN 37203
FDA Number: 1000475598
   Fax: 615-386-6661

HEALTHCARE MANAGEMENT SYSTEMS, INC.   800-383-3317
(cont'd)
E-mail: marketing@hmstn.com
Web site: www.hmstn.com
Ownership: Private
Produces/Sells CE-marked Devices: N

Software, Blood Bank (Stand-Alone Products)	Hematology

HEALTHCARE SERVICE AND SUPPLY   714-669-8803
10602 Mira Vista Drive, Santa Ana, CA 92705
FDA Number: 2030561   Fax: 626-303-2947
E-mail: rickroeder@curriemedical.com
Year Founded: 1990
Total Employees: 1   *Marketing Staff:* 1   *Sales Staff:* 1
Ownership: Private
Produces/Sells CE-marked Devices: N
Federal Procurement Eligibility: Small Business
Distribution: Manufacturer Through Distributor

Sleeve, Compressible Limb	Cardiovascular

HEALTHCARE-ID, INC.   847-465-9935
1635 Barclay Blvd., Buffalo Grove, IL 60089
FDA Number: 3003770140   Fax: 847-465-9940
Ownership: Private
Produces/Sells CE-marked Devices: N

Software, Blood Bank (Stand-Alone Products)	Hematology

HEALTHCO INTERNATIONAL, LLC   603-255-4200
2000 Cold Spring Road, Dixville Notch, Colebrook, NH 03576
FDA Number: 3004355758
Ownership: Private
Produces/Sells CE-marked Devices: N

Glove, Patient Examination, Latex	General
Glove, Patient Examination, Poly	General
Glove, Surgical, Plastic Surgery	Surgery

HEALTHCRAFT PRODUCTS INC.   888-619-9992   613-822-1885
2790 Fenton Road, Unit 411,
Ottawa, ONT K1T 3 Canada
FDA Number: n/a   Fax: 613-822-1886
E-mail: info@healthcraftprroducts.com
Web site: www.healthcraftproducts.com
Year Founded: 1994
Total Employees: 10
Ownership: Private
Produces/Sells CE-marked Devices: N
Distribution: Manufacturer Direct

HEALTHDENT'L L.L.C.   800-845-5172   630-851-0088
1355 S. Route 59, Ste. 202, Naperville, IL 60564
FDA Number: 1422728   Fax: 630-851-8899
E-mail: info@healthdentl.com
Web site: http://www.healthdentl.com
Medical Products Sales Volume: $3,500,000
Annual Revenue: $5-$10 Million
Total Employees: 7   *Marketing Staff:* 2   *Sales Staff:* 4
Ownership: Private
Quality System Registration Information: ISO9002
Produces/Sells CE-marked Devices: Y
Federal Procurement Eligibility: Small Business
Distribution: Manufacturer Direct, Manufacturer Through Distributor, OEM
General Admin.: Dreana Olver/Office Manager
         Bob Bevilacqua/President, Chief Executive Officer
Mktg./Adv.: Steve Bevilacqua/Manager International Marketing & Sales
         Steve Bevilacqua/Vice President Marketing & Sales

Cement, Dental	Dental And Oral
Desensitizer	Anesthesiology
Material, Acrylic, Dental	Dental And Oral

HEALTHDRIVE AG   617-964-6681
25 Needham St, Newton, MA 02461
FDA Number: 3005643732

Hearing-Aid	Ear/Nose/Throat

HEALTHDYNE CARDIOVASCULAR
See St. Jude Medical Neuromodulation Division

HEALTHDYNE HOME CARE PRODUCTS
See Respironics Georgia, Inc.

HEALTHDYNE OXYGEN CONCENTRATOR DIV.
See Respironics Georgia, Inc.

HEALTHDYNE TECHNOLOGIES
See Respironics Georgia, Inc.

HEALTHFIRST CORP.   425-771-5733
22316 70th Ave. West, Unit A, Mountlake Terrace, WA 98043
FDA Number: 3014534

Cart, Emergency, Cardiopulmonary Resuscitation (Crash)	Anesthesiology

MANUFACTURER PROFILES

HEALTHLINE MEDICAL IMAGING 704-655-0447
705 Northeast Drive, Suite 17, Davidson, NC 28036
FDA Number: 3004497134
Ownership: Private
Produces/Sells CE-marked Devices: N
  Device, Storage, Image, Digital   Radiology
  Image Processing System   Radiology

HEALTHLINE MEDICAL PRODUCTS, INC. 1-800-987-3577
1065 E Story Rd., Oakland, FL 34787   407-656-0704
FDA Number: 3005878604   Fax: 407-656-5641
E-mail: pvcdmeds1@aol.com
Ownership: Private
Produces/Sells CE-marked Devices: N
  Chair, Geriatric   General
  Chair, With Casters   Physical Med
  Stretcher, Wheeled (Mobile)   General
  Walker, Mechanical   Physical Med

HEALTHLINK 800-288-6580
3611 St Johns Bluff Rd. South, Suite 1,   904 996 7758
Jacksonville, FL 32224
FDA Number: 1059020   Fax: 904 996 7078
E-mail: custsvc@hlk.cc
Web site: www.frayproducts.com
Total Employees: 8
Ownership: Private
Produces/Sells CE-marked Devices: N
Federal Procurement Eligibility: Small Business
Distribution: Manufacturer Through Distributor, Exporter
  Culture Media, Enriched   Microbiology
  Culture Media, General Nutrient Broth   Microbiology
  Culture Media, Non-Selective And Non-Differential   Microbiology
  Culture Media, Selective And Differential   Microbiology
  Culture Media, Selective And Non-Differential   Microbiology
  Curette, Ear   Ear/Nose/Throat
  General Purpose Microbiology Diagnostic Device   Microbiology
  Instrument, Manual, General Surgical   Surgery
  Kit, Quality Control   Microbiology
  Punch, Biopsy   Gastroenterology/Urology

HEALTHLINK 904-996-7758
3611 St. Johns Bluff Rd. South, Suite 1, Jacksonville, FL 32224
FDA Number: 1059020
  Culture Media, Enriched   Microbiology
  Culture Media, For Isolation Of Pathogenic Neisseria   Microbiology
  Culture Media, General Nutrient Broth   Microbiology
  Culture Media, Mueller Hinton Agar Broth   Microbiology
  Culture Media, Non-Selective And Differential   Microbiology
  Culture Media, Non-Selective And Non-Differential   Microbiology
  Culture Media, Selective And Differential   Microbiology
  Culture Media, Selective And Non-Differential   Microbiology
  Culture Media, Selective Broth   Microbiology
  General Purpose Microbiology Diagnostic Device   Microbiology
  Kit, Quality Control   Microbiology

HEALTHMARK INDUSTRIES 800-521-6224
33671 Doreka, Fraser, MI 48026   810-774-7600
FDA Number: 1834190   Fax: 810-774-6473
E-mail: healthmark@hmark.com
Web site: www.hmark.com
Medical Products Sales Volume: $3,000,000
Annual Revenue: $1-$5 Million
Total Employees: 28   *Marketing Staff:* 5   *Sales Staff:* 36
Ownership: Private
Produces/Sells CE-marked Devices: N
Federal Procurement Eligibility: Small Business
Distribution: Manufacturer Direct, Manufacturer Through Distributor, OEM, Importer, Exporter
General Admin.: Mark Basile/President
              Ralph Basile/Vice President
Mktg./Adv.: Steven Basile/Director National Accounts
              Steve Basile/Vice President Sales
Production: Julie Clubertson/Manager Warehouse
              Mark Basile/Vice President Production
  Bin, Storage   General
  Brush, Other   General
  Cart, Instrument   Surgery
  Cart, Multipurpose   General
  Casters, Hospital Equipment   General
  Container, Surgical Instrument   Surgery
  Cover, Cart   General
  Instrument Guard   Surgery
  Labware, Basic, Reusable   Chemistry
  Rack, Test Tube   Chemistry
  Security Equipment/Supplies   General
  Stand, Operating Room Instrument (Mayo)   Surgery
  System, Transport, In-House   General
  Tray, Blood Collection   Hematology

HEALTHMARK INDUSTRIES 800-521-6224 *(cont'd)*
  Tray, Medicine   General
  Tray, Surgical Instrument   Surgery

HEALTHMARK LTD. 800-665-5492
8827 Henri-Bourassa O. Blvd.,   514-336-0012
MontrAcal, QUE H4S-1 Canada
FDA Number: n/a   Fax: 514-336-7111
Year Founded: 1990
Total Employees: 25
Ownership: Private
Produces/Sells CE-marked Devices: N
Distribution: Exclusive Distributor

HEALTHMARK, INC. 971-236-9171
8440 Se Sunnybrook Blvd #210, Clackamas, OR 97015
FDA Number: 3004424236
Ownership: Private
Produces/Sells CE-marked Devices: N
  Computer and Software, Medical   General

HEALTHONICS, INC. 770-955-2006
903 Main St. South, New Ellenton, SC 29809
FDA Number: 1067152
Ownership: Private
Produces/Sells CE-marked Devices: N
  Stimulator, Nerve, Transcutaneous (Pain Relief, TENS)   Cns/Neurology

HEALTHPOSTURES, LLC 800-277-1841
125 East Main Street, Belle Plaine, MN 56011   320-864-4359
FDA Number: 3004594123
E-mail: info@healthpostures.com
Ownership: Private
Produces/Sells CE-marked Devices: N
  Chair, Adjustable, Mechanical   Physical Med

HEALTHSCAN PRODUCTS, INC.
See Respironics New Jersey, Inc.

HEALTHSENSE INC. 952-400-7300
1191 Northland Dr., Suite 100, Mendota Heights, MN 55120
FDA Number: n/a   Fax: 800-576-1779
E-mail: 952-400-7299
Web site: http://www.healthsense.com
Ownership: Private
Produces/Sells CE-marked Devices: N
General Admin.: Mr. Brian Bischoff/President, Chief Executive Officer
Mktg./Adv.: Mr. Bryan Fuhr/Vice President Business Development
Research: Mr. Dean Anderson/Vice President Engineering
Finance: Mr. Terry Bark/Chief Financial Officer

HEALTHSHIELD TECHNOLOGIES LLC
See Agion Technologies Inc.

HEALTHSONIX INC. 949-417-8880
14252 Culver Drive, Suite 107, Irvine, CA 92604-0317
FDA Number: 3005799371
Ownership: Private
Produces/Sells CE-marked Devices: N
  Vibrator, Therapeutic   Physical Med

HEALTHSOUTH CORPORATION 888-476-8849
3660 Grandview Parkway, Suite 200,   800-765-4772
Birmingham, AL 35243
FDA Number: n/a
Web site: www.healthsouth.com
Annual Revenue: More than $1 Billion
Total Employees: 22000
Ownership: Public
Stock Symbol: HLS
Traded On: NYSE
Produces/Sells CE-marked Devices: N
General Admin.: John L. Workman/Chief Financial Officer, Executive Vice President
        John P. Whittington/Executive Vice President, General Manager
        Jay Grinney/President, Chief Executive Officer
Production: Mark J. Tarr/Executive Vice President Operations
  Computer and Software, Medical   General
  Exerciser, Powered   Anesthesiology
  Orthosis, Truncal/Limb   Physical Med
  Prosthesis Alignment Device   Physical Med

HEALTHSTREAM, INC. 800-521-0574
209 10th Avenue S., #450, Nashville, TN 37203   800-933-9293
FDA Number: n/a   Fax: 615-301-3200
E-mail: contact@healthstream.com
Web site: www.healthstream.com
Medical Products Sales Volume: $31,780,000
Year Founded: 1990
Total Employees: 160

HEALTHSTREAM, INC.   800-521-0574 *(cont'd)*
Ownership: Public
Stock Symbol: HSTM
Traded On: NASDAQ
Produces/Sells CE-marked Devices: N
Federal Procurement Eligibility: Small Business
Distribution: Manufacturer Direct, Service Direct
Mktg./Adv.: Tammy Wise Rutherford/Manager Market Development
  Office Product   General

HEALTHTRONICS INC.   888-252-6575
9825 Spectrum Dr., Building B, Austin, TX 78717   512-328-2892
FDA Number: n/a   *Fax:* 512-439-8303
E-mail: Sales@HealthTronics.com
Web site: www.healthtronics.com
Total Employees: 293
Ownership: Public
Stock Symbol: HTRN
Traded On: NASDAQ
Produces/Sells CE-marked Devices: N
General Admin.: Mr. James Whittenburg/President, Chief Executive Officer
Mktg./Adv.: Mr. Scott Herz/Vice President Corporate Development
Finance: Mr. Richard Rusk/Chief Financial Officer
  Catheter, Urological   Gastroenterology/Urology
  Cryosurgical Unit   Surgery
  Surgical Device, For Ablation Of Cardiac Tissue   Surgery
  Transducer, Ultrasonic, Diagnostic   Radiology

HEAR EAR INC   574-256-0000
3718 Lincolnway East, Mishawaka, IN 46544
FDA Number: 3006269084
  Hearing-Aid   Ear/Nose/Throat

HEAR SAVER LIMITED   905-690-6277
60 Innovation Dr., Flamborough, ONT L9H-7P3 Canada
FDA Number: n/a   *Fax:* 905-690-6281
E-mail: info@hearsaver.com
Web site: www.hearsaver.com
Year Founded: 1969
Total Employees: 25
Ownership: Private
Produces/Sells CE-marked Devices: N
Distribution: Manufacturer Direct, Exporter

HEARING AID CENTER   808-973-1551
615 Piikoi St., Suite 1111, Honolulu, HI 96814
FDA Number: n/a
Web site: www.familyhearingaidcenter.com
Ownership: Private
Produces/Sells CE-marked Devices: N
  Hearing-Aid   Ear/Nose/Throat

HEARING AID EXPRESS   713-666-1704
11888 Marsh Ln., Suite 111, Dallas, TX 75234
FDA Number: 1643921
  Hearing-Aid   Ear/Nose/Throat

HEARING AID EXPRESS   713-666-1704
5201 Bellaire Blvd., Bellaire, TX 77401
FDA Number: 1649872
Ownership: Private
Produces/Sells CE-marked Devices: N
  Hearing-Aid   Ear/Nose/Throat

HEARING AID FACTORY   409-883-3010
105 Camellia, P.o. Box 61, Orange, TX 77631
FDA Number: 1642941
  Hearing-Aid   Ear/Nose/Throat

HEARING COMPONENTS INC.   800-872-8986
420 Hayward Ave., N., Oakdale, MN 55128   651-739-9427
FDA Number: n/a   *Fax:* 651-735-2790
E-mail: info@hearingcomponents.com
Web site: www.hearingcomponents.com
Year Founded: 1990
Total Employees: 20
Ownership: Private
Produces/Sells CE-marked Devices: Y
Federal Procurement Eligibility: Small Business, Minority Owned
Distribution: Manufacturer Direct, OEM, Exporter
General Admin.: Bob Oliveira/President, Chief Executive Officer
           Barbara Hoeker/Vice President Human Resources
Mktg./Adv.: Joe Romeo/Vice President Marketing & Sales
Production: John Dolin/Vice President Manufacturing
  Protector, Hearing (Insert)   Ear/Nose/Throat

HEARING CRAFTERS OF AMERICA   417-466-4085
708 E. Mount Vernon Blvd., Mt. Vernon, MO 65712
FDA Number: 1931637

HEARING CRAFTERS OF AMERICA   417-466-4085 *(cont'd)*
Ownership: Private
Produces/Sells CE-marked Devices: N
  Hearing-Aid   Ear/Nose/Throat

HEARING IMPROVEMENT   801-392-4310
1961 Washington Blvd., Ogden, UT 84401-0433
FDA Number: 1722258
Ownership: Private
Produces/Sells CE-marked Devices: N
  Hearing-Aid   Ear/Nose/Throat

HEARING TECH, INC.   520-297-7555
7225 North Oracle Rd. #111, Tucson, AZ 85704
FDA Number: 2028973
E-mail: hearingtech@aol.com
Web site: www.hearingtechtucson.com
Ownership: Private
Produces/Sells CE-marked Devices: N
  Hearing-Aid   Ear/Nose/Throat

HEARING TECHNOLOGIES   727-525-7770
6251 44th St 109, Pinellas Park, FL 33781
FDA Number: 1052213
Medical Products Sales Volume: $4,000,000
Year Founded: 1976
Total Employees: 4
Ownership: Bar-Ray Products, Inc.
Produces/Sells CE-marked Devices: N
Federal Procurement Eligibility: Small Business
  Hearing-Aid   Ear/Nose/Throat

HEARING TODAY LABORATORY, INC.   877-888-6336
11954 West 95th St., Lenexa, KS 66215   913-888-6336
FDA Number: 1933217
E-mail: info@hearingtodaylaboratory.com
Web site: www.hearingtodaylaboratory.com
Ownership: Private
Produces/Sells CE-marked Devices: N
  Hearing-Aid   Ear/Nose/Throat

HEARING TODAY LABORATORY, INC.   800-567-0088
14473 W. Center Rd., Omaha, NE 68144   913-888-6336
FDA Number: 1933947
Ownership: Private
Produces/Sells CE-marked Devices: N
  Hearing-Aid   Ear/Nose/Throat

HEARMORE CO., INC.   651-771-4019
1445 White Bear Ave., St. Paul, MN 55106
FDA Number: 2184021
Ownership: Private
Produces/Sells CE-marked Devices: N
  Hearing-Aid   Ear/Nose/Throat

HEARMORE COMPANY INC.   800-881-4327
75 W Baseline Rd. #9, Gilbert, AZ 85233   480-633-1830
FDA Number: 2030615   *Fax:* 631-752-0689
Web site: www.hearmore.com
Ownership: Private
Produces/Sells CE-marked Devices: N
  Hearing-Aid   Ear/Nose/Throat

HEART FORCE MEDICAL INC.   604-566-8200
1818 Cornwall Avenue, Suite 305,
Vancouver, BC V6J 1 Canada
FDA Number: n/a   *Fax:* 604-566-8201
E-mail: info@heartforcemedical.com
Web site: www.heartforcemedical.com
Ownership: Private
Produces/Sells CE-marked Devices: N

HEART IMAGING TECHNOLOGIES, LLC   919-384-5044
5003 Southpark Dr., Suite 140, Durham, NC 27713
FDA Number: 3005107869
  Image Processing System   Radiology
  System, Communication, Image, Digital   Radiology

HEART RATE, INC.   800-237-2271
3190 E Airport Loop,   714-850-9716
Costa Mesa, CA 92626
FDA Number: 2024189   *Fax:* 714-755-4973
E-mail: email@heartrateinc.com
Web site: www.versaclimber.com (or) www.heartrateinc.com
Medical Products Sales Volume: $1,800,000
Annual Revenue: $1-$5 Million
Year Founded: 1978
Total Employees: 23   *Marketing Staff:* 1   *Sales Staff:* 3
Ownership: Private

HEART RATE, INC.   800-237-2271 (cont'd)
Produces/Sells CE-marked Devices: N
Federal Procurement Eligibility: Small Business, GSA Contract
Distribution: Manufacturer Direct, Manufacturer Through Distributor, Manufacturer Through Manufacturer Reps, Service Direct, Exclusive Distributor, Exporter
General Admin.: Dan Charnitski/General Manager
         Richard D. Charnitski/President
Mktg./Adv.: Brett Collins/Director Marketing
         Dan Charnitski/Manager International & National Sales
         Brett Collins/Managing Director Marketing
   Exerciser, Other   Physical Med
   Monitor, Heart Rate, Other   Cardiovascular

HEARTBEAT MEDICAL CORP.   505-823-1990
8917 Adams St., N.e., Albuquerque, NM 87113
FDA Number: 1722395
Ownership: Private
Produces/Sells CE-marked Devices: N
   Pacemaker, Cardiac, External Transcutaneous (Non-Invasive)   Cardiovascular

HEARTLAND TANNING, INC.   816-795-1414
4251 Ne Port Dr., Lee's Summit, MO 64064
FDA Number: 1932879
   Booth, Sun Tan   Physical Med
   Light, Ultraviolet, Dermatologic   Surgery

HEARTPORT   888-478-7678
700 Bay Road, Redwood City, CA 94063   650-306-7900
FDA Number: n/a   Fax: 415-306-7905
E-mail: jgw@heartport.com
Web site: www.heartport.com
Annual Revenue: $0-$1 Million
Total Employees: 250
Ownership: Public
Stock Symbol: HPRT
Traded On: NASDAQ
Federal Procurement Eligibility: Small Business
Distribution: Manufacturer Direct, Importer, Exporter
General Admin.: Casey M. Tansey/President, Chief Executive Officer
Mktg./Adv.: Christopher A. Hubbard/Vice President Sales
Production: Steven E. Johnson/Senior Vice President Operations
Research: Casy Punsi/Vice President Research & Development
Finance: Rebecca L. Kuhn/Director Finance
         Rebecca L. Kuhn/Treasurer
   Catheter, Cardiovascular   Surgery

HEARTSINE TECHNOLOGIES, INC.   866-478-7463
121 Friends Lane, Suite 400,   215-860-8100
Newtown, PA 18940
FDA Number: 2032757   Fax: 215-860-8192
E-mail: info@heartsine.com
Web site: www.heartsine.com
Ownership: Private
Produces/Sells CE-marked Devices: N
General Admin.: Mr. John Anderson/Chief Technology Officer
         Mr. Gregory Cash/President, Chief Executive Officer
         Mr. Volker Brand/Vice President
Finance: Mr. Ian McRoberts/Chief Financial Officer
   Defibrillator, External, Automatic   Cardiovascular

HEARTSOUNDS CORP.   416-383-1520
314-801 York Mills Rd, Don Mills M3B 1X7 Canada
FDA Number: 9615238
   Stethoscope, Electronic (Auscultoscope)   Cardiovascular

HEARTWARE INTERNATIONAL, INC.   877-367-4823
205 Newbury Street, Suite 101,   508-739-0950
Framingham, MA 01701
FDA Number: 3007042319   Fax: 508-739-0948
E-mail: enquiries@heartware.com.au
Web site: www.heartware.com.au
Ownership: Public
Stock Symbol: HTWR
Traded On: NASDAQ
Produces/Sells CE-marked Devices: N
General Admin.: Douglas Godshall/Chief Executive Officer
         David McIntyre/Chief Operating Officer, Chief Financial Officer
         Jeffrey A. LaRose/Chief Scientific Officer
Medical Admin.: Dr. David Hathaway/Chief Medical Officer
Mktg./Adv.: Mr. James Schuermann/Vice President Marketing & Sales

HEAT SYSTEMS ULTRASONICS, INC.
See Misonix, Inc.

HEATMAX, INC.   800-533-7349
505 Hill Rd., Dalton, GA 30722
FDA Number: 1054358

HEATMAX, INC.   800-533-7349 (cont'd)
   Pack, Hot Or Cold, Disposable   Physical Med

HEATRON, INC.   913-651-4420
3000 Wilson Ave., Leavenworth, KS 66048
FDA Number: n/a   Fax: 913-651-5352
E-mail: heatron1@heatron.com
Web site: www.heatron.com
Annual Revenue: $25-$50 Million
Total Employees: 300
Ownership: Private
Quality System Registration Information: ISO9001
Produces/Sells CE-marked Devices: N
Federal Procurement Eligibility: Small Business
Distribution: Manufacturer Direct, Manufacturer Through Distributor, Manufacturer Through Manufacturer Reps
General Admin.: Mr. HB Turner/President
Mktg./Adv.: Mr. Robert Doyle/Vice President Marketing & Sales
   Contract Manufacturing   General
   Heat Exchanger, Extracorporeal Perfusion   Surgery
   Heat Exchanger, Heart-Lung Bypass   Cardiovascular
   Heat Exchanger, Heart-Lung Bypass, AC-Powered   Cardiovascular
   Heat Exchanger, Regional Perfusion   Surgery
   Heater, Electrical Instrument   General
   Monitor, Temperature, Dialysis   Gastroenterology/Urology
   Service, Engineering/Design   General

HEDY CANADA   403-571-2277
4535 É_, 104 Avenue S.E., Calga ALB T2C 5C6   Canada
FDA Number: N   Fax: 1-800-661-HEDY
Web site: info@hedycanada.com
Medical Products Sales Volume: $50
Total Employees: 403-287
Ownership: I
Stock Symbol: N
Distribution: Manufacturer Through Distributor, Service Direct

HEFCO
See Airguard

HEIDELBERG MEDICAL, INC.   706-745-9698
627 Gainesville Highway, Suite B, Blairsville, GA 30512
FDA Number: 1031128
   Electrode, pH   Gastroenterology/Urology

HEINE INSTRUMENTS CANADA LTD.   519-895-1020
20 Steckle Place, Unit 3, Kitchener, ONT N2E-2C3 Canada
FDA Number: n/a   Fax: 519-895-1022
E-mail: mgrundy@heineweb.com
Web site: www.heineweb.com
Year Founded: 1946
Total Employees: 10
Ownership: Private
Produces/Sells CE-marked Devices: N
Distribution: Importer

HEINE USA LTD.   800-367-4872
10 Innovation Way, Dover, NH 03820-3831   603-742-7103
FDA Number: n/a   Fax: 603-742-7217
E-mail: service@heine-na.com
Web site: www.heine.com
Total Employees: 25   *Marketing Staff:* 3   *Sales Staff:* 12
Ownership: HEINE OPTOTECHNIK
Quality System Registration Information: ISO9000
Produces/Sells CE-marked Devices: Y
Distribution: Manufacturer Through Distributor
General Admin.: Ben St. Jean/General Manager
Mktg./Adv.: Christian Berling/Director Marketing
         Richard James/Manager National Sales
   Telescope, Hand-Held, Low-Vision   Ophthalmology
   Telescope, Laryngeal-Bronchial   Ear/Nose/Throat

HEINKE TECHNOLOGY, INC.
See Heinke Technoogy, Inc. (Hti Plastics)

HEINKE TECHNOOGY, INC. (HTI PLASTICS)   800-824-0607
5120 N.W. 38th St., Lincoln, NE 68524   402-470-2600
FDA Number: 1925276   Fax: 402-470-2929
E-mail: jdobbs@htiplastic.com
Web site: www.htiplastic.com
Medical Products Sales Volume: $8,500,000
Annual Revenue: $5-$10 Million
Year Founded: 1985
Total Employees: 130   *Marketing Staff:* 2   *Sales Staff:* 4
Ownership: PLASTIC COMPANIES ENTERPRISES
Quality System Registration Information: ISO9001
Produces/Sells CE-marked Devices: Y
Federal Procurement Eligibility: Small Business
Distribution: Manufacturer Through Manufacturer Reps, OEM, Exporter
General Admin.: Paul Almburg/President, Chief Executive Officer

HEINKE TECHNOOGY, INC. (HTI PLASTICS)   800-824-0607
(cont'd)
Mktg./Adv.: Debora L. Wilcox/Director Marketing
     Judy Grant/Manager Market Research
     Cathy Hietbrink/Manager National Sales
Finance: Sheli Carpenter/Manager Finance
   Applicator, Vaginal   Obstetrics/Gynecology

HELENA LABORATORIES   409-842-3714
Point of Care Division, PO Box 752, Beaumont, TX 77704-0752
FDA Number: 1618982   *Fax:* 409-842-2703
E-mail: pointofcare@helena.com
Web site: www.helena.com
Medical Products Sales Volume: $84,100,000
Year Founded: 1966
Total Employees: 1000   *Marketing Staff:* 10   *Sales Staff:* 30
Ownership: Private
Stock Symbol: ASD
Traded On: NYSE
Quality System Registration Information: ISO9001
Produces/Sells CE-marked Devices: Y
Federal Procurement Eligibility: GSA Contract
Distribution: Manufacturer Direct, Manufacturer Through Distributor, Manufacturer Through Manufacturer Reps
General Admin.: Tipton Golias/Chief Executive Officer
Mktg./Adv.: Sharon Mathews/Director Marketing
     Terry Falgeut/Director National Accounts
     Joe Golias/Vice President Marketing
Production: Marc Barclay/Manager Regulatory Affairs
     Eric Petersen/Vice President Manufacturing

2, 4-dinitrophenylhydrazine, Lactate Dehydrogenase	Chemistry
Analyzer, Chemistry, Enzyme	Chemistry
Analyzer, Chemistry, Multi-Channel, Programmable	Chemistry
Analyzer, Chemistry, Single Channel, Programmable	Chemistry
Analyzer, Coagulation	Hematology
Antigen, Antiserum, Control, Haptoglobin	Immunology
Antigen, Antiserum, Control, IGA	Immunology
Antigen, Antiserum, Control, IGD	Immunology
Antigen, Antiserum, Control, IGE	Immunology
Antigen, Antiserum, Control, IGG (Gamma Chain Specific)	Immunology
Antigen, Antiserum, Control, IGM (Mu Chain Specific)	Immunology
Antigen, Antiserum, Control, Kappa	Immunology
Antigen, Antiserum, Control, Lambda	Immunology
Antigen, Antiserum, Control, Prealbumin	Immunology
Antigen, Antiserum, Control, Whole Human Serum	Immunology
Buffer, pH	Hematology
Chart, Anatomical Training	General
Chromatographic Separation, Lecithin-Sphingomyelin Ratio	Chemistry
Chromatography Equipment, Thin Layer	Toxicology
Control, Analyte (Assayed And Unassayed)	Chemistry
Control, Coagulation, Plasma	Hematology
Control, Enzyme (Assayed And Unassayed)	Chemistry
Control, Hemoglobin, Abnormal	Hematology
Control, Multi Analyte, All Kinds (Assayed And Unassayed)	Chemistry
Control, Plasma, Abnormal	Hematology
Densitometer	Cardiovascular
Densitometer, Laboratory	Chemistry
Densitometer/Scanner (Integrating, Reflectance, TLC, Radio)	Chemistry
Electrophoresis Equipment, Cellulose Acetate Membrane	Chemistry
Electrophoresis Equipment, Gel	Chemistry
Electrophoresis Instrumentation	Immunology
Electrophoretic Separation, Alkaline Phosphatase Isoenzymes	Chemistry
Electrophoretic Separation, Lipoproteins	Chemistry
Electrophoretic, Glucose-6-Phosphate Dehydrogenase	Hematology
Electrophoretic, Lactate Dehydrogenase Isoenzymes	Chemistry
Electrophoretic, Protein Fractionation	Chemistry
Enzymatic Method, Blood, Occcult, Fecal	Chemistry
Equipment, Immunoelectrophoresis, Rocket	Immunology
Fluorometric Method, CPK Or Isoenzymes	Chemistry
Glucose-6-Phosphate Dehydrogenase (Erythrocytic), Electro	Hematology
Hemoglobin A2 Quantitation	Hematology
Immundiffusion Equipment (Agar Cutter)	Chemistry
Immunoelectrophoretic, Immunoglobulins, (G, A, M)	Chemistry
Pipette Tip	Chemistry
Pipette, Micro	Chemistry
Plasma, Control, Normal	Hematology
Plate, Agar, Ouchterlony	Immunology
Plate, Radial Immunodiffusion	Immunology
Prothrombin Time	Hematology
Quantitation, Hemoglobin, Abnormal	Hematology
Reagent, Cholesterol (Total Test System)	Chemistry
Stain, Other	Pathology
Stain, Ponceau, Hematology	Hematology
Standard/Control, Fibrinogen Determination	Hematology
Standard/Control, Hemoglobin, Normal/Abnormal	Hematology
System, Determination, Fibrinogen	Hematology
Test, Heparin (Clotting Time)	Hematology

Medical Product Subsidiaries (Listed Separately)
   Helena Plastics

HELENA LABORATORIES   409-842-3714 *(cont'd)*
Labcon North America

HELENA PLASTICS   800-227-1727
3700 Lakeville Highway, Suite 200,   707-766-2103
Petaluma, CA 94954
FDA Number: n/a   *Fax:* 707-766-2199
E-mail: tmoulton@labcon.com
Web site: www.helenaplastics.com
Medical Products Sales Volume: $2,000,000
Ownership: Helena Laboratories
Quality System Registration Information: ISO9001
Produces/Sells CE-marked Devices: N
Federal Procurement Eligibility: Small Business
Distribution: Manufacturer Through Distributor, Manufacturer Through Manufacturer Reps
Mktg./Adv.: Tom Moulton/Director Marketing

Container, Urine Specimen	General
Labware, Basic, Disposable	Chemistry
Pipette Tip	Chemistry

HELICOS BIOSCIENCES CORPORATION   877-243-5426
One Kendall Square, Ste. 7301,   617-264-1800
Cambridge, MA 02139
FDA Number: n/a   *Fax:* 617-264-1700
Web site: www.helicosbio.com
Ownership: Private
Produces/Sells CE-marked Devices: N
General Admin.: Mr. Jeffrey Moore/Chief Financial Officer, Senior Vice President
     Dr. Patrice Milos/Chief Scientific Officer
     Dr. William Efcavitch/Chief Technology Officer
     Mr. Ivan Trifunovich/President, Chief Executive Officer, Chairman
Mktg./Adv.: Mr. Marc Levine/Senior Vice President Product Development

HELIO BALANCE   425-453-9849
13000 Bel-red Rd., #207, Bellevue, WA 98005
FDA Number: 3033031
   Booth, Sun Tan   Physical Med

HELIO MEDICAL SUPPLIES, INC.   408-433-3355
606 Charcot Ave., San Jose, CA 95131
FDA Number: 2950885

Applier, Pressure, Physical Medicine	Physical Med
Needle, Acupuncture, Single Use	General

HELITREX
See Integra Lifesciences Holdings Corp.

HELIX MEDICAL, INC.   800-266-4421
1110 Mark Avenue, Carpinteria, CA 93013-2918   805-684-3304
FDA Number: 2025182   *Fax:* 805-684-1934
E-mail: sales@helixmed.com
Web site: www.helixmed.com
Medical Products Sales Volume: $20,000,000
Annual Revenue: $10-$25 Million
Year Founded: 1984
Total Employees: 150   *Marketing Staff:* 5   *Sales Staff:* 4
Ownership: Private
Quality System Registration Information: ISO9001
Produces/Sells CE-marked Devices: N
Federal Procurement Eligibility: Small Business
Distribution: Manufacturer Direct, Manufacturer Through Distributor, OEM, Exporter
General Admin.: Ed Jesle/Chief Financial Officer, Executive Vice President
     Ed Seder/President, Chief Executive Officer
     Monetta Williams/Vice President Human Resources
Mktg./Adv.: Sean McPherson/Director National Accounts
     Cathy Fletcher/Manager Advertising
     Tom Vassallo/Manager International & National Sales
     Tom Vassallo/Vice President Marketing & Sales
Production: Carol Gauthier/Vice President Manufacturing
     Cindy Anderson/Vice President Quality Assurance
Research: Dan Pasterick/Vice President Research & Development & Engineering

Component, Silicone	General
Contract Manufacturing	General
Molding, Custom	General
Prosthesis, Laryngeal (Taub)	Ear/Nose/Throat
Service, Engineering/Design	General
Tubing, Silicone	General

HELLIGE INC.
See Orbeco Analytical Systems, Inc.

HELMER, INC.   800-743-5637
15425 Herriman Blvd., Noblesville, IN 46060   317-773-9073
FDA Number: 2182537   *Fax:* 317-773-9082
E-mail: sales@helmerinc.com
Web site: www.helmerinc.com
Medical Products Sales Volume: $6,500,000

HELMER, INC.   800-743-5637 *(cont'd)*

Year Founded: 1977
Total Employees: 85
Ownership: Private
Produces/Sells CE-marked Devices: Y
Federal Procurement Eligibility: Small Business, GSA Contract
Distribution: Manufacturer Direct, Exporter

Centrifuge, Cell Washing, Automated, Immuno-Hematology	Hematology
Centrifuge, General (Up to 5,000 rpm)	Pathology
Chamber, Environmental, Platelet Storage	Hematology
Freezer, Blood Storage	Hematology
Freezer, Laboratory, Biological	Chemistry
Refrigerator, Blood Bank	Hematology
Refrigerator, Laboratory	General
Refrigerator, Pharmacy	General

HELP U LIFT   702-435-9001

5653 Wheatfield Drive, Las Vegas, NV 89120
FDA Number: 3005950956
Ownership: Private
Produces/Sells CE-marked Devices: N

Lift, Patient	General

HELPING HAND TRAYS   303-781-4019

4351 S. Galapago, Englewood, CO 80110-5624
FDA Number: 5233256   *Fax:* 303-781-4019
E-mail: kanolhht@uswest.net
Web site: www.inmax.com (password 1121)
Year Founded: 1968
Total Employees: 1   *Sales Staff:* 1
Ownership: Private
Produces/Sells CE-marked Devices: N
Federal Procurement Eligibility: Small Business, Female Owned
Distribution: Manufacturer Direct, Manufacturer Through Distributor, Service Direct, Exclusive Distributor
General Admin.: Kay Kohler/Owner

Accessories, Wheelchair	Physical Med
Tray, Walker	General

HELVETIA DEVELOPMENT CO. LLC.   269-345-1620

225 Parson's St., Kalamazoo, MI 49007
FDA Number: 1835834

Accessories, Wheelchair	Physical Med

HELVOET PHARMA, INC.   856-663-2202

9012 Pennsauken Hwy., Pennsauken, NJ 08110
FDA Number: n/a   *Fax:* 856-663-2636
E-mail: info@helvoetpharma.be
Web site: helvoetpharma.com
Year Founded: 1970
Total Employees: 1250
Ownership: Helvoet Pharma Del Yium Nv
Traded On: Switzerland
Quality System Registration Information: ISO9002
Produces/Sells CE-marked Devices: N
Federal Procurement Eligibility: Small Business
General Admin.: Guido Wallraff/President

Cover, Other	General
Dropper, Medicine	General
Equipment, Device Coating, Protective	General
Molding, Custom	General
Nipple, Feeding	General
Stopper	General
Syringe, Piston	General

HELY AND WEBER   800-221-5465

1185 East Main St., Santa Paula, CA 93060
FDA Number: 2031466   *Fax:* 800-559-5975
E-mail: info@hely-weber.com
Web site: www.hely-weber.com
Annual Revenue: $10-$25 Million
Year Founded: 1987
Total Employees: 40   *Marketing Staff:* 3   *Sales Staff:* 100
Ownership: Private
Produces/Sells CE-marked Devices: N
Federal Procurement Eligibility: Small Business
Distribution: Manufacturer Direct, Manufacturer Through Manufacturer Reps
General Admin.: John Hely/Chief Executive Officer
     Jim Weber/President
Mktg./Adv.: Mike Bellio/Director Product Development
     Rose Gregory/Manager Advertising
     Jim Buckhout/Manager International & National Sales

Orthosis, Limb Brace	Physical Med

HEMA DIAGNOSTIC SYSTEMS, LLC   954-919-5123

10102 USA Today Way, Miramar, FL 33025
FDA Number: n/a   *Fax:* 954-374-6345
E-mail: info@rapid123.com
Web site: http://www.rapid123.com

HEMA DIAGNOSTIC SYSTEMS, LLC   954-919-5123 *(cont'd)*

Medical Products Sales Volume: $4,600,000
Year Founded: 2000
Total Employees: 11   *Marketing Staff:* 3   *Sales Staff:* 2
Ownership: Private
Produces/Sells CE-marked Devices: N
Federal Procurement Eligibility: Small Business
Distribution: Manufacturer Direct, Manufacturer Through Distributor, Manufacturer Through Manufacturer Reps, OEM
General Admin.: Lawrence Salvo/Chief Executive Officer, Chairman
     Dr. Paul Slowey/Executive Vice President
Production: Ashley Gidley/Coord. Regulatory Affairs
Finance: Luis Agudelo/Director Finance

Hepatitis B Test (B Core, BE Antigen & Antibody, B Core IGM)	Microbiology
Kit, Gonorrhoeae Test (Male Use)	Microbiology
Kit, Mycobacteria Identification	Microbiology
Pipette, Quantitative, Hematology	Hematology
Test, Antibody, Acquired Immune Deficiency Syndrome (AIDS)	Hematology
Test, Syphilis (RPR or VDRL)	Microbiology

Medical Product Subsidiaries (Listed Separately)
International Diagnostic And Medical Supply Corp.

HEMACARE CORPORATION   888-481-1538

15350 Sherman Way,, Suite 350,   818-226-1968
Van Nuys, CA 91406
FDA Number: n/a   *Fax:* 818-251-5300
E-mail: mailroom@hemacare.com
Web site: www.hemacare.com
Medical Products Sales Volume: $12,000,000
Annual Revenue: $10-$25 Million
Total Employees: 150   *Sales Staff:* 2
Ownership: Public
Stock Symbol: HEMA
Traded On: OTC Bulletin
Produces/Sells CE-marked Devices: N
Federal Procurement Eligibility: Small Business
Distribution: Service Direct
General Admin.: Alan C. Darlington/Chairman
     William D. Nicely/Chief Executive Officer
     JoAnn R. Stover/Director Admin.
     Hal I. Lieberman/President, Chief Executive Officer
     Linda McDermott/Vice President Human Resources
Medical Admin.: Joshua Levy/Medical Director
Mktg./Adv.: Richard Cupp/Manager Market Research
     Julie Harris/Manager Marketing & Sales
Production: Rosemary Tsuneta/Director Regulatory Affairs
Finance: Sharon C. Kaiser/Chief Financial Officer

Kit, Blood Donor	Hematology

HEMAGEN DIAGNOSTICS, INC.   800-436-2436

9033 Red Branch Rd., Columbia, MD 21045   443-367-5500
FDA Number: 1181055   *Fax:* 410-997-7812
E-mail: sales@hemagen.com
Web site: www.hemagen.com
Medical Products Sales Volume: $9,000,000
Annual Revenue: $10-$25 Million
Year Founded: 1985
Total Employees: 50   *Marketing Staff:* 2   *Sales Staff:* 6
Ownership: Public
Stock Symbol: HMGN
Traded On: OTC Bulletin
Produces/Sells CE-marked Devices: Y
Distribution: Manufacturer Direct, Manufacturer Through Distributor, Manufacturer Through Manufacturer Reps
General Admin.: William P. Hales/President, Chief Executive Officer

Analyzer, Chemistry, Centrifuge	Chemistry
Anti-DNA Indirect Immunofluorescent Solid Phase	Immunology
Antibody Igm, If, Cytomegalovirus Virus	Microbiology
Antibody, Anti-Smooth Muscle, Indirect Immunofluorescent	Immunology
Antibody, Antimitochondrial, Indirect Immunofluorescent	Immunology
Antibody, Antinuclear, Indirect Immunofluorescent, Antigen	Immunology
Antigen, Antiserum, Control, IGG, FITC	Immunology
Antigen, CF, (Including CF Control), Varicella-Zoster	Microbiology
Antigen, IF, Toxoplasma Gondii	Microbiology
Antigen, Indirect Hemagglutination, Herpes Simplex Virus	Microbiology
Antiparietal Antibody, Immunofluorescent, Antigen, Control	Immunology
Antisera, Fluorescent, Herpesvirus Hominis 1, 2	Microbiology
Antiserum, Fluorescent Antibody For FTA-ABS Test	Microbiology
Antiserum, Fluorescent, Chlamydia Trachomatis	Microbiology
Antiserum, Fluorescent, Mumps Virus	Microbiology
Antiserum, Fluorescent, Rubeola	Microbiology
Calibrator, Primary, Clinical Chemistry	Chemistry
Calibrator, Secondary, Clinical Chemistry	Chemistry
Catalytic Method, Amylase	Chemistry
Colorimetric Method, Lipoproteins	Chemistry
Complexone, Cresolphthalein, Calcium	Chemistry
Control, Multi Analyte, All Kinds (Assayed And Unassayed)	Chemistry
Enzymatic Esterase-Oxidase, Cholesterol	Chemistry

HEMAGEN DIAGNOSTICS, INC.   800-436-2436 *(cont'd)*

Enzymatic Method, Bilirubin	Chemistry
Enzymatic Method, Creatinine	Chemistry
Enzyme Immunoassay, Non-Radiolabeled, Total Thyroxine	Chemistry
Hexokinase, Glucose	Chemistry
Kinetic Method, Gamma-Glutamyl Transpeptidase	Chemistry
Lipase Hydrolysis/Glycerol Kinase Enzyme, Triglycerides	Chemistry
Multi Analyte Mixture, Calibrator	Chemistry
NADH Oxidation/NAD Reduction, AST/SGOT	Chemistry
Nitrophenylphosphate, Alkaline Phosphatase Or Isoenzymes	Chemistry
Radioassay, Triiodothyronine Uptake	Chemistry
Reagent, General Purpose	Pathology
Reagent, Protein, Total	Chemistry
Respiratory Syncytial Virus, Antigen, Antibody, IFA	Microbiology
Rubella, Other Assays	Microbiology
SGPT, Ultraviolet	Chemistry
Test System, Antineutrophil Cytoplasmic Antibodies (ANCA)	Immunology
Test, Infectious Mononucleosis	Immunology
Thyroglobulin, FITC, Antigen, Antiserum, Control	Immunology
U.V. Spectrometry, Theophylline	Toxicology
Urease And Glutamic Dehydrogenase, Urea Nitrogen	Chemistry
Uricase (Coulometric), Uric Acid	Chemistry

HEMATECHNOLOGIES, INC.   877-436-2835
291 Rte. 22, Suite 12, Lebanon, NJ 08833   908-823-9430
FDA Number: n/a   *Fax:* 908-823-9428
E-mail: hematek@hematek.com
Web site: www.hematek.com
Medical Products Sales Volume: $2,000,000
Annual Revenue: $1-$5 Million
Year Founded: 1980
Total Employees: 12   *Marketing Staff:* 1   *Sales Staff:* 3
Ownership: Private
Produces/Sells CE-marked Devices: Y
Federal Procurement Eligibility: Small Business
Distribution: Manufacturer Through Distributor, Manufacturer Through Manufacturer Reps
General Admin.: Stephen M. Shoemaker/President, Chief Executive Officer
Production: Ian Hunter/Manager Manufacturing
Research: Ian Hunter/Vice President Research & Development

Analyzer, Sedimentation Rate, Erythrocyte	Hematology
Bilirubinometer	Chemistry

HEMATRONIX
  See Bio-Rad Laboratories, Diagnostic Group

HEMCO CORP.   816-796-2900
111 Powell Road, Independence, MO 64056-2602
FDA Number: n/a   *Fax:* 816-796-3333
E-mail: info@HEMCOcorp.com
Web site: www.hemcocorp.com
Medical Products Sales Volume: $2,400,000
Annual Revenue: $1-$5 Million
Year Founded: 1958
Total Employees: 50   *Marketing Staff:* 1   *Sales Staff:* 22
Ownership: Private
Quality System Registration Information: ISO9001
Produces/Sells CE-marked Devices: Y
Federal Procurement Eligibility: Small Business
Distribution: Manufacturer Direct, Manufacturer Through Distributor, Manufacturer Through Manufacturer Reps, OEM, Exporter
General Admin.: Ronald E. Hill/President, Chief Executive Officer
Mktg./Adv.: David R. Campbell/Director National Accounts
  Mark Teig/Manager Advertising & Media
  David R. Campbell/Vice President Marketing & Sales
Production: Kyle Macrander/Manager Regulatory Affairs
  Walt Hatley/Vice President Manufacturing

Cabinet Casework, Laboratory	Chemistry
Cabinet, Laboratory	Chemistry
Cleanroom Equipment	General
Fountain, Eye Wash	Chemistry
Hood, Chemical	Chemistry
Hood, Fume	Toxicology
Hood, Fume, Chemical	Chemistry
Shower, Emergency	Chemistry
Table, Other	General

HEMCON MEDICAL TECHNOLOGIES, INC.   877-247-0196
10575 SW Cascade Blvd., Suite 130,   503-245-0459
Portland, OR 97223
FDA Number: 3004050854   *Fax:* 503-245-1326
E-mail: info@hemcon.com
Web site: www.hemcon.com
Medical Products Sales Volume: $12,000,000
Year Founded: 2001
Total Employees: 85
Ownership: Private
Produces/Sells CE-marked Devices: N
Federal Procurement Eligibility: Small Business

HEMCON MEDICAL TECHNOLOGIES, INC.   877-247-0196 *(cont'd)*
Distribution: Manufacturer Direct
General Admin.: Mr. Nick Hart/President
Research: Dr. Simon McCarthy/Chief Scientist
  Dr. Keith Real/Executive Vice President Research & Development

Bandage, Liquid	Surgery
Dressing, Other	General
Dressing, Wound and Burn, Hydrogel	Surgery

HEMEDEX INCORPORATED   866-436-3339
222 Third Street, Suite 0123,   617-577-1759
Cambridge, MA 02142
FDA Number: 3003730855
E-mail: info@hemedex.com   *Fax:* 617-577-9328
Web site: www.hemedex.com
Medical Products Sales Volume: $1,400,000
Year Founded: 2000
Total Employees: 14
Ownership: Private
Quality System Registration Information: ISO9001
Produces/Sells CE-marked Devices: Y
Federal Procurement Eligibility: Small Business
Distribution: Manufacturer Direct, OEM, Exporter
IS: Dr. Gregory Martin/Chief Technologist

Catheter, Biliary	Gastroenterology/Urology
Flowmeter, Blood, Intravenous	Cardiovascular
Flowmeter, Blood, Other	Cardiovascular
Monitor, Intracranial Pressure	Cns/Neurology
Probe, Blood Flow, Extravascular	Cardiovascular

HEMERUS MEDICAL, LLC.   651-635-0070
5000 Township Parkway, St. Paul, MN 55110
FDA Number: 3004405714

Kit, Administration, Intravenous	General

HEMO SAPIENS, INC.   928-202-4453
325 Lookout Dr., Sedona, AZ 86351
FDA Number: 2029373

Computer, Diagnostic, Pre-Programmed, Single-Function	Cardiovascular
Computer, Diagnostic, Programmable	Cardiovascular
Plethysmograph, Impedance	Cardiovascular

HEMO-DE, INC.   800-355-3689
2000 Whitley Rd., Keller, TX 76248   817-379-7328
FDA Number: 2023536   *Fax:* 817-431-5611
E-mail: info@hemo-de.com
Web site: www.hemo-de.com
Ownership: Private
Produces/Sells CE-marked Devices: N

Clearing Agent	Pathology

HEMOCARE
  See Mediware Information Systems, Inc.

HEMOKINETICS, INC.
  See Intellectual Property, Llc

HEMOSENSE, INC.   877-436-6444
651 River Oaks Parkway, San Jose, CA 95134   408-719-1393
FDA Number: 2954730   *Fax:* 408-719-1184
E-mail: moreinfo@hemosense.com
Web site: www.hemosense.com
Annual Revenue: $0-$1 Million
Total Employees: 20
Ownership: Alere, Inc.
Produces/Sells CE-marked Devices: Y
General Admin.: Jim Merselis/Chief Executive Officer
  Judith Blunt/Director Clinical Affairs
Mktg./Adv.: Dale Clendon/Vice President Business Development
  David Phillips/Vice President Marketing
Production: Joe Widunas/Director Engineering
  Mike Acosta/Director Quality Assurance
  Mike Acosta/Manager Regulatory Affairs
  Gary Hewett/Vice President Manufacturing

Prothrombin Time	Hematology

HEMOSTATIX MEDICAL TECHNOLOGIES, LLC   901-261-0012
8400 Wolf Lake Dr., Ste. 109, Bartlett, TN 38133
FDA Number: 3006119098

Electrosurgical Unit, Cutting & Coagulation Device	Surgery

HEMOTEC, INC.
  See Medtronic Perfusion Systems

HENDRICKS ORTHOTIC PROSTHETIC ENTERPRISES, INC.   407-850-0411
6439 Milner Blvd., Suite 6, Orlando, FL 32809
FDA Number: 3004192103

Joint, Hip, External Brace	Physical Med

MANUFACTURER PROFILES

HENDRICKS ORTHOTIC PROSTHETIC 407-850-0411 *(cont'd)*
Orthosis, Truncal/Limb — Physical Med

HENDRICKSON, INC.
See Otto Bock Heathcare

HENKE SASS WOLF OF AMERICA, INC.
See Henke Sass Wolf Of America, Inc.

HENLEY BOARD, INC. 800-874-0552
P.O. Box 92, Damascus, MD 20872 301-831-6662
FDA Number: 1121574 *Fax:* 301-865-1799
E-mail: henleyboard92@msn.com
Web site: www.henleyboard.com
Ownership: Private
Produces/Sells CE-marked Devices: N
Stretcher, Hand-Carried — General

HENNESSY DENTAL LABORATORY 800-694-6862
3709 Interstate Park Road South, Riviera Beach, FL 33404
FDA Number: n/a *Fax:* 561-844-5910
E-mail: mike@hennessydental.com
Web site: www.hdlinc.com
Medical Products Sales Volume: $1,300,000
Annual Revenue: $1-$5 Million
Year Founded: 1983
Total Employees: 24
Ownership: Private
Produces/Sells CE-marked Devices: N
Federal Procurement Eligibility: Small Business
Distribution: Manufacturer Direct, Manufacturer Through Distributor, Manufacturer Through Manufacturer Reps
General Admin.: Mr. Michael Hennessey/President, Chief Executive Officer
Crown And Bridge, Temporary, Resin — Dental And Oral
Crown, Preformed — Dental And Oral
Denture, Gold — Dental And Oral
Denture, Preformed — Dental And Oral
Teeth, Porcelain — Dental And Oral

HENRY G. DIETZ CO., INC. 718-726-7270
1426 28th Ave., Long Island City, NY 11102
FDA Number: 2435543 *Fax:* 718-728-3976
E-mail: hgdietz@lowpressure.com
Web site: www.lowpressure.com
Year Founded: 1947
Ownership: Private
Produces/Sells CE-marked Devices: N
Ventilator, Non-Continuous (Respirator) — Anesthesiology

HENRY SCHEIN ARCONA INC. 800-668-5558
345 Townline Road, PO Box 6000, 905-646-1711
Niagara-on-the-Lake, ONT L0S 1 Canada
FDA Number: n/a *Fax:* 1-905-646-4201
E-mail: info@has.ca
Web site: www.has.ca
Year Founded: 1980
Total Employees: 100
Ownership: Private
Produces/Sells CE-marked Devices: N
Distribution: Service Direct

HENRY SCHEIN, INC. 631-843-5500
135 Duryea Rd., Melville, NY 11747
FDA Number: 3004065985
Web site: www.henryschein.com
Annual Revenue: $1-$5 Million
Year Founded: 1932
Total Employees: 12500
Ownership: Private
Stock Symbol: HSIC
Traded On: NASDAQ
Quality System Registration Information: ISO9000; ISO9001
Produces/Sells CE-marked Devices: Y
Federal Procurement Eligibility: Small Business
Distribution: Manufacturer Direct, Exporter
General Admin.: Stanley M. Bergman/Chief Executive Officer, Chairman
Steven Paladino/Chief Financial Officer, Executive Vice President
Furniture, General — General

HENRY'S ACUPUNCTURE EQUIPMENT 415-337-8290
241 Leland Ave., San Francisco, CA 94134
FDA Number: 2919386
Ownership: Private
Produces/Sells CE-marked Devices: N
Needle, Acupuncture, Single Use — General

HENTHORN OCULAR PROSTHETICS 316-688-5235
744 South Hillside, Wichita, KS 67211
FDA Number: 1933222
Conformer, Ophthalmic — Ophthalmology

HENTHORN OCULAR PROSTHETICS 316-688-5235 *(cont'd)*
Eye, Artificial, Non-Custom — Ophthalmology
Shell, Scleral — Ophthalmology

HEPTEST LABORATORIES, INC. 888-314-6008
1431 Hanley Industrial Court, 314-962-3527
St. Louis, MO 63144
FDA Number: 3005021886
E-mail: info@heptest.com
Web site: www.heptest.com
Ownership: Private
Produces/Sells CE-marked Devices: N
Test, Heparin (Clotting Time) — Hematology
Test, Qualitative And Quantitative Factor Deficiency — Hematology
Test, Thrombin Time — Hematology

HER-MAR, INC. 800-327-8209
8550 N.W. 30th Terr., Miami, FL 33122 305-482-9912
FDA Number: 1042716 *Fax:* 305-482-9922
E-mail: rmayer@hermar.com
Web site: www.hermar.com
Annual Revenue: $0-$1 Million
Year Founded: 1971
Total Employees: 3 *Marketing Staff:* 1 *Sales Staff:* 1
Ownership: Private
Produces/Sells CE-marked Devices: Y
Federal Procurement Eligibility: Small Business
Distribution: Manufacturer Through Distributor, Importer, Exporter
General Admin.: Ron Mayer/President, Chief Executive Officer
Blade, Scalpel — Surgery
Cover, Thermometer — General
Cuff, Blood Pressure — Cardiovascular
Cutter, Cast, AC-Powered — Orthopedics
Electrocardiograph, Single Channel — Cardiovascular
Electrocautery Unit, Line-Powered — Surgery
Hammer, Neurological — Cns/Neurology
Hammer, Percussion — Cns/Neurology
Laryngoscope, Rigid — Anesthesiology
Monitor, Blood Pressure, Indirect, Automatic — Cardiovascular
Monitor, Fetal Doppler Ultrasound — Obstetrics/Gynecology
Monitor, Pulse Rate — Anesthesiology
Ophthalmoscope, Battery-Powered — Ophthalmology
Otoscope — Ear/Nose/Throat
Speculum, Vaginal, Metal — Obstetrics/Gynecology
Sphygmomanometer, Electronic, Automatic — General
Sphygmomanometer, Electronic, Manual — General
Sphygmomanometer, Mercury (Arterial Pressure) — General
Sterilizer, Dry Heat, Dental — Dental And Oral
Stethoscope, Electronic (Auscultoscope) — Cardiovascular
Stethoscope, Mechanical — General
Surgical Instrument, Disposable — Surgery
Surgical Instrument, Manual (General Use) — Surgery

HERAEUS KULZER, INC. 800-431-1785
99 Business Park Drive, 914-273-8600
Armonk, NY 10504
FDA Number: 2428288 *Fax:* 914-273-9379
E-mail: info@kulzer.com
Web site: www.heraeus-kulzer-us.com
Medical Products Sales Volume: $90,500,000
Annual Revenue: $50-$100 Million
Year Founded: 1851
Total Employees: 210 *Marketing Staff:* 4 *Sales Staff:* 48
Ownership: Heraeus GmbH
Stock Symbol: LANZ
Quality System Registration Information: ISO9001
Produces/Sells CE-marked Devices: Y
Federal Procurement Eligibility: Small Business, GSA Contract, VA Contract
Distribution: Manufacturer Through Distributor
General Admin.: Gerrit Steen/President
Mktg./Adv.: Warren Rogers/Vice President Sales
Alloy, Gold Based, For Clinical Use — Dental And Oral
Alloy, Precious Metal, For Clinical Use — Dental And Oral
Attachment, Precision — Dental And Oral
Material, Acrylic, Dental — Dental And Oral
Material, Investment — Dental And Oral
Powder, Porcelain — Dental And Oral
Wax, Dental — Dental And Oral

HERAEUS KULZER, INC., DENTAL PRODUCTS DIVISION 574-299-6662
4315 South Lafayette Blvd., South Bend, IN 46614
FDA Number: 1925223
Ownership: Private
Produces/Sells CE-marked Devices: N
Clamp, Rubber Dam — Dental And Oral
Cleaner, Medical Device — General
Dam, Rubber — Dental And Oral
Disk, Abrasive — Dental And Oral

HERAEUS KULZER, INC., DENTAL PRODUCTS   574-299-6662
(cont'd)

Forceps, Rubber Dam Clamp	Dental And Oral
Material, Investment	Dental And Oral
Mouthpiece, Saliva Ejector	Dental And Oral
Paper, Articulation	Dental And Oral
Wax, Dental	Dental And Oral
Wheel, Polishing Agent	Dental And Oral

HERAEUS LASERSONICS, INC.
See Ams Innovative Center-San Jose

HERAEUS SURGICAL, INC.
See Ams Innovative Center-San Jose

HERB WINSTON ASSOCIATES, INC.
See All Pro Exercise Products, Inc.

HERBSTHELP, CORP.   702-245-6958
2917 Linkview Dr., Las Vegas, NV 89134
FDA Number: 3003526424
Ownership: Private
Produces/Sells CE-marked Devices: N

Bracket, Metal, Orthodontic	Dental And Oral
Retainer, Screw Expansion, Orthodontic	Dental And Oral

HERCEG INC., T.F.
See Surehands Lift & Care Systems

HERCON LABORATORIES CORP.   717-764-1191
101 Sinking Springs Ln., Emigsville, PA 17318
                  Fax: 717-764-5395
FDA Number: 2522638
E-mail: info@herconlabs.com
Web site: www.granardrx.com
Medical Products Sales Volume: $9,700,000
Annual Revenue: $10-$25 Million
Year Founded: 1985
Total Employees: 50   *Marketing Staff:* 2
Ownership: Hercon Laboratories Corp.
Stock Symbol: hclc
Traded On: NASDAQ
Produces/Sells CE-marked Devices: N
Federal Procurement Eligibility: Small Business
Distribution: Manufacturer Through Manufacturer Reps
General Admin.: Mr. Ken Brody/Chief Executive Officer

Dressing, Other	General

Medical Product Subsidiaries (Listed Separately)
Hercon Laboratories Corp.

HERCULITE PRODUCTS, INC.   800-772-0036
P.O. Box 435, Emigsville, PA 17318   717-764-1192
                  Fax: 717-764-5211
FDA Number: 9200533
E-mail: customercare@hercullite.com
Web site: www.herculite.com
Annual Revenue: $25-$50 Million
Total Employees: 100   *Marketing Staff:* 2   *Sales Staff:* 20
Ownership: Private
Produces/Sells CE-marked Devices: N
Federal Procurement Eligibility: Small Business
Distribution: Manufacturer Through Manufacturer Reps
General Admin.: Peter F. McKernan/President, Chief Executive Officer
Mktg./Adv.: William O. Wanner/Vice President Sales

Cover, Cart	General
Cover, Laundry Hamper	General
Cover, Mattress	General
Cover, Mattress, Conductive	General
Cover, Mattress, Waterproof	General
Curtain, Cubicle	General
Curtain, Shower	General
Mattress, Bed	General
Mattress, Operating Table	General
Pillow	General
Pillow, Cervical	Orthopedics
Screen, Bedside	General

HERITAGE LABS INTL., LLC   913-764-1045
1111 West Old 56 Hwy., Olathe, KS 66061
                  Fax: 913-764-3372
FDA Number: 1932057
E-mail: heritagethelab@heritagelabs.com
Web site: www.heritagelabs.com
Medical Products Sales Volume: $5,800,000
Year Founded: 1998
Total Employees: 150   *Marketing Staff:* 2   *Sales Staff:* 3
Ownership: Private
Stock Symbol: HH
Traded On: AMEX
Produces/Sells CE-marked Devices: N
Federal Procurement Eligibility: Small Business
Distribution: Manufacturer Direct, Service Direct

Container, Specimen Mailer And Storage	Pathology

HERITAGE LABS INTL., LLC   913-764-1045 *(cont'd)*

Container, Specimen Mailer And Storage, Temperature Control	Pathology

HERITAGE MEDCALL   800-396-6157
202 E. Virginia Ave., Tampa, FL 33603   813-221-1000
                  Fax: 813-223-1405
FDA Number: n/a
E-mail: email@heritagemedcall.com
Web site: www.heritagemedcall.com
Annual Revenue: $1-$5 Million
Total Employees: 5   *Marketing Staff:* 1   *Sales Staff:* 1
Ownership: Private
Produces/Sells CE-marked Devices: N
Federal Procurement Eligibility: Small Business
Distribution: Manufacturer Through Distributor
General Admin.: Donald R. Musselman/President
Mktg./Adv.: John Thomas/Director Product Development
         Garrison Collins/Manager National Sales
Production: John Thomas/Vice President Manufacturing

Communication System, Emergency Alert, Personal	General

HERITAGE MEDICAL PRODUCTS, INC   417-256-3628
10380 Cr 6310, Lanton, MO 65775
FDA Number: 3003881889

Bed, Electric	General

HERMAN MILLER FOR HEALTHCARE
See Herman Miller, Inc.

HERMAN MILLER, INC.   616-654-3000
855 East Main Ave., P.O. Box 302, Zeeland, MI 49464
FDA Number: n/a
Web site: www.hermanmiller.com
Medical Products Sales Volume: $109,000,000
Annual Revenue: More than $1 Billion
Total Employees: 6292
Ownership: Public
Stock Symbol: MLHR
Traded On: NASDAQ
Produces/Sells CE-marked Devices: N
Distribution: Manufacturer Direct
General Admin.: Michael A. Volkema/Chairman
         Curtis S. Pullen/Chief Financial Officer, Executive Vice President
         Andrew J. Lock/Executive Vice President
         Charles J. Vranian/Executive Vice President
         Elizabeth A. Nickels/Executive Vice President
         Gary S. Miller/Executive Vice President
         John P. Portlock/Executive Vice President
         Kristen L. Manos/Executive Vice President
         Brian C. Walker/President, Chief Executive Officer
         James E. Christenson/Senior Vice President
Production: Kenneth L. Goodson/Executive Vice President Operations
Research: Donald D. Goeman/Executive Vice President Research & Development
Finance: Joseph M. Nowicki/Vice President, Treasurer

Bin, Storage	General
Cabinet Casework, Laboratory	Chemistry
Cabinet Casework, Modular	General
Cabinet Casework, Pharmacy	General
Cabinet, Storage, Endoscope	Gastroenterology/Urology
Cart, Anesthetist's	Anesthesiology
Cart, Emergency, Cardiopulmonary Resuscitation (Crash)	Anesthesiology
Cart, Equipment, Video	General
Cart, Isolation	General
Cart, Medicine	General
Cart, Multipurpose	General
Cart, Orthopedic Supply (Cast)	Orthopedics
Cart, Other	General
Cart, Supply	General
Cart, Supply, Operating Room	Surgery
Chair, Other	General
Furniture, Patient Room	General
Station, Nursing	General

HERMANSON DENTAL   800-328-9648
1055 Highway 36 East, Saint Paul, MN 55109   651-483-6611
                  Fax: 651-415-0275
FDA Number: 3005840237
E-mail: hermanson@dtidental.com
Web site: www.hermansondti.com
Year Founded: 1950
Ownership: DENTAL TECHNOLOGIES, INC.
Produces/Sells CE-marked Devices: N

Denture, Plastic, Teeth	Dental And Oral
Denture, Preformed	Dental And Oral
Retainer, Dental	Dental And Oral
Teeth, Porcelain	Dental And Oral

HERMELL PRODUCTS, INC.   800-233-2342
9 Britton Drive, PO Box 7345,   860-242-6550
Bloomfield, CT 06002
FDA Number: 1217997   Fax: 860-243-0361

HERMELL PRODUCTS, INC. 800-233-2342 (cont'd)
E-mail: hermell@hermell.com
Web site: www.hermell.com
Medical Products Sales Volume: $4,200,000
Annual Revenue: $1-$5 Million
Year Founded: 1969
Total Employees: 38   *Marketing Staff:* 1   *Sales Staff:* 2
Ownership: Private
Produces/Sells CE-marked Devices: N
Federal Procurement Eligibility: Small Business
Distribution: Manufacturer Direct, Manufacturer Through Manufacturer Reps
General Admin.: Ronald Pollack/President, Chief Executive Officer
Mktg./Adv.: Ron Perrott/Manager Contract Sales
Production: Pierre Z/Manager Materials

Bandage, Other	General
Belt, Rib (Support)	Orthopedics
Binder, Wrist	Orthopedics
Collar, Cervical Neck	Orthopedics
Cushion, Other	General
Cushion, Ring, Foam Rubber	General
Cushion, Ring, Inflatable	General
Cushion, Wheelchair (Pad)	Physical Med
Extrication Equipment	General
Immobilizer, Shoulder	Orthopedics
Leg Rest	General
Linen	General
Pad, Pressure, Air	General
Pad, Pressure, Foam (Elbow, Heel)	General
Pad, Pressure, Foam Convoluted	General
Pillow	General
Pillow, Cervical	Orthopedics
Protector, Heel	General
Shield, Bunion	Orthopedics
Sling, Arm	Physical Med
Stockinette	Orthopedics
Stocking, Support (Anti-Embolic)	General
Support, Ankle	Orthopedics
Support, Elbow	Orthopedics
Support, Hand	Orthopedics
Support, Knee	Physical Med
Support, Leg	Physical Med
Support, Thigh	Physical Med
Support, Wrist	Physical Med

HERRCO ENTERPRISES, INC.
See Concepts International, Inc.

HERSCO ARCH PRODUCTS CORP.
See Hersco Ortho Labs

HERSCO ORTHO LABS 718-391-0416
39-28 Crescent St., Long Island City, NY 11101
FDA Number: n/a   *Fax:* 718-391-0406
E-mail: seamus@hersco.com
Web site: www.hersco.com
Annual Revenue: $1-$5 Million
Total Employees: 20   *Marketing Staff:* 1   *Sales Staff:* 1
Ownership: Private
Produces/Sells CE-marked Devices: N
Federal Procurement Eligibility: Small Business
Distribution: Manufacturer Direct
General Admin.: Cathal Kennedy/Chief Executive Officer, Chief Operating Officer
James Kennedy/President

Orthosis, Other	Physical Med

HESKA CORPORATION 800-GO HESKA
3760 Rocky Mountain Ave, Loveland, CO 80538 970-493-7272
FDA Number: n/a   *Fax:* 970-619-3008
E-mail: market@heska.com
Web site: www.heska.com
Total Employees: 299
Ownership: Public
Stock Symbol: HSKA
Traded On: NASDAQ
Produces/Sells CE-marked Devices: N
General Admin.: Robert B. Grieve/Chief Executive Officer, Chairman
Jason A. Napolitano/Chief Financial Officer, Executive Vice President
Dr. Michael McGinley/Chief Operating Officer
Mktg./Adv.: Ms. Claudine Zachara,/Vice President Marketing & Communications
G. Lynn Snodgrass/Vice President Sales

HESSLER ENTERPRISES, INC.
See Hessler Forms & Labels

HESSLER FORMS & LABELS 800-346-1304
106 Susan Dr., Unit #1, Elkins Park, PA 19027 215-379-2300
FDA Number: n/a   *Fax:* 215-663-8839
E-mail: info@hessler.com
Web site: www.hessler.com
Annual Revenue: $1-$5 Million

HESSLER FORMS & LABELS 800-346-1304 (cont'd)
Total Employees: 7
Ownership: HESSLER ENTERPRISES, INC.
Produces/Sells CE-marked Devices: N
Federal Procurement Eligibility: Small Business
Distribution: Exclusive Distributor
General Admin.: Edwin S. Hessler/President
Brian D. Hessler/Vice President
Mktg./Adv.: Sharon Mancuso/Manager National Sales
Jackie Zandlli/Sales Representative

Forms, Medical And Patient	General
Office Equipment	General
Office Product	General

HETCO
See Omni International, Inc.

HETTICH ZENTRIFUGEN
See Omni International, Inc.

HEUMANN & ASSOCIATES DENTAL LAB 800-255-2412
520 East Fifth St., Topeka, KS 66607 785-235-9293
FDA Number: 1981041   *Fax:* 785-235-0978
E-mail: ddittmer@dentalservices.net
Web site: www.dentalservices.net
Ownership: Private
Produces/Sells CE-marked Devices: N

Crown, Preformed	Dental And Oral
Device, Anti-Snoring	Ear/Nose/Throat
Device, Repositioning, Jaw	Dental And Oral
Mouthguard	Dental And Oral

HEWLETT-PACKARD CO., LITTLE FALLS SITE
See Agilent Technologies, Inc.

HEWLETT-PACKARD COMPANY 408-472-2702
20555 State Highway 249, Houston, TX 77070
FDA Number: 3004098813
Ownership: Hewlett-Packard Co.

Device, Storage, Image, Digital	Radiology

HEX FF INC.
See Hex Laboratory Systems

HEX LABORATORY SYSTEMS 800-729-2085
1042B El Camino Real, Ste. 308, 336-584-4010
Encinitas, CA 92024
FDA Number: n/a   *Fax:* 800-959-5696
E-mail: info@hexlab.com
Web site: www.hexlab.com
Medical Products Sales Volume: $1,000,000
Annual Revenue: $0-$1 Million
Total Employees: 15   *Marketing Staff:* 2   *Sales Staff:* 2
Ownership: Private
Produces/Sells CE-marked Devices: N
Distribution: Manufacturer Direct, Manufacturer Through Distributor, Service Direct, Exporter
General Admin.: Mel Brandel/President, Chief Executive Officer
Susan Bollinger/Vice President, General Manager
Mktg./Adv.: Susan Bollinger/Director Marketing
Dan Simmons/Director Product Development
Susan Bollinger/Vice President Sales
Production: Phillip Rois/Director Quality Assurance

Computer Software	General

HEYER AMERICA, INC. 703-506-0040
1320 Old Chain Bridge Rd., Suite 405, Mclean, VA 22101
FDA Number: 1122990
Ownership: Private
Produces/Sells CE-marked Devices: N

Pump, Nebulizer, Electric	Ear/Nose/Throat

HEYER-SCHULTE MED. OPTICS
See Allergan

HF PURE WATER 800-421-5000
203 W. Artesia Blvd., Compton, CA 90220-5550 310-605-0755
FDA Number: n/a   *Fax:* 310-608-1181
E-mail: support@houstonfearless.com
Web site: www.hfpurewater.com
Annual Revenue: $0-$1 Million
Ownership: Private
Produces/Sells CE-marked Devices: Y
Federal Procurement Eligibility: Small Business
Distribution: Manufacturer Through Distributor
General Admin.: James Lee/President
Production: Richard Choi/Chemical Engineer
Vince Jose/Process Engineer

Processor, Radiographic Film, Automatic	Radiology

HGM MEDICAL LASER SYSTEMS, INC.
See Lumenis Inc.

HI-TECH RUBBER, INC.
800-924-4832
714-632-7710
3191 E. La Palma Avenue, Anaheim, CA 92806
Fax: 714-632-5647
FDA Number: 2027934
E-mail: techteam@hitech1.com
Web site: www.hitechrubber.com
Medical Products Sales Volume: $64,600,000
Year Founded: 2004
Total Employees: 400 *Marketing Staff:* 1 *Sales Staff:* 7
Ownership: Private
Quality System Registration Information: ISO9002
Produces/Sells CE-marked Devices: N
Federal Procurement Eligibility: Small Business
Distribution: Manufacturer Direct
General Admin.: Ken Lester/Chairman
        Jim Brown/Executive Vice President
        Bill Sherman/President

Bag, Breathing	Anesthesiology
Component, Rubber	General
Component, Silicone	General
Contract Manufacturing	General
Molding, Custom	General
Nipple, Feeding	General
Tubing, Silicone	General

HIATT METAL PRODUCTS
765-284-8351
720 West Willard St., Muncie, IN 47302
FDA Number: 1836115
Ownership: Private
Produces/Sells CE-marked Devices: N

Orthopedic Manual Surgical Instrument	Orthopedics

HICKMAN INC., DOW. B.
See Mylan Pharmaceuticals Inc

HIGA MANUFACTURING LTD.
604-922-5261
Po Box 91160 Stn West Vancouver,
West Vancouver V7V 3 Canada
FDA Number: 8022001

Remover, Crown	Dental And Oral

HIGGS MEDICAL PRODUCTS, LLC
973-625-4424
21 Pine St., Suite 109, Rockaway, NJ 07866
FDA Number: 3002864376
Ownership: Private
Produces/Sells CE-marked Devices: N

Adapter, Hygiene	Physical Med

HIGH EFFICIENCY FILTER CORP.
See Airguard

HIGH FREQUENCY TECHNOLOGY CO., INC.
800-342-3020
631-242-3020
172 Brook Ave., Deer Park, NY 11729
Fax: 631-242-4823
FDA Number: n/a
E-mail: Info@HFTInc.com
Web site: www.hftinc.com
Medical Products Sales Volume: $2,500,000
Annual Revenue: $1-$5 Million
Total Employees: 25 *Sales Staff:* 3
Ownership: Private
Produces/Sells CE-marked Devices: N
Federal Procurement Eligibility: Small Business
Distribution: OEM
General Admin.: Andrew Amabile/President

Buffer, pH	Hematology
Production Equipment	General

HIGH PHOENIX, INC.
886-422-5567
1124 Wrigley Way, Milpitas, CA 95035
FDA Number: n/a
Ownership: Private
Produces/Sells CE-marked Devices: N

Accessories, Wheelchair	Physical Med
Attachment, Commode, Wheelchair	Physical Med
Band, Support, Pelvic	Physical Med
Brace, Joint, Ankle (External)	Physical Med
Cane	Physical Med
Crutch	Physical Med
Insoles, Medical	General
Splint, Hand, And Component	Physical Med
Support, Column, GLC	Toxicology
Walker, Mechanical, Poly Vinyl Chloride (pvc)	Physical Med

HIGH RISE RECYCLING
See Wilkinson Hi-Rise

HIGH TECHNOLOGY SYSTEMS INC.
See Peregrine Pharmaceuticals, Inc.

HIGH TECHSPLANATIONS
See Immersion Medical

HIGHLAND LABS, INC.
508-429-2918
42 B Pope Road, Holliston, MA 01746-2218
Fax: 508-429-6282
FDA Number: 1217664
E-mail: info@highlandlabs.com
Web site: www.highlandlabs.com
Annual Revenue: $1-$5 Million
Year Founded: 1953
Total Employees: 30 *Marketing Staff:* 1 *Sales Staff:* 3
Ownership: Private
Produces/Sells CE-marked Devices: N
Federal Procurement Eligibility: Small Business, GSA Contract, VA Contract
Distribution: Manufacturer Direct, OEM, Exporter
General Admin.: Mr. Peter Lewis/President
Mktg./Adv.: Mr. Jim Bengiovanni/Vice President Sales
Production: Mr. Peter Lewis/General Manager Operations

Dispenser, Fluid	General
Dispenser, Soap	General
Scale, Blood	Hematology
Sink, Hospital	General

HIGHLAND METALS, INC.
800-368-6484
408-271-2955
419 Perrymont Drive, San Jose, CA 95125
Fax: 408-271-2962
FDA Number: 2939494
E-mail: info@highlandmetals.com
Web site: http://highlandmetals.com/
Medical Products Sales Volume: $15,000,000
Annual Revenue: $1-$5 Million
Year Founded: 1979
Total Employees: 60
Ownership: Private
Produces/Sells CE-marked Devices: Y
Federal Procurement Eligibility: Small Business
Distribution: Manufacturer Direct

Band, Elastic, Orthodontic	Dental And Oral
Clamp, Wire, Orthodontic	Dental And Oral
Spring, Orthodontic	Dental And Oral
Wire, Orthodontic	Dental And Oral

HIGHRES BIOSOLUTIONS, INC.
781.932.1912
299 Washington Street, Woburn, MA 01801
Fax: 781.938.0813
FDA Number: n/a
E-mail: sales@highresbio.com
Web site: http://www.highresbio.com
Year Founded: 2004
Ownership: Private
Produces/Sells CE-marked Devices: N
Research: Dr. Chris Pacheco/Director Technology

HILCO
800-955-6544
508-699-4406
33 W. Bacon St., Plainville, MA 02762
FDA Number: 1218954
Web site: www.hilco.com
Annual Revenue: $1-$5 Million
Year Founded: 1993
Total Employees: 180 *Marketing Staff:* 5 *Sales Staff:* 26
Ownership: Private
Produces/Sells CE-marked Devices: Y
Distribution: Manufacturer Direct, OEM, Importer, Exporter

Case, Contact Lens	Ophthalmology
Frame, Spectacle (Eyeglasses)	Ophthalmology
Goggles, Protective, Eye	Ophthalmology
Patch, Eye	Ophthalmology
Screwdriver	Orthopedics
Spectacle, Magnifier	Ophthalmology
Sunglasses (Including Photosensitive)	Ophthalmology

HILL LABORATORIES CO.
877-445-5020
610-644-2867
3 N. Bacton Hill Road, PO Box 2028,
Frazer, PA 19355
Fax: 610-647-6297
FDA Number: 2510425
E-mail: info@hilllabs.com
Web site: www.hilllabs.com
Medical Products Sales Volume: $3,100,000
Annual Revenue: $5-$10 Million
Year Founded: 1938
Total Employees: 40
Ownership: Private
Produces/Sells CE-marked Devices: Y
Federal Procurement Eligibility: Small Business, GSA Contract
Distribution: Manufacturer Direct, Manufacturer Through Distributor, Exclusive Distributor, Exporter
General Admin.: Howard A. Hill/President
Mktg./Adv.: Jim Gemmell/Manager Advertising
        Brady Aller/Vice President Marketing & Sales
Production: Brian Rickards/Executive Production

Stimulator, Ultrasound, Muscle	Physical Med
Table, Examination/Treatment	General
Table, Physical Medicine, Powered	Physical Med

MANUFACTURER PROFILES

HILL LABORATORIES CO.   877-445-5020 *(cont'd)*
Table, Physical Therapy	Physical Med
Table, Traction	Orthopedics

HILL TOP RESEARCH CORP   513-831-3114
P.o. Box 138, 6088 Main & Mill Streets, Miamiville, OH 45147
FDA Number: 1521654   *Fax:* 513-831-1217
E-mail: abrady@hill-top.com
Web site: www.hill-top.com
Ownership: Private
Produces/Sells CE-marked Devices: N
Delivery System, Allergen And Vaccine	General

HILL-MED, INC.   305-594-7474
7217 N.W. 46th St., Miami, FL 33166
FDA Number: ÿ1056771   *Fax:* 305-477-0699
E-mail: support@hillusa.com
Web site: www.hillusa.com
Medical Products Sales Volume: $370,000
Annual Revenue: $1-$5 Million
Year Founded: 1980
Total Employees: 3
Ownership: Hillusa Corp.
Produces/Sells CE-marked Devices: N
Federal Procurement Eligibility: Small Business
Distribution: Exclusive Distributor
Mktg./Adv.: Gisela Ackerman/Director Marketing
Colposcope	Obstetrics/Gynecology
Cryosurgical Unit	Surgery
Electrosurgical Unit, Cutting & Coagulation Device	Surgery
Microscope, Operating, AC-Powered, Ophthalmic	Ophthalmology
Monitor, Blood Pressure, Indirect, Automatic	Cardiovascular

HILL-ROM (LONG-TERM CARE DIVISION)
See Hill-Rom Manufacturing, Inc.

HILL-ROM COMPANY, INC.
See Hill-Rom Holdings, Inc.

HILL-ROM HOLDINGS, INC.   800-445-3730
1069 State Route 46 East, Batesville, IN 47006   812-934-7777
FDA Number: 1824206   *Fax:* 812-934-8189
Web site: www.hill-rom.com
Medical Products Sales Volume: $2,194,000,000
Annual Revenue: More than $1 Billion
Year Founded: 1929
Total Employees: 6500
Ownership: Public
Stock Symbol: HRC
Traded On: NYSE
Produces/Sells CE-marked Devices: N
Distribution: Manufacturer Direct
General Admin.: Mr. Abel Ang/Chief Technology Officer
     Mr. John Greisch/President, Chief Executive Officer
     Ms. Martha Goldberg Aronson/Senior Vice President
Mktg./Adv.: Dr. Phillip Settimi/Senior Vice President Marketing
     Ms. Susan Lichtenstein/Vice President Corporate Affairs
Finance: Mr. Gregory Miller/Chief Financial Officer
     Mr. Richard Keller/Director Accounting
Bassinet (Infant Bed)	General
Bed, Birthing	General
Bed, Electric	General
Bed, Flotation Therapy, Powered	Physical Med
Bed, Manual	General
Bed, Patient Rotation, Powered	Physical Med
Cabinet Casework, Modular	General
Cabinet, Bedside	General
Cart, Multipurpose	General
Chair, Adjustable, Mechanical	Physical Med
Chair, Other	General
Console, Patient Service	General
Furniture, Patient Room	General
Headwall System (Patient Room)	General
Infusion Stand	General
Lamp, Examination (Light)	General
Mattress, Bed	General
Mattress, Reduction, Pressure	General
Stretcher, Hydraulic	General
Stretcher, Transfer	Surgery
Table, Obstetrical	Obstetrics/Gynecology
Table, Overbed	General
Warmer, Radiant, Infant	General

Medical Product Subsidiaries (Listed Separately)
Allen Medical Systems, Inc.
Hill-Rom Manufacturing, Inc.
Hill-Rom, Inc

HILL-ROM MANUFACTURING, INC.   800-445-3730
1225 Crescent Green Dr., Suite 200,   919-854-3600
Cary, NC 27511
FDA Number: 2027454   *Fax:* 812-934-8189
E-mail: us.customerservice@hill-rom.com
Web site: www.hill-rom.com
Year Founded: 1929
Ownership: Hill-Rom Holdings, Inc.
Stock Symbol: HRC
Traded On: NYSE
Produces/Sells CE-marked Devices: N
General Admin.: Peter Soderberg/President, Chief Executive Officer
Mktg./Adv.: Lauren Green-Caldwell/Director Corporate Communications & Public Affairs
Communication System, Powered	Physical Med
Monitor, Bed Patient	General
Monitor, Perinatal	Obstetrics/Gynecology

HILL-ROM MANUFACTURING, INC.   800-638-2546
4349 Corporate Rd., Charleston, SC 29405   843-740-8000
FDA Number: 1045510   *Fax:* 843-740-8418
E-mail: us.customerservice@hill-rom.com
Web site: www.hill-rom.com
Year Founded: 1929
Ownership: Hill-Rom Holdings, Inc.
Stock Symbol: HRC
Traded On: NYSE
Quality System Registration Information: ISO9001
Produces/Sells CE-marked Devices: N
Distribution: Manufacturer Direct
General Admin.: Walt Rosebrough/Chief Executive Officer
     Mark Liebetrau/Vice President, General Manager
Mktg./Adv.: Mike Mutka/Director Marketing
     Brett Bennett/Vice President Marketing
     Joe Tallariti/Vice President Sales
Bed, Air Fluidized	Physical Med
Bed, Electric	General
Bed, Flotation Therapy, Powered	Physical Med
Bed, Patient Rotation, Powered	Physical Med
Cover, Mattress	General
Lift, Patient	General
Mattress, Air Flotation	General
Mattress, Bed	General
Mattress, Non-Powered Flotation Therapy	Physical Med
Mattress, Reduction, Pressure	General
Pad, Incontinence (Underpad)	General
Percussor, Powered	Anesthesiology
Service, Consulting	General

HILL-ROM, INC   812-934-7777
1069 State Route 46 East, Batesville, IN 47006
FDA Number: n/a   *Fax:* 812-934-8189
E-mail: us.customerservice@hill-rom.com
Web site: www.hill-rom.com
Ownership: Hill-Rom Holdings, Inc.
Stock Symbol: HRC
Traded On: NYSE
Produces/Sells CE-marked Devices: N
General Admin.: Mr. Mark Guinan/Chief Financial Officer, Executive Vice President
     Mr. Gregory Miller/Chief Financial Officer, Senior Vice President
     Mr. Abel Ang/Chief Technology Officer
     Mr. John Greisch/President, Chief Executive Officer
Finance: Mr. Richard Keller/Chief Accountant

HILL-ROM, INC.
See Hill-Rom Holdings, Inc.

HILL-ROM, INC.   812-934-7777
4115 Dorchester Rd., Unit 600, North Charleston, SC 29405
FDA Number: n/a
Web site: www.hill-rom.com
Ownership: Private
Stock Symbol: HB
Traded On: NYSE
Produces/Sells CE-marked Devices: N
Bed, Electric	General
Bed, Flotation Therapy, Powered	Physical Med
Bed, Manual	General
Bed, Pediatric (Crib)	General
Chair, Adjustable, Mechanical	Physical Med
Chair/Table, Medical	General
Environmental Control System, Powered	Physical Med
Examination Device, AC-Powered	General
Infusion Stand	General
Linen, Bed	General
Mattress, Air Flotation	General
Stool, Operating Room, Adjustable	Surgery
Stretcher, Wheeled (Mobile)	General
Table, Obstetrical, AC-Powered	Obstetrics/Gynecology

HILL-ROM, INC.   812-934-7777 *(cont'd)*
Traction Unit, Non-Powered   Orthopedics

HILLCREST BIOLOGICALS
See Focus Technologies

HILLMOR PRODUCTS   734-721-3485
39292 Montana Dr., Romulus, MI 48174
FDA Number: 3003767605
Ownership: Private
Produces/Sells CE-marked Devices: N
Transfer Aid   Physical Med

HILLUSA CORP.   305-594-7474
7215 N.W. 46th St., Miami, FL 33166-6422
FDA Number: 1036399   *Fax:* 305-477-0699
E-mail: sales@hillusa.com
Web site: www.hillusa.com
Annual Revenue: $1-$5 Million
Year Founded: 1983
Total Employees: 10   *Marketing Staff:* 3   *Sales Staff:* 7
Ownership: Private
Quality System Registration Information: ISO9002
Produces/Sells CE-marked Devices: N
Federal Procurement Eligibility: Minority Owned
Distribution: OEM, Exporter
General Admin.: Mr. Ernesto Ackerman/President, Chief Executive Officer
Mktg./Adv.: Giselle Plata/Sales Representative
            Gisela Ackerman/Vice President Sales
Finance: Ramon Granja/Controller
          Pedro Chau/Manager Acctg.
IS: Mrs. Maria LLanes/Manager Tech. Support
Computer, Stress Exercise   Cardiovascular
Electrocardiograph, Single Channel   Cardiovascular
Ergometer, Treadmill   Cardiovascular
Monitor, Blood Pressure, Indirect, Automatic   Cardiovascular
Paper, Recording, ECG/EEG   General
Recorder, Long-Term, Trend   General
Scanner, Ultrasonic (Pulsed Echo)   Radiology
Scanner, Ultrasonic, Abdominal   Radiology
Scanner, Ultrasonic, Obstetrical/Gynecological   Obstetrics/Gynecology
Scanner, Ultrasonic, Obstetrical/Gynecological, Mobile Obstetrics/Gynecology
Service, Import/Export   General
Medical Product Subsidiaries (Listed Separately)
Hill-Med, Inc.

HILLYARD CHEMICAL CO.
See Hillyard, Inc.

HILLYARD, INC.   816-233-1321
302 North 4th St., P.O. Box 909, St. Joseph, MO 64501
FDA Number: n/a   *Fax:* 800-861-0256
Web site: www.hillyard.com
Year Founded: 1891
Ownership: Private
Produces/Sells CE-marked Devices: N
Distribution: Manufacturer Direct, Manufacturer Through Distributor, Manufacturer
Through Manufacturer Reps, Importer, Exporter
Solution, Antibacterial Cleaner   General

HILSINGER COMPANY, THE
See Hilco

HIMMELSTEIN & CO., S.   800-632-7873
2490 Pembroke Ave.,   847-843-3300
Hoffman Estates, IL 60169
FDA Number: n/a   *Fax:* 847-843-8488
E-mail: sales@himmelstein.com
Web site: www.himmelstein.com
Ownership: Private
Produces/Sells CE-marked Devices: Y
Federal Procurement Eligibility: Small Business
Distribution: Manufacturer Direct
General Admin.: S. Himmelstein/President
Mktg./Adv.: S. E. Tveter/Manager Sales
Production: R. S. Tveter/Vice President Production
Detector, Leakage, Medical Gas   General
Transducer, Force   General

HIPCO., INC.
See Fallgard Llc

HIPGRAPHICS, INC.   410-821-7040
100 West Road, Suite 302, Towson, MD 21204
FDA Number: 1122593
System, Communication, Image, Digital   Radiology

HIPSAVERS, INC.   800-358-4477
7 Hubbard St., Canton, MA 02021
FDA Number: 1225916   *Fax:* 781-821-6514
E-mail: hipsavers@msn.com

HIPSAVERS, INC.   800-358-4477 *(cont'd)*
Web site: www.hipsavers.com
Annual Revenue: $0-$1 Million
Ownership: Private
Produces/Sells CE-marked Devices: N
Distribution: Manufacturer Direct
Band, Support, Pelvic   Physical Med
Clothing, Protective   General
Cover, Limb   Physical Med

HIRSCH & CO., G.
See G. Hirsch & Co.

HISTORX, INC.   877-654-2345
35 Northeast Industrial Road,   203-498-7500
Branford, CT 06405
FDA Number: n/a   *Fax:* 203-498-7501
E-mail: info@historx.com
Web site: http://www.historx.com
Ownership: Private
Produces/Sells CE-marked Devices: N
General Admin.: Mr. Ranka Gupta/Chief Executive Officer
Mktg./Adv.: Ms. Kathleen Adams/Vice President Marketing
Research: Dr. Richard Carroll/Vice President Clinical Research
           Ms. Wendy Davis/Vice President Diagnostics

HISTORX, INC.   203-498-7500
35 Northeast Industrial Road, Bradford, CT 06405
FDA Number: n/a   *Fax:* 203-498-7501
E-mail: info@historx.com
Web site: http://www.historx.com
Ownership: Private
Produces/Sells CE-marked Devices: N
General Admin.: Rana Gupta/Chief Executive Officer
Research: Dr. Richard Carroll/Vice President Clinical Research
           Kathleen Adams/Vice President Diagnostics
           Ms. Wendy Davis/Vice President Diagnostics

HITACHI ALOKA MEDICAL   203-269-5088
10 Fairfield Boulevard, Wallingford, CT 06492
FDA Number: 9610865   *Fax:* 203-269-6075
E-mail: mail@aloka.com
Web site: www.hitachi-aloka.com
Ownership: Private
Produces/Sells CE-marked Devices: N
General Admin.: Mr. Akimitsu Harada/Director
                Mr. Hiroaki Tanaka/Executive Managing Director
                Mr. Minoru Yoshizumi/President
Image Processing System   Radiology
Scanner, Ultrasonic (Pulsed Doppler)   Radiology
Scanner, Ultrasonic (Pulsed Echo)   Radiology
Station Pipetting   Chemistry
Transducer, Ultrasonic, Diagnostic   Radiology

HITACHI AMERICA, LTD., POWER SYSTEMS   713-792-1804
DIVISION
1840 Old Spanish Trail, Houston, TX 77054
FDA Number: 3003993895
Radiotherapy Unit, Charged-Particle   Radiology

HITACHI CHEMICAL DIAGNOSTICS, INC.   650-961-5501
630 Clyde Ct., Mountain View, CA 94043
FDA Number: 2936856
Test, Radio-Allergen Absorbent (RAST)   Immunology

HITACHI DENSHI CANADA LTD.   800-268-3597
1 Select Ave., Unit 14,   416-299-5900
Scarborough, ONT M1V-5 Canada
FDA Number: n/a   *Fax:* 416-299-0450
E-mail: nanos_f@hitachidenshi.ca
Web site: www.hitachidenshi.ca
Year Founded: 1974
Total Employees: 10
Ownership: Private
Produces/Sells CE-marked Devices: N
Distribution: Exclusive Distributor

HITACHI HIGH TECHNOLOGIES AMERICA   925-218-2800
5100 Franklin Dr., Pleasanton, CA 94588-3355
FDA Number: n/a
Web site: www.hitachi-hhta.com
Year Founded: 2002
Ownership: Nissei Sangyo Co. Ltd.
Quality System Registration Information: ISO9001
Produces/Sells CE-marked Devices: N
Distribution: Exclusive Distributor
Microscope, Laboratory, Electron   Microbiology

HITACHI HIGH TECHNOLOGIES AMERICA, INC. 800-548-9001
3100 N. First St., San Jose, CA 95134 408-432-0520
FDA Number: n/a   Fax: 408-432-0704
E-mail: sales-LS@hitachi-hta.com
Web site: www.hitachi-hta.com/LSHome/
Annual Revenue: $1-$5 Million
Total Employees: 500   Marketing Staff: 5   Sales Staff: 10
Ownership: Private
Quality System Registration Information: ISO9000
Produces/Sells CE-marked Devices: Y
Distribution: Manufacturer Direct, Manufacturer Through Distributor
Mktg./Adv.: Dr. Peter Grosshans/Director Sales
    Dr. Chad Ostrander/Manager Market Development
    David Skiados/Manager Sales
    David Skiados/Vice President Business Development

Analyzer, Amino Acid	Microbiology
Chromatography, Liquid, Performance, High	Toxicology
Fluorometer	Immunology
Mass Spectrometer, Clinical Use	Toxicology
Spectrophotometer, Fluorescence	Chemistry
Spectrophotometer, U.V./Visible	Chemistry

HITACHI KOKUSAI ELECTRIC AMERICA, LTD. 516-921-7200
150 Crossways Park Drive, Woodbury, NY 11797-2028
FDA Number: n/a   Fax: 516-496-3718
E-mail: ivsinfo@hdal.com
Web site: www.hitachikokusai.com
Medical Products Sales Volume: $23,500,000
Annual Revenue: $25-$50 Million
Year Founded: 2001
Total Employees: 21   Marketing Staff: 5   Sales Staff: 15
Ownership: Private
Stock Symbol: RADN.
Traded On: NASDAQ
Quality System Registration Information: ISO9002
Produces/Sells CE-marked Devices: Y
Federal Procurement Eligibility: GSA Contract
Distribution: Manufacturer Through Distributor, OEM
Mktg./Adv.: Mr. Rob Johnston/Vice President Marketing & Sales

Camera, Microscope	Microbiology
Camera, Television, Surgical (With Audio)	Surgery
Camera, Video	General
Camera, Videotape, Surgical	Surgery
Monitor, Video, Endoscope	General
Printer, Image, Video	General

HITACHI MEDICAL SYSTEMS AMERICA, INC. 800-800-3106
1959 Summit Commerce Park, 330-425-1313
Twinsburg, OH 44087
FDA Number: 1528028   Fax: 330-425-1410
E-mail: info@hitachimed.com
Web site: www.hitachimed.com
Medical Products Sales Volume: $55,000,000
Year Founded: 1989
Total Employees: 370
Ownership: Hitachi Medical Corp.
Traded On: NYSE
Produces/Sells CE-marked Devices: N
Federal Procurement Eligibility: Small Business
Distribution: Manufacturer Direct
General Admin.: Richard L. Ernst/President, Chief Executive Officer
    Sheldon I. Schaffer/Vice President, General Manager
Mktg./Adv.: Bill Valters/Vice President Sales
Production: Doug Thistlehwaite/Manager Quality Assurance

Guide, Surgical, Needle	Surgery
Nuclear Magnetic Resonance Imaging System	Radiology
Scanner, Computed Tomography, X-Ray, Full Body	Radiology
Scanner, Positron Emission Tomography (PET)	Radiology
Scanner, Ultrasonic, General Purpose	Radiology

HITACHI NSA
See Hitachi High Technologies America

HITEC GROUP INTL. 800-288-8303
1743 Quincy Ave., Unit 155, Naperville, IL 60540 630-654-9200
FDA Number: n/a   Fax: 630-654-9219
E-mail: info@hitec.com
Web site: www.hitec.com
Medical Products Sales Volume: $3,200,000
Year Founded: 1982
Total Employees: 25   Marketing Staff: 2   Sales Staff: 7
Ownership: Private
Traded On: Oslo
Produces/Sells CE-marked Devices: Y
Federal Procurement Eligibility: Small Business, Female Owned, GSA Contract
Distribution: Manufacturer Direct, Manufacturer Through Distributor, Manufacturer Through Manufacturer Reps
General Admin.: Madeline Uzuanis/President

HITEC GROUP INTL. 800-288-8303 (cont'd)
Richard Uzuanis/Vice President
Production: Ms. Michele Ahlman/Vice President Operations

Amplifier, Voice	Ear/Nose/Throat
Battery, Hearing-Aid	Ear/Nose/Throat
Hearing-Aid	Ear/Nose/Throat
Telephone Equipment	General

HMB ENDOSCOPY PRODUCTS 800-659-5743
3746 SW 30th Avenue, Hollywood, FL 33312 954-792-6522
FDA Number: n/a   Fax: 954-792-6535
E-mail: sales@hmbendoscopy.com
Web site: www.hmbendoscopy.com
Medical Products Sales Volume: $2,800,000
Annual Revenue: $1-$5 Million
Year Founded: 1991
Total Employees: 11   Marketing Staff: 1   Sales Staff: 2
Ownership: Private
Produces/Sells CE-marked Devices: N
Federal Procurement Eligibility: Small Business, Female Owned
Distribution: Manufacturer Through Distributor, Service Direct
General Admin.: Victor Rugama/General Manager
    Harvey Buxbaum/President

Accessories, Cleaning Brushes (For Endoscope)	Gastroenterology/Urology
Accessories, Cleaning, Endoscopic	Gastroenterology/Urology
Accessories, Photographic, Endoscopic	Gastroenterology/Urology
Endoscope, Flexible	Gastroenterology/Urology
Light Source, Fiberoptic, Routine	Gastroenterology/Urology
Service, Repair, Endoscopic	General

HMI INDUSTRIES, INC. 440-846-7873
13325 Darice Pkwy., Unit A, Strongsville, OH 44149
FDA Number: 3003007759
Ownership: Private
Produces/Sells CE-marked Devices: N

Equipment, Cleaning, Air	General

HOBBS MEDICAL, INC. 860-684-5875
8 Spring St., Stafford Springs, CT 06076
FDA Number: 1220592

Brush, Cytology, Endoscopic	Gastroenterology/Urology
Cannula, Injection	Gastroenterology/Urology
Catheter, Balloon (Foley Type)	Surgery
Catheter, Biliary	Gastroenterology/Urology
Culture Media, Non-Propagating Transport	Microbiology
Dislodger, Stone, Basket, Ureteral, Metal	Gastroenterology/Urology
Electrosurgical Unit, Gastroenterology	Gastroenterology/Urology
Needle, Endoscopic	Gastroenterology/Urology
Splint, Ureteral	Gastroenterology/Urology

HODGE MANUFACTURING CO.
See DURHAM MANUFACTURING COMPANY

HODGES & CO., WM.
See Falcon Products, Inc.

HOEFER PHARMACIA BIOTECH, INC. 800-227-4750
84 October Hill Road, Holliston, MA 01746 508-893-8999
FDA Number: n/a   Fax: 508-429-5732
E-mail: sales@hoeferinc.com
Web site: www.Hoeferinc.com
Total Employees: 90
Ownership: AMERSHAM PHARMACIA BIOTECH
Quality System Registration Information: ISO9000
Produces/Sells CE-marked Devices: Y
Distribution: Manufacturer Direct, Manufacturer Through Distributor, Importer, Exporter
Mktg./Adv.: Mindy Lee/Director Marketing
    Terry Landers/Manager Business Development
Production: John Kelley/Manager Production
    Mindy Lee/Product Manager

Computer Software	General
Densitometer, Laboratory	Chemistry
Dialyzer, Laboratory	Chemistry
Electrofocusing Equipment	Chemistry
Electrophoresis Equipment, Cellulose Acetate Membrane	Chemistry
Electrophoresis Equipment, Gel	Chemistry
Electrophoresis Instrumentation	Immunology
Electrophoretic Separation, Vanilmandelic Acid	Chemistry
Fluorometer, Chemistry	Chemistry
Incubator, Test Tube, Portable	Microbiology
Test, Agar Plate	Microbiology
Washer, Labware	Chemistry

HOGGAN HEALTH INDUSTRIES, INC. 800-678-7888
8020 South 1300 West, West Jordan, UT 84088 801-572-6500
FDA Number: n/a   Fax: 801-572-6514
E-mail: marvas@hogganhealth.com
Web site: www.hogganhealth.com
Medical Products Sales Volume: $200,000
Annual Revenue: $5-$10 Million

HOGGAN HEALTH INDUSTRIES, INC.   800-678-7888 *(cont'd)*

Total Employees: 40	*Marketing Staff:* 1	*Sales Staff:* 6

Ownership: Private
Produces/Sells CE-marked Devices: N
Federal Procurement Eligibility: Small Business, GSA Contract
Distribution: Manufacturer Direct, Manufacturer Through Distributor, Exporter
General Admin.: Lynn D. Hoggan/Chief Executive Officer, Chairman
    Marva Sadler/President
Mktg./Adv.: Cynthia McKenna/Vice President Sales

Exercise Stair	Physical Med
Exerciser, Arm	Physical Med
Exerciser, Bicycle	Physical Med
Exerciser, Other	Physical Med
Transducer, Force	General
Treadmill, Powered	Physical Med

HOKANSON INC., D.E.   800-999-8251
12840 N.E. 21st Pl., Bellevue, WA 98005-1910   425-882-1689
FDA Number: 3019130   *Fax:* 425-881-1636
E-mail: info@deh-inc.com
Web site: www.hokanson.cc
Annual Revenue: $1-$5 Million
Year Founded: 1973
Total Employees: 15
Ownership: Private
Quality System Registration Information: ISO9001
Produces/Sells CE-marked Devices: Y
Federal Procurement Eligibility: Small Business, Female Owned
Distribution: Manufacturer Direct, Manufacturer Through Manufacturer Reps, Exporter
General Admin.: Kyra Gray/President
Mktg./Adv.: Sigrid Hokanson/Manager International Business
    Molly Ciliberti/Manager Marketing & Sales

Computer Software	General
Cuff, Blood Pressure	Cardiovascular
Detector, Blood Flow, Ultrasonic (Doppler)	Cardiovascular
Equipment, Ultrasound, Doppler, Evaluation, Fetal	Obstetrics/Gynecology
Gauge, Strain	General
Inflator, Cuff	General
Monitor, Heart Rate, R-Wave (ECG)	Cardiovascular
Plethysmograph, Photo-Electric, Pneumatic Or Hydraulic	Cardiovascular
Recorder, Chart, Laboratory	Chemistry
Sphygmomanometer, Aneroid (Arterial Pressure)	General
Support, Patient Position, Radiographic	Radiology
Transducer, Ultrasonic	Cardiovascular

HOLABIRD & ROOT LLC   312-357-1771
140 South Dearborn Street, Chicago, IL 60603
FDA Number: n/a   *Fax:* 312-357-1909
E-mail: holabird@holabird.com
Web site: www.holabird.com
Medical Products Sales Volume: $8,200,000
Annual Revenue: $5-$10 Million
Year Founded: 1880
Total Employees: 88   *Marketing Staff:* 3
Ownership: Private
Federal Procurement Eligibility: Small Business
Distribution: Service Direct
General Admin.: Gerald Horn/Chief Executive Officer
    Elisabeth Brandt/Director Admin.
Mktg./Adv.: Deborah Kirsner/Director Marketing

Service, Architectural	General

HOLBURN BIOMEDICAL CORPORATION   905-623-1484
1100 Bennett Road, Bowmanville, ONT L1C 3K5 Canada
FDA Number: n/a   *Fax:* 905-623-6702
E-mail: mail@holburn.com
Web site: www.holburn.com
Year Founded: 1996
Ownership: Private
Produces/Sells CE-marked Devices: N
Distribution: Manufacturer Direct

HOLCO
    See Aesculap Implant Systems Inc.

HOLL MEDITRONICS INC.   800-387-0563
4 Marconi Court, Bolton, ONT L7E-1E7 Canada   905-857-6867
FDA Number: n/a   *Fax:* 905-857-8550
E-mail: hollmedi@netcom.ca
Web site: www.hollmed.com
Year Founded: 1988
Total Employees: 10
Ownership: Private
Produces/Sells CE-marked Devices: N
Distribution: Exclusive Distributor, Exporter

HOLLES LABORATORIES, INC.   800-356-4015
30 Forest Notch, Cohasset, MA 02025   781-383-0741
FDA Number: 1250073   *Fax:* 781-383-0005
E-mail: Orders@HollesLabs.com
Web site: www.holleslabs.com
Medical Products Sales Volume: $100,000
Year Founded: 1975
Total Employees: 4
Ownership: Private
Produces/Sells CE-marked Devices: N
Federal Procurement Eligibility: Small Business
Distribution: Manufacturer Direct, Manufacturer Through Distributor

Strip, Fluorescein	Ophthalmology

HOLLISTER INCORPORATED   888-740-8999
2000 Hollister Dr., Libertyville, IL 60048-3746
FDA Number: 1480288
Web site: www.hollister.com
Year Founded: 1921
Ownership: Private
Quality System Registration Information: ISO9002
Produces/Sells CE-marked Devices: Y
Distribution: Manufacturer Direct, Manufacturer Through Distributor, Service Direct
General Admin.: Alan F. Herbert/President, Chief Executive Officer, Chairman

Amniotome	Obstetrics/Gynecology
Appliance, Incontinence, Urosheath Type	Gastroenterology/Urology
Bag, Collection, Urine, Newborn	General
Bag, Drainage (Incontinence)	Gastroenterology/Urology
Bag, Drainage, Ostomy (With Adhesive)	General
Bag, Leg	Gastroenterology/Urology
Bag, Stomal	Surgery
Bag, Urinary Collection	General
Bag, Urinary Collection, Ureterostomy	Gastroenterology/Urology
Bag, Urinary, Ileostomy	Gastroenterology/Urology
Bandage, Elastic	General
Bedpan	General
Bell, Circumcision	Gastroenterology/Urology
Bracelet, Identification	General
Catheter, Irrigation	Surgery
Catheter, Urinary, Condom	Gastroenterology/Urology
Catheter, Urological	Gastroenterology/Urology
Cement, Stomal Appliance, Ostomy	Gastroenterology/Urology
Clamp, Umbilical	Obstetrics/Gynecology
Collector, Ostomy	Gastroenterology/Urology
Collector, Urine	Gastroenterology/Urology
Collector, Urine, Disposable	Gastroenterology/Urology
Colostomy Appliance, Disposable	Gastroenterology/Urology
Cushion, Flotation	Physical Med
Device, Incontinence, Paste-On	Gastroenterology/Urology
Dressing, Other	General
Dressing, Universal	General
Dressing, Wound and Burn, Hydrogel	Surgery
Dressing, Wound and Burn, Occlusive	Surgery
Endoscope	Gastroenterology/Urology
Irrigator, Ostomy	Gastroenterology/Urology
Kit, Catheterization, Sterile Urethral	Gastroenterology/Urology
Kit, Circumcision, Disposable Tray	Obstetrics/Gynecology
Kit, Enema (For Cleaning Purposes)	Gastroenterology/Urology
Kit, Wound Drainage	General
Lotion, Skin Care	General
Ostomy Appliance (Ileostomy, Colostomy)	Gastroenterology/Urology
Pack, Hot Or Cold, Water Circulating	Physical Med
Pad, Incontinence (Underpad)	General
Pad, Pressure, Foam (Elbow, Heel)	General
Perforator, Amniotic Membrane	Obstetrics/Gynecology
Perineometer	Obstetrics/Gynecology
Pouch, Colostomy	Gastroenterology/Urology
Protector, Ostomy	Gastroenterology/Urology
Rod, Colostomy	Gastroenterology/Urology
Sign, Hospital	General
Sponge, External	Surgery
Sponge, External, Synthetic	Surgery
Stimulator, Incontinence (Non-Implantable), Electrical	Gastroenterology/Urology
Tube, Gastrointestinal	Gastroenterology/Urology
Wristlet, Patient Return	Gastroenterology/Urology

Medical Product Subsidiaries (Listed Separately)
    Dansac A/S
    Thames Valley Medical Ltd.

HOLLISTER LIMITED   800-263-7400
95 Mary St., Aurora, ONT L4G-1G3 Canada   905-727-4344
FDA Number: n/a   *Fax:* 800-432-8846
E-mail: sales&admin.holcan@hollister.com
Web site: www.hollister.com
Year Founded: 1958
Total Employees: 50
Ownership: Private
Produces/Sells CE-marked Devices: N

HOLLISTER LIMITED
800-263-7400 (cont'd)
Distribution: Exclusive Distributor

HOLLISTER, INC.
1-888-740-8999.
2000 Hollister Drive, Libertyville, IL 60048
FDA Number: 1119193
Ownership: Private
Produces/Sells CE-marked Devices: N

Bag, Leg	Gastroenterology/Urology
Bag, Stomal	Surgery
Bag, Urinary Collection, Ureterostomy	Gastroenterology/Urology
Bag, Urine Collection, Leg, For External Use, Non-sterile	Gastroenterology/Urology
Catheter, Irrigation	Surgery
Cement, Stomal Appliance, Ostomy	Gastroenterology/Urology
Collector, Ostomy	Gastroenterology/Urology
Device, Incontinence, Urosheath Type, Non-sterile	Gastroenterology/Urology
Device, Paste-on For Incontinence, Non-sterile	Gastroenterology/Urology
Dressing, Wound, Hydrophilic	Surgery
Dressing, Wound, Occlusive	Surgery
Fixation Device, Tracheal Tube	Anesthesiology
Irrigator, Ostomy	Gastroenterology/Urology
Protector, Ostomy	Gastroenterology/Urology
Rod, Colostomy	Gastroenterology/Urology

HOLLISTER-STIER LABORATORIES, LLC
800-992-1120
3525 North Regal St., Spokane, WA 99207-5788
509-489-5656
FDA Number: 3010477
Fax: 509-484-4320
E-mail: fill@hollister-stier.com
Web site: www.Hollister-Stier.com
Medical Products Sales Volume: $32,700,000
Year Founded: 1921
Total Employees: 400
Ownership: Private
Produces/Sells CE-marked Devices: N
Federal Procurement Eligibility: Small Business
Distribution: Manufacturer Direct, Manufacturer Through Distributor, Manufacturer Through Manufacturer Reps, Exporter
Mktg./Adv.: Mr. Anthony Kiepe/Director National Sales

Delivery System, Allergen And Vaccine	General
Vial, Other	General

HOLLYWOOD TANNING SYSTEMS, INC.
856-914-9090
11 Enterprise Ct., Sewell, NJ 08080
FDA Number: 2249199
Ownership: Private
Produces/Sells CE-marked Devices: N

Booth, Sun Tan	Physical Med

HOLMED CORPORATION
508-238-3351
40 Norfolk Avenue, South Easton, MA 02375
FDA Number: 1219518
Fax: 508-238-3807
E-mail: Sales-CustomerSupport@holmed.net
Web site: www.holmed.net
Medical Products Sales Volume: $5,000,000
Annual Revenue: $5-$10 Million
Year Founded: 1979
Total Employees: 55   Marketing Staff: 1   Sales Staff: 1
Ownership: Private
Produces/Sells CE-marked Devices: Y
Federal Procurement Eligibility: Small Business
Distribution: OEM, Exporter
General Admin.: Russell P. Holmes/President
Mktg./Adv.: Peter Randall/Vice President Sales
Production: Mr. Frank Slauenwhite/Director Engineering
Mr. Richard Devine/Manager Quality Assurance

Accessories, Fixation, Orthopedic	Orthopedics
Accessories, Fixation, Spinal Interlaminal	Orthopedics
Accessories, Fixation, Spinal Intervertebral Body	Orthopedics
Bender	Orthopedics
Chisel (Osteotome)	Surgery
Chisel, Orthopedic	Orthopedics
Contract Manufacturing	General
Curette	Orthopedics
Cutter, Bone, Ultrasonic	Cns/Neurology
Cutter, Orthopedic	Orthopedics
Cutter, Wire And Pin	Orthopedics
Driver/Extractor, Bone Nail/Pin	Orthopedics
Driver/Extractor, Bone Plate	Orthopedics
Elevator, Orthopedic	Orthopedics
Goniometer, Orthopedic	Orthopedics
Gouge, Surgical, General & Plastic Surgery	Surgery
Guide	Orthopedics
Guide, Drill	Orthopedics
Holder, Leg	Surgery
Holder, Needle, Other	Surgery
Hook, Bone	Surgery
Impactor	Orthopedics
Implant, Fixation Device, Spinal	Orthopedics
Instrument, Manual, General Surgical	Surgery
Instrument, Needle Holder/Knot Tying	Surgery

HOLMED CORPORATION
508-238-3351 (cont'd)

Mallet, Bone	Orthopedics
Orthopedic Manual Surgical Instrument	Orthopedics
Osteotome (Orthopedic)	Surgery
Plate, Bone, Skull (Cranioplasty)	Cns/Neurology
Plate, Fixation, Bone	Orthopedics
Pliers, Surgical	Orthopedics
Prosthesis Implantation Instrument, Orthopedic	Orthopedics
Reamer	Orthopedics
Retractor, Other	Surgery
Screw, Fixation, Bone	Orthopedics
Screwdriver	Orthopedics
Service, Design, Implant, Custom	Orthopedics
Spreader, Other	Surgery
Staple, Fixation, Bone	Orthopedics
Tap, Bone	Orthopedics
Wrench	Orthopedics

HOLMES DENTAL CORP.
800-322-5577
50 S. Penn St., Hatboro, PA 19040-3246
215-675-2877
FDA Number: n/a
Fax: 215-675-7147
E-mail: ssage@aol.com
Web site: www.holmesdental.com
Annual Revenue: $0-$1 Million
Total Employees: 3
Ownership: Private
Produces/Sells CE-marked Devices: N
Federal Procurement Eligibility: Small Business
Distribution: Manufacturer Direct
General Admin.: Dr. Shelly M. Greene/President

Chemical, Film Processor	Radiology
Forceps, Dressing, Dental	Dental And Oral
Material, Acrylic, Dental	Dental And Oral
Material, Impression	Dental And Oral
Reliner, Denture, OTC	Dental And Oral

HOLOGIC, INC.
888-773-8376
1240 Elko Drive, Sunnyvale, CA 94089
408-745-0975
FDA Number: 2939852
Ownership: Hologic, Inc.
Stock Symbol: HOLX
Traded On: NASDAQ
Produces/Sells CE-marked Devices: N

Collector, Specimen	Microbiology
Enzyme Immunoassay, Fetal Fibronectin	Chemistry
Sampler, Amniotic Fluid (Amniocentesis Tray)	Obstetrics/Gynecology

HOLOGIC, INC.
800-442-9892
250 Campus Drive, Marlborough, MA 01752
508-263-2900
FDA Number: 1222780
Fax: 508-229-2795
Web site: www.cytyc.com
Ownership: Hologic, Inc.
Stock Symbol: HOLX
Traded On: NASDAQ
Produces/Sells CE-marked Devices: N
General Admin.: Mr. Patrick J. Sullivan/Chairman
Mr. Jack Cumming/Chief Executive Officer

Applicator, Radionuclide, Manual	Radiology
Applicator, Radionuclide, Remote-Controlled	Radiology
Bandage, Adhesive	Surgery
Biopsy Instrument	Gastroenterology/Urology
Contraceptive Tubal Occlusion Device, Male	Obstetrics/Gynecology
Cytocentrifuge	Pathology
Device, Ablation, Thermal, Endometrial	Obstetrics/Gynecology
Enzyme Immunoassay, Fetal Fibronectin	Chemistry
Equipment, Laboratory, Gen. Purpose (Specific Medical Use)	Chemistry
Filter, Cell Collection, Tissue Processing	Pathology
Instrument, Manual, General Surgical	Surgery
Kit, Smear, Cervical	Obstetrics/Gynecology
Kit, Surgical Instrument, Disposable	Surgery
Kit, Wound Dressing	Surgery
Melting Point Apparatus, Paraffin	Pathology
Needle, Hypodermic, Single Lumen With Syringe	General
Preservative, Cytological	Pathology
Processor, Slide, Cytology, Automated	Pathology
Reader, Slide, Cytology, Cervical, Automated	Pathology
Reagent, General Purpose	Pathology
Sampler, Amniotic Fluid (Amniocentesis Tray)	Obstetrics/Gynecology
Slide, Microscope	Pathology
Sound, Uterine	Obstetrics/Gynecology
Source, Brachytherapy, Radionuclide	Radiology
Stain, Papanicolau	Pathology
Station Pipetting	Chemistry
Tray, Surgical	Surgery

HOLOGIC, INC.
800-343-9729
35 Crosby Drive, Bedford, MA 01730
781-999-7300
FDA Number: 1221300
Fax: 781-280-0669
E-mail: info@hologic.com
Web site: www.hologic.com

HOLOGIC, INC.   800-343-9729 *(cont'd)*
Medical Products Sales Volume: $100,000,000
Annual Revenue: More than $1 Billion
Year Founded: 1986
Total Employees: 3580
Ownership: Public
Stock Symbol: HOLX
Traded On: NASDAQ
Quality System Registration Information: ISO9001
Produces/Sells CE-marked Devices: Y
Distribution: Manufacturer Direct
General Admin.: Mr. John W. Cumming/Chairman
     Glenn P. Muir/Chief Financial Officer, Executive Vice President
     Dr. Jay A. Stein/Chief Technology Officer
     Mr. Robert A. Cascella/President, Chief Executive Officer
     Dr. Peter Soltani/Vice President, General Manager

Coil, Magnetic Resonance, Specialty	Radiology
Densitometer, Bone, Dual Photon	Radiology
Densitometer, Bone, Single Photon	Radiology
Image Processing System	Radiology
Mount, X-Ray Tube, Diagnostic	Radiology
Phantom, Anthropomorphic, Radiographic	Radiology
Radiographic Unit, Diagnostic	Radiology
Sonometer, Bone	Radiology
Table, Radiographic	Radiology
Tube, X-Ray	Radiology

Medical Product Subsidiaries (Listed Separately)
   Direct Radiography
   HOLOGIC, INC.
   Hologic, Inc.
   Hologic|r2, Inc
   Lorad, A Hologic Company
   Suros Surgical Systems, Inc

HOLOGIC, INC.   800-442-9892
445 Simarano Drive, Marlboro, MA 01752   **508-263-2900**
FDA Number: 3006330030
Web site: www.cytyc.com
Medical Products Sales Volume: $230,000,000
Total Employees: 554   *Marketing Staff:* 20   *Sales Staff:* 175
Ownership: Hologic, Inc.
Stock Symbol: HOLX
Traded On: NASDAQ
Quality System Registration Information: ISO9000; ISO9001
Produces/Sells CE-marked Devices: Y
Distribution: Manufacturer Direct
General Admin.: Mr. Patrick J. Sullivan/Chairman
     Mr. Jack Cumming/Chief Executive Officer
     Daniel J. Levangie/Chief Operating Officer
     A. Suzanne Meszner-Eltrich/Vice President Human Resources
Medical Admin.: James Linder/Medical Director
Mktg./Adv.: Victoria Robinson/Vice President Business Development
     Craig Sands/Vice President Marketing & Sales
Research: David Zahniser/Vice President Scientific Affairs
Finance: Robert Bowen/Chief Financial Officer

Applicator, Radionuclide, Remote-Controlled	Radiology
Cytocentrifuge	Pathology
Kit, Smear, Cervical	Obstetrics/Gynecology
Processor, Slide, Cytology, Automated	Pathology

HOLOGIC|R2, INC   866-243-2533
2585 Augustine Drive, Santa Clara, CA 95054   **408-352-0100**
FDA Number: 2953690   *Fax:* 408-352-0101
E-mail: r2info@hologic.com
Web site: www.r2tech.com
Ownership: Hologic, Inc.
Stock Symbol: HOLX
Traded On: NASDAQ
Produces/Sells CE-marked Devices: N
General Admin.: John W. Cumming/Chief Executive Officer, Chairman
     Glenn P. Muir/Chief Financial Officer, Executive Vice President
     David R. LaVance/President, Chief Executive Officer
     Robert Cascella/President, Chief Operating Officer
     C. William McDaniel/Principal
     Wayne Wilson/Principal

Analyzer, Medical Image	Radiology
Image Processing System	Radiology

HOLOPACK INTL. CORP.   803-806-3300
1 Technology Circle, Columbia, SC 29203
FDA Number: 1063407

Nebulizer, Direct Patient Interface	Anesthesiology

HOLORAD LLC   801-983-6075
2929 South Main St., Salt Lake City, UT 84115
FDA Number: 3005475993

Film, X-Ray, Special Purpose	Radiology

HOLORAD LLC   801-983-6075 *(cont'd)*

Illuminator, Radiographic Film	Radiology

HOMAK MANUFACTURING COMPANY INC.   800-874-6625
1605 Old Route 18, Suite 4-36,   **724-535-1080**
Wampum, PA 16157
FDA Number: n/a   *Fax:* 724-535-1081
E-mail: bmiller@homakmfg.com
Web site: www.homakmfg.com
Total Employees: 4
Ownership: Private
Produces/Sells CE-marked Devices: N
Federal Procurement Eligibility: Small Business, Female Owned, GSA Contract
Distribution: Manufacturer Through Distributor
General Admin.: Gertrude Danziger/President
Mktg./Adv.: John Dopak/Director Marketing & Sales

Accessories, Cart, Multipurpose	General
Board, Cardiopulmonary Resuscitation	General
Cabinet Casework, General Purpose	General
Cabinet, Narcotic Control	General
Cart, Anesthetist's	Anesthesiology
Cart, Emergency, Cardiopulmonary Resuscitation (Crash)	Anesthesiology
Cart, Instrument	Surgery
Cart, Isolation	General
Cart, Medicine	General
Cart, Multipurpose	General
Cart, Other	General
Cart, Supply	General
Cart, Supply, Operating Room	Surgery
Infusion Stand	General
Tray, Medicine	General

HOME ACCESS HEALTH CORP.   800-HIV-TEST
2401 W. Hassell Rd.,, Ste. 1510,   **847-781-2500**
Hoffman Estates, IL 60169
FDA Number: 1423455   *Fax:* 847-781-2560
E-mail: info@homeaccess.com
Web site: www.homeaccess.com
Total Employees: 60   *Marketing Staff:* 5   *Sales Staff:* 10
Ownership: Private
Quality System Registration Information: ISO9000; ISO9001
Produces/Sells CE-marked Devices: N
Distribution: Manufacturer Direct
General Admin.: Tracy T. Powell/Chief Executive Officer
     Mike Wandell/Chief Scientific Officer
     Richard Quattrocchi/President
     Michele Crown/Vice President Human Resources
Mktg./Adv.: Jeff Clouse/Director National Accounts
     Richard Brown/Director Product Development
     Joe Smith/Vice President Business Development
     Joe Smith/Vice President Marketing & Sales
Production: Richard Brown/Manager Regulatory Affairs
     Barb Godsey/Vice President Manufacturing
Finance: Ben Crown/Chief Financial Officer

Antibody, Other	General
Assay, Enzyme Linked Immunosorbent, Hepatitis C Virus	Microbiology
Colorimetric Method, Triglycerides	Chemistry
Container, Specimen Mailer And Storage	Pathology
Enzymatic Esterase-Oxidase, Cholesterol	Chemistry
LDL & VLDL Precipitation, Cholesterol Via Esterase-Oxidase	Chemistry
Reagent, Cholesterol (Total Test System)	Chemistry
System, Test, Home, Hiv-1	Hematology
Test, Antibody, Acquired Immune Deficiency Syndrome (AIDS)	Hematology

HOME CARE EXPRESS & MASS BAY RESPIRATORY   781-740-9797
85 Research Rd., Hingham, MA 02043
FDA Number: 3003671203
Ownership: Private
Produces/Sells CE-marked Devices: N

Canister, Liquid Oxygen, Portable	Anesthesiology

HOME DIAGNOSTICS, INC.
See Nipro Diagnostics, Inc.

HOME GYM CANADA INC.   416-762-7920
9 Brockhouse Rd., Toronto, ONT M8W-2W8 Canada
FDA Number: n/a   *Fax:* 416-762-4968
Year Founded: 1991
Total Employees: 25
Ownership: Private
Produces/Sells CE-marked Devices: N
Distribution: Manufacturer Direct, Exporter

HOME HEALTH   800-445-7137
2100 Smithtown Ave, Ronkonkoma, NY 11772   **631-244-2021**
FDA Number: n/a   *Fax:* 631-244-1777
E-mail: info@homehealthus.com
Web site: www.homehealthus.com

HOME HEALTH 800-445-7137 *(cont'd)*
Annual Revenue: $0-$1 Million
Total Employees: 50   *Marketing Staff:* 1   *Sales Staff:* 1
Ownership: NBTY, INC.
Produces/Sells CE-marked Devices: N
Distribution: Manufacturer Through Distributor
Mktg./Adv.: Kim Nagel/Director Marketing
Theresa Ierardi/Manager Contract Sales
Lotion, Skin Care .... General
Soap .... General

HOME HEALTH PRODUCTS INC.
See Home Health

HOME HOSPITAL EQUIPMENT COMPANY
See Ez Way, Inc.

HOME MEDICAL OF AMERICA
See JACE SYSTEMS, INC

HOME SOLUTIONS, INC.
See Pyramid Industries, Llc

HOME STRETCH PRODUCTS, INC. 847-816-1852
536 W. Mckinley Ave., Libertyville, IL 60048
FDA Number: 3004934209
Ownership: Private
Produces/Sells CE-marked Devices: N
Component, Exercise .... Physical Med

HOME-AID-HEALTHCARE, INC. 888-297-9109
PO Box 801764, Santa Clarita, CA 91380-1764 661-294-9509
FDA Number: n/a   *Fax:* 661-294-9837
E-mail: info@homeaid.com
Web site: www.homeaid.com
Medical Products Sales Volume: $1,000,000
Annual Revenue: $1-$5 Million
Year Founded: 1994
Total Employees: 4   *Marketing Staff:* 4   *Sales Staff:* 4
Ownership: Private
Produces/Sells CE-marked Devices: N
Federal Procurement Eligibility: Small Business, Minority Owned
Distribution: Manufacturer Through Distributor, Exclusive Distributor, Importer
General Admin.: Roland A. Hinds/President
Bandage, Elastic .... General
Bandage, Gauze .... General
Support, Back .... Orthopedics
Support, Elbow .... Orthopedics
Support, Knee .... Physical Med
Support, Wrist .... Physical Med
Medical Product Subsidiaries (Listed Separately)
Dr.'s Page

HOMECARE CLINICAL EMERGENCIES, INC. 416-665-7373
21-1111 Flint Rd, North York M3J 3C7 Canada
FDA Number: 9681401
Bandage, Adhesive .... Surgery

HOMECARE PRODUCTS, INC. 800-451-1903
1704 B STREET NW SUITE 110, Auburn, WA 98001 253-249-1108
FDA Number: 3032368   *Fax:* 800-630-2350
E-mail: customerservice@ezaccess.com
Web site: www.homecareproducts.com
Medical Products Sales Volume: $9,200,000
Annual Revenue: $1-$5 Million
Year Founded: 1984
Total Employees: 90
Ownership: Private
Produces/Sells CE-marked Devices: Y
Federal Procurement Eligibility: Small Business, Female Owned
Distribution: Manufacturer Through Distributor, Manufacturer Through
Manufacturer Reps, Importer, Exporter
General Admin.: Don Everard/Chief Executive Officer
Madonna Akard/Office Manager
Glenda Everard/President
Deanne Sandvold/Vice President
Mktg./Adv.: Don Everard/Director Marketing
Lee Sandvold/Director Product Development
Norm Alexander/Manager International & National Sales
Lloyd Everard/Manager Product Development
Production: Norm Alexander/Manager Materials
Lee Sandvold/Production Engineer
Accessories, Wheelchair .... Physical Med
Basin, Wash .... General
Bathtub, Portable .... General
Ramp, Wheelchair .... General

HOMEDICS INC. 800-333-8282
3000 Pontiac Trail, 248-863-3000
Commerce Township, MI 48390
FDA Number: 1832894   *Fax:* 248-863-3100

HOMEDICS INC. 800-333-8282 *(cont'd)*
E-mail: cservice@homedics.com
Web site: www.homedics.com/
Medical Products Sales Volume: $50,600,000
Annual Revenue: $0-$1 Million
Year Founded: 1987
Total Employees: 1020   *Marketing Staff:* 3   *Sales Staff:* 3
Ownership: Private
Federal Procurement Eligibility: GSA Contract
Distribution: Manufacturer Direct, Manufacturer Through Manufacturer Reps
General Admin.: Ron Ferber/President, Chief Executive Officer
Mktg./Adv.: Alon Kaufman/Vice President Marketing & Sales
Mike Matthews/Vice President Sales
Bath, Hydro-Massage (Whirlpool) .... Physical Med
Clipper, Hair .... General
Cushion, Other .... General
Magnetic Unit, Therapeutic .... Physical Med
Massager, Therapeutic .... Physical Med
Orthosis, Lumbar .... Physical Med
Pack, Hot Or Cold, Reusable .... Physical Med
Prosthesis, Sensory .... Cns/Neurology
Toothbrush, Powered .... Dental And Oral

HON COMPANY, THE
See Allsteel Inc.

HONEYWELL BURDICK & JACKSON 800-368-0050
1953 S. Harvey St., Muskegon, MI 49442-6101 231-726-3171
FDA Number: 7000071   *Fax:* 231-725-6297
E-mail: linda.jones2@honeywell.com
Web site: www.burdickandjackson.com
Year Founded: 1959
Total Employees: 125   *Marketing Staff:* 2   *Sales Staff:* 9
Ownership: Public
Quality System Registration Information: ISO9001
Produces/Sells CE-marked Devices: N
Distribution: Manufacturer Through Distributor
General Admin.: Michael Willerer/Vice President Human Resources
Whitney Erickson/Vice President, General Manager
Mktg./Adv.: Mike Andre/Director Marketing & Sales
Production: James Przybytek/Director Quality Assurance
Michael Sale/Vice President Manufacturing
Research: James Przybytek/Vice President Research & Development
Acetone .... Chemistry
Chromatography, Liquid, Performance, High ...... Toxicology
Solvent .... Chemistry
Solvent, Spectrophotometer .... Chemistry

HONEYWELL HOMMED, LLC 888-353-5440
3400 Intertech Dr., Suite 200, Brookfield, WI 53045
FDA Number: 3004183721   *Fax:* 262-252-5795
Web site: www.hommed.com
Ownership: Private
Produces/Sells CE-marked Devices: N
Production: Michael Leigh/Director Regulatory Affairs
Communication System, Powered .... Physical Med
Dispenser, Solid Medication .... Physical Med
Monitor, Blood Pressure, Indirect, Semi-Automatic .... Cardiovascular
Oximeter, Intracardiac .... Cardiovascular
Scale, Stand-On .... General
Transmitter/Receiver System, Physiological, Radiofrequency .... Cardiovascular

HONG KONG DENTAL LAB 415-330-9099
9 Silliman Street, Suite C, San Francisco, CA 94134
FDA Number: 3005905638
Ownership: Private
Produces/Sells CE-marked Devices: N
Alloy, Gold Based, For Clinical Use .... Dental And Oral
Denture, Gold .... Dental And Oral
Denture, Plastic, Teeth .... Dental And Oral
Metal, Base .... Dental And Oral

HOOD LABORATORIES
See E. Benson Hood Laboratories, Inc.

HOOD THERMO-PAD CANADA LTD. 800-665-9555
5918 Kennedy St., 250-494-5002
Summerland, BC V0H-1 Canada
FDA Number: n/a   *Fax:* 250-494-5003
E-mail: admin@thermo-pad.com
Web site: www.thermo-pad.com
Year Founded: 1984
Total Employees: 10
Ownership: Private
Produces/Sells CE-marked Devices: N
Distribution: Manufacturer Direct, Exporter

HOOSIER, INC. 951-272-3070
1152 California Ave., Corona, CA 92881
FDA Number: 2032093   *Fax:* 951-272-8090

HOOSIER, INC.   951-272-3070 (cont'd)
E-mail: info@hoosierinc.com
Ownership: Private
Produces/Sells CE-marked Devices: N

Appliance, Fixation, Spinal Interlaminal	Orthopedics
Orthosis, Fixation, Pedicle, Spinal	Orthopedics
Orthosis, Fixation, Spinal, Spondylolisthesis	Orthopedics

HOOVER PRECISION PRODUCTS
See Hoover Precision Products, Inc

HOOVER PRECISION PRODUCTS, INC   906-632-7310
1390 Industrial Park Drive, Sault St. Marie, MI 49783
FDA Number: n/a   *Fax:* 906-632-7555
E-mail: Sales@hooverprecision.com
Web site: www.hooverprecision.com
Medical Products Sales Volume: $4,000,000
Annual Revenue: $10-$25 Million
Year Founded: 1913
Total Employees: 40
Ownership: Tsubaki Nakashima Co., Ltd.
Quality System Registration Information: ISO9002
Produces/Sells CE-marked Devices: N
Federal Procurement Eligibility: Small Business
Distribution: Manufacturer Direct, Manufacturer Through Distributor, Manufacturer Through Manufacturer Reps
General Admin.: Eric L. Sturdy/Vice President, General Manager
Mktg./Adv.: Nancy Whitworth/Manager National Sales
    Gary Bos/Vice President Sales

Cap, Tip, Syringe	General
Component, Other	General
Component, Plastic	General

HOPE LABORATORIES   650-591-6271
409-a Old County Rd., Belmont, CA 94002
FDA Number: 2954357

Radioimmunoassay, Prolactin (Lactogen)	Chemistry

HOPKINS IMAGING   951-302-8416
34721 El Mirador Corte, Temecula, CA 92592
FDA Number: 2030864

System, Communication, Image, Digital	Radiology

HOPPECKE BATTERY SYSTEMS, INC.   856-616-0032
1960 Old Cuthbert Road, Suite 130, Cherry Hill, NJ 08034
FDA Number: n/a   *Fax:* 856-616-0132
E-mail: info@hoppecke-us.com
Web site: www.hoppecke-us.com
Annual Revenue: $0-$1 Million
Ownership: Private
Quality System Registration Information: ISO9000
Produces/Sells CE-marked Devices: N
Federal Procurement Eligibility: Small Business
Distribution: Manufacturer Through Distributor

Battery	General

HORCHER LIFTING SYSTEMS, INC.   800-582-8732
1884 NW 57th Street, Ocala, FL 34475   352-687-8020
FDA Number: 9001625   *Fax:* 866-378-3318
E-mail: Cecil.Rider@Horcher.com
Web site: www.horcher.com
Annual Revenue: $5-$10 Million
Year Founded: 1990
Total Employees: 12   *Marketing Staff:* 3   *Sales Staff:* 3
Ownership: Private
Produces/Sells CE-marked Devices: Y
Federal Procurement Eligibility: Small Business
Distribution: Manufacturer Through Distributor, Exclusive Distributor, Importer
General Admin.: Mr. Cecil Rider/President

Lift, Patient	General
Patient Transfer Unit, Powered	General

HORIBA ABX   888-903-5001
34 Bunsen Drive, Irvine, CA 92618-4210   949-453-0500
FDA Number: 2086725   *Fax:* 949-453-0600
E-mail: abxinc@us.abx.fr
Web site: www.horiba-abx.com
Medical Products Sales Volume: $21,000,000
Annual Revenue: $10-$25 Million
Year Founded: 1983
Total Employees: 108   *Marketing Staff:* 2   *Sales Staff:* 14
Ownership: Horiba Ltd.
Produces/Sells CE-marked Devices: N
Federal Procurement Eligibility: Small Business
Distribution: Service Direct, Exclusive Distributor, Exporter

Calibrator, Cell Indices	Hematology
Calibrator, Hemoglobin And Hematocrit Measurement	Hematology
Calibrator, Platelet Counting	Hematology
Calibrator, Red Cell And White Cell Counting	Hematology

HORIBA ABX   888-903-5001 (cont'd)

Computer, Hematology Analyzer	Hematology
Counter, Cell Or Particle, Automated	Hematology
Counter, Cell, Differential Classifier, Automated	Hematology
Diluent, Blood Cell	Hematology
Fluid, Red Cell Lysing	Hematology
Hematology Quality Control Mixture	Hematology
Reagent, General Purpose	Pathology
Stainer, Slide, Hematology, Automated	Hematology

HORIBA JOBIN YVON INC   866-JOBINYVON
3880 Park Avenue, Edison, NJ 08820-3012   732-494-8660
FDA Number: 7000342   *Fax:* 732-549-5125
E-mail: info@jobinyvon.com
Web site: www.jobinyvon.com
Medical Products Sales Volume: $50,000,000
Annual Revenue: $1-$5 Million
Year Founded: 1819
Total Employees: 211
Ownership: Horiba Ltd.
Quality System Registration Information: ISO9001
Produces/Sells CE-marked Devices: Y
Federal Procurement Eligibility: Small Business, GSA Contract
Distribution: Manufacturer Direct
General Admin.: Neil Stein/President
    Ray Kaminski/Vice President
Mktg./Adv.: Diane Madrid/Manager Advertising

Fluorometer	Immunology
Monochromator, for Clinical Use	Chemistry
Spectrophotometer, Infrared	Chemistry
Spectrophotometer, Ultraviolet	Chemistry
Spectrophotometer, Visible	Chemistry

HORIZON HEALTHCARE TECHNOLOGIES   800-477-5827
PO Box 27809, St. Louis, MO 63146   314-569-5995
FDA Number: n/a   *Fax:* 314-569-3388
E-mail: info@e-hht.com
Web site: www.e-hht.com
Total Employees: 50   *Marketing Staff:* 3   *Sales Staff:* 10
Ownership: Briggs Corporation
Produces/Sells CE-marked Devices: N
Distribution: Service Direct
General Admin.: Geoff Marsh/President
Mktg./Adv.: Bob Finnegan/Director Sales
Production: David Robbins/Director Operations

Computer Software	General
Computer Software, Hospital/Nursing Management	General

HORIZON MEDICAL
See Scanlan International, Inc.

HORIZON MEDICAL PRODUCTS, INC.
See Angiodynamics, Inc.

HORN & BROTHERS INC., WM. H.
See Bell-Horn, Inc.

HORTON AUTOMATICS   800-531-3111
4242 Baldwin Blvd., Corpus Christi, TX 78405   361-888-5591
FDA Number: n/a   *Fax:* 361-888-6510
Web site: http://www.hortondoors.com
Medical Products Sales Volume: $3,000,000
Annual Revenue: $1-$5 Million
Total Employees: 50   *Sales Staff:* 6
Ownership: HORTON AUTOMATICS - TEXAS
Produces/Sells CE-marked Devices: Y
Distribution: Manufacturer Direct, OEM

Cleanroom Equipment	General

HORTON EMERGENCY VEHICLES   614-539-8181
3800 McDowell Rd., Grove City, OH 43123
FDA Number: n/a   *Fax:* 614-539-8165
E-mail: info@hortonambulance.com
Web site: www.hortonambulance.com
Annual Revenue: $50-$100 Million
Total Employees: 265
Ownership: IMPAX LABORATORIES, INC.
Produces/Sells CE-marked Devices: N
Distribution: Manufacturer Direct, Manufacturer Through Distributor
General Admin.: Mike Grimes/President
Mktg./Adv.: David M. Lamon/Director Marketing

Ambulance	General

HOS-PILLOW CORP.   800-468-7874
1011 Campus Drive, Mundelein, IL 60060   847-680-7040
FDA Number: n/a   *Fax:* 847-680-7160
E-mail: ed@justdoit.net
Web site: www.bedsandbeyond.com
Medical Products Sales Volume: $940,000
Annual Revenue: $1-$5 Million

MANUFACTURER PROFILES

HOS-PILLOW CORP.   800-468-7874 (cont'd)
Year Founded: 1999
Total Employees: 16   Marketing Staff: 3   Sales Staff: 3
Ownership: Private
Produces/Sells CE-marked Devices: N
Federal Procurement Eligibility: Small Business, Female Owned, GSA Contract, VA Contract
Distribution: Manufacturer Direct, Exporter
General Admin.: Edward Halpern/Chairman
     Gregory Halpern/President
     Dianne Halpern/Secretary Treasurer
     Robert H. Givens/Vice President Human Resources
Mktg./Adv.: Gregory Halpern/Director Marketing
     Pearl Smith/Manager Sales Training
     John Betts/Vice President Marketing & Sales
Research: Lindsey H. Givens/Manager Research

Bib	General
Cart, Other	General
Cover, Bedrail	General
Cover, Cart	General
Cover, Laundry Hamper	General
Cover, Mattress	General
Cover, Mattress, Waterproof	General
Cover, Other	General
Curtain, Shower	General
Hypo/Hyperthermia Blanket	General
Laundry Hamper	General
Linen, Bed	General
Pillow	General
Stand, Laundry Hamper	General

HOSHIZAKI AMERICA, INC.   800-438-6087
618 Hwy. 74 S., Peachtree City, GA 30269-3002   **770-487-2331**
FDA Number: n/a   Fax: 770-487-1325
E-mail: marketing@hoshizaki.com
Web site: www.hoshizaki.com
Medical Products Sales Volume: $130,000,000
Year Founded: 1981
Total Employees: 350   Marketing Staff: 7   Sales Staff: 15
Ownership: Hoshizaki America, Inc.
Quality System Registration Information: ISO9001
Produces/Sells CE-marked Devices: Y
Federal Procurement Eligibility: Small Business, GSA Contract
Distribution: Manufacturer Through Distributor, Exporter
General Admin.: Mr. Youki Suzuki/Executive Vice President
Mktg./Adv.: Mr. Estuardo Herrera/Director International Marketing & Sales
     Mrs. Julie Strain/Manager Marketing
     Mr. Keith Black/Manager National Sales
     Mr. Mickey Gardner/Manager National Sales
     Mr. Carter Davis/Vice President Marketing & Sales
Production: Mrs. Barbara Harrison/Director Operations
     Mr. Tom Machingo/Vice President Manufacturing

Dispenser, Ice	General
Refrigerator, Foodservice	General

Medical Product Subsidiaries (Listed Separately)
   Hoshizaki America, Inc.

HOSMER DORRANCE CORP.   408-379-5151
561 Division St., Campbell, CA 95008
FDA Number: 2917184

Ankle/Foot, External Limb Component	Physical Med
Assembly, Shoulder/Elbow/Forearm/Wrist/Hand, Mechanical	Physical Med
Assembly, Shoulder/Elbow/Forearm/Wrist/Hand, Powered	Physical Med
Brace, Joint, Ankle (External)	Physical Med
Glove, Patient Examination, Specialty	General
Hand, External Limb Component, Mechanical	Physical Med
Hook, External Limb Component, Mechanical	Physical Med
Hook, External Limb Component, Powered	Physical Med
Joint, Elbow, External Limb Component, Mechanical	Physical Med
Joint, Elbow, External Limb Component, Powered	Physical Med
Joint, Hip, External Brace	Physical Med
Joint, Hip, External Limb Component	Physical Med
Joint, Knee, External Brace	Physical Med
Joint, Knee, External Limb Component	Physical Med
Joint, Shoulder, External Limb Component	Physical Med
Joint, Wrist, External Limb Component, Mechanical	Physical Med
Orthosis, Limb Brace	Physical Med
Prosthesis Alignment Device	Physical Med
Prosthesis, Thigh Socket, External Component	Physical Med
Valve, Prosthesis	Physical Med

HOSMER-DORRANCE CORP.   800-827-0070
561 Division St., Campbell, CA 95008-6952   **408-379-5151**
FDA Number: n/a   Fax: 408-379-5263
E-mail: jbradford@hosmer.com
Web site: www.hosmer.com
Annual Revenue: $10-$25 Million
Total Employees: 60   Marketing Staff: 2   Sales Staff: 2
Ownership: Fillauer Companies, Inc.

HOSMER-DORRANCE CORP.   800-827-0070 (cont'd)
Quality System Registration Information: ISO9001
Produces/Sells CE-marked Devices: N
Federal Procurement Eligibility: Small Business
Distribution: Manufacturer Through Distributor
General Admin.: Judy Wehle/Manager Human Resources
     Carl Karlvohand/President, Chief Executive Officer
Mktg./Adv.: Elida Travis/Director Marketing
     Jackie Bradford/Director Marketing
     Gerald Stark/Director Product Development
     Jackie Bradford/Manager International & National Sales
Production: Karl Hovland/Director Quality Assurance
     Karl Hovland/Manager Engineering

Ankle/Foot, External Limb Component	Physical Med
Hand, External Limb Component, Mechanical	Physical Med
Hook, External Limb Component, Mechanical	Physical Med
Joint, Elbow, External Limb Component, Mechanical	Physical Med
Joint, Elbow, External Limb Component, Powered	Physical Med
Joint, Knee, External Limb Component	Physical Med
Joint, Wrist, External Limb Component, Mechanical	Physical Med
Orthosis, Limb Brace	Physical Med
Prosthesis, Arm	Orthopedics
Prosthesis, Foot	Orthopedics
Prosthesis, Leg	Orthopedics

HOSPI-TEL MANUFACTURING CORP.   973-678-7100
545 N. Arlington Ave., East Orange, NJ 07017
FDA Number: n/a   Fax: 973-678-1482
E-mail: info@hospitel.com
Web site: www.hospitel.com
Annual Revenue: $5-$10 Million
Total Employees: 96
Ownership: Private
Produces/Sells CE-marked Devices: N
Federal Procurement Eligibility: Small Business
Distribution: Manufacturer Through Distributor
General Admin.: D. L. Freedland/President
Mktg./Adv.: R. Damiano/Executive Vice President Marketing
     M. Genaro/Manager International & National Sales
Production: J. Freedland/Vice President Operations

Curtain, Cubicle	General
Curtain, Shower	General
Track And Carrier, Cubicle Curtain	General

HOSPIRA   800-441-4100
268 E. Fourth St., Ashland, OH 44805-2494   **419-289-3555**
FDA Number: 1520456   Fax: 419-281-3970
E-mail: hpdashlandsales@abbott.com
Web site: www.hospira.com
Medical Products Sales Volume: $2,800,000,000
Year Founded: 1930
Total Employees: 16000
Ownership: Abbott Laboratories
Stock Symbol: HSP
Traded On: NYSE
Quality System Registration Information: ISO9002
Produces/Sells CE-marked Devices: N
Distribution: Manufacturer Direct
Mktg./Adv.: Greg Talese/Director Sales
Production: Robert Whites/Manager Manufacturing

Applicator, Tipped, Absorbent	General
Aspirator, Infant	General
Aspirator, Wound Suction Pump	General
Bag, Breathing	Anesthesiology
Bag, Ice	General
Bottle, Hot/Cold Water	General
Clamp, Tubing	General
Component, Rubber	General
Contract Sterilization	General
Douche, Vaginal	Obstetrics/Gynecology
Finger Cot	General
Fitting, Luer	General
Glove, Other	General
Glove, Patient Examination, Specialty	General
Hanger, Intravenous	General
Nipple, Feeding	General
Pump, Breast, Non-Powered	Obstetrics/Gynecology
Stopper	General
Syringe, Bulb, Air Or Water	Dental And Oral
Tip, Enema	General
Tubing, Polyvinyl Chloride	General

HOSPIRA INC.   877-946-7747
275 N. Field Drive, Lake forest, IL 60045   **224-212-2000**
FDA Number: 3005579246
Web site: www.hospira.com
Medical Products Sales Volume: $2,262,315,000
Annual Revenue: More than $1 Billion
Total Employees: 14000

HOSPIRA INC.   877-946-7747 *(cont'd)*

Ownership: Public
Stock Symbol: HSP
Traded On: NYSE
Produces/Sells CE-marked Devices: N
Distribution: OEM
General Admin.: Mr. Christopher B. Begley/Chief Executive Officer, Chairman
         Mr. Thomas E. Werner/Chief Financial Officer, Senior Vice President
         Ms. Daphne Jones/Chief Information Officer
         Mr. Terrence C. Kearney/Chief Operating Officer
         Dr. Sumant Ramachandra/Chief Scientific Officer
         Mr. Brian J. Smith/Senior Vice President, General Counsel, Secretary
Mktg./Adv.: Mr. Rob Squarer/Commercial Director
         Mr. Anil D'Sousa/Vice President Global Marketing

Adapter, Syringe	General
Catheter, Intravascular, Therapeutic, Short-term Less Than 30 Days	General
Container, IV	General
Filter, Infusion Line	General
Infusion Stand	General
Needle, Other	General
Pump, Infusion	General
Set, Administration, Intravenous, Needle-Free	General
Stopcock	General
Surgical Instrument, Disposable	Surgery
Syringe, Piston	General
Transfer Unit, IV Fluid	General
Tube, Connecting	General
Tubing, Fluid Delivery	General

Medical Product Subsidiaries (Listed Separately)
Hospira Sedation, Inc.
Hospira, Inc
Hospira, Inc.

HOSPIRA SEDATION, INC.   877-946-7747
Five Billerica Park, 101 Billerica Avenue, North Billerica, MA 01862
FDA Number: 1224640
Web site: www.hospira.com
Total Employees: 40
Ownership: Hospira Inc.
Stock Symbol: HSP
Traded On: NYSE
Quality System Registration Information: ISO9001
Produces/Sells CE-marked Devices: N
Distribution: Manufacturer Through Distributor

Amplifier, Physiological Signal	Cns/Neurology
Electrode, Cutaneous	Cns/Neurology

HOSPIRA, INC   877-946-7747
13520 Evening Creek Drive, Suite 200, San Diego, CA 92128
FDA Number: 2024064
Web site: www.hospira.com
Ownership: Hospira Inc.
Stock Symbol: HSP
Traded On: NYSE
Produces/Sells CE-marked Devices: Y
Distribution: Manufacturer Direct, Manufacturer Through Manufacturer Reps
General Admin.: Miles D. White/Chief Executive Officer
         Robert L. Parkinson/Chief Operating Officer

Pump, Infusion, Ambulatory	General

HOSPIRA, INC.   877-946-7747
1776 North Centennial Drive, Mcpherson, KS 67460
FDA Number: 1925262
Web site: www.hospira.com
Ownership: Hospira Inc.
Stock Symbol: HSP
Traded On: NYSE
Produces/Sells CE-marked Devices: N

Adapter, Holder, Syringe	Physical Med
Controller, Injector, Angiographic	Cardiovascular
Syringe, Piston	General
Transfer Device, Patient, Manual	General

HOSPIRA, INC.   877-946-7747
755 Jarvis Drive, Morgan Hill, CA 95037
FDA Number: 2921482
Web site: www.hospira.com
Ownership: Hospira Inc.
Stock Symbol: HSP
Traded On: NYSE
Quality System Registration Information: ISO9000
Produces/Sells CE-marked Devices: Y
Distribution: Manufacturer Direct, Importer, Exporter

Cardiac Output Unit, Indicator Dilution (Thermal)	Cardiovascular
Catheter, Arterial	Cardiovascular
Catheter, Cardiovascular	Surgery

HOSPIRA, INC.   877-946-7747 *(cont'd)*

Catheter, Continuous Flush	Cardiovascular
Catheter, Flow Directed	Cardiovascular
Catheter, Infusion	Surgery
Catheter, Intravascular, Diagnostic	Cardiovascular
Catheter, Intravascular, Therapeutic, Short-term Less Than 30 Days	General
Catheter, Light, Fiberoptic, Glass, Ureteral	Gastroenterology/Urology
Catheter, Multiple Lumen	Surgery
Catheter, Oximeter, Fiberoptic	Cardiovascular
Catheter, Subclavian	Cardiovascular
Cautery, Radiofrequency, AC-Powered	Ophthalmology
Cautery, Thermal, AC-Powered	Ophthalmology
Cautery, Thermal, Battery-Powered	Ophthalmology
Computer, Diagnostic, Pre-Programmed, Single-Function	Cardiovascular
Cutter, Surgical	Surgery
Dome, Pressure Transducer	General
Electrocautery Unit, Battery-Powered	Surgery
Electrocautery Unit, Line-Powered	Surgery
Flushing Device, Automatic	Anesthesiology
Guidewire	Cardiovascular
Introducer, Catheter	Cardiovascular
Kit, Administration, Intravenous	General
Kit, Blood Pressure, Central Venous	Cardiovascular
Kit, Pressure Monitoring (Air/Gas)	General
Labeling Equipment	General
Oximeter, Intracardiac	Cardiovascular
Pump, Infusion	General
Stopcock	General
Transducer, Blood Flow, Invasive	Anesthesiology
Transducer, Blood Pressure	General
Valve, Catheter Flush	Cardiovascular
Valve, Catheter Flush, Continuous	Cardiovascular

HOSPIRA, INC.   877-946-7747
8484 U.S 70 West, Clayton, NC 27520   224-212-2000
FDA Number: 1048698
Web site: www.hospira.com
Total Employees: 170
Ownership: Hospira Inc.
Stock Symbol: HSP
Traded On: NYSE
Produces/Sells CE-marked Devices: N
Distribution: Importer, Exporter

Standard, Amino Acid	Chemistry
Standard, Lipid	Chemistry

HOSPIRA, INC.   877-946-7747
Hwy. 301 North, Rocky Mount, NC 27801   224-212-2000
FDA Number: 1021343
Web site: www.hospira.com
Ownership: Hospira Inc.
Stock Symbol: HSP
Traded On: NYSE
Produces/Sells CE-marked Devices: N

Adapter, Catheter	Surgery
Container, IV	General
Hysteroscopy Fluid	Obstetrics/Gynecology
Kit, Administration, Intravenous	General
Kit, Administration, Peritoneal Dialysis, Disposable	Gastroenterology/Urology
Kit, Anesthesia, Conduction	Anesthesiology
Kit, Urinary Drainage Collection	Gastroenterology/Urology
Pump, Infusion, Patient Controlled Analgesia (PCA)	General
Transfer Aid	Physical Med

HOSPITAL COMM. & ELECTRONICS, INC.   800-558-8957
7915 North 81st Street,, Milwaukee, WI 53223   414-351-4660
FDA Number: n/a   *Fax:* 414-351-4657
E-mail: sales@cornell.com
Web site: www.cornell.com
Medical Products Sales Volume: $1,000,000
Annual Revenue: $1-$5 Million
Year Founded: 1986
Total Employees: 25   *Marketing Staff:* 1   *Sales Staff:* 1
Ownership: Private
Produces/Sells CE-marked Devices: N
Federal Procurement Eligibility: Small Business, Female Owned, GSA Contract
Distribution: Manufacturer Direct, Manufacturer Through Manufacturer Reps
General Admin.: Maryanne Dwyer/President
Mktg./Adv.: Suzanne Rahall/Director Marketing
         Suzanne Rahall/Vice President Sales

Nurse Call System	General

HOSPITAL COMPUTER SYSTEMS, INC.
See Health Care Software, Inc. (Hcs)

HOSPITAL LAUNDRY SERVICES - STERILE RECOVERY DIVISION   847-229-0900
45 West Hintz Road, Wheeling, IL 60090
FDA Number: 1424436   *Fax:* 847-537-9138
E-mail: tgarcia@hlschicago.com

HOSPITAL LAUNDRY SERVICES - STERILE 847-229-0900 (cont'd)

Web site: www.hlschicago.com
Medical Products Sales Volume: $30,400,000
Annual Revenue: $5-$10 Million
Year Founded: 1996
Total Employees: 400   *Marketing Staff:* 1   *Sales Staff:* 1
Ownership: Private
Quality System Registration Information: ISO9002
Produces/Sells CE-marked Devices: N
Federal Procurement Eligibility: Small Business
Distribution: Manufacturer Direct
General Admin.: Don Pedder/President, Chief Executive Officer
     Gary Vanderlinden/Vice President Human Resources
Mktg./Adv.: Rosemary Burke/Director Marketing & Advertising
     Donna Swenson/Director Product Development
     Therese Gacki/Manager Contract Sales
     Rosemary Burke/Manager Market Research
     Rosemary Burke/Manager Sales Training
     Bill Jones/Vice President Business Development
Production: Mr. Gary Vanderlinden/Director Materials Management
     Donna Swenson/Director Quality Assurance
     Donna Swenson/Manager Regulatory Affairs
     Bill Jones/Vice President Manufacturing

Kit, Surgical (General)	Surgery

HOSPITAL MARKETING SVCS. COMPANY, INC.   800-786-5094
162 Great Hill Rd., Naugatuck, CT 06770   **203-723-1466**
FDA Number: 1216030   *Fax:* 203-723-7248
E-mail: info@hmsmedical.com
Web site: www.hmsmedical.com
Total Employees: 50   *Marketing Staff:* 4   *Sales Staff:* 42
Ownership: Private
Produces/Sells CE-marked Devices: Y
Federal Procurement Eligibility: Small Business, Female Owned, GSA Contract, VA Contract
Distribution: Manufacturer Through Distributor, Manufacturer Through Manufacturer Reps, OEM, Exporter
General Admin.: Barbara A. Strachan/Office Manager
     Brian C. Hurley/President, Chief Executive Officer
     Mildred Hurley/Vice President
Mktg./Adv.: Edward Cooney/Vice President Sales
Production: Barbara A. Strachan/Customer Service Representative
     Nancy A. Capizzi/Director Customer Services
     Judson Doyle/Vice President Manufacturing
IS: Dennis Talarino/Manager Information Systems

Bag, Ice	General
Bandage, Compression	General
Bandage, Elastic	General
Bandage, Other	General
Belt, Abdominal	Gastroenterology/Urology
Belt, Lumbosacral	Orthopedics
Belt, Rib (Support)	Orthopedics
Belt, Support, Pelvic	Physical Med
Belt, Traction, Pelvic	Physical Med
Belt, Traction, Pelvic, Orthopedic	Orthopedics
Binder, Abdominal	General
Binder, Abdominal, OB/GYN	Obstetrics/Gynecology
Binder, Ankle	Orthopedics
Binder, Breast	Obstetrics/Gynecology
Binder, Chest	General
Binder, Elastic	General
Binder, Perineal	General
Binder, Wrist	Orthopedics
Blade, Scalpel	Surgery
Collar, Ice	General
Contract Manufacturing, Product, Disposable	General
Contract Packaging	General
Heater, Hot Pack	Physical Med
Heater, Perineal	Obstetrics/Gynecology
Heater, Perineal, Direct Contact	Obstetrics/Gynecology
Kit, Maternity	Obstetrics/Gynecology
Knife, Other	Surgery
Knife, Scalpel	Surgery
Knife, Surgical	Dental And Oral
Marker, Skin	Surgery
Marker, X-Ray	Radiology
Needle, Other	General
Needle, Suture, Disposable	Surgery
Needle, Suture, Reusable	Surgery
Orthosis, Rib Fracture, Soft	Physical Med
Orthosis, Thoracic	Physical Med
Pack, Cold	General
Pack, Cold, Chemical	General
Pack, Hot Or Cold, Disposable	Physical Med
Pack, Hot Or Cold, Reusable	Physical Med
Pack, Hot, Chemical	General
Pack, Moist Heat	Physical Med
Pen, Marking, Surgical	Ophthalmology
Pin, Safety	General

HOSPITAL MARKETING SVCS. COMPANY, INC.   800-786-5094
(cont'd)

Scalpel, One-Piece (Knife)	Surgery
Support, Abdominal	Physical Med
Support, Ankle	Orthopedics
Support, Arm	Physical Med
Support, Back	Orthopedics
Support, Hot/Cold Pack	Physical Med
Support, Knee	Physical Med
Support, Thigh	Physical Med
Support, Wrist	Physical Med
Waste Disposal Unit, Surgical Instrument (Sharps)	Surgery

HOSPITAL SPECIALTY COMPANY   800-321-9832
26301 Curtiss-Wright Parkway, Cleveland, OH 44143
FDA Number: 1034584   *Fax:* 800-362-0073
E-mail: Hospecomarketing@tranzonic.com
Web site: www.hospeco.com
Annual Revenue: $50-$100 Million
Year Founded: 1919
Total Employees: 420   *Marketing Staff:* 5   *Sales Staff:* 10
Ownership: Hospital Specialty Co. Division Of Tranzonic
Stock Symbol: TRNZ
Traded On: AMEX
Produces/Sells CE-marked Devices: N
Federal Procurement Eligibility: Small Business
Distribution: Manufacturer Through Distributor, OEM, Exclusive Distributor, Importer, Exporter
General Admin.: William Hemann/President
     Kathy Metzger/Vice President, General Manager
Medical Admin.: Ernest Clarke/Vice President Health Care
Mktg./Adv.: Mark Prosser/Director National Accounts
     Rob Lippucci/Director Product Development
     Susan Cole/Manager Advertising
     Nobie Reed/Manager Contract Sales
     Tony Startup/Manager National Sales
     Paul Marion/Vice President Marketing
     Beth Richman/Vice President Sales
Production: Chester Ritter/Director Quality Assurance
     Robert May/Manager Regulatory Affairs

Condom	Obstetrics/Gynecology
Diaper, Adult	General
Diaper, Pediatric	General
Kit, First Aid	Surgery
Pad, Incontinence (Underpad)	General

HOSPITAL SYSTEMS, INC.   925-427-7800
750 Garcia Ave., Pittsburg, CA 94565
FDA Number: n/a   *Fax:* 925-427-0800
E-mail: info@hospitalsystems.com
Web site: www.hospitalsystems.com
Annual Revenue: $5-$10 Million
Year Founded: 1970
Total Employees: 65
Ownership: Private
Produces/Sells CE-marked Devices: N
Federal Procurement Eligibility: Small Business
Distribution: Manufacturer Direct, Manufacturer Through Distributor, Manufacturer Through Manufacturer Reps, Exporter
General Admin.: David Miller/President
Production: Seye Louie/Manager Materials
     Russell Weng/Vice President Manufacturing

Furniture, Patient Room	General
Headwall System (Patient Room)	General

HOSPITAL THERAPY PRODUCTS, INC.   630-766-7101
757 North Central Ave., Wood Dale, IL 60191
FDA Number: 1419182

Adapter, Hygiene	Physical Med
Bath, Hydro-Massage (Whirlpool)	Physical Med
Bath, Sitz, Physical Medicine	Physical Med
Glove, Patient Examination	General
Pack, Hot Or Cold, Water Circulating	Physical Med
Plinth	Physical Med

HOSPITECNICA, S.A. DE C.V.   800 003-3400
Ave. Universidad 771, DF cp. 03100 Mexico   **55 5688-5422**
FDA Number: n/a   *Fax:* 5-688-5649
E-mail: ventas@hospitecnica.com.mx
Web site: www.hospitecnica.com.mx
Medical Products Sales Volume: $1,000,000
Total Employees: 30   *Marketing Staff:* 2   *Sales Staff:* 10
Ownership: Private
Produces/Sells CE-marked Devices: N
Federal Procurement Eligibility: Small Business
Distribution: Manufacturer Through Distributor, Service Direct, Exclusive Distributor, Importer

HOSUK AMERICA CO.
303-750-3829
1583 South Tucson Street, Aurora, CO 80012
FDA Number: 1724738   Fax: 303-750-4139
E-mail: hoamco@msn.com
Ownership: Private
Produces/Sells CE-marked Devices: N
General Admin.: Mr. Chang Han/President
           Mr. Timothy Han/Vice President

Lancet, Blood	General
Syringe, Piston	General

HOT CELL SERVICES
800-562-2439
253-854-4945
22626 85th Place South, Kent, WA 98031
FDA Number: n/a   Fax: 253-854-4947
E-mail: hotcell@hotcell.com
Web site: www.hotcell.com
Annual Revenue: $1-$5 Million
Year Founded: 1979
Total Employees: 50   Marketing Staff: 1   Sales Staff: 3
Ownership: Private
Produces/Sells CE-marked Devices: N
Federal Procurement Eligibility: Small Business
Distribution: Manufacturer Direct, Manufacturer Through Manufacturer Reps, Service Direct
Mktg./Adv.: Zbigniew Tomalik/Sales Representative

Service, Maintenance/Repair	General

HOTPACK
800-523-3608
215-824-1700
10940 Dutton Rd., Philadelphia, PA 19154-3286
FDA Number: 9200547   Fax: 215-637-0519
E-mail: hotpack@hotpack.com
Web site: www.hotpack.com
Annual Revenue: $0-$1 Million
Total Employees: 100   Marketing Staff: 2   Sales Staff: 4
Ownership: SP INDUSTRIES, INC.
Produces/Sells CE-marked Devices: Y
Federal Procurement Eligibility: Small Business
Distribution: Manufacturer Through Manufacturer Reps
General Admin.: Chuck Grant/Chief Executive Officer
           Jill Strauss/Human Resources Associate
           Yury Zlobinsky/President
Mktg./Adv.: Vadim Klauberg/Director Product Development
           Allen Spector/Manager Contract Sales
           Sofia Morales/Manager International & National Sales
           Cesar Montalvo/Manager International Marketing & Sales
           Ed Carroll/Manager Sales
           Ken Clary/Manager Sales Training
           Ken Clary/Vice President Marketing & Sales
Production: Barbara Lewis/Director Quality Assurance
           Jaak Kusma/Manager Materials
           Yury Langer/Vice President Manufacturing
Research: Vadim klauberg/Vice President Research & Development
Finance: Christopher Byers/Controller

Chamber, Constant Temperature (Environmental)	Microbiology
Incubator, Aerobic	Microbiology
Incubator, Anaerobic	Microbiology
Incubator, Test Tube, Stationary	Microbiology
Oven	Chemistry
Refrigerator, Biological	Microbiology
Refrigerator, Morgue, Walk-In	Pathology
Washer, Labware	Chemistry

HOTSPUR TECHNOLOGIES INC.
650-969-3150
880 Maude Avenue, Suite A, Mountain View, CA 94043
FDA Number: 3008513522   Fax: 408-608-1597
E-mail: info@hotspur-inc.com
Web site: http://www.hotspur-inc.com
Year Founded: 2008
Ownership: Private
Produces/Sells CE-marked Devices: N
General Admin.: Ms. Gwen Watanabe/President, Chief Executive Officer

Catheter, Angioplasty, Peripheral, Transluminal, Dual-balloon	Cardiovascular
Catheter, Embolectomy (Fogarty Type)	Cardiovascular

HOUDAILLE INDUSTRIES INC.
See Tyco Valves and Controls

HOUSE OF HEARING
480-649-9609
4020 E. Main St., Mesa, AZ 85205
FDA Number: 3004900330

Hearing-Aid, Plate, Face	Ear/Nose/Throat

HOUSTON FEARLESS 76, INC.
See Hf Pure Water

HOVEROUND CORPORATION
800-964-6837
941-739-6200
2151 Whitfield Industrial Way, Sarasota, FL 34243
FDA Number: 1056601   Fax: 941-782-1475

HOVEROUND CORPORATION
800-964-6837 (cont'd)
E-mail: marketing@hoveround.com
Web site: www.hoveround.com
Medical Products Sales Volume: $42,400,000
Annual Revenue: $25-$50 Million
Total Employees: 556   Marketing Staff: 5   Sales Staff: 130
Ownership: Private
Quality System Registration Information: ISO9001
Produces/Sells CE-marked Devices: N
Federal Procurement Eligibility: VA Contract
Distribution: Manufacturer Direct
General Admin.: Dave Thayer/Chief Operating Officer, Vice President
           Erica Dow/Director Human Resources
           Thomas Kruse/President
Mktg./Adv.: Cheryl Ferreira/Director Marketing & Advertising
           Calvin L. Cole/Manager National Sales
Production: Tim Adwell/Manager Materials

Scooter (Motorized 3-Wheeled Vehicle)	Physical Med
Wheelchair, Powered	Physical Med

HOVERTECH INTERNATIONAL
800-471-2776
610-694-9600
513 S. Clewell St., Bethlehem, PA 18015
FDA Number: n/a   Fax: 610-694-9601
E-mail: info@hoovermatt.com
Web site: www.hovermatt.com
Annual Revenue: $10-$25 Million
Year Founded: 1997
Total Employees: 20   Marketing Staff: 3   Sales Staff: 25
Ownership: Private
Produces/Sells CE-marked Devices: Y
Federal Procurement Eligibility: Small Business
Distribution: Manufacturer Direct, Manufacturer Through Distributor, Manufacturer Through Manufacturer Reps
General Admin.: David T. Davis/Owner, Chief Executive Officer
           Mr. Jerry Silvertooth/President, Chief Operating Officer
Mktg./Adv.: Richard Eveld/Manager International & National Sales

Lift, Patient	General
Mattress, Air Flotation	General
Patient Transfer Unit	General

HOWARD INSTRUMENTS, INC.
205-758-9083
4749 Appletree, Tuscaloosa, AL 35405-5747
FDA Number: 1039865   Fax: 205-758-9083
E-mail: howard@howardinstruments.com
Web site: www.howardinstruments.com
Medical Products Sales Volume: $1,000,000
Annual Revenue: $1-$5 Million
Year Founded: 1981
Total Employees: 4   Marketing Staff: 1   Sales Staff: 1
Ownership: Private
Quality System Registration Information: ISO9001
Produces/Sells CE-marked Devices: Y
Federal Procurement Eligibility: Small Business, Minority Owned
Distribution: Manufacturer Direct, Manufacturer Through Distributor, Manufacturer Through Manufacturer Reps, Importer, Exporter
General Admin.: Jack Howard/President, Chief Executive Officer

Cannula, Surgical, General & Plastic Surgery	Surgery
Catheter, Balloon, Reattachment, Retinal	Ophthalmology
Clip, Iris Retractor	Ophthalmology
Clip, Other	Surgery
Drape, Patient, Ophthalmic	Ophthalmology
Lens, Intraocular	Ophthalmology
Phacofragmentation Unit	Ophthalmology
Scissors, Iris	Ophthalmology
Tubing, Silicone	General

HOWARD MEDICAL COMPANY
800-443-1444
773-278-1440
1690 N. Elston, Chicago, IL 60622-1530
FDA Number: 1451041   Fax: 773-278-9513
E-mail: info@howardmedical.com
Web site: www.howardmedical.com
Medical Products Sales Volume: $2,000,000
Annual Revenue: $1-$5 Million
Year Founded: 1978
Total Employees: 10   Marketing Staff: 1   Sales Staff: 4
Ownership: Private
Produces/Sells CE-marked Devices: N
Federal Procurement Eligibility: Small Business
Distribution: Manufacturer Direct, Manufacturer Through Distributor
General Admin.: Ross Litton/President
           Bernie Litton/Vice President

Bed, Flotation Therapy, Neonatal	General
Computer Software	General
Diaper, Adult	General
Diaper, Pediatric	General
Glove, Autopsy	Pathology
Glove, Surgical	General
Glove, Surgical, Powder-Free	Surgery

HOWARD MEDICAL COMPANY   800-443-1444 *(cont'd)*

Gown, Patient, Disposable	General
Holder, Medical Chart	General
Mattress, Air Flotation	General
Mattress, Water	General
Pad, Incontinence (Underpad)	General
Reader, Bar Code	General
Sheet, Examination Table, Disposable	General
Stand/Holder, Equipment, Laboratory	Chemistry
Toothbrush, Manual	Dental And Oral

HOWARD/MCCRAY REFRIGERATOR, INC.   800-344-8222
831 East Cayuga St, Philadelphia, PA 19124   215-464-6800
FDA Number: n/a   Fax: 215-969-4890
E-mail: sales@howardmccray.com
Web site: www.howardmccray.com
Annual Revenue: $5-$10 Million
Year Founded: 1887
Ownership: Private
Produces/Sells CE-marked Devices: N
Federal Procurement Eligibility: Small Business
Distribution: Manufacturer Direct

Refrigerator, Foodservice	General

HOWELL VENTURES LTD.   888-370-5050
4850 Route 102,   506-363-5289
Upper Kingsclear, NB E3E- Canada
FDA Number: n/a   Fax: 800-506-6666
E-mail: keith@suregrip-hvl.com
Web site: www.suregrip-hvl.com
Year Founded: 1986
Total Employees: 10
Ownership: Private
Produces/Sells CE-marked Devices: N
Distribution: Manufacturer Direct, Exclusive Distributor, Exporter

HOWMEDICA INC., DENTAL DIVISION
See Dentsply Prosthetics

HOWMEDICA LEIBINGER, INC.
See Striker Corp.

HOWMEDICA, INC.
See Stryker Spine

HOWMEDICA, INC. UNITED DIV.
See Smith & Nephew, Inc.

HOYLE PRODUCTS, INC.   800-345-1950
10675 Highway 155, Glennville, CA 93226   661-536-8063
FDA Number: n/a   Fax: 661-536-8067
Web site: http://acu-arc.com
Annual Revenue: $0-$1 Million
Ownership: Private
Produces/Sells CE-marked Devices: N
Federal Procurement Eligibility: Small Business
Distribution: Manufacturer Direct, Exporter

Utensil, Handicapped Aid	Physical Med

HOYT CORP.   800-343-9411
251 Forge Road, Westport, MA 02790-0217   508-636-8811
FDA Number: 9330049   Fax: 508-636-2088
E-mail: ramsey@hoytcorp.com
Web site: www.hoytcorp.com
Medical Products Sales Volume: $5,700,000
Annual Revenue: $0-$1 Million
Year Founded: 1949
Total Employees: 65
Ownership: Private
Federal Procurement Eligibility: Small Business, Female Owned, GSA Contract
Distribution: Manufacturer Direct, Manufacturer Through Manufacturer Reps
General Admin.: John Olinger/President, Chief Executive Officer
Mktg./Adv.: Pat King/Vice President Marketing
      Cary Becknell/Vice President Sales

Laundry Equipment	General
Washer, Laundry	General

HPG INTERNATIONAL, INC.   800-242-3909
755 Oakhill Rd, Crestwood Ind Park,   800-221-1356x36
Mountain Top, PA 18707
FDA Number: n/a   Fax: 570-474-0998
E-mail: info@i2M.us.com
Web site: www.hpg-intl.com
Medical Products Sales Volume: $4,000,000
Annual Revenue: $1-$5 Million
Year Founded: 1994
Total Employees: 623   *Marketing Staff:* 6   *Sales Staff:* 9
Ownership: Private
Produces/Sells CE-marked Devices: Y
Federal Procurement Eligibility: Small Business

HPG INTERNATIONAL, INC.   800-242-3909 *(cont'd)*
Distribution: Manufacturer Through Distributor, Manufacturer Through
Manufacturer Reps

Building Material	General
Component, Plastic	General
Floor, Conductive	General
Flooring	General
Packaging Material	General

HPK INDUSTRIES LLC   315-724-0196
1208 Broad St., Utica, NY 13501
FDA Number: 3005006384

Gown, Examination	General
Gown, Isolation, Surgical	Surgery
Wrap, Sterilization	General

HPLC TECHNOLOGY
See Phenomenex, Inc.

HQ, INC.
See Hq, Inc.

HR, INC.
See Cenorin

HT MEDICAL SYSTEMS, INC.
See Immersion Medical

HTI PLASTIC
See Heinke Technoogy, Inc. (Hti Plastics)

HTI TECHNOLOGIES
See Hq, Inc.

HTI, INC.   800-685-2997
500 West Wilson Bridge Road, Suite 105,   614-885-2997
Worthington, OH 43085
FDA Number: 1527668   Fax: 614-885-4337
E-mail: webmaster@htiinc.com
Web site: www.htiinc.com
Medical Products Sales Volume: $910,000
Year Founded: 1977
Total Employees: 21
Ownership: Private
Produces/Sells CE-marked Devices: N
Federal Procurement Eligibility: Small Business
General Admin.: Dr. Timothy Rink/Chief Executive Officer

Audiometer	Ear/Nose/Throat

HTL-STREFA, INC.   770-528-0410
3005 Chastain Meadows Pkwy, Suite 300, Marietta, GA 30066
FDA Number: 3006142663   Fax: 770-528-0411
E-mail: info@htl-strefa.com
Web site: www.htl-strefa.com
Ownership: HTL-STREFA S.A.
Stock Symbol: HTL
Quality System Registration Information: ISO9001
Produces/Sells CE-marked Devices: Y
Distribution: Manufacturer Through Distributor, OEM
General Admin.: Mr. Wojciech Wyszogrodzki/President

Lancet, Blood	General

HU-FRIEDY MANUFACTURING CO., INC.   800-483-7433
3232 N. Rockwell, Chicago, IL 60618-5982
FDA Number: 1416605   Fax: 773-975-1683
E-mail: info@hufriedy.com
Web site: www.hufriedy.com
Year Founded: 1908
Ownership: Private
Quality System Registration Information: ISO9001
Produces/Sells CE-marked Devices: Y
Federal Procurement Eligibility: Small Business
Distribution: Manufacturer Through Distributor
General Admin.: Richard Saslow/Chairman
      Ronald Saslow/President, Chief Executive Officer

Awl	Orthopedics
Band, Matrix	Dental And Oral
Blade, Scalpel	Surgery
Burnisher, Operative, Dental	Dental And Oral
Burr, Dental	Dental And Oral
Carrier, Amalgam, Operative	Dental And Oral
Carver, Dental Amalgam, Operative	Dental And Oral
Carver, Wax, Dental	Dental And Oral
Chisel, Bone, Surgical	Dental And Oral
Chisel, Osteotome, Surgical	Dental And Oral
Clamp, Rubber Dam	Dental And Oral
Cleaner, Ultrasonic, Dental Laboratory	Dental And Oral
Condenser, Amalgam And Foil, Operative	Dental And Oral
Curette, Operative	Dental And Oral
Curette, Periodontic	Dental And Oral
Curette, Surgical, Dental	Dental And Oral
Cutter, Operative	Dental And Oral
Elevator, Surgical, Dental	Dental And Oral

HU-FRIEDY MANUFACTURING CO., INC.   800-483-7433 *(cont'd)*

Excavator, Dental, Operative	Dental And Oral
Explorer, Operative	Dental And Oral
File, Bone, Surgical	Dental And Oral
File, Margin Finishing, Operative	Dental And Oral
File, Periodontic	Dental And Oral
Filling, Instrument Plastic, Dental	Dental And Oral
Forceps, Articulation Paper	Dental And Oral
Forceps, Rongeur, Surgical	Dental And Oral
Forceps, Tooth Extractor, Surgical	Dental And Oral
Gag, Mouth	Ear/Nose/Throat
Hand Instrument, Calculus Removal	Dental And Oral
Handle, Instrument, Dental	Dental And Oral
Hemostat, Surgical	Dental And Oral
Hoe, Periodontic	Dental And Oral
Holder, Needle, Other	Surgery
Instrument, Forming, Material, Cranioplasty	Cns/Neurology
Knife, Margin Finishing, Operative	Dental And Oral
Knife, Periodontic	Dental And Oral
Mirror, Mouth	Dental And Oral
Pliers, Operative	Dental And Oral
Pliers, Orthodontic	Dental And Oral
Plugger, Root Canal, Endodontic	Dental And Oral
Probe, Periodontic	Dental And Oral
Pusher, Band, Orthodontic	Dental And Oral
Retractor, All Types	Dental And Oral
Rongeur, Dental	Dental And Oral
Scaler, Periodontic	Dental And Oral
Scaler, Ultrasonic	Dental And Oral
Scissors, Surgical Tissue, Dental (Oral)	Dental And Oral
Sharpener, Dental	Dental And Oral
Sharpener, Microtome Blade	Pathology
Spatula, Cement	Dental And Oral
Spreader, Pulp Canal Filling Material, Endodontic	Dental And Oral
Sterilization Process Indicator, Physical/Chemical	General
Suture, Absorbable, Natural	Surgery
Suture, Absorbable, Synthetic, Polyglycolic Acid	Surgery
Suture, Non-Absorbable	Surgery
Suture, Non-Absorbable, Silk	Surgery
Suture, Non-Absorbable, Synthetic, Polyester	Surgery
Suture, Non-Absorbable, Synthetic, Polypropylene	Surgery
Syringe, Irrigating, Dental	Dental And Oral
Tester, Pulp	Dental And Oral
Tucker, Ligature, Orthodontic	Dental And Oral
Well, Amalgam	Dental And Oral
Wrap, Sterilization	General

Medical Product Subsidiaries (Listed Separately)
   Hu-Friedy Mfg. Co., Inc. - Deutschland

HUBINGER CO., THE
   See Roquette America

HUDSON CONTROL GROUP, INC.   973-376-7400
10 Stern Ave., Springfield, NJ 07081
FDA Number: 2248226
Ownership: Private
Produces/Sells CE-marked Devices: N

Equipment, Laboratory, Gen. Purpose (Specific Medical Use)	Chemistry

HUEBSCH ORIGINATORS
   See Huebsch Sales

HUEBSCH SALES   800-553-5120
PO Box 990, Shepard Street,   920-748-3121
Ripon, WI 54971
FDA Number: n/a   *Fax:* 920-748-4456
E-mail: kevin.hietpas@alliancels.com
Web site: www.huebsch.com
Medical Products Sales Volume: $101,100,000
Year Founded: 1998
Total Employees: 890
Ownership: Private
Quality System Registration Information: ISO9001
Produces/Sells CE-marked Devices: Y
Federal Procurement Eligibility: GSA Contract
Distribution: Manufacturer Through Distributor
Mktg./Adv.: Kevin Hietpas/Manager National Sales

Laundry Equipment	General
Washer, Laundry	General

HUESTIS MACHINE CORP.
   See Huestis Medical

HUESTIS MEDICAL   800-972-9222
68 Buttonwood St., Bristol, RI 02809-3600   401-253-5500
FDA Number: 1219183   *Fax:* 401-253-7350
E-mail: sales@huestis.com
Web site: www.huestismedical.com
Year Founded: 1975
Total Employees: 75   *Marketing Staff:* 2   *Sales Staff:* 9
Ownership: HMC HOLDING CORPORATION
Quality System Registration Information: ISO9001

HUESTIS MEDICAL   800-972-9222 *(cont'd)*
Produces/Sells CE-marked Devices: N
Federal Procurement Eligibility: Small Business
Distribution: Manufacturer Direct, OEM
General Admin.: Mike Doherty/Chairman
           Peter C. Martin/President
Mktg./Adv.: Terry Chwalk/Executive Vice President Marketing
Production: Randy White/Plant & Production Manager

Accelerator, Linear, Medical	Radiology
Block, Beam Shaping, Radionuclide	Radiology
Cassette, Radiographic Film	Radiology
Collimator, Radiographic, Manual	Radiology
Holder, X-Ray Film	Dental And Oral
Shield, X-Ray	Radiology
Simulator, Radiotherapy	Radiology
Therapeutic X-Ray System	Radiology

HUHTAMAKI   484-527-2011
2400 Continental Blvd., Malvern, PA 19355
FDA Number: 1528730   *Fax:* 484 527 2100
Ownership: Private
Produces/Sells CE-marked Devices: N

Container, Specimen, All Types	General

HUHTAMAKI CONSUMER PACKAGING, INC.   913-583-3025
100 State St., Fulton, NY 13069-2599
FDA Number: 1317269
Ownership: Private
Produces/Sells CE-marked Devices: N

Container, Specimen, All Types	General

HULL ANESTHESIA, INC.   800-400-4484
7521 Talbert Avenue,   714-375-2651
Huntington Beach, CA 92648
FDA Number: 2081107   *Fax:* 714-375-2658
E-mail: info@hullanesthesia.com
Web site: www.hullanesthesia.com
Medical Products Sales Volume: $17,000,000
Year Founded: 1971
Total Employees: 14
Ownership: Private
Produces/Sells CE-marked Devices: Y
Federal Procurement Eligibility: Small Business
Distribution: Exclusive Distributor

HULS AMERICA, INC.
   See Hpg International, Inc.

HUMAGEN FERTILITY DIAGNOSTICS, INC.   800-937-3210
2400 Hunter's Way,   434-979-4000
Charlottesville, VA 22911
FDA Number: 1122330   *Fax:* 434-295-5912
E-mail: humagen@humagenivf.com
Web site: www.humagenivf.com
Medical Products Sales Volume: $34,620,000
Year Founded: 1992
Total Employees: 45
Ownership: Private
Produces/Sells CE-marked Devices: Y
Federal Procurement Eligibility: Small Business, Female Owned
Distribution: Manufacturer Direct, Manufacturer Through Distributor, Manufacturer Through Manufacturer Reps, Importer, Exporter
General Admin.: Debra Bryant/President, Chief Executive Officer
Production: Cindy Showalter/Director Quality Assurance
Finance: Kathy Bias/Chief Financial Officer

Counter, Cell	Microbiology
Device, Semen Analysis	Obstetrics/Gynecology
Pipette, Micro	Chemistry

HUMAN MEASUREMENT SYSTEMS   626-201-2437
1159 N. Conwell Ave. # 311, P.o. Box 2442, Covina, CA 91722
FDA Number: 2032854
Ownership: Private
Produces/Sells CE-marked Devices: N

Biofeedback Device	Cns/Neurology

HUMANE RESTRAINT CO INC   800-356-7472
912 Bethel Circle, Waunakee, WI 53597   608-849-6313
FDA Number: 2126660   *Fax:* 608-849-6315
E-mail: schultz1@chorus.net
Web site: www.humanerestraint.com
Medical Products Sales Volume: $21,900,000
Annual Revenue: $1-$5 Million
Year Founded: 1876
Total Employees: 9
Ownership: Private
Produces/Sells CE-marked Devices: N
Federal Procurement Eligibility: Small Business
Distribution: Manufacturer Direct, Manufacturer Through Distributor, Exporter

HUMANE RESTRAINT CO INC   800-356-7472 (cont'd)

General Admin.: Stacy Schultz/General Manager
David Schultz/President

Belt, Wheelchair	Physical Med
Immobilizer, Ankle	Orthopedics
Immobilizer, Wrist/Hand	Orthopedics
Restraint, Ankle/Foot	General
Restraint, Protective (Body)	General
Restraint, Wrist/Hand	General

HUMANICARE INTERNATIONAL, INC.   800-631-5270
9 Elkins Road, East Brunswick, NJ 08816   **888-232-7000**
FDA Number: 2243664   *Fax:* 732-432-5475
E-mail: info@humanicare.com
Web site: www.humanicare.com
Medical Products Sales Volume: $101,100,000
Year Founded: 1980
Total Employees: 50
Ownership: Private
Produces/Sells CE-marked Devices: N
Federal Procurement Eligibility: Small Business
Distribution: Manufacturer Through Distributor, Manufacturer Through Manufacturer Reps, Exporter
General Admin.: Anthony A. Gegelys/Chief Executive Officer
Chris Gegelys/President
Mktg./Adv.: Elaine Austin/Vice President Marketing
Jack C. Fehrenback/Vice President Sales
Production: Daniel Sivilich/Manager Regulatory Affairs
Daniel Sivilich/Vice President Operations

Diaper, Adult	General
Garment, Protective, For Incontinence	Gastroenterology/Urology
Pad, Incontinence (Underpad)	General
Pant, Incontinence	General
Solution, Ostomy, Odor Control	Gastroenterology/Urology

HUMANOID SYSTEMS
See Radiology Support Devices

HUMANTRONIC, INC   866-340-1648
1103 Leeland Hgts Blvd E,   **239-368-7767**
Lehigh Acres, FL 33936
FDA Number: n/a   *Fax:* 239-368-3854
E-mail: office@humantronic.com
Web site: http://humantronic.com
Medical Products Sales Volume: $4,500,000
Annual Revenue: $1-$5 Million
Year Founded: 1999
Total Employees: 5   *Sales Staff:* 2
Ownership: Private
Produces/Sells CE-marked Devices: N
Federal Procurement Eligibility: Small Business
Distribution: Manufacturer Direct, Manufacturer Through Distributor, Manufacturer Through Manufacturer Reps, OEM, Exclusive Distributor, Importer
General Admin.: Mr. Ernst Heinrich/President
Mr. Oliver Gruenwald/Vice President

Stimulator, Neuromuscular, External Functional	Cns/Neurology

HUMANWARE   800-722-3393
175 Mason Circle, Concord, CA 94520   **925-680-7100**
FDA Number: 1420070   *Fax:* 925-681-4630
E-mail: us.info@humanware.com
Web site: www.humanware.com
Medical Products Sales Volume: $17,000,000
Annual Revenue: $10-$25 Million
Year Founded: 2005
Total Employees: 21   *Marketing Staff:* 4   *Sales Staff:* 16
Ownership: Hearing Oasis
Produces/Sells CE-marked Devices: N
Federal Procurement Eligibility: Small Business
Distribution: Exclusive Distributor
General Admin.: Philip Rance/President, Chief Executive Officer
Mktg./Adv.: Jim Halliday/Director Marketing
Sharon Spiker/Manager Business

Computer Equipment	General
Vision Aid, Braille	General

HUMBOLDT PRODUCTS CORP.
See Microtek Medical, Inc

HUNT'S CONVALESCENT EQUIPMENT CO. INC.   800-838-5146
7-109 Woodbine Downs Blvd.,   **416-798-1303**
Toronto, ONT M9W-6 Canada
FDA Number: n/a   *Fax:* 416-798-1290
E-mail: hunts@idirect.com
Web site: www.huntshealthcare.com
Year Founded: 1979
Total Employees: 10
Ownership: Private
Produces/Sells CE-marked Devices: N

HUNT'S CONVALESCENT EQUIPMENT CO. INC.   800-838-5146
(cont'd)
Distribution: Service Direct

HUNTER ASSOCIATES LAB., INC.   703-471-6870
11491 Sunset Hills Road, Reston, VA 20190-5280
FDA Number: 7000182   *Fax:* 703-471-4237
E-mail: info@hunterlab.com
Web site: www.hunterlab.com
Medical Products Sales Volume: $101,100,000
Annual Revenue: $10-$25 Million
Year Founded: 1952
Total Employees: 100
Ownership: Private
Quality System Registration Information: ISO9001
Produces/Sells CE-marked Devices: Y
Distribution: Manufacturer Direct, Manufacturer Through Manufacturer Reps, Exporter
General Admin.: P. S. Hunter/President, Chief Executive Officer
Mktg./Adv.: Hal Good/Director Marketing
Lore Potoker/Manager Marketing Communications
Paul Barnes/Manager National Sales
Bob Weaver/Vice President Marketing & Sales

Colorimeter, General Use	Chemistry
Spectrophotometer, Visible	Chemistry

HUNTER RESEARCH LABORATORIES, INC.   888-764-5463
2225 sierra heights drive, Las Vegas, NV 89134   **303-696-8888**
FDA Number: 1724807   *Fax:* 303-744-8998
E-mail: saferneedle@yahoo.com
Web site: www.saferneedle.com
Medical Products Sales Volume: $4,500,000
Annual Revenue: $10-$25 Million
Year Founded: 1999
Ownership: Private
Produces/Sells CE-marked Devices: Y
Federal Procurement Eligibility: Small Business, Minority Owned, Female Owned
Distribution: Manufacturer Direct, Manufacturer Through Distributor, OEM, Exporter
General Admin.: Dr. Carl Brownd/Chief Executive Officer
Mktg./Adv.: Barbara Pedigo/Director Marketing
Barbara Pedigo/Manager International & National Sales
Barbara Pedigo/Manager Market Research
Research: Dr. Carl Brownd/Director Professional Research

Instrument Guard	Surgery

HUNTINGTON MECHANICAL LABORATORIES, INC.   800-227-8059
1040 La Avenida Street,   **650-964-3323**
Mountain View, CA 94043
FDA Number: n/a   *Fax:* 650-964-6153
E-mail: vacman@huntvac.com
Web site: www.huntvac.com
Medical Products Sales Volume: $500,000
Annual Revenue: $5-$10 Million
Year Founded: 1969
Ownership: Private
Produces/Sells CE-marked Devices: N
Federal Procurement Eligibility: Small Business
Distribution: Manufacturer Direct, Manufacturer Through Manufacturer Reps, Importer, Exporter
General Admin.: Ron Hooper/President
Mktg./Adv.: Tom Frantz/Vice President Sales

Bottle, Collection, Vacuum (Aspirator)	General
Lamp, Infrared	Physical Med
Micrometer, Microscope	Pathology

HUNTINGTON MEDICAL PRODUCTS
See Great Midwest Packaging, Llc

HUOT INSTRUMENTS, LLC   262-373-1700
N50 W13740 Overview Dr., Suite A,
Menomonee Falls, WI 53051
FDA Number: 3005934371

Punch, Surgical	Surgery

HURLEY MAT COMPANY, B.F.   800-274-6287
5601 Bayshore Blvd., P.O. Box 13217,   **813-837-0616**
Tampa, FL 33681
FDA Number: n/a   *Fax:* 813-837-2527
E-mail: mats@hurleymat.com
Web site: www.hurleymat.com
Annual Revenue: $0-$1 Million
Total Employees: 30   *Marketing Staff:* 2
Ownership: Private
Produces/Sells CE-marked Devices: N
Federal Procurement Eligibility: Small Business

HURLEY MAT COMPANY, B.F.　　800-274-6287 (cont'd)
Distribution: Manufacturer Direct
General Admin.: Richard Hurley/President
Mktg./Adv.: John Hurley/Vice President Marketing
　　Mike Hurley/Vice President Marketing & Sales
Production: Mike Hurley/Vice President Manufacturing
Research: Mike Hurley/Vice President Research & Development

Floor Mat	General

HURRICANE MEDICAL　　941-751-0588
5315 Lena Road, Bradenton, FL 34211
FDA Number: 1064005

Cannula, Ophthalmic	Ophthalmology
Cystotome, Ophthalmic	Ophthalmology
Guide, Intraocular Lens	Ophthalmology
Knife, Ophthalmic	Ophthalmology
Marker, Sclera (Ocular)	Ophthalmology
Needle, Aspiration And Injection, Disposable	Surgery
Probe, Lacrimal	Ophthalmology
Shield, Eye, Ophthalmic	Ophthalmology
Sponge, Ophthalmic	Ophthalmology
Tubing, Fluid Delivery	General
Tubing, Replacement, Phacofragmentation Unit	Ophthalmology
Unit, Filter, Membrane	Chemistry

HUSSMAN/SECO PRODUCTS
See Piper Products, Inc.

HUTCHINSON TECHNOLOGY, INC.　　320-587-3797
40 West Highland Park, Hutchinson, MN 55350
FDA Number: 2184064

Oximeter, Tissue Saturation	Cardiovascular

HVO　　1-800-789-0416
56 Scates St., Waynesville, NC 28786　　828-456-4455
FDA Number: 1043549　　Fax: 828-456-8639
E-mail: HVOSales@hvoinc.com
Web site: www.hvoinc.com
Annual Revenue: $25-$50 Million
Year Founded: 1972
Total Employees: 475
Ownership: Private
Quality System Registration Information: ISO9001
Produces/Sells CE-marked Devices: N
Federal Procurement Eligibility: Small Business
Distribution: Manufacturer Direct, Manufacturer Through Distributor, Manufacturer Through Manufacturer Reps, Exporter

Drape, Patient, Ophthalmic	Ophthalmology
Drape, Surgical	Surgery
Immunoassay, Placental Alpha-1 Microglobulin (pamg-1)	Chemistry
Kit, Surgical Instrument, Disposable	Surgery
Lancet, Blood	General
Needle, Aspiration And Injection, Disposable	Surgery
System, Blood Collection, Vacuum-assisted, Automated	Hematology

HY-MARK CYLINDERS, INC.　　757-245-7331
305 E St., Hampton, VA 23661
FDA Number: 3003987352
Ownership: Private
Produces/Sells CE-marked Devices: N

Cylinder, Gas (Empty)	Anesthesiology

HY-TAPE CORP.
See Hy-Tape International

HY-TAPE INTERNATIONAL　　800-248-0101
70 John Barrett Road　　845-878-4848
Robin Hill Corporate Park
Patterson, NY 12563
FDA Number: 2417991　　Fax: 875-878-4104
E-mail: info@hytape.com
Web site: www.hytape.com
Ownership: Private
Produces/Sells CE-marked Devices: Y
Federal Procurement Eligibility: Small Business
Distribution: OEM, Exclusive Distributor
General Admin.: Sarah Higgins/President
Mktg./Adv.: Mr. Sean Higgins/Manager Sales

Pant, Incontinence	General
Tape, Adhesive, Waterproof	General

HY-TAPE SURGICAL PRODUCTS CORP.
See Hy-Tape International

HYCLONE LABORATORIES, INC.　　435-792-8000
925 West 1800 South, Logan, UT 84321
FDA Number: 1718427

Culture Media, Synthetic Cell And Tissue	Pathology
Serum, Animal	Pathology

HYCOR BIOMEDICAL, INC.　　800-382-2527
7272 Chapman Ave., Garden Grove, CA 92841
FDA Number: 2016473　　Fax: 714-933-3222
Web site: http://www.hycorbiomedical.com
Year Founded: 1981
Ownership: Private
Produces/Sells CE-marked Devices: N

Anti-DNA Antibody (Enzyme-Labeled), Antigen, Control	Immunology
Anti-RNP-Antibody, Antigen And Control	Immunology
Anti-SM-Antibody, Antigen And Control	Immunology
Antibody, Antimitochondrial, Indirect Immunofluorescent	Immunology
Antigen, Antiserum, Control, Spinal Fluid, Total	Immunology
Antinuclear Antibody (Enzyme-Labeled), Antigen, Controls	Immunology
Antinuclear Antibody, Antigen, Control	Immunology
Campylobacter Pylori	Microbiology
Computer, Chemistry Analyzer	Chemistry
Container, Specimen Mailer And Storage	Pathology
Control, Analyte (Assayed And Unassayed)	Chemistry
Control, Cell Counter, Normal And Abnormal	Hematology
Control, Drug Mixture	Toxicology
Control, Hemoglobin	Hematology
Control, Urinalysis (Assayed And Unassayed)	Chemistry
Extractable Antinuclear Antibody (Rnp/Sm), Antigen/Control	Immunology
Hematocrit Control	Hematology
Hematology Quality Control Mixture	Hematology
Immunochemical, Thyroglobulin Autoantibody	Immunology
Kit, Screening, Urine	Microbiology
Kit, Urinary Drainage Collection	Gastroenterology/Urology
Labware, Blood Collection	Chemistry
Multi Analyte Mixture, Calibrator	Chemistry
Pipetting And Diluting System, Automated	Chemistry
Slide, Microscope	Pathology
Stain, Crystal Violet, Histology	Pathology
Test, Radio-Allergen Absorbent (RAST)	Immunology
Test, Rheumatoid Factor	Immunology

HYDOR THERME
See Hotpack

HYDRO SERVICE & SUPPLIES, INC.　　800-950-7426
PO Box 12197,　　919-544-3744
Research Triangle Park, NC 27709
FDA Number: n/a　　Fax: 919-544-5852
E-mail: info@hydroservice.com
Web site: www.hydroservice.com
Medical Products Sales Volume: $17,000,000
Year Founded: 1967
Total Employees: 30
Ownership: Private
Produces/Sells CE-marked Devices: N
Federal Procurement Eligibility: Small Business, GSA Contract
Distribution: OEM
General Admin.: Charles Atwater/President
Mktg./Adv.: Christine Sorrell/Executive Marketing
　　Dave Currin/Manager Sales
Research: C. D. Riley/Vice President Research & Development
Finance: Dave Currin/Chief Financial Officer
IS: Darrell Baber/Manager Tech. Services

Purification System, Water	Gastroenterology/Urology
Purification System, Water, Deionization	Chemistry
Reverse Osmosis Membrane Equipment	Chemistry
Ultrafiltration Equipment	Chemistry

HYDRO-MED PRODUCTS, INC.　　214-350-5100
3400 Royalty Row, Irving, TX 75062
FDA Number: 1625657

Bandage, Elastic	General
Container, Frozen Donor Tissue Storage	General
Cushion, Flotation	Physical Med
Drape, Surgical	Surgery
Tourniquet, Non-Pneumatic, Surgical	Surgery

HYDROCISION, INC.　　888-747-7470
267 Boston Road, Suite 28, Billerica, MA 01821　　978-474-9300
FDA Number: 1226424　　Fax: 978-474-5037
E-mail: info@hydrocision.com
Web site: www.hydrocision.com
Medical Products Sales Volume: $34,620,000
Annual Revenue: $25-$50 Million
Year Founded: 1996
Total Employees: 30　　Marketing Staff: 2　　Sales Staff: 5
Ownership: Private
Quality System Registration Information: ISO9001
Produces/Sells CE-marked Devices: Y
Federal Procurement Eligibility: Small Business
Distribution: Manufacturer Direct, Manufacturer Through Distributor, Manufacturer Through Manufacturer Reps, OEM, Exporter
General Admin.: Ms. Patricia Van Blarcom/Chief Financial Officer, Vice President
　　Mr. Howard Donnelly/President, Chief Executive Officer

MANUFACTURER PROFILES

HYDROCISION, INC. 888-747-7470 *(cont'd)*
Mktg./Adv.: Mr. Paul Kowalski/Vice President Marketing & Sales
Research: Mr. Kevin Staid/Vice President Engineering

Burr, Orthopedic	Orthopedics
Lavage Unit, Water Jet	General
Surgical Instrument, Disposable	Surgery
Surgical Instrument, Orthopedic, AC-Powered Motor	Orthopedics

HYDRODOT, INC. 978-399-0206
238 Littleton Road, Suite 202, Westford, MA 01886
FDA Number: 3006315274

Electrode, Cutaneous	Cns/Neurology
Electroencephalograph	Cns/Neurology

HYDROFERA LLC 866-861-7548
322 Main St., Willimantic, CT 06226 860-456-0677
Fax: 860-456-0898
E-mail: hydrofera@aol.com
Web site: www.hydrofera.com
Medical Products Sales Volume: $21,900,000
Annual Revenue: $10-$25 Million
Year Founded: 1996
Total Employees: 20
Ownership: Private
Produces/Sells CE-marked Devices: N
Federal Procurement Eligibility: Small Business
Distribution: Manufacturer Through Distributor, OEM
General Admin.: Tom Rallo/Chief Executive Officer
　　　Tom Drury/President
Mktg./Adv.: Heather Bond/Vice President Business Development
　　　Heather Bond/Vice President Marketing & Sales
Production: Joretta Ortiz/Manager Materials

Balloon, Epistaxis (Nasal)	Ear/Nose/Throat
Bandage, Liquid	Surgery
Cleanroom Equipment	General
Contract Manufacturing	General
Dressing, Wound and Burn, Hydrogel	Surgery
Gauze/sponge, Nonresorbable For External Use	Surgery
Sponge, Ophthalmic	Ophthalmology

HYDROGEL VISION CORPORATION 877-336-2482
7575 Commerce Ct, Sarasota, FL 34243-9825 941-739-1382
Fax: 888-612-6379
FDA Number: 3005184723
E-mail: customercare@extreme-h2o.com
Web site: www.extreme-h2o.com
Medical Products Sales Volume: $4,200,000
Year Founded: 1999
Total Employees: 67　　　*Sales Staff:* 11
Ownership: Private
Produces/Sells CE-marked Devices: N
Federal Procurement Eligibility: Small Business
General Admin.: Mr. Steve Schuster/Chief Executive Officer
Mktg./Adv.: Mr. Frankie Romo/Manager Distribution
　　　Mr. James Massa/Manager National Sales
　　　Mr. Gary Galliher/Manager Regional Sales
　　　Ms. Nancy Leland/Senior Sales Manager
Production: Mr. Jeff Curhan/Chief Engineer
　　　Mr. Tung Nguyen/Director Manufacturing & Engineering
　　　Mrs. Michelle Blackstone/Director Operations
　　　Ms. Hue Tran/Manager Production
　　　Mrs. Donna Hovanec/Manager Quality Systems
IS: Mr. Joshua Hu/Systems Engineer

Lenses, Soft Contact, Daily Wear	Ophthalmology

HYDROL CHEMICAL CO. 610-622-3603
520 Commerce Dr., Yeadon, PA 19050
FDA Number: 2530966

Fluid, Bouin's	Pathology
Formaldehyde (Formalin, Formol)	Pathology
Formalin, Neutral Buffered	Pathology
Glutaraldehyde (Fixative)	Pathology
Solution, Formalin/Sodium Acetate	Pathology
Solution, Pathology, Carnoy's	Pathology
Solution, Pathology, Decalcifier, Acid Containing	Pathology
Solution, Pathology, Formalin-Alcohol-Acetic Acid	Pathology

HYDROMER, INC. 877-493-7663
35 Industrial Pky., Branchburg, NJ 08876 908-722-5000
Fax: 908-526-3633
FDA Number: n/a
E-mail: sales@hydromer.com
Web site: www.hydromer.com
Medical Products Sales Volume: $4,500,000
Annual Revenue: $5-$10 Million
Year Founded: 1980
Ownership: Public
Stock Symbol: HYDI
Traded On: OTC Bulletin
Quality System Registration Information: ISO9000; ISO9001

HYDROMER, INC. 877-493-7663 *(cont'd)*
Produces/Sells CE-marked Devices: Y
Federal Procurement Eligibility: Small Business
Distribution: Manufacturer Direct, OEM, Service Direct, Exporter
General Admin.: Manfred Dyck/Chief Executive Officer
　　　Robert Moravsik/Senior Vice President, General Counsel
Production: Martin Dyck/Executive Vice President Operations
　　　Rainer Gruening/Vice President Quality Assurance & Quality Control
Research: Rainer Gruening/Vice President Research & Development
Finance: Robert Y. Lee/Vice President Finance

Biofeedback Device	Cns/Neurology
Catheter, Jejunostomy	Gastroenterology/Urology
Equipment, Device Coating, Protective	General
Guidewire	Cardiovascular
Lubricant, Instrument	General
Probe	Orthopedics
Service, Device Coating, Protective	General
Solution, Instrument, Laparoscopic, Anti-Fog	General
Stent, Other	Obstetrics/Gynecology

HYGIENE SPECIALTIES, INC./ANDERMAC, INC. 800-824-0214
2626 Live Oak Hwy., Yuba City, CA 95991-8810 530-674-8450
Fax: 530-674-1806
FDA Number: n/a
E-mail: info@hygenique.com
Web site: www.hygenique.com
Medical Products Sales Volume: $17,000,000
Annual Revenue: $10-$25 Million
Year Founded: 1961
Total Employees: 15　　*Marketing Staff:* 8　　*Sales Staff:* 6
Ownership: Andermac, Inc.
Produces/Sells CE-marked Devices: Y
Federal Procurement Eligibility: Small Business, GSA Contract
Distribution: Manufacturer Direct, Manufacturer Through Distributor, Manufacturer Through Manufacturer Reps, Exporter
General Admin.: Mick Anderson/President, Chief Executive Officer
Mktg./Adv.: C.M. Anderson/Director National Accounts
　　　Randy Mower/Director Product Development
　　　Rosa Ramos/Manager Advertising
　　　Cathy Zmuda/Manager Contract Sales
　　　Dana Daniels/Manager International & National Sales
Production: Laurie Graves/Customer Service Representative
　　　Dan Meringa/Director Quality Assurance
　　　Dave Brune/Manager Materials

Bath, Hydro-Massage (Whirlpool)	Physical Med
Mirror, Posture	Physical Med
System, Transport, In-House	General

HYGIENICS INDUSTRIES DIV.OF KLEINERT'S, INC. 800-498-7051
3968 194 Trail, Miami, FL 33160 305-937-0824
Fax: 305-937-0825
FDA Number: 7000573
E-mail: yourkleinerts@aol.com
Web site: www.hygienics.com
Medical Products Sales Volume: $34,620,000
Annual Revenue: $25-$50 Million
Year Founded: 1869
Total Employees: 14　　*Marketing Staff:* 3　　*Sales Staff:* 6
Ownership: Private
Quality System Registration Information: ISO9000
Produces/Sells CE-marked Devices: N
Federal Procurement Eligibility: Small Business
Distribution: Manufacturer Direct, Manufacturer Through Distributor, Manufacturer Through Manufacturer Reps, Exclusive Distributor, Importer, Exporter
General Admin.: Michael Brier/President, Chief Executive Officer

Pad, Incontinence (Underpad)	General
Pant, Incontinence	General

HYGINET CORP. OF AMERICA 800-245-1036
505 North Drive, 79 North Industrial Park, 412-741-0100
Sewickley, PA 15143
Fax: 412-741-0140
FDA Number: 2522775
E-mail: info@jetnetcorp.com
Web site: www.jetnetcorp.com
Annual Revenue: $0-$1 Million
Total Employees: 70
Ownership: Private
Produces/Sells CE-marked Devices: N
Distribution: Manufacturer Direct
General Admin.: Donald Sartore/President

Bandage, Elastic	General
Retainer, Bandage (Elastic Net)	General

HYGO PLASTIC, INC. 414-375-4011
1376 Cheyenne Ave., Grafton, WI 53024
FDA Number: 2132604
Ownership: Private
Produces/Sells CE-marked Devices: N

HYGO PLASTIC, INC. 414-375-4011 *(cont'd)*
Catheter, Suction, With Tip General
Evacuator, Oral Cavity Dental And Oral
Toothbrush, Manual Dental And Oral

HYGOLET USA 800-494-6538
349 S.E. 2nd Avenue, Deerfield Beach, FL 33441 954-481-8601
FDA Number: n/a *Fax:* 954-481-8669
E-mail: hygolet@hygolet.com
Web site: www.hygolet.com
Medical Products Sales Volume: $21,900,000
Annual Revenue: $5-$10 Million
Year Founded: 1983
Total Employees: 10 *Marketing Staff:* 2 *Sales Staff:* 1
Ownership: Private
Produces/Sells CE-marked Devices: N
Federal Procurement Eligibility: Small Business
Distribution: Manufacturer Direct, Manufacturer Through Distributor, Manufacturer Through Manufacturer Reps
General Admin.: Mr. Chris Van Leare/Director International Operations
  Ms. Dorothy Jordan/Executive Vice President
  Mr. Andre O. Stucki/President, Chief Executive Officer
Mktg./Adv.: Ms. Lori McCarron/Director Marketing & Sales
Production: Mr. Carlos Garcia/Manager Production
Brush, Other General
Cover, Seat, Toilet, Sanitary General
Housekeeping Equipment General
Waste Receptacle, General Purpose General

HYLAND DIAGNOSTICS
See Biomerieux Inc.

HYPERBARIC TECHNOLOGIES, INC. 619-336-2022
3224 Hoover Ave., National City, CA 91950
FDA Number: 2029408
Chamber, Hyperbaric Anesthesiology

HYPERBARIC THERAPY SYSTEMS INC.
See Perry Baromedical Corp.

HYPERION, INC. 305-238-3020
14100 S.W. 136th St., Miami, FL 33186-5598
FDA Number: 1028110 *Fax:* 305-232-7375
E-mail: hyperion@hyperionclinical.com
Web site: www.hyperionclinical.com
Medical Products Sales Volume: $101,100,000
Total Employees: 54 *Marketing Staff:* 1 *Sales Staff:* 7
Ownership: Private
Federal Procurement Eligibility: Small Business, GSA Contract
Distribution: Manufacturer Direct, Manufacturer Through Distributor
General Admin.: William P. Murphy/Chairman, Chief Executive Officer
  Mary Ann Gleason/Manager Human Resources
  Edward J. Botz/President
  David Chesterfield/Vice President
Production: Radha Goolabsingh/Director Quality Assurance
  Radha Goohbsingh/Director Regulatory Affairs
  Victor Rana/Vice President Operations
Colorimeter, General Use Chemistry
Photometer Chemistry
Pipetting And Diluting System, Automated Chemistry
Washer, Microplate General

HYPERMED, INC 781-229-5900
41 Second Avenue, Burlington, MA 01803
FDA Number: 3006129921
Oximeter, Tissue Saturation Cardiovascular

HYPERTEC, INC. 800-218-3588
301B East Main Street, Olney, TX 76374 940-564-5600
FDA Number: 1651406 *Fax:* 940-564-5609
E-mail: ppjanca@aol.com
Web site: www.hypertec-o2.com
Medical Products Sales Volume: $5,500,000
Year Founded: 1989
Total Employees: 17
Ownership: Private
Produces/Sells CE-marked Devices: N
Federal Procurement Eligibility: Small Business
Chamber, Hyperbaric Anesthesiology

HYPERTENSION DIAGNOSTICS, INC. 888-785-7392
2915 Waters Road, Suite 108, 651-687-9999
Eagan, MN 55121
FDA Number: 2134830 *Fax:* 651-687-0485
E-mail: info@HDII.com
Web site: www.CVProfilor.com
Medical Products Sales Volume: $1,900,000
Annual Revenue: $1-$5 Million
Year Founded: 1988
Total Employees: 10 *Marketing Staff:* 2 *Sales Staff:* 6

HYPERTENSION DIAGNOSTICS, INC. 888-785-7392 *(cont'd)*
Ownership: Public
Stock Symbol: HDII
Traded On: OTC Bulletin
Quality System Registration Information: ISO9001
Produces/Sells CE-marked Devices: Y
Federal Procurement Eligibility: Small Business
Distribution: Manufacturer Direct, Manufacturer Through Distributor, Manufacturer Through Manufacturer Reps, Service Direct, Exporter
General Admin.: Dr. Charles F. Chesney/Chief Technology Officer, Executive Vice President
  Mr. Greg H. Guettler/President
Mktg./Adv.: Ms. Julie Radosevich/Director Marketing
  Mr. Frank Tappen/Director Sales
Production: Mr. E. Paul Maloney/Vice President, Engineer
Finance: Mr. James S. Murphy/Chief Financial Officer, Senior Vice President Finance
Monitor, Blood Pressure, Indirect, Semi-Automatic Cardiovascular

HYTECH BIOMEDICAL INC.
See Nuclear Pharmacy Services

I-BEAM WALKING MACHINE 248-477-9808
21755 Ruth St, Farmington Hills, MI 48336
FDA Number: 3005019884
Ownership: Private
Produces/Sells CE-marked Devices: N
Lift, Patient General

I-FLOW CORPORATION 800-448-3569
20202 Windrow Dr., Lake Forest, CA 92630 949-206-2700
FDA Number: 2026095 *Fax:* 949-206-2600
E-mail: info@I-flowcorp.com
Web site: www.I-flowcorp.com
Medical Products Sales Volume: $30,000,000
Annual Revenue: $25-$50 Million
Year Founded: 1985
Total Employees: 70
Ownership: Public
Stock Symbol: IFLO
Traded On: NASDAQ
Quality System Registration Information: ISO9000; ISO9001
Produces/Sells CE-marked Devices: Y
Federal Procurement Eligibility: Small Business, GSA Contract, VA Contract
Distribution: Manufacturer Direct, Manufacturer Through Distributor, Manufacturer Through Manufacturer Reps, OEM, Exclusive Distributor, Importer, Exporter
General Admin.: James Telarich/Chief Financial Officer, Treasurer
  James J. Dal Porto/Chief Operating Officer
  Evangelina Vargas/Director Human Resources
  Donald M. Earhart/President, Chief Executive Officer
Medical Admin.: Barbara Lorenzen/Director Clinical Affairs
Mktg./Adv.: Eric Mabry/Vice President International Marketing & Sales
  Roger Massengale/Vice President Marketing & Business Development
Production: Stanley E. Fry/Vice President Regulatory Affairs
Research: Bill Porter/Vice President Engineering
Catheter, Conduction, Anesthesia Anesthesiology
Pump, Infusion, Ambulatory General
Pump, Infusion, Elastomeric General
System, Delivery, Drug, Unit-Dose General

I-MED PHARMA INC. 800-463-1008
1601 St. Regis Blvd., 514-685-8118
Montreal, QUE H9B-3 Canada
FDA Number: n/a *Fax:* 514-685-8998
E-mail: info@imedpharma.com
Web site: www.imedpharma.com
Year Founded: 1989
Total Employees: 10
Ownership: Private
Produces/Sells CE-marked Devices: N
Distribution: Manufacturer Direct, Exclusive Distributor, Importer

I-REP, INC. 800-828-0852
508 Chaney Street #B, Lake Elsinore, CA 92530 951-674-7628
FDA Number: 2023645 *Fax:* 909-674-8126
E-mail: btwilhelm@juno.com
Web site: www.irepinc.net
Medical Products Sales Volume: $1,800,000
Annual Revenue: $1-$5 Million
Year Founded: 1982
Total Employees: 11 *Marketing Staff:* 2 *Sales Staff:* 3
Ownership: Private
Produces/Sells CE-marked Devices: N
Federal Procurement Eligibility: Small Business
Distribution: Manufacturer Direct, Manufacturer Through Distributor, Manufacturer Through Manufacturer Reps, Exclusive Distributor, Importer, Exporter
General Admin.: Bradley T. Wilhelm/President
Mktg./Adv.: Greg Harris/Manager Marketing

I-REP, INC. — 800-828-0852 (cont'd)

Exerciser, Other	Physical Med
Exerciser, Wrist	Physical Med
General Medical Device	General
Pack, Cold	General
Pack, Hot, Chemical	General
Stimulator, Muscle, Electrical-Powered (EMS)	Physical Med
Support, Ankle	Orthopedics
Support, Thigh	Physical Med
Support, Wrist	Physical Med
Table, Examination/Treatment	General
Table, Physical Medicine, Powered	Physical Med
Table, Physical Therapy	Physical Med
Traction Unit, Powered, Mobile	Orthopedics

Medical Product Subsidiaries (Listed Separately)
Body Therapeutics, Div. Of I-Rep, Inc.

I.B.F. CORPORATION — 800-423-3456
44 Plauderville Avenue, Garfield, NJ 07026-0278 — 973-546-0055
FDA Number: 2246647 — *Fax:* 973-546-1048
E-mail: msouto@ibfcorp.com
Web site: www.ibfcorp.com
Medical Products Sales Volume: $101,100,000
Annual Revenue: $10-$25 Million
Year Founded: 1970
Total Employees: 23
Ownership: Private
Quality System Registration Information: ISO9001
Produces/Sells CE-marked Devices: N
Federal Procurement Eligibility: Small Business, Minority Owned
Distribution: Manufacturer Through Distributor
General Admin.: Mr. Marcal Souto/Vice President

Film, X-Ray	Radiology

I.B.S. (ICE BAG SUPPORT) — 270-443-0443
1117 North 8th St., Suite 201, Paducah, KY 42001
FDA Number: 1037460
Ownership: Private
Produces/Sells CE-marked Devices: N

Pack, Hot Or Cold, Reusable	Physical Med

I.C. MEDICAL, INC. — 623-780-0700
2002 W. Quail Ave., Phoenix, AZ 85027
FDA Number: 2027757

Electrosurgical Unit, Cutting & Coagulation Device	Surgery
Exhaust System, Surgical	Surgery
Laparoscope, General & Plastic Surgery	Surgery
Laser, Surgical	Surgery

I.C.E. DOWN, INC.
See Icd, Inc.

I.D.C. TECTONICS LTD. — 905-646-6335
P.O. Box 2104, St. Catharines, ONT L2R 7R7 Canada
FDA Number: n/a — *Fax:* 905-646-6338
E-mail: shauck@idctectonics.on.ca
Web site: www.idctectonics.on.ca
Year Founded: 1981
Total Employees: 10
Ownership: Private
Produces/Sells CE-marked Devices: N
Distribution: Manufacturer Direct, Exclusive Distributor

I.F. OPTICAL, INC. — 773-761-3323
2812 West Touhy Ave., Chicago, IL 60645
FDA Number: 1460659
Ownership: Private
Produces/Sells CE-marked Devices: N

Lens, Spectacle/Eyeglasses, Non-Custom	Ophthalmology

I.F.S. INDUSTRIAL & FINANCIAL SYSTEMS — 888-437-4968
300 Park Boulevard, Suite 555, — 847-592-0200
Suite 555, IL 60143
FDA Number: n/a
E-mail: request@ifsworld.com
Web site: www.ifsworld.com
Annual Revenue: $100-$500 Million
Year Founded: 1983
Total Employees: 2723
Ownership: I.F.S. AB
Stock Symbol: IFS
Produces/Sells CE-marked Devices: N

Computer Software	General

I.M.A. ELECTRONICS, INC. — 352-378-7551
6614 N.w. 26th Terrace, Gainesville, FL 32653
FDA Number: 3006371990

Electroencephalograph	Cns/Neurology

I.M.K. DISTRIBUTORS, INC. — 800-878-5552
19 W. 34th St., Ste. 915, New York, NY 10001 — 212-967-7591
FDA Number: 2433126 — *Fax:* 212-967-7592
E-mail: info@herniainstitute.com
Web site: www.herniainstitute.com
Annual Revenue: $0-$1 Million
Year Founded: 1973
Total Employees: 10
Ownership: Private
Produces/Sells CE-marked Devices: N
Distribution: Manufacturer Through Manufacturer Reps, Exclusive Distributor
General Admin.: Joseph Pauler/President, Chief Executive Officer
Mktg./Adv.: Joseph Pauler/Director Marketing

Brace, Joint, Ankle (External)	Physical Med
Support, Hernia	Gastroenterology/Urology

I.P.I.-INTERNATIONAL PRODUCTS, INC. — 703-237-2774
1929 Poole Lane, McLean, VA 22101
FDA Number: n/a — *Fax:* 703-237-6687
E-mail: sales@intproducts.com
Web site: www.intproducts.com
Medical Products Sales Volume: $700,000
Annual Revenue: $0-$1 Million
Year Founded: 1992
Total Employees: 3
Ownership: Private
Produces/Sells CE-marked Devices: Y
Federal Procurement Eligibility: Small Business, Female Owned
Distribution: Exclusive Distributor
General Admin.: Uwe Klotz/President

Monitor, ECG	Cardiovascular

I.T.I., INC. — 406-251-7000
6150 Hwy. 93 South, Missoula, MT 59804
FDA Number: 3026458
Ownership: Private
Produces/Sells CE-marked Devices: N

Knife, Orthopedic	Orthopedics

I.V. HOUSE, INC. — 800-530-0400
418 Seven Gables Court, — (314) 453-9200
Chesterfield, MO 63017
FDA Number: 1954553 — *Fax:* (314) 453-9576
E-mail: lisa@ivhouse.com
Web site: www.ivhouse.com
Year Founded: 1991
Total Employees: 3 — *Marketing Staff:* 1 — *Sales Staff:* 1
Ownership: Private
Produces/Sells CE-marked Devices: N
Federal Procurement Eligibility: Female Owned
Distribution: Manufacturer Direct, Manufacturer Through Distributor
General Admin.: Betty Rozier/President, Chief Executive Officer
Medical Admin.: Lisa Vallino/Vice President Clinical Affairs

Holder, Intravascular Catheter	General

I.V. LEAGUE MEDICAL — 805-988-1010
460 S. Lombard St., Oxnard, CA 93030
FDA Number: 2025766

Infusion Stand	General

I.W. TREMONT CO. — 973-427-3800
79 Fourth Ave., Hawthorne, NJ 07506
FDA Number: n/a — *Fax:* 973-427-3778
E-mail: custserv@iwtremont.com
Web site: www.iwtremont.com
Year Founded: 1979
Ownership: Private
Produces/Sells CE-marked Devices: N
Federal Procurement Eligibility: Small Business
Distribution: Manufacturer Direct, OEM
Mktg./Adv.: Mr. Jim Averso/Vice President Marketing & Sales

Contract Manufacturing	General
Media, Filter	General

I.Z.I. MEDICAL PRODUCTS, INC. — 800-231-1499
7020 Tudsbury Road, Baltimore, MD 21244 — 410-594-9403
FDA Number: n/a — *Fax:* 410-594-0540
E-mail: info@izimed.com
Web site: www.izimed.com
Medical Products Sales Volume: $320,000
Year Founded: 1993
Total Employees: 4
Ownership: Private
Produces/Sells CE-marked Devices: Y
Federal Procurement Eligibility: Small Business

Bandage, Adhesive	Surgery
Marker, Skin	Surgery
Nuclear Magnetic Resonance Imaging System	Radiology

I.Z.I. MEDICAL PRODUCTS, INC. 800-231-1499 *(cont'd)*
Radiographic Unit, Diagnostic — Radiology
Radiographic/Fluoroscopic Unit, Image-Intensified — Radiology
Simulator, Radiotherapy, Special Purpose — Radiology
Stereotaxy Equipment — Cns/Neurology
System, Marking, Film, Radiographic — Radiology

IATROMED, INC.
See Capstone Therapeutics

IBA-RDI 516-254-6800
151 Heartland Blvd., New York, NY 11717
FDA Number: n/a
E-mail: iba.us@iba-group.com
Web site: www.iba-worldwide.com
Annual Revenue: $100-$500 Million
Year Founded: 1986
Total Employees: 2067
Ownership: Iba
Stock Symbol: IBAB
Quality System Registration Information: ISO9001
Produces/Sells CE-marked Devices: N
Federal Procurement Eligibility: Small Business
Distribution: Service Direct
General Admin.: Pierre Mottet/Chief Executive Officer
Contract Sterilization — General
Sterilizer, Ethylene-Oxide Gas — General

IBC INT'L, INC. 727-551-2087
100 4th Ave. South #412, St. Petersburg, FL 33701
FDA Number: 3006306405
Web site: southern-tier-pumking ale
Ownership: Private
Produces/Sells CE-marked Devices: N
Pack, Hot Or Cold, Reusable — Physical Med

IBIOM INSTRUMENTS LTD. 450-678-5468
1065 Pacific Street, suite 403,
Sherbrooke, QUE J1H 2 Canada
FDA Number: n/a   *Fax:* 450-445-9837
E-mail: info@ibiom.com
Web site: www.ibiom.com
Medical Products Sales Volume: $350,000
Year Founded: 1978
Total Employees: 4   *Marketing Staff:* 1   *Sales Staff:* 1
Ownership: Private
Produces/Sells CE-marked Devices: N
Federal Procurement Eligibility: Small Business
Distribution: Manufacturer Direct, Exporter

IBM INTEGRATED TOOL TECHNOLOGY CENTER 507-253-5215
3605 Hwy 52 N, Rochester, MN 55901
FDA Number: 3004743815
Ownership: Private
Produces/Sells CE-marked Devices: N
Biofeedback Device — Cns/Neurology
Coil, Magnetic Resonance, Specialty — Radiology

IBS CORP.
See Industrial & Biomedical Sensors Corp.

ICAD INC. 866-280-2239
98 Spit Brook Rd,, Suite 100, Nashua, NH 03062 603-882-5200
FDA Number: 1225671   *Fax:* 603-880-3843
E-mail: sales@icadmed.com
Web site: www.icadmed.com
Year Founded: 1984
Total Employees: 106
Ownership: Public
Stock Symbol: ICAD
Traded On: NASDAQ
Produces/Sells CE-marked Devices: N
General Admin.: Darlene Deptula-Hicks/Chief Financial Officer, Executive Vice President

Ken Ferry/President, Chief Executive Officer
Mktg./Adv.: Stacey Stevens/Senior Vice President Marketing
Production: Jeffrey Barnes/Executive Vice President Operations
Research: Jonathan Go/Senior Vice President Research & Development
Finance: Mr. Kevin Burns/Chief Financial Officer
Analyzer, Medical Image — Radiology
Image Digitizer — Radiology
Image Processing System — Radiology
Nuclear Magnetic Resonance Imaging System — Radiology
Scanner, Computed Tomography, X-Ray (CAT, CT) — Cns/Neurology

ICARDIOGRAM, INCORPORATED 919-534-2150
333 Six Forks Road,, Raleigh, NC 27609
FDA Number: 3006191323
Ownership: Private
Produces/Sells CE-marked Devices: N

ICARDIOGRAM, INCORPORATED 919-534-2150 *(cont'd)*
Image Processing System — Radiology

ICD, INC. 866-791-2503
2232 Verus Street, Suite C, San Diego, CA 92154
FDA Number: n/a   *Fax:* 619-661-1235
E-mail: contacticd@icedown.com
Web site: www.icedown.com
Annual Revenue: $0-$1 Million
Total Employees: 25
Ownership: Private
Produces/Sells CE-marked Devices: N
Federal Procurement Eligibility: Small Business
Distribution: Manufacturer Through Distributor
General Admin.: Chris Kirkman/President
Pack, Cold — General
Wrap, Sterilization — General

ICN BIOMEDICALS, INC.
See Mirion Technologies

ICN ISO-DATA
See Titertek Instruments, Inc.

ICN PHARMACEUTICALS INC., DIV. ICN DOSIMETRY SERV.
See Mirion Technologies

ICON INTERVENTIONAL SYSTEMS, INC. 216-382-3119
1414 South Green Rd., Suite 309, Cleveland, OH 44121
FDA Number: 3003955704
Ownership: Private
Produces/Sells CE-marked Devices: N
Stent, Coronary, Drug-eluting — Cardiovascular

ICON LLC 501-374-2929
8 Ten Tee Circle, Maumelle, AR 72113
FDA Number: 3006451793
Handle, Instrument, Dental — Dental And Oral
Pick, Massaging — Dental And Oral

ICP MEDICAL 314-429-1000
10486 Baur Blvd., St. Louis, MO 63132
FDA Number: 1933975   *Fax:* 314-429-8626
Web site: www.icpproducts.com
Annual Revenue: $5-$10 Million
Year Founded: 1991
Total Employees: 16   *Marketing Staff:* 1   *Sales Staff:* 6
Ownership: Private
Produces/Sells CE-marked Devices: N
Federal Procurement Eligibility: Small Business
Distribution: Manufacturer Direct, Manufacturer Through Distributor, Manufacturer Through Manufacturer Reps, Importer, Exporter
Applicator, Tipped, Absorbent, Non-Sterile — General
Detector/Remover, Lice — General
Gown, Other — General

ICRCO INC. 310-921-9559
2580 West 237th Street, Torrance, CA 90505
FDA Number: 2030510
Image Digitizer — Radiology
Image Processing System — Radiology

ICS MEDICAL
See Gn Otometrics

ICU MEDICAL (UT), INC 949-366-2183
4455 Atherton Dr., Salt Lake City, UT 84123
FDA Number: 1713468
Ownership: Icu Medical, Inc.
Stock Symbol: ICUI
Traded On: NASDAQ
Produces/Sells CE-marked Devices: N
Adapter, Stopcock, Manifold, Cardiopulmonary Bypass — Cardiovascular
Autotransfusion Unit (Blood) — Anesthesiology
Cannula, AV Shunt — Gastroenterology/Urology
Catheter, Continuous Flush — Cardiovascular
Catheter, Flow Directed — Cardiovascular
Catheter, Intravascular, Diagnostic — Cardiovascular
Catheter, Multiple Lumen — Surgery
Catheter, Oximeter, Fiberoptic — Cardiovascular
Computer, Diagnostic, Pre-Programmed, Single-Function — Cardiovascular
Container, Specimen, All Types — General
Cuff, Blood Pressure — Cardiovascular
Infusion Stand — General
Injector, Angiographic (Cardiac Catheterization) — Cardiovascular
Introducer, Catheter — Cardiovascular
Kit, Administration, Intravenous — General
Kit, Sampling, Arterial Blood — Anesthesiology
Microfilter, Blood Transfusion — Anesthesiology
Monitor, Blood Pressure, Indirect, Semi-Automatic — Cardiovascular
Needle, Hypodermic, Single Lumen With Syringe — General
Pressure Infusor, IV Container — General
Probe, Thermodilution — Cardiovascular

ICU MEDICAL (UT), INC
949-366-2183 *(cont'd)*
Pump, Infusion	General
Regulator, Thermal, Cardiopulmonary Bypass	Cardiovascular
Regulator, Vacuum	General
Stopcock	General
Suction Apparatus, Operating Room, Wall Vacuum-Powered	Surgery
Syringe, Piston	General
Transducer, Blood Pressure, Extravascular	Cardiovascular
Transfer Aid	Physical Med
Tube, Drainage	Gastroenterology/Urology
Tube, Gastrointestinal	Gastroenterology/Urology
Tubing, Fluid Delivery	General
Tubing, Non-Invasive	Surgery

ICU MEDICAL, INC
See Icu Medical (Ut), Inc

ICU MEDICAL, INC.
951 Calle Amanecer,
San Clemente, CA 92673
800-824-7890
949-366-2183

FDA Number: n/a
Fax: 949-366-8368
Web site: www.icumed.com
Year Founded: 1984
Total Employees: 1696
Ownership: Public
Stock Symbol: ICUI
Traded On: NASDAQ
Quality System Registration Information: ISO9001; ISO9002
Produces/Sells CE-marked Devices: Y
Distribution: Manufacturer Through Distributor, OEM, Exclusive Distributor, Exporter
General Admin.: George Lopez/President, Chief Executive Officer
Mktg./Adv.: Mr. Tom McCall/Vice President Marketing
　　　　　Richard Costello/Vice President Sales
Production: Steven Riggs/Vice President Operations
Research: Alison Burcar/Vice President Product Development
Finance: Mr. Scott Lamb/Chief Financial Officer
Kit, Administration, Intravenous	General
Needle, Hypodermic, Single Lumen With Syringe	General
Stopcock	General
Supplies, Blood Bank	Hematology
Syringe, Piston	General
Tube, Gastrointestinal	Gastroenterology/Urology
Tubing, Non-Invasive	Surgery

Medical Product Subsidiaries (Listed Separately)
　Icu Medical (Ut), Inc

IDAHO TECHNOLOGY, INC.
390 Wakara Way, Salt Lake City, UT 84108
1-800-735-6544
801-736-6354

FDA Number: 3002773840
Fax: 801-588-0507
E-mail: it@idahotech.com
Web site: http://www.idahotech.com
Ownership: Private
Produces/Sells CE-marked Devices: N
Analyzer, Chemistry, Micro	Chemistry
Joint Biological Agent Identification And Diagnostic System (jbaids) Tularemia Detection Kit	Microbiology
Reagents, Specific, Analyte	Hematology

IDEA SCIENTIFIC CO.
PO Box 13210, Minneapolis, MN 55414-5210
800-433-2535
651-331-4612

FDA Number: n/a
Fax: 612-331-4217
Web site: www.ideascientific.com
Medical Products Sales Volume: $730,000
Year Founded: 1979
Total Employees: 10
Ownership: Private
Federal Procurement Eligibility: Small Business
Distribution: Manufacturer Direct
General Admin.: Gregory Ide/President
Electrophoresis Equipment, Gel	Chemistry
Electrophoresis Instrumentation	Immunology

IDEA, INC.
3755 Boettler Oaks Dr., Green, OH 44685
330-896-2300

FDA Number: n/a
Fax: 330-896-2301
E-mail: ideas@ideasincweb.com
Web site: www.ideasincweb.com
Year Founded: 1993
Ownership: Private
Produces/Sells CE-marked Devices: N
Federal Procurement Eligibility: Small Business
Distribution: Exclusive Distributor
Radiographic Unit, Diagnostic	Radiology
Radiographic Unit, Diagnostic, Photofluorographic	Radiology
Radiographic Unit, Digital	Radiology

IDEAL BRANDS, INC.
1513 Mirasol St., Commerce, CA 90023
213-422-8526

FDA Number: 3006125195
Ownership: Private
Produces/Sells CE-marked Devices: N
Garment, Protective, For Incontinence	Gastroenterology/Urology

IDEAL MEDICAL SOURCE, INC.
2805 East. Oakland Blvd, Suite 352,
Fort Lauderdale, FL 33306
800-537-0739
954-563-7856

FDA Number: n/a
Fax: 954-563-5769
E-mail: info@idealmed.com
Web site: www.idealmed.com
Medical Products Sales Volume: $1,500,000
Annual Revenue: $1-$5 Million
Ownership: Private
Produces/Sells CE-marked Devices: N
Federal Procurement Eligibility: Small Business
Distribution: Exclusive Distributor, Exporter
Gel, Ultrasonic Transmission	General
Holder, Medical Chart	General
Printer, Image, Video	General
Scanner, Ultrasonic, Other	Radiology
Service, Used Equipment	General
Transducer, Ultrasonic	Cardiovascular

IDEAL OPTICS, INC.
2775 Premiere Parkway, Suite 600, Duluth, GA 30097
612-520-6000

FDA Number: 1042064
Ownership: Private
Produces/Sells CE-marked Devices: N
Lens, Contact (Other Material)	Ophthalmology
Lens, Contact, Polymethylmethacrylate	Ophthalmology
Lens, Contact, Polymethylmethacrylate, Diagnostic	Ophthalmology
Lenses, Soft Contact, Daily Wear	Ophthalmology

IDEAL PRODUCTS
1287 County Road 623, Broseley, MO 63932
800-321-5490
573-686-0003

FDA Number: 1641802
Fax: 800-532-4691
E-mail: help@idealproducts.com
Web site: www.idealproducts.com
Medical Products Sales Volume: $1,800,000
Year Founded: 1987
Total Employees: 25
Ownership: Private
Produces/Sells CE-marked Devices: N
Federal Procurement Eligibility: Small Business
Distribution: Manufacturer Through Distributor
General Admin.: Dan Duvall/Chief Executive Officer
　　　　　Mike Hohn/President
Bin, Storage	General
Cart, Housekeeping	General
Cart, Instrument	Surgery
Cart, Other	General
Cart, Supply	General
Component, Exercise	Physical Med
Warmer, Gel	General

IDEAS FOR LIVING
1285 North Cedarbrook Rd., Boulder, CO 80304
303-440-8517

FDA Number: 1722222
Alarm, Enuresis	Gastroenterology/Urology

IDEATRICS, INC.
4845 Pearl East Circle, Suite 101, Boulder, CO 80301
303-417-6353

FDA Number: 1723325
Fax: 303-417-6301
E-mail: info@ideatrics.com
Web site: www.ideatrics.com
Medical Products Sales Volume: $21,900,000
Ownership: Private
Produces/Sells CE-marked Devices: N
Distribution: Manufacturer Through Distributor
General Admin.: James Heller/President
Wire, Fixation, Intraosseous	Dental And Oral

IDENTITECH CORP.
See Sensormatic Electronics

IDESCO CORP.
37 W. 26th St., New York, NY 10010-1097
800-336-1383
212-889-2530

FDA Number: 9200571
Fax: 212-889-7033
E-mail: marketing@idesco.com
Web site: www.idesco.com
Medical Products Sales Volume: $7,300,000
Annual Revenue: $5-$10 Million
Year Founded: 1943
Total Employees: 40　　*Marketing Staff:* 3　　*Sales Staff:* 4
Ownership: Private
Produces/Sells CE-marked Devices: N

IDESCO CORP.   800-336-1383 (cont'd)
Federal Procurement Eligibility: Small Business, GSA Contract
Distribution: Manufacturer Direct
General Admin.: Andrew Schonzeit/Chief Executive Officer
     Andrew Schonzeit/President
Mktg./Adv.: Joel Hershkowitz/Director Marketing
     Joel Hershkowitz/Manager Market Research
     Andy Goldstone/Vice President Sales
Production: Gerald Brodsky/Executive Vice President Production

Security Equipment/Supplies	General
Sign, Hospital	General
Tag, Device Status	General

IDEV TECHNOLOGIES, INC.   866-806-4338
253 Medical Center Blvd., Webster, TX 77598   **281-525-2000**
FDA Number: 3005325609   *Fax:* 281-525-2001
E-mail: sales@idevmd.com
Web site: www.idevmd.com.
Ownership: Private
Produces/Sells CE-marked Devices: N
General Admin.: Mr. William Burke/Chief Financial Officer, Executive Vice President
     Mr. Christopher Owens/President, Chief Executive Officer
Medical Admin.: Dr. Dennis Donohoe/Chief Medical Officer
Mktg./Adv.: Mr. Eric Schlote/Vice President International Sales
Production: Mr. Charles Tribie/Senior Vice President Operations
     Mr. Kenneth Beuche/Vice President Process Development

Catheter, Biliary	Gastroenterology/Urology
Catheter, Peripheral, Atherectomy	Cardiovascular
Device, Retrieval, Percutaneous	Cardiovascular
Stent, Other	Obstetrics/Gynecology

IDEXX LABORATORIES, INC.   800-548-6733
1 Idexx Dr., Westbrook, ME 04092   **207-856-0300**
FDA Number: n/a   *Fax:* 207-856-0346
Web site: www.idexx.com
Annual Revenue: $500 Million-$1 Billion
Total Employees: 4500
Ownership: Public
Stock Symbol: IDXX
Traded On: NASDAQ
Produces/Sells CE-marked Devices: N
Distribution: Manufacturer Through Distributor
General Admin.: David Shaw/Chief Executive Officer
     Irvin Workman/President
Mktg./Adv.: Dean Layton/Director Marketing
     Brad MacKinnon/Vice President Sales
Research: Quentin Tonelli/Vice President Research & Development

Contract Laboratory	General
Kit, Admission (Patient Utensil)	General

IDM PLASTICS   904-734-4740
1813 Patterson Ave., Deland, FL 32724
FDA Number: 1063827

Airway, Oropharyngeal, Anesthesia	Anesthesiology

IDT, INC.
See Viacirq, Inc.

IDX SYSTEMS CORPORATION   802-862-1022
1400 Shelburne Rd., Burlington, VT 05402-1070
FDA Number: n/a   *Fax:* 802-862-9591
E-mail: info@idx.com
Web site: www.idx.com
Total Employees: 2250   *Marketing Staff:* 50   *Sales Staff:* 170
Ownership: Private
Produces/Sells CE-marked Devices: N
Distribution: Manufacturer Direct
General Admin.: Robert H. Hoehl/Chairman
     John A. Kane/Chief Financial Officer, Vice President
     Jim Crook/Chief Operating Officer, Executive Vice President
     Kathy Dellplain/Director Human Resources
     Kathy Dellplain/Manager Human Resources
     Richard E. Tarrant/President, Chief Executive Officer
     Robert Baker/Vice President Legal Services
Mktg./Adv.: Lisa Howe/Director Marketing
     Tracey Moran/Manager Communications
     Robert Galin/Senior Vice President Sales
     Pamela Pure/Vice President Marketing

Computer Software	General
Computer Software, Hospital/Nursing Management	General
Computer, Patient Data Management	General

IEC & LABSYSTEMS
See Thermo Fisher Scientific - Laboratory Equipment Division Headquarters

IET LABS, INC.   800-899-8438
534 Main St., Westbury, NY 11590-4806   **516-334-5959**
FDA Number: n/a   *Fax:* 516-334-5988

IET LABS, INC.   800-899-8438 (cont'd)
E-mail: sales@ietlabs.com
Web site: www.ietlabs.com
Annual Revenue: $1-$5 Million
Year Founded: 1976
Total Employees: 19
Ownership: Private
Federal Procurement Eligibility: Small Business, GSA Contract
Distribution: Manufacturer Direct
General Admin.: Sam Sheena/General Manager

Voltmeter	Chemistry

IGS GENERON AMERICAS   713-937-5200
11985 Fm 529, Houston, TX 77041
FDA Number: 3004153309
Ownership: Private
Produces/Sells CE-marked Devices: N

Generator, Oxygen, Portable	Anesthesiology

IGUS, INC.   800-521-2747
PO Box 14349, East Providence, RI 02914   **401-438-2200**
FDA Number: n/a   *Fax:* 401-438-7270
E-mail: sales@igus.com
Web site: www.igus.com
Annual Revenue: $50-$100 Million
Total Employees: 60   *Marketing Staff:* 1   *Sales Staff:* 30
Ownership: Private
Produces/Sells CE-marked Devices: N
Distribution: Manufacturer Direct, Manufacturer Through Manufacturer Reps, OEM, Service Direct
General Admin.: Frank Blas,/Chief Executive Officer
     Carsten Blas,/President
     Cartsen Blas,/Vice President Human Resources
Mktg./Adv.: Halley Lavenstein/Director Marketing & Communications
     C. Blas,/Director National Accounts
     Carsten Blas,/Manager Advertising
     C. Blas,/Manager Business Development
     Carsten Blas,/Manager Contract Sales
     F. Blas,/Manager International Marketing & Sales
     F. Blas,/Manager Market Research
     Halley Lavenstein/Manager Marketing & Communications
     C. Blas,/Manager National Sales
Production: C. Blas,/Manager Regulatory Affairs
     Carsten Blas,/Vice President Manufacturing
Research: Frank Blas,/Vice President Research & Development

Component, Plastic	General

IHC AFFILIATED SERVICES INC.
See Siemens Medical Solutions Health Services Corp.

IHN, INC.   517-706-0060
4572 Ottawa Dr., Suite 105, Okemos, MI 48864
FDA Number: 3004012851
Ownership: Private
Produces/Sells CE-marked Devices: N

Traction Unit, Non-Powered	Orthopedics

II-VI, INC.   724-352-4455
375 Saxonburg Blvd., Saxonburg, PA 16056-9499
FDA Number: n/a   *Fax:* 724-352-5284
E-mail: info@ii-vi.com
Web site: www.ii-vi.com
Annual Revenue: $100-$500 Million
Year Founded: 1971
Total Employees: 2342
Ownership: Public
Stock Symbol: IIVI
Traded On: NASDAQ
Produces/Sells CE-marked Devices: N
Distribution: Manufacturer Direct, OEM
General Admin.: Craig A. Creaturo/Chief Financial Officer, Treasurer
     Carl J. Johnson/Director
     Herman E. Reedy/Executive Vice President
     Francis J. Kramer/President, Chief Executive Officer
     Vincent D. Mattera/Vice President, General Manager
Production: James Martinelli/Vice President Materials & Development

Accessories, Laser	General

IIT RESEARCH INSTITUTE   312.567.4924
10 W. 35th St., Chicago, IL 60616-3799
FDA Number: n/a   *Fax:* 312.567.4106
E-mail: info@iitri.org
Web site: www.iitri.com
Medical Products Sales Volume: $130,000,000
Total Employees: 1300
Ownership: Public
Produces/Sells CE-marked Devices: N
Distribution: OEM

IIT RESEARCH INSTITUTE
312.567.4924 *(cont'd)*
General Admin.: Dr. Sid Firstman/Corporate Director
Dr. Bahman Ateti/President
Mktg./Adv.: John Navarrete/Director Corporate Marketing
Terry Buckner/Manager Corporate Affairs
Research: randy Crawford/Vice President Engineering
IS: Barry Watson/Vice President Tech. Services
Kerry Rowe/Vice President Technology
Contract R&D, Equipment — General

IKA-WORKS, INC.
800-733-3037
2635 N. Chase Pkwy. S.E.,
910-452-7059
Wilmington, NC 28405
FDA Number: 1061025
Fax: 910-452-7693
E-mail: usa@ika.net
Web site: www.ika.net
Medical Products Sales Volume: $4,500,000
Year Founded: 1985
Total Employees: 77 *Sales Staff:* 10
Ownership: IKA-LABORTECHNIQUE
Produces/Sells CE-marked Devices: Y
Federal Procurement Eligibility: Small Business
Distribution: Manufacturer Direct, Manufacturer Through Distributor
General Admin.: Rene Stiegelmann/Chief Executive Officer
Bob Hardin/Vice President, General Manager
Mktg./Adv.: Elmo Amaya/Manager International Sales
Davis Thompson/Manager Lab. Sales
Blair Polanski/Marketing Coordinator
Research: Victor Press/Vice President Research & Development

Bone Mill	Orthopedics
Calorimeter	Chemistry
Dispenser, Microbiology Media	Microbiology
Equipment, Laboratory, Gen. Purpose (Specific Medical Use)	Chemistry
Mixer, Clinical Laboratory	Chemistry
Plate, Hot	Chemistry
Stirrer	Chemistry

IKI MFG. CO, INC.
608-884-3411
116 N. Swift St., Edgerton, WI 53534
FDA Number: 3003616479
Fax: 608-884-4712
E-mail: cjmoline@ikimfg.com
Web site: www.ikimfg.com
Ownership: Private
Produces/Sells CE-marked Devices: N
Refrigerant, Topical (Vapocoolant) — Physical Med

IKONISYS, INC
203-776-0791
5 Science Park, Suite 1000, New Haven, CT 06511
FDA Number: 3005566046
Fax: 203.776.0795
E-mail: questions@ikonisys.com
Ownership: Private
Produces/Sells CE-marked Devices: N
General Admin.: Paul White/President
Locator, Cell, Automated — Hematology
Reagents, Specific, Analyte — Hematology
System, Automated Scanning Microscope And Image Analysis For Fluorescence In Situ
Hybridization (fish) Assays — Immunology

ILLUMINA, INC.
1-800-809-4566
9865 Towne Centre Drive, San Diego, CA 92121
FDA Number: 3003218906
Fax: 1-858-202-4766
E-mail: info@illumina.com
Web site: www.illumina.com
Year Founded: 1998
Ownership: Public
Stock Symbol: ILMN
Traded On: NASDAQ
Produces/Sells CE-marked Devices: N
General Admin.: Dr. Mostafa Ronaghi/Chief Technology Officer, Senior Vice President
Mr. Jay Flatley/President, Chief Executive Officer
Dr. Gregory Heath/Senior Vice President
Mr. Tristan Orphan/Senior Vice President
Mktg./Adv.: Mr. Nicholas Naclerio/Senior Vice President Corporate Development
Ms. Laura Lauman/Vice President Marketing
Finance: Mr. Christian Henry/Chief Financial Officer
Analyzer, Karyotype — Pathology
Instrumentation For Clinical Multiplex Test Systems — Chemistry

ILLUMINATION INDUSTRIES
See Uvp, Llc

IMA NOVA
1-800-851-1518
7 New Lancaster, Leominster, MA 01453
978-537-8534
FDA Number: n/a
Fax: 978-840-0730
Web site: www.kalishdti.com
Medical Products Sales Volume: $26,000,000
Annual Revenue: $25-$50 Million
Total Employees: 100 *Marketing Staff:* 2 *Sales Staff:* 9

IMA NOVA
1-800-851-1518 *(cont'd)*
Ownership: D. T. INDUSTRIES, INC.
Produces/Sells CE-marked Devices: Y
Distribution: Manufacturer Direct, Manufacturer Through Manufacturer Reps
General Admin.: Jim Ririe/President
Mktg./Adv.: Mike Cameron/Manager International & National Sales
Lisa Barbieri/Manager Marketing
Counter, Pill — General
Dispenser, Liquid, Unit-Dose — General

IMA NOVA
978-537-8534
7 New Lancaster Road, Leominster, MA 01453-2962
FDA Number: n/a
Fax: 978-840-0730
E-mail: novasales@imanova.com
Web site: www.imanova.com
Medical Products Sales Volume: $9,500,000
Annual Revenue: $25-$50 Million
Total Employees: 100 *Marketing Staff:* 2 *Sales Staff:* 9
Ownership: DT INDUSTRIES
Produces/Sells CE-marked Devices: N
Federal Procurement Eligibility: Small Business
Distribution: Manufacturer Direct
General Admin.: Mr. James Ririe/President
Mr. Jeff Scheminger/Vice President, General Manager
Mktg./Adv.: Mr. Dan Doret/Manager International Sales
Mr. Ed Mazur/Vice President Marketing & Advertising
IS: Mr. Jim Hills/Vice President Application Development
Packaging Equipment — General
Thermoforming, Extrusion, Custom — General

IMACOR LLC.
516-393-0970
839 Stewart Avenue, Suite #3, Garden City, NY 11530
FDA Number: 300638218
Fax: 516-393-0969
E-mail: info@imacormonitoring.com
Web site: www.imacormonitoring.com
Ownership: Private
Produces/Sells CE-marked Devices: N
General Admin.: Mr. Peter Pellerito/President, Chief Executive Officer
Echocardiograph (Ultrasonic Scanner) — Cardiovascular
Scanner, Ultrasonic (Pulsed Doppler) — Radiology
Scanner, Ultrasonic (Pulsed Echo) — Radiology
Transducer, Ultrasonic, Diagnostic — Radiology

IMAGE ANALYSIS, INC.
800-548-4849
1380 Burkesville St., Columbia, KY 42728
270-384-6400
FDA Number: 2027364
Fax: 270-384-6405
E-mail: info@image-analysis.com
Web site: www.image-analysis.com
Medical Products Sales Volume: $34,620,000
Annual Revenue: $25-$50 Million
Year Founded: 1984
Total Employees: 8 *Marketing Staff:* 1 *Sales Staff:* 6
Ownership: Private
Produces/Sells CE-marked Devices: N
Federal Procurement Eligibility: Small Business
Distribution: Manufacturer Direct, Manufacturer Through Distributor, OEM, Exporter
General Admin.: Ben Arnold/President, Chief Executive Officer
Mktg./Adv.: Roger Schulte/Vice President Marketing & Sales
Computer Software — General
Computer, Radiographic Image Analysis — Radiology
Densitometer, Radiographic — Radiology
Densitometer, Radiography, Digital, Quantitative — Radiology
Phantom, Anthropomorphic, Radiographic — Radiology
Phantom, Computed Axial Tomography (CAT, CT) — Radiology

IMAGE DIAGNOSTICS, INC.
978-422-8601
98 Pratts Junction Rd., Sterling, MA 01564
FDA Number: 1223864
Radiographic/Fluoroscopic Unit, Image-Intensified — Radiology
Table, Radiographic, Stationary Top — Radiology
Table, Radiographic, Tilting — Radiology

IMAGE MARKETING CORP.
800-466-7032
1636 N. 24th St., PO Box 30935, Mesa, AZ 85275
480-969-7032
FDA Number: n/a
Fax: 480-969-0939
E-mail: info@image4u.com
Web site: www.image4u.com
Medical Products Sales Volume: $21,900,000
Annual Revenue: $0-$1 Million
Year Founded: 1980
Total Employees: 3
Ownership: Private
Produces/Sells CE-marked Devices: Y
Federal Procurement Eligibility: Small Business
Distribution: Manufacturer Direct, Importer, Exporter
General Admin.: Rik Beimfohr/President
Chemical, Film Processor — Radiology

IMAGE MARKETING CORP.　800-466-7032 (cont'd)
Illuminator, Radiographic Film　Radiology
Viewer/Magnifier　Hematology

IMAGE MOLDING, INC.　800-525-1875
4525 Kingston St., Denver, CO 80239-3016　**303-371-3338**
FDA Number: n/a　*Fax:* 303-371-3299
E-mail: iminc@qwest.net
Web site: http://www.imagemolding.com
Medical Products Sales Volume: $2,700,000
Annual Revenue: $1-$5 Million
Year Founded: 1997
Total Employees: 25　*Marketing Staff:* 1　*Sales Staff:* 1
Ownership: Private
Quality System Registration Information: ISO9001
Produces/Sells CE-marked Devices: N
Federal Procurement Eligibility: Small Business
Distribution: Manufacturer Direct, OEM, Importer, Exporter
General Admin.: Ewan R. Grantham/President
Production: Dan Thornton/Manager Engineering
　Ewan R. Grantham/Manager Quality Assurance
Finance: Tony Lonardo/Controller
　Chromatography Equipment, Ion Exchange　Toxicology
　Collector, Urine, Disposable　Gastroenterology/Urology
　Column, Ion Exchange With Colorimetry, Delta-Aminolevulinic　Chemistry
　Container, Specimen Mailer And Storage　Pathology
　Container, Urine Specimen　General
　Control, Urinalysis (Assayed And Unassayed)　Chemistry
　Coverslip, Microscope Slide　Pathology
　Labware, Basic, Disposable　Chemistry
　Labware, Blood Collection　Chemistry
　Pipette　Chemistry
　Rack, Test Tube　Chemistry
　Slide And Coverslip　Hematology
　Slide, Microscope　Pathology
　Stain, Hematology　Pathology
　Tube, Centrifuge　Chemistry

IMAGE TECHNOLOGY LABORATORIES, INC.　845-338-3366
602 Enterprise Dr., Kingston, NY 12401
FDA Number: 3004572316　*Fax:* 866-931-9409
E-mail: dedwards@imagetechlabs.com
Web site: www.imagetechlabs.com
Ownership: Private
Produces/Sells CE-marked Devices: N
　Device, Communications, Images, Ophthalmic　Ophthalmology

IMAGE TECHNOLOGY, INC.　800-554-6243
1380 N. Knollwood Circle, Anaheim, CA 92801　**714-252-0160**
FDA Number: n/a　*Fax:* 714-252-9436
E-mail: itsales@imagetechnology.com
Web site: www.imagetechnology.com
Annual Revenue: $1-$5 Million
Ownership: Private
Produces/Sells CE-marked Devices: N
Distribution: Service Direct
General Admin.: Marshall Shannon/Chief Executive Officer
Mktg./Adv.: Marshall Shannon/Director Marketing
　Jamey Hodges/Manager Sales Training
Production: Jamey Hodges/Manager Regulatory Affairs
　Service, Maintenance/Repair　General

IMAGEDERM, INC.　866-462-4334
632 W Elk Ave, Glendale, CA 91204　**818-500-9034**
FDA Number: n/a　*Fax:* 818-507-7506
E-mail: sales@imagederm.com
Web site: www.imagederm.com
Annual Revenue: $0-$1 Million
Total Employees: 10　*Marketing Staff:* 1　*Sales Staff:* 2
Ownership: Private
Produces/Sells CE-marked Devices: N
Federal Procurement Eligibility: Small Business
Distribution: Manufacturer Direct
Mktg./Adv.: Nancy Stillwell/Sales Specialist
　Brush, Dermabrasion　Surgery

IMAGEFLOW INC.　408-569-3860
730 Bantry Court, Sunnyvale, CA 94087
FDA Number: 3003900408
Ownership: Private
Produces/Sells CE-marked Devices: N
　Device, Storage, Image, Digital　Radiology

IMAGEMAX
See X-Ray Support, Inc

IMAGEN (AN EX ONE COMPANY)　724-863-9663
8075 Pennsylvania Avenue, Irwin, PA 15642
FDA Number: 3005970520

IMAGEN (AN EX ONE COMPANY)　724-863-9663 (cont'd)
Alloy, Gold Based, For Clinical Use　Dental And Oral

IMAGEPATH SYSTEMS, INC.　269-699-7182
23126 South Shore Rd., Edwardsburg, MI 49112
FDA Number: 1226014
Ownership: Private
Produces/Sells CE-marked Devices: N
　Stain, Cresyl Violet Acetate　Pathology

IMAGES-ON-CALL　214-902-8337
10290 Monroe Drive, Suite 202, Dallas, TX 75229
FDA Number: 1643795　*Fax:* 214-902-8303
E-mail: Sales@IOC.bz
Web site: www.imagesoncall.com
Medical Products Sales Volume: $4,500,000
Annual Revenue: $5-$10 Million
Year Founded: 1977
Total Employees: 18　*Marketing Staff:* 2　*Sales Staff:* 12
Ownership: Private
Produces/Sells CE-marked Devices: N
Federal Procurement Eligibility: Small Business
Distribution: Manufacturer Through Manufacturer Reps
General Admin.: Charlie Moore/President
Mktg./Adv.: Bob Maher/Director Marketing
　Bob Maher/Director National Accounts
　Patrick W. Barr/Director Product Development
Production: Jenean Pritzkow/Director Quality Assurance
　Ann Swenson/Manager Materials
　Transmitter, Image & Data, Radiographic　Radiology

IMAGING 3, INC.
See Imaging3, Inc.

IMAGING ARCHIVE INTERNATIONAL, LLC.　770-565-6166
5966 Exeter Circle, Norcross, GA 30071
FDA Number: 1066034
　Device, Storage, Image, Digital　Radiology

IMAGING ASSOCIATES, INC.　800-821-3230
11110 Westlake Dr., Charlotte, NC 28273　**704-522-8094**
FDA Number: 1064265　*Fax:* 704-522-8098
Web site: www.imaginga.com
Medical Products Sales Volume: $30,000,000
Annual Revenue: $25-$50 Million
Ownership: Private
Produces/Sells CE-marked Devices: N
Federal Procurement Eligibility: Small Business
Distribution: OEM, Service Direct, Exclusive Distributor, Exporter
　Computer Software　General
　Computer, Ultrasound　Radiology
　Condom　Obstetrics/Gynecology
　Equipment, Ultrasound, Doppler, Evaluation, Fetal　Obstetrics/Gynecology
　Equipment, Ultrasound, Intravascular, 3-Dimensional　Cardiovascular
　Media, Contrast, Ultrasound　Radiology

IMAGING DIAGNOSTIC SYSTEMS, INC.　800-992-9008
5307 NW 35th Terrace, Ft. Lauderdale, FL 33309　**954-581-9800**
FDA Number: 3001452873　*Fax:* 954-581-0555
E-mail: info@imds.com
Web site: www.imds.com
Medical Products Sales Volume: $17,000,000
Annual Revenue: $10-$25 Million
Year Founded: 1993
Total Employees: 40　*Marketing Staff:* 2　*Sales Staff:* 1
Ownership: Public
Stock Symbol: IMDS
Traded On: OTC Bulletin
Quality System Registration Information: ISO9001
Produces/Sells CE-marked Devices: Y
Federal Procurement Eligibility: Small Business
Distribution: Manufacturer Direct, Manufacturer Through Distributor, Exporter
General Admin.: Ms. Linda Grable/Chief Executive Officer
　Mr. Allan L. Schwartz/Chief Financial Officer, Vice President
　Deborah O'Brien/Senior Vice President
Production: Mr. Donovan Brown/Director Quality Assurance & Regulatory Affairs
　Scanner, Computed Tomography, X-Ray, Special Procedure　Radiology
　Scanner, Ultrasonic, Breast (Mammographic)　Obstetrics/Gynecology

IMAGING DYNAMICS CORPORATION　866-975-6737
2340 Pegasus Way N.E., Suite 151, Unit 14,　**403-251-9939**
Calgary, ALB T2E-8 Canada
FDA Number: 9616853　*Fax:* 403-251-1771
E-mail: info@imagingdynamics.com
Web site: www.imagingdynamics.com
Year Founded: 1995
Total Employees: 10
Ownership: Public
Stock Symbol: IDL

IMAGING DYNAMICS CORPORATION — 866-975-6737 (cont'd)
Traded On: Toronto
Produces/Sells CE-marked Devices: N
Distribution: Manufacturer Direct

IMAGING SCIENCES INTERNATIONAL, LLC — 215-997-5666
1910 North Penn Rd., Hatfield, PA 19440
FDA Number: 2530069
Ownership: Danaher Corporation
Image Processing System	Radiology
Radiographic Unit, Diagnostic, Dental, Extraoral	Dental And Oral
Scanner, Computed Tomography, X-Ray, Special Procedure	Radiology
System, X-Ray, Mobile	Radiology
System, X-ray, Extraoral Source, Digital	Radiology

IMAGING3, INC. — 800-900-9729
3200 W. Valhalla Dr., Burbank, CA 91505
FDA Number: 2030565
E-mail: dean@imaging3.com
Web site: www.imaging3.com
Year Founded: 1993
Ownership: Public
Stock Symbol: IMGG
Traded On: OTC Bulletin
Produces/Sells CE-marked Devices: N
General Admin.: Dean Janes/Chief Executive Officer, Chairman
Xavier Aguilera/Chief Financial Officer, Senior Vice President
Christopher Sohn/President, Chief Operating Officer
Michele Janes/Vice President Admin.
Mktg./Adv.: Mike Nessen/Vice President Business Development
| System, X-Ray, Mobile | Radiology |

IMAK PRODUCTS CORP. — 619-291-9990
2515 Camino Del Rio South,#240, San Diego, CA 92108
FDA Number: 2032529
Ownership: Private
Produces/Sells CE-marked Devices: N
| Orthosis, Cervical | Physical Med |
| Splint, Hand, And Component | Physical Med |

IMALUX CORPORATION — 216-502-0755
11000 Cedar Avenue, Suite 250, Cleveland, OH 44106
FDA Number: 3003883695
| Drape, Surgical | Surgery |
| System, Imaging, Optical Coherence Tomography (oct) | Radiology |

IMBIOTECHNOLOGIES LTD. — 780-945-6609
9650 - 20th Avenue, Suite 113,
Edmonton, ALBER T6N 1 Canada
FDA Number: n/a   *Fax:* 780-987-0941
E-mail: mstewart@tbwifi.ca
Web site: http://www.imbiotechnologies.com
Ownership: Private
Produces/Sells CE-marked Devices: N

IMCO TECHNOLOGIES — 800-300-7734 / 262-523-4445
N27 W23957 Paul Road,Suite 101,
Pewaukee, WI 53072
FDA Number: 2184004   *Fax:* 262-523-1141
E-mail: info@imco-tech.com
Web site: www.imco-tech.com
Medical Products Sales Volume: $34,620,000
Year Founded: 1990
Total Employees: 15
Ownership: Private
Produces/Sells CE-marked Devices: N
Federal Procurement Eligibility: Small Business
Distribution: Exclusive Distributor
General Admin.: Mr. Mark Schwartz/President, Chief Executive Officer
| System, Communication, Image, Digital | Radiology |

IMEB
See International Medical Equipment

IMED MOBILITY INC. — 800-788-7479 / 651-635-0655
1915 W. County Rd. C, Roseville, MN 55113-1320
FDA Number: n/a   *Fax:* 651-635-9237
E-mail: cms1@usinternet.com
Web site: http://www.imedmobility.com
Annual Revenue: $1-$5 Million
Total Employees: 13   *Marketing Staff:* 1   *Sales Staff:* 2
Ownership: Private
Produces/Sells CE-marked Devices: N
Federal Procurement Eligibility: Small Business
General Admin.: William Snyder/President, Chief Executive Officer
S. Mattson/Vice President, General Manager
Mktg./Adv.: William Snyder/Director Marketing
Dave Eckstrom/Manager International & National Sales
| Control, Hand Driving, Automobile, Mechanical | Physical Med |

IMED MOBILITY INC. — 800-788-7479 (cont'd)
Lift, Wheelchair	General
Restraint, Wheelchair	General
Scooter (Motorized 3-Wheeled Vehicle)	Physical Med
Vehicle, Handicapped	Physical Med

IMED TECHNOLOGY, INC. — 972-732-7333
17408 Tamaron Drive, Dallas, TX 75287
FDA Number: 3003813437
| Bag, Urinary Collection, Ureterostomy | Gastroenterology/Urology |
| Collector, Urine | Gastroenterology/Urology |

IMETRA, INC. — 914-592-2800
200 Clearbrook Rd., Elmsford, NY 10523-1396
FDA Number: n/a   *Fax:* 914-592-1637
E-mail: info@imetra.com
Web site: www.imetra.com
Medical Products Sales Volume: $4,000,000
Annual Revenue: $1-$5 Million
Total Employees: 3
Ownership: Private
Produces/Sells CE-marked Devices: N
Distribution: Manufacturer Through Distributor
| Component, Metal, Other | General |

IMETRIKUS, INC.
See Numera

IMI CORNELIUS, INC. — 800-551-4423 / 630-539-6911
500 Regency Drive,
Glendale Heights, IL 60139
FDA Number: n/a   *Fax:* 800-519-4423
E-mail: karloneb@cornlius.com
Web site: www.imiremcor.com
Medical Products Sales Volume: $21,900,000
Total Employees: 800
Ownership: Private
Produces/Sells CE-marked Devices: Y
Distribution: Manufacturer Direct
Mktg./Adv.: Thomas Best/Manager Business Development
Chilling Unit	Physical Med
Dispenser, Ice	General
Foodservice Product/Equipment	General

IMMCO DIAGNOSTICS, INC. — 800-537-8378 / 716-691-0091
60 Pineview Drive, Buffalo, NY 14228-2120
FDA Number: 1315336   *Fax:* 716-691-0466
E-mail: info@immcodiagnostics.com
Web site: www.immcodiagnostics.com
Medical Products Sales Volume: $101,100,000
Annual Revenue: $100-$500 Million
Year Founded: 1980
Total Employees: 50   *Marketing Staff:* 2   *Sales Staff:* 2
Ownership: Private
Quality System Registration Information: ISO9001
Produces/Sells CE-marked Devices: N
Federal Procurement Eligibility: Small Business
Distribution: Manufacturer Direct, Manufacturer Through Distributor, OEM, Service Direct
General Admin.: Vijay Kumar/President, Chief Executive Officer
Raj Mittal/Vice President Human Resources
Mktg./Adv.: Raul Saona/Manager Marketing & Sales
Production: Vince Ramsperger/Manager Materials
Kevin Lawson/Manager Regulatory Affairs
Vince Ramsperger/Vice President Manufacturing
Antibody, Antinuclear, Indirect Immunofluorescent, Antigen	Immunology
Antigen, Antiserum, Control, IGG, FITC	Immunology
Antiparietal Antibody, Immunofluorescent, Antigen, Control	Immunology
Enzyme Immunoassay, Other	Chemistry
Media, Mounting, Water Soluble	Pathology

IMMERSION MEDICAL — 800-929-4709 / 301-984-3706
55 West Watkins Mill Rd.,
Gaithersburg, MD 20878
FDA Number: n/a   *Fax:* 301-984-2104
E-mail: tnewak@immersion.com
Web site: www.immersion.com
Total Employees: 30
Ownership: Public
Produces/Sells CE-marked Devices: Y
Federal Procurement Eligibility: Small Business
Distribution: Manufacturer Direct, Service Direct
General Admin.: Richard Stacey/General Manager
Mktg./Adv.: Thomas Newak/Director Marketing
Ralph Stever/Director National Accounts
Research: Richard Cunningham/Vice President Research & Development
| Computer, Image, Endoscopic | General |

2013 MEDICAL DEVICE REGISTER

IMMERSION MEDICAL 800-929-4709 *(cont'd)*
Training Aid Orthopedics

IMMUCELL CORP. 800-466-8235
56 Evergreen Dr., Portland, ME 04103-5907
FDA Number: n/a
E-mail: info@immucell.com
Web site: www.immucell.com
Annual Revenue: $5-$10 Million
Year Founded: 1982
Ownership: Public
Stock Symbol: ICCC
Traded On: NASDAQ
Produces/Sells CE-marked Devices: Y
Federal Procurement Eligibility: Small Business
Distribution: Manufacturer Direct, Manufacturer Through Distributor, Manufacturer Through Manufacturer Reps, Exclusive Distributor, Exporter
General Admin.: Micheal F. Brigham/Chief Financial Officer, Vice President
Joseph H. Crabb/Chief Scientific Officer, Vice President
Micheal F. Brigham/President, Chief Executive Officer
Mktg./Adv.: Samuel A. Bond/Director Marketing
Antibody, Other General
Antigen, Antiserum, Control, Lactoferrin Immunology
Purification System, Water Gastroenterology/Urology

IMMUCOR CANADA INC. 800-661-9993
9703 45th Ave., Edmonton, ONT T6E 5Z8 Canada 403-437-5842
FDA Number: n/a Fax: 780-438-6595
Web site: www.immucan.com
Total Employees: 25 Marketing Staff: 2 Sales Staff: 12
Ownership: Private
Produces/Sells CE-marked Devices: N
Distribution: Exclusive Distributor, Exporter

IMMUCOR, INC. 800-829-2553
3130 Gateway Drive, PO Box 5625, 770-441-2051
Norcross, GA 30091
FDA Number: 1034569 Fax: 770-441-3807
E-mail: immucor@immucor.com
Web site: www.immucor.com
Medical Products Sales Volume: $4,500,000
Annual Revenue: $100-$500 Million
Year Founded: 1982
Total Employees: 610 Marketing Staff: 5 Sales Staff: 23
Ownership: Public
Stock Symbol: BLUD
Traded On: NASDAQ
Quality System Registration Information: ISO9001
Produces/Sells CE-marked Devices: Y
Distribution: Manufacturer Direct, Importer, Exporter
General Admin.: Joseph Rosen/Chairman
Richard Flynt/Chief Financial Officer, Vice President
Gioacchino DeChirico/President, Chief Executive Officer
Jean-Jacques De Jaegher/Vice President International Operations
Mktg./Adv.: Noel Brown/Vice President Sales
Research: Ralph Eatz/Senior Vice President Scientific Affairs
Lyle Sinor/Vice President Research & Development
IS: Carolyn Gambino/Vice President Tech. Services
Analyzer, Blood Grouping/Antibody, Automated Hematology
Antigen, Antiserum, Control, Albumin Immunology
Antigen, Antiserum, Control, Other Immunology
Antigen, Antiserum, Control, Prealbumin Immunology
Antigen, Antiserum, Control, Prothrombin Immunology
Antigen, Antiserum, Control, Red Cells Hematology
Antigen, IHA, Cytomegalovirus Microbiology
Buffer, pH Hematology
Diluent, Blood Cell Hematology
Kit, Quality Control, Blood Banking Hematology
Lectins/Protectins Hematology
Media, Potentiating Hematology
Pipette, Micro Chemistry
Processor, Frozen Blood Hematology
Rickettsia Serological Reagents, Other Microbiology
Solution, Stabilized Enzyme Hematology
Substance, Grouping, Blood (Non-Human Origin) Hematology
Supplies, Blood Bank Hematology
Test, D Positive Fetal Rbc Hematology
Test, Platelet Antibody Hematology
Medical Product Subsidiaries (Listed Separately)
Dominion Biologicals Ltd.
Gamma Biologicals - Netherlands

IMMUNA CARE CORP. 610-941-2167
13654 N. 12th St., Suite 3, Tampa, FL 33613
FDA Number: 2529061
Radioimmunoassay, Estrone Chemistry

IMMUNA CARE CORP. 610-941-2167 *(cont'd)*
Radioimmunoassay, Total Estrogen, Other Chemistry

IMMUNALYSIS CORPORATION 909-482-0840
829 Towne Center Drive, Pomona, CA 91767
FDA Number: 2020952
Radioimmunoassay, Dehydroepiandrosterone (Free And Sulfate) Chemistry
Radioimmunoassay, Estriol Chemistry
Radioimmunoassay, Follicle Stimulating Hormone Chemistry
Radioimmunoassay, Luteinizing Hormone Chemistry
Radioimmunoassay, Phencyclidine Toxicology
Test, Tetrahydrocannabinol Toxicology

IMMUNETECH PHARMACEUTICALS
See Elan

IMMUNETECH, INC. 650-470-7420
888 Oak Grove Ave., Suite 4, Menlo Park, CA 94025
FDA Number: 3004091547
Labware, Blood Collection Chemistry

IMMUNETICS, INC. 800-227-4765
27 Drydock Avenue, 6th Floor, 617-896-9100
Boston, MA 02210
FDA Number: 1226144 Fax: 617-896-9110
E-mail: info@immunetics.com
Web site: www.immunetics.com
Medical Products Sales Volume: $17,000,000
Annual Revenue: $1-$5 Million
Year Founded: 1987
Total Employees: 4 Marketing Staff: 1 Sales Staff: 1
Ownership: Private
Produces/Sells CE-marked Devices: N
Distribution: Manufacturer Direct, Manufacturer Through Distributor, Exporter
General Admin.: Andrew E. Levin/Chief Technology Officer
Inna Radzihovsky/Office Manager
Andrew Levin/President, Chief Executive Officer
Mktg./Adv.: Larry Fava/Director Marketing & Sales
Peter Condon/Director Product Development
Equipment, Test, Western Blot Microbiology
Reagent, Cysticercosis Microbiology
Test, DNA-Probe, Other Microbiology
Test, Disease, Lyme Immunology

IMMUNO CONCEPTS N.A. LTD. 800-251-5115
9825 Goethe Road, Suite 350, 916-363-2649
Sacramento, CA 95827
FDA Number: 2918768 Fax: 916-363-2843
E-mail: bert@immunoconcepts.com
Web site: www.immunoconcepts.com
Total Employees: 46
Ownership: Private
Quality System Registration Information: ISO9001
Produces/Sells CE-marked Devices: N
Federal Procurement Eligibility: Small Business
Distribution: Manufacturer Through Distributor
General Admin.: Bert R. Williams/President
Bob Boyes/Senior Vice President, General Manager
Bob Boyes/Vice President
Mktg./Adv.: Napolean Monce/Director Product Development
Production: Eric Hoy/Manager Regulatory Affairs
Anti-DNA Indirect Immunofluorescent Solid Phase Immunology
Antibody IGM, IF, Epstein-Barr Virus Microbiology
Antibody, Antinuclear, Indirect Immunofluorescent, Antigen Immunology
Antinuclear Antibody, Antigen, Control Immunology
Antiserum, CF, Epstein-Barr Virus Microbiology
Epstein-Barr Virus, Other Microbiology
Extractable Antinuclear Antibody (Rnp/Sm), Antigen/Control Immunology
Slide, Microscope Pathology
System, Test, Anticardiolipin, Immunological Immunology
Test System, Antineutrophil Cytoplasmic Antibodies (ANCA) Immunology
Test, DNA-Probe, Other Microbiology

IMMUNO DIAGNOSTIC CENTER, INC. 214-351-1231
9978 Monroe Dr., Ste. 303, Dallas, TX 75220-1498
FDA Number: 1644972 Fax: 775-924-4989
E-mail: idcdallas@aol.com
Medical Products Sales Volume: $500,000
Annual Revenue: $0-$1 Million
Total Employees: 4 Sales Staff: 3
Ownership: Private
Produces/Sells CE-marked Devices: N
Federal Procurement Eligibility: Small Business
Distribution: Manufacturer Through Manufacturer Reps, OEM
General Admin.: Amal Mukherjee/President
Mktg./Adv.: Subrata Roy/Manager Market Research
Analyzer, Chemistry, ELISA Chemistry
Antigen, Antiserum, Control, Albumin Immunology
Antigen, Antiserum, Control, Myoglobin Immunology

MANUFACTURER PROFILES

IMMUNO DIAGNOSTIC CENTER, INC. 214-351-1231 *(cont'd)*
- Kit, RIA, Basic Protein, Myelin — Immunology
- Myoglobin, FITC, Antigen, Antiserum, Control — Immunology
- Reagent, Kinase, Phosphate, Creatine — Chemistry
- Strip, HAMA IGG, ELISA, In Vitro Test System — Immunology
- Whole Human Plasma, Antigen, Antiserum, Control — Immunology

IMMUNO DIAGNOSTIC CENTER, INC. 214-351-1231
9978 Monroe Dr., Suite 303, Dallas, TX 75220
FDA Number: 1644972
- Antigen, Antiserum, Control, Albumin — Immunology
- Biosensor, Immunoassay, Myoglobin — Immunology

IMMUNO NUCLEAR CORP.
See Diasorin Inc

IMMUNO PHARMACEUTICALS
See Qed Bioscience, Inc.

IMMUNO RESOURCES, INC. 830-537-6199
415 Sisterdale Rd., Boerne, TX 78006
FDA Number: 1649983
Ownership: Private
Produces/Sells CE-marked Devices: N
- Antigen, (Febrile), Agglutination, Brucella SPP. — Microbiology
- Antigen, Febrile — Microbiology
- Antigen, Febrile, Slide And Tube, Salmonella — Microbiology
- Antigen, Salmonella SPP. — Microbiology
- Antigen, Slide And Tube, Francisella Tularensis — Microbiology
- Antigen, Streptococcus SPP. — Microbiology
- Antisera, Fluorescent, All Globulins, Proteus SPP. — Microbiology
- Antiserum, Escherichia Coli — Microbiology
- Antiserum, Fluorescent, Brucella SPP. — Microbiology
- Antiserum, Francisella Tularensis — Microbiology
- Antiserum, Listeria Monocytogenes — Microbiology
- Antiserum, Positive And Negative Febrile Antigen Control — Microbiology
- Antiserum, Salmonella SPP. — Microbiology
- Antiserum, Shigella SPP. — Microbiology
- Antiserum, Streptococcus SPP. — Microbiology
- Antiserum, Vibrio Cholerae — Microbiology

IMMUNO VISION, INC. 800-541-0960
1820 Ford Ave., Springdale, AR 72764
FDA Number: n/a   *Fax:* 479-751-7002
E-mail: cusserv@immunovision.com
Web site: www.immunovision.com
Annual Revenue: $1-$5 Million
Ownership: IVAX CORP.
Produces/Sells CE-marked Devices: N
Federal Procurement Eligibility: Small Business
Distribution: Manufacturer Direct
General Admin.: Kevin Clark/Chief Operating Officer
- Antibody, Antinuclear, Indirect Immunofluorescent, Antigen — Immunology
- Antigen, Antiserum, Control, Whole Human Serum — Immunology
- Antinuclear Antibody (Enzyme-Labeled), Antigen, Controls — Immunology
- Extractable Antinuclear Antibody (Rnp/Sm), Antigen/Control — Immunology
- Reagent, Other — General
- Test, DNA-Probe, Other — Microbiology
- Test, Thyroid Autoantibody — Immunology

IMMUNO-MYCOLOGICS, INC. 800-654-3639
2700 Technology Pl, Norman, OK 73071 405-360-4669
FDA Number: 1627497   *Fax:* 405-364-1058
E-mail: immy@immy.com
Web site: www.immy.com
Annual Revenue: $0-$1 Million
Year Founded: 1979
Total Employees: 12   *Marketing Staff:* 1
Ownership: Private
Produces/Sells CE-marked Devices: N
Federal Procurement Eligibility: Small Business, Female Owned
Distribution: Manufacturer Direct, Manufacturer Through Distributor, OEM, Exporter
General Admin.: David S. Bauman/Chief Executive Officer
             Sharon Bauman/President
Mktg./Adv.: Sean Bauman/Director Product Development
             Toby Branum/Manager Marketing
Production: Sharon Harris/Manager Quality Assurance
- Antigen, CF And/Or ID, Coccidioides Immitis — Microbiology
- Antigen, CF, Aspergillus SPP. — Microbiology
- Antigen, CF, B. Dermatitidis — Microbiology
- Antigen, Histoplasma Capsulatum, All — Microbiology
- Antigen, ID, Candida Albicans — Microbiology
- Antigen, Latex Agglutination, Coccidioides Immitis — Microbiology
- Antiserum, Latex Agglutination, Cryptococcus Neoformans — Microbiology
- Antiserum, Positive Control, Blastomyces Dermatitidis — Microbiology
- Antiserum, Positive Control, Coccidioides Immitis — Microbiology
- Antiserum, Positive Control, Histoplasma Capsulatum — Microbiology
- Enzyme Immunoassay, Other — Chemistry
- Plate, Radial Immunodiffusion — Immunology

IMMUNO-REAGENTS ASSOCIATES, INC.
See Consolidated Technologies, Inc.

IMMUNOGENETICS
See Hemacare Corporation

IMMUNOMEDICS, INC. 973-605-8200
300 American Road, Morris Plains, NJ 07950
FDA Number: n/a   *Fax:* 973-605-8282
E-mail: info@immunomedics.com
Web site: www.immunomedics.com
Medical Products Sales Volume: $34,620,000
Annual Revenue: $25-$50 Million
Year Founded: 1982
Total Employees: 106
Ownership: Public
Stock Symbol: IMMU
Traded On: NASDAQ
Produces/Sells CE-marked Devices: N
Federal Procurement Eligibility: Small Business
Distribution: OEM
General Admin.: Dr. David Goldenberg/Chairman
             Alfred Aronson/Director Human Resources
             Cynthia L. Sullivan/President, Chief Executive Officer
Production: Dr. Thomas Eckhardt/Vice President Regulatory Affairs
Research: Dr. Ivan Horak/Vice President Research & Development
Finance: Gerard Gorman/Chief Financial Officer, Vice President Finance
- Strip, HAMA IGG, ELISA, In Vitro Test System — Immunology
- Test, Cancer Detection, Other — Hematology

IMMUNOSCIENCE, INC. 925-460-8111
7066-d Commerce Cir., Pleasanton, CA 94588
FDA Number: 2953155
- Enzyme Linked Immunoabsorbent Assay, Treponema Pallidum — Microbiology
- Hepatitis B Test (B Core, BE Antigen & Antibody, B Core IGM) — Microbiology
- Kit, Mycobacteria Identification — Microbiology
- Kit, Test, Multiple, Drugs Of Abuse, Over The Counter — Toxicology

IMMUNOSPEC CORPORATION 818-717-1840
9428 Eton Avenue, Unit O, Chatsworth, CA 91311
FDA Number: 3005823191
- Campylobacter Pylori — Microbiology
- Radioimmunoassay, Cortisol — Chemistry
- Radioimmunoassay, Follicle Stimulating Hormone — Chemistry
- Radioimmunoassay, Free Thyroxine — Chemistry
- Radioimmunoassay, Human Chorionic Gonadotropin — Chemistry
- Radioimmunoassay, Prolactin (Lactogen) — Chemistry
- Radioimmunoassay, Thyroid Stimulating Hormone — Chemistry
- Test, Rheumatoid Factor — Immunology

IMMUNOSTICS, INC. 800-722-7505
3505 Sunset Avenue, Ocean, NJ 07712 732-918-0770
FDA Number: 2244821   *Fax:* 732-918-0618
E-mail: sales@immunostics.com
Web site: www.immunostics.com
Medical Products Sales Volume: $21,900,000
Annual Revenue: $10-$25 Million
Year Founded: 1983
Total Employees: 30   *Marketing Staff:* 2   *Sales Staff:* 4
Ownership: Private
Produces/Sells CE-marked Devices: N
Federal Procurement Eligibility: Small Business
Distribution: Manufacturer Through Distributor, OEM, Exporter
General Admin.: Kenn Kupits/President
Mktg./Adv.: Andrea Geffon/Manager Exports
             Andrea Geffon/Marketing & Sales Representative
- Agglutination Method, Human Chorionic Gonadotropin — Chemistry
- Anti-Streptokinase — Microbiology
- Antigen, (Febrile), Agglutination, Brucella SPP. — Microbiology
- Antigen, All Groups, Shigella SPP. — Microbiology
- Antigen, Febrile — Microbiology
- Antigen, Febrile, Slide And Tube, Salmonella — Microbiology
- Antigen, Non-Treponemal, All — Microbiology
- Antigen, Salmonella SPP. — Microbiology
- Antiserum, Control For Non-Treponemal Test — Microbiology
- Antiserum, Positive And Negative Febrile Antigen Control — Microbiology
- Kit, Pregnancy Test — Obstetrics/Gynecology
- Kit, Pregnancy Test, Over The Counter, HCG — Chemistry
- Reagent, Occult Blood — Hematology
- Serum, Animal — Pathology
- Test, C-Reactive Protein — Immunology
- Test, Direct Agglutination, Toxoplasma Gondii — Microbiology
- Test, Human Chorionic Gonadotropin — Immunology
- Test, Human Chorionic Gonadotropin, Serum — Immunology
- Test, Infectious Mononucleosis — Immunology
- Test, Rheumatoid Factor — Immunology
- Test, Syphilis (RPR or VDRL) — Microbiology
- Test, Systemic Lupus Erythematosus — Immunology

IMONTI AND ASSOCIATES INC., M. 949-248-1058
25707 Compass Way, San Juan Capistrano, CA 92675-4003
FDA Number: 2028042 *Fax:* 949-248-1874
E-mail: imonti12@cox.net
Web site: www.vitcutter.com
Medical Products Sales Volume: $101,100,000
Annual Revenue: $100-$500 Million
Total Employees: 3 *Marketing Staff:* 2 *Sales Staff:* 2
Ownership: Private
Produces/Sells CE-marked Devices: N
Federal Procurement Eligibility: Small Business
Distribution: Manufacturer Direct, Manufacturer Through Manufacturer Reps, OEM, Exporter
General Admin.: Maurice Imonti/President, Chief Executive Officer
Mktg./Adv.: Marcia Imonti/Manager International & National Sales
    Marcia Imonti/Vice President Business Development
    Marcia Imonti/Vice President Marketing & Sales

Cutter, Vitreous Aspiration, AC-Powered	Ophthalmology
Dressing, Other	General
Phacofragmentation Unit	Ophthalmology

IMP GROUP LTD. 902-453-2400
400-2651 Dutch Village Rd, Halifax B3L 4T1 Canada
FDA Number: 8020320

Kit, Administration, Intravenous	General

Medical Product Subsidiaries (Listed Separately)
Can-Med Surgical Supplies Limited

IMPAC MEDICAL SYSTEMS, INC. 888-464-6722
100 W. Evelyn Avenue, 650-623-8800
Mountain View, CA 94041
FDA Number: 2950347 *Fax:* 650-428-0721
E-mail: pr@impac.com
Web site: www.impac.com
Medical Products Sales Volume: $4,500,000
Annual Revenue: $25-$50 Million
Year Founded: 1990
Total Employees: 430
Ownership: ELEKTA AB
Quality System Registration Information: ISO9001
Produces/Sells CE-marked Devices: N
Federal Procurement Eligibility: Small Business
Distribution: Manufacturer Direct
General Admin.: Jay Hoey/Chief Operating Officer
    Joe Jachinowski/President, Chief Executive Officer
Mktg./Adv.: George Rugg/Vice President Business Development
    Suzanne Hoey/Vice President Marketing
    Scott Soehl/Vice President Sales
Production: Thom Faris/Director Quality Assurance & Regulatory Affairs
Research: Todd Powell/Vice President Research & Development

Accelerator, Linear, Medical	Radiology
Accessories, Radiotherapy	Radiology
Computer Software, Hospital/Nursing Management	General
Computer and Software, Medical	General
Paper, Chart, Record, Medical	General

IMPACT DIAGNOSTIC INTERNATIONAL 888-628-5118
748 E. Bonita Ave., Unit 211, Pomona, CA 91767 909-621-5118
FDA Number: 3004877011 *Fax:* 909-621-6866
E-mail: sales@impactdiagnostic.com
Web site: www.impactdiagnostic.com
Ownership: Private
Produces/Sells CE-marked Devices: N

Culture Media, Selective And Differential	Microbiology

IMPACT INSTRUMENTATION, INC. 800-969-0750
27 Fairfield Place, West Caldwell, NJ 07006-6206 973-882-1212
FDA Number: 2242630 *Fax:* 973-882-4993
E-mail: sales@impactii.com
Web site: www.impactii.com
Medical Products Sales Volume: $10,000,000
Annual Revenue: $10-$25 Million
Year Founded: 1977
Total Employees: 135 *Marketing Staff:* 2 *Sales Staff:* 2
Ownership: Private
Quality System Registration Information: ISO9001
Produces/Sells CE-marked Devices: Y
Federal Procurement Eligibility: Small Business
Distribution: Manufacturer Direct, Manufacturer Through Distributor, Manufacturer Through Manufacturer Reps
General Admin.: L. H. Sherman/President
    Melvin L. Chettum/Secretary, Treasurer
Mktg./Adv.: Anthony J. Altamore/Coord. Marketing & Sales
    Greg Grubaugh/Manager National Sales
Production: George Beck/Manager Engineering
    Gloria Bernstein/Manager Quality Systems
    Alan Giordano/Manager Regulatory Affairs

IMPACT INSTRUMENTATION, INC. 800-969-0750 *(cont'd)*

Pump, Aspiration, Portable	Anesthesiology
Suction Apparatus, Ward Use, Portable, AC-Powered	Surgery
Ventilator, Continuous (Respirator)	Anesthesiology
Ventilator, Volume (Critical Care)	Anesthesiology

IMPACT MEDICAL TECHNOLOGIES, LLC 770-817-3300
311 Curie Drive, Alpharetta, GA 30005
FDA Number: 3005257817
Ownership: Private
Produces/Sells CE-marked Devices: N

Catheter, Continuous Flush	Cardiovascular

IMPEL NEUROPHARMA 206-695-5817
720 Broadway Ave, Suite 413, Seattle, WA 98122
FDA Number: n/a
E-mail: hite@impelneuropharma.com
Web site: www.impelneuropharma.com
Ownership: Private
Produces/Sells CE-marked Devices: N
General Admin.: Mr. Michael Hite/Chief Executive Officer
    Mr. John Hoekman/Chief Scientific Officer

IMPERIAL FASTENER CO., INC. 954-782-7130
1400 S.W. 8th St., Pompano Beach, FL 33069
FDA Number: n/a *Fax:* 954-782-0089
E-mail: info@imperialfastener.com
Web site: www.imperialfastener.com
Medical Products Sales Volume: $5,500,000
Annual Revenue: $5-$10 Million
Year Founded: 1967
Ownership: Private
Produces/Sells CE-marked Devices: N
Federal Procurement Eligibility: Small Business
Distribution: Manufacturer Through Distributor

Cover, Laundry Hamper	General
Curtain, Cubicle	General
Curtain, Shower	General
Hanger, Intravenous	General
Track And Carrier, Cubicle Curtain	General
Track And Carrier, Intravenous	General

IMPERIAL ORTHOFLEX MANUFACTURING LTD. 800-667-3442
5920 No. 6 Rd., Ste. 205, 604-273-2836
Richmond, BC V6V-1 Canada
FDA Number: n/a *Fax:* 604-270-4512
E-mail: info@anatechinc.com
Web site: www.anatechinc.com
Year Founded: 1985
Total Employees: 25
Ownership: Private
Produces/Sells CE-marked Devices: N
Distribution: Manufacturer Direct, Exclusive Distributor

IMPERIAL SUPPLIES LLC 800-558-2808
789 Armed Forces Dr., PO Box 11008,
Green Bay, WI 54307
FDA Number: n/a *Fax:* 800-553-8769
Web site: www.imperialinc.com
Annual Revenue: $0-$1 Million
Year Founded: 1958
Ownership: Private
Produces/Sells CE-marked Devices: N
Federal Procurement Eligibility: Small Business
Distribution: Manufacturer Through Distributor, Manufacturer Through Manufacturer Reps, Exclusive Distributor, Importer
General Admin.: Clifton Kipe/President
Mktg./Adv.: Pauline Kipe/Vice President Marketing

Cabinet Casework, General Purpose	General

IMPERIAL SURGICAL LTD. 800-661-5432
850 Halpern Ave, Dorval, ONT H9P 1G6 Canada 514-631-7988
FDA Number: 9681599 *Fax:* 514-631-9083
E-mail: info@surgmed.com
Web site: www.surgmed.com
Year Founded: 1935
Total Employees: 25 *Marketing Staff:* 2 *Sales Staff:* 10
Ownership: Private
Quality System Registration Information: ISO9002
Produces/Sells CE-marked Devices: N
Federal Procurement Eligibility: Small Business
Distribution: Manufacturer Direct, Manufacturer Through Manufacturer Reps, Exporter

IMPERIAL, INC.
See Imperial Supplies Llc

MANUFACTURER PROFILES

IMPLADENT LTD.   800-526-9343   718-465-1810
198-45 Foothill Avenue,
Holliswood, NY 11423
FDA Number: 2431866   *Fax:* 718-464-9620
E-mail: ImpladentLtd@ImpladentLtd.com
Web site: www.Impladentltd.com
Medical Products Sales Volume: $34,620,000
Annual Revenue: $1-$5 Million
Year Founded: 1985
Total Employees: 8   *Marketing Staff:* 2   *Sales Staff:* 2
Ownership: Private
Quality System Registration Information: ISO9000; ISO9001; ISO9002; ISO9003
Produces/Sells CE-marked Devices: N
Federal Procurement Eligibility: Small Business
Distribution: Manufacturer Direct, Manufacturer Through Distributor, Manufacturer Through Manufacturer Reps, Importer, Exporter
General Admin.: Maurice Valen/President
     V. G. Valen/Vice President
Mktg./Adv.: Stephanie Georgi/Director Marketing & Advertising
     Virginia Scott/Director National Accounts & Sales
     Andrew Valen/Director Product Marketing
     Joe Torres/Manager Customer Services & Sales
     Maurice Valen/Market Research Analyst
Production: Barry Sands/Director Quality Assurance
     Nelson Vinuya/Quality Control, Product Engineer
Research: Dr. Joe Bowden/Vice President, Director Research & Development

Burr, Dental	Dental And Oral
Graft, Bone	Orthopedics
Implant, Endosseous	Dental And Oral

IMPLANT CENTER OF THE PALM BEACHES   561-627-5560
824 U.S. Hwy. 1, Ste. 370, North Palm Beach, FL 33408
FDA Number: n/a   *Fax:* 561-627-4214
Web site: www.jacktkrauser.com
Annual Revenue: $0-$1 Million
Ownership: Private
Produces/Sells CE-marked Devices: N
Distribution: Manufacturer Through Distributor
General Admin.: Jack T. Krauser/President

Implant, Endosseous	Dental And Oral

IMPLANT DEVELOPMENT CORP.
     See Surgical Implants, Inc.

IMPLANT DIRECT LLC   818-444-3300
27030 Malibu Hills Rd., Calabasas Hills, CA 91301
FDA Number: 3001617766

Abutment, Implant, Dental, Endosseous	Dental And Oral

IMPLANT LOGIC SYSTEMS, LTD.   516-295-1121
76 Spruce St., Cedarhurst, NY 11516
FDA Number: 3003508226

Image Processing System	Radiology

IMPLANT SCIENCES CORP.   781-246-0700
107 Audubon Road, #5, Wakefield, MA 01880-1246
FDA Number: 1226547   *Fax:* 781-246-1167
E-mail: info@implantsciences.com
Web site: www.implantsciences.com
Annual Revenue: $5-$10 Million
Year Founded: 1984
Total Employees: 112   *Marketing Staff:* 2   *Sales Staff:* 6
Ownership: Public
Stock Symbol: IMX
Traded On: AMEX
Quality System Registration Information: ISO9001
Produces/Sells CE-marked Devices: Y
Federal Procurement Eligibility: Small Business
Distribution: Manufacturer Through Distributor, Service Direct
General Admin.: Anthony J. Armini/President, Chief Executive Officer
Mktg./Adv.: Richard Sahagian/Director Product Development
     Robert Hayward/Manager Sales Training
     Alan Lucas/Vice President Business Development
     Alan Lucas/Vice President Marketing & Sales
Production: Jeff Gibbs/Director Quality Assurance
     Jeff Gibbs/Manager Regulatory Affairs
Research: Steven N, Bunker/Vice President Research & Development

Equipment, Device Coating, Protective	General
Service, Device Coating, Protective	General
Service, Modification, Product	General

IMPLANTECH ASSOCIATES, INC.   800-733-0833   805-339-9415
6025 Nicolle Street, Suite B, Ventura, CA 93003
FDA Number: 2028924   *Fax:* 805-339-9414
E-mail: info@impantech.com
Web site: www.implantech.com
Medical Products Sales Volume: $101,100,000
Annual Revenue: $1-$5 Million

IMPLANTECH ASSOCIATES, INC.   800-733-0833 *(cont'd)*
Year Founded: 1989
Total Employees: 30
Ownership: Private
Quality System Registration Information: ISO9001
Produces/Sells CE-marked Devices: Y
Federal Procurement Eligibility: Small Business
Distribution: Manufacturer Direct, Manufacturer Through Distributor, Manufacturer Through Manufacturer Reps
General Admin.: Ed Leicht/General Manager

Catheter, Suction, With Tip	General
Malar Implant	Surgery
Prosthesis, Facial, Mandibular Implant	Ear/Nose/Throat
Prosthesis, Nasal, Dorsal	Surgery

Medical Product Subsidiaries (Listed Separately)
     Allied Biomedical

IMPLEX CORP.   800-613-6131   866-688-7656
1800 West Center Street,
Warsaw, IN 46581
FDA Number: n/a   *Fax:* 201-818-0567
E-mail: info@implex.com
Web site: www.zimmer.com
Medical Products Sales Volume: $4,500,000
Year Founded: 1991
Ownership: Private
Quality System Registration Information: ISO9001
Produces/Sells CE-marked Devices: Y
Distribution: Manufacturer Through Distributor
General Admin.: Mr. Alex Khowaylo/President, Chief Executive Officer, Chairman
Research: Mr. Robert Cohen/Vice President Research & Development & Quality Control
Finance: Mr. Dave Washburn/Vice President Finance & Operations

Accessories, Fixation, Spinal Intervertebral Body	Orthopedics
Device, Spinal Vertebral Body Replacement	Orthopedics
Orthopedic Implant Material	Orthopedics
Prosthesis, Hip, Semi-Const., Metal/Poly., Porous Uncemented	Orthopedics
Prosthesis, Hip, Semi-Const., Uncem., Non-P., M/P, Ca./Phos.	Orthopedics
Prosthesis, Hip, Semi-Constrained (Cemented Acetabular)	Orthopedics
Prosthesis, Hip, Semi-Constrained, Metal/Polymer	Orthopedics
Prosthesis, Knee, Femorotibial, Constrained, Metal	Orthopedics
Prosthesis, Knee, Femorotibial, Constrained, Metal/Polymer	Orthopedics
Prosthesis, Knee, Total	Orthopedics
Prosthesis, Spine, Intervertebral Disc	Orthopedics
Prosthesis, Tibial	Orthopedics

IMRIS INCORPORATED   888-304-0114   204-480-7070
100 - 1370 Sony Place,
Winnepeg, MAN R3T 1 Canada
FDA Number: 3003807210
E-mail: info@imris.com   *Fax:* 204-480-7071
Web site: www.imris.com
Year Founded: 1997
Total Employees: 25
Ownership: Public
Stock Symbol: IM
Traded On: Toronto
Produces/Sells CE-marked Devices: N

IMS, INC.   847-956-1940
600 Bonnie Ln., Elk Grove Village, IL 60007
FDA Number: 1424423
E-mail: info@intmeasys.com
Web site: www.intmeasys.com
Ownership: Private
Produces/Sells CE-marked Devices: N

Scale, Infant	General

IMS-ESS   951-676-2751
27449 Colt Court, Temecula, CA 92590
FDA Number: 2027537   *Fax:* 951-694-0097
Web site: www.ims-ess.com
Annual Revenue: $0-$1 Million
Year Founded: 1977
Ownership: Private
Produces/Sells CE-marked Devices: N
Federal Procurement Eligibility: Small Business, Female Owned
Distribution: Manufacturer Direct, Manufacturer Through Manufacturer Reps
General Admin.: Mark Bridgeford/Chief Financial Officer, Secretary
     Richard Olson/President, Chairman

Contract Assembly	General
Contract Manufacturing, Product, Durable	General

IMSI, INTEGRATED MODULAR SYSTEMS INC.   800-220-9729   610-789-7000
2500 Township Line Road, PO Box 616,
Havertown, PA 19083
FDA Number: 3004561695   *Fax:* 610-789-7730
E-mail: info@imsimed.com

IMSI, INTEGRATED MODULAR SYSTEMS INC. 800-220-9729
(cont'd)
Web site: www.imsimed.com
Medical Products Sales Volume: $17,000,000
Year Founded: 1980
Total Employees: 10   *Marketing Staff:* 1   *Sales Staff:* 3
Ownership: Private
Produces/Sells CE-marked Devices: Y
Federal Procurement Eligibility: Small Business
Distribution: Manufacturer Direct, Manufacturer Through Distributor, Manufacturer Through Manufacturer Reps, OEM, Service Direct, Exclusive Distributor, Importer, Exporter
General Admin.: John Mazur/President
     Mr. Geoff Mazur/Vice President
Mktg./Adv.: Mrs. Helen Mazur/Director Marketing & Sales

Analyzer, Bone, Sonic, Non-Invasive	Orthopedics
Analyzer, Motility, Gastrointestinal, Electrical	Gastroenterology/Urology
Computer Equipment	General
Computer Software	General
Computer and Software, Medical	General
Computer, Diagnostic, Programmable	Cardiovascular
Computer, Image, Endoscopic	General
Computer, Imaging, Presurgery	Surgery
Computer, Patient Data Management	General
Computer, Radiographic Image Analysis	Radiology
Computer, Ultrasound	Radiology
Device, Storage, Image, Digital	Radiology
Image Digitizer	Radiology
Service, Consulting	General
Storage Device, Fluoroscopic Image	Radiology
Storage Unit, X-Ray Film	Radiology
System, Communication, Image, Digital	Radiology
System, Network And Communication, Physiological Monitors	Cardiovascular
System, X-Ray, Mobile	Radiology

IMTEC IMAGING L.L.C. 800-226-3220
2401 North Commerce, Ardmore, OK 73401
FDA Number: 3005779915

Scanner, Computed Tomography, X-Ray, Special Procedure	Radiology

IMTEC, A 3M COMPANY 800-879-9799
IMTEC Plaza, 2401 N. Commerce,   **580-223-4456**
Ardmore, OK 73401
FDA Number: 1645158   *Fax:* 800-986-9574
E-mail: imtec@imtec.com
Web site: www.imtec.com
Medical Products Sales Volume: $34,620,000
Year Founded: 1990
Total Employees: 150
Ownership: 3m Co.
Stock Symbol: MMM
Traded On: NYSE
Quality System Registration Information: ISO9001
Produces/Sells CE-marked Devices: Y
Federal Procurement Eligibility: Small Business
Distribution: Manufacturer Direct, Manufacturer Through Distributor
General Admin.: Dr. Ronald A. Bulard/Chairman
     Dr. Victor I. Sendax/Director
     Mr. Timothy M. Ott/Director
     Mr. Tim Thompson/President, Chief Executive Officer
     Mr. Steven J. Hadwin/Vice President
Production: Mr. Brad Vance/Director Quality Assurance & Regulatory Affairs

Implant, Endosseous	Dental And Oral
Implant, Endosseous (Bone Filling and/or Augmentation)	Dental And Oral

IMTEK ENVIRONMENTAL CORP. 770-667-8621
P.O. Box 2066, Alpharetta, GA 30023
FDA Number: n/a   *Fax:* 770-667-8683
E-mail: imtek@noodor.com
Web site: www.noodor.com
Annual Revenue: $5-$10 Million
Year Founded: 1989
Total Employees: 200   *Marketing Staff:* 5   *Sales Staff:* 6
Ownership: Private
Produces/Sells CE-marked Devices: N
Federal Procurement Eligibility: Small Business, Minority Owned
Distribution: Manufacturer Direct, Manufacturer Through Distributor, Manufacturer Through Manufacturer Reps, OEM, Exclusive Distributor, Exporter
General Admin.: D.J. Keller/President, Chief Executive Officer

Equipment, Control, Pollution	General
Media, Filter	General
Pack, Hot Or Cold, Reusable	Physical Med
Solution, Ostomy, Odor Control	Gastroenterology/Urology

IN DISPOSABLES INC. 800-269-4568
P.O. Box 528, Stratford, CT 06615   **203-332-7678**
FDA Number: 1646760   *Fax:* 203-384-1932
E-mail: info@indisposables.com

IN DISPOSABLES INC. 800-269-4568 *(cont'd)*
Web site: www.indisposables.com
Medical Products Sales Volume: $5,000,000
Annual Revenue: $5-$10 Million
Total Employees: 9   *Marketing Staff:* 1
Ownership: Private
Produces/Sells CE-marked Devices: N
Federal Procurement Eligibility: Small Business
Distribution: Exclusive Distributor
General Admin.: Thomas Carpenter/President
     William Lichtenberger/Vice President, General Manager
Mktg./Adv.: William Lichtenberger/Vice President Sales

Cover, Shoe, Operating Room	Surgery
Glove, Patient Examination, Latex	General
Glove, Patient Examination, Vinyl	General
Gown, Isolation, Surgical	Surgery
Mask, Face	General

IN HOME PRODUCTS, INC. 800-810-8475
12015 Shiloh Rd., Ste. 158-B, Dallas, TX 75228   **214-319-7772**
FDA Number: n/a   *Fax:* 214-319-9411
E-mail: globalron@aol.com
Web site: www.inhomeproducts.com
Medical Products Sales Volume: $2,500,000
Annual Revenue: $1-$5 Million
Year Founded: 1994
Total Employees: 19   *Marketing Staff:* 2   *Sales Staff:* 7
Ownership: Private
Produces/Sells CE-marked Devices: Y
Distribution: Manufacturer Direct, Manufacturer Through Distributor, Exporter
General Admin.: Gina Gardner/Office Manager
     Mr. Ron Schnier/President, Owner

Cane, Safety Walk	Physical Med
Exerciser, Powered	Anesthesiology

IN VIVO METRIC 707-433-2949
PO Box 397, Healdsburg, CA 95448
FDA Number: 2916286   *Fax:* 707-433-2407
E-mail: ivm@invivometric.com
Web site: www.invivometric.com
Annual Revenue: $0-$1 Million
Year Founded: 1965
Ownership: Private
Produces/Sells CE-marked Devices: Y
Federal Procurement Eligibility: Small Business
Distribution: Manufacturer Direct, OEM, Exporter

Component, Other	General
Electrode, Biopotential, Surface, Composite	Physical Med
Occluder, Cardiovascular	Cardiovascular

IN'TECH MEDICAL, INCORPORATED 757-224-0177
2851 Lamb Place, Suite 15,, Memphis, TN 38118
FDA Number: 3004627597

Caliper	Orthopedics
Curette, Surgical	Surgery
Elevator, Orthopedic	Orthopedics
Orthopedic Manual Surgical Instrument	Orthopedics

IN-SIGHT 401-434-1211
750 Narragansett Park Dr., Rumford, RI 02916
FDA Number: 1222291
Ownership: Private
Produces/Sells CE-marked Devices: N

Kit, Surgical (General)	Surgery

IN-STEP MOBILITY 800-558-7837
8027 N. Monticiello Ave., Skokie, IL 60076   **847-676-1275**
FDA Number: 3004361304   *Fax:* 847-676-1202
E-mail: walkers@ustep.com
Web site: www.ustep.com
Ownership: Private
Produces/Sells CE-marked Devices: N

Cane	Physical Med
Walker, Mechanical	Physical Med

IN/US SYSTEMS, INC. 800-875-4687
5809 N. 50th St., Tampa, FL 33610-4809   **813-626-6848**
FDA Number: n/a   *Fax:* 813-620-3708
E-mail: fl@inus.com
Web site: www.inus.com.
Medical Products Sales Volume: $3,000,000
Annual Revenue: $1-$5 Million
Year Founded: 1990
Total Employees: 12   *Marketing Staff:* 1   *Sales Staff:* 5
Ownership: Private
Produces/Sells CE-marked Devices: Y
Federal Procurement Eligibility: Small Business
Distribution: Manufacturer Direct, Manufacturer Through Manufacturer Reps

IN/US SYSTEMS, INC.   800-875-4687 (cont'd)
General Admin.: Edward Rapkin/President, Chief Executive Officer
Mktg./Adv.: John E. Hnizdil/Vice President Sales
Production: Russell Schavey/Vice President Manufacturing
Detector, Beta/Gamma   Chemistry
Detector, Radioisotope   Radiology

INAMED
See Allergan

INBIOS INTL., INC.   866-INBIOS1
562 1st. Avenue South, Suite 600,   **206-344-5821**
Seattle, WA 98104
FDA Number: 3032562
E-mail: info@inbios.com   *Fax:* 206-344-5823
Web site: www.inbios.com
Medical Products Sales Volume: $17,000,000
Year Founded: 1996
Total Employees: 18
Ownership: Private
Produces/Sells CE-marked Devices: N
Federal Procurement Eligibility: Small Business
Distribution: Manufacturer Direct, Manufacturer Through Distributor, OEM, Exclusive Distributor
Reagent, Leishmanii Serological   Microbiology

INC RESEARCH   866-462-7373
4700 Falls of Neuse Road, Suite 400,   **919-876-9300**
Raleigh, NC 27609
FDA Number: n/a
E-mail: tvonder@incresearch.com   *Fax:* 919-876-9360
Web site: www.incresearch.com
Medical Products Sales Volume: $34,620,000
Annual Revenue: $100-$500 Million
Year Founded: 1980
Total Employees: 700   *Marketing Staff:* 3
Ownership: Private
Produces/Sells CE-marked Devices: N
Distribution: Service Direct
General Admin.: James Ogle/Chief Executive Officer
    Dr. John Potthoff/Chief Operating Officer
    Dr. Michael Corrado/Chief Scientific Officer
Medical Admin.: Dr. Malcom Fletcher/Chief Medical Officer
Research: Dr. Kevin Keim/Director Development
Finance: Mr. Dan Hartnett/Chief Financial Officer
Service, Consulting   General

INCAPPE, INC.   601-638-2345
9 Ashland Ave., Brandon, MS 39047
FDA Number: 3003996345
Ownership: Private
Produces/Sells CE-marked Devices: N
Stocking, Support (Anti-Embolic)   General

INCARE ORTHOPAEDIC/PROTECTAIR, INC.
See Protectair Inc.

INCELL CORPORATION, LLC   210-877-0100
12734 Cimarron Path, San Antonio, TX 78249
FDA Number: 3004107906
Culture Media, Enriched   Microbiology
Culture Media, Supplements   Microbiology
Culture Media, Synthetic Cell And Tissue   Pathology

INCELLDX INC.   650-777-7630
1700 El Camino Real, Menlo Park, CA 94027
FDA Number: 3008272746
E-mail: info@incelldx.com   *Fax:* 650-587-1528
Web site: http://incelldx.com
Ownership: Private
Produces/Sells CE-marked Devices: N
General Admin.: Dr. Bruce Patterson/Chief Executive Officer
    Mr. Eric Hass/Chief Operating Officer
Mktg./Adv.: Mr. Brandon Steele/Vice President Commercial Operations
    Ms. Carol Penfold-Patterson/Vice President Marketing
Research: Ms. Grace Knutson/Vice President Product Development
Fixative, Formalin Containing   Pathology
Reagent, General Purpose   Pathology
Reagents, Specific, Analyte   Hematology

INCEPTIO MEDICAL TECHNOLOGIES, LC   801-447-7000
1401 north 1075, west suite 230, farmington, UT 84025
FDA Number: 3003736665
E-mail: info@punctsure.com   *Fax:* 801-447-3625
Web site: www.punctsure.com
Year Founded: 1999
Ownership: Private
Produces/Sells CE-marked Devices: N
General Admin.: Bradley Stringer/Chief Executive Officer

INCEPTIO MEDICAL TECHNOLOGIES, LC   801-447-7000 (cont'd)
Mktg./Adv.: Michael Russell/Vice President Marketing & Sales
Production: Judy Dyreng/Director Operations
Scanner, Ultrasonic (Pulsed Doppler)   Radiology
Transducer, Ultrasonic, Diagnostic   Radiology

INCISIVE SURGICAL, INC.   877-246-7672
14405 - 21st Avenue North, Suite 130,   **952-591-2543**
Plymouth, MN 55447
FDA Number: 3004028675
E-mail: custserv@insorb.com   *Fax:* 952-591-5989
Web site: www.insorb.com
Medical Products Sales Volume: $21,900,000
Annual Revenue: $25-$50 Million
Year Founded: 1999
Total Employees: 31   *Marketing Staff:* 1   *Sales Staff:* 10
Ownership: Private
Quality System Registration Information: ISO9001
Produces/Sells CE-marked Devices: Y
Federal Procurement Eligibility: Small Business
Distribution: Manufacturer Through Manufacturer Reps
General Admin.: Mr. John Shannon/President, Chief Executive Officer, Director
Production: Mr. David Stoen/Vice President Operations
Research: Mr. James Peterson/Vice President Development
    Mr. David Herridge/Vice President Engineering
Finance: Mr. Ronald McClurg/Chief Financial Officer
Forceps, General & Plastic Surgery   Surgery
Staple, Implantable   Surgery

INCISIVE, LLC.   510-669-9401
3095 Richmond Pkwy., Suite 213, Richmond, CA 94806
FDA Number: 2954939
Laser, Surgical   Surgery

INCITE INTERNATIONAL, INC.   816-220-7533
2749 Hunter Dr, Nw, Blue Springs, MO 64015
FDA Number: 1954164
Ownership: Private
Produces/Sells CE-marked Devices: N
Frame, Spectacle (Eyeglasses)   Ophthalmology

INCLINATOR CO. OF AMERICA   800-343-9007
601 Gibson Boulevard,   **717-939-8420**
Harrisburg, PA 17104
FDA Number: n/a
E-mail: isales@inclinator.com   *Fax:* 717-939-8075
Web site: www.inclinator.com
Annual Revenue: $10-$25 Million
Year Founded: 1923
Ownership: Private
Quality System Registration Information: ISO9000
Produces/Sells CE-marked Devices: Y
Federal Procurement Eligibility: Small Business
Distribution: Manufacturer Through Distributor, Manufacturer Through Manufacturer Reps
Elevator, Other   General
Lift, Stair Climbing   General
Lift, Wheelchair   General
System, Transport, In-House   General

INCONTROL, INC.
See Boston Scientific Corp.

INCREDIBLE SCENTS, INC.   (877) 233- 94
1009 Glen Cove Avenue, Glen Head, NY 11545
FDA Number: 3003563086
E-mail: Info@incrediblescents.com
Ownership: Private
Produces/Sells CE-marked Devices: N
Dilator, Nasal   Ear/Nose/Throat

INCSTAR CORP.
See Diasorin Inc

INDEC SYSTEMS, INC.   408-986-1600
2210 Martin Avenue, Santa Clara, CA 95050
FDA Number: n/a
E-mail: info@imagingworkbench.com   *Fax:* 408-986-1605
Web site: www.indecsystems.com
Medical Products Sales Volume: $101,100,000
Annual Revenue: $1-$5 Million
Total Employees: 15   *Marketing Staff:* 2   *Sales Staff:* 2
Ownership: Private
Produces/Sells CE-marked Devices: Y
Federal Procurement Eligibility: Small Business, Female Owned
Distribution: Manufacturer Direct, Manufacturer Through Distributor
General Admin.: Kal Hubler/President, Chief Executive Officer
    Carol Hubler/Vice President
Mktg./Adv.: Carol Anderson/Vice President Marketing

INDEC SYSTEMS, INC.   408-986-1600 *(cont'd)*
Production: Robert Brackett/Vice President Manufacturing
Research: Richard Didday/Vice President Research & Development

Computer Software	General
Computer, Clinical Laboratory	Chemistry
Computer, Nuclear Medicine	Radiology
Computer, Radiographic Image Analysis	Radiology
Computer, Ultrasound	Radiology
Contract R&D, Equipment	General
Radiographic Picture Archiving/Communication System (PACS)	Radiology
Radiographic Unit, Digital Subtraction Angiographic (DSA)	Radiology
Radiotherapy Treatment Planning Unit	Radiology

INDELPA, S.A. DE C.V.   609-983-8006
Carlos B. Zetina No. 22, Xalostoc Mexico
FDA Number: 9616080

Pad, Menstrual, Scented	Obstetrics/Gynecology
Pad, Menstrual, Unscented	Obstetrics/Gynecology

INDEPENDENCE CHAIR COMPANY, THE
See Ortho-Kinetics, Inc.

INDEPENDENT BRACE, INC.   863-647-5559
3633 Century Blvd, Ste 1, Lakeland, FL 33811
FDA Number: 1063842

Orthosis, Limb Brace	Physical Med

INDEPENDENT CARE PRODUCTS, INC.   866-357-0353
P.O. Box 6258, Abilene, TX 79608   325-698-8151
FDA Number: 1650735   *Fax:* 325-695-9561
E-mail: ind-care@swbell.net
Web site: www.medmarket.com/indcare
Medical Products Sales Volume: $100,000
Total Employees: 15   *Marketing Staff:* 4   *Sales Staff:* 4
Ownership: Private
Produces/Sells CE-marked Devices: N
Distribution: Manufacturer Direct, Manufacturer Through Manufacturer Reps

Chair, Shower	General

INDEPENDENT NEEDS CENTRE   905-479-1448
3415 Fourteenth Ave., Unit #2,, Markham, ONT L3R 0H3 Canada
FDA Number: n/a   *Fax:* 905-479-7618
E-mail: info@independentneeds.com
Web site: www.independentneeds.com
Year Founded: 1980
Total Employees: 10
Ownership: Private
Produces/Sells CE-marked Devices: N
Distribution: Manufacturer Direct, Exclusive Distributor

INDEPENDENT SOLUTIONS, INC.   847-498-0500
900 Skokie Blvd., Suite 118, Northbrook, IL 60062-4014
FDA Number: n/a   *Fax:* 847-498-9319
E-mail: conspecinc@aol.com
Medical Products Sales Volume: $5,000,000
Annual Revenue: $5-$10 Million
Year Founded: 2003
Total Employees: 5   *Marketing Staff:* 1   *Sales Staff:* 3
Ownership: Private
Produces/Sells CE-marked Devices: N
Federal Procurement Eligibility: Small Business
Distribution: Manufacturer Direct, Manufacturer Through Distributor, Manufacturer Through Manufacturer Reps, Service Direct, Exclusive Distributor, Importer, Exporter
General Admin.: William L. Glass/President, Chief Executive Officer
Mktg./Adv.: Steve Zima/Manager Contract Sales
    William L. Glass/Manager Market Research
Production: William L. Glass/Manager Regulatory Affairs

Bumper Guard, Corner	General
Cabinet Casework, General Purpose	General
Cabinet Casework, Laboratory	Chemistry
Cabinet Casework, Modular	General
Cabinet Casework, Patient Room	General
Cabinet Casework, Pharmacy	General
Cabinet, Bedside	General
Cabinet, Dental	Dental And Oral
Cabinet, Instrument	General
Cabinet, Laboratory	Chemistry
Cabinet, Narcotic Control	General
Cabinet, Other	General
Cabinet, Pass Through	General
Cabinet, Warming	General
Cabinet, X-Ray Transfer	Radiology
Cleaner, Bedpan (Sterilizer)	General
Clock, Elapsed Time	General
Column, Life Support (Electrical/Gas)	General
Console, Patient Service	General
Curtain, Cubicle	General
Curtain, Shower	General
Hanger, Intravenous	General

INDEPENDENT SOLUTIONS, INC.   847-498-0500 *(cont'd)*

Headwall System (Patient Room)	General
Illuminator, Radiographic Film	Radiology
Lamp, Examination (Light)	General
Lamp, Examination, Ceiling Mounted (Light)	General
Light, Overbed	General
Mount, Monitor (Support)	General
Mount, Television Set	General
Ophthalmoscope, AC-Powered	Ophthalmology
Ophthalmoscope, Battery-Powered	Ophthalmology
Ophthalmoscope, Direct	Ophthalmology
Ophthalmoscope, Indirect	Ophthalmology
Rail, Wall Side	General
Rails, Equipment	General
Sanitizer	General
Service, Consulting	General
Sink, Hospital	General
Station, Nourishment	General
Station, Nursing	General
Sterilizer, Steam, Table Top	General
System, Pipeline, Gas	General
Track And Carrier, Cubicle Curtain	General
Track And Carrier, Intravenous	General
Warmer, Bedpan	General
Warmer, Blanket	General
Warmer, Solution	Chemistry
Washer, Cart	General
Washer, Utensil	General

INDEX INSTRUMENTS U.S. INC.   407-932-3688
3305 Commerce Blvd., Kissimmee, FL 34741
FDA Number: n/a   *Fax:* 407-932-3686
E-mail: IndexUS@aol.com
Web site: www.indexinstrumentsus.com
Year Founded: 1990
Total Employees: 5   *Marketing Staff:* 1   *Sales Staff:* 2
Ownership: INDEX INSTRUMENTS LTD. & OPTICAL ACTIVITY LTD.
Produces/Sells CE-marked Devices: N
Federal Procurement Eligibility: Small Business, Female Owned
Distribution: Manufacturer Direct, Service Direct, Importer, Exporter
General Admin.: Dr. J. L. Horn/President, Chief Executive Officer
    Jennifer L. Horn/Vice President
Mktg./Adv.: Linnell Oakes/Manager Customer Services & Sales
    Ian Allison/Manager National Sales
    Linnell Oakes/Vice President Sales
Production: June Bork/Manager Materials
IS: Darrell L. Wayman/Manager Tech. Services

Polarimeter	Chemistry
Refractometer	Chemistry

INDIANA TECHNOLOGY DEVELOPMENT, INC.   317-814-6194
4181 E. 96th St., Suite 200, Indianapolis, IN 46240
FDA Number: 1831083
Ownership: Private
Produces/Sells CE-marked Devices: N

Scanner, Ultrasonic (Pulsed Echo)	Radiology

INDIGENOUS PEOPLES TECHNOLOGY AND EDUCATION CENTER   352-465-4545
10575 Sw 147th Circle, Dunnellon, FL 34432
FDA Number: 3004015784

Chair/Table, Medical	General

INDIGO MICRO TECHNOLOGIES, INC.   815-874-3557
3220 Gunflint Trail, Rockford, IL 61109
FDA Number: 1064491

Pupillometer, AC-Powered	Ophthalmology

INDIGO ORB, INC.   949-784-0303
2454 Alton Parkway, Irvine, CA 92606
FDA Number: 3006018131

Syringe, Piston	General

INDILAB, INC.   800-441-5000
10367 Franklin Avenue, Franklin Park, IL 60131   847-928-1050
FDA Number: 1450962   *Fax:* 847-928-1052
E-mail: rgavrick@indilab.com
Web site: www.indilab.com
Medical Products Sales Volume: $17,000,000
Annual Revenue: $10-$25 Million
Year Founded: 1987
Total Employees: 20   *Marketing Staff:* 2
Ownership: Private
Quality System Registration Information: ISO9001
Produces/Sells CE-marked Devices: Y
Federal Procurement Eligibility: Small Business
Distribution: Manufacturer Direct, OEM
General Admin.: Robert Gavrick/President, Chief Executive Officer
Production: Mark Espenscheid/Director Quality Assurance & Regulatory Affairs

INDILAB, INC.   800-441-5000 *(cont'd)*
Thomas Griffin/Vice President Operations
Sterilization Process Indicator, Physical/Chemical   General

INDIVIDUAL MONITORING SYSTEMS, INC.   410-296-7723
1055 Taylor Ave., Suite 300, Baltimore, MD 21286
FDA Number: 1125605

Electroencephalograph	Cns/Neurology
Recorder, Ventilatory Effort	Anesthesiology

INDO LENS US, INC.   800-729-1959
224 W. James St, Bensenville, IL 60106
FDA Number: 2032595
Ownership: Private
Produces/Sells CE-marked Devices: N

Lens, Spectacle/Eyeglasses, Non-Custom   Ophthalmology

INDOOR SUN SYSTEMS, INC.
See Tan America-Indoor Sunsystem

INDUSTRIA BRASILEIRA DE FILMES CORP.
See I.B.F. Corporation

INDUSTRIAL & BIOMEDICAL SENSORS CORP.   781-891-4201
1377 Main St., Waltham, MA 02451-1624
FDA Number: 1218924   *Fax:* 781-891-6408
E-mail: ibsma@ibs-corp.com
Web site: www.ibs-corp.com
Medical Products Sales Volume: $1,000,000
Annual Revenue: $0-$1 Million
Year Founded: 1975
Total Employees: 12
Ownership: Private
Produces/Sells CE-marked Devices: N
Federal Procurement Eligibility: Small Business, Minority Owned, Female Owned
Distribution: Manufacturer Direct, Exclusive Distributor
General Admin.: S. Chang/President, Chief Executive Officer

Biofeedback Device	Cns/Neurology
Monitor, Blood Pressure, Indirect, Anesthesiology	Anesthesiology
Monitor, Blood Pressure, Indirect, Automatic	Cardiovascular
Monitor, Pulse Rate	Anesthesiology

INDUSTRIAL ACOUSTICS CO., INC.   718-931-8000
1160 Commerce Avenue, Bronx, NY 10462-5506
FDA Number: 9200575   *Fax:* 718-863-1138
E-mail: info@industrialacoustics.com
Web site: www.industrialacoustics.com
Medical Products Sales Volume: $55,800,000
Annual Revenue: $5-$10 Million
Year Founded: 1949
Total Employees: 500   *Marketing Staff:* 3   *Sales Staff:* 3
Ownership: Public
Stock Symbol: IACI
Traded On: NASDAQ
Produces/Sells CE-marked Devices: N
Federal Procurement Eligibility: Small Business
Distribution: Manufacturer Direct, Manufacturer Through Manufacturer Reps
General Admin.: Dominick Nardi/Manager
     Robert Schmitt/President
Mktg./Adv.: Melvyn A. Romero/Manager Advertising
     Ken DeLasho/Vice President Marketing
     Bob Schmidt/Vice President Sales
Production: Ron Spineli/Vice President Production

Chamber, Acoustic, Testing   Ear/Nose/Throat

INDUSTRIAL COMPUTER SOURCE   800-523-2320   619-677-0877
6260 Sequence Dr., San Diego, CA 92121-4371
FDA Number: n/a   *Fax:* 858-677-0895
E-mail: salesteam@industrial-computer-source.com
Web site: www.indcompsrc.com
Medical Products Sales Volume: $5,000,000
Total Employees: 350   *Sales Staff:* 23
Ownership: Private
Quality System Registration Information: ISO9001
Produces/Sells CE-marked Devices: N
Distribution: Manufacturer Direct
General Admin.: Jim Jameson/President, Chief Executive Officer
Mktg./Adv.: Marty Kleine/Director Marketing & Communications
     Mike Dickey/Director National Accounts

Computer Equipment   General

INDUSTRIAL MUNICIPAL EQUIPMENT, INC.   410-795-0500
1430 Progress Way, Suite 105, Eldersburg, MD 21784
FDA Number: 3001226865

Monitor, Microbial Growth   Microbiology

INDUSTRIAL SPECIALITIES MANUFACTURING, INC.   800-781-8487   303-781-8486
4091 So. Eliot Street, Englewood, CO 80110
FDA Number: n/a   *Fax:* 303-761-7939
E-mail: sales@industrialspec.com
Web site: www.industrialspec.com
Medical Products Sales Volume: $1,000,000
Annual Revenue: $1-$5 Million
Year Founded: 1980
Total Employees: 10   *Sales Staff:* 4
Ownership: Private
Produces/Sells CE-marked Devices: N
Federal Procurement Eligibility: Small Business
Distribution: Manufacturer Direct
General Admin.: John Curzon/President

Component, Electrical	General
Dryer, Labware	Chemistry
Dryer, Respiratory/Anesthesia Equipment	General
Filter, Air	General
Fitting, Other	General
Kit, Intravenous Extension Tubing	General
Valve, Other	Chemistry

INDUSTRIAL SUPPORT SERVICES, INC.   217-223-6180
2600 North 42th St., Quincy, IL 62305-5066
FDA Number: 3003699646   *Fax:* 217-223-6470
E-mail: info@issquincy.com
Web site: www.issquincy.com
Ownership: Private
Produces/Sells CE-marked Devices: N

Pack, Hot Or Cold, Disposable   Physical Med

INDUSTRIAL WELDING SUPPLIES OF HATTIESBURG, INC.   601-545-1800
1924 Byron St., Hattiesburg, MS 39402
FDA Number: 2318311

Analyzer, Gas, Argon, Gaseous Phase	Anesthesiology
Analyzer, Gas, Carbon-Monoxide, Gaseous Phase	Anesthesiology
Laser, Gastroenterology/Urology	Gastroenterology/Urology

INDUSTRIAS MEDISON, S.A. DE C.V.   800-851-4431
Lote 7 Manzana 3 Parque, Industrial De Cananea,km.5, Carretera a Inuris, Sonora Mexico
FDA Number: 9616830

Gown, Surgical   Surgery

INDUSTRIAS TUK, S.A. DE C.V.   8-313-7421-2
Antigua Carretera a Roma, Km 7 5‾, Apodaca 66632 Mexico
FDA Number: 9611592

Sterilization Process Indicator, Physical/Chemical   General

INFAB CORP.   805-987-5255
3651 Via Pescador, Camarillo, CA 93012-5050
FDA Number: n/a   *Fax:* 805-482-8424
E-mail: xray@infab.org
Web site: www.infab.org
Medical Products Sales Volume: $21,900,000
Annual Revenue: $10-$25 Million
Year Founded: 1981
Total Employees: 26   *Marketing Staff:* 4   *Sales Staff:* 8
Ownership: Private
Produces/Sells CE-marked Devices: N
Federal Procurement Eligibility: Small Business
Distribution: Manufacturer Through Distributor, OEM, Importer, Exporter
General Admin.: L. S. Cusick/President, Chief Financial Officer
Mktg./Adv.: Brittany Ryniewicz/Director Sales
Production: Doug Cusick/Vice President Manufacturing

Apron, Lead, Radiographic	Radiology
Cart, Other	General
Eyeglasses, Safety	Ophthalmology
Glove, Protective, Radiographic	Radiology
Support, Patient Position, Radiographic	Radiology

INFECTIO DIAGNOSTIC INC. (I.D.I.)   418-681-4343
2050 boul. Rene-Levesque Ouest, 4th Floor, Sainte-Foy, QUE G1V-2 Canada
FDA Number: n/a   *Fax:* 418-681-5254
E-mail: jacquesmilette@infectio.com
Web site: www.infectio.com
Year Founded: 1996
Total Employees: 100
Ownership: Private
Produces/Sells CE-marked Devices: N
Distribution: Manufacturer Direct

INFECTION CONTROL SYSTEMS INC.
888-235-4569
905-318-8334
402 Concession St.,
Hamilton, ONT L9A-1 Canada
FDA Number: n/a   Fax: 905-648-2217
E-mail: info@infectioncontrol.on.ca
Web site: www.infectioncontrol.on.ca
Year Founded: 1997
Total Employees: 10
Ownership: Private
Produces/Sells CE-marked Devices: N
Distribution: Manufacturer Direct, Exclusive Distributor

INFECTION LAB., INC.
See Specialty Laboratories, Inc.

INFICON LEYBOLD-HERAEUS
See Infimed, Inc.

INFIMED, INC.
315-453-4545
121 Metropolitan Dr., Liverpool, NY 13088-5335
FDA Number: 1318879   Fax: 315-453-4550
E-mail: customercare@infimed.com
Web site: www.infimed.com
Total Employees: 90
Ownership: Private
Quality System Registration Information: ISO9001
Produces/Sells CE-marked Devices: Y
Federal Procurement Eligibility: Small Business
Distribution: Manufacturer Direct, Manufacturer Through Distributor, OEM, Exporter
General Admin.: Amy Ryan/Executive Vice President
Brian Fleming/President
Production: Dave Klementowski/Director Quality Assurance
Research: Oscar Khutoryansky/Vice President Research & Engineering
Computer, Cardiac Catheterization Laboratory   Cardiovascular
Radiographic Unit, Digital Subtraction Angiographic (DSA)   Radiology
Radiographic/Fluoroscopic Unit, Angiographic, Digital   Radiology
Radiographic/Fluoroscopic Unit, Special Procedure   Radiology

INFOMETRIX, INC.
425-402-1450
10634 E. Riverside Dr., Suite 250, Bothell, WA 98011
FDA Number: n/a   Fax: 425-402-1040
E-mail: info@infometrix.com
Web site: www.infometrix.com
Annual Revenue: $1-$5 Million
Total Employees: 15   Marketing Staff: 2   Sales Staff: 3
Ownership: Private
Produces/Sells CE-marked Devices: N
Federal Procurement Eligibility: Small Business
Distribution: Manufacturer Direct, Manufacturer Through Manufacturer Reps, Service Direct
General Admin.: Brian G. Rohrback/Chief Executive Officer
Mktg./Adv.: Paul J. Bailey/Director Marketing
Paul J. Bailey/Manager International & National Sales
Computer Software   General

INFORMATION DATA MANAGEMENT, INC.
800-249-4276
847-588-0453
6231 W. Howard Street, Niles,, IL 60714
FDA Number: 1421202   Fax: 847-588-0455
E-mail: idmsales@idm.com
Web site: www.haemoscope.com
Medical Products Sales Volume: $4,500,000
Annual Revenue: $5-$10 Million
Year Founded: 1977
Total Employees: 65   Marketing Staff: 1   Sales Staff: 2
Ownership: HAEMONETICS CORP.
Stock Symbol: HAE
Traded On: NYSE
Produces/Sells CE-marked Devices: N
Federal Procurement Eligibility: Small Business
Distribution: Manufacturer Direct
General Admin.: Emanuel Yonan/Chief Executive Officer
Timothy Coburn/President
Mktg./Adv.: Sue McBride/Manager Business Development
Production: Vicki Moore/Manager Regulatory Affairs
Computer Software   General
Computer, Patient Data Management   General

INFORMATION HEALTH NETWORK
800-443-0613
517-706-0060
PO Box 23056, Lansing, MI 48909-3056
FDA Number: n/a   Fax: 517-706-0065
E-mail: info@InfoHealthNet.com
Web site: www.infohealthnet.com
Medical Products Sales Volume: $17,000,000
Year Founded: 1982
Total Employees: 10   Marketing Staff: 2   Sales Staff: 4
Ownership: Private
Produces/Sells CE-marked Devices: N

INFORMATION HEALTH NETWORK
800-443-0613 *(cont'd)*
Federal Procurement Eligibility: Small Business, Female Owned
Distribution: Manufacturer Direct
Mktg./Adv.: Autumn Johnson/Manager Marketing
Jeannie Cleary/Manager National Sales
Computer, Patient Data Management   General
Immobilizer, Knee   Orthopedics

INFOSYS, INC.
800-978-4636
888-463-6797
1821 Walden Office Square, Suite 350,
Schaumburg, IL 60173
FDA Number: n/a   Fax: 847-925-9421
E-mail: sales@infosysusa.com
Web site: www.infosysusa.com
Medical Products Sales Volume: $34,620,000
Annual Revenue: $25-$50 Million
Ownership: Private
Produces/Sells CE-marked Devices: N
Federal Procurement Eligibility: Minority Owned
Distribution: Manufacturer Direct, Manufacturer Through Distributor
General Admin.: K. Pasupathy/President, Chief Executive Officer
Janice Kahl/Vice President Human Resources
Vernon Mathias/Vice President, General Manager
Mktg./Adv.: Dave Hammonds/Manager National Sales
Sharon Harder/Manager Sales Training
Kelly Ace/Marketing Associate
Vernon Mathias/Vice President Marketing & Sales
Research: K. Challappan/Vice President Research & Development
Computer Software, Home Healthcare   General
Computer and Software, Medical   General

INFOWORLD MANAGEMENT SYSTEMS
See Great Valley Technologies

INFOWORLD MANAGEMENT SYSTEMS, DIV OF GREAT VALLEY TECH
See Great Valley Technologies

INFOWORLD MEDICAL SYSTEMS, INC.
See Great Valley Technologies

INFRAMETRICS INC.
See Sea Horse Bio Science

INFRARED FIBER SYSTEMS, INC.
301-622-7131
2301-A Broadbirch Dr., Silver Spring, MD 20904
FDA Number: n/a   Fax: 301-622-7136
E-mail: fiber@infraredfibersystems.com
Web site: www.infraredfibersystems.com
Annual Revenue: $1-$5 Million
Total Employees: 11   Marketing Staff: 2   Sales Staff: 1
Ownership: Private
Produces/Sells CE-marked Devices: N
Federal Procurement Eligibility: Small Business
Distribution: Manufacturer Through Distributor
General Admin.: Danh Tran/Chief Executive Officer
Mktg./Adv.: Ken Levin/Vice President Marketing
Production: Danh Tran/Vice President Manufacturing
Accessories, Laser   General
Spectrophotometer, Infrared   Chemistry

INFRARED SCIENCES CORP.
516-482-9001
213 Hallock Rd., Suite 5, Stony Brook, NY 11790
FDA Number: 3004513841
Telethermographic System (Adjunctive Use)   Radiology

INFRAREDRX
888-680-7339
781-221-0053
34 3rd. Avenue, Burlington, MA 01803
FDA Number: 3004722468
E-mail: info@infraredx.com
Web site: http://www.infraredx.com
Ownership: Private
Produces/Sells CE-marked Devices: N
General Admin.: Dr. James Muller/Chief Executive Officer
Mr. Steven Nakashige/President, Chief Operating Officer
Mktg./Adv.: Mr. Grant Frazier/Vice President Marketing
Mr. Jim Dillon/Vice President Sales
Production: Ms. Deborah Thurston/Director Quality Assurance
Mr. Steve Chartier/Vice President Regulatory & Clinical Affairs
Research: Mr. Robert Silva/Vice President Product Development
Catheter, Intravascular, Plaque Morphology Evaluation   Cardiovascular

INFRAREDX INC.
888-680-7339
781-221-0053
34 Third Ave., Burlington, MA 01803
FDA Number: 3004722468
E-mail: info@infraredx.com
Web site: www.infraredx.com
Ownership: Private
Produces/Sells CE-marked Devices: N
General Admin.: Mr. Donald Southard/President, Chief Executive Officer

INFRAREDX INC.   888-680-7339 *(cont'd)*
Mr. Steve Nakashige/President, Chief Operating Officer
Medical Admin.: Dr. James Muller/Chief Medical Officer
Mktg./Adv.: Mr. Grant Frazier/Vice President Marketing
Mr. James Dillon/Vice President Sales
Production: Mr. Steve Chartier/Vice President Regulatory & Clinical Affairs
Research: Mr. Robert Silva/Vice President Product Development
Finance: Mr. Jeffrey Mazur/Vice President Finance
Catheter, Intravenous   Cardiovascular

INGEN TECHNOLOGIES, INC.   757-224-0177
35193 Avenue A, Suite C, Yucaipa, CA 92399
FDA Number: 3005686889
Ownership: Public
Stock Symbol: ITEC
Traded On: OTC Bulletin
Produces/Sells CE-marked Devices: N
Tube, Thorpe, Uncompensated   Anesthesiology

INGENIOUS TECHNOLOGIES CORP.   941-966-0690
1109 Millpond Ct, Osprey, FL 34229
FDA Number: 1528558
Needle, Hypodermic, Single Lumen With Syringe   General

INGLIS FOUNDATION   215-581-0725
2600 Belmont Ave., Phila, PA 19131
FDA Number: 2531571
Accessories, Wheelchair   Physical Med
Utensil, Food   Physical Med

INGMAR MEDICAL, LTD.   800-583-9910
P.O. Box 10106, Pittsburgh, PA 15232   412-683-8228
FDA Number: n/a   *Fax:* 412-683-8404
E-mail: info@ingmarmed.com
Web site: www.ingmarmed.com
Medical Products Sales Volume: $1
Annual Revenue: $1-$5 Million
Year Founded: 1993
Ownership: Private
Produces/Sells CE-marked Devices: Y
Federal Procurement Eligibility: Small Business
Distribution: Manufacturer Direct
General Admin.: Dr. Stefan Frembgen/Chief Executive Officer
Mktg./Adv.: Ms. Susan Petersen/Vice President Market Development
Mr. Nick Coniglio/Vice President Sales
Simulator, Lung   Anesthesiology

INGOLD ELECTRODES, INC.
See Mettler-Toledo Process Analytical, Inc.

INLAND DENTAL DISTRIBUTORS LTD.   800-661-6569
10569 111 St., Edmonton, ALB T5H-3E8 Canada   780-420-6901
FDA Number: n/a   *Fax:* 780-425-2241
Year Founded: 1975
Ownership: Private
Produces/Sells CE-marked Devices: N
Distribution: Manufacturer Direct, Exclusive Distributor

INLET MEDICAL, INC.   800-969-0269
10340 Vilking Drive, Suite 125,   952-942-5034
Eden Prairie, MN 55344
FDA Number: K923528   *Fax:* 952-829-7112
E-mail: info@inletmedical.com
Web site: www.inletmedical.com
Medical Products Sales Volume: $101,100,000
Annual Revenue: $1-$5 Million
Total Employees: 12   *Marketing Staff:* 2   *Sales Staff:* 6
Ownership: Private
Produces/Sells CE-marked Devices: N
Federal Procurement Eligibility: Small Business
Distribution: Manufacturer Direct, Manufacturer Through Distributor
General Admin.: Lee Jones/President, Chief Executive Officer
Mktg./Adv.: Susan Lazar/Vice President Marketing
Ralph Germscheid/Vice President Sales
Instrument, Passing, Suture, Laparoscopic   Surgery

INMAN ORTHODONTIC LABORATORIES, INC.   954-340-8477
9381 W. Sample Rd., Coral Springs, FL 33065
FDA Number: 3005663102
Clamp, Wire, Orthodontic   Dental And Oral
Clasp, Wire   Dental And Oral
Tray, Fluoride, Disposable   Dental And Oral

INMARK CORPORATION   800-899-7947
4 Byington Place, Norwalk, CT 06850-3309   203-866-8474
FDA Number: 9000494   *Fax:* 203-866-0918
E-mail: xray@inmarkcorp.com
Web site: inmarkcorp.com
Medical Products Sales Volume: $4,500,000

INMARK CORPORATION   800-899-7947 *(cont'd)*
Annual Revenue: $1-$5 Million
Total Employees: 4   *Marketing Staff:* 1   *Sales Staff:* 2
Ownership: Private
Quality System Registration Information: ISO9002
Produces/Sells CE-marked Devices: Y
Federal Procurement Eligibility: Small Business
Distribution: Manufacturer Through Distributor, Exporter
General Admin.: Lars Giers/President
Production: Carol J. Castellano/Manager Operations & Services
IS: Peter Taylor/Tech. Specialist
Tube, X-Ray   Radiology

INMARK, INC.   800-646-6275
675 Hartman Road, Suite 100, Austell, GA 30168   770-373-3300
FDA Number: n/a   *Fax:* 770-373-3301
E-mail: service@inmarkinc.com
Web site: www.inmarkinc.com
Medical Products Sales Volume: $17,000,000
Annual Revenue: $25-$50 Million
Year Founded: 1975
Total Employees: 70
Ownership: Private
Produces/Sells CE-marked Devices: N
Federal Procurement Eligibility: Small Business
Distribution: Manufacturer Through Distributor, OEM, Exclusive Distributor, Exporter
Production: Jay Johnson/Manager Regulatory Services
Packaging Equipment   General

INNERCOOL THERAPIES, INC.- A DELAWARE CORPORATION   858-713-5904
6740 Top Gun Street, San Diego, CA 92121
FDA Number: 2032640
Regulator, Thermal, Cardiopulmonary Bypass   Cardiovascular

INNERPULSE INC.   919-287-4100
4025 Stirrup Creek Dr., Suite 200,
Research Triangle Park, NC 27703
FDA Number: n/a   *Fax:* 919-287-4109
E-mail: info@Inner-Pulse.com
Web site: www.Inner-Pulse.com
Year Founded: 2003
Ownership: Private
Produces/Sells CE-marked Devices: N
General Admin.: Steve Mason/Chief Technology Officer
Dan Palek/President

INNERSPACE, INC.   877.HUM.BIRD
1622 Edinger Avenue, Suite C,   714-259-7900
Tustin, CA 92780
FDA Number: 2084683   *Fax:* 714-259-7999
E-mail: info@innerspacemedical.com
Web site: www.innerspacemedical.com
Annual Revenue: $1-$5 Million
Year Founded: 1991
Total Employees: 3
Ownership: Private
Produces/Sells CE-marked Devices: N
General Admin.: Mr. Don Bobo/Chief Executive Officer
Mrs. Elise Vazquez/Coord. Admin.
Mktg./Adv.: Mr. Ben Bobo/Vice President Marketing & Sales
Cannula, Ventricular   Cns/Neurology
Catheter, Ventricular   Cns/Neurology
Monitor, Pressure, Intracranial, Implantable   Cns/Neurology

INNERVISION INC.   901-682-0417
6258 Shady Grove Rd. E., Memphis, TN 38120
FDA Number: n/a   *Fax:* 901-682-1846
Annual Revenue: $0-$1 Million
Total Employees: 4   *Marketing Staff:* 2
Ownership: Private
Produces/Sells CE-marked Devices: Y
Federal Procurement Eligibility: Small Business
Distribution: Manufacturer Direct, Importer, Exporter
General Admin.: Frank M. Lewis/Chief Executive Officer
Camera, Video, Endoscopic   General
Electrosurgical Unit, Cutting & Coagulation Device   Surgery
Endoscope   Gastroenterology/Urology
Insufflator, Hysteroscopic   Obstetrics/Gynecology
Insufflator, Laparoscopic   Obstetrics/Gynecology
Laparoscope, General & Plastic Surgery   Surgery
Laparoscope, Gynecologic   Obstetrics/Gynecology
Printer, Image, Video   General
Probe   Orthopedics
Retractor, Surgical   Surgery

INNERVISION INC.　901-682-0417 *(cont'd)*
Sleeve, Trocar　Surgery

INNOCURE, LLC　480-966-0980
1045 East Sandpiper Dr., Tempe, AZ 85283
FDA Number: 3005254469
　Block, Beam Shaping, Radionuclide　Radiology

INNOMED CHRISTIE GROUP LTD.　780-483-6177
18208 102 Ave., Edmonton, ALB T5S-1S7 Canada
FDA Number: n/a　*Fax:* 780-483-6343
E-mail: info@christieinnomed.com
Web site: www.christieinnomed.com
Year Founded: 1988
Total Employees: 100
Ownership: Private
Produces/Sells CE-marked Devices: N
Distribution: Exclusive Distributor

INNOMEDICA
　See Greatbach Medical

INNOMINATA DBA GENBIO　800-288-4368
15222 Ave. Of Science, Suite A,　858-592-9300
San Diego, CA 92128
FDA Number: 2027113
Web site: www.genbio.com　*Fax:* 858-592-9400
Annual Revenue: $1-$5 Million
Year Founded: 1994
Ownership: Private
Produces/Sells CE-marked Devices: N
Federal Procurement Eligibility: Small Business
Distribution: Manufacturer Direct, Manufacturer Through Distributor, OEM, Service Direct, Importer
　Anti-DNA Antibody (Enzyme-Labeled), Antigen, Control　Immunology
　Anti-RNP-Antibody, Antigen And Control　Immunology
　Anti-SM-Antibody, Antigen And Control　Immunology
　Antibody IGM, IF, Epstein-Barr Virus　Microbiology
　Antigen, CF (Including CF Control), Cytomegalovirus　Microbiology
　Antigen, CF (Including CF Control), Epstein-Barr Virus　Microbiology
　Antigen, Cf (including Cf Control), Herpesvirus Hominis 1, 2　Microbiology
　Antigen, HA (Including HA Control), Rubella　Microbiology
　Antigen, IF, Toxoplasma Gondii　Microbiology
　Antinuclear Antibody (Enzyme-Labeled), Antigen, Controls　Immunology
　Antinuclear Antibody, Antigen, Control　Immunology
　Enzyme Linked Immunoabsorbent Assay, Mycoplasma SPP.　Microbiology
　Enzyme Linked Immunoabsorbent Assay, Rubella　Microbiology
　Enzyme Linked Immunoabsorbent Assay, Treponema Pallidum　Microbiology
　Epstein-Barr Virus, Other　Microbiology
　Extractable Antinuclear Antibody (Rnp/Sm), Antigen/Control　Immunology
　Reagent, Borrelia, Serological　Microbiology
　System, Test, Anticardiolipin, Immunological　Immunology
　Test, Nuclear Antigen, Epstein-Barr Virus　Microbiology
　Test, Thyroid Autoantibody　Immunology

INNOPHARMA LLC　732-885-2939
10 Knightsbridge Road, Piscataway, NJ 08854
FDA Number: n/a　*Fax:* 732-885-2939
E-mail: info@innopharmallc.com
Web site: http://www.innopharmallc.com
Ownership: Private
Produces/Sells CE-marked Devices: N
General Admin.: Dr. Navneet Puri/Chief Executive Officer
　　Sriram Ramanathan/Chief Operating Officer
　　Dr. Satish Pejaver/Chief Scientific Officer

INNOTECH REHABILITATION PRODUCTS INC.　800-361-0228
P.O. Box 534, Orillia, ONT L3V-6K2 Canada　705-325-8940
FDA Number: n/a　*Fax:* 705-325-8695
E-mail: info@embraceairbackrests.com
Web site: www.embraceairbackrests.com
Year Founded: 1992
Ownership: Private
Produces/Sells CE-marked Devices: N
Distribution: Manufacturer Direct, Exporter

INNOTRON DIAGNOSTICS
　See Oxis International, Inc.

INNOTRON OF OREGON INC.
　See Oxis International, Inc.

INNOVA CORP.　860-728-3210
29 Industrial Rd., New Hartford, CT 06057
FDA Number: n/a　*Fax:* 860-738-6590
E-mail: innova@innovausa.com
Web site: www.innovausa.com
Medical Products Sales Volume: $34,620,000
Annual Revenue: $25-$50 Million
Year Founded: 1998
Total Employees: 10　*Marketing Staff:* 2　*Sales Staff:* 2

INNOVA CORP.　860-728-3210 *(cont'd)*
Ownership: Private
Quality System Registration Information: ISO9001
Produces/Sells CE-marked Devices: N
Federal Procurement Eligibility: Small Business
Distribution: Manufacturer Direct, Manufacturer Through Distributor, Manufacturer Through Manufacturer Reps, OEM
General Admin.: Curt Rutsky/President, Chief Executive Officer
　　Aaron Rutsky/Vice President, General Manager
Production: Mr. Terry Davis/Manager Quality Systems
　Bandage, Adhesive　Surgery
　Bandage, Elastic　General
　Bandage, Gauze　General
　Bandage, Other　General
　Contract Manufacturing　General
　Drape, Surgical　Surgery
　Drape, Surgical, Disposable　Surgery
　Dressing, Foam　General
　Dressing, Gel　General
　Dressing, Non-Adherent　General
　Dressing, Other　General
　Dressing, Permeable, Moisture　General
　Dressing, Universal　General
　Dressing, Wound and Burn, Hydrogel　Surgery
　Dressing, Wound and Burn, Occlusive　Surgery
　Electrode, Electrosurgical, Return (Ground, Dispersive)　Surgery
　Electrode, Gel　Cardiovascular
　Electrode, Neuromuscular Stimulator　Cns/Neurology
　Electrode, Other　General
　Electrode, TENS　Cns/Neurology
　Gel, Electrode, Electrosurgical　Surgery
　Gel, Electrode, TENS　Physical Med

INNOVA MEDICAL OPHTHALMICS INC.　800-461-1200
1430 Birchmount Rd.,　416.615.0185
Toronto, ONT M1P 2 Canada
FDA Number: n/a　*Fax:* 416-631-8272
E-mail: info@innovamed.com
Web site: www.innovamed.com
Year Founded: 1986
Ownership: Private
Produces/Sells CE-marked Devices: N
Distribution: Service Direct, Exclusive Distributor

INNOVACON, INC.　858-535-2030
4106 Sorrento Valley Blvd., San Diego, CA 92121
FDA Number: 3005689981　*Fax:* 858-430-3132
E-mail: info@innovaconinc.com
Web site: www.innovaconinc.com
Ownership: Alere, Inc.
Stock Symbol: IMA
Traded On: AMEX
Produces/Sells CE-marked Devices: N
　Antigen, Streptococcus SPP.　Microbiology
　Campylobacter Pylori　Microbiology
　Enzyme Immunoassay, Amphetamine　Toxicology
　Enzyme Immunoassay, Barbiturate　Toxicology
　Enzyme Immunoassay, Benzodiazepine　Toxicology
　Enzyme Immunoassay, Cannabinoids　Toxicology
　Enzyme Immunoassay, Cocaine And Cocaine Metabolites　Toxicology
　Enzyme Immunoassay, Methadone　Toxicology
　Enzyme Immunoassay, Opiates　Toxicology
　Enzyme Immunoassay, Phencyclidine　Toxicology
　Enzyme Immunoassay, Propoxyphene　Toxicology
　Gas Chromatography, Methamphetamine　Toxicology
　Kit, Pregnancy Test, Over The Counter, HCG　Chemistry
　Radioimmunoassay, Follicle Stimulating Hormone　Chemistry
　Radioimmunoassay, Human Chorionic Gonadotropin　Chemistry
　Radioimmunoassay, Luteinizing Hormone　Chemistry
　Radioimmunoassay, Tricyclic Antidepressant Drugs　Toxicology
　Reagent, Occult Blood　Hematology
　Test, Infectious Mononucleosis　Immunology

INNOVAMED, INC.　801-885-9085
13524 Oakridge Dr., Alpine, UT 84004
FDA Number: 3005844491
　Accessories, Apparel, Surgical　Surgery
　Diathermy, Shortwave, Pulsed　Physical Med

INNOVASIS, INC.　801-261-2236
614 East 3900 South, Salt Lake City, UT 84107
FDA Number: 3004719693
　Appliance, Fixation, Spinal Intervertebral Body　Orthopedics
　Orthosis, Fixation, Pedicle, Spinal　Orthopedics
　Prosthesis, Hip, Cement Restrictor　Orthopedics

INNOVASIVE DEVICES, INC.　800-435-6001
734 Forest St., Marlborough, MA 01752　508-460-8229
FDA Number: n/a　*Fax:* 508-460-6661
Medical Products Sales Volume: $4,500,000

MANUFACTURER PROFILES

INNOVASIVE DEVICES, INC.   800-435-6001 (cont'd)
Annual Revenue: $1-$5 Million
Total Employees: 125
Ownership: Public
Stock Symbol: IDEA
Traded On: NASDAQ
Distribution: Manufacturer Direct
General Admin.: Alan Chervitz/Chief Operating Officer, Executive Vice President
Richard Randall/President, Chief Executive Officer
Mktg./Adv.: Rick Simmons/Vice President Marketing & Sales
Production: Rocky Kahler/Vice President Manufacturing

Electrosurgical Equipment, General Purpose	Surgery
Fastener, Fixation, Non-Biodegradable, Soft Tissue	Orthopedics
Kit, Surgical Instrument, Disposable	Surgery
Laparoscope, General & Plastic Surgery	Surgery
Peritoneoscope	Gastroenterology/Urology
Staple, Fixation, Bone	Orthopedics

INNOVATE MEDICAL, L.L.C.   866-839-7874
2210 Buffalo Road, Johnson City, TN 37604   423-854-9694
FDA Number: 2321034
E-mail: info@innovatemed.com
Web site: www.innovatemed.com
Ownership: Private
Produces/Sells CE-marked Devices: N

Bandage, Elastic	General
Dam, Rubber	Dental And Oral
Exerciser, Non-Measuring	Physical Med
Support, Patient Position	Anesthesiology
Tourniquet, Non-Pneumatic, Surgical	Surgery

INNOVATEK MEDICAL INC.   604-522-8303
#3 - 1600 Derwent Way, Delta, BC V3M 6M5 Canada
FDA Number: n/a   *Fax:* 604-522-8318
E-mail: info@innovatekmed.com
Web site: www.innovatekmed.com
Year Founded: 1990
Total Employees: 25
Ownership: Private
Produces/Sells CE-marked Devices: N
Distribution: Manufacturer Direct, Exclusive Distributor

INNOVATION GENESIS, LLC   617-234-0070
One Canal Park, Cambridge, MA 02141
FDA Number: n/a   *Fax:* 617-354-8304
E-mail: info@productgenesis.com
Web site: www.productgenesis.com
Medical Products Sales Volume: $2,000,000
Year Founded: 1986
Total Employees: 15
Ownership: Private
Produces/Sells CE-marked Devices: N
Federal Procurement Eligibility: Small Business
General Admin.: Mr. Chuck Brunner/Director
Mr. Jeff Hovis/Principal

Contract R&D, Diagnostics	General
Contract R&D, Equipment	General
Service, Design, Implant, Custom	Orthopedics
Service, Engineering/Design	General

INNOVATIONS FOR ACCESS, INC.   800-297-8485
1815 Nw 169th Place,, Suite #6030, Beaverton, OR 97006
FDA Number: 3004202080

Accessories, Blood Circuit, Hemodialysis	Gastroenterology/Urology

INNOVATIVE CHEMISTRY, INC.   781-837-6709
PO Box 578, Marshfield, MA 02050-0090
FDA Number: n/a   *Fax:* 781-834-7325
E-mail: nfpatterson@earthlink.net
Web site: www.innovativechem.com
Medical Products Sales Volume: $400,000
Annual Revenue: $1-$5 Million
Year Founded: 1985
Total Employees: 6
Ownership: Private
Produces/Sells CE-marked Devices: Y
Federal Procurement Eligibility: Small Business
Distribution: Manufacturer Direct, Exporter
General Admin.: James Ziegenmeyer/Chief Executive Officer
Mktg./Adv.: Dr. Nancy Patterson/Director Marketing
Nancy Patterson/Vice President Marketing & Sales

Identification Panel, Blood Cell	Hematology
Reagent, Other	General

INNOVATIVE CHOICES, INC.   315-482-2583
700 Progress Ave, Scarborough M1H 2Z7 Canada
FDA Number: 9615401

Orthosis, Cervical-Thoracic, Rigid	Physical Med

INNOVATIVE CONCEPTS   800-676-5030
300 N. State St., Girard, OH 44420   330-545-6390
FDA Number: n/a   *Fax:* 330-545-6389
E-mail: sales@icrehab.com
Web site: www.icrehab.com
Medical Products Sales Volume: $34,620,000
Annual Revenue: $0-$1 Million
Total Employees: 6   *Marketing Staff:* 2   *Sales Staff:* 2
Ownership: BOARDMAN MEDICAL SUPPLIES
Produces/Sells CE-marked Devices: N
Distribution: Manufacturer Direct
General Admin.: Robert Garwood/General Manager
Sam Savon/President, Chief Executive Officer
Mktg./Adv.: Eric Behnke/Manager National Accounts
Production: Eric Behnke/Manager Operations

Belt, Wheelchair	Physical Med
Support, Head And Trunk, Wheelchair	Physical Med
Tray, Wheelchair	Physical Med

INNOVATIVE DIAGNOSTIC ELECTRNCS OF AMER.
See Idea, Inc.

INNOVATIVE DIAGNOSTIC SYSTEMS, L. P.
See Remel Atlanta, Div. Of Remel, Inc.

INNOVATIVE DISPOSABLES   908-222-7111
3611 Kennedy Rd., South Plainfield, NJ 07080
FDA Number: 3004524293

Linen, Bed	General

INNOVATIVE EXCIMER SOLUTIONS, INC.   416-410-1868
3340a Yonge St, Toronto M4N 2M4 Canada
FDA Number: 8043867

Burr, Corneal, Battery-Powered	Ophthalmology
Speculum, Ophthalmic	Ophthalmology

INNOVATIVE HEALTH CARE PRODUCTS, INC.   678-320-0009
6850 Peachtree-Dunwoody Road, Suite #402, Atlanta, GA 30328
FDA Number: n/a   *Fax:* 678-320-0050
E-mail: info@sunzyme.com
Web site: www.sunzyme.com
Medical Products Sales Volume: $101,100,000
Year Founded: 1991
Total Employees: 2   *Marketing Staff:* 4   *Sales Staff:* 10
Ownership: Private
Produces/Sells CE-marked Devices: N
Federal Procurement Eligibility: Small Business
Distribution: Manufacturer Through Distributor
General Admin.: Mark M. Fowls/President, Chief Executive Officer

Bath, Portable	General
Pad, Pressure, Gel	General
Purifier, Air, Ultraviolet	General
Sanitizer	General
Solution, Ostomy, Odor Control	Gastroenterology/Urology
Sterilizer, Steam (Autoclave)	General
Sterilizer, Steam, Table Top	General
Washer/Sterilizer	General

INNOVATIVE HEALTHCARE PRODUCTS, LLC   231-755-0277
3120 South Getty St., Muskegon, MI 49444
FDA Number: 3003845039
Ownership: Private
Produces/Sells CE-marked Devices: N

Table, Mechanical	Physical Med

INNOVATIVE IMAGING, INC.   800-765-7226
**9940 Business Park Drive, Suite 155,   916-363-0774
Sacramento, CA 95827**
FDA Number: 2950189   *Fax:* 916-363-3815
E-mail: contact@eye-imaging.com
Web site: www.eye-imaging.com
Medical Products Sales Volume: $960,000
Annual Revenue: $1-$5 Million
Year Founded: 1988
Total Employees: 15
Ownership: Private
Produces/Sells CE-marked Devices: Y
Federal Procurement Eligibility: Small Business, Female Owned, GSA Contract, VA Contract
Distribution: Manufacturer Direct
General Admin.: Cynthia Kendall/President, Chief Executive Officer
Research: Rainer Nikel/Director Research & Development

Laboratory Equipment, Ophthalmic	Ophthalmology

INNOVATIVE MACHINERY PACKAGING AND   503-581-3239
CONVERTING INC.
PO Box 535, Salem, OR 97308
FDA Number: 3027939   *Fax:* 503-364-7754

INNOVATIVE MACHINERY PACKAGING AND
503-581-3239
(cont'd)
E-mail: edmiller@impacinc.net
Web site: www.impacinc.net
Medical Products Sales Volume: $350,000
Year Founded: 1982
Total Employees: 4
Ownership: Private
Produces/Sells CE-marked Devices: N
Federal Procurement Eligibility: Small Business

Plunger-Like Joint Manipulator	Physical Med
Vibrator, Therapeutic	Physical Med

INNOVATIVE MED INC.
877-779-9492
4 Autry, Suite B, Irvine, CA 92618
949-458-1897
FDA Number: 300411262
Fax: 949-458-7416
E-mail: info@imibeauty.com
Web site: www.imiimi.com
Medical Products Sales Volume: $1,000,000
Annual Revenue: $1-$5 Million
Year Founded: 1999
Ownership: Private
Produces/Sells CE-marked Devices: N
Federal Procurement Eligibility: Small Business
Distribution: Manufacturer Direct
Mktg./Adv.: Ms. Sonya Khalaj/Vice President Marketing & Advertising

Accessories, Catheter	Surgery
Binder, Abdominal	General
Bottle, Collection, Vacuum (Aspirator)	General
Brush, Dermabrasion	Surgery
Cannula, Surgical, General & Plastic Surgery	Surgery
Dermabrasion Unit	Surgery
Dermatome	Surgery
Guide, Surgical, Instrument	Surgery
Injector, Syringe	General
Light, Fiberoptic, Dental	Dental And Oral
Light, Other	General
Massager, Therapeutic, Manual	Physical Med
Regulator, Pressure, Gas Cylinder	Anesthesiology
Source, Heat, Bleaching, Teeth, Dental	Dental And Oral
Suture, Polypropylene Monofilament	Surgery

INNOVATIVE MEDICAL DESIGNS
317-421-0308
130 West Rampart Rd., Shelbyville, IN 46176
FDA Number: 3005575651

Infusion Stand	General

INNOVATIVE MEDICAL DEVICES, INC.
516-766-3800
3571 Hargale Road, Oceanside, NY 11572
FDA Number: 3006295485

Stylet, Tracheal Tube	Anesthesiology

INNOVATIVE MEDICAL PRODUCTS, INC.
800-467-4944
87 Spring Lane, Plainville Industrial Pk,
860-793-0391
Plainville, CT 06062
FDA Number: 1223419
Fax: 860-793-8975
E-mail: impinc@worldnet.att.net
Web site: www.innovativemedical.com
Year Founded: 1983
Total Employees: 6 *Marketing Staff:* 2 *Sales Staff:* 2
Ownership: Private
Produces/Sells CE-marked Devices: Y
Federal Procurement Eligibility: Small Business
Distribution: Manufacturer Direct, Manufacturer Through Distributor, Manufacturer Through Manufacturer Reps, Exporter
General Admin.: Alan Wasley/Chief Executive Officer
Alan A. Wasley/President
James R. Bailey/Vice President
Mktg./Adv.: James Baiky/Director International & National Sales
James Baiky/Director Marketing
Alan Wasley/Director Product Development
Nancy Wasley/Manager Advertising
James Bailey/Vice President Marketing & Sales
Production: Nancy Wasley/Manager Regulatory Affairs
Alan Wasley/Vice President Manufacturing

Accessories, Operating Room, Table	Surgery
Cushion, Wheelchair (Pad)	Physical Med
Guide, Surgical, Instrument	Surgery
Splint, Abduction, Congenital Hip Dislocation	Physical Med
Stand, Casting	Orthopedics
Support, Patient Position	Anesthesiology
System, X-Ray, Mobile	Radiology
Tray, Surgical Instrument	Surgery

INNOVATIVE MEDICAL PRODUCTS-PJC,LLC
216-961-8735
3510 Chatham Road, Cleveland, OH 44113
FDA Number: 3003967891
Ownership: Private
Produces/Sells CE-marked Devices: N

INNOVATIVE MEDICAL PRODUCTS-PJC,LLC
216-961-8735
(cont'd)

Splint, Extermity, Non-inflatable, External, Non-sterile	Surgery

INNOVATIVE MEDICAL SOLUTIONS, INC.
414-774-7614
N2462 W. Miner Dr., Waupaca, WI 54981
FDA Number: 2134851
Ownership: Private
Produces/Sells CE-marked Devices: N

Image Processing System	Radiology

INNOVATIVE MEDICAL SYSTEMS, INC.
See Sleepnet Corporation

INNOVATIVE MEDICAL TECHNOLOGIES, INC.
866-560-1820
15059 Cedar St., Leawood, KS 66224
913-685-2972
FDA Number: 1933913
Fax: 800-768-2825
E-mail: support@innovativemedtech.com
Web site: innovativemedtech.com
Medical Products Sales Volume: $250,000
Annual Revenue: $0-$1 Million
Year Founded: 1992
Total Employees: 1 *Marketing Staff:* 1 *Sales Staff:* 1
Ownership: Private
Produces/Sells CE-marked Devices: Y
Federal Procurement Eligibility: Small Business
Distribution: Manufacturer Direct, Manufacturer Through Distributor, Importer
General Admin.: Mr. Brad Brown/President, Chief Executive Officer

Tube, Capillary Blood Collection	Hematology

INNOVATIVE MEDICAL VISIONS, INC.
516-766-3800
3571 Hargale Road, Oceanside, NY 11572
FDA Number: 3006413834
Ownership: Private
Produces/Sells CE-marked Devices: N

Stylet, Tracheal Tube	Anesthesiology

INNOVATIVE ORTHOTICS & REHABILITATION, INC.
404-222-9998
13oo Dekalb Ave., Atlanta, GA 30006
FDA Number: 1065995

Orthosis, Lumbosacral	Physical Med

INNOVATIVE PRODUCTS UNLIMITED, INC.
800-833-2826
2120 Industrial Drive, Niles, MI 49120
269-684-5050
FDA Number: 1833497
Fax: 888-757-2826
E-mail: ipu@ipu.com
Web site: www.ipu.com
Medical Products Sales Volume: $15,000,000
Annual Revenue: $10-$25 Million
Year Founded: 1985
Total Employees: 35
Ownership: Private
Produces/Sells CE-marked Devices: N
Federal Procurement Eligibility: Small Business, VA Contract
Distribution: Manufacturer Through Distributor, Exporter
General Admin.: Fritz Heerdt/President
Mktg./Adv.: Bill Becker/Vice President Marketing & Sales
Production: Arthur Fochs/Vice President Manufacturing

Cart, Laundry	General
Cart, Other	General
Chair, Other	General
Chair, Shower	General
Laundry Hamper	General
Stretcher, Wheeled (Mobile)	General
Walker, Mechanical	Physical Med

INNOVATIVE SURGICAL PRODUCTS, INC.
714-836-4474
2761 Walnut Avenue, Tustin, CA 92780
FDA Number: 2022502
Fax: 714-836-3506
E-mail: chris.mazelin@innovativesurgical.com
Web site: www.innovativesurgical.com
Year Founded: 1987
Total Employees: 100
Ownership: Private
Produces/Sells CE-marked Devices: Y
Federal Procurement Eligibility: Small Business
Distribution: Manufacturer Direct, OEM
General Admin.: William Reising/President
Mktg./Adv.: Chris Mazelin/Manager Product Development
Production: An Le/Director Quality Assurance

Contract Assembly	General
Contract Manufacturing	General
Contract Packaging	General
Contract Sterilization	General

INNOVATIVE SWAB TECHNOLOGIES
See Great Midwest Packaging, Llc

INNOVATIVE TECHNOLOGY, INC.   877-462-4415
2 New Pasture Road, Newburyport, MA 01950   **978-462-4415**
FDA Number: n/a   *Fax:* 978-462-3338
E-mail: gloveboxes@gloveboxes.com
Web site: www.gloveboxes.com
Medical Products Sales Volume: $1,100,000
Annual Revenue: $1-$5 Million
Year Founded: 1981
Total Employees: 10   *Marketing Staff:* 1   *Sales Staff:* 1
Ownership: Private
Produces/Sells CE-marked Devices: Y
Federal Procurement Eligibility: Small Business
Distribution: Manufacturer Direct, OEM, Exporter
General Admin.: Glen Cleaver/Vice President, General Manager
  Patient Isolation Chamber   General
  Solvent   Chemistry

INNOVATIVE THERAPIES, INC.   866-484-6798
8-2 Metropolitan Court, Darnestown, MD 20878
FDA Number: 3006367520
  Pump, Aspiration, Portable   Anesthesiology

INNOVATIVE WOUND MANAGEMENT, LLC   866-527-3706
29001 Cedar Rd, Suite 325, Cleveland, OH 44124   **440-461-1295**
FDA Number: 1531173
E-mail: info@laser-seal.net
Web site: www.laser-seal.net
Ownership: Private
Produces/Sells CE-marked Devices: N
  Dressing, Wound and Burn, Occlusive   Surgery
  Dressing, Wound, Occlusive   Surgery

INNOVENTIONS, INC.   800-854-6554
9593 Corsair Dr., Conifer, CO 80433-9317   **303-797-6554**
FDA Number: n/a   *Fax:* 303-727-4940
E-mail: magnicam@magnicam.com
Web site: http://www.magnicam.com
Ownership: Private
Produces/Sells CE-marked Devices: N
  Reading System, Closed-Circuit Television   Ophthalmology

INNOVENTOR, INC.   314-785-0900
3600 Rider Trail South, Bridgeton, MO 63045
FDA Number: 3006058848   *Fax:* 314.785.0044
Ownership: Private
Produces/Sells CE-marked Devices: N
  Treadmill, Powered   Physical Med

INNOVIA LLC   305-378-2651
12415 S.w. 136th Ave., Unit 3, Miami, FL 33186
FDA Number: 3004444223
  Expander, Tissue, Orbital   Ophthalmology

INNOVISION MEDICAL TECHNOLOGIES, LLC   410-694-9450
1302 Concourse Dr., Ste. 302, Linthicum, MD 21090
FDA Number: 3005545408
  Ventilator, Continuous (Respirator), Accessory   Anesthesiology

INNOVISION, INC.   402-558-3000
3125 South 61st Ave., Omaha, NE 68106
FDA Number: 1933291
  Lens, Contact (Other Material)   Ophthalmology

INNTEC, INC.   608-742-1188
401 E. Edgewater St., Portage, WI 53901
FDA Number: 98958
Ownership: Private
Produces/Sells CE-marked Devices: N
  Catheter, Assisted Reproduction   Obstetrics/Gynecology
  Needle, Assisted Reproduction   Obstetrics/Gynecology

INOCRAFT, INC.   678-985-2926
478 Northdale Rd. Nw, Suite 706, Lawrenceville, GA 30045
FDA Number: 1055891
  Illuminator, Radiographic Film   Radiology

INOGEN, INC.   805-562-0500
326 Bollay Drive, Goleta, CA 93117
FDA Number: 3004672275
  Generator, Oxygen, Portable   Anesthesiology

INOTECH BIOSYSTEMS INTERNATIONAL, INC.   800-635-4070
15713 Crabbs Branch Way, #110,   **301-670-2850**
Rockville, MD 20855
FDA Number: 1832416   *Fax:* 301-670-2859
E-mail: inotech@inotechintl.com
Web site: www.inotechintl.com
Medical Products Sales Volume: $100,000
Annual Revenue: $0-$1 Million

INOTECH BIOSYSTEMS INTERNATIONAL, INC.   800-635-4070
(cont'd)
Year Founded: 1987
Total Employees: 4   *Marketing Staff:* 1   *Sales Staff:* 1
Ownership: Private
Stock Symbol: ABI
Traded On: NYSE
Produces/Sells CE-marked Devices: Y
Federal Procurement Eligibility: Small Business
Distribution: Exclusive Distributor
Mktg./Adv.: David Mines/Manager National Sales
  Encapsulator, Fluid   General
  Extractor, Plasma   Hematology

INOVA DIAGNOSTICS, INC.   800-545-9495
9900 Old Grove Rd, San Diego, CA 92131-1638   **858-586-9900**
FDA Number: 2026994   *Fax:* 858-586-9911
E-mail: info@inovadx.com
Web site: www.inovadx.com
Annual Revenue: $10-$25 Million
Year Founded: 1987
Ownership: Private
Produces/Sells CE-marked Devices: N
Federal Procurement Eligibility: Small Business
Distribution: Manufacturer Direct
  Antibody, Anti-Smooth Muscle, Indirect Immunofluorescent   Immunology
  Antibody, Antimitochondrial, Indirect Immunofluorescent   Immunology
  Antibody, Antinuclear, Indirect Immunofluorescent, Antigen   Immunology
  Antigen, Antiserum, Control, IGE   Immunology
  Antinuclear Antibody, Antigen, Control   Immunology
  Antiparietal Antibody, Immunofluorescent, Antigen, Control   Immunology
  Extractable Antinuclear Antibody (Rnp/Sm), Antigen/Control   Immunology
  Strip, Test   Chemistry
  System, Test, Anticardiolipin, Immunological   Immunology
  Test, Systemic Lupus Erythematosus   Immunology
  Test, Thyroid Autoantibody   Immunology
  Thyroglobulin, Antigen, Antiserum, Control   Immunology

INOVA LABS   800-220-9977
3500 Comsouth Rd, Suite 100, Austin, TX 78744   **512-814-0063**
FDA Number: 3008185181
E-mail: info@lifechoiceoxygen.com
Web site: www.lifechoiceoxygen.com
Ownership: Private
Produces/Sells CE-marked Devices: N
  Generator, Oxygen, Portable   Anesthesiology

INOVAR, INC.   866-898-4949
1073 West 1700 North, Logan, UT 84321   **435-792-4949**
FDA Number: 3003743956   *Fax:* 435-792-4950
E-mail: sales@inovar-inc.com
Web site: www.inovar-inc.com/
Ownership: Private
Produces/Sells CE-marked Devices: N
  Analyzer, Chemistry, Micro   Chemistry
  Stimulator, Nerve, Transcutaneous (Pain Relief, TENS)   Cns/Neurology

INOVEL LLC   866-546-6835
10111 W. Jefferson Blvd., Culver City, CA 90232
FDA Number: 3004785874
  Respirator, Surgical, Combination Product   General

INOVEON CORP.   405-271-9025
800 North Research Pkwy., Suite 370,
Oklahoma City, OK 73104
FDA Number: 1651093
  Device, Communications, Images, Ophthalmic   Ophthalmology

INOVISE MEDICAL, INC.   503-431-3800
10565 Sw Nimbus Ave., Suite 100, Portland, OR 97223
FDA Number: 3033850
  Electrocardiograph, Ambulatory(without Analysis)   Cardiovascular
  Electrocardiograph, Single Channel   Cardiovascular
  Electrode, Electrocardiograph   Cardiovascular
  Stethoscope, Electronic (Auscultoscope)   Cardiovascular

INOVO, INC.   239-643-6577
2975 S. Horseshoe Drive, Suite 600, Naples, FL 34104
FDA Number: 1062191
  Canister, Liquid Oxygen, Portable   Anesthesiology
  Conserver, Oxygen   Anesthesiology
  Regulator, Pressure, Gas Cylinder   Anesthesiology

INPRO CORPORATION   800-222-5556
S80 W18766 Apollo Drive, Muskego, WI 53150   **262-679-5521**
FDA Number: n/a   *Fax:* 888-715-8407
E-mail: service@inprocorp.com
Web site: www.inprocorp.com
Medical Products Sales Volume: $66,000,000

INPRO CORPORATION 800-222-5556 (cont'd)
Annual Revenue: $25-$50 Million
Year Founded: 1979
Total Employees: 340   *Marketing Staff:* 12   *Sales Staff:* 60
Ownership: Private
Quality System Registration Information: ISO9001
Produces/Sells CE-marked Devices: N
Federal Procurement Eligibility: Small Business
Distribution: Manufacturer Direct, Manufacturer Through Distributor, Exporter
General Admin.: Steve Ziegler/President, Chief Executive Officer
Laurie O'Laughlin/Vice President Human Resources
Mktg./Adv.: Jennifer Moreau/Marketing Communications Specialist
Larry Dronek/Vice President Marketing
Phil Ziegler/Vice President Sales
Production: Glenn Kennedy/Vice President Manufacturing
Research: Matt Bennett/Vice President Research & Development
Rail, Wall Side   General

INRAD 800-558-4647
4375 Donker Court S.E., Kentwood, MI 49512   616-301-7800
FDA Number: 1835568   *Fax:* 616-301-7799
E-mail: inrad-inc@inrad-inc.com
Web site: http://inrad-inc.com/
Medical Products Sales Volume: $810,000
Annual Revenue: $5-$10 Million
Year Founded: 1981
Total Employees: 10
Ownership: Private
Quality System Registration Information: ISO9001
Produces/Sells CE-marked Devices: Y
Federal Procurement Eligibility: Small Business
Distribution: Manufacturer Direct, Manufacturer Through Distributor, Manufacturer Through Manufacturer Reps, OEM, Importer, Exporter
General Admin.: Diane Lambrix/Office Manager
Steve Field/President
Mktg./Adv.: Patrick Smiggen/Manager Marketing & Sales
Biopsy Instrument   Gastroenterology/Urology
Biopsy Instrument, Mechanical, Gastrointestinal   Gastroenterology/Urology
Guide, Surgical, Instrument   Surgery
Guide, Surgical, Needle   Surgery
Holder, Syringe, Leaded   Radiology
Introducer, Catheter   Cardiovascular
Introducer, Syringe Needle   General
Kit, Surgical Instrument, Disposable   Surgery
Needle, Aspiration And Injection, Disposable   Surgery
Staple, Implantable   Surgery
Transfer Unit, IV Fluid   General

INREACH CORPORATION 888-517-3224
2017 Cardinal Circle, Anderson, SC 29621-1503
FDA Number: 1067144
Ownership: Private
Produces/Sells CE-marked Devices: N
Software, Blood Bank (Stand-Alone Products)   Hematology

INRO MEDICAL DESIGNS, INC. 800-527-1093
P.O. Box 9, De Soto, TX 75115   972-296-3224
FDA Number: n/a   *Fax:* 972-296-3575
Web site: www.inro.com
Annual Revenue: $0-$1 Million
Ownership: Private
Produces/Sells CE-marked Devices: N
Federal Procurement Eligibility: Small Business
Distribution: Manufacturer Direct
Prosthesis, Nail   Surgery

INSIGHT BIODESIGN LLC 775-250-0267
1065 Waverly Drive, Reno, NV 89519
FDA Number: 3006074149
Ownership: Private
Produces/Sells CE-marked Devices: N
Holder, Catheter   Gastroenterology/Urology
Urological Irrigation System   Gastroenterology/Urology

INSIGHT INSTRUMENTS, INC. 800-255-8354
2580 S.E. Willoughby Blvd., Stuart, FL 34994   772-219-9393
FDA Number: 1052234   *Fax:* 772-219-9342
Web site: www.insightinstruments.com
Annual Revenue: $1-$5 Million
Ownership: Private
Produces/Sells CE-marked Devices: N
Federal Procurement Eligibility: Small Business
Distribution: Manufacturer Direct, Manufacturer Through Distributor, Manufacturer Through Manufacturer Reps, Exclusive Distributor, Importer
Cannula, Ophthalmic   Ophthalmology
Endoscope, Ophthalmic   Gastroenterology/Urology
Forceps, Ophthalmic   Ophthalmology
Irrigator, Ocular Surgery   Ophthalmology

INSIGHT INSTRUMENTS, INC. 800-255-8354 (cont'd)
Lens, Condensing, Diagnostic   Ophthalmology
Lens, Contact, Polymethacrylate   Ophthalmology
Lens, Other   Ophthalmology
Loupe, Diagnostic/Surgical   Surgery
Microscope, Surgical   Ear/Nose/Throat
Probe   Orthopedics
Punch, Corneo-Scleral   Ophthalmology

INSIGHT MEDICAL PRODUCTS, LLC 561-742-3650
710 Ne 7th St. Bld# 403, Boynton Beach, FL 33435-3930
FDA Number: 3003768894
Ownership: Private
Produces/Sells CE-marked Devices: N
Fixation Device, Tracheal Tube   Anesthesiology

INSIPHIL (US) LLC 408-616-8700
650 Vaqueros Avenue, Suite F, Sunnyvale, CA 94085-3533
FDA Number: 2916582   *Fax:* 408-616-8720
E-mail: info@insiphil.com
Web site: www.telesensory.com
Medical Products Sales Volume: $8,700,000
Annual Revenue: $10-$25 Million
Year Founded: 1970
Total Employees: 92
Ownership: Private
Federal Procurement Eligibility: Small Business
Distribution: Manufacturer Through Distributor
General Admin.: Patty Regalado/Director Human Resources
Edward Long/President, Chief Executive Officer
Mktg./Adv.: Art Bookbinder/Director National Sales
Marc Stenzel/Vice President Sales
Production: Barbara Sorensen/Director Materials
Larry Meyer/Vice President Operations
Research: Timothy Couture/Vice President Product Development
Communication System, Non-Powered   Physical Med
Communication System, Powered   Physical Med
Computer Equipment   General
Reading System, Closed-Circuit Television   Ophthalmology
Tactile Hearing-Aid   Ear/Nose/Throat
Telephone, Handicapped Use   Physical Med
Vision Aid, Image Intensification, Battery-Powered   Ophthalmology

INSITE CLINICAL TRIALS
See Unitedhealthcare

INSITE CLINICAL TRIALS/KERN MCNEILL INTERNATIONAL
See Unitedhealthcare

INSITE ONE, INC. 800-441-0091
135 North Plains Industrial Rd,   203-265-6111
Wallingford, CT 06492
FDA Number: 1226580   *Fax:* 203-265-1144
Web site: www.insiteone.com
Year Founded: 1999
Ownership: Private
Produces/Sells CE-marked Devices: N
General Admin.: Henry Schaffer/Chief Financial Officer, Executive Vice President
Paul Dandrow/Chief Operating Officer, Executive Vice President
Jim Champagne/President, Chief Executive Officer
Device, Storage, Image, Digital   Radiology

INSITU TECHNOLOGIES, INC. 651-389-1017
539 Phalen Blvd., St. Paul, MN 55130
FDA Number: 2134244   *Fax:* 651-305-1089
E-mail: sales@insitu-tech.com
Web site: www.insitu-tech.com
Ownership: Private
Produces/Sells CE-marked Devices: N
Angiography/angioplasty Kit   Cardiovascular
Cannula, Catheter   Cardiovascular
Catheter, Angioplasty, Coronary, Transluminal, Percut. Oper.   Cardiovascular
Catheter, Angioplasty, Transluminal, Peripheral   Cardiovascular
Catheter, Intravascular, Diagnostic   Cardiovascular
Endoscope, Fiberoptic   Surgery
Guidewire, Catheter   Cardiovascular
Guidewire, Catheter, Reprocessed   Cardiovascular
Light, Fiberoptic, Dental   Dental And Oral
Stent, Cardiovascular   Cardiovascular
Stent, Coronary, Drug-eluting   Cardiovascular
Tube, Gastrointestinal   Gastroenterology/Urology

INSOUND MEDICAL INC. 510-792-4000
39660 Eureka Drive, Newark, CA 94560
FDA Number: 3003793405
Hearing-Aid   Ear/Nose/Throat

INSOURCE, INC. 800-366-3829
PO Box 9, Bastian, VA 24314   540-688-4121
FDA Number: n/a   *Fax:* 800-869-8895
E-mail: customersfirst@insourceonline.com

INSOURCE, INC.
800-366-3829 *(cont'd)*
Web site: www.insourceonline.com
Medical Products Sales Volume: $1,500,000
Year Founded: 1991
Total Employees: 12
Ownership: American Greetings
Stock Symbol: HSIC
Produces/Sells CE-marked Devices: N
Federal Procurement Eligibility: Small Business
General Admin.: James Short/Vice President, General Manager
Mktg./Adv.: Kim Crabtree/Director Marketing
    Gary Blankenship/Manager Business
Finance: Leslie Wellman/Director Finance
    Delivery System, Allergen And Vaccine   General

INSOURCE/WILLIAMS, INC.
See Insource, Inc.

INSPIRE MEDICAL SYSTEMS
763-205-7970
9700 63rd Avenue North, Suite 200, Maple Grove, MN 55369
FDA Number: n/a   *Fax:* 763-537-4310
E-mail: info@inspiresleep.com
Web site: http://www.inspiresleep.com
Year Founded: 1994
Ownership: Private
Produces/Sells CE-marked Devices: N
General Admin.: Mr. Tim Herbert/President, Chief Executive Officer
Production: Mr. Randy Ban/Senior Vice President Operations
Research: Mr. Mark Christopherson/Vice President Product Development
    Mr. Quan Ni/Vice President Research

INSPIRE PHARMACEUTICALS, INC.
919-941-9777
8081 Arco Corporate Drive,, Suite 400, Raleigh, NC 27617
FDA Number: n/a   *Fax:* 919-941-9797
E-mail: info@inspirepharm.com
Web site: www.inspirepharm.com
Ownership: Public
Produces/Sells CE-marked Devices: N
Distribution: Service Direct
General Admin.: Christy Shaffer/President, Chief Executive Officer
Production: Mary Bennett/Vice President Operations
    Airway, Esophageal (Obturator)   Anesthesiology
    Contract R&D, Diagnostics   General

INSPIRED TECHNOLOGIES INC
724-861-5510
1061 Main Street, #24, North Huntingdon, PA 15642
FDA Number: 3006791269
E-mail: info@inspiredtechnologiesinc.com
Ownership: Private
Produces/Sells CE-marked Devices: N
    Generator, Oxygen, Portable   Anesthesiology
    Recorder, Ventilatory Effort   Anesthesiology

INSTACOOL, INC.
See Thermogenesis Corp.

INSTANT SYSTEMS, INC.
757-200-5494
965 Denison Avenue, Norfolk, VA 23513
FDA Number: 3004096738   *Fax:* 757-200-5711
E-mail: info@instantsystems.com
Web site: www.instantsystems.com
Ownership: Private
Produces/Sells CE-marked Devices: N
    Container, Frozen Donor Tissue Storage   General

INSTANTEL INC.
800-267-9111
309 Legget Dr., Kanata, ON K2K 3A3 Canada
613-592-4642
FDA Number: n/a   *Fax:* 613-592-4296
E-mail: info@instantel.com
Web site: www.instantel.com
Year Founded: 1982
Total Employees: 70
Ownership: Private
Quality System Registration Information: ISO9001
Produces/Sells CE-marked Devices: N
Federal Procurement Eligibility: Small Business
Distribution: Manufacturer Through Distributor, Exporter

INSTANTRON
401-433-6800
3712 Pawtucket Ave., Riverside, RI 02915
FDA Number: 1211132
    Epilator, High-Frequency, Needle-Type   Surgery

INSTITUTIONAL PRODUCTS CORP.
See Inpro Corporation

INSTRATEK, INC.
281-890-8020
210 Spring Hill Drive, Suite 130, Spring, TX 77386
FDA Number: 1645311   *Fax:* 281-890-8068
E-mail: manny@instratek.com

INSTRATEK, INC.
281-890-8020 *(cont'd)*
Web site: www.instratek.com
Medical Products Sales Volume: $3,200,000
Annual Revenue: $1-$5 Million
Year Founded: 1993
Total Employees: 10   *Marketing Staff:* 2   *Sales Staff:* 2
Ownership: Private
Quality System Registration Information: ISO9001
Produces/Sells CE-marked Devices: Y
Federal Procurement Eligibility: Small Business, VA Contract
Distribution: Manufacturer Direct, Exporter
General Admin.: Mrs. Leigh Wagner/Compliance Officer
    Manny Guyot/Vice President

Arthroscope	Orthopedics
Endoscope	Gastroenterology/Urology
Instrument, Manual, General Surgical	Surgery
Screw, Fixation, Bone	Orthopedics

INSTROMEDIX, A CARD GUARD CO.
800-633-3361
10255 West Higgins Road, Suite 100,
847-720-2295
Rosemont, IL 60018
FDA Number: n/a   *Fax:* 800-954-2375
E-mail: webmaster@instromedix.com
Web site: www.instromedix.com
Annual Revenue: $10-$25 Million
Year Founded: 1969
Total Employees: 40   *Marketing Staff:* 1   *Sales Staff:* 12
Ownership: GOODFELLOW CAMBRIDGE LIMITED
Traded On: Switzerland
Quality System Registration Information: ISO9001
Produces/Sells CE-marked Devices: N
Federal Procurement Eligibility: Small Business, GSA Contract
Distribution: Manufacturer Direct, Manufacturer Through Distributor, Manufacturer Through Manufacturer Reps, OEM
General Admin.: Robert White/President, Chief Executive Officer

Analyzer, Pacemaker Generator Function, Indirect	Cardiovascular
Computer Software	General
Electrocardiograph, Single Channel	Cardiovascular
Electrode, Electrocardiograph	Cardiovascular
Magnet, Test, Pacemaker	Cardiovascular
Monitor, ECG, Arrhythmia	Cardiovascular
Monitor, Heart Rate, R-Wave (ECG)	Cardiovascular
Recorder, Long-Term, Blood Pressure, Portable	Cardiovascular
Recorder, Long-Term, ECG	Cardiovascular
Transmitter/Receiver System, ECG, Telephone Single-Channel	Cardiovascular
Transmitter/Receiver System, Physiological, Telephone	Cardiovascular

INSTROMEDIX, INC.
See Instromedix, A Card Guard Co.

INSTRU-MED, CO.
404-252-6188
5775 Glenridge Drive, East Building Suite 360,
Atlanta, GA 30328
FDA Number: 1063670   *Fax:* 404-252-5653
E-mail: info@instrumed.com
Web site: www.instrumed.com
Medical Products Sales Volume: $1,100,000
Annual Revenue: $5-$10 Million
Year Founded: 1982
Total Employees: 8   *Marketing Staff:* 15   *Sales Staff:* 15
Ownership: Private
Produces/Sells CE-marked Devices: N
Federal Procurement Eligibility: Small Business
Distribution: Manufacturer Through Distributor, Exclusive Distributor
General Admin.: Mario Oves/President, Chief Executive Officer
Mktg./Adv.: Carolina Hoyos/Manager Advertising Sales
    Juan P. Zuluaga/Manager International Marketing & Sales
IS: Henry Patino/Web Master
    Service, Used Equipment   General

INSTRUMED OEM
800-368-1301
2801 S. Vallejo St., Englewood, CO 80110
303-761-2801
FDA Number: 1721185   *Fax:* 303-762-8213
E-mail: service@instrumedeom.com
Web site: www.instrumedoem.com
Medical Products Sales Volume: $6,000,000
Annual Revenue: $10-$25 Million
Total Employees: 56   *Marketing Staff:* 3   *Sales Staff:* 7
Ownership: Private
Produces/Sells CE-marked Devices: Y
Federal Procurement Eligibility: Small Business, GSA Contract
Distribution: Manufacturer Direct, Manufacturer Through Manufacturer Reps
General Admin.: Peter J. Niedecker/Chief Executive Officer
Mktg./Adv.: Thomas K. Richey/Director Marketing
Production: James R. Chambers/Director Engineering
    Robert L. Brown/Manager Operations
    Jerry Bauman/Manager Regulatory Affairs
    Coagulator, Laparoscopic, Unipolar   Obstetrics/Gynecology

INSTRUMED OEM
800-368-1301 *(cont'd)*

Coagulator/Cutter, Endoscopic, Unipolar	Obstetrics/Gynecology
Electrode, Electrosurgical, Active (Blade)	Surgery

INSTRUMED SURGICAL
800-667-5653
2180 Dunwin Dr., Units 5 & 6, **905-820-0902**
Mississauga, ONT L5L 5 Canada
FDA Number: n/a *Fax:* 905-820-0983
E-mail: instramedsurgical@on.aibn.com
Web site: www.instrumedsurgical.com
Year Founded: 1978
Total Employees: 10
Ownership: Private
Produces/Sells CE-marked Devices: N
Distribution: Exclusive Distributor

INSTRUMENT SPECIALISTS, INC.
800-537-1945
32390 IH-10 West, Boerne, TX 78006
FDA Number: 1642835 *Fax:* 830-249- 9433
E-mail: isi@isisurgery.com
Web site: www.isisurgery.com
Medical Products Sales Volume: $2,000,000
Annual Revenue: $1-$5 Million
Year Founded: 1978
Ownership: Private
Quality System Registration Information: ISO9001
Produces/Sells CE-marked Devices: N
Federal Procurement Eligibility: Small Business, Female Owned
Distribution: Manufacturer Direct

Accessories, Traction	Physical Med
Brush, Other	General
Immobilizer, Wrist/Hand	Orthopedics
Infusion Stand	General
Service, Maintenance/Repair	General
Solution, Instrument Cleaner	General
Support, Patient Position	Anesthesiology
Table, Other	General
Table, Surgical, Orthopedic	Orthopedics

INSTRUMENT TECHNOLOGY, INC.
413-562-3606
33 Airport Rd., Westfield, MA 01085
FDA Number: n/a *Fax:* 413-568-9809
E-mail: phils@scopes.com
Web site: www.scopes.com
Annual Revenue: $10-$25 Million
Year Founded: 1967
Total Employees: 52 *Sales Staff:* 6
Ownership: Private
Produces/Sells CE-marked Devices: N
Federal Procurement Eligibility: Small Business, GSA Contract
Distribution: Manufacturer Through Manufacturer Reps, OEM
General Admin.: Mr. Gregory K. Carignan/President
Mktg./Adv.: Mr. Philip Samson/Product & Sales Manager

Contract Manufacturing	General
Endoscope	Gastroenterology/Urology
Endoscope, Direct Vision	Surgery
Endoscope, Electronic (Videoendoscope)	Surgery
Endoscope, Fiberoptic	Surgery
Endoscope, Flexible	Gastroenterology/Urology
Endoscope, Rigid	Surgery

INSTRUMENTARIUM IMAGING, INC.
800-558-6120
1245 W. Canal St., Milwaukee, WI 53233 **414-747-1030**
FDA Number: 1219099 *Fax:* 414-481-8665
E-mail: usainfo@instrudental.com
Web site: www.instrumentariumdental.Aùcomusa
Medical Products Sales Volume: $11,600,000
Annual Revenue: $10-$25 Million
Year Founded: 1989
Total Employees: 75 *Marketing Staff:* 2 *Sales Staff:* 25
Ownership: Ge Medical Systems Information Technologies
Stock Symbol: INMRY
Traded On: NASDAQ
Quality System Registration Information: ISO9002
Produces/Sells CE-marked Devices: Y
Federal Procurement Eligibility: Small Business
Distribution: Manufacturer Direct, Manufacturer Through Distributor, Importer
General Admin.: Mike Palazzola/President
Vicki Lemberger/Vice President Human Resources
Mktg./Adv.: John Rater/Admin. Sales
Chris Rohde/Director Marketing
Max Lindert/Director Product Development
Don Blomatrom/Manager National Sales

Radiographic Unit, Diagnostic, Dental (X-Ray)	Dental And Oral
Radiographic Unit, Diagnostic, Dental, Extraoral	Dental And Oral
Radiographic Unit, Diagnostic, Mammographic	Radiology

INSTRUMENTARIUM INC.
800-361-1502
1273 St-Louis St., **450-471-1379**
Terrebonne, QUE J6W-3 Canada
FDA Number: n/a *Fax:* 450-471-1030
E-mail: info@instrumentarium-online.com
Web site: instrumentarium-online.com
Year Founded: 1977
Total Employees: 50
Ownership: Private
Produces/Sells CE-marked Devices: N
Distribution: Manufacturer Direct, Exclusive Distributor, Importer

INSTRUMENTATION & CONTROL SYS.
See Gn Otometrics

INSTRUMENTATION FOR MEDICINE, INC.
203-637-8377
31 Macarthur Dr., Old Greenwich, CT 06870
FDA Number: 1217914
Ownership: Private
Produces/Sells CE-marked Devices: N

Plethysmograph, Impedance	Cardiovascular

INSTRUMENTATION INDUSTRIES, INC.
800-633-8577
2990 Industrial Blvd., **412-854-1133**
Bethel Park, PA 15102
FDA Number: 2518436 *Fax:* 412-854-5668
E-mail: iiimed@iiirespiratory.com
Web site: www.iiiMedical.com
Medical Products Sales Volume: $2,300,000
Annual Revenue: $1-$5 Million
Year Founded: 1967
Total Employees: 32 *Marketing Staff:* 1 *Sales Staff:* 1
Ownership: Private
Quality System Registration Information: ISO9003
Produces/Sells CE-marked Devices: N
Federal Procurement Eligibility: Small Business
Distribution: Manufacturer Direct, Manufacturer Through Distributor, OEM
General Admin.: Edward Horey/Chief Executive Officer
Mktg./Adv.: Lawrence Slattery/Director Marketing & Advertising
Lawrence Slattery/Director National Accounts
Steven Reiner/Director Product Development
Production: Ms. Doris Walter/Director Quality Assurance & Regulatory Affairs
Finance: Robert Ralph/Controller

Adapter, Anesthesia	Anesthesiology
Adapter, Tube, Tracheal	Anesthesiology
Attachment, Breathing, Positive End Expiratory Pressure	Anesthesiology
Attachment, Intermittent Mandatory Ventilation (IMV)	Anesthesiology
Bag, Breathing	Anesthesiology
Bottle, Blow (Exerciser)	Anesthesiology
Changer, Tube, Endotracheal	Anesthesiology
Circuit, Breathing (W Connector, Adapter, Y Piece)	Anesthesiology
Circuit, Breathing, Ventilator	Anesthesiology
Clip, Nose	Anesthesiology
Component, Exercise	Physical Med
Connector, Airway (Extension)	Anesthesiology
Drain, Tee (Water Trap)	Anesthesiology
Kit, Cricothyrotomy	Anesthesiology
Laryngoscope, Rigid	Anesthesiology
Monitor, Airway Pressure (Gauge/Alarm)	Anesthesiology
Monitor, Airway Pressure (Inspiratory Force)	Anesthesiology
Needle, Emergency Airway	Anesthesiology
Support, Breathing Tube	Anesthesiology
Tubing, Flexible, Medical Gas, Low-Pressure	Anesthesiology
Valve, Non-Rebreathing	Anesthesiology
Ventilator, Emergency, Powered (Resuscitator)	Anesthesiology

INSTRUMENTATION LABORATORY COMPANY
800-955-9525
180 Hartwell Road, Bedford, MA 02421 **781-861-0710**
FDA Number: 1217183 *Fax:* 781-861-1908
E-mail: customerservice@ilww.com
Web site: www.ilus.com
Medical Products Sales Volume: $50,400,000
Year Founded: 1959
Ownership: C. H. WERFEN
Produces/Sells CE-marked Devices: N
Federal Procurement Eligibility: Small Business
Distribution: Manufacturer Direct
General Admin.: Mr. Ramon Benet/Chief Executive Officer

Analyzer, Blood Gas pH	Anesthesiology
Analyzer, Chemistry, Electrolyte	Chemistry
Analyzer, Coagulation, Automated	Hematology
Analyzer, Coagulation, Whole Blood	Hematology
Co-Oximeter	Hematology
Electrode, Ion Specific, Potassium	Chemistry
Electrode, Ion Specific, Sodium	Chemistry
Photometer, Flame, Lithium, Toxicology	Toxicology
Standard, Fibrinogen	Toxicology
Test, Systemic Lupus Erythematosus	Immunology

INSTRUMENTATION LABORATORY COMPANY   800-955-9525
(cont'd)

Timer, Coagulation, Automated	Hematology

INSTRUMENTS S.A. INC./JOBIN YVON/SPEX
See Horiba Jobin Yvon Inc

INSULET CORPORATION   800-591-3455
9 Oak Park Dr., Bedford, MA 01730   **781-457-5098**
FDA Number: 3004464228   *Fax:* 781-457-5011
E-mail: international@insulet.com
Web site: www.myomnipod.com
Year Founded: 2000
Ownership: Public
Stock Symbol: PODD
Traded On: NASDAQ
Produces/Sells CE-marked Devices: N
General Admin.: Luis J. Malave/Chief Operating Officer
    Duane DeSisto/President, Chief Executive Officer
Finance: Brian K. Roberts/Chief Financial Officer

Glucose Dehydrogenase, Glucose	Chemistry
Infusion Pump, Insulin	General

INTARSIA LTD.   203-355-1357
14 Martha Ln., Gaylordsville, CT 06755
FDA Number: 1221552
Ownership: Private
Produces/Sells CE-marked Devices: N

Accessories, Wheelchair	Physical Med
Belt, Wheelchair	Physical Med
Chair, Adjustable, Mechanical	Physical Med
Cushion, Wheelchair (Pad)	Physical Med
Support, Head And Trunk, Wheelchair	Physical Med
Transfer Device, Patient, Manual	General
Tray, Wheelchair	Physical Med

INTEC INDUSTRIES, INC.   205-251-5600
2024 12th Avenue N., Birmingham, AL 35234
FDA Number: 1057495   *Fax:* 205-251-5699
E-mail: jsandel@intecind.com
Web site: http://intecind.com/
Medical Products Sales Volume: $2,000,000
Annual Revenue: $1-$5 Million
Year Founded: 1994
Total Employees: 10   *Marketing Staff:* 1   *Sales Staff:* 1
Ownership: Private
Produces/Sells CE-marked Devices: Y
Federal Procurement Eligibility: Small Business
Distribution: Manufacturer Direct, Manufacturer Through Distributor, OEM
General Admin.: Frank Lee/President, Chief Executive Officer

Eyeglasses, Safety	Ophthalmology
Mask, Face	General
Mask, Surgical	Surgery
Shield, Protective, Personnel	Radiology

INTEGRA BIOTECHNICAL LLC   760-597-9878
2755 Dos Aarons Way, Suite B, Vista, CA 92081
FDA Number: 2030116   *Fax:* 760-597-9879
Web site: www.integrabio.com
Ownership: Private
Stock Symbol: IART
Traded On: NASDAQ
Produces/Sells CE-marked Devices: Y
Federal Procurement Eligibility: Small Business
Distribution: OEM

Kit, Administration, Intravenous	General
Kit, Intravenous Extension Tubing	General

INTEGRA ENVIRONMENTAL INC.   800-661-6678
5035 n. Service Rd., Unit C7,   **905-336-2096**
Burlington, ONT L7L-5 Canada
FDA Number: n/a   *Fax:* 888-336-8694
Year Founded: 1983
Total Employees: 25
Ownership: Private
Produces/Sells CE-marked Devices: N
Distribution: Exclusive Distributor

INTEGRA LIFE   1-800-654-2873
311 Enterprise Drive, Plainsboro, NJ 08536   **609-275-0500**
FDA Number: 1121308   *Fax:* 609-799-3297
E-mail: custsvcnj@integralife.com
Web site: http://integralife.com
Ownership: Private
Produces/Sells CE-marked Devices: N
General Admin.: Mr. Stuart Essig/Chief Executive Officer
    Mr. Simon Archibald/Chief Scientific Officer
    Mr. Kevin Breeden/Senior Vice President
Mktg./Adv.: Mr. Jerry Corbin/Vice President Corporate Accounts

INTEGRA LIFE   1-800-654-2873 *(cont'd)*
Finance: Mr. John Henneman III/Executive Vice President Finance
    Mr. Peter Arduini/President
    Mr. John Bostjancic/Senior Vice President Finance
    Ms. Nora Brennan/Vice President Treasury

Accessories, Catheter	Surgery
Agent, Hemostatic, Absorbable, Collagen-Based	Surgery
Beads, Hydrophilic, Wound Exudate Absorption	Surgery
Cuff, Nerve	Cns/Neurology
Dura-Substitute	Cns/Neurology
Material, Dressing, Surgical, Acid, Polylactic	Dental And Oral
Mesh, Surgical, Polymeric	Surgery

INTEGRA LIFESCIENCES CORP.   609-275-0500
311 Enterprise Drive, Plainsboro, NJ 08536
FDA Number: 3003418325   *Fax:* 609-275-5363
E-mail: custsvcnj@integra-ls.com
Web site: www.integra-ls.com
Ownership: Private
Produces/Sells CE-marked Devices: N

Accessories, Pump, Infusion	General
Cabinet, Table And Tray, Anesthesia	Anesthesiology
Dispenser, Cement	Orthopedics
Dressing, Wound, Occlusive	Surgery
Introducer, Catheter	Cardiovascular
Needle, Aspiration And Injection, Disposable	Surgery
Needle, Aspiration And Injection, Reusable	Surgery
Pump, Infusion, Patient Controlled Analgesia (PCA)	General
Syringe, Piston	General
Tubing, Fluid Delivery	General

INTEGRA LIFESCIENCES CORP.   801-886-9505
3395 West 1820 South, Salt Lake City, UT 84104
FDA Number: 1722447
Ownership: Integra Lifesciences Holdings Corp.
Stock Symbol: IART
Traded On: NASDAQ
Produces/Sells CE-marked Devices: N
General Admin.: Brian Baker/President

Kit, Anesthesia, Conduction	Anesthesiology
Syringe, Piston	General

INTEGRA LIFESCIENCES CORPORATION
See Integra Lifesciences Holdings Corp.

INTEGRA LIFESCIENCES CORPORATION   800-654-2873
311 Enterprise Drive, Plainsboro, NJ 08536   **609-275-0500**
FDA Number: 1121308   *Fax:* 609-799-3297
E-mail: custsvcnj@integralife.com
Web site: www.integra-ls.com
Medical Products Sales Volume: $8,400,000
Annual Revenue: $10-$25 Million
Total Employees: 150   *Marketing Staff:* 8   *Sales Staff:* 8
Ownership: Integra Lifesciences Holdings Corp.
Stock Symbol: IART
Traded On: NASDAQ
Produces/Sells CE-marked Devices: N
Distribution: Manufacturer Direct, Manufacturer Through Distributor, Manufacturer Through Manufacturer Reps, OEM, Service Direct, Exporter
General Admin.: Richard E. Caruso/President, Chief Executive Officer
Mktg./Adv.: Andre Decarie/Senior Vice President Marketing & Sales
    Robert G. Runckel/Vice President International Marketing
Production: Robert J. Towarnicki/Executive Vice President Development
    John R. Emery/Senior Vice President Operations
    Judith E. O'Grady/Vice President Regulatory Affairs
Research: Frederick Cahn/Senior Vice President Research
    Michael D. Pierschbacher/Senior Vice President Research & Development
    Surendra P. Batra/Vice President Product Development

Cuff, Nerve	Cns/Neurology
Device, Dermal Replacement	Surgery
Graft, Bone	Orthopedics

INTEGRA LIFESCIENCES HOLDINGS CORP.   800-654-2873
311 Enterprise Drive, Plainsboro, NJ 08536-3339   **609-275-0500**
FDA Number: 1121308   *Fax:* 609-275-5363
E-mail: custsvcnj@integra-ls.com
Web site: www.integra-ls.com
Medical Products Sales Volume: $550,459,000
Annual Revenue: $500 Million-$1 Billion
Year Founded: 1989
Total Employees: 2500   *Marketing Staff:* 2   *Sales Staff:* 45
Ownership: Public
Stock Symbol: IART
Traded On: NASDAQ
Produces/Sells CE-marked Devices: Y
Federal Procurement Eligibility: Small Business
Distribution: Manufacturer Direct, Manufacturer Through Distributor, Manufacturer Through Manufacturer Reps, Exporter

INTEGRA LIFESCIENCES HOLDINGS CORP. 800-654-2873
(cont'd)

General Admin.: Mr. Richard E. Caruso/Chairman
Mr. John B. Henneman III/Chief Financial Officer, Executive Vice President
Mr. Gerard S. Carlozzi/Chief Operating Officer, Executive Vice President
Mr. Stuart M. Essig/President, Chief Executive Officer, Director
James Oti/Senior Vice President International Operations
Wilma Davis/Senior Vice President, Chief Information Officer
Richard Gorelick/Senior Vice President, General Counsel
Medical Admin.: Dr. Carlos Blanco/Vice President, Medical Director
Mktg./Adv.: Keith Johnson/Senior Vice President Business Development
Debbie Leonetti/Vice President Marketing
Robert Paltridge/Vice President Sales
Production: Debbie Lindenmuth/Director Quality Assurance
Ms. Judith E. O'Grady/Senior Vice President Regulatory Affairs
Don Nociolo/Vice President Manufacturing
Research: Fred Cahn/Senior Vice President Research
Michael Pierschbacher/Senior Vice President Research & Development

Accessories, Catheter	Surgery
Agent, Hemostatic, Absorbable, Collagen-Based	Surgery
Beads, Hydrophilic, Wound Exudate Absorption	Surgery
Cuff, Nerve	Cns/Neurology
Dressing, Other	General
Dressing, Wound and Burn, Occlusive	Surgery
Sponge, Hemostatic, Absorbable Collagen	Surgery
Sponge, Neuro	Cns/Neurology

Medical Product Subsidiaries (Listed Separately)
Integra Lifesciences Corp.
Integra Lifesciences Corporation
Integra Lifesciences Of Ohio
Integra Luxtec, Inc.
Integra Neurosciences
Integra Neurosciences Pr
Integra Radionics
J. Jamner Surgical Instruments, Inc
Miltex Inc.

INTEGRA LIFESCIENCES OF OHIO 800-654-2873
4900 Charlemar Drive, Building A, Cincinnati, OH 45227
FDA Number: 3004608878
E-mail: ohiohr@integra-ls.com
Ownership: Integra Lifesciences Holdings Corp.
Stock Symbol: IART
Traded On: NASDAQ
Produces/Sells CE-marked Devices: N

Accessories, Operating Room, Table	Surgery
Appliance, Fixation, Spinal Interlaminal	Orthopedics
Bit, Drill	Orthopedics
Cover, Burr Hole (Cranial)	Cns/Neurology
Expander, Surgical, Skin Graft	Surgery
Head Rest, Neurosurgical	Cns/Neurology
Holder, Head, Neurosurgical (Skull Clamp)	Cns/Neurology
Infusion Stand	General
Plate, Fixation, Bone	Orthopedics
Retractor, Self-Retaining, Neurology	Cns/Neurology
Screw, Fixation, Bone	Orthopedics
Tray, Surgical Instrument	Surgery

INTEGRA LUXTEC INC.
See Integra Luxtec, Inc.

INTEGRA LUXTEC, INC. 800-325-8966 / 508-835-9700
99 Hartwell St., West Boylston, MA 01583
FDA Number: 1221336   *Fax:* 508-835-9976
E-mail: info@luxtec.com
Web site: www.luxtec.com
Annual Revenue: $10-$25 Million
Year Founded: 1981
Total Employees: 143   *Marketing Staff:* 3   *Sales Staff:* 5
Ownership: Integra Lifesciences Holdings Corp.
Stock Symbol: IART
Traded On: NASDAQ
Quality System Registration Information: ISO9001
Produces/Sells CE-marked Devices: Y
Federal Procurement Eligibility: Small Business
Distribution: Manufacturer Through Distributor, Exporter
General Admin.: Mr. Samuel Stein/Vice President, General Manager
Mktg./Adv.: Mr. Craig Stevens/Vice President Export Sales
Production: Mrs. Rita Wadleigh/Manager Quality Assurance & Regulatory Affairs
Research: Mr. William Perry/Vice President Engineering

Cable, Fiberoptic	General
Camera, Video	General
Camera, Video, Endoscopic	General
Fiberoptic Light Source & Carrier	Ear/Nose/Throat
Headlight, ENT	Ear/Nose/Throat
Headlight, Fiberoptic Focusing	Gastroenterology/Urology
Light Source, Endoscope, Xenon Arc	Surgery

INTEGRA LUXTEC, INC. 800-325-8966 *(cont'd)*

Light Source, Endoscopic	Obstetrics/Gynecology
Light Source, Fiberoptic, Routine	Gastroenterology/Urology
Light, Surgical Headlight	Dental And Oral
System, Camera, 3-Dimensional	Surgery

INTEGRA NEUROCARE LLC
See Integra Neurosciences

INTEGRA NEUROSCIENCES 800-762-1574
5955 Pacific Center Boulevard, San Diego, CA 92121-4309
FDA Number: 2023988
Web site: http://www.integralife.com
Ownership: Integra Lifesciences Holdings Corp.
Stock Symbol: IART
Traded On: NASDAQ
Produces/Sells CE-marked Devices: N

Bag, Reservoir (Blood)	Anesthesiology
Electrode, Cortical	Cns/Neurology
Monitor, Intracranial Pressure, Continuous	Cns/Neurology
Shunt, Central Nerve, With Component	Cns/Neurology

INTEGRA NEUROSCIENCES PR 800-654-2873
Road 402 North, Km 1.2, Anasco, PR 00610
FDA Number: 2648988
Web site: www.integra-ls.com
Ownership: Integra Lifesciences Holdings Corp.
Stock Symbol: IART
Traded On: NASDAQ
Produces/Sells CE-marked Devices: Y

Agent, Hemostatic, Absorbable, Collagen-Based	Surgery
Cannula, Ventricular	Cns/Neurology
Catheter, Peritoneal	Surgery
Catheter, Vascular, Cardiopulmonary Bypass	Cardiovascular
Catheter, Ventricular	Cns/Neurology
Cover, Burr Hole (Cranial)	Cns/Neurology
Cuff, Nerve	Cns/Neurology
Dressing, Other	General
Dura-Substitute	Cns/Neurology
Instrument, Implantation, Shunt	Cns/Neurology
Material, Dressing, Surgical, Acid, Polylactic	Dental And Oral
Retractor, Surgical	Surgery
Shunt, Central Nerve, With Component	Cns/Neurology
Strip, Craniosynostosis, Preformed	Cns/Neurology
Tape, Measuring, Ruler And Caliper	Surgery

INTEGRA RADIONICS 800-466-6814 / 781-272-1233
22 Terry Avenue, Burlington, MA 01803
FDA Number: 1222895   *Fax:* 781-272-2428
E-mail: info@radionics.com
Web site: www.radionics.com
Medical Products Sales Volume: $22,800,000
Annual Revenue: $25-$50 Million
Year Founded: 1938
Total Employees: 135   *Marketing Staff:* 6   *Sales Staff:* 10
Ownership: Integra Lifesciences Holdings Corp.
Stock Symbol: IART
Traded On: NASDAQ
Quality System Registration Information: ISO9001
Produces/Sells CE-marked Devices: Y
Federal Procurement Eligibility: Small Business
Distribution: Manufacturer Direct, Service Direct
Mktg./Adv.: Rob Ascoli/Director Sales

Accelerator, Linear, Medical	Radiology
Camera, Television, Surgical (With Audio)	Surgery
Electrocautery Unit, Line-Powered	Surgery
Electrode, Other	General
Endoscope	Gastroenterology/Urology
Light Source, Fiberoptic, Routine	Gastroenterology/Urology
Light, Headband, Surgical	Surgery
Light, Surgical, Fiberoptic	Surgery
Loupe, Diagnostic/Surgical	Surgery
Monitor, Intracranial Pressure	Cns/Neurology
Monitor, Intracranial Pressure, Continuous	Cns/Neurology
Needle, Biopsy, Cardiovascular	Cardiovascular
Probe, Radiofrequency Lesion	Cns/Neurology
Splint, Traction	Orthopedics
Stereotaxy Equipment	Cns/Neurology
Sterotaxic Unit	Cns/Neurology
Stimulator, Electrical, Evoked Response	Cns/Neurology
Stimulator, Neurological	Surgery
Surgical Instrument, Ultrasonic	Surgery
System, Planning, Radiation Therapy Treatment	Radiology
Transducer, Ultrasonic	Cardiovascular

INTEGRA SPINE 330-475-8600
1800 Triplett Blvd., Akron, OH 44306
FDA Number: 3004155681   *Fax:* 330-773-7697
E-mail: spine.info@integra-ls.com
Web site: www.therics.com
Year Founded: 1996

INTEGRA SPINE   **330-475-8600** *(cont'd)*
Ownership: Private
Produces/Sells CE-marked Devices: N

Filler, Calcium Sulfate Preformed Pellets	Orthopedics
Implant, Endosseous (Bone Filling and/or Augmentation)	Dental And Oral

INTEGRAL DESIGN INC.   **781-740-2036**
52 Burr Road, Hingham, MA 02043
FDA Number: 1222026   Fax: 781-741-5771
E-mail: rich@integral-design.com
Web site: www.integral-design.com
Medical Products Sales Volume: $600,000
Annual Revenue: $1-$5 Million
Total Employees: 6   Marketing Staff: 1   Sales Staff: 1
Ownership: Private
Quality System Registration Information: ISO9001
Produces/Sells CE-marked Devices: N
Federal Procurement Eligibility: Small Business
Distribution: Manufacturer Direct, Service Direct
General Admin.: Richard Beane/Chief Executive Officer

Accessories, Arthroscope	Orthopedics
Awl	Orthopedics
Bit, Drill	Orthopedics
Cannula, Drainage, Arthroscopy	Orthopedics
Carrier, Ligature	Surgery
Coagulator/Cutter, Endoscopic, Bipolar	Obstetrics/Gynecology
Cutter, Orthopedic	Orthopedics
Electrode, Biopotential, Surface, Composite	Physical Med
Electrode, Electro-Oculograph	Ophthalmology
Electrode, Electroencephalographic	Cns/Neurology
Electrode, Electromyographic	Cns/Neurology
Electrode, Neurological	Cns/Neurology
Electrode, Other	General
Electrode, Surface	Anesthesiology
Electrosurgical Unit, Cutting & Coagulation Device	Surgery
Electrosurgical Unit, General Purpose (ESU)	Surgery
File	Orthopedics
Forceps, Dressing	Surgery
Forceps, Electrosurgical	Surgery
Forceps, General & Plastic Surgery	Surgery
Forceps, Suction	Surgery
Forceps, Tissue	Surgery
Forceps, Tonsil	Ear/Nose/Throat
Hook, Ophthalmic	Ophthalmology
Instrument, Microsurgical	Cns/Neurology
Instrument, Passing, Ligature, Knot Tying	Cns/Neurology
Introducer, Sphere	Ophthalmology
Mallet, Bone	Orthopedics
Needle, Other	General
Osteotome (Orthopedic)	Surgery
Rasp, Bone	Orthopedics
Service, Consulting	General
Service, Engineering/Design	General
Skid, Bone	Orthopedics
Surgical Instrument, Non-Powered, Neurosurgical	Cns/Neurology

INTEGRAMED AMERICA, INC.   **212-835-8500**
2 Manhattanville Rd., Purchase, NY 10577-2113
FDA Number: 3004059998
E-mail: doug.weiss@integramed.com
Web site: www.integramed.com
Ownership: Private
Produces/Sells CE-marked Devices: N

Computer, Chemistry Analyzer	Chemistry

INTEGRATED BIOMEDICAL CORP.   **702-450-1005**
5030 S. Decatur Blvd. #e, Las Vegas, NV 89118
FDA Number: 3004413879

Stimulator, Muscle, Electrical-Powered (EMS)	Physical Med
Stimulator, Nerve, Transcutaneous (Pain Relief, TENS)	Cns/Neurology

INTEGRATED BIOMEDICAL TECHNOLOGY, INC.   **574-264-0025**
2931 Moose Trail, Elkhart, IN 46514
FDA Number: 1833983

Dialysate Delivery System, Single Patient	Gastroenterology/Urology
Dialyzer Reprocessing System	Gastroenterology/Urology
Strip, Test, Reagent, Residuals For Dialysate, Disinfectant	Gastroenterology/Urology

INTEGRATED MEDICAL DEVICES, INC.   **888-486-6900**
549 Electronics Parkway, Liverpool, NY 13088   **315-457-4200**
FDA Number: 1318742   Fax: 315-457-4222
E-mail: sales@integrated-medical.com
Web site: www.integrated-medical.com
Medical Products Sales Volume: $720,000
Year Founded: 1992
Total Employees: 7
Ownership: Private
Produces/Sells CE-marked Devices: N
Federal Procurement Eligibility: Small Business

INTEGRATED MEDICAL DEVICES, INC.   **888-486-6900** *(cont'd)*
Distribution: Manufacturer Direct, Manufacturer Through Distributor, Manufacturer Through Manufacturer Reps, OEM, Service Direct

Electrocardiograph, Single Channel	Cardiovascular
Transmitter/Receiver System, ECG, Telephone Single-Channel	Cardiovascular
Transmitter/Receiver System, Physiological, Telephone	Cardiovascular

INTEGRATED MEDICAL SYSTEMS, INC.   **800-783-9251**
1823 27th Ave. S., Birmingham, AL 35209   **205-879-3840**
FDA Number: n/a   Fax: 205-803-4057
E-mail: info@imsready.com
Web site: www.imsrepair.com
Annual Revenue: $10-$25 Million
Ownership: Private
Produces/Sells CE-marked Devices: N
Distribution: Service Direct, Exclusive Distributor
General Admin.: Gene Robinson/Chief Executive Officer
    Debra Robinson/Vice President, General Manager
Mktg./Adv.: Ellen Henderson/Director Marketing
    James Monday/Manager Sales Training
    Bo Mundy/Vice President Sales

Service, Repair, Endoscopic	General

INTEGRATED MEDICAL SYSTEMS, INC.   **562-498-1776**
1984 Obispo Avenue, Signal Hill, CA 90755
FDA Number: 2030911   Fax: 562-597-6423
E-mail: info@LSTAT.com
Web site: www.LSTAT.com
Medical Products Sales Volume: $8,000,000
Annual Revenue: $5-$10 Million
Year Founded: 1999
Total Employees: 24   Marketing Staff: 2   Sales Staff: 2
Ownership: Private
Produces/Sells CE-marked Devices: Y
Federal Procurement Eligibility: Small Business
Distribution: Manufacturer Direct, Manufacturer Through Distributor, Manufacturer Through Manufacturer Reps, Exporter
General Admin.: Steve Alexander/President, Chief Operating Officer
    Todd Kneale/Program Manager
Mktg./Adv.: Dr. Matthew E. Hanson/Vice President Sales

Patient Transfer Unit	General

INTEGRATED MEDICAL TECHNOLOGIES   **518-368-2400**
157 First St., Troy, NY 12180
FDA Number: 3005616556

Tester, Radiology	Radiology

INTEGRATED MEDICAL TECHNOLOGIES, INC.
    See Compass International, Inc.

INTEGRATED NEUROSCIENCE CONSORTIUM, INC.
    See Inc Research

INTEGRATED ORBITAL IMPLANTS, INC.   **800-424-6537**
12625 High Bluff Drive, Suite 314,   **858-259-4355**
San Diego, CA 92130
FDA Number: 2027377   Fax: 858-259-6277
E-mail: haimplants@aol.com
Web site: www.ioi.com
Medical Products Sales Volume: $410,000
Year Founded: 1990
Total Employees: 7   Marketing Staff: 2   Sales Staff: 5
Ownership: Private
Quality System Registration Information: ISO9003
Produces/Sells CE-marked Devices: Y
Federal Procurement Eligibility: Small Business
Distribution: Manufacturer Through Distributor, Service Direct
Medical Admin.: Arthur Perry/Medical Director
Mktg./Adv.: Clifton Hawley/Manager Business Development

General Medical Device	General
Implant, Orbital, Extra-Ocular	Ophthalmology

INTEGRATED SOFTWARE DESIGN, INC.   **800-600-2242**
171 Forbes Blvd Suite 3000,   **508-339-4928**
Mansfield, MA 02048
FDA Number: n/a   Fax: 508-339-2257
E-mail: info@isdweb.com
Web site: www.isdweb.com
Medical Products Sales Volume: $2,500,000
Annual Revenue: $1-$5 Million
Year Founded: 1982
Total Employees: 26   Marketing Staff: 2   Sales Staff: 8
Ownership: Private
Produces/Sells CE-marked Devices: N
Federal Procurement Eligibility: Small Business
Distribution: Manufacturer Direct, Service Direct
General Admin.: Mr. Ramin Khoshatefeh/President
Mktg./Adv.: Mr. Kenneth Legault/Director Business Development
    Ms. Phyllis Zaiger/Director Marketing

INTEGRATED SOFTWARE DESIGN, INC. 800-600-2242 (cont'd)
IS: Ms. Alis Ourouj/Director Tech. Services

Computer Software	General
Computer, Bar Code	General
Label, Bar Code	General

INTEGRATED SURGICAL SYSTEMS 530-792-2600
1850 Research Park Drive, Davis, CA 95616
FDA Number: n/a   Fax: 530-792-2690
E-mail: info@robodoc.com
Web site: www.robodoc.com
Year Founded: 1992
Total Employees: 30
Ownership: Public
Stock Symbol: ISSM
Traded On: OTC Bulletin
Quality System Registration Information: ISO9001
Produces/Sells CE-marked Devices: Y
Distribution: Manufacturer Direct
General Admin.: Ramesh C. Trivedi/President, Chief Executive Officer
Finance: Chuck Novak/Chief Financial Officer

Assistant, Surgical, Orthopedic, Automated	Orthopedics
Drill, Cranial	Cns/Neurology

INTEGRITI SYSTEMS, LLC 206-652-4700
80 South Jackson, Suite 407, Seattle, WA 98104
FDA Number: 3004160088
Ownership: Private
Produces/Sells CE-marked Devices: N

Monitor, Physiological, Patient(without Arrhythmia Detection Or Alarms)	Cardiovascular

INTEGRITY MEDICAL DEVICES INC 609-567-8175
360 Fairview Ave., Hammonton, NJ 08037
FDA Number: 2249550

Dressing, Wound And Burn, Occlusive, Heated	Surgery
Dressing, Wound, Hydrogel W/out Drug And/or Biologic	Surgery
Dressing, Wound, Hydrophilic	Surgery
Dressing, Wound, Occlusive	Surgery

INTEGRITY PRODUCTS, INC. 816-965-0308
P.O. Box 4411, Grandview, MO 64030-0844
FDA Number: 1933015   Fax: 816-761-1070
E-mail: jeff@integrityproductsinc.com
Year Founded: 1993
Total Employees: 6   Sales Staff: 2
Ownership: Private
Produces/Sells CE-marked Devices: N
Federal Procurement Eligibility: Small Business
Distribution: Manufacturer Direct

Colorimeter, General Use	Chemistry

INTEL CORP. DIGITAL HEALTH GROUP 916-356-8080
1900 Prairie City Rd., FM7-197, Folsom, CA 95630
FDA Number: 3006785459
Ownership: Private
Produces/Sells CE-marked Devices: N

Glucose Dehydrogenase, Glucose	Chemistry
Transmitter/Receiver System, Physiological, Radiofrequency	Cardiovascular

INTELERAD 514-931-6222
895 de la GauchetiAüí'A,A, re Street W.,   Canada
Suite 400, Montr QC H3B 4G1
FDA Number: N   Fax: 866-951-6222
Web site: info@intelerad.com
Total Employees: 514-931
Ownership: I
Stock Symbol: N

INTELIFUSE, INC. 504-561-1100
1515 Poydras St. Suite 1490, New Orleans, LA 70112
FDA Number: 3005509435

Staple, Fixation, Bone	Orthopedics

INTELLA INTERVENTIONAL SYSTEMS, INC. 408-737-7121
870 Hermosa Drive, Sunnyvale, CA 94086
FDA Number: 2953691   Fax: 408-737-1214
E-mail: info@iisi.com
Medical Products Sales Volume: $5,900,000
Total Employees: 62
Ownership: Private
Produces/Sells CE-marked Devices: N
Federal Procurement Eligibility: Small Business

Catheter, Angioplasty, Coronary, Transluminal, Percut. Oper.	Cardiovascular
Guidewire, Catheter	Cardiovascular

INTELLECTUAL PROPERTY, LLC 608-798-0904
8030 Stagecoach Road, Cross Plains, WI 53528
FDA Number: n/a   Fax: 608-798-0914
E-mail: reining@ipllc.cc

INTELLECTUAL PROPERTY, LLC 608-798-0904 (cont'd)
Web site: www.ipllc.cc
Annual Revenue: $0-$1 Million
Year Founded: 1999
Total Employees: 2
Ownership: Private
Produces/Sells CE-marked Devices: N
Federal Procurement Eligibility: Small Business
Distribution: Manufacturer Direct
General Admin.: William N. Reining/General Manager

Cardiac Output Unit, Other	Cardiovascular
Monitor, Bed Occupancy	General
Monitor, Physiological, Patient	Cardiovascular

INTELLIGENT HEARING SYSTEMS, CORP. 800-447-9783
6860 SW 81st street, Miami, FL 33143 305-668-6102
FDA Number: 1052723   Fax: 305-668-6103
E-mail: ihs@ihsys.com
Web site: www.ihsys.com
Medical Products Sales Volume: $5,000,000
Annual Revenue: $1-$5 Million
Year Founded: 1983
Total Employees: 15   Marketing Staff: 5   Sales Staff: 8
Ownership: Private
Produces/Sells CE-marked Devices: Y
Federal Procurement Eligibility: Small Business
Distribution: Manufacturer Direct, Manufacturer Through Distributor, OEM
General Admin.: Edward Miskiel/President, Chief Executive Officer
          Rafael Delgado/Vice President, General Manager
Mktg./Adv.: Carlos Lopez/Director Product Development
Production: Octavio Garrastacho/Manager Manufacturing
          Kavita Thombre/Manager Regulatory Affairs
          Carlos Lopez/Vice President Manufacturing
IS: Rafael Delgado/Director Software
          Marra Lashbrook/Director Tech. Services

Audiometer	Ear/Nose/Throat
Computer, Audiometry	Ear/Nose/Throat
Evoked Potential Unit, Audiometric	Cns/Neurology
Evoked Response Unit, Auditory	Ear/Nose/Throat
Speech Training Aid, AC-Powered	Ear/Nose/Throat
Stimulator, Auditory, Evoked Response	Cns/Neurology
Stimulator, Photic, Evoked Response	Cns/Neurology
Tester, Auditory Impedance	Ear/Nose/Throat

INTELLINETX 877-370-0477
2301 West 205th St., # 102, Torrance, CA 90501
FDA Number: 2028047

Nystagmograph	Cns/Neurology

INTELSOURCE GROUP, INC 602-790-8034
15953 N Greenway Hayden Loop Suit I, Scottsdale, AZ 85260
FDA Number: 3006791967
Ownership: Private
Produces/Sells CE-marked Devices: N

Stimulator, Nerve, Transcutaneous (Pain Relief, TENS)	Cns/Neurology

INTELWAVE, LLC 732-738-8800
1090 King Georges Post Road, Suite 1004, Edison, NJ 08837
FDA Number: 3006173899

Electrocardiograph, Single Channel	Cardiovascular

INTEMPO WOOD FURNITURE, INC. 888-232-4809
P.O. Box 82816, Oklahoma City, OK 73148-0816 405-232-4805
FDA Number: n/a   Fax: 405-232-4816
Web site: http://www.intempowood.com
Annual Revenue: $1-$5 Million
Total Employees: 15
Ownership: Private
Produces/Sells CE-marked Devices: N
Federal Procurement Eligibility: Small Business, Female Owned
Distribution: Manufacturer Direct
General Admin.: Marla Roth/President
Mktg./Adv.: Joshua Goodman/Manager Marketing
          Linda Valentine/Marketing Assistant

Chair, Other	General
Furniture, General	General
Furniture, Patient Room	General
Mattress, Bed	General
Table, Other	General

INTER MEDICO 800-387-9643
50 Valleywood Dr., 905-470-2520
Markham, ONT L3R-6 Canada
FDA Number: n/a   Fax: 905-470-2381
E-mail: info@inter-medico.com
Web site: www.inter-medico.com
Year Founded: 1979
Total Employees: 50

INTER MEDICO

800-387-9643 *(cont'd)*

Ownership: Private
Produces/Sells CE-marked Devices: N
Distribution: Exclusive Distributor, Importer

INTER V MEDICAL INC.

800-667-1073
514-955-3410

5179 Metropolitain East,
Montreal, QUE H1R 1 Canada

FDA Number: n/a
E-mail: info@intervmedical.com
Web site: http://www.intervmedical.com/
Year Founded: 1991
Total Employees: 10
Ownership: Private
Produces/Sells CE-marked Devices: N
Distribution: Exclusive Distributor

Fax: 514-955-3411

INTER-APPAREL CORPORATION

See Pfb Inter-Apparel Corp.

INTER-MED, INC.

877-418-4782
262-636-9755

2200 Northwestern Ave., Racine, WI 53404

FDA Number: 2133714
E-mail: inquiries@vista-dental.com
Web site: www.vista-dental.com
Ownership: Private
Produces/Sells CE-marked Devices: Y
General Admin.: Mr. Tony Martell/Vice President

Fax: 262-636-9760

Applicator, Tipped, Absorbent, Non-Sterile	General
Depressor, Tongue	General
Dispenser, Medication, Liquid	General
Evacuator, Oral Cavity	Dental And Oral
Irrigator, Oral	Dental And Oral
Mirror, Mouth	Dental And Oral
Needle, Dental	Dental And Oral
Preparer, Root Canal, Endodontic	Dental And Oral
Scraper, Tongue	Dental And Oral
Syringe Unit, Air And/Or Water	Dental And Oral
Syringe, Antistick	General
Syringe, Periodontic, Endodontic	Dental And Oral
Syringe, Restorative And Impression Material	Dental And Oral
Toothbrush, Manual	Dental And Oral
Tray, Fluoride, Disposable	Dental And Oral
Tray, Impression	Dental And Oral
Unit, Filter, Membrane	Chemistry
Warmer, Irrigation Solution	General

INTERACOUSTICS-USA

See Medi

INTERACT PLUS

800-944-8002
256-704-8787

2225 Drake Avenue, Suite 2,
Huntsville, AL 35805

FDA Number: 1066222
E-mail: info@interactplus.com
Web site: www.interactplus.com
Total Employees: 15
Ownership: Private
Produces/Sells CE-marked Devices: Y
Federal Procurement Eligibility: Small Business
Distribution: Manufacturer Direct, Manufacturer Through Manufacturer Reps

Fax: 256-880-8785

Environmental Control System, Powered	Physical Med

INTERACTION CHROMATOGRAPHY

See Trans-Genomic

INTERACTIVE MOTION TECHNOLOGIES, INC.

617-497-6330

37 Spinelli Place, Cambridge, MA 02138

FDA Number: 1226192

Exerciser, Powered	Anesthesiology
Isokinetic Testing And Evaluation System	Physical Med

INTERACTIVE PERFORMANCE MONITORING, INC. (IPM)

509-334-6363

1230 Ne Hickman Ct., Pullman, WA 99163

FDA Number: 3033029
Ownership: Private
Produces/Sells CE-marked Devices: N

Isokinetic Testing And Evaluation System	Physical Med

INTERCALL SYSTEMS INC.

516-294-4524

150 Herricks Road, Mineola, NY 11501

FDA Number: n/a
E-mail: sales@intercallsystems.com
Web site: www.intercallsystems.com
Medical Products Sales Volume: $2,000,000
Annual Revenue: $1-$5 Million
Year Founded: 1971
Total Employees: 25   *Marketing Staff:* 1
Ownership: Private

Fax: 516-294-4526

INTERCALL SYSTEMS INC.

516-294-4524 *(cont'd)*

Produces/Sells CE-marked Devices: N
Federal Procurement Eligibility: Small Business, Female Owned
Distribution: Manufacturer Through Distributor
General Admin.: Elias Gurman/President
          Mary Greene/Vice President
Mktg./Adv.: Therese Dessauce/Manager Advertising
          Philip Cibrano/Vice President Sales
Research: Jack Jacobs/Vice President Research & Development

Nurse Call System	General

INTERCARE DX, INC.

310-242-5634

6080 Center Drive Suite 640, Los Angeles, CA 90045

FDA Number: 3005735282
Ownership: Public
Stock Symbol: ICCO
Traded On: OTC Bulletin
Produces/Sells CE-marked Devices: N

Monitor, Blood Pressure, Indirect, Semi-Automatic	Cardiovascular

INTERCON CHEMICAL

800-325-9218
314-771-6600

1100 Central Industrial Dr., St. Louis, MO 63110

FDA Number: 3000246414
E-mail: inter001@aol.com
Total Employees: 75   *Marketing Staff:* 3   *Sales Staff:* 15
Ownership: Private
Produces/Sells CE-marked Devices: N
Distribution: Manufacturer Through Distributor, OEM
General Admin.: James Epstein/President
Mktg./Adv.: Nick Mahan/Director Marketing
Production: Jeff Huber/Vice President Manufacturing

Fax: 314-771-6608

Disinfector, Liquid	General
Disinfector, Medical Device	General
Solution, Antibacterial Cleaner	General

INTERCON CHEMICAL CO.

800-325-9218

1100 Central Industrial Dr., St. Louis, MO 63110

FDA Number: 3000246414

Medical Disinfectants/Cleaners for Instruments	General

INTERCURE INC.

646-652-5800

589 8th Avenue, 6th Floor, New York, NY 10018

FDA Number: 3005105254
Web site: www.intercure.com
Year Founded: 1994
Ownership: INTERCURE LTD.
Stock Symbol: INCR
Produces/Sells CE-marked Devices: N
Distribution: Manufacturer Direct
General Admin.: Dr. Benjamin Gavish/Chief Scientific Officer
          Erez Gavish/President, Chief Executive Officer
Medical Admin.: Dr. Ariela Alter/Director Clinical Affairs
Mktg./Adv.: Ofer Ben Arad/Vice President Products
          Scot DubAc/Vice President Sales
Production: Ari Sabah/Vice President Operations
Finance: ARik Kleinstein/Chief Financial Officer

Fax: 212-967-5060

INTEREX CORP.

See Interex Div. Of Industrial Safety & Supply

INTEREX DIV. OF INDUSTRIAL SAFETY & SUPPLY

800-671-5080
-

176 Newington Rd., Hartford, CT 06110-2320

FDA Number: n/a
E-mail: info@industrialsafety.com
Web site: www.industrialsafety.com
Medical Products Sales Volume: $200,000
Annual Revenue: $1-$5 Million
Total Employees: 100   *Marketing Staff:* 2   *Sales Staff:* 98
Ownership: INDUSTRIAL SAFETY & SUPPLY CO., INC.
Quality System Registration Information: ISO9001
Produces/Sells CE-marked Devices: N
Federal Procurement Eligibility: Small Business
Distribution: Exclusive Distributor
General Admin.: William Bonk/President, Chief Executive Officer
          Gene Knorr/Vice President Human Resources
Mktg./Adv.: Neal Reading/Director Marketing
          Richard Dickensen/Director Product Development
          Neal Reading/Manager Advertising
          Mark Anton/Manager Business Development
          Neal Reading/Manager National Sales
          Bruce Aiken/Manager Sales Training
          Mark Anton/Vice President Sales
Production: Dennis Farraday/Director Quality Assurance

Fax: 860-371-2166

Labware, Basic, Disposable	Chemistry
Pipetter	Hematology
Solution, Antibacterial Cleaner	General

INTEREX DIV. OF INDUSTRIAL SAFETY 800-671-5080 (cont'd)
Waste Receptacle, General Purpose — General

INTERFERON SCIENCES, INC. 888-728-4372
783 Jersey Avenue, New Brunswick, NJ 08901 732-249-3250
FDA Number: n/a — Fax: 732-249-6895
E-mail: info@interferonsciences.com
Web site: www.interferonsciences.com
Medical Products Sales Volume: $14,300,000
Annual Revenue: $1-$5 Million
Year Founded: 2004
Total Employees: 40
Ownership: Public
Stock Symbol: IFSC
Traded On: NASDAQ
Quality System Registration Information: ISO9000
Produces/Sells CE-marked Devices: N
Federal Procurement Eligibility: Small Business
Distribution: Manufacturer Direct, Importer, Exporter
General Admin.: Lawrence Gordon/Chief Executive Officer
    Stan Schutzbank/President
Production: Bob Hansen/Vice President Manufacturing
Genetic Engineering — Microbiology

INTERGRAPH CORPORATION 800-345-4856
P.O. Box 240000, Huntsville, AL 35894-0001 256-730-2000
FDA Number: n/a — Fax: 256-730-2048
Web site: http://www.intergraph.com/
Annual Revenue: $0-$1 Million
Ownership: Public
Stock Symbol: INGR
Traded On: NASDAQ
Quality System Registration Information: ISO9002
Produces/Sells CE-marked Devices: N
Distribution: Manufacturer Through Distributor, Manufacturer Through Manufacturer Reps, OEM
General Admin.: Jim Meadlock/President
Mktg./Adv.: Harriet Polskoy/Marketing Representative
Computer Equipment — General
Computer Software — General

INTERGRAPH PUBLIC SAFETY 800-345-4856
19 Interpro Road, Madison, AL 35758 256-730-2000
FDA Number: n/a — Fax: 256-730-2048
Web site: www.intergraph.com
Annual Revenue: $0-$1 Million
Ownership: FONG BROTHERS PRINTING
Traded On: NASDAQ
Produces/Sells CE-marked Devices: N
Federal Procurement Eligibility: Small Business
Distribution: Manufacturer Direct
Security Equipment/Supplies — General

INTERGRATED DENTAL SOLUTIONS, INC. 858-643-1143
6195 Cornerstone Court East, Suite 108, San Diego, CA 92121
FDA Number: 3005931737
Ownership: Private
Produces/Sells CE-marked Devices: N
Crown, Preformed — Dental And Oral
Cusp, Gold And Stainless Steel — Dental And Oral
Teeth, Artificial, Backing And Facing — Dental And Oral
Teeth, Artificial, Posterior With Metal Insert — Dental And Oral

INTERLECTRIC CORP. 800-722-2184
1401 Lexington Avenue, Warren, PA 16365-2849 814-723-6061
FDA Number: 2523544 — Fax: 814-723-6069
E-mail: ic@interlectric.com
Web site: www.interlectric.com
Medical Products Sales Volume: $13,700,000
Year Founded: 1973
Total Employees: 130 — Marketing Staff: 1 — Sales Staff: 14
Ownership: Private
Produces/Sells CE-marked Devices: N
Federal Procurement Eligibility: Small Business, Female Owned
Distribution: Manufacturer Direct, Manufacturer Through Distributor
Mktg./Adv.: Mr. Jared Villella/Marketing Coordinator
Light, Ultraviolet, Dermatologic — Surgery
Phototherapy Unit (Bilirubin Lamp) — General

INTERMARK (USA), INC. 408-971-2055
1310 Tully Road, Suite 117, San Jose, CA 95122
FDA Number: n/a — Fax: 408-971-6033
E-mail: sales@intermark-usa.com
Web site: www.intermark-usa.com
Medical Products Sales Volume: $2,100,000
Annual Revenue: $5-$10 Million
Year Founded: 1990
Total Employees: 13 — Marketing Staff: 1 — Sales Staff: 3

INTERMARK (USA), INC. 408-971-2055 (cont'd)
Ownership: Kitagawa Industries, Co. Ltd.
Stock Symbol: 6896
Quality System Registration Information: ISO9000
Produces/Sells CE-marked Devices: Y
Federal Procurement Eligibility: Small Business
Distribution: Manufacturer Direct
General Admin.: Klyoto Kitagawa/President
    Masaharu Hatakeyama/Vice President, General Manager
Shield Radio Frequency — Radiology
Shield, Magnetic Field — Radiology

INTERMED GROUP, INC. 561-586-3667
3550 23rd Ave. South, Suite #1, Lake Worth, FL 33461
FDA Number: 1061811
Colposcope — Obstetrics/Gynecology
Electrosurgical Unit, Anesthesiology Accessories — Surgery
Speculum, Vaginal, Non-Metal — Obstetrics/Gynecology

INTERMED LABORATORIES
See Intermed Supplies

INTERMED SUPPLIES 800-766-3131
7115 Belgold Street Suite E, Houston, TX 77066 281-587-0300
FDA Number: 1644015 — Fax: 832-201-7443
E-mail: glovespecialist@intermedgloves.com
Web site: www.intermedgloves.com
Medical Products Sales Volume: $70,000
Annual Revenue: $0-$1 Million
Year Founded: 1986
Ownership: Private
Federal Procurement Eligibility: Small Business
Distribution: Importer
Glove, Patient Examination — General
Glove, Patient Examination, Latex — General

INTERMED VIDEO TECHNOLOGIES INC. 203-270-0677
18 Commerce Road, Newtown, CT 06470
FDA Number: n/a — Fax: 203-270-9619
E-mail: sales@intermedvideo.com
Web site: www.intermedvideo.com
Medical Products Sales Volume: $1,500,000
Year Founded: 1990
Total Employees: 11 — Sales Staff: 2
Ownership: Private
Produces/Sells CE-marked Devices: N
Federal Procurement Eligibility: Small Business
Distribution: OEM
General Admin.: Mr. Harry Davies/President
IS: Mr. Robert Strong/Tech. Specialist
Recorder, Videotape/Videodisc — General
Recorder, X-Ray Image — Radiology

INTERMEDICS INC.
See Zimmer Dental, Inc.

INTERMEDICS ORTHOPEDICS, INC.
See Centerpulse Orthopedics Inc.

INTERMETRA CORP. 305-889-1194
10100 N.W. 116th Way, Suite 11, Miami, FL 33178-1154
FDA Number: n/a — Fax: 305-888-1900
E-mail: info@intermetra.com
Web site: www.intermetra.com
Medical Products Sales Volume: $400,000
Year Founded: 1973
Total Employees: 5
Ownership: Private
Federal Procurement Eligibility: Small Business
Distribution: Exporter
General Admin.: Michael Maidan/Vice President
Mktg./Adv.: Michael Maiden/Director Product Development
Finance: Ira Hartzman/Treasurer
Service, Import/Export — General

INTERMETRO INDUSTRIES CORP. 800-441-2714
651 N. Washington St., 570-825-2741
Wilkes Barre, PA 18705
FDA Number: 2531463 — Fax: 570-823-0250
E-mail: moreinfo-hc@intermetro.com
Web site: www.metro.com
Medical Products Sales Volume: $97,600,000
Year Founded: 1929
Total Employees: 1400
Ownership: Emerson Electric Company
Stock Symbol: EMR
Traded On: NYSE
Quality System Registration Information: ISO9000; ISO9001; ISO9002; ISO9003
Produces/Sells CE-marked Devices: N
Federal Procurement Eligibility: GSA Contract, VA Contract

INTERMETRO INDUSTRIES CORP.   800-441-2714 *(cont'd)*
Distribution: Manufacturer Direct, Manufacturer Through Distributor, Manufacturer Through Manufacturer Reps, OEM
General Admin.: Mr. John Nackley/President, Chief Executive Officer
           Theo Sonnenberg/Vice President International Operations
Mktg./Adv.: Carl Dymond/Director Marketing
           Mr. Edward Thompson/Director Sales
           Joseph Sokirka/Manager Advertising
           Mr. David Salus/Manager Marketing
           Karin Orrson/Manager Sales Training
           Kent Droppers/Vice President Sales
Production: Steve Yodoff/Vice President Manufacturing
Research: Jack Welsch/Vice President Product Development

Bin, Storage	General
Cabinet Casework, General Purpose	General
Cabinet Casework, Modular	General
Cabinet Casework, Pharmacy	General
Cabinet, Bedside	General
Cabinet, Instrument	General
Cabinet, Other	General
Cabinet, Storage, Catheter	General
Cabinet, Storage, Endoscope	Gastroenterology/Urology
Cart, Dressing	General
Cart, Emergency, Cardiopulmonary Resuscitation (Crash)	Anesthesiology
Cart, Equipment, Video	General
Cart, Foodservice	General
Cart, Gas Cylinder (Carrier)	Anesthesiology
Cart, Housekeeping	General
Cart, Instrument	Surgery
Cart, Instrument/Equipment, Laparoscopy	Surgery
Cart, Isolation	General
Cart, Laundry	General
Cart, Monitor	General
Cart, Multipurpose	General
Cart, Orthopedic Supply (Cast)	Orthopedics
Cart, Other	General
Cart, Supply	General
Cart, Supply, Operating Room	Surgery
Cart, Tissue	General
Cover, Cart	General
Foodservice Product/Equipment	General
Holder, Catheter	Gastroenterology/Urology
Rack, Surgical Instrument	Surgery
Station, Nourishment	General
Station, Nursing	General
Table, Other	General

INTERMEX TRADING & SUPPORTS SA DE CV.   52-553-58953
Rio Neva 33 Col.cuauthemoc, Mexico City Of, Df Mexico
FDA Number: 9616565

Container, Sharpes	General

INTERMOUNTAIN OCULAR PROSTHETICS, INC.   208-378-8200
2995 North Cole Rd., Suite 115, Boise, ID 83704-5965
FDA Number: 3031012
Ownership: Private
Produces/Sells CE-marked Devices: N

Eye, Artificial, Non-Custom	Ophthalmology

INTERNAL FIXATION SYSTEMS, INC.   305-491-9133
10100 N.w. 116th Way, Ste. 18, Miami, FL 33178
FDA Number: 3005960102
Ownership: Private
Produces/Sells CE-marked Devices: N

Bit, Drill	Orthopedics
Countersink	Orthopedics
Forceps, General & Plastic Surgery	Surgery
Gauge, Depth	Orthopedics
Orthopedic Manual Surgical Instrument	Orthopedics
Reamer	Orthopedics
Screw, Fixation, Bone	Orthopedics
Screwdriver	Orthopedics
Tray, Surgical Instrument	Surgery

INTERNATIONAL BIOCLINICAL, INC.
See Oxis International, Inc.

INTERNATIONAL BIOMEDICAL, LTD.   512-873-0033
2725 North Main St., Cleburne, TX 76033
FDA Number: 1629497

Glove, Protective, Radiographic	Radiology
Glove, Surgical, Plastic Surgery	Surgery
Incubator, Neonatal Transport	General

INTERNATIONAL BIOPHYSICS CORP.   512-326-3244
2101 East St. Elmo Rd., Suite 275, Austin, TX 78744
FDA Number: 1645362

Accessories, Cardiopulmonary Bypass	Cardiovascular
Laser, Surgical	Surgery
Monitor, Blood Gas, On-Line, Cardiopulmonary Bypass	Cardiovascular
Probe, Blood Flow, Extravascular	Cardiovascular

INTERNATIONAL BIOPHYSICS CORP.   512-326-3244 *(cont'd)*

Pump, Blood, Cardiopulmonary Bypass, Non-Roller Type	Cardiovascular
Sensor, Blood Gas, In-Line, Cardiopulmonary Bypass	Cardiovascular
Sucker, Cardiotomy Return, Cardiopulmonary Bypass	Cardiovascular
Surgical Instrument, Cardiovascular	Cardiovascular

INTERNATIONAL BRACHYTHERAPY, INC.   770-582-0662
6000 Live Oak Pkwy., #107, Norcross, GA 30093
FDA Number: 1065226
Ownership: Private
Produces/Sells CE-marked Devices: N

Applicator, Radionuclide, Manual	Radiology
Source, Brachytherapy, Radionuclide	Radiology

INTERNATIONAL BUSINESS SOLUTIONS, INC.   901-861-7144
350 Poplar View, Collierville, TN 38017
FDA Number: 2320857

Brush, Dermabrasion	Surgery

INTERNATIONAL CRYOGENICS, INC.   800-886-2796
**4040 Championship Drive,   317-297-4777
Indianapolis, IN 46268**
FDA Number: n/a   *Fax:* 317-297-7988
E-mail: ic@intlcryo.com
Web site: www.intlcryo.com
Medical Products Sales Volume: $1,300,000
Year Founded: 1980
Total Employees: 16   *Marketing Staff:* 2   *Sales Staff:* 4
Ownership: Private
Federal Procurement Eligibility: Small Business
Distribution: Manufacturer Direct, Manufacturer Through Distributor, Service Direct, Exporter
General Admin.: Rex Leonard/President
Mktg./Adv.: Donna Jung/Director Marketing & Sales
Production: Scott Randall/Manager Materials
Research: Rex Leonard/Vice President Research & Development

Flask, Dewar	Chemistry

INTERNATIONAL CRYSTAL LABORATORIES   973-478-8944
11 Erie St., Garfield, NJ 07026-2307
FDA Number: n/a   *Fax:* 973-478-4201
E-mail: iclmail@internationalcrystal.net
Web site: www.internationalcrystal.net
Medical Products Sales Volume: $2,700,000
Annual Revenue: $1-$5 Million
Year Founded: 1982
Total Employees: 22   *Marketing Staff:* 3   *Sales Staff:* 4
Ownership: Private
Produces/Sells CE-marked Devices: Y
Federal Procurement Eligibility: Small Business, Female Owned
Distribution: Manufacturer Direct, OEM, Exporter
General Admin.: Robert D. Herpst/Chairman
           Irene Ascuitto/Vice President, General Manager
Mktg./Adv.: Jill Levine/Manager Advertising
           Irene Ascuitto/Manager National Sales
           Theresa M. Herpst/Manager Product Development
           Theresa M. Herpst/President Marketing

Cell, Spectrophotometer	Chemistry
Component, Optical	General
Crusher, Pill	General

INTERNATIONAL DESIGN & MARKETING INCORPORATED   978-921-0638
140 Elliot St., Rt. 62 Business Center, Bldg E, Beverly, MA 01915
FDA Number: 3004136266
Ownership: Private
Produces/Sells CE-marked Devices: N

Booth, Sun Tan	Physical Med

INTERNATIONAL ENZYMES, INC.
See Cliniqa Corporation

INTERNATIONAL EQUIPMENT CO.
See Thermo Fisher Scientific - Laboratory Equipment Division Headquarters

INTERNATIONAL HEARING AIDS LTD.   800-387-7943
5041 Mainway, Burlington, ONT L7L 5H9 Canada   905 315 8303
FDA Number: n/a   *Fax:* 905 315 8176
E-mail: info@widexcanada.com
Web site: www.widex.com
Year Founded: 1962
Ownership: Private
Produces/Sells CE-marked Devices: N
Distribution: Manufacturer Direct, Exclusive Distributor

INTERNATIONAL HOSPITAL PRODUCTS, INC.   732-842-1246
38 Winding Way, P.O. Box 158, Little Silver, NJ 07739-0158
FDA Number: n/a

INTERNATIONAL HOSPITAL PRODUCTS, INC.   732-842-1246
(cont'd)
Ownership: Private
Produces/Sells CE-marked Devices: N
Federal Procurement Eligibility: Small Business
Distribution: Manufacturer Direct, Manufacturer Through Distributor, Manufacturer Through Manufacturer Reps

Tube, Decompression	General
Tube, Double Lumen For Intestinal Decompression	Gastroenterology/Urology
Tube, Gastrointestinal Decompression, Baker Jejunostomy	Gastroenterology/Urology

INTERNATIONAL HOSPITAL SUPPLY CO.   800-398-9450
6914 Canby Ave., Ste. 105,   818-996-0600
Reseda, CA 91335
FDA Number: 2083617   *Fax:* 818-996-0603
E-mail: info@internationalhospitalsupply.com
Web site: www.internationalhospitalsupply.com
Medical Products Sales Volume: $3,000,000
Annual Revenue: $1-$5 Million
Year Founded: 1977
Total Employees: 5   *Marketing Staff:* 2   *Sales Staff:* 2
Ownership: Private
Quality System Registration Information: ISO9002
Produces/Sells CE-marked Devices: N
Federal Procurement Eligibility: Small Business
Distribution: Manufacturer Direct, Exclusive Distributor, Importer, Exporter
General Admin.: Michael D Harris/President
Mktg./Adv.: Mike Harris/Manager International & National Sales
          Michael D Harris/Vice President Marketing & Sales
Production: Russell Bennett/Manager Materials
          Michael D Harris/Manager Regulatory Affairs
Finance: Karen Norton/Treasurer

Bed, Electric	General
Biopsy Instrument, Mechanical, Gastrointestinal	Gastroenterology/Urology
Cabinet, Instrument	General
Clamp, Surgical, General & Plastic Surgery	Surgery
Clamp, Uterine	Obstetrics/Gynecology
Clamp, Vascular	Cardiovascular
Component, Cast	Orthopedics
Curette, Biopsy, Bronchoscope (Non-Rigid)	Anesthesiology
Drill, Bone	Orthopedics
ENT Manual Surgical Instrument	Ear/Nose/Throat
Electrosurgical Equipment, General Purpose	Surgery
Endoscope	Gastroenterology/Urology
Equipment, Laboratory, Gen. Purpose (Specific Medical Use)	Chemistry
Foodservice Product/Equipment	General
Forceps, Biopsy, Bronchoscope (Non-Rigid)	Anesthesiology
Forceps, Biopsy, Bronchoscope (Rigid)	Anesthesiology
Forceps, General & Plastic Surgery	Surgery
Forceps, Ophthalmic	Ophthalmology
Forceps, Surgical, Gynecological	Obstetrics/Gynecology
Furniture, General	General
Gas-Machine, Anesthesia	Anesthesiology
General Use Surgical Scissors	Surgery
Glove, Other	General
Gown, Operating Room, Disposable	Surgery
Gown, Operating Room, Reusable	Surgery
Gown, Patient	Surgery
Instrument, Manual, General Surgical	Surgery
Instrument, Microsurgical	Cns/Neurology
Lamp, Operating Room	General
Laryngoscope	Ear/Nose/Throat
Laser, Gynecologic	Obstetrics/Gynecology
Light, Surgical, Instrument	Surgery
Mask, Gas, Anesthesia	Anesthesiology
Microscope, Surgical, General & Plastic Surgery	Surgery
Molding, Custom	General
Nail, Fixation, Bone	Orthopedics
Needle, Gastro-Urology	Gastroenterology/Urology
Phototherapy Unit, Neonatal	General
Pin, Fixation, Smooth	Orthopedics
Punch, Biopsy, Surgical	Dental And Oral
Retractor	Orthopedics
Retractor, All Types	Dental And Oral
Retractor, Laminectomy	Surgery
Retractor, Manual	Cns/Neurology
Retractor, Ophthalmic	Ophthalmology
Retractor, Self-Retaining	Gastroenterology/Urology
Retractor, Self-Retaining, Neurology	Cns/Neurology
Retractor, Surgical	Surgery
Retractor, Vaginal	Obstetrics/Gynecology
Service, Import/Export	General
Stand, Operating Room Instrument (Mayo)	Surgery
Staple, Fixation, Bone	Orthopedics
Sterilizer, Ethylene-Oxide Gas, Operating Room	Surgery
Sterilizer, Laboratory	Microbiology
Stretcher, Collapsible	General
Stretcher, Transfer	Surgery
Suction Apparatus, Operating Room, Wall Vacuum-Powered	Surgery
Surgical Instrument, Cardiovascular	Cardiovascular

INTERNATIONAL HOSPITAL SUPPLY CO.   800-398-9450 *(cont'd)*

Surgical Instrument, Disposable	Surgery
Surgical Instrument, Obstetric/Gynecologic, General	Obstetrics/Gynecology
System, Laser, Excimer, Ophthalmic	Ophthalmology
Table, Surgical, Manual	General
Tray, Custom/Special Procedure	General
Warmer, Radiant, Infant	General
Wheelchair, Manual	Physical Med

INTERNATIONAL IMMUNOLOGY CORP.   800-843-2853
PO Box 972, Murrieta, CA 92564-0972   951-677-5629
FDA Number: n/a   *Fax:* 951-677-6752
E-mail: iic.sales@iicsera.com
Web site: www.iicsera.com
Medical Products Sales Volume: $4,000,000
Year Founded: 1982
Total Employees: 42   *Marketing Staff:* 2   *Sales Staff:* 3
Ownership: Nitto Boseki Co., Ltd.
Quality System Registration Information: ISO9001
Produces/Sells CE-marked Devices: N
Federal Procurement Eligibility: Small Business, Minority Owned
Distribution: Manufacturer Direct, Manufacturer Through Distributor, Manufacturer Through Manufacturer Reps, OEM
General Admin.: Mr. K. Tani/President
          Alice Kleiss/Vice President, General Manager
Mktg./Adv.: Leo Valdez/Manager Product Development
Production: Eduardo Vanella/Manager Materials
          Marlena Murray/Manager Production
          Janell Cole/Manager Quality Assurance

Alpha-1-Acid-Glycoprotein, Antigen, Antiserum, Control	Immunology
Antigen, Antiserum, Control, Albumin	Immunology
Antigen, Antiserum, Control, Alpha-1-Antitrypsin	Immunology
Antigen, Antiserum, Control, Alpha-2-Macroglobulin	Immunology
Antigen, Antiserum, Control, Antithrombin III	Immunology
Antigen, Antiserum, Control, Complement C3	Immunology
Antigen, Antiserum, Control, Complement C4	Immunology
Antigen, Antiserum, Control, Haptoglobin	Immunology
Antigen, Antiserum, Control, IGA	Immunology
Antigen, Antiserum, Control, IGD	Immunology
Antigen, Antiserum, Control, IGE	Immunology
Antigen, Antiserum, Control, IGG (Fc Fragment Specific)	Immunology
Antigen, Antiserum, Control, IGM (Mu Chain Specific)	Immunology
Antigen, Antiserum, Control, Kappa	Immunology
Antigen, Antiserum, Control, Lambda	Immunology
Antigen, Antiserum, Control, Myoglobin	Immunology
Antigen, Antiserum, Control, Other	Immunology
Antigen, Antiserum, Control, Transferrin	Immunology
Antigen, Antiserum, Control, Whole Human Serum	Immunology
Contract Manufacturing, Reagent	General

INTERNATIONAL ISOTOPES IDAHO, INC.
See International Isotopes Inc.

INTERNATIONAL ISOTOPES INC.   800-699-3108
4137 Commerce Circle, Idaho Falls, ID 83401   208-524-5300
FDA Number: 3034521   *Fax:* 208-524-1411
Web site: http://www.intisoid.com
Year Founded: 1995
Ownership: Private
Produces/Sells CE-marked Devices: N
General Admin.: Steve Laflin/President, Chief Executive Officer
Finance: Laurie McKenzie-Carter/Chief Financial Officer

Calibrator Source, Nuclear Sealed	Radiology
Phantom, Flood Source, Nuclear	Radiology
Source, Teletherapy, Radionuclide	Radiology

INTERNATIONAL LIGHT TECHNOLOGIES, INC.   978-818-6180
10 Technology Drive, Peabody, MA 01960
FDA Number: n/a   *Fax:* 978-818-6181
E-mail: ilsales@intl-lighttech.com
Web site: www.intl-lighttech.com
Ownership: Private
Produces/Sells CE-marked Devices: N
Federal Procurement Eligibility: Small Business
Distribution: Manufacturer Direct, Manufacturer Through Manufacturer Reps, OEM, Exporter
General Admin.: Thomas Connolly/President
Mktg./Adv.: Jill Fowler/Manager Advertising & Sales

Bilirubinometer	Chemistry
Photometer	Chemistry
Radiometer, Laser	General
Radiometer, Phototherapy	General
Radiometer, Ultraviolet	General

INTERNATIONAL MEDICAL ELECTRONICS LTD.   800-432-8003
1319 Central Ave., PO BOX 45030,   913-342-3629
Kansas City, MO 64111
FDA Number: 1921974   *Fax:* 913-371-7324
E-mail: magnatherm@aol.com
Web site: http://magnatherm.net

INTERNATIONAL MEDICAL ELECTRONICS LTD. 800-432-8003
(cont'd)
Annual Revenue: $1-$5 Million
Ownership: Private
Produces/Sells CE-marked Devices: N
Federal Procurement Eligibility: Small Business
Distribution: Manufacturer Direct, Exporter
General Admin.: Eugene C. Lipsky/President
Mktg./Adv.: Jeffrey H. Lipsky/Vice President Marketing

Diathermy, Shortwave	Physical Med
Equipment, Management, Pain, Radiofrequency, Non-Invasive	General

INTERNATIONAL MEDICAL EQUIP. BROKERS, INC.
See International Medical Equipment

INTERNATIONAL MEDICAL EQUIPMENT 800.543.8496
170 Vallecitos De Oro, San Marcos, CA 92069 **760-761-0836**
FDA Number: n/a *Fax:* 760.761.0859
E-mail: Info@imebinc.com
Web site: www.imebinc.com
Annual Revenue: $0-$1 Million
Ownership: Private
Produces/Sells CE-marked Devices: N
Distribution: Service Direct

Gas-Machine, Anesthesia	Anesthesiology
Microtome, Cryostat	Pathology
Microtome, Rotary	Pathology
Service, Used Equipment	General
Tissue Processor (Infiltrator)	Pathology

INTERNATIONAL MEDICAL INDUSTRIES 800-344-2554
2881 West McNab Road, **954-917-9570**
Pompano Beach, FL 33069
FDA Number: 1217831 *Fax:* 954-917-9244
E-mail: sales@imiweb.com
Web site: www.imiweb.com
Annual Revenue: $0-$1 Million
Ownership: Private
Produces/Sells CE-marked Devices: N
Federal Procurement Eligibility: Small Business
Distribution: Manufacturer Direct

Cap, Tip, Syringe	General
Check Valve, Retrograde Flow (In-Line)	General
Dispenser, Medication, Liquid	General
Filter, Infusion Line	General
Kit, Administration, Intravenous	General
Needle, Hypodermic, Single Lumen With Syringe	General
Scanner, Nuclear, Rectilinear	Radiology
Set, Administration, Intravenous, Needle-Free	General
Syringe, Piston	General
Transfer Unit, Radioisotope	Radiology

INTERNATIONAL MEDICAL INSTRUMENTS 905-882-8181
(IMI) INC.

1600 Steeles Ave. W,, Concord, ONT L4K 4M2 Canada
FDA Number: n/a
E-mail: imi@interlog.com
Web site: www.interlog.com/~imi
Year Founded: 1986
Total Employees: 10
Ownership: Private
Produces/Sells CE-marked Devices: N
Distribution: Manufacturer Direct, Service Direct, Exclusive Distributor

INTERNATIONAL MEDICAL PROSTHETICS RESEAR
See Bard Peripheral Vascular, Inc.

INTERNATIONAL MEDICAL SYSTEMS INC
See Medical Technology Products, Inc.

INTERNATIONAL MEDICAL SYSTEMS, INC.
See Ziehm Imaging, Inc.

INTERNATIONAL MEDICATION SYSTEMS, LTD. 800-423-4136
1886 Santa Anita Ave., South El Monte, CA 91733
FDA Number: n/a *Fax:* 909-909-5726
E-mail: info@ims-limited.com
Web site: www.ims-limited.com
Ownership: Private
Produces/Sells CE-marked Devices: N

Kit, Anesthesia, Pudendal	Obstetrics/Gynecology
Kit, Sampling, Arterial Blood	Anesthesiology
Needle, Hypodermic, Single Lumen With Syringe	General
Pump, Infusion	General
Splint, Extremity, Non-Inflatable, External	Surgery
Transfer Aid	Physical Med

INTERNATIONAL MYO-KLEBER, INC
See I.M.K. Distributors, Inc.

INTERNATIONAL NEWTECH 877-463-8885
DEVELOPMENT INC.

1629 Fosters Way, Delta, BC V3M-6S7 Canada **604-522-1619**
FDA Number: n/a *Fax:* 604-522-6331
E-mail: info@ind.ca
Web site: www.ind.ca
Year Founded: 1992
Total Employees: 100
Ownership: Private
Produces/Sells CE-marked Devices: N
Distribution: Manufacturer Direct, Exclusive Distributor, Exporter

INTERNATIONAL OPHTHALMIC INDUSTRIES CORP.
See Surgical Tools, Inc.

INTERNATIONAL PLASTICS, LLC 800-665-3464
4965 N. Campbell Dr., **262-781-2270**
Menomonee Falls, WI 53051
FDA Number: 3006369204
E-mail: sales@internationalplasticsllc.com
Web site: www.internationalplasticsllc.com
Ownership: Private
Produces/Sells CE-marked Devices: N

Applier, Surgical, Clip	Surgery
File, Pulp Canal, Endodontic	Dental And Oral
Stimulator, Nerve, Transcutaneous (Pain Relief, TENS)	Cns/Neurology
System, Orientation, Identification, Specimen/Tissue	Pathology

INTERNATIONAL PROJECT ASSISTANCE SVS.
See Ipas

INTERNATIONAL PURIFICATION SYSTEMS, INC.
See Isopure Corp.

INTERNATIONAL RADIOGRAPHIC, INC. 1-504-455-8311
395 Grand Teton Circle, Fayetteville, GA 30215
FDA Number: n/a *Fax:* 404-806-8218
E-mail: dtortorich@hotmail.com
Web site: http://meddevinternational.com
Medical Products Sales Volume: $1,500,000
Annual Revenue: $1-$5 Million
Year Founded: 1985
Total Employees: 6 *Marketing Staff:* 1 *Sales Staff:* 1
Ownership: Private
Produces/Sells CE-marked Devices: Y
Federal Procurement Eligibility: Small Business, Female Owned
Distribution: Exclusive Distributor, Importer, Exporter
General Admin.: David Tortorich/Executive Vice President
Linda Tortorich/President
Mktg./Adv.: Christian Tortorich/Director Marketing

Accelerator, Linear, Medical	Radiology
Radiographic Picture Archiving/Communication System (PACS)	Radiology
Service, Used Equipment	General

INTERNATIONAL SCIENCE AND 800-867-8081
TECHNOLOGY, LP

1544 Sawdust Road, Suite 502, Spring, TX 77380
FDA Number: 1651405 *Fax:* 281-292-5480
Ownership: Private
Produces/Sells CE-marked Devices: N

Caliper, Ophthalmic	Ophthalmology
Cannula, Ophthalmic	Ophthalmology
Cystotome, Ophthalmic	Ophthalmology
Forceps, Ophthalmic	Ophthalmology
Hook, Ophthalmic	Ophthalmology
Knife, Ophthalmic	Ophthalmology
Marker, Ocular	Ophthalmology
Scissors, Ophthalmic	Ophthalmology

INTERNATIONAL STEEL, PLASTIC & GLASS, INC.
See Ispg, Inc.

INTERNATIONAL STRETCHER SYSTEMS 800-229-4180
1605 Hwy #3 West, R.R. 5, **905-774-7766**
Dunnville, ONT N1A-2 Canada
FDA Number: n/a *Fax:* 905-774-7703
E-mail: iss@rescuestretchers.com
Web site: www.rescuestretchers.com
Year Founded: 1983
Total Employees: 10
Ownership: Private
Produces/Sells CE-marked Devices: N
Distribution: Manufacturer Direct, Exporter

INTERNATIONAL TANNING TECHNOLOGIES 800-832-8267
5225 W 140th St., Brook Park, OH 44142
FDA Number: 1527620
Ownership: Private
Produces/Sells CE-marked Devices: N

INTERNATIONAL TANNING TECHNOLOGIES 800-832-8267
(cont'd)

Light, Ultraviolet, Dermatologic	Surgery

INTERNATIONAL TECHNIDYNE CORP. 800-631-5945
23 Nevsky St, Edison, NJ 08820 **732-548-5700**
FDA Number: 2250033 *Fax: 732-548-9824*
Web site: www.itcmed.com
Annual Revenue: $25-$50 Million
Ownership: Thoratec Corporation
Quality System Registration Information: ISO9001
Produces/Sells CE-marked Devices: Y
Distribution: Manufacturer Through Distributor
General Admin.: Lawrence Cohen/President
Mktg./Adv.: Brett Giffin/Vice President Marketing & Sales
Research: Gregory Colella/Vice President Research & Development
Finance: Larry Wojcik/Vice President Finance

Activated Whole Blood Clotting Time	Hematology
Analyzer, Coagulation, Automated	Hematology
Analyzer, Coagulation, Multipurpose	Hematology
Bleeding Time Device	Hematology
Control, Coagulation, Plasma	Hematology
Kit, Sampling, Blood	General
Labware, Blood Collection	Chemistry
Lancet, Blood	General
Needle, Blood Collection	General
Protamine Sulphate	Hematology
Prothrombin Time	Hematology
System, Determination, Fibrinogen	Hematology
Test, Heparin (Clotting Time)	Hematology
Test, Thrombin Time	Hematology
Thromboplastin, Activated Partial	Hematology
Timer, Clot, Automated	Hematology
Timer, Coagulation	Hematology
Tube, Vacuum Sample, With Anticoagulant	Hematology

Medical Product Subsidiaries (Listed Separately)
  International Technidyne Corporation

INTERNATIONAL TECHNIDYNE CORPORATION 732-548-5700
8 Olson Ave., Edison, NJ 08820
FDA Number: 3005234525 *Fax: 732-548-9824*
E-mail: customerservice@itcmed.com
Web site: http://www.itcmed.com
Ownership: International Technidyne Corp.
Produces/Sells CE-marked Devices: N
General Admin.: Mr. Lawrence Cohen/President
Mktg./Adv.: Mr. Brett Giffin/Vice President Marketing & Sales
Production: Mr. Alex Bourdon/Vice President Manufacturing
      Ms. Lesley Traver/Vice President Quality Assurance & Regulatory
Affairs
Research: Mr. Gregory Colella/Vice President Research & Development
Finance: Mr. Larry Wojcik/Vice President Finance

Activated Whole Blood Clotting Time	Hematology
Analyzer, Coagulation, Multipurpose	Hematology
Analyzer, Coagulation, Semi-Automated	Hematology
Bleeding Time Device	Hematology
Computer, Diagnostic, Programmable	Cardiovascular
Control, Coagulation, Plasma	Hematology
Fiber, Absorbent	General
Hemoglobinometer, Automated	Hematology
Labware, Blood Collection	Chemistry
Lancet, Blood	General
Oximeter, Intracardiac	Cardiovascular
Oxyhemoglobin/Carboxyhemoglobin Curve, Carbon-Monoxide	Toxicology
Prothrombin Time	Hematology
System, Determination, Fibrinogen	Hematology
Test, Heparin (Clotting Time)	Hematology
Test, Qualitative And Quantitative Factor Deficiency	Hematology
Test, Thrombin Time	Hematology
Thromboplastin, Activated Partial	Hematology
Timer, Clot, Automated	Hematology

INTERNATIONAL TOOL SPECIALTIES CO.
  See Bestway Products Co.

INTERNATIONAL WEX TECHNOLOGIES INC. 800-722-7549
Suite 1601 - 700 West Pender Street, **604-683-8880**
Vancouver, BC V6C 1 Canada
FDA Number: n/a *Fax: 604-683-8868*
E-mail: wex@wexpharma.com
Web site: www.wextech.ca
Year Founded: 1992
Ownership: Private
Produces/Sells CE-marked Devices: N
Distribution: Manufacturer Direct, Exclusive Distributor

INTERPHASE IMPLANTS, INC. 248-442-1460
19928 Farmington Road, Livonia, MI 48152
FDA Number: 1833828 *Fax: 248-477-4338*
E-mail: interpha@mich.com

INTERPHASE IMPLANTS, INC. 248-442-1460 *(cont'd)*
Web site: www.interphase-implants.com
Year Founded: 1991
Ownership: Private
Produces/Sells CE-marked Devices: N
Distribution: Manufacturer Direct

Bit, Drill	Orthopedics
Guide, Surgical, Instrument	Surgery
Plate, Bone, Orthodontic	Dental And Oral
Screwdriver, Surgical	Surgery

INTERPLEX MEDICAL, LLC 513-248-5120
25 Whitney Dr. Ste 114, Milford, OH 45150
FDA Number: 3005221616

Headlamp, Operating, Battery-Operated	Ophthalmology

INTERPORE CROSS INTERNATIONAL 800-722-4489
181 Technology Dr., Irvine, CA 92618 **949-453-3200**
FDA Number: 2029012 *Fax: 949-453-3225*
Web site: www.interpore.com
Medical Products Sales Volume: $51,000,000
Annual Revenue: $50-$100 Million
Year Founded: 1975
Total Employees: 150 Marketing Staff: 14 Sales Staff: 30
Ownership: Public
Stock Symbol: BONZ
Traded On: NASDAQ
Quality System Registration Information: ISO9001
Produces/Sells CE-marked Devices: Y
Federal Procurement Eligibility: Small Business
Distribution: Manufacturer Direct, Manufacturer Through Distributor, Manufacturer Through Manufacturer Reps
General Admin.: David Mercer/Chairman, Chief Executive Officer
      Joseph Mussey/Chief Operating Officer
      Joe Mussey/President
  Medical Admin.: Michael Hughes/Vice President Health Care
Mktg./Adv.: Mike Soloway/Director Sales Training
      Chris MacDoff/Manager Contract Sales
      Michael Hughes/Vice President International Sales
      M. Ross Simmonds/Vice President Marketing & Sales
      Tom Boyd/Vice President Sales
Production: Prosie Rey-Fessler/Director Quality Assurance & Regulatory Affairs
      Stacy Doty/Manager Materials
      Lynn Rodarti/Manager Regulatory Affairs
      Park Carmon/Vice President Manufacturing
      Park Carmon/Vice President Operations
Research: Phil Mellinger/Vice President Product Development
      Edwin Shors/Vice President Research & Development
Finance: Richard Harrison/Chief Financial Officer, Vice President Finance

Bone Grafting Material, Dental, With Biologic Component	Dental And Oral
Dialyzer, Capillary, Hollow Fiber (Hemodialysis)	Gastroenterology/Urology
Filler, Bone Void, Osteoinduction	Physical Med
Methyl Metacrylate	Cns/Neurology
Stopcock	General
Syringe, Piston	General

INTERPORE ORTHOPAEDICS, INC.
  See Exogen, Inc.

INTERPRETIVE DATA SYSTEMS
  See Idx Systems Corporation

INTERRAD MEDICAL 763-225-6699
181 Cheshire Lane, Suite 100, Plymouth, MN 55441
FDA Number: 3007795799 *Fax: 763-225-6695*
Web site: http://interradmedical.com
Ownership: Private
Produces/Sells CE-marked Devices: N
General Admin.: Mr. Joe Goldberger/President, Chief Executive Officer
  Medical Admin.: Dr. Michael Rosenberg/Chief Medical Officer
Mktg./Adv.: Mr. Jeff Killion/Director Marketing
Production: Dr. Sew-Wah Tay/Vice President Regulatory & Clinical Affairs
Finance: Ms. Nancy Ness/Chief Financial Officer

Implanted Subcutaneous Securement Catheter	General

INTERSCAN CORP. 800-458-6153
21700 Nordhoff Street, PO Box 2496, **818-882-2331**
Chatsworth, CA 91313
FDA Number: n/a *Fax: 818-341-0642*
E-mail: info@gasdetection.com
Web site: www.gasdetection.com
Annual Revenue: $25-$50 Million
Year Founded: 1975
Total Employees: 25 Marketing Staff: 2 Sales Staff: 3
Ownership: Private
Quality System Registration Information: ISO9001
Produces/Sells CE-marked Devices: Y
Federal Procurement Eligibility: Small Business, GSA Contract

INTERSCAN CORP.
800-458-6153 *(cont'd)*

Distribution: Manufacturer Direct, Manufacturer Through Distributor, Manufacturer Through Manufacturer Reps, OEM, Exclusive Distributor, Exporter
General Admin.: Richard Shaw/President, Chief Executive Officer
Mktg./Adv.: Michael Shaw/Executive Vice President Marketing & Sales
  Chrisi Saje/Sales Assistant
  Lori Shaw/Sales Associate
Production: Grant McClure/Production Engineer
  Luis Porres/Production Engineer
Research: Gitty Gilani/Chemist
IS: Scott Richards/Systems Engineer

Analyzer, Ethylene-Oxide	General
Detector, Ethylene-Oxide Leakage	General
Monitor, Biological (Contamination Testing)	General
Monitor, Contamination, Environmental, Personal	General
Monitor, Gas, Atmospheric, Environmental	General

INTERSCIENCE DIAGNOSTICS
See PerkinElmer

INTERSCIENCES INC.
800-661-6431
169 Idema Rd., Markham, ONT L3R 1A9 Canada **905-940-1831**
FDA Number: n/a Fax: 905-940-1832
E-mail: marketing@interscience.com
Web site: www.interscience.com
Year Founded: 1991
Total Employees: 20 *Marketing Staff:* 5 *Sales Staff:* 10
Ownership: Private
Produces/Sells CE-marked Devices: N
Federal Procurement Eligibility: Small Business
Distribution: Manufacturer Direct, Exclusive Distributor, Importer, Exporter

INTERSIGN CORP.
800-322-8426
2156 Amnicola Highway, Chattanooga, TN 37406 **423-698-3085**
FDA Number: n/a Fax: 423-698-2864
E-mail: emailus@intersigncorp.com
Web site: www.intersigncorp.com
Medical Products Sales Volume: $3,400,000
Annual Revenue: $1-$5 Million
Year Founded: 1987
Total Employees: 53 *Marketing Staff:* 4 *Sales Staff:* 35
Ownership: Private
Federal Procurement Eligibility: Small Business
Distribution: Manufacturer Direct
General Admin.: Hank McMahon/Chief Executive Officer
  Mitch McGrath/Chief Executive Officer

Labeling Equipment	General
Sign, Hospital	General

INTERSPEC FABRICS
800-526-2800
P.O. Box 705, Allenwood, NJ 08720 **732-938-4114**
FDA Number: n/a Fax: 732-938-9083
Web site: www.interspec.com
Ownership: Private
Produces/Sells CE-marked Devices: N
Distribution: Manufacturer Direct, Manufacturer Through Distributor, Manufacturer Through Manufacturer Reps, Exporter

Curtain, Cubicle	General
Linen	General

INTERSTATE BATTERY SYSTEM OF AMERICA
800-730-7868
12770 Merit Drive, Suite 1000, Dallas, TX 75251
FDA Number: n/a
E-mail: generalinfo@interstatebatteries.com
Web site: www.interstatebatteries.com
Year Founded: 1952
Total Employees: 1400
Ownership: Private
Produces/Sells CE-marked Devices: N
Distribution: Service Direct, Exclusive Distributor
General Admin.: Norm Miller/Chairman
  Carlos Sepulveda/President, Chief Executive Officer
  Chris Willis/Vice President Human Resources
  Merv Tarde/Vice President Information Technology
Mktg./Adv.: Scott Miller/Vice President Advertising
  Dennis Brown/Vice President International Marketing
  Billy Norris/Vice President National Accounts
Finance: Lisa Huntsberry/Vice President Accounting

Battery	General

INTERSTATE BLOOD BANK, INC.
800-258-9557
5700 Pleasant View Road, Memphis, TN 38134 **901-384-6200**
FDA Number: 173 Fax: 901-384-6210
E-mail: smoss@interstatebloodbank.com
Web site: www.interstatebloodbank.com
Annual Revenue: $50-$100 Million
Year Founded: 1949
Total Employees: 400

INTERSTATE BLOOD BANK, INC.
800-258-9557 *(cont'd)*

Ownership: Private
Produces/Sells CE-marked Devices: N
Federal Procurement Eligibility: Small Business
Distribution: Manufacturer Direct
General Admin.: Mr. Matt Moss/Executive Manager
  Larry Moss/President
  Stephen D. Moss/Vice President
Mktg./Adv.: Randy Hirsh/Manager Sales

Contract Laboratory	General
Serum, Human	Pathology
Supplies, Blood Bank	Hematology

INTERSTATE DENTAL COMPANY INC.
See Temrex Corporation

INTERSURGICAL INC.
315-451-2900
417 Electronics Pkwy., Liverpool, NY 13088
FDA Number: 1319447 Fax: 315-451-3696
E-mail: support@intersurgicalinc.com
Web site: www.intersurgical.com
Medical Products Sales Volume: $240,000
Annual Revenue: $1-$5 Million
Year Founded: 1991
Total Employees: 2 *Marketing Staff:* 2 *Sales Staff:* 5
Ownership: Private
Quality System Registration Information: ISO9002
Produces/Sells CE-marked Devices: N
Federal Procurement Eligibility: Small Business
Distribution: Manufacturer Direct, Manufacturer Through Distributor, OEM, Importer, Exporter
General Admin.: Thomas R. Gunerman/President, Chief Executive Officer
Mktg./Adv.: Mary Sweeney/Manager Marketing
  Kevin J. Flaherty/Vice President Sales
Production: Michael Zalewski/Manager Regulatory Affairs

Absorbent, Carbon-Dioxide	Anesthesiology
Accessories, Catheter	Surgery
Adapter, Anesthesia	Anesthesiology
Airway, Oropharyngeal, Anesthesia	Anesthesiology
Bag, Breathing	Anesthesiology
Circuit, Breathing (W Connector, Adapter, Y Piece)	Anesthesiology
Circuit, Breathing, Ventilator	Anesthesiology
Condenser, Heat And Moisture (Artificial Nose)	Anesthesiology
Connector, Airway (Extension)	Anesthesiology
Contract Assembly	General
Contract Manufacturing, Product, Disposable	General
Drain, Tee (Water Trap)	Anesthesiology
Filter, Bacterial, Breathing Circuit	Anesthesiology
Filter, Ventilator	Anesthesiology
Fitting, Luer	General
Fitting, Other	General
Fixation Device, Tracheal Tube	Anesthesiology
Humidifier, Heat/Moisture Exchange	Anesthesiology
Mask, Oxygen, Aerosol Administration	Anesthesiology
Mask, Oxygen, Low Concentration, Venturi	Anesthesiology
Mask, Oxygen, Non-Rebreathing	Anesthesiology
Mask, Oxygen, Other	General
Mask, Oxygen, Partial Rebreathing	General
Mount, Equipment	General
Mouthpiece, Breathing	Anesthesiology
Nebulizer, Direct Patient Interface	Anesthesiology
Nebulizer, Medicinal	Ear/Nose/Throat
Nebulizer, Non-Heated	General
Support, Breathing Tube	Anesthesiology
Tubing, Corrugated	General
Tubing, Flexible, Medical Gas, Low-Pressure	Anesthesiology
Tubing, Oxygen Connecting	General
Tubing, Plastic	General
Tubing, Ventilator	Anesthesiology
Valve, Breathing	Anesthesiology
Valve, Non-Rebreathing	Anesthesiology

INTERVENTIONAL HEMOSTASIS PRODUCTS, INC.
503-638-9743
1815 Nw 169th Place, Suite 6030, Beaverton, OR 97006
FDA Number: 3005058817

Accessories, Blood Circuit, Hemodialysis	Gastroenterology/Urology
Clamp, Vascular	Cardiovascular

INTERVENTIONAL SPINE, INC.
800-497-0484
13700 Alton Pkwy., Suite 160, Irvine, CA 92618 **949-472-0006**
FDA Number: 2032499 Fax: 949-472-0016
E-mail: cs@i-spineinc.com
Web site: www.i-spineinc.com
Ownership: Private
Produces/Sells CE-marked Devices: N
General Admin.: Walter A. Cuevas/Chief Executive Officer
Mktg./Adv.: Ms. Rebecca Price/Director Business
  Mr. Stephen Colaiezzi/Senior Vice President Marketing
  Mr. Klaus Dahmen/Vice President U.S. Sales

INTERVENTIONAL SPINE, INC.　800-497-0484 *(cont'd)*

Bit, Drill	Orthopedics
Bolt, Nut, Washer	Orthopedics
Compression Instrument	Orthopedics
Countersink	Orthopedics
Cutter, Wire And Pin	Orthopedics
Device, Biopsy, Percutaneous	Surgery
Extractor, Nail	Orthopedics
Gauge, Depth	Orthopedics
Guide, Surgical, Instrument	Surgery
Hammer, Surgical	Surgery
Implant, Fixation Device, Spinal	Orthopedics
Passer, Wire, Orthopedic	Orthopedics
Retractor, Surgical	Surgery
Screw, Fixation, Bone	Orthopedics
Screwdriver	Orthopedics
System, Facet Screw Spinal Device	Orthopedics
Tap, Bone	Orthopedics

INTERVENTIONAL TECHNOLOGIES, INC.　858-268-4488
30590 Cochise Circle, Murrieta, CA 92563
FDA Number: 2030666
Web site: www.bostonscientific.com
Ownership: BOSTON SCIENTIFIC CORPORATION
Stock Symbol: BSX
Traded On: NYSE
Produces/Sells CE-marked Devices: N

Guidewire, Catheter	Cardiovascular

INTERVENTIONAL THERAPIES, LLC.　203-291-4893
One Gorham Island, Suite 9, Westport, CT 06880-3217
FDA Number: 1226550　　*Fax:* 203-341-9800
E-mail: melissa.mazzoni@it-llc.com
Medical Products Sales Volume: $540,000
Total Employees: 7
Ownership: Private
Produces/Sells CE-marked Devices: N
Federal Procurement Eligibility: Small Business

INTL. MEDICAL, INC.　952-890-6547
14470 Burnsville Pkwy., Burnsville, MN 55306
FDA Number: 2120123
Ownership: Private
Produces/Sells CE-marked Devices: N

Meter, Peak Flow, Spirometry	Anesthesiology
Tube, Tracheostomy (W/Wo Connector)	Anesthesiology

INTL. MEDSURG CONNECTION, INC.　847-619-9926
935 N. Plum Grove Road, Suite V, Schaumburg, IL 60173-4770
FDA Number: 1423625　　*Fax:* 847-619-9927
E-mail: info@intlmedsurg.com
Web site: www.intlmedsurg.com
Medical Products Sales Volume: $12,000,000
Year Founded: 1996
Total Employees: 7　　*Sales Staff:* 2
Ownership: Private
Produces/Sells CE-marked Devices: N
Federal Procurement Eligibility: Small Business, Minority Owned
Distribution: Importer
General Admin.: Dr. Omi Bhati/President
　　　　Mr. Dave Fliss/Vice President
　　　　Mr. Manny Gupta/Vice President, General Manager
Mktg./Adv.: Mr. Rory Rochester/Vice President Sales

Cover, Barrier, Protective	General
Drape, Surgical	Surgery
Gauze/sponge, Nonresorbable For External Use	Surgery
Sponge, Internal	Cns/Neurology
Syringe, Irrigating	General

INTOUCH TECHNOLOGIES, INC.　805-562-8686
90 Castilian Dr., Ste. 200, Santa Barbara, CA 93117
FDA Number: n/a　　*Fax:* 805-562-8663
Web site: www.intouchhealth.com
Year Founded: 2002
Ownership: Private
Produces/Sells CE-marked Devices: N
General Admin.: Yulun Wang/Chief Executive Officer, Chairman
　　　　David Adornetto/Chief Financial Officer, Vice President
Operations
Mktg./Adv.: Micheal Chan/Executive Vice President Marketing & Sales
　　　　Charlie Hunier/Vice President Business Development
　　　　Tim Wright/Vice President Strategic Marketing & Communications
　　　　Herb von Winckelmann/Vice President U.S. Sales
Research: Steve Jordan/Executive Vice President Research & Development

Transmitter/Receiver System, Physiological, Radiofrequency	Cardiovascular

INTOXIMETERS, INC.　800-451-8639
8110 Lackland Road, St. Louis, MO 63114　314-429-4000
FDA Number: 1933078　　*Fax:* 314-429-4170

INTOXIMETERS, INC.　800-451-8639 *(cont'd)*
E-mail: sales@intox.com
Web site: www.intox.com
Medical Products Sales Volume: $3,600,000
Annual Revenue: $10-$25 Million
Year Founded: 1945
Total Employees: 50
Ownership: Private
Produces/Sells CE-marked Devices: Y
Federal Procurement Eligibility: Small Business, GSA Contract
Distribution: Manufacturer Direct, Manufacturer Through Manufacturer Reps
General Admin.: M. Rankine Forrester/Chief Executive Officer
　　　　Christopher H. Dalton/President
Mktg./Adv.: Mark E. Gilmer/Manager National Sales

Alcohol Breath Trapping Device	Toxicology
Test, Ethyl Alcohol	Toxicology

INTRA-LOCK INTERNATIONAL　561-447-8282
6560 West Rogers Circle, Suite 24, Boca Raton, FL 33487
FDA Number: 3003631996

Implant, Endosseous	Dental And Oral

INTRACEL CORPORATION　301-668-8400
93 Monocacy Blvd., Unit A8, Frederick, MD 21701
FDA Number: n/a　　*Fax:* 301-668-6317
E-mail: info@intracel.com
Web site: www.intracel.com
Annual Revenue: $1-$5 Million
Total Employees: 500　　*Marketing Staff:* 1　　*Sales Staff:* 1
Ownership: Intracel Corporation
Quality System Registration Information: ISO9000
Produces/Sells CE-marked Devices: N
Distribution: Manufacturer Direct, Manufacturer Through Distributor, Exclusive Distributor
General Admin.: Dr. Michael G. Hanna/President
　　　　Leslie Ivy/Vice President Human Resources
　　　　Peter R. Nardin/Vice President, General Manager
Mktg./Adv.: John Borger/Manager International & National Sales
Production: Maysoon Hassan/Director Quality Assurance
　　　　Barry Phelps/Manager Materials
　　　　Nicholas Pomaro/Vice President Manufacturing
Research: Martin V. Haspel/Vice President Product Development

Antibody, Monoclonal	Microbiology
Contract R&D, Diagnostics	General

Medical Product Subsidiaries (Listed Separately)
　Intracel Corporation

INTRALASE CORP.　714-247-8200
9701 Jeronimo Road, Irvine, CA 92618-1916
FDA Number: 2032002
Ownership: Private
Produces/Sells CE-marked Devices: N

Laser, Surgical	Surgery

INTRALUMINAL THERAPEUTICS, INC.　800-513-4458
6354 Corte Del Abeto, Suite A,　760-918-1820
Carlsbad, CA 92009
FDA Number: 2031958　　*Fax:* 760-918-1823
E-mail: ahedrick@intraluminal.com
Web site: www.intraluminal.com
Year Founded: 1997
Ownership: Private
Produces/Sells CE-marked Devices: Y
Distribution: Manufacturer Direct, Manufacturer Through Distributor

Catheter, Steerable	Cardiovascular
Control System, Catheter, Steerable	Cardiovascular
Guidewire, Catheter	Cardiovascular

INTRAMEDICAL IMAGING LLC　800-519-3959
12340 Santa Monica Blvd., Suite 227,　310-826-9834
Los Angeles, CA 90025
FDA Number: 2031874　　*Fax:* 310-826-9854
E-mail: fd@intra-medical.com
Web site: www.intra-medical.com
Medical Products Sales Volume: $2,000,000
Annual Revenue: $1-$5 Million
Year Founded: 1998
Total Employees: 6　　*Marketing Staff:* 2　　*Sales Staff:* 5
Ownership: Private
Quality System Registration Information: ISO9002
Produces/Sells CE-marked Devices: Y
Federal Procurement Eligibility: Small Business
Distribution: Manufacturer Direct, Manufacturer Through Distributor, Manufacturer Through Manufacturer Reps, Service Direct, Exclusive Distributor, Importer, Exporter
General Admin.: Dr. Farhad Daghighian/President
Mktg./Adv.: Terry Groome/Vice President Marketing & Sales

MANUFACTURER PROFILES

INTRAMEDICAL IMAGING LLC   800-519-3959 *(cont'd)*
Production: Dr. Mike Loloyan/Director Product Development & Customer Support
     Mrs. Azita Sach/Vice President Customer Support
Probe, Detector, Flow, Blood, Laparoscopy, Ultrasonic   Surgery
Probe, Uptake, Nuclear   Radiology

INTRAOP MEDICAL CORP.   408-636-1020
570 Del Rey Ave, Sunnyvale, CA 94085
FDA Number: 2953704   *Fax:* 408-636-0022
Web site: http://www.intraopmedical.com
Year Founded: 1993
Ownership: Public
Stock Symbol: IOPM
Traded On: OTC Bulletin
Produces/Sells CE-marked Devices: N
General Admin.: Mr. John Powers/Chief Executive Officer
Mktg./Adv.: Mr. Wink Jones/Vice President Marketing
Production: Mr. Andy Merrill/Vice President Operations
     Mr. Richard Belford/Vice President Quality Assurance & Regulatory
Affairs
Research: Dr. Donald Goer/Chief Scientist
Finance: Mr. J.K. Hullet/Chief Financial Officer
Radiotherapy Unit, Charged-Particle   Radiology

INTRAPACE INC.   650-316 4070
967 N. Shoreline Blvd., Mountain View, CA 94043
FDA Number: n/a
Web site: http://www.intrapace.com
Year Founded: 2001
Ownership: Private
Produces/Sells CE-marked Devices: N
General Admin.: Mr. Chuck Brynelsen/President, Chief Executive Officer
Production: Mr. Steve Schellenberg/Vice President Operations
     Mr. Robert Nardelli/Vice President Quality Assurance & Regulatory
Affairs
Research: Mr. Vince Kapral/Director Research & Development
Finance: Mr. Gary Castro/Vice President Admin., Finance
Implant, Intragastric, Obesity, Morbid   Gastroenterology/Urology

INTRAVASCULAR INCORPORATED   800-917-3234
3600 Bur Wood Drive, Waukegan, IL 60085   847-596-7700
FDA Number: n/a   *Fax:* 847-596-7710
E-mail: contactus@intravascularinc.com
Web site: www.intravascularinc.com
Year Founded: 2001
Total Employees: 7   *Marketing Staff:* 3   *Sales Staff:* 3
Ownership: Private
Produces/Sells CE-marked Devices: N
Distribution: Exclusive Distributor
General Admin.: Mr. David Sanders/Chief Executive Officer, Chairman
     Mr. Steven Aperavich/President
Mktg./Adv.: Mr. Joseph Scully/Vice President Sales
Production: Ms. Diana Fitzgibbons/Design Engineer
     Mr. Douglas Bulgrin/Vice President Operations
Accessories, Catheter   Surgery
Catheter, Infusion   Surgery
Connector, Catheter   Surgery
Set, Administration, Intravenous, Needle-Free   General

INTRICON CORPORATION   651-636-9770
1260 Red Fox Rd., Arden Hills, MN 55112
FDA Number: 2134850   *Fax:* 651-636-9503
Web site: www.intricon.com
Year Founded: 1977
Total Employees: 625
Ownership: Public
Stock Symbol: IIN
Traded On: NASDAQ
Produces/Sells CE-marked Devices: N
General Admin.: Scott Longval/Chief Financial Officer, Treasurer
     Mark Gorder/President, Chief Executive Officer
Mktg./Adv.: Mike Geraci/Vice President Marketing & Sales
     Michael Geraci/Vice President Sales
Production: Greg Gruenhagen/Vice President Quality Assurance & Regulatory
Affairs
Research: Chris Conger/Vice President Research & Development
Hearing Aid, Air Conduction, Transcutaneous System   Ear/Nose/Throat

INTRINSIC THERAPEUTICS INC.   781-932-0222
30 Commerce Way, Woburn, MA 01801
FDA Number: 3006232063   *Fax:* 781-932-0252
Web site: http://www.intrinsic-therapeutics.com
Year Founded: 2000
Ownership: Private
Produces/Sells CE-marked Devices: N
General Admin.: Mr. Greg Lambrecht/Executive Director
     Mr. Cary Hagan/President, Chief Executive Officer
Production: Mr. Noel Rolon/Vice President Regulatory & Clinical Affairs

INTRINSIC THERAPEUTICS INC.   781-932-0222 *(cont'd)*
Research: Mr. Jacob Einhorn/Vice President Research & Development
Finance: Mr. Scott LeBlanc/Director Finance
Gauge, Depth   Orthopedics
Orthopedic Implant Material   Orthopedics
Orthopedic Manual Surgical Instrument   Orthopedics

INTRIQUIP INSTRUMENTS   800-361-3777
1862 Angus St., Regina, SK S4T-1Z4 Canada   306-584-3993
FDA Number: n/a   *Fax:* 306-525-5112
E-mail: info@intriquip.com
Web site: http://www.intriquip.com/
Year Founded: 1989
Total Employees: 10
Ownership: Private
Produces/Sells CE-marked Devices: N
Distribution: Importer

INTRONIX TECHNOLOGIES CORPORATION   800-819-9996
26 McEwan Dr., Unit 15,   905-951-3361
Bolton, ONT L7E-1 Canada
FDA Number: n/a   *Fax:* 905-951-3192
E-mail: inx@intronixtech.com
Web site: www.intronix.com
Year Founded: 1984
Ownership: Private
Produces/Sells CE-marked Devices: N
Distribution: Manufacturer Direct, Exporter

INTUBATION PLUS, INC.   814-663-4688
1524 Enterprise Rd., Corry, PA 16407
FDA Number: 3003789461
E-mail: info@intubationplus.com
Web site: www.intubationplus.com
Ownership: Private
Produces/Sells CE-marked Devices: N
Laryngoscope, Rigid   Anesthesiology

INTUITIVE SURGICAL, INC.   888-409-4774
1266 Kifer Road, Sunnyvale, CA 94086-5304   408-523-2100
FDA Number: 2955842   *Fax:* 408-523-1390
Web site: www.intuitivesurgical.com
Year Founded: 1995
Total Employees: 859
Ownership: Public
Stock Symbol: ISRG
Traded On: NASDAQ
Produces/Sells CE-marked Devices: N
General Admin.: Lonnie M. Smith/Chief Executive Officer, Chairman
     Mr. Gary S. Guthart/President, Chief Operating Officer
Cannula, Manipulator/Injector, Uterine   Obstetrics/Gynecology
Electrosurgical Unit, Cutting & Coagulation Device   Surgery
Laparoscope, General & Plastic Surgery   Surgery
Sizer, Heart Valve Prosthesis   Cardiovascular
System, Surgical, Computer Controlled Instrument   Surgery
Table, Operating Room, AC-Powered   Surgery
Wrap, Sterilization   General
Medical Product Subsidiaries (Listed Separately)
Computer Motion, Inc.

INTUITY MEDICAL INC.   408-530-1700
350 Potrero Avenue, Sunnyvale, CA 94085
FDA Number: n/a   *Fax:* 408-530-1717
Web site: http://www.presspogo.com
Ownership: Private
Produces/Sells CE-marked Devices: N
General Admin.: Mr. Emory Anderson/President, Chief Executive Officer
Mktg./Adv.: Ms. Kelley Lipman/Vice President Marketing
Production: Mr. Nelson Lam/Vice President Quality Control & Regulatory Affairs
Research: Mr. John Howard/Vice President Research & Development

INTUSOFT   310-833-0710
P.O. Box 710, San Pedro, CA 90733-9918
FDA Number: n/a   *Fax:* 310-833-9658
E-mail: info@intusoft.com
Web site: www.intusoft.com
Ownership: Private
Produces/Sells CE-marked Devices: N
Computer Software   General

INVACARE CANADA   800-668-5324
16769 Boul Hymus, Kirkland H9H 3L4 Canada   440 3296356
FDA Number: 3002416487   *Fax:* 440 3263458
E-mail: brogers@invacare.com
Web site: www.invacare.com
Medical Products Sales Volume: $3,300,000
Total Employees: 170   *Marketing Staff:* 3   *Sales Staff:* 12
Ownership: Invacare Corporation

INVACARE CANADA   800-668-5324 *(cont'd)*

Traded On: NASDAQ
Quality System Registration Information: ISO9002
Produces/Sells CE-marked Devices: Y
Federal Procurement Eligibility: Small Business
Distribution: Manufacturer Direct, Exporter

INVACARE CORPORATION   800-327-9438
2101 East Lake Mary Blvd., Sanford, FL 32773   407-321-5630
FDA Number: 1031452
E-mail: info@invacare.com
Web site: www.invacare.com
Ownership: Invacare Corporation
Stock Symbol: IVC
Traded On: NYSE
Produces/Sells CE-marked Devices: N

Bed, Manual	General
Chair/Table, Medical	General
Generator, Oxygen, Portable	Anesthesiology
Humidifier, Respiratory Gas, (Direct Patient Interface)	Anesthesiology
Mask, Oxygen, Other	General
Mattress, Air Flotation	General
Ventilator, Non-Continuous (Respirator)	Anesthesiology

INVACARE CORPORATION   800-333-6900
One Invacare Way, Elyria, OH 44035   440-329-6000
                  Fax: 877-619-7996
FDA Number: 1525712
E-mail: info@invacare.com
Web site: http://www.invacare.com
Medical Products Sales Volume: $1,490,000,000
Annual Revenue: More than $1 Billion
Year Founded: 1979
Total Employees: 5700   *Marketing Staff:* 40   *Sales Staff:* 130
Ownership: Public
Stock Symbol: IVC
Traded On: NYSE
Quality System Registration Information: ISO9001
Produces/Sells CE-marked Devices: N
Distribution: Manufacturer Through Distributor, Manufacturer Through Manufacturer Reps, Exporter
General Admin.: Mr. A. Malachi Mixon/Chief Executive Officer
        Mr. Robert K Gudbranson/Chief Financial Officer, Senior Vice President
        Mr. Gerry B. Blouch/Chief Operating Officer
        Mr. Doug Newlin/Compliance Officer
        J. B. Richey/President
Mktg./Adv.: Lou Slangen/Senior Vice President Marketing & Sales

Accessories, Walker	General
Accessories, Wheelchair	Physical Med
Analyzer, Gas, Oxygen, Gaseous Phase	Anesthesiology
Arm Rest	Physical Med
Aspirator, Nasal	Ear/Nose/Throat
Aspirator, Tracheal	Ear/Nose/Throat
Bed, Electric	General
Bed, Electric, Home-Use	General
Bed, Flotation Therapy, Powered	Physical Med
Bed, Manual	General
Bedrail	General
Cane, Safety Walk	Physical Med
Cannula, Nasal	General
Chair, Adjustable, Mechanical	Physical Med
Chair, Bath	General
Chair, Geriatric	General
Chair, Pediatric	General
Chair, Position, Electric	Physical Med
Chair, Rehabilitation	General
Chair, Shower	General
Chair, With Casters	Physical Med
Commode (Toilet)	General
Commode Seat	General
Component, Wheelchair	Physical Med
Compressor, Air, Portable	Anesthesiology
Concentrator, Oxygen	Anesthesiology
Continuous Positive Airway Pressure Unit (CPAP, CPPB)	Anesthesiology
Crutch	Physical Med
Cushion, Other	General
Cushion, Ring, Foam Rubber	General
Cushion, Wheelchair (Pad)	Physical Med
Footrest, Wheelchair	Physical Med
Frame, Traction	Orthopedics
Generator, Oxygen, Portable	Anesthesiology
Holder, Needle, Other	Surgery
Humidifier, Respiratory Gas, (Direct Patient Interface)	Anesthesiology
Lift, Patient	General
Mask, Other	General
Mattress, Bed	General
Nebulizer, Medicinal	Ear/Nose/Throat
Oximeter, Pulse	General
Rail, Bath	General
Scooter (Motorized 3-Wheeled Vehicle)	Physical Med

INVACARE CORPORATION   800-333-6900 *(cont'd)*

Support, Back	Orthopedics
Tips And Pads, Cane, Crutch And Walker	Physical Med
Transfer Aid	Physical Med
Tray, Walker	General
Ventilator, Non-Continuous (Respirator)	Anesthesiology
Wheelchair, Manual	Physical Med
Wheelchair, Powered	Physical Med

Medical Product Subsidiaries (Listed Separately)
   Adaptive Switch Laboratories, Inc.
   Altimate Medical, Inc.
   Champion Mfg. Inc.
   Garden City Medical, Inc.
   Invacare Canada
   Invacare Corporation
   Invacare Supply Group
   Invacare Supply Group, Inc
   Invacare Top End
   The Aftermarket Group

INVACARE SUPPLY GROUP   440-329-6356
111 Interstate Blvd., Jamesburg, NJ 08831
FDA Number: 3004635535
E-mail: service.isg@invacare.com
Web site: www.invacaresg.com
Year Founded: 1975
Ownership: Invacare Corporation
Stock Symbol: IVC
Traded On: NYSE
Produces/Sells CE-marked Devices: N

INVACARE SUPPLY GROUP   508-429-1000
11231 Jersey Blvd, Suite 101, Cucamonga, CA 91730
FDA Number: 2085237
E-mail: service.isg@invacare.com
Web site: www.invacaresg.com
Year Founded: 1975
Ownership: Invacare Corporation
Stock Symbol: IVC
Traded On: NYSE
Produces/Sells CE-marked Devices: N

INVACARE SUPPLY GROUP   508-429-1000
1825 West Park Dr., Suite 200, Grand Prairie, TX 75050
FDA Number: 1647140
E-mail: service.isg@invacare.com
Web site: www.invacaresg.com
Year Founded: 1975
Ownership: Invacare Corporation
Stock Symbol: IVC
Traded On: NYSE
Produces/Sells CE-marked Devices: N

INVACARE SUPPLY GROUP, AN INVACARE CO.   800-225-4792
75 October Hill Road, Holliston, MA 01746   508-893-1200
FDA Number: 1223502   *Fax:* 508-429-1581
E-mail: service.isg@invacare.com
Web site: www.invacaresupplygroup.com
Medical Products Sales Volume: $37,300,000
Annual Revenue: $100-$500 Million
Year Founded: 1975
Total Employees: 125   *Marketing Staff:* 10   *Sales Staff:* 45
Ownership: Public
Stock Symbol: IVC
Traded On: NYSE
Produces/Sells CE-marked Devices: N
Federal Procurement Eligibility: Small Business
Distribution: Exclusive Distributor
General Admin.: Michael A. Perry/Vice President, General Manager
Mktg./Adv.: Greg Bosco/Director Marketing
        Bill Leonard/Manager Contract Sales
        Florence Newcum/Services Manager
        Rick Safarz/Vice President, Manager Sales

Catheter, Urinary	Gastroenterology/Urology
Chair, Bath	General
Collector, Ostomy	Gastroenterology/Urology
Diaper, Adult	General
Drainage Unit, Urinary	General
Dressing, Other	General
Glove, Patient Examination	General
Irrigator, Ostomy	Gastroenterology/Urology
Kit, Administration, Enteral	Gastroenterology/Urology
Monitor, Blood Glucose (Test)	Gastroenterology/Urology
Ostomy Appliance (Ileostomy, Colostomy)	Gastroenterology/Urology
Protector, Ostomy	Gastroenterology/Urology
Sphygmomanometer, Aneroid (Arterial Pressure)	General
Stimulator, Nerve, Transcutaneous (Pain Relief, TENS)	Cns/Neurology
Surgical Instrument, Disposable	Surgery

INVACARE SUPPLY GROUP, AN INVACARE CO.   800-225-4792
(cont'd)

     Surgical Instrument, Non-Powered, Neurosurgical   Cns/Neurology

INVACARE SUPPLY GROUP, INC   508-429-1000
     3507 N. Olive Rd, South Bend, IN 46628
     FDA Number: 1834090
     E-mail: service.isg@invacare.com
     Web site: www.invacaresg.com
     Year Founded: 1975
     Ownership: Invacare Corporation
     Stock Symbol: IVC
     Traded On: NYSE
     Produces/Sells CE-marked Devices: N

INVACARE TOP END   800-532-8677
     4501 63rd Circle North,   727-522-8677
     Pinellas Park, FL 33781
     FDA Number: 1056571
     E-mail: info@topendwheelchair.com
     Web site: www.topendwheelchair.com
     Year Founded: 1986
     Ownership: Invacare Corporation
     Stock Symbol: IVC
     Traded On: NYSE
     Produces/Sells CE-marked Devices: N
     Wheelchair, Manual   Physical Med
     Wheelchair, Powered   Physical Med

INVACARE TOP END SPORTS AND   800-532-8677
RECREATION PRODUCTS

     4501 63rd Circle N., Pinellas Park, FL 33781
        727-522-8677
     FDA Number: n/a   *Fax:* 727-522-1007
     E-mail: askinvacare@invacare.com
     Web site: www.invacare.com
     Medical Products Sales Volume: $2,000,000
     Annual Revenue: $1-$5 Million
     Total Employees: 25   *Marketing Staff:* 4
     Ownership: Invacare Corporation
     Stock Symbol: IVCR
     Traded On: NASDAQ
     Quality System Registration Information: ISO9000
     Produces/Sells CE-marked Devices: N
     Mktg./Adv.: Mary Carol Peterson/Director Marketing
     Production: Jim Rivers/Manager Materials
         Al Crisp/Plant Manager
     Research: Christopher Peterson/Manager Research & Development
     Wheelchair, Special Grade   Physical Med

INVAMEX S.A. DE C.V.   440-329-6595
     Carretera Reynosa-Matamros,, Km#1,
     Reynosa Tamaulipas Mexico
     FDA Number: 9616091
     Wheelchair, Manual   Physical Med

INVAQUEST   406-543-4228
     3116 Old Pond Rd., Missoula, MT 59802-1420
     FDA Number: 3030747
     Ownership: Private
     Produces/Sells CE-marked Devices: N
     Accessories, Wheelchair   Physical Med

INVATEC   +1 877 446 8283
     3101 Emrick Blvd, Suite 113, Bethlehem, PA 18020
     FDA Number: 3006466080   *Fax:* +1 610 694 8115
     E-mail: info@invatec-us.com
     Web site: www.invatec.com
     Year Founded: 1996
     Ownership: Medtronic, Inc.
     Produces/Sells CE-marked Devices: N
     Catheter, Percutaneous   Cardiovascular

INVECARE   800-333-6900
     39400 Taylor St., North Ridgeville, OH 44039
         440-329-6990
     FDA Number: 9200369   *Fax:* 440-329-6270
     Medical Products Sales Volume: $10,000,000
     Ownership: Private
     Produces/Sells CE-marked Devices: N
     Federal Procurement Eligibility: Small Business
     Distribution: Manufacturer Through Manufacturer Reps, Exporter
     General Admin.: Wally Reams/Vice President, General Manager
     Mktg./Adv.: Brad Moore/Director Marketing
         Brig Carr/Director Sales
     Chair, Bath   General
     Chair, Shower   General
     Commode Seat   General
     Rail, Bath   General
     Rail, Commode   General

INVECARE   800-333-6900 *(cont'd)*
     Rail, Wall Side   General

INVENEX LABORATORIES
     See Astellas Pharma Us, Inc.

INVENSYS PROCESS SYSTEMS   866-746-6477
     5601 Granite Parkway III, Suite 1000,   1.469.365.6400
     Plano, TX 75024
     FDA Number: n/a
     E-mail: support@invensys.com
     Web site: ips.invensys.com
     Annual Revenue: $1-$5 Million
     Ownership: Foxboro Company, The
     Quality System Registration Information: ISO9001
     Produces/Sells CE-marked Devices: N
     Distribution: Manufacturer Through Distributor, Manufacturer Through
     Manufacturer Reps
     Cell, Spectrophotometer   Chemistry
     Chromatography Equipment, Gas   Chemistry
     Chromatography Equipment, Liquid   Chemistry
     Monitor, Gas, Atmospheric, Environmental   General
     Photometer, Flame, General Use   Toxicology
     Solvent, Spectrophotometer   Chemistry
     Spectrometer, Infrared   Chemistry

INVENTIVE PRODUCTS, INC.
     See Wright Products, Inc.

INVENTIVE RESOURCES, INC.   209-545-1663 É_
     5038 Salida Blvd., Salida, CA 95368
     FDA Number: n/a
     Ownership: Private
     Produces/Sells CE-marked Devices: N
     Device, Repositioning, Jaw   Dental And Oral

INVERNESS CORP.   800) 423-2060
     6 Hazel Street, PO Box 2973,   (774) 203-1130
     Aattleboro, MA 02703
     FDA Number: 2243569
     Ownership: Private
     Stock Symbol: IMA
     Traded On: AMEX
     Produces/Sells CE-marked Devices: N
     Perforator, Ear-Lobe   Ear/Nose/Throat

INVERNESS MEDICAL   800-257-9525
     2 Research Way, Princeton, NJ 08540   609-627-8038
     FDA Number: 3004011380
     Web site: www.invernessmedicalpd.com
     Ownership: Alere, Inc.
     Stock Symbol: IMA
     Traded On: AMEX
     Produces/Sells CE-marked Devices: Y
     Enzymatic Esterase-Oxidase, Cholesterol   Chemistry
     Enzyme Immunoassay, Cannabinoids   Toxicology
     Enzyme Immunoassay, Cocaine And Cocaine Metabolites   Toxicology
     Kit, Pregnancy Test, Over The Counter, HCG   Chemistry
     Radioimmunoassay, Luteinizing Hormone   Chemistry

INVERNESS MEDICAL INC.
     See Inverness Medical Inc.

INVERNESS MEDICAL INNOVATIONS NORTH   (877) 441-7440
AMERICA, INC
     30 S. Keller Road, Suite 100, Lockhart, FL 32810
     FDA Number: 3006984151
     Web site: www.invernessmedical.com
     Ownership: Alere, Inc.
     Stock Symbol: IMA
     Traded On: AMEX
     Produces/Sells CE-marked Devices: Y

INVERNESS MEDICAL INNOVATIONS, INC.
     See Alere, Inc.

INVERNESS MEDICAL PROFESSIONAL   858-535-2030
DIAGNOSTICS-SAN DIE
     4106 Sorrento Valley Boulevard, San Diego, CA 92121
     FDA Number: 3005758701   *Fax:* 858-430-3132
     E-mail: info@innovaconinc.com
     Web site: www.innovaconinc.com
     Ownership: Alere, Inc.
     Stock Symbol: IMA
     Traded On: AMEX
     Produces/Sells CE-marked Devices: Y
     Antigen, Streptococcus SPP.   Microbiology
     Campylobacter Pylori   Microbiology
     Kit, Pregnancy Test, Over The Counter, HCG   Chemistry
     Radioimmunoassay, Follicle Stimulating Hormone   Chemistry
     Radioimmunoassay, Human Chorionic Gonadotropin   Chemistry

INVERNESS MEDICAL PROFESSIONAL 858-535-2030 (cont'd)
Radioimmunoassay, Luteinizing Hormone	Chemistry
Reagent, Occult Blood	Hematology
Test, Infectious Mononucleosis	Immunology

INVERNESS MEDICAL, INC
See Alere, Inc.

INVERSE TECHNOLOGY CORP. 800-222-5778
1000 West O St., Suite B, Lincoln, NE 68528
FDA Number: 1933001
Stirrup, External Brace Component	Physical Med

INVIA, LLC 734-205-1231
3025 Boardwalk Street, Suite 200, Ann Arbor, MI 48108
FDA Number: 3004993756 Fax: 734-205-1537
E-mail: web@inviasolutions.com
Web site: www.inviasolutions.com
Ownership: Private
Produces/Sells CE-marked Devices: N
Scanner, Emission Computed Tomography	Radiology

INVINCIBLE OFFICE FURNITURE CO. 800-558-4417
PO Box 1117, Manitowoc, WI 54221 920-682-4601
FDA Number: n/a Fax: 920-683-2970
E-mail: tmeissner@invincible.cc
Web site: www.invinciblefurniture.com
Medical Products Sales Volume: $9,200,000
Annual Revenue: $1-$5 Million
Year Founded: 1913
Total Employees: 100 Marketing Staff: 6 Sales Staff: 82
Ownership: Private
Produces/Sells CE-marked Devices: N
Federal Procurement Eligibility: Small Business, GSA Contract
Distribution: Exclusive Distributor
General Admin.: John A. Schuette/President
Mktg./Adv.: Brett Bogin/Vice President Sales
Production: Tina M. Meissner/Manager Customer Services
Mark Hatenbeller/Plant Manager
Cabinet Casework, General Purpose	General
Cabinet Casework, Modular	General
Chair, Adjustable, Mechanical	Physical Med

INVIRION, INC. 866-231-8378
2350 Pilgrim Hwy., Frankfort, MI 49635
FDA Number: n/a
Ownership: Private
Produces/Sells CE-marked Devices: N
Reagents, Specific, Analyte	Hematology

INVITROGEN CANADA INC. 800-263-6236
5250 Mainway, Burlington, ONT L7L 5Z1 Canada
FDA Number: n/a Fax: 800-387-1007
E-mail: caorders@invitrogen.com
Web site: www.invitrogen.com
Total Employees: 9500
Ownership: LIFE TECHNOLOGIES CORPORATION
Stock Symbol: LIFE
Traded On: NASDAQ
Produces/Sells CE-marked Devices: N
Distribution: Exclusive Distributor

INVITROGEN CORPORATION 800-955-6288
101 Lincoln Centre Drive, Foster City, CA 94404
FDA Number: n/a
Web site: www.invitrogen.com
Annual Revenue: $25-$50 Million
Ownership: LIFE THERAPEUTICS INC.
Produces/Sells CE-marked Devices: N
Distribution: Manufacturer Direct
2nd Antibody (Species Specific Anti-Animal Gamma Globulin)	Immunology
Analyzer, Chromosome, Automated	Pathology
Antibody, Other	General
Antigen, Antiserum, Control, Bence-Jones Protein	Immunology
Antigen, Antiserum, Control, FAB	Immunology
Antigen, Antiserum, Control, FAB, FITC	Immunology
Antigen, Antiserum, Control, FAB, Rhodamine	Immunology
Antigen, Antiserum, Control, IGA	Immunology
Antigen, Antiserum, Control, IGA, FITC	Immunology
Antigen, Antiserum, Control, IGA, Peroxidase	Immunology
Antigen, Antiserum, Control, IGD	Immunology
Antigen, Antiserum, Control, IGD, FITC	Immunology
Antigen, Antiserum, Control, IGD, Peroxidase	Immunology
Antigen, Antiserum, Control, IGE	Immunology
Antigen, Antiserum, Control, IGE, FITC	Immunology
Antigen, Antiserum, Control, IGE, Peroxidase	Immunology
Antigen, Antiserum, Control, IGG (FAB Fragment Specific)	Immunology
Antigen, Antiserum, Control, IGG (Gamma Chain Specific)	Immunology
Antigen, Antiserum, Control, IGG, FITC	Immunology
Antigen, Antiserum, Control, IGG, Peroxidase	Immunology

INVITROGEN CORPORATION 800-955-6288 (cont'd)
Antigen, Antiserum, Control, IGG, Rhodamine	Immunology
Antigen, Antiserum, Control, IGM (Mu Chain Specific)	Immunology
Antigen, Antiserum, Control, IGM, FITC	Immunology
Antigen, Antiserum, Control, IGM, Peroxidase	Immunology
Antigen, Antiserum, Control, IGM, Rhodamine	Immunology
Antigen, Antiserum, Control, Kappa	Immunology
Antigen, Antiserum, Control, Kappa, FITC	Immunology
Antigen, Antiserum, Control, Lambda	Immunology
Antigen, Antiserum, Control, Lambda, FITC	Immunology
Antigen, Antiserum, Control, Lymphocyte Typing	Immunology
Plate, Radial Immunodiffusion	Immunology
Stain, Dye Solution	Pathology
Test, Cancer Detection, Monoclonal Antibody	Immunology
Test, Receptor, Interleukin, Serum	Immunology

INVITROGEN CORPORATION
See Life Technologies Corporation

INVITROGEN CORPORATION
See Life Technologies Corporation

INVITRON
See Centocor, Inc.

INVITRX, INC. 877-468-4879
101 Theory, suite 100, Irvine, CA 92617 949-856-3142
FDA Number: 2032826 Fax: 888-389-7949
E-mail: info@invitrx.com
Web site: www.invitrx.com
Ownership: Private
Produces/Sells CE-marked Devices: N
General Admin.: Mr. Habib Torfi/Chief Executive Officer
Dressing, Wound and Burn, Interactive	Surgery

INVIVO 800-331-3220
12501 Research Parkway, Orlando, FL 32826 407-275-3220
FDA Number: 1056069 Fax: 407-249-2022
E-mail: info@invivocorp.com
Web site: http://www.invivocorp.com
Annual Revenue: $10-$25 Million
Year Founded: 1987
Ownership: Private
Quality System Registration Information: ISO9001
Produces/Sells CE-marked Devices: Y
Federal Procurement Eligibility: Small Business
Distribution: Manufacturer Through Manufacturer Reps, OEM
General Admin.: Stuart Baumgarten/President
Mr. James B. Hawkins/President, Chief Executive Officer
Mktg./Adv.: Cathy Yudzevich/Manager Investor Relations
Leon Lumens/Manager Sales
Terence Yip/Manager Sales
Coil, Magnetic Resonance, Specialty	Radiology
Component, Other	General
Nuclear Magnetic Resonance Imaging System	Radiology

INVIVO 352-336-0010
3650 N.E. 53rd Ave., Gainesville, FL 32608
FDA Number: 3005722672 Fax: 352-336-1401
E-mail: info@invivocorp.com
Web site: www.invivocorp.com
Year Founded: 1987
Ownership: Private
Produces/Sells CE-marked Devices: N
General Admin.: Stuart Baumgarten/President
James B. Hawkins/President, Chief Executive Officer
Mktg./Adv.: Cathy Yudzevich/Manager Investor Relations
Leon Lumens/Manager Sales
Terence Yip/Manager Sales

INVIVO CORPORATION 425-487-7000
12151 Research Pkwy., Orlando, FL 32826
FDA Number: 1051786
Ownership: Private
Produces/Sells CE-marked Devices: N
Analyzer, Gas, Carbon-Dioxide, Gaseous Phase (Capnograph)	Anesthesiology
Analyzer, Gas, Nitrous-Oxide, Gaseous Phase	Anesthesiology
Cable, Electrode	Physical Med
Computer, Blood Pressure	Cardiovascular
Connector, Airway (Extension)	Anesthesiology
Cuff, Blood Pressure	Cardiovascular
Detector, Arrhythmia Alarm	Cardiovascular
Electrode, Cutaneous	Cns/Neurology
Monitor, Bed Patient	General
Monitor, Blood Pressure, Indirect, Semi-Automatic	Cardiovascular
Monitor, Cardiac (Cardiotachometer & Rate Alarm)	Cardiovascular
Monitor, Physiological, Patient(without Arrhythmia Detection Or Alarms)	Cardiovascular
Monitor, Ventilatory Frequency	Anesthesiology
Oximeter, Intracardiac	Cardiovascular
Pacemaker, Cardiac, External Transcutaneous (Non-Invasive)	Cardiovascular
Recorder, Paper Chart	Cardiovascular

INVIVO CORPORATION   425-487-7000 *(cont'd)*
   Thermometer, Electronic, Continuous   General
   Tubing, Non-Invasive   Surgery

INVIVO CORPORATION   262-524-1402
N27 W23676 Paul Road, Pewaukee, WI 53072
FDA Number: 2183683
E-mail: info@invivocorp.com   *Fax:* 262-524-1403
Web site: www.invivocorp.com
Year Founded: 1987
Ownership: Private
Produces/Sells CE-marked Devices: N
General Admin.: Stuart Baumgarten/President
    James B. Hawkins/President, Chief Executive Officer
Mktg./Adv.: Cathy Yudzevich/Manager Investor Relations
    Leon Lumens/Manager Sales
    Terence Yip/Manager Sales
   Coil, Magnetic Resonance, Specialty   Radiology
   Nuclear Magnetic Resonance Imaging System   Radiology

INVIVO CORPORATION (INSTRUMENTS GROUP)
   See Linear Laboratories Corporation

INVIVO THERAPEUTICS   617-475-1520
One Broadway, 14th Floor, Cambridge, MA 02142
FDA Number: n/a
E-mail: info@invivotherapeutics.com
Web site: www.invivotherapeutics.com
Ownership: Private
Produces/Sells CE-marked Devices: N
General Admin.: Mr. Frank Reynolds/Chief Executive Officer
    Dr. Edward Wirth/Chief Scientific Officer
Medical Admin.: Dr. Eric Woodard/Chief Medical Officer
Finance: Mr. Sean Moran/Chief Financial Officer

INVIVOSCRIBE TECHNOLOGIES, LLC   1 858 224-6601
6330 Nancy Ridge Drive, Suite 106,   858 224-6600
San Diego, CA 92121
FDA Number: 3004774989
E-mail: sales@invivoscribe.com   *Fax:* 1 858 224-6601
Web site: www.invivoscribe.com
Ownership: Private
Produces/Sells CE-marked Devices: N
   DNA-Probe, Chromosome, Human   Hematology
   DNA-Probe, Lymphocyte, B & T   Hematology
   Reagents, Specific, Analyte   Hematology

INVOKE IMAGING, INC.   630-271-8111
1250 Palmer St., Downers Grove, IL 60516
FDA Number: 3004153797
Ownership: Private
Produces/Sells CE-marked Devices: N
   Device, Storage, Image, Digital   Radiology
   System, Communication, Image, Digital   Radiology

INVOTEC INTL.   800-998-8580
6833 Phillips Industrial Blvd.,   904-880-1229
Jacksonville, FL 32256
FDA Number: 1052728   *Fax:* 904-886-9517
E-mail: jaull@invotec.net
Web site: www.invotec.net
Medical Products Sales Volume: $190,000
Annual Revenue: $5-$10 Million
Year Founded: 1990
Total Employees: 3
Ownership: Private
Quality System Registration Information: ISO9001; ISO9002
Produces/Sells CE-marked Devices: Y
Federal Procurement Eligibility: Small Business
Distribution: Manufacturer Direct, Manufacturer Through Distributor, Importer, Exporter
   Balloon, Epistaxis (Nasal)   Ear/Nose/Throat
   Button, Nasal Septal   Ear/Nose/Throat
   Curette, Nasal   Ear/Nose/Throat
   Drape, Surgical, ENT   Ear/Nose/Throat
   Forceps, ENT   Ear/Nose/Throat
   Knife, Nasal   Ear/Nose/Throat
   Pack, Hot Or Cold, Reusable   Physical Med
   Prosthesis, Chin, Internal   Surgery
   Prosthesis, Nose, Internal   Surgery
   Punch, Nasal   Ear/Nose/Throat
   Scissors, Nasal   Ear/Nose/Throat
   Splint, Nasal   Ear/Nose/Throat
   Tube, Tracheal (Endotracheal)   Anesthesiology
   Tube, Tympanostomy   Ear/Nose/Throat

INVUITY, INC.   760-744-4447
334 Via Vera Cruz, Suite 255, San Marcos, CA 92078
FDA Number: 3006158343

INVUITY, INC.   760-744-4447 *(cont'd)*
   Accessories, Operating Room, Table   Surgery
   Cannula, Surgical, General & Plastic Surgery   Surgery
   Curette   Orthopedics
   Dissector, Surgical, General & Plastic Surgery   Surgery
   Elevator, Surgical, General & Plastic Surgery   Surgery
   Fiberoptic Light Source & Carrier   Ear/Nose/Throat
   Forceps, General & Plastic Surgery   Surgery
   Orthopedic Manual Surgical Instrument   Orthopedics
   Probe   Orthopedics
   Retractor, Fiberoptic   Gastroenterology/Urology
   Retractor, Surgical   Surgery
   Rongeur, Rib   Orthopedics
   Tray, Surgical Instrument   Surgery

INVUITY, INC.   866-711-7768
39 Stillman Street, San Francisco, CA 94107   -
FDA Number: 3007037347
E-mail: info@invuity.com
Ownership: Private
Produces/Sells CE-marked Devices: N
   Accessories, Operating Room, Table   Surgery
   Cannula, Surgical, General & Plastic Surgery   Surgery
   Curette   Orthopedics
   Dissector, Surgical, General & Plastic Surgery   Surgery
   Elevator, Surgical, General & Plastic Surgery   Surgery
   Fiberoptic Light Source & Carrier   Ear/Nose/Throat
   Forceps, General & Plastic Surgery   Surgery
   Light, Surgical, Fiberoptic   Surgery
   Orthopedic Manual Surgical Instrument   Orthopedics
   Probe   Orthopedics
   Retractor, All Types   Dental And Oral
   Retractor, Fiberoptic   Gastroenterology/Urology
   Retractor, Surgical   Surgery
   Rongeur, Rib   Orthopedics
   Tray, Surgical Instrument   Surgery

INWELD CORP.   317-248-0651
5353 West Southern Avenue, Indianapolis, IN 46242
FDA Number: 1825418   *Fax:* 317-248-0079
E-mail: fred@inweld.com
Web site: www.inweld.com
Medical Products Sales Volume: $9,500,000
Annual Revenue: $10-$25 Million
Year Founded: 1992
Total Employees: 23
Ownership: Private
Produces/Sells CE-marked Devices: N
Federal Procurement Eligibility: Small Business
   Gas, Calibrated (Specified Concentration)   Anesthesiology
   Laser, Surgical   Surgery

IO LASER, INC.   407-296-0544
6140-b Edgewater Dr., Orlando, FL 32810-4860
FDA Number: 3004735249
Ownership: Private
Produces/Sells CE-marked Devices: N
   Lamp, Infrared   Physical Med

IOMED, INC.   800-621-3347
2441 South 3850 West, Suite A,   801-975-1191
Salt Lake City, UT 84120
FDA Number: 1718048   *Fax:* 801-972-9072
E-mail: cs@iomed.com
Web site: www.iomed.com
Medical Products Sales Volume: $10,800,000
Annual Revenue: $10-$25 Million
Year Founded: 1974
Total Employees: 48   *Marketing Staff:* 2   *Sales Staff:* 5
Ownership: Private
Quality System Registration Information: ISO9001
Produces/Sells CE-marked Devices: Y
Federal Procurement Eligibility: Small Business
Distribution: Manufacturer Through Distributor, Manufacturer Through Manufacturer Reps, Exporter
General Admin.: Robert Lollini/President, Chief Executive Officer
Mktg./Adv.: Jessica Barrett/Director National Marketing & Sales
Production: Curtis Jensen/Manager Quality Assurance
    Roger Anderson/Product Manager
Research: Greg Fischer/Vice President Product Development
   Electrode, Other   General
   Iontophoresis Unit, Physical Medicine   Physical Med
   System, Delivery, Drug, Non-invasive   General
   System, Delivery, Drug, Unit-Dose   General

ION VISION, INC.   760-450-4548
7933 Paseo Membrillo, Carlsbad, CA 92009
FDA Number: 3004363219

ION VISION, INC.   760-450-4548 (cont'd)
Lens, Condensing, Diagnostic   Ophthalmology

ION-TRACE INC.   905-640-0295
5649 Concession 2, Stouffville, ONT L4A-7X4 Canada
FDA Number: n/a   *Fax:* 905-640-0297
E-mail: ionpaul@aol.com
Web site: www.iontrace.com
Year Founded: 1985
Total Employees: 10
Ownership: Private
Produces/Sells CE-marked Devices: N
Distribution: Manufacturer Direct, Exporter

IOPI NORTHWEST COMPANY, LLC   425-333-5721
5901 Tolt River Rd. N.e., Carnation, WA 98014
FDA Number: 3003857800
Dynamometer, Non-Powered   Orthopedics

IOTRON TECHNOLOGIES, INC.   604-945-8838
1425 Kebet Way, Port Coquitlam, BC V3C 6L3 Canada
FDA Number: 9680579   *Fax:* 604-945-8827
E-mail: iotron@iotron.com
Web site: www.iotron.com
Year Founded: 1989
Total Employees: 20   *Marketing Staff:* 2   *Sales Staff:* 2
Ownership: IOTRON INDUSTRIES, INC.
Quality System Registration Information: ISO9002
Produces/Sells CE-marked Devices: N
Federal Procurement Eligibility: Small Business
Distribution: Service Direct

IPAS   919-967-7052
PO Box 5027, Chapel Hill, NC 27514
FDA Number: 1047838   *Fax:* 919-929-0258
E-mail: ipas@ipas.org
Web site: www.ipas.org
Medical Products Sales Volume: $18,000,000
Annual Revenue: $10-$25 Million
Year Founded: 1973
Total Employees: 110   *Marketing Staff:* 12   *Sales Staff:* 8
Ownership: Private
Quality System Registration Information: ISO9002
Produces/Sells CE-marked Devices: Y
Federal Procurement Eligibility: Small Business
Distribution: Manufacturer Direct, Manufacturer Through Distributor, Importer, Exporter
General Admin.: Mr. Terence Kominski/Executive Vice President
Mktg./Adv.: Ms. Fen Zhang/Associate Manager Marketing
    Nadine Burton/Director Marketing
    Jerry Lazarus/Project Manager Marketing
Aspirator, Endocervical   Obstetrics/Gynecology
Aspirator, Endometrial   Obstetrics/Gynecology
Cannula, Suction, Uterine   Obstetrics/Gynecology
Dilator, Cervical, Fixed Size   Obstetrics/Gynecology
Kit, Biopsy   General
Syringe, Other   General

IPAX, INC.   303-975-2444
2700 South Raritan Street, Englewood, CO 80110
FDA Number: 1720734   *Fax:* 303-975-2882
E-mail: sales@ipaxinc.com
Web site: www.ipaxinc.com
Medical Products Sales Volume: $500,000
Annual Revenue: $0-$1 Million
Year Founded: 1983
Total Employees: 10   *Marketing Staff:* 1   *Sales Staff:* 1
Ownership: Private
Quality System Registration Information: ISO9001
Produces/Sells CE-marked Devices: Y
Federal Procurement Eligibility: Small Business
Distribution: Manufacturer Direct, Manufacturer Through Distributor, OEM
General Admin.: KEVIN HORKY/Manager
    Kevin Horky/President, Chief Executive Officer
Contract Assembly   General
Service, Engineering/Design   General
Tubing, Plastic   General

IPC - INPRO CORPORATION
See Inpro Corporation

IPC DOOR AND WALL PROTECTION SYSTEMS, INPRO CORP.
See Inpro Corporation

IPCO CORP.
See Sterling Vision, Inc.

IPCO HOSPITAL SUPPLY CORPORATION
See Mckesson General Medical

IPI MEDICAL PRODUCTS
See I.P.I.-International Products, Inc.

IPSO USA, INC.   800-872-4776
PO Box 990, Shepard Street, Ripon, WI 54971   920-748-3121
FDA Number: 5218788   *Fax:* 850-271-1109
E-mail: beisenberg@ipsousa.com
Web site: www.ipsousa.com
Medical Products Sales Volume: $10,000,000
Annual Revenue: $10-$25 Million
Total Employees: 35   *Marketing Staff:* 1   *Sales Staff:* 4
Ownership: IPSO
Produces/Sells CE-marked Devices: Y
Distribution: Manufacturer Through Distributor, Exclusive Distributor
General Admin.: B. Bruce/President
Mktg./Adv.: Robert F. Eisenberg/Director National Sales
    D. Kelly/Manager Regional Sales
    R. Carson/Manager Regional Sales
Washer, Laundry   General

IQUIRE, LLC   845-277-1846
2 Fallsview Lane, Brewster, NY 10509
FDA Number: 3005112581
Device, Storage, Image, Digital   Radiology

IQUUM, INC.   508-970-0099
700 Nickerson Road, Marlborough, MA 01752
FDA Number: n/a   *Fax:* 508-970-0119
E-mail: info@IQuum.com
Web site: www.IQuum.com
Year Founded: 1998
Ownership: Private
Produces/Sells CE-marked Devices: N
General Admin.: Dr. Shuqi Chen/Chairman, Chief Executive Officer
Production: Mr. Keith Greenfield/Executive Vice President Development
Finance: Mr. Daniel Sutherby/Chief Financial Officer

IR THERAPIES, LLC   602-595-3426
19827 North 20th Way, Phoenix, AZ 85024
FDA Number: 3005823198
Ownership: Private
Produces/Sells CE-marked Devices: N
Pad, Heating, Powered   Physical Med

IRADIMED CORPORATION   407-677-8022
7457 Aloma Ave., Suite 201, Winter Park, FL 32792
FDA Number: 3005053560
Infusion Stand   General
Kit, Administration, Intravenous   General
Pump, Infusion   General

IRENDA CORP.   323-770-4222
14131 South Avalon Blvd., Los Angeles, CA 90061
FDA Number: 2050154
Ownership: Private
Produces/Sells CE-marked Devices: N
Cleaner, Lens, Contact   Ophthalmology

IREX TECHNOLOGY GROUP
See Johnson & Johnson

IRHYTHM TECHNOLOGIES, INC.   415-632-5700
650 Townsend Street, Suite 350, San Francisco, CA 94103
FDA Number: n/a   *Fax:* 415-632-5701
E-mail: info@irhythmtech.com
Web site: http://www.irhythmtech.com
Ownership: Private
Produces/Sells CE-marked Devices: N
General Admin.: Mr. Bill Willis/Chief Executive Officer
    Ms. Judy Lenane/Chief Operating Officer
Medical Admin.: Dr. Uday Kumar/Chief Medical Officer
Mktg./Adv.: Mr. Jon Darsee/Executive Vice President Business Development
Research: Dr. Mark Day/Vice President Research & Development
Finance: Ms. Shelly Guyer/Chief Financial Officer

IRIDEX
See Iridex Corporation

IRIDEX CORPORATION   800-388-4747
1212 Terra Bella Avenue,   650-962-8100
Mountain View, CA 94043
FDA Number: 2939653   *Fax:* 650-962-0486
E-mail: info@iridex.com
Web site: www.iridex.com
Annual Revenue: $50-$100 Million
Year Founded: 1989
Ownership: Public
Stock Symbol: IRIX
Traded On: NASDAQ
Quality System Registration Information: ISO9001

IRIDEX CORPORATION 800-388-4747 *(cont'd)*
Produces/Sells CE-marked Devices: Y
Federal Procurement Eligibility: Small Business
Distribution: Manufacturer Through Distributor
General Admin.: Theodore A. Boutacoff/President, Chief Executive Officer
Mktg./Adv.: Eduardo Arias/Senior Vice President International Sales
James Donovan/Vice President Business Development
Finance: James Mackaness/Chief Financial Officer

Accessories, Laser	General
Cannula, Ophthalmic	Ophthalmology
Endoilluminator	Ophthalmology
Lamp, Slit	Ophthalmology
Laser, Ophthalmic	Ophthalmology
Laser, Surgical	Surgery
Lens, Contact, Polymethylmethacrylate	Ophthalmology
Ophthalmoscope, Laser	Ophthalmology

IRIS
See Iris International, Inc.

IRIS DIAGNOSTICS 800-776-4747
9172 Eton Ave., Chatsworth, CA 91311 **818-709-1244**
FDA Number: 2023446 Fax: 818-700-9661
E-mail: irisdiag@proiris.com
Web site: www.irisdiagnostics.com
Ownership: IRIS INTERNATIONAL, INC.
Stock Symbol: IRIS
Traded On: NASDAQ
Produces/Sells CE-marked Devices: N

Analyzer, Chemistry, Urinalysis	Chemistry
Computer, Chemistry Analyzer	Chemistry
Control, Urinalysis (Assayed And Unassayed)	Chemistry
Counter, Cell Or Particle, Automated	Hematology
Counter, Urine Particle	Pathology
Diazonium Colorimetry, Urobilinogen (Urinary, Non-Quant.)	Chemistry
Diluent, Blood Cell	Hematology
Enzymatic Method, Glucose (Urinary, Non-Quantitative)	Chemistry
Fluid, Red Cell Lysing	Hematology
Hematology Quality Control Mixture	Hematology
Indicator, pH, Dye (Urinary, Non-Quantitative)	Chemistry
Reagent, General Purpose	Pathology
Stain, Microbiological	Microbiology
Urinometer, Electrical	Gastroenterology/Urology

IRIS INTERNATIONAL, INC. 800-776-4747
9162 Eton Avenue, Chatsworth, CA 91311-5805 **818-709-1244**
FDA Number: 2023446 Fax: 818-700-9661
E-mail: irisinc@proiris.com
Web site: www.proiris.com
Medical Products Sales Volume: $70,500,000
Annual Revenue: $50-$100 Million
Year Founded: 1979
Total Employees: 90
Ownership: Public
Stock Symbol: IRIS
Traded On: NASDAQ
Produces/Sells CE-marked Devices: Y
Federal Procurement Eligibility: Small Business
Distribution: Manufacturer Direct, Manufacturer Through Distributor
General Admin.: Peter Donato/Chief Financial Officer, Vice President
Cesar Garcia/President, Chief Executive Officer
Robert Mello/Vice President, General Manager
Mktg./Adv.: Alan E. Koontz/Vice President Marketing & Business Development
Production: Michael Zachariash/Vice President Manufacturing
John Yi/Vice President Operations
Research: Harvey Kasdan/Vice President Research & Development

Acid, Ascorbic, 2, 4-dinitrophenylhydrazine (spectrophotometric)	Chemistry
Analyzer, Chemistry, Urinalysis, Automated	Chemistry
Azo-Dyes, Colorimetric, Bilirubin And Conjugates	Chemistry
Colorimetric, Occult Blood in Urine	Hematology
Control, Urinalysis (Assayed And Unassayed)	Chemistry
Counter, Cell Or Particle, Automated	Hematology
Counter, Urine Particle	Pathology
Diazo (Colorimetric), Nitrite (Urinary, Non-Quantitative)	Chemistry
Diazonium Colorimetry, Urobilinogen (Urinary, Non-Quant.)	Chemistry
Diluent, Blood Cell	Hematology
Enzymatic Method, Glucose (Urinary, Non-Quantitative)	Chemistry
Fluid, Red Cell Lysing	Hematology
Hematology Quality Control Mixture	Hematology
Indicator Method, Protein Or Albumin (Urinary, Non-Quant.)	Chemistry
Indicator, pH, Dye (Urinary, Non-Quantitative)	Chemistry
Nitroprusside, Ketones (Urinary, Non-Quantitative)	Chemistry
Photometer	Chemistry
Reagent, General Purpose	Pathology
Test, Urine Leukocyte	Hematology

Medical Product Subsidiaries (Listed Separately)
Leica Microsystems (San Jose) Corporation
Statspin, Inc.

IRIS MEDICAL DIODE LASERS, INC.
See Iridex Corporation

IRIS MEDICAL INSTRUMENTS, INC.
See Iridex Corporation

IRIS SAMPLE PROCESSING 800-782-8774
60 Glacier Drive, Westwood, MA 02090-1825 **781-551-0100**
FDA Number: 1221015 Fax: 781-551-0036
E-mail: sales1@proiris.com
Web site: www.statspin.com
Ownership: IRIS INTERNATIONAL, INC.
Stock Symbol: IRIS
Traded On: NASDAQ
Produces/Sells CE-marked Devices: N

Block, Heating	Chemistry
Centrifuge, Cell Washing	Hematology
Centrifuge, Hematocrit	Hematology
Cytocentrifuge	Pathology
Hematocrit Tube, Rack, Sealer, Holder	Hematology
Hematocrit, Manual	Hematology
Labware, Blood Collection	Chemistry
Refractometer	Chemistry
Slide, Microscope	Pathology
Spinner, Slide, Automated	Hematology
Tube, Capillary Blood Collection	Hematology

IRITECH, INC. 703-787-7680
459 Herndon Pkwy Suite 21, Herndon, VA 20170
FDA Number: 2954967

Pupillometer, AC-Powered	Ophthalmology
Pupillometer, Manual	Ophthalmology

IRON DUCK, A DIV. OF FLEMING INDUSTRIES, INC. 800-669-6900
20 Veterans Drive, Chicopee, MA 01022 **413-593-3300**
FDA Number: 7000483 Fax: 413-593-5800
E-mail: idinfo@ironduck.com
Web site: www.ironduck.com
Medical Products Sales Volume: $500,000
Annual Revenue: $5-$10 Million
Year Founded: 1976
Total Employees: 8 *Marketing Staff:* 3 *Sales Staff:* 4
Ownership: Private
Produces/Sells CE-marked Devices: Y
Federal Procurement Eligibility: Small Business, GSA Contract, VA Contract
Distribution: Manufacturer Through Distributor
General Admin.: Tina Borcea/Manager Human Resources
Michael J. Fleming/President, Chief Executive Officer
Mktg./Adv.: Sharon Glaszcz/Manager Contract Sales
Sharon Glaszcz/Manager International Marketing & Sales
Mr. Brooke A. Lawrence/Vice President Sales
Production: Linda Gasperini/Director Quality Assurance

Bag, Laundry, Infection Control	General
Bag, Medical, Physician	General
Board, Spine	Orthopedics
Bumper Guard, Corner	General
Cover, Cart	General
Liner, Laundry Hamper	General
Rescue Equipment	General
Stretcher, Emergency, Other	General

IRONWOOD INDUSTRIES, INC. 847-362-8681
115 S. Bradley Road, Libertyville, IL 60048-9509
FDA Number: 1420088 Fax: 847-362-9190
E-mail: ggrant@ironind.com
Web site: www.ironind.com
Medical Products Sales Volume: $4,800,000
Total Employees: 78 *Sales Staff:* 4
Ownership: Private
Quality System Registration Information: ISO9002
Produces/Sells CE-marked Devices: N
Federal Procurement Eligibility: Small Business
General Admin.: Robert Grala/President
Mktg./Adv.: Gary Grant/Manager Sales

Contract Manufacturing	General
Molding, Custom	General
Molding, Injection	General

IRONWOOD PLASTICS, INC. 906-932-5025
1235 Wall St., Ironwood, MI 49938
FDA Number: 3003651519 Fax: 906-932-4356
E-mail: iwp@ironwood.com
Web site: www.ironwood.com
Ownership: Private
Produces/Sells CE-marked Devices: N

Stapler, Surgical	Surgery

IRRADIA AB
736 W. Double Shaols Rd, Lawndale, NC 28090
800-300-5558
704-538-7780
FDA Number: 3006297489
Fax: 704-538-7781
E-mail: info@irradia.us
Web site: http://www.irradia.us
Total Employees: 10   *Marketing Staff:* 2   *Sales Staff:* 1
Ownership: Private
Produces/Sells CE-marked Devices: Y
Distribution: Manufacturer Direct, Manufacturer Through Distributor, OEM, Exporter
General Admin.: Lars Hode/President
Research: Stefan Jordison/Manager Technology
   Laser, Combination   General
   Laser, Surgical   Surgery

IRVINE BIOMEDICAL, INC.
2375 Morse Avenue, Irvine, CA 92614-6234
888-IBI-9876
949-851-3053
FDA Number: 2030404
Fax: 949-851-3062
E-mail: sales@ibiep.com
Web site: www.ibiep.com
Medical Products Sales Volume: $19,200,000
Year Founded: 1995
Total Employees: 200   *Marketing Staff:* 2   *Sales Staff:* 4
Ownership: St. Jude Medical, Inc.
Quality System Registration Information: ISO9001
Produces/Sells CE-marked Devices: Y
Federal Procurement Eligibility: Small Business, VA Contract
Distribution: Manufacturer Through Distributor
General Admin.: Dr. Peter Chen/President, Chief Executive Officer
     Dr. Raymond Chia/Vice President
Mktg./Adv.: Mr. Peter van der Sluis/Director International Marketing & Sales
Production: Ms. Bonnie Bishop/Director Quality Assurance & Regulatory Affairs
Research: Caroline Burk/Director Clinical Research
Finance: Mr. Brett Scott/Chief Financial Officer
   Catheter, Intravascular, Diagnostic   Cardiovascular

IS2 RESEARCH INC.
3 6-20 Gurdwara Rd, Nepean K2E 8B3 Canada
613-228-8755
FDA Number: 9615403
   Scanner, Emission Computed Tomography   Radiology

ISCHEMIA TECHNOLOGIES, INC.
4600 West 60th Ave., Arvada, CO 80003
720-540-0200
FDA Number: 3003434025
Ownership: Private
Produces/Sells CE-marked Devices: N
   Test, Albumin Cobalt Binding   Chemistry

ISCIENCE INTERVENTIONAL
4055 Campbell Avenue, Menlo Park, CA 94025
650-421-2700
FDA Number: 3005641545
E-mail: info@iscienceinterventional.com
Web site: www.iscienceinterventional.com
Ownership: Private
Produces/Sells CE-marked Devices: N
   Cannula, Ophthalmic   Ophthalmology
   Endoilluminator   Ophthalmology
   Pump, Infusion, Ophthalmic   Ophthalmology
   Scanner, Ultrasonic (Pulsed Echo)   Radiology
   Transducer, Ultrasonic, Diagnostic   Radiology

ISEE 3D, INC.
100-4 Car Westmount, Westmount H3Z 2S6 Canada
514-908-2233
FDA Number: 9680440
   Endoscope   Gastroenterology/Urology

ISEE3D, INC.
759 Victoria Square, Ste. 200, Montreal, QUE H2Y-2J7 Canada
514-908-2234
FDA Number: n/a
Fax: 514-289-8609
E-mail: info@isee3d.com
Web site: www.isee3d.com
Total Employees: 30
Ownership: Public
Stock Symbol: V.ICT
Traded On: Toronto
Produces/Sells CE-marked Devices: N

ISL NORTH AMERICA, INC.
   See Pac

ISLAND BIOSURGICAL, LLC
18 Meadow Lane, Mercer Island, WA 98040
425-251-3455
FDA Number: 3028027
Fax: 206-656-5002
E-mail: islandbio@attbi.com
Annual Revenue: $0-$1 Million
Total Employees: 4
Ownership: Private
Produces/Sells CE-marked Devices: N
Federal Procurement Eligibility: Small Business

ISLAND BIOSURGICAL, LLC
425-251-3455 *(cont'd)*
Distribution: Manufacturer Through Manufacturer Reps, Exclusive Distributor
General Admin.: Hunter A. McKay/Manager
   Carrier, Ligature   Surgery
   Endoscope   Gastroenterology/Urology
   Spreader, Bladder Neck   Gastroenterology/Urology

ISO-SCIENCE LABORATORIES INC.
   See Isotope Products Laboratories, Inc.

ISOAID, L.L.C.
7824 Clark Moody Blvd., Port Richey, FL 34668
727-815-3262
FDA Number: 3003440305
   Source, Brachytherapy, Radionuclide   Radiology

ISOCOMFORTER, INC.
3531 SW Corporate Pkwy., Palm City, FL 34990
877-277-0367
772-220-2350
FDA Number: 1834248
Fax: 772-220-6645
E-mail: esesack@bellsouth.net
Web site: www.isocomforter.com
Medical Products Sales Volume: $490,000
Annual Revenue: $0-$1 Million
Year Founded: 2001
Total Employees: 4   *Marketing Staff:* 2   *Sales Staff:* 12
Ownership: Private
Produces/Sells CE-marked Devices: N
Federal Procurement Eligibility: Small Business
Distribution: Manufacturer Direct, Manufacturer Through Distributor, Manufacturer Through Manufacturer Reps
General Admin.: Eric Sesack/President
   Chilling Unit   Physical Med

ISOLUX LLC
1045 Collier Center Way, Suite #6, Naples, FL 34110
239-514-7475
FDA Number: 1064515
   Camera, Television, Surgical (Without Audio)   Surgery
   Headlamp, Operating, Battery-Operated   Ophthalmology
   Illuminator, Fiberoptic (For Endoscope)   Gastroenterology/Urology
   Illuminator, Fiberoptic, Surgical Field   Cns/Neurology
   Light, Surgical Operating, Dental   Dental And Oral
   Light, Surgical, Fiberoptic   Surgery

ISOMEDIX, INC.
   See Steris Isomedix Services

ISOPAD
300 Constitution Drive, Menlo Park, CA 940025-1164
800-545-6258
FDA Number: n/a
Fax: 800-596-5004
E-mail: info@tycothermal.com
Web site: www.tycothermal.com
Annual Revenue: $0-$1 Million
Total Employees: 60   *Marketing Staff:* 2   *Sales Staff:* 8
Ownership: Private
Quality System Registration Information: ISO9001
Produces/Sells CE-marked Devices: Y
Distribution: Manufacturer Direct, Importer, Exporter
General Admin.: P. Dunnage/Partner
Mktg./Adv.: P. Dunnage/Manager Marketing
     Jan Cain/Manager Marketing & Sales
   Heating Mantle   Microbiology
   Heating Unit, Powered   Physical Med

ISOPURE CORP.
141 Citizens Blvd., Simpsonville, KY 40067
800-280-7873
502-722-1000
FDA Number: 3003768032
Fax: 502-722-2244
E-mail: Info@isopure.com
Web site: www.isopure.com
Medical Products Sales Volume: $3,500,000
Annual Revenue: $1-$5 Million
Year Founded: 1996
Total Employees: 12   *Marketing Staff:* 1   *Sales Staff:* 1
Ownership: Private
Produces/Sells CE-marked Devices: N
Federal Procurement Eligibility: Small Business
Distribution: Manufacturer Direct, Manufacturer Through Distributor, Manufacturer Through Manufacturer Reps, OEM, Exporter
General Admin.: Kevin Gillespie/President, Chief Executive Officer
Mktg./Adv.: Sarah Gillespie/Manager Market Research
Production: Tom Justice/Design Engineer
     Joe Piorkowski/Quality Control, Product Engineer
   Purification System, Water   Gastroenterology/Urology
   Purification System, Water, Reverse Osmosis   Chemistry
   Reverse Osmosis Membrane Equipment   Chemistry
   Ultrafiltration Equipment   Chemistry

ISORAY, INC
350 Hills Street Suite 106, Richland, WA 99354
877-447-6729
509-375-1202
FDA Number: 3005520039
Fax: 509-267-3670
E-mail: info@isoray.com
Web site: www.isoray.com

MANUFACTURER PROFILES

ISORAY, INC   877-447-6729 *(cont'd)*
Year Founded: 1998
Ownership: Public
Stock Symbol: ISR
Traded On: AMEX
Produces/Sells CE-marked Devices: N
General Admin.: Mr. Dwight Babcock/Chief Executive Officer, Chairman
Production: Mr. Fred Swindler/Vice President Quality Assurance & Regulatory Affairs
Research: Mr. William Cavanaugh/Vice President Research & Development
Source, Brachytherapy, Radionuclide   Radiology

ISOTECHNIKA INC.   888-487-9944
5120 75th St., Edmonton, ALB T6E 6W2 Canada   780-487-1600
FDA Number: n/a   *Fax:* 780-484-4105
E-mail: sgillis@isotechnika.com
Web site: www.isotechnika.com
Year Founded: 1993
Total Employees: 74
Ownership: Public
Stock Symbol: ISA
Traded On: TSX Venture Exchange
Produces/Sells CE-marked Devices: N
Distribution: Manufacturer Direct, Exclusive Distributor, Exporter

ISOTOPE PRODUCTS LABORATORIES, INC.   661-309-1010
24937 Ave Tibbitts, Valencia, CA 91355
FDA Number: 2020604   *Fax:* 661-257-8303
E-mail: sales@isotopeproducts.com
Web site: www.isotopeproducts.com
Medical Products Sales Volume: $8,900,000
Annual Revenue: $10-$25 Million
Year Founded: 1999
Total Employees: 45   *Marketing Staff:* 2   *Sales Staff:* 10
Ownership: ECKERT & ZIEGLER ISOTOPE PRODUCTS
Quality System Registration Information: ISO9001
Produces/Sells CE-marked Devices: Y
Federal Procurement Eligibility: Small Business
Distribution: Manufacturer Direct
General Admin.: Len Hendrickson/Chief Executive Officer
Leonard Hendrickson/President, Chief Executive Officer
Pete Nilson/Vice President, General Manager
Mktg./Adv.: Ruth Amlauer/Manager International Sales
Peter Nilson/Vice President Business Development
Production: Robert David/Manager Materials
Lloyd Flowers/Manager Regulatory Affairs
Calibrator Source, Nuclear Sealed   Radiology
Camera, Other   General
Needle, Isotope, Gold, Titanium, Platinum   Radiology
Source, Radioisotope Reference   Chemistry

ISOVAC PRODUCTS LLC   630-679-1740
1306 Enterprise Dr., Unit C, Romeoville, IL 60446
FDA Number: 3006076009
Chamber, Isolation, Patient Transport   General

ISP
See Innovative Surgical Products, Inc.

ISPG, INC.   860-355-8511
517 Litchfield Road, New Milford, CT 06776-2008
FDA Number: 1221435   *Fax:* 860-355-8533
E-mail: office@ispg.com
Web site: www.ispg.com
Annual Revenue: $10-$25 Million
Total Employees: 18
Ownership: Private
Produces/Sells CE-marked Devices: N
Federal Procurement Eligibility: Small Business, Female Owned
Distribution: OEM, Importer, Exporter
General Admin.: James Fitzgibbons/President, Chief Executive Officer
Mktg./Adv.: Rosalie Fitzgibbons/Manager Advertising
Gerald Luhman/Manager International & National Sales
Loretta F. Luhman/Vice President Sales
Production: Chris Young/Director Quality Assurance
Cannula, Arterial   Cardiovascular
Cannula, Aspirating   Cardiovascular
Cannula, Catheter   Cardiovascular
Cannula, Epidural   Obstetrics/Gynecology
Cannula, Injection   Gastroenterology/Urology
Cannula, Other   General
Cannula, Venous   Cardiovascular
Component, Metal, Other   General
Contract Manufacturing   General
Needle, Aspiration And Injection, Disposable   Surgery
Needle, Other   General
Needle, Spinal, Short-Term   General
Syringe, Anesthesia   Anesthesiology
Syringe, Hypodermic   General

ISPG, INC.   860-355-8511 *(cont'd)*
Syringe, Other   General
Syringe, Piston   General
Tubing, Hypodermic   General
Tubing, Other   General

ISS
See Integrated Surgical Systems

ISURGICAL   847-949-9744
26625 Countryside Lake Drive, Countryside Lake, IL 60060
FDA Number: 3004153905
Ownership: Private
Produces/Sells CE-marked Devices: N
Electrode, Needle   Cns/Neurology

ITA-MED CO.   888-9IT-AMED
310 Littlefield Ave.,   650-873-7900
South San Francisco, CA 94080
FDA Number: 2951599   *Fax:* 650-873-6900
E-mail: infohealth@itamed.com
Web site: www.itamed.com
Annual Revenue: $1-$5 Million
Year Founded: 1992
Total Employees: 50   *Marketing Staff:* 4   *Sales Staff:* 4
Ownership: Private
Produces/Sells CE-marked Devices: Y
Federal Procurement Eligibility: Small Business
Distribution: Manufacturer Direct, Manufacturer Through Distributor, Manufacturer Through Manufacturer Reps, Exporter
General Admin.: Lev Tripolsky/President, Chief Executive Officer
Mktg./Adv.: Yury Yuger/Vice President Sales
Accessories, Wheelchair   Physical Med
Band, Support, Pelvic   Physical Med
Bandage, Elastic   General
Belt, Abdominal   Gastroenterology/Urology
Belt, Support, Pelvic   Physical Med
Binder, Elastic   General
Brace, Joint, Ankle (External)   Physical Med
Cane   Physical Med
Collar, Cervical Neck   Orthopedics
Joint, Knee, External Brace   Physical Med
Orthosis, Abdominal   Physical Med
Orthosis, Cervical   Physical Med
Orthosis, Lumbosacral   Physical Med
Orthosis, Thoracic   Physical Med
Splint, Hand, And Component   Physical Med
Splint, Other   Orthopedics
Stocking, Elastic   General
Support, Arm   Physical Med
Support, Hernia   Gastroenterology/Urology

ITEC/EMS LLP   903-365-6390
400 Allstar Dr., Winnsboro, TX 75494
FDA Number: 3005168210
Splint, Extermity, Non-inflatable, External, Non-sterile   Surgery
Transfer Device, Patient, Manual   General

ITM INSTRUMENTS INC.   800-361-1042
20800 Industriel Boulevard,   514-457-7280
Ste-Anne-de-Bellevue, QUE H9X 0 Canada
FDA Number: n/a   *Fax:* 514-457-4329
E-mail: info@itm-ins.com
Web site: www.itm-ins.com
Year Founded: 1983
Total Employees: 50
Ownership: Private
Produces/Sells CE-marked Devices: N
Distribution: Exclusive Distributor

ITM PARTNERS, LTD.   210-651-9066
5925 Corridor Pkwy., Schertz, TX 78154
FDA Number: n/a   *Fax:* 210-651-9067
E-mail: mail@itm-texas.com
Web site: www.itm-texas.com
Annual Revenue: $1-$5 Million
Year Founded: 1929
Total Employees: 25   *Marketing Staff:* 3   *Sales Staff:* 3
Ownership: Avakian DBA DataTran
Produces/Sells CE-marked Devices: N
Federal Procurement Eligibility: Small Business
Distribution: Manufacturer Direct, OEM
General Admin.: Klaus D. Weiswurm/President, Chief Executive Officer
Production: Mr. John Dewey/Vice President Operations
Research: Andrew Pettersson/Vice President Engineering
Camera, Other   General
Component, Electronic   General
Shield, X-Ray   Radiology

ITT ELECTRO OPTICAL PRODUCTS DIV.
See Itt Night Vision

ITT NIGHT VISION
7635 Plantation Road, Roanoke, VA 24019-3257   **800-448-8678**
   540-563-0371
FDA Number: 1118984   *Fax:* 540-366-9015
E-mail: nv.orderadmin@itt.com
Web site: www.nightvision.com
Total Employees: 1100
Ownership: ITT INDUSTRIES
Quality System Registration Information: ISO9001
Produces/Sells CE-marked Devices: N
Distribution: Manufacturer Direct, Manufacturer Through Manufacturer Reps
General Admin.: Gary Aicher/President
     John Hertzog/Vice President Human Resources
Mktg./Adv.: Jim Harris/Director Product Development
     Courtney Reynolds/Manager Advertising & Promotions
     Harry Montoro/Manager International & National Sales
     Laurel Holder/Manager PR
     Richard Hall/Manager Sales Training
     Larry Curfiss/Vice President Business Development
     Larry Curfiss/Vice President Marketing & Sales
Production: Kacy Litzy/Vice President Manufacturing
Research: Jim Harris/Vice President Research & Development
   Vision Aid, Image Intensification, Battery-Powered   Ophthalmology

ITT PNEUMOTIVE
See Thomas Products Division

IVACO INDUSTRIES
See Diamedix Corp.

IVALON, INC.
1015 Cordova Street, San Diego, CA 92107   **800-948-2566**
   619-224-2921
FDA Number: 2028294   *Fax:* 619-299-8320
E-mail: ivalon@cox.net
Web site: www.ivalon.com
Medical Products Sales Volume: $360,000
Year Founded: 1991
Total Employees: 4
Ownership: Private
Produces/Sells CE-marked Devices: N
Federal Procurement Eligibility: Small Business, Female Owned
Distribution: Manufacturer Direct, Manufacturer Through Distributor
General Admin.: Elizabeth J. Melaragno/President
Mktg./Adv.: Lisa Malachowski/Manager Product Development
Research: Mitchell R. Malachowski/Vice President Research
   Agent, Embolization/Occlusion   Surgery
   Device, Embolization, Artificial   Cns/Neurology
   Embolization Device   Cardiovascular

IVAX DIAGNOSTICS INC.
2140 North Miami Avenue, Miami, FL 33127   **800-327-4565**
   305-324-2338
FDA Number: n/a   *Fax:* 305-324-2395
E-mail: investor_relations@ivaxdiagnostics.com
Web site: www.ivaxdiagnostics.com
Ownership: Public
Stock Symbol: IVD
Traded On: AMEX
Produces/Sells CE-marked Devices: N

IVD RESEARCH, INC.
5909 Sea Lion Place, Suite D,   **866-794-2126**
Carlsbad, CA 92010   **760-929-7744**
FDA Number: n/a   *Fax:* 760-431-7759
E-mail: ivd@ivdresearch.com
Web site: www.ivdresearch.com
Medical Products Sales Volume: $650,000
Annual Revenue: $1-$5 Million
Year Founded: 1996
Total Employees: 10
Ownership: Private
Produces/Sells CE-marked Devices: Y
Federal Procurement Eligibility: Small Business
Distribution: Manufacturer Direct, Manufacturer Through Distributor, OEM, Exporter
   Antigen, All Types, Escherichia Coli   Microbiology
   Antigen, C. Difficile   Microbiology
   Antigen, Fluorescent Antibody Test, Echinococcus Granulosus   Microbiology
   Antigen, Latex Agglutination, Entamoeba Histolytica & Rel.   Microbiology
   Antiserum, Escherichia Coli   Microbiology
   Antiserum, Fluorescent, Adenovirus 1-33   Microbiology
   Cryptosporidium Spp.   Microbiology
   Enzyme Linked Immunoabsorbent Assay, Rotavirus   Microbiology
   Enzyme Linked Immunoabsorbent Assay, Trichinella Spiralis   Microbiology
   Giardia Spp.   Microbiology
   Immunofluorescent Assay, T. Cruzi   Microbiology
   Indirect Fluorescent Antibody Test, Entamoeba Histolytica   Microbiology
   Legionella, Spp., ELISA   Microbiology
   Reagent, Cysticercosis   Microbiology

IVD RESEARCH, INC.   866-794-2126 *(cont'd)*
   Reagent, Leishmanii Serological   Microbiology

IVD TECHNOLOGIES   714-549-5050
2002 S. Grand Ave Ste A, Cowan Heights, CA 92705
FDA Number: 3005916611   *Fax:* 714- 549-5055
E-mail: sales@ivdtechnologies.com
Ownership: Private
Produces/Sells CE-marked Devices: N
   Radioimmunoassay, Immunoreactive Insulin   Chemistry

IVM
See In Vivo Metric

IVOCLAR NORTH AMERICA
See Ivoclar Vivadent, Inc.

IVOCLAR VIVADENT, INC.
175 Pineview Drive, Amherst, NY 14228-2231   **800-533-6825**
   716-691-0010
FDA Number: 3003310824   *Fax:* 716-691-2285
E-mail: Donna.Hartnett@ivoclarvivadent.us.com
Web site: www.ivoclarvivadent.us.com
Medical Products Sales Volume: $125,000,000
Annual Revenue: More than $100 Million
Year Founded: 1986
Total Employees: 150   *Marketing Staff:* 7   *Sales Staff:* 40
Ownership: Ivoclar Vivadent, Inc.
Quality System Registration Information: ISO9001
Produces/Sells CE-marked Devices: Y
Federal Procurement Eligibility: Small Business
Distribution: Manufacturer Direct, Exclusive Distributor
General Admin.: Alan S. Korman/General Counsel
     Robert A. Ganley/President
Mktg./Adv.: Brian Allen/Director Marketing
     Micheal F. Brennan/Vice President Marketing
     Patrick M. Segnere/Vice President Sales
     Pierre Lamoure/Vice President Sales
Production: Donna M. Hartnett/Director Quality Assurance
     Anderjeet Gulati/Manager Quality Assurance & Regulatory Affairs
Research: George W. Tysowsky/Vice President Research & Development
Finance: Thomas Kingston/Vice President Finance
   Activator, Ultraviolet, Polymerization   Dental And Oral
   Adhesive, Bracket And Conditioner, Resin   Dental And Oral
   Agent, Polishing, Abrasive, Oral Cavity   Dental And Oral
   Alloy, Gold Based, For Clinical Use   Dental And Oral
   Alloy, Precious Metal, For Clinical Use   Dental And Oral
   Amalgam, Dental, Powder   Dental And Oral
   Amalgamator, Dental, AC-Powered   Dental And Oral
   Articulators   Dental And Oral
   Base, Denture, Relining, Repairing, Rebasing, Resin   Dental And Oral
   Capsule, Dental, Amalgam   Dental And Oral
   Cement, Dental   Dental And Oral
   Coating, Filling Material, Resin   Dental And Oral
   Crown And Bridge, Temporary, Resin   Dental And Oral
   Culture Media, Selective And Differential   Microbiology
   Denture, Plastic, Teeth   Dental And Oral
   Denture, Preformed   Dental And Oral
   Disk, Abrasive   Dental And Oral
   Face Bow   Dental And Oral
   Foil, Dental   Dental And Oral
   Liner, Cavity, Calcium Hydroxide   Dental And Oral
   Material, Impression   Dental And Oral
   Material, Impression Tray, Resin   Dental And Oral
   Material, Investment   Dental And Oral
   Material, Tooth Shade, Resin   Dental And Oral
   Matrix, Dental   Dental And Oral
   Metal, Base   Dental And Oral
   Mixing Slab   Dental And Oral
   Mouthguard   Dental And Oral
   Point, Abrasive   Dental And Oral
   Post, Root Canal   Dental And Oral
   Powder, Porcelain   Dental And Oral
   Primer, Cavity, Resin   Dental And Oral
   Probe, Periodontic   Dental And Oral
   Reamer, Pulp Canal, Endodontic   Dental And Oral
   Sealant, Pit And Fissure, And Conditioner, Resin   Dental And Oral
   Spatula, Cement   Dental And Oral
   Teeth, Artificial, Backing And Facing   Dental And Oral
   Teeth, Porcelain   Dental And Oral
   Tooth Bonding Agent, Resin Restoration   Dental And Oral
   Varnish, Cavity   Dental And Oral
   Wheel, Polishing Agent   Dental And Oral
Medical Product Subsidiaries (Listed Separately)
Ivoclar Vivadent, Inc.

IVORY DENTAL LABORATORY   323-663-6422
4205 Santa Monica Blvd., Los Angeles, CA 90029
FDA Number: 2032262   *Fax:* 323-663-0345
Medical Products Sales Volume: $600,000
Year Founded: 1978
Total Employees: 16

IVORY DENTAL LABORATORY
323-663-6422 *(cont'd)*
Ownership: Private
Produces/Sells CE-marked Devices: N
Federal Procurement Eligibility: Small Business
Teeth, Artificial, Posterior With Metal Insert — Dental And Oral

IVY BIOMEDICAL SYSTEMS, INC.
800-247-4614
11 Business Park Drive, Branford, CT 06405 **203-481-4183**
FDA Number: 1221108 — Fax: 203-481-8734
E-mail: info@ivybiomedical.com
Web site: www.ivybiomedical.com
Medical Products Sales Volume: $4,500,000
Annual Revenue: $5-$10 Million
Year Founded: 1984
Total Employees: 43 — *Marketing Staff:* 2 — *Sales Staff:* 3
Ownership: Private
Quality System Registration Information: ISO9001
Produces/Sells CE-marked Devices: Y
Federal Procurement Eligibility: Small Business
Distribution: Manufacturer Direct, Manufacturer Through Distributor, Manufacturer Through Manufacturer Reps, OEM, Exporter
General Admin.: Thomas Abbenante/President, Chief Executive Officer
 Donald Golan/Vice President, General Manager
Mktg./Adv.: Sandy Eames/Director Marketing
 Richard Menteles/Director Product Development
 Chris Sheridan/Vice President Marketing
 Chris Sheridan/Vice President Sales
Production: Richard Listro/Director Quality Assurance
 Richard Listro/Manager Regulatory Affairs
 Joseph Narciso/Production Engineer
Finance: Ronald Johnson/Accountant
Monitor, Bed Patient — General
Monitor, ECG — Cardiovascular
Monitor, ECG, Ambulatory, Real-Time — Cardiovascular
Monitor, Neonatal — Obstetrics/Gynecology
Monitor, Neonatal, Heart Rate — General
Monitor, Neonatal, Physiological — Obstetrics/Gynecology
Oximeter, Intracardiac — Cardiovascular
Pressure Measurement, System, Intermittent — Physical Med

IWORX SYSTEMS, INC.
800-234-1757
One Washington Street, Suite 404, Dover, NH 03820
FDA Number: n/a — Fax: 603-742-2455
E-mail: info@iworks.com
Web site: www.iworx.com
Medical Products Sales Volume: $3,000,000
Annual Revenue: $1-$5 Million
Ownership: Private
Produces/Sells CE-marked Devices: Y
Federal Procurement Eligibility: Small Business
Distribution: Manufacturer Direct, Exclusive Distributor
Recorder, Chart, Laboratory — Chemistry

IYIA TECHNOLOGIES, INC.
760-752-1036
1195 Linda Vista Drive, Suite C, San Marcos, CA 92078
FDA Number: 3004661310
Ownership: Private
Produces/Sells CE-marked Devices: N
Chamber, Oxygen, Topical, Extremity — Surgery

IZI MEDICAL PRODUCTS
800-231-1499
7020 Tudsbury Road, Baltimore, MD 21244 **410-594-9403**
FDA Number: 1123169 — Fax: 410-9594-0540
E-mail: info@izimed.com
Web site: http://www.izimed.com
Ownership: Private
Produces/Sells CE-marked Devices: N
Distribution: Manufacturer Direct
General Admin.: Ms. Helen Shafer/Chief Executive Officer
Mktg./Adv.: Mr. Jovie Soriano/Vice President Sales
Finance: Mr. David Zinreich/Chief Financial Officer
Simulator, Radiotherapy — Radiology
Tape, Adhesive — General

J & H BERGE, INC.
800-684-1234
4111 S. Clinton Avenue, **908-561-1234**
South Plainfield, NJ 07080
FDA Number: n/a — Fax: 908-561-3002
E-mail: sales@labmart.com
Web site: www.jhberge.com
Year Founded: 1850
Ownership: Private
Produces/Sells CE-marked Devices: N
Federal Procurement Eligibility: Small Business, Female Owned
Distribution: Exclusive Distributor
Mktg./Adv.: Rob Gardner/Vice President Marketing & Sales
Equipment, Laboratory, Gen. Purpose (Specific Medical Use) — Chemistry

J & J
See Johnson & Johnson

J E MEINHARD ASSOCIATES
See Meinhard Glass Products

J TECH MEDICAL INDUSTRIES
See JTECH Medical

J&B PRODUCTS, LTD.
800-556-3201
2201 S. Michigan, Saginaw, MI 48602-1275 **989-792-6119**
FDA Number: n/a — Fax: 989-792-2491
E-mail: info@itehex.com
Web site: www.itehex.com
Annual Revenue: $0-$1 Million
Total Employees: 7
Ownership: Private
Produces/Sells CE-marked Devices: N
Federal Procurement Eligibility: Small Business
Distribution: Manufacturer Direct
General Admin.: Joe Bommarito/President
Mktg./Adv.: Joe Bommarito/Vice President Marketing & Sales
Booth, Sun Tan — Physical Med

J&J ENGINEERING INC.
888-550-8300
22797 Holgar Ct. N.E., Poulsbo, WA 98370 **360-779-3853**
FDA Number: 3018871 — Fax: 360-697-4435
E-mail: sales@jjengineering.com
Web site: www.jjengineering.com
Medical Products Sales Volume: $9,000,000
Annual Revenue: $5-$10 Million
Year Founded: 1971
Total Employees: 10 — *Sales Staff:* 2
Ownership: Private
Produces/Sells CE-marked Devices: N
Federal Procurement Eligibility: Small Business
Distribution: Manufacturer Direct, Manufacturer Through Distributor
General Admin.: J.C. Hoover/President, Chief Executive Officer
 Robin Hoover/Vice President, General Manager
Biofeedback Device — Cns/Neurology

J&J ENGINEERING LLC
503-626-7812
11791 SW Crater LP, Beaverton, OR 97008
FDA Number: n/a — Fax: 503-626-7813
E-mail: j.schaeff@verizon.net
Web site: www.QuantumRunner.com
Annual Revenue: $0-$1 Million
Year Founded: 2000
Total Employees: 2
Ownership: Private
Produces/Sells CE-marked Devices: N
Federal Procurement Eligibility: Small Business
Distribution: Manufacturer Direct
Production: Jon Schaeffer/Product Executive
Wheelchair, Manual — Physical Med

J&J ENTERPRISES
See J&J Engineering Inc.

J&J HEALTHCARE PRODUCTS DIV MCNEIL-PPC, INC
866-565-2229
199 Grandview Rd, Skillman, NJ 08558
FDA Number: 2214133
Web site: www.jnj.com
Annual Revenue: $0-$1 Million
Total Employees: 1200
Ownership: Johnson & Johnson
Stock Symbol: JNJ
Traded On: NYSE
Produces/Sells CE-marked Devices: Y
Distribution: Manufacturer Through Distributor, Service Direct
General Admin.: Patrick Mutchler/President
Condom — Obstetrics/Gynecology
Floss, Dental — Dental And Oral
Lubricant, Patient — General
Pad, Menstrual, Scented — Obstetrics/Gynecology
Pad, Menstrual, Unscented — Obstetrics/Gynecology
Tampon, Menstrual, Scented — Obstetrics/Gynecology
Tampon, Menstrual, Unscented — Obstetrics/Gynecology
Toothbrush, Manual — Dental And Oral

J&S MEDICAL ASSOCIATES
800-229-6000
35 Tripp St., Bldg. 1, Framingham, MA 01702 **508-370-9797**
FDA Number: n/a — Fax: 508-370-4554
Web site: www.jsmed.com
Annual Revenue: $5-$10 Million
Year Founded: 1970
Ownership: Private
Produces/Sells CE-marked Devices: N
Federal Procurement Eligibility: Small Business

J&S MEDICAL ASSOCIATES 800-229-6000 *(cont'd)*

Distribution: Manufacturer Direct, Manufacturer Through Distributor, Manufacturer Through Manufacturer Reps, OEM, Service Direct, Exclusive Distributor, Importer, Exporter

Antigen, Latex Agglutination, Coccidioides Immitis	Microbiology
Antigen, Streptococcus SPP.	Microbiology
Computer Software	General
Contract Laboratory	General
Fluid, Manual Cell Diluting	Hematology
Fluid, Red Cell Lysing	Hematology
General Purpose Microbiology Diagnostic Device	Microbiology
Hematology Quality Control Mixture	Hematology
Kit, Screening, Staphylococcus Aureus	Microbiology
Kit, Screening, Urine	Microbiology
Reagent, Iron (Test System)	Chemistry
Reagent, Occult Blood	Hematology
Reagent, Streptolysin O/Antistreptolysin-Titer	Microbiology
Service, Used Equipment	General
System, Test, Drugs of Abuse	Chemistry
Test, C-Reactive Protein	Immunology
Test, Human Chorionic Gonadotropin	Immunology
Test, Infectious Mononucleosis	Immunology
Test, Rheumatoid Factor	Immunology
Test, Syphilis (RPR or VDRL)	Microbiology
Test, Systemic Lupus Erythematosus	Immunology

J-PAC, LLC 603-692-9955

25 Centre Road, Somersworth, NH 03878-2927
FDA Number: 1221051   *Fax:* 603-692-0909
E-mail: Sales@J-PAC.com
Web site: www.j-pac.com
Medical Products Sales Volume: $14,300,000
Annual Revenue: $5-$10 Million
Year Founded: 1983
Total Employees: 90   *Marketing Staff:* 2   *Sales Staff:* 3
Ownership: Doyen Medipharm, Inc.
Produces/Sells CE-marked Devices: N
Federal Procurement Eligibility: Small Business
Distribution: Manufacturer Direct
General Admin.: William J. McLaughlin/President, Chief Executive Officer
Mktg./Adv.: Norm Brown/Director Product Development
  Steve Sousa/Manager National Sales
  Richard S. Crane/Vice President Business Development
Production: Lori Gosselin/Director Quality Assurance
  Paul Shaw/Director Tech. Operations
  Betty Ryan/Manager Regulatory Affairs
  Richard Howard/Vice President Manufacturing

Contract Assembly	General
Contract Manufacturing	General
Contract Manufacturing, Product, Disposable	General
Contract Packaging	General
Contract Sterilization	General
Service, Engineering/Design	General
Thermoforming, Extrusion, Custom	General

J. BAROT & ASSOC. 321-383-7574

1125 White Dr., P.o. Box 5293, Titusville, FL 32780
FDA Number: 1063747
Ownership: Private
Produces/Sells CE-marked Devices: N

Clip, Iris Retractor	Ophthalmology

J. E. HANGER LTD. 888-592-3433
514-489-8213

5545 St. Jacques St. W.,
Montreal, QUE H4A-2 Canada
FDA Number: 8043617
E-mail: info@jehanger.ca   *Fax:* 514-489-9599
Web site: www.jehanger.ca
Year Founded: 1952
Ownership: Private
Produces/Sells CE-marked Devices: N
Distribution: Manufacturer Direct

J. G. FINNERAN ASSOCIATES, INC. 800-552-3696
856-696-3605

3600 Reilly Ct., Vineland, NJ 08360
FDA Number: n/a   *Fax:* 856-696-9002
E-mail: dnelson@jgfinneran.com
Web site: www.jgfinneran.com
Year Founded: 1977
Total Employees: 75   *Marketing Staff:* 2   *Sales Staff:* 2
Ownership: Private
Quality System Registration Information: ISO9001
Produces/Sells CE-marked Devices: N
Federal Procurement Eligibility: Small Business
Distribution: Manufacturer Through Distributor
General Admin.: James G. Finneran/Chief Executive Officer
  Josephine Finneran/President
  Sandy F. Hitchner/Vice President
Mktg./Adv.: Dawn C. Nelson/Manager Marketing & Sales

J. G. FINNERAN ASSOCIATES, INC. 800-552-3696 *(cont'd)*

Production: Steve McKishen/Manager Materials
  Sharon DaSilva/Manager Quality Assurance

Ampule	Gastroenterology/Urology
Packaging Material	General
Vial, Other	General

J. H. EMERSON CO. 800-252-1414

22 Cottage Park Avenue, Cambridge, MA 02140 617-864-1414
FDA Number: 1216146   *Fax:* 617-868-0841
E-mail: info@jhemerson.com
Web site: www.jhemerson.com
Medical Products Sales Volume: $10,000,000
Annual Revenue: $5-$10 Million
Year Founded: 1928
Total Employees: 17
Ownership: Private
Quality System Registration Information: ISO9001
Produces/Sells CE-marked Devices: Y
Federal Procurement Eligibility: Small Business
Distribution: Manufacturer Through Distributor

Bottle, Collection, Vacuum (Aspirator)	General
Lamp, Infrared	Physical Med
Suction Apparatus, Ward Use, Portable, AC-Powered	Surgery
Ventilator, Non-Continuous (Respirator)	Anesthesiology
Warmer, Radiant, Infant	General

J. HEWITT INCORPORATED 800-543-9488
949-855-8104

6 Faraday, Unit B, Irvine, CA 92618
FDA Number: 7000544   *Fax:* 949-855-8104
E-mail: administration@jhewitt.com
Web site: www.jhewitt.com
Medical Products Sales Volume: $300,000
Annual Revenue: $1-$5 Million
Total Employees: 2   *Sales Staff:* 10
Ownership: Private
Produces/Sells CE-marked Devices: Y
Federal Procurement Eligibility: Small Business
Distribution: Manufacturer Direct, Exporter
General Admin.: Mr. James Hewitt/Chief Executive Officer, Chairman
  Mr. Jason Hewitt/Chief Financial Officer, Controller

Perforator, Ear-Lobe	Ear/Nose/Throat
Solution, Patient Preparation	General

J. JAMNER SURGICAL INSTRUMENTS, INC 800-431-1123
877-468-5572

9 Skyline Dr., Hawthorne, NY 10532
FDA Number: 2430952   *Fax:* 609-750-4257
E-mail: info@jarit.com
Web site: www.jarit.com
Ownership: Integra Lifesciences Holdings Corp.
Stock Symbol: IART
Traded On: NASDAQ
Quality System Registration Information: ISO9001
Produces/Sells CE-marked Devices: Y
Federal Procurement Eligibility: Small Business
Distribution: Manufacturer Through Distributor
General Admin.: Howard Jamner/President
Mktg./Adv.: Robert Rogowski/Vice President Sales

Coagulator/Cutter, Endoscopic, Unipolar	Obstetrics/Gynecology
Electrosurgical Equipment, General Purpose	Surgery
Electrosurgical Unit, Cutting & Coagulation Device	Surgery
Endoscope And Accessories, AC-Powered	Surgery
Forceps	Orthopedics
Forceps, Endoscopic	Gastroenterology/Urology
Forceps, General & Plastic Surgery	Surgery
Forceps, Hemostatic	Surgery
Forceps, Ophthalmic	Ophthalmology
Forceps, Tissue	Surgery
Forceps, Wire Holding	Orthopedics
Instrument, Manual, General Surgical	Surgery
Kit, Cholecystectomy	Gastroenterology/Urology
Kit, Instruments and Accessories, Surgical	Surgery
Laparoscope, General & Plastic Surgery	Surgery
Nasopharyngoscope (Flexible Or Rigid)	Ear/Nose/Throat
Scissors, Cardiovascular	Cardiovascular
Scissors, Corneal	Ophthalmology
Scissors, Enucleation	Ophthalmology
Scissors, General Dissecting	General
Scissors, Iris	Ophthalmology
Scissors, Neurosurgical (Dura)	Cns/Neurology
Scissors, Orthopedic	Orthopedics
Scissors, Plastic Surgery (Dissecting)	Surgery
Surgical Instrument, Cardiovascular	Cardiovascular

J. L. SHEPHERD AND ASSOC. 818-898-2361

1010 Arroyo Ave., San Fernando, CA 91340
FDA Number: 2028419

Irradiator, Blood to Prevent Graft Vs Host Disease	Radiology

MANUFACTURER PROFILES

J. LAMB, INC. A DIVISION OF THE STRONGWATER GROUP   **888-379-6453**

250 Moonachie Avenue, Moonachie, NJ 07074
FDA Number: 2249296
E-mail: diane@jlamb.com   Fax: 201-440-2899
Web site: www.philmontmfg.com
Ownership: Private
Produces/Sells CE-marked Devices: N
Federal Procurement Eligibility: Female Owned
Distribution: Manufacturer Direct, Manufacturer Through Distributor, Manufacturer Through Manufacturer Reps, Importer, Exporter
General Admin.: Mr. Bruce Strongwater/Chief Executive Officer, Chairman

Cover, Mattress	General

J. MORITA USA, INC.   **888-566-7482**
9 Mason, Irvine, CA 92618   **949-581-9600**
FDA Number: 2081055   Fax: 949-465-1095
E-mail: info@jmoritausa.com
Web site: www.jmoritausa.com
Medical Products Sales Volume: $15,000,000
Year Founded: 1964
Total Employees: 34   Marketing Staff: 4   Sales Staff: 20
Ownership: J. MORITA CORPORATION, JAPAN
Quality System Registration Information: ISO9001
Produces/Sells CE-marked Devices: Y
Federal Procurement Eligibility: Small Business
Distribution: Manufacturer Direct, Manufacturer Through Distributor, Exclusive Distributor, Importer, Exporter
General Admin.: Mr. Junichi Miyata/President
Mktg./Adv.: Ms. Cheri Booth/Manager Marketing
    Mr. Walid Wardaki/Vice President Sales
Production: Mr. Phil Moen/Vice President Operations

Adhesive, Dental	Dental And Oral
Base, Denture, Relining, Repairing, Rebasing, Resin	Dental And Oral
Cement, Dental	Dental And Oral
Chair, Dental	Dental And Oral
Endodontic Instrument	Dental And Oral
Light, Dental	Dental And Oral
Locator, Apex, Root	Dental And Oral
Material, Dental Filling	Dental And Oral
Material, Impression	Dental And Oral
Post, Root Canal	Dental And Oral
Processor, Radiographic Film, Automatic, Dental	Dental And Oral
Remover, Crown	Dental And Oral
Retractor, All Types	Dental And Oral
Tooth Bonding Agent, Resin Restoration	Dental And Oral

J. POHLER   **305-757-7733**
8740 Sw 21st Street, Ft. Lauderdale, FL 33324
FDA Number: 1038610
Ownership: Private
Produces/Sells CE-marked Devices: N

Pack, Hot Or Cold, Water Circulating	Physical Med

J. SLAWNER LTD.   **514-735-6565**
5713 Cote des Neiges, Montreal, QUE H3S-1Y7 Canada
FDA Number: n/a   Fax: 514-735-6565
E-mail: info@slawner.com
Web site: www.slawner.com
Year Founded: 1952
Total Employees: 50
Ownership: Private
Produces/Sells CE-marked Devices: N
Distribution: Manufacturer Direct

J. STERLING INDUSTRIES LTD.   **(905) 264-6657**
405 Rowntree Dairy Road, Woodbridge, ONT L4L 8H1 Canada
FDA Number: n/a   Fax: (905) 264-5571
E-mail: info@sterlingindustries.com
Web site: www.sterlingindustries.com
Year Founded: 1983
Total Employees: 10
Ownership: Private
Produces/Sells CE-marked Devices: N
Distribution: Manufacturer Direct, Exporter

J. T. POSEY CO.   **800-447-6739**
5635 Peck Rd., Arcadia, CA 91006-5851   **626-443-3143**
FDA Number: 2020362   Fax: 626-443-5014
Web site: www.posey.com
Year Founded: 1937
Total Employees: 250   Marketing Staff: 8   Sales Staff: 15
Ownership: Private
Produces/Sells CE-marked Devices: N
Federal Procurement Eligibility: Small Business
Distribution: Manufacturer Direct, Manufacturer Through Manufacturer Reps, OEM
General Admin.: J.T. Posey/Chief Executive Officer
    Mike Keefe/General Manager

J. T. POSEY CO.   **800-447-6739** (cont'd)
    Molly Aragon/Manager Personnel
    Ernest Posey/President
Mktg./Adv.: Jeffrey Yates/Director Marketing
Production: Janet Lidikay/Director Quality Assurance

Accessories, Wheelchair	Physical Med
Bag, Leg	Gastroenterology/Urology
Bed Cradle	General
Bed, Electric	General
Bed, Manual	General
Belt, Wheelchair	Physical Med
Board, Arm	Anesthesiology
Board, Foot	Orthopedics
Collar, Cervical Neck	Orthopedics
Component, Exercise	Physical Med
Cuff, Tracheal Tube, Inflatable	Anesthesiology
Cushion, Flotation	Physical Med
Cushion, Foot	Orthopedics
Cushion, Wheelchair (Pad)	Physical Med
Exerciser, Hand	Physical Med
Fixation Device, Tracheal Tube	Anesthesiology
Garment, Protective, For Incontinence	Gastroenterology/Urology
Gown, Examination	General
Mask, Eye, Phototherapy	Ophthalmology
Monitor, Bed Patient	General
Orthosis, Limb Brace	Physical Med
Pad, Neonatal Eye	General
Pad, Pressure, Foam (Elbow, Heel)	General
Pad, Pressure, Foam Convoluted	General
Protector, Skin Pressure	General
Restraint, Ankle/Foot	General
Restraint, Arm	General
Restraint, Patient, Conductive	Anesthesiology
Restraint, Protective (Body)	General
Restraint, Vest	General
Restraint, Wheelchair	General
Restraint, Wrist/Hand	General
Sling, Arm	Physical Med
Splint, Extremity, Non-Inflatable, External	Surgery
Strap, Head, Gas Mask	Anesthesiology
Stretcher, Hand-Carried	General
Support, Foot	Orthopedics
Support, Head And Trunk, Wheelchair	Physical Med
Traction Unit, Non-Powered	Orthopedics
Transfer Aid	Physical Med

J.B.C AND CO.   **702-914-8842**
7980 West Torino Ave, Las Vegas, NV 89113
FDA Number: 2954315

Base, Denture, Relining, Repairing, Rebasing, Resin	Dental And Oral

J.E.M. SALES LTD.   **416-663-7313**
6-110 Norfinch Dr, Toronto M3N 1X1 Canada
FDA Number: 9681417

Shield, Eye, Ophthalmic	Ophthalmology

J.G. LENS CORPORATION
    See J.G. Optical

J.G. OPTICAL   **718-891-1414**
1424 Sheepshead Bay Rd., Brooklyn, NY 11235-3814
FDA Number: n/a   Fax: 718-332-6398
Web site: www.jgoptical.com
Annual Revenue: $0-$1 Million
Ownership: Private
Produces/Sells CE-marked Devices: N
Distribution: Manufacturer Through Distributor, Importer, Exporter

Lens, Spectacle/Eyeglasses, Custom (Prescription)	Ophthalmology

J.M. BARAGANO BIOMEDICAL P.M. AND CONSULTING, INC.   **787-722-4007**
808 Fernandez Juncos Avenue, San Juan, PR 00907
FDA Number: n/a   Fax: 787-722-4491
E-mail: info@bioclinic.com
Web site: www.bioclinic.com
Medical Products Sales Volume: $1,600,000
Annual Revenue: $1-$5 Million
Year Founded: 1990
Total Employees: 24   Marketing Staff: 2   Sales Staff: 7
Ownership: Private
Produces/Sells CE-marked Devices: N
Federal Procurement Eligibility: Small Business
Distribution: Service Direct, Exclusive Distributor, Importer, Exporter
General Admin.: Ing Jorge M. Baragano/Chief Executive Officer
    Jorge M. Baragano/President
Mktg./Adv.: Carliany Reyes/Director Marketing
    Jorge M. Baragaşo/Manager International & National Sales
Production: Francisco J. Oms/Director Quality Assurance
Finance: Ms. Nereida Lopez/Director Finance

Analyzer, ECG	Cardiovascular

J.M. BARAGANO BIOMEDICAL P.M. AND   787-722-4007 *(cont'd)*
Monitor, ECG	Cardiovascular
Security Equipment/Supplies	General
Service, Maintenance/Repair	General

J.M. MURRAY CENTER, INC.   800-566-8772
823 NYS Rte. 13, Cortland, NY 13045   **607-756-9913**
FDA Number: 1319147   *Fax:* 607-753-6954
Web site: www.jmmurray.com
Annual Revenue: $1-$5 Million
Ownership: Private
Produces/Sells CE-marked Devices: N
Distribution: Manufacturer Direct, Service Direct
Floss, Dental	Dental And Oral
Toothbrush, Manual	Dental And Oral
Unit, Sanitation/Sterilization, Toothbrush, Ultraviolet	Dental And Oral

J.P. GILBERT CO.   610-367-7457
548 Mountain Rd., Boyertown, PA 19512
FDA Number: 2531191   *Fax:* 610-369-9288
E-mail: ironstone4@dejazzd.com
Web site: www.hemaprep.com
Ownership: Private
Produces/Sells CE-marked Devices: N
Spinner, Slide, Automated	Hematology

J.R. RAND CORP.   800-526-7111
100 S. Jeffryn Blvd. E., Deer Park, NY 11729   **631-253-0101**
FDA Number: 2418518   *Fax:* 631-253-0505
E-mail: ckelly@jrrand.com
Web site: www.jrrand.com
Medical Products Sales Volume: $600,000
Annual Revenue: $1-$5 Million
Year Founded: 1964
Total Employees: 10
Ownership: Private
Produces/Sells CE-marked Devices: N
Federal Procurement Eligibility: Small Business
Distribution: Manufacturer Direct
General Admin.: Richard Stenn/President, Chief Executive Officer
Mktg./Adv.: Cynthia Kelly/Vice President Marketing
Band, Matrix	Dental And Oral

J.S. ASSOCIATES   813-975-4354
8403 Ridgebrook Cir, Odessa, FL 33556
FDA Number: 1066500
Ownership: Private
Produces/Sells CE-marked Devices: N
Component, Exercise	Physical Med

J.W. WESTMAN INC.   800-387-8204
5-2800 Argentia Road,   **905-821-3166**
Mississauga, ONT L5N 8 Canada
FDA Number: n/a   *Fax:* 905-821-3168
E-mail: info@jwwestman.com
Year Founded: 1978
Total Employees: 25
Ownership: Private
Produces/Sells CE-marked Devices: N
Distribution: Exclusive Distributor

JABIL GLOBAL SERVICES   502-240-1000
11201 Electron Dr., Louisville, KY 40299
FDA Number: 1531264   *Fax:* 502-240-1193
Web site: www.jabil.com
Annual Revenue: $10-$25 Million
Year Founded: 1966
Total Employees: 85000
Ownership: Private
Produces/Sells CE-marked Devices: N
General Admin.: Mark Mondello/Chief Operating Officer
　　　　　Timothy L. Main/President, Chief Executive Officer
Finance: Forbes I.J. Alexander/Chief Financial Officer
Electrocardiograph, Single Channel	Cardiovascular
Monitor, Blood Pressure, Indirect, Semi-Automatic	Cardiovascular
Oximeter, Intracardiac	Cardiovascular
Scale, Infant	General
Transmitter/Receiver System, Physiological, Radiofrequency	Cardiovascular

JACE SYSTEMS   800-800-4276
5 Rockhill Rd, Suite 2, Cherry Hill, NJ 08003   **856-470-2100**
FDA Number: 2246559   *Fax:* 800-236-2308
E-mail: salesinfo@jacesystems.com
Web site: www.jacesystems.com
Medical Products Sales Volume: $4,000,000
Annual Revenue: $1-$5 Million
Year Founded: 1989
Total Employees: 22   *Sales Staff:* 8

JACE SYSTEMS   800-800-4276 *(cont'd)*
Ownership: Private
Quality System Registration Information: ISO9001
Produces/Sells CE-marked Devices: Y
Federal Procurement Eligibility: Small Business
Distribution: OEM, Service Direct, Exclusive Distributor, Exporter
General Admin.: Mr. Thomas Zieser/Owner, Chief Executive Officer
Production: Mr. Wayne Maurer/Director Operations
Exerciser, Finger, Powered	Physical Med
Exerciser, Other	Physical Med
Exerciser, Passive, Non-Measuring (CPM Machine)	Physical Med
Joint, Knee, External Brace	Physical Med
Stimulator, Electrical, Muscle	Physical Med
Wrist, External Limb Component, Powered	Physical Med

JACE SYSTEMS, INC   (856) 470-2100
55 Carnegie Plaza, Cherry Hill, NJ 08003   **(856) 470-2100**
FDA Number: 2246559   *Fax:* 800-236-2308
E-mail: info@homemedical.com
Web site: www.homemedical.com
Annual Revenue: $25-$50 Million
Total Employees: 900   *Marketing Staff:* 5   *Sales Staff:* 150
Ownership: JACE SYSTEMS, INC
Produces/Sells CE-marked Devices: N
Federal Procurement Eligibility: Small Business
Distribution: Manufacturer Direct, Exclusive Distributor
General Admin.: Craig Porter/President, Chief Executive Officer
　　　　　Ganine Weiss/Vice President Human Resources
　　　　　Greg Butler/Vice President, Assistant Secretary
Mktg./Adv.: Mary Webb/Director Education
　　　　　Jerry Bodie/Director National Accounts
　　　　　Jerry Bodie/Manager National Sales
　　　　　Richard Buck/Vice President Marketing & Communications
　　　　　Dan O'Grady/Vice President Sales
Production: Don Linske/Director Manufacturing
　　　　　Bob Kaiser/Vice President Manufacturing
　　　　　Julia Melendez/Vice President Regulatory Affairs
Finance: Jack Brown/Chief Financial Officer
Exerciser, Passive, Non-Measuring (CPM Machine)	Physical Med
Exerciser, Powered	Anesthesiology
Splint, Other	Orthopedics
Stimulator, Muscle, Electrical-Powered (EMS)	Physical Med
Support, Knee	Physical Med
Medical Product Subsidiaries (Listed Separately)
　JACE SYSTEMS, INC

JACE SYSTEMS, INC.
See JACE SYSTEMS, INC

JACK JONES HEARING AID CENTERS, INC.   800-722-8534
400 South Henderson, Ft. Worth, TX 76104   **817-335-2583**
FDA Number: 1643698   *Fax:* 817-335-2597
E-mail: sales@jonesaudiology.com
Web site: www.jonesaudiology.com
Medical Products Sales Volume: $1,300,000
Year Founded: 1959
Total Employees: 18   *Sales Staff:* 29
Ownership: Private
Produces/Sells CE-marked Devices: N
Federal Procurement Eligibility: Small Business
Distribution: Manufacturer Direct
Hearing-Aid, Master	Ear/Nose/Throat

JACKSON COUNTY SHELTERED WORKS
　See Webster Enterprises, Inc.

JACKSON INC., S.
　See S Jackson Inc.

JACO MEDICAL EQUIPMENT INC.   858-278-7743
4848 Ronson Ct., Suite E, San Diego, CA 92111
FDA Number: 2084727   *Fax:* 858-278-5472
E-mail: info@jacomed.com
Web site: www.jacomed.com
Medical Products Sales Volume: $1,000,000
Annual Revenue: $1-$5 Million
Year Founded: 1991
Total Employees: 3   *Marketing Staff:* 1   *Sales Staff:* 4
Ownership: Private
Produces/Sells CE-marked Devices: N
Federal Procurement Eligibility: Small Business, Minority Owned
Distribution: Service Direct, Exporter
General Admin.: Jaime Munoz/President, Chief Executive Officer
Mktg./Adv.: Rosa L. Larrano/Manager International Marketing & Sales
Echocardiograph (Ultrasonic Scanner)	Cardiovascular
Radiographic Unit, Diagnostic	Radiology
Scanner, Ultrasonic (Pulsed Doppler)	Radiology
Scanner, Ultrasonic, General Purpose	Radiology
Scanner, Ultrasonic, Obstetrical/Gynecological	Obstetrics/Gynecology
Scanner, Ultrasonic, Obstetrical/Gynecological, Mobile	Obstetrics/Gynecology

JACO MEDICAL EQUIPMENT INC.   858-278-7743 *(cont'd)*
Scanner, Ultrasonic, Other   Radiology

JACUZZI, BATH DIVISION   800-288-4002
14880 Monte Vista Avenue, Suite 550,   909-548-7732
Chino, CA 91710
FDA Number: 9330054   *Fax:* 909-606-2913
E-mail: custserv@jacuzzi.com
Web site: www.jacuzzi.com
Total Employees: 500   *Marketing Staff:* 50   *Sales Staff:* 50
Ownership: JACUZZI BRANDS
Stock Symbol: JJZ
Traded On: NYSE
Produces/Sells CE-marked Devices: N
Federal Procurement Eligibility: Small Business
Distribution: Manufacturer Direct, Manufacturer Through Distributor, Manufacturer Through Manufacturer Reps, Service Direct, Exporter
General Admin.: Jan Jerger-Stevens/Director Human Resources
Mktg./Adv.: Melissa Gosling/Director Corporate Communications
Production: Jim Barry/Vice President Manufacturing
   Bath, Hydro-Massage (Whirlpool)   Physical Med

JADE HEARING INSTRUMENTS   248-922-5600
6803 Dixie Hwy., Suite #2, Clarkston, MI 48346
FDA Number: 1831353
   Hearing-Aid   Ear/Nose/Throat

JAECE INDUSTRIES, INC.   716-694-2811
908 Niagara Falls Boulevard, North Tonawanda, NY 14120-2020
FDA Number: n/a   *Fax:* 716-694-2811
E-mail: sales@jaece.com
Web site: www.jaece.com
Medical Products Sales Volume: $4,500,000
Annual Revenue: $0-$1 Million
Year Founded: 1982
Total Employees: 5   *Marketing Staff:* 1   *Sales Staff:* 1
Ownership: Private
Produces/Sells CE-marked Devices: N
Federal Procurement Eligibility: Small Business
Distribution: Manufacturer Through Distributor
General Admin.: Joseph M. Palka/Chief Executive Officer
     Vicki Zimmerman/Office Manager
     Judith A. Palka/President
   Cabinet Casework, General Purpose   General
   Cabinet, Storage, Slide   General
   Cover, Other   General
   Pen, Marking, Surgical   Ophthalmology
   Stand/Holder, Equipment, Laboratory   Chemistry
   Stopper   General
   Tube, Centrifuge   Chemistry

JAECO ORTHOPEDIC SPECIALTIES, INC.   501-623-5944
214 Drexel Street, Hot Springs, AR 71901
FDA Number: n/a   *Fax:* 501-623-0159
E-mail: info@jaecoorthopedic.com
Web site: www.jaecoorthopedic.com
Annual Revenue: $0-$1 Million
Year Founded: 1953
Ownership: Private
Produces/Sells CE-marked Devices: N
Federal Procurement Eligibility: Small Business
Distribution: Manufacturer Direct, Manufacturer Through Distributor
General Admin.: Randall Sims/Business Manager
     Mark Conry/President
   Attachment, Narrowing, Wheelchair   Physical Med
   Support, Arm   Physical Med
   Support, Hand   Orthopedics

JAISONS INTERNATIONAL, INC.   203-261-1653
22 Bittersweet Lane, Trumbull, CT 06611
FDA Number: n/a
E-mail: jaisons@sprynet.com
Medical Products Sales Volume: $2,000,000
Annual Revenue: $1-$5 Million
Total Employees: 2
Ownership: Private
Quality System Registration Information: ISO9002; ISO9003
Produces/Sells CE-marked Devices: Y
Federal Procurement Eligibility: Minority Owned
Distribution: Manufacturer Direct, Manufacturer Through Distributor, Manufacturer Through Manufacturer Reps, Importer, Exporter
Mktg./Adv.: Niraj Gupta/Director Marketing
   Blade, Scalpel   Surgery
   Collector, Urine   Gastroenterology/Urology
   Condom With Nonoxynol-9   Obstetrics/Gynecology
   Glove, Patient Examination, Latex   General
   Glove, Patient Examination, Vinyl   General

JAISONS INTERNATIONAL, INC.   203-261-1653 *(cont'd)*
Glove, Surgical   General

JAMES CONSOLIDATED, INC.   800-884-3317
PO Box 3483, 1867 Ygnacio Valley Rd,   925-691-5117
Walnut Creek, CA 94598
FDA Number: n/a   *Fax:* 925-691-4200
E-mail: jamescon@astound.net
Web site: www.volkner.com
Medical Products Sales Volume: $900,000
Annual Revenue: $1-$5 Million
Year Founded: 1983
Total Employees: 4
Ownership: Private
Quality System Registration Information: ISO9001
Produces/Sells CE-marked Devices: Y
Federal Procurement Eligibility: Small Business, Female Owned
Distribution: Manufacturer Direct, Manufacturer Through Distributor, Manufacturer Through Manufacturer Reps, OEM, Exporter
General Admin.: Ingrid James/Executive President
     Brian James/President, Chief Executive Officer
   Mattress, Air Flotation   General

JAMES MEDICAL INDUSTRIES
See King Pharmaceuticals, Inc.

JAMESTOWN METAL PRODUCTS   716-665-5313
178 Blackstone Avenue, Jamestown, NY 14701-2297
FDA Number: 9330055   *Fax:* 716-665-5121
E-mail: sales@jamestown.com
Web site: www.jamestown.com
Medical Products Sales Volume: $10,400,000
Annual Revenue: $25-$50 Million
Year Founded: 1943
Total Employees: 105   *Marketing Staff:* 8   *Sales Staff:* 50
Ownership: Private
Produces/Sells CE-marked Devices: N
Federal Procurement Eligibility: Small Business, Female Owned, GSA Contract
Distribution: Manufacturer Through Distributor
General Admin.: Jeff Christie/President
     Chip Wiseman/Regional Manager
     Michael Cook/Regional Manager
     Warren Sieber/Regional Manager
Mktg./Adv.: David Weber/Vice President Marketing & Sales
Finance: Chuck Papia/Vice President Finance
   Cabinet Casework, Laboratory   Chemistry
   Cabinet Casework, Modular   General
   Cabinet Casework, Patient Room   General
   Cabinet Casework, Pharmacy   General
   Hood, Fume   Toxicology
   Station, Nursing   General

JAMIESAN COMPANY   781-444-1026
1492 Highland Ave, Needham, MA 02492
FDA Number: n/a
Ownership: Private
Produces/Sells CE-marked Devices: N
Federal Procurement Eligibility: Small Business
Distribution: Manufacturer Direct
   Component, Metal, Other   General
   Contract Manufacturing   General
   Molding, Injection   General

JAMNER SURGICAL INSTRUMENTS
See J. Jamner Surgical Instruments, Inc

JANCO PAC CORP.
See J-Pac, Llc

JANIN GROUP, INC.   800-323-5389
14A Stonehill Road, Oswego, IL 60543-9400   630-554-5533
FDA Number: 1450420   *Fax:* 630-554-5535
E-mail: jnavis@medigroupinc.com
Web site: www.medigroupinc.com
Medical Products Sales Volume: $300,000
Annual Revenue: $1-$5 Million
Year Founded: 1979
Total Employees: 4   *Marketing Staff:* 1   *Sales Staff:* 2
Ownership: Private
Quality System Registration Information: ISO9001
Produces/Sells CE-marked Devices: Y
Federal Procurement Eligibility: Small Business
Distribution: Manufacturer Direct, Manufacturer Through Distributor, Manufacturer Through Manufacturer Reps, OEM, Exporter
General Admin.: John A. Navis/President
Mktg./Adv.: John A. Navis/Director Marketing
Finance: Irene K. Navis/Manager Finance
   Catheter, Other   Gastroenterology/Urology
   Catheter, Peritoneal   Surgery
   Cover, Shoe, Non-Conductive   General

JANIN GROUP, INC.   800-323-5389 *(cont'd)*

Cover, Shoe, Operating Room	Surgery
Drape, Surgical, Disposable	Surgery
Peritoneal Dialysis Unit (CAPD)	Gastroenterology/Urology

JANLER CORPORATION   773-774-0166
6545 N. Avondale Avenue, Chicago, IL 60631
FDA Number: 90069
Ownership: Private
Produces/Sells CE-marked Devices: N

Applicator, Vaginal	Obstetrics/Gynecology

JANNX MEDICAL SYSTEMS INC.   800-325-4334
12166 Old Big Bend Blvd., Ste. 300,   314-822-7799
St. Louis, MO 63122
FDA Number: n/a
Web site: jannx.com
Annual Revenue: $0-$1 Million
Ownership: Rsti (Radiological Service Training Institute)
Produces/Sells CE-marked Devices: N
Distribution: Service Direct

Contract R&D, Diagnostics	General

JANNX MEDICAL SYSTEMS INC., DIAG. IMAGING DIV.
See Jannx Medical Systems Inc.

JANSSEN-ORTHO INC.   1 (800) 387-87
19 Green Belt Dr,   416-449-9444
North York, ON M3C 1 Canada
FDA Number: 9200828   *Fax:* 416-449-2658
Web site: www.janssen-ortho.com
Total Employees: 400
Ownership: Private
Quality System Registration Information: ISO9001
Produces/Sells CE-marked Devices: N
Distribution: Manufacturer Through Distributor

JANT PHARMACAL CORP.   800-676-5565
16255 Ventura Blvd., Suite 505,   818-986-8530
Encino, CA 91436
FDA Number: 2030633   *Fax:* 818-986-0235
E-mail: info@accutest.net
Web site: www.accutest.net
Medical Products Sales Volume: $1,600,000
Annual Revenue: $5-$10 Million
Year Founded: 1986
Total Employees: 10
Ownership: Private
Produces/Sells CE-marked Devices: N
Federal Procurement Eligibility: Small Business, GSA Contract
Distribution: Manufacturer Through Manufacturer Reps, OEM, Service Direct, Exporter
Mktg./Adv.: Kristi Beck/Manager Marketing
           Jack C. Tawfik/Vice President Sales

Antiserum, Streptococcus SPP.	Microbiology
Enzyme Immunoassay, Amphetamine	Toxicology
Enzyme Immunoassay, Benzodiazepine	Toxicology
Enzyme Immunoassay, Cannabinoids	Toxicology
Enzyme Immunoassay, Methadone	Toxicology
Enzyme Immunoassay, Phencyclidine	Toxicology
Fluorometry, Morphine	Toxicology
Gas Chromatography, Methamphetamine	Toxicology
Kit, Pregnancy Test, Over The Counter, HCG	Chemistry
Radioimmunoassay, Luteinizing Hormone	Chemistry
System, Test, Drugs of Abuse	Chemistry
Test, Fertility Monitoring	Obstetrics/Gynecology
Test, Human Chorionic Gonadotropin, Serum	Immunology
Test, Infectious Mononucleosis	Immunology
Thin Layer Chromatography, Benzoylecgnonine	Toxicology

JANUS DEVELOPMENT GROUP, INC.   866-551-9042
112 Staton Rd., Greenville, NC 27834   252-551-9042
FDA Number: 1066749   *Fax:* 252-413-0950
E-mail: customerserv@janusdevelopment.com
Web site: www.janusdevelopment.com
Year Founded: 2001
Total Employees: 12
Ownership: Private
Produces/Sells CE-marked Devices: Y
Distribution: Manufacturer Through Distributor

Anti-Stammering Device	Ear/Nose/Throat

JARDON EYE PROSTHETICS, INC.   248-424-8560
15920 W 12 Mile Road, Southfield, MI 48076-2115
FDA Number: 1824736   *Fax:* 248-424-8561
E-mail: jardoneye@aol.com
Web site: http://jardoneye.com/
Medical Products Sales Volume: $200,000
Total Employees: 4

JARDON EYE PROSTHETICS, INC.   248-424-8560 *(cont'd)*
Ownership: Private
Produces/Sells CE-marked Devices: N
Federal Procurement Eligibility: Small Business
Distribution: Manufacturer Direct
General Admin.: Paul Jardon/Chief Executive Officer

Conformer, Ophthalmic	Ophthalmology
Eye, Artificial, Custom	Ophthalmology
Implant, Subperiosteal	Dental And Oral
Ring, Symblepharon	Ophthalmology
Shield, Eye, Ophthalmic	Ophthalmology
Sphere, Ophthalmic (Implant)	Ophthalmology
Tray, Impression	Dental And Oral

JARDON INSTITUTE FOR EYE CARE, INC.
See Jardon Eye Prosthetics, Inc.

JARI ELECTRODE SUPPLY   800-745-1934
380 Tomkins Ct., Gilroy, CA 95020   408-847-1895
FDA Number: n/a   *Fax:* 408-847-3620
E-mail: sales@jarisupply.com
Web site: www.jarisupply.com
Medical Products Sales Volume: $2,100,000
Annual Revenue: $1-$5 Million
Total Employees: 4   *Marketing Staff:* 3   *Sales Staff:* 3
Ownership: Private
Produces/Sells CE-marked Devices: N
Federal Procurement Eligibility: Small Business, Female Owned
Distribution: Manufacturer Direct, Exporter
General Admin.: RICHARD KAISER/President
           RICHARD KAISER/Vice President
Mktg./Adv.: Sonja Lujan/Manager National Sales

Electrode, Needle	Cns/Neurology
Electrode, Surface	Anesthesiology

JARO, INC.   610-527-1889
1111 Lancaster Ave., Rosemont, PA 19010
FDA Number: 2522272
Ownership: Private
Produces/Sells CE-marked Devices: N

Handpiece, Belt and/or Gear Driven, Dental	Dental And Oral

JARRELL-ASH
See Fisher Scientific Co., Llc.

JARVIS SURGICAL, INC.   413-562-6659
53 Airport Rd., Westfield, MA 01085
FDA Number: n/a
Web site: www.jarvissurgical.com
Annual Revenue: $0-$1 Million
Ownership: Private
Quality System Registration Information: ISO9000
Produces/Sells CE-marked Devices: N
Federal Procurement Eligibility: Small Business
Distribution: Manufacturer Direct

Contract Manufacturing	General
Service, Design, Implant, Custom	Orthopedics

JAS DIAGNOSTICS, INC.   305-418-2320
14100 n.w. 57th court, Miami Lakes, FL 33014
FDA Number: 1064608   *Fax:* 305-418-2321
E-mail: d.johnston@jasdiagnostics.com
Web site: www.jasdiagnostics.com
Medical Products Sales Volume: $2,000,000
Annual Revenue: $1-$5 Million
Ownership: Drew Scientific Ltd.
Produces/Sells CE-marked Devices: N
General Admin.: David Johnston/President

Analyzer, Chemistry, Photometric, Discrete	Chemistry
Antigen, Antiserum, Control, Prealbumin	Immunology
Azo-Dye, Calcium	Chemistry
Calibrator, Ethyl Alcohol	Toxicology
Calibrator, Primary, Clinical Chemistry	Chemistry
Calibrator, Secondary, Clinical Chemistry	Chemistry
Catalytic Method, Amylase	Chemistry
Colorimetric Method, Lipoproteins	Chemistry
Complexone, Cresolphthalein, Calcium	Chemistry
Control, Analyte (Assayed And Unassayed)	Chemistry
Control, Multi Analyte, All Kinds (Assayed And Unassayed)	Chemistry
Dye-Binding, Albumin, Bromcresol, Green	Chemistry
Electrode, Ion Specific, Potassium	Chemistry
Electrode, Ion Specific, Sodium	Chemistry
Enzymatic Esterase-Oxidase, Cholesterol	Chemistry
Enzymatic, Carbon-Dioxide	Chemistry
Ferrozine (Colorimetric) Iron Binding Capacity	Chemistry
Hemoglobin F Quantitation	Hematology
Hexokinase, Glucose	Chemistry
Kinetic Method, Gamma-Glutamyl Transpeptidase	Chemistry
LDL & VLDL Precipitation, Cholesterol Via Esterase-Oxidase	Chemistry
LDL & VLDL Precipitation, HDL	Chemistry
Lipase Hydrolysis/Glycerol Kinase Enzyme, Triglycerides	Chemistry

MANUFACTURER PROFILES

JAS DIAGNOSTICS, INC. 305-418-2320 *(cont'd)*

Lipase-Esterase, Enzymatic, Photometric, Lipase	Chemistry
Multi Analyte Mixture, Calibrator	Chemistry
NAD Reduction/NADH Oxidation, CPK Or Isoenzymes	Chemistry
NAD Reduction/NADH Oxidation, Lactate Dehydrogenase	Chemistry
NADH Oxidation/NAD Reduction, AST/SGOT	Chemistry
Naphthyl Phosphate, Acid Phosphatase	Chemistry
Nitrophenylphosphate, Alkaline Phosphatase Or Isoenzymes	Chemistry
Phosphorus Reagent (Test System)	Chemistry
Photometric Method, Magnesium	Chemistry
Radioimmunoassay, Human Chorionic Gonadotropin	Chemistry
Reagent, Antistreptolysin-Titer/Streptolysin O	Microbiology
Reagent, Bilirubin (Total Or Direct Test System)	Chemistry
Reagent, Chloride (Test System)	Chemistry
Reagent, Creatinine (Test System)	Chemistry
Reagent, Glucose (Test System)	Chemistry
Reagent, Protein, Total	Chemistry
SGPT, Ultraviolet	Chemistry
Test, C-Reactive Protein, FITC	Immunology
Test, Glycosylated Hemoglobin Assay	Hematology
Test, Rheumatoid Factor	Immunology
Turbidimetric Method, Protein Or Albumin (Urinary)	Chemistry
Turbidimetric, Total Protein	Chemistry
Urease And Glutamic Dehydrogenase, Urea Nitrogen	Chemistry
Uricase (Colorimetric), Uric Acid	Chemistry
Urinary Homocystine (Non-Quantitative) Test System	Chemistry

JASCO, INC. 800-333-5272
28600 Mary's Court, Easton, MD 21601 410-822-1220
FDA Number: n/a   *Fax:* 410-822-7526
E-mail: sales@jascoinc.com
Web site: www.jascoinc.com
Medical Products Sales Volume: $9,200,000
Annual Revenue: $5-$10 Million
Year Founded: 1972
Total Employees: 35
Ownership: Private
Quality System Registration Information: ISO9001
Produces/Sells CE-marked Devices: N
Federal Procurement Eligibility: Small Business, GSA Contract
Distribution: Manufacturer Direct, Manufacturer Through Manufacturer Reps, OEM
General Admin.: Frank Mason/President
Mktg./Adv.: Kristen Miller/Marketing Coordinator
　　　　　Harriet Mills/National Director Marketing

Analyzer, Chromatography Infrared	Chemistry
Cell, Spectrophotometer	Chemistry
Chromatography Equipment, Liquid	Chemistry
Chromatography, Liquid, Performance, High	Toxicology
Injector, Sample	Chemistry
Polarimeter	Chemistry
Spectrophotometer, Fluorescence	Chemistry
Spectrophotometer, Infrared	Chemistry
Spectrophotometer, U.V./Visible	Chemistry
Spectrophotometer, Ultraviolet	Chemistry
Spectrophotometer, Visible	Chemistry

JASINS & SAYLES ASSOCIATES, INC.
See J&S Medical Associates

JASON MARINE ENTERPRISES, INC. 954-346-5240
4311 Northwest 64th Avenue, Coral Springs, FL 33067
FDA Number: 3004021087   *Fax:* 954-346-5240
E-mail: seeker1097@aol.com
Web site: www.jmeseeker.com
Ownership: Private
Produces/Sells CE-marked Devices: N

Wheelchair, Manual	Physical Med
Wheelchair, Powered	Physical Med

JASON NATURAL PRODUCTS INC., PERSONAL 310-945-4308
CARE DIVISIO
8468 Warner Dr., Culver City, CA 90232
FDA Number: 2020572
Web site: www.jason-natural.com
Ownership: Private
Produces/Sells CE-marked Devices: N

Lubricant, Vaginal, Patient	General

JAY-Y ENTERPRISE CO. 909-469-4898
632 New York Drive, Pomona, CA 91768
FDA Number: 2082436   *Fax:* 909-469-4896
E-mail: info@jay-ysunglasses.com
Web site: www.jay-ysunglasses.net
Medical Products Sales Volume: $9,100,000
Annual Revenue: $5-$10 Million
Year Founded: 1983
Total Employees: 16   *Sales Staff:* 6
Ownership: Private
Federal Procurement Eligibility: Small Business
Distribution: Importer, Exporter

JAY-Y ENTERPRISE CO. 909-469-4898 *(cont'd)*

Sunglasses (Including Photosensitive)	Ophthalmology

JAYPRO CORPORATION 800-243-0533
976 Hartford Tpke., Waterford, CT 06385-4002 860-447-3001
FDA Number: n/a   *Fax:* 800-988-3363
E-mail: info@jaypro.com
Web site: www.jaypro.com
Annual Revenue: $0-$1 Million
Year Founded: 1953
Ownership: Private
Produces/Sells CE-marked Devices: N
Federal Procurement Eligibility: Small Business
Distribution: Manufacturer Direct

Bars, Parallel, Exercise	Physical Med
Exerciser, Other	Physical Med
Floor Mat	General

JAYZA CORP. 305-477-1136
7215 NW 41ST, Bay A, Miami, FL 33166-6701
FDA Number: 1034187   *Fax:* 305-477-4078
E-mail: jazyzacorp@aol.com
Medical Products Sales Volume: $1,000,000
Annual Revenue: $0-$1 Million
Year Founded: 1980
Total Employees: 5   *Sales Staff:* 3
Ownership: Private
Produces/Sells CE-marked Devices: N
Federal Procurement Eligibility: Small Business, Minority Owned
Distribution: Exclusive Distributor, Importer, Exporter
General Admin.: Javier Zapata/Chief Executive Officer
　　　　　Ana Maria Brierton/General Manager
　　　　　July Galvez/President
Mktg./Adv.: Javier Zapata/Manager Exports

Balance, Mechanical	Chemistry
Electrocardiograph, Single Channel	Cardiovascular
Electrocautery Unit, Line-Powered	Surgery
Generator, Pulsatile Flow, Cardiopulmonary Bypass	Cardiovascular
Lancet, Blood	General
Monitor, Blood Pressure, Indirect, Automatic	Cardiovascular
Nebulizer, Medicinal	Ear/Nose/Throat
Slide And Coverslip	Hematology
Stethoscope, Manual	Cardiovascular
Thermometer, Electronic, Continuous	General
Thermometer, Mercury	General
Tube, Capillary	Chemistry
Tube, Capillary Blood Collection	Hematology

JB MEDICAL DEVELOPMENT INC. 813-645-2855
3000-10 N.w. 25th Ave., Pompano Beach, FL 33069
FDA Number: 3006019086

Orthopedic Manual Surgical Instrument	Orthopedics

JEDMED INSTRUMENTS CO. 314-845-3770
5416 Jedmed Ct., St. Louis, MO 63129-2221
FDA Number: 1926681   *Fax:* 314-845-3771
E-mail: info@jedmed.com
Web site: www.jedmed.com
Annual Revenue: $0-$1 Million
Total Employees: 44   *Marketing Staff:* 3   *Sales Staff:* 18
Ownership: Private
Produces/Sells CE-marked Devices: N
Federal Procurement Eligibility: Small Business
Distribution: Manufacturer Direct, OEM, Exclusive Distributor, Importer, Exporter
Mktg./Adv.: Tom Williams/Manager National Sales
　　　　　James Lankford/President, Chief Executive Officer, Marketing Manager
Production: Thomas E. Schreiber/Manager Customer Services
　　　　　Craig Parks/Manager Regulatory Affairs
Finance: Daniel C. Kroupa/Vice President Finance

Accessories, Surgical Camera	Surgery
Applicator, Ocular Pressure	Ophthalmology
Aspirator, Surgical	Surgery
Bottle, Collection, Vacuum (Aspirator)	General
Cabinet, ENT Treatment	Ear/Nose/Throat
Camera, Cine, Microsurgical (With Audio)	Surgery
Camera, Television, Microsurgical (With Audio)	Surgery
Camera, Television, Microsurgical (Without Audio)	Surgery
Camera, Video	General
Camera, Video, Endoscopic	General
Cannula, Ear	Ear/Nose/Throat
Cannula, Lacrimal (Eye)	Ophthalmology
Cannula, Ophthalmic	Ophthalmology
Chair, Examination And Treatment	General
Chisel, Middle Ear	Ear/Nose/Throat
Clip, Iris Retractor	Ophthalmology
Colposcope	Obstetrics/Gynecology
Dilator, Lacrimal	Ophthalmology
Drape, Patient, Ophthalmic	Ophthalmology
Drill, Bone, Powered	Dental And Oral

JEDMED INSTRUMENTS CO.
314-845-3770 *(cont'd)*

Drill, Middle Ear Surgery	Ear/Nose/Throat
Drill, Surgical, ENT (Electric Or Pneumatic)	Ear/Nose/Throat
ENT Manual Surgical Instrument	Ear/Nose/Throat
Electrocautery Unit, Line-Powered	Surgery
Examination Device, AC-Powered	General
Fiberoptic Light Source & Carrier	Ear/Nose/Throat
Forceps, Electrosurgical	Surgery
Forceps, Epilation	Surgery
Forceps, Hemostatic	Surgery
Forceps, Ophthalmic	Ophthalmology
Forceps, Tissue	Surgery
Fork, Tuning, ENT	Ear/Nose/Throat
Headlight, ENT	Ear/Nose/Throat
Illuminator, Radiographic Film	Radiology
Implant, Cochlear	Ear/Nose/Throat
Infusion Stand	General
Instrument, Microsurgical	Cns/Neurology
Irrigator, Powered Nasal	Ear/Nose/Throat
Irrigator, Sinus	Ear/Nose/Throat
Irrigator, Suction	General
Knife, Ear	Ear/Nose/Throat
Lamp, Examination (Light)	General
Lamp, Surgical, Incandescent	Surgery
Laryngoscope	Ear/Nose/Throat
Laryngostroboscope	Ear/Nose/Throat
Light Source, Fiberoptic, Routine	Gastroenterology/Urology
Loop, Lens	Ophthalmology
Loupe, Diagnostic/Surgical	Surgery
Microscope, Ear	Ear/Nose/Throat
Microscope, Surgical	Ear/Nose/Throat
Microscope, Surgical, General & Plastic Surgery	Surgery
Mirror, ENT	Ear/Nose/Throat
Mirror, Headband, Ophthalmic	Ophthalmology
Mirror, Laryngeal	Ophthalmology
Mount, Surgical Microscope	Surgery
Nasopharyngoscope (Flexible Or Rigid)	Ear/Nose/Throat
Needle, Ophthalmic	Ophthalmology
Ophthalmoscope, Battery-Powered	Ophthalmology
Otoscope	Ear/Nose/Throat
Photokeratoscope	Ophthalmology
Pick, Microsurgical Ear	Ear/Nose/Throat
Probe, Lacrimal	Ophthalmology
Probe, Ophthalmic	Ophthalmology
Prosthesis, Cochlear	Ear/Nose/Throat
Prosthesis, Ossicular	Ear/Nose/Throat
Prosthesis, Ossicular (Total), Absorbable Gelatin Material	Ear/Nose/Throat
Prosthesis, Ossicular, Incus And Stapes	Ear/Nose/Throat
Prosthesis, Ossicular, Porous Polyethylene	Ear/Nose/Throat
Prosthesis, Ossicular, Total, Porous Polyethylene	Ear/Nose/Throat
Pump, Aspiration, Portable	Anesthesiology
Punch, Corneo-Scleral	Ophthalmology
Retractor, Ophthalmic	Ophthalmology
Scissors, Nasal	Ear/Nose/Throat
Scissors, Ophthalmic	Ophthalmology
Scissors, Plastic Surgery (Dissecting)	Surgery
Scissors, Tenotomy	Ophthalmology
Shield, Eye, Ophthalmic	Ophthalmology
Spatula, Middle Ear	Ear/Nose/Throat
Spatula, Ophthalmic	Ophthalmology
Spatula, Surgical, General & Plastic Surgery	Surgery
Spectacle, Operating (Loupe), Ophthalmic	Ophthalmology
Speculum, Ear	Ear/Nose/Throat
Speculum, Nasal	Ear/Nose/Throat
Speculum, Ophthalmic	Ophthalmology
Splint, Septal, Intranasal	Ear/Nose/Throat
Sponge, Ophthalmic	Ophthalmology
Stand, Instrument, Ophthalmic	Ophthalmology
Stand, Operating Room Instrument (Mayo)	Surgery
Stimulator, Caloric Air	Ear/Nose/Throat
Stimulator, Caloric Water	Ear/Nose/Throat
Stool, Operating Room, Adjustable	Surgery
Syringe, Ear	Ear/Nose/Throat
Table, Examination/Treatment	General
Teaching Attachment, Endoscopic	Gastroenterology/Urology
Telescope, Laryngeal-Bronchial	Ear/Nose/Throat
Television Monitor, Operating Room	General
Tip, Suction Tube (Yankauer, Poole, Etc.)	Surgery
Tip, Suction, Electrosurgical	Surgery
Transilluminator, Fiber Optic	Ear/Nose/Throat
Tray, Surgical Instrument	Surgery
Trephine, Manual, Ophthalmic (Corneal)	Ophthalmology
Trocar, Sinus	Ear/Nose/Throat
Unit, Examining/Treatment, ENT	Ear/Nose/Throat
Weights, Eyelid, External	Ophthalmology

JELCO
See Ge Medical Systems Information Technologies

JELENKO & CO., J.F.
See Heraeus Kulzer, Inc.

JEMO SPINE, LLC
801-266-4811
6170 South 380 West, Suite 200, Murray, UT 84107
FDA Number: 3006431090

Orthosis, Fixation, Pedicle, Spinal	Orthopedics

JENAVALVE TECHNOLOGY INC.
302-295-4897
1000 N. West St., Suite 1200, Wilmington, DE 19801
FDA Number: n/a   *Fax:* 302-295-4801
E-mail: info@jenavalve.de
Web site: www.jenavalve.de
Year Founded: 2006
Ownership: Private
Produces/Sells CE-marked Devices: N
General Admin.: Helmut Straubinger/Chief Executive Officer
Medical Admin.: Dr. Katrin Leadley/Chief Medical Officer
Finance: Stephan Wehselau/Chief Financial Officer

JENERIC INDUSTRIES INC., RX JENERIC GOLD
See Pentron Laboratory Technologies

JENERIC/PENTRON, INC.
See Pentron Laboratory Technologies

JENEX CORPORATION
800-496-4682
733 Overlook Drive, Alliance, OH 44601
330-823-4705
FDA Number: 1531043   *Fax:* 905-632-3774
E-mail: jenex@sprint.ca
Web site: www.jenexcorp.com
Annual Revenue: $0-$1 Million
Year Founded: 1999
Total Employees: 4
Ownership: Private
Stock Symbol: JEN
Traded On: Toronto
Produces/Sells CE-marked Devices: N
General Admin.: Mr. Michael Jenkins/Chief Executive Officer
    Mr. Donald Felice/Vice President International Operations

Lamp, Infrared	Physical Med

JENLINE INDUSTRIES, INC.
734-451-0020
92 Blackburn Center, Gloucester, MA 01930
FDA Number: 1225996
Ownership: Private
Produces/Sells CE-marked Devices: N

Elastomer, Silicone (Scar Management)	Surgery

JENSEN INDUSTRIES, INC.
203-239-2090
50 Stillman Rd., North Haven, CT 06473
FDA Number: 1219645

Alloy, Gold Based, For Clinical Use	Dental And Oral
Alloy, Precious Metal, For Clinical Use	Dental And Oral
Metal, Base	Dental And Oral
Powder, Porcelain	Dental And Oral

JEOL USA, INC.
978-536-2270
11 Dearborn Road, Peabody, MA 01960-3823
FDA Number: 7000202   *Fax:* 978-536-2205
E-mail: hamilton@jeol.com
Web site: www.jeol.com
Medical Products Sales Volume: $125,500,000
Annual Revenue: $50-$100 Million
Year Founded: 1962
Total Employees: 320   *Marketing Staff:* 7   *Sales Staff:* 25
Ownership: JEOL LTD.
Federal Procurement Eligibility: Small Business
Distribution: Manufacturer Direct, Importer
General Admin.: Fran J. Murphy/Manager Human Resources
    K. Yasutake/President, Chief Executive Officer
Mktg./Adv.: Robert Santorelli/Director National Accounts
    Steven Hamilton/Manager Advertising
    Peter A. Genovese/Manager Contract Sales
    Robert Santorelli/Vice President Marketing & Sales
Production: William Balletti/Director Quality Assurance
    Nick Giordano/Manager Materials
    Tom Huber/Manager Regulatory Affairs
    Peter Newell/Vice President Manufacturing
Research: Peter Newell/Vice President Research & Development

Calibrator, Mass Spectrometer	General
Mass Spectrometer, Clinical Use	Toxicology
Microscope, Laboratory, Electron	Microbiology
Nuclear Magnetic Resonance Equipment, Laboratory	Chemistry

JEREMY ETHAN INDUSTRIES, INC.
954-772-9779
809 N.w. 57th St., Fort Lauderdale, FL 33309
FDA Number: 3003000040
Ownership: Private
Produces/Sells CE-marked Devices: N

Operative Dental Treatment Unit	Dental And Oral

JERO MEDICAL EQUIPMENT & SUPPLIES, INC.   800-457-0644
1701 W. 13th St., Chicago, IL 60608-1207   312-829-5376
FDA Number: 1424292   *Fax:* 312-829-5671
E-mail: juliabowens@jeromedical.com
Web site: www.jeromedical.com
Medical Products Sales Volume: $1,800,000
Annual Revenue: $1-$5 Million
Year Founded: 1987
Total Employees: 12   *Marketing Staff:* 2   *Sales Staff:* 3
Ownership: Private
Produces/Sells CE-marked Devices: N
Federal Procurement Eligibility: Small Business, Minority Owned, GSA Contract, VA Contract
Distribution: Manufacturer Through Distributor
General Admin.: Obie Wordlaw/Chief Executive Officer
       Dr. Julia Bowens/President

Bag, Body	General
Cap, Surgical	Surgery
Casters, Hospital Equipment	General
Clip, Bandage	General
Clipper, Nail	General
Clothing, Protective	General
Container, Specimen, All Types	General
Contract Manufacturing, Product, Disposable	General
Cover, Barrier, Protective	General
Cover, Cart	General
Cover, Seat, Toilet, Sanitary	General
Facial Tissue	General
Gown, Examination	General
Kit, Admission (Patient Utensil)	General
Mitt/Washcloth, Patient	General
Sheet, Examination Table, Disposable	General
Shoe And Shoe Cover, Conductive	Anesthesiology

JEROME GROUP INC.
See Jerome Medical

JEROME MEDICAL   800-257-8440
305 Harper Drive, Moorestown, NJ 08057-3239   856-234-8600
FDA Number: n/a   *Fax:* 856-778-5333
E-mail: jeromemail@jeromemedical.com
Web site: www.jeromemedical.com
Medical Products Sales Volume: $4,000,000
Year Founded: 1970
Ownership: Public
Quality System Registration Information: ISO9000; ISO9002
Produces/Sells CE-marked Devices: Y
Distribution: Manufacturer Direct, Manufacturer Through Distributor, Exporter
General Admin.: Bernard Tatro/Director International Management
       Lisa Tweardy/General Manager
Mktg./Adv.: Bernard Tatro/Director National Accounts

Immobilizer, Cervical	Orthopedics
Orthosis, Cervical	Physical Med
Support, Patient Position	Anesthesiology

JERON ELECTRONIC SYSTEMS, INC.   800-621-1903
1743-55 W. Rosehill Dr., Chicago, IL 60660-3921   -
FDA Number: n/a   *Fax:* 773-275-0283
E-mail: sales@jeron.com
Web site: www.jeron.com
Year Founded: 1965
Total Employees: 100
Ownership: Private
Produces/Sells CE-marked Devices: N
Federal Procurement Eligibility: Small Business
Distribution: Manufacturer Direct, Manufacturer Through Distributor, Exclusive Distributor

Communication Equipment	General
Light Source, Flash	Chemistry
Nurse Call System	General

JETCOR, INC.   206-243-2230
15001 8th Ave. Sw, Suite #16, Burien, WA 98166
FDA Number: 3032507

Transducer, Blood Pressure, Extravascular	Cardiovascular

JETER SYSTEMS CORP.   877-252-0220
The National City Center, Suite #110, One Cascade Plaza,
Akron, OH 44308
FDA Number: n/a   *Fax:* 800-336-3453
E-mail: info@jetersystems.com
Web site: www.jetersystems.com
Annual Revenue: $1-$5 Million
Year Founded: 1971
Ownership: Private
Produces/Sells CE-marked Devices: N
Federal Procurement Eligibility: Small Business
Distribution: Manufacturer Direct, OEM

Cabinet, Other	General

JETER SYSTEMS CORP.   877-252-0220 *(cont'd)*

Chart, Posture	Orthopedics
Office Equipment	General
Storage Unit, X-Ray Film	Radiology

JETTA CORPORATION   800-288-7771
425 Centennial Blvd., Edmond, OK 73013-3714   405-340-6661
FDA Number: n/a   *Fax:* 405-348-9745
E-mail: sales@jettacorp.com
Web site: www.jettacorp.com
Annual Revenue: $10-$25 Million
Total Employees: 100   *Marketing Staff:* 2   *Sales Staff:* 6
Ownership: Private
Produces/Sells CE-marked Devices: N
Federal Procurement Eligibility: Small Business
Distribution: Manufacturer Direct, Manufacturer Through Distributor, Manufacturer Through Manufacturer Reps
General Admin.: Jerry Conners/President, Chief Executive Officer
Mktg./Adv.: Terry Sorrells/Director National Sales
       Lea Sevier/Market Manager
       Tony Rhodes/Marketing Coordinator

Bathtub	General

JETTA PRODUCTS
See Jetta Corporation

JEUNIQUE INTERNATIONAL, INC.   800-732-9289
10528 Pioneer Blvd., Santa Fe Springs, CA 90670
FDA Number: 2032778   *Fax:* 800-508-8359
E-mail: support@jeunique.com
Web site: www.jeunique.com
Ownership: Private
Produces/Sells CE-marked Devices: N

Binder, Abdominal	General
Orthosis, Lumbosacral	Physical Med

JIFFY MIXER CO., INC.   800-560-2903
1691 California Avenue, Corona, CA 92881   951-272-0838
FDA Number: n/a   *Fax:* 951-279-7651
E-mail: jiffymixer@jiffymixer.com
Web site: www.jiffymixer.com
Medical Products Sales Volume: $500,000
Annual Revenue: $0-$1 Million
Year Founded: 1957
Ownership: Private
Produces/Sells CE-marked Devices: N
Federal Procurement Eligibility: Small Business, Female Owned
Distribution: Manufacturer Through Distributor

Mixer, Clinical Laboratory	Chemistry

JILSON CASTERS, INC.
See Jilson Group, Inc.

JILSON GROUP, INC.   800-969-5400
20 Industrial Road, Lodi, NJ 07644-2608   973-471-2400
FDA Number: 5000001   *Fax:* 973-471-3993
E-mail: info@jilson.com
Web site: www.jilson.com
Medical Products Sales Volume: $2,000,000
Annual Revenue: $1-$5 Million
Year Founded: 1974
Total Employees: 12   *Marketing Staff:* 1   *Sales Staff:* 5
Ownership: Magnus Mobility Systems
Produces/Sells CE-marked Devices: N
Federal Procurement Eligibility: Small Business
Distribution: Manufacturer Direct, Manufacturer Through Manufacturer Reps, Importer
General Admin.: David Baughn/Vice President, General Manager
Production: Tony Alfano/Manager Materials
       Ronald Fulmore/Manager Production

Casters, Hospital Equipment	General

JIM'S INSTRUMENT MFG., INC.   319-351-3429
1910 South Gilbert St., Iowa City, IA 52240
FDA Number: 1937420   *Fax:* 319-354-8901
Web site: www.plexicraft.com
Ownership: Private
Produces/Sells CE-marked Devices: N

Trephine, Manual, Ophthalmic (Corneal)	Ophthalmology

JK PRODUCTS & SERVICES, INC.   870-268-2852
1 Walter Kratz Dr., Jonesboro, AR 72401
FDA Number: 2311923

Booth, Sun Tan	Physical Med

JKRUZ INC.   410-444-2944
7315 Harford Rd., Baltimore, MD 21234
FDA Number: 3006226543
Ownership: Private
Produces/Sells CE-marked Devices: N

JKRUZ INC. 410-444-2944 *(cont'd)*
Sunglasses (Including Photosensitive) — Ophthalmology

JMAR PRECISION SYSTEMS, INC.
See Pacific Precision Laboratories, Inc.

JMM DISTRIBUTING, INC 360-308-9841
10332 Central Valley Rd., Poulsbo, WA 98370
FDA Number: 3004067951
Ownership: Private
Produces/Sells CE-marked Devices: N
Elastomer, Silicone (Scar Management) — Surgery

JMP
See Jamestown Metal Products

JOBAR INTL., INC. 310-222-8682
21022 Figueroa St., Carson, CA 90745-1937
FDA Number: 2081036 Fax: 310-222-8657
E-mail: Info@jobar.com
Web site: www.jobar.com
Year Founded: 1972
Ownership: Private
Produces/Sells CE-marked Devices: Y
Distribution: Importer
Monitor, Blood Pressure, Indirect, Semi-Automatic — Cardiovascular
Orthosis, Lumbar — Physical Med
Pack, Hot Or Cold, Reusable — Physical Med

JOBRI LLC 800-432-2225
520 N Division St, Konawa, OK 74849 580-925-3500
FDA Number: 2027936 Fax: 580-925-3501
E-mail: support@jobri.com
Web site: www.jobri.com
Medical Products Sales Volume: $2,800,000
Annual Revenue: $5-$10 Million
Year Founded: 1997
Total Employees: 40 *Marketing Staff:* 2 *Sales Staff:* 6
Ownership: Private
Quality System Registration Information: ISO9002
Produces/Sells CE-marked Devices: Y
Federal Procurement Eligibility: Small Business
Distribution: Manufacturer Through Distributor, Manufacturer Through
Manufacturer Reps, OEM, Exclusive Distributor, Importer, Exporter
General Admin.: Mr. Brian Gourley/Chief Executive Officer
Mr. Mike Deaton/Office Manager
Mktg./Adv.: Mr. John Biddle/International Sales Representative
Finance: Mrs. Joan Gourley/Chief Financial Officer
Bed, Orthopedic — Orthopedics
Belt, Rib (Support) — Orthopedics
Belt, Traction, Pelvic, Orthopedic — Orthopedics
Collar, Cervical Neck — Orthopedics
Immobilizer, Knee — Orthopedics
Pillow, Cervical — Orthopedics
Shoe, Cast — Physical Med
Sling, Arm — Physical Med
Support, Arm — Physical Med
Support, Back — Orthopedics
Support, Leg — Physical Med

JODEE BRA, INC.
See Jodee, Inc.

JODEE, INC. 800-423-9038
3100 N. 29th Ave., Hollywood, FL 33020 954-926-1900
FDA Number: 1039386
Web site: retail.jodee.com
Annual Revenue: $10-$25 Million
Year Founded: 1971
Ownership: Private
Produces/Sells CE-marked Devices: N
Federal Procurement Eligibility: Small Business
Distribution: Manufacturer Direct, Manufacturer Through Manufacturer Reps
Prosthesis, Breast, External — Surgery

JOERNS HEALTHCARE, INC 800-826-0270
5001 Joerns Dr., Stevens Point, WI 54481
FDA Number: 2182305
E-mail: info@joerns.com
Web site: www.joerns.com
Medical Products Sales Volume: $40,000,000
Annual Revenue: $25-$50 Million
Year Founded: 1889
Ownership: Sunrise Medical, Inc.
Quality System Registration Information: ISO9001
Produces/Sells CE-marked Devices: N
Distribution: Manufacturer Direct
Bed, Electric — General
Bed, Manual — General
Chair, Geriatric — General
Furniture, General — General

JOERNS HEALTHCARE, INC 800-826-0270 *(cont'd)*
Lift, Bath, Non-AC-Powered — General
Mattress, Bed — General
Table, Overbed — General

JOERNS HEALTHCARE, INC. 715-341-3600
1032 North 4th Street, Baldwyn, MS 38824
FDA Number: 1034630
Cover, Mattress — General
Holder, Infant Position — General
Mattress, Non-Powered Flotation Therapy — Physical Med
Orthosis, Truncal/Limb — Physical Med
Protector, Skin Pressure — General
Wheelchair, Manual — Physical Med
Wheelchair, Powered — Physical Med

JOERNS HEALTHCARE, INC.
See Joerns Healthcare, Inc

JOHN CUDIA AND ASSOCIATES, INC. 408-782-2628
18440 Technology Dr., #110, Morgan Hill, CA 95037-2844
FDA Number: n/a Fax: 408-782-2619
E-mail: sales@jcamedical.com
Web site: http://jcamedical.com
Annual Revenue: $0-$1 Million
Year Founded: 1976
Ownership: Private
Produces/Sells CE-marked Devices: N
Federal Procurement Eligibility: Small Business
Distribution: Manufacturer Direct, Service Direct
General Admin.: John Cudia/President
Accessories, Light, Surgical — Surgery
Service, Consulting — General
Service, Used Equipment — General

JOHN EVANS SONS, INC. 215-368-7700
1 Spring Ave., Lansdale, PA 19446
FDA Number: 2522941 Fax: 215-368-9019
E-mail: ales@springcompany.com
Web site: www.springcompany.com
Ownership: Private
Produces/Sells CE-marked Devices: N
Accessories, Traction — Physical Med

JOHN GOODMAN & ASSOCIATES, INC. 310-828 - 504
1734 Colorado Ave., Santa Monica, CA 90404
FDA Number: n/a
Web site: www.jgoodman.net
Annual Revenue: $1-$5 Million
Ownership: Private
Produces/Sells CE-marked Devices: N
Federal Procurement Eligibility: Small Business
Distribution: Service Direct
General Admin.: Angel Zepeda/Executive Vice President
John Goodman/President, Chief Executive Officer
Michelle Alva/Senior Vice President
Service, Consulting — General

JOHN H. PRUSAITIS MANUFACTURING CO.
See Pru-Dent Manufacturing Co.

JOHN J. BROGAN, INC. 908-859-2300
1161 Third Ave., Alpha, NJ 08865
FDA Number: 2249758
Ownership: Private
Produces/Sells CE-marked Devices: N
Glove, Patient Examination, Poly — General

JOHN J. KELLEY ASSOCIATES LTD. 215-567-1377
1528 Walnut Street, Suite 1801, Mid City East, PA 19102
FDA Number: 2519200
Conformer, Ophthalmic — Ophthalmology
Implant, Eye Valve — Ophthalmology
Implant, Orbital, Extra-Ocular — Ophthalmology
Shell, Scleral — Ophthalmology
Sphere, Ophthalmic (Implant) — Ophthalmology

JOHN WHITMAN AND ASSOCIATES
See Whitman Group, The

JOHNS MANVILLE 800-654-3103
P.O. Box 5108, Denver, CO 80217-5108 303-978-2000
FDA Number: n/a
Web site: www.jm.com
Annual Revenue: $50-$100 Million
Year Founded: 1858
Total Employees: 7500
Ownership: Public
Stock Symbol: BRK.A
Traded On: NYSE
Produces/Sells CE-marked Devices: N

MANUFACTURER PROFILES

JOHNS MANVILLE   **800-654-3103** *(cont'd)*

Distribution: Manufacturer Direct, Manufacturer Through Manufacturer Reps, Exporter

Chromatography Equipment, Liquid	Chemistry
Filter, Air	General
Filter, Aspirator	Surgery

JOHNSON & JOHNSON   **800-526-2459**

1 Johnson & Johnson Plaza,   **732-524-0400**
New Brunswick, NJ 08933
FDA Number: 2249557
Web site: www.jnj.com   *Fax:* 732-214-0332
Annual Revenue: More than $1 Billion
Total Employees: 120500
Ownership: Public
Stock Symbol: JNJ
Traded On: NYSE
Produces/Sells CE-marked Devices: N
General Admin.: Brian Perkins/Chairman
     Colleen Goggins/Chairman
     James T. Lenehan/Chairman
     W. C. Weldon/Chairman
     Ralph S. Larsen/Chief Executive Officer
     JoAnn H. Heisen/Corporate Vice President
     Lesley Fishman/Director
     Stan Panasewicz/Director
     Tina Pinto/Director
     Roger Fine/General Counsel
     Robert N. Wilson/Vice Chairman
     Louise Mehrotra/Vice President
     Russ Deyo/Vice President Admin.
     Jean Messina/Vice President Human Resources
Mktg./Adv.: Andrea Alstrup/Vice President Advertising
     Larry Pickering/Vice President Business Development
     Willard D. Nielsen/Vice President Public Relations
Research: Raymond Rudden/Vice President Science & Technology
Finance: Robert J. Daretta/Chief Financial Officer
     Robert J. Darretta/Treasurer

Catheter, Biliary	Gastroenterology/Urology
Stent, Coronary, Drug-eluting	Cardiovascular

Medical Product Subsidiaries (Listed Separately)
Advanced Sterilization Products
Animas Corp.
Biosense Webster
Biosense Webster, Inc
Closure Medical
Codman & Shurtleff, Inc
Codman And Shurtleff, Inc
Cordis Corporation
Cordis Endovascular
Cordis Llc
Cordis Neurovascular, Inc.
Depuy Bridgewater
Depuy Mitek, A Johnson & Johnson Company
Depuy Mitek, Inc.
Depuy Orthopaedics, Inc.
Depuy Spine, Inc.
Depuy-Raynham, A Div. Of Depuy Orthopaedics
Ethicon Endo-Surgery, Inc.
Ethicon Endo-Surgery, Llc
Ethicon, Inc
Ethicon, Inc.
Ethicon, Llc.
Hand Innovations, Llc.
J&J Healthcare Products Div Mcneil-Ppc, Inc
Johnson & Johnson Consumer Products, Inc.
Johnson & Johnson Healthcare Products Div Mcneil-Ppc, Inc.
Johnson & Johnson Hemisferica, S.A.
Johnson & Johnson International
Johnson & Johnson Vision Care, Inc.
Lifescan Llc.
Lifescan Products, Llc
Lifescan, Inc.
Mcneil Healthcare, Inc.
Mcneil-Ppc, Inc.
Micrus Corporation
Noramco, Inc.
Orapharma, Inc.
Ortho Dermatologics
Ortho Mcneil Janssen Pharmaceuticals, Inc.
Ortho-Clinical Diagnostics, Inc.
Ortho-Mcneil-Janssen Pharmaceuticals, Inc.

JOHNSON & JOHNSON CONSUMER   **908-874-1402**
PRODUCTS, INC.
185 Tabor Road, Morris plains, NJ 07950
FDA Number: 2246407
Web site: www.jnjsportsmed.com
Ownership: Johnson & Johnson
Stock Symbol: JNJ
Traded On: NYSE
Produces/Sells CE-marked Devices: N

Accessories, Solution, Lens, Contact	Ophthalmology
Pick, Massaging	Dental And Oral

JOHNSON & JOHNSON CONSUMER   **800-526-3967**
PRODUCTS, INC.
199 Grandview Rd., Skillman, NJ 08558-9417   **908-874-1000**
FDA Number: 2243656   *Fax:* 908-874-1090
Web site: www.jnjsportsmed.com
Annual Revenue: $0-$1 Million
Total Employees: 1200
Ownership: Johnson & Johnson
Stock Symbol: JNJ
Traded On: NYSE
Produces/Sells CE-marked Devices: N
Distribution: Manufacturer Direct, Manufacturer Through Distributor, Service Direct, Exclusive Distributor
General Admin.: Neal Matheson/Vice President

Bandage, Adhesive	Surgery
Bandage, Elastic	General
Care Kit, Baby	General
Dressing, Wound and Burn, Hydrogel	Surgery
Dressing, Wound and Burn, Occlusive	Surgery
Fiber, Absorbent	General
Gauze/sponge, Nonresorbable For External Use	Surgery
Jelly, Lubricating	General
Kit, First Aid	Surgery
Pack, Hot Or Cold, Disposable	Physical Med
Sponge, Gauze	Dental And Oral
Tape, Adhesive, Waterproof	General

JOHNSON & JOHNSON DE MONTERREY,   **817-262-5211**
SA DE CV
Carretera Miguel Aleman,km21.7,
Apodaca, Monterrey Mexico
FDA Number: 9616567

Accessories, Catheter	Surgery
Catheter, Intravascular, Therapeutic, Long-term Greater Than 30 Days	General
Catheter, Intravascular, Therapeutic, Short-term Less Than 30 Days	General

JOHNSON & JOHNSON HEALTHCARE   **973-385-6546**
PRODUCTS DIV MCNEIL-PPC, INC.
185 Tabor Rd, Morris Plains, NJ 07950
FDA Number: 2214133
Web site: www.jnj.com
Ownership: Johnson & Johnson
Stock Symbol: JNJ
Traded On: NYSE
Produces/Sells CE-marked Devices: N

JOHNSON & JOHNSON HEMISFERICA, S.A.   **868-640-3772**
Calle C # 475, Los Frailes Ind. Park, Guaynabo, PR 00969
FDA Number: 2617561
Web site: www.jnj.com
Ownership: Johnson & Johnson
Stock Symbol: JNJ
Traded On: NYSE
Produces/Sells CE-marked Devices: N

Pad, Menstrual, Scented	Obstetrics/Gynecology
Pad, Menstrual, Unscented	Obstetrics/Gynecology

JOHNSON & JOHNSON INTERNATIONAL   **787-272-1900**
Calle C #475, Suite 200; Los Frailes Industrial Park,
Guaynabo, PR 00969
FDA Number: 3005273611
Web site: www.jnj.com
Ownership: Johnson & Johnson
Stock Symbol: JNJ
Traded On: NYSE
Produces/Sells CE-marked Devices: N

JOHNSON & JOHNSON INTERVTL. SYS.-CORDIS
     See Cordis Endovascular

JOHNSON & JOHNSON MEDICAL DIVISION OF   **800-423-4018**
ETHICON, INC.
2500 E. Arbrook Blvd., Arlington, TX 76014   **817-262-3900**
FDA Number: 1618732
Total Employees: 5000

JOHNSON & JOHNSON MEDICAL DIVISION OF   800-423-4018
(cont'd)

Ownership: Public
Stock Symbol: JNJ
Traded On: NYSE
Quality System Registration Information: ISO9001
Produces/Sells CE-marked Devices: Y
Distribution: Manufacturer Through Distributor, Exclusive Distributor
General Admin.: Steven J. Fanning/President
     Shelly Carpenter/Vice President Human Resources
Mktg./Adv.: Donna Fernandez/Vice President Sales
Production: Bill Griffin/Vice President Operations
     Susan Hevey/Vice President Regulatory Affairs

Adhesive Strip, Hypoallergenic	General
Adhesive Strip, Waterproof	General
Agent, Hemostatic, Absorbable, Collagen-Based	Surgery
Agent, Hemostatic, Non-Absorbable, Collagen-Based	Surgery
Bag, Reservoir (Blood)	Anesthesiology
Bandage, Adhesive	Surgery
Bandage, Elastic	General
Bandage, Gauze	General
Bandage, Liquid	Surgery
Barrier, Adhesion, Absorbable	Obstetrics/Gynecology
Beads, Hydrophilic, Wound Exudate Absorption	Surgery
Cap, Surgical	General
Container, Sterilization (Tray)	General
Container, Surgical Instrument	Surgery
Cover, Head, Surgical	Surgery
Cuff, Blood Pressure	Cardiovascular
Disinfector, Liquid	General
Drape, Incision, Surgical	Surgery
Drape, Patient, Ophthalmic	Ophthalmology
Drape, Surgical, Disposable	Surgery
Drape, Surgical, ENT	Ear/Nose/Throat
Drape, Surgical, Reusable	Surgery
Dressing, Gel	General
Dressing, Non-Adherent	General
Dressing, Other	General
Dressing, Permeable, Moisture	General
Dressing, Universal	General
Dressing, Wound and Burn, Occlusive	Surgery
Gauze, Non-Absorbable, X-Ray Detectable (Internal Sponge)	Surgery
Glove, Other	General
Glove, Patient Examination	General
Glove, Patient Examination, Latex	General
Glove, Surgical	General
Glove, Surgical, Hypoallergenic	General
Glove, Surgical, Plastic Surgery	Surgery
Goggles, Protective, Eye	Ophthalmology
Gown, Operating Room, Disposable	Surgery
Gown, Patient, Reusable	General
Gown, Surgical	Surgery
Hemostat	Orthopedics
Hood, Surgical	Surgery
Jelly, Lubricating	General
Kit, First Aid	Surgery
Kit, Wound Drainage	General
Kit, Wound Dressing	Surgery
Mask, Face	General
Mask, Surgical	General
Pack, Custom/Special Procedure	Surgery
Pack, Surgical (Drape)	Surgery
Packing, Surgical	Surgery
Pad, Dressing	General
Sheet, Drape, Disposable	Surgery
Sheet, Operating Room	Surgery
Sheet, Operating Room, Disposable	Surgery
Sponge, External	Surgery
Sponge, Hemostatic, Absorbable Collagen	Surgery
Stockinette	Orthopedics
Strip, Adhesive	Surgery
Suit, Scrub, Disposable	Surgery
Tape, Adhesive	General
Tape, Adhesive, Hypoallergenic	General
Tape, Adhesive, Waterproof	General
Tape, Gauze, Adhesive	General
Test, Equipment, Sterilization	General
Tray, Custom/Special Procedure	General
Tubing, Silicone	General
Waste Disposal Unit, Sharps	General

JOHNSON & JOHNSON MEDICAL, INC.
See Johnson & Johnson Medical Division Of Ethicon, Inc.

JOHNSON & JOHNSON MEDICAL, INC.
See Ge Medical Systems Information Technologies

JOHNSON & JOHNSON ORTHOPEDICS
See Codman & Shurtleff, Inc

JOHNSON & JOHNSON VISION CARE, INC.   800-843-2020
7500 Centurion Pkwy, Suite 100,   904-443-1763
Jacksonville, FL 32256
FDA Number: 1057985
E-mail: vpiweb@visus.jnj.com
Web site: www.jnjvisioncare.com
Ownership: Johnson & Johnson
Stock Symbol: JNJ
Traded On: NYSE
Produces/Sells CE-marked Devices: N
General Admin.: Sheila B. Hickson-Curran/Director
Mktg./Adv.: Silja Schiller/Market Manager

Lens, Contact, Disposable	Ophthalmology
Lenses, Soft Contact, Daily Wear	Ophthalmology
Lenses, Soft Contact, Extended Wear	Ophthalmology

JOHNSON & JOHNSON, PROFESSIONAL DENTAL
See Dentsply International, Inc.

JOHNSON INC., M.C.
See M.C. Johnson Co., Inc.

JOHNSON ORTHOPEDICS, INC.
See Core Products International, Inc.

JOHNSONDIVERSEY, INC.   262-631-4001
8310 16th St, P.O. Box 902, Sturtevant, WI 53177-0902
FDA Number: 2135168
Web site: www.johnsondiversey.com
Annual Revenue: $0-$1 Million
Ownership: Private
Produces/Sells CE-marked Devices: N
Distribution: Manufacturer Through Distributor
General Admin.: Joseph F. Smorada/Chief Financial Officer, Executive Vice President
     Edward F. Lonergan/President, Chief Executive Officer, Director

Disinfector, Liquid	General
Solution, Antibacterial Cleaner	General

JOHNSONDIVERSEY, INC.   262-631-4101
8311 16th Street, Bldg. 65c, Sturtevant, WI 53177
FDA Number: 2135168

Medical Disinfectants/Cleaners for Instruments	General

JOHNSTON DEVELOPMENTAL EQUIPMENT, INC.
See Don Johnston Incorporated

JOHNSTON, INC., DON
See Don Johnston Incorporated

JOIMAX USA INC.   949-859-3472
14 Goodyear, Suite 145, Irvine, CA 92618
FDA Number: 3005042595   Fax: 949-859-3473
Web site: http://www.joimax.com
Ownership: Private
Produces/Sells CE-marked Devices: N
General Admin.: Mr. Rodney Kellogg/President

JOINT VENTURE DEVELOPMENT, INC.   713-501-0075
1628 Beaconshire, Houston, TX 77077
FDA Number: 3006104245
Ownership: Private
Produces/Sells CE-marked Devices: N

Massager, Therapeutic, Manual	Physical Med

JOINTSMART LLC   231-920-7329
801 S. Garfield Ave, Traverse City, MI 49686
FDA Number: n/a
E-mail: betsy@rotatoreliever.com
Web site: www.bejointsmart.org
Ownership: Private
Produces/Sells CE-marked Devices: N
General Admin.: Mr. Michael Carroll/Chief Executive Officer

JOLDON DIAGNOSTICS   800-661-4556
233 Linwood Crescent, Unit 12,   905-634-8691
Burlington, ONT L7L-3 Canada
FDA Number: n/a   Fax: 905-634-8719
E-mail: info@joldon.com
Web site: www.joldon.com
Year Founded: 1995
Total Employees: 10
Ownership: Private
Produces/Sells CE-marked Devices: N
Distribution: Exclusive Distributor

JONES MEDICAL INSTRUMENT CO.   800-323-7336
200 Windsor Drive, Oak Brook, IL 60523   630-571-1980
FDA Number: 1416588   Fax: 630-571-2023
E-mail: info@jonesmedical.com
Web site: www.jonesmedical.com

JONES MEDICAL INSTRUMENT CO.   800-323-7336 *(cont'd)*
Medical Products Sales Volume: $1,600,000
Year Founded: 1919
Total Employees: 20
Ownership: Private
Produces/Sells CE-marked Devices: Y
Federal Procurement Eligibility: Small Business, GSA Contract, VA Contract
Distribution: Manufacturer Through Distributor
General Admin.: Bill Jones/Chief Executive Officer
         Scott Jones/President

Calibrator, Respiratory Therapy Unit	Anesthesiology
Computer, Pulmonary Function Laboratory	Anesthesiology
Spirometer, Diagnostic (Respirometer)	Anesthesiology
Spirometer, Monitoring (Volumeter)	Anesthesiology

JONES SPECIALITY PRODUCTS   314-845-6850
4010 Nottingham Est Dr., St. Louis, MO 63129
FDA Number: 3004150915
Ownership: Private
Produces/Sells CE-marked Devices: N

Bandage, Adhesive	Surgery

JONES-ZYLON COMPANY   800-848-8160
P.O. Box 149, West Lafayette, OH 43845-1224   **740-545-6341**
FDA Number: n/a   Fax: 740-545-6671
E-mail: kathy@joneszylon.com
Web site: www.joneszylon.com
Medical Products Sales Volume: $5,000,000
Annual Revenue: $5-$10 Million
Total Employees: 50
Ownership: Private
Produces/Sells CE-marked Devices: N
Distribution: Manufacturer Through Distributor
General Admin.: Todd Kohl/President
Mktg./Adv.: Michael Robertson/Manager National Sales
Production: Steven Loos/Manager Materials

Basin, Emesis	General
Basin, Wash	General
Bedpan	General
Foodservice Product/Equipment	General
Kit, Admission (Patient Utensil)	General
Kit, Maternity	Obstetrics/Gynecology
Urinal	General

JORDCO, INC.   800-752-2812
595 N.W. 167th Ave., Beaverton, OR 97006   **503-531-3904**
FDA Number: 3026760   Fax: 503-531-3757
E-mail: dealers@jordco.com
Web site: www.jordco.com
Year Founded: 1980
Total Employees: 5   Marketing Staff: 2   Sales Staff: 2
Ownership: Private
Produces/Sells CE-marked Devices: Y
Federal Procurement Eligibility: Small Business
Distribution: Manufacturer Through Distributor
General Admin.: James Johnsen/President, Owner
         Hal Oien/Vice President

Cleanser, Root Canal	Dental And Oral
Dental Laboratory Equipment	Dental And Oral
Disk, Abrasive	Dental And Oral
Endodontic Instrument	Dental And Oral
Gauge, Depth, Instrument, Dental	Dental And Oral
Handle, Instrument, Dental	Dental And Oral

JORDI ASSOCIATES, FLP   877-337-9589
4 Mill St., Bellingham, MA 02019   **508-966-1301**
FDA Number: n/a   Fax: 508-966-4063
E-mail: info@jordilabs.com
Web site: www.jordiflp.com
Annual Revenue: $1-$5 Million
Total Employees: 12   Marketing Staff: 2
Ownership: Private
Produces/Sells CE-marked Devices: N
Federal Procurement Eligibility: Small Business
Distribution: Manufacturer Direct, Manufacturer Through Manufacturer Reps
General Admin.: Howard Jordi/President
Mktg./Adv.: Pam Jordi/Vice President Sales

Column, Liquid Chromatography	Toxicology
Oven	Chemistry

JORGENSEN LABORATORIES   970-669-2500
1450 N. Van Buren Avenue, Loveland, CO 80538-3683
FDA Number: n/a   Fax: 970-663-5042
E-mail: info@jorvet.com
Web site: www.jorvet.com
Medical Products Sales Volume: $5,000,000
Year Founded: 1965
Total Employees: 35   Marketing Staff: 3   Sales Staff: 8

JORGENSEN LABORATORIES   970-669-2500 *(cont'd)*
Ownership: Private
Federal Procurement Eligibility: Small Business
Distribution: Manufacturer Through Distributor
General Admin.: Hans Jorgensen/President, Chief Executive Officer
Mktg./Adv.: Norm Jorgensen/Director Product Development
         Earl Sethre/Vice President Marketing
Research: Norm Jorgensen/Vice President Research & Development

Container, IV	General
Needle, Aspiration And Injection, Disposable	Surgery
Suture, Other	Surgery
Syringe, Hypodermic	General

JORI MEDICAL CO.
See Arista Surgical Supply Co. Inc.

JOSLIN DIABETES CENTER   617-226-5808
1 Joslin Place, Boston, MA 02215
FDA Number: 3005280257

Device, Communications, Images, Ophthalmic	Ophthalmology

JOSTRA BENTLEY, INC.   302-454-9959
Rd. 402 N. Km 1.4, Industrial Park, Anasco, PR 00610-1577
FDA Number: 72189
Ownership: Private
Produces/Sells CE-marked Devices: N

Accessories, Cardiopulmonary Bypass	Cardiovascular
Autotransfusion Unit (Blood)	Anesthesiology
Catheter, Vascular, Cardiopulmonary Bypass	Cardiovascular
Filter, Bacterial, Breathing Circuit	Anesthesiology
Filter, Blood, Cardiopulmonary Bypass, Arterial Line	Cardiovascular
Filter, Infusion Line	General
Heat Exchanger, Heart-Lung Bypass	Cardiovascular
Kit, Administration, Intravenous	General
Kit, Sampling, Arterial Blood	Anesthesiology
Oximeter, Intracardiac	Cardiovascular
Oxygenator, Cardiopulmonary Bypass	Cardiovascular
Reservoir, Blood, Cardiopulmonary Bypass	Cardiovascular
Separator, Blood Cell, Automated	Hematology
Sucker, Cardiotomy Return, Cardiopulmonary Bypass	Cardiovascular
Tube, Pump, Cardiopulmonary Bypass	Cardiovascular

JOSTRA USA
See Origen Biomedical, Inc.

JPB ENTERPRISES, INC.
See Courion

JPL ELECTRONICS CORP.   631-345-9700
22A Unit#4 Industrial Blvd., Medford, NY 11763
FDA Number: n/a   Fax: 631-345-6954
E-mail: info@jplelectronics.com
Web site: www.jplelectronics.com
Ownership: Private
Produces/Sells CE-marked Devices: N

Bed, Scanning, Nuclear/Fluoroscopic	Radiology

JR SCIENTIFIC, INC.   530-666-9868
1242-d Commerce Ave., Woodland, CA 95776
FDA Number: 2954349

Serum, Animal	Pathology

JS DENTAL MFG., INC.   800-284-3368
196 North Salem Rd., P.O. Box 904,   **203-438-8832**
Ridgefield, CT 06877
FDA Number: 2432966   Fax: 203-431-8485
E-mail: info@jsdental.com
Web site: www.jsdental.com
Year Founded: 1982
Total Employees: 7
Ownership: Private
Produces/Sells CE-marked Devices: N
General Admin.: Gunnar Engstrom/Chief Executive Officer
         Mats Engstrom/President

Broach, Endodontic	Dental And Oral
Disinfector, Medical Device	General
Elevator, Surgical, Dental	Dental And Oral
File, Pulp Canal, Endodontic	Dental And Oral
Gutta Percha	Dental And Oral
Instrument, Dental, Manual	Dental And Oral
Light, Surgical Operating, Dental	Dental And Oral
Liner, Cavity, Calcium Hydroxide	Dental And Oral
Medical Disinfectants/Cleaners for Instruments	General
Plugger, Root Canal, Endodontic	Dental And Oral
Powder, Porcelain	Dental And Oral
Reamer, Pulp Canal, Endodontic	Dental And Oral
Spreader, Pulp Canal Filling Material, Endodontic	Dental And Oral
Syringe, Periodontic, Endodontic	Dental And Oral

JT USA   800-854-2188
515 Otay Valley Rd., Chula Vista, CA 91911-6059   **619-421-2660**
FDA Number: 2027469   Fax: 619-421-8160

JT USA   800-854-2188 *(cont'd)*
Web site: www.jtusa.com
Annual Revenue: $0-$1 Million
Total Employees: 100
Ownership: Private
Produces/Sells CE-marked Devices: N
General Admin.: John Gregory/President
        Rita Gregory/Vice President
Mktg./Adv.: Rita Gregory/Director Marketing
  Sunglasses (Including Photosensitive)   Ophthalmology

JTECH MEDICAL   801-478-0680
470 Lawndale Dr., Ste. G, Salt Lake City, UT 84115
FDA Number: 3004904656
  Dynamometer, Non-Powered   Orthopedics
  Goniometer, AC-powered   Orthopedics
  Plunger-Like Joint Manipulator   Physical Med

JTECH MEDICAL   800-985-8324
470 West Longdale Dr., Suite G,   **801-478-0680**
Salt Lake City, UT 84115
FDA Number: 3004904656   *Fax:* 801-478-0674
E-mail: support@jtechmedical.com
Web site: www.jtechmedical.com
Medical Products Sales Volume: $30,000,000
Annual Revenue: $25-$50 Million
Ownership: Private
Quality System Registration Information: ISO9001
Produces/Sells CE-marked Devices: Y
Federal Procurement Eligibility: Small Business
Distribution: Manufacturer Direct, Manufacturer Through Manufacturer Reps,
Exporter
  Dynamometer, AC-Powered   Orthopedics
  Dynamometer, Non-Powered   Orthopedics
  Goniometer, AC-powered   Orthopedics
  Monitor, Spine Curvature   Physical Med

JTL ENTERPRISES   800-699-1008
15395 Roosevelt Blvd, Clearwater, FL 33760   **727-536-5566**
FDA Number: 1055758   *Fax:* 727-536-6633
E-mail: info@aquamed.com
Web site: www.aquamed.com
Medical Products Sales Volume: $4,700,000
Year Founded: 1989
Total Employees: 35
Ownership: Private
Produces/Sells CE-marked Devices: N
Federal Procurement Eligibility: Small Business
  Massager, Therapeutic   Physical Med

JUDAH MFG. CORP.   800-618-9792
13657 Jupiter Road, #100, Dallas, TX 65238   **214-340-6200**
FDA Number: 1651179   *Fax:* 214-340-2204
E-mail: lynnt@judahmanufacturing.com
Web site: www.judahmanufacturing.com
Medical Products Sales Volume: $2,800,000
Annual Revenue: $1-$5 Million
Year Founded: 1997
Total Employees: 20
Ownership: Private
Produces/Sells CE-marked Devices: N
Federal Procurement Eligibility: Small Business, VA Contract
Distribution: Manufacturer Direct, Manufacturer Through Manufacturer Reps, OEM,
Importer, Exporter
  Bandage, Elastic   General
  Binder, Medical, Therapeutic   General
  Joint, Knee, External Brace   Physical Med
  Orthosis, Lumbosacral   Physical Med

JULIE ASSOCIATES, INC.
  See Julie Industries, Inc

JULIE INDUSTRIES, INC   978-276-0820
PO Box 153, North Reading, MA 01864
FDA Number: n/a   *Fax:* 978-276-0821
E-mail: jerry@staticsmart.com
Web site: www.julieindustries.com
Medical Products Sales Volume: $300,000
Annual Revenue: $5-$10 Million
Year Founded: 1973
Total Employees: 10   *Marketing Staff:* 2   *Sales Staff:* 6
Ownership: Private
Produces/Sells CE-marked Devices: Y
Federal Procurement Eligibility: Small Business, Female Owned
Distribution: Manufacturer Direct, Manufacturer Through Distributor, Manufacturer
Through Manufacturer Reps, Importer, Exporter
General Admin.: Audrey Giuliano/Chief Executive Officer
        Jerry M. Giuliano/President

JULIE INDUSTRIES, INC   978-276-0820 *(cont'd)*
        James Patterson/Vice President, General Manager
Mktg./Adv.: Jay MacKay/Director Marketing
        Steve Parker/Director National Accounts
        Jerry R. Giuliano/Director Product Development
        David H. Long/Vice President Business Development
Production: Steve Acquaviva/Manager Materials
  Detector, Electrostatic Voltage   General
  Generator, Ionized Air   Anesthesiology

JULY SOFT   800-350-7693
610 East Knox Drive, Tucson, AZ 85705   **520-797-1844**
FDA Number: n/a   *Fax:* 520-797-0552
E-mail: sales@julysoft.com
Web site: www.julysoft.com
Medical Products Sales Volume: $1,000,000
Annual Revenue: $1-$5 Million
Year Founded: 1990
Total Employees: 10
Ownership: Private
Produces/Sells CE-marked Devices: N
Federal Procurement Eligibility: Small Business
Distribution: Manufacturer Direct, Manufacturer Through Distributor, Manufacturer
Through Manufacturer Reps, Exporter
Mktg./Adv.: Donna S. Lepley/Vice President Customer Relations
  Communication Equipment   General
  Computer and Software, Medical   General

JUMAR CORP.   928-442-0038
329 N. Alarcon St., Prescott, AZ 86301
FDA Number: 1420333
  Device, Repositioning, Jaw   Dental And Oral

JUN-AIR USA,INC.   jun-air.usa@ide
2300 Highway M-139, Benton Harbor, MI 49022   **269-934-1216**
FDA Number: n/a   *Fax:* 269-927-5725
E-mail: info@jun-air.com
Web site: www.jun-air.com
Annual Revenue: $5-$10 Million
Year Founded: 1958
Ownership: JUN-AIR INTERNATIONAL A/S
Produces/Sells CE-marked Devices: Y
Federal Procurement Eligibility: Small Business
Distribution: Manufacturer Direct, Manufacturer Through Distributor, OEM
General Admin.: Tomas Torp/President
  Compressor, Air, Portable   Anesthesiology

JUNE R.R. NICHOLS, OCULARIST LTD.   847-803-5050
1767 E. Oakton Street, Des Plaines, IL 60018
FDA Number: 3006342671
  Eye, Artificial, Non-Custom   Ophthalmology
  Shell, Scleral   Ophthalmology

JUNKIN SAFETY APPLIANCE CO., INC.   502-775-8303
3121 Millers Ln., Louisville, KY 40216
FDA Number: 1043584
  Stretcher, Hand-Carried   General

JURGAN DEVELOPMENT & MFG.   800-587-4262
6018 S. Highlands Avenue, Madison, WI 53705   **608-231-1742**
FDA Number: n/a   *Fax:* 608-231-2119
E-mail: George@Jurgan.com
Web site: www.Jurgan.com
Medical Products Sales Volume: $600,000
Year Founded: 1981
Total Employees: 9
Ownership: Private
Produces/Sells CE-marked Devices: Y
Federal Procurement Eligibility: Small Business, Female Owned
Distribution: Manufacturer Direct, Manufacturer Through Distributor, Manufacturer
Through Manufacturer Reps, Exporter
General Admin.: Erika Plzak/Chief Executive Officer
Mktg./Adv.: Faith Bajema/Director Marketing
        Erika Plzak/Vice President Marketing & Sales
Research: Erika Plzak/Vice President Research & Development
  Protector, Finger   Orthopedics

JURGAN DEVELOPMENT & MFG., LTD.   608-231-1742
6018 South Highlands Ave., Madison, WI 53705
FDA Number: 2183463
  Pin, Fixation, Smooth   Orthopedics

JUST PACKAGING INC.   908-753-6700
450 Oak Tree Ave., South Plainfield, NJ 07080
FDA Number: 2245519
  Bandage, Cast   Physical Med
  Brace, Joint, Ankle (External)   Physical Med
  Component, Cast   Orthopedics
  Joint, Knee, External Brace   Physical Med

JUST PACKAGING INC. 908-753-6700 *(cont'd)*
  Orthosis, Limb Brace — Physical Med
  Orthosis, Sacroiliac, Soft — Physical Med
  Orthosis, Thoracic — Physical Med
  Splint, Hand, And Component — Physical Med

JUSTCO INC.
  See Beck-Lee

JUSTMAN BRUSH CO. 800-800-6940
828 Crown Point Avenue, Omaha, NE 68110 402-451-4420
  FDA Number: 7000563   Fax: 402-451-1473
  E-mail: john@justmanbrush.com
  Web site: www.justmanbrush.com
  Medical Products Sales Volume: $1,700,000
  Annual Revenue: $1-$5 Million
  Year Founded: 1929
  Total Employees: 25   *Marketing Staff:* 2   *Sales Staff:* 2
  Ownership: Private
  Produces/Sells CE-marked Devices: N
  Federal Procurement Eligibility: Small Business
  Distribution: Manufacturer Direct, Manufacturer Through Distributor, OEM
  General Admin.: John S. Matthews/President
  Mktg./Adv.: Ms. Spring Madsen/Admin. Marketing
  Production: Mr. Nathan Griffith/Director Manufacturing & Engineering
  Accessories, Cleaning, Endoscopic — Gastroenterology/Urology
  Brush, Centrifuge — Hematology
  Brush, Cleaning, Tracheal Tube — Ear/Nose/Throat
  Brush, Other — General

JUSTMED, INC. 877-390-1799
8152 SW Hall Blvd., Suite 512, 503-524-4223
Beaverton, OR 97008
  FDA Number: 3005056817   Fax: 503-524-2697
  Web site: www.justmed.com
  Ownership: Private
  Produces/Sells CE-marked Devices: N
  Larynx, Artificial Battery-Powered — Ear/Nose/Throat

JUSTRITE MANUFACTURING CO., L.L.C. 800-798-9250
2454 Dempster Street, 847-298-9250
Des Plaines, IL 60016
  FDA Number: n/a   Fax: 847-298-3429
  E-mail: justrite@justritemfg.com
  Web site: www.justritemfg.com
  Year Founded: 1906
  Total Employees: 200
  Ownership: FEDERAL SIGNAL CORP.
  Stock Symbol: FSS
  Traded On: NYSE
  Produces/Sells CE-marked Devices: N
  Federal Procurement Eligibility: Small Business, GSA Contract
  Distribution: Manufacturer Through Distributor
  Mktg./Adv.: Michael Baldwin/Director National Sales
      Patricia M. Maruszak/Manager Marketing Communications
  Cabinet, Other — General
  Cabinet, Pass Through — General
  High Performance Liquid Chromatography, Cyclosporine — Chemistry
  Safety Equipment, Laboratory — Chemistry
  Waste Receptacle, General Purpose — General

JUVENT INC. 732-748-8866
300 Atrium Drive, Somerset, NJ 08873
  FDA Number: 3005765729
  Exerciser, Powered — Anesthesiology

JUZO 800-222-4999
80 Chart Road, PO Box 1088, 330-923-4999
Cuyahoga Falls, OH 44223
  FDA Number: 1527846   Fax: 800-645-2519
  E-mail: support@juzousa.com
  Web site: www.juzousa.com
  Medical Products Sales Volume: $5,200,000
  Year Founded: 1912
  Total Employees: 75
  Ownership: Private
  Produces/Sells CE-marked Devices: N
  Federal Procurement Eligibility: Small Business, Female Owned
  Cover, Limb — Physical Med
  Orthosis, Limb Brace — Physical Med
  Stocking, Elastic — General

JVC AMERICAS CORP. 973-315-5000
1700 Valley Rd., Wayne, NJ 07470
  FDA Number: 2443110   Fax: 973-315-5030
  Web site: http://pro.jvc.com
  Ownership: Private
  Produces/Sells CE-marked Devices: N
  Distribution: Manufacturer Through Distributor

JVC AMERICAS CORP. 973-315-5000 *(cont'd)*
  Camera, Cine, Endoscopic (Without Audio) — Surgery
  Camera, Cine, Surgical (Without Audio) — Surgery
  Camera, Microscope — Microbiology
  Camera, Videotape, Surgical — Surgery
  Monitor, Bed Patient — General
  Monitor, Video, Endoscope — General
  Recorder, Videotape/Videodisc — General
  Television Monitor, Microscope — General

JVC COMPANY OF AMERICA
  See JVC Americas Corp.

JVC PROFESSIONAL PRODUCTS CO.
  See JVC Americas Corp.

JVS SOLUTIONS 800-325-3303
1200 Switzer Ave., St. Louis, MO 63147
  FDA Number: n/a
  Web site: www.jamesvarley.com
  Annual Revenue: $0-$1 Million
  Ownership: DALEY INTERNATIONAL, LTD., J. F.
  Produces/Sells CE-marked Devices: N
  Federal Procurement Eligibility: Small Business
  Distribution: Manufacturer Through Distributor
  Disinfector, Liquid — General
  Solution, Antibacterial Cleaner — General

JWP & ASSOCIATES, INC. 636-536-5055
15259 Kingsman Circle, Chesterfield, MO 63017
  FDA Number: 1930927
  Ownership: Private
  Produces/Sells CE-marked Devices: N
  Table, Mechanical — Physical Med
  Table, Physical Medicine, Powered — Physical Med
  Table, Physical Therapy — Physical Med

K & R PRODUCTS, INC. 831-426-6061
33170 Central Avenue, Union City, CA 94587
  FDA Number: 2939104
  Kit, Earmold Impression — Ear/Nose/Throat

K & W MEDICAL SPECIALTIES, INC. 215-675-4653
115 Pritchard Hollow Rd., Westfield, PA 16950
  FDA Number: 2523802
  Ownership: Private
  Produces/Sells CE-marked Devices: N
  Syringe, Piston — General

K + A MEDICAL
  See Kem Medical Products Corp.

K MEDICAL 800-478-5633
PO Box 5224, Fort Lauderdale, FL 33310 954-974-3078
  FDA Number: n/a   Fax: 954-974-7437
  E-mail: kmed@hotmail.com
  Web site: www.Face-Shields.com/
  Medical Products Sales Volume: $100,000
  Annual Revenue: $0-$1 Million
  Ownership: Private
  Produces/Sells CE-marked Devices: Y
  Federal Procurement Eligibility: Small Business, VA Contract
  Distribution: Manufacturer Direct, Manufacturer Through Distributor, Importer, Exporter
  Mask, Face — General
  Shield, Eye, Ophthalmic — Ophthalmology
  Shield, Ophthalmic, Radiological — Radiology
  Shield, Protective, Personnel — Radiology

K W GRIFFEN COMPANY 800-424-5556
100 Pearl St., Norwalk, CT 06850-1629 203-846-1923
  FDA Number: n/a   Fax: 203-849-0077
  E-mail: biomed@biomedsystemsinc.com
  Medical Products Sales Volume: $4,800,000
  Annual Revenue: $1-$5 Million
  Year Founded: 1962
  Total Employees: 65   *Marketing Staff:* 5   *Sales Staff:* 5
  Ownership: Private
  Quality System Registration Information: ISO9000
  Produces/Sells CE-marked Devices: Y
  Federal Procurement Eligibility: Small Business
  Distribution: Manufacturer Direct, Manufacturer Through Manufacturer Reps, OEM, Service Direct, Exporter
  General Admin.: James B. Brown/President, Chief Executive Officer
  Mktg./Adv.: James B. Brown/Vice President Marketing
  Production: Jamie Brown/Vice President Manufacturing
  Research: David Beghum/Vice President Research & Development
  Brush, Other — General
  Dispenser, Soap — General
  Dressing, Other — General
  Gauze, Absorbable — Surgery

K W GRIFFEN COMPANY   800-424-5556 *(cont'd)*
Lancet, Blood	General
Sling, Arm	Physical Med
Suction Apparatus, Single Patient, Portable, Non-Powered	Surgery

K&S ASSOC., INC.   615-883-9760
1926 Elm Tree Dr., Nashville, TN 37210
FDA Number: 1054249
Accelerator, Linear, Medical	Radiology
Radiotherapy Unit, Charged-Particle	Radiology

K-10 ENTERPRIZES, INC.
See K-10 Inc.

K-10 INC.   800-531-7496
PO Drawer 1170 Mission, Mission, TX 78573   956-584-0114
FDA Number: 9310035   *Fax:* 956-584-0120
E-mail: sales@k-10.com
Web site: www.k-10.com
Medical Products Sales Volume: $1,100,000
Annual Revenue: $1-$5 Million
Year Founded: 1979
Total Employees: 10   *Marketing Staff:* 2   *Sales Staff:* 5
Ownership: Private
Quality System Registration Information: ISO9002
Produces/Sells CE-marked Devices: N
Federal Procurement Eligibility: Small Business, Female Owned
Distribution: Manufacturer Direct, Manufacturer Through Distributor, OEM, Exporter
General Admin.: Lorraine Kolenda/Chief Executive Officer
     Robert Kolenda/President
     Lorraine Kolenda/Vice President, General Manager
Mktg./Adv.: Dennis Dahlquist/Director Marketing
     Robert Kolenda/Director National Accounts
     Joel Geshay/Director Product Development
     Robert Kolenda/Manager International & National Sales
Production: Joel Geshay/Director Quality Assurance
     Joel Geshay/Vice President Manufacturing
Mirror, Corridor Safety	General
Mirror, Obstetrical	Obstetrics/Gynecology

K-ALPHA X-RAY   630-860-1864
175 Hansen Ct., Suite 108, Wood Dale, IL 60191
FDA Number: 3006264635
Housing, X-Ray Tube, Diagnostic	Radiology

K-FIT ORTHOTICS LLC   516-293-6400
1464 Old Country Rd., Plainview, NY 11803
FDA Number: 3005426352
Ownership: Private
Produces/Sells CE-marked Devices: N
Brace, Joint, Ankle (External)	Physical Med
Insoles, Medical	General

K-MED
See Medegen

K-SERA, INC.   661-775-5988
27525 Newhall Ranch Rd, Unit 8, Valencia, CA 91355
FDA Number: 3005735395
Ownership: Private
Produces/Sells CE-marked Devices: N
Pipette, Pasteur	Hematology

K-STAT, L.L.C.   702-262-1044
11126 Olivia Pkwy., Henderson, NV 89011
FDA Number: 3003890348
Ownership: Private
Produces/Sells CE-marked Devices: N
Holder, X-Ray Film	Dental And Oral

K. W. GRIFFEN CO.   203-846-1923
100 Pearl St., Norwalk, CT 06850
FDA Number: 1211177
Adhesive, Wound Closure	Surgery
Airway, Esophageal (Obturator)	Anesthesiology
Bandage, Adhesive	Surgery
Bandage, Elastic	General
Brush, Scrub, Operating Room	Surgery
Cushion, Denture, OTC	Dental And Oral
Device, Assist, CPR	Anesthesiology
Dressing, Other	General
Dressing, Wound and Burn, Hydrogel	Surgery
Electrode, Needle	Cns/Neurology
Fiber, Absorbent	General
Forceps	Orthopedics
Gas, Collecting Vessel	Anesthesiology
Gauze/sponge, Nonresorbable For External Use	Surgery
Holder, Intravascular Catheter	General
Jelly, Contact (For Transurethral Surgical Instrument)	Gastroenterology/Urology
Kit, Suture Removal	Surgery

K. W. GRIFFEN CO.   203-846-1923 *(cont'd)*
Lancet, Blood	General
Pad, Alcohol	General
Pen, Marking, Surgical	Ophthalmology
Retainer, Surgical	Surgery
Scissors, Disposable	General
Sling, Arm	Physical Med
Sponge, Gauze	Dental And Oral
Tourniquet, Non-Pneumatic, Surgical	Surgery

K.O.L. ISLAND RETAINER, LLC.   808-871-8577
360 Papa Place #203, Kahului, HI 96732
FDA Number: 2954754
Ownership: Private
Produces/Sells CE-marked Devices: N
Retainer, Screw Expansion, Orthodontic	Dental And Oral

K2M, INC.   866-526-4171
751 Miller Dr., SE, Leesburg, VA 20175
FDA Number: 3004774118
E-mail: info@K2M.com
Web site: www.k2m.com
Ownership: Private
Produces/Sells CE-marked Devices: N
General Admin.: Luke Miller/Corporate Counsel
     Mr. Eric Major/President, Chief Executive Officer
     Mr. Larry Found/Senior Vice President Human Resources
Medical Admin.: Dr. John Kostuik/Chief Medical Officer
Mktg./Adv.: Ms. Carol Pinto/Area Manager
     Mr. Andrew Rock/Senior Vice President Business Development
     Mr. Gianluca Iasci/Senior Vice President International Sales
     Mr. Joe Chaudoin/Senior Vice President Marketing & Business Development
     Mr. Lane Major/Vice President Global Marketing
     Mr. John Ulmer/Vice President Sales
Production: Mr. Dave MacDonald/Senior Vice President Operations
Research: Mr. Richard Woods/Senior Vice President Research & Development
Finance: Mr. Gregory Cole/Chief Financial Officer
Appliance, Fixation, Spinal Interlaminal	Orthopedics
Appliance, Fixation, Spinal Intervertebral Body	Orthopedics
Awl	Orthopedics
Bender	Orthopedics
Bit, Drill	Orthopedics
Brace, Drill	Orthopedics
Caliper	Orthopedics
Compression Instrument	Orthopedics
Cutter, Wire And Pin	Orthopedics
Device, Spinal Vertebral Body Replacement	Orthopedics
Extractor, Nail	Orthopedics
Fork	Orthopedics
Gauge, Depth	Orthopedics
Instrument, Bending (Contouring)	Orthopedics
Orthopedic Manual Surgical Instrument	Orthopedics
Orthosis, Fixation, Pedicle, Spinal	Orthopedics
Orthosis, Fixation, Spinal, Spondylolisthesis	Orthopedics
Probe	Orthopedics
Reamer	Orthopedics
Screwdriver	Orthopedics
Tamp	Orthopedics
Tap, Bone	Orthopedics
Template	Orthopedics
Wrench	Orthopedics

KABIVITRUM, INC.
See Hospira, Inc.

KADA RESEARCH, INC.   281-385-9951
21218 Kingsland Blvd, Katy, TX 77450
FDA Number: 75809   *Fax:* 281-437-6387
E-mail: wcpaske@kadamedical.com
Web site: www.kadamedical.com
Year Founded: 2000
Ownership: Private
Produces/Sells CE-marked Devices: N
Dynamometer, AC-Powered	Orthopedics

KADAN CO. INC., D.A.   800-325-2326
1 Brigadoon Lane, Waxhaw, NC 28173-8574   704-843-1144
FDA Number: 2431018   *Fax:* 704-843-1180
E-mail: rkadan@dakadan.com
Web site: www.dakadan.com
Medical Products Sales Volume: $1,000,000
Annual Revenue: $1-$5 Million
Year Founded: 1936
Total Employees: 5
Ownership: Private
Produces/Sells CE-marked Devices: N
Federal Procurement Eligibility: Small Business
Distribution: Manufacturer Through Distributor, Exclusive Distributor
General Admin.: Ronald N. Kadan/President, Chief Executive Officer

KADAN CO. INC., D.A.　　　　800-325-2326 *(cont'd)*
Production: Paul Marino/Vice President Manufacturing

Cabinet, Other	General
Cart, Instrument	Surgery
Lamp, Examination (Light)	General
Lamp, Other	General
Sterilizer, Dry Heat, Dental	Dental And Oral
Sterilizer, Steam (Autoclave)	General
Sterilizer, Steam (Autoclave), Surgical	Surgery
Table, Examination/Treatment	General
Table, Obstetrical, Manual	Obstetrics/Gynecology
Table, Other	General
Table, Physical Therapy	Physical Med

KAESER COMPRESSORS, INC.　　800-777-7873
P.O. Box 946, Fredericksburg, VA 22404　　540-898-5500
FDA Number: n/a　　　　　　　　　*Fax:* 540-898-5520
E-mail: info.usa@kaeser.com
Web site: http://www.kaesercompressors.com
Year Founded: 1919
Total Employees: 4000
Ownership: Private
Quality System Registration Information: ISO9001
Produces/Sells CE-marked Devices: N
Distribution: Manufacturer Direct

Compressor, Air, Portable	Anesthesiology
Compressor, External, Cardiac, Powered	General
Pump, Vacuum, Central	Anesthesiology

KAGAWA SHEARS.COM, LLC.　　404-931-0258
3605 Swiftwater Park Dr., Suwanee, GA 30024
FDA Number: 1058386
E-mail: Info@KagawaTechnologies.com
Web site: www.kagawatechnologies.com
Ownership: Private
Produces/Sells CE-marked Devices: N

Retractor, Self-Retaining	Gastroenterology/Urology

KAHN & CO., INC.
See The Kahn Companies

KAHN INSTRUMENTS, INC.
See The Kahn Companies

KAINOS DENTAL LABORATORY　　925-943-2332
1844 San Miguel Drive, #308b, Walnut Creek, CA 94596
FDA Number: 3005738041

Teeth, Artificial, Posterior With Metal Insert	Dental And Oral

KALE RESEARCH AND TECHNOLOGY　　864-574-4800
1211 Park West Blvd., Mt. Pleasant, SC 29466
FDA Number: 1039626　　　　　　　*Fax:* 864-208-5500
Web site: www.kale.com
Ownership: Private
Produces/Sells CE-marked Devices: N

Monitor, Temperature, Neurosurgery, Direct Contact, Powered	Cns/Neurology

KALISH CO. INC., H.G.
See IMA Nova

KAMIYA BIOMEDICAL COMPANY　　206-575-8068
12779 Gateway Drive, Seattle, WA 98168
FDA Number: 2084025　　　　　　　*Fax:* 206-575-8094
E-mail: kassays@kamiyabiomedical.com
Web site: www.kamiyabiomedical.com
Medical Products Sales Volume: $1,300,000
Annual Revenue: $1-$5 Million
Year Founded: 1983
Total Employees: 8　　*Marketing Staff:* 3　　*Sales Staff:* 5
Ownership: Private
Produces/Sells CE-marked Devices: N
Federal Procurement Eligibility: Small Business, Minority Owned
Distribution: Manufacturer Direct, Manufacturer Through Distributor, OEM, Exclusive Distributor, Importer, Exporter
General Admin.: Kohji Kamiya/President, Chief Executive Officer
Mktg./Adv.: Brian Schliesman/Manager International & National Sales
　　Colin Getty/Vice President Marketing & Business Development
Production: Nell Lund/Manager Regulatory Affairs

Antibody, Monoclonal	Microbiology
Indicator Method, Protein Or Albumin (Urinary, Non-Quant.)	Chemistry
Material, Raw, Production	General
Nephelometric Method, Immunoglobulins (G, A, M)	Chemistry
Reagent, Other	General
Serum, Screening, Blood	Hematology
Service, Import/Export	General
Test, C-Reactive Protein, FITC	Immunology

KANE BIOTECH INC.　　204-453-1301
5-1250 Waverley St., Winnipeg, MB R3T 6C6 Canada
FDA Number: n/a　　　　　　　　　*Fax:* 204-453-1314
E-mail: info@kanebiotech.com

KANE BIOTECH INC.　　204-453-1301 *(cont'd)*
Web site: www.kanebiotech.com
Year Founded: 2001
Ownership: Public
Stock Symbol: KNE
Traded On: TSX Venture Exchange
Produces/Sells CE-marked Devices: N

KANE MAY MEASURING INSTRUMENTS
See Uei

KANEKA AMERICA CORP.
See Kaneka Pharma America Llc

KANEKA PHARMA AMERICA LLC　　800-526-3522
546 Fifth Avenue, 21st Floor,　　212-705-4340
New York, NY 10036
FDA Number: 2435151　　　　　　　*Fax:* 212-705-4350
E-mail: info@liposorber.com
Web site: www.liposorber.com
Total Employees: 6　　*Sales Staff:* 3
Ownership: Private
Produces/Sells CE-marked Devices: Y
General Admin.: Mr. Masaaki Fukunishi/Business Manager
　　　　Mr. Kiyoshi Nagai/President
　　　　Hiroyasu Higuchi/Vice President
　　　　Masaharu Inoue/Vice President
Medical Admin.: Ms. Renee Alexander/Manager Clinical Affairs
Mktg./Adv.: Mr. Mike Shine/Manager Sales
IS: Mr. Mark Quick/Tech. Specialist

Column, Adsorption, Lipid	Cardiovascular
Column, Adsorption, Lipoprotein, Low Density	General
Equipment, Apheresis	Hematology

KAP MEDICAL　　951-340-4360
1395 Pico St., Corona, CA 92881
FDA Number: 2032121

Bed, Flotation Therapy, Powered	Physical Med
Bed, Patient Rotation, Powered	Physical Med
Mattress, Air Flotation	General

KAPCO (KENT ADHESIVE PRODUCTS CO.)　　800-791-8964
1000 Cherry St., Kent, OH 44240-7520　　330-678-1626
FDA Number: 1528169　　　　　　　*Fax:* 800-451-3724
E-mail: converting@kapco.com
Web site: www.kapco.com
Annual Revenue: $10-$25 Million
Year Founded: 1974
Total Employees: 113　　*Marketing Staff:* 3　　*Sales Staff:* 6
Ownership: Private
Quality System Registration Information: ISO9002
Produces/Sells CE-marked Devices: N
Federal Procurement Eligibility: Small Business
Distribution: Manufacturer Direct
General Admin.: N/A N/A/Chief Executive Officer
　　　　Ed Small/President
Mktg./Adv.: Dan Bartlett/Director National Accounts
　　　　Steve Davis/Manager National Sales
　　　　Steve Davis/Manager Sales
Production: Phil Zavracky/Vice President Manufacturing

Contract Manufacturing	General

KAPP SURGICAL INSTRUMENT, INC.　　800-282-5277
4919 Warrensville Center Rd.,　　216-587-4400
Cleveland, OH 44128
FDA Number: 1522875　　　　　　　*Fax:* 216-587-0411
E-mail: info@kappsurgical.com
Web site: www.kappsurgical.com
Medical Products Sales Volume: $1,500,000
Annual Revenue: $1-$5 Million
Year Founded: 1927
Total Employees: 7　　*Marketing Staff:* 1　　*Sales Staff:* 1
Ownership: Private
Produces/Sells CE-marked Devices: Y
Federal Procurement Eligibility: Small Business
Distribution: Manufacturer Direct, Manufacturer Through Distributor, Manufacturer Through Manufacturer Reps
General Admin.: NICOLE MERRIFIELD/Office Manager
　　　　Albert Santilli/President, Chief Executive Officer
Production: Jim Zmina/Vice President Manufacturing

Hook, Surgical, General & Plastic Surgery	Surgery
Implant, Fixation Device, Spinal	Orthopedics
Instrument, Microsurgical	Cns/Neurology
Kit, Instruments and Accessories, Surgical	Surgery
Plate, Fixation, Bone	Orthopedics
Retractor	Orthopedics
Retractor, Cardiac	Cardiovascular
Retractor, Other	Surgery
Service, Parts, Repair	General

KAPP SURGICAL INSTRUMENT, INC.   800-282-5277 (cont'd)
Stand/Holder, Equipment, Laboratory	Chemistry
Strip, Adhesive	Surgery
Surgical Instrument, Orthopedic, AC-Powered Motor	Orthopedics

KAPPA MEDICAL, INC.   800-634-0880
P.O. Box 11808, Prescott, AZ 86304-1808   928-778-0840
FDA Number: 2245344   *Fax:* 928-776-9250
E-mail: kappamedical@gmail.com
Web site: www.kappamedical.com
Annual Revenue: $0-$1 Million
Total Employees: 10
Ownership: Private
Produces/Sells CE-marked Devices: N
Federal Procurement Eligibility: Small Business, Female Owned
General Admin.: Linda Bethanis/Chief Executive Officer
Mktg./Adv.: James F. Bethanis/Manager Sales

Electrode, Electrocardiograph	Cardiovascular
Gel, Electrode, Electrocardiograph	Cardiovascular
Paper, Recording, ECG/EEG	General
Recorder, Long-Term, ECG, Portable (Holter Monitor)	Cardiovascular

KAPPLER PROTECTIVE APPAREL & FABRICS   800-600-4019
115 Grimes Drive, Guntersville, AL 35976-9480   256-505-4005
FDA Number: 1038119   *Fax:* 256-505-4151
E-mail: usa@kappler.com
Web site: www.kappler.com
Medical Products Sales Volume: $46,900,000
Annual Revenue: $50-$100 Million
Year Founded: 1986
Total Employees: 300   *Marketing Staff:* 50   *Sales Staff:* 65
Ownership: Private
Quality System Registration Information: ISO9001
Produces/Sells CE-marked Devices: Y
Federal Procurement Eligibility: Small Business, GSA Contract
Distribution: Manufacturer Through Distributor
General Admin.: George Kappler/Chief Executive Officer
        George Kappler/President
Mktg./Adv.: John Langley/Director Product Development
        Philip Mann/Manager Sales Training
        Craig Woodward/Senior Vice President Marketing & Sales

Clothing, Protective	General
Coat, Laboratory	General
Cover, Shoe, Operating Room	Surgery
Gown, Examination	General
Gown, Isolation, Surgical	Surgery
Gown, Operating Room, Disposable	Surgery
Gown, Other	General
Gown, Surgical	Surgery
Suit, Scrub, Disposable	Surgery

KAPPLER USA
See Kappler Protective Apparel & Fabrics

KARDEX SYSTEMS, INC.   800-234-3654
114 Westview Avenue, Marietta, OH 45750-0171   740-374-9300
FDA Number: n/a   *Fax:* 740-374-9953
E-mail: sales@kardex.com
Web site: www.kardex.com
Medical Products Sales Volume: $1,000,000
Annual Revenue: $10-$25 Million
Total Employees: 120   *Marketing Staff:* 6
Ownership: Rem Systems
Produces/Sells CE-marked Devices: N
Federal Procurement Eligibility: Small Business
Distribution: Manufacturer Direct, Manufacturer Through Distributor
General Admin.: Mr. Ronald Miller/Chief Executive Officer
        Joe Compitello/President
        Richard Hersman/Vice President Human Resources
Mktg./Adv.: Mr. Alan Bartlett/Director National Accounts
        Bill Bennett/Manager Advertising
        Mr. Alan Bartlett/Vice President Business Development
Production: Richard Hersman/Vice President Manufacturing
Purchasing: Mr. Alan Bartlett/Vice President Contracts

Bin, Storage	General
Office Equipment	General
Office Product	General

KARECO INTERNATIONAL, INC.   800-8KA-RECO
299 Rte. 22 E., Green Brook, NJ 08812-1714   732-752-9292
FDA Number: 2244724   *Fax:* 732-752-9636
E-mail: kareco@earthlink.net
Medical Products Sales Volume: $300,000
Annual Revenue: $0-$1 Million
Year Founded: 1983
Total Employees: 2   *Sales Staff:* 30
Ownership: Private
Produces/Sells CE-marked Devices: N
Federal Procurement Eligibility: Small Business

KARECO INTERNATIONAL, INC.   800-8KA-RECO (cont'd)
Distribution: Manufacturer Direct, Manufacturer Through Distributor, Manufacturer Through Manufacturer Reps, Importer
General Admin.: Kevin O'Neil/President

Accessories, Wheelchair	Physical Med
Attachment, Bag (Crutch, Walker, Wheelchair)	Physical Med
Attachment, Oxygen Canister/IV Pole, Wheelchair	General
Belt, Wheelchair	Physical Med
Footrest, Wheelchair	Physical Med
Pad, Incontinence (Underpad)	General
Ramp, Wheelchair	General
Wheelchair, Manual	Physical Med

KARETECH, LLC   415-824-3769
3573 22nd St., San Francisco, CA 94114
FDA Number: 2953703   *Fax:* 415-824-3769
E-mail: msnopper@aol.com
Year Founded: 1996
Total Employees: 5
Ownership: Private
Produces/Sells CE-marked Devices: N
Federal Procurement Eligibility: Small Business

Curette, Ear	Ear/Nose/Throat

KARL HAGER LIMB & BRACE & THE KNEE CENTRE   800-387-5053
10733 124 St., Edmonton, ALB T5M-0H2 Canada   780-452-5771
FDA Number: n/a   *Fax:* 780-452-2752
E-mail: reception@khager.com
Web site: www.khager.com
Year Founded: 1979
Total Employees: 25
Ownership: Private
Produces/Sells CE-marked Devices: N
Distribution: Manufacturer Direct, Exclusive Distributor

KARL STORZ ENDOSCOPIA LATINO AMERICA   305-262-8980
815 N.W. 57th Ave. Ste. 480, Miami, FL 33126-2042
FDA Number: 1038749   *Fax:* 305-262-8986
E-mail: info@ksela.com
Web site: www.karlstorz.com
Year Founded: 1986
Ownership: Storz Gmbh & Co., Karl
Quality System Registration Information: ISO9001
Produces/Sells CE-marked Devices: N
Distribution: Manufacturer Direct, Manufacturer Through Distributor, Manufacturer Through Manufacturer Reps

Accessories, Arthroscope	Orthopedics
Accessories, Cleaning, Endoscopic	Gastroenterology/Urology
Accessories, Photographic, Endoscopic	Gastroenterology/Urology
Applier, Surgical, Clip	Surgery
Arthroscope	Orthopedics
Endoscope	Gastroenterology/Urology
Endoscope And Accessories, AC-Powered	Surgery
Endoscope And Accessories, Battery-Powered	Surgery
Endoscope, Direct Vision	Surgery
Endoscope, Rigid	Surgery

KARL STORZ ENDOSCOPY-AMERICA INC.   800-421-0837
600 Corporate Pointe,   310-338-8100
Culver City, CA 90230
FDA Number: 2020550   *Fax:* 310-410-5527
E-mail: info@ksea.com
Web site: www.karlstorz.com
Ownership: Private
Quality System Registration Information: ISO9000
Produces/Sells CE-marked Devices: Y
Distribution: Manufacturer Direct
General Admin.: Mrs. Sybill Storz/Managing Director
        Charles H. Wilhelm/President, Chief Operating Officer
Mktg./Adv.: Kelly Allard/Communication Specialist
        Susan Jaffy/Director Marketing Communications
        Eric Partlow/Director Marketing Services
        Simon Solingen/Director Product Development
        Kevin Condrin/Director Sales Training
        Jeff Lersch/Executive Director Sales
        Ali Amiri/Vice President Marketing & Product Development
Production: Susie Chen/Director Regulatory Affairs
        Frances Ridlehoover/Vice President Production Operations
Finance: Mark Green/Chief Financial Officer, Vice President Finance
IS: Brian Kern/Manager Tech. Support

Accessories, Arthroscope	Orthopedics
Accessories, Cleaning, Endoscopic	Gastroenterology/Urology
Accessories, Photographic, Endoscopic	Gastroenterology/Urology
Applier, Surgical, Clip	Surgery
Arthroscope	Orthopedics
Bougie, Esophageal, ENT	Ear/Nose/Throat
Bougie, Urological	Gastroenterology/Urology

MANUFACTURER PROFILES

KARL STORZ ENDOSCOPY-AMERICA INC. 800-421-0837 *(cont'd)*

Bronchoscope, Non-Rigid	Ear/Nose/Throat
Bronchoscope, Rigid	Ear/Nose/Throat
Bronchoscope, Rigid, Non-Ventilating	Anesthesiology
Bronchoscope, Rigid, Ventilating	Anesthesiology
Brush, Cytology, Endoscopic	Gastroenterology/Urology
Cable, Fiberoptic	General
Camera, Still, Endoscopic	Surgery
Camera, Television, Endoscopic (Without Audio)	Surgery
Camera, Television, Surgical (With Audio)	Surgery
Camera, Video, Endoscopic	General
Cannula, Drainage, Arthroscopy	Orthopedics
Cannula, Suprapubic, With Trocar	Gastroenterology/Urology
Cart, Equipment, Video	General
Choledochoscope, Flexible Or Rigid	Gastroenterology/Urology
Coagulator/Cutter, Endoscopic, Bipolar	Obstetrics/Gynecology
Coagulator/Cutter, Endoscopic, Unipolar	Obstetrics/Gynecology
Culdoscope	Obstetrics/Gynecology
Curette, Uterine	Obstetrics/Gynecology
Cutter, Orthopedic	Orthopedics
Cystoscope	Gastroenterology/Urology
Cystourethroscope	Gastroenterology/Urology
Dispenser, Thorascopic	Cardiovascular
Dissector, Surgical, General & Plastic Surgery	Surgery
Drill, Surgical, ENT (Electric Or Pneumatic)	Ear/Nose/Throat
Electrode, Cystoscopic	Gastroenterology/Urology
Electrode, Electrosurgical, Active (Blade)	Surgery
Electrode, Electrosurgical, Return (Ground, Dispersive)	Surgery
Electrosurgical Unit, Cutting & Coagulation Device	Surgery
Endoscope	Gastroenterology/Urology
Endoscope And Accessories, AC-Powered	Surgery
Endoscope And Accessories, Battery-Powered	Surgery
Endoscope, Direct Vision	Surgery
Endoscope, Neurological	Cns/Neurology
Endoscope, Rigid	Surgery
Esophagoscope (Flexible Or Rigid)	Ear/Nose/Throat
Fastener, Fixation, Biodegradable, Soft Tissue	Orthopedics
Fiberoptic Light Source & Carrier	Ear/Nose/Throat
Forceps	Orthopedics
Forceps, Biopsy, Bronchoscope (Rigid)	Anesthesiology
Forceps, Biopsy, Electric	Gastroenterology/Urology
Forceps, Biopsy, Gynecological	Obstetrics/Gynecology
Forceps, ENT	Ear/Nose/Throat
Forceps, Electrosurgical	Surgery
Forceps, Endoscopic	Gastroenterology/Urology
Forceps, Grasping, Flexible Endoscopic	Gastroenterology/Urology
Forceps, Stone Manipulation	Gastroenterology/Urology
Handle, Instrument, Laparoscopic (Electrocautery)	Surgery
Headlight, ENT	Ear/Nose/Throat
Holder, Needle	Gastroenterology/Urology
Hysteroscope	Obstetrics/Gynecology
Illuminator, Fiberoptic (For Endoscope)	Gastroenterology/Urology
Injector & Accessories, Manipulator, Uterine	Obstetrics/Gynecology
Instrument, Removal, Myoma, Laparoscopic	Surgery
Insufflator, Carbon-Dioxide, Uterotubal	Obstetrics/Gynecology
Insufflator, Hysteroscopic	Obstetrics/Gynecology
Insufflator, Laparoscopic	Obstetrics/Gynecology
Kit, Cholecystectomy	Gastroenterology/Urology
Lamp, Endoscopic, Incandescent	Surgery
Laparoscope, General & Plastic Surgery	Surgery
Laparoscope, Gynecologic	Obstetrics/Gynecology
Laryngoscope	Ear/Nose/Throat
Laryngoscope, Surgical	Surgery
Light Source, Endoscope, Xenon Arc	Surgery
Light Source, Endoscopic	Obstetrics/Gynecology
Light Source, Fiberoptic, Routine	Gastroenterology/Urology
Light Source, Flash	Chemistry
Light Source, Photographic, Fiberoptic	Gastroenterology/Urology
Light, Surgical, Fiberoptic	Surgery
Lithotriptor	Gastroenterology/Urology
Lithotriptor, Electro-Hydraulic, Percutaneous	Gastroenterology/Urology
Lithotriptor, Ultrasonic	Gastroenterology/Urology
Mediastinoscope	Surgery
Monitor, Video, Endoscope	General
Nasopharyngoscope (Flexible Or Rigid)	Ear/Nose/Throat
Needle, Cholangiography	Cardiovascular
Needle, Endoscopic	Gastroenterology/Urology
Needle, Pneumoperitoneum, Simple	Gastroenterology/Urology
Needle, Pneumoperitoneum, Spring Loaded	Gastroenterology/Urology
Nephroscope Set	Gastroenterology/Urology
Nephroscope, Rigid	Gastroenterology/Urology
Observerscope	General
Obturator, Endoscopic	Gastroenterology/Urology
Otoscope	Ear/Nose/Throat
Peritoneoscope	Gastroenterology/Urology
Pneumoperitoneum Apparatus, Automatic	Gastroenterology/Urology
Printer, Image, Video	General
Probe	Orthopedics
Probe, Ultrasonic	Radiology
Proctoscope	Surgery
Pump, Air, Non-Manual, Endoscopic	Gastroenterology/Urology
Pump, Withdrawal/Infusion	Cardiovascular

KARL STORZ ENDOSCOPY-AMERICA INC. 800-421-0837 *(cont'd)*

Punch, Biopsy	Gastroenterology/Urology
Recorder, Videotape/Videodisc	General
Resectoscope	Gastroenterology/Urology
Resectoscope Working Element	Gastroenterology/Urology
Retractor	Orthopedics
Retractor, Ophthalmic	Ophthalmology
Rhinoscope	Ear/Nose/Throat
Saw, Surgical, ENT (Electric Or Pneumatic)	Ear/Nose/Throat
Scissors, Cystoscopic	Gastroenterology/Urology
Scissors, Orthopedic	Orthopedics
Scissors, Thoracic	Cardiovascular
Service, Maintenance/Repair	General
Sheath, Endoscopic	Gastroenterology/Urology
Sigmoidoscope, Rigid, Non-Electrical	Gastroenterology/Urology
Sleeve, Trocar	Surgery
Snare, Endoscopic	Surgery
Snare, Polyp	Surgery
Spreader, Rib	Orthopedics
Tape, Television & Video, Endoscopic	Gastroenterology/Urology
Teaching Attachment, Endoscopic	Gastroenterology/Urology
Telescope, Laryngeal-Bronchial	Ear/Nose/Throat
Telescope, Rigid, Endoscopic	Gastroenterology/Urology
Tenaculum, Uterine	Obstetrics/Gynecology
Thoracoscope	Cardiovascular
Tray, Surgical Instrument	Surgery
Trocar, Abdominal	Gastroenterology/Urology
Trocar, Antrum	Ear/Nose/Throat
Trocar, Cardiovascular	Cardiovascular
Trocar, Laryngeal	Ear/Nose/Throat
Trocar, Other	General
Trocar, Sinus	Ear/Nose/Throat
Ureteroscope	Gastroenterology/Urology
Ureterotome	Gastroenterology/Urology
Urethroscope	Gastroenterology/Urology
Urethrotome	Gastroenterology/Urology
Urological Irrigation System	Gastroenterology/Urology
Vaginoscope	Obstetrics/Gynecology

Medical Product Subsidiaries (Listed Separately)
Karl Storz Lithotripsy-America, Inc.

KARL STORZ ENDOVISION, INC.   800-421-0837
91 Carpenter Hill Rd., Charlton, MA 01507   **508-248-9011**
FDA Number: 1221826   *Fax:* 508-248-6490
Web site: www.karlstorz.com
Year Founded: 1945
Ownership: Storz Gmbh & Co., Karl
Quality System Registration Information: ISO9001
Produces/Sells CE-marked Devices: Y
Distribution: Manufacturer Direct

Bronchoscope, Non-Rigid	Ear/Nose/Throat
Bronchoscope, Rigid	Ear/Nose/Throat
Camera, Video, Endoscopic	General
Choledochoscope, Flexible Or Rigid	Gastroenterology/Urology
Endoscope And Accessories, Battery-Powered	Surgery
Illuminator, Fiberoptic (For Endoscope)	Gastroenterology/Urology
Insufflator, Laparoscopic	Obstetrics/Gynecology
Light Source, Fiberoptic, Routine	Gastroenterology/Urology
Nasopharyngoscope (Flexible Or Rigid)	Ear/Nose/Throat
Service, Repair, Endoscopic	General

KARL STORZ IMAGING   805-968-5563
175 Cremona Dr., Golita, CA 93117-5502
FDA Number: 2027009
Web site: www.karlstorz.com
Annual Revenue: $25-$50 Million
Year Founded: 1945
Ownership: Storz Gmbh & Co., Karl
Quality System Registration Information: ISO9001
Produces/Sells CE-marked Devices: Y
Federal Procurement Eligibility: Small Business
Distribution: OEM, Exclusive Distributor

Camera, Ophthalmic, AC-Powered (Fundus)	Ophthalmology
Camera, Video, Endoscopic	General
Device, Storage, Image, Digital	Radiology
Endoscope	Gastroenterology/Urology
Hysteroscope	Obstetrics/Gynecology
Lamp, Slit, Biomicroscope, AC-Powered	Ophthalmology
Laparoscope, General & Plastic Surgery	Surgery
Laparoscope, General & Plastic Surgery, Reprocessed	Gastroenterology/Urology
Microscope, Surgical, General & Plastic Surgery	Surgery

KARL STORZ LITHOTRIPSY-AMERICA, INC.   800-965-4846
1000 Cobb Place Blvd., Building 400, Suite 450,   **678-354-6229**
Kennesaw, GA 30144
FDA Number: 1061158   *Fax:* 678-354-6943
Web site: www.storzmedical.com
Annual Revenue: $10-$25 Million
Ownership: Karl Storz Endoscopy-America Inc.
Produces/Sells CE-marked Devices: N

KARL STORZ LITHOTRIPSY-AMERICA, INC.   800-965-4846
(cont'd)
Federal Procurement Eligibility: Small Business
Distribution: Service Direct, Exclusive Distributor
Lithotriptor	Gastroenterology/Urology
Lithotriptor, Ultrasonic	Gastroenterology/Urology

KARMA INC.   800-558-9565
500 Milford St., Box 433, Watertown, WI 53094   **920-261-1424**
FDA Number: n/a   *Fax:* 920-261-3302
E-mail: karma@karma-inc.com
Web site: http://www.karma-inc.com/
Annual Revenue: $1-$5 Million
Total Employees: 135   *Marketing Staff:* 5   *Sales Staff:* 20
Ownership: Private
Produces/Sells CE-marked Devices: Y
Federal Procurement Eligibility: Small Business
Distribution: Manufacturer Direct, Manufacturer Through Distributor, Manufacturer Through Manufacturer Reps, OEM, Service Direct, Exporter
General Admin.: Chris Gorski/Chief Executive Officer
     Suzzanne Schuett/Manager Human Resources
Mktg./Adv.: Elizabeth Bergmann/Vice President Marketing
     Jerry Scheider/Vice President Sales
Research: Pat Vandenberg/Vice President Engineering
Foodservice Product/Equipment	General

KARMAN HEALTHCARE, INC.   800-805-2762
19255 San Jose Ave., City of Industry, CA 91748   **626-581-2235**
FDA Number: 2085336   *Fax:* 626-581-2335
E-mail: karmanhc@yahoo.com
Web site: www.karmanhealthcare.com
Annual Revenue: $1-$5 Million
Year Founded: 1994
Ownership: Private
Produces/Sells CE-marked Devices: Y
Federal Procurement Eligibility: Small Business, Minority Owned
Distribution: Manufacturer Through Distributor, Manufacturer Through Manufacturer Reps, OEM, Exclusive Distributor, Importer, Exporter
General Admin.: Alex Horng/President, General Manager
Mktg./Adv.: David Chen/Manager National Sales
Walker, Mechanical	Physical Med
Wheelchair, Manual	Physical Med

KARWOSKI DENTAL   925-938-8977
418 Iron Hill St., Pleasant Hill, CA 94523
FDA Number: 2954732
Ownership: Private
Produces/Sells CE-marked Devices: N
Protector, Dental	Anesthesiology

KATECHO, INC.   515-244-1212
4020 Gannett Ave., Des Moines, IA 50321
FDA Number: 1930027   *Fax:* 515-244-4912
E-mail: katecho@katecho.net
Web site: katecho.com
Annual Revenue: $25-$50 Million
Year Founded: 1984
Total Employees: 250
Ownership: Private
Quality System Registration Information: ISO9002
Produces/Sells CE-marked Devices: Y
Federal Procurement Eligibility: Small Business
Distribution: OEM
General Admin.: Lorne Scharnberg/President, Chief Executive Officer
     Warren R. Walters/Vice President
Finance: Kathleen Scharnberg/Chief Financial Officer
Defibrillator, Battery-Powered, Low Energy	Cardiovascular
Defibrillator, External, Automatic	Cardiovascular
Dressing, Gel	General
Electrode, Cutaneous	Cns/Neurology
Electrode, Defibrillator	Cardiovascular
Electrode, Neuromuscular Stimulator	Cns/Neurology
Electrode, Other	General
Electrode, Pacemaker, External	Cardiovascular
Electrode, TENS	Cns/Neurology
Pacemaker, Cardiac, External Transcutaneous (Non-Invasive)	Cardiovascular
Pad, Defibrillator Paddle	Cardiovascular

KATENA PRODUCTS, INC.   800-225-1195
4 Stewart Ct., Denville, NJ 07834-1028   **973-989-1600**
FDA Number: 2242450   *Fax:* 973-989-8175
E-mail: globe@katena.com
Web site: www.katena.com
Annual Revenue: $10-$25 Million
Total Employees: 25
Ownership: Private
Quality System Registration Information: ISO9002
Produces/Sells CE-marked Devices: Y

KATENA PRODUCTS, INC.   800-225-1195 *(cont'd)*
Federal Procurement Eligibility: Small Business, Female Owned
Distribution: Manufacturer Direct
General Admin.: Kate Tiedemann/Chief Executive Officer, Chairman
     Michael Vedral/President, General Manager
Mktg./Adv.: Gordon Dahl/Vice President Sales
Production: Bryan Weinmann/Vice President Regulatory Affairs
Accessories, Operating Room, Table	Surgery
Blade, Scalpel	Surgery
Burr, Corneal, Manual	Ophthalmology
Caliper, Ophthalmic	Ophthalmology
Cannula, Ophthalmic	Ophthalmology
Clamp, Eyelid, Ophthalmic	Ophthalmology
Clamp, Muscle, Ophthalmic	Ophthalmology
Container, Sterilization (Tray)	General
Curette, Ophthalmic	Ophthalmology
Curette, Surgical	Surgery
Cystotome, Ophthalmic	Ophthalmology
Depressor, Orbital	Ophthalmology
Dilator, Lacrimal	Ophthalmology
Electrosurgical Unit, Cutting & Coagulation Device	Surgery
Forceps, Dressing	Surgery
Forceps, Epilation	Surgery
Forceps, Fixation	Surgery
Forceps, Hemostatic	Surgery
Forceps, Ophthalmic	Ophthalmology
Forceps, Tissue	Surgery
Forceps, Utility	Surgery
Guide, Needle	Surgery
Handle, Scalpel	Surgery
Holder, Needle	Gastroenterology/Urology
Hook, Ophthalmic	Ophthalmology
Hook, Other	Surgery
Hook, Scleral Fixation	Ophthalmology
Hook, Skin	Surgery
Hook, Strabismus	Ophthalmology
Instrument, Microsurgical	Cns/Neurology
Keratome, AC-Powered	Ophthalmology
Knife, Ophthalmic	Ophthalmology
Knife, Other	Surgery
Loop, Lens	Ophthalmology
Needle, Aspiration And Injection, Disposable	Surgery
Probe, Lacrimal	Ophthalmology
Punch, Corneo-Scleral	Ophthalmology
Retractor, Ophthalmic	Ophthalmology
Ring, Ophthalmic (Flieringa)	Ophthalmology
Scissors, Corneal	Ophthalmology
Scissors, Enucleation	Ophthalmology
Scissors, Iris	Ophthalmology
Scissors, Ophthalmic	Ophthalmology
Scissors, Tenotomy	Ophthalmology
Spatula, Ophthalmic	Ophthalmology
Speculum, Ophthalmic	Ophthalmology
Sponge, Rayon Cellulose	General
Spoon, Ophthalmic	Ophthalmology
Spud, Ophthalmic	Ophthalmology
Surgical Instrument, Disposable	Surgery
Trephine, Manual, Ophthalmic (Corneal)	Ophthalmology
Tubing, Non-Invasive	Surgery

KATIE HEALTHCARE SYSTEMS
See New Laser Science, Inc.

KAULSON LABORATORIES, INC.   973-226-9494
693 Bloomfield Ave., Caldwell, NJ 07006-7539
FDA Number: n/a   *Fax:* 973-226-3244
E-mail: kaulsonlab@aol.com
Web site: www.kaulsonlab.com
Annual Revenue: $0-$1 Million
Total Employees: 7
Ownership: Private
Produces/Sells CE-marked Devices: N
Federal Procurement Eligibility: Small Business
Distribution: Manufacturer Direct, Service Direct
General Admin.: Balkrishena Kaul/President
Control, Drug Mixture	Toxicology
Control, Heavy Metals	Toxicology
Fluorometric Measurement, Porphyrins	Chemistry
Reagent, Iron (Test System)	Chemistry

KAULSON LABORATORIES, INC.   973-226-9494
693 Bloomfield Ave., West Caldwell, NJ 07006
FDA Number: 2244591
Control, Drug Mixture	Toxicology
Control, Heavy Metals	Toxicology
Fluorometric Measurement, Porphyrins	Chemistry

KAVO DENTAL CORP.   800-323-8029
340 East Route 22, Lake Zurich, IL 60047   **847-550-6800**
FDA Number: 1419798   *Fax:* 847-550-6825
E-mail: info.us@kavo.com

KAVO DENTAL CORP.   800-323-8029 *(cont'd)*

Web site: www.kavousa.com
Medical Products Sales Volume: $4,500,000
Year Founded: 1909
Total Employees: 105   *Marketing Staff:* 6   *Sales Staff:* 60
Ownership: Private
Stock Symbol: DHR
Quality System Registration Information: ISO9001
Produces/Sells CE-marked Devices: Y
Federal Procurement Eligibility: Small Business
Distribution: Manufacturer Through Distributor
General Admin.: John Franz/President, Chief Executive Officer
Mktg./Adv.: Angelika Goeppel/Director Communications
    Richard Maynard/Vice President National Sales
    Teresa May/Vice President, Director Marketing
    Tom Perlitz/Vice President, Director Marketing
Finance: Dave Strehl/Vice President Finance
IS: Dale Peterson/Manager Tech. Services

Airbrush	Dental And Oral
Drill, Dental, Intraoral	Dental And Oral
Laser, Laboratory	Chemistry
Light Source, Fiberoptic, Routine	Gastroenterology/Urology
Sterilizer, Steam (Autoclave)	General

KAVO DENTAL MANUFACTURING INC   202-828-0850

901 West Oakton St., Des Plaines, IL 60018-1884
FDA Number: 3004115000
Ownership: Danaher Corporation
Produces/Sells CE-marked Devices: N

Chair, Dental (With Unit)	Dental And Oral
Light, Surgical Operating, Dental	Dental And Oral
Unit, Operative Dental, Accessories	Dental And Oral

KAWASUMI LABORATORIES

See Medisystems Corporation

KAWASUMI LABORATORIES AMERICA, INC.   800-529-2786   813-630-5554

4723 Oakfair Blvd, Tampa, FL 33610
FDA Number: 1055927   Fax: 813-630-5033
E-mail: info@kawasumiamerica.com
Web site: www.kawasumiamerica.com
Annual Revenue: $10-$25 Million
Year Founded: 1991
Total Employees: 19   *Marketing Staff:* 2   *Sales Staff:* 12
Ownership: Public
Stock Symbol: 7703
Traded On: Tokyo
Quality System Registration Information: ISO9000
Produces/Sells CE-marked Devices: Y
Distribution: Manufacturer Through Distributor, Manufacturer Through Manufacturer Reps, Importer, Exporter
General Admin.: Ronald Lamb/President
Mktg./Adv.: Scott Horowitz/Manager Marketing
    Bob Passamano/Manager National Sales
Production: Jack Pavlo/Manager Regulatory Affairs

Cannula, Hemodialysis	Gastroenterology/Urology
Contract Manufacturing	General
IV Start Kit	Surgery
Kit, Administration, Blood	General
Kit, Administration, Intravenous	General
Kit, Blood Collection, Phlebotomy	Cardiovascular
Kit, Catheterization, Intravenous, Winged	Cardiovascular
Kit, Hemodialysis Tubing	Gastroenterology/Urology
Kit, Intravenous Extension Tubing	General
Monitor, Infusion, Gravity Flow	General
Needle, Dialysis	Gastroenterology/Urology
Needle, Intravenous	General
Needle, Other	General
Shield, Wound, Injection Site	General
System, Infusion, Administration, Drug, Implantable	General
Transfer Unit, Blood	Hematology
Transfer Unit, IV Fluid	General
Tubing, Other	General

KAY SEE DENTAL MFG. CO.   800-842-8844   816-842-2817

124 East Missouri Ave.,
Kansas City, MO 64106
FDA Number: 1914596   Fax: 816-842-3402
Ownership: Private
Produces/Sells CE-marked Devices: N

Base, Denture, Relining, Repairing, Rebasing, Resin	Dental And Oral
Cement, Dental	Dental And Oral
Crown And Bridge, Temporary, Resin	Dental And Oral
Device, Incontinence, Mechanical/Hydraulic	Gastroenterology/Urology
Operative Dental Treatment Unit	Dental And Oral
Sealant, Pit And Fissure, And Conditioner, Resin	Dental And Oral
Wax, Dental	Dental And Oral

KAYE PRODUCTS, INC.   919-732-6444

535 Dimmocks Mill Rd., Hillsborough, NC 27278-2352
FDA Number: 1047834   Fax: 919-732-1444
Web site: www.kayeproducts.com
Ownership: Private
Produces/Sells CE-marked Devices: Y
Federal Procurement Eligibility: Small Business
Distribution: Manufacturer Direct, Manufacturer Through Distributor, Importer, Exporter
General Admin.: Andrew Howle/President
    Edward Howle/Vice President
Mktg./Adv.: Janet Wilson/Vice President Marketing

Accessories, Walker	General
Adaptor, Recreational	Physical Med
Cane	Physical Med
Chair, Adjustable, Mechanical	Physical Med
Chair, Pediatric	General
Chair, With Casters	Physical Med
Component, Exercise	Physical Med
Crutch	Physical Med
Exerciser, Non-Measuring	Physical Med
Holder, Infant Position	General
Support, Patient Position	Anesthesiology
Table, Mechanical	Physical Med
Tips And Pads, Cane, Crutch And Walker	Physical Med
Vehicle, Handicapped	Physical Med
Walker, Mechanical	Physical Med
Wheelchair, Powered	Physical Med

KAYJAE MFG. CO. INC.   888-452-9523   804-725-9664

Rte. 198 at Chapel Creek Road, PO Box 95, Cobbs Creek, VA 23035
FDA Number: 1125739   Fax: 804-725-0166
E-mail: sales@kayjae.com
Web site: www.kayjae.com
Medical Products Sales Volume: $34,620,000
Annual Revenue: $0-$1 Million
Year Founded: 1992
Ownership: Private
Produces/Sells CE-marked Devices: N
Federal Procurement Eligibility: Small Business
Distribution: Manufacturer Direct
General Admin.: Mr. Donald Jaeger/President
Mktg./Adv.: Mrs. Lynn Jaeger/Vice President Marketing

Accessories, Wheelchair	Physical Med
Tray, Wheelchair	Physical Med

KAYLINE INC.   423-472-7118

606 18th St., Cleveld, TN 37311
FDA Number: 3004868417   Fax: 423-478-3502
Ownership: Private
Produces/Sells CE-marked Devices: N

Chair, Position, Electric	Physical Med

KAYPENTAX   800-289-5297   973-628-6200

3 Paragon Drive, Montvale, NJ 07645
FDA Number: 2245496   Fax: 201-391-2063
E-mail: sales@kaypentax.com
Web site: www.kaypentax.com
Annual Revenue: $10-$25 Million
Total Employees: 50   *Marketing Staff:* 4   *Sales Staff:* 17
Ownership: Public
Produces/Sells CE-marked Devices: Y
Federal Procurement Eligibility: Small Business
Distribution: Manufacturer Direct, Manufacturer Through Manufacturer Reps
General Admin.: John Crump/General Manager
Mktg./Adv.: Robert McClurkin/Director Marketing
    Stephen Crump/Director Sales
    Jerilynn Prokop/Manager Advertising
    Paul Arcell/Manager Sales

Analyzer, Audio Spectrum	Ear/Nose/Throat
Computer Equipment	General
Electroglottograph	Ear/Nose/Throat
Image Processing System	Radiology
Laryngostroboscope	Ear/Nose/Throat
Monitor, Esophageal Motility, And Tube	Gastroenterology/Urology
Rhinoscope	Ear/Nose/Throat
Speech Therapy Unit (Trainer)	Ear/Nose/Throat

KAYSER-ROTH CORP.   800-575-3497   336-547-4603

102 Corporate Center Blvd., Greensboro, NC 27408
FDA Number: 1065454
Web site: www.kayser-roth.com
Ownership: Private
Produces/Sells CE-marked Devices: N

Stocking, Elastic	General

KAYSER-ROTH CORP.   800-575-3497 *(cont'd)*
Stocking, Support (Anti-Embolic)   General

KAZ USA, INC.   518-828-0450
4755 Southpoint Drive, Memphis, TN 38118
FDA Number: 3004169268
Humidifier, Non-Direct Patient Interface (Home-Use)   Anesthesiology
Pad, Heating, Powered   Physical Med

KAZ, INC.   518-828-0450
One Vapor Trail, Hudson, NY 12534
FDA Number: 1314800
Filter, Bacterial, Breathing Circuit   Anesthesiology
Humidifier, Non-Direct Patient Interface (Home-Use)   Anesthesiology
Nebulizer, Direct Patient Interface   Anesthesiology
Pad, Heating, Powered   Physical Med

KBD, INC.   800-544-3757
2550 American Ct, Crescent Springs, KY 41017   859-331-0800
FDA Number: 1022129   *Fax:* 859-331-0802
E-mail: sales@sperti.com
Web site: www.sperti.com
Medical Products Sales Volume: $1,000,000
Annual Revenue: $1-$5 Million
Total Employees: 18   *Marketing Staff:* 1   *Sales Staff:* 2
Ownership: Private
Produces/Sells CE-marked Devices: N
Federal Procurement Eligibility: Small Business
Distribution: Manufacturer Direct, Manufacturer Through Distributor, Exporter
General Admin.: James Shepherd/President
    Kathy Shepherd/Vice President
Production: Elaine Scherder/Plant Manager
Lamp, Infrared   Physical Med
Lamp, Sun, Incandescent   General
Lamp, Ultraviolet, Physical Medicine   Physical Med
Light, Ultraviolet, Dermatologic   Surgery
Shield, Eye, Ophthalmic   Ophthalmology

KBD, INC.   859-331-0800
2550 American Ct., Crescent Springs, KY 41017
FDA Number: 1022129
Lamp, Infrared   Physical Med
Lamp, Ultraviolet, Physical Medicine   Physical Med

KC PHARMACAL, INC.
See Kc Pharmaceuticals, Inc.

KC PHARMACEUTICALS, INC.   909-598-9499
3201 Producer Way, Pomona, CA 91768-3915
FDA Number: n/a
Annual Revenue: $1-$5 Million
Ownership: Private
Produces/Sells CE-marked Devices: N
Federal Procurement Eligibility: Small Business
Distribution: Manufacturer Direct, Exporter
Cleaner, Lens, Contact   Ophthalmology
Dropper, Eye   Ophthalmology

KCI USA, INC.   210-255-6137
6203 Farinon Dr., San Antonio, TX 78249
FDA Number: 3005178245
Web site: www.kci1.com
Ownership: KINETIC CONCEPTS, INC.
Stock Symbol: KCI
Traded On: NYSE
Produces/Sells CE-marked Devices: N
Production: Edward Newton/Director Regulatory Affairs
Bed, Adjustable Hospital   General
Bed, Pediatric (Crib)   General
Lift, Patient   General
Mattress, Air Flotation   General
Mesh, Surgical, Polymeric   Surgery

KCK INDUSTRIES   888-800-1967
14941 Calvert St., Van Nuys, CA 91411   818-997-8574
FDA Number: n/a   *Fax:* 818-997-6770
E-mail: info@kckind.com
Web site: www.kckind.com
Medical Products Sales Volume: $101,100,000
Annual Revenue: $1-$5 Million
Year Founded: 1982
Total Employees: 14   *Marketing Staff:* 4   *Sales Staff:* 4
Ownership: Private
Produces/Sells CE-marked Devices: N
Federal Procurement Eligibility: Small Business, GSA Contract, VA Contract
Distribution: Exclusive Distributor
General Admin.: Bruce R. Sather/President, Chief Executive Officer
    Clark Sather/Vice President, General Manager
Mktg./Adv.: Kyle Sather/Vice President Sales
Connector, Catheter   Surgery

KCK INDUSTRIES   888-800-1967 *(cont'd)*
Cuff, Blood Pressure   Cardiovascular
Dressing, Roller Gauze   General
Garment, Protective, For Incontinence   Gastroenterology/Urology
Kit, Administration, Enteral   Gastroenterology/Urology
Kit, Skin Scrub   General
Kit, Wound Drainage   General
Lotion, Skin Care   General
Mask, Oxygen, Other   General
Monitor, Blood Glucose (Test)   Gastroenterology/Urology
Needle, Other   General
Stethoscope, Manual   Cardiovascular
Stimulator, Wound Healing   Physical Med
Tape, Adhesive   General

KEBO HEALTH SYSTEMS, INC.
See Ferno-Washington, Inc.

KEELER INSTRUMENTS INC.   800-523-5620
456 Parkway, Broomall, PA 19008   610-353-4350
FDA Number: n/a   *Fax:* 610-353-7814
E-mail: keeler@keelerusa.com
Web site: www.keelerusa.com
Year Founded: 1917
Total Employees: 20   *Marketing Staff:* 1   *Sales Staff:* 5
Ownership: HALMA HOLDINGS, INC.
Produces/Sells CE-marked Devices: Y
Federal Procurement Eligibility: Small Business, GSA Contract, VA Contract
Distribution: Exclusive Distributor
General Admin.: David J. Keeler/President, Chief Executive Officer
Mktg./Adv.: Eugene Van Arsdale/Director Marketing
    Doug Black/Manager Contract Sales
Production: Eugene Van Arsdale/Manager Regulatory Affairs
Finance: Daniel J. Delaney/Controller
Cable, Fiberoptic   General
Cryophthalmic Unit   Ophthalmology
Cryotherapy, Unit, Ophthalmic   Ophthalmology
Drape, Patient, Ophthalmic   Ophthalmology
Fixation Device, Extra-Cranial (Head Frame)   Orthopedics
Forceps, Ophthalmic   Ophthalmology
Grid, Amsler   Ophthalmology
Light, Surgical Headlight   Dental And Oral
Loupe, Diagnostic/Surgical   Surgery
Ophthalmoscope, AC-Powered   Ophthalmology
Ophthalmoscope, Direct   Ophthalmology
Ophthalmoscope, Indirect   Ophthalmology
Retinoscope, AC-Powered   Ophthalmology
Stool, Operating Room, Adjustable   Surgery
Surgical Instrument, Manual (General Use)   Surgery
Tonometer, Manual   Ophthalmology
Transilluminator, AC-Powered, Ophthalmic   Ophthalmology
Vision Aid, Image Intensification, Battery-Powered   Ophthalmology

KEELER OPTICAL PRODUCTS, INC
See Keeler Instruments Inc.

KEEN MOBILITY COMPANY   503-285-9090
6500 Ne Halsey St Bldg B, Portland, OR 97213
FDA Number: 3003908950   *Fax:* 503.223.9488
E-mail: info@keenmobility.com
Ownership: Private
Produces/Sells CE-marked Devices: N
Attachment, Commode, Wheelchair   Physical Med
Cane, Safety Walk   Physical Med
Crutch   Physical Med
Cushion, Flotation   Physical Med
Cushion, Wheelchair (Pad)   Physical Med
Mattress, Non-Powered Flotation Therapy   Physical Med
Tips And Pads, Cane, Crutch And Walker   Physical Med
Walker, Mechanical   Physical Med
Wheelchair, Powered   Physical Med

KEENE MEDICAL PRODUCTS, INC.   800 447-0028
240 Meriden Rd. No. 439, PO Box 439,   603-448-5290
Lebanon, NH 03766
FDA Number: 1219063
Web site: www.keenemedicalproducts.com
Ownership: Private
Produces/Sells CE-marked Devices: N
Analyzer, Gas, Oxygen, Gaseous Phase   Anesthesiology
Cylinder, Compressed Gas, With Valve   Anesthesiology
Cylinder, Gas (Empty)   Anesthesiology

KEEPERS!, INC.   503-546-5696
PO Box 12648, Portland, OR 97212
FDA Number: 3032370   *Fax:* 503-284-9883
E-mail: info@gladrags.com
Web site: www.gladrags.com
Medical Products Sales Volume: $17,000,000
Year Founded: 1993
Total Employees: 6

KEEPERS!, INC. 503-546-5696 *(cont'd)*
Ownership: Private
Produces/Sells CE-marked Devices: N
Federal Procurement Eligibility: Female Owned
Distribution: Manufacturer Direct, Manufacturer Through Distributor
Pad, Menstrual, Unscented — Obstetrics/Gynecology

KEES GOEBEL MEDICAL SPECIALTIES, INC. 800-354-0445
9663 Glades Drive, Hamilton, OH 45011 **513-874-2201**
FDA Number: 7000568 *Fax:* 513-874-5827
E-mail: info@keesgoebel.com
Web site: www.keesgoebel.com
Medical Products Sales Volume: $34,620,000
Year Founded: 1977
Total Employees: 15
Ownership: Private
Produces/Sells CE-marked Devices: N
Federal Procurement Eligibility: Small Business
Distribution: Manufacturer Direct, Exclusive Distributor
General Admin.: Skip Warm/President
　　　　　　　　Bert Goebel/Vice President, General Manager
Mktg./Adv.: John Kuprionis/Manager National Sales
　　　　　　　　Bert Goebel/Vice President Sales
Cushion, Wheelchair (Pad) — Physical Med
Equipment, Therapy, Handicapped/Physical — Physical Med
Pack, Hot Or Cold, Reusable — Physical Med
Pad, Pressure, Foam (Elbow, Heel) — General
Splint, Padded Stays — Orthopedics

KEGELMASTER INC. 352-625-2156
4125 Se Hwy 314a, Ocklawaha, FL 32179
FDA Number: 3006336965 *Fax:* 352-625-2158
E-mail: Kegelmaster@earthlink.net
Web site: www.kegelmaster.com
Ownership: Private
Produces/Sells CE-marked Devices: N
Perineometer — Obstetrics/Gynecology

KEILEI INTERNATIONAL
See Dukal Corporation

KEIR SURGICAL LTD. 800.663.4525
126-408 East Kent Avenue South, **604-261-9596**
Vancouver, BC V5X 2 Canada
FDA Number: n/a *Fax:* 604-261-9549
E-mail: info@keirsurgical.com
Web site: www.keirsurgical.com
Year Founded: 1923
Total Employees: 25
Ownership: Private
Produces/Sells CE-marked Devices: N
Distribution: Exclusive Distributor

KELKOM SYSTEMS 800-985-3556
418 MacArthur Avenue, **650-366-3877**
Redwood City, CA 94063
FDA Number: n/a *Fax:* 650-366-4226
E-mail: dkellems@pacbell.net
Web site: www.kelkom.com
Medical Products Sales Volume: $21,900,000
Annual Revenue: $0-$1 Million
Year Founded: 1974
Ownership: Private
Produces/Sells CE-marked Devices: N
Federal Procurement Eligibility: Small Business
Distribution: Manufacturer Direct, Manufacturer Through Manufacturer Reps
General Admin.: Dave Kellems/President, Chief Executive Officer
Communication System, Room Status — General
Nurse Call System — General
Pager, Non-Radio — General
Physician Registry — General

KELLEHER MEDICAL, INC. 804-378-9956
3049 St. Marys Way, Powhatan, VA 23139-5322
FDA Number: 1120846 *Fax:* 804-378-9958
E-mail: kellmed@kellehermedical.com
Web site: www.kellehermedical.com
Medical Products Sales Volume: $101,100,000
Year Founded: 1988
Ownership: Private
Produces/Sells CE-marked Devices: N
Federal Procurement Eligibility: Small Business
Distribution: Service Direct, Importer, Exporter
General Admin.: Francis J. Kelleher/President
Accessories, Surgical Camera — Surgery
Camera, Video — General
Chamber, Acoustic, Testing — Ear/Nose/Throat
Computer Software — General
Fiberoptic Light Source & Carrier — Ear/Nose/Throat

KELLEHER MEDICAL, INC. 804-378-9956 *(cont'd)*
Headlight, Fiberoptic Focusing — Gastroenterology/Urology
Laryngoscope — Ear/Nose/Throat
Laryngoscope, Rigid — Anesthesiology
Laryngostroboscope — Ear/Nose/Throat
Nasopharyngoscope (Flexible Or Rigid) — Ear/Nose/Throat
Nasoscope — Ear/Nose/Throat
Otoscope — Ear/Nose/Throat
Unit, Examining/Treatment, ENT — Ear/Nose/Throat

KELLER CRESCENT 508-478-7641
1072 Boulder Road, Greensboro, NC 27409
FDA Number: n/a
Web site: www.kellercrescent.com
Annual Revenue: $1-$5 Million
Ownership: NORTHSTATE PACKAGING
Quality System Registration Information: ISO9002
Produces/Sells CE-marked Devices: N
Distribution: Manufacturer Direct
Contract Packaging — General

KELLER ENGINEERING, INC. 310-326-6291
3203 Kashiwa St., Torrance, CA 90505
FDA Number: 2030893 *Fax:* 310-326-0417
E-mail: steve@kellereng.com
Web site: www.kellereng.com
Medical Products Sales Volume: $4,500,000
Year Founded: 1972
Total Employees: 28
Ownership: Private
Produces/Sells CE-marked Devices: N
Federal Procurement Eligibility: Small Business, Female Owned
Implant, Fixation Device, Proximal Femoral — Orthopedics
Nail, Fixation, Bone — Orthopedics
Plate, Fixation, Bone — Orthopedics

KELLY HEARING AID 702-309-3724
150 South Decatur Blvd., Las Vegas, NV 89107
FDA Number: 2090044
Ownership: Private
Produces/Sells CE-marked Devices: N
Hearing-Aid — Ear/Nose/Throat

KELSAR, S.A. 508-261-8000
Blvd. Insurgentes, Libriamento a La, Tijuana 22450 Mexico
FDA Number: 9610849
Appliance, Incontinence, Urosheath Type — Gastroenterology/Urology
Applier, Surgical, Clip — Surgery
Bag, Leg — Gastroenterology/Urology
Bottle, Collection, Vacuum (Aspirator) — General
Brush, Cleaning, Tracheal Tube — Ear/Nose/Throat
Cannula, Nasal, Oxygen — Anesthesiology
Carrier, Ligature — Surgery
Catheter, Aspiration — Surgery
Catheter, Intravascular, Diagnostic — Cardiovascular
Catheter, Rectal — Surgery
Catheter, Retention Type, Balloon — Gastroenterology/Urology
Catheter, Suction (Tracheal Aspirating Tube) — Anesthesiology
Catheter, Suction, With Tip — General
Catheter, Urethral — Gastroenterology/Urology
Catheter, Urological — Gastroenterology/Urology
Catheter, Vascular, Cardiopulmonary Bypass — Cardiovascular
Chamber, Decompression, Abdominal — Obstetrics/Gynecology
Clamp, Vascular — Cardiovascular
Clip, Implantable — Surgery
Collector, Urine — Gastroenterology/Urology
Connector, Catheter — Surgery
Cuff, Tracheostomy Tube — Ear/Nose/Throat
Drainage System, Urine, Closed — Gastroenterology/Urology
Dressing, Other — General
Guide, Surgical, Needle — Surgery
Instrument, Manual, General Surgical — Surgery
Kit, Administration, Intravenous — General
Kit, Anesthesia, Conduction — Anesthesiology
Kit, Anesthesia, Pudendal — Obstetrics/Gynecology
Kit, Catheterization, Sterile Urethral — Gastroenterology/Urology
Kit, Collection/Transfusion, Marrow, Bone — General
Kit, Enema (For Cleaning Purposes) — Gastroenterology/Urology
Kit, Irrigation, Sterile — Gastroenterology/Urology
Kit, Urinary Drainage Collection — Gastroenterology/Urology
Light Source, Fiberoptic, Routine — Gastroenterology/Urology
Manometer, Spinal Fluid — General
Mesh, Surgical, Polymeric — Surgery
Needle, Catheter — Surgery
Needle, Suture, Disposable — Surgery
Oral Administration Set — General
Pump, Infusion — General
Punch, Surgical — Surgery
Retractor, Surgical — Surgery
Rod, Colostomy — Gastroenterology/Urology
Sampler, Blood, Fetal — Obstetrics/Gynecology

KELSAR, S.A.   508-261-8000 *(cont'd)*

Staple, Removable (Skin)	Surgery
Stapler, Surgical	Surgery
Surgical Instrument, Cardiovascular	Cardiovascular
Suture, Absorbable, Natural	Surgery
Suture, Absorbable, Ophthalmic	Ophthalmology
Suture, Absorbable, Synthetic, Polyglycolic Acid	Surgery
Suture, Cardiovascular	Cardiovascular
Suture, Non-Absorbable	Surgery
Suture, Non-Absorbable, Ophthalmic	Ophthalmology
Suture, Non-Absorbable, Silk	Surgery
Suture, Non-Absorbable, Steel, Monofilament & Multifilament	Surgery
Suture, Non-Absorbable, Synthetic, Polyamide	Surgery
Suture, Non-Absorbable, Synthetic, Polyester	Surgery
Suture, Non-Absorbable, Synthetic, Polypropylene	Surgery
Syringe, Irrigating	General
Syringe, Piston	General
Thermometer, Electronic, Continuous	General
Tourniquet, Non-Pneumatic, Surgical	Surgery
Trap, Sterile Specimen	Anesthesiology
Tray, Blood Collection	Hematology
Tray, Surgical Instrument	Surgery
Trocar, Cardiovascular	Cardiovascular
Tube, Aspirating, Flexible, Connecting	Anesthesiology
Tube, Aspirating, Rigid Bronchoscope Aspirating	Ear/Nose/Throat
Tube, Feeding	General
Tube, Nasogastric	Anesthesiology
Urinometer, Non-Electrical	Gastroenterology/Urology

KELYNIAM GLOBAL, INC   800-280-8192
97 River Road, Canton, CT 60619
FDA Number: n/a
E-mail: Inventivepr@att.net
Web site: www.kelyniam.com
Ownership: Private
Produces/Sells CE-marked Devices: N

Plate, Bone, Skull, Preformed, Non-Alterable	Cns/Neurology

KEM ENT., INC.   888-562-8802
PO Box 6342, Grand Rapids, MI 49516   616-452-8802
FDA Number: 1835573   *Fax:* 616-452-9177
E-mail: info@kemonline.com
Web site: www.kemOnline.com
Medical Products Sales Volume: $17,000,000
Year Founded: 1997
Total Employees: 4
Ownership: Private
Produces/Sells CE-marked Devices: N
Federal Procurement Eligibility: Small Business, Female Owned
Distribution: Manufacturer Through Distributor

Collector, Ostomy	Gastroenterology/Urology

KEM MEDICAL PRODUCTS CORP.   800-553-0330
75 Price Parkway, Farmingdale, NY 11735   631-454-6565
FDA Number: 2432141   *Fax:* 631-454-8083
E-mail: mail@kemmed.com
Web site: www.kemmed.com
Medical Products Sales Volume: $34,620,000
Annual Revenue: $1-$5 Million
Year Founded: 1980
Total Employees: 3   *Marketing Staff:* 2   *Sales Staff:* 6
Ownership: Private
Produces/Sells CE-marked Devices: N
Federal Procurement Eligibility: Small Business, GSA Contract
Distribution: Manufacturer Direct, Manufacturer Through Distributor
General Admin.: Joseph Ebenstein/Executive Vice President
    Douglas A. Kruger/President, Chief Executive Officer

Analyzer, Ethylene-Oxide	General
Computer Equipment	General
Formaldehyde (Formalin, Formol)	Pathology
Glutaraldehyde (Fixative)	Pathology
Sterilization Process Indicator, Chemical	General

KEMBLE INSTRUMENTS
See Mgm Instruments

KEMPF   800-255-6174
1245 Lakeside Dr., #3005, Sunnyvale, CA 94086   408-773-0219
FDA Number: n/a   *Fax:* 408-773-0524
E-mail: info@kempf-usa.com
Web site: www.kempf-usa.com
Ownership: Private
Produces/Sells CE-marked Devices: N
Federal Procurement Eligibility: Small Business, Female Owned
Distribution: Manufacturer Direct
General Admin.: Martine Kempf/Chief Executive Officer

Environmental Control System, Powered	Physical Med
Wheelchair, Powered	Physical Med

KEN-A-VISION MANUFACTURING CO., INC.   800-627-1953
5615 Raytown Road, Kansas City, MO 64133   816-353-4787
FDA Number: 7000215   *Fax:* 816-358-5072
E-mail: info@ken-a-vision.com
Web site: www.ken-a-vision.com
Medical Products Sales Volume: $21,900,000
Annual Revenue: $10-$25 Million
Year Founded: 1968
Total Employees: 25   *Marketing Staff:* 2   *Sales Staff:* 4
Ownership: Private
Produces/Sells CE-marked Devices: Y
Federal Procurement Eligibility: Small Business
Distribution: Manufacturer Through Distributor, Importer, Exporter
General Admin.: Steve Dunn/President
    Mr. Mike Mathews/Vice President
Mktg./Adv.: Steve Dunn/Manager International & National Sales
    Ben Hoke/Manager Sales

Camera, Video	General
Microscope	Hematology
Microscope, Laboratory, Optical	Microbiology

KENAD SG MEDICAL, INC.   800-825-0606
2692 Huntley Dr., Memphis, TN 38132   901-345-0606
FDA Number: 1054236   *Fax:* 901-345-0608
E-mail: celmore@kenad.com
Web site: www.kenad.com
Year Founded: 1991
Ownership: Private
Produces/Sells CE-marked Devices: N

Belt, Traction, Pelvic, Orthopedic	Orthopedics
Binder, Abdominal	General
Brace, Joint, Ankle (External)	Physical Med
Component, Exercise	Physical Med
Joint, Knee, External Brace	Physical Med
Orthosis, Cervical	Physical Med
Orthosis, Lumbar	Physical Med
Orthosis, Lumbosacral	Physical Med
Orthosis, Rib Fracture, Soft	Physical Med
Protector, Skin Pressure	General
Restraint, Protective (Body)	General
Scissors, Orthopedic	Orthopedics
Shoe, Cast	Physical Med
Sling, Arm	Physical Med
Splint, Clavicle	Physical Med
Splint, Hand, And Component	Physical Med

KENDA AMERICAN AIRLESS   800-248-4737
7120 Americana Parkway, Reynoldsburg, OH 43068   614-552-0146
FDA Number: n/a   *Fax:* 614-866-9805
E-mail: americanairless@kendausa.com
Annual Revenue: $1-$5 Million
Year Founded: 1983
Total Employees: 15   *Sales Staff:* 15
Ownership: Private
Produces/Sells CE-marked Devices: Y
Federal Procurement Eligibility: Small Business
Distribution: Manufacturer Direct, Manufacturer Through Distributor, Manufacturer Through Manufacturer Reps, OEM, Service Direct, Exclusive Distributor, Exporter
General Admin.: B. J. Hoesman/Chief Executive Officer
    Brent Hoesman/Vice President, General Manager

Accessories, Wheelchair	Physical Med
Component, Wheelchair	Physical Med

KENDALL DE MEXICO, S.A. DE C.V.   508-261-8000
Piniente 44, No. 3401, 16 D.f, Co. San Salvador Xochimanca, Mexico City Mexico
FDA Number: 8030602

Bandage, Cast	Physical Med

KENDALL KENMEX, A DIVISION OF TYCO HEALTHCARE GROUP LP   (01152) 664-623
Calle 9 Sur No. 125, Tijuana CP 22500 Mexico
FDA Number: 9612030   *Fax:* (01152) 664-62
Web site: www.tycohealthcare.com
Ownership: Private
Produces/Sells CE-marked Devices: N

KENDALL SHERWOOD-DAVIS & GECK
See Covidien Lp

KENDRO LABORATORY PRODUCTS   800-252-7100
308 Ridgefield Court, Asheville, NC 28806   828-658-2711
FDA Number: 7000305   *Fax:* 828-645-3368
E-mail: info.labequipment@thermo.com
Web site: www.kendro.com
Medical Products Sales Volume: $101,100,000
Total Employees: 867

KENDRO LABORATORY PRODUCTS 800-252-7100 (cont'd)

Ownership: SPX
Traded On: NYSE
Quality System Registration Information: ISO9001
Produces/Sells CE-marked Devices: Y
Federal Procurement Eligibility: GSA Contract
Distribution: Manufacturer Direct, Manufacturer Through Distributor, Manufacturer Through Manufacturer Reps, Exporter

Alarm, Refrigerator	Hematology
Centrifuge, Cell Washing	Hematology
Centrifuge, Floor	Pathology
Centrifuge, General (Over 5,000 rpm)	Toxicology
Centrifuge, General (Up to 5,000 rpm)	Pathology
Centrifuge, Refrigerated	Pathology
Centrifuge, Tabletop	Pathology
Chamber, Constant Temperature (Environmental)	Microbiology
Freezer, Blood Storage	Hematology
Freezer, Bone	Orthopedics
Freezer, Laboratory, Biological	Chemistry
Freezer, Laboratory, General Purpose	Chemistry
Freezer, Laboratory, Ultra-Low Temperature	Chemistry
Meter, pH, General Use	Toxicology
Microtome, Cryostat	Pathology
Microtome, Rotary	Pathology
Regulator, Temperature	Chemistry
Ultracentrifuge	Chemistry

KENLOR INDUSTRIES, INC. 800-899-9371
1560 East Edinger Ave., Suite A-1, 714-647-0770
Santa Ana, CA 92705
FDA Number: 2027370
E-mail: kamales@kenlor.com   Fax: 714-647-0770
Web site: www.kenlor.com
Medical Products Sales Volume: $1,500,000
Annual Revenue: $1-$5 Million
Ownership: Private
Produces/Sells CE-marked Devices: N
Federal Procurement Eligibility: Small Business
Distribution: Manufacturer Direct, Manufacturer Through Distributor, Manufacturer Through Manufacturer Reps, OEM, Exclusive Distributor, Exporter

Antigen, Antiserum, Control, Spinal Fluid, Total	Immunology
Contract Manufacturing, Pharmaceuticals/Chemicals	General
Control, Urinalysis (Assayed And Unassayed)	Chemistry
Disinfector, Liquid	General
Reagent, Iron (Test System)	Chemistry
Reagent, Other	General
Reagent, Protein, Total	Chemistry
Solution, Antibacterial Cleaner	General
Stick, Urinalysis Test	Chemistry

KENLOR INDUSTRIES, INC. 714-647-0770
1560 East Edinger Ave.,, Suite A-1, Santa Ana, CA 92705
FDA Number: 2027370

Antigen, Antiserum, Control, Spinal Fluid, Total	Immunology
Campylobacter Pylori	Microbiology
Control, Urinalysis (Assayed And Unassayed)	Chemistry

KENNEDY CENTER, INC. 203-365-8522
2440 Reservoir Ave., Trumbull, CT 06611
FDA Number: 1221436
E-mail: info@kennedyctr.org
Web site: www.thekennedycenterinc.org
Ownership: Private
Produces/Sells CE-marked Devices: N
General Admin.: Mr. Martin Schwartz/President, Chief Executive Officer
         Ms. Lynn Pellegrino/Vice President Human Resources
Finance: Mr. Stuart Gordon/Vice President Finance

Bandage, Elastic	General
Gown, Patient	Surgery

KENNEX DEVELOPMENT INC 626-458-0598
533 S. Atlantic Blvd, Suite 301, Monterey Park, CA 91754
FDA Number: 3006391782
Ownership: Private
Produces/Sells CE-marked Devices: N

Heating Unit, Powered	Physical Med
Orthosis, Cervical	Physical Med
Pack, Moist Heat	Physical Med
Splint, Hand, And Component	Physical Med

KENSEY NASH CORPORATION 484-713-2100
735 Pennsylvania Drive, Exton, PA 19341
FDA Number: 2530154   Fax: 484-713-2900
E-mail: info@kenseynash.com
Web site: www.kenseynash.com
Medical Products Sales Volume: $70,900,000
Annual Revenue: $50-$100 Million
Year Founded: 1984
Total Employees: 358   Marketing Staff: 6   Sales Staff: 23

KENSEY NASH CORPORATION 484-713-2100 (cont'd)

Ownership: Public
Stock Symbol: KNSY
Traded On: NASDAQ
Quality System Registration Information: ISO9001
Produces/Sells CE-marked Devices: Y
Distribution: Manufacturer Direct, Manufacturer Through Distributor, OEM
General Admin.: Mr. Douglas Evans/Chief Operating Officer
         Mr. Joseph Kaufman/President, Chief Executive Officer
Production: Mr. Thomas Maguire/Vice President Regulatory & Clinical Affairs
Finance: Mr. Michael Celano/Chief Financial Officer

Appliance, Fixation, Spinal Intervertebral Body	Orthopedics
Catheter, Angioplasty, Transluminal, Peripheral	Cardiovascular
Collagen, Platelet Aggregation And Adhesion	Hematology
Contract R&D, Equipment	General
Device, Closure, Puncture, Hemostatic	Cardiovascular
Fastener, Fixation, Biodegradable, Soft Tissue	Orthopedics
Mesh, Surgical (Steel Gauze)	Surgery
Orthopedic Manual Surgical Instrument	Orthopedics
Plate, Fixation, Bone	Orthopedics
Polymer, Synthetic, Other	General
Prosthesis, Membrane	Surgery
Screw, Fixation, Bone	Orthopedics
Sponge, Other	General
Tamp	Orthopedics

KENSHIN TRADING CORP. 800-766-1313
22353 South Western Avenue, Suite 201, 310-212-3199
Torrance, CA 90501
FDA Number: 2027975   Fax: 310-212-3299
E-mail: sales@kenshin.com
Web site: www.kenshin.com
Medical Products Sales Volume: $21,900,000
Year Founded: 1990
Ownership: Private
Produces/Sells CE-marked Devices: N
Distribution: Importer, Exporter

Needle, Acupuncture	Anesthesiology
Needle, Acupuncture, Single Use	General
Traction Unit, Non-Powered	Orthopedics

KENT ADHESIVE PRODUCTS CO. (KAPCO)
See Kapco (Kent Adhesive Products Co.)

KENT ELASTOMER PRODUCTS, INC 330-628-1802
3890 Mogadore Industrial Prkwy, Mogadore, OH 44260
FDA Number: 3004995608

Catheter, Peritoneal	Surgery
Tourniquet, Non-Pneumatic, Surgical	Surgery

KENT ELASTOMER PRODUCTS, INC. 800-331-4762
1500 St. Clair Avenue, PO Box 668, 330-673-1011
Kent, OH 44240
FDA Number: 3002303166   Fax: 330-673-1351
E-mail: info@kentelastomer.com
Web site: www.kentelastomer.com
Medical Products Sales Volume: $101,100,000
Annual Revenue: $100-$500 Million
Year Founded: 1960
Total Employees: 45   Marketing Staff: 1   Sales Staff: 3
Ownership: Private
Produces/Sells CE-marked Devices: N
Federal Procurement Eligibility: Small Business
Distribution: Manufacturer Direct, Manufacturer Through Distributor, OEM, Importer, Exporter
General Admin.: M. VanEpp/President
Mktg./Adv.: Cindy Harry/Director Marketing
         Cindy Harry/Director National Accounts
         Cindy Harry/Manager International & National Sales
         Cindy Harry/Manager National Sales
Production: Jim Houser/Director Quality Assurance
         R. Oborn/Vice President Manufacturing
Finance: D. Leeper/Controller
IS: T. Harrington/Director Tech. Services

Bag, Breathing	Anesthesiology
Component, Rubber	General
Contract Manufacturing	General
Polymer, Synthetic, Other	General
Tourniquet	General
Tubing, Latex	General
Tubing, Other	General
Tubing, Plastic	General
Tubing, Polyvinyl Chloride	General
Tubing, Vinyl	General

KENT LABORATORIES, INC. 360-398-8641
777 Jorgensen Pl., Bellingham, WA 98226
FDA Number: 3019906   Fax: 603-954-6333
E-mail: kent@kentlabs.com

KENT LABORATORIES, INC.   360-398-8641 (cont'd)

Web site: www.kentlabs.com
Medical Products Sales Volume: $1,000,000
Annual Revenue: $0-$1 Million
Year Founded: 1974
Total Employees: 10
Ownership: Private
Produces/Sells CE-marked Devices: N
Federal Procurement Eligibility: Small Business, Female Owned
Distribution: Manufacturer Direct, Manufacturer Through Distributor, OEM, Exporter
General Admin.: Allan H. Jorgensen/Chief Executive Officer
　　　　　Donald A. Jorgensen/President
Mktg./Adv.: Mary P. Jorgensen/Manager International & National Sales

Antibody, Other	General
Antigen, Antiserum, Complement C1 Inhibitor (Inactivator)	Immunology
Antigen, Antiserum, Control, Alpha-1-Antitrypsin	Immunology
Antigen, Antiserum, Control, Antithrombin III	Immunology
Antigen, Antiserum, Control, Bence-Jones Protein	Immunology
Antigen, Antiserum, Control, Complement C1q	Immunology
Antigen, Antiserum, Control, Complement C3	Immunology
Antigen, Antiserum, Control, Complement C4	Immunology
Antigen, Antiserum, Control, Complement C5	Immunology
Antigen, Antiserum, Control, FAB, Rhodamine	Immunology
Antigen, Antiserum, Control, Factor B	Immunology
Antigen, Antiserum, Control, Ferritin	Immunology
Antigen, Antiserum, Control, Haptoglobin	Immunology
Antigen, Antiserum, Control, IGA	Immunology
Antigen, Antiserum, Control, IGD	Immunology
Antigen, Antiserum, Control, IGE	Immunology
Antigen, Antiserum, Control, IGG	Immunology
Antigen, Antiserum, Control, IGM	Immunology
Antigen, Antiserum, Control, Kappa	Immunology
Antigen, Antiserum, Control, Lambda	Immunology
Antigen, Antiserum, Control, Other	Immunology
Antigen, Antiserum, Control, Transferrin	Immunology
Antigen, Antiserum, Control, Whole Human Serum	Immunology
Control, Antiserum, Antigen, Activator, C3, Complement	Immunology
IGA, Ferritin, Antigen, Antiserum, Control	Immunology
IGE, Ferritin, Antigen, Antiserum, Control	Immunology
IGG, Ferritin, Antigen, Antiserum, Control	Immunology
IGM, Ferritin, Antigen, Antiserum, Control	Immunology
Immunodiffusion, Protein Fractionation	Chemistry
Plate, Radial Immunodiffusion	Chemistry
Radial Immunodiffusion, Albumin	Chemistry
Test, C-Reactive Protein	Immunology
Test, Fibrinogen	Hematology

KENTEC MEDICAL INC.   800-825-5996
17871 Fitch, Irvine, CA 92614   **949-863-0810**
FDA Number: 2080225   *Fax:* 949-833-9730
E-mail: sales@kentecmedical.com
Web site: www.kentecmedical.com
Medical Products Sales Volume: $1,900,000
Annual Revenue: $10-$25 Million
Year Founded: 1975
Total Employees: 40   *Marketing Staff:* 3   *Sales Staff:* 17
Ownership: Private
Quality System Registration Information: ISO9001
Produces/Sells CE-marked Devices: Y
Federal Procurement Eligibility: Small Business
Distribution: Manufacturer Direct, Manufacturer Through Distributor, Service Direct, Exclusive Distributor, Importer, Exporter
General Admin.: Kent Wilken/Chief Executive Officer
　　　　　Steve Becsi/President
Mktg./Adv.: Bryan Flaherty/Vice President Marketing & Sales

Board, Arm	Anesthesiology
Cover, Probe, Transducer	Surgery
Electrode, Electrocardiograph	Cardiovascular
Oximeter, Finger	General
Probe, Temperature	General
Scale, Infant	General
Splint, Extremity, Non-Inflatable, External	Surgery
Tape, Gauze, Adhesive	General
Transducer, Ultrasonic, Obstetrical	Obstetrics/Gynecology
Tube, Feeding	General
Warmer, Radiant, Infant	General

KENTEK CORP.   800-432-2323
1 Elm St., Pittsfield, NH 03263   **603-435-5580**
FDA Number: n/a   *Fax:* 603-435-7441
E-mail: info@kenteklaserstore.com
Web site: www.kenteklaserstore.com
Annual Revenue: $1-$5 Million
Ownership: Private
Produces/Sells CE-marked Devices: N
Federal Procurement Eligibility: Small Business, Minority Owned
Distribution: Manufacturer Direct, OEM

Curtain, Protective, Radiographic	Radiology

KENTEK CORP.   800-432-2323 (cont'd)

Eyeglasses, Safety	Ophthalmology
Laser, Argon, Surgical	Surgery
Laser, Dental	Dental And Oral
Laser, Nd:YAG, Laparoscopy	Surgery
Laser, Nd:YAG, Surgical	Surgery
Sign, Hospital	General
Viewer/Magnifier	Hematology

KENTRON HEALTH CARE, INC.   615-384-0573
3604 Kelton Jackson Road, P.o. Box 120, Springfield, TN 37172
FDA Number: 1062671

Accessories, Apparel, Surgical	Surgery
Accessories, Catheter	Surgery
Airway, Nasopharyngeal (Breathing Tube)	Anesthesiology
Airway, Oropharyngeal, Anesthesia	Anesthesiology
Applicator, Tipped, Absorbent, Non-Sterile	General
Applicator, Tipped, Absorbent, Sterile	General
Bag, Ice	General
Bag, Leg	Gastroenterology/Urology
Bandage, Adhesive	Surgery
Bandage, Elastic	Surgery
Bandage, Liquid	Surgery
Basin, Emesis	General
Bedpan	General
Binder, Abdominal	General
Board, Arm	Anesthesiology
Cannula, Nasal, Oxygen	Anesthesiology
Cap, Surgical	Surgery
Catheter, Irrigation	Surgery
Catheter, Retention Type, Balloon	Gastroenterology/Urology
Catheter, Suction (Tracheal Aspirating Tube)	Anesthesiology
Catheter, Suction, With Tip	General
Container, Specimen, All Types	General
Container, Specimen, Non-sterile	General
Cotton, Roll	Dental And Oral
Cover, Mattress	General
Cover, Shoe, Operating Room	Surgery
Cuff, Blood Pressure	Cardiovascular
Cutter, Ring	General
Depressor, Tongue	General
Dispenser, Medication, Liquid	General
Dressing, Wound, Hydrophilic	Surgery
Electrode, Electrocardiograph	Cardiovascular
Forceps	Orthopedics
Gauze/sponge, Nonresorbable For External Use	Surgery
Gown, Isolation, Surgical	Surgery
Hemostat	Orthopedics
Holder, Catheter	Gastroenterology/Urology
Instrument, Manual, General Surgical	Surgery
Kit, Suctioning, Tracheostomy and Nasal	Surgery
Kit, Surgical (General)	Surgery
Kit, Suture Removal	Surgery
Kit, Urinary Drainage Collection	Gastroenterology/Urology
Lancet, Blood	General
Laryngoscope, Rigid	Anesthesiology
Light, Examination, Battery-Powered	General
Light, Wood's, Fluorescence	Microbiology
Linen, Bed	General
Mask, Oxygen, Aerosol Administration	Anesthesiology
Mask, Oxygen, Non-Rebreathing	Anesthesiology
Mask, Surgical	Surgery
Nebulizer, Direct Patient Interface	Anesthesiology
Nebulizer, Medicinal, Non-Ventilatory (Atomizer)	Anesthesiology
Needle, Catheter	Surgery
Needle, Fistula	Gastroenterology/Urology
Needle, Hypodermic, Single Lumen With Syringe	General
Occluder, Umbilical	General
Pack, Hot Or Cold, Disposable	Physical Med
Pack, Hot Or Cold, Reusable	Physical Med
Pad, Eye	Ophthalmology
Percussor	Cns/Neurology
Protector, Skin Pressure	General
Scissors, Orthopedic	Orthopedics
Sheet, Burn	General
Sling, Arm	Physical Med
Spatula, Cervical, Cytology	Obstetrics/Gynecology
Speculum, Vaginal, Non-Metal	Obstetrics/Gynecology
Sponge, Gauze	Dental And Oral
Stethoscope, Esophageal	Anesthesiology
Stethoscope, Manual	Cardiovascular
Stopcock	General
Stretcher, Hand-Carried	General
Stylet, Tracheal Tube	Anesthesiology
Syringe, Irrigating	General
Syringe, Piston	General
Thermometer, Electronic, Continuous	General
Thermometer, Mercury	General
Tourniquet, Non-Pneumatic, Surgical	Surgery
Tube, Tracheal (Endotracheal)	Anesthesiology
Tubing, Flexible, Medical Gas, Low-Pressure	Anesthesiology
Tubing, Non-Invasive	Surgery

KENTRON HEALTH CARE, INC.   615-384-0573 (cont'd)
Ventilator, Emergency, Manual (Resuscitator)   Anesthesiology

KENYON INDUSTRIES, INC.   973-962-4844
235 Margaret King Ave., Ringwood, NJ 07456
FDA Number: 2248188   Fax: 973-962-6252
E-mail: kenyon@warwick.com
Medical Products Sales Volume: $1,000,000
Total Employees: 8   Marketing Staff: 1   Sales Staff: 2
Ownership: Private
Quality System Registration Information: ISO9002
Produces/Sells CE-marked Devices: N
Federal Procurement Eligibility: Small Business
Distribution: Exclusive Distributor, Importer, Exporter
General Admin.: Martin Delin/President

Contract Manufacturing	General
Forceps	Orthopedics
Scissors, Disposable	General
Toothbrush, Manual	Dental And Oral

KERAVISION, INC.
See Addition Technology, Inc.

KERMA MEDICAL PRODUCTS, INC.   757-398-8400
400 Port Centre Parkway, Portsmouth, VA 23704
FDA Number: 1123029

Accessories, Apparel, Surgical	Surgery
Bag, Ice	General
Bandage, Elastic	General
Cuff, Blood Pressure	Cardiovascular
Drape, Surgical	Surgery
Dressing, Other	General
Holder, Infant Position	General
Linen, Bed	General
Mask, Surgical	Surgery
Protector, Hearing (Insert)	Ear/Nose/Throat
Sponge, External	Surgery
Stethoscope, Manual	Cardiovascular
Stocking, Elastic	General
Sunglasses (Including Photosensitive)	Ophthalmology
Thermometer, Electronic, Continuous	General

KERN SURGICAL SUPPLY, INC.   800-582-3939
2823 Gibson St., Bakersfield, CA 93308-6105   661-716-2700
FDA Number: n/a   Fax: 661-716-2757
E-mail: sales@kernsurgical.com
Web site: www.kernsurgical.com
Medical Products Sales Volume: $9,000,000
Annual Revenue: $5-$10 Million
Year Founded: 1961
Total Employees: 36   Marketing Staff: 2   Sales Staff: 12
Ownership: Private
Produces/Sells CE-marked Devices: N
Federal Procurement Eligibility: GSA Contract, VA Contract
Distribution: Manufacturer Through Distributor
General Admin.: Richard Haverstock/President
Mktg./Adv.: Marc Haverstock/Vice President Business Development

Bandage, Adhesive	Surgery
Brace, Joint, Ankle (External)	Physical Med
Glove, Patient Examination	General
Joint, Knee, External Brace	Physical Med
Kit, First Aid	Surgery
Scissors, Bandage/Gauze/Plaster	General
Support, Ankle	Orthopedics
Support, Back	Orthopedics
Support, Knee	Physical Med
Walker, Mechanical	Physical Med
Wheelchair, Manual	Physical Med

KERNCO INSTRUMENTS CO., INC.   800-325-3875
420 Kenazo Ave., El Paso, TX 79928-7338   915-852-3375
FDA Number: n/a   Fax: 915-852-4084
E-mail: nfo@rwctesting.com
Web site: www.kerncoinstr.com
Medical Products Sales Volume: $1,000,000
Annual Revenue: $25-$50 Million
Total Employees: 11   Marketing Staff: 3   Sales Staff: 4
Ownership: Private
Produces/Sells CE-marked Devices: Y
Federal Procurement Eligibility: Small Business
Distribution: Exclusive Distributor
General Admin.: John Kelly/General Manager
    John Kelly/President, Chief Executive Officer
Mktg./Adv.: Chris Huizar/Vice President Marketing & Sales

Meter, Conductivity	Chemistry
Meter, pH, Portable	Chemistry
Plate, Hot	Chemistry
Refractometer	Chemistry
Refractometric, Total Protein	Chemistry
Stirrer	Chemistry

KERNCO INSTRUMENTS CO., INC.   800-325-3875 (cont'd)
Tachometer   General

KERR CORP.   949-255-8766
1717 West Collins Ave., Orange, CA 92867
FDA Number: 2024312
Ownership: Sybron Dental Specialties, Inc.
Produces/Sells CE-marked Devices: N

Adhesive, Bracket And Conditioner, Resin	Dental And Oral
Agent, Polishing, Abrasive, Oral Cavity	Dental And Oral
Bandage, Adhesive	Surgery
Crown And Bridge, Temporary, Resin	Dental And Oral
Implant, Endosseous (Bone Filling and/or Augmentation)	Dental And Oral
Material, Tooth Shade, Resin	Dental And Oral
Sealant, Pit And Fissure, And Conditioner, Resin	Dental And Oral
Tooth Bonding Agent, Resin Restoration	Dental And Oral
Varnish, Cavity	Dental And Oral

KERR CORP.   800-537-7123
28200 Wick Rd., Romulus, MI 48174   714-516-7400
FDA Number: 1815757   Fax: 800-537-7345
Web site: www.kerrdental.com
Ownership: Sybron Dental Specialties, Inc.
Produces/Sells CE-marked Devices: N

Agent, Polishing, Abrasive, Oral Cavity	Dental And Oral
Alloy, Amalgam	Dental And Oral
Amalgamator, Dental, AC-Powered	Dental And Oral
Capsule, Dental, Amalgam	Dental And Oral
Cement, Dental	Dental And Oral
Denture, Plastic, Teeth	Dental And Oral
Disk, Abrasive	Dental And Oral
Dispenser, Mercury And/Or Alloy	Dental And Oral
File, Pulp Canal, Endodontic	Dental And Oral
Gutta Percha	Dental And Oral
Handpiece, Contra- And Right-Angle Attachment, Dental	Dental And Oral
Liner, Cavity, Calcium Hydroxide	Dental And Oral
Material, Impression	Dental And Oral
Material, Impression Tray, Resin	Dental And Oral
Material, Tooth Shade, Resin	Dental And Oral
Mirror, Mouth	Dental And Oral
Operative Dental Treatment Unit	Dental And Oral
Paper, Articulation	Dental And Oral
Plugger, Root Canal, Endodontic	Dental And Oral
Reamer, Pulp Canal, Endodontic	Dental And Oral
Resin, Root Canal Filling	Dental And Oral
Spreader, Pulp Canal Filling Material, Endodontic	Dental And Oral
Syringe, Restorative And Impression Material	Dental And Oral
Tooth Bonding Agent, Resin Restoration	Dental And Oral
Tray, Fluoride, Disposable	Dental And Oral
Wax, Dental	Dental And Oral
Zinc Oxide Eugenol	Dental And Oral

KERR CORP.   949-255-8766
3225 Deming Way, Suite 190, Middleton, WI 53562
FDA Number: 3003848022
Ownership: Sybron Dental Specialties, Inc.
Produces/Sells CE-marked Devices: N

Activator, Ultraviolet, Polymerization	Dental And Oral
Amalgamator, Dental, AC-Powered	Dental And Oral
Light, Surgical Headlight	Dental And Oral
Loupe, Diagnostic/Surgical	Surgery
Plugger, Root Canal, Endodontic	Dental And Oral
Tester, Pulp	Dental And Oral

KERR GROUP   800-524-3577
1400 Holcomb Bridge Road,   770-587-8000
Roswell, GA 30076
FDA Number: 1033422
E-mail: kchealthcare@kcc.com   Fax: 770-587-7752
Web site: www.kchealthcare.com
Annual Revenue: More than $1 Billion
Year Founded: 1903
Total Employees: 30
Ownership: Kimberly Clark Corp.
Produces/Sells CE-marked Devices: Y
Federal Procurement Eligibility: Small Business
Distribution: Manufacturer Direct, Manufacturer Through Distributor, Manufacturer Through Manufacturer Reps, Importer, Exporter
General Admin.: Thomas Falk/Chief Executive Officer
    J. Bauer/President
Mktg./Adv.: Tim Jones/Associate Director Marketing

Accessories, Fixation, Orthopedic	Orthopedics
Adhesive, Wound Closure	Surgery
Apron, Laboratory	Chemistry
Apron, Surgical	Surgery
Bag, Ice	General
Cap, Surgical	Surgery
Cover, Head, Surgical	Surgery
Cover, Shoe, Conductive	General
Cover, Shoe, Non-Conductive	General

KERR GROUP

800-524-3577 *(cont'd)*

Cuff, Blood Pressure	Cardiovascular
Diaper, Pediatric	General
Drape, Patient, Ophthalmic	Ophthalmology
Drape, Surgical, Disposable	Surgery
Drape, Surgical, ENT	Ear/Nose/Throat
Drape, Urological, Disposable	Gastroenterology/Urology
Dressing, Permeable, Moisture	General
Facial Tissue	General
Gown, Isolation, Surgical	Surgery
Gown, Operating Room, Disposable	Surgery
Gown, Patient, Disposable	General
Gown, Surgical	Surgery
Mask, Face	General
Material, PTFE/Carbon, Maxillofacial	Surgery
Pack, Sterilization Wrapper (Bag And Accessories)	Surgery
Pack, Surgical (Drape)	Surgery
Restraint, Protective (Body)	General
Sheet, Drape, Disposable	Surgery
Sheet, Operating Room	Surgery
Sheeting, Examination Table	General
Stockinette	Orthopedics
Suit, Scrub, Disposable	Surgery
Towel, Surgical	Surgery
Wrap, Sterilization	General

KESAIR TECHNOLOGIES, LLC

800-236-1846
770-427-6500

3625 Kennesaw N. Ind. Pkwy.,
Kennesaw, GA 30144
FDA Number: 3002959861   *Fax:* 770-425-0837
E-mail: request@kesair.com
Web site: www.kesair.com
Year Founded: 2003
Ownership: Private
Produces/Sells CE-marked Devices: Y
Federal Procurement Eligibility: Small Business, Female Owned
Distribution: Manufacturer Direct, Manufacturer Through Distributor, Manufacturer Through Manufacturer Reps, OEM, Exclusive Distributor

Purifier, Air, Ultraviolet	General

KESNER C.R.

630-232-4945

2520 Kaneville Ct., Geneva, IL 60134-2506
FDA Number: 1419501   *Fax:* 630-232-7042
E-mail: dynawave@inil.com
Web site: http://my.inil.com/~dynawave/
Annual Revenue: $0-$1 Million
Total Employees: 8   *Marketing Staff:* 2   *Sales Staff:* 2
Ownership: Private
Produces/Sells CE-marked Devices: N
Federal Procurement Eligibility: Small Business
Distribution: Manufacturer Direct
General Admin.: Clarence R. Kesner/Chief Executive Officer
Keith D. Kesner/Vice President
Production: Erwin Stark/Manager Production

Diathermy, Ultrasonic (Non-Beep Heat)	Physical Med
Diathermy, Ultrasonic (Physical Therapy)	Physical Med
Stimulator, Muscle, Electrical-Powered (EMS)	Physical Med
Stimulator, Muscle, Powered, Invasive	Physical Med
Stimulator, Ultrasound, Muscle	Physical Med

KESTREL

See Atrion Medical Products, Inc.

KETEMA/RODAN DIVISION

See Rti Electronics, Inc.

KETTLER INTERNATIONAL

757-427-2400

PO Box 2747, 1355 London Bridge Rdÿ,
Virginia Beach, VA 23453
FDA Number: n/a   *Fax:* 757-427-0183
E-mail: info@kettlerusa.com
Web site: www.kettlerusa.com
Medical Products Sales Volume: $7,400,000
Year Founded: 1981
Total Employees: 35   *Marketing Staff:* 1   *Sales Staff:* 3
Ownership: Private
Produces/Sells CE-marked Devices: Y
Federal Procurement Eligibility: Small Business
Distribution: Manufacturer Through Distributor, Manufacturer Through Manufacturer Reps, Importer
General Admin.: Ludger Busche/Chief Executive Officer
Heinz Kettler/President
Mktg./Adv.: Isabelle Kintziger/Director Marketing
David Selfe/Manager Contract Sales
Scott Kramer/Manager International & National Sales
Frank Mansfield/Manager National Sales

Computer Software	General
Exerciser, Bicycle	Physical Med
Exerciser, Other	Physical Med

KEWAUNEE SCIENTIFIC CORP.

704-873-7202

2700 West Front Street, PO Box 1842, Statesville, NC 28677
FDA Number: 9330062   *Fax:* 800-932-3296
E-mail: marketing@kewaunee.com
Web site: www.kewaunee.com
Medical Products Sales Volume: $2,000,000
Annual Revenue: $50-$100 Million
Year Founded: 1906
Total Employees: 200   *Marketing Staff:* 4
Ownership: Public
Stock Symbol: KEQU
Traded On: NASDAQ
Produces/Sells CE-marked Devices: N
Federal Procurement Eligibility: Small Business
Distribution: Manufacturer Direct, Manufacturer Through Distributor, Manufacturer Through Manufacturer Reps
General Admin.: William A. Shumaker/President, Chief Executive Officer
Mktg./Adv.: Dana L. Dahlgren/Vice President Marketing & Sales
Production: Keith D. Smith/Vice President Manufacturing
Research: Kurt P. Rindoks/Vice President Engineering & Development
Finance: D. Michael Parker/Chief Financial Officer

Cabinet Casework, Laboratory	Chemistry
Cabinet Casework, Patient Room	General
Cabinet, Laboratory	Chemistry
Enclosure, Bacteriological Safety	Chemistry
Furniture, Patient Room	General
Hood, Fume	Toxicology
Hood, Microbiological	Microbiology
Sink, Laboratory	Chemistry

KEY / SUN MEDICAL SERVICES, INC.

847-546-4795

5483 North Northwest Hwy., Chicago, IL 60630-1133
FDA Number: 1058218   *Fax:* 847-546-4780
E-mail: keysun91@sbcglobal.net
Annual Revenue: $5-$10 Million
Year Founded: 1991
Total Employees: 100   *Marketing Staff:* 7   *Sales Staff:* 5
Ownership: Private
Quality System Registration Information: ISO9002
Produces/Sells CE-marked Devices: Y
Federal Procurement Eligibility: Small Business, VA Contract
Distribution: Manufacturer Direct, Manufacturer Through Distributor
General Admin.: Mr. Robert. Gore/President, Chief Executive Officer
Mktg./Adv.: Mr. M. Gore/Vice President Sales

Drainage System, Urine, Closed	Gastroenterology/Urology

KEY ELEMENT DENTAL LABORATORY LLC

866 446 1833
757-644-3355

2006 Old Greenbrier Rd, Suite 8,
Chesapeake, VA 23320
FDA Number: n/a   *Fax:* 866 831 4153
E-mail: Keyelementdental@hotmail.com
Web site: www.keyelementdental.com
Ownership: Private
Produces/Sells CE-marked Devices: N

KEY INSTRUMENTS

215-357-6488

250 Andrews Rd., Trevose, PA 19053
FDA Number: 2528975

Diazo, P-Nitroaniline/Vanillin, Vanilmandelic Acid	Chemistry

KEY SCIENTIFIC PRODUCTS

325-773-3918

1113 East Reynolds St, Stamford, TX 79553
FDA Number: 2016672

Culture Media, Non-Selective And Non-Differential	Microbiology
Culture Media, Selective And Differential	Microbiology
Disc, Strip And Reagent, Microorganism Differentiation	Microbiology

KEY SURGICAL, INC.

800-541-7995
952-914-9789

8101 Wallace Road, Suite 100,
Eden Prairie, MN 55344
FDA Number: 2183785   *Fax:* 952-914-9866
E-mail: info@keysurgical.com
Web site: www.keysurgical.com
Medical Products Sales Volume: $1,600,000
Year Founded: 1988
Total Employees: 11
Ownership: Private
Quality System Registration Information: ISO9002
Produces/Sells CE-marked Devices: Y
Federal Procurement Eligibility: Small Business
Distribution: Manufacturer Direct, OEM
General Admin.: Peter S. Huck/General Manager

Brush, Burr Cleaning	Dental And Oral
Brush, Other	General
Cutter, Wire And Pin	Orthopedics
Loop, Vascular	Cardiovascular
Mask, Face	General
Pliers, Surgical	Orthopedics

KEY SURGICAL, INC.   800-541-7995 *(cont'd)*
  Protector, Surgical Instrument   Surgery
  Suture, Other   Surgery
  System, Coding, Color, Instrument   Dental And Oral
  Tag, Device Status   General
  Tape, Adhesive   General

KEY TECHNOLOGIES INC.
  See Bovie Medical Corp.

KEY-BAK   800-685-2403
4245 Pacific Privado, Ontario, CA 91761-7609   **909-923-7800**
  FDA Number: 3980154   *Fax:* 909-923-0024
  E-mail: mikew@keybak.com
  Web site: www.keybak.com/
  Medical Products Sales Volume: $2,700,000
  Annual Revenue: $0-$1 Million
  Year Founded: 1997
  Total Employees: 45   *Marketing Staff:* 2   *Sales Staff:* 7
  Ownership: Key-Bak
  Produces/Sells CE-marked Devices: N
  Federal Procurement Eligibility: Small Business
  Distribution: Exclusive Distributor, Importer, Exporter
  General Admin.: Craig Paugh/President, Chief Executive Officer
       Boake Paugh/Vice President, General Manager
  Mktg./Adv.: Ms. Tonya Willis/Coord. Sales
       Tom Ngo/Manager International Sales
       Tom Ngo/Manager Marketing
       Tom Ngo/Manager National Sales
  Security Equipment/Supplies   General
  Medical Product Subsidiaries (Listed Separately)
    Key-Bak

KEYES MANUFACTURING & SUPPLY LLC.   316-284-2200
2015 West 1st, Newton, KS 67114
  FDA Number: n/a
  Annual Revenue: $1-$5 Million
  Ownership: Private
  Produces/Sells CE-marked Devices: N
  Support, Head And Trunk, Wheelchair   Physical Med

KEYSTONE LABS
  See Invitrogen Corporation

KEYSTONE VIEW CO.
  See Mast/Keystone View

KEZAR ENTERPRISES, INC.   541-334-6100
747 Blair Blvd., Eugene, OR 97402
  FDA Number: 3004756964
  Ownership: Private
  Produces/Sells CE-marked Devices: N
  Hearing Aid, Air Conduction, Transcutaneous System   Ear/Nose/Throat

KFX MEDICAL   866-883-8718
5845 Avenida Encinas, Suite 128,   **760-444-8846**
Carlsbad, CA 92008
  FDA Number: 3005887059
  Ownership: Private
  Produces/Sells CE-marked Devices: N
  Fastener, Fixation, Non-Biodegradable, Soft Tissue   Orthopedics
  Screw, Fixation, Bone   Orthopedics

KHI INC.
  See Kmi Surgical Ltd.

KHL, INC.   206-915-2115
18300 N.e. 146th Way, Woodinville, WA 98072
  FDA Number: 3029784
  Ownership: Private
  Produces/Sells CE-marked Devices: N
  Stretcher, Wheeled (Mobile)   General
  Unit, Examining/Treatment, ENT   Ear/Nose/Throat

KI   800-424-2432
1330 Bellevue St., Green Bay, WI 54302   **920-468-8100**
  FDA Number: n/a   *Fax:* 920-468-0280
  Web site: www.ki.com
  Annual Revenue: $1-$5 Million
  Year Founded: 1941
  Total Employees: 3000
  Ownership: Private
  Produces/Sells CE-marked Devices: N
  Distribution: Manufacturer Through Distributor, Manufacturer Through Manufacturer Reps
  Chair, Other   General
  Computer Equipment   General
  Furniture, General   General
  Office Equipment   General
  Office Product   General
  Medical Product Subsidiaries (Listed Separately)

KI   800-424-2432 *(cont'd)*
  Spacesaver Corporation

KI-ADD SPECIALIZED SUPPORT TECHNOLOGY, INC.   920-468-8100
6500 South Avalon Blvd., Los Angeles, CA 90003-1934
  FDA Number: 2024063
  Ownership: Private
  Produces/Sells CE-marked Devices: N
  Chair, Adjustable, Mechanical   Physical Med

KIDDIE PRODUCTS, INC.
  See Learning Curve Brands Inc. THE FIRST YEARS

KIDSNEB, INC.   630-930-9412
310 N. Villa Ave., Villa Park, IL 60181
  FDA Number: 3006026623
  Mouthpiece, Breathing   Anesthesiology

KIEL LABORATORIES, INC.   678-450-9187
2225 Centennial Dr., Gainesville, GA 30504
  FDA Number: 1055270   *Fax:* 770-534-0229
  Web site: www.kielpharm.com
  Ownership: Private
  Produces/Sells CE-marked Devices: N
  Detector/Remover, Lice   General

KIGRE, INC.   843-651-5800
100 Marshland Rd., Hilton Head Island, SC 29926
  FDA Number: n/a   *Fax:* 843-681-4559
  E-mail: info@kigre.com
  Web site: info@kigre.com
  Annual Revenue: $0-$1 Million
  Total Employees: 35   *Marketing Staff:* 2   *Sales Staff:* 5
  Ownership: Private
  Produces/Sells CE-marked Devices: Y
  Federal Procurement Eligibility: Small Business
  Distribution: Manufacturer Direct
  General Admin.: John D. Myers/Chief Executive Officer
       John D. Myers/President
  Component, Other   General

KIK CUSTOM PRODUCTS   800-479-6603
1 West Hegeler Lane, Danville, IL 61832-8398   **217-442-1400**
  FDA Number: n/a   *Fax:* 217-431-0038
  Web site: www.kikcorp.com
  Ownership: Private
  Produces/Sells CE-marked Devices: N
  Disinfector, Liquid   General
  Solution, Antibacterial Cleaner   General

KIK CUSTOM PRODUCTS   574-295-0000
1919 Superior Street, PO Box 2988, Elkhart, IN 46515
  FDA Number: 9615332   *Fax:* 574-296-1700
  E-mail: helpdesk@kikcorp.com
  Web site: www.kikcorp.com
  Medical Products Sales Volume: $28,200,000
  Year Founded: 1955
  Total Employees: 189
  Ownership: Private
  Produces/Sells CE-marked Devices: N
  Federal Procurement Eligibility: Small Business
  Adhesive, Aerosol   General

KILGORE INTERNATIONAL, INC.   800-892-9999
36 W. Pearl St., Coldwater, MI 49036-0098   **517-279-9000**
  FDA Number: 9330063   *Fax:* 517-278-2956
  E-mail: tthomas@cbpu.com
  Web site: www.kilgoreinternational.com
  Medical Products Sales Volume: $800,000
  Annual Revenue: $1-$5 Million
  Year Founded: 1955
  Total Employees: 9   *Sales Staff:* 3
  Ownership: Private
  Produces/Sells CE-marked Devices: N
  Federal Procurement Eligibility: Small Business
  General Admin.: Craig W. Kilgore/President, Chief Executive Officer
  Mktg./Adv.: Craig W. Kilgore/Director Marketing
       Michael Gregory/Manager National Sales
  Anatomical Training Model   General
  Chart, Anatomical Training   General
  Training Aid   Orthopedics

KILTEX CORP.   330-644-6746
2064 Killian Road, Akron, OH 44312
  FDA Number: 1527493
  Scanner, Ultrasonic (Pulsed Echo)   Radiology

KIMBALL ELECTRONICS TAMPA   813-814-8114
13750 Reptron Blvd., Tampa, FL 33626
FDA Number: 3004577621
Defibrillator, Battery-Powered, Low Energy   Cardiovascular
Stimulator, Neuromuscular, External Functional   Cns/Neurology
Transmitter/Receiver System, Physiological, Radiofrequency   Cardiovascular

KIMBALL INTERNATIONAL   800-482-1616
1600 Royal Street, Jasper, IN 47549   812-482-8255
FDA Number: n/a
E-mail: PublicRelations@kimball.com
Web site: http://www.kimball.com
Year Founded: 1950
Ownership: Public
Stock Symbol: KBALB
Traded On: NASDAQ
Produces/Sells CE-marked Devices: N
General Admin.: Mr. Robert Schneider/Chief Financial Officer, Executive Vice President
        Mr. Gary Schwartz/Chief Information Officer
        Mr. Donald Charron/Executive Vice President
        Mr. James Thyen/President, Chief Executive Officer

KIMBERLY-CLARK CORP.   888-525-8388
1300 Orchard Hill Rd., Lagrange, GA 30240
FDA Number: 1038181
Web site: www.kimberly-clark.com
Ownership: Public
Stock Symbol: KMB
Traded On: NYSE
Produces/Sells CE-marked Devices: N
Gown, Examination   General
Gown, Other   General
Linen, Bed   General

KIMBERLY-CLARK CORP.   770-587-7835
14 Finegan Rd., Del Rio, TX 78840
FDA Number: n/a
Web site: www.kimberly-clark.com
Ownership: Public
Stock Symbol: KMB
Traded On: NYSE
Produces/Sells CE-marked Devices: N
Accessories, Operating Room, Table   Surgery
Tourniquet, Gastro-Urology   Surgery

KIMBERLY-CLARK CORP.   888-525-8388
2100 Winchester Rd., PO Box 2020, Neenah, WI 54957-2020
FDA Number: 3003701733
Web site: www.kimberly-clark.com
Ownership: Public
Stock Symbol: KMB
Traded On: NYSE
Produces/Sells CE-marked Devices: N
Distribution: Manufacturer Direct, Manufacturer Through Distributor
Cover, Shoe, Operating Room   Surgery
Diaper, Adult   General
Drape, Surgical   Surgery
Garment, Protective, For Incontinence   Gastroenterology/Urology
Pad, Incontinence (Underpad)   General
Pad, Menstrual, Unscented   Obstetrics/Gynecology
Pant, Incontinence   General
Tampon, Menstrual, Unscented   Obstetrics/Gynecology
Tray, Surgical   Surgery
Wrap, Sterilization   General
Wrapper, Surgical Instrument (Sterile)   General
Medical Product Subsidiaries (Listed Separately)
KIMBERLY-CLARK CORP. CONWAY MILL
Kimberly-Clark Gmbh

KIMBERLY-CLARK CORP.   888-525-838
3461 County Road 100, Corinth, MS 38834
FDA Number: 1031395
Web site: www.kimberly-clark.com
Ownership: Public
Stock Symbol: KMB
Traded On: NYSE
Produces/Sells CE-marked Devices: N
Wrap, Sterilization   General

KIMBERLY-CLARK CORP.   888-525-8388
389 Clyde Fitzgerald Rd, Linwood, NC 27299
FDA Number: 1054380
Web site: www.kimberly-clark.com
Ownership: Public
Stock Symbol: KMB
Traded On: NYSE
Produces/Sells CE-marked Devices: N

KIMBERLY-CLARK CORP.   888-525-8388 *(cont'd)*
Wrap, Sterilization   General

KIMBERLY-CLARK CORP. (BEECH ISLAND MILL)   888-525-8388
246 Old Jackson Highway, Beech Island, SC 29842
FDA Number: 3005682435
Web site: www.kimberly-clark.com
Ownership: Public
Stock Symbol: KMB
Traded On: NYSE
Produces/Sells CE-marked Devices: N
Garment, Protective, For Incontinence   Gastroenterology/Urology

KIMBERLY-CLARK CORP. CONWAY MILL   501-329-2973
480 Exchange Ave., Conway, AR 72032
FDA Number: 2381757   *Fax:* 501-336-6214
Ownership: Kimberly-Clark Corp.
Produces/Sells CE-marked Devices: N
Distribution: Manufacturer Direct
Garment, Protective, For Incontinence   Gastroenterology/Urology
Pad, Menstrual, Unscented   Obstetrics/Gynecology
Pads, Menstrual, Scented-deodorized   Obstetrics/Gynecology
Tampon, Menstrual, Unscented   Obstetrics/Gynecology

KIMBERLY-CLARK CORP., LAKEVIEW FEMININE CARE PLANT   888-525-8388
1050 Cold Spring Rd., Neenah, WI 54956
FDA Number: 2184163
Web site: www.kimberly-clark.com
Ownership: Public
Stock Symbol: KMB
Traded On: NYSE
Produces/Sells CE-marked Devices: N
Garment, Protective, For Incontinence   Gastroenterology/Urology
Pad, Menstrual, Unscented   Obstetrics/Gynecology
Pads, Menstrual, Scented-deodorized   Obstetrics/Gynecology

KIMBERLY-CLARK CORP., PARIS CHILD CARE PLANT   888-525-8388
2466 Farm Road 137, Paris, TX 75460
FDA Number: 1650783
Web site: www.kimberly-clark.com
Ownership: Public
Stock Symbol: KMB
Traded On: NYSE
Produces/Sells CE-marked Devices: N
General Admin.: Mr. Thomas Falk/Chairman, Chief Executive Officer
        Mr. Mark Buthman/Chief Financial Officer, Senior Vice President
        Ms. Lizanne Gottung/Senior Vice President Human Resources
Mktg./Adv.: Mr. Anthony Palmer/Senior Vice President Marketing
Garment, Protective, For Incontinence   Gastroenterology/Urology

KIMBLE CHASE LIFE SCIENCE AND RESEARCH PRODUCTS LLC   888-546-2531
234 Cardiff Valley Road, Ozone, TN 37854   856-692-8500
FDA Number: 3006808300   *Fax:* 856-794-9762
E-mail: cs@kimkon.com
Web site: www.kimble-kontes.com
Ownership: Private
Quality System Registration Information: ISO9001
Produces/Sells CE-marked Devices: N
Federal Procurement Eligibility: Small Business
Distribution: Manufacturer Through Distributor
Hematocrit Tube, Rack, Sealer, Holder   Hematology
Pipette, Pasteur   Hematology
Tube, Capillary Blood Collection   Hematology
Tube, Sedimentation Rate   Hematology
Tube, Tissue Culture   Pathology
Vial, Other   General

KIMBLE GLASS, INC.   888-546-2531
537 Crystal Avenue, Vineland, NJ 08360-3200   856-692-3600
FDA Number: 2241693   *Fax:* 856-692-0280
E-mail: R.Hasenauer@gerresheimer.com
Web site: http://kimble.com/
Medical Products Sales Volume: $64,400,000
Annual Revenue: $50-$100 Million
Year Founded: 1901
Total Employees: 767   *Marketing Staff:* 8   *Sales Staff:* 40
Ownership: Private
Stock Symbol: AMC
Traded On: AMEX
Quality System Registration Information: ISO9001; ISO9002
Produces/Sells CE-marked Devices: N
Federal Procurement Eligibility: GSA Contract
Distribution: Manufacturer Through Distributor
General Admin.: Uwe Roehrhoff/Chief Executive Officer

KIMBLE GLASS, INC.   888-546-2531 *(cont'd)*
Richard Hasenaurer/Vice President Personnel
Mktg./Adv.: Doug Grady/Director Marketing
Dave Fenili/Manager Advertising

Beaker (Laboratory)	Chemistry
Buret	Chemistry
Coverslip, Microscope Slide	Pathology
Labware, Basic, Disposable	Chemistry
Labware, Basic, Reusable	Chemistry
Manifold, Liquid	Chemistry
Packaging Equipment	General
Pipette, Micro	Chemistry
Still, Solvent Recovery	Chemistry
Tissue Embedding Equipment/Reagent	Pathology
Tube, Capillary Blood Collection	Hematology
Tube, Culture	Microbiology
Tube, Test	Chemistry
Vial, Liquid Scintillation Counting	Chemistry

KIMBLE TERUMO INC.
See Terumo Medical Corp.

KIMCHUK, INC.   203-790-7800
Corporate Drive, Danbury, CT 06810-4130
FDA Number: 1226008   Fax: 203-797-8976
E-mail: sales@kimchuk.com
Web site: www.kimchuk.com
Medical Products Sales Volume: $12,400,000
Year Founded: 1957
Total Employees: 150
Ownership: Private
Produces/Sells CE-marked Devices: N
Federal Procurement Eligibility: Small Business

Container, Sharpes	General

KINAMED, INC.   800-827-5775
820 Flynn Road, Camarillo, CA 93012-8701   805-384-2748
FDA Number: 2027148   Fax: 805-384-2792
E-mail: contact@kinamed.com
Web site: www.kinamed.com
Medical Products Sales Volume: $1,700,000
Annual Revenue: $5-$10 Million
Year Founded: 1987
Total Employees: 20   *Marketing Staff:* 2   *Sales Staff:* 2
Ownership: Private
Stock Symbol: SMA
Traded On: NASDAQ
Quality System Registration Information: ISO9001
Produces/Sells CE-marked Devices: Y
Federal Procurement Eligibility: Small Business
Distribution: Manufacturer Direct, Manufacturer Through Distributor, Manufacturer Through Manufacturer Reps, OEM, Service Direct, Importer, Exporter
General Admin.: Clyde R. Pratt/Chief Executive Officer
Mktg./Adv.: Bob Bruce/Vice President Marketing
Production: Marguerite Demeter/Manager Regulatory Affairs
William Pratt/Vice President Operations

Plate, Bone, Skull (Cranioplasty)	Cns/Neurology
Prosthesis, Femoral Head	Orthopedics
Prosthesis, Knee, Patellofemoral, Semi-Constrained	Orthopedics
Prosthesis, Knee, Total	Orthopedics
Surgical Instrument, Orthopedic, AC-Powered Motor	Orthopedics

KINDT COLLINS CO.   800-321-3170
12651 Elmwood Ave., Cleveland, OH 44111   216-252-4122
FDA Number: 1526785   Fax: 216-252-5639
E-mail: info@kindt-collins.com
Web site: www.kindt-collins.com
Annual Revenue: $0-$1 Million
Year Founded: 1914
Ownership: Private
Quality System Registration Information: ISO9001
Produces/Sells CE-marked Devices: N
Federal Procurement Eligibility: Small Business
Distribution: Manufacturer Direct, Exclusive Distributor

Component, Plastic	General
Wax, Dental	Dental And Oral

KINEDYNE CORP.
See Sure-Lok, Inc.

KINEMED, INC.   855-546-3633
5980 Horton Street, Suite 400,   510-655-6525
Emeryville, CA 94608
FDA Number: n/a   Fax: 510-655-6506
E-mail: service@kinemed.com
Web site: http://kinemed.com
Year Founded: 2001
Ownership: Private
Produces/Sells CE-marked Devices: N
General Admin.: Mr. David Fineman/President, Chief Executive Officer

KINEMED, INC.   855-546-3633 *(cont'd)*
Production: Dr. Alexander Glass/Vice President Operations
Research: Dr. Scott Turner/Vice President Research & Development
Finance: Ms. Karen Carothers/Vice President Finance

Electromyograph, Diagnostic	Physical Med

KINETIC CONCEPTS, INC.   800-275-4524
8023 Vantage Drive, San Antonio, TX 78230   210-524-9000
FDA Number: 3005178245
Web site: www.kci1.com
Annual Revenue: More than $1 Billion
Year Founded: 1976
Ownership: Private
Stock Symbol: KCI
Traded On: NYSE
Produces/Sells CE-marked Devices: N
General Admin.: Ronald W. Dollens/Chairman
Martin J. Landon/Chief Financial Officer, Executive Vice President
Mr. John Bibb/General Counsel
Catherine M Burzik/President, Chief Executive Officer
Mr. Michael Franz/Vice President
Mr. David Lillbeck/Vice President Human Resources
Mktg./Adv.: Mr. Kevin Belgrade/Communication Specialist
Production: Mr. Michael Schneider/Senior Vice President Operations

Accessories, Operating Room, Table	Surgery
Bed, Air Fluidized	Physical Med
Bed, Electric	General
Bed, Flotation Therapy, Powered	Physical Med
Bed, Patient Rotation, Powered	Physical Med
Bed, Pediatric (Crib)	General
Cushion, Flotation	Physical Med
Environmental Control System, Powered	Physical Med
Mattress, Air Flotation	General
Mattress, Non-Powered Flotation Therapy	Physical Med
Sleeve, Compressible Limb	Cardiovascular
Suction Apparatus, Ward Use, Portable, AC-Powered	Surgery
Support, Breathing Tube	Anesthesiology

Medical Product Subsidiaries (Listed Separately)
Lifecell Corp.

KINETIC DIVERSIFIED INDUSTRIES, INC.   858-566-0550
7746 Arjons Dr., San Diego, CA 92126   858-566-4850
FDA Number: 2027143
E-mail: info@tushcush.com
Web site: www.tushcush.com
Ownership: Private
Produces/Sells CE-marked Devices: N

Orthosis, Lumbar	Physical Med

KINETIC INSTRUMENTS, INC.   800-233-2346
17 Berkshire Blvd., Bethel, CT 06801   203-743-0080
FDA Number: 1294153   Fax: 203-790-1227
E-mail: sales@kineticinc.com
Web site: www.kineticinc.com
Medical Products Sales Volume: $1,900,000
Annual Revenue: $1-$5 Million
Year Founded: 1977
Total Employees: 25   *Marketing Staff:* 2   *Sales Staff:* 6
Ownership: Private
Stock Symbol: LIA
Traded On: AMEX
Produces/Sells CE-marked Devices: Y
Federal Procurement Eligibility: Small Business
Distribution: Manufacturer Direct, Manufacturer Through Distributor, Manufacturer Through Manufacturer Reps, OEM, Service Direct, Exporter
General Admin.: William Becker/President
Mktg./Adv.: Bruce Green/Manager Sales
Louis Memoli/Vice President Marketing
Frank Barbera/Vice President Sales
Production: Jeanne Kozlowski/Manager Customer Services

Curing Unit, Acrylic	Dental And Oral
Handpiece, Air-Powered, Dental	Dental And Oral
Scaler, Ultrasonic	Dental And Oral

KINETIC MUSCLES, INC.   480-557-0448
2103 E Cedar St, #3, Tempe, AZ 85281-7432
FDA Number: 84998   Fax: 480-557-0449
E-mail: info@kineticmuscles.com
Web site: www.kineticmuscles.com
Medical Products Sales Volume: $500,000
Annual Revenue: $0-$1 Million
Year Founded: 2001
Total Employees: 4
Ownership: Private
Produces/Sells CE-marked Devices: N
Federal Procurement Eligibility: Small Business, GSA Contract
Distribution: Manufacturer Direct
General Admin.: Edward Koeneman/Chief Operating Officer

KINETIC MUSCLES, INC. 480-557-0448 (cont'd)
James Koeneman/President, Chief Executive Officer
Exerciser, Finger, Powered Physical Med

KINETIC SYSTEMS CO., LLC 800-DATA-NOW
900 N. State St., Lockport, IL 60441 815-838-0005
FDA Number: n/a Fax: 815-838-4424
E-mail: sales@kscorp.com
Web site: www.kscorp.com
Medical Products Sales Volume: $10,000,000
Annual Revenue: $5-$10 Million
Year Founded: 1970
Ownership: Private
Quality System Registration Information: ISO9000
Produces/Sells CE-marked Devices: Y
Distribution: Manufacturer Direct, Manufacturer Through Manufacturer Reps, OEM, Exporter
General Admin.: Patricia Ramazinski/Director Human Resources
William A. Boston/President, Chief Executive Officer
Production: Steven Krebs/Director Engineering
Wayne G. Coppe/Director Manufacturing
Finance: Eric Schroeder/Chief Financial Officer
Computer Equipment General

KINETIKOS MEDICAL, INC. 800-546-3845
6005 Hidden Valley Road, Suite 180, 760-448-1700
Carlsbad, CA 92009
FDA Number: 2028840 Fax: 760-448-1739
E-mail: JpKMI@aol.com
Web site: www.VisitKMI.com
Medical Products Sales Volume: $1,700,000
Year Founded: 1992
Total Employees: 20 Marketing Staff: 11
Ownership: Private
Quality System Registration Information: ISO9001
Produces/Sells CE-marked Devices: Y
Federal Procurement Eligibility: Small Business
Distribution: Manufacturer Through Distributor
General Admin.: Paul Kammann/Chief Financial Officer, Vice President Operations
James F. Ham/President
Mktg./Adv.: Jill Pflieger/Vice President Marketing
Research: Rob Ball/Vice President Product Development
Implant, Fixation Device, Proximal Femoral Orthopedics
Knife, Other Surgery
Support, Wrist Physical Med

KINEXUS BIOINFORMATICS CORPORATION 1-866-546-3987
8755 Ash Street, Suite 1, 604-323-2547
Vancouver, BRITI V6P 6 Canada
FDA Number: n/a Fax: 604-323-2548
E-mail: info@kinexus.ca
Web site: www.kinexus.ca
Ownership: Private
Produces/Sells CE-marked Devices: N

KING KOIL SLEEP PRODUCTS 1-800-899-5645
752 30th Avenue Southeast, Minneapolis, MN 55414
FDA Number: n/a
E-mail: sleepbetter@kingkoil.com
Web site: www.kingkoil.com
Annual Revenue: $50-$100 Million
Ownership: Private
Produces/Sells CE-marked Devices: N
Distribution: Manufacturer Direct, Manufacturer Through Manufacturer Reps
General Admin.: Ernie Friedman/President
Mary Ann Michaels/Vice President
Mktg./Adv.: E. Friedman/Manager International Sales
Mary Ann Michaels/Manager Market Research
Michael V. Kehnast/Vice President Marketing & Sales
Mattress, Bed General

KING MANUFACTURING CO.
See Onyx Medical Corp.

KING PHARMACEUTICALS, INC. 800-525-8466
501 Fifth Street, Bristol, TN 37620 423-989-8000
FDA Number: n/a Fax: 866-990-0545
E-mail: info@jmeopharma.com
Web site: www.jmedpharma.com
Medical Products Sales Volume: $1,980,000,000
Annual Revenue: More than $100 Million
Year Founded: 1994
Total Employees: 204 Marketing Staff: 6 Sales Staff: 125
Ownership: Public
Stock Symbol: KG
Traded On: NASDAQ
Produces/Sells CE-marked Devices: N
Federal Procurement Eligibility: Small Business, VA Contract

KING PHARMACEUTICALS, INC. 800-525-8466 (cont'd)
Distribution: Manufacturer Direct, Manufacturer Through Distributor, Exclusive Distributor
General Admin.: Drew Franz/Chief Operating Officer
Kelley Rushin/Director Human Resources
Judy Jones/Executive Vice President
Mike Bramblett/Executive Vice President
Dennis Jones/President, Chief Executive Officer
Mktg./Adv.: Tom Lewandowski/Manager International & National Sales
Larry Chaffin/Vice President Marketing
Tom Lewandowski/Vice President National Accounts
Production: Nancy Cafmeyer/Director Quality Assurance
David McLaughlin/Senior Vice President Operations
Contract Manufacturing, Pharmaceuticals/Chemicals General
Medical Product Subsidiaries (Listed Separately)
Gentrac, Inc.
Jmi - Canton
Jmi - St. Petersburg
Meridian Medical Technologies

KING SYSTEMS CORP. 800-642-5464
15011 Herriman Blvd., Noblesville, IN 46060 317-776-6823
FDA Number: 1824226 Fax: 317-776-6827
E-mail: kingsystems@iquest.net
Web site: www.kingsystems.com
Annual Revenue: $25-$50 Million
Year Founded: 1977
Ownership: Private
Quality System Registration Information: ISO9001
Produces/Sells CE-marked Devices: Y
Federal Procurement Eligibility: Small Business
Distribution: Manufacturer Through Distributor
Airway, Oropharyngeal, Anesthesia Anesthesiology
Circuit, Breathing (W Connector, Adapter, Y Piece) Anesthesiology
Condenser, Heat And Moisture (Artificial Nose) Anesthesiology
Connector, Airway (Extension) Anesthesiology
Filter, Bacterial, Breathing Circuit Anesthesiology
Laryngoscope, Rigid Anesthesiology
Mask, Gas, Anesthesia Anesthesiology
Tubing, Corrugated General
Tubing, Flexible, Medical Gas, Low-Pressure Anesthesiology
Tubing, Other General
Ventilator, Continuous (Respirator) Anesthesiology

KING TOOL, INC. 800-587-9445
5350 Love Ln, Bozeman, MT 59718 406-586-1541
FDA Number: n/a Fax: 406-585-9028
E-mail: sales@king-tool.com
Web site: www.king-tool.com
Ownership: Private
Produces/Sells CE-marked Devices: N
Forceps Orthopedics
Stripper, Surgical Orthopedics
Surgical Instrument, Non-Powered, Neurosurgical Cns/Neurology

KING'S MEDICAL 330-653-3968
1894 Georgetown Rd., Hudson, OH 44236-4065
FDA Number: n/a Fax: 330-656-0600
Web site: www.kingsmedical.com
Medical Products Sales Volume: $60,000,000
Annual Revenue: $50-$100 Million
Year Founded: 1981
Ownership: Private
Produces/Sells CE-marked Devices: N
Federal Procurement Eligibility: Small Business
Distribution: Service Direct
General Admin.: Albert C. Van Kirk/President, Chief Executive Officer
Cineangiograph (Cardiac Catheterization) Radiology
Scanner, Computed Tomography, X-Ray, Full Body Radiology
Scanner, Magnetic Resonance (NMR/MRI) Radiology
Service, Consulting General
Service, Licensing, Device, Medical General

KING'S SPECIALTY COMPANY
See Young Innovations, Inc.

KINGSLEY MFG. CO. 800-854-3479
1984 Placentia Ave., Costa Mesa, CA 92627 949-645-4401
FDA Number: 2021683 Fax: 949-646-0805
E-mail: info@kingsleymfg.com
Web site: www.kingsleymfg.com
Annual Revenue: $0-$1 Million
Ownership: Private
Quality System Registration Information: ISO9002
Produces/Sells CE-marked Devices: Y
Federal Procurement Eligibility: Small Business
Distribution: Manufacturer Direct
General Admin.: Jeffrey Kingsley/President, Chief Executive Officer
Prosthesis, Foot Orthopedics

KINGSLEY MFG. CO.   800-854-3479 *(cont'd)*
Stockinette, Cast   Orthopedics

KINGSTEC MEDICAL PRODUCTS   905-712-2171
175 Traders Blvd. E, Mississauga, ONT L4Z 3S8 Canada
FDA Number: n/a   Fax: 905-712-2484
E-mail: sales@kingstec.com
Web site: www.kingstec.com
Year Founded: 1987
Total Employees: 25
Ownership: Private
Produces/Sells CE-marked Devices: N
Distribution: Manufacturer Direct, Exclusive Distributor

KINGSWOOD LABORATORIES, INC.   800-968-7772
10375 Hague Rd., Indianapolis, IN 46256   317-849-9513
FDA Number: 1827405   Fax: 317-849-9514
E-mail: sales@kingswood-labs.com
Web site: www.kingswood-labs.com
Annual Revenue: $0-$1 Million
Total Employees: 14
Ownership: Private
Produces/Sells CE-marked Devices: N
Federal Procurement Eligibility: Small Business
Distribution: Manufacturer Direct, Manufacturer Through Distributor
General Admin.: Ross Deardorff/General Manager
    Carol Deardorff/Office Manager
    Ross Deardorff/President, Chief Executive Officer
Swabs, Oral Care   General

KINGSWOOD TECHNOLOGY, INC.   203-386-1839
44 Rachel Drive, Stratford, CT 06615
FDA Number: 1221260
E-mail: kingswood.tech@snet.net
Medical Products Sales Volume: $900,000
Year Founded: 1985
Total Employees: 12
Ownership: Private
Produces/Sells CE-marked Devices: N
Federal Procurement Eligibility: Small Business, Minority Owned
Inserter, Sacculotomy Tack   Ear/Nose/Throat

KINMAN OF INDIANAPOLIS, INC.   800-444-8891
1401 Harding Ct., Suite K,   317-787-6303
Indianapolis, IN 46217
FDA Number: n/a   Fax: 317-783-9328
E-mail: rogerkinman@spitfire.net
Web site: www.kinman-inc.com
Annual Revenue: $0-$1 Million
Total Employees: 3
Ownership: Private
Produces/Sells CE-marked Devices: N
Federal Procurement Eligibility: Small Business
Distribution: Manufacturer Direct, Manufacturer Through Distributor
General Admin.: Ross Kinman/President
    Roger L. Kinman/Secretary, Treasurer
Rescue Equipment   General

KINO MOBILITY INC.   4166355873
1140 Sheppard Ave. West Unit #3,
Toronto, ON M3K 2 Canada
FDA Number: n/a   Fax: 4166355910
Ownership: Private
Produces/Sells CE-marked Devices: N

KINTECH ORTHOPAEDICS LTD.   1 (888) 793-044
360 Revus Avenue, Unit #13,   (905) 278-6534
Mississauga, ONT L5G 4 Canada
FDA Number: 8022273   Fax: (905) 278-8943
Year Founded: 1988
Total Employees: 10
Ownership: Private
Produces/Sells CE-marked Devices: N
Distribution: Manufacturer Direct

KIPP & ZONEN   631-589-2065
125 Wilbur Place, Bohemia, NY 11716
FDA Number: n/a   Fax: 631-589-2068
E-mail: kipp.usa@kippzonen.com
Web site: www.kippzonen.com
Annual Revenue: $1-$5 Million
Ownership: Private
Quality System Registration Information: ISO9000
Produces/Sells CE-marked Devices: Y
Distribution: Manufacturer Direct, OEM, Importer, Exporter
Recorder, Chart, Laboratory   Chemistry

KIPP & ZONEN   631-589-2065 *(cont'd)*
Recorder, Paper Chart   Cardiovascular

KIPPMED
See Medegen

KIPS BAY MEDICAL, INC   763-235-3540
3405 Annapolis Ln N Ste 200, Minneapolis, MN 55447-5346
FDA Number: 3007319005   Fax: 763-235-3545
E-mail: info@kipsbaymedical.com
Web site: Kips Bay Medical, Inc
Ownership: Private
Produces/Sells CE-marked Devices: N
General Admin.: Mr. Manny Villafana/Chairman, Chief Executive Officer
    Mr. Scott Kellen/Chief Financial Officer, Vice President
Mktg./Adv.: Mr. Michael Reinhardt/Vice President Marketing & Sales
Production: Mr. Randy LaBounty/Vice President Regulatory & Clinical Affairs
Research: Mr. Eric Solien/Director Research & Development
Pledget And Intracardiac Patch, PETP, PTFE, Polypropylene   Cardiovascular

KIRWAN SURGICAL PRODUCTS, INC.   888-547-9267
180 Enterprise Drive, PO Box 427Aÿ,   781-834-9500
Marshfield, MA 02050
FDA Number: 1219619   Fax: 781-834-0022
E-mail: sales@kirwans.com
Web site: www.kirwans.com
Year Founded: 1979
Total Employees: 175   Marketing Staff: 1
Ownership: Private
Stock Symbol: ULGX
Traded On: NASDAQ
Quality System Registration Information: ISO9001
Produces/Sells CE-marked Devices: Y
Federal Procurement Eligibility: Small Business, Female Owned
Distribution: Manufacturer Direct, Manufacturer Through Distributor, Manufacturer Through Manufacturer Reps, OEM
General Admin.: Mrs. Jean M. Kirwan/President
    Mr. Lawrence T. Kirvwan/Vice President, General Manager
Mktg./Adv.: Ms. Kate Ward/Marketing Associate
Production: Mr. Kevin Prario/Manager Regulatory Affairs
Adapter, Electrosurgical Unit, Cable   Surgery
Awl   Orthopedics
Bit, Surgical   Surgery
Cable, Electrosurgical Unit   Surgery
Carrier, Ligature   Surgery
Cautery, Thermal, Battery-Powered   Ophthalmology
Coagulator/Cutter, Endoscopic, Bipolar   Obstetrics/Gynecology
Cord, Electric, Endoscope   Gastroenterology/Urology
Drill, Cranial   Cns/Neurology
Electrode, Other   General
Electrosurgical Unit, Cutting & Coagulation Device   Surgery
Electrosurgical Unit, General Purpose (ESU)   Surgery
Forceps   Orthopedics
Forceps, Dressing   Surgery
Forceps, Electrosurgical   Surgery
Forceps, Endoscopic   Gastroenterology/Urology
Forceps, General & Plastic Surgery   Surgery
Forceps, Suction   Surgery
Forceps, Tissue   Surgery
Forceps, Tonsil   Ear/Nose/Throat
Instrument, Microsurgical   Cns/Neurology
Instrument, Passing, Ligature, Knot Tying   Cns/Neurology
Mallet, Bone   Orthopedics
Osteotome (Orthopedic)   Surgery
Rasp, Bone   Orthopedics
Skid, Bone   Orthopedics
Surgical Instrument, Non-Powered, Neurosurgical   Cns/Neurology

KISTLER INSTRUMENT CORP.   716-691-5100
75 John Glenn Drive, Amherst, NY 14228-2171
FDA Number: 9330064   Fax: 716-691-5226
E-mail: biomech@kistler.com
Web site: www.kistler.com
Medical Products Sales Volume: $8,100,000
Annual Revenue: $10-$25 Million
Year Founded: 1955
Total Employees: 85   Marketing Staff: 3   Sales Staff: 12
Ownership: Private
Stock Symbol: MSS
Traded On: NASDAQ
Quality System Registration Information: ISO9001
Produces/Sells CE-marked Devices: Y
Federal Procurement Eligibility: Small Business, GSA Contract
Distribution: Manufacturer Direct, Manufacturer Through Manufacturer Reps
General Admin.: John Kubler/President, Chief Executive Officer
Mktg./Adv.: Don Beehler/Director Advertising
    Jerry Lisowski/Manager Sales
Production: Paul Bussman/Product Manager
    Klaus Koeller/Vice President Manufacturing

KISTLER INSTRUMENT CORP.   716-691-5100 *(cont'd)*
Accelerometer — Chemistry
Calibrator, Pressure Transducer — Anesthesiology
Ergometer, Treadmill — Cardiovascular
Scale, Platform, Wheelchair — Physical Med

KLARMANN RULINGS, INC.   800-252-2401
480 Charles Bancroft Hwy., Litchfield, NH 03052   603-424-2401
FDA Number: n/a   *Fax:* 603-424-0970
E-mail: sales@reticles.com
Web site: www.reticles.com
Medical Products Sales Volume: $1,000,000
Annual Revenue: $0-$1 Million
Year Founded: 1964
Total Employees: 15   *Marketing Staff:* 3   *Sales Staff:* 3
Ownership: Private
Produces/Sells CE-marked Devices: N
Federal Procurement Eligibility: Small Business, Female Owned
Distribution: Manufacturer Direct, OEM, Service Direct, Exporter
General Admin.: Christopher Wilmot/President
　　Kathy Lawrence/Vice President, General Manager
Mktg./Adv.: Kathy Lawrence/Manager International & National Sales
　　Dawna Morin/Manager Marketing
Production: Keith Kurowski/Director Quality Assurance
Component, Optical — General

KLEAN N KONSTANT DENTAL WATER COMPANY, LLC   205-422-3904
2204 Longleaf Blvd., Birmingham, AL 35243
FDA Number: 3005080495
Ownership: Private
Produces/Sells CE-marked Devices: N
Chair, Dental, Without Operative Unit — Dental And Oral

KLEEN LAUNDRY & DRYCLEANING SERVICES, INC.   603-448-1134
1 Foundry St., Lebanon, NH 03766-1594
FDA Number: 3003643802
Ownership: Private
Produces/Sells CE-marked Devices: N
Gown, Surgical — Surgery
Homopolymer, Karaya and Ethylene-Oxide — Dental And Oral
Wrap, Sterilization — General

KLEEN TEST PRODUCTS CORPORATION   330-878-5586
216 12th St. NE, Strasburg, OH 44680
FDA Number: 1526481
Ownership: Private
Produces/Sells CE-marked Devices: N
Dental Cement w/out Zinc-Oxide Eugenol as an Ulcer Covering for Pain Relief — Dental And Oral
Floss, Dental — Dental And Oral
Toothbrush, Manual — Dental And Oral

KLEIN BAKER MEDICAL, INC.
See Neo-Care Arrow International

KLEINERT'S INC.
See Hygienics Industries Div.Of Kleinert's, Inc.

KLI CORP.   317-846-7452
1119 Third Ave SW, Carmel, IN 46032
FDA Number: 1833694   *Fax:* 317-846-1676
E-mail: info@entertainers-secret.com
Web site: www.entertainers-secret.com
Ownership: Private
Produces/Sells CE-marked Devices: N
Federal Procurement Eligibility: Small Business
Distribution: Manufacturer Direct, Manufacturer Through Distributor
Dressing, Other — General
Pump, Nebulizer, Manual — Ear/Nose/Throat

KLINGER EYE SHIELDS, INC.   800-848-1244
1108A Singleton Drive, Selma, AL 36701   334-875-7906
FDA Number: 1052871   *Fax:* 334-875-7302
E-mail: dave@klingereyeshields.com
Web site: www.klingereyeshields.com
Annual Revenue: $0-$1 Million
Year Founded: 1994
Ownership: Private
Produces/Sells CE-marked Devices: N
Federal Procurement Eligibility: Small Business
Distribution: Manufacturer Direct, Manufacturer Through Distributor, Manufacturer Through Manufacturer Reps
General Admin.: Mr. David Brooks/President
Sunglasses (Including Photosensitive) — Ophthalmology

KLM LABORATORIES, INC.   800-556-3668
28280 Alta Vista, Valencia, CA 91355   805-294-2446
FDA Number: 2028483   *Fax:* 800-556-3338
E-mail: tdelgado@klmlabs.com
Medical Products Sales Volume: $5,200,000
Year Founded: 1973
Total Employees: 75   *Marketing Staff:* 1   *Sales Staff:* 2
Ownership: Private
Produces/Sells CE-marked Devices: N
Federal Procurement Eligibility: Small Business
Distribution: Manufacturer Direct, Exporter
Mktg./Adv.: Mr. Thomas Delgado/Director Marketing & Sales
Immobilizer, Ankle — Orthopedics
Insoles, Medical — General

KLN STEEL PRODUCTS COMPANY   800-624-9101
Two Winnco Dr., P.O. Box 34690,   210-227-4747
San Antonio, TX 78218
FDA Number: n/a   *Fax:* 210-227-4747
Web site: www.kln.com
Medical Products Sales Volume: $500,000
Annual Revenue: $10-$25 Million
Ownership: Private
Produces/Sells CE-marked Devices: N
Federal Procurement Eligibility: Small Business
Distribution: Manufacturer Direct, Manufacturer Through Manufacturer Reps
Cabinet, Bedside — General
Furniture, Patient Room — General
Table, Autopsy — Pathology

KLOEHN CO., LTD.   800-358-4342
10000 Banburry Cross Drive,   702-243-7727
Las Vegas, NV 89144
FDA Number: n/a   *Fax:* 702-243-6036
E-mail: info@kloehn.com
Web site: www.kloehn.com
Medical Products Sales Volume: $200,000
Annual Revenue: $10-$25 Million
Year Founded: 1970
Total Employees: 150   *Sales Staff:* 4
Ownership: Private
Quality System Registration Information: ISO9001
Produces/Sells CE-marked Devices: N
Federal Procurement Eligibility: Small Business
Distribution: Manufacturer Direct, OEM
General Admin.: Garth Kloehn/President, Chief Executive Officer
　　Christy Rowley/Vice President Human Resources
Mktg./Adv.: Jim Sostarich/Manager National Sales
Production: Walter Kish/Manager Engineering
　　Mike Marshall/Vice President Manufacturing
Component, Electrical — General
Diluter — Chemistry
Dispenser, Syringe And Needle — General
Fitting, Other — General
Pipette, Micro — Chemistry
Syringe, Other — General
Valve, Other — Chemistry

KLS MARTIN LP   800-625-1557
11239-1 st. johns ind. pkwy. 5,   904-641-7746
Jacksonville, FL 32246
FDA Number: n/a   *Fax:* 604-641-7378
Web site: www.klsmartinusa.com
Year Founded: 1994
Ownership: Private
Produces/Sells CE-marked Devices: N
Electrosurgical Unit, Cutting & Coagulation Device — Surgery

KLS-MARTIN L.P.   800-625-1557
11239-1 St. John`s Industrial, Parkway South,   904-641-7746
Jacksonville, FL 32250
FDA Number: 1057946   *Fax:* 904-641-7378
E-mail: sburke@klsmartin.com
Web site: www.klsmartin.com
Medical Products Sales Volume: $15,600,000
Year Founded: 1993
Total Employees: 98   *Marketing Staff:* 8   *Sales Staff:* 45
Quality System Registration Information: ISO9001
Produces/Sells CE-marked Devices: N
Federal Procurement Eligibility: Small Business
Distribution: Manufacturer Direct
General Admin.: Karl Leibinger/Chief Executive Officer
　　Mike Teague/President
Mktg./Adv.: Jeff Ashby/Manager Advertising
　　Tammi Keithan/Project Manager
　　Jeff Ashby/Vice President Marketing
　　Michael Greene/Vice President Sales

MANUFACTURER PROFILES

KLS-MARTIN L.P.
800-625-1557 (cont'd)

Production: Jennifer Damato/Manager Regulatory Affairs
Research: Michael Greene/Vice President Research & Development

Awl	Orthopedics
Bit, Drill	Orthopedics
Container, Sterilization (Tray)	General
Cover, Burr Hole (Cranial)	Cns/Neurology
Drill, Bone	Orthopedics
Forceps, Wire Holding	Orthopedics
Gauge, Depth	Orthopedics
Guide, Drill	Orthopedics
Instrument, Bending (Contouring)	Orthopedics
Instrument, Dental, Manual	Dental And Oral
Plate, Bone, Orthodontic	Dental And Oral
Plate, Fixation, Bone	Orthopedics
Retractor, Manual	Cns/Neurology
Screw, Cranioplasty Plate	Cns/Neurology
Screw, Fixation, Bone	Orthopedics
Screwdriver	Orthopedics
Screwdriver, Surgical	Surgery
Starter, Bone Screw	Orthopedics
Surgical Instrument, Manual (General Use)	Surgery
Template	Orthopedics
Tray, Surgical Instrument	Surgery
Twister, Wire	Orthopedics
Wire, Bone	Orthopedics
Wire, Surgical	Orthopedics

KM INSTRUMENTS, LLC
520-529-8455

5941 East Fort Crittendon, Tucson, AZ 85750
FDA Number: 2032337

Blade, Scalpel	Surgery

KMA REMARKETING CORP.
814-371-5242

302 Aspen Way, Dubois, PA 15801
FDA Number: 3004215244

Bed, Electric	General
Bed, Hydraulic	General
Bed, Manual	General
Light, Surgical, Ceiling Mounted	Surgery
Light, Surgical, Floor Standing	Surgery
Table, Operating Room, AC-Powered	Surgery
Table, Operating Room, Mechanical	Surgery
Table, Surgical, Electrical	Surgery
Table, Surgical, Hydraulic	Surgery
Table, Surgical, Manual	General

KMEDIC
800-955-0559
201-767-4002

190 Veterans Drive, Northvale, NJ 07647
FDA Number: n/a
Fax: 201-768-0494
E-mail: oeminfo@kmedic.com
Web site: www.kmedic.com
Medical Products Sales Volume: $100,000
Year Founded: 1986
Total Employees: 2
Ownership: TELEFLEX, INC.
Produces/Sells CE-marked Devices: N
Federal Procurement Eligibility: Small Business
Distribution: Manufacturer Through Distributor, Manufacturer Through
Manufacturer Reps, OEM, Exclusive Distributor
General Admin.: Blair Engelken/President
Mktg./Adv.: Liz Ostrow/Director Marketing
      Holger Gruenert/Director Product Development
      David Barwick/Manager Product Development
      Lourdes Figueroa/Manager Sales
Production: Ken Casazza/Director Quality Assurance
Purchasing: Patrice Schmitz/Manager Purchasing

Applier, Hemostatic Clip	Cns/Neurology
Awl	Orthopedics
Bender	Orthopedics
Bit, Drill	Orthopedics
Caliper, Orthopedic	Orthopedics
Chisel (Osteotome)	Surgery
Chisel, Bone, Surgical	Dental And Oral
Chisel, Osteotome, Surgical	Dental And Oral
Chisel, Surgical, Manual	Surgery
Clamp, Bone	Orthopedics
Clamp, Carotid Artery	Cns/Neurology
Clamp, Surgical, General & Plastic Surgery	Surgery
Countersink	Orthopedics
Curette	Orthopedics
Curette, Ear	Ear/Nose/Throat
Curette, Nasal	Ear/Nose/Throat
Curette, Surgical, Dental	Dental And Oral
Curette, Uterine	Obstetrics/Gynecology
Cutter, Operative	Dental And Oral
Cutter, Orthopedic	Orthopedics
Cutter, Ring	General
Cutter, Wire And Pin	Orthopedics
Dilator, Vaginal	Obstetrics/Gynecology

KMEDIC
800-955-0559 (cont'd)

Driver, Surgical, Pin	Surgery
Driver, Wire	Orthopedics
Driver, Wire, And Bone Drill, Manual	Dental And Oral
Elevator, Orthopedic	Orthopedics
Elevator, Surgical, General & Plastic Surgery	Surgery
Extractor, Nail	Orthopedics
File	Orthopedics
File, Bone, Surgical	Dental And Oral
File, Surgical, General & Plastic Surgery	Surgery
Forceps	Orthopedics
Forceps, Dressing	Surgery
Forceps, General & Plastic Surgery	Surgery
Forceps, Hemostatic	Surgery
Forceps, Obstetrical	Obstetrics/Gynecology
Forceps, Ophthalmic	Ophthalmology
Forceps, Rongeur, Surgical	Dental And Oral
Forceps, Sponge	Surgery
Forceps, Surgical, Gynecological	Obstetrics/Gynecology
Forceps, Tissue	Surgery
Forceps, Wire Holding	Orthopedics
Fork, Tuning	Cns/Neurology
Gag, Mouth	Ear/Nose/Throat
Gauge, Depth	Orthopedics
Goniometer, Orthopedic	Orthopedics
Gouge, Surgical, General & Plastic Surgery	Surgery
Hammer, Surgical	Surgery
Handle, Scalpel	Surgery
Hemostat	Orthopedics
Hemostat, Surgical	Dental And Oral
Holder, Needle	Gastroenterology/Urology
Holder, Needle, Orthopedic	Orthopedics
Hook, Other	Surgery
Hook, Surgical, General & Plastic Surgery	Surgery
Impactor	Orthopedics
Implant, Fixation Device, Condylar Plate	Orthopedics
Implant, Fixation Device, Proximal Femoral	Orthopedics
Instrument, Microsurgical	Cns/Neurology
Knife, Amputation	Surgery
Knife, Orthopedic	Orthopedics
Laparoscope, General & Plastic Surgery	Surgery
Mallet, Bone	Orthopedics
Mallet, Surgical, General & Plastic Surgery	Surgery
Needle, Spinal, Short-Term	General
Osteotome (Orthopedic)	Surgery
Passer, Wire, Orthopedic	Orthopedics
Pin, Fixation, Smooth	Orthopedics
Pin, Fixation, Threaded	Orthopedics
Pinwheel	Cns/Neurology
Plate, Bone, Orthodontic	Dental And Oral
Plate, Fixation, Bone	Orthopedics
Pliers, Operative	Dental And Oral
Pliers, Surgical	Orthopedics
Punch, Biopsy	Gastroenterology/Urology
Punch, Biopsy, Surgical	Dental And Oral
Punch, Dermal	Surgery
Rack, Surgical Instrument	Surgery
Rasp, Bone	Orthopedics
Rasp, Nasal	Ear/Nose/Throat
Rasp, Other	Surgery
Rasp, Surgical, General & Plastic Surgery	Surgery
Retractor	Orthopedics
Retractor, All Types	Dental And Oral
Retractor, Manual	Cns/Neurology
Retractor, Other	Surgery
Retractor, Self-Retaining	Gastroenterology/Urology
Retractor, Surgical	Surgery
Rongeur, Other	Surgery
Rongeur, Rib	Orthopedics
Saw, Bone Cutting	Orthopedics
Saw, Other	Surgery
Scissors, Bandage/Gauze/Plaster	General
Scissors, Collar And Crown	Dental And Oral
Scissors, Disposable	General
Scissors, Episiotomy	Obstetrics/Gynecology
Scissors, Iris	Ophthalmology
Scissors, Ophthalmic	Ophthalmology
Scissors, Orthopedic	Orthopedics
Scissors, Surgical Tissue, Dental (Oral)	Dental And Oral
Scissors, Suture	Surgery
Scissors, Wire Cutting, ENT	Ear/Nose/Throat
Screw, Fixation, Bone	Orthopedics
Screw, Fixation, Intraosseous	Dental And Oral
Screwdriver	Orthopedics
Speculum, Other	General
Speculum, Rectal	Gastroenterology/Urology
Speculum, Vaginal, Metal	Obstetrics/Gynecology
Spreader, Plaster (Cast)	Orthopedics
Surgical Instrument, Cardiovascular	Cardiovascular
Surgical Instrument, Manual (General Use)	Surgery
Surgical Instrument, Non-Powered, Neurosurgical	Cns/Neurology
Surgical Instrument, Orthopedic, AC-Powered Motor	Orthopedics

KMEDIC   800-955-0559 (cont'd)

Tap, Bone	Orthopedics
Tonometer, Manual	Ophthalmology
Trephine, Bone	Orthopedics
Twister, Wire	Orthopedics
Wire, Bone	Orthopedics
Wire, Fixation, Intraosseous	Dental And Oral
Wire, Orthodontic	Dental And Oral
Wire, Surgical	Orthopedics

KMI KOLSTER METHODS, INC.   909-737-5476
3185 Palisades Dr., Corona, CA 92880
FDA Number: 2027739

Accessories, Catheter	Surgery
Bandage, Compression	General
Binder, Abdominal	General
Cannula, Suction, Uterine	Obstetrics/Gynecology
Cannula, Suprapubic, With Trocar	Gastroenterology/Urology
Cannula, Surgical, General & Plastic Surgery	Surgery
Diathermy, Ultrasonic (Physical Therapy)	Physical Med
Dissector, Surgical, General & Plastic Surgery	Surgery
Endoscope	Gastroenterology/Urology
Holder, Needle	Gastroenterology/Urology
Pump, Infusion	General
Retractor, Fiberoptic	Gastroenterology/Urology
Speculum, Non-Illuminated	Surgery
Suction Apparatus, Ward Use, Portable, AC-Powered	Surgery
Suture, Non-Absorbable, Synthetic, Polypropylene	Surgery
System, Suction, Lipoplasty	Surgery

KMI SURGICAL LTD.   800-528-2900
Laird Professional Building, 110 Hopewell Rd,   610-518-7114
Downingtown, PA 19335
FDA Number: 2521978
E-mail: contact@kmisurgical.com
Web site: www.kmisurgical.com
Annual Revenue: $5-$10 Million
Total Employees: 25
Ownership: Private
Produces/Sells CE-marked Devices: N
Federal Procurement Eligibility: Small Business, Female Owned
Distribution: Manufacturer Direct, Manufacturer Through Manufacturer Reps, OEM

Cannula, Cyclodialysis (Eye)	Ophthalmology
Cannula, Lacrimal (Eye)	Ophthalmology
Cannula, Ophthalmic	Ophthalmology
Container, Sterilization (Tray)	General
Cystotome, Ophthalmic	Ophthalmology
Instrument, Microsurgical	Cns/Neurology
Knife, Cataract	Ophthalmology
Knife, Keratome	Ophthalmology
Knife, Ophthalmic	Ophthalmology
Knife, Surgical	Dental And Oral
Surgical Instrument, Radial Keratotomy	Ophthalmology

KMI, INC.
See Kmi Surgical Ltd.

KNEEBOURNE THERAPEUTIC, LLC   317-776-2770
15299 Stony Creek Way, Noblesville, IN 46060
FDA Number: 3005109974

Exerciser, Non-Measuring	Physical Med
Orthosis, Limb Brace	Physical Med

KNIT-RITE, INC.   800-821-3094
120 Osage Avenue, Kansas City, KS 66105   913-281-4600
FDA Number: 1922710   Fax: 800-462-4707
E-mail: customerservice@knitrite.com
Web site: www.knitrite.com
Medical Products Sales Volume: $25,000,000
Annual Revenue: $10-$25 Million
Year Founded: 1923
Total Employees: 90   Marketing Staff: 3   Sales Staff: 4
Ownership: Private
Quality System Registration Information: ISO9000
Produces/Sells CE-marked Devices: Y
Federal Procurement Eligibility: Small Business
Distribution: Manufacturer Direct, Manufacturer Through Distributor, OEM, Importer, Exporter
General Admin.: Perry H. Bacon/President, Chief Executive Officer
    Ron Hercules/Senior Vice President
    Lisa Trussel/Vice President Human Resources
Mktg./Adv.: Linda Shelton/Manager Advertising
    Les Chubick/Manager Marketing
    Jeff Dalbey/Manager Product Development
    Matt Stengenga/Vice President Marketing
Production: Gail Hawkins/Manager Materials
Research: Martha Field/Manager Research
Purchasing: Gail Hawkins/Buyer

Bandage, Tubular	General
Orthosis, Other	Physical Med

KNIT-RITE, INC.   800-821-3094 (cont'd)

Sock, Fracture	Orthopedics
Sock, Protective, Skin	General
Sock, Stump Cover	General
Stockinette	Orthopedics

Medical Product Subsidiaries (Listed Separately)
    Paramedical Distributors

KNOGO CORP.
See Sentry Technology Corp.

KNOGO NORTH AMERICA
See Sentry Technology Corp.

KNOGO NORTH AMERICA INC.
See Sentry Technology Corp.

KNOLL GROUP
See Knoll, Inc.

KNOLL MUSKEGON
See Knoll, Inc.

KNOLL, INC.   800-343-5665
2800 Estes St., Muskegon, MI 49441-1697   215 679-7991
FDA Number: n/a
E-mail: info@knoll.com
Web site: www.knoll.com
Annual Revenue: More than $1 Billion
Year Founded: 1938
Total Employees: 3838
Ownership: Public
Stock Symbol: KNL
Traded On: NYSE
Produces/Sells CE-marked Devices: N
Distribution: Manufacturer Direct, Manufacturer Through Distributor, Service Direct
General Admin.: Burton B. Staniar/Chairman
    Andrew B. Cogan/Chief Executive Officer
Finance: Barry L. McCabe/Chief Financial Officer

Computer Equipment	General
Furniture, General	General
Linen	General

KNOX COMPANY   800-552-5669
1601 W Deer Valley Road, Phoenix, AZ 85027   866-625-4563
FDA Number: n/a   Fax: 623-687-2290
Web site: www.knoxbox.com
Annual Revenue: $5-$10 Million
Ownership: Private
Produces/Sells CE-marked Devices: N
Distribution: Manufacturer Direct

Cabinet, Other	General
Equipment, Building Security	General
Rescue Equipment	General

KNÄRR USA INC.   800-465-6877
1890 N. Voyager Avenue, Simi Valley, CA 93063   805-526-7733
FDA Number: n/a   Fax: 805-584-8371
E-mail: info@knurr.com
Web site: www.knurr.com
Medical Products Sales Volume: $100,000
Annual Revenue: $5-$10 Million
Year Founded: 1931
Total Employees: 22
Ownership: Knurr - Mechanik Fur Die Elektronik Ag
Traded On: Munich
Quality System Registration Information: ISO9001; ISO9002
Produces/Sells CE-marked Devices: Y
Federal Procurement Eligibility: Small Business, GSA Contract
Distribution: Manufacturer Direct, Manufacturer Through Distributor, Manufacturer Through Manufacturer Reps
Mktg./Adv.: Mr. Paul Costa/Vice President Sales
Finance: Mr. Adam Steadman/Vice President Finance & Operations

Cart, Instrument	Surgery

KOAMAN INTERNATIONAL   909-983-4888
656 E. D St., Ontario, CA 91764-4250
FDA Number: n/a   Fax: 909-986-3121
E-mail: koaman@unitel.co.kr
Medical Products Sales Volume: $2,000,000
Annual Revenue: $1-$5 Million
Year Founded: 1984
Total Employees: 8
Ownership: Private
Produces/Sells CE-marked Devices: N
Federal Procurement Eligibility: Small Business, Minority Owned
Distribution: Manufacturer Through Distributor, Service Direct, Exclusive Distributor, Exporter
General Admin.: Frank Hwang/President, Chief Executive Officer
Mktg./Adv.: Steve Kim/Director Marketing
    Bob Eaken/Manager International Marketing & Sales

KOAMAN INTERNATIONAL   909-983-4888 (cont'd)
Ron Bout/Vice President Marketing

Analyzer, Cell Size	Microbiology
Analyzer, Chromosome, Automated	Pathology
Analyzer, Karyotype	Pathology
Computer, Image, Endoscopic	General
DNA-Probe, Chromosome, Human	Hematology
Electrosurgical Unit, General Purpose (ESU)	Surgery
Extractor, Vacuum, Fetal	Obstetrics/Gynecology
Genetic Engineering	Microbiology
Monitor, Blood Pressure, Indirect (Arterial)	Cardiovascular
Monitor, Pulse Rate	Anesthesiology
Service, Consulting	General
Service, Import/Export	General

KOCH SYSTEMS
See Koch X-Ray Systems Inc

KOCH X-RAY SYSTEMS INC   305-252-8770
10500 S.W. 184 Terrace, Miami, FL 33157-6760
FDA Number: n/a
Fax: 305-662-7393
E-mail: kochx@netrox.net
Web site: www.kochxray.com
Medical Products Sales Volume: $900,000
Year Founded: 1952
Total Employees: 7   Sales Staff: 2
Ownership: Private
Produces/Sells CE-marked Devices: N
Federal Procurement Eligibility: Small Business
Distribution: Manufacturer Direct, Service Direct, Exclusive Distributor
General Admin.: Thad Koch/Chief Executive Officer
Mktg./Adv.: Robert Koch/Vice President Sales

Radiographic Unit, Diagnostic	Radiology

KODAK CANADA INC., HEALTH IMAGING DIVISION   800-465-6325
6 Monogram Place, Suite 200,   416-766-8233
Toronto, ONT M9R 0 Canada
FDA Number: n/a
Fax: (416) 761-4371
E-mail: kciinternet@kodak.com
Web site: www.kodak.ca
Year Founded: 1899
Total Employees: 1600   Marketing Staff: 6   Sales Staff: 20
Ownership: Public
Produces/Sells CE-marked Devices: N
Distribution: Manufacturer Direct, Exclusive Distributor

KODENT INC.   562-404-8466
13340 E. Firestone Blvd., Suite J, Santa Fe Springs, CA 90670
FDA Number: 3006158523
Ownership: Private
Produces/Sells CE-marked Devices: N

Alloy, Gold Based, For Clinical Use	Dental And Oral

KOEHLER INSTRUMENT CO., INC.   800-878-9070
1595 Sycamore Avenue,   631-589-3800
Bohemia, NY 11716
FDA Number: 2431764
Fax: 631-589-3815
E-mail: info@koehlerinstrument.com
Web site: www.koehlerinstrument.com
Medical Products Sales Volume: $5,100,000
Annual Revenue: $5-$10 Million
Year Founded: 1982
Total Employees: 55
Ownership: Private
Produces/Sells CE-marked Devices: Y
Federal Procurement Eligibility: Small Business
Distribution: Manufacturer Direct, Manufacturer Through Distributor, Manufacturer Through Manufacturer Reps, OEM, Exporter
Mktg./Adv.: Dr. Wayne Goldenberg/Director Marketing
                    Dr. Raj Shah/Director Marketing & Sales

Balance, Analytical	Chemistry
Bath, Kinematic Viscosity	Chemistry
Colorimeter, General Use	Chemistry
Penetrometer	Radiology
Viscometer	Chemistry

KOENIGKRAMER, F & F
See HAAG-STREIT USA, INC.

KOHLER CO.   800-456-4537
444 Highland Dr., Kohler, WI 53044   920-457-4441
FDA Number: 2182295
Web site: www.kohler.com
Annual Revenue: $10-$25 Million
Year Founded: 1973
Total Employees: 35500
Ownership: Private
Produces/Sells CE-marked Devices: N

KOHLER CO.   800-456-4537 (cont'd)
Distribution: Manufacturer Through Distributor
General Admin.: Herbert V. Kohler/Chairman, Chief Executive Officer

Bath, Hydro-Massage (Whirlpool)	Physical Med
Bath, Sitz, Physical Medicine	Physical Med

KOL BIO-MEDICAL INSTRUMENTS, INC.   800-336-5018
13901 Willard Rd., P.O. Box 220630,   703-378-8600
Chantilly, VA 20153
FDA Number: n/a
Fax: 703-266-2447
E-mail: requests@kolbio.com
Web site: www.kolbio.com
Medical Products Sales Volume: $30,000,000
Total Employees: 30
Ownership: Private
Produces/Sells CE-marked Devices: N
Federal Procurement Eligibility: Small Business
Distribution: Exclusive Distributor
General Admin.: Roger S. Kolasinski/Chief Executive Officer
                    Timothy D. C. McInerney/President
Mktg./Adv.: Michael C. Whitaker/Vice President Marketing & Sales
Finance: Philip M. Reilly/Vice President Finance

Surgical Instrument, Cardiovascular	Cardiovascular
Surgical Instrument, Obstetric/Gynecologic, General	Obstetrics/Gynecology

KOLBERG OCULAR PRODUCTS, INC.   858-695-2021
9663 Tierra Grande St.,, Suite 201, San Diego, CA 92126
FDA Number: 2029308

Conformer, Ophthalmic	Ophthalmology

KOLD-DRAFT   800-840-9577
1525 E. Lake Road, Erie, PA 16511   814-453-6761
FDA Number: 9330129
Fax: 814-548-9392
E-mail: info@kold-draft.com
Web site: www.kold-draft.com
Medical Products Sales Volume: $2,500,000
Annual Revenue: $5-$10 Million
Year Founded: 1920
Total Employees: 7   Sales Staff: 4
Ownership: Private
Produces/Sells CE-marked Devices: Y
Federal Procurement Eligibility: Small Business, GSA Contract
Distribution: Manufacturer Through Distributor, Exporter
General Admin.: Randy Lachowski/President, Chief Executive Officer
Mktg./Adv.: John Collins/Vice President Marketing & Sales
Production: Linda Prescott/Customer Service Representative
                    Clarke Kuebler/Vice President Manufacturing

Foodservice Product/Equipment	General

KOLLSMAN, INC.   603-886-7500
220 Daniel Webster Hwy., Merrimack, NH 03054
FDA Number: 1219738
Ownership: Private
Produces/Sells CE-marked Devices: N

Software, Blood Bank (Stand-Alone Products)	Hematology

KOLLSUT SCIENTIFIC CORPORATION   630-290-5746
3286 North 29th Court, Hollywood, FL 33020
FDA Number: 3005953126

Catheter, Intravascular, Therapeutic, Short-term Less Than 30 Days	General
Mesh, Surgical, Polymeric	Surgery
Suture, Absorbable, Synthetic, Polyglycolic Acid	Surgery
Suture, Non-Absorbable, Silk	Surgery
Suture, Non-Absorbable, Synthetic, Polyamide	Surgery
Suture, Non-Absorbable, Synthetic, Polyethylene	Surgery
Suture, Non-Absorbable, Synthetic, Polypropylene	Surgery

KONICA MINOLTA MEDICAL IMAGING USA, INC.   800-934-1034
411 Newark Pompton Tpke., Wayne, NJ 07470   973-633-1500
FDA Number: 2241281
Fax: 973-523-7408
Web site: www.konicaminolta.com/medicalusa/
Medical Products Sales Volume: $17,400,000
Annual Revenue: More than $1 Billion
Year Founded: 1963
Total Employees: 31800
Ownership: Konica Minolta
Stock Symbol: 4902
Traded On: Tokyo
Quality System Registration Information: ISO9001
Produces/Sells CE-marked Devices: N
Distribution: Manufacturer Direct, OEM
General Admin.: Yoshikatsu Ota/Chairman
                    Masatoshi Matsuzaki/President, Chief Executive Officer

Cassette, Radiographic Film	Radiology
Chemical, Film Processor	Radiology
Densitometer	Cardiovascular
Film, X-Ray	Radiology
Film, X-Ray, Special Purpose	Radiology

KONICA MINOLTA MEDICAL IMAGING USA, INC. 800-934-1034
(cont'd)

Handling Unit, Automatic Daylight X-Ray Film	Radiology
Processor, Radiographic Film, Automatic	Radiology
Radiographic Unit, Digital	Radiology
Screen, Intensifying, Radiographic	Radiology
Sensitometer, Radiographic	Radiology

KONICA MINOLTA SENSING AMERICAS, INC. 888-473-2656
101 Williams Dr., Ramsey, NJ 07446   **201-236-4300**
FDA Number: 2247797   *Fax:* 201-785-2480
E-mail: color@se.konicaminolta.us
Web site: www.konicaminolta.com/sensingusa/
Annual Revenue: More than $1 Billion
Total Employees: 31800
Ownership: Public
Stock Symbol: 4902
Traded On: Tokyo
Quality System Registration Information: ISO9001
Produces/Sells CE-marked Devices: N
Distribution: Manufacturer Direct, Importer, Exporter
General Admin.: Yoshikatsu Ota/Chairman
      Masatoshi Matsuzaki/President, Chief Executive Officer

KONICA-MINOLTA CORP.
See Konica Minolta Sensing Americas, Inc.

KONIGSBERG INSTRUMENTS, INC. 626-449-0016
2000 East Foothill Blvd., Pasadena, CA 91107
FDA Number: 2020337   *Fax:* 626-585-4068
E-mail: kiinfo@konigsberginc.com
Web site: www.konigsberginc.com
Medical Products Sales Volume: $4,400,000
Annual Revenue: $1-$5 Million
Year Founded: 1968
Total Employees: 55   *Marketing Staff:* 4   *Sales Staff:* 4
Ownership: Private
Stock Symbol: KGBC
Traded On: NYSE
Produces/Sells CE-marked Devices: Y
Federal Procurement Eligibility: Small Business
Distribution: Manufacturer Direct, OEM, Service Direct, Exporter
General Admin.: William Mills/General Manager
      Eph Konigsberg/President
Production: Zaiga Alksnitis/Manager Quality Assurance

Contract Manufacturing	General
Contract R&D, Equipment	General
Electrode, pH	Gastroenterology/Urology
Monitor, Blood Pressure, Invasive (Arterial)	Cardiovascular
Monitor, Blood Pressure, Venous	Cardiovascular
Monitor, Cardiac Output, Flowmeter	Cardiovascular
Monitor, Esophageal Pressure	Gastroenterology/Urology
Monitor, Eye Movement	Ophthalmology
Recorder, Long-Term, Respiration	Anesthesiology
Telemetry Unit, Physiological, ECG	Cardiovascular
Telemetry Unit, Physiological, EEG	Cns/Neurology
Telemetry Unit, Physiological, EMG	Physical Med
Telemetry Unit, Physiological, EOG	Cns/Neurology
Telemetry Unit, Physiological, Multiple Channel	General
Telemetry Unit, Physiological, Neurological	Cns/Neurology
Telemetry Unit, Physiological, Pressure	General
Telemetry Unit, Physiological, Temperature	General
Tonograph	Ophthalmology
Transducer, Blood Pressure	General
Transmitter/Receiver System, Physiological, Radiofrequency	Cardiovascular

KONSYL PHARMACEUTICALS, INC. 800-356-6795
8050 Industrial Park Road, Easton, MD 21601   **410-822-5192**
FDA Number: 1119033   *Fax:* 410-820-7032
E-mail: contact@konsyl.com
Web site: www.konsyl.com
Medical Products Sales Volume: $8,200,000
Total Employees: 60
Ownership: ICC Industries
Produces/Sells CE-marked Devices: N
Federal Procurement Eligibility: Small Business

Analyzer, Motility, Gastrointestinal, Electrical	Gastroenterology/Urology

KONTES GLASS CO. 888-546-2531
1022 Spruce St., Vineland, NJ 08360-2841   **856-692-8500**
FDA Number: 2240956   *Fax:* 856-794-9762
E-mail: cs@kimkon.com
Web site: www.kontes.com
Medical Products Sales Volume: $22,000,000
Year Founded: 1993
Total Employees: 150
Ownership: GERRESHEIMER
Quality System Registration Information: ISO9001
Produces/Sells CE-marked Devices: N

KONTES GLASS CO. 888-546-2531 *(cont'd)*
Federal Procurement Eligibility: Small Business
Distribution: Manufacturer Direct, Manufacturer Through Distributor
General Admin.: Uwe Roehrhoff/Chief Executive Officer
Mktg./Adv.: Doug Grady/Director Marketing
      David Fenili/Manager Advertising

Accessories, Chromatography (Gas, Gel, Liquid, Thin Layer)	Chemistry
Buret	Chemistry
Chromatography Equipment, Liquid	Chemistry
Chromatography Equipment, Paper	Chemistry
Chromatography Equipment, Thin Layer	Toxicology
Column, Chromatography	Chemistry
Densitometer, Laboratory	Chemistry
Densitometer/Scanner (Integrating, Reflectance, TLC, Radio)	Chemistry
Distilling Unit	Chemistry
Distilling Unit, Molecular	Chemistry
Evaporator	Chemistry
Flowmeter, Gas (Oxygen), Calibrated	Anesthesiology
Homogenizer, Tissue	Microbiology
Labware, Basic, Reusable	Chemistry
Nuclear Magnetic Resonance Equipment, Laboratory	Chemistry
Pipette, Micro	Chemistry
Still, Solvent Recovery	Chemistry
Still, Water	Chemistry
Stirrer	Chemistry
Stopcock	General
Tissue Culture Apparatus	Microbiology
Valve, Other	Chemistry

KONTUR KONTACT LENS CO., INC. 800-227-1320
642 Alfred Nobel Drive,   **510-964-9760**
Hercules, CA 94547
FDA Number: 2919245   *Fax:* 800-650-6525
E-mail: danaewell@aol.com
Medical Products Sales Volume: $1,400,000
Annual Revenue: $1-$5 Million
Year Founded: 1958
Total Employees: 13   *Marketing Staff:* 1   *Sales Staff:* 1
Ownership: Private
Produces/Sells CE-marked Devices: N
Federal Procurement Eligibility: Small Business
Distribution: Manufacturer Direct
General Admin.: Dana Ewell/General Manager
      Dana Ewell/President, Chief Executive Officer

Lens, Contact, Hydrophilic	Ophthalmology

KORCHEK TECHNOLOGIES, LLC 203-452-8295
115 Technology Drive, Suite B 206, Trumbull, CT 06611
FDA Number: 3004587266

Software, Blood Bank (Stand-Alone Products)	Hematology

KOROS USA, INC. 805-529-0825
610 Flinn Ave., Moorpark, CA 93021
FDA Number: 2023918

Bolt, Nut, Washer	Orthopedics
Cannula, Suprapubic, With Trocar	Gastroenterology/Urology
Chisel, Middle Ear	Ear/Nose/Throat
Cover, Biopsy Forceps	Gastroenterology/Urology
Curette, Surgical	Surgery
Cutter, Wire And Pin	Orthopedics
Endoscope, Neurological	Cns/Neurology
Forceps, General & Plastic Surgery	Surgery
Holder, Needle	Gastroenterology/Urology
Kit, Laparoscopy	Gastroenterology/Urology
Pump, Suction Operatory	Dental And Oral
Retractor, Self-Retaining	Gastroenterology/Urology
Rongeur, Rib	Orthopedics
Scissors, Surgical Tissue, Dental (Oral)	Dental And Oral
Sling, Overhead Suspension, Wheelchair	Physical Med
Surgical Instrument, Disposable	Surgery
Wire, Surgical	Orthopedics

KORR MEDICAL TECHNOLOGIES, INC. 801-483-2080
2463 South 3850 West #200, Salt Lake City, UT 84120
FDA Number: 1724967

Computer, Oxygen-Uptake	Anesthesiology

KORR MEDICAL TECHNOLOGIES, INC. 800-895-4048
3487 W 2100 South, Bldg #300,   **801-483-2080**
Salt Lake City, UT 84119
FDA Number: n/a   *Fax:* 801-483-2123
E-mail: sales@korr.com
Web site: www.korr.com
Year Founded: 1993
Ownership: Private
Produces/Sells CE-marked Devices: N
Federal Procurement Eligibility: Small Business
Distribution: Manufacturer Direct

KORR MEDICAL TECHNOLOGIES, INC. 800-895-4048 *(cont'd)*
    Meter, Peak Flow, Spirometry   Anesthesiology

KOSMA-KARE CANADA INC.   450-679-6380
    2044, de la Province, Longueuil, QUE J4G-1Z1 Canada
    FDA Number: n/a   *Fax:* 450-679-6362
    E-mail: kosmakare@msn.com
    Year Founded: 1989
    Total Employees: 100
    Ownership: Private
    Produces/Sells CE-marked Devices: N
    Distribution: Manufacturer Direct, Exporter

KOTNER MEDICAL SYSTEMS, INC.
    See Val Med

KOTTLER RESEARCH CORP.   850-983-0552
    2000 Garcon Point Road, Milton, FL 32583
    FDA Number: 2027760
    E-mail: INFO@KOTTLER.COM
    Ownership: Private
    Produces/Sells CE-marked Devices: N
    Material, Impression   Dental And Oral

KOVEN AND ASSOCIATES, INC.
    See Koven Technology, Inc.

KOVEN TECHNOLOGY, INC.   800-521-8342
    12125 Woodcrest Executive Dr., Suite 320,   314-542-2101
    St. Louis, MO 63141
    FDA Number: 1937397
    E-mail: info@koven.com   *Fax:* 314-542-6020
    Web site: www.koven.com
    Ownership: Private
    Produces/Sells CE-marked Devices: N
    Federal Procurement Eligibility: Small Business, Female Owned
    Distribution: Exclusive Distributor, Importer
    General Admin.: Heather Koven Bell/President
    Flowmeter, Blood, Intravenous   Cardiovascular
    Monitor, Blood Flow, Ultrasonic   Obstetrics/Gynecology
    Monitor, Blood Pressure, Indirect, Semi-Automatic   Cardiovascular
    Plethysmograph, Photo-Electric, Pneumatic Or Hydraulic Cardiovascular
    Sleep Assessment Equipment   Cns/Neurology
    Transducer, Ultrasonic, Diagnostic   Radiology
    Valvulotome   Cardiovascular

KPMG LLP   416-777-8500
    333 Bay Street, Suite 4600, Toronto, ONT M5H 2S5 Canada
    FDA Number: n/a   *Fax:* 416-777-8818
    E-mail: jerling@kpmg.ca
    Web site: www.kpmg.ca
    Year Founded: 1994
    Total Employees: 250
    Ownership: Private
    Produces/Sells CE-marked Devices: N

KRAMER SCIENTIFIC LABORATORY   201-767-8505
PRODUCTS CORP.
    50 Maple St., Norwood, NJ 07648
    FDA Number: 2434936
    Ownership: Private
    Produces/Sells CE-marked Devices: N
    Kit, Sampling, Arterial Blood   Anesthesiology

KRATOS ANALYTICAL INC.   800-935-0213
    100 Red Schoolhouse Road #Bldg.-A,   845-426-6700
    Spring Valley, NY 10977
    FDA Number: 7000219   *Fax:* 845-426-6192
    E-mail: jd@kratos.com
    Web site: www.kratos.com
    Medical Products Sales Volume: $12,000,000
    Annual Revenue: $0-$1 Million
    Year Founded: 1986
    Total Employees: 19   *Marketing Staff:* 4   *Sales Staff:* 4
    Ownership: SHIMADZU CORP.
    Traded On: Tokyo
    Quality System Registration Information: ISO9000
    Produces/Sells CE-marked Devices: N
    Federal Procurement Eligibility: GSA Contract
    Distribution: Manufacturer Direct, Exclusive Distributor, Importer, Exporter
    General Admin.: David Surman/Vice President, General Manager
    Mktg./Adv.: Jeannette De Gennaro/Vice President Marketing
    Calibrator, Mass Spectrometer   General
    Mass Spectrometer, Clinical Use   Toxicology

KRAUSE SURGICAL INSTRUMENT CORP. 314-842-0327
    5544 Robertwood Dr., St. Louis, MO 63128
    FDA Number: 1931304
    Ownership: Private

KRAUSE SURGICAL INSTRUMENT CORP. 314-842-0327 *(cont'd)*
    Produces/Sells CE-marked Devices: N
    Forceps, Ophthalmic   Ophthalmology

KREBS INSTRUMENTS   201-871-6969
    195 Redneck Ave, Little Ferry, NJ 07643
    FDA Number: n/a
    Web site: krebsinstruments.com
    Annual Revenue: $0-$1 Million
    Ownership: Private
    Produces/Sells CE-marked Devices: N
    Federal Procurement Eligibility: Small Business
    Distribution: Exclusive Distributor
    Camera, Ophthalmic, AC-Powered (Fundus)   Ophthalmology
    Chair, Ophthalmic, Manual   Ophthalmology
    Keratometer   Ophthalmology
    Lamp, Slit   Ophthalmology
    Lens, Set, Trial, Ophthalmic   Ophthalmology
    Lensometer   Ophthalmology
    Ophthalmoscope, Direct   Ophthalmology
    Ophthalmoscope, Indirect   Ophthalmology
    Perimeter, Manual   Ophthalmology
    Projector, Ophthalmic   Ophthalmology
    Refractor, Ophthalmic   Ophthalmology
    Stand, Instrument, Ophthalmic   Ophthalmology

KREBS OPHTHALMIC INSTRUMENTS INC.
    See Krebs Instruments

KREE TECHNOLOGIES USA, INC.   450-676-9444
    11429 53rd Street North, Clearwater, FL 33760
    FDA Number: 1321241
    Ownership: Private
    Produces/Sells CE-marked Devices: N
    Bandage, Adhesive   Surgery

KREG MEDICAL, INC.   312-275-7002
    2240 W. Walnut St., Chicago, IL 60612
    FDA Number: 3005179379
    Cover, Mattress   General
    Mattress, Non-Powered Flotation Therapy   Physical Med

KREISERS INC.   800-843-7948
    2200 West 46th St., Sioux Falls, SD 57105 605-336-1155
    FDA Number: 1716765   *Fax:* 605-336-1157
    E-mail: info@kreisers.com
    Web site: www.kreisers.com
    Medical Products Sales Volume: $25,000,000
    Annual Revenue: $25-$50 Million
    Year Founded: 1905
    Total Employees: 8   *Marketing Staff:* 15   *Sales Staff:* 15
    Ownership: Private
    Produces/Sells CE-marked Devices: N
    Federal Procurement Eligibility: Small Business, GSA Contract, VA Contract
    Distribution: Manufacturer Through Distributor, Manufacturer Through Manufacturer Reps, Exclusive Distributor
    General Admin.: David H. Larson/President, Chief Executive Officer
    Mktg./Adv.: Gary Hembree/Executive Marketing
            Phil Johnson/Manager Advertising
            Ron Roehl/Vice President Sales
            Phil Johnson/Vice President, General Manager Marketing
    Production: John Schuety/Manager Materials
            Phil Johnson/Vice President Production
    Labware, Basic, Reusable   Chemistry
    Slide, Microscope   Pathology

KRESS MEDICAL SUPPLY, INC.
    See Total Titanium

KRESS U.S.A.
    See Total Titanium

KRISHNA EYE INSTRUMENTS
    See Stephens Instruments, Inc.

KRISTI-CARE, INC.   207-637-2672
    110 Millturn Rd., Limington, ME 04049
    FDA Number: 1226713
    Ownership: Private
    Produces/Sells CE-marked Devices: N
    Accessories, Wheelchair   Physical Med

KRISTOFOAM INDUSTRIES INC.   905-669-6616
    120 Planchet Rd, Concord, ON L4K 2C7 Canada
    FDA Number: n/a   *Fax:* 905-669-6235
    Total Employees: 60   *Marketing Staff:* 10   *Sales Staff:* 10
    Ownership: Private
    Produces/Sells CE-marked Devices: N
    Distribution: Manufacturer Direct, Exporter

KROHN-HITE CORPORATION
877-549-7781
508-580-1660
15 Jonathan Drive, Unit 4,
Brockton, MA 02301
FDA Number: n/a   *Fax:* 508-583-8989
E-mail: info@krohn-hite.com
Web site: www.krohn-hite.com
Medical Products Sales Volume: $2,000,000
Annual Revenue: $1-$5 Million
Year Founded: 1949
Total Employees: 21
Ownership: KROHN-HITE CORPORATION
Produces/Sells CE-marked Devices: Y
Federal Procurement Eligibility: Small Business
Distribution: Manufacturer Direct, Manufacturer Through Distributor, OEM, Service Direct, Exclusive Distributor, Exporter
General Admin.: Richard Haddad/President, Chief Executive Officer
Mktg./Adv.: Robert B. Ross/Director Marketing
Mr. Joe Inglis/Manager Sales Admin.
Analyzer, Electrical Safety   General
Potentiometer   Chemistry

KRONNER MEDICAL
800-706-3533
541-672-2543
1443 Upper Cleveland Rapids Rd.,
Roseburg, OR 97470
FDA Number: 3018984
E-mail: kronner@rosenet.net   *Fax:* 541-672-1074
Web site: www.kronner.com
Annual Revenue: $0-$1 Million
Total Employees: 5
Ownership: Private
Produces/Sells CE-marked Devices: N
Federal Procurement Eligibility: Small Business, Female Owned
Distribution: Manufacturer Direct
General Admin.: Richard F. Kronner/President
Mktg./Adv.: Crystal Kronner/Manager Advertising
Accessories, Traction (Cart, Frame, Cord, Weight)   Orthopedics
Endoscope   Gastroenterology/Urology
Holder, Instrument, Laparoscopic   Surgery
Holder, Laparoscope   Obstetrics/Gynecology
Laparoscope, General & Plastic Surgery   Surgery
Stand, Casting   Orthopedics
Support, Foot   Orthopedics

KRONUS, INC.
See Kronus, Inc.

KROWN MANUFACTURING, INC.
800-366-9950
817-738-2485
3408 Indale Rd., Fort Worth, TX 76116
FDA Number: n/a   *Fax:* 817-738-1970
E-mail: info@krownmfg.com
Web site: www.krownmfg.com
Medical Products Sales Volume: $1,500,000
Annual Revenue: $1-$5 Million
Year Founded: 1995
Ownership: COMPU-TTY, INC.
Produces/Sells CE-marked Devices: N
Federal Procurement Eligibility: Small Business, Minority Owned, Female Owned
Distribution: Manufacturer Direct, Manufacturer Through Distributor
Telephone, Handicapped Use   Physical Med

KROY MEDICAL, INC.
See Enova Medical Technologies

KROY SIGN SYSTEMS
See Kroy, Llc

KROY, INC.
See Kroy, Llc

KROY, LLC
888-888-5769
216-426-5600
3830 Kelly Avenue, Cleveland, OH 44114
FDA Number: n/a   *Fax:* 216-426-5601
E-mail: hall@kroy.com
Web site: www.kroy.com
Medical Products Sales Volume: $23,300,000
Annual Revenue: $25-$50 Million
Year Founded: 1998
Total Employees: 255   *Marketing Staff:* 2   *Sales Staff:* 7
Ownership: Private
Quality System Registration Information: ISO9001
Produces/Sells CE-marked Devices: N
Federal Procurement Eligibility: Small Business
Distribution: Manufacturer Through Distributor, Manufacturer Through Manufacturer Reps, OEM
General Admin.: Bill Dillingham/President
Benny Bonanno/Vice President
Mktg./Adv.: Ed Hall/Manager Sales
Benny Bonanno/Vice President Marketing
Production: Ed Hall/Manager Regulatory Affairs
Label, Bar Code   General

KROY, LLC
888-888-5769 *(cont'd)*
Labeling Equipment   General
Sign, Hospital   General

KRUEGER INTERNATIONAL
See Ki

KRUSE TOOL AND DIE INC.
215-674-1730
P.O. Box 2247, Warminster, PA 18974
FDA Number: n/a   *Fax:* 215-674-4938
E-mail: info@krusetool.com
Web site: www.krusetool.com
Annual Revenue: $0-$1 Million
Total Employees: 60
Ownership: Private
Produces/Sells CE-marked Devices: N
Federal Procurement Eligibility: Small Business
Distribution: OEM
General Admin.: Juergen Kruse/President
Mktg./Adv.: Juergen Kruse/Manager Advertising
Juergen Kruse/Vice President Marketing & Sales
Component, Plastic   General
Molding, Custom   General

KS MANUFACTURING, INC.
508-427-5727
254 Bodwell St., Unit E, Avon, MA 02322
FDA Number: 3004959302
Gauze/sponge, Nonresorbable For External Use   Surgery

KT MEDICAL CORP.
800-633-3757
423-843-5120
P.O. Box 50876, Knoxville, TN 37950-0876
FDA Number: 1053670
E-mail: loumd@hiwaay.net   *Fax:* 423-843-5101
Web site: www.ktmedical.com
Medical Products Sales Volume: $1,000,000
Annual Revenue: $1-$5 Million
Total Employees: 35   *Marketing Staff:* 2   *Sales Staff:* 10
Ownership: Private
Produces/Sells CE-marked Devices: N
Federal Procurement Eligibility: Small Business, Minority Owned
Distribution: Manufacturer Direct, OEM, Exporter
General Admin.: Marcos A. More/President
Mktg./Adv.: Marcos A. Lepchitz/Director National Accounts
Marcos A. More/Manager Marketing & Sales
Production: Marcos A. More/Vice President Manufacturing
Bandage, Elastic   General
Brace, Joint, Ankle (External)   Physical Med
Support, Ankle   Orthopedics
Support, Back   Orthopedics
Support, Elbow   Orthopedics
Support, Knee   Physical Med
Support, Wrist   Physical Med

KUBLY OCULAR PROSTHETICS INC.
813-977-7676
3500 East Fletcher Ave.,, Suite 509, Tampa, FL 33613
FDA Number: 1045058   *Fax:* 813-977-1999
E-mail: sales@ocularist.com
Web site: www.ocularist.com
Year Founded: 1978
Total Employees: 3   *Sales Staff:* 3
Ownership: Private
Produces/Sells CE-marked Devices: N
Distribution: Manufacturer Direct
Button, Iris, Eye, Artificial   Ophthalmology
Conformer, Ophthalmic   Ophthalmology
Eye, Artificial, Non-Custom   Ophthalmology
Material, Impression   Dental And Oral
Shell, Scleral   Ophthalmology

KURI TEC CORPORATION
519-753-6717
140 Roy Blvd, Brantford, ONT N3R-7K2 Canada
FDA Number: n/a   *Fax:* 519-753-7737
E-mail: sales@kuritec.com
Web site: www.kuritec.com
Year Founded: 1985
Ownership: Private
Produces/Sells CE-marked Devices: N
Distribution: Manufacturer Direct, Exporter

KURT MANUFACTURING CO., A DIVISION OF THERADYNE HEALTHCARE
See Theradyne Products Division

KUSCH USA INC.
See Thompson Contract Inc.

KVB MANUFACTURING
800-565-9845
613-283-3196
62 Maple Ave.,
Smith Falls, ONT K7A-2 Canada
FDA Number: n/a   *Fax:* 613-283-7216

KVB MANUFACTURING 800-565-9845 (cont'd)
E-mail: seawolf888@aol.com
Web site: http://www.kvb.com
Year Founded: 1990
Total Employees: 10
Ownership: Private
Produces/Sells CE-marked Devices: N
Distribution: Manufacturer Direct

KYOCERA INDUSTRIAL CERAMICS CORP. 800-826-0527
472 Kato Terrace, Fremont, CA 94539 510-257-0112
FDA Number: 3007208876
E-mail: joe.maurer@kyocera.com
Web site: americas.kyocera.com/kicc
Year Founded: 1969
Ownership: KYOCERA CORP.
Stock Symbol: KYO
Traded On: NYSE
Produces/Sells CE-marked Devices: N
Federal Procurement Eligibility: Small Business
Distribution: Manufacturer Through Distributor
  Pump, Vacuum, Central   Anesthesiology

KYPHON, INC.
See Medtronic Spine Llc

KYRO MFG. CO. 817-336-1319
2601 Weisenberger St., Fort Worth, TX 76107
FDA Number: 1625539
  Table, Mechanical   Physical Med

L & G MEDICAL SOFTWARE 503-924-2429
15685 Nw Melody Ln, Aloha, OR 97006
FDA Number: 3007063018
E-mail: info@lgmds.com
Ownership: Private
Produces/Sells CE-marked Devices: N

L&L SPECIAL FURNACE CO., INC. 888-808-3676
20 Kent Road, Aston, PA 19014 610-459-9216
FDA Number: n/a   *Fax:* 610-459-3689
E-mail: sales@hotfurnace.com
Web site: www.hotfurnace.com
Medical Products Sales Volume: $2,000,000
Annual Revenue: $1-$5 Million
Year Founded: 1948
Total Employees: 18   *Marketing Staff:* 1   *Sales Staff:* 3
Ownership: Private
Produces/Sells CE-marked Devices: N
Federal Procurement Eligibility: Small Business
Distribution: Manufacturer Direct, Manufacturer Through Manufacturer Reps
General Admin.: Ms. Nancy Kester/Office Manager
      Gregory Lewicki/President
      Stephen Lewicki/Secretary Treasurer
Mktg./Adv.: Mr. Thomas Schultz/Sales Specialist
  Oven   Chemistry
  System, Hyperthermia, Rf/microwave (benign Prostatic Hyperplasia), Thermotherapy
  Gastroenterology/Urology

L&R MANUFACTURING CO. 201-991-5330
577 Elm St., PO Box 607, Kearny, NJ 07032-0607
FDA Number: 2244004   *Fax:* 201-991-5870
E-mail: info@LRultrasonics.com
Web site: www.LRultrasonics.com
Medical Products Sales Volume: $10,000,000
Annual Revenue: $10-$25 Million
Year Founded: 1930
Total Employees: 150   *Marketing Staff:* 3   *Sales Staff:* 9
Ownership: Private
Quality System Registration Information: ISO9001
Produces/Sells CE-marked Devices: Y
Federal Procurement Eligibility: Small Business
Distribution: Manufacturer Direct, Manufacturer Through Distributor, Manufacturer Through Manufacturer Reps, Exporter
General Admin.: James Lazarus/Chairman
      Robert Lazarus/President
Mktg./Adv.: Lenny Shapiro/Manager Contract Sales
      Bruce Letsch/Manager International & National Sales
      Brian McGrath/Manager Marketing
      Pattie Faul-Burnett/Marketing Coordinator
Production: Joanne Vander Fliet/Manager Customer Services
      Ralph DeVito/Manager Quality Assurance
      Ralph Devito/Product Manager
Finance: David Romanok/Chief Financial Officer
  Cleaner, Ultrasonic, Medical Instrument   General
  Lubricant, Instrument   General
  Solution, Instrument Cleaner   General

L'AMY, INC. 800-USA-LAMY
37 Danbury Road, Wilton, CT 06897-4405 203-761-0611
FDA Number: 1049017   *Fax:* 203-761-9262
E-mail: lamyamerica@lamygroup.com
Web site: www.lamygroup.com
Medical Products Sales Volume: $7,400,000
Annual Revenue: $10-$25 Million
Year Founded: 1987
Total Employees: 83   *Marketing Staff:* 3   *Sales Staff:* 55
Ownership: L'AMY GROUP
Produces/Sells CE-marked Devices: N
Federal Procurement Eligibility: Small Business
Distribution: Manufacturer Direct, Service Direct
General Admin.: Marc Lamy/Chief Executive Officer
      Stephen Rappopport/President
      Carol Interlandi/Vice President Human Resources
Mktg./Adv.: Beatrice Querel/Manager Advertising
      Cheryl Canning/Manager Marketing
      Tom Phillips/Manager National Sales
  Frame, Spectacle (Eyeglasses)   Ophthalmology

L'NARD ASSOCIATES, INC.
See Restorative Care Of America Inc

L'NARD RESTORATIVE CONCEPTS
See Restorative Care Of America Inc

L-3 COMMUNICATIONS ELECTRON DEVICES 650-591-8411
960 Industrial Road, San Carlos, CA 94070-4194
FDA Number: 2920853   *Fax:* 650-508-1956
E-mail: msweeney@littonedd.com
Year Founded: 1959
Ownership: Private
Stock Symbol: NOC
Traded On: NYSE
Quality System Registration Information: ISO9001
Produces/Sells CE-marked Devices: N
Distribution: Manufacturer Through Distributor
General Admin.: Michael Sweeney/Program Manager
  Accelerator, Linear, Medical   Radiology

L.A.B. INSTRUMENTS, LTD. 775-883-1205
3692 Green Acres Dr., Carson City, NV 89705
FDA Number: 2939819
  Knife, Ophthalmic   Ophthalmology

L.A.K. ENTERPRISES, INC. 800-824-3112
423 Broadway, Suite 501, 650-344-6830
Millbrae, CA 94030
FDA Number: 2937820   *Fax:* 650-375-0511
E-mail: cs@lakdental.com
Web site: www.lakdental.com
Year Founded: 1987
Ownership: Private
Produces/Sells CE-marked Devices: N
  Articulators   Dental And Oral
  Floss, Dental   Dental And Oral
  Pick, Massaging   Dental And Oral
  Toothbrush, Manual   Dental And Oral

L.D. TECHNOLOGY, LLC 305-777-0336
100 N. Biscayne Boulevard, Miami, FL 33132
FDA Number: 3006146787
  Biofeedback Device   Cns/Neurology

L.J. GREINER & SONS, INC. 973-977-9441
63-69 Danforth Avenue, Paterson, NJ 07501
FDA Number: 2247666   *Fax:* 973-278-9766
E-mail: cscllc@aol.com
Medical Products Sales Volume: $100,000
Year Founded: 1978
Total Employees: 2
Ownership: Private
Produces/Sells CE-marked Devices: N
Distribution: Exclusive Distributor
General Admin.: Mr. Lothar J. Greiner/President
Finance: Mr. Michael E. Greiner/Vice President, Treasurer
  Eye, Artificial, Non-Custom   Ophthalmology

L.L. DENTAL 541-822-3839
91780 Mill Creek Rd., Blue River, OR 97413
FDA Number: 2918321
  Syringe Unit, Air And/Or Water   Dental And Oral

L.P. SYSTEMS CORP. 718-805-6926
116-08 Myrtle Ave., Suite 330, Richmond Hill, NY 11418
FDA Number: 2435083
  Epilator, High-Frequency, Needle-Type   Surgery

L.P.A. MEDICAL, INC.
460 Desrochers,
Vanier, QUEBE G1M 1 Canada
800-663-4863
418-681-1313
FDA Number: 9680035   *Fax:* 418-681-4488
E-mail: lpa@lpamedical.com
Web site: lpa@lpamedical.com
Year Founded: 1989
Total Employees: 25   *Marketing Staff:* 4   *Sales Staff:* 46
Ownership: Private
Produces/Sells CE-marked Devices: N
Federal Procurement Eligibility: Small Business
Distribution: Manufacturer Through Manufacturer Reps, Exclusive Distributor

LA CALHENE
1325 Field Avenue S., PO Box 567, Rush City, MN 55069
320-358-4713
FDA Number: n/a   *Fax:* 320-358-3549
E-mail: info@lacalhene.com
Web site: www.lacalhene.com
Medical Products Sales Volume: $6,000,000
Annual Revenue: $5-$10 Million
Year Founded: 1984
Total Employees: 45   *Marketing Staff:* 2   *Sales Staff:* 5
Ownership: Brooks-PRI Automation, Inc.
Stock Symbol: GETIB
Quality System Registration Information: ISO9001
Produces/Sells CE-marked Devices: N
Federal Procurement Eligibility: Small Business
Distribution: Manufacturer Direct, Manufacturer Through Manufacturer Reps, Service Direct
General Admin.: Steve Jones/Chief Executive Officer
Mktg./Adv.: Paul Olson/Vice President Marketing & Sales

Cleanroom Equipment	General
Filter, Air	General
Laminar Air Flow Unit	General
Table, Other	General

LA CHARME LLC
45 Main St., Ste. 309 #22, Brooklyn, NY 11201
718-816-1347
FDA Number: 3005313219
Ownership: Private
Produces/Sells CE-marked Devices: N

Prosthesis, Breast, External	Surgery
Prosthesis, Breast, External, No Adhesive	Surgery

LA CROIX OPTICAL CO.
PO Box 2556, Batesville, AR 72501
870-698-1881
FDA Number: n/a   *Fax:* 870-698-1880
E-mail: lacroix@lacroixoptical.com
Web site: www.lacroixoptical.com
Annual Revenue: $5-$10 Million
Year Founded: 1947
Total Employees: 100   *Marketing Staff:* 1   *Sales Staff:* 2
Ownership: Private
Stock Symbol: ZIGO
Traded On: NASDAQ
Quality System Registration Information: ISO9002
Produces/Sells CE-marked Devices: N
Federal Procurement Eligibility: Small Business
Distribution: Manufacturer Direct
General Admin.: Raymond La Croix/President
Mktg./Adv.: Dennis Whitener/Manager Customer Services & Sales
         Karen Palmer/Marketing Officer
Production: Tom Cox/Manager Engineering

Lens, Other	Ophthalmology

LA LABS
7334 Hollister Ave., Suite H, Goleta, CA 93117
805-562-9889
FDA Number: 2030885
Ownership: Private
Produces/Sells CE-marked Devices: N

Viscoelastic Surgical Aid	Ophthalmology

LA MONT MEDICAL, INC.
555 D'Onofrio Drive,
Madison, WI 53719
888-452-6688
608-827-9000
FDA Number: 2134214   *Fax:* 608-827-8600
E-mail: inquiry@lamontmedical.com
Web site: www.lamontmedical.com
Medical Products Sales Volume: $400,000
Annual Revenue: $1-$5 Million
Year Founded: 1994
Total Employees: 4   *Marketing Staff:* 1   *Sales Staff:* 1
Ownership: Private
Stock Symbol: VITL
Traded On: NASDAQ
Quality System Registration Information: ISO9001
Produces/Sells CE-marked Devices: Y

LA MONT MEDICAL, INC.
888-452-6688 *(cont'd)*
Federal Procurement Eligibility: Small Business
Distribution: Manufacturer Direct, OEM, Service Direct, Exporter
General Admin.: Tony Montgomery/President, Chief Executive Officer
Mktg./Adv.: Peter Montgomery/Director New Product Development
Production: Ernest Jacobs/Director Quality Assurance

Electroencephalograph	Cns/Neurology

LA-Z-BOY INCORPORATED
1284 North Telegraph Rd., Monroe, MI 48162
734-242-1444
FDA Number: 1831673
Ownership: Private
Produces/Sells CE-marked Devices: N

Chair, Adjustable, Mechanical	Physical Med

LAB CORP OF AMERICA
1904 Alexander Drive, Durham, NC 27709-2652
800-833-3984
919-549-8263
FDA Number: n/a   *Fax:* 919-248-6462
E-mail: webmaster@labcorp.com
Medical Products Sales Volume: $3,600,000
Year Founded: 1971
Ownership: Lab Corp.
Stock Symbol: LH
Traded On: NYSE
Produces/Sells CE-marked Devices: N
Distribution: Manufacturer Direct
General Admin.: Thomas P. MacMahon/President
Mktg./Adv.: Stevan Stark/Vice President Sales

Contract Laboratory	General
Kit, Forensic Evidence	Pathology

LAB CORP.
430 S. Spring St., Burlington, NC 27215
800-222-7566
336-584-5171
FDA Number: n/a   *Fax:* 336-513-4121
E-mail: slaughl@labcorp.com
Web site: www.labcorp.com
Medical Products Sales Volume: $431,600,000
Annual Revenue: More than $100 Million
Year Founded: 1971
Total Employees: 20000
Ownership: Private
Stock Symbol: LH
Traded On: NYSE
Produces/Sells CE-marked Devices: N
Distribution: Manufacturer Direct
General Admin.: Thomas P. Mac Mahon/Chief Executive Officer
         Brad Smith/Executive Vice President
Mktg./Adv.: Steven Stark/Executive Vice President Sales
         Bill Bucher/Vice President Marketing
Production: Lesley Slaughter/Project Coord.

Contract Laboratory	General

Medical Product Subsidiaries (Listed Separately)
   Lab Corp Of America

LAB FABRICATORS COMPANY
1802 E. 47th St., Cleveland, OH 44103-2468
888-431-5444
216-431-5444
FDA Number: 9330065   *Fax:* 216-431-5447
E-mail: sales@labfabricators.com
Web site: www.labfabricators.com
Medical Products Sales Volume: $9,000,000,000
Annual Revenue: $1-$5 Million
Year Founded: 1956
Total Employees: 30   *Marketing Staff:* 2   *Sales Staff:* 3
Ownership: Private
Produces/Sells CE-marked Devices: N
Federal Procurement Eligibility: Small Business
Distribution: Manufacturer Direct, Exporter
General Admin.: Mr. Alex S. Moskovits/President
Mktg./Adv.: Ms. Carol A. Reynolds/Manager Advertising
         Mr. David M. Sajna/Manager International & National Sales
         Mr. David M. Sajna/Vice President Sales

Cabinet Casework, Laboratory	Chemistry
Cabinet, Laboratory	Chemistry
Hood, Fume	Toxicology
Hood, Fume, Chemical	Chemistry
Sink, Laboratory	Chemistry

LAB SAFETY SUPPLY, INC.
401 S. Wright Rd., Janesville, WI 53546-1368
800-356-0783
FDA Number: n/a   *Fax:* 800-543-9910
E-mail: custsvc@labsafety.com
Web site: www.labsafety.com
Year Founded: 1967
Ownership: W. W. GRAINGER, INC.
Produces/Sells CE-marked Devices: N
Distribution: Manufacturer Direct, Manufacturer Through Distributor, Manufacturer Through Manufacturer Reps

Cabinet Casework, General Purpose	General

LAB SAFETY SUPPLY, INC.　800-356-0783 *(cont'd)*

Cabinet Casework, Laboratory	Chemistry
Cabinet, Laboratory	Chemistry
Environmental Control System, Powered	Physical Med
Floor Mat, Antibacterial	General
Fountain, Eye Wash	Chemistry
Glove, Patient Examination	General
Glove, Surgical	General
Kit, First Aid	Surgery
Label, Bar Code	General
Labeling Equipment	General
Material, Training, Audiovisual	General
Monitor, Contamination, Environmental, Personal	General
Monitor, Gas, Atmospheric, Environmental	General
Safety Equipment, Laboratory	Chemistry
Shower, Emergency	Chemistry
Sign, Hospital	General
Support, Back	Orthopedics
Ventilator, Continuous (Respirator)	Anesthesiology

LAB VISION CORP.　510-991-2800
47777 Warm Springs Blvd., Fremont, CA 94539
FDA Number: 2953151

Immunohistochemistry Reagents And Kits	Pathology
Reagents, Specific, Analyte	Hematology
Stainer, Slide, Automated	Pathology

LAB-INTERLINK, INC.　705-860-1220
8950 J Street, Omaha, NE 68127
FDA Number: 1933725
Ownership: Private
Produces/Sells CE-marked Devices: N

Analyzer, Chemistry, Photometric, Discrete	Chemistry
Equipment, Laboratory, Gen. Purpose (Specific Medical Use)	Chemistry

LAB. & ENVIR. DIV., THE
See Invensys Process Systems

LABAC SYSTEMS
See Labac Systems, Inc.

LABAC SYSTEMS, INC.　800-445-4402　303-914-9914
4965 Kingston Street, Denver, CO 80239
FDA Number: n/a　　　*Fax:* 303-914-9880
Web site: www.falconrehab.com
Annual Revenue: $0-$1 Million
Year Founded: 1978
Total Employees: 100
Ownership: PHOENIX GROUP, THE
Produces/Sells CE-marked Devices: N
Federal Procurement Eligibility: Small Business
Distribution: Manufacturer Through Distributor

Accessories, Wheelchair	Physical Med
Wheelchair, Manual	Physical Med
Wheelchair, Powered	Physical Med

LABCHEM, INC.　412-826-5230
200 William Pitt Way, Pittsburgh, PA 15238
FDA Number: 2523642　　　*Fax:* 412-826-5234
E-mail: info@labchem.net
Web site: www.labchem.net
Year Founded: 1986
Total Employees: 40
Ownership: Private
Quality System Registration Information: ISO9001
Produces/Sells CE-marked Devices: N
Federal Procurement Eligibility: Small Business
General Admin.: Al Beraner/Chief Executive Officer
　　　Mike Semon/Executive Vice President
　　　A.G. Craske/President

Buffer, pH	Hematology
Diluent, Blood Cell	Hematology
Fluid, Bouin's	Pathology
Reagent, General Purpose	Pathology
Solution, Pathology, Formalin-Alcohol-Acetic Acid	Pathology
Solution, Pathology, Lugol's	Pathology
Stain, Carbol Fuchsin	Pathology
Stain, Eosin Y	Pathology
Stain, Giemsa	Pathology
Stain, Grams Iodine	Pathology
Stain, Hematology	Pathology
Stain, Methylene Blue	Pathology
Stain, Safranin	Pathology
Turbidimetric Method, Protein Or Albumin (Urinary)	Chemistry

LABCON NORTH AMERICA　800-227-1466　707-766-2100
3700 Lakeville Highway, Suite 200,
Petaluma, CA 94954
FDA Number: n/a　　　*Fax:* 707-766-2199
E-mail: info@labcon.com
Web site: www.labcon.com

LABCON NORTH AMERICA　800-227-1466 *(cont'd)*
Medical Products Sales Volume: $15,000,000
Annual Revenue: $10-$25 Million
Total Employees: 150　　*Marketing Staff:* 1　　*Sales Staff:* 6
Ownership: Helena Laboratories
Quality System Registration Information: ISO9001
Produces/Sells CE-marked Devices: N
Distribution: Manufacturer Through Distributor, Exporter
General Admin.: Jim Happ/President
Mktg./Adv.: Tom Moulton/Director Marketing
　　　Ed Browning/Director Product Development
　　　Tom Moulton/Director Product Development
　　　Aaron Barnard/Manager Customer Services & Sales
Production: Lily Remennik/Director Quality Assurance
　　　Diane Kavantjas/Manager Regulatory Affairs

Labware, Basic, Disposable	Chemistry
Pipette Tip	Chemistry
Pipette, Quantitative, Hematology	Hematology
Rack, Test Tube	Chemistry
Tube, Centrifuge	Chemistry
Tube, Culture	Microbiology
Vial, Hematology	General

LABCONCO CORP.　800-821-5525　816-333-8811
8811 Prospect Avenue,
Kansas City, MO 64132
FDA Number: 1928389　　　*Fax:* 816-363-0130
E-mail: labconco@labconco.com
Web site: www.labconco.com
Annual Revenue: $25-$50 Million
Year Founded: 1925
Total Employees: 220　　*Marketing Staff:* 10　　*Sales Staff:* 17
Ownership: Private
Quality System Registration Information: ISO9001
Produces/Sells CE-marked Devices: Y
Federal Procurement Eligibility: Small Business, GSA Contract
Distribution: Manufacturer Through Distributor
General Admin.: John McConnell/Chairman
　　　Stephen Gound/President
　　　Mike Wyckoff/Vice President Human Resources
Mktg./Adv.: Nancy Simonds/Coord. Advertising & Promotions
　　　Mr. Pat Anderson/Vice President International Marketing & Sales
　　　Debbie Kenny/Vice President Marketing
　　　Mr. Tom Schwaller/Vice President National Sales
Production: Dick Rosewicz/Vice President Manufacturing
Research: Mark Schmitz/Vice President Engineering & Development

Box, Glove	Microbiology
Cart, Instrument	Surgery
Cart, Multipurpose	General
Chair, Blood Drawing	General
Chloridimeter	Gastroenterology/Urology
Desiccator	Chemistry
Distilling Unit	Chemistry
Enclosure, Bacteriological Safety	Chemistry
Evaporator	Chemistry
Freeze Drying Equipment	Chemistry
Hood, Chemical	Chemistry
Hood, Fume	Toxicology
Hood, Isolation, Laminar Air Flow	General
Laminar Air Flow Unit, Fixed (Air Curtain)	Chemistry
Purification Filter, Water, Charcoal	Chemistry
Purification Filter, Water, Particulate	Chemistry
Tissue Culture Apparatus	Microbiology
Washer, Labware	Chemistry

LABCYTE INC.　1.408.747.2000
1190 Borregas Avenue, Sunnyvale, CA 94089
FDA Number: n/a　　　*Fax:* 1.408.747.2010
E-mail: info@labcyte.com
Web site: http://labcyte.com
Ownership: Private
Produces/Sells CE-marked Devices: N

LABEQUIP LTD.　905-475-5880
170 Shields Ct.,, Unit 2, Markham, ONT L3R9T5 Canada
FDA Number: n/a　　　*Fax:* 905-475-1231
E-mail: info@labequip.com
Web site: www.labequip.com
Year Founded: 1974
Total Employees: 25
Ownership: Private
Produces/Sells CE-marked Devices: N
Distribution: Service Direct, Exclusive Distributor

LABFUSIONS　909-592-8131
437 S. Cataract Ave., Suite 5, San Dimas, CA 91773-2979
FDA Number: n/a
Annual Revenue: $0-$1 Million

LABFUSIONS 909-592-8131 (cont'd)
Ownership: Keane Inc.
Produces/Sells CE-marked Devices: N
Distribution: Manufacturer Direct
Computer, Clinical Laboratory — Chemistry

LABNET INTERNATIONAL 888-522-6381
P.O. Box 841, Woodbridge, NJ 07095-0841 — 732-417-0700
FDA Number: n/a
E-mail: labnet@labnetlink.com
Web site: www.labnetlink.com
Annual Revenue: $10-$25 Million
Ownership: Private
Produces/Sells CE-marked Devices: Y
Federal Procurement Eligibility: Small Business
Distribution: Manufacturer Through Distributor, Manufacturer Through Manufacturer Reps, Importer, Exporter
Pipette — Chemistry
Service, Import/Export — General
Shaker, Waterbath — Chemistry

LABO AMERICA, INC. 510-445-1257
920 Auburn Ct., Fremont, CA 94538
FDA Number: n/a — Fax: 510-991-9862
E-mail: sales@laboamerica.com
Web site: www.laboamerica.com
Ownership: Private
Quality System Registration Information: ISO9000; ISO9001
Produces/Sells CE-marked Devices: Y
Federal Procurement Eligibility: Minority Owned, Female Owned
Distribution: Manufacturer Through Distributor, Exclusive Distributor
Immunofluorescence Equipment — Immunology
Microscope — Hematology
Microscope, Fluorescence/U.V. — Pathology
Microscope, Inverted Stage, Tissue Culture — Pathology
Microscope, Laboratory, Optical — Microbiology
Microscope, Light — Pathology
Microscope, Phase Contrast — Pathology
Microscope, Tissue Culture — Microbiology

LABORATOIRE M.P. LANGELIER INC. 450.467.0762
675 Laurier Blvd., Rte. 116, Beloeil, QUE J3G-4J1 Canada
FDA Number: n/a — Fax: 450.467.4109
E-mail: info@labmpl.com
Web site: www.labmpl.com
Year Founded: 1960
Ownership: Private
Produces/Sells CE-marked Devices: N
Distribution: Manufacturer Direct, Exclusive Distributor, Importer

LABORATOIRE MAT INC. 800-890-8666
610 Adanac St., Beauport, QUE G1C-7B7 Canada — 418-660-8666
FDA Number: n/a — Fax: 418-660-8998
E-mail: labmat@labmat.com
Year Founded: 1979
Total Employees: 25
Ownership: Private
Produces/Sells CE-marked Devices: N
Distribution: Manufacturer Direct, Exclusive Distributor

LABORATOIRE POULIOT INC. 800-363-6172
2990 chemin Ste-Foy, — 418-652-0100
Sainte-Foy, QUE G1X-1 Canada
FDA Number: n/a — Fax: 418-652-7115
Year Founded: 1968
Total Employees: 25
Ownership: Private
Produces/Sells CE-marked Devices: N
Distribution: Manufacturer Direct

LABORATORIOS JALOMA, S.A. DE C.V. 3-617-5010
Aquiles Serdan No. 438, Guadalajara, Jalisco Mexico
FDA Number: 9616518
Bandage, Elastic — General
Gauze/sponge, Nonresorbable For External Use — Surgery

LABORATORY CORPORATION OF AMERICA 336-584-5171
358 South Main St., Burlington, NC 27215
FDA Number: n/a — Fax: 336-436-1569
Web site: https://www.labcorp.com
Total Employees: 28000
Ownership: Private
Produces/Sells CE-marked Devices: N
General Admin.: Mr. David King/Chairman, Chief Executive Officer
Ms. Lidia Fonseca/Chief Information Officer
Dr. Mark Brecher/Chief Medical Officer, Vice President
Mr. James Boyle/Chief Operating Officer, Executive Vice President

LABORATORY CORPORATION OF AMERICA 336-584-5171
(cont'd)
Dr. Andrew Conrad/Chief Scientific Officer & Executive Vice President

LABORATORY DISPOSABLE PRODUCTS 973-335-2966
PO Box 2239, Wayne, NJ 07474-2239
FDA Number: n/a — Fax: 973-335-2466
E-mail: mail@labdisposable.com
Web site: www.labdisposable.com
Annual Revenue: $0-$1 Million
Ownership: Private
Produces/Sells CE-marked Devices: N
Federal Procurement Eligibility: Female Owned
Distribution: Manufacturer Through Distributor
Labware, Basic, Disposable — Chemistry

LABORATORY ENVIRONMENT SUPPORT SERVICES
See Laboratory Environment Support Systems, Inc.

LABORATORY ENVIRONMENT SUPPORT 800-621-6404
SYSTEMS, INC.
7755 E. Evans, Scottsdale, AZ 85260 — 480-951-0911
FDA Number: n/a — Fax: 480-951-4456
E-mail: admin@lessinc.net
Web site: www.lessinc.net
Medical Products Sales Volume: $800,000
Annual Revenue: $1-$5 Million
Year Founded: 1982
Total Employees: 17 — Marketing Staff: 2 — Sales Staff: 5
Ownership: Private
Quality System Registration Information: ISO9002
Produces/Sells CE-marked Devices: Y
Federal Procurement Eligibility: Small Business, VA Contract
Distribution: Service Direct, Importer, Exporter
General Admin.: Jim Westhoff/President, Chief Executive Officer
Production: Corky Harbison/Director Customer Services
Dave Westhoff/Vice President Operations
Finance: Nancy Bill/Chief Financial Officer
Cuvette, Spectrophotometer — Chemistry
Cuvette, Thermostated — Chemistry
Service, Used Equipment — General

LABORATORY PRODUCTS CO. INC.
See Pml Microbiologicals

LABORATORY TECHNOLOGIES, INC. 800-542-1123
43 W 900 Rte. 64, Maple Park, IL 60151 — 630-365-1000
FDA Number: n/a — Fax: 630-365-9687
E-mail: customerservice@labtechinc.com
Web site: www.labtechinc.com
Annual Revenue: $1-$5 Million
Year Founded: 1983
Ownership: Private
Produces/Sells CE-marked Devices: Y
Federal Procurement Eligibility: Small Business
Distribution: Manufacturer Direct, Manufacturer Through Distributor, Manufacturer Through Manufacturer Reps, Exporter
ATP Release (Luminescence) — Hematology
Counter, Gamma, General Use — Toxicology
Decontamination Kit — Surgery
Reagent, Calibration — General
Solution, Antibacterial Cleaner — General

LABORIE MEDICAL TECHNOLOGIES INC. 888-522-6743
6415 Northwest Dr., Units 7-14, — 905-612-1170
Mississauga, ONT L4V-1 Canada
FDA Number: n/a — Fax: 905-612-0481
E-mail: igoping@laborie.ca
Web site: www.laborie.com
Year Founded: 1977
Total Employees: 50 — Marketing Staff: 4
Ownership: Private
Quality System Registration Information: ISO9000; ISO9001
Produces/Sells CE-marked Devices: Y
Distribution: Manufacturer Direct

LABOTIX AUTOMATION INC. 800-661-5229
2097 Whittington Drive Unit B, — 705-876-1220
Peterborough, ONT K9J 6 Canada
FDA Number: n/a — Fax: 705-876-1499
E-mail: info@labotix.com
Web site: www.labotix.ca
Year Founded: 1990
Ownership: Private
Produces/Sells CE-marked Devices: N
Distribution: Manufacturer Direct, Exporter

LABRON MOBILITY AIDS LTD.   604-270-1117
8385 Saint George St., Vancouver, BC V5X-4P3 Canada
FDA Number: n/a   *Fax:* 604-270-1147
E-mail: oh_systems@bc.sympatico.ca
Year Founded: 1981
Total Employees: 10
Ownership: Private
Produces/Sells CE-marked Devices: N
Distribution: Manufacturer Direct, Exclusive Distributor, Importer

LABSPHERE, INC.   603-927-4266
231 Shaker St., North Sutton, NH 03260-9986
FDA Number: n/a   *Fax:* 603-927-4694
E-mail: blai@labsphere.com
Web site: www.labsphere.com
Medical Products Sales Volume: $66,600,000
Annual Revenue: $50-$100 Million
Year Founded: 1979
Total Employees: 75   *Marketing Staff:* 1   *Sales Staff:* 12
Ownership: X-Rite, Inc.
Stock Symbol: xrit
Traded On: NASDAQ
Quality System Registration Information: ISO9001
Produces/Sells CE-marked Devices: Y
Distribution: Manufacturer Direct, Manufacturer Through Manufacturer Reps, OEM
General Admin.: Tim Kardish/General Manager
Mktg./Adv.: Greg McKee/Manager Product Marketing
 Fred Conroy/Manager Regional Sales
 Hugh Convery/Manager Regional Sales
 Richard Corbyn/Manager Sales
 Kenneth Johnson/Vice President Sales
Production: Bill Miller/Director Quality Assurance
 Chris Donnelly/Manager Customer Services
 Blaine Flores/Vice President Operations
Research: Dante D'Amato/Vice President Research & Development

Accessories, Laser	General
Camera, Other	General
Camera, Video, Endoscopic	General
Photometer	Chemistry
Photometer, Reflectance	Chemistry
Radiometer, Laser	General
Service, Device Coating, Protective	General
Spectrometer, Infrared	Chemistry
Spectrophotometer, Infrared	Chemistry
Spectrophotometer, U.V./Visible	Chemistry
Standard/Control, All Types	Chemistry

LABSYSTEMS
See Thermo Fisher Scientific - Laboratory Equipment Division Headquarters

LABTHERMICS TECHNOLOGIES   217-351-7722
701 Devonshire Dr., Champaign, IL 61820-7328
FDA Number: n/a   *Fax:* 217-351-7705
E-mail: johnston@labthermics.com
Web site: www.labthermics.com
Annual Revenue: $1-$5 Million
Total Employees: 20   *Marketing Staff:* 4   *Sales Staff:* 5
Ownership: Private
Produces/Sells CE-marked Devices: Y
Federal Procurement Eligibility: Small Business
Distribution: Manufacturer Direct, Manufacturer Through Manufacturer Reps, OEM, Exporter
General Admin.: Peter Taylor/Chief Executive Officer
 Melissa Bilentschuk/Chief Financial Officer, Treasurer
 Ronald Johnston/President
 Robin Ruhlan/Vice President, General Manager
Mktg./Adv.: Eric Landau/Vice President Business Development
Production: David Blight/Director Operations
 David Blight/Vice President Manufacturing
Research: Jeff Kouzmanoff/Vice President Research & Development

Gel, Ultrasonic Coupling	Physical Med
Hyperthermia Unit, Microwave	Radiology
System, Cancer Treatment, Hyperthermia, RF/Microwave	Radiology
Thermometer, Electronic, Continuous	General
Ultrasound, Hyperthermia, Cancer Treatment	Radiology

LABTICIAN OPHTHALMICS, INC.   800-265-8391
            905-829-0055
2140 Winston Park Dr., Unit 6,
Oakville, ONTAR L6H 5 Canada
FDA Number: 9612327   *Fax:* 905-829-0056
E-mail: info@labtician.com
Web site: www.labtician.com
Year Founded: 1988
Total Employees: 25
Ownership: Private
Quality System Registration Information: ISO9001
Produces/Sells CE-marked Devices: Y
Federal Procurement Eligibility: Small Business

LABTICIAN OPHTHALMICS, INC.   800-265-8391 *(cont'd)*
Distribution: Manufacturer Direct, Manufacturer Through Distributor, OEM, Exclusive Distributor, Importer, Exporter

LABTRONICS, INC.   519-767-1061
546 Governors Rd, Guelph, ONT N1K-1E3 Canada
FDA Number: n/a   *Fax:* 519-836-4431
E-mail: sales@labtronics.com
Web site: www.labtronics.com
Total Employees: 42   *Marketing Staff:* 3   *Sales Staff:* 6
Ownership: Private
Produces/Sells CE-marked Devices: N
Federal Procurement Eligibility: Small Business
Distribution: Manufacturer Direct, Exporter

LABWORLD, INC.   800-447-2428
471 Page St., Bldg 4, Stoughton, MA 02072   781-341-1733
FDA Number: n/a   *Fax:* 781-341-3732
E-mail: markl@labworld1.com
Web site: www.labworld1.com
Annual Revenue: $5-$10 Million
Total Employees: 10
Ownership: Labworld, Inc.
Produces/Sells CE-marked Devices: Y
Distribution: Exclusive Distributor
General Admin.: David Klayman/Chief Executive Officer
 Mark Levine/Vice President, General Manager
Mktg./Adv.: Mark Levine/Director Marketing
 Mark Levine/Manager International & National Sales

Analyzer, Chemistry, Micro	Chemistry
Service, Used Equipment	General

LAC MAC, LTD.   519-432-2616
425 Rectory St, London N5W 3W5 Canada
FDA Number: 8022129

Dress, Surgical	Surgery
Gown, Surgical	Surgery
Suit, Surgical	Surgery

LAC-MAC LTD.   519-432-2616
847 Highbury Ave. N, Building 2 É_,   Canada
, Londo ONT ON N5Y 5B8
FDA Number: N   *Fax:* 888.452.2622
E-mail: Guy Spence/VP Mktg.
Web site: gspence@mail.lac-mac.com
Medical Products Sales Volume: $130
Total Employees: 519-432
Ownership: I
Stock Symbol: N
Federal Procurement Eligibility: Small Business
Distribution: Manufacturer Through Distributor

LACEY MANUFACTURING CO., LLC   203-336-0121
1146 Barnum Avenue, PO Box 5156, Bridgeport, CT 06610-0156
FDA Number: 1218017   *Fax:* 203-336-1774
E-mail: laceysales@laceymfg.com
Web site: www.laceymfg.com
Year Founded: 1921
Total Employees: 311   *Marketing Staff:* 2   *Sales Staff:* 3
Ownership: Precision Engineered Products, LLC
Quality System Registration Information: ISO9001
Produces/Sells CE-marked Devices: Y
Distribution: Manufacturer Direct
General Admin.: Ken Lisk/President
Mktg./Adv.: Mr. Matt Oravetz/Manager Marketing & Sales
Production: Craig Mikita/Director Manufacturing
 Jim Rodgers/Manager Regulatory Affairs

Cleanroom Equipment	General
Contract Manufacturing	General
Contract Packaging	General
Equipment/Service, Quality Control	General
Labeling Equipment	General
Molding, Injection	General
Service, Engineering/Design	General
Stapler, Surgical	Surgery

LACLEDE PROFESSIONAL PRODUCTS, INC
See Laclede, Inc.

LACLEDE RESEARCH LABORATORY, INC.
See Laclede, Inc.

LACLEDE, INC.   877-522-5333
2103 E. University Dr., Rancho Dominguez, CA 90220
FDA Number: 2022474
Web site: www.laclede.com
Annual Revenue: $10-$25 Million
Ownership: Private
Produces/Sells CE-marked Devices: N
Federal Procurement Eligibility: Small Business

LACLEDE, INC.   877-522-5333 (cont'd)

Distribution: Manufacturer Through Distributor

Adhesive, Dental	Dental And Oral
Dentifrice	Dental And Oral
Saliva, Artificial	Dental And Oral
Toothbrush, Manual	Dental And Oral

LACRIMEDICS   800-367-8327

P.O. Box 1209, 9 Hope Lane,   **360-376-7095**
Eastsound, WA 98245

FDA Number: 2024818   *Fax:* 360-376-7085
E-mail: info@lacrimedics.com
Web site: www.lacrimedics.com
Annual Revenue: $1-$5 Million
Total Employees: 12   *Marketing Staff:* 2   *Sales Staff:* 4
Ownership: HERRICK FAMILY L.P.
Quality System Registration Information: ISO9001
Produces/Sells CE-marked Devices: Y
Federal Procurement Eligibility: Small Business
Distribution: Manufacturer Direct, Manufacturer Through Distributor, Manufacturer Through Manufacturer Reps, Exporter
General Admin.: Janice Meyers/Vice President Human Resources
    Brian Logan/Vice President, General Manager
Mktg./Adv.: Gordon McGilton/Director Product Development
    David Wamsley/Manager National Sales

Cannula, Lacrimal (Eye)	Ophthalmology
Dilator, Lacrimal	Ophthalmology
Forceps, Ophthalmic	Ophthalmology
Plug, Punctum	Ophthalmology
Syringe, Ophthalmic	Ophthalmology

LACRIMEDICS, INC.   360-376-7095

#9 Hope Lane, Eastsound, WA 98245

FDA Number: 2024818

Implant, Collagen (Non-Aesthetic Use)	Surgery
Plug, Punctum	Ophthalmology

LACT-AID INTERNATIONAL   866-866-1239

PO Box 1066, Athens, TN 37371-1066   **423-744-9090**

FDA Number: n/a   *Fax:* 423-744-9116
E-mail: orders@lact-aid.com
Web site: www.lact-aid.com
Medical Products Sales Volume: $130,000
Year Founded: 1971
Total Employees: 2
Ownership: Private
Produces/Sells CE-marked Devices: N
Federal Procurement Eligibility: Small Business
Distribution: Manufacturer Direct
General Admin.: J. R. Avery/President
Mktg./Adv.: J. L. Avery/Vice President Marketing & Sales
Production: J. L. Avery/Vice President Manufacturing

Kit, Feeding, Pediatric (Enteral)	General

LACTONA CORP.

See Univac Dental Company

LACTONA CORPORATION   1 - 888 - 522 -

1669 School Road, P.o. Box 428,   **215-692-9000**
Hatfield, PA 19440

FDA Number: 2522258   *Fax:* 1 - 215 - 215 -
E-mail: lactona@comcast.net
Ownership: Private
Produces/Sells CE-marked Devices: N

Floss, Dental	Dental And Oral
Teeth, Artificial, Backing And Facing	Dental And Oral
Toothbrush, Manual	Dental And Oral

LADIES FIRST, INC.   800-497-8285

P.O. Box 4400, Salem, OR 97302   **503-363-3980**

FDA Number: n/a   *Fax:* 503-363-1985
E-mail: info@ladiesfirst.com
Web site: www.ladiesfirst.com
Year Founded: 1990
Ownership: Private
Produces/Sells CE-marked Devices: N
Federal Procurement Eligibility: Small Business, Female Owned
Distribution: Manufacturer Direct, Manufacturer Through Distributor
General Admin.: Linda Jackson/President
Mktg./Adv.: Julie Harris/Director Marketing

Brassiere, Surgical	Surgery
Prosthesis, Breast, External	Surgery

LAERDAL MEDICAL CORPORATION   800-227-1143

167 Myers Corners Rd., PO Box 1840,   **845-297-7770**
Wappingers Falls, NY 12590

FDA Number: 2425852   *Fax:* 845-298-4555
Web site: www.laerdal.com

LAERDAL MEDICAL CORPORATION   800-227-1143 (cont'd)

Total Employees: 200   *Marketing Staff:* 16   *Sales Staff:* 50
Ownership: Private
Quality System Registration Information: ISO9001
Produces/Sells CE-marked Devices: N
Federal Procurement Eligibility: Small Business
Distribution: Manufacturer Direct, Manufacturer Through Distributor, Manufacturer Through Manufacturer Reps, OEM, Service Direct
General Admin.: W. Clive Patrickson/President, Chief Executive Officer
Mktg./Adv.: George Walls/Director Product Development
    Dan Preniszni/Manager Corporate Communications
    Bill Lyon/Vice President Marketing & Sales
Production: Eileen Cranney/Manager Materials
    Ron Weyhrauch/Manager Regulatory Affairs
    John Kuphal/Vice President Regulatory Affairs

Aspirator, Emergency Suction	General
Defibrillator, Battery-Powered	Cardiovascular
Defibrillator/Monitor, Battery-Powered	Cardiovascular
Fixation Device, Spinal (External)	Orthopedics
Kit, Emergency, Cardiopulmonary Resuscitation	General
Mask, Gas, Anesthesia	Anesthesiology
Mask, Other	General
Mask, Oxygen, Non-Rebreathing	Anesthesiology
Resuscitator, Emergency Oxygen	Dental And Oral
Resuscitator, Pulmonary, Manual (Demand Valve)	General
Simulator, ECG	Cardiovascular
Training Manikin, CPR (Resuscitation)	General
Training Manikin, Intravenous Arm	General
Training Manikin, Other	General

LAFAYETTE DENTAL LAB., INC.   765-447-9341

2211 South St., PO Box 5479, Lafayette, IN 47904-2968

FDA Number: n/a   *Fax:* 765-447-9343
Annual Revenue: $0-$1 Million
Ownership: Private
Produces/Sells CE-marked Devices: N
Federal Procurement Eligibility: Small Business
Distribution: Manufacturer Direct
General Admin.: Joe Rock/Owner
    Randy Jackson/Owner
    Rick Jackson/Owner

Denture, Plastic, Teeth	Dental And Oral
Prosthesis, Dental	Dental And Oral

LAFAYETTE INSTRUMENT COMPANY   800-428-7545

3700 Sagamore Pkwy., PO Box 5729,   **765-423-1505**
Lafayette, IN 47903

FDA Number: 1816267   *Fax:* 765-423-4111
E-mail: info@lafayetteinstrument.com
Web site: www.lafayetteinstrument.com
Medical Products Sales Volume: $5,100,000
Annual Revenue: $1-$5 Million
Year Founded: 1947
Total Employees: 53   *Marketing Staff:* 2   *Sales Staff:* 9
Ownership: Private
Quality System Registration Information: ISO9001
Produces/Sells CE-marked Devices: Y
Federal Procurement Eligibility: Small Business
Distribution: Manufacturer Direct, Manufacturer Through Distributor, Manufacturer Through Manufacturer Reps, Exclusive Distributor, Importer, Exporter
General Admin.: Sheryl Cohen/Manager Human Resources
    Roger B. McClellan/President, Chief Executive Officer
Mktg./Adv.: Chris Fausett/Vice President Marketing & Sales
    Terry Echard/Vice President Sales
Production: Todd Hooker/Manager Materials
    Terry Echard/Manager Regulatory Affairs
    Mike Greene/Vice President Manufacturing
Research: Mark Lane/Director Research & Development

Biofeedback Device	Cns/Neurology
Chart, Anatomical Training	General
Dynamometer, Grip-Strength (Squeeze)	Anesthesiology
Esthesiometer	Cns/Neurology
Exerciser, Other	Physical Med
Goniometer, Orthopedic	Orthopedics
Isokinetic Testing And Evaluation System	Physical Med
Monitor, Spine Curvature	Physical Med

LAFAYETTE INSTRUMENT COMPANY   800-428-7545

3700 Sagamore Pkwy. North, PO Box 5729,   **765-423-1505**
Lafayette, IN 47903

FDA Number: 1816267   *Fax:* 765-423-4111
E-mail: sales@lafayetteinstrument.com
Web site: www.lafayetteinstrument.com
Ownership: Private
Produces/Sells CE-marked Devices: N
General Admin.: Mr. Roger McClellan/President, General Manager
    Mr. Terry Echard/Vice President
Mktg./Adv.: Mr. Chris Fausett/Vice President Sales

MANUFACTURER PROFILES

LAFAYETTE INSTRUMENT COMPANY   800-428-7545 *(cont'd)*
Production: Mr. Brent Smitley/Manager Engineering
        Mr. Mike Greene/Manager Operations
  Goniometer, Non-Powered   Orthopedics

LAGUNA TETRIX, INC.
See CYBEX INTERNATIONAL, INC.

LAKE REGION MANUFACTURING, INC.   952-448-5111
340 Lake Hazeltine Dr., Chaska, MN 55318-1034
FDA Number: 2126666
E-mail: mktgsales@lakergn.com   *Fax:* 952-448-7012
Web site: www.lakergn.com
Year Founded: 1947
Ownership: Private
Quality System Registration Information: ISO9001
Produces/Sells CE-marked Devices: N
Distribution: OEM, Exclusive Distributor
General Admin.: Joseph Fleischhacker/Chief Executive Officer
        Mark Fleischhacker/President, Chief Operating Officer
Mktg./Adv.: John Schreiner/Director Product Development
        Tom Kleist/Vice President Marketing & Sales
Production: Jim Klosterman/Director Quality Assurance & Regulatory Affairs
  Cable   Physical Med
  Contract Manufacturing   General
  Guide, Wire, Angiographic (And Accessories)   Cns/Neurology
  Guidewire   Cardiovascular
  Lead, Pacemaker (Catheter)   Cardiovascular
  Lead, Pacemaker, Implantable Endocardial   Cardiovascular
  Lead, Pacemaker, Implantable Myocardial   Cardiovascular
  Phacoemulsification System   Ophthalmology

LAKE SHORE CRYOTRONICS, INC.   614-891-2243
575 McCorkle Blvd., Westerville, OH 43082
FDA Number: 7000226
E-mail: sales@lakeshore.com   *Fax:* 614-818-1600
Web site: www.lakeshore.com
Medical Products Sales Volume: $9,000,000
Year Founded: 1968
Total Employees: 110
Ownership: Private
Quality System Registration Information: ISO9001
Produces/Sells CE-marked Devices: Y
Federal Procurement Eligibility: Small Business
Distribution: Manufacturer Direct
General Admin.: Dr. John Swartz/President, Chief Executive Officer
Mktg./Adv.: Michael Swartz/Director Product Development
Research: Philip Swinehart/Vice President Development
  Controller, Temperature, Other   General
  Gaussmeter   General
  Monitor, Temperature (Self-Contained)   General
  Power System, Isolated   General

LAKELAND DE MEXICO S.A. DE C.V.   516-981-9700
Rancho La Soledad Lote No. 2, Fracc. Poniente C.p.,
Celaya, Guajuato Mexico
FDA Number: 9617595
  Accessories, Apparel, Surgical   Surgery
  Cap, Surgical   Surgery
  Cover, Mattress   General
  Cover, Shoe, Operating Room   Surgery
  Drape, Surgical   Surgery
  Gown, Examination   General
  Gown, Isolation, Surgical   Surgery
  Gown, Patient   Surgery
  Gown, Surgical   Surgery
  Linen, Bed   General

LAKESHORE TECHNOLOGIES INC.   315-699-2975
7536 Murray Dr., Cicero, NY 13039
FDA Number: 1320194
  Imager, X-Ray, Solid State (Flat Panel/Digital)   Radiology
  Radiographic/Fluoroscopic Unit, Image-Intensified   Radiology

LAKESIDE MANUFACTURING CO., INC.   800-558-8565
                       414-902-6400
4900 W. Electric Avenue,
West Milwaukee, WI 53219
FDA Number: 7000580
E-mail: info@elakeside.com   *Fax:* 414-902-6446
Web site: www.elakeside.com
Medical Products Sales Volume: $8,900,000
Annual Revenue: $10-$25 Million
Total Employees: 120   *Marketing Staff:* 3   *Sales Staff:* 8
Ownership: Private
Produces/Sells CE-marked Devices: N
Federal Procurement Eligibility: Small Business, GSA Contract
Distribution: Manufacturer Through Distributor
General Admin.: Lawrence Moon/Chief Executive Officer
        Joseph Carlson/President

LAKESIDE MANUFACTURING CO., INC.   800-558-8565 *(cont'd)*
Mktg./Adv.: Mary Jo Vasarella/Coord. Marketing
        Bill Scallon/Director Marketing
        Alex Carayannopoulos/Director National Accounts
        Alex Carayannopoulos/Manager International & National Sales
        Alex Carayannopoulos/Manager Marketing
  Cart, Housekeeping   General
  Cart, Multipurpose   General
  Cart, Supply   General

LAKEVIEW CENTER, INC.   850-595-1330
1221 W. Lakeview Ave., Pensacola, FL 32501-1836
FDA Number: 1066310
E-mail: rwhite@bhcpns.org   *Fax:* 850-595-1340
Web site: elakeviewcenter.org
Medical Products Sales Volume: $100,000
Annual Revenue: $100-$500 Million
Year Founded: 1950
Total Employees: 1900   *Marketing Staff:* 3   *Sales Staff:* 1
Ownership: Baptist Health Care, Inc.
Produces/Sells CE-marked Devices: N
Federal Procurement Eligibility: Small Business
Distribution: Manufacturer Through Distributor
Production: Mr. Reuben White/Manager Production
        Mr. Richard Gilmartin/Vice President Services
  Wheelchair, Manual   Physical Med

LAMBRECHT, KARL CORP.   773-472-5442
4204 N. Lincoln Ave., Chicago, IL 60618-2902
FDA Number: 7000227
E-mail: sales@klccgo.com   *Fax:* 773-472-2724
Web site: www.klccgo.com
Medical Products Sales Volume: $3,500,000
Annual Revenue: $1-$5 Million
Total Employees: 28   *Marketing Staff:* 2   *Sales Staff:* 3
Ownership: Private
Produces/Sells CE-marked Devices: N
Federal Procurement Eligibility: Small Business
Distribution: Manufacturer Direct
General Admin.: Raymond Lambrecht/President
Mktg./Adv.: Raymond Lambrecht/Vice President Sales
Production: Alvin Lambrecht/Vice President Manufacturing
  Service, Engineering/Design   General

LAMICO, INC.   920-231-1672
474 Marion Rd., Oshkosh, WI 54901
FDA Number: 2182304
  Crutch   Physical Med

LAMINAR FLOW, INC.   800-553-FLOW
102 Richard Road, PO Box 2427,   215-672-0232
Warminster, PA 18974
FDA Number: 9200635
E-mail: info@laminarflowinc.com   *Fax:* 215-441-0426
Web site: www.laminarflowinc.com
Medical Products Sales Volume: $3,800,000
Annual Revenue: $10-$25 Million
Year Founded: 1969
Total Employees: 52   *Marketing Staff:* 3   *Sales Staff:* 6
Ownership: Private
Federal Procurement Eligibility: Small Business
Distribution: Manufacturer Direct, Manufacturer Through Distributor, Manufacturer Through Manufacturer Reps, Exclusive Distributor, Importer, Exporter
General Admin.: Anthony Diccianni/President
        Doreen Novi/Vice President Human Resources
        Eric Dicciani/Vice President, General Manager
  Desiccator   Chemistry
  Hood, Fume   Toxicology
  Hood, Isolation, Laminar Air Flow   General
  Laminar Air Flow Unit   General
  Laminar Air Flow Unit, Fixed (Air Curtain)   Chemistry
  Laminar Air Flow Unit, Mobile   Chemistry

LAMINEX, INC.   800-438-8850
9900 Brookford Street, Charlotte, NC 28273   704-679-4170
FDA Number: n/a   *Fax:* 704-679-8453
E-mail: info@laminex.com
Web site: www.laminex.com
Medical Products Sales Volume: $3,900,000
Total Employees: 30
Ownership: Private
Produces/Sells CE-marked Devices: N
Federal Procurement Eligibility: Small Business, GSA Contract
Distribution: Manufacturer Through Distributor, Service Direct
General Admin.: Tim Long/President
  Camera, Identification   General
  Cover, Film, X-Ray   Radiology

LAMOTTE CHEMICAL PRODUCTS COMPANY 800-344-3100
802 Washington Ave., Chestertown, MD 21620 410-778-3100
FDA Number: 3000303483   Fax: 410-778-6394
Ownership: Private
Produces/Sells CE-marked Devices: N
Nitroprusside, Ketones (Urinary, Non-Quantitative)   Chemistry

LAMOTTE CO. 800-344-3100
802 Washington Avenue, PO Box 329, 410-778-3100
Chestertown, MD 21620
FDA Number: n/a   Fax: 410-778-6394
E-mail: mkt@lamotte.com
Web site: www.lamotte.com
Annual Revenue: $10-$25 Million
Year Founded: 1919
Total Employees: 15   Marketing Staff: 7   Sales Staff: 8
Ownership: Thomas Scientific
Produces/Sells CE-marked Devices: N
Federal Procurement Eligibility: Small Business, GSA Contract
Distribution: Manufacturer Through Distributor, Manufacturer Through
Manufacturer Reps, OEM, Exclusive Distributor, Importer, Exporter
General Admin.: David La Motte/President
Mktg./Adv.: Richard La Motte/Director Marketing
            Margaret P. Hill/Manager Marketing
Buret	Chemistry
Colorimeter, General Use	Chemistry
Formaldehyde (Formalin, Formol)	Pathology
Meter, pH, Portable	Chemistry
Nephelometer	Chemistry
Strip, Test	Chemistry

LAMP TECHNOLOGY, INC. 800-533-7548
1645 Sycamore Avenue, 631-567-1800
Bohemia, NY 11716
FDA Number: n/a   Fax: 631-567-1806
E-mail: info@lamptech.com
Web site: www.lamptech.com
Medical Products Sales Volume: $2,900,000
Annual Revenue: $5-$10 Million
Year Founded: 1979
Total Employees: 15   Marketing Staff: 2   Sales Staff: 13
Ownership: Private
Federal Procurement Eligibility: Small Business, Female Owned, GSA Contract
Distribution: Manufacturer Direct, Manufacturer Through Distributor, Manufacturer
Through Manufacturer Reps, Service Direct, Importer, Exporter
General Admin.: Neal Shupak/President, Chief Executive Officer
Mktg./Adv.: Kevin McBrien/Director Marketing
Lamp, Endoscopic, Incandescent	Surgery
Lamp, Microscope	Pathology
Lamp, Other	General
Lamp, Surgical, Incandescent	Surgery
Lamp, Surgical, Xenon	Surgery

LAMPAC INTERNATIONAL LTD. 636-797-3659
230 North Lake Drive, Hillsboro, MO 63050
FDA Number: 1928036   Fax: 636-789-3582
E-mail: rdm@lampac.com
Web site: www.lampac.com
Medical Products Sales Volume: $650,000
Annual Revenue: $0-$1 Million
Year Founded: 1980
Total Employees: 2   Marketing Staff: 1
Ownership: Private
Produces/Sells CE-marked Devices: Y
Distribution: Service Direct, Exclusive Distributor, Importer, Exporter
General Admin.: Ruthven D. Maddox/President
Mktg./Adv.: Ruthven D. Maddox/Director Marketing
Blade, Scalpel	Surgery
Brush, Scrub, Operating Room	Surgery
Cannula, Nasal, Oxygen	Anesthesiology
Catheter, Balloon (Foley Type)	Surgery
Circuit, Breathing (W Connector, Adapter, Y Piece)	Anesthesiology
Cuff, Blood Pressure	Cardiovascular
Mask, Oxygen, Aerosol Administration	Anesthesiology
Mask, Surgical	Surgery
Scalpel, One-Piece (Knife)	Surgery
Service, Import/Export	General
Thermometer, Electronic	General
Thermometer, Mercury	General
Tube, Tracheal (Endotracheal)	Anesthesiology
Waste Disposal Unit, Sharps	General

LAMPIRE BIOLOGICAL LABORATORIES 215-795-2838
PO Box 270, Pipersville, PA 18947
FDA Number: 2531564   Fax: 215-795-0237
E-mail: lampire@lampire.com
Web site: www.lampire.com
Annual Revenue: $1-$5 Million

LAMPIRE BIOLOGICAL LABORATORIES 215-795-2838 (cont'd)
Year Founded: 1977
Total Employees: 60
Ownership: Private
Produces/Sells CE-marked Devices: N
Federal Procurement Eligibility: Small Business
Distribution: Manufacturer Direct
General Admin.: Gregory F. Krug/President, Chief Executive Officer
Cultured Animal And Human Cells	Pathology
Serum, Biological, General	Toxicology

LAMPIRE BIOLOGICAL LABORATORIES, INC. 215-795-2838
405 South Main St., Coopersburg, PA 18036
FDA Number: 2550014
Serum, Animal	Pathology

LANCER
See Covidien Lp

LANCER ORTHODONTICS, INC. 760-304-2705
253 Pawnee St., San Marcos, CA 92078
FDA Number: 2020397
Adhesive, Bracket And Conditioner, Resin	Dental And Oral
Band, Elastic, Orthodontic	Dental And Oral
Band, Preformed, Orthodontic	Dental And Oral
Bracket, Metal, Orthodontic	Dental And Oral
Cement, Dental	Dental And Oral
Driver, Band, Orthodontic	Dental And Oral
Face Bow	Dental And Oral
Headgear, Extraoral, Orthodontic	Dental And Oral
Material, Impression	Dental And Oral
Pliers, Orthodontic	Dental And Oral
Pusher, Band, Orthodontic	Dental And Oral
Retainer, Screw Expansion, Orthodontic	Dental And Oral
Spring, Orthodontic	Dental And Oral
Toothbrush, Manual	Dental And Oral
Tray, Impression	Dental And Oral
Tube, Orthodontic	Dental And Oral
Wax, Dental	Dental And Oral
Wire, Orthodontic	Dental And Oral

LANCER USA, INC. 800-332-1855
3543 State Rd 419, Winter Springs, FL 32708 407-327-8488
FDA Number: n/a   Fax: 407-327-1229
E-mail: sales@lancer.com
Web site: www.lancer.com
Annual Revenue: $5-$10 Million
Total Employees: 13   Marketing Staff: 2   Sales Staff: 5
Ownership: Private
Quality System Registration Information: ISO9002
Produces/Sells CE-marked Devices: Y
Federal Procurement Eligibility: Small Business
Distribution: Manufacturer Through Manufacturer Reps
General Admin.: Lore Cronin/Office Manager
            James T. Fry/President, Chief Executive Officer
Mktg./Adv.: Mike Martin/Manager National Sales
Production: Kevin Kyle/Manager Production Services
Washer, Labware	Chemistry
Washer/Disinfector	General

LANDAUER, INC. 800-323-8830
2 Science Road, Glenwood, IL 60425-1586 708-755-7000
FDA Number: 7000837   Fax: 708-755-7016
E-mail: custserv@landauerinc.com
Web site: www.landauerinc.com
Medical Products Sales Volume: $79,000,000
Annual Revenue: $50-$100 Million
Year Founded: 1954
Total Employees: 300   Sales Staff: 8
Ownership: Public
Stock Symbol: LDR
Traded On: NYSE
Produces/Sells CE-marked Devices: N
Federal Procurement Eligibility: Small Business
Distribution: Service Direct
General Admin.: William Saxelby/President, Chief Executive Officer
Mktg./Adv.: Inid Deneau/Manager Marketing
            Bill Megale/Manager National Sales
            Craig Yoder/Vice President Marketing
Dosimeter, Radiation	Radiology
Monitor, Gas, Atmospheric, Environmental	General
Monitor, Radiation	Radiology

LANDEC CORP. 650-306-1650
3603 Haven Ave., Menlo Park, CA 94025
FDA Number: n/a   Fax: 650-368-9818
E-mail: sskinner@landec.com
Web site: www.landec.com
Total Employees: 110
Ownership: Public

LANDEC CORP. 650-306-1650 (cont'd)
Stock Symbol: LNDC
Traded On: NASDAQ
Produces/Sells CE-marked Devices: N
Federal Procurement Eligibility: Small Business
General Admin.: Nicholas Tompkins/Chairman
    Gary T. Steele/President, Chief Executive Officer
Finance: Gregory S. Skinner/Chief Financial Officer, Vice President Finance
Laboratory Equipment, Ophthalmic	Ophthalmology
Occluder, Ophthalmic	Ophthalmology

Medical Product Subsidiaries (Listed Separately)
  Lifecore Biomedical, Inc.

LANDICE, INC. 800-LANDICE
111 Canfield Ave., Suite A1, Randolph, NJ 07869   **973-927-9010**
FDA Number: 2243082   Fax: 973-927-0630
E-mail: sales@landice.com
Web site: www.landice.com
Year Founded: 1968
Total Employees: 40   Sales Staff: 4
Ownership: Private
Produces/Sells CE-marked Devices: Y
Federal Procurement Eligibility: Small Business
Distribution: Exclusive Distributor, Exporter
General Admin.: Greg Savttiere/President
Mktg./Adv.: Chuck Alchermes/Director Marketing
    Chuck Alchermes/Director Sales
Treadmill, Powered	Physical Med

LANDON LENS MANUFACTURING CORP. 800-793-6687
301 East 69th St., New York, NY 10021   **212-348-4020**
FDA Number: 2434057   Fax: 212-348-4373
Ownership: Private
Produces/Sells CE-marked Devices: N
Lens, Spectacle/Eyeglasses, Non-Custom	Ophthalmology

LANG DENTAL MANUFACTURING CO., INC. 800-222-5264
175 Messner Drive, Wheeling, IL 60090   **847-215-6622**
FDA Number: 1417322   Fax: 847-215-6678
E-mail: dlang@langdental.com
Web site: www.langdental.com
Medical Products Sales Volume: $4,600,000
Annual Revenue: $1-$5 Million
Year Founded: 1929
Total Employees: 18   Marketing Staff: 1
Ownership: Private
Quality System Registration Information: ISO9002
Produces/Sells CE-marked Devices: Y
Federal Procurement Eligibility: Small Business, GSA Contract
Distribution: Manufacturer Through Distributor
General Admin.: David J. Lang/President, Chief Executive Officer
    Daniel W. Beck/Vice President, General Manager
Mktg./Adv.: Gladys Ferrer/Manager International & National Sales
Production: Joanne Lang/Director Quality Assurance
    Daniel W. Beck/Vice President Operations
Research: Chah Shen/Vice President Product Development
    Chah Shen/Vice President Research & Development
Base, Denture, Relining, Repairing, Rebasing, Resin	Dental And Oral
Coating, Filling Material, Resin	Dental And Oral
Cup, Denture	Dental And Oral
Curing Unit, Acrylic	Dental And Oral
Material, Impression Tray, Resin	Dental And Oral
Material, Tooth Shade, Resin	Dental And Oral

LANG HEARING INSTRUMENTS
See Argosy

LANGER BIOMECHANICS GROUP, INC.
See Langer, Inc.

LANGER, INC. 800-645-5520
450 Commack Road, Deer Park, NY 11729   **631-667-1200**
FDA Number: 2432963   Fax: 661-667-1203
E-mail: info@langerinc.com
Web site: www.langerbiomechanics.com
Medical Products Sales Volume: $35,200,000
Year Founded: 2001
Total Employees: 135   Marketing Staff: 4   Sales Staff: 2
Ownership: Private
Produces/Sells CE-marked Devices: N
Federal Procurement Eligibility: Small Business
Distribution: Exclusive Distributor
General Admin.: CPO Andrew H. Meyers/Chief Executive Officer
    CPO Andrew H. Meyers/President, Chief Executive Officer
    Steven Goldstein/Vice President
Mktg./Adv.: Linda Grassia/Manager Communications
Production: Tyrone Jackson/Manager Materials
Cushion, Foot	Orthopedics
Cushion, Other	General

LANGER, INC. 800-645-5520 (cont'd)
Orthosis, Other	Physical Med
Prosthesis, Foot Arch	Orthopedics
Splint, Other	Orthopedics
Support, Arch	Physical Med
Support, Foot	Orthopedics

LANGFORD IC SYSTEMS, INC. 520-745-6201
310 S. Williams Blvd., Suite 270, Tucson, AZ 85711
FDA Number: 3005480485
Washer, Cleaner, Automated, Endoscope	Gastroenterology/Urology

LANGLEY OPTICAL
See Duffens Optical

LANHERNE TECHNOLOGY LTD. 613-376-3100
4567 Bedford Rd., P.O. Box 410,
Sydenham, ONT K0H-2 Canada
FDA Number: n/a   Fax: 613-376-3102
E-mail: lobbrlt@adan.kingston.net
Year Founded: 1973
Total Employees: 10
Ownership: Private
Produces/Sells CE-marked Devices: N
Distribution: Manufacturer Direct

LANIER BUSINESS PRODUCTS, INC.
See Lanier Worldwide, Inc.

LANIER WORLDWIDE, INC. 800-727-1885
2300 Parklake Dr. N.E., Atlanta, GA 30345
FDA Number: n/a   Fax: 770-495-4199
E-mail: info@ricoh-usa.com
Web site: www.lanier.com
Total Employees: 10000   Marketing Staff: 25   Sales Staff: 3500
Ownership: HARRIS CORPORATION
Produces/Sells CE-marked Devices: N
Distribution: Manufacturer Through Distributor, Manufacturer Through Manufacturer Reps
General Admin.: Wes Cartell/Chief Executive Officer
    Harley Ostis/Director Human Resources
Mktg./Adv.: Susan Melum/Director Marketing
    Yvonne Jordan/Director Marketing Communications
    Charlie Cobb/Director Sales
Office Equipment	General
Office Product	General

LANSINOH LABORATORIES 800-292-4794
333 North Fairfax Street, Suite 400, Fairfax, VA 22314
FDA Number: 2032361   Fax: 865-481-0799
E-mail: customerservice@lansinoh.com
Web site: http://www.lansinoh.com
Ownership: Private
Produces/Sells CE-marked Devices: N
General Admin.: Mr. Richard Thorne/Chief Operating Officer
Lotion, Skin Care	General

LANTHEUS MEDICAL IMAGING 800-362-2668
331 Treble Cove Rd., Bldg. 200-2,   **978-671-8350**
Billerica, MA 01862
FDA Number: 1216602   Fax: 978-436-7501
E-mail: bi.webadmin@lantheus.com
Web site: www.lantheus.com
Ownership: Private
Produces/Sells CE-marked Devices: N
Amalgamator, Dental, AC-Powered	Dental And Oral
Calibrator Source, Nuclear Sealed	Radiology

LANTHEUS MEDICAL IMAGING, INC. 1-800-362-2668
331 Treble Cove Rd., Bldg. 200-2,   **978-667-9531**
N. Billerica, MA 01862
FDA Number: 1216602   Fax: 1-978-436-7501
E-mail: bi.webadmin@lantheus.com
Web site: www.lantheus.com
Year Founded: 1956
Ownership: Private
Produces/Sells CE-marked Devices: N
General Admin.: Don Kiepert/President, Chief Executive Officer
Mktg./Adv.: Mr. Peter Card/Vice President Corporate Development
    Mr. Robert Spurr/Vice President Marketing & Sales
Research: Dr. Simon Robinson/Vice President Research & Development
Finance: Mr. Robert Gaffey/Chief Financial Officer
Amalgamator, Dental, AC-Powered	Dental And Oral
Calibrator Source, Nuclear Sealed	Radiology

LANTISEPTIC
See Lantiseptic Division, Summit Industries, Inc.

LANTISEPTIC DIVISION, SUMMIT INDUSTRIES, INC.
800-241-6996

P.O. Box 7329, Marietta, GA 30065-0329 **770-590-0600**
FDA Number: n/a   Fax: 770-590-0714
E-mail: sdayal@summitinds.com
Web site: www.Lantiseptic.com
Annual Revenue: $10-$25 Million
Year Founded: 1920
Total Employees: 50   *Marketing Staff:* 4   *Sales Staff:* 25
Ownership: Private
Produces/Sells CE-marked Devices: N
Federal Procurement Eligibility: Small Business
Distribution: Manufacturer Through Distributor, Manufacturer Through Manufacturer Reps, Exporter
General Admin.: Mike Franchot/President
Mktg./Adv.: Carolyn Gray/Admin. Sales
    Mark Higgins/Director National Accounts
    Dan Brooks/Manager Advertising
    Mark Higgins/Manager Contract Sales
    Mark Higgins/Product & Sales Manager
    Phil Meyers/Vice President Sales
Production: Nancy Muzik/Director Quality Assurance & Regulatory Affairs
Purchasing: Ron Teat/Director Purchasing

Lotion, Skin Care	General

LANTZ DENTAL PROSTHETICS, INC.
419-866-1515

6490 Wheatstone Ct., Maumee, OH 43537
FDA Number: 3005703661
E-mail: lantzdental@gmail.com
Web site: www.lantzdental.comÉ_Z
Ownership: Private
Produces/Sells CE-marked Devices: N

Device, Anti-Snoring	Ear/Nose/Throat

LANX INC.
303-443-7500

390 Interlocken Crescent, Broomfield, CO 80021
FDA Number: 3004485144   Fax: 303-443-7501
E-mail: info@lanx.com
Web site: http://www.lanx.com
Year Founded: 2003
Ownership: Private
Produces/Sells CE-marked Devices: N

Appliance, Fixation, Spinal Interlaminal	Orthopedics
Appliance, Fixation, Spinal Intervertebral Body	Orthopedics
Device, Spinal Vertebral Body Replacement	Orthopedics
Intervertebral Fusion Device With Bone Graft, Cervical	Orthopedics
Orthosis, Fixation, Pedicle, Spinal	Orthopedics
Orthosis, Fixation, Spinal, Spondylolisthesis	Orthopedics

LANX, LLC
See Lanx Inc.

LAPROSTOP, LLC
858-705-3838

1845 Newport Avenue, San Diego, CA 92107
FDA Number: 3005867375

Cannula, Bronchial	Ear/Nose/Throat
Cannula, Surgical, General & Plastic Surgery	Surgery
Instrument, Manual, General Surgical	Surgery
Surgical Instrument, G-U, Manual	Gastroenterology/Urology
Surgical Instrument, Obstetric/Gynecologic, General	Obstetrics/Gynecology

LAR MFG., LLC.
727-846-7860

6828 Commerce Ave., Port Richey, FL 34668
FDA Number: 1064395
Ownership: Private
Produces/Sells CE-marked Devices: N

Bracket, Plastic, Orthodontic	Dental And Oral

LARADA SCIENCES INC.
801-533-5423

350 West 800 North, Suite 203, Salt Lake City, UT 84103
FDA Number: n/a   Fax: 801-355-5423
Web site: http://www.lousebuster.com
Year Founded: 1996
Ownership: Private
Produces/Sells CE-marked Devices: N
General Admin.: Mr. Larry Rigby/Chairman, Chief Executive Officer
    Mr. Randall Block/Chief Operating Officer
Mktg./Adv.: Ms. Marleen De Winter/Director Marketing

Detector/Remover, Lice	General

LARC INTERNATIONAL
See Integra Lifesciences Holdings Corp.

LARES RESEARCH
800-347-3289

295 Lockheed Avenue, Chico, CA 95973   **530-345-1767**
FDA Number: 2916440   Fax: 530-345-1870
E-mail: laser_sales_careers@laresdental.com
Web site: www.laresdental.com
Medical Products Sales Volume: $7,000,000

LARES RESEARCH
800-347-3289 *(cont'd)*

Annual Revenue: $10-$25 Million
Year Founded: 1956
Total Employees: 90   *Marketing Staff:* 1   *Sales Staff:* 7
Ownership: Private
Quality System Registration Information: ISO9000
Produces/Sells CE-marked Devices: N
Federal Procurement Eligibility: Small Business
Distribution: Manufacturer Direct, Manufacturer Through Distributor, Manufacturer Through Manufacturer Reps, OEM, Service Direct, Exporter
General Admin.: Craig Lares/President, Chief Executive Officer
Mktg./Adv.: Stanley Perkins/Manager Advertising
    Stanley Perkins/Vice President Marketing & Sales
Research: Jason Orgain/Vice President Research & Development
Finance: Richard Mounkes/Controller

Airbrush	Dental And Oral
Handpiece, Air-Powered, Dental	Dental And Oral
Handpiece, Fiberoptic	Dental And Oral
Laser, Dental	Dental And Oral
Light, Dental, Intraoral	Dental And Oral
Light, Fiberoptic, Dental	Dental And Oral
Purification System, Water	Gastroenterology/Urology

LARKOTEX COMPANY
800-972-3037

1002 Olive St., Texarkana, TX 75501-0449   **903-793-4647**
FDA Number: 1616494   Fax: 903-793-4650
Total Employees: 16
Ownership: Private
Federal Procurement Eligibility: Small Business
Distribution: Manufacturer Through Distributor
General Admin.: Fred R. Norton/President

Accessories, Traction	Physical Med
Accessories, Traction (Cart, Frame, Cord, Weight)	Orthopedics
Bedrail	General
Belt, Abdominal	Gastroenterology/Urology
Belt, Lumbosacral	Orthopedics
Belt, Rib (Support)	Orthopedics
Belt, Traction, Pelvic, Orthopedic	Orthopedics
Binder, Abdominal	General
Binder, Ankle	Orthopedics
Binder, Wrist	Orthopedics
Cane	Physical Med
Chair, Shower	General
Chair, With Casters	Physical Med
Collar, Cervical Neck	Orthopedics
Commode (Toilet)	General
Compress, Cold	General
Corset	Orthopedics
Crutch	Physical Med
Footstool, Non-Conductive	General
Halter, Head, Traction	Physical Med
Halter, Head, Traction, Orthopedic	Orthopedics
Immobilizer, Knee	Orthopedics
Orthosis, Cervical	Physical Med
Orthosis, Cervical-Thoracic, Rigid	Physical Med
Orthosis, Limb Brace	Physical Med
Orthosis, Lumbar	Physical Med
Orthosis, Lumbosacral	Physical Med
Orthosis, Other	Physical Med
Orthosis, Rib Fracture, Soft	Physical Med
Orthosis, Sacroiliac, Soft	Physical Med
Protector, Heel	General
Protector, Skin Pressure	General
Screen, Bedside	General
Sling, Arm	Physical Med
Splint, Abduction, Congenital Hip Dislocation	Physical Med
Splint, Clavicle	Physical Med
Splint, Denis Brown	Physical Med
Splint, Hand, And Component	Physical Med
Splint, Molded, Plastic	Orthopedics
Support, Abdominal	Physical Med
Support, Ankle	Orthopedics
Support, Arm	Physical Med
Support, Back	Orthopedics
Support, Clavicle	Orthopedics
Support, Elbow	Orthopedics
Support, Foot	Orthopedics
Support, Hand	Orthopedics
Support, Hernia	Gastroenterology/Urology
Support, Knee	Physical Med
Support, Leg	Physical Med
Support, Wrist	Physical Med
Tips And Pads, Cane, Crutch And Walker	Physical Med
Truss, Hernia (Belt)	Gastroenterology/Urology
Truss, Umbilical	Gastroenterology/Urology

LARSON MEDICAL PRODUCTS, INC.
614-235-9100

2844 Banwick Rd., Columbus, OH 43232
FDA Number: 1530561

Accelerator, Linear, Medical	Radiology

MANUFACTURER PROFILES

LARSON MEDICAL PRODUCTS, INC.   614-235-9100 (cont'd)
  Holder, Head, Radiographic   Radiology
  Orthosis, Moldable, Supportive, Skin Protective   Physical Med
  Restraint, Patient, Conductive   Anesthesiology
  Splint, Extremity, Non-Inflatable, External   Surgery
  Splint, Hand, And Component   Physical Med
  Splint, Nasal   Ear/Nose/Throat

LASALLE SCIENTIFIC INC.   519 824 7301
121 Malcolm Road, Guelph, ON N1K 1A8 Canada
FDA Number: n/a   *Fax:* 519 824 9576
E-mail: info@lasallescientific.com
Web site: www.lasallescientific.com
Year Founded: 1985
Total Employees: 10
Ownership: Private
Produces/Sells CE-marked Devices: N
Distribution: Exclusive Distributor

LASCHAL SURGICAL, INC.   800-352-7242
     914-949-8577
4 Baltusrol Dr., Purchase, NY 10577
FDA Number: 2431425   *Fax:* 914-683-3938
E-mail: service@laschalsurgical.com
Web site: www.laschalsurgical.com
Ownership: Private
Produces/Sells CE-marked Devices: N
  Forceps, General & Plastic Surgery   Surgery
  General Use Surgical Scissors   Surgery

LASCO DIAMOND PRODUCTS   800-621-4726
     818-882-2423
9950 Canoga Avenue, Unit A-8, PO Box 4657, Chatsworth, CA 91311
FDA Number: 2020356   *Fax:* 818-882-3550
E-mail: info@lascodiamond.com
Web site: www.lascodiamond.com
Medical Products Sales Volume: $800,000
Annual Revenue: $1-$5 Million
Year Founded: 1963
Total Employees: 12
Ownership: Private
Produces/Sells CE-marked Devices: N
Federal Procurement Eligibility: Small Business
Distribution: Manufacturer Direct, Manufacturer Through Distributor, Manufacturer Through Manufacturer Reps, OEM
General Admin.: Raymond A. Schultze/President
  Burr   Ear/Nose/Throat
  Burr, Dental   Dental And Oral
  Burr, Surgical, General & Plastic Surgery   Surgery
  Instrument, Diamond, Dental   Dental And Oral

LASE-R SHIELD, A BACOU USA COMPANY
See Lase-R Shield, A Bacou-Dalloz Company

LASE-R SHIELD, A BACOU-DALLOZ COMPANY   800-288-1164
     505-872-3400
7011 Prospect Pl. NE, Albuquerque, NM 87110
FDA Number: n/a   *Fax:* 505-872-3500
E-mail: arthur@highfiber.com
Web site: www.lase-rshield.com
Medical Products Sales Volume: $1,000,000
Annual Revenue: More than $100 Million
Total Employees: 3   *Marketing Staff:* 1   *Sales Staff:* 2
Ownership: BACOU USA
Quality System Registration Information: ISO9001
Produces/Sells CE-marked Devices: Y
Federal Procurement Eligibility: Small Business
Distribution: Manufacturer Direct
General Admin.: Will Arthur/General Manager
  Accessories, Laser   General
  Eyeglasses, Safety   Ophthalmology
  Goggles, Protective, Eye   Ophthalmology

LASER BAND   800-238-0870
     314 726.1060
120 S Central Ave, Ste. 450, St. Louis, MI 63105
FDA Number: n/a   *Fax:* 314-726-1028
E-mail: info@laserband.com
Ownership: Private
Produces/Sells CE-marked Devices: N

LASER DENTAL INNOVATIONS   877-753-5054
     408-832-7617
745 Dubanski Drive, San Jose, CA 95123
FDA Number: 3003610527   *Fax:* 408-528-3544
E-mail: howard_ldi@hotmail.com
Web site: http://www.lazertips.com
Annual Revenue: $0-$1 Million
Year Founded: 1999
Total Employees: 4   *Marketing Staff:* 1   *Sales Staff:* 1
Ownership: Private
Quality System Registration Information: ISO9000
Produces/Sells CE-marked Devices: N

LASER DENTAL INNOVATIONS   877-753-5054 (cont'd)
Federal Procurement Eligibility: Small Business
Distribution: Manufacturer Direct, Manufacturer Through Manufacturer Reps, OEM
  Laser, Surgical   Surgery

LASER ENDO TECHNIC, INC.
See Biolase Technology, Inc.

LASER FARE, INC.
See Lfi, Inc-Laser Fare, Inc.

LASER MEDICAL TECHNOLOGY, INC.
See Biolase Technology, Inc.

LASER NEUROTHERAPY DEVELOPMENT LABS, INC.   719-264-7632
3855 Interpark Drive, Colorado Springs, CO 80907
FDA Number: 3004828609   *Fax:* 719-548-8289
Ownership: Private
Produces/Sells CE-marked Devices: N
  Lamp, Infrared   Physical Med

LASER PROBE, INC.   315-797-4492
23 Wells Avenue, Utica, NY 13502
FDA Number: n/a   *Fax:* 315-797-0696
E-mail: sales@laserprobeinc.com
Web site: laserprobeinc.com
Annual Revenue: $1-$5 Million
Year Founded: 1992
Total Employees: 15
Ownership: Private
Produces/Sells CE-marked Devices: Y
Federal Procurement Eligibility: Small Business
Distribution: Manufacturer Direct
General Admin.: Charles Carpenter/President, Chief Executive Officer
Mktg./Adv.: Mark Proulx/Vice President Marketing & Sales
  Radiometer, Laser   General

LASER SOLUTIONS, INC.   800-230-7705
     908-696-0404
44 Bullion Road, Basking Ridge, NJ 07920
FDA Number: n/a   *Fax:* 908-696-0405
E-mail: info@lasersolutions.net
Web site: www.lasersolutions.net
Medical Products Sales Volume: $100,000
Annual Revenue: $0-$1 Million
Year Founded: 1992
Total Employees: 2
Ownership: Private
Produces/Sells CE-marked Devices: N
Federal Procurement Eligibility: Small Business
Distribution: Service Direct
IS: Richard Cook/Technical Director
  Service, Maintenance/Repair   General

LASER, INC.   800-367-5694
27831 Commercial Park Lane, Tomball, TX 77375
FDA Number: n/a   *Fax:* 281-255-3024
E-mail: laser@ams-source.com
Web site: www.ams-source.com
Medical Products Sales Volume: $1,000,000
Annual Revenue: $1-$5 Million
Total Employees: 5   *Marketing Staff:* 3   *Sales Staff:* 15
Ownership: Private
Produces/Sells CE-marked Devices: N
Federal Procurement Eligibility: Small Business, Female Owned
Distribution: Manufacturer Through Distributor, Manufacturer Through Manufacturer Reps, OEM, Exclusive Distributor, Importer, Exporter
General Admin.: Mr. Keith Pizybyia/President
     William J. Przybyla/President, Chief Executive Officer
  Accessories, Laser   General
  Laparoscope, Gynecologic   Obstetrics/Gynecology
  Sleeve, Trocar   Surgery

LASERCARD SYSTEMS CORPORATION   650-969-4428
1875 N. Shoreline Blvd., Mountain View, CA 94043-1601
FDA Number: n/a   *Fax:* 650-969-3140
E-mail: sales@lasercard.com
Web site: www.lasercard.com
Medical Products Sales Volume: $1,000,000
Annual Revenue: $25-$50 Million
Total Employees: 227
Ownership: DREXA TECHNOLOGY
Stock Symbol: LCRD
Traded On: NASDAQ
Produces/Sells CE-marked Devices: N
Federal Procurement Eligibility: Small Business
Distribution: Manufacturer Direct, Importer, Exporter
  Card, Identification   General
  Computer Software   General
  Identification, Alert, Medical   General

LASERCARD SYSTEMS CORPORATION 650-969-4428 *(cont'd)*
Paper, Recording, Data   General

LASERCRAFT INC.
See Macken Instruments, Inc.

LASERSIGHT TECHNOLOGIES, INC. 407-678-9900 ex
931 S. Semoran Blvd, Unit 204, Winter Park, FL 32792
FDA Number: 1064221   *Fax:* 407-678-9981
Ownership: Private
Produces/Sells CE-marked Devices: N
Blade, Surgical, Saw, General & Plastic Surgery   Surgery
Keratome, AC-Powered   Ophthalmology
Keratoscope, AC-Powered   Ophthalmology
System, Laser, Excimer, Ophthalmic   Ophthalmology
Topographer, Corneal   Ophthalmology

LASERVISION USA 1-800-393-5565
595 Phalen Blvd., Saint Paul, MN 55101 651-357-1800
FDA Number: 2133450   *Fax:* 651-357-1830
Web site: www.lasersafety.com
Ownership: Private
Produces/Sells CE-marked Devices: N
Spectacle, Operating (Loupe), Ophthalmic   Ophthalmology

LASZLO CORP. 314-830-3222
2573 Millvalley Drive, Florissant, MO 63031
FDA Number: 1938172   *Fax:* 314-830-3222
E-mail: suhayda@mc-usa.com
Web site: www.mc-usa.com
Year Founded: 1989
Total Employees: 4
Ownership: Private
Produces/Sells CE-marked Devices: N
Federal Procurement Eligibility: Small Business
Distribution: Manufacturer Direct, Importer
General Admin.: Mr. Leslie Suhayda/Chief Executive Officer
Aid, Living, Handicapped   General
Attachment, Commode, Wheelchair   Physical Med
Chair, Adjustable, Mechanical   Physical Med
Chair, With Casters   Physical Med
Lift, Bath, Non-AC-Powered   General
Lift, Patient   General

LATAM MEDICAL 1-877-989-4040
400 Belleville Ave., Bloomfield, NJ 07003-2604 973-259-1400
FDA Number: n/a   *Fax:* 973-259-1711
E-mail: info@latam-medical.com
Web site: http://latam-medical.com
Total Employees: 2
Ownership: Private
Produces/Sells CE-marked Devices: N
Distribution: Manufacturer Through Distributor, Service Direct, Exporter
General Admin.: Kevin Sullivan/Chief Executive Officer
Kevin Sullivan/General Manager
Service, Maintenance/Repair   General

LAUNDERCENTER EQUIPMENT CO.
See Ipso Usa, Inc.

LAVOPTIK CO. INC.
See H.L. Bouton Company, Inc.

LAWLER MANUFACTURING CORP. 732-777-2040
7 Kilmer Ct., Edison, NJ 08817
FDA Number: n/a   *Fax:* 732-777-4828
E-mail: info@lawlercorp.com
Web site: www.lawler-mfg.com
Medical Products Sales Volume: $1,500,000
Annual Revenue: $1-$5 Million
Total Employees: 15   *Marketing Staff:* 1   *Sales Staff:* 3
Ownership: Private
Produces/Sells CE-marked Devices: Y
Federal Procurement Eligibility: Small Business
Distribution: Manufacturer Direct, Manufacturer Through Distributor, Manufacturer Through Manufacturer Reps, OEM, Service Direct
General Admin.: J. Cekada/President, Chief Executive Officer
Mktg./Adv.: Anthony Romano/Manager National Sales
Research: J. Aruldoss/Vice President Research & Development
Equipment, Laboratory, Gen. Purpose (Specific Medical Use)   Chemistry

LAWRENCE-NELSON, LLC 859-252-0335
325 Virginia Ave., Lexington, KY 40504
FDA Number: n/a   *Fax:* 859-253-7621
E-mail: lawrence-nelson@insightbb.com
Web site: www.lawrence-nelson.com
Year Founded: 2002
Ownership: Private
Produces/Sells CE-marked Devices: N
Brake, Extension, Wheelchair   Physical Med

LAYTECH, INC. 1.847.254.9295
1771 RFD, Lake Zurich, IL 60047-7317
FDA Number: n/a
E-mail: tnl@laytechinc.com
Web site: tnl@laytechinc.com
Total Employees: 5
Ownership: Private
Produces/Sells CE-marked Devices: N
Federal Procurement Eligibility: Small Business, Female Owned
Distribution: Manufacturer Direct
General Admin.: Terry Layton/Chief Technology Officer
Catherine Layton/President
Flowmeter, Urine, Disposable   Gastroenterology/Urology

LAZAR RESEARCH LABORATORIES, INC. 800-824-2066
509 N. Fairfax Avenue, Suite 219, 323-931-1204
Los Angeles, CA 90036
FDA Number: n/a   *Fax:* 323-931-1434
E-mail: service@lazarlab.com
Web site: www.lazarlab.com
Medical Products Sales Volume: $100,000
Annual Revenue: $0-$1 Million
Year Founded: 1976
Total Employees: 4
Ownership: Private
Produces/Sells CE-marked Devices: N
Federal Procurement Eligibility: Small Business
Distribution: Manufacturer Direct, Manufacturer Through Distributor, OEM, Exporter
General Admin.: Dan Altura/Chief Executive Officer
Susan Cavanaugh/Office Manager
Research: Michael Altura/Manager Research
Microelectrode   General

LBA TECHNOLOGY, INC. 252-757-0279
3400 Tupper Dr., Greenville, NC 27834
FDA Number: 1055799
Bed, Patient Rotation, Powered   Physical Med

LCI MEDICAL, INC.
See Airpal Patient Transfer Systems Inc.

LCR HALLCREST 800-527-1419
1911 Pickwick Lane, Glenview, IL 60026-1307 847-998-8580
FDA Number: 1424489   *Fax:* 847-998-8051
E-mail: info@lcr-usa.com
Web site: www.hallcrest.com
Medical Products Sales Volume: $1,000,000
Annual Revenue: $10-$25 Million
Total Employees: 45   *Marketing Staff:* 4   *Sales Staff:* 10
Ownership: Private
Quality System Registration Information: ISO9002
Produces/Sells CE-marked Devices: Y
Federal Procurement Eligibility: Small Business
Distribution: Manufacturer Direct, Manufacturer Through Distributor, Manufacturer Through Manufacturer Reps, OEM, Exclusive Distributor, Exporter
General Admin.: Patrick Van Minnen/President, Chief Executive Officer
Mktg./Adv.: Peggy Froiz/Director Marketing
Tom Knesel/Director National Accounts
Finder, Vein   General
System, Thermographic, Liquid Crystal   Obstetrics/Gynecology
Temperature Strip, Forehead, Liquid Crystal   General
Thermometer, Chemical Color Change   General
Thermometer, Liquid Crystals   Surgery

LCR-HALLCREST--FLORIDA 847-998-8580
6705 Parke East Blvd., Unit A, Tampa, FL 33610
FDA Number: 1051420
Equipment, Laboratory, Gen. Purpose (Specific Medical Use)   Chemistry
Temperature Strip, Forehead, Liquid Crystal   General
Thermometer, Chemical Color Change   General

LDB MEDICAL, INC. 800-243-2554
2909 Langford Road, Suite 500B, 770-446-2554
Norcross, GA 30071
FDA Number: 1053487   *Fax:* 770-446-5229
E-mail: info@ldbmedical.com
Web site: www.ldbmedical.com
Medical Products Sales Volume: $600,000
Year Founded: 1990
Total Employees: 8
Ownership: Private
Produces/Sells CE-marked Devices: N
Federal Procurement Eligibility: Small Business
Distribution: Manufacturer Direct, Manufacturer Through Distributor, OEM, Importer, Exporter
General Admin.: L. Derryl Breazeale/Chief Executive Officer
Mktg./Adv.: L. Nolan Breazeale/Vice President Marketing

LDB MEDICAL, INC.   800-243-2554 (cont'd)

Production: L. Adam Breazeale/Vice President Operations

Adhesive, Liquid	General
Adhesive, Prosthesis, External	Surgery
Appliance, Incontinence, Urosheath Type	Gastroenterology/Urology
Bag, Drainage (Incontinence)	Gastroenterology/Urology
Bag, Leg	Gastroenterology/Urology
Bag, Urinary Collection	General
Bag, Urinary, Ileostomy	Gastroenterology/Urology
Belt, Abdominal	Gastroenterology/Urology
Cement, Stomal Appliance, Ostomy	Gastroenterology/Urology
Collector, Ostomy	Gastroenterology/Urology
Collector, Urine	Gastroenterology/Urology
Kit, Urinary Drainage Collection	Gastroenterology/Urology
Ostomy Appliance (Ileostomy, Colostomy)	Gastroenterology/Urology
Pad, Incontinence (Underpad)	General
Solvent, Adhesive Tape	Surgery
Tube, Drainage	Gastroenterology/Urology

LDR SPINE USA   512-344-3333
4030 West Braker Lane, Suite 360, Austin, TX 78759

FDA Number: 3004903783
Web site: www.ldrspine.com
Ownership: LDR Medical
Produces/Sells CE-marked Devices: N
General Admin.: James Burrows/Chief Operating Officer
Mktg./Adv.: Mr. Joe Brown/Vice President Marketing
       Andre Potgiete/Vice President Sales
Finance: Dennis Hynson/Chief Financial Officer

LDS LIFE SCIENCE (FORMERLY GOULD INSTRUMENT SYSTEMS INC.)   216-328-7000
5525 Cloverleaf Parkway, Valley View, OH 44125-6100

FDA Number: 9009862   *Fax:* 216-328-7400
E-mail: lifescience@LDS.SPX.com
Web site: www.LDS-group.com
Total Employees: 50   *Marketing Staff:* 4   *Sales Staff:* 6
Ownership: SPX CORPORATION
Quality System Registration Information: ISO9001
Produces/Sells CE-marked Devices: Y
Distribution: Manufacturer Direct, Manufacturer Through Distributor, Manufacturer Through Manufacturer Reps
General Admin.: Mr. Bob Dakes/Vice President, General Manager
Mktg./Adv.: Mr. David Soper/Manager National Sales
       Mr. John Kroehle/Managing Director Marketing & Sales

Amplifier, Biopotential (W Signal Conditioner)	Cardiovascular
Amplifier, Transducer Signal (W Signal Conditioner)	Cardiovascular
Analyzer, ECG	Cardiovascular
Computer Software	General
Computer, Pulmonary Function Data	Anesthesiology
Detector, Strain	General
Electroencephalograph	Cns/Neurology
Monitor, Blood Pressure, Invasive (Arterial)	Cardiovascular
Monitor, Blood Pressure, Venous	Cardiovascular
Monitor, Heart Rate, Other	Cardiovascular
Monitor, Heart Rate, R-Wave (ECG)	Cardiovascular
Pneumotachograph	Anesthesiology
Polygraph	General
Rack, Surgical Instrument	Surgery
Recorder, Chart, Laboratory	Chemistry
Recorder, Long-Term, Trend	General
Recorder, Paper Chart	Cardiovascular

LEAD ENTERPRISES INC.   800-253-4249   305-635-8644
3300 N.W. 29 St., Miami, FL 33142-6310

FDA Number: n/a   *Fax:* 305-635-8645
E-mail: info@leadenterprises.com
Web site: www.leadenterprises.com
Medical Products Sales Volume: $1,000,000
Annual Revenue: $0-$1 Million
Year Founded: 1961
Total Employees: 18   *Marketing Staff:* 3   *Sales Staff:* 4
Ownership: Private
Produces/Sells CE-marked Devices: N
Federal Procurement Eligibility: Small Business
Distribution: Manufacturer Direct, OEM, Importer, Exporter
General Admin.: Thomas T. Taylor/Chief Executive Officer
       Roger Lara/Vice President

Shield, X-Ray	Radiology
Shield, X-Ray, Door	Radiology
Shield, X-Ray, Leaded	Dental And Oral
Shield, X-Ray, Transparent	Radiology

LEAD-LOK, INC.   208-263-5071
500 Airport Way, Sandpoint, ID 83864

FDA Number: 3023164

Electrode, Cutaneous	Cns/Neurology
Electrode, Electrocardiograph	Cardiovascular

LEAD-LOK, INC.   800-201-3958   208-263-5071
814 Airport Way, Sandpoint, ID 83864-9222

FDA Number: 3023164   *Fax:* 208-263-9654
E-mail: leadlok@mindspring.com
Web site: www.leadlok.com
Medical Products Sales Volume: $3,000,000
Annual Revenue: $1-$5 Million
Total Employees: 30
Ownership: Private
Quality System Registration Information: ISO9001
Produces/Sells CE-marked Devices: Y
Federal Procurement Eligibility: Small Business
Distribution: Manufacturer Direct, Manufacturer Through Distributor, Manufacturer Through Manufacturer Reps, OEM, Exporter
General Admin.: James W. Healy/President, Chief Executive Officer
       Chris Healy/Vice President

Electrode, Cutaneous	Cns/Neurology
Electrode, Electrocardiograph	Cardiovascular
Electrode, Electrocardiograph, Long-Term	Cardiovascular
Electrode, Holter	Cardiovascular
Electrode, Ion Specific, Chloride	Chemistry
Electrode, Other	General

LEADER INDUSTRIES INC.   800-847-2001   514-334-3611
3585 Ashby, St. Laurent, Montreal, QUE H4R 2 Canada

FDA Number: n/a   *Fax:* 514-334-7997
E-mail: kpeever@zleader.com
Web site: www.zleader.com
Year Founded: 1972
Total Employees: 100
Ownership: Private
Produces/Sells CE-marked Devices: N
Distribution: Manufacturer Direct, Exporter

LEADER INSTRUMENTS CORP.   800-645-5104   714-527-9300
6484 Commerce Dr., Cypress, CA 90630

FDA Number: 9200639   *Fax:* 714-527-7490
E-mail: sales@leaderusa.com
Web site: www.leaderusa.com
Total Employees: 21
Ownership: Private
Produces/Sells CE-marked Devices: N
Distribution: Manufacturer Through Distributor
General Admin.: M. Sawa/President
Mktg./Adv.: G. Gonos/Director Marketing

Cart, Other	General
Oscilloscope	General
Voltmeter	Chemistry

LEADING EDGE INNOVATIONS   805-388-7669
699 Mobil Ave, Camarillo, CA 93010

FDA Number: 2032738   *Fax:* 805-389-8142
E-mail: Info@urinedevice.com
Web site: www.urinedevice.com
Ownership: Private
Quality System Registration Information: ISO9002
Produces/Sells CE-marked Devices: N
Federal Procurement Eligibility: Small Business
Distribution: Manufacturer Direct
General Admin.: Paul Dwork/President
IS: Edward E. Elson/Vice President Technology

Appliance, Incontinence, Urosheath Type	Gastroenterology/Urology
Catheter, Urinary, Condom	Gastroenterology/Urology

LEADING LADY, INC.   216-464-5490
24050 Commerce Park Dr., Beachwood, OH 44122

FDA Number: 3004024638

Binder, Abdominal	General
Binder, Breast	Obstetrics/Gynecology

LEANDER HEALTH TECHNOLOGIES/HEALTHCARE DIVISION   1-800-532-6337
315 N E Industrial Lane, Suite A, Lawrence, KS 66044   1

FDA Number: 3023805   *Fax:* 785-856-3456
E-mail: sales@theleader.com
Web site: www.theleader.com
Medical Products Sales Volume: $2,120,000
Annual Revenue: $5-$10 Million
Year Founded: 1982
Total Employees: 50   *Marketing Staff:* 2   *Sales Staff:* 4
Ownership: Private
Produces/Sells CE-marked Devices: Y
Federal Procurement Eligibility: Small Business
Distribution: Manufacturer Direct, Manufacturer Through Distributor, Exclusive Distributor, Exporter

LEANDER HEALTH
1-800-532-6337 *(cont'd)*
General Admin.: Richard A. Flaherty/President, Chief Executive Officer
Cathy A. Flaherty/Vice President Admin.
Mktg./Adv.: Anne Brown/Manager International & National Sales
Research: Michael Coffey/Vice President Research & Development
Finance: Peggy Haugen, CPA/Controller

Contract R&D, Equipment	General
Solution, Instrument Cleaner	General
Support, Back	Orthopedics
Table, Mechanical	Physical Med
Table, Other	General

LEANDER RESEARCH MANUFACTURING & DISTRIB
See Leander Health Technologies/Healthcare Division

LEAP TECHNOLOGIES
800-229-8814
919-929-8814
PO Box 969, Carrboro, NC 27510
FDA Number: n/a
Fax: 919-929-8956
E-mail: info@leaptec.com
Web site: www.leaptec.com
Medical Products Sales Volume: $2,900,000
Annual Revenue: $1-$5 Million
Year Founded: 1989
Total Employees: 30
Ownership: Private
Stock Symbol: LPTC
Quality System Registration Information: ISO9000
Produces/Sells CE-marked Devices: N
Federal Procurement Eligibility: Small Business
Distribution: Manufacturer Direct, Manufacturer Through Distributor, Manufacturer Through Manufacturer Reps, OEM, Importer, Exporter
General Admin.: Warner Martin/Chief Executive Officer
Mktg./Adv.: Susie Martin/Manager Advertising
Susie Martin/Vice President Marketing & Sales
Research: Warner Martin/Vice President Research & Development

Applicator, Sample	Chemistry
Injector, Sample	Chemistry
Kit, Prep	General

LEARNING CURVE BRANDS INC. THE
FIRST YEARS
800-225-0382
100 Technology Center Drive, Suite 2A, Stoughton, MA 02072
FDA Number: 1217805
Web site: www.learningcurve.com
Ownership: RC2 Corporation
Produces/Sells CE-marked Devices: N
Distribution: Manufacturer Direct, Manufacturer Through Distributor, Manufacturer Through Manufacturer Reps, Exporter

Syringe, Hypodermic	General
Thermometer, Liquid Crystals	Surgery
Thermometer, Mercury	General

LEASING INNOVATIONS INCORPORATED
800-532-7388
858-259-4794
437 S. Highway 101, Suite 104,
Solana Beach, CA 92075
FDA Number: n/a
Fax: 858-259-7076
E-mail: info@leasing123.com
Web site: www.leasing123.com
Medical Products Sales Volume: $1,300,000
Annual Revenue: $25-$50 Million
Year Founded: 1989
Total Employees: 12   *Sales Staff:* 3
Ownership: Private
Produces/Sells CE-marked Devices: N
Federal Procurement Eligibility: Small Business, Minority Owned, Female Owned
Distribution: Service Direct
General Admin.: Heather G. Fritz/President, Chief Executive Officer
Charles Grysell/Vice President, General Manager
Mktg./Adv.: Heather G. Fritz/Director Marketing
Chris Conlee/Director National Accounts
Cameron Bushell/Director Product Development
Lisa Stahley/Manager Contract Sales
Chris Conlee/Vice President Business Development

Service, Equipment Leasing	General
Service, Used Equipment	General

LEASING SERVICES, INC.
See Leasing Innovations Incorporated

LEBANON CORP., THE
800-428-2310
765-482-7273
1700 Lebanon St., Lebanon, IN 46052-1501
FDA Number: 1824818
Fax: 765-482-5660
E-mail: david@honanballoon.com
Web site: www.honanballoon.com
Annual Revenue: $0-$1 Million
Year Founded: 1976
Total Employees: 3   *Marketing Staff:* 1   *Sales Staff:* 1
Ownership: Private
Produces/Sells CE-marked Devices: Y

LEBANON CORP., THE
800-428-2310 *(cont'd)*
Federal Procurement Eligibility: Small Business
Distribution: Manufacturer Direct
General Admin.: Paul R. Honan/Chief Executive Officer
David A. Honan/Vice President
Mktg./Adv.: David A. Honan/Manager Marketing

Applicator, Ocular Pressure	Ophthalmology
Reducer, Pressure, Intraocular	Ophthalmology

LEBANON COUNTY WORKSHOP, INC.
See Quest Inc.

LEBERCO CELSIS TESTING
See Celsis Laboratory Group

LEBERCO TESTING, INC.
See Celsis Laboratory Group

LECHNOLOGIES RESEARCH, INC..
866-321-2342
262-246-7374
N64 W24801 Main Street, Suite 107,
Sussex, WI 53089
FDA Number: 2183422
Fax: 262-432-0271
E-mail: tadler@lechnologies.com
Web site: www.lechnologies.com
Year Founded: 2004
Total Employees: 4   *Marketing Staff:* 1   *Sales Staff:* 2
Ownership: Private
Produces/Sells CE-marked Devices: N
Federal Procurement Eligibility: Small Business
Distribution: Manufacturer Direct
General Admin.: Mr. Timothy Lohman/President
Mktg./Adv.: Mr. Thomas Adler/Director Marketing
Ms. Sue Wendland/Vice President Marketing & Sales
IS: Mr. Dan Gomoll/Director Information Systems

Amplifier, Biopotential (W Signal Conditioner)	Cardiovascular
Monitor, ECG	Cardiovascular
Monitor, ECG, Arrhythmia	Cardiovascular
Tester, Electrode, Surface, Electrocardiograph	Cardiovascular
Transmitter/Receiver System, ECG, Telephone Multi-Channel	Cardiovascular
Transmitter/Receiver System, ECG, Telephone Single-Channel	Cardiovascular

LECROY CORP.
800-553-2769
845-425-2000
700 Chestnut Ridge Rd.,
Chestnut Ridge, NY 10977
FDA Number: n/a
Fax: 845-578-5985
E-mail: contract.corp@lecroy.com
Web site: www.lecroy.com
Medical Products Sales Volume: $15,000,000
Year Founded: 1964
Total Employees: 389
Ownership: Public
Stock Symbol: LCRY
Traded On: NASDAQ
Produces/Sells CE-marked Devices: Y
Federal Procurement Eligibility: Small Business
Distribution: Manufacturer Direct
General Admin.: Thomas H. Reslewic/President, Chief Executive Officer
Mktg./Adv.: Roberto Petrillo/Vice President Sales

Oscilloscope	General

LECTEC CORP.
903-832-0993
1407 South Kings Highway, Texarkana, TX 75501
FDA Number: n/a
Fax: 763-559-7593
E-mail: info@lectec.com
Web site: http://www.lectec.com
Year Founded: 1977
Ownership: Public
Stock Symbol: LECT
Traded On: OTC Bulletin
Produces/Sells CE-marked Devices: N
General Admin.: Mr. Gregory Freitag Jr./Chief Executive Officer, Chief Financial Officer

Bandage, Adhesive	Surgery
Electrode, Electrocardiograph	Cardiovascular

LEDTRONICS
800-579-4875
310-534-1505
23105 Kashiwa Court, Torrance, CA 90505
FDA Number: n/a
Fax: 310-534-1424
E-mail: webmaster@ledtronics.com
Web site: www.ledtronics.com
Medical Products Sales Volume: $10,800,000
Annual Revenue: $10-$25 Million
Year Founded: 1983
Total Employees: 130   *Marketing Staff:* 4   *Sales Staff:* 12
Ownership: Private
Quality System Registration Information: ISO9001
Produces/Sells CE-marked Devices: N
Federal Procurement Eligibility: Small Business, Minority Owned, Female Owned
Distribution: Manufacturer Direct, Manufacturer Through Manufacturer Reps, OEM

MANUFACTURER PROFILES

LEDTRONICS   **800-579-4875** *(cont'd)*
General Admin.: Pervaiz Lodhie/President
          Adil Gandhi/Vice President, General Manager
Mktg./Adv.: Jordon Papanier/Director Marketing
          Gary Peterson/Manager Contract Sales
Monitor, Bed Patient	General
Nurse Call System	General
Service, Engineering/Design	General

LEE LABORATORIES, INC.   **1-800-732-9150**
1475 Athens Highway, Grayson, GA 30017
FDA Number: 1025402   *Fax:* 580-762-6176
E-mail: LeeLabs@bd.com
Web site: http://www.bd.com/leelabs
Annual Revenue: $0-$1 Million
Total Employees: 8
Ownership: Private
Produces/Sells CE-marked Devices: Y
Distribution: Manufacturer Through Distributor, Importer, Exporter
Antigen, (Febrile), Agglutination, Brucella SPP.	Microbiology
Antigen, All Groups, Shigella SPP.	Microbiology
Antigen, B. Pertussis	Microbiology
Antigen, Febrile	Microbiology
Antigen, Febrile, Slide And Tube, Salmonella	Microbiology
Antigen, Slide And Tube, Francisella Tularensis	Microbiology
Antigen, Slide And Tube, Listeria Monocytogenes	Microbiology
Antiserum, Agglutinating, B. Parapertussis	Microbiology
Antiserum, Francisella Tularensis	Microbiology
Antiserum, N. Meningitidis	Microbiology
Antiserum, Positive And Negative Febrile Antigen Control	Microbiology
Antiserum, Salmonella SPP.	Microbiology
Antiserum, Vibrio Cholerae	Microbiology
Headgear, Extraoral, Orthodontic	Dental And Oral
Plasma, Coagulase, Human/Horse/Rabbit	Microbiology

LEE MEDICAL INTERNATIONAL, INC.   **800-433-8950**
612 Distributors Row, Harahan, LA 70123   **504-734-9336**
FDA Number: 2316883   *Fax:* 504-734-9232
E-mail: jeffb@eleemedical.com
Web site: www.eleemedical.com
Medical Products Sales Volume: $3,800,000
Annual Revenue: $10-$25 Million
Total Employees: 22   *Marketing Staff:* 1   *Sales Staff:* 15
Ownership: Private
Produces/Sells CE-marked Devices: N
Federal Procurement Eligibility: Small Business
Distribution: OEM, Importer
General Admin.: Jerry Tauzier/President
Mktg./Adv.: Jeff Boudreaux/Manager National Marketing & Sales
Production: Bruce Anzalone/Manager Operations
Accessories, Blood Circuit, Hemodialysis	Gastroenterology/Urology
Catheter, Hemodialysis	Gastroenterology/Urology
Chair, Dialysis, Unpowered (Without Scale)	Gastroenterology/Urology
Disinfector, Liquid	General
Glove, Other	General
Kit, Administration, Peritoneal Dialysis, Disposable	Gastroenterology/Urology
Kit, Dialysis, Single Needle (Co-Axial Flow)	Gastroenterology/Urology
Lotion, Skin Care	General
Mask, Face	General
Pack, Custom/Special Procedure	General
Purifier, Air, Ultraviolet	General
Scales, Dialysis	General
Tray, Start/Stop (Including Contents), Dialysis	Gastroenterology/Urology
Waste Receptacle, Contaminated	General

LEE PHARMACEUTICALS   **626-442-3141**
1434 Santa Anita Ave., El Monte, CA 91733
FDA Number: 2016608
Band, Elastic, Orthodontic	Dental And Oral
Bracket, Metal, Orthodontic	Dental And Oral
Bracket, Plastic, Orthodontic	Dental And Oral
Material, Tooth Shade, Resin	Dental And Oral
Wire, Orthodontic	Dental And Oral

LEE PLASTIC
See Leeco Industries, Inc.

LEECO INDUSTRIES, INC.   **662-551-1025**
540 S Industrial Park Road, Holly Springs, MS 38635
FDA Number: n/a   *Fax:* 662-551-1014
E-mail: customerservice@leecoindustries.com
Web site: www.leecoindustries.com
Annual Revenue: $1-$5 Million
Total Employees: 16   *Marketing Staff:* 4   *Sales Staff:* 4
Ownership: Private
Produces/Sells CE-marked Devices: N
Federal Procurement Eligibility: Small Business
Distribution: Manufacturer Direct, Manufacturer Through Distributor, Importer
General Admin.: Scott D. Smith/President
Mktg./Adv.: Keith Smith/Manager International & National Sales

LEECO INDUSTRIES, INC.   **662-551-1025** *(cont'd)*
Cart, Other	General

LEEDAL, INC.   **847-498-0111**
3453 Commercial Ave., Northbrook, IL 60062
FDA Number: n/a   *Fax:* 847-498-0198
E-mail: sink@leedal.com
Web site: www.leedal.com
Annual Revenue: $1-$5 Million
Year Founded: 1946
Total Employees: 30   *Marketing Staff:* 1   *Sales Staff:* 2
Ownership: Private
Produces/Sells CE-marked Devices: N
Federal Procurement Eligibility: Small Business
Distribution: Manufacturer Direct
General Admin.: Sheldon L. Levin/President, Chief Executive Officer
Mktg./Adv.: A.J. Levin/Vice President Sales
Component, Other	General
Foodservice Product/Equipment	General
Illuminator, Radiographic Film	Radiology
Purification Filter, Water, Particulate	Chemistry

LEEDER GROUP, INC.   **305-436-5030**
8508 N.w. 66th St., Miami, FL 33166
FDA Number: 1062848
Armrest, Wheelchair	Physical Med
Brace, Joint, Ankle (External)	Physical Med
Cushion, Flotation	Physical Med
Cushion, Flotation, Therapeutic	Physical Med
Mattress, Non-Powered Flotation Therapy	Physical Med
Orthosis, Limb Brace	Physical Med
Splint, Hand, And Component	Physical Med
Stirrup, External Brace Component	Physical Med
Transfer Aid	Physical Med

LEEGIN CREATIVE LEATHER PRODUCTS, INC.
See Brighton Collectibles Inc.

LEEMAH ELECTRONICS, INC.   **415-394-1288**
1088 Sansome St., --, San Francisco, CA 94111
FDA Number: 2939492   *Fax:* (415) 433-2560
E-mail: inquiry@leemah.com
Web site: www.leemah.com
Ownership: Private
Produces/Sells CE-marked Devices: N
Oximeter, Ear	Cardiovascular
Pack, Hot Or Cold, Water Circulating	Physical Med

LEEMAH ELECTRONICS, INC.   **415-394-1288**
1301 Folsom Street, --, San Francisco, CA 94103
FDA Number: 3004769169
Ownership: Private
Produces/Sells CE-marked Devices: N
Pack, Hot Or Cold, Water Circulating	Physical Med

LEEMING/PACQUIN
See Pfizer, Inc.

LEESAN MAQUILAS S.A. DE C.V.   **52-5-561-526**
Enrique Dunant No., 12 Centro,
Tlalnepantla,edo.de Mexico Cp Mexico
FDA Number: 9615143
Pack, Hot Or Cold, Reusable	Physical Med

LEGACY INTEGRATORS, LLC   **800-272-5169**
68 Forman St., Fair Haven, NJ 07704
FDA Number: n/a   *Fax:* 800-272-5169
E-mail: info@legacyintegrators.com
Ownership: Private
Produces/Sells CE-marked Devices: N
General Admin.: Mr. Francis Cheh/President
Service, Computer	General

LEGEND AEROSPACE, INC.   **305-883-8804**
8292 NW South River Drive, Medley, FL 33166
FDA Number: 3003770530   *Fax:* 305-883-8664
E-mail: sales@legendaerospace.com
Ownership: Private
Produces/Sells CE-marked Devices: N
Bandage, Adhesive	Surgery
Bandage, Elastic	General
Emergency Response Safety Kit	Surgery
First Aid Kit Without Drug	Surgery
Tape, Adhesive	General

LEGGETT & PLATT INC.   **417-358-8131**
P.O. Box 757, 1 Leggett Road, Carthage, MO 64836-0757
FDA Number: n/a   *Fax:* 417-358-8773
E-mail: beddinggroup@leggett.com
Web site: www.leggett.com
Annual Revenue: More than $1 Billion

LEGGETT & PLATT INC. 417-358-8131 *(cont'd)*
Year Founded: 1883
Total Employees: 20600
Ownership: Public
Stock Symbol: LEG
Traded On: NYSE
Quality System Registration Information: ISO9003
Produces/Sells CE-marked Devices: Y
Federal Procurement Eligibility: Small Business
Distribution: Manufacturer Direct
General Admin.: Karl G. Glassman/Chief Operating Officer, Executive Vice President
David S. Haffner/President, Chief Executive Officer

Bed, Electric	General
Component, Plastic	General
Mattress, Non-Powered Flotation Therapy	Physical Med

LEGRAND ASSOC. 800-523-4314
1601 Walnut Street, Suite 616, 215-496-1307
Philadelphia, PA 19102
FDA Number: 2519029 *Fax:* 215-496-1693
E-mail: joelegrand@gmail.com
Web site: www.legrandeyes.com
Annual Revenue: $0-$1 Million
Ownership: Private
Produces/Sells CE-marked Devices: N
Federal Procurement Eligibility: Small Business
Distribution: Manufacturer Direct
General Admin.: Joseph A. LeGrand/President

Eye, Artificial, Custom	Ophthalmology
Eye, Artificial, Non-Custom	Ophthalmology

LEHRER BRILLENPERFEKTION WERKS, INC. 818-407-1890
3908 North Fifth St., North Las Vegas, NV 89030
FDA Number: 2953169

Frame, Spectacle (Eyeglasses)	Ophthalmology
Spectacle, Magnifier	Ophthalmology
Sunglasses (Including Photosensitive)	Ophthalmology

LEIBINGER & FISCHER
See Striker Corp.

LEIBINGER L.P.
See Striker Corp.

LEICA BIOSYSTEMS - ST. LOUIS, LLC 847-317-7209
12100a Prichard Farm Rd., Maryland Heights, MO 63043
FDA Number: 3005314894
Ownership: Danaher Corporation
Produces/Sells CE-marked Devices: N

Cassette, Tissue	Pathology
Paraffin, All Formulations	Pathology

LEICA INC.
See Leica Microsystems Inc.

LEICA MICROSYSTEMS (CANADA) INC. 800-248-0123
111 Granton Dr., 800 248 0123
Richmond Hill, ONT L4B 1 Canada
FDA Number: n/a *Fax:* 847-405-0164
E-mail: charles.boelens@leica-microsystems.com
Web site: www.leica-microsystems.com
Year Founded: 1997
Total Employees: 25 *Marketing Staff:* 3 *Sales Staff:* 15
Ownership: Leica Microsystems Inc.
Produces/Sells CE-marked Devices: Y
Distribution: Manufacturer Direct, Manufacturer Through Distributor, Manufacturer Through Manufacturer Reps, OEM, Service Direct, Exclusive Distributor

LEICA MICROSYSTEMS (SAN JOSE) 800-634-3622
CORPORATION
120 Baytech Drive, San Jose, CA 95134-2302 408-719-6400
FDA Number: 2939903 *Fax:* 408-719-6401
E-mail: sales@genetix.com
Web site: www.genetix.com
Annual Revenue: $25-$50 Million
Total Employees: 161
Ownership: Iris International, Inc.
Produces/Sells CE-marked Devices: N
Federal Procurement Eligibility: Small Business
Distribution: Manufacturer Direct
General Admin.: Charles de Rohan/Chief Executive Officer
Research: Dr. Julian Burke/Director Scientific Affairs
Finance: Andrew Kellett/Director Finance

Analyzer, Chromosome, Automated	Pathology
Analyzer, Karyotype	Pathology
Computer, Radiographic Image Analysis	Radiology
Genetic Engineering	Microbiology
Safety Equipment, Laboratory	Chemistry

LEICA MICROSYSTEMS (SAN JOSE) 800-634-3622 *(cont'd)*
Test, DNA-Probe, Other Microbiology

LEICA MICROSYSTEMS INC. 800-248-0123
2345 Waukegan Road, Bannockburn, IL 60015 847-405-0123
FDA Number: 1423337 *Fax:* 847-405-0164
E-mail: info@leica-microsystems.com
Web site: www.leica-microsystems.com
Medical Products Sales Volume: $17,500,000
Year Founded: 1986
Total Employees: 150
Ownership: Danaher Corporation
Quality System Registration Information: ISO9000
Produces/Sells CE-marked Devices: Y
Federal Procurement Eligibility: Small Business, GSA Contract
Distribution: Manufacturer Direct, Manufacturer Through Distributor, Exporter
General Admin.: Mr. Ludger Althoff/Executive Vice President
Mr. David Martyr/President
Mktg./Adv.: Mr. Arnd Kaldowski/Executive Vice President Marketing & Sales

Coverslip, Microscope Slide	Pathology
Microscope	Hematology
Microscope, Laboratory, Optical	Microbiology
Microtome, Rotary	Pathology
Microtome, Ultra	Pathology
Tissue Processor, Automated	Pathology

Medical Product Subsidiaries (Listed Separately)
Leica Microsystems (Canada) Inc.

LEICA MICROSYSTEMS INC., OPTHALMIC INSTRUMENTS DIV.
See Reichert, Inc.

LEICA MICROSYSTEMS, INC., EDUCATIONAL & 800-346-4560
ANALYTICAL DIVISION
P.O. Box 123, Buffalo, NY 14240-0123 716-686-3000
FDA Number: 1315334 *Fax:* 716-686-3085
E-mail: analytical@leica-microsystems.com
Web site: www.analytical-refractometers.com
Ownership: Private
Quality System Registration Information: ISO9001
Produces/Sells CE-marked Devices: Y
Distribution: Manufacturer Through Distributor
General Admin.: Art Alix/President
Mktg./Adv.: Tom Ryan/Director Marketing
Production: Thor Roalsvig/Product Manager

Bilirubinometer	Chemistry
Counter, Colony	Microbiology
Microscope, Fluorescence/U.V.	Pathology
Microscope, Laboratory, Optical	Microbiology
Microscope, Light	Pathology
Microscope, Phase Contrast	Pathology
Oximeter, Whole Blood	Hematology
Refractometer	Chemistry

LEICA, INC., OPTICAL PRODUCTS DIV.
See Leica Microsystems, Inc., Educational & Analytical Division

LEINCO TECHNOLOGIES INC. 800-538-1145
410 Axminister Drive, St. Louis, MO 63026 636-230-9477
FDA Number: n/a *Fax:* 636-527-5545
E-mail: leincoglobal@leinco.com
Web site: www.leinco.com
Annual Revenue: $0-$1 Million
Year Founded: 1992
Ownership: Private
Produces/Sells CE-marked Devices: N
Federal Procurement Eligibility: Small Business
Distribution: Manufacturer Through Distributor, OEM, Service Direct

Antibodies, Anti-Ribosomal P	Immunology
Azo-Dyes, Colorimetric, Bilirubin And Conjugates	Chemistry
Contract Manufacturing	General

LEINER ASSOCIATES, INC.
See Lighthouse Imaging Corp.

LEISEGANG MEDICAL, INC.
See Coopersurgical, Inc.

LEISURE TIME 440-934-1032
1284 Miller Rd., Avon, OH 44011-0276
FDA Number: n/a
Annual Revenue: $0-$1 Million
Ownership: Private
Produces/Sells CE-marked Devices: N
Federal Procurement Eligibility: Small Business
Distribution: Manufacturer Direct

Component, Other	General
Restraint, Wheelchair	General

LEISURE-LIFT, INC. 800-255-0285
1800 Merriam Lane, Kansas City, KS 66106-4714 913-722-5658
FDA Number: 1919278 *Fax:* 913-722-2614

LEISURE-LIFT, INC.   800-255-0285 (cont'd)
E-mail: leisurelift@kc.rr.com
Web site: www.pacesaver.com
Medical Products Sales Volume: $4,500,000
Total Employees: 63   *Marketing Staff:* 4   *Sales Staff:* 51
Ownership: Private
Produces/Sells CE-marked Devices: Y
Federal Procurement Eligibility: Small Business, GSA Contract, VA Contract
Distribution: Manufacturer Through Distributor, Manufacturer Through Manufacturer Reps
General Admin.: Jim Ernst/General Manager
     DuWayne Kramer/President
     Ron Kruse/Vice President, General Manager
Mktg./Adv.: Tammy Stewart/Coord. Communications
     DuWayne Kramer/Director Marketing
     DuWayne Kramer/Director National Accounts
     Steve Allee/Manager International Sales
     Mike Wade/Manager Sales Training
Production: Steve Stephens/Director Product Development & Regulatory Affairs
     Fred Shirley/Manager Materials

Cart, Other	General
Chair, Other	General
Chair, Position, Electric	Physical Med
Scooter (Motorized 3-Wheeled Vehicle)	Physical Med
Vehicle, Handicapped	Physical Med
Wheelchair, Powered	Physical Med
Wheelchair, Special Grade	Physical Med

LELAND MANUFACTURING LLC   812-367-1761
1300 North Broad Street, Leland, Bourbon, MS 38756
FDA Number: 3005290141
Ownership: Private
Produces/Sells CE-marked Devices: N

Chair, Adjustable, Mechanical	Physical Med
Chair, Dialysis, Unpowered (Without Scale)	Gastroenterology/Urology
Chair, With Casters	Physical Med
Chair/Table, Medical	General

LEMAITRE VASCULAR, INC.   781-221-2266
63 Second Avenue, Burlington, MA 01803
FDA Number: 1220948   *Fax:* 781-425-5049
E-mail: lemaitre@lemaitre.com
Web site: www.lemaitre.com
Medical Products Sales Volume: $34,620,000
Annual Revenue: $25-$50 Million
Year Founded: 1983
Total Employees: 251   *Sales Staff:* 91
Ownership: Public
Stock Symbol: LMAT
Traded On: NASDAQ
Quality System Registration Information: ISO9001
Produces/Sells CE-marked Devices: Y
Federal Procurement Eligibility: Small Business
Distribution: Manufacturer Direct
General Admin.: George W. LeMaitre/Chief Executive Officer, Chairman
     Nobuhiro Okabe/General Manager
     David B. Roberts/President
     Peter R. Gebauer/President International Operations
     Cornelia W. LeMaitre/Vice President Human Resources
     Jonathon W. Ngau/Vice President Information Technology
     Aaron M. Grossman/Vice President, General Counsel
Medical Admin.: Andrew Hodgkinson/Director Clinical Affairs
Mktg./Adv.: Kimberly L. Cieslak/Vice President Marketing
     Maik D. Helmers/Vice President Sales
     Robert V. Linden/Vice President Sales
Production: Trent G. Kamke/Senior Vice President Operations
Research: Ryan H. Connelly/Director Research & Development
Finance: Joseph P. Pellegrino/Chief Financial Officer

Bandage, Adhesive	Surgery
Catheter, Arterial	Cardiovascular
Catheter, Cholangiography	Surgery
Catheter, Occlusion	Cardiovascular
Clip, Vascular	Cardiovascular
Material, Training, Audiovisual	General
Needle, Suture, Disposable	Surgery
Shunt, Carotid	Cardiovascular
Stent, Vascular	Cardiovascular
Stripper, Artery, Intraluminal	Cardiovascular
Stripper, Vein, External	Cardiovascular
Valvulotome	Cardiovascular

LEMANS INDUSTRIES CORP.   800-289-5667
79 Express St., Plainview, NY 11803-2404   **516-942-9800**
FDA Number: n/a   *Fax:* 516-942-7556
E-mail: sales@lemansind.com
Web site: www.lemansind.com
Ownership: Private
Produces/Sells CE-marked Devices: N

LEMANS INDUSTRIES CORP.   800-289-5667 (cont'd)
Distribution: Manufacturer Direct, Exclusive Distributor
General Admin.: Glenn Mandler/President

Component, Plastic	General
Cover, Other	General

LEMARGO INC.   800-469-3932
259 Traders Blvd., Unit 8,   **905-949-4939**
Mississauga, ONT L4Z 2 Canada
FDA Number: n/a   *Fax:* 905-949-4606
E-mail: biomed@lemargo.com
Web site: www.lemargo.com
Year Founded: 1994
Total Employees: 10
Ownership: Private
Produces/Sells CE-marked Devices: N
Distribution: Exclusive Distributor, Importer

LEMCO ENTERPRISES, INC.   580-226-7808
3204 Hale Rd., Ardmore, OK 73401
FDA Number: 1644312   *Fax:* 580-226-6395
E-mail: lemco@brightok.net
Web site: www.lemcoenterprises.com
Medical Products Sales Volume: $5,000,000
Annual Revenue: $1-$5 Million
Year Founded: 1990
Total Employees: 20
Ownership: Private
Produces/Sells CE-marked Devices: N
Federal Procurement Eligibility: Small Business
Distribution: Service Direct
General Admin.: Steven Wells/Chief Executive Officer
     Aaron W. Midden/President
Mktg./Adv.: Barry Guffey/Marketing Representative

Bandage, Cast	Physical Med
Contract Sterilization	General

LENDELL MFG., INC.   800-566-8569
5301 South Graham Road, St. Charles, MI 48655   **989-865-8200**
FDA Number: 1835085   *Fax:* 989-865-8118
E-mail: info@lendell.com
Web site: www.LENDELL.com
Medical Products Sales Volume: $1,800,000
Year Founded: 1994
Total Employees: 25
Ownership: Private
Quality System Registration Information: ISO9001
Produces/Sells CE-marked Devices: N
Federal Procurement Eligibility: Small Business

Beads, Hydrophilic, Wound Exudate Absorption	Surgery

LENJOY MEDICAL ENGINEERING, INC.   310-353-2481
13112 Crenshaw Blvd., Gardena, CA 90249-2466
FDA Number: 2025918   *Fax:* 310-353-2484
E-mail: custserv@comfysplints.com
Web site: www.comfysplints.com
Annual Revenue: $0-$1 Million
Year Founded: 1992
Ownership: Private
Produces/Sells CE-marked Devices: N
Federal Procurement Eligibility: Female Owned

Bandage, Compression	General
Binder, Breast	Obstetrics/Gynecology
Binder, Elastic	General
Brace, Joint, Ankle (External)	Physical Med
Communication System, Non-Powered	Physical Med
Monitor, Bed Patient	General
Pin, Retentive And Splinting	Dental And Oral
Tips And Pads, Cane, Crutch And Walker	Physical Med
Wheelchair, Manual	Physical Med

LENOX HILL BRACE / SEATTLE SYSTEMS   360-697-5656
26296 Twelve Trees Ln NW, Poulsbo, WA 98370
FDA Number: n/a   *Fax:* 360-697-5876
E-mail: customerservice@seattlesystems.com
Web site: www.seattlesystems.com
Total Employees: 25
Ownership: Seattle Systems
Produces/Sells CE-marked Devices: N
Federal Procurement Eligibility: Small Business
Distribution: Manufacturer Direct
General Admin.: Patricia Perez/Manager Human Resources
     Calvin Andre/President, Chief Executive Officer
Mktg./Adv.: David Adams/Vice President Marketing
     Patrick Patterson/Vice President Sales
Production: Meg Hall/Product Manager
     Ryan Terry/Product Manager
     Dick Winslow/Vice President Manufacturing

LENOX HILL BRACE / SEATTLE SYSTEMS 360-697-5656 (cont'd)
Research: Jeremy Adelson/Manager Research & Development
Finance: Laurence Leslie/Chief Financial Officer
  Joint, Knee, External Brace   Physical Med

LENOX LASER   800-494-6537
12530 Manor Road, Glen Arm, MD 21057   410-592-3106
FDA Number: n/a   *Fax:* 410-592-3362
E-mail: lenox@lenoxlaser.com
Web site: www.lenoxlaser.com
Medical Products Sales Volume: $1,900,000
Annual Revenue: $1-$5 Million
Year Founded: 1980
Total Employees: 28   *Marketing Staff:* 2   *Sales Staff:* 2
Ownership: Private
Produces/Sells CE-marked Devices: N
Federal Procurement Eligibility: Small Business
Distribution: Manufacturer Direct
General Admin.: Joe d'Entremont/President
     Gary Thornton/Vice President, General Manager
Mktg./Adv.: Gary Thornton/Manager Contract Sales
     Rachel Loper/Manager Market Research
Production: Joshua Gray/Director Quality Assurance
     Robert Gidner/Senior Engineer
     John Demed/Vice President Manufacturing
Research: Tom Cardock/Vice President Research & Development
  Gas Mixtures, Laboratory   General
  Microplate   General
  Service, Consulting   General
  Service, Used Equipment   General

LENOX-MACLAREN SURGICAL CORP.   720-890-9660
657 S. Taylor Avenue, Suite A, Colorado Technology Center,
Louisville, CO 80027
FDA Number: 1722824   *Fax:* 720-890-9868
E-mail: lenoxmaclaren@ aol.com
Web site: www.lenoxmaclaren.com
Medical Products Sales Volume: $3,800,000
Annual Revenue: $1-$5 Million
Year Founded: 1983
Total Employees: 3
Federal Procurement Eligibility: Small Business, Female Owned
Distribution: Manufacturer Direct
General Admin.: Linda Lenox/President, Chief Executive Officer
  Awl   Orthopedics
  Bone Mill   Orthopedics
  Chisel, Bone, Surgical   Dental And Oral
  Compression Instrument   Orthopedics
  Curette, Surgical   Surgery
  Elevator, Surgical, General & Plastic Surgery   Surgery
  Expander, Surgical, Skin Graft   Surgery
  Gouge, Surgical, General & Plastic Surgery   Surgery
  Impactor   Orthopedics
  Mallet, Surgical, General & Plastic Surgery   Surgery
  Osteotome, Manual (Plastic Surgery)   Surgery
  Retractor, All Types   Dental And Oral
  Tap, Bone   Orthopedics
  Tray, Surgical Instrument   Surgery
  Twister, Wire   Orthopedics

LENS DYNAMICS, INC.   303-237-6927
14998 W. 6th Ave, #830, Golden, CO 80401
FDA Number: 1718651
  Cleaner, Lens, Contact   Ophthalmology
  Lens, Contact (Other Material)   Ophthalmology
  Lens, Contact, Polymethylmethacrylate   Ophthalmology
  Lenses, Soft Contact, Extended Wear   Ophthalmology

LENS EXPRESS, INC.   800-536-7397
350 S.W. 12th Avenue,   954-421-5800
Deerfield Beach, FL 33442
FDA Number: n/a   *Fax:* 954-480-8505
E-mail: customerservice@lensexpress.com
Web site: www.lensexpress.com
Medical Products Sales Volume: $1,000,000
Total Employees: 25
Ownership: Private
Produces/Sells CE-marked Devices: N
Federal Procurement Eligibility: Small Business
Distribution: Service Direct
  Lens, Contact (Other Material)   Ophthalmology

LENS MODE, INC.   800-852-5880
150 Main St., Millburn, NJ 07041-1114
FDA Number: n/a   *Fax:* 888-852-5880
E-mail: info@lensmodecontacts.com
Web site: www.lensmodecontacts.com
Annual Revenue: $0-$1 Million

LENS MODE, INC.   800-852-5880 (cont'd)
Ownership: Private
Produces/Sells CE-marked Devices: N
Federal Procurement Eligibility: Small Business
Distribution: Manufacturer Direct
General Admin.: Daniel Strulowitz/President
  Lens, Contact, Gas-Permeable   Ophthalmology

LENSCRAFTERS, INC.   770-305-7352
9926 International Blvd., Cincinnati, OH 45246
FDA Number: 1527326
  Frame, Spectacle (Eyeglasses)   Ophthalmology
  Lens, Spectacle/Eyeglasses, Non-Custom   Ophthalmology

LENSTEC, INC.   727-571-2272
1765 Commerce Ave. N, Saint Petersburg, FL 33716
FDA Number: 1063199   *Fax:* 1 727-571-1792
E-mail: lenstec@lenstec.com
Ownership: Private
Produces/Sells CE-marked Devices: N
  Folders and Injectors, Intraocular Lens (IOL)   Ophthalmology
  Hook, Ophthalmic   Ophthalmology
  Lens, Intraocular   Ophthalmology
  Phacofragmentation Unit   Ophthalmology

LENZING FIBERS INC.   251-679-2811
12950 US Highway 43 North, Axis, AL 36505
FDA Number: 1055132   *Fax:* 251-679-2880
E-mail: m.griffith@lenzing.com
Web site: www.tencel.com
Year Founded: 1992
Total Employees: 110
Ownership: Private
Produces/Sells CE-marked Devices: N
Federal Procurement Eligibility: Small Business
Mktg./Adv.: Mr. Nick Simpson/Market Manager
  Sponge, External, Neurological   Cns/Neurology

LEPCO
  See Luwa Lepco

LES EQUIPEMENTS ADAPTES PHYSIPRO INC.   800-668-2252
370, 10e Avenue South,   819-823-2252
Sherbrooke, QUE J1G 2 Canada
FDA Number: n/a   *Fax:* 819-565-3337
E-mail: physipro@abacom.com
Web site: www.physipro.com
Year Founded: 1988
Total Employees: 25
Ownership: Private
Produces/Sells CE-marked Devices: N
Distribution: Manufacturer Direct, Exporter

LES ESCALATEURS ATLAS INC.   888-773-6708
8255 Boul. Laframboise,   450-796-5708
St-Hyacinthe, QUE J2R 1 Canada
FDA Number: n/a   *Fax:* 450-796-5110
Year Founded: 1979
Ownership: Private
Produces/Sells CE-marked Devices: N
Distribution: Manufacturer Direct

LES LABORATOIRES QUELAB INC.   1 (800) 579-099
5615, Fullum, Montreal, QUE H2G 2H6 Canada   514-277-2558
FDA Number: n/a   *Fax:* 514-277-4714
E-mail: info@quelab.qc.ca
Web site: www.quelab.qc.ca
Year Founded: 1974
Total Employees: 50
Ownership: Private
Produces/Sells CE-marked Devices: N
Distribution: Manufacturer Direct, Exclusive Distributor

LESCO OPTICAL   520-323-1538
4444 East Grant Rd, Tucson, AZ 85712
FDA Number: n/a
Annual Revenue: $0-$1 Million
Ownership: Private
Produces/Sells CE-marked Devices: N
Federal Procurement Eligibility: Small Business
Distribution: Manufacturer Direct
  Eyeglasses   Ophthalmology

LESTER ELECTRICAL OF NEBRASKA, INC.   402-477-8988
625 West A St., Lincoln, NE 68522-1706
FDA Number: n/a   *Fax:* 402-441-3727
E-mail: sales@lesterelectrical.com
Web site: www.lesterelectrical.com
Medical Products Sales Volume: $2,000,000

LESTER ELECTRICAL OF NEBRASKA, INC.   402-477-8988
(cont'd)
  Annual Revenue: $25-$50 Million
  Total Employees: 540   *Marketing Staff:* 2   *Sales Staff:* 3
  Ownership: Private
  Quality System Registration Information: ISO9001
  Produces/Sells CE-marked Devices: Y
  Distribution: Manufacturer Direct, OEM
  General Admin.: James L. Carrier/President
  Mktg./Adv.: K.R. Jeffcoat/Director Marketing & Sales
  Production: Michael L. Schukar/Vice President Production
    Accessories, Wheelchair   Physical Med
    Charger, Battery   General

LETO MEDICAL LLC.   904-261-8218
1886 S. 14th Street, Suite 6, Fernandina Beach, FL 32034
  FDA Number: n/a
  E-mail: info@letomedical.com
  Web site: http://www.letomedical.com
  Year Founded: 2010
  Ownership: Private
  Produces/Sells CE-marked Devices: N
  General Admin.: Dr. John Minasi/Chief Scientific Officer
    Mr. Jim Schneider/President

LETOURNEAU LIFELIKE ORTHOTICS & PROSTHETICS, INC.
  See Letourneau Prosthetics

LETOURNEAU PROSTHETICS   800-609-5005
2452 Calder Ave., Beaumont, TX 77702   **409-832-5005**
  FDA Number: n/a   *Fax:* 409-832-5015
  Web site: www.orthotics-prosthetics.com
  Ownership: Private
  Produces/Sells CE-marked Devices: N
  Federal Procurement Eligibility: Small Business
  Distribution: Manufacturer Direct
    Custom Prosthesis   Orthopedics
    Prosthesis, Arm   Orthopedics
    Prosthesis, Leg   Orthopedics
    Support, Arch   Physical Med

LEVEL 1 TECHNOLOGIES, INC.
  See Smiths Medical Asd, Inc.

LEVERTEC THERAPY EQUIPMENT LTD.   1 888 261-6341
P.O. Box 907,   **250-396-7406**
100 Mile House, BC V0K-2 Canada
  FDA Number: n/a   *Fax:* 250-396-7506
  E-mail: info@levertec.com
  Web site: www.levertec.com
  Year Founded: 10
  Total Employees: 10
  Ownership: Private
  Produces/Sells CE-marked Devices: N
  Distribution: Manufacturer Direct, Exclusive Distributor

LEVINE HEALTH PRODUCTS   800-426-6763
21101 N.E. 108th St., Redmond, WA 98053-2116   **425-836-3309**
  FDA Number: 3014823   *Fax:* 425-868-5393
  E-mail: levhealth@aol.com
  Web site: www.levinehealth.com
  Medical Products Sales Volume: $870,000
  Annual Revenue: $0-$1 Million
  Year Founded: 1974
  Total Employees: 7
  Ownership: Private
  Produces/Sells CE-marked Devices: N
  Federal Procurement Eligibility: Small Business
  Distribution: Manufacturer Direct, Service Direct, Exclusive Distributor, Exporter
  General Admin.: Bill Levine/Chief Executive Officer
    Bandage, Elastic   General
    Bracelet, Identification   General
    Dispenser, Medication, Liquid   General
    Otoscope   Ear/Nose/Throat

LEVITRONIX LLC   1 (866) 487 - 2
45 First Ave., North Waltham, MA 02451   **781-622-5075**
  FDA Number: 1226752   *Fax:* 1 (781) 622 509
  E-mail: info@levitronix.com
  Ownership: Private
  Produces/Sells CE-marked Devices: N
    Controller, Pump Speed, Cardiopulmonary Bypass   Cardiovascular

LEVO USA   888-538-6872
7105 Northland Terrace, Brooklyn Park,   **763-544-7779**
Minneapolis, MN 55428
  FDA Number: n/a   *Fax:* 763-544-4234
  E-mail: request@levousa.com
  Web site: www.levousa.com

LEVO USA   888-538-6872 *(cont'd)*
  Medical Products Sales Volume: $11,000,000
  Year Founded: 1975
  Total Employees: 63   *Marketing Staff:* 1   *Sales Staff:* 3
  Ownership: None
  Produces/Sells CE-marked Devices: N
  Federal Procurement Eligibility: Small Business, VA Contract
  Distribution: Exclusive Distributor
  General Admin.: Dr. Kurt Fischer/Chief Executive Officer
    Rick Klusovsky/General Manager
    Thomas Raeber/President
  Production: Brandi Jones/Manager Customer Services
    Fred Rodes/Manager Materials
    Wade Holley/Managing Director Production
    Wheelchair, Standup   Physical Med

LEW JAN TEXTILE   800-899-0531
366 Veterans Memorial Hwy. Suite 4,   **631-543-0531**
Commack, NY 11725
  FDA Number: n/a   *Fax:* 631-543-0561
  E-mail: sjanicola@lewjan.com
  Web site: www.lewjan.com
  Ownership: Private
  Produces/Sells CE-marked Devices: N
  Distribution: Manufacturer Through Distributor
  General Admin.: Scott Janicola/President, Chief Executive Officer
    Bib   General
    Diaper, Adult   General
    Pad, Incontinence (Underpad)   General

LEWIS BINS+   877-97L-EWIS
PO BOX 389, Oconomowoc, WI 53066   **262-560-5700**
  FDA Number: n/a   *Fax:* 262-560-5533
  E-mail: info@lewisbins.com
  Web site: www.lewisbins.com
  Annual Revenue: $50-$100 Million
  Ownership: Private
  Quality System Registration Information: ISO9001
  Produces/Sells CE-marked Devices: N
  Distribution: Manufacturer Through Distributor, Manufacturer Through Manufacturer Reps
  Production: Joni Sterwald/Product Manager
    Bin, Storage   General
    Carrier, Container, Oxygen, Portable   General
    Tray, Medicine   General

LEWIS CORP.
  See Stoelting

LEWIS PHARMACEUTICAL INFORMATION, LLC   423-942-9445
534 Spears Road, Kimball, TN 37347
  FDA Number: 1037361
  Ownership: Private
  Produces/Sells CE-marked Devices: N
    Calculator, Drug Dose   Surgery

LEWISYSTEMS
  See Orbis Corporation

LEX-TON ORTHOPEDICS   615-890-6969
1133 White Cliff Rd., Lawrenceburg, TN 38464
  FDA Number: 1037142
  Ownership: Private
  Produces/Sells CE-marked Devices: N
    Accessories, Operating Room, Table   Surgery

LEXAMED   419-693-5307
705 Front St., Northwood, OH 43605
  FDA Number: 1525897
    Accessories, Apparel, Surgical   Surgery
    Dressing, Other   General
    Kit, Administration, Intravenous   General
    Kit, Surgical (General)   Surgery
    Kit, Surgical Instrument, Disposable   Surgery
    Needle, Hypodermic, Single Lumen With Syringe   General

LEXICON BRANDING, INC.   415-332-1811
30 Liberty Ship Way, Suite 3360, Sausalito, CA 94965
  FDA Number: n/a   *Fax:* 415-332-2528
  E-mail: information@lexiconbranding.com
  Web site: www.lexiconbranding.com
  Annual Revenue: $0-$1 Million
  Year Founded: 1982
  Total Employees: 20
  Ownership: Private
  Produces/Sells CE-marked Devices: N
  Federal Procurement Eligibility: Small Business
  Distribution: Service Direct
  General Admin.: J. David Placek/President

LEXICON BRANDING, INC.
415-332-1811 *(cont'd)*
Service, Consulting
General

LEXICON NAMING
See Lexicon Branding, Inc.

LEXICOR MEDICAL TECHNOLOGY, INC.
303-443-9944
2840 Wilderness Pl, Suite E, Boulder, CO 80301
FDA Number: 1721975
Fax: 303-443-0591
Web site: www.lexicor.com
Ownership: Private
Produces/Sells CE-marked Devices: N
Analyzer, Spectrum, EEG Signal	Cns/Neurology
Biofeedback Device	Cns/Neurology
Computer, Chemistry Analyzer	Chemistry
Electroencephalograph	Cns/Neurology

LEXINGTON INTERNATIONAL, LLC
800-973-4769
561-417-0200
777 Yamato Rd., Suite 105, Boca Raton, FL 33431
FDA Number: 3006182775
Fax: 561-892-0747
E-mail: info@hairmax.com
Web site: www.hairmax.com
Ownership: Private
Produces/Sells CE-marked Devices: N
Laser, Comb, Hair
Physical Med

LEXION MEDICAL, LLC.
651-635-0000
5000 Township Pkwy, Saint Paul, MN 55110
FDA Number: 2135348
Insufflator, Laparoscopic
Obstetrics/Gynecology

LEYBOLD INFICON INC., MED. PROD. DIV.
See Infimed, Inc.

LEYSHON MILLER INDUSTRIES
740-432-2969
534 N 1st St., Cambridge, OH 43725
FDA Number: 3004634242
Fax: 740-432-8865
E-mail: Info@LMIDesign.com
Web site: www.LMIDesign.com
Ownership: Private
Produces/Sells CE-marked Devices: N
Kit, Enema (For Cleaning Purposes)
Gastroenterology/Urology

LFI, INC-LASER FARE, INC.
(401) 278-9100
315 Iron Horse Way,, Suite 101, Providence, RI 02908
FDA Number: 1287338
Fax: (401) 273-8270
E-mail: info@lfiinc.com
Web site: www.riedc.com
Medical Products Sales Volume: $4,000,000
Annual Revenue: $5-$10 Million
Year Founded: 1978
Total Employees: 50   Marketing Staff: 1   Sales Staff: 3
Ownership: Private
Quality System Registration Information: ISO9001
Produces/Sells CE-marked Devices: Y
Federal Procurement Eligibility: Small Business
Distribution: Manufacturer Direct, Service Direct
General Admin.: Mr. Clifford Brockmyre/Chief Executive Officer, Chairman
        Tyler Smith/General Manager
        Clifford Brockmyre/President
        Ms. Beth Blackburn/Program Manager
Production: Mr. Kevin Costa/Manager Engineering
        Mrs. Rachel Pouliot/Manager Quality Assurance
Finance: Roland Benjamin/Vice President, Secretary Treasurer
Cannula, Sinus	Ear/Nose/Throat
Instrument, Microsurgical	Cns/Neurology
Instrument, Surgical, Powered, Pneumatic	Orthopedics
Suture, Other	Surgery
System, Marking, Laser	General

LG ELECTRONICS U.S.A., INC.
800-884-1742
847-941-8181
2000 Millbrook Drive, Lincolnshire, IL 60069
FDA Number: n/a
Fax: 847-941-8405
E-mail: timothy.wright@lge.com
Web site: www.lgusa.com
Year Founded: 1958
Ownership: Saint-Gobain
Produces/Sells CE-marked Devices: N
Federal Procurement Eligibility: GSA Contract, VA Contract
Distribution: Manufacturer Direct, Importer, Exporter
General Admin.: Michael Ahn/Chief Executive Officer
        Gary Bonomolo/Vice President Human Resources
Mktg./Adv.: Sam Caputo/Director Advertising
        Mike Kosla/Director Sales
        Tim Wright/Manager National Sales
        Ron Snaidauf/Vice President Commercial Products
        John Taylor/Vice President Public Affairs
Research: Richard Lewis/Vice President Research & Development
Finance: John Taylor/Vice President Public Communications & Investor Relations
Recorder, Videotape/Videodisc
General

LG ELECTRONICS U.S.A., INC.
800-884-1742 *(cont'd)*
Television, Patient Room
General

LG MEDICAL TECHNOLOGY, LLC
360-668-0803
22529 39th Ave Se, Bothell, WA 98021
FDA Number: 3006137931
Ownership: Private
Produces/Sells CE-marked Devices: N
Pack, Hot Or Cold, Reusable
Physical Med

LGM INTERNATIONAL INC.
410-472-9930
3030 Venture Lane,suite 106, Melbourne, FL 32934
FDA Number: 3004421347
Fixative, Alcohol Containing	Pathology
Media, Mounting	Pathology
Reagent, General Purpose	Pathology

LHASA MEDICAL, INC.
See Lhasa Oms, Inc.

LHASA OMS, INC.
800-722-8775
781-340-1071
230 Libbey Parkway, Weymouth, MA 02189
FDA Number: 1222811
Fax: 781-335-5779
E-mail: info@lhasaoms.com
Web site: www.lhasaoms.com
Annual Revenue: $1-$5 Million
Ownership: Private
Produces/Sells CE-marked Devices: N
Federal Procurement Eligibility: Small Business, Female Owned
Distribution: Exclusive Distributor, Importer, Exporter
Chart, Acupuncture	Surgery
Needle, Acupuncture	Anesthesiology
Stimulator, Electro/Acupuncture	Anesthesiology
Stimulator, Muscle, Electrical-Powered (EMS)	Physical Med
Stimulator, Nerve, Transcutaneous (Pain Relief, TENS)	Cns/Neurology

LHB INDUSTRIES
800-542-3697
314-423-7955
10440 Trenton Avenue, St. Louis, MO 63132
FDA Number: 1925025
Fax: 314-423-0139
E-mail: customerservice@lhbindustries.com
Web site: www.lhbindustries.com
Year Founded: 1940
Total Employees: 55
Ownership: Private
Produces/Sells CE-marked Devices: N
Federal Procurement Eligibility: Small Business
Production: Mr. Angelo Vangel/Quality Control, Product Engineer
Kit, First Aid
Surgery

LI-COR, INC.
800-645-4267
402-467-0700
4647 Superior Street Lincoln,
Lincoln, NE 68504
FDA Number: n/a
Fax: 402-467-0819
E-mail: biohelp@licor.com
Web site: www.licor.com
Annual Revenue: $10-$25 Million
Ownership: Private
Quality System Registration Information: ISO9001
Produces/Sells CE-marked Devices: Y
Federal Procurement Eligibility: Small Business
Distribution: Manufacturer Direct
Photometer
Chemistry

LIBERATING TECHNOLOGIES, INC.
800-437-0024
508-893-6363
325 Hopping Brook Road, Suite A,
Holliston, MA 01746
FDA Number: 1220851
Fax: 508-893-9966
E-mail: info@liberatingtech.com
Web site: www.liberatingtechnologies.com
Medical Products Sales Volume: $1,800,000
Year Founded: 2001
Total Employees: 8
Ownership: Private
Produces/Sells CE-marked Devices: Y
Federal Procurement Eligibility: Small Business
Distribution: Manufacturer Direct
Joint, Hip, External Brace
Physical Med

LIBERTY ENTERPRISES
518-842-5080
43 Liberty Dr, Amsterdam, NY 12010
FDA Number: n/a
Fax: 518-842-0143
E-mail: info@libertyarc.org
Web site: www.libertyarc.org
Medical Products Sales Volume: $5,500,000
Annual Revenue: $10-$25 Million
Year Founded: 1954
Ownership: Private
Produces/Sells CE-marked Devices: N
Federal Procurement Eligibility: Small Business

LIBERTY ENTERPRISES
518-842-5080 (cont'd)
Distribution: Manufacturer Direct, Manufacturer Through Distributor

Detergent	Hematology
Disinfector, Liquid	General
Encapsulator, Fluid	General
Kit, Prep	General
Pack, Cold	General
Pack, Hot, Chemical	General
Soap	General

LIBERTY INDUSTRIES, INC.
800-828-5656
133 Commerce St., East Berlin, CT 06023
860-828-6361
FDA Number: 9200647
Fax: 860-828-8879
E-mail: libind@liberty-ind.com
Web site: www.liberty-ind.com
Medical Products Sales Volume: $3,000,000
Annual Revenue: $5-$10 Million
Year Founded: 1953
Total Employees: 30   *Marketing Staff:* 2   *Sales Staff:* 8
Ownership: Private
Produces/Sells CE-marked Devices: Y
Federal Procurement Eligibility: Small Business
Distribution: Manufacturer Direct, Manufacturer Through Distributor, Manufacturer Through Manufacturer Reps, Exporter
General Admin.: John Nappi/Chief Executive Officer
        Robert Kaiser/President
Mktg./Adv.: George Pollick/Director Product Development
        Greg Bunnell/Manager Sales Training
        Mrs. Cathy Albano/Product & Sales Manager

Cabinet, Pass Through	General
Cleanroom Equipment	General
Filter, Air	General
Finger Cot	General
Floor Mat, Antibacterial	General
Glove, Other	General
Hood, Isolation, Laminar Air Flow	General
Laminar Air Flow Unit	General
Laminar Air Flow Unit, Fixed (Air Curtain)	Chemistry
Laminar Air Flow Unit, Mobile	Chemistry

LIBERTY MEDICAL LLC
888-257-2408
10 Acacia Lane, Sterling, VA 20166
FDA Number: 3004982143

Applicator, Radionuclide, Manual	Radiology

LIDCO LTD. USA
877-543-2611
500 Park Avenue, Suite 103, Lake Villa, IL 60046
847-265-3700
FDA Number: n/a
Fax: 847-265-3737
E-mail: usorders@lidco.com
Web site: www.lidco.com
Year Founded: 1991
Total Employees: 39
Ownership: Lidco Ltd.
Quality System Registration Information: ISO9001
Produces/Sells CE-marked Devices: N
Federal Procurement Eligibility: Small Business
Distribution: Manufacturer Through Distributor
General Admin.: Dr. Terence O'Brien/Chief Executive Officer

Cardiac Output Unit, Other	Cardiovascular

LIDE LABORATORIES, INC.
952-758-9760
401 4th. Ave.sw, New Prague, MN 56071
FDA Number: 1924632
Fax: 952-758-9760
E-mail: lidelabs@aol.com
Web site: www.lidelabs.com
Annual Revenue: $0-$1 Million
Year Founded: 1948
Ownership: Private
Produces/Sells CE-marked Devices: N
Federal Procurement Eligibility: Small Business
Distribution: Manufacturer Direct, Manufacturer Through Distributor

Stain, Giemsa	Pathology
Stain, Microbiological	Microbiology

LIEBEL-FLARSHEIM
See Mallinckrodt, Inc.

LIF-O-GEN INC.
See Allied Healthcare Products, Inc.

LIFE BACK ENTERPRISES, INC.
727-641-9042
416 Admiral Cove, Tarpon Springs, FL 34689
FDA Number: 3006208405

Orthosis, Lumbosacral	Physical Med

LIFE CARE TECHNOLOGIES, INC.
800-671-0580
4710 Eisenhower Boulevard, Suite A-10,
813-886-7500
Tampa, FL 33634
FDA Number: 2950326
Fax: 813-881-0700
E-mail: Info@lifecaretech.com

LIFE CARE TECHNOLOGIES, INC.
800-671-0580 (cont'd)
Web site: www.lifecaretech.com
Medical Products Sales Volume: $5,900,000
Year Founded: 1999
Total Employees: 70
Ownership: Mts Medication Technologies
Produces/Sells CE-marked Devices: N
Federal Procurement Eligibility: Small Business
Distribution: Manufacturer Direct, Manufacturer Through Distributor, Service Direct
General Admin.: Kenny Grewal/Chief Operating Officer, Vice President

Computer Software	General
Computer Software, Hospital/Nursing Management	General
Computer, Clinical Laboratory	Chemistry
Computer, Patient Data Management	General
Dispenser, Narcotic	General
System, Drug Dispensing, Pharmacy, Automated	General

LIFE CENTERS, INC.
See Sterion, Incorporated

LIFE CORPORATION
800-700-0202
1776 North Water Street,
414-272-4000
Milwaukee, WI 53202
FDA Number: 2183615
E-mail: email@LIFEcorporation.com
Fax: 414-272-0000
Web site: www.LIFEcorporation.com
Year Founded: 1985
Total Employees: 12   *Marketing Staff:* 3   *Sales Staff:* 3
Ownership: Private
Stock Symbol: N/A
Produces/Sells CE-marked Devices: Y
Federal Procurement Eligibility: Small Business, GSA Contract, VA Contract
Distribution: Manufacturer Through Distributor, Manufacturer Through Manufacturer Reps, OEM, Exporter
General Admin.: Sarah Finnessy/Business Manager
        Mark Veenendaal/General Manager
        John Kirchgeorg/President, Chief Executive Officer
Mktg./Adv.: Amy Carroll/Director Marketing

Canister, Oxygen	Anesthesiology
Cannula, Nasal, Oxygen	Anesthesiology
Carrier, Container, Oxygen, Portable	General
Cart, Emergency, Cardiopulmonary Resuscitation (Crash)	Anesthesiology
Cart, Gas Cylinder (Carrier)	Anesthesiology
Cylinder, Compressed Gas, With Valve	Anesthesiology
Cylinder, Gas (Empty)	Anesthesiology
Cylinder, Oxygen	Anesthesiology
Flowmeter, Back-Pressure Compensated, Thorpe Tube	Anesthesiology
Flowmeter, Gas (Oxygen), Calibrated	Anesthesiology
Flowmeter, Gas, Non-Back-Pressure Compensated, Bourdon Gauge	Anesthesiology
Gauge, Gas Pressure, Cylinder/Pipeline	Anesthesiology
Holder, Gas Cylinder	Anesthesiology
Kit, Administration, Oxygen	Anesthesiology
Mask, Oxygen, Aerosol Administration	Anesthesiology
Mask, Oxygen, Low Concentration, Venturi	Anesthesiology
Mask, Oxygen, Non-Rebreathing	Anesthesiology
Mask, Oxygen, Other	General
Mask, Oxygen, Partial Rebreathing	General
Oxygen	Anesthesiology
Regulator, Oxygen, Mechanical	General
Regulator, Pressure, Gas Cylinder	Anesthesiology
Rescue Equipment	General
Resuscitator, Cardiac, Mechanical, Compressor	Anesthesiology
Resuscitator, Emergency Oxygen	Dental And Oral
Resuscitator, Emergency, Protective, Infection	General
Resuscitator, Pulmonary, Gas	General
Resuscitator, Pulmonary, Manual (Demand Valve)	General
Stand, Gas Cylinder	Anesthesiology
Tubing, Flexible, Medical Gas, Low-Pressure	Anesthesiology
Tubing, Oxygen Connecting	General
Valve, Breathing	Anesthesiology
Valve, Non-Rebreathing	Anesthesiology
Ventilator, Emergency, Manual (Resuscitator)	Anesthesiology
Ventilator, Emergency, Powered (Resuscitator)	Anesthesiology
Ventilator, Other	Anesthesiology

LIFE ENHANCEMENT TECHNOLOGIES, INC.
408-330-6940
807 Aldo Ave., Suite 101, Santa Clara, CA 95054
FDA Number: 2954778

Pack, Hot Or Cold, Water Circulating	Physical Med

LIFE FITNESS
800-735-3867
10601 W. Belmont Avenue,
847-288-3300
Franklin Park, IL 60131
FDA Number: n/a
Fax: 847-288-3703
E-mail: commercialsales@lifefitness.com
Web site: www.lifefitness.com
Year Founded: 1968
Total Employees: 786   *Marketing Staff:* 30   *Sales Staff:* 100
Ownership: BRUNSWICK
Quality System Registration Information: ISO9000

LIFE FITNESS · 800-735-3867 (cont'd)
Produces/Sells CE-marked Devices: Y
Federal Procurement Eligibility: Small Business, GSA Contract
Distribution: Manufacturer Direct
Mktg./Adv.: Ms. Cheryl Jasinski/National Sales Representative

Exercise Stair	Physical Med
Exerciser, Bicycle	Physical Med
Exerciser, Other	Physical Med
Treadmill, Powered	Physical Med

LIFE GUARD · 626-965-1588
18400 San Jose Avenue, City of Industry, CA 91748
FDA Number: 2086535 · *Fax:* 626-965-3599
E-mail: nick@lifeguardgloves.com
Web site: www.LifeGuardGloves.com
Medical Products Sales Volume: $3,600,000
Annual Revenue: $10-$25 Million
Year Founded: 1987
Total Employees: 12 · *Marketing Staff:* 3 · *Sales Staff:* 7
Ownership: Private
Quality System Registration Information: ISO9002
Produces/Sells CE-marked Devices: Y
Federal Procurement Eligibility: Small Business, Minority Owned, Female Owned, GSA Contract
Distribution: Manufacturer Direct, Manufacturer Through Distributor, Manufacturer Through Manufacturer Reps, OEM, Service Direct, Exclusive Distributor
General Admin.: Nicholas Hung/Vice President
Mktg./Adv.: Mr. Stephen Wang/Director Marketing

Glove, Patient Examination	General
Glove, Patient Examination, Latex	General
Glove, Patient Examination, Vinyl	General

Medical Product Subsidiaries (Listed Separately)
  A Plus Intl., Inc.
  American Dental Supply, Inc.
  Ansell Healthcare Products, Inc.

LIFE GUARD SUPPLY, INC.
See Life Guard

LIFE MEASUREMENT, INC. · 925-676-6002
1850 Bates Ave., Concord, CA 94520
FDA Number: 3003873943

Analyzer, Body Composition	Cardiovascular

LIFE MEDICAL EQUIPMENT · 800-749-4646 · 305-594-0000
7874 N.W. 64 St., Miami, FL 33166
FDA Number: n/a · *Fax:* 305-594-2020
E-mail: lme@lifemedicalequipment.com
Web site: www.lifemedicalequipment.com
Medical Products Sales Volume: $1,700,000
Annual Revenue: $1-$5 Million
Year Founded: 1980
Total Employees: 14 · *Marketing Staff:* 1 · *Sales Staff:* 4
Ownership: LIFE MEDICAL
Produces/Sells CE-marked Devices: N
Federal Procurement Eligibility: Small Business
Distribution: Service Direct, Exporter
General Admin.: Ari Lipson/President, Chief Executive Officer
Mktg./Adv.: Ari Lipson/Manager Advertising

Service, Import/Export	General
Service, Maintenance/Repair	General
Service, Used Equipment	General

LIFE MEDICAL LLC · 317-840-3816
10424 Snapper Ct., Indianapolis, IN 46256
FDA Number: n/a · *Fax:* 317-570-5831
E-mail: aelsbury@LifeMedicalLLC.com
Web site: www.LifeMedicalLLC.com/
Year Founded: 2003
Ownership: Private
Produces/Sells CE-marked Devices: N
Federal Procurement Eligibility: Small Business
Distribution: Manufacturer Direct
General Admin.: Mr. Andrew Elsbury/Chief Executive Officer

Implant, Fixation Device, Spinal	Orthopedics

LIFE PLUS INTERNATIONAL · 800-572-8446
P.O. Box 3749, Batesville, AR 72503
FDA Number: 208523 · *Fax:* 870-698-2379
E-mail: info.us@lifeplus.com
Web site: www.lifeplus.com
Medical Products Sales Volume: $18,000,000
Total Employees: 500 · *Marketing Staff:* 8 · *Sales Staff:* 400000
Ownership: V.M. NUTRI
Quality System Registration Information: ISO9001
Produces/Sells CE-marked Devices: N
Federal Procurement Eligibility: Small Business
Distribution: Manufacturer Through Distributor, Manufacturer Through Manufacturer Reps, Exporter

LIFE PLUS INTERNATIONAL · 800-572-8446 (cont'd)
General Admin.: J. Robert Lemon/Chief Executive Officer

Colposcope	Obstetrics/Gynecology
Lotion, Skin Care	General

LIFE RECOVERY SYSTEMS HD, LLC. · 973-283-2800
170 Kinnelon Road, Kinnelon, NJ 07405
FDA Number: 3006059109 · *Fax:* 973-283-2910
E-mail: info@life-recovery.com
Ownership: Private
Produces/Sells CE-marked Devices: N
General Admin.: Russel VanZandt/Chief Operating Officer

Hypothermia System, Hyperthermia	Cardiovascular

LIFE SCIENCE INSTRUMENTATION
See Midmark Diagnostics Group

LIFE SCIENCE TECHNOLOGIES, LTD. · 828-295-3821
1145 Flat Top Road, Blowing Rock, NC 28607
FDA Number: n/a · *Fax:* 828-295-7149
E-mail: lifesciencesltd@columbine-enterprises.com
Web site: www.Life-ScienceTech.com
Medical Products Sales Volume: $300,000
Annual Revenue: $0-$1 Million
Year Founded: 1994
Total Employees: 5
Ownership: Private
Quality System Registration Information: ISO9000
Produces/Sells CE-marked Devices: Y
Federal Procurement Eligibility: Small Business
Distribution: Manufacturer Direct, Manufacturer Through Distributor, Manufacturer Through Manufacturer Reps, OEM, Exclusive Distributor

Analyzer, Sedimentation Rate, Erythrocyte	Hematology

LIFE SCIENCES INTERNATIONAL
See Day & Zimmermann Validation Services

LIFE SENSING INSTRUMENT COMPANY, INC. · 800-624-2732 · 931-455-9019
329 W. Lincoln St., Tullahoma, TN 37388
FDA Number: 1037137 · *Fax:* 931-455-9093
E-mail: sales@lsimed.com
Web site: www.lsimed.com
Medical Products Sales Volume: $5,000,000
Annual Revenue: $1-$5 Million
Year Founded: 1984
Total Employees: 20 · *Marketing Staff:* 2 · *Sales Staff:* 1
Ownership: Private
Quality System Registration Information: ISO9000
Produces/Sells CE-marked Devices: N
Federal Procurement Eligibility: Small Business
Distribution: OEM, Exporter
General Admin.: B. Custshaw/President
Mktg./Adv.: Roger Caldwell/Director Product Development
    Steve Poteef/Manager Sales
    Charlie Rogers/Vice President Marketing
Production: Theresa Lemmon/Manager Regulatory Affairs
    Tommy Hayes/Vice President Manufacturing
Research: Gene Money/Vice President Research & Development

Monitor, ECG, Arrhythmia	Cardiovascular
Monitor, Hemodynamic	Anesthesiology
Station, Nursing	General
Telemetry Unit, Physiological, ECG	Cardiovascular

LIFE SPINE INC. · 847-884-6117
2401 W. Hassell Road, Suite 1535, Hoffman Estates, IL 60169
FDA Number: 3004499989 · *Fax:* 847-884-6118
E-mail: Info@Lifespine.com
Ownership: Private
Produces/Sells CE-marked Devices: N

Appliance, Fixation, Spinal Interlaminal	Orthopedics
Orthosis, Fixation, Pedicle, Spinal	Orthopedics
Orthosis, Fixation, Spinal, Spondylolisthesis	Orthopedics
Prosthesis, Hip, Cement Restrictor	Orthopedics

LIFE SUPPORT PRODUCTS, INC.
See Allied Healthcare Products, Inc.

LIFE TECHNOLOGIES CORPORATION · 716-774-6700
3175 Staley Rd., Grand Island, NY 14072
FDA Number: 1317268 · *Fax:* 716-774-6694
Web site: www.lifetechnologies.com
Total Employees: 9500
Ownership: LIFE TECHNOLOGIES CORPORATION
Stock Symbol: LIFE
Traded On: NASDAQ
Produces/Sells CE-marked Devices: Y
General Admin.: Gregory T. Lucier/Chief Executive Officer, Chairman
    David F. Hoffmeister/Chief Financial Officer, Senior Vice President
    Mark P. Stevenson/President, Chief Operating Officer

Culture Media, Supplements	Microbiology

LIFE TECHNOLOGIES CORPORATION   716-774-6700 *(cont'd)*
Solution, Balanced Salt   Pathology

LIFE TECHNOLOGIES CORPORATION   760-603-7200
5791 Van Allen Way, Carlsbad, CA 92008
FDA Number: 2917132   *Fax:* 760-602-6500
Web site: http://www.lifetechnologies.com
Medical Products Sales Volume: $126,350,000
Annual Revenue: More than $1 Billion
Year Founded: 1987
Total Employees: 9500
Ownership: Public
Stock Symbol: LIFE
Traded On: NASDAQ
Produces/Sells CE-marked Devices: N
Federal Procurement Eligibility: Small Business, Minority Owned
Distribution: Manufacturer Direct, OEM, Exporter
General Admin.: Gregory T. Lucier/Chief Executive Officer, Chairman
     David F. Hoffmeister/Chief Financial Officer, Senior Vice President
     Mr. Joe Beery/Chief Information Officer
     Dr. Brian Pollak/Chief Scientific Officer
     Mark P. Stevenson/President, Chief Operating Officer
Mktg./Adv.: Mr. Bernd Brust/Commercial Director
     Ms. Farnaz Khadem/Director Corporate Communications
     Ms. Amanda Clardy/Director Marketing

Counter, Cell, Differential Classifier, Automated	Hematology
Cytokeratins	Immunology
Fixative, Formalin Containing	Pathology
Immunohistochemical Reagent, Antibody (monoclonal Or Polyclonal) To P63 Protein In Nucleus Of Prostatic Basal Cells	Hematology
Reagent, General Purpose	Pathology
Reagent, Virus, General	Pathology
Stain, Hematology	Pathology

LIFE TECHNOLOGIES CORPORATION   760-603-7200
5791 Van Allen Way, Carlsbad, CA 92008
FDA Number: 2917132   *Fax:* 760-602-650
Web site: www.lifetechnologies.com
Ownership: Private
Produces/Sells CE-marked Devices: N
General Admin.: Dr. Ora Hirsch Pescovitz/Executive Vice President

Counter, Cell	Microbiology
Cytokeratins	Immunology
Fixative, Formalin Containing	Pathology
Reagent, General Purpose	Pathology
Reagents, Specific, Analyte	Hematology
Stain, Fetal Hemoglobin	Hematology

LIFE TECHNOLOGIES CORPORATION   301-840-8000
7300 Governors Way, Frederick, MD 21704
FDA Number: 3003335080
Web site: www.lifetechnologies.com
Medical Products Sales Volume: $306,000,000
Total Employees: 9500
Ownership: LIFE TECHNOLOGIES CORPORATION
Stock Symbol: LIFE
Traded On: NASDAQ
Quality System Registration Information: ISO9001
Produces/Sells CE-marked Devices: N
Distribution: Manufacturer Through Distributor, Exclusive Distributor
General Admin.: Gregory T. Lucier/Chief Executive Officer, Chairman
     David F. Hoffmeister/Chief Financial Officer, Senior Vice President
     Mark P. Stevenson/President, Chief Operating Officer

Kit, DNA Detection, Human Papillomavirus	Microbiology
Production Equipment	General
Reagent, Virus, General	Pathology

LIFE TECHNOLOGIES CORPORATION   414-214-4048
9099 North Deerbrook Trail, Brown Deer, WI 53223
FDA Number: 2244574
Web site: www.lifetechnologies.com
Total Employees: 9500
Ownership: LIFE TECHNOLOGIES CORPORATION
Stock Symbol: LIFE
Traded On: NASDAQ
Produces/Sells CE-marked Devices: N
General Admin.: Gregory T. Lucier/Chief Executive Officer, Chairman
     David F. Hoffmeister/Chief Financial Officer, Senior Vice President
     Mark P. Stevenson/President, Chief Operating Officer

Antigen, Antiserum, Control, Whole Human Serum	Immunology
Complement	Immunology
Test, Leukocyte Typing	Hematology
Test, Quantitative, For Hla, Non-diagnostic	Hematology

LIFE THERAPEUTICS INC.   404-300-5000
780 Park North Blvd., Suite 100, Clarkston, GA 30021
FDA Number: 3004737529

Control, Plasma, Abnormal	Hematology
Partial Thromboplastin Time	Hematology

LIFE THERAPEUTICS INC.   404-300-5000 *(cont'd)*
Reagent, Russel Viper Venom   Hematology

LIFE WITHOUT PAIN, LLC   954-786-0007
4600 140th Ave. North, Suite 190, Clearwater, FL 33762
FDA Number: 3004604022
Ownership: Private
Produces/Sells CE-marked Devices: N

Lamp, Infrared	Physical Med

LIFE-LIKE LABORATORY   972-620-0203
1544 Valwood Pkwy., Suite 104, Carrollton, TX 75006
FDA Number: n/a   *Fax:* 972-620-0204
E-mail: silconarm@aol.com
Web site: www.lifelikelab.com
Year Founded: 1980
Ownership: MARMICK, INC.
Produces/Sells CE-marked Devices: N
Federal Procurement Eligibility: Small Business
Distribution: Manufacturer Direct, Service Direct

Component, Silicone	General
Prosthesis, Facial, Mandibular Implant	Ear/Nose/Throat
Prosthesis, Foot	Orthopedics
Prosthesis, Hand	Orthopedics

LIFE-LIKE PROSTHETICS, LLC   310-320-5777
1319 W. Carson St., Torrance, CA 90501
FDA Number: n/a   *Fax:* 310-320-6341
E-mail: lifelike1@earthlink.net
Web site: www.lifelikeprosthetics.com
Medical Products Sales Volume: $800,000
Year Founded: 1993
Total Employees: 5
Ownership: Private
Federal Procurement Eligibility: Small Business

Orthosis, Limb Brace	Physical Med
Prosthesis, Foot	Orthopedics
Prosthesis, Hand	Orthopedics

LIFE-TECH, INC.   800-231-9841
13235 N. Promenade Blvd., Stafford, TX 77477   281-491-6600
FDA Number: 1625424   *Fax:* 281-491-6646
E-mail: nkc@life-tech.com
Web site: www.life-tech.com
Medical Products Sales Volume: $12,800,000
Annual Revenue: $10-$25 Million
Year Founded: 1970
Total Employees: 120   *Marketing Staff:* 1   *Sales Staff:* 10
Ownership: Private
Quality System Registration Information: ISO9001
Produces/Sells CE-marked Devices: Y
Federal Procurement Eligibility: Small Business, GSA Contract, VA Contract
Distribution: Manufacturer Direct, Manufacturer Through Distributor, Manufacturer Through Manufacturer Reps, OEM, Exporter
General Admin.: Alfred C. Coats/President, Chief Executive Officer
Mktg./Adv.: Al Coats/Director Marketing
     Lee McLeod/Director National Sales
     Howard V. Wimberly/Vice President Business Development
     Howard V. Wimberly/Vice President International Sales
     Katherine Hughey/Vice President Special Product Development
Production: Jeff Kasoff/Director Regulatory Affairs
     Steve Crow/Vice President Manufacturing
Research: Bill Hardin/Director Research & Development
Finance: Jeannine Jiral/Controller

Biofeedback Device	Cns/Neurology
Catheter, Urethral	Gastroenterology/Urology
Catheter, Urinary	Gastroenterology/Urology
Catheter, Urological	Gastroenterology/Urology
Device, Dysfunction, Erectile	Gastroenterology/Urology
Electrode, Neuromuscular Stimulator	Cns/Neurology
Electrode, Other	General
Gel, Ultrasonic Transmission	General
Iontophoresis Unit, Physical Medicine	Physical Med
Irrigator, Caloric	Ear/Nose/Throat
Kit, Catheterization, Sterile Urethral	Gastroenterology/Urology
Needle, Conduction, Anesthesia (W/Wo Introducer)	Anesthesiology
Stimulator, Nerve, Battery-Powered	Anesthesiology
Stimulator, Peripheral Nerve, Blockade Monitor	Anesthesiology
Table, Urological (Cystological)	Gastroenterology/Urology
Urodynamic Measurement System	Gastroenterology/Urology
Uroflowmeter	Gastroenterology/Urology

LIFECARE IMAGING INTL., LTD.   815-477-1291
8411 Pyott Rd., Lake In The Hills 60102
FDA Number: 1420853
Ownership: Private
Produces/Sells CE-marked Devices: N

Radiographic/Fluoroscopic Unit, Image-Intensified	Radiology

LIFECARE INTERNATIONAL, INC.
See Respironics Colorado

LIFECELL CORP.   800-367-5737
One Millennium Way,   908-947-1100
Branchburg, NJ 08876
FDA Number: 1647098
E-mail: custserv@lifecell.com   *Fax:* 908-947-1089
Web site: www.lifecell.com
Year Founded: 1986
Total Employees: 335   *Marketing Staff:* 4   *Sales Staff:* 25
Ownership: Kinetic Concepts, Inc.
Produces/Sells CE-marked Devices: N
Federal Procurement Eligibility: Small Business
Distribution: Exclusive Distributor
General Admin.: Carrie Falcone/Compliance Officer
     Stephen A. Livesey/Executive Vice President
     Lisa Colleran/President

Allograft, Processed	Surgery
Dressing, Skin Graft, Donor Site	General
Filler, Bone Void, Osteoinduction	Physical Med
Graft, Skin	Surgery

LIFECLINIC INTERNATIONAL, INC.   301-476-9888
4032 Blackburn Lane, Burtonsville, MD 20866
FDA Number: n/a   *Fax:* 301-476-9388
E-mail: salesteam@lifeclinic.com
Web site: www.lifeclinic.com
Annual Revenue: $1-$5 Million
Year Founded: 1976
Ownership: Private
Produces/Sells CE-marked Devices: N
Federal Procurement Eligibility: Small Business
Distribution: Manufacturer Direct, Manufacturer Through Distributor, Exporter
General Admin.: David J. Horne/Chief Technology Officer
     Phil Claxton/President
Medical Admin.: Dr. John T. Kelly/Chief Medical Officer
Mktg./Adv.: Michael A. Cavotta/Senior Vice President Product Development
Finance: Jim R. Evans/Chief Financial Officer

Monitor, Blood Pressure, Indirect, Anesthesiology	Anesthesiology

LIFECLINIC INTERNATIONAL, LTD.   800-543-2787
511 Creasman Dr., Winchester, TN 37398   931-967-4879
FDA Number: 1037371   *Fax:* 931-967-4891
E-mail: service@lifeclinic.com
Web site: www.lifeclinic.com
Year Founded: 1976
Ownership: LIFECLINIC INTERNATIONAL, INC.
Produces/Sells CE-marked Devices: N

Monitor, Blood Pressure, Indirect, Semi-Automatic	Cardiovascular
Turbidimetric Method, Myoglobin	Chemistry

LIFECORE BIOMEDICAL, INC.   952-368-4300
3515 Lyman Blvd., Chaska, MN 55318
FDA Number: 2184002   *Fax:* 952-368-3411
E-mail: info@lifecore.com
Web site: www.lifecore.com
Medical Products Sales Volume: $69,600,000
Annual Revenue: $50-$100 Million
Year Founded: 1965
Total Employees: 205   *Marketing Staff:* 12   *Sales Staff:* 27
Ownership: Landec Corp.
Quality System Registration Information: ISO9001
Produces/Sells CE-marked Devices: Y
Federal Procurement Eligibility: Small Business
Distribution: Manufacturer Direct, Manufacturer Through Distributor, Manufacturer Through Manufacturer Reps, OEM, Exporter
General Admin.: Mr. Dennis J. Allingham/President, Chief Executive Officer
     Larry D. Hiebert/Vice President, General Manager
Mktg./Adv.: Dr. Kipling Thacker/Vice President New Business
Production: James G. Hall/Vice President Tech. Operations

Acid, Hyaluronic	Dental And Oral
Acid, Hyaluronic, Intraarticular	Physical Med
Contract Manufacturing	General
Fixation Device, Jaw Fracture	Orthopedics
Graft, Bone	Orthopedics
Implant, Endosseous (Bone Filling and/or Augmentation)	Dental And Oral
Prosthesis, Dental	Dental And Oral
Viscoelastic Surgical Aid	Ophthalmology

LIFEGAS LLC   866-543-3427
1500 Indian Trail Road,   678-380-4402
Norcross, GA 30093
FDA Number: n/a   *Fax:* 770-806-8532
E-mail: atlanta@lifegas.com
Web site: www.lifegas.com
Year Founded: 1986
Ownership: Biocentric Solutions

LIFEGAS LLC   866-543-3427 *(cont'd)*
Quality System Registration Information: ISO9001
Produces/Sells CE-marked Devices: N
Distribution: Manufacturer Direct, Manufacturer Through Distributor, Service Direct
General Admin.: Penny Wermescher/Human Resources Associate
Mktg./Adv.: Kim Marks/Manager Marketing & Communications
     Chris White/National Accounts Representative
Production: Greg Reppar/Director Quality Control & Regulatory Affairs

Analyzer, Gas, Carbon-Dioxide, Gaseous Phase (Capnograph)	Anesthesiology
Analyzer, Gas, Helium, Gaseous Phase	Anesthesiology
Detector, Leakage, Medical Gas	General
Gas Mixtures, Sterilization	General
Material, Training, Audiovisual	General
Oxygen	Anesthesiology
Regulator, Intake, Oxygen	Anesthesiology
Regulator, Oxygen, Mechanical	General

Medical Product Subsidiaries (Listed Separately)
Aga Linde Healthcare P.R. Inc.

LIFELINE MEDICAL, INC.   800-452-4566
22 Shelter Rock Ln., Danbury, CT 06810
FDA Number: 1226143

Brush, Dermabrasion	Surgery
Diazonium Colorimetry, Urobilinogen (Urinary, Non-Quant.)	Chemistry

LIFELINE PRODUCTS, INC.   203-265-2846
3 Marshall St., Wallingford, CT 06492
FDA Number: n/a   *Fax:* 203-284-8831
Web site: www.lifelineproductsinc.com
Annual Revenue: $1-$5 Million
Year Founded: 1976
Ownership: Private
Quality System Registration Information: ISO9002
Produces/Sells CE-marked Devices: N
Federal Procurement Eligibility: Small Business, Female Owned
Distribution: OEM

Needle, Hypodermic	General

LIFELINE SOFTWARE, INC.   903-894-9923
311 Hines Crossing, Bullard, TX 75757
FDA Number: 1651102

Radiotherapy Unit, Charged-Particle	Radiology

LIFELINE SYSTEMS CANADA INC.   800-387-8120
95 Barber Greene Rd., Ste. 105,   416-445-0742
Toronto, ONT M3C-3 Canada
FDA Number: n/a   *Fax:* 416-445-1208
E-mail: inquiries@lifelinecanada.com
Web site: www.lifelinecanada.com
Year Founded: 1974
Total Employees: 25
Ownership: Private
Produces/Sells CE-marked Devices: N
Distribution: Exclusive Distributor, Importer

LIFELINE USA   800-553-6633
3201 Syene Road, Madison, WI 53713   608-288-9252
FDA Number: 2132523   *Fax:* 608-288-9294
E-mail: info@lifelineusa.com
Web site: www.lifelineusa.com
Medical Products Sales Volume: $3,600,000
Year Founded: 1973
Total Employees: 25   *Marketing Staff:* 1   *Sales Staff:* 1
Ownership: Private
Produces/Sells CE-marked Devices: N
Federal Procurement Eligibility: Small Business
Distribution: Manufacturer Direct, Manufacturer Through Distributor, Manufacturer Through Manufacturer Reps, OEM
General Admin.: Mr. Bobby Hinds/Chief Executive Officer
Mktg./Adv.: Mr. John Maloney/Director Marketing

Ankle/Foot, External Limb Component	Physical Med
Assembly, Knee/Shank/Ankle/Foot, External	Physical Med
Component, Exercise	Physical Med
Equipment, Therapy, Handicapped/Physical	Physical Med
Exerciser, Measuring	Physical Med
Exerciser, Wrist	Physical Med

LIFEMED OF CALIFORNIA   800-543-3633
1216 So. Allec St., Anaheim, CA 92805-6301   714-517-6900
FDA Number: 2018692   *Fax:* 714-517-6911
E-mail: info@lifemedofcalifornia.com
Web site: www.lifemedofcalifornia.com
Annual Revenue: $1-$5 Million
Total Employees: 20
Ownership: Private
Quality System Registration Information: ISO9001
Produces/Sells CE-marked Devices: N
Federal Procurement Eligibility: Small Business

LIFEMED OF CALIFORNIA
800-543-3633 *(cont'd)*

Distribution: Manufacturer Direct, Manufacturer Through Distributor, Manufacturer Through Manufacturer Reps, OEM, Importer, Exporter
General Admin.: Tom Hamon/President, Chief Executive Officer
Production: Patricia Brinker/Vice President Quality Assurance & Quality Control

Accessories, AV Shunt	Gastroenterology/Urology
Accessories, Catheter	Surgery
Adapter, Shunt	Gastroenterology/Urology
Catheter, Peritoneal Dialysis, Single-Use	Gastroenterology/Urology
Catheter, Peritoneal, Indwelling, Long-Term	Gastroenterology/Urology
Catheter, Tenckhoff	Gastroenterology/Urology
Clamp, Cannula	Gastroenterology/Urology
Component, Plastic	General
Component, Rubber	General
Component, Silicone	General
Connector, Shunt	Gastroenterology/Urology
Connector, Tubing, Blood, Infusion, T-Type	Gastroenterology/Urology
Contract Assembly	General
Contract Manufacturing	General
Contract Manufacturing, Product, Disposable	General
Contract Packaging	General
Introducer, Catheter	Cardiovascular
Kit, Administration, Intravenous	General
Kit, Hemodialysis Tubing	Gastroenterology/Urology
Kit, Intravenous Extension Tubing	General
Kit, Intravenous, Administration, Buret	General
Tip, Vessel	Gastroenterology/Urology
Transfer Unit, IV Fluid	General
Tubing, Other	General

LIFENET HEALTH
800-847-7831
757-464-4761
1864 Concert Drive,
Virginia Beach, VA 23453
FDA Number: 3005064037
E-mail: doug_wilson@lifenet.org
Fax: 757-301-6582
Web site: www.lifenet.org
Medical Products Sales Volume: $18,000,000
Annual Revenue: $100-$500 Million
Year Founded: 1982
Total Employees: 375   *Marketing Staff:* 8   *Sales Staff:* 18
Ownership: Private
Quality System Registration Information: ISO9001
Produces/Sells CE-marked Devices: N
Federal Procurement Eligibility: Small Business
Distribution: Manufacturer Direct, Manufacturer Through Manufacturer Reps
General Admin.: Dr. Richard Hurwitz/Chief Executive Officer
Mktg./Adv.: Doug Wilson/Senior Vice President Corporate Development
    Perry Lange/Vice President Sales
Research: Lloyd Wolfinbarger/Vice President Research & Development

Service, Tissue Bank	General

LIFESAVING SYSTEMS CORP.
813-645-2748
220 Elsberry Rd., Apollo Beach, FL 33572-2289
FDA Number: 1036458
E-mail: info@lifesavingsystems.com
Fax: 813-645-2768
Web site: www.lifesavingsystems.com
Ownership: Private
Produces/Sells CE-marked Devices: N

Stretcher, Hand-Carried	General

LIFESCAN CANADA LTD.
800-663-5521
604-293-2266
4170 Still Creek Dr. #234,
Burnaby, BC V5C-6 Canada
FDA Number: n/a
E-mail: jagraham@lfsca.jnj.com
Fax: 604-293-1619
Web site: www.lifescan.com
Year Founded: 1981
Ownership: Private
Produces/Sells CE-marked Devices: N
Distribution: Exclusive Distributor

LIFESCAN LLC.
408-263-9789
Rd. 308 Km 0.8, Pedernales Industrial Park,
Cabo Rojo, PR 00623
FDA Number: 2648724
Web site: www.lifescan.com
Ownership: Johnson & Johnson
Stock Symbol: JNJ
Traded On: NYSE
Produces/Sells CE-marked Devices: N

Reagent, Glucose (Test System)	Chemistry
System, Test, Blood Glucose, Over-The-Counter	Chemistry

LIFESCAN PRODUCTS, LLC
408-942-3589
San Antonio Industrial Park, Extension, Rd. 110 Km. 5.9,
Aguadilla, PR 00603
FDA Number: 3006791677
Web site: www.jnj.com

LIFESCAN PRODUCTS, LLC
408-942-3589 *(cont'd)*
Ownership: Johnson & Johnson
Produces/Sells CE-marked Devices: N

LIFESCAN, INC.
800-227-8862
408-263-9789
1000 Gibraltar Dr, Milpitas, CA 95035-6314
FDA Number: 2939301
Fax: 408-942-6070
E-mail: CustomerService@LifeScan.com
Web site: www.lifescan.com
Annual Revenue: $0-$1 Million
Total Employees: 1398   *Marketing Staff:* 150   *Sales Staff:* 150
Ownership: Johnson & Johnson
Produces/Sells CE-marked Devices: N
Federal Procurement Eligibility: Small Business
Distribution: Manufacturer Direct
General Admin.: John Hughes/Manager
    Richard Wiesner/President
Mktg./Adv.: Lloyce Jaunkelnietis/Manager Marketing

Colorimeter, General Use	Chemistry
Control, Analyte (Assayed And Unassayed)	Chemistry
Lancet, Blood	General
Monitor, Blood Glucose (Test)	Gastroenterology/Urology
Pump, Infusion	General
Reagent, Glucose (Test System)	Chemistry
Strip, Test	Chemistry
System, Test, Blood Glucose, Over-The-Counter	Chemistry

LIFESCIENCE PLUS, INC.
650-565-8172
473 Sapena Ct., Suite # 7, Santa Clara, CA 95054
FDA Number: 3004957256

Bandage, Adhesive	Surgery
Drape, Adhesive, Aerosol	Surgery
Gauze, Non-Absorbable, X-Ray Detectable (Internal Sponge)	Surgery
Gauze/sponge, Nonresorbable For External Use	Surgery

LIFESIGN
800-526-2125
732-246-3366
71 Veronica Avenue, Somerset, NJ 08873
FDA Number: 2249224
Fax: 732-246-0570
E-mail: lifesign@lifesignmed.com
Web site: www.lifesignmed.com
Medical Products Sales Volume: $5,900,000
Annual Revenue: $5-$10 Million
Year Founded: 1998
Total Employees: 30   *Marketing Staff:* 3   *Sales Staff:* 10
Ownership: Princeton Biomeditech Corp.
Quality System Registration Information: ISO9001
Produces/Sells CE-marked Devices: N
Federal Procurement Eligibility: Small Business, Minority Owned
Distribution: Manufacturer Direct, Manufacturer Through Distributor, Exclusive Distributor
General Admin.: L. Porter/President
Mktg./Adv.: S. Przybylski/Vice President Marketing & Sales

Antigen, Streptococcus SPP.	Microbiology
Antiserum, Streptococcus SPP.	Microbiology
Assay, Agglutination, Latex, Rubella	Microbiology
Enzyme Immunoassay, Other	Chemistry
Incubator, Test Tube, Portable	Microbiology
Incubator, Test Tube, Stationary	Microbiology
Kit, Pregnancy Test	Obstetrics/Gynecology
Kit, Screening, Urine	Microbiology
Kit, Test, Coagglutinin	Hematology
Radioimmunoassay, Infectious Mononucleosis	Microbiology
System, Test, Drugs of Abuse	Chemistry
Test, Rotavirus	Microbiology

LIFESTREAM MEDICAL CORPORATION
407-529-9920
12024 Green Emerald Court, Orlando, FL 32837
FDA Number: 3005054309
Ownership: Private
Produces/Sells CE-marked Devices: N

Fixation Device, Tracheal Tube	Anesthesiology

LIFESTREAM PURIFICATION SYSTEMS, LLC
877-564-3185
512-707-8383
2001 S. Lamar Boulevard, Suite G,
Austin, TX 78704
FDA Number: 3003860916
Fax: 512-707-8484
E-mail: info@angelofwater.com
Web site: www.angelofwater.com
Annual Revenue: $0-$1 Million
Year Founded: 2000
Total Employees: 10   *Marketing Staff:* 3   *Sales Staff:* 8
Ownership: Private
Produces/Sells CE-marked Devices: Y
Distribution: Manufacturer Direct
General Admin.: Amy Heilman/General Manager
Mktg./Adv.: Gary Russ/Vice President Marketing & Sales
Production: Rocco Bruno/Designer

Douche, Vaginal	Obstetrics/Gynecology
Irrigator, Colonic	Gastroenterology/Urology

LIFESTREAM PURIFICATION SYSTEMS, LLC 877-564-3185
(cont'd)
Kit, Enema (For Cleaning Purposes) Gastroenterology/Urology

LIFESTYLE CO. INC., THE
See The Lifestyle Co. Inc.

LIFESTYLE MEDICAL MFG 520-323-0099
6479 E. 22nd St, Tucson, AZ 85710
FDA Number: 2029177
Ownership: Private
Produces/Sells CE-marked Devices: N
Hearing-Aid Ear/Nose/Throat

LIFESYNC CORPORATION 866-324-3888
One East Broward Blvd,, Suite 1701, 954-745-3509
Fort Lauderdale, FL 33301
FDA Number: 3003829651
E-mail: customerservice@lifesynccorp.com
Web site: www.lifesynccorp.com
Year Founded: 2000
Ownership: Private
Produces/Sells CE-marked Devices: N
Cable Physical Med
Transmitter/Receiver System, Physiological, Radiofrequency Cardiovascular

LIFETECHNIQUES INC., MEDSIGNALS 210-222-2067
CORP. DIV.
217 Alamo Plaza,suite 200, San Antonio, TX 78205
FDA Number: 3006412413
Dispenser, Solid Medication Physical Med

LIFEWATCH SERVICES, INC. 877-774-9846
O'hare International Center II 847.720.2100
10255 West Higgins Rd., Ste. 100
Rosemont, IL 60018
FDA Number: 3027765 *Fax:* 847-720-2111
Web site: www.lifewatch.com
Year Founded: 1993
Ownership: LIFEWATCH AG
Produces/Sells CE-marked Devices: N
General Admin.: Roger Richardson/President, Chief Operating Officer
Mktg./Adv.: Brent Atwood/Executive Vice President Marketing & Sales
Detector, Arrhythmia Alarm Cardiovascular
Meter, Peak Flow, Spirometry Anesthesiology
Monitor, Perinatal Obstetrics/Gynecology
Oximeter, Intracardiac Cardiovascular
Recorder, Magnetic Tape/Disc Cardiovascular
Recorder, Ventilatory Effort Anesthesiology
Transmitter/Receiver System, ECG, Telephone Multi-Channel Cardiovascular
Transmitter/Receiver System, Physiological, Telephone Cardiovascular

LIFTABILITY INC. 800-267-8883
2600 Lancaster Road, 613-738-2721
Ottawa, ONT K1B 4 Canada
FDA Number: n/a *Fax:* 613-738-2704
E-mail: Liftability@conval-aid.com
Web site: www.conval-aid.com
Year Founded: 1990
Ownership: Private
Produces/Sells CE-marked Devices: N

LIFTNWALK LP 972-837-4615
P.O. Box 742855, Dallas, TX 75374-2855
FDA Number: n/a *Fax:* 214-343-6496
E-mail: sales@liftnwalk.com
Web site: www.liftnwalk.com
Year Founded: 2003
Ownership: Private
Produces/Sells CE-marked Devices: N
Federal Procurement Eligibility: Small Business
Distribution: Manufacturer Through Distributor
Chair/Table, Medical General
Tray, Foodservice General
Walker, Mechanical Physical Med

LIFTSEAT CORPORATION 630-424-2840
158 Eisenhower Lane South, Lombard, IL 60148
FDA Number: 3006270986
Adapter, Hygiene Physical Med

LIFTVEST U.S.A, LLC 800-300-5671
35 W. 83 St., New York, NY 10024-5201 212-874-4159
FDA Number: 2438608 *Fax:* 212-874-2499
E-mail: info@liftvest.com
Web site: www.liftvest.com
Medical Products Sales Volume: $800,000
Year Founded: 2000
Total Employees: 3

LIFTVEST U.S.A, LLC 800-300-5671 *(cont'd)*
Ownership: Private
Produces/Sells CE-marked Devices: Y
Federal Procurement Eligibility: Small Business, Female Owned
Distribution: Manufacturer Direct, Exporter
General Admin.: Dr. Cynthia Price Cohen/Director, General Manager
Mr. Joseph Cohen/Director, General Manager
Transfer Aid Physical Med
Transfer Device, Patient, Manual General

LIGHT AGE INC. 732-563-0600
500 Apgar Drive, Somerset, NJ 08873
FDA Number: 2246844 *Fax:* 732-563-1571
E-mail: sales@lightage.com
Web site: www.lightage.com
Medical Products Sales Volume: $4,000,000
Annual Revenue: $5-$10 Million
Total Employees: 40 *Marketing Staff:* 4 *Sales Staff:* 6
Ownership: Private
Produces/Sells CE-marked Devices: N
Federal Procurement Eligibility: Small Business
Distribution: Manufacturer Direct, Manufacturer Through Distributor, Manufacturer Through Manufacturer Reps, OEM
General Admin.: Dr. Don Heller/Chief Executive Officer
Dr. John Walling/President
Mktg./Adv.: Ms. Myla Papariello/Director Development & Sales
Contract Manufacturing, Product, Durable General
Laser, Angioplasty, Coronary Cardiovascular
Laser, Combination General
Laser, Dental Dental And Oral
Laser, Surgical Surgery
Lithotriptor Gastroenterology/Urology

LIGHT SOURCES, INC. 203-234-7338
37 Robinson Blvd., Orange, CT 06477
FDA Number: 1221013
Booth, Sun Tan Physical Med

LIGHTHOUSE IMAGING CORP. 207-253-5350
477 Congress St., Portland, ME 04101
FDA Number: 1226499 *Fax:* 207-253-5603
E-mail: dcleiner@lighthouseoptics.com
Web site: www.lighthouseoptics.com
Year Founded: 1984
Total Employees: 5
Ownership: Private
Quality System Registration Information: ISO9001
Produces/Sells CE-marked Devices: Y
Federal Procurement Eligibility: Small Business
Distribution: Manufacturer Direct, Manufacturer Through Distributor, OEM, Service Direct
General Admin.: Mr. Mark Waite/Chief Executive Officer
Mr. Dennis Leiner/Chief Technology Officer
Accessories, Surgical Camera Surgery
Component, Optical General

LIGHTHOUSE INDUSTRIES 219-879-1550
107 Eastwood Rd., Po Box 8905, Michigan City, IN 46360
FDA Number: 3004057261 *Fax:* 219.879.1509
E-mail: info@lighthouseindustries.com
Web site: www.lighthouseindustries.com
Ownership: Private
Produces/Sells CE-marked Devices: N
Bone Mill Orthopedics
Joint, Wrist, External Limb Component, Mechanical Physical Med

LIGHTLAB IMAGING INC. 978-399-1000
One Technology Park Drive, Westford, MA 01886
FDA Number: 3004672267 *Fax:* 978-692-1409
Web site: http://www.lightlabimaging.com
Year Founded: 1998
Ownership: Private
Produces/Sells CE-marked Devices: N
General Admin.: Mr. Kevin Librett/Chief Operating Officer
Dr. Joseph Schmitt/Chief Technology Officer
Mr. David Kolstad/President, Chief Executive Officer
Mktg./Adv.: Mr. Nathan Harris/Vice President Marketing & Sales
Production: Mr. Doug Woodruff/Vice President Regulatory & Clinical Affairs
Finance: Mr. Warren Clark III/Chief Financial Officer
Catheter, Intravascular, Diagnostic Cardiovascular
System, Imaging, Optical Coherence Tomography (oct) Radiology

LIGHTNIN MIXERS 888-MIX-BEST
135 Mt. Read Blvd., Rochester, NY 14611 585-436-5550
FDA Number: n/a *Fax:* 585-527-1742
Web site: www.lightninmixers.com
Year Founded: 1923
Ownership: SPX

LIGHTNIN MIXERS 888-MIX-BEST (cont'd)
Quality System Registration Information: ISO9001
Produces/Sells CE-marked Devices: Y
Distribution: Manufacturer Through Manufacturer Reps
  Stirrer — Chemistry

LIGHTOLIER A GENLYTE CO. 978-657-7600
45 Industrial Way, Wilmington, MA 01887
FDA Number: 2023273
Ownership: Private
Produces/Sells CE-marked Devices: N
  Light Source, Incandescent, Diagnostic — Gastroenterology/Urology

LIGHTPATH TECHNOLOGIES 407-382-4003
2603 Challenger Tech Ct., Suite 100, Orlando, FL 32826
FDA Number: n/a   Fax: 407-382-4007
Web site: www.lightpath.com
Annual Revenue: $5-$10 Million
Year Founded: 1985
Total Employees: 171   Marketing Staff: 10   Sales Staff: 10
Ownership: Public
Stock Symbol: LPTH
Traded On: NASDAQ
Quality System Registration Information: ISO9001
Produces/Sells CE-marked Devices: N
Federal Procurement Eligibility: Small Business
Distribution: OEM
General Admin.: Dorothy Cipolla/Chief Financial Officer, Treasurer
    Joseph Gaynor/President, Chief Executive Officer
  Lens, Other — Ophthalmology

LIGHTSPEED TECHNOLOGY, INC. 210-495-4942
403 E. Ramsey, Suite 205, San Antonio, TX 78216
FDA Number: 1646920
  Handle, Instrument, Dental — Dental And Oral
  Needle, Dental — Dental And Oral
  Plugger, Root Canal, Endodontic — Dental And Oral
  Reamer, Pulp Canal, Endodontic — Dental And Oral

LIGHTWAVE TECHNOLOGIES LLC 302-356-2717
121 Continental Drive, Suite 110, Newark, DE 19713
FDA Number: 3005110836   Fax: 302-356-2737
E-mail: info@lightwavelogic.com
Ownership: Private
Produces/Sells CE-marked Devices: N
General Admin.: Dr. David Eaton/Chief Technology Officer
    Mr. James Marcelli/President, Chief Executive Officer
    Mr. Federick Goetz/Senior Vice President
Mktg./Adv.: Mr. Steven Cordovano/Director Corporate Communications
Finance: Mr. Andrew Ashton/Treasurer, Assistant Secretary
  Laser, Surgical — Surgery

LIKO NORTH AMERICA 888-545-6671
122 Grove Street, Franklin, MA 02038
FDA Number: 3006252983   Fax: 508-528-6642
E-mail: lorrie.spencer@liko.com
Ownership: Liko Ab
Produces/Sells CE-marked Devices: N
Distribution: Manufacturer Through Distributor
  Lift, Bath, Non-AC-Powered — General
  Lift, Patient — General

LIMERICK INCORPORATE 818-566-3060
2150 N. Glenoaks Blvd., Burbank, CA 91504
FDA Number: 3002297831
  Pump, Breast, Powered — Obstetrics/Gynecology

LIN-ZHI INTERNATIONAL, INC. 408-732-3856
670 Almanor Avenue, Sunnyvale, CA 94085
FDA Number: 3003610499   Fax: 408-732-3849
E-mail: drcilin@aol.com
Web site: lin-zhi.com
Annual Revenue: $1-$5 Million
Year Founded: 2001
Total Employees: 10
Ownership: Private
Produces/Sells CE-marked Devices: N
Federal Procurement Eligibility: Small Business, Minority Owned
Distribution: Manufacturer Direct, Manufacturer Through Manufacturer Reps, OEM, Exporter
  Calibrator, Drug Specific — Toxicology
  Control, Drug Specific — Toxicology
  Enzyme Immunoassay, Amphetamine — Toxicology
  Enzyme Immunoassay, Cannabinoids — Toxicology
  Enzyme Immunoassay, Cocaine And Cocaine Metabolites — Toxicology
  Enzyme Immunoassay, Methadone — Toxicology
  Enzyme Immunoassay, Opiates — Toxicology
  Enzyme Immunoassay, Phencyclidine — Toxicology

LIN-ZHI INTERNATIONAL, INC. 408-732-3856 (cont'd)
Enzyme Immunoassay, Propoxyphene — Toxicology

LINAK U.S. INC. 502-253-5595
2200 Stanley Gault Pkwy., Louisville, KY 40223
FDA Number: n/a   Fax: 502-253-5596
E-mail: info@linak-us.com
Web site: www.linak-us.com
Medical Products Sales Volume: $11,700,000
Annual Revenue: $10-$25 Million
Year Founded: 1907
Total Employees: 62   Marketing Staff: 3   Sales Staff: 12
Ownership: LINAK A/S
Quality System Registration Information: ISO9002
Produces/Sells CE-marked Devices: Y
Federal Procurement Eligibility: Small Business
Distribution: Manufacturer Direct, Manufacturer Through Manufacturer Reps, OEM
General Admin.: Soren Stig-Nielsen/President
    Lisa Tabler/Vice President Human Resources
Mktg./Adv.: Ann Hall/Director Marketing
    Rob Tupman/Director National Accounts
Production: Derek Manz/Manager Regulatory Affairs
    Jan Petersen/Vice President Manufacturing
  Component, Electrical — General
  Lift, Patient — General
  Unit, Control, Bed, Patient, Powered — General
  Unit, Evaluation, Height, Lift — Orthopedics

LINC QUANTUM ANALYTICS 800-992-4199
363 Vintage Park Dr., 650-312-0900
Foster City, CA 94404
FDA Number: n/a   Fax: 650-312-0313
E-mail: lqa@lqa.com
Web site: www.lqa.com
Annual Revenue: $0-$1 Million
Total Employees: 45   Marketing Staff: 4   Sales Staff: 10
Ownership: Private
Produces/Sells CE-marked Devices: N
Federal Procurement Eligibility: Small Business
Distribution: Exclusive Distributor
General Admin.: Bert Laing/President
    Gerard Farren/Vice President, General Manager
Mktg./Adv.: Lissa Shope/Manager Advertising
  Spectrophotometer, U.V./Visible — Chemistry

LINCARE HOLDINGS, INC. 727-530-7700
19387 U.S. 19 North, Clearwater, FL 33764
FDA Number: n/a   Fax: 727-532-9692
E-mail: 1nfo@lincare.com
Web site: www.lincare.com
Annual Revenue: More than $1 Billion
Year Founded: 1990
Total Employees: 9957
Ownership: Public
Stock Symbol: LNCR
Traded On: NASDAQ
Produces/Sells CE-marked Devices: Y
Distribution: Service Direct
General Admin.: Jenna Pedersen/Compliance Officer
    John P. Byrnes/President, Chief Executive Officer
    Shawn Schabel/President, Chief Operating Officer
Finance: Paul G. Gabos/Chief Financial Officer
  Bed, Manual — General
  Cart, Gas Cylinder (Carrier) — Anesthesiology
  Concentrator, Oxygen — Anesthesiology
  Monitor, Oxygen (Ventilatory) W/Wo Alarm — Anesthesiology
  Stand, Gas Cylinder — Anesthesiology
  Ventilator, Volume (Critical Care) — Anesthesiology
  Walker, Mechanical — Physical Med
  Wheelchair, Manual — Physical Med

LINCARE, INC.
See Lincare Holdings, Inc.

LINCO RESEARCH,INC. 866-441-8400
6 Research Park Dr., St. Charles, MO 63304 636-441-8400
FDA Number: 1954434   Fax: 636-441-8050
Web site: www.millipore.com
Ownership: Private
Produces/Sells CE-marked Devices: N
  Radioimmunoassay, Immunoreactive Insulin — Chemistry

LINCOLN DIAGNOSTICS, INC. 800-537-1336
PO Box 1128, Decatur, IL 62525-1139 217-877-2531
FDA Number: 1450391   Fax: 217-877-5645
E-mail: jlenski@lincolndiagnostics.com
Web site: www.lincolndiagnostics.com
Annual Revenue: $5-$10 Million
Year Founded: 1978

LINCOLN DIAGNOSTICS, INC.   800-537-1336 *(cont'd)*
Total Employees: 31   *Marketing Staff:* 1   *Sales Staff:* 2
Ownership: Private
Produces/Sells CE-marked Devices: N
Federal Procurement Eligibility: Small Business
Distribution: Manufacturer Direct, Manufacturer Through Distributor, Manufacturer Through Manufacturer Reps, Exclusive Distributor, Exporter
General Admin.: Gary Hein/President
Mktg./Adv.: John Lenski, Jr./Director Marketing & Sales
   Test, Allergy   Immunology

LINCOLN ELECTRIC CO.   216-481-8100
22801 St. Clair Ave., Cleveland, OH 44117-1199
FDA Number: n/a   *Fax:* 216-486-1751
Web site: www.lincolnelectric.com
Annual Revenue: $50-$100 Million
Total Employees: 3500   *Marketing Staff:* 12
Ownership: Public
Stock Symbol: LECOA
Traded On: NASDAQ
Produces/Sells CE-marked Devices: N
Distribution: Manufacturer Through Distributor
General Admin.: Anthony Massaro/President, Chief Executive Officer
     Raymond S. Vogt/Vice President Human Resources
Production: Richard C. Ulstad/Senior Vice President Manufacturing
     Charles H, Murray/Vice President Materials Management.
     Paul Fantelli/Vice President Quality Assurance
   Component, Electrical   General
Medical Product Subsidiaries (Listed Separately)
   Harris Products Group

LINDBERG/BLUE M   800-216-7725
2121 Reach Rd., Williamsport, PA 17701   **920-261-7000**
FDA Number: 9999999   *Fax:* 570-326-7304
Web site: www.blue-m.com
Annual Revenue: $1-$5 Million
Total Employees: 200   *Marketing Staff:* 30
Ownership: Private
Quality System Registration Information: ISO9000
Produces/Sells CE-marked Devices: N
Federal Procurement Eligibility: Small Business
Distribution: Manufacturer Direct, Manufacturer Through Distributor, Manufacturer Through Manufacturer Reps, OEM, Service Direct, Exporter
General Admin.: Ed Osborn/President
     Walt Ninkovich/Vice President Human Resources
     Joe Lyons/Vice President, General Manager
Mktg./Adv.: Keith Itsell/Manager International & National Sales
     Ed Osborne/Manager Marketing
   Oven   Chemistry

LINDBURG ENTERPRISES INC.
   See Chrontrol Corporation

LINDE GAS NORTH AMERICA LLC   800-262-4273
7390 Graham Fairborn Rd., Fairburn, GA 30213   **770-590-6200**
FDA Number: 1054077
Web site: www.lindeus.com
Year Founded: 1877
Total Employees: 51000
Ownership: Private
Quality System Registration Information: ISO9001
Produces/Sells CE-marked Devices: N
   Gas, Calibrated (Specified Concentration)   Anesthesiology

LINDE GAS PUERTO RICO INC.   908-771-1669
Carr 869 Km 1 Hm 8s Flamboya, Catano, PR 00962
FDA Number: 3004575922
   Gas, Calibrated (Specified Concentration)   Anesthesiology

LINDE GAS USA LLC   216-642-6600
3930 Michigan Street, Hammond, IN 46323
FDA Number: 1828043
Ownership: Private
Produces/Sells CE-marked Devices: N
   Gas, Calibrated (Specified Concentration)   Anesthesiology

LINDE HOMECARE MEDICAL SYSTEMS, INC.
   See Lincare Holdings, Inc.

LINDE MEDICAL GASES
   See Praxair, Inc.

LINE ONE LABORATORIES INC.   800-222-9848
21230 Lassen St., Chatsworth, CA 91311   **818-886-2288**
FDA Number: 2084739   *Fax:* 818-886-2818
E-mail: info@lineonelabsusa.com
Web site: www.lineonelabsusa.com
Ownership: Private
Produces/Sells CE-marked Devices: N
   Condom   Obstetrics/Gynecology

LINE ONE LABORATORIES INC.   800-222-9848 *(cont'd)*
   Dam, Rubber   Dental And Oral
   Massager, Therapeutic   Physical Med

LINEAGEN INC.   801-931-6200
423 Wakara Way, Suite 200, Salt Lake City, UT 84108
FDA Number: n/a   *Fax:* 801-931-6176
E-mail: info@lineagen.com
Web site: http://www.lineagen.com
Year Founded: 2002
Ownership: Private
Produces/Sells CE-marked Devices: N
General Admin.: Mr. Gayland Moffat/Chief Operating Officer
     Dr. Mark Leppert/Chief Scientific Officer
     Mr. Michael Paul/President, Chief Executive Officer
Mktg./Adv.: Mr. Alex Lindell/Director Corporate Development

LINEAR LABORATORIES CORPORATION   800-536-0262
42025 Osgood Road, Fremont, CA 94539   **510-226-0488**
FDA Number: n/a   *Fax:* 510-226-1112
E-mail: info@linearlabs.com
Web site: www.linearlabs.com/productdis.html
Medical Products Sales Volume: $800,000
Annual Revenue: $25-$50 Million
Year Founded: 1980
Total Employees: 9   *Marketing Staff:* 1   *Sales Staff:* 5
Ownership: INVIVO CORPORATION
Produces/Sells CE-marked Devices: N
Federal Procurement Eligibility: Small Business
Distribution: Manufacturer Direct, Manufacturer Through Distributor, Manufacturer Through Manufacturer Reps, Importer, Exporter
General Admin.: James Hawkins/President
Mktg./Adv.: Rick Foley/Vice President Marketing & Sales
   Thermographic Device, Infrared   Obstetrics/Gynecology

LINEAR MEDICAL CORPORATION   303-962-5730
1130 West 124th Avenue,, Suite 400, Westminster, CO 80234
FDA Number: 3006266622
   Generator, Diagnostic X-Ray, High Voltage, Single Phase   Radiology
   Radiographic Unit, Diagnostic, Mammographic   Radiology

LINEAR TONOMETERS, INC.   800-786-2163
PO Box 322, Commack, NY 11725-0322   **631-864-2113**
FDA Number: 2433600   *Fax:* 631-864-5927
E-mail: fineprint@msn.com
Web site: http://lineartonometers.com
Medical Products Sales Volume: $500,000
Total Employees: 5   *Marketing Staff:* 2   *Sales Staff:* 4
Ownership: Private
Produces/Sells CE-marked Devices: N
Federal Procurement Eligibility: Small Business
Distribution: Manufacturer Direct
Mktg./Adv.: Carl Klass/Director National Sales
   Tonometer (Calibration And Q.C. Of Blood Gas Instruments)   Chemistry

LINGPRODUCTS/APPLIED TECHNOLOGY
   See Tidi Products, Llc

LINGRAPHICARE AMERICA, INC.   888-274-2742
103 Carnegie Center, Suite 204,   **609-275-1300**
Princeton, NJ 08540
FDA Number: 2950167   *Fax:* 609-275-1311
E-mail: info@lingraphicare.com
Web site: www.aphasia.com
Year Founded: 1990
Ownership: Private
Produces/Sells CE-marked Devices: N
Federal Procurement Eligibility: Small Business
Distribution: Manufacturer Direct
General Admin.: Andrew Gomory/Chief Executive Officer
   Communication System, Powered   Physical Med

LINK AMERICA, INC.
   See LinkBio Corp.

LINK ERGONOMICS CORP.   800-424-5465
902 E. 4th Street, Joplin, MO 64801
FDA Number: n/a   *Fax:* 417-206-4622
E-mail: contact@linkdental.com
Web site: www.linkdental.com
Annual Revenue: $0-$1 Million
Year Founded: 1977
Ownership: Private
Produces/Sells CE-marked Devices: N
Federal Procurement Eligibility: Small Business
Distribution: Manufacturer Direct
   Chair, Dental   Dental And Oral
   Chair, Ophthalmic, Manual   Ophthalmology

LINK ERGONOMICS CORP.   800-424-5465 *(cont'd)*
Chair, Other   General

LINK ORTHOPAEDICS
See LinkBio Corp.

LINKBIO CORP.   800-932-0616
300 Roundhill Dr, Rockaway, NJ 07866   973-625-1333
FDA Number: 3006721341   Fax: 973-625-4445
E-mail: info@linkbio.com
Web site: www.linkbio.com
Year Founded: 1948
Ownership: Link Gmbh & Co., Waldemar
Quality System Registration Information: ISO9001; ISO9002
Produces/Sells CE-marked Devices: Y
Distribution: Manufacturer Through Manufacturer Reps
   Equipment, Shaving, Disc, Spinal   Orthopedics
   Implant, Fixation Device, Proximal Femoral   Orthopedics
   Instrument, Microsurgical   Cns/Neurology
   Splint, Hand, And Component   Physical Med
   Stripper, Tendon   Surgery
   Surgical Instrument, Orthopedic, AC-Powered Motor   Orthopedics

LINOS PHOTONICS, INC   800-334-5678
459 Fortune Blvd., Milford, MA 01757-1723   508-478-6200
FDA Number: n/a   Fax: 508-478-5980
E-mail: info@linos-photonics.com
Web site: www.linos-photonics.com
Medical Products Sales Volume: $1,700,000
Total Employees: 18   Marketing Staff: 1   Sales Staff: 6
Ownership: HALMA HOLDINGS PLC.
Quality System Registration Information: ISO9000
Produces/Sells CE-marked Devices: N
Federal Procurement Eligibility: Small Business
Distribution: Manufacturer Direct
General Admin.: Dan Nagle/Chief Operating Officer
   Accessories, Laser   General
   Fiberoptic Light Source & Carrier   Ear/Nose/Throat
   Laser, Combination   General

LINSCAN ULTRASOUND   800-533-7226
202 W. 9th. St., Suite 301, Rolla, MO 65402-1217   573-364-6631
FDA Number: n/a   Fax: 573-364-2517
E-mail: linscan@linscan.com
Web site: www.linscan.com
Medical Products Sales Volume: $200,000
Annual Revenue: $0-$1 Million
Year Founded: 1982
Total Employees: 3   Marketing Staff: 1
Ownership: Public
Produces/Sells CE-marked Devices: N
Federal Procurement Eligibility: Small Business
Distribution: Manufacturer Direct, Manufacturer Through Distributor, Manufacturer Through Manufacturer Reps, OEM
General Admin.: William A. Lindgren/President
   Scanner, Ultrasonic, Other   Radiology
   Scanner, Ultrasonic, Surgical   Surgery

LINSEIS, INC.   800-732-6733
PO Box 666, Princeton Junction, NJ 08550-0666   609-799-6282
FDA Number: n/a   Fax: 609-799-7739
E-mail: info@linseis.com
Web site: www.linseis.com
Medical Products Sales Volume: $1,500,000
Annual Revenue: $1-$5 Million
Year Founded: 1978
Total Employees: 7   Marketing Staff: 2   Sales Staff: 3
Ownership: Private
Produces/Sells CE-marked Devices: Y
Federal Procurement Eligibility: Small Business
Distribution: Manufacturer Direct, Manufacturer Through Manufacturer Reps, OEM
General Admin.: Michael Bissell/Chief Executive Officer
Mktg./Adv.: Michael Bissell/Manager Marketing
   Calorimeter   Chemistry
   Computer Software   General
   Hygrometer (Humidity Indicator)   Anesthesiology
   Recorder, Chart, Laboratory   Chemistry
   Recorder, Paper Chart   Cardiovascular
   Thermometer, Electronic   General
   Thermometer, Electronic, Continuous   General
   Thermometer, Infrared   General
   Thermometer, Laboratory   Chemistry
   Thermometer, Laboratory, Recording   General

LINVATEC/HALL SURGICAL
See Conmed Linvatec

LINWELD INC.   402-323-8450
9920 deer park road, Waverly, NE 68462
FDA Number: 1950212   Fax: 402-323-8456

LINWELD INC.   402-323-8450 *(cont'd)*
E-mail: mbell@linweld.com
Web site: www.linweld.com
Medical Products Sales Volume: $54,100,000
Year Founded: 1945
Total Employees: 350   Marketing Staff: 1   Sales Staff: 90
Ownership: Private
Quality System Registration Information: ISO9001
Produces/Sells CE-marked Devices: N
Federal Procurement Eligibility: Small Business, GSA Contract, VA Contract
Distribution: Manufacturer Direct, Exclusive Distributor
General Admin.: Greg Vasek/President
Mktg./Adv.: Mark C. Bell/Director Sales
     Mark C. Bell/Manager Regional Affairs
   Cylinder, Gas (Empty)   Anesthesiology

LIONVILLE SYSTEMS, INC.   800-523-7114
501 Gunnard Carlson Drive,   610-363-9100
Coatesville, PA 19341
FDA Number: 3006042862   Fax: 610-423-4523
E-mail: lionville@lionville.com
Web site: www.lionville.com
Year Founded: 1960
Total Employees: 100
Ownership: Private
Produces/Sells CE-marked Devices: N
Federal Procurement Eligibility: Small Business, GSA Contract, VA Contract
Distribution: Manufacturer Direct, Exporter
General Admin.: E. Ford Williams/President
Mktg./Adv.: Tobin Williams/Vice President Marketing & Sales
Production: Jane F. Laycock/Product Manager
     Joel Craig/Product Manager
   Cabinet Casework, Modular   General
   Cabinet, Medicine   General
   Cabinet, Other   General
   Cart, Medicine   General
   Cart, Multipurpose   General
   Cart, Other   General
   Computer Equipment   General
   Forms, Medical And Patient   General

LIPOMAX MFG., INC.   562-623-9364
13055 Tom White Way, Suite G, Norwalk, CA 90650
FDA Number: 3005032396
   Kit, Instruments and Accessories, Surgical   Surgery

LIQUI-MARK CORP.   800-486-9005
30 Davids Dr., P.o. Box 18015,   631-236-4333
Hauppauge, NY 11788
FDA Number: 3005706445   Fax: 631-236-4334
E-mail: info@liquimark.com
Web site: www.liquimark.com
Ownership: Private
Produces/Sells CE-marked Devices: N
   Marker, Skin   Surgery

LIQUID AIR CORP SPECIALTY GASES DIV.
See Air Liquide America Corporation, Cambridge Div.

LIQUID CRYSTAL RESOURCES, L.L.C.
See LCR Hallcrest

LIQUID CRYSTAL TECHNOLOGY, INC.
See LCR Hallcrest

LIQUIDMETAL TECHNOLOGIES, INC.   949-635-2100
30452 Esperanza, Rancho Santa Margarita, CA 92688
FDA Number: 3003557555   Fax: 949-635-2188
Web site: www.liquidmetal.com
Ownership: Private
Produces/Sells CE-marked Devices: N
General Admin.: Mr. Ricardo Salas/Executive Vice President, Managing Director
     Mr. Tom Steipp/President, Chief Executive Officer
Finance: Mr. Tony Chung/Chief Financial Officer
   Knife, Ophthalmic   Ophthalmology

LIQUIPAK CORP.   989-463-5510
2205 Michigan Ave., Alma, MI 48801
FDA Number: 1815703
Web site: www.liquipak.com
Ownership: Private
Produces/Sells CE-marked Devices: N
   Cement, Dental   Dental And Oral
   Medical Disinfectants/Cleaners for Instruments   General
   Zinc Oxide Eugenol   Dental And Oral

LISADENT CORP.   516-822-9393
35 Broadway, Hicksville, NY 11801
FDA Number: 2429457
Ownership: Private

LISADENT CORP.
516-822-9393 *(cont'd)*

Produces/Sells CE-marked Devices: N
Denture, Plastic, Teeth — Dental And Oral

LISTA INTERNATIONAL CORP.
(877-465-4782)

106 Lowland St., Holliston, MA 01746-2094
508-429-1350

FDA Number: n/a
Fax: 508-626-0353
E-mail: sales@listaintl.com
Web site: www.listaintl.com
Annual Revenue: $50-$100 Million
Year Founded: 1968
Total Employees: 275   Marketing Staff: 3   Sales Staff: 27
Ownership: Lista B&L Holding
Quality System Registration Information: ISO9001
Produces/Sells CE-marked Devices: N
Distribution: Manufacturer Through Distributor
General Admin.: Don Brown/President
Mktg./Adv.: Anne Smagorinsky/Manager Marketing & Communications
John Alfieri/Vice President Sales
Production: Aaron Tessitore/Plant Manager
Finance: Debera Falcone/Chief Financial Officer
Cabinet Casework, Laboratory — Chemistry
Cabinet Casework, Modular — General
Cart, Other — General
Furniture, General — General

LISTEN TECHNOLOGIES CORP.
800-330-0891

14912 S. Heritagecrest Way,
801-233-8992
Bluffdale, UT 84065

FDA Number: 1724770
Fax: 801-233-8995
E-mail: info@listentech.com
Web site: www.listentech.com
Ownership: Private
Produces/Sells CE-marked Devices: N
Hearing-Aid, Group, Or Auditory Trainer — Ear/Nose/Throat

LITE TECH, INC.
610-650-8690

975 Madison Ave., Norristown, PA 19403

FDA Number: 2529886
Apron, Lead, Dental — Dental And Oral
Apron, Lead, Radiographic — Radiology
Curtain, Protective, Radiographic — Radiology
Shield, Protective, Personnel — Radiology

LITECURE, LLC
302-709-0408

930 Old Harmony Rd., Suite A, Newark, DE 19713

FDA Number: 3006268867
Lamp, Infrared — Physical Med

LITTLE SHEPHERD INDUSTRIES
870-453-4874

316 River Run Lane, Flippin, AR 72634

FDA Number: 3005289268
Ownership: Private
Produces/Sells CE-marked Devices: N
Component, Exercise — Physical Med

LITTLEFIELD CO.
801-485-1441

1441 East 2100 South, Salt Lake City, UT 84105

FDA Number: 1721443
Hearing-Aid — Ear/Nose/Throat

LITTLEFORD DAY, INC.
800-365-8555

PO Box 128, Florence, KY 41042
859-525-7600

FDA Number: n/a
Fax: 859-525-1446
E-mail: sales@littleford.com
Web site: www.littleford.com
Medical Products Sales Volume: $50,000,000
Annual Revenue: $25-$50 Million
Year Founded: 1882
Total Employees: 500   Marketing Staff: 3   Sales Staff: 10
Ownership: Private
Produces/Sells CE-marked Devices: N
Federal Procurement Eligibility: Small Business
Distribution: Manufacturer Direct
General Admin.: Donald L. Steedman/President, Chief Executive Officer
Mktg./Adv.: William R. Barker/Market Manager
Production: Don Schreck/Plant Manager
Charles Kroeger/Vice President Manufacturing
Research: Glenn Vice/Vice President Research & Development
Production Equipment — General

LITTON DENTAL PRODUCTS
See Engler Engineering Corp.

LIV INTERNATIONAL USA, INC.
909-931-1719

2335 West Foothill Blvd., Suite 14 And 15, Upland, CA 91784

FDA Number: 3004865539
Ownership: Private
Produces/Sells CE-marked Devices: N

LIV INTERNATIONAL USA, INC.
909-931-1719 *(cont'd)*

Radiographic Unit, Diagnostic, Mammographic — Radiology

LIVEDO USA, INC.
252-237-1373

4925 Livedo Dr., Wilson, NC 27893

FDA Number: 3004780365
Garment, Protective, For Incontinence — Gastroenterology/Urology

LIVENGOOD ENGINEERING INC.
970-493-2569

1112 Oakridge Dr., #104 Pmb 51, Fort Collins, CO 80525

FDA Number: 3005801809
Infusion Stand — General

LIVING EARTH CRAFTS
800-358-8292

3210 Executive Dr, Viats, CA 92081
760-597-2155

FDA Number: n/a
E-mail: sales@livingearthcrafts.com
Web site: www.livingearthcrafts.com
Annual Revenue: $5-$10 Million
Year Founded: 1973
Ownership: EVERETT ASSOCIATES, INC.
Produces/Sells CE-marked Devices: Y
Federal Procurement Eligibility: Small Business
Distribution: Manufacturer Direct, Manufacturer Through Distributor, Manufacturer Through Manufacturer Reps, OEM, Exporter
Chair, Examination And Treatment — General
Equipment, Therapy, Handicapped/Physical — Physical Med
Table, Examination/Treatment — General
Table, Mechanical — Physical Med
Table, Other — General
Table, Physical Medicine, Powered — Physical Med
Table, Physical Therapy — Physical Med

LIVING INFORMATION SYSTEMS LLC
315-469-7399

886 East Brighton Ave., Syracuse, NY 13205

FDA Number: 3005196642
Biofeedback Device — Cns/Neurology

LIVINGSTON PRODUCTS, INC.
800-822-2156

1377 Barclay Blvd., Buffalo Grove, IL 60089
847-808-0900

FDA Number: 1422581
Fax: 847-808-0904
E-mail: lpi@lpicorp.net
Web site: www.livingstonproducts.com
Ownership: Private
Quality System Registration Information: ISO9001
Produces/Sells CE-marked Devices: N
Federal Procurement Eligibility: Small Business, VA Contract
Distribution: Manufacturer Direct, Manufacturer Through Distributor, OEM
Accessories, Cart, Multipurpose — General
Needle, Biopsy, Mammary — Obstetrics/Gynecology
System, Marking, Film, Radiographic — Radiology

LIXI, INC.
847-961-6666

11980 Oak Creek Parkway, Huntley, IL 60142

FDA Number: 1419514
Web site: www.lixi.com
Ownership: Private
Produces/Sells CE-marked Devices: N
Radiographic/Fluoroscopic Unit, Image-Intensified — Radiology

LKB DIAGNOSTICS INC.
See Perkin Elmer Wallac, Inc.

LKC TECHNOLOGIES, INC.
800-638-7055

2 Professional Drive, Suite 222,
301-840-1992
Gaithersburg, MD 20879

FDA Number: 1119189
Fax: 301-330-2237
E-mail: Info@lkc.com
Web site: www.lkc.com
Medical Products Sales Volume: $10,000,000
Annual Revenue: $1-$5 Million
Year Founded: 1976
Total Employees: 50   Marketing Staff: 1   Sales Staff: 2
Ownership: Private
Quality System Registration Information: ISO9001
Produces/Sells CE-marked Devices: Y
Federal Procurement Eligibility: Small Business
Distribution: Manufacturer Direct, Manufacturer Through Manufacturer Reps, Exporter
General Admin.: James Datovech/President, Chief Executive Officer
Mktg./Adv.: Dr. Yang Tsau/Director Product Development
David Scheraga/Manager International & National Sales
George Barstis/Vice President Strategic Development
Production: Lin Gao/Director Quality Assurance
Mr. Russ Eicher/Manager Operations
Adaptometer (Biophotometer) — Ophthalmology
Electro-Oculograph — Ophthalmology
Electroretinograph (ERG) — Ophthalmology
Evoked Response Unit — Cns/Neurology

LKC TECHNOLOGIES, INC.
800-638-7055 *(cont'd)*

Photostimulator	General
Recorder, Analog/Digital, Ophthalmic	Ophthalmology
Stimulator, Photic, Evoked Response	Cns/Neurology
Tester, Color Vision	Ophthalmology

LLOYD HEARING AID CORP.
800-323-4212
4435 Manchester Drive, Rockford, IL 61109 **815-964-4191**
FDA Number: n/a *Fax:* 815-964-8378
Total Employees: 21
Ownership: Private
Produces/Sells CE-marked Devices: N

Hearing-Aid	Ear/Nose/Throat

LLOYD TABLE CO.
319-455-2110
102-122 West Main St., Lisbon, IA 52253
FDA Number: 1925206

Chair/Table, Medical	General

LM AIR TECHNOLOGY, INC.
866-381-8200
1467 Pinewood St., Rahway, NJ 07065-5697 **732-381-8200**
FDA Number: n/a *Fax:* 732-381-4091
E-mail: sales@LMAIRTECH.com
Web site: www.LMAIRTECH.com
Medical Products Sales Volume: $2,000,000
Annual Revenue: $5-$10 Million
Total Employees: 48   *Marketing Staff:* 1   *Sales Staff:* 5
Ownership: Private
Quality System Registration Information: ISO9001
Produces/Sells CE-marked Devices: N
Federal Procurement Eligibility: Small Business, GSA Contract
Distribution: Manufacturer Direct, Manufacturer Through Manufacturer Reps, OEM, Exclusive Distributor
General Admin.: Pete Daniele/Owner

Cabinet, Pass Through	General
Cart, Other	General
Cleanroom Equipment	General
Equipment, Filtering, Air, ETO	General
Filter, Air	General
Laminar Air Flow Unit	General
Table, Other	General

LMI
714-349-5386
2324 Rain Tree Drive, Brea, CA 92821
FDA Number: 3005837180
Ownership: Private
Produces/Sells CE-marked Devices: N

Accessories, Retractor, Dental	Dental And Oral

LMS MEDICAL SYSTEMS LTD.
514-488-3461
314-5252 Boul De Maisonneuve O, Montreal H4A 3S5 Canada
FDA Number: 9615396

Monitor, Perinatal	Obstetrics/Gynecology

LND, INC.
516-678-6141
3230 Lawson Blvd., Oceanside, NY 11572-3724
FDA Number: n/a *Fax:* 516-678-6704
E-mail: info@lndinc.com
Web site: www.lndinc.com
Medical Products Sales Volume: $7,000,000
Annual Revenue: $5-$10 Million
Year Founded: 1964
Total Employees: 45   *Marketing Staff:* 1   *Sales Staff:* 2
Ownership: Private
Quality System Registration Information: ISO9001
Produces/Sells CE-marked Devices: N
Federal Procurement Eligibility: Small Business
Distribution: Manufacturer Direct, OEM, Exporter
General Admin.: Peter T. Neyland/Chief Executive Officer
Mktg./Adv.: Robert W. Lehnert/Director Marketing
    Robert W. Lehnert/Vice President Marketing
Production: Joseph W. Keller/Director Quality Assurance

Calibrator, Radioisotope	Radiology
Counter, Radiation	Radiology
Detector, Beta/Gamma	Chemistry
Diffractometer, X-Ray	Chemistry
Dosimeter, Radiation	Radiology
Monitor, Radiation	Radiology

LOBOB LABORATORIES, INC.
800-83-LOBOB
1440 Atteberry Lane, San Jose, CA 95131-1410 **408-432-0580**
FDA Number: 2915925 *Fax:* 408-432-8253
E-mail: loboblabs@aol.com
Web site: www.loboblabs.com
Medical Products Sales Volume: $4,500,000
Annual Revenue: $1-$5 Million
Total Employees: 35
Ownership: Private
Produces/Sells CE-marked Devices: N

LOBOB LABORATORIES, INC.
800-83-LOBOB *(cont'd)*
Federal Procurement Eligibility: Small Business
Distribution: Manufacturer Direct, Manufacturer Through Distributor, Manufacturer Through Manufacturer Reps, Importer, Exporter
General Admin.: Robert M. Lohr/President
    Jerry Uy/Vice President, General Manager
Mktg./Adv.: Thomas R. Pominville/Manager National Sales
    James H. McCreary/Manager Product Development
Production: M. Alan Maxfield/Manager Regulatory Affairs

Cleaner, Lens, Contact	Ophthalmology
Lens, Contact (Other Material)	Ophthalmology

LOCIN INDUSTRIES LTD.
800-663-8270
#200-18 Gostick Pk., **604-980-9318**
North Vancouver, BC V7M- Canada
FDA Number: 8022089 *Fax:* 604-980-7090
E-mail: andrew@locin.com
Annual Revenue: $0-$1 Million
Total Employees: 4
Federal Procurement Eligibility: Small Business
Distribution: Importer
General Admin.: David C. Nicol/Chief Executive Officer
    Diane Nicol/Chief Executive Officer

Floss, Dental	Dental And Oral

LOGIC PRODUCT DEVELOPMENT
952-941-8071
6201 Bury Drive, Eden Prairie, MN 55346
FDA Number: n/a *Fax:* 952-941-8065
E-mail: sales@logicpd.com
Web site: www.logicpd.com
Medical Products Sales Volume: $10,000,000
Annual Revenue: $5-$10 Million
Year Founded: 1960
Total Employees: 50   *Marketing Staff:* 1   *Sales Staff:* 1
Ownership: Private
Produces/Sells CE-marked Devices: N
Federal Procurement Eligibility: Small Business
Distribution: Manufacturer Through Distributor, Manufacturer Through Manufacturer Reps, OEM, Service Direct, Exporter
General Admin.: Danny Cunagin/President

Computer Software	General
Service, Engineering/Design	General

LOGICAL TECHNICAL SERVICES CORP.
See Peripheral Dynamics Inc.

LOGICAL TECHNOLOGY, INC.
800-266-7591
6907 N. Knoxville, Peoria, IL 61614-4868 **309-689-2900**
FDA Number: n/a *Fax:* 309-218-0189
E-mail: info@comply1.com
Web site: www.comply1.com/
Medical Products Sales Volume: $4,900,000
Annual Revenue: $1-$5 Million
Year Founded: 1987
Total Employees: 65   *Marketing Staff:* 2   *Sales Staff:* 4
Ownership: Private
Produces/Sells CE-marked Devices: N
Federal Procurement Eligibility: Small Business
Distribution: Manufacturer Direct
General Admin.: J. M. Krakowiecki/President
Production: Jerry R. Webber/Vice President Manufacturing & Development
IS: Greg Schroeder/Manager Tech. Support

Computer Software	General

LOGOS SCIENTIFIC, INC.
See Volu-Sol, Inc.

LOGOVOX SYSTEMS, INC.
925-253-8303
128 Diablo View Dr., Orinda, CA 94563
FDA Number: 3004145462
Ownership: Private
Produces/Sells CE-marked Devices: N

Communication System, Powered	Physical Med

LOHMANN & RAUSCHER, INC.
800-279-3863
6001 SW Sixth Avenue, Suite #101, **785-862-1100**
Topeka, KS 66615
FDA Number: 1933439 *Fax:* 785-862-2860
E-mail: office@us.LRmed.com
Web site: www.lohmann-rauscher.com
Ownership: Private
Quality System Registration Information: ISO9001
Produces/Sells CE-marked Devices: Y
Federal Procurement Eligibility: Small Business
Distribution: Manufacturer Through Distributor, Manufacturer Through Manufacturer Reps, OEM, Importer, Exporter
General Admin.: Mr. Michael R. Hall/President
Mktg./Adv.: Ms. Lisa G. Phlegar/Manager Marketing
    Mr. Dave W. Lob/Vice President Marketing & Sales

LOHMANN & RAUSCHER, INC. 800-279-3863 (cont'd)

Purchasing: Mr. Ryan G. Rochelle/Director Purchasing
Mr. Charlie R. Gray/Purchasing Agent

Bandage, Adhesive	Surgery
Bandage, Cast	Physical Med
Bandage, Compression	General
Bandage, Elastic	General
Bandage, Gauze	General
Bandage, Other	General
Bandage, Tubular	General
Belt, Abdominal	Gastroenterology/Urology
Belt, Lumbosacral	Orthopedics
Belt, Rib (Support)	Orthopedics
Belt, Traction, Pelvic	Physical Med
Belt, Traction, Pelvic, Orthopedic	Orthopedics
Binder, Abdominal	General
Binder, Abdominal, OB/GYN	Obstetrics/Gynecology
Binder, Elastic	General
Brace, Joint, Ankle (External)	Physical Med
Clothing, Protective	General
Collar, Cervical Neck	Orthopedics
Cushion, Other	General
Dressing, Gel	General
Dressing, Non-Adherent	General
Dressing, Other	General
Dressing, Permeable, Moisture	General
Dressing, Universal	General
Dressing, Wound and Burn, Hydrogel	Surgery
Dressing, Wound and Burn, Occlusive	Surgery
Glove, Other	General
Halter, Head, Traction, Orthopedic	Orthopedics
Immobilizer, Knee	Orthopedics
Insoles, Medical	General
Legging, Compression, Non-Inflatable	General
Pack, Hot Or Cold, Reusable	Physical Med
Pillow	General
Pillow, Cervical	Orthopedics
Sleeve, Compressible Limb	Cardiovascular
Splint, Other	Orthopedics
Stockinette	Orthopedics
Support, Abdominal	Physical Med
Support, Ankle	Orthopedics
Support, Back	Orthopedics
Support, Elbow	Orthopedics
Support, Hot/Cold Pack	Physical Med
Support, Knee	Physical Med
Support, Thigh	Physical Med
Support, Wrist	Physical Med
Traction Unit, Non-Powered	Orthopedics

LOHMANN CORPORATION 1 859 334 4900

3000 Earhart Court, Ste. 155, Hebron, KY 41048
FDA Number: n/a   Fax: 1 859 334 4903
Web site: www.lohmanncorp.com
Annual Revenue: $10-$25 Million
Total Employees: 2   Sales Staff: 1
Ownership: Lohmann & Rauscher Int'L Gmbh & Co. Kg
Quality System Registration Information: ISO9001
Produces/Sells CE-marked Devices: Y
Distribution: Manufacturer Direct, Manufacturer Through Manufacturer Reps
General Admin.: Steven J. De Jong/Chief Executive Officer
Jan Roberts/Vice President Human Resources
Mktg./Adv.: Stan Riches/Manager National Sales
Production: Bernie Darling/Vice President Manufacturing

Service, Device Coating, Protective	General

LOHMANN TECHNOLOGIES CORP.

See Lohmann Corporation

LOMBART INSTRUMENTS 800-831-1194

1312 Marquette Drive, Suite N, Romeo, IL 60446 630-759-7666
FDA Number: n/a   Fax: 630-759-1744
E-mail: customer@lombartinstrument.com
Web site: www.lombartinstruments.com
Annual Revenue: $10-$25 Million
Total Employees: 35   Marketing Staff: 23   Sales Staff: 23
Ownership: Public
Stock Symbol: FKLN
Traded On: NASDAQ
Quality System Registration Information: ISO9000
Produces/Sells CE-marked Devices: N
Distribution: Manufacturer Through Manufacturer Reps
General Admin.: Mike Carroll/President, Chief Financial Officer
Mktg./Adv.: Mike Carroll/Vice President Marketing & Sales
Production: Mike Carroll/Vice President Manufacturing

Office Equipment	General
Service, Consulting	General
Service, Maintenance/Repair	General

LONDON COMPANY

See Radiometer America, Inc.

LONDON HEALTH CARE & OSTOMY CENTRE 800-265-0410

675 Adelaide St. N, 519-858-2300
London, ONT N5Y-2 Canada
FDA Number: n/a   Fax: 519-858-2170
E-mail: lhostaff@londonostomy.com
Web site: http://www.londonostomy.com
Year Founded: 1971
Total Employees: 10
Ownership: Private
Produces/Sells CE-marked Devices: N

LONDON SCIENTIFIC LIMITED 800-270-5665

833 Consortium Ct., 519-681-2239
London, ONT N6E-2 Canada
FDA Number: n/a   Fax: 519-681-0553
E-mail: londonscientific@lsl.ca
Web site: http://lsl.ca/index.shtml
Year Founded: 1995
Total Employees: 25
Ownership: Private
Produces/Sells CE-marked Devices: N
Distribution: Exclusive Distributor, Exporter

LONE OAK MEDICAL TECHNOLOGIES 267-221-0661

3805 Old Easton Road, Doylestown, PA 18901
FDA Number: 3006442319

Densitometer, Bone, Single Photon	Radiology

LONE STAR MEDICAL PRODUCTS, INC. 800-331-7427

11211 Cash Road, Stafford, TX 77477 281-340-6010
FDA Number: 1627186   Fax: 281-340-6091
E-mail: sales@medicalblue.com
Web site: www.lsmp.com
Medical Products Sales Volume: $3,700,000
Annual Revenue: $5-$10 Million
Year Founded: 1979
Total Employees: 50   Marketing Staff: 2   Sales Staff: 4
Ownership: Private
Quality System Registration Information: ISO9001
Produces/Sells CE-marked Devices: Y
Federal Procurement Eligibility: Small Business
Distribution: Manufacturer Direct, Exporter
General Admin.: James Fowler/President
Sean Self/Vice President, General Manager
Mktg./Adv.: Barbara Smith/Director Marketing & Sales

Isolation Unit, Surgical	General
Retractor, Other	Surgery
Retractor, Self-Retaining	Gastroenterology/Urology
Retractor, Vaginal	Obstetrics/Gynecology
Surgical Instrument, G-U, Manual	Gastroenterology/Urology

LONG AND ROSSI PRODUCTS 303-233-9581

895 Field St., Lakewood, CO 80215
FDA Number: 1724315
Ownership: Private
Produces/Sells CE-marked Devices: N

Forceps, Tooth Extractor, Surgical	Dental And Oral

LONGTERM COMPUTER SYSTEMS

See Horizon Healthcare Technologies

LONZA ROCKLAND, INC. 207-594-3400

191 Thomaston St., Rockland, ME 04841
FDA Number: 1219614

Electrophoresis Equipment, Liquid	Chemistry

LONZA WALKERSVILLE, INC. 201-316-9200

8830 Biggs Ford Rd., Walkersville, MD 21793
FDA Number: 1114298   Fax: 301-845-4024
E-mail: contact.walkersville@lonza.com
Web site: www.lonza.com
Year Founded: 1984
Ownership: Private
Quality System Registration Information: ISO9001
Produces/Sells CE-marked Devices: N

Antigen, CF (Including CF Control), Coxsackievirus A 1-24	Microbiology
Antigen, CF (Including CF Control), Influenza Virus	Microbiology
Antigen, CF (Including CF Control), Parainfluenza Virus	Microbiology
Antigen, CF, Mycoplasma SPP.	Microbiology
Antiserum, CF, Coxsackievirus A 1-24, B 1-6	Microbiology
Antiserum, CF, Influenza Virus A, B, C	Microbiology
Antiserum, CF, Parainfluenza Virus 1-4	Microbiology
Antiserum, Mycoplasma SPP.	Microbiology
Culture Media, Synthetic Cell And Tissue	Pathology
Neuramininase (Sialidase)	Pathology
Serum, Animal	Pathology
Solution, Balanced Salt	Pathology

LOOPS, L.L.C.   360-366-3009
7152 Everett Rd., P. O. Box 2936, Ferndale, WA 98248
FDA Number: 2087362

Floss, Dental	Dental And Oral
Toothbrush, Manual	Dental And Oral

LORAD, A HOLOGIC CO.
See Lorad, A Hologic Company

LORAD, A HOLOGIC COMPANY   800-321-4659
36 Apple Ridge Road, Danbury, CT 06810   203-207-4500
FDA Number: 1220984   *Fax:* 781-280-0672
E-mail: sales@hologic.com
Web site: www.hologic.com
Ownership: Hologic, Inc.
Stock Symbol: HOLX
Traded On: NASDAQ
Produces/Sells CE-marked Devices: N
General Admin.: Mr. John W. Cumming/Chief Executive Officer, Chairman
    Mr. Glenn P. Muir/Chief Financial Officer, Executive Vice President
    David R. LaVance/President, Chief Executive Officer
    Robert Cascella/President, Chief Operating Officer
    Wayne Wilson/Principal

Full Field Digital, System, X-ray, Mammographic	Radiology
Radiographic Unit, Diagnostic, Mammographic	Radiology
System, Marking, Film, Radiographic	Radiology
System, X-Ray, Mobile	Radiology

LORD CUSTOM MOLDED SHOES, INC.   631-471-3090
1395-1 Lakeland Ave., Bohemia, NY 11716
FDA Number: 2434559
Ownership: Private
Produces/Sells CE-marked Devices: N

Shoe, Cast	Physical Med

LORDEX, INC.   281-395-9512
32357 Morton Rd., Bldg. 3, Brookshire, TX 77423
FDA Number: 3004171292

Equipment, Traction, Powered	Physical Med
Exerciser, Non-Measuring	Physical Med

LORON INC.
See Katecho, Inc.

LORVIC CORP.   800-325-1881
13705 Shoreline Ct. East, Earth City, MO 63045   314-344-0010
FDA Number: 1941138   *Fax:* 314-344-0021
E-mail: info@youngdental.com
Web site: www.youngdental.com
Ownership: YOUNG INNOVATIONS, INC.
Stock Symbol: YDNT
Traded On: NASDAQ
Quality System Registration Information: ISO9001
Produces/Sells CE-marked Devices: Y
Distribution: Manufacturer Through Distributor
Mktg./Adv.: Ms. Elizabeth Bowen/Admin. National Sales

Absorber, Saliva, Paper	Dental And Oral
Evacuator, Oral Cavity	Dental And Oral
Liner, Cavity, Calcium Hydroxide	Dental And Oral
Matrix, Dental	Dental And Oral
Protector, Silicate	Dental And Oral
Sterilization Process Indicator, Physical/Chemical	General
Tooth Bonding Agent, Resin Restoration	Dental And Oral
Tray, Fluoride, Disposable	Dental And Oral
Wrap, Sterilization	General

LOTS CORP.   520-730-6068
10977 E. Tanque Verde Road, Tucson, AZ 85749
FDA Number: 3027784
Ownership: Private
Produces/Sells CE-marked Devices: N

Splint, Clavicle	Physical Med
Splint, Traction	Orthopedics

LOTUS HYGIENE SYSTEMS INC.   714-259-8805
15042 Parkway Loop, #b, Tustin, CA 92780
FDA Number: 3005596594
Ownership: Private
Produces/Sells CE-marked Devices: N

Adapter, Hygiene	Physical Med

LOTUS TECHNOLOGY, INC.   704-658-0406
110 Talbert Pointe Drive, Mooresville, NC 28117
FDA Number: 2135153   *Fax:* 704-658-0409
E-mail: cyoung@lotustechnology.net
Web site: www.lotustechnology.net
Medical Products Sales Volume: $10,000,000
Year Founded: 1999
Total Employees: 125
Ownership: Private

LOTUS TECHNOLOGY, INC.   704-658-0406 *(cont'd)*
Produces/Sells CE-marked Devices: N
Federal Procurement Eligibility: Small Business

Hearing-Aid	Ear/Nose/Throat

LOUISVILLE APL DIAGNOSTICS, INC.   800-624-3192
2622 Nasa Parkway, Suite G2,   770-455-7129
Seabrook, TX 77586
FDA Number: 1529254   *Fax:* 770-455-6499
E-mail: feedback@louisvilleapl.com
Web site: www.louisvilleapl.com
Annual Revenue: $0-$1 Million
Year Founded: 1993
Ownership: Private
Produces/Sells CE-marked Devices: Y
Distribution: Manufacturer Direct, Manufacturer Through Distributor, OEM, Exporter

System, Test, Anticardiolipin, Immunological	Immunology

LOVE IMPORTS   800-944-5523
PO Box 759, Grapeland, TX 75844   800-944-5523
FDA Number: 1055767   *Fax:* 770-684-6778
E-mail: love@loveimports.com
Web site: www.loveimports.com
Medical Products Sales Volume: $250,000
Annual Revenue: $0-$1 Million
Year Founded: 1991
Total Employees: 7
Ownership: Private
Produces/Sells CE-marked Devices: Y
Federal Procurement Eligibility: Small Business, Minority Owned, Female Owned
Distribution: Manufacturer Direct, Exclusive Distributor, Importer, Exporter
General Admin.: Charles Love/President

Glove, Other	General
Glove, Patient Examination	General
Glove, Patient Examination, Latex	General
Glove, Utility	General

LPA MEDICAL INC.   800-663-4863
460 Desrochers #150,   418-681-1313
Vanier, QUE G1M-1 Canada
FDA Number: n/a   *Fax:* 418-681-4488
E-mail: lpa@lpamedical.qc.ca
Web site: www.lpamedical.qc.ca
Year Founded: 1989
Total Employees: 25
Ownership: Private
Produces/Sells CE-marked Devices: N
Distribution: Manufacturer Direct, Exclusive Distributor

LPS INDUSTRIES, INC.   800-275-4577
10 Caesar Place, Moonachie, NJ 07074   201-438-3515
FDA Number: n/a   *Fax:* 201-438-0040
E-mail: info@lpsind.com
Web site: www.lpsind.com
Annual Revenue: $25-$50 Million
Total Employees: 225   *Marketing Staff:* 6   *Sales Staff:* 26
Ownership: Private
Quality System Registration Information: ISO9001
Produces/Sells CE-marked Devices: N
Federal Procurement Eligibility: Female Owned
Distribution: Manufacturer Direct, Manufacturer Through Manufacturer Reps
General Admin.: Madeleine D. Robinson/Chief Executive Officer
Mktg./Adv.: Ann McHenry/Manager Marketing
    Jack Cunneen/Vice President Sales
Production: Tim Fletcher/Vice President Production

Collector, Specimen	Microbiology
Packaging Material	General

LRL LOGIX   800-800-3650
1301 W. Hwy 407 # 201, Lewisville, TX 75077   972-691-7447
FDA Number: 1651097   *Fax:* 972-691-7557
E-mail: Info@lrldirect.com
Web site: www.lrldirect.com
Medical Products Sales Volume: $100,000
Year Founded: 1995
Total Employees: 4
Ownership: Lrl Logix
Produces/Sells CE-marked Devices: N
Federal Procurement Eligibility: Small Business

Monitor, Patient Position, Light Beam	Radiology

Medical Product Subsidiaries (Listed Separately)
Lrl Logix

LSI INTL., INC.   913-894-4493
11529 W. 79th St, Lenexa, KS 66214
FDA Number: 1932354

LSI INTL., INC.   913-894-4493 *(cont'd)*
Ownership: Private
Produces/Sells CE-marked Devices: N

Stimulator, Muscle, Electrical-Powered (EMS)	Physical Med
Stimulator, Nerve, Transcutaneous (Pain Relief, TENS)	Cns/Neurology

LSI SOLUTIONS INC.   585-869-6641
7796 Victor-mendon Rd., Victor, NY 14564
FDA Number: 1320468

Endoscope	Gastroenterology/Urology
Instrument, Passing, Ligature, Knot Tying	Cns/Neurology
Laparoscope, General & Plastic Surgery	Surgery
Suture, Absorbable, Synthetic, Polyglycolic Acid	Surgery
Suture, Non-Absorbable, Synthetic, Polyester	Surgery
Suture, Non-Absorbable, Synthetic, Polyethylene	Surgery
Suture, Non-Absorbable, Synthetic, Polypropylene	Surgery
Suture, Surgical, Absorbable, Polydioxanone	Surgery

LSL INDUSTRIES, INC.   888-225-5575   773-878-1100
5535 N. Wolcott Avenue, Chicago, IL 60640
FDA Number: 1420054
Fax: 773-878-9100
E-mail: sales@LSLIND.com
Web site: www.LSLIND.com
Medical Products Sales Volume: $2,600,000
Annual Revenue: $10-$25 Million
Year Founded: 1981
Total Employees: 35   *Marketing Staff:* 5   *Sales Staff:* 15
Ownership: Private
Produces/Sells CE-marked Devices: N
Federal Procurement Eligibility: Small Business, Minority Owned, GSA Contract, VA Contract
Distribution: Manufacturer Through Distributor, Manufacturer Through Manufacturer Reps, OEM, Exporter
General Admin.: Ash Luthra/President, Chief Executive Officer
Mktg./Adv.: Artis Carroll/Director National Accounts
　　　　　Roger Drozd/Director Sales
　　　　　Robert Luetzow/Manager National Sales
Production: V. Hussain/Director Quality Assurance

Basin, Emesis	General
Basin, Wash	General
Bedpan	General
Bedpan, Fracture	General
Bowl, Solution	General
Brush, Scrub, Operating Room	Surgery
Catheter, Central Venous	General
Catheter, Urinary	Gastroenterology/Urology
Container, Specimen, All Types	General
Cup, Denture	Dental And Oral
Drainage System, Urine, Closed	Gastroenterology/Urology
Drainage Unit, Urinary	General
IV Start Kit	Surgery
Kit, Admission (Patient Utensil)	General
Kit, Catheter Care	General
Kit, Catheterization, Sterile Urethral	Gastroenterology/Urology
Kit, Enema	General
Kit, Irrigation, Sterile	Gastroenterology/Urology
Kit, Mid-Stream Collection	General
Kit, Prep	General
Kit, Sitz Bath	Physical Med
Kit, Suture Removal	Surgery
Kit, Tracheostomy Care	Anesthesiology
Kit, Urinary Drainage Collection	Gastroenterology/Urology
Slippers	General
Syringe, Bulb	General
Syringe, Ear	Ear/Nose/Throat
Syringe, Irrigating	General
Syringe, Piston	General
Tray, Custom/Special Procedure	General
Urinal	General
Urological Irrigation System	Gastroenterology/Urology

LSVP INTERNATIONAL, INC.   866-969-0100   650-969-1000
4692 El Camino Real, Unit 126, Los Altos, CA 94022
FDA Number: n/a
Fax: 650-969-2300
E-mail: info@lsvpusa.com
Web site: www.lsvpusa.com
Annual Revenue: $1-$5 Million
Year Founded: 1992
Ownership: Private
Produces/Sells CE-marked Devices: Y
Federal Procurement Eligibility: Small Business, Female Owned
Distribution: Manufacturer Through Distributor, OEM, Importer
General Admin.: Sophia Pesotchinsky/Senior Vice President

Endoscope, Flexible	Gastroenterology/Urology
Forceps, Biopsy, Bronchoscope (Non-Rigid)	Anesthesiology
Forceps, Biopsy, Electric	Gastroenterology/Urology
Forceps, Biopsy, Gynecological	Obstetrics/Gynecology
Forceps, Biopsy, Non-Electric	Gastroenterology/Urology
Forceps, Endoscopic	Gastroenterology/Urology

LSVP INTERNATIONAL, INC.   866-969-0100 *(cont'd)*

Forceps, Grasping, Flexible Endoscopic	Gastroenterology/Urology

LT ACQUISITION, INC.   616-698-1830
4489 East Paris Ave., Grand Rapids, MI 49512
FDA Number: 1835044

Shield, Eye, Ophthalmic	Ophthalmology
Shield, Ophthalmic, Radiological	Radiology

LTC SOLUTIONS
See Horizon Healthcare Technologies

LUCAS MEDICAL, INC.   714-938-0233
1751 South Douglass Rd., Anaheim, CA 92806
FDA Number: 2029386

Catheter, Biliary	Gastroenterology/Urology
Catheter, Embolectomy (Fogarty Type)	Cardiovascular
Catheter, Intravascular, Diagnostic	Cardiovascular
Catheter, Irrigation	Surgery

LUCENT MEDICAL SYSTEMS, INC.   425-822-3310
811 Kirkland Avenue, Suite 100, Kirkland, WA 98033
FDA Number: n/a
Fax: 425-822-3486
E-mail: mail@lucentmedical.com
Web site: www.lucentmedical.com
Medical Products Sales Volume: $500,000
Annual Revenue: $1-$5 Million
Year Founded: 1994
Total Employees: 7
Ownership: Private
Quality System Registration Information: ISO9001
Produces/Sells CE-marked Devices: N
Federal Procurement Eligibility: Small Business
Distribution: Manufacturer Direct, Manufacturer Through Distributor, OEM
General Admin.: Robert Golden/President, Chief Executive Officer
Production: Steve Vincent/Director Engineering
　　　　　Cynthia Pestka/Director Quality Assurance & Regulatory Affairs

Locator, Magnetic	Surgery

LUCENT SPECIALTY FIBER TECHNOLOGIES
See Ofs, Specialty Photonics Division

LUCID, INC.   585-239-9800
2320 Brighton Henrietta Townline Rd., Rochester, NY 14623
FDA Number: 1320925
Fax: 585-239-9806
Web site: www.lucid-tech.com
Ownership: Private
Produces/Sells CE-marked Devices: N

Device, Storage, Image, Digital	Radiology
Examination Device, AC-Powered	General
Light, Surgical, Floor Standing	Surgery
Microscope, Phase Contrast	Pathology

LUCKMAN CORPORATION   215-659-1664
1930 Old York Road, Abington, PA 19001
FDA Number: n/a
Fax: 215-659-5506
E-mail: info@luckmancorp.com
Web site: www.luckmancorp.com
Medical Products Sales Volume: $600,000
Year Founded: 1977
Total Employees: 4   *Marketing Staff:* 2   *Sales Staff:* 2
Ownership: Private
Produces/Sells CE-marked Devices: N
Federal Procurement Eligibility: Small Business
Distribution: Manufacturer Direct, Manufacturer Through Distributor, OEM, Importer, Exporter
General Admin.: Frank Luckman/President
Mktg./Adv.: Frank Luckman/Manager Advertising
　　　　　Frank Luckman/Vice President Marketing & Sales

Compression Instrument	Orthopedics
Instrument, Dental, Manual	Dental And Oral

LUCOMED INC.   800-633-7877   973-575-0614
45 Kulick Rd., Fairfield, NJ 07004
FDA Number: 2244060
Fax: 973-227-0151
E-mail: wghelfi@lucomedinc.com
Web site: www.lucomedinc.com
Medical Products Sales Volume: $6,000,000
Annual Revenue: $5-$10 Million
Year Founded: 1991
Total Employees: 7   *Marketing Staff:* 1   *Sales Staff:* 3
Ownership: Lucomed SpA
Quality System Registration Information: ISO9002
Produces/Sells CE-marked Devices: Y
Distribution: OEM, Exclusive Distributor, Importer
General Admin.: Willer Ghelfi/Chief Executive Officer, Vice President
　　　　　Silvio Eruzzi/President
Mktg./Adv.: Willer Ghelfi/Director Marketing
Production: Ms. Candi Longo/Customer Service Representative

LUCOMED INC.   800-633-7877 *(cont'd)*
Finance: Thomas Karwacki/Controller

Component, Plastic	General
Container, IV	General
Contract Assembly	General
Contract Manufacturing, Product, Disposable	General
Kit, Administration, Intravenous	General
Kit, Administration, Parenteral	Gastroenterology/Urology
Kit, Hemodialysis Tubing	Gastroenterology/Urology
Kit, Intravenous, Administration, Buret	General
Molding, Injection	General
Service, Engineering/Design	General
Tube, Dialysate	Gastroenterology/Urology
Tubing, Polyvinyl Chloride	General

LUDL ELECTRONIC PRODUCTS LTD. (LEP LTD.)   888-769-6111
171 Brady Ave., Hawthorne, NY 10532   **914-769-6111**
FDA Number: n/a   Fax: 914-769-4759
E-mail: cust-service@ludl.com
Web site: www.ludl.com
Total Employees: 40
Ownership: Private
Quality System Registration Information: ISO9001
Produces/Sells CE-marked Devices: Y
Federal Procurement Eligibility: Small Business
Distribution: Manufacturer Direct, OEM
General Admin.: Helmot Ludl/Chief Executive Officer
         David Dumneli/Vice President, General Manager
Mktg./Adv.: Marrillyn Graham/Manager Advertising

Media, Filter	General

LUDLUM MEASUREMENTS, INC.   800-622-0828
501 Oak St., Sweetwater, TX 79556-3209   **325-235-5494**
FDA Number: n/a   Fax: 325-235-4672
E-mail: ludlum@ludlums.com
Web site: www.ludlums.com
Annual Revenue: $10-$25 Million
Year Founded: 1962
Total Employees: 300   *Sales Staff:* 5
Ownership: Private
Produces/Sells CE-marked Devices: Y
Federal Procurement Eligibility: Small Business
Distribution: Manufacturer Direct, Manufacturer Through Manufacturer Reps
General Admin.: Donald G. Ludlum/President
Mktg./Adv.: Patricia Ramsey/Coord. Sales
         Dwane Stevens/Manager Sales
         Bill Huckabee/Sales Associate
         Brenda Ramey/Sales Associate
         Dru Carson/Sales Associate
         Heather Gesin/Sales Associate
         Mike Miller/Sales Associate

Alarm, Radiation	Radiology
Cable	Physical Med
Counter, Radiation	Radiology
Counter, Scintillation	Chemistry
Counter, Scintillation, Liquid, Toxicology	Toxicology
Monitor, Biological (Contamination Testing)	General
Monitor, Radiation	Radiology
Probe, Other	General
Spectrometer, Nuclear	Chemistry

LUDWIG MEDICAL, INC.   217-342-6570
1010 Parkview St., P.o. Box 207, Effingham, IL 62401
FDA Number: 1419537

Trap, Sterile Specimen	Anesthesiology

LUITPOLD PHARMACEUTICALS, INC.   631-924-4000
One Luitpold Drive, Shirley, NY 11967
FDA Number: 2410375   Fax: 631-924-1731
E-mail: inquiry@luitpold.com
Web site: www.luitpold.com
Medical Products Sales Volume: $358,000,000
Year Founded: 1991
Total Employees: 400
Ownership: Private
Produces/Sells CE-marked Devices: N
Federal Procurement Eligibility: Small Business

Implant, Endosseous (Bone Filling and/or Augmentation)	Dental And Oral

LUKE INDUSTRIES INC.
See Precision Dynamics Corp.

LUMALITE, INC.   800-400-2262
2830 Via Orange Way, Suite B,   **619-660-5410**
Spring Valley, CA 91978
FDA Number: 2031820   Fax: 619-660-5459
E-mail: info@luma-lite.com
Web site: www.luma-lite.com
Medical Products Sales Volume: $610,000

LUMALITE, INC.   800-400-2262 *(cont'd)*
Annual Revenue: $1-$5 Million
Year Founded: 1999
Total Employees: 7
Ownership: Private
Quality System Registration Information: ISO9000
Produces/Sells CE-marked Devices: Y
Federal Procurement Eligibility: Small Business
Distribution: Manufacturer Through Distributor, OEM, Exporter
General Admin.: Mr. Mike Jackson/President

Source, Heat, Bleaching, Teeth, Dental	Dental And Oral

LUMASENSE TECHNOLOGIES INC.   408-727-1600
3301 Leonard Court, Santa Clara, CA 95054
FDA Number: 2936522   Fax: 408-727-1677
E-mail: info@lumasenseinc.com
Web site: http://www.lumasenseinc.com
Year Founded: 2005
Ownership: Private
Produces/Sells CE-marked Devices: N
Distribution: OEM

Analyzer, Gas, Carbon-Dioxide, Gaseous Phase (Capnograph)	Anesthesiology
Thermometer, Electronic	General

LUMEDX CORP.   800-966-0669
110 110th Ave. NE, Bellevue, WA 98004   **510-419-1000**
FDA Number: 3008012314   Fax: 510-419-3699
E-mail: sales@lumedx.com
Web site: www.lumedx.com
Annual Revenue: $1-$5 Million
Total Employees: 100   *Marketing Staff:* 4   *Sales Staff:* 10
Ownership: Private
Produces/Sells CE-marked Devices: N
Federal Procurement Eligibility: Small Business
Distribution: Manufacturer Direct, Manufacturer Through Manufacturer Reps, Exporter
General Admin.: Mr. Chris Winquist/Chief Operating Officer
         Dr. David McAuley/Chief Technology Officer
         Laurel Shearer/Executive Vice President
         Dr. Allyn McAuley/President, Chief Executive Officer
Finance: Mr. Jay Soni/Chief Financial Officer

Computer Software	General
Image Processing System	Radiology

LUMEN BIOMEDICAL, INC.   763-577-9600
10900 73rd Ave N. #150, Maple Grove, MN 55369
FDA Number: 3005522028   Fax: 763-577-1044
E-mail: info@lumenbio.com
Web site: www.lumenbio.com
Ownership: Private
Produces/Sells CE-marked Devices: N

Catheter, Carotid, Temporary, For Embolization Capture	Cardiovascular
Catheter, Embolectomy (Fogarty Type)	Cardiovascular
Device, Coronary Saphenous Vein Bypass Graft, Temporary, For Embolization Protection	Cardiovascular

LUMENIS INC.   800-447-0234
3959 W. 1820 S., Salt Lake City, UT 84104-4951   **801-656-2300**
FDA Number: 1720381   Fax: 801-972-4884
E-mail: laserbeam@hgmmedical.com
Web site: www.lumenis.com
Annual Revenue: $10-$25 Million
Total Employees: 100   *Marketing Staff:* 6   *Sales Staff:* 30
Ownership: Private
Quality System Registration Information: ISO9000
Produces/Sells CE-marked Devices: Y
Federal Procurement Eligibility: Small Business, GSA Contract, VA Contract
Distribution: Manufacturer Direct, Exporter
General Admin.: William McMahan/Chief Executive Officer
         Shelby Gann/Vice President Human Resources
Mktg./Adv.: Polly Peckham/Admin. Marketing
         Walt Slazinski/Manager Sales Training
Production: Brian Sandberg/Manager Materials
         Doug Kane/Manager Regulatory Affairs

Laser, Ophthalmic	Ophthalmology

LUMIGEN, INC.
See Beckman Coulter, Inc.

LUMINAUD, INC.   800-255-3408
8688 Tyler Blvd., Mentor, OH 44060-4348   **440-255-9082**
FDA Number: n/a   Fax: 440-255-2250
E-mail: info@luminaud.com
Web site: www.luminaud.com
Medical Products Sales Volume: $700,000
Annual Revenue: $0-$1 Million
Year Founded: 1972
Total Employees: 6   *Marketing Staff:* 5   *Sales Staff:* 5

LUMINAUD, INC.   800-255-3408 (cont'd)

Ownership: Private
Produces/Sells CE-marked Devices: N
Federal Procurement Eligibility: Small Business
Distribution: Manufacturer Direct, Manufacturer Through Distributor, Importer, Exporter
General Admin.: Thomas Lennox/President
Mktg./Adv.: Tom Lennox/Manager Contract Sales
         Dorothy Lennox/Vice President Marketing

Amplifier, Voice	Ear/Nose/Throat
Cuff, Tracheostomy Tube	Ear/Nose/Throat
Irrigator, Oral	Dental And Oral
Larynx, Artificial Battery-Powered	Ear/Nose/Throat

LUMINESCENT DENTAL SUPPLY CO.   866-33D-ENTA
64 Creekview Dr., Buffalo, NY 14224   **716-674-9990**

FDA Number: n/a   *Fax:* 716-677-4047
E-mail: luminescent@adelphia.net
Annual Revenue: $0-$1 Million
Total Employees: 4   *Marketing Staff:* 1   *Sales Staff:* 3
Ownership: Private
Produces/Sells CE-marked Devices: N
Federal Procurement Eligibility: Small Business, Female Owned
Distribution: Service Direct, Exclusive Distributor
General Admin.: Diane M. Zubricky/President
Mktg./Adv.: Denice Devlin/Manager Marketing & Sales

Lamp, Examination (Light)	General
Light, Dental	Dental And Oral

LUMINEX CORP.   888-219-8020
12212 Technology Blvd., Austin, TX 78727-6115   **512-219-8020**

FDA Number: 1650733   *Fax:* 512-219-5195
E-mail: info@luminexcorp.com
Web site: http://www.luminexcorp.com
Year Founded: 1995
Ownership: Public
Stock Symbol: LMNX
Traded On: NASDAQ
Produces/Sells CE-marked Devices: N
General Admin.: Mr. Patrick Balthrop/President, Chief Executive Officer
Production: Mr. Michael Pintek/Senior Vice President Operations
Research: Mr. Timothy Dehne/Vice President Research & Development
Finance: Mr. Harriss Currie/Chief Financial Officer

Exoenzyme, Multiple, Streptococcal	Microbiology
Fluorometer, Chemistry	Chemistry
Instrumentation For Clinical Multiplex Test Systems	Chemistry

LUMITEX, INC.   800-969-5483
8443 Dow Circle, Strongsville, OH 44136-1759   **440-243-8401**

FDA Number: 1528108   *Fax:* 440-243-8402
E-mail: info@lumitex.com
Web site: www.LumitexMD.com
Medical Products Sales Volume: $16,000,000
Total Employees: 79   *Marketing Staff:* 2   *Sales Staff:* 5
Ownership: Private
Quality System Registration Information: ISO9000; ISO9001
Produces/Sells CE-marked Devices: N
Federal Procurement Eligibility: Small Business
Distribution: Manufacturer Direct, Manufacturer Through Distributor, Manufacturer Through Manufacturer Reps, OEM, Exclusive Distributor, Exporter
General Admin.: Peter Broer/President, Chief Executive Officer
Mktg./Adv.: Mr. Mike Diroff/Manager Sales
         Sales Inquirey/Sales Associate
Production: Mr. Jeffrey Williams/Manager Engineering

Light, Other	General
Phototherapy Unit, Neonatal	General
Retractor, Fiberoptic	Gastroenterology/Urology
Transilluminator, Battery-Powered	Ophthalmology

LUNA INNOVATIONS INCORPORATED   540-769-8400
1 Riverside Circle, Suite 400, Roanoke, VA 24016

FDA Number: 3004473905   *Fax:* 540-769-8401
E-mail: solutions@lunainnovations.com
Web site: http://www.lunainnovations.com
Ownership: Public
Stock Symbol: LUNA
Traded On: NASDAQ
Produces/Sells CE-marked Devices: N
General Admin.: Dr. Mark Froggatt/Chief Technology Officer
         Mr. Dale Messick/President, Chief Operating Officer
Finance: Mr. Scott Graeff/Chief Financial Officer

Detector, Bubble, Cardiopulmonary Bypass	Cardiovascular

LUNAX CORP.   800-355-8629
6669 Westridge, Brighton, MI 48116

FDA Number: 1834342
Ownership: Private
Produces/Sells CE-marked Devices: N

LUNAX CORP.   800-355-8629 (cont'd)
    Shoe, Cast   Physical Med

LUNDY MEDICAL PRODUCT, LLC   480-473-7330
9376 East Bahia, Suite D-101, Scottsdale, AZ 85260

FDA Number: n/a   *Fax:* 480-315-1790
E-mail: sschramm@lundymedical.com
Web site: www.lundymedical.com
Annual Revenue: $0-$1 Million
Year Founded: 1978
Total Employees: 8   *Marketing Staff:* 6
Ownership: Private
Produces/Sells CE-marked Devices: N
Federal Procurement Eligibility: Small Business, Female Owned
Distribution: Manufacturer Direct
General Admin.: Sara Lundy-Schramm/President
Mktg./Adv.: Steven Schramm/Vice President Marketing

Board, Arm	Anesthesiology
Cushion, Ring, Foam Rubber	General

LUSYS LABORATORIES INC.   888-898-3909
10054 Mesa Ridge Court, Suite 118, San Diego, CA 92121

FDA Number: 3004473533   *Fax:* 858-866-1688
E-mail: onestep@lusyslab.com
Web site: www.lusyslab.com
Ownership: Private
Produces/Sells CE-marked Devices: N

Enzymatic Method, Troponin Subunit	Chemistry
Enzyme Immunoassay, Phencyclidine	Toxicology

LUTONIX, INC   763-445-2352
7351 Kirkwood Lane North, Suite 138, Maple Grove, MN 55369

FDA Number: n/a   *Fax:* 763-445-2353
E-mail: info@lutonix.com.
Web site: www.lutonix.com
Ownership: C. R. BARD, INC.
Produces/Sells CE-marked Devices: N
General Admin.: Mr. Shawn McCormick/Chief Operating Officer
         Mr. Lixiao Wang/Chief Technology Officer
         Mr. Dennis Wahr/President, Chief Executive Officer
Mktg./Adv.: Ms. Leslie Trigg/Executive Vice President Marketing
Research: Dr. Scott Naisbitt/Director Scientific Affairs
Finance: Mr. Chris Barry/Vice President Finance
         Mr. kari Kubesh/Vice President Finance

LUTRONIC INC.   888-588-7644
51 Everett Dr., Unit A 50, Unit A-50,   **609-275-1565**
Princeton Junction, NJ 08550

FDA Number: 3006247712   *Fax:* 609-275-3800
E-mail: office@lutronic.com
Web site: http://www.lutronic.com
Year Founded: 1997
Total Employees: 61
Ownership: Public
Produces/Sells CE-marked Devices: Y

LUWA LEPCO   713-461-1131
1750 Stebbins Drive, Houston, TX 77043

FDA Number: n/a   *Fax:* 713-464-1148
E-mail: sschleisman@luwalepco.com
Web site: www.luwalepco.com
Medical Products Sales Volume: $7,000,000
Annual Revenue: $25-$50 Million
Year Founded: 1969
Total Employees: 50   *Marketing Staff:* 2   *Sales Staff:* 20
Ownership: Private
Federal Procurement Eligibility: Small Business
Distribution: Manufacturer Direct, Manufacturer Through Manufacturer Reps
General Admin.: Gary Devloo/President
Mktg./Adv.: Sara Schleisman/Manager Marketing
         Ray Schneider/Vice President Marketing & Sales
Production: Tom Patton/Vice President Production

Controller, Temperature, Other	General
Equipment/Service, Quality Control	General
Hood, Isolation, Laminar Air Flow	General
Service, Engineering/Design	General

LUXFER GAS CYLINDERS   800-764-0366
3016 Kansas Avenue, Riverside, CA 92507   **951-684-5110**

FDA Number: n/a   *Fax:* 951-328-1117
E-mail: orion.goe@luxfer.net
Web site: www.luxfercylinders.com
Medical Products Sales Volume: $42,700,000
Annual Revenue: $100-$500 Million
Year Founded: 1898
Total Employees: 511
Ownership: Luxfer Group Ltd.
Quality System Registration Information: ISO9001

LUXFER GAS CYLINDERS — 800-764-0366 (cont'd)
Produces/Sells CE-marked Devices: N
Distribution: Manufacturer Through Distributor
General Admin.: John S. Rhodes/President
Mktg./Adv.: Mr. Dan Stracner/Director Marketing & Communications
　　　　　Mr. Rob DuPuis/Director Sales
　　　　　Ms. Lisa Stano/Market Manager
Research: H. Holroyd/Vice President Research & Development
　Cylinder, Oxygen　　　　　　　　　　　　　　　Anesthesiology

LUXO CORPORATION — 800-222-5896
Five Westchester Plaza, Elmsford, NY 10523 — 914-345-0067
FDA Number: 9200663
E-mail: office@luxous.com　　　　　　　　　　Fax: 914-345-0068
Web site: www.luxous.com
Annual Revenue: $10-$25 Million
Ownership: Luxo AS
Quality System Registration Information: ISO9001
Produces/Sells CE-marked Devices: N
Federal Procurement Eligibility: Small Business
Distribution: Manufacturer Through Distributor, Manufacturer Through Manufacturer Reps
General Admin.: Sam Gumins/President, Chief Executive Officer
Mktg./Adv.: Philip Matsen/Vice President Sales
　Lamp, Other　　　　　　　　　　　　　　　　　General

LUXO LAMP LTD. — (800) 361-3993
1904 St. Regis, Dorval, QUE H9P 1H6 Canada — (514) 685-5896
FDA Number: n/a　　　　　　　　　　　　　　Fax: (514) 685-7912
E-mail: office@luxo.ca
Web site: www.luxo.com
Year Founded: 1953
Total Employees: 25
Ownership: Private
Produces/Sells CE-marked Devices: N
Distribution: Manufacturer Direct, Exporter

LW SCIENTIFIC — 800-726-7345
865 Marathon Parkway, — 770-270-1394
Lawrenceville, GA 30045
FDA Number: n/a　　　　　　　　　　　　　Fax: 770-270-2389
E-mail: sales@lwscientific.com
Web site: www.lwscientific.com
Medical Products Sales Volume: $7,000,000
Annual Revenue: $5-$10 Million
Year Founded: 1994
Total Employees: 25　　　　Marketing Staff: 2　　　　Sales Staff: 7
Ownership: Private
Quality System Registration Information: ISO9001
Produces/Sells CE-marked Devices: Y
Federal Procurement Eligibility: Small Business, Minority Owned, GSA Contract
Distribution: Manufacturer Through Distributor, Manufacturer Through Manufacturer Reps, OEM, Exporter
General Admin.: Ernie Tai/President
Mktg./Adv.: Mike Thomas/Director Marketing
　　　　　Laura Templeton/Manager International & National Sales
　　　　　Mike Thomas/Manager National Sales
　　　　　Phillip Walker/National Sales Representative
Production: Tim Chambers/Director Quality Assurance
　Camera, Video　　　　　　　　　　　　　　　General
　Centrifuge, General (Up to 5,000 rpm)　　　　　Pathology
　Centrifuge, Hematocrit　　　　　　　　　　　Hematology
　Centrifuge, Tabletop　　　　　　　　　　　　Pathology
　Counter, Cell　　　　　　　　　　　　　　Microbiology
　Microscope　　　　　　　　　　　　　　　Hematology
　Refractometer　　　　　　　　　　　　　　Chemistry
　Rotator, Transverse　　　　　　　　　　　　Physical Med

LYDALL FILTRATION / SEPARATION GROUP
See Lydall, Inc.

LYDALL TECHNICAL PAPERS
See Lydall, Inc.

LYDALL, INC. — 860-646-1233
One Colonial Road, Manchester, CT 06042
FDA Number: n/a　　　　　　　　　　　　Fax: 860-646-4917
E-mail: info@lydall.com
Web site: www.lydall.com
Medical Products Sales Volume: $4,000,500
Annual Revenue: $1-$5 Million
Ownership: Public
Stock Symbol: LDL
Traded On: NYSE
Quality System Registration Information: ISO9002
Produces/Sells CE-marked Devices: Y
Federal Procurement Eligibility: Small Business
Distribution: Manufacturer Direct
　Filter, Air　　　　　　　　　　　　　　　　General

LYDALL, INC. — 860-646-1233 (cont'd)
Filter, Membrane　　　　　　　　　　　　　Chemistry

LYDIA'S PROFESSIONAL UNIFORMS — 800-942-3378
2500 E Beltline Ave SE #K, — 616.954.1445
Grand Rapids, MI 49546
FDA Number: n/a　　　　　　　　　　　　Fax: 616-453-8629
E-mail: mail@lydiasuniforms.com
Web site: www.lydiasuniforms.com
Year Founded: 1971
Total Employees: 140
Ownership: Private
Produces/Sells CE-marked Devices: N
Federal Procurement Eligibility: Minority Owned, Female Owned
Distribution: Manufacturer Through Distributor, Exclusive Distributor, Importer
General Admin.: Ms. Natacha Fahey/Executive Assistant
Production: Mr. Jim Fotis/Vice President Operations
　Scissors, Bandage/Gauze/Plaster　　　　　　　General
　Sphygmomanometer, Aneroid (Arterial Pressure)　　General
　Sphygmomanometer, Electronic (Arterial Pressure)　General
　Stethoscope, Amplified　　　　　　　　　　　General
　Stethoscope, Manual　　　　　　　　　　　Cardiovascular

LYNE LABORATORIES, INC. — 508-583-8700
10 Burke Dr., Brockton, MA 02301
FDA Number: 1219639
Ownership: Private
Produces/Sells CE-marked Devices: N
　Elastomer, Silicone (Scar Management)　　　　　Surgery
　Sterilant, Medical Device　　　　　　　　　　General

LYNELL MEDICAL TECHNOLOGY
See Staar Surgical Co.

LYNN MEDICAL — 888-596-6633
764 Denison Ct., Bloomfield Hills, MI 48302-0300 — 248-338-4571
FDA Number: n/a　　　　　　　　　　　　Fax: 248-338-6242
E-mail: customerservice@lynnmed.com
Web site: www.lynnmed.com
Medical Products Sales Volume: $20,000,000
Annual Revenue: $10-$25 Million
Total Employees: 47　　　Marketing Staff: 4　　　Sales Staff: 17
Ownership: Private
Produces/Sells CE-marked Devices: N
Federal Procurement Eligibility: Small Business
Distribution: Manufacturer Through Distributor, Service Direct, Exclusive Distributor, Exporter
General Admin.: Brian G. Fagnani/President, Chief Executive Officer
Mktg./Adv.: Russell Green/Manager National Sales
Production: Pam Vandekerkhove/Manager Regulatory Affairs
Finance: Frank Gerds/Controller
　Electrode, Other　　　　　　　　　　　　　General
　Oximeter, Pulse　　　　　　　　　　　　　General
　Printer, Image, Video　　　　　　　　　　　General
　Recorder, Long-Term, ECG, Portable (Holter Monitor)　Cardiovascular

LYNN PEAVEY CO. — 800-255-6499
10749 West 84th Terrace, P.O. Box 14100, — 913-888-0600
Lenexa, KS 66215
FDA Number: 1932350
Web site: www.lynnpeavey.com/　　　　　　Fax: 913-495-6787
Ownership: Private
Produces/Sells CE-marked Devices: N
　Applicator, Tipped, Absorbent, Sterile　　　　　General
　Chamber, Slide Culture　　　　　　　　　　Pathology
　Collector, Blood, Vacuum-Assisted　　　　　　Hematology
　Iodine (Tincture)　　　　　　　　　　　　Pathology
　Kit, Screening, Urine　　　　　　　　　　　Microbiology
　Lancet, Blood　　　　　　　　　　　　　　General
　Needle, Aspiration And Injection, Disposable　　Surgery

LYONS COMPANY, H.L.
See The Lyons Companies

LYONS TOOL AND DIE COMPANY — 800-422-9363
185 Research Pkwy., Meriden, CT 06450 — 203-238-2689
FDA Number: 3004047479　　　　　　　Fax: 203-237-8769
E-mail: will.lyons@lyons.com
Web site: www.lyons.com
Medical Products Sales Volume: $10,000,000
Annual Revenue: $10-$25 Million
Year Founded: 1951
Total Employees: 38　　　Marketing Staff: 1　　　Sales Staff: 4
Ownership: Private
Quality System Registration Information: ISO9001; ISO9002
Produces/Sells CE-marked Devices: Y
Federal Procurement Eligibility: Small Business
Distribution: Manufacturer Direct, Service Direct, Exporter
General Admin.: Mr. Will Lyons/President

LYONS TOOL AND DIE COMPANY   800-422-9363 (cont'd)
Mr. David Brown/Vice President
Production: Mr. Michael Malo/Director Engineering

Blade, Knife, Laparoscopic	Surgery
Component, Metal, Other	General
Component, Other	General
Contract Assembly	General
Contract Manufacturing	General
Contract Manufacturing, Product, Disposable	General
Contract Manufacturing, Product, Durable	General
Contract Packaging	General
Knife, Laparoscopic	Surgery
Knife, Other	Surgery
Knife, Surgical	Dental And Oral
Scissors, Disposable	General
Scissors, Laparoscopy	Surgery
Service, Consulting	General
Service, Engineering/Design	General
Stapler, Laparoscopic	Surgery
Stapler, Surgical	Surgery

LYTRON, INC.   781-933-7300
55 Dragon Ct., Woburn, MA 01801-1039
FDA Number: n/a   Fax: 781-935-4529
E-mail: info@lytron.com
Web site: www.lytron.com
Total Employees: 50
Ownership: Private
Quality System Registration Information: ISO9001
Produces/Sells CE-marked Devices: Y
Federal Procurement Eligibility: Small Business, GSA Contract
Distribution: Manufacturer Direct
Mktg./Adv.: Kathryn Whitenack/Director Marketing

Heat Exchanger, Regional Perfusion	Surgery
Plate, Cooling	Chemistry
Refrigerator, Laboratory	General
Transfer Aid	Physical Med

M & CC LTD.   800-388-6236
10721 Keele St. N, Maple, ONT L6A-1S5 Canada   905-832-8311
FDA Number: n/a   Fax: 905-832-0732
E-mail: info@mccdentalcabinets.com
Web site: www.mccdentalcabinets.com
Year Founded: 1969
Total Employees: 50
Ownership: Private
Produces/Sells CE-marked Devices: N
Distribution: Manufacturer Direct, Exporter

M & I MEDICAL SALES, INC.   305-663-6444
4711 S.W. 72 Ave., Miami, FL 33155
FDA Number: n/a   Fax: 305-663-6201
E-mail: contact@mimedical.com
Web site: www.mimedical.com
Medical Products Sales Volume: $4,000,000
Annual Revenue: $1-$5 Million
Total Employees: 4   Marketing Staff: 2   Sales Staff: 2
Ownership: Private
Produces/Sells CE-marked Devices: Y
Federal Procurement Eligibility: Small Business
Distribution: Service Direct, Exclusive Distributor, Importer
General Admin.: Mr. Isam Tahoun/Chief Executive Officer

Accessories, Catheter	Surgery
Balloon, Angioplasty, Peripheral, Heated	Cardiovascular
Catheter, Balloon, Dilatation, Vessel	Gastroenterology/Urology
Catheter, Cardiac Thermodilution	Cardiovascular
Catheter, Cardiovascular	Surgery
Cineangiograph (Cardiac Catheterization)	Radiology
Electrocardiograph, Interpretive	Cardiovascular
Electrosurgical Equipment, General Purpose	Surgery
Filter, Vena Cava	Cardiovascular
Guide, Catheter	Cardiovascular
Guidewire	Cardiovascular
Image Intensification System	Radiology
Manifold, Gas	Chemistry
Oximeter, Finger	General
Oximeter, Pulse	General
Radiographic/Fluoroscopic Unit, Mobile C-Arm	Radiology
Scanner, Computed Tomography, Cine	Radiology
Stent, Cardiovascular	Cardiovascular
Tube, X-Ray	Radiology
Ventilator, Other	Anesthesiology

M & M INDUSTRIES   800-331-5305
316 Corporate Place,   423-821-3302
Chattanooga, TN 37419
FDA Number: n/a   Fax: 423-821-9017
E-mail: pails@m-m-industries.com
Web site: www.mmcontainer.com

M & M INDUSTRIES   800-331-5305 (cont'd)
Medical Products Sales Volume: $18,300,000
Annual Revenue: $10-$25 Million
Year Founded: 1986
Total Employees: 115   Marketing Staff: 6   Sales Staff: 6
Ownership: Private
Quality System Registration Information: ISO9001
Produces/Sells CE-marked Devices: N
Federal Procurement Eligibility: Small Business
Distribution: Manufacturer Direct, Manufacturer Through Distributor
General Admin.: Glenn Morris/Chief Operating Officer, Vice President
Mktg./Adv.: Janet Rogers/Vice President Sales
Production: Brenda Walker/Director Quality Assurance
     Dennis Walker/Vice President Manufacturing

Waste Receptacle, Contaminated	General

M & Q PACKAGING CORP.   877-726-7287
Earl Street, Schuylkill Haven, PA 17972   570-385-4991
FDA Number: 2523664   Fax: 570-385-4954
E-mail: info@mqplastics.com
Web site: www.mqplasticproducts.com
Medical Products Sales Volume: $7,700,000
Year Founded: 1979
Total Employees: 100
Ownership: M & Q Packaging Corp.
Quality System Registration Information: ISO9000
Produces/Sells CE-marked Devices: N
Federal Procurement Eligibility: Small Business, GSA Contract
Distribution: Manufacturer Direct, Manufacturer Through Distributor, Manufacturer Through Manufacturer Reps
Mktg./Adv.: Mr. Tim Blucher/Vice President Sales

Wrap, Sterilization	General

Medical Product Subsidiaries (Listed Separately)
   M & Q Packaging Corp.
   M & Q Plastic Products

M & S SPECIALTIES CO. A DIV. OF RITEWAY PRECISION
See Bolt Bethel, Llc

M .W. MOONEY & CO., INC.   800-230-5770
415 Williamson Way, Ste. 9, Ashland, OR 97520   541-488-2381
FDA Number: 2950889   Fax: 541-488-2396
E-mail: mike@ringcutter.com
Web site: www.ringcutter.com
Medical Products Sales Volume: $2,000,000
Annual Revenue: $1-$5 Million
Total Employees: 4   Marketing Staff: 2   Sales Staff: 2
Ownership: Private
Produces/Sells CE-marked Devices: N
Federal Procurement Eligibility: Small Business
Distribution: Manufacturer Direct, Service Direct, Exclusive Distributor, Importer, Exporter
General Admin.: Michael Mooney/President, Chief Executive Officer
     Katherine Mooney/Vice President, General Manager

Cutter, Ring	General

M D TECHNOLOGIES, INC.   800-201-3060
PO BOX 60, Galena, IL 61036   815-598-3143
FDA Number: 1422374   Fax: 815-598-3110
E-mail: sales@mdtechnologiesinc.com
Web site: www.mdtechnologiesinc.com
Annual Revenue: $0-$1 Million
Year Founded: 1993
Ownership: Private
Quality System Registration Information: ISO9001
Produces/Sells CE-marked Devices: N
Federal Procurement Eligibility: Small Business
Distribution: Manufacturer Direct, Manufacturer Through Distributor, Manufacturer Through Manufacturer Reps

Bottle, Collection, Vacuum (Aspirator)	General
Trap, Sterile Specimen	Anesthesiology
Washer, Receptacle, Waste, Body	General

M&C SPECIALTIES CO.   800-441-6996
90 James Way, Southampton, PA 18966-3816   215-322-1600
FDA Number: 2523928   Fax: 215-322-1620
E-mail: info@mcspecialties.com
Web site: www.mcspecialties.com
Medical Products Sales Volume: $22,400,000
Annual Revenue: $10-$25 Million
Year Founded: 1945
Total Employees: 1000   Marketing Staff: 2   Sales Staff: 11
Ownership: Private
Quality System Registration Information: ISO9001
Produces/Sells CE-marked Devices: N
Federal Procurement Eligibility: Small Business
Distribution: Manufacturer Direct, OEM
General Admin.: Donald Rauch/President, Chief Executive Officer

M&C SPECIALTIES CO.   800-441-6996 *(cont'd)*
Mktg./Adv.: Pamela Lipschutz/Manager Marketing & Advertising
    David R. Cornelison/Vice President Marketing & Sales
Production: Donna Dimitri/Manager Materials
    Joe Benincasa/Manager Operations
    David Lee/Manager Quality Control
    Mike Boyle/Vice President Manufacturing
Finance: Don Nichols/Controller
    Daniel Cistone/Vice President Finance
IS: John Donnelly/Manager Tech. Services

Contract Assembly	General
Contract Manufacturing	General
Contract Manufacturing, Product, Disposable	General
Drape, Adhesive, Aerosol	Surgery
Dressing, Gel	General
Dressing, Wound and Burn, Occlusive	Surgery
Sterilization Process Indicator, Chemical	General
Strip, Adhesive	Surgery
Tape, Adhesive	General
Tape, Adhesive, Hypoallergenic	General
Tape, Adhesive, Waterproof	General
Tape, Gauze, Adhesive	General

M&R PRINTING EQUIPMENT, INC.   630-858-6101
1 N 372 Main Street, Glen Ellyn, IL 60137
FDA Number: 89789
Ownership: Private
Produces/Sells CE-marked Devices: N

Booth, Sun Tan	Physical Med

M&S TECHNOLOGIES, INC. / MARINO   1-877-225-6101
5557 W Howard St, Skokie, IL 60077
FDA Number: 1000431353
Ownership: Private
Produces/Sells CE-marked Devices: N

Projector, Ophthalmic	Ophthalmology

M-CON TECHNOLOGIES
See Microstat Laboratories, Inc.

M-E MANUFACTURING AND SERVICES, INC.   763-268-4500
5010 Cheshire Lane North, Plymouth, MN 55446
FDA Number: 2135129
Web site: www.memsi.com
Ownership: Siemens Ag
Stock Symbol: SI
Traded On: NYSE
Produces/Sells CE-marked Devices: N

Hearing-Aid, Bone-Conduction, Percutaneous	Ear/Nose/Throat

M-P MFG., INC.   815-334-1112
13802 Washington St. #b, Woodstock, IL 60098
FDA Number: 1424141   *Fax:* 815-334-1113
E-mail: mp@mpmfg.com
Web site: www.mpmfg.com
Ownership: Private
Produces/Sells CE-marked Devices: N

Rongeur, Rib	Orthopedics

M. & I.E.
See Mercury Medical

M. BRAUN INC.   603-773-9333
14 Marin Way, Stratham, NH 03885
FDA Number: n/a   *Fax:* 603-773-0008
E-mail: info@mbraunusa.com
Web site: www.mbraunusa.com
Medical Products Sales Volume: $5,000,000
Annual Revenue: $10-$25 Million
Ownership: M. BRAUN GMBH
Quality System Registration Information: ISO9001
Produces/Sells CE-marked Devices: Y
Federal Procurement Eligibility: Small Business
Distribution: Manufacturer Direct, OEM, Service Direct, Exporter

Box, Glove	Microbiology
Cover, Barrier, Protective	General
Oven	Chemistry

M.B. INDUSTRIES, INC.   (419) 738-4769
11158 Infirmary Road, Wapakoneta, OH 45895
FDA Number: n/a   *Fax:* (419) 738-5316
E-mail: mborges@mbind.com
Web site: www.mbind.com
Medical Products Sales Volume: $500,000
Annual Revenue: $0-$1 Million
Total Employees: 10   *Marketing Staff:* 1   *Sales Staff:* 1
Ownership: Private
Produces/Sells CE-marked Devices: N
Federal Procurement Eligibility: Small Business
Distribution: Manufacturer Direct

M.B. INDUSTRIES, INC.   (419) 738-4769 *(cont'd)*
General Admin.: William Buttermore/President
Mktg./Adv.: Chuck Weed/Vice President Marketing & Sales
Production: Linda Clutts/Manager Operations

Aspirator, Ophthalmic	Ophthalmology
Illuminator, Fiberoptic (For Endoscope)	Gastroenterology/Urology
Illuminator, Ultraviolet	Dental And Oral
Instrument, Manual, General Surgical	Surgery

M.B.S. FABRICATING & COATING, INC.   704-871-1830
174a Crawford Rd, Po Box 249, Statesville, NC 28687
FDA Number: 1064842

Protector, Skin Pressure	General
Splint, Hand, And Component	Physical Med

M.C. HEALTHCARE PRODUCTS, INC.   800-268-8671 / 905-563-8264
4658 Ontario St., Beamsville, ONT L0R 1 Canada
FDA Number: n/a   *Fax:* 905-563-8680
E-mail: beds@mchealthcare.com
Web site: www.mchealthcare.com
Medical Products Sales Volume: $15,000,000
Year Founded: 1912
Total Employees: 60   *Marketing Staff:* 2   *Sales Staff:* 8
Ownership: Private
Produces/Sells CE-marked Devices: Y
Federal Procurement Eligibility: Small Business
Distribution: Manufacturer Direct, Manufacturer Through Manufacturer Reps, Exporter

M.C. JOHNSON CO., INC.   800-553-8483 / 239-591-2600
2037 J & C Blvd., Naples, FL 34109-6213
FDA Number: n/a   *Fax:* 239-591-2133
E-mail: mcjohnson5445@earthlink.net
Web site: www.mcjohnson.com
Ownership: Private
Produces/Sells CE-marked Devices: N
Federal Procurement Eligibility: Small Business, Female Owned
Distribution: Manufacturer Direct, Manufacturer Through Distributor
General Admin.: Susan L. LeBlanc/Chief Executive Officer
    Susan L. LeBlanc/President
Mktg./Adv.: Philip Baker/Director Marketing

Holder, Catheter	Gastroenterology/Urology
Mask, Face	General

M.D. ENGINEERING
See Medical Device Resource Corporation

M.D. RESOURCES, INC.
See Life Plus International

M.E.D. SERVI-SYSTEMS CANADA LTD.   800-267-6868 / 613-836-3004
8 Sweetnam Dr., Stittsville, ONT K2S 1 Canada
FDA Number: n/a   *Fax:* 613-831-0240
E-mail: sales@medserv.ca
Web site: www.medserv.ca
Medical Products Sales Volume: $720,000
Total Employees: 6
Ownership: Private
Produces/Sells CE-marked Devices: N
Federal Procurement Eligibility: Small Business, Female Owned
Distribution: Service Direct, Exclusive Distributor, Importer, Exporter

M.E.E.I. MFG.   941-492-2560
Claes H Dohlman, Md Room 550l, Meei, 5th Floor, Boston, MA 02114
FDA Number: 1222945

Keratoprosthesis, Non-Custom	Ophthalmology

M.J. THIESEN CO. INC.   800-443-8773 / 559-591-0839
151 S N ST, Dinuba, CA 93618
FDA Number: n/a   *Fax:* 559-591-0848
E-mail: service@mjthiesen.com
Web site: mjthiesen.com
Medical Products Sales Volume: $700,000
Annual Revenue: $0-$1 Million
Year Founded: 1956
Ownership: Private
Produces/Sells CE-marked Devices: N
Federal Procurement Eligibility: Small Business
Distribution: Manufacturer Direct, Exporter

Bed, Pediatric (Crib)	General

M.O.S. PLASTICS, INC.
See MOS Plastics Inc.

M.W. SALES AND SERVICE, INC.   830-303-2508
2549 O'daniel Rd., Seguin, TX 78155
FDA Number: 1651489

M.W. SALES AND SERVICE, INC.
830-303-2508 *(cont'd)*
Exerciser, Non-Measuring — Physical Med

MA BIOSERVICES INC.
See Bioreliance

MABIS HEALTHCARE INC.
800-526-4753
1931 Norman Drive, Waukegan, IL 60085
FDA Number: 1422443
Fax: 800-479-7968
Web site: www.mabisdmi.com
Medical Products Sales Volume: $11,600,000
Annual Revenue: $25-$50 Million
Year Founded: 1992
Ownership: Private
Produces/Sells CE-marked Devices: N
Federal Procurement Eligibility: Small Business
Distribution: Manufacturer Through Distributor

Accessories, Wheelchair	Physical Med
Adaptor, Dressing	Physical Med
Amniotome	Obstetrics/Gynecology
Attachment, Commode, Wheelchair	Physical Med
Bag, Urinary Collection	General
Bandage, Adhesive	Surgery
Bandage, Elastic	General
Basin, Emesis	General
Bedpan	General
Bell, Circumcision	Gastroenterology/Urology
Binder, Medical, Therapeutic	General
Bottle, Hot/Cold Water	General
Cane	Physical Med
Connector, Tubing, Blood, Infusion, T-Type	Gastroenterology/Urology
Container, Medication, Graduated Liquid	General
Cover, Thermometer	General
Crutch	Physical Med
Cuff, Blood Pressure	Cardiovascular
Cutter, Ring	General
Douche, Vaginal	Obstetrics/Gynecology
Forceps, General & Plastic Surgery	Surgery
General Use Surgical Scissors	Surgery
Hemostat, Surgical	Dental And Oral
Laryngoscope	Ear/Nose/Throat
Light, Examination, Battery-Powered	General
Nebulizer, Direct Patient Interface	Anesthesiology
Restraint, Protective (Body)	General
Restraint, Wheelchair	General
Scissors, Disposable	General
Stethoscope, Fetal	Obstetrics/Gynecology
Stethoscope, Manual	Cardiovascular
Syringe, Cartridge	Dental And Oral
Tape, Measuring, Ruler And Caliper	Surgery
Thermometer, Electronic	General
Thermometer, Liquid Crystals	Surgery
Thermometer, Mercury	General
Tray, Surgical Instrument	Surgery
Walker, Mechanical	Physical Med

MAC MEDICAL
618-476-3550
820 S. Mulberry, Millstadt, IL 62260
FDA Number: 3006342679
Stretcher, Wheeled (Mobile) — General

MAC'S LIFT GATE, INC.
800-795-6227
562-634-5962
2715 Seaboard Lane,
Long Beach, CA 90805
FDA Number: n/a
Fax: 562-634-4120
E-mail: macslift@blvd.com
Web site: www.macslift.com
Medical Products Sales Volume: $2,000,000
Annual Revenue: $1-$5 Million
Total Employees: 25   *Marketing Staff:* 2   *Sales Staff:* 5
Ownership: Private
Produces/Sells CE-marked Devices: N
Federal Procurement Eligibility: Small Business
Distribution: Manufacturer Through Distributor, OEM
General Admin.: Gerald MacDonald/Chief Executive Officer, Vice President
     Richard MacDonald/President
Mktg./Adv.: Betty Haskins/Director Marketing
     Michael MacDonald/Director Marketing & Sales
     George Clark/Director National Accounts
     James MacDonald/Vice President Sales
Production: Lawrence MacDonald/Vice President Manufacturing

Ambulance	General
Lift, Wheelchair	General

MACAN ENGINEERING COMPANY
302-645-8068
21 Shay Lane, P.O. BOX 166 Milton, Milton, DE 19968
FDA Number: 1418975
Fax: 302-645-7049
E-mail: info@macanmanufacturing.com
Web site: www.macanengineering.com
Medical Products Sales Volume: $1,000,000

MACAN ENGINEERING COMPANY
302-645-8068 *(cont'd)*
Annual Revenue: $1-$5 Million
Ownership: Private
Quality System Registration Information: ISO9001
Produces/Sells CE-marked Devices: N
Federal Procurement Eligibility: Small Business, Female Owned
Distribution: Manufacturer Through Manufacturer Reps, Exporter

Electrosurgical Unit, Dental	Dental And Oral
Electrosurgical Unit, General Purpose (ESU)	Surgery

MACDEE, INC.
See Orchid Macdee Inc.

MACHIDA, INC.
800-431-5420
914-365-0600
40 Ramland Rd. South, Orangeburg, NY 10962
FDA Number: 2242464
Fax: 845-365-0620
Web site: http://www.machidascope.com
Annual Revenue: $5-$10 Million
Year Founded: 1987
Total Employees: 72   *Marketing Staff:* 6   *Sales Staff:* 6
Ownership: VISION-SCIENCES, INC.
Produces/Sells CE-marked Devices: N
Federal Procurement Eligibility: Small Business
Distribution: Manufacturer Direct, Manufacturer Through Distributor, OEM, Importer, Exporter

Bronchoscope, Rigid	Ear/Nose/Throat
Camera, Cine, Endoscopic (Without Audio)	Surgery
Choledochoscope, Flexible Or Rigid	Gastroenterology/Urology
Cystoscope	Gastroenterology/Urology
Esophagoscope (Flexible Or Rigid)	Ear/Nose/Throat
Hysteroscope	Obstetrics/Gynecology
Illuminator, Fiberoptic (For Endoscope)	Gastroenterology/Urology
Nasopharyngoscope (Flexible Or Rigid)	Ear/Nose/Throat
Vibration Threshold Measurement Device	Cns/Neurology

MACK MOLDING CO.
802-375-2511
608 Warm Brook Rd., Arlington, VT 05250
FDA Number: 3000236920
Fax: 802-375-9419
E-mail: salesnorth@mack.com
Web site: www.mack.com
Annual Revenue: $100-$500 Million
Year Founded: 1920
Total Employees: 1850
Ownership: Private
Quality System Registration Information: ISO9001
Produces/Sells CE-marked Devices: N
Distribution: Manufacturer Direct
General Admin.: Kevin Dailey/Director Human Resources
     Jeff Somple/President
     Don Kendall/President, Chief Executive Officer
Mktg./Adv.: Julie Horst/Communications Director
     Larry Walck/Director Business Development
     Joan Magrath/Vice President Sales
Production: Wanda Knowles/Director Quality Assurance
Purchasing: Bruce Bixler/Vice President Purchasing

Contract Assembly	General
Molding, Injection	General

MACKEN INSTRUMENTS, INC.
707-566-2110
3186 Coffee Lane., Santa Rosa, CA 95403
FDA Number: n/a
Fax: 707-566-2119
E-mail: info@macken.com
Web site: www.macken.com
Medical Products Sales Volume: $750,000
Annual Revenue: $0-$1 Million
Ownership: Private
Produces/Sells CE-marked Devices: Y
Federal Procurement Eligibility: Small Business
Distribution: Manufacturer Direct, Exporter

Accessories, Laser	General

MACMILLAN RESEARCH, LTD.
See North American Science Associates, Inc.

MACO BAG
315-226-1000
412 Van Buren St., Newark, NY 14513
FDA Number: 2438932
Fax: 315-226-1050
Web site: www.macobag.com
Ownership: Private
Produces/Sells CE-marked Devices: N

Orthosis, Limb Brace	Physical Med

MACPHERSON MEDICAL INC.
800-699-9751
905-670-1008
5775 Atlantic Dr., Unit 10,
Mississauga, ONT L4W-4 Canada
FDA Number: n/a
Fax: 905-670-1422
E-mail: sales@macphersonmedical.com
Web site: www.macphersonmedical.com
Year Founded: 1990

MANUFACTURER PROFILES

MACPHERSON MEDICAL INC.　　800-699-9751 (cont'd)
Total Employees: 10
Ownership: Private
Produces/Sells CE-marked Devices: N
Distribution: Exclusive Distributor, Importer, Exporter

MACROPORE BIOSURGERY, INC.
See Cytori Therapeutics, Inc.

MADA, INC.　　800-526-6370
625 Washington Avenue,　　**201-460-0454**
Carlstadt, NJ 07072
FDA Number: 2225311
E-mail: jeffadam@mail.madamedical.com　　Fax: 201-460-3509
Web site: www.madamedical.com
Medical Products Sales Volume: $18,300,000
Annual Revenue: $10-$25 Million
Year Founded: 1969
Total Employees: 90　　*Marketing Staff:* 4　　*Sales Staff:* 30
Ownership: Private
Produces/Sells CE-marked Devices: N
Federal Procurement Eligibility: Small Business
Distribution: Manufacturer Through Distributor, Manufacturer Through
Manufacturer Reps, Importer
General Admin.: Jeffrey W. Adam/Chief Executive Officer
　　　　Frances Adam/Secretary, Treasurer
　　　　Bob Chasmar/Vice President Human Resources
Mktg./Adv.: Mike Longo/Director Advertising
　　　　Mike Longo/Director Marketing
　　　　Jeffrey W. Adam/Director Product Development
　　　　Joel Filipowicz/Manager Advertising
　　　　Robert Sorbello/Manager Marketing & Sales
　　　　Robert Sorbello/Vice President Sales
Production: Jim Havas/Manager Materials
　　　　David Nina/Manager Production
　　　　Jeffrey W. Adam/Manager Regulatory Affairs
　　　　Jeffrey W. Adam/Vice President Manufacturing
　　　　Jeffrey W. Adam/Vice President Regulatory Affairs
Research: Jeffrey W. Adam/Vice President Product Development

Anti-Choke Device, Suction	Ear/Nose/Throat
Aspirator, Emergency Suction	General
Canister, Oxygen	Anesthesiology
Cannula, Nasal, Oxygen	Anesthesiology
Cart, Emergency, Cardiopulmonary Resuscitation (Crash)	Anesthesiology
Cart, Gas Cylinder (Carrier)	Anesthesiology
Catheter, Nasal, Oxygen (Tube)	Anesthesiology
Compressor, Air, Portable	Anesthesiology
Cylinder, Compressed Gas, With Valve	Anesthesiology
Disinfector, Liquid	General
Flowmeter, Gas (Oxygen), Calibrated	Anesthesiology
Flowmeter, Pulmonary Function	Anesthesiology
Injector, Jet, Mechanical-Powered	Dental And Oral
Injector, Medication (Inoculator)	General
Kit, Administration, Oxygen	Anesthesiology
Mask, Oxygen, Aerosol Administration	Anesthesiology
Mask, Oxygen, Partial Rebreathing	General
Nebulizer, Medicinal	Ear/Nose/Throat
Regulator, Pressure, Gas Cylinder	Anesthesiology
Resuscitator, Emergency Oxygen	Dental And Oral
Resuscitator, Pulmonary, Gas	General
Resuscitator, Pulmonary, Manual (Demand Valve)	General
Suction Apparatus, Single Patient, Portable, Non-Powered	Surgery
Tubing, Oxygen Connecting	General
Ventilator, Emergency, Manual (Resuscitator)	Anesthesiology
Ventilator, Emergency, Powered (Resuscitator)	Anesthesiology
Ventilator, Other	Anesthesiology

MADDAK INC.　　800-443-4926
661 Route 23 South, Wayne, NJ 07470　　**973-628-7600**
FDA Number: 2242757　　Fax: 973-305-0841
E-mail: CustService@Maddak.com
Web site: www.maddak.com
Medical Products Sales Volume: $50,000,000
Annual Revenue: $25-$50 Million
Year Founded: 1971
Total Employees: 14　　*Marketing Staff:* 2　　*Sales Staff:* 5
Ownership: Bel-Art Products
Quality System Registration Information: ISO9000
Produces/Sells CE-marked Devices: N
Federal Procurement Eligibility: Small Business
Distribution: Manufacturer Direct, Manufacturer Through Distributor
General Admin.: Kurt Landsberger/Chief Executive Officer
　　　　Charles Silkwood/General Manager
　　　　David Landsberger/President
Mktg./Adv.: Susan Tulanowski/Coord. Marketing
　　　　Joe Kelly/Manager International Marketing & Sales
　　　　Steve Levine/Vice President Marketing
Research: G. McClure/Vice President Engineering

Accessories, Wheelchair	Physical Med

MADDAK INC.　　800-443-4926 (cont'd)

Adapter, Hygiene	Physical Med
Adaptor, Grooming	Physical Med
Adaptor, Recreational	Physical Med
Apron, Laboratory	Chemistry
Bedrail	General
Bib	General
Chair, Bath	General
Chair, With Casters	Physical Med
Commode Seat	General
Cup, Denture	Dental And Oral
Cup, Eye	Ophthalmology
Exerciser, Hand	Physical Med
Exerciser, Non-Measuring	Physical Med
Mirror, Speech	Ear/Nose/Throat
Page Turner (Handicapped)	General
Plug, Catheter	Gastroenterology/Urology
Rail, Bath	General
Rail, Wall Side	General
Reacher (Handicapped)	General
Sling, Arm	Physical Med
Tray, Medicine	General
Tray, Wheelchair	Physical Med
Tubing, Vinyl	General
Utensil, Food	Physical Med
Utensil, Handicapped Aid	Physical Med

MADE ON EARTH　　831-475-7352
5044-b Wilder Dr., Soquel, CA 95073
FDA Number: 2916775
Ownership: Private
Produces/Sells CE-marked Devices: N

Biofeedback Device	Cns/Neurology

MADE RITE ROCKER INC.　　203-723-5600
44 Gorman St., Naugatuck, CT 06770
FDA Number: 84138
Ownership: Private
Produces/Sells CE-marked Devices: N

Chair, Adjustable, Mechanical	Physical Med

MADELON LOUDEN CO.INC.
See Finebrand Co.

MADENTEC LIMITED　　877-623-3682
4664 - 99 Street,　　**780-450-8926**
Edmonton, ALB T6E 5 Canada
FDA Number: n/a　　Fax: 780-988-6182
E-mail: sales@madentec.com
Web site: www.madentec.com
Year Founded: 1988
Total Employees: 10
Ownership: Private
Produces/Sells CE-marked Devices: N
Distribution: Manufacturer Direct, Exclusive Distributor

MADORECO INC.
See Shielding International, Inc.

MAGELLAN BIOSCIENCES　　978-856-2345
22 Alpha Road, Chemsford, MA 01824
FDA Number: 1218996　　Fax: 978-856-2335
E-mail: info@magellanbio.com
Web site: http://www.magellanbio.com
Year Founded: 2004
Ownership: Private
Produces/Sells CE-marked Devices: N
General Admin.: Mr. Adrian Brunce/Executive Vice President
　　　　Mr. Edward Sztukowski/Executive Vice President
　　　　Mr. Hiroshi Uchida/President, Chief Executive Officer
　　　　Mr. Jefrey Cohen/Vice President Information Technology
Mktg./Adv.: Mr. Joel de Jesus/Vice President Business Development
　　　　Ms. Nancy Sandy/Vice President International Marketing
　　　　Mr. Simon Price/Vice President International Sales
Production: Mr. Douglas Kaspar/Vice President Operations
Finance: Ms. Pam Gornall/Chief Financial Officer

Absorption, Atomic, Lead	Toxicology

MAGELLAN BIOSCIENCES INC.　　978-856-2345
22 alpha Road, Chelmsford, MA 01824
FDA Number: 1218996　　Fax: 978-856-2335
E-mail: Info@magellanbio.com
Web site: www.magellanbio.com
Year Founded: 2004
Ownership: Private
Produces/Sells CE-marked Devices: N
General Admin.: Mr. Adrian Bunce/Executive Vice President
　　　　Mr. Hiroshi Uchida/President, Chief Executive Officer
Mktg./Adv.: Mr. Chris Destro/Vice President Sales

MAGELLAN BIOSCIENCES INC.   978-856-2345 *(cont'd)*
Production: Ms. Andrea MacGillivray/Vice President Quality Assurance &
Regulatory Affairs
Finance: Ms. Pam Gornall/Chief Financial Officer
  Absorption, Atomic, Lead   Toxicology

MAGIC WALK, INC.   408-435-7380
2372 Qume Dr., Suite E, San Jose, CA 95131-1843
FDA Number: 76399
Ownership: Private
Produces/Sells CE-marked Devices: N
  Orthosis, Corrective Shoe   Physical Med

MAGIC WHEELS, INC.   206-282-0760
3837 13th Ave W., Suite 104, Interbay, WA 98119
FDA Number: 3004626622
  Component, Wheelchair   Physical Med

MAGISTER CORPORATION   800-396-3130
310 Sylvan St., Chattanooga, TN 37405   423-265-3574
FDA Number: 1058442   *Fax:* 423-265-4581
E-mail: sales@magistercorp.com
Web site: www.magistercorp.com
Annual Revenue: $1-$5 Million
Year Founded: 1995
Total Employees: 15
Ownership: Private
Produces/Sells CE-marked Devices: Y
Distribution: Manufacturer Through Distributor, Importer, Exporter
General Admin.: David Maley/President, Chief Executive Officer
            Becky Coveney/Vice President
  Equipment, Therapy, Handicapped/Physical   Physical Med
  Exerciser, Hand   Physical Med
  Exerciser, Non-Measuring   Physical Med
  Exerciser, Other   Physical Med
  Floor Mat   General
  Insoles, Medical   General

MAGNA-LAB, INC.   516-393-5874
6800 Jericho Turnpike, Suite 120w, Syosset, NY 11791
FDA Number: 2435891
Ownership: Private
Produces/Sells CE-marked Devices: N
  Coil, Magnetic Resonance, Specialty   Radiology
  Nuclear Magnetic Resonance Imaging System   Radiology

MAGNAPLAN CORP.   800-361-1192
1320 Rte. 9, Champlain, NY 12919-5007   518-298-8404
FDA Number: n/a   *Fax:* 518-298-2368
E-mail: info@visualplanning.com
Web site: www.visualplanning.com
Annual Revenue: $5-$10 Million
Year Founded: 1967
Total Employees: 40   *Marketing Staff:* 3   *Sales Staff:* 10
Ownership: Private
Produces/Sells CE-marked Devices: N
Federal Procurement Eligibility: Small Business, Female Owned
Distribution: Manufacturer Direct
General Admin.: Joseph Josephson/Chief Executive Officer
            Helen Josephson/President
Mktg./Adv.: Boris Polanski/Manager Advertising
  Blade, Scalpel   Surgery
  Knife, Scalpel   Surgery
  Projector, X-Ray Film   Radiology

MAGNATONE HEARING AID CORP.   800-789-6543
170 N. Cypress Way, Casselberry, FL 32707   407-339-2422
FDA Number: 1044692   *Fax:* 407-260-6438
E-mail: sales@magnatone.com
Web site: www.magnatone.com
Medical Products Sales Volume: $8,100,000
Annual Revenue: $10-$25 Million
Year Founded: 1967
Total Employees: 125   *Marketing Staff:* 4   *Sales Staff:* 13
Ownership: Private
Quality System Registration Information: ISO9001
Produces/Sells CE-marked Devices: Y
Federal Procurement Eligibility: Small Business, Female Owned
Distribution: Manufacturer Through Distributor, Exporter
General Admin.: Beverly J. Campbell/Chief Executive Officer
            Donald Campbell/General Manager
            Donald Campbell/President
Production: Sagar Chari/Director Engineering
            Edith Alfaro/Manager Materials
            Donald Campbell/Vice President Manufacturing
  Hearing-Aid   Ear/Nose/Throat

MAGNE VU   760-929-8000
1916 Palomar Oaks Way, Suite 150, Carlsbad, CA 92008
FDA Number: 2032105
Ownership: Private
Produces/Sells CE-marked Devices: N
  Nuclear Magnetic Resonance Imaging System   Radiology

MAGNET SALES & MANUFACTURING   800-421-6692
11248 Playa Ct., Culver City, CA 90230   310-391-7213
FDA Number: n/a   *Fax:* 310-391-7463
E-mail: info@magnetsales.com
Web site: www.magnetsales.com
Medical Products Sales Volume: $1,000,000
Annual Revenue: $10-$25 Million
Year Founded: 1955
Ownership: Private
Quality System Registration Information: ISO9001; ISO9002
Produces/Sells CE-marked Devices: N
Federal Procurement Eligibility: Small Business, Minority Owned
Distribution: Manufacturer Direct
  Magnetic Unit, Therapeutic   Physical Med

MAGNETECS   310-670-7700
10524 La Cienega Blvd, Inglewood, CA 90304
FDA Number: n/a
E-mail: dsaks@magnetecs.com
Web site: http://www.magnetecs.com
Ownership: Private
Produces/Sells CE-marked Devices: N
General Admin.: Mr. Josh Shachar/Chief Executive Officer
            Mr. Daniel Saks/Senior Vice President
Medical Admin.: Mr. Eli Gang/Chief Medical Officer
Mktg./Adv.: Mr. Frank Adell/Executive Vice President Business Development
Finance: Mr. Clive Zickel/Chief Financial Officer

MAGNETIC RADIATION LABORATORIES   888-251-5942
690 Hilltop Dr., Itasca, IL 60143   630-285-0800
FDA Number: n/a   *Fax:* 630-285-0807
Web site: www.magrad.com
Year Founded: 1960
Ownership: Private
Produces/Sells CE-marked Devices: N
Federal Procurement Eligibility: Small Business
Distribution: Service Direct
  Contract Manufacturing   General
  Shield, Magnetic Field   Radiology

MAGNEVU   760-929-8000
2225 Faraday Avenue, Suite F, Carlsbad, CA 92008
FDA Number: n/a   *Fax:* 760-929-8100
E-mail: mvsales@magnevu.com
Web site: www.magnevu.com
Medical Products Sales Volume: $5,600,000
Annual Revenue: $1-$5 Million
Year Founded: 1990
Total Employees: 20
Ownership: Private
Produces/Sells CE-marked Devices: N
Federal Procurement Eligibility: Small Business
Distribution: Manufacturer Direct, Manufacturer Through Distributor
General Admin.: Freeman H. Rose/Chief Executive Officer
Mktg./Adv.: Mr. Michael Barry/Vice President Marketing & Sales
IS: Timothy W. James, PhD./Vice President Application Development
  Scanner, Magnetic Resonance (NMR/MRI)   Radiology

MAGNISIGHT, INC.   800-753-4767
3631 N. Stone Avenue,
Colorado Springs, CO 80907
FDA Number: 79404   *Fax:* 719-578-9887
E-mail: info@magnisight.com
Web site: www.magnisight.com
Year Founded: 1990
Ownership: Private
Produces/Sells CE-marked Devices: N
Federal Procurement Eligibility: Small Business, VA Contract
Distribution: Manufacturer Through Manufacturer Reps
Mktg./Adv.: Garry Greenspan/Project Manager
  Reading System, Closed-Circuit Television   Ophthalmology

MAGNIVISION, INC.   954-986-9000
3700 Commerce Parkway, Hollywood, FL 33025
FDA Number: 1045828   *Fax:* 954-986-3217
E-mail: eleanor.chilson@amgreetings.com
Total Employees: 250   *Marketing Staff:* 6
Ownership: ThyssenKrupp
Quality System Registration Information: ISO9001
Produces/Sells CE-marked Devices: N
Distribution: Manufacturer Direct, Exclusive Distributor

MAGNIVISION, INC.　954-986-9000 *(cont'd)*
Production: Eleanor Chilson/Manager Quality Assurance & Customer Services
　Spectacle, Magnifier　Ophthalmology

MAGNUM MEDICAL　800-336-9710
3265 N. Nevada St., Chandler, AZ 85225　**480-633-2777**
FDA Number: 1421307　Fax: 480-633-2525
E-mail: magnummed@earthlink.net
Web site: www.magnummed.com/1984.htm
Annual Revenue: $1-$5 Million
Year Founded: 1984
Total Employees: 10　*Marketing Staff:* 3
Ownership: Private
Produces/Sells CE-marked Devices: N
Federal Procurement Eligibility: Small Business, Minority Owned, VA Contract
Distribution: Manufacturer Through Distributor, OEM, Importer
General Admin.: Mark Hamid/Vice President, General Manager
Mktg./Adv.: Omar Hameed/Director Marketing & Sales
　ENT Manual Surgical Instrument　Ear/Nose/Throat
　Instrument, Manual, General Surgical　Surgery
　Kit, Surgical Instrument, Disposable　Surgery
　Laryngoscope　Ear/Nose/Throat
　Surgical Instrument, Disposable　Surgery

MAGNUM PLASTICS, INC.　303-828-3156
425 Bonnell Ave., Erie, CO 80516
FDA Number: 3003865400
E-mail: sales@magnum-plastics.com
Web site: www.magnum-plastics.com
Ownership: Private
Produces/Sells CE-marked Devices: N
General Admin.: Mr. Dave MIller/President
Production: Ms. Julie Miller/Vice President Operations
　Syringe, Antistick　General

MAGNUS MOBILITY SYSTEMS　800-858-7801
1912 W. Business Center Drive,　**714-771-2630**
Orange, CA 92867
FDA Number: n/a　Fax: 714-744-0134
E-mail: heretohelp@magnusinc.com
Web site: www.magnusinc.com
Medical Products Sales Volume: $3,400,000
Annual Revenue: $10-$25 Million
Year Founded: 1978
Total Employees: 16　*Marketing Staff:* 2　*Sales Staff:* 10
Ownership: Private
Quality System Registration Information: ISO9001
Produces/Sells CE-marked Devices: N
Federal Procurement Eligibility: Small Business
Distribution: Manufacturer Direct, Manufacturer Through Distributor, Manufacturer Through Manufacturer Reps, OEM, Importer, Exporter
General Admin.: R. E. VerWayne/President
Mktg./Adv.: Jonathan Cuyler/General Manager Sales
Production: Jim Griffen/Manager Materials
　Casters, Hospital Equipment　General
Medical Product Subsidiaries (Listed Separately)
　Jilson Group, Inc.

MAGUIRE ENTERPRISES, INC.　800-548-9686
10289 NW 46th Street,　**954-572-6000**
Fort Lauderdale, FL 33351
FDA Number: 1049754　Fax: 954-578-7100
E-mail: ceo@hackettgroup.org
Web site: www.hackettgroup.org
Medical Products Sales Volume: $1,100,000
Annual Revenue: $1-$5 Million
Year Founded: 1969
Total Employees: 8　*Marketing Staff:* 2　*Sales Staff:* 1
Ownership: Private
Produces/Sells CE-marked Devices: N
Federal Procurement Eligibility: Small Business
Distribution: Manufacturer Direct
General Admin.: Mr. Paul Ashby/Compliance Officer
　　　Mr. William R. Hackett/President, Chief Executive Officer
　　　Mr. Kenneth A. Hackett/Vice President Corporate Operations
Production: Mr. Jeff Stoll/Vice President Manufacturing
Finance: Mrs. Linda Hackett/Treasurer
　Cable　Physical Med
　Cable, Electrode　Physical Med
　Cable/Lead, ECG　Cardiovascular
　Paper, Recording, ECG/EEG　General
　Telemetry Unit, Physiological, ECG　Cardiovascular

MAHE INTERNATIONAL INC.　800-294-7946
928 5th Ave, Nashville, TN 37204　**615-269-7526**
FDA Number: 1057358　Fax: 615-269-4605
E-mail: info@maheinternational.com

MAHE INTERNATIONAL INC.　800-294-7946 *(cont'd)*
Web site: www.maheinternational.com
Medical Products Sales Volume: $1,200,000
Annual Revenue: $5-$10 Million
Year Founded: 1993
Total Employees: 8　*Marketing Staff:* 5　*Sales Staff:* 50
Ownership: Private
Quality System Registration Information: ISO9001
Produces/Sells CE-marked Devices: Y
Federal Procurement Eligibility: Small Business
Distribution: Manufacturer Direct, Manufacturer Through Distributor, Manufacturer Through Manufacturer Reps, OEM, Exclusive Distributor, Importer, Exporter
General Admin.: Winfried W. Reich/President, Chief Executive Officer
Mktg./Adv.: John Soroko/Vice President Marketing & Sales
Research: Ralf Rotter/Vice President Research & Development
　Accessories, Cleaning, Endoscopic　Gastroenterology/Urology
　Accessories, Light, Surgical　Surgery
　Accessories, Photographic, Endoscopic　Gastroenterology/Urology
　Amnioscope, Transabdominal (Fetoscope)　Obstetrics/Gynecology
　Angioscope　Cardiovascular
　Anoscope, Non-Powered　Gastroenterology/Urology
　Biopsy Instrument, Mechanical, Gastrointestinal　Gastroenterology/Urology
　Biopsy Instrument, Suction　Gastroenterology/Urology
　Bronchoscope, Non-Rigid　Ear/Nose/Throat
　Bronchoscope, Rigid　Ear/Nose/Throat
　Bronchoscope, Rigid, Ventilating　Anesthesiology
　Camera, Still, Endoscopic　Surgery
　Camera, Television, Endoscopic (With Audio)　Surgery
　Camera, Video, Endoscopic　General
　Cannula, Drainage, Arthroscopy　Orthopedics
　Cannula, Suprapubic, With Trocar　Gastroenterology/Urology
　Cannula, Tracheostomy　Ear/Nose/Throat
　Choledochoscope, Flexible Or Rigid　Gastroenterology/Urology
　Coagulator/Cutter, Endoscopic, Bipolar　Obstetrics/Gynecology
　Colposcope　Obstetrics/Gynecology
　Culdoscope　Obstetrics/Gynecology
　Cutter, Orthopedic　Orthopedics
　Cystoscope　Gastroenterology/Urology
　Cystourethroscope　Gastroenterology/Urology
　Electrode, Cystoscopic　Gastroenterology/Urology
　Electrode, Electrosurgical, Active (Blade)　Surgery
　Electrosurgical Equipment, Special Purpose　Surgery
　Endoscope　Gastroenterology/Urology
　Endoscope And Accessories, AC-Powered　Surgery
　Endoscope And Accessories, Battery-Powered　Surgery
　Endoscope, Direct Vision　Surgery
　Endoscope, Rigid　Surgery
　Endoscope, Transcervical (Amnioscope)　Obstetrics/Gynecology
　Esophagoscope (Flexible Or Rigid)　Ear/Nose/Throat
　Eyepiece, Lens, Non-Prescription, Endoscopic　Gastroenterology/Urology
　Eyepiece, Lens, Prescription, Endoscopic　Gastroenterology/Urology
　Fiberoptic Light Source & Carrier　Ear/Nose/Throat
　Forceps　Orthopedics
　Forceps, Biopsy　Surgery
　Forceps, Biopsy, Bronchoscope (Non-Rigid)　Anesthesiology
　Forceps, Biopsy, Bronchoscope (Rigid)　Anesthesiology
　Forceps, Electrosurgical　Surgery
　Forceps, Endoscopic　Gastroenterology/Urology
　Forceps, Gallbladder (Biliary Duct)　Gastroenterology/Urology
　Forceps, Grasping, Flexible Endoscopic　Gastroenterology/Urology
　Forceps, Stone Manipulation　Gastroenterology/Urology
　Gastroscope, General & Plastic Surgery　Gastroenterology/Urology
　Gown, Operating Room, Reusable　Surgery
　Headlight, ENT　Ear/Nose/Throat
　Hysteroscope　Obstetrics/Gynecology
　Illuminator, Fiberoptic (For Endoscope)　Gastroenterology/Urology
　Instrument, Electrosurgery, Laparoscopic　Surgery
　Insufflator, Carbon-Dioxide, Automatic (For Endoscope)　Gastroenterology/Urology
　Insufflator, Carbon-Dioxide, Uterotubal　Obstetrics/Gynecology
　Insufflator, Laparoscopic　Obstetrics/Gynecology
　Insufflator, Other　Surgery
　Kit, Tracheotomy　Anesthesiology
　Lamp, Endoscopic, Incandescent　Surgery
　Laparoscope, General & Plastic Surgery　Surgery
　Laparoscope, Gynecologic　Obstetrics/Gynecology
　Laryngoscope　Ear/Nose/Throat
　Laryngoscope, Rigid　Anesthesiology
　Laryngoscope, Surgical　Surgery
　Light Source, Endoscope, Xenon Arc　Surgery
　Light Source, Endoscopic　Obstetrics/Gynecology
　Light Source, Fiberoptic, Routine　Gastroenterology/Urology
　Light Source, Flash　Chemistry
　Light Source, Photographic, Fiberoptic　Gastroenterology/Urology
　Lithotriptor　Gastroenterology/Urology
　Loupe, Binocular, Low Power　Ophthalmology
　Mediastinoscope, ENT　Ear/Nose/Throat
　Mirror, ENT　Ear/Nose/Throat
　Monitor, Video, Endoscope　General
　Nasopharyngoscope (Flexible Or Rigid)　Ear/Nose/Throat
　Needle, Cholangiography　Cardiovascular
　Needle, Endoscopic　Gastroenterology/Urology

MAHE INTERNATIONAL INC. 800-294-7946 *(cont'd)*

Needle, Pneumoperitoneum, Simple	Gastroenterology/Urology
Needle, Pneumoperitoneum, Spring Loaded	Gastroenterology/Urology
Nephroscope Set	Gastroenterology/Urology
Nephroscope, Rigid	Gastroenterology/Urology
Observerscope	General
Obturator, Endoscopic	Gastroenterology/Urology
Otoscope	Ear/Nose/Throat
Peritoneoscope	Gastroenterology/Urology
Pharyngoscope	Ear/Nose/Throat
Pneumoperitoneum Apparatus, Automatic	Gastroenterology/Urology
Power Supply, Endoscopic, Battery-Operated	General
Probe, Ultrasonic	Radiology
Proctoscope	Surgery
Punch, Biopsy	Gastroenterology/Urology
Recorder, Videotape/Videodisc	General
Remover, Foreign Body, Bronchoscope (Non-Rigid)	Anesthesiology
Resectoscope	Gastroenterology/Urology
Resectoscope Working Element	Gastroenterology/Urology
Rhinoscope	Ear/Nose/Throat
Scissors, Cystoscopic	Gastroenterology/Urology
Scissors, Orthopedic	Orthopedics
Sheath, Endoscopic	Gastroenterology/Urology
Sigmoidoscope, Rigid, Non-Electrical	Gastroenterology/Urology
Snare, Endoscopic	Surgery
Snare, Polyp	Surgery
Teaching Attachment, Endoscopic	Gastroenterology/Urology
Telescope, Rigid, Endoscopic	Gastroenterology/Urology
Thoracoscope	Cardiovascular
Tonsillectome	Ear/Nose/Throat
Tray, Surgical Instrument	Surgery
Trocar, Abdominal	Gastroenterology/Urology
Trocar, Amniotic	Obstetrics/Gynecology
Trocar, Antrum	Ear/Nose/Throat
Trocar, Laryngeal	Ear/Nose/Throat
Trocar, Sinus	Ear/Nose/Throat
Trocar, Thoracic	Cardiovascular
Ureteroscope	Gastroenterology/Urology
Ureterotome	Gastroenterology/Urology
Urethroscope	Gastroenterology/Urology
Urethrotome	Gastroenterology/Urology
Vaginoscope	Obstetrics/Gynecology

MAICO DIAGNOSTICS 888-941-4201 / 952-941-4200

**7625 Golden Triangle Drive,
Eden Prairie, MN 55344**
FDA Number: 3002504821 *Fax:* 952-903-4200
E-mail: info@maico-diagnostics.com
Web site: www.maico-diagnostics.com
Medical Products Sales Volume: $2,100,000
Annual Revenue: $5-$10 Million
Year Founded: 1937
Total Employees: 27 *Marketing Staff:* 1 *Sales Staff:* 4
Ownership: Private
Quality System Registration Information: ISO9003
Produces/Sells CE-marked Devices: Y
Federal Procurement Eligibility: Small Business
Distribution: Manufacturer Through Distributor, Manufacturer Through Manufacturer Reps, Exporter
General Admin.: Ron Perlt/Vice President, General Manager
Mktg./Adv.: David Adlin/Manager Sales

Audiometer	Ear/Nose/Throat
Tester, Auditory Impedance	Ear/Nose/Throat

MAILHAWK MANUFACTURING COMPANY 800-331-5070 / 706-655-3849

**Hwy. 85-W, 5292 White House Pkwy.,
Warm Springs, GA 31830**
FDA Number: n/a *Fax:* 706-538-4722
E-mail: mailhawk@alltel.net
Web site: www.mailhawkmfg.com
Annual Revenue: $0-$1 Million
Year Founded: 1958
Total Employees: 10 *Marketing Staff:* 1 *Sales Staff:* 1
Ownership: Private
Produces/Sells CE-marked Devices: N
Federal Procurement Eligibility: Small Business
Distribution: Manufacturer Direct, Manufacturer Through Distributor
General Admin.: Jeff Hill/President
Mktg./Adv.: Lucy Hill/Director Marketing

Reacher (Handicapped)	General

MAIN LINE INTERNATIONAL, INC. 800-397-9020 / 706-227-1800

**151 Ben Burton Circle, Coggins Park,
Bogart, GA 30622**
FDA Number: n/a *Fax:* 706-227-3633
E-mail: info@mlimedical.com
Web site: www.mlimedical.com
Medical Products Sales Volume: $4,000,000
Annual Revenue: $1-$5 Million

MAIN LINE INTERNATIONAL, INC. 800-397-9020 *(cont'd)*

Year Founded: 1988
Total Employees: 6 *Marketing Staff:* 2 *Sales Staff:* 2
Ownership: Private
Produces/Sells CE-marked Devices: N
Federal Procurement Eligibility: Small Business

Scanner, Ultrasonic, Obstetrical/Gynecological, Mobile	Obstetrics/Gynecology
Transducer, Ultrasonic	Cardiovascular

MAINE ANTI-GRAVITY SYSTEMS, INC. 207-775-3800

98 Gray St., Portland, ME 04102
FDA Number: 1223006
E-mail: MAGS1992@aol.com
Web site: www.magsvest.com
Ownership: Private
Produces/Sells CE-marked Devices: N

Transfer Device, Patient, Manual	General

MAINE BIOTECHNOLOGY SERVICES, INC. 207-797-5454

1037 R Forest Ave., Portland, ME 04103
FDA Number: 1226802

Stimulator, Vagus Nerve, Implanted, Tremor	Cns/Neurology

MAINE MOLECULAR QUALITY CONTROLS, INC. 207-885-1072

10 Southgate Road, Suite 170, Scarborough, ME 04074
FDA Number: 3005959679 *Fax:* 207-885-1079
E-mail: info@mmqci.com
Web site: www.mmqci.com
Year Founded: 2000
Ownership: Private
Produces/Sells CE-marked Devices: N
General Admin.: Joan H. Gordon/President
Research: Clark A. Rundell/Vice President Research

Quality Control Material, Genetics, Dna	Microbiology

MAINE OXY-ACETYLENE SUPPLY CO. 207-784-5788

22 Albiston Way, Auburn, ME 04210
FDA Number: 1218978

Analyzer, Gas, Carbon-Dioxide, Blood Phase, Indwelling	Anesthesiology
Analyzer, Oxyhemoglobin Concentration, Blood Phase, Indwell.	Anesthesiology

MAINE STANDARDS COMPANY, LLC 800-377-9684 / 207-892-1300

**765 Roosevelt Trail, Suite 9A,
Windham, ME 04062**
FDA Number: 1226774 *Fax:* 207-892-2266
E-mail: info@mainestandards.com
Web site: www.mainestandards.com
Medical Products Sales Volume: $1,800,000
Year Founded: 2001
Total Employees: 22
Ownership: Private
Produces/Sells CE-marked Devices: N
Federal Procurement Eligibility: Small Business

Calibrator, Primary, Clinical Chemistry	Chemistry
Control, Multi Analyte, All Kinds (Assayed And Unassayed)	Chemistry
Multi Analyte Mixture, Calibrator	Chemistry

MAINLINE MEDICAL, INC. 800-366-2084 / 770-409-2800

**3250-J Peachtree Corners Circle,
Norcross, GA 30092**
FDA Number: 1066013 *Fax:* 800-261-3066
E-mail: service@mainlinemedical.com
Web site: www.mainlinemedical.com
Medical Products Sales Volume: $1,600,000
Year Founded: 1991
Total Employees: 10
Ownership: Private
Produces/Sells CE-marked Devices: N
Federal Procurement Eligibility: Small Business, Female Owned, GSA Contract, VA Contract
Distribution: Manufacturer Direct, Manufacturer Through Distributor, OEM
General Admin.: Liz Wall/Chief Executive Officer, Chief Financial Officer
Mktg./Adv.: Nancy Meyer/Manager International & National Sales
Production: Mrs. Linda Pulley/Manager Materials

Airway, Oropharyngeal, Anesthesia	Anesthesiology
Laryngoscope, Rigid	Anesthesiology
Protector, Dental	Anesthesiology

MAJESTIC DRUG CO., INC. 845-436-0011

4996 Main St., Route 42, Pob 490, S Fallsburg, NY 12779
FDA Number: 2411564

Cement, Dental	Dental And Oral

MAJOR LAB. MANUFACTURING 800-598-2621 / 405-524-2281

**4408 N. Sewell St.,
Oklahoma City, OK 73118**
FDA Number: 1622935 *Fax:* 405-524-2282
E-mail: major@aol.com

MAJOR LAB. MANUFACTURING
800-598-2621 (cont'd)
Annual Revenue: $0-$1 Million
Total Employees: 7 — Marketing Staff: 2 — Sales Staff: 2
Ownership: Private
Produces/Sells CE-marked Devices: N
Federal Procurement Eligibility: Small Business
Distribution: Manufacturer Through Distributor
General Admin.: DeLisa Mingee/Office Manager
Mktg./Adv.: Martha A. Mitchell/Manager Marketing

Bed, Pediatric (Crib)	General
Cart, Emergency, Cardiopulmonary Resuscitation (Crash)	Anesthesiology
Chair, Blood Donor	General
Table, Physical Therapy	Physical Med

MAKITA USA INC. - DRAPERY OPENER DIV.
800-462-5482
14930 Northam St., La Mirada, CA 90638-5753 — **714-522-8088**
FDA Number: n/a — Fax: 714-522-8133
E-mail: plilly@makitausa.com
Web site: www.makitatools.com
Medical Products Sales Volume: $310,200,000
Year Founded: 1970
Total Employees: 1561 — Marketing Staff: 2
Ownership: Private
Produces/Sells CE-marked Devices: N
Distribution: Manufacturer Through Distributor
General Admin.: Gary Morikawa/President
Mktg./Adv.: Porter Lilly/Coord. Marketing
    Bill Austin/Manager Advertising

Track And Carrier, Cubicle Curtain	General

MAKO SURGICAL CORP.
954-927-2044
2555 Davie Rd., Suite 110, Ft. Lauderdale, FL 33317
FDA Number: 3005985723 — Fax: 954.927.0446
E-mail: contactus@makosurgical.com
Web site: www.makosurgical.com
Total Employees: 130
Ownership: Public
Stock Symbol: MAKO
Traded On: NASDAQ
Produces/Sells CE-marked Devices: N
General Admin.: Fritz LaPorte/Chief Financial Officer, Treasurer
    Rony Abovitz/Chief Technology Officer, Senior Vice President
    Maurice Ferre/President, Chief Executive Officer, Chairman
    Menashe Frank/Senior Vice President, General Counsel
Mktg./Adv.: Steven Nunes/Senior Vice President Marketing & Sales
    Benny Hagag/Vice President Business Development
Production: Duncan Moffat/Senior Vice President Operations
    William Tapia/Vice President Quality Assurance & Regulatory Affairs

Prosthesis, Knee, Femorotibial, Non-Constrained	Orthopedics
Prosthesis, Knee, Femorotibial, Semi-Constrained	Orthopedics
Prosthesis, Knee, Femorotibial, Semi-Constrained, Metal	Orthopedics
Prosthesis, Knee, Patellofemoral, Semi-Constrained	Orthopedics
Stereotaxy Equipment	Cns/Neurology

MALCOMTECH INTERNATIONAL
510-293-0580
26200 Industrial Blvd., Hayward, CA 94545
FDA Number: 3006162735

Traction Unit, Non-Powered	Orthopedics

MALLARD MEDICAL, INC.
530-226-0727
20268 Skypark Dr., Redding, CA 96002
FDA Number: 2084342 — Fax: 530-226-0713
E-mail: info@mallaardmedical.net
Web site: www.mallardmedical.com
Annual Revenue: $0-$1 Million
Year Founded: 1986
Total Employees: 6 — Marketing Staff: 1 — Sales Staff: 1
Ownership: Private
Produces/Sells CE-marked Devices: N
Federal Procurement Eligibility: Small Business
Distribution: Manufacturer Direct
General Admin.: Robert M. Pearson/Chief Executive Officer
    Robert M. Pearson/President

Ventilator, Anesthesia Unit	Anesthesiology
Ventilator, Volume (Critical Care)	Anesthesiology

MALLINCKRODT BAKER, INC.
See Avantor Performance Materials

MALLINCKRODT BAKER, INC.
See AVANTOR PERFORMANCE MATERIALS, INC.

MALLINCKRODT MEDICAL INC.
866-885-5988
7500 Trans Canada Highway,
Pointe Claire, QUE H9R-5 Canada
FDA Number: n/a — Fax: 866-511-4567
Web site: www.mallinckrodt.com
Year Founded: 1867
Total Employees: 3500

MALLINCKRODT MEDICAL INC.
866-885-5988 (cont'd)
Ownership: Public
Stock Symbol: COV
Traded On: NYSE
Produces/Sells CE-marked Devices: N
Distribution: Manufacturer Direct, Exporter

MALLINCKRODT, INC.
800-325-8888
675 McDonnell Blvd, Hazelwood, MO 63042
FDA Number: 1946929
Web site: www.mallinckrodt.com
Total Employees: 3500
Ownership: Covidien Ltd.
Stock Symbol: COV
Traded On: NYSE
Produces/Sells CE-marked Devices: N

Nebulizer, Direct Patient Interface	Anesthesiology
Nebulizer, Medicinal, Non-Ventilatory (Atomizer)	Anesthesiology
Shield, Vial	Radiology

MALLINCKRODT, INC.
800-325-8888
675 McDonnell Blvd., Hazelwood, MO 63042 — **314-654-2000**
FDA Number: n/a
Web site: www.mallinckrodt.com
Year Founded: 1867
Total Employees: 3500
Ownership: Covidien Ltd.
Stock Symbol: COV
Traded On: NYSE
Produces/Sells CE-marked Devices: Y
Distribution: Manufacturer Direct, Manufacturer Through Distributor, Manufacturer Through Manufacturer Reps, Importer, Exporter

Bag, Drainage (Incontinence)	Gastroenterology/Urology
Collector, Urine, Disposable	Gastroenterology/Urology
Guidewire, Catheter, Radiological	Radiology
Injector, Contrast Medium, Automatic	Radiology
Media, Contrast, Radiologic	Radiology
Media, Gastroenterographic Contrast (Barium Sulfate)	Radiology
Media, Radioactive Isotope Contrast	Radiology
Table, Urological (Cystological)	Gastroenterology/Urology
Table, Urological, Radiographic	Gastroenterology/Urology

MALLINCKRODT, INC.
800-325-8888
8800 Durant Rd., Raleigh, NC 27616
FDA Number: 1028892
Web site: www.mallinckrodt.com
Total Employees: 3500
Ownership: Covidien Ltd.
Stock Symbol: COV
Traded On: NYSE
Produces/Sells CE-marked Devices: N

Set, Administration, Intravenous, Needle-Free	General

MALONEY'S CUSTOM OCULAR PROSTHETICS, INC.
503-675-1320
4035 S.w. Mercantile Dr., #208, Lake Oswego, OR 97035
FDA Number: 3030716

Eye, Artificial, Non-Custom	Ophthalmology

MALVERN/INSITEC
See Process Metrix

MAMMATECH CORP.
800-626-2273
930 NW 8th Avenue, Gainesville, FL 32601-5071 — **352-375-0607**
FDA Number: n/a — Fax: 352-375-6111
E-mail: information@mammacare.com
Web site: www.mammacare.com
Medical Products Sales Volume: $340,000
Annual Revenue: $0-$1 Million
Year Founded: 1974
Total Employees: 11 — Marketing Staff: 4 — Sales Staff: 4
Ownership: Public
Stock Symbol: MAMM
Traded On: OTC Bulletin
Produces/Sells CE-marked Devices: N
Federal Procurement Eligibility: Small Business
Distribution: Manufacturer Direct, Service Direct, Exporter
General Admin.: M. K. Goldstein/Chairman
    H. S. Pennypacker/President, Chief Executive Officer
Finance: Mary Bailey Sellers/Chief Financial Officer

Anatomical Training Model	General
Kit, Breast Cancer Detection	Obstetrics/Gynecology
Material, Training, Audiovisual	General
Training Manikin, Other	General

MANAN TECHNOLOGIES, INC.
800-416-2434
102 Northfield Drive East, Bainbridge, IN 46105 — **765-522-1774**
FDA Number: 104219
Web site: www.manantechnologies.com

MANAN TECHNOLOGIES, INC.   800-416-2434 *(cont'd)*
Ownership: Private
Produces/Sells CE-marked Devices: N
| Hearing-Aid | Ear/Nose/Throat |

MANDEL SCIENTIFIC COMPANY   **(888) 883-3636**
2 Admiral Place, Guelph, ONT N1G-4N4 Canada   **(519) 763-9292**
FDA Number: n/a   *Fax: 519) 763-2005*
E-mail: info@mandel.ca
Web site: www.mandel.ca
Year Founded: 1969
Total Employees: 100
Ownership: Private
Produces/Sells CE-marked Devices: N
Distribution: Manufacturer Direct, Exclusive Distributor

MANEXIM MULTICORP, LTD.   **416-955-0737**
62 Harrington Cres, Willowdale M2M 2Y5 Canada
FDA Number: 8022048
| Condom | Obstetrics/Gynecology |

MANHATTAN INSTRUMENTS
See Varian Sample Preparation Products

MANICO BLOOMINGTON   **812-336-2567**
515 Woodscrest Medical Bldg.,, Suite 001, P.o. Box 5504, Bloomington, IN 47407
FDA Number: n/a
Ownership: Private
Produces/Sells CE-marked Devices: N
| Attachment, Binocular, Endoscopic | Gastroenterology/Urology |

MANREX LIMITED   **800-665-7652**
1036 Waverly St.,   **204-453-6247**
Winnepeg, MAN R3T-0 Canada
FDA Number: n/a   *Fax: 204-453-6350*
E-mail: info@manrex.com
Web site: www.manrex.com
Year Founded: 1973
Ownership: Private
Produces/Sells CE-marked Devices: N
Distribution: Manufacturer Direct, Exclusive Distributor

MANSFIELD MEDICAL DISTRIBUTORS LTD.   **800-361-6240**
5775 Andover, Montreal, QUE H4T-1H6 Canada   **514-739-3633**
FDA Number: n/a   *Fax: 514-342-1632*
E-mail: info@mansfieldmedical.com
Web site: www.mansfieldmedical.com
Year Founded: 1959
Total Employees: 50
Ownership: Private
Produces/Sells CE-marked Devices: N
Distribution: Exclusive Distributor, Importer

MANSFIELD ORTHOTIC & PROSTHETIC CENTER, INC.   **419-522-4171**
240 Marion Ave., Mansfield, OH 44903
FDA Number: 1526766
| Stirrup, External Brace Component | Physical Med |

MANUFACTURERA DENTAL CONTINENTAL   **523-633-8329**
2113 Calle Indust Del Plastico
269 Fracc Zapopan Indust Norte
Zapopan, Jalisco Mexico
FDA Number: 9616065
| Dam, Rubber | Dental And Oral |
| Frame, Rubber Dam | Dental And Oral |

MANUFACTURING & RESEARCH, INC.(DBA MRI MEDICAL)   **520-882-7794**
4700 S. Overland Drive, Tucson, AZ 85714
FDA Number: 2025851   *Fax: 520-882-6849*
E-mail: mriinfo@mrimedical.com
Web site: www.mrimedical.com
Medical Products Sales Volume: $15,700,000
Annual Revenue: $10-$25 Million
Year Founded: 1986
Total Employees: 40   *Marketing Staff:* 3   *Sales Staff:* 2
Ownership: Private
Quality System Registration Information: ISO9001
Produces/Sells CE-marked Devices: N
Federal Procurement Eligibility: Small Business
Distribution: OEM
General Admin.: Robert Kelliher/Chief Executive Officer
     Ms. Stella Myers-Rosas/Manager Human Resources
     John McCambridge/President, Chief Operating Officer
Mktg./Adv.: Ms. Renee Moomjian/Vice President Business Development
Production: Ms. Suzanne Dew/Director Engineering

MANUFACTURING & RESEARCH, INC.(DBA MRI   **520-882-7794**
(cont'd)
     Mr. James Daugherty/Director Quality Assurance & Regulatory Affairs
     Debra Patrone/Manager Materials
     Suzanne Dew/Vice President Operations
Finance: Gabe Quiroz/Controller
Catheter, Balloon (Foley Type)	Surgery
Catheter, Cardiovascular, Balloon Type	Cardiovascular
Catheter, Embolectomy (Fogarty Type)	Cardiovascular
Catheter, Multiple Lumen	Surgery
Catheter, Nephrostomy	Gastroenterology/Urology
Catheter, Other	Gastroenterology/Urology
Catheter, Retention Type, Balloon	Gastroenterology/Urology
Catheter, Retention, Barium Enema With Bag	Gastroenterology/Urology
Catheter, Suprapubic	Gastroenterology/Urology
Catheter, Thermal Dilution	Cardiovascular
Catheter, Urinary	Gastroenterology/Urology
Catheter, Urinary, Irrigation	Gastroenterology/Urology
Catheter, Urological	Gastroenterology/Urology
Tube, Feeding	General
Tube, Gastro-Enterostomy	Gastroenterology/Urology
Tube, Gastrointestinal Decompression, Baker Jejunostomy	Gastroenterology/Urology
Tube, Nasogastric	Anesthesiology
Tube, Rectal	Gastroenterology/Urology

MANUFACTURING TECHNOLOGY, INC.   **850-664-6070**
70 Ready Ave., N.w., Fort Walton Beach, FL 32548
FDA Number: n/a
Ownership: Private
Produces/Sells CE-marked Devices: N
Biofeedback Device	Cns/Neurology
Electroencephalograph	Cns/Neurology
Isokinetic Testing And Evaluation System	Physical Med

MANVILLE CORP.
See Johns Manville

MAPLE LEAF WHEELCHAIR MFG., INC.   **905-602-0566**
12/13-1655 Sismet Rd, Mississauga L4W 1Z4 Canada
FDA Number: 9680932
| Wheelchair, Manual | Physical Med |

MAQUET   **800-288-2121**
15 Law Drive, Fairfield, NJ 07004   **201-391-8100**
FDA Number: 2248146   *Fax: 201-307-5400*
Web site: www.datascope.com
Medical Products Sales Volume: $325,000,000
Year Founded: 1964
Total Employees: 1400   *Sales Staff:* 400
Ownership: Public
Stock Symbol: DSCP
Traded On: NASDAQ
Quality System Registration Information: ISO9000; ISO9001; ISO9002; ISO9003
Produces/Sells CE-marked Devices: Y
Distribution: Manufacturer Direct, Manufacturer Through Distributor, Service Direct
General Admin.: Lawrence Saper/Chairman
     Lawrence Saper/Chief Executive Officer
     William Friedberg/General Manager
     Murray Pitkowsky/Senior Vice President
     James Cooper/Vice President Human Resources
Mktg./Adv.: Thomas Dugan/Vice President Business Development
Production: Tim Krauskopf/Vice President Regulatory & Clinical Affairs
     S. Arieh Zak/Vice President Regulatory Affairs
Analyzer, Gas, Oxygen, Continuous Monitor	Anesthesiology
Catheter and Accessories, Urological	Gastroenterology/Urology
Catheter, Intra-Aortic Balloon	Cardiovascular
Circulatory Assist Unit, Intra-Aortic Balloon	Cardiovascular
Computer Equipment	General
Computer, Patient Monitor	Anesthesiology
Defibrillator/Monitor, Battery-Powered	Cardiovascular
Device, Hemostasis, Vascular	Cardiovascular
Graft, Vascular, Synthetic/Biological Composite	Cardiovascular
Guide, Catheter	Cardiovascular
Introducer, Catheter	Cardiovascular
Monitor, Bed Patient	General
Monitor, Blood Pressure, Indirect, Automatic	Cardiovascular
Monitor, Blood Pressure, Indirect, Surgery	Surgery
Monitor, Blood Pressure, Invasive (Arterial)	Cardiovascular
Monitor, Heart Rate, Other	Cardiovascular
Monitor, Physiological, Acute Care	Anesthesiology
Monitor, Pulse Rate	Anesthesiology
Monitor, Respiratory	Surgery
Monitor, Temperature (With Probe)	Anesthesiology
Oximeter, Pulse	General
Sphygmomanometer, Electronic, Automatic	General
Transducer, Blood Pressure	General
Medical Product Subsidiaries (Listed Separately)
     Datascope Gmbh

MAQUET CARDIOVASCULAR LLC   888-880-2874
45 Barbour Pond Dr., Wayne, NJ 07470
FDA Number: 2242352
E-mail: info@maquet.com   Fax: 973-709-7699
Web site: www.maquet.com
Year Founded: 2003
Total Employees: 5019
Ownership: Private
Produces/Sells CE-marked Devices: N
General Admin.: Dr. Chima Abuba/Chief Executive Officer
Mktg./Adv.: Mr. Christophe Lenze/Vice President Marketing
         Mr. Joseph Knight/Vice President Sales

Catheter, Irrigation	Surgery
Clamp, Vascular	Cardiovascular
Cutter, Surgical	Surgery
Device, Embolization, Artificial	Cns/Neurology
Electrosurgical Unit, Cutting & Coagulation Device	Surgery
Graft, Vascular, Synthetic/Biological Composite	Cardiovascular
Laparoscope, General & Plastic Surgery, Reprocessed	Gastroenterology/Urology
Mesh, Surgical, Polymeric	Surgery
Pledget And Intracardiac Patch, PETP, PTFE, Polypropylene	Cardiovascular
Prosthesis, Vascular Graft, Less Than 6mm Diameter	Cardiovascular
Prosthesis, Vascular Graft, Of 6mm And Greater Diameter	Cardiovascular
Stabilizer, Heart, Non-compression, Reprocessed	Cardiovascular
Surgical Instrument, Cardiovascular	Cardiovascular

Medical Product Subsidiaries (Listed Separately)
Maquet Puerto Rico Inc.

MAQUET PUERTO RICO INC.   408-635-3900
No. 12, Rd. #698, Dorado, PR 00646
FDA Number: 3006976022
Web site: www.bostonscientific.com
Ownership: Maquet Cardiovascular LLC
Stock Symbol: BSX
Traded On: NYSE
Produces/Sells CE-marked Devices: N

Adapter, Lead, Pacemaker	Cardiovascular
Catheter, Steerable	Cardiovascular
Defibrillator, Implantable, Automatic	Cardiovascular
Device, Stabilizer, Heart	Cardiovascular
Dilator, Vessel, Percutaneous Catheterization	Cardiovascular
Electrosurgical Unit, Cutting & Coagulation Device	Surgery
Guidewire, Catheter	Cardiovascular
Kit, Repair, Pacemaker	Cardiovascular
Laparoscope, General & Plastic Surgery	Surgery
Laparoscope, Gynecologic	Obstetrics/Gynecology
Lead, Pacemaker, Implantable Myocardial	Cardiovascular
Stylet, Catheter	Cardiovascular
Surgical Instrument, Cardiovascular	Cardiovascular
System, Ablation, Microwave And Accessories	Surgery

MAQUET, INC.   1-888-MAQUET3
45 Barbour Pond Drive, Wayne, NJ 07470
FDA Number: 1225700
E-mail: info@maquet-inc.com
Web site: www.maquet.com
Ownership: ArjoHuntleigh
Produces/Sells CE-marked Devices: N

Accessories, Light, Surgical	Surgery
Accessories, Operating Room, Table	Surgery
Cabinet, Table And Tray, Anesthesia	Anesthesiology
Compressor, Air, Portable	Anesthesiology
Infusion Stand	General
Light, Surgical, Ceiling Mounted	Surgery
Light, Surgical, Fiberoptic	Surgery
Light, Surgical, Floor Standing	Surgery
Syringe, Irrigating, Dental	Dental And Oral
Table, Obstetrical, Manual	Obstetrics/Gynecology
Table, Operating Room, AC-Powered	Surgery

MAQUET, INC.   843-552-8652
7371 Spartan Blvd. East, N Charleston, SC 29418
FDA Number: 3019090
Ownership: Private
Produces/Sells CE-marked Devices: N

Accessories, Light, Surgical	Surgery
Accessories, Operating Room, Table	Surgery
Bottle, Collection, Vacuum (Aspirator)	General
Cabinet, Table And Tray, Anesthesia	Anesthesiology
Examination Device, AC-Powered	General
Infusion Stand	General
Light, Surgical, Ceiling Mounted	Surgery
Light, Surgical, Floor Standing	Surgery
Regulator, Vacuum	General
Suction Apparatus, Operating Room, Wall Vacuum-Powered	Surgery
Table, Obstetrical, Manual	Obstetrics/Gynecology
Table, Operating Room, AC-Powered	Surgery
Tube, Smoke Removal, Endoscopic	Gastroenterology/Urology

MAQUILAS TETA-KAWI, S.A. DE C.V.   413-593-6400
Carretera Internacional, Km 1969, Enpalme, Sonora Mexico
FDA Number: 8044184

Cap, Surgical	Surgery
Cover, Shoe, Operating Room	Surgery
Drape, Surgical	Surgery
Gown, Surgical	Surgery
Hood, Surgical	Surgery
Pack, Sterilization Wrapper (Bag And Accessories)	Surgery

MAR COR PURIFICATION   800-346-0365
4450 Township Line Road,   484-991-0220
Skippack, PA 19474
FDA Number: 3019131
E-mail: info@mcpur.com   Fax: 484-991-0230
Web site: http://www.mcpur.com
Medical Products Sales Volume: $30,000,000
Annual Revenue: $25-$50 Million
Year Founded: 1970
Total Employees: 50   Marketing Staff: 5   Sales Staff: 18
Ownership: Charter Oak Partners
Stock Symbol: CMN
Traded On: NYSE
Produces/Sells CE-marked Devices: N
Federal Procurement Eligibility: Small Business
Distribution: Manufacturer Direct, OEM, Service Direct
Mktg./Adv.: Mr. Michael Verguldi/Vice President Marketing
Production: Mr. Jim Bowman/Director Operations
Finance: Mr. Andrew Stitzinger/Vice President Finance & Operations
IS: Mr. Don Bechtel/Director Tech. Services

Dialysate Delivery System, Central Multiple Patient	Gastroenterology/Urology
Purification System, Water	Gastroenterology/Urology
Tank, Holding, Dialysis	Gastroenterology/Urology

MAR COR PURIFICATION, INC.   (800) 633-3080
14550 28th Avenue North, Plymouth, MN 55447   (484) 991-0220
FDA Number: 3019131   Fax: (763) 210-3868
Web site: www.mcpur.com
Ownership: Private
Produces/Sells CE-marked Devices: N

System, Water Purification, General Medical Use	Gastroenterology/Urology
Tank, Holding, Dialysis	Gastroenterology/Urology

MAR-LEE COMPANIES   978-343 9600
190 Authority Dr., Fitchburg, MA 01420
FDA Number: n/a
Ownership: Private
Produces/Sells CE-marked Devices: N

Fastener, Fixation, Biodegradable, Soft Tissue	Orthopedics

MAR-MED CO.   800-369-3434
345 Fuller Ave. NE, Grand Rapids, MI 49503
FDA Number: 1832653   Fax: 616-459-5119
E-mail: info@marmedco.com
Web site: www.marmedco.com
Annual Revenue: $0-$1 Million
Ownership: Private
Produces/Sells CE-marked Devices: N
Federal Procurement Eligibility: Small Business, Female Owned
Distribution: Manufacturer Direct, Service Direct

Bottle, Medicine Spray	General
Cover, Cast	General
Legging, Compression, Non-Inflatable	General
Protector, Finger	Orthopedics
Tourniquet	General

MARAMED ORTHOPEDIC SYSTEMS   800-327-5830
2480 W. 82nd St., No. 8, Hialeah, FL 33016-2753   305-823-8300
FDA Number: 1047125   Fax: 305-823-8304
E-mail: maramed@oandp.com
Web site: www.maramed.com
Medical Products Sales Volume: $1,500,000
Annual Revenue: $1-$5 Million
Year Founded: 1972
Total Employees: 20   Marketing Staff: 1   Sales Staff: 2
Ownership: Private
Produces/Sells CE-marked Devices: Y
Federal Procurement Eligibility: Small Business
Distribution: Manufacturer Direct, Manufacturer Through Distributor, OEM, Exporter
General Admin.: Alan R. Finniaston/President
         Mark Mazloff/Vice President, General Manager
Mktg./Adv.: Mark Mazloff/Director Product Development
Production: Paul Spencer/Manager Materials

Brace, Joint, Ankle (External)	Physical Med
Custom Prosthesis	Orthopedics
Holder, Leg, Arthroscopy	Orthopedics
Immobilizer, Wrist/Hand	Orthopedics

MARAMED ORTHOPEDIC SYSTEMS   800-327-5830 *(cont'd)*

Joint, Knee, External Brace	Physical Med
Material, Training, Audiovisual	General
Orthosis, Limb Brace	Physical Med
Orthosis, Other	Physical Med
Shoe, Cast	Physical Med
Sling, Arm, Overhead Supported	Physical Med
Splint, Hand, And Component	Physical Med
Splint, Molded, Plastic	Orthopedics
Stockinette	Orthopedics
Support, Ankle	Orthopedics
Support, Arm	Physical Med
Support, Leg	Physical Med
Support, Wrist	Physical Med

MARAMED PRECISION CORPORATION
See Maramed Orthopedic Systems

MARATHON EQUIPMENT COMPANY   800-269-7237
P.O. Box 1798, Vernon, AL 35592   **205-695-9105**
FDA Number: n/a   *Fax:* 205-695-8813
E-mail: marketing@marathonequipment.com
Web site: www.MarathonEquipment.com
Annual Revenue: $100-$500 Million
Year Founded: 1967
Ownership: Private
Produces/Sells CE-marked Devices: N
Distribution: Manufacturer Direct, Manufacturer Through Distributor, Manufacturer Through Manufacturer Reps
Mktg./Adv.: Renee Boman/Coord. Marketing Communications

Paper, Chart, Record, Medical	General
Waste Receptacle, General Purpose	General

MARATHON MEDICAL EQUIPMENT CORP.
See Caire, Inc.

MARCAL MEDICAL, INC.   800-628-9214
1114 Benfield Blvd., Suite H,   **410-987-4001**
Millersville, MD 21108
FDA Number: 1122814   *Fax:* 410-987-4004
E-mail: customerservice@marcalmedical.com
Web site: www.marcalmedical.com
Medical Products Sales Volume: $2,200,000
Annual Revenue: $1-$5 Million
Ownership: Private
Produces/Sells CE-marked Devices: N
Federal Procurement Eligibility: Small Business, Female Owned
Distribution: Manufacturer Through Distributor, Manufacturer Through Manufacturer Reps, Service Direct, Exclusive Distributor, Importer
General Admin.: Candace Keaton/Chief Executive Officer

Pump, Infusion, Syringe	General

MARCH & GREEN   800-447-6004
P.O. Box 155, Wayne, IL 60184-0155   **630-377-6004**
FDA Number: 9200680   *Fax:* 630-377-6005
E-mail: marchgren@aol.com
Web site: www.marchandgreen.com
Total Employees: 10
Ownership: Private
Produces/Sells CE-marked Devices: N
Federal Procurement Eligibility: Small Business, Female Owned
Distribution: Manufacturer Direct
General Admin.: Carolyn G. Anderson/Chief Executive Officer
Mktg./Adv.: Douglas Anderson/Vice President, General Manager Marketing

Forms, Medical And Patient	General
Holder, X-Ray Film	Dental And Oral

MARCO EQUIPMENT, INC.
See Marco Ophthalmic, Inc.

MARCO OPHTHALMIC, INC.   800-874-5274
11825 Central Pkwy., Jacksonville, FL 32224   **904-642-9330**
FDA Number: 1041845   *Fax:* 904-642-9338
E-mail: dgutzwiller@marcooph.com
Web site: www.marcooph.com
Medical Products Sales Volume: $2,900,000
Annual Revenue: $25-$50 Million
Year Founded: 1962
Total Employees: 45   *Marketing Staff:* 4   *Sales Staff:* 20
Ownership: Private
Produces/Sells CE-marked Devices: N
Federal Procurement Eligibility: Small Business, GSA Contract, VA Contract
Distribution: Manufacturer Direct, Manufacturer Through Distributor, Manufacturer Through Manufacturer Reps
General Admin.: David Marco/President
    Gene Ricks/Vice President Personnel
    David Gurvis/Vice President, General Manager
Mktg./Adv.: Robert Kalapp/Director Marketing
    Robert Kalapp/Vice President Sales
Production: Mr. David Gutzwiller/Production Engineer

MARCO OPHTHALMIC, INC.   800-874-5274 *(cont'd)*

Chair, Ophthalmic, AC-Powered	Ophthalmology
Keratometer	Ophthalmology
Lamp, Slit, Biomicroscope, AC-Powered	Ophthalmology
Lens, Other	Ophthalmology
Lens, Set, Trial, Ophthalmic	Ophthalmology
Lensometer	Ophthalmology
Microscope, Surgical	Ear/Nose/Throat
Perimeter, Automatic, AC-Powered	Ophthalmology
Perimeter, Manual	Ophthalmology
Projector, Ophthalmic	Ophthalmology
Refractometer, Ophthalmic	Ophthalmology
Refractor, Ophthalmic	Ophthalmology
Stand, Instrument, Ophthalmic	Ophthalmology
Table, Ophthalmic, Instrument, Manual	Ophthalmology
Table, Ophthalmic, Instrument, Powered	Ophthalmology

MARCO PRODUCTS COMPANY   800-572-USA1
12860 San Fernando Road, Sylmar, CA 91342   **818-367-2227**
FDA Number: 2025810   *Fax:* 818-367-5380
E-mail: info@marcosnakes.com
Web site: www.marcosnakes.com
Medical Products Sales Volume: $3,200,000
Year Founded: 1924
Total Employees: 45
Ownership: ACTEON GROUP
Produces/Sells CE-marked Devices: N
Federal Procurement Eligibility: Small Business
Distribution: Manufacturer Through Distributor
General Admin.: Charles Chao/Vice President Admin.

Aid, Resuscitation, Cardiopulmonary	Cardiovascular

MARCO-MED U.S.A.   305-661-7046
1521 Zuleta Ave., Coral Gables, FL 33146
FDA Number: n/a   *Fax:* 305-661-9553
E-mail: medmarco@bellsouth.net
Web site: www.marco-med.net
Medical Products Sales Volume: $600,000
Annual Revenue: $0-$1 Million
Ownership: Private
Produces/Sells CE-marked Devices: N
Federal Procurement Eligibility: Small Business
Distribution: Manufacturer Through Distributor

Handpiece, Water-Powered	Dental And Oral

MARCOLIN USA   888-627-2654
7543 E. Tierra Buena Lane,   **480-951-7174**
Scottsdale, AZ 85260
FDA Number: 2249128   *Fax:* 888-627-2671
E-mail: info@marcolinusa.com
Web site: www.marcolinusa.com
Medical Products Sales Volume: $45,000,000
Annual Revenue: $50-$100 Million
Year Founded: 1961
Total Employees: 130   *Marketing Staff:* 5   *Sales Staff:* 100
Ownership: MARCOLIN SPA
Produces/Sells CE-marked Devices: N
Federal Procurement Eligibility: Small Business
Distribution: Manufacturer Direct, Manufacturer Through Distributor, Manufacturer Through Manufacturer Reps, Exclusive Distributor, Importer, Exporter
General Admin.: Mr. Richard Babboni/Chief Operating Officer
Finance: Mr. Joseph Ivenz/Vice President Finance

Frame, Spectacle (Eyeglasses)	Ophthalmology
Spectacle, Magnifier	Ophthalmology
Sunglasses (Including Photosensitive)	Ophthalmology

MARCON GROUP, INC.   800-547-5021
655 Du Bois Street, Suite D,   **415-259-0530**
San Rafael, CA 94901
FDA Number: 2952598   *Fax:* 415-259-0540
E-mail: infoUsa@marcolin.com
Web site: www.marcongroup.com
Medical Products Sales Volume: $400,000
Annual Revenue: $1-$5 Million
Year Founded: 1995
Total Employees: 6   *Marketing Staff:* 1   *Sales Staff:* 3
Ownership: Private
Produces/Sells CE-marked Devices: N
Federal Procurement Eligibility: Small Business, Female Owned
Distribution: Manufacturer Direct, Manufacturer Through Distributor

Mattress, Air Flotation	General

MARCONI MEDICAL SYSTEMS CANADA INC.   800-668-5211
7956 Torbam Rd.,   **905-791-1494**
Brampton, ONT L6T-5 Canada
FDA Number: n/a   *Fax:* 905-791-7297
E-mail: rod.sykes@marconimed.com
Web site: www.marconimed.com

MARCONI MEDICAL SYSTEMS CANADA INC.   800-668-5211
(cont'd)
- Year Founded: 1948
- Total Employees: 100
- Ownership: Private
- Produces/Sells CE-marked Devices: N
- Distribution: Exclusive Distributor

MARCOOP MOLDING   787-863-3952
Puerto Real Ind'l. Park Rd. 195, Km. 2.9, Fajardo, PR 00738
- FDA Number: n/a
- Ownership: Private
- Produces/Sells CE-marked Devices: N

Component, Plastic	General
Contract Packaging	General
Molding, Custom	General
Molding, Injection	General
Thermoforming, Extrusion, Custom	General
Tube, Suction	General

MARCOR DEVELOPMENT CORP.   201-935-2111
341 Michelle Pl, Carlstadt, NJ 07072-2304
- FDA Number: n/a   Fax: 201-935-5223
- E-mail: sales@marcordev.com
- Web site: www.marcordev.com
- Annual Revenue: $25-$50 Million
- Ownership: Private
- Produces/Sells CE-marked Devices: N
- Federal Procurement Eligibility: Small Business
- Distribution: Service Direct, Importer

Culture Media, General Nutrient Broth	Microbiology

MARCOTE, LLC   907-345-1377
1120 E. Huffman Rd. Pmb 348, Anchorage, AK 99516
- FDA Number: n/a
- Ownership: Private
- Produces/Sells CE-marked Devices: N

Sling, Arm	Physical Med

MARDX DIAGNOSTICS, INC.   760-929-0500
5919 Farnsworth Ct., Carlsbad, CA 92008
- FDA Number: 2245544
- Web site: www.mardx.com
- Medical Products Sales Volume: $8,000,000
- Annual Revenue: $5-$10 Million
- Ownership: Trinity Biotech Plc
- Produces/Sells CE-marked Devices: N
- Distribution: Manufacturer Direct, Exporter

Antibody, Anti-Smooth Muscle, Indirect Immunofluorescent	Immunology
Antibody, Anti-Thyroid, Indirect Immunofluorescent	Immunology
Antibody, Antimitochondrial, Indirect Immunofluorescent	Immunology
Antibody, Antinuclear, Indirect Immunofluorescent, Antigen	Immunology
Antibody, Multiple Auto, Indirect Immunofluorescent	Immunology
Antibody, Other	General
Antibody, Treponema Pallidum	Microbiology
Reagent, Legionella Detection	Microbiology
Reagent, Other	General
Test, Disease, Lyme	Immunology
Test, Nuclear Antigen, Epstein-Barr Virus	Microbiology

MAREL CORPORATION   203-934-8187
5 Sawmill Rd., West Haven, CT 06516
- FDA Number: 1225801   Fax: 203-934-7488
- E-mail: krice@marelcorp.com
- Medical Products Sales Volume: $3,500,000
- Annual Revenue: $1-$5 Million
- Year Founded: 1998
- Total Employees: 20
- Ownership: Private
- Produces/Sells CE-marked Devices: N
- Federal Procurement Eligibility: Female Owned
- Distribution: Manufacturer Through Distributor

Dressing, Other	General
Gauze, Non-Absorbable, X-Ray Detectable (Internal Sponge)	Surgery
Sponge, External	Surgery
Sponge, Gauze	Dental And Oral

MARENA GROUP, INC.   770-822-6925
650 Progress Industrial Blvd, Lawrenceville, GA 30043
- FDA Number: 1062379   Fax: 770-822-1058
- E-mail: info@marenagroup.com
- Web site: www.marenagroup.com
- Medical Products Sales Volume: $4,300,000
- Year Founded: 1994
- Total Employees: 26
- Ownership: Private
- Produces/Sells CE-marked Devices: N
- Federal Procurement Eligibility: Small Business

MARENA GROUP, INC.   770-822-6925 *(cont'd)*
Orthosis, Abdominal	Physical Med

MARGRAF DENTAL MANUFACTURING, INC.   800-762-2641
611 Harper Ave., Jenkintown, PA 19046-3206   **215-884-0369**
- FDA Number: 2585044   Fax: 215-884-9116
- E-mail: info@margrafcorp.com
- Web site: www.margrafcorp.com
- Annual Revenue: $0-$1 Million
- Year Founded: 1967
- Total Employees: 10   Marketing Staff: 1   Sales Staff: 2
- Ownership: Private
- Produces/Sells CE-marked Devices: N
- Federal Procurement Eligibility: Small Business
- Distribution: Manufacturer Direct, Manufacturer Through Distributor, Manufacturer Through Manufacturer Reps
- General Admin.: Amanda Alesch/Administrator
  - Barry R. Margraf/President, Chief Executive Officer
- Mktg./Adv.: James W. Margraf/Vice President Marketing & Sales
- Production: Barry R. Margraf/Director Product Development & Regulatory Affairs
  - James W. Margraf/Vice President Engineering & Operations

Aligner, Beam, X-Ray (Collimator)	Dental And Oral
Cephalometer	Dental And Oral
Collimator, Radiographic, Automatic	Radiology
Collimator, X-Ray	Dental And Oral
Cone, Radiographic	Radiology
Cone, Radiographic, Lead-Lined	Dental And Oral
Holder, X-Ray Film	Dental And Oral

MARGUS ENTERPRISES, INC.
See Akorn, Inc.

MARINA MEDICAL INSTRUMENTS, INC.   800-697-1119
955 Shotgun Road, Sunrise, FL 33326   **954-924-4418**
- FDA Number: 2084346   Fax: 954-924-4419
- E-mail: alexbarron@marinamedical.com
- Web site: www.marinamedical.com
- Medical Products Sales Volume: $4,500,000
- Annual Revenue: $1-$5 Million
- Year Founded: 1998
- Total Employees: 26   Sales Staff: 9
- Ownership: Private
- Produces/Sells CE-marked Devices: N
- Federal Procurement Eligibility: Small Business
- Distribution: Manufacturer Through Distributor, Manufacturer Through Manufacturer Reps
- General Admin.: Mr. Anthony Zinnanti, Jr./Chairman
  - Mr. Alexander H. Barron/Chief Executive Officer, General Manager
  - Marina C. Zinnanti/President
- Mktg./Adv.: Scott Clelland/Vice President Business Development

Carrier, Ligature	Surgery
Curette	Orthopedics
Curette, Suction, Endometrial	Obstetrics/Gynecology
Curette, Uterine	Obstetrics/Gynecology
Dilator, Cervical, Fixed Size	Obstetrics/Gynecology
Forceps	Orthopedics
Forceps, Biopsy, Gynecological	Obstetrics/Gynecology
Forceps, Surgical, Gynecological	Obstetrics/Gynecology
General Use Surgical Scissors	Surgery
Holder, Needle	Gastroenterology/Urology
Retractor, Fiberoptic	Gastroenterology/Urology
Retractor, Surgical	Surgery
Retractor, Vaginal	Obstetrics/Gynecology
Speculum, Vaginal, Metal	Obstetrics/Gynecology
Speculum, Vaginal, Non-Metal	Obstetrics/Gynecology
Tenaculum, Uterine	Obstetrics/Gynecology

MARINCO SPECIALTY WIRING DEVICES   800-767-8541
2655 Napa Valley Corporate Drive, Napa, CA 94558   **707-226-8600**
- FDA Number: n/a   Fax: 707-226-9670
- E-mail: info@marinco.com
- Web site: www.marinco.com
- Medical Products Sales Volume: $13,700,000
- Annual Revenue: $50-$100 Million
- Year Founded: 1972
- Total Employees: 150
- Ownership: Public
- Traded On: NYSE
- Quality System Registration Information: ISO9001
- Produces/Sells CE-marked Devices: N
- Federal Procurement Eligibility: Small Business
- Distribution: Manufacturer Direct, Manufacturer Through Distributor, Manufacturer Through Manufacturer Reps
- General Admin.: J. Marty O'Donohue/President
- Mktg./Adv.: Phil Fram/Vice President Marketing

Component, Electrical	General

MARINE DYNAMICS CORP. 951-699-4299
6475 E. Pch, #412, Long Beach, CA 90803
FDA Number: 2025758
Ownership: Private
Produces/Sells CE-marked Devices: N
  Chamber, Hyperbaric   Anesthesiology

MARINE MEDICAL INTL., INC. 954-523-1404
1414 South Andrews Avenue, Fort Lauderdale, FL 33316
FDA Number: 1057979   *Fax:* 954-523-1403
E-mail: renee@marmed.com
Web site: www.marmed.com
Medical Products Sales Volume: $300,000
Year Founded: 1998
Total Employees: 2
Ownership: Private
Produces/Sells CE-marked Devices: N
Federal Procurement Eligibility: Small Business
  Kit, First Aid   Surgery

MARINE POLYMER TECHNOLOGIES, INC. 888-666-2560
461 Boston St., Unit B5, Topsfield, MA 01983
FDA Number: 1225598
  Bandage, Adhesive   Surgery
  Bandage, Liquid   Surgery
  Clamp, Vascular   Cardiovascular
  Dressing, Other   General
  Dressing, Wound, Hydrophilic   Surgery
  Fiber, Absorbent   General

MARIVAC LIMITED 800-565-5821
5821 Russell St., Halifax, NS B3K-1X5 Canada   902-454-5544
FDA Number: n/a   *Fax:* 902-455-4007
E-mail: marivac@ns.sympatico.ca
Web site: www.marivac.com
Year Founded: 1977
Total Employees: 10
Ownership: Private
Produces/Sells CE-marked Devices: N
Distribution: Exclusive Distributor, Exporter

MARK MEDICAL MANUFACTURING, INC. 610-269-4420
530 Brandywine Ave., Downingtown, PA 19335-2608
FDA Number: 2531099   *Fax:* 610-269-4428
E-mail: sales@markmed.com
Web site: www.markmed.com
Annual Revenue: $0-$1 Million
Total Employees: 8   *Marketing Staff:* 1   *Sales Staff:* 2
Ownership: Private
Produces/Sells CE-marked Devices: Y
Federal Procurement Eligibility: Small Business, Female Owned
Distribution: Manufacturer Through Distributor
General Admin.: Diana L. McBrinn/President
Mktg./Adv.: Mark T. McBrinn/Vice President Marketing & Sales
  Electrosurgical Equipment, General Purpose   Surgery
  Electrosurgical Unit, Cutting & Coagulation Device   Surgery
  Forceps   Orthopedics
  Forceps, Biopsy, Gynecological   Obstetrics/Gynecology
  General Use Surgical Scissors   Surgery
  Holder, Needle   Gastroenterology/Urology
  Instrument, Microsurgical   Cns/Neurology
  Knife, Ophthalmic   Ophthalmology
  Knife, Scalpel   Surgery
  Laparoscope, General & Plastic Surgery   Surgery
  Orthopedic Manual Surgical Instrument   Orthopedics
  Rack, Surgical Instrument   Surgery
  Retractor, Vaginal   Obstetrics/Gynecology
  Scissors, Rectal   Gastroenterology/Urology
  Service, Maintenance/Repair   General
  Service, Parts, Repair   General
  Speculum, Vaginal, Metal   Obstetrics/Gynecology
  Surgical Instrument, Cardiovascular   Cardiovascular
  Surgical Instrument, Obstetric/Gynecologic, General   Obstetrics/Gynecology
  System, Coding, Color, Instrument   Dental And Oral
  Tray, Surgical Instrument   Surgery

MARK TWO ENGINEERING 305-889-3280
8324 NW 74th Ave., Miami, FL 33166
FDA Number: n/a   *Fax:* 305-889-3281
E-mail: info@marktwo.com
Web site: www.marktwo.com
Year Founded: 1996
Ownership: Private
Produces/Sells CE-marked Devices: N
Federal Procurement Eligibility: Small Business, Minority Owned
Distribution: Service Direct
  Component, Metal, Other   General
  Contract Manufacturing   General

MARK TWO ENGINEERING 305-889-3280 *(cont'd)*
Contract R&D, Equipment   General

MARKEL INDUSTRIES, INC. 860-646-5303
PO Box 1388, 135A Sheldon Road,   860-646-5303
Manchester, CT 06040
FDA Number: n/a   *Fax:* 860-646-6108
E-mail: info@markelind.com
Web site: www.markelind.com
Annual Revenue: $1-$5 Million
Year Founded: 1982
Total Employees: 10   *Marketing Staff:* 1   *Sales Staff:* 1
Ownership: Private
Produces/Sells CE-marked Devices: N
Federal Procurement Eligibility: Small Business
Distribution: Manufacturer Direct, Manufacturer Through Distributor, Manufacturer Through Manufacturer Reps, Exporter
General Admin.: Marcel Lussier/President
          Marc Lussier/Vice President, General Manager
Mktg./Adv.: Dawn Bird/Manager International & National Sales
  Floor Mat   General
  Monitor, Biological (Contamination Testing)   General

MARKET-FORGE
  See Getinge Usa, Inc.

MARKET-TIERS, INC. D/B/A WISAP AMERICA
  See Wisap America

MARKETING INTERNATIONAL, INC. 800-447-0173
P.O. Box 4835, Topeka, KS 66604-0835   785-272-4773
FDA Number: 1925290   *Fax:* 785-272-4273
E-mail: mktgintl@inlandnet.net
Web site: www.marketing-international.net
Annual Revenue: $0-$1 Million
Total Employees: 2   *Marketing Staff:* 1   *Sales Staff:* 2
Ownership: Private
Produces/Sells CE-marked Devices: N
Federal Procurement Eligibility: Small Business
Distribution: Manufacturer Direct, Manufacturer Through Distributor, Importer, Exporter
General Admin.: Candace Becker/President, Chief Executive Officer
Mktg./Adv.: Kristy Harvey/Director Marketing Operations
          Kristy Harvey/Director National Marketing & Sales
  Board, Dissecting   Pathology
  Glove, Patient Examination, Specialty   General
  Knife, Surgical   Dental And Oral

MARKPERI INTERNATIONAL ENTERPRISES 888-627-5737
180 Oval Dr., Islandia, NY 11772   516-342-8900
FDA Number: n/a   *Fax:* 516-342-9711
E-mail: sales@markperi.com
Web site: www.markperi.com
Annual Revenue: $1-$5 Million
Total Employees: 21
Ownership: Private
Produces/Sells CE-marked Devices: N
Federal Procurement Eligibility: Small Business
Distribution: Manufacturer Direct
General Admin.: Mark Greenspecht/Chief Executive Officer
          James Bohorodzaner/President
Mktg./Adv.: Robert J. Wasilko/Director Marketing
          Lori Battell/Vice President Business Development
  Heat-Sealing Device   Hematology
  Production Equipment   General

MARLEN MANUFACTURING & DEVELOPMENT CO. 216-292-7060
5150 Richmond Rd., Bedford, OH 44146
FDA Number: 1520020   *Fax:* 216-292-9196
E-mail: info@marlenmfg.com
Web site: www.marlenmfg.com
Annual Revenue: $5-$10 Million
Year Founded: 1952
Ownership: Private
Produces/Sells CE-marked Devices: N
Federal Procurement Eligibility: Small Business
Distribution: Manufacturer Through Manufacturer Reps
  Bag, Bile Collection   Gastroenterology/Urology
  Bag, Drainage, Ostomy (With Adhesive)   General
  Bag, Leg   Gastroenterology/Urology
  Bag, Stomal   Surgery
  Bag, Urinary Collection, Ureterostomy   Gastroenterology/Urology
  Bag, Urinary, Ileostomy   Gastroenterology/Urology
  Bandage, Adhesive   Surgery
  Colostomy Appliance, Disposable   Gastroenterology/Urology
  Irrigator, Ostomy   Gastroenterology/Urology
  Kit, Enema   General
  Kit, Incision And Drainage   Surgery

MARLEN MANUFACTURING & 216-292-7060 (cont'd)

Kit, Urinary Drainage Collection	Gastroenterology/Urology
Kit, Wound Drainage	General
Ostomy Appliance (Ileostomy, Colostomy)	Gastroenterology/Urology
Pouch, Colostomy	Gastroenterology/Urology
Rod, Colostomy	Gastroenterology/Urology

MARLENE C. ROCHE 519-658-4519
96 Grey Abbey Trail, Cambridge N3C 3G1 Canada
FDA Number: 9616388

Pack, Hot Or Cold, Reusable	Physical Med

MARPAC INC. 800-334-6413
8430 Washington Place NE, 505-344-4740
Albuquerque, NM 87113
FDA Number: 1722095
Fax: 505-344-4169
E-mail: sales@marpac.biz
Web site: www.marpac.biz
Medical Products Sales Volume: $1,600,000
Annual Revenue: $1-$5 Million
Year Founded: 1992
Total Employees: 20 *Marketing Staff:* 1 *Sales Staff:* 1
Ownership: Private
Quality System Registration Information: ISO9001
Produces/Sells CE-marked Devices: Y
Federal Procurement Eligibility: Small Business
Distribution: Manufacturer Direct, Manufacturer Through Distributor, Manufacturer Through Manufacturer Reps, OEM, Exporter
General Admin.: John E. Rockwell/President, Chief Executive Officer
Mktg./Adv.: John Kiegel/Director Marketing & Sales
Evelyn Trujillo/Director Product Development
Production: Evelyn Trujillo/Director Quality Assurance

Fixation Device, Tracheal Tube	Anesthesiology
Holder, Tracheostomy Tube	Anesthesiology
Strap, Tracheostomy Tube	Anesthesiology

MARQUEST MEDICAL PRODUCTS, INC.
See Vital Signs Colorado

MARQUETTE MEDICAL SYSTEMS (WORLD HEADQUARTERS)
See Ge Medical Systems Information Technologies

MARQUETTE MEDICAL, INC. 800-296-2134
2600 Cabover Drive, Suite J, Hanover, MD 21076 -
FDA Number: 1120886 *Fax:* 410-987-2998
E-mail: marquette@toad.net
Web site: www.pilotmedicalproducts.com
Medical Products Sales Volume: $2,500,000
Annual Revenue: $1-$5 Million
Year Founded: 1985
Total Employees: 6 *Sales Staff:* 3
Ownership: Private
Produces/Sells CE-marked Devices: N
Federal Procurement Eligibility: Small Business
General Admin.: Mr. Earl Marquette Jr./President

Needle, Hypodermic, Single Lumen With Syringe	General
Tubing, Fluid Delivery	General

MARQUIS DENTAL MANUFACTURING CO. 800-359-3206
15370 Smith Rd., Unit H, Aurora, CO 80011 303-344-5222
FDA Number: 1718461 *Fax:* 303-344-5232
Web site: www.perio-aid.net
Annual Revenue: $0-$1 Million
Year Founded: 1953
Ownership: Private
Produces/Sells CE-marked Devices: N
Federal Procurement Eligibility: Small Business
Distribution: Manufacturer Direct

Pick, Massaging	Dental And Oral
Probe, Periodontic	Dental And Oral

MARQUIS DENTAL MFG. CO. 303-344-5222
15370-h Smith Rd., Aurora, CO 80011
FDA Number: 1718461

Pick, Massaging	Dental And Oral
Probe, Periodontic	Dental And Oral

MARS AIR DOORS 800-421-1266
14716 S. Broadway, Gardena, CA 90248-1814 310-532-1555
FDA Number: n/a *Fax:* 310-324-3030
E-mail: info@marsair.com
Web site: www.marsair.com
Medical Products Sales Volume: $3,000,000
Annual Revenue: $10-$25 Million
Year Founded: 1962
Total Employees: 55 *Marketing Staff:* 3 *Sales Staff:* 6
Ownership: Private
Produces/Sells CE-marked Devices: N
Federal Procurement Eligibility: Small Business, Female Owned, GSA Contract

MARS AIR DOORS 800-421-1266 (cont'd)
Distribution: Manufacturer Through Distributor, Manufacturer Through Manufacturer Reps, Exporter
General Admin.: Martin Smilo/President, Chief Executive Officer
Juliette Smilo/Vice President
Steve Rosol/Vice President Human Resources
Steve Rosol/Vice President, General Manager
Mktg./Adv.: Martin Smilo/Director Product Development
Shelly Thrower/Manager Advertising
Dana Agens/Manager Contract Sales
Dana Agens/Manager International & National Sales
Shelly Thrower/Manager International Marketing & Sales
Steve Rosol/Manager Market Research
Steve Rosol/Manager Sales Training
Juliette Smilo/Vice President Marketing
Production: Frank Cuaderno/Director Quality Assurance
Martin Smilo/Manager Materials
Juliette Smilo/Manager Regulatory Affairs
Frank Cuaderno/Plant Manager

Filter, Air	General
Laminar Air Flow Unit, Fixed (Air Curtain)	Chemistry

MARSH BELLOFRAM 800-727-5646
8019 Ohio River Blvd., Newell, WV 26050 304-387-1200
FDA Number: n/a *Fax:* 304-387-1212
E-mail: info@marshbellofram.com
Web site: www.marshbellofram.com
Medical Products Sales Volume: $5,000,000
Annual Revenue: $25-$50 Million
Total Employees: 500 *Marketing Staff:* 3 *Sales Staff:* 17
Ownership: Private
Quality System Registration Information: ISO9001
Produces/Sells CE-marked Devices: N
Distribution: Manufacturer Direct, Manufacturer Through Distributor, Manufacturer Through Manufacturer Reps, Exporter
General Admin.: Joe Colletti/President
Mktg./Adv.: Jeff Gamble/Manager Sales
Dwight Nafziger/Vice President Marketing & Sales

Gauge, Pressure	General
Regulator, Oxygen, Mechanical	General
Thermometer, Laboratory	Chemistry

MARSH/MARSHALLTOWN INSTRUMENTS
See Marsh Bellofram

MARSHALL MATTRESS COMPANY LIMITED 800-682-6861
83 Bakersfield St., 416-633-5543
North York, ONT M3J-1 Canada
FDA Number: n/a *Fax:* 416-633-9262
Year Founded: 1900
Total Employees: 25
Ownership: Private
Produces/Sells CE-marked Devices: N
Distribution: Manufacturer Direct, Exporter

MARTEC INC.
See Maxtec, Inc.

MARTECH MEDICAL PRODUCTS 215-256-8833
1500 Delp Dr., Harleysville, PA 19438
FDA Number: 2527072
Ownership: Private
Produces/Sells CE-marked Devices: N

Catheter, Hemodialysis	Gastroenterology/Urology
Catheter, Intravascular, Therapeutic, Long-term Greater Than 30 Days	General
Catheter, Peritoneal, Indwelling, Long-Term	Gastroenterology/Urology
Dilator, Vessel, Percutaneous Catheterization	Cardiovascular
Guidewire, Catheter	Cardiovascular
Introducer, Catheter	Cardiovascular
Stent, Ureteral	Gastroenterology/Urology
Stethoscope, Esophageal	Anesthesiology

MARTEK POWER 310-202-8820
1111 Knox Street, Torrance, CA 90503
FDA Number: n/a *Fax:* 310-836-4926
E-mail: sales@martekpower.com
Web site: www.martekpower.com
Annual Revenue: $10-$25 Million
Total Employees: 45 *Marketing Staff:* 5 *Sales Staff:* 5
Ownership: Private
Quality System Registration Information: ISO9002
Produces/Sells CE-marked Devices: Y
Federal Procurement Eligibility: Small Business
Distribution: Manufacturer Direct, Manufacturer Through Manufacturer Reps, OEM, Importer, Exporter
General Admin.: Angelo Lowprest/President
Mktg./Adv.: Mike Hesketh/Manager Advertising
Mike Hesketh/Vice President Marketing & Sales

Component, Electrical	General

MARTEK POWER   310-202-8820 *(cont'd)*
Computer Software   General

MARTIN TECHNOLOGY, LLC   901-682-1006
1505 South Perkins, Memphis, TN 38117-6530
FDA Number: 3006365733
Ownership: Private
Produces/Sells CE-marked Devices: N
Cap, Bone   Orthopedics

MARTIN USA INC.
See Berchtold Corp.

MARTIN WORLDWIDE INC.
See Bsn Medical, Inc

MARTIN-MARS, INC.   985-438-4402
415 Camelia Drive, Thibodaux, LA 70301-6508
FDA Number: 2320597   Fax: 985-868-1525
E-mail: davemarse@charter.net
Annual Revenue: $0-$1 Million
Year Founded: 1997
Ownership: Private
Produces/Sells CE-marked Devices: N
Federal Procurement Eligibility: Small Business
Distribution: Manufacturer Direct
Holder, Intravascular Catheter   General

MARVEL SCIENTIFIC   800-223-3900
PO Box 400, Greenville, MI 48838   616-754-5601
FDA Number: n/a   Fax: 616-754-9690
E-mail: emoore@marvelindustries.com
Web site: www.marvelscientific.com
Total Employees: 70   *Marketing Staff:* 3   *Sales Staff:* 3
Ownership: Northland Corporation
Produces/Sells CE-marked Devices: N
Federal Procurement Eligibility: Small Business, GSA Contract
Distribution: Manufacturer Through Distributor, OEM
General Admin.: Gordon Stauffer/Chief Executive Officer
    Richard Detrick/General Manager
Mktg./Adv.: Larry Ferguson/Director Marketing & Sales
    Ann Rohe/Manager Contract Sales
Dispenser, Ice   General
Freezer, Laboratory, General Purpose   Chemistry
Refrigerator, Biological   Microbiology

MASEL CO., INC.   800-423-8227
2701 Bartram Road, Bristol, PA 19007-6810   215-785-1600
FDA Number: n/a   Fax: 215-785-1680
E-mail: sales@masel.net
Web site: www.maselortho.com
Medical Products Sales Volume: $9,000,000
Year Founded: 1977
Total Employees: 50
Ownership: Private
Quality System Registration Information: ISO9002
Produces/Sells CE-marked Devices: Y
Federal Procurement Eligibility: Small Business
Distribution: Manufacturer Direct, Manufacturer Through Distributor
General Admin.: Ron Baron/General Manager
Mktg./Adv.: Kathy Perini/Manager Marketing
Aligner, Bracket, Orthodontic   Dental And Oral
Band, Elastic, Orthodontic   Dental And Oral
Denture, Gold   Dental And Oral
Face Bow   Dental And Oral
Headgear, Extraoral, Orthodontic   Dental And Oral
Mirror, Mouth   Dental And Oral
Mixer, Alginate   Dental And Oral
Mouthguard   Dental And Oral
Pliers, Orthodontic   Dental And Oral
Protector, Mouth Guard   Dental And Oral
Pusher, Band, Orthodontic   Dental And Oral
Wire, Orthodontic   Dental And Oral

MASIMO CORP.   800-326-4890
40, 50 & 60 Parker, Irvine, CA 92618   949-297-7000
FDA Number: 2031172   Fax: 949-297-7499
E-mail: tech@masimo.com
Web site: www.masimo.com
Medical Products Sales Volume: $80,000,000
Year Founded: 1989
Total Employees: 1000
Ownership: Public
Stock Symbol: MASI
Traded On: NASDAQ
Produces/Sells CE-marked Devices: Y
Distribution: Manufacturer Direct, Manufacturer Through Distributor, Manufacturer Through Manufacturer Reps, OEM, Exclusive Distributor, Importer, Exporter
General Admin.: Mr. Joe Kiani/Chief Executive Officer, Chairman
    Mr. Tony Allan/Chief Operating Officer

MASIMO CORP.   800-326-4890 *(cont'd)*
Rick Fishel/President
Mr. Jon Coleman/Vice President
Medical Admin.: Dr. Michael O'Reilly/Vice President Medical Affairs
Mktg./Adv.: Mr. Paul Jansen/Executive Vice President Marketing
Production: Mr. Yongsam Lee/Executive Vice President Quality Assurance & Regulatory Affairs
Research: Mr. Anand Sampath/Vice President Engineering
Finance: Mr. Mark de Raad/Chief Financial Officer
Cable/Lead, ECG, With Transducer And Electrode   Cardiovascular
Oximeter, Ear   Cardiovascular
Oximeter, Intracardiac   Cardiovascular
Oxyhemoglobin/Carboxyhemoglobin Curve, Carbon-Monoxide   Toxicology
System, Network And Communication, Physiological Monitors   Cardiovascular

MASON CHEMICAL   800-362-1855
721 W. Algonquin Rd.,   847-290-1621
Arlington Heights, IL 60005
FDA Number: n/a   Fax: 847-290-1625
E-mail: mason@maquat.com
Web site: www.maquat.com
Annual Revenue: $0-$1 Million
Total Employees: 10   *Marketing Staff:* 7   *Sales Staff:* 7
Ownership: Private
Produces/Sells CE-marked Devices: N
Federal Procurement Eligibility: Small Business
Distribution: Manufacturer Direct, Service Direct
General Admin.: Mark Mason/President
Disinfector, Liquid   General
Solution, Antibacterial Cleaner   General

MASON DENTAL MIDWEST, INC.   734-525-1070
12752 Stark Road, Livonia, MI 48150
FDA Number: 87390
Ownership: Private
Produces/Sells CE-marked Devices: N
Crown, Preformed   Dental And Oral
Teeth, Porcelain   Dental And Oral

MAST BIOSURGERY USA INC.   858-550-8050
6749 Top Gun St., Suite 108, San Diego, CA 92121
FDA Number: 3004661493
Ownership: Private
Produces/Sells CE-marked Devices: N
Mesh, Surgical, Polymeric   Surgery
Pledget And Intracardiac Patch, PETP, PTFE, Polypropylene   Cardiovascular

MAST/KEYSTONE VIEW   800-806-6569
2200 Dickerson Rd., Reno, NV 89503   775-324-2799
FDA Number: 1926420   Fax: 775-324-5375
E-mail: sales@keystoneview.com
Web site: www.keystoneview.com
Medical Products Sales Volume: $3,000,000
Total Employees: 50   *Marketing Staff:* 1   *Sales Staff:* 2
Ownership: Private
Produces/Sells CE-marked Devices: Y
Federal Procurement Eligibility: Small Business, Female Owned
Distribution: Manufacturer Direct, Manufacturer Through Distributor, Manufacturer Through Manufacturer Reps
General Admin.: G. Mast/Chief Executive Officer
Mktg./Adv.: Eric Mast/Director Marketing
    Eric Mast/Manager International & National Sales
Analyzer, Visual Function   Ophthalmology
Chart, Visual Acuity   Ophthalmology
Measurer, Stereopsis   Ophthalmology
Perimeter, AC-Powered   Ophthalmology
Perimeter, Manual   Ophthalmology
Stereoscope, AC-Powered   Ophthalmology
Target, Fusion/Stereoscopic   Ophthalmology
Tester, Color Vision   Ophthalmology

MASTEL PRECISION, INC.   800-657-8057
2843 Samco Road, Suite A,   605-341-4595
Rapid City, SD 57702
FDA Number: 9005641   Fax: 605-343-3631
E-mail: mastel@mastel.com
Web site: www.mastel.com
Medical Products Sales Volume: $820,000
Year Founded: 1991
Total Employees: 11
Ownership: Private
Produces/Sells CE-marked Devices: N
Federal Procurement Eligibility: Small Business
Distribution: Manufacturer Direct, Service Direct
Knife, Ophthalmic   Ophthalmology
Marker, Ocular   Ophthalmology
Spectacle Microscope, Low-Vision   Ophthalmology

MASTER BOND INC.   201-343-8983
154 Hobart Street, Hackensack, NJ 07601
FDA Number: n/a   *Fax:* 201-343-2132
E-mail: technical@masterbond.com
Web site: www.masterbond.com
Year Founded: 1976
Ownership: Private
Produces/Sells CE-marked Devices: N
Distribution: Service Direct

Adhesive, Liquid	General
Encapsulator, Fluid	General

MASTER BOND, INC.   201-343-8983
154 Hobart St., Hackensack, NJ 07601
FDA Number: n/a   *Fax:* 201-343-2132
E-mail: main@masterbond.com
Web site: www.masterbond.com
Annual Revenue: $1-$5 Million
Ownership: Private
Produces/Sells CE-marked Devices: N
Federal Procurement Eligibility: Small Business
Distribution: Manufacturer Direct
General Admin.: David Mushabac/Chief Executive Officer
         Walter Brenner/President
         Susan Carol/Vice President Human Resources
Mktg./Adv.: Marvin Goldman/Manager Advertising
         James Brenner/Vice President Marketing
         Robert Michaels/Vice President Sales
Production: John Policht/Vice President Manufacturing
Research: Sam Rahman/Vice President Research & Development

Adhesive, Liquid	General
Component, Other	General
Component, Silicone	General
Packaging Equipment	General

MASTER CRAFT LABS   800-233-1413
102 Main St., P.o. Box 11, Bethel, MN 55005
FDA Number: 2182344

Hearing-Aid, Plate, Face	Ear/Nose/Throat

MASTER MEDICAL CORP., THE
    See Conmed Corporation

MASTER SALES CORP.
    See Stinson Manufacturing

MASTERCARE PATIENT EQUIPMENT, INC.   800-798-5867
2071 14th Ave., PO Box 1435,   402-564-5867
Columbus, NE 68601
FDA Number: 3003336913   *Fax:* 402-563-9102
E-mail: mastercarepeinc@frontiernet.net
Web site: www.mastercarebath.net
Ownership: Private
Produces/Sells CE-marked Devices: N

Lift, Bath, Non-AC-Powered	General
Scale, Infant	General
Transfer Device, Patient, Manual	General

MASTERCRAFT DENTAL CO. OF TEXAS   972-775-8757
880 Eastgate Rd., PO Box 882, Midlothian, TX 76065
FDA Number: 1625854
Annual Revenue: $1-$5 Million
Ownership: Private
Produces/Sells CE-marked Devices: N
Federal Procurement Eligibility: Small Business
Distribution: Manufacturer Through Distributor, Manufacturer Through
Manufacturer Reps, OEM, Service Direct, Exclusive Distributor

Cabinet, Dental	Dental And Oral
Chair, Dental	Dental And Oral
Operative Dental Treatment Unit	Dental And Oral

MASTERCRAFT DIV., LANCER PACIFIC
    See Mastercraft Dental Co. Of Texas

MASTERCRAFT MEDICAL & INDUSTRIAL CORP.
    See Mastercraft Products Corporation

MASTERCRAFT OF SEATTLE   206-768-1297
300 South Bennett St., Seattle, WA 98108
FDA Number: 3006138110   *Fax:* 206-768-1301
E-mail: info@mastercraftofseattle.com
Web site: www.mastercraftofseattle.com
Ownership: Private
Produces/Sells CE-marked Devices: N

Pack, Hot Or Cold, Reusable	Physical Med

MASTERCRAFT PRODUCTS CORPORATION   800-874-6094
5797 Lake Winona Rd,   386-985-4667
De Leon Springs, FL 32130
FDA Number: n/a   *Fax:* 386-985-0202
E-mail: office@mastercraftplastics.com

MASTERCRAFT PRODUCTS CORPORATION   800-874-6094
(cont'd)
Web site: www.mastercraftplastics.com
Annual Revenue: $1-$5 Million
Year Founded: 1944
Total Employees: 20
Ownership: Private
Stock Symbol: MPCP
Traded On: OTC Bulletin
Produces/Sells CE-marked Devices: N
Federal Procurement Eligibility: Small Business, Female Owned
Distribution: Manufacturer Through Distributor
General Admin.: A. David Logan/President
         Joyce Monaco/Vice President Human Resources

Bassinet (Infant Bed)	General

MASTERMAN'S   800-525-3313
11 C Street, PO BOX 411, Auburn, MA 01501-0411
FDA Number: n/a   *Fax:* 800-525-0396
E-mail: cs@mastermans.com
Web site: www.mastermans.com
Year Founded: 1961
Ownership: Private
Quality System Registration Information: ISO9000
Produces/Sells CE-marked Devices: N
Federal Procurement Eligibility: Small Business
Distribution: Manufacturer Through Distributor

Apron, Laboratory	Chemistry
Clothing, Protective	General
Eyeglasses, Safety	Ophthalmology
Glove, Utility	General
Housekeeping Equipment	General
Mask, Face	General
Protector, Hearing (Insert)	Ear/Nose/Throat
Sign, Hospital	General
Towel/Towelette, Paper	General
Ventilator, Other	Anesthesiology

MASTERQUEST INTERNATIONAL   315-298-2904
801 Hammond Street Suite 200, Coppell, TX 75019
FDA Number: 1000634072
Ownership: Private
Produces/Sells CE-marked Devices: N

Equipment, Cleaning, Air	General

MAT AUTOMOTIVE   847-821-9630
625 Barclay Boulevard, Lincolnshire, IL 60069
FDA Number: n/a   *Fax:* 847-821-9644
Ownership: Private
Produces/Sells CE-marked Devices: N

Bed, Electric	General
Bed, Manual	General

MATAMATIC INC.   888-696-5678
230 Westec Drive, Mount Pleasant, PA 15666
FDA Number: n/a   *Fax:* 888-696-5661
Web site: www.matamatic.com
Ownership: Private
Produces/Sells CE-marked Devices: N

Accessories, Wheelchair	Physical Med
Monitor, Bed Patient	General

MATEC INSTRUMENT COMPANIES, INC.   508-393-0155
56 Hudson St., Northborough, MA 01532
FDA Number: n/a   *Fax:* 508-393-5476
E-mail: sales@matec.com
Web site: www.matec.com
Medical Products Sales Volume: $6,000,000
Annual Revenue: $1-$5 Million
Total Employees: 30   *Marketing Staff:* 2   *Sales Staff:* 4
Ownership: Private
Produces/Sells CE-marked Devices: Y
Federal Procurement Eligibility: Small Business
Distribution: Manufacturer Direct, Exporter
General Admin.: Kenneth Bishop/President
         Gene Murray/Vice President Human Resources
         Gabriel Des Ramos/Vice President, General Manager
Mktg./Adv.: Michael Bliss/Coord. Marketing

Analyzer, Particle	Chemistry

MATECH   818-991-8500
31304 Via Colinas, Suite 102, Westlake, CA 91362
FDA Number: 2031831

Fluorometer, Chemistry	Chemistry

MATECH, INC.   818-367-2472
13000 San Fernando Rd., Sylmar, CA 91342
FDA Number: 2022626

Alloy, Precious Metal, For Clinical Use	Dental And Oral

MATECH, INC.
818-367-2472 *(cont'd)*
Material, Impression	Dental And Oral
Metal, Base	Dental And Oral

MATERIALS DEVELOPMENT CORPORATION
781-391-0400
81 Hicks Avenue, Medford, MA 02155-6318
FDA Number: n/a
Fax: 781-391-7964
E-mail: info@materialsdevelopment.com
Web site: www.materialsdevelopment.com
Annual Revenue: $0-$1 Million
Total Employees: 5   *Marketing Staff:* 1   *Sales Staff:* 2
Ownership: Private
Produces/Sells CE-marked Devices: N
Federal Procurement Eligibility: Small Business, Minority Owned
Distribution: Manufacturer Through Distributor, Importer, Exporter
General Admin.: Richard Y. S. Chen/President, Chief Executive Officer
Mktg./Adv.: Richard Y. S. Chen/Vice President Marketing & Sales
Production: Richard Y. S. Chen/Vice President Manufacturing
Research: Wei Gu/Research Scientist
    Wei Gu/Vice President Research & Development
Lens, Contact (Other Material)	Ophthalmology

MATERNAL CARE, INC.
678-770-4355
11585 Jones Bridge Rd., Suite 420-216, Alpharetta, GA 30022
FDA Number: n/a
Ownership: Private
Produces/Sells CE-marked Devices: N
Pack, Hot Or Cold, Reusable	Physical Med

MATHESON TRI-GAS, INC.
972-893-5600
8200 Washington N.E., Albuquerque, NM 87113
FDA Number: 1619650
Ownership: Private
Produces/Sells CE-marked Devices: N
Box, Glove	Microbiology
Gas, Calibrated (Specified Concentration)	Anesthesiology
Laser, Surgical	Surgery

MATHESON TRI-GAS, INC.
713-869-7351
2200 Houston Ave., Houston, TX 77007
FDA Number: 1625735
Fax: 713-869-4929
Web site: www.mathesongas.com
Ownership: Private
Produces/Sells CE-marked Devices: N
Gas, Calibrated (Specified Concentration)	Anesthesiology
Gas, Laser Generating	Surgery

MATHISON INDUSTRIES, INC.
775-284-1020
220 Coney Island Drive, Sparks, NV 89431
FDA Number: 2020491
Ownership: Private
Produces/Sells CE-marked Devices: N
Band, Elastic, Orthodontic	Dental And Oral
Chair, With Casters	Physical Med

MATLOCK ENDOSCOPIC REPAIRS, SALES, AND SERVICE, INC.
800-394-9822
4320 Kenilwood Drive,, Suite 107, Nashville, TN 37204
615-831-5268
FDA Number: n/a
Fax: 615-831-5271
E-mail: info@matlockendo.com
Web site: www.matlockendo.com
Medical Products Sales Volume: $670,000
Annual Revenue: $0-$1 Million
Year Founded: 1991
Total Employees: 7
Ownership: Private
Produces/Sells CE-marked Devices: N
Federal Procurement Eligibility: Small Business
Distribution: Manufacturer Direct, Manufacturer Through Manufacturer Reps, Importer, Exporter
General Admin.: Nichole Hawkins/Office Manager
    William Matlock/President
Mktg./Adv.: Doyle Merhoff/Vice President Sales
Endoscope	Gastroenterology/Urology
Endoscope, Flexible	Gastroenterology/Urology
Service, Repair, Endoscopic	General

MATREYA LLC
800-342-3595
168 Tressler St., Pleasant Gap, PA 16823-3218
814-359-5060
FDA Number: n/a
Fax: 814-359-5062
E-mail: customerservice@matreya.com
Web site: www.matreya.com
Total Employees: 10   *Marketing Staff:* 1   *Sales Staff:* 1
Ownership: Private
Produces/Sells CE-marked Devices: N
Federal Procurement Eligibility: Small Business
Distribution: Manufacturer Direct

MATREYA LLC
800-342-3595 *(cont'd)*
Chromatographic Derivative, Total Lipids	Chemistry

MATRITECH, INC.
617-928-0820
330 Nevada St., Newton, MA 02460
FDA Number: n/a
Fax: 617-928-0821
Web site: www.matritech.com
Medical Products Sales Volume: $2,000,000
Annual Revenue: $1-$5 Million
Year Founded: 1987
Ownership: Private
Produces/Sells CE-marked Devices: N
Federal Procurement Eligibility: Small Business
Distribution: Manufacturer Direct, Manufacturer Through Distributor
General Admin.: Stephen D. Chubb/Chief Executive Officer, Chairman
    Richard A. Sandberg/Chief Financial Officer, Vice President
    David L. Corbet/President, Chief Operating Officer
    Patricia Randall/Vice President General Counsel & Secretary
Medical Admin.: Melodie R. Domurad/Vice President Clinical Affairs
Mktg./Adv.: John E. Quigley/Vice President Marketing
    David G. Kolasinski/Vice President Sales
Research: Gary Fagan/Vice President Research & Development
Test, Cancer Detection, Other	Hematology

MATRIX INSTRUMENTS, INC.
See Agfa Corp.

MATRIX TECHNOLOGIES CORPORATION
1 800 345 0206
22 Friars Drive, Hudson, NH 03051
1 603 595 0505
FDA Number: 3004419158
Fax: 1 603 595 0106
Ownership: Private
Produces/Sells CE-marked Devices: N
Block, Heating	Chemistry
Equipment, Laboratory, Gen. Purpose (Specific Medical Use)	Chemistry
Pipette, Micro	Chemistry
Pipetting And Diluting System, Automated	Chemistry
Station Pipetting	Chemistry

MATROX ELECTRONIC SYSTEMS, LTD.
800-804-6243
1055 St. Regis Blvd.,
514-685-2630
Dorval, QUE H9P 2 Canada
FDA Number: n/a
Fax: 514-822-6273
E-mail: imaging.info@matrox.com
Web site: www.matrox.com/imaging
Total Employees: 1300
Ownership: Private
Produces/Sells CE-marked Devices: N
Distribution: Manufacturer Through Manufacturer Reps

MATRX
716-662-6650
145 Mid County Dr., Orchard Park, NY 14127
FDA Number: 1381607
Attachment, Breathing, Positive End Expiratory Pressure	Anesthesiology
Bag, Reservoir (Blood)	Anesthesiology
Bottle, Collection, Vacuum (Aspirator)	General
Dressing, Other	General
Gas-Machine, Anesthesia	Anesthesiology
Mask, Oxygen, Aerosol Administration	Anesthesiology
Mask, Scavenging	Anesthesiology
Regulator, Pressure, Gas Cylinder	Anesthesiology
Scavenger, Gas	Anesthesiology
Ventilator, Emergency, Manual (Resuscitator)	Anesthesiology
Ventilator, Emergency, Powered (Resuscitator)	Anesthesiology
Yoke, Medical Gas	Anesthesiology

MATRX BY MIDMARK
800-847-1000
145 Mid County Drive,
716-662-6650
Orchard Park, NY 14127
FDA Number: 9915004
Fax: 716-662-8440
E-mail: matrx@matrxmedical.com
Web site: www.matrxmedical.com
Annual Revenue: $10-$25 Million
Total Employees: 100   *Marketing Staff:* 2   *Sales Staff:* 35
Ownership: Midmark Corporation
Quality System Registration Information: ISO9001
Produces/Sells CE-marked Devices: Y
Federal Procurement Eligibility: Small Business
Distribution: Manufacturer Through Distributor, Exporter
General Admin.: John Young/General Manager
Mktg./Adv.: William Hogan/Director Marketing & Sales
    Sandi Burgess/Manager Communications
Production: Mike Peccia/Manager Engineering
Finance: George Brunecz/Manager Finance
Bag, Breathing	Anesthesiology
Evacuator, Oral Cavity	Dental And Oral
Gas-Machine, Analgesia	Anesthesiology
Holder, Gas Cylinder	Anesthesiology
Regulator, Pressure, Gas Cylinder	Anesthesiology
Resuscitator, Emergency Oxygen	Dental And Oral

MATRX BY MIDMARK
800-847-1000 *(cont'd)*

Resuscitator, Pulmonary, Manual (Demand Valve) — General Anesthesiology
Yoke, Medical Gas

MATRX MEDICAL, INC.
See Matrx By Midmark

MAUCH LABORATORIES, INC.
See Mauch, Inc.

MAUCH, INC.
800-622-8742
937-299-8751

3035 Dryden Road, Dayton, OH 45439-1619
FDA Number: 1522546
Fax: 937-299-9694
E-mail: info@mauchinc.com
Web site: www.mauchinc.com
Total Employees: 50 — *Marketing Staff:* 2 — *Sales Staff:* 2
Ownership: FLEX-FOOT, INC.
Quality System Registration Information: ISO9001
Produces/Sells CE-marked Devices: Y
Federal Procurement Eligibility: Small Business
Distribution: Manufacturer Direct, Manufacturer Through Distributor, Exporter
General Admin.: William Phillips/President, Chief Executive Officer
Mktg./Adv.: Jon F. Bork/Director Marketing
Production: Mike Carroll/Director Quality Assurance
Chuck Jewell/Manager Customer Services
Finance: Patrick Pritchett/Chief Financial Officer
Joint, Knee, External Limb Component — Physical Med
Prosthesis, Joint, Other — Orthopedics

MAUI JIM SUNGLASSES INC.
See Rlisys Practice Solutions, Inc.

MAVEN MEDICAL MANUFACTURING, INC.
800-562-7326
727-518-0555

2250 Lake Ave. S.E., Largo, FL 33771
FDA Number: n/a
Fax: 727-518-0444
E-mail: mavenmed2@aol.com
Web site: /www.mavenmedical.us
Annual Revenue: $1-$5 Million
Total Employees: 24 — *Marketing Staff:* 2 — *Sales Staff:* 2
Ownership: Private
Produces/Sells CE-marked Devices: N
Federal Procurement Eligibility: Small Business
Distribution: Manufacturer Direct
General Admin.: Paul R. Vaughan/President
Pamela J. Vaughan/Vice President
Mktg./Adv.: Victoria Miller/Director Marketing
Victoria Miller/Manager Sales
Amy Vaughan/Marketing Representative
Pad, Pressure, Animal Skin — General

MAVERICK TECHNOLOGIES, INC.
727-791-6151

1754 Grove Drive, Clearwater, FL 33759
FDA Number: 1062919
Ownership: Private
Produces/Sells CE-marked Devices: N
Shield, Eye, Ophthalmic — Ophthalmology

MAVIDON MEDICAL PRODUCTS
800-654-0385
561-585-2227

1820 2nd Ave N, Lake Worth, FL 33461
FDA Number: 1064095
Fax: 888-913-4311
Web site: www.mavidon.com
Ownership: Private
Produces/Sells CE-marked Devices: N
Collodion — Pathology
Degreaser, Skin, Surgical — Surgery
Gel, Electrode, Stimulator — Cns/Neurology
Pack, Hot Or Cold, Reusable — Physical Med
Solution, Cement Dissolving — Dental And Oral
Solvent, Adhesive Tape — Surgery

MAX BLOOM, M.D.
401-785-9671

111 Roger Williams Cir., Cranston, RI 02905-1128
FDA Number: 1220610
Fax: 401-785-9671
E-mail: mbloom3@cox.net
Ownership: Private
Produces/Sells CE-marked Devices: N
Distribution: Manufacturer Direct
Stethoscope, Manual — Cardiovascular

MAX ENDOSCOPY INC.
330-425-7041

1410 Highland Road, Suite 6, Macedonia, OH 44056
FDA Number: 3006457890
Ownership: Private
Produces/Sells CE-marked Devices: N
Accessories, Cleaning Brushes (For Endoscope) — Gastroenterology/Urology

MAXANT TECHNOLOGIES, INC.
800-307-4190
847-588-2280

7540 Caldwell Avenue, Niles, IL 60714
FDA Number: 9914043
Fax: 847-588-1920
E-mail: info@maxant.com
Web site: www.maxant.com

MAXANT TECHNOLOGIES, INC.
800-307-4190 *(cont'd)*

Medical Products Sales Volume: $2,500,000
Annual Revenue: $5-$10 Million
Year Founded: 1984
Total Employees: 31 — *Marketing Staff:* 2 — *Sales Staff:* 2
Ownership: Private
Quality System Registration Information: ISO9002
Produces/Sells CE-marked Devices: N
Federal Procurement Eligibility: Small Business
Distribution: Manufacturer Through Distributor
General Admin.: Mr. Lars Wilhelm/Chairman
Mr. John Patterson/Chief Operating Officer, Executive Vice President
Mr. R. F. Sturgis/President, Chief Executive Officer
Mktg./Adv.: Mr. Andy Hansen/National Sales Representative
Mrs. Karla Forster/Sales Associate
Production: Mrs. Linda Niewierowski/Customer Service Representative
Mr. Romero Patino/Product Manager
Mrs. Marie Brown/Supervisor Customer Service
Purchasing: Mr. Rick Wilhelm/Purchasing Agent
Illuminator, Radiographic Film — Radiology

MAXCOR INC
(877) ENDO MAX
(330) 425-7041

17517 Fabrica Way, Suite H,
Artesia, CA 90703
FDA Number: 3007009425
Fax: (330) 425-7040
E-mail: info@maxendoscopy.com
Web site: www.maxendoscopy.com
Ownership: Private
Produces/Sells CE-marked Devices: N
Stent, Cardiovascular — Cardiovascular

MAXCYTE INC.
301-944-1700

22 Firstfield Road, Suite 110, Gaithersburg, MD 20878
FDA Number: n/a
Fax: 301-944-1703
E-mail: info@maxcyte.com
Web site: http://www.maxcyte.com
Year Founded: 1999
Ownership: Private
Produces/Sells CE-marked Devices: N
General Admin.: Mr. Douglas Doerfler/President, Chief Executive Officer
Mktg./Adv.: Dr. Karen Donato/Executive Vice President Marketing & Sales
Finance: Mr. Ronald Holtz/Chief Financial Officer

MAXIFLEX, LLC
866-629-4359
(504) 265-8972

1516 Thalia St, New Orleans, LA 70130
FDA Number: 3006812215
Fax: 504) 265-8977
E-mail: customerservice@maxiflexllc.com
Ownership: Private
Produces/Sells CE-marked Devices: N
Ureteroscope — Gastroenterology/Urology

MAXILL INC.
1-800-268-8633
519-631-7370

80 Elm St., St. Thomas, ONT N5R-6C8 Canada
FDA Number: n/a
Fax: 519-631-3388
E-mail: info@maxill.com
Web site: www.maxill.com
Year Founded: 1988
Total Employees: 25
Ownership: Private
Produces/Sells CE-marked Devices: N
Distribution: Manufacturer Direct, Exporter

MAXILON LABORATORIES, INC.
603-594-9300

105 State Rt. 101a, Unit 8, Amherst, NH 03031
FDA Number: 1225686
Rasp, Surgical, General & Plastic Surgery — Surgery

MAXIM BIOMEDICAL INCORPORATED
301-251-0800

1500 East Gude Dr., Suite A, Rockville, MD 20850
FDA Number: 1122236
Fax: 301-217-9080
E-mail: info_mbi@mbidiagnostic.com
Web site: www.mbidiagnostic.com
Ownership: Private
Produces/Sells CE-marked Devices: N
Kit, Western Blot, Hiv-1 — Hematology
Test, Hiv Detection — Immunology

MAXIMUM DENTAL, INC.
631-245-2176

600 Meadowlands Parkway, Suite 269, Secaucus, NJ 07094
FDA Number: 3006251816
Fax: 201 955 3300
E-mail: info@dentalmaximum.com
Ownership: Private
Produces/Sells CE-marked Devices: N
File, Pulp Canal, Endodontic — Dental And Oral
Gutta Percha — Dental And Oral
Motor, Surgical Instrument, AC-Powered — Surgery
Pump, Suction Operatory — Dental And Oral

MAXIMUM DENTAL, INC.   **631-245-2176** *(cont'd)*
Scaler, Periodontic   Dental And Oral

MAXPAK, LLC   **863-682-0123**
2808 New Tampa Hwy., Lakeland, FL 33815
FDA Number: 3006227415
Bandage, Adhesive	Surgery
Bandage, Elastic	General
Gauze/sponge, Nonresorbable For External Use	Surgery
Protectant, Skin	Surgery
Strip, Adhesive	Surgery

MAXTEC, INC.   **800-748-5355**
6526 S. Cottonwood St.,   **801-266-5300**
Salt Lake City, UT 84107
FDA Number: 1722070   *Fax:* 801-270-5590
E-mail: sales@maxtecinc.com
Web site: www.maxtecinc.com
Medical Products Sales Volume: $8,700,000
Annual Revenue: $5-$10 Million
Year Founded: 1991
Total Employees: 44   *Marketing Staff:* 6   *Sales Staff:* 6
Ownership: Private
Quality System Registration Information: ISO9001
Produces/Sells CE-marked Devices: Y
Federal Procurement Eligibility: Small Business, GSA Contract
Distribution: Manufacturer Direct, Manufacturer Through Distributor, Manufacturer Through Manufacturer Reps, OEM, Service Direct, Importer, Exporter
General Admin.: Mr. Bruce Brierly/Chief Executive Officer
Production: Mr. Alan Boardman/Manager Manufacturing & Engineering
     Ms. Tammy Lavery/Manager Quality Assurance & Regulatory Affairs
Finance: Ms. Mary Brierly/Chief Financial Officer
Analyzer, Gas, Oxygen, Continuous Controller	Anesthesiology
Analyzer, Gas, Oxygen, Continuous Monitor	Anesthesiology
Mixer, Breathing Gases, Anesthesia Inhalation	Anesthesiology
Sensor, Oxygen	Anesthesiology

MAXWELL TECHNOLOGIES POWER SYSTEMS   **877-511-4324**
9244 Balboa Avenue, San Diego, CA 92123   **858-503-3300**
FDA Number: n/a   *Fax:* 858-503-3301
E-mail: sales@maxwell.com
Web site: www.maxwell.com
Medical Products Sales Volume: $53,900,000
Annual Revenue: $50-$100 Million
Year Founded: 1965
Total Employees: 241   *Marketing Staff:* 5   *Sales Staff:* 10
Ownership: MAXWELL TECHNOLOGIES, INC.
Stock Symbol: MXWL
Traded On: NASDAQ
Quality System Registration Information: ISO9001
Produces/Sells CE-marked Devices: Y
Federal Procurement Eligibility: Small Business
Distribution: Manufacturer Direct, Exporter
General Admin.: Richard Balanson/Chief Executive Officer
     Pam Nichols/Vice President Human Resources
Mktg./Adv.: Gary Jasinski/Director New Business Development
     Robert Tressler/Executive Vice President Marketing & Sales
     Deb Buckley/Manager Advertising
Battery	General
Control System, Energy	General
Power System, Isolated	General
Power Systems, Uninterruptible (UPS)	General

MAXXVISION, LLC   **1-877-340-6483**
2800 Aurora Avenue, Suite E,   **321-752-5578**
Melbourne, FL 32935
FDA Number: n/a   *Fax:* 352-378-0273
Web site: www.maxxvisionmedical.com
Medical Products Sales Volume: $350,000
Annual Revenue: $0-$1 Million
Year Founded: 1989
Total Employees: 6   *Marketing Staff:* 1
Ownership: Private
Quality System Registration Information: ISO9002
Produces/Sells CE-marked Devices: N
Federal Procurement Eligibility: Small Business
Distribution: Manufacturer Through Distributor
General Admin.: Mr. Fredric Derwitsch/President, Chief Operating Officer
Mktg./Adv.: Mrs. Rose Cauchon/Director Marketing
Image Digitizer	Radiology

MAY CORP.   **218-294-6700**
103 E. Espelee Street, Grygla, MN 56727
FDA Number: n/a
Ownership: Private
Produces/Sells CE-marked Devices: N
Chair, With Casters	Physical Med

MAYCLIN DENTAL STUDIO, INC.   **952-926-1809**
7505 Hwy 7, Suite 100, St. Louis Park, MN 55426
FDA Number: 3004894612
Crown, Preformed	Dental And Oral

MAYO MEDICAL, S.A. DE C.V.   **800-715-3872**
Edison 1141 Nte., Col. Talleres,   **52 8 123-0005**
Monterrey N.L. 64480 Mexico
FDA Number: n/a   *Fax:* 52 8 333-8009
E-mail: mayomedical@infosel.com
Web site: www.mayomedical.com.mx
Medical Products Sales Volume: $700,000
Total Employees: 6   *Marketing Staff:* 2   *Sales Staff:* 4
Ownership: Private
Federal Procurement Eligibility: Small Business
Distribution: Manufacturer Through Distributor, Manufacturer Through Manufacturer Reps, Importer, Exporter

MAYON PLASTICS, INC.   **612-935-2187**
1595 K Tel Dr, Hopkins, MN 55343-7280
FDA Number: 2120149   *Fax:* 612-935-2188
E-mail: rayjohnson@qwest.net
Web site: www.mayonplastics.com
Medical Products Sales Volume: $1,000,000
Annual Revenue: $0-$1 Million
Total Employees: 10   *Marketing Staff:* 1   *Sales Staff:* 1
Ownership: Private
Produces/Sells CE-marked Devices: N
Federal Procurement Eligibility: Small Business
Distribution: Manufacturer Direct, Manufacturer Through Distributor, OEM, Exporter
General Admin.: Ray D. Johnson/President, Chief Executive Officer
Mktg./Adv.: Ray D. Johnson/Director Marketing
     Ray D. Johnoson/Director National Accounts
     Ray D. Hohnson/Director Product Development
     Ray D. Johnson/Manager Sales
Production: Ray D. Johnson/Director Quality Assurance
Tube, Pump, Cardiopulmonary Bypass	Cardiovascular
Tubing, Flexible, Medical Gas, Low-Pressure	Anesthesiology
Tubing, Polyvinyl Chloride	General
Tubing, Vinyl	General

MAYTEX CORP.   **800-462-9839**
23521 Foley Street, Hayward, CA 94545   **510-887-4888**
FDA Number: 2939286   *Fax:* 510-786-0209
E-mail: sales@maytexcorp.com
Web site: www.maytexcorp.com
Medical Products Sales Volume: $1,200,000
Year Founded: 1988
Total Employees: 7   *Marketing Staff:* 1   *Sales Staff:* 2
Ownership: Private
Quality System Registration Information: ISO9002
Produces/Sells CE-marked Devices: N
Federal Procurement Eligibility: Small Business, Minority Owned
Distribution: Manufacturer Through Distributor, Importer
Mktg./Adv.: Joseph Tung/Vice President Marketing & Sales
Cap, Surgical	Surgery
Coat, Laboratory	General
Cover, Shoe, Operating Room	Surgery
Glove, Patient Examination, Latex	General
Glove, Patient Examination, Vinyl	General
Gown, Surgical	Surgery
Mask, Face	General

MAZOR ROBOTICS LTD.   **800-706-2967**
4361 Shackleford Rd., Norcross, GA 30093   **770-564-5790**
FDA Number: 3006046610   *Fax:* 770-564-5791
E-mail: usa@mazorst.com
Web site: www.mazorst.com
Year Founded: 2001
Ownership: Private
Produces/Sells CE-marked Devices: N
General Admin.: Ori Hadomi/Chief Executive Officer
     Nancy Sousa/Chief Operating Officer
     Moshe Shoham/Chief Technology Officer
Mktg./Adv.: Ave Posen/Vice President International Marketing & Sales
     Dr. Doron Dinstein/Vice President Marketing
Finance: Ms. Sharon Levita/Chief Financial Officer

MAZOR SURGICAL TECHNOLOGIES INC.
See Mazor Robotics Ltd.

MBF SALES, LLC   **480-422-6742**
7025 E Greenway Parkway, #250, Scottsdale, AZ 85254
FDA Number: 2032642
Ownership: Private
Produces/Sells CE-marked Devices: N

MANUFACTURER PROFILES

MBF SALES, LLC   **480-422-6742** *(cont'd)*
Radiographic Unit, Diagnostic, Mammographic   Radiology

MBI FERMENTAS INC.   **800-340-9026**
830 Harrington Ct.,   **905-690-0800**
Burlington, ONT L7N-3 Canada
FDA Number: n/a   *Fax:* 905-690-0802
E-mail: fermentas.info@thermofisher.com
Web site: www.fermentas.com
Year Founded: 1996
Ownership: Private
Produces/Sells CE-marked Devices: N
Distribution: Manufacturer Direct, Exclusive Distributor

MBI, INC.   **702-259-1999**
1353 Arville St., Las Vegas, NV 89102-1608
FDA Number: 2937892
Ownership: Private
Produces/Sells CE-marked Devices: N
  Radiographic Unit, Diagnostic   Radiology

MCAIRLAID'S INC.   **540-352-5050**
180 Corporate Drive, Rocky Mount, VA 24151
FDA Number: 3005975572   *Fax:* 1 540 352 5053
Ownership: Private
Produces/Sells CE-marked Devices: N
  Linen, Bed   General

MCARTHUR MEDICAL SALES INC.   **800-996-6674**
1846 5th Concession W., P.O. Box 7,   **519-622-4030**
Rockton, ONT L0R-1 Canada
FDA Number: n/a   *Fax:* 519-622-1142
E-mail: mmsi@mcarthurmedical.com
Web site: www.mcarthurmedical.com
Year Founded: 1984
Total Employees: 10
Ownership: Private
Produces/Sells CE-marked Devices: N
Distribution: Exclusive Distributor, Importer

MCCARTY'S SACRO-EASE LLC   **800-635-3557**
3329 Industrial Avenue,   **208-765-8408**
Coeur D'Alene, ID 83815
FDA Number: 2912738   *Fax:* 208-664-6891
E-mail: sacroease@aol.com
Web site: www.mccartys.com
Medical Products Sales Volume: $2,100,000
Annual Revenue: $1-$5 Million
Year Founded: 1940
Total Employees: 20   *Marketing Staff:* 1   *Sales Staff:* 2
Ownership: Private
Produces/Sells CE-marked Devices: N
Federal Procurement Eligibility: Small Business
Distribution: Manufacturer Direct, Manufacturer Through Manufacturer Reps, Exporter
General Admin.: Michele Dirks/President
Mktg./Adv.: Kerry Standish/Director Marketing
       Kerry Standish/Director National Accounts
  Back Rest   General
  Cushion, Other   General
  Pillow, Cervical   Orthopedics
  Support, Back   Orthopedics
  Support, Patient Position   Anesthesiology

MCCLURE INDUSTRIES, INC.   **800-752-2821**
9051 S.E. 55th Ave., Portland, OR 97206-0605   **503-777-2821**
FDA Number: n/a   *Fax:* 503-775-2828
E-mail: sanitrux@aol.com
Web site: www.mcclureindustries.com
Annual Revenue: $5-$10 Million
Total Employees: 30   *Marketing Staff:* 3   *Sales Staff:* 3
Ownership: Private
Produces/Sells CE-marked Devices: N
Federal Procurement Eligibility: Small Business
Distribution: Manufacturer Direct
General Admin.: Delmar McClure/President
Mktg./Adv.: Tom Mac Laren/Director Marketing
  Accessories, Cart, Multipurpose   General
  Cart, Housekeeping   General
  Cart, Laundry   General
  Cart, Multipurpose   General
  Cart, Other   General
  Cart, Waste   General
  Unloader, Cart   General
  Washer, Cart   General

MCCONNELL ORTHOPEDIC MFG. CO.   **513-573-0085**
1324 East Interstate 30 Bldg. B, Floyd, TX 75401
FDA Number: 1641643
  Accessories, Operating Room, Table   Surgery
  Support, Arm   Physical Med
  Support, Patient Position   Anesthesiology

MCCRONE MICROSCOPES & ACCESSORIES   **800-622-8122**
850 Pasquinelli Drive, Westmont, IL 60559   **630-887-7100**
FDA Number: n/a   *Fax:* 630-887-7764
E-mail: mma@mccrone.com
Web site: www.mccronemicroscopes.com
Medical Products Sales Volume: $2,500,000
Annual Revenue: $0-$1 Million
Year Founded: 1956
Ownership: MCCRONE ASSOCIATES, INC.
Produces/Sells CE-marked Devices: N
Federal Procurement Eligibility: Small Business
Distribution: Manufacturer Direct, Importer, Exporter
General Admin.: Don Brooks/President
Mktg./Adv.: David Wiley/Vice President Marketing & Sales
Production: Chuck Zona/Director Operations
       Charles Zona/Manager Operations
  Cabinet, Storage, Slide   General
  Coverslip, Microscope Slide   Pathology
  Equipment, Laboratory, Gen. Purpose (Specific Medical Use)   Chemistry
  Television Monitor, Microscope   General

MCDALT MEDICAL CORP.   **800-841-5774**
2225 Prestonwood Drive,, SUite 100-A,   **817-461-8558**
Arlington, TX 76012
FDA Number: 1646952   *Fax:* 817-801-0330
E-mail: info@McDaltMedical.com
Web site: www.mcdalemedical.com
Medical Products Sales Volume: $900,000
Annual Revenue: $1-$5 Million
Year Founded: 1992
Total Employees: 7   *Marketing Staff:* 2   *Sales Staff:* 6
Ownership: Private
Produces/Sells CE-marked Devices: N
Federal Procurement Eligibility: Small Business
Distribution: Exclusive Distributor, Importer
General Admin.: T. S. McDonald/President, Chief Executive Officer
Mktg./Adv.: J. Campbell/Manager Contract Sales
Production: D. Brown/Manager Materials
       D. Walden/Manager Regulatory Affairs
  Analyzer, Concentration, Oxyhemoglobin, BP, Transcutaneous   Cardiovascular
  Applicator, Radionuclide, Manual   Radiology
  Apron, Lead, Radiographic   Radiology
  Biopsy Instrument   Gastroenterology/Urology
  Device, Closure, Puncture, Hemostatic   Cardiovascular
  Guidewire   Cardiovascular
  Needle, Biopsy, Mammary   Obstetrics/Gynecology
  Storage Unit, X-Ray Film   Radiology
  Telemetry Unit, Physiological, ECG   Cardiovascular
  Warmer, Infusion Fluid, Thermal   General

MCGHAN MEDICAL CORP.
  See Allergan

MCGILL AIRPRESSURE CORP.   **614-829-1200**
1777 Refugee Road, Columbus, OH 43207-2119
FDA Number: n/a   *Fax:* 614-445-8759
E-mail: sales@mcgillairpressure.com
Web site: www.mcgillairpressure.com
Medical Products Sales Volume: $360,000
Annual Revenue: $10-$25 Million
Year Founded: 1951
Total Employees: 5
Ownership: UNITED MCGILL CORPORATION
Produces/Sells CE-marked Devices: Y
Distribution: Manufacturer Direct, Manufacturer Through Manufacturer Reps
General Admin.: James D. McGill/President, Chief Executive Officer
       James Besst/Vice President, General Manager
Mktg./Adv.: Henry Philips/Manager Advertising
       Mr. Don B. Crockett/Manager National Sales
  Dryer, Labware   Chemistry
  Sterilizer, Steam (Autoclave)   General

MCI OPTONIX, DIV. OF USR OPTONIX INC.   **800-678-6649**
253 E Washington avenue,   **908-835-0004**
Washington, NJ 07882
FDA Number: 2244584   *Fax:* 908-835-0380
E-mail: mcio@mcio.com
Web site: www.mcio.com
Medical Products Sales Volume: $3,000,000
Annual Revenue: $1-$5 Million
Total Employees: 14   *Marketing Staff:* 1   *Sales Staff:* 2

MCI OPTONIX, DIV. OF USR OPTONIX INC. 800-678-6649 (cont'd)
Ownership: USR OPTONICS, INC.
Produces/Sells CE-marked Devices: Y
Distribution: Manufacturer Through Distributor, OEM, Exporter
General Admin.: Dr. Oguri/President
    John Da Forno/Senior Vice President

Cassette, Radiographic Film	Radiology
Screen, Intensifying, Radiographic	Radiology
Screen, Intensifying, Radiographic, Dental	Dental And Oral

MCKELOR TECHNOLOGIES, LTD. 800-273-5233
6312 Seeds Road, Grove City, OH 43123   **614-871-1470**
FDA Number: 1530917   *Fax:* 614-871-9353
E-mail: sales@mckelor.com
Web site: www.mckelor.com
Annual Revenue: $1-$5 Million
Year Founded: 1997
Total Employees: 15
Ownership: Private
Produces/Sells CE-marked Devices: Y
Distribution: Manufacturer Direct, Manufacturer Through Distributor
General Admin.: Andy J. Furniss/President, Owner
Mktg./Adv.: Sherri Perry/National Sales Representative

Exerciser, Powered	Anesthesiology

MCKEON PRODUCTS, INC. 586-427-7560
25460 Guenther, Warren, MI 48091
FDA Number: 1818945

Protector, Hearing (Insert)	Ear/Nose/Throat

MCKEON PRODUCTS, INC. 810-427-7560
25460 Guenther Rd., Warren, MI 48091
FDA Number: 1818945   *Fax:* 810-427-7204
E-mail: mckeon@ameritech.net
Web site: www.macksearplugs.com
Medical Products Sales Volume: $3,000,000
Annual Revenue: $1-$5 Million
Total Employees: 35   *Marketing Staff:* 3
Ownership: Private
Quality System Registration Information: ISO9002
Produces/Sells CE-marked Devices: Y
Federal Procurement Eligibility: Small Business, Female Owned
Distribution: Manufacturer Direct, Manufacturer Through Distributor, Manufacturer Through Manufacturer Reps, Importer, Exporter
General Admin.: Raymond Benner/Chief Executive Officer
    Devin Benner/President
    Marian Green/Vice President Human Resources
Mktg./Adv.: Devin Benner/Director Marketing
    Devin Benner/Director Product Development
    Jim Leumer/Manager National Sales
Production: Marian Green/Director Quality Assurance
    Cecilia Benner/Vice President Production

Plug, Ear	Ear/Nose/Throat
Protector, Hearing (Insert)	Ear/Nose/Throat

MCKESSON 800-826-9360
One Post Street, San Francisco, CA 94104   **415-983-8300**
FDA Number: n/a
E-mail: corp.communications@mckesson.com
Web site: www.mckesson.com
Annual Revenue: $500 Million-$1 Billion
Total Employees: 32900
Ownership: Public
Stock Symbol: MCK
Traded On: NYSE
Produces/Sells CE-marked Devices: N
Federal Procurement Eligibility: Small Business
Distribution: Manufacturer Direct
General Admin.: Jeffrey C. Campbell/Chief Financial Officer, Executive Vice President
    Laureen E. Seeger/Executive Vice President
    Marc E. Owen/Executive Vice President
    Pamela J. Pure/Executive Vice President
    Paul C. Julian/Executive Vice President
    Paul E. Kirincic/Executive Vice President Human Resources
    Randall N. Spratt/Executive Vice President, Chief Information Officer
    John H. Hammergren/President, Chief Executive Officer, Chairman

Armrest, Wheelchair	Physical Med
System, Drug Dispensing, Pharmacy, Automated	General
Wheelchair, Manual	Physical Med

MCKESSON DRUG CO. 856-461-7800
400 Delray Pkwy., Riverside, NJ 08075   **609-764-6333**
FDA Number: n/a   *Fax:* 609-764-9717
Web site: www.mckesson.com
Annual Revenue: $0-$1 Million

MCKESSON DRUG CO. 856-461-7800 (cont'd)
Total Employees: 852
Ownership: MCKESSION CORPORATION
Stock Symbol: MCK
Traded On: NYSE
Produces/Sells CE-marked Devices: N
Distribution: Exclusive Distributor
General Admin.: Alan Seelenfreund/Chairman
    Mark Pudulo/President

Cane	Physical Med
Walker, Mechanical	Physical Med

MCKESSON GENERAL MEDICAL 800-446-3008
8741 Landmark Road, Richmond, VA 23228   **804-264-7500**
FDA Number: 2210875   *Fax:* 804-264-7679
E-mail: webmail@mckgenmed.com
Web site: www.mckesson.com
Medical Products Sales Volume: $498,800,000
Annual Revenue: $5-$10 Million
Year Founded: 1997
Total Employees: 350
Ownership: Public
Stock Symbol: MCK
Traded On: NYSE
Produces/Sells CE-marked Devices: N
Federal Procurement Eligibility: GSA Contract, VA Contract
Distribution: Exclusive Distributor
General Admin.: F. DeWight Titus/Vice Chairman

Aspirator, Emergency Suction	General
Computer Software	General
Container, Specimen, All Types	General
Container, Urine Specimen	General
Disinfector, Liquid	General
Drape, Surgical	Surgery
Glove, Patient Examination	General
Gown, Examination	General
Gown, Patient	Surgery
Kit, Catheterization, Sterile Urethral	Gastroenterology/Urology
Kit, Disposable Procedure	Cardiovascular
Kit, Irrigation, Sterile	Gastroenterology/Urology
Kit, Prep	General
Kit, Surgical (General)	Surgery
Lift, Bath, Non-AC-Powered	General
Lotion, Skin Care	General
Media, Radiographic Injectable Contrast	Radiology
Pack, Custom/Special Procedure	General
Restraint, Patient, Conductive	Anesthesiology
Sheeting, Examination Table	General
Sponge, Other	General
Surgical Instrument, Disposable	Surgery
Swabs, Alcohol	General
Tray, Surgical	Surgery
Tray, Surgical Instrument	Surgery
Tube, Capillary	Chemistry
Tube, Culture	Microbiology

MCKESSON HBOC AUTOMATED HEALTHCARE
See Mckesson

MCKESSON JENKINTOWN
See Mckesson Drug Co.

MCKESSON MEDICAL IMAGING 800-826-9360
130-10711 Cambie Rd,   **604-279-5422**
Richmond, BC V6X 3 Canada
FDA Number: 8022257
E-mail: corp.communications@mckesson.com
Web site: www.mckesson.com
Medical Products Sales Volume: $25,439,000
Year Founded: 1985
Total Employees: 32900
Ownership: MCKESSON
Stock Symbol: MCK
Traded On: NYSE
Produces/Sells CE-marked Devices: Y
Distribution: Manufacturer Direct, Exporter

MCKIE SPLINTS, LLC 888-477-5468
P. O. Box 16046, Duluth, MN 55816
FDA Number: 2133983   *Fax:* 218-720-2844
E-mail: info@mckiesplints.com
Web site: www.mckiesplints.com
Annual Revenue: $0-$1 Million
Year Founded: 1988
Total Employees: 1
Ownership: Private
Produces/Sells CE-marked Devices: Y
Federal Procurement Eligibility: Small Business, Female Owned
Distribution: Manufacturer Direct
General Admin.: Ann McKie/Owner

MCKIE SPLINTS, LLC   888-477-5468 *(cont'd)*
Splint, Hand, And Component   Physical Med

MCLEAN MEDICAL AND SCIENTIFIC, INC.   800-777-9987
292 E. Lafayette Frontage Road,   651-227-9953
St. Paul, MN 55107
FDA Number: n/a   Fax: 651-227-7859
E-mail: info@mcleanmedical.com
Web site: www.mcleanmedical.com
Ownership: Private
Quality System Registration Information: ISO9001
Produces/Sells CE-marked Devices: N
Federal Procurement Eligibility: Small Business
Distribution: OEM, Service Direct
General Admin.: Timothy M. Scanlan/President, Chief Executive Officer
Mktg./Adv.: Mark J. Anderson/Manager Marketing
Research: Kenneth R. Blake/Vice President Research & Development

General Medical Device	General
Kit, Surgical (General)	Surgery
Laparoscope, General & Plastic Surgery	Surgery

MCMERLIN DENTAL PRODUCTS, LP   972-602-3746
1610 W. Polo Rd., Grand Prairie, TX 75052
FDA Number: 3006253843

Dressing, Wound and Burn, Hydrogel	Surgery

MCNEIL HEALTHCARE, INC.   203-932-6263
5 saw mill rd, West Haven, CT 06516
FDA Number: 1223924   Fax: 203-934-7488
E-mail: tmcneil@mcneilhealthcare.com
Web site: www.mcneilhealthcare.com
Ownership: Johnson & Johnson
Stock Symbol: JNJ
Traded On: NYSE
Produces/Sells CE-marked Devices: N

Dissector, Surgical, General & Plastic Surgery	Surgery
Dissector, Tonsil	Ear/Nose/Throat
Dressing, Other	General
Gauze, Non-Absorbable, Non-Medicated (Internal Sponge)	Surgery
Gauze, Non-Absorbable, X-Ray Detectable (Internal Sponge)	Surgery
Restraint, Protective (Body)	General
Sponge, External	Surgery
Sponge, Gauze	Dental And Oral
Sponge, Internal	Cns/Neurology

MCNEIL-PPC, INC.   908-874-1402
100 Jefferson Rd., Parsippany, NJ 07054
FDA Number: 3006185173
Web site: www.jnj.com
Ownership: Johnson & Johnson
Stock Symbol: JNJ
Traded On: NYSE
Produces/Sells CE-marked Devices: N

Cleaner, Lens, Contact	Ophthalmology

MCP SYSTEMS
See Mcp Systems

MCPHERSON ENTERPRISES, INC.   813-931-4201
3851 62nd Ave. N., Suite A, Pinellas Park, FL 33781
FDA Number: 1033972

Biopsy Instrument	Gastroenterology/Urology
Catheter, Eustachian, General & Plastic Surgery	Surgery
Clamp, Vascular	Cardiovascular
Elevator, Surgical, General & Plastic Surgery	Surgery
Pacemaker, Heart, External	Cardiovascular

MCRIGHT SUPPLIES INC., KEN   918-492-9657
7456 S. Oswego, Tulsa, OK 74136-5903
FDA Number: 1642153   Fax: 918-492-9694
E-mail: bbd4@busprod.com
Web site: www.expresspages.com
Total Employees: 10   Marketing Staff: 10   Sales Staff: 10
Ownership: Private
Produces/Sells CE-marked Devices: N
Federal Procurement Eligibility: Small Business
Distribution: Manufacturer Direct, Manufacturer Through Manufacturer Reps, Exclusive Distributor
General Admin.: Ken McRight/President
Production: J. R. Barker/Assistant Manager Production
Research: W. Darryl McRight/Vice President Research

Cover, Mattress	General
Cushion, Wheelchair (Pad)	Physical Med
Mattress, Air Flotation	General
Mattress, Bed	General
Pad, Pressure, Air	General

MD COMPONENTS INC.   954-565-5328
3560 NW 53rd Ct., Fort Lauderdale, FL 33309
FDA Number: n/a

MD COMPONENTS INC.   954-565-5328 *(cont'd)*
Annual Revenue: $0-$1 Million
Year Founded: 2000
Total Employees: 5   Sales Staff: 2
Ownership: Private
Produces/Sells CE-marked Devices: N
Federal Procurement Eligibility: Small Business
Distribution: Manufacturer Through Distributor, OEM, Importer, Exporter

Light, Surgical Operating, Dental	Dental And Oral

MD INTERNATIONAL, INC.   305-669-9003
11300 N.W. 41st St., Miami, FL 33178
FDA Number: n/a   Fax: 305-669-8951
E-mail: e-sales@mdint.com
Web site: www.mdinternational.com
Medical Products Sales Volume: $28,000,000
Annual Revenue: $25-$50 Million
Year Founded: 1987
Total Employees: 65   Marketing Staff: 3   Sales Staff: 40
Ownership: Private
Quality System Registration Information: ISO9000
Produces/Sells CE-marked Devices: Y
Federal Procurement Eligibility: Small Business
Distribution: Manufacturer Through Distributor, Exclusive Distributor, Importer, Exporter
General Admin.: Al Merritt/Chief Executive Officer
     Pedro Infante/President
Mktg./Adv.: Ann Doucette/Director Marketing

Analyzer, Doppler Spectrum	General
Analyzer, Middle Ear	Ear/Nose/Throat
Audiometer	Ear/Nose/Throat
Bed, Electric	General
Bed, Manual	General
Bed, Pediatric (Crib)	General
Cabinet Casework, Modular	General
Cabinet, Instrument	General
Camera, Video, Endoscopic	General
Cardiac Output Unit, Other	Cardiovascular
Cart, Instrument	Surgery
Chair, Examination And Treatment	General
Chair, Podiatric	Orthopedics
Chair, Surgical, AC-Powered	Surgery
Cleaner, Ultrasonic, Medical Instrument	General
Coagulator, Laparoscopic, Unipolar	Obstetrics/Gynecology
Coagulator/Cutter, Endoscopic, Bipolar	Obstetrics/Gynecology
Coagulator/Cutter, Endoscopic, Unipolar	Obstetrics/Gynecology
Colposcope	Obstetrics/Gynecology
Computer, Patient Data Management	General
Computer, Stress Exercise	Cardiovascular
Controller, Foot, Handpiece And Cord	Dental And Oral
Controller, Temperature, Cardiopulmonary Bypass	Cardiovascular
Cryophthalmic Unit	Ophthalmology
Cryosurgical Unit	Surgery
Cryosurgical Unit, Gynecologic	Obstetrics/Gynecology
Cuff, Blood Pressure	Cardiovascular
Defibrillator, External, Automatic	Cardiovascular
Defibrillator/Monitor, Battery-Powered	Cardiovascular
Defibrillator/Monitor, Line-Powered	Cardiovascular
Detector, Air Bubble	Gastroenterology/Urology
Detector, Blood Flow, Ultrasonic (Doppler)	Cardiovascular
Diathermy, Shortwave	Physical Med
Diathermy, Ultrasonic (Physical Therapy)	Physical Med
Doppler, Blood Flow, Transcranial	Cardiovascular
Electrocardiograph, Ambulatory (With Analysis Algorithm)	Cardiovascular
Electrocardiograph, Multi-Channel	Cardiovascular
Electrocardiograph, Single Channel	Cardiovascular
Electrocautery Unit, Endoscopic	Obstetrics/Gynecology
Electrocautery Unit, Line-Powered	Surgery
Electrode, Electrocardiograph	Cardiovascular
Electrode, Electrosurgery, Laparoscopic	Surgery
Electrode, Electrosurgical, Active (Blade)	Surgery
Electrode, Electrosurgical, Active, Foot Controlled	Surgery
Electrode, Electrosurgical, Return (Ground, Dispersive)	Surgery
Electrosurgical Equipment, General Purpose	Surgery
Electrosurgical Equipment, Special Purpose	Surgery
Electrosurgical Unit, Cutting & Coagulation Device	Surgery
Electrosurgical Unit, General Purpose (ESU)	Surgery
Endoscope, Fiberoptic	Surgery
Endoscope, Rigid	Surgery
Equipment, Suction/Irrigation, Laparoscopic	Surgery
Evoked Response Unit	Cns/Neurology
Forceps, Endoscopic	Gastroenterology/Urology
Forceps, Grasping, Atraumatic	Surgery
Forceps, Grasping, Traumatic	Surgery
Gas-Machine, Anesthesia	Anesthesia
Gel, Electrode, Electrocardiograph	Cardiovascular
Gel, Ultrasonic Transmission	General
Generator, Power, Electrosurgical	Surgery
Headlight, ENT	Ear/Nose/Throat
Holder, Needle, Laparoscopic	Surgery

MD INTERNATIONAL, INC.   305-669-9003 (cont'd)

Hypo/Hyperthermia Blanket	General
Hypo/Hyperthermia Unit, Mobile	General
Hypothermia Unit	General
Hypothermic Equipment	Microbiology
Instrument, Dissecting, Laparoscopic	Surgery
Lamp, Examination (Light)	General
Lamp, Surgical	Surgery
Laparoscope, General & Plastic Surgery	Surgery
Laparoscope, Gynecologic	Obstetrics/Gynecology
Laryngoscope	Ear/Nose/Throat
Laser, Argon, Surgical	Surgery
Light, Surgical Headlight	Dental And Oral
Mattress, Bed	General
Microscope	Hematology
Microscope, Operating, AC-Powered, Ophthalmic	Ophthalmology
Microscope, Surgical, General & Plastic Surgery	Surgery
Mirror, ENT	Ear/Nose/Throat
Monitor, Blood Pressure, Indirect, Transducer	Anesthesiology
Monitor, ECG	Cardiovascular
Monitor, Fetal Doppler Ultrasound	Obstetrics/Gynecology
Nystagmograph, ENT	Ear/Nose/Throat
Ophthalmoscope, Battery-Powered	Ophthalmology
Ophthalmoscope, Direct	Ophthalmology
Otoscope	Ear/Nose/Throat
Pad, Electrode	Cardiovascular
Probe, Electrocauterization, Multi-Use	Surgery
Probe, Electrocauterization, Single-Use	Surgery
Proctoscope	Surgery
Proctosigmoidoscope	Gastroenterology/Urology
Recorder, Long-Term, Trend	General
Retinoscope, AC-Powered	Ophthalmology
Retinoscope, Battery-Powered	Ophthalmology
Retractor, Fan-Type, Laparoscopy	Surgery
Scale, Bed	General
Scale, Chair	General
Scale, Infant	General
Scale, Laboratory	Chemistry
Scale, Stand-On	General
Security Equipment/Supplies	General
Sigmoidoscope, Rigid, Electrical	Gastroenterology/Urology
Sigmoidoscope, Rigid, Non-Electrical	Gastroenterology/Urology
Solution, Instrument Cleaner	General
Speculum, Ear	Ear/Nose/Throat
Speculum, Nasal	Ear/Nose/Throat
Speculum, Vaginal, Metal	Obstetrics/Gynecology
Speculum, Vaginal, Non-Metal	Obstetrics/Gynecology
Sphygmomanometer, Aneroid (Arterial Pressure)	General
Sphygmomanometer, Electronic, Automatic	General
Sphygmomanometer, Mercury (Arterial Pressure)	General
Sterilizer, Steam (Autoclave)	General
Stethoscope, Amplified	General
Stethoscope, Direct (Acoustic), Ultrasonic	General
Stethoscope, Fetal	Obstetrics/Gynecology
Stethoscope, Manual	Cardiovascular
Stethoscope, Mechanical	General
Stimulator, Muscle, Electrical-Powered (EMS)	Physical Med
Stimulator, Neurological	Surgery
Stimulator, Ultrasound, Muscle	Physical Med
Stretcher, Transfer	Surgery
Stretcher, Wheeled (Mobile)	General
Table, Examination/Treatment	General
Table, Obstetrical, AC-Powered	Obstetrics/Gynecology
Table, Operating Room, AC-Powered	Surgery
Table, Surgical, Orthopedic	Orthopedics
Table, Urological (Cystological)	Gastroenterology/Urology
Telescope, Rigid, Endoscopic	Gastroenterology/Urology
Tester, Auditory Impedance	Ear/Nose/Throat
Thermometer, Electronic	General
Thermometer, Electronic, Continuous	General
Thoracoscope	Cardiovascular
Transducer, Ultrasonic, Diagnostic	Radiology
Transilluminator, AC-Powered, Other	Ophthalmology
Transilluminator, Battery-Powered	Ophthalmology
Treadmill, Powered	Physical Med

MD ORTHOPAEDICS   877-766-7384
604 North Parkway St, Wayland, IA 52654
FDA Number: 3005663580

Orthosis, Corrective Shoe	Physical Med
Splint, Denis Brown	Physical Med

MD PRODUCTS, LLC   843-971-2684
506 Hickory Cove, Mt. Pleasant, SC 29464
FDA Number: 3006450293
Ownership: Private
Produces/Sells CE-marked Devices: N

Depressor, Tongue	General

MD SCIENTIFIC LLC   704-335-1300
2815 Coliseum Centre Drive, --suite 250, Charlotte, NC 28217
FDA Number: 3005214420

MD SCIENTIFIC LLC   704-335-1300 (cont'd)

Calculator, Drug Dose	Surgery

MD SYSTEMS, INC.   614-818-3000
P.O. Box 1647, Westerville, OH 43086
FDA Number: n/a   Fax: 614-818-3182
E-mail: masmyser@mdsystems.com.
Web site: www.mdsystems.com
Ownership: Private
Produces/Sells CE-marked Devices: N

Exerciser, Powered	Anesthesiology

MD WORKS, INC.   770-409-9639
1895-i Beaver Ridge Cir., Suite 410, Norcross, GA 30071
FDA Number: 1066012   Fax: 770-446-3086
E-mail: hbaker@mdworks.net
Web site: www.mdworks.net
Annual Revenue: $0-$1 Million
Year Founded: 1997
Ownership: Private
Quality System Registration Information: ISO9001
Produces/Sells CE-marked Devices: N
Federal Procurement Eligibility: Small Business
Distribution: Manufacturer Direct, Manufacturer Through Distributor, Manufacturer Through Manufacturer Reps

Needle, Hypodermic	General
Shield, X-Ray, Portable	Radiology

MDC CORP.
See H.L. Bouton Co., Inc.

MDH
See Radcal Corp.

MDL INFORMATION SYSTEMS, INC.
See Symyx Technologies, Inc.

MDRNA, INC.   425-908-3600
3830 Monte Villa Parkway, Bothell, WA 98021
FDA Number: n/a
Web site: www.mdrnainc.com
Annual Revenue: $1-$5 Million
Total Employees: 16   Marketing Staff: 3
Ownership: Public
Stock Symbol: MRNA
Traded On: NASDAQ
Produces/Sells CE-marked Devices: N
Federal Procurement Eligibility: Small Business
General Admin.: Barry Polisky/Chief Scientific Officer
       J. Michael French/President, Chief Executive Officer
Mktg./Adv.: June D. Ameen/Vice President Corporate Development
Finance: Peter S. Garcia/Chief Financial Officer

System, Delivery, Drug, Unit-Dose	General

MDS NORDION   800-267-6211
447 March Rd., Kanata, ON K2K 1X8 Canada   613-592-2790
FDA Number: 8022247   Fax: 613-592-6937
E-mail: emartell@mds.nordion.com
Web site: www.mds.nordion.com
Year Founded: 1946
Total Employees: 750   Marketing Staff: 12   Sales Staff: 15
Ownership: Mds, Inc.
Stock Symbol: MHG
Traded On: Toronto
Produces/Sells CE-marked Devices: N
Distribution: Manufacturer Direct, Exclusive Distributor, Exporter

MDS PRODUCTS, INC.   800-637-2330
22991 La Cadena Drive,   949-330-0140
Laguna Hills, CA 92653
FDA Number: 2020496   Fax: 949-330-0145
E-mail: info@mdsadds.com
Web site: www.mdsadds.com
Year Founded: 1975
Ownership: Private
Produces/Sells CE-marked Devices: N
Federal Procurement Eligibility: Small Business
Distribution: Manufacturer Direct, Manufacturer Through Distributor

Adhesive, Dental	Dental And Oral
Airbrush	Dental And Oral
Articulators	Dental And Oral
Base, Denture, Relining, Repairing, Rebasing, Resin	Dental And Oral
Carver, Wax, Dental	Dental And Oral
Casting Unit, Dental	Dental And Oral
Dental Laboratory Equipment	Dental And Oral
Disk, Abrasive	Dental And Oral
Material, Casting	Dental And Oral
Paper, Articulation	Dental And Oral

Medical Product Subsidiaries (Listed Separately)

MDS PRODUCTS, INC.　800-637-2330 (cont'd)
American Diversified Dental Systems

MDS SCIEX　416-675-6777
71 Four Valley Dr, Concord L4K 4V8 Canada
FDA Number: 9616622
　Mass Spectrometer, Clinical Use　　　　Toxicology

MDS SCIEX　905-660-9005
71 Four Valley Dr., Concord, ON L4K 4V8 Canada
FDA Number: n/a　　　　　*Fax:* 905-660-2600
E-mail: bori@sciex.com
Web site: www.sciex.com
Year Founded: 1974
Total Employees: 475
Ownership: MDS, INC.
Stock Symbol: MDS
Traded On: Toronto
Quality System Registration Information: ISO9002
Produces/Sells CE-marked Devices: Y
Distribution: Manufacturer Through Distributor, Exporter

MDS, INC.　416-675-6777
2700 Matheson Blvd. E., Suite 300, West Tower,
Mississauga, ON L4W 4 Canada
FDA Number: n/a　　　　　*Fax:* 416-213-4220
E-mail: info.mds@mdsinc.com
Web site: www.mdsinc.com
Year Founded: 1969
Total Employees: 5500　　*Marketing Staff:* 6
Ownership: Public
Stock Symbol: MDZ
Traded On: NYSE
Produces/Sells CE-marked Devices: N
Distribution: Service Direct, Exclusive Distributor

MDT BIOLOGIC CO.
See Getinge Usa, Inc.

MDT CORPORATION
See Getinge Usa, Inc.

MDT DIAGNOSTIC CO.
See Getinge Usa, Inc.

MDT TECHNIONIC CO.
See Getinge Usa, Inc.

MDXHEALTH INC.　919-281-0980
2505 Meridian Parkway, Suite 310, DURHAM, NC 27713
FDA Number: n/a　　　　　*Fax:* 919-281-0981
E-mail: info@mdxhealth.com
Web site: http://mdxhealth.com/company
Ownership: Public
Stock Symbol: MDXH
Traded On: NYSE
Produces/Sells CE-marked Devices: N
General Admin.: Dr. Jan Groan/Chief Executive Officer
　Medical Admin.: Mr. Joseph Bigley/Vice President Clinical Affairs
Mktg./Adv.: Mr. Christopher Thibodeau/Vice President Commercial Operations
Production: Dr. Melissa Thompson/Vice President Quality Assurance & Regulatory Affairs
Research: Dr. James Clark/Vice President Research & Development
Finance: Mr. Philip Devine/Chief Financial Officer

MEADVILLE PRECISION TOOL & MOLD INC.
See C&J Industries, Inc.

MEALTIME PARTNERS, INC.　817-237-9991
1137 S. E. Parkway, Azle, TX 76020
FDA Number: 3006137761
　Utensil, Food　　　　　　　Physical Med

MECANAIDS CO., INC.　800-227-0877
21 Hampden Drive, South Easton, MA 02375　508-238-2163
FDA Number: n/a　　　　　*Fax:* 508-238-1752
E-mail: customerservice@mecanaids.com
Web site: www.Mecanaids.com
Medical Products Sales Volume: $500,000
Annual Revenue: $0-$1 Million
Year Founded: 1981
Total Employees: 7
Ownership: Private
Produces/Sells CE-marked Devices: N
Federal Procurement Eligibility: Small Business
Distribution: Manufacturer Through Distributor
General Admin.: Jay Luippold/President, Chief Executive Officer
　Adaptor, Dressing　　　　　Physical Med
　Adaptor, Grooming　　　　　Physical Med
　Reacher (Handicapped)　　　　General

MECANAIDS CO., INC.　800-227-0877 (cont'd)
Utensil, Handicapped Aid　　　　Physical Med

MECTA CORPORATION　503-612-6780
19799 SW 95th Avenue, Suite B, Bldg. D, Tualatin, OR 97062
FDA Number: 965070　　　　*Fax:* 503-612-6542
E-mail: sales@mectacorp.com
Year Founded: 1973
Total Employees: 12　　*Sales Staff:* 5
Ownership: Private
Quality System Registration Information: ISO9001
Produces/Sells CE-marked Devices: Y
Federal Procurement Eligibility: Small Business, Female Owned
Distribution: Manufacturer Direct, Manufacturer Through Distributor, Exporter
General Admin.: Robin H. Nicol/President
Mktg./Adv.: Brienna K. Finke/General Manager Marketing & Sales
　　　　Ms. Orrada Somboondee/Manager International Sales
　Electroconvulsive Therapy Unit (Electroshock)　Cns/Neurology

MECTRA LABS, INC.　800-323-3968
Two Quality Way, Bloomfield, IN 47424　812-384-3521
FDA Number: 1833052　　　　*Fax:* 812-384-8518
E-mail: mectrasales@mectralabs.com
Web site: www.mectralabs.com
Medical Products Sales Volume: $1,500,000
Annual Revenue: $1-$5 Million
Year Founded: 1988
Total Employees: 20　　*Marketing Staff:* 6　　*Sales Staff:* 6
Ownership: Private
Quality System Registration Information: ISO9001
Produces/Sells CE-marked Devices: Y
Federal Procurement Eligibility: Small Business, Minority Owned, VA Contract
Distribution: Manufacturer Direct, Manufacturer Through Distributor, Manufacturer Through Manufacturer Reps, OEM, Exporter
General Admin.: Thomas P. Clement/Chief Executive Officer
　　　　Teresa English/Office Manager
Mktg./Adv.: Thomas P. Clement/Vice President Sales
Production: Deni Baker/Manager Materials
　　　　Charles Allgood/Manager Regulatory Affairs
　Accessories, Solution, Lens, Contact　Ophthalmology
　Electrocautery Unit, Battery-Powered　Surgery
　Filter, Air　　　　　　　　General
　Filter, Gas　　　　　　　Anesthesiology
　Irrigator, Suction　　　　　General
　Kit, Trocar　　　　　　　Surgery
　Needle, Insufflation, Laparoscopic　Surgery
　Probe　　　　　　　　Orthopedics
　Probe, Suction, Irrigator/Aspirator, Laparoscopic　Surgery
　Retainer, Surgical　　　　　Surgery

MED LABS INC.　800-968-2486
28 Vereda Cordillera, Goleta, CA 93117-5300　805-968-2486
FDA Number: 2026803　　　　*Fax:* 805-968-2486
E-mail: medlabsinc@aol.com
Web site: www.hometown.aol.com/medlabsinc
Medical Products Sales Volume: $600,000
Annual Revenue: $0-$1 Million
Year Founded: 1969
Total Employees: 4
Ownership: Private
Produces/Sells CE-marked Devices: N
Federal Procurement Eligibility: Small Business
Distribution: Manufacturer Through Distributor
General Admin.: Philip D. Norvell/President, Chief Executive Officer
Mktg./Adv.: Gloria G. Norvell/Manager Marketing
Production: Jeff Shuck/Manager Production
　Component, Other　　　　　General
　Nurse Call System　　　　　General
　Stimulator, Muscle, Electrical-Powered (EMS)　Physical Med

MED SYSTEMS　800-345-9061
2631 Ariane Drive, San Diego, CA 92117　858-483-9671
FDA Number: 2022691　　　　*Fax:* 858-483-9827
E-mail: jamesepdavis@earthlink.net
Web site: www.medsystems.com
Medical Products Sales Volume: $600,000
Total Employees: 6
Ownership: Private
Produces/Sells CE-marked Devices: N
Federal Procurement Eligibility: Small Business, Female Owned
Distribution: Manufacturer Direct, Manufacturer Through Distributor
General Admin.: James E. P. Davis/Chief Executive Officer
　Compressor, Air, Portable　　　Anesthesiology
　Mask, Face　　　　　　　General
　Mask, Gas, Anesthesia　　　　Anesthesiology
　Percussor, Powered　　　　　Anesthesiology

MED X CHANGE, INC.   941-794-9977
525 8th Street West, Bradenton, FL 34205
FDA Number: 3006341616
Accessories, Surgical Camera — Surgery

MED-AESTHETIC SOLUTIONS, INC.   505-341-2577
6808 Academy Pkwy., East N.e., Bldg. A Suite 1, Albuquerque, NM 87109
FDA Number: 1724657
Dermatome — Surgery

MED-ASSIST TECHNOLOGY, INC.   801-296-6848
2441 South 1560 West, Woods Cross, UT 84087
FDA Number: 1724347
Ownership: Private
Produces/Sells CE-marked Devices: N
Urinal — General

MED-COM SYSTEMS CORP.   800-324-3283   918-749-0423
1519 S. Lewis Ave., Tulsa, OK 74104-4919
FDA Number: n/a   *Fax:* 918-749-3023
E-mail: hugh@cme-usa.com
Web site: www.cme-usa.com
Annual Revenue: $0-$1 Million
Total Employees: 11   *Marketing Staff:* 2   *Sales Staff:* 3
Ownership: Private
Produces/Sells CE-marked Devices: N
Federal Procurement Eligibility: Small Business
Distribution: Manufacturer Direct
General Admin.: Hugh Holly/President
Production: William Ninke/Director Quality Assurance
Research: Carl Osborne/Vice President Engineering
Transmitter/Receiver System, ECG, Telephone Multi-Channel — Cardiovascular
Transmitter/Receiver System, ECG, Telephone Single-Channel — Cardiovascular

MED-CON, INC.   800-366-1366   847-395-8844
PO Box 244, Antioch, IL 60002
FDA Number: n/a   *Fax:* 847-395-8858
E-mail: info@med-con.net
Web site: www.med-con.net
Medical Products Sales Volume: $200,000
Annual Revenue: $0-$1 Million
Year Founded: 1984
Total Employees: 4   *Sales Staff:* 2
Ownership: Private
Quality System Registration Information: ISO9002
Produces/Sells CE-marked Devices: Y
Federal Procurement Eligibility: Small Business
Distribution: Service Direct
General Admin.: Edward Piet/President
Sheli Burdick/Vice President, General Manager
Service, Consulting — General

MED-DYNE   502-429-4140
2775 South Floyd Street, Louisville, KY 40209-1817
FDA Number: 1531159   *Fax:* 502-429-6759
E-mail: ew@med-dyne.com
Web site: www.med-dyne.com
Ownership: Private
Produces/Sells CE-marked Devices: N
Federal Procurement Eligibility: Small Business, Female Owned
Distribution: Manufacturer Through Distributor
Cable/Lead, ECG, With Transducer And Electrode — Cardiovascular
Electrode, Electrocardiograph — Cardiovascular
Electrode, Gel — Cardiovascular
Monitor, ECG — Cardiovascular

MED-EDGE, INC.   800-360-3682   336-945-3682
1843 Pinehurst Drive, Clemmons, NC 27012
FDA Number: 1039684   *Fax:* 336-945-6038
E-mail: jowenby@triad.rr.com
Medical Products Sales Volume: $220,000
Year Founded: 1995
Total Employees: 4
Ownership: Private
Produces/Sells CE-marked Devices: N
Federal Procurement Eligibility: Small Business, Female Owned
Distribution: Manufacturer Direct, Manufacturer Through Manufacturer Reps
Marker, Cardiopulmonary Bypass (Vein Marker) — Cardiovascular

MED-FIT SYSTEMS, INC.   800-831-7665   760-723-9618
3553 Rosa Way, Fallbrook, CA 92028
FDA Number: 2085371   *Fax:* 760-723-5396
E-mail: medfit@aol.com
Web site: www.medfitsystems.com
Medical Products Sales Volume: $900,000
Annual Revenue: $5-$10 Million
Year Founded: 1993

MED-FIT SYSTEMS, INC.   800-831-7665 *(cont'd)*
Total Employees: 6   *Marketing Staff:* 1   *Sales Staff:* 3
Ownership: Private
Produces/Sells CE-marked Devices: N
Federal Procurement Eligibility: Small Business
Distribution: Manufacturer Direct, Exclusive Distributor, Importer
General Admin.: Dean Sbragia/Chief Executive Officer
Juergan Kopf/Vice President, General Manager
Mktg./Adv.: Alex Marquez/Director Marketing
Diathermy, Ultrasonic (Physical Therapy) — Physical Med
Equipment, Therapy, Handicapped/Physical — Physical Med
Exerciser, Bicycle — Physical Med
Exerciser, Chest — Physical Med
Rowing Unit — Physical Med
Table, Physical Medicine, Powered — Physical Med
Treadmill, Powered — Physical Med

MED-GENERAL USA LLC   239-597-9967
1045 Collier Center Way, Unit #1, Naples, FL 34110
FDA Number: 3004552902
Ownership: Private
Produces/Sells CE-marked Devices: N
Headlamp, Operating, AC-Powered — Ophthalmology
Light, Surgical, Fiberoptic — Surgery

MED-LAB SUPPLY CO., INC.   800-330-5144   305-642-5144
923 N.W. 27th Ave., Miami, FL 33125
FDA Number: n/a   *Fax:* 305-541-0832
Web site: www.med-lab.com
Medical Products Sales Volume: $8,000,000
Annual Revenue: $10-$25 Million
Year Founded: 1964
Ownership: Siemens Medical Solutions USA, Inc.
Produces/Sells CE-marked Devices: N
Federal Procurement Eligibility: Small Business, Minority Owned
Distribution: Manufacturer Direct
Service, Maintenance/Repair — General

MED-LIFT & MOBILITY, INC.   800-748-9438
310 S. Madison, Calhoun City, MS 38916
FDA Number: 2318456   *Fax:* 800-628-8709
E-mail: medlift@tycom.net
Web site: www.medlift.com
Medical Products Sales Volume: $10,000,000
Annual Revenue: $10-$25 Million
Year Founded: 1990
Total Employees: 45   *Marketing Staff:* 2   *Sales Staff:* 7
Ownership: Private
Produces/Sells CE-marked Devices: Y
Distribution: Manufacturer Direct, Manufacturer Through Distributor, Manufacturer Through Manufacturer Reps, Importer, Exporter
General Admin.: A. D. Blount/Chief Executive Officer
A. D. Blount/President
Mktg./Adv.: Alison Blount Nichols/Vice President Marketing
Ronald Harville/Vice President Sales
Production: Ron Pollan/Director Quality Assurance
David Crocker/Vice President Manufacturing
Purchasing: Judy Tedford/Credit Manager
Chair, Other — General
Chair, Seat Lifting (Standing Aid) — General
Scooter (Motorized 3-Wheeled Vehicle) — Physical Med

MED-LOGICS, INC.   800-651-2962   949-582-3891
26061 Merit Circle, Suite 102, Laguna Hills, CA 92653
FDA Number: 2085081   *Fax:* 949-582-2676
E-mail: info@mlogics.com
Web site: www.mlogics.com
Year Founded: 1992
Ownership: Private
Produces/Sells CE-marked Devices: N
Federal Procurement Eligibility: Small Business
Distribution: Manufacturer Through Distributor
Irrigator, Ocular Surgery — Ophthalmology
Keratome, AC-Powered — Ophthalmology
Sponge, Ophthalmic — Ophthalmology
Tubing, Other — General

MED-LOGICS, INC.   949-582-3891
26061 Merit Circle, Suite #102, Laguna Hills, CA 92653
FDA Number: 2085081   *Fax:* 949-582-2676
E-mail: info@mlogics.com
Web site: www.mlogics.com
Medical Products Sales Volume: $600,000
Year Founded: 1992
Total Employees: 9
Ownership: Private
Produces/Sells CE-marked Devices: Y

MED-LOGICS, INC.   949-582-3891 *(cont'd)*

Federal Procurement Eligibility: Small Business

Irrigator, Ocular Surgery	Ophthalmology
Keratome, AC-Powered	Ophthalmology
Sponge, Ophthalmic	Ophthalmology

MED-MIZER, INC   812-932-2345
80 Commerce Drive, Batesville, IN 47006
FDA Number: 3004976058

Bed, Electric	General

MED-ORTHO DESIGN & MANUFACTURING LTD.   905-837-7789
900 Brock Rd. S, Unit 6, Pickering, ONT L1W-1Z9 Canada
FDA Number: n/a   *Fax:* 905-837-7790
Year Founded: 1980
Total Employees: 25
Ownership: Private
Produces/Sells CE-marked Devices: N
Distribution: Manufacturer Direct, Exclusive Distributor

MED-OX DIAGNOSTICS INC. (MDI)   800-818-8335
1-57 Iber Rd., Ottawa, ONT K2S-1E7 Canada   613-271-1144
FDA Number: n/a   *Fax:* 613-271-1148
E-mail: jroberts@medox.net
Web site: www.medox.com
Year Founded: 1998
Total Employees: 25
Ownership: Private
Produces/Sells CE-marked Devices: N
Distribution: Exclusive Distributor, Importer, Exporter

MED-PLAST   800-567-1108
161 Oneida Drive,   514.694.9835
Pointe Claire, QUE H9R 1 Canada
FDA Number: n/a   *Fax:* 514.697.7012
E-mail: sales@medplas.com
Web site: http://www.medplas.com
Year Founded: 1990
Total Employees: 50
Ownership: Private
Produces/Sells CE-marked Devices: N
Distribution: Manufacturer Direct, Exporter

MED-SAVER, INC.
See Msi Precision, Specialty Instrument

MED-STOR, A DIVISION OF THE GRATES CORPORATION   800-952-7775

25701 Jefferson Rd.,   586-777-7775
Saint Clair Shores, MI 48081
FDA Number: n/a   *Fax:* 800-952-0140
E-mail: customerservices@medstor.com
Web site: stores.medstor.com
Annual Revenue: $1-$5 Million
Year Founded: 1992
Ownership: Private
Produces/Sells CE-marked Devices: N
Federal Procurement Eligibility: Small Business
Distribution: Manufacturer Direct

Container, Sterilization (Tray)	General
Cover, Cart	General

MED-SURGICAL SERVICES INC.   408-617-2000
465 E. Evelyn Ave., Sunnyvale, CA 94086
FDA Number: 2954952

Stereotaxy Equipment	Cns/Neurology

MED-WORLD MARKETING
See Marketing International, Inc.

MEDAC INC.
See Conmed Corporation

MEDAIR, INC.   800-325-7780
PO Box 635, East Bridgewater, MA 02333   508-823-7780
FDA Number: n/a   *Fax:* 508-822-7799
E-mail: info@medairinc.com
Web site: www.medair.com
Medical Products Sales Volume: $160,000
Year Founded: 1992
Total Employees: 2
Ownership: Private
Produces/Sells CE-marked Devices: N
Federal Procurement Eligibility: Small Business
Distribution: Manufacturer Direct, Manufacturer Through Manufacturer Reps, Service Direct, Exclusive Distributor
General Admin.: Seth Grady/Chief Technology Officer
Mktg./Adv.: Kevin Whittington/Director National Marketing & Sales

MEDAIR, INC.   800-325-7780 *(cont'd)*

Equipment, Cleaning, Air	General

MEDAN INC.   541-231-4141
131 Nw 4th Street, Suite 395, Corvallis, OR 97330
FDA Number: 3003643920

Device, Cystometric, Hydraulic	Gastroenterology/Urology

MEDCARE PRODUCTS, INC.   800-695-4479
151 E. Cliff Road, Suite #40,   952-894-7076
Burnsville, MN 55337
FDA Number: 2135150   *Fax:* 952-894-7153
E-mail: medcare@medcarelifts.com
Web site: www.medcarelifts.com
Medical Products Sales Volume: $440,000
Year Founded: 1998
Total Employees: 8
Ownership: Private
Produces/Sells CE-marked Devices: N
Federal Procurement Eligibility: Small Business, Female Owned, GSA Contract
Distribution: Manufacturer Through Distributor, Manufacturer Through Manufacturer Reps
Mktg./Adv.: Glenn VanHulzen/Manager National Sales

Computer Software, Hospital/Nursing Management	General
Lift, Patient	General

MEDCARE TECHNOLOGIES   800-388-6235
850 St. Paul St., Rochester, NY 14605-1095   716-232-5560
FDA Number: 1318903   *Fax:* 716-454-3604
E-mail: sales@scissorsusa.com
Web site: www.scissorsusa.com
Medical Products Sales Volume: $270,000
Annual Revenue: $0-$1 Million
Year Founded: 1999
Total Employees: 3
Ownership: Private
Produces/Sells CE-marked Devices: N
Federal Procurement Eligibility: Small Business
Distribution: Manufacturer Through Distributor
General Admin.: Anthony G. Heiner/President
Mktg./Adv.: Lori M. Heiner/Vice President Marketing

Forceps, Tissue	Surgery
Scissors, Bandage/Gauze/Plaster	General

MEDCASTER INC.   866-462-9700
800 N. Clark Street, Albion, MI 49224
FDA Number: n/a   *Fax:* 517-686-1072
E-mail: info@medcaster.com
Web site: www.medcaster.com
Ownership: Private
Produces/Sells CE-marked Devices: N
Distribution: OEM

Casters, Hospital Equipment	General

MEDCENTER CORP. ADVANCED SUPPLEMENTS
See Vitamedics Corporation

MEDCHANNEL LLC   617-314-9861
1241 Adams St, Ste 110, Boston, MA 02124
FDA Number: n/a
Ownership: Private
Produces/Sells CE-marked Devices: N

Brush, Biopsy, General & Plastic Surgery	Surgery
Catheter, Cholangiography	Surgery
Container, Specimen, All Types	General
Instrument, Manual, General Surgical	Surgery
Ligator, Hemorrhoidal	Gastroenterology/Urology
Locator, Magnetic	Surgery
Scanner, Ultrasonic (Pulsed Echo)	Radiology
Staple, Implantable	Surgery

MEDCHEM PRODUCTS, INC.   800-451-4716
160 New Boston St., Woburn, MA 01801-6333   781-932-5900
FDA Number: 1223089   *Fax:* 401-946-5379
Medical Products Sales Volume: $13,000,000
Annual Revenue: $25-$50 Million
Total Employees: 125   *Marketing Staff:* 3   *Sales Staff:* 20
Ownership: Private
Quality System Registration Information: ISO9001
Produces/Sells CE-marked Devices: Y
Distribution: Manufacturer Direct, Manufacturer Through Manufacturer Reps
General Admin.: Janice Valliere/Manager Human Resources
Mktg./Adv.: Dennis D'Oria/Manager International Marketing & Sales
    M. McCartin/Manager Marketing
Production: Matthew Nowland/Director Regulatory Affairs
Research: James Wilkie/Executive Vice President Research & Development
Finance: Ray Guilbault/Controller

Agent, Hemostatic, Absorbable, Collagen-Based	Surgery
Hemostat	Orthopedics

MEDCHEM PRODUCTS, INC.
800-451-4716 *(cont'd)*
Mesh, Surgical (Steel Gauze) — Surgery

MEDCHEM PRODUCTS, INC.
908-277-8000
160 New Boston St., Woburn, MA 01801
FDA Number: 1223089
Ownership: C. R. Bard, Inc.
Stock Symbol: BCR
Traded On: NYSE
Produces/Sells CE-marked Devices: N
Agent, Hemostatic, Absorbable, Collagen-Based — Surgery
Bandage, Liquid — Surgery
Mesh, Surgical (Steel Gauze) — Surgery

MEDCO EQUIPMENT, INC.
800-717-3626
105 Old Hwy 8, Unit 3, New Brighton, MN 55112
651-639-8684
FDA Number: n/a
Fax: 651-639-8685
E-mail: medcoequipment@email.msn.com
Web site: www.medcoequipment.com
Medical Products Sales Volume: $710,000
Year Founded: 1993
Total Employees: 9
Ownership: Public
Federal Procurement Eligibility: Small Business
Washer/Sterilizer — General

MEDCO MFG.
281-379-3100
8319 Thora #a1, Spring, TX 77379
FDA Number: 1649660
Pump, Aspiration, Portable — Anesthesiology

MEDCO SCHOOL FIRST AID
See Medco Supply Company

MEDCO SPORTS MEDICINE
See Medco Supply Company

MEDCO SUPPLY COMPANY
800-556-3326
500 Fillmore Avenue, Tonawanda, NY 14150
716-695-3244
FDA Number: 1319486
Fax: 800-222-1934
E-mail: customersupport@medcosupply.com
Web site: www.medcomedical.com
Medical Products Sales Volume: $1,100,000
Year Founded: 1998
Total Employees: 11
Marketing Staff: 12
Sales Staff: 50
Ownership: AbilityOne Products Corp.
Produces/Sells CE-marked Devices: N
Federal Procurement Eligibility: Small Business, GSA Contract
Distribution: Service Direct
General Admin.: Mark Ladouceur/President
Mktg./Adv.: Don Laux/Director Marketing
Karen Blaha/Director Product Development
Kate Kennedy/Manager Advertising
Paul DeMartinis/Manager International & National Sales
Applicator, Antiseptic — General
Chart, Anatomical Training — General
Dispenser, Medication, Liquid — General
Eyeglasses, Safety — Ophthalmology
Glove, Other — General
Kit, First Aid — Surgery
Kit, Irrigation, Wound — General
Lotion, Skin Care — General
Pack, Hot Or Cold, Disposable — Physical Med

MEDCOM, INC.
See Creative Medical Technologies

MEDCOM, INC.
800-877-1443
6060 Phyllis Drive, Cypress, CA 90630
714-891-1443
FDA Number: 9330124
Fax: 714-891-3140
E-mail: customerservice@medcominc.com
Web site: www.medcominc.com
Medical Products Sales Volume: $7,500,000
Annual Revenue: $5-$10 Million
Year Founded: 1986
Total Employees: 50
Marketing Staff: 4
Sales Staff: 25
Ownership: Private
Produces/Sells CE-marked Devices: N
Federal Procurement Eligibility: Small Business
Distribution: Manufacturer Direct
General Admin.: L. Gorum/President, Chief Executive Officer
Mktg./Adv.: M. Zoradi/Director Marketing
M. Zoradi/Director National Accounts
M. Zoradi/Vice President Business Development
Mike Zoradi/Vice President Sales
Production: T. Armstrong/Vice President Production
Finance: P. Muecke/Vice President Finance
Anatomical Training Model — General
Material, Training, Audiovisual — General

MEDCOMP (MEDICAL COMPONENTS, INC.)
800-220-3791
1499 Delp Dr., Harleysville, PA 19438-2936
215-256-4201
FDA Number: 2518902
Fax: 215-256-9191
E-mail: medcomp@medcompnet.com
Web site: www.medcompnet.com
Ownership: Private
Produces/Sells CE-marked Devices: Y
Federal Procurement Eligibility: Small Business
Distribution: Manufacturer Through Distributor, Service Direct, Exporter
General Admin.: David Markel/Chief Executive Officer
Tim Schweikert/President
Mktg./Adv.: Michael I. Basta/Director International Sales
William Cassium/Director National Sales
Ron Plummer/Manager Advertising
Production: Kevin Sanford/Director Engineering
David Kunin/Director Regulatory Affairs
Terry Morgan/Manager Production
Purchasing: Dennis Gawronski/Manager Purchasing
Catheter, Femoral — Gastroenterology/Urology
Catheter, Hemodialysis — Gastroenterology/Urology
Catheter, Peritoneal, Indwelling, Long-Term — Gastroenterology/Urology
Catheter, Subclavian — Cardiovascular

MEDCOVERS, INC
800-948-8917
500 W. Goldsboro Street, Kenly, NC 27542
919-284-6628
FDA Number: n/a
Fax: 919-779-3555
E-mail: medteam@medcovers.com
Web site: www.medcovers.com
Medical Products Sales Volume: $1,000,000
Annual Revenue: $1-$5 Million
Total Employees: 21
Marketing Staff: 3
Sales Staff: 3
Ownership: Private
Produces/Sells CE-marked Devices: N
Federal Procurement Eligibility: Small Business
Distribution: Manufacturer Direct
General Admin.: David M. Sutherland/Chief Executive Officer
Mktg./Adv.: Jeanie Falkie/Manager Sales
Jack Van Schoor/Vice President Marketing & Sales
Attachment, Bag (Crutch, Walker, Wheelchair) — Physical Med
Bag, Breathing — Anesthesiology
Canister, Liquid Oxygen, Portable — Anesthesiology
Carrier, Container, Oxygen, Portable — General
Component, Other — General
Continuous Positive Airway Pressure Unit (CPAP, CPPB) — Anesthesiology
Cover, Mattress — General

MEDCREST TEXTILES
See Medline Industries, Inc.

MEDDEV CORPORATION
800-543-2789
730 N. Pastoria Avenue, Sunnyvale, CA 94085
408-730-9702
FDA Number: 2921577
Fax: 408-730-9732
E-mail: info@meddev-corp.com
Web site: www.meddev-corp.com
Medical Products Sales Volume: $1,500,000
Annual Revenue: $1-$5 Million
Year Founded: 1971
Total Employees: 10
Marketing Staff: 2
Sales Staff: 3
Ownership: Private
Produces/Sells CE-marked Devices: N
Federal Procurement Eligibility: Small Business
Distribution: Manufacturer Direct, Manufacturer Through Distributor, Manufacturer Through Manufacturer Reps, Service Direct, Exclusive Distributor, Exporter
General Admin.: Suzanne Grey/President
Mktg./Adv.: Mark Wilson/Marketing Coordinator
Production: Mauro Salazar/Manager Materials
Adhesive Strip, Hypoallergenic — General
Equipment, Therapy, Handicapped/Physical — Physical Med
Exerciser, Finger, Powered — Physical Med
Exerciser, Hand — Physical Med
Headlamp, Operating, Battery-Operated — Ophthalmology
Lamp, Examination (Light) — General
Prosthesis, Eyelid — Ophthalmology
Weights, Eyelid, External — Ophthalmology

MEDDEX, S.A.
5-581-8022
Calz. Ermita Iztapalapa, #855,, Col. Sta. Isabel Industrial,
Cd. Mexico, D.f. Mexico
FDA Number: 8030609
Cuff, Blood Pressure — Cardiovascular

MEDEC
866-586-3332
405 The West Mal, Suite 900,
416-620-1915
Toronto, ONTAR M9C 5 Canada
FDA Number: n/a
Web site: www.medec.org
Ownership: Private

MEDEC   866-586-3332 *(cont'd)*
Produces/Sells CE-marked Devices: N

MEDECON   954-742-6300
10001 NW 50th St., Suite W-2, Sunrise, FL 33351-8061
FDA Number: 1064484   *Fax:* 954-742-6518
E-mail: zoyahaji1@aol.com
Medical Products Sales Volume: $10,000,000
Total Employees: 25
Ownership: Private
Produces/Sells CE-marked Devices: N
Federal Procurement Eligibility: Small Business

Vibrator, Therapeutic	Physical Med

MEDEFFICIENCY, INC.   303-321-7755
8620 Wolff Court, Suite 120, Denver, CO 80031
FDA Number: 3003924847

Orthosis, Limb Brace	Physical Med

MEDEFIL, INC.   630-682-4600
250 Windy Point Drive, Glendale Heights, IL 60139
FDA Number: 1423982   *Fax:* 630-681-9100
E-mail: info@medefil.com
Web site: www.medefil.com
Medical Products Sales Volume: $5,000,000
Year Founded: 1998
Total Employees: 30
Ownership: Private
Produces/Sells CE-marked Devices: N
Federal Procurement Eligibility: Small Business, Minority Owned
Distribution: Manufacturer Through Distributor
General Admin.: Mr. Pradeep Aggarwal/President, Chief Executive Officer
     Mr. Sandeep Aggarwal/Vice President

Catheter, Intravascular, Therapeutic, Short-term Less Than 30 Days	General

MEDEGEN   800-520-7999   909-390-9080
4501 Wall Street, Ontario, CA 91761-8151
FDA Number: 2031055   *Fax:* 909-390-9081
E-mail: mms.email@medegen.com
Web site: www.medegen.com
Medical Products Sales Volume: $35,000,000
Year Founded: 2001
Total Employees: 180   *Marketing Staff:* 2   *Sales Staff:* 5
Ownership: Private
Traded On: NASDAQ
Quality System Registration Information: ISO9001
Produces/Sells CE-marked Devices: N
Federal Procurement Eligibility: Small Business
Distribution: OEM, Exclusive Distributor
General Admin.: Jeff Goble/Chief Executive Officer
Mktg./Adv.: Janice Tarwater/Manager Marketing
Production: Joleen Kennelley/Customer Service Representative
     Richard Rambaud/Vice President Operations, General Manager
Research: Tim Truitt/Manager Research & Development

Contract Manufacturing	General
Contract R&D, Equipment	General
Fitting, Luer	General
Molding, Custom	General
Molding, Injection	General
Service, Printing	General
Set, Administration, Intravenous, Needle-Free	General
Tubing, Connecting	General

MEDEGEN MEDICAL PRODUCTS, LLC   800-233-1987   901-867-2951
209 Medegen Drive, Gallaway, TN 38036-0228
FDA Number: 1043646   *Fax:* 901-867-8954
E-mail: email@medegen.com
Web site: www.medegen.com
Annual Revenue: $50-$100 Million
Year Founded: 1874
Total Employees: 440   *Marketing Staff:* 2   *Sales Staff:* 40
Ownership: Medical Action Industries, Inc
Produces/Sells CE-marked Devices: N
Federal Procurement Eligibility: Small Business, GSA Contract, VA Contract
Distribution: Manufacturer Direct, Manufacturer Through Distributor, Manufacturer Through Manufacturer Reps
General Admin.: Mr. Mark Dorris/President
     Jim Jenkins/Vice President Human Resources
Mktg./Adv.: John Penhollow/Director National Accounts
     Jim Trautschold/Vice President Business Development
     Jim Trautschold/Vice President Corporate Development
     Phil Royston/Vice President Marketing & Sales
Production: Bob Koenig/Director Materials Management
     Judy Thun/Vice President Customer Service
     Mr. Paul Ellis/Vice President Manufacturing & Operations
     Jim Bennett/Vice President Manufacturing & Production

Basin, Emesis	General
Basin, Sponge	General

MEDEGEN MEDICAL PRODUCTS, LLC   800-233-1987 *(cont'd)*

Basin, Wash	General
Bath, Sitz, Physical Medicine	Physical Med
Beaker (Laboratory)	Chemistry
Bedpan	General
Bedpan, Fracture	General
Bowl, Solution	General
Bowl, Sponge	General
Cart, Housekeeping	General
Commode Seat	General
Container, Specimen, All Types	General
Container, Sterilization (Tray)	General
Container, Urine Specimen	General
Contract Manufacturing	General
Cup, Denture	Dental And Oral
Cup, Geriatric Feeding	General
Cup, Medicine	General
Foodservice Product/Equipment	General
Jar, Dressing	Surgery
Jar, Forceps	Surgery
Kit, Sitz Bath	Physical Med
Shield, Eye, Ophthalmic	Ophthalmology
Tray, Surgical Instrument	Surgery
Urinal	General
Waste Receptacle, Kick Bucket	General

MEDELA, INC.   800-435-8316   815-363-1166
1101 Corporate Drive, McHenry, IL 60050
FDA Number: 3002807523   *Fax:* 815-363-1246
E-mail: customer.service@medela.com
Web site: www.medela.com
Medical Products Sales Volume: $45,300,000
Year Founded: 1961
Total Employees: 300
Ownership: Medela Ag
Quality System Registration Information: ISO9000; ISO9001
Produces/Sells CE-marked Devices: Y
Federal Procurement Eligibility: Small Business, GSA Contract
General Admin.: Carr Lane Quackenbush/President
     Joe Hoffman/Vice President Human Resources
Mktg./Adv.: Carolin Archibald/Vice President Marketing
     Peter Host/Vice President Sales
Production: Scott Baxter/Vice President Operations
     Christopher Peterson/Vice President Quality Assurance
Research: Sam Levey/Vice President Engineering
     Brian Silver/Vice President Research
Finance: Rick Dettman/Chief Financial Officer
IS: Rick Russell/Chief Tech. Manager

Aspirator, Low Volume (Gastric Suction)	Gastroenterology/Urology
Aspirator, Surgical	Surgery
Aspirator, Thoracic (Suction Unit)	Cardiovascular
Aspirator, Tracheal	Ear/Nose/Throat
Aspirator, Wound Suction Pump	General
Bag, Plastic	General
Canister, Suction	Cardiovascular
Collector, Specimen	Microbiology
Component, Other	General
Drain, Thoracic, Water Seal	Anesthesiology
Filter, Aspirator	Surgery
Lotion, Skin Care	General
Pad, Breast	Obstetrics/Gynecology
Phototherapy Unit (Bilirubin Lamp)	General
Pump, Breast, Non-Powered	Obstetrics/Gynecology
Pump, Breast, Powered	Obstetrics/Gynecology
Scale, Infant	General
Shield, Breast	Obstetrics/Gynecology
Shield, Nipple	Obstetrics/Gynecology
Timer, Apgar	General
Wipe, Instrument	General

MEDELCO LTD.   800-268-7927   905-673-2108
6469 Northam Drive,
Mississauga, ONT L4V 1 Canada
FDA Number: n/a   *Fax:* 905-673-3109
E-mail: sales@medelco.ca
Web site: www.medelco.ca
Year Founded: 1974
Total Employees: 25   *Marketing Staff:* 1   *Sales Staff:* 6
Ownership: Private
Produces/Sells CE-marked Devices: N
Distribution: Exclusive Distributor, Importer

MEDELEC INDUSTRIES   888-522-6452
6800 S.w. 40th St., Pmb-700, Miami, FL 33155
FDA Number: 1052962
Ownership: Private
Produces/Sells CE-marked Devices: N

Electrosurgical Unit, Cutting & Coagulation Device	Surgery

MEDELEX, INC.   800-644-0692   408-481-9100
3012 Lawrence Expressway,
Santa Clara, CA 95051
FDA Number: n/a   *Fax:* 408-481-9199
E-mail: medelex@medelex.com
Web site: www.medelex.com
Ownership: Private
Produces/Sells CE-marked Devices: N
   Imager, X-Ray, Solid State (Flat Panel/Digital)   Radiology

MEDENNIUM, INC.   949-789-5385
9 Parker, Suite 150, Irvine, CA 92618
FDA Number: 2031959
   Lens, Intraocular   Ophthalmology

MEDENTAL INTL.   760-727-5889
3008 Palm Hill Dr., Vista, CA 92084
FDA Number: 1723973
Ownership: Private
Produces/Sells CE-marked Devices: N
   Adhesive, Bracket And Conditioner, Resin   Dental And Oral
   Cement, Dental   Dental And Oral
   Material, Impression   Dental And Oral
   Material, Tooth Shade, Resin   Dental And Oral
   Sealant, Pit And Fissure, And Conditioner, Resin   Dental And Oral
   Varnish, Cavity   Dental And Oral

MEDERI THERAPEUTICS INC   203-930-9900
8 Sound Shore Drive, Suite 304, Greenwich, CT 06830
FDA Number: 3007729452
E-mail: info@mederitherapeutics.com
Web site: www.mederitherapeutics.com
Ownership: Private
Produces/Sells CE-marked Devices: N
   Electrosurgical Unit, Cutting & Coagulation Device   Surgery

MEDEVICES, INC.   847-548-8499
888 E. Belvidere Rd., Suite 212, Grayslake, IL 60030
FDA Number: 1424558   *Fax:* 817-346-9326
E-mail: sales@sightsure.com
Web site: www.medevices.org
Ownership: Private
Produces/Sells CE-marked Devices: N
   Tube, Gastrointestinal   Gastroenterology/Urology

MEDEX CARDIO-PULMONARY
   See Smiths Medical Asd, Inc.

MEDEX PARA-MEDICAL EQUIPMENT INC.   450-581-3966
275 Boul Pierre-Legardeur, Le Gardeur J5Z 3A7 Canada
FDA Number: 9617546
   Stretcher, Hand-Carried   General
   Transfer Device, Patient, Manual   General

MEDEX SYSTEMS INTERNATIONAL INC.   604-607-7008
25990 48th Ave., Aldergrove, BC V4W-1J2 Canada
FDA Number: n/a   *Fax:* 604-857-8942
Year Founded: 1981
Total Employees: 50
Ownership: Private
Produces/Sells CE-marked Devices: N
Distribution: Manufacturer Direct

MEDEX, INC.
   See Smiths Medical OEM

MEDEXCEL   716-438-0132
5444 Leete Rd., Lockport, NY 14094
FDA Number: n/a   *Fax:* 716-433-3183
E-mail: dgrabow@aol.com
Medical Products Sales Volume: $2,000,000
Annual Revenue: $1-$5 Million
Total Employees: 3   *Marketing Staff:* 1   *Sales Staff:* 2
Ownership: Private
Quality System Registration Information: ISO9000
Produces/Sells CE-marked Devices: Y
Federal Procurement Eligibility: Small Business
Distribution: Manufacturer Direct
General Admin.: Dan Grabowski/President
     John C. Anain/Vice President
   Electrocardiograph, Single Channel   Cardiovascular
   Electrode, Holter   Cardiovascular
   Monitor, Bed Patient   General
   Monitor, Blood Pressure, Indirect, Automatic   Cardiovascular
   Monitor, Cardiac Output, Thermal (Balloon Type Catheter)   Surgery
   Monitor, ECG   Cardiovascular
   Monitor, ECG, Anesthesia   Anesthesiology
   Monitor, Neonatal   Obstetrics/Gynecology
   Monitor, Physiological, Acute Care   Anesthesiology
   Oximeter, Pulse   General

MEDEXCEL   716-438-0132 *(cont'd)*
   Scanner, Long-Term, ECG, Recording   Cardiovascular
   Telemetry Unit, Physiological, ECG   Cardiovascular

MEDFILMS, INC.   800-535-5593   520-575-8900
4910 W. Monte Carlo Drive, Tucson, AZ 85745
FDA Number: n/a   *Fax:* 520-742-6052
E-mail: info@medfilms.com
Web site: www.medfilms.com
Medical Products Sales Volume: $400,000
Year Founded: 1982
Total Employees: 3
Ownership: Private
Federal Procurement Eligibility: Small Business
Distribution: Manufacturer Direct
General Admin.: Alan K. Reeter/President
Mktg./Adv.: Kim Ohl/Manager Marketing
   Material, Training, Audiovisual   General

MEDGE PLATFORMS, INC.   212-351-5029
100 Park Ave., Ste. 1600, New York, NY 10017
FDA Number: 2438941
   Scanner, Ultrasonic (Pulsed Echo)   Radiology

MEDGENESIS
   See Arkray Usa

MEDGYN PRODUCTS, INC.   800-451-9667   630-627-4105
328 N. Eisenhower Lane, Lombard, IL 60148
FDA Number: 1450908   *Fax:* 630-627-0127
E-mail: medgyn@medgyn.com
Web site: www.medgyn.com
Medical Products Sales Volume: $7,300,000
Annual Revenue: $5-$10 Million
Year Founded: 1975
Total Employees: 55   *Marketing Staff:* 3   *Sales Staff:* 7
Ownership: Private
Quality System Registration Information: ISO9002
Produces/Sells CE-marked Devices: Y
Federal Procurement Eligibility: Small Business, Minority Owned
Distribution: Manufacturer Direct, Manufacturer Through Distributor, OEM, Exporter
General Admin.: Brenda Gousset/Office Manager
     Lakshman Agadi/President, Chief Executive Officer
     Ramesh Vyas/Vice President, General Manager
Mktg./Adv.: Lakshman Agadi/Director Product Development
     Ramesh Vyas/Manager Contract Sales
     John Jaresko/Manager National Sales
     Lakshman Agadi/Vice President Marketing & Sales
Production: Srini Muthuswamy/Director Quality Assurance
   Colposcope   Obstetrics/Gynecology
   Curette   Orthopedics
   Curette, Uterine   Obstetrics/Gynecology
   Dilator, Cervical, Hygroscopic-Laminaria   Obstetrics/Gynecology
   Dilator, Other   Surgery
   Electrosurgical Equipment, General Purpose   Surgery
   Hysteroscope   Obstetrics/Gynecology
   Laparoscope, Gynecologic   Obstetrics/Gynecology
   Monitor, Fetal Doppler Ultrasound   Obstetrics/Gynecology
   Punch, Biopsy   Gastroenterology/Urology
   Speculum, Vaginal, Metal   Obstetrics/Gynecology
   Tube, Aspirating, Flexible, Connecting   Anesthesiology

MEDI   800-947-6334
4814 E. 2nd St., Benicia, CA 94510
FDA Number: n/a   *Fax:* 707-746-6374
E-mail: info@interacoustics.com
Web site: www.interacoustics.com
Medical Products Sales Volume: $101,100,000
Annual Revenue: $0-$1 Million
Total Employees: 200   *Marketing Staff:* 1   *Sales Staff:* 1
Ownership: Private
Produces/Sells CE-marked Devices: Y
Federal Procurement Eligibility: Small Business, GSA Contract
Distribution: Manufacturer Through Manufacturer Reps
General Admin.: Donna Ward/Chief Executive Officer
     Philip Korbas/President
Mktg./Adv.: James Taber/Director Marketing
     James Tabar/Manager Sales Training
Production: James Tabar/Manager Regulatory Affairs
   Chamber, Acoustic, Testing   Ear/Nose/Throat
   General Medical Device   General

MEDI MFG., INC.   336-449-4440
6481 Franz Warner Pkwy., Whitsett, NC 27377
FDA Number: 1063312
Ownership: Private
Produces/Sells CE-marked Devices: N

MEDI MFG., INC.   336-449-4440 *(cont'd)*

Stocking, Support (Anti-Embolic)	General

MEDI USA   800-633-6334
6481 Franz Warner Parkway, Whitsett, NC 27377   **336-449-4440**

FDA Number: 1450371
E-mail: bruceg@mediusa.com
Web site: www.mediusa.com
Annual Revenue: $10-$25 Million
Year Founded: 1984
Total Employees: 159   *Marketing Staff:* 4   *Sales Staff:* 29
Ownership: Private
Quality System Registration Information: ISO9000
Produces/Sells CE-marked Devices: Y
Distribution: Manufacturer Through Distributor
General Admin.: D. Bruce Guynn/President, Chief Executive Officer
Mktg./Adv.: John Cody/Director Marketing
    Tonya Bradshear/Director National Accounts
    Craig Garrison/Director Product Development
    Ed Wilbourne/Manager Advertising
    Michal Canon/Manager Sales Training
Production: Craig Garrison/Vice President Manufacturing

Brace, Joint, Ankle (External)	Physical Med
Joint, Knee, External Brace	Physical Med
Sleeve, Compressible Limb	Cardiovascular
Stocking, Elastic	General
Support, Arm	Physical Med

MEDI-CRUSH COMPANY   800-262-6334
P.O. BOX 321381, Flowood, MS 39232   **800-262-6334**

FDA Number: n/a   *Fax:* 601-898-3249
E-mail: medicrush@c-gate.net
Medical Products Sales Volume: $500,000
Annual Revenue: $0-$1 Million
Total Employees: 4   *Marketing Staff:* 2   *Sales Staff:* 2
Ownership: Private
Produces/Sells CE-marked Devices: N
Federal Procurement Eligibility: Small Business
Distribution: Manufacturer Through Distributor
General Admin.: Rita Dudley/General Manager
    Bill W. Elkins/President

Apron, Laboratory	Chemistry
Apron, Surgical	Surgery
Box, Glove	Microbiology
Breaker, Ampule	General
Cabinet Casework, General Purpose	General
Cabinet, Narcotic Control	General
Container, Medication, Home-Use	General
Cover, Head, Surgical	Surgery
Cover, Shoe, Operating Room	Surgery
Crusher, Pill	General
Depressor, Tongue	General
Dispenser, Narcotic	General
Goggles, Protective, Eye	Ophthalmology
Holder, Catheter	Gastroenterology/Urology
Holder, Medical Chart	General
Infusion Stand	General
Kit, First Aid	Surgery
Mask, Face	General
Packaging System, Unit-Dose	General
Paper, Chart, Record, Medical	General
Rack, Test Tube	Chemistry
Screen, Bedside	General
Suit, Scrub, Reusable	Surgery
Tray, Medicine	General
Tray, Wheelchair	Physical Med
Waste Disposal Unit, Syringe	General

MEDI-DOSE, INC.   800-523-8966
70 Industrial Drive, Ivyland, PA 18974   **215-396-8600**

FDA Number: 2521373   *Fax:* 800-323-8966
E-mail: info@medi-dose.com
Web site: www.medi-dose.com
Year Founded: 1971
Total Employees: 25
Ownership: Private
Produces/Sells CE-marked Devices: N
Federal Procurement Eligibility: Small Business
Distribution: Manufacturer Direct, Manufacturer Through Distributor, Manufacturer Through Manufacturer Reps, Exclusive Distributor
General Admin.: Robert Braverman/General Manager
    Mark Braverman/President
Mktg./Adv.: Robert Braverman/Director Marketing
Production: Mark Bea/Director Operations

Bag, Plastic	General
Bottle, Medicine Spray	General
Bottle, Nursing	Obstetrics/Gynecology
Cabinet, Narcotic Control	General
Cap, Tip, Syringe	General

MEDI-DOSE, INC.   800-523-8966 *(cont'd)*

Container, IV	General
Container, Medication, Graduated Liquid	General
Container, Specimen, All Types	General
Crusher, Pill	General
Cup, Medicine	General
Dispenser, Fluid	General
Dispenser, Liquid, Unit-Dose	General
Dispenser, Syringe And Needle	General
Filter, Air	General
Filter, Infusion Line	General
Filter, Intravenous Tubing	General
Fitting, Luer	General
Holder, Medical Chart	General
Label, Device	General
Labeling Equipment	General
Labware, Basic, Disposable	Chemistry
Lancet, Blood	General
Packaging System, Unit-Dose	General
Port, Vascular Access	Cardiovascular
Rack, Medical Chart	General
Syringe, Other	General
Unit, Filter, Membrane	Chemistry

MEDI-DYN, INC.
See Crothall

MEDI-DYNE HEALTHCARE PRODUCTS, L.L.C.   800-810-1740
1812 Industrial Boulevard, Colleyville, TX 76034   **817-251-8660**

FDA Number: 3003175285   *Fax:* 817-488-6616
Web site: www.medi-dyne.com
Medical Products Sales Volume: $1,100,000
Ownership: Private
Produces/Sells CE-marked Devices: N
Federal Procurement Eligibility: Small Business
Distribution: Manufacturer Through Distributor, Exclusive Distributor

Cushion, Wheelchair (Pad)	Physical Med
Insoles, Medical	General
Pillow, Cervical	Orthopedics

MEDI-GARB CO., INC.   800-233-2463
216 W. Broad St., Statesville, NC 28687   **704-873-7888**

FDA Number: 1067140   *Fax:* 704-873-7899
E-mail: info@breastbinder.com
Web site: www.breastbinder.com
Medical Products Sales Volume: $200,000
Annual Revenue: $0-$1 Million
Year Founded: 1991
Total Employees: 3   *Marketing Staff:* 1
Ownership: Private
Produces/Sells CE-marked Devices: N
Federal Procurement Eligibility: Small Business, Female Owned
Distribution: Manufacturer Direct
General Admin.: Bonita W. Eisele/President
Mktg./Adv.: Alan Eisele/Vice President Marketing & Sales

Binder, Breast	Obstetrics/Gynecology

MEDI-GLOBE CORPORATION   800-966-1431
110 W. Orion St., Suite 136, Tempe, AZ 85283   **480-897-2772**

FDA Number: 2084263   *Fax:* 480-897-2878
E-mail: info@mediglobe.com
Web site: www.mediglobe.com
Medical Products Sales Volume: $37,800,000
Annual Revenue: $25-$50 Million
Year Founded: 1985
Ownership: Private
Quality System Registration Information: ISO9001
Produces/Sells CE-marked Devices: Y
Federal Procurement Eligibility: Small Business
Distribution: Manufacturer Direct, Manufacturer Through Distributor, Manufacturer Through Manufacturer Reps, OEM, Exclusive Distributor, Importer
General Admin.: Stefan Wohnhas/President, Chief Executive Officer
Mktg./Adv.: Scott Karler/Manager National Sales
Production: Brian Karler/Vice President Operations

Basket, Biliary Stone Retrieval	Gastroenterology/Urology
Catheter, Other	Gastroenterology/Urology
Endoscope, Flexible	Gastroenterology/Urology
Forceps, Biopsy	Surgery
Forceps, Biopsy, Non-Electric	Gastroenterology/Urology
Guidewire	Cardiovascular
Lithotriptor, Mechanical, Biliary	Gastroenterology/Urology
Needle, Other	General
Papillotome	Surgery
Probe, Other	General
Snare, Polyp	Surgery

MEDI-HUT CO., INC.   800-882-0139
1935 Swarthmore Avenue,   **732-901-0606**
Lakewood, NJ 08701

FDA Number: n/a   *Fax:* 732-901-1177

MEDI-HUT CO., INC.   800-882-0139 *(cont'd)*

E-mail: medihut@aol.com
Web site: www.medihutonline.com
Annual Revenue: $10-$25 Million
Year Founded: 1982
Total Employees: 50   *Marketing Staff:* 2   *Sales Staff:* 2
Ownership: Public
Stock Symbol: MHUT
Traded On: NASDAQ
Produces/Sells CE-marked Devices: N
Federal Procurement Eligibility: Small Business
Distribution: Manufacturer Direct, Manufacturer Through Distributor, Manufacturer Through Manufacturer Reps
General Admin.: Mr. Laurence Simon/Chief Financial Officer, Treasurer
    Mr. Joseph A. Sanpietro/President, Chief Executive Officer
    Mr. Vincent Sanpietro/Secretary

Condom	Obstetrics/Gynecology
Label, Bar Code	General
Pad, Alcohol	General
Syringe, Insulin	General
Syringe, Other	General

MEDI-INN INC.   888-633-4466   (705) 359-1900

6-6150 Highway 7, Suite 491, Woodbridge, ONT L4H 0 Canada
FDA Number: n/a   Fax: (705) 359-1955
E-mail: pphillips@medi-inn.com
Web site: http://www.medi-inn.com
Year Founded: 1996
Total Employees: 25
Ownership: Private
Produces/Sells CE-marked Devices: N
Distribution: Manufacturer Direct, Exclusive Distributor

MEDI-KID CO.   888-463-3543   951-925-8800

P.O. Box 5398, Hemet, CA 92544
FDA Number: n/a   Fax: 951-925-0686
Web site: www.medi-kid.com
Medical Products Sales Volume: $500,000
Annual Revenue: $1-$5 Million
Year Founded: 1984
Ownership: Private
Produces/Sells CE-marked Devices: N
Federal Procurement Eligibility: Small Business, Female Owned
Distribution: Manufacturer Direct, Manufacturer Through Distributor

Immobilizer, Arm	Orthopedics
Restraint	Physical Med

MEDI-PART,INC.   715-476-7600

5844 North Rice Lake Rd., P.o. Box 276, Mercer, WI 54547
FDA Number: 1420751
E-mail: sales@medi-part.com
Web site: www.medi-part.com
Ownership: Private
Produces/Sells CE-marked Devices: N

Circuit, Breathing (W Connector, Adapter, Y Piece)	Anesthesiology

MEDI-PHYSICS, INC., DBA GE HEALTHCARE   800-633-4123   847-398-8400

3350 N Ridge Ave., Arlington Heights, IL 60004
FDA Number: 2915056
Web site: www.gehealthcare.com
Ownership: Ge Healthcare
Stock Symbol: GE
Traded On: NYSE
Produces/Sells CE-marked Devices: N
General Admin.: Laurence J. Steudle/President, Chief Executive Officer
    M. Kenneth Oboz/Vice President, General Counsel
Mktg./Adv.: James F. Rogers/Vice President Marketing
    Lawrence W. Sarokin/Vice President Sales
Production: Daniel H. Schumann/Vice President Product Engineering Development

Seed, Isotope, Gold, Titanium, Platinum	Radiology
Source, Brachytherapy, Radionuclide	Radiology
Source, Isotope, Sealed, Gold, Titanium, Platinum	Radiology

MEDI-SIM

See Educational Software Concepts, Inc.

MEDI-SOURCE, INC.   740-524-0358

7719 State Route 656, Sunbury, OH 43074
FDA Number: 1531212

Electrode, Cutaneous	Cns/Neurology

MEDI-SPAN, INC.   800-388-8884   317-735-5300

8425 Woodfield Crossing Blvd., Suite 490, Indianapolis, IN 46240
FDA Number: n/a
E-mail: medispan-support@wolterskluwer.com

MEDI-SPAN, INC.   800-388-8884 *(cont'd)*

Web site: www.medispan.com
Ownership: Private
Produces/Sells CE-marked Devices: N
Distribution: Manufacturer Direct

Computer Software	General

MEDI-TECH HOLDINGS, INC.   714-841-8603

15209 Springdale Ave., Huntington Beach, CA 92649
FDA Number: 2032795
Ownership: Private
Produces/Sells CE-marked Devices: N

Disc, Strip And Reagent, Microorganism Differentiation	Microbiology

MEDI-TECH INTERNATIONAL CORP.   800-333-0109   718-875-4535

26 Court St., Brooklyn, NY 11242-1102
FDA Number: 2430583   Fax: 718-855-1618
E-mail: mtiorderdesk@aol.com
Web site: www.medi-techintl.com/
Medical Products Sales Volume: $800,000
Annual Revenue: $1-$5 Million
Year Founded: 1973
Total Employees: 6   *Marketing Staff:* 5   *Sales Staff:* 12
Ownership: Private
Produces/Sells CE-marked Devices: N
Federal Procurement Eligibility: Small Business, GSA Contract, VA Contract
Distribution: Manufacturer Direct, Manufacturer Through Distributor, Manufacturer Through Manufacturer Reps, OEM
General Admin.: H. A. Perry/Chief Executive Officer
    George Fortunato/President
    Herbert Perry/Vice President, General Manager
Mktg./Adv.: H. A. Perry/Executive Vice President Marketing & Sales
    H. A. Perry/Manager International & National Sales
    Herbert Perry/Vice President Business Development
Production: Herbert Perry/Manager Regulatory Affairs
Research: Herbert Perry/Executive Vice President, Director Research & Development

Bandage, Cast	Physical Med
Bandage, Elastic	General
Bandage, Other	General
Bandage, Tubular	General
Dressing, Non-Adherent	General
Dressing, Other	General
Dressing, Skin Graft, Donor Site	General
Dressing, Universal	General
Dressing, Wound and Burn, Hydrogel	Surgery
Dressing, Wound and Burn, Occlusive	Surgery
Kit, Wound Dressing	Surgery
Lotion, Skin Care	General
Retainer, Bandage (Elastic Net)	General

MEDI-TECH INTERNATIONAL, INC.   305-593-9373

2924 N.W. 109th Avenue, Miami, FL 33172
FDA Number: n/a   Fax: 305-599-1951
E-mail: orders@meditechintl.com
Web site: www.meditechintl.com
Medical Products Sales Volume: $2,900,000
Annual Revenue: $1-$5 Million
Year Founded: 1979
Total Employees: 6   *Sales Staff:* 6
Ownership: Private
Produces/Sells CE-marked Devices: Y
Federal Procurement Eligibility: Small Business
Distribution: Manufacturer Through Distributor, Manufacturer Through Manufacturer Reps, Exporter
General Admin.: Al Perrini/Chief Executive Officer
Mktg./Adv.: Joe Fernandez/President Marketing & Sales
    Diego Grave de Peralta/Vice President Marketing & Sales

Accessories, Operating Room, Table	Surgery
Anatomical Training Model	General
Aspirator, Emergency Suction	General
Aspirator, Infant	General
Aspirator, Wound Suction Pump	General
Bag, Body	General
Bassinet (Infant Bed)	General
Bath, Hydro-Massage (Whirlpool)	Physical Med
Bed, Obese	General
Bilirubinometer, Cutaneous (Jaundice Meter)	General
Blanket, Fire	General
Refrigerator, Blood Bank	Hematology
Refrigerator, Laboratory	General
Refrigerator, Morgue, Walk-In	Pathology
Sterilizer, Laboratory	Microbiology
Stretcher, Wheeled (Mobile)	General
Table, Autopsy	Pathology
Washer/Sterilizer	General

MANUFACTURER PROFILES

MEDI-TEK, INC.　　　　　　　　661-940-0030
4555 W. Avenue G, Suite # 6, Lancaster, CA 93536
FDA Number: n/a　　　　　　　　*Fax:* 661-940-3447
E-mail: meditek@as.net
Web site: www.medi-tek.net
Medical Products Sales Volume: $300,000
Annual Revenue: $0-$1 Million
Year Founded: 1988
Total Employees: 3　　　　　*Sales Staff:* 1
Ownership: Private
Produces/Sells CE-marked Devices: N
Federal Procurement Eligibility: Small Business
Distribution: Service Direct
General Admin.: Robert Hania/Chief Executive Officer
Mktg./Adv.: Morris Hania/Manager Sales
　Service, Maintenance/Repair　　　　　　　　General
　Service, Used Equipment　　　　　　　　　　General

MEDI-TEMP TECHNOLOGY INTL., LLC　888-669-0600
14131 N. Rio Vista Blvd. # 8, Peoria, AZ 85381　623-878-8400
FDA Number: 2031638　　　　　*Fax:* 623-878-8403
E-mail: info@medi-temp.com
Web site: www.medi-temp.com
Annual Revenue: $1-$5 Million
Year Founded: 1993
Total Employees: 10
Ownership: Private
Produces/Sells CE-marked Devices: N
Federal Procurement Eligibility: Small Business
Distribution: Manufacturer Direct, Manufacturer Through Distributor, Manufacturer Through Manufacturer Reps
General Admin.: Randy Evans/President, Chief Executive Officer
Mktg./Adv.: Greig Derry/Director Marketing & Product Development
Production: Brent Ewasiuk/Vice President Manufacturing
　Pack, Hot Or Cold, Disposable　　　　　Physical Med
　Pack, Hot Or Cold, Reusable　　　　　　Physical Med

MEDI-TONIC PERFUSION SYSTEM
See Medtronic Perfusion Systems

MEDI/NUCLEAR CORP.　　　　　　800-321-5981
4610 Littlejohn St., Baldwin Park, CA 91706　626-960-9822
FDA Number: 2050098　　　　　*Fax:* 626-960-8700
E-mail: info@medinuclear.com
Web site: www.medinuclear.com
Medical Products Sales Volume: $3,800,000
Annual Revenue: $1-$5 Million
Year Founded: 1973
Total Employees: 14　　*Marketing Staff:* 1　　*Sales Staff:* 2
Ownership: Private
Produces/Sells CE-marked Devices: N
Federal Procurement Eligibility: Small Business
Distribution: Manufacturer Direct, Exporter
General Admin.: Lyman Newton/Chief Executive Officer
　　　　　　Russell King/President
Mktg./Adv.: Glenn Samford/Director Marketing
　　　　　Leslie McLeod/Manager Advertising
Production: Shari Fuhst/Manager Materials
　　　　　Ross Potter/Manager Regulatory Affairs
　Nebulizer, Direct Patient Interface　　　　Anesthesiology
　Protector, Mouth Guard　　　　　　Dental And Oral
　Xenon System　　　　　　　　　　Anesthesiology

MEDIA CYBERNETICS INC.　　　　301-495-3305
4340 East-West Hwy, Suite 400, Bethesda, MD 20814
FDA Number: n/a　　　　　　　　*Fax:* 301-495-5964
E-mail: customerservice@mediacy.com
Web site: http://www.mediacy.com
Year Founded: 1981
Ownership: Private
Produces/Sells CE-marked Devices: N

MEDIAID INC.　　　　　　　　　714-367-2848
17517 Fabrica Way, Suite H, Cerritos, CA 90703
FDA Number: 2087439
　Oximeter, Intracardiac　　　　　　　Cardiovascular

MEDIANA TECHNOLOGIES CORP　　800-829-6427
5850 Farinon Drive, San Antonio, TX 78249　210-690-6200
FDA Number: 2245530　　　　　*Fax:* 210-696-8808
E-mail: info@medianatech.com
Web site: http://www.medianatech.com
Medical Products Sales Volume: $2,700,000
Annual Revenue: $10-$25 Million
Total Employees: 35　　*Marketing Staff:* 3　　*Sales Staff:* 8
Ownership: Colin Corporation
Quality System Registration Information: ISO9000; ISO9001
Produces/Sells CE-marked Devices: N

MEDIANA TECHNOLOGIES CORP　　800-829-6427 *(cont'd)*
Federal Procurement Eligibility: Small Business, GSA Contract, VA Contract
Distribution: Manufacturer Direct, Manufacturer Through Distributor, Manufacturer Through Manufacturer Reps, OEM
General Admin.: Dr. MJ Khil/Chief Executive Officer, Chairman
　　　　　Mr. Peter Hsu/President, Chief Executive Officer
　Monitor, Blood Pressure, Indirect, Automatic　Cardiovascular
　Monitor, ECG　　　　　　　　　　Cardiovascular
　Monitor, ECG, Ambulatory, Real-Time　　Cardiovascular
　Monitor, Neonatal　　　　　　Obstetrics/Gynecology
　Monitor, Physiological, Patient　　　　Cardiovascular
　Monitor, Physiological, Stress Exercise　Cardiovascular
　Monitor, Pulse Rate　　　　　　　　Anesthesiology
　Monitor, Temperature (Self-Contained)　　　General

MEDIATECH, INC.　　　　　　　800-235-5476
9345 Discovery Blvd., Manassas, VA 20109　703-471-5955
FDA Number: 1121482　　　　　*Fax:* 703-471-0363
E-mail: custserv@cellgro.com
Web site: www.cellgro.com
Annual Revenue: $10-$25 Million
Year Founded: 1984
Total Employees: 90　　*Marketing Staff:* 5　　*Sales Staff:* 20
Ownership: Private
Produces/Sells CE-marked Devices: N
Federal Procurement Eligibility: Small Business
Distribution: Manufacturer Direct, Manufacturer Through Distributor, Manufacturer Through Manufacturer Reps, OEM
General Admin.: John Elliott/Executive Vice President
　　　　　James Deolden/President
Mktg./Adv.: Jason Laufer/Vice President Sales
Production: Matt Maupin/Manager Manufacturing
　Culture Media, Synthetic Cell And Tissue　　Pathology
　Solution, Balanced Salt　　　　　　　Pathology

MEDIC ALERT FOUNDATION UNITED STATES
See Medicalert Foundation International

MEDIC COMPUTER SYSTEMS
See Allscripts-Misys Healthcare Solutions

MEDIC ID'S INTERNATIONAL　　　800-926-3342
PO Box 571687, Tarzana, CA 91357　　818-705-0595
FDA Number: n/a　　　　　　　　*Fax:* 818-705-0773
E-mail: medicid@medicid.org
Web site: www.medicid.com
Medical Products Sales Volume: $700,000
Annual Revenue: $1-$5 Million
Year Founded: 1990
Total Employees: 10　　*Marketing Staff:* 4　　*Sales Staff:* 15
Ownership: Private
Produces/Sells CE-marked Devices: N
Federal Procurement Eligibility: Small Business
Distribution: Manufacturer Direct, Manufacturer Through Distributor, Manufacturer Through Manufacturer Reps, Exporter
General Admin.: M. Silverstein/President
Mktg./Adv.: M.J. Silverstein/Director Marketing
　Bracelet, Identification　　　　　　　　General

MEDIC UNIQUE　　　　　　　　310-698-0739
2962 Mindanao Dr., Costa Mesa, CA 92626
FDA Number: 2029174
Ownership: Private
Produces/Sells CE-marked Devices: N
　Marker, Periodontic　　　　　　Dental And Oral

MEDIC-AIR, A DIVISION OF CORFLEX, INC.　800-426-7353
669 E. Industrial Park Dr.,　　　　603-623-3344
Manchester, NH 03109
FDA Number: n/a　　　　　　　　*Fax:* 603-623-4111
E-mail: sales@corflex.com
Web site: www.corflex.com
Annual Revenue: $5-$10 Million
Total Employees: 50
Ownership: Private
Produces/Sells CE-marked Devices: N
Federal Procurement Eligibility: Small Business
Distribution: Manufacturer Through Distributor, Manufacturer Through Manufacturer Reps
General Admin.: Paul Lorenzetti/Chief Executive Officer
Mktg./Adv.: Ted Lorenzetti/Vice President Sales
　Pillow　　　　　　　　　　　　　General
　Pillow, Cervical　　　　　　　　　Orthopedics
　Support, Back　　　　　　　　　　Orthopedics

MEDICA CORP.　　　　　　　　800-777-5983
5 Oak Park Drive, Bedford, MA 01730　781-275-4892
FDA Number: 1220972　　　　　*Fax:* 781-275-2731
E-mail: sales@medicacorp.com

MEDICA CORP.   800-777-5983 *(cont'd)*

Web site: www.medicacorp.com
Medical Products Sales Volume: $10,000,000
Annual Revenue: $10-$25 Million
Year Founded: 1984
Total Employees: 100   *Marketing Staff:* 3   *Sales Staff:* 6
Ownership: Private
Produces/Sells CE-marked Devices: Y
Federal Procurement Eligibility: Small Business, GSA Contract
Distribution: Manufacturer Through Distributor, OEM, Exclusive Distributor
General Admin.: Robert W. Hagopian/President, Chief Executive Officer
Mktg./Adv.: Steve Rettew/Director Product Development
     Kevin McCollum/Manager International & National Sales
     Steve Rettew/Vice President Advertising
     Douglas A. Moe/Vice President Business Development
Production: Richard Kruszynski/Director Operations
     Photios Makris/Director Quality Assurance
Research: Richard Rodgers/Vice President Research & Development

Analyzer, Blood Gas pH	Anesthesiology
Analyzer, Chemistry, Electrolyte	Chemistry
Electrode, Ion Selective (Non-Specified)	Chemistry
Electrode, Ion Specific, Calcium	Chemistry
Electrode, Ion Specific, Chloride	Chemistry
Electrode, Ion Specific, Potassium	Chemistry
Electrode, Ion Specific, Sodium	Chemistry
Electrode, Other	General

MEDICA, INC.   800-845-6496
336 Encinitas Blvd., Suite 200,   760-634-5440
Encinitas, CA 92024

FDA Number: 2021875   *Fax:* 760-634-5442
E-mail: medica@medica-dx.com
Web site: http://www.medica-dx.com
Medical Products Sales Volume: $900,000
Annual Revenue: $0-$1 Million
Year Founded: 1979
Total Employees: 11   *Marketing Staff:* 1   *Sales Staff:* 1
Ownership: Private
Produces/Sells CE-marked Devices: Y
Federal Procurement Eligibility: Small Business, Female Owned
Distribution: Manufacturer Direct, Manufacturer Through Distributor, OEM, Exporter
General Admin.: Jarka Bartl/President, Chief Executive Officer
Production: Rhodora Chapoco/Director Quality Assurance & Product Development
     Rhodora Chapoco/Manager Production & RA

Anti-DNA Antibody, Antigen and Control	Immunology
Antibody, Anti-Smooth Muscle, Indirect Immunofluorescent	Immunology
Antibody, Anti-Thyroid, Indirect Immunofluorescent	Immunology
Antibody, Antimitochondrial, Indirect Immunofluorescent	Immunology
Antibody, Antinuclear, Indirect Immunofluorescent, Antigen	Immunology
Antibody, Multiple Auto, Indirect Immunofluorescent	Immunology
Antibody, Other	General
Antiparietal Antibody, Immunofluorescent, Antigen, Control	Immunology
Autoantibodies, Endomysial(tissue Transglutaminase)	Immunology

MEDICAL & CLINICAL CONSORTIUM (MCC)   877-622-8378
13740 East Nelson Ave.,   626-934-9364
City of Industry, CA 91746

FDA Number: 2032252   *Fax:* 626-934-9384
E-mail: info@mcctest.com
Web site: www.mcctest.com
Annual Revenue: $1-$5 Million
Year Founded: 1999
Ownership: Private
Produces/Sells CE-marked Devices: N
Federal Procurement Eligibility: Minority Owned, Female Owned
Distribution: Manufacturer Direct, Manufacturer Through Distributor, Manufacturer Through Manufacturer Reps, Exporter

Antigen, Salmonella SPP.	Microbiology
Kit, Forensic Evidence	Pathology
Kit, Screening, Urine	Microbiology
Kit, Test, Multiple, Drugs Of Abuse, Over The Counter	Toxicology
Test, Ethyl Alcohol	Toxicology

MEDICAL & INDUSTRIAL EQUIPMENT
See Mercury Medical

MEDICAL ACCESSORIES, INC.   800-275-1624
92 Youngs Rd., Trenton, NJ 08619-1013   609-890-8304

FDA Number: 2242454   *Fax:* 609-890-0638
E-mail: medicalacc@aol.com
Web site: www.medicalacc.com
Year Founded: 1976
Ownership: Private
Produces/Sells CE-marked Devices: N
Federal Procurement Eligibility: Small Business
Distribution: Manufacturer Direct
General Admin.: Janis G. Ziedonis/Chief Executive Officer

MEDICAL ACCESSORIES, INC.   800-275-1624 *(cont'd)*
     Igor E. Ziedonis/President

Cuff, Blood Pressure	Cardiovascular
Electrode, Fetal Scalp	Obstetrics/Gynecology
Electrode, Other	General
Paper, Chart, Record, Medical	General
Service, Maintenance/Repair	General
Support, Abdominal	Physical Med
Transducer, Ultrasonic	Cardiovascular
Transducer, Ultrasonic, Obstetrical	Obstetrics/Gynecology

MEDICAL ACTION
See Medical Action Industries, Inc

MEDICAL ACTION INDUSTRIES, INC   828-681-8820
10 Columbia Blvd, Clarksburg, WV 26301

FDA Number: 1123871
Ownership: Medical Action Industries, Inc
Stock Symbol: MDCI
Traded On: NASDAQ
Produces/Sells CE-marked Devices: N

MEDICAL ACTION INDUSTRIES, INC   800-645-7042
500 Expressway Drive South,   631-231-4600
Brentwood, NY 11717

FDA Number: 3004755266   *Fax:* 631-231-3075
E-mail: mdci@medical-action.com
Web site: www.medical-action.com
Medical Products Sales Volume: $217,328,000
Annual Revenue: $100-$500 Million
Year Founded: 1977
Total Employees: 716
Ownership: Public
Stock Symbol: MDCI
Traded On: NASDAQ
Produces/Sells CE-marked Devices: N
Federal Procurement Eligibility: Small Business
Distribution: Manufacturer Through Distributor
General Admin.: Paul Meringolo/President, Chief Executive Officer
Mktg./Adv.: Mr. Rick Setian/Vice President Marketing & Sales
Production: Eric Liu/Vice President Operations
Finance: Charles L. Kelly/Chief Financial Officer

Box, Transportation, Container, Specimen	General
Cover, Other	General
Locator, Magnetic	Surgery
Packaging Material	General
Packaging, Sterilization	General
Sterilization Process Indicator, Physical/Chemical	General

Medical Product Subsidiaries (Listed Separately)
Medegen Medical Products, Llc
Medical Action Industries, Inc
Medical Action Industries, Inc.

MEDICAL ACTION INDUSTRIES, INC.   800-645-7042
25 Heywood Rd, Arden, NC 28704

FDA Number: 1030451   *Fax:* 631-231-3075
Web site: www.medical-action.com
Year Founded: 1977
Ownership: Medical Action Industries, Inc
Stock Symbol: MDCI
Traded On: NASDAQ
Produces/Sells CE-marked Devices: N
General Admin.: Paul D. Meringolo/Chief Executive Officer
     Eric Liu/Vice President
     Richard G Satin/Vice President, General Counsel
Mktg./Adv.: Manuel B. Losada/Vice President Sales
Finance: Charles L. Kelly, Jr./Chief Financial Officer

Accessories, Light, Surgical	Surgery
Adapter, Catheter	Surgery
Airway, Oropharyngeal, Anesthesia	Anesthesiology
Applicator, Tipped, Absorbent, Non-Sterile	General
Bandage, Adhesive	Surgery
Brush, Cleaning, Tracheal Tube	Ear/Nose/Throat
Cap, Surgical	Surgery
Container, Sharpes	General
Container, Specimen, All Types	General
Counter, Sponge, Surgical	Surgery
Cover, Shoe, Operating Room	Surgery
Device, Assist, CPR	Anesthesiology
Dressing, Other	General
Electrosurgical Unit, Cutting & Coagulation Device	Surgery
Glove, Patient Examination, Latex	General
Gown, Isolation, Surgical	Surgery
Kit, Administration, Intravenous	General
Kit, Surgical Instrument, Disposable	Surgery
Kit, Suture Removal	Surgery
Labware, Blood Collection	Chemistry
Lubricant, Patient	General
Mask, Surgical	Surgery
Needle, Hypodermic, Single Lumen With Syringe	General

MEDICAL ACTION INDUSTRIES, INC.   800-645-7042 *(cont'd)*

Pack, Sterilization Wrapper (Bag And Accessories)	Surgery
Pen, Marking, Surgical	Ophthalmology
Protector, Skin Pressure	General
Surgical Instrument, Disposable	Surgery
Syringe, Antistick	General
System, Skin Closure	Surgery
Tourniquet, Non-Pneumatic, Surgical	Surgery
Trap, Sterile Specimen	Anesthesiology
Tubing, Non-Invasive	Surgery
Wrap, Sterilization	General

MEDICAL AIR TECHNOLOGIES CORP.
See Medair, Inc.

MEDICAL ALIGNMENT SYSTEMS   801-733-6787
3656 Macintosh Ln., Salt Lake City, UT 84121-4515
FDA Number: 1721412   *Fax:* 801-943-1091
E-mail: info@maslasers.com
Web site: www.maslasers.com
Annual Revenue: $0-$1 Million
Year Founded: 1990
Ownership: Private
Produces/Sells CE-marked Devices: N
Federal Procurement Eligibility: Small Business, Female Owned
Distribution: Service Direct
General Admin.: Margo McDonald/President

Monitor, Patient Position, Light Beam	Radiology

MEDICAL ART RESOURCES, INC.   877-203-7829
3400 S. 103rd St., Suite 200,   **414-543-1002**
Greenfield, WI 53227
FDA Number: 2132778   *Fax:* 414-543-0137
E-mail: info@medicalartresources.com
Ownership: Private
Produces/Sells CE-marked Devices: N

Prosthesis, Breast, External	Surgery
Prosthesis, Maxillofacial	Ear/Nose/Throat

MEDICAL ARTS PRESS   800-328-2179
8500 Wyoming Ave. N., P.O. Box 43200, Minneapolis, MN 55445
FDA Number: n/a   *Fax:* 800-328-0023
Web site: www.medicalartspress.com
Year Founded: 1950
Total Employees: 600
Ownership: Private
Produces/Sells CE-marked Devices: N
Distribution: Manufacturer Direct

Accessories, Apparel, Surgical	Surgery
Cabinet, Other	General
Cart, Supply	General
Computer Software	General
Fountain, Eye Wash	Chemistry
Furniture, General	General
Illuminator, Radiographic Film	Radiology
Scale, Stand-On	General
Waste Disposal Unit, Sharps	General
Waste Disposal Unit, Surgical Instrument (Sharps)	Surgery
Waste Receptacle, General Purpose	General

MEDICAL ASSOCIATES INTERNATIONAL
See Marketing International, Inc.

MEDICAL ASSOCIATES NETWORK   818-500-7711
801 N. Brand Blvd., #690, Glendale, CA 91203
FDA Number: 1528245   *Fax:* 818-500-7745
E-mail: mednetca@aol.com
Annual Revenue: $5-$10 Million
Ownership: Private
Quality System Registration Information: ISO9001
Produces/Sells CE-marked Devices: Y
Federal Procurement Eligibility: Small Business
Distribution: Manufacturer Direct, Manufacturer Through Distributor, OEM
General Admin.: Phil Wyatt/President, Chief Executive Officer
Mktg./Adv.: Gary Schaeffer/Director Product Development
    Jim Mullin/Manager Business Development
    Jim Mullin/Manager International & National Sales

Transfer Device, Patient, Manual	General
Vial, Other	General

Medical Product Subsidiaries (Listed Separately)
Elcam Medical

MEDICAL AUTOMATION SYSTEMS   434-971-7953
2000 Holiday Drive; Suite 500, Charlottesville, VA 22901
FDA Number: 3005332178

Computer, Chemistry Analyzer	Chemistry

MEDICAL CABLES, INC.   800-314-51111
1365 Logan Ave., Costa Mesa, CA 92626-4023   **714-641-3395**
FDA Number: n/a   *Fax:* 714-545-7212

MEDICAL CABLES, INC.   800-314-51111 *(cont'd)*
E-mail: info@cphginc.com
Web site: www.medicalcables.com
Medical Products Sales Volume: $5,500,000
Annual Revenue: $5-$10 Million
Total Employees: 40   Marketing Staff: 2   Sales Staff: 6
Ownership: Private
Quality System Registration Information: ISO9002
Produces/Sells CE-marked Devices: N
Federal Procurement Eligibility: Small Business
Distribution: Manufacturer Direct, Manufacturer Through Distributor, Manufacturer Through Manufacturer Reps, Service Direct, Exporter
General Admin.: Pete Bonin/President, Chief Executive Officer
    Kristen Demedenko/Vice President Human Resources
    Christopher Fontana/Vice President, General Manager
Mktg./Adv.: Christopher Fontana/Director National Accounts
    Andrew Bonin/Director Product Development
    Kathleen Steck/Manager National Sales
Production: Dr. Robert Hilman/Director Quality Assurance
    Dr. Robert Hilman/Manager Regulatory Affairs
    Andy Bonin/Vice President Manufacturing
Research: Greg Fontana/Vice President Research & Development

Cable	Physical Med
Cable/Lead, ECG, With Transducer And Electrode	Cardiovascular
Monitor, Apnea	General
Monitor, Fetal, Cardiac	Obstetrics/Gynecology
Oximeter, Pulse	General
Phacofragmentation Unit	Ophthalmology
Service, Maintenance/Repair	General

MEDICAL CARBON RESEARCH INSTITUTE, LLC - MCRI   512-339-8000
8200 Cameron Road, Suite A-196, Austin, TX 78754-3823
FDA Number: 1649833   *Fax:* 512-339-3636
E-mail: onx@mcritx.com
Web site: www.mcritx.com
Medical Products Sales Volume: $10,000,000
Year Founded: 1994
Total Employees: 69   Marketing Staff: 4   Sales Staff: 10
Ownership: Private
Produces/Sells CE-marked Devices: Y
Federal Procurement Eligibility: Small Business
Distribution: Manufacturer Direct, Manufacturer Through Distributor, Manufacturer Through Manufacturer Reps
General Admin.: Jack Bokros/Chairman
    Jonathan Stupka/Chief Operating Officer, Vice President Operations
    Clyde Baker/President
Mktg./Adv.: Catheran Burnett/Director Education
    Regina Creekmore/Director International Sales
    Scott Peters/Director International Sales
Production: John Ely/Senior Vice President Regulatory Affairs
Finance: Bill McClellan/Chief Financial Officer, Vice President Finance

Orthopedic Implant Material	Orthopedics
Prosthesis, Cardiac Valve	Cardiovascular

MEDICAL CHEMICAL CORP.   800-424-9394
19430 Van Ness Avenue, Torrance, CA 90501   **310-787-6800**
FDA Number: 2013736   *Fax:* 310-787-4464
E-mail: christinagomez@med-chem.com
Web site: www.med-chem.com
Medical Products Sales Volume: $6,000,000
Annual Revenue: $1-$5 Million
Year Founded: 1954
Total Employees: 45   Marketing Staff: 2   Sales Staff: 12
Ownership: Private
Quality System Registration Information: ISO9001
Produces/Sells CE-marked Devices: Y
Federal Procurement Eligibility: Small Business
Distribution: Manufacturer Direct, Manufacturer Through Distributor, Manufacturer Through Manufacturer Reps
General Admin.: Mr. Emmanuel Didier/President, Chief Executive Officer
Mktg./Adv.: Mr. Andrew Rocha/Vice President Marketing & Sales
Production: Mr. Jose Arias/Director Quality Assurance & Regulatory Affairs
Research: Mr. Patrick Braden/Vice President Research & Development & Production

Brilliant Cresyl Blue	Hematology
Crystal Violet	Hematology
Cyanomethemoglobin	Hematology
Disinfector, Liquid	General
Dye-Binding, Albumin, Bromcresol, Green	Chemistry
Fluid, Bouin's	Pathology
Formaldehyde (Formalin, Formol)	Pathology
Kit, Pap Smear	Obstetrics/Gynecology
Kit, Screening, Urine	Microbiology
Mercuric Nitrate And Diphenyl Carbazone (Titrimetric)	Chemistry
Mounting Media, Oil Soluble	Pathology

MEDICAL CHEMICAL CORP.   800-424-9394 *(cont'd)*

Phosphorus Reagent (Test System)	Chemistry
Phosphotungstate Reduction, Uric Acid	Chemistry
Reagent, Cyanomethemoglobin, With Standard	Hematology
Reagent, Protein, Total	Chemistry
Solution, Antibacterial Cleaner	General
Solution, Pathology, Lugol's	Pathology
Solution, Surgical Scrub	General
Stain, Biological, General	Pathology
Stain, Carbol Fuchsin	Pathology
Stain, Eosin Y	Pathology
Stain, Giemsa	Pathology
Stain, Giemsa, Hematology	Hematology
Stain, Grams Iodine	Pathology
Stain, Hematoxylin, Harris's	Pathology
Stain, Hematoxylin, Mayer's	Pathology
Stain, Methylene Blue, New	Hematology
Stain, Microbiological	Microbiology
Stain, Other	Pathology
Stain, Papanicolau	Pathology
Stain, Reticulocyte	Hematology
Stain, Safranin	Pathology
Stain, Toluidine Blue	Pathology
Stain, Wright's	Pathology
Sulfophosphovanillin, Colorimetry, Total Lipids	Chemistry
Titrimetric Phenol Red, Carbon-Dioxide	Chemistry

MEDICAL COACHES, INC.   607-432-1333

399 County Highway 58, Oneonta, NY 13820-0129
FDA Number: 9320126   *Fax:* 607-432-8190
E-mail: gsmith@medcoach.com
Web site: www.medcoach.com
Annual Revenue: $10-$25 Million
Year Founded: 1952
Total Employees: 70   *Marketing Staff:* 5   *Sales Staff:* 5
Ownership: Private
Quality System Registration Information: ISO9001
Produces/Sells CE-marked Devices: N
Federal Procurement Eligibility: Small Business
Distribution: Manufacturer Direct, Manufacturer Through Distributor, Manufacturer Through Manufacturer Reps, Exporter
General Admin.: Geoffrey A. Smith/President, Chief Executive Officer
    Leonard W. Marsh/Vice President, General Manager
Mktg./Adv.: Al Collins/Director Marketing
    Chad W. Smith/Director National Accounts
    Brett Buzzy/Director Product Development
    Chad Smith/Manager Advertising
    James Bazan/Manager Contract Sales
    Geoffrey A. Smith/Manager International & National Sales
    Chad W. Smith/Manager National Sales
    James Bazan/Vice President Business Development
    Al Collins/Vice President Sales
Production: Gary Allen/Director Quality Assurance
    John P. Janitz/Manager Materials
    Leonard W. Marsh/Vice President Manufacturing
    Leonard W. Marsh/Vice President Operations
Research: Richard E. Mattice/Vice President Engineering

Ambulance	General
Facility, Equipment, Medical, Mobile	General
Radiographic Unit, Diagnostic, Mammographic	Radiology

MEDICAL COLLAR COVERS, INC.   606-836-2575

600 Greenup Ave. Suite 101, Raceland, KY 41169
FDA Number: 1531172
Ownership: Private
Produces/Sells CE-marked Devices: N

Orthosis, Cervical	Physical Med

MEDICAL COMPONENTS, INC.

See Medcomp (Medical Components, Inc.)

MEDICAL CONCEPTS DEVELOPMENT   800-345-0644

2500 Ventura Dr., St. Paul, MN 55125-3927   651-735-0498
FDA Number: 2129617   *Fax:* 651-735-7197
E-mail: sales@medconceptsdev.com
Web site: www.medconceptsdev.com
Total Employees: 115   *Marketing Staff:* 1   *Sales Staff:* 8
Ownership: Private
Quality System Registration Information: ISO9001
Produces/Sells CE-marked Devices: Y
Federal Procurement Eligibility: Small Business
Distribution: Manufacturer Direct, Manufacturer Through Distributor, OEM
General Admin.: Leland W. Annett/Chief Executive Officer
    Mark St. Michel/President
    Jolie Nisbet/Vice President Human Resources
    David Padget/Vice President, General Manager
Mktg./Adv.: Jeanne Berg/Director National Accounts
    Mr. Mark Benjamin/Marketing Communications Specialist
    David Padget/Vice President Marketing

MEDICAL CONCEPTS DEVELOPMENT   800-345-0644 *(cont'd)*

Production: Mark St Michel/Manager Regulatory Affairs
    Timothy Smalstig/Vice President Manufacturing
Finance: Stephanie Thoreson/Chief Financial Officer

Bag, Intestine	Surgery
Contract Manufacturing	General
Contract Manufacturing, Product, Disposable	General
Drape, Adhesive, Aerosol	Surgery
Drape, Patient, Ophthalmic	Ophthalmology
Drape, Surgical	Surgery
Drape, Surgical, Disposable	Surgery
Drape, Surgical, ENT	Ear/Nose/Throat
Material, Raw, Production	General
Ring Drape Retention, Internal (Wound Protector)	Surgery

MEDICAL CONCEPTS, INC.

See Karl Storz Imaging

MEDICAL DATA TECHNOLOGIES, INC.   866-643-7424

1421 Oakfield Dr., Brandon, FL 33511
FDA Number: 3003886479

Device, Storage, Image, Digital	Radiology
System, Communication, Image, Digital	Radiology

MEDICAL DECISIONS NETWORK   434-971-7953

2000 Holiday Drive, Suite 200, Charlottesville, VA 22901
FDA Number: 3005906905

Computer, Chemistry Analyzer	Chemistry

MEDICAL DEPOT   516-998-4600

99 Seaview Blvd., Port Washington, NY 11050
FDA Number: 2438477
Ownership: Private
Produces/Sells CE-marked Devices: N

Accessories, Traction	Physical Med
Accessories, Wheelchair	Physical Med
Adapter, Hygiene	Physical Med
Bath, Hydro-Massage (Whirlpool)	Physical Med
Bath, Sitz, Non-Powered	Physical Med
Bed, Electric	General
Bed, Hydraulic	General
Bed, Manual	General
Board, Bed	General
Cane	Physical Med
Catheter, Suction, With Tip	General
Chair, With Casters	Physical Med
Chair/Table, Medical	General
Component, Exercise	Physical Med
Cover, Mattress	General
Crutch	Physical Med
Cushion, Wheelchair (Pad)	Physical Med
Examination Device, AC-Powered	General
Infusion Stand	General
Lift, Bath, Non-AC-Powered	General
Massager, Therapeutic	Physical Med
Mattress, Air Flotation	General
Mattress, Non-Powered Flotation Therapy	Physical Med
Monitor, Bed Patient	General
Nebulizer, Direct Patient Interface	Anesthesiology
Nebulizer, Medicinal, Non-Ventilatory (Atomizer)	Anesthesiology
Orthosis, Cervical	Physical Med
Pad, Heating, Powered	Physical Med
Regulator, Pressure, Gas Cylinder	Anesthesiology
Scooter (Motorized 3-Wheeled Vehicle)	Physical Med
Sling, Overhead Suspension, Wheelchair	Physical Med
Table, Mechanical	Physical Med
Tips And Pads, Cane, Crutch And Walker	Physical Med
Traction Unit, Non-Powered	Orthopedics
Tray, Wheelchair	Physical Med
Walker, Mechanical	Physical Med
Wheelchair, Manual	Physical Med
Wheelchair, Powered	Physical Med

MEDICAL DESIGN CONCEPTS, INC.   951-296-2600

41980 Winchester Rd., Temecula, CA 92590-3666
FDA Number: 2025245   *Fax:* 951-296-2628
E-mail: info@phsyes.com
Web site: www.phsyes.com
Year Founded: 1981
Total Employees: 950   *Sales Staff:* 58
Ownership: Private
Produces/Sells CE-marked Devices: N
Distribution: Manufacturer Direct, Manufacturer Through Distributor
General Admin.: John H. Luttgens/Vice President
Mktg./Adv.: John H. Luttgens/President Marketing
Finance: Jenise M. Luttgens/Treasurer

Tray, Custom/Special Procedure	General

MEDICAL DESIGN SYSTEMS, INC.   800-593-1900

14560 W. 99th St., Lenexa, KS 66215   913-438-8835
FDA Number: n/a   *Fax:* 913-438-2275

MEDICAL DESIGN SYSTEMS, INC.   800-593-1900 *(cont'd)*
E-mail: info@masscabinets.com
Web site: www.masscabinets.com
Medical Products Sales Volume: $2,000,000
Annual Revenue: $1-$5 Million
Year Founded: 1994
Total Employees: 11   *Marketing Staff:* 3   *Sales Staff:* 2
Ownership: Private
Produces/Sells CE-marked Devices: N
Federal Procurement Eligibility: Small Business, VA Contract
Distribution: Manufacturer Through Distributor, Manufacturer Through Manufacturer Reps, OEM
General Admin.: Gary Simmons/President, Chief Executive Officer
Mktg./Adv.: Patricia List/Director National Accounts
     Barbara Lynd/Manager Advertising
     Patricia List/Manager Sales Training
     Patricia List/Vice President Marketing & Sales
Production: Greg Bulmer/Manager Manufacturing
     Greg Bulmer/Manager Materials

Cabinet Casework, General Purpose	General
Cabinet, Other	General
Cabinet, Storage, Catheter	General
Cart, Monitor	General
Cart, Other	General

MEDICAL DEVICE CONCEPTS, LLC.   201-446-6691
4 Lawrence Way, Cedar Grove, NJ 07009
FDA Number: 2249309
Ownership: Private
Produces/Sells CE-marked Devices: N

Orthopedic Manual Surgical Instrument	Orthopedics

MEDICAL DEVICE RESOURCE CORPORATION   800-633-8423
5981 Graham Ct, Livermore, CA 94550   510-732-9950
FDA Number: 2938001   *Fax:* 510-785-8182
E-mail: mel@mdresource.com
Web site: www.mdresource.com
Medical Products Sales Volume: $1,000,000
Annual Revenue: $0-$1 Million
Year Founded: 1985
Total Employees: 5
Ownership: Private
Produces/Sells CE-marked Devices: N
Federal Procurement Eligibility: Small Business
Distribution: Manufacturer Direct, Manufacturer Through Distributor, Manufacturer Through Manufacturer Reps, Importer, Exporter
General Admin.: Melbourne Kimsey/President
Mktg./Adv.: Mr. Ryan Kimsey/Sales Engineer
Production: Brennan Nicks/Manager Production

Aspirator, Surgical	Surgery
Bottle, Collection, Vacuum (Aspirator)	General
Cannula, Surgical, General & Plastic Surgery	Surgery
Dermabrasion Unit	Surgery
Insufflator, Other	Surgery
Pump, Aspiration, Portable	Anesthesiology
Suction Apparatus, Ward Use, Portable, AC-Powered	Surgery

Medical Product Subsidiaries (Listed Separately)
   Reliance Medical Corp.

MEDICAL DEVICE TECHNOLOGIES, INC. (MD TECH)   800-338-0440
3600 S.W. 47th Avenue, Gainesville, FL 32608   352-338-0440
FDA Number: 1036710   *Fax:* 352-338-0662
E-mail: Customer_Service@angio.com
Web site: www.interv.net
Medical Products Sales Volume: $11,400,000
Annual Revenue: $25-$50 Million
Year Founded: 2003
Total Employees: 150   *Marketing Staff:* 4   *Sales Staff:* 42
Ownership: Marmon Group, Inc., The
Quality System Registration Information: ISO9001
Produces/Sells CE-marked Devices: Y
Federal Procurement Eligibility: Small Business, GSA Contract
Distribution: Manufacturer Direct, Manufacturer Through Distributor
General Admin.: Karl Swartz/President
Mktg./Adv.: George leondis/Director Marketing
     Michael C. Ryan/Vice President Marketing & Sales
Production: Karl Swartz/Director Quality Assurance & Regulatory Affairs

Biopsy Instrument	Gastroenterology/Urology
Guidewire, Catheter	Cardiovascular
Guidewire, Catheter, Radiological	Radiology
Needle, Aspiration And Injection, Disposable	Surgery
Needle, Biopsy, Mammary	Obstetrics/Gynecology
Needle, Blunt	General

MEDICAL DEVICES INTERNATIONAL, INC.
See International Radiographic, Inc.

MEDICAL DEVICES, INC.
See Compex Technologies, Inc.

MEDICAL DIAGNOSTIC TECHNOLOGIES, INC.
See Remel

MEDICAL DIAGNOSTICS CALIFORNIA
See Medica, Inc.

MEDICAL DIGITAL DEVELOPERS LLC   508-393-3100
767 Lexington Ave., Suite 505, New York, NY 10065
FDA Number: 3005439497

Device, Storage, Image, Digital	Radiology

MEDICAL DOSIMETRY SERVICES, INC.   405-680-5222
1601 Sw 89th, Suite E-100, Oklahoma City, OK 73159
FDA Number: 1649665

Accelerator, Linear, Medical	Radiology

MEDICAL ELECTRONIC DEVICES, INC.   310-618-0306
2807 Oregon Ct. #d6, Torrance, CA 90503
FDA Number: 2025586
Ownership: Private
Produces/Sells CE-marked Devices: N

Conserver, Oxygen	Anesthesiology
Ventilator, Non-Continuous (Respirator)	Anesthesiology

MEDICAL ELECTRONICS LABORATORIES
See Analogic Corporation

MEDICAL ENERGY, INC.   8806 Paul Starr
8806 Paul Starr Drive, Pensacola, FL 32514
FDA Number: 1038823   *Fax:* 850-469-1746
E-mail: medenergy@aol.com
Web site: www.medicalenergy.com
Medical Products Sales Volume: $1,500,000
Annual Revenue: $1-$5 Million
Year Founded: 1987
Ownership: Medical Energy, Inc.
Quality System Registration Information: ISO9000
Produces/Sells CE-marked Devices: Y
Federal Procurement Eligibility: Small Business
Distribution: Manufacturer Direct, Service Direct, Exporter
General Admin.: David P. Lewing/President, Chief Executive Officer
Mktg./Adv.: Michael McGinn/Director Product Development
     Michelle B. Scott/Manager International & National Sales
     Michelle B. Scott/Vice President Marketing & Sales
Production: Michael McGinn/Director Quality Assurance
     Jason Lewing/Manager Materials
     David P. Lewing/Manager Regulatory Affairs
Research: Michael McGinn/Vice President Research & Development

Accessories, Laser	General
Cable, Laser, Fiberoptic	Surgery
Laser, Gynecologic	Obstetrics/Gynecology
Laser, Surgical	Surgery

Medical Product Subsidiaries (Listed Separately)
   Medical Energy, Inc.

MEDICAL ENGINEERING LABORATORY, INC.   704-487-0166
108 West Warren St., Suite 207, Shelby, NC 28150
FDA Number: 1037861
Ownership: Private
Produces/Sells CE-marked Devices: N

Accessories, Cleaning, Endoscopic	Gastroenterology/Urology
Forceps, Biopsy, Non-Electric	Gastroenterology/Urology

MEDICAL EQUIPMENT DEVELOPMENT CO., INC.
See Best Nomos Corp.

MEDICAL EQUIPMENT DEVELOPMENT, INC.   520-743-7874
PO Box 85820, Tucson, AZ 85754-5820
FDA Number: n/a   *Fax:* 520-743-7863
E-mail: medinc@aol.com
Annual Revenue: $0-$1 Million
Year Founded: 1982
Total Employees: 3
Ownership: Private
Produces/Sells CE-marked Devices: N
Federal Procurement Eligibility: Small Business
Distribution: Service Direct
General Admin.: Terence A. Torzala/President
     Kathleen McCormack/Vice President

Service, Consulting	General

MEDICAL EQUIPMENT SPECIALISTS, INC.   800-795-6641
107 Otis Street, Northborough, MA 01532   508-393-1255
FDA Number: 1224667   *Fax:* 508-393-1663
E-mail: mesinc@mes-usa.com
Web site: www.mes-usa.com
Annual Revenue: $1-$5 Million
Year Founded: 1992
Total Employees: 4   *Marketing Staff:* 1   *Sales Staff:* 2

MEDICAL EQUIPMENT SPECIALISTS, INC. 800-795-6641 *(cont'd)*

Ownership: Private
Produces/Sells CE-marked Devices: N
Federal Procurement Eligibility: Small Business, Minority Owned
Distribution: Exclusive Distributor, Importer, Exporter
General Admin.: Eduardo Paredes/President, Chief Executive Officer
Mktg./Adv.: Eduardo Paredes/Manager International & National Sales
　　　　Yolanda Paredes/Vice President Marketing & Sales

Bandage, Tubular	General
Gel, Ultrasonic Transmission	General

MEDICAL EVALUATION DEVICES & INSTRU. COR

See Epimed International, Inc.

MEDICAL EXTRUSION TECHNOLOGIES, INC. 800-618-4346

26608 Pierce Circle, Murrieta, CA 92562 **951-698-4346**
FDA Number: n/a *Fax:* 951-698-4347
Web site: http://www.medicalextrusion.com
Ownership: Private
Quality System Registration Information: ISO9002
Produces/Sells CE-marked Devices: N
Distribution: Manufacturer Direct
General Admin.: Tom E. Baur/President
　　　　Rikki Baur/Vice President

Contract R&D, Equipment	General
Service, Consulting	General
Tubing, Nylon	General

MEDICAL FITTINGS 800-331-2685

300 Held Dr., Northampton, PA 18067 **610-262-6020**
FDA Number: 2523851 *Fax:* 800-352-1240
E-mail: tdeuerling@precisionmedical.com
Web site: www.medicalfittings.com
Medical Products Sales Volume: $3,000,000
Annual Revenue: $1-$5 Million
Total Employees: 20 *Marketing Staff:* 1 *Sales Staff:* 8
Ownership: Private
Produces/Sells CE-marked Devices: N
Distribution: Manufacturer Direct, Manufacturer Through Distributor
Mktg./Adv.: Tim Deuerling/Director National Marketing & Sales
　　　　Suzanne Moyer/International Sales Representative
Production: Jim Parker/Director Quality Assurance

Fitting, Other	General
Fitting, Quick Connect (Gas Connector)	General

MEDICAL GRAPHICS CORPORATION 800-950-5597

350 Oak Grove Pkwy., St. Paul, MN 55127-8536 **651-484-4874**
FDA Number: 2183022 *Fax:* 651-484-8941
E-mail: rod.young@medgraphics.com
Web site: www.medgraphics.com
Annual Revenue: $25-$50 Million
Year Founded: 1977
Total Employees: 130 *Marketing Staff:* 10 *Sales Staff:* 25
Ownership: ANGEION CORPORATION
Quality System Registration Information: ISO9001
Produces/Sells CE-marked Devices: Y
Distribution: Manufacturer Direct, Manufacturer Through Distributor, Service Direct
General Admin.: Rod Young/President, Chief Executive Officer
　　　　Sheryl Rapheal/Vice President Human Resources
Mktg./Adv.: Terrance Kapsen/Marketing Representative
　　　　Jim Gaul/Vice President Sales
Production: Tim Fitzgerald/Vice President Manufacturing
　　　　Michael Snow/Vice President Regulatory Affairs
Research: Michael Snow/Vice President Research & Development
Finance: Dale Johnson/Chief Financial Officer

Computer Software	General
Computer, Pulmonary Function Data	Anesthesiology
Computer, Pulmonary Function Interpretator (Diagnostic)	Anesthesiology
Computer, Pulmonary Function Laboratory	Anesthesiology
Computer, Stress Exercise	Cardiovascular
Exerciser, Powered	Anesthesiology
Plethysmograph, Pressure (Body)	Anesthesiology

MEDICAL ID SYSTEMS INC. 800-262-2399

3954 44th Street S.E., **616-698-0535**
Grand Rapids, MI 49512
FDA Number: n/a *Fax:* 616-698-0603
E-mail: medidxry@aol.com
Web site: www.medid.com
Annual Revenue: $0-$1 Million
Year Founded: 1985
Ownership: Private
Produces/Sells CE-marked Devices: N
Federal Procurement Eligibility: Small Business
Distribution: Manufacturer Direct, Manufacturer Through Distributor, Manufacturer Through Manufacturer Reps, Importer, Exporter

Labeler, X-Ray Film	Radiology

MEDICAL ID SYSTEMS INC. 800-262-2399 *(cont'd)*

Marker, X-Ray	Radiology

MEDICAL ILLUMINATION INTERNATIONAL 800-831-1222

547 Library St., San Fernando, CA 91340 **818-838-3025**
FDA Number: 2028295 *Fax:* 818-838-3725
E-mail: cs@medillum.com
Web site: www.medillum.com
Year Founded: 1978
Total Employees: 74
Ownership: Private
Produces/Sells CE-marked Devices: Y
Federal Procurement Eligibility: Small Business, GSA Contract
Distribution: Manufacturer Through Distributor
General Admin.: Mr. Bill Schellenberg/Chairman
　　　　Mr. Alan Kiviat/President, General Manager
Mktg./Adv.: Mr. Ben Binegar/Manager National Sales
　　　　Mr. Larry Debord/Vice President Marketing & Sales
Production: Mr. Mike Alcala/Director Quality Assurance & Regulatory Affairs
　　　　Mr. David Glover/Manager Engineering
　　　　Mr. Richard Davis/Manager Manufacturing

Accessories, Light, Surgical	Surgery
Lamp, Examination (Light)	General
Lamp, Operating Room	General
Lamp, Other	General
Lamp, Surgical	Surgery
Light Source, Endoscopic	Obstetrics/Gynecology
Light, Examination, Battery-Powered	General
Light, Other	General
Light, Surgical, Ceiling Mounted	Surgery
Light, Surgical, Endoscopic	Surgery

Medical Product Subsidiaries (Listed Separately)
Nuvo, Inc.

MEDICAL IMAGING APPLICATIONS, LLC 319-358-1529

832 Forest Hill Drive, Coralville, IA 52241
FDA Number: 3004201331

Computer, Diagnostic, Programmable	Cardiovascular

MEDICAL IMAGING SOLUTIONS, INC. 504-733-9729

800 Central Ave., Jefferson, LA 70121
FDA Number: 1055563
Ownership: Private
Produces/Sells CE-marked Devices: N

Radiographic/Fluoroscopic Unit, Angiographic	Radiology

MEDICAL INCORPORATED

See Medicalcv, Inc.

MEDICAL INDICATORS, INC. 609-737-1600

1589 Reed Rd., Pennington, NJ 08534
FDA Number: 2246308 *Fax:* 609-737-0588
E-mail: sales@medicalindicators.com
Web site: www.medicalindicators.com
Annual Revenue: $1-$5 Million
Year Founded: 1985
Total Employees: 15 *Marketing Staff:* 2 *Sales Staff:* 2
Ownership: Private
Produces/Sells CE-marked Devices: Y
Federal Procurement Eligibility: Small Business
Distribution: Manufacturer Direct, Manufacturer Through Distributor, Manufacturer Through Manufacturer Reps
Mktg./Adv.: Bill Burnham/Manager International Sales
　　　　Bill Burnham/Vice President, General Manager Marketing
Production: Tim Ursell/Manager Regulatory Affairs
Finance: Ms. Carole Tucker/Controller

Thermometer, Chemical Color Change	General
Thermometer, Electronic, Continuous	General
Thermometer, Liquid Crystals	Surgery

MEDICAL INDUSTRIAL SCIENTIFIC PROD.

See Rismed Oncology Systems

MEDICAL INDUSTRIES AMERICA INC. 800-759-3038

2636 289th Place, Adel, IA 50003 **515-993-5001**
FDA Number: 1931654 *Fax:* 515-993-4172
E-mail: cusserv@medindustries.com
Web site: www.medindustries.com
Medical Products Sales Volume: $4,600,000
Annual Revenue: $5-$10 Million
Year Founded: 1987
Total Employees: 40 *Marketing Staff:* 3 *Sales Staff:* 52
Ownership: Private
Quality System Registration Information: ISO9001
Produces/Sells CE-marked Devices: N
Federal Procurement Eligibility: Small Business
Distribution: Manufacturer Through Manufacturer Reps
General Admin.: Bryan Hansel/President
　　　　Marilyn Bird/Vice President
　　　　Vanessa Saltmarsh/Vice President Human Resources

MEDICAL INDUSTRIES AMERICA INC.   800-759-3038 *(cont'd)*
Production: Randy Pellham/Manager Materials
     Anne Carlson/Manager Regulatory Affairs
Research: Edward Simonds/Vice President Research & Development

Compressor, Air, Portable	Anesthesiology
Generator, Aerosol	Ear/Nose/Throat
Nebulizer, Direct Patient Interface	Anesthesiology
Suction Apparatus, Single Patient, Portable, Non-Powered	Surgery
Ventilator, Non-Continuous (Respirator)	Anesthesiology

MEDICAL INDUSTRIES OF AMERICA LLC.   203-254-8080
1735 Post Road, Unit 6, Fairfield, CT 06824
FDA Number: 3004126850

Brace, Joint, Ankle (External)	Physical Med
Prosthesis Alignment Device	Physical Med

MEDICAL INFORMATION TECHNOLOGY, INC.   781-821-3000
Meditech Circle, Westwood, MA 02090
FDA Number: 1222805

Software, Blood Bank (Stand-Alone Products)	Hematology

MEDICAL INFORMATION TECHNOLOGY, INC.   781-821-3000
(MEDITECH)
Meditech Circle, Westwood, MA 02090
FDA Number: 1222805   *Fax:* 781-821-2199
Web site: www.meditech.com
Medical Products Sales Volume: $204,000,000
Total Employees: 2700
Ownership: Private
Produces/Sells CE-marked Devices: N
Distribution: Exclusive Distributor
General Admin.: A. Neil Pappalardo/Chairman, Chief Executive Officer
     Barbara Manzolillo/Chief Financial Officer, Treasurer
     Howard Messing/President, Chief Operating Officer
     Lawrence Polimeno/Vice Chairman

Computer, Clinical Laboratory	Chemistry
Computer, Diagnostic, Programmable	Cardiovascular
Computer, Patient Data Management	General
Software, Blood Bank (Stand-Alone Products)	Hematology

MEDICAL INNOVATIONS INTERNATIONAL INC.   507-289-0761
6256 N.W. 34th Avenue, Rochester, MN 55901
FDA Number: n/a   *Fax:* 507-288-8888
E-mail: info@medicalinnovations.com
Web site: www.medicalinnovations.com
Medical Products Sales Volume: $1,800,000
Annual Revenue: $1-$5 Million
Year Founded: 2000
Total Employees: 12
Ownership: Private
Produces/Sells CE-marked Devices: Y
Federal Procurement Eligibility: Small Business
Distribution: Manufacturer Direct, Manufacturer Through Distributor, Manufacturer Through Manufacturer Reps, OEM, Exclusive Distributor, Exporter
General Admin.: Paul Sadler/Executive Vice President

Adapter, Bulb, Endoscope, Miscellaneous	Gastroenterology/Urology
Analyzer, Coagulation, Manual	Hematology
Button, Nasal Septal	Ear/Nose/Throat
Button, Tracheostomy Tube	Anesthesiology
Clamp, Cannula	Gastroenterology/Urology
Lamp, Examination (Light)	General
Trephine, Bone	Orthopedics

MEDICAL INNOVATORS, INC.   888-422-7717
9277 E. Star Hill Lane, Lone Tree, CO 80124
FDA Number: 3005155526

Orthopedic Manual Surgical Instrument	Orthopedics

MEDICAL INSTILL TECHNOLOGIES, INC.   860-350-1900
201 Housatonic Avenue, New Milford, CT 06776
FDA Number: 3003645082

Dispenser, Medication, Liquid	General

MEDICAL INSTRUMENT DEVELOPMENT CO.
See Varitronics, Inc.

MEDICAL INSTRUMENT SUPPLY CO.
See Misc Inc.

MEDICAL INSTRUMENTATION & DIAGNOSTICS   858-635-2230
CORP.(MIDCO)
7964 Arjons Drive #e, Suite E, San Diego, CA 92126
FDA Number: 1721849   *Fax:* 858-635-2234
E-mail: support@stereotaxybymidco.com
Web site: www.stereotaxybymidco.com
Ownership: Private
Produces/Sells CE-marked Devices: N

Accelerator, Linear, Medical	Radiology
Phantom, Anthropomorphic, Radiographic	Radiology
Source, Brachytherapy, Radionuclide	Radiology

MEDICAL INSTRUMENTATION & DIAGNOSTICS   858-635-2230
(cont'd)

Stereotaxy Equipment	Cns/Neurology

MEDICAL INSTRUMENTATION   800-929-5227
DEVELOPMENT LABS
557 McCormick Street, San Leandro, CA 94577   **510-357-3952**
FDA Number: 2935428   *Fax:* 510-357-1582
E-mail: info@midlabs.com
Web site: www.midlabs.com
Medical Products Sales Volume: $3,200,000
Annual Revenue: $1-$5 Million
Year Founded: 1981
Total Employees: 35   *Marketing Staff:* 3
Ownership: Private
Quality System Registration Information: ISO9001
Produces/Sells CE-marked Devices: N
Federal Procurement Eligibility: Small Business, Minority Owned
Distribution: Manufacturer Direct, Manufacturer Through Distributor, Service Direct, Exclusive Distributor, Exporter
General Admin.: Peter Hyde/Chief Executive Officer
     Carl Wang/President
Mktg./Adv.: Steve Smith/Director Marketing
Production: Linda Upton/Director Regulatory Affairs
Research: Erik Peterson/Vice President Research & Development
Finance: Linda Upton/Vice President Admin., Finance

Cutter, Vitreous Aspiration, AC-Powered	Ophthalmology

MEDICAL INTERNATIONAL TECHNOLOGY INC.   514-339-9355
1872 Beaulac Ville St-Laurent,
Montreal, QUEBE H4R 2 Canada
FDA Number: n/a   *Fax:* 514-339-2885
Web site: http://www.mitneedlefree.com
Year Founded: 1971
Ownership: Public
Stock Symbol: MDLH
Traded On: OTC Bulletin
Produces/Sells CE-marked Devices: N

MEDICAL LASER SYSTEMS INC   203-481-2395
20 Baldwin Dr., Branford, CT 06405
FDA Number: 3006157902

Lamp, Non-heating, For Adjunctive Use In Pain Therapy	Physical Med

MEDICAL LASER TECHNOLOGIES, LLC   512-626-6267
3708 Ebony Hollow Cove, Austin, TX 78739
FDA Number: 3005053838

Laser, Surgical	Surgery

MEDICAL MANAGER HEALTH SYSTEMS, INC.   800-222-7701
516 Clyde Avenue, Mountain View, CA 94043   **650-567-6999**
FDA Number: n/a   *Fax:* 650-969-0118
E-mail: info@mdmgr.com
Web site: www.medicalmanager.com
Medical Products Sales Volume: $200,000,000
Total Employees: 1200   *Marketing Staff:* 20   *Sales Staff:* 200
Ownership: WEB MD
Produces/Sells CE-marked Devices: N
Distribution: Service Direct
General Admin.: Mickey Singer/Chief Executive Officer
     John Sessions/President
Mktg./Adv.: Nanci Adams/Director Marketing
     David Ward/Director National Accounts
     Julie DeSantis/Manager Marketing Communications
     Deveny Bywaters/Manager Sales Training
     Sam Omron/Vice President Sales

Computer Software	General

MEDICAL MANAGER RESEARCH &   386-462-2148
DEVELOPMENT, LLC
15151 Nw 99th St., Alachua, FL 32615
FDA Number: 1064739

Image Processing System	Radiology

MEDICAL MARKETING SERVICES   800-927-0791
2322 Nazareth Rd., Kalamazoo, MI 49048   **269-381-1953**
FDA Number: n/a   *Fax:* 269-381-2079
E-mail: medmarkser@aol.com
Annual Revenue: $0-$1 Million
Total Employees: 5   *Marketing Staff:* 2   *Sales Staff:* 3
Ownership: Private
Produces/Sells CE-marked Devices: N
Federal Procurement Eligibility: Small Business
Distribution: Manufacturer Through Distributor
General Admin.: Frank Murphy/President
Mktg./Adv.: Ms. Rong Lin/International Sales Representative
     Karen Bomar/Manager Advertising

MEDICAL MARKETING SERVICES 800-927-0791 (cont'd)
Frank Murphy/Manager International & National Sales
Kevin Ruddy/Manager Sales Training
Bill Parker/Vice President Business Development
Service, Consulting   General

MEDICAL MARKETPLACE 760-242-4171
18737 Hwy. 18, Suite 5A, Apple Valley, CA 92307-2311
FDA Number: n/a   Fax: 760-242-3301
E-mail: medmkpl@aol.com
Medical Products Sales Volume: $4,400,000
Year Founded: 1994
Total Employees: 4   Marketing Staff: 3   Sales Staff: 3
Ownership: Private
Stock Symbol: MKPL
Traded On: NASDAQ
Produces/Sells CE-marked Devices: N
Federal Procurement Eligibility: Small Business
Distribution: Manufacturer Direct
General Admin.: Justin Gatewood/Assistant Manager
Brian Hintergardt/President, Owner
Mauri Lathouwers/President, Owner
Computer Equipment   General

MEDICAL MART SUPPLIES LTD. 800-268-2848
5875 Chedworth Way, 905-624-6200
Mississauga, ONT L5R 3 Canada
FDA Number: n/a   Fax: 905-624-2848
E-mail: kkirby@medimart.com
Web site: www.medimart.com
Year Founded: 1978
Total Employees: 100
Ownership: Private
Produces/Sells CE-marked Devices: N
Distribution: Exclusive Distributor

MEDICAL MEASUREMENTS, INC. 201-489-9400
56 Linden St, Hackensack, NJ 07601
FDA Number: 2243491
Annual Revenue: $1-$5 Million
Ownership: Private
Produces/Sells CE-marked Devices: Y
Federal Procurement Eligibility: Small Business
Distribution: Manufacturer Through Distributor, Manufacturer Through
Manufacturer Reps, Exclusive Distributor, Importer, Exporter
Analyzer, Motility, Gastrointestinal, Electrical   Gastroenterology/Urology
Biopsy Instrument, Suction   Gastroenterology/Urology
Monitor, Esophageal Motility, And Tube   Gastroenterology/Urology
Monitor, Intracranial Pressure   Cns/Neurology
Monitor, Pressure, Intrauterine   Obstetrics/Gynecology
Transducer, Blood Pressure, Catheter Tip   Cardiovascular
Transducer, Gas Pressure, Differential   Anesthesiology
Urodynamic Measurement System   Gastroenterology/Urology

MEDICAL MEDIA LABORATORY, INC.
See Mml Diagnostics Packaging, Inc.

MEDICAL MEDIA SYSTEMS, INC.
See Medical Metrx Solutions

MEDICAL MEDICAL
See Thermo Biostar, Inc.

MEDICAL METRICS, INC. 713-850-7500
4600 Post Oak Place, Ste. 359, Houston, TX 77027
FDA Number: 1651903
Image Processing System   Radiology
Radiographic/Fluoroscopic Unit, Image-Intensified   Radiology

MEDICAL METRX SOLUTIONS 603-298-5509
12 Commerce Ave., West Lebanon, NH 03784
FDA Number: 1225988   Fax: 603-298-5055
Web site: www.medicalmetrx.com
Medical Products Sales Volume: $15,000
Annual Revenue: $5-$10 Million
Total Employees: 80   Marketing Staff: 3   Sales Staff: 7
Ownership: Private
Quality System Registration Information: ISO9000; ISO9001
Produces/Sells CE-marked Devices: N
Distribution: Manufacturer Direct
General Admin.: Mr. Greg Lange/President, Chief Executive Officer
Medical Admin.: Mrs. Jack Cronenwett/Chief Medical Officer
Finance: Mr. Ed York/Chief Financial Officer
Image Processing System   Radiology
System, Communication, Image, Digital   Radiology

MEDICAL MFG., INC. 415-282-5580
1290 Sanchez St., #2, San Francisco, CA 94114
FDA Number: 2950795
Ownership: Private
Produces/Sells CE-marked Devices: N

MEDICAL MFG., INC. 415-282-5580 (cont'd)
Circuit, Breathing (W Connector, Adapter, Y Piece)   Anesthesiology

MEDICAL MODELING INC 303-273-5344
17301 W. Colfax Ave., Suite 300, Golden, CO 80401
FDA Number: 1724955
Template   Orthopedics

MEDICAL MONOFILAMENT MANUFACTURING 508-746-7877
116 Long Pond Rd., Plymouth, MA 02360
FDA Number: 1226347
Esthesiometer   Cns/Neurology

MEDICAL MURRAY INC. 847-620-7990
400 N. Rand Rd., North Barrington, IL 60010
FDA Number: 1424778   Fax: 847-620-7995
Web site: http://www.medicalmurray.com
Year Founded: 1980
Ownership: Private
Produces/Sells CE-marked Devices: N
General Admin.: Mr. Andrew Leopold/Vice President
Mktg./Adv.: Mr. Brent Roland/Vice President Marketing & Sales
Catheter, Continuous Flush   Cardiovascular
Catheter, Percutaneous   Cardiovascular

MEDICAL PACKAGING CORPORATION 800-792-0600
941 Avenida Acaso, Camarillo, CA 93012-8700 805-388-2383
FDA Number: 2023790   Fax: 805-388-5531
E-mail: taylorschultz@medicalpackaging.com
Web site: www.medicalpackaging.com
Medical Products Sales Volume: $7,300,000
Annual Revenue: $10-$25 Million
Year Founded: 1974
Total Employees: 100   Marketing Staff: 2   Sales Staff: 2
Ownership: Private
Quality System Registration Information: ISO9002
Produces/Sells CE-marked Devices: Y
Federal Procurement Eligibility: Small Business, GSA Contract
Distribution: Manufacturer Through Distributor, OEM
General Admin.: Frederic L. Nason/President, Chief Executive Officer
Susan Nason/Vice President
Mktg./Adv.: Richard Geiszler/Director Marketing & Sales
Taylor Schultz/Director National Accounts
Neil Percy/Director Product Development
Production: Kim Garcia/Director Customer Services
Darren Davidson/Director Operations
Research: Neil Percy/Vice President Research & Development
Applicator, Tipped, Absorbent   General
Bin, Storage   General
Brush, Cytology   General
Culture Media, Non-Propagating Transport   Microbiology
Fixative, Alcohol Containing   Pathology
Kit, Pap Smear   Obstetrics/Gynecology
Slide, Microscope   Pathology
Swabs, Cotton   General
Swabs, Specimen Collection   General

MEDICAL PACKAGING INC. 800-257-5282
470 Rte. 31, PO Box 500, Ringoes, NJ 08551-1409 609-466-8991
FDA Number: n/a   Fax: 609-466-3775
E-mail: medpak@medpak.com
Web site: www.medpak.com
Medical Products Sales Volume: $2,900,000
Annual Revenue: $1-$5 Million
Year Founded: 1970
Total Employees: 15   Marketing Staff: 2   Sales Staff: 2
Ownership: Private
Produces/Sells CE-marked Devices: Y
Federal Procurement Eligibility: Small Business, GSA Contract
Distribution: Manufacturer Direct, Manufacturer Through Distributor, Manufacturer
Through Manufacturer Reps, Service Direct, Importer, Exporter
General Admin.: Emily Petillo/Office Manager
George Bartels/President, Chief Executive Officer
Mktg./Adv.: Rich Bennett/Director Marketing
Ron Kavchok/Director Product Development
Rich Bennett/Manager International & National Sales
Rich Bennett/Manager Market Research
Derek Spalter/Manager Product Development
Contract Packaging   General
Dispenser, Liquid, Unit-Dose   General
Labeling Equipment   General
Packaging System, Unit-Dose   General

MEDICAL PHYSICS INSTRUMENTATION, INC.
See Scanditronix - Wellhofer North America

MEDICAL PLASTIC DEVICES (MPD), INC.   866-633-7527
161 Oneida Dr.,   514-694-9835
Pointe Claire, QUE H9R 1 Canada
FDA Number: 9615384   *Fax:* 514-697-7012
E-mail: sales@medplas.com
Web site: www.medplas.com
Year Founded: 1984
Total Employees: 100
Ownership: Private
Produces/Sells CE-marked Devices: N
Federal Procurement Eligibility: Small Business
Distribution: Manufacturer Direct, OEM, Exporter

MEDICAL PLASTICS LABORATORY, INC.   800-433-5539
226 FM 116, Industrial Air Park, PO Box 38,   254-865-7221
Gatesville, TX 76528
FDA Number: n/a   *Fax:* 254-865-8011
E-mail: services@mpltx.com
Web site: www.medicalplastics.com
Medical Products Sales Volume: $12,300,000
Annual Revenue: $10-$25 Million
Year Founded: 1951
Total Employees: 141   *Marketing Staff:* 3   *Sales Staff:* 30
Ownership: Private
Produces/Sells CE-marked Devices: Y
Federal Procurement Eligibility: Small Business, GSA Contract
Distribution: Manufacturer Direct, Manufacturer Through Distributor, Manufacturer Through Manufacturer Reps, Service Direct, Exclusive Distributor
General Admin.: Deirdre Champ/Manager Human Resources
     David N. Broussard/President, Chief Executive Officer
Mktg./Adv.: Susan Snoddy/Manager International & National Sales
     Marion Young/Manager Marketing
     Sam Rhudy/Manager Regional Sales
     Rosie Patterson/Vice President Marketing & Sales
Production: Mark Mc Carver/Manager Operations
     Kellie Hendrickson/Manager Production
     Aage Hoejmark/Vice President Logistics
     Clint Evans/Vice President Manufacturing
Research: Danny Smith/Vice President Research & Development
Finance: Marcia Hoge/Controller

Anatomical Training Model	General
Chart, Anatomical Training	General
Simulator, Arrhythmia	Cardiovascular
Simulator, Blood Pressure	Cardiovascular
Simulator, Heart Sound	Cardiovascular
Training Manikin, Intravenous Arm	General
Training Manikin, Other	General
Training Manikin, Wound Moulage	General

MEDICAL PLASTICS/DUPACO, INC.
See Dupaco, Inc.

MEDICAL POSITIONING, INC.   800-593-3246
1717 Washington, Kansas City, MO 64108   816-474-1555
FDA Number: 9033862   *Fax:* 816-474-7755
E-mail: support@kcmpi.net
Web site: www.medicalpositioning.com
Medical Products Sales Volume: $6,200,000
Annual Revenue: $1-$5 Million
Year Founded: 1990
Total Employees: 25   *Marketing Staff:* 2   *Sales Staff:* 12
Ownership: Private
Produces/Sells CE-marked Devices: N
Federal Procurement Eligibility: Small Business, GSA Contract
Distribution: Manufacturer Direct
General Admin.: Martin Smoler/President
Mktg./Adv.: Marilyn Wiesehan/Director Marketing
Research: Michael G. Falbo/Vice President Product Development
Finance: John Gordon/Chief Financial Officer

Support, Patient Position	Anesthesiology
Table, Examination/Treatment	General
Table, Other	General
Table, Radiographic, Tilting	Radiology

MEDICAL PRODUCT SPECIALISTS
See Mps Acacia

MEDICAL PRODUCTS LABORATORIES, INC.   215-677-2700
9990 Global Rd., Philadelphia, PA 19115
FDA Number: 2513595

Agent, Polishing, Abrasive, Oral Cavity	Dental And Oral
Cleanser, Root Canal	Dental And Oral
Cord, Retraction	Dental And Oral
Preparer, Root Canal, Endodontic	Dental And Oral
Varnish, Cavity	Dental And Oral

MEDICAL PRODUCTS OF MILWAUKEE, LLC.   414-281-8713
2500 W. Layton Avenue, Suite 250, Milwaukee, WI 53221
FDA Number: 3004022327

MEDICAL PRODUCTS OF MILWAUKEE, LLC.   414-281-8713
(cont'd)
Ownership: Private
Produces/Sells CE-marked Devices: N

Adapter, Hygiene	Physical Med

MEDICAL PRODUCTS, INC.   800-638-0489
511 E. Walnut St., PO Box 207,   662-837-8522
Ripley, MS 38663
FDA Number: 2318499   *Fax:* 800-837-8572
E-mail: mhobson@med-pro.com
Web site: www.med-pro.com
Medical Products Sales Volume: $10,000,000
Annual Revenue: $5-$10 Million
Year Founded: 1984
Total Employees: 16
Ownership: Private
Produces/Sells CE-marked Devices: N
Federal Procurement Eligibility: Small Business
Distribution: Exclusive Distributor
General Admin.: Eddie McCafferty/President, Chief Executive Officer
Mktg./Adv.: Mimi Hobson/Director Marketing
Production: Christy Vandygriff/Manager Materials
Finance: Dustin McCafferty/Chief Financial Officer

Contract Manufacturing, Product, Disposable	General

MEDICAL RECORDS UNLIMITED INC.
See Suppleyes, Inc.

MEDICAL RESEARCH LABORATORIES, INC.
See Welch Allyn Protocol, Inc.

MEDICAL RESOURCES, INC.
See Medical Resources, Inc.

MEDICAL SAFETY SYSTEMS INC.   888-803-9303
230 White Pond Drive, Akron, OH 44313   330-865-4383
FDA Number: n/a   *Fax:* 330-865-4393
E-mail: info@ms2inc.com
Web site: www.ms2inc.com
Medical Products Sales Volume: $500,000
Annual Revenue: $1-$5 Million
Year Founded: 2001
Total Employees: 4   *Marketing Staff:* 1   *Sales Staff:* 4
Ownership: Private
Produces/Sells CE-marked Devices: N
Federal Procurement Eligibility: Small Business
Distribution: Manufacturer Direct, Manufacturer Through Distributor, Manufacturer Through Manufacturer Reps
General Admin.: Mr. Patrick Meridieth/President, Owner
Mktg./Adv.: Ms. Melissa Packard/Manager Customer Services & Sales
Purchasing: Mr. Dewayne Greene/Manager Purchasing

Bag, Garbage	General
Bag, Laundry, Infection Control	General
Cart, Multipurpose	General
Device, Assist, CPR	Anesthesiology
Eyeglasses, Safety	Ophthalmology
Fountain, Eye Wash	Chemistry
Glove, Utility	General
Goggles, Protective, Eye	Ophthalmology
Holder, Needle	Gastroenterology/Urology
Kit, First Aid	Surgery
Labeling Equipment	General
Manual, Policies	General
Mask, Other	General
Material, Training, Audiovisual	General
Monitor, Contamination, Environmental, Personal	General
Plug, Ear	Ear/Nose/Throat
Protector, Puncture, Needle	General
Remover, Blade, Scalpel	General
Resuscitator, Emergency, Protective, Infection	Anesthesiology
Service, Consulting	General
Stand, Laundry Hamper	General
Support, Back	Orthopedics
Support, Wrist	Physical Med
Tag, Device Status	General
Waste Disposal Unit, Sharps	General
Waste Disposal Unit, Surgical Instrument (Sharps)	Surgery
Waste Receptacle, Kick Bucket	General

MEDICAL SAFETY TECHNOLOGIES, INC.   1-866-403-6784
5412 N. 10th St, McAllen, TX 78596   956-687-6784
FDA Number: 3007067175   *Fax:* (956) 687-6787
E-mail: info@medicalsafetytechnologies.com
Ownership: Private
Produces/Sells CE-marked Devices: N

MEDICAL SALES
See Icd, Inc.

MEDICAL SALES & SERVICE GROUP — 888-357-6520
10 Woodchester Drive, Acton, MA 01720 — 508-357-6520
FDA Number: n/a — *Fax:* 508-357-6521
E-mail: mssg@mssg.com
Web site: www.mssg.com
Annual Revenue: $1-$5 Million
Total Employees: 15 — *Marketing Staff:* 5 — *Sales Staff:* 4
Ownership: Private
Produces/Sells CE-marked Devices: N
Federal Procurement Eligibility: Small Business
General Admin.: Ed Pasquarosa/President, Chief Executive Officer
    Bill Walker/Vice President
Mktg./Adv.: Arthur Winner/Manager Advertising
    Patricia Nicholas/Market Manager
    Al Jordan/Vice President Business Development
    Al Jordan/Vice President Marketing & Sales

Analyzer, Blood Gas pH	Anesthesiology
Analyzer, Chemistry, Electrolyte	Chemistry
Analyzer, Chemistry, Multi-Channel, Fixed	Chemistry
Analyzer, Chemistry, Radioimmunoassay	Chemistry
Analyzer, Chemistry, Single Channel, Programmable	Chemistry
Analyzer, Chemistry, Urine	Chemistry
Centrifuge, Cell Washing	Hematology
Centrifuge, General (Over 5,000 rpm)	Toxicology
Centrifuge, General (Up to 5,000 rpm)	Pathology
Centrifuge, Tabletop	Pathology
Chromatography, Liquid, Performance, High	Toxicology
Counter, Cell	Microbiology
Counter, Gamma, General Use	Toxicology
Flame Photometer, Pesticides (Dedicated Instruments)	Toxicology
Light, Surgical Headlight	Dental And Oral
Microtome, Cryostat	Pathology
Microtome, Rotary	Pathology
Service, Maintenance/Repair	General
Service, Used Equipment	General
Stainer, Slide, Automated	Pathology
Stainer, Slide, Histology	Microbiology
Sterilizer, Steam (Autoclave)	General
System, Automated, Microbiological	Microbiology
Timer, Coagulation, Automated	Hematology
Tissue Processor, Automated	Pathology

MEDICAL SCIENCE PRODUCTS, INC. — 800-456-1971
517 Elm Ridge Ave., Canal Fulton, OH 44614 — 330-854-4060
FDA Number: 1526822 — *Fax:* 330-854-1953
E-mail: info@medsciencepro.com
Web site: www.medsciencepro.com
Total Employees: 20
Ownership: Private
Produces/Sells CE-marked Devices: N
Federal Procurement Eligibility: Small Business, Female Owned
Distribution: Manufacturer Direct, Manufacturer Through Distributor, OEM
General Admin.: Gary Smith/President
    B. J. Smith/Vice President, General Manager
Mktg./Adv.: Gary Smith/Manager Advertising
    Joann Armstrong/Manager International & National Sales
    B. J. Smith/Vice President Marketing
Production: Gary Smith/Vice President Manufacturing
Research: Gary Smith/Vice President Research & Development

Cable/Lead, TENS	Cns/Neurology
Electrode, Cutaneous	Cns/Neurology
Electrode, Neurological	Cns/Neurology
Electrode, TENS	Cns/Neurology
Lotion, Skin Care	General

MEDICAL SCIENTIFIC, INC. — 508-880-7313
725 Myles Standish Blvd., Taunton, MA 02780
FDA Number: 1221941 — *Fax:* 508-880-7347
E-mail: info@medicalscientificinc.com
Web site: www.medicalscientificinc.com
Total Employees: 10
Ownership: Private
Quality System Registration Information: ISO9001
Produces/Sells CE-marked Devices: N
Distribution: OEM
General Admin.: Paul Nardella/President

Electrosurgical Unit, Gastroenterology	Gastroenterology/Urology
Urological Irrigation System	Gastroenterology/Urology

MEDICAL SKYHOOK COMPANY — 801-262-1471
PO Box 17213, Salt Lake City, UT 84117-0213
FDA Number: 9310042 — *Fax:* 801-254-8470
E-mail: skyhook@mstar2.net
Medical Products Sales Volume: $100,000
Annual Revenue: $0-$1 Million
Total Employees: 3
Federal Procurement Eligibility: Small Business
Distribution: Manufacturer Direct, Manufacturer Through Manufacturer Reps,
Exporter

MEDICAL SKYHOOK COMPANY — 801-262-1471 *(cont'd)*
General Admin.: Alicia S. Clayton/President
Mktg./Adv.: James R. Clayton/Vice President Marketing

Hanger, Intravenous	General
Track And Carrier, Intravenous	General

MEDICAL SOFT, INC. — 937-293-2575
1800 Southwood Ln. West, Dayton, OH 45419
FDA Number: 2248006

Computer and Software, Medical	General

MEDICAL SOFTWARE SYSTEMS, INC.
See SourceMedical

MEDICAL SOFTWARE SYSTEMS, INC.,DIV OF SOURCE MEDICAL
See SourceMedical

MEDICAL SOLUTIONS DISTRIBUTION GROUP — 501-450-9063
535 Enterprise Ave., Conway, AR 72032
FDA Number: 3005860657

Orthosis, Corrective Shoe	Physical Med

MEDICAL SOLUTIONS INTERNATIONAL, INC. — 757-224-0177
5646 Merriam Drive, Merriam, KS 66203
FDA Number: 3005021818

Tank, Holding, Dialysis	Gastroenterology/Urology

MEDICAL SPECIALTIES, INC. — 800-582-4040
4600 Lebanon Road, Charlotte, NC 28227 — 704-573-4040
FDA Number: 1016498 — *Fax:* 704-573-4047
E-mail: request@medspec.com
Web site: www.medspec.com
Annual Revenue: $5-$10 Million
Total Employees: 100
Ownership: Private
Produces/Sells CE-marked Devices: Y
Federal Procurement Eligibility: Small Business
Distribution: Manufacturer Through Distributor, Manufacturer Through
Manufacturer Reps, OEM, Exporter
General Admin.: John F. Gaylord/Chief Executive Officer
    Rick Gaylord/Vice President
Mktg./Adv.: Scott Gaylord/Vice President Business Development

Binder, Abdominal	General
Binder, Chest	General
Collar, Cervical Neck	Orthopedics
Immobilizer, Ankle	Orthopedics
Immobilizer, Arm	Orthopedics
Immobilizer, Wrist/Hand	Orthopedics
Shoe, Cast	Physical Med

MEDICAL STERILE PRODUCTS, INC. — 800-292-2887
Rd. 115. Km. 12.9, Rincon, PR 00743 — 787-823-2595
FDA Number: 2618676 — *Fax:* 787-823-8665
Year Founded: 1963
Total Employees: 75 — *Marketing Staff:* 2 — *Sales Staff:* 4
Ownership: Private
Quality System Registration Information: ISO9001
Produces/Sells CE-marked Devices: Y
Federal Procurement Eligibility: Small Business
Distribution: Manufacturer Through Distributor, OEM
General Admin.: David H. Wishinsky/President, Chief Executive Officer
Mktg./Adv.: Theresa Caro/Manager Advertising
    Gary C. Dionne/Vice President Marketing & Sales
Production: Javier Caro/Manager Production
Research: Harry Wishinsky/Vice President Research & Development

Blade, Saw, Surgical, Cardiovascular	Cardiovascular
Blade, Scalpel	Surgery
Contract Packaging	General
Forceps, Ophthalmic	Ophthalmology
Handle, Knife Blade	Surgery
Handle, Scalpel	Surgery
Molding, Injection	General
Packaging, Sterilization	General
Service, Engineering/Design	General

MEDICAL STERILIZATION, INC.
See Specialty Care

MEDICAL SUPPLIES CORPORATION T/A.ROBERTS MANUFACTURING CO., — 800-451-9951
4002 Dillon Street, Baltimore, MD 21224 — 410-366-2700
FDA Number: 1119234 — *Fax:* 410-467-4065
E-mail: info@robertsmedical.com
Web site: www.robertsmedical.com
Year Founded: 1921
Ownership: Private
Produces/Sells CE-marked Devices: N
Federal Procurement Eligibility: Small Business

MEDICAL SUPPLIES CORPORATION 800-451-9951 *(cont'd)*
Distribution: Manufacturer Direct, Manufacturer Through Distributor, Manufacturer Through Manufacturer Reps
General Admin.: Mr. Rohit Patel/President

Moist Therapy Pack	Physical Med
Pack, Moist Heat	Physical Med
Pad, Heating, Electrical	Physical Med

MEDICAL SYSTEMS LTD. 310-445-8590
11444 W. Olympic Blvd., Los Angeles, CA 90064
FDA Number: n/a — *Fax:* 310-445-4269
E-mail: Reggie@mirthless.com
Web site: www.medicalsystems.com
Total Employees: 12
Ownership: Private
Quality System Registration Information: ISO9001
Produces/Sells CE-marked Devices: N
Federal Procurement Eligibility: Small Business, Female Owned
Distribution: Service Direct
Mktg./Adv.: Larry Fata/Director Sales

Computer Software	General

MEDICAL SYSTEMS SUPPORT, INC. 800-239-2778
2301 Moody Pkwy., Suite 1, Moody, AL 35004 205-640-1080
FDA Number: n/a
E-mail: support@mssus.com
Web site: www.mssus.com
Year Founded: 1982
Ownership: Private
Produces/Sells CE-marked Devices: N
Federal Procurement Eligibility: Small Business
Distribution: Manufacturer Direct

Computer Software	General
Form, Computer	General

MEDICAL SYSTEMS, INC. 800-441-1973
30 Winter Sport Lane, PO Box 966, 802-862-1017
Williston, VT 05495
FDA Number: 1225121 — *Fax:* 802-862-3767
E-mail: michel@selectmedical.com
Web site: www.selectmedical.com
Year Founded: 1995
Ownership: Private
Produces/Sells CE-marked Devices: N

Aspirator, Endocervical	Obstetrics/Gynecology
Cannula, Intrauterine Insemination	Obstetrics/Gynecology
Curette, Suction, Endometrial	Obstetrics/Gynecology

MEDICAL TACTILE, INC. 310-641-8228
5757 W. Century Blvd #600, Los Angeles, CA 90045
FDA Number: 3005735227 — *Fax:* 310-507-0229
E-mail: info@medicaltactile.com
Web site: www.medicaltactile.com
Medical Products Sales Volume: $1,500,000
Total Employees: 15
Ownership: Private
Produces/Sells CE-marked Devices: N
Federal Procurement Eligibility: Small Business
Mktg./Adv.: Ms. Randee Wood/Vice President Market Development

Paper, Chart, Record, Medical	General
Scanner, Breast, Thermographic, Ultrasonic, Computer-Asstd.	Obstetrics/Gynecology
Sensor, Optical Contour, Physical Medicine	Physical Med

MEDICAL TECHNICAL PRODUCTS 949-551-4762
14980 Sand Canyon Avenue, Suite 200, Irvine, CA 92618-2102
FDA Number: 2025303 — *Fax:* 949-551-4764
E-mail: sales@medtechprods.com
Web site: www.medtechprods.com
Medical Products Sales Volume: $1,000,000
Annual Revenue: $1-$5 Million
Year Founded: 1984
Total Employees: 5
Ownership: Private
Quality System Registration Information: ISO9000
Produces/Sells CE-marked Devices: N
Federal Procurement Eligibility: Small Business
Distribution: Manufacturer Direct, Manufacturer Through Distributor, Manufacturer Through Manufacturer Reps, OEM, Exporter
General Admin.: Jim Bakos/President

Phacoemulsification System	Ophthalmology
Phacofragmentation Unit	Ophthalmology

MEDICAL TECHNIQUES USA 801-936-4501
125 North 400 West, Suite C, North Salt Lake, UT 84054
FDA Number: 1721368 — *Fax:* 801-936-4601
E-mail: email@medicaltechniquesusa.com
Web site: www.medicaltechniquesusa.com
Medical Products Sales Volume: $1,000,000

MEDICAL TECHNIQUES USA 801-936-4501 *(cont'd)*
Annual Revenue: $1-$5 Million
Year Founded: 1980
Total Employees: 8 — *Sales Staff:* 2
Ownership: Private
Produces/Sells CE-marked Devices: Y
Federal Procurement Eligibility: Small Business, Female Owned, GSA Contract, VA Contract
Distribution: Manufacturer Direct, Manufacturer Through Distributor, Manufacturer Through Manufacturer Reps, OEM, Exporter
Mktg./Adv.: Thor B. Roundy/Director National Accounts
 Michael Thompson/Manager International Marketing & Sales
Production: Teri McRae/Director Customer Services
 JoAnn Sokol/Manager Production
 Michael L. Thompon/Manager Quality Assurance & Regulatory Affairs

Kit, Angiographic, Digital	Radiology
Kit, Angiographic, Special Procedure	Radiology
Kit, Biopsy	General
Kit, Catheterization, Cardiac	Cardiovascular
Kit, Disposable Procedure	Cardiovascular
Kit, Maternity	Obstetrics/Gynecology
Kit, Myelogram	Cns/Neurology
Kit, Prep	General
Kit, Surgical (General)	Surgery
Kit, Surgical Instrument, Disposable	Surgery
Pack, Custom/Special Procedure	General
Pack, Surgical (Drape)	Surgery
Packaging, Sterilization	General
Syringe, Angioplasty	Cardiovascular
Syringe, Piston	General
Tray, Custom/Special Procedure	General
Tray, Surgical	Surgery
Tray, Surgical Instrument	Surgery

MEDICAL TECHNOLOGIES CO. 800-280-3220
1728A West Park Center Dr, Fenton, MO 63026 636-343-8928
FDA Number: 1937823 — *Fax:* 636-349-2262
E-mail: medtech1@primary.net
Web site: www.medical-technologies.com
Medical Products Sales Volume: $1,200,000
Annual Revenue: $1-$5 Million
Year Founded: 1997
Total Employees: 10 — *Marketing Staff:* 1 — *Sales Staff:* 1
Ownership: Private
Produces/Sells CE-marked Devices: N
Federal Procurement Eligibility: Small Business
Distribution: Manufacturer Direct, Service Direct
General Admin.: Mr. Jeff Fitzgerald/President

Cabinet, Warming	General
Cleaner, Ultrasonic, Medical Instrument	General
Light, Surgical Headlight	Dental And Oral
Scrub Machine, Surgical	Surgery
Service, Maintenance/Repair	General
Sterilizer, Steam (Autoclave), Surgical	Surgery
Table, Operating Room, Mechanical	Surgery
Washer, Labware	Chemistry

MEDICAL TECHNOLOGIES OF GEORGIA, INC. 404-394-2478
15151 Prater Drive, Covington, GA 30014
FDA Number: 1063732

Kit, Administration, Intravenous	General

MEDICAL TECHNOLOGY INDUSTRIES, INC. 800-924-4655
3555 W. Ninigret Drive, Salt Lake City, UT 84104 801-887-5114
FDA Number: 1724810 — *Fax:* 801-952-0548
E-mail: info@mti-inc.us
Web site: www.mti-inc.us
Ownership: Private
Produces/Sells CE-marked Devices: N
Federal Procurement Eligibility: Small Business, VA Contract
Distribution: Manufacturer Direct, Manufacturer Through Distributor, OEM, Exporter
General Admin.: Mr. Jeff Baker/President
Mktg./Adv.: Mr. David Andersen/Manager International & National Sales
 Mr. Brad Baker/Manager Sales
Production: Mr. Michael Bradfield/Chief Engineer
 Mr. Dee Truong/Manager Production
Purchasing: Wilson Svedin/Manager Purchasing

Cabinet, ENT Treatment	Ear/Nose/Throat
Cabinet, Instrument, AC-Powered, Ophthalmic	Ophthalmology
Chair, Examination And Treatment	General
Stool, Operating Room, Adjustable	Surgery

MEDICAL TECHNOLOGY PRODUCTS, INC. 800-314-0210
2221-16 5th Avenue, Ronkonkoma, NY 11779 631-285-6640
FDA Number: 2244732 — *Fax:* 631-285-6641
E-mail: Service@Medtechproducts.Com
Web site: www.medtechproducts.com
Annual Revenue: $1-$5 Million

MEDICAL TECHNOLOGY PRODUCTS, INC. 800-314-0210 *(cont'd)*
Year Founded: 1982
Ownership: Private
Produces/Sells CE-marked Devices: N
Distribution: Manufacturer Through Distributor
General Admin.: Thomas J. Hartnett/President, Chief Executive Officer
  Pump, Infusion   General
  Pump, Infusion, Ambulatory   General

MEDICAL TECHNOLOGY, INC.
See Bledsoe Brace Systems

MEDICAL TECHONOLOGY CORP.
See Lifesign

MEDICAL TITANIUM CORP.
See Akorn, Inc.

MEDICAL TRONIK LTEE   800-361-0877
190 boul. St-Elzear Quest,   450-669-8985
laval, QUE H7L-3 Canada
FDA Number: n/a   *Fax:* 450-669-9532
E-mail: info@medicaltronik.ca
Web site: http://www.medicaltronik.ca
Year Founded: 1985
Total Employees: 25
Ownership: Private
Produces/Sells CE-marked Devices: N
Distribution: Exclusive Distributor

MEDICAL VISION INDUSTRIES, INC.   800-775-2088
3117 Mchenry Ave., Suite B, Modesto, CA 95350
FDA Number: 3006435260
Ownership: Private
Produces/Sells CE-marked Devices: N
  Headlamp, Operating, Battery-Operated   Ophthalmology
  Illuminator, Non-Remote   Surgery

MEDICALCV, INC.   800-328-2060
9725 S. Robert Trail,   651-452-3000
Inver Grove Heights, MN 55077
FDA Number: 2124529   *Fax:* 651-452-4948
E-mail: info@medcvinc.com
Web site: www.medcvinc.com
Medical Products Sales Volume: $2,400,000
Total Employees: 2
Ownership: Private
Stock Symbol: MCVI
Traded On: OTC Bulletin
Quality System Registration Information: ISO9001
Produces/Sells CE-marked Devices: Y
Federal Procurement Eligibility: Small Business, Female Owned, VA Contract
Distribution: Manufacturer Direct, Manufacturer Through Distributor, Manufacturer Through Manufacturer Reps
General Admin.: Dr. Adel Mikhail/Chairman
    Mr. Blair Mowery/President
Medical Admin.: Shelly Johnson/Vice President Medical Affairs
Mktg./Adv.: Mr. Richard Kramp/President New Product Development
    Allan Seck/Vice President Marketing
Finance: Mr. John (Jack) Jungbauer/Chief Financial Officer
    Mr. Jeff Etten/Controller
  Filter, Blood, Cardiopulmonary Bypass, Arterial Line   Cardiovascular
  Filter, Blood, Cardiotomy Suction Line, Cardiopulmonary   Cardiovascular
  Filter, Pre-Bypass, Cardiopulmonary Bypass   Cardiovascular
  Microfilter, Blood Transfusion   Anesthesiology
  Prosthesis, Cardiac Valve   Cardiovascular

MEDICALERT FOUNDATION INTERNATIONAL   800-432-5378
2323 Colorado Avenue, Turlock, CA 95382   209-668-3333
FDA Number: 1906755   *Fax:* 209-669-2450
E-mail: customerservice@medicalert.org
Web site: www.medicalert.org
Year Founded: 1956
Total Employees: 100   *Marketing Staff:* 7
Ownership: Private
Produces/Sells CE-marked Devices: N
Federal Procurement Eligibility: Small Business
Distribution: Manufacturer Direct
General Admin.: Tanya Glazebrook/President, Chief Executive Officer
Mktg./Adv.: Mr. Ramesh Srinivasan/Vice President Market Development
Production: Long Doan/Vice President Operations
Finance: David Camp/Vice President Finance
IS: David Harrington/Chief Technologist
  Identification, Alert, Medical   General

MEDICALIBRATION PHYSICS CONSULTANT   209-524-6789
SERVICES, INC.
558 Van Dyken Way, Ripon, CA 95366
FDA Number: 2938059

MEDICALIBRATION PHYSICS CONSULTANT   209-524-6789
(cont'd)
Ownership: Private
Produces/Sells CE-marked Devices: N
  Accelerator, Linear, Medical   Radiology
  Simulator, Radiotherapy, Special Purpose   Radiology

MEDICANA INC.   800-361-9496
2261 Guenette St.,   514-335-2677
St-Laurent, QUE H4R-2 Canada
FDA Number: n/a   *Fax:* 514-745-2983
E-mail: SALES@MEDICANA.COM
Web site: www.medicana.com
Year Founded: 1963
Ownership: Private
Produces/Sells CE-marked Devices: N
Distribution: Exclusive Distributor

MEDICATION MANAGEMENT SYSTEMS, INC.
See Life Care Technologies, Inc.

MEDICEPT, INC.   508-231-8842
200 Homer Ave., Ashland, MA 01721
FDA Number: 1226526
Ownership: Private
Produces/Sells CE-marked Devices: N
  Instrument, Manual, General Surgical   Surgery

MEDICHAIR LTD.   800-667-0087
500 - 1121 Centre St NW,   403-204-1419
Calgary, ALB T2E 7 Canada
FDA Number: n/a   *Fax:* 403-204-1409
E-mail: medichair@medichair.com
Web site: www.medichair.com
Year Founded: 1985
Total Employees: 100
Ownership: Private
Produces/Sells CE-marked Devices: N
Distribution: Exclusive Distributor, Importer

MEDICOM   800-361-2862
1200, 55th Avenue,   514-636-6262
Lachine, QUE H8T 1 Canada
FDA Number: 9680179   *Fax:* 514-636-6266
E-mail: olevy@medicom.ca
Web site: www.medicom.ca
Total Employees: 121   *Marketing Staff:* 4   *Sales Staff:* 20
Ownership: Private
Quality System Registration Information: ISO9002
Produces/Sells CE-marked Devices: Y
Distribution: Manufacturer Through Distributor, Exclusive Distributor

MEDICOMP   763-389-4473
12535 316th Ave., Princeton, MN 55371
FDA Number: 2183585
  Cannula, Nasal, Oxygen   Anesthesiology
  Condenser, Heat And Moisture (Artificial Nose)   Anesthesiology
  Filter, Bacterial, Breathing Circuit   Anesthesiology
  Hood, Oxygen, Infant   General

MEDICOMP, INC.   800-23-HEART
7845 Ellis Rd., Melbourne, FL 32904-1117   321-676-0010
FDA Number: 1033601   *Fax:* 321-676-2282
E-mail: sales1@medicompinc.com
Web site: www.medicompinc.com
Annual Revenue: $5-$10 Million
Year Founded: 1981
Ownership: United Therapeutics Corporation
Stock Symbol: UTHR
Produces/Sells CE-marked Devices: N
Distribution: Manufacturer Direct, Manufacturer Through Manufacturer Reps
General Admin.: Dr. Dan Balda/President, Chief Operating Officer
Mktg./Adv.: Tony Balda/Director Marketing
    Patrick McVicker/Vice President Sales
Research: Michael Thomas/Vice President Engineering
Finance: Kimberly Collins/Controller
  Computer, Diagnostic, Programmable   Cardiovascular
  Detector, Arrhythmia Alarm   Cardiovascular
  Electrocardiograph, Ambulatory (With Analysis Algorithm)   Cardiovascular
  Transmitter/Receiver System, Physiological, Radiofrequency   Cardiovascular
  Transmitter/Receiver System, Physiological, Telephone   Cardiovascular

MEDICONTROL
See Microfluidics International Corporation

MEDICOOL, INC.   800-426-3227
20460 Gramercy Place, Torrance, CA 90501   310-782-2200
FDA Number: 2027434   *Fax:* 310-782-8900
E-mail: stevew@medicool.com

MEDICOOL, INC. 800-426-3227 (cont'd)
Web site: www.medicool.com
Ownership: Private
Produces/Sells CE-marked Devices: Y
Distribution: Manufacturer Direct, Manufacturer Through Distributor, Manufacturer Through Manufacturer Reps, Exporter
General Admin.: Steve Yeager/President
Mktg./Adv.: Mr. Steve Wallace/Vice President Sales

General Medical Device	General

MEDICOR IMAGING, DIV. OF LEAD TECHNOLOGIES INC. 704-227-2642
1201 Greenwood Cliff, Ste 400, Charlotte, NC 28204
FDA Number: 3004915908

Device, Storage, Image, Digital	Radiology

MEDICORE, INC. 800-327-8894
2647 West 81 St., Hialeah, FL 33016 305-556-5084
FDA Number: 1031058 *Fax:* 305-557-1163
E-mail: info@medicore.com
Web site: www.medicore.com
Medical Products Sales Volume: $41,700,000
Total Employees: 304
Ownership: Private
Produces/Sells CE-marked Devices: N
Federal Procurement Eligibility: Small Business
Mktg./Adv.: Bonnie Kaplan/Vice President Marketing & Sales

Lancet, Blood	General

MEDICORP, INC. 514-733-1900
5800 Royalmount, Montreal, QUE H4P 1K5 Canada
FDA Number: n/a *Fax:* 514-733-1212
E-mail: pdr@medicorp.com
Web site: www.medicorp.com
Year Founded: 1987
Total Employees: 20 *Marketing Staff:* 5 *Sales Staff:* 5
Ownership: Private
Quality System Registration Information: ISO9001
Produces/Sells CE-marked Devices: N
Distribution: Manufacturer Direct, Manufacturer Through Manufacturer Reps, OEM, Exclusive Distributor, Importer

MEDICOS LABORATORIES, INC. (MDT) 800-724-4003
801 Montrose Avenue, 908-754-4880
South Plainfield, NJ 07080
FDA Number: n/a *Fax:* 908-754-5181
E-mail: cs@inamco.com
Web site: www.inamco.com
Medical Products Sales Volume: $300,000
Annual Revenue: $1-$5 Million
Year Founded: 1987
Ownership: Private
Produces/Sells CE-marked Devices: N
Federal Procurement Eligibility: Small Business, Minority Owned
Distribution: Manufacturer Through Distributor, OEM, Exporter
General Admin.: Varges George/Chief Executive Officer, Chairman
　　　　　　 Dr. Padam Bansal/President

Analyzer, Coagulation	Hematology
Calorimeter	Chemistry
Contract Manufacturing, Pharmaceuticals/Chemicals	General
Fluorometer	Immunology
Glove, Patient Examination, Latex	General
Mask, Face	General
Microscope, Ear	Ear/Nose/Throat
Spectrophotometer, U.V./Visible	Chemistry
Sterilizer, Steam (Autoclave)	General

Medical Product Subsidiaries (Listed Separately)
Advanced Diagnostics, Inc.

MEDICUS TECHNOLOGIES 800-762-1574
105 Morgan Lane, Plainsboro, NJ 08536 609-275-0500
FDA Number: n/a *Fax:* 609-799-3297
Web site: http://www.medicus-tech.com
Ownership: Private
Produces/Sells CE-marked Devices: N

Accessories, Catheter	Surgery
Agent, Hemostatic, Absorbable, Collagen-Based	Surgery
Beads, Hydrophilic, Wound Exudate Absorption	Surgery

MEDICUS USA
See Rea Incorporated

MEDIDENTA DENTAL SUPPLY CORP.
See Medidenta International, Inc.

MEDIDENTA INTERNATIONAL, INC. 800-221-0750
3923 62nd Street, PO Box 409, 718-672-4670
Woodside, NY 11377
FDA Number: 2427609 *Fax:* 718-565-6208

MEDIDENTA INTERNATIONAL, INC. 800-221-0750 (cont'd)
E-mail: Boba@Medidenta.com
Web site: www.medidenta.com
Medical Products Sales Volume: $5,100,000
Year Founded: 1944
Total Employees: 26 *Sales Staff:* 29
Ownership: Private
Quality System Registration Information: ISO9000; ISO9002
Produces/Sells CE-marked Devices: Y
Federal Procurement Eligibility: Small Business, VA Contract
Distribution: Manufacturer Direct, Manufacturer Through Distributor, OEM, Service Direct, Exclusive Distributor, Importer, Exporter
General Admin.: Robert J. Achtziger/President, Chief Executive Officer
　　　　　　 Leonard B. Shaoul/Vice President
Mktg./Adv.: Kenneth Coyne/Manager Contract Sales
Production: Kevin Dresch/Director Quality Assurance

Broach, Endodontic	Dental And Oral
Cement, Dental	Dental And Oral
Drill, Oral Surgery	Dental And Oral
Endodontic Instrument	Dental And Oral
Gutta Percha	Dental And Oral
Handpiece, Contra- And Right-Angle Attachment, Dental	Dental And Oral
Reamer, Pulp Canal, Endodontic	Dental And Oral

MEDIFIX, INC 847-965-1898
8727 Narragansett Ave, Morton Grove, IL 60053
FDA Number: 1424786

Arthroscope	Orthopedics
Cystoscope	Gastroenterology/Urology
Endoscope	Gastroenterology/Urology

MEDIFLEX SURGICAL PRODUCTS 800-879-7575
250 Gibbs Road, Islandia, NY 11749 631-582-8440
FDA Number: 2424366 *Fax:* 631-582-8487
E-mail: sales@mediflex.com
Web site: www.mediflex.com
Medical Products Sales Volume: $5,000,000
Annual Revenue: $10-$25 Million
Year Founded: 1965
Total Employees: 30 *Marketing Staff:* 4 *Sales Staff:* 8
Ownership: FLEXBAR MACHINE CORPORATION
Quality System Registration Information: ISO9001
Produces/Sells CE-marked Devices: Y
Federal Procurement Eligibility: Small Business
Distribution: Manufacturer Direct, Manufacturer Through Distributor, OEM, Service Direct, Importer
General Admin.: Jonathan S. Adler/President, Chief Executive Officer
Mktg./Adv.: Al Fischer/Director Sales
Production: Larry Derrig/Manager Quality Assurance
　　　　　 Bernie Ascher/Product Manager
　　　　　 Steve Culver/Production Engineer

Cannula, Ophthalmic	Ophthalmology
Cannula, Suction/Irrigation, Laparoscopic	Surgery
Clamp, Laparoscopy	Surgery
Clamp, Surgical, General & Plastic Surgery	Surgery
Device, Suturing, Endoscopic	Surgery
Electrode, Electrosurgery, Laparoscopic	Surgery
Elevator, Surgical, General & Plastic Surgery	Surgery
Endoscope	Gastroenterology/Urology
Forceps, Grasping, Atraumatic	Surgery
Forceps, Grasping, Traumatic	Surgery
Forceps, Laparoscopy, Electrosurgical	Surgery
Handle, Instrument, Laparoscopic (Electrocautery)	Surgery
Holder, Camera, Surgical	Surgery
Holder, Instrument, Laparoscopic	Surgery
Holder, Laparoscope	Obstetrics/Gynecology
Holder, Retractor	Surgery
Holder/Scissors, Needle, Laparoscopic	Surgery
Laparoscope, General & Plastic Surgery	Surgery
Laparoscope, Gynecologic	Obstetrics/Gynecology
Light Source, Endoscope, Xenon Arc	Surgery
Light, Surgical, Fiberoptic	Surgery
Printer, Image, Video	General
Probe, Suction, Irrigator/Aspirator, Laparoscopic	Surgery
Retractor	Orthopedics
Retractor, Abdominal	Surgery
Retractor, Other	Surgery
Retractor, Self-Retaining, Neurology	Cns/Neurology
Retractor, Surgical	Surgery
Scissors, Laparoscopy	Surgery
Service, Engineering/Design	General
Sleeve, Trocar	Surgery
Trocar, Laparoscopic	Surgery

MEDIFOCUS, INC. 866-322-8354
5500 North Service Road, Suite 905, 905-319-7070
Burlington, ONTAR L7L 6 Canada
FDA Number: n/a
E-mail: gwalsh@walshdeltagroup.com

MEDIFOCUS, INC. 866-322-8354 *(cont'd)*
Web site: http://medifocusinc.com
Ownership: Private
Produces/Sells CE-marked Devices: N

MEDIGAS INC. 866-446-6302
4 - 55 Frid Street, Hamilton, ON L8P 4M3 Canada
FDA Number: n/a *Fax:* 905-312-0639
E-mail: info@praxair.com
Web site: www.medigas.com
Year Founded: 1907
Total Employees: 26396
Ownership: PRAXAIR, INC.
Stock Symbol: PX
Traded On: NYSE
Produces/Sells CE-marked Devices: N
Distribution: Exclusive Distributor

MEDIKMARK INC. 800-424-8520
3600 Bur Wood, Waukegan, IL 60085-8399 847-887-8400
FDA Number: 1450943 *Fax:* 847-887-0766
E-mail: sales@medikmark.com
Web site: www.medikmark.com
Medical Products Sales Volume: $15,200,000
Annual Revenue: $10-$25 Million
Year Founded: 1987
Total Employees: 100 *Marketing Staff:* 3 *Sales Staff:* 3
Ownership: Private
Produces/Sells CE-marked Devices: N
Federal Procurement Eligibility: Small Business, GSA Contract, VA Contract
Distribution: Manufacturer Direct, Manufacturer Through Distributor, Manufacturer Through Manufacturer Reps, OEM
General Admin.: Mr. Dave Sanders/Chief Executive Officer, Chairman
　　　Mr. Ken Maltas/Executive Vice President
　　　Mr. Jim Ronk/President
Mktg./Adv.: Mr. Dan Schaffnit/Sales Representative
Production: Mr. Doug Bulgrin/Manager Materials

Bandage, Elastic	General
Cart, Dressing	General
Catheter, Ureteral, Gastro-Urology	Gastroenterology/Urology
Dressing, Universal	General
General Medical Device	General
Glove, Other	General
IV Start Kit	Surgery
Kit, Dental Prophylaxis	Dental And Oral
Kit, Tracheostomy Care	Anesthesiology
Kit, Wound Drainage	General
Needle, Other	General
Training Aid	Orthopedics
Transfer Unit, IV Fluid	General
Tray, Custom/Special Procedure	General
Tray, Surgical Instrument	Surgery

MEDIMAGE, INC. 734-665-5400
6276 Jackson Rd. Ste. G, Ann Arbor, MI 48103
FDA Number: 1833124

Scanner, Emission Computed Tomography	Radiology

MEDIMAGING TECNOLOGY, INC. 800-244-9035
49 Herb Hill Road, Glen Cove, NY 11542 516-674-8900
FDA Number: n/a *Fax:* 516-674-8040
Annual Revenue: $10-$25 Million
Total Employees: 100 *Marketing Staff:* 1 *Sales Staff:* 5
Ownership: Swissray International, Inc.
Produces/Sells CE-marked Devices: N
Distribution: Manufacturer Through Distributor, Exclusive Distributor
General Admin.: E.R. Parker/President
　　　J.F. Krieger/Vice President, General Manager

Generator, Diagnostic X-Ray, High Voltage, Single Phase	Radiology
Radiographic Unit, Diagnostic	Radiology
System, Communication, Image, Digital	Radiology

MEDIN CORPORATION 800-922-0476
90 Dayton Avenue, Bldg. 16 C, Passaic, NJ 07055 973-779-2400
FDA Number: 2246425 *Fax:* 973-779-2463
E-mail: info@medin.com
Web site: www.medin.com
Medical Products Sales Volume: $6,000,000
Annual Revenue: $10-$25 Million
Year Founded: 1966
Total Employees: 75 *Marketing Staff:* 2 *Sales Staff:* 5
Ownership: Private
Quality System Registration Information: ISO9001
Produces/Sells CE-marked Devices: Y
Federal Procurement Eligibility: Small Business
Distribution: Manufacturer Direct, Manufacturer Through Distributor, Manufacturer Through Manufacturer Reps, OEM, Service Direct, Exporter
General Admin.: Mr. Jay Schainholz/President

MEDIN CORPORATION 800-922-0476 *(cont'd)*
Mktg./Adv.: Mr. Michael Librot/Vice President Sales
Production: Mr. Ariel Mazer/Director Operations
　　　Mr. Mark DiSilvestro/Vice President Quality Engineering

Cart, Other	General
Container, Sterilization (Tray)	General

MEDINOTES CORPORATION 877-633-6683
1025 Ashworth Road, Suite 222, 515-327-8850
West Des Moines, IA 50265
FDA Number: n/a *Fax:* 515-327-8856
E-mail: info@medinotes.com
Web site: www.medinotes.com
Medical Products Sales Volume: $7,600,000
Year Founded: 1995
Total Employees: 98 *Marketing Staff:* 4 *Sales Staff:* 10
Ownership: Private
Produces/Sells CE-marked Devices: N
Federal Procurement Eligibility: Small Business
Distribution: Manufacturer Direct, Manufacturer Through Distributor, Manufacturer Through Manufacturer Reps
General Admin.: Mr. Donald G. Schoen/Chief Executive Officer
Mktg./Adv.: Mr. Scott Riedel/Director Marketing Operations
　　　Mr. Tom Edgeton/Vice President Sales
Research: Mr. Davin Hills/Vice President Product Development

Computer Software	General
Computer and Software, Medical	General

MEDIONICS INTERNATIONAL INC. 800-463-6087
114 Anderson Ave., 905-472-6544
Markham, ONT L6E 1 Canada
FDA Number: 9611088 *Fax:* 905-472-6549
E-mail: info@medionics.com
Web site: www.medionics.com
Year Founded: 1976
Total Employees: 35 *Marketing Staff:* 2 *Sales Staff:* 2
Ownership: Private
Quality System Registration Information: ISO9001
Produces/Sells CE-marked Devices: Y
Federal Procurement Eligibility: Small Business
Distribution: Manufacturer Direct, Exporter

MEDIPOINT, INC. 800-445-0525
72 E. 2nd St., Mineola, NY 11501-3591 516-294-8822
FDA Number: 2416465 *Fax:* 516-746-6693
E-mail: medipoint1@aol.com
Web site: www.medipoint.com
Medical Products Sales Volume: $1,000,000
Annual Revenue: $1-$5 Million
Year Founded: 1957
Total Employees: 12
Ownership: Private
Quality System Registration Information: ISO9002
Produces/Sells CE-marked Devices: Y
Federal Procurement Eligibility: Small Business
Distribution: Manufacturer Direct, Manufacturer Through Distributor, OEM, Exporter
General Admin.: Peter Gollobin/President, Chief Executive Officer

Contract R&D, Diagnostics	General
Kit, First Aid	Surgery
Lancet, Blood	General
Tourniquet	General

MEDIPURPOSE INC. 770-448-9493
3850 Holcomb BridgeÉ_, Road, United States
Suite 350, Norcr GA 30092
FDA Number: N
Total Employees: 770-559
Ownership: I
Stock Symbol: N
General Admin.: Mr. Patrick Yi/Chief Executive Officer
　　　Mr. Randy Prather/President, Chief Operating Officer
Mktg./Adv.: Mr. Mark Stoppenbach/Vice President Marketing & Sales

MEDIQ/PRN 800-222-4776
1 Mediq Plaza, Pennsauken, NJ 08110 609-662-3200
FDA Number: n/a *Fax:* 856-661-0223
E-mail: contactus@mediq.net
Web site: www.mediq.net
Total Employees: 1150 *Marketing Staff:* 5 *Sales Staff:* 100
Ownership: MEDIQ, INC.
Stock Symbol: MED
Produces/Sells CE-marked Devices: N
Federal Procurement Eligibility: Small Business
Distribution: Manufacturer Direct, Service Direct, Exclusive Distributor, Importer
General Admin.: Regis Farrell/President, Chief Executive Officer
　　　Lynne Shapiro/Vice President Human Resources

MEDIQ/PRN
800-222-4776 *(cont'd)*

Mktg./Adv.: Kevin Farrell/Director Marketing
Karen Malin/Director National Accounts
Production: Binseng Wang/Director Quality Assurance
Ron Sokol/Manager Materials

Pump, Infusion	General
Service, Equipment Leasing	General

MEDIQUE
800-793-6210
514-342-4294

5900 Andover Ave.,
Mount-Royal, QUE H4T-1 Canada
FDA Number: n/a — *Fax:* 514-342-2294
E-mail: customerservice@mediquemed.com
Web site: www.mediquemed.com
Year Founded: 1991
Total Employees: 50
Ownership: Private
Produces/Sells CE-marked Devices: N
Distribution: Exclusive Distributor, Importer

MEDIQUIP/ A DIVISION OF STRYKER SERVICE
See Medical Technologies Co.

MEDIREX SYSTEMS LTD.
800-387-9848
416-363-9313

P.O. Box 40 Station F,
Toronto, ONT M4Y 2 Canada
FDA Number: n/a — *Fax:* 416-363-9016
E-mail: medirex@medirexsys.com
Web site: www.medirexsys.com
Total Employees: 10 — *Sales Staff:* 5
Ownership: Private
Produces/Sells CE-marked Devices: N
Federal Procurement Eligibility: Small Business
Distribution: Manufacturer Direct

MEDISAV SERVICES, INC.
905-201-1313

B-56 Elson St, Markham L3S 1Y7 Canada
FDA Number: 9614492

Adhesive, Soft Tissue Approximation	Surgery

MEDISEARCH P.R., INC.
787-864-0684

Machete Industrial Center, Guayama, PR 00784
FDA Number: 2649783

Cushion, Flotation	Physical Med
Mattress, Air Flotation	General
Mattress, Non-Powered Flotation Therapy	Physical Med
Mattress, Water, Temperature Regulated	General
Regulator, Thermal, Cardiopulmonary Bypass	Cardiovascular

MEDISISS
866-866-7477

2747 Sw 6th Street, Redmond, OR 97756
FDA Number: 3032391
E-mail: customer.service@medisiss.com
Web site: www.medisiss.com
Year Founded: 1994
Ownership: Private
Produces/Sells CE-marked Devices: N

Accessories, Arthroscopic	Orthopedics
Applier, Hemostatic Clip	Cns/Neurology
Applier, Surgical Staple	Surgery
Arthroscope	Orthopedics
Bit, Drill	Orthopedics
Blade, Saw, Surgical, Cardiovascular	Cardiovascular
Blade, Scalpel	Surgery
Blade, Surgical, Saw, General & Plastic Surgery	Surgery
Brush, Biopsy, General & Plastic Surgery	Surgery
Burr, Orthopedic	Orthopedics
Burr, Surgical, General & Plastic Surgery	Surgery
Chisel, Surgical, Manual	Surgery
Cutter, Surgical	Surgery
Driver, Bone Staple, Powered	Orthopedics
Electrosurgical Unit, Cutting & Coagulation Device	Surgery
Forceps, Biopsy, Electric, Reprocessed	Gastroenterology/Urology
Forceps, Biopsy, Non-electric, Reprocessed	Gastroenterology/Urology
Forceps, General & Plastic Surgery	Surgery
General Use Surgical Scissors	Surgery
Guide, Surgical, Needle	Surgery
Handle, Scalpel	Surgery
Knife, Nasal	Ear/Nose/Throat
Knife, Orthopedic	Orthopedics
Knife, Tonsil	Ear/Nose/Throat
Laparoscope, General & Plastic Surgery	Surgery
Motor, Surgical Instrument, AC-Powered	Surgery
Motor, Surgical Instrument, Pneumatic-Powered	Surgery
Needle, Phacoemulsification, Reprocessed	Ophthalmology
Orthopedic Manual Surgical Instrument	Orthopedics
Osteotome (Orthopedic)	Surgery
Rasp, Bone	Orthopedics
Reamer	Orthopedics
Retractor, Surgical	Surgery

MEDISISS
866-866-7477 *(cont'd)*

Scalpel, One-Piece (Knife)	Surgery
Scalpel, Ultrasonic, Reprocessed	Surgery
Scissors, Orthopedic	Orthopedics
Sleeve, Compressible Limb	Cardiovascular
Snare, Surgical	Surgery
Stapler, Surgical	Surgery
Surgical Instrument, Cardiovascular	Cardiovascular
Suture Apparatus, Stomach And Intestinal	Gastroenterology/Urology
Tap, Bone	Orthopedics
Tourniquet, Pneumatic	Surgery

MEDISOL U.S.A., INC.
626-350-6662

9713 Factorial Way, South El Monte, CA 91733
FDA Number: 2032379 — *Fax:* 626-350-0057
E-mail: MEDISOL@pacbell.net
Web site: www.medisol.com
Medical Products Sales Volume: $100,000
Year Founded: 1979
Total Employees: 25
Ownership: Private
Produces/Sells CE-marked Devices: N
Federal Procurement Eligibility: Small Business

Wheelchair, Manual	Physical Med

MEDISON AMERICA, INC.
800-829-SONO
714-889-3000

11075 Knott Ave, Suite C, Cypress, CA 90630
FDA Number: 2951220 — *Fax:* 714-889-3030
E-mail: info@medisonusa.com
Web site: www.medisonusa.com
Annual Revenue: $10-$25 Million
Year Founded: 1985
Total Employees: 422
Ownership: Private
Produces/Sells CE-marked Devices: N
Distribution: Manufacturer Direct, Exclusive Distributor
General Admin.: Sohn Won-gihl/Chief Executive Officer

Equipment, Ultrasound, Doppler, Evaluation, Fetal	Obstetrics/Gynecology
Gel, Ultrasonic Transmission	General
Scanner, Ultrasonic, Other	Radiology

MEDISPEC LTD. - USA
888-663-3477
301-944-1575

20410 Observation Drive, Suite # 102,
Germantown, MD 20876
FDA Number: 1123459 — *Fax:* 301-972-6098
E-mail: info@medispec.com
Web site: www.medispec.com
Medical Products Sales Volume: $7,000,000
Annual Revenue: $10-$25 Million
Year Founded: 1991
Total Employees: 28 — *Sales Staff:* 10
Ownership: Private
Quality System Registration Information: ISO9001; ISO9002
Produces/Sells CE-marked Devices: Y
Federal Procurement Eligibility: Small Business
Distribution: Manufacturer Direct, Manufacturer Through Distributor, Manufacturer Through Manufacturer Reps
General Admin.: Avner Spector/President, Chief Executive Officer
Anil Dhingra/Vice President, General Manager
Mktg./Adv.: Walt Reichert/Manager National Sales
Production: Sheryl Skinner/Manager Regulatory Affairs

Flowmeter, Urine, Disposable	Gastroenterology/Urology
Hyperthermia System, Automatic Control	Radiology
Lithotriptor, Extracorporeal Shock-wave, Urological	Gastroenterology/Urology
Locator, Intracorporeal Device, Ultrasonic	Obstetrics/Gynecology

MEDISPEC/SONTEC INSTRUMENTS INC.
See Sontec Instruments Inc.

MEDISPECTRA INC
781-372-2430

45 Hartwell Ave., Lexington, MA 02421
FDA Number: 3002634893
Ownership: Private
Produces/Sells CE-marked Devices: N

Sensor, Electro-optical(for Cervical Cancer)	Obstetrics/Gynecology

MEDIST INTERNATIONAL
901-380-9411

9160 HWY 64, Suite 12, Lakeland, TN 38002
FDA Number: 2320830 — *Fax:* 901-380-8412
E-mail: medist1@aol.com
Web site: www.medist.com
Ownership: Private
Produces/Sells CE-marked Devices: N

System, Skin Closure	Surgery
Tape, Orthopedic	Orthopedics

MEDISURG RESEARCH AND MANAGEMENT CORP.   610-277-3937

100 West Fornance St., Norristown, PA 19401
FDA Number: 2532084
E-mail: john@medisurg.com
Web site: www.medisurg.com
Year Founded: 2002
Ownership: Private
Produces/Sells CE-marked Devices: N
  Apparatus, Cutting, Radiofrequency, Electrosurgical, Battery-powered   Ophthalmology

MEDISYSTEMS CORPORATION   800-369-6334

439 South Union St., 5th Floor, Lawrence, MA 01843
FDA Number: 2919260   *Fax:* 888-372-8459
E-mail: medisystems@hotmail.com
Web site: www.medisystems.com
Annual Revenue: $1-$5 Million
Year Founded: 1981
Ownership: Nxstage Medical, Inc.
Quality System Registration Information: ISO9000
Produces/Sells CE-marked Devices: N
Federal Procurement Eligibility: Small Business, Minority Owned
Distribution: Manufacturer Direct, Manufacturer Through Manufacturer Reps
  Accessories, Blood Circuit, Hemodialysis   Gastroenterology/Urology
  Cannula, Hemodialysis   Gastroenterology/Urology
  Catheter, Hemodialysis, Single-Needle   Gastroenterology/Urology
  Detector, Hemodialysis Unit Air Bubble-Foam   Gastroenterology/Urology
  Dialyzer, Capillary, Hollow Fiber (Hemodialysis)   Gastroenterology/Urology
  Dialyzer, Parallel Flow (Hemodialysis)   Gastroenterology/Urology
  Kit, Administration, Peritoneal Dialysis, Disposable   Gastroenterology/Urology
  Kit, Catheterization, Intravenous, Winged   Cardiovascular
  Kit, Hemodialysis Tubing   Gastroenterology/Urology
  Kit, Intravenous Extension Tubing   General
  Kit, Tubing, Dialysis, Peritoneal   Gastroenterology/Urology
  Needle, Dialysis   Gastroenterology/Urology
  Syringe, Antistick   General

MEDITECH

  See Medical Information Technology, Inc. (Meditech)

MEDITECH INTERNATIONAL INC.   416-251-1055

411 Horner Ave., Unit 1, Toronto, ONT M8W-4W3 Canada
FDA Number: n/a   *Fax:* 416-251-2446
E-mail: info@meditech-bioflex.com
Web site: www.meditech-bioflex.com
Year Founded: 1993
Total Employees: 25
Ownership: Private
Produces/Sells CE-marked Devices: N
Distribution: Manufacturer Direct, Exclusive Distributor, Exporter

MEDITHERM INC.   503-639-8496

400 Front Street, Unit 8, Beaufort, NC 28516
FDA Number: 3006111110
  Telethermographic System (Adjunctive Use)   Radiology

MEDITRACK PRODUCTS, LLC   800-863-9633   978-567-9412

433 Main St., Hudson, MA 01749
FDA Number: 1223961   *Fax:* 978-567-9421
E-mail: info@doser.com
Web site: www.doser.com
Medical Products Sales Volume: $1,500,000
Annual Revenue: $1-$5 Million
Year Founded: 1997
Total Employees: 15   *Marketing Staff:* 2   *Sales Staff:* 6
Ownership: Private
Quality System Registration Information: ISO9000
Produces/Sells CE-marked Devices: Y
Federal Procurement Eligibility: Small Business
Distribution: Manufacturer Direct
General Admin.: Mr. David Urbanus/President, Chief Executive Officer
  Nebulizer, Direct Patient Interface   Anesthesiology

MEDIVANCE, INC.   303-926-1917

1172 Century Dr., Suite 240, Louisville, CO 80027
FDA Number: 1725056
  Regulator, Thermal, Cardiopulmonary Bypass   Cardiovascular

MEDIVISION ENDOSCOPY   800-349-5367   714-563-2772

1210 N. Jefferson St, Suite D, Anaheim, CA 92807
FDA Number: n/a   *Fax:* 714-563-2711
E-mail: endoscopy@medivisionusa.com
Web site: www.medivisionusa.com
Medical Products Sales Volume: $1,000,000
Annual Revenue: $1-$5 Million
Year Founded: 1994
Total Employees: 20   *Marketing Staff:* 2   *Sales Staff:* 3
Ownership: Private

MEDIVISION ENDOSCOPY   800-349-5367 *(cont'd)*

Quality System Registration Information: ISO9000; ISO9001
Produces/Sells CE-marked Devices: Y
Federal Procurement Eligibility: Small Business
Distribution: Manufacturer Through Distributor, Manufacturer Through Manufacturer Reps, OEM
General Admin.: Alex Vayser/President, Chief Executive Officer
Production: Betty Rangel/Manager Regulatory Affairs
    Kevin May/Vice President Operations
  Arthroscope   Orthopedics
  Cystoscope   Gastroenterology/Urology
  Endoscope, Rigid   Surgery
  Laparoscope, General & Plastic Surgery   Surgery
  Service, Maintenance/Repair   General
Medical Product Subsidiaries (Listed Separately)
  Ophthalmic Imaging Systems

MEDIVISION SCOPE SERVICE CENTER, INC.

  See Medivision Endoscopy

MEDIWARE CHICAGO SERVICE CENTER   630-218-2700

1900 Spring Rd., Suite 450, Oak Brook, IL 60523
FDA Number: 3004548718
Ownership: Private
Produces/Sells CE-marked Devices: N
  Software, Blood Bank (Stand-Alone Products)   Hematology

MEDIWARE DALLAS SERVICE CENTER   913-307-1000

4545 Fuller Dr., Suite 320, Irving, TX 75038
FDA Number: 1651376
Ownership: Private
Produces/Sells CE-marked Devices: N
  Software, Blood Bank (Stand-Alone Products)   Hematology

MEDIWARE INFORMATION SYSTEMS, INC.   800-255-0026   913-307-1000

11711 W 79th Street, Lenexa, KS 66214
FDA Number: 2437251   *Fax:* 913-307-1111
E-mail: info@mediware.com
Web site: www.mediware.com
Medical Products Sales Volume: $41,200,000
Annual Revenue: $10-$25 Million
Year Founded: 1980
Total Employees: 202   *Marketing Staff:* 2   *Sales Staff:* 10
Ownership: Public
Stock Symbol: MEDW
Traded On: NASDAQ
Produces/Sells CE-marked Devices: N
Federal Procurement Eligibility: Small Business
Distribution: Manufacturer Direct, Service Direct
General Admin.: Mr. George Barry/President, Chief Executive Officer
    Mr. Don Jackson/Vice President, General Manager
Mktg./Adv.: Mr. Gary Correll/Director Marketing
    Mr. Joe Tehan/Director National Sales
  Computer Software   General
  Computer, Patient Data Management   General

MEDIX PHARMACEUTICALS AMERICAS, INC.   888-242-3463   727-507-9844

12505 Starkey Road, Suite M, Largo, FL 33773
FDA Number: 9028685   *Fax:* 866-257-5267
E-mail: cservice@biafine.com
Web site: www.medix.homestead.com/files
Medical Products Sales Volume: $1,900,000
Annual Revenue: $1-$5 Million
Year Founded: 1994
Total Employees: 7   *Marketing Staff:* 1   *Sales Staff:* 15
Ownership: Laboratoire Medix
Produces/Sells CE-marked Devices: N
Federal Procurement Eligibility: Small Business
Distribution: Exclusive Distributor, Importer
General Admin.: Mr. Timothy Kost/President
Production: Mr. George Hudak/Vice President Operations
  Dressing, Wound and Burn, Occlusive   Surgery

MEDLAB CO., THE

  See 3m Health Information Systems

MEDLINE INDUSTRIES DYNACOR DIVISION

  See Medline Industries, Inc.

MEDLINE INDUSTRIES HOLDINGS, L.P.   847-837-2759

7267 Schantz Rd., Allentown, PA 18106
FDA Number: 2529859
Ownership: Private
Produces/Sells CE-marked Devices: N
  Patient Personal Hygiene Kit   Dental And Oral

MEDLINE INDUSTRIES HOLDINGS, L.P.   847-837-2759

9303 Stoneview Dr., Dallas, TX 75237
FDA Number: 1646422

MANUFACTURER PROFILES

MEDLINE INDUSTRIES HOLDINGS, L.P.   **847-837-2759** *(cont'd)*
Patient Personal Hygiene Kit   Dental And Oral

MEDLINE INDUSTRIES, INC.   **800-633-5463**
1 Medline Place, Mundelein, IL 60060
FDA Number: 1417592   *Fax:* 800-351-1512
E-mail: info@medline.com
Web site: www.medline.com
Year Founded: 1910
Ownership: Medline Industries, Inc.
Quality System Registration Information: ISO9000
Produces/Sells CE-marked Devices: N
Distribution: Manufacturer Direct

Bag, Drainage (Incontinence)	Gastroenterology/Urology
Catheter, Balloon (Foley Type)	Surgery
Catheter, Suction, With Tip	General
Catheter, Urological	Gastroenterology/Urology
Douche, Vaginal	Obstetrics/Gynecology
Kit, Enema (For Cleaning Purposes)	Gastroenterology/Urology
Kit, Feeding, Adult (Enteral)	General
Pump, Food (Enteral Feeding)	General
Tube, Feeding	General
Urological Irrigation System	Gastroenterology/Urology

MEDLINE INDUSTRIES, INC.   **800-633-5886**
1 Medline Place, Mundelein, IL 60060-4486   **847-949-5500**
FDA Number: 1417592   *Fax:* 847-949-3126
E-mail: service@medline.com
Web site: www.medlineinc.com
Annual Revenue: $0-$1 Million
Total Employees: 3000   *Marketing Staff:* 15   *Sales Staff:* 630
Ownership: Private
Produces/Sells CE-marked Devices: N
Distribution: Manufacturer Direct, Importer
General Admin.: Andy Mills/President
Mktg./Adv.: Tom Pawlik/Vice President Marketing
     Ray Swaback/Vice President Sales
Finance: Bill Abbington/Chief Financial Officer

Airway, Oropharyngeal, Anesthesia	Anesthesiology
Appliance, Incontinence, Urosheath Type	Gastroenterology/Urology
Bag, Laundry, Infection Control	General
Bag, Leg	Gastroenterology/Urology
Binder, Abdominal	General
Cannula, Nasal, Oxygen	Anesthesiology
Catheter, Continuous Irrigation	Surgery
Catheter, Nasal, Oxygen (Tube)	Anesthesiology
Catheter, Nasopharyngeal	Ear/Nose/Throat
Catheter, Retention Type, Balloon	Gastroenterology/Urology
Catheter, Suction (Tracheal Aspirating Tube)	Anesthesiology
Chair, Position, Electric	Physical Med
Circuit, Breathing (W Connector, Adapter, Y Piece)	Anesthesiology
Circulator, Breathing Circuit	Anesthesiology
Container, Specimen, All Types	General
Container, Surgical Instrument	Surgery
Cover, Laundry Hamper	General
Cover, Mattress, Waterproof	General
Cover, Shoe, Conductive	General
Cover, Shoe, Non-Conductive	General
Crutch	Physical Med
Curtain, Cubicle	General
Douche, Vaginal	Obstetrics/Gynecology
Drainage System, Urine, Closed	Gastroenterology/Urology
Drape, Surgical, Reusable	Surgery
Dress, Scrub, Reusable	Surgery
Filter, Bacterial, Breathing Circuit	Anesthesiology
Finger Cot	General
Gauze, Non-Absorbable, X-Ray Detectable (Internal Sponge)	Surgery
Gown, Isolation, Surgical	Surgery
Gown, Operating Room, Reusable	Surgery
Gown, Patient, Reusable	General
Humidifier, Heat/Moisture Exchange	Anesthesiology
Kit, Catheterization, Sterile Urethral	Gastroenterology/Urology
Kit, Catheterization, Urinary	Gastroenterology/Urology
Kit, Enema (For Cleaning Purposes)	Gastroenterology/Urology
Kit, Irrigation, Sterile	Gastroenterology/Urology
Kit, Prep	General
Kit, Sitz Bath	Physical Med
Kit, Surgical Instrument, Disposable	Surgery
Mask, Gas, Anesthesia	Anesthesiology
Mask, Surgical	Surgery
Pad, Incontinence (Underpad)	General
Restraint, Arm	General
Speculum, Vaginal, Non-Metal	Obstetrics/Gynecology
Suit, Scrub, Reusable	Surgery
Syringe, Ear	Ear/Nose/Throat
Thermometer, Mercury	General
Tip, Suction	Anesthesiology
Tips And Pads, Cane, Crutch And Walker	Physical Med
Towel, Surgical	Surgery
Tube, Tonsil Suction	Ear/Nose/Throat
Tube, Tracheal (Endotracheal)	Anesthesiology

MEDLINE INDUSTRIES, INC.   **800-633-5886** *(cont'd)*

Tubing, Oxygen Connecting	General
Urinal	General
Ventilator, Other	Anesthesiology
Wrap, Sterilization	General

Medical Product Subsidiaries (Listed Separately)
Medline Industries, Inc.

MEDLINE MANUFACTURING AND SERVICES LLC   **847-837-2759**
One Medline Place, Mundelein, IL 60060
FDA Number: 97712
Ownership: Private
Produces/Sells CE-marked Devices: N

Airway, Oropharyngeal, Anesthesia	Anesthesiology
Bag, Leg	Gastroenterology/Urology
Bandage, Elastic	General
Catheter, Retention Type, Balloon	Gastroenterology/Urology
Catheter, Suction (Tracheal Aspirating Tube)	Anesthesiology
Catheter, Suction, With Tip	General
Catheter, Ureteral, Gastro-Urology	Gastroenterology/Urology
Catheter, Urethral	Gastroenterology/Urology
Component, Cast	Orthopedics
Connector, Catheter	Surgery
Dispenser, Medication, Liquid	General
Douche, Vaginal	Obstetrics/Gynecology
Drainage System, Urine, Closed	Gastroenterology/Urology
Instrument, Manual, General Surgical	Surgery
Kit, Catheterization, Sterile Urethral	Gastroenterology/Urology
Kit, Irrigation, Sterile	Gastroenterology/Urology
Kit, Surgical (General)	Surgery
Speculum, Vaginal, Non-Metal	Obstetrics/Gynecology
Syringe, Ear	Ear/Nose/Throat
Syringe, Irrigating	General
Syringe, Piston	General
Thermometer, Mercury	General
Tourniquet, Non-Pneumatic, Surgical	Surgery
Trap, Sterile Specimen	Anesthesiology
Tube, Aspirating, Flexible, Connecting	Anesthesiology
Tube, Levine	General

MEDLINE SYSTEMS INC.
See Quality Software Systems

MEDLINK IMAGING, INC.   **800-456-7800**
200 Clearbrook Road, Elmsford, NY 10523   **914-347-0102**
FDA Number: 2433615   *Fax:* 888-437-9729
E-mail: jose.rodriguez@medlinkimaging.com
Web site: www.medlinkimaging.com
Medical Products Sales Volume: $6,800,000
Annual Revenue: $25-$50 Million
Year Founded: 2005
Total Employees: 35   *Marketing Staff:* 5   *Sales Staff:* 7
Ownership: Cine Magnetics, Inc.
Quality System Registration Information: ISO9002
Produces/Sells CE-marked Devices: Y
Federal Procurement Eligibility: Small Business
Distribution: Exclusive Distributor, Importer, Exporter
General Admin.: Mr. John Garcia/Vice President Chief Information Officer
Mktg./Adv.: Mr. Paul Joyce/Director Sales
     Mr. Eddie Massetti/Manager International & National Sales
IS: Mr. Bill Raccioppi/Manager Tech. Support

Apron, Lead, Radiographic	Radiology
Cassette, Radiographic Film	Radiology
Chemical, Film Processor	Radiology
Computer, Radiographic Image Analysis	Radiology
Film, X-Ray	Radiology
Film, X-Ray, Special Purpose	Radiology
Generator, Diagnostic X-Ray, High Voltage, 3-Phase	Radiology
Radiographic Unit, Diagnostic	Radiology
Radiographic Unit, Diagnostic, Chest	Radiology
Shield, X-Ray	Radiology

MEDLOGIC GLOBAL CORPORATION   **800-625-6442**
4815 List Dr., Colorado Springs, CO 80919   **719-540-8200**
FDA Number: n/a   *Fax:* 719-535-8999
E-mail: info@medlogic.com
Web site: www.medlogic.com
Ownership: Private
Produces/Sells CE-marked Devices: Y
General Admin.: Donald H. McLean/Chief Financial Officer, Vice President
     Michael M. Byram/President, Chief Executive Officer
Mktg./Adv.: Edward F. Coghlan/Vice President Marketing & Communications

Adhesive, Wound Closure	Surgery

MEDLOGIX, INC.   **804-530-2906**
9409 Burge Avenue, Richmond, VA 23236
FDA Number: 3007033496
E-mail: sales@medlogixinc.com
Ownership: Private
Produces/Sells CE-marked Devices: N

MEDLOGIX, INC.   804-530-2906 *(cont'd)*
Pack, Hot Or Cold, Disposable   Physical Med

MEDLON INC.
See Codan Us Corporation

MEDMARK TECHNOLOGIES, LLC   215-249-1540
724 H West Rt 313 Dublin Park, Perkasie, PA 18944
FDA Number: 99135   Fax: 215-249-1029
E-mail: info@medmarktechnologies.com
Web site: www.medmarktechnologies.com
Ownership: Private
Produces/Sells CE-marked Devices: N
Sleeve, Compressible Limb   Cardiovascular

MEDMETRIC CORP.   800-995-6066
7542 Trade St., San Diego, CA 92121-2412   858-536-9122
FDA Number: 2022004   Fax: 858-536-9303
E-mail: info@medmetric.com
Web site: www.medmetric.com
Medical Products Sales Volume: $1,000,000
Annual Revenue: $1-$5 Million
Year Founded: 1977
Total Employees: 11   *Marketing Staff:* 1   *Sales Staff:* 1
Ownership: Private
Produces/Sells CE-marked Devices: Y
Federal Procurement Eligibility: Small Business
Distribution: Manufacturer Direct, Exporter
General Admin.: Dick Watkins/President, Chief Executive Officer
Arthrometer   Orthopedics
Holder, Leg   Surgery
Protractor   Orthopedics

MEDMIRA LABORATORIES INC.   1-877-MEDMIRA
155 Chain Lake Dr, Unit 1,   902-450-1588
Halifax, NS B3S 1 Canada
FDA Number: 9616225   Fax: 902-450-1580
E-mail: sales@medmira.com
Web site: www.medmira.com
Year Founded: 1992
Total Employees: 55
Ownership: Private
Stock Symbol: MIR
Traded On: Vancouver
Quality System Registration Information: ISO9001
Produces/Sells CE-marked Devices: N
Distribution: Manufacturer Direct

MEDNET HEALTHCARE TECHNOLOGIES, INC.   800-606-5511
100 Ludlow Drive, Ewing, NJ 08638   609-671-1790
FDA Number: n/a   Fax: 800-889-5415
E-mail: info@mednethealth.net
Web site: www.mednethealth.net
Annual Revenue: $10-$25 Million
Year Founded: 1989
Total Employees: 15   *Marketing Staff:* 1   *Sales Staff:* 10
Ownership: MEDNET HEALTHCARE TECHNOLOGIES
Quality System Registration Information: ISO9000
Produces/Sells CE-marked Devices: N
Federal Procurement Eligibility: Small Business
Distribution: Manufacturer Direct, Manufacturer Through Distributor, Manufacturer Through Manufacturer Reps, OEM
General Admin.: Frank Movizzo/Chief Executive Officer
   Steve Adamsky/Vice President, General Manager
Mktg./Adv.: Mr. Brian Pike/Vice President National Marketing & Sales
Monitor, Cardiac (Cardiotachometer & Rate Alarm)   Cardiovascular
Transmitter/Receiver System, ECG, Telephone Single-Channel   Cardiovascular
Medical Product Subsidiaries (Listed Separately)
Universal Medical, Inc.

MEDNET LOCATOR, INC.   800-754-5070
7000 Shadow Oaks, Memphis, TN 38125
FDA Number: 1034684
Brush, Dermabrasion   Surgery
Drill, Surgical, ENT (Electric Or Pneumatic)   Ear/Nose/Throat
Inserter, Myringotomy Tube   Ear/Nose/Throat
Knife, Myringotomy   Ear/Nose/Throat
Light, Surgical, Fiberoptic   Surgery
Prosthesis, Ossicular   Ear/Nose/Throat

MEDNET SERVICES, INC.   612-788-6228
2855 Anthony Ln. South, #b10, Minneapolis, MN 55418
FDA Number: 2134073
Stimulator, Muscle, Electrical-Powered (EMS)   Physical Med
Stimulator, Nerve, Transcutaneous (Pain Relief, TENS)   Cns/Neurology
Unit, Therapy, Current, Interferential   Cns/Neurology

MEDONE SURGICAL, INC.   941-359-3129
670 Tallevast Road, Sarasota, FL 34243
FDA Number: 1064371
Cannula, Ophthalmic   Ophthalmology
Cystotome, Ophthalmic   Ophthalmology
Forceps, Ophthalmic   Ophthalmology
Instrument, Manual, General Surgical   Surgery
Instrument, Microsurgical   Cns/Neurology
Knife, Ear   Ear/Nose/Throat
Knife, Myringotomy   Ear/Nose/Throat
Knife, Ophthalmic   Ophthalmology
Needle, Aspiration And Injection, Disposable   Surgery
Scissors, Ear   Ear/Nose/Throat
Scissors, Ophthalmic   Ophthalmology
Shield, Eye, Ophthalmic   Ophthalmology
Spatula, Ophthalmic   Ophthalmology

MEDOVATIONS, INC.   800-558-6408
102 E. Keefe Avenue, Milwaukee, WI 53212   414-265-7620
FDA Number: 2183446   Fax: 414-265-7628
E-mail: medo@medovations.com
Web site: www.medovations.com
Medical Products Sales Volume: $6,000,000
Annual Revenue: $5-$10 Million
Year Founded: 1986
Total Employees: 40
Ownership: Private
Quality System Registration Information: ISO9002
Produces/Sells CE-marked Devices: Y
Federal Procurement Eligibility: Small Business
Distribution: Manufacturer Direct, Manufacturer Through Distributor, OEM, Exporter
General Admin.: Brant Stanford/President, Chief Executive Officer, Chief Operating Officer
   Meg Vierling/Vice President, General Manager
Production: Holly Kersting/Product Specialist
Accessories, Catheter   Surgery
Accessories, Catheter, G-U   Gastroenterology/Urology
Aspirator, Low Volume (Gastric Suction)   Gastroenterology/Urology
Bougie, Esophageal, And Gastrointestinal, Gastro-Urology   Gastroenterology/Urology
Bougie, Esophageal, ENT   Ear/Nose/Throat
Cannula, Aspirating   Cardiovascular
Cannula, Catheter   Cardiovascular
Cannula, Surgical, General & Plastic Surgery   Surgery
Catheter, Cardiovascular   Surgery
Catheter, Other   Gastroenterology/Urology
Connector, Catheter   Surgery
Connector, Suction/Irrigation   Surgery
Contract Manufacturing   General
Contract Manufacturing, Product, Disposable   General
Dilator, Esophageal   Gastroenterology/Urology
Dilator, Esophageal, ENT   Ear/Nose/Throat
Drain, Sump   Gastroenterology/Urology
Drain, Thoracic (Chest)   Anesthesiology
Evacuator, Gastro-Urology   Gastroenterology/Urology
Guidewire   Cardiovascular
Irrigator, Suction   General
Tip, Suction Tube (Yankauer, Poole, Etc.)   Surgery
Trocar, Other   General
Trocar, Thoracic   Cardiovascular
Tube, Decompression   General
Tube, Double Lumen For Intestinal Decompression   Gastroenterology/Urology
Tube, Drainage   Gastroenterology/Urology
Tube, Gastrointestinal   Gastroenterology/Urology
Tube, Suction   General
Tubing, Connecting   General
Tubing, Other   General
Tubing, Oxygen Connecting   General
Tubing, Plastic   General

MEDPORT, LLC   800-299-5704
23 Acorn St., Providence, RI 02903   978-927-3808
FDA Number: 3000218795
Ownership: Private
Produces/Sells CE-marked Devices: N
Monitor, Blood Pressure, Indirect, Semi-Automatic   Cardiovascular
Thermometer, Electronic, Continuous   General

MEDPRO IMAGING   877-846-8818
821 Corporate Court, Suite 101,   262-522-6740
Waukesha, WI 53189
FDA Number: n/a   Fax: 262-522-6770
Web site: http://medproimaging.com
Ownership: Private
Produces/Sells CE-marked Devices: N
General Admin.: Mr. Charlie Jahnke/President, Chief Executive Officer
Mktg./Adv.: Mr. Keith Rubenstein/Senior Vice President Sales

MEDPRO IMGAING INC.
877-846-8818
262-522-6740
821 Corporate Court, Suite 101,
Waukesha, WI 53189
FDA Number: n/a
E-mail: info@medproimaging.com   *Fax:* 262-522-6770
Web site: http://www.medproimaging.com/
Year Founded: 2005
Ownership: Private
Produces/Sells CE-marked Devices: N
General Admin.: Charlie Jahnke/President, Chief Executive Officer

MEDPRO SAFETY PRODUCTS, INC.
859-225-5375
145 Rose Street, Lexington, KY 40507
FDA Number: 1531258
Web site: http://www.medprosafety.com   *Fax:* 859-225-5347
Ownership: Public
Stock Symbol: MPSP
Traded On: OTC Bulletin
Produces/Sells CE-marked Devices: N
General Admin.: Mr. Gregory Schupp/Chief Operating Officer

Needle, Dental	Dental And Oral
Needle, Hypodermic, Single Lumen With Syringe	General
Serum Separation System	Hematology
Syringe, Antistick	General

MEDPRO, INC.
See Medpro Safety Products, Inc.

MEDRAD INC.
724-940-7940
625 Alpha Dr., Pittsburgh, PA 15238
FDA Number: 3004056159
Ownership: Medrad, Inc.
Produces/Sells CE-marked Devices: N

Probe, Rectal, Non-Powered	Gastroenterology/Urology

MEDRAD SAXONBURG, INC.
724-940-7940
150 Victory Road, Saxonburg, PA 16056
FDA Number: 3006791331
Ownership: Medrad, Inc.
Produces/Sells CE-marked Devices: N

Injector, Syringe	General

MEDRAD, INC.
800-633-7231
724-940-6800
100 Global View Dr., Warrendale, PA 15086
FDA Number: 2520313   *Fax:* 412-767-4120
E-mail: info@medrad.com
Web site: www.medrad.com
Medical Products Sales Volume: $343,600,000
Annual Revenue: $500 Million-$1 Billion
Year Founded: 1964
Total Employees: 1700   *Marketing Staff:* 35   *Sales Staff:* 50
Ownership: Private
Stock Symbol: MDRD
Traded On: OTC Bulletin
Quality System Registration Information: ISO9001; ISO9002
Produces/Sells CE-marked Devices: Y
Distribution: Manufacturer Direct, Manufacturer Through Distributor, OEM, Service Direct, Exclusive Distributor, Exporter
General Admin.: Gary Bucciarelli/Chief Administrative Officer
    Joe Havrilla/Chief Technology Officer
    Julio Rivera/Compliance Officer
    Mr. Sam Liang/President, Chief Executive Officer
Mktg./Adv.: John R. Tedeschi/Senior Vice President International & National Sales
Production: Jeff Owoc/Senior Vice President Operations
    Jim Kessing/Vice President Manufacturing

Canister, Coil	Gastroenterology/Urology
Component, Other	General
Injector, Angiographic (Cardiac Catheterization)	Cardiovascular
Injector, Syringe	General
Probe, Other	General
Syringe, Angiographic	Cns/Neurology

Medical Product Subsidiaries (Listed Separately)
Medrad Inc.
Medrad Saxonburg, Inc.
Possis Medical, Inc.

MEDRECON, INC.
877-526-4323
908-789-2050
257 South Avenue, Garwood, NJ 07027-1341
FDA Number: 2246649   *Fax:* 908-789-3275
E-mail: ortables@medrecon.com
Web site: www.medrecon.com
Medical Products Sales Volume: $1,400,000
Annual Revenue: $1-$5 Million
Year Founded: 1972
Total Employees: 19   *Marketing Staff:* 2   *Sales Staff:* 3
Ownership: Private
Produces/Sells CE-marked Devices: N
Federal Procurement Eligibility: Small Business

MEDRECON, INC.
877-526-4323 *(cont'd)*
Distribution: Service Direct
General Admin.: Mr. Gary P. Sitcer/President, Chief Executive Officer
    Ms. Nicole Jackson/Senior Admin.
    Ms. Wende Sitcer/Senior Admin.
Production: Mr. Andy Kroszczynski/Vice President Production

Accessories, Operating Room, Table	Surgery
Board, Arm	Anesthesiology
Holder, Leg	Surgery
Holder, Leg, Arthroscopy	Orthopedics
Holder, X-Ray Film	Dental And Oral
Mattress, Operating Table	General
Screen, Anesthesia	Anesthesiology
Service, Equipment Leasing	General
Service, Maintenance/Repair	General
Service, Used Equipment	General
Stirrup	Gastroenterology/Urology
Support, Arm	Physical Med
Synchronizer, ECG/Respirator, Radiographic	Radiology
Table, Cystometric, Non-Electrical	Gastroenterology/Urology
Table, Examination/Treatment	General
Table, Obstetrical	Obstetrics/Gynecology
Table, Obstetrical, AC-Powered	Obstetrics/Gynecology
Table, Obstetrical, Manual	Obstetrics/Gynecology
Table, Operating Room, AC-Powered	Surgery
Table, Operating Room, Mechanical	Surgery
Table, Operating Room, Pneumatic	Surgery
Table, Surgical With Orthopedic Accessories, AC-Powered	Surgery
Table, Surgical, Electrical	Surgery
Table, Surgical, Hydraulic	Surgery
Table, Surgical, Manual	General
Table, Surgical, Orthopedic	Orthopedics
Table, Urological (Cystological)	Gastroenterology/Urology
Table, Urological, Non-Electrical	Gastroenterology/Urology
Table, Urological, Radiographic	Gastroenterology/Urology

MEDRO SYSTEMS, INC.
972-542-8200
416 E. Industrial Blvd., McKinney, TX 75069-7323
FDA Number: 1641306   *Fax:* 972-542-8220
E-mail: joanstivers@medrosystems.com
Web site: www.medrosystems.com
Medical Products Sales Volume: $1,000,000
Annual Revenue: $1-$5 Million
Year Founded: 1975
Total Employees: 6   *Sales Staff:* 2
Ownership: Private
Produces/Sells CE-marked Devices: N
Federal Procurement Eligibility: Small Business
Distribution: Manufacturer Direct, Manufacturer Through Manufacturer Reps, OEM
General Admin.: Lewis E. Stivers/President, Chief Executive Officer
    Joan Stivers/Vice President, Corporate Secretary

Demineralizer	Chemistry
Purification Filter, Water, Charcoal	Chemistry
Purification Filter, Water, Particulate	Chemistry
Purification System, Water	Gastroenterology/Urology
Purification System, Water, Reverse Osmosis	Chemistry

MEDRON, INC.
801-974-3010
1518 S. Gladiola St., Salt Lake City, UT 84104
FDA Number: 1722746   *Fax:* 801-974-3063
E-mail: medron@medroninc.com
Web site: http://www.medroninc.com/
Annual Revenue: $1-$5 Million
Year Founded: 1994
Total Employees: 35   *Marketing Staff:* 2   *Sales Staff:* 1
Ownership: Private
Quality System Registration Information: ISO9002
Produces/Sells CE-marked Devices: N
Distribution: OEM
General Admin.: Ron Wortley/President, Chief Executive Officer
Mktg./Adv.: Eric King/Director Product Development
Production: Dave Wortley/Vice President Manufacturing

Catheter, Femoral	Gastroenterology/Urology
Kit, Administration, Intravenous	General

MEDRX, INC.
727-584-9600
1200 Starkey Rd., #105, Largo, FL 33771
FDA Number: 1058264

Audiometer	Ear/Nose/Throat
Otoscope	Ear/Nose/Throat

MEDSCI, INC.
336-274-3496
201 Pine St., Greensboro, NC 27401
FDA Number: 1066018
Ownership: Private
Produces/Sells CE-marked Devices: N

Sterilant, Medical Device	General

MEDSEP CORP., A SUBSIDIARY OF PALL CORP. 516-484-5400
1630 Industrial Park St., Covina, CA 91722
FDA Number: 2013342
Ownership: PALL CORPORATION
Stock Symbol: PLL
Traded On: NYSE
Produces/Sells CE-marked Devices: N

Bag, Blood, Collection	Hematology
Cover, Barrier, Protective	General
Microfilter, Blood Transfusion	Anesthesiology
System, Detection, Bacterial, For Platelet Transfusion Products	Immunology
Transfer Unit, Blood	Hematology

MEDSERV BIOLOGICALS, LLC 631-757-8401
1019 Fort Salonga Rd., Suite 109, Northport, NY 11768
FDA Number: 3003449393

Software, Blood Bank (Stand-Alone Products)	Hematology

MEDSHAPE SOLUTIONS INC. 877-343-7016
1575 Northside Drive, Suite 440, 404-249-9155
Atlanta, GA 30318
FDA Number: 3007593722 Fax: 404-249-9158
E-mail: info@medshape.com
Web site: http://www.medshape.com
Ownership: Private
Produces/Sells CE-marked Devices: N
General Admin.: Dr. Kenneth Gall/Chief Technology Officer
Mr. J. Kurt Jacobus/President, Chief Executive Officer, Chairman

Fastener, Fixation, Non-Biodegradable, Soft Tissue	Orthopedics
Screw, Fixation, Bone	Orthopedics
Suture, Non-Absorbable, Synthetic, Polyethylene	Surgery

MEDSIM-EAGLE SIMULATION INC. 607-779-6000
151 Court St., Binghamton, NY 13901
FDA Number: n/a Fax: 607-779-6049
E-mail: marketing@eaglesim.com
Web site: www.eaglesim.com
Medical Products Sales Volume: $10,000,000
Annual Revenue: $5-$10 Million
Total Employees: 50 Marketing Staff: 2 Sales Staff: 5
Ownership: Private
Federal Procurement Eligibility: Small Business
Distribution: Manufacturer Direct, Manufacturer Through Distributor, Manufacturer Through Manufacturer Reps
General Admin.: Christopher Paulsen/President
Nimrod Goor/President, Chief Executive Officer
Mktg./Adv.: Christopher Paulsen/Director Marketing & Sales
Charles Dispenza/Manager Marketing & Sales
John Archbold/Manager Marketing & Sales

Anatomical Training Model	General
Training Aid	Orthopedics
Training Manikin, Other	General

MEDSONIC U.S.A., INC. 716-565-1700
8865 Sheridan Drive, Clarence, NY 14031-2002
FDA Number: 1319309 Fax: 716-565-1559
Annual Revenue: $0-$1 Million
Ownership: Private
Federal Procurement Eligibility: Small Business
Distribution: Manufacturer Direct, Manufacturer Through Manufacturer Reps, Exporter
General Admin.: Don Trainer/President

Compressor, Air, Portable	Anesthesiology
Meter, Ultrasonic Power	General
Nebulizer, Ultrasonic	Anesthesiology
Regulator, Intake, Oxygen	Anesthesiology

MEDSONIC, INC.
See Misonix, Inc.

MEDSONIX 702-873-3700
2626 S. Rainbow Blvd., Suite 109, Las Vegas, NV 89146
FDA Number: 3004573517

Massager, Therapeutic	Physical Med

MEDSPHERE INTERNATIONAL, INC 510-656-8232
48531 Warm Springs Blvd., Suite 417, Fremont, CA 94539
FDA Number: n/a
Ownership: Private
Produces/Sells CE-marked Devices: N

Electrosurgical Unit, Cutting & Coagulation Device	Surgery

MEDSPRING GROUP, INC. 801-295-9750
533 West 2600 South, Suite 105, Bountiful, UT 84010
FDA Number: 1724377
Ownership: Private
Produces/Sells CE-marked Devices: N

Bandage, Adhesive	Surgery
Gauze/sponge, Nonresorbable For External Use	Surgery
Glove, Patient Examination	General

MEDSPRING GROUP, INC. 801-295-9750 (cont'd)

Light, Examination, Battery-Powered	General
Mask, Surgical	Surgery
Protectant, Skin	Surgery
Sponge, Gauze	Dental And Oral

MEDSTAT INC. 901-452-5697
3251 Poplar Ave., Memphis, TN 38111
FDA Number: n/a
Medical Products Sales Volume: $2,500,000
Annual Revenue: $1-$5 Million
Ownership: Medstat Inc.
Produces/Sells CE-marked Devices: Y
Federal Procurement Eligibility: Small Business
Distribution: Manufacturer Direct, Exporter

Brace, Joint, Ankle (External)	Physical Med
Orthosis, Other	Physical Med

Medical Product Subsidiaries (Listed Separately)
Medstat Inc.

MEDSTONE INTERNATIONAL, INC. 949-367-1238
229 Arnold Mill Rd., Suite 200, Woodstock, GA 30188
FDA Number: 3004968068
Ownership: Private
Produces/Sells CE-marked Devices: N

Table, Radiographic, Tilting	Radiology

MEDSTRAT, INC. 800-882-4224
1901 Butterfield Rd., Suite 600, 630-960-8700
Downers Grove, IL 60515
FDA Number: 3003574171 Fax: 630-960-9787
E-mail: sales@medstrat.com
Web site: www.medstrat.com
Ownership: Private
Produces/Sells CE-marked Devices: N

Device, Storage, Image, Digital	Radiology
System, Communication, Image, Digital	Radiology

MEDTEC 800-445-6741
102 First Street South, Kalona, IA 52247 319-656-4447
FDA Number: 1932738 Fax: 319-656-4451
E-mail: int@civco.com
Web site: www.medtec.com
Annual Revenue: $25-$50 Million
Year Founded: 1983
Total Employees: 84 Marketing Staff: 4 Sales Staff: 18
Ownership: Private
Quality System Registration Information: ISO9001
Produces/Sells CE-marked Devices: Y
Federal Procurement Eligibility: Small Business
Distribution: Manufacturer Direct, Manufacturer Through Distributor, OEM, Service Direct, Exclusive Distributor, Importer, Exporter
General Admin.: Bryan Kooi/Director Human Resources
Dave Van Gorp/President, Chief Executive Officer, Director
Mktg./Adv.: Kim Einerwold/Manager International Sales
Patrick Dammekens/Manager International Sales
Stephanie Jurgens/Manager Marketing
Larry Schmitzer/Manager National Sales
Production: John Milroy/Director Quality Assurance
Ren Eide/Manager Materials
Don Riibe/Manager Regulatory Affairs

Accelerator, Linear, Medical	Radiology
Couch, Radiation Therapy, Powered	Radiology
Holder, Head, Radiographic	Radiology
Phantom, Anthropomorphic, Radiographic	Radiology
Table, Mechanical	Physical Med
Table, Radiographic	Radiology

MEDTEC AMBULANCE CORP. 866-263-3832
2429 Lincoln Way East, Goshen, IN 46526 574-534-2631
FDA Number: 9201045 Fax: 574-534-3629
E-mail: salesmed@medtecambulance.com
Web site: www.medtecambulance.com
Medical Products Sales Volume: $21,500,000
Annual Revenue: $25-$50 Million
Year Founded: 1974
Total Employees: 120 Marketing Staff: 9 Sales Staff: 9
Ownership: Private
Produces/Sells CE-marked Devices: N
Federal Procurement Eligibility: Small Business
Distribution: Manufacturer Through Distributor
General Admin.: Tim McDonald/General Manager
Jean Allen/Manager Human Resources
Mktg./Adv.: Kevin Noble/Assistant Manager Sales
Denny Neff/Manager Sales
Production: David Hill/Director Operations

MEDTEC AMBULANCE CORP.   866-263-3832 *(cont'd)*
Finance: Ross Munn/Director Finance
Ambulance   General

MEDTEC APPLICATIONS, INC.   630-628-0444
50 West Fay Ave., Addison, IL 60101
FDA Number: 1483278
Arthroscope   Orthopedics
Catheter, Aspiration   Surgery
Insufflator, Laparoscopic   Obstetrics/Gynecology
Laparoscope, General & Plastic Surgery   Surgery
Laparoscope, Gynecologic   Obstetrics/Gynecology
Light Source, Endoscope, Xenon Arc   Surgery

MEDTEC, INC.   919-241-1400
600 Meadowland Drive, Hillsborough, NC 27278
FDA Number: 1062273   Fax: 919-241-1420
E-mail: info@medtecbiolab.com
Web site: www.medtecbiolab.com
Year Founded: 1994
Total Employees: 21   *Marketing Staff:* 2
Ownership: Private
Produces/Sells CE-marked Devices: Y
Distribution: Manufacturer Direct, OEM
General Admin.: Mr. Eric Paul/Chief Executive Officer
Microplate   General
Reader, Microplate   General
Stainer, Slide, Automated   Pathology

MEDTECH
See Buffalo Filter, A Division Of Medtek Devices Inc.

MEDTECH GROUP INC., THE   800-348-2759
6 Century Road, South Plainfield, NJ 07080   908-561-0717
FDA Number: 2244012   Fax: 908-561-3811
E-mail: info@medtech-grp.com
Web site: www.medtech-grp.com
Medical Products Sales Volume: $27,900,000
Year Founded: 1979
Total Employees: 170   *Sales Staff:* 7
Ownership: Private
Quality System Registration Information: ISO9002
Produces/Sells CE-marked Devices: N
Federal Procurement Eligibility: Small Business
Distribution: Manufacturer Direct, OEM
General Admin.: Mr. Dan Croteau/Chief Executive Officer
   George W. Blank/President
   Edwin P. Murray/Vice President Admin.
   John Pfaff/Vice President, General Manager
Mktg./Adv.: Ms. Harriet Blank/Admin. Marketing & Sales
   Gil Reich/Vice President Marketing & Sales
Production: Mary Aldridge/Director Quality Assurance
Cannula, Injection   Gastroenterology/Urology
Contract Manufacturing, Product, Disposable   General
Molding, Custom   General
Molding, Injection   General
Packaging, Sterilization   General
Service, Engineering/Design   General
Syringe, Other   General

MEDTECH SYSTEMS   903-504-5001
221 Pine St., Florence, MA 01062
FDA Number: n/a   Fax: 866-350-8015
E-mail: info@medtechsystems.com
Web site: info@medtechsystems.com
Total Employees: 4   *Marketing Staff:* 2   *Sales Staff:* 2
Ownership: Private
Produces/Sells CE-marked Devices: N
Federal Procurement Eligibility: Small Business
Distribution: Manufacturer Through Distributor
General Admin.: Dan Cherry/President, Chief Executive Officer
Mktg./Adv.: Barry Charland/Manager Advertising
   Barry Charland/Vice President Marketing & Sales
Applier, Cast   Orthopedics

MEDTEK DEVICES, INC.   716-835-7000
595 Commerce Dr., 155 Pineview Dr., Amherst, NY 14228
FDA Number: 1319774
Bottle, Collection, Vacuum (Aspirator)   General
Exhaust System, Surgical   Surgery
Laser, Surgical   Surgery
Mask, Surgical   Surgery
Regulator, Vacuum   General
Tubing, Non-Invasive   Surgery

MEDTEK DEVICES, INC.
See Buffalo Filter, A Division Of Medtek Devices Inc.

MEDTEK INC.
See St. Jude Medical Neuromodulation Division

MEDTOX DIAGNOSTICS INC.   800-334-1116
1238 Anthony Rd., Burlington, NC 27215-8831   336-226-6311
FDA Number: 1050155   Fax: 336-229-4471
E-mail: sales@medtox.com
Web site: www.medtox.com
Medical Products Sales Volume: $4,000,000
Annual Revenue: $1-$5 Million
Total Employees: 300
Ownership: Medtox Scientific Inc.
Produces/Sells CE-marked Devices: N
Distribution: Manufacturer Direct, Manufacturer Through Manufacturer Reps
General Admin.: Harry McCoy/President
Production: Mitch Owens/Vice President Operations
Finance: Peter Heath/Chief Financial Officer, Vice President Finance
Enzyme Immunoassay, Amphetamine   Toxicology
Enzyme Immunoassay, Barbiturate   Toxicology
Enzyme Immunoassay, Cannabinoids   Toxicology
Enzyme Immunoassay, Cocaine   Toxicology
Enzyme Immunoassay, Cocaine And Cocaine Metabolites   Toxicology
Enzyme Immunoassay, Opiates   Toxicology
Enzyme Immunoassay, Phencyclidine   Toxicology
Gas Chromatography, Cocaine   Toxicology
Gas Chromatography, Opiates   Toxicology
Radioimmunoassay, Tricyclic Antidepressant Drugs   Toxicology
Test, Tetrahydrocannabinol   Toxicology
Thin Layer Chromatography, Metamphetamine   Toxicology

MEDTOX DIAGNOSTICS, INC.   800-334-1116
1640 Nova Lane, Burlington, NC 27215
FDA Number: 3004175381
Web site: www.medtox.com
Ownership: Medtox Scientific Inc.
Produces/Sells CE-marked Devices: N
Colorimeter, General Use   Chemistry
Enzyme Immunoassay, Amphetamine   Toxicology
Enzyme Immunoassay, Barbiturate   Toxicology
Enzyme Immunoassay, Benzodiazepine   Toxicology
Enzyme Immunoassay, Cocaine And Cocaine Metabolites   Toxicology
Enzyme Immunoassay, Methadone   Toxicology
Enzyme Immunoassay, Opiates   Toxicology
Enzyme Immunoassay, Phencyclidine   Toxicology
Enzyme Immunoassay, Propoxyphene   Toxicology
Radioimmunoassay, Tricyclic Antidepressant Drugs   Toxicology
Test, Tetrahydrocannabinol   Toxicology
Thin Layer Chromatography, Metamphetamine   Toxicology

MEDTOX SCIENTIFIC INC.   800-832-3244
402 West County Road D, St. Paul, MN 55112   651-636-7466
FDA Number: n/a
E-mail: clientservices@medtox.com
Web site: www.medtox.com
Annual Revenue: $50-$100 Million
Year Founded: 1984
Total Employees: 523
Ownership: Public
Stock Symbol: MTOX
Traded On: NASDAQ
Produces/Sells CE-marked Devices: N
General Admin.: Kevin J. Wiersma/Chief Financial Officer, Vice President
   B. Mitchell Owens/Chief Operating Officer, Vice President
   Richard J. Braun/President, Chief Executive Officer
   Susan E. Puskas/Vice President
Mktg./Adv.: James A. Schoonover/Vice President Sales
Medical Product Subsidiaries (Listed Separately)
Medtox Diagnostics Inc.
Medtox Diagnostics, Inc.

MEDTROL, INC.   1-800-647-7180
7157 N. Austin, Niles, IL 60714
FDA Number: n/a   Fax: 1-800-255-3027
E-mail: sales@medtrol.com
Web site: www.medtrol.com
Annual Revenue: $1-$5 Million
Total Employees: 30   *Marketing Staff:* 4   *Sales Staff:* 4
Ownership: Private
Produces/Sells CE-marked Devices: N
Federal Procurement Eligibility: Small Business
Distribution: Manufacturer Direct, Manufacturer Through Distributor, Manufacturer Through Manufacturer Reps
General Admin.: Jospeh G. Martorano/President
Mktg./Adv.: Ray Gorgzynski/Vice President Sales
Production: Jan Gorzynski/Manager Customer Services
   Paul W. Stiffler/Manager Regulatory Affairs
Bag, Laundry, Infection Control   General
Disinfector, Medical Device   General
Glove, Patient Examination   General
Glove, Patient Examination, Vinyl   General
Mask, Surgical   Surgery

MEDTROL, INC.   1-800-647-7180 *(cont'd)*
Wipe, Instrument   General

MEDTROL, INC.   847-647-6555
7157 North Austin, Niles, IL 60714
FDA Number: 1424233
Glove, Patient Examination, Vinyl   General

MEDTRONIC
See Avalon Laboratories, Inc.

MEDTRONIC BLOOD MANAGEMENT   612-514-4000
18501 East Plaza Dr., Parker, CO 80134
FDA Number: 1718389
Web site: www.medtronic.com
Ownership: Medtronic, Inc.
Stock Symbol: MDT
Traded On: NYSE
Produces/Sells CE-marked Devices: N

Activated Whole Blood Clotting Time	Hematology
Analyzer, Heparin, Automated	Hematology
Autotransfusion Unit (Blood)	Anesthesiology
Bag, Blood, Collection	Hematology
Catheter, Urethral	Gastroenterology/Urology
Catheter, Vascular, Cardiopulmonary Bypass	Cardiovascular
Collector, Urine	Gastroenterology/Urology
Control, Coagulation, Plasma	Hematology
Filter, Blood, Cardiopulmonary Bypass, Arterial Line	Cardiovascular
Heat Exchanger, Heart-Lung Bypass	Cardiovascular
Protamine Sulphate	Hematology
Reservoir, Blood, Cardiopulmonary Bypass	Cardiovascular
Stethoscope, Electronic (Auscultoscope)	Cardiovascular
Sucker, Cardiotomy Return, Cardiopulmonary Bypass	Cardiovascular
Thermometer, Electronic	General
Thermometer, Electronic, Continuous	General
Tourniquet, Pneumatic	Surgery
Transducer, Miniature Pressure	Physical Med
Trocar, Cardiovascular	Cardiovascular
Tube, Pump, Cardiopulmonary Bypass	Cardiovascular
Tubing, Non-Invasive	Surgery

MEDTRONIC BLOOD MANAGEMENT
See Medtronic Perfusion Systems

MEDTRONIC CARDIAC SURGERY TECHNOLOGIES   877-526-7890
8200 coral sea street, moundsview, MN 55112   763-391-9030
FDA Number: 2135394
Web site: www.medtronic.com
Ownership: Medtronic, Inc.
Stock Symbol: MDT
Traded On: NYSE
Produces/Sells CE-marked Devices: N

Electrode, Pacemaker, Temporary	Cardiovascular
Electrosurgical Unit, Cutting & Coagulation Device	Surgery
Holder, Heart Valve Prosthesis	Cardiovascular
Laparoscope, General & Plastic Surgery	Surgery
Sizer, Heart Valve Prosthesis	Cardiovascular
Valve, Heart, Mechanical	Cardiovascular

MEDTRONIC CARDIAC SURGICAL PRODUCTS
See Atek Medical

MEDTRONIC CARDIOVASCULAR SURGERY, THE HEART VALVE DIV.   800-328-2518
1851 East Deere Ave., Santa Ana, CA 92705
FDA Number: 2025587
Web site: www.medtronic.com
Annual Revenue: More than $1 Billion
Ownership: Medtronic, Inc.
Stock Symbol: MDT
Traded On: NYSE
Produces/Sells CE-marked Devices: N

Circulatory Assist Unit, Left Ventricular	Cardiovascular
Conduit, Valved, Pulmonic	Cardiovascular
Holder, Heart Valve Prosthesis	Cardiovascular
Patch, Pericardial	Cardiovascular
Prosthesis, Cardiac Valve, Biological	Cardiovascular
Ring, Annuloplasty	Cardiovascular
Sizer, Heart Valve Prosthesis	Cardiovascular
Surgical Instrument, Cardiovascular	Cardiovascular
Trocar, Cardiovascular	Cardiovascular
Valve, Heart, Tissue	Cardiovascular

MEDTRONIC DLP   616-643-5200
620 Watson St., S.W., Grand Rapids, MI 49504-6450
FDA Number: 1833441   *Fax:* 616-643-1017
Annual Revenue: $1-$5 Million
Total Employees: 11
Ownership: Public
Stock Symbol: MDT

MEDTRONIC DLP   616-643-5200 *(cont'd)*
Traded On: NYSE
Produces/Sells CE-marked Devices: N

Adapter, Stopcock, Manifold, Cardiopulmonary Bypass	Cardiovascular
Cannula, Surgical, General & Plastic Surgery	Surgery
Catheter, Vascular, Cardiopulmonary Bypass	Cardiovascular
Contract Sterilization	General

MEDTRONIC ELECTROMEDICS HEMOTEC, INC.
See Medtronic Perfusion Systems

MEDTRONIC EP SYSTEMS   763-514-4000
Spring Lake Park, 8299 Central Ave. Ne, Minneapolis, MN 55432
FDA Number: 2183572
Ownership: Private
Produces/Sells CE-marked Devices: N

Bandage, Adhesive	Surgery
Bandage, Liquid	Surgery
Catheter, Electrode Recording, Or Probe	Cardiovascular
Catheter, Percutaneous	Cardiovascular
Computer, Diagnostic, Programmable	Cardiovascular
Electrode, Ablation, Tissue, Conduction, Percutaneous	Cardiovascular
Holder, Intravascular Catheter	General

MEDTRONIC HEART VALVES   800-227-3191
8299 Central Ave., N.e., Spring Lake Park, MN 55432-3576
FDA Number: 2127690
Web site: http://www.medtronic.com
Ownership: MEDTRONIC, INC.
Produces/Sells CE-marked Devices: N

Cautery, Thermal, Battery-Powered	Ophthalmology
Circulatory Assist Unit, Left Ventricular	Cardiovascular
Electrode, Pacemaker, Temporary	Cardiovascular
Holder, Heart Valve Prosthesis	Cardiovascular
Patch, Pericardial	Cardiovascular
Prosthesis, Cardiac Valve, Biological	Cardiovascular
Ring, Annuloplasty	Cardiovascular
Sizer, Heart Valve Prosthesis	Cardiovascular
Surgical Instrument, Cardiovascular	Cardiovascular
Trocar, Cardiovascular	Cardiovascular

MEDTRONIC IMAGE-GUIDED NEUROLOGICS, INC.   800-707-0933
2290 West Eau Gallie Blvd., Melbourne, FL 32935   763-505-0604
FDA Number: 1064128
Web site: www.igneurologics.com
Ownership: Medtronic, Inc.
Stock Symbol: MDT
Traded On: NYSE
Produces/Sells CE-marked Devices: N

Catheter, Ventricular	Cns/Neurology
Cover, Burr Hole (Cranial)	Cns/Neurology
Holder, Head, Neurosurgical (Skull Clamp)	Cns/Neurology
Motor, Drill, Pneumatic	Cns/Neurology
Nuclear Magnetic Resonance Imaging System	Radiology
Screwdriver, Skullplate	Cns/Neurology
Stereotaxy Equipment	Cns/Neurology

MEDTRONIC INC, PACEART   763-514-4000
4265 Lexington Avenue North, Arden Hills, MN 55126
FDA Number: 2246356
Ownership: Private
Produces/Sells CE-marked Devices: N

Analyzer, Pacemaker Generator Function, Indirect	Cardiovascular
Electrode, Electrocardiograph	Cardiovascular
Transmitter/Receiver System, Physiological, Telephone	Cardiovascular

MEDTRONIC INC., BRADYCARDIA DIV.
See Medtronic, Inc.

MEDTRONIC MINIMED   800-933-3322
18000 Devonshire, Northridge, CA 91325   818-362-5958
FDA Number: 2032227   *Fax:* 818-576-6534
Web site: www.minimed.com
Year Founded: 1983
Total Employees: 2000   *Marketing Staff:* 15   *Sales Staff:* 80
Ownership: Medtronic, Inc.
Quality System Registration Information: ISO9001
Produces/Sells CE-marked Devices: Y
Federal Procurement Eligibility: Small Business
Distribution: Manufacturer Direct

Accessories, Pump, Infusion	General
Catheter, Infusion	Surgery
Infusion Pump, Insulin	General
Introducer, Syringe Needle	General
Kit, Administration, Intravenous	General
Kit, Intravenous Extension Tubing	General
Pump, Infusion	General

MANUFACTURER PROFILES

MEDTRONIC MINIMED
800-933-3322 *(cont'd)*

Sensor, Glucose, Invasive	General
Set, Administration, Intravenous, Needle-Free	General
Syringe, Piston	General
System, Test, Blood Glucose, Over-The-Counter	Chemistry
Tubing, Fluid Delivery	General
Warmer, Infusion Fluid, Thermal	General

MEDTRONIC NAVIGATION, INC.
888-580-8860
826 Coal Creek Cir., Louisville, CO 80027 **720-890-3200**
FDA Number: 1723170 Fax: 720-890-3500
E-mail: rs.navceiregistrar@medtronic.com
Web site: www.medtronicnavigation.com
Ownership: Medtronic, Inc.
Stock Symbol: MDT
Traded On: NYSE
Produces/Sells CE-marked Devices: N
General Admin.: Mr. Jim Cloar/Vice President, General Manager

Infusion Stand	General
Stereotaxy Equipment	Cns/Neurology
Wrap, Sterilization	General

MEDTRONIC NAVIGATION, INC. (LITTLETON)
720-890-3325
300 Foster Street, Harwood Station, Littleton, MA 01460
FDA Number: 3004785967
Web site: www.medtronicnavigation.com
Ownership: Medtronic, Inc.
Stock Symbol: MDT
Traded On: NYSE
Produces/Sells CE-marked Devices: N

System, Planning, Radiation Therapy Treatment	Radiology
System, X-Ray, Mobile	Radiology

MEDTRONIC NEUROLOGICAL
See Medtronic Neuromodulation

MEDTRONIC NEUROMODULATION
1-800-633-8766
710 Medtronic Parkway, **763) 514-4000**
Minneapolis, MN 55432
FDA Number: 2182207
Web site: www.medtronic.com Fax: (763) 514-4879
Ownership: Medtronic, Inc.
Stock Symbol: MDT
Traded On: NYSE
Produces/Sells CE-marked Devices: N

Pump, Infusion, Implantable, General	General
Stimulator, Electrical, Implanted (Parkinsonian Tremor)	Cns/Neurology
Stimulator, Peripheral Nerve, Implantable (Pain Relief)	Cns/Neurology
Stimulator, Sacral Nerve, Implanted	Cns/Neurology
Stimulator, Spinal Cord, Implantable (Pain Relief)	Cns/Neurology

MEDTRONIC NEUROMODULATION
800-633-8766
710 Medtronic Parkway NE, **763-514-4000**
Minneapolis, MN 55459
FDA Number: 2950887
Web site: www.medtronic.com Fax: 763-505-0130
Ownership: MEDTRONIC, INC.
Produces/Sells CE-marked Devices: N
General Admin.: Mr. Jean-Luc Butel/President
Mr. William A. Hawkins/President, Chief Executive Officer

Analyzer, Motility, Gastrointestinal, Electrical	Gastroenterology/Urology
Cable, Electrode	Physical Med
Cystometric Gas (Carbon-Dioxide) Or Hydraulic Device	Gastroenterology/Urology
Device, Cystometric, Hydraulic	Gastroenterology/Urology
Device, Measurement, Velocity, Conduction, Nerve	Cns/Neurology
Electrode, Cutaneous	Cns/Neurology
Electrode, Needle	Cns/Neurology
Electrode, Needle, Diagnostic Electromyograph	Physical Med
Electrode, pH	Gastroenterology/Urology
Electrosurgical Unit, Cutting & Coagulation Device	Surgery
Electrosurgical, Unit, Gastroenterology	Gastroenterology/Urology
Endoscope	Gastroenterology/Urology
Monitor, Esophageal Motility, And Tube	Gastroenterology/Urology
Monitor, Ventilatory Frequency	Anesthesiology
Recorder, External, Pressure, Amplifier & Transducer	Gastroenterology/Urology
Spirometer, Diagnostic (Respirometer)	Anesthesiology
System, Electrogastrography(egg)	Gastroenterology/Urology
Uroflowmeter	Gastroenterology/Urology

MEDTRONIC NEUROSURGERY
800-468-9710
125 Cremona Dr.,, Goleta, CA 93117
FDA Number: 2021898
Web site: www.medtronic.com/neurosurgery Fax: 800-468-9713
Ownership: Medtronic, Inc.
Stock Symbol: MDT
Traded On: NYSE
Produces/Sells CE-marked Devices: N

Catheter, Intraspinal, Percutaneous, Short-Term	General
Catheter, Intravascular, Therapeutic, Long-term Greater Than 30 Days	General
Catheter, Subcutaneous Intravascular, Implanted	General

MEDTRONIC NEUROSURGERY
800-468-9710 *(cont'd)*

Catheter, Ventricular	Cns/Neurology
Clip, Implantable	Surgery
Clip, Scalp	Cns/Neurology
Cover, Burr Hole (Cranial)	Cns/Neurology
Drill, Manual (With Burr, Trephine & Accessories)	Cns/Neurology
Dura-Substitute	Cns/Neurology
Electrosurgical Unit, Cutting & Coagulation Device	Surgery
Endoscope, Neurological	Cns/Neurology
Instrument, Implantation, Shunt	Cns/Neurology
Mesh, Metal	Gastroenterology/Urology
Mesh, Surgical (Steel Gauze)	Surgery
Monitor, Intracranial Pressure	Cns/Neurology
Monitor, Intracranial Pressure, Continuous	Cns/Neurology
Plate, Bone, Skull, Preformed, Alterable	Cns/Neurology
Shunt, Central Nerve, With Component	Cns/Neurology

MEDTRONIC NORTECH DIV.
See Empi, Inc.

MEDTRONIC OF CANADA LTD.
800-268-5346
6733 Kitimat Rd., **905-826-6020**
Mississauga, ON L5N 1 Canada
FDA Number: n/a Fax: 905-826-6620
Year Founded: 1968
Total Employees: 95
Ownership: Public
Stock Symbol: MDT
Traded On: NYSE
Produces/Sells CE-marked Devices: N
Distribution: Exclusive Distributor, Importer

MEDTRONIC PERFUSION SYSTEM
See Medtronic Perfusion Systems

MEDTRONIC PERFUSION SYSTEMS
1-800-633-8766
710 Medtronic Parkway, Mail Stop: L100, **(763) 514-4000**
Minneapolis, MN 55432
FDA Number: 2184009
Web site: www.medtronic.com Fax: (763) 514-4879
Medical Products Sales Volume: $39,000,000
Annual Revenue: $25-$50 Million
Total Employees: 500
Ownership: Public
Stock Symbol: MDT
Traded On: NYSE
Quality System Registration Information: ISO9002
Produces/Sells CE-marked Devices: Y
Distribution: Manufacturer Through Distributor, Manufacturer Through Manufacturer Reps
General Admin.: Michelle Light/Director Human Resources
Mktg./Adv.: Dick Reid/Director Media
John Keaveny/Director National Sales
John Rivera/Manager International & National Sales

Adapter, Stopcock, Manifold, Cardiopulmonary Bypass	Cardiovascular
Analyzer, Coagulation, Automated	Hematology
Analyzer, Heparin, Automated	Hematology
Autotransfusion Unit (Blood)	Anesthesiology
Bag, Reservoir (Blood)	Anesthesiology
Bleeding Time Device	Hematology
Catheter, Electrode Recording, Or Probe	Cardiovascular
Catheter, Percutaneous	Cardiovascular
Catheter, Steerable	Cardiovascular
Device, Hemostasis, Vascular	Cardiovascular
Dilator, Vessel	Gastroenterology/Urology
Equipment, Apheresis	Hematology
Filter, Blood, Cardiopulmonary Bypass, Arterial Line	Cardiovascular
Heat Exchanger, Heart-Lung Bypass	Cardiovascular
Kit, Administration, Cardioplegia Solution	Cardiovascular
Kit, Wound Drainage	General
Monitor, Temperature (With Probe)	Anesthesiology
Occluder, Catheter Tip	Cardiovascular
Oxygenator, Cardiopulmonary Bypass	Cardiovascular
Probe, Blood Flow, Extravascular	Cardiovascular
Probe, Temperature	General
Reservoir, Blood, Cardiopulmonary Bypass	Cardiovascular
Sensor, Blood Gas, In-Line, Cardiopulmonary Bypass	Cardiovascular
Sucker, Cardiotomy Return, Cardiopulmonary Bypass	Cardiovascular
Tourniquet, Air Pressure	Orthopedics

MEDTRONIC PERFUSION SYSTEMS
800-854-3570
7611 Northland Dr., Brooklyn Park, MN 55428 **763-391-9000**
FDA Number: 2184009 Fax: 763-391-9100
Web site: www.perfusionsystems.com
Annual Revenue: $1-$5 Million
Ownership: Medtronic, Inc.
Stock Symbol: MXR
Traded On: NYSE
Quality System Registration Information: ISO9001
Produces/Sells CE-marked Devices: Y

MEDTRONIC PERFUSION SYSTEMS   800-854-3570 *(cont'd)*

Distribution: Manufacturer Direct, Manufacturer Through Manufacturer Reps
General Admin.: Anthony Badolato/Chief Executive Officer
               Gregory Melsen/Chief Financial Officer, Vice President
               Glenn Taylor/President, Chief Operating Officer
Mktg./Adv.: Al Seck/Vice President Marketing
Research: Bill Haworth/Vice President Research & Development

Accessories, Cardiopulmonary Bypass	Cardiovascular
Adapter, Stopcock, Manifold, Cardiopulmonary Bypass	Cardiovascular
Filter, Pre-Bypass, Cardiopulmonary Bypass	Cardiovascular
Heat Exchanger, Heart-Lung Bypass	Cardiovascular
Lung, Membrane (For Long-Term Respiratory Support)	Anesthesiology
Oxygenator, Cardiopulmonary Bypass	Cardiovascular
Reservoir, Blood, Cardiopulmonary Bypass	Cardiovascular
Tube, Pump, Cardiopulmonary Bypass	Cardiovascular

MEDTRONIC PHYSIO-CONTROL

See Physio-Control, Inc.

MEDTRONIC POWERED SURGICAL SOLUTIONS   800-643-2773

4620 North Beach St., Fort Worth, TX 76137   **817-788-6400**
FDA Number: 1625507   *Fax:* 817-788-6489
E-mail: midasrexinstitute@medtronic.com
Web site: www.medtronic.com/neuro/midasrex
Ownership: Medtronic, Inc.
Stock Symbol: MDT
Traded On: NYSE
Produces/Sells CE-marked Devices: N

Accessories, Powered Drill	Cns/Neurology
Blade, Saw, Surgical, Cardiovascular	Cardiovascular
Burr	Ear/Nose/Throat
Burr, Surgical, General & Plastic Surgery	Surgery
Drill, Surgical, ENT (Electric Or Pneumatic)	Ear/Nose/Throat
Instrument, Surgical, Powered, Pneumatic	Orthopedics
Motor, Drill, Electric	Cns/Neurology
Motor, Drill, Pneumatic	Cns/Neurology
Motor, Surgical Instrument, AC-Powered	Surgery
Motor, Surgical Instrument, Pneumatic-Powered	Surgery
Saw, Pneumatically Powered	Surgery
Surgical Instrument, Orthopedic, Battery-Powered	Surgery

MEDTRONIC PUERTO RICO OPERATIONS   763-514-4000
CO., JUNCOS

Road 31, Km. 24, Hm 4, Ceiba Norte Industrial Park,
Juncos, PR 00777
FDA Number: 3004209178
Web site: www.medtronic.com
Ownership: Medtronic, Inc.
Stock Symbol: MDT
Traded On: NYSE
Produces/Sells CE-marked Devices: N

Defibrillator, Automatic Implantable Cardioverter, With Cardiac Resynchronization	
Cardiovascular	
Defibrillator, Implantable, Automatic	Cardiovascular
Dual Chamber, Implantable Pulse Generator	Cardiovascular
Infusion Pump, Insulin	General
Pacemaker, Heart, Implantable, Programmable	Cardiovascular
Pump, Infusion, Implantable, General	General
Recorder, Event, Implantable Cardiac, (without Arrhythmia Detection)	Cardiovascular
Stimulator, Cerebellar, Full Implant (Pain Relief)	Cns/Neurology
Stimulator, Electrical, For Incontinence	Gastroenterology/Urology
Stimulator, Intestinal	Gastroenterology/Urology
Stimulator, Spinal Cord, Implantable (Pain Relief)	Cns/Neurology

MEDTRONIC PUERTO RICO OPERATIONS CO.,   763-514-4000
VILLALBA

Rd. 149, Km. 56.3, Call Box 6001, Villalba, PR 00766
FDA Number: 2649622
Web site: www.medtronic.com
Ownership: Medtronic, Inc.
Stock Symbol: MDT
Traded On: NYSE
Produces/Sells CE-marked Devices: N

Catheter, Electrode Recording, Or Probe	Cardiovascular
Electrode, Ablation, Tissue, Conduction, Percutaneous	Cardiovascular
Electrosurgical Unit, Cutting & Coagulation Device	Surgery
Lead, Pacemaker, Implantable Myocardial	Cardiovascular
Stimulator, Cerebellar, Full Implant (Pain Relief)	Cns/Neurology
Stimulator, Electrical, Implanted (Parkinsonian Tremor)	Cns/Neurology
Stimulator, Peripheral Nerve, Implantable (Pain Relief)	Cns/Neurology
Stimulator, Spinal Cord, Implantable (Pain Relief)	Cns/Neurology

MEDTRONIC PUERTO RICO OPERATIONS   763-514-4000
CO.,MED REL

Road 909, Km. 0.4., Barrio Mariana, Humacao, PR 00792
FDA Number: 2647346
Web site: www.medtronic.com
Ownership: Medtronic, Inc.
Stock Symbol: MDT

MEDTRONIC PUERTO RICO OPERATIONS   763-514-4000 *(cont'd)*

Traded On: NYSE
Produces/Sells CE-marked Devices: N

Appliance, Fixation, Spinal Intervertebral Body	Orthopedics
Bit, Drill	Orthopedics
Catheter, Electrode Recording, Or Probe	Cardiovascular
Defibrillator, Implantable, Automatic	Cardiovascular
Dispenser, Cement	Orthopedics
Forceps	Orthopedics
Implant, Fixation Device, Proximal Femoral	Orthopedics
Implant, Fixation Device, Spinal	Orthopedics
Knife, Orthopedic	Orthopedics
Light, Surgical, Carrier	Surgery
Orthopedic Manual Surgical Instrument	Orthopedics
Orthosis, Spine, Plate, Laminoplasty, Metal	Orthopedics
Pacemaker, Heart, Implantable, Programmable	Cardiovascular
Plate, Bone, Orthodontic	Dental And Oral
Probe	Orthopedics
Stimulator, Electrical, Implanted (Parkinsonian Tremor)	Cns/Neurology
Stimulator, Peripheral Nerve, Implantable (Pain Relief)	Cns/Neurology
Stimulator, Spinal Cord, Implantable (Pain Relief)	Cns/Neurology
Stylet, Catheter	Cardiovascular

MEDTRONIC SOFAMOR DANEK

See Medtronic Sofamor Danek Usa, Inc

MEDTRONIC SOFAMOR DANEK CANADA   1-800-268-5346

99 Hereford Street,   **(905) 460-3800**
Brampton, ONT L6Y 0 Canada
FDA Number: n/a   *Fax:* (905) 826-6620
E-mail: lhardy@sofamordanek.ca
Web site: www.sofamordanek.com
Year Founded: 1996
Total Employees: 50
Ownership: Private
Produces/Sells CE-marked Devices: N
Distribution: Exclusive Distributor

MEDTRONIC SOFAMOR DANEK INSTRUMENT   901-396-3133
MANUFACTURING

7375 Adrianne Place, Bartlett, TN 38133
FDA Number: 3004564008
Web site: www.sofamordanek.com
Ownership: Medtronic, Inc.
Stock Symbol: MDT
Traded On: NYSE
Produces/Sells CE-marked Devices: N

Accessories, Arthroscopic	Orthopedics
Bit, Drill	Orthopedics
Chisel (Osteotome)	Surgery
Clamp, Bone	Orthopedics
Compression Instrument	Orthopedics
Countersink	Orthopedics
Crimper, Pin	Orthopedics
Curette	Orthopedics
Cutter, Orthopedic	Orthopedics
Cutter, Wire And Pin	Orthopedics
Electrosurgical Unit, Cutting & Coagulation Device	Surgery
Elevator, Orthopedic	Orthopedics
Extractor, Nail	Orthopedics
Forceps	Orthopedics
Gauge, Depth	Orthopedics
Guide, Surgical, Instrument	Surgery
Holder, Needle, Orthopedic	Orthopedics
Instrument, Bending (Contouring)	Orthopedics
Mallet, Bone	Orthopedics
Motor, Surgical Instrument, AC-Powered	Surgery
Orthopedic Manual Surgical Instrument	Orthopedics
Osteotome (Orthopedic)	Surgery
Pliers, Surgical	Orthopedics
Rasp, Bone	Orthopedics
Reamer	Orthopedics
Retractor, Surgical	Surgery
Rongeur, Rib	Orthopedics
Scissors, Orthopedic	Orthopedics
Screwdriver	Orthopedics
Surgical Instrument, Orthopedic, AC-Powered Motor	Orthopedics
Table, Surgical, Electrical	Surgery
Tamp	Orthopedics
Template	Orthopedics
Tray, Surgical Instrument	Surgery
Wrench	Orthopedics

MEDTRONIC SOFAMOR DANEK USA, INC   901-399-2346

1800 Pyramid Pl, Memphis, TN 38132
FDA Number: 1030489   *Fax:* 901-332-3920
E-mail: cathy.polk@medtronic.com
Web site: www.sofamordanek.com
Annual Revenue: $0-$1 Million
Total Employees: 250

MANUFACTURER PROFILES

MEDTRONIC SOFAMOR DANEK USA, INC 901-399-2346 *(cont'd)*
Ownership: Medtronic, Inc.
Stock Symbol: MDT
Traded On: NYSE
Produces/Sells CE-marked Devices: Y
Federal Procurement Eligibility: Small Business
Distribution: Manufacturer Direct
General Admin.: Gene Sponseller/Chief Executive Officer
Mktg./Adv.: Lori Brunson/Senior Manager Accounts

Equipment, Shaving, Disc, Spinal	Orthopedics
General Medical Device	General
Intervertebral Fusion Device With Bone Graft, Cervical	Orthopedics
Orthosis, Spine, Plate, Laminoplasty, Metal	Orthopedics

MEDTRONIC SOFAMOR DANEK USA, INC.   901-396-3133
4340 Swinnea Rd., Memphis, TN 38118
FDA Number: 3003120897
Web site: www.sofamordanek.com
Ownership: Medtronic, Inc.
Stock Symbol: MDT
Traded On: NYSE
Produces/Sells CE-marked Devices: N
Mktg./Adv.: Lori Brunson/Senior Manager Accounts

Accessories, Arthroscopic	Orthopedics
Agent, Hemostatic, Absorbable, Collagen-Based	Surgery
Appliance, Fixation, Spinal Interlaminal	Orthopedics
Appliance, Fixation, Spinal Intervertebral Body	Orthopedics
Awl	Orthopedics
Bender	Orthopedics
Bit, Drill	Orthopedics
Chisel (Osteotome)	Surgery
Clamp, Bone	Orthopedics
Compression Instrument	Orthopedics
Countersink	Orthopedics
Crimper, Pin	Orthopedics
Curette	Orthopedics
Cutter, Orthopedic	Orthopedics
Cutter, Wire And Pin	Orthopedics
Dispenser, Cement	Orthopedics
Electromyograph, Diagnostic	Physical Med
Electrosurgical Unit, Cutting & Coagulation Device	Surgery
Elevator, Orthopedic	Orthopedics
Extractor, Nail	Orthopedics
Filler, Bone Cement (for Vertebroplasty)	Orthopedics
Filler, Bone Void, Non-Osteoinduction	Physical Med
Filler, Calcium Sulfate Preformed Pellets	Orthopedics
Filler, Recombinant Human Bone Morphogenetic Protein, Collagen Scaffold With Metal	
Prosthesis, Osteoinduction	Orthopedics
Forceps	Orthopedics
Fork	Orthopedics
Gauge, Depth	Orthopedics
Guide, Surgical, Instrument	Surgery
Impactor	Orthopedics
Implant, Endosseous (Bone Filling and/or Augmentation)	Dental And Oral
Implant, Fixation Device, Proximal Femoral	Orthopedics
Instrument, Bending (Contouring)	Orthopedics
Instrument, Microsurgical	Cns/Neurology
Light, Surgical, Carrier	Surgery
Mallet, Bone	Orthopedics
Motor, Surgical Instrument, AC-Powered	Surgery
Orthopedic Manual Surgical Instrument	Orthopedics
Orthosis, Fixation, Spinal, Spondylolisthesis	Orthopedics
Orthosis, Fusion, Intervertebral, Spinal	Orthopedics
Orthosis, Spinal Pedicle Fixation, For Degenerative Disc Disease	Orthopedics
Orthosis, Spine, Plate, Laminoplasty, Metal	Orthopedics
Osteotome (Orthopedic)	Surgery
Plate, Bone, Orthodontic	Dental And Oral
Pliers, Surgical	Orthopedics
Prosthesis, Hip, Cement Restrictor	Orthopedics
Prosthesis, Hip, Femoral Component, Cemented, Metal	Orthopedics
Prosthesis, Hip, Semi-constrained, Metal/ceramic/polymer, Cemented Or Non-porous Cemented, Osteophilic Finish	Orthopedics
Prosthesis, Spine, Intervertebral Disc	Orthopedics
Pusher, Socket	Orthopedics
Rasp, Bone	Orthopedics
Reamer	Orthopedics
Retractor, Surgical	Surgery
Rongeur, Rib	Orthopedics
Scissors, Orthopedic	Orthopedics
Screw, Fixation, Bone	Orthopedics
Screwdriver	Orthopedics
Stimulator, Electrical, Evoked Response	Cns/Neurology
Stimulator, Nerve, ENT	Ear/Nose/Throat
Surgical Instrument, Orthopedic, AC-Powered Motor	Orthopedics
Syringe, Piston	General
Table, Surgical, Electrical	Surgery
Tamp	Orthopedics
Template	Orthopedics
Tray, Surgical Instrument	Surgery
Trephine, Bone	Orthopedics

MEDTRONIC SOFAMOR DANEK USA, INC. 901-396-3133 *(cont'd)*
Wrench	Orthopedics

**MEDTRONIC SPINAL AND BIOLOGICS NEW   901-396-3133
YORK DISTRIBUTION CENTER**
699 kapkowksi road, Suite 3, elizabeth,, NJ 07201
FDA Number: 3007026906
Web site: www.medtronicspine.com
Ownership: Medtronic, Inc.
Stock Symbol: MDT
Traded On: NYSE
Produces/Sells CE-marked Devices: N

Arthroscope	Orthopedics
Dissector, Surgical, General & Plastic Surgery	Surgery
Elevator, Orthopedic	Orthopedics
Endoscope, Neurological	Cns/Neurology
Forceps	Orthopedics
Guide, Surgical, Instrument	Surgery
Hook, Surgical, General & Plastic Surgery	Surgery
Light, Surgical, Instrument	Surgery
Mesh, Surgical (Steel Gauze)	Surgery
Motor, Surgical Instrument, AC-Powered	Surgery
Pliers, Surgical	Orthopedics
Retractor, Mastoid	Ear/Nose/Throat
Saw, Other	Surgery
Scissors, Orthopedic	Orthopedics
Tape, Measuring, Ruler And Caliper	Surgery
Tray, Surgical Instrument	Surgery

MEDTRONIC SPINE LLC   877-690-5353
1221 Crossman Ave., Sunnyvale, CA 94089   408-548-6500
FDA Number: 2953769
E-mail: spinalcodingmd@medtronic.com
Web site: www.medtronicspine.com
Year Founded: 1994
Ownership: Medtronic, Inc.
Stock Symbol: MDT
Traded On: NYSE
Produces/Sells CE-marked Devices: N

Arthroscope	Orthopedics
Bit, Drill	Orthopedics
Cannula, Surgical, General & Plastic Surgery	Surgery
Container, Specimen, All Types	General
Device, Biopsy, Percutaneous	Surgery
Dispenser, Cement	Orthopedics
Dispenser, Medication, Liquid	General
Dissector, Surgical, General & Plastic Surgery	Surgery
Filler, Bone Cement (for Vertebroplasty)	Orthopedics
Forceps	Orthopedics
Gauge, Depth	Orthopedics
Guide, Surgical, Instrument	Surgery
Injector, Syringe	General
Instrument, Manual, General Surgical	Surgery
Mixing Equipment, Cement	Orthopedics
Needle, Aspiration And Injection, Disposable	Surgery
Needle, Conduction, Anesthesia (W/Wo Introducer)	Anesthesiology
Orthopedic Manual Surgical Instrument	Orthopedics
Syringe, Balloon Inflation	Cardiovascular
Tamp	Orthopedics

MEDTRONIC VASCULAR   978-777-0042
35-37A Cherry Hill Dr, Danvers, MA 01923
FDA Number: 1220452
Web site: www.medtronic.com
Ownership: Medtronic, Inc.
Stock Symbol: MDT
Traded On: NYSE
Produces/Sells CE-marked Devices: N

Adapter, Stopcock, Manifold, Cardiopulmonary Bypass	Cardiovascular
Bandage, Adhesive	Surgery
Catheter, Embolectomy (Fogarty Type)	Cardiovascular
Catheter, Percutaneous	Cardiovascular
Catheter, Septostomy	Cardiovascular
Device, Hemostasis, Vascular	Cardiovascular
Guidewire, Catheter	Cardiovascular
Introducer, Catheter	Cardiovascular
Syringe, Balloon Inflation	Cardiovascular

MEDTRONIC VASCULAR   707-566-1548
5345 Skylane Blvd, Santa Rosa, CA 95403
FDA Number: 3003311129
Web site: www.medtronic.com
Ownership: Medtronic, Inc.
Stock Symbol: MDT
Traded On: NYSE
Produces/Sells CE-marked Devices: N

System, Treatment, Aortic Aneurysm, Endovascular Graft	Cardiovascular

MEDTRONIC VASCULAR

1-800-633-8766
(763) 514-4000

710 Medtronic Parkway, L100,
Minneapolis,, MN 55432
FDA Number: 2953200   Fax: (763) 514-487
Web site: www.medtronic.com
Ownership: Medtronic, Inc.
Stock Symbol: MDT
Traded On: NYSE
Produces/Sells CE-marked Devices: N
General Admin.: Lucinda Fox/Manager

Adapter, Stopcock, Manifold, Cardiopulmonary Bypass	Cardiovascular
Bandage, Adhesive	Surgery
Catheter, Biliary	Gastroenterology/Urology
Catheter, Embolectomy (Fogarty Type)	Cardiovascular
Catheter, Intravascular, Diagnostic	Cardiovascular
Catheter, Percutaneous	Cardiovascular
Catheter, Septostomy	Cardiovascular
Device, Coronary Saphenous Vein Bypass Graft, Temporary, For Embolization Protection	Cardiovascular
Guidewire, Catheter	Cardiovascular
Introducer, Catheter	Cardiovascular
Syringe, Balloon Inflation	Cardiovascular
Transducer, Ultrasonic, Diagnostic	Radiology
Trocar, Cardiovascular	Cardiovascular

MEDTRONIC XOMED, INC.

800-874-5797
904-296-9600

6743 Southpoint Drive North,
Jacksonville, FL 32216
FDA Number: 1045254   Fax: 904-296-9666
E-mail: rs.jaxcustomerservice@medtronic.com
Web site: www.xomed.com
Medical Products Sales Volume: $500,000,000
Year Founded: 1999
Ownership: Medtronic, Inc.
Quality System Registration Information: ISO9001
Produces/Sells CE-marked Devices: Y
Distribution: Manufacturer Direct, Manufacturer Through Distributor, Manufacturer Through Manufacturer Reps, Service Direct

Balloon, Epistaxis (Nasal)	Ear/Nose/Throat
Burr	Ear/Nose/Throat
Button, Nasal Septal	Ear/Nose/Throat
Cautery, Thermal, Battery-Powered	Ophthalmology
Drill, Surgical, ENT (Electric Or Pneumatic)	Ear/Nose/Throat
ENT Manual Surgical Instrument	Ear/Nose/Throat
Electromyograph, Diagnostic	Physical Med
Forceps, Ophthalmic	Ophthalmology
Knife, Ophthalmic	Ophthalmology
Motor, Surgical Instrument, AC-Powered	Surgery
Nasopharyngoscope (Flexible Or Rigid)	Ear/Nose/Throat
Paddie, Cottonoid	Cns/Neurology
Prosthesis, Ossicular	Ear/Nose/Throat
Prosthesis, Ossicular, Incus And Stapes	Ear/Nose/Throat
Prosthesis, Ossicular, Total	Ear/Nose/Throat
Splint, Nasal	Ear/Nose/Throat
Sponge, Ophthalmic	Ophthalmology
Stimulator, Nerve, ENT	Ear/Nose/Throat
Tube, Myringotomy	Ear/Nose/Throat
Tube, Tracheal (Endotracheal)	Anesthesiology
Tube, Tympanostomy	Ear/Nose/Throat

MEDTRONIC XOMED, INC.

800-637-6235

950 Flanders Rd., Mystic, CT 06355
FDA Number: 1219071
Web site: www.merocel.com
Year Founded: 1974
Ownership: Public
Quality System Registration Information: ISO9001
Produces/Sells CE-marked Devices: Y
Distribution: Manufacturer Direct

Balloon, Epistaxis (Nasal)	Ear/Nose/Throat
Button, Nasal Septal	Ear/Nose/Throat
Drill, Surgical, ENT (Electric Or Pneumatic)	Ear/Nose/Throat
ENT Manual Surgical Instrument	Ear/Nose/Throat
Electromyograph, Diagnostic	Physical Med
Gauze/sponge, Nonresorbable For External Use	Surgery
Knife, Ophthalmic	Ophthalmology
Nasopharyngoscope (Flexible Or Rigid)	Ear/Nose/Throat
Paddie, Cottonoid	Cns/Neurology
Prosthesis, Ossicular	Ear/Nose/Throat
Prosthesis, Ossicular, Incus And Stapes	Ear/Nose/Throat
Prosthesis, Ossicular, Total	Ear/Nose/Throat
Splint, Nasal	Ear/Nose/Throat
Sponge, Ophthalmic	Ophthalmology
Stimulator, Nerve, ENT	Ear/Nose/Throat
Tube, Myringotomy	Ear/Nose/Throat
Tube, Tracheal (Endotracheal)	Anesthesiology
Tube, Tympanostomy	Ear/Nose/Throat
Wick, Ear	Ear/Nose/Throat

MEDTRONIC, INC.

800-633-8766
763-514-4000

710 Medtronic Parkway, Mail Stop: L100,
Minneapolis, MN 55432
FDA Number: 2182208   Fax: 763-514-4879
Web site: www.medtronic.com
Annual Revenue: More than $1 Billion
Year Founded: 1949
Ownership: Public
Stock Symbol: MDT
Traded On: NYSE
Quality System Registration Information: ISO9000; ISO9001
Produces/Sells CE-marked Devices: Y
Distribution: Manufacturer Direct, OEM, Exporter
General Admin.: Gary L. Ellis/Chief Financial Officer, Senior Vice President
Richard Kuntz/Chief Scientific Officer, Senior Vice President
Christopher O'Connell/Executive Vice President
Jean-Luc Butel/Executive Vice President
William Hawkins/President, Chief Executive Officer, Chairman
Catherine Szyman/Senior Vice President
Pat Mackin/Senior Vice President
Scott Ward/Senior Vice President
Stephen La Neve/Senior Vice President
Stephen Oesterle/Senior Vice President
Mktg./Adv.: Mr. joe shmo/Account Specialist
Production: H. James Dallas/Senior Vice President Operations
Susan Alpert/Senior Vice President Regulatory Affairs

Adapter, Lead, Pacemaker	Cardiovascular
Adapter, Stopcock, Manifold, Cardiopulmonary Bypass	Cardiovascular
Biopsy Instrument	Gastroenterology/Urology
Cable, Electrode	Physical Med
Cannula, Catheter	Cardiovascular
Catheter, Angioplasty, Coronary, Transluminal, Percut. Oper.	Cardiovascular
Catheter, Cardiac Thermodilution	Cardiovascular
Catheter, Percutaneous	Cardiovascular
Catheter, Ventricular, General & Plastic Surgery	Surgery
Curette, Surgical	Surgery
Defibrillator, Implantable, Automatic	Cardiovascular
Dual Chamber, Implantable Pulse Generator	Cardiovascular
Electrocardiograph, Single Channel	Cardiovascular
Electrode, Defibrillator	Cardiovascular
Generator, Pulsatile Flow, Cardiopulmonary Bypass	Cardiovascular
Guidewire, Catheter	Cardiovascular
Introducer, Catheter	Cardiovascular
Kit, Biopsy	General
Lead, Pacemaker (Catheter)	Cardiovascular
Monitor, ECG, Arrhythmia	Cardiovascular
Needle, Biopsy, Cardiovascular	Cardiovascular
Occluder, Cardiovascular	Cardiovascular
Oxygenator, Cardiopulmonary Bypass	Cardiovascular
Perfusion Apparatus	Pathology
Plate, Fixation, Bone	Orthopedics
Prosthesis, Cardiac Valve	Cardiovascular
Pulse Generator, Pacemaker, Implantable, With Cardiac Resynchronization	Cardiovascular
Pump, Blood, Cardiopulmonary Bypass, Roller Type	Cardiovascular
Pump, Infusion, Implantable, General	General
Ring, Annuloplasty	Cardiovascular
Rod, Fixation, Intramedullary And Accessories, Metallic And Non-collapsible	Orthopedics
Sensor, Glucose, Invasive	General
Stent, Cardiovascular	Cardiovascular
Stimulator, Spinal Cord, Implantable (Pain Relief)	Cns/Neurology
Stylet, Catheter	Cardiovascular
Surgical Instrument, Cardiovascular	Cardiovascular
System, Pacing, Anti-Tachycardia	Cardiovascular
Tools, Pacemaker Service	Cardiovascular
Transmitter/Receiver System, ECG, Telephone Multi-Channel	Cardiovascular
Valve, Heart, Mechanical	Cardiovascular

Medical Product Subsidiaries (Listed Separately)
Arizona Device Manufacturing
Cryocath Technologies Inc.
Invatec
Medtronic Blood Management
Medtronic Cardiac Surgery Technologies
Medtronic Cardiovascular Surgery, The Heart Valve Div.
Medtronic Image-Guided Neurologics, Inc.
Medtronic Minimed
Medtronic Navigation, Inc.
Medtronic Navigation, Inc. (Littleton)
Medtronic Neuromodulation
Medtronic Neurosurgery
Medtronic Perfusion Systems
Medtronic Powered Surgical Solutions
Medtronic Puerto Rico Operations Co., Juncos
Medtronic Puerto Rico Operations Co., Villalba
Medtronic Puerto Rico Operations Co.,Med Rel
Medtronic Sofamor Danek Instrument Manufacturing
Medtronic Sofamor Danek Usa, Inc

MANUFACTURER PROFILES

MEDTRONIC, INC. 800-633-8766 *(cont'd)*
Medtronic Sofamor Danek Usa, Inc.
Medtronic Spinal And Biologics New York Distribution Center
Medtronic Spine Llc
Medtronic Vascular
Medtronic Xomed, Inc.
Ndi Medical, Inc.
Physio-Control, Inc.
Restore Medical Inc.

MEDVED PRODUCTS, INC. 651-482-8413
P.O. Box 120883, St. Paul, MN 55112-0883
FDA Number: n/a *Fax:* 651-482-8413
E-mail: mdr@medvedproducts.com
Web site: www.medvedproducts.com
Year Founded: 1989
Total Employees: 6
Ownership: Private
Produces/Sells CE-marked Devices: N
Federal Procurement Eligibility: Small Business
Distribution: Manufacturer Direct, Manufacturer Through Distributor, OEM
General Admin.: Charles W. Medved/President
Analyzer, Infusion Pump	General
Cart, Monitor	General
Infusion Stand	General
Mount, Monitor (Support)	General

MEDVENTURE TECHNOLOGY CORP. (812) 280-2400
2301 Centennial Blvd., Jeffersonville,, IN 47130
FDA Number: 1222140
Ownership: Private
Produces/Sells CE-marked Devices: N
General Admin.: Kevin Bramer/President, Chief Executive Officer

MEDWAVES, INCORPORATED (858) 946-0015
16760 West Bernardo Drive, San Diego, CA 92127
FDA Number: 3005382058 *Fax:* (858) 946-0016
E-mail: tedormsby@avecure.com
Web site: www.medwaves.com
Ownership: Private
Produces/Sells CE-marked Devices: N

MEDWEB 800-863-3932
667 Folsom St., San Francisco, CA 94107 415-541-9980
FDA Number: 2953193 *Fax:* 415-541-9984
E-mail: sales@medweb.com
Web site: www.medweb.com
Medical Products Sales Volume: $100,000
Annual Revenue: $5-$10 Million
Year Founded: 1992
Total Employees: 2 *Marketing Staff:* 6 *Sales Staff:* 5
Ownership: Private
Produces/Sells CE-marked Devices: N
Federal Procurement Eligibility: Small Business, GSA Contract
Distribution: Service Direct
System, Communication, Image, Digital	Radiology

MEDWORKS INSTRUMENTS 800-323-9790
PO Box 581, Chatham, IL 62629 217-698-3935
FDA Number: 1925213 *Fax:* 775-255-8668
E-mail: info@medexamtools.com
Web site: www.medexamtools.com
Medical Products Sales Volume: $300,000
Annual Revenue: $0-$1 Million
Year Founded: 1971
Total Employees: 4 *Marketing Staff:* 1 *Sales Staff:* 4
Ownership: Private
Produces/Sells CE-marked Devices: N
Federal Procurement Eligibility: Small Business, Female Owned
Distribution: Exclusive Distributor
General Admin.: Cynthia Heise-Swartz/President, Chief Executive Officer
Chart, Visual Acuity	Ophthalmology
Cuff, Blood Pressure	Cardiovascular
Discriminator, Two-point	Cns/Neurology
Forceps, Dressing	Surgery
Forceps, Hemostatic	Surgery
Forceps, Tissue	Surgery
Fork, Tuning	Cns/Neurology
Goniometer, Orthopedic	Orthopedics
Hammer, Neurological	Cns/Neurology
Hammer, Percussion	Cns/Neurology
Handle, Scalpel	Surgery
Holder, Needle, Other	Surgery
Probe, Other	General
Scissors, Bandage/Gauze/Plaster	General
Scissors, General Dissecting	General
Stethoscope, Mechanical	General

MEDWORLD, INC.
See Labworld, Inc.

MEDX CORPORATION
See Medx Corporation

MEDX HEALTH CORP. 888-363-3112
220 Superior Blvd., 905-670-4428
Mississauga, ON L5T 2 Canada
FDA Number: 3003725190 *Fax:* 905-826-0086
E-mail: info@medxhealth.com
Web site: www.medxhealth.com
Year Founded: 1999
Ownership: Public
Stock Symbol: MDX
Traded On: TSX Venture Exchange
Quality System Registration Information: ISO9001
Produces/Sells CE-marked Devices: N

MEDX INCORPORATED 800-323-6339
3456 N. Ridge Ave. #100, 847-463-2020
Arlington Heights, IL 60004
FDA Number: 1419459 *Fax:* 847-463-2019
E-mail: sales@medx-inc.com
Web site: www.medx-inc.com
Medical Products Sales Volume: $6,000,000
Annual Revenue: $5-$10 Million
Year Founded: 1973
Total Employees: 35 *Marketing Staff:* 2 *Sales Staff:* 5
Ownership: Private
Produces/Sells CE-marked Devices: N
Federal Procurement Eligibility: Small Business
Distribution: Manufacturer Direct, Manufacturer Through Distributor
General Admin.: Eric Ellingson/Chief Executive Officer, Chairman
Production: Floyd R. Rowan/Executive Vice President Operations
Camera, Gamma (Nuclear/Scintillation)	Radiology
Scanner, Emission Computed Tomography	Radiology

MEDX, INC. 847-463-2020
3456 North Ridge Ave., #100, Arlington Heights, IL 60004
FDA Number: 1419459
Camera, Gamma (Nuclear/Scintillation)	Radiology
Scanner, Emission Computed Tomography	Radiology
Table, Radiographic	Radiology

MEENA MEDICAL EQUIPMENT, INC. 888-225-2502
1905 Bedford Rd |, Ste. 105, Bedford,, TX 76021 817-251-9772
FDA Number: 1473915 *Fax:* 817-251-9281
E-mail: sales@meenamedical.com
Web site: www.meenamedical.com
Annual Revenue: $0-$1 Million
Total Employees: 3 *Marketing Staff:* 1 *Sales Staff:* 1
Ownership: Private
Produces/Sells CE-marked Devices: N
Federal Procurement Eligibility: Small Business
Distribution: Service Direct
General Admin.: George Girgis/Owner
Service, Maintenance/Repair	General

MEESE ORBITRON DUNNE CO. 800-829-3230
535 N. Midland Ave., 201-796-4667
Saddle Brook, NJ 07663
FDA Number: n/a *Fax:* 201-796-5820
E-mail: papemod@aol.com
Web site: www.meeseinc.com
Medical Products Sales Volume: $10,000,000
Annual Revenue: $10-$25 Million
Total Employees: 150
Ownership: TINGUE BROWN
Produces/Sells CE-marked Devices: N
Federal Procurement Eligibility: Small Business
Distribution: Manufacturer Through Distributor
General Admin.: R. Midili/President
Mktg./Adv.: J. Pape/Vice President Sales
Production: Michael Dorsey/Vice President Manufacturing
Cart, Housekeeping	General
Cart, Laundry	General
Cart, Supply	General
Cart, Supply, Operating Room	Surgery
Stand, Laundry Hamper	General
Washer, Cart	General

MEESE, INC.
See Meese Orbitron Dunne Co.

MEGADYNE MEDICAL PRODUCTS, INC. 800-747-6110
11506 S. State St., Draper, UT 84020 801-576-9669
FDA Number: 1721194 *Fax:* 801-576-9698
E-mail: mhintze@megadyne.com

MEGADYNE MEDICAL PRODUCTS, INC.   800-747-6110 (cont'd)

Web site: www.megadyne.com
Annual Revenue: $25-$50 Million
Year Founded: 1985
Total Employees: 95   *Marketing Staff:* 4   *Sales Staff:* 35
Ownership: Private
Quality System Registration Information: ISO9001
Produces/Sells CE-marked Devices: Y
Federal Procurement Eligibility: Small Business
Distribution: Manufacturer Direct, Manufacturer Through Distributor, Manufacturer Through Manufacturer Reps, OEM, Exclusive Distributor, Importer, Exporter
General Admin.: Robert Farnsworth/President, Chief Executive Officer
   Robert Farnsworth/President, Chief Operating Officer
   Theresa Vonk/Secretary
   Robert Farnsworth/Vice President, General Manager
Mktg./Adv.: Michael Hintze/Director Business Development
   Wayne Chappell/Director International Sales
   Robert Brosseau/Manager Sales Training
   Michael Hintze/Vice President Marketing
   Rob Brosseau/Vice President Sales
Production: Ronda Magneson/Director Quality Assurance
   Tara Rogers/Manager Materials
   Ronda Magneson/Manager Regulatory Affairs
Finance: Michael Facer/Chief Financial Officer

Cover, Tip, Probe, Cauterization	Surgery
Electrode, Electrosurgical, Return (Ground, Dispersive)	Surgery
Electrode, Other	General
Electrosurgical Unit, Cutting & Coagulation Device	Surgery
Equipment, Suction/Irrigation, Laparoscopic	Surgery
Probe, Suction, Irrigator/Aspirator, Laparoscopic	Surgery
Shield, Eye, Ophthalmic	Ophthalmology
System, Evacuation, Smoke, Laser	Surgery
Tube, Smoke Removal, Endoscopic	Gastroenterology/Urology

MEGAMED CORPORATION   305-665-6876

7432 SW 48th St., Miami, FL 33155
FDA Number: 9613213   *Fax:* 305-665-6357
E-mail: megamed@bellsouth.net
Web site: www.CyberOfficeUSA.com
Annual Revenue: $0-$1 Million
Year Founded: 1993
Ownership: Private
Produces/Sells CE-marked Devices: N
Federal Procurement Eligibility: Small Business
Distribution: Service Direct, Exclusive Distributor, Importer, Exporter

Kit, Hemodialysis Tubing	Gastroenterology/Urology
Tray, Start/Stop (Including Contents), Dialysis	Gastroenterology/Urology

MEGASUN   800-229-7432
          314-772-7000

4515 Miami Street, St. Louis, MO 63116
FDA Number: n/a   *Fax:* 314-533-6891
E-mail: sales@megasun.com
Web site: www.megasun.com
Annual Revenue: $0-$1 Million
Year Founded: 1991
Total Employees: 60
Ownership: Private
Produces/Sells CE-marked Devices: N
Federal Procurement Eligibility: Small Business
Distribution: Manufacturer Through Distributor, Manufacturer Through Manufacturer Reps, Importer, Exporter
General Admin.: Ron Poe/President

Booth, Sun Tan	Physical Med
Eyeglasses, Safety	Ophthalmology

MEGGER INC. (FORMERLY AVO INTERNATIONAL)   800-723-2861

2621 Van Buren Avenue, Norristown, PA 19403   610-676-8500
FDA Number: 9200117   *Fax:* 610-676-8610
E-mail: sales@megger.com
Web site: www.megger.com
Annual Revenue: $25-$50 Million
Total Employees: 140   *Marketing Staff:* 18   *Sales Staff:* 25
Ownership: Private
Quality System Registration Information: ISO9001
Produces/Sells CE-marked Devices: N
Federal Procurement Eligibility: Small Business
Distribution: Manufacturer Direct, Manufacturer Through Distributor, Manufacturer Through Manufacturer Reps
General Admin.: Arthur Stine/Vice President, General Manager
Mktg./Adv.: Gary Guthrie/Director Marketing
   Peg Houck/Manager Marketing Communications
Production: Richard Brown/Manager Engineering
   Art Stine/Manager Manufacturing

Regulator, Line Voltage	General
Tester, Grounding System	General

MEHLROSE ASSOCIATES   410-730-0263

11660-304 Little Patuxent Pkwy, Columbia, MD 21044
FDA Number: 3002970902
Ownership: Private
Produces/Sells CE-marked Devices: N

Balance, Analytical	Chemistry

MEI BEAUTY PRODUCTS, INC.   909-861-7575

1971 West Holt Ave., Pomona, CA 91768
FDA Number: 3004846413

Brush, Dermabrasion	Surgery

MEI CORPORATION   402-339-3300

4907 South 90th St., Omaha, NE 68127
FDA Number: 1954551   *Fax:* 402-339-1333
E-mail: meicorp@cox.net
Web site: www.meicorp.net
Ownership: Private
Produces/Sells CE-marked Devices: N
Distribution: Manufacturer Direct, Manufacturer Through Distributor
General Admin.: Mr. Loyd Messerli/President

Infusion Stand	General

MEIJI TECHNO AMERICA   800-832-0060
          408-970-4799

3010 Olcott Street, Santa Clara, CA 95054
FDA Number: n/a   *Fax:* 408-970-5054
E-mail: Sales@meijitechno.com
Web site: www.meijitechno.com
Year Founded: 1986
Total Employees: 10   *Sales Staff:* 137
Ownership: Private
Quality System Registration Information: ISO9003
Produces/Sells CE-marked Devices: Y
Distribution: Exclusive Distributor, Importer
General Admin.: Mr. Jim Dutkiewicz/General Manager
   Mr. Z. Sato/President
Mktg./Adv.: Mr. Anthony Peter Rivero/Sales Specialist

Microscope, Laboratory, Optical	Microbiology

MEINHARD GLASS PRODUCTS   303-277-9776

700 Corporate Circle, Suite A, Golden, CO 80401-5636
FDA Number: n/a   *Fax:* 303-216-2649
E-mail: sales@meinhard.com
Web site: www.meinhard.com
Medical Products Sales Volume: $1,300,000
Annual Revenue: $1-$5 Million
Total Employees: 10
Ownership: Private
Produces/Sells CE-marked Devices: N
Federal Procurement Eligibility: Small Business, Female Owned
Distribution: Manufacturer Direct, Manufacturer Through Distributor, Manufacturer Through Manufacturer Reps, OEM, Importer, Exporter
General Admin.: Patricia Kacsir/President

Nebulizer, Medicinal	Ear/Nose/Throat

MEKANIKA, INC.   561-417-7244

3998 Fau Blvd., Suite 210, Boca Raton, FL 33431
FDA Number: 1052987
Ownership: Private
Produces/Sells CE-marked Devices: N

Bit, Drill	Orthopedics
Burr, Surgical, General & Plastic Surgery	Surgery
Dynamometer, AC-Powered	Orthopedics

MEL R. MANUFACTURAS   956-655-1380

417 East Coma Street, Suite 534, Hidalgo, TX 78557
FDA Number: n/a   *Fax:* 956-843-9632
E-mail: jorgeselvera@melretrabajadora.com
Web site: www.melretrabajadora.com
Medical Products Sales Volume: $250,000
Annual Revenue: $0-$1 Million
Year Founded: 1992
Total Employees: 50   *Marketing Staff:* 2   *Sales Staff:* 8
Ownership: Private
Stock Symbol: NA
Quality System Registration Information: ISO9000
Produces/Sells CE-marked Devices: Y
Federal Procurement Eligibility: Small Business, Minority Owned
Distribution: Manufacturer Direct, Importer, Exporter
General Admin.: Mr. Jorge Selvera/President, Chief Executive Officer
Mktg./Adv.: Ms. Brenda Selvera/Admin. Contract Sales

Accessories, Cart, Multipurpose	General
Kit, Laryngeal Injection	Ear/Nose/Throat

MELCO ENGINEERING CORP.   888-635-2688

P.O. Box 8907, Calabasas, CA 91372-8907
FDA Number: n/a   *Fax:* 818-591-1073
E-mail: websales@melcowire.com

MELCO ENGINEERING CORP.   888-635-2688 *(cont'd)*
Web site: http://melcowire.com
Annual Revenue: $1-$5 Million
Year Founded: 1946
Total Employees: 10
Ownership: Private
Produces/Sells CE-marked Devices: N
Federal Procurement Eligibility: Small Business
Distribution: Manufacturer Direct, Exporter
General Admin.: Henry David/President, Chief Executive Officer
  Stripper, Donor Tube   Hematology

MELCOR TECHNOLOGIES, INC.   408-247-0350
1030 E. El Camino Real #435, Sunnyvale, CA 94087
FDA Number: n/a   *Fax:* 408-247-0350
E-mail: melvinebeling@email.msn.com
Annual Revenue: $0-$1 Million
Year Founded: 1991
Ownership: Private
Produces/Sells CE-marked Devices: N
Federal Procurement Eligibility: Small Business
Distribution: Manufacturer Direct
General Admin.: Melvin E. Ebeling/President, Chief Executive Officer
Mktg./Adv.: Melvin E. Ebeling/Director Marketing
Production: Darlene Florek/Director Quality Assurance & Regulatory Affairs
  Column, Liquid Chromatography   Toxicology

MELET PLASTICS, INC.   204-667-6635
34 De Baets St, Winnipeg R2J 3S9 Canada
FDA Number: 8022025
  Cane   Physical Med

MELLEN AIR MANUFACTURING, INC.   800-770-6264
2601 East 28th Street, Suite 307,   **562-595-8004**
Signal Hill, CA 90755
FDA Number: 2028696   *Fax:* 562-595-5924
E-mail: billing@mellenair.com
Web site: www.mellenair.com
Annual Revenue: $0-$1 Million
Year Founded: 1992
Total Employees: 9   *Sales Staff:* 4
Ownership: Private
Produces/Sells CE-marked Devices: N
Federal Procurement Eligibility: Small Business, Female Owned
Distribution: Manufacturer Through Distributor
  Mattress, Air Flotation   General

MELROSE MATTRESS, INC.   800-500-0233
8241 Lankersheim Blvd.,   **818-982-2234**
North Hollywood, CA 91605
FDA Number: n/a   *Fax:* 818-504-2788
E-mail: melmatt@pacbell.net
Medical Products Sales Volume: $500,000
Year Founded: 1936
Total Employees: 6   *Sales Staff:* 1
Ownership: Private
Produces/Sells CE-marked Devices: N
Federal Procurement Eligibility: Small Business
Distribution: Manufacturer Through Manufacturer Reps
General Admin.: Greg Myers/Chief Executive Officer
Mktg./Adv.: Greg Myers/Manager Marketing
Production: Greg Myers/Manager Production
  Mattress, Bed   General

MELYX CORPORATION   888-886-3599
21830 Industrial Blvd., Rogers, MN 55374   **763-428-6000**
FDA Number: n/a   *Fax:* 763-428-7585
E-mail: sales@melyx.com
Web site: www.melyx.com
Medical Products Sales Volume: $2,000,000
Annual Revenue: $1-$5 Million
Year Founded: 1978
Total Employees: 25
Ownership: Private
Produces/Sells CE-marked Devices: N
Federal Procurement Eligibility: Small Business
Distribution: Manufacturer Direct
General Admin.: Rick Johnston/President
Mktg./Adv.: Richard Johnston/Director Marketing
      Doreen Arlandson/Manager Sales Training
      Doreen Arlandson/Vice President Sales
  Computer Software, Hospital/Nursing Management   General

MEMPHIS DENTAL MFG. CO., INC.   901-526-6328
402 South Second St., Memphis, TN 38103
FDA Number: 1049722

MEMPHIS DENTAL MFG. CO., INC.   901-526-6328 *(cont'd)*
Wax, Dental   Dental And Oral

MEMRY CORP.
  See Saes Memry

MEMTEC CORP.   603-893-8080
68 Stiles Rd. Unit D, Salem, NH 03079
FDA Number: n/a   *Fax:* 603-893-8699
E-mail: info@memteccorp.com
Web site: www.memteccorp.com
Annual Revenue: $0-$1 Million
Total Employees: 10
Ownership: Private
Produces/Sells CE-marked Devices: Y
Federal Procurement Eligibility: Small Business
Distribution: Manufacturer Direct, Manufacturer Through Distributor, Manufacturer Through Manufacturer Reps, OEM
General Admin.: Val Dell/Human Resources Representative
      Dennis Garboski/President
Mktg./Adv.: Harold Sanford/Vice President Sales
  Recorder, Analog/Digital, Ophthalmic   Ophthalmology
  Recorder, Magnetic Tape/Disc   Cardiovascular

MEMTEC CORP.   603-893-8080
68 Stiles Rd. Unit D, Salem, NH 03079
FDA Number: 1225818
  Electrocardiograph, Ambulatory (With Analysis Algorithm)   Cardiovascular
  Recorder, Magnetic Tape/Disc   Cardiovascular

MENLO TOOL CO., INC.   810-756-6010
22760 Dequindre Road, Warren, MI 48091-2199
FDA Number: n/a   *Fax:* 586-756-1821
E-mail: Menlo.Service@imcousa.com
Web site: www.menlo-usa.com
Medical Products Sales Volume: $5,200,000
Annual Revenue: $5-$10 Million
Year Founded: 1962
Total Employees: 45   *Marketing Staff:* 2   *Sales Staff:* 3
Ownership: Private
Quality System Registration Information: ISO9002
Produces/Sells CE-marked Devices: N
Federal Procurement Eligibility: Small Business
Distribution: Manufacturer Through Distributor
General Admin.: John E. Falk/Chief Executive Officer
      John E. Falk/Executive Vice President
      Frank M. Kostelic/President
Mktg./Adv.: John E. Falk/Director Marketing
      John E. Falk/Manager International & National Sales
      Erich P. Wester/Vice President Marketing
      Ronald Lee/Vice President Marketing & Sales
  Burr, Dental   Dental And Oral
  Burr, Podiatric   Orthopedics
  Dental Laboratory Equipment   Dental And Oral

MENNEN MEDICAL CORP.   800-223-2201
2540 Metropolitan Drive,   **215-322-9997**
Trevose, PA 19053
FDA Number: 1315366   *Fax:* 215-322-0199
E-mail: info@menenmedical.com
Web site: www.mennenmedical.com
Medical Products Sales Volume: $5,000,000
Annual Revenue: $1-$5 Million
Year Founded: 1963
Total Employees: 20   *Sales Staff:* 4
Ownership: Mennen Medical Ltd. Israel
Quality System Registration Information: ISO9000; ISO9001
Produces/Sells CE-marked Devices: Y
Federal Procurement Eligibility: Small Business
Distribution: Manufacturer Direct, Importer
General Admin.: Mr. Danny Harel/President
Finance: Tom Triolo/Controller
  Cardiac Output Unit, Indicator Dilution (Thermal)   Cardiovascular
  Computer, Cardiac Catheterization Laboratory   Cardiovascular
  Computer, Patient Monitor   Anesthesiology
  Detector, Arrhythmia Alarm   Cardiovascular
  Kit, Angiographic, Special Procedure   Radiology
  Monitor, Apnea   General
  Monitor, Blood Pressure, Indirect (Arterial)   Cardiovascular
  Monitor, Blood Pressure, Indirect, Anesthesiology   Anesthesiology
  Monitor, Blood Pressure, Indirect, Automatic   Cardiovascular
  Monitor, Blood Pressure, Invasive (Arterial)   Cardiovascular
  Monitor, Blood Pressure, Venous   Cardiovascular
  Monitor, Cardiac (Cardiotachometer & Rate Alarm)   Cardiovascular
  Monitor, Cardiac Output, Thermal (Balloon Type Catheter)   Surgery
  Monitor, ECG   Cardiovascular
  Monitor, ECG, Anesthesia   Anesthesiology
  Monitor, ECG, Arrhythmia   Cardiovascular
  Monitor, EEG   Cns/Neurology

MENNEN MEDICAL CORP.   800-223-2201 *(cont'd)*

Monitor, Heart Rate, R-Wave (ECG)	Cardiovascular
Monitor, Impedance Pneumograph	Anesthesiology
Monitor, Neonatal	Obstetrics/Gynecology
Monitor, Neonatal, Blood Pressure, Invasive	General
Monitor, Neonatal, Heart Rate	General
Monitor, Neonatal, Physiological	Obstetrics/Gynecology
Monitor, Physiological, Acute Care	Anesthesiology
Monitor, Physiological, Cardiac Catheterization	Cardiovascular
Monitor, Physiological, Patient	Cardiovascular
Monitor, Pulse Rate	Anesthesiology
Monitor, Respiratory	Surgery
Monitor, Temperature (With Probe)	Anesthesiology
Mount, Monitor (Support)	General
Probe, Temperature	General
Recorder, Paper Chart	Cardiovascular
Sphygmomanometer, Electronic, Automatic	General

MENNEN-GREATBATCH, INC.

See Mennen Medical Corp.

MENTOR CORP.   800-525-0245

201 Mentor Drive, Santa Barbara, CA 93111   805-879-6000
FDA Number: 1222091   *Fax:* 805-964-2712
E-mail: gfriedrich@mentorcorp.com
Web site: www.mentorcorp.com
Medical Products Sales Volume: $301,974,000
Annual Revenue: $100-$500 Million
Year Founded: 1969
Total Employees: 1190   *Marketing Staff:* 288   *Sales Staff:* 288
Ownership: Public
Stock Symbol: MNT
Traded On: NYSE
Quality System Registration Information: ISO9000; ISO9001
Produces/Sells CE-marked Devices: Y
Federal Procurement Eligibility: Small Business
Distribution: Manufacturer Direct, Manufacturer Through Distributor, Manufacturer Through Manufacturer Reps, Exclusive Distributor
General Admin.: Mr. Michael O'Neill/Chief Financial Officer, Vice President
   Mr. Edward S. Northup/Chief Operating Officer, Vice President
   Mr. Joshua H. Levine/President, Chief Executive Officer
   Mr. Vicki S. Chuck/Vice President Human Resources
Mktg./Adv.: Mr. John Anderson/Director Marketing
   John VanDenburgh/Director National Accounts
   Mr. Joel Morrell/Director National Accounts
   Mr. Grant Friedrich/Marketing Coordinator
   Ms. Kathleen Beauchamp/Senior Vice President Marketing & Sales
   Mr. Udo W. Graf/Vice President Marketing & Sales
Production: Mr. Kevin O'Donnell/Product Manager
   Mrs. Teena Broumand/Product Manager

Appliance, Incontinence, Urosheath Type	Gastroenterology/Urology
Bag, Drainage, Ostomy (With Adhesive)	General
Bag, Urinary Collection	General
Catheter, Balloon (Foley Type)	Surgery
Catheter, Urethral, Diagnostic	Gastroenterology/Urology
Catheter, Urinary	Gastroenterology/Urology
Catheter, Urological	Gastroenterology/Urology
Drainage System, Urine, Closed	Gastroenterology/Urology
Drainage Unit, Urinary	General
Ostomy Appliance (Ileostomy, Colostomy)	Gastroenterology/Urology
Pack, Custom/Special Procedure	General
Tray, Custom/Special Procedure	General

MENTOR O&O, INC.

See Mentor Ophthalmics, Inc.

MENTOR OPHTHALMICS, INC.   800-525-0245

201 Mentor Dr., Santa Barbara, CA 93111   805-879-6000
FDA Number: n/a
Web site: www.mentorcorp.com
Medical Products Sales Volume: $24,000,000
Year Founded: 1969
Ownership: MENTOR CORP.
Quality System Registration Information: ISO9000; ISO9001
Produces/Sells CE-marked Devices: Y
Distribution: Manufacturer Direct, Manufacturer Through Distributor, Manufacturer Through Manufacturer Reps, Exclusive Distributor, Exporter
General Admin.: Joshua H. Levine/President

Applicator, Ocular Pressure	Ophthalmology
Aspirator, Ophthalmic	Ophthalmology
Cautery, Radiofrequency, AC-Powered	Ophthalmology
Cautery, Radiofrequency, Battery-Powered	Ophthalmology
Cutter, Vitreous Aspiration, AC-Powered	Ophthalmology
Forceps, Ophthalmic	Ophthalmology
Pachometer	Surgery
Phacoemulsification System	Ophthalmology
Tonometer, AC-Powered	Ophthalmology
Tonometer, Manual	Ophthalmology
Vision Aid, Electronic, AC-Powered	Ophthalmology

MENTOR OPHTHALMICS, INC.   800-525-0245 *(cont'd)*

Wipe, Instrument	General

MENTOR TEXAS, INC.   972-252-6060

3041 Skyway Circle North, Irving, TX 75038
FDA Number: 1645337
Web site: www.mentorcorp.com
Year Founded: 1969
Ownership: MENTOR CORP.
Stock Symbol: MNT
Traded On: NYSE
Produces/Sells CE-marked Devices: N
General Admin.: Joshua H. Levine/President

Expander, Skin, Inflatable	Surgery
Instrument, Manual, General Surgical	Surgery
Kit, Instruments and Accessories, Surgical	Surgery
Prosthesis, Breast, Inflatable, Internal	Surgery
Prosthesis, Breast, Non-Inflatable, Internal	Surgery
Prosthesis, Chin, Internal	Surgery
Prosthesis, Nose, Internal	Surgery
Pump, Infusion	General
Sizer, Mammary, Breast Implant Volume	Surgery

MENTOR UROLOGY

See Mentor Corp.

MERCATOR MEDSYSTEMS, INC.   510-614-4550

1670 Alvarado Street, Suite 4, San Leandro, CA 94577
FDA Number: 3004142795   *Fax:* 510-614-4560
E-mail: info@mercatormed.com
Web site: http://www.mercatormed.com
Ownership: Private
Produces/Sells CE-marked Devices: N
General Admin.: Thomas Loarie/Chief Executive Officer, Chairman

Catheter, Continuous Flush	Cardiovascular

MERCER SCIENTIFIC INTERNATIONAL

See Peripheral Dynamics Inc.

MERCURY COMPUTER SYSTEMS, INC.   978-256-1300

201 Riverneck Road, Chelmsford, MA 01824
FDA Number: n/a   *Fax:* 978-256-3599
E-mail: jflannery@mc.com
Web site: www.mc.com
Medical Products Sales Volume: $236,110,000
Year Founded: 1981
Total Employees: 211
Ownership: Public
Stock Symbol: MRCY
Traded On: NASDAQ
Quality System Registration Information: ISO9001
Produces/Sells CE-marked Devices: N
Federal Procurement Eligibility: Small Business
Distribution: Manufacturer Direct
General Admin.: James R. Bratelli/Chief Executive Officer
   Didier Thibaud/Vice President, General Manager
Production: John M. Flannery/Director Operations

Computer Equipment	General

MERCURY ENTERPRISES INC.

See Mercury Medical

MERCURY MEDICAL   800-237-6418

11300 49th St. N., Clearwater, FL 33762-4800   727-573-0088
FDA Number: 1024404   *Fax:* 727-573-6040
E-mail: mercury@mercurymed.com
Web site: www.mercurymed.com
Medical Products Sales Volume: $31,000,000
Annual Revenue: $25-$50 Million
Year Founded: 1963
Total Employees: 170   *Marketing Staff:* 5   *Sales Staff:* 25
Ownership: Private
Quality System Registration Information: ISO9001
Produces/Sells CE-marked Devices: Y
Federal Procurement Eligibility: Small Business
Distribution: Manufacturer Direct, Manufacturer Through Distributor, Importer, Exporter
General Admin.: Stanley G. Tangalakis/Chief Executive Officer
   George E. Howe/Executive Vice President
   Deanna Russell/Manager Human Resources
   Al Sousa/President
Mktg./Adv.: Deborah Olson/Director Marketing
   Garry P. Blount/Director National Sales
   Sally Barlowe/Manager Advertising
   Gary French/Manager International Sales
   David Tyson/Vice President Sales
Production: Karen Seltzer/Manager Regulatory Affairs
Finance: Bill Brown/Vice President Finance

Adapter, Anesthesia	Anesthesiology
Adapter, Catheter	Surgery

MANUFACTURER PROFILES

MERCURY MEDICAL   800-237-6418 *(cont'd)*

Adapter, Tube, Tracheal	Anesthesiology
Airway, Oropharyngeal, Anesthesia	Anesthesiology
Analyzer, Gas, Oxygen, Gaseous Phase	Anesthesiology
Attachment, Breathing, Positive End Expiratory Pressure	Anesthesiology
Bag, Breathing	Anesthesiology
Clip, Nose	Anesthesiology
Connector, Airway (Extension)	Anesthesiology
Detector, Leakage, Medical Gas	General
Fitting, Other	General
Forceps, Tube Introduction	Anesthesiology
Laryngoscope	Ear/Nose/Throat
Laryngoscope, Rigid	Anesthesiology
Laryngoscope, Surgical	Surgery
Manometer, Laboratory	Chemistry
Mask, Gas, Anesthesia	Anesthesiology
Mask, Oxygen, Other	General
Mouthpiece, Breathing	Anesthesiology
Protector, Dental	Anesthesiology
Receptacle, Electrical	General
Resuscitator, Pulmonary, Gas	General
Resuscitator, Pulmonary, Manual (Demand Valve)	General
Spirometer, Therapeutic (Incentive)	Anesthesiology
Stimulator, Nerve, Anesthesia	Anesthesiology
Stylet, Tracheal Tube	Anesthesiology
Support, Breathing Tube	Anesthesiology
Tube, Aspirating, Flexible, Connecting	Anesthesiology
Tubing, Braided	General
Tubing, Conductive	General
Tubing, Corrugated	General
Tubing, Flexible, Medical Gas, Low-Pressure	Anesthesiology
Valve, Positive End Expiratory Pressure (PEEP)	Anesthesiology
Ventilator, Emergency, Manual (Resuscitator)	Anesthesiology
Ventilator, Emergency, Powered (Resuscitator)	Anesthesiology

MERGE EMED
See GE Healthcare

MERGE HEALTHCARE
See GE Healthcare

MERGENET MEDICAL INC.   888-925-2526
6601 Lyons Road, Suite B1-B4,   **561-208-3770**
Coconut Creek, FL 33073
FDA Number: 3003619538
Web site: http://www.mergenetmedical.com
Year Founded: 2004
Ownership: Private
Produces/Sells CE-marked Devices: N

Connector, Airway (Extension)	Anesthesiology
Ventilator, Non-Continuous (Respirator)	Anesthesiology

MERIAM PROCESS TECHNOLOGIES   216-281-1100
10920 Madison Avenue, Cleveland, OH 44102-2599
FDA Number: 7000254   *Fax:* 216-281-0228
E-mail: meriam@meriam.com
Annual Revenue: $10-$25 Million
Year Founded: 1911
Total Employees: 63   *Marketing Staff:* 2   *Sales Staff:* 13
Ownership: Scott Fetzer Company
Stock Symbol: BRK
Quality System Registration Information: ISO9000
Produces/Sells CE-marked Devices: Y
Federal Procurement Eligibility: Small Business
Distribution: Manufacturer Through Manufacturer Reps
General Admin.: Rick D'angelo/Chief Executive Officer
Mktg./Adv.: Dave Thomas/Manager Advertising
       Rick D'angelo/Manager Business Development
       Dave Thomas/Manager Market Research
       Dave Thomas/Manager Marketing & Sales
       Kelly O'Brien/Manager Sales Training
       Carol French/Manager Services & Sales
       Linda Welker/Sales Associate
Production: Jason Dewar/Director Quality Assurance
       Steve Szcecinski/Manager Materials

Manometer, Laboratory	Chemistry

MERIDIAN AMERICA MEDICALS, INC.   800-638-8093
2691 Richter Ave., Suite 104, Irvine, CA 92606
FDA Number: 2087359
E-mail: info@meridianmt.com   *Fax:* 443-259-7801
Web site: www.meridianmeds.com
Year Founded: 1988
Ownership: Meridian Co., Ltd.
Stock Symbol: MTEC
Traded On: NASDAQ
Produces/Sells CE-marked Devices: N
General Admin.: Geoffrey Ritson/Manager
       Ted Marcuccio/Vice President
Mktg./Adv.: Ireatha Woods/Account Services Representative

MERIDIAN AMERICA MEDICALS, INC.   800-638-8093 *(cont'd)*
    Sean Cowherd/Account Services Representative
    Paul Lippner/Sales Specialist

MERIDIAN BIOSCIENCE, INC.   800-696-0739
3471 River Hills Dr., Cincinnati, OH 45244-3023   **513-271-3700**
FDA Number: 1524213   *Fax:* 513-271-3762
E-mail: mdi@meridianbioscience.com
Web site: www.meridianbioscience.com
Medical Products Sales Volume: $122,963,000
Annual Revenue: $100-$500 Million
Year Founded: 1977
Total Employees: 250   *Marketing Staff:* 10   *Sales Staff:* 36
Ownership: Public
Stock Symbol: VIVO
Traded On: NASDAQ
Produces/Sells CE-marked Devices: N
Federal Procurement Eligibility: Small Business
Distribution: Manufacturer Direct, Manufacturer Through Manufacturer Reps, OEM
General Admin.: Mr. John Kraeutler/Chief Executive Officer
       Ms. Melissa Lueke/Chief Financial Officer, Executive Vice
President
Mktg./Adv.: Mr. Todd Motto/Vice President Business Development
       Mr. James Barter/Vice President Marketing & Sales
Production: Mr. Lawrence Baldini/Executive Vice President Operations
       Ms. Susan Rolih/Vice President Quality Assurance & Regulatory
Affairs
Research: Mr. Steve Elagin/Vice President Research & Development

Analyzer, Chemistry, ELISA	Chemistry
Analyzer, Chemistry, Enzyme Immunoassay	Chemistry
Analyzer, Parasite Concentration	Microbiology
Antibody IGM, IF, Epstein-Barr Virus	Microbiology
Antibody, Monoclonal	Microbiology
Antibody, Multiple Auto, Indirect Immunofluorescent	Immunology
Antigen, Antiserum, Control, IGG	Immunology
Antigen, CF And/Or ID, Coccidioides Immitis	Microbiology
Antigen, CF, Mycoplasma SPP.	Microbiology
Antigen, Enzyme Linked Immunoabsorbent Assay, Cryptococcus	Microbiology
Antigen, Latex Agglutination, Coccidioides Immitis	Microbiology
Antigen, Streptococcus SPP.	Microbiology
Antisera, Conjugated Fluorescent, Cytomegalovirus	Microbiology
Antisera, Fluorescent, Chlamydia SPP.	Microbiology
Antiserum, Escherichia Coli	Microbiology
Antiserum, Fluorescent, Chlamydia Trachomatis	Microbiology
Antiserum, Fluorescent, Cryptococcus Neoformans	Microbiology
Antiserum, Latex Agglutination, Cryptococcus Neoformans	Microbiology
Antiserum, Streptococcus SPP.	Microbiology
Campylobacter Pylori	Microbiology
Collector, Specimen	Microbiology
Container, Specimen Mailer And Storage	Pathology
Cryptosporidium Spp.	Microbiology
Enzyme Linked Immunoabsorbent Assay, Chlamydia Group	Microbiology
Enzyme Linked Immunoabsorbent Assay, Coccidioides Immitis	Microbiology
Enzyme Linked Immunoabsorbent Assay, Herpes Simplex Virus	Microbiology
Enzyme Linked Immunoabsorbent Assay, Mycoplasma SPP.	Microbiology
Enzyme Linked Immunoabsorbent Assay, Resp. Syncytial Virus	Microbiology
Enzyme Linked Immunoabsorbent Assay, Rotavirus	Microbiology
Fixative, Formalin Containing	Pathology
Fixative, Metallic Containing	Pathology
Formalin, Neutral Buffered	Pathology
Immunodiffusion Method, Immunoglobulins (G, A, M)	Chemistry
Kit, Identification, Enterobacteriaceae	Microbiology
Kit, Screening, Urine	Microbiology
Media, Mounting, Water Soluble	Pathology
Plate, Radial Immunodiffusion	Immunology
Pneumocystis Carinii	Microbiology
Reagent, Clostridium Difficile Toxin	Microbiology
Respiratory Syncytial Virus, Antigen, Antibody, IFA	Microbiology
Solution, Formalin/Sodium Acetate	Pathology
Stain, Microbiological	Microbiology
Test, Bacterial Diagnostic	Microbiology
Test, Infectious Mononucleosis	Immunology
Test, Rotavirus	Microbiology

Medical Product Subsidiaries (Listed Separately)
   Meridian Life Science, Inc.

MERIDIAN DIAGNOSTICS, INC.
See Meridian Bioscience, Inc.

MERIDIAN LIFE SCIENCE, INC.   800-327-6299
5171 Wilfong Road, Memphis, TN 38134   **901-382-8716**
FDA Number: 1060964   *Fax:* 901-382-0027
E-mail: cGMP@meridianlifescience.com
Web site: www.meridianlifescience.com
Year Founded: 1982
Total Employees: 55   *Marketing Staff:* 3
Ownership: Meridian Life Science, Inc.
Stock Symbol: VIVO
Traded On: NASDAQ
Quality System Registration Information: ISO9001

MERIDIAN LIFE SCIENCE, INC.   800-327-6299 *(cont'd)*

Produces/Sells CE-marked Devices: N
Federal Procurement Eligibility: Small Business
Distribution: OEM
Mktg./Adv.: Mrs. Donna Wright/Manager Marketing
     Mr. Robert M. Studholme/Vice President Marketing

Antigen, Epstein-Barr Virus, Capsid	Microbiology
Antigen, Rubella, Other	Microbiology
Contract Manufacturing, Pharmaceuticals/Chemicals	General
Respiratory Syncytial Virus, Antigen, Antibody, IFA	Microbiology

MERIDIAN LIFE SCIENCE, INC.   888-530-0140
60 Industrial Park Road, Saco, ME 04072   207-283-6500

FDA Number: 1226080   *Fax:* 207-283-4800
E-mail: info@biodesign.com
Web site: http://www.meridianlifescience.com
Year Founded: 1983
Total Employees: 25
Ownership: Meridian Bioscience, Inc.
Stock Symbol: VIVO
Traded On: NASDAQ
Quality System Registration Information: ISO9001
Produces/Sells CE-marked Devices: N
Federal Procurement Eligibility: Small Business
Distribution: Manufacturer Direct, Manufacturer Through Distributor, OEM
General Admin.: Linda Diou/General Director
Mktg./Adv.: Rick Whetstone/Director Sales
Production: Andrew Snyder/Director Manufacturing
     Jim Champlin/Manager Regulatory Affairs

Antibody, Other	General
Reagents, Specific, Analyte	Hematology

Medical Product Subsidiaries (Listed Separately)
   Meridian Life Science, Inc.

MERIDIAN MEDICAL TECHNOLOGIES   800-638-8093
501 Fifth Street, Bristol, TN 37620   443-259-7800

FDA Number: n/a   *Fax:* 443-259-7801
E-mail: info@meridianmt.com
Web site: www.meridianmeds.com
Medical Products Sales Volume: $82,000,000
Annual Revenue: $50-$100 Million
Total Employees: 32   *Marketing Staff:* 3   *Sales Staff:* 3
Ownership: King Pharmaceuticals, Inc.
Produces/Sells CE-marked Devices: N
Federal Procurement Eligibility: Small Business
Distribution: Manufacturer Direct, Manufacturer Through Distributor, OEM, Importer, Exporter
General Admin.: James H. Miller/President, Chief Executive Officer
     Peter Garbis/Vice President Human Resources
     Robert J. Kilgore/Vice President, General Manager
Mktg./Adv.: Geoffrey Ritson/Director National Accounts
     Robert Hill/Director Product Development
     Greg Gonzales/Manager Contract Sales
     Peter Charalambous/Manager International Accounts
     Thomas Mandel/Vice President Sales
Production: Clint Lawson/Director Quality Assurance
     Monica Chiu/Manager Regulatory Affairs
     Don Ferry/Vice President Manufacturing
     Gerald Wannarka/Vice President Regulatory Affairs
Finance: Dennis O'Brien/Chief Financial Officer

Analyzer, Pacemaker Generator Function	Cardiovascular
Injector, Medication (Inoculator)	General
Injector, Syringe	General
Set, Administration, Intravenous, Needle-Free	General
Syringe, Hypodermic	General
Transmitter/Receiver System, ECG, Telephone Single-Channel	Cardiovascular

MERISCO, INC.   414-365-3522
5400 W. Brown Deer Rd., Milwaukee, WI 53223

FDA Number: n/a   *Fax:* 414-365-3537
Web site: meriscowipes.com
Year Founded: 1988
Ownership: Private
Produces/Sells CE-marked Devices: N
Distribution: Manufacturer Direct
General Admin.: William Sauer/President
     Ed Sauer/Vice President
Production: Randy Schmitt/Director Operations
     Jack Davis/Director Quality Assurance

Contract Manufacturing	General

MERIT CABLES, INC.   877-637-4848
830 N. Poinsettia St., Santa Ana, CA 92701   714-918-1932

FDA Number: 2027281   *Fax:* 714-918-1933
E-mail: info@meritcables.com
Web site: www.meritcables.com
Medical Products Sales Volume: $1,700,000
Annual Revenue: $1-$5 Million

MERIT CABLES, INC.   877-637-4848 *(cont'd)*

Year Founded: 1983
Total Employees: 25   *Marketing Staff:* 3   *Sales Staff:* 6
Ownership: Merit Medical Systems, Inc.
Quality System Registration Information: ISO9001
Produces/Sells CE-marked Devices: Y
Federal Procurement Eligibility: Small Business, GSA Contract
Distribution: Manufacturer Direct, Manufacturer Through Distributor, Manufacturer Through Manufacturer Reps, OEM, Exporter
General Admin.: Mr. Ted Hendrickson/Chief Executive Officer
     Mr. David Greenwald/Chief Operating Officer
     Darrell Garland/President
     Jose Cortez/Vice President, General Manager
Mktg./Adv.: Andrea Bohl/Vice President Marketing & Sales
Production: Mark Neeley/Manager Quality Assurance & Regulatory Affairs
Finance: Mr. Ruben Mauricio/Chief Financial Officer

Component, Electrical	General

MERIT MEDICAL SYSTEMS INC.   804-416-1030
12701 Kingston Ave, Chesterfield, VA 23837

FDA Number: 1125782   *Fax:* 804-416-1031
Web site: http://www.merit.com/
Year Founded: 1997
Total Employees: 27   *Sales Staff:* 10
Ownership: Merit Medical Systems, Inc.
Stock Symbol: MMSI
Traded On: NASDAQ
Produces/Sells CE-marked Devices: N
Federal Procurement Eligibility: Small Business
Distribution: Manufacturer Direct, Manufacturer Through Distributor, Manufacturer Through Manufacturer Reps, OEM
General Admin.: Bob Hale/Chief Executive Officer
     Gary Kazee/Chief Operating Officer
     Jon Chase/Vice President
Mktg./Adv.: Sheryl Duncan/Manager Sales Admin.
Finance: Charles Long/Chief Financial Officer

Kit, Administration, Intravenous	General
Kit, Biopsy	General
Kit, Disposable Procedure	Cardiovascular
Kit, Incision And Drainage	Surgery
Kit, Prep	General
Kit, Surgical Instrument, Disposable	Surgery
Kit, Wound Dressing	Surgery
Tray, Blood Collection	Hematology
Tray, Custom/Special Procedure	General
Tray, Start/Stop (Including Contents), Dialysis	Gastroenterology/Urology
Tray, Surgical	Surgery

MERIT MEDICAL SYSTEMS LTD.   800-667-5720
2209-A Dunwin Dr.,   905-828-7511
Mississauga, ONT L5L-1 Canada

FDA Number: n/a   *Fax:* 905-828-9344
E-mail: merit@netrover.com
Web site: www.meritmedsyst.com
Year Founded: 1976
Total Employees: 10
Ownership: Merit Medical Systems, Inc.
Produces/Sells CE-marked Devices: N
Distribution: Exclusive Distributor, Importer

MERIT MEDICAL SYSTEMS, INC.   1-800-35-MERIT
1111 South Velasco, Angleton, TX 77515   801-253-1600

FDA Number: 1628221   *Fax:* 1-801-253-1652
Ownership: Merit Medical Systems, Inc.
Stock Symbol: MMSI
Traded On: NASDAQ
Produces/Sells CE-marked Devices: N

Catheter, Balloon (Foley Type)	Surgery
Catheter, Intravascular, Diagnostic	Cardiovascular
Catheter, Percutaneous	Cardiovascular
Cleaner, Needle	General
Dilator, Vessel, Percutaneous Catheterization	Cardiovascular
Guidewire, Catheter	Cardiovascular
Introducer, Catheter	Cardiovascular
Kit, Administration, Intravenous	General
Regulator, Thermal, Cardiopulmonary Bypass	Cardiovascular
Stopcock	General
Syringe, Balloon Inflation	Cardiovascular
Trocar, Cardiovascular	Cardiovascular

MERIT MEDICAL SYSTEMS, INC.   800-356-3748
1600 W. Merit Pkwy., South Jordan, UT 84095   801-253-1600

FDA Number: 1721504   *Fax:* 801-253-1652
E-mail: awright@merit.com
Web site: www.merit.com
Medical Products Sales Volume: $116,000,000
Annual Revenue: $100-$500 Million
Year Founded: 1987

MERIT MEDICAL SYSTEMS, INC.   800-356-3748 (cont'd)

Total Employees: 1700	Marketing Staff: 11	Sales Staff: 72

Ownership: Public
Stock Symbol: MMSI
Traded On: NASDAQ
Quality System Registration Information: ISO9001
Produces/Sells CE-marked Devices: Y
Distribution: Manufacturer Direct
General Admin.: Mr. Arlin Nelson/Chief Operating Officer
     Fred P Lampropoulos/President, Chief Executive Officer
Mktg./Adv.: Mr. Martin Stephens/Executive Vice President Marketing & Sales
Finance: Kent Stanger/Chief Financial Officer

Adapter, Stopcock, Manifold, Cardiopulmonary Bypass	Cardiovascular
Catheter, Continuous Flush	Cardiovascular
Catheter, Intravascular, Diagnostic	Cardiovascular
Guidewire, Catheter	Cardiovascular
Introducer, Catheter	Cardiovascular
Kit, Administration, Intravenous	General
Needle, Angiographic	Cns/Neurology
Syringe, Balloon Inflation	Cardiovascular
Syringe, Piston	General
Transducer, Blood Pressure, Extravascular	Cardiovascular
Tubing, Fluid Delivery	General

Medical Product Subsidiaries (Listed Separately)
   Ameritek Usa, Inc.
   Merit Cables, Inc.
   Merit Medical Systems Inc.
   Merit Medical Systems Ltd.
   Merit Medical Systems, Inc.
   Prestige Ameritech

MERITECH, INC.   800-932-7707
600 Corporate Circle, Suite H, Golden, CO 80401   303-790-4670

FDA Number: n/a   Fax: 303-790-4859
E-mail: cleantech@meritech.com
Web site: www.meritech.com
Medical Products Sales Volume: $200,000
Annual Revenue: $5-$10 Million
Year Founded: 1986

Total Employees: 2	Marketing Staff: 1	Sales Staff: 6

Ownership: Private
Produces/Sells CE-marked Devices: N
Federal Procurement Eligibility: Small Business
Distribution: Manufacturer Direct
General Admin.: Paul Barnhill/President
Mktg./Adv.: Michele Colbert/Marketing Coordinator
Production: Chris Maybach/Design Engineer

Sanitizer	General
Sink, Hospital	General
Soap	General

MERLIN LABS, INC.   760-804-1782
6082 Corte Del Cedro, Carlsbad, CA 92011

FDA Number: 3004955131

Kit, Test, Malaria	Toxicology

MERLIN'S MEDICAL SUPPLY   800-639-9322
699 Mobil Avenue, Camarillo, CA 93010   805-388-7669

FDA Number: n/a   Fax: 805-389-8142
E-mail: merlinpaul@aol.com
Medical Products Sales Volume: $400,000
Annual Revenue: $1-$5 Million
Year Founded: 1985

Total Employees: 6	Marketing Staff: 3	Sales Staff: 2

Ownership: Merlin's Medical Supply
Quality System Registration Information: ISO9002
Produces/Sells CE-marked Devices: N
Federal Procurement Eligibility: Small Business
Distribution: Manufacturer Direct, Manufacturer Through Distributor, Manufacturer Through Manufacturer Reps, Exclusive Distributor, Exporter
General Admin.: Paul Dwork/President, Chief Executive Officer

Accessories, Catheter	Surgery
Catheter, Urinary, Condom	Gastroenterology/Urology
Contract R&D, Diagnostics	General

Medical Product Subsidiaries (Listed Separately)
   Leading Edge Innovations
   Merlin's Medical Supply

MERLO CO., LLC.   800-290-9199
62038 MN Highway 24, PO Box 570,   320-593-4006
Litchfield, MN 55355

FDA Number: 2135131
E-mail: info@cuddleewe.com   Fax: 320-693-2288
Web site: www.cuddleewe.com
Medical Products Sales Volume: $300,000
Annual Revenue: $0-$1 Million
Year Founded: 2003

Total Employees: 5	Marketing Staff: 1	Sales Staff: 1

MERLO CO., LLC.   800-290-9199 (cont'd)

Ownership: Private
Produces/Sells CE-marked Devices: N
Federal Procurement Eligibility: Small Business
Distribution: Manufacturer Direct
General Admin.: Mr. John Merrill/Partner

Mattress, Non-Powered Flotation Therapy	Physical Med

MERLYN PHARMACEUTICALS, INC.   513-831-3005
8175 Kroger Farm Rd., Cincinnati, OH 45243-1639

FDA Number: n/a   Fax: 513-831-5237
E-mail: merlynp@yahoo.com
Web site: merlynp.homestead.com
Total Employees: 20
Ownership: Private
Quality System Registration Information: ISO9001
Produces/Sells CE-marked Devices: N
Federal Procurement Eligibility: Small Business, Minority Owned, Female Owned
Distribution: OEM
General Admin.: Mary Ann Baker/Chief Financial Officer, Vice President
     James Baker/President
Production: Tom Hart/Manager Production

Airway, Nasopharyngeal (Breathing Tube)	Anesthesiology
Balloon, Epistaxis (Nasal)	Ear/Nose/Throat
Blade, Electrosurgery, Laparoscopic	Surgery
Bougie, Esophageal, And Gastrointestinal, Gastro-Urology	Gastroenterology/Urology
Camera, Television, Endoscopic (With Audio)	Surgery
Camera, Video, Endoscopic	General
Catheter, Balloon (Foley Type)	Surgery
Catheter, Continuous Irrigation	Surgery
Catheter, Coude	Gastroenterology/Urology
Catheter, Depezzer	Gastroenterology/Urology
Catheter, Irrigation	Surgery
Catheter, Jejunostomy	Gastroenterology/Urology
Catheter, Malecot (Gastrostomy Tube)	Gastroenterology/Urology
Catheter, Multiple Lumen	Surgery
Catheter, Nelaton	Gastroenterology/Urology
Catheter, Nephrostomy, General & Plastic Surgery	Surgery
Catheter, Pediatric, General & Plastic Surgery	Surgery
Catheter, Retention Type, Balloon	Gastroenterology/Urology
Catheter, Suction (Tracheal Aspirating Tube)	Anesthesiology
Catheter, Suprapubic, With Tube	Gastroenterology/Urology
Catheter, Ureteral, Gastro-Urology	Gastroenterology/Urology
Catheter, Ureteral, General & Plastic Surgery	Surgery
Catheter, Urethral	Gastroenterology/Urology
Catheter, Urinary	Gastroenterology/Urology
Catheter, Urinary, Condom	Gastroenterology/Urology
Catheter, Urinary, Irrigation	Gastroenterology/Urology
Clamp, Bone	Orthopedics
Clamp, Other	Surgery
Cutter, Ring	General
Cutter, Wire And Pin	Orthopedics
Dislodger, Stone, Basket, Ureteral, Metal	Gastroenterology/Urology
Dislodger, Stone, Flexible	Gastroenterology/Urology
Drain, T	Gastroenterology/Urology
Drill, Bone	Orthopedics
Driver, Bone Staple	Orthopedics
Elevator, Surgical, Dental	Dental And Oral
Excavator, Dental, Operative	Dental And Oral
Extractor, Nail	Orthopedics
File, Bone, Surgical	Dental And Oral
Fixation Device, Jaw Fracture	Orthopedics
Forceps	Orthopedics
Forceps, Biopsy	Surgery
Forceps, Disconnect	Gastroenterology/Urology
Forceps, Dressing	Surgery
Forceps, Dressing, Dental	Dental And Oral
Forceps, Endoscopic	Gastroenterology/Urology
Forceps, Epilation	Surgery
Forceps, Fixation	Surgery
Forceps, Hemostatic	Surgery
Forceps, Intestinal (Clamps)	Gastroenterology/Urology
Forceps, Obstetrical	Obstetrics/Gynecology
Forceps, Ophthalmic	Ophthalmology
Forceps, Rubber Dam Clamp	Dental And Oral
Forceps, Sponge	Surgery
Forceps, Tissue	Surgery
Forceps, Tonsil	Ear/Nose/Throat
Forceps, Utility	Surgery
Glove, Surgical	General
Glove, Surgical, Hypoallergenic	General
Hammer, Neurological	Cns/Neurology
Hammer, Percussion	Cns/Neurology
Handle, Knife Blade	Surgery
Holder, Needle	Gastroenterology/Urology
Instrument, Dental, Manual	Dental And Oral
Insufflator, Laparoscopic	Obstetrics/Gynecology
Kit, Administration, Intravenous	General
Knife, Amputation	Surgery
Knife, Cataract	Ophthalmology
Knife, Ear	Ear/Nose/Throat

MERLYN PHARMACEUTICALS, INC.   513-831-3005 *(cont'd)*

Knife, Meniscus	Surgery
Knife, Other	Surgery
Knife, Scalpel	Surgery
Knife, Sternum	Surgery
Knife, Tonsil	Ear/Nose/Throat
Laparoscope, Flexible	Surgery
Laparoscope, General & Plastic Surgery	Surgery
Mallet, Bone	Orthopedics
Mallet, Dental	Dental And Oral
Osteotome (Orthopedic)	Surgery
Plate, Fixation, Bone	Orthopedics
Punch, Bone	Orthopedics
Punch, Dental, Rubber Dam	Dental And Oral
Rasp, Bone	Orthopedics
Retractor, Abdominal	Surgery
Retractor, Brain	Cns/Neurology
Retractor, Laminectomy	Surgery
Retractor, Other	Surgery
Retractor, Rib	Orthopedics
Retractor, Self-Retaining	Gastroenterology/Urology
Rongeur, Dental	Dental And Oral
Rongeur, Intervertebral Disk	Orthopedics
Rongeur, Other	Surgery
Rongeur, Rib	Orthopedics
Saw, Bone Cutting	Orthopedics
Saw, Bone, Pneumatic	Orthopedics
Saw, Electric Bone	Dental And Oral
Saw, Other	Surgery
Scissors, Bandage/Gauze/Plaster	General
Scissors, Cardiovascular	Cardiovascular
Scissors, Corneal	Ophthalmology
Scissors, Orthopedic	Orthopedics
Scissors, Pediatric	General
Scissors, Plastic Surgery (Dissecting)	Surgery
Scissors, Suture	Surgery
Screw, Fixation, Bone	Orthopedics
System, Appliance, Fixation, Spinal Pedicle Screw	Orthopedics
Tube, Colon	Gastroenterology/Urology
Tube, Connecting	General
Tube, Feeding	General
Tube, Levine	General
Tube, Rectal	Gastroenterology/Urology
Tube, Tracheal (Endotracheal)	Anesthesiology
Tubing, Braided	General
Tubing, Conductive	General
Tubing, Latex	General
Tubing, Multi-Lumen	General
Tubing, Non-Conductive	General
Tubing, Non-Invasive	Surgery
Tubing, Nylon	General
Tubing, Oxygen Connecting	General
Tubing, Plastic	General
Tubing, Polyethylene	General
Tubing, Polyvinyl Chloride	General
Tubing, Radiopaque	General
Tubing, Silicone	General
Tubing, Urethane	General
Tubing, Vinyl	General

MEROCEL SURGICAL PRODUCTS
See Medtronic Xomed, Inc.

MERRY WALKER CORP.   847-837-9580
21350 S. Sylvan Drive, Unit 9 Box P, Mundelein, IL 60060
FDA Number: 1422355   *Fax: 847-837-9582*
E-mail: customerservice@merrywalker.com
Web site: www.merrywalker.com
Medical Products Sales Volume: $500,000
Annual Revenue: $0-$1 Million
Year Founded: 1990
Total Employees: 2   *Marketing Staff: 2*   *Sales Staff: 2*
Ownership: Private
Produces/Sells CE-marked Devices: Y
Federal Procurement Eligibility: Small Business, Female Owned, VA Contract
Distribution: Manufacturer Direct, Manufacturer Through Distributor, Manufacturer Through Manufacturer Reps, Service Direct, Exporter
General Admin.: Kathy Thoma/General Manager
      Mary M. Harroun/President, Chief Executive Officer
Mktg./Adv.: Mary M. Harroun/Director Product Development
      Heather Brauer/Vice President Marketing & Sales
Production: Mark Clark/Director Quality Assurance
      Mary M. Harroun/Manager Regulatory Affairs

Cane, Safety Walk	Physical Med
Walker, Mechanical	Physical Med

MERUS LABS INTERNATIONAL INC.   604-221-0595
1177 West Hastings Street, Suite 2007,
Vancouver, B.C. V6E 2 Canada
FDA Number: n/a   *Fax: 604-225-0588*
E-mail: adoroudian@meruslabs.com

MERUS LABS INTERNATIONAL INC.   604-221-0595 *(cont'd)*
Ownership: Private
Produces/Sells CE-marked Devices: N

MES, INC.   800-423-2215
1968 E US Hwy 90, Seguin, TX 78155   **830-372-5913**
FDA Number: n/a   *Fax: 830-372-3015*
E-mail: info@mymesinc.com
Web site: www.mesinc.cc
Year Founded: 1967
Ownership: Private
Produces/Sells CE-marked Devices: N
Federal Procurement Eligibility: Small Business
Distribution: Manufacturer Direct, Manufacturer Through Distributor, Service Direct, Importer, Exporter
General Admin.: James Borre/President
Production: Mr. Jeremy Ward/Customer Service Representative

Bag, Plastic	General
Cart, Gas Cylinder (Carrier)	Anesthesiology
Cover, Mattress	General
Cover, Mattress, Waterproof	General
Cover, Other	General
Fixation Device, Tracheal Tube	Anesthesiology
Sealer, Packaging	General
Tent, Pediatric Aerosol	General

MESA LABORATORIES, INC.   800-992-6372
12100 W. 6th Avenue, Lakewood, CO 80228   **303-987-8000**
FDA Number: 1720309   *Fax: 303-987-8989*
E-mail: InvestorRelations@mesalabs.com
Web site: www.mesalabs.com
Medical Products Sales Volume: $21,929,000
Annual Revenue: $10-$25 Million
Year Founded: 1982
Total Employees: 112   *Marketing Staff: 2*   *Sales Staff: 4*
Ownership: Public
Stock Symbol: MLAB
Traded On: NASDAQ
Produces/Sells CE-marked Devices: Y
Federal Procurement Eligibility: Small Business
Distribution: Manufacturer Direct, Manufacturer Through Distributor, Manufacturer Through Manufacturer Reps
General Admin.: Luke R. Schmieder/President, Chief Executive Officer
Mktg./Adv.: John Sullivan/Director Marketing & Sales
      John Sullivan/Director National Accounts
Finance: Steve Peterson/Chief Financial Officer, Vice President Finance

Dialysis Unit Test Equipment	Gastroenterology/Urology
Dialyzer Reprocessing System	Gastroenterology/Urology
General Medical Device	General
Monitor, Hemodialysis Unit Conductivity	Gastroenterology/Urology
Reprocessing Unit, Dialyzer	Gastroenterology/Urology

MESA MEDICAL
See Mesa Laboratories, Inc.

MESA, INC.   210-699-6911
9807 Fredericksburg Rd., San Antonio, TX 78240
FDA Number: 1651561
Ownership: Private
Produces/Sells CE-marked Devices: N

Lift, Bath, Non-AC-Powered	General

MESSER GRIESHAM INDUSTRIES
See Praxair Distribution Mid-Atlantic LLC

MESSERLI ENTERPRISES, INC.
See MEI Corporation

MESTAMED
See Carecentric, Inc.

MET LABORATORIES, INC.   800-638-6057
914 W. Patapsco Avenue,   **410-354-3300**
Baltimore, MD 21230
FDA Number: n/a   *Fax: 410-354-3313*
E-mail: info@metlabs.com
Web site: www.metlabs.com
Medical Products Sales Volume: $200,000,000
Annual Revenue: $10-$25 Million
Year Founded: 1959
Total Employees: 100   *Marketing Staff: 2*   *Sales Staff: 5*
Ownership: Private
Stock Symbol: LARD
Traded On: London
Federal Procurement Eligibility: Small Business
General Admin.: Robert Frier/President
Mktg./Adv.: Jim McDonald/Manager Advertising
      Kevin Harbarger/Manager National Sales
      Troy Franklin/Vice President Business Development
      Kevin Harbarger/Vice President Sales

MET LABORATORIES, INC.
800-638-6057 (cont'd)
Service, Licensing, Device, Medical
General

MET-PRO CORP., SETHCO DIV.
See Met-Pro Corporation

MET-PRO CORPORATION
215-723-6751
160 Cassell Road, P.O. Box 144, Harleysville, PA 19438
FDA Number: n/a
Fax: 215-723-6758
E-mail: mpr@met-pro.com
Web site: www.met-pro.com
Annual Revenue: $5-$10 Million
Total Employees: 50   Marketing Staff: 3   Sales Staff: 10
Ownership: MET-PRO CORPORATION
Stock Symbol: MPR
Traded On: NYSE
Produces/Sells CE-marked Devices: N
Federal Procurement Eligibility: Small Business
Distribution: Manufacturer Through Distributor
General Admin.: William Kacin/President
         Mark Betchader/Vice President, General Manager
Mktg./Adv.: Ernest Carman/Manager Advertising
         James Cascro/Manager National Sales
Pump, Laboratory   Chemistry
Unit, Filter, Membrane   Chemistry

META FUSION, INC.
408-345-0500
15209 Blue Gum Court, Saratoga, CA 95070
FDA Number: 101133
Ownership: Private
Produces/Sells CE-marked Devices: N
Device, Storage, Image, Digital   Radiology

META HEALTH TECHNOLOGY INC.
800-334-6840
212-695-5870
330 Seventh Avenue, New York, NY 10001-3904
FDA Number: n/a
Fax: 212-643-2913
E-mail: brosenberg@metahealth.com
Web site: www.metahealth.com
Medical Products Sales Volume: $3,200,000
Year Founded: 1978
Total Employees: 20   Marketing Staff: 3   Sales Staff: 5
Ownership: Private
Produces/Sells CE-marked Devices: N
Federal Procurement Eligibility: Small Business
Distribution: Manufacturer Direct
General Admin.: Eli Nahmias/President
Mktg./Adv.: Bob Rosenberg/Vice President Sales
Computer Software   General
Service, Consulting   General

META SOFTWARE, INC.
See Meta Health Technology Inc.

METABOLIC SOLUTIONS, INC.
866-302-1998
603-598-6960
460 Amherst St., Nashua, NH 03063-1220
FDA Number: 1223869
Fax: 603-598-6973
E-mail: info@metsol.com
Web site: www.metsol.com
Medical Products Sales Volume: $400,000
Annual Revenue: $1-$5 Million
Year Founded: 1990
Total Employees: 7
Ownership: Private
Produces/Sells CE-marked Devices: N
Federal Procurement Eligibility: Small Business
Distribution: Manufacturer Direct, Manufacturer Through Distributor, Service Direct
Production: Martin Baker/Executive Vice President Operations
General Purpose Microbiology Diagnostic Device   Microbiology
Probe, Gastrointestinal   Gastroenterology/Urology
Test, Urea (Breath or Blood)   Microbiology

METABOLON INC.
919-572-1711
617 Davis Drive, Suite 400, Durham, NC 27713
FDA Number: n/a
Fax: 919-572-1721
E-mail: info@metabolon.com
Web site: www.metabolon.com
Ownership: Private
Produces/Sells CE-marked Devices: N
General Admin.: Dr. Mike Milburn/Chief Scientific Officer
         Dr. John Ryals/President, Chief Executive Officer
Mktg./Adv.: Mr. Chris Bernard/Senior Vice President Marketing & Sales
Finance: Mr. S. Todd Lynch/Chief Financial Officer

METAL TECHOLOGY, INC.
800-394-9979
541-926-9968
173 Queen Ave., S.E., Albany, OR 97321-9905
FDA Number: n/a
Fax: 541-928-0596
E-mail: sales@mtialbany.com
Web site: www.mtialbany.com
Annual Revenue: $1-$5 Million

METAL TECHOLOGY, INC.
800-394-9979 (cont'd)
Year Founded: 1971
Total Employees: 14   Marketing Staff: 1   Sales Staff: 2
Ownership: MT HOLDINGS, INC.
Produces/Sells CE-marked Devices: N
Federal Procurement Eligibility: Small Business, Female Owned
Distribution: Manufacturer Direct
General Admin.: Patrick Coffey/General Manager
         Michael L. DeBonny/President, Chief Executive Officer
Mktg./Adv.: Pam Montellano/Manager Marketing
Production: Patrick Coffey/Vice President Operations
Labware, Basic, Reusable   Chemistry

METAL-FAB INC.
See Micro Air Air Cleaners By Metal-Fab

METALCRAFT INDUSTRIES, INC.
608-835-3232
399 North Burr Oak Ave, Fitchburg, WI 53575
FDA Number: 2134716
Accessories, Wheelchair   Physical Med

METALOR TECHNOLOGIES USA
800-554-5504
011-413-2720
255 John L. Dietsch Blvd., PO Box 255,
North Attleborough, MA 02761
FDA Number: 2435711
Fax: 508-695-1603
E-mail: denta.us@metalor.com
Web site: www.metalor.com
Medical Products Sales Volume: $45,400,000
Year Founded: 1852
Total Employees: 150
Ownership: METALOR TECHNOLOGIES INTERNATIONAL SA
Quality System Registration Information: ISO9002
Produces/Sells CE-marked Devices: N
Federal Procurement Eligibility: Small Business
Production: Mike Davis/Director Operations
Alloy, Gold Based, For Clinical Use   Dental And Oral
Alloy, Precious Metal, For Clinical Use   Dental And Oral
Attachment, Precision   Dental And Oral
Metal, Base   Dental And Oral
Post, Root Canal   Dental And Oral

METAMARK GENETICS INC.
617-583-1400
245 First Street, Suite 150, Cambridge, MA 02142
FDA Number: n/a
E-mail: info@metamarkgenetics.com
Web site: http://www.metamarkgenetics.com
Year Founded: 2007
Ownership: Private
Produces/Sells CE-marked Devices: N
General Admin.: Mr. Kenneth Weg/Chief Executive Officer
         Dr. Peter Blume-Jensen/Chief Scientific Officer
Mktg./Adv.: Dr. Eric Devroe/Director Business Development
Finance: Mr. David Cordo/Chief Financial Officer

METICO INSTRUMENTS
See Akorn, Inc.

METREX INFECTION CONTROL PRODUCTS
See Metrex Research Corp.

METREX RESEARCH CORP.
800-841-1428
714-516-7788
28210 Wick Rd., Romulus, MI 48174
FDA Number: 1722021
Fax: 714-516-7581
E-mail: info@metrex.com
Web site: www.metrex.com
Annual Revenue: $10-$25 Million
Year Founded: 1985
Total Employees: 150   Marketing Staff: 4   Sales Staff: 22
Ownership: Sybron Dental Specialties, Inc.
Quality System Registration Information: ISO9002
Produces/Sells CE-marked Devices: Y
Distribution: Manufacturer Through Distributor, Exporter
General Admin.: Todd Norbe/President
         Jason Harris/Regional Manager
         Patrick Kiley/Regional Manager
         Thomas Restuccia/Regional Manager
Mktg./Adv.: Marcus Browne/National Accounts Manager
         Rob Starcher/Vice President Advertising & Sales
Aligner, Beam, X-Ray (Collimator)   Dental And Oral
Cover, Barrier, Protective   General
Disinfector, Liquid   General
Disinfector, Medical Device   General
Handpiece, Air-Powered, Dental   Dental And Oral
Holder, X-Ray Film   Dental And Oral
Lubricant, Instrument   General
Solution, Antibacterial Cleaner   General
Sterilant, Medical Device   General
Washer/Disinfector   General

METRIKA, INC.
See Bayer Healthcare, Llc

METRO CAD, INC
612-302-8056
2277-49th Avenue North, Minneapolis, MN 55430
FDA Number: n/a
E-mail: pauls@metro-cad.com
Fax: 612-302-7672
Web site: www.metro-cad.com
Annual Revenue: $0-$1 Million
Year Founded: 1988
Total Employees: 4   *Sales Staff:* 3
Ownership: Private
Produces/Sells CE-marked Devices: Y
Federal Procurement Eligibility: Small Business
Distribution: Manufacturer Direct, Manufacturer Through Manufacturer Reps, Exclusive Distributor
Mktg./Adv.: Mr. Paul Sullivan/Sales Specialist
   Security Equipment/Supplies   General

METRO EQUIPMENT CORP.
See Yamato Corporation

METRO MEDICAL EQUIPMENT, INC.
734-522-8400
12985 Wayne Road, Livonia, MI 48150
FDA Number: 1834250
E-mail: metromedical@sbcglobal.net
Fax: 734-522-9380
Medical Products Sales Volume: $2,700,000
Year Founded: 1986
Total Employees: 45
Ownership: Private
Produces/Sells CE-marked Devices: N
Federal Procurement Eligibility: Small Business
General Admin.: Paul Mocur/President
   Accessories, Wheelchair   Physical Med

METRO MEDICAL SUPPLY WHOLESALE
800-768-2002
200 Cumberland Bend, Nashville, TN 37228
615-329-2002
FDA Number: n/a
E-mail: customersvc@metromedical.com
Fax: 615-256-4194
Web site: www.metromedical.com
Year Founded: 1985
Total Employees: 68   *Marketing Staff:* 1   *Sales Staff:* 10
Ownership: Private
Produces/Sells CE-marked Devices: N
Distribution: Manufacturer Through Distributor
General Admin.: F.H. Tompkins/Chief Operating Officer
   Bart Ashley/President, Chief Executive Officer
Mktg./Adv.: Mike Tigert/Director Marketing & Sales
   Collector, Ostomy   Gastroenterology/Urology
   Concentrator, Oxygen   Anesthesiology
   Ostomy Appliance (Ileostomy, Colostomy)   Gastroenterology/Urology
   Walker, Mechanical   Physical Med
   Wheelchair, Manual   Physical Med

METRO OPTICS OF AUSTIN, LTD.
512-251-2382
15802 Vision Dr., Pflugerville, TX 78660
FDA Number: 1627258
   Lenses, Soft Contact, Daily Wear   Ophthalmology

METRON OPTICS, INC.
858-755-4477
813 Academy Drive, Solana Beach, CA 92075-0690
FDA Number: n/a
E-mail: mail@metronusa.com
Fax: 858-755-4752
Web site: www.metronusa.com
Medical Products Sales Volume: $2,500,000
Annual Revenue: $1-$5 Million
Year Founded: 1971
Total Employees: 8   *Marketing Staff:* 1   *Sales Staff:* 1
Ownership: Private
Produces/Sells CE-marked Devices: N
Federal Procurement Eligibility: Small Business, Minority Owned, Female Owned
Distribution: Manufacturer Direct, Manufacturer Through Distributor, Manufacturer Through Manufacturer Reps, OEM, Exporter
General Admin.: Charles Kempf/Chief Executive Officer
   Charles Kempf/President
   Pilar Kempf/Vice President
Mktg./Adv.: Dany C. Starr/Manager National Sales
   Endoscope, Flexible   Gastroenterology/Urology
   Endoscope, Rigid   Surgery
   Mirror, Mouth   Dental And Oral
   System, Marking, Laser   General

METRONIX
813-972-1212
12421 N. Florida Avenue, Suite D-201, Tampa, FL 33612-4201
FDA Number: 1051091
E-mail: metronix@att.net
Fax: 813-932-4200
Web site: www.metronixinc.com
Medical Products Sales Volume: $1,100,000
Annual Revenue: $1-$5 Million

METRONIX
813-972-1212 *(cont'd)*
Year Founded: 1980
Total Employees: 8   *Marketing Staff:* 2   *Sales Staff:* 4
Ownership: Private
Stock Symbol: MDT
Traded On: NYSE
Quality System Registration Information: ISO9002
Produces/Sells CE-marked Devices: N
Federal Procurement Eligibility: Small Business
Distribution: Manufacturer Through Distributor, Exclusive Distributor, Exporter
General Admin.: Dr. A. R. Tashkandi/Chief Executive Officer
   Adrien Ragazzi/Office Manager
   Mathew Ninan/President, Chief Executive Officer
   James Orvis/Vice President Human Resources
   Molly Ninan/Vice President, General Manager
Mktg./Adv.: Tony Abraham/Director Marketing
   Tony Abraham/Director National Accounts
   A. B. Dike/Director Product Development
   Maria Abraham/Manager Advertising
   Mathew Ninan/Manager Contract Sales
   Mathew Ninan/Manager International & National Sales
   Tony Abraham/Manager Market Research
   Mathew Ninan/Manager Sales Training
   James Orvis/Vice President Business Development
   Mathew Ninan/Vice President Sales
Production: A. B. Dike/Director Quality Assurance
   Adrienne Ragazzi/Manager Materials
   Thomas Mathew/Manager Regulatory Affairs
Research: Mathew Ninan/Vice President Research & Development
   Ambulance   General
   Cart, Medicine   General
   Contract Assembly   General
   Contract Manufacturing   General
   Kit, First Aid   Surgery
   Service, Import/Export   General
   System, Test, Drugs of Abuse   Chemistry

METROPOLITAN WIRE CORP.
See Intermetro Industries Corp.

METTLER ELECTRONICS CORP.
800-854-9305
1333 S. Claudina Street,
714-533-2221
Anaheim, CA 92805
FDA Number: 2013558
E-mail: mail@mettlerelectronics.com
Fax: 714-635-7539
Web site: www.mettlerelectronics.com
Annual Revenue: $5-$10 Million
Year Founded: 1957
Total Employees: 50   *Marketing Staff:* 1   *Sales Staff:* 6
Ownership: Private
Produces/Sells CE-marked Devices: Y
Federal Procurement Eligibility: Small Business
Distribution: Manufacturer Through Distributor, Manufacturer Through Manufacturer Reps, OEM, Importer, Exporter
General Admin.: Stephen C. Mettler/Chairman
   Mark Mettler/President
Mktg./Adv.: Jennifer Rohl/Manager Marketing
   Matt Mettler/Vice President Marketing & Sales
Production: Aftab Kapadya/Manager Engineering
   Stacy Mclean/Manager Manufacturing
   Rob Fleming/Manager Regulatory Affairs
Finance: Matthew Ferrari/Chief Controller
   Cleaner, Ultrasonic, Medical Instrument   General
   Diathermy, Shortwave   Physical Med
   Diathermy, Ultrasonic (Physical Therapy)   Physical Med
   Gel, Ultrasonic Transmission   General
   Lamp, Infrared   Physical Med
   Pump, Infusion   General
   Solution, Instrument Cleaner   General
   Stimulator, Muscle, Electrical-Powered (EMS)   Physical Med
   Stimulator, Ultrasound, Muscle   Physical Med

METTLER INSTRUMENT CORP.
See Mettler-Toledo, Inc.

METTLER TOLEDO LASENTEC PRODUCTS (LASENTEC)
425-881-7117
14833 Ne 87th St, Redmond, WA 98052
FDA Number: n/a
E-mail: info@lasentec.com
Fax: 425-881-8964
Web site: www.lasentec.com
Medical Products Sales Volume: $2,800,000
Annual Revenue: $1-$5 Million
Year Founded: 1981
Total Employees: 30   *Marketing Staff:* 4   *Sales Staff:* 6
Ownership: Mettler-Toledo, Inc.
Quality System Registration Information: ISO9001
Produces/Sells CE-marked Devices: Y
Federal Procurement Eligibility: Small Business

MANUFACTURER PROFILES

METTLER TOLEDO LASENTEC PRODUCTS   425-881-7117
(cont'd)

Distribution: Manufacturer Direct, Service Direct
Mktg./Adv.: Rich Becker/Vice President Marketing
Production: John Hokanson/Vice President Manufacturing
Research: John Hokanson/Vice President Research & Development

Analyzer, Coagulation   Hematology

METTLER-TOLEDO GROUP   800 METTLER (80
1900 Polaris Parkway, Columbus, OH 43240   **(614) 438-4972**
FDA Number: n/a   *Fax:* :(614) 985-8122
E-mail: Matt.Wilson@mt.com
Total Employees: 6000
Ownership: Private
Quality System Registration Information: ISO9001
Produces/Sells CE-marked Devices: Y
Distribution: Manufacturer Direct, Importer, Exporter
Mktg./Adv.: Mrs. Lynch/Corporate Communications Specialist
     Thomar Khehr/Director Marketing

Balance, Electronic	Chemistry
Balance, Macro (0.1 mg Accuracy)	Chemistry
Balance, Semimicro (0.01 mg Accuracy)	Chemistry
Balance, Ultramicro (0.0001 mg Accuracy)	Chemistry
Reaction Apparatus	Microbiology
Titrator	Chemistry
Unit, Imaging, Thermal	Radiology

Medical Product Subsidiaries (Listed Separately)
Mettler-Toledo Gmbh

METTLER-TOLEDO PROCESS ANALYTICAL, INC.   800-352-8763

36 Middlesex Turnpike, Bedford, MA 01730   **781-939-6300**
FDA Number: n/a   *Fax:* 781-939-6390
E-mail: mark.ecker@mt.com
Web site: www.mt.com
Medical Products Sales Volume: $12,000
Annual Revenue: $5-$10 Million
Total Employees: 80   *Marketing Staff:* 3   *Sales Staff:* 5
Ownership: Mettler-Toledo, Inc.
Quality System Registration Information: ISO9001
Produces/Sells CE-marked Devices: Y
Federal Procurement Eligibility: Small Business
Distribution: Manufacturer Through Distributor

Electrofocusing Equipment	Chemistry
Fermentation Equipment	Microbiology

METTLER-TOLEDO, INC.   800-638-8537
1900 Polaris Pkwy., Columbus, OH 43240   **614-438-4511**
FDA Number: 7000256   *Fax:* 614-438-4900
E-mail: TellMeMore@mt.com
Web site: www.mt.com
Annual Revenue: $50-$100 Million
Year Founded: 1945
Total Employees: 702
Ownership: Public
Stock Symbol: MTD
Traded On: NYSE
Quality System Registration Information: ISO9000; ISO9001
Produces/Sells CE-marked Devices: Y
Distribution: Manufacturer Direct, Manufacturer Through Distributor, Manufacturer Through Manufacturer Reps
General Admin.: Robert Spoerry/Chief Executive Officer
     Ken Peters/President
     Alexis Street/Vice President Human Resources
     Kia Serajfar/Vice President, General Manager
Mktg./Adv.: Michael Ross/Director National Accounts
     George McLean/Manager Product Marketing
     Ian Ciesniewski/Manager Product Marketing
Production: Hans Joerg Burkhard/Director Quality Assurance

Balance, Electronic	Chemistry
Balance, Macro (0.1 mg Accuracy)	Chemistry
Balance, Micro (0.001 mg Accuracy)	Chemistry
Balance, Semimicro (0.01 mg Accuracy)	Chemistry
Balance, Ultramicro (0.0001 mg Accuracy)	Chemistry
Contract Manufacturing	General
Densitometer, Laboratory	Chemistry
Refractometer	Chemistry
Thermogravimetric Analysis Equipment	Chemistry
Titrator	Chemistry

Medical Product Subsidiaries (Listed Separately)
Mettler Toledo Lasentec Products (Lasentec)
Mettler-Toledo Process Analytical, Inc.

MEVION MEDICAL SYSTEMS   978-540-1500
300 Foster St, Littleton, MA 01460
FDA Number: n/a   *Fax:* 978 540 1501
Web site: http://www.stillriversystems.com
Ownership: Private

MEVION MEDICAL SYSTEMS   978-540-1500 *(cont'd)*
Produces/Sells CE-marked Devices: N
General Admin.: Mr. Joseph Jachinowski/Chief Executive Officer
     Dr. Kenneth Gall/Chief Technology Officer
     Mr. Marc Buntaine/President
Medical Admin.: Dr. Stanley Rosenthal/Vice President Clinical Affairs
Production: Mr. Bill Alvord/Vice President Operations
Research: Mr. Earl Cleveland/Vice President Engineering

MEXICANA DE EQUIPOS DENTALES, S,A,   523-684-8110
Guillermo Baca 3738, Lomas De Polanco,
Guadalajara 44960 Mexico
FDA Number: 8030641

Mercury	Dental And Oral
Sterilizer, Dry Heat, Dental	Dental And Oral

MEXPO INTERNATIONAL, INC.   800-838-8299
2695B McCone Ave., Hayward, CA 94545   **510-293-6800**
FDA Number: 2939935   *Fax:* 510-293-9056
E-mail: mexpoglove@aol.com
Web site: www.blossom-disposables.com
Annual Revenue: $1-$5 Million
Year Founded: 1989
Total Employees: 6   *Marketing Staff:* 2   *Sales Staff:* 3
Ownership: CYPRO ENVIRONMENTAL
Quality System Registration Information: ISO9001
Produces/Sells CE-marked Devices: Y
Federal Procurement Eligibility: Small Business, Minority Owned
Distribution: Manufacturer Direct, Manufacturer Through Distributor, Exclusive Distributor, Importer, Exporter
General Admin.: Mr. Tim Thai/Chief Executive Officer
     Mr. Ben Loh/General Manager
Production: Mr. Ken Loh/Manager Materials

Glove, Patient Examination	General
Glove, Patient Examination, Latex	General
Gown, Isolation, Surgical	Surgery
Mask, Face	General

MEYLAN CORPORATION   888-769-9667
543 Valley Road,   **973-744-6400**
Upper Montclair, NJ 07043
FDA Number: 7000650   *Fax:* 973-744-1011
E-mail: meylan1@aol.com
Web site: www.meylan.com
Medical Products Sales Volume: $1,000,000
Year Founded: 1984
Total Employees: 6
Ownership: Private
Federal Procurement Eligibility: Small Business
Distribution: Service Direct
General Admin.: C. M. Prinaris/President
Mktg./Adv.: A. Prinaris/Manager National Sales

Clock, Elapsed Time	General
Counter, Differential Hand Tally	Hematology
Recorder, Paper Chart	Cardiovascular
Tachometer	General
Timer, General Laboratory	Hematology

MEZA MEDICAL EQUIPMENT   888-308-7116
108 W. Nakoma Drive, San Antonio, TX 78216   **210-308-7116**
FDA Number: n/a   *Fax:* 210-308-5925
E-mail: rodolfo@meza-medical.com
Web site: www.meza-medical.com
Medical Products Sales Volume: $300,000
Annual Revenue: $0-$1 Million
Year Founded: 1990
Total Employees: 3   *Marketing Staff:* 1   *Sales Staff:* 2
Ownership: Private
Stock Symbol: MME
Produces/Sells CE-marked Devices: N
Federal Procurement Eligibility: Small Business, Minority Owned, GSA Contract
Distribution: Manufacturer Direct, Exclusive Distributor, Exporter
Mktg./Adv.: Rodolfo Meza/Director Marketing

Computer, Ultrasound	Radiology
Electrocardiograph, Interpretive	Cardiovascular
Light, Surgical, Ceiling Mounted	Surgery
Light, Surgical, Floor Standing	Surgery
Monitor, ECG	Cardiovascular
Printer, Image, Video	General
Service, Used Equipment	General
Spirometer, Diagnostic (Respirometer)	Anesthesiology
Stretcher, Hand-Carried	General

MFG ONE, LLC   703-437-9838
3900 Skyhawk Dr., Chantilly, VA 20151
FDA Number: 3004167615

Freezer, Laboratory, General Purpose	Chemistry
Pressure Infusor, IV Container	General

MFG ONE, LLC   703-437-9838 *(cont'd)*
Warmer, Infusion Fluid, Thermal   General
Warmer, Irrigation Solution   General

MFI
See Faxitron X-Ray, Llc

MFI MEDICAL EQUIPMENT INC   800-633-1558
7929 Silverton Avenue, #610,   **858-831-7718**
San Diego, CA 92126
FDA Number: n/a   *Fax:* 858-831-7721
E-mail: drsdeal@mfimedical.com
Web site: www.mfimedical.com
Medical Products Sales Volume: $1,600,000
Annual Revenue: $0-$1 Million
Year Founded: 1982
Total Employees: 10   *Marketing Staff:* 6   *Sales Staff:* 6
Ownership: Private
Produces/Sells CE-marked Devices: N
Federal Procurement Eligibility: Small Business
Distribution: Manufacturer Direct
General Admin.: Arnold Wiesel/President
Mktg./Adv.: Annette Wiesel/Manager Marketing
    Service, Used Equipment   General

MG INDUSTRIES
See Praxair Distribution Mid-Atlantic LLC

MG SCIENTIFIC, INC.   800-343-8338
8500 107th St., Pleasant Prairie, WI 53158   **262-947-7000**
FDA Number: n/a   *Fax:* 262-947-7007
E-mail: customerservice@mgscientific.com
Web site: www.mgscientific.com
Medical Products Sales Volume: $7,000,000
Annual Revenue: $5-$10 Million
Total Employees: 20   *Marketing Staff:* 2   *Sales Staff:* 5
Ownership: Private
Produces/Sells CE-marked Devices: N
Federal Procurement Eligibility: Small Business
Distribution: Exclusive Distributor
General Admin.: Jim McKeown/President
    Balance, Analytical   Chemistry
    Buffer, pH   Hematology
    Buret   Chemistry
    Burner   Chemistry
    Calorimeter   Chemistry
    Dispenser, Pipette   Chemistry
    Pipette   Chemistry
    Pipette Tip   Chemistry
    Pipette, Micro   Chemistry
    Pipetter   Hematology
    Spectrophotometer, U.V./Visible   Chemistry
    Sterilizer, Steam (Autoclave)   General
    Vial, Liquid Scintillation Counting   Chemistry

MGE UPS SYTEMS, INC.   800-523-0142
1660 Scenic Avenue,   **714-557-1636**
Costa Mesa, CA 92626
FDA Number: n/a   *Fax:* 714-557-9788
E-mail: info@mgeups.com
Web site: www.mgeups.com
Medical Products Sales Volume: $1,000,000
Annual Revenue: $500 Million-$1 Billion
Year Founded: 1996
Total Employees: 325   *Marketing Staff:* 9   *Sales Staff:* 50
Ownership: Private
Stock Symbol: CYN
Traded On: Toronto
Quality System Registration Information: ISO9001; ISO9002
Produces/Sells CE-marked Devices: Y
Federal Procurement Eligibility: Small Business, GSA Contract
Distribution: Manufacturer Direct, Manufacturer Through Distributor, Manufacturer Through Manufacturer Reps, OEM, Service Direct, Exporter
General Admin.: Claude Graff/Chief Executive Officer
       Ray Prince/President
       Nina Kazmarek/Vice President Human Resources
Mktg./Adv.: David McNulty/Director National Accounts
       Jonna Quintana/Manager Marketing
       Mike Chmura/Vice President Sales
Production: Jeff Weiderkehr/Director Operations
       Monty Jones/Director Quality Assurance
    Power System, Isolated   General
    Power Systems, Uninterruptible (UPS)   General

MGM INSTRUMENTS   800-551-1415
925 Sherman Avenue, Hamden, CT 06514-1117   **203-248-4008**
FDA Number: 1220293   *Fax:* 203-288-2621
E-mail: sales@mgminstruments.com
Web site: www.mgminstruments.com

MGM INSTRUMENTS   800-551-1415 *(cont'd)*
Annual Revenue: $1-$5 Million
Year Founded: 1972
Total Employees: 35   *Marketing Staff:* 2   *Sales Staff:* 2
Ownership: Private
Produces/Sells CE-marked Devices: Y
Federal Procurement Eligibility: Small Business
Distribution: Manufacturer Direct, Manufacturer Through Manufacturer Reps, OEM, Exporter
General Admin.: G. Mismas/Chief Executive Officer
       N. Rydzy/General Manager
Mktg./Adv.: Steve Meyer/Director Marketing
Production: T. Calderoni/Director Engineering
    Analyzer, Chemistry, Photometric, Discrete   Chemistry
    Counter, Gamma, General Use   Toxicology
    Luminometer   Chemistry

MGR EQUIPMENT CORP.   516-239-3030
22 Gates Ave., Inwood, NY 11096
FDA Number: 2433731   *Fax:* 516-239-3602
E-mail: info@mgrequip.com
Web site: www.mgrequip.com
Ownership: Private
Produces/Sells CE-marked Devices: N
    Freezer, Blood Storage   Hematology

MIAMI MEDICAL EQUIPMENT & SUPPLY CORP.   305-592-0111
2150 N.W. 93 Ave., Miami, FL 33172
FDA Number: 1035817   *Fax:* 305-591-4004
E-mail: sales@miamimedical.com
Annual Revenue: $1-$5 Million
Total Employees: 15
Ownership: Private
Produces/Sells CE-marked Devices: N
Federal Procurement Eligibility: Small Business
Distribution: Exporter
General Admin.: Mrs. Tere Zapata/General Manager
       Mr. Rene Teran/President
Mktg./Adv.: Ms. Renata Teran/Vice President Marketing & Sales
    Bandage, Adhesive   Surgery
    Glove, Patient Examination   General
    Glove, Surgical   General
    Kit, Pregnancy Test   Obstetrics/Gynecology
    Speculum, Vaginal, Non-Metal   Obstetrics/Gynecology
    Swabs, Alcohol   General

MICARDIA CORPORATION   949-951-4888
30 Hughes, Suite 206, Irvine, CA 92618
FDA Number: 3006265015   *Fax:* 949-951-4812
E-mail: info@micardia.com
Web site: http://www.micardia.com
Year Founded: 2004
Ownership: Private
Produces/Sells CE-marked Devices: N
General Admin.: Mr. Donald Rohrbaugh/Chief Executive Officer
       Mr. Samuel Shaolian/Chief Technology Officer
Mktg./Adv.: Ms. Robin Gibbs/Director Marketing
Production: Mr. Bart Navarro/Director Operations
       Mr. John Mcintyre/Director Regulatory Affairs
Research: Mr. Ross Tsukashima/Director Research & Engineering
    Ring, Annuloplasty   Cardiovascular

MICELL TECHNOLOGIES INC.   919-313-2102
801 Capitola Drive, Suite 1, Durham, NC 27713
FDA Number: n/a   *Fax:* 919-313-2103
E-mail: info@micell.com
Web site: www.micell.com
Ownership: Private
Produces/Sells CE-marked Devices: N
General Admin.: Mr. Arthur Benvenuto/Chairman, Chief Executive Officer
       Mr. Jack Herman/Chief Operating Officer
       Dr. James McClain/Senior Vice President
Finance: Mr. James Klein, Jr./Chief Financial Officer

MICHAEL D. WARREN SERVICES LTD.   905-455-1915
211-338 Queen St E, Brampton L6V 1C4 Canada
FDA Number: 9617852
    Epilator, High-Frequency, Needle-Type   Surgery

MICHCLONE ASSOCIATES, INC.   248-583-1150
680 Ajax Dr, Madison Heights, MI 48071
FDA Number: 1831312
Ownership: Private
Produces/Sells CE-marked Devices: N
    Fixative, Formalin Containing   Pathology
    Fixative, Metallic Containing   Pathology
    Hemoglobin M   Hematology
    Test, Sickle Cell   Hematology

MANUFACTURER PROFILES

MICHEL CULLEN MEDICAL INC. 888-438-9544
1040 boul. Michele-Bohec., Ste. 100, 450-434-1920
Blainville, QUE J7C-5 Canada
FDA Number: n/a Fax: 450-434-1738
E-mail: admin@michel-cullen.com
Web site: www.michel-cullen.com
Year Founded: 1972
Total Employees: 10
Ownership: Private
Produces/Sells CE-marked Devices: N
Distribution: Manufacturer Direct, Exclusive Distributor, Importer

MICHIGAN AIRGAS
See Airgas Great Lakes, Inc.

MICHIGAN INSTRUMENTS, INC. 800-530-9939
4717 Talon Ct. S.E., Grand Rapids, MI 49512-5409 616-554-9696
FDA Number: 1821850 Fax: 616-554-3067
E-mail: mii@michiganinstruments.com
Web site: www.michiganinstruments.com
Medical Products Sales Volume: $200,000
Annual Revenue: $1-$5 Million
Year Founded: 1964
Total Employees: 20 *Marketing Staff:* 2 *Sales Staff:* 3
Ownership: Private
Quality System Registration Information: ISO9001
Produces/Sells CE-marked Devices: Y
Federal Procurement Eligibility: Small Business
Distribution: Manufacturer Direct, Manufacturer Through Manufacturer Reps, OEM, Exporter
General Admin.: Mr. Ruben Derderian/President
Mktg./Adv.: Ms. Maureen Oostendorp/Director Marketing
    Ms. Jaclyn Karsten/Marketing Coordinator
    Mr. Jason Ulanowicz/Sales Representative

Carrier, Container, Oxygen, Portable	General
Compressor, Cardiac, External	Cardiovascular
Flowmeter, Gas (Oxygen), Calibrated	Anesthesiology
Resuscitator, Cardiopulmonary	Cardiovascular
Simulator, Lung	Anesthesiology
Yoke, Medical Gas	Anesthesiology

MICK RADIO-NUCLEAR INSTRUMENTS 877-597-6764
521 Homestead Ave., Mount Vernon, NY 10550 914-667-3999
FDA Number: 2431392 Fax: 914-665-8834
E-mail: sales@micknuclear.com
Web site: www.micknuclear.com
Annual Revenue: $0-$1 Million
Ownership: Private
Produces/Sells CE-marked Devices: N
Federal Procurement Eligibility: Small Business
Distribution: Manufacturer Direct

Accelerator, Linear, Medical	Radiology
Afterloader, Radiotherapy	Radiology
Applicator, Radionuclide, Manual	Radiology
Applicator, Radionuclide, Remote-Controlled	Radiology
Block, Beam Shaping, Radionuclide	Radiology
Phantom, Anthropomorphic, Nuclear	Radiology
Tape, Measuring, Ruler And Caliper	Surgery

MICOR, INC. 412-487-1113
2855 Oxford Blvd., Allison Park, PA 15101-2455
FDA Number: 2523449 Fax: 412-487-1747
E-mail: info@micorinc.com
Web site: www.micorinc.com
Medical Products Sales Volume: $3,000,000
Annual Revenue: $1-$5 Million
Year Founded: 1984
Total Employees: 35 *Sales Staff:* 1
Ownership: Private
Produces/Sells CE-marked Devices: N
Federal Procurement Eligibility: Small Business
Distribution: OEM, Exporter
General Admin.: Stephen Brushey/President
Production: Mrs. Diane Smith/Customer Service Representative
    Susan Forgrave/Manager Regulatory Affairs
    Mr. Dave Graner/Product Manager

Accessories, Catheter	Surgery
Catheter, Conduction, Anesthesia	Anesthesiology
Catheter, Epidural	Obstetrics/Gynecology
Molding, Custom	General
Protector, Puncture, Needle	General

MICRA SCIENTIFIC, INC.
See Eprogen, Inc.

MICRAD, INC. 865-690-6389
312 Trossachs Lane, Knoxville, TN 37922
FDA Number: n/a Fax: 865-670-8559
E-mail: ron@micrad.com

MICRAD, INC. 865-690-6389 *(cont'd)*
Medical Products Sales Volume: $400,000
Annual Revenue: $0-$1 Million
Total Employees: 1
Ownership: Private
Produces/Sells CE-marked Devices: N
Federal Procurement Eligibility: Small Business
Distribution: Manufacturer Through Manufacturer Reps
General Admin.: Ron Baldry/President

Counter, Radiation	Radiology

MICRINS SURGICAL INSTRUMENTS, INC. 800-833-3380
28438 Ballard Drive, Lake Forest, IL 60045 847-549-1410
FDA Number: 1450863 Fax: 847-549-1510
E-mail: micrins@micrins.com
Web site: www.micrins.com
Year Founded: 1987
Ownership: Private
Produces/Sells CE-marked Devices: N
Federal Procurement Eligibility: Small Business
Distribution: Manufacturer Direct, Manufacturer Through Manufacturer Reps, Exclusive Distributor
General Admin.: Bernhard Teitz/President
Mktg./Adv.: George Torres/Director Sales

Clamp, Surgical, General & Plastic Surgery	Surgery
Cutter, Orthopedic	Orthopedics
Dilator, Vessel, Surgical	Cardiovascular
Dissector, Surgical, General & Plastic Surgery	Surgery
ENT Manual Surgical Instrument	Ear/Nose/Throat
Electrosurgical Unit, Anesthesiology Accessories	Surgery
Elevator, Surgical, General & Plastic Surgery	Surgery
Forceps, ENT	Ear/Nose/Throat
Forceps, General & Plastic Surgery	Surgery
General Use Surgical Scissors	Surgery
Hemostat	Orthopedics
Hemostat, Surgical	Dental And Oral
Hook, Surgical, General & Plastic Surgery	Surgery
Instrument Guard	Surgery
Instrument, Manual, General Surgical	Surgery
Instrument, Microsurgical	Cns/Neurology
Laboratory Equipment, Ophthalmic	Ophthalmology
Osteotome, Manual (Plastic Surgery)	Surgery
Prosthesis, Arterial Graft, Synthetic, Less Than 6mm	Surgery
Scissors, Ophthalmic	Ophthalmology
Scissors, Plastic Surgery (Dissecting)	Surgery
Speculum, Ear	Ear/Nose/Throat
Suture, Non-Absorbable	Surgery
Tray, Surgical	Surgery
Tray, Surgical Instrument	Surgery

MICRO & INFARED
See Mikron Infrared, Inc.

MICRO AIR AIR CLEANERS BY METAL-FAB 800-835-2830
PO Box 1138, Wichita, KS 67201-1138 316-943-2351
FDA Number: n/a Fax: 316-943-2717
E-mail: info@mtlfab.com
Web site: www.microaironline.com
Total Employees: 300 *Marketing Staff:* 2 *Sales Staff:* 7
Ownership: Private
Produces/Sells CE-marked Devices: Y
Federal Procurement Eligibility: Small Business
Distribution: Manufacturer Through Distributor, Manufacturer Through Manufacturer Reps, OEM, Importer, Exporter
General Admin.: Ken Shannon/Chief Executive Officer
Mktg./Adv.: Jim Orr/Manager General Sales

Equipment, Cleaning, Air	General

MICRO AUDIOMETRICS CORP. 800-729-9509
655 Keller Road, Murphy, NC 28906-5890 828-644-0771
FDA Number: 1220135 Fax: 828-644-0772
E-mail: sales@microaud.com
Web site: www.microaud.com
Medical Products Sales Volume: $900,000
Year Founded: 1980
Total Employees: 11 *Marketing Staff:* 2 *Sales Staff:* 2
Ownership: Private
Produces/Sells CE-marked Devices: N
Federal Procurement Eligibility: Small Business
Distribution: Manufacturer Through Distributor
Mktg./Adv.: Jason R. Keller/Account Services Representative
    Lance Ralph/Director Marketing
    Jim Keller/Director Product Development
    Kathy Keller/Manager Advertising
Production: Jim Keller/Chief Engineering Officer
Research: Larry Robinette/Director Research

Analyzer, Middle Ear	Ear/Nose/Throat
Audiometer	Ear/Nose/Throat
Computer, Audiometry	Ear/Nose/Throat

MICRO AUDIOMETRICS CORP. 800-729-9509 *(cont'd)*
Tester, Auditory Impedance — Ear/Nose/Throat

MICRO BIO-MEDICS, INC.
See Caligor

MICRO BIO-PHYSIC LABORATORY, INC. 626-451-6813
5917 Oak Avenue, #357, Temple City, CA 91780
FDA Number: 3004860201
Ownership: Private
Produces/Sells CE-marked Devices: N
Computer, Diagnostic, Programmable — Cardiovascular

MICRO CARE CORP. 800-638-0125
595 John Downey Drive, New Britain, CT 06051 — 860-827-0626
FDA Number: n/a — Fax: 860-827-8105
E-mail: techsupport@microcare.com
Web site: www.microcare.com
Medical Products Sales Volume: $1,600,000
Year Founded: 1983
Total Employees: 15
Ownership: Private
Produces/Sells CE-marked Devices: N
Federal Procurement Eligibility: Small Business
Distribution: Manufacturer Direct, Manufacturer Through Distributor, Manufacturer Through Manufacturer Reps
Mktg./Adv.: Heather Gombos/Manager General Sales
Cleanroom Equipment — General
Lubricant, Instrument — General

MICRO CURRENT TECHNOLOGY, INC. 206-778-5717
2244 1st. Ave. S., Seattle, WA 98134
FDA Number: 3026264
Dermatome — Surgery
Massager, Therapeutic — Physical Med
Stimulator, Nerve, Transcutaneous (Pain Relief, TENS) — Cns/Neurology

MICRO DETECT, INC. 714-832-8234
2852 Walnut Ave., Suite H-1, Tustin, CA 92780
FDA Number: 2031341
Anti-DNA Antibody (Enzyme-Labeled), Antigen, Control — Immunology
Antibodies, Gliadin — Immunology
Antinuclear Antibody (Enzyme-Labeled), Antigen, Controls — Immunology
Campylobacter Pylori — Microbiology
Extractable Antinuclear Antibody (Rnp/Sm), Antigen/Control — Immunology
Test, Rheumatoid Factor — Immunology

MICRO DIAGNOSTICS, INC.
See Biomerieux Industry

MICRO ESSENTIAL LABORATORY, INC. 718-338-3618
4224 Avenue H, P.O. Box 100824, Brooklyn, NY 11210
FDA Number: n/a — Fax: 718-692-4491
E-mail: customerservice@microessentiallab.com
Web site: www.microessentiallab.com
Year Founded: 1934
Total Employees: 10
Ownership: Private
Produces/Sells CE-marked Devices: N
Federal Procurement Eligibility: Small Business
Distribution: Manufacturer Direct, Importer, Exporter
Buffer, pH — Hematology
Pump, Infusion, Laboratory — Chemistry
Solution, pH Buffer — Chemistry

MICRO HEARING AIDS 480-895-2153
10440 East Riggs Rd.,suite 120, Sun Lakes, AZ 85248
FDA Number: 2032851
Ownership: Private
Produces/Sells CE-marked Devices: N
Hearing-Aid — Ear/Nose/Throat

MICRO MED, INC.
See Disetronic Sterile Products

MICRO MEDICAL DEVICES, INC. 818-874-0000
23945 Calabasas Rd., Suite 110, Calabasas, CA 91302
FDA Number: 3004574050
Scanner, Ultrasonic (Pulsed Echo) — Radiology

MICRO POWER ELECTRONICS, INC. 800-576-6177
13955 SW Millikan Way, Beaverton, OR 97005 — 503-693-7600
FDA Number: 3032867 — Fax: 503-648-9625
E-mail: powerexpert@micro-power.com
Web site: www.micro-power.com
Medical Products Sales Volume: $20,400,000
Annual Revenue: $25-$50 Million
Total Employees: 250 — Marketing Staff: 2 — Sales Staff: 7
Ownership: Private
Stock Symbol: CBAK.
Traded On: NASDAQ

MICRO POWER ELECTRONICS, INC. 800-576-6177 *(cont'd)*
Quality System Registration Information: ISO9001
Produces/Sells CE-marked Devices: N
Federal Procurement Eligibility: Small Business
Distribution: OEM
General Admin.: Mr. Mike DuBose/Chief Executive Officer, Chairman
Mktg./Adv.: Mr. Jeffrey VanZwol/Vice President Marketing
    Mr. Greg Webster/Vice President Sales
Production: Mr. Sam Ishizaka/Manager Operations
Research: Mr. Ron Pitchel/Vice President Engineering
Finance: Mr. Paul Brown/Chief Financial Officer, Senior Vice President Finance
Battery — General

MICRO SENSORS, INC.
See Northern Technologies Intl. Corp.

MICRO STAMPING CORP. 513-573-0085
140 Belmont Dr., Somerset, NJ 08873
FDA Number: 2248148
General Use Surgical Scissors — Surgery

MICRO TOOL ENGINEERING, INC. 561-842-7381
7575 Central Industrial Drive, West Palm Beach, FL 33404
FDA Number: 3003925093 — Fax: (561) 842-7401
E-mail: info@mte-fl.com
Web site: www.mte-fl.com
Ownership: Private
Produces/Sells CE-marked Devices: N
Applicator, Radionuclide, Manual — Radiology
Source, Brachytherapy, Radionuclide — Radiology
Transducer, Ultrasonic, Diagnostic — Radiology

MICRO TYPING SYSTEMS, INC. 908-218-8177
1295 S.w. 29th Ave., Pompano Beach, FL 33069
FDA Number: 1056600
Analyzer, Blood Grouping/Antibody, Automated — Hematology
Bag, Blood, Collection — Hematology
Centrifuge, Blood Bank, Diagnostic — Hematology
Media, Potentiating — Hematology
Reagent, General Purpose — Pathology
Supplies, Blood Bank — Hematology
View Box, Blood Grouping — Hematology

MICRO-AIRE SURGICAL INSTRUMENTS, INC. 800-722-0822
1641 Edlich Dr., Charlottesville, VA 22911-1278 — 434-975-8000
FDA Number: 2020601 — Fax: 804-975-4144
Web site: http://www.microaire.com
Medical Products Sales Volume: $28,000,000
Annual Revenue: $25-$50 Million
Year Founded: 1977
Total Employees: 115 — Marketing Staff: 5 — Sales Staff: 8
Ownership: Private
Produces/Sells CE-marked Devices: Y
Federal Procurement Eligibility: GSA Contract, VA Contract
Distribution: Manufacturer Through Manufacturer Reps, OEM
General Admin.: Frank Altenhofen/President
Mktg./Adv.: Ann Cooper/Director Marketing
    Boli Emch/Manager International Sales
    Craig Johnson/Manager National Sales
    Mike Fard/Vice President Business Development
    John Lauer/Vice President International Marketing & Sales
    John Lauer/Vice President Marketing & Sales
Production: Judy Wimmer/Director Operations
    Chris Spofford/Manager Quality Assurance & Regulatory Affairs
Research: Mike Fard/Vice President Research & Development
Finance: Paul Skolnick/Vice President Finance
Blade, Bone Cutting — Orthopedics
Blade, Saw, Cast Cutting — Orthopedics
Blade, Surgical, Saw, General & Plastic Surgery — Surgery
Burr, Orthopedic — Orthopedics
Burr, Other — Surgery
Burr, Podiatric — Orthopedics
Chisel (Osteotome) — Surgery
Compress, Cold — General
Compress, Moist Heat — Physical Med
Contract Manufacturing, Product, Durable — General
Drill, Bone — Orthopedics
Drill, Middle Ear Surgery — Ear/Nose/Throat
Drill, Oral Surgery — Dental And Oral
Driver, Wire — Orthopedics
Gouge, Surgical, General & Plastic Surgery — Surgery
Instrument, Microsurgical — Cns/Neurology
Instrument, Surgical, Powered, Pneumatic — Orthopedics
Lavage Unit, Surgical — Surgery
Osteotome (Orthopedic) — Surgery
Osteotome, Other — Surgery
Prosthesis Implantation Instrument, Orthopedic — Orthopedics
Regulator, Pressure, Gas Cylinder — Anesthesiology
Saw, Bone Cutting, Micro — Orthopedics
Saw, Bone, Pneumatic — Orthopedics

MANUFACTURER PROFILES

MICRO-AIRE SURGICAL INSTRUMENTS, INC. 800-722-0822
(cont'd)
- Service, Engineering/Design — General
- Surgical Instrument, Orthopedic, AC-Powered Motor — Orthopedics
- System, Extraction, Cement Removal — Orthopedics

MICRO-ASEPTIC INDUSTRIES, INC.
See Micro-Scientific Industries, Inc.

MICRO-BIO-LOGICS.INC 800-599-2847
217 Osseo Avenue N., St. Cloud, MN 56303-4452 320-253-1640
FDA Number: n/a Fax: 320-253-6250
E-mail: info@mbl2000.com
Web site: www.microbiologics.com
Medical Products Sales Volume: $7,100,000
Annual Revenue: $1-$5 Million
Year Founded: 1971
Total Employees: 32 *Marketing Staff:* 3
Ownership: Private
Quality System Registration Information: ISO9001
Produces/Sells CE-marked Devices: Y
Federal Procurement Eligibility: Small Business, GSA Contract
Distribution: Manufacturer Direct, Manufacturer Through Distributor
General Admin.: Bob Coborn/President
   Sharon Rausch/Vice President, General Manager
Mktg./Adv.: RaNae Alcorn/Director Marketing
   Robert Coborn/Vice President Marketing
Production: Donna Scholer/General Manager Production
IS: Marilyn Lueck/Director Tech. Services
- Kit, Quality Control — Microbiology
- Tube, Culture — Microbiology

MICRO-DENT INC. 866-526-1166
379 Hollow Hill Rd., Wauconda, IL 60084
FDA Number: 1450714
Ownership: Private
Produces/Sells CE-marked Devices: N
- Burnisher, Operative, Dental — Dental And Oral
- Carver, Dental Amalgam, Operative — Dental And Oral
- Condenser, Amalgam And Foil, Operative — Dental And Oral
- Curette, Periodontic — Dental And Oral
- Elevator, Surgical, Dental — Dental And Oral
- Excavator, Dental, Operative — Dental And Oral
- Explorer, Operative — Dental And Oral
- File, Margin Finishing, Operative — Dental And Oral
- Handle, Instrument, Dental — Dental And Oral
- Plugger, Root Canal, Endodontic — Dental And Oral
- Probe, Periodontic — Dental And Oral
- Scaler, Periodontic — Dental And Oral

MICRO-EAR TECHNOLOGY, INC. 952-995-8800
6425 Flying Cloud Dr., Eden Prairie, MN 55344
FDA Number: 2183674
Ownership: Private
Produces/Sells CE-marked Devices: N
- Hearing-Aid — Ear/Nose/Throat
- Masker, Tinnitus — Ear/Nose/Throat

MICRO-MEDIA SYSTEMS INC.
See Beckman Coulter, Inc.

MICRO-SCIENTIFIC INDUSTRIES, INC. 888-253-2536
1225 Carnegie Street, Ste. 101, 847-454-0835
Rolling Meadows, IL 60008
FDA Number: n/a Fax: 847-454-0837
E-mail: msi@opticide.com
Web site: www.opticide.com
Medical Products Sales Volume: $1,200,000
Annual Revenue: $1-$5 Million
Year Founded: 1996
Total Employees: 12 *Marketing Staff:* 3 *Sales Staff:* 25
Ownership: Private
Produces/Sells CE-marked Devices: N
Federal Procurement Eligibility: Small Business
Distribution: Manufacturer Direct, Manufacturer Through Distributor, Manufacturer Through Manufacturer Reps, Importer, Exporter
General Admin.: Jack Wagner/Chief Executive Officer
- Detergent — Hematology
- Disinfector, Liquid — General
- Lubricant, Instrument — General

MICRO-SELECT INSTRUMENTS, INC. 636-273-5227
165 Duckworth St., Saint Clair, MO 63077
FDA Number: 3005672949
- Forceps, Ophthalmic — Ophthalmology

MICRO-TECH 952-995-8800
6425 Flying Cloud Dr., Eden Prairie, MN 55344
FDA Number: n/a
Web site: www.mthearing.com

MICRO-TECH 952-995-8800 *(cont'd)*
Year Founded: 1986
Ownership: Private
Produces/Sells CE-marked Devices: N
- Hearing-Aid — Ear/Nose/Throat

MICRO-VAC, INC. 800-729-1020
5905 E. 5th St., Tucson, AZ 85711-4522 520-750-1200
FDA Number: 2027794 Fax: 520-750-0001
E-mail: microvac1@aol.com
Medical Products Sales Volume: $100,000
Annual Revenue: $0-$1 Million
Year Founded: 1986
Total Employees: 5 *Marketing Staff:* 2 *Sales Staff:* 2
Ownership: Private
Stock Symbol: IFMX
Traded On: NASDAQ
Produces/Sells CE-marked Devices: N
Federal Procurement Eligibility: Small Business, Female Owned
Distribution: Exclusive Distributor
General Admin.: Cheryl Henderson/President
Mktg./Adv.: Ronen Ben-Dov/Vice President Sales
- Agent, Polishing, Abrasive, Oral Cavity — Dental And Oral
- Forceps, Dressing, Dental — Dental And Oral
- Tubing, Other — General

MICROAIRE SURGICAL INSTRUMENTS, LLC 800-722-0822
1641 Edlich Dr., Charlottesville, VA 22911 434-975-8000
FDA Number: 2020601 Fax: 434-975-4134
Web site: www.microaire.com
Ownership: Private
Produces/Sells CE-marked Devices: N
- Arthroscope — Orthopedics
- Blade, Surgical, Saw, General & Plastic Surgery — Surgery
- Burr, Orthopedic — Orthopedics
- Burr, Surgical, General & Plastic Surgery — Surgery
- Dissector, Surgical, General & Plastic Surgery — Surgery
- Instrument, Surgical, Powered, Pneumatic — Orthopedics
- Lavage Unit, Water Jet — General
- Motor, Drill, Pneumatic — Cns/Neurology
- Motor, Surgical Instrument, AC-Powered — Surgery
- Orthodontic Instrument — Dental And Oral
- Pin, Fixation, Smooth — Orthopedics
- Rasp, Surgical, General & Plastic Surgery — Surgery
- Screw, Fixation, Bone — Orthopedics
- Suction Apparatus, Single Patient, Portable, Non-Powered — Surgery
- Surgical Instrument, Orthopedic, AC-Powered Motor — Orthopedics
- Suture, Absorbable, Synthetic — Surgery

MICROBAN GERMICIDE CO.
See Surco Products

MICROBICS CORPORATION
See Strategic Diagnostics Inc.

MICROBIOLOGICAL ASSOCIATES, INC.
See Bioreliance

MICROBIOLOGICAL SPECIALTIES 602-867-7323
3311 East Charter Oak Rd., Phoenix, AZ 85032
FDA Number: 2022130
Ownership: Private
Produces/Sells CE-marked Devices: N
- Culture Media, Multiple Biochemical Test — Microbiology
- Culture Media, Single Biochemical Test — Microbiology

MICROBIOLOGICS, INC. 800-599-BUGS
217 Osseo Ave. North, 320-253-1640
St. Cloud, MN 56303
FDA Number: 2150138 Fax: 320-229-7599
E-mail: info@microbiologics.com
Web site: www.microbiologics.com
Annual Revenue: $5-$10 Million
Year Founded: 1971
Total Employees: 45 *Marketing Staff:* 3 *Sales Staff:* 5
Ownership: Private
Quality System Registration Information: ISO9001
Produces/Sells CE-marked Devices: Y
Federal Procurement Eligibility: Small Business
Distribution: Manufacturer Direct, Manufacturer Through Distributor
Mktg./Adv.: Mrs. RaNae Alcorn/Director Marketing
Production: Mrs. Delene Axeen/Supervisor Customer Service
- Kit, Quality Control — Microbiology
- Slide, Control, Quality — Microbiology

MICROBIOLOGY REFERENCE LABORATORY
See Focus Technologies

MICROBIX BIOSYSTEMS, INC.
800-794-6694
416-234-1624
115 Skyway Ave,
Toronto, ONT M9W 4 Canada
FDA Number: n/a   *Fax:* 416-234-1626
E-mail: microbix@microbix.com
Web site: www.microbix.com
Total Employees: 35   *Marketing Staff:* 2   *Sales Staff:* 2
Ownership: Public
Stock Symbol: MBX
Traded On: Toronto
Produces/Sells CE-marked Devices: N
Federal Procurement Eligibility: Small Business
Distribution: Manufacturer Direct, Exporter

MICROCAL, LLC
800-633-3115
413-586-7720
22 Industrial Dr. E.,
Northampton, MA 01060
FDA Number: n/a   *Fax:* 413-586-0149
E-mail: info@microcalorimetry.com
Web site: www.microcalorimetry.com
Annual Revenue: $10-$25 Million
Ownership: Private
Quality System Registration Information: ISO9001
Produces/Sells CE-marked Devices: N
Federal Procurement Eligibility: Small Business
Distribution: Manufacturer Direct, Manufacturer Through Distributor
General Admin.: John Brandts/Chief Executive Officer
    William Gelb/President
Mktg./Adv.: Matt Potter/Director Marketing
Production: Mike Brandts/Director Quality Assurance
Research: Valerian Plotinikov/Vice President Research & Development
IS: Verna Frasca/Manager Tech. Support
Calorimeter	Chemistry
Computer Software	General

MICROCHECK, INC.
877-934-3284
802-485-6600
142 Gould Road, Northfield, VT 05663
FDA Number: 1225729   *Fax:* 802-485-6100
E-mail: microcheck@microcheck.com
Web site: www.microcheck.com
Medical Products Sales Volume: $1,000,000
Annual Revenue: $0-$1 Million
Year Founded: 1988
Total Employees: 15   *Marketing Staff:* 1   *Sales Staff:* 1
Ownership: Private
Quality System Registration Information: ISO9002
Federal Procurement Eligibility: Small Business, Female Owned
Distribution: Service Direct
General Admin.: Mary Dolenmaier/President, General Manager
Mktg./Adv.: Mary Sinclair/Manager Advertising
    Cindy Glidden/Manager Business
Chromatographic Bacterial Identification	Microbiology
Contract Laboratory	General

MICROCISION LLC
800-264-3811
215-744-0770
5805 Keystone St., Philadelphia, PA 19135-4293
FDA Number: 2530808   *Fax:* 215-744-3787
E-mail: microcision@microcision.com
Web site: www.microcision.com
Year Founded: 1955
Total Employees: 76   *Marketing Staff:* 2   *Sales Staff:* 2
Ownership: Private
Quality System Registration Information: ISO9001
Produces/Sells CE-marked Devices: N
Federal Procurement Eligibility: Small Business
Distribution: Manufacturer Direct
General Admin.: Luda Pevzner/Office Manager
    Robert Kramer/President, Chief Executive Officer
    Don Labowsky/Vice President, General Manager
Mktg./Adv.: Terry Oreszko/Director Sales
Production: Anatoli Krivoruk/Director Engineering
    Christina Shannon/Director Quality Control & Regulatory Affairs
    George Chamberlin/Manager Materials
    Steve Hogan/Vice President Operations
Accessories, Catheter, G-U	Gastroenterology/Urology
Component, Electronic	General
Component, Metal, Other	General
Connector, Catheter	Surgery
Connector, Hydrocephalic	Cns/Neurology
Connector, Shunt	Gastroenterology/Urology
Contract Manufacturing	General
Fitting, Luer	General
Fixation Device, Spinal (External)	Orthopedics
Implant, Endosseous	Dental And Oral
Implant, Fixation Device, Spinal	Orthopedics
Implant, Subperiosteal	Dental And Oral
Instrument, Implantation, Shunt	Cns/Neurology

MICROCISION LLC
800-264-3811 *(cont'd)*
Pin, Fixation, Threaded	Orthopedics
Reservoir, Hydrocephalic Catheter	Cns/Neurology
Screw, Fixation, Bone	Orthopedics
Screwdriver	Orthopedics
Screwdriver, Surgical	Surgery

MICROCOPY, DIV. NEO-FLO, INC.
800-235-1863
770-425-5715
3120 Moon Station Rd.,
Kennesaw, GA 30144
FDA Number: 2023633   *Fax:* 770-423-4996
Web site: www.microcopydental.com
Annual Revenue: $0-$1 Million
Year Founded: 1970
Ownership: Private
Produces/Sells CE-marked Devices: N
Federal Procurement Eligibility: Small Business
Distribution: Manufacturer Direct, Importer, Exporter
General Admin.: Thomas Maass/President
    Perry L. Parke/Vice President
Absorber, Saliva, Paper	Dental And Oral
Dental Laboratory Equipment	Dental And Oral
Holder, X-Ray Film	Dental And Oral
Instrument, Diamond, Dental	Dental And Oral

MICROELECTRODES, INC.
603-668-0692
40 Harvey Road, Bedford, NH 03110-6805
FDA Number: 1219434   *Fax:* 603-668-7926
E-mail: info@microelectrodes.com
Web site: www.microelectrodes.com
Medical Products Sales Volume: $800,000
Annual Revenue: $0-$1 Million
Year Founded: 1970
Total Employees: 6
Ownership: Private
Produces/Sells CE-marked Devices: N
Federal Procurement Eligibility: Small Business
Distribution: Manufacturer Direct
General Admin.: Normand C. Hebert/President, Chief Executive Officer
    Marc Hebert/Vice President, General Manager
Research: Marc Hebert/Vice President Research & Development
Electrode, Esophageal	Gastroenterology/Urology
Electrode, Laboratory pH	Chemistry
Electrode, Specific Ion	Chemistry
Electrode, pH	Gastroenterology/Urology

MICROFIT, INC.
650-969-7296
1077-b Independence Ave., Mountain View, CA 94043
FDA Number: 2936523
Monitor, Blood Pressure, Indirect, Semi-Automatic	Cardiovascular

MICROFLEX CORPORATION
800-876-6866
775-746-6600
PO Box 32000, 2301 Robb Drive,,
Reno, NV 89533
FDA Number: n/a   *Fax:* 775-746-6577
E-mail: marketing@microflex.com
Web site: www.microflex.com
Medical Products Sales Volume: $7,200,000
Year Founded: 1987
Total Employees: 97
Ownership: Private
Quality System Registration Information: ISO9001
Produces/Sells CE-marked Devices: Y
Federal Procurement Eligibility: Small Business
Distribution: Manufacturer Direct, Importer
General Admin.: Lloyd Rogers/Chief Executive Officer
    Rich Todd/Vice President International Operations
Mktg./Adv.: Russ Vossen/Director Sales
    Gene Barbera/Market Manager
    Bob Cramer/Vice President Marketing
Production: Don Cronk/Manager Regulatory Affairs
Glove, Other	General
Glove, Patient Examination, Latex	General

MICROFLUIDICS INTERNATIONAL CORPORATION
800-370-5452
617-969-5452
30 Ossipee Rd.,
Newton Upper Falls, MA 02464
FDA Number: n/a   *Fax:* 617-965-1213
Web site: www.microfluidicscorp.com
Medical Products Sales Volume: $7,000,000
Annual Revenue: $10-$25 Million
Year Founded: 1984
Ownership: IDEX CORPORATION
Produces/Sells CE-marked Devices: Y
Federal Procurement Eligibility: Small Business

MICROFLUIDICS INTERNATIONAL   800-370-5452 *(cont'd)*

Distribution: Manufacturer Direct, Manufacturer Through Distributor, Manufacturer Through Manufacturer Reps
General Admin.: Michael C. Ferrara/Chief Executive Officer
       Thomai Panagiotou/Chief Technology Officer
Production: William J. Conroy/Vice President Operations
Finance: Peter F. Byczko/Vice President Finance

Mixer, Clinical Laboratory	Chemistry

MICROGENESYS, INC.
See Protein Sciences Corp.

MICROGENICS CORPORATION   800-232-3342
46360 Fremont Blvd., Fremont, CA 94538   510-979-5000
FDA Number: 2937369   *Fax:* 510-979-5002
Web site: www.microgenics.com
Total Employees: 240   *Marketing Staff:* 5
Ownership: APOGENT TECHNOLOGIES, INC.
Quality System Registration Information: ISO9001
Produces/Sells CE-marked Devices: Y
Distribution: Manufacturer Direct, OEM
General Admin.: Maryanne Allen/Director Human Resources
       Dr. Yuh-Geng Tsay/President, Chief Executive Officer
       Bob Wolf/Vice President International Operations
Mktg./Adv.: Paula Stonemetz/Director Business Development
       Lorenzo Ajel/Director Marketing Operations
       Kathy Ruzich/Manager Advertising
       Mr. Azeem Syed/Vice President Marketing & Sales
Production: Bill Picht/Vice President Manufacturing & Operations
       Parisa Khosropour/Vice President Operations
       Andy Morozovsky/Vice President Regulatory Affairs
Finance: Linda Lechner/Chief Financial Officer

Control, Drug Specific	Toxicology
Enzyme Immunoassay, Amphetamine	Toxicology
Enzyme Immunoassay, Barbiturate	Toxicology
Enzyme Immunoassay, Benzodiazepine	Toxicology
Enzyme Immunoassay, Carbamazepine	Toxicology
Enzyme Immunoassay, Digitoxin	Toxicology
Enzyme Immunoassay, Digoxin	Toxicology
Enzyme Immunoassay, Diphenylhydantoin	Toxicology
Enzyme Immunoassay, Gentamicin	Toxicology
Enzyme Immunoassay, Methadone	Toxicology
Enzyme Immunoassay, N-Acetylprocainamide	Toxicology
Enzyme Immunoassay, Non-Radiolabeled, Total Thyroxine	Chemistry
Enzyme Immunoassay, Other	Chemistry
Enzyme Immunoassay, Phencyclidine	Toxicology
Enzyme Immunoassay, Phenobarbital	Toxicology
Enzyme Immunoassay, Theophylline	Toxicology
Enzyme Immunoassay, Valproic Acid	Toxicology
Thyroid Uptake System	Radiology

MICROGON, INC.
See Spectrum Laboratories, Inc.

MICROGROUP   800-255-8823
7 Industrial Park Road, Medway, MA 02053   508-533-4925
FDA Number: n/a   *Fax:* 508-533-5691
E-mail: info@microgroup.com
Web site: www.microgroup.com
Medical Products Sales Volume: $52,700,000
Annual Revenue: $50-$100 Million
Year Founded: 1971
Total Employees: 150   *Marketing Staff:* 3   *Sales Staff:* 12
Ownership: Private
Quality System Registration Information: ISO9002
Produces/Sells CE-marked Devices: N
Federal Procurement Eligibility: Small Business
Distribution: Manufacturer Direct, Manufacturer Through Manufacturer Reps, OEM
General Admin.: Bill Hulbig/Chief Executive Officer
       William Hulbig/President, Chief Executive Officer
Mktg./Adv.: Bob Lamson/Vice President Business Development
Production: Jim Owens/Director Quality Assurance
       Thomas Hayes/Manager Materials

Adapter, Holder, Syringe	Physical Med
Adapter, Needle	Cardiovascular
Adapter, Stopcock, Manifold, Cardiopulmonary Bypass	Cardiovascular
Adapter, Syringe	General
Component, Metal, Other	General
Component, Other	General
Dispenser, Fluid	General
Dispenser, Syringe And Needle	General
Fitting, Luer	General
Fitting, Other	General
Fitting, Quick Connect (Gas Connector)	General
Manifold, Gas	Chemistry
Manifold, Liquid	Chemistry
Needle, Hypodermic	General
Needle, Hypodermic, Single Lumen With Syringe	General
Needle, Other	General
Needle, Spinal, Short-Term	General

MICROGROUP   800-255-8823 *(cont'd)*

Pipette	Chemistry
Pipette Tip	Chemistry
Stopcock	General
Syringe, Drug, Luer-Lock	Dental And Oral
Syringe, Laboratory	Chemistry
Syringe, Other	General
Syringe, Piston	General
Tube, Capillary	Chemistry
Tubing, Connecting	General
Valve, Other	Chemistry

MICROGUIDE, INC.   630-964-3368
1635 Plum Ct., Downers Grove, IL 60515-1325
FDA Number: 1422301   *Fax:* 630-964-8368
E-mail: sales@eyemove.com
Web site: www.eyemove.com
Medical Products Sales Volume: $200,000
Annual Revenue: $0-$1 Million
Year Founded: 1981
Total Employees: 3   *Marketing Staff:* 1   *Sales Staff:* 1
Ownership: Private
Stock Symbol: VAS
Traded On: NYSE
Quality System Registration Information: ISO9000
Produces/Sells CE-marked Devices: N
Federal Procurement Eligibility: Small Business
Distribution: Manufacturer Direct
General Admin.: Glenn Krol/President

Monitor, Eye Movement, Diagnostic	Ophthalmology

MICROLIFE MEDICAL HOME SOLUTIONS, INC.   1-800-968-1378
2801 Youngfield Street, Suite 241,   303-274-2277
Golden, CO 80401
FDA Number: 3003288989   *Fax:* 303-274-2244
E-mail: info@MiMHS.com
Ownership: Private
Produces/Sells CE-marked Devices: N

Computer, Oxygen-Uptake	Anesthesiology

MICROLIFE USA, INC.   888-314-2599
424 Skinner Blvd.,,, Suite C, Dunedin, FL 34698   727-451-0484
FDA Number: 3003719302   *Fax:* 727-451-0492
E-mail: info@microlifeusa.com
Web site: www.microlifeusa.com
Medical Products Sales Volume: $50,000,000
Year Founded: 1997
Total Employees: 20
Ownership: Private
Produces/Sells CE-marked Devices: Y
Federal Procurement Eligibility: Small Business
Distribution: Manufacturer Direct, Manufacturer Through Distributor, Exporter

Computer, Oxygen-Uptake	Anesthesiology

MICROLIGHT CORPORATION OF AMERICA   281-433-4648
2935 Highland Lakes Dr., Missouri City, TX 77459
FDA Number: 3003654318
E-mail: m.barbour@sbcglobal.net
Web site: www.microlightcorp.com
Ownership: Private
Produces/Sells CE-marked Devices: N

MICROLINE PENTAX, INC.   978-922-9810
800 Cummings Center, Suite # 166t, Beverly, MA 01915
FDA Number: 1223422   *Fax:* 978-922-9209
E-mail: info@microlinesurgical.com
Web site: www.microlinesurgical.com
Year Founded: 1987
Total Employees: 140
Ownership: Private
Produces/Sells CE-marked Devices: Y
General Admin.: Dr. Jean-Luc Boulnois/President, Chief Executive Officer

Clip, Implantable	Surgery
Electrosurgical Unit, Cutting & Coagulation Device	Surgery
Electrosurgical, Cutting & Coagulation Accessories, Laparoscopic & Endoscopic, Reprocessed	Surgery
Laparoscope, General & Plastic Surgery	Surgery

MICROMACHINING TECHNOLOGIES, INC.   314-785-6800
2345 Millpark Dr., Suite A, Maryland Heights, MO 63043
FDA Number: 3004864805
Ownership: Private
Produces/Sells CE-marked Devices: N

Cystotome, Ophthalmic	Ophthalmology

MICROMANIPULATOR CO., INC., THE   800-972-4032
1555 Forrest Way, Carson City, NV 89706-0448   775-882-2400
FDA Number: n/a   *Fax:* 775-882-7694
E-mail: sales@micromanipulator.com

MICROMANIPULATOR CO., INC., THE   800-972-4032 *(cont'd)*

Web site: www.micromanipulator.com
Annual Revenue: $5-$10 Million
Year Founded: 1956
Total Employees: 50
Ownership: Private
Stock Symbol: SCP
Traded On: NASDAQ
Produces/Sells CE-marked Devices: N
Federal Procurement Eligibility: Small Business
Distribution: Manufacturer Direct, Manufacturer Through Distributor, Manufacturer Through Manufacturer Reps
General Admin.: Kenneth F. Hollman/President

Camera, Microscope	Microbiology
Contract R&D, Equipment	General
Contrast Enhancement Unit, Microscope	Microbiology
General Purpose Microbiology Diagnostic Device	Microbiology
Instrument, Microsurgical	Cns/Neurology
Micro-Injector, Transplant, Gene	Microbiology
Micromanipulator	General
Microscope	Hematology
Microscope, Laboratory, Optical	Microbiology
Microscope, Light	Pathology
Probe	Orthopedics
Television Monitor, Microscope	General

MICROMED TECHNOLOGY, INC.   713-838-9210

8965 Interchange Dr., Houston, TX 77054
FDA Number: 1651839   *Fax:* 713-828-9214
Web site: www.micromedtech.com
Year Founded: 1996
Ownership: Private
Produces/Sells CE-marked Devices: N
General Admin.: Mr. Robert J. Benkowski/Chief Executive Officer
Mktg./Adv.: Mr. Don Isaacs/Director Communications
Production: Mr. Bryan E. Lynch/Director Operations
Finance: Ms. Deanne Yartz/Chief Financial Officer

Circulatory Assist Unit, Left Ventricular	Cardiovascular

MICROMEDEX, INC.   303-486-6400

6200 S. Syracuse Way, Suite 300,
Greenwood Village, CO 80111
FDA Number: n/a   *Fax:* 303-486-6464
E-mail: info@mdx.com
Web site: www.micromedex.com
Year Founded: 1944
Total Employees: 450   *Marketing Staff:* 20   *Sales Staff:* 50
Ownership: The Thomson Corporation
Stock Symbol: TOC
Traded On: NYSE
Produces/Sells CE-marked Devices: N
Distribution: Manufacturer Direct
General Admin.: Rick Noble/Chief Executive Officer
          Jeff Reihl/Chief Operating Officer
Mktg./Adv.: Phil Bird/Executive Vice President Marketing & Sales

Computer Software	General

MICROMEDICAL TECHNOLOGIES, INC.   800-334-4154

10 Kemp Drive, Chatham, IL 62629   217-483-2122
FDA Number: 1450721   *Fax:* 217-483-4533
E-mail: mminfo@micromedical.com
Web site: www.micromedical.com
Medical Products Sales Volume: $50,000,000
Annual Revenue: $25-$50 Million
Year Founded: 1985
Total Employees: 13   *Marketing Staff:* 3   *Sales Staff:* 3
Ownership: Private
Produces/Sells CE-marked Devices: N
Federal Procurement Eligibility: Small Business
Distribution: Manufacturer Direct, Manufacturer Through Distributor, Manufacturer Through Manufacturer Reps, OEM, Importer, Exporter
General Admin.: Richard Miles/President, Chief Executive Officer
Mktg./Adv.: Diane Miles/Vice President Sales
Production: Joe Cannella/Director Quality Assurance
          Julie Chapman/Manager Materials
IS: Amjad Malki/Manager Software

Analyzer, Apparatus, Vestibular	Ear/Nose/Throat
Chair, Rotating	Cns/Neurology
Electronystagmograph (ENG)	Ophthalmology
Goggles, Protective, Eye	Ophthalmology
Monitor, Eye Movement	Ophthalmology
Stimulator, Caloric Air	Ear/Nose/Throat
Stimulator, Caloric Water	Ear/Nose/Throat

MICROMEDICS   800-624-5662

1270 Eagan Industrial Road,   651-452-1977
St. Paul, MN 55121
FDA Number: 2183425   *Fax:* 651-452-1787

MICROMEDICS   800-624-5662 *(cont'd)*

E-mail: customerservice@micromedics.com
Web site: www.micromedics.com
Medical Products Sales Volume: $9,800,000
Annual Revenue: $5-$10 Million
Year Founded: 1982
Total Employees: 70   *Marketing Staff:* 5   *Sales Staff:* 5
Ownership: Nordson Corporation
Quality System Registration Information: ISO9001
Produces/Sells CE-marked Devices: Y
Federal Procurement Eligibility: Small Business
Distribution: Manufacturer Direct, Manufacturer Through Distributor, Manufacturer Through Manufacturer Reps, OEM

Applicator, ENT	Ear/Nose/Throat
Applicator, Other	General
Atomizer And Tip, ENT	Ear/Nose/Throat
Burr	Ear/Nose/Throat
Button, Nasal Septal	Ear/Nose/Throat
Catheter, Nasopharyngeal	Ear/Nose/Throat
Container, Sterilization (Tray)	General
Device, Inflation, Middle Ear	Ear/Nose/Throat
Glue, Surgical Tissue	Surgery
Inserter, Myringotomy Tube	Ear/Nose/Throat
Knife, Myringotomy	Ear/Nose/Throat
Protector, Surgical Instrument	Surgery
Rack, Surgical Instrument	Surgery
Splint, Nasal	Ear/Nose/Throat
Splint, Septal, Intranasal	Ear/Nose/Throat
Tray, Sterilization, Instrument	Surgery
Tray, Surgical	Surgery
Tube, Myringotomy	Ear/Nose/Throat
Tube, Tympanostomy	Ear/Nose/Throat
Wick, Ear	Ear/Nose/Throat

MICROMERITICS INSTRUMENT CORP.

See GP Instruments

MICROMRI, INC.   267-212-1100

580 Middletown Boulevard,, #D-150, Langhorne, PA 19047
FDA Number: 3005871119   *Fax:* 267-212-1101
E-mail: info@micromri.com
Web site: www.micromri.com
Ownership: Private
Produces/Sells CE-marked Devices: N

Coil, Magnetic Resonance, Specialty	Radiology

MICRON MEDICAL PRODUCTS, INC.

See Micron Products, Inc.

MICRON PRECISION ENGINEERING, INC.   310-874-4963

939 Evening Shade Dr, San Pedro, CA 90731
FDA Number: 2031762
Ownership: Private
Produces/Sells CE-marked Devices: N

Implant, Fixation Device, Spinal	Orthopedics
Orthosis, Fixation, Pedicle, Spinal	Orthopedics
Orthosis, Fusion, Intervertebral, Spinal	Orthopedics

MICRON PRODUCTS, INC.   800-370-5500

25 Sawyer Passway, Fitchburg, MA 01420   978-345-5000
FDA Number: n/a   *Fax:* 978-342-0168
E-mail: info@micronproducts.com
Web site: www.micronproducts.com
Medical Products Sales Volume: $19,300,000
Annual Revenue: $5-$10 Million
Year Founded: 1978
Total Employees: 65   *Marketing Staff:* 2   *Sales Staff:* 2
Ownership: Public
Stock Symbol: HRT
Traded On: AMEX
Quality System Registration Information: ISO9001
Produces/Sells CE-marked Devices: N
Federal Procurement Eligibility: Small Business
Distribution: Manufacturer Direct, Manufacturer Through Manufacturer Reps
General Admin.: David Garrison/Chief Financial Officer, Treasurer
          James E. Rouse/President, Chief Executive Officer
          N/A N/A/Vice President, General Manager
Mktg./Adv.: Frederick Lane/Director Product Development
          Mark R. LaViolette/Vice President Marketing & Sales
Production: Karen Rokes/Plant Manager
          Peter Pignone/Vice President, Director Engineering
Research: Frederick Lane/Vice President Research & Development & Quality Control

Electrode, Electrocardiograph	Cardiovascular

MICRON SEPARATIONS PRODUCTS/OSMONICS

See Ge Infrastructure Water & Process Technologies

MICRON VIDEO INTERNATIONAL, INC.   800-564-2766

18585 Coastal Highway,, Suite 149, Rehoboth, DE 19971
FDA Number: n/a   *Fax:* 302-258-0880

MANUFACTURER PROFILES

MICRON VIDEO INTERNATIONAL, INC.   800-564-2766 *(cont'd)*
E-mail: mvi-usa@mvitraining.com
Web site: www.mvitraining.com
Ownership: Private
Produces/Sells CE-marked Devices: N
Distribution: Exclusive Distributor, Exporter
Material, Training, Audiovisual   General

MICRONICS, INC.   425-895-9197
8463 154th Avenue NE, Building G, Redmond, WA 98052
FDA Number: n/a   *Fax:* 425-895-1183
Web site: http://www.micronics.net
Year Founded: 1996
Ownership: Private
Produces/Sells CE-marked Devices: N
General Admin.: Mr. John Gerdes/Chief Scientific Officer
    Dr. Fred Battrell/Chief Technology Officer
    Ms. Karen Hedine/President, Chief Executive Officer
Mktg./Adv.: Mr. Larry Hambleton/Vice President Marketing & Sales
Production: Mr. Reed Simmons/Vice President Manufacturing
    Dr. Diane Wierzbicki/Vice President Regulatory Affairs
Finance: Mr. Manu Talwar/Chief Financial Officer
Kit, Test, Periodontal, In Vitro   Dental And Oral

MICRONOVA   888-816-4876
3431 W. Lomita Blvd., Torrance, CA 90505-5010   310-784-6990
FDA Number: n/a   *Fax:* 310-784-6980
E-mail: micronv100@aol.com
Web site: www.micronova-mfg.com
Medical Products Sales Volume: $1,800,000
Year Founded: 1984
Total Employees: 30
Ownership: Private
Quality System Registration Information: ISO9001
Federal Procurement Eligibility: Small Business, Female Owned
Distribution: Manufacturer Through Distributor
General Admin.: Deborah Leonard/General Manager
    Audrey Reynolds/President, Chief Executive Officer
Mktg./Adv.: Deborah Leonard/Vice President Marketing & Sales
Component, Other   General
Detergent   Hematology

MICRONOVA TECHNOLOGY, INC.   615-662-1304
914 Harpeth Valley Place, Nashville, TN 37221
FDA Number: n/a   *Fax:* 615-662-1226
E-mail: info@micronovatech.com
Web site: www.micronovatech.com
Medical Products Sales Volume: $2,700,000
Year Founded: 1991
Total Employees: 25
Ownership: Private
Produces/Sells CE-marked Devices: N
General Admin.: Mr. Roland Keistler, Jr./President, Chief Executive Officer
IS: Mr. Robert V. Allen/Chief Technologist
Communication Equipment   General

MICROPATENT   800-648-6787
250 Dodge Ave., East Haven, CT 06512   203-466-5055
FDA Number: n/a   *Fax:* 203-466-5054
E-mail: info@micropat.com
Web site: www.micropat.com
Annual Revenue: $1-$5 Million
Ownership: Public
Produces/Sells CE-marked Devices: N
General Admin.: Steve Wolfson/President, Chief Executive Officer
Mktg./Adv.: Laura Glaze/Director Marketing
    Judy Hickey/Director Product Development
    Laryssa Kaiser/Manager Advertising
    Taka Nakashima/Manager National Sales
Service, Licensing, Device, Medical   General

MICROPHAGE INC.   303-652-5200
2400 Trade Centre Avenue, Longmont, CO 80503
FDA Number: 3008501195   *Fax:* 303-652-5080
Web site: http://www.microphage.com
Year Founded: 2002
Ownership: Private
Produces/Sells CE-marked Devices: N
Production: Mr. Preston Brown/Director Manufacturing
    Ms. Michelle Dowling/Director Quality Assurance
Research: Dr. J. Drew Smith/Vice President Research & Development
Staphylococcus Aureus Protein A Insoluble   Microbiology

MICROPLASTICS, INC.   630-513-2900
406 38th Avenue, St. Charles, IL 60174
FDA Number: n/a   *Fax:* 630-513-2901
E-mail: sales@microplasticsinc.com
Web site: www.microplasticsinc.com

MICROPLASTICS, INC.   630-513-2900 *(cont'd)*
Year Founded: 1989
Ownership: Private
Quality System Registration Information: ISO9001
Produces/Sells CE-marked Devices: N
Injector, Pen   General
Syringe, Insulin   General

MICROSCOPY/MICROSCOPY EDUCATION   413-746-6931
125 Paridon St., Suite 102, Springfield, MA 01108-2140
FDA Number: n/a   *Fax:* 413-746-9311
E-mail: mme@map.com
Web site: www.mme-microscopy.com/education
Medical Products Sales Volume: $2,000,000
Annual Revenue: $0-$1 Million
Year Founded: 1981
Total Employees: 27   *Marketing Staff:* 3   *Sales Staff:* 3
Ownership: Private
Federal Procurement Eligibility: Small Business, Female Owned
Distribution: Service Direct
General Admin.: Kenneth Piel/Chief Operating Officer, Chief Financial Officer
    Barbara Foster/President
Microscope   Hematology
Training Aid   Orthopedics

MICROSPECIALTIES, INC.   877-874-1933
264 Quarry Road, PO Box 3030,   203-874-1832
Milford, CT 06460
FDA Number: 1226074   *Fax:* 203-877-3762
E-mail: microspecialties@usa.com
Web site: www.microspecialties.com
Annual Revenue: $1-$5 Million
Year Founded: 1984
Ownership: Private
Quality System Registration Information: ISO9001
Produces/Sells CE-marked Devices: Y
Federal Procurement Eligibility: Small Business
Distribution: Manufacturer Direct, Manufacturer Through Distributor, Manufacturer Through Manufacturer Reps
Blade, Surgical, Saw, General & Plastic Surgery   Surgery

MICROSTAT LABORATORIES, INC.   877-204-2007
PO Box 115, Dover, MN 55929   507-932-3968
FDA Number: n/a   *Fax:* 507-932-3979
E-mail: carl@microstatlabs.com
Web site: www.microstatlabs.com
Medical Products Sales Volume: $33,000,000
Annual Revenue: $0-$1 Million
Year Founded: 1998
Total Employees: 2   *Sales Staff:* 2
Ownership: RIVERS EDGE TECHNICAL SERVICE, INC.
Produces/Sells CE-marked Devices: N
Federal Procurement Eligibility: Small Business
Distribution: Service Direct
General Admin.: Carl Newberg/President
Equipment/Service, Quality Control   General

MICROSTIM TECHNOLOGY, INC.   772-283-0235
3879 NE Skyline Drive, Jensen Beach, FL 34957
FDA Number: 2939358
E-mail: jrossen@microstim.com
Web site: www.microstim.com
Ownership: Private
Produces/Sells CE-marked Devices: N
Bandage, Adhesive   Surgery
Electrode, Cutaneous   Cns/Neurology
Massager, Therapeutic   Physical Med
Stimulator, Nerve, Transcutaneous (Pain Relief, TENS)   Cns/Neurology

MICROSTOMIA PREVENTION APPLIANCE
See Life-Like Laboratory

MICROSURGICAL LABORATORIES   800-414-1076
11333 Chimney Rock Road, Suite 120,   713-723-6900
Houston, TX 77035
FDA Number: 1646747   *Fax:* 713-723-6906
E-mail: micro@wexlersurgical.com
Web site: www.wexlersurgical.com
Medical Products Sales Volume: $1,600,000
Year Founded: 1991
Total Employees: 11
Ownership: Private
Produces/Sells CE-marked Devices: Y
Federal Procurement Eligibility: Small Business
Distribution: OEM
Mktg./Adv.: Danny Fishman/Director Marketing
Contract Manufacturing   General
Contract R&D, Equipment   General

MICROSURGICAL LABORATORIES 800-414-1076 *(cont'd)*
Kit, Instruments and Accessories, Surgical — Surgery
Retractor — Orthopedics

MICROSURGICAL TECHNOLOGY, INC. 425-556-0544
8415 154th Ave NE, Redmond, WA 98052
FDA Number: 3019924 — Fax: 425-556-0437
E-mail: info@microsurgical.com
Web site: www.microsurgical.com
Year Founded: 1976
Total Employees: 50 — Marketing Staff: 2 — Sales Staff: 2
Ownership: Private
Quality System Registration Information: ISO9001
Produces/Sells CE-marked Devices: Y
Federal Procurement Eligibility: Small Business
Distribution: Manufacturer Through Distributor, Manufacturer Through Manufacturer Reps, OEM, Exporter
General Admin.: Mr. Larry Laks/President
Mktg./Adv.: Mr. Mark Anderson/Vice President Sales
Production: Mr. Bob May/Vice President Operations
Finance: Ms. Marie Lanese/Controller
Applicator, Ocular Pressure	Ophthalmology
Cannula, Ophthalmic	Ophthalmology
Controller, Infusion	Cardiovascular
Cystotome, Ophthalmic	Ophthalmology
Forceps, Ophthalmic	Ophthalmology
Hook, Ophthalmic	Ophthalmology
Irrigator, Ocular Surgery	Ophthalmology
Kit, Irrigation, Eye	Ophthalmology
Knife, Ophthalmic	Ophthalmology
Phacofragmentation Unit	Ophthalmology
Spatula, Ophthalmic	Ophthalmology

MICROTECH 714-966-1645
3633 West Macarthur Blvd., Suite 410, Santa Ana, CA 92704
FDA Number: 2032725
Handpiece, Air-Powered, Dental — Dental And Oral

MICROTECH MEDICAL SYSTEMS 303-363-0007
401 Laredo St. - Unit I, Aurora, CO 80011-9207
FDA Number: 1720153
Medical Products Sales Volume: $550,000
Annual Revenue: $0-$1 Million
Ownership: Private
Produces/Sells CE-marked Devices: N
Federal Procurement Eligibility: Small Business
Distribution: Manufacturer Direct
Production: Jerry Kilgore/President Production
Computer, Clinical Laboratory	Chemistry
Contract Laboratory	General
Kit, Identification, Enterobacteriaceae	Microbiology
Test, Antibiotic Susceptibility	Microbiology

MICROTEK MEDICAL, INC 800-936-9248
512 Lehmberg Road, Columbus, MS 39704 662-327-1863
FDA Number: 1043582 — Fax: 800-642-0255
E-mail: Microtek-Info@ecolab.com
Web site: www.microtekmed.com
Medical Products Sales Volume: $1,392,120
Annual Revenue: $100-$500 Million
Year Founded: 1983
Total Employees: 1829 — Marketing Staff: 3 — Sales Staff: 38
Ownership: Public
Stock Symbol: MTMD
Traded On: NASDAQ
Produces/Sells CE-marked Devices: Y
Distribution: Manufacturer Direct, Manufacturer Through Distributor, OEM, Exporter
General Admin.: Dan R Lee/Chairman
　　　　　Kenneth F Davis/Director
　　　　　Marc R Sarni/Director
　　　　　Michael E Glasscock/Director
　　　　　Rosdon Hendrix/Director
Accessories, Apparel, Surgical	Surgery
Accessories, Arthroscope	Orthopedics
Accessories, Laser	General
Accessories, Photographic, Endoscopic	Gastroenterology/Urology
Ambulance	General
Bag, Collection, Urine, Newborn	General
Contract Manufacturing	General
Cover, Camera	Surgery
Cover, Microscope	Microbiology
Cover, Other	General
Drape, Surgical	Surgery
Encapsulator, Fluid	General

MICROTELE LABORATORIES INC.
See Physitemp Instruments, Inc.

MICROTEST, INC. (800) 631-1680
104 Gold Street, Agawam, MA 01001-3807 (413) 786-1680
FDA Number: n/a — Fax: (413) 789-4334
E-mail: info@microtestlabs.com
Web site: www.microtestlabs.com
Medical Products Sales Volume: $1,500,000
Total Employees: 7 — Marketing Staff: 2 — Sales Staff: 1
Ownership: Private
Produces/Sells CE-marked Devices: N
Federal Procurement Eligibility: Small Business
Distribution: Manufacturer Direct, Manufacturer Through Distributor
General Admin.: Steve Racioppi/President, Chief Executive Officer
Transport System, Aerobic — Microbiology

MICROTRONICS CORP. OF CHAPEL HILL 919-929-2657
88 Vilcom Center, Ste. 165, Chapel Hill, NC 27516
FDA Number: n/a — Fax: 919-968-0074
E-mail: csupport@microtronics-bit.com
Web site: www.microtonics-nc.com
Ownership: Private
Produces/Sells CE-marked Devices: N
Federal Procurement Eligibility: Small Business
Distribution: Manufacturer Direct
General Admin.: J. S. Hutcheson/Chief Executive Officer
Mktg./Adv.: Richard W. Lutz/Manager Advertising
　　　　　R. W. Lutz/Manager Marketing
　　　　　Richard W. Lutz/Vice President Marketing & Sales
Production: Richard W. Lutz/Vice President Manufacturing
Research: Richard W. Lutz/Vice President Research & Development
Speech Therapy Unit (Trainer) — Ear/Nose/Throat

MICROVENTION, INC. 949-461-3314
1311 valencia avenue, tustin, CA 92780
FDA Number: 2032493 — Fax: 949-461-3329
Web site: www.terumomedical.com
Ownership: Terumo Corporation
Produces/Sells CE-marked Devices: N
Catheter, Percutaneous	Cardiovascular
Device, Embolization, Artificial	Cns/Neurology
Embolization Device	Cardiovascular
Guidewire, Catheter	Cardiovascular

MICROVISION, INC. 603-474-5566
34 Folly Mill Rd., Seabrook, NH 03874
FDA Number: 1226011
Cannula, Ophthalmic	Ophthalmology
Clip, Iris Retractor	Ophthalmology
Cutter, Vitreous Aspiration, AC-Powered	Ophthalmology
Laser, Ophthalmic	Ophthalmology
Light, Surgical, Fiberoptic	Surgery
Phacofragmentation Unit	Ophthalmology

MICROWAVE RESEARCH & APPLICATIONS, INC. 866-953-1771
8685 Cherry Ln., Laurel, MD 20707-6302 301-953-1771
FDA Number: 3004869321 — Fax: 301-369-0523
E-mail: info@microwaveresearch.com
Web site: www.microwaveresearch.com
Medical Products Sales Volume: $200,000
Annual Revenue: $1-$5 Million
Year Founded: 1999
Total Employees: 3 — Sales Staff: 2
Ownership: Private
Produces/Sells CE-marked Devices: N
Federal Procurement Eligibility: Small Business, GSA Contract, VA Contract
Distribution: Manufacturer Direct, Manufacturer Through Distributor, Manufacturer Through Manufacturer Reps, OEM
General Admin.: Wayne Love/President
　　　　　James C. Stratton/Vice President
Research: Randy Hill/Director Tech. Affairs
Oven	Chemistry
Tissue Processor, Automated	Pathology

MICROWAVE SPECIALTIES INC.
See Microwave Research & Applications, Inc.

MICROWORLD MEDICAL INSTRUMENTS, INC. 510-534-7401
4640 Malat St., Oakland, CA 94601
FDA Number: 9058259 — Fax: 510-534-7403
E-mail: microworld@sbcglobal.net
Annual Revenue: $0-$1 Million
Year Founded: 2002
Total Employees: 7 — Marketing Staff: 1 — Sales Staff: 1
Ownership: Private
Produces/Sells CE-marked Devices: N
Federal Procurement Eligibility: Small Business
Distribution: Manufacturer Through Distributor

MANUFACTURER PROFILES

MICROWORLD MEDICAL INSTRUMENTS, INC.   510-534-7401
(cont'd)
  General Admin.: Mr. Semyon Gambarin/Chief Executive Officer, Chief Financial
Officer
    Cutter, Vitreous Aspiration, AC-Powered   Ophthalmology

MICROZONE CORPORATION   877-252-7710
86 Harry Douglas Drive,   613-831-8318
Ottawa, ONT K2S 2 Canada
  FDA Number: n/a   Fax: 613-831-8321
  E-mail: sales@microzone.com
  Web site: www.microzone.com
  Year Founded: 1968
  Total Employees: 45   Marketing Staff: 2   Sales Staff: 6
  Ownership: Canadian Erectors Ltd.
  Produces/Sells CE-marked Devices: Y
  Distribution: Manufacturer Direct, Manufacturer Through Distributor, Manufacturer
Through Manufacturer Reps, OEM, Exporter

MICRUS CORPORATION   408-830-5900
610 Palomar Avenue, Sunnyvale, CA 94085
  FDA Number: 9042070   Fax: 408-830-5910
  E-mail: kaw@micruscorp.com
  Web site: www.micruscorp.com
  Ownership: Johnson & Johnson
  Produces/Sells CE-marked Devices: Y
    Device, Embolization, Artificial   Cns/Neurology

MICRUS DESIGN TECHNOLOGY, INC.   408-433-1460
9344 N.w. 13th St., Miami, FL 33172
  FDA Number: 3004107186
    Catheter, Percutaneous   Cardiovascular

MICRUS ENDOVASCULAR CORPORATION   888-550-4120
821 Fox Lane, San Jose, CA 95131   408-433-1400
  FDA Number: 2954740   Fax: 408-433-1401
  E-mail: customerservice@micruscorp.com
  Web site: www.micruscorp.com
  Year Founded: 1996
  Total Employees: 287
  Ownership: JOHNSON & JOHNSON
  Produces/Sells CE-marked Devices: N
  General Admin.: Mr. John Kilcyone/Chairman, Chief Executive Officer
         Mr. Robert Stern/President, Chief Operating Officer
  Mktg./Adv.: Mr. Robert Colloton/Vice President Marketing & Sales
  Finance: Mr. Gordon Sangster/Chief Financial Officer
    Catheter, Intravascular, Diagnostic   Cardiovascular
    Device, Embolization, Artificial   Cns/Neurology
    Guidewire, Catheter   Cardiovascular

MICTRON, INC.   941-371-6659
8130 Fruitville Rd., Sarasota, FL 34240
  FDA Number: 1055443   Fax: 941-379-2345
  E-mail: mictron@mictron.net
  Web site: www.mictron.net
  Ownership: Private
  Produces/Sells CE-marked Devices: N
    Traction Unit, Non-Powered   Orthopedics

MID-ATLANTIC DIAGNOSTICS INC., CUSTOM   856-762-2000
PRODUCTS DIV
  77 Elbo Lane, Mount Laurel, NJ 08054
  FDA Number: 2249709
    Accessory, Assisted Reproduction   Obstetrics/Gynecology

MID-ATLANTIC MEDICAL SERVICES
  See Pyramid Industries, Llc

MID-CONTINENTAL DENTAL SUPPLY CO., LTD.   204-888-5031
242 Alboro St, Headingley R4J 1A4 Canada
  FDA Number: 9615151
    Cleaner, Denture   Dental And Oral

MID-DELTA HOME HEALTH & HOSPICE   800-543-9055
405 North Hayden St., Belzoni, MS 39038   662-247-1254
  FDA Number: 2320745   Fax: 662-247-4924
  E-mail: creed@mail.middelta.com
  Web site: www.middelta.com
  Year Founded: 1978
  Total Employees: 354   Marketing Staff: 17   Sales Staff: 17
  Ownership: Private
  Produces/Sells CE-marked Devices: N
  Federal Procurement Eligibility: Small Business, Minority Owned, Female Owned
  Distribution: Manufacturer Direct
  General Admin.: Mrs. Clara Reed/Chief Executive Officer
  Purchasing: Mr. Henry Reed/Vice President Purchasing
    DI (O-Hydroxyphenylimine) Ethane, Calcium   Chemistry

MID-STATES LABORATORIES, INC.   800-247-3669
600 N Saint Francis, Wichita, KS 67202-2102   316-262-7013
  FDA Number: n/a   Fax: 316-262-7724
  E-mail: info@mid-stateslabs.com
  Web site: www.mid-stateslabs.com
  Medical Products Sales Volume: $1,100,000
  Annual Revenue: $0-$1 Million
  Year Founded: 1951
  Total Employees: 3   Marketing Staff: 2   Sales Staff: 2
  Ownership: Private
  Produces/Sells CE-marked Devices: Y
  Federal Procurement Eligibility: Small Business, GSA Contract
  Distribution: Manufacturer Direct, Manufacturer Through Distributor
  General Admin.: Woodrow Rice/President
  Mktg./Adv.: Sherry Rice DuPerier, M.S./Director Marketing
  Production: W. R. Rice/Vice President Manufacturing
    Material, Impression   Dental And Oral
    Mold, Middle Ear   Ear/Nose/Throat
    Plug, Ear   Ear/Nose/Throat

MIDBROOK, INC.   1-800-966-WASH
2080 Brooklyn Rd., Jackson, MI 49203   517-787-3481
  FDA Number: 3000232301   Fax: 517-787-2349
  E-mail: sales@midbrook.com
  Web site: www.midbrook.com
  Ownership: Private
  Produces/Sells CE-marked Devices: N
    Hot Water Pasteurization Device   General
    Tray, Surgical Instrument   Surgery

MIDDLESEX GASES & TECHNOLOGIES, INC.   617-387-5050
292 Second St., Everett, MA 02149
  FDA Number: 1225722
    Gas, Calibrated (Specified Concentration)   Anesthesiology

MIDI, INC.   302-737-4297
125 Sandy Dr., Newark, DE 19713
  FDA Number: 3005786028
    Chromatographic Bacterial Identification   Microbiology

MIDLAND MANUFACTURING CO., INC.   803-776-5398
802 Universal Dr., Columbia, SC 29209
  FDA Number: 1048003
  Annual Revenue: $1-$5 Million
  Ownership: Private
  Produces/Sells CE-marked Devices: N
  Federal Procurement Eligibility: Small Business
    Bars, Parallel, Exercise   Physical Med
    Bars, Parallel, Powered   Physical Med
    Exercise Stair   Physical Med
    Exerciser, Non-Measuring   Physical Med
    Plinth   Physical Med
    Table, Mechanical   Physical Med
    Table, Other   General
    Table, Physical Medicine, Powered   Physical Med
    Table, Physical Therapy   Physical Med
    Table, Traction   Orthopedics
    Transfer Aid   Physical Med
    Wheelchair, Standup   Physical Med

MIDMARK CORPORATION   800-643-6275
60 Vista Dr., P.O. Box 286, Versailles, OH 45380   937-526-3662
  FDA Number: 1523530   Fax: 937-526-8384
  E-mail: webmaster@midmark.com
  Web site: www.midmark.com
  Medical Products Sales Volume: $100,000,000
  Annual Revenue: $100-$500 Million
  Year Founded: 1915
  Total Employees: 500
  Ownership: Private
  Quality System Registration Information: ISO9001
  Produces/Sells CE-marked Devices: Y
  Distribution: Manufacturer Through Distributor, Exporter
  General Admin.: Anne Eiting Klamar/President, Chief Executive Officer
         Mickey Scherer/Vice President Human Resources
  Mktg./Adv.: Bill Zulauf/Director Marketing
         Jon Wells/Director Marketing
         Bill Hogan/Director Marketing & Sales
         Jerry Stahl/Director National Accounts
         Eric Shirley/Vice President Marketing & Sales
         Joseph Rothstein/Vice President Marketing & Sales
         Dick Moorman/Vice President Sales
  Production: Gene Harshbarger/Manager Regulatory Affairs
         Karl Weidner/Vice President Manufacturing
    Bracket, Table Assembly, N2O Delivery System   Dental And Oral
    Cabinet Casework, Modular   General
    Cabinet, Instrument   General
    Cart, Instrument   Surgery

MIDMARK CORPORATION 800-643-6275 *(cont'd)*

Chair, Blood Donor	General
Chair, Dental	Dental And Oral
Chair, Dental (With Unit)	Dental And Oral
Chair, Dental, Without Operative Unit	Dental And Oral
Chair, Examination And Treatment	General
Chair, Operative	Dental And Oral
Chair, Podiatric	Orthopedics
Chair, Surgical, AC-Powered	Surgery
Cleaner, Ultrasonic, Dental Laboratory	Dental And Oral
Cuspidor	Dental And Oral
Furniture, General	General
Lamp, Examination (Light)	General
Light, Dental	Dental And Oral
Light, Surgical Operating, Dental	Dental And Oral
Light, Surgical, Floor Standing	Surgery
Operative Dental Treatment Unit	Dental And Oral
Sterilizer, Steam (Autoclave)	General
Sterilizer, Steam (Autoclave), Dental	Dental And Oral
Sterilizer, Steam, Table Top	General
Stool, Dental	Dental And Oral
Stool, Operating Room, Adjustable	Surgery
Syringe Unit, Air And/Or Water	Dental And Oral
Table, Examination/Treatment	General
Table, Obstetrical, AC-Powered	Obstetrics/Gynecology
Table, Physical Medicine, Powered	Physical Med
Unit, Anesthesia, Dental, Electric	Dental And Oral

Medical Product Subsidiaries (Listed Separately)
Matrx By Midmark
Midmark Diagnostics Group

MIDMARK DIAGNOSTICS GROUP 800-643-6275
1125 W 90th Street, Gardena, CA 90248 937-526-3662
FDA Number: 2081230
E-mail: info@midmarkdiagnostics.com
Web site: www.midmarkdiagnostics.com
Medical Products Sales Volume: $9,000,000
Annual Revenue: $5-$10 Million
Year Founded: 1978
Total Employees: 45   *Marketing Staff:* 2   *Sales Staff:* 8
Ownership: Midmark Corporation
Quality System Registration Information: ISO9001
Produces/Sells CE-marked Devices: Y
Federal Procurement Eligibility: Small Business, GSA Contract
Distribution: Manufacturer Direct, Manufacturer Through Distributor, Manufacturer Through Manufacturer Reps, OEM, Importer, Exporter
General Admin.: Ruomei Zhang/Chief Technology Officer
Mktg./Adv.: Anthony Capparelli/Director Product Development
Mr. Michael Paquin/President, Director Sales
Production: Maria Cervantes/Manager Quality Assurance
Y. H. Teng/Senior Product Manager

Analyzer, ECG	Cardiovascular
Analyzer, Pulmonary Function	Anesthesiology
Computer, ECG Interpretation (Arrhythmia)	Cardiovascular
Computer, Pulmonary Function Interpretator (Diagnostic)	Anesthesiology
Computer, Pulmonary Function, Predicted Values	Anesthesiology
Electrocardiograph, Interpretive	Cardiovascular
Electrocardiograph, Multi-Channel	Cardiovascular
Recorder, Long-Term, ECG, Portable (Holter Monitor)	Cardiovascular
Spirometer, Diagnostic (Respirometer)	Anesthesiology

MIDSHORE INDUSTRIES, INC. 410-822-8622
29526 Canvasback Drive, Easton, MD 21601
FDA Number: 1120110   *Fax:* 410-822-8622
E-mail: gibb@goeaston.net
Medical Products Sales Volume: $100,000
Annual Revenue: $0-$1 Million
Year Founded: 1975
Total Employees: 2
Ownership: Private
Produces/Sells CE-marked Devices: N
Federal Procurement Eligibility: Small Business
Distribution: Manufacturer Direct

Hammer, Surgical	Surgery

MIDWEST CITY HEARING AID CENTER 405-732-8682
1401 South Midwest Blvd., Midwest City, OK 73110
FDA Number: 1648179
Ownership: Private
Produces/Sells CE-marked Devices: N

Hearing-Aid	Ear/Nose/Throat
Hearing-Aid, Plate, Face	Ear/Nose/Throat

MIDWEST CO.
See Del Medical Systems

MIDWEST DENTAL SUPPLY CORP.
See Del Medical Systems

MIDWEST EYE LABORATORIES, INC. 800-543-7936
1600 South Western, Suite C, Park Ridge Mall, 715-833-2277
Sioux Falls, SD 57105
FDA Number: 2183957
E-mail: info@MidwestEyeLab.com   *Fax:* 715-833-2295
Web site: www.midwesteyelab.com
Year Founded: 1986
Ownership: MIDWEST EYE LABORATORIES, INC.
Produces/Sells CE-marked Devices: N
General Admin.: Michael R. Barrett/President, Chief Executive Officer
Timothy J. Barrett/Vice President

Conformer, Ophthalmic	Ophthalmology
Eye, Artificial, Non-Custom	Ophthalmology
Shell, Scleral	Ophthalmology

MIDWEST EYE LABORATORIES, INC. 800-543-7936
20 2nd Ave., S.w., Suite 223, 715-833-2277
Rochester, MN 55901
FDA Number: 2183958
E-mail: Tim@MidwestEyeLab.com   *Fax:* 715-833-2295
Web site: www.midwesteyelab.com
Year Founded: 1986
Ownership: MIDWEST EYE LABORATORIES, INC.
Produces/Sells CE-marked Devices: N
General Admin.: Michael R. Barrett/President, Chief Executive Officer
Timothy J. Barrett/Vice President

Eye, Artificial, Non-Custom	Ophthalmology
Shell, Scleral	Ophthalmology

MIDWEST EYE LABORATORIES, INC. 800-543-7936
4606 Commerce Valley Rd, Suite 201, 715-833-2277
Eau Claire, WI 54701
FDA Number: 2183955   *Fax:* 715-833-2295
E-mail: info@MidwestEyeLab.com
Web site: www.midwesteyelab.com
Medical Products Sales Volume: $1,000,000
Annual Revenue: $0-$1 Million
Year Founded: 1986
Ownership: Private
Produces/Sells CE-marked Devices: N
Federal Procurement Eligibility: Small Business
Distribution: Exclusive Distributor
General Admin.: Michael R. Barrett/President, Chief Executive Officer
Timothy J. Barrett/Vice President

Conformer, Ophthalmic	Ophthalmology
Eye, Artificial, Custom	Ophthalmology
Eye, Artificial, Non-Custom	Ophthalmology
Prosthesis, Eye, Internal (Sphere)	Surgery
Shell, Scleral	Ophthalmology

MIDWEST EYE LABORATORIES, INC. 800-543-7936
7582 Currell Blvd., Suite 109, 715-833-2277
Woodbury, MN 55125
FDA Number: 2183831
E-mail: info@MidwestEyeLab.com   *Fax:* 715-833-2295
Web site: www.midwesteyelab.com
Year Founded: 1986
Ownership: MIDWEST EYE LABORATORIES, INC.
Produces/Sells CE-marked Devices: N
General Admin.: Michael R. Barrett/President, Chief Executive Officer
Timothy J. Barrett/Vice President

Conformer, Ophthalmic	Ophthalmology
Eye, Artificial, Non-Custom	Ophthalmology
Shell, Scleral	Ophthalmology

MIDWEST HEALTH CARE CONSULTANTS INC. 231-354-7482
154 Southern Shores, Brooklyn, MI 49230
FDA Number: 3006012338
Ownership: Private
Produces/Sells CE-marked Devices: N

Traction Unit, Non-Powered	Orthopedics

MIDWEST LASER PRODUCTS 815-462-9500
PO Box 262, Frankfort, IL 60423
FDA Number: n/a   *Fax:* 815-462-8955
E-mail: mlp@midwest-laser.com
Web site: www.midwest-laser.com
Medical Products Sales Volume: $300,000
Year Founded: 1988
Total Employees: 2
Ownership: Private
Produces/Sells CE-marked Devices: N
Federal Procurement Eligibility: Small Business
Distribution: Manufacturer Direct, Importer, Exporter
General Admin.: Steve Garrett/President

Service, Used Equipment	General

MANUFACTURER PROFILES

MIDWEST MEDICAL SOLUTIONS, LLC   800-451-6244
1310 Michigan St., Gary, IN 46402-3034
FDA Number: 103858
Ownership: Private
Produces/Sells CE-marked Devices: N
   Needle, Hypodermic, Single Lumen With Syringe   General

MIDWEST ORTHOTIC SERVICES, LLC   574-233-3352
17530 Dugdale Dr., South Bend, IN 46635
FDA Number: 3003895329
   Orthosis, Limb Brace   Physical Med

MIDWEST PRODUCTS & ENGINEERING, INC.   800-266-1687
10597 W. Glenbrook Court,   414-355-0310
Milwaukee, WI 53224
FDA Number: n/a   *Fax:* 414-355-5259
E-mail: sales@mpe-inc.com
Web site: www.mpe-inc.com.
Medical Products Sales Volume: $9,200,000
Annual Revenue: $25-$50 Million
Year Founded: 1985
Total Employees: 130   *Marketing Staff:* 1   *Sales Staff:* 6
Ownership: Private
Quality System Registration Information: ISO9001; ISO9002
Produces/Sells CE-marked Devices: N
Federal Procurement Eligibility: Small Business
Distribution: OEM, Exporter
General Admin.: Dennis L. Wenger/President, Chief Executive Officer
   David A. Barta/Vice President
Mktg./Adv.: David A. Barta/Director National Accounts
Production: Keith Chaudoir/Product Specialist
   Gary Pfannerstill/Vice President Manufacturing
Research: David Bongard/Vice President Research & Development
   Cart, Anesthetist's   Anesthesiology
   Cart, Emergency, Cardiopulmonary Resuscitation (Crash)   Anesthesiology
   Cart, Instrument   Surgery
   Cart, Monitor   General
   Cart, Multipurpose   General
   Cart, Other   General

MIDWEST RF, LLC   262-367-8254
535 Norton Drive, PO Box 350, Hartland, WI 53029
FDA Number: 2134565   *Fax:* 262-367-7684
E-mail: info@midwestrf.com
Web site: www.midwestrf.com
Year Founded: 1998
Total Employees: 8   *Marketing Staff:* 1   *Sales Staff:* 1
Ownership: Cleaning Technologies Group
Quality System Registration Information: ISO9001
Produces/Sells CE-marked Devices: N
Distribution: Manufacturer Direct
General Admin.: Bobbie Keidl/Manager Admin.
   Helmut Keidl/President
Mktg./Adv.: Chris Keidl/Director Product Development
   Lee Taylor/Sales Specialist
   Coil, Magnetic Resonance, Specialty   Radiology

MIDWEST SCIENTIFIC   800-227-9997
280 Vance Road, St. Louis, MO 63088   636-225-9997
FDA Number: n/a   *Fax:* 636-225-9998
E-mail: custserv@midsci.com
Web site: www.midsci.com
Medical Products Sales Volume: $4,200,000
Year Founded: 1983
Total Employees: 27   *Marketing Staff:* 4   *Sales Staff:* 11
Ownership: Private
Produces/Sells CE-marked Devices: N
Federal Procurement Eligibility: Small Business, GSA Contract
Distribution: Exclusive Distributor
General Admin.: Larry Degenhart/President
Mktg./Adv.: Amy Bitz/Director Marketing
   Dave Guile/Manager Advertising
   Robyn Degenhart/Manager Business
   Michael Degenhart/Manager Sales
   Glove, Patient Examination, Latex   General
   Liner, Glove   General
   Tube, Centrifuge   Chemistry
   Tube, Test   Chemistry

MIDWEST STERILIZATION CORP.   573-243-8456
1204 Lenco Ave., Jackson, MO 63755-0411
FDA Number: 1928237   *Fax:* 573-243-3799
E-mail: audry@midweststerilization.com
Medical Products Sales Volume: $10,000,000
Annual Revenue: $5-$10 Million
Total Employees: 120
Ownership: Private
Quality System Registration Information: ISO9002

MIDWEST STERILIZATION CORP.   573-243-8456 *(cont'd)*
Produces/Sells CE-marked Devices: N
Federal Procurement Eligibility: Female Owned
Distribution: Service Direct
General Admin.: Audry E. Eldridge/President
   Contract Sterilization   General

MIDWEST X-RAY EQUIPMENT CO.   630-892-2414
701 West Illinois Ave., Aurora, IL 60506
FDA Number: 1419105
   Holder, Radiographic Cassette, Wall-Mounted   Radiology
   Holder, X-Ray Film   Dental And Oral

MIE AMERICA, INC.   847-981-6100
420 Bennett Rd., Elk Grove Village, IL 60007
FDA Number: 1423348
Ownership: Private
Produces/Sells CE-marked Devices: N
   Bed, Scanning, Nuclear/Fluoroscopic   Radiology
   Camera, Gamma (Nuclear/Scintillation)   Radiology
   Scanner, Emission Computed Tomography   Radiology

MIELE APPLIANCES
   See Miele Professional Products Group

MIELE PROFESSIONAL PRODUCTS GROUP   800-843-7231
9 Independence Way, Princeton, NJ 08540   609-419-9898
FDA Number: 2248632   *Fax:* 609-419-4241
E-mail: products@mieleusa.com
Web site: www.miele.com
Total Employees: 150   *Marketing Staff:* 2   *Sales Staff:* 5
Ownership: Private
Quality System Registration Information: ISO9000
Produces/Sells CE-marked Devices: N
Distribution: Manufacturer Direct, Manufacturer Through Manufacturer Reps
General Admin.: Dan Mc Dougall/President
Mktg./Adv.: Ken Austin/Manager Marketing
   Michael A. Saperstein/Marketing Representative
   Accessories, Cleaning, Endoscopic   Gastroenterology/Urology
   Washer/Disinfector   General

MIGLIARA/KAPLAN ASSOCIATES   410-581-8188
9 Park Center Ct., Owings Mills, MD 21117-4200
FDA Number: n/a   *Fax:* 410-581-9998
E-mail: jmigliara@migkap.com
Medical Products Sales Volume: $7,100,000
Annual Revenue: $10-$25 Million
Year Founded: 1996
Total Employees: 100
Ownership: NFO WORLDWIDE
Produces/Sells CE-marked Devices: N
Federal Procurement Eligibility: Small Business
Distribution: Service Direct
General Admin.: Harris Kaplan/Executive Vice President
   Sheryl Olitzky/President, Chief Executive Officer
Mktg./Adv.: Susan Newlin/Vice President Marketing
   Service, Consulting   General

MIKI, INC.   808-943-6454
1450 Ala Moana Blvd #1247, Hon, HI 96814
FDA Number: 2938170
   Lens, Spectacle/Eyeglasses, Non-Custom   Ophthalmology

MIKRON DIGITAL IMAGING, INC.   800-925-3905
30425 Eight Mile Road, Livonia, MI 48152   248-888-1003
FDA Number: n/a   *Fax:* 248-888-1004
E-mail: sales@mikrondigital.com
Web site: www.mikrondigital.com
Medical Products Sales Volume: $400,000
Annual Revenue: $1-$5 Million
Year Founded: 1986
Total Employees: 12   *Marketing Staff:* 1   *Sales Staff:* 2
Ownership: Private
Produces/Sells CE-marked Devices: N
Federal Procurement Eligibility: Small Business
Distribution: Manufacturer Direct
General Admin.: Mike Harvey/Chief Executive Officer
   Tim Colling/President
Mktg./Adv.: Don Dotson/Director Marketing
   Computer, Cardiac Catheterization Laboratory   Cardiovascular
   Image Intensification System   Radiology
   Service, Maintenance/Repair   General
   Tube, X-Ray   Radiology

MIKRON INFRARED, INC.   805-644-9544
3033 Scott Blvd., Santa Clara, CA 95054
FDA Number: n/a   *Fax:* 805-644-9584
E-mail: info@lumasenseinc.com
Web site: www.mikroninfrared.com

MIKRON INFRARED, INC.   805-644-9544 *(cont'd)*
Medical Products Sales Volume: $1,800,000
Annual Revenue: $1-$5 Million
Year Founded: 1969
Ownership: LumaSense Technologies, Inc
Produces/Sells CE-marked Devices: Y
Distribution: Manufacturer Through Manufacturer Reps
   Thermometer, Electronic   General

MIKRON PRECISION, INC.   310-515-6221
1558-c West 139th St., Gardena, CA 90249
FDA Number: 2027170
   Applier, Surgical, Clip   Surgery
   Clip, Removable (Skin)   Surgery
   Instrument, Clip Removal   Cns/Neurology

MILCARE, INC.
See Herman Miller, Inc.

MILES AHEAD PRODUCTS   615-834-0195
3137 Glencliff Rd., Nashville, TN 37211
FDA Number: 3003661346
Ownership: Private
Produces/Sells CE-marked Devices: N
   Exerciser, Non-Measuring   Physical Med

MILES DIAGNOSTICS
See Siemens Healthcare Diagnostics Inc.

MILESTONE SCIENTIFIC INC.   800-862-1125
220 South Orange Ave., Livingston, NJ 07039
FDA Number: 3004082685
Web site: www.milestonescientific.com
Ownership: Milestone Scientific Inc.
Stock Symbol: MLSS
Traded On: OTC Bulletin
Produces/Sells CE-marked Devices: N
General Admin.: Mr. Leonard Osser/Chief Executive Officer
   Medical Admin.: Mr. MIke Hochman/Director Clinical Affairs
Production: Mr. Stephen Soloman/Director Engineering
Finance: Mr. Joseph DÉ_TAgostino/Chief Financial Officer
   Activator, Ultraviolet, Polymerization   Dental And Oral
   Pump, Infusion   General
   Syringe, Cartridge   Dental And Oral
   Syringe, Piston   General

MILEX PRODUCTS, INC.   800-621-1278
4311 N. Normandy, Chicago, IL 60634-1403   773-736-5500
FDA Number: 1413139   *Fax:* 800-972-0696
E-mail: Bobs@milexproducts.com
Web site: www.milexproducts.com
Medical Products Sales Volume: $14,700,000
Year Founded: 1937
Total Employees: 150   *Sales Staff:* 100
Ownership: Private
Quality System Registration Information: ISO9001
Produces/Sells CE-marked Devices: Y
Federal Procurement Eligibility: Small Business
Distribution: Manufacturer Direct, Manufacturer Through Distributor, Exporter
General Admin.: Richard Gross/Office Manager
           H. T. Milgrom/President, Chief Executive Officer
           Robert Shaw/Vice President
Mktg./Adv.: R. E. Shaw/Vice President Marketing
Production: Cara Furlong/Director Quality Assurance
           Steve McCarty/Manager Materials
IS: Ruth Cogan/Vice President, Tech. Director
   Aspirator, Endocervical   Obstetrics/Gynecology
   Aspirator, Endometrial   Obstetrics/Gynecology
   Brush, Other   General
   Cap, Cervical   Obstetrics/Gynecology
   Catheter, Other   Gastroenterology/Urology
   Curette   Orthopedics
   Curette, Suction, Endometrial   Obstetrics/Gynecology
   Curette, Uterine   Obstetrics/Gynecology
   Diaphragm, Contraceptive   Obstetrics/Gynecology
   Dilator, Cervical, Hygroscopic-Laminaria   Obstetrics/Gynecology
   Dilator, Rectal   Gastroenterology/Urology
   Dilator, Vaginal   Obstetrics/Gynecology
   Needle, Biopsy, Mammary   Obstetrics/Gynecology
   Pessary, Vaginal   Obstetrics/Gynecology
   Pump, Suction Operatory   Dental And Oral
   Spatula, Cervical, Cytology   Obstetrics/Gynecology

MILIAN USA   614-416-1600
1000-B Taylor Staion Rd, Gahanna, OH 43230
FDA Number: n/a   *Fax:* 614-416-1636
E-mail: usa@milian.com
Web site: www.milian.com
Annual Revenue: $0-$1 Million
Ownership: Private

MILIAN USA   614-416-1600 *(cont'd)*
Produces/Sells CE-marked Devices: N
Federal Procurement Eligibility: Small Business
Distribution: Manufacturer Through Distributor, Importer
General Admin.: Heather Kegg/General Manager
           Pierre-Olivier Chisten/President
Mktg./Adv.: Christopher Dillon/Sales Manager
   Labware, Basic, Disposable   Chemistry

MILL-ROSE COMPANY   800-321-3533
7995 Tyler Blvd., Mentor, OH 44060   440-255-9171
FDA Number: n/a   *Fax:* 440-255-5039
E-mail: info@millrose.com
Web site: www.millrose.com
Medical Products Sales Volume: $200,000
Annual Revenue: $10-$25 Million
Year Founded: 1919
Ownership: Private
Produces/Sells CE-marked Devices: N
   Accessories, Cleaning Brushes (For Endoscope)   Gastroenterology/Urology

MILLAR INSTRUMENTS, INC.   800.669.2343
6001-A Gulf Freeway, Houston, TX 77023-5417   832-667-7000
FDA Number: 1625382   *Fax:* 832-667-7001
E-mail: info@millarmail.com
Web site: www.millarinstruments.com
Medical Products Sales Volume: $9,100,000
Annual Revenue: $5-$10 Million
Year Founded: 1971
Total Employees: 85
Ownership: Private
Quality System Registration Information: ISO9001
Produces/Sells CE-marked Devices: Y
Federal Procurement Eligibility: Small Business
Distribution: Manufacturer Direct, Manufacturer Through Distributor, OEM
General Admin.: Huntly D. Millar/Chief Executive Officer
           Guy Robertson/Chief Operating Officer
           Craig Thummel/President
Mktg./Adv.: Tim Daugherty/Director Marketing & Sales
           Michael Ellis/Manager Marketing
Production: William Redmond/Manager Materials
           William Redmond/Vice President Operations
   Catheter, Cardiovascular   Surgery
   Catheter, Cardiovascular, Balloon Type   Cardiovascular
   Catheter, Electrode Recording, Or Probe   Cardiovascular
   Catheter, Intravascular, Diagnostic   Cardiovascular
   Catheter, Intravascular, Therapeutic, Short-term Less Than 30 Days   General
   Catheter, Percutaneous   Cardiovascular
   Catheter, Ureteral, Gastro-Urology   Gastroenterology/Urology
   Catheter, Vascular, Long-Term   Cardiovascular
   Catheter, Ventricular   Cns/Neurology
   Detector, Blood Flow, Ultrasonic (Doppler)   Cardiovascular
   Flowmeter, Blood, Other   Cardiovascular
   Transducer, Blood Pressure   General
   Transducer, Blood Pressure, Catheter Tip   Cardiovascular
   Transducer, Blood Pressure, Extravascular   Cardiovascular
   Transducer, Flow, Catheter Tip   Cardiovascular
   Transducer, Miniature Pressure   Physical Med
   Transmitter/Receiver System, Physiological, Radiofrequency   Cardiovascular
   Transmitter/Receiver System, Physiological, Telephone   Cardiovascular

MILLENIA DIAGNOSTICS   858-626-2777
9380 Waples Street Suite 101, San Diego, CA 92121
FDA Number: n/a   *Fax:* 858-587-8118
E-mail: mdx@milleniadiagnostics.com
Web site: www.milleniadiagnostics.com
Ownership: Private
Produces/Sells CE-marked Devices: N
   Quantitation, Antithrombin III   Hematology

MILLENIUM LABORATORIES   877-451-3534
16981 Via Tazon, San Diego, CA 92127
FDA Number: n/a   *Fax:* 585-451-3636
Web site: http://www.becausepainmatters.com
Ownership: Private
Produces/Sells CE-marked Devices: N
General Admin.: Mr. James Slattery/Chief Executive Officer
           Mr. David Cohen/Chief Operating Officer
           Dr. Charles Mikel/Chief Scientific Officer
           Mr. Howard Appel/President
Medical Admin.: Dr. Murray Rosenthal/Chief Medical Officer
           Dr. Marvin Retsky/Medical Director
Mktg./Adv.: Ms. Renee Bryan/Vice President Marketing & Planning
           Ms. Elizabeth Peacock/Vice President Sales

MANUFACTURER PROFILES

MILLENIUM SURGICAL CORP.   877-771-0850
822 Montgomery Ave., Suite 205,   610-771-0850
Narberth, PA 19072
FDA Number: n/a   *Fax:* 800-600-0429
E-mail: info@surgicalinstruments.com
Ownership: Private
Produces/Sells CE-marked Devices: N

MILLENIUM TECHNOLOGY INC.   604-273-6736
Suite 305, South Tower, 5811 Cooney Road,
Richmond, BC V6X 3 Canada
FDA Number: n/a   *Fax:* 604-278-3180
E-mail: info-mti@millennium.ca
Web site: www.millenium.ca
Year Founded: 1994
Total Employees: 50
Ownership: Private
Produces/Sells CE-marked Devices: N
Distribution: Manufacturer Direct, Exporter

MILLENNIA TECHNOLOGY, INC.   724-274-7741
1105 Pittsburgh St., Cheswick, PA 15024
FDA Number: 2529524   *Fax:* 724-274-2234
E-mail: sales@the-millennia-group.com
Web site: www.the-millennia-group.com
Medical Products Sales Volume: $8,400,000
Year Founded: 1980
Total Employees: 125
Federal Procurement Eligibility: Small Business
  Ventilator, Non-Continuous (Respirator)   Anesthesiology

MILLENNIUM DENTAL TECHNOLOGIES, INC.   562-860-2908
10945 South St., Suite 104-A, Cerritos, CA 90703
FDA Number: 2031763   *Fax:* 562-860-2429
E-mail: dmccarthy@millenniumdental.com
Web site: www.lanap.com
Year Founded: 1994
Total Employees: 12   *Sales Staff:* 8
Ownership: Private
Produces/Sells CE-marked Devices: N
Distribution: Manufacturer Through Manufacturer Reps
General Admin.: Dr. Delwin McCarthy/Chief Operating Officer
            Dr. Robert Gregg, II/President
  Laser, Dental   Dental And Oral
  Laser, Surgical   Surgery

MILLENNIUM DEVICES, INC.   631-582-6424
250 Gibbs Rd., Islandia, NY 11749-2697
FDA Number: 2438167
Ownership: Private
Produces/Sells CE-marked Devices: N
  Screwdriver, Surgical   Surgery
  Splint, Extremity, Non-Inflatable, External   Surgery

MILLENNIUM MEDICAL TECHNOLOGIES, INC.   505-988-7595
460 St. Michael's Dr., #901, Santa Fe, NM 87505
FDA Number: 1724527
Ownership: Private
Produces/Sells CE-marked Devices: N
  Fixation Appliance, Multiple Component   Orthopedics
  Monitor, Pressure, Intracompartmental   Orthopedics
  Screw, Fixation, Bone   Orthopedics

MILLER ARTIFICIAL EYE LABORATORY, INC.   419-474-3939
3030 W. Sylvania Ave., Suite 13, Toledo, OH 43613
FDA Number: 3006194072
  Conformer, Ophthalmic   Ophthalmology
  Eye, Artificial, Non-Custom   Ophthalmology
  Shell, Scleral   Ophthalmology

MILLER COACH CO., INC.   800-824-9643
1744 W COLLEGE ST, SPRINGFIELD, MO 65806   417-353-2408
FDA Number: n/a   *Fax:* 417-581-8839
E-mail: al@millercoach.com
Web site: www.millercoach.com
Medical Products Sales Volume: $2,000,000
Year Founded: 1974
Total Employees: 8
Ownership: Private
Produces/Sells CE-marked Devices: N
Federal Procurement Eligibility: Small Business
Distribution: Manufacturer Direct, Manufacturer Through Manufacturer Reps
General Admin.: Al Miller/President
  Ambulance   General

MILLER EQUIPMENT
  See Sperian Protection

MILLER INC., HERMAN
  See Herman Miller, Inc.

MILLER'S ADAPTIVE TECHNOLOGIES   800-837-4544
2023 Romig Road, Akron, OH 44320-3819   330-753-9799
FDA Number: 1527742   *Fax:* 330-572-2603
E-mail: dmi@millers.com
Web site: www.millersadaptive.com
Medical Products Sales Volume: $16,000,000
Annual Revenue: $5-$10 Million
Year Founded: 1949
Total Employees: 60   *Marketing Staff:* 1   *Sales Staff:* 1
Ownership: Private
Produces/Sells CE-marked Devices: N
Federal Procurement Eligibility: Small Business
Distribution: Manufacturer Through Distributor
General Admin.: John J. Miller/President, Chief Executive Officer
Mktg./Adv.: David M. Iammarino/Director Marketing
Production: Matt McCourry/Manager Materials
  Accessories, Wheelchair   Physical Med
  Footrest, Wheelchair   Physical Med
  Support, Head And Trunk, Wheelchair   Physical Med

MILLER'S SPECIAL PRODUCTS
  See Miller's Adaptive Technologies

MILLER-STEPHENSON CHEMICAL   800-992-2424
COMPANY, INC.
George Washington Highway,   203-743-4447
Danbury, CT 06810
FDA Number: 9310044   *Fax:* 203-791-8702
E-mail: ct.sales@miller-stephenson.com
Web site: www.miller-stephenson.com
Year Founded: 1955
Ownership: Private
Produces/Sells CE-marked Devices: N
Federal Procurement Eligibility: Small Business
Distribution: Manufacturer Direct, Service Direct, Importer, Exporter
Mktg./Adv.: George M. Stephenson/Director Marketing
          Dr. John Skewis/Director Product Development
          Belinda Gardner/Manager Advertising
Production: Joanna Saffo/Director Quality Assurance
          Mourad Fahmi/Plant General Manager
  Degreaser, Skin, Surgical   Surgery
  Solution, Patient Preparation   General
  Solvent, Adhesive Tape   Surgery

MILLERS FORGE, INC.   972-422-2145
1411 Capital Ave., Plano, TX 75074-8198
FDA Number: n/a   *Fax:* 972-881-0639
E-mail: info@millersforge.com
Web site: info@millersforge.com
Medical Products Sales Volume: $5,000,000
Annual Revenue: $1-$5 Million
Total Employees: 25   *Marketing Staff:* 4   *Sales Staff:* 4
Ownership: Private
Produces/Sells CE-marked Devices: N
Federal Procurement Eligibility: Small Business
Distribution: Exclusive Distributor
General Admin.: Trudy Gress/Office Manager
          Ted Hughes/President
Mktg./Adv.: Ted Hughes/Director Product Development
          Ted Hughes/Manager Marketing
          Mike Engels/Vice President Marketing
Production: Ted Hughes/Director Quality Assurance
  Animal, Laboratory   Microbiology
  Instrument, Manual, General Surgical   Surgery

MILLIGEN BIOSEARCH
  See Millipore Corporation

MILLIKEN & COMPANY   864-503-2844
920 Milliken Road, PO Box 1926, Spartanburg, SC 29303
FDA Number: 3001186500
Web site: www.milliken.com
Ownership: Private
Produces/Sells CE-marked Devices: N
  Dressing, Wound, Hydrophilic   Surgery
  Dressing, Wound, Occlusive   Surgery
  Sheet, Burn   General

MILLIKEN & COMPANY, ANTICON PRODUCTS   800-762-3472
201 Lukken Industrial Drive West M-836,   706-880-5639
LaGrange, GA 30240
FDA Number: n/a   *Fax:* 706-880-3140
E-mail: anticon@milliken.com
Web site: www.anticonwipers.com
Year Founded: 1850
Total Employees: 10000

MILLIKEN & COMPANY, ANTICON PRODUCTS 800-762-3472
(cont'd)
Ownership: Milliken & Company
Quality System Registration Information: ISO9001
Produces/Sells CE-marked Devices: N
Distribution: Manufacturer Through Distributor
Mktg./Adv.: Mr. Archie Booker/Area Manager
Equipment/Service, Quality Control — General

MILLIPORE CORP. (603) 532-8711
Prescott Rd., Jaffrey, NH 03452
FDA Number: 1218884   *Fax:* (603) 532-7602
Ownership: Private
Produces/Sells CE-marked Devices: N
Purifier, Water — Chemistry
Unit, Filter, Membrane — Chemistry

MILLIPORE CORPORATION 877-246-2247
290 Concord Road, Billerica, MA 01821   978-715-4321
FDA Number: 1216103   *Fax:* 800-645-5439
E-mail: biobagsales@shasta.com
Web site: www.millipore.com
Medical Products Sales Volume: $1,250,000,000
Year Founded: 1954
Total Employees: 1000
Ownership: Private
Stock Symbol: MIL
Traded On: NYSE
Quality System Registration Information: ISO9001
Produces/Sells CE-marked Devices: N
Federal Procurement Eligibility: Small Business
Distribution: Manufacturer Direct, Manufacturer Through Distributor, Manufacturer Through Manufacturer Reps, OEM
Bag, Blood — Hematology
Concentrator, Clinical Sample — Chemistry
Container, IV — General
Contract Assembly — General
Culture Media, Synthetic Cell And Tissue — Pathology
Filter, Membrane — Chemistry
Kit, Administration, Peritoneal Dialysis, Disposable — Gastroenterology/Urology
Purifier, Water — Chemistry
Vial, Other — General

MILLIPORE CORPORATION 800-MILLIPORE
80 Ashby Road, Bedford, MA 01730   781-533-2383
FDA Number: 1216103   *Fax:* 781-533-3110
E-mail: tech-service@millipore.com
Web site: www.millipore.com
Medical Products Sales Volume: $700,000,000
Total Employees: 200
Ownership: MILLIPORE CORPORATION
Quality System Registration Information: ISO9002
Produces/Sells CE-marked Devices: N
Federal Procurement Eligibility: Small Business
Distribution: Manufacturer Direct, Manufacturer Through Manufacturer Reps, OEM
General Admin.: Fran Lunger/Chief Operating Officer
    Kathy Stearns/Vice President Human Resources
    Susan Vogt/Vice President, General Manager
Mktg./Adv.: William McKenzie/Director Marketing
    Thomas Taylor/Manager International & National Sales
    Jeorgiann Lelecas/Manager Marketing Communications
Production: Thomas Borrows/Director Quality Assurance
Equipment/Service, Quality Control — General
Filter, Air — General
Filter, Bacterial, Breathing Circuit — Anesthesiology
Filter, Bacteriological, Laboratory — Chemistry
Filter, Blood, Cardiopulmonary Bypass, Arterial Line — Cardiovascular
Filter, Blood, Cardiotomy Suction Line, Cardiopulmonary — Cardiovascular
Filter, Blood, Dialysis — Gastroenterology/Urology
Filter, Cell Collection, Tissue Processing — Pathology
Filter, Conduction, Anesthesia — Anesthesiology
Filter, Gas — Anesthesiology
Filter, Infusion Line — General
Filter, Intravascular, Cardiovascular — Cardiovascular
Filter, Intravenous Tubing — General
Filter, Membrane — Chemistry
Filter, Syringe — General
Filter, Vena Cava — Cardiovascular
Filter, Ventilator — Anesthesiology
Protector, Transducer, Dialysis — Gastroenterology/Urology
Purification Filter, Water, Particulate — Chemistry
Purification System, Water — Gastroenterology/Urology
Purification System, Water, Deionization — Chemistry
Purification System, Water, Reverse Osmosis — Chemistry
Purification System, Water, Reverse Osmosis, Reagent Grade — Chemistry
Purifier, Water — Chemistry
Reverse Osmosis Membrane Equipment — Chemistry
Sampler, Air — General
Tissue Culture Apparatus — Microbiology

MILLIPORE CORPORATION 800-MILLIPORE (cont'd)
Ultrafiltration Equipment — Chemistry
Unit, Filter, Membrane — Chemistry
Medical Product Subsidiaries (Listed Separately)
Millipore S.A.

MILLS BIOPHARMACEUTICALS, LLC 405-523-1868
120 N.e. 26th St., Oklahoma City, OK 73105
FDA Number: 1650923
Applicator, Radionuclide, Manual — Radiology
Applicator, Radionuclide, Remote-Controlled — Radiology
Calibrator, Dose, Radionuclide — Radiology
Source, Brachytherapy, Radionuclide — Radiology

MILLSTONE MEDICAL OUTSOURCING 508-679-8384
1565 N. Main St., Suite 408, Fall River, MA 02720
FDA Number: 1226544   *Fax:* 508-679-8414
E-mail: sales@millstonemedical.com
Web site: www.millstonemedical.com
Medical Products Sales Volume: $6,000,000
Annual Revenue: $5-$10 Million
Year Founded: 2000
Total Employees: 85   *Marketing Staff:* 1   *Sales Staff:* 2
Ownership: Private
Quality System Registration Information: ISO9001
Produces/Sells CE-marked Devices: Y
Federal Procurement Eligibility: Small Business
General Admin.: Shannon Tillman/President
Mktg./Adv.: Jonathan Tillman/Director Sales
Production: William Tillman/Vice President Quality Systems
Hip, Hemi-, Femoral, Metal Ball — Orthopedics
Implant, Fixation Device, Spinal — Orthopedics
Kit, Instruments and Accessories, Surgical — Surgery
Kit, Surgical Instrument, Disposable — Surgery
Orthopedic Manual Surgical Instrument — Orthopedics
Syringe, Dental — Dental And Oral
System, Appliance, Fixation, Spinal Pedicle Screw — Orthopedics

MILTENBERG INC.
See Miltex Inc.

MILTEX DENTAL TECHNOLOGIES, INC. 516-576-6022
589 Davies Dr., York, PA 17402
FDA Number: 2523190
Ownership: Private
Produces/Sells CE-marked Devices: N
Accessories, Retractor, Dental — Dental And Oral
Agent, Polishing, Abrasive, Oral Cavity — Dental And Oral
Broach, Endodontic — Dental And Oral
Burr, Dental — Dental And Oral
Carrier, Amalgam, Operative — Dental And Oral
Clamp, Rubber Dam — Dental And Oral
Cleanser, Root Canal — Dental And Oral
Cup, Prophylaxis — Dental And Oral
Curette, Endodontic — Dental And Oral
Disk, Abrasive — Dental And Oral
Drill, Dental, Intraoral — Dental And Oral
Excavator, Dental, Operative — Dental And Oral
Explorer, Operative — Dental And Oral
File, Pulp Canal, Endodontic — Dental And Oral
Forceps, Articulation Paper — Dental And Oral
Forceps, Dressing, Dental — Dental And Oral
Forceps, Rubber Dam Clamp — Dental And Oral
Frame, Rubber Dam — Dental And Oral
General Use Surgical Scissors — Surgery
Gutta Percha — Dental And Oral
Handle, Instrument, Dental — Dental And Oral
Handpiece, Contra- And Right-Angle Attachment, Dental — Dental And Oral
Hemostat, Surgical — Dental And Oral
Instrument, Diamond, Dental — Dental And Oral
Locator, Apex, Root — Dental And Oral
Mallet, Surgical, General & Plastic Surgery — Surgery
Matrix, Dental — Dental And Oral
Mirror, ENT — Ear/Nose/Throat
Mirror, Mouth — Dental And Oral
Operative Dental Treatment Unit — Dental And Oral
Paper, Articulation — Dental And Oral
Plate, Base, Shellac — Dental And Oral
Pliers, Operative — Dental And Oral
Pliers, Orthodontic — Dental And Oral
Plugger, Root Canal, Endodontic — Dental And Oral
Plunger-Like Joint Manipulator — Physical Med
Point, Paper, Endodontic — Dental And Oral
Point, Silver, Endodontic — Dental And Oral
Post, Root Canal — Dental And Oral
Probe, Periodontic — Dental And Oral
Reamer, Pulp Canal, Endodontic — Dental And Oral
Remover, Crown — Dental And Oral
Retainer, Matrix — Dental And Oral
Scissors, Collar And Crown — Dental And Oral
Scissors, Surgical Tissue, Dental (Oral) — Dental And Oral

MANUFACTURER PROFILES

MILTEX DENTAL TECHNOLOGIES, INC.   516-576-6022 *(cont'd)*

Source, Heat, Bleaching, Teeth, Dental	Dental And Oral
Spreader, Pulp Canal Filling Material, Endodontic	Dental And Oral
Strip, Polishing Agent	Dental And Oral
Syringe Unit, Air And/Or Water	Dental And Oral
Syringe, Cartridge	Dental And Oral
Syringe, Periodontic, Endodontic	Dental And Oral
Tape, Measuring, Ruler And Caliper	Surgery
Tester, Pulp	Dental And Oral
Tray, Impression	Dental And Oral
Wax, Dental	Dental And Oral
Zinc Oxide Eugenol	Dental And Oral

MILTEX INC.   800-645-8000

589 Davies Drive, York, PA 17402   717-840-9335

FDA Number: 2523190   *Fax:* 717-840-9347
E-mail: customerservice.miltex@integralife.com
Web site: www.miltex.com
Year Founded: 1950
Total Employees: 200   *Marketing Staff:* 7   *Sales Staff:* 22
Ownership: Integra Lifesciences Holdings Corp.
Stock Symbol: IART
Traded On: NASDAQ
Quality System Registration Information: ISO9001
Produces/Sells CE-marked Devices: Y
Distribution: Manufacturer Through Distributor, Exporter
General Admin.: Mr. Bob Perrett/President, Chief Executive Officer
Mktg./Adv.: Mr. Kevin Hays/Director National Sales
    Mr. Sean E. Browne/Executive Vice President Marketing & Sales
    Mr. Bill Aab/Vice President International Sales
    Mr. Robert Regan/Vice President Marketing

Anoscope, Non-Powered	Gastroenterology/Urology
Band, Matrix	Dental And Oral
Blade, Scalpel	Surgery
Blade, Surgical, Saw, General & Plastic Surgery	Surgery
Brush, Other	General
Burr, Dental	Dental And Oral
Burr, Dental Excavating	Dental And Oral
Cannula, Brain	Cns/Neurology
Cannula, Ear	Ear/Nose/Throat
Cannula, Sinus	Ear/Nose/Throat
Catheter, Urethral	Gastroenterology/Urology
Chisel, Bone, Surgical	Dental And Oral
Chisel, Nasal	Ear/Nose/Throat
Clamp, Aorta	Cardiovascular
Clamp, Bronchus	Ear/Nose/Throat
Clamp, Bulldog	Surgery
Clamp, Umbilical	Obstetrics/Gynecology
Clamp, Vascular	Cardiovascular
Clip, Suture	Surgery
Clip, Towel	Surgery
Container, Sterilization (Tray)	General
Curette, Ear	Ear/Nose/Throat
Curette, Uterine	Obstetrics/Gynecology
Cystotome, Ophthalmic	Ophthalmology
Depressor, Tongue	General
Dilator, Urethral, Mechanical	Gastroenterology/Urology
Dilator, Uterine	Obstetrics/Gynecology
Drill, Bone	Orthopedics
Drill, Perforator	Cns/Neurology
Driver/Extractor, Bone Nail/Pin	Orthopedics
Elevator, Uterine	Obstetrics/Gynecology
File, Bone, Surgical	Dental And Oral
Forceps, Biopsy, Gynecological	Obstetrics/Gynecology
Forceps, Fixation	Surgery
Forceps, Lung	Surgery
Forceps, Obstetrical	Obstetrics/Gynecology
Forceps, Stone Manipulation	Gastroenterology/Urology
Forceps, Tissue	Surgery
Forceps, Tooth Extractor, Surgical	Dental And Oral
Fork, Tuning	Cns/Neurology
Gag, Mouth	Ear/Nose/Throat
Goniometer, Orthopedic	Orthopedics
Gouge, Nasal	Ear/Nose/Throat
Hammer, Neurological	Cns/Neurology
Hammer, Percussion	Cns/Neurology
Handle, Scalpel	Surgery
Handpiece, Belt and/or Gear Driven, Dental	Dental And Oral
Holder, Needle, Other	Surgery
Hook, Other	Surgery
Hook, Rhinoplastic	Surgery
Hook, Scleral Fixation	Ophthalmology
Hook, Skin	Surgery
Hook, Strabismus	Ophthalmology
Hook, Sympathectomy	Cns/Neurology
Hook, Tracheal	Ear/Nose/Throat
Instrument, Dental, Manual	Dental And Oral
Instrument, Diamond, Dental	Dental And Oral
Instrument, Microsurgical	Cns/Neurology
Knife, Amputation	Surgery
Knife, Ear	Ear/Nose/Throat

MILTEX INC.   800-645-8000 *(cont'd)*

Knife, Meniscus	Surgery
Knife, Plaster	Orthopedics
Knife, Scalpel	Surgery
Knife, Skin Grafting	Surgery
Knife, Sternum	Surgery
Knife, Tonsil	Ear/Nose/Throat
Ligator, Hemorrhoidal	Gastroenterology/Urology
Lubricant, Instrument	General
Magnet, Permanent	Ophthalmology
Mallet, Bone	Orthopedics
Mallet, Dental	Dental And Oral
Mandrel	Dental And Oral
Mirror, Laryngeal	Ear/Nose/Throat
Needle, Knife	Surgery
Needle, Ophthalmic	Ophthalmology
Needle, Suture, Reusable	Surgery
Osteotome (Orthopedic)	Surgery
Osteotome, Manual (Plastic Surgery)	Surgery
Osteotome, Other	Surgery
Otoscope	Ear/Nose/Throat
Packer, Gauze	General
Pelvimeter	Obstetrics/Gynecology
Perforator, Ear-Lobe	Ear/Nose/Throat
Periodontal Instrument	Dental And Oral
Probe, Common Duct	Gastroenterology/Urology
Probe, Fistula	Gastroenterology/Urology
Probe, Lacrimal	Ophthalmology
Probe, Sinus	Ear/Nose/Throat
Proctoscope	Surgery
Punch, Biopsy	Gastroenterology/Urology
Punch, Corneo-Scleral	Ophthalmology
Rasp, Nasal	Ear/Nose/Throat
Rasp, Surgical, General & Plastic Surgery	Surgery
Raspatory	Surgery
Retainer, Dental	Dental And Oral
Retractor, Abdominal	Surgery
Retractor, All Types	Dental And Oral
Retractor, Bladder	Gastroenterology/Urology
Retractor, ENT (Thoracic)	Ear/Nose/Throat
Retractor, Laminectomy	Surgery
Retractor, Ophthalmic	Ophthalmology
Retractor, Rectal	Gastroenterology/Urology
Retractor, Rib	Orthopedics
Retractor, Surgical	Surgery
Retractor, Vaginal	Obstetrics/Gynecology
Rongeur, Manual, Neurosurgical	Cns/Neurology
Rongeur, Rib	Orthopedics
Saw, Manual, And Accessories	Surgery
Scalpel, One-Piece (Knife)	Surgery
Scissors, Bandage/Gauze/Plaster	General
Scissors, Cardiovascular	Cardiovascular
Scissors, Corneal	Ophthalmology
Scissors, Cystoscopic	Gastroenterology/Urology
Scissors, Enucleation	Ophthalmology
Scissors, General Dissecting	General
Scissors, Gynecological	Obstetrics/Gynecology
Scissors, Iris	Ophthalmology
Scissors, Nasal	Ear/Nose/Throat
Scissors, Neurosurgical (Dura)	Cns/Neurology
Scissors, Pediatric	General
Scissors, Plastic Surgery (Dissecting)	Surgery
Scissors, Rectal	Gastroenterology/Urology
Scissors, Surgical Tissue, Dental (Oral)	Dental And Oral
Scissors, Suture	Surgery
Scissors, Tenotomy	Ophthalmology
Scissors, Thoracic	Cardiovascular
Sclerotome	Ophthalmology
Scoop, Gallstone	Gastroenterology/Urology
Separator, Dural	Cns/Neurology
Separator, Pylorus	Gastroenterology/Urology
Sleeve, Trocar	Surgery
Snare, Polyp	Surgery
Snare, Tonsil	Ear/Nose/Throat
Solution, Instrument Cleaner	General
Sound, Urethral, Metal Or Plastic	Gastroenterology/Urology
Sound, Uterine	Obstetrics/Gynecology
Spatula, Brain	Cns/Neurology
Spatula, Cement	Dental And Oral
Spatula, Middle Ear	Ear/Nose/Throat
Spatula, Ophthalmic	Ophthalmology
Spatula, Other	Surgery
Speculum, Ear	Ear/Nose/Throat
Speculum, Nasal	Ear/Nose/Throat
Speculum, Ophthalmic	Ophthalmology
Speculum, Rectal	Gastroenterology/Urology
Speculum, Vaginal, Metal	Obstetrics/Gynecology
Spreader, Plaster (Cast)	Orthopedics
Stethoscope, Mechanical	General
Stripper, Tendon	Surgery
Stripper, Vein, Reusable	Surgery
Syringe, Dental	Dental And Oral

MILTEX INC.   800-645-8000 *(cont'd)*

Syringe, Ear	Ear/Nose/Throat
Tip, Suction	Anesthesiology
Tip, Suction Tube (Yankauer, Poole, Etc.)	Surgery
Tongs, Skull	Cns/Neurology
Tonometer, Manual	Ophthalmology
Tray, Sterilization, Instrument	Surgery
Trephine, Manual, Ophthalmic (Corneal)	Ophthalmology
Trephine, Skull	Cns/Neurology
Trocar, Antrum	Ear/Nose/Throat
Trocar, Cardiovascular	Cardiovascular
Trocar, Thoracic	Cardiovascular
Trocar, Tracheal	Ear/Nose/Throat
Tube, Tracheal (Endotracheal)	Anesthesiology
Tweezers	General
Well, Amalgam	Dental And Oral
Wire, Ligature	Surgery

MILTEX INSTRUMENT CO., INC.
See Miltex Inc.

MILVELLA LIMITED   952-746-1369
12100 Singletree Lane, Eden Prairie, MN 55344
FDA Number: 3004531715

Clip, Iris Retractor	Ophthalmology
Phacofragmentation Unit	Ophthalmology

MILWAUKEE MATTRESS & FURNITURE   800-373-1462
423 N. 3rd St., Milwaukee, WI 53203-3001   **414-271-7335**
FDA Number: 9200740   *Fax:* 414-271-8670
E-mail: kenmichaels@ameritech.net
Web site: http://www.kenmichaelsfurniture.com
Medical Products Sales Volume: $300,000
Annual Revenue: $0-$1 Million
Year Founded: 1960
Total Employees: 40   *Marketing Staff:* 1   *Sales Staff:* 1
Ownership: Private
Produces/Sells CE-marked Devices: N
Federal Procurement Eligibility: Small Business
Distribution: Manufacturer Direct
General Admin.: Michael E. Dethloff/President
Mktg./Adv.: Frank R. Dethloff/Manager Contract Sales

Mattress, Bed	General
Mattress, Reduction, Pressure	General

MIMEDX GROUP INC.   866-477-4219
60 Chastain Center Blvd, Suite 60, Suite B,
Kennesaw, GA 30144
FDA Number: 3006731846   *Fax:* 678-384-6720
Web site: http://www.mimedx.com
Ownership: Private
Produces/Sells CE-marked Devices: N
General Admin.: Mr. Parker Petit/Chairman, Chief Executive Officer
     Mr. Michael Senken/Chief Financial Officer, Vice President
     Dr. Thomas Koob/Chief Scientific Officer
     Mr. Robert Shaw/General Counsel
     Mr. William Taylor/President, Chief Operating Officer
     Mr. Thorton Kuntz/Vice President Human Resources
Mktg./Adv.: Mr. Randall Spencer/Director Product Development
     Mr. Michael Carlton/Vice President Marketing & Sales
Production: Mr. William Jackson/Vice President Quality Assurance & Regulatory Affairs
Research: Dr. Rebeccah Brown/Vice President Product Development

MIMOSA ACOUSTICS, INC.   217-367-9740
60 Hazelwood Dr., Suite #209, Champaign, IL 61820
FDA Number: 2249246

Audiometer	Ear/Nose/Throat

MIMVISTA CORP.   216-896-9798
25200 Chagrin Blvd. Suite 200, Cleveland, OH 44122
FDA Number: 3004363352

Image Processing System	Radiology
Scanner, Emission Computed Tomography	Radiology

MINATRONICS CORP.   412-488-6435
1 Trimont Lane, 850C, Pittsburgh, PA 15211
FDA Number: n/a
E-mail: protector@minatronics.com
Web site: www.minatronics.com
Medical Products Sales Volume: $200,000
Annual Revenue: $0-$1 Million
Year Founded: 1961
Total Employees: 4   *Marketing Staff:* 2   *Sales Staff:* 2
Ownership: Private
Produces/Sells CE-marked Devices: N
Federal Procurement Eligibility: Small Business
Distribution: Manufacturer Direct, Manufacturer Through Distributor, Exporter
General Admin.: Edwin P. Wilson/President

Equipment, Building Security	General

MINATRONICS CORP.   412-488-6435 *(cont'd)*

Security Equipment/Supplies	General

MINCO PRODUCTS, INC.   763-571-3121
7300 Commerce Lane, Minneapolis, MN 55432
FDA Number: 7000257
E-mail: sales@minco.com   *Fax:* 763-571-0927
Web site: www.minco.com
Medical Products Sales Volume: $44,000,000
Annual Revenue: $50-$100 Million
Total Employees: 700
Ownership: Private
Quality System Registration Information: ISO9001
Produces/Sells CE-marked Devices: N
Distribution: Manufacturer Direct, Manufacturer Through Manufacturer Reps
Mktg./Adv.: Sue Espeseth/Advertising Assistant
     Brian Williams/Manager Product Marketing

Heater, Electrical Instrument	General
Heating Mantle	Microbiology
Probe, Temperature	General
Thermistor	General
Thermometer, Laboratory	Chemistry

MIND ALIVE INC.   800-661-6463
9008 51 Avenue,   **780-450-6463**
Edmonton, ALBER T6E-5 Canada
FDA Number: n/a   *Fax:* 780-450-9551
E-mail: info@mindalive.com
Web site: www.mindalive.com
Year Founded: 1981
Total Employees: 10   *Marketing Staff:* 1
Ownership: Private
Produces/Sells CE-marked Devices: N
Distribution: Manufacturer Direct, Manufacturer Through Distributor, Exporter

MINDFRAME INC   949-204-0800
12 Goodyear, Suite 125, Irvine, CA 92618
FDA Number: 3007098640
E-mail: info@MindFrameInc.com
Web site: www.mindframeinc.com
Ownership: Private
Produces/Sells CE-marked Devices: N
General Admin.: Mr. Steve Sosnowski/Chief Technology Officer
     Mr. Kenneth Charhut/President, Chief Executive Officer
Research: Mr. Joshua Benjamin/Manager Research & Development

MINDWAYS SOFTWARE, INC.   512-912-0871
3001 South Lamar, Suite 302, Austin, TX 78704
FDA Number: 2939827

Computer and Software, Medical	General
Densitometer, Bone, Single Photon	Radiology

MINE SAFETY APPLIANCES CO., INC.
See Mine Safety Appliances Company

MINE SAFETY APPLIANCES COMPANY   866-MSA-1001
1000 Cranberry Woods Drive,   **724-776-8600**
Cranberry Township, PA 16066
FDA Number: 3000127635
E-mail: info@msa.com   *Fax:* 412-967-3367
Web site: www.msanet.com
Medical Products Sales Volume: $913,700,000
Year Founded: 1914
Total Employees: 6200   *Marketing Staff:* 20   *Sales Staff:* 10
Ownership: Public
Stock Symbol: MSA
Traded On: NYSE
Quality System Registration Information: ISO9002
Produces/Sells CE-marked Devices: Y
Distribution: Manufacturer Direct, Manufacturer Through Distributor, Manufacturer Through Manufacturer Reps, OEM
General Admin.: J. T. Ryan/Chief Executive Officer
     William Lambert/President
     Kerry Bove/Vice President, General Manager
Mktg./Adv.: Steve Bayer/Manager Marketing
Production: Ron Campbell/Director Quality Assurance

Analyzer, Gas, Oxygen, Gaseous Phase	Anesthesiology
Bandage, Adhesive	Surgery
Bandage, Gauze	General
Forceps, Dressing	Surgery
Forceps, Utility	Surgery
Kit, Administration, Oxygen	Anesthesiology
Kit, First Aid	Surgery
Mask, Other	General
Pack, Cold	General
Pad, Eye	Ophthalmology
Splint, Pneumatic	Orthopedics
Sponge, Gauze	Dental And Oral
Stretcher, Hand-Carried	General

MANUFACTURER PROFILES

MINE SAFETY APPLIANCES COMPANY 866-MSA-1001 *(cont'd)*
Tourniquet	General
Ventilator, Continuous (Respirator)	Anesthesiology

MINI-MITTER COMPANY, INC. 800-685-2999
20300 Empire Ave., Bldg. B-3, Bend, OR 97701 541-598-3800
FDA Number: 3032377 Fax: 541-322-7277
E-mail: respironics.minimitter@philips.com
Web site: www.minimitter.com
Annual Revenue: $5-$10 Million
Year Founded: 1971
Ownership: Private
Quality System Registration Information: ISO9001
Produces/Sells CE-marked Devices: Y
Federal Procurement Eligibility: Small Business, Female Owned
Distribution: Manufacturer Direct, Manufacturer Through Distributor, Manufacturer Through Manufacturer Reps
General Admin.: Corey Schmid/Business Manager
  Mr. David Motley/Vice President
Mktg./Adv.: Dr. Jack McKenzie/Director Sales
  Dennis Dalangin/Vice President Marketing
Production: Bill Littlefield/Director Operations
  Dr. Dan Burns/Manager Quality Systems
Research: Dr. Florian Bell/Vice President Engineering
Finance: Scott Satko/Controller
General Medical Device	General
Sleep Assessment Equipment	Cns/Neurology
Thermometer, Laboratory, Recording	General

MINIMAX COMPANY 800-292-2620
100 West Industry Court, Deer Park, NY 11729 631-925-5000
FDA Number: 1419190 Fax: 631-925-5001
E-mail: info@minimaxco.com
Web site: www.minimaxco.com
Medical Products Sales Volume: $2,000,000
Annual Revenue: $1-$5 Million
Year Founded: 1925
Total Employees: 15
Ownership: Private
Quality System Registration Information: ISO9001
Produces/Sells CE-marked Devices: Y
Federal Procurement Eligibility: Small Business
Distribution: Manufacturer Through Distributor
General Admin.: M. Wolf/President
  C. Price/Vice President, General Manager
Film, X-Ray, Dental, Intraoral	Dental And Oral

MINIMAX CORPORATION
See Minimax Company

MINIMED INC.
See Medtronic Minimed

MINISUN, LLC 559-439-4600
935 Mill Creek Drive, Fresno, CA 93720
FDA Number: 2954729 Fax: 559-439-4641
E-mail: minisun@comcast.net
Web site: www.MiniSun.com
Medical Products Sales Volume: $300,000
Year Founded: 2000
Total Employees: 4
Ownership: Private
Produces/Sells CE-marked Devices: N
Federal Procurement Eligibility: Small Business
Distribution: Manufacturer Direct, Manufacturer Through Distributor
General Admin.: Dr. Ming Sun/President
Analyzer, Gait	Orthopedics
Device, Measurement, Velocity, Conduction, Nerve	Cns/Neurology
Lamp, Ultraviolet, Physical Medicine	Physical Med

MINITOOL, INC. 888-395-1599
634 University Ave., Los Gatos, CA 95032-4416 408-395-1585
FDA Number: n/a Fax: 408-395-1605
E-mail: info@minitool.com
Web site: www.minitoolinc.com
Annual Revenue: $0-$1 Million
Total Employees: 10 Sales Staff: 3
Ownership: Private
Produces/Sells CE-marked Devices: N
Federal Procurement Eligibility: Small Business
Distribution: Manufacturer Direct
General Admin.: David H. Healey/General Manager
  Heinz Reich/President
Micromanipulator, Laboratory	Microbiology
Microscope	Hematology

MINITUBE OF AMERICA, INC 608-845-1502
P.O. Box 930187, 419 Venture Court, Verona, WI 53593
FDA Number: 3004181177 Fax: 608 845 1522

MINITUBE OF AMERICA, INC 608-845-1502 *(cont'd)*
E-mail: usa@minitube.com
Web site: www.minitube.us
Ownership: Private
Produces/Sells CE-marked Devices: N
Counter, Cell Or Particle, Automated	Hematology
Labware, Assisted Reproduction	Obstetrics/Gynecology
Media, Reproductive	Obstetrics/Gynecology

MINIVATOR
See Sunrise Medical, Inc.

MINNESOTA BRAMSTEDT SURGICAL, INC. 800-456-5052
1835 Energy Park Drive, St. Paul, MN 55108 651-644-7519
FDA Number: n/a Fax: 651-642-9201
E-mail: jbramstedt@mnwire.com
Web site: http://mnwire.com
Medical Products Sales Volume: $400,000
Year Founded: 1939
Total Employees: 7
Ownership: Private
Produces/Sells CE-marked Devices: Y
Federal Procurement Eligibility: Small Business
Distribution: Manufacturer Through Distributor, Manufacturer Through Manufacturer Reps, OEM, Service Direct
General Admin.: Mr. Paul Wagner/Chief Executive Officer
Mktg./Adv.: Mr. Lane Beard/Director Sales
Blade, Surgical, Saw, General & Plastic Surgery	Surgery
Drill, Bone	Orthopedics
Driver/Extractor, Bone Nail/Pin	Orthopedics
Extractor, Nail	Orthopedics
Holder, Needle	Gastroenterology/Urology
Instrument, Surgical, Powered, Pneumatic	Orthopedics
Rack, Surgical Instrument	Surgery
Service, Maintenance/Repair	General
Tray, Surgical Instrument	Surgery

MINNESOTA MEDICAL DEVELOPMENT, INC. 763-354-7105
14305 21st Ave. North, Suite 100, Minneapolis, MN 55447
FDA Number: 3005770977
Mesh, Surgical, Polymeric	Surgery

MINNESOTA MINING AND MANUFACTURING CO.
See 3m Co.

MINNESOTA RUBBER & QMR PLASTICS 952-927-1400
1100 xenium lane north, Minneapolis, MN 55441
FDA Number: 3006339918 Fax: 952-927-1470
E-mail: webmaster@mnrubber.com
Web site: www.mnrubber.com
Medical Products Sales Volume: $100,000,000
Year Founded: 1946
Total Employees: 1070 Marketing Staff: 2 Sales Staff: 13
Ownership: Private
Quality System Registration Information: ISO9003
Produces/Sells CE-marked Devices: N
Federal Procurement Eligibility: Small Business
Distribution: Manufacturer Direct, Manufacturer Through Manufacturer Reps, Service Direct, Exclusive Distributor
General Admin.: Pete Peterson/Vice President Human Resources
Mktg./Adv.: Bill Pederson/Director Marketing & Advertising
Production: Craig Swanberg/Director Engineering
  Tim Reski/Director Materials
  Mark Riedel/Director Quality Assurance
Finance: Mark Kocon/Controller
Component, Plastic	General
Component, Rubber	General
Molding, Custom	General

MINNESOTA RUBBER COMPANY
See Minnesota Rubber & Qmr Plastics

MINNESOTA SCIENTIFIC, INC.
See Omni-Tract Surgical, A Div. Of Minnesota Scientific, Inc.

MINNESOTA WIRE & CABLE CO. 800-258-6922
1835 Energy Park Drive, St. Paul, MN 55108 651-642-1800
FDA Number: n/a Fax: 651-642-9201
E-mail: info@mnwire.com
Web site: www.mnwire.com
Medical Products Sales Volume: $17,000,000
Year Founded: 1968
Total Employees: 82
Ownership: Private
Quality System Registration Information: ISO9001
Produces/Sells CE-marked Devices: N
Federal Procurement Eligibility: Small Business
Distribution: OEM
General Admin.: Fred Wagner/Chairman
  Joan Thompson/Chief Financial Officer, Executive Vice President
  Paul Wagner/President, Chief Executive Officer

MINNESOTA WIRE & CABLE CO. 800-258-6922 (cont'd)

Mktg./Adv.: Eric Chalgren/Director Marketing
Marge Andre/Manager Accounts
Lane F. Beard/Manager Marketing & Sales
Production: Eric Wagner/Director Manufacturing & Quality Assurance

Cable	Physical Med
Cable, Electric	General
Cable, Electrode	Physical Med
Cable, Electrosurgical Unit	Surgery
Cable/Lead, ECG	Cardiovascular
Cable/Lead, ECG, Radiolucent	Cardiovascular
Cable/Lead, ECG, With Transducer And Electrode	Cardiovascular
Cable/Lead, EEG	Cns/Neurology
Cable/Lead, EMG	Cns/Neurology
Cable/Lead, TENS	Cns/Neurology
Component, Electrical	General
Component, Electronic	General
Component, Other	General
Contract Manufacturing	General
Contract Manufacturing, Product, Disposable	General
Hearing-Aid	Ear/Nose/Throat
Molding, Custom	General

Medical Product Subsidiaries (Listed Separately)
Farrand Optical Components & Instruments, Div. Of Ruhle Co.

MINNETONKA INC.

See King Pharmaceuticals, Inc.

MINNETRONIX INC. 888-301-1025

1635 Energy Park Drive, St. Paul, MN 55108 651-917-4060
FDA Number: 2133810
E-mail: info@minnetronix.com
Web site: http://www.minnetronix.com
Year Founded: 1996
Ownership: Private
Produces/Sells CE-marked Devices: N
General Admin.: Mr. Joe Renzetti/Chief Operating Officer
Ms. Diane Richard/Director Human Resources
Mr. Rich Nazarian/President, Chief Executive Officer
Mktg./Adv.: Ms. Lynn Ihlenfeldt/Vice President Business Development
Mr. Mike Schreiber/Vice President Marketing & Sales
Production: Mr. Stan Crossett/Vice President Manufacturing
Mr. Steve Strong/Vice President Quality Assurance & Regulatory
Affairs
Research: Mr. Dirk Smith/Vice President Engineering

Biopsy Instrument	Gastroenterology/Urology
Catheter, Coronary, Atherectomy	Cardiovascular
Catheter, Peripheral, Atherectomy	Cardiovascular
Controller, Pump Speed, Cardiopulmonary Bypass	Cardiovascular
Electromyograph, Diagnostic	Physical Med
Electrosurgical Unit, Cutting & Coagulation Device	Surgery
Laser, Surgical	Surgery
Surgical Device, For Ablation Of Cardiac Tissue	Surgery
System, Ablation, Ultrasound And Accessories	Surgery

MINNOW MEDICAL INC.

See Vessix Vascular, Inc.

MINNTECH CORPORATION 800-328-3345

14605 28th Avenue N., Minneapolis, MN 55447 763-553-3300
FDA Number: 2150060   Fax: 763-553-3387
E-mail: info@minntech.com
Web site: www.minntech.com
Medical Products Sales Volume: $41,600,000
Annual Revenue: $25-$50 Million
Year Founded: 1974
Total Employees: 400
Ownership: Cantel Medical
Quality System Registration Information: ISO9001
Produces/Sells CE-marked Devices: Y
Distribution: Manufacturer Direct
General Admin.: Paul E. Helms/Executive Vice President
Roy Malkin/President, Chief Executive Officer
Kevin Finkle/Senior Vice President Admin. & Finance
Denise Bauer/Vice President Human Resources
Production: Jim McMillen/Vice President Manufacturing
Craig Smith/Vice President Quality Assurance & Regulatory Affairs
Research: Michael Petersen/Vice President, Director Research & Development

Accessories, Blood Circuit, Hemodialysis	Gastroenterology/Urology
Accessories, Cardiopulmonary Bypass	Cardiovascular
Accessories, Cleaning, Endoscopic	Gastroenterology/Urology
Bulb, Inflation (Endoscope)	Gastroenterology/Urology
Concentrate, Dialysis, Hemodialysis (Liquid or Powder)	Gastroenterology/Urology
Detector, Air Bubble	Gastroenterology/Urology
Dialysate Delivery System, Central Multiple Patient	Gastroenterology/Urology
Dialyzer Reprocessing System	Gastroenterology/Urology
Dialyzer, High Permeability	Gastroenterology/Urology
Disinfector, Medical Device	General
Electrode, Electrosurgical, Active (Blade)	Surgery
Endoscope	Gastroenterology/Urology

MINNTECH CORPORATION 800-328-3345 (cont'd)

Meter, Conductivity, Non-Remote	Gastroenterology/Urology
Oxygenator, Cardiopulmonary Bypass	Cardiovascular
Pump, Blood, Extra-Luminal	Gastroenterology/Urology
Purification System, Water	Gastroenterology/Urology
Sterilant, Medical Device	General
Sterilization Process Indicator, Physical/Chemical	General

MINOGUE MEDICAL INC. 800-665-6466
514-287-1644
180 Peel, Ste. 300,
Montreal, QUE H3C-2 Canada
FDA Number: n/a   Fax: 514-287-0853
E-mail: info@minogue-med.com
Web site: http://www.minogue-med.com
Year Founded: 1986
Total Employees: 25
Ownership: Private
Produces/Sells CE-marked Devices: N
Distribution: Exclusive Distributor, Importer, Exporter

MINRAD, INC. 716-855-1068
50 Cobham Dr., Orchard Park, NY 14127
FDA Number: 1320909

Arthroscope	Orthopedics
Biopsy Instrument	Gastroenterology/Urology
Drape, Surgical	Surgery
Hysteroscope	Obstetrics/Gynecology
Instrument, Manual, General Surgical	Surgery
Laparoscope, General & Plastic Surgery	Surgery
Laryngoscope, Rigid	Anesthesiology
Light, Examination, Battery-Powered	General
Monitor, Patient Position, Light Beam	Radiology
Nasopharyngoscope (Flexible Or Rigid)	Ear/Nose/Throat
Radiographic/Fluoroscopic Unit, Image-Intensified	Radiology
Syringe, Piston	General
System, X-Ray, Mobile	Radiology
Tape, Television & Video, Endoscopic	Gastroenterology/Urology

MINSURG INTERNATIONAL, INC. 727-466-4550
611 Druid Road Eas, Suite 200, Clearwater, FL 33756
FDA Number: 3005953162   Fax: 727-441-2089
Web site: www.trufuse.com
Ownership: Private
Produces/Sells CE-marked Devices: N

Bit, Surgical	Surgery
Orthopedic Manual Surgical Instrument	Orthopedics
Reamer	Orthopedics

MINTO R&D, INC. 530-222-2373
20270 Charlanne Drive, Redding, CA 96002
FDA Number: 2936686   Fax: 530-222-0679
E-mail: mintord@aol.com
Web site: www.sagersplints.com
Medical Products Sales Volume: $1,000,000
Annual Revenue: $0-$1 Million
Year Founded: 1979
Total Employees: 8   Marketing Staff: 1   Sales Staff: 1
Ownership: Private
Produces/Sells CE-marked Devices: Y
Federal Procurement Eligibility: Small Business, Female Owned
Distribution: Manufacturer Through Distributor, Exporter
General Admin.: Gloria M. Borschneck/President, Chief Executive Officer
Mktg./Adv.: Anne L. Borschneck/Vice President Marketing & Sales
Production: John T. Gordon/Director Quality Assurance
John T. Gordon/Manager Materials
Anthony G. Borschneck/Vice President Production
Research: Anthony G. Borschneck/Vice President Research & Development

Splint, Extremity, Non-Inflatable, External	Surgery
Splint, Traction	Orthopedics
Stretcher, Hand-Carried	General

MINXRAY, INC. 800-221-2245
847-564-0323
3611 Commercial Avenue,
Northbrook, IL 60062
FDA Number: 1418960   Fax: 847-564-9040
E-mail: info@minxray.com
Web site: www.minxray.com
Medical Products Sales Volume: $17,000,000
Annual Revenue: $0-$1 Million
Year Founded: 1967
Total Employees: 8
Ownership: Kretchmer Corp., The
Quality System Registration Information: ISO9001
Produces/Sells CE-marked Devices: N
Federal Procurement Eligibility: Small Business
Distribution: Manufacturer Through Distributor, Importer, Exporter
General Admin.: Keith R. Kretchmer/President, Chief Executive Officer

MINXRAY, INC. 800-221-2245 (cont'd)
Radiographic Unit, Diagnostic Radiology

MIP INC. 800-361-4964
9100 Ray Lawson Blvd., 514-356-1224
Montreal, QC H1J-1 Canada
FDA Number: n/a Fax: 514-356-0055
E-mail: info@mip.ca
Web site: www.mipinc.com
Year Founded: 1977
Total Employees: 120 Marketing Staff: 5 Sales Staff: 50
Ownership: Private
Quality System Registration Information: ISO9001
Produces/Sells CE-marked Devices: Y
Distribution: Manufacturer Through Distributor, Manufacturer Through Manufacturer Reps, Exclusive Distributor, Exporter

MIRA, INC. 508-278-7877
414 Quaker Highway, Uxbridge, MA 01569
FDA Number: 1218813
Cannula, Ophthalmic Ophthalmology
Cautery, Radiofrequency, AC-Powered Ophthalmology
Cautery, Radiofrequency, Battery-Powered Ophthalmology
Cryophthalmic Unit Ophthalmology
Cryotherapy, Unit, Ophthalmic Ophthalmology
Implant, Absorbable (Scleral Buckling Method) Ophthalmology
Implant, Orbital, Extra-Ocular Ophthalmology
Ophthalmoscope, AC-Powered Ophthalmology
Retractor, Ophthalmic Ophthalmology
Transilluminator, AC-Powered, Ophthalmic Ophthalmology

MIRACLE HOUSE 713-433-0333
5 Broadhurst St., Houston, TX 77047
FDA Number: n/a Fax: 713-433-7836
Web site: www.miraclehouse.net
Ownership: Private
Produces/Sells CE-marked Devices: N
Kit, Enema (For Cleaning Purposes) Gastroenterology/Urology

MIRACLE-EAR 877-268-4264
5000 Cheshire Lane North, 763-268-4000
Minneapolis, MN 55446
FDA Number: n/a Fax: 763-268-4365
Web site: www.miracle-ear.com
Annual Revenue: $50-$100 Million
Ownership: AMPLIFON
Quality System Registration Information: ISO9000
Produces/Sells CE-marked Devices: N
Distribution: Exclusive Distributor
General Admin.: Jeff Bilas/President
Hearing-Aid Ear/Nose/Throat

MIRION TECHNOLOGIES 925-543-0800
Bishop Ranch 8, 3000 Executive Parkway Suite 222,
San Ramon, CA 94583
FDA Number: n/a
E-mail: Info@mirion.com
Web site: www.mirion.com
Medical Products Sales Volume: $6,600,000
Year Founded: 1947
Ownership: Private
Produces/Sells CE-marked Devices: Y
Distribution: Manufacturer Direct, Service Direct
General Admin.: Mrs. Sandi Nemecek/President
Mktg./Adv.: Mr. Lou Biacchi/Director National Sales
　　　　　Mr. Lou Biacchi/Manager International & National Sales
Production: Mr. Al Mandelblatt/Product Manager
　　　　　Ms. Nancy Ronquillo/Vice President Customer Service
　　　　　Mr. Luis Espada/Vice President Manufacturing
　　　　　Mr. Sander Perle/Vice President Tech. Affairs
IS: Mr. Malcolm Smith/Vice President Information Systems
Dosimeter, Radiation Radiology
Monitor, Radiation Radiology

MIROLIN INDUSTRIES INC. 800-463-2236
60 Shorncliffe Rd., 416-231-9030
Toronto, ONT M8Z-5 Canada
FDA Number: n/a Fax: 416-231-0929
E-mail: info@mirolin.com
Web site: www.mirolin.com
Year Founded: 1991
Total Employees: 100
Ownership: Private
Produces/Sells CE-marked Devices: N

MISC INC. 800-524-1155
1889-97 Route 9, Toms River, NJ 08755 732-240-0178
FDA Number: n/a Fax: 732-240-1979

MISC INC. 800-524-1155 (cont'd)
E-mail: marketing@miscpaper.com
Web site: www.miscpaper.com
Annual Revenue: $0-$1 Million
Year Founded: 1983
Total Employees: 6 Marketing Staff: 3
Ownership: Private
Produces/Sells CE-marked Devices: N
Federal Procurement Eligibility: Small Business
Distribution: Manufacturer Direct, Manufacturer Through Manufacturer Reps
General Admin.: Joel Gardner/President
Mktg./Adv.: Irwin Klar/Vice President Marketing
Finance: Anne Turtora/Vice President Finance
Paper, Recording, Data General

MISCO PRODUCTS CORP. 800-548-4568
1048 Stinson Dr., Reading, PA 19605 610-926-4106
FDA Number: n/a Fax: 610-926-1194
E-mail: david.james@miscoproducts.com
Web site: www.miscoprod.com
Ownership: Private
Produces/Sells CE-marked Devices: N
Distribution: Manufacturer Direct, Manufacturer Through Manufacturer Reps, Service Direct
General Admin.: Steve Gable/Chief Executive Officer, Chairman
　　　　　Larry Fry/Information Technology Administrator
　　　　　Audra Donato/Manager Human Resources
Mktg./Adv.: Ben Gable/Product & Sales Manager
Production: Todd Northey/Vice President Operations
　　　　　Jeff Gable/Vice President Quality Systems
Research: Joe Zhou/Vice President, Director Research & Development
Disinfector, Liquid General
Solution, Antibacterial Cleaner General

MISCO PRODUCTS DIV.
See Misco Refractometer

MISCO REFRACTOMETER 866-831-1999
3401 Virginia Rd., Cleveland, OH 44122-4218 216-831-1000
FDA Number: n/a Fax: 216-831-1195
E-mail: sales@misco.com
Web site: www.misco.com
Annual Revenue: $0-$1 Million
Year Founded: 1954
Ownership: Private
Quality System Registration Information: ISO9000
Produces/Sells CE-marked Devices: N
Federal Procurement Eligibility: Small Business
Distribution: Manufacturer Direct, Manufacturer Through Distributor, Manufacturer Through Manufacturer Reps, Importer, Exporter
Refractometer Chemistry

MISONIX, INC. 800-694-9612
1938 New Hwy., Farmingdale, NY 11735 631-694-9555
FDA Number: 2435119 Fax: 631-694-9412
E-mail: bberger@misonix.com
Web site: www.misonix.com
Medical Products Sales Volume: $42,400,000
Annual Revenue: $25-$50 Million
Year Founded: 1959
Total Employees: 80 Marketing Staff: 6 Sales Staff: 16
Ownership: Public
Stock Symbol: MSON
Traded On: NASDAQ
Quality System Registration Information: ISO9001; ISO9002
Produces/Sells CE-marked Devices: Y
Federal Procurement Eligibility: Small Business
Distribution: Manufacturer Direct, Manufacturer Through Distributor, Manufacturer Through Manufacturer Reps, OEM, Service Direct, Importer, Exporter
General Admin.: Mike Mc Manus/President, Chief Executive Officer
　Medical Admin.: Mr. Michael Ryan/Senior Vice President Medical Affairs
Production: Mr. Frank Napoli/Vice President Operations
　　　　　Ronald Manna/Vice President Regulatory Affairs
Research: Mr. Dan Voic/Vice President Research & Development & Engineering
Finance: Rich Zaremba/Chief Financial Officer
Aspirator, Ultrasonic Obstetrics/Gynecology
Cleaner, Ultrasonic, Dental Laboratory Dental And Oral
Cleaner, Ultrasonic, Medical Instrument General
Cutter, Bone, Ultrasonic Cns/Neurology
Electrosurgical Unit, Cutting & Coagulation Device Surgery
Equipment, Control, Pollution General
Hood, Fume Toxicology
Hood, Isolation, Laminar Air Flow General
Lithotriptor, Ultrasonic Gastroenterology/Urology
Surgical Instrument, Ultrasonic Surgery
System, Suction, Lipoplasty Surgery
Medical Product Subsidiaries (Listed Separately)

MISONIX, INC. 800-694-9612 *(cont'd)*
Sonora Medical Systems, Inc.

MISSION DIAGNOSTICS 508-429-0450
333 Fiske St., Holliston, MA 01746
FDA Number: 3003656721
Calibrator, Secondary, Clinical Chemistry Chemistry

MISSION PHARMACAL CO. 210-696-8400
10999 IH-10 West, Suite 1000, San Antonio, TX 78230-1355
FDA Number: 1649184 *Fax:* 210-696-6010
E-mail: customerservice@missionpharmacal.com
Web site: www.missionpharmacal.com
Medical Products Sales Volume: $97,700,000
Year Founded: 1946
Total Employees: 110
Ownership: Private
Produces/Sells CE-marked Devices: Y
Federal Procurement Eligibility: Small Business
Distribution: Manufacturer Direct, Manufacturer Through Manufacturer Reps, Exporter
Mktg./Adv.: Susan Breidenbach/Director Media
　　　　　　Dan Kibbe/Manager National Sales
　　　　　　Jim Foody/Vice President International Sales
Chromatographic, Cystine Chemistry
Container, Specimen, All Types General
Impotence Device, Mechanical/Hydraulic Gastroenterology/Urology
Qualitative Chemical Reactions, Urinary Calculi (Stone) Chemistry

MISSION X-RAY 800-676-8718
45459 Industrial Pllace, Suite 1, 510-656-6739
Fremont, CA 94538
FDA Number: n/a *Fax:* 510-683-9242
E-mail: mark@missionxray.com
Web site: www.missionxray.com
Medical Products Sales Volume: $300,000
Annual Revenue: $0-$1 Million
Year Founded: 1990
Total Employees: 4 *Marketing Staff:* 1 *Sales Staff:* 1
Ownership: Private
Produces/Sells CE-marked Devices: N
Federal Procurement Eligibility: Small Business, Female Owned
Distribution: Manufacturer Direct
General Admin.: Mark Graham/General Manager
　　　　　　　　Laura Graham/Owner
Chair, Other General
Clamp, Other Surgery
Component, Metal, Other General

MIT POLY-CART CORP. 800-234-7659
211 Central Park W., New York, NY 10024-6020 212-724-7290
FDA Number: n/a *Fax:* 212-721-9022
E-mail: info@mitpolycart.com
Web site: www.mitpolycart.com
Annual Revenue: $0-$1 Million
Total Employees: 10
Ownership: Private
Produces/Sells CE-marked Devices: N
Federal Procurement Eligibility: Small Business
Distribution: Manufacturer Direct
General Admin.: Daniel Moss/President
Mktg./Adv.: Irwin Perton/Manager Advertising
　　　　　　Marty Winnick/Manager National Sales
　　　　　　Sandra Divak/Vice President Marketing
Production: Carol Keller/Manager Customer Services
Research: Isaac Rinkowich/Vice President Engineering
Cart, Housekeeping General
Cart, Laundry General
Cart, Other General

MIT SERVICE, INC. 800-343-8828
1354 Swallow Drive, Suite 104, 619-596-9859
El Cajon, CA 92020
FDA Number: n/a *Fax:* 619-596-9860
E-mail: info@mitservice.com
Web site: www.mitservice.com
Medical Products Sales Volume: $200,000
Annual Revenue: $1-$5 Million
Year Founded: 1982
Total Employees: 3
Ownership: Private
Produces/Sells CE-marked Devices: N
Federal Procurement Eligibility: Small Business
Distribution: Manufacturer Direct, Manufacturer Through Distributor, Manufacturer Through Manufacturer Reps, Service Direct, Exporter
General Admin.: Charles K. Adkins/President, Chief Executive Officer
Production: Charles Osbrink/Vice President Operations

MIT SERVICE, INC. 800-343-8828 *(cont'd)*
Service, Used Equipment General

MITEK PRODUCTS 800-356-4835
325 Paramount Drive, Raynham, MA 02767 (800) 227-6633
FDA Number: n/a *Fax:* 781-961-9166
E-mail: DePuySpine@dpyus.jnj.com
Web site: www.mitek.com
Ownership: Ethicon, Inc.
Produces/Sells CE-marked Devices: N
Prosthesis, Knee, Total Orthopedics
Screw, Fixation, Bone Orthopedics

MITER CORP.
See University Of Miami Tissue Bank

MITSUI / MAM-A 888-626-3472
10045 Federal Dr., Colorado Springs, CO 80908 719-262-2430
FDA Number: 2438114 *Fax:* 719-592-0057
E-mail: lora.swenson@mam-a.com
Web site: www.mam-a.com
Ownership: Private
Produces/Sells CE-marked Devices: N
Device, Storage, Image, Digital Radiology

MIV THERAPEUTICS, INC. 604-301-9545
8765 Ash St., Unit #1, Vancouver, BC V6P-6T3 Canada
FDA Number: n/a *Fax:* 604-301-9546
E-mail: contact@mivtherapeutics.com
Web site: www.mivtherapeutics.com
Year Founded: 1999
Total Employees: 10
Ownership: Public
Stock Symbol: MIVI
Traded On: OTC Bulletin
Produces/Sells CE-marked Devices: N
Distribution: Manufacturer Direct

MIXING EQUIPMENT CO. INC.
See Lightnin Mixers

MIZUHO AMERICA INC. 800-699-2547
133 Brimbal Avenue, Beverly, MA 01915 978-921-1718
FDA Number: 1223656 *Fax:* 978-921-4003
E-mail: mizuho@mizuho.com
Web site: www.mizuho.com
Medical Products Sales Volume: $8,000,000
Annual Revenue: $5-$10 Million
Year Founded: 1939
Total Employees: 10 *Marketing Staff:* 2 *Sales Staff:* 24
Ownership: Private
Produces/Sells CE-marked Devices: Y
Federal Procurement Eligibility: Small Business
Distribution: Manufacturer Through Distributor, Exclusive Distributor
General Admin.: Mr. Russ Hanson/President
Mktg./Adv.: Mark Swanson/Vice President Marketing & Sales
Production: Jonathan Wilber/Product Manager
Applier, Aneurysm Clip Cns/Neurology
Clip, Aneurysm (Intracranial) Cns/Neurology
Doppler, Flow Mapping Radiology
Head Rest, Neurosurgical Cns/Neurology
Instrument, Microsurgical Cns/Neurology
Remover, Clip Surgery

MIZUHO OSI 800-777-4674
30031 Ahern Avenue, Union City, CA 94587-1234 510-429-1500
FDA Number: 2921578 *Fax:* 510-429-8500
E-mail: CustSvc@mizuhosi.com
Web site: www.osiosi.com
Medical Products Sales Volume: $50,000,000
Annual Revenue: $50-$100 Million
Year Founded: 1978
Total Employees: 268 *Marketing Staff:* 7 *Sales Staff:* 44
Ownership: Private
Quality System Registration Information: ISO9001
Produces/Sells CE-marked Devices: Y
Federal Procurement Eligibility: Small Business, GSA Contract, VA Contract
Distribution: Manufacturer Direct
General Admin.: Stephanie Jones/Manager Human Resources
　　　　　　　　Steve Lamb/President
Mktg./Adv.: Roxane Hunry/Admin. International Sales
　　　　　　Mark Lane/Vice President Marketing & Sales
Production: Larry Waters/Vice President Manufacturing
Research: Steve Lamb/Vice President Research & Development
Accessories, Arthroscope Orthopedics
Accessories, Traction Physical Med
Accessories, Traction (Cart, Frame, Cord, Weight) Orthopedics
Bandage, Cast Physical Med
Belt, Traction, Pelvic Physical Med

MIZUHO OSI
800-777-4674 *(cont'd)*

Belt, Traction, Pelvic, Orthopedic	Orthopedics
Board, Arm	Anesthesiology
Brace, Joint, Ankle (External)	Physical Med
Cast Walking Heel	Orthopedics
Clamp, Other	Surgery
Equipment, Screening, Scoliosis	Orthopedics
Frame, Traction	Orthopedics
Goniometer, Orthopedic	Orthopedics
Halter, Head, Traction, Orthopedic	Orthopedics
Holder, Leg, Arthroscopy	Orthopedics
Immobilizer, Arm	Orthopedics
Immobilizer, Shoulder	Orthopedics
Orthosis, Cervical	Physical Med
Orthosis, Limb Brace	Physical Med
Orthosis, Lumbosacral	Physical Med
Orthosis, Other	Physical Med
Orthosis, Rib Fracture, Soft	Physical Med
Pad, Pressure, Foam (Elbow, Heel)	General
Passer	Orthopedics
Protector, Finger	Orthopedics
Protector, Skin Pressure	General
Roller, Patient	General
Sling, Arm, Overhead Supported	Physical Med
Sling, Knee	Orthopedics
Splint, Clavicle	Physical Med
Splint, Hand, And Component	Physical Med
Splint, Molded, Aluminum	Orthopedics
Splint, Padded Stays	Orthopedics
Splint, Traction	Orthopedics
Stand, Casting	Orthopedics
Strap, Clavicle	Orthopedics
Strap, Restraining	General
Support, Ankle	Orthopedics
Support, Arm	Physical Med
Support, Elbow	Orthopedics
Support, Knee	Physical Med
Support, Patient Position	Anesthesiology
Table, Other	General
Table, Radiographic	Radiology
Table, Radiographic, Stationary Top	Radiology
Table, Surgical, Manual	General
Table, Surgical, Orthopedic	Orthopedics
Traction Unit, Static, Other	Orthopedics
Transfer Aid	Physical Med
Transfer Device, Patient, Manual	General

MIZUHO USA, INC.
858-679-0555

12131 Community Road, Poway, CA 92064
FDA Number: 2028977   *Fax:* 858-547-3937
E-mail: bzin@mizuhousa.com
Annual Revenue: $5-$10 Million
Total Employees: 25
Ownership: MIZUHO MEDY CO. Ltd.
Quality System Registration Information: ISO9001
Produces/Sells CE-marked Devices: N
Federal Procurement Eligibility: Small Business
Distribution: Manufacturer Direct, Manufacturer Through Distributor, OEM, Exporter
General Admin.: Benedict Zin/President

Kit, Pregnancy Test	Obstetrics/Gynecology
Kit, Pregnancy Test, Over The Counter, HCG	Chemistry

MIZZY, INC. OF NATIONAL KEYSTONE
800-333-3131
856-663-4700

616 Hollywood Avenue,
Cherry Hill, NJ 08002
FDA Number: 2280629   *Fax:* 856-663-0381
E-mail: skatz@keystoneind.com
Web site: ww.keystoneind.com
Total Employees: 80   *Marketing Staff:* 3   *Sales Staff:* 25
Ownership: KEYSTONE INDUSTRIES
Quality System Registration Information: ISO9001
Produces/Sells CE-marked Devices: Y
Federal Procurement Eligibility: Small Business
Distribution: Manufacturer Through Distributor, Exporter
General Admin.: Fred Robinson/Chief Executive Officer
　　　　　　Cary B. Robinson/Chief Operating Officer
Mktg./Adv.: Steve Katz/Manager International Sales
　　　　Michael Prozzillo/Vice President, Director Marketing

Cement, Dental	Dental And Oral
Disk, Abrasive	Dental And Oral
Injector, Jet, Mechanical-Powered	Dental And Oral
Mask, Analgesia	Dental And Oral
Material, Acrylic, Dental	Dental And Oral
Material, Dental Filling	Dental And Oral
Saw, Other	Surgery
Wax, Dental	Dental And Oral

MJM INTERNATIONAL CORPORATION
956-781-5000

2003 N. I Rd., Ste. 10, San Juan, TX 78589
FDA Number: 3004499949

Bed, Manual	General
Cart, Emergency, Cardiopulmonary Resuscitation (Crash)	Anesthesiology
Chair, Adjustable, Mechanical	Physical Med
Chair, Geriatric	General
Chair, With Casters	Physical Med
Device, Anti-Tip, Wheelchair	Physical Med
Stretcher, Wheeled (Mobile)	General
Transfer Device, Patient, Manual	General
Walker, Mechanical	Physical Med

MJS BIOLYNX INC.
888-593-5969
613-498-2126

300 Laurier Blvd., P.O. Box 1150,
Brockville, ONT K6V-5 Canada
FDA Number: n/a   *Fax:* 613-342-1341
E-mail: sales@biolynx.ca
Web site: www.biolynx.ca
Year Founded: 1998
Total Employees: 10
Ownership: Private
Produces/Sells CE-marked Devices: N
Distribution: Exclusive Distributor

MK BATTERY
800-372-9253
714-937-1033

1645 S. Sinclair St., Anaheim, CA 92806
FDA Number: n/a   *Fax:* 714-937-0818
E-mail: info@mkbattery.com
Web site: www.mkbattery.com
Medical Products Sales Volume: $58,000,000
Annual Revenue: $50-$100 Million
Year Founded: 1983
Total Employees: 25   *Marketing Staff:* 6   *Sales Staff:* 40
Ownership: East Penn Mfg.
Quality System Registration Information: ISO9001
Produces/Sells CE-marked Devices: N
Federal Procurement Eligibility: Small Business
Distribution: Manufacturer Through Distributor, OEM, Exporter
General Admin.: Mark Wels/President
Mktg./Adv.: Dennis Sharpe/Manager National Sales
　　　　　David Brunelle/Vice President Sales
Production: Kathy Couture/Customer Service Representative
Purchasing: Rick Spiegel/Vice President Purchasing

Battery	General
Charger, Battery	General

MKM HEALTHCARE CORP.
　See Gentell

ML LIFESCIENCES
949-699-3800

17 Hammond, Suite 408, Irvine, CA 92618
FDA Number: 3006793669   *Fax:* (949) 699-3888
Ownership: Private
Produces/Sells CE-marked Devices: N

Culture Media, General Nutrient Broth	Microbiology
Culture Media, Non-Selective And Non-Differential	Microbiology
Culture Media, Selective And Differential	Microbiology

MLA/STRETCHAIR PATIENT TRANSFER SYSTEMS
　See Stretchair Patient Transfer Systems, Inc,

MLW INC.
970-434-2222

510 Fruitvale Ct., Suite C, Grand Junction, CO 81504
FDA Number: 2022026
Ownership: Private
Produces/Sells CE-marked Devices: N

Cover, Cast	General

MMAR MEDICAL GROUP, INC.
800-662-7633

9619 Yupondale Dr., Houston, TX 77080-7233
FDA Number: n/a   *Fax:* 713-465-2818
E-mail: service@mmarmedical.com
Web site: www.mmarmedical.com
Year Founded: 1990
Ownership: Private
Produces/Sells CE-marked Devices: N
Federal Procurement Eligibility: Small Business
Distribution: Manufacturer Through Distributor

Exerciser, Finger, Powered	Physical Med
Immobilizer, Ankle	Orthopedics
Immobilizer, Arm	Orthopedics
Immobilizer, Elbow	Orthopedics
Immobilizer, Knee	Orthopedics
Orthosis, Limb Brace	Physical Med
Orthosis, Other	Physical Med

MMI
800-999-4664
847-816-1009

P.O. Box 5396, Vernon Hills, IL 60061
FDA Number: n/a   *Fax:* 866-816-6646

MMI
800-999-4664 *(cont'd)*

E-mail: John.Froemke@mmimedical.com
Web site: www.offthemall.com/mmi
Medical Products Sales Volume: $2,000,000
Annual Revenue: $1-$5 Million
Year Founded: 1998
Ownership: JAL LLC
Produces/Sells CE-marked Devices: N
Distribution: Service Direct
General Admin.: John Froemke/Chief Executive Officer
　　　　　　　John Froemke/Owner
　Catheter, Angiographic ... Cns/Neurology

MMI OF MISSISSIPPI, INC.
800-448-5918
PO Box 488, Crystal Springs, MS 39059-0488
601-892-1105
FDA Number: n/a ... *Fax:* 601-892-1150
E-mail: mmiofms@mmiofms.com
Medical Products Sales Volume: $5,300,000
Annual Revenue: $5-$10 Million
Year Founded: 1956
Total Employees: 62
Ownership: Private
Produces/Sells CE-marked Devices: N
Federal Procurement Eligibility: Small Business, GSA Contract, VA Contract
Distribution: Exclusive Distributor
General Admin.: William Reeves/President
Mktg./Adv.: Marianne Defever/Vice President Marketing
Finance: Billy Sullivan/Treasurer
　Cabinet Casework, General Purpose ... General
　Defroster, Drug, Frozen ... General

MMI-USA
866-682-7577
6060 Poplar Ave., Suite 254, Memphis, TN 38119
FDA Number: n/a ... *Fax:* 901-683-7077
Web site: http://www.mmi-usa.com
Year Founded: 1992
Ownership: Private
Produces/Sells CE-marked Devices: N

MMJ S.A. DE C.V.
314-654-2000
716 Ponciano Arriaga, Cd. Juarez, Chih. Mexico
FDA Number: 9680580
　Accessories, Cardiopulmonary Bypass ... Cardiovascular
　Cable, Electrode ... Physical Med
　Catheter, Retention Type, Balloon ... Gastroenterology/Urology
　Catheter, Ureteral, Gastro-Urology ... Gastroenterology/Urology
　Catheter, Urological ... Gastroenterology/Urology
　Pressure Infusor, IV Container ... General
　Probe, Thermodilution ... Cardiovascular
　Regulator, Thermal, Cardiopulmonary Bypass ... Cardiovascular
　Stethoscope, Esophageal, With Electrical Conductors ... Anesthesiology
　Thermometer, Electronic, Continuous ... General
　Tube, Levine ... General
　Warmer, Blood, Non-Electromagnetic Radiation ... Anesthesiology

MML DIAGNOSTICS PACKAGING, INC.
800-826-7186
1625 N.W. Sundial Rd., P.O. Box 458,
503-666-8398
Troutdale, OR 97060
FDA Number: 3018348 ... *Fax:* 503-666-8510
Web site: www.mmldiagnostics.com
Ownership: Private
Produces/Sells CE-marked Devices: N
Federal Procurement Eligibility: Small Business
Distribution: Manufacturer Direct
General Admin.: Carrie Schwartzenberger/Office Manager
　　　　　　　Dale Pestes/President
Production: Larry Bullock/Manager Materials
　　　　　　Lynn Creitz/Vice President Operations
　Applicator, Other ... General
　Culture Media, Non-Propagating Transport ... Microbiology

MMSI
503-538-3270
PO Box 3005, Newberg, OR 97132
FDA Number: n/a ... *Fax:* 507-538-5767
E-mail: sales@mmsieng.com
Web site: www.mmsieng.com
Year Founded: 1993
Ownership: Private
Produces/Sells CE-marked Devices: N
Distribution: Manufacturer Through Manufacturer Reps
General Admin.: Richard Meissner/President
　Catheter, Angioplasty, Coronary, Ultrasonic ... Cardiovascular

MNEMONICS, INC.
800-842-5333
3900 Dow Road, Suite J, Melbourne, FL 32934
321-254-7300
FDA Number: 1063120 ... *Fax:* 321-255-4697
E-mail: CS@Mnemonics-inc.com
Web site: http://mnemonics-inc.com/

MNEMONICS, INC.
800-842-5333 *(cont'd)*

Medical Products Sales Volume: $17,000,000
Year Founded: 1979
Total Employees: 100 ... *Marketing Staff:* 3
Ownership: Public
Quality System Registration Information: ISO9001
Produces/Sells CE-marked Devices: N
Distribution: Manufacturer Direct, Manufacturer Through Manufacturer Reps, OEM

MOBILE DENTAL EQUIPMENT CORP.(M-DEC)
425-747-5424
13300 S.E. 30th St.# 101, Bellevue, WA 98005
FDA Number: 3021504 ... *Fax:* 425-746-6332
E-mail: m-dec@earthlink.com
Web site: www.portabledentistry.com
Medical Products Sales Volume: $500,000
Annual Revenue: $0-$1 Million
Year Founded: 1983
Total Employees: 6 ... *Marketing Staff:* 3 ... *Sales Staff:* 3
Ownership: Private
Produces/Sells CE-marked Devices: N
Federal Procurement Eligibility: Small Business, GSA Contract
Distribution: Manufacturer Direct, Manufacturer Through Distributor, Manufacturer Through Manufacturer Reps, Service Direct
General Admin.: Peter E. Moore/President, Chief Executive Officer
Mktg./Adv.: Alex Garcia/Manager Sales
　Case, Protection, Equipment ... General
　Chair, Dental ... Dental And Oral
　Headlamp, Operating, AC-Powered ... Ophthalmology
　Operative Dental Treatment Unit ... Dental And Oral
　Radiographic Unit, Diagnostic, Dental (X-Ray) ... Dental And Oral
　Stool, Operating Room, Adjustable ... Surgery

MOBILE DESIGNS, INC.
530-244-1050
4650 Caterpillar Rd., Redding, CA 96003
FDA Number: 3004841377
　Chair, Blood Donor ... General
　Chair/Table, Medical ... General

MOBILE I.V. SYSTEMS, LLC
623-434-3136
23630 N. 35th Dr, Glendale, AZ 85310
FDA Number: 3006990582
Ownership: Private
Produces/Sells CE-marked Devices: N
　Pressure Infusor, IV Container ... General

MOBILE INSTRUMENT SERVICE AND REPAIR, INC.
800-722-3675
333 Water Ave., Bellefontaine, OH 43311
937-592-5025
FDA Number: 1527797 ... *Fax:* 937-592-7004
E-mail: mobileinstrument@logannet
Web site: mobileinstrument.com
Annual Revenue: $25-$50 Million
Year Founded: 1978
Total Employees: 74 ... *Marketing Staff:* 7 ... *Sales Staff:* 121
Ownership: Private
Quality System Registration Information: ISO9002
Produces/Sells CE-marked Devices: N
Federal Procurement Eligibility: Small Business
Distribution: Manufacturer Through Manufacturer Reps, Service Direct
General Admin.: Mick Reed/Chief Executive Officer
　　　　　　　Dwight E. Reed/President, Chief Executive Officer
　　　　　　　Kelley Hooper/Vice President Human Resources
Mktg./Adv.: Beverly Young/Director Marketing
　　　　　　Mike Berryman/Director National Accounts
　　　　　　Beverly Young/Manager Advertising
　　　　　　Mick Reed/Manager Contract Sales
　　　　　　Beverly Young/Vice President Marketing
　　　　　　Mick Reed/Vice President Sales
Production: Curtis Champion/Director Quality Assurance
　　　　　　Lew Tracey/Vice President Manufacturing
　Coagulator, Laparoscopic, Unipolar ... Obstetrics/Gynecology
　Endoscope, Flexible ... Gastroenterology/Urology
　Endoscope, Rigid ... Surgery
　Service, Maintenance/Repair ... General

MOBILE MEDICAL INTERNATIONAL CORPORATION
800-748-2322
2176 Portland St., Suite 4, PO Box 672,
802-748-2322
St. Johnsbury, VT 05819
FDA Number: n/a ... *Fax:* 802-748-2323
E-mail: mmic@mobile-medical.com
Web site: www.mobile-medical.com
Medical Products Sales Volume: $11,200,000
Annual Revenue: $10-$25 Million
Year Founded: 1994
Total Employees: 30 ... *Marketing Staff:* 5 ... *Sales Staff:* 6
Ownership: Public

MOBILE MEDICAL INTERNATIONAL   800-748-2322 *(cont'd)*
Produces/Sells CE-marked Devices: N
Federal Procurement Eligibility: Small Business, VA Contract
Distribution: Manufacturer Direct, Manufacturer Through Distributor, Manufacturer Through Manufacturer Reps, OEM, Exporter
General Admin.: Rick Cochran/President, Chief Executive Officer
Mktg./Adv.: Randy North/Vice President Design
         Mark Munroe/Vice President Marketing & Sales
Production: Kyle Affeldt/Senior Vice President Operations
Research: Ted Cantin/Vice President Engineering
Finance: Lou Silvestre/Chief Financial Officer
   Facility, Equipment, Medical, Mobile   General

MOBILE-TRONICS CO., INC.   800-368-8181
28570 Marguerite Pkwy. #227,   **949-347-1557**
Mission Viejo, CA 92692
FDA Number: 9200749
Fax: 800-259-0064
E-mail: sales@mobile-tronics.com
Web site: www.mobile-tronics.com
Annual Revenue: $0-$1 Million
Total Employees: 8   *Sales Staff:* 3
Ownership: Private
Produces/Sells CE-marked Devices: N
Federal Procurement Eligibility: Small Business
Distribution: Manufacturer Direct
General Admin.: Brian Somodi/President
Mktg./Adv.: Carol Crowell/Admin. Marketing & Sales
   Cart, Housekeeping   General
   Cart, Instrument   Surgery
   Cart, Other   General
   Cart, Supply   General

MOBILECTRICS
See Gould Discount Medical

MOBILIFE, LLC   262-646-5433
78 Enterprise Road, Unit D, Delafield, WI 53018
FDA Number: 3006369740
   Wheelchair, Powered   Physical Med

MOBILITE CORP.
See Invacare Corporation

MOBILITY CONCEPTS, L.L.C.   660-668-3918
16999 Boyer Ave, Cole Camp, MO 65325
FDA Number: 3004365769
Ownership: Private
Produces/Sells CE-marked Devices: N
   Crutch   Physical Med

MOBILITY INC.   858-456-8121
5726 La Jolla Blvd., Suite 104, La Jolla, CA 92037
FDA Number: 2031718
Fax: 858-456-8139
E-mail: info@mobilityinc.net
Web site: www.mobilityinc.net
Year Founded: 1997
Ownership: Public
Produces/Sells CE-marked Devices: Y
Distribution: Manufacturer Through Distributor, Manufacturer Through Manufacturer Reps
Mktg./Adv.: Ms. Michelle Norsten/Marketing Coordinator
   Adapter, Hygiene   Physical Med
   Transfer Aid   Physical Med

MOBILITY MATTERS INCORPORATED   812-459-4584
3588 Katalla, Newburgh, IN 47630
FDA Number: n/a
Fax: 812-490-2677
E-mail: mobility4you@aol.com
Medical Products Sales Volume: $100,000
Year Founded: 1962
Ownership: Private
Produces/Sells CE-marked Devices: N
Federal Procurement Eligibility: Small Business
General Admin.: Mr. Paul Medcalf/President, Chief Executive Officer, Chairman
   Cart, Supply, Operating Room   Surgery

MOBILITY RESEARCH   800.332.WALK
P.O. Box 3141, Tempe, AZ 85280   **480-829-1727**
FDA Number: 2029188
Fax: 480.829.0737
E-mail: sales@litegait.com
Web site: www.litegait.com
Ownership: Private
Produces/Sells CE-marked Devices: N
   Lift, Bath, Non-AC-Powered   General
   Walker, Mechanical   Physical Med

MOBILITY TRANSFER SYSTEMS   888-854-4687
34 Sullivan Road , Unit 32,   **781-306-1570**
North Billerica, MA 01862
FDA Number: n/a
Fax: 781-306-1573

MOBILITY TRANSFER SYSTEMS   888-854-4687 *(cont'd)*
E-mail: thomasmts@aol.com
Web site: www.bedhandle.com
Ownership: Private
Produces/Sells CE-marked Devices: N
Distribution: Manufacturer Direct
General Admin.: Thomas Leoutsakos/Chief Executive Officer
   Accessories, Walker   General
   Bedrail   General
   Orthosis, Lumbar   Physical Med
   Urinal   General

MOBILSONIC, INC.   408-390-4002
19 North 2nd Street, Ste. 206, San Jose, CA 95113
FDA Number: 3004506358
Fax: 408-292-7050
E-mail: info@mobilsonic.com
Web site: www.mobilsonic.com
Ownership: Private
Produces/Sells CE-marked Devices: N
   Scanner, Ultrasonic (Pulsed Echo)   Radiology

MODELS PLUS   800-522-4044
605 Grayton Road, PO Box 600,   **219-393-5591**
Kingsford Heights, IN 46346
FDA Number: 1834209
Fax: 219-393-5593
E-mail: info@dentalmodelsplus.com
Web site: www.dentalmodelsplus.com
Medical Products Sales Volume: $2,900,000
Year Founded: 1988
Total Employees: 40
Ownership: Private
Produces/Sells CE-marked Devices: N
Federal Procurement Eligibility: Small Business
   Wire, Orthodontic   Dental And Oral

MODERN AIDS, INC.   847-437-8600
201 Bond St., Elk Grove Village, IL 60007
FDA Number: 1418457
   Tape, Orthopedic   Orthopedics

MODERN AIDS, INC.   800-437-1063
201 Bond St., Elk Grove Village, IL 60007-1220   **847-437-8600**
FDA Number: 9200752
Fax: 847-437-8602
Annual Revenue: $0-$1 Million
Total Employees: 20
Ownership: Private
Produces/Sells CE-marked Devices: N
Federal Procurement Eligibility: Small Business
Distribution: Importer, Exporter
General Admin.: D. E. Croft/President
   Bandage, Other   General
   Tape, Orthopedic   Orthopedics

MODERN PLASTICS CORP.   570-822-1124
152 Horton St., Wilkes Barre, PA 18702-3499
FDA Number: n/a
Fax: 570-823-9666
E-mail: mp152@epix.net
Medical Products Sales Volume: $250,000
Annual Revenue: $1-$5 Million
Total Employees: 40   *Marketing Staff:* 1   *Sales Staff:* 6
Ownership: Private
Produces/Sells CE-marked Devices: N
Federal Procurement Eligibility: Small Business
Distribution: Manufacturer Direct, Manufacturer Through Distributor
General Admin.: Bernadette Murphy/Chief Executive Officer
                 Larry I. Taren/President
   Cabinet Casework, Laboratory   Chemistry
   Furniture, General   General
   Station, Nursing   General

MODERN PLASTICS, INC.   800.243.9696
Modern Plastics, Inc., Shelton, CT 06484   **203.333.3128**
FDA Number: n/a
Fax: 203.333.4625
E-mail: customerservice@modernplastics.com
Web site: www.modernplastics.com
Ownership: Private
Produces/Sells CE-marked Devices: N

MODERN WAY IMMOBILIZERS, INC.   866-694-7444
100 Johnson St, PO Box 660, Clifton, TN 38425   **931-676-5274**
FDA Number: n/a
Fax: 931-676-3860
E-mail: info@piggostat.com
Web site: www.piggostat.com
Medical Products Sales Volume: $1,200,000
Annual Revenue: $0-$1 Million
Year Founded: 1960
Total Employees: 15
Ownership: Private

MODERN WAY IMMOBILIZERS, INC.   866-694-7444 *(cont'd)*
Produces/Sells CE-marked Devices: N
Federal Procurement Eligibility: Small Business
Distribution: Manufacturer Direct, Manufacturer Through Distributor, Exporter
General Admin.: Cindy H. Pigg/Corporate Secretary
     Jimmy Pigg/President
   Support, Patient Position, Radiographic   Radiology

MODULAR CUTTING SYSTEMS, INC.   203-336-3526
650 Clinton Ave., Bridgeport, CT 06605
FDA Number: 1226077
Ownership: Private
Produces/Sells CE-marked Devices: N
   Accessories, Operating Room, Table   Surgery
   Osteotome (Orthopedic)   Surgery
   Rod, Fixation, Intramedullary   Orthopedics
   Surgical Instrument, Orthopedic, AC-Powered Motor   Orthopedics

MODULAR PACKAGING SYSTEM, INC.   973-882-0633
45 Rte. 46, Pine Brook, NJ 07058
FDA Number: n/a   *Fax:* 973-882-4665
E-mail: info@modularpackaging.com
Web site: www.modularpackaging.com
Annual Revenue: $5-$10 Million
Ownership: Private
Produces/Sells CE-marked Devices: N
Distribution: Exclusive Distributor
   Contract Packaging   General

MODULAR SERVICES COMPANY   405-521-9923
109 N.e. 38th St., Oklahoma City, OK 73105
FDA Number: 1640663
   Infusion Stand   General

MODULATION OPTICS, INC.   516-609-000
40 Garvies Point Rd., Glen Cove, NY 11542
FDA Number: 9200755   *Fax:* 516-609-0093
E-mail: rick@modulationoptics.com
Web site: www.modulationoptics.com
Annual Revenue: $1-$5 Million
Total Employees: 10
Ownership: Private
Produces/Sells CE-marked Devices: N
Distribution: Manufacturer Direct, Manufacturer Through Distributor, Manufacturer Through Manufacturer Reps
General Admin.: Donald Brown/President
     Bruce Phillips/Vice President, General Manager
Mktg./Adv.: Sel Steinberg/Vice President Marketing
Production: Rick Graziosi/Product Manager
   Contrast Enhancement Unit, Microscope   Microbiology

MODULUS DATA SYSTEMS, INC.   888-663-8547
386 MAIN STREET, SUITE 200,   650-365-3111
REDWOOD CITY, CA 94063
FDA Number: 2921591   *Fax:* 650-365-6111
E-mail: info@modulusdatasystems.com
Web site: www.modulusdatasystems.com
Medical Products Sales Volume: $400,000
Annual Revenue: $1-$5 Million
Year Founded: 1972
Total Employees: 4   *Marketing Staff:* 2   *Sales Staff:* 1
Ownership: Private
Produces/Sells CE-marked Devices: N
Federal Procurement Eligibility: Small Business, VA Contract
Distribution: Manufacturer Direct, Manufacturer Through Distributor, Exporter
General Admin.: George J. Liviakis/President, Chief Executive Officer
Mktg./Adv.: Mary Halkos/Director Marketing
     Steven Waites/Director Product Development
     Burt Miller/Manager Sales Training
     Mary Liviakis/Vice President Marketing
Production: George Jordan/Program Director Production
     Steve Waites/Vice President Manufacturing
   Computer Equipment   General
   Computer, Clinical Laboratory   Chemistry
   Counter, Cell   Microbiology
   Counter, Cell, Differential Classifier, Automated   Hematology
   Counter, Differential Hand Tally   Hematology

MODUS MEDICAL DEVICES INC.   519-438-2409
17 Masonville Cres, London N5X 3T1 Canada
FDA Number: 9616855
   Tester, Radiology   Radiology

MOLDED PRODUCTS INC.   800-435-8957
1112 Chatburn Ave., Harlan, IA 51537   712-755-5557
FDA Number: 1932668   *Fax:* 712-755-7089
E-mail: moldprod@harlannet.com
Web site: www.moldedproducts.com

MOLDED PRODUCTS INC.   800-435-8957 *(cont'd)*
Year Founded: 1986
Ownership: Private
Produces/Sells CE-marked Devices: N
Federal Procurement Eligibility: Small Business, Female Owned
Distribution: Manufacturer Direct, Manufacturer Through Distributor, Manufacturer Through Manufacturer Reps, OEM
Mktg./Adv.: Ms. Sheri Bissen/Director Marketing & Sales
   Accessories, Blood Circuit, Hemodialysis   Gastroenterology/Urology
   Cannula, Injection   Gastroenterology/Urology
   Cap, Tip, Syringe   General
   Clamp, Hemodialysis Unit Blood Line   Gastroenterology/Urology
   Clamp, Non-Electrical   Gastroenterology/Urology
   Connector, Tubing, Blood   Cardiovascular
   Dialyzer Reprocessing System   Gastroenterology/Urology
   Dialyzer, Capillary, Hollow Fiber (Hemodialysis)   Gastroenterology/Urology
   Forceps, General & Plastic Surgery   Surgery
   Holder, Needle   Gastroenterology/Urology
   Molding, Injection   General
   Protector, Transducer, Dialysis   Gastroenterology/Urology
   Set, Holder, Dialyzer   Gastroenterology/Urology
   Shield, Protective, Personnel   Radiology
   Tourniquet, Non-Pneumatic, Surgical   Surgery
   Tubing, Dialysate (And Connector)   Gastroenterology/Urology

MOLDEX-METRIC, INC.   800-421-0668
10111 West Jefferson Blvd.,   310-837-6500
Culver City, CA 90232
FDA Number: 2023299   *Fax:* 310-837-9563
E-mail: sales@moldex.com
Web site: www.moldex.com
Medical Products Sales Volume: $38,100,000
Year Founded: 1960
Total Employees: 500
Ownership: Private
Quality System Registration Information: ISO9000
Produces/Sells CE-marked Devices: N
Federal Procurement Eligibility: Small Business
Distribution: Manufacturer Through Distributor
Mktg./Adv.: Mr. Fred Ryan/Vice President Marketing & Sales
   Mask, Surgical   Surgery

MOLDING SOLUTIONS   859-231-0031
781 Enterprise Dr., Lexington, KY 40510
FDA Number: n/a   *Fax:* 859-254-8884
E-mail: solutions@molders.com
Web site: www.molders.com
Total Employees: 35   *Marketing Staff:* 2
Ownership: Private
Quality System Registration Information: ISO9002
Produces/Sells CE-marked Devices: N
Distribution: Manufacturer Direct, OEM
General Admin.: Michael Necessary/General Manager
     Paul Heflin/President, Chief Executive Officer
     Sheri Heflin/Vice President
Mktg./Adv.: Paul Price/Sales Associate
   Molding, Custom   General

MOLDPRO, INC.   603-721-6286
36 Denman Thompson Hwy., West Swanzey, NH 03446
FDA Number: n/a   *Fax:* 603-357-5061
E-mail: info@moldproinc.com
Web site: www.moldproinc.com
Medical Products Sales Volume: $1,000,000
Annual Revenue: $1-$5 Million
Year Founded: 1989
Total Employees: 25   *Sales Staff:* 1
Ownership: Private
Produces/Sells CE-marked Devices: N
Distribution: Manufacturer Direct
General Admin.: Mr. Gary Barnard/President
Mktg./Adv.: Mr. Chip Southgate/Manager New Business Development
   Connector, Suction/Irrigation   Surgery
   Labware, Basic, Disposable   Chemistry
   Tip, Suction Tube (Yankauer, Poole, Etc.)   Surgery

MOLECTRON CORPORATION
See Ams Innovative Center-San Jose

MOLECULAR DETECTION INC.   610-590-1974
400 East Lancaster Avenue, Suite 300, Wayne, PA 19087
FDA Number: n/a
E-mail: corporate@detect-ready.com
Web site: http://www.detect-ready.com
Year Founded: 2007
Ownership: Private
Produces/Sells CE-marked Devices: N
General Admin.: Mr. Todd Wallach/Chief Executive Officer
     Dr. Aryeh Gassel/President

MOLECULAR DETECTION INC.
610-590-1974 *(cont'd)*

Production: Mr. Fredi Kleinman/Director Production
Mr. Avraham Harris/Director Quality Assurance & Regulatory Affairs
Research: Dr. Tzvi Tzubery/Director Research & Development

MOLECULAR DEVICES CORP.
800-635-5577
1311 Orleans Drive, Sunnyvale, CA 94089-1136
408-747-1700
FDA Number: n/a
Fax: 408-747-3602
E-mail: info@moldev.com
Web site: www.moldev.com
Medical Products Sales Volume: $186,400,000
Annual Revenue: $100-$500 Million
Year Founded: 1983
Total Employees: 125   *Marketing Staff:* 15   *Sales Staff:* 35
Ownership: Public
Stock Symbol: MDCC
Traded On: NASDAQ
Quality System Registration Information: ISO9001
Produces/Sells CE-marked Devices: Y
Federal Procurement Eligibility: Small Business
Distribution: Manufacturer Direct, Exclusive Distributor
General Admin.: Jan Dahlin/Director Human Resources
Joseph Keegan/President, Chief Executive Officer
Mktg./Adv.: John Senaldi/Vice President Marketing
Tony Lima/Vice President Sales
Production: Richard Armenta/Manager Regulatory Affairs
Bob Murray/Vice President Manufacturing
Finance: Tim Harkness/Chief Financial Officer
IS: Gill Humphries/Vice President Application Development

Microplate	General
Reader, Microplate	General
Spectrophotometer, U.V./Visible	Chemistry

MOLECULAR METALLURGY, INC.
619-596-7444
11649 Riverside Drive, Suite 139, Lakeside, CA 92040
FDA Number: 2032803

Blade, Scalpel	Surgery
Blade, Surgical, Saw, General & Plastic Surgery	Surgery

MOLEX
800-786-6539
2222 Wellington Ct., Lisle, IL 60532
630-969-4550
FDA Number: n/a
Fax: 630-968-8356
E-mail: amerinfo@molex.com
Web site: www.molex.com
Ownership: Private
Produces/Sells CE-marked Devices: N
Distribution: Manufacturer Direct, OEM, Service Direct

MOLL INDUSTRIES, INC.
972-663-6900
13455 Noel Rd, Suite 1310, Dallas, TX 75240
FDA Number: 1047423
Fax: 972-663-6950
E-mail: info@mollindustries.com
Web site: www.mollindustries.com
Medical Products Sales Volume: $41,500,000
Year Founded: 1945
Total Employees: 20   *Marketing Staff:* 5   *Sales Staff:* 15
Ownership: Private
Stock Symbol: WMX
Traded On: NYSE
Quality System Registration Information: ISO9000; ISO9001; ISO9002
Produces/Sells CE-marked Devices: N
Federal Procurement Eligibility: Small Business
Distribution: Manufacturer Direct
Mktg./Adv.: Dana Gecker/Marketing & Communications Officer
Joe Pack/Vice President Sales

Analyzer, Cell Size	Microbiology
Contract Manufacturing	General

MOLNLYCKE HEALTH CARE INC.
678-250-7900
5550 Peachtree Parkway, Suite 500, Norcross, GA 30092
FDA Number: 3004763499
Fax: 678-250-7984
E-mail: info.hq@molnlycke.com
Web site: www.molnlycke.com
Medical Products Sales Volume: $1,100,000
Year Founded: 1951
Ownership: Regent Medical Ltd.
Quality System Registration Information: ISO9002
Produces/Sells CE-marked Devices: Y
Federal Procurement Eligibility: Small Business
Distribution: Manufacturer Through Distributor

Disinfector, Liquid	General
Glove, Patient Examination	General
Glove, Patient Examination, Latex	General
Glove, Patient Examination, Specialty	General
Glove, Surgical	General
Glove, Surgical, Plastic Surgery	Surgery
Glove, Surgical, Powder-Free	Surgery

MOLNLYCKE HEALTH CARE INC.
678-250-7900 *(cont'd)*

Solution, Antimicrobial	Microbiology

MOLTECH POWER SYSTEMS INC
800-677-6937
1908 Nw 67th Pl, Gainesville, FL 32614-7114
904-462-3911
FDA Number: n/a
Fax: 904-462-6210
E-mail: sales@moltech.com
Web site: www.moltech.com
Medical Products Sales Volume: $82,800,000
Year Founded: 1999
Total Employees: 595
Ownership: Public
Produces/Sells CE-marked Devices: N
Distribution: Manufacturer Direct, Service Direct, Importer, Exporter

Battery	General

MOMENTUM MEDICAL
208-523-3600
1330 Enterprise Street, Idaho Falls, ID 83402
FDA Number: 1723193
Ownership: Private
Produces/Sells CE-marked Devices: N

Cane	Physical Med
Cane, Safety Walk	Physical Med
Catheter, Urethral	Gastroenterology/Urology

MONAGHAN MEDICAL CORP.
800-833-9653
5 Latour Ave., Ste. 1600,
518-561-7330
Plattsburgh, NY 12901
FDA Number: n/a
Fax: 518-561-5660
E-mail: monaghan@westelcom.com
Total Employees: 100
Ownership: Trudell Medical Marketing Ltd.
Quality System Registration Information: ISO9001
Produces/Sells CE-marked Devices: Y
Distribution: Manufacturer Through Distributor
General Admin.: Mitchell A. Baran/Chief Executive Officer
M. T. Amato/Senior Vice President
Mktg./Adv.: Jon Schoeler/Vice President Marketing & Sales
Production: Liz Lonegan/Manager Operations

Generator, Aerosol	Ear/Nose/Throat
Meter, Peak Flow, Spirometry	Anesthesiology
Nebulizer, Direct Patient Interface	Anesthesiology
Ventilator, Other	Anesthesiology

MONARCH ART PLASTICS, LLC.
856-235-5151
3838 Church Road, Mt. Laurel, NJ 08054
FDA Number: 3003712559
Fax: 856-778-9032
E-mail: apepitone@monarchplastics.com
Web site: www.monarchplastics.com
Medical Products Sales Volume: $7,600,000
Annual Revenue: $5-$10 Million
Year Founded: 1960
Total Employees: 60
Ownership: Private
Produces/Sells CE-marked Devices: N
Federal Procurement Eligibility: Small Business
Distribution: Manufacturer Direct, Manufacturer Through Distributor
General Admin.: Mr. William Shanley/Chief Executive Officer
Mr. Thomas Shanley/President
Mktg./Adv.: Ms. Anita Pepitone/Director Marketing
Mr. Gary Brown/Vice President Sales
Mr. Robert Jozaitis/Vice President Sales

Analyzer, Composition, Weight, Patient	General
Device, Fertility, Contraceptive, Diagnostic	Obstetrics/Gynecology
Electrocardiograph, Single Channel	Cardiovascular

MONARCH LABS, LLC.
949-679-3000
17875 Sky Park Circle, Suite K, Irvine, CA 92614
FDA Number: 3005735989

MONARCH MOLDING INC.
888-767-5116
120 Liberty St., Council Grove, KS 66846-1218
620-767-5115
FDA Number: 1925197
Fax: 620-767-6500
E-mail: mmonarch@tctelco.net
Web site: www.monarchmoldinginc
Medical Products Sales Volume: $400,000
Annual Revenue: $0-$1 Million
Year Founded: 1968
Total Employees: 10   *Marketing Staff:* 1   *Sales Staff:* 2
Ownership: Private
Produces/Sells CE-marked Devices: N
Federal Procurement Eligibility: Small Business, Minority Owned, Female Owned
Distribution: Manufacturer Direct, Manufacturer Through Distributor, Exclusive Distributor, Exporter
General Admin.: Judy Scott/President
Denise Chaney/Secretary
Production: Roy DeHoff/Vice President Manufacturing

Sigmoidoscope, Rigid, Non-Electrical	Gastroenterology/Urology

MONARCH MOLDING INC.   888-767-5116 *(cont'd)*
Speculum, Rectal	Gastroenterology/Urology
Speculum, Vaginal, Non-Metal	Obstetrics/Gynecology
Vaginoscope	Obstetrics/Gynecology

MONCHIS S.A.DE. D.U.   336-292-8877
Bustamente 514 Col., Arboledas, Montemorelos, N.I Mexico
FDA Number: 9613802
Gown, Examination	General

MONEBO TECHNOLOGIES, INC.   512-732-0235
1800 Barton Creek Blvd., Austin, TX 78735-1606
FDA Number: 3005407853   *Fax:* 512-732-0285
E-mail: sales@monebo.com
Web site: www.monebo.com
Ownership: Private
Produces/Sells CE-marked Devices: N
Electrocardiograph, Single Channel	Cardiovascular

MONITOR INSTRUMENTS INC.   800-853-6785   919-732-5400
437 Dimmocks Mill Road,
Hillsborough, NC 27278
FDA Number: 1043912   *Fax:* 919-732-6153
E-mail: info@monitorinstrumentsinc.com
Web site: www.monitorinstrumentsinc.com
Medical Products Sales Volume: $400,000
Annual Revenue: $0-$1 Million
Year Founded: 1996
Total Employees: 3   *Marketing Staff:* 1   *Sales Staff:* 1
Ownership: Private
Produces/Sells CE-marked Devices: N
Federal Procurement Eligibility: Small Business
Distribution: Manufacturer Through Distributor, Service Direct, Exporter
General Admin.: Mack Preslar/General Manager
           Van Anderson/President
Mktg./Adv.: Mack J. Preslar/Manager Marketing
           Mack Preslar/Vice President Marketing & Sales
Production: N/A N/A/Director Manufacturing
Apparatus, Audiometric, Reinforcement, Visual	Ear/Nose/Throat
Audiometer	Ear/Nose/Throat
Calibrator, Audiometer	Ear/Nose/Throat

MONMOUTH EQUIPMENT & SERVICE CO. INC.   732-919-1444
5105 Rts. 33/34, Farmingdale, NJ 07727
FDA Number: 3004163323
Ownership: Private
Produces/Sells CE-marked Devices: N
Control, Hand Driving, Automobile, Mechanical	Physical Med

MONO RESEARCH LAB LTD.   716-634-6800
5436 Main St., Ste. 4, Buffalo, NY 14231
FDA Number: 8020428   *Fax:* 716-634-6869
E-mail: info@monoresearch.com
Annual Revenue: $0-$1 Million
Total Employees: 10
Ownership: Private
Quality System Registration Information: ISO9002
Produces/Sells CE-marked Devices: Y
Federal Procurement Eligibility: Small Business
Distribution: Exclusive Distributor, Exporter
General Admin.: Nigel H. K. Armstrong/President
Mktg./Adv.: Janice Brown/Vice President Marketing
General Medical Device	General

MONOBIND, INC.   800-854-6265   949-951-2665
100 North Pointe Drive, Lake Forrest, CA 92630
FDA Number: 2020726   *Fax:* 949-951-3539
E-mail: info@monobind.com
Web site: www.monobind.com
Medical Products Sales Volume: $3,500,000
Annual Revenue: $1-$5 Million
Year Founded: 1978
Ownership: Private
Quality System Registration Information: ISO9001
Produces/Sells CE-marked Devices: N
Federal Procurement Eligibility: Small Business, Minority Owned
Distribution: Manufacturer Direct, Manufacturer Through Manufacturer Reps, OEM, Exclusive Distributor, Exporter
General Admin.: Dr. Frederick R. Jerome/President, Chief Executive Officer
Radioimmunoassay, Digoxin	Toxicology
Radioimmunoassay, Follicle Stimulating Hormone	Chemistry
Radioimmunoassay, Human Chorionic Gonadotropin	Chemistry
Radioimmunoassay, Luteinizing Hormone	Chemistry
Radioimmunoassay, Other	Chemistry
Radioimmunoassay, Prolactin (Lactogen)	Chemistry
Radioimmunoassay, T3 Uptake	Chemistry
Radioimmunoassay, T4	Chemistry
Radioimmunoassay, Thyroid Stimulating Hormone	Chemistry
Radioimmunoassay, Total Thyroxine	Chemistry

MONOBIND, INC.   800-854-6265 *(cont'd)*
Radioimmunoassay, Total Triiodothyronine	Chemistry
Thyroid Function Unit	Chemistry

MONOCLONAL ANTIBODIES INC.
See Quidel Corporation

MONOCLONAL TECHNOLOGIES INC.   888-683-2414   770-521-1960
16335 New Bullpen Road, Alpharetta, GA 30004
FDA Number: 1037677   *Fax:* 770-521-1930
E-mail: m-tech@mindspring.com
Web site: www.4m-tech.com
Year Founded: 1984
Ownership: Private
Produces/Sells CE-marked Devices: N
Federal Procurement Eligibility: Small Business
Distribution: Manufacturer Direct
Legionella Direct & Indirect Fluorescent Antibody Regents	Microbiology

MONOGEN, INC.   847-573-6700
3630 Bur Wood Dr., Waukegan, IL 60085
FDA Number: 1125077   *Fax:* 847-758-4273
E-mail: info@monogen.com
Web site: www.monogen.com
Year Founded: 1996
Ownership: Public
Stock Symbol: MOG
Traded On: TSX Venture Exchange
Produces/Sells CE-marked Devices: N
General Admin.: Ted Geiselman/President, Chief Executive Officer
   Medical Admin.: Juan Felix/Medical Director
Mktg./Adv.: James Cureton/Vice President Marketing & Sales
Production: John Witkowski/Vice President Operations
             Jan Zorn/Vice President Quality Control & Regulatory Affairs
Research: Matthew Zelinski/Vice President Research & Development
Finance: James Boyle/Chief Financial Officer, Vice President Finance
Computer, Chemistry Analyzer	Chemistry
Container, Specimen, All Types	General
Container, Specimen, Non-sterile	General
Cytocentrifuge	Pathology
Filter, Cell Collection, Tissue Processing	Pathology
Fixative, Alcohol Containing	Pathology
Kit, Smear, Cervical	Obstetrics/Gynecology
Processor, Slide, Cytology, Automated	Pathology
Tubing, Fluid Delivery	General
Unit, Filter, Membrane	Chemistry

MONOJECT
See Covidien Lp

MONROE ELECTRONICS, INC.   800-821-6001   585-765-2254
100 Housel Avenue, Lyndonville, NY 14098
FDA Number: 9200763   *Fax:* 585-765-9330
E-mail: electrostatics@monroe-electronics.com
Web site: www.monroe-electronics.com
Annual Revenue: $1-$5 Million
Year Founded: 1952
Total Employees: 31
Ownership: Private
Produces/Sells CE-marked Devices: Y
Federal Procurement Eligibility: Small Business
Distribution: Manufacturer Direct, Manufacturer Through Manufacturer Reps, Exporter
General Admin.: William E. Vosteen/President
           Mr. James F. Heminway/Vice President, General Manager
Detector, Electrostatic Voltage	General

MONROE MFG., INC.   318-338-3172
3030 Aurora Ave., 2nd Fl., Monroe, LA 71201
FDA Number: 2319386
Ownership: Private
Produces/Sells CE-marked Devices: N
Dispenser, Medication, Liquid	General
Nipple, Feeding	General
Ring, Teething, Non-Fluid-Filled	Dental And Oral

MONTEREY MEDICAL SOLUTIONS, INC.   831-210-5514
455 Canyon Del Rey Blvd., Suite #411, Monterey, CA 93940
FDA Number: 3004967992
Computer, Chemistry Analyzer	Chemistry

MOOG INC.   716-652-2000
Jamison Rd., East Aurora, NY 14052
FDA Number: 3008058400   *Fax:* 716-687-4457
E-mail: info.usa@moog.com
Web site: www.moog.com
Medical Products Sales Volume: $103,000,000
Year Founded: 1951
Ownership: Public
Stock Symbol: MOG.A

MOOG INC.   716-652-2000 *(cont'd)*
Traded On: NYSE
Produces/Sells CE-marked Devices: N

Pump, Infusion	General
Tube, Gastrointestinal	Gastroenterology/Urology

Medical Product Subsidiaries (Listed Separately)
Ethox International
Zevex Incorporated

MOORE DIVERSIFIED SERVICES, INC.   817-731-4266
3001 Halloran St., Ste. C, Fort Worth, TX 76107
FDA Number: n/a   *Fax:* 817-738-2031
E-mail: JimMoore@m-d-s.com
Web site: www.m-d-s.com
Annual Revenue: $0-$1 Million
Year Founded: 1971
Ownership: Private
Produces/Sells CE-marked Devices: N
Federal Procurement Eligibility: Small Business
Distribution: Manufacturer Direct
General Admin.: Sue Bregenzer/Business Manager
         Jim Moore/President
         Lynne Moore/President, General Manager

Service, Consulting	General

MOORE INDUSTRIES INC.
See Thermionics Corp.

MOORE PRODUCTS, A SALE PROPRIETORSHIP   650-592-1822
596 Teredo Dr., Redwood City, CA 94065
FDA Number: 2918010
Ownership: Private
Produces/Sells CE-marked Devices: N

Binder, Abdominal	General

MOORE PUSH-PIN CO.   800-289-6667
1300 East Mermaid Lane,   215-233-5700
Wyndmoor, PA 19038
FDA Number: 2529845   *Fax:* 215-233-0660
E-mail: sales@push-pin.com
Web site: www.push-pin.com
Medical Products Sales Volume: $3,200,000
Year Founded: 1900
Total Employees: 53
Ownership: Private
Produces/Sells CE-marked Devices: N
Federal Procurement Eligibility: Small Business, GSA Contract
Distribution: Manufacturer Direct, Manufacturer Through Distributor, Manufacturer Through Manufacturer Reps, OEM, Importer, Exporter

MOR-LOC CORPORATION
See Jobri Llc

MORE DIAGNOSTICS, INC.   800-758-0978
2020 11th St, PO Box 6714, Los Osos, CA 93412   805-528-6005
FDA Number: 2085085   *Fax:* 805-528-3532
E-mail: info@morediagnostics.com
Web site: www.morediagnostics.com
Medical Products Sales Volume: $800,000
Annual Revenue: $1-$5 Million
Year Founded: 1993
Total Employees: 10   *Marketing Staff:* 1   *Sales Staff:* 3
Ownership: Private
Quality System Registration Information: ISO9001
Produces/Sells CE-marked Devices: Y
Federal Procurement Eligibility: Small Business
Distribution: Manufacturer Direct, Manufacturer Through Distributor, OEM
General Admin.: James Snipes/President
Mktg./Adv.: Mr. Peter Bennett/Manager International & National Sales
Production: Wayne Hamari/Director Quality Assurance & Regulatory Affairs
         Thad Tuck/Manager Operations

Antigen, Antiserum, Fibrinogen And Fibrin Split Products	Immunology
Calibrator, Primary, Clinical Chemistry	Chemistry
Control, Analyte (Assayed And Unassayed)	Chemistry
Control, Multi Analyte, All Kinds (Assayed And Unassayed)	Chemistry

MORETZ MILLS, INC.
See Moretz, Inc.

MORETZ, INC.   800-438-9127
514 W. 21st St., PO Box 580,   828-464-0751
Newton, NC 28658
FDA Number: n/a
Web site: www.moretzsports.com
Medical Products Sales Volume: $144,000,000
Annual Revenue: $100-$500 Million
Year Founded: 1946
Total Employees: 1100
Ownership: Private
Produces/Sells CE-marked Devices: N

MORETZ, INC.   800-438-9127 *(cont'd)*
Distribution: Manufacturer Through Distributor
General Admin.: John Moretz/President, Chief Executive Officer

Bandage, Adhesive	Surgery
Bandage, Elastic	General
Bandage, Gauze	General
Pack, Cold	General
Pack, Hot Or Cold, Disposable	Physical Med

MORGAN ADVANCE CERAMICS   800-433-0638
26 Madison Rd., Fairfield, NJ 07004
FDA Number: n/a   *Fax:* 973-808-2257
E-mail: sales@morganadvancedceramics.com
Web site: www.wesgoduramic.com
Annual Revenue: $0-$1 Million
Ownership: MORGAN-CRUCIBLE, PLC
Produces/Sells CE-marked Devices: N
General Admin.: Ray Santos/Vice President, General Manager
Mktg./Adv.: Kevin McAloon/Manager International & National Sales

Component, Ceramic	General

MORGAN INSTRUMENTS INC., P.K.
See Morgan Scientific Inc.

MORGAN MEDESIGN, INC.   888-799-4633
947 Piner Place, Santa Rosa, CA 95403   707-568-2929
FDA Number: n/a   *Fax:* 707-568-2925
E-mail: sales@morganmedesign.com
Web site: www.morganmedesign.com
Medical Products Sales Volume: $3,700,000
Year Founded: 1985
Total Employees: 11
Ownership: Private
Quality System Registration Information: ISO9001
Produces/Sells CE-marked Devices: N
Federal Procurement Eligibility: Small Business
Distribution: Manufacturer Direct, Manufacturer Through Distributor, Manufacturer Through Manufacturer Reps, OEM, Exporter
Mktg./Adv.: Nancy Leon/Sales Specialist

Shield, Protective, Personnel	Radiology
Table, Radiographic, Tilting	Radiology
Table, Surgical, Electrical	Surgery

MORGAN SCIENTIFIC INC.   800-525-5002
151 Essex St., Haverhill, MA 01832-5528   978-521-4440
FDA Number: 1219775   *Fax:* 978-521-4445
E-mail: support@morgansci.com
Web site: www.morgansci.com
Medical Products Sales Volume: $2,000,000
Annual Revenue: $1-$5 Million
Year Founded: 1980
Total Employees: 9   *Marketing Staff:* 2   *Sales Staff:* 14
Ownership: Private
Produces/Sells CE-marked Devices: Y
Federal Procurement Eligibility: Small Business, GSA Contract
Distribution: Manufacturer Direct
General Admin.: Mr. Patrick F. Morgan/Chief Executive Officer
         Mrs. Christina Morgan/Vice President Human Resources
Mktg./Adv.: Mr. Ronald Schmader/Manager International Marketing & Sales
         Mr. Michael Callahan/Manager Marketing
Research: Mr. Phillip Stanway/Product Development Specialist
IS: Mr. Michael Farrington/Programmer
         Mrs. Kelly Farrington/Web Master

Analyzer, Pulmonary Function	Anesthesiology
Plethysmograph, Pressure (Body)	Anesthesiology
Pneumotachograph	Anesthesiology

MORGAN-GALLACHER, INC.   562-695-1232
8707 Millergrove Dr., Santa Fe Springs, CA 90670
FDA Number: 2022194

Medical Disinfectants/Cleaners for Instruments	General

MORMAC CORP
See Mormac Tube Guard Co.

MORMAC TUBE GUARD CO.   800-445-2868
Main St., P.O. Box 40, North Loup, NE 68859-0040   308-496-4781
FDA Number: 1926453   *Fax:* 308-496-4786
E-mail: mormac3@nctc.net
Web site: ngtubeholder.com
Medical Products Sales Volume: $55,000
Annual Revenue: $0-$1 Million
Total Employees: 2   *Marketing Staff:* 1   *Sales Staff:* 1
Ownership: Private
Produces/Sells CE-marked Devices: N
Federal Procurement Eligibility: Small Business, Female Owned
Distribution: Manufacturer Direct
General Admin.: Claire Brush/President
         William Brush/Vice President

MORMAC TUBE GUARD CO.
800-445-2868 *(cont'd)*
Mktg./Adv.: Pam Soper/Manager Marketing
Finance: Pam Soper/Treasurer
Tube, Nasogastric   Anesthesiology

MORRIS DESIGNS, INC.
757-463-9400
2212 Commerce Pkwy, Virginia Beach, VA 23454
FDA Number: 1121306
Web site: www.morrisdesigns.com
Ownership: Private
Produces/Sells CE-marked Devices: N
Binder, Abdominal   General
Binder, Breast   Obstetrics/Gynecology
Support, Head, Surgical, ENT   Ear/Nose/Throat

MORRIS INNOVATIVE RESEARCH
812-355-0450
907 W.second St, Blmgtn, IN 47403
FDA Number: 3004534947
Ownership: Private
Produces/Sells CE-marked Devices: N
Device, Hemostasis, Vascular   Cardiovascular

MORRISON MEDICAL
800-438-6677
3735 Paragon Drive, Columbus, OH 43228
614-461-4400
FDA Number: 1523622   *Fax:* 614-469-9696
E-mail: morr@morrisonmed.com
Web site: www.morrisonmed.com
Annual Revenue: $5-$10 Million
Year Founded: 1970
Total Employees: 35   *Marketing Staff:* 2   *Sales Staff:* 5
Ownership: Private
Produces/Sells CE-marked Devices: Y
Federal Procurement Eligibility: Small Business, GSA Contract, VA Contract
Distribution: Manufacturer Through Distributor, OEM
General Admin.: Donald Evans/Vice President
Accessories, Traction (Cart, Frame, Cord, Weight)   Orthopedics
Bandage, Other   General
Board, Arm   Anesthesiology
Cart, Patient (Stretcher)   Anesthesiology
Cleanroom Equipment   General
Collar, Cervical Neck   Orthopedics
Halter, Head, Traction   Physical Med
Housekeeping Equipment   General
Immobilizer, Cervical   Orthopedics
Kit, Labor and Delivery   Obstetrics/Gynecology
Pack, Cold, Chemical   General
Pillow   General
Restraint, Ankle/Foot   General
Restraint, Protective (Body)   General
Restraint, Wrist/Hand   General
Sand Bag   Radiology
Splint, Other   Orthopedics
Splint, Padded Stays   Orthopedics
Strap, Restraining   General

MORTAN, INC.
800-423-8659
329 E. Pine Street, Missoula, MT 59802
406-728-2522
FDA Number: 1718285   *Fax:* 406-728-9332
E-mail: mortan@morganlens.com
Web site: www.morganlens.com
Medical Products Sales Volume: $1,900,000
Total Employees: 5
Ownership: Private
Quality System Registration Information: ISO9001
Produces/Sells CE-marked Devices: Y
Federal Procurement Eligibility: Small Business
Distribution: Manufacturer Direct, Manufacturer Through Distributor, Exporter
General Admin.: Dr. Loran B. Morgan/Chairman, Vice President
    Mr. Daniel T. Morgan/President, Chief Executive Officer
Mktg./Adv.: Mr. Steve Bixby/Manager International Accounts
Production: Ms. Judy Devine/Director Quality Assurance
    Ms. Judy Devine/Manager Regulatory Affairs
Irrigator, Ocular Surgery   Ophthalmology
Irrigator, Ocular, Emergency   Ophthalmology
Kit, Irrigation, Eye   Ophthalmology

MORTARA INSTRUMENT INC., CARDIODATA DIV.
See Mortara Instrument, Inc.

MORTARA INSTRUMENT, INC.
800-231-7437
7865 N. 86th St., Milwaukee, WI 53224-3431
414-354-1600
FDA Number: 2183461   *Fax:* 414-354-4760
E-mail: mentzer@mortara.com
Web site: www.mortara.com
Medical Products Sales Volume: $14,000,000
Annual Revenue: $10-$25 Million
Year Founded: 1982
Total Employees: 180
Ownership: Private

MORTARA INSTRUMENT, INC.
800-231-7437 *(cont'd)*
Quality System Registration Information: ISO9001
Produces/Sells CE-marked Devices: Y
Federal Procurement Eligibility: Small Business
Distribution: Manufacturer Direct, OEM
General Admin.: David W. Mortara/President
Mktg./Adv.: Mark Mentzel/Director Marketing
    Linda Carota/Director Product Development
    Justin Mortara/Vice President Marketing & Sales
Research: Maurizio Fumagalli/Vice President Engineering
Finance: Brian Brenegan/Vice President Finance
Computer, ECG Interpretation (Arrhythmia)   Cardiovascular
Computer, Stress Exercise   Cardiovascular
Electrocardiograph, Interpretive   Cardiovascular
Electrocardiograph, Multi-Channel   Cardiovascular
Monitor, ECG   Cardiovascular
Monitor, ECG, Anesthesia   Anesthesiology
Monitor, ECG, Surgery   Surgery
Monitor, Physiological, Acute Care   Anesthesiology
Recorder, Long-Term, ECG, Portable (Holter Monitor)   Cardiovascular
Transmitter/Receiver System, ECG, Telephone Multi-Channel   Cardiovascular
Transmitter/Receiver System, Physiological, Telephone   Cardiovascular
Treadmill, Powered   Physical Med

MORTECH MANUFACTURING COMPANY
800) 410-0100
411 N. Aerojet Avenue, Azusa, CA 91702
757-224-0177
FDA Number: 2087564   *Fax:* (626) 334-1471
E-mail: info@mortechmfg.com
Web site: www.mortechmfg.com
Ownership: Private
Produces/Sells CE-marked Devices: N
Container, Specimen Mailer And Storage, Non-sterile   Pathology

MORTECH, LLC.
406-542-7040
323 Sw Higgins Ave., Missoula, MT 59803
FDA Number: 3031065
Ownership: Private
Produces/Sells CE-marked Devices: N
Irrigator, Ocular Surgery   Ophthalmology

MOS PLASTICS INC.
408-944-9407
2308 Zanker Rd., San Jose, CA 95131
FDA Number: n/a   *Fax:* 408-944-9439
Web site: www.mosinc.com
Annual Revenue: $0-$1 Million
Year Founded: 1974
Ownership: Private
Quality System Registration Information: ISO9001
Produces/Sells CE-marked Devices: N
Federal Procurement Eligibility: Small Business
Distribution: Manufacturer Direct, Importer, Exporter
General Admin.: Deanna Musil/Program Manager
Mktg./Adv.: Rick Cameron/Director Business Development
Production: Pete Yager/Manager Operations
    Earnest Harper/Manager Production
    Sunil Behl/Manager Quality Assurance
Component, Plastic   General
Computer and Software, Medical   General

MOSAIC INDUSTRIES, INC.
510-790-8222
5437 Central Avenue, Suite 1, Newark, CA 94560
FDA Number: n/a   *Fax:* 510-790-0925
E-mail: info@mosaic-industries.com
Web site: www.mosaic-industries.com
Medical Products Sales Volume: $1,000,000
Annual Revenue: $0-$1 Million
Year Founded: 1985
Total Employees: 50   *Marketing Staff:* 3   *Sales Staff:* 4
Ownership: Private
Produces/Sells CE-marked Devices: N
Federal Procurement Eligibility: Small Business
Distribution: Manufacturer Direct, OEM
Mktg./Adv.: Elena Belkine/Director Tech. Marketing
Production: Karen Fillmore/Engineer
Service, Engineering/Design   General

MOSS TUBES, INC.
800-827-0470
749 Columbia Turnpike,
518-674-3109
East Greenbush, NY 12061
FDA Number: 1320599   *Fax:* 518-674-8067
E-mail: mosstube@nycap.rr.com
Web site: www.mosstubesinc.com
Medical Products Sales Volume: $1,400,000
Annual Revenue: $0-$1 Million
Total Employees: 4
Ownership: Private
Produces/Sells CE-marked Devices: N
Federal Procurement Eligibility: Small Business, Female Owned

MOSS TUBES, INC.   800-827-0470 *(cont'd)*
Distribution: Manufacturer Direct
General Admin.: Kathryn Moss/Chief Executive Officer
    Mrs. Maureen Dorr/Office Manager
Finance: Michael Moss/Treasurer
Anchor, Preformed	Dental And Oral
Tube, Feeding	General
Tube, Gastro-Enterostomy	Gastroenterology/Urology

MOTION ANALYSIS CORP.   707-579-6500
3617 West Wind Blvd., Santa Rosa, CA 95403
FDA Number: 3008172891
E-mail: info@motionanalysis.com   *Fax:* 707-578-8473
Web site: www.motionanalysis.com
Ownership: Private
Produces/Sells CE-marked Devices: N
Optical Position/Movement Recording System	Physical Med

MOTION CONCEPTS   905-695-0134
84 Citation Dr., Concord, ONTAR L4K 3C1 Canada
FDA Number: 9615350
E-mail: info@motionconcepts.com   *Fax:* 905-695-0138
Web site: www.motionconcepts.com
Year Founded: 1997
Total Employees: 50   *Marketing Staff:* 3
Ownership: Private
Produces/Sells CE-marked Devices: N
Distribution: Manufacturer Through Distributor

MOTION CONTROL, INC.   888-696-2767
115 N. Wright Brothers Drive,   **801-326-3434**
Salt Lake City, UT 84116
FDA Number: 1723997   *Fax:* 801-978-0848
E-mail: info@UtahArm.com
Web site: www.UtahArm.com
Year Founded: 1981
Total Employees: 28   *Marketing Staff:* 2   *Sales Staff:* 2
Ownership: Fillauer Companies, Inc.
Quality System Registration Information: ISO9001
Produces/Sells CE-marked Devices: Y
Federal Procurement Eligibility: Small Business
Distribution: Manufacturer Through Distributor
General Admin.: Harold Sears/President
Mktg./Adv.: Joanna Rendi/Director Marketing
Production: Caesar Rivera/Director Quality Assurance
    Caesar Rivera/Production Engineer
Research: Ed Iversen/Vice President Research & Development
Ankle/Foot, External Limb Component	Physical Med
Biofeedback Device	Cns/Neurology
Driver, Prosthesis	Orthopedics
Hand, External Limb Component, Powered	Physical Med
Joint, Knee, External Limb Component	Physical Med
Prosthesis, Arm	Orthopedics
Prosthesis, Hand	Orthopedics
Stimulator, Muscle, Diagnostic	Physical Med

MOTION SPECIALTIES INC.   800-267-2920
82 Carnforth Road,   **416-751-0400**
Toronto, ONT M4A 2 Canada
FDA Number: n/a   *Fax:* 416-751-2716
E-mail: toronto@motionspecialties.com
Web site: www.motionspecialties.com
Year Founded: 1985
Total Employees: 50
Ownership: Private
Produces/Sells CE-marked Devices: N
Distribution: Manufacturer Direct, Exclusive Distributor

MOTLOID COMPANY   800-662-5021
300 N. Elizabeth St., Chicago, IL 60607   **312-226-2454**
FDA Number: 1416675   *Fax:* 312-226-2480
E-mail: sales@yates-motloid.com
Web site: www.yates-motloid.com
Annual Revenue: $1-$5 Million
Total Employees: 50   *Marketing Staff:* 2   *Sales Staff:* 4
Ownership: Private
Quality System Registration Information: ISO9002
Produces/Sells CE-marked Devices: Y
Federal Procurement Eligibility: Small Business
Distribution: Manufacturer Direct, Manufacturer Through Distributor
General Admin.: Richard Seid/Chairman
    Ronald I. Schwarcz/President
Mktg./Adv.: Mona Zemsky/Vice President Marketing
    Joe Seid/Vice President Sales
Agent, Polishing, Abrasive, Oral Cavity	Dental And Oral
Alloy, Gold Based, For Clinical Use	Dental And Oral
Buffer, pH	Hematology
Burnisher, Operative, Dental	Dental And Oral

MOTLOID COMPANY   800-662-5021 *(cont'd)*
Burr	Ear/Nose/Throat
Caliper	Orthopedics
Cleaner, Ultrasonic, Dental Laboratory	Dental And Oral
Component, Electrical	General
Component, Plastic	General
Crown And Bridge, Temporary, Resin	Dental And Oral
Instrument, Dental, Manual	Dental And Oral
Material, Acrylic, Dental	Dental And Oral
Saw, Other	Surgery
Tooth Bonding Agent, Resin Restoration	Dental And Oral
Wax, Dental	Dental And Oral

MOTOROLA COMM. AND ELECTRONICS INC.   847-576-5000
1303 E. Algonquin Rd.,   **-**
Schaumburg, IL 60196
FDA Number: n/a
Annual Revenue: $1-$5 Million
Total Employees: 2500   *Marketing Staff:* 15   *Sales Staff:* 50
Ownership: Public
Stock Symbol: MOT
Traded On: NYSE
Quality System Registration Information: ISO9002
Produces/Sells CE-marked Devices: N
Distribution: Manufacturer Direct, Importer, Exporter
General Admin.: Gary Tooker/Chief Executive Officer
Mktg./Adv.: Chris Galvan/Manager Contract Sales
    Pat Schod/Vice President Marketing
Communication System, Powered	Physical Med
Pager, Radio	General
Pager, Visual	General
Telephone Equipment	General
Transmitter/Receiver System, ECG, Telephone Multi-Channel	Cardiovascular

Medical Product Subsidiaries (Listed Separately)
    Motorola Gmbh

MOTOROLA INC. COMMUNICATIONS SECTOR
See Motorola Comm. And Electronics Inc.

MOTUS BIOENGINEERING INC.   707-745-4194
133 Carlisle Way, Benicia, CA 94510
FDA Number: 3005597075
Goniometer, AC-powered	Orthopedics

MOUNT OLIVE MANUFACTURING, INC.   317-834-8525
3304 Hancel Circle, Mooresville, IN 46158
FDA Number: 3006192859   *Fax:* 317-834-8535
E-mail: info@mtolivemfg.com
Web site: www.mtolivemfg.com
Ownership: Private
Produces/Sells CE-marked Devices: N
Bag, Reservoir (Blood)	Anesthesiology

MOUNTAIN MEDICAL EQUIPMENT INC.
See Caire, Inc.

MOUNTAIN MEDICO, INC.   909-931-0688
600 North Mountain Ave., #d204, Upland, CA 91786
FDA Number: 2086103   *Fax:* 909-931-0908
E-mail: info@mountainmedico.com
Web site: www.mountainmedico.com
Ownership: Private
Produces/Sells CE-marked Devices: N
Alloy, Gold Based, For Clinical Use	Dental And Oral
Alloy, Precious Metal, For Clinical Use	Dental And Oral
Metal, Base	Dental And Oral

MOUNTAIN PRECISION MFG. LTD. CO.   208-322-1111
11000 Executive Dr., Boise, ID 83713
FDA Number: 3029791
Larynx, Artificial Battery-Powered	Ear/Nose/Throat

MOVINCOOL, NIPPONDENSO OF LOS ANGELES
See Movincool/Denso Sales California, Inc.

MOVINCOOL/DENSO SALES CALIFORNIA, INC.   800-264-9573
3900 Via Oro Avenue, Long Beach, CA 90810
FDA Number: n/a   *Fax:* 310-835-8724
E-mail: info2@movincool.com
Web site: www.movincool.com
Medical Products Sales Volume: $64,000,000
Annual Revenue: More than $100 Million
Year Founded: 1982
Total Employees: 504
Ownership: DENSO CORPORATION JAPAN
Produces/Sells CE-marked Devices: N
Federal Procurement Eligibility: GSA Contract
Distribution: Manufacturer Through Distributor
Mktg./Adv.: Eddie Stevenson/Manager Product Marketing
Controller, Temperature, Other	General

MOVINGPEOPLE.NET CANADA, INC.   416-739-8333
500 Norfinch Dr, Downsview M3N 1Y4 Canada
FDA Number: 9680744

Chair, With Casters	Physical Med
Wheelchair, Powered	Physical Med

MOWBRAY CO., INC.   800-325-5787
706 Sheridan Road, Waterloo, IA 50701   319-234-5119
FDA Number: 1921196   Fax: 319-234-5119
E-mail: contact@mowbraycompany.com
Web site: www.mowbraycompany.com
Medical Products Sales Volume: $100,000
Year Founded: 1984
Ownership: Private
Produces/Sells CE-marked Devices: N
Federal Procurement Eligibility: Small Business

Bandage, Adhesive	Surgery

MOYCO INDUSTRIES INC.
See Moyco Technologies, Inc.

MOYCO TECHNOLOGIES, INC.   800-331-8837
200 Commerce Drive,   215-855-4300
Montgomeryville, PA 18936
FDA Number: 2518040   Fax: 215-362-3809
E-mail: moyco@moycotech.com
Web site: www.moycotech.com
Medical Products Sales Volume: $6,500,000
Annual Revenue: $10-$25 Million
Year Founded: 1893
Total Employees: 43   *Marketing Staff:* 2   *Sales Staff:* 6
Ownership: Public
Stock Symbol: MOYC
Traded On: NASDAQ
Produces/Sells CE-marked Devices: Y
Federal Procurement Eligibility: Small Business
Distribution: Manufacturer Through Distributor, Importer, Exporter
General Admin.: M.E. Sternberg/Chief Executive Officer
    M. E. Sternberg/President
    Jerry Lipkin/Vice President, General Manager
Mktg./Adv.: Tom Thompson/Director National Accounts
    Frank Palm/Director Product Development
    Drew Lipkin/Manager Advertising
    Toula Royster/Manager Contract Sales
    Walt Wiltschek/Manager International Marketing & Sales
    Drew Lipkin/Manager Marketing & Sales
    Tom Thompson/Manager National Sales
    Drew Lipkin/Manager Sales Training
    Mark Sternberg/Vice President Business Development
Production: Wayne Morris/Director Quality Assurance
    Joseph Stenberg/Manager Regulatory Affairs
    Lonnie Graybill/Vice President Manufacturing
Research: Charles Weaver/Vice President Research & Development
Finance: William Woodhead/Controller

Adhesive, Denture, OTC	Dental And Oral
Agent, Polishing, Abrasive, Oral Cavity	Dental And Oral
Alloy, Precious Metal, For Clinical Use	Dental And Oral
Band, Matrix	Dental And Oral
Broach, Endodontic	Dental And Oral
Brush, Other	General
Cabinet, Dental	Dental And Oral
Carrier, Amalgam, Operative	Dental And Oral
Cement, Dental	Dental And Oral
Cleaner, Denture	Dental And Oral
Clip, Towel	Surgery
Component, Plastic	General
Component, Rubber	General
Component, Silicone	General
Cup, Denture	Dental And Oral
Dam, Rubber	Dental And Oral
Disk, Abrasive	Dental And Oral
Endodontic Instrument	Dental And Oral
File, Pulp Canal, Endodontic	Dental And Oral
Forceps, Rubber Dam Clamp	Dental And Oral
Frame, Rubber Dam	Dental And Oral
Gauge, Depth, Instrument, Dental	Dental And Oral
Gutta Percha	Dental And Oral
Instrument, Diamond, Dental	Dental And Oral
Kit, Endodontic	Dental And Oral
Mandrel	Dental And Oral
Matrix, Dental	Dental And Oral
Mercury	Dental And Oral
Mirror, Mouth	Dental And Oral
Mixing Slab	Dental And Oral
Mouth Prop	Dental And Oral
Paper, Articulation	Dental And Oral
Pipette	Chemistry
Plugger, Root Canal, Endodontic	Dental And Oral
Point, Paper, Endodontic	Dental And Oral

MOYCO TECHNOLOGIES, INC.   800-331-8837 *(cont'd)*

Point, Silver, Endodontic	Dental And Oral
Post, Root Canal	Dental And Oral
Punch, Dental, Rubber Dam	Dental And Oral
Reamer, Pulp Canal, Endodontic	Dental And Oral
Retainer, Matrix	Dental And Oral
Sharpener, Dental	Dental And Oral
Spatula, Cement	Dental And Oral
Spreader, Pulp Canal Filling Material, Endodontic	Dental And Oral
Stand/Holder, Equipment, Laboratory	Chemistry
Strip, Polishing Agent	Dental And Oral
Syringe, Bulb, Air Or Water	Dental And Oral
Syringe, Cartridge	Dental And Oral
Syringe, Periodontic, Endodontic	Dental And Oral
Tester, Pulp	Dental And Oral
Tray, Impression	Dental And Oral
Tray, Sterilization, Instrument	Surgery
Wax, Dental	Dental And Oral
Well, Amalgam	Dental And Oral
Zinc Oxide Eugenol	Dental And Oral

Medical Product Subsidiaries (Listed Separately)
    Moyco Union Broach

MPA
See Life-Like Laboratory

MPE-INC   800-266-1687
10597 W. Glenbrook Court,   414-355-0310
Milwaukee, WI 53224
FDA Number: n/a   Fax: 414-355-5259
E-mail: sales@mpe-inc.com
Web site: http://www.mpe-inc.com
Ownership: Private
Produces/Sells CE-marked Devices: N
Distribution: OEM

Accessories, Cart, Multipurpose	General
Cart, Multipurpose	General
Chair/Table, Medical	General
Console, Patient Service	General
Contract Manufacturing	General
Metal, Medical	General
Service, Engineering/Design	General

MPI MEDICAL PRODUCTS, INC.   321-676-1299
1631 Elmhurst Circle, S.e., Palm Bay, FL 32909
FDA Number: 1055939

Accelerator, Linear, Medical	Radiology
Applicator, Radionuclide, Manual	Radiology
Applicator, Radionuclide, Remote-Controlled	Radiology

MPI, INC.
See Scanditronix - Wellhofer North America

MPI/DUPACO, INC.
See Dupaco, Inc.

MPM MEDICAL, INC.   800-232-5512
2301 Crown Ct., Irving, TX 75038   972-893-4090
FDA Number: 1646434   Fax: 972-893-4092
E-mail: info@mpmmedicalinc.com
Web site: www.mpmmedicalinc.com
Medical Products Sales Volume: $3,000,000
Annual Revenue: $1-$5 Million
Total Employees: 20   *Marketing Staff:* 5   *Sales Staff:* 15
Ownership: Public
Stock Symbol: ROBE
Traded On: OTC Bulletin
Produces/Sells CE-marked Devices: N
Federal Procurement Eligibility: Small Business
Distribution: Manufacturer Through Distributor, Manufacturer Through Manufacturer Reps, OEM
General Admin.: Paul Miller/President, Chief Executive Officer
    Scott Miller/Regional Manager
Mktg./Adv.: Paul Miller/Director Product Development
    Twiggy Wadley/Manager Sales Support
Production: Rita Rains/Manager Operations

Bandage, Adhesive	Surgery
Dressing, Foam	General
Dressing, Gel	General
Dressing, Other	General
Dressing, Wound and Burn, Hydrogel	Surgery
Solution, Antibacterial Cleaner	General

MPP HAND DRILL COMPANY LLC.   715-294-3400
807 Prospect Ave., Osceola, WI 54020
FDA Number: 3003668121
Ownership: Private
Produces/Sells CE-marked Devices: N

Drill, Manual (With Burr, Trephine & Accessories)	Cns/Neurology

MPS ACACIA
785 Challenger St., Brea, CA 92821
800-486-6677
714-257-0470
FDA Number: 2084012
Fax: 714-257-0513
E-mail: info@mpsacacia.com
Web site: www.mpsacacia.com
Medical Products Sales Volume: $5,000,000
Annual Revenue: $5-$10 Million
Year Founded: 1990
Total Employees: 50   *Marketing Staff:* 1   *Sales Staff:* 4
Ownership: Private
Produces/Sells CE-marked Devices: N
Distribution: Manufacturer Direct, Manufacturer Through Distributor, Manufacturer Through Manufacturer Reps, Exclusive Distributor
General Admin.: Dan Hyun/President
Mktg./Adv.: Dan Hyun/Director Product Development
    Cathleen Eckhart/Vice President Marketing & Sales
Production: Fergie Ferguson/Director Quality Assurance
    Jim Shilo/Vice President Manufacturing

Calibrator, Drug Mixture	Toxicology
Container, Medication, Graduated Liquid	General
Dispenser, Medication, Liquid	General
Dropper, Eye	Ophthalmology
Filter, Infusion Line	General
Filter, Intravenous Tubing	General
Fitting, Luer	General
Kit, Intravenous Extension Tubing	General
Needle, Other	General
Pump, Infusion, Ambulatory	General
Pump, Infusion, Patient Controlled Analgesia (PCA)	General
Stopcock	General
System, Delivery, Drug, Non-invasive	General
System, Delivery, Drug, Unit-Dose	General
Transfer Unit, IV Fluid	General
Tubing, Connecting	General
Tubing, Fluid Delivery	General
Tubing, Non-Invasive	Surgery

MR INSTRUMENTS, INC.
5610 Rowland Rd., Suite 145, Minnetonka, MN 55343
952-746-1435
FDA Number: 3003852428

Coil, Magnetic Resonance, Specialty	Radiology

MR. AMERICA MANUFACTURING, INC.
See Ooltewah Manufacturing

MRC INDUSTRIES INC.
85 Denton Ave, New Hyde Park, NY 11040
516-328-6900
FDA Number: 2434435

Board, Bed	General
Component, Wheelchair	Physical Med
Lift, Bath, Non-AC-Powered	General
Mattress, Air Flotation	General
Mattress, Non-Powered Flotation Therapy	Physical Med

MRI
See Manufacturing & Research, Inc.(Dba Mri Medical)

MRI CARDIAC SERVICES, INCORPORATED
8 West Third St. Suite M-9, Winston-Salem, NC 27101
336-831-1908
FDA Number: 1067139
Fax: 336-727-0919
E-mail: dwight.ball@provaimages.com
Year Founded: 2002
Total Employees: 3
Ownership: Private
Produces/Sells CE-marked Devices: N
Distribution: Manufacturer Direct
General Admin.: Scott Huber/President
Production: Mr. Dwight Ball/Vice President Operations

Image Processing System	Radiology

MRI DEVICES CORP.
See Invivo

MRL DIAGNOSTICS
See Focus Technologies

MRLB INTL., INC.
2450 College Way, Fergus Falls, MN 56537
715-425-8180
FDA Number: 2134071

Operative Dental Treatment Unit	Dental And Oral

MSA
See Mine Safety Appliances Company

MSA BASELINE INDUSTRIES, INC.
See Baseline - Mocon, Inc.

MSI
See Ge Infrastructure Water & Process Technologies

MSI PRECISION, INC.
See Msi Precision, Specialty Instrument

MSI PRECISION, SPECIALTY INSTRUMENT
1220 Valley Forge Rd., Bldg. 34, Phoenixville, PA 19460
800-322-4674
610-935-8181
FDA Number: n/a
Fax: 610-935-5844
E-mail: sales@msiprecision.com
Web site: www.msiprecision.com
Annual Revenue: $1-5 Million
Total Employees: 9   *Marketing Staff:* 1   *Sales Staff:* 4
Ownership: Private
Produces/Sells CE-marked Devices: N
Federal Procurement Eligibility: Small Business
Distribution: OEM, Exclusive Distributor
General Admin.: Donald A. Seavey/President, Chief Executive Officer
Mktg./Adv.: Donald A. Seavey/Director Marketing & Advertising
    Donald A. Seavey/Director Product Development
    Patrick Conway/Manager Contract Sales
    Kris Chikotas/Manager International & National Sales
Production: Chris Cheesman/Director Quality Assurance
    Andria McCarther/Manager Materials
Purchasing: Lois Jones/Credit Manager

Knife, Scalpel	Surgery
Knife, Surgical	Dental And Oral

MTC
See Lifesign

MTD, INC.
24 Slabtown Creek Rd, Blairstown, NJ 07871
908-362-6807
FDA Number: 2242692
Fax: 908-362-5068
E-mail: info@mtdmed.com
Web site: www.mtdmed.com
Annual Revenue: $0-$1 Million
Year Founded: 1977
Ownership: Private
Produces/Sells CE-marked Devices: Y
Federal Procurement Eligibility: Small Business
Distribution: Manufacturer Direct

Holder, Head, Neurosurgical (Skull Clamp)	Cns/Neurology
Support, Patient Position, Radiographic	Radiology

MTI PRECISION PRODUCTS
175 Oberlin North Ave., Lakewood, NJ 08701
732-905-7440
FDA Number: 2246821

Handpiece, Air-Powered, Dental	Dental And Oral
Scaler, Ultrasonic	Dental And Oral

MTI-MEDICAL TECHNIQUE, INC.
8060 E. research Court., Tucson, AZ 85710
800-426-9053
520-733-7999
FDA Number: 3024615
Fax: 520-733-7474
E-mail: info@mtidrape.com
Web site: http://mtidrape.com/
Medical Products Sales Volume: $1,700,000
Annual Revenue: $5-$10 Million
Year Founded: 1974
Total Employees: 33   *Marketing Staff:* 2   *Sales Staff:* 125
Ownership: Private
Quality System Registration Information: ISO9002
Produces/Sells CE-marked Devices: Y
Federal Procurement Eligibility: Small Business
Distribution: Manufacturer Direct, Manufacturer Through Distributor, OEM, Exclusive Distributor
General Admin.: Mr. Paul Bistline/Manager Admin.
    Mr. Lou Castagna/President, Owner

Bandage, Elastic	General
Drape, Microscope, Ophthalmic	Ophthalmology
Patient Transfer Unit	General

MTM HEALTH PRODUCTS LTD.
2349 Fairview St., Burlington, ONT L7R 2 Canada
800-263-8253
905-333-0720
FDA Number: 8020427
Fax: 905-333-6880
E-mail: mtm@worldchat.com
Web site: http://web.idirect.com/~mtm
Year Founded: 1985
Total Employees: 4
Ownership: Private
Quality System Registration Information: ISO9002
Produces/Sells CE-marked Devices: Y
Federal Procurement Eligibility: Small Business
Distribution: Manufacturer Through Distributor, Exclusive Distributor, Exporter

MTM LABORATORIES INC.
One Research Drive, Suite 120c, Westborough, MA 01581
866-686-5227
FDA Number: 3006074790
Fax: 508-366-8511
Web site: http://www.mtmlabs.com/us
Ownership: Private
Produces/Sells CE-marked Devices: N
General Admin.: Mr. Robert Silverman/Chief Executive Officer

MTM LABORATORIES INC.   866-686-5227 (cont'd)
Dr. Rudiger Ridder/Chief Scientific Officer

MTP INC.
See Medical Technology Products, Inc.

MTS MEDICATION TECHNOLOGIES   800-671-0508
2003 Gandy Blvd., Suite 800,   727-576-6311
St. Petersburg, FL 33702
FDA Number: n/a   Fax: 727-579-8067
Web site: www.mtsp.com
Annual Revenue: $0-$1 Million
Total Employees: 110   Marketing Staff: 5   Sales Staff: 25
Ownership: Public
Stock Symbol: MTSI
Traded On: NASDAQ
Quality System Registration Information: ISO9000
Produces/Sells CE-marked Devices: N
Federal Procurement Eligibility: Small Business
Distribution: Manufacturer Direct, Manufacturer Through Manufacturer Reps
General Admin.: Todd E. Siegel/President
Mktg./Adv.: Dennis H. Ayo/Senior Vice President Marketing & Sales
　　　　　Perry Larson/Vice President Marketing & Sales
Finance: Michael P. Conroy/Chief Financial Officer
IS: Ronald M. Rosenbaum/Vice President Technology
　Labeling Equipment   General
　Packaging Equipment   General
　Packaging System, Unit-Dose   General
Medical Product Subsidiaries (Listed Separately)
　Life Care Technologies, Inc.
　Mts Packaging Systems, Inc.

MUELLER SPORTS MEDICINE   800-356-9522
One Quench Dr., P.O. Box 99,   608-643-8530
Prairie Du Sac, WI 53578
FDA Number: 2110420   Fax: 608-643-2568
E-mail: sportcare@muellersportsmed.com
Web site: www.muellersportsmed.com
Medical Products Sales Volume: $45,000,000
Annual Revenue: $50-$100 Million
Year Founded: 1961
Total Employees: 116   Marketing Staff: 22   Sales Staff: 22
Ownership: Private
Produces/Sells CE-marked Devices: Y
Federal Procurement Eligibility: Small Business
Distribution: Manufacturer Direct, Manufacturer Through Manufacturer Reps,
Exporter
General Admin.: Curt Mueller/Chief Executive Officer
　　　　　Brett Mueller/President
　　　　　John Swafford/Senior Vice President
Mktg./Adv.: Herbert Raschka/Vice President Marketing & Sales
　　　　　Ginger Mueller-Mann/Vice President Sales
Production: Gina Accola/Director Quality Control & Regulatory Affairs
Finance: Stanley Johnston/Controller
　Bag, Ice   General
　Bandage, Elastic   General
　Bandage, Liquid   Surgery
　Cast   Orthopedics
　Depressor, Tongue   General
　Dressing, Wound and Burn, Hydrogel   Surgery
　Gauze/sponge, Nonresorbable For External Use   Surgery
　Kit, First Aid   Surgery
　Orthosis, Limb Brace   Physical Med
　Orthosis, Lumbosacral   Physical Med
　Pack, Cold, Chemical   General
　Pack, Hot Or Cold, Disposable   Physical Med
　Pack, Hot Or Cold, Reusable   Physical Med
　Refrigerant, Topical (Vapocoolant)   Physical Med
　Sling, Arm   Physical Med
　Solvent, Adhesive Tape   Surgery
　Splint, Extremity, Inflatable, External   Surgery
　Splint, Extremity, Non-Inflatable, External   Surgery
　Splint, Nasal   Ear/Nose/Throat
　Support, Scrotal, Therapeutic   General
　Tape, Adhesive   General

MUFFIN ENTERPRISES, INC.   800-338-9041
2 Brenneman Circle, Suite 2,   717-691-9800
Mechanicsburg, PA 17050
FDA Number: n/a   Fax: 717-691-9803
E-mail: muffin@pa.net
Web site: www.muffinenterprises.com
Medical Products Sales Volume: $300,000
Annual Revenue: $0-$1 Million
Year Founded: 1990
Total Employees: 4   Marketing Staff: 1   Sales Staff: 1
Ownership: Private
Produces/Sells CE-marked Devices: N

MUFFIN ENTERPRISES, INC.   800-338-9041 (cont'd)
Federal Procurement Eligibility: Small Business, Female Owned
Distribution: Exclusive Distributor
General Admin.: Scott Shirey/President
Mktg./Adv.: Debbie Vogel/Manager National Sales
Production: Crystal Gordon/Manager Materials
　Pillow   General

MUI SCIENTIFIC   800-303-6611
145 Traders Blvd. E., Unit 34,   905-890-5525
Mississauga, ONT L4Z 3 Canada
FDA Number: 8020403   Fax: 905-890-3523
E-mail: mail@muiscientific.com
Web site: www.muiscientific.com
Medical Products Sales Volume: $1,000,000
Year Founded: 1979
Total Employees: 10   Marketing Staff: 1   Sales Staff: 3
Ownership: H & A MUI ENTERPRISES INC.
Quality System Registration Information: ISO9002
Produces/Sells CE-marked Devices: Y
Federal Procurement Eligibility: Small Business, Minority Owned
Distribution: Manufacturer Direct, Manufacturer Through Distributor, Manufacturer
Through Manufacturer Reps, Service Direct, Exclusive Distributor, Importer,
Exporter

MULTI BIOSENSORS, INC.   915-581-9684
4944 Vista Grande, El Paso, TX 79922
FDA Number: 1640699   Fax: 915-772-2034
E-mail: harold@multibiosensors.com
Web site: www.multibiosensors.com
Medical Products Sales Volume: $280,000
Year Founded: 1984
Total Employees: 5
Ownership: Private
Produces/Sells CE-marked Devices: Y
Federal Procurement Eligibility: Small Business
Distribution: Manufacturer Direct, Manufacturer Through Distributor, OEM
　Electrode, Electrocardiograph   Cardiovascular

MULTI FOCAL RX LENS LABORATORIES, INC.   800-241-9030
216 Valley Hill Rd., Riverdale, GA 30274   770-478-2121
FDA Number: n/a   Fax: 800-448-0078
E-mail: multifocal@aol.com
Medical Products Sales Volume: $10,700,000
Annual Revenue: $10-$25 Million
Total Employees: 30   Marketing Staff: 11   Sales Staff: 5
Ownership: Private
Quality System Registration Information: ISO9000
Produces/Sells CE-marked Devices: N
Federal Procurement Eligibility: Small Business
Distribution: Manufacturer Direct, Manufacturer Through Manufacturer Reps,
Exclusive Distributor, Exporter
General Admin.: Gloria Leach/Vice President Human Resources
　　　　　Dennis Tindall/Vice President, General Manager
Mktg./Adv.: Carolyn Stockton/Manager National Sales
　　　　　Sylvia Mosel/Manager Sales Training
Production: Doug Nagle/Director Quality Assurance
　　　　　Lesliy Lambert/Manager Materials
　　　　　Glorian Kossowski/Manager Regulatory Affairs
　　　　　Rick Johnson/Vice President Manufacturing
　Lens, Other   Ophthalmology
　Lens, Set, Trial, Ophthalmic   Ophthalmology

MULTI IMAGER SERVICE, INC   800-400-4549
990 E. Cedar Street, Ontario, CA 91761   909-591-6444
FDA Number: n/a   Fax: 909-591-5293
E-mail: sales@multiimager.com
Web site: www.multiimager.com
Medical Products Sales Volume: $2,300,000
Annual Revenue: $1-$5 Million
Total Employees: 9   Marketing Staff: 2   Sales Staff: 3
Ownership: Private
Produces/Sells CE-marked Devices: Y
Federal Procurement Eligibility: Small Business
Distribution: OEM, Service Direct, Exclusive Distributor, Exporter
General Admin.: Klaus Kraemer/President, Chief Executive Officer
Mktg./Adv.: Dan Moretti/Director Marketing & Sales
　Camera, Multi Format   Radiology
　Camera, Multi-Image   Radiology
　Camera, Video   General
　Camera, Video, Multi-Image   General
　Changer, Radiographic Film/Cassette   Radiology
　Computer, Radiographic Data   Radiology
　Image Digitizer   Radiology
　Image Processing System   Radiology
　Laser, Combination   General
　Radiographic Picture Archiving/Communication System (PACS)   Radiology
　Service, Used Equipment   General

MANUFACTURER PROFILES

MULTI IMAGER SERVICE, INC   800-400-4549 *(cont'd)*
System, Marking, Laser   General

MULTI MARKETING & MANUFACTURING, INC.   303-794-5955
PO Box 1070, 5401 Prince Street, Littleton, CO 80160-1070
FDA Number: n/a   *Fax:* 303-795-6946
E-mail: Multimarketing@comcast.net
Web site: www.penlane.com/multimktg
Annual Revenue: $0-$1 Million
Year Founded: 1977
Total Employees: 10
Ownership: Private
Federal Procurement Eligibility: Small Business, Female Owned
Distribution: Manufacturer Direct, Manufacturer Through Manufacturer Reps
General Admin.: Janet Lane/President
Mktg./Adv.: Dugg Holmes/Director Marketing
     Janet Lane/Manager Advertising
Production: John R. Penaligon/Manager Production
Foodservice Product/Equipment   General
Housekeeping Equipment   General
Utensil, Handicapped Aid   Physical Med

MULTI-AMP
See Cardionics, Inc.

MULTI-MED, INC.   603-357-8733
Winchester St., P.O. Box 660, West Swanzey, NH 03469
FDA Number: 1221765   *Fax:* 603-357-0732
E-mail: info@multimedinc.com
Web site: www.multimedinc.com
Annual Revenue: $0-$1 Million
Ownership: Private
Produces/Sells CE-marked Devices: N
Federal Procurement Eligibility: Small Business
Distribution: Manufacturer Through Distributor, Manufacturer Through Manufacturer Reps
Contract Manufacturing, Product, Disposable   General
Needle, Biopsy, Cardiovascular   Cardiovascular
Set, Administration, Intravenous, Needle-Free   General
Tube, Gastrointestinal   Gastroenterology/Urology

MULTI-PURE DRINKING WATER SYSTEM   800-622-9206
7251 Cathedral Rock Drive,   702-360-8880
Las Vegas, NV 89128
FDA Number: n/a   *Fax:* 702-360-8575
E-mail: headquarters@multipure.com
Web site: www.multipure.com
Annual Revenue: $25-$50 Million
Total Employees: 400   *Marketing Staff:* 14
Ownership: Private
Produces/Sells CE-marked Devices: N
Federal Procurement Eligibility: Small Business
Distribution: Manufacturer Direct, Manufacturer Through Distributor, Exporter
General Admin.: Allen Rice/Chief Executive Officer
     Alvin Rice/President
     Jim Cantrell/Vice President
Mktg./Adv.: Edward Fagan/Vice President Marketing
     Alvin Rice/Vice President Marketing & Sales
     Edward Fagan/Vice President Marketing & Sales
     Paula Rice/Vice President Public Relations
Research: Ken Smith/Manager Research & Development
     Alvin Rice/Vice President Research & Development
Purifier, Water   Chemistry

MULTI-TRONICS CORP.   817-246-5821
8400 White Settlement, Fort Worth, TX 76108
FDA Number: 1646830
Ownership: Private
Produces/Sells CE-marked Devices: N
Anomaloscope   Ophthalmology

MULTIDATA SYSTEMS INTERNATIONAL CORP.   314-968-6880
10816 Indian Head Ind Blvd, St. Louis, MO 63119
FDA Number: 1938060
Ownership: Private
Produces/Sells CE-marked Devices: N
Accelerator, Linear, Medical   Radiology
Simulator, Radiotherapy, Special Purpose   Radiology
Tester, Radiology   Radiology

MULTIFORM DESICCANTS, INC.
See Multisorb Technologies, Inc.

MULTIGON INDUSTRIES, INC.   800-289-6858
One Odell Plaza, Yonkers, NY 10701   914-376-5200
FDA Number: 2434117   *Fax:* 914-376-5565
E-mail: tcdinfo@multigon.com
Web site: www.multigon.com
Medical Products Sales Volume: $22,500,000
Annual Revenue: $10-$25 Million

MULTIGON INDUSTRIES, INC.   800-289-6858 *(cont'd)*
Year Founded: 1985
Total Employees: 85   *Marketing Staff:* 6   *Sales Staff:* 42
Ownership: Private
Quality System Registration Information: ISO9001
Produces/Sells CE-marked Devices: Y
Federal Procurement Eligibility: Small Business
Distribution: Manufacturer Direct, Manufacturer Through Distributor, Manufacturer Through Manufacturer Reps, Exclusive Distributor
General Admin.: A. Frum/Chief Executive Officer
     William Stern/President
     A. Abela/Vice President Human Resources
     J. Davis/Vice President, General Manager
Mktg./Adv.: S. Rand/Director Marketing
     J. Hennesy/Director National Accounts
     S. Gilles/Manager Advertising
     D. Handal/Manager Business Development
     M. Tonow/Manager International Marketing & Sales
     K. Janoka/Manager Market Research
     J. Lefkoa/Manager National Sales
     M. Muzab/Manager Sales
     W. Markowitz/Vice President Marketing
     Emily Incitti/Vice President Sales
Production: G. Miller/Manager Materials
     S. Silverstein/Manager Regulatory Affairs
     R. Costa/Vice President Manufacturing
Research: H. Fidel/Vice President Research & Development
Doppler, Blood Flow, Transcranial   Cardiovascular
Scanner, Ultrasonic, Other   Radiology
Scanner, Ultrasonic, Vascular   Radiology
Unit, Imaging, Thermal   Radiology

MULTIPERM LTD.
See The Lifestyle Co. Inc.

MULTIPLEX STIMULATOR LTD.   800-663-8576
2-1750 McLean Ave.,   604-941-0551
Port Coquitlam, BC V3C 1 Canada
FDA Number: 8022052   *Fax:* 604-941-5659
E-mail: info@multiplexstimulator.com
Web site: www.multiplexstimulator.com
Medical Products Sales Volume: $750,000
Year Founded: 1982
Total Employees: 5
Ownership: Private
Produces/Sells CE-marked Devices: N
Distribution: Manufacturer Direct, Exporter

MULTIPLIER INDUSTRIES CORP.   800-642-2424
2195 Britannia Blvd, Suite 104,   619-661-7992
San Diego, CA 92154
FDA Number: n/a   *Fax:* 619-661-5096
E-mail: sales@multiplier.com
Web site: www.multiplier.com
Medical Products Sales Volume: $20,000,000
Annual Revenue: $10-$25 Million
Total Employees: 140   *Marketing Staff:* 5   *Sales Staff:* 12
Ownership: Private
Quality System Registration Information: ISO9001
Produces/Sells CE-marked Devices: N
Federal Procurement Eligibility: Small Business
Distribution: Manufacturer Direct
General Admin.: Elaine Ullrich/Executive Vice President
     Walter Ullrich/President, Chief Executive Officer
Research: Danny Amato/Vice President Research & Development
Battery   General

MULTISORB TECHNOLOGIES, INC.   800-445-9890
325 Harlem Road, Buffalo, NY 14224   716-824-8900
FDA Number: 1314490   *Fax:* 716-824-4128
E-mail: info@multisorb.com
Web site: www.multisorb.com
Medical Products Sales Volume: $50,000,000
Annual Revenue: $25-$50 Million
Year Founded: 1961
Total Employees: 300   *Marketing Staff:* 1   *Sales Staff:* 10
Ownership: Private
Quality System Registration Information: ISO9001
Produces/Sells CE-marked Devices: N
Federal Procurement Eligibility: Small Business
Distribution: Manufacturer Direct, Manufacturer Through Distributor, Importer, Exporter
Mktg./Adv.: Mr. Steven Lloyd/Director Tech. Sales
     Mr. Mike Morelli/Sales Specialist
Production: Greg Fronczak/Manager Materials
Desiccator   Chemistry
Packaging Material   General
Sponge, Other   General

MULTISORB TECHNOLOGIES, INC. 800-445-9890 *(cont'd)*
Washer, Receptacle, Waste, Body General

MUNCHKIN, INC. 800-247-2223
16689 Schoenborn, North Hills, CA 91343 818-893-5000
FDA Number: 3000215556 *Fax:* 818-893-6343
E-mail: mark.hatherill@munchkin.com
Year Founded: 1991
Ownership: Private
Produces/Sells CE-marked Devices: N
Research: Mr. Mark Hatherill/Vice President Product Development
Container, Medication, Graduated Liquid General
Dispenser, Medication, Liquid General

MUNTERS CORP. - CARGOCAIRE DIVISION 800-843-5360
79 Monroe St., Amesbury, MA 01913 978-241-1100
FDA Number: n/a *Fax:* 978-241-1214
E-mail: dhinfo@munters.com
Web site: www.munters.com
Medical Products Sales Volume: $25,000,000
Annual Revenue: $25-$50 Million
Total Employees: 2000 *Marketing Staff:* 25 *Sales Staff:* 15
Ownership: Munters Corp. - Cargocaire Division
Quality System Registration Information: ISO9000
Produces/Sells CE-marked Devices: Y
Distribution: Manufacturer Through Distributor, Manufacturer Through Manufacturer Reps
General Admin.: Mike McDonald/General Manager
Sven Lundin/President
Mktg./Adv.: Courtney Perkins/Coord. Marketing
Courtney Perkins/Director Marketing
Dave McDougall/Manager National Sales
Dehumidifier General
Medical Product Subsidiaries (Listed Separately)
Munters Corp. - Cargocaire Division

MURDOCK LABORATORIES, INC. 800 439-2497
123 Primrose Rd., Burlingame, CA 94010 650-579-1352
FDA Number: 2435708 *Fax:* 650-579-1351
E-mail: info@purebrush.com
Web site: www.purebrush.com
Medical Products Sales Volume: $2,500,000
Annual Revenue: $1-$5 Million
Year Founded: 1985
Total Employees: 5 *Marketing Staff:* 5 *Sales Staff:* 5
Ownership: Private
Produces/Sells CE-marked Devices: Y
Federal Procurement Eligibility: Small Business
Distribution: Manufacturer Direct, Manufacturer Through Manufacturer Reps
General Admin.: Mr. James O. Murdock III/Chief Executive Officer
Sterilizer, Dry Heat, Dental Dental And Oral
Unit, Sanitation/Sterilization, Toothbrush, Ultraviolet Dental And Oral

MUSCULOSKELETAL TRANSPLANT FOUNDATION 800-433-6576
125 May St, Ste 300, Edison Corp Ctr, Edison, NJ 08837 732-661-0202
FDA Number: 2249062 *Fax:* 731-661-2298
E-mail: information@mtf.org
Web site: www.mtf.org
Ownership: Private
Produces/Sells CE-marked Devices: N
Bone Grafting Material, Human Source Dental And Oral
Filler, Calcium Sulfate Preformed Pellets Orthopedics
Gauge, Depth Orthopedics
Orthopedic Manual Surgical Instrument Orthopedics
Suture, Non-Absorbable, Synthetic, Polyethylene Surgery
Wax, Bone Surgery

MUSCULOSKELETAL TRANSPLANT FOUNDATION 1-800-433-6576
125 May Street, Edison, PA 18434 732-661-0202
FDA Number: 1000307092 *Fax:* 732-661-2298
E-mail: Information@mtf.org
Web site: www.mtf.org
Ownership: Private
Produces/Sells CE-marked Devices: N
Bit, Surgical Surgery
Burr, Surgical, General & Plastic Surgery Surgery
Elevator, Orthopedic Orthopedics
Elevator, Other General
Forceps Orthopedics
Gauge, Depth Orthopedics
Instrument, Bending (Contouring) Orthopedics
Knife, Orthopedic Orthopedics
Punch, Surgical Surgery
Reamer Orthopedics

MUSCULOSKELETAL TRANSPLANT 1-800-433-6576 *(cont'd)*
Screw, Fixation, Bone Orthopedics
Staple, Fixation, Bone Orthopedics
Syringe, Irrigating General

MUSHIELD COMPANY, INC., THE 888-669-3539
9 Ricker Avenue, Londonderry, NH 03053 603-666-4433
FDA Number: n/a *Fax:* 603-666-4013
E-mail: info@mushield.com
Web site: www.mushield.com
Medical Products Sales Volume: $1,000,000
Annual Revenue: $1-$5 Million
Year Founded: 1989
Total Employees: 27 *Marketing Staff:* 2 *Sales Staff:* 3
Ownership: Private
Quality System Registration Information: ISO9001
Produces/Sells CE-marked Devices: N
Federal Procurement Eligibility: Small Business
Distribution: Manufacturer Direct
General Admin.: David Grilli/President, Chief Executive Officer
Mktg./Adv.: David Grilli/Marketing & Sales Representative
Production: David Grilli/Applications Engineer
Robert Joy/Manager Materials
Edward Nordengren/Manager Operations
Robert Joy/Vice President Manufacturing
Finance: Karen Baer/Controller, Credit Manager
Case, Protection, Equipment General
Computer, Nuclear Medicine Radiology
Display, Cathode-Ray Tube Cardiovascular
Magnet, Permanent, MRI (Magnetic Resonance Imaging) Radiology
Magnet, Superconducting, MRI (Magnetic Resonance Imaging) Radiology

MUSTANG MACHINERY
See Star Industries

MUSTARD TREE INSTRUMENTS 919-972-7920
PO Box 14527, 10 Laboratory Drive, Bldg 2, Suite 200, Research Triangle Park, NC 27709
FDA Number: n/a
E-mail: info@mustardtree.com
Web site: www.mustardtree.com
Ownership: Private
Produces/Sells CE-marked Devices: N
General Admin.: Mr. Todd Blonshine/Chief Executive Officer
Mr. Brian Garrett/Chief Technology Officer
Mktg./Adv.: Mr. Joseph Colamarino/Vice President Sales
Production: Mr. Stan Ayers/Manager Engineering
Mr. Peter Cregger/Product Director
Finance: Mr. Robert Povlock/Chief Financial Officer

MUSTER ASSOCIATES, INC. 800-274-3619
135 E. 3rd St., Calhoun, KY 42327 -
FDA Number: n/a *Fax:* 270-273-3964
E-mail: jmuster47@aol.com
Web site: www.mustercoaches.com
Medical Products Sales Volume: $12,000,000
Annual Revenue: $10-$25 Million
Total Employees: 15 *Marketing Staff:* 3 *Sales Staff:* 5
Ownership: Private
Produces/Sells CE-marked Devices: N
Distribution: Exclusive Distributor
General Admin.: John W. Muster/President
Mktg./Adv.: Michael Muster/Vice President Sales
Ambulance General

MUTH & MUMMA DENTAL LAB 952-541-9622
6360 Flank Drive, Suite 500, Harrisburg, PA 17112
FDA Number: 3004142419
Ownership: Private
Produces/Sells CE-marked Devices: N
Base, Denture, Relining, Repairing, Rebasing, Resin Dental And Oral
Crown, Preformed Dental And Oral
Device, Anti-Snoring Ear/Nose/Throat
Device, Repositioning, Jaw Dental And Oral
Mouthguard Dental And Oral

MW INSTRUMENTS, INC.
See Drew Scientific, Inc.

MWF, INC.
See Drew Scientific, Inc.

MWI VETERINARY SUPPLY 800-824-3703
651 S. Stratford Drive, Suite 100, Meridian, ID 83642 888-562-3405
FDA Number: n/a
E-mail: sweepteam@mwivet.com.
Web site: www.mwivet.com
Medical Products Sales Volume: $664,351,000
Annual Revenue: More than $1 Billion

MWI VETERINARY SUPPLY   800-824-3703 *(cont'd)*
Year Founded: 1976
Total Employees: 850
Ownership: Private
Stock Symbol: MWIV
Traded On: NASDAQ
Produces/Sells CE-marked Devices: N
General Admin.: Mr. James S. Hay/Chief Information Officer
　　　　Mr. James F. Cleary/President, Chief Executive Officer
Mktg./Adv.: Mr. Mick Wells/Director Sales
　　　　Mr. Jhon R. Ryan/Vice President Marketing
　　　　Mr. Jeffrey W. Culpepper/Vice President Sales
Production: Mr. Bryan P. Mooney/Vice President Operations
Finance: Ms. Mary Patricia B. Thomson/Chief Financial Officer, Senior Vice President Finance

MWI, INC./DANAM ELECTRONICS
　　See Drew Scientific, Inc.

MWT MATERIALS, INC.   973-472-5161
90 Dayton Ave., Suite 6 E, Passaic, NJ 07055
FDA Number: 3004863903

Shield, Protective, Personnel	Radiology

MXE, INC.   800-252-1801
12107 W. Jefferson Blvd.,   310-823-0799
Culver City, CA 90230
FDA Number: n/a   Fax: 310-823-2349
E-mail: mxe@mxe.com
Web site: www.mxe.com
Medical Products Sales Volume: $1,500,000
Annual Revenue: $1-$5 Million
Year Founded: 1974
Total Employees: 10   *Marketing Staff:* 2   *Sales Staff:* 4
Ownership: Private
Quality System Registration Information: ISO9002
Produces/Sells CE-marked Devices: N
Federal Procurement Eligibility: Small Business, Minority Owned
Distribution: Manufacturer Direct, Manufacturer Through Distributor, Manufacturer Through Manufacturer Reps, OEM, Service Direct, Exporter
General Admin.: Carol Gellner/Office Manager
　　　　Henry Cortez/President

Chair, Other	General
Grid, Radiographic	Radiology
Holder, X-Ray Film Cassette, Vertical	Radiology
Patient Transfer Unit	General
Service, Maintenance/Repair	General
Table, Ultrasound	General

MY TRUE IMAGE MFG.   510-231-5253
999 Marina Way South, Richmond, CA 94804
FDA Number: 3004511024

Binder, Abdominal	General
Binder, Breast	Obstetrics/Gynecology
Binder, Elastic	General
Binder, Medical, Therapeutic	General

MY WATER HOUSE, INC.   407-428-9377
3319 Bartlett Blvd., Orlando, FL 32817
FDA Number: 3003793543   Fax: 407-648-0817
E-mail: bprice@mywaterhouse.net
Ownership: Private
Produces/Sells CE-marked Devices: N

Purification System, Water	Gastroenterology/Urology

MYCO INSTRUMENTATION SOURCE, INC.   425-228-4239
PO Box 354, Renton, WA 98057
FDA Number: 3024605   Fax: 425-271-8270
E-mail: myco@nwlink.com
Web site: www.medstore.com/myco
Medical Products Sales Volume: $5,000,000
Annual Revenue: $1-$5 Million
Year Founded: 1978
Total Employees: 7   *Marketing Staff:* 1   *Sales Staff:* 4
Ownership: Private
Produces/Sells CE-marked Devices: N
Federal Procurement Eligibility: Small Business
Distribution: Importer, Exporter
General Admin.: Philip Johnson/President, Owner
Mktg./Adv.: Bryan Biddulph/Sales Representative
Finance: Kyle Biddulph/Associate Business Support

Analyzer, Blood Gas pH	Anesthesiology
Analyzer, Chemistry, Multi-Channel, Fixed	Chemistry
Analyzer, Chemistry, Single Channel, Programmable	Chemistry
Analyzer, Gas, Oxygen, Sampling	Anesthesiology
Camera, Gamma (Nuclear/Scintillation)	Radiology
Chromatography, Liquid, Performance, High	Toxicology
Counter, Cell	Microbiology
Counter, Gamma, General Use	Toxicology

MYCO INSTRUMENTATION SOURCE, INC.   425-228-4239 *(cont'd)*

Diffractometer, X-Ray	Chemistry
Fluorometer	Immunology
Microscope, Laboratory, Electron	Microbiology
Microtome, Cryostat	Pathology
Photometer, Flame, General Use	Toxicology
Scanner, Computed Tomography, X-Ray (CAT, CT)	Cns/Neurology
Service, Used Equipment	General
Spectrograph, Mass	Chemistry
Tissue Processor, Automated	Pathology

MYCO MEDICAL   800-454-6926
158 Towerview Court, Cary, NC 27513   919-460-2535
FDA Number: 1058382   Fax: 919-460-2536
E-mail: sales@mycomedical.com
Web site: www.mycomedical.com
Year Founded: 1993
Total Employees: 11   *Marketing Staff:* 2   *Sales Staff:* 6
Ownership: Private
Quality System Registration Information: ISO9001
Produces/Sells CE-marked Devices: Y
Federal Procurement Eligibility: Small Business, Minority Owned
Distribution: Manufacturer Through Distributor, OEM
General Admin.: Sanjiv Kumar/President, Chief Executive Officer
Mktg./Adv.: Michael Taylor/Director National Accounts

Blade, Scalpel	Surgery
Catheter, Intravenous	Cardiovascular
Kit, Administration, Intravenous	General
Needle, Dental	Dental And Oral
Needle, Hypodermic	General
Needle, Scalp	Cns/Neurology
Needle, Spinal, Short-Term	General
Needle, Suture, Disposable	Surgery
Scalpel, One-Piece (Knife)	Surgery
Suture, Absorbable	Surgery
Suture, Dental	Dental And Oral
Syringe, Hypodermic	General

MYCOAL PRODUCTS CORPORATION OF USA   678-765-4000
475 Horizon Drive, Suwanee, GA 30024
FDA Number: 3005893229

Pack, Hot Or Cold, Disposable	Physical Med

MYCONE DENTAL SUPPLY CO. INC. T/A KEYSTONE IND-MYERSTOWN   717-866-7571
52 West King St., Myerstwn, PA 17067
FDA Number: 2523320

Articulators	Dental And Oral
Material, Impression Tray, Resin	Dental And Oral
Pump, Suction Operatory	Dental And Oral

MYCOSCIENCE, INC.   860-684-0030
25 Village Hill Rd., Willington, CT 06279
FDA Number: 1222747   Fax: 860-684-0040
E-mail: mycosci@mindspring.com
Web site: www.mycoscience.com
Annual Revenue: $0-$1 Million
Total Employees: 7
Ownership: Private
Quality System Registration Information: ISO9002
Produces/Sells CE-marked Devices: N
Federal Procurement Eligibility: Small Business
Distribution: OEM
General Admin.: Robert G. Whalen/Chief Executive Officer
　　　　Richard Arsenault/Vice President, General Manager

Campylobacter Pylori	Microbiology
Contract Manufacturing	General
Contract R&D, Diagnostics	General

MYDENT INTERNATIONAL   800-275-0020
80 Suffolk Court, Hauppauge, NY 11788   631-434-3190
FDA Number: 2435126   Fax: 631-434-7750
E-mail: mrieders@defend.com
Web site: www.defend.com
Medical Products Sales Volume: $5,000,000
Annual Revenue: $5-$10 Million
Year Founded: 1985
Total Employees: 10   *Marketing Staff:* 1   *Sales Staff:* 5
Ownership: Private
Produces/Sells CE-marked Devices: Y
Federal Procurement Eligibility: Small Business
Distribution: Manufacturer Through Distributor, Exporter
General Admin.: Andrew Parker/Chief Executive Officer
　　　　Mitchell Rieders/President
Mktg./Adv.: Mitchell Rieders/Vice President Marketing & Sales

Aspirator, Ultrasonic	Obstetrics/Gynecology
Caliper	Orthopedics
Coat, Laboratory	General
Cotton, Roll	Dental And Oral

MYDENT INTERNATIONAL   800-275-0020 *(cont'd)*

Cover, Barrier, Protective	General
Gauze, Absorbable	Surgery
Glove, Patient Examination, Latex	General
Glove, Patient Examination, Vinyl	General
Glove, Surgical, Powder-Free	Surgery
Goggles, Protective, Eye	Ophthalmology
Mask, Face	General
Material, Impression	Dental And Oral
Mirror, Mouth	Dental And Oral
Packaging, Sterilization	General
Sponge, Other	General
Tubing, Other	General
Wrap, Sterilization	General

MYELOTEC, INC.   770-664-4656
4000 Northfield Way, Suite 900, Roswell, GA 30076
FDA Number: 1062474

Arthroscope	Orthopedics

MYERS-STEVENS GROUP, INC.   903-566-6696
2931 Vail Ave,, Commerce, CA 90040
FDA Number: 2025932

Antiserum, Streptococcus SPP.	Microbiology
Colorimetric Method, CPK Or Isoenzymes	Chemistry
Control, Enzyme (Assayed And Unassayed)	Chemistry
Control, Urinalysis (Assayed And Unassayed)	Chemistry
Densitometer/Scanner (Integrating, Reflectance, TLC, Radio)	Chemistry
Enzyme Immunoassay, Amphetamine	Toxicology
Enzyme Immunoassay, Cannabinoids	Toxicology
Enzyme Immunoassay, Digoxin	Toxicology
Enzyme Immunoassay, Non-Radiolabeled, Total Thyroxine	Chemistry
Enzyme Immunoassay, Opiates	Toxicology
Kit, Pregnancy Test, Over The Counter, HCG	Chemistry
Pipetting And Diluting System, Automated	Chemistry
Radioimmunoassay, Cocaine Metabolite	Toxicology
Radioimmunoassay, Human Chorionic Gonadotropin	Chemistry
Radioimmunoassay, Thyroid Stimulating Hormone	Chemistry
Stain, Dye Solution	Pathology

MYERSON TOOTH CORP.
See Dentsply Prosthetics

MYHEAL TECHNOLOGIES   201-703-9059
34-14 Linwood Rd., Fair Lawn, NJ 07410-4012
FDA Number: n/a
Total Employees: 1
Ownership: Private
Produces/Sells CE-marked Devices: N
Distribution: Manufacturer Direct

Component, Electronic	General

MYLAN INC.   724-514-1800
1500 Corporate Drive, Canonsburg, PA 15317
FDA Number: n/a
Web site: www.mylan.com
Year Founded: 1970
Ownership: Public
Stock Symbol: MYL
Traded On: NASDAQ
Produces/Sells CE-marked Devices: N
General Admin.: Robert J. Coury/Chairman, Chief Executive Officer
         Rodney L. Piatt/Vice Chairman

MYLAN PHARMACEUTICALS INC   888-523-7835
Research Triangle Pa, Morgantown, NC 27709   919-991-9800
FDA Number: n/a   Fax: 919-993-5907
E-mail: info@bertek.com
Web site: www.mylanpharms.com
Medical Products Sales Volume: $4,800,000
Year Founded: 1961
Total Employees: 50   Marketing Staff: 10   Sales Staff: 220
Ownership: MYLAN INC.
Quality System Registration Information: ISO9000
Produces/Sells CE-marked Devices: Y
Federal Procurement Eligibility: Small Business
Distribution: Manufacturer Through Distributor, Manufacturer Through Manufacturer Reps
General Admin.: Michael Marquaro/Chief Executive Officer
         David Satter/Chief Financial Officer, Vice President
Mktg./Adv.: Ross Whitfield/Director Marketing
         Sean Spears/Director National Accounts
         Wes Kench/Manager Sales Training
         Julie Ward Crocker/Vice President Business Development
         Bill Richardson/Vice President Sales
Production: Dewayne Dickey/Executive Production
         Andrea Miller/Vice President Regulatory Affairs

Dressing, Aerosol	General
Dressing, Foam	General
Dressing, Universal	General

MYLAN PHARMACEUTICALS INC   888-523-7835 *(cont'd)*

Dressing, Wound and Burn, Occlusive	Surgery

MYLAN TECHNOLOGIES, INC.   800-532-5226
110 Lake St., St. Albans, VT 05478   802-527-7792
FDA Number: 1220747   Fax: 802-527-8151
E-mail: mtisales@mylanlabs.com
Web site: www.mylantech.com
Medical Products Sales Volume: $18,400,000
Annual Revenue: $50-$100 Million
Year Founded: 1961
Total Employees: 250   Marketing Staff: 10   Sales Staff: 10
Ownership: MYLAN INC.
Quality System Registration Information: ISO9001
Produces/Sells CE-marked Devices: N
Federal Procurement Eligibility: Small Business
Distribution: Manufacturer Direct, Manufacturer Through Distributor
General Admin.: Mr. Mike Tardugno/Chief Operating Officer, Vice President
         Dr. Sharad Govil/President
Mktg./Adv.: Mr. Martin Flethcher/Director Business
         Mr. Thomas Campbell/Sales Associate
Production: Kirk Cullen/Director Manufacturing

Drape, Surgical, Disposable	Surgery
Drape, Surgical, ENT	Ear/Nose/Throat
Drape, Urological, Disposable	Gastroenterology/Urology
Dress, Scrub, Disposable	Surgery
Dress, Surgical	Surgery
Dressing, Foam	General
Dressing, Gel	General
Dressing, Germicidal	General
Dressing, Other	General
Dressing, Permeable, Moisture	General
Dressing, Wound and Burn, Occlusive	Surgery
Material, Raw, Production	General
Pad, Dressing	General
Pad, Medicated	General
Patch, Transdermal	General
Protector, Ostomy	Gastroenterology/Urology
Service, Consulting	General
Service, Engineering/Design	General
Suit, Scrub, Disposable	Surgery
Tape, Gauze, Adhesive	General

MYLIN MEDICAL SYSTEMS, INC.   630-321-1450
11904 Heritage Drive, Burr Ridge, IL 60527-7123
FDA Number: n/a   Fax: 630-321-1459
E-mail: mylinmedical@comcast.net
Medical Products Sales Volume: $3,500,000
Annual Revenue: $1-$5 Million
Year Founded: 1983
Total Employees: 2   Marketing Staff: 2   Sales Staff: 2
Ownership: Private
Produces/Sells CE-marked Devices: N
Federal Procurement Eligibility: Small Business
Distribution: Service Direct, Exporter
General Admin.: Michael F. Glynn/President

Service, Used Equipment	General

MYO/KINETIC SYSTEMS, INC.   414-255-1005
North 84 West 13562 Leon Rd., Menomonee Falls, WI 53051
FDA Number: 2184032
Ownership: Private
Produces/Sells CE-marked Devices: N

Device, Cystometric, Hydraulic	Gastroenterology/Urology
Stimulator, Muscle, Electrical-Powered (EMS)	Physical Med
Stimulator, Nerve, Transcutaneous (Pain Relief, TENS)	Cns/Neurology
Uroflowmeter	Gastroenterology/Urology

MYODERM   610-272-8660
48 East Main Street, Norristown, PA 19401
FDA Number: n/a   Fax: 610-272-4604
E-mail: sales@myoderm.com
Web site: www.myoderm.com
Annual Revenue: $0-$1 Million
Ownership: Private
Produces/Sells CE-marked Devices: N
Federal Procurement Eligibility: Small Business
Distribution: Exclusive Distributor
General Admin.: Mike Cohen/Managing Director
Mktg./Adv.: Lorann Morse/Director Business Development
Production: Dave Caccavo/Director Operations

Analyzer, Gas, Carbon-Dioxide, Gaseous Phase (Capnograph)	Anesthesiology
Cable/Lead, ECG	Cardiovascular
Cable/Lead, ECG, With Transducer And Electrode	Cardiovascular
Defibrillator, Line-Powered	Cardiovascular
Glove, Surgical	General
Monitor, Blood Pressure, Indirect, Automatic	Cardiovascular
Monitor, ECG	Cardiovascular
Monitor, Pulse Rate	Anesthesiology

MYODERM   610-272-8660 *(cont'd)*
     Monitor, Respiratory   Surgery
     Oximeter, Pulse   General
     Sleep Assessment Equipment   Cns/Neurology
     Suture, Other   Surgery

MYOMO, INC.   1-877-736-9666
     1 Broadway,, 14th Floor,   617-996-9058
     Cambridge, MA 02142
     FDA Number: 3006240003
     E-mail: info@myomo.com   *Fax:* 617-886-0333
     Ownership: Private
     Produces/Sells CE-marked Devices: N
     Biofeedback Device   Cns/Neurology
     Orthosis, Limb Brace   Physical Med

MYOTRONICS-NOROMED, INC.   206-243-4214
     5870 S 194th Street, Kent, WA 98032
     FDA Number: 3014732   *Fax:* 206-243-3625
     E-mail: myotronics@aol.com
     Web site: www.myotronics-noromed.com
     Medical Products Sales Volume: $1,100,000
     Annual Revenue: $1-$5 Million
     Year Founded: 1964
     Total Employees: 18   *Marketing Staff:* 1   *Sales Staff:* 2
     Ownership: Private
     Quality System Registration Information: ISO9001
     Produces/Sells CE-marked Devices: Y
     Federal Procurement Eligibility: Small Business
     Distribution: Manufacturer Through Distributor, Service Direct, Exclusive Distributor
     General Admin.: Fray Adib/President
     Analyzer, Motion   General
     Articulators   Dental And Oral
     Biofeedback Device   Cns/Neurology
     Biofeedback Equipment, Myoelectric, Powered   Physical Med
     Kinesthesiometer   Orthopedics
     Monitor, Muscle, Dental   Dental And Oral
     Stimulator, Nerve, Transcutaneous (Pain Relief, TENS)   Cns/Neurology

MYRON L COMPANY   760-438-2021
     2450 Impala Drive, Carlsbad, CA 92010-7226
     FDA Number: 2020976   *Fax:* 760-931-9189
     E-mail: info@myronl.com
     Web site: www.myronl.com
     Year Founded: 1957
     Total Employees: 70
     Ownership: Private
     Produces/Sells CE-marked Devices: Y
     Federal Procurement Eligibility: Small Business
     Distribution: Manufacturer Through Distributor
     General Admin.: GARY Robinson/President
       JERRY ADAMS/Vice President, General Manager
     Mktg./Adv.: Kathryn Robinson/Director Marketing & Sales
     Meter, Conductivity   Chemistry
     Meter, Conductivity, Non-Remote   Gastroenterology/Urology
     Meter, Dialysate Conductivity   Gastroenterology/Urology
     Meter, pH, Portable   Chemistry
     Solution, pH Buffer   Chemistry
     Solution-Test, Standard-Conductivity, Dialysis   Gastroenterology/Urology

MYTREX, INC.   1-800-688-9576
     10321 South Beckstead Ln., South Jordan, UT 84095
     FDA Number: 3005167695   *Fax:* 1-877-571-4606
     E-mail: info@rescuealert.com
     Web site: www.rescuealert.com
     Medical Products Sales Volume: $1,000,000
     Annual Revenue: $0-$1 Million
     Ownership: Private
     Produces/Sells CE-marked Devices: N
     Federal Procurement Eligibility: Small Business
     Distribution: Manufacturer Direct
     Communication System, Emergency Alert, Personal   General

N SPINE, INC.
     See Synthes San Diego

N-K PRODUCTS COMPANY, DIV. OF I-REP,INC.   800-462-6509
     508 Chaney Street #B, Lake Elsinore, CA 92530   951-471-0588
     FDA Number: 2083287   *Fax:* 888-584-8126
     E-mail: nkproducts@yahoo.com
     Web site: www.nkproducts.net
     Medical Products Sales Volume: $1,800,000
     Annual Revenue: $0-$1 Million
     Year Founded: 1956
     Total Employees: 11   *Marketing Staff:* 2   *Sales Staff:* 3
     Ownership: Private
     Produces/Sells CE-marked Devices: N
     Federal Procurement Eligibility: Small Business

N-K PRODUCTS COMPANY, DIV. OF I-REP,INC.   800-462-6509
(cont'd)
     Distribution: Manufacturer Direct, Manufacturer Through Distributor, Manufacturer Through Manufacturer Reps, Exporter
     General Admin.: Bradley Wilhelm/President
       Greg Harris/Vice President, General Manager
     Mktg./Adv.: Bradley Wilhelm/Vice President Marketing & Sales
     Bars, Parallel, Walking   Physical Med
     Table, Mechanical   Physical Med
     Table, Other   General
     Training Aid   Orthopedics

N-TECH ENDOSCOPY, INC.   480-348-7861
     14255 N. 79th St., Suite 3, Scottsdale, AZ 85260
     FDA Number: 1424161
     Endoscope   Gastroenterology/Urology

N.I.T., INC.
     See Avid Medical

N.M. BEALE CO. INC.   978-456-6990
     89 Old Shirley Road, PO Box 494, Harvard, MA 01451-1309
     FDA Number: 1222219   *Fax:* 978-456-3927
     E-mail: sales@nmbco.com
     Web site: www.nmbco.com
     Medical Products Sales Volume: $100,000
     Year Founded: 1985
     Ownership: Private
     Produces/Sells CE-marked Devices: N
     Federal Procurement Eligibility: Small Business
     Distribution: Manufacturer Direct, Manufacturer Through Distributor, Manufacturer Through Manufacturer Reps
     General Admin.: Mr. Nathaniel Beale/President
     Accessories, Cleaning, Endoscopic   Gastroenterology/Urology

NADA-CONCEPTS   800-722-2587
     2448 Larpenteur Ave. W., St. Paul, MN 55113   651-644-4466
     FDA Number: 2183656   *Fax:* 651-644-4488
     E-mail: info@nadachair.com
     Web site: www.nadachair.com
     Medical Products Sales Volume: $1,500,000
     Annual Revenue: $1-$5 Million
     Total Employees: 4   *Marketing Staff:* 1   *Sales Staff:* 1
     Ownership: Private
     Produces/Sells CE-marked Devices: N
     Federal Procurement Eligibility: Small Business
     Distribution: Manufacturer Direct, Manufacturer Through Distributor, Manufacturer Through Manufacturer Reps, Service Direct, Exclusive Distributor, Exporter
     General Admin.: Victor Toso/Chief Executive Officer
     Support, Back   Orthopedics

NAGL MANUFACTURING CO.   423-587-2199
     3626 Martha St., Omaha, NE 68105
     FDA Number: 3004183541
     Applicator, Resin   Dental And Oral
     Applicator, Tipped, Absorbent, Non-Sterile   General
     Toothbrush, Manual   Dental And Oral

NAI TECH PRODUCTS   866-342-6629
     12919 Earhart Avenue, Auburn, CA 95602   530-887-1008
     FDA Number: 2938727   *Fax:* 530-887-1108
     E-mail: sales@dicombox.com
     Web site: www.dicombox.com
     Medical Products Sales Volume: $10,000,000
     Annual Revenue: $10-$25 Million
     Total Employees: 22   *Marketing Staff:* 2   *Sales Staff:* 4
     Ownership: North American Imaging, Inc.
     Quality System Registration Information: ISO9000
     Produces/Sells CE-marked Devices: Y
     Federal Procurement Eligibility: Small Business
     Distribution: Manufacturer Direct, OEM
     Production: Mr. Gordon Smith/Regulatory Affairs Engineer
     Image Digitizer   Radiology
     Radiographic Picture Archiving/Communication System (PACS)   Radiology

NAIMCO, INC.   423-648-7730
     4120 South Creek Road, Chattanooga, TN 37406
     FDA Number: 3004750362
     Electrode, Cutaneous   Cns/Neurology
     Heating Unit, Powered   Physical Med
     Iontophoresis Device, Dental   Dental And Oral
     Pack, Hot Or Cold, Reusable   Physical Med
     Pack, Moist Heat   Physical Med
     Pad, Heating, Powered   Physical Med
     Stimulator, Nerve, Transcutaneous (Pain Relief, TENS)   Cns/Neurology

NALGE COMPANY
     See Nalge Nunc International

NALGE NUNC INTERNATIONAL
800-625-4327
585-586-8800

75 Panorama Creek Drive,
Rochester, NY 14625
FDA Number: n/a
Fax: 585-586-3294
E-mail: nnitech@nalgenunc.com
Web site: www.NALGENE.com
Medical Products Sales Volume: $114,400,000
Annual Revenue: $100-$500 Million
Year Founded: 1949
Total Employees: 903   *Marketing Staff:* 70   *Sales Staff:* 50
Ownership: Fisher Scientific Co., Llc.
Produces/Sells CE-marked Devices: Y
Distribution: Manufacturer Through Distributor, OEM
General Admin.: Craig Jack/President
Mktg./Adv.: Liz Reagan/Manager Marketing
     Karen Dally/Vice President Marketing
     Steve Zegas/Vice President Sales
Production: Marty Launer/Manager Regulatory Affairs
     Roman Siryk/Vice President Manufacturing

Adapter, Centrifuge Tube	Chemistry
Beaker (Laboratory)	Chemistry
Bottle, Sterile Solution	General
Buret	Chemistry
Cage, Animal	Microbiology
Container, Sterilization (Tray)	General
Desiccator	Chemistry
Dish, Petri	Chemistry
Dispenser, Fluid	General
Dispenser, Liquid, Laboratory	Chemistry
Filter, Cell Collection, Tissue Processing	Pathology
Filter, Membrane	Chemistry
Filter, Syringe	General
Flask, Dewar	Chemistry
Labware, Basic, Reusable	Chemistry
Mixer, Clinical Laboratory	Chemistry
Pipette, Diluting	Hematology
Rack, Test Tube	Chemistry
Sink, Laboratory	Chemistry
Stirrer	Chemistry
Tissue Culture Apparatus	Microbiology
Tube, Centrifuge	Chemistry
Tubing, Fluid Delivery	General
Tubing, Polyethylene	General
Tubing, Polyvinyl Chloride	General
Unit, Filter, Membrane	Chemistry
Valve, Other	Chemistry
Washer, Pipette	Chemistry

NAMIC/VA
See Navilyst Medical

NANO MASK INC.
888-656-3697
702-558-5164

175 Cassia Way, Suite A115,
Henderson, NV 89014
FDA Number: 2953736
Fax: 702-567-1893
E-mail: contactus@emergencyfiltration.com
Web site: www.emergencyfiltration.com
Medical Products Sales Volume: $600,000
Year Founded: 1991
Total Employees: 25
Ownership: Public
Stock Symbol: EMFP
Traded On: OTC Bulletin
Quality System Registration Information: ISO9001
Produces/Sells CE-marked Devices: N
Federal Procurement Eligibility: Small Business
Distribution: Manufacturer Through Distributor, Manufacturer Through
Manufacturer Reps, OEM
Mktg./Adv.: Pete Clark/Vice President Marketing & Sales

Bag, Breathing	Anesthesiology
Collagen, Platelet Aggregation And Adhesion	Hematology
Filter, Bacterial, Breathing Circuit	Anesthesiology
Mask, Face	General
Valve, Non-Rebreathing	Anesthesiology

NANO-DITECH CORPORATION
609-409-0700

7 Clarke Drive, Cranbury, NJ 08512
FDA Number: 3005174594

Antigen, Antiserum, Control, Myoglobin	Immunology
Chromatographic Separation, CPK Isoenzymes	Chemistry
Enzymatic Method, Troponin Subunit	Chemistry
Enzyme Immunoassay, Cannabinoids	Toxicology
Enzyme Immunoassay, Cocaine And Cocaine Metabolites	Toxicology
Enzyme Immunoassay, Opiates	Toxicology
Enzyme Immunoassay, Phencyclidine	Toxicology
Thin Layer Chromatography, Metamphetamine	Toxicology

NANO-WRITE CORPORATION
925-606-1388

2021 Las Positas Court, Suite 121, Livermore, CA 94551
FDA Number: 3004573454

NANO-WRITE CORPORATION
925-606-1388 *(cont'd)*

Ownership: Private
Produces/Sells CE-marked Devices: N

Metal, Base	Dental And Oral

NANODETECTION TECHNOLOGY, INC
937-550-4502

301 Industrial Drive, Suite B, Franklin, OH 45005
FDA Number: n/a
Fax: 937-550-4503
E-mail: Joel@NanoDetectionTechnology.com
Web site: www.nanodetectiontechnology.com
Ownership: Private
Produces/Sells CE-marked Devices: N

NANOGEN INC.
See Nanogen Molecular Research Products Division

NANOGEN MOLECULAR RESEARCH PRODUCTS DIVISION
800-526-5544

21720 23rd Drive, Suite 150, Bothell, WA 98021
425-482-5555
FDA Number: 3003540236
Fax: 425-482-5550
E-mail: technicalassistance@epochbio.com
Web site: www.nanogen.com
Ownership: Nanogen, Inc.
Stock Symbol: NGEN
Traded On: NASDAQ
Produces/Sells CE-marked Devices: N

Reagent, General Purpose	Pathology
Reagents, Specific, Analyte	Hematology

NANOGEN, INC.
877-626-6436
848-410-4600

10398 Pacific Center Ct.,
San Diego, CA 92121
FDA Number: 2032530
Fax: 858-410-4952
E-mail: technicalassistance@nanogen.com
Web site: www.nanogen.com
Year Founded: 1993
Ownership: Public
Stock Symbol: NGEN
Traded On: NASDAQ
Produces/Sells CE-marked Devices: N

Equipment, Laboratory, Gen. Purpose (Specific Medical Use)	Chemistry
Reagent, General Purpose	Pathology
Reagents, Specific, Analyte	Hematology

Medical Product Subsidiaries (Listed Separately)
Nanogen Molecular Research Products Division

NANOINK INC.
847-679-6266

8025 Lamon Ave., Skokie, IL 60077
FDA Number: n/a
Fax: 847-679-8767
E-mail: info@nanoink.net
Web site: www.nanoink.net
Ownership: Private
Produces/Sells CE-marked Devices: N
General Admin.: Mr. James Hussey/Chief Executive Officer
     Mr. Robert Janosky/Chief Operating Officer
Mktg./Adv.: Mr. Dean Hart/Vice President Commercial Operations
Research: Mr. Michael Nelson/Vice President Engineering
Finance: Mr. Ben Pothast/Chief Financial Officer

NANOMATERIALS, INC.
401-433-7022

9 Preston Drive, Barrington, RI 02806
FDA Number: n/a
Fax: 401-433-7001
E-mail: sales@nanomaterials.biz
Web site: www.nanomaterials.biz
Annual Revenue: $1-$5 Million
Year Founded: 1996
Total Employees: 18172   *Sales Staff:* 3
Ownership: Private
Quality System Registration Information: ISO9001
Produces/Sells CE-marked Devices: N
Federal Procurement Eligibility: Small Business, Female Owned
Distribution: Manufacturer Direct, Importer, Exporter
General Admin.: Emily S. Reade/President, Chief Executive Officer
Mktg./Adv.: Charles Reade/Manager International & National Sales
     Steve Munson/Manager Marketing & Sales
Production: Karen Ramos/Manager Materials

Component, Metal, Other	General
Component, Other	General
Zinc Oxide Eugenol	Dental And Oral

NANOMED DEVICES, INC.
518-862-0151

116 Kennewyck Circle, Slingerlands, NY 12159
FDA Number: 3005280613
Ownership: Private
Produces/Sells CE-marked Devices: N

Instrument, Manual, General Surgical	Surgery
Needle, Aspiration And Injection, Disposable	Surgery

NANOMETRICS, INC.   408-545-6000
1550 Buckeye Drive, Milpitas, CA 95035
FDA Number: n/a   *Fax:* 408-232-5910
E-mail: service@nanometrics.com
Web site: www.nanometrics.com
Year Founded: 1975
Total Employees: 465   *Sales Staff:* 39
Ownership: Private
Stock Symbol: NANO
Traded On: NASDAQ
Produces/Sells CE-marked Devices: N
Federal Procurement Eligibility: Small Business
Distribution: Manufacturer Direct
General Admin.: Bruce A. Crawford/Chief Operating Officer, Chief Financial Officer
     Timothy J. Stultz/President, Chief Executive Officer
     Microscope, Laboratory, Optical   Microbiology

NANOPROBES, INC.   877-447-6266
95 Horseblock Rd., Yaphank, NY 11980   631-205-9490
FDA Number: n/a   *Fax:* 631-205-9493
E-mail: nano@nanoprobes.com
Web site: www.nanoprobes.com
Total Employees: 8
Ownership: Private
Produces/Sells CE-marked Devices: N
Federal Procurement Eligibility: Small Business
Distribution: Manufacturer Direct
General Admin.: James Hainfeld/President
     Frederic Fuyura/Vice President, General Manager
Research: Richard D. Powell/Research & Development Associate
     Antibody, Monoclonal   Microbiology
     Antibody, Polyclonal   Microbiology
     Metal, Medical   General

NANOPTICS, INC.   352-378-6620
3014 NE 21st Way, Gainesville, FL 32609-3307
FDA Number: 1063754   *Fax:* 352-378-0273
E-mail: info@nanoptics.com
Web site: www.nanoptics.com
Medical Products Sales Volume: $900,000
Annual Revenue: $1-$5 Million
Year Founded: 1987
Total Employees: 12
Ownership: Private
Produces/Sells CE-marked Devices: N
Federal Procurement Eligibility: Small Business
Distribution: Manufacturer Direct
General Admin.: Dr. James Walker/President
Mktg./Adv.: Mrs. Barbara Hall/Director Sales
Production: Dr. Young Noh/Vice President, Director Operations
     Component, Optical   General
     Component, Plastic   General
     Contract R&D, Equipment   General
     Endoscope   Gastroenterology/Urology

NANOSPHERE INC   888-837-4436
4088 Commercial Ave, Northbrook, IL 60062   847-400-9000
FDA Number: 3006028115
E-mail: info@nanosphere.us
Web site: www.nanosphere.us
Ownership: Private
Produces/Sells CE-marked Devices: N
General Admin.: Mr. Tim Patno/Chief Technology Officer, Vice President
     Mr. William Moffitt/President, Chief Executive Officer
Medical Admin.: Dr. Greg Shipp/Chief Medical Officer
Mktg./Adv.: Mr. Winton Gibbons/Senior Vice President Business Development
     Mr. Bill Athenson/Vice President International Marketing & Sales
     Mr. Michael McGarrity/Vice President Marketing & Sales
Production: Mr. Mark Del Vecchio/Vice President Regulatory Affairs
Finance: Mr. Roger Moody/Chief Financial Officer, Vice President Finance
     Cytochrome P450 2c9 (cyp450 2c9) Drug Metabolizing Enzyme Genotyping System
     Toxicology
     Instrumentation For Clinical Multiplex Test Systems   Chemistry
     System, Cystic Fibrosis Transmembrane Conductance Regulator, Gene Mutation
     Detection   Immunology
     Test, Factor Ii G20210a Mutations, Genomic Dna Pcr   Hematology
     Test, Factor V Leiden Mutations, Genomic Dna Pcr   Hematology

NANOSTRING TECHNOLOGIES INC   1-888-358-NANO
530 Fairview Avenue N, Suite 2000, Seattle, WA 98109
FDA Number: n/a   *Fax:* 206-378-6288
E-mail: info@nanostring.com
Web site: www.NanoString.com
Ownership: Private
Produces/Sells CE-marked Devices: N
General Admin.: Mr. William Young/Executive Chairman
     Mr. Brad Gray/President, Chief Executive Officer
Medical Admin.: Dr. J. Wayne Cowens/Chief Medical Officer

NANOSTRING TECHNOLOGIES INC   1-888-358-NANO *(cont'd)*
Mktg./Adv.: Mr. Chris Grimley/Vice President Marketing
Production: Dr. Mary Allen/Vice President Manufacturing
Research: Dr. Philippa Webster/Senior Scientist
Finance: Mr. Wayne Burns/Chief Financial Officer

NANOTHERAPEUTICS, INC.   386-462-9663
13859 Progress Blvd, Suite 300, Alachua, FL 32615
FDA Number: 3005565760
     Filler, Calcium Sulfate Preformed Pellets   Orthopedics

NANZEE DENTAL PRODUCTS   717-792-9795
2916 Robin Road, York, PA 17404-5768
FDA Number: 2529021   *Fax:* 717-792-9795
E-mail: cleanerdenture@cs.com
Web site: www.cleanerdenture.com
Medical Products Sales Volume: $100,000
Annual Revenue: $0-$1 Million
Year Founded: 1960
Total Employees: 2   *Marketing Staff:* 1   *Sales Staff:* 1
Ownership: Private
Produces/Sells CE-marked Devices: Y
Federal Procurement Eligibility: Small Business
Distribution: Manufacturer Direct
     Cleaner, Denture, Mechanical   Dental And Oral
     Pin, Retentive And Splinting   Dental And Oral

NARCO SCIENTIFIC, PILLING DIVISION
     See Teleflex Medical

NARDA MICROWAVE CORP., THE
     See Narda Safety Test Solutions

NARDA SAFETY TEST SOLUTIONS   631-231-1700
435 Moreland Road, Hauppauge, NY 11788
FDA Number: 9200776   *Fax:* 631-231-1711
E-mail: nardasts@l-3com.com
Web site: www.narda-sts.com
Medical Products Sales Volume: $10,000,000
Annual Revenue: $25-$50 Million
Year Founded: 1983
Total Employees: 300   *Marketing Staff:* 5   *Sales Staff:* 15
Ownership: L-3 Communications Corporation
Stock Symbol: LLL
Traded On: NYSE
Quality System Registration Information: ISO9001
Produces/Sells CE-marked Devices: Y
Federal Procurement Eligibility: Small Business, GSA Contract
Distribution: Manufacturer Through Distributor, Manufacturer Through
     Manufacturer Reps
General Admin.: John Mega/President
Mktg./Adv.: William Reich/Manager Corporate Publications
     Mr. Robert Johnson/Manager Product Sales
     Detector, Microwave Leakage   General
     Monitor, Radiation   Radiology

NARISHIGE INTERNATIONAL USA, INC.   800-445-7914
1710 Hempstead Tpke., East Meadow, NY 11554   516-794-8000
FDA Number: 2438595   *Fax:* 516-794-0066
E-mail: info@narishige-usa.com
Web site: www.narishige.co.jp
Ownership: Private
Produces/Sells CE-marked Devices: N
Distribution: Manufacturer Through Distributor, Manufacturer Through
     Manufacturer Reps
General Admin.: Shinji Yoneyama/President
     Yuki Yoneyama/Vice President, General Manager
     Micromanipulators and Microinjectors, Assisted Reproduction   Obstetrics/Gynecology

NARRAGANSETT IMAGING   401-767-4462
51 Industrial Drive, North Smithfield, RI 02896
FDA Number: n/a   *Fax:* 401-767-4407
E-mail: sales@nimaging.com
Web site: www.nimaging.com
Total Employees: 65
Ownership: Private
Quality System Registration Information: ISO9002
Produces/Sells CE-marked Devices: N
Distribution: Manufacturer Through Distributor, OEM
Mktg./Adv.: Dawn Poirier/Director Product Management
     Tube, X-Ray   Radiology

NASA TECH MEMORY FOAM SLEEP SYSTEMS   727-447-0957
8300 Ulmerton Rd., Ste. 100, Largo, FL 33771
FDA Number: 3003947078
Ownership: Private
Produces/Sells CE-marked Devices: N
     Mattress, Non-Powered Flotation Therapy   Physical Med

NASA TECH MEMORY FOAM SLEEP SYSTEMS   727-447-0957
(cont'd)
Pillow, Cervical(for Mild Sleep Apnea)	Ear/Nose/Throat

NASCO   800-558-9595
4825 Stoddard Road, PO Box 3837,   **209-545-1600**
Modesto, CA 95356
FDA Number: n/a   Fax: 209-545-1669
E-mail: info@enasco.com
Web site: www.enasco.com
Annual Revenue: $10-$25 Million
Year Founded: 1941
Total Employees: 75
Ownership: Public
Stock Symbol: ARTL
Traded On: NASDAQ
Produces/Sells CE-marked Devices: N
Federal Procurement Eligibility: Small Business
Distribution: Manufacturer Direct, Manufacturer Through Distributor
General Admin.: Tom Swafford/Executive Vice President
Mktg./Adv.: Jim Felt/Director Sales
Purchasing: Eldon Williams/Director Purchasing
Training Aid	Orthopedics
Training Manikin, CPR (Resuscitation)	General
Training Manikin, Intravenous Arm	General

NASCO   800-558-9595
901 Janesville Avenue, PO Box 901,   **920-563-2446**
Fort Atkinson, WI 53538
FDA Number: n/a   Fax: 920-563-8296
E-mail: info@enasco.com
Web site: www.enasco.com
Year Founded: 1941
Total Employees: 500
Ownership: The Ultimate Companies, Inc.
Stock Symbol: ARTL
Traded On: NASDAQ
Produces/Sells CE-marked Devices: Y
Federal Procurement Eligibility: GSA Contract
Distribution: Manufacturer Direct, Manufacturer Through Distributor, Exclusive Distributor, Importer, Exporter
General Admin.: Mike Wagner/Executive Vice President
Mktg./Adv.: Kent Parks/Director Advertising
    Dan Christianson/Director Sales
Simulator, Blood Pressure	Cardiovascular
Simulator, ECG	Cardiovascular
Simulator, Heart Sound	Cardiovascular
Training Manikin, Intravenous Arm	General
Training Manikin, Other	General
Transducer, Force	General

NASHVILLE MEDICAL ELECTRONICS, INC.   800-966-1001
319 Fesslers Lane, Suite A, Nashville, TN 37210   **615-320-1001**
FDA Number: n/a   Fax: 615-320-1057
E-mail: dguffey@nashmed.com
Web site: www.nashmed.com
Medical Products Sales Volume: $1,000,000
Annual Revenue: $0-$1 Million
Year Founded: 1986
Total Employees: 9   Marketing Staff: 1   Sales Staff: 2
Ownership: Private
Produces/Sells CE-marked Devices: N
Federal Procurement Eligibility: Small Business
Distribution: Service Direct
General Admin.: Daryl E. Guffey/President, Chief Executive Officer
    Alisa Guffey/Vice President Human Resources
    Alisa Guffey/Vice President, General Manager
Mktg./Adv.: Alisa Guffey/Director Marketing
    Daryl Guffey/Manager Contract Sales
    Brad Guffey/Vice President Business Development
Service, Maintenance/Repair	General
Service, Used Equipment	General

NASIFF ASSOC., INC.   315-676-2346
841-1 County Route 37, Central Square, NY 13036
FDA Number: 1319390
Analyzer, ECG	Cardiovascular
Echocardiograph (Ultrasonic Scanner)	Cardiovascular
Electrocardiograph, Single Channel	Cardiovascular
Monitor, Blood Pressure, Indirect, Semi-Automatic	Cardiovascular
Monitor, Cardiac (Cardiotachometer & Rate Alarm)	Cardiovascular

NASORCAP ENTERPRISES, INC.
See Nasorcap Medical, Inc.

NASORCAP MEDICAL, INC.   412-466-1412
1077 Huston Drive, West Mifflin, PA 15122-3101
FDA Number: 2529489   Fax: 412-466-1412
E-mail: sderrick@icubed.com

NASORCAP MEDICAL, INC.   412-466-1412 (cont'd)
Web site: www.nauticom.net/www/tfc/CAPNOGRAPHY/nasorcap.html
Medical Products Sales Volume: $200,000
Annual Revenue: $0-$1 Million
Year Founded: 1991
Total Employees: 2   Marketing Staff: 2   Sales Staff: 2
Ownership: Private
Federal Procurement Eligibility: Small Business
Distribution: Manufacturer Direct, Manufacturer Through Distributor, Exclusive Distributor, Exporter
General Admin.: Steven J. Derrick/President, Chief Executive Officer
    Joyce A. Derrick/Secretary, Treasurer
Sampler, Gas	Chemistry

NASORCAP MEDSPEC, INC.
See Nasorcap Medical, Inc.

NASTECH PHARMACEUTICAL COMPANY INC.
See Mdrna, Inc.

NATIONAL AIR AMBULANCE   800-327-3710
3495 S.W. 9th Avenue,   **954-359-9900**
Fort Lauderdale, FL 33315
FDA Number: n/a   Fax: 954-359-9500
E-mail: inquiry@nationalairambulance.com
Web site: www.nationalairambulance.com
Medical Products Sales Volume: $19,000,000
Annual Revenue: $10-$25 Million
Year Founded: 1976
Total Employees: 108   Marketing Staff: 1   Sales Staff: 2
Ownership: CAROLINA AIRCRAFT
Produces/Sells CE-marked Devices: N
Federal Procurement Eligibility: Small Business
Distribution: Service Direct
General Admin.: Thomas E. Boy/President, Chief Executive Officer
    Sam Robbin/Vice President, General Manager
Mktg./Adv.: Sam Robbin/Director Marketing
Production: George Martinez/Manager Operations
Ambulance, Air	General

NATIONAL AMBULANCE BUILDERS, INC.   800-747-0064
230 N. Ortman Drive, Orlando, FL 32805   **407-299-0064**
FDA Number: n/a   Fax: 407-291-2224
Medical Products Sales Volume: $15,000,000
Total Employees: 125   Sales Staff: 4
Ownership: Private
Produces/Sells CE-marked Devices: N
Federal Procurement Eligibility: Small Business
Distribution: Manufacturer Through Distributor
General Admin.: Philip Lai/Chief Executive
    Philip Lai/President, Chief Executive Officer
    Phil Chapman/Vice President Human Resources
    Philip Lai/Vice President, General Manager
Mktg./Adv.: Idus Willis/Executive Marketing
    Idus Willis/Vice President Marketing
Production: Chuck Brandenburg/Manager Production
Research: Joe Oettinger/Vice President Research & Development
Ambulance	General

NATIONAL BIOLOGICAL CORP.   800-338-5045
1532 Enterprise Pkwy.,   **330-425-3535**
Twinsburg, OH 44087
FDA Number: 1521608   Fax: 330-425-9614
E-mail: nbc@natbiocorp.com
Web site: www.natbiocorp.com
Medical Products Sales Volume: $3,700,000
Annual Revenue: $5-$10 Million
Year Founded: 1967
Total Employees: 45   Marketing Staff: 2   Sales Staff: 5
Ownership: Private
Produces/Sells CE-marked Devices: N
Federal Procurement Eligibility: Small Business
Distribution: Manufacturer Direct
General Admin.: Mark Friddman/President, Chief Executive Officer
Mktg./Adv.: Ken Oif/Director Marketing
Production: Fran Lamm/Manager Regulatory Affairs
Cabinet, Phototherapy (PUVA)	Surgery
Cabinet, Treatment, Ultraviolet	General
Goggles, Protective, Eye	Ophthalmology
Lamp, Other	General
Lamp, Ultraviolet, Physical Medicine	Physical Med
Light, Ultraviolet, Dermatologic	Surgery
Radiometer, Ultraviolet	General

NATIONAL BUSINESS SYSTEMS, INC.
See Nbs Technologies Inc.

NATIONAL CABLE MOLDING 323-225-5611
136 N. San Fernando Rd., Los Angeles, CA 90031
FDA Number: 2020439 *Fax:* 323-225-4630
E-mail: info@nationalwire.com
Web site: www.nationalwire.com
Ownership: Spectris, Inc.
Quality System Registration Information: ISO9001
Produces/Sells CE-marked Devices: N
Distribution: OEM
  Cable, Electrode Physical Med

NATIONAL DENTEX CORP 508-907-7800
2 Vision Drive, 3rd Floor, N Natick, MA 01760
FDA Number: 3003643785
Ownership: Public
Stock Symbol: NADX
Traded On: NASDAQ
Produces/Sells CE-marked Devices: N
  Device, Repositioning, Jaw Dental And Oral
  Splint, Temporary Training Physical Med

NATIONAL DRAEGER, INC.
See Draeger Safety, Inc.

NATIONAL ELECTRONIC ATTACHMENT, INC. 800-782-5150
3577 Parkway Lane, Suite 250, Norcross, GA 30092
FDA Number: 1066683 *Fax:* 770-441-3204
E-mail: tom.hughes@nea-fast.com
Web site: www.nea-fast.com
Medical Products Sales Volume: $350,000
Annual Revenue: $1-$5 Million
Year Founded: 1997
Total Employees: 22 *Marketing Staff:* 1 *Sales Staff:* 5
Ownership: Private
Produces/Sells CE-marked Devices: N
  System, Communication, Image, Digital Radiology

NATIONAL FELT CO.
See National Nonwovens

NATIONAL GRAPHIC SUPPLY 800-223-7130
226 N. Allen St., Albany, NY 12206 518-438-8411
FDA Number: n/a *Fax:* 518-438-0940
E-mail: mail@ngscorp.com
Web site: www.ngscorp.com
Medical Products Sales Volume: $8,000,000
Year Founded: 1927
Total Employees: 55 *Marketing Staff:* 1 *Sales Staff:* 15
Ownership: Private
Produces/Sells CE-marked Devices: N
Federal Procurement Eligibility: Small Business
Distribution: Exclusive Distributor
General Admin.: Roberta Berkowitz/Executive Vice President
Mktg./Adv.: Renee Carmen/Director Marketing
  Component, Electronic General
  Paper, Photographic General

NATIONAL HANSEN'S DISEASE PROGRAMS 225-756-3740
1770 Physicians Park Drive, Baton Rouge, LA 70816
FDA Number: 2317053
  Esthesiometer Cns/Neurology

NATIONAL HEALTHCARE MANUFACTURING CORP.
See Great Midwest Packaging, Llc

NATIONAL HOME PRODUCTS LTD. 416-661-2770
188 Limestone Crescent, Toronto, ONT M3J 2S4 Canada
FDA Number: 9680262 *Fax:* 416-661-8807
E-mail: nhp@nathome.com
Year Founded: 1960
Total Employees: 24 *Sales Staff:* 2
Ownership: Private
Produces/Sells CE-marked Devices: N
Distribution: Manufacturer Direct, Exclusive Distributor, Importer

NATIONAL IMPLANT REGISTRY, THE
See Medicalert Foundation International

NATIONAL INSTITUTE OF STANDARDS & TECHNOLOGY 301-975-6776
100 Bureau Drive, Stop 2322, Bldg. 202, Rm. 204, Gaithersburg, MD 20899
FDA Number: n/a *Fax:* 301-948-3730
E-mail: inquiries@nist.gov
Web site: http://www.nist.gov/public_affairs/contact.htm
Annual Revenue: $0-$1 Million
Total Employees: 3500 *Marketing Staff:* 5 *Sales Staff:* 5
Ownership: Private
Produces/Sells CE-marked Devices: N
Distribution: Manufacturer Direct, Service Direct, Exporter

NATIONAL INSTITUTE OF STANDARDS & 301-975-6776 *(cont'd)*
Mktg./Adv.: Lee Best/Manager Advertising
  Lee Best/Vice President Marketing
Research: Nancy Trahey/Vice President Research & Development
  Buffer, pH Hematology

NATIONAL INSTRUMENT CO., INC. 866-258-1914
4119 Fordleigh Rd., Baltimore, MD 21215-2214 410-764-0900
FDA Number: 9200779 *Fax:* 410-764-7719
E-mail: www.info@filamatic.com
Web site: www.filamatic.com
Annual Revenue: $5-$10 Million
Total Employees: 95 *Marketing Staff:* 5 *Sales Staff:* 9
Ownership: Private
Quality System Registration Information: ISO9002
Produces/Sells CE-marked Devices: Y
Federal Procurement Eligibility: Small Business
Distribution: Manufacturer Direct, Manufacturer Through Manufacturer Reps
General Admin.: Robert Rosen/President, Chief Executive Officer
  Dispenser, Fluid General
  General Medical Device General
  Pipetting And Diluting System, Automated Chemistry
  Sealer, Packaging General

NATIONAL INSTRUMENT LLC 866-258-1914
4119 Fordleigh Road, Baltimore, MD 21215 410-764-0900
FDA Number: 1120551 *Fax:* 410-764-7719
E-mail: info@filamatic.com
Web site: www.filamatic.com
Medical Products Sales Volume: $4,500,000
Annual Revenue: $5-$10 Million
Year Founded: 1950
Total Employees: 60
Ownership: Private
Produces/Sells CE-marked Devices: Y
Federal Procurement Eligibility: Small Business
Distribution: Manufacturer Direct
Mktg./Adv.: Ms. Mary Burchard/Supervisor Marketing & Sales
  Dispenser, Other General
  Packaging Equipment General
  Production Equipment General

NATIONAL KEYSTONE 856-663-4700
616 Hollywood Ave., Cherry Hill, NJ 08002-2821
FDA Number: n/a *Fax:* 856-663-0381
E-mail: lkramer@keystoneind.com
Web site: www.keystoneind.com
Total Employees: 70 *Marketing Staff:* 3
Ownership: Private
Quality System Registration Information: ISO9000
Produces/Sells CE-marked Devices: N
Distribution: Manufacturer Through Distributor
General Admin.: Fred Robinson/Chief Executive Officer
  Cary Robinson/President
Mktg./Adv.: Michael B. Prozzillo/Manager International & National Sales
  Gloria Berger/Vice President Sales
  Injector, Hand-Held Radiology

NATIONAL LABNET COMPANY
See Labnet International

NATIONAL LABS, INC.
See Medstat Inc.

NATIONAL MEDICAL PRODUCTS 800-940-6262
9775 Mining Drive, #104, Jacksonville, FL 32257 904-288-8509
FDA Number: 7000667 *Fax:* 904-288-8501
E-mail: julienatmed@aol.com
Web site: www.posiblock.com
Year Founded: 1978
Total Employees: 5 *Marketing Staff:* 2 *Sales Staff:* 2
Ownership: Private
Produces/Sells CE-marked Devices: N
Federal Procurement Eligibility: Small Business, VA Contract
Distribution: Manufacturer Direct, Manufacturer Through Distributor, Manufacturer Through Manufacturer Reps, Service Direct
General Admin.: Larry Thigpen/President
  Julie Thigpen/Vice President, General Manager
Mktg./Adv.: Julie Thigpen/Director Marketing
  Julie Thigpen/Director Product Development
  Julie Thigpen/Manager National Sales
Production: Dale Schock/Director Quality Assurance & Regulatory Affairs
  Dale Schock/Manager Materials
  Contract Manufacturing General
  Elevator, Other General
  Pad, Pressure, Foam (Elbow, Heel) General
  Support, Patient Position Anesthesiology

NATIONAL MEDICAL PRODUCTS, INC.   949-768-1147
57 Parker St., Irvine, CA 92618
FDA Number: 2027063
  Injector, Fluid, Non-Electric   General

NATIONAL NONWOVENS   800-333-3469
P.O. Box 150, Easthampton, MA 01027-0150   413-527-3445
FDA Number: n/a   Fax: 413-527-9570
Web site: www.nationalnonwovens.com
Year Founded: 1905
Total Employees: 500
Ownership: Private
Produces/Sells CE-marked Devices: N
Federal Procurement Eligibility: Small Business
Distribution: Manufacturer Direct
General Admin.: Anthony J. Centofanti/President, Chief Executive Officer
Mktg./Adv.: Conrad D'Elie/Director Product Development
  Felt   Surgery
  Floor Mat   General
  Floor Mat, Antibacterial   General
  Formalin, Neutral Buffered   Pathology
  Table, Autopsy   Pathology

NATIONAL OPTICAL CO.
See Marcolin Usa

NATIONAL OPTRONICS   434-295-9126
100 Avon St., Charlottesville, VA 22902
FDA Number: 3004285005
Ownership: Private
Produces/Sells CE-marked Devices: N
  Chart, Visual Acuity   Ophthalmology
  Tester, Color Vision   Ophthalmology

NATIONAL OPTRONICS, INC.   800-247-9796
100 Avon St., Charlottesville, VA 22902   800-866-5640
FDA Number: n/a   Fax: 804-295-7799
E-mail: mfries@nationaloptronics.com
Web site: www.nationaloptronics.com
Ownership: Private
Produces/Sells CE-marked Devices: N
  System, Identification, Lens, Contact   Ophthalmology

NATIONAL ORTHOTIC LABORATORIES, INC.
See Medstat Inc.

NATIONAL PATIENT CARE SYSTEMS, INC.
See Pyramid Industries, Llc

NATIONAL PRECISION INSTRUMENTS   215-355-7525
1621 Loretta Ave., Unit #4, Feasterville, PA 19053
FDA Number: 3004755041
  Pliers, Orthodontic   Dental And Oral

NATIONAL REFRIG. & AIR CONDITIONING PRODUCTS, INC
See Continental Scientific

NATIONAL STARCH & CHEMICAL CO.   317-656-2227
1001 Bedford Ave., North Kansas City, MO 64116
FDA Number: 1912227
Web site: www.nationalstarch.com
Ownership: Private
Produces/Sells CE-marked Devices: N
  Dusting Powder, Surgical   Surgery

NATIONAL SUPER SERVICE CO.
See Nss Enterprises, Inc.

NATIONAL SYSTEMS CO.   877-672-4278
31B Durward Pl., Waterloo N2J 3Z9 Canada   519-884-0270
FDA Number: n/a   Fax: 519-884-0279
E-mail: wpearen@attglobal.net
Web site: /www.nationalsystems.ca
Medical Products Sales Volume: $500,000
Total Employees: 4   Marketing Staff: 1   Sales Staff: 3
Ownership: Private
Produces/Sells CE-marked Devices: N
Federal Procurement Eligibility: Small Business
Distribution: Manufacturer Through Distributor, Exporter

NATIONAL VIDEO SERVICES, INC.   203-270-0677
18 Commerce Road, Newtown, CT 06470-1607
FDA Number: n/a   Fax: 203-270-9619
E-mail: sales@intermedvideo.com
Web site: www.intermedvideo.com
Medical Products Sales Volume: $670,000
Year Founded: 1990
Total Employees: 7   Sales Staff: 2
Ownership: Private
Produces/Sells CE-marked Devices: N
Federal Procurement Eligibility: Small Business
Distribution: OEM

NATIONAL VIDEO SERVICES, INC.   203-270-0677 *(cont'd)*
IS: Bob Strong/Tech. Specialist
  Recorder, Radiographic Video Tape   Radiology

NATIONAL VISION, INC.   800-637-3597
296 Grayson Hwy., Attn: Legal/C. Mingle,   770-822-3600
Lawrenceville, GA 30045
FDA Number: 1062202   Fax: 770-822-3601
E-mail: nve@nationalvision.com
Web site: www.nationalvision.com
Medical Products Sales Volume: $216,700,000
Annual Revenue: $100-$500 Million
Year Founded: 1990
Total Employees: 2547   Marketing Staff: 6
Ownership: Private
Produces/Sells CE-marked Devices: N
General Admin.: Mr. Reade Fass/Chief Executive Officer
     Mr. Chuck Criscillis/Chief Financial Officer, Senior Vice President
     Mr. L. Reade Fahs, Jr./President
     Mr. Mitchell Goodman/Senior Vice President, General Counsel
Production: Mr. Desmond Taylor/Senior Vice President Manufacturing
Finance: Mr. Bob Schnelle/Vice President Finance, Treasurer
  Lens, Spectacle/Eyeglasses, Non-Custom   Ophthalmology

NATIONAL WELDERS   919-544-3772
630 United Dr., Durham, NC 27713
FDA Number: 1054016
  Console, Heart-Lung Machine, Cardiopulmonary Bypass   Cardiovascular
  Electrode, Blood pH   Chemistry

NATIONAL WIRE & STAMPING, INC.
See Instrumed Oem

NATIONWIDE FLASHING SIGNAL SYSTEMS, INC.
See Assisted Access-Nfss, Inc.

NATRACARE, LLC   303-617-3476
14901 E. Hampden Avenue, Suite 190, Aurora, CO 80014
FDA Number: 1722618   Fax: 303-617-3495
E-mail: info@natracare.com
Web site: www.natracare.com
Annual Revenue: $1-$5 Million
Year Founded: 1989
Total Employees: 1
Ownership: Private
Produces/Sells CE-marked Devices: N
Federal Procurement Eligibility: Small Business, Female Owned
Distribution: Manufacturer Through Distributor
  Pad, Menstrual, Unscented   Obstetrics/Gynecology
  Tampon, Menstrual, Unscented   Obstetrics/Gynecology

NATURAL WONDERS CA INC.   818-341-7007
21011 Itasca Street, Suite E, Chatsworth, CA 91311
FDA Number: 3005723288
  Pack, Hot Or Cold, Reusable   Physical Med
  Pack, Moist Heat   Physical Med

NATURE'S WAY THERAPEUTIC PRODUCTS, INC.   604-921-2601
91021-1427 Bellevue Ave, West Vancouver V7T 1C3 Canada
FDA Number: 9613750
  Pack, Hot Or Cold, Reusable   Physical Med

NATUS MEDICAL INC.   800-255-3901
1501 Industrial Road, San Carlos, CA 94070   650-802-0400
FDA Number: 2938854   Fax: 650-802-0401
E-mail: customer_service@natus.com
Web site: www.natus.com
Medical Products Sales Volume: $89,900,000
Year Founded: 1987
Total Employees: 364   Marketing Staff: 7   Sales Staff: 21
Ownership: Public
Stock Symbol: BABY
Traded On: NASDAQ
Quality System Registration Information: ISO9001
Produces/Sells CE-marked Devices: Y
Federal Procurement Eligibility: Small Business
Distribution: Manufacturer Direct
General Admin.: James Hawkins/President, Chief Executive Officer
  Medical Admin.: Dr. D. Christopher Chung/Vice President Medical Affairs
Mktg./Adv.: Kenneth Traverso/Vice President Sales
Production: William Mince/Vice President Operations
Finance: Steven Murphy/Chief Financial Officer, Vice President Finance
  Analyzer, Gas, Carbon-Monoxide, Gaseous Phase   Anesthesiology
  Evoked Response Unit, Auditory   Ear/Nose/Throat
  Light, Bilirubin (Phototherapy)   General
  Protector, Hearing (Circumaural)   Ear/Nose/Throat
Medical Product Subsidiaries (Listed Separately)
  Excel Tech. Ltd.
  Neometrics, A Division Of Natus

NATUS MEDICAL INC.   800-255-3901 (cont'd)
Olympic Medical Corp.

NAUTILUS SPORTS/MEDICAL INDUSTRIES
See Nautilus, Inc.

NAUTILUS, INC.   360-859-2900
16400 SE Nautilus Drive, Vancouver, WA 98683
FDA Number: n/a   Fax: 360-694-7755
E-mail: sales@nautilus.com
Web site: www.nautilus.com
Medical Products Sales Volume: $680,300,000
Year Founded: 1986
Total Employees: 1500
Ownership: The Nautilus Group, Inc.
Stock Symbol: NLS
Traded On: NYSE
Produces/Sells CE-marked Devices: N
Federal Procurement Eligibility: GSA Contract
Distribution: Manufacturer Direct, Manufacturer Through Distributor, Manufacturer Through Manufacturer Reps, Service Direct
Mktg./Adv.: Ms. Caroline Howe/Vice President Marketing
Finance: Mr. Kenneth Fish/Chief Financial Officer

Component, Exercise	Physical Med
Equipment, Therapy, Handicapped/Physical	Physical Med
Exercise Stair	Physical Med
Exerciser, Bicycle	Physical Med
Exerciser, Chest	Physical Med
Exerciser, Isorobic	Physical Med
Exerciser, Measuring	Physical Med
Exerciser, Non-Measuring	Physical Med
Monitor, Physiological, Stress Exercise	Cardiovascular

NAVILYST MEDICAL   877.658.7990
26 Forest Street, Marlborough, MA 01752   508.658.7990
FDA Number: 1317056
Web site: www.navilystmedical.com
Year Founded: 2008
Total Employees: 800
Ownership: Private
Produces/Sells CE-marked Devices: N
General Admin.: Ron Sparks/Chief Executive Officer

Accessories, Catheter	Surgery
Adapter, Stopcock, Manifold, Cardiopulmonary Bypass	Cardiovascular
Cable, Electrode	Physical Med
Catheter, Angioplasty, Transluminal, Peripheral	Cardiovascular
Catheter, Balloon (Foley Type)	Surgery
Catheter, Cholangiography	Surgery
Catheter, Hemodialysis, Implanted	Gastroenterology/Urology
Catheter, Intravascular, Diagnostic	Cardiovascular
Catheter, Intravascular, Therapeutic, Long-term Greater Than 30 Days	General
Catheter, Intravascular, Therapeutic, Short-term Less Than 30 Days	General
Catheter, Subcutaneous Intravascular, Implanted	General
Catheter, Urological	Gastroenterology/Urology
Dilator, Vessel, Percutaneous Catheterization	Cardiovascular
Electrode, Pacemaker, Temporary	Cardiovascular
Endoscope	Gastroenterology/Urology
Filter, Intravascular, Cardiovascular	Cardiovascular
Grid, Radiographic	Radiology
Guide, Catheter	Cardiovascular
Guidewire, Catheter	Cardiovascular
Injector, Angiographic (Cardiac Catheterization)	Cardiovascular
Introducer, Catheter	Cardiovascular
Kit, Administration, Intravenous	General
Kit, Biopsy Needle	Gastroenterology/Urology
Kit, Biopsy, Gastro-Urology	Gastroenterology/Urology
Monitor, Line Isolation	Cardiovascular
Needle, Hypodermic, Single Lumen With Syringe	General
Oxygenator, Cardiopulmonary Bypass	Cardiovascular
Radiographic/Fluoroscopic Unit, Angiographic	Radiology
Set, Administration, Intravenous, Needle-Free	General
Surgical Instrument, Cardiovascular	Cardiovascular
Syringe, Balloon Inflation	Cardiovascular
Transducer, Blood Pressure, Extravascular	Cardiovascular

NAVISCAN INC.   858-587-3641
6865 Flanders Dr., Suite B, San Diego, CA 92121
FDA Number: 3005945241   Fax: 858-587-2596
E-mail: inquiries@naviscan.com
Web site: www.naviscan.com
Year Founded: 1995
Ownership: Private
Produces/Sells CE-marked Devices: N
General Admin.: Paul Mirabella/Chief Executive Officer, Chairman
　　Larry Lugo/Chief Operating Officer
Medical Admin.: Judy Kalinyak/Chief Medical Officer
Mktg./Adv.: Mr. Gary Seelhorst/Vice President Business Development
　　Guillaume Bailliard/Vice President Marketing
　　Skip Mendelson/Vice President Sales

NAVISCAN INC.   858-587-3641 (cont'd)
Finance: Mr. R. Gary Gilmore/Chief Financial Officer
　　Kathleen Winer/Vice President Finance

Scanner, Emission Computed Tomography	Radiology
System, Communication, Image, Digital	Radiology

NAVISCAN PET SYSTEMS
See Naviscan Inc.

NAVITAR, INC.   800-828-6778
200 Commerce Drive, Rochester, NY 14623   585-359-4000
FDA Number: n/a   Fax: 585-359-4999
E-mail: info@navitar.com
Web site: www.navitar.com/
Medical Products Sales Volume: $23,300,000
Annual Revenue: $10-$25 Million
Year Founded: 1994
Total Employees: 56
Ownership: Private
Federal Procurement Eligibility: Small Business
Distribution: Manufacturer Through Manufacturer Reps
General Admin.: Tom McCune/Chief Operating Officer
　　Jeremy Goldstein/President
Mktg./Adv.: Rosemary Kelly/Director Marketing
　　Rosemary Kelly/Manager Advertising

Camera, Microscope	Microbiology
Lens, Other	Ophthalmology

NBC PRODUCTS, INC.   952-226-1112
16873 Fish Point Road, Prior Lake, MN 55372
FDA Number: 3004531513
Ownership: Private
Produces/Sells CE-marked Devices: N

Purifier, Air, Ultraviolet	General

NBM LLC   502-895-7503
2604 River Green Circle, Louisville, KY 40206
FDA Number: 3005893095
Ownership: Private
Produces/Sells CE-marked Devices: N

Brush, Scrub, Operating Room	Surgery

NBN PRODUCTS, L.L.C.   800-792-9795
1310 Amesbury Avenue, Liberty, MO 64068
FDA Number: 3004129952

Pick, Microsurgical Ear	Ear/Nose/Throat

NBS MEDICAL PRODUCTS INC.   888-800-8192
257 Livingston Ave., New Brunswick, NJ 08901   732-745-8192
FDA Number: 2249651   Fax: 732-745-1192
E-mail: info@nbsmedical.com
Web site: www.nbsmedical.com
Medical Products Sales Volume: $2,000,000
Annual Revenue: $1-$5 Million
Total Employees: 50   *Marketing Staff:* 4   *Sales Staff:* 4
Ownership: NBS GROUP SUPPLY
Quality System Registration Information: ISO9002
Produces/Sells CE-marked Devices: N
Federal Procurement Eligibility: Small Business
Distribution: Importer
General Admin.: Osman Boraie/President, Chief Executive Officer
Mktg./Adv.: Sam Owen/Manager Market Research
　　Charles E. Meisch/Vice President Marketing & Sales
Production: Tom Enns/Vice President Operations
Research: Charles E. Meisch/Vice President Research & Development

Accessories, Catheter, G-U	Gastroenterology/Urology
Dressing, Wound and Burn, Hydrogel	Surgery
Endoscope And Accessories, AC-Powered	Surgery
Media, Filter	General

NBS TECHNOLOGIES INC.   800-524-0419
70 Eisenhower Drive, Paramus, NJ 07652   201-845-7373
FDA Number: n/a   Fax: 201-845-3337
E-mail: info@nbstech.com
Web site: www.nbstech.com
Medical Products Sales Volume: $56,600,000
Annual Revenue: $25-$50 Million
Year Founded: 1974
Total Employees: 222   *Marketing Staff:* 3   *Sales Staff:* 32
Ownership: NBS TECHNOLOGIES, INC.
Stock Symbol: NBS
Traded On: Toronto
Produces/Sells CE-marked Devices: N
Federal Procurement Eligibility: Small Business, GSA Contract
Distribution: Manufacturer Direct, Manufacturer Through Distributor
Mktg./Adv.: Dianne Rychlewski/Director Marketing & Public Relations
　　Mike Utsal/Executive Vice President Sales
　　Joe Gulics/Vice President Sales

Bracelet, Identification	General

NBS TECHNOLOGIES INC.   800-524-0419 *(cont'd)*

Image Processing System	Radiology
Labeling Equipment	General
Printer, Bar Code	General

NCH CORPORATION   1-800-527-9929

ATTN: Marketing Department, 5N   **972-438-0211**
P.O. Box 152170
Irving, TX 75015
FDA Number: n/a   *Fax:* 972-438-0634
Web site: www.nch.com
Year Founded: 1919
Total Employees: 8500
Ownership: Private
Produces/Sells CE-marked Devices: N
Cleaner, Medical Device   General

NCONTACT INC.   919-466-9810

1001 Aviation Parkway, Suite 400, Morrisville, NC 27560
FDA Number: 3006142617   *Fax:* 919-466-9811
E-mail: info@ncontactsurgical.com
Web site: www.ncontactinc.com
Year Founded: 2005
Ownership: Private
Produces/Sells CE-marked Devices: N
General Admin.: Dr. Michael S. Estes/Chairman
     John P. Funkhouser/President, Chief Executive Officer
Mktg./Adv.: Mr. Edgar Rey/Vice President Marketing & Sales
Production: Ms. Jane Ricupero/Director Quality Control & Regulatory Affairs
Research: Mr. Sidney Fleischman/Vice President Development
     Mr. Jim Whayne/Vice President Research
Finance: Ms. Nathalie Greene/Vice President Finance

Cannula, Surgical, General & Plastic Surgery	Surgery
Electrosurgical Unit, Cutting & Coagulation Device	Surgery
Surgical Device, For Ablation Of Cardiac Tissue	Surgery

NCONTACT SURGICAL, INC.

See nContact Inc.

NCR CORP.   800-225-5627

1700 S. Patterson Blvd., Dayton, OH 45479-0001   **937-445-1936**
FDA Number: n/a
Web site: www.ncr.com
Annual Revenue: More than $1 Billion
Year Founded: 1884
Total Employees: 22400
Ownership: Public
Stock Symbol: NCR
Traded On: NYSE
Quality System Registration Information: ISO9002
Produces/Sells CE-marked Devices: Y
Distribution: Manufacturer Direct, Importer, Exporter
General Admin.: Lars Nyberg/President
Computer Equipment   General

NCR CORP./MED. SYSTEMS DEPT.

See Ncr Corp.

NCS MEDICAL INCORPORATED   800-661-5005

5421 8B Ave., Delta, BC V4M-1V5 Canada   **604-948-0779**
FDA Number: n/a   *Fax:* 604-948-0116
E-mail: ncs@ncsmedical.com
Web site: www.ncsmedical.com
Year Founded: 1989
Total Employees: 10
Ownership: Private
Produces/Sells CE-marked Devices: N
Distribution: Exclusive Distributor, Importer

NDI MEDICAL, INC.   216-378-9106

22901 Millcreek Blvd.,, Suite 110, Cleveland, OH 44122
FDA Number: 3004061992
E-mail: info@ndimedical.com
Web site: www.ndimedical.com
Year Founded: 2002
Ownership: Medtronic, Inc.
Stock Symbol: MDT
Traded On: NYSE
Produces/Sells CE-marked Devices: N
General Admin.: Robert Blankenship/Executive Vice President
     Geoffrey Thrope/President, Chief Executive Officer
Medical Admin.: Maria Bennett/Vice President Clinical Affairs
Production: Julie H. Grill/Vice President Regulatory Affairs
Research: Bob Strother/Vice President Engineering
Stimulator, Nerve, ENT   Ear/Nose/Throat

NDO SURGICAL, INC.   877-337-8887

125 High St.,, Suite 7, Mansfield, MA 02048
FDA Number: 1226693

NDO SURGICAL, INC.   877-337-8887 *(cont'd)*

Ownership: Private
Produces/Sells CE-marked Devices: N
Endoscope   Gastroenterology/Urology

NDS SURGICAL IMAGING, INC.   866-637-5237

5750 Hellyer Ave, San Jose, CA 95138   **408-776-0085**
FDA Number: 2954921   *Fax:* 408-776-9878
E-mail: info@ndssi.com
Web site: www.ndssi.com
Annual Revenue: $50-$100 Million
Year Founded: 1996
Ownership: Private
Quality System Registration Information: ISO9001; ISO9002
Produces/Sells CE-marked Devices: Y
Distribution: Manufacturer Direct, Manufacturer Through Distributor, OEM, Service Direct
General Admin.: Mr. Daniel Berry/Chief Executive Officer
     Mr. Sam Brown/Chief Financial Officer, Executive Vice President
     Ron Hansen/Chief Technology Officer
     Katia Bejan/Vice President Human Resources
     Kees Poot/Vice President, General Manager
Mktg./Adv.: Mr. Brent Michaels/Vice President Sales
Production: Trina Ciraulo/Vice President Operations
Finance: Steve Tomei/Controller

Accessories, Operating Room, Table	Surgery
Accessories, Surgical Camera	Surgery
Camera, Television, Endoscopic (With Audio)	Surgery
Camera, Television, Surgical (With Audio)	Surgery
Camera, Television, Surgical (Without Audio)	Surgery
Computer, Radiographic Image Analysis	Radiology
Drape, Surgical, Disposable	Surgery
Image Processing System	Radiology
System, Communication, Image, Digital	Radiology

NEARLY ME

See Spenco Medical Corp.

NEARLY ME TECHNOLOGIES, INC.   800-887-3370

3630 South I 35, Suite A, Waco, TX 76706   **254-662-1752**
FDA Number: 1650562   *Fax:* 254-662-1760
E-mail: info@nearlymetech.com
Web site: www.nearlyme.org
Medical Products Sales Volume: $3,750,000
Year Founded: 1976
Total Employees: 44
Ownership: Private
Produces/Sells CE-marked Devices: Y
Federal Procurement Eligibility: Small Business
Distribution: Manufacturer Direct, OEM

Adhesive, Prosthesis, External	Surgery
Bandage, Adhesive	Surgery
Elastomer, Silicone (Scar Management)	Surgery
Prosthesis, Breast, External	Surgery
Protector, Skin Pressure	General
Shield, Nipple	Obstetrics/Gynecology

NEEDLE AID, LTD.   902-895-8015

23 Lower Truro Rd, Truro B2N 5A9 Canada
FDA Number: 9615825
Transfer Aid   Physical Med

NEEDLE TECHNOLOGIES, INC.

See Avid Medical

NEGAFILE SYSTEMS   800-523-5474

1560 Industry Road, Hatfield, PA 19440   **215-412-8400**
FDA Number: 2094042   *Fax:* 215-412-8450
E-mail: sgkcck@aol.com
Web site: www.negafile.com
Medical Products Sales Volume: $1,000,000
Annual Revenue: $0-$1 Million
Year Founded: 1998
Total Employees: 100
Ownership: Private
Federal Procurement Eligibility: Small Business
Distribution: Manufacturer Direct, Service Direct
General Admin.: Peter Goodman/President
Mktg./Adv.: Peter Goodman/Vice President Marketing & Sales
Production: Christopher Goodman/Vice President Manufacturing

Cabinet, Storage, Slide	General
Storage Unit, X-Ray Film	Radiology

NEKTAR THERAPEUTICS   650-631-3100

150 Industrial Road, San Carlos, CA 94070
FDA Number: 3003905156   *Fax:* 650-631-3150
E-mail: NektarSC@nektar.com
Web site: www.nektar.com
Year Founded: 1990
Total Employees: 793

NEKTAR THERAPEUTICS   650-631-3100 (cont'd)
Ownership: Public
Stock Symbol: NKTR
Traded On: NASDAQ
Produces/Sells CE-marked Devices: N
General Admin.: Bharatt Chowrira/Chief Operating Officer
    Gil M Labrucherie/General Counsel
    Howard W Robin/President, Chief Executive Officer
    Nevan Elam/Senior Vice President
Mktg./Adv.: Rinko Ghosh/Senior Vice President Business Development
Inhaler, Nasal   Ear/Nose/Throat

NELLCOR AND PURITAN BENNETT/TYCO HEALTHCARE
See Covidien (Formerly Nellcor Puritan Bennett / Tyco Healthcare)

NELLCOR INC.
See Covidien (Formerly Nellcor Puritan Bennett / Tyco Healthcare)

NELLCOR PURITAN BENNETT
See Covidien (Formerly Nellcor Puritan Bennett / Tyco Healthcare)

NELLCOR PURITAN BENNETT
See Mallinckrodt, Inc.

NELLCOR PURITAN BENNETT (MELVILLE) LTD.   613-238-1840
700-141 Laurier Ave W, Ottawa K1P 5J3 Canada
FDA Number: 9680138
Amplifier, Physiological Signal   Cns/Neurology
Conditioner, Signal, Physiological   Cns/Neurology

NELLCOR PURITAN-BENNETT
See Covidien (Formerly Nellcor Puritan Bennett / Tyco Healthcare)

NELLCOR, INC.
See Mallinckrodt, Inc.

NELSON ENVIRONMENTAL TECHNOLOGIES, INC.   956-618-0375
813 E. Fir, Mcallen, TX 78501
FDA Number: 1651434   *Fax:* 956-618-4330
E-mail: Info@nelsonenvironmentaltechnologies.com
Web site: www.nelsonenvironmentaltechnologies.com
Year Founded: 1994
Ownership: Private
Produces/Sells CE-marked Devices: N
Purification System, Water   Gastroenterology/Urology

NELSON INC., A.R.   800-377-6625
35-55 Scarlett Oak Blvd., St. Louis, MO 63122   **636-225-4700**
FDA Number: n/a   *Fax:* 636-225-9090
Web site: www.arnelson.com
Medical Products Sales Volume: $1,000,000
Total Employees: 8
Ownership: Private
Produces/Sells CE-marked Devices: N
General Admin.: Ned Golterman/President
Curtain, Cubicle   General
Curtain, Shower   General
Track And Carrier, Cubicle Curtain   General
Track And Carrier, Intravenous   General

NELSON PROSTHETIC & ORTHOTIC LABORATORY   716-894-6666
2959 Genesee St., Cheektowaga, NY 14225-2653
FDA Number: n/a   *Fax:* 716-894-1858
E-mail: info@nelsonpando.com
Web site: www.nelsonpando.com
Annual Revenue: $0-$1 Million
Ownership: Private
Produces/Sells CE-marked Devices: Y
Federal Procurement Eligibility: Small Business
Distribution: Manufacturer Direct
General Admin.: John Helper/Vice President
Medical Admin.: Donald House/CO
    Joyelle Krysztof/CO
    Daniel J. Wojcik/CPO
    Christopher Van Dusen/President, CPO
Mktg./Adv.: Lisa Marek/Admin. Advertising
Custom Prosthesis   Orthopedics
Insoles, Medical   General
Orthosis, Limb Brace   Physical Med
Orthosis, Lumbar   Physical Med
Support, Arch   Physical Med

NELSON RESEARCH & DEVELOPMENT CO.
See UCB Inc.

NEMCO INC.
See Nemcomed

NEMCOMED   800-255-4576
8727 Clinton Park Drive, Fort Wayne, IN 46825   **419-542-7743**
FDA Number: 3006128100   *Fax:* 419-542-8931

NEMCOMED   800-255-4576 (cont'd)
E-mail: jpritchard@nemcomedical.com
Web site: www.nemcomed.com
Medical Products Sales Volume: $8,600,000
Annual Revenue: $10-$25 Million
Year Founded: 1976
Total Employees: 125   *Marketing Staff:* 3   *Sales Staff:* 3
Ownership: Advantis Medical
Produces/Sells CE-marked Devices: Y
Federal Procurement Eligibility: Small Business
Distribution: Manufacturer Direct, OEM
General Admin.: Kevin Countryman/President, Chief Executive Officer
    Janis Edwards/Vice President Human Resources
Mktg./Adv.: Greg Stalcup/Director Product Development
    Jim Pritchard/Manager International & National Sales
    Jim Pritchard/Vice President Marketing
    Jim Pritchard/Vice President Sales
Production: Charles Miller/Director Quality Assurance
    Mark Bissell/Vice President Manufacturing
Research: Greg Stalcup/Vice President Research & Development
Contract Manufacturing   General
Contract R&D, Equipment   General
Driver, Prosthesis   Orthopedics
Orthopedic Manual Surgical Instrument   Orthopedics
Prosthesis Implantation Instrument, Orthopedic   Orthopedics
Retractor   Orthopedics
Splint, Molded, Aluminum   Orthopedics

NEMOTO MEDICAL U.S., INC.   949-863-9395
24992 Del Monte St, Laguna Hills, CA 92653-5617
FDA Number: n/a   *Fax:* 949-863-9399
E-mail: info@nemotous.com
Web site: www.nemotous.com/
Medical Products Sales Volume: $1,000,000
Total Employees: 5
Ownership: Private
Produces/Sells CE-marked Devices: N
Federal Procurement Eligibility: Small Business
Injector, Angiographic (Cardiac Catheterization)   Cardiovascular

NEO MEDICAL INC.   888-450-3334
42514 Albrea Street, Fremont, CA 94538
FDA Number: 2925153
Ownership: Private
Produces/Sells CE-marked Devices: N
Accessories, Catheter   Surgery
Catheter, Intraspinal, Percutaneous, Short-Term   General
Catheter, Intravascular, Therapeutic, Long-term Greater Than 30 Days   General
Catheter, Intravascular, Therapeutic, Short-term Less Than 30 Days   General
Catheter, Percutaneous   Cardiovascular
Catheter, Rectal   Surgery
Catheter, Subcutaneous Intravascular, Implanted   General
Collector, Specimen   Microbiology
Condom   Obstetrics/Gynecology
Dilator, Vessel, Surgical   Cardiovascular
Fertility Diagnostic Device   Obstetrics/Gynecology
Introducer, Catheter   Cardiovascular
Introducer, Syringe Needle   General
Kit, Anesthesia, Conduction   Anesthesiology
Locator, Bleeding, Gastrointestinal, String And Tube   Gastroenterology/Urology
Needle, Conduction, Anesthesia (W/Wo Introducer)   Anesthesiology
Port & Catheter, Infusion, Implanted, Subcut., Intraperit.   General
Stimulator, Nerve, Battery-Powered   Anesthesiology
Stimulator, Nerve, ENT   Ear/Nose/Throat
Tube, Double Lumen For Intestinal Decompression   Gastroenterology/Urology
Tube, Drainage   Gastroenterology/Urology
Tube, Feeding   General
Tube, Gastrointestinal   Gastroenterology/Urology

NEO METRICS, INC.   763-559-4440
Fernbrook Lane N, Suite J, Minneapolis, MN 55447
FDA Number: 2135342
Guidewire, Catheter   Cardiovascular

NEO PHARM INC.   714-226-0070
10532 Walker St., Suite #b, Cypress, CA 90630
FDA Number: 2090154
Ownership: Private
Produces/Sells CE-marked Devices: N
Enzymatic Method, Glucose (Urinary, Non-Quantitative)   Chemistry
Enzyme Immunoassay, Cocaine And Cocaine Metabolites   Toxicology
Enzyme Immunoassay, Opiates   Toxicology
Kit, Pregnancy Test, Over The Counter, HCG   Chemistry
Nitroprusside, Ketones (Urinary, Non-Quantitative)   Chemistry

NEO-CARE ARROW INTERNATIONAL   800-640-6428
5714 Epsilon Rd., San Antonio, TX 78249-3407   **210-696-4061**
FDA Number: n/a   *Fax:* 210-696-1305
E-mail: neocarekb@aol.com
Web site: www.neocare.com

NEO-CARE ARROW INTERNATIONAL 800-640-6428 (cont'd)
Annual Revenue: $5-$10 Million
Year Founded: 1994
Total Employees: 40
Ownership: Private
Produces/Sells CE-marked Devices: N
Federal Procurement Eligibility: Small Business
Distribution: Manufacturer Through Distributor, Manufacturer Through Manufacturer Reps
General Admin.: Clyde Baker/Executive Vice President
James K. Klein/President

Catheter, Intravascular, Therapeutic, Long-term Greater Than 30 Days	General
Catheter, Intravascular, Therapeutic, Short-term Less Than 30 Days	General
Catheter, Straight	Gastroenterology/Urology
Tube, Gastrointestinal	Gastroenterology/Urology

NEO-FLO, INC.
See Microcopy, Div. Neo-Flo, Inc.

NEO-GENESIS, A DIVISION OF NATUS 503-657-8000
15140 SE 82nd Drive, Suite 270, Clackamas, OR 97015
FDA Number: 3026271
Ownership: NATUS MEDICAL INC.
Stock Symbol: BABY
Traded On: NASDAQ
Produces/Sells CE-marked Devices: N

Enzymatic Method, Galactose	Chemistry
Enzyme Immunoassay, Non-Radiolabeled, Total Thyroxine	Chemistry
Ninhydrin And L-Leucyl-L-Alanine (Fluorimetric)	Chemistry
Radioimmunoassay, 17-Hydroxyprogesterone	Chemistry
Radioimmunoassay, Thyroid Stimulating Hormone	Chemistry
Radioimmunoassay, Total Thyroxine	Chemistry

NEOCOIL, LLC 262-347-1250
N27 W23910a Paul Rd., Pewaukee, WI 53072
FDA Number: 3006369484

Coil, Magnetic Resonance, Specialty	Radiology

NEOGEMICS LABORATIES 866-776-5907
12701 Commonwealth Drive, Suite 5, 239-768-0600
Fort Myers, FL 33913
FDA Number: n/a   *Fax:* 239-768-0711
Ownership: Public
Stock Symbol: NGNM
Traded On: OTC Bulletin
Produces/Sells CE-marked Devices: N
General Admin.: Mr. Douglas Van Oort/Chief Executive Officer
Mr. Robert Gasparini/Chief Scientific Officer
Mktg./Adv.: Mr. Grant Carlson/Vice President Marketing & Sales
Finance: Mr. George Cardoza/Chief Financial Officer
Mr. Steven Jones/Executive Vice President Finance

NEOGEN CORPORATION 800-234-5333
620 Lesher Place, Lansing, MI 48912 517-372-9200
FDA Number: n/a   *Fax:* 517-372-2006
E-mail: foodsafety@neogen.com
Web site: http://www.neogen.com
Annual Revenue: $50-$100 Million
Year Founded: 1982
Total Employees: 447
Ownership: Public
Stock Symbol: NEOG
Traded On: NASDAQ
Quality System Registration Information: ISO9001
Produces/Sells CE-marked Devices: N
Federal Procurement Eligibility: Small Business
Distribution: Manufacturer Through Distributor
General Admin.: James L. Herbert/Chief Executive Officer, Chairman
Lon M. Bohannon/President, Chief Operating Officer
Edward L. Bradley/Vice President
Terri A. Morrical/Vice President
Mktg./Adv.: Anthony E. Maltese/Vice President Corporate Development
Production: Kenneth V. Kodilla/Vice President Manufacturing
Research: Paul S. Satoh/Vice President Research
Joseph M. Madden/Vice President Scientific Affairs
Mark A. Mozola/Vice President, Director Research & Development
Finance: Richard R. Current/Vice President Admin., Chief Financial Officer

Forceps, General & Plastic Surgery	Surgery
Glove, Patient Examination	General
Knife, Other	Surgery
Monitor, Heart Rate, Other	Cardiovascular
Needle, Other	General
Syringe, Other	General

NEOGUIDE SYSTEMS, INC. 408-321-8844
2712 Orchard Parkway, San Jose, CA 95134
FDA Number: 3005620008

Colonoscope, Gastro-Urology	Gastroenterology/Urology

NEOMATRIX, LLC 877-425-6727
19800 MacArthur Blvd.,, Suite 690, 949-753-7844
Irvine, CA 92612
FDA Number: 3005030604
E-mail: info@neomatrix.com   *Fax:* 949-753-7845
Web site: /www.neomatrix.com
Ownership: Private
Produces/Sells CE-marked Devices: N
General Admin.: John Stroh/Chief Executive Officer
Matthew Heindel/Chief Operating Officer
Mktg./Adv.: Rob Thornhill/Vice President Sales

Biopsy Instrument	Gastroenterology/Urology

NEOMED
See Conmed Corporation

NEOMEDIX CORP. 949-258-8355
15042 Parkwary Loop, Suite A, Tustin, CA 92780
FDA Number: 2032569

Cautery, Radiofrequency, AC-Powered	Ophthalmology
Electrosurgical Unit, Cutting & Coagulation Device	Surgery
Irrigator, Ocular Surgery	Ophthalmology
Suction Apparatus, Ward Use, Portable, AC-Powered	Surgery
Trabeculotome	Ophthalmology

NEOMEND, INC. 888-776-4351
60 Technology Drive, Irvine, CA 92618 949-916-1630
FDA Number: 2953195   *Fax:* 949-916-1635
Web site: http://www.neomend.com
Ownership: Private
Produces/Sells CE-marked Devices: N
General Admin.: Mr. David Renzi/President, Chief Executive Officer
Mktg./Adv.: Mr. Wade King/Executive Vice President Business Development
Mr. Mike Nagel/Vice President Marketing & Sales

Clamp, Vascular	Cardiovascular
Electrode, Electrosurgical, Return (Ground, Dispersive)	Surgery
Introducer, Syringe Needle	General

NEOMETRICS, A DIVISION OF NATUS 800-645-3616
150 Motor Parkway, Suite #203, 631-457-4430
Hauppauge, NY 11788
FDA Number: n/a   *Fax:* 650-802-0401
Web site: www.natus.com
Medical Products Sales Volume: $1,000,000
Annual Revenue: $5-$10 Million
Year Founded: 1978
Total Employees: 25
Ownership: Natus Medical Inc.
Stock Symbol: BABY
Traded On: NASDAQ
Produces/Sells CE-marked Devices: N
Federal Procurement Eligibility: Small Business
Distribution: Manufacturer Direct
General Admin.: Mr. Robert Gunst/Chairman
Mr. James Hawkins/Chief Executive Officer
Mr. Kenneth Ludlum/Director
Mr. Mark Michael/Director
Mr. William Moore/Director
Ms. Doris Enqibous/Director
Mr. John Buhler/President, Chief Operating Officer
Medical Admin.: Mr. Christopher Chung/Vice President Medical Affairs
Mktg./Adv.: Mr. Kenneth Traverso/Vice President Marketing & Sales
Finance: Mr. Steven Murphy/Chief Financial Officer, Senior Vice President Finance

Enzyme Immunoassay, Other	Chemistry
Radioimmunoassay, 17-Hydroxyprogesterone	Chemistry
Radioimmunoassay, Thyroid Stimulating Hormone	Chemistry
Radioimmunoassay, Thyroxine Binding Globulin	Chemistry

NEOMETRICS, INC.
See Neometrics, A Division Of Natus

NEONATAL, INFANT, PEDIATRIC, AND ADULT 305-267-8885
ADVANCED HE
815 N.w. 57th Ave., Suite 110, Miami, FL 33126
FDA Number: 3005278558

Mattress, Non-Powered Flotation Therapy	Physical Med
Protector, Skin Pressure	General

NEOPROBE CORPORATION 800-793-0079
425 Metro Place North, Suite 300, 614-793-7500
Dublin, OH 43017
FDA Number: 1527245   *Fax:* 614-793-7520
E-mail: info@neoprobe.com
Web site: www.neoprobe.com
Medical Products Sales Volume: $6,100,000
Annual Revenue: $5-$10 Million
Year Founded: 1983
Ownership: Public

NEOPROBE CORPORATION — 800-793-0079 (cont'd)

Stock Symbol: NEOP
Traded On: OTC Bulletin
Quality System Registration Information: ISO9001
Produces/Sells CE-marked Devices: Y
Federal Procurement Eligibility: Small Business
Distribution: Manufacturer Through Distributor, Manufacturer Through Manufacturer Reps, Exporter
General Admin.: David C. Bupp/President, Chief Executive Officer
Mktg./Adv.: Mr. Douglas Rash/Vice President Marketing
Production: Mr. Anthony Blair/Vice President Manufacturing & Operations
    Mr. Rodger Brown/Vice President Regulatory Affairs
Research: Dr. Frederick Cope/Vice President Research
Finance: Brent L. Larson/Chief Financial Officer, Vice President Finance

Device, Measurement, Velocity, Conduction, Nerve	Cns/Neurology
Doppler, Blood Flow, Transcranial	Cardiovascular
Flowmeter, Blood, Other	Cardiovascular
Probe, Detector, Flow, Blood, Laparoscopy, Ultrasonic	Surgery
Probe, Uptake, Nuclear	Radiology
Test, Cancer Detection, Other	Hematology

NEOSTAR MEDICAL TECHNOLOGIES, INC.

See Angiodynamics, Inc.

NEOTECH PRODUCTS, INC. — 800-966-0500 / 661-775-7466

27822 Fremont Ct, Valencia, CA 91355
FDA Number: 2025917   *Fax:* 800-966-0585
E-mail: info@neotechproducts.com
Web site: www.neotechproducts.com
Year Founded: 1986
Ownership: Private
Produces/Sells CE-marked Devices: Y
Federal Procurement Eligibility: Small Business
Distribution: Manufacturer Direct, Manufacturer Through Distributor, Manufacturer Through Manufacturer Reps, Exporter
General Admin.: Tom Thornbury/Chief Executive Officer
    Craig McCrary/General Manager
Mktg./Adv.: Ms. Cindy Cisneros/Sales Specialist
Research: Arnold M. Heyman/Vice President Research & Development

Airway, Bi-Nasopharyngeal (With Connector)	Anesthesiology
Airway, Nasopharyngeal (Breathing Tube)	Anesthesiology
Catheter, Suction, With Tip	General
Changer, Tube, Endotracheal	Anesthesiology
Cover, Other	General
Electrode, Gel	Cardiovascular
Electrode, Other	General
Holder, Catheter	Gastroenterology/Urology
Kit, Suction, Airway (Tracheal)	Anesthesiology
Pad, Neonatal Eye	General
Pouch, Telemetry	General
Shield, Eye, Ophthalmic	Ophthalmology
Stethoscope, Manual	Cardiovascular
Support, Breathing Tube	Anesthesiology
Tubing, Other	General

NEOTRACT INC. — 925-401-0700

4473 Willow Road, Suite 100, Pleasanton, CA 94588
FDA Number: 3005791775   *Fax:* 925-401-0699
E-mail: info@neotract.com
Web site: http://www.neotract.com
Year Founded: 2004
Ownership: Private
Produces/Sells CE-marked Devices: N
General Admin.: Dr. Ted Lamson/Chief Technology Officer
    Mr. Christopher Rowland/President, Chief Executive Officer
Production: Mr. Douglas Fraits/Vice President Operations
    Ms. Nancy Isaac/Vice President Quality Assurance & Regulatory Affairs
Research: Dr. Joseph Catanese/Vice President Research & Development

Staple, Implantable	Surgery
Suture, Non-Absorbable, Synthetic, Polyethylene	Surgery

NEOVASC INC — 1.866.760.7131 / 604-270-4344

13700 Mayfield Pl. #2135,
Richmond, BC V6V 2 Canada
FDA Number: 3003555689   *Fax:* 604-270-4384
E-mail: info@neovasc.com
Web site: www.neovasc.com
Year Founded: 1999
Total Employees: 25
Ownership: Private
Produces/Sells CE-marked Devices: N
Distribution: Manufacturer Direct, Exclusive Distributor, Importer

NEOVASC, INC. — 604-270-4344

13700 Mayfield Place, Suite 2135,
Richmond, BC V6V 2 Canada
FDA Number: 3003555689   *Fax:* 604-270-4384
E-mail: info@neovasc.com

NEOVASC, INC. — 604-270-4344 (cont'd)

Web site: www.neovasc.com
Year Founded: 2008
Ownership: Private
Stock Symbol: NVC
Traded On: TSX Venture Exchange
Produces/Sells CE-marked Devices: N

NEPHROS, INC. — 201-343-5202

41 Grand Ave., Suite 200, Rivers Edge, NJ 07661
FDA Number: 3003337893   *Fax:* 201-343-5207
Web site: www.nephros.com
Year Founded: 1997
Ownership: Public
Stock Symbol: NEPH
Traded On: OTC Bulletin
Produces/Sells CE-marked Devices: N
General Admin.: Dr. Paul Mieyal/Chief Executive Officer
Finance: Mr. Gerald Kochanski/Chief Financial Officer

Dialyzer, High Permeability	Gastroenterology/Urology
Purification System, Water	Gastroenterology/Urology

NEPSCO INC., BACKSAVER PRODUCTS DIV.

See Backsaver

NERL DIAGNOSTICS LLC. — 401-824-2046

14 Almeida Ave., East Providence, RI 02914
FDA Number: 1215667

Buffer, pH	Hematology
Calibrator, Ethyl Alcohol	Toxicology
Calibrator, Primary, Clinical Chemistry	Chemistry
Calibrator, Secondary, Clinical Chemistry	Chemistry
Colorimetric, Xylose	Chemistry
Diluent, Blood Cell	Hematology
Disc, Strip And Reagent, Microorganism Differentiation	Microbiology
Kit, Screening, Staphylococcus Aureus	Microbiology
Multi Analyte Mixture, Calibrator	Chemistry
Purifier, Water	Chemistry
Reagent, Antistreptolysin-Titer/Streptolysin O	Microbiology
Reagent, General Purpose	Pathology
Solution, Isotonic	Hematology
Supplies, Blood Bank	Hematology
Test, C-Reactive Protein, FITC	Immunology
Test, Glycosylated Hemoglobin Assay	Hematology
Test, Infectious Mononucleosis	Immunology
Test, Rheumatoid Factor	Immunology
Test, Systemic Lupus Erythematosus	Immunology

NESAR SYSTEMS, INC. — 724-827-8172

420 Ashwood Road, Darlington, PA 16115-2910
FDA Number: 3004106781
Ownership: Private
Produces/Sells CE-marked Devices: N

Exerciser, Non-Measuring	Physical Med

NESLAB INSTRUMENTS, INC.

See Thermo Fisher Scientific

NESPA ENTERPRISES, INC. — 888-479-4677 / 530-534-9910

2800 Richter Ave.ste. C, Oroville, CA 95966
FDA Number: n/a   *Fax:* 530-534-9915
E-mail: info@tiledspas.com
Web site: www.tiledspas.com
Ownership: Private
Produces/Sells CE-marked Devices: N

Exerciser, Powered	Anesthesiology

NEST GROUP INC., THE — 800-347-6378 / 508-481-6223

45 Valley Rd., Southborough, MA 01772
FDA Number: n/a   *Fax:* 508-485-5736
E-mail: info@nestgrp.com
Web site: www.nestgrp.com
Annual Revenue: $1-$5 Million
Year Founded: 1984
Total Employees: 3   *Marketing Staff:* 1   *Sales Staff:* 1
Ownership: Private
Produces/Sells CE-marked Devices: N
Federal Procurement Eligibility: Small Business
Distribution: Exclusive Distributor
General Admin.: Connie Nicolas/Office Manager
    Amos Heckendorf/President
IS: Amos Heckendorf/Director Tech. Services

Chromatography Equipment, Liquid	Chemistry
Dialyzer, Laboratory	Chemistry

NESTOR MACHINE CO INC — 818-707-1678

5537 Fairview Pl, Agoura Hills, CA 91301
FDA Number: 2029098
Ownership: Private
Produces/Sells CE-marked Devices: N

NESTOR MACHINE CO INC   818-707-1678 *(cont'd)*
Wheelchair, Standup   Physical Med

NETECH CORP.
See Netech, Corp.

NETECH, CORP.   800-547-6557
110 Toledo Street, Farmingdale, NY 11735   631-531-0100
FDA Number: 2436826   *Fax:* 631-531-0101
E-mail: info@netech.org
Web site: www.gonetech.com
Medical Products Sales Volume: $1,100,000
Annual Revenue: $1-$5 Million
Year Founded: 1986
Total Employees: 11
Ownership: Private
Quality System Registration Information: ISO9001
Produces/Sells CE-marked Devices: Y
Federal Procurement Eligibility: Small Business, Minority Owned
Distribution: Manufacturer Direct, Manufacturer Through Distributor, Service Direct, Importer, Exporter
General Admin.: Mohan Das/President
Mktg./Adv.: Ron Shepard/Vice President Marketing & Sales
  Analyzer, Electrical Safety   General
  Calibrator, Gas, Pressure   Anesthesiology
  Meter, Ultrasonic Power   General
  Monitor, Cardiac Output, Trend (Arterial Pressure Pulse)   Surgery
  Simulator, Arrhythmia   Cardiovascular
  Tester, Defibrillator   Cardiovascular
  Tester, Pacemaker Electrode Function   Cardiovascular

NETECH, DIV. OF TESTRONIX CORP.
See Netech, Corp.

NETWAL DENTAL LABORATORY   800-991-8111
115 5th Ave. South, Suite 307,   608-782-1724
La Crosse, WI 54602
FDA Number: 3006264111   *Fax:* 608-782-4249
Ownership: Private
Produces/Sells CE-marked Devices: N
  Device, Anti-Snoring   Ear/Nose/Throat

NETZSCH INSTRUMENTS, INC.   800-688-6738
37 North Avenue, Burlington, MA 01803   781-272-5353
FDA Number: n/a   *Fax:* 781-272-5225
E-mail: NIB-Sales@netzsch.com
Web site: www.nib.netzsch.us
Medical Products Sales Volume: $2,400,000
Year Founded: 1952
Total Employees: 20   *Marketing Staff:* 5   *Sales Staff:* 8
Ownership: Netzsch-Geratebau Gmbh
Produces/Sells CE-marked Devices: N
Federal Procurement Eligibility: Small Business
Distribution: Manufacturer Direct, Manufacturer Through Manufacturer Reps, Exclusive Distributor
Research: Dr. Jack Henderson/Vice President Scientific Affairs
  Calorimeter   Chemistry
  Thermogravimetric Analysis Equipment   Chemistry

NEU-ION, INC.   800-678-4360
7200 Rutherford Rd., Suite 100,   410-944-5200
Baltimore, MD 21244
FDA Number: 1125781   *Fax:* 410-944-5289
E-mail: info@neu-ion.com
Web site: www.neu-ion.com
Ownership: Private
Produces/Sells CE-marked Devices: N
  Purification System, Water   Gastroenterology/Urology

NEUMED INC.   800-367-1238
800 Silvia Street, West Trenton, NJ 08628   609-896-3444
FDA Number: n/a   *Fax:* 609-896-2798
E-mail: info@neumedinc.com
Web site: www.neumedinc.com
Total Employees: 15
Ownership: Private
Produces/Sells CE-marked Devices: Y
Federal Procurement Eligibility: Small Business
Distribution: Manufacturer Direct, Manufacturer Through Distributor, Manufacturer Through Manufacturer Reps
General Admin.: Mr. Eric Guldalian/Managing Director
  Brace, Joint, Ankle (External)   Physical Med
  Device, Measurement, Velocity, Conduction, Nerve   Cns/Neurology
  Electrode, Cutaneous   Cns/Neurology
  Electrode, TENS   Cns/Neurology

NEURAL SIGNALS,INC.   770-220-9964
3688 Clearview Ave Ste 110, Atlanta, GA 30340
FDA Number: 3004890020

NEURAL SIGNALS,INC.   770-220-9964 *(cont'd)*
Communication System, Powered   Physical Med

NEURALSTEM, INC.   301-366-4960
9700 Great Seneca Highway, Rockville, MD 20850
FDA Number: n/a
Ownership: Private
Produces/Sells CE-marked Devices: N

NEURO DIAGNOSTIC DEVICES   888-SHUNT-OK
3701 Market St, 3rd Floor,   215-966-6104
Philadelphia, PA 19104
FDA Number: 3004082659
E-mail: ffritz@neurodx.com   *Fax:* 856-672-0670
Web site: www.ShuntCheck.com
Annual Revenue: $0-$1 Million
Year Founded: 2003
Total Employees: 5   *Marketing Staff:* 2   *Sales Staff:* 2
Ownership: Private
Produces/Sells CE-marked Devices: Y
Federal Procurement Eligibility: Small Business
Distribution: Manufacturer Through Manufacturer Reps
General Admin.: Mr. Alan Neff/Chief Executive Officer
Research: Dr. Samuel Neff/Chief Scientist
  Shunt, Central Nerve, With Component   Cns/Neurology

NEURO DIAGNOSTIC SYSTEMS
See Telediagnostic Systems

NEURO KINETICS   412-963-6649
128 Gamma Dr., Pittsburgh, PA 15238
FDA Number: 2519945
Web site: http://www.neuro-kinetics.com
Ownership: Private
Produces/Sells CE-marked Devices: N
  Analyzer, Apparatus, Vestibular   Ear/Nose/Throat

NEURO RESOURCE GROUP, INC.   972-665-1810
1100 Jupiter Rd., Ste. 190, Plano, TX 75074
FDA Number: 3004786509
  Biofeedback Device   Cns/Neurology
  Stimulator, Nerve, Transcutaneous (Pain Relief, TENS)   Cns/Neurology

NEURO VASX, INC.   763-315-0013
7351 Kirkwood Lane, Suite 112, Maple Grove, MN 55369
FDA Number: 2134714
  Catheter, Intravascular, Diagnostic   Cardiovascular

NEURO-DIAGNOSTIC ASSOC.   949-497-1207
2514 Temple Hills Drive, Laguna Beach, CA 92651
FDA Number: 2031209
  Vibration Threshold Measurement Device   Cns/Neurology

NEUROCARE, INC.   877-571-3599
6252 Skyline Road S., Salem, OR 97306   503-371-6605
FDA Number: 3030875   *Fax:* 503-763-8727
E-mail: ems@neurocare.com
Web site: www.neurocare.com
Annual Revenue: $0-$1 Million
Year Founded: 1989
Total Employees: 9   *Marketing Staff:* 3   *Sales Staff:* 3
Ownership: Private
Quality System Registration Information: ISO9002
Produces/Sells CE-marked Devices: Y
Federal Procurement Eligibility: Small Business, Minority Owned, Female Owned
Distribution: Manufacturer Direct, Manufacturer Through Distributor, Manufacturer Through Manufacturer Reps, Service Direct, Exclusive Distributor, Exporter
General Admin.: Mrs. Debra Oliver/Chief Executive Officer, General Manager
  Stimulator, Muscle, Electrical-Powered (EMS)   Physical Med

NEUROCOM INTERNATIONAL, INC.   503-653-2144
9570 S.e. Lawnfield Rd., Clackamas, OR 97015
FDA Number: 3023102
  Analyzer, Apparatus, Vestibular   Ear/Nose/Throat
  Electromyograph, Diagnostic   Physical Med
  Platform, Force-Measuring   Physical Med
  Tester, Auditory Impedance   Ear/Nose/Throat

NEUROCYBERNETICS, INC.   516-482-9001
21601 Vanowen St., Suite 100, Canoga Park, CA 91303
FDA Number: 2032366
  Biofeedback Device   Cns/Neurology
  Electroencephalograph   Cns/Neurology

NEURODYNE MEDICAL CORP.   800-963-8633
186 Alewife Brook Parkway,   617-234-1100
Cambridge, MA 02138
FDA Number: n/a   *Fax:* 617-234-1108
E-mail: neumed@neumed.com
Web site: www.neumed.com

NEURODYNE MEDICAL CORP.   800-963-8633 *(cont'd)*
Annual Revenue: $0-$1 Million
Year Founded: 1993
Total Employees: 16   *Marketing Staff:* 2   *Sales Staff:* 2
Ownership: Private
Produces/Sells CE-marked Devices: Y
Federal Procurement Eligibility: Small Business, Minority Owned, GSA Contract, VA Contract
Distribution: Manufacturer Direct, Manufacturer Through Distributor, Manufacturer Through Manufacturer Reps, Service Direct, Exporter
General Admin.: Tahir H. Chaudhry/President, Chief Executive Officer
Mktg./Adv.: Ann Johnson/Admin. Sales
     Tahir H. Chaudhry/Director Marketing
Production: Rudolph Johnson/Manager Manufacturing
     Tahira Nasreen/Manager Materials
     Bruce L. Mehler/Vice President Operations
Research: Bruce L. Mehler/Director Application & Clinical Research

Biofeedback Device	Cns/Neurology
Device, Incontinence, Mechanical/Hydraulic	Gastroenterology/Urology
Electrode, Electromyographic	Cns/Neurology
Meter, Skin Resistance, Battery-Powered	Physical Med
Myograph	Physical Med
Plethysmograph, Photo-Electric, Pneumatic Or Hydraulic	Cardiovascular

NEUROGNOSTICS, INC.   414-727-7950
10437 Innovation Dr., Suite 309, Milwaukee, WI 53226
FDA Number: 94256
Ownership: Private
Produces/Sells CE-marked Devices: N

Nuclear Magnetic Resonance Imaging System	Radiology

NEUROLOGICA CORPORATION   877-564-8520
14 Electronics Avenue, Danvers, MA 01923   **978-564-8500**
FDA Number: 3004938766   *Fax:* 978-560-0602
E-mail: info@neurologica.com
Web site: http://www.NeuroLogica.com
Ownership: Private
Produces/Sells CE-marked Devices: N
General Admin.: Dr. Eric Bailey/President, Chief Executive Officer
   Medical Admin.: Dr. Colin Timothy McDonald/Chief Medical Officer
Mktg./Adv.: Mr. David Webster/Vice President Marketing & Sales
Production: Mr. Philip Sullivan/Vice President Operations
     Mr. Don Fickett/Vice President Quality Control & Regulatory Affairs
Research: Mr. Andrew Tybinkowski/Vice President Engineering

Scanner, Computed Tomography, X-Ray, Special Procedure	Radiology
Scanner, Emission Computed Tomography	Radiology

NEUROLOGICAL RESEARCH
   See The Neurological Research And Development Group

NEUROMECHANICAL INNOVATIONS, LLC   480-785-8448
11011 South 48th St., Ste. 220, Phoenix, AZ 85044
FDA Number: 3004620782

Plunger-Like Joint Manipulator	Physical Med

NEUROMETRIX, INC.   888-786-7287
62 Fourth Ave., Waltham, MA 02451   **781-890-9989**
FDA Number: 1225994
E-mail: info@neurometrix.com
Web site: www.neurometrix.com
Year Founded: 1996
Total Employees: 143
Ownership: Public
Stock Symbol: NURO
Traded On: NASDAQ
Produces/Sells CE-marked Devices: N
General Admin.: Shai Gozani/President, Chief Executive Officer, Director
     Guy Daniello/Senior Vice President
     Krishnamurthy Balachandra/Senior Vice President, General Manager
   Medical Admin.: Mr. Kenneth Snow/Chief Medical Officer
Mktg./Adv.: Michael MacDonald/Vice President Marketing
Production: Charles Fendrock/Vice President Manufacturing
Research: Xuan Kong/Vice President Research
Finance: Thomas T. Higgins/Chief Financial Officer

Amplifier, Physiological Signal	Cns/Neurology
Device, Measurement, Velocity, Conduction, Nerve	Cns/Neurology
Electrode, Needle	Cns/Neurology
Electrode, Needle, Diagnostic Electromyograph	Physical Med
Electromyograph, Diagnostic	Physical Med

NEUROMONICS INC.   484-821-1260
2810 Emrick Blvd., Bethlehem, PA 18020
FDA Number: 3005777056

Masker, Tinnitus	Ear/Nose/Throat

NEURONETICS, INC.   877-600-7555
31 General Warren Blvd., Malvern, PA 19355   **877-600-7555**
FDA Number: 3004824012   *Fax:* 610-640-4206

NEURONETICS, INC.   877-600-7555 *(cont'd)*
E-mail: info@neuornetics.com
Web site: http://www.neurostartms.com
Ownership: Private
Produces/Sells CE-marked Devices: N
General Admin.: Bruce Shook/President, Chief Executive Officer
Mktg./Adv.: Peter Anastasiou/Vice President Marketing
     Jim Breidenstein/Vice President Sales
Production: Mark Riehl/Vice President Product Development & Operations
     Judy Ways/Vice President Quality Assurance & Regulatory Affairs
Finance: Mark Bausinger/Chief Financial Officer

NEUROPTICS, INC.   949-250-9792
1001 Avenida Pico, Suite C495, San Clemente, CA 92673
FDA Number: 2032833

Pupillometer, AC-Powered	Ophthalmology

NEUROS MEDICAL INC.   440-951-2565
4230 Route 306, Suite 305, Willoughby, OH 44094
FDA Number: n/a   *Fax:* 440-951-1470
Web site: http://neurosmedical.com
Ownership: Private
Produces/Sells CE-marked Devices: N
General Admin.: Mr. Mark Teague/Chief Operating Officer
     Dr. Zi-Ping Fang/Chief Technology Officer
     Mr. Jon Snyder/President, Chief Executive Officer

NEUROSIGMA INC.   310-479-3100
10960 Wilshire Boulevard, Suite 1230, Los Angeles, CA 90024
FDA Number: n/a
E-mail: info@neurosigma.com
Web site: http://www.neurosigma.com
Ownership: Private
Produces/Sells CE-marked Devices: N
General Admin.: Mr. Lodwrick Cook/Chairman
     Dr. Leon Ekchian/President, Chief Executive Officer
Finance: Mr. Charles Winckler/Chief Financial Officer

NEUROSTAR SOLUTIONS, INC.   866-809-4746
6 Concourse Parkway NE, Suite 1625,   **404-575-4222**
Atlanta, GA 30328
FDA Number: 1067108   *Fax:* 404-526-6099
E-mail: sales_info@accelarad.com
Web site: www.accelarad.com
Ownership: Private
Produces/Sells CE-marked Devices: N

Device, Storage, Image, Digital	Radiology
Image Processing System	Radiology

NEUROSYNC LLC   425-605-8694
12215 Ne 39th St., Bellevue, WA 98005
FDA Number: 3005523715

Biofeedback Device	Cns/Neurology

NEUROTHERM INC.   978-777-3916
2 Debush Ave., Middleton, MA 01949
FDA Number: 1226344

Generator, Radiofrequency Lesion	Cns/Neurology
Probe, Radiofrequency Lesion	Cns/Neurology

NEUROTONE SYSTEMS, INC.   972-271-1978
510 Nesbit Dr., Garland, TX 75041
FDA Number: 1619885
Ownership: Private
Produces/Sells CE-marked Devices: N
General Admin.: Mr. Gerry Kearby/Chief Executive Officer
     Mr. Hank Barry/Director
Research: Dr. Earl Levine/Vice President Engineering

Biofeedback Device	Cns/Neurology
Stimulator, Cranial Electrotherapy	Cns/Neurology
Stimulator, Nerve, Transcutaneous (Pain Relief, TENS)	Cns/Neurology

NEUROTRON MEDICAL   609-896-3444
800 Silvia St., Ewing, NJ 08628
FDA Number: 2245302

Computer and Software, Medical	General
Device, Measurement, Velocity, Conduction, Nerve	Cns/Neurology
Electrode, Cutaneous	Cns/Neurology
Splint, Extremity, Non-Inflatable, External	Surgery

NEUROTRON MEDICAL, INC.
   See Neumed Inc.

NEUROTRONICS, INC.   352-372-9955
912 NE 2nd Street, Suite 5, Gainesville, FL 32601
FDA Number: 1063925   *Fax:* 815-550-2871
E-mail: dawn@neurotronics.com
Web site: www.neurotronics.com
Medical Products Sales Volume: $570,000
Total Employees: 7

NEUROTRONICS, INC.   352-372-9955 *(cont'd)*

Ownership: Private
Produces/Sells CE-marked Devices: N
Federal Procurement Eligibility: Small Business
Recorder, Ventilatory Effort   Anesthesiology

NEUROVIGIL INC.   858-454-5134
7606 Fay Avenue, La Jolla, CA 92037
FDA Number: n/a   *Fax:* 858-454-5164
E-mail: info@neurovigil.com
Web site: http://www.neurovigil.com
Ownership: Private
Produces/Sells CE-marked Devices: N
General Admin.: Dr. Philip Low/Chairman, Chief Executive Officer

NEUROWAVE MEDICAL TECHNOLOGIES   312-334-2505
200 East Randolph Suite, Suite 2200, Chicago, IL 60601
FDA Number: 3006614152
Web site: http://www.neurowavemedical.com
Ownership: Private
Produces/Sells CE-marked Devices: N
General Admin.: Mr. Farhan Hussain/President, Chief Executive Officer
Mktg./Adv.: Mr. Chris Littel/Vice President Marketing
Finance: Mr. Jeffrey Whitnell/Vice President Finance
Stimulator, Nerve, Transcutaneous (Pain Relief, TENS)   Cns/Neurology

NEUTRAL POSTURE, INC.   979-778-0502
3904 North Texas Ave., Bryan, TX 77803
FDA Number: 1644461
Chair, Posture, For Cardiac And Pulmonary Treatment   Anesthesiology

NEUTROGENA CORPORATION
See Ortho Dermatologics

NEUTRON PRODUCTS INC   800-424-8169
22301 Mt. Ephraim Road, Box 68,   301-349-5001
Dickerson, MD 20842
FDA Number: 1121502   *Fax:* 301-349-5007
E-mail: neutronprod@erols.com
Web site: neutronproducts.com
Medical Products Sales Volume: $5,000,000
Annual Revenue: $5-$10 Million
Year Founded: 1959
Total Employees: 50   *Sales Staff:* 2
Ownership: Private
Produces/Sells CE-marked Devices: N
Federal Procurement Eligibility: Small Business
Distribution: Manufacturer Direct, Manufacturer Through Manufacturer Reps, OEM, Service Direct, Exporter
General Admin.: Mr. Marvin Turkanis/Vice President
Mktg./Adv.: Mr. Edmond J. DeRosa/Sales Engineer
Source, Teletherapy, Radionuclide   Radiology
Teletherapy System, Radionuclide   Radiology

NEUTRON PRODUCTS, INC.   301-349-5001
22301 Mt. Ephraim Rd., Dickerson, MD 20842
FDA Number: n/a   *Fax:* 301-349-5007
E-mail: neutronprod@erols.com
Web site: http://www.neutronprod.com
Medical Products Sales Volume: $125,000
Annual Revenue: $5-$10 Million
Total Employees: 50   *Marketing Staff:* 4   *Sales Staff:* 3
Ownership: Private
Produces/Sells CE-marked Devices: N
Federal Procurement Eligibility: Small Business
Distribution: Manufacturer Direct, Manufacturer Through Distributor, Manufacturer Through Manufacturer Reps, Service Direct, Exclusive Distributor, Importer, Exporter
General Admin.: Jackson A. Ransohoff/President, Chief Executive Officer
Mktg./Adv.: Edmond J. DeRosa/Manager Marketing
Finance: James W. Jordan/Treasurer
Couch, Radiation Therapy, Powered   Radiology
Device, Limiting, Beam, Teletherapy   Radiology
Device, Limiting, Beam, Teletherapy, Radionuclide   Radiology
Source, Teletherapy, Radionuclide   Radiology
Sterilizer, Radiation   General
Teletherapy System, Radionuclide   Radiology

NEVIN LABORATORIES, INC   800-544-5337
5000 S. Halsted Street, Chicago, IL 60609-5130   773-624-4330
FDA Number: n/a   *Fax:* 773-624-7337
E-mail: robertlnevin@cs.com
Web site: www.nevinlabs.com
Annual Revenue: $1-$5 Million
Year Founded: 1987
Total Employees: 25
Ownership: Private
Produces/Sells CE-marked Devices: N
Federal Procurement Eligibility: Small Business, GSA Contract, VA Contract

NEVIN LABORATORIES, INC   800-544-5337 *(cont'd)*
Distribution: Manufacturer Through Distributor
General Admin.: Robert L. Nevin/President
Mktg./Adv.: R. Grano/Manager Marketing
Production: D. M. Sexton/Manager Production
       J. W. Wood/Manager Production
Finance: James Creek/Vice President Finance
Cabinet Casework, Modular   General
Cabinet, Other   General
Fountain, Eye Wash   Chemistry
Furniture, General   General
Monitor, Gas, Atmospheric, Environmental   General

NEW BRUNSWICK SCIENTIFIC CO., INC.   800-631-5417
44 Talmadge Rd.,,, P.O. Box 4005,   732-287-1200
Edison, NJ 08818
FDA Number: n/a   *Fax:* 732-287-4222
E-mail: bioinfo@nbsc.com
Web site: www.nbsc.com
Annual Revenue: $50-$100 Million
Total Employees: 350   *Marketing Staff:* 7   *Sales Staff:* 35
Ownership: EPPENDORF AG
Produces/Sells CE-marked Devices: Y
Federal Procurement Eligibility: Small Business
Distribution: Manufacturer Direct
General Admin.: Jim Orcutt/President, Chief Executive Officer
Mktg./Adv.: Mike Sattan/Director Marketing
       Suzy Kedzierski/Manager Advertising
       William J. Dunne/Vice President Worldwide sales and service
Research: Yinliang Chen/Director Research
Finance: Tom Bocchino/Chief Financial Officer
Counter, Cell   Microbiology
Fermentation Equipment   Microbiology
Freezer, Laboratory, Biological   Chemistry
Freezer, Laboratory, Ultra-Low Temperature   Chemistry
Incubator, Aerobic   Microbiology
Incubator/Water Bath, Microbiology   Microbiology
Monitor, Microbial Growth   Microbiology
Sampler, Air   General
Shaker/Stirrer   Chemistry
Sterilizer, Laboratory   Microbiology
Suspension System, Cell Culture   Pathology
Test, Agar Plate   Microbiology
Tissue Culture Apparatus   Microbiology

NEW DEANTRONICS, LTD.   925-280-8388
1990 N. California Blvd., Suite 1040, Walnut Creek, CA 94596
FDA Number: 2031569   *Fax:* 925-280-1788
E-mail: sales@newdean.com
Web site: http://www.newdean.com.tw
Medical Products Sales Volume: $7,000,000
Year Founded: 1985
Total Employees: 5   *Marketing Staff:* 2   *Sales Staff:* 6
Ownership: Private
Quality System Registration Information: ISO9000; ISO9001
Produces/Sells CE-marked Devices: Y
Federal Procurement Eligibility: Small Business
Distribution: Manufacturer Through Distributor, OEM
Electrosurgial Unit, Cutting & Coagulation Device   Surgery

NEW ENGLAND BIOLABS, INC.   800-632-5227
240 County Rd., Ipswich, MA 01938-2723   978-927-5054
FDA Number: n/a   *Fax:* 978-921-1350
E-mail: info@neb.com
Web site: www.neb.com
Year Founded: 1970
Ownership: Private
Quality System Registration Information: ISO9001
Produces/Sells CE-marked Devices: N
Federal Procurement Eligibility: Small Business
Distribution: Manufacturer Direct, Manufacturer Through Distributor, Service Direct, Exclusive Distributor, Exporter
General Admin.: Jim Ellard/Chief Executive Officer
       Dr. Richard Roberts/Chief Scientific Officer
Mktg./Adv.: Dr. Peter Nathan/Director Business Development
Control, Enzyme (Assayed And Unassayed)   Chemistry
Genetic Engineering   Microbiology
Test, DNA-Probe, Other   Microbiology

NEW ENGLAND MEDICAL CORP.   845-778-4200
2274 Albany Post Road, Walden, NY 12586
FDA Number: 1320371   *Fax:* 845-778-4199
E-mail: sigmanet@frontiernet.net
Web site: www.conefor.com
Medical Products Sales Volume: $100,000
Year Founded: 1995
Ownership: Private
Produces/Sells CE-marked Devices: N

NEW ENGLAND MEDICAL CORP.   845-778-4200 *(cont'd)*

Electrode, Electrosurgical, Active (Blade)	Surgery
Knife, Cervical Cone	Obstetrics/Gynecology

NEW ENGLAND SURGICAL INSTRUMENT CORP.
See Kirwan Surgical Products, Inc.

NEW FSI, INC.
See Focus Surgery, Inc.

NEW HORIZONS DIAGNOSTICS CORPORATION   410-992-9357
9110 Red Branch Road, Suite B, Columbia, MD 21045
FDA Number: 1120832   Fax: 410-992-0328
E-mail: nhdiag@aol.com
Web site: www.nhdiag.com
Medical Products Sales Volume: $1,000,000
Annual Revenue: $1-$5 Million
Ownership: Private
Quality System Registration Information: ISO9001
Produces/Sells CE-marked Devices: Y
Federal Procurement Eligibility: Small Business
Distribution: Manufacturer Direct, Manufacturer Through Distributor, OEM, Exporter

Antibody, Monoclonal	Microbiology
Antibody, Polyclonal	Microbiology
Antigen, Streptococcus SPP.	Microbiology
Antiserum, Coagglutination (Direct) Neisseria Gonorrhoeae	Microbiology
Antiserum, Control For Non-Treponemal Test	Microbiology
Antiserum, Vibrio Cholerae	Microbiology
Kit, Identification, Neisseria Gonorrhoeae	Microbiology
Luminometer	Chemistry
Monitor, Biological (Contamination Testing)	General
Test, Bacteria Characterization	General

NEW INNOVATIONS INC.   765-668-7470
125 E. Bradford St., Marion, IN 46952
FDA Number: 3003884516
Ownership: Private
Produces/Sells CE-marked Devices: N

Cannula, Suprapubic, With Trocar	Gastroenterology/Urology

NEW LASER SCIENCE, INC.   858-487-5880
16776 Bernardo Center Drive, #203, San Diego, CA 92128
FDA Number: n/a   Fax: 858-487-0662
E-mail: sales@newlaserscience.com
Web site: http://www.newlaserscience.com/
Medical Products Sales Volume: $2,000,000
Annual Revenue: $5-$10 Million
Year Founded: 1998
Total Employees: 6   *Marketing Staff:* 4   *Sales Staff:* 10
Ownership: Private
Produces/Sells CE-marked Devices: Y
Distribution: OEM, Exclusive Distributor
General Admin.: John P. Clark/Chief Executive Officer

Dermabrasion Unit	Surgery
Laser, Surgical	Surgery
Laser, Surgical, Holmium	Surgery
Scanner, Ultrasonic, Other	Radiology
Service, Used Equipment	General

NEW LIFE SYSTEMS, INC.   954-972-4600
PO Box 8767, Coral Springs, FL 33075
FDA Number: n/a   Fax: 954-974-6646
E-mail: nulifesys@aol.com
Annual Revenue: $1-$5 Million
Total Employees: 10   *Marketing Staff:* 3   *Sales Staff:* 7
Ownership: Private
General Admin.: Edgar Bentolila/President
Mktg./Adv.: Claude de Monterry/Manager Advertising

Analyzer, Doppler Spectrum	General
Analyzer, Pulmonary Function	Anesthesiology
Defibrillator, Line-Powered	Cardiovascular
Defibrillator/Monitor, Line-Powered	Cardiovascular
Doppler, Blood Flow, Transcranial	Cardiovascular
Echocardiograph (Ultrasonic Scanner)	Cardiovascular
Electrocardiograph, Multi-Channel	Cardiovascular
Electrocardiograph, Single Channel	Cardiovascular
Electrode, Electrocardiograph	Cardiovascular
Endoscope	Gastroenterology/Urology
Monitor, Blood Pressure, Indirect, Automatic	Cardiovascular
Monitor, Physiological, Stress Exercise	Cardiovascular
Monitor, Pulse Rate	Anesthesiology
Recorder, Long-Term, ECG	Cardiovascular
Recorder, Long-Term, ECG, Portable (Holter Monitor)	Cardiovascular
Scanner, Long-Term, ECG, Recording	Cardiovascular
Scanner, Ultrasonic, Abdominal	Radiology
Scanner, Ultrasonic, Obstetrical/Gynecological, Mobile	Obstetrics/Gynecology
Scanner, Ultrasonic, Other	Radiology
Scanner, Ultrasonic, Small Parts	Radiology
Scanner, Ultrasonic, Vascular	Radiology
Service, Consulting	General

NEW LIFE SYSTEMS, INC.   954-972-4600 *(cont'd)*

Service, Import/Export	General
Service, Maintenance/Repair	General
Service, Used Equipment	General
Spirometer, Diagnostic (Respirometer)	Anesthesiology
Telemetry Unit, Physiological, ECG	Cardiovascular
Treadmill, Mechanical	Physical Med
Treadmill, Powered	Physical Med

NEW OPTIONS, INC.   214-638-6422
2545 Merrell Rd., Dallas, TX 75229
FDA Number: 1648709

Orthosis, Limb Brace	Physical Med

NEW PRODUCT DEVELOPMENT, INC.   315-434-9000
6700 Old Collamer Road, East Syracuse, NY 13057
FDA Number: 1320512

Computer, Diagnostic, Programmable	Cardiovascular

NEW PX IMAGING
See Brotherston Homecare Inc., Pxi Div.

NEW STAR LASERS, INC.   916-677-1900
9085 Foothills Blvd., Roseville, CA 95747
FDA Number: 2951571   Fax: 916-677-1901
E-mail: info@newstarlasers.com
Web site: www.newstarlasers.com
Medical Products Sales Volume: $9,500,000
Annual Revenue: $10-$25 Million
Year Founded: 1994
Total Employees: 42   *Marketing Staff:* 3   *Sales Staff:* 10
Ownership: Private
Quality System Registration Information: ISO9001
Produces/Sells CE-marked Devices: Y
Federal Procurement Eligibility: Small Business
Distribution: Manufacturer Direct, Manufacturer Through Distributor, OEM, Exporter
General Admin.: Mr. David Hennings/Chief Executive Officer
                 Ms. Nina Davis/President
Mktg./Adv.: Ms. Kathy Van Velzer/Director Marketing
Production: Mr. Donald Johnson/Vice President Operations

Lamp, Infrared	Physical Med
Laser, Surgical	Surgery

NEW WORLD IMPORTS   800-329-1903
160 Athens Way, Nashville, TN 37228   **615-329-1906**
FDA Number: 1044117   Fax: 615-329-3816
E-mail: tammy@newworldimports.org
Web site: www.newworldimports.org
Medical Products Sales Volume: $1,000,000
Year Founded: 1971
Total Employees: 10
Ownership: Private
Produces/Sells CE-marked Devices: N
Federal Procurement Eligibility: Small Business, GSA Contract
Distribution: Manufacturer Through Distributor
General Admin.: Randoph M. Lagasse/President, Chief Executive Officer

Bag, Plastic	General
Brush, Other	General
Dentifrice	Dental And Oral
Kit, Admission (Patient Utensil)	General
Soap	General
Toothbrush, Manual	Dental And Oral

NEW WORLD MEDICAL, INC.   800-832-5327
10763 Edison Ct.,   **909-466-4304**
Rancho Cucamonga, CA 91730
FDA Number: 2028380   Fax: 909-466-4305
E-mail: info@ahmedvalve.com
Web site: www.ahmedvalve.com
Medical Products Sales Volume: $900,000
Annual Revenue: $1-$5 Million
Year Founded: 1990
Total Employees: 10   *Marketing Staff:* 4   *Sales Staff:* 32
Ownership: Private
Produces/Sells CE-marked Devices: Y
Federal Procurement Eligibility: Small Business, Minority Owned
Distribution: Manufacturer Direct
General Admin.: Dr. A. MATEEN AHMED/President, Chief Executive Officer, Chairman

Implant, Eye Valve	Ophthalmology

Medical Product Subsidiaries (Listed Separately)
Cpac Equipment, Inc.

NEW YORK HOSPITAL DISPOSABLES, INC.   718-384-1620
101 Richardson Street, Brooklyn, NY 11211-1310
FDA Number: 2433094   Fax: 718-599-1183
E-mail: nyhdi@aol.com
Medical Products Sales Volume: $900,000

NEW YORK HOSPITAL DISPOSABLES, INC.   718-384-1620
(cont'd)
Year Founded: 1981
Total Employees: 20
Federal Procurement Eligibility: Small Business, Minority Owned
Distribution: Manufacturer Direct
General Admin.: Victor Cora/President
Mktg./Adv.: Raymond Cora/Vice President Sales

Cap, Surgical	Surgery
Cover, Head, Surgical	Surgery
Cover, Shoe, Operating Room	Surgery
Dress, Scrub, Disposable	Surgery
Gown, Isolation, Surgical	Surgery
Mask, Surgical	Surgery
Suit, Scrub, Disposable	Surgery

NEWBOLD CORPORATION   800-552-3282
450 Weaver St., Rocky Mount, VA 24151   **540-489-4400**
FDA Number: n/a   *Fax:* 540-489-4393
E-mail: mark@newboldcorp.com
Web site: www.newboldcorp.com
Medical Products Sales Volume: $5,000,000
Annual Revenue: $10-$25 Million
Year Founded: 1994
Total Employees: 100   *Marketing Staff:* 2   *Sales Staff:* 9
Ownership: Private
Produces/Sells CE-marked Devices: N
Federal Procurement Eligibility: Small Business
Distribution: Manufacturer Direct, Manufacturer Through Distributor, Manufacturer Through Manufacturer Reps, Exporter
Mktg./Adv.: Mark Hathaway/Director Sales
     Don Zeppenfeld/Vice President Sales

Card, Identification	General
Computer, Patient Data Management	General
Forms, Medical And Patient	General

NEWCARDIO INC.   408-516-5000
2350 Mission College Blvd, Suite 1175, Santa Clara, CA 95054
FDA Number: n/a   *Fax:* 408-516-5005
E-mail: info@newcardio.com
Web site: www.newcardio.com
Ownership: Public
Stock Symbol: NWCI
Traded On: OTC Bulletin
Produces/Sells CE-marked Devices: N
General Admin.: Patrick Maguire/Chairman
     Dr. Ihor Gussak/Chief Medical Officer, Vice President
     Mr. Dorin Panescu/Chief Technology Officer, Vice President
     Mr. Vincent Renz/President, Chief Executive Officer
Finance: Mr. Richard Brounstein/Chief Financial Officer

NEWPORT CORPORATION   949-863-3144
1791 Deere Avenue, Irvine, CA 92606
FDA Number: n/a   *Fax:* 949-253-1680
E-mail: sales@newport.com
Web site: www.newport.com
Year Founded: 1969
Ownership: Public
Stock Symbol: NEWP
Traded On: NASDAQ
Produces/Sells CE-marked Devices: N

NEWPORT FRANKLIN, INC.   800-598-6783
1791 Deere Avenue, Irvine, CA 92606   **508-528-4411**
FDA Number: n/a   *Fax:* 508-520-7583
E-mail: filters.sales@newport.com
Web site: www.newport.com
Medical Products Sales Volume: $15,000,000
Annual Revenue: $10-$25 Million
Year Founded: 1969
Total Employees: 100   *Marketing Staff:* 1   *Sales Staff:* 7
Ownership: NEWPORT CORPORATION
Quality System Registration Information: ISO9001
Produces/Sells CE-marked Devices: Y
Federal Procurement Eligibility: Small Business
Distribution: Manufacturer Direct, OEM
General Admin.: Don McLeod/General Manager
Mktg./Adv.: David Montgomery/Director Marketing & Sales
     Jamie Knapp/Director Product Development
Production: Debra Bricault/Director Quality Assurance
     Michael Carta/Vice President Manufacturing

Component, Optical	General
Filter, Lens	Ophthalmology

NEWPORT GLASS WORKS, LTD.   714-484-8100
PO Box 127, 10564 Fern Avenue, Stanton, CA 90680
FDA Number: n/a   *Fax:* 714-484-8181
E-mail: ngw@newportglass.com

NEWPORT GLASS WORKS, LTD.   714-484-8100 *(cont'd)*
Web site: www.newportglass.com
Medical Products Sales Volume: $900,000
Annual Revenue: $0-$1 Million
Year Founded: 1979
Total Employees: 13
Ownership: Private
Stock Symbol: 4042
Traded On: Tokyo
Produces/Sells CE-marked Devices: N
Federal Procurement Eligibility: Small Business, Minority Owned
Distribution: Manufacturer Direct
General Admin.: Ray Larsen/President
Mktg./Adv.: Ray Larsen/Manager Sales

Component, Other	General
Equipment, Device Coating, Protective	General
Filter, Lens	Ophthalmology
Laboratory Equipment, Ophthalmic	Ophthalmology
Lens, Camera, Surgical	Surgery
Lens, Set, Trial, Ophthalmic	Ophthalmology

NEWPORT INSTRUMENTS INC.
See Allen Medical Instruments Corp.

NEWPORT MEDICAL INSTRUMENTS, INC.   800-451-3111
1620 Sunflower Ave, Costa Mesa, CA 92626   **714-427-5811**
FDA Number: 7000674   *Fax:* 714-427-0489
E-mail: info@ventilators.com
Web site: www.ventilators.com
Medical Products Sales Volume: $12,000,000
Annual Revenue: $10-$25 Million
Year Founded: 1981
Total Employees: 100
Ownership: Private
Produces/Sells CE-marked Devices: Y
Distribution: Manufacturer Direct, Manufacturer Through Distributor, Manufacturer Through Manufacturer Reps
General Admin.: Jay Nash/Executive Vice President
Mktg./Adv.: Janus Baker/Manager Marketing Communications
Production: Cindi Davis/Manager Customer Services
IS: Robert Rodriguez/Manager Tech. Services

Ventilator, Other	Anesthesiology
Ventilator, Volume (Critical Care)	Anesthesiology

NEWPORT OPTICAL INDUSTRIES
See Newport Glass Works, Ltd.

NEWPORT OPTICAL LABORATORIES, INC.   714-484-3200
10564-C Fern Ave., Stanton, CA 90680
FDA Number: n/a   *Fax:* 714-484-7600
E-mail: newportlab@hotmail.com
Total Employees: 10   *Marketing Staff:* 1   *Sales Staff:* 2
Ownership: Private
Produces/Sells CE-marked Devices: N
Federal Procurement Eligibility: Small Business, Minority Owned
Distribution: Manufacturer Direct, OEM, Exporter
General Admin.: Ray Larson/President, Chief Executive Officer
Mktg./Adv.: Chris Gomez/Vice President Marketing & Sales
Production: Operto Nelson/Vice President Manufacturing

Bar, Prism, Ophthalmic	Ophthalmology
Endoscope	Gastroenterology/Urology
Goggles, Protective, Eye	Ophthalmology
Laboratory Equipment, Ophthalmic	Ophthalmology
Microscope, Surgical, General & Plastic Surgery	Surgery

NEWSCHOFF CHAIRS, INC.   800-203-8916
909 North 8 St., Sheboygan, WI 53081   **920-457-7726**
FDA Number: n/a   *Fax:* 920-459-1284
Web site: www.nemschoff.com
Annual Revenue: $1-$5 Million
Total Employees: 350
Ownership: Private
Produces/Sells CE-marked Devices: N
Federal Procurement Eligibility: Small Business, GSA Contract, VA Contract
Distribution: Manufacturer Through Manufacturer Reps, OEM, Exporter
General Admin.: Mark S. Nemschoff/President, Chief Executive Officer
Mktg./Adv.: Mark Nemschoff/Senior Vice President Marketing & Sales
     David Stinson/Vice President Sales

Cabinet Casework, Patient Room	General
Cabinet, Bedside	General
Chair, Geriatric	General
Chair, Pediatric	General
Chair, Shower	General
Furniture, General	General
Furniture, Patient Room	General
Mattress, Bed	General

NEWTECH DENTAL LABORATORIES   866-635-5227
1141 Smile Ln., Lansdale, PA 19446   **215-699-8861**
FDA Number: 2529794   *Fax:* 215-699-8862

NEWTECH DENTAL LABORATORIES — 866-635-5227 (cont'd)
E-mail: info@ndlsmile.com
Web site: www.ndlsmile.com
Year Founded: 1979
Total Employees: 50
Ownership: Private
Produces/Sells CE-marked Devices: N
Federal Procurement Eligibility: Small Business

Crown And Bridge, Temporary, Resin	Dental And Oral

NEWTEX INDUSTRIES, INC. — 800-836-1001
8050 Victor-Mendon Rd., Victor, NY 14564 — **585-924-9135**
FDA Number: n/a — Fax: 585-924-4645
E-mail: sales@newtex.com
Web site: www.newtex.com
Ownership: Private
Quality System Registration Information: ISO9001
Produces/Sells CE-marked Devices: Y
Federal Procurement Eligibility: Small Business, Minority Owned
Distribution: Manufacturer Direct, Manufacturer Through Distributor, Manufacturer Through Manufacturer Reps
General Admin.: Bal Dixit/Chief Executive Officer
Mktg./Adv.: Skip Mattox/Director Marketing
David Gisbourne/Director Product Development
Skip Mattox/Manager International & National Sales
Production: Siresh Deshpande/Director Quality Assurance

Blanket, Fire	General
Clothing, Protective	General
Glove, Other	General

NEWTRON PRODUCTS — 513-561-7373
3874 Virginia Ave, PO BOX 27175, Cincinnati, OH 45227
FDA Number: n/a — Fax: 513-561-3673
Web site: www.newtronproducts.com
Total Employees: 7
Ownership: Private
Produces/Sells CE-marked Devices: N
Federal Procurement Eligibility: Small Business
Distribution: Manufacturer Direct

Equipment, Cleaning, Air	General

NEWWAVE MEDICAL LLC — 888-513-9283
1239 Durham Road, Whitewright, TX 75491 — **903-364-2087**
FDA Number: 1651161 — Fax: 903-364-1522
E-mail: info@newwavemed.com
Web site: www.newwavemed.com
Medical Products Sales Volume: $300,000
Year Founded: 1992
Total Employees: 4
Ownership: Private
Produces/Sells CE-marked Devices: N
Federal Procurement Eligibility: Small Business
Distribution: Manufacturer Through Distributor

Electrode, Cutaneous	Cns/Neurology
Stimulator, Muscle, Electrical-Powered (EMS)	Physical Med
Unit, Therapy, Current, Interferential	Cns/Neurology

NEXAIR, LLC. — 901-729-5547
1211 North Mclean Blvd., Mem, TN 38108
FDA Number: 1020303

Gas, Calibrated (Specified Concentration)	Anesthesiology
Laser, Surgical	Surgery

NEXSTIM OY — +358 9 2727 171
ElimAüAenkatu 9 B, Helsinki FI-00510
FDA Number: 3007147067 — Fax: +358 9 2727 171
Web site: http://www.nexstim.com
Ownership: Private
Produces/Sells CE-marked Devices: N
General Admin.: Mr. Richard Karroum/Chief Executive Officer
Medical Admin.: Dr. Jari Karhu/Chief Medical Officer
Mktg./Adv.: Mr. Henri Hannula/Director Marketing & Sales
Production: Mr. Ville Lappi/Manager Operations
Mr. Rainer Harjunpaa/Manager Quality Assurance & Regulatory Affairs
Research: Mr. Gustaf Jarnefelt/Director Research & Development
Finance: Mr. Janne Huhtala/Chief Financial Officer

Electromyograph, Diagnostic	Physical Med
Stimulator, Electrical, Evoked Response	Cns/Neurology

NEXT GENERATION CO. — 800-598-4303
41740 Enterprise Cir., North, #108, — **909-296-1990**
Temecula, CA 92590
FDA Number: 2029389 — Fax: 909-296-1993
E-mail: mnextgenco@aol.com
Medical Products Sales Volume: $3,200,000
Annual Revenue: $1-$5 Million
Year Founded: 1988
Total Employees: 10 — Sales Staff: 10

NEXT GENERATION CO. — 800-598-4303 (cont'd)
Ownership: Private
Produces/Sells CE-marked Devices: N
Federal Procurement Eligibility: Small Business

Cushion, Wheelchair (Pad)	Physical Med

NEXTGEN SCIENCES INC — 1-866-973-7914
401 Varsity Drive, Suite E, — **734-973-7914**
Ann Arbor, MI 48108
FDA Number: n/a — Fax: 734-973-7932
E-mail: info@nextgensciences.com
Web site: www.nextgensciences.com
Ownership: Private
Produces/Sells CE-marked Devices: N
General Admin.: Mr. Klaus Rosenau/Chairman, Chief Executive Officer
Mr. Barry McAleer/Director
Finance: Mr. Leif Hamo/Chief Financial Officer

NEXUS MEDICAL, LLC — 913-451-2234
11315 Strang Line Road, Lenexa, KS 66215
FDA Number: 3004194523

Holder, Intravascular Catheter	General
Kit, Administration, Intravenous	General
Urological Irrigation System	Gastroenterology/Urology

NFOCUS NEUROMEDICAL INC. — 888-483-6287
2191 E. Bayshore Rd., Suite 100, — **650-845-3040**
Palo Alto, CA 94303
FDA Number: 3007289509 — Fax: 650-813-1869
E-mail: info@nfocusneuro.com
Web site: www.nfocusneuro.com
Year Founded: 2007
Ownership: Private
Produces/Sells CE-marked Devices: N
General Admin.: Mr. Eric Milledge/Chief Executive Officer
Martin Dieck/President, Chief Operating Officer
Production: Ms. Kelly Roberts/Vice President Quality Assurance
Mr. Robert O'Halla/Vice President Regulatory Affairs
Research: Mr. Frank Becking/Vice President Engineering
Finance: Ms. JIll Papp/Chief Financial Officer

NIAGARA PHARMACEUTICALS DIV. — 905-690-6277
60 Innovation Dr., Flamborough, ONT L9H-7P3 Canada
FDA Number: n/a — Fax: 905-690-6281
E-mail: edmaloney@hearsaver.com
Web site: www.hearsaver.com
Total Employees: 30
Ownership: Private
Quality System Registration Information: ISO9002
Produces/Sells CE-marked Devices: Y
Federal Procurement Eligibility: Small Business
Distribution: Manufacturer Direct, Manufacturer Through Distributor, Manufacturer Through Manufacturer Reps, OEM, Importer, Exporter

NICA-POWER BATTERY CORP. — 800-565-6422
5155 Spectrum Way, — **905-624-0000**
Mississauga, ON L4W 5 Canada
FDA Number: n/a — Fax: 905-624-5060
E-mail: sales@nicapowr.com
Web site: www.nicapower.com
Year Founded: 1983
Total Employees: 10 — Marketing Staff: 2 — Sales Staff: 2
Ownership: Private
Produces/Sells CE-marked Devices: N
Federal Procurement Eligibility: Small Business
Distribution: Manufacturer Direct, Exclusive Distributor

NICHE MEDICAL, INC. — 800-633-1055
55 Access Rd., Warwick, RI 02886 — **401-732-3321**
FDA Number: 1224874 — Fax: 401-739-8095
E-mail: info@nichemedical.com
Web site: www.nichemedical.com
Year Founded: 1995
Ownership: NORTEK, INC.
Produces/Sells CE-marked Devices: N
Distribution: Manufacturer Direct, Manufacturer Through Distributor, Manufacturer Through Manufacturer Reps, OEM, Service Direct, Exclusive Distributor
General Admin.: Ms. Tammy Healey/Manager
Mr. Dennis Sleister/President

Evacuator, Vapor, Cement Monomer	Orthopedics
Exhaust System, Surgical	Surgery
Filter, Air	General
Mask, Surgical	Surgery
System, Evacuation, Smoke, Laser	Surgery
Tubing, Corrugated	General

NICHOLE MEDICAL EQUIPMENT & SUPPLY, INC. 888-673-6335
2200 Michener St., Suite #4,   215-673-6333
Philadelphia, PA 19115
FDA Number: 2529773   *Fax:* 215-673-7181
E-mail: dominic@nicholemedical.com
Web site: www.nicholemedical.com
Medical Products Sales Volume: $600,000
Annual Revenue: $1-$5 Million
Year Founded: 1986
Total Employees: 7   *Sales Staff:* 2
Ownership: Private
Produces/Sells CE-marked Devices: N
Federal Procurement Eligibility: Small Business
   Regulator, Pressure, Gas Cylinder   Anesthesiology

NICHOLS INSTITUTE DIAGNOSTICS   949-940-7200
1311 Calle Batido, San Clemente, CA 92673
FDA Number: 2050095
Ownership: Private
Produces/Sells CE-marked Devices: N
   Control, Hemoglobin, Abnormal   Hematology
   Immunochemical, Thyroglobulin Autoantibody   Immunology
   Immunochemical, Transferrin   Immunology
   Radioimmunoassay, ACTH   Chemistry
   Radioimmunoassay, Angiotensin I And Renin   Chemistry
   Radioimmunoassay, Calcitonin   Chemistry
   Radioimmunoassay, Cortisol   Chemistry
   Radioimmunoassay, Dehydroepiandrosterone (Free And Sulfate)   Chemistry
   Radioimmunoassay, Ferritin   Microbiology
   Radioimmunoassay, Follicle Stimulating Hormone   Chemistry
   Radioimmunoassay, Free Thyroxine   Chemistry
   Radioimmunoassay, Human Chorionic Gonadotropin   Chemistry
   Radioimmunoassay, Human Growth Hormone   Chemistry
   Radioimmunoassay, Luteinizing Hormone   Chemistry
   Radioimmunoassay, Parathyroid Hormone   Chemistry
   Radioimmunoassay, Prolactin (Lactogen)   Chemistry
   Radioimmunoassay, Thyroid Stimulating Hormone   Chemistry
   Radioimmunoassay, Total Triiodothyronine   Chemistry
   Reagent, General Purpose   Pathology
   System, Test, Thyroglobulin   Immunology
   System, Test, Vitamin D   Chemistry
   Test, Erythropoietin   Hematology
   Test, Thyroid Autoantibody   Immunology
   Thyroglobulin, Antigen, Antiserum, Control   Immunology

NICORE EQUIPMENT & LEASING, INC.
See Scottcare Corporation

NIDACON CANADA INC.   613-260-0886
250-600 Peter Morand Cres, Ottawa K1G 5Z3 Canada
FDA Number: 9613749
   Media, Reproductive   Obstetrics/Gynecology

NIDEK INC.   800-223-9044
47651 Westinghouse Drive,   510-353-7710
Fremont, CA 94539
FDA Number: 8030392   *Fax:* 510-226-5750
E-mail: info@nidek.com
Web site: www.nidek.com
Medical Products Sales Volume: $1,200,000
Annual Revenue: $50-$100 Million
Year Founded: 1987
Total Employees: 50   *Marketing Staff:* 5   *Sales Staff:* 15
Ownership: Private
Quality System Registration Information: ISO9001
Produces/Sells CE-marked Devices: Y
Federal Procurement Eligibility: Small Business, Minority Owned, GSA Contract, VA Contract
Distribution: Manufacturer Direct, Manufacturer Through Distributor, Manufacturer Through Manufacturer Reps, OEM, Service Direct, Exclusive Distributor, Importer, Exporter
General Admin.: Mr. Kio Iwase/Assistant Vice President, Controller
     Mr. Hideo Ozawa/President
     Mr. Ted Shimomura/Vice President, General Manager
Mktg./Adv.: Mr. Kuntal Joshi/Director Marketing
     Mr. David Yeh/Director Sales
     Mr. Jim Potter/Manager National Sales
     Mr. Hiro Matsuzaki/Manager Product Development
   Camera, Ophthalmic, AC-Powered (Fundus)   Ophthalmology
   Camera, Other   General
   Keratome, AC-Powered   Ophthalmology
   Keratoscope, AC-Powered   Ophthalmology
   Laser, Ophthalmic   Ophthalmology
   Laser, Surgical   Surgery
   Monitor, Eye Movement   Ophthalmology
   Pachometer   Ophthalmology
   Refractometer, Ophthalmic   Ophthalmology
   Scanner, Ultrasonic, Ophthalmic   Radiology

NIDEK INC.   800-223-9044 *(cont'd)*
   System, Laser, Excimer, Ophthalmic   Ophthalmology

NIDEK MEDICAL PRODUCTS INC.   800-822-9255
3949 Valley E. Industrial Dr.,   205-856-7200
Birmingham, AL 35217
FDA Number: 1039215   *Fax:* 205-856-0533
E-mail: info@nidekmedical.com
Web site: www.nidekmedical.com
Annual Revenue: $10-$25 Million
Year Founded: 1987
Total Employees: 70   *Marketing Staff:* 4   *Sales Staff:* 35
Ownership: Private
Quality System Registration Information: ISO9002
Produces/Sells CE-marked Devices: Y
Federal Procurement Eligibility: Small Business, Minority Owned
Distribution: Manufacturer Through Distributor, Manufacturer Through Manufacturer Reps, Exporter
General Admin.: Anand Chitlangia/President, Chief Executive Officer
     Len Suelter/Vice President
     Gregg Gaskins/Vice President, General Manager
Mktg./Adv.: Debbie A. Moore/Manager Marketing
     Joe Krawczyk/Manager Sales
Production: Jennifer McWilliams/Director Quality Assurance
   Compressor, Air, Portable   Anesthesiology
   Concentrator, Oxygen   Anesthesiology
   Generator, Oxygen, Portable   Anesthesiology
   Nebulizer, Direct Patient Interface   Anesthesiology

NIDEK, INC.   510-226-5700
47651 Westinghouse Dr., Fremont, CA 94539
FDA Number: 2936921
Ownership: Private
Produces/Sells CE-marked Devices: N
   Camera, Ophthalmic, AC-Powered (Fundus)   Ophthalmology
   Device, Analysis, Anterior Segment   Ophthalmology
   Device, Storage, Images, Ophthalmic   Ophthalmology
   Fluidic, Phacoemulsification/fragmentation   Ophthalmology
   Keratome, AC-Powered   Ophthalmology
   Keratoscope, AC-Powered   Ophthalmology
   Lamp, Slit, Biomicroscope, AC-Powered   Ophthalmology
   Laser, Neodymium:YAG, Ophthalmic (Post. Capsulotomy)   Ophthalmology
   Laser, Ophthalmic   Ophthalmology
   Laser, Surgical   Surgery
   Perimeter, Automatic, AC-Powered   Ophthalmology
   Phacofragmentation Unit   Ophthalmology
   Photocoagulator   Ophthalmology
   Scanner, Ultrasonic (Pulsed Echo)   Radiology
   System, Laser, Excimer, Ophthalmic   Ophthalmology

NIGHTHAWK MANUFACTURING INC.   1-800-661-6247
3204 - 121 Avenue NE,   780-457-2937
Edmonton, ALB T6S-1 Canada
FDA Number: n/a   *Fax:* 780-457-7814
E-mail: info@nthawk.com
Web site: www.nthawk.com
Year Founded: 1986
Total Employees: 10
Ownership: Private
Produces/Sells CE-marked Devices: N
Distribution: Manufacturer Direct, Importer, Exporter

NIGHTINGALE LENS LABS   800-561-0034
387 Sunset Dr., Fredericton, NB E3A-1J2 Canada   506-453-1063
FDA Number: n/a   *Fax:* 506-457-0919
E-mail: nightingale@brunnet.net
Year Founded: 1979
Ownership: Private
Produces/Sells CE-marked Devices: N
Distribution: Manufacturer Direct

NIGHTINGALE UNIFORM CO., INC.   334-376-2296
210 E. Mill St., P.O. Box 578, Georgiana, AL 36033-0578
FDA Number: n/a   *Fax:* 334-376-2478
E-mail: nightingale@alaweb.com
Web site: www.nightingaleuniform.com
Annual Revenue: $0-$1 Million
Year Founded: 1933
Total Employees: 30
Ownership: Private
Produces/Sells CE-marked Devices: N
Federal Procurement Eligibility: Small Business
Distribution: Manufacturer Direct
   Gown, Other   General

NIHON KOHDEN AMERICA, INC.   800-325-0283
90 Icon St., Foothill Ranch, CA 92610   949-580-1555
FDA Number: 2080783   *Fax:* 949-580-1550

NIHON KOHDEN AMERICA, INC.   800-325-0283 *(cont'd)*

E-mail: info@nkusa.com
Web site: www.nkusa.com
Annual Revenue: $50-$100 Million
Year Founded: 1979
Ownership: Nihon Kohden Corp.
Quality System Registration Information: ISO9001
Produces/Sells CE-marked Devices: Y
Distribution: Manufacturer Direct, Manufacturer Through Manufacturer Reps
General Admin.: E. Tanaka/President
         Y. Nakajima/Vice President
Mktg./Adv.: G. Reasoner/Director Sales
         M. Dashefsky/Vice President Marketing & Sales
Production: M. Ohsawa/Director Operations

Computer and Software, Medical	General
Computer, Patient Monitor	Anesthesiology
Conditioner, Signal, Physiological	Cns/Neurology
Electrocardiograph, Multi-Channel	Cardiovascular
Electrocardiograph, Single Channel	Cardiovascular
Electroencephalograph	Cns/Neurology
Evoked Response Unit	Cns/Neurology
Monitor, ECG	Cardiovascular
Monitor, Neonatal	Obstetrics/Gynecology
Monitor, Neonatal, Physiological	Obstetrics/Gynecology
Monitor, Physiological, Acute Care	Anesthesiology
Monitor, Physiological, Patient	Cardiovascular
Monitor, Physiological, Stress Exercise	Cardiovascular
Oximeter, Pulse	General
Recorder, Paper Chart	Cardiovascular
Sleep Assessment Equipment	Cns/Neurology
Stimulator, Neurological	Surgery
Telemetry Unit, Physiological, ECG	Cardiovascular
Telemetry Unit, Physiological, EEG	Cns/Neurology
Telemetry Unit, Physiological, Multiple Channel	General
Transmitter/Receiver System, Physiological, Radiofrequency	Cardiovascular

NIKE, INC.   800-344-6453
One Bowerman Drive,   **503-671-2872**
Beaverton, OR 97005
FDA Number: 3032111   Fax: 503-671-6397
E-mail: christy.miller@nike.com
Web site: www.nike.com
Medical Products Sales Volume: $14,950,000,000
Year Founded: 1964
Total Employees: 6000
Ownership: Private
Stock Symbol: NKE
Traded On: NYSE
Produces/Sells CE-marked Devices: N
Sunglasses (Including Photosensitive)   Ophthalmology

NIKOMED U.S.A., INC.   800-355-6456
2000 Pioneer Rd.,   **215-443-8989**
Huntington Valley, PA 19006
FDA Number: 2245574   Fax: 215-443-8990
Web site: www.nikomedusa.com
Year Founded: 1986
Total Employees: 12   Marketing Staff: 4   Sales Staff: 4
Ownership: Private
Produces/Sells CE-marked Devices: N
Federal Procurement Eligibility: Small Business
Distribution: Manufacturer Through Distributor, OEM
General Admin.: Donald Epstein/Chief Executive Officer
         Steve Epstein/Vice President, General Manager
Mktg./Adv.: Neil Epstein/Director Marketing

Electrode, Electrocardiograph	Cardiovascular
Electrosurgical Unit, Neurological	Cns/Neurology
Stimulator, Muscle, Low Intensity	Physical Med

NIKON CANADA INC., INSTRUMENT DIV.   905-625-9910
1366 Aerowood Dr., Mississauga, ONT L4W-1C1 Canada
FDA Number: n/a   Fax: (905) 602-9953
E-mail: info@nikon.ca
Web site: www.nikon.ca
Year Founded: 1978
Total Employees: 25
Ownership: NIKON CORP.- JAPAN
Produces/Sells CE-marked Devices: N
Distribution: Exclusive Distributor

NIKON INSTRUMENTS INC.   800-52-Nikon
1300 Walt Whitman Road,   **631-547-8500**
Melville, NY 11747
FDA Number: n/a   Fax: 631-547-4025
E-mail: biosales@nikon.net
Web site: www.nikonusa.com
Medical Products Sales Volume: $17,400,000
Year Founded: 1975

NIKON INSTRUMENTS INC.   800-52-Nikon *(cont'd)*

Total Employees: 85   Marketing Staff: 10   Sales Staff: 100
Ownership: NIKON CORP.- JAPAN
Traded On: Tokyo
Quality System Registration Information: ISO9000; ISO9002
Produces/Sells CE-marked Devices: Y
Federal Procurement Eligibility: Small Business, GSA Contract
Distribution: Manufacturer Direct, Manufacturer Through Distributor, Manufacturer Through Manufacturer Reps, OEM, Service Direct, Exclusive Distributor, Importer
General Admin.: Lee Shuett/Executive Vice President
         Lee Shuett/General Manager
Mktg./Adv.: Stanley Schwartz/Manager Marketing

Camera, Identification	General
Camera, Microscope	Microbiology
Camera, Still, Surgical	Surgery
Lamp, Microscope	Pathology
Micromanipulator	General
Microscope, Inverted Stage, Tissue Culture	Pathology
Microscope, Laboratory, Optical	Microbiology
Microscope, Light	Pathology

NIKON OPTICAL CANADA, INC.   011-813-5600
100-5075 Rue Fullum, Montreal H2H 2K3 Canada
FDA Number: 8043497
Lens, Spectacle/Eyeglasses, Non-Custom   Ophthalmology

NILAN TOOL & MOLD CORP.   630-543-7114
1215 National Ave., Addison, IL 60101-3180
FDA Number: n/a   Fax: 630-543-6727
E-mail: herman@nilantool.com
Web site: www.nilantool.com
Annual Revenue: $1-$5 Million
Total Employees: 35
Ownership: Private
Produces/Sells CE-marked Devices: N
General Admin.: Herman Grabenstetter/Chief Executive Officer
         Glen Pari/President
Mktg./Adv.: Louis Turilli/Vice President Sales
Production: Glen Pari/Vice President Manufacturing
         Lou Turilli/Vice President, Engineer
Molding, Custom   General

NILODOR, INC.   800-443-4321
10966 Industrial Pkwy., N.W., Bolivar, OH 44612   **330-874-1017**
FDA Number: n/a   Fax: 330-874-3366
E-mail: info@nilodor.com
Web site: www.nilodor.com
Medical Products Sales Volume: $3,800,000
Annual Revenue: $1-$5 Million
Total Employees: 35   Sales Staff: 4
Ownership: Private
Produces/Sells CE-marked Devices: N
Federal Procurement Eligibility: Small Business
Distribution: Manufacturer Through Distributor
General Admin.: Les W. Mitson/President
Mktg./Adv.: Todd Sauser/Director Marketing
         Kurt Peterson/Manager International & National Sales
         Kurt Peterson/Vice President Sales
Production: Robert Bemis/Manager Regulatory Affairs
Sanitizer   General

NIMBIC SYSTEMS, LLC   281-565-5700
4910 Wright Road, Suite 170, Stafford, TX 77477
FDA Number: 3006412720
Accessories, Operating Room, Table   Surgery

NINEPOINT MEDICAL INC.   617-250-7190
One Kendall Square, Suite B7501, Cambridge, MA 02139
FDA Number: n/a   Fax: 617-250-7199
E-mail: info@ninepointmedical.com
Web site: www.ninepointmedical.com
Ownership: Private
Produces/Sells CE-marked Devices: N

NIPRO DIABETES SYSTEMS, INC.   888-651-7867
3361 Enterprise Way, Miramar, FL 33025   **816-637-2233**
FDA Number: 1066380   Fax: 954-435-9295
Web site: www.nipro.com
Ownership: Nipro Corp.
Produces/Sells CE-marked Devices: N

Infusion Pump, Insulin	General
Kit, Administration, Intravenous	General
Syringe, Piston	General

NIPRO DIAGNOSTICS, INC.   800-342-7226
2400 N.W. 55th Ct., Fort Lauderdale, FL 33309   **954-677-9201**
FDA Number: 1052693
E-mail: professionals@hdidiabetes.com

NIPRO DIAGNOSTICS, INC.   800-342-7226 *(cont'd)*
Web site: www.niprodiagnostics.com
Ownership: Public
Stock Symbol: HDIX
Traded On: NASDAQ
Produces/Sells CE-marked Devices: N
General Admin.: Mr. Scott Verner/President

Control, Analyte (Assayed And Unassayed)	Chemistry
Lancet, Blood	General
Nitroprusside, Ketones (Urinary, Non-Quantitative)	Chemistry
Reagent, Glucose (Test System)	Chemistry
System, Test, Blood Glucose, Over-The-Counter	Chemistry

NITE TRAIN'R   503-626-8833
9735 S.W. Sunshine Ct., Suite 100, Beaverton, OR 97005
FDA Number: 3019107   *Fax:* 503-644-1366
E-mail: info@nitetrain-r.com
Web site: www.nitetrain-r.com
Year Founded: 1988
Ownership: Private
Produces/Sells CE-marked Devices: N
Federal Procurement Eligibility: Minority Owned
Distribution: Manufacturer Direct
General Admin.: H. J. Park/President, Chief Executive Officer

Alarm, Enuresis	Gastroenterology/Urology
Conditioner, Signal, Physiological	Cns/Neurology

NITINOL DEVICES & COMPONENTS, INC.   510-683-2000
47533 Westinghouse Dr., Fremont, CA 94539
FDA Number: 3007635982
E-mail: sales@nitinol.com
Web site: www.nitinol.com
Year Founded: 1991
Total Employees: 125
Ownership: Private
Quality System Registration Information: ISO9000
Produces/Sells CE-marked Devices: N
General Admin.: Tom Dureig/Chief Executive Officer
     Mr. Alan Pelton/Chief Technology Officer
Mktg./Adv.: Ms. Atilla Meretei/Vice President Business Development
     Mr. David Niedermaier/Vice President Marketing & Sales
Production: Mr. Chuck Faris/Vice President Quality Assurance & Regulatory Affairs
Finance: Mr. Chun Tam/Chief Financial Officer

Contract Manufacturing	General
Guidewire, Catheter	Cardiovascular

NITRIC BIO, INC.   866-957-6200
2 Canal's End Road, Suite 201-A,   215-788-6200
Bristol, PA 19007
FDA Number: 3007135529   *Fax:* 215-788-6345
E-mail: info@nitricbio.com
Web site: www.nitricbio.com
Ownership: Cardinal Health Inc.
Produces/Sells CE-marked Devices: N
General Admin.: Frank McCaney/Chief Executive Officer
     Mr. James A. Ratigan/Chief Financial Officer, Vice President
     Tanya Rhodes/Chief Technology Officer
     Mr. Frank McCaney/President, Chief Executive Officer
Medical Admin.: Dr. Joel S. Lippman/Vice President Medical Affairs
Mktg./Adv.: Clare McKune/Market Manager

NK BIOTECHNICAL CORP.   612-541-0411
701 Decatur Avenue North, Suite 111a,
Golden Valley, MN 55427
FDA Number: 2183999

Caliper	Orthopedics
Goniometer, AC-powered	Orthopedics

NK MEDICAL PRODUCTS INC.   800-274-2742
10123 Main St, PO Box 627, Clarence, NY 14031   716-759-7200
FDA Number: 1318843   *Fax:* 716-759-0700
E-mail: info@nkmedicalproducts.com
Web site: www.nkmedicalproducts.com
Annual Revenue: $1-$5 Million
Year Founded: 1985
Total Employees: 25   *Marketing Staff:* 2   *Sales Staff:* 40
Ownership: Private
Produces/Sells CE-marked Devices: Y
Federal Procurement Eligibility: Small Business, GSA Contract
Distribution: Manufacturer Direct, Manufacturer Through Distributor, Manufacturer Through Manufacturer Reps, OEM, Importer, Exporter
General Admin.: Norman V. Kurlander/President, Chief Executive Officer
Production: SUSAN PLONKA/Manager Operations

Bassinet (Infant Bed)	General
Bed, Electric	General
Bed, Manual	General
Bed, Pediatric (Crib)	General
Chair, Other	General

NK MEDICAL PRODUCTS INC.   800-274-2742 *(cont'd)*

Furniture, Patient Room	General
Lift, Patient	General
Mattress, Bed	General
Stretcher, Emergency, Other	General
Stretcher, Transfer	Surgery
Table, Examination/Treatment	General
Table, Overbed	General

NKUS LAB   949-474-9207
2446 Dupont Dr., Irvine, CA 92612-1523
FDA Number: 2032233
Ownership: Private
Produces/Sells CE-marked Devices: N

Monitor, Physiological, Patient	Cardiovascular
Transmitter/Receiver System, Physiological, Radiofrequency	Cardiovascular

NMS PHARMACEUTICALS, DIAGN. DIV.
See Biomerica, Inc.

NMT MEDICAL, INC.   617-737-0930
27-43 Wormwood St., Boston, MA 02210
FDA Number: 1222632
Ownership: Public
Stock Symbol: NMTI
Traded On: NASDAQ
Produces/Sells CE-marked Devices: N

Clip, Aneurysm (Intracranial)	Cns/Neurology
Device, Occlusion, Cardiac, Transcatheter	Cardiovascular
Filter, Intravascular, Cardiovascular	Cardiovascular
Introducer, Catheter	Cardiovascular

NO RINSE LABORATORIES, LLC.   800-223-9348
868 Pleasant Valley Drive,   937-746-7357
Springboro, OH 45066
FDA Number: n/a   *Fax:* 937-746-7621
E-mail: gdavis@norinse.com
Web site: www.norinse.com
Medical Products Sales Volume: $2,000,000
Annual Revenue: $1-$5 Million
Total Employees: 9   *Sales Staff:* 2
Ownership: Private
Produces/Sells CE-marked Devices: N
Federal Procurement Eligibility: Small Business
Distribution: Manufacturer Direct, Manufacturer Through Distributor, Exporter
General Admin.: Greg Davis/President
Mktg./Adv.: Greg Davis/Manager Advertising
     Robert J. Laravie/Manager Sales

Sanitizer	General
Soap	General

NOA MEDICAL INDUSTRIES   800-633-6068
801 Terry Lane, Washington, MO 63090   636-239-7600
FDA Number: 1931947   *Fax:* 636-239-6900
E-mail: info@noamedical.com
Web site: www.noamedical.com
Medical Products Sales Volume: $1,600,000
Annual Revenue: $5-$10 Million
Year Founded: 1988
Total Employees: 30   *Marketing Staff:* 2   *Sales Staff:* 6
Ownership: Private
Produces/Sells CE-marked Devices: N
Federal Procurement Eligibility: Small Business, Female Owned
Distribution: Manufacturer Direct, Manufacturer Through Distributor, Manufacturer Through Manufacturer Reps
General Admin.: Michael W. Megown/Chief Executive Officer
Mktg./Adv.: Douglas Proffitt/Director Marketing & Sales

Bed, Electric	General
Bed, Manual	General
Bedrail	General
Table, Other	General
Table, Overbed	General

NOBEL BIOCARE PROCERA LLC.   714-282-5074
800 Corporate Dr., Mahwah, NJ 07430
FDA Number: 3005031178
Ownership: Private
Produces/Sells CE-marked Devices: N

Teeth, Porcelain	Dental And Oral

NOBEL BIOCARE PROCERA, INC.   201-828-9268
800 Corporate Drive, Mahwah, NJ 07410-2812
FDA Number: 2249603   *Fax:* 201-398-7435
E-mail: jan.kvist@procerasandvik.com
Ownership: Dental Advancements, Inc.
Produces/Sells CE-marked Devices: N

Teeth, Porcelain	Dental And Oral

NOBEL BIOCARE USA, LLC
800-579-6515
714-282-5074
22715/22725 Savi Ranch Parkway,
Yorba Linda, CA 92887
FDA Number: 2027971
Fax: 714-998-9236
E-mail: info.usa@nobelbiocare.com
Web site: www.nobelbiocare.com/us
Ownership: Private
Produces/Sells CE-marked Devices: N

Abutment, Implant, Dental, Endosseous	Dental And Oral
Accessories, Implant, Dental, Endosseous	Dental And Oral
Base, Denture, Relining, Repairing, Rebasing, Resin	Dental And Oral
Burr, Dental	Dental And Oral
Cement, Dental	Dental And Oral
Clamp, Bone	Orthopedics
Drill, Bone, Powered	Dental And Oral
Extractor, Nail	Orthopedics
Gauge, Depth, Instrument, Dental	Dental And Oral
Handle, Instrument, Dental	Dental And Oral
Impactor	Orthopedics
Implant, Endosseous	Dental And Oral
Point, Abrasive	Dental And Oral
Powder, Porcelain	Dental And Oral
Punch, Surgical	Surgery
Reamer	Orthopedics
Scaler, Periodontic	Dental And Oral
Screwdriver	Orthopedics
System, Optical Impression, Computer Assisted Design And Manufacturing (cad/cam) Of Dental Restorations	Dental And Oral
Teeth, Porcelain	Dental And Oral
Tray, Surgical Instrument	Surgery
Wrench	Orthopedics

NOBELPHARMA
See Dentsply Prosthetics

NOBILE CONSULTING USA LLC
866-500-7463
1555 Jupiter Park Dr., Ste. 11, Jupiter, FL 33468
FDA Number: 3003744879
Ownership: Private
Produces/Sells CE-marked Devices: N

Orthosis, Corrective Shoe	Physical Med

NOBLE ANESTHESIA-AIR, INC.
772-225-2711
4637Nw 6th Street, Gainesville, FL 32609
FDA Number: 3004904578
Web site: www.anesthesia-air.com
Ownership: Private
Produces/Sells CE-marked Devices: N

Batteries, Rechargeable, Class Ii Devices	Cardiovascular
Cannula, Nasal, Oxygen	Anesthesiology
Circuit, Breathing (W Connector, Adapter, Y Piece)	Anesthesiology
Stethoscope, Electronic (Auscultoscope)	Cardiovascular
Transducer, Stethoscope	Anesthesiology
Tubing, Flexible, Medical Gas, Low-Pressure	Anesthesiology

NOBLE PINE PRODUCTS CO.
800-359-4913
914-664-5877
Centuck Station, PO Box 41,
Yonkers, NY 10710
FDA Number: n/a
Fax: 914-664-9383
E-mail: sterifab@sterifab.com
Web site: www.sterifab.com
Annual Revenue: $10-$25 Million
Year Founded: 1920
Ownership: CASTOLEUM CORPORATION
Produces/Sells CE-marked Devices: N
Federal Procurement Eligibility: Small Business, Female Owned
Distribution: Manufacturer Direct, Manufacturer Through Distributor, Manufacturer Through Manufacturer Reps, OEM
General Admin.: S. V. Goldrich/President
E. Brito/Vice President Human Resources
Mktg./Adv.: E. Familia/Director National Accounts
L. Brown/Manager Contract Sales
B. SIMON/Manager National Sales
E. Bryan/Vice President Marketing
M. HOUSE/Vice President Marketing
S. Neil/Vice President Sales

Disinfector, Liquid	General

NOBLE-MET, LTD., DIV. OF UTI
See Accellent Inc.

NOBLES INDUSTRIES, INC.
See Nobles Manufacturing, Inc.

NOBLES MANUFACTURING, INC.
715-483-3079
1105 East Pine St., St. Croix Falls, WI 54024
FDA Number: n/a
Fax: 715-483-1884
Web site: www.noblesmfg.com
Medical Products Sales Volume: $4,000,000
Annual Revenue: $5-$10 Million
Ownership: Private

NOBLES MANUFACTURING, INC.
715-483-3079 *(cont'd)*
Produces/Sells CE-marked Devices: N
Federal Procurement Eligibility: Small Business
Distribution: Manufacturer Direct, Manufacturer Through Distributor

Centrifuge, Floor	Pathology
Cleaner, Medical Device	General

NOBLES MEDICAL TECHNOLOGIES, INC.
714-751-8332
17080 Newhope St., Fountain Valley, CA 92708
FDA Number: n/a
Web site: http://www.noblesmedical.com
Annual Revenue: $5-$10 Million
Ownership: Private
Quality System Registration Information: ISO9001
Produces/Sells CE-marked Devices: N
Federal Procurement Eligibility: Small Business
Distribution: OEM
General Admin.: Tony Nobles/President, Chief Executive Officer
Production: Tom Schroeder/Vice President Regulatory Affairs

Instrument, Knot Tying, Suture, Laparoscopic	Surgery
Punch, Aortic	Cardiovascular
Suture, Absorbable, Synthetic, Polyglycolic Acid	Surgery
Unit, Ultraviolet Sanitation/sterilization (for Toothbrushes), Non-sterile	Dental And Oral

NOBLES-LAI ENGINEERING
See Nobles Medical Technologies, Inc.

NOCWATCH INTERNATIONAL, INC.
775-833-4142
288 Village Blvd., Suite 5, Incline Village, NV 89451
FDA Number: 3005705595
Ownership: Private
Produces/Sells CE-marked Devices: N

Monitor, Bed Patient	General

NOCWATCH INTERNATIONAL, INC./FALLSAVER
877-614-5616
775-833-4142
PO Box 1367, Crystal Bay, NV 89402
FDA Number: 9086623
Fax: 775-833-0270
E-mail: info@fallsaver.net
Web site: www.fallsaver.net
Year Founded: 2004
Ownership: NOCwatch International, Inc.
Produces/Sells CE-marked Devices: Y
Federal Procurement Eligibility: Small Business, Female Owned
Distribution: Manufacturer Direct, Manufacturer Through Distributor

Monitor, Bed Occupancy	General

NOIR LASERSHIELD
See Noir Manufacturing

NOIR MANUFACTURING
800-521-9746
734-769-5565
10125 Colonial Industrial Dr.,
South Lyon, MI 48178
FDA Number: n/a
Fax: 734-769-1708
E-mail: david.bothner@noir-medical.com
Web site: www.noir-medical.com
Annual Revenue: $1-$5 Million
Total Employees: 25   *Marketing Staff:* 13   *Sales Staff:* 9
Ownership: Private
Produces/Sells CE-marked Devices: Y
Federal Procurement Eligibility: Small Business
Distribution: Manufacturer Direct, Exporter
General Admin.: Brooks Gleichert/President
Mktg./Adv.: David W. Bothner/Director Marketing
Marc Gleichert/Director Product Development
David W. Bothner/Manager International & National Sales
Production: Marc Gleichert/Vice President Manufacturing

Goggles, Protective, Eye	Ophthalmology
Sunglasses (Including Photosensitive)	Ophthalmology

NOKIA SIEMENS NETWORKS
561-923-9590
900 Broken Sound Pkwy., Boca Raton, FL 33487
FDA Number: n/a
E-mail: zeljko.bulut@siemens.com
Web site: www.nokiasiemensnetworks.com
Annual Revenue: $0-$1 Million
Ownership: Siemens Medical
Produces/Sells CE-marked Devices: N
Federal Procurement Eligibility: Small Business
Distribution: Manufacturer Direct
General Admin.: Susan Spradley/President

Communication Equipment	General

NOMAX, INC.
314-961-2500
40 North Rock Hill Rd., St. Louis, MO 63119
FDA Number: 1937310

Agent, Polishing, Abrasive, Oral Cavity	Dental And Oral
Case, Contact Lens	Ophthalmology
Cleaner, Lens, Contact	Ophthalmology
Strip, Schirmer	Ophthalmology

NOMAX, INC.   314-961-2500 (cont'd)
Sunglasses (Including Photosensitive)   Ophthalmology

NOMIR MEDICAL TECHNOLOGIES INC.   718.676.1502
3021 avenue j, Brooklyn, NY 11210
FDA Number: n/a
E-mail: r.burtt@nomirmedical.com
Web site: www.nomirmedical.com
Year Founded: 2005
Total Employees: 3
Ownership: Private
Produces/Sells CE-marked Devices: N
Federal Procurement Eligibility: Small Business
General Admin.: Richard Burtt/President, Chief Executive Officer
Laser, Surgical   Surgery

NOMOS CORPORATION
See Best Nomos Corp.

NON-INVASIVE MONITORING SYSTEMS, INC.   305-575-4200
4400 Biscayne Blvd., Miami, FL 33137
FDA Number: 2431353   *Fax:* 305-575-4201
E-mail: info@nims-inc.com
Web site: http://www.nims-us.com
Ownership: Public
Stock Symbol: NIMU
Traded On: OTC Bulletin
Produces/Sells CE-marked Devices: N
General Admin.: Dr. Marvin Sackner/Chief Executive Officer
    Mr. Joshua Weingard/Chief Legal Officer
    Mr. Stephen Mrha/Chief Operating Officer
Production: Mr. Emmerance Gummels/Director Quality Assurance & Quality Control
Finance: Mr. Adam Jackson/Chief Financial Officer
Computer, Diagnostic, Programmable   Cardiovascular
Exerciser, Powered   Anesthesiology
Monitor, Ventilatory Frequency   Anesthesiology
Rod, Measuring Ear   Ear/Nose/Throat
Spirometer, Monitoring (Volumeter)   Anesthesiology

NONIN MEDICAL, INC.   800-356-8874
    763-553-9968
13700 1st Avenue North, Plymouth, MN 55441
FDA Number: 2183646   *Fax:* 763-553-7807
E-mail: info@nonin.com
Web site: http://www.nonin.com
Medical Products Sales Volume: $15,400,000
Year Founded: 1986
Total Employees: 180   *Marketing Staff:* 5   *Sales Staff:* 11
Ownership: Private
Quality System Registration Information: ISO9001
Produces/Sells CE-marked Devices: Y
Federal Procurement Eligibility: Small Business
Distribution: Manufacturer Through Distributor, OEM
General Admin.: Gary Tschautscher/Chief Executive Officer
    Steve Bucholz/Chief Operating Officer
    Kevin McGowan, OEM Sales/Director
    Philip Isaacson/Managing Director
Mktg./Adv.: Don Giroux/Manager International Marketing & Sales
    Holly Larkin/Manager Marketing
    Bill Kalb/Manager Sales
Production: Rick Bennett/Manager Regulatory Affairs
Finance: Andy Rusinko/Director Finance
Analyzer, Gas, Carbon-Dioxide, Gaseous Phase (Capnograph)   Anesthesiology
Magnet, Superconducting, MRI (Magnetic Resonance Imaging)   Radiology
Monitor, Blood Pressure, Indirect, Automatic   Cardiovascular
Oximeter, Ear   Cardiovascular
Oximeter, Finger   General
Oximeter, Pulse   General
Oximeter, Tissue Saturation   Cardiovascular

NOR CAL DESIGN   800-525-5402
3600 Haven Ave., #1, Redwood City, CA 94063
FDA Number: n/a   *Fax:* 650-364-0860
E-mail: sales@norcaldesign.com
Web site: www.norcaldesign.com
Ownership: Private
Produces/Sells CE-marked Devices: N
Federal Procurement Eligibility: Small Business
Distribution: Manufacturer Direct
Orthosis, Fixation, Cervical Intervertebral Body, Spinal   Orthopedics
Orthosis, Other   Physical Med
Prosthesis, Ankle, Tibial Component   Orthopedics

NOR-LAKE INC., NOR-LAKE SCIENTIFIC   800-955-5253
    715-386-2323
891 County Road U, Hudson, WI 54016
FDA Number: 9921044   *Fax:* 15-386-6149
E-mail: sales@norlake.com
Web site: www.norlake.com
Ownership: Private

NOR-LAKE INC., NOR-LAKE SCIENTIFIC   800-955-5253 (cont'd)
Produces/Sells CE-marked Devices: N
Freezer, Blood Storage   Hematology
Freezer, Laboratory, General Purpose   Chemistry

NORA-DALL   919-942-2592
111 Glosson Circle, Carrboro, NC 27510
FDA Number: 3004824712
Ownership: Private
Produces/Sells CE-marked Devices: N
Pack, Hot Or Cold, Reusable   Physical Med

NORAM SEATING, INC.   866-236-7328
18 Market Street, Union City, PA 16438
FDA Number: 3004595445
Ownership: Private
Produces/Sells CE-marked Devices: N
Transfer Aid   Physical Med
Utensil, Handicapped Aid   Physical Med

NORAM SOLUTIONS   800-387-7103
    716-285-7548
PO Box 543, Lewiston, NY 14092-0543
FDA Number: 1318912   *Fax:* 905-336-1708
E-mail: sales@noramsolutions.com
Web site: www.noramsolutions.com
Year Founded: 1979
Total Employees: 28   *Marketing Staff:* 5   *Sales Staff:* 5
Ownership: Private
Produces/Sells CE-marked Devices: N
Federal Procurement Eligibility: Small Business
Distribution: Manufacturer Direct, Manufacturer Through Distributor, Service Direct, Exclusive Distributor, Importer, Exporter
General Admin.: Mr. Wim Van Voorst/President, Chief Executive Officer
Mktg./Adv.: Mrs. Tracy White/Director Marketing
    Mr. Kevin Klipfel/Manager National Marketing
Production: Mr. Manny Alves/Manager Materials
Finance: Mr. Paul A. Jones/Vice President Finance & Operations
IS: Mr. Alexei Nalbandyan/Systems Engineer
Bath, Hydro-Massage (Whirlpool)   Physical Med
Bath, Portable   General
Exerciser, Other   Physical Med
Lift, Patient   General
Table, Physical Therapy   Physical Med

NORAMCO, INC.   706-353-4400
1440 Olympic Dr., Athens, GA 30601
FDA Number: 1033845   *Fax:* 706-353-3205
Web site: www.noramco.com
Ownership: Johnson & Johnson
Produces/Sells CE-marked Devices: N
Agent, Hemostatic, Absorbable, Collagen-Based   Surgery
Agent, Hemostatic, Non-Absorbable, Collagen-Based   Surgery
Barrier, Adhesion, Absorbable   Obstetrics/Gynecology

NORAXON USA, INC.   800-364-8985
    480-443-3413
13430 N. Scottsdale Road, Suite #104, Scottsdale, AZ 85254
FDA Number: 2084126   *Fax:* 480-443-4327
E-mail: info@noraxon.com
Web site: www.noraxon.com
Medical Products Sales Volume: $1,500,000
Annual Revenue: $1-$5 Million
Year Founded: 1989
Total Employees: 10   *Sales Staff:* 3
Ownership: Private
Produces/Sells CE-marked Devices: Y
Federal Procurement Eligibility: Small Business, GSA Contract
Distribution: Manufacturer Direct, Manufacturer Through Distributor, Manufacturer Through Manufacturer Reps, Exclusive Distributor, Exporter
General Admin.: Randy Raisanen/President, Chief Executive Officer
Mktg./Adv.: Jeff Dooley/Admin. National Sales
    Todd Shewman/Admin. National Sales
    Randy Raisanen/Manager International & National Sales
Production: Frank Hosner/Director Quality Assurance & Product Development
    Frank Hosner/Vice President Manufacturing & Operations
Biofeedback Device   Cns/Neurology
Biofeedback Equipment, Myoelectric, Powered   Physical Med
Computer Software   General
Myograph   Physical Med

NORCO   800-657-6672
    208-336-1643
1125 W. Amity, Boise, ID 83705
FDA Number: 3020756   *Fax:* 208-331-9843
E-mail: jimk@norco-inc.com
Web site: www.norco-inc.com
Medical Products Sales Volume: $77,200,000
Annual Revenue: $50-$100 Million
Year Founded: 1989

NORCO
800-657-6672 *(cont'd)*

Total Employees: 205   Sales Staff: 39
Ownership: Private
Quality System Registration Information: ISO9002
Produces/Sells CE-marked Devices: N
Federal Procurement Eligibility: Small Business, VA Contract
Distribution: Exclusive Distributor
General Admin.: Jim Kissler/Chief Executive Officer
   Ned Pontious/President

Holder, Gas Cylinder	Anesthesiology
Humidifier, Respiratory Gas, (Direct Patient Interface)	Anesthesiology
Kit, Anesthesia, Epidural	Anesthesiology
Monitor, Oxygen	General
Nebulizer, Ultrasonic	Anesthesiology
Oximeter, Pulse	General
Oxygen	Anesthesiology
Regulator, Pressure, Gas Cylinder	Anesthesiology
Spirometer, Diagnostic (Respirometer)	Anesthesiology

NORCO MEDICAL
386-734-9080
1501 Lexington Ave., Deland, FL 32724-2117
FDA Number: 3004632053
Ownership: Private
Produces/Sells CE-marked Devices: N

Lancet, Blood	General

NORCROSS CORP.
617-969-7020
255 Newtonville Avenue, Newton, MA 02458
FDA Number: 7000272   Fax: 617-969-3260
E-mail: sales@viscosity.com
Web site: www.viscosity.com
Medical Products Sales Volume: $1,300,000
Annual Revenue: $1-$5 Million
Total Employees: 12   Sales Staff: 4
Ownership: Private
Produces/Sells CE-marked Devices: N
Federal Procurement Eligibility: Small Business
Distribution: Manufacturer Direct, Manufacturer Through Manufacturer Reps, Exporter
General Admin.: Robert A. Norcross/Chief Executive Officer

Viscometer	Chemistry

NORDENT MANUFACTURING, INC.
800-966-7336
610 Bonnie Lane,
847-437-4780
Elk Grove Village, IL 60007
FDA Number: 1419489   Fax: 847-437-4786
E-mail: btatum@nordent.com
Web site: http://www.nordent.com
Annual Revenue: $5-$10 Million
Year Founded: 1969
Total Employees: 28   Marketing Staff: 4   Sales Staff: 14
Ownership: Private
Quality System Registration Information: ISO9001
Produces/Sells CE-marked Devices: Y
Federal Procurement Eligibility: Small Business, VA Contract
Distribution: Manufacturer Through Distributor, OEM, Service Direct, Importer
General Admin.: Robert Tatum/President
   Joe Martin/Vice President Admin.
Mktg./Adv.: Tim Irwin/Vice President Sales
Production: Joseph Martin/Director Quality Assurance
   Dave Schero/Manager Materials

Burnisher, Operative, Dental	Dental And Oral
Carrier, Amalgam, Operative	Dental And Oral
Carver, Dental Amalgam, Operative	Dental And Oral
Chisel, Bone, Surgical	Dental And Oral
Condenser, Amalgam And Foil, Operative	Dental And Oral
Curette, Periodontic	Dental And Oral
Curette, Surgical, Dental	Dental And Oral
Cutter, Operative	Dental And Oral
Elevator, Surgical, Dental	Dental And Oral
Excavator, Dental, Operative	Dental And Oral
Explorer, Operative	Dental And Oral
File, Bone, Surgical	Dental And Oral
File, Periodontic	Dental And Oral
Filling, Instrument Plastic, Dental	Dental And Oral
Forceps, Hemostatic	Surgery
Forceps, Tissue	Surgery
Forceps, Tooth Extractor, Surgical	Dental And Oral
Hand Instrument, Calculus Removal	Dental And Oral
Handle, Instrument, Dental	Dental And Oral
Hemostat, Surgical	Dental And Oral
Holder, Needle, Orthopedic	Orthopedics
Holder, Needle, Other	Surgery
Knife, Periodontic	Dental And Oral
Mirror, Mouth	Dental And Oral
Probe, Periodontic	Dental And Oral
Rongeur, Dental	Dental And Oral
Scaler, Periodontic	Dental And Oral
Scissors, General Dissecting	General

NORDENT MANUFACTURING, INC.
800-966-7336 *(cont'd)*

Scissors, Iris	Ophthalmology
Scissors, Plastic Surgery (Dissecting)	Surgery
Scissors, Surgical Tissue, Dental (Oral)	Dental And Oral
Scissors, Suture	Surgery

NORDSON CORPORATION
440-892-1580
28601 Clemens Road, Westlake, OH 44145
FDA Number: n/a
Web site: http://www.nordson.com
Ownership: Private
Produces/Sells CE-marked Devices: N
General Admin.: Mr. Gregory Thaxton/Chief Financial Officer, Vice President
   Ms. Shelly Peet/Chief Information Officer
   Mr. Michael Hilton/President, Chief Executive Officer

NORELL, INC.
800-519-3688
314 E. Arbor Avenue, P. O. Box 307,
609-697-0020
Landisville, NJ 08326
FDA Number: 7000273   Fax: 800-245-5932
E-mail: customerservice@nmrtubes.com
Web site: www.norellinc.com
Annual Revenue: $0-$1 Million
Total Employees: 11
Ownership: Private
Produces/Sells CE-marked Devices: N
Federal Procurement Eligibility: Small Business
Distribution: Manufacturer Direct
General Admin.: Mark W. Norell/President
   Gregory B. Norell/Vice President, General Manager

Labware, Basic, Reusable	Chemistry
M. Lysodeikticus Cells (Spectrophotometric), Lysozyme	Chemistry
Nuclear Magnetic Resonance Equipment, Laboratory	Chemistry

NORFOLK MEDICAL PRODUCTS, INC.
847-674-7075
7350 North Ridgeway, Skokie, IL 60076
FDA Number: 1450392

Catheter, Angioplasty, Transluminal, Peripheral	Cardiovascular
Catheter, Subcutaneous Intravascular, Implanted	General
Needle, Aspiration And Injection, Disposable	Surgery
Tubing, Fluid Delivery	General

NORFOLK SCIENTIFIC, INC.
See Statspin, Inc.

NORMED
800-288-8200
PO Box 3644, Seattle, WA 98124-3644
206-242-8228
FDA Number: 3013226   Fax: 206-242-3315
E-mail: sales@normed.com
Web site: www.normed.com
Medical Products Sales Volume: $1,000,000
Year Founded: 1974
Total Employees: 50
Ownership: Private
Produces/Sells CE-marked Devices: N
Federal Procurement Eligibility: Small Business

Bandage, Adhesive	Surgery
Bandage, Elastic	General
Cutter, Ring	General
Forceps, General & Plastic Surgery	Surgery
General Use Surgical Scissors	Surgery
Glove, Patient Examination, Latex	General
Glove, Patient Examination, Poly	General
Handle, Scalpel	Surgery
Kit, First Aid	Surgery
Linen, Bed	General
Mouthpiece, Breathing	Anesthesiology
Orthosis, Limb Brace	Physical Med
Orthosis, Lumbosacral	Physical Med
Pack, Hot Or Cold, Disposable	Physical Med
Splint, Extremity, Inflatable, External	Surgery
Splint, Extremity, Non-Inflatable, External	Surgery
Sponge, Gauze	Dental And Oral
Strip, Adhesive	Surgery
Tourniquet, Non-Pneumatic, Surgical	Surgery

NORTECH
See Northgate Technologies Inc.

NORTECH LABORATORIES, INC.
888-265-3725
125 Sherwood Ave.,
631-501-1452
Farmingdale, NY 11735
FDA Number: 2415591   Fax: 631-501-1453
E-mail: info@nortechlabs.com
Web site: www.nortechlabs.com
Medical Products Sales Volume: $2,000,000
Annual Revenue: $1-$5 Million
Year Founded: 1961
Total Employees: 10
Ownership: Private

NORTECH LABORATORIES, INC.   888-265-3725 (cont'd)
Produces/Sells CE-marked Devices: N
Federal Procurement Eligibility: Small Business
Distribution: Manufacturer Direct
General Admin.: Sandy Spencer/Office Manager
     Karen Nazirikh/President, Chief Executive Officer
Mktg./Adv.: David Nazarieh/Vice President Marketing & Sales
Production: David Nazarieh/Vice President Manufacturing

Exerciser, Hand	Physical Med
Pack, Cold	General
Pack, Hot Or Cold, Reusable	Physical Med
Washer, Utensil	General

NORTECH SYSTEMS INCORPORATED   952-345-2244
1120 Wayzata Blvd E., Suite 201, Wayzata, MN 55391
FDA Number: 2183613
E-mail: sales@nortechsys.com
Web site: www.nortechsys.com
Ownership: Public
Stock Symbol: NSYS
Traded On: NASDAQ
Quality System Registration Information: ISO9001; ISO9002
Produces/Sells CE-marked Devices: N
Federal Procurement Eligibility: Small Business
Distribution: Manufacturer Direct
General Admin.: Mr. Michael Degen/Chief Executive Officer
Mktg./Adv.: Mr. Curtis Steichen/Vice President Commercial Operations
Production: Mr. Peter Kucera/Senior Vice President Quality Assurance
Finance: Mr. Richard Wasielewski/Chief Financial Officer

Contract Manufacturing	General
Probe, Uptake, Nuclear	Radiology
Warmer, Blood and Plasma	Hematology

NORTECH SYSTEMS, ZERCOM DIVISION
    See Nortech Systems Incorporated

NORTH AMERICA MATTRESS CORP.   800-448-6163
                                                503-655-6163
10768 SE Hwy. 212, Clackamas, OR 97015
FDA Number: 3031027   Fax: 503-655-6227
E-mail: Johnny@namattress.com
Web site: www.northamericamattress.com
Ownership: Private
Produces/Sells CE-marked Devices: N

Cover, Mattress	General

NORTH AMERICAN IMAGING, INC.   800-288-8823
924 Via Alondra, Camarillo, CA 93012   805-383-2200
FDA Number: 1122823   Fax: 805-383-2212
E-mail: info@northamericanimaging.com
Web site: www.naimaging.com
Ownership: Private
Produces/Sells CE-marked Devices: N

Housing, X-Ray Tube, Diagnostic	Radiology

NORTH AMERICAN LATEX CORP.   812-268-6608
049 East Industrial Park Drive, Lake Sullivan, IN 47882
FDA Number: 1832931

Bag, Urinary, Ileostomy	Gastroenterology/Urology
Collector, Ostomy	Gastroenterology/Urology
Tubing, Non-Invasive	Surgery

NORTH AMERICAN MARKETING, INC.   (410) 721-8803
2127 Espey Court, Suite 220, Crofton, MD 21114
FDA Number: 3025109   Fax: (410) 721-0079
E-mail: kz750b@srv.net
Annual Revenue: $0-$1 Million
Year Founded: 1988
Total Employees: 4   Sales Staff: 4
Ownership: Private
Produces/Sells CE-marked Devices: N
Federal Procurement Eligibility: Small Business
Distribution: Manufacturer Through Distributor, Manufacturer Through Manufacturer Reps
General Admin.: Karen Wright/President

Accessories, Cleaning, Endoscopic	Gastroenterology/Urology

NORTH AMERICAN MEDICAL CORP (NAM)   770-541-0012
1649 Sands Pl SE, Suite A, Marietta, GA 30067
FDA Number: 9049276   Fax: 770-541-0032
E-mail: office@namcorporation.com
Web site: www.namcorporation.com
Ownership: Private
Produces/Sells CE-marked Devices: N

Equipment, Traction, Powered	Physical Med

NORTH AMERICAN MEDICAL CORPORATION   770-541-0012
1649 Sands Place S.e., Suite A, Marietta, GA 30067
FDA Number: 1067107   Fax: 770-541-0032
E-mail: office@namcorporation.com

NORTH AMERICAN MEDICAL CORPORATION   770-541-0012
(cont'd)
Web site: www.namcorporation.com
Year Founded: 2000
Total Employees: 60   Marketing Staff: 4   Sales Staff: 65
Ownership: Private
Stock Symbol: AMMD
Traded On: NASDAQ
Quality System Registration Information: ISO9001
Produces/Sells CE-marked Devices: Y
Federal Procurement Eligibility: Small Business
Distribution: Manufacturer Through Distributor, Manufacturer Through Manufacturer Reps
General Admin.: Mr. Gidgette Rubin/Senior Vice President

Equipment, Traction, Powered	Physical Med
Pad, Heating, Powered	Physical Med
Scanner, Ultrasonic (Pulsed Doppler)	Radiology
Transducer, Ultrasonic, Diagnostic	Radiology
Unit, Therapy, Current, Interferential	Cns/Neurology
Vibrator, Therapeutic	Physical Med

NORTH AMERICAN MEDICAL PRODUCTS, INC.   800-488-6267
6- British American Blvd. Suite B,   518-218-0402
Latham, NY 12110
FDA Number: n/a   Fax: 518-218-0405
E-mail: namp1inc@aol.com
Web site: www.nampinc.com
Annual Revenue: $0-$1 Million
Year Founded: 1984
Total Employees: 12   Marketing Staff: 4   Sales Staff: 1
Ownership: Private
Produces/Sells CE-marked Devices: N
Federal Procurement Eligibility: Small Business, GSA Contract, VA Contract
Distribution: Manufacturer Direct, Manufacturer Through Distributor, Manufacturer Through Manufacturer Reps, Exclusive Distributor, Exporter
General Admin.: Arthur Gianakos/President, Chief Executive Officer
Mktg./Adv.: Art Gianakos/Manager Contracts

Laryngoscope	Ear/Nose/Throat
Ophthalmoscope, AC-Powered	Ophthalmology
Otoscope	Ear/Nose/Throat
Protector, Puncture, Needle	General
Scope, Fiberoptic Intubation	Anesthesiology
System, Blood Culturing	Microbiology

NORTH AMERICAN SCIENCE ASSOCIATES, INC.   866-666-9455
6750 Wales Road, Northwood, OH 43619   419-666-9455
FDA Number: 1521876   Fax: 419-662-4386
E-mail: info@namsa.com
Web site: www.namsa.com
Medical Products Sales Volume: $12,900,000
Year Founded: 1967
Total Employees: 200   Marketing Staff: 3   Sales Staff: 10
Ownership: Private
Quality System Registration Information: ISO9001
Produces/Sells CE-marked Devices: Y
Federal Procurement Eligibility: Small Business, Female Owned
Distribution: Manufacturer Direct, Manufacturer Through Distributor, Exclusive Distributor, Importer, Exporter
General Admin.: Dr. Richard A. Wallin/Chairman
     Jeff Blair/President, Chief Executive Officer
Mktg./Adv.: Dr. Joel Gorski/Director Business Development
     Terry Langenderfer/Director Marketing
     Ms. Rachael Lanning/Marketing Assistant
     Dennis Nevins/Vice President Sales
Production: Matt Sliva/Director Quality Assurance & Regulatory Affairs
     John Bommorito/Manager Materials

Service, Consulting	General
Sterilization Indicator	Surgery
Sterilization Process Indicator, Biological	General
Suspension System, Cell Culture	Pathology

NORTH AMERICAN SCIENTIFIC, INC.   818-734-8600
8300 Aurora Ave North, Seattle, WA 98103
FDA Number: 87068
Ownership: Private
Produces/Sells CE-marked Devices: N

Accessories, Operating Room, Table	Surgery
Applicator, Radionuclide, Manual	Radiology
Shield, Protective, Personnel	Radiology

NORTH AMERICAN STERILIZATION & PACKAGING   800-392-6310
19 Park Dr., Franklin, NJ 07416   973-209-4388
FDA Number: 2244478   Fax: 973-209-6374
E-mail: info@naspco.com
Web site: www.naspco.com
Medical Products Sales Volume: $6,000,000

NORTH AMERICAN STERILIZATION & 800-392-6310 *(cont'd)*
Annual Revenue: $5-$10 Million
Year Founded: 1996
Ownership: Private
Produces/Sells CE-marked Devices: N
Federal Procurement Eligibility: Small Business
Distribution: OEM
General Admin.: Edward J. Gumpy/Chief Operating Officer

Contract Manufacturing	General
Contract Packaging	General
Contract Sterilization	General
Endoscope And Accessories, AC-Powered	Surgery
Service, Engineering/Design	General
Service, Licensing, Device, Medical	General
Surgical Instrument, Disposable	Surgery

NORTH COAST MEDICAL, INC. 800-821-9319
8100 Camino Arroyo, Gilroy, CA 95020 **408-776-5000**
FDA Number: 2939821 *Fax:* 877-213-9300
E-mail: custserv@ncmedical.com
Web site: www.ncmedical.com
Annual Revenue: $25-$50 Million
Year Founded: 1976
Total Employees: 130 *Marketing Staff:* 6 *Sales Staff:* 15
Ownership: Private
Produces/Sells CE-marked Devices: Y
Federal Procurement Eligibility: Small Business
Distribution: Manufacturer Direct, Manufacturer Through Distributor
General Admin.: Jeselle Foster/Human Resources Representative
　　　　　Mark Biehl/President, Chief Executive Officer
Mktg./Adv.: Tom Ciccone/Director Marketing
　　　　　Barbara Boling/Director Product Development
　　　　　Roy Beckham/Manager Advertising
　　　　　Micheal Jensen/Manager International & National Sales
　　　　　Adam Buglio/Manager National Sales
Production: Rich Chaboya/Manager Materials
　　　　　Dan Lynch/Manager Quality Assurance
　　　　　Jeff Kamimoto/Manager Regulatory Affairs

Bath, Sitz, Physical Medicine	Physical Med
Bathtub	General
Equipment, Therapy, Handicapped/Physical	Physical Med
Reacher (Handicapped)	General
Restraint, Wrist/Hand	General
Splint, Extremity, Non-Inflatable, External	Surgery
Strap, Restraining	General

NORTH EAST CRYOGENICS INC.
See Andonian Cryogenics, Inc.

NORTH HEALTH CARE
See North Safety Products

NORTH PACIFIC DENTAL, INC.
See Aseptico, Inc.

NORTH SAFETY PRODUCTS 401-943-4400
1101 B Calle Neutron, Parque Industrial Maran,
Mexicali, B.c. Mexico
FDA Number: 9616064

Bandage, Adhesive	Surgery
Binder, Medical, Therapeutic	General
Cover, Shoe, Operating Room	Surgery
Decontamination Kit	Surgery
Depressor, Tongue	General
Device, Assist, CPR	Anesthesiology
Fiber, Absorbent	General
Glove, Patient Examination, Latex	General
Gown, Surgical	Surgery
Kit, First Aid	Surgery
Kit, Snake Bite, Suction	General
Lancet, Blood	General
Mask, Surgical	Surgery
Needle, Hypodermic, Single Lumen With Syringe	General
Pack, Hot Or Cold, Disposable	Physical Med
Pad, Eye	Ophthalmology
Regulator, Thermal, Cardiopulmonary Bypass	Cardiovascular
Scissors, Disposable	General
Sheet, Burn	General
Sling, Arm	Physical Med
Stethoscope, Manual	Cardiovascular
Syringe, Piston	General
Tourniquet, Non-Pneumatic, Surgical	Surgery

NORTH SAFETY PRODUCTS 800-430-4110
2000 Plainfield Pike, Cranston, RI 02921-2012 **401-943-4400**
FDA Number: 1217998 *Fax:* 401-946-7560
E-mail: marketing@northsafety.com
Web site: www.northsafety.com
Medical Products Sales Volume: $7,000,000
Year Founded: 1973
Ownership: North Safety Products

NORTH SAFETY PRODUCTS 800-430-4110 *(cont'd)*
Quality System Registration Information: ISO9001
Produces/Sells CE-marked Devices: N
Distribution: Manufacturer Through Manufacturer Reps, OEM, Service Direct
General Admin.: John Zuleger/General Manager
Mktg./Adv.: John Friend/Director Sales
Production: Sonny Hayes/Senior Vice President Manufacturing
Finance: Mark Sheehan/Vice President Finance

Ampule	Gastroenterology/Urology
Bandage, Adhesive	Surgery
Bandage, Butterfly	General
Bandage, Gauze	General
Cover, Shoe, Non-Conductive	General
Eyeglasses	Ophthalmology
Eyeglasses, Safety	Ophthalmology
Finger Cot	General
Glove, Utility	General
Kit, First Aid	Surgery
Kit, Snake Bite	General
Kit, Snake Bite, Suction	General
Lens, Spectacle/Eyeglasses, Non-Custom	Ophthalmology
Plug, Ear	Ear/Nose/Throat
Protector, Hearing (Circumaural)	Ear/Nose/Throat
Protector, Hearing (Insert)	Ear/Nose/Throat
Safety Equipment, Laboratory	Chemistry
Strip, Adhesive	Surgery

Medical Product Subsidiaries (Listed Separately)
　North Safety Products

NORTH TEXAS CIRCUIT BOARD 800-466-6822
1501 W. Shady Grove Rd., **972-790-7610**
Grand Prairie, TX 75053
FDA Number: n/a *Fax:* 972-986-2381
E-mail: ntcb@ntcb.com
Web site: www.ntcb.com
Medical Products Sales Volume: $100,000
Annual Revenue: $10-$25 Million
Total Employees: 89 *Marketing Staff:* 1 *Sales Staff:* 10
Ownership: Private
Quality System Registration Information: ISO9002
Produces/Sells CE-marked Devices: N
Federal Procurement Eligibility: Small Business, Female Owned
Distribution: Manufacturer Direct, Manufacturer Through Manufacturer Reps
General Admin.: Michael Wetzel/President, Chief Executive Officer
　　　　　Andy White/Vice President, General Manager
Mktg./Adv.: Paul Olson/Director National Accounts
　　　　　Andy White/Director Product Development
　　　　　Larry Andrews/Manager Advertising
　　　　　Paul Olson/Manager Contract Sales
　　　　　Paul Olson/Manager International & National Sales
　　　　　Paul Olson/Manager Market Research
Production: Wendell Goodson/Director Quality Assurance
　　　　　Jim Pierce/Manager Materials
　　　　　Paul Baber/Manager Regulatory Affairs

Contract Manufacturing	General

NORTH VALLEY PRECISION PRODUCTS, LLC 775-829-2566
4750 Turbo Cr, Reno, NV 89502
FDA Number: 3005302337
Ownership: Private
Produces/Sells CE-marked Devices: N

Laser, Surgical	Surgery

NORTHEAST AIRGAS, INC.
See Airgas East, Inc.

NORTHEAST LABORATORY SERVICES, INC. 800-244-8378
227 China Road, Winslow, ME 04901 **207-873-7711**
FDA Number: 1210083 *Fax:* 207-873-7022
E-mail: info@nelabservices.com
Web site: www.nelabservices.com
Medical Products Sales Volume: $5,600,000
Year Founded: 1972
Total Employees: 67
Ownership: Private
Produces/Sells CE-marked Devices: N
Federal Procurement Eligibility: Small Business
Distribution: Manufacturer Direct, Manufacturer Through Distributor

Culture Media, For Isolation Of Pathogenic Neisseria	Microbiology
Culture Media, General Nutrient Broth	Microbiology
Culture Media, Mueller Hinton Agar Broth	Microbiology
Culture Media, Multiple Biochemical Test	Microbiology
Culture Media, Non-Selective And Differential	Microbiology
Culture Media, Non-Selective And Non-Differential	Microbiology
Culture Media, Selective And Non-Differential	Microbiology
Culture Media, Selective Broth	Microbiology
Culture Media, Single Biochemical Test	Microbiology
Culture Media, Supplements	Microbiology

NORTHEAST MEDICAL SYSTEMS CORP.   856-910-8111
901 Beechwood Ave., Cherry Hill, NJ 08002-3405
FDA Number: 2249018   *Fax:* 856-910-8112
E-mail: NMSC901@aol.com
Web site: www.Northeastmedicalsystems.com
Annual Revenue: $1-$5 Million
Year Founded: 1988
Total Employees: 6   *Marketing Staff:* 1   *Sales Staff:* 2
Ownership: Private
Produces/Sells CE-marked Devices: N
Federal Procurement Eligibility: Small Business
Distribution: Manufacturer Through Distributor
General Admin.: Joseph M. Conte/President
         David C. Oberg/Vice President

Cart, Equipment, Video	General
Holder, Transducer	Anesthesiology
Stirrup	Gastroenterology/Urology
Support, Foot	Orthopedics
Table, Ultrasound	General
Tray, Surgical Instrument	Surgery
Weight, IV Pole	General

NORTHEAST MONITORING, INC.   866-346-5837
     978-461-3992
Two Clock Tower Place, Suite 555,
Maynard, MA 01754
FDA Number: 1224919   *Fax:* 978-461-5991
E-mail: sstrickland@nemon.com
Web site: www.nemon.com
Year Founded: 1997
Total Employees: 6   *Marketing Staff:* 1   *Sales Staff:* 1
Ownership: Private
Produces/Sells CE-marked Devices: Y
Distribution: Exclusive Distributor
General Admin.: Sherrie Strickland/Office Manager

Computer, Diagnostic, Programmable	Cardiovascular
Electrocardiograph, Ambulatory(without Analysis)	Cardiovascular
Recorder, Magnetic Tape/Disc	Cardiovascular
Transmitter/Receiver System, ECG, Telephone Multi-Channel	Cardiovascular

NORTHEAST RESINS & SILICONES, LLC.   860-620-9547
     203-272-4931
122 Spring St., Unit C-1, Southington, CT 06489
FDA Number: 1226099   *Fax:* 860-620-9576
Ownership: Private
Produces/Sells CE-marked Devices: N

Kit, Earmold Impression	Ear/Nose/Throat
Material, Impression	Dental And Oral

NORTHEASTERN BIOMECHANICAL MANUFACTURING CORP.   716-692-9585
81 Penarrow Dr., Tonawanda, NY 14150
FDA Number: 3005667555
Ownership: Private
Produces/Sells CE-marked Devices: N

Walker, Mechanical	Physical Med

NORTHEASTERN SONICS   800-243-2452
     203-348-8088
130 Lenox Ave., Ste. #23, Stamford, CT 06906
FDA Number: n/a   *Fax:* 203-961-1823
E-mail: tom.m-nesonics@worldnet.att.net
Annual Revenue: $0-$1 Million
Ownership: Private
Quality System Registration Information: ISO9000
Produces/Sells CE-marked Devices: N
Federal Procurement Eligibility: Small Business
Distribution: Service Direct
General Admin.: Fred Lorenzen/Chief Executive Officer
Mktg./Adv.: Thomas Martinez/Manager Marketing

Cleaner, Ultrasonic, Medical Instrument	General

NORTHERN CALIFORNIA TRANSPLANT BANK
     See Tissue Banks International

NORTHERN FALLS, LLC   616-975-0733
4460 44th Se, Suite A, Kentwood, MI 49512
FDA Number: 3004974194
Ownership: Private
Produces/Sells CE-marked Devices: N

Bottle, Hot/Cold Water	General

NORTHERN HOSPITAL SUPPLIES LTD.   867-668-5083
4200 4th Avenue, Whitehorse, YT Y1A 1K1 Canada
FDA Number: n/a   *Fax:* 867-668-6155
E-mail: info@nh-supplies
Web site: http://www.norhosp.com
Year Founded: 1998
Total Employees: 10
Ownership: Private
Produces/Sells CE-marked Devices: N

NORTHERN HOSPITAL SUPPLIES LTD.   867-668-5083 *(cont'd)*
Distribution: Manufacturer Direct, Exclusive Distributor

NORTHERN LIGHT TECHNOLOGIES   800-263-0066
     514-335-1763
8971 Henri-Bourassa W,
Montreal, QUE H4S-1 Canada
FDA Number: n/a   *Fax:* 514-335-7764
E-mail: info@northernlight-tech.com
Web site: www.NorthernLightTechnologies.ca
Year Founded: 1990
Total Employees: 25
Ownership: Private
Produces/Sells CE-marked Devices: N
Distribution: Manufacturer Direct, Exclusive Distributor, Exporter

NORTHERN SCIENTIFIC CORPORATION   800-465-8377
     416-247-8787
418-2895 Derry Rd E,,
Mississauga, ONT L4T 1 Canada
FDA Number: n/a   *Fax:* 416-247-6141
E-mail: northern@sprint.ca
Web site: www.northernsc.com
Year Founded: 1989
Total Employees: 25
Ownership: Private
Produces/Sells CE-marked Devices: N
Distribution: Exclusive Distributor, Importer

NORTHERN TECHNOLOGIES INC.   509-927-0401
23123 E. Mission Avenue, Liberty Lake, WA 99019
FDA Number: n/a   *Fax:* 509-927-0435
E-mail: karrie.thomson@emersonnetworkpower.com
Web site: www.northern-tech.com
Medical Products Sales Volume: $3,300,000
Annual Revenue: $25-$50 Million
Year Founded: 1985
Total Employees: 30   *Marketing Staff:* 3   *Sales Staff:* 10
Ownership: Emerson Network Power
Stock Symbol: EMR
Traded On: NYSE
Quality System Registration Information: ISO9001
Produces/Sells CE-marked Devices: Y
Federal Procurement Eligibility: Small Business, GSA Contract
Distribution: Manufacturer Direct
General Admin.: Steve Baker/President
   Medical Admin.: John Jensen/Director Medical Div.

Power Systems, Uninterruptible (UPS)	General
Regulator, Line Voltage	General

NORTHERN TECHNOLOGIES INTL. CORP.   800-328-2433
     651-784-1250
6680 N. Hwy. 49, Lino Lakes, MN 55014
FDA Number: n/a   *Fax:* 651-784-2902
E-mail: sales@ntic.com
Web site: www.ntic.com
Medical Products Sales Volume: $16,600,000
Annual Revenue: $5-$10 Million
Year Founded: 1970
Total Employees: 41   *Marketing Staff:* 4   *Sales Staff:* 15
Ownership: Northern Technologies Intl. Corp.
Stock Symbol: NTI
Traded On: AMEX
Quality System Registration Information: ISO9001
Produces/Sells CE-marked Devices: N
Federal Procurement Eligibility: Small Business, GSA Contract
Distribution: Manufacturer Through Manufacturer Reps
General Admin.: Philip Lynch/Chief Executive Officer
       Patrick Lynch/President, Chairman
Mktg./Adv.: Ik Hau Ng/Director Marketing
       Lance Trepper/Manager National Sales

General Medical Device	General

Medical Product Subsidiaries (Listed Separately)
Northern Technologies Intl. Corp.

NORTHGATE RESEARCH CORPORATION
     See Northgate Technologies Inc.

NORTHGATE TECHNOLOGIES INC.   800-348-0424
     847-608-8900
1591 Scottsdale Ct., Elgin, IL 60123
FDA Number: 1450997   *Fax:* 847-608-9405
E-mail: customerservice@northgate-tech.com
Web site: www.northgate-tech.com
Medical Products Sales Volume: $2,700,000
Year Founded: 1972
Total Employees: 40   *Marketing Staff:* 1   *Sales Staff:* 1
Ownership: Trudell Medical Marketing Ltd.
Quality System Registration Information: ISO9001; ISO9002
Produces/Sells CE-marked Devices: Y
Federal Procurement Eligibility: Small Business
Distribution: Manufacturer Direct, Manufacturer Through Distributor, OEM

NORTHGATE TECHNOLOGIES INC.   800-348-0424 *(cont'd)*

General Admin.: Debi Pope/Coord. Admin.
    Robert Mantell/Vice President, General Manager
Mktg./Adv.: Peter Manzie/Director Product Marketing
    Chuck Zander/Manager Product Development
    Peter Manzie/Marketing & Sales Specialist
Production: Chuck Zander/Manager Engineering
    Julio Morejon/Manager Manufacturing
    Chris DeGrane/Manager Operations
    Casey Kurek/Manager Regulatory Affairs
Finance: Dan Washburn/Chief Financial Officer

Endoscope	Gastroenterology/Urology
Evacuator, Gastro-Urology	Gastroenterology/Urology
Insufflator, Laparoscopic	Obstetrics/Gynecology
Lithotriptor, Electro-Hydraulic, Extracorporeal	Gastroenterology/Urology
Tubing, Other	General
Urological Irrigation System	Gastroenterology/Urology

NORTHLAND HEALTHCARE PRODUCTS LTD.   204-786-3345
865 Bradford St., Winnipeg, MAN R3E-0G5 Canada
FDA Number: n/a
E-mail: wileen@nhcp.com   *Fax:* 204-783-7496
Web site: www.nhcp.com
Year Founded: 1980
Total Employees: 25
Ownership: Private
Produces/Sells CE-marked Devices: N
Distribution: Exclusive Distributor

NORTHSTAR MEDICAL. INC,   800-457-3217
38 Buckingham Drive, Rogers, AR 72758
FDA Number: n/a
E-mail: sales@northstar-medical.com   *Fax:* 479-271-6139
Web site: www.northstar-medical.com
Year Founded: 1997
Ownership: Private
Produces/Sells CE-marked Devices: N
Federal Procurement Eligibility: Small Business, Minority Owned
Distribution: Manufacturer Through Distributor
Mktg./Adv.: Charyl Olander/Manager Contract Sales

Positioner, Spine, Surgical	Orthopedics

NORTHSTATE CARTONS
See Keller Crescent

NORTHWEST BEDDING CO.   509-244-3000
6102 South Hayford Rd., Spokane, WA 99224
FDA Number: 3019820
Web site: www.nwbedding.com   *Fax:* 509-244-9905
Ownership: Private
Produces/Sells CE-marked Devices: N

Mattress, Air Flotation	General

NORTHWEST MEDICAL PHYSICS EQUIPMENT, INC.   319-656-4447
21031 67th Ave. West, Lynnwood, WA 98036
FDA Number: 3025265
Ownership: Private
Produces/Sells CE-marked Devices: N

Accelerator, Linear, Medical	Radiology

NORTHWEST STAMPING & PRECISION, INC.   541-747-4269
86365 College View Rd., Eugene, OR 97405
FDA Number: 1000234188
E-mail: tmoore@nwstamping.com   *Fax:* 541-747-1169
Web site: www.nwstamping.com
Year Founded: 1965
Total Employees: 26   *Marketing Staff:* 1   *Sales Staff:* 1
Ownership: Private
Quality System Registration Information: ISO9000
Produces/Sells CE-marked Devices: N
Federal Procurement Eligibility: Small Business
Distribution: Manufacturer Direct
General Admin.: Jim Creech/General Manager
    Niles Hanson/President
Mktg./Adv.: Tom Moore/Director Sales

Retractor, Self-Retaining, Neurology	Cns/Neurology
Retractor, Surgical	Surgery

NORTON PERFORMANCE PLASTICS CORP., FLUID SYSTEMS
See Saint-Gobain Performance Plastics--Akron

NORWOOD PROMOTIONAL PRODUCTS, INC.   651-388-1298
5151 Moundview Drive, Red Wing, MN 55066
FDA Number: 2111760
E-mail: BJLeitner@Norwood.com   *Fax:* 651-388-2298
Web site: www.norwood.com
Year Founded: 1989
Total Employees: 320

NORWOOD PROMOTIONAL PRODUCTS, INC.   651-388-1298
(cont'd)
Ownership: Private
Produces/Sells CE-marked Devices: N
Federal Procurement Eligibility: Small Business
Distribution: Manufacturer Through Distributor
IS: Mrs. Barbara Leitner/Tech. Specialist

Applicator, Tipped, Absorbent, Sterile	General
Bandage, Adhesive	Surgery
Dispenser, Medication, Liquid	General
Floss, Dental	Dental And Oral
Glove, Patient Examination, Latex	General
Kit, First Aid	Surgery
Mask, Other	General
Pack, Hot Or Cold, Disposable	Physical Med
Plug, Ear	Ear/Nose/Throat
Sunglasses (Including Photosensitive)	Ophthalmology
Thermometer, Electronic, Continuous	General
Thermometer, Mercury	General
Toothbrush, Manual	Dental And Oral

NOSE BREATHE   808-949-8876
2065 S. King St., #304, Honolulu, HI 96826
FDA Number: 3003463830
E-mail: steven@nosebreathe.com   *Fax:* 808-949-8878
Web site: www.nosebreathe.com
Ownership: Private
Produces/Sells CE-marked Devices: N

Device, Anti-Snoring	Ear/Nose/Throat
Retainer, Screw Expansion, Orthodontic	Dental And Oral
Ring, Teething, Non-Fluid-Filled	Dental And Oral

NOSHOK, INC.   440-243-0888
1010 W. Bagley Rd., Berea, OH 44017
FDA Number: n/a
E-mail: jdillen@noshok.com   *Fax:* 440-243-3472
Web site: http://www.noshok.com
Annual Revenue: $10-$25 Million
Year Founded: 1967
Total Employees: 49   *Marketing Staff:* 2   *Sales Staff:* 13
Ownership: Private
Produces/Sells CE-marked Devices: Y
Federal Procurement Eligibility: Small Business
Distribution: Manufacturer Direct, Manufacturer Through Distributor
General Admin.: James B. Cole/Chief Executive Officer
    Jeff N. Scott/President
    Chrisitian F. L. Cole/Vice President Admin.
Mktg./Adv.: Ms. Sheryl Pritt/Manager Marketing
    Robert Torsiello/Manager National Sales

Gauge, Pressure	General
Gauge, Pressure, Coronary, Cardiopulmonary Bypass	Cardiovascular
Thermometer, Laboratory	Chemistry
Transducer, Ultrasonic, Diagnostic	Radiology
Valve, Other	Chemistry

NOTOCO LLC.   707-786-4400
660 Berding St., P.o. Box 300, Ferndale, CA 95536
FDA Number: 2918126

Otoscope	Ear/Nose/Throat

NOVA BIOMEDICAL   800-458-5813 781-894-0800
200 Prospect St., Waltham, MA 02454-9141
FDA Number: 1219029
E-mail: info@novabio.com   *Fax:* 781-894-5915
Web site: www.novabiomedical.com
Medical Products Sales Volume: $152,000,000
Annual Revenue: $100-$500 Million
Year Founded: 1976
Total Employees: 621   *Marketing Staff:* 6   *Sales Staff:* 42
Ownership: Public
Quality System Registration Information: ISO9001
Produces/Sells CE-marked Devices: Y
Federal Procurement Eligibility: Small Business, GSA Contract, VA Contract
Distribution: Manufacturer Direct, Manufacturer Through Distributor, OEM, Service Direct, Exporter
General Admin.: John J. Wallace/Chief Operating Officer
    Frank Manganaro/President, Chief Executive Officer
    Kathy Nicholson/Vice President Human Resources
    John J. Wallace/Vice President, General Manager
Mktg./Adv.: Ron Newby/Director Marketing
    Scot Fine/Director National Accounts
    Lloyd Adams/Director Product Development
    Cliff Larsson/Manager Advertising
    Lloyd Adams/Manager Market Research
    Harlan Polishook/Manager Marketing & Communications
    Howard Deahr/Manager National Sales
    Ron Newby/Manager Sales Training
    Jeffrey A. DuBois/Vice President Business Development

NOVA BIOMEDICAL 800-458-5813 *(cont'd)*

Charles Kircher/Vice President International Sales
Howard Deahr/Vice President National Sales
Production: Paul MacDonald/Manager Regulatory Affairs
Paul MacDonald/Vice President Quality Assurance
Research: Jeff Chien/Vice President Research & Development
Purchasing: Robert Laflamme/Manager Materials, Director Purchasing

Analyzer, Blood Gas pH	Anesthesiology
Analyzer, Chemistry, Electrolyte	Chemistry
Analyzer, Glucose	Chemistry
Contract Manufacturing	General
Contract R&D, Equipment	General
Control, Blood Gas	Chemistry
Control, Electrolyte (Assayed And Unassayed)	Chemistry
Electrode, Ion Specific, Ammonia	Chemistry
Electrode, Ion Specific, Calcium	Chemistry
Electrode, Ion Specific, Chloride	Chemistry
Electrode, Ion Specific, Potassium	Chemistry
Electrode, Ion Specific, Sodium	Chemistry
Enzymatic Method, Lactic Acid	Chemistry
Oximeter, Whole Blood	Hematology
Retainer, Matrix	Dental And Oral

NOVA BIOMEDICAL CORPORATION DIABETES PRODUCTS 781-894-0800

205 Burlington Road, Bedford, MA 01730
FDA Number: 3004193489

Reagent, Glucose (Test System)	Chemistry
System, Test, Blood Glucose, Over-The-Counter	Chemistry

NOVA CARE SABOLICH

See Hanger Orthopedic Group, Inc.

NOVA CENTURY SCIENTIFIC LTD. 800-615-5072
 (800) 615-5072

5022 South Service Rd.,
Burlington, ONT L7L 5 Canada
FDA Number: n/a   *Fax:* (800) 639-9006
E-mail: ncssale@aol.com
Year Founded: 1989
Total Employees: 10
Ownership: Private
Produces/Sells CE-marked Devices: N
Distribution: Manufacturer Direct, Exclusive Distributor, Importer

NOVA COMPANIES 217-763-4041

209 E South St., Po Box 139, Cerro Gordo, IL 61818
FDA Number: 3003691143
Ownership: Private
Produces/Sells CE-marked Devices: N

Booth, Sun Tan	Physical Med

NOVA HEALTH PRODUCTS, LLC 843-673-0702

1138 Annelle Dr., Florence, SC 29505
FDA Number: 1067154
Ownership: Private
Produces/Sells CE-marked Devices: N

Component, Wheelchair	Physical Med
Glove, Patient Examination	General
Wheelchair, Manual	Physical Med

NOVA HEALTH SYSTEMS, INC. 800-225-NOVA
 315-798-9018

1001 Broad St., Utica, NY 13501   *Fax:* 315-798-9337
FDA Number: 2246737
E-mail: info@novahealthsystems.com
Web site: www.novahealthsystems.com
Medical Products Sales Volume: $400,000
Annual Revenue: $0-$1 Million
Year Founded: 1977
Total Employees: 6
Ownership: Private
Produces/Sells CE-marked Devices: N
Federal Procurement Eligibility: Small Business, VA Contract
Distribution: Manufacturer Direct
General Admin.: Wade Abraham/President
Mktg./Adv.: Maryanne Marsh/Manager Marketing

Cuff, Blood Pressure	Cardiovascular
Hood, Oxygen, Infant	General
Mattress, Air Flotation	General
Pressure Pad, Alternating, Disposable	General
Pump, Alternating Pressure Pad	General
Support, Breathing Tube	Anesthesiology
Tent, Oxygen (Canopy)	Anesthesiology

NOVA PACKAGING SYSTEMS

See IMA Nova

NOVA RANGER, INC. 760-274-6344

9885 Mesa Rim Rd., Suite 127, San Diego, CA 92121
FDA Number: 3005149692
E-mail: jmost@novaranger.com

NOVA RANGER, INC. 760-274-6344 *(cont'd)*

Web site: www.novaranger.com
Ownership: Private
Produces/Sells CE-marked Devices: N

Activator, Ultraviolet, Polymerization	Dental And Oral

NOVA-TECH, INC. 308-381-8841

Central Ne. Regional Airport, 1982 East Citation Way,
Grand Island, NE 68801
FDA Number: 1931182

Culture Media, Synthetic Cell And Tissue	Pathology
Serum, Animal	Pathology

NOVABONE PRODUCTS, LLC 386-462-7660

13631 Progress Blvd, Suite #600, Alachua, FL 32615
FDA Number: 3003768919   *Fax:* 386-418-1636
E-mail: sales@novabone.com
Web site: www.novabone.com
Year Founded: 2002
Ownership: Private
Produces/Sells CE-marked Devices: Y
Distribution: Manufacturer Through Distributor

Filler, Bone Void, Osteoinduction	Physical Med
Filler, Calcium Sulfate Preformed Pellets	Orthopedics
Graft, Bone	Orthopedics
Implant, Endosseous (Bone Filling and/or Augmentation)	Dental And Oral

NOVACARE ORTHODICS 800-272-2464
 516-481-9670

151 Hempstead Tpke., Hempstead, NY 11552   *Fax:* 516-481-3725
FDA Number: n/a
Annual Revenue: $1-$5 Million
Total Employees: 175
Ownership: Private
Produces/Sells CE-marked Devices: N
Distribution: Manufacturer Direct, Service Direct
General Admin.: Andrew Meyers/President, Chief Executive Officer
Mktg./Adv.: Bonnie H. Mosher/Director National Accounts
Research: Jesse Fink/Vice President Research & Development

Orthosis, Other	Physical Med

NOVADAQ TECHNOLOGIES INC. 888-728-4368
 905-629-3822

2585 Skymark Ave., Suite 306,
Mississauga, ON L4W 4 Canada
FDA Number: 3004957274   *Fax:* 905-629-0282
E-mail: feedback@novadaq.com
Web site: www.novadaq.com
Year Founded: 2000
Ownership: Public
Stock Symbol: NDQ
Traded On: TSX Venture Exchange
Produces/Sells CE-marked Devices: N

NOVALIS MEDICAL, LLC 813-645-2855

813 S. Westshore Blvd, Tampa, FL 33609
FDA Number: 1066382

Laser, Surgical	Surgery

NOVAMED, LLC 800-425-3535
 914-789-2100

4 Westchester Plaza, Elmsford, NY 10523   *Fax:* 914-789-2102
FDA Number: 2432320
E-mail: info@novamed-usa.com
Web site: www.novamed-usa.com
Medical Products Sales Volume: $2,300,000
Annual Revenue: $10-$25 Million
Year Founded: 1988
Total Employees: 25   *Marketing Staff:* 5   *Sales Staff:* 20
Ownership: Private
Quality System Registration Information: ISO9000; ISO9001; ISO9002
Produces/Sells CE-marked Devices: Y
Federal Procurement Eligibility: Small Business
Distribution: Manufacturer Direct, Manufacturer Through Distributor, Manufacturer Through Manufacturer Reps, OEM, Service Direct, Exclusive Distributor, Exporter
General Admin.: Mr. Peter M. Derrico/President, Chief Executive Officer
Mktg./Adv.: Ms. Rebecca Hermann/Director Marketing & Sales
Ms. Carol Schuler/Executive Vice President Marketing & Sales
Production: Mr. Robert Gates/Director Product Development & Regulatory Affairs

Catheter, Balloon (Foley Type)	Surgery
Laryngoscope	Ear/Nose/Throat
Laryngoscope, Flexible	Anesthesiology
Laryngoscope, Rigid	Anesthesiology
Monitor, Temperature (With Probe)	Anesthesiology
Monitor, Temperature, Surgery	Surgery
Stethoscope, Electronic-Amplified	Surgery
Stethoscope, Esophageal	Anesthesiology
Thermometer, Liquid Crystals	Surgery

NOVAMIN TECHNOLOGY INC.
386-418-1551
13859 Progress Blvd., #600, Alachua, FL 32615
FDA Number: 3004465436

Floss, Dental	Dental And Oral
Toothbrush, Manual	Dental And Oral
Varnish, Cavity	Dental And Oral

NOVARAY, INC.
510-619-9200
39655 Eureka Dr., Newark, CA 94560
FDA Number: n/a   *Fax:* 510-291-3001
E-mail: marketing@novaraymedical.com
Web site: www.novaraymedical.com
Year Founded: 2005
Ownership: Private
Produces/Sells CE-marked Devices: N
General Admin.: Marc Whyte/Chief Operating Officer
　　　　　Edward Solomon/Chief Technology Officer
　　　　　Jack Price/President, Chief Executive Officer

NOVARE SURGICAL SYSTEMS, INC.
408-873-3161
10440 Bubb Road, Suite A, Cupertino, CA 95014
FDA Number: 2954739   *Fax:* 408-873-3167
E-mail: kpope@novaresurgical.com
Web site: www.novaresurgical.com
Medical Products Sales Volume: $5,000,000
Annual Revenue: $1-$5 Million
Year Founded: 1999
Total Employees: 19   *Marketing Staff:* 1   *Sales Staff:* 3
Ownership: Private
Quality System Registration Information: ISO9001
Produces/Sells CE-marked Devices: Y
Federal Procurement Eligibility: Small Business
Distribution: Manufacturer Direct, Manufacturer Through Distributor, OEM, Exporter

Clamp, Bulldog	Surgery
Clamp, Other	Surgery
Clamp, Vascular	Cardiovascular
Device, Anastomotic, Microvascular	Cardiovascular

NOVARTIS NUTRITION
800-333-3785
1600 Utica Ave S Suite 600, PO Box 370,
952-848-6000
Minneapolis, MN 55416
FDA Number: n/a   *Fax:* 952-593-7990
E-mail: ann.erickson@ch.novartis.com
Web site: www.novartis.com
Medical Products Sales Volume: $72,800,000
Year Founded: 1973
Total Employees: 470
Ownership: NOVARTIS
Quality System Registration Information: ISO9001
Produces/Sells CE-marked Devices: Y
Federal Procurement Eligibility: Small Business
Distribution: Manufacturer Through Distributor
General Admin.: Joe Heron/Chief Executive Officer
　　　　　Jerry Armstrong/Vice President Human Resources
Mktg./Adv.: Nena Haetman/Director Marketing
　　　　　Bill Pwinica/Vice President Corporate Accounts
　　　　　Hank O'Brian/Vice President Marketing
　　　　　Rob Harrington/Vice President Sales
Production: Bob Lang/Director Quality Assurance
　　　　　Bob Lang/Manager Regulatory Affairs
　　　　　Ann Erickson/Product Manager
　　　　　David Egberg/Vice President Manufacturing
Research: David Egberg/Vice President Research & Development

Catheter, Malecot (Gastrostomy Tube)	Gastroenterology/Urology
Infusion Pump, Enteral	General
Kit, Administration, Enteral	Gastroenterology/Urology
Kit, Feeding, Pediatric (Enteral)	General
Solution, Nutrition, Enteral	Gastroenterology/Urology
Tube, Feeding	General
Tube, Gastrointestinal	Gastroenterology/Urology
Tube, Nasogastric	Anesthesiology

NOVASOM
See NovaSom, Inc.

NOVASOM, INC.
1-877-753-3775
801 Cromwell Park Drive, Suite 108, Glen Burnie, MD 21061
FDA Number: 3005908471
E-mail: info@novasom.com
Ownership: Private
Produces/Sells CE-marked Devices: N
General Admin.: Michael Thomas/President, Chief Executive Officer
Mktg./Adv.: Kevin Quinn/Vice President Sales
Production: Roger Richardson/Vice President Operations

Monitor, Apnea	General
Recorder, Ventilatory Effort	Anesthesiology

NOVASONIC
800-843-0133
4565 Panther Place, Charlotte,, NC 28269
651-554-8113
FDA Number: 2184043   *Fax:* 651-455-4166
E-mail: novasonic.carol@gmail.com
Web site: www.novasonic.us
Annual Revenue: $0-$1 Million
Year Founded: 1990
Total Employees: 5   *Marketing Staff:* 2   *Sales Staff:* 2
Ownership: Private
Produces/Sells CE-marked Devices: N
Federal Procurement Eligibility: Small Business, Female Owned
Distribution: Service Direct
General Admin.: Carol Slavick/President

Hearing-Aid	Ear/Nose/Throat

NOVASYS MEDICAL, INC.
866-784-4777
39684 Eureka Dr., Newark, CA 94560-4805
510-226-4060
FDA Number: 3003647794   *Fax:* 510-353-0524
E-mail: info@novasysmedical.com
Web site: www.novasysmedical.com
Ownership: Private
Produces/Sells CE-marked Devices: N
General Admin.: Mr. Scott Cramer/President, Chief Executive Officer
Medical Admin.: Mr. Damian Alagia/Vice President Medical Affairs
Mktg./Adv.: Ms. Lauri Campbell/Vice President Marketing
　　　　　Mr. Eric Heil/Vice President Sales
Finance: Mr. Michael Gandy/Chief Financial Officer

Electrosurgical Unit, Cutting & Coagulation Device	Surgery

NOVAVISION, INC.
561-558-2040
3651 Fau Blvd., Suite 300, Boca Raton, FL 33431
FDA Number: 3004594297
Ownership: Private
Produces/Sells CE-marked Devices: N
General Admin.: Holger Weiss/Chief Financial Officer, Vice President
　　　　　Rudy Mazzochi/President, Chief Executive Officer

Perimeter, Automatic, AC-Powered	Ophthalmology
Recorder, Attention Task Performance	Cns/Neurology

NOVEL PRODUCTS, INC.
800-323-5143
PO Box 408, Rockton, IL 61072-0408
815-624-4888
FDA Number: 7000540   *Fax:* 815-624-4866
E-mail: Info@NovelProducts.com
Web site: www.novelproductsinc.com
Medical Products Sales Volume: $600,000
Annual Revenue: $0-$1 Million
Year Founded: 1975
Total Employees: 3
Ownership: Private
Produces/Sells CE-marked Devices: N
Federal Procurement Eligibility: Small Business, Female Owned
Distribution: Manufacturer Through Distributor
General Admin.: Carol J. Muehlenbein/President
Mktg./Adv.: James A. Muehlenbein/Manager Marketing

Analyzer, Composition, Weight, Patient	General
Caliper, Skinfold	General
Clock, Elapsed Time	General
Component, Exercise	Physical Med
Gauge, Measuring	Ear/Nose/Throat
Tape, Measuring, Ruler And Caliper	Surgery
Timer, Diagnostic Use	General

NOVEN PHARMACEUTICALS, INC.
305-253-5099
11960 SW 144th Street, Miami, FL 33186
FDA Number: n/a
Web site: www.noven.com
Year Founded: 1988
Total Employees: 610
Ownership: Public
Stock Symbol: NOVN
Traded On: NASDAQ
Produces/Sells CE-marked Devices: N
Federal Procurement Eligibility: Small Business
Distribution: Manufacturer Direct
General Admin.: Wayne P. Yetter/Chairman
　　　　　Michael D. Price/Chief Financial Officer, Vice President
　　　　　Jeffrey F. Eisenberg/Executive Vice President

Contract R&D, Diagnostics	General
Packaging Equipment	General

NOVO NORDISK CANADA, INC.
800-465-4334
300-2680 Skymark Avenue,,
905-629-4222
Mississauga, ONT L4W 5 Canada
FDA Number: n/a   *Fax:* 905-629-8662
E-mail: sdm@novonordisk.com
Web site: http://www.novonordisk.ca
Total Employees: 100

NOVO NORDISK CANADA, INC. 800-465-4334 (cont'd)

Ownership: Novo Nordisk A/S
Stock Symbol: NVO
Traded On: NYSE
Produces/Sells CE-marked Devices: Y
Distribution: Manufacturer Direct, Exclusive Distributor, Importer

NOVO NORDISK PHARMACEUTICALS, INC. 800-727-6500
100 College Road West, 609-987-5800
Princeton, NJ 08540
FDA Number: 2244771 Fax: 609-921-8082
E-mail: sspv@novonordisk.com
Web site: www.novonordisk-us.com
Year Founded: 1950
Total Employees: 350 Marketing Staff: 15 Sales Staff: 200
Ownership: Public
Stock Symbol: NVO
Traded On: NYSE
Produces/Sells CE-marked Devices: N
Distribution: Manufacturer Direct
General Admin.: Mr. Jerzy Gruhn/President
    Sarajane Machersic/Vice President Human Resources
  Medical Admin.: John Wisnart/Vice President Medical Affairs
Mktg./Adv.: Lars Barfod/Vice President Marketing
Research: Ms. Anne Phillips/Vice President Clinicial Development

Enzyme, Cell (Erythrocytic And Leukocytic)	Hematology
IV Start Kit	Surgery
Injector, Insulin	Gastroenterology/Urology
Needle, Aspiration And Injection, Disposable	Surgery
Needle, Hypodermic, Single Lumen With Syringe	General
Transfer Unit, IV Fluid	General

NOVOCOL, INC. 303-665-7535
416 South Taylor Ave., Louisville, CO 80027
FDA Number: 1721729
Ownership: Private
Produces/Sells CE-marked Devices: N

Adhesive, Bracket And Conditioner, Resin	Dental And Oral
Cement, Dental	Dental And Oral
Dam, Rubber	Dental And Oral
Detector, Caries	Dental And Oral
Disinfector, Medical Device	General
Material, Impression	Dental And Oral
Material, Tooth Shade, Resin	Dental And Oral
Medical Disinfectants/Cleaners for Instruments	General
Polyvinyl Methylether Maleic Acid/Carboxymethylcellulose	Dental And Oral
Resin, Other	General
Resin, Root Canal Filling	Dental And Oral
Sealant, Pit And Fissure, And Conditioner, Resin	Dental And Oral
Solution, Cement Dissolving	Dental And Oral
Tooth Bonding Agent, Resin Restoration	Dental And Oral
Tray, Impression	Dental And Oral
Zinc Oxide Eugenol	Dental And Oral

NOVOCURE 215-854-4095
170 West Road, Unit #9, Portsmouth, NH 03801
FDA Number: n/a
E-mail: generalinfo@novocure.com
Web site: www.novocure.com
Ownership: Private
Produces/Sells CE-marked Devices: N
General Admin.: Mr. Asaf Danzigner/Chief Executive Officer
    Mr. Mike Anbrogi/Chief Operating Officer
    Dr. Yoram Palti/Chief Technology Officer
    Mr. William Doyle/Executive Chairman
    Mr. Gabriel Leung/Vice Chairman
  Medical Admin.: Dr. Eilon Kirson/Chief Medical Officer
Finance: Mr. Wilco Groenhuysen/Chief Financial Officer

NOVOSCI CORP. 281-363-4949
2828 N. Crescent Ridge Drive, The Woodlands, TX 77381
FDA Number: 1625519 Fax: 888-570-4009
E-mail: Info@novosci.us
Web site: www.novosci.us
Medical Products Sales Volume: $2,300,000
Annual Revenue: $50-$100 Million
Year Founded: 2003
Total Employees: 23 Marketing Staff: 5
Ownership: Private
Quality System Registration Information: ISO9000; ISO9001
Produces/Sells CE-marked Devices: Y
Federal Procurement Eligibility: Small Business
Distribution: Manufacturer Direct, Manufacturer Through Distributor, Manufacturer Through Manufacturer Reps, OEM, Service Direct
General Admin.: Sherry Darden/Manager Human Resources
    Robert W. Kleinert/President, Chief Executive Officer
    Dan L. Cox/Vice President, General Manager
  Mktg./Adv.: Michael D. Dawson/Vice President International Marketing & Sales

NOVOSCI CORP. 281-363-4949 (cont'd)
Production: David Huff/Director Manufacturing
    Todd A. Tetreault/Director Materials
    Lynda Wargo/Manager Customer Services

Accessories, Catheter	Surgery
Accessories, Laser	General
Accessories, Laser, Endoscopic	Surgery
Cable, Laser, Fiberoptic	Surgery
Cannula, Aspirating	Cardiovascular
Cannula, Femoral	Gastroenterology/Urology
Cannula, Vena Cava	Cardiovascular
Cannula, Venous	Cardiovascular
Catheter, Cholangiography	Surgery
Catheter, Hydrocephalic, Atrial	Cns/Neurology
Centrifuge, Blood Bank, Diagnostic	Hematology
Clamp, Vascular	Cardiovascular
Connector, Tubing, Blood, Infusion, T-Type	Gastroenterology/Urology
Contract Assembly	General
Contract Packaging	General
Drain, Sump	Gastroenterology/Urology
Equipment, Cleaning, Air	General
Equipment/Service, Quality Control	General
Eyeglasses	Ophthalmology
Eyeglasses, Safety	Ophthalmology
Filter, Air	General
Filter, Blood, Cardiopulmonary Bypass, Arterial Line	Cardiovascular
Filter, Gas	Anesthesiology
Fitting, Luer	General
Gauge, Pressure	General
Kit, Administration, Cardioplegia Solution	Cardiovascular
Needle, Aspiration And Injection, Disposable	Surgery
Oxygenator, Cardiopulmonary Bypass	Cardiovascular
Oxygenator, Intravascular	Anesthesiology
Pack, Surgical (Drape)	Surgery
Perfusion Apparatus	Pathology
Reservoir, Blood, Cardiopulmonary Bypass	Cardiovascular
Stopcock	General
Suction Apparatus, Operating Room, Wall Vacuum-Powered	Surgery
System, Evacuation, Smoke, Laser	Surgery
Tip, Suction	Anesthesiology
Tip, Suction Tube (Yankauer, Poole, Etc.)	Surgery
Tube, Centrifuge	Chemistry
Tube, Pump, Cardiopulmonary Bypass	Cardiovascular
Tube, Tonsil Suction	Ear/Nose/Throat
Tubing, Connecting	General
Tubing, Plastic	General

NOVOZYMES BIOLOGICALS, INC. 540-389-9361
111 Kessler Mill Rd., Salem, VA 24153
FDA Number: 3004315006 Fax: 540-389-2688
Web site: www.novozymes.com
Ownership: Private
Produces/Sells CE-marked Devices: N

Cleaner, Ultrasonic, Medical Instrument	General

NOVUM INC. 412-363-3300
5900 Penn Ave., Pittsburgh, PA 15206-3817
FDA Number: n/a Fax: 412-362-5783
E-mail: businessdevelopment@novumprs.com
Web site: www.novumprs.com
Year Founded: 1972
Ownership: Private
Produces/Sells CE-marked Devices: N
Federal Procurement Eligibility: Small Business
Distribution: Service Direct

Contract R&D, Diagnostics	General

NOYES CO. INC., P.J.
See P. J. Noyes Company, Inc.

NP MEDICAL, INC. 978-368-4514
101 Union St., Clinton, MA 01510
FDA Number: 1000304305 Fax: 978-365-4025
E-mail: sales@npmedical.com
Web site: www.npmedical.com
Medical Products Sales Volume: $1,023,000,000
Annual Revenue: $25-$50 Million
Year Founded: 1955
Total Employees: 1000 Marketing Staff: 3 Sales Staff: 4
Ownership: Nypro Inc.
Produces/Sells CE-marked Devices: N
Distribution: OEM
General Admin.: Boris Levin/President
Mktg./Adv.: Donna Gasper/Manager Product Marketing
    Gary MacEachern/Manager Product Marketing
Research: Jeff Kane/Director Research & Development

Check Valve, Retrograde Flow (In-Line)	General
Connector, Tubing, Blood, Infusion, T-Type	Gastroenterology/Urology
Kit, Administration, Intravenous	General

NSA HITACHI
See Hitachi High Technologies America

NSG PRECISION CELLS, INC.   631-249-7474
195 G Central Avenue, Farmingdale, NY 11735-6904
FDA Number: 9320139
E-mail: nsgpciny@aol.com   Fax: 631-249-8575
Web site: www.nsgpci.com
Medical Products Sales Volume: $1,200,000
Total Employees: 5
Ownership: Private
Quality System Registration Information: ISO9002
Produces/Sells CE-marked Devices: N
Federal Procurement Eligibility: Small Business
Distribution: Manufacturer Direct
General Admin.: Elsa Garcia/General Manager
     Seymour Schoenfeld/President
Mktg./Adv.: E. Garcia/Manager Marketing
     S. Schoenfeld/Vice President Marketing
     E. Garcia/Vice President Sales

Cell, Spectrophotometer	Chemistry
Refractometer	Chemistry

NSK AMERICA CORPORATION   800-585-4675
700B Cooper Ct., Schaumburg, IL 60173
FDA Number: 1422375
E-mail: info@nskamericacorp.com   Fax: 847-843-7622
Web site: www.nskamericacorp.com
Medical Products Sales Volume: $5,000,000
Annual Revenue: $1-$5 Million
Total Employees: 20
Ownership: NAKANISHI, INC.
Traded On: Tokyo
Quality System Registration Information: ISO9000; ISO9001
Produces/Sells CE-marked Devices: N
Federal Procurement Eligibility: Small Business
Distribution: Manufacturer Direct, Manufacturer Through Distributor, OEM
Mktg./Adv.: Masayuki Onoguchi/Manager Marketing

Equipment, Laboratory, Gen. Purpose (Specific Medical Use)	Chemistry
Handpiece, Air-Powered, Dental	Dental And Oral
Handpiece, Direct Drive, AC-Powered	Dental And Oral

NSPIRE HEALTH, INC   800-574-7374
1830 Lefthand Circle, Longmont, CO 80501   303-666-5555
FDA Number: 1722076   Fax: 303-666-5588
E-mail: sales@nspirehealth.com
Web site: www.nspirehealth.com
Medical Products Sales Volume: $5,400,000
Annual Revenue: $10-$25 Million
Year Founded: 1990
Total Employees: 65   *Marketing Staff:* 5   *Sales Staff:* 170
Ownership: FERRARIS GROUP PLC
Stock Symbol: FER
Traded On: London
Quality System Registration Information: ISO9002
Produces/Sells CE-marked Devices: Y
Federal Procurement Eligibility: Small Business, GSA Contract, VA Contract
Distribution: Manufacturer Direct, Manufacturer Through Distributor, OEM, Exporter
General Admin.: Mr. Mike Sims/President
Mktg./Adv.: Mr. Tom Carpenter/Director Sales
     Ms. Krystanne Borgen/Manager Corporate Communications
     Mr. Larry Murdock/Vice President, Director Marketing
Production: Wendy Greenberg/Director Customer Services
     Mr. David Jackson/Vice President, Director Operations
     Mr. Ed Chu/Vice President, Engineer

Analyzer, Pulmonary Function	Anesthesiology
Dosimeter, Nitrous-Oxide	Anesthesiology
Filter, Bacterial, Breathing Circuit	Anesthesiology
Meter, Peak Flow, Spirometry	Anesthesiology
Nebulizer, Direct Patient Interface	Anesthesiology
Nebulizer, Medicinal, Non-Ventilatory (Atomizer)	Anesthesiology
Plethysmograph, Pressure (Body)	Anesthesiology
Spirometer, Diagnostic (Respirometer)	Anesthesiology
Spirometer, Monitoring (Volumeter)	Anesthesiology

NSS ENTERPRISES, INC.   419-531-2121
3115 Frenchmens Rd., Toledo, OH 43607-2958
FDA Number: n/a   Fax: 419-531-3761
E-mail: mailus@nss
Web site: www.nss.com
Total Employees: 180   *Marketing Staff:* 3   *Sales Staff:* 26
Ownership: Private
Quality System Registration Information: ISO9001
Produces/Sells CE-marked Devices: N
Distribution: Manufacturer Direct, Manufacturer Through Distributor
General Admin.: Mark J. Bevington/President
Mktg./Adv.: Diane Kornowa/Manager Marketing

NSS ENTERPRISES, INC.   419-531-2121 *(cont'd)*
     Tom Dyszkiewicz/Manager National Sales
     Bob Daniels/Vice President, Director Marketing
Housekeeping Equipment   General

NTI-TSS, INC.   574-258-5963
2303 Blue Smoke Trail, Mishawaka, IN 46546
FDA Number: 3005841560
Device, Repositioning, Jaw   Dental And Oral

NU GYN, INC   763-398-0108
1633 County Hwy. 10 N.e., Suite 15,
Spring Lake Park, MN 55432
FDA Number: 2134152
Ownership: Private
Produces/Sells CE-marked Devices: N

Device, Engorgement, Clitoral	Obstetrics/Gynecology
Plethysmograph, Impedance	Cardiovascular
Scanner, Ultrasonic (Pulsed Doppler)	Radiology

NU-BACK   262-695-1660
140 Sussex St., Pewaukee, WI 53072
FDA Number: 3003697995
E-mail: webmaster@nu-back.com
Web site: www.nu-back.com
Ownership: Private
Produces/Sells CE-marked Devices: N
Exerciser, Non-Measuring   Physical Med

NU-EAR ELECTRONICS   800-626-8327
6769 Mesa Ridge Rd., Ste. 100,   858-450-9972
San Diego, CA 92121
FDA Number: 2021333
Web site: www.nu-ear.com   Fax: 858-450-1947
Medical Products Sales Volume: $15,000,000
Annual Revenue: $10-$25 Million
Total Employees: 122   *Marketing Staff:* 12   *Sales Staff:* 15
Ownership: Starkey Laboratories, Inc.
Produces/Sells CE-marked Devices: N
Federal Procurement Eligibility: Small Business
Distribution: Manufacturer Through Distributor
General Admin.: William Austin/Chief Executive Officer
     Chao Jorgenson/President
Mktg./Adv.: Diana Prat/Director Marketing
     Debbie Kastor/Manager National Sales
     Bill Noel/Manager Sales Training
Production: Jerry Ruczika/Vice President Manufacturing

Battery, Hearing-Aid	Ear/Nose/Throat
Hearing-Aid	Ear/Nose/Throat

NU-EAR ELECTRONICS   952-947-4734
6769 Mesa Ridge Rd. Suite 100, San Diego, CA 92121
FDA Number: 2021333
Hearing-Aid   Ear/Nose/Throat

NU-HOPE LABORATORIES, INC.   800-899-5017
12640 Branford St., Pacoima, CA 91331   818-899-7711
FDA Number: 2014640   Fax: 818-899-2079
E-mail: info@nu-hope.com
Web site: www.nu-hope.com
Medical Products Sales Volume: $3,000,000
Annual Revenue: $1-$5 Million
Year Founded: 1959
Ownership: Private
Produces/Sells CE-marked Devices: Y
Federal Procurement Eligibility: Small Business, Minority Owned
Distribution: Manufacturer Through Distributor

Adhesive, Liquid	General
Bag, Drainage (Incontinence)	Gastroenterology/Urology
Bag, Drainage, Ostomy (With Adhesive)	General
Bag, Urinary Collection	General
Cement, Stomal Appliance, Ostomy	Gastroenterology/Urology
Collector, Ostomy	Gastroenterology/Urology
Pouch, Colostomy	Gastroenterology/Urology
Selector, Size, Ostomy	Gastroenterology/Urology
Support, Hernia	Gastroenterology/Urology
Tubing, Latex	General

NUAIRE, INC.   800-328-3352
2100 Fernbrook Lane,   763-553-1270
Plymouth, MN 55447
FDA Number: 9200805   Fax: 763-553-0459
E-mail: nuaire@nuaire.com
Web site: www.nuaire.com
Medical Products Sales Volume: $14,100,000
Annual Revenue: $25-$50 Million
Year Founded: 1971
Total Employees: 200

NUAIRE, INC.　800-328-3352 (cont'd)

Ownership: Private
Quality System Registration Information: ISO9001
Produces/Sells CE-marked Devices: Y
Federal Procurement Eligibility: Small Business, GSA Contract
Distribution: Manufacturer Direct, Manufacturer Through Manufacturer Reps, Importer, Exporter
General Admin.: Richard Peters/President
Mktg./Adv.: Buck Richerson/Manager International Marketing & Sales
　　　　Scott Christensen/Manager National Sales

Box, Glove	Microbiology
Cabinet Casework, Laboratory	Chemistry
Cabinet, Laboratory	Chemistry
Enclosure, Bacteriological Safety	Chemistry
Freezer, Laboratory, Ultra-Low Temperature	Chemistry
Hood, Fume, Chemical	Chemistry
Hood, Isolation, Laminar Air Flow	General
Hood, Microbiological	Microbiology
Incubator/Water Bath	Chemistry
Laminar Air Flow Unit, Fixed (Air Curtain)	Chemistry
Tissue Culture Apparatus	Microbiology

NUALINE LASER　801-304-9678

1213 Twelve Pines Cir., Sandy, UT 84094
FDA Number: 3003603929　　　　　*Fax:* 801-304-5926
E-mail: sales@nualinelaser.com
Web site: www.nualinelaser.com
Medical Products Sales Volume: $100,000
Year Founded: 1992
Total Employees: 2
Ownership: Private
Produces/Sells CE-marked Devices: N
Federal Procurement Eligibility: Small Business, Minority Owned
Distribution: Manufacturer Direct
General Admin.: Dr. Roger Lee/President

Monitor, Patient Position, Light Beam	Radiology

NUBENCO ENT., INC.　800-633-1322　201-967-9000

One Kalisa Way, Ste. 207, Paramus, NJ 07652
FDA Number: 2434060　　　　　*Fax:* 201-960-9444
E-mail: info@nubenco.com
Web site: www.nubenco.com
Ownership: Private
Produces/Sells CE-marked Devices: N

Enzyme Immunoassay, Benzodiazepine	Toxicology
Enzyme Immunoassay, Cannabinoids	Toxicology
Enzyme Immunoassay, Cocaine And Cocaine Metabolites	Toxicology
Enzyme Immunoassay, Opiates	Toxicology
Radioimmunoassay, Human Chorionic Gonadotropin	Chemistry

NUCLEAR CARDIOLOGY SYSTEMS, INC.　303-541-0044

5660 Airport Blvd., Suite 101, Boulder, CO 80301
FDA Number: 1722659

Computer and Software, Medical	General
Scanner, Emission Computed Tomography	Radiology

NUCLEAR DATA SYSTEMS
See Canberra Industries

NUCLEAR MED.,INC.
See Theragenics Corp.

NUCLEAR MEDICAL LABORATORIES
See Biomerieux Inc.

NUCLEAR MEDICAL SYSTEMS
See Biomerica, Inc.

NUCLEAR METALS, INC.
See Starmet Corporation

NUCLEAR PHARMACY SERVICES　614-757-5000

7000 Cardinal Place, Dublin, OH 43017
FDA Number: n/a
E-mail: npsinfo@cardinal.com
Web site: www.cardinalhealth.com
Ownership: CARDINAL HEALTH
Produces/Sells CE-marked Devices: N
Distribution: Manufacturer Through Distributor, Service Direct, Exclusive Distributor

Calibrator, Radioisotope	Radiology
Xenon System	Anesthesiology

NUCLEAR RESEARCH CORP.
See Canberra

NUCLETRON CORPORATION　800-336-2249　410-312-4100

8671A,AÿRobertA,AÿFultonA,AÿDrive, Columbia, MD 21046
FDA Number: 1121753　　　　　*Fax:* 410-312-4199
E-mail: info@nucletron.com
Web site: www.nucletron.com
Medical Products Sales Volume: $25,000,000
Annual Revenue: $10-$25 Million

NUCLETRON CORPORATION　800-336-2249 (cont'd)

Year Founded: 1975
Ownership: Private
Traded On: Amsterdam
Quality System Registration Information: ISO9000; ISO9001
Produces/Sells CE-marked Devices: N
Federal Procurement Eligibility: Small Business
Distribution: Manufacturer Direct
General Admin.: Jos Lamers, MSc/Chief Executive Officer
　　　　Jeroen Cammeraat, DDS, MSc, MBA/Chief Operating Officer
Finance: Jan Sigger, MSc/Chief Financial Officer

Afterloader, Radiotherapy	Radiology
Radiographic Unit, Diagnostic, Chest	Radiology
Radiotherapy Treatment Planning Unit	Radiology
Simulator, Radiotherapy	Radiology
Simulator, Radiotherapy, Special Purpose	Radiology
Therapeutic X-Ray System	Radiology

NUCLETRON-OLDELFT CORPORATION
See Nucletron Corporation

NUCLIN DIAGNOSTICS, INC.　847-498-5210

3322 Commercial Ave., Northbrook, IL 60062
FDA Number: n/a　　　　　*Fax:* 847-498-5211
Ownership: Private
Quality System Registration Information: ISO9001
Produces/Sells CE-marked Devices: Y
Federal Procurement Eligibility: Small Business
Distribution: Manufacturer Direct

Analyzer, Chemistry, Enzyme Immunoassay	Chemistry
Enzyme Immunoassay, Other	Chemistry
Radioimmunoassay, Other	Chemistry

NUCON INTERNATIONAL, INC.　800-992-5192　614-846-5710

7000 Huntley Rd., Columbus, OH 43229
FDA Number: n/a　　　　　*Fax:* 614-431-0858
E-mail: sales@nucon-int.com
Web site: www.nucon-int.com
Annual Revenue: $5-$10 Million
Year Founded: 1972
Total Employees: 45　　*Marketing Staff:* 4　　*Sales Staff:* 4
Ownership: Private
Produces/Sells CE-marked Devices: N
Federal Procurement Eligibility: Small Business
Distribution: Manufacturer Direct
General Admin.: J. L. Korach/President, Chief Executive Officer
Mktg./Adv.: C. E. Graves/Manager National Sales
　　　　J. C. Enneking/Vice President Marketing
Production: P. E. Kovach/Director Quality Assurance

Equipment, Control, Pollution	General
Recovery Equipment, Gas	General

NUCRO-TECHNICS INCORPORATED　416-438-6727

2000 Ellesmere Rd. #16, Scarborough, ONT M1H-2W4 Canada
FDA Number: n/a　　　　　*Fax:* 416-438-3463
E-mail: info@nucro-technics.com
Web site: www.nucro-technics.com
Year Founded: 1971
Total Employees: 100
Ownership: Private
Produces/Sells CE-marked Devices: N
Distribution: Manufacturer Direct, Exclusive Distributor, Exporter

NUCRYST PHARMACEUTICALS CORP.　781-224-1444

50 Audobon Rd., Suite B, Wakefield, MA 01880
FDA Number: 1226019　　　　　*Fax:* 781-246-6002
E-mail: info@nucryst.com
Web site: www.nucryst.com
Year Founded: 1993
Total Employees: 133
Ownership: Public
Stock Symbol: NCST
Traded On: NASDAQ
Produces/Sells CE-marked Devices: N
General Admin.: David Holtz/Chief Financial Officer, Vice President
　　　　Thomas Gardner/President, Chief Executive Officer, Chairman
　　　　Carol Amelio/Vice President General Counsel & Secretary
Mktg./Adv.: Ed Gaj. Jr./Vice President Corporate Development
Production: David McDowell/Vice President Manufacturing

NUELL AIR EQUIPMENT & HOSPITAL SUPPLIES, INC.
See Nuell, Inc.

NUELL, INC.　800-829-7694　574-453-4900

312 East Van Buren St., PO Box 55, Leesburg, IN 46538
FDA Number: 1827813　　　　　*Fax:* 574-453-3797
E-mail: audra@nuellinc.com
Web site: www.nuell.com

NUELL, INC.   800-829-7694 *(cont'd)*

Medical Products Sales Volume: $2,700,000
Year Founded: 1968
Total Employees: 55   *Sales Staff:* 3
Ownership: Private
Produces/Sells CE-marked Devices: N
Federal Procurement Eligibility: Small Business, Female Owned
Distribution: Manufacturer Through Manufacturer Reps, Service Direct
General Admin.: David Holsclaw/President, Chief Executive Officer
Mktg./Adv.: Jamie Slone/Manager Marketing
Production: Stephanie Holsclaw/Vice President Customer Service

Blade, Surgical, Saw, General & Plastic Surgery	Surgery
Burr, Surgical, General & Plastic Surgery	Surgery
Contract Manufacturing	General
Service, Maintenance/Repair	General

NUMA CORP.   800-327-2212
2290 North CR 427, Unit 136,   **407-331-1666**
Longwood, FL 32750
FDA Number: 1034190   *Fax:* 407-331-1883
E-mail: info@numacorporation.com
Web site: www.numacorporation.com
Year Founded: 1977
Ownership: Private
Produces/Sells CE-marked Devices: Y
Federal Procurement Eligibility: Small Business
Distribution: Manufacturer Direct, OEM

Sterilizer, Tonometer	Ophthalmology

NUMA, INC.   603-883-1909
10 Northern Blvd., Unit 12, Amherst, NH 03031
FDA Number: 9008963   *Fax:* 603-883-0839
E-mail: info@numa-inc.com
Web site: www.numa-inc.com
Medical Products Sales Volume: $2,200,000
Year Founded: 1992
Total Employees: 19
Federal Procurement Eligibility: Small Business

Scanner, Magnetic Resonance (NMR/MRI)	Radiology
Scanner, Nuclear, Tomographic	Radiology

NUMASK, INC.   866-686-2751
6320 Canoga Avenue, Suite#1500,   **818-596-2100**
Woodland Hills, CA 91367
FDA Number: 3005872389   *Fax:* 818-227-5099
Web site: www.numask.com
Ownership: Private
Produces/Sells CE-marked Devices: N

Airway, Oropharyngeal, Anesthesia	Anesthesiology
Mouthpiece, Breathing	Anesthesiology

NUMED CANADA, INC.   613-936-2592
45 Second Street West, Cornwall, ONT K6J 1G3 Canada
FDA Number: 9618000   *Fax:* 613-936-2593
E-mail: catheters@numed.on.ca
Web site: www.numed.on.ca
Medical Products Sales Volume: $3,000,000
Total Employees: 35
Ownership: Numed, Inc.
Quality System Registration Information: ISO9002
Produces/Sells CE-marked Devices: Y
Distribution: OEM, Exclusive Distributor

NUMED, INC.   315-328-4491
2880 Main St., Hopkinton, NY 12965
FDA Number: 1318694   *Fax:* 315-328-4941
E-mail: numedorders@slic.com
Web site: www.numedforchildren.com
Medical Products Sales Volume: $50,000,000
Year Founded: 1982
Total Employees: 25
Ownership: Private
Quality System Registration Information: ISO9001
Produces/Sells CE-marked Devices: Y
Federal Procurement Eligibility: Small Business
Distribution: Manufacturer Direct, Manufacturer Through Distributor, Manufacturer Through Manufacturer Reps
General Admin.: Mr. Allen Tower/President, Chief Executive Officer
    Mr. Michael Martin/Vice President
Production: Ms. Cyndie Richards/Manager Quality Assurance & Quality Control
    Ms. Alicia Sutton/Manager Quality Systems
    Ms. Nichelle LaFlesh/Manager Regulatory Affairs
    Mr. Allen Tower, Jr./Vice President, Product Manager
Research: Mr. Doug Villnave/Vice President Research
Finance: Mr. John Southwick/Vice President, Controller

Catheter, Angioplasty, Transluminal, Peripheral	Cardiovascular
Catheter, Electrode Recording, Or Probe	Cardiovascular
Catheter, Intravascular Occluding, Temporary	Cardiovascular

NUMED, INC.   315-328-4491 *(cont'd)*

Catheter, Intravascular, Diagnostic	Cardiovascular
Catheter, Percutaneous	Cardiovascular
Catheter, Percutaneous (Valvuloplasty)	Cardiovascular
Catheter, Septostomy	Cardiovascular
Probe, Blood Flow, Extravascular	Cardiovascular

NUMERA   800-233-4323
1511 3rd Avenue, Suite 808, Seattle, WA 98101   **260-876-1200**
FDA Number: 2032583
Ownership: Private
Produces/Sells CE-marked Devices: N

Meter, Peak Flow, Spirometry	Anesthesiology
Monitor, Blood Pressure, Indirect, Semi-Automatic	Cardiovascular
Spirometer, Therapeutic (Incentive)	Anesthesiology

NUMOTECH, INC.   818-772-1579
9420 Reseda Blvd., Suite 504, Northridge, CA 91324
FDA Number: 2030595
Ownership: Private
Produces/Sells CE-marked Devices: N

Bed, Flotation Therapy, Powered	Physical Med
Chamber, Oxygen, Topical, Extremity	Surgery
Cushion, Flotation	Physical Med
Support, Head And Trunk, Wheelchair	Physical Med

NUPRODX, INC.   888-288-5653
4 Malone Lane, San Rafael, CA 94903
FDA Number: 2954747   *Fax:* 415-492-1396
E-mail: info.nuprodx@comcast.net
Web site: www.nuprodx.com
Annual Revenue: $0-$1 Million
Year Founded: 1998
Total Employees: 3
Ownership: Private
Produces/Sells CE-marked Devices: N
Federal Procurement Eligibility: Small Business
Distribution: Manufacturer Direct, Manufacturer Through Manufacturer Reps

Attachment, Commode, Wheelchair	Physical Med

NURAD MEDICAL SOLUTIONS LLC   949-737-7523
396 Cliffwood Park St., Brea, CA 92821
FDA Number: 3005034497
Ownership: Private
Produces/Sells CE-marked Devices: N

Table, Radiographic, Tilting	Radiology

NURSE ASSIST ,INC.   800-649-6800
3400 Northern Cross Blvd.,   **817-231-1300**
Fort Worth, TX 76137
FDA Number: 1650927   *Fax:* 817-231-1500
E-mail: sales@nurseassist.com
Web site: www.nurseassist.com
Medical Products Sales Volume: $15,400,000
Annual Revenue: $10-$25 Million
Year Founded: 1999
Total Employees: 85   *Marketing Staff:* 2   *Sales Staff:* 14
Ownership: Private
Quality System Registration Information: ISO9001
Produces/Sells CE-marked Devices: Y
Federal Procurement Eligibility: Small Business, GSA Contract
Distribution: Manufacturer Direct, Manufacturer Through Distributor, Manufacturer Through Manufacturer Reps, OEM
General Admin.: Kevin W. Kile/President
Mktg./Adv.: Cary Terry/Director Marketing
    Dave Riedl/Vice President Sales
Production: William J. Kanewske/Vice President Operations

Accessories, Wheelchair	Physical Med
Cable	Physical Med
Monitor, Bed Occupancy	General
Monitor, Bed Patient	General

NURSES CHOICE SPECIALTY TEXTILES   910-452-1500
6611 Amsterdam Wy., Wilmington, NC 28405
FDA Number: 1053445
Web site: www.nurses-choice.com
Annual Revenue: $0-$1 Million
Ownership: Private
Produces/Sells CE-marked Devices: N
Federal Procurement Eligibility: Small Business, Female Owned
Distribution: Manufacturer Direct

Clothing, Protective	General
Garment, Protective, For Incontinence	Gastroenterology/Urology
Pad, Incontinence (Underpad)	General

NURSING CARE CURTAIN CO.   215-723-8166
114 W. Broad St., Telford, PA 18969-1922
FDA Number: n/a
Medical Products Sales Volume: $2,000,000

NURSING CARE CURTAIN CO.   215-723-8166 *(cont'd)*
Annual Revenue: $1-$5 Million
Ownership: Private
Produces/Sells CE-marked Devices: N
Federal Procurement Eligibility: Small Business
Distribution: Manufacturer Direct
Curtain, Cubicle	General
Track And Carrier, Cubicle Curtain	General

NURTURE BIOTECH INC.
See Nurture Inc.

NURTURE INC.   406-728-0260
5840 Express Way, Missoula, MT 59802
FDA Number: n/a
Ownership: Private
Produces/Sells CE-marked Devices: Y
Federal Procurement Eligibility: Small Business
Distribution: Manufacturer Direct, Manufacturer Through Distributor, Service Direct
Solution, Nutrition, Parenteral	Gastroenterology/Urology

NUTECH MOLDING CORPORATION   1-800-423-5278
2024 Broad St., PO Box 840,   **410-957-9500**
Pocomoke City, MD 21851
FDA Number: 9005144   *Fax:* 410-957-4995
E-mail: gsmith@belart.com
Year Founded: 1986
Total Employees: 100
Ownership: Bel-Art Products
Produces/Sells CE-marked Devices: Y
Federal Procurement Eligibility: Small Business, GSA Contract
Distribution: Manufacturer Direct, OEM
Colorimeter, General Use	Chemistry
Desiccator	Chemistry
Dish, Petri	Chemistry
Dispenser, Liquid, Laboratory	Chemistry
Dispenser, Pipette	Chemistry
Dispenser, Slide	Chemistry
Dryer, Labware	Chemistry
Electrophoresis Equipment, Gel	Chemistry
Equipment, Laboratory, Gen. Purpose (Specific Medical Use)	Chemistry
Fountain, Eye Wash	Chemistry
Labware, Basic, Disposable	Chemistry
Labware, Basic, Reusable	Chemistry
Pipette	Chemistry
Rack, Drying	Chemistry
Rack, Test Tube	Chemistry
Sink, Laboratory	Chemistry
Stirrer	Chemistry
Support, Tube, Test	Chemistry

NUTEK ORTHOPAEDICS, LLC   954-779-1400
301 SW 7th Street, Ft. Lauderdale, FL 33301
FDA Number: 3005893246   *Fax:* 949-779-7300
E-mail: info@nutekortho.com
Web site: www.nutekortho.com
Ownership: Private
Produces/Sells CE-marked Devices: N
Appliance, Fix., Nail/Blade/Plate Comb., Multiple Component	Orthopedics
Fixation Appliance, Multiple Component	Orthopedics

NUTOPES CO.
See Nuclear Pharmacy Services

NUTRA LUXE MD, LLC   877-241-0459
6835 International Center Blvd, Unit 5,   **239-561-9699**
Fort Myers, FL 33912
FDA Number: 3005680967
E-mail: info@nutraluxemd.com
Web site: www.nutraluxe.net
Ownership: Private
Produces/Sells CE-marked Devices: N
Massager, Therapeutic	Physical Med

NUTRACEUTICAL INTERNATIONAL CORP.   800-669-8877
1400 Kearns Blvd., Second Floor, Park City, UT 84060
FDA Number: n/a   *Fax:* 800-767-8514
E-mail: info@nutraceutical.com
Web site: www.nutraceutical.com
Year Founded: 1932
Ownership: Public
Stock Symbol: NUTR
Traded On: NASDAQ
Produces/Sells CE-marked Devices: N
General Admin.: Frank W. Gay/Chief Executive Officer, Chairman
    Cory J. McQueen/Chief Financial Officer, Vice President
    Jeffrey A. Hinrichs/Chief Operating Officer, Executive Vice President
    Gary M. Hume/Executive Vice President

NUTRACEUTICAL INTERNATIONAL CORP. 800-669-8877 *(cont'd)*
    Bruce R. Hough/President

NUTRITION-ENDOCRINE-METABOLIC LABORATORI
See Specialty Laboratories, Inc.

NUVASIVE, INC.   800-475-9131
7475 Lusk Blvd., San Diego, CA 92121   **858-909-1800**
FDA Number: 2031966   *Fax:* 800-475-9134
E-mail: customerservice@nuvasive.com
Web site: www.nuvasive.com
Year Founded: 1997
Ownership: Public
Stock Symbol: NUVA
Traded On: NASDAQ
Produces/Sells CE-marked Devices: N
General Admin.: Mr. Alexis V. Lukianov/Chief Executive Officer, Chairman
    Michael J. Lambert/Chief Financial Officer, Executive Vice President
    Keith C. Valentine/President, Chief Operating Officer
Accessories, Arthroscopic	Orthopedics
Appliance, Fixation, Spinal Interlaminal	Orthopedics
Appliance, Fixation, Spinal Intervertebral Body	Orthopedics
Arthroscope	Orthopedics
Cable, Electrode	Physical Med
Device, Spinal Vertebral Body Replacement	Orthopedics
Electrode, Cutaneous	Cns/Neurology
Filler, Calcium Sulfate Preformed Pellets	Orthopedics
Light, Surgical, Fiberoptic	Surgery
Mesh, Metal	Gastroenterology/Urology
Orthopedic Manual Surgical Instrument	Orthopedics
Orthosis, Fixation, Pedicle, Spinal	Orthopedics
Orthosis, Fixation, Spondylolisthesis	Orthopedics
Prosthesis, Hip, Cement Restrictor	Orthopedics
Stimulator, Electrical, Evoked Response	Cns/Neurology
Stimulator, Nerve, AC-Powered	Anesthesiology
Stimulator, Nerve, ENT	Ear/Nose/Throat
System, Facet Screw Spinal Device	Orthopedics

NUVISION, INC.
See Pearle Vision

NUVO, INC.   814-899-4220
5368 Kuhl Rd., Corry, PA 16407
FDA Number: 2531685
Endoscope	Gastroenterology/Urology
Light, Surgical, Ceiling Mounted	Surgery
Table, Surgical With Orthopedic Accessories, AC-Powered	Surgery

NUVON INC.   215-966-6142
3624 Market Street, Suite 5E, Philadelphia, PA 19104
FDA Number: 3008517660
Web site: http://nuvon.com
Ownership: Private
Produces/Sells CE-marked Devices: N
General Admin.: Ms. Cathleen Asch/Chief Executive Officer
  Medical Admin.: Dr. John Zaleski/Vice President Clinical Affairs
Computer Software	General

NXSTAGE MEDICAL, INC.   866-697-8243
439 South Union St., 5th Floor,   **978-687-4700**
Lawrence, MA 01843
FDA Number: 3003464075   *Fax:* 978-687-4809
Web site: http://www.nxstage.com
Ownership: Public
Stock Symbol: NXTM
Traded On: NASDAQ
Produces/Sells CE-marked Devices: N
General Admin.: Mr. Jeffrey Burbank/Chief Executive Officer
    Mr. Joseph Turk/President
Production: Mr. Gus Azel/Senior Vice President Manufacturing
    Mr. Michael Webb/Senior Vice President Quality Assurance
Finance: Mr. Robert Brown/Chief Financial Officer
Accessories, Blood Circuit, Hemodialysis	Gastroenterology/Urology
Concentrate, Dialysis, Hemodialysis (Liquid or Powder)	Gastroenterology/Urology
Dialysate Delivery System, Single Patient	Gastroenterology/Urology
Dialyzer, High Permeability	Gastroenterology/Urology
Kit, Tubing, Blood, Anti-Regurgitation	Gastroenterology/Urology
Needle, Fistula	Gastroenterology/Urology
Needle, Hypodermic, Single Lumen With Syringe	General
Plasma, Coagulase, Human/Horse/Rabbit	Microbiology
Proportioning Apparatus	Gastroenterology/Urology
Protector, Transducer, Dialysis	Gastroenterology/Urology
Purification System, Water	Gastroenterology/Urology
System, Hemodialysis, Remote Accessories	Gastroenterology/Urology
Warmer, Infusion Fluid, Thermal	General
Medical Product Subsidiaries (Listed Separately)
Medisystems Corporation

NY ORTHOPEDIC USA, INC. — 718-852-5330
63 Flushing Ave, Unit #333, Bldg #77, Brooklyn, NY 11205
FDA Number: 3006336810
Fax: 718-852-4095
E-mail: customerservice@nyorthousa.com
Web site: www.nyorthousa.com
Ownership: Private
Produces/Sells CE-marked Devices: N

Binder, Abdominal	General
Orthosis, Lumbosacral	Physical Med
Sling, Arm	Physical Med

NYCO PRODUCTS CO. — 800-752-4754
5332 Dansher Rd., Countryside, IL 60525
FDA Number: n/a
Fax: 708-579-9898
E-mail: customerservice@nycoproducts.com
Web site: www.nycoproducts.com
Annual Revenue: $1-$5 Million
Ownership: Private
Produces/Sells CE-marked Devices: N
General Admin.: Robert Stahurski/Chief Executive Officer
Mktg./Adv.: Jim Shae/Vice President Marketing & Sales
Production: Bob Houston/Vice President Manufacturing

Disinfector, Liquid	General
Solution, Antibacterial Cleaner	General

NYPRO INC. — 978-365-9721
101 Union St., Clinton, MA 01510-2005
FDA Number: 1219365
Fax: 978-368-0236
E-mail: information@nypro.com
Web site: www.nypro.com
Medical Products Sales Volume: $225,000,000
Year Founded: 1955
Total Employees: 10000
Ownership: Private
Quality System Registration Information: ISO9001; ISO9002
Produces/Sells CE-marked Devices: N
Federal Procurement Eligibility: Minority Owned
Distribution: OEM, Service Direct
General Admin.: Brian Jones/President, Chief Executive Officer
Greg Adams/Vice President
James Buonomo/Vice President
Mktg./Adv.: Barry Potter/Manager International Sales
Angelo Sabatalo/Manager Sales Training
Randall Barko/Vice President Marketing
Ken Branham/Vice President Sales
Production: Eric Pettes/Director Quality Assurance
Research: Richard Hoeske/Vice President Engineering
Finance: Nick Aznoian/Chief Financial Officer
IS: Mike MacKenty/Vice President Information Systems

Cleanroom Equipment	General
Component, Plastic	General
Contract Manufacturing	General
Equipment, Extruding/Molding	General
Production Equipment	General

Medical Product Subsidiaries (Listed Separately)
Np Medical, Inc.

NYSARC, COLUMBIA COUNTY CHAPTER, INC. — 518-672-4451
Po Box 2 Rt 217, Mellenville, NY 12544
FDA Number: 1319722
Ownership: Private
Produces/Sells CE-marked Devices: N

Floss, Dental	Dental And Oral
Toothbrush, Manual	Dental And Oral

NYSTROM — 800-621-8086
4719 W. 62nd St., Indianapolis, IN 46268-2593 -
FDA Number: n/a
Fax: 317-329-3305
Web site: www.nystromnet.com
Total Employees: 80
Ownership: HERFF JONES, INC.
Produces/Sells CE-marked Devices: N
Federal Procurement Eligibility: Small Business
Distribution: Manufacturer Through Distributor
General Admin.: J. J. Cerza/President, Chief Executive Officer
Production: Rich Barcachewski/Manager Production

Anatomical Training Model	General
Chart, Anatomical Training	General

NYTONE MEDICAL PRODUCTS — 801-973-4090
2424 S. 900 W., Salt Lake City, UT 84119-1518
FDA Number: 1718047
Fax: 801-973-0176
E-mail: info@nytone.com
Web site: www.nytone.com
Medical Products Sales Volume: $900,000
Annual Revenue: $0-$1 Million
Year Founded: 1972
Total Employees: 6
Marketing Staff: 1
Sales Staff: 1

NYTONE MEDICAL PRODUCTS — 801-973-4090 *(cont'd)*
Ownership: NYTONE, INC.
Produces/Sells CE-marked Devices: N
Federal Procurement Eligibility: Small Business, Female Owned, GSA Contract
Distribution: Manufacturer Direct, Service Direct
General Admin.: Darlene Balding/Corporate Secretary
George Balding/President

Alarm, Enuresis	Gastroenterology/Urology

O'RYAN INDUSTRIES, INC. — 800-426-4311 / 360-892-0447
12711 N.E. 95th St., PO Box 1736,
Vancouver, WA 98682
FDA Number: 3024622
Fax: 360-892-6742
E-mail: info@oryanindustries.com
Web site: www.oryanindustries.com
Medical Products Sales Volume: $2,300,000
Annual Revenue: $1-$5 Million
Year Founded: 1982
Total Employees: 25
Marketing Staff: 2
Sales Staff: 4
Ownership: Private
Produces/Sells CE-marked Devices: Y
Federal Procurement Eligibility: Small Business
Distribution: Manufacturer Direct, Manufacturer Through Manufacturer Reps, OEM, Importer, Exporter
General Admin.: Rick Grant/President
Sharon Grant/Vice President

Endoscope And Accessories, AC-Powered	Surgery

O'SULLIVAN CORP.
See O'sullivan Corp.

O-TWO SYSTEMS INTERNATIONAL INC. — 800-387-3405 / 905-677-9410
7575 Kimbel St.,
Mississauga, ONT L5S 1 Canada
FDA Number: 38186
Fax: 905-677-2035
E-mail: resuscitation@otwo.com
Web site: www.otwo.com
Year Founded: 1971
Total Employees: 50
Marketing Staff: 4
Sales Staff: 8
Ownership: Private
Quality System Registration Information: ISO9001
Produces/Sells CE-marked Devices: Y
Federal Procurement Eligibility: Small Business
Distribution: Manufacturer Direct, Manufacturer Through Distributor, Manufacturer Through Manufacturer Reps, OEM, Exclusive Distributor, Exporter

O.O.S. MEDICAL — 800-387-5150 / 416-298-8500
60 Shorting Rd.,
Scarborough, ONT M1S-3 Canada
FDA Number: n/a
Fax: 416-298-0476
E-mail: oos@oosmedical.com
Web site: www.oosmedical.com
Year Founded: 1983
Total Employees: 10
Ownership: Private
Produces/Sells CE-marked Devices: N
Distribution: Exclusive Distributor, Importer

O.R. COMFORT, LLC — 973-239-1950
28 Appleton Rd., Glen Ridge, NJ 07028-2204
FDA Number: 2249310
Fax: 973-239-1808
E-mail: sales@orcomfort.com
Web site: www.orcomfort.com
Annual Revenue: $0-$1 Million
Year Founded: 1998
Ownership: Private
Produces/Sells CE-marked Devices: Y
Federal Procurement Eligibility: Small Business
Distribution: Manufacturer Through Distributor, OEM

Support, Patient Position	Anesthesiology

O2 TECHNOLOGIES, INC. — 804-897-8555
11341-c Business Center Drive, Richmond, VA 23236
FDA Number: 1125588
Fax: 804-897-9549
E-mail: o2tech@comcast.net
Web site: www.o2technologies.com
Medical Products Sales Volume: $270,000
Year Founded: 1997
Total Employees: 3
Ownership: Private
Quality System Registration Information: ISO9001
Produces/Sells CE-marked Devices: N
Federal Procurement Eligibility: Small Business
Distribution: Manufacturer Direct, Manufacturer Through Distributor, Manufacturer Through Manufacturer Reps, OEM

Analyzer, Gas, Oxygen, Gaseous Phase	Anesthesiology

OAK FREQUENCY CONTRACT GROUP
See Vectron International

OAK GLOVES DIVISION OF OMAR MEDICAL SUPPLIES, INC.
800-823-2289

208 Industrial Blvd, Tullahoma, TN 37388   **708-534-8200**
FDA Number: 3007366674   *Fax:* 708-534-8271
Web site: www.oakgloves.com
Annual Revenue: $25-$50 Million
Year Founded: 1997
Ownership: Private
Quality System Registration Information: ISO9002
Produces/Sells CE-marked Devices: Y
Federal Procurement Eligibility: Small Business
Distribution: Manufacturer Through Distributor
Glove, Patient Examination   General
Glove, Patient Examination, Vinyl   General
Glove, Utility   General
Medical Product Subsidiaries (Listed Separately)
Oak Technical, Inc.

OAK RIDGE PRODUCTS
888-650-7444

4612 Century Court, McHenry, IL 60050   **815-363-4700**
FDA Number: n/a   *Fax:* 815-344-6070
E-mail: comalley@OakridgeProducts.com
Web site: www.oakridgeproducts.com
Medical Products Sales Volume: $1,500,000
Annual Revenue: $1-$5 Million
Total Employees: 10   *Marketing Staff:* 1   *Sales Staff:* 3
Ownership: Private
Produces/Sells CE-marked Devices: N
Federal Procurement Eligibility: Small Business
Distribution: Manufacturer Direct
General Admin.: Andy Kovari/Partner
    Conor O' Malley/President, Chief Executive Officer, Chief Financial Officer
Mktg./Adv.: Andrew Kovari/Manager National Sales
    Wayne Kalis/Manager Sales
Cup, Medicine   General
Depressor, Tongue   General

OAK RUBBER COMPANY
See Oak Gloves Division Of Omar Medical Supplies, Inc.

OAK TECHNICAL, INC.
See Oak Gloves Division Of Omar Medical Supplies, Inc.

OAK TECHNICAL, LLC
423-587-0690

208 Industrial Blvd., Tullahoma, TN 37388
FDA Number: 1065336
Web site: www.oakgloves.com
Ownership: Private
Produces/Sells CE-marked Devices: N
Glove, Patient Examination, Vinyl   General

OAKLEY, INC.
800-431-1439

One Icon, Foothill Ranch, CA 92610   **949-951-0991**
FDA Number: 2083323   *Fax:* 949-699-3500
E-mail: info@oakley.com
Web site: www.oakley.com
Medical Products Sales Volume: $761,900,000
Year Founded: 1975
Total Employees: 900
Ownership: Private
Stock Symbol: OO
Traded On: NYSE
Produces/Sells CE-marked Devices: N
Federal Procurement Eligibility: Small Business, GSA Contract
Distribution: Manufacturer Direct, Manufacturer Through Distributor
Lens, Spectacle/Eyeglasses, Non-Custom   Ophthalmology
Sunglasses (Including Photosensitive)   Ophthalmology

OAKWORKS, INC.
800-558-8850

923 East Wellspring Road,   **717-235-6807**
New Freedom, PA 17349
FDA Number: 2529571   *Fax:* 717-235-6798
E-mail: information@oakworks.com
Web site: www.oakworks.com
Medical Products Sales Volume: $26,200,000
Annual Revenue: $10-$25 Million
Year Founded: 1977
Total Employees: 150
Ownership: Private
Produces/Sells CE-marked Devices: Y
Federal Procurement Eligibility: Small Business, Female Owned, GSA Contract
Distribution: Manufacturer Direct, Manufacturer Through Distributor
General Admin.: Ms. Linda Riach/Chief Executive Officer
    Mr. Jeff Riach/Chief Operating Officer
Mktg./Adv.: Mr. Rich Elsen/Director Medical Marketing

OAKWORKS, INC.
800-558-8850 *(cont'd)*

Chair/Table, Medical   General
Cradle, Patient, Radiographic   Radiology
Orthosis, Thoracic   Physical Med
Support, Patient Position   Anesthesiology
Table, Mechanical   Physical Med
Table, Radiographic, Tilting   Radiology

OASIS MEDICAL, INC.
800-528-9786

510-528 S. Vermont Ave., Glendora, CA 91741   **909-305-5400**
FDA Number: 2083373   *Fax:* 909-305-9987
E-mail: sales@oasismedical.com
Web site: http://www.oasismedical.com
Annual Revenue: $10-$25 Million
Year Founded: 1987
Total Employees: 65   *Marketing Staff:* 2   *Sales Staff:* 8
Ownership: Private
Quality System Registration Information: ISO9001
Produces/Sells CE-marked Devices: Y
Federal Procurement Eligibility: Small Business
Distribution: Manufacturer Through Distributor, Manufacturer Through Manufacturer Reps, OEM
General Admin.: Craig Delgado/President
Mktg./Adv.: Travis Delgado/Director International Sales
Production: Michael Ekinaka/Director Production
    Robyn Scopis/Director Quality Assurance & Regulatory Affairs
    Tommy Craig/Manager Materials
Aspirator, Ophthalmic   Ophthalmology
Astigmometer   Ophthalmology
Cannula, Lacrimal (Eye)   Ophthalmology
Cannula, Ophthalmic   Ophthalmology
Cautery, Thermal, Battery-Powered   Ophthalmology
Cystotome, Ophthalmic   Ophthalmology
Dilator, Lacrimal   Ophthalmology
Fluid, Intraocular   Ophthalmology
Forceps, Ophthalmic   Ophthalmology
Knife, Cataract   Ophthalmology
Knife, Ophthalmic   Ophthalmology
Laboratory Equipment, Ophthalmic   Ophthalmology
Needle, Ophthalmic   Ophthalmology
Plug, Punctum   Ophthalmology
Pupillometer   Ophthalmology
Shield, Corneal   Ophthalmology
Tissue, Corneal   Ophthalmology

OB SCIENTIFIC, INC.
888-530-4561

N 112 W18741, Mequon Rd., P.O. Box 787,   **262-532-8200**
Germantown, WI 53022
FDA Number: 2135142   *Fax:* 262-532-8201
E-mail: sherri.huff@obscientific.com
Web site: www.obscientific.com
Ownership: Private
Produces/Sells CE-marked Devices: N
Extractor, Vacuum, Fetal   Obstetrics/Gynecology
Oximeter, Pulse, Fetal   Obstetrics/Gynecology

OBAGI MEDICAL PRODUCTS, INC.
800-636-7546

3760 Kilroy Airport Way, Suite 500,   **562-628-1007**
Long Beach, CA 90806
FDA Number: n/a   *Fax:* 562-628-1008
E-mail: webmaster@obagi.com
Web site: http://www.obagi.com
Year Founded: 1988
Ownership: Public
Stock Symbol: OMPI
Traded On: NASDAQ
Produces/Sells CE-marked Devices: N
General Admin.: Mr. Albert Hummel/Chief Executive Officer
    Mr. Preston Romm/Chief Financial Officer, Executive Vice President
Mktg./Adv.: Mr. David Goldstein/Executive Vice President Marketing & Sales
    Mr. James Hartman/Vice President International Marketing & Sales

OBERON COMPANY ,DIV OF THE PARAMOUNT CORP.
800-322-3348

22 Logan St., PO Box 61008,   **508-999-4442**
New Bedford, MA 02746
FDA Number: n/a   *Fax:* 508-999-4443
E-mail: sales@oberoncompany.com
Web site: www.oberoncompany.com
Annual Revenue: $5-$10 Million
Year Founded: 1978
Total Employees: 50
Ownership: PARAMOUNT CORPORATION
Produces/Sells CE-marked Devices: N
Federal Procurement Eligibility: Small Business
Distribution: Manufacturer Through Distributor, OEM, Exporter

OBERON COMPANY ,DIV OF THE
800-322-3348 *(cont'd)*
General Admin.: Jack B. Hirschmann/Chief Executive Officer
Mktg./Adv.: Mr. Randell Hirschmann/Director Marketing

Goggles, Protective, Eye	Ophthalmology
Mask, Face	General
Shield, Ophthalmic, Radiological	Radiology
Shield, Protective, Personnel	Radiology

OBS MEDICAL
866-424-6744
Two Meridian Plaza
10401 N Meridian St., Ste. 300
Indianapolis, IN 46290
317-581-9236
FDA Number: 3005768010   *Fax:* 317-581-8941
Web site: www.obsmedical.com
Ownership: Private
Produces/Sells CE-marked Devices: N

Monitor, Physiological, Patient	Cardiovascular

OBSIDIAN DENTAL INC.
541-617-0129
62915 Ne 18th St., Suite 4, Bend, OR 97701
FDA Number: 3004184125

Operative Dental Treatment Unit	Dental And Oral

OBSIDIAN MEDICAL TECHNOLOGY, INC.
832-767-9606
5108 Corona Covet, Pleasanton, CA 94588
FDA Number: 3003692377
Ownership: Private
Produces/Sells CE-marked Devices: N

Illuminator, Radiographic Film	Radiology
Image Processing System	Radiology

OBTURA SPARTAN
800-344-1321
13729 Shoreline Ct. East, Earth City, MO 63045
FDA Number: n/a   *Fax:* 636-343-5794
E-mail: enhancingendo@obtura.com
Web site: www.obtura.com
Medical Products Sales Volume: $1,500,000
Annual Revenue: $1-$5 Million
Year Founded: 1979
Ownership: Private
Produces/Sells CE-marked Devices: N
Federal Procurement Eligibility: Small Business
Distribution: Manufacturer Direct, OEM

Controller, Foot, Handpiece And Cord	Dental And Oral
Handpiece, Air-Powered, Dental	Dental And Oral
Scaler, Ultrasonic	Dental And Oral

OBUS FORME LTD.
888-225-7378
344 Consumers Road,
Toronto, ON M2J 1 Canada
416-785-1386
FDA Number: 7000682   *Fax:* 416-785-5862
E-mail: cservice@homedicsgroup.ca
Web site: www.obusforme.com
Year Founded: 1980
Total Employees: 150   *Marketing Staff:* 25   *Sales Staff:* 90
Ownership: Private
Produces/Sells CE-marked Devices: N
Distribution: Manufacturer Direct, Manufacturer Through Distributor, Manufacturer Through Manufacturer Reps, Exclusive Distributor, Importer, Exporter

OCCK, INC.
800-526-9731
1710 West Schilling Road, Salina, KS 67401
785-857-9383
FDA Number: 9051942   *Fax:* 785-823-2015
E-mail: occk@occk.com
Web site: www.occk.com
Medical Products Sales Volume: $14,260,000
Annual Revenue: $10-$25 Million
Year Founded: 1970
Total Employees: 210
Ownership: Private
Produces/Sells CE-marked Devices: N
Federal Procurement Eligibility: Small Business
Distribution: Manufacturer Through Distributor, Manufacturer Through Manufacturer Reps, OEM

Apron, Lead, Radiographic	Radiology
Bag, Ice	General
Hemorrhoid Cushion	Gastroenterology/Urology

OCCLUTECH AB
+46 42 33 65 21
RAnnowsgatan 8, Helsingborg S-252 25
FDA Number: n/a   *Fax:* +46 42 311 09 7
E-mail: order@occlutech.net
Web site: http://www.occlutech.com
Year Founded: 2003
Ownership: Private
Produces/Sells CE-marked Devices: N

OCCUPATIONAL HEARING SERVICES
800-622-3277
300 South Chester Road, Suite 301,
Swarthmore, PA 19081
610-544-7700
FDA Number: 9000746   *Fax:* 610-543-2802
E-mail: dahst@aol.com
Medical Products Sales Volume: $340,000
Year Founded: 1983
Total Employees: 4
Ownership: Private
Produces/Sells CE-marked Devices: N
Federal Procurement Eligibility: Small Business

Audiometer	Ear/Nose/Throat

OCEANIC MEDICAL PRODUCTS, INC.
913-874-2000
8005 Shannon Industrial Park, Ln., Atchison, KS 66002
FDA Number: 1933971

Gas-Machine, Anesthesia	Anesthesiology
Ventilator, Continuous (Respirator)	Anesthesiology
Ventilator, Non-Continuous (Respirator)	Anesthesiology

OCEANS SEVEN INT'L.
502-634-3221
Hughes Airport Center, 6620 Escondido, Las Vegas, NV 89119
FDA Number: 9040682   *Fax:* 502-634-3221
E-mail: theyfit@theyfit.com
Web site: www.THEYFIT.COM
Ownership: Private
Produces/Sells CE-marked Devices: N
General Admin.: Frank C Sadlo/Chief Executive Officer, Chairman
         Klaus Richter/President

Condom	Obstetrics/Gynecology

OCELCO, INC.
800-328-5343
1111 Industrial Park Road, Brainerd, MN 56401
218-828-7788
FDA Number: n/a   *Fax:* 866-829-9744
E-mail: customerservice@ocelco.com
Web site: www.ocelco.com
Medical Products Sales Volume: $2,400,000
Annual Revenue: $1-$5 Million
Year Founded: 1974
Total Employees: 19   *Marketing Staff:* 1   *Sales Staff:* 1
Ownership: Private
Produces/Sells CE-marked Devices: N
Federal Procurement Eligibility: Small Business, Minority Owned, Female Owned
Distribution: Service Direct
General Admin.: Diana Bean/President
         Mark Ocel/Vice President

Accessories, Wheelchair	Physical Med
Belt, Wheelchair	Physical Med
Crusher, Pill	General
Wheelchair, Manual	Physical Med
Wheelchair, Powered	Physical Med

OCG TECHNOLOGY, INC.
914-576-8457
56 Harisson St., New Rochelle, NY 10801-6555
FDA Number: 9200812   *Fax:* 914-576-7821
E-mail: jnelson@octg.com
Medical Products Sales Volume: $300,000
Annual Revenue: $0-$1 Million
Total Employees: 3   *Marketing Staff:* 4   *Sales Staff:* 4
Ownership: Private
Produces/Sells CE-marked Devices: N
Federal Procurement Eligibility: Small Business
Distribution: Manufacturer Through Distributor
General Admin.: Edward C. Levine/President

Computer Software	General
Computer Software, Industrial	General
Omnicardiograph (Cardiointegraph)	Cardiovascular

OCKIOBEL, INC.
305-261-6144
777 NW 72 Avenue, Suite 2K20, Miami, FL 33126-3009
FDA Number: 1064536   *Fax:* 305-847-0742
E-mail: mail@ockiobel.com
Web site: www.ockiobel.com
Medical Products Sales Volume: $400,000
Annual Revenue: $0-$1 Million
Year Founded: 2000
Total Employees: 4
Ownership: Private
Produces/Sells CE-marked Devices: Y
Federal Procurement Eligibility: Small Business
Distribution: Exclusive Distributor, Importer, Exporter

Frame, Spectacle (Eyeglasses)	Ophthalmology
Sunglasses (Including Photosensitive)	Ophthalmology

OCO BIOMEDICAL
See OCO Biomedical

OCO INC.
See OCO Biomedical

OCT USA, INC. — 720-962-5412
17 Hammond, Suite 411, Irvine, CA 92618
FDA Number: 3004859950
Ownership: Private
Produces/Sells CE-marked Devices: N
Implant, Endosseous (Bone Filling and/or Augmentation) — Dental And Oral

OCTOMED SYSTEMS
See Vitamedics Corporation

OCTOSTOP INC. — 888-422-7151 / 450-978-9805
1675 boul. Saint Elzear, Ouest,
Laval, QUE H7L-3 Canada
FDA Number: 8022065 — Fax: 450-978-9766
E-mail: octostop@octostop.com
Web site: www.octostop.com
Year Founded: 1964
Total Employees: 7 — Marketing Staff: 1 — Sales Staff: 1
Ownership: Private
Produces/Sells CE-marked Devices: Y
Distribution: Manufacturer Direct, Exporter

OCU-EASE OPTICAL PRODUCTS, INC. — 800-521-8984 / 510-724-0384
920 San Pablo Ave, Pinole, CA 94564-1630
FDA Number: 2916547 — Fax: 510-724-4842
E-mail: sandyl@ocuease.com
Web site: www.ocuease.com
Medical Products Sales Volume: $1,000,000
Annual Revenue: $0-$1 Million
Total Employees: 17 — Marketing Staff: 1 — Sales Staff: 1
Ownership: Private
Produces/Sells CE-marked Devices: N
Federal Procurement Eligibility: Small Business
Distribution: Manufacturer Direct
General Admin.: Charles R. Vermette/President, Chief Executive Officer
Ronald Fujii/Vice President
Research: Troy Bolin/Manager Laboratories
Lens, Contact (Other Material) — Ophthalmology

OCU-LABS, INC. — 952-854-6702
7851 Metro Parkway #225, Bloomington, MN 55425
FDA Number: 2131669
Eye, Artificial, Non-Custom — Ophthalmology

OCULAR CONCEPTS LLC. — 503-699-7700
4035 Sw Mercantile Dr., Suite #208, Lake Grove, OR 97035
FDA Number: 3033510
Button, Iris, Eye, Artificial — Ophthalmology
Conformer, Ophthalmic — Ophthalmology

OCULAR INNOVATIONS, INC. — 813-645-2855
1121 Lewis Ave., Sarasota, FL 34237
FDA Number: 3005603852
Fornixscope — Ophthalmology

OCULAR INSTRUMENTS, INC. — 800-888-6616 / 425-455-5200
2255-116th Avenue NE, Bellevue, WA 98004-3039
FDA Number: 3014865 — Fax: 425-462-6669
E-mail: ocular@ocular-instruments.com
Web site: www.ocular-instruments.com
Medical Products Sales Volume: $4,300,000
Year Founded: 1960
Total Employees: 55 — Marketing Staff: 2 — Sales Staff: 2
Ownership: Private
Quality System Registration Information: ISO9001
Produces/Sells CE-marked Devices: Y
Federal Procurement Eligibility: Small Business
Distribution: Manufacturer Direct, Manufacturer Through Distributor, OEM, Exporter
General Admin.: James P. Erickson/Chairman, Chief Executive Officer
Phillip J. Erickson/President
Mktg./Adv.: Phillip J. Erickson/Director Marketing
Raymond Graham/Director Product Development
Production: Raymond Graham/Manager Regulatory Affairs
Accessories, Laser — General
Lens, Contact, Polymethylmethacrylate, Diagnostic — Ophthalmology
Lens, Set, Trial, Ophthalmic — Ophthalmology
Lens, Surgical, Laser — Ophthalmology
Table, Ophthalmic, Instrument, Manual — Ophthalmology
Table, Ophthalmic, Instrument, Powered — Ophthalmology

OCULAR INSTRUMENTS, NORTH FACILITY — 800-888-6616 / 425-455-5200
2255 116th Ave NE, Bellevue, WA 98004
FDA Number: 3004067900 — Fax: 425-462-6669
Ownership: Private
Produces/Sells CE-marked Devices: N
Gauge, Lens, Ophthalmic — Ophthalmology
Gonioscope (Prism) — Ophthalmology
Keratoprosthesis, Temporary Implant, Surgical — Ophthalmology

OCULAR INSTRUMENTS, NORTH FACILITY — 800-888-6616
(cont'd)
Lens, Condensing, Diagnostic — Ophthalmology
Lens, Contact, Polymethylmethacrylate — Ophthalmology
Lens, Fundus, Hruby, Diagnostic — Ophthalmology
Lens, Surgical, Laser — Ophthalmology
Ring, Ophthalmic (Flieringa) — Ophthalmology
Stand, Instrument, AC-Powered, Ophthalmic — Ophthalmology

OCULAR PROSTHETICS, INC. — 323-462-6004
321 N. Larchmont Blvd., Suite # 711, Los Angeles, CA 90004
FDA Number: 3005690771 — Fax: 323.462.4939
E-mail: Stephen at info@ocularpro.com.
Ownership: Private
Produces/Sells CE-marked Devices: N
Eye, Artificial, Non-Custom — Ophthalmology

OCULAR TECHNOLOGIES
See Materials Development Corporation

OCULARVISION, INC. — 800-964-9433 / 805-688-4400
687 Alisa Rd, Solvang, CA 93463
FDA Number: n/a — Fax: 805-688-5126
E-mail: info@ocularvision.com
Web site: www.ocularvision.com
Annual Revenue: $0-$1 Million
Ownership: Private
Produces/Sells CE-marked Devices: Y
Distribution: Manufacturer Direct, OEM, Exporter
General Admin.: Jerry Wilson/President
Ann Wilson/Vice President
Accessories, Chromatography (Gas, Gel, Liquid, Thin Layer) — Chemistry
Lens, Intraocular — Ophthalmology

OCULO PLASTIK INC. — 888-381-3292 / 514-381-3292
200 Sauve West, Montreal, QUE H3L-1Y9 Canada
FDA Number: 8022166 — Fax: 514-381-1164
E-mail: sales@oculoplastik.com
Web site: www.oculoplastik.com
Medical Products Sales Volume: $900,000
Total Employees: 12 — Marketing Staff: 1 — Sales Staff: 3
Ownership: Private
Produces/Sells CE-marked Devices: Y
Federal Procurement Eligibility: Small Business
Distribution: Manufacturer Direct

OCULO-PLASTIK INC. — 888-381-3292 / 514-381-3292
200 Suave West, Montreal, QUE H3L-1Y9 Canada
FDA Number: n/a — Fax: 514-381-1164
E-mail: sales@oculoplastik.com
Web site: www.oculoplastik.com
Year Founded: 1985
Total Employees: 25
Ownership: Private
Produces/Sells CE-marked Devices: N
Distribution: Manufacturer Direct, Exclusive Distributor, Importer, Exporter

OCULUS INNOVATIVE SCIENCES, INC. — 707-283-0550
1135 N. Mc Dowell Blvd, Petaluma, CA 94954
FDA Number: 3004554409 — Fax: 707-283-0551
E-mail: ir@oculisis.com
Ownership: Private
Produces/Sells CE-marked Devices: N
General Admin.: Mr. James Shutz/Chief Operating Officer
Mr. Bruce Thornton/Executive Vice President
Mr. Hoji Alimi/President, Chief Executive Officer, Chairman
Research: Dr. Robert Northey/Director Research & Development
Finance: Mr. Robert Miller/Chief Financial Officer
Dressing, Wound, Occlusive — Surgery
Solution, Saline(wound Dressing) — Surgery

OCULUS OF AMERICA
See Insight Instruments, Inc.

OCUMETRICS, INC. — 650-960-3955
2224-c Old Middlefield Way, Mountain View, CA 94043
FDA Number: 2951269
Lamp, Slit, Biomicroscope, AC-Powered — Ophthalmology

OCUSERV
See Ocuserv Instruments, Inc.

OCUSERV INSTRUMENTS, INC. — 800-628-5272 / 718-656-1105
147-39 175th St., Jamaica, NY 11434
FDA Number: n/a — Fax: 718-656-1107
E-mail: ocuserv@verizon.net
Web site: www.ocuserv.com
Total Employees: 10
Ownership: Private
Produces/Sells CE-marked Devices: Y

OCUSERV INSTRUMENTS, INC.　800-628-5272 (cont'd)
Federal Procurement Eligibility: Small Business
Distribution: Manufacturer Direct, Manufacturer Through Distributor, Manufacturer Through Manufacturer Reps
General Admin.: Moishe Fuchs/President
　Scanner, Ultrasonic, Ophthalmic　Radiology

OCUSOFT, INC.　281-342-3350
P.O Box 429, Richmond, TX 77406-0429
FDA Number: 1641445
　　　　　　　　　Fax: 281-232-6015
E-mail: ocusoft@ocusoft.com
Web site: www.ocusoft.com
Medical Products Sales Volume: $9,500,000
Year Founded: 1986
Total Employees: 85
Ownership: Private
Produces/Sells CE-marked Devices: N
Federal Procurement Eligibility: Small Business, Female Owned
Distribution: Manufacturer Direct, Manufacturer Through Distributor, Manufacturer Through Manufacturer Reps
　Cannula, Ophthalmic　Ophthalmology
　Marker, Ocular　Ophthalmology
　Sponge, Ophthalmic　Ophthalmology

ODYSSEY MEDICAL EQUIPMENT　604-524-9446
331 Columbia St. E, New Westminster, BC V3L 3W8 Canada
FDA Number: n/a
　　　　　　　　　Fax: 604-524-4202
Year Founded: 1992
Total Employees: 10
Ownership: Private
Produces/Sells CE-marked Devices: N

ODYSSEY MEDICAL, INC.　901-383-7777
5828 Shelby Oaks Dr., Memphis, TN 38134
FDA Number: 1060840
　Drape, Surgical　Surgery
　Forceps　Orthopedics
　Plug, Punctum　Ophthalmology

ODYSSEY THERA INC.　925-242-5000
4550 Norris Canyon Road, Suite 140, San Ramon, CA 94583
FDA Number: n/a
　　　　　　　　　Fax: 925-242-1936
E-mail: info@odysseythera.com
Web site: www.odysseythera.com
Ownership: Private
Produces/Sells CE-marked Devices: N
General Admin.: Dr. John Westwick/President, Chief Executive Officer

OEC DIASONICS INC.
See Ge Oec Medical Systems Inc.

OEMEDIC INTERNATIONAL, INC.　886-2-22903959
No. 162, Atlantic Street, Pomona, CA 91768
FDA Number: 3005803978
Ownership: Private
Produces/Sells CE-marked Devices: N
　Ventilator, Emergency, Manual (Resuscitator)　Anesthesiology

OERLIKON LEYBOLD VACUUM USA INC.　800-433-4021
5700 Mellon Road, Export, PA 15632-8900　724-327-5700
FDA Number: n/a
　　　　　　　　　Fax: 724-325-3577
E-mail: info.vacuum.ex@oerlikon.com
Web site: www.leyboldvacuum.com
Medical Products Sales Volume: $71,600,000
Annual Revenue: $50-$100 Million
Year Founded: 1994
Total Employees: 90　*Marketing Staff:* 10　*Sales Staff:* 25
Ownership: LEYBOLD VACUUM GMBH
Quality System Registration Information: ISO9001
Produces/Sells CE-marked Devices: Y
Federal Procurement Eligibility: Small Business
Distribution: Manufacturer Direct, Importer, Exporter
General Admin.: V. Mooney/Manager Human Resources
　　　　　Dennis Pellegrino/President
Mktg./Adv.: B. Chapman/Manager National Sales
　　　　　Kim Matvey/Marketing Communications Specialist
　　　　　P. Albert/National Director Marketing
Production: B. Carbaugh/Manager Quality Assurance & Engineering
　Pump, Laboratory　Chemistry
　Pump, Vacuum, Central　Anesthesiology

OFS, SPECIALTY PHOTONICS DIVISION　888-438-9936
55 Darling Drive, Avon, CT 06001　860-678-0371
FDA Number: 1221275
　　　　　　　　　Fax: 860-674-8818
E-mail: info@specialtyphotonics.com
Web site: www.SpecialtyPhotonics.com
Medical Products Sales Volume: $90,400,000
Year Founded: 2000
Total Employees: 120

OFS, SPECIALTY PHOTONICS DIVISION　888-438-9936 (cont'd)
Ownership: Private
Quality System Registration Information: ISO9001
Produces/Sells CE-marked Devices: N
Federal Procurement Eligibility: Small Business
Distribution: OEM
General Admin.: Timothy Murray/President, General Manager
Mktg./Adv.: Mick Speciale/Manager Product Marketing
　　　　　Julie Rodriguez/Marketing Communications Specialist
　　　　　Michael Fortin/Vice President Marketing & Sales
　Communication Equipment　General

OGGS BRANCH INC.
See Thermionics Corp.

OHIO LATEX CO.
See Chagrin Safety Supply, Inc.

OHIO MEDICAL CORP.　800-662-5822
1111 Lakeside Dr., Gurnee, IL 60031-4099　847-855-0500
FDA Number: 1419185
　　　　　　　　　Fax: 847-855-6300
E-mail: customer.service@ohiomedical.com
Web site: www.ohiomedical.com
Medical Products Sales Volume: $12,000,000
Year Founded: 2005
Total Employees: 130　*Marketing Staff:* 3　*Sales Staff:* 14
Ownership: SQUIRE-COGSWELL /Aeros Instruments, Inc.
Produces/Sells CE-marked Devices: N
Federal Procurement Eligibility: Small Business
Distribution: Manufacturer Direct, Manufacturer Through Distributor
General Admin.: Craig R. Schifter/Chief Executive Officer
　　　　　Sue Koppa/Manager Human Resources
　　　　　Jim Koppa/President
Mktg./Adv.: Christine Drewry/Manager Marketing
　　　　　Marty Jindra/Vice President Sales
Production: Luis Morales/Director Manufacturing
　　　　　Hoby Chae/Engineer
　　　　　Andrew Grom/Manager Quality Assurance
　　　　　Eric Baum/Vice President, General Manager Production
Finance: Carol Lewis/Chief Financial Officer
　　　　　Mike Klug/Controller
　Analyzer, Gas, Oxygen, Gaseous Phase　Anesthesiology
　Aspirator, Emergency Suction　General
　Aspirator, Low Volume (Gastric Suction)　Gastroenterology/Urology
　Aspirator, Nasal　Ear/Nose/Throat
　Aspirator, Surgical　Surgery
　Aspirator, Thoracic (Suction Unit)　Cardiovascular
　Aspirator, Tracheal　Ear/Nose/Throat
　Bottle, Collection, Vacuum (Aspirator)　General
　Canister, Suction　Cardiovascular
　Drain, Thoracic, Water Seal　Anesthesiology
　Flowmeter, Back-Pressure Compensated, Thorpe Tube　Anesthesiology
　Gas-Machine, Analgesia　Anesthesiology
　Generator, Oxygen, Portable　Anesthesiology
　Pump, Aspiration, Portable　Anesthesiology
　Regulator, Vacuum　General
　Suction Apparatus, Ward Use, Portable, AC-Powered　Surgery
Medical Product Subsidiaries (Listed Separately)
　Amvex Corporation

OHIO WILLOW WOOD COMPANY　800-848-4930
15441 Scioto Darby Rd.,　740-869-3377
Mount Sterling, OH 43143
FDA Number: 1522166
　　　　　　　　　Fax: 740-869-4374
E-mail: customerservice@owwco.com
Web site: www.owwco.com
Annual Revenue: $10-$25 Million
Year Founded: 1907
Total Employees: 140　*Marketing Staff:* 15　*Sales Staff:* 15
Ownership: Private
Produces/Sells CE-marked Devices: Y
Federal Procurement Eligibility: Small Business
Distribution: Manufacturer Direct, Manufacturer Through Distributor, OEM, Exporter
General Admin.: Robert Arbogast/President
　　　　　Joe Arbogast/Vice President
Mktg./Adv.: Mark Ford/Director Marketing
　　　　　James Colvin/Director Product Development
Production: Mitch Neff/Manager Regulatory Affairs
　Ankle/Foot, External Limb Component　Physical Med
　Joint, Knee, External Limb Component　Physical Med
　Prosthesis, Foot　Orthopedics
　Prosthesis, Leg　Orthopedics
　Prosthesis, Thigh Socket, External Component　Physical Med

OHLENDORF COMPANY　314-533-3440
2840 Clark Avenue, St. Louis, MO 63103
FDA Number: 1000380364

OHLENDORF COMPANY　314-533-3440 *(cont'd)*
Tray, Fluoride, Disposable　Dental And Oral

OHMEDA MEDICAL　800-345-2700
8880 Gorman Road, Laurel, MD 20723　410-888-5200
FDA Number: 1121732　Fax: 301-483-8340
E-mail: icss@ohmedamedical.com
Web site: www.gehealthcare.com
Total Employees: 250
Ownership: Ge Healthcare
Quality System Registration Information: ISO9001
Produces/Sells CE-marked Devices: Y
Federal Procurement Eligibility: Small Business
Distribution: Manufacturer Direct, Manufacturer Through Distributor, Manufacturer Through Manufacturer Reps, Service Direct
General Admin.: Mr. Richard Smith/General Manager
Mktg./Adv.: Mr. Chris Burton/General Manager Sales
Production: Alberto Profumo/Director Quality Assurance & Regulatory Affairs
Research: Matt Severns/Vice President Research & Development

Bassinet (Infant Bed)	General
Bottle, Collection, Vacuum (Aspirator)	General
Canister, Suction	Cardiovascular
Examination Device, AC-Powered	General
Flowmeter, Back-Pressure Compensated, Thorpe Tube	Anesthesiology
Incubator, Neonatal	General
Infusion Stand	General
Mattress, Air Flotation	General
Monitor, Perinatal	Obstetrics/Gynecology
Phototherapy Unit, Neonatal	General
Regulator, Pressure, Gas Cylinder	Anesthesiology
Regulator, Suction, Thoracic	Anesthesiology
Regulator, Vacuum	General
Scale, Infant	General
Suction Apparatus, Operating Room, Wall Vacuum-Powered	Surgery
Tent, Oxygen (Canopy)	Anesthesiology
Tent, Oxygen, Electric	Anesthesiology
Transilluminator, AC-Powered, Other	Ophthalmology
Ventilator, Emergency, Powered (Resuscitator)	Anesthesiology
Warmer, Radiant, Infant	General

OHMEDA, INC.
See Matrx By Midmark

OHMEDA, INC. (MEDICAL SYSTEMS/SPECIAL PRODUCTS DIVISION)
See Datex-Ohmeda, Inc. (Madison)

OHMEDA/FRASER HARLAKE DIV.
See Matrx By Midmark

OIS ORTHODONTICS
See Sc/Ois Orthodontics

OISMUELLER & PARTNER, INC.　770-874-1767
1968 Sixes Rd., Canton, GA 30114
FDA Number: 1064840
Ownership: Private
Produces/Sells CE-marked Devices: N
Massager, Therapeutic　Physical Med

OK-1 MANUFACTURING CO., INC.　800-654-9873
709 S. Veterans Drive, PO Box 736,　580-482-0891
Altus, OK 73522
FDA Number: 1644454　Fax: 580-482-2760
E-mail: frogers@altusok1.com
Web site: www.ok-1safety.com
Medical Products Sales Volume: $8,500,000
Year Founded: 1975
Total Employees: 150　Marketing Staff: 2　Sales Staff: 5
Ownership: Private
Produces/Sells CE-marked Devices: Y
Federal Procurement Eligibility: Small Business, VA Contract
Distribution: Manufacturer Through Distributor, Manufacturer Through Manufacturer Reps, Importer, Exporter
Mktg./Adv.: Jim Teigen/Manager Business
　　　Felicia Rogers/Manager International Marketing & Sales
　　　Jeff Huff/Manager National Sales
Support, Back　Orthopedics

OKAMOTO U.S.A., INC.　800-283-7546
18 King St., Stratford, CT 06615-5827　203-378-0003
FDA Number: 2431332　Fax: 203-375-2040
E-mail: okamotousa@okamotoUSA.com
Web site: www.okamotousa.com
Medical Products Sales Volume: $1,500,000
Annual Revenue: $10-$25 Million
Total Employees: 6　Marketing Staff: 1　Sales Staff: 3
Ownership: Private
Quality System Registration Information: ISO9002
Produces/Sells CE-marked Devices: Y

OKAMOTO U.S.A., INC.　800-283-7546 *(cont'd)*
Distribution: Manufacturer Direct, Manufacturer Through Distributor, Manufacturer Through Manufacturer Reps, Importer, Exporter
General Admin.: Hisayuki Naito/President
Production: Jennifer Jordan/Product Manager
Condom　Obstetrics/Gynecology

OKAY INDUSTRIES, INC.　860-225-8707
200 Ellis St., P.O. Box 2470, New Britain, CT 06050-2470
FDA Number: n/a　Fax: 860-225-7047
E-mail: stamp@okayind.com
Web site: www.okayind.com
Medical Products Sales Volume: $20,000,000
Annual Revenue: $25-$50 Million
Total Employees: 150　Sales Staff: 2
Ownership: Private
Quality System Registration Information: ISO9002
Produces/Sells CE-marked Devices: N
Federal Procurement Eligibility: Small Business
Distribution: Manufacturer Direct
General Admin.: Gregory B. Howey/President, Chief Executive Officer
　　　Donna Lasher/Vice President
Mktg./Adv.: Mr. Jason Howey/Manager Business Development
Research: Mr. Shawn Russell/Vice President Engineering & Development

Applier, Ligature Clip	Surgery
Applier, Surgical, Clip	Surgery
Blade, Electrosurgery, Laparoscopic	Surgery
Blade, Knife, Laparoscopic	Surgery
Component, Metal, Other	General
Contract R&D, Equipment	General
Cutter, Linear, Laparoscopic	Surgery
Cutter, Surgical	Surgery
Forceps, Biopsy	Surgery
Forceps, Laparoscopy, Bipolar, Electrosurgical	Surgery
Knife, Laparoscopic	Surgery
Remover, Clip	Surgery
Scissors, Laparoscopy	Surgery
Scissors, Laparoscopy, Bipolar, Electrosurgical	Surgery
Staple, Implantable	Surgery
Stapler, Laparoscopic	Surgery
Stapler, Surgical	Surgery

OLD 97 CO.　813-247-6677
2306 North 35th St., Tampa, FL 33605
FDA Number: 1010294
Cement, Stomal Appliance, Ostomy　Gastroenterology/Urology

OLIGOS ETC., INC.　503-682-1814
9775 S.w. Commerce Cir., Bldg. C-6, Wilsonville, OR 97070
FDA Number: 3032540
Reagents, Specific, Analyte　Hematology

OLIN CONDUCTIVE MATERIALS
See Acheson Colloids Company

OLIS: ON-LINE INSTRUMENT SYSTEMS, INC.　800-852-3504
130 Conway Drive, Suite A & B,　706-353-6547
Bogart, GA 30622
FDA Number: n/a　Fax: 706-353-1972
E-mail: sales@olisweb.com
Web site: www.olisweb.com
Medical Products Sales Volume: $1,500,000
Annual Revenue: $1-$5 Million
Year Founded: 1974
Total Employees: 25　Marketing Staff: 1　Sales Staff: 1
Ownership: Private
Produces/Sells CE-marked Devices: N
Federal Procurement Eligibility: Small Business
Distribution: Manufacturer Direct, Manufacturer Through Manufacturer Reps
General Admin.: Richard J. DeSa/President, Chief Executive Officer
　　　Julie D. Lorenz/Vice President
Mktg./Adv.: Julie D. Lorenz/Director National Accounts
　　　Richard J. DeSa/Director Product Development
　　　Julie D. Lorenz/Vice President Marketing & Sales
Research: Richard J. DeSa/Director Research & Development

Fluorometer	Immunology
Polarimeter	Chemistry
Spectrometer, Infrared	Chemistry
Spectrophotometer, U.V./Visible	Chemistry

OLIVER MEDICAL　800-253-3893
445 Sixth St. N.W., Grand Rapids, MI 49504-5253　616-456-7711
FDA Number: 1000396174　Fax: 616-456-5820
E-mail: info@olivermedical.com
Web site: www.olivermedical.com
Medical Products Sales Volume: $26,700,000
Annual Revenue: $25-$50 Million
Total Employees: 250　Sales Staff: 10
Ownership: Oliver Products Company

MANUFACTURER PROFILES

OLIVER MEDICAL
800-253-3893 *(cont'd)*

Quality System Registration Information: ISO9001
Produces/Sells CE-marked Devices: N
Federal Procurement Eligibility: Small Business
Distribution: Manufacturer Direct
General Admin.: Jeff Murak/Director International Management
    John R. Green/President, Chief Executive Officer
Mktg./Adv.: Marv Snedeker/Director Business
    Jeff Murak/Director Marketing & Sales
Production: Lora Keena/Director Quality Assurance

Contract Assembly	General
Packaging Equipment	General
Packaging Material	General
Packaging, Sterilization	General

OLSEN MEDICAL
800-297-6344
3001 W. Kentucky St., Louisville, KY 40211-1505
502-772-4280
FDA Number: 1530493
Fax: 502-772-4282
E-mail: info@olsenmedical.com
Web site: www.olsenmedical.com
Year Founded: 1880
Total Employees: 54   *Marketing Staff:* 1   *Sales Staff:* 4
Ownership: Ercon Associates
Quality System Registration Information: ISO9001
Produces/Sells CE-marked Devices: Y
Federal Procurement Eligibility: Small Business, GSA Contract, VA Contract
Distribution: Manufacturer Direct, Manufacturer Through Distributor, OEM, Exclusive Distributor, Exporter
General Admin.: Larry Potts/President
Mktg./Adv.: Mike Hand/Vice President, Manager Sales
Production: David Self/Customer Service Representative
    Doug McWhorter/Director Quality Assurance & Regulatory Affairs
    Nunie Tabermejo/Engineer
Purchasing: Phyllis Huber/Purchasing Agent

Accessories, Speculum	Surgery
Adapter, Electrosurgical Unit, Cable	Surgery
Blade, Electrosurgery, Laparoscopic	Surgery
Electrode, Electrosurgery, Laparoscopic	Surgery
Electrode, Electrosurgical, Active (Blade)	Surgery
Electrode, Electrosurgical, Active, Foot Controlled	Surgery
Electrode, Other	General
Electrosurgical Equipment, General Purpose	Surgery
Electrosurgical Equipment, Special Purpose	Surgery
Equipment, Suction/Irrigation, Laparoscopic	Surgery
Equipment, Suction/Irrigation/Electrocautery, Laparoscopic	Surgery
Equipment/Accessories, Laser, Laparoscopy	Surgery
Forceps, Electrosurgical	Surgery
Forceps, General & Plastic Surgery	Surgery
Forceps, Tissue	Surgery
Kit, Surgical Instrument, Disposable	Surgery
Marker, Skin	Surgery
Pen, Marking, Surgical	Ophthalmology
Safety Equipment, Laboratory	Chemistry
Speculum, Non-Illuminated	Surgery
Stylet, Surgical	Surgery
Surgical Instrument, Disposable	Surgery

OLSON CORP., BILL
See Zefon International

OLYMPIC MEDICAL CORP.
206-767-3500
5900 First Avenue S., Seattle, WA 98108
FDA Number: 3018859
Fax: 206-762-4200
E-mail: Oly_Customer_Service@olympicmedical.com
Web site: www.OlympicMedical.com
Annual Revenue: $5-$10 Million
Year Founded: 1959
Total Employees: 100   *Marketing Staff:* 2   *Sales Staff:* 5
Ownership: Natus Medical Inc.
Quality System Registration Information: ISO9001
Produces/Sells CE-marked Devices: Y
Federal Procurement Eligibility: Small Business, GSA Contract
Distribution: Manufacturer Direct
General Admin.: Jay Jones/President, Chief Executive Officer
Mktg./Adv.: Joe Reback/Director Marketing
    Brian McNair/Manager National Sales
Production: George Biggins/Director Quality Assurance
    Ed Bateman/Vice President Manufacturing & Operations

Accessories, Operating Room, Table	Surgery
Button, Tracheostomy Tube	Anesthesiology
Dryer, Respiratory/Anesthesia Equipment	General
Hood, Oxygen, Infant	General
Immobilizer, Infant (Circumcision Board)	Orthopedics
Light, Bilirubin (Phototherapy)	General
Mask, Eye, Phototherapy	Ophthalmology
Meter, Patient Height	General
Monitor, Cerebral Function	Cns/Neurology
Pad, Vacuum Stabilized	General
Phototherapy Unit (Bilirubin Lamp)	General
Radiometer, Phototherapy	General

OLYMPIC MEDICAL CORP.
206-767-3500 *(cont'd)*

Restraint, Protective (Body)	General
Ring, Suture	Surgery
Scale, Infant	General
Splint, Vacuum	Orthopedics
Table, Examination/Treatment	General
Timer, Phototherapy	General
Transilluminator, Battery-Powered	Ophthalmology

OLYMPIC SPORT, INC.
914-347-4737
500 Executive Blvd., Elmsford, NY 10523
FDA Number: 3006052451
Ownership: Private
Produces/Sells CE-marked Devices: N

Exerciser, Non-Measuring	Physical Med

OLYMPUS AMERICA, INC.
800-645-8160
3500 Corporate Parkway, PO Box 610,
484-896-5000
Center Valley, PA 18034
FDA Number: 2429304
Fax: 484-896-7121
E-mail: mail@olympus.com
Web site: www.olympusamerica.com
Medical Products Sales Volume: $299,400,000
Annual Revenue: More than $1 Billion
Year Founded: 1919
Total Employees: 700
Ownership: OLYMPUS MEDICAL SYSTEMS CORP
Produces/Sells CE-marked Devices: N
Federal Procurement Eligibility: GSA Contract
Distribution: Manufacturer Direct
Research: David Barlow/Vice President Research & Development

Accessories, Surgical Camera	Surgery
Analyzer, Chemistry, Enzyme	Chemistry
Analyzer, Chemistry, Multi-Channel, Fixed	Chemistry
Analyzer, Chemistry, Single Channel, Programmable	Chemistry
Angioscope	Cardiovascular
Arthroscope	Orthopedics
Bronchoscope, Non-Rigid	Ear/Nose/Throat
Brush, Biopsy, Bronchoscope (Non-Rigid)	Anesthesiology
Brush, Cytology, Endoscopic	Gastroenterology/Urology
Camera, Video, Endoscopic	General
Choledochoscope, Flexible Or Rigid	Gastroenterology/Urology
Choledochoscope, Mini-Diameter (5mm or Less)	Gastroenterology/Urology
Colonoscope, Gastro-Urology	Gastroenterology/Urology
Cystoscope	Gastroenterology/Urology
Cystourethroscope	Gastroenterology/Urology
Duodenoscope, Esophago/Gastro	Gastroenterology/Urology
Electrophoresis Equipment, Cellulose Acetate Membrane	Chemistry
Electrophoresis Instrumentation	Immunology
Electrosurgical Equipment, General Purpose	Surgery
Electrosurgical Unit, General Purpose (ESU)	Surgery
Endoscope	Gastroenterology/Urology
Endoscope, Fiberoptic	Surgery
Esophagoscope (Flexible Or Rigid)	Ear/Nose/Throat
Forceps, Endoscopic	Gastroenterology/Urology
Gastroscope, Flexible	Gastroenterology/Urology
Hysteroscope	Obstetrics/Gynecology
Lamp, Microscope	Pathology
Laparoscope, General & Plastic Surgery	Surgery
Laparoscope, Gynecologic	Obstetrics/Gynecology
Laryngoscope	Ear/Nose/Throat
Laryngoscope, Flexible	Anesthesiology
Laryngoscope, Rigid	Anesthesiology
Laser, Excimer, Surgical	Surgery
Light Source, Endoscopic	Obstetrics/Gynecology
Light Source, Fiberoptic, Routine	Gastroenterology/Urology
Microscope, Ear	Ear/Nose/Throat
Microscope, Laboratory, Optical	Microbiology
Microscope, Surgical, General & Plastic Surgery	Surgery
Monitor, Video, Endoscope	General
Nasopharyngoscope (Flexible Or Rigid)	Ear/Nose/Throat
Nephroscope, Flexible	Gastroenterology/Urology
Panendoscope (Gastroduodenoscope)	Gastroenterology/Urology
Resectoscope	Gastroenterology/Urology
Sigmoidoscope, Flexible	Gastroenterology/Urology
System, Camera, 3-Dimensional	Surgery
Tape, Television & Video, Endoscopic	Gastroenterology/Urology
Telescope, Rigid, Endoscopic	Gastroenterology/Urology
Thoracoscope	Cardiovascular
Ureteroscope	Gastroenterology/Urology
Ureterotome	Gastroenterology/Urology

OLYMPUS BIOTECH CORPORATION
603-298-3000
9 Technology Dr., W. Lebanon, NH 03784
FDA Number: 1284048
Ownership: Stryker Corp.
Stock Symbol: SYK
Traded On: NYSE
Produces/Sells CE-marked Devices: N

OLYMPUS BIOTECH CORPORATION   603-298-3000 *(cont'd)*
Filler, Bovine Protein Mixture, Bone Morphogenetic Proteins, Collagen Scaffold,
Osteoinduction
    Physical Med

OLYMPUS CANADA, INC.   800-387-0437
151 Telson Road, Markham, ON L3R 1E7 Canada
FDA Number: n/a   *Fax:* 905-479-2595
E-mail: sales@circoncorp.com
Web site: www.olympuscanada.com
Total Employees: 100
Ownership: OLYMPUS CORPORATION
Quality System Registration Information: ISO9000; ISO9001; ISO9002
Produces/Sells CE-marked Devices: Y
Distribution: Manufacturer Direct, Manufacturer Through Manufacturer Reps, OEM

OLYMPUS MEDICAL EQUIPMENT SERVICES   484-896-5000
AMERICA, INC.
3500 Corporate Parkway, Center valley, PA 18034
FDA Number: 3006219967
E-mail: oemsales@pixela.co.jp
Web site: www.olympus.co.jp
Year Founded: 1999
Ownership: OLYMPUS AMERICA, INC.
Stock Symbol: OCPN
Traded On: London
Produces/Sells CE-marked Devices: N
General Admin.: Masatoshi Kishimoto/Chairman
     Haruhito Morishima/President
     Tsuyoshi Kikukawa/President
     Mark Gumz/President, Chief Operating Officer
     Dave McKinley/Vice President
     Daisuke Okada/Vice President, General Manager

OLYMPUS SURGICAL & INDUSTRIAL   845-398-9400
AMERICA, INC.
One Corporate Drive, Orangeburg, NY 10962
FDA Number: 3005087031
E-mail: oemsales@pixela.co.jp
Web site: www.olympus.co.jp/en
Year Founded: 1999
Ownership: OLYMPUS AMERICA, INC.
Stock Symbol: OCPN
Traded On: London
Produces/Sells CE-marked Devices: N
General Admin.: Toshiro Shimoyama/Chairman
     Haruhito Morishima/President
     Reni L. Witt/President
     Ronald Reagan/President
     Tsuyoshi Kikukawa/President
     Mark Gumz/President, Chief Operating Officer
     Daisuke Okada/Vice President, General Manager

OMAR INDUSTRIES LTD.
    See Sunnydale Industries, Inc.

OMED SYSTEMS, INC.
    See Ardus Medical, Inc.

OMEGA ENGINEERING, INC.   800-848-4286
1 Omega Drive, Stamford, CT 06907-0047   203-359-1660
FDA Number: 9200823   *Fax:* 203-359-7700
E-mail: info@omega.com
Web site: www.omega.com
Medical Products Sales Volume: $48,600,000
Year Founded: 1962
Total Employees: 565
Ownership: Private
Quality System Registration Information: ISO9001
Produces/Sells CE-marked Devices: Y
Federal Procurement Eligibility: Female Owned
Distribution: Manufacturer Direct
General Admin.: Betty Ruth Hollander/President
Mktg./Adv.: Kathy Kwiat/Manager Advertising
   Bath, Dry (Constant Temperature)   Chemistry
   Controller, pH   Chemistry
   Electrode, Laboratory pH   Chemistry
   Electrode, pH   Gastroenterology/Urology
   Meter, Conductivity   Chemistry
   Meter, Oxygen   Anesthesiology
   Meter, pH, Portable   Chemistry
   Plate, Hot   Chemistry
   Pyrometer   General
   Recorder, Chart, Laboratory   Chemistry
   Regulator, Temperature   Chemistry
   Spectrophotometer, U.V./Visible   Chemistry
   Thermistor   General
   Thermometer, Laboratory   Chemistry
   Thermometer, Laboratory, Recording   General

OMEGA ENGINEERING, INC.   800-848-4286 *(cont'd)*
   Voltmeter   Chemistry

OMEGA MEDICAL ELECTRONICS LTD.   910-763-9331
725 Wellington Avenue, Wilmington, NC 28401
FDA Number: n/a   *Fax:* 910-763-6442
E-mail: service@omegamed.net
Web site: http://omegamed.net
Medical Products Sales Volume: $280,000
Annual Revenue: $0-$1 Million
Year Founded: 1979
Total Employees: 5   *Marketing Staff:* 1   *Sales Staff:* 1
Ownership: Private
Produces/Sells CE-marked Devices: Y
Federal Procurement Eligibility: Small Business
Distribution: Service Direct, Exclusive Distributor, Exporter
General Admin.: Mr. A. William D'Emilio/President, Chief Executive Officer
Production: George Hassinger/Director Services
   Service, Maintenance/Repair   General

OMEGA MEDICAL IMAGING, INC.   407-323-9400
675 Hickman Circle, Sanford, FL 32771
FDA Number: 1052701   *Fax:* 407-323-9331
E-mail: info@omegamedicalimaging.com
Web site: www.omegamedicalimaging.com
Ownership: Private
Produces/Sells CE-marked Devices: N
   Radiographic/Fluoroscopic Unit, Image-Intensified   Radiology

OMEGA MEDICAL PRODUCTS CORP.   888-837-TAPE
494 Saw Mill River Rd., Yonkers, NY 10701   914-375-4500
FDA Number: 2438416   *Fax:* 914-375-7780
E-mail: info@omegamedicalproducts.com
Web site: www.omegamedicalproducts.com
Ownership: Private
Produces/Sells CE-marked Devices: N
Federal Procurement Eligibility: Small Business, Female Owned
Distribution: Manufacturer Through Distributor
   Bandage, Adhesive   Surgery

OMEGA POSTURE SYSTEMS   800-665-4839
846 Marion St. #4,   204-237-6724
Winnipeg, MAN R2J-0 Canada
FDA Number: n/a   *Fax:* 204-237-0994
E-mail: omega@caribou.mb.ca
Web site: www.mbnet.mb.ca/~omega/
Year Founded: 1983
Total Employees: 10
Ownership: Private
Produces/Sells CE-marked Devices: N
Distribution: Manufacturer Direct, Exclusive Distributor

OMEGA SURGICAL INSTRUMENTS   800-656-6342
G-8305 Saginaw St., Suite 6,   810-695-9800
Grand Blanc, MI 48439
FDA Number: 1834251   *Fax:* 810-695-7800
E-mail: omega@sysmatrix.net
Web site: www.omegasurgical.com
Medical Products Sales Volume: $1,500,000
Annual Revenue: $1-$5 Million
Year Founded: 1993
Total Employees: 3   *Marketing Staff:* 2   *Sales Staff:* 29
Ownership: Private
Produces/Sells CE-marked Devices: N
Federal Procurement Eligibility: Small Business
Distribution: Manufacturer Through Distributor, Manufacturer Through
Manufacturer Reps, Exporter
General Admin.: Gary L. Adam/President, Chief Executive Officer
Mktg./Adv.: David R Miller/Manager Marketing & Quality Assurance
   Blade, Surgical, Saw, General & Plastic Surgery   Surgery
   Burr, Surgical, General & Plastic Surgery   Surgery

OMEGA-MED INT'L., INC.
    See Sterion, Incorporated

OMEGAPOINT SYSTEMS, LLC   513-241-7540
1077 Celestial St., Suite 400, Cincinnati, OH 45202
FDA Number: 3005205089
   Alcohol Breath Trapping Device   Toxicology

OMEX TECHNOLOGIES, INC.   847-564-0206
3665 Woodhead Drive, Northbrook, IL 60062-1816
FDA Number: 3002258067   *Fax:* 847-564-0306
E-mail: alz@omextech.com
Web site: www.omextech.com
Medical Products Sales Volume: $17,900,000
Annual Revenue: $0-$1 Million
Year Founded: 1988

MANUFACTURER PROFILES

OMEX TECHNOLOGIES, INC.   847-564-0206 *(cont'd)*
Total Employees: 5   *Marketing Staff:* 1   *Sales Staff:* 1
Ownership: Private
Produces/Sells CE-marked Devices: N
Federal Procurement Eligibility: Small Business
Distribution: Manufacturer Direct, Manufacturer Through Distributor, OEM
   Accessories, Photographic, Endoscopic   Gastroenterology/Urology

OMI SURGICAL PRODUCTS
See Schaerer Mayfield Usa

OMIDERM LTD.   415-753-9989
One Oakwood Blvd., #50, Hollywood, FL 33020
FDA Number: 3004477045
Ownership: Private
Produces/Sells CE-marked Devices: N
   Dressing, Other   General

OMNI INTERNATIONAL, INC.   540-347-5331
P.O. Box 861455, Warrenton, VA 20187-1455
FDA Number: n/a   Fax: 540-347-5352
E-mail: omni@omni.com
Web site: www.omni-inc.com
Annual Revenue: $1-$5 Million
Year Founded: 1985
Total Employees: 20   *Sales Staff:* 5
Ownership: Private
Produces/Sells CE-marked Devices: Y
Federal Procurement Eligibility: Small Business
Distribution: Manufacturer Direct, Manufacturer Through Distributor, Manufacturer
Through Manufacturer Reps, OEM, Service Direct
General Admin.: Karl H. Jahn/President, Chief Executive Officer
Mktg./Adv.: Paula Hicks/Manager National Sales
    Jim Partridge/Vice President Marketing & Sales
   Homogenizer, Tissue   Microbiology

OMNI LIFE SCIENCE, INC   800-448-6664
50 O'Connell Way, East Taunton, MA 02718   508-824-2444
FDA Number: 1226188   Fax: 508-822-6030
E-mail: support@omnils.com
Web site: www.omnils.com
Year Founded: 1999
Ownership: Private
Produces/Sells CE-marked Devices: Y
Federal Procurement Eligibility: Small Business
Distribution: Manufacturer Direct, Manufacturer Through Distributor, Manufacturer
Through Manufacturer Reps
Bit, Drill	Orthopedics
Clamp, Other	Surgery
Curette	Orthopedics
Driver, Prosthesis	Orthopedics
Driver, Surgical, Pin	Surgery
Gauge, Depth	Orthopedics
Orthopedic Manual Surgical Instrument	Orthopedics
Osteotome (Orthopedic)	Surgery
Prosthesis, Hip, Semi-Const., Metal/Poly., Porous Uncemented	Orthopedics
Prosthesis, Hip, Semi-Constr., Metal/Ceramic, Cemented/NC	Orthopedics
Prosthesis, Knee, Patellofemorotibial, Semi-Constrained	Orthopedics
Punch, Femoral Neck	Orthopedics
Rasp, Other	Surgery
Reamer	Orthopedics
Template	Orthopedics
Wrench	Orthopedics

OMNI LIFE SCIENCE, INC.   800-448-OMNI
1390 Decision Street, Vista, CA 92081   760-734-1550
FDA Number: 2918697   Fax: 760-734-1577
E-mail: support@bw-omni.com
Web site: www.omnils.com
Medical Products Sales Volume: $3,800,000
Year Founded: 1998
Total Employees: 35
Ownership: Private
Produces/Sells CE-marked Devices: N
Federal Procurement Eligibility: Small Business
Distribution: Manufacturer Through Distributor, Manufacturer Through
Manufacturer Reps, OEM, Exporter
General Admin.: Dr. Robert Gilmour/President, Chief Executive Officer
Mktg./Adv.: Shamus Fairhaul/Director Product Development
    Terry O'Donnell/Manager International & National Sales
Production: Eeuwout Hoogendijk/Director Operations
    Colin Heald/Director Quality Assurance
    Robin McMahon/Manager Customer Services
Immobilizer, Shoulder	Orthopedics
Joint, Knee, External Brace	Physical Med
Orthosis, Limb Brace	Physical Med
Orthosis, Other	Physical Med
Support, Ankle	Orthopedics
Support, Foot	Orthopedics

OMNI LIFE SCIENCE, INC.   800-448-OMNI *(cont'd)*
   Support, Knee   Physical Med

OMNI MEASUREMENT SYSTEMS, INC.   802-865-5223
1150 Airport Drive, South Burlington, VT 05403-6000
FDA Number: 3005105203   Fax: 802-865-6789
Ownership: Private
Produces/Sells CE-marked Devices: N
   Collector, Urine, Powered, Non Indwelling Catheter   Gastroenterology/Urology

OMNI MEDICAL SUPPLY INC.   800-860-6664
4153 Pioneer Drive, Walled Lake, MI 48390   248-360-8000
FDA Number: n/a   Fax: 248-360-9375
E-mail: omni@omnimedicalsupply.com
Web site: www.omnimedicalsupply.com
Medical Products Sales Volume: $5,100,000
Annual Revenue: $1-$5 Million
Year Founded: 1992
Total Employees: 20   *Marketing Staff:* 5   *Sales Staff:* 5
Ownership: Private
Produces/Sells CE-marked Devices: N
Federal Procurement Eligibility: Small Business
Distribution: Exclusive Distributor
General Admin.: Bill Pierce/President
    Greta Delabbio/Vice President
Mktg./Adv.: Mrs. Vicki Nelson/Senior Sales Manager
Analyzer, Coagulation, Whole Blood	Hematology
Analyzer, ECG	Cardiovascular
Analyzer, Pacemaker Generator Function, Indirect	Cardiovascular
Analyzer, Pulmonary Function	Anesthesiology
Bag, Enteral Feeding	General
Bandage, Elastic	General
Bandage, Gauze	General
Blade, Saw, Cast Cutting	Orthopedics
Block, Bite	Cns/Neurology
Brush, Cytology, Endoscopic	Gastroenterology/Urology
Brush, Other	General
Cannula, Nasal, Oxygen	Anesthesiology
Cast	Orthopedics
Catheter, Malecot (Gastrostomy Tube)	Gastroenterology/Urology
Cover, Probe, Transducer	Surgery
Curette, Ear	Ear/Nose/Throat
Electrocardiograph, Interpretive	Cardiovascular
Electrocardiograph, Single Channel	Cardiovascular
Electrode, Electrocardiograph	Cardiovascular
Equipment, Therapy, Apnea	Anesthesiology
Glove, Patient Examination	General
Infusion Pump, Enteral	General
Infusion Stand	General
Kit, Administration, Intravenous	General
Kit, Catheterization, Sterile Urethral	Gastroenterology/Urology
Kit, Pregnancy Test	Obstetrics/Gynecology
Moleskin	General
Monitor, Apnea	General
Monitor, Blood Pressure, Indirect, Anesthesiology	Anesthesiology
Monitor, ECG	Cardiovascular
Monitor, ECG, Ambulatory, Real-Time	Cardiovascular
Oximeter, Finger	General
Oximeter, Pulse	General
Paper, Chart, Record, Medical	General
Paper, Recording, Data	General
Paper, Recording, ECG/EEG	General
Pump, Infusion	General
Recorder, Long-Term, ECG	Cardiovascular
Recorder, Long-Term, ECG, Portable (Holter Monitor)	Cardiovascular
Solution, Antimicrobial	Microbiology
Surgical, Razor	Surgery
Swabs, Alcohol	General
Table, Physical Therapy	Physical Med
Tube, Capillary Blood Collection	Hematology
Tube, Nasogastric	Anesthesiology

OMNI SCIENTIFIC, INC.
See Omni Life Science, Inc.

OMNI-TRACT SURGICAL, A DIV. OF MINNESOTA SCIENTIFIC, INC.   800-367-8657
4849 White Bear Parkway, St. Paul, MN 55110   651-287-4300
FDA Number: 2125289   Fax: 651-287-4400
E-mail: info@omni-tract.com
Web site: www.omni-tract.com
Medical Products Sales Volume: $10,000,000
Annual Revenue: $5-$10 Million
Year Founded: 1971
Total Employees: 40   *Marketing Staff:* 2   *Sales Staff:* 8
Ownership: MINNESOTA SCIENTIFIC, INC.
Quality System Registration Information: ISO9001
Produces/Sells CE-marked Devices: Y
Federal Procurement Eligibility: Small Business, GSA Contract

OMNI-TRACT SURGICAL, A DIV. OF MINNESOTA   800-367-8657
(cont'd)
   Distribution: Manufacturer Direct, OEM
   General Admin.: Steve LeVahn/President
   Mktg./Adv.: Bob Ballantine/Director Marketing
       Bob Ballantine/Director Product Development
       Kirk Larson/Manager National Sales
   Production: Ron Tollefson/Director Quality Assurance
       Cathy LeVahn/Manager Regulatory Affairs

Instrument, Manual, General Surgical	Surgery
Retractor	Orthopedics
Retractor, Self-Retaining	Gastroenterology/Urology
Retractor, Surgical	Surgery

OMNIA TECHNOLOGY AN OPTIMATION COMPANY   585-321-2300
2550 Grayfalls Dr., Ste. 207, Houston, TX 77077
   FDA Number: 3006115116

Electromyograph, Diagnostic	Physical Med

OMNIA, INC.   863-619-8100
3125 Drane Field Rd.,suite 29, Lakeland, FL 33811
   FDA Number: 1035837

Cotton, Roll	Dental And Oral
Fiber, Absorbent	General
Gauze, Non-Absorbable, X-Ray Detectable (Internal Sponge)	Surgery
Gauze/sponge, Nonresorbable For External Use	Surgery
Sponge, External	Surgery
Sponge, Gauze	Dental And Oral

OMNICAL, INC.   818-837-7531
557 Jessie St., San Fernando, CA 91340
   FDA Number: 2023276   *Fax:* 818-837-9871
   E-mail: info@omnical.com
   Web site: www.omnical.com
   Medical Products Sales Volume: $1,000,000
   Annual Revenue: $1-$5 Million
   Year Founded: 1994
   Total Employees: 12   *Marketing Staff:* 2   *Sales Staff:* 2
   Ownership: Private
   Produces/Sells CE-marked Devices: N
   Federal Procurement Eligibility: Small Business
   Distribution: Manufacturer Through Distributor
   General Admin.: Ron Tinero/Chief Executive Officer

Cover, Head, Surgical	Surgery
Cover, Other	General
Cover, Shoe, Operating Room	Surgery
Mask, Face	General
Swabs, Cotton	General

OMNICELL   800-850-6664
1201 Charleston Road,   650-251-6100
Mountain View, CA 94043
   FDA Number: n/a   *Fax:* 650-251-6266
   E-mail: info@omnicell.com
   Web site: http://www.omnicell.com
   Year Founded: 1992
   Ownership: Private
   Produces/Sells CE-marked Devices: N
   General Admin.: Mr. Randall Lipps/Chief Executive Officer
   Mktg./Adv.: Mr. Nhat Ngo/Vice President Business Development
       Mr. Marga Ortigas-Wedekind/Vice President Global Marketing
   Production: Mr. J. Christopher Drew/Senior Vice President Operations
   Finance: Mr. Rob Seim/Chief Financial Officer

OMNIGUIDE, INC.   888-666-4484
One Kendall Square, Bldg 100, 3rd Floor,   617-551-8444
Cambridge, MA 02139
   FDA Number: 3005350457   *Fax:* 617-551-8472
   E-mail: CustomerService@Omni-Guide.com
   Web site: www.omni-guide.com
   Year Founded: 2000
   Total Employees: 30
   Ownership: Private
   Produces/Sells CE-marked Devices: N
   General Admin.: Yoel Fink/Chief Executive Officer
       Mr. Scott Flora/President, Chief Executive Officer

Laser, Ophthalmic	Ophthalmology
Laser, Surgical	Surgery

OMNIMED, INC. (BEAM PRODUCTS)   800-257-2326
800 Glen Avenue, Moorestown, NJ 08057   856-359-2231
   FDA Number: n/a   *Fax:* 856-359-2249
   E-mail: info@omnimedbeam.com
   Web site: www.omnimedbeam.com
   Medical Products Sales Volume: $3,200,000
   Year Founded: 1972
   Total Employees: 35

OMNIMED, INC. (BEAM PRODUCTS)   800-257-2326 *(cont'd)*
   Ownership: Private
   Produces/Sells CE-marked Devices: N
   Federal Procurement Eligibility: Small Business
   Distribution: Manufacturer Through Distributor
   Mktg./Adv.: Joe Clarke/Director Marketing & Sales
       Ed Morris/Director Product Development
   Production: Steve Heffernen/Director Operations
       Larry Godfrey/Plant Manager

Box, Glove	Microbiology
Bracelet, Identification	General
Cabinet Casework, General Purpose	General
Cabinet, Narcotic Control	General
Cabinet, Other	General
Cart, Housekeeping	General
Cart, Other	General
Holder, Medical Chart	General
Rack, Medical Chart	General
Screen, Bedside	General
Stand, Operating Room Instrument (Mayo)	Surgery

OMNIQUR, INC.   626-336-9737
15342-b East Valley Blvd., City Of Industry, CA 91746
   FDA Number: 2032378
   Ownership: Private
   Produces/Sells CE-marked Devices: N

Pack, Hot Or Cold, Reusable	Physical Med

OMNISONICS MEDICAL TECHNOLOGIES   978-657-9980
66 Concord Street, Suite A, Wilmington, MA 01887
   FDA Number: 3003043897

Catheter, Embolectomy (Fogarty Type)	Cardiovascular

OMNISYS, INC.   800-448-6891
2824 Terrell Road, Suite 602,   903-455-0461
Greenville, TX 75402
   FDA Number: n/a   *Fax:* 903-455-7910
   E-mail: tcsales@omnisys-inc.com
   Web site: www.omnisys-inc.com
   Medical Products Sales Volume: $5,300,000
   Year Founded: 1988
   Total Employees: 65   *Marketing Staff:* 2   *Sales Staff:* 6
   Ownership: Private
   Federal Procurement Eligibility: Small Business
   Distribution: Manufacturer Direct, OEM
   General Admin.: Todd Airhart/Chief Operating Officer
       Jerry J. Ranson/President
   Mktg./Adv.: Heather Benzi/Manager International & National Sales
       Heather Benzi/Manager Marketing

Computer Software, Home Healthcare	General

OMNITECH ELECTRONICS, INC.
   See Accu Scan Instruments, Inc.

OMNITECH SYSTEMS, INC.   866-266-9490
450 S. Campbell St., Ste. 2, Valparaiso, IN 46385   219-531-5532
   FDA Number: 1835241   *Fax:* 219-464-0380
   E-mail: info@omnitechsystems.com
   Web site: www.omnitechsystems.com
   Medical Products Sales Volume: $2,800,000
   Annual Revenue: $1-$5 Million
   Year Founded: 1995
   Total Employees: 50
   Ownership: Private
   Produces/Sells CE-marked Devices: N
   Federal Procurement Eligibility: Small Business
   Distribution: OEM
   General Admin.: Mr. Gregg VanDusseldorp/President, Chief Executive Officer
   Mktg./Adv.: Mr. Kelly Pickering/Vice President Sales

Accessories, Cleaning Brushes (For Endoscope)	Gastroenterology/Urology
Coagulator/Cutter, Endoscopic, Unipolar	Obstetrics/Gynecology
Dislodger, Stone, Basket, Ureteral, Metal	Gastroenterology/Urology
Electrode, Electrosurgical, Active (Blade)	Surgery
Electrode, Electrosurgical, Active, Foot Controlled	Surgery
Electrode, Electrosurgical, Return (Ground, Dispersive)	Surgery
Surgical Instrument, G-U, Manual	Gastroenterology/Urology
Surgical Instrument, Obstetric/Gynecologic	Obstetrics/Gynecology

OMNIVATIONS   714-990-0904
445 Capricorn St., Brea, CA 92821
   FDA Number: n/a   *Fax:* 714-990-0907
   E-mail: sales@omnivations.com
   Web site: www.omnivations.com
   Ownership: Private
   Produces/Sells CE-marked Devices: N
   Distribution: Manufacturer Direct

Service, Engineering/Design	General

OMNYX LLC
412-894-2100
30 Isabella Street, Suite 301, Pittsburgh, PA 15212
FDA Number: n/a
E-mail: contact@omnyx.com
Web site: www.omnyx.com
Ownership: Private
Produces/Sells CE-marked Devices: N
General Admin.: Mr. Gene Cartwright/Chief Executive Officer
Mktg./Adv.: Mr. Rajiv Enand/Senior Vice President Business Development
Mr. Tony Melanson/Vice President Strategic Marketing & Communications
Research: Mr. Mike Montalto/Vice President Research
Finance: Mr. Andrew Chomos/Vice President Finance & Operations
IS: Mr. Michael Meissner/Vice President Software

OMRON ELECTRONICS, INC.
800-55-OMRON
One E. Commerce Dr., Schaumburg, IL 60173
847-843-7900
FDA Number: n/a
Fax: 847-843-7787
Total Employees: 150
Ownership: Private
Produces/Sells CE-marked Devices: N
General Admin.: Shingo Akechi/President
Mktg./Adv.: Marsha Ruck/Director Marketing
  Component, Electronic   General

OMRON HEALTHCARE, INC.
847-680-6200
1925 W. Field Court, Lake Forest, IL 60045
FDA Number: 1450057   *Fax:* 847-680-6269
Year Founded: 1990
Total Employees: 118   *Marketing Staff:* 12   *Sales Staff:* 22
Ownership: Private
Quality System Registration Information: ISO9002
Produces/Sells CE-marked Devices: N
Distribution: Manufacturer Direct, Manufacturer Through Distributor, Manufacturer Through Manufacturer Reps
  Nebulizer, Direct Patient Interface   Anesthesiology
  Shield, Nipple   Obstetrics/Gynecology

OMS, 177108 CANADA INC.
800-461-6637
97 Columbus,
514-426-3055
Pointe Claire, QUE H9R-4 Canada
FDA Number: 8020420   *Fax:* 514-426-1138
E-mail: oms_optical@yahoo.com
Web site: www.optochemicals.com
Medical Products Sales Volume: $800,000
Year Founded: 1981
Total Employees: 8
Ownership: Private
Produces/Sells CE-marked Devices: N
Federal Procurement Eligibility: Small Business
Distribution: Manufacturer Direct, Manufacturer Through Distributor, Service Direct, Exporter

ON SITE GAS SYSTEMS, INC.
888-748-3429
35 Budney Road, Newington, CT 06111
860-667-8888
FDA Number: 3003637574   *Fax:* 860-667-2222
E-mail: info@onsitegas.com
Web site: www.onsitegas.com
Medical Products Sales Volume: $10,000,000
Year Founded: 1987
Total Employees: 50
Ownership: Private
Produces/Sells CE-marked Devices: N
Federal Procurement Eligibility: Small Business
Distribution: Manufacturer Direct, Manufacturer Through Manufacturer Reps
Mktg./Adv.: Mr. Wayne Heist/Sales Specialist
Ms. Laurie Burt/Sales Specialist
  Generator, Oxygen, Portable   Anesthesiology

ON-X LIFE TECHNOLOGIES, INC.
888-339-8000
1300 East Anderson Lane, Building-B,
512-339-8000
Austin, TX 78752
FDA Number: 1649833   *Fax:* 512-339-3636
E-mail: cs@onxlti.com
Web site: http://www.onxlti.com
Ownership: Private
Produces/Sells CE-marked Devices: N
General Admin.: Mr. Clyde Baker/President, Chief Executive Officer
Mktg./Adv.: Mr. Michael Cox/Vice President Marketing & Sales
Production: Mr. Derek Southard/Executive Vice President Engineering
Mr. John Ely/Executive Vice President Quality Assurance & Regulatory Affairs
  Insufflator, Laparoscopic   Obstetrics/Gynecology
  Sizer, Heart Valve Prosthesis   Cardiovascular
  Valve, Heart, Mechanical   Cardiovascular

ONCOBIONIC
518-798-1215
30211 Avenida De Las Banderas, Suite 200,
Rancho Santa Margarita, CA 92688
FDA Number: 3007009552
Ownership: Angiodynamics, Inc.
Stock Symbol: ANGO
Traded On: NASDAQ
Produces/Sells CE-marked Devices: N

ONCOGENE RESEARCH PRODUCTS
800-854-3417
10394 Pacific Center Court,
858-450-9600
San Diego, CA 92121
FDA Number: n/a   *Fax:* 858-453-3552
E-mail: technical@apoptosis.com
Web site: www.emdbiosciences.comhtmlcbcintermediatepage.htm
Total Employees: 150   *Marketing Staff:* 6   *Sales Staff:* 8
Ownership: MERCK KGAA
Stock Symbol: CNBSC
Traded On: NASDAQ
Produces/Sells CE-marked Devices: N
Federal Procurement Eligibility: Small Business
Distribution: Manufacturer Direct, Manufacturer Through Distributor, OEM
General Admin.: Octavio Diaz/President
Mktg./Adv.: Kim Harris/Director Sales
  Analyzer, Chemistry, ELISA   Chemistry
  Contract R&D, Diagnostics   General

ONCOLAB, INC.
800-922-8378
36 The Fenway, Boston, MA 02215
617-536-0850
FDA Number: n/a   *Fax:* 617-536-0657
Annual Revenue: $0-$1 Million
Total Employees: 10
Ownership: Private
Produces/Sells CE-marked Devices: N
Federal Procurement Eligibility: Small Business, Female Owned
Distribution: Manufacturer Direct
General Admin.: Elenore Bogoch/President
  Test, Cancer Detection, Other   Hematology

ONCOLOGY AUTOMATION, INC.
337-998-6837
105 Water Oaks Dr., Lafayette, LA 70503
FDA Number: 2321015
Ownership: Private
Produces/Sells CE-marked Devices: N
  Shield, Protective, Personnel   Radiology

ONCOLOGY SERVICES INTERNATIONAL
800-445-4516
400 Rella Boulevard, Suite 123,
845 357 6560
Montebello, NY 10901
FDA Number: 3007204455   *Fax:* 845 357 6599
E-mail: inquiry@thinkosi.com
Web site: www.thinkosi.com
Medical Products Sales Volume: $8,000,000
Annual Revenue: $10-$25 Million
Total Employees: 98
Ownership: Private
Produces/Sells CE-marked Devices: N
Distribution: Manufacturer Direct, Service Direct
  Accelerator, Linear, Medical   Radiology

ONCOLOGY TECH, LLC
210-497-2100
5608 Business Park, San Antonio, TX 78218
FDA Number: 3006404247
  Block, Beam Shaping, Radionuclide   Radiology

ONCOSEC MEDICAL INC.
775-562-0504
200 South Virginia Street, 8th Floor, Reno, NV 89501
FDA Number: n/a
E-mail: investors@oncosec.com
Web site: www.oncosec.com
Ownership: Private
Produces/Sells CE-marked Devices: N
General Admin.: Mr. Avtar Dhillon/Chairman
Dr. James DeMesa/Director
Mr. Punit Dhillon/President, Chief Executive Officer
Finance: Veronica Vallejo/Vice President Finance, Controller

ONCOTECH
  See Exiqon Inc.

ONCOTHYREON INC.
520-622-5552
221 East 6th Street, Tucson, AZ 85705
FDA Number: n/a   *Fax:* 520-622-5553
Web site: www.oncothyreon.com
Total Employees: 18
Ownership: Oncothyreon Inc.
Produces/Sells CE-marked Devices: N
General Admin.: Robert L. Kirkman/President, Chief Executive Officer

ONCOTHYREON INC.   520-622-5552 *(cont'd)*
     Test, Cancer Detection, Monoclonal Antibody   Immunology
     Test, Cancer Detection, Other   Hematology

ONCOTHYREON INC.   206-801-2100
     2601 Fourth Ave, Suite 500, Seattle, WA 98121
     FDA Number: n/a   Fax: 206) 801-2111
     E-mail: ir@oncothyreon.com
     Web site: www.oncothyreon.com
     Ownership: Public
     Stock Symbol: ONTY
     Traded On: NASDAQ
     Produces/Sells CE-marked Devices: N
     General Admin.: Robert L. Kirkman/President, Chief Executive Officer
     Test, Cancer Detection, Monoclonal Antibody   Immunology
     Test, Cancer Detection, Other   Hematology
     Medical Product Subsidiaries (Listed Separately)
     Oncothyreon Inc.

ONDA CORPORATION   408-745-0383
     592 Weddell Drive, Suite 7, Sunnyvale, CA 94089
     FDA Number: n/a   Fax: 408-745-0956
     E-mail: info@ondacorp.com
     Web site: http://www.ondacorp.com
     Year Founded: 1990
     Ownership: Private
     Produces/Sells CE-marked Devices: N

ONE LAMBDA, INC.   800-822-8824
     21001 Kittridge St., Canoga Park, CA 91303   818-702-0042
     FDA Number: 2024375   Fax: 818-702-6904
     E-mail: sales@onelambda.com
     Web site: www.onelambda.com
     Medical Products Sales Volume: $26,500,000
     Annual Revenue: $0-$1 Million
     Total Employees: 200   *Marketing Staff:* 6   *Sales Staff:* 10
     Ownership: Private
     Quality System Registration Information: ISO9001
     Produces/Sells CE-marked Devices: Y
     Federal Procurement Eligibility: Small Business, Minority Owned
     Distribution: Manufacturer Direct, Manufacturer Through Distributor
     General Admin.: Dennis Morrison/Chief Executive Officer
     Mktg./Adv.: Paul Tausch/Director Sales
         Stewart Han/Manager Marketing Operations
     Antibody, Monoclonal   Microbiology
     Coverslip, Microscope Slide   Pathology
     Dispenser, Other   General
     Medium, Lymphocyte Separation   Hematology
     Reagent, Other   General
     Stage, Microscope   Pathology
     Stain, Other   Pathology
     Test, Leukocyte Typing   Hematology

ONE ZONE DEVICES   858-350-9284
     3525 Del Mar Hts. Road #366, San Diego, CA 92130
     FDA Number: 1933510
     Shield, X-Ray, Leaded   Dental And Oral

ONEAC CORPORATION   800-327-8801
     27944 N. Bradley Road,   847-816-6000
     Libertyville, IL 60048
     FDA Number: n/a   Fax: 847-680-5124
     E-mail: info@oneac.com
     Web site: www.oneac.com
     Medical Products Sales Volume: $10,000,000
     Annual Revenue: $25-$50 Million
     Year Founded: 1979
     Total Employees: 25   *Marketing Staff:* 10   *Sales Staff:* 30
     Ownership: Chloride Group PLC
     Traded On: London
     Quality System Registration Information: ISO9001
     Produces/Sells CE-marked Devices: Y
     Federal Procurement Eligibility: Small Business, GSA Contract
     Distribution: Manufacturer Direct, Manufacturer Through Distributor, Manufacturer
     Through Manufacturer Reps, OEM
     General Admin.: Ted Antonitis/President, Chief Executive Officer
     Mktg./Adv.: Maureen Janosch/Director Product Marketing
         Lori Pasenelli/Manager Marketing Communications
         Louis Pace/Vice President Marketing & Sales
     Power System, Isolated   General
     Power Systems, Uninterruptible (UPS)   General

ONGOING CARE SOLUTIONS, INC.   800-375-0207
     6545 44th St., N., Ste. 4007,   727-526-0707
     Pinellas Park, FL 33781
     FDA Number: 1056683   Fax: 727-525-1424
     E-mail: ongoingcare@algxmail.com
     Web site: www.ongoingcare.com

ONGOING CARE SOLUTIONS, INC.   800-375-0207 *(cont'd)*
     Annual Revenue: $1-$5 Million
     Year Founded: 2000
     Total Employees: 50   *Marketing Staff:* 4
     Ownership: Private
     Produces/Sells CE-marked Devices: N
     Federal Procurement Eligibility: Small Business
     Distribution: Manufacturer Direct, Manufacturer Through Manufacturer Reps
     General Admin.: Harold Covert/Chief Executive Officer
     Mktg./Adv.: Bill Warning/Director Marketing
         Lara Mosley/Director National Accounts
         Linda Lee/Director Product Development
     Cushion, Flotation, Therapeutic   Physical Med
     Cushion, Wheelchair (Pad)   Physical Med
     Mattress, Non-Powered Flotation Therapy   Physical Med
     Orthosis, Limb Brace   Physical Med

ONI MEDICAL SYSTEMS, INC.   978-658-0020
     301 Ballardvale Street, Suite 4, Wilmington, MA 01887-4405
     FDA Number: 1226563   Fax: 978-658-0898
     E-mail: info@onicorp.com
     Web site: www.onicorp.com
     Medical Products Sales Volume: $8,900,000
     Year Founded: 1997
     Total Employees: 46
     Ownership: Private
     Produces/Sells CE-marked Devices: Y
     Federal Procurement Eligibility: Small Business
     Nuclear Magnetic Resonance Imaging System   Radiology

ONLINE POWER, INC.   800-227-8899
     5701 Smithway St.,   323-721-5017
     Los Angeles, CA 90040
     FDA Number: n/a   Fax: 323-721-3929
     E-mail: tech@onlinepower.com
     Web site: www.onlinepower.com
     Medical Products Sales Volume: $8,900,000
     Annual Revenue: $10-$25 Million
     Year Founded: 1975
     Total Employees: 100   *Marketing Staff:* 1   *Sales Staff:* 20
     Ownership: Private
     Quality System Registration Information: ISO9001
     Federal Procurement Eligibility: Small Business
     Distribution: Manufacturer Direct, Manufacturer Through Distributor, Manufacturer
     Through Manufacturer Reps, OEM
     General Admin.: Abbie Gougerchian/President
     Mktg./Adv.: Jan Visser/Director Marketing & Sales
         Marc Lepesant/Director Marketing & Sales
     Power Systems, Uninterruptible (UPS)   General
     Regulator, Line Voltage   General

ONSET MEDICAL CORPORATION   949-716-1100
     13900 Alton Parkway, Suite 120, Irvine, CA 92618
     FDA Number: 3004672932
     Web site: http://www.onsetmedical.com
     Year Founded: 2003
     Ownership: Private
     Produces/Sells CE-marked Devices: N
     Dilator, Catheter, Ureteral   Gastroenterology/Urology
     Introducer, Catheter   Cardiovascular

ONTARIO MEDICAL SUPPLY LIMITED   800-267-1069
     1100 Algoma Road,,   613-244-8620
     Ottawa, ONT K1B 0 Canada
     FDA Number: n/a   Fax: 613-244-3826
     E-mail: jdesjardins@ontariomedicalsupply.com
     Web site: www.oms.ca
     Year Founded: 1947
     Total Employees: 100
     Ownership: Private
     Produces/Sells CE-marked Devices: N
     Distribution: Exclusive Distributor

ONYX INDUSTRIES, INC./QUADRTECH   310-851-6161
     521 West Rosecrans Ave., Gardena, CA 90248
     FDA Number: 2025291
     Perforator, Ear-Lobe   Ear/Nose/Throat

ONYX MEDICAL CORP.   800.238.6981
     1800 North Shelby Oaks Drive,   901-323-6699
     Memphis, TN 38134
     FDA Number: 1043653   Fax: 901-454-0295
     E-mail: sales@onyxmedical.net
     Web site: www.onyxmedical.net
     Annual Revenue: $1-$5 Million
     Year Founded: 1990
     Total Employees: 40
     Ownership: Private

ONYX MEDICAL CORP.   800.238.6981 *(cont'd)*

Quality System Registration Information: ISO9002
Produces/Sells CE-marked Devices: Y
Federal Procurement Eligibility: Small Business, Female Owned
Distribution: OEM
General Admin.: Lorri Allen Moore/Manager Human Resources
      Laraine B. Gilmore/President
      Roger E. Gilmore/Vice President, General Manager
Mktg./Adv.: Jodie Gilmore/Vice President Marketing & Sales
Production: Harlan Stillions/Manager Quality Assurance
      Patrick Gilmore/Vice President Manufacturing

Bit, Drill	Orthopedics
Nail, Fixation, Bone	Orthopedics
Pin, Fixation, Smooth	Orthopedics
Pin, Fixation, Threaded	Orthopedics
Plate, Fixation, Bone	Orthopedics
Tap, Bone	Orthopedics
Wire, Bone	Orthopedics

ONYX MEDICAL INC./FACE-IT   800-333-5773
16 Digital Drive, Suite 120, Novato, CA 94949   **415-884-4412**

FDA Number: 2951557   *Fax:* 415-884-4415
E-mail: info@onyxmedical.com
Web site: www.onyxmedical.com
Annual Revenue: $1-$5 Million
Year Founded: 1986
Ownership: Private
Quality System Registration Information: ISO9001
Produces/Sells CE-marked Devices: N
Federal Procurement Eligibility: Small Business
Distribution: Manufacturer Through Distributor
General Admin.: Roger Machson/President, Chief Executive Officer
Research: Roger Machson/Vice President Research & Development

Accessories, Apparel, Surgical	Surgery
Accessories, Solution, Lens, Contact	Ophthalmology
Mask, Face	General

OOLTEWAH MANUFACTURING   800-251-6040x25
5722 Main St., P.O. Box 587, Ooltewah, TN 37363

FDA Number: n/a
Web site: www.ooltewah.com
Annual Revenue: $1-$5 Million
Ownership: Private
Produces/Sells CE-marked Devices: N
Federal Procurement Eligibility: Small Business
Distribution: Manufacturer Through Distributor, OEM, Service Direct, Exclusive Distributor

Exerciser, Other	Physical Med
Moist Therapy Pack	Physical Med
Pillow, Cervical	Orthopedics
Strap, Restraining	General
Support, Back	Orthopedics

OP-D-OP, INC.   916-783-5741
8559 Washington Blvd., Roseville, CA 95678-6435

FDA Number: n/a   *Fax:* 916-783-5765
E-mail: info@opdop.com
Web site: www.opdop.com
Medical Products Sales Volume: $2,000,000
Total Employees: 10   *Marketing Staff:* 3   *Sales Staff:* 3
Ownership: Private
Produces/Sells CE-marked Devices: Y
Federal Procurement Eligibility: Small Business
Distribution: Manufacturer Through Distributor, Exporter
General Admin.: Tim Landis/President
Mktg./Adv.: Laura Craig/Manager International & National Sales
      Julie Ervin/Manager National Sales

Shield, Protective, Personnel	Radiology

OPAP, INC.   831-458-5626
3523 Deanes Ln., Capitola, CA 95010

FDA Number: 2954297

Mouthpiece, Breathing	Anesthesiology

OPCO LABORATORY, INC.   978-345-2522
704 River St., Fitchburg, MA 01420

FDA Number: n/a   *Fax:* 978-345-5515
E-mail: info@opcolab.com
Web site: www.opcolab.com
Medical Products Sales Volume: $2,800,000
Annual Revenue: $1-$5 Million
Year Founded: 1976
Total Employees: 20   *Marketing Staff:* 1   *Sales Staff:* 1
Ownership: Private
Produces/Sells CE-marked Devices: N
Federal Procurement Eligibility: Small Business
Distribution: Manufacturer Direct
General Admin.: Mario Maldari/President, Chief Executive Officer

OPCO LABORATORY, INC.   978-345-2522 *(cont'd)*

      Linda Sheehan/Vice President Human Resources
Mktg./Adv.: Linda Sheehan/Director Marketing
      Saverio Maldari/Manager International Marketing & Sales
      Richard Donnelly/Manager National Sales
Production: Janice Kemp/Director Quality Assurance
      David Maldari/Manager Materials
      David Maldari/Vice President Manufacturing

Envelope, Film, X-Ray	Radiology
Lens, Other	Ophthalmology
Mirror, General & Plastic Surgery	Surgery

OPENMED TECHNOLOGIES CORPORATION   877-717-6215
256 West Cummings Park,   **781-938-4210**
Woburn, MA 01801

FDA Number: 9038301
E-mail: info@openmed.com   *Fax:* 781-938-4782
Web site: www.openmed.com
Medical Products Sales Volume: $2,500,000
Annual Revenue: $5-$10 Million
Year Founded: 1992
Total Employees: 15   *Marketing Staff:* 1   *Sales Staff:* 7
Ownership: Openmed Technologies Corporation
Produces/Sells CE-marked Devices: N
Federal Procurement Eligibility: Small Business
Distribution: Manufacturer Direct, Manufacturer Through Distributor, OEM, Exporter
General Admin.: Mr. Albert Kelley/President, Chief Executive Officer
Production: Mr. Daniel Harris/Manager Application Engineering
      Dr. Andrew Kirik/Managing Engineer
      Mr. Boris Grinberg/Managing Engineer
      Mr. Murat Kumykov/Managing Engineer
      Mr. Bernard Maury/Vice President, Director Engineering
IS: Ms. Miranda Wolfe/Manager Tech. Support

Computer, Radiographic Data	Radiology
Computer, Radiographic Image Analysis	Radiology
Device, Storage, Image, Digital	Radiology
Image Digitizer	Radiology
Radiographic Picture Archiving/Communication System (PACS)	Radiology
System, Communication, Image, Digital	Radiology

Medical Product Subsidiaries (Listed Separately)
    Openmed Technologies Corporation

OPHARDT HYGIENE TECHNOLOGIES INC.   905-563-4987
4743 Christie Dr., Beamsville, ONT L0R 1B4 Canada

FDA Number: n/a   *Fax:* 905-563-6266
E-mail: info@gotoHTI.com
Web site: www.hygienetechnik.com
Ownership: Ophardt Hygiene Technik GmbH & Co. KG
Quality System Registration Information: ISO9002
Produces/Sells CE-marked Devices: N
Distribution: Manufacturer Through Distributor, OEM

OPHIR OPTRONICS, INC.   800-820-0814
260A Fordham Road, Wilmington, MA 01887   **978-657-6410**

FDA Number: n/a   *Fax:* 978-657-6056
E-mail: optics@ophiropticsinc.com
Web site: www.ophiropt.com
Medical Products Sales Volume: $2,400,000
Year Founded: 1976
Total Employees: 13
Ownership: Ophir Optronics Ltd.
Quality System Registration Information: ISO9001
Produces/Sells CE-marked Devices: Y
Federal Procurement Eligibility: Small Business
Distribution: Exclusive Distributor
General Admin.: Carl G. Burns/President
Mktg./Adv.: Dick Rieley/Manager Sales
Production: Motti Shemesh/Customer Service Representative

Accessories, Laser	General
Radiometer, Laser	General

OPHTEC USA, INC.   561-989-8767
6421 Congress Avenue, Suite 112, Boca Raton, FL 33487

FDA Number: 1062939   *Fax:* 661-989-9744
E-mail: ophtecusa@aol.com
Web site: www.ophtec.com/
Medical Products Sales Volume: $400,000
Annual Revenue: $0-$1 Million
Year Founded: 1983
Total Employees: 7   *Marketing Staff:* 1   *Sales Staff:* 1
Ownership: Private
Quality System Registration Information: ISO9001
Produces/Sells CE-marked Devices: Y
Federal Procurement Eligibility: Small Business
Distribution: Manufacturer Direct
General Admin.: Rick McCarley/President, Chief Executive Officer

Contract Manufacturing	General

OPHTEC USA, INC. 561-989-8767 *(cont'd)*
Lens, Intraocular — *Ophthalmology*

OPHTHALMED LLC 770-777-6613
11660 Alpharetta Hwy., Suite 205, Roswell, GA 30076
FDA Number: 3004497289
Laser, Ophthalmic — *Ophthalmology*
Laser, Surgical — *Surgery*

OPHTHALMIC IMAGING SYSTEMS 800-338-8436
221 Lathrop Way, Ste. I, 916-646-2020
Sacramento, CA 95815
FDA Number: n/a — *Fax:* 916-646-0207
E-mail: info@oisi.com
Web site: www.oisi.com
Annual Revenue: $5-$10 Million
Total Employees: 55
Ownership: Luxo AS
Stock Symbol: OISI
Traded On: OTC Bulletin
Produces/Sells CE-marked Devices: Y
Distribution: Manufacturer Direct, Manufacturer Through Distributor
General Admin.: Gil Allon/Chief Executive Officer
Mktg./Adv.: Mr. Marc Hollingworth/Vice President, Director Marketing
  Mr. Tony Migon/Vice President, Manager Sales
Camera, Ophthalmic, AC-Powered (Fundus) — *Ophthalmology*
Camera, Other — *General*
Ophthalmoscope, AC-Powered — *Ophthalmology*

OPHTHALMIC INNOVATIONS INTL., INC. 909-937-1033
4290 E. Brickell St., Bldg-a, Ontario, CA 91761
FDA Number: 2027748
Lens, Intraocular — *Ophthalmology*

OPHTHALMIC INTL. 480-837-6165
16857 E. Saguaro Blvd, Fountain Hills, AZ 85268
FDA Number: 2030755 — *Fax:* 480-837-6870
E-mail: inquiries@oi-pnt.com
Web site: www.oi-pnt.com
Medical Products Sales Volume: $500,000
Total Employees: 6
Ownership: Ophthalmic Intl.
Stock Symbol: CDIK
Traded On: OTC Bulletin
Quality System Registration Information: ISO9002
Produces/Sells CE-marked Devices: Y
Federal Procurement Eligibility: Small Business
Distribution: Manufacturer Through Distributor, OEM, Exporter
General Admin.: Mr. Richard Smith/Chief Executive Officer, Chairman
  Mr. Gary Smith/President
Production: Dr. John Sharkey/Director Operations
Fixation Device, AC-Powered, Ophthalmic — *Ophthalmology*
Medical Product Subsidiaries (Listed Separately)
Ophthalmic Intl.

OPHTHALMIC TECHNOLOGIES, INC. 416-631-9123
12-37 Kodiak Cres, Downsview M3J 3E5 Canada
FDA Number: 9681722
Cautery, Radiofrequency, AC-Powered — *Ophthalmology*
Endoscope, Ophthalmic — *Gastroenterology/Urology*
Scanner, Ultrasonic (Pulsed Echo) — *Radiology*

OPHTHONIX INC. 760-842-5772
1491 Poinsettia Avenue, Vista, CA 92081
FDA Number: 3003981661
Aberrometer, Ophthalmic — *Ophthalmology*
Lens, Spectacle/Eyeglasses, Non-Custom — *Ophthalmology*

OPI, INC. 260-248-4414
700 South Main Street, Columbia City, IN 46725
FDA Number: 1836545 — *Fax:* (260) 248-8571
Ownership: Private
Produces/Sells CE-marked Devices: N
Orthopedic Manual Surgical Instrument — *Orthopedics*

OPKO HEALTH INC. 305-575-4100
4400 Biscayne Blvd., Suite 1180, Miami, FL 33137
FDA Number: n/a
E-mail: info@opko.com
Web site: www.opko.com
Ownership: Public
Stock Symbol: OPK
Traded On: AMEX
Produces/Sells CE-marked Devices: N
IS: Jane Hsiao/Chief Tech. Manager
Scanner, Ultrasonic (Pulsed Echo) — *Radiology*
Transducer, Ultrasonic, Diagnostic — *Radiology*

OPNEXT INC. 510-580-8828
46429 Landing Parkway, Fremont, CA 94538
FDA Number: n/a — *Fax:* 510-580-8819
E-mail: info@opnext.com
Web site: http://www.opnext.com
Year Founded: 2000
Ownership: Private
Produces/Sells CE-marked Devices: N
General Admin.: Mr. Harry Bosco/President, Chief Executive Officer
Mktg./Adv.: Mr. James Horiuchi/Vice President Sales
Production: Mr. Scott Clark/Vice President Operations
Finance: Mr. Robert Nobile/Chief Financial Officer

OPSALES, INC.
4217 Austin Blvd., Island Park, NY 11558
FDA Number: 2431442
Sunglasses (Including Photosensitive) — *Ophthalmology*

OPSENS 418-682-9996
2014 Cyrille-Duquet Street, Suite 125,
Quebec, QUEBE G1N 4 Canada
FDA Number: n/a — *Fax:* 418-682-9939
E-mail: INFO@OPSENS.COM
Web site: www.opsens.com
Ownership: Public
Stock Symbol: OPS
Traded On: Toronto
Quality System Registration Information: ISO9001
Produces/Sells CE-marked Devices: N

OPTACRYL INC.
See Optikem International, Inc.

OPTEC SPECIALTIES, INC. 770-513-7380
975 Progress Circle, Lawrenceville, GA 30043
FDA Number: 1063727
Insoles, Medical — *General*
Orthosis, Lumbosacral — *Physical Med*

OPTELEC U.S., INC. 800-828-1056
3030 Enterprise Court, Suite C, Vista, CA 92081 760-741-0767
FDA Number: n/a — *Fax:* 978-692-6073
E-mail: optelec@optelec.com
Web site: www.optelec.com
Medical Products Sales Volume: $6,600,000
Year Founded: 1985
Total Employees: 30
Ownership: Private
Federal Procurement Eligibility: Small Business
Distribution: Manufacturer Direct, Manufacturer Through Manufacturer Reps,
Exclusive Distributor
General Admin.: Alan Rabin/President
  Dave Dutton/Vice President Human Resources
Mktg./Adv.: Paul Shibley/Vice President Marketing
  Mike Callahan/Vice President Sales
Container, Medication, Home-Use — *General*
Monitor, Blood Pressure, Finger — *Cardiovascular*
Viewer/Magnifier — *Hematology*
Vision Aid, Electronic, AC-Powered — *Ophthalmology*

OPTELECOM-NKF, INC 800-293-4237
12920 Cloverleaf Center Drive, 301-444-2200
Germantown, MD 20874
FDA Number: n/a — *Fax:* 301-444-2299
E-mail: sales.us@optelecom-nkf.com
Web site: www.optelecom-nkf.com
Medical Products Sales Volume: $39,500,000
Annual Revenue: $10-$25 Million
Year Founded: 1972
Total Employees: 53
Ownership: Public
Stock Symbol: OPTC
Traded On: NASDAQ
Quality System Registration Information: ISO9001
Produces/Sells CE-marked Devices: Y
Federal Procurement Eligibility: Small Business
Distribution: Manufacturer Direct, Manufacturer Through Distributor, Manufacturer
Through Manufacturer Reps, Service Direct
General Admin.: Edmund Ludwig/President
Mktg./Adv.: Leonard May/Vice President Marketing & Sales
Communication Equipment — *General*
Contract R&D, Equipment — *General*
Laser, Laboratory — *Chemistry*

OPTI MEDICAL SYSTEMS INC. 770-510-4444
235 Hembree Park Drive, Roswell, GA 30076
FDA Number: 3004102403
Computer, Chemistry Analyzer — *Chemistry*
Control, Multi Analyte, All Kinds (Assayed And Unassayed) — *Chemistry*

OPTI MEDICAL SYSTEMS INC.   770-510-4444 (cont'd)

Electrode, Blood pH	Chemistry
Electrode, Ion Specific, Calcium	Chemistry
Electrode, Ion Specific, Chloride	Chemistry
Electrode, Ion Specific, Potassium	Chemistry
Electrode, Ion Specific, Sodium	Chemistry
Electrode, Ion Specific, Urea Nitrogen	Chemistry
Hemoglobinometer, Automated	Hematology
Kit, Sampling, Arterial Blood	Anesthesiology
Oximeter, Whole Blood	Hematology
Reagent, Glucose (Test System)	Chemistry

OPTI-QUIP, INC.   845-928-2254
548 Route 32, Box 469, Highland Mills, NY 10930
FDA Number: 7000279   Fax: 845-928-6206
E-mail: optiquip@warwick.net
Annual Revenue: $0-$1 Million
Total Employees: 12
Ownership: Private
Produces/Sells CE-marked Devices: N
Federal Procurement Eligibility: Small Business
Distribution: Manufacturer Direct, Manufacturer Through Manufacturer Reps
General Admin.: Melvin L. Decker/Chief Executive Officer
Mktg./Adv.: Melvin L. Decker/Manager Advertising
     Melvin L. Decker/Vice President Marketing
Production: Lawrence Decker/Manager Production

Microscope	Hematology

OPTICAL DYNAMICS CORPORATION   800-587-2743
1950 Production Ct, Louisville, KY 40299   **502-671-2020**
FDA Number: 3002707783   Fax: 888-900-5504
E-mail: domsales@opticaldynamics.com
Web site: www.opticaldynamics.com
Ownership: Private
Produces/Sells CE-marked Devices: N

Lens, Spectacle/Eyeglasses, Non-Custom	Ophthalmology

OPTICAL ELECTRONICS, INC.   520-889-8811
4455 S. Park Ave #106, Tucson, AZ 85714
FDA Number: n/a   Fax: 520-889-8575
E-mail: info@oei-az.com
Web site: www.oei-az.com
Annual Revenue: $0-$1 Million
Year Founded: 1964
Ownership: Private
Produces/Sells CE-marked Devices: N
Federal Procurement Eligibility: Small Business, Female Owned
Distribution: OEM, Exporter

Image Processing System	Radiology

OPTICAL ENGINEERING, INC.
See Macken Instruments, Inc.

OPTICAL INTEGRITY, INC.   850-233-5512
8317 Front Beach Rd., Suite 21, Panama City Beach, FL 32407
FDA Number: 3003708273

Laser, Surgical	Surgery

OPTICAL LABORATORY, INC.   508-993-8665
14 S. Sixth St., New Bedford, MA 02740-5911
FDA Number: n/a
Annual Revenue: $0-$1 Million
Ownership: Private
Produces/Sells CE-marked Devices: N
Distribution: Manufacturer Direct

Eyeglasses	Ophthalmology

OPTICAL POLYMER RESEARCH, INC.   352-378-1027
5921 N.e. 38th St., Gainesville, FL 32609
FDA Number: 1036035

Lens, Contact (Other Material)	Ophthalmology

OPTICAL SHOP OF ASPEN   800-647-2345
25 Brookline, Aliso Viejo, CA 92656   **949-360-1010**
FDA Number: 2084270   Fax: 949-425-4785
E-mail: info@osainternational.com
Web site: www.osainternational.com
Medical Products Sales Volume: $400,000
Annual Revenue: $10-$25 Million
Year Founded: 1988
Total Employees: 3   Marketing Staff: 1   Sales Staff: 6
Ownership: Private
Produces/Sells CE-marked Devices: N
Federal Procurement Eligibility: Small Business
Distribution: Manufacturer Direct, Manufacturer Through Distributor, Manufacturer Through Manufacturer Reps, Exclusive Distributor, Importer, Exporter
General Admin.: Ms. Vicki Davis/Chief Financial Officer, Treasurer
     Mr. Troy Schmidt/Chief Operating Officer
     Mr. Larry Sands/President, Chief Executive Officer

OPTICAL SHOP OF ASPEN   800-647-2345 (cont'd)
Mktg./Adv.: Mr. Troy Schmidt/Director Product Development
     Mrs. Michelle Arena/General Manager Sales
     Mr. Trent Graham/Manager International Sales & Exports
     Ms. Alice Chun/Manager Marketing & Advertising

Frame, Spectacle (Eyeglasses)	Ophthalmology

OPTICAL SUPPLIERS, INC.   808-486-2933
99-1253 Halawa Valley St., Aiea, HI 96701
FDA Number: 2920760
Ownership: Private
Produces/Sells CE-marked Devices: N

Frame, Spectacle (Eyeglasses)	Ophthalmology
Lens, Spectacle/Eyeglasses, Non-Custom	Ophthalmology

OPTICAL TECHNOLOGY - USA
See Insight Instruments, Inc.

OPTICAL VENTURES, INC.   626-915-1533
150 N. Grand Ave., Suite 203, West Covina, CA 91791
FDA Number: 2032707

Sunglasses (Including Photosensitive)	Ophthalmology

OPTICON MEDICAL   614-336-2000
7001 Post Road, Suite 100, Dublin, OH 43016
FDA Number: 1932267

Catheter, Retention Type, Balloon	Gastroenterology/Urology

OPTICON, INC.   800-636-0090
8 Olympic Drive, Orangeburg, NY 10962   **845-365-0090**
FDA Number: n/a   Fax: 845-365-1251
E-mail: sales@opticonusa.com
Web site: www.opticonusa.com
Medical Products Sales Volume: $20,000,000
Annual Revenue: $10-$25 Million
Year Founded: 1976
Total Employees: 20
Ownership: OPTO ELECTRONIC COMPANY, LTD.
Quality System Registration Information: ISO9002
Produces/Sells CE-marked Devices: Y
Federal Procurement Eligibility: Small Business
Distribution: Manufacturer Direct, OEM
General Admin.: Masami Tawara/Chief Executive Officer
Mktg./Adv.: Hank Weber/Director Marketing
     Mike Howell/Director National Accounts
     Charley Patkochis/Vice President Marketing & Sales
Production: Dean Spacht/Product Manager
     David Bewig/Vice President Manufacturing

Reader, Bar Code	General

OPTICOTE INC.   847-678-8900
10455 Seymour Ave., Franklin Park, IL 60131
FDA Number: 3002838042

Sunglasses (Including Photosensitive)	Ophthalmology

OPTIKEM INTERNATIONAL, INC.   800-525-1752
2172 S. Jason St., Denver, CO 80223   **303-936-1137**
FDA Number: 1720129   Fax: 303-936-7320
E-mail: optikemint@aol.com
Medical Products Sales Volume: $3,100,000
Annual Revenue: $5-$10 Million
Year Founded: 1976
Total Employees: 10
Ownership: Private
Produces/Sells CE-marked Devices: N
Federal Procurement Eligibility: Small Business, Female Owned
Distribution: Manufacturer Direct
General Admin.: Sally Cook/President
     Camille Zehnder/Vice President
Production: Betty Medina/Director Quality Assurance

Accessories, Solution, Lens, Contact	Ophthalmology
Lens, Contact, Hydrophilic	Ophthalmology
Lens, Contact, Polymethylmethacrylate	Ophthalmology

OPTIM INCORPORATED   800-225-7486
64 Technology Park Road,   **508-347-5100**
Sturbridge, MA 01566
FDA Number: 1218141   Fax: 508-347-2380
E-mail: sales@optimnet.com
Web site: www.optimnet.com
Medical Products Sales Volume: $1,000,000
Annual Revenue: $5-$10 Million
Year Founded: 1971
Total Employees: 50   Marketing Staff: 2   Sales Staff: 7
Ownership: Private
Quality System Registration Information: ISO9001
Produces/Sells CE-marked Devices: Y
Federal Procurement Eligibility: Small Business, GSA Contract

OPTIM INCORPORATED · 800-225-7486 *(cont'd)*
Distribution: Manufacturer Direct, Manufacturer Through Distributor, Manufacturer Through Manufacturer Reps, OEM, Exporter
General Admin.: Thomas V. Root/President, Chief Executive Officer
Robert V. Griffin/Vice President, General Manager
Mktg./Adv.: Anna Melander/Manager Contract Sales
Production: Mark Fuller/Director Quality Assurance & Regulatory Affairs

Endoscope	Gastroenterology/Urology
Endoscope, Neurological	Cns/Neurology
Nasopharyngoscope (Flexible Or Rigid)	Ear/Nose/Throat

OPTIMA, INC. · 203-377-8835
111 Research Dr., Stratford, CT 06615
FDA Number: 1221837
Ownership: Private
Produces/Sells CE-marked Devices: N

Lens, Spectacle/Eyeglasses, Non-Custom	Ophthalmology

OPTIMED TECHNOLOGIES, INC. · 973-575-9911
20 New Dutch Lane, Fairfield, NJ 07004
FDA Number: 2248956 — Fax: 973-575-9722
E-mail: Marketing@optimed.com
Web site: www.optimed.com
Medical Products Sales Volume: $4,100,000
Year Founded: 1993
Total Employees: 38
Ownership: Private
Produces/Sells CE-marked Devices: N
Federal Procurement Eligibility: Small Business
Distribution: Manufacturer Through Manufacturer Reps
General Admin.: Mr. Efraim Landa/Chairman, Chief Executive Officer
Mr. Ben Noy/President
Finance: Mr. Michael Winer/Chief Financial Officer
IS: Mr. Moshe Zchut/Vice President Technology

Computer, Nuclear Medicine	Radiology
Computer, Patient Data Management	General
Radiographic/Fluoroscopic Unit, Angiographic	Radiology
System, Network And Communication, Physiological Monitors	Cardiovascular

OPTIMEDICA CORPORATION · 888-850-1230
3100 Coronado Drive, Santa Clara, CA 95054 · 408-850-8600
FDA Number: 3005675890 — Fax: 408-850-8595
E-mail: info@optimedica.com
Web site: www.optimedica.com
Ownership: Private
Produces/Sells CE-marked Devices: N
General Admin.: Mr. Mark Forchette/President, Chief Executive Officer
Mktg./Adv.: Mr. Robert Eno/Vice President Global Marketing
Mr. Greg Anderson/Vice President Sales
Production: Mr. Robert Haddad/Vice President Operations
Mr. Alan Marquardt/Vice President Regulatory & Clinical Affairs
Research: Dr. George Marcellino/Vice President Clinical Development
Mr. David Scott/Vice President Research & Development
Finance: Mr. Mark Murray/Chief Financial Officer

Laser, Ophthalmic	Ophthalmology
Laser, Surgical	Surgery

OPTIMIZE MFG. CO. · 520-287-4605
**Apdo Postal 205-A,, Parque Industrial San Ramon,
Nogales, Sonora Mexico**
FDA Number: 8030632

Absorbent, Carbon-Dioxide	Anesthesiology
Absorber, Carbon-Dioxide	Anesthesiology
Circuit, Breathing (W Connector, Adapter, Y Piece)	Anesthesiology

OPTIQUE DU MONDE LTD./SAFILO USA
See Safilo Usa

OPTIVIA BIOTECHNOLOGY, INC. · 650-324-3177 ex
115 Constitution Drive, Suite 7, Menlo Park, CA 94025
FDA Number: n/a — Fax: 650-324-1855
E-mail: sales@optiviabio.com
Web site: http://www.optiviabio.com/
Ownership: Private
Produces/Sells CE-marked Devices: N
General Admin.: Dr. Yong Huang/Chief Executive Officer
Mr. Alan Mendelson/General Counsel
Mktg./Adv.: Mr. Chuck Boggs/Director Corporate Development
Dr. David Lustig/Vice President Business Development

OPTIVUS PROTON THERAPY, INC · 888-PROTONS
PO Box 608, Loma Linda, CA 92354 · 909-799-8300
FDA Number: 2032229 — Fax: 909-799-8348
E-mail: optivus@optivus.com
Web site: www.optivus.com
Medical Products Sales Volume: $7,500,000
Year Founded: 1993
Total Employees: 75
Ownership: Private

OPTIVUS PROTON THERAPY, INC · 888-PROTONS *(cont'd)*
Quality System Registration Information: ISO9001
Produces/Sells CE-marked Devices: N
Federal Procurement Eligibility: Small Business

Synchrotron, Medical	Radiology

OPTIWAY INC. · 800-514-7061
500 Norfinch Dr., · 416-739-8333
Downsview, ONT M3N-1 Canada
FDA Number: n/a — Fax: 416-739-6622
E-mail: sales@optiway.com
Web site: www.optiway.com
Year Founded: 1994
Total Employees: 50
Ownership: Private
Produces/Sells CE-marked Devices: N
Distribution: Manufacturer Direct, Exporter

OPTOMETRICS LLC · 978-772-1700
8 Nemco Way, Stony Brook Ind. Pk., Ayer, MA 01432
FDA Number: 2554740 — Fax: 978-772-0017
E-mail: websales@optometrics.com
Web site: www.optometrics.com
Medical Products Sales Volume: $3,200,000
Year Founded: 2005
Total Employees: 30 · Marketing Staff: 1 · Sales Staff: 2
Ownership: Private
Produces/Sells CE-marked Devices: Y
Federal Procurement Eligibility: Small Business
Distribution: Manufacturer Direct, OEM, Importer, Exporter
General Admin.: Frank Denton/President
Mktg./Adv.: Laura Lunardo/Vice President Marketing & Sales
Production: Richard Tennyson/Director Quality Assurance
Purchasing: Erin Mahoney/Director Purchasing

Contract Manufacturing	General
Spectrophotometer, Visible	Chemistry

OPTOS, INC. · 441-383-8433
67 Forest St., Marlboro, MA 01752
FDA Number: 1226140
Ownership: Private
Produces/Sells CE-marked Devices: N

Ophthalmoscope, AC-Powered	Ophthalmology
Ophthalmoscope, Laser, Scanning	Ophthalmology

OPTOVUE, INC. · 866-344-8948
45531 Northport Loop West, Fremont, CA 94538 · 510-623-8868
FDA Number: 3005950902 — Fax: 510-623-8668
E-mail: info@optovue.com
Web site: http://www.optovue.com
Year Founded: 2003
Ownership: Private
Produces/Sells CE-marked Devices: N
General Admin.: Dr. Tom Zhao/Chief Technology Officer
Mr. Jay Wei/President, Chief Executive Officer
Mktg./Adv.: Mr. Paul Kealey/Vice President Marketing
Production: Mr. John Talarico/Vice President Regulatory & Clinical Affairs
Finance: Mr. Gordon Wong/Vice President Finance

Ophthalmoscope, AC-Powered	Ophthalmology
Tomography, Optical Coherence	Ophthalmology

OPTP · 888-819-0121
3800 Annapolis Lane, Suite 165, PO Box 47009, · 763-553-0452
Minneapolis, MN 55447
FDA Number: n/a — Fax: 763-553-9355
E-mail: customerservice@optp.com
Web site: www.optp.com
Medical Products Sales Volume: $10,000,000
Total Employees: 20
Ownership: Private
Produces/Sells CE-marked Devices: N
Federal Procurement Eligibility: Small Business, Female Owned
Distribution: Exclusive Distributor
General Admin.: Shari Schroeder/President
Clare Cahill/Vice President Personnel
Mktg./Adv.: Deanna Watson/Director Marketing
Production: Karen Klingel/Vice President Operations

Exerciser, Arm	Physical Med
Exerciser, Leg And Ankle	Physical Med
Material, Training, Audiovisual	General
Orthosis, Cervical	Physical Med
Orthosis, Lumbar	Physical Med
Orthosis, Sacroiliac, Soft	Physical Med
Strap, Restraining	General
Support, Patient Position	Anesthesiology
Support, Wrist	Physical Med
Training Aid	Orthopedics

OPTRONICS INTERNATIONAL, INC.
See Intergraph Public Safety

OPUS DIAGNOSTICS, INC.   **877-944-1777**
One Parker Plaza, Fort Lee, NJ 07024   **201-944-1777**
FDA Number: 2249761   *Fax:* 201-592-0393
E-mail: sales@opusdiagnostics.com
Web site: www.opusdiagnostics.com
Medical Products Sales Volume: $200,000
Total Employees: 3
Ownership: Caprius, Inc.
Quality System Registration Information: ISO9001
Produces/Sells CE-marked Devices: N
Federal Procurement Eligibility: Small Business
Distribution: Manufacturer Through Distributor, OEM

Calibrator, Drug Specific	Toxicology
Control, Drug Specific	Toxicology
Enzyme Immunoassay, Carbamazepine	Toxicology
Enzyme Immunoassay, Digitoxin	Toxicology
Enzyme Immunoassay, Quinidine	Toxicology
Enzyme Immunoassay, Valproic Acid	Toxicology
Fluorescence Polarization Immunoassay, Diphenylhydantoin	Toxicology
Fluorescence Polarization Immunoassay, Phenobarbital	Toxicology
Fluorescence Polarization Immunoassay, Theophylline	Toxicology
Fluorescence Polarization Immunoassay, Tobramycin	Toxicology
System, Test, Topiramatee	Toxicology

ORACEUTICAL LLC   **413-528-5070**
815 Pleasant St., Lee, MA 01238
FDA Number: 1226386

Accessories, Retractor, Dental	Dental And Oral
Dam, Rubber	Dental And Oral
Toothbrush, Manual	Dental And Oral

ORACLE LENS MFG. CORP.   **401-736-9600**
30 Jefferson Park Rd., Warwick, RI 02888
FDA Number: 1225528

Lens, Spectacle/Eyeglasses, Non-Custom	Ophthalmology

ORAL BIOTECH   **541-928-4445**
812 Water St. Ne, Albany, OR 97321
FDA Number: 3005686375
Ownership: Private
Produces/Sells CE-marked Devices: N

Culture Media, Non-Selective And Differential	Microbiology
Culture Media, Selective And Differential	Microbiology
Kit, Screening, Urine	Microbiology
Saliva, Artificial	Dental And Oral
Varnish, Cavity	Dental And Oral

ORAL DESIGNS, INC.   **800-292-5516**
1259 Jackson Keller, San Antonio, TX 78213   **210-828-8102**
FDA Number: n/a   *Fax:* 210-824-1550
E-mail: services@oraldesigns.com
Web site: www.oraldesigns.com
Year Founded: 1975
Ownership: Private
Produces/Sells CE-marked Devices: N

ORAL HEALTH PRODUCTS, INC.   **918-622-9412**
6847 East 40th St., Tulsa, OK 74145
FDA Number: 1622044

Culture Media, Synthetic Cell And Tissue	Pathology
Floss, Dental	Dental And Oral
Toothbrush, Manual	Dental And Oral

ORAL OSTEODISTRACTION, L.P.
See Yan Razdolsky Ltd

ORAL-B LABORATORIES, INC.   **800-566-7252**
1832 Lower Muscantine Rd, Iowa City, IA 52240
FDA Number: 1910469
Web site: www.oralb.com
Annual Revenue: $0-$1 Million
Ownership: PROCTER & GAMBLE GMBH
Produces/Sells CE-marked Devices: N
Distribution: Manufacturer Direct

Dentifrice	Dental And Oral
Floss, Dental	Dental And Oral
Toothbrush, Manual	Dental And Oral
Toothbrush, Powered	Dental And Oral
Tray, Fluoride	Dental And Oral

ORAL-TX, LLC   **580-832-3058**
121 South Market, Cordell, OK 73632
FDA Number: 3004153280

Exerciser, Non-Measuring	Physical Med

ORALBOTIC RESEARCH, INC.   **760-743-5160**
701 South Andreasen Dr., Suite C, Escondido, CA 92029
FDA Number: 2032814

ORALBOTIC RESEARCH, INC.   **760-743-5160** *(cont'd)*

Toothbrush, Manual	Dental And Oral
Toothbrush, Powered	Dental And Oral

ORALGIENE USA, INC.   **800-933-6725**
8460 Higuera St., Culver City, CA 90232   **310-204-7888**
FDA Number: 2086150   *Fax:* 310-204-7893
E-mail: oralgiene@oralgiene.com
Web site: www.timemachinetoothbrush.com
Medical Products Sales Volume: $2,100,000
Annual Revenue: $10-$25 Million
Year Founded: 1999
Total Employees: 12   *Marketing Staff:* 2   *Sales Staff:* 10
Ownership: Private
Quality System Registration Information: ISO9001; ISO9002
Produces/Sells CE-marked Devices: Y
Federal Procurement Eligibility: Small Business
Distribution: Manufacturer Direct, Manufacturer Through Manufacturer Reps, Exporter
General Admin.: Paul Krok/President, Chief Executive Officer
Mktg./Adv.: Loren Krok/Director Product Development
    Ian Ellis/Manager National Sales
    Ian Ellis/Vice President Sales
Production: Marie Guirairdio/Manager Materials
    Paul Krok/Vice President Manufacturing

Scraper, Tongue	Dental And Oral
Toothbrush, Powered	Dental And Oral

ORAMAAX DENTAL PRODUCTS,INC.   **800-672-6229**
216 North Main St., Bldg A-1, Freeport, NY 11520   **516-771-8514**
FDA Number: 2436068   *Fax:* 516-771-8518
Web site: www.flosscard.com
Ownership: Private
Produces/Sells CE-marked Devices: N

Floss, Dental	Dental And Oral

ORAMETRIX INC.   **493-024-3091**
2350 Campbell Creek Blvd., Suite 400, Richardson, TX 75082
FDA Number: 1649995

Operative Dental Treatment Unit	Dental And Oral

ORANGE-SOL MEDICAL PRODUCTS, INC.   **800-877-7771**
1400 N. Fiesta Blvd. #100, Gilbert, AZ 85233   **480-497-8822**
FDA Number: n/a   *Fax:* 480-497-0444
E-mail: jerry@orange-sol.com
Web site: www.orange-sol.com
Annual Revenue: $10-$25 Million
Total Employees: 60   *Marketing Staff:* 4   *Sales Staff:* 4
Ownership: Private
Produces/Sells CE-marked Devices: N
Federal Procurement Eligibility: Small Business
Distribution: Manufacturer Direct, Manufacturer Through Distributor, Manufacturer Through Manufacturer Reps
General Admin.: A. Stephen Farnsworth/President, Chief Executive Officer
Mktg./Adv.: Mr. Jerry White/Vice President Sales
Production: Jack Farnsworth/Vice President Manufacturing

Bandage, Adhesive	Surgery
Bandage, Elastic	General
Dressing, Universal	General
Solution, Ostomy, Odor Control	Gastroenterology/Urology

ORAPHARMA, INC.   **215-956-2200**
732 Louis Drive, Warminster, PA 18974
FDA Number: 3003150799
Web site: www.jnj.com
Year Founded: 1996
Ownership: Johnson & Johnson
Produces/Sells CE-marked Devices: N
General Admin.: Russell Secter/President
    James Charnetski/Vice President
Production: John Lenart/Product Director

ORASURE TECHNOLOGIES, INC.   **610-882-1820**
1745 Eaton Ave., Bethlehem, PA 18018
FDA Number: 2528909   *Fax:* 503-643-2781
Web site: www.orasure.com
Medical Products Sales Volume: $4,819,000
Annual Revenue: $1-$5 Million
Year Founded: 2000
Total Employees: 85   *Marketing Staff:* 4   *Sales Staff:* 10
Ownership: ORASURE TECHNOLOGIES, INC.
Produces/Sells CE-marked Devices: N
Federal Procurement Eligibility: Small Business
Distribution: Manufacturer Direct, Manufacturer Through Distributor
General Admin.: J. Richard George/Chief Scientific Officer
    John Morgan/President, Chief Executive Officer
Mktg./Adv.: Ronald Mink/Director Product Development
    Angelica Nacrelli/Manager International & National Sales

ORASURE TECHNOLOGIES, INC.   610-882-1820 (cont'd)
Andrew S. Goldstein/Senior Vice President Product Development
Edward Collom/Vice President Marketing & Sales
Production: Michelle Rahm/Director Quality Assurance
     Quoc Pham/Manager Materials
     Joni Shimabukuro/Manager Regulatory Affairs
Finance: Charles Bergeron/Chief Financial Officer

Alcohol Dehydrogenase, Spec. Reagent - Ethanol Enzyme	Toxicology
Collector, Sputum	Anesthesiology
Cryosurgical Unit	Surgery
Enzyme Immunoassay, Amphetamine	Toxicology
Enzyme Immunoassay, Barbiturate	Toxicology
Enzyme Immunoassay, Benzodiazepine	Toxicology
Enzyme Immunoassay, Cannabinoids	Toxicology
Enzyme Immunoassay, Cocaine And Cocaine Metabolites	Toxicology
Enzyme Immunoassay, Methadone	Toxicology
Enzyme Immunoassay, Nicotine and Nicotine Metabolites	Toxicology
Enzyme Immunoassay, Opiates	Toxicology
Enzyme Immunoassay, Phencyclidine	Toxicology
Equipment, Test, Western Blot	Microbiology
Hexokinase, Glucose	Chemistry
Monitor, Test, Hiv-1	Hematology

ORASURE TECHNOLOGIES, INC.   800-869-3538
220 East First Street, Bethlehem, PA 18015   610-882-1820
FDA Number: 3004142665   Fax: 610-882-3572
E-mail: customerservice@orasure.com
Web site: www.orasure.com
Medical Products Sales Volume: $68,200,000
Annual Revenue: $50-$100 Million
Year Founded: 2000
Total Employees: 240
Ownership: Public
Stock Symbol: OSUR
Traded On: NASDAQ
Quality System Registration Information: ISO9000
Produces/Sells CE-marked Devices: Y
Federal Procurement Eligibility: Small Business
Distribution: Manufacturer Direct, Manufacturer Through Manufacturer Reps, Exporter
General Admin.: Ronald H. Spair/Chief Operating Officer, Chief Financial Officer
     Stephen R. Lee/Executive Vice President
     Douglas A. Michels/President, Chief Executive Officer
     Michael Gausling/President, Chief Executive Officer
     Wade Smedley/Vice President Human Resources
Mktg./Adv.: Lisa Botteri/Communication Specialist
     Brian Feeley/Director Sales
     William Zack/Executive Vice President Marketing
     Joseph E. Zack/Executive Vice President Marketing & Sales
     William Bruckner/Vice President Marketing
Production: P. Michael Formica/Executive Vice President Operations
Research: R. Sam Niedbala/Executive Vice President Research

Analyzer, Chemistry, Sequential Multiple, Continuous Flow	Chemistry
Container, Specimen, All Types	General
Cryosurgical Unit	Surgery
Enzyme Immunoassay, Amphetamine	Toxicology
Enzyme Immunoassay, Benzodiazepine	Toxicology
Enzyme Immunoassay, Cocaine And Cocaine Metabolites	Toxicology
Enzyme Immunoassay, Methadone	Toxicology
Enzyme Immunoassay, Nicotine and Nicotine Metabolites	Toxicology
Enzyme Immunoassay, Opiates	Toxicology
Enzyme Immunoassay, Other	Chemistry
Enzyme Immunoassay, Phencyclidine	Toxicology
Hexokinase, Glucose	Chemistry
Kit, Test, Saliva, Hiv-1&2	Hematology
Monitor, Test, Hiv-1	Hematology
System, Test, Drugs of Abuse	Chemistry
System, Test, Home, Hiv-1	Hematology

ORATECH, LLC   801-553-4493
475 West 10200 South, Salt Lake City, UT 84095
FDA Number: 3004977131

Cement, Dental	Dental And Oral
Cleanser, Root Canal	Dental And Oral
Detector, Caries	Dental And Oral
Liner, Cavity, Calcium Hydroxide	Dental And Oral
Material, Tooth Shade, Resin	Dental And Oral
Sealant, Pit And Fissure, And Conditioner, Resin	Dental And Oral
Zinc Oxide Eugenol	Dental And Oral

ORATRONICS, INC.   212-986-0050
405 Lexington Ave., New York, NY 10174
FDA Number: 2443020
Ownership: Private
Produces/Sells CE-marked Devices: N

Burr, Dental	Dental And Oral
Chisel, Osteotome, Surgical	Dental And Oral
Drill, Bone, Powered	Dental And Oral
Elevator, Surgical, Dental	Dental And Oral

ORATRONICS, INC.   212-986-0050 (cont'd)

Extractor, Nail	Orthopedics
Forceps, Rongeur, Surgical	Dental And Oral
Gauge, Depth, Instrument, Dental	Dental And Oral
Handle, Scalpel	Surgery
Hemostat, Surgical	Dental And Oral
Implant, Endosseous	Dental And Oral
Marker, Skin	Surgery
Pin, Retentive And Splinting	Dental And Oral
Pliers, Operative	Dental And Oral
Punch, Biopsy, Surgical	Dental And Oral
Retractor, Surgical	Surgery
Scalpel, One-Piece (Knife)	Surgery
Scissors, Surgical Tissue, Dental (Oral)	Dental And Oral
Splint, Endodontic Stabilizer	Dental And Oral

ORBECO ANALYTICAL SYSTEMS, INC.   800-922-5242
185 Marine St., Farmingdale, NY 11735-5609   631-293-4110
FDA Number: 9200529   Fax: 631-293-8258
E-mail: service@orbeco.com
Web site: www.orbeco.com
Annual Revenue: $1-$5 Million
Year Founded: 1985
Total Employees: 20
Ownership: Private
Produces/Sells CE-marked Devices: Y
Federal Procurement Eligibility: Small Business
General Admin.: John Esposito/Vice President, General Manager
Mktg./Adv.: Kay Patamapongse/Director Marketing
Production: Joe Del Casino/Manager Production

Colorimeter, General Use	Chemistry
Counter, Cell	Microbiology
Counter, Colony	Microbiology
Electrode, pH	Gastroenterology/Urology
Meter, pH, Portable	Chemistry
Nephelometer	Chemistry
Photometer	Chemistry
Solution, pH Buffer	Chemistry
Stain, Other	Pathology

ORBIS CORPORATION   800-890-7292
1055 Corporate Center Drive, PO Box 389,   262-560-5000
Oconomowoc, WI 53066
FDA Number: 9200646   Fax: 262-560-5841
E-mail: info@orbiscorporation.com
Web site: www.orbiscorporation.com
Medical Products Sales Volume: $63,800,000
Annual Revenue: $100-$500 Million
Year Founded: 2000
Total Employees: 150   Marketing Staff: 20   Sales Staff: 50
Ownership: Menasha Corp.
Quality System Registration Information: ISO9001
Produces/Sells CE-marked Devices: N
Federal Procurement Eligibility: Small Business, GSA Contract
Distribution: Manufacturer Direct, Manufacturer Through Distributor, Manufacturer Through Manufacturer Reps, Importer, Exporter
General Admin.: Jim Kotek/President
Mktg./Adv.: Jill Christian/Manager Health Care Marketing
     Samantha Goetz/Market Manager

Bin, Storage	General
Carrier, Container, Oxygen, Portable	General
Tray, Medicine	General

Medical Product Subsidiaries (Listed Separately)
Lewis Bins+

ORBITAL ENTERPRISES LLC   440-349-5100
6850 Cochran Rd., Solon, OH 44139
FDA Number: 3005128428

Exerciser, Powered	Anesthesiology

ORBUSNEICH MEDICAL, INC.   852-280-2228
5363 N.W. 35th Ave., Ft. Lauderdale, FL 33309-6315
FDA Number: 1064498   Fax: 954-730-7601
Web site: http://www.OrbusNeich.com
Ownership: Private
Produces/Sells CE-marked Devices: Y
General Admin.: Mr. Wayne Johnson/Chief Operating Officer
     Mr. Al Novak/President, Chief Executive Officer
Mktg./Adv.: Mr. David Camp/Vice President Corporate Development
     Mr. Samuel Rassmussen/Vice President Marketing & Sales
Production: Mr. Jim Clossick/Director Quality Assurance & Regulatory Affairs
Research: Dr. Steve Rowland/Vice President Research & Development

Catheter, Biliary	Gastroenterology/Urology
Stent, Cardiovascular	Cardiovascular

ORCHID DENTAL STUDIO, INC   469-619-2368
1101 E Plano Parkway, Suite J, Plano, TX 75074
FDA Number: 3005939057

ORCHID DENTAL STUDIO, INC
469-619-2368 *(cont'd)*
Teeth, Artificial, Posterior With Metal Insert
Dental And Oral

ORCHID MACDEE INC.
734-475-9165
13800 Luick Drive, Chelsea, MI 48118-9588
FDA Number: n/a
Fax: 734-475-3825
E-mail: info@macdeeinc.com
Web site: www.macdeeinc.com
Medical Products Sales Volume: $5,200,000
Annual Revenue: $5-$10 Million
Year Founded: 1987
Total Employees: 70
Ownership: Private
Quality System Registration Information: ISO9002
Produces/Sells CE-marked Devices: N
Federal Procurement Eligibility: Small Business
Distribution: OEM
General Admin.: Maynard Wellman/President
Mktg./Adv.: Bill Vrabel/Director Marketing & Sales
Mark Wellman/Vice President Marketing & Sales
Component, Other
General
Implant, Fixation Device, Proximal Femoral
Orthopedics

ORCHID STEALTH ORTHOPEDIC SOLUTIONS
517-694-2300
1489 Cedar St., Holt, MI 48842
FDA Number: n/a
Fax: 517-694-2340
E-mail: mike.miller@orchid-orthopedics.com
Web site: www.stealth-medical.com
Medical Products Sales Volume: $6,200,000
Annual Revenue: $25-$50 Million
Year Founded: 1992
Total Employees: 70
Marketing Staff: 2
Sales Staff: 2
Ownership: AbilityOne Products Corp.
Quality System Registration Information: ISO9001
Produces/Sells CE-marked Devices: N
Federal Procurement Eligibility: Small Business
Distribution: Manufacturer Direct
General Admin.: William Frey/Chief Operating Officer
Mr. Michael Miller/President, General Manager
Mktg./Adv.: Joe Zuzula/Director Sales
Prosthesis, Hip, Acetabular Component, Metal, Non-Cemented
Orthopedics
Prosthesis, Hip, Femoral Component, Cemented, Metal
Orthopedics
Prosthesis, Knee, Total
Orthopedics

ORCHID UNIQUE
989-746-0780
6688 Dixie Hwy., Bridgeport, MI 48722
FDA Number: n/a
Fax: 989-746-9004
E-mail: UniqueSales@orchid-orthopedics.com
Web site: www.orchid-orthopedics.com
Medical Products Sales Volume: $15,000,000
Annual Revenue: $10-$25 Million
Ownership: Private
Produces/Sells CE-marked Devices: N
Federal Procurement Eligibility: Small Business
Distribution: OEM
Contract Manufacturing
General
Kit, Instruments and Accessories, Surgical
Surgery

OREC CORP.
800-624-5517
7747 South West Citrrus Dr,
503-924-1945
Beaverton, OR 97008
FDA Number: n/a
Fax: 503-924-2032
E-mail: info@orec.com
Web site: www.orecpmsi.com
Annual Revenue: $1-$5 Million
Ownership: Private
Produces/Sells CE-marked Devices: N
Federal Procurement Eligibility: Small Business
Distribution: Manufacturer Through Distributor
Accessories, Apparel, Surgical
Surgery
Bracket, Metal, Orthodontic
Dental And Oral
Computer Software
General
Orthodontic Instrument
Dental And Oral

ORGAN RECOVERY SYSTEMS, INC.
847-824-2600
1 Pierce Place, Ste 475w, Itasca, IL 60143
FDA Number: 3004068499
Fax: 847-824-0234
E-mail: info@organ-recovery.com
Web site: www.organ-recovery.com
Ownership: Private
Produces/Sells CE-marked Devices: N
Kit, Perfusion, Kidney, Disposable
Gastroenterology/Urology
Perfusion System, Kidney
Gastroenterology/Urology

ORGANIC ESSENTIALS
800-765-6491
822 Baldridge St., O'Donnell, TX 79351
806-428-3486
FDA Number: 1648563
Fax: 806-428-3475
E-mail: info@organicessentials.com

ORGANIC ESSENTIALS
800-765-6491 *(cont'd)*
Web site: www.organicessentials.com
Medical Products Sales Volume: $400,000
Year Founded: 1995
Total Employees: 6
Ownership: Private
Produces/Sells CE-marked Devices: N
Federal Procurement Eligibility: Small Business
Tampon, Menstrual, Unscented
Obstetrics/Gynecology

ORGANICS CORPORATION OF AMERICA
973-890-9002
55 West End Road, Paterson, NJ 07512
FDA Number: 2218854
Bag, Drainage, Ostomy (With Adhesive)
General
Polyvinyl Methylether Maleic Acid-Calcium-Sodium Dbl. Salt
Dental And Oral

ORGANOGENESIS INC.
888-432-5232
150 Dan Road, Canton, MA 02021-2820
781-575-0775
FDA Number: 9008375
Fax: 781-575-1570
E-mail: hkeeping@organo.com
Web site: www.organogenesis.com
Medical Products Sales Volume: $13,700,000
Annual Revenue: $10-$25 Million
Year Founded: 1985
Total Employees: 300
Marketing Staff: 2
Sales Staff: 24
Ownership: Private
Produces/Sells CE-marked Devices: N
Federal Procurement Eligibility: Small Business
Distribution: Manufacturer Through Distributor
General Admin.: Geoff MacKay/President, Chief Executive Officer
Finance: Gary S. Gillheeney/Chief Financial Officer, Vice President Finance
Accessories, Extracorporeal System
Gastroenterology/Urology
Graft, Skin
Surgery
Graft, Vascular, Biological
Cardiovascular

ORGANOMATION ASSOCIATES, INC.
978-838-7300
266 River Road West, Berlin, MA 01503-1699
FDA Number: 2490343
Fax: 978-838-2786
E-mail: organomation@worldnet.att.net
Web site: www.organomation.com
Medical Products Sales Volume: $1,100,000
Annual Revenue: $1-$5 Million
Year Founded: 1959
Total Employees: 7
Marketing Staff: 1
Sales Staff: 2
Ownership: Private
Produces/Sells CE-marked Devices: Y
Federal Procurement Eligibility: Small Business
Distribution: Manufacturer Direct, Manufacturer Through Distributor, Manufacturer Through Manufacturer Reps
General Admin.: Andrew McNiven/President, General Manager
Mktg./Adv.: Heather King/Vice President, Manager Business
Production: Jeffrey King/Vice President Manufacturing
Bath, Portable
General
Evaporator
Chemistry
Extractor, Plasma
Hematology

ORGANON TEKNIKA CORP.
See Biomerieux Inc.

ORIDION MEDICAL INC.
888-674-3466
140 Towne& Country Drive, SuiteB,
925-362-0440
Danville, CA 94526
FDA Number: n/a
Fax: 925-362-0444
E-mail: luann.joy@oridion.com
Web site: www.oridion.com
Annual Revenue: $10-$25 Million
Total Employees: 150
Marketing Staff: 3
Sales Staff: 5
Ownership: ORIDION SYSTEMS LTD.
Quality System Registration Information: ISO9001
Produces/Sells CE-marked Devices: Y
Distribution: Manufacturer Direct, Manufacturer Through Distributor, OEM, Service Direct, Exporter
General Admin.: George Yariv/Chief Executive Officer
Walter Tabachnik/Chief Financial Officer, Vice President
Yacov Bubis/Chief Operating Officer, Vice President Operations
Pat Hennessey/General Manager
Mktg./Adv.: Tom Millonig/Director Marketing & Sales
Ephraim Carlebach/Director Product Development
Al Weirenga/Manager Marketing Research
LuAnn Joy/Vice President Marketing
Production: Chava Shamir/Director Quality Assurance
Shlomo Rvach/Manager Materials
Sandy Brown/Manager Regulatory Affairs
Research: Ron Shifron/Director Research & Development
Analyzer, Gas, Carbon-Dioxide, Gaseous Phase (Capnograph)
Anesthesiology
Computer, Patient Monitor
Anesthesiology

ORIEL INSTRUMENTS
See Thermo Oriel

ORIGEN BIOMEDICAL, INC.   512-474-7278
7000 Burleson Rd, Bldg D, Austin, TX 78744-3202
FDA Number: n/a   *Fax:* 512-708-8522
E-mail: dmartin@origen.com
Web site: www.origen.com
Annual Revenue: $1-$5 Million
Year Founded: 1990
Total Employees: 15
Ownership: Private
Quality System Registration Information: ISO9000
Produces/Sells CE-marked Devices: Y
Federal Procurement Eligibility: Small Business
Distribution: Manufacturer Direct, Manufacturer Through Distributor, OEM
General Admin.: Richard Martin/Managing Director
Production: Bo Johnson/Director Quality Assurance
Bag, Plastic   General
Catheter, Vascular, Cardiopulmonary Bypass   Cardiovascular
Equipment, Cryotherapy   Physical Med

ORIGINATOR CORPORATION   888-859-5031
832 NW First St., Fort Lauderdale, FL 33311   954-463-7231
FDA Number: n/a
E-mail: info@originatorcorp.com
Web site: www.originatorcorp.com
Annual Revenue: $0-$1 Million
Year Founded: 1974
Ownership: Private
Produces/Sells CE-marked Devices: N
Federal Procurement Eligibility: Small Business
Distribution: Manufacturer Direct, Importer, Exporter
Control, Foot Driving, Automobile, Mechanical   Physical Med
Control, Hand Driving, Automobile, Mechanical   Physical Med
Lift, Wheelchair   General

ORION DIAGNOSTICA, INC.
See Lifesign

ORION RESEARCH, INC.   800-225-1480
166 Cummings Center, Beverly, MA 01915   978-232-6000
FDA Number: n/a   *Fax:* 978-232-6015
E-mail: webmaster@orionres.com
Web site: www.thermo.com
Medical Products Sales Volume: $3,790,000
Annual Revenue: $50-$100 Million
Total Employees: 60   *Marketing Staff:* 15   *Sales Staff:* 40
Ownership: Private
Quality System Registration Information: ISO9001
Produces/Sells CE-marked Devices: N
Federal Procurement Eligibility: Small Business
Distribution: Manufacturer Through Distributor
General Admin.: Jim Barbookles/Chief Executive Officer
    Jim Barbookles/President, Chief Executive Officer
Mktg./Adv.: Jeff Cohen/Director Marketing
    Nick Toussi/Director Product Development
    Dave Ingalls/Manager Advertising
    Ron Breaux/Manager National Sales
    Richard Gentile/Vice President Business Development
    Jeff Cohen/Vice President Marketing
Production: Tom Paquette/Director Quality Assurance
    Tom Paquette/Manager Regulatory Affairs
    Chris McIntire/Vice President Manufacturing
Research: Steve West/Vice President Research & Development
Balance, Micro (0.001 mg Accuracy)   Chemistry
Buffer, pH   Hematology
Electrode, Ion Selective (Non-Specified)   Chemistry
Electrode, Ion Specific, Calcium   Chemistry
Electrode, Ion Specific, Chloride   Chemistry
Electrode, Ion Specific, Potassium   Chemistry
Electrode, Ion Specific, Sodium   Chemistry
Electrode, Ion Specific, Urea Nitrogen   Chemistry
Electrode, Laboratory pH   Chemistry
Electrode, Specific Ion   Chemistry
Electrode, pH   Gastroenterology/Urology
Meter, Conductivity   Chemistry
Meter, pH, Portable   Chemistry
Pump, Infusion, Laboratory   Chemistry
Pump, Infusion, Syringe   General
Solution, pH Buffer   Chemistry

ORMANTINE USA LTD.   321-676-7003
1740 Convair St, Palm-Bay, FL 32909
FDA Number: n/a   *Fax:* 321-676-7699
E-mail: sales@ormantineusa.com
Web site: www.ormantineusa.com
Annual Revenue: $0-$1 Million
Ownership: Gradko International Ltd.
Produces/Sells CE-marked Devices: N
Federal Procurement Eligibility: Small Business
Distribution: Manufacturer Through Distributor

ORMANTINE USA LTD.   321-676-7003 *(cont'd)*
Tubing, Connecting   General

ORMCO CORP.   800-672-5068
1332 S. Lone Hill Ave., Glendora, CA 91740   909-596-0100
FDA Number: 2024258   *Fax:* 909-962-5717
Ownership: Sybron Dental Specialties, Inc.
Produces/Sells CE-marked Devices: N
Band, Preformed, Orthodontic   Dental And Oral
Bracket, Metal, Orthodontic   Dental And Oral
Headgear, Extraoral, Orthodontic   Dental And Oral
Retainer, Screw Expansion, Orthodontic   Dental And Oral
Setter, Band, Orthodontic   Dental And Oral
Wire, Orthodontic   Dental And Oral

ORMCO CORP.
See Sybron Dental Specialties, Inc.

ORMED CORPORATION   800-440-2784
599 Cardigan Road, St. Paul, MN 55126
FDA Number: 2247872   *Fax:* 800-242-8329
E-mail: r.suddendorf@ormedusa.com
Web site: www.ormedusa.com
Annual Revenue: $1-$5 Million
Year Founded: 1992
Total Employees: 130
Ownership: ORMED GMBH
Produces/Sells CE-marked Devices: N
Federal Procurement Eligibility: Small Business
Distribution: Manufacturer Through Distributor
General Admin.: Phillip Vierling/Chief Executive Officer
    Rudiger Hausherr/President, Director
Mktg./Adv.: Frank Boemers/Director Marketing
    Rick Suddendorf/Manager National Sales
Exerciser, Passive, Measuring   Physical Med
Kit, Wound Dressing   Surgery

ORNIM INC.   866-811-6384
23462 Thornewood Dr, Santa Clara, CA 91321   661-310-0240
FDA Number: n/a
E-mail: info@ornim.com
Web site: http://www.ornim.com/
Year Founded: 2004
Ownership: Private
Produces/Sells CE-marked Devices: N
General Admin.: Mr. Yitzhak Zilberman/Chief Executive Officer
    Dr. Michal Balberg/Chief Technology Officer
Medical Admin.: Dr. Moshe Kamar/Vice President Medical Affairs
Research: Dr. Revital Shechter/Vice President Research & Development

OROX CORP.
See Merlyn Pharmaceuticals, Inc.

ORREX MEDICAL TECHNOLOGIES, LLP   940-458-7150
403 Acker St., Sanger, TX 76266
FDA Number: 3003962148
Ownership: Private
Produces/Sells CE-marked Devices: N
Saw, Powered, And Accessories   Cns/Neurology

ORTEC - (ADVANCED MEASUREMENT   800-251-9750
TECHNOLOGY)
801 S. Illinois Avenue, Oak Ridge, TN 37831   865-482-4411
FDA Number: n/a   *Fax:* 865-425-1380
E-mail: ortec.info@ametek.com
Web site: www.ortec-online.com
Annual Revenue: $50-$100 Million
Year Founded: 1960
Total Employees: 250   *Marketing Staff:* 3
Ownership: Ametek
Quality System Registration Information: ISO9002
Produces/Sells CE-marked Devices: Y
Federal Procurement Eligibility: Small Business
Distribution: Manufacturer Direct
General Admin.: Jon Kidder/President
Mktg./Adv.: Richard Bly/Director Marketing
    Sam Hitch/Director Product Development
    Barry Stanner/Manager National Sales
Counter, Radiation   Radiology

ORTHEON MEDICAL, LLC.   866-836-6349
777 West Swan Street, Columbus, OH 43212   407-671-2944
FDA Number: 3003745909   *Fax:* 407-671-2231
E-mail: sales@ortheon.com
Web site: www.ortheon.com
Medical Products Sales Volume: $5,000,000
Annual Revenue: $1-$5 Million
Year Founded: 1997
Total Employees: 13   *Marketing Staff:* 2   *Sales Staff:* 5

ORTHEON MEDICAL, LLC. 866-836-6349 (cont'd)
Ownership: Private
Quality System Registration Information: ISO9001
Produces/Sells CE-marked Devices: Y
Distribution: Manufacturer Direct, Manufacturer Through Distributor, Exporter
Suture, Non-Absorbable, Steel, Monofilament & Multifilament   Surgery

ORTHESE PROTHESE RIVE SUD INC. 450-672-0078
127 rue St-Louis, Ville Lemoyne, QUE J4R-2L3 Canada
FDA Number: n/a   *Fax:* 450-672-9144
E-mail: info@oprivesud.com
Web site: www.oprivesud.com
Year Founded: 1981
Total Employees: 25
Ownership: Private
Produces/Sells CE-marked Devices: N
Distribution: Manufacturer Direct, Exclusive Distributor

ORTHO ACTIVE APPLIANCES LTD. 800-663-1254
103-250 Schoolhouse St.,   604-520-3414
Coquitlam, BC V3K 6 Canada
FDA Number: 8022022
E-mail: sales@orthoactive.com   *Fax:* 604-520-1193
Web site: www.orthoactive.com
Year Founded: 1983
Total Employees: 23   *Marketing Staff:* 2   *Sales Staff:* 4
Ownership: Private
Produces/Sells CE-marked Devices: N
Federal Procurement Eligibility: Small Business
Distribution: Manufacturer Direct, Manufacturer Through Distributor, Exclusive
Distributor, Importer, Exporter

ORTHO CLINICAL DIAGNOSTICS, INC. 800-828-6316
100 Indigo Creek Dr., Rochester, NY 14650   716-453-3000
FDA Number: 1319681
Web site: www.orthoclinical.com   *Fax:* 585-453-3660
Annual Revenue: $0-$1 Million
Year Founded: 1937
Total Employees: 1000
Ownership: JOHNSON & JOHNSON
Stock Symbol: JNJ
Traded On: NYSE
Produces/Sells CE-marked Devices: N
General Admin.: Elaine J. Thibodeau/General Manager
                 Clifford E. Holland/President
                 Stuart J. Magloff/Vice President
Production: John Gethin/Plant Manager
            Paul J. Testa/Plant Manager
Calibrator, Secondary, Clinical Chemistry   Chemistry
Enzyme Immunoassay, Diphenylhydantoin   Toxicology
System, Automated, Microbiological   Microbiology

ORTHO CONCEPT INC. 450-973-6700
2101, boul Le Carrefour, suite 100, Laval, QUE H7S 2J7 Canada
FDA Number: n/a   *Fax:* 450-973-3848
E-mail: info@orthoconcept
Web site: www.orthoconcept.com
Year Founded: 1988
Ownership: Private
Produces/Sells CE-marked Devices: N
Distribution: Manufacturer Direct, Exclusive Distributor

ORTHO DERMATOLOGICS 310-642-1150
5760 W. 96th St., Los Angeles, CA 90045-5544
FDA Number: 3004950073   *Fax:* 310-337-5556
Web site: www.orthoneutrogena.com
Year Founded: 1930
Ownership: Johnson & Johnson
Produces/Sells CE-marked Devices: N
General Admin.: Leela Petrakis/General Manager
                 Jim Colleran/President
Lotion, Skin Care   General

ORTHO DEVELOPMENT CORP. 800-429-8339
12187 S. Business Park. Drive, Draper, UT 84020 801-553-9991
FDA Number: 1722511   *Fax:* 801-553-9993
E-mail: info@orthodevelopment.com
Web site: www.orthodevelopment.com
Medical Products Sales Volume: $26,800,000
Annual Revenue: $10-$25 Million
Year Founded: 1994
Total Employees: 65   *Marketing Staff:* 5   *Sales Staff:* 9
Ownership: Japan Medical Dynamic Marketing, Inc.
Quality System Registration Information: ISO9000; ISO9001
Produces/Sells CE-marked Devices: N
Federal Procurement Eligibility: Small Business

ORTHO DEVELOPMENT CORP. 800-429-8339 (cont'd)
Distribution: Manufacturer Direct, Manufacturer Through Distributor, OEM,
Exclusive Distributor, Exporter
General Admin.: Masao Okawa/President, Chief Executive Officer
Mktg./Adv.: Mike Kaufman/Vice President Marketing & Product Development
            Ross Chamberlain/Vice President Sales
Production: Randy Wheeland/Director Quality Assurance & Regulatory Affairs
Finance: Brent Bartholomew/Chief Financial Officer
Board, Bed   General
Holder, Needle, Other   Surgery
Instrument, Microsurgical   Cns/Neurology
Joint, Hip, External Limb Component   Physical Med
Prosthesis, Hip, Hemi-, Femoral, Metal/Polymer   Orthopedics
Prosthesis, Knee, Total   Orthopedics
Stereotaxy Equipment   Cns/Neurology
Surgical Instrument, Orthopedic, AC-Powered Motor   Orthopedics
System, Appliance, Fixation, Spinal Pedicle Screw   Orthopedics

ORTHO DIAGNOSTICS
See Meridian Bioscience, Inc.

ORTHO INNOVATIONS, INC. 507-269-2895
121 23rd Ave. Southwest, Rochester, MN 55902
FDA Number: 3006337256
Joint, Knee, External Brace   Physical Med
Lift, Bath, Non-AC-Powered   General
Orthosis, Limb Brace   Physical Med
Pylon, Post Surgical   Physical Med
Splint, Abduction, Congenital Hip Dislocation   Physical Med

ORTHO KINETICS CORP. 512-334-5490
7004 Bee Cave Road, Building III, Suite 315, Austin, TX 78746
FDA Number: 2029096
Web site: http://www.orthokinematics.com
Ownership: Private
Produces/Sells CE-marked Devices: N
General Admin.: Mr. Adam Deitz/Chief Executive Officer
Medical Admin.: Mr. Ken Walker/Director Clinical Affairs
Mktg./Adv.: Mr. David Muller/Vice President Sales
Finance: Mr. John Rodakis/Chief Financial Officer
Band, Elastic, Orthodontic   Dental And Oral
Headgear, Extraoral, Orthodontic   Dental And Oral

ORTHO MCNEIL JANSSEN 800-526-7736
PHARMACEUTICALS, INC.
1125 Trenton-Harbourton Road, P.O. Box 200,   908-218-6811
Titusville, NJ 08560
FDA Number: 3007024659   *Fax:* 732-302-0425
Web site: www.orthomcneil.com
Total Employees: 1300
Ownership: Johnson & Johnson
Produces/Sells CE-marked Devices: N
General Admin.: Jeffrey N. Smith/President
                 Seth H.Z. Fischer/President

ORTHO ORGANIZERS, INC. 760-448-8730
1822 Aston Avenue, Carlsbad, CA 92008
FDA Number: 2081322
Adhesive, Bracket And Conditioner, Resin   Dental And Oral
Band, Elastic, Orthodontic   Dental And Oral
Band, Preformed, Orthodontic   Dental And Oral
Bracket, Ceramic, Orthodontic   Dental And Oral
Bracket, Metal, Orthodontic   Dental And Oral
Bracket, Plastic, Orthodontic   Dental And Oral
Clamp, Wire, Orthodontic   Dental And Oral
Face Bow   Dental And Oral
Headgear, Extraoral, Orthodontic   Dental And Oral
Implant, Endosseous   Dental And Oral
Pliers, Orthodontic   Dental And Oral
Retainer, Screw Expansion, Orthodontic   Dental And Oral
Spring, Orthodontic   Dental And Oral
Tray, Impression   Dental And Oral
Tube, Orthodontic   Dental And Oral
Tucker, Ligature, Orthodontic   Dental And Oral
Wax, Dental   Dental And Oral
Wire, Orthodontic   Dental And Oral

ORTHO PHARMACEUTICAL CORPORATION
See Ortho-Mcneil-Janssen Pharmaceuticals, Inc.

ORTHO-CLINICAL DIAGNOSTICS, INC. 585-453-3768
100 Indigo Creek Dr., Rochester, NY 14626
FDA Number: 1319681
Web site: www.orthoclinical.com
Year Founded: 1937
Total Employees: 1000
Ownership: Johnson & Johnson
Produces/Sells CE-marked Devices: N
General Admin.: Elaine J. Thibodeau/General Manager
                 Clifford E. Holland/President

ORTHO-CLINICAL DIAGNOSTICS, INC.   585-453-3768 *(cont'd)*
Stuart J. Magloff/Vice President
Production: John Gethin/Plant Manager
Paul J. Testa/Plant Manager

Analyzer, Chemistry, Photometric, Discrete	Chemistry
Fluorometer, Chemistry	Chemistry

ORTHO-CLINICAL DIAGNOSTICS, INC.   800-828-6316
100 Indigo Creek Dr., Room 350,   **716-453-3000**
Rochester, NY 14650
FDA Number: 3003935657   Fax: 585-453-3660
Web site: www.orthoclinical.com
Year Founded: 1937
Ownership: Johnson & Johnson
Produces/Sells CE-marked Devices: N
General Admin.: Elaine J. Thibodeau/General Manager
Clifford E Holland/President
Stuart J. Magloff/Vice President
Production: John Gethin/Plant Manager
Paul J. Testa/Plant Manager

Reagents, Specific, Analyte	Hematology

ORTHO-CLINICAL DIAGNOSTICS, INC.   585-453-3768
1000 Lee Rd., Rochester, NY 14606
FDA Number: 1319808
Web site: www.orthoclinical.com
Year Founded: 1937
Total Employees: 1000
Ownership: Johnson & Johnson
Produces/Sells CE-marked Devices: N
General Admin.: Elaine J. Thibodeau/General Manager
Clifford E. Holland/President
Stuart J. Magloff/Vice President
Production: John Gethin/Plant Manager
Paul J. Testa/Plant Manager

Analyzer, Chemistry, Photometric, Discrete	Chemistry
Electrode, Ion Specific, Potassium	Chemistry
Enzymatic Esterase-Oxidase, Cholesterol	Chemistry
Fluorometer, Chemistry	Chemistry
Nephelometric Method, Immunoglobulins (G, A, M)	Chemistry
Vanillin Pyruvate, AST/SGOT	Chemistry

ORTHO-CLINICAL DIAGNOSTICS, INC.   800-828-6316
513 Technology Blvd., Rochester, NJ 14626   **716-453-3000**
FDA Number: 1319809   Fax: 585-453-3660
Web site: www.orthoclinical.com
Year Founded: 1937
Ownership: Johnson & Johnson
Produces/Sells CE-marked Devices: N
General Admin.: Elaine J. Thibodeau/General Manager
Elaine J. Holland/President
Stuart J. Magloff/Vice President
Production: John Gethin/Plant Manager
Paul J. Testa/Plant Manager

Analyzer, Chemistry, Photometric, Discrete	Chemistry
Antigen, Antiserum, Control, Whole Human Serum	Immunology
Centrifuge, Blood Bank, Diagnostic	Hematology
Centrifuge, Cell Washing, Automated, Immuno-Hematology	Hematology
Colorimeter, General Use	Chemistry
Diluent, Blood Cell	Hematology
Electrode, Ion Specific, Potassium	Chemistry
Fluid, Red Cell Diluting	Hematology
Incubator/Water Bath, Microbiology	Microbiology
Kit, Quality Control, Blood Banking	Hematology
Labware, Blood Collection	Chemistry
Lectins/Protectins	Hematology
Lipase Hydrolysis/Glycerol Kinase Enzyme, Triglycerides	Chemistry
Media, Potentiating	Hematology
NAD Reduction/NADH Oxidation, Lactate Dehydrogenase	Chemistry
Pipetting And Diluting System, Automated	Chemistry
Software, Blood Bank (Stand-Alone Products)	Hematology
Supplies, Blood Bank	Hematology
System, Surgical, Computer Controlled Instrument	Surgery
Test, Fetal Hemoglobin	Hematology
Test, Sickle Cell	Hematology
Urease, Photometric, Urea Nitrogen	Chemistry

ORTHO-CLINICAL DIAGNOSTICS, INC.   908-218-8177
Route 202, Raritan, NJ 08869
FDA Number: 2250051
Web site: www.orthoclinical.com
Annual Revenue: $0-$1 Million
Year Founded: 1937
Total Employees: 1000
Ownership: Johnson & Johnson
Produces/Sells CE-marked Devices: N
General Admin.: Elaine J. Thibodeau/General Manager
Clifford E. Holland/President
Charlie Raffin/Vice President

ORTHO-CLINICAL DIAGNOSTICS, INC.   908-218-8177 *(cont'd)*
Stuart J. Magloff/Vice President
Production: John Gethin/Plant Manager
Paul J. Testa/Plant Manager

Analyzer, Chemistry, Photometric, Discrete	Chemistry
Fluorometer, Chemistry	Chemistry

ORTHO-CYCLE CO., INC.   800-82-CYCLE
2026 Scott St., Hollywood, FL 33020   **954-920-9074**
FDA Number: 1052235   Fax: 954-921-4174
E-mail: OrthoCycle@aol.com
Web site: www.OrthoCycle.com
Year Founded: 1976
Total Employees: 33   *Marketing Staff:* 1   *Sales Staff:* 2
Ownership: Private
Quality System Registration Information: ISO9002
Produces/Sells CE-marked Devices: Y
Federal Procurement Eligibility: Small Business
Distribution: Service Direct
General Admin.: Claude Matasa/Owner
Eugenia Matasa/Owner

Service, Maintenance/Repair	General

ORTHO-KINETICS, INC.   800-824-1068
W194 N11301 McCormick Drive,   **262.250.7740**
Germantown, WI 53022
FDA Number: n/a   Fax: 262.250.7741
E-mail: Sales@EK-Tech.com
Web site: http://www.orthokinetics.com
Medical Products Sales Volume: $11,000,000
Annual Revenue: $10-$25 Million
Ownership: Private
Produces/Sells CE-marked Devices: N
Distribution: Manufacturer Direct, Manufacturer Through Distributor, Manufacturer Through Manufacturer Reps, OEM, Service Direct, Exclusive Distributor, Importer, Exporter

Chair, Rehabilitation	General
Component, Electrical	General
Scooter (Motorized 3-Wheeled Vehicle)	Physical Med

ORTHO-MCNEIL-JANSSEN PHARMACEUTICALS, INC.   800-526-7736
1000 U.S. Route 202 South, Raritan, NJ 08869   **(908) 722-5393**
FDA Number: 2211100   Fax: 732-302-0425
Web site: www.orthmcneil.com
Annual Revenue: $0-$1 Million
Total Employees: 1300   *Marketing Staff:* 26   *Sales Staff:* 32
Ownership: Johnson & Johnson
Produces/Sells CE-marked Devices: Y
Distribution: Manufacturer Direct
General Admin.: Jeffrey N. Smith/President
Seth H.Z. Fischer/President

Applicator, Vaginal	Obstetrics/Gynecology
Diaphragm, Contraceptive	Obstetrics/Gynecology
Intrauterine Device, Contraceptive (IUD) And Introducer	Obstetrics/Gynecology

ORTHO-MED INTL., INC.   760-357-5040
357-a West 2nd St., Calexico, CA 92231-2114
FDA Number: 2031967
Ownership: Private
Produces/Sells CE-marked Devices: N

Pliers, Orthodontic	Dental And Oral
Tucker, Ligature, Orthodontic	Dental And Oral

ORTHO-MED, INC.   800-547-5571
3208 S.E. 13th Ave., Portland, OR 97202-2407   **503-234-9691**
FDA Number: 3019455   Fax: 503-234-8629
E-mail: custserv@orthomedinc.com
Web site: www.orthomedinc.com
Annual Revenue: $1-$5 Million
Year Founded: 1970
Total Employees: 11
Ownership: Private
Produces/Sells CE-marked Devices: N
Federal Procurement Eligibility: Small Business, Female Owned
Distribution: Manufacturer Direct, Manufacturer Through Distributor, Manufacturer Through Manufacturer Reps
General Admin.: Ronald S. Dyches/Chief Executive Officer

Applier, Cast	Orthopedics
Bandage, Elastic	General
Cane	Physical Med
Cast	Orthopedics
Crutch	Physical Med
Instrument, Microsurgical	Cns/Neurology
Material, Casting	Dental And Oral
Orthopedic Manual Surgical Instrument	Orthopedics
Orthosis, Other	Physical Med
Pack, Hot Or Cold, Disposable	Physical Med

ORTHO-MED, INC.   800-547-5571 *(cont'd)*

Sphygmomanometer, Aneroid (Arterial Pressure)	General
Spreader, Plaster (Cast)	Orthopedics
Stand, Casting	Orthopedics
Surgical Instrument, Cardiovascular	Cardiovascular

ORTHO-TAIN, INC.   800-541-6612

Carr 861, K.m. 5.0, Barrio, Pinas,   **847-446-7601**
Toa Alta, PR 00953
FDA Number: 2649784
Fax: 847-446-7606
E-mail: info@orthotain.com
Web site: www.orthotain.com
Ownership: Private
Produces/Sells CE-marked Devices: N

Band, Material, Orthodontic	Dental And Oral
Band, Preformed, Orthodontic	Dental And Oral
Wire, Orthodontic	Dental And Oral

ORTHO-TEC LIMITED   905-571-3633

585 Wentworth St. E #31, Oshawa, ONT L1H-3V8 Canada
FDA Number: n/a
Fax: 905-571-7364
Year Founded: 1978
Ownership: Private
Produces/Sells CE-marked Devices: N
Distribution: Manufacturer Direct

ORTHO/MCNEIL PHARM.

See Ortho-Mcneil-Janssen Pharmaceuticals, Inc.

ORTHOACCEL TECHNOLOGIES INC.   832-631-1659

8275 El Rio, Suite 100, Houston, TX 77054
FDA Number: n/a
Fax: 713-583-9972
E-mail: info@orthoaccel.com
Web site: www.orthoaccel.com
Ownership: Private
Produces/Sells CE-marked Devices: N
General Admin.: Mr. Michael Lowe/Chief Executive Officer
Mktg./Adv.: Mr. Michael Kauffman/Vice President Business Development
Production: Mr. Lawrance Swol/Vice President Operations
Finance: Ms. Pamela Westbrook/Chief Financial Officer

Orthodontic Instrument	Dental And Oral

ORTHOBAND COMPANY, INC.   800-325-9973

3690 Hwy. M, Imperial, MO 63052   **314-942-3133**
FDA Number: 9320123
Fax: 636-948-3152
E-mail: anna@barnhartindustries.com
Web site: www.orthoband.com
Medical Products Sales Volume: $400,000
Annual Revenue: $0-$1 Million
Year Founded: 1957
Total Employees: 15   *Marketing Staff:* 2   *Sales Staff:* 2
Ownership: Private
Produces/Sells CE-marked Devices: Y
Federal Procurement Eligibility: Small Business
Distribution: Manufacturer Through Distributor, Exporter
General Admin.: Anna Boehm/President, General Manager
Production: Brenda Marler/Vice President Manufacturing

Band, Elastic, Orthodontic	Dental And Oral
Headgear, Extraoral, Orthodontic	Dental And Oral
Orthodontic Instrument	Dental And Oral
Pad, Pressure, Foam (Elbow, Heel)	General
Restraint, Patient, Conductive	Anesthesiology
Safety Equipment, Laboratory	Chemistry
Spring, Orthodontic	Dental And Oral

ORTHOCANADA MEDICAL PRODUCTS   800-561-0310

37 Katimavik Rd.,   **819-671-3399**
Val-des-Monts, QUE J8N-5 Canada
FDA Number: n/a
Fax: 819-671-7847
E-mail: mail@orthocanada.com
Web site: www.orthocanada.com
Year Founded: 1989
Total Employees: 25
Ownership: Private
Produces/Sells CE-marked Devices: N
Distribution: Manufacturer Direct, Exclusive Distributor, Importer

ORTHOCARE INNOVATIONS, LLC   425-771-0797

6405 218th Ave. Sw, Suite 100, Mountlake Ter, WA 98043
FDA Number: 3004623408
E-mail: info@orthocareinnovations.com
Web site: www.orthocareinnovations.com
Ownership: Private
Produces/Sells CE-marked Devices: N
General Admin.: Mr. Doug McCormack/Chief Executive Officer
     Mr. David Adams/Chief Operating Officer
     Dr. David Boone/Chief Technology Officer
Mktg./Adv.: Mr. Stephen Jacobs/Vice President Marketing & Sales

ORTHOCARE INNOVATIONS, LLC   425-771-0797 *(cont'd)*

Isokinetic Testing And Evaluation System	Physical Med

ORTHOCON, INC.   888-445-6784

1 Bridge Street, Suite 121, Irvington, NY 10533
FDA Number: 3005972619
Fax: 914-231-7884
E-mail: info@ORTHOCON.com
Web site: http://www.orthocon.com
Ownership: Private
Produces/Sells CE-marked Devices: N
General Admin.: Dr. Richard Kronenthal/Chief Scientific Officer
     Mr. John Pacifico/President, Chief Executive Officer
Production: Mr. Brian Kunst/Vice President Quality Assurance & Regulatory Affairs
Research: Dr. David Knaack/Vice President Product Development

Wax, Bone	Surgery

ORTHODENTAL INTL., INC   760-357-8070

280 avenida campillo ste m, Calexico, CA 92231
FDA Number: 2086211
Web site: www.dentsply.com
Ownership: Dentsply International, Inc.
Stock Symbol: XRAY
Traded On: NASDAQ
Produces/Sells CE-marked Devices: N

ORTHODENTAL S.A. DE C.V.   011-526-5611

Calle Industria Del Acero 18, Parque Industrial El Vigia,
Mexicali 21397 Mexico
FDA Number: 9680786

Pliers, Orthodontic	Dental And Oral

ORTHODONTIC DESIGN AND PRODUCTION, INC. 760-734-3995

1370 Decision Street, Suite D, Vista, CA 92081
FDA Number: 2029191

Adhesive, Bracket And Conditioner, Resin	Dental And Oral
Aligner, Bracket, Orthodontic	Dental And Oral
Band, Elastic, Orthodontic	Dental And Oral
Band, Preformed, Orthodontic	Dental And Oral
Bracket, Ceramic, Orthodontic	Dental And Oral
Bracket, Metal, Orthodontic	Dental And Oral
Headgear, Extraoral, Orthodontic	Dental And Oral
Material, Impression	Dental And Oral
Pliers, Orthodontic	Dental And Oral
Pusher, Band, Orthodontic	Dental And Oral
Setter, Band, Orthodontic	Dental And Oral
Spring, Orthodontic	Dental And Oral
Tube, Orthodontic	Dental And Oral
Tucker, Ligature, Orthodontic	Dental And Oral
Wire, Orthodontic	Dental And Oral

ORTHODONTIC INTERNATIONAL SERVICES

See Sc/Ois Orthodontics

ORTHODONTIC SUPPLY & EQUIPMENT   800-638-4003
CO., INC.

7851 Airpark Road, Unit 202,   **301-869-3801**
Gaithersburg, MD 20879
FDA Number: 1121924
Fax: 301-869-3800
E-mail: osecoinc@aol.com
Web site: http://osecompany.com/
Medical Products Sales Volume: $2,500,000
Annual Revenue: $1-$5 Million
Year Founded: 1975
Total Employees: 11   *Sales Staff:* 6
Ownership: Private
Produces/Sells CE-marked Devices: N
Federal Procurement Eligibility: Small Business, GSA Contract
Distribution: Manufacturer Through Distributor, Importer, Exporter
General Admin.: C. Richard McAlister/President, Chief Executive Officer
     Richard R. McAlister/Vice President, General Manager
Mktg./Adv.: Richard R. McAlister/Vice President Sales

Bracket, Metal, Orthodontic	Dental And Oral
Disinfector, Liquid	General
Film, X-Ray, Dental, Extraoral	Dental And Oral
Film, X-Ray, Dental, Intraoral	Dental And Oral
Orthodontic Instrument	Dental And Oral
Protector, Mouth Guard	Dental And Oral
Soap	General
Toothbrush, Manual	Dental And Oral
Wire, Orthodontic	Dental And Oral

ORTHODONTIC TECHNOLOGIES, INC.   800-346-5133

5524 Cornish, Houston, TX 77007   **713-861-0033**
FDA Number: 3003065956
Fax: 713-861-0273
E-mail: custserv@orthodontictechnologies.com
Web site: www.orthodontictechnologies.com
Ownership: Private
Produces/Sells CE-marked Devices: N

ORTHODONTIC TECHNOLOGIES, INC.   800-346-5133 *(cont'd)*
Device, Anti-Snoring   Ear/Nose/Throat

ORTHOFAB INC.   800-463-5293
2160 rue de Celles,   **418-847-5225**
Quebec, QUE G2C-1 Canada
FDA Number: n/a   Fax: 418-847-5378
E-mail: admini@orthofab.com
Year Founded: 1986
Total Employees: 100
Ownership: Private
Produces/Sells CE-marked Devices: N
Distribution: Manufacturer Direct

ORTHOFIX
See Orthofix Inc.

ORTHOFIX INC.   1.800.527.0404
3451 Plano Parkway, Lewisville, TX 75056   **1.214.937.2000**
FDA Number: 3008524126
E-mail: customerservice@orthofix.com
Web site: www.orthofix.com
Year Founded: 1980
Total Employees: 200   *Marketing Staff:* 20   *Sales Staff:* 140
Ownership: Public
Stock Symbol: OFIX
Traded On: NASDAQ
Produces/Sells CE-marked Devices: N
Federal Procurement Eligibility: Small Business
Distribution: Manufacturer Through Distributor, Manufacturer Through Manufacturer Reps
General Admin.: Charlie Federico/Chief Executive Officer
Mktg./Adv.: Ellen Worsham/Director Marketing Communications
     Eric Brown/Senior Vice President Marketing & Sales

Accessories, Operating Room, Table	Surgery
Appliance, Fix., Nail/Blade/Plate Comb., Multiple Component	Orthopedics
Appliance, Fixation, Spinal Interlaminal	Orthopedics
Appliance, Fixation, Spinal Intervertebral Body	Orthopedics
Arthroscope	Orthopedics
Awl	Orthopedics
Belt, Traction, Pelvic, Orthopedic	Orthopedics
Bender	Orthopedics
Bit, Drill	Orthopedics
Cannula, Surgical, General & Plastic Surgery	Surgery
Catheter, Suction, With Tip	General
Component, Traction, Invasive	Orthopedics
Curette, Surgical	Surgery
Cutter, Surgical	Surgery
Dissector, Surgical, General & Plastic Surgery	Surgery
Driver, Prosthesis	Orthopedics
Electrotherapeutic Unit	General
Elevator, Surgical, General & Plastic Surgery	Surgery
Fixation Appliance, Multiple Component	Orthopedics
Fixation Device, Spinal (External)	Orthopedics
Guide, Surgical, Instrument	Surgery
Hammer, Surgical	Surgery
Handle, Scalpel	Surgery
Hook, Surgical, General & Plastic Surgery	Surgery
Impactor	Orthopedics
Mallet, Other	Surgery
Orthopedic Manual Surgical Instrument	Orthopedics
Orthosis, Fixation, Pedicle, Spinal	Orthopedics
Orthosis, Fixation, Spinal, Spondylolisthesis	Orthopedics
Orthosis, Fusion, Intervertebral, Spinal	Orthopedics
Pin, Fixation, Threaded	Orthopedics
Plate, Fixation, Bone	Orthopedics
Probe	Orthopedics
Pusher, Socket	Orthopedics
Rasp, Other	Surgery
Retractor	Orthopedics
Rod, Fixation, Intramedullary	Orthopedics
Rongeur, Other	Surgery
Screw, Fixation, Bone	Orthopedics
Screwdriver	Orthopedics
Spatula, Orthopedic	Orthopedics
Stimulator, Growth, Bone, Non-Invasive	Orthopedics
Stimulator, Osteogenesis, Electric, Non-Invasive	Orthopedics
Stylet, Surgical	Surgery
Surgical Instrument, Sonic	Orthopedics
System, Extraction, Cement Removal	Orthopedics
Tamp	Orthopedics
Tap, Bone	Orthopedics
Tape, Measuring, Ruler And Caliper	Surgery
Template	Orthopedics
Tray, Surgical	Surgery
Wrench	Orthopedics

ORTHOGENESIS, INC.   530-672-8560
4315 Product Drive, #c, Cameron Park, CA 95682
FDA Number: 3004490114
Ownership: Private

ORTHOGENESIS, INC.   530-672-8560 *(cont'd)*
Produces/Sells CE-marked Devices: N
Impactor   Orthopedics
Reamer   Orthopedics

ORTHOHELIX SURGICAL DESIGNS, INC.   1-866-90-HELIX
1065 Medina Rd, Ste 500, Medina, OH 44256   **330-869-9582**
FDA Number: 3005039508
E-mail: info@orthohelix.com
Web site: www.orthohelix.com
Ownership: Private
Produces/Sells CE-marked Devices: N
Orthopedic Manual Surgical Instrument   Orthopedics
Plate, Fixation, Bone   Orthopedics
Screw, Fixation, Bone   Orthopedics

ORTHOLINE   800-243-3351
13 Chapel St., Norwalk, CT 06850-4113   **203-854-0400**
FDA Number: 1220853   Fax: 203-854-9141
E-mail: ortholinemail@aol.com
Web site: ortholine.net
Annual Revenue: $1-$5 Million
Year Founded: 1979
Total Employees: 10   *Sales Staff:* 6
Ownership: Private
Produces/Sells CE-marked Devices: N
Federal Procurement Eligibility: Small Business
Distribution: Manufacturer Through Manufacturer Reps, Exclusive Distributor
General Admin.: Paul Hefele/President, Chief Operating Officer

Accessories, Traction	Physical Med
Bandage, Elastic	General
Belt, Traction, Pelvic	Physical Med
Binder, Abdominal	General
Collar, Cervical Neck	Orthopedics
Compress, Cold	General
Halter, Head, Traction	Physical Med
Immobilizer, Knee	Orthopedics
Joint, Knee, External Brace	Physical Med
Orthosis, Limb Brace	Physical Med
Orthosis, Other	Physical Med
Shoe, Cast	Physical Med
Shoe, Operating Room	Surgery
Shoe, Orthopedic	Orthopedics
Sling, Arm	Physical Med
Splint, Clavicle	Physical Med
Splint, Hand, And Component	Physical Med
Splint, Other	Orthopedics
Stocking, Elastic	General
Support, Arm	Physical Med
Support, Back	Orthopedics
Traction Unit, Non-Powered	Orthopedics

ORTHOLOGIC CANADA   602-286-5520
901 Dillingham Rd, Pickering L1W 2Y5 Canada
FDA Number: 9615317
Exerciser, Finger, Powered   Physical Med
Exerciser, Powered   Anesthesiology

ORTHOLOGIC CORP.
See Capstone Therapeutics

ORTHOMED PRODUCTS, INC.   800-338-8512
12150 Charles Drive, #5, Grass Valley, CA 95945   **530-477-8450**
FDA Number: n/a   Fax: 530-477-8349
E-mail: aquashield@orthomed.net
Web site: www.aquashieldusa.com
Medical Products Sales Volume: $400,000
Annual Revenue: $0-$1 Million
Total Employees: 6
Ownership: Private
Produces/Sells CE-marked Devices: Y
Federal Procurement Eligibility: Small Business
Distribution: Manufacturer Direct, Manufacturer Through Distributor, Manufacturer Through Manufacturer Reps, OEM
General Admin.: Bruce Renfrew/Chief Executive Officer
Mktg./Adv.: Caryn McQueen/Vice President Marketing
Cover, Cast   General

ORTHOMERICA PRODUCTS, INC.   800-446-6770
6333 N. Orange Blossom Trl., Suite 220,   **407-290-6592**
Orlando, FL 32810
FDA Number: 1058152   Fax: 407-290-2419
E-mail: custserv@orthomerica.com
Web site: www.orthomerica.com
Annual Revenue: $10-$25 Million
Year Founded: 1989
Total Employees: 90
Ownership: Private
Quality System Registration Information: ISO9001

MANUFACTURER PROFILES

ORTHOMERICA PRODUCTS, INC.　800-446-6770 (cont'd)
Produces/Sells CE-marked Devices: Y
Federal Procurement Eligibility: Small Business
Distribution: Manufacturer Direct, Manufacturer Through Distributor, Manufacturer Through Manufacturer Reps
General Admin.: David Kerr/Chief Executive Officer
Mktg./Adv.: Bill Gustanson/Director Marketing
　　　　Jack Walker/Manager National Sales
Production: Shannon Schwenn/Vice President Manufacturing
　Orthosis, Cranial　　　　　　　　　Cns/Neurology
　Orthosis, Lumbar　　　　　　　　　Physical Med

ORTHOMOTION INC.　800-387-5139
901 Dillingham Rd.,　905-420-3303
Pickering, ONT L1W 2 Canada
FDA Number: n/a　　　　　　　　Fax: 905-420-3970
E-mail: olcanada@olcanada.com
Web site: www.orthorehab.com
Year Founded: 1979
Total Employees: 100　*Marketing Staff:* 4　*Sales Staff:* 2
Ownership: ORTHOREHAB
Stock Symbol: OLGC
Traded On: NASDAQ
Quality System Registration Information: ISO9001
Produces/Sells CE-marked Devices: Y
Federal Procurement Eligibility: Small Business
Distribution: Manufacturer Direct, Manufacturer Through Distributor, OEM, Service Direct, Exclusive Distributor

ORTHONETX, INC.　877-370-0477
2301 W. 205th Street #102, Torrance, CA 90501
FDA Number: 3003933484
　External Mandibular Fixator And/or Distractor　Dental And Oral
　Fixation Appliance, Multiple Component　Orthopedics

ORTHONEUTROGENA
See Ortho Dermatologics

ORTHOPAEDIC DEVELOPMENT, LLC　561-827-8006
1300 Corporate Center Way, Wellington, FL 33414
FDA Number: 3005267806
Ownership: Private
Produces/Sells CE-marked Devices: N
　Cannula, Surgical, General & Plastic Surgery　Surgery

ORTHOPAEDIC SERVICES　905-529-0395
280 Barton St. E, Hamilton, ONT L8L-2X3 Canada
FDA Number: n/a　　　　　　　　Fax: 905-529-0342
Year Founded: 1951
Total Employees: 25
Ownership: Private
Produces/Sells CE-marked Devices: N
Distribution: Manufacturer Direct, Exclusive Distributor

ORTHOPAX
See Pedifix, Inc.

ORTHOPEDIC IMPLANT COMPANY
See Zimmer Holdings, Inc.

ORTHOPEDIC PHYSICAL THERAPY PRODUCTS
See Optp

ORTHOPEDIC SCIENCES, INC　562-799-5550
3020 Old Ranch Parkway, Suite 325, Seal Beach, CA 90740
FDA Number: 2032830
　Plate, Fixation, Bone　　　　　　　Orthopedics
　System, Appliance, Fixation, Spinal Pedicle Screw　Orthopedics
　Trephine, Bone　　　　　　　　　Orthopedics

ORTHOPEDIC TECHNOLOGY, INC.
See DJO Inc.

ORTHOPLI CORP.
10061 Sandmeyer Ln., Philadelphia, PA 19116
FDA Number: 2518634
　Handle, Instrument, Dental　　　　Dental And Oral
　Pliers, Orthodontic　　　　　　　Dental And Oral
　Tray, Impression　　　　　　　　Dental And Oral

ORTHOPRO ENR.　800-267-4344
30 Rue De L'artisan,　819-758-4344
Victoriaville, QUE G6P 7 Canada
FDA Number: n/a　　　　　　　　Fax: 819-758-7181
E-mail: drolet@ivic.qc.ca
Year Founded: 1986
Total Employees: 10
Ownership: Private
Produces/Sells CE-marked Devices: N

ORTHORX, INC.　858-457-3545
8929 University Center Ln.,, Suite 200, San Diego, CA 92122
FDA Number: 2029376
Ownership: Private
Produces/Sells CE-marked Devices: N
　Joint, Knee, External Brace　　　　Physical Med

ORTHOSCAN, INC.　866-996-0472
8212 E. Evans Road, Scottsdale, AZ 85260　480-503-8010
FDA Number: 3005254598　　　　Fax: 480-503-8011
E-mail: nfo@orthoscan.com
Web site: www.orthoscan.com
Ownership: Private
Produces/Sells CE-marked Devices: N
　System, X-Ray, Mobile　　　　　　Radiology

ORTHOSONICS, LTD.　973-665-0001
71 Passaic Ave., Chatham, NJ 07928
FDA Number: 3003563329
Ownership: Private
Produces/Sells CE-marked Devices: N
　Surgical Instrument, Sonic　　　　Orthopedics
　System, Extraction, Cement Removal　Orthopedics

ORTHOSOURCE, INC.　800-649-5525
17374 Sunset Blvd., Pacific Palisades, CA 90272　310-573-4116
FDA Number: 2031448　　　　　Fax: 310-573-3709
E-mail: info@orthosourceinc.com
Web site: www.orthosourceinc.com
Medical Products Sales Volume: $200,000
Year Founded: 1996
Total Employees: 2
Ownership: Private
Produces/Sells CE-marked Devices: N
Federal Procurement Eligibility: Small Business, Female Owned
Mktg./Adv.: Wendy Magur/Director Sales
　Belt, Lumbosacral　　　　　　　Orthopedics
　Belt, Rib (Support)　　　　　　　Orthopedics
　Joint, Knee, External Brace　　　　Physical Med

ORTHOSPEC
See Exogen, Inc.

ORTHOTEC, LLC　800-557-2988
9595 Wilshire Blvd., Suite 502,　310-273-1500
Beverly Hills, CA 90212
FDA Number: 2031734　　　　　Fax: 310-273-4448
E-mail: info@orthotec.net
Web site: www.orthotec.net
Medical Products Sales Volume: $200,000
Year Founded: 1998
Total Employees: 2
Ownership: Private
Produces/Sells CE-marked Devices: N
Federal Procurement Eligibility: Small Business
Distribution: Manufacturer Through Distributor
General Admin.: Dr. Patrick Bertranou/Chief Executive Officer
　Appliance, Fixation, Spinal Interlaminal　Orthopedics
　Appliance, Fixation, Spinal Intervertebral Body　Orthopedics
　Orthosis, Fixation, Pedicle, Spinal　Orthopedics
　Orthosis, Fixation, Spinal, Spondylolisthesis　Orthopedics

ORTHOTIC & PROSTHETIC LAB, INC.　314-968-8555
748 Marshall Ave., Webster Groves, MO 63119
FDA Number: 1953038
Ownership: Private
Produces/Sells CE-marked Devices: N
　Brace, Joint, Ankle (External)　　　Physical Med
　Cage, Knee　　　　　　　　　　Physical Med
　Joint, Knee, External Brace　　　　Physical Med
　Orthosis, Cervical　　　　　　　Physical Med
　Orthosis, Cranial　　　　　　　　Cns/Neurology
　Orthosis, Limb Brace　　　　　　Physical Med
　Orthosis, Lumbar　　　　　　　　Physical Med
　Orthosis, Lumbosacral　　　　　　Physical Med
　Orthosis, Truncal/Limb　　　　　Physical Med
　Prosthesis, Thigh Socket, External Component　Physical Med
　Splint, Hand, And Component　　　Physical Med
　Support, Arm　　　　　　　　　Physical Med
　Valve, Prosthesis　　　　　　　Physical Med

ORTHOTIC MOBILITY SYSTEMS, INC.　301-949-2444
10421 Metropolitan Ave., Kensington, MD 20895
FDA Number: 1123742
Ownership: Private
Produces/Sells CE-marked Devices: N
　Cane, Safety Walk　　　　　　　Physical Med
　Crutch　　　　　　　　　　　　Physical Med

ORTHOTIC MOBILITY SYSTEMS, INC.   301-949-2444 *(cont'd)*
Orthosis, Limb Brace   Physical Med

ORTHOTIC REHABILITATION PRODUCTS, INC.   813-620-0035
7002 East Broadway, Tampa, FL 33619
FDA Number: 1055445
Orthosis, Limb Brace   Physical Med
Orthosis, Thoracic   Physical Med

ORTHOTIC SOLUTIONS, LLC.   877-849-9201   703-849-9200
2802 Merrilee Dr. Suite 100,
Fairfax, VA 22031
FDA Number: 1126198   Fax: 703-849-8499
Ownership: Private
Produces/Sells CE-marked Devices: N
Orthosis, Cranial   Cns/Neurology

ORTHOTIC TECHNICAL SUPPLY CORP.
See Ots Corp.

ORTHOTICS CHOICE LLC.   407-321-0454
451 E. Airport Blvd., Sanford, FL 32773
FDA Number: 3006139201
Brace, Joint, Ankle (External)   Physical Med
Orthosis, Limb Brace   Physical Med
Orthosis, Lumbar   Physical Med
Orthosis, Thoracic   Physical Med

ORTHOVATION, LLC   979-885-2012
2060 Highway 90 W., Sealy, TX 77474
FDA Number: 3006084165
Ownership: Private
Produces/Sells CE-marked Devices: N
Retractor, Surgical   Surgery

ORTHOVITA, INC.   610-640-1775
45 Great Valley Pwy., Malvern, PA 19355
FDA Number: 2530131   Fax: 610-640-2603
E-mail: investorrelations@orthovita.com
Web site: www.orthovita.com
Year Founded: 1992
Ownership: Public
Stock Symbol: VITA
Traded On: NASDAQ
Produces/Sells CE-marked Devices: N
General Admin.: Maarten Persenaire/Chief Medical Officer, Vice President
     Antony Koblish/President, Chief Executive Officer
Mktg./Adv.: Christopher Smith/Senior Vice President Marketing & Sales
Finance: Ms. Nancy Broadbent/Chief Financial Officer
Agent, Hemostatic, Absorbable, Collagen-Based   Surgery
Biopsy Instrument   Gastroenterology/Urology
Bone Cement   Orthopedics
Device, Biopsy, Percutaneous   Surgery
Device, Spinal Vertebral Body Replacement   Orthopedics
Dispenser, Cement   Orthopedics
Filler, Calcium Sulfate Preformed Pellets   Orthopedics
Needle, Catheter   Surgery
Orthopedic Manual Surgical Instrument   Orthopedics
Reamer   Surgery
Stylet, Surgical   Surgery
Syringe, Piston   General

ORTIVUS   800-537-3927   563-387-3191
2324 Sweet Parkway Road, PO Box 276,
Decorah, IA 52101
FDA Number: n/a   Fax: 563-387-9333
E-mail: sales@ortivusna.com
Web site: www.ortivus.com
Medical Products Sales Volume: $8,200,000
Annual Revenue: $10-$25 Million
Year Founded: 2001
Total Employees: 45   Marketing Staff: 3   Sales Staff: 7
Ownership: Private
Stock Symbol: OMX
Traded On: NYSE
Produces/Sells CE-marked Devices: N
Federal Procurement Eligibility: Small Business
Distribution: Manufacturer Direct
General Admin.: Walter Young/President, Chief Executive Officer
Mktg./Adv.: TBA TBA/Director Marketing
     Ellen Manning-Puffer/Director Product Development
     Pam Matt/Vice President Sales
Production: Teresa Ruroden Sweet/Vice President Operations
Computer Software   General
Computer and Software, Medical   General

OSADA, INC.   800-426-7232   310-841-2220
3000 S. Robertson Blvd., Suite 130,
Los Angeles, CA 90034
FDA Number: 2020943   Fax: 310-841-2221
E-mail: info@osadausa.com
Web site: osadausa.com
Medical Products Sales Volume: $1,500,000
Annual Revenue: $1-$5 Million
Year Founded: 1972
Total Employees: 8
Ownership: OSADA ELECTRIC CO., LTD.
Quality System Registration Information: ISO9001
Produces/Sells CE-marked Devices: N
Federal Procurement Eligibility: Small Business, Minority Owned
Distribution: Manufacturer Direct, Manufacturer Through Distributor
General Admin.: Koji Osada/President
     Y. Charlene Hara/Vice President, General Manager
Mktg./Adv.: Emiko Ota/Coord. Marketing
Controller, Foot, Handpiece And Cord   Dental And Oral
Drill, Bone, Powered   Dental And Oral
Drill, Dental, Intraoral   Dental And Oral
Drill, Oral Surgery   Dental And Oral
Endodontic Instrument   Dental And Oral
Handpiece, Contra- And Right-Angle Attachment, Dental   Dental And Oral
Handpiece, Direct Drive, AC-Powered   Dental And Oral
Irrigator, Oral   Dental And Oral
Locator, Apex, Root   Dental And Oral
Preparer, Root Canal, Endodontic   Dental And Oral
Scaler, Ultrasonic   Dental And Oral

OSBORN MEDICAL CORP.   800-535-5865   507-932-5028
100 West Main, PO Box 324, Utica, MN 55979
FDA Number: 2184046   Fax: 507-932-5044
E-mail: info@osbornmedical.com
Web site: http://osbornmedical.com/
Medical Products Sales Volume: $1,300,000
Annual Revenue: $1-$5 Million
Year Founded: 1987
Total Employees: 20
Ownership: Private
Produces/Sells CE-marked Devices: Y
Federal Procurement Eligibility: Small Business
Distribution: Manufacturer Direct, Manufacturer Through Distributor, Manufacturer Through Manufacturer Reps
Immobilizer, Knee   Orthopedics
Orthosis, Limb Brace   Physical Med
Plethysmograph, Photo-Electric, Pneumatic Or Hydraulic   Cardiovascular
Protector, Skin Pressure   General

OSCAR, INC.   317-849-2618
11793 Technology Dr., Fishers, IN 46038
FDA Number: 1828631
Accessories, Retractor, Dental   Dental And Oral
Aligner, Bracket, Orthodontic   Dental And Oral
Band, Elastic, Orthodontic   Dental And Oral
Band, Material, Orthodontic   Dental And Oral
Bracket, Metal, Orthodontic   Dental And Oral
Face Bow   Dental And Oral
Headgear, Extraoral, Orthodontic   Dental And Oral
Pliers, Orthodontic   Dental And Oral
Spring, Orthodontic   Dental And Oral
Tray, Impression   Dental And Oral
Tube, Orthodontic   Dental And Oral
Wire, Orthodontic   Dental And Oral

OSCOR, INC.   800-726-7267   727-937-2511
3816 De Soto Blvd., Palm Harbor, FL 34683-1618
FDA Number: 1035166   Fax: 727-934-9835
E-mail: tosypka@oscor.com
Web site: http://www.oscor.com/
Medical Products Sales Volume: $10,400,000
Annual Revenue: $10-$25 Million
Year Founded: 1982
Total Employees: 130   Marketing Staff: 4   Sales Staff: 8
Ownership: Private
Quality System Registration Information: ISO9001
Produces/Sells CE-marked Devices: Y
Federal Procurement Eligibility: Small Business, VA Contract
Distribution: Manufacturer Direct, Manufacturer Through Manufacturer Reps, OEM, Service Direct, Exclusive Distributor, Importer, Exporter
General Admin.: Mary Ellen Palinkas/Manager Personnel
     Thomas Osypka/President, Chief Executive Officer
Mktg./Adv.: Bethania Tavarez/Director Marketing
Production: Dorit Segal/Director Quality Assurance
     Ronald Van Den Nieuwenhof/Director Tech. Operations
     Vicki Haakinson/Manager Manufacturing
     Mila Doskocil/Manager Regulatory Affairs
Adapter, Lead, Pacemaker   Cardiovascular

OSCOR, INC.   800-726-7267 *(cont'd)*

Analyzer, Pacemaker Generator Function	Cardiovascular
Catheter, Cardiovascular, Balloon Type	Cardiovascular
Catheter, Steerable	Cardiovascular
Electrode, Pacemaker, Temporary	Cardiovascular
Generator, Radiofrequency Lesion	Cns/Neurology
Guide, Wire, Angiographic (And Accessories)	Cns/Neurology
Introducer, Catheter	Cardiovascular
Lead, Pacemaker, Implantable Myocardial	Cardiovascular
Pacemaker, Heart, External	Cardiovascular
Probe, Radiofrequency Lesion	Cns/Neurology

OSHKOSH SPECIALTY VEHICLES   800-596-aksv
16745 S. Lathrop Avenue, Harvey, IL 60426   708-596-5066
FDA Number: 1418996   *Fax:* 708-596-2480
E-mail: info@aksv.com
Web site: www.aksv.com
Medical Products Sales Volume: $12,200,000
Annual Revenue: $50-$100 Million
Year Founded: 1991
Total Employees: 88   *Marketing Staff:* 1   *Sales Staff:* 6
Ownership: Prime Medical Services, Inc.
Quality System Registration Information: ISO9001
Produces/Sells CE-marked Devices: N
Federal Procurement Eligibility: Small Business
Distribution: Manufacturer Direct, OEM, Exporter
General Admin.: Brad Hummel/Chief Executive Officer
　　　　Phillip J. Supple/President
　　　　Larry Sodomire/Vice President, General Manager
Mktg./Adv.: Michael Mitchell/Director Marketing & Advertising
　　　　Martijn Gevers/Manager International & National Sales
　　　　Tom Biwan/Manager National Sales
　　　　Bob Bachman/Vice President Sales
Production: Ryan Loeffler/Director Quality Assurance
　　　　Bernadette Cwik/Manager Materials
　　　　Ed Wajda/Vice President Manufacturing

Facility, Equipment, Medical, Mobile	General

OSI
See Mizuho Osi

OSI ELECTRONICS BOSTON   978.552.7099
25 Commerce Way, North Andover, MA 01845
FDA Number: 3003515080   *Fax:* 978.657.7105
Web site: www.osielectronics.com
Ownership: Private
Produces/Sells CE-marked Devices: N

OSI SYSTEMS, INC.   310-978-0516
12525 Chadron Avenue, Hawthorne, CA 90250
FDA Number: n/a   *Fax:* 310-644-7213
Web site: www.osi-systems.com
Year Founded: 1987
Ownership: Public
Stock Symbol: OSIS
Traded On: NASDAQ
Produces/Sells CE-marked Devices: N
Distribution: Manufacturer Through Manufacturer Reps
General Admin.: Mr. Deepak Chopra/Chief Executive Officer, Chairman
　　　　Mr. Alan Edrick/Chief Financial Officer, Executive Vice President
　　　　Mr. Ajay Mehra/Executive Vice President
　　　　Mr. Victor Sze/Vice President, Corporate Secretary

OSMETECH, INC.   800-373-6767
5964 La Place Court, Carlsbad, CA 92008   (760) 448-4300
FDA Number: 3003344507   *Fax:* 760) 448-4301
E-mail: info@genmarkdx.com
Web site: /www.genmarkdx.com
Year Founded: 1993
Ownership: Public
Stock Symbol: OMH
Traded On: London
Produces/Sells CE-marked Devices: N
General Admin.: Dan Bowman/Vice President International Operations
　　　　Edward Kreusser/Vice President Legal Affairs, Corporate Counsel
Mktg./Adv.: Alina Hakopyan/Project Manager
　　　　Mathew Longiaru/Senior Vice President Product Development
Production: Pankaj Singhal/Vice President Operations
　　　　Robert Dicheck/Vice President Quality Assurance & Regulatory Affairs
Research: Bill Coty/Vice President Research & Development
IS: Gary Gust/Vice President Systems

Control, Multi Analyte, All Kinds (Assayed And Unassayed)	Chemistry
Electrode, Blood pH	Chemistry
Electrode, Ion Specific, Calcium	Chemistry
Electrode, Ion Specific, Chloride	Chemistry
Electrode, Ion Specific, Potassium	Chemistry
Electrode, Ion Specific, Sodium	Chemistry
Hemoglobinometer, Automated	Hematology
Oximeter, Whole Blood	Hematology

OSMETECH, INC.   800-373-6767 *(cont'd)*

Reagent, Glucose (Test System)	Chemistry

OSRAM DE MEXICO   52 55 58 99 19
Av. de la Industria, Lote 9,10,11, Tepotzotlan 54600 Mexico
FDA Number: 9614040   *Fax:* 52 55 58 99 19
Web site: www.osram.com
Ownership: OSRAM SYLVANIA INC.
Produces/Sells CE-marked Devices: N

OSRAM SYLVANIA INC.   978-777-1900
100 Endicott St., Danvers, MA 01923
FDA Number: n/a   *Fax:* 978-750-2152
Web site: www.osram.com
Annual Revenue: More than $1 Billion
Year Founded: 1901
Total Employees: 43500
Ownership: OSRAM GMBH
Quality System Registration Information: ISO9000; ISO9001; ISO9002
Produces/Sells CE-marked Devices: N
Distribution: OEM, Importer, Exporter
General Admin.: Charlie Jerabek/Chief Executive Officer
　　　　Martin Goetzeler/Chief Executive Officer
　　　　Kurt Gerl/Chief Human Resources
　　　　Claus Regitz/Chief Technology Officer
Mktg./Adv.: Frank Santiago/Product & Sales Manager
Finance: Thomas Schaffer/Chief Financial Officer

Lamp, Infrared	Physical Med

OSRAM SYLVANIA LTD./LTEE   905 673 61 71
1 Sylvan St., Drummondville, QUEBE J2C 2S8 Canada
FDA Number: 9615321   *Fax:* 905 673 62 90
Ownership: OSRAM SYLVANIA INC.
Produces/Sells CE-marked Devices: N

OSSEON THERAPEUTICS, INC.   877-567-7366
2330 Circadian Way, Santa Rosa, CA 95407   707-636-5940
FDA Number: 3007111981   *Fax:* 707-636-5941
E-mail: info@osseon.com
Web site: http://www.osseon.com
Ownership: Private
Produces/Sells CE-marked Devices: N
General Admin.: Dr. John Stalcup/Chief Executive Officer
　　　　Dr. Y. King Liu/Chief Scientific Officer
Medical Admin.: Dr. Micheal Lyster/Chief Medical Officer
Mktg./Adv.: Mr. Michael Bivens/Director Business Development
Finance: Mr. James Bielenberg/Chief Financial Officer

Accessories, Arthroscopic	Orthopedics
Cannula, Surgical, General & Plastic Surgery	Surgery
Cement, Bone, Vertebroplasty, Pre-formed, Modular	Orthopedics
Device, Biopsy, Percutaneous	Surgery
Dispenser, Cement	Orthopedics
Injector, Vertebroplasty (does Not Contain Cement)	Orthopedics
Needle, Aspiration And Injection, Disposable	Surgery
Stylet, Surgical	Surgery
Tamp	Orthopedics

OSSUR AMERICAS   800-257-8440
1414 Metropolitan Avenue, Paulsboro, NJ 08066   856-345-6000
FDA Number: 2242474   *Fax:* 856-848-0531
E-mail: spine@ossur.com
Web site: www.ossur.com
Ownership: Ossur Hf
Produces/Sells CE-marked Devices: Y
Distribution: Manufacturer Direct, Manufacturer Through Distributor, Importer, Exporter
General Admin.: Bernie Tatro/Director

Collar, Cervical Neck	Orthopedics
Collar, Extrication	General
Immobilizer, Cervical	Orthopedics
Orthosis, Cervical	Physical Med
Protector, Skin Pressure	General
Tongs, Skull, Traction	Cns/Neurology

OSSUR AMERICAS   800-233-6263
742 Pancho Rd., Camarillo, CA 93012   949-268-3155
FDA Number: 2020250   *Fax:* 800-821-3160
E-mail: ossurusa@ossur.com
Web site: http://ossur.com
Ownership: Private
Produces/Sells CE-marked Devices: N

Bandage, Adhesive	Surgery
Bandage, Cast	Physical Med
Bandage, Elastic	General
Binder, Abdominal	General
Brace, Joint, Ankle (External)	Physical Med
Component, Cast	Orthopedics
Component, Traction, Non-Invasive	Orthopedics
Crutch	Physical Med

OSSUR AMERICAS   800-233-6263 *(cont'd)*

Insoles, Medical	General
Orthosis, Cervical	Physical Med
Orthosis, Limb Brace	Physical Med
Orthosis, Lumbar	Physical Med
Orthosis, Lumbosacral	Physical Med
Orthosis, Rib Fracture, Soft	Physical Med
Pack, Hot Or Cold, Water Circulating	Physical Med
Shoe, Cast	Physical Med
Sling, Arm	Physical Med
Splint, Clavicle	Physical Med
Splint, Hand, And Component	Physical Med
Support, Arm	Physical Med
Tape, Orthopedic	Orthopedics

OSSUR AMERICAS   517-629-8890
910 Burstein Dr., Albion, MI 49224
FDA Number: 1836248
Ownership: Private
Produces/Sells CE-marked Devices: N

Ankle/Foot, External Limb Component	Physical Med
Joint, Knee, External Limb Component	Physical Med
Tongs, Skull, Traction	Cns/Neurology

OSSUR AMERICAS, INC   800-222-4284
19762 Pauling, Foothill Ranch, CA 92610   949-859-4407
FDA Number: 2023821   Fax: 800-453-4567
E-mail: ossurusa@ossur.com
Web site: www.ossur.com
Medical Products Sales Volume: $8,100,000
Year Founded: 1983
Total Employees: 99
Ownership: Private
Produces/Sells CE-marked Devices: Y
Federal Procurement Eligibility: Small Business, VA Contract
Distribution: Manufacturer Direct, Manufacturer Through Manufacturer Reps, OEM, Exporter
General Admin.: Mr. John Turnbull/Chief Operating Officer
    Jim Castillo/President, Chief Executive Officer
Mktg./Adv.: Mr. Brian Kendrick/Director International Sales
    Liddy Lind/Director Marketing
    Murali Sreeramagiri/Director Product Development
    Mrs. Trish Terena/Director Sales
    Ms. Karen McCarty/Manager Customer Support
    Mrs. Trish Terena/Manager National Sales
    Mr. Brett Guerin/Market Manager
Production: Sherry Castillo/Director Quality Assurance
    Mr. George Douglas/Manager Materials
    Ms. Sherry Castillo/Manager Regulatory Affairs
Finance: Mrs. Carol Anne Harves/Chief Financial Officer
IS: Mr. John Kendrick/Technical Manager

Joint, Knee, External Limb Brace	Physical Med
Pack, Hot Or Cold, Water Circulating	Physical Med
Support, Ankle	Orthopedics
Support, Back	Orthopedics
Support, Clavicle	Orthopedics
Support, Foot	Orthopedics
Support, Hand	Orthopedics
Table, Traction	Orthopedics
Training Aid	Orthopedics

OST MEDICAL INC.   401-737-3774
11 Knight St., Bldg F-23, Warwick, RI 02886
FDA Number: n/a   Fax: 401-737-4519
E-mail: asles@ostmedical.com
Web site: www.ostmedical.com
Ownership: Private
Produces/Sells CE-marked Devices: N

Infusion Pump, Enteral	General

OSTEOGENICS BIOMEDICAL, INC.   806-796-1923
4620 71st St., Bldg. 78-79, Lubbock, TX 79424
FDA Number: 1650372

Implant, Endosseous (Bone Filling and/or Augmentation)	Dental And Oral
Material, PTFE/Carbon, Maxillofacial	Surgery
Plate, Bone, Orthodontic	Dental And Oral
Suture, Surgical, Nonabsorbable, Expanded, Polytetraflouroethylene	Surgery

OSTEOIMPLANT TECHNOLOGY, INC.   410-785-0700
11201 Pepper Road, Hunt Valley, MD 21031
FDA Number: 2245518   Fax: 410-785-0748
E-mail: rmurray@oti-global.com
Web site: www.osteoimplant.com
Medical Products Sales Volume: $6,000,000
Annual Revenue: $5-$10 Million
Year Founded: 1985
Total Employees: 41   Marketing Staff: 4   Sales Staff: 4
Ownership: Private
Stock Symbol: OITN

OSTEOIMPLANT TECHNOLOGY, INC.   410-785-0700 *(cont'd)*
Traded On: Stockholm
Quality System Registration Information: ISO9001
Produces/Sells CE-marked Devices: Y
Federal Procurement Eligibility: Small Business, GSA Contract, VA Contract
Distribution: Manufacturer Through Manufacturer Reps, Importer, Exporter
General Admin.: Stephanie Coyne/Manager Human Resources
    Ian P. Murray/President, Chief Executive Officer
    Robyn J. Murray/Vice President, General Manager
Mktg./Adv.: Mark Jenkins/Director Marketing & Sales
    Leonard Ariff/Director National Accounts
    Mark Jenkins/Director Product Management
    Mark Jenkins/Manager Sales Training
Production: Tom Shabinaw/Director Manufacturing
    Andrew Hardin/Director Quality Assurance
    Lee Yancey/Manager Materials
    Sam Son/Manager Regulatory Affairs
    Sam Son/Vice President Tech. Affairs
Research: Sam Son/Vice President Product Development

Prosthesis, Hip, Semi-Const., Metal/Poly., Porous Uncemented	Orthopedics
Prosthesis, Hip, Semi-Const., Uncem., Non-P., M/P, Ca./Phos.	Orthopedics
Prosthesis, Joint, Other	Orthopedics
Prosthesis, Knee, Femorotibial, Non-Constrained	Orthopedics
Prosthesis, Knee, Femorotibial, Non-Constrained, Metal	Orthopedics
Prosthesis, Knee, Total	Orthopedics

OSTEOMED L.P.   800-456-7779
3880 Arapaho Road, Addison, TX 75001-4311   972-677-4600
FDA Number: 2027754   Fax: 972-677-4601
E-mail: webinfo@osteomed.com
Web site: www.osteomedcorp.com
Medical Products Sales Volume: $45,000,000
Year Founded: 2002
Total Employees: 180
Ownership: Colson Associates, INC.
Produces/Sells CE-marked Devices: N
Federal Procurement Eligibility: Small Business

Kit, Instruments and Accessories, Surgical	Surgery

OSTEOMETER MEDITECH, INC.   866-421-7762
12515 Chadron Avenue, Hawthorne, CA 90250   310-978-3073
FDA Number: 3002935476   Fax: 310-676-0948
E-mail: info@osteometer.com
Web site: www.osteometer.com
Medical Products Sales Volume: $532,300,000
Year Founded: 1989
Total Employees: 2580
Ownership: OSI Systems
Stock Symbol: OSIS
Traded On: NASDAQ
Quality System Registration Information: ISO9001
Produces/Sells CE-marked Devices: Y
Distribution: Manufacturer Direct, Manufacturer Through Distributor, Manufacturer Through Manufacturer Reps, Exporter
General Admin.: Jim Roop/General Manager
Mktg./Adv.: Jim Roop/Director Sales
Production: Christian Wulff Pedersen/Director Production
Research: Ms. Tanja Schulz/Director Research & Development

Densitometer, Radiography, Digital, Quantitative	Radiology

OSTEOSECURE   1-877-734-8338
23230 Chagrin Blvd, Beachwood, OH 44122   216-360-8103
FDA Number: 3005372870   Fax: 216-360-7333
E-mail: support@osteosecure.com
Web site: www.osteosecure.com
Ownership: Private
Produces/Sells CE-marked Devices: N

OSTER PROFESSIONAL PRODUCTS, INC.   800-830-3678
904 Red Rd, McMinnville, TN 37110
FDA Number: 2120612
E-mail: vallind@sunbeam.com
Web site: www.osterpro.com
Total Employees: 3000   Marketing Staff: 8   Sales Staff: 35
Ownership: SUNBEAM CORPORATION
Stock Symbol: SOC
Traded On: NYSE
Produces/Sells CE-marked Devices: Y
Distribution: Manufacturer Through Distributor, Manufacturer Through Manufacturer Reps
General Admin.: Andy Hill/President
    Joe Tadeo/Vice President, General Manager
Mktg./Adv.: David Vallin/Director Marketing
    Dan Parsons/Director National Accounts
    Kevin Dealy/Director Product Development
    Peggy Stevens/Manager Advertising
    Cesar Chujoy/Manager International & National Sales

OSTER PROFESSIONAL PRODUCTS, INC. 800-830-3678 (cont'd)

John Davenport/Vice President Marketing & Sales
Production: Phil Tuggle/Director Quality Assurance
Art Oxley/Manager Facilities

Disinfector, Liquid	General
Kit, Prep	General
Massager, Therapeutic	Physical Med

OSYPKA MEDICAL, INC. 858-454-0021
7855 Ivanhoe Ave., Suite 226, La Jolla, CA 92037
FDA Number: 2032836

Pacemaker, Heart, External	Cardiovascular

OT/BIOTECHNOLOGY RESEARCH INSTITUTE
See Intracel Corporation

OTICON, INC. 800-526-3921
29 Schoolhouse Rd., Somerset, NJ 08873-1212 732-560-1220
FDA Number: 2240713 Fax: 732-560-0029
E-mail: webmaster@oticonusa.com
Web site: www.oticonusa.com
Total Employees: 350 Marketing Staff: 9 Sales Staff: 50
Ownership: Private
Quality System Registration Information: ISO9000; ISO9001
Produces/Sells CE-marked Devices: Y
Federal Procurement Eligibility: Small Business
Distribution: Manufacturer Through Distributor, Exclusive Distributor, Importer
General Admin.: Maureen Alcino/Director Human Resources
Peer Lauritsen/President
Don Schum/Vice President
Mktg./Adv.: Henning Falster/Manager Marketing
Gordon Wilson/Vice President Marketing
Jim Kothe/Vice President Sales
Production: Therese Velde/Manager Quality Assurance & Regulatory Affairs
Tom Falvey/Vice President Operations

Hearing-Aid	Ear/Nose/Throat
Kit, Earmold Impression	Ear/Nose/Throat

OTISMED CORPORATION 888-684-7633
1600 Harbor Bay Pwy., Alameda, CA 94502 510-887-3171
FDA Number: 3005738134
E-mail: marketing@otismed.com
Web site: www.otismed.com
Year Founded: 2005
Ownership: Private
Produces/Sells CE-marked Devices: N
General Admin.: Charlie Chi/Chief Executive Officer
Ilwhan Park/Chief Technology Officer
Mktg./Adv.: Wilson Constantine/Vice President Corporate Affairs

Template	Orthopedics

OTIX GLOBAL, INC. 888-678-4327
4246 S. Riverboat Road, Suite 300, 801-312-1717
Salt Lake City, UT 84123
FDA Number: n/a
Web site: http://www.otixglobal.com
Ownership: William Demant Holding A/S
Stock Symbol: OTIX
Traded On: NASDAQ
Produces/Sells CE-marked Devices: N
General Admin.: Mr. Samuel Westover/Chairman, Chief Executive Officer
Mr. Paul Wennerholm/Chief Operating Officer
Mr. Brent Shimada/Vice President Admin.
Finance: Mr. Michael Halloran/Chief Financial Officer

OTO HEARING PRODUCTS LTD. 800-661-7723
12837 76th Ave., Unit 214, 604-590-1211
Surrey, BC V3W-2 Canada
FDA Number: n/a Fax: 604-590-0331
E-mail: info@otohearing.com
Web site: www.otohearing.com
Year Founded: 1958
Ownership: Private
Produces/Sells CE-marked Devices: N
Distribution: Manufacturer Direct, Exclusive Distributor

OTO-MED, INC. 800-433-7703
1090 Empire Dr., Lake Havasu City, AZ 86404 928-453-1022
FDA Number: 2021687 Fax: 928-453-3809
E-mail: info@otomed.com
Web site: www.otomed.com
Annual Revenue: $1-$5 Million
Year Founded: 1972
Total Employees: 9 Marketing Staff: 2 Sales Staff: 4
Ownership: Private
Produces/Sells CE-marked Devices: N
Federal Procurement Eligibility: Small Business
Distribution: Manufacturer Direct

OTO-MED, INC. 800-433-7703 (cont'd)
General Admin.: Charlene Fisher/President, Chief Executive Officer

Accessories, Apparel, Surgical	Surgery
Accessories, Laser, Endoscopic	Surgery
Block, Cutting, ENT	Ear/Nose/Throat
Blower, Powder, ENT	Ear/Nose/Throat
Catheter, Irrigation	Surgery
Drape, Surgical, ENT	Ear/Nose/Throat
Evacuator, Oral Cavity	Dental And Oral
Inserter, Myringotomy Tube	Ear/Nose/Throat
Instrument, Manual, General Surgical	Surgery
Kit, Irrigation, Ear	Ear/Nose/Throat
Plug, Ear	Ear/Nose/Throat
Suction Apparatus, Operating Room, Wall Vacuum-Powered	Surgery
Support, Head, Surgical, ENT	Ear/Nose/Throat
Tube, Myringotomy	Ear/Nose/Throat
Wick, Ear	Ear/Nose/Throat

OTOVATION, LLC 866-OTOVATION
1001 W. Ninth Avenue, Suite A, 610-768-9300
King of Prussia, PA 19406
FDA Number: 3004052117 Fax: 610-992-2316
E-mail: info@otovation.com
Web site: www.otovation.com
Year Founded: 2003
Total Employees: 5
Ownership: Private
Produces/Sells CE-marked Devices: N
Federal Procurement Eligibility: Small Business
Distribution: Manufacturer Through Distributor, Manufacturer Through Manufacturer Reps, OEM, Exporter
General Admin.: Mr. Dave Davis/President, Chief Executive Officer, Chairman
Mktg./Adv.: Mr. Brett Strouss/Vice President Business Development

Audiometer	Ear/Nose/Throat

OTS CORP. 800-221-4769
220 Merrimon Avenue, Weaverville, NC 28787 828-658-8330
FDA Number: 1036132 Fax: 828-658-8363
E-mail: info@ots-corp.com
Web site: www.ots-corp.com
Medical Products Sales Volume: $4,000,000
Annual Revenue: $1-$5 Million
Total Employees: 40 Marketing Staff: 1
Ownership: Private
Produces/Sells CE-marked Devices: Y
Federal Procurement Eligibility: Small Business
Distribution: Manufacturer Direct, Manufacturer Through Distributor, Exclusive Distributor, Exporter
General Admin.: Timothy T. Pansiera/President
Richard Anderson/Vice President
Mktg./Adv.: Steve Hill/Director Marketing & Sales

Molding, Custom	General
Orthosis, Limb Brace	Physical Med

OTTAWA DENTAL LABORATORY, LTD 800-851-8239
1304 Starfire Dr., Ottawa, IL 61350 815-434-0655
FDA Number: 3004590965
E-mail: odl@ottawadentallab.com
Web site: www.ottawadentallab.com
Ownership: Private
Produces/Sells CE-marked Devices: N

Device, Anti-Snoring	Ear/Nose/Throat

OTTAWA INSTRUMENTATION LTD. 613-563-8159
169 Fifth Ave., Ottawa, ONT K1S-2MS Canada
FDA Number: n/a Fax: 613-563-8781
Year Founded: 1991
Total Employees: 10
Ownership: Private
Produces/Sells CE-marked Devices: N
Distribution: Manufacturer Direct, Exporter

OTTO BOCK HEALTHCARE 763-489-5106
3820 West Great Lakes Dr., Salt Lake City, UT 84120
FDA Number: 1721652
Ownership: Private
Produces/Sells CE-marked Devices: N

Ankle/Foot, External Limb Component	Physical Med
Orthosis, Corrective Shoe	Physical Med
Orthosis, Cranial	Cns/Neurology

OTTO BOCK HEALTHCARE, LP 763-489-5106
9420 Delegates Drive, Ste.100, Orlando, FL 32837
FDA Number: 3004067443
Ownership: Private
Produces/Sells CE-marked Devices: N

Ankle/Foot, External Limb Component	Physical Med
Brace, Joint, Ankle (External)	Physical Med
Joint, Knee, External Limb Component	Physical Med

OTTO BOCK HEALTHCARE, LP
763-489-5106 *(cont'd)*

Orthosis, Abdominal	Physical Med
Orthosis, Cervical	Physical Med
Orthosis, Corrective Shoe	Physical Med
Orthosis, Limb Brace	Physical Med
Orthosis, Lumbar	Physical Med
Orthosis, Lumbosacral	Physical Med
Orthosis, Thoracic	Physical Med
Orthosis, Truncal/Limb	Physical Med

OTTO BOCK HEATHCARE
800-328-4058
Two Carlson Parkway, Suite 100,
763-553-9464
Minneapolis, MN 55447
FDA Number: 2087517 — Fax: 763-519-6153
E-mail: info@ottobockus.com
Web site: www.ottobockus.com
Medical Products Sales Volume: $18,300,000
Year Founded: 1958
Total Employees: 90
Ownership: Private
Quality System Registration Information: ISO9001
Produces/Sells CE-marked Devices: Y
Federal Procurement Eligibility: Small Business
Distribution: Manufacturer Through Manufacturer Reps, Exporter
General Admin.: Bert Harman/President, Chief Executive Officer
　　　　Joan McIntosh/Vice President Human Resources
Mktg./Adv.: Pat Chelf/Vice President Marketing
　　　　Brad Ruhl/Vice President Sales
Production: Dave Wall/Vice President Manufacturing & Engineering
Research: Bill Clover/Vice President Research & Engineering
Finance: Rick Schmidt/Chief Financial Officer

Contract Manufacturing	General
Custom Prosthesis	Orthopedics

OTTO BOCK TECHNICAL CENTER
(800) 810-7994
14800 28th Ave. N. #110,
(763) 519-9000
Minneapolis, MN 55447
FDA Number: 2135126 — Fax: (763) 519-6151
Ownership: Private
Produces/Sells CE-marked Devices: N

Ankle/Foot, External Limb Component	Physical Med
Orthosis, Limb Brace	Physical Med

OUTWIN INSTRUMENTS
See Hermell Products, Inc.

OVAGENE ONCOLOGY
949-748-6415
10 Pasteur, Suite 150, Irvine, CA 92618
FDA Number: n/a
E-mail: info@ovagene.com
Web site: http://www.ovagene.com
Ownership: Private
Produces/Sells CE-marked Devices: N
General Admin.: Mr. Frank Kiesner/Chief Executive Officer
　　　　Dr. William Ricketts/Chief Scientific Officer
Medical Admin.: Dr. Neil Finkler/Chief Medical Officer
Mktg./Adv.: Mr. Douglas Stone/Vice President Marketing & Sales
　　　　Dr. Jay Coonan/Vice President Strategic Development

OVEN INDUSTRIES, INC.
1-877-766-6836
5060 Ritter Rd., Bldg C, Suite 8,
717-766-0721
Mechanicsburg, PA 17055
FDA Number: 2523566 — Fax: 717-766-4786
E-mail: sales@ovenind.com
Web site: ovenind.com
Annual Revenue: $1-$5 Million
Year Founded: 1971
Total Employees: 30 — *Marketing Staff:* 1 — *Sales Staff:* 6
Ownership: Private
Produces/Sells CE-marked Devices: N
Federal Procurement Eligibility: Small Business
Distribution: Manufacturer Direct, Manufacturer Through Manufacturer Reps, Exclusive Distributor
General Admin.: Mrs. Ann Fagan/General Manager

Controller, Temperature, Humidifier	General
Controller, Temperature, Other	General
Probe, Temperature	General

OVERLY MANUFACTURING CO.
800-979-7300
574 W. Otterman St., PO Box 70,
724-834-7300
Greensburg, PA 15601
FDA Number: n/a — Fax: 724-830-2871
Web site: www.overly.com
Annual Revenue: $0-$1 Million
Year Founded: 1888
Ownership: Private
Quality System Registration Information: ISO9000; ISO9001
Produces/Sells CE-marked Devices: N

OVERLY MANUFACTURING CO.
800-979-7300 *(cont'd)*
Federal Procurement Eligibility: Small Business
Distribution: Manufacturer Direct
General Admin.: Terry Reese/Chief Executive Officer
　　　　John Brooks/General Manager

Security Equipment/Supplies	General
Shield, X-Ray, Door	Radiology

OVERSEAS EXPORT
See Medical Marketing Services

OVONIC BATTERY COMPANY
248-293-0440
2983 Waterview Dr., Rochester Hills, MI 48309
FDA Number: n/a — Fax: 248-853-4296
E-mail: OMD@ovonic.com
Web site: http://www.energyconversiondevices.com
Annual Revenue: $0-$1 Million
Total Employees: 100 — *Marketing Staff:* 3 — *Sales Staff:* 9
Ownership: Private
Produces/Sells CE-marked Devices: N
Federal Procurement Eligibility: Small Business
Distribution: Manufacturer Direct
General Admin.: S. K. Dhar/President
Mktg./Adv.: Paul Gifford/Director Corporate Development
　　　　Laura McCallahan/Manager Advertising
Production: Larry Conway/Manager Materials
　　　　Ed Dunwoody/Vice President Manufacturing
Research: Ven Katesan/Vice President Research & Development

Battery	General

OVUSOFT, LLC.
757-722-0991
120 W. Queens Way, Suite 202, Hampton, VA 23669
FDA Number: 1126201
Ownership: Private
Produces/Sells CE-marked Devices: N

Fertility Diagnostic Device	Obstetrics/Gynecology

OWEN MUMFORD USA, INC.
800-421-6936
1755-A West Oak, Commons Court,
770-977-2226
Marietta, GA 30062
FDA Number: 1058602 — Fax: 770-977-2866
E-mail: info@owenmumfordinc.com
Web site: www.owenmumford.com
Medical Products Sales Volume: $27,100,000
Total Employees: 31
Ownership: OWEN MUMFORD, LTD.
Quality System Registration Information: ISO9001
Produces/Sells CE-marked Devices: Y
Federal Procurement Eligibility: Small Business, GSA Contract
Distribution: Manufacturer Through Distributor

Dropper, Eye	Ophthalmology
Injector, Insulin	Gastroenterology/Urology
Injector, Medication (Inoculator)	General
Kit, Sampling, Blood	General
Lancet, Blood	General
Syringe, Insulin	General

OWENS SCIENTIFIC INC.
281-394-2311
23230 Sand Sage Lane, Katy, TX 77494-4207
FDA Number: n/a — Fax: 281-394-2522
E-mail: sales@owensscientific.com
Web site: www.owensscientific.com
Annual Revenue: $0-$1 Million
Total Employees: 3 — *Sales Staff:* 3
Ownership: Private
Produces/Sells CE-marked Devices: N
Federal Procurement Eligibility: Small Business, Female Owned
Distribution: Exclusive Distributor
General Admin.: Betty Hail/President, Chief Executive Officer
Mktg./Adv.: Jack Owens/Director Marketing
　　　　Jack A. Owens/Vice President Marketing & Sales

Accessories, Radiotherapy	Radiology
Apron, Lead, Radiographic	Radiology
Calibrator, Radioisotope	Radiology
Counter, Radiation	Radiology
Densitometer, Radiographic	Radiology
Detector, Beta/Gamma	Chemistry
Dosimeter, Radiation	Radiology
Monitor, Radiation	Radiology
Phantom, Mammographic	Radiology
Radiographic Unit, Diagnostic	Radiology
Sensitometer, Radiographic	Radiology
Shield, X-Ray, Lead-Plastic	Radiology
Shield, X-Ray, Portable	Radiology
Table, Nuclear Medicine	Radiology
Test Pattern, Radiographic	Radiology
Thyroid Uptake System	Radiology

OXAIR LTD.
8320 Quarry Road, Niagara Falls, NY 14304-1068   **716-298-8288**
FDA Number: 3002650806   *Fax:* 716-298-8889
E-mail: info@oxair.com
Web site: www.oxair.com
Ownership: Private
Produces/Sells CE-marked Devices: N
  Generator, Oxygen, Portable   Anesthesiology

OXFORD INSTRUMENTS
300 Baker Avenue, Suite 150,   **800-438-8322**
Concord, MA 01742   **978-369-9933**
FDA Number: 2410848   *Fax:* 978-369-6616
E-mail: info@ma.oxinst.com
Web site: www.oxford-instruments.com
Medical Products Sales Volume: $25,700,000
Total Employees: 50
Ownership: OXFORD INSTRUMENTS PLC
Stock Symbol: OXIG
Traded On: London
Quality System Registration Information: ISO9001
Produces/Sells CE-marked Devices: Y
Federal Procurement Eligibility: Small Business, GSA Contract, VA Contract
Distribution: Manufacturer Direct, Manufacturer Through Manufacturer Reps, OEM, Exclusive Distributor, Importer
General Admin.: Michael Pattinson/President
Finance: Keri Page/Treasurer
  Electrode, Biopotential, Surface, Composite   Physical Med
  Electrode, Electroencephalographic   Cns/Neurology
  Electrode, Electromyographic   Cns/Neurology
  Electrode, Needle   Cns/Neurology
  Electrode, Needle, Diagnostic Electromyograph   Physical Med
  Electromyograph, Diagnostic   Physical Med
  Gel, Electrode, Stimulator   Cns/Neurology

OXIA U.S. LTD.
665 Industrial Avenue, Unit B, Hartland, WI 53029   **262-369-1978**
FDA Number: 3004474388
  Cylinder, Compressed Gas, With Valve   Anesthesiology
  Mask, Oxygen, Aerosol Administration   Anesthesiology
  Regulator, Pressure, Gas Cylinder   Anesthesiology

OXIGRAF, INC.
1170 Terra Bella Ave., Mountain View, CA 94043   **650-237-0155**
FDA Number: 2953744
  Analyzer, Gas, Oxygen, Gaseous Phase   Anesthesiology

OXIMETRIX, INC.
  See Hospira, Inc.

OXIS INTERNATIONAL, INC.
468 N. Camden Dr., 2nd Floor,   **800-547-3686**
Beverly Hills, CA 90210   **310-860-5184**
FDA Number: n/a
E-mail: info@oxis.com
Web site: www.oxis.com
Medical Products Sales Volume: $5,100,000
Annual Revenue: $5-$10 Million
Total Employees: 5
Ownership: Public
Stock Symbol: OXISE
Traded On: OTC Bulletin
Quality System Registration Information: ISO9000
Produces/Sells CE-marked Devices: N
Federal Procurement Eligibility: Small Business
Distribution: Manufacturer Direct, Manufacturer Through Distributor, OEM, Exporter
General Admin.: Anthony J. Cataldo/Chief Executive Officer, Chairman
       Mr. Bernard Landes/President
Finance: Michael D. Handelman, CPA/Chief Financial Officer
  Calibrator, Drug Specific   Toxicology
  Enzyme Immunoassay, Other   Chemistry
  Enzyme Immunoassay, Quinidine   Toxicology
  Enzyme Immunoassay, Valproic Acid   Toxicology
  Fluorescence Polarization Immunoassay, Carbamazepine   Toxicology
  Fluorescence Polarization Immunoassay, Diphenylhydantoin   Toxicology
  Fluorescence Polarization Immunoassay, Phenobarbital   Toxicology
  Fluorescence Polarization Immunoassay, Theophylline   Toxicology
  Fluorescence Polarization Immunoassay, Tobramycin   Toxicology
  Fluorescent Immunoassay Gentamicin   Toxicology
  Immunoassay, Other   Toxicology
Medical Product Subsidiaries (Listed Separately)
  Oxis International S.A.

OXLIFE LLC
141 Twin Springs Rd., Hendersonville, NC 28792   **828-684-7353**
FDA Number: 1052940
  Generator, Oxygen, Portable   Anesthesiology

OXOID, INC.
800 Proctor Avenue,   **800-567-8378**
Ogdensburg, NY 13669   **315-394-1727**
FDA Number: 1119969
E-mail: sales@oxoid.ca   *Fax:* 613-226-3728
Web site: www.oxoid.com
Annual Revenue: $1-$5 Million
Total Employees: 970   *Marketing Staff:* 3   *Sales Staff:* 8
Ownership: Private
Stock Symbol: TMO
Traded On: NYSE
Produces/Sells CE-marked Devices: N
Federal Procurement Eligibility: GSA Contract
Distribution: Manufacturer Direct, Manufacturer Through Distributor, Manufacturer Through Manufacturer Reps, OEM, Exclusive Distributor, Importer
General Admin.: Stephane Perreault/Director Admin. & Finance
       Greg Nyman/President
Mktg./Adv.: Jeff Crawford/Manager National Sales
  Antigen, All Types, Escherichia Coli   Microbiology
  Antigen, Somatic, Staphylococcus Aureus   Microbiology
  Antigen, Streptococcus SPP.   Microbiology
  Culture Media, Anaerobic Transport   Microbiology
  Culture Media, Antibiotic Assay   Microbiology
  Culture Media, For Isolation Of Pathogenic Neisseria   Microbiology
  Culture Media, General Nutrient Broth   Microbiology
  Culture Media, Multiple Biochemical Test   Microbiology
  Culture Media, Non-Selective And Differential   Microbiology
  Culture Media, Non-Selective And Non-Differential   Microbiology
  Culture Media, Selective And Differential   Microbiology
  Culture Media, Selective And Non-Differential   Microbiology
  Culture Media, Selective Broth   Microbiology
  Generator, Gas, Microbiology   Microbiology
  Kit, Screening, Urine   Microbiology
  Reagent, Clostridium Difficile Toxin   Microbiology
  System, Blood Culturing   Microbiology

OXUS ENVIRONMENTAL, LLC
264 Industrial Park Street, Pittsfield, ME 04967   **207-487-5300**
FDA Number: 3006367446
  Container, Sharpes   General

OXY-SURE COMPANY, LLC
13930 2nd Avenue West, Orofino, ID 83544-9410   **866-476-3800**
  208-476-3800
FDA Number: 3034609   *Fax:* 877-699-7873
E-mail: oxy-sure@oxy-sure.com
Web site: www.oxy-sure.com
Year Founded: 2000
Total Employees: 2
Ownership: Private
Produces/Sells CE-marked Devices: N
Federal Procurement Eligibility: Small Business, Female Owned
Distribution: Manufacturer Direct, Manufacturer Through Distributor
General Admin.: Roberta McGlothen/Owner
       Mr. Darryl McGlothen/Owner
  Support, Patient Position   Anesthesiology

OXY-VIEW, INC.
109 Inverness Dr. East, Ste. C,   **877-699-8439**
Englewood, CO 80112   **877-699-8439**
FDA Number: 1725011   *Fax:* 303-790-4588
E-mail: lpeterson@oxyview.com
Web site: www.oxyview.com
Annual Revenue: $0-$1 Million
Total Employees: 5
Ownership: Private
Quality System Registration Information: ISO9001
Produces/Sells CE-marked Devices: Y
Distribution: Manufacturer Direct, Manufacturer Through Distributor
General Admin.: Les Peterson/President, Chief Executive Officer
Mktg./Adv.: Shawn Gillespie/Manager Contract Sales
       Les Peterson/Manager National Sales
Production: Scott Durkop/Director Quality Assurance
       Dan Baird/Manager Materials
  Cannula, Nasal, Oxygen   Anesthesiology
  Eyeglasses   Ophthalmology

OXYBEC MEDICAL
981 King Street West,   **800 361 9911**
Sherbrooke, QUE 981 K Canada   **819-566-8711**
FDA Number: n/a   *Fax:* 819-566-0371
E-mail: llemay@oxybec.com
Year Founded: 1988
Total Employees: 25
Ownership: Private
Produces/Sells CE-marked Devices: N
Distribution: Exclusive Distributor, Importer

OXYGEN THERAPY INSTITUTE   989-752-9891
106 West Johnson, Saginaw, MI 48604
FDA Number: 1823393
Ventilator, Emergency, Powered (Resuscitator)   Anesthesiology

OXYRASE, INC.   419-589-8800
175 South Illinois Ave., Mansfield, OH 44905
FDA Number: 1530248
Culture Media, Enriched   Microbiology
Culture Media, Non-Selective And Non-Differential   Microbiology
Culture Media, Selective And Non-Differential   Microbiology

OZARK SYSTEMS MANUFACTURING, LLC.   479-524-9778
501 North Lincoln Street, Siloam Springs, AR 72761
FDA Number: 3003985569   Fax: 479-524-6913
Ownership: Private
Produces/Sells CE-marked Devices: N
Exerciser, Powered   Anesthesiology

P AND G ENGINEERING, INCORPORATED   978-263-6254
20 Main St. Unit E, Acton, MA 01720
FDA Number: 3004361359
Accessories, Operating Room, Table   Surgery

P M ASSOC.   828-324-5739
826 Airport Road, Hickory, NC 28601
FDA Number: 1064854   Fax: 828-324-5739
E-mail: jpjohnson@charter.net
Annual Revenue: $0-$1 Million
Year Founded: 1992
Total Employees: 3
Ownership: Private
Produces/Sells CE-marked Devices: N
Bandage, Adhesive   Surgery

P-RYTON CORP.   800-221-9840
5-04 50th Ave., Long Island City, NY 11709   718-937-7052
FDA Number: n/a   Fax: 718-729-1795
E-mail: pryton@worldnet.att.net
Web site: www.p-ryton.com
Medical Products Sales Volume: $1,000,000
Annual Revenue: $0-$1 Million
Total Employees: 8
Ownership: Private
Produces/Sells CE-marked Devices: Y
Federal Procurement Eligibility: Small Business
Distribution: Manufacturer Through Distributor
General Admin.: Joseph C. Palumbo/President
Mktg./Adv.: Linda Palumbo/Vice President Marketing
Production: Sergio Palumbo/Vice President Manufacturing
Bath, Portable   General
Brush, Dermabrasion   Surgery
Vaporizer   General

P. J. NOYES COMPANY, INC.
See P. J. Noyes Company, Inc.

P. W. MINOR   585-815-0659
3 Treadeasy Avenue, Batavia, NY 14020
FDA Number: 1000230596
Orthosis, Corrective Shoe   Physical Med

P.B. CONNECTIONS, INC.   412-825-6095
341 Marguerite Ave., Wilmerding, PA 15148
FDA Number: 3005482702
Ownership: Private
Produces/Sells CE-marked Devices: N
Chair/Table, Medical   General

P.R.I.D.E. FOUNDATION   800-332-9122
391 Long Hill Road, Groton, CT 06340-1293   860-445-7320
FDA Number: n/a   Fax: 860-445-1448
E-mail: Sewtique@aol.com
Web site: www.sewtiqueonline.com
Medical Products Sales Volume: $3,000
Annual Revenue: $0-$1 Million
Year Founded: 1978
Ownership: Private
Produces/Sells CE-marked Devices: N
Federal Procurement Eligibility: Small Business, Minority Owned, Female Owned
Distribution: Service Direct
General Admin.: Evelyn S. Kennedy/President
C. Siefert/Vice President
Adaptor, Grooming   Physical Med

PAAR USA, ANTON
See Anton Paar Usa

PAC   281-580-0339
300 Bammel Westfield, Houston, TX 77090-3533
FDA Number: n/a   Fax: 281-580-0719
E-mail: sales@paclp.com
Web site: www.paclp.com
Total Employees: 300   Marketing Staff: 2   Sales Staff: 10
Ownership: ROPER INDUSTRIES
Quality System Registration Information: ISO9002
Produces/Sells CE-marked Devices: N
Distribution: Manufacturer Direct, Manufacturer Through Distributor, Manufacturer Through Manufacturer Reps
General Admin.: Tom McMullen/President
Jim Hepp/Vice President, General Manager
Mktg./Adv.: Didier Pigeon/Director Marketing
Andre Yves Cottereau/Manager International & National Sales
Didier Pigeon/Manager Market Research
Viscometer   Chemistry

PAC KIT SAFETY EQUIPMENT CO.   800-243-5050
57 Chestnut St., South Norwalk, CT 06854   203-857-5361
FDA Number: 1219245   Fax: 203-857-5368
E-mail: info@pac-kit.com
Web site: www.pac-kit.com
Medical Products Sales Volume: $1,500,000
Ownership: Private
Produces/Sells CE-marked Devices: N
Federal Procurement Eligibility: Small Business
Distribution: Manufacturer Direct, Manufacturer Through Distributor, Manufacturer Through Manufacturer Reps, Service Direct, Exclusive Distributor
Bandage, Elastic   General
Dressing, Other   General
Gauze/sponge, Nonresorbable For External Use   Surgery
Kit, Burn   General
Kit, First Aid   Surgery
Kit, Snake Bite   General
Kit, Snake Bite, Suction   General
Mouthpiece, Breathing   Anesthesiology
Pack, Hot Or Cold, Disposable   Physical Med
Pad, Eye   Ophthalmology
Sheet, Burn   General
Sling, Arm   Physical Med
Solution, Isotonic   Hematology
Splint, Extremity, Non-Inflatable, External   Surgery
Splint, Hand, And Component   Physical Med
Splint, Wire Board   Orthopedics
Swabs, Antiseptic   General
Tape, Adhesive   General
Tourniquet   General
Tourniquet, Non-Pneumatic, Surgical   Surgery

PAC-DENT INTL., INC.   909-839-0888
21078 Commerce Pointe Dr., Walnut, CA 91789
FDA Number: 2086043
Accessories, Retractor, Dental   Dental And Oral
Activator, Ultraviolet, Polymerization   Dental And Oral
Agent, Polishing, Abrasive, Oral Cavity   Dental And Oral
Burnisher, Operative, Dental   Dental And Oral
Burr, Dental   Dental And Oral
Cannula, Surgical, General & Plastic Surgery   Surgery
Carver, Wax, Dental   Dental And Oral
Cement, Dental   Dental And Oral
Chisel, Bone, Surgical   Dental And Oral
Chisel, Osteotome, Surgical   Dental And Oral
Crown And Bridge, Temporary, Resin   Dental And Oral
Cup, Prophylaxis   Dental And Oral
Curette, Endodontic   Dental And Oral
Curette, Operative   Dental And Oral
Curette, Periodontic   Dental And Oral
Curette, Surgical, Dental   Dental And Oral
Elevator, Surgical, Dental   Dental And Oral
Eraser, Dental Stain   Dental And Oral
Evacuator, Oral Cavity   Dental And Oral
Excavator, Dental, Operative   Dental And Oral
Frame, Rubber Dam   Dental And Oral
Gauze/sponge, Nonresorbable For External Use   Surgery
Handle, Instrument, Dental   Dental And Oral
Handpiece, Air-Powered, Dental   Dental And Oral
Handpiece, Contra- And Right-Angle Attachment, Dental   Dental And Oral
Heat-Sealing Device   Hematology
Holder, X-Ray Film   Dental And Oral
Instrument, Manual, General Surgical   Surgery
Mask, Surgical   Surgery
Material, Impression   Dental And Oral
Material, Tooth Shade, Resin   Dental And Oral
Mixing Equipment, Cement   Orthopedics
Needle, Dental   Dental And Oral
Operative Dental Treatment Unit   Dental And Oral
Scaler, Periodontal   Dental And Oral
Source, Heat, Bleaching, Teeth, Dental   Dental And Oral
Sponge, Gauze   Dental And Oral

PAC-DENT INTL., INC.   909-839-0888 (cont'd)

Syringe Unit, Air And/Or Water	Dental And Oral
Syringe, Periodontic, Endodontic	Dental And Oral
Syringe, Restorative And Impression Material	Dental And Oral
Tape, Measuring, Ruler And Caliper	Surgery
Tooth Bonding Agent, Resin Restoration	Dental And Oral
Tray, Impression	Dental And Oral
Tray, Surgical Instrument	Surgery

PACE MEDICAL, INC.   781-890-5656
391 Totten Pond Rd., Waltham, MA 02451
FDA Number: n/a   Fax: 781-890-4894
Web site: www.pacemedicalinc.com
Medical Products Sales Volume: $2,500,000
Annual Revenue: $1-$5 Million
Year Founded: 1985
Total Employees: 14
Ownership: Public
Stock Symbol: PMDL
Traded On: OTC Bulletin
Quality System Registration Information: ISO9001
Produces/Sells CE-marked Devices: Y
Federal Procurement Eligibility: Small Business
Distribution: Manufacturer Through Distributor, OEM, Importer, Exporter
General Admin.: Ralph Hanson/Chairman
    Steven Hanson/President, Chief Executive Officer
    Drusilla F. Hays/Vice President, Corporate Secretary

Analyzer, Pacemaker Generator Function	Cardiovascular
Cable/Lead, ECG, With Transducer And Electrode	Cardiovascular
Lead, Pacemaker, Implantable Myocardial	Cardiovascular
Pacemaker, Heart, External	Cardiovascular

Medical Product Subsidiaries (Listed Separately)
Apc Medical Ltd.

PACE TECH, INC.   800-722-3024
    727-442-8118
510 Garden Avenue N., Clearwater, FL 33755
FDA Number: 1051088   Fax: 727-443-7257
E-mail: pacetech@pacetech-med.com
Web site: www.pacetech-med.com
Medical Products Sales Volume: $1,100,000
Annual Revenue: $5-$10 Million
Year Founded: 1987
Total Employees: 15   Marketing Staff: 1   Sales Staff: 2
Ownership: Private
Quality System Registration Information: ISO9001
Produces/Sells CE-marked Devices: Y
Federal Procurement Eligibility: Small Business, GSA Contract, VA Contract
Distribution: Manufacturer Through Distributor, Manufacturer Through Manufacturer Reps, Exclusive Distributor, Exporter
General Admin.: Ilhan Bilgutay/President
Mktg./Adv.: Jim Arnold/Vice President Marketing & Sales

Analyzer, ECG	Cardiovascular
Analyzer, Gas, Carbon-Dioxide, Gaseous Phase (Capnograph)	Anesthesiology
Analyzer, Gas, Enflurane, Gaseous Phase (Anesthetic Conc.)	Anesthesiology
Analyzer, Gas, Halothane, Gaseous Phase (Anesthetic Conc.)	Anesthesiology
Analyzer, Gas, Nitrous-Oxide, Gaseous Phase	Anesthesiology
Analyzer, Gas, Oxygen, Gaseous Phase	Anesthesiology
Monitor, Bed Patient	General
Monitor, Blood Pressure, Indirect, Anesthesiology	Anesthesiology
Monitor, Blood Pressure, Invasive (Arterial)	Cardiovascular
Monitor, Blood Pressure, Invasive (Arterial), Anesthesia	Anesthesiology
Monitor, ECG, Anesthesia	Anesthesiology
Monitor, Neonatal, Blood Pressure, Invasive	General
Monitor, Pulse Rate	Anesthesiology
Monitor, Temperature (With Probe)	Anesthesiology
Monitor, Ventilatory Frequency	Anesthesiology
Oximeter, Pulse	General
Paper, Chart, Record, Medical	General
Ventilator, Continuous (Respirator)	Anesthesiology

PACESETTER, INC.
See St. Jude Medical Cardiac Rhythm Management Div.

PACESETTER, INC., A ST. JUDE MEDICAL CO.
See St. Jude Medical Cardiac Rhythm Management Div.

PACIFIC BIOMETRICS, INC.   206-298-0068
220 West Harrison Street, Seattle, WA 98119
FDA Number: n/a   Fax: 206.298.9838
E-mail: contact@pacbio.com
Web site: www.pacbio.com
Annual Revenue: $1-$5 Million
Ownership: Public
Stock Symbol: PBMIW
Traded On: NASDAQ
Produces/Sells CE-marked Devices: Y
Distribution: Manufacturer Through Distributor
General Admin.: Ellen A. Rudnick/Chairman
    Ronald Helm/Chief Executive Officer, Chairman
Mktg./Adv.: Sayed M. Badrawi/Vice President Marketing

PACIFIC BIOMETRICS, INC.   206-298-0068 (cont'd)
Finance: Peter B. Ludlum/Vice President Finance

Collector, Sweat	Chemistry

PACIFIC BIOTECH, INC.
See Quidel Corporation

PACIFIC COAST MFG., INC.   425-485-8866
15604 163nd Ave., Ne, Woodinville, WA 98072
FDA Number: 3025143
Ownership: Private
Produces/Sells CE-marked Devices: N

Headgear, Extraoral, Orthodontic	Dental And Oral
Spring, Orthodontic	Dental And Oral

PACIFIC CONSOLIDATED INDUSTRIES, LLC   951-479-0872
12201 Magnolia Ave., Riverside, CA 92503
FDA Number: 2032532

Generator, Oxygen, Portable	Anesthesiology

PACIFIC ELECTRONICS   800-281-7782
    815-206-5450
10200 US Route 14, Woodstock, IL 60098
FDA Number: 3001632425   Fax: 815-206-5460
E-mail: jim@pacificelectronicscorp.com
Web site: www.pacificelectronicscorp.com
Medical Products Sales Volume: $38,000,000
Annual Revenue: $5-$10 Million
Year Founded: 1984
Total Employees: 15   Marketing Staff: 2   Sales Staff: 5
Ownership: Private
Quality System Registration Information: ISO9001
Produces/Sells CE-marked Devices: N
Federal Procurement Eligibility: Small Business
Distribution: Manufacturer Direct, Importer
General Admin.: Jim Gorman/President
    Cris Schauer/Vice President Human Resources
Mktg./Adv.: Jim Gorman/Manager International & National Sales
Production: Patty Salgado/Customer Service Representative
    Brian Hagen/Project Director
IS: Ms. Jennifer Stohr/Tech. Specialist

Nurse Call System	General

PACIFIC HEMOSTASIS
See Fisher Diagnostics

PACIFIC IMPLANT, INC.   800-336-2282
    707-764-5602
920 Rio Dell Ave., Rio Dell, CA 95562
FDA Number: 2935740   Fax: 707-764-2620
E-mail: robertspac@sbcglobal.net
Ownership: Private
Produces/Sells CE-marked Devices: N

Implant, Endosseous	Dental And Oral
Point, Silver, Endodontic	Dental And Oral

PACIFIC INTEGRATED MFG., INC.   619-921-3464
4364 Bonita Rd., #454, Bonita, CA 91902
FDA Number: 2032383   Fax: 619-934-5811
Ownership: Private
Produces/Sells CE-marked Devices: N

Kit, Pregnancy Test, Over The Counter, HCG	Chemistry

PACIFIC INTL. CO.   715-886-4550
555 Birch St., Nekoosa, WI 54457
FDA Number: 2124257
Ownership: Private
Produces/Sells CE-marked Devices: N

Alarm, Enuresis	Gastroenterology/Urology

PACIFIC PAPER PRODUCTS, INC.
See Graham Medical Products/Div. Of Little Rapids Corp

PACIFIC PRECISION LABORATORIES, INC.
See Pacific Precision Laboratories, Inc.

PACIFIC PRECISION SYSTEMS, INC.
See Pacific Precision Laboratories, Inc.

PACIFIC RESEARCH LABORATORIES, INC.   206-463-5551
10221 S.W. 188th St., PO Box 409, Vashon, WA 98070-0409
FDA Number: 7000872   Fax: 206-463-2526
E-mail: info@sawbones.com
Web site: www.sawbones.com
Medical Products Sales Volume: $5,000,000
Annual Revenue: $1-$5 Million
Year Founded: 1976
Total Employees: 68   Marketing Staff: 4   Sales Staff: 4
Ownership: Private
Produces/Sells CE-marked Devices: N
Federal Procurement Eligibility: Small Business
Distribution: Manufacturer Direct, Exporter
General Admin.: Forrest Miller/President
    Denzil Miller/Secretary, Treasurer

PACIFIC RESEARCH LABORATORIES, INC. 206-463-5551 *(cont'd)*
Mktg./Adv.: Denzil Miller/Director Product Development
    Joanne McGinnis/Manager International & National Sales
Production: Thomas N. Porro/Director Operations
    Thomas Beall/Manager Materials
  Anatomical Training Model   General
  Table, Autopsy   Pathology
  Training Aid   Orthopedics

PACIFICA GLOVES   800-635-4430
West Coast Distribution, 1709 E. Del Amo Blvd.,   **310-604-7711**
Carson, CA 90746
FDA Number: 2084811   *Fax:* 310-763-1016
E-mail: info@pacifica.com
Web site: www.pacifica.com
Medical Products Sales Volume: $10,000,000
Annual Revenue: $10-$25 Million
Year Founded: 1992
Total Employees: 14   *Marketing Staff:* 10   *Sales Staff:* 4
Ownership: Private
Quality System Registration Information: ISO9002
Produces/Sells CE-marked Devices: Y
Federal Procurement Eligibility: Small Business
Distribution: Exclusive Distributor
General Admin.: R. Mattice/Chief Executive Officer
    J. Mattice/President
Mktg./Adv.: B. Edwards/Manager Sales
    R. Briggs/Manager Sales
    G Ng/Marketing Assistant
Production: G. Wu/Manager Materials
  Glove, Patient Examination   General
  Glove, Patient Examination, Specialty   General
  Glove, Surgical, Powder-Free   Surgery

PACIFIQ SYSTEMS LLC   949-442-2454
5015 Birch St., Newport Beach, CA 92660-2216
FDA Number: n/a   *Fax:* 949-442-7686
E-mail: info@pacifiqsystems.com
Web site: www.pacifiqsystems.com
Annual Revenue: $1-$5 Million
Total Employees: 40   *Marketing Staff:* 2   *Sales Staff:* 3
Ownership: Private
Produces/Sells CE-marked Devices: N
Federal Procurement Eligibility: Female Owned
Distribution: Service Direct
General Admin.: Virginia Colwell/Chief Executive Officer
    Denise Moon/President
    Dave Wright/Vice President, General Manager
  Service, Computer   General

PACKAGE MACHINERY CO.   413-732-4000
380 Union St. #58, West Springfield, MA 01089
FDA Number: n/a   *Fax:* 413-732-1163
E-mail: customerservice@packagemachinery.com
Web site: www.packagemachinery.com
Annual Revenue: $5-$10 Million
Total Employees: 25   *Marketing Staff:* 5   *Sales Staff:* 5
Ownership: Private
Produces/Sells CE-marked Devices: N
Federal Procurement Eligibility: Female Owned
Distribution: OEM, Service Direct
General Admin.: Katherine E. Putnam/President, Chairman
    Paul Striebel/Vice President, General Manager
Mktg./Adv.: Timothy Seltzer/Manager International & National Sales
    Meg Cook/Vice President Marketing
    Mikal Johansen/Vice President Sales
  Packaging Equipment   General

PACKAGING ALTERNATIVES CORP.   714-662-0277
1685 Toronto Way, Costa Mesa, CA 92626
FDA Number: n/a   *Fax:* 714-662-2718
E-mail: sales@pacfoam.com
Web site: www.pacfoam.com
Medical Products Sales Volume: $3,800,000
Annual Revenue: $5-$10 Million
Year Founded: 1977
Total Employees: 50   *Marketing Staff:* 1   *Sales Staff:* 5
Ownership: Private
Quality System Registration Information: ISO9001; ISO9002
Produces/Sells CE-marked Devices: N
Federal Procurement Eligibility: Small Business
Distribution: Manufacturer Direct
General Admin.: Richard Tunila/President
Mktg./Adv.: Richard Tunila/Director Marketing
  Dressing, Foam   General

PACKAGING PLUS LLC   714-522-5400
14450 Industry Circle, La Mirada, CA 90638
FDA Number: 2032691   *Fax:* 714-522-5544
E-mail: lminfo@packagingplus.com
Web site: www.berkleyindustries.com
Medical Products Sales Volume: $150,800,000
Annual Revenue: $5-$10 Million
Year Founded: 1983
Total Employees: 2000   *Marketing Staff:* 3   *Sales Staff:* 5
Ownership: Private
Quality System Registration Information: ISO9001
Produces/Sells CE-marked Devices: N
Distribution: Manufacturer Direct
General Admin.: Jeff Berkley/President, Chief Executive Officer
Mktg./Adv.: Dave Jacobs/Director New Business Development
    Sue Van Wagenen/Vice President Business Development
Production: Randy Samples/Manager Quality Systems
    John Kelly/Vice President Manufacturing & Operations
Research: Steve Milburn/Manager Design
Finance: Craig Sannom/Chief Financial Officer
  Molding, Custom   General
  Tray, Custom/Special Procedure   General

PACKAGING PLUS, INC.   763-566-8808
6840 Shingle Creek Pkwy., Minneapolis, MN 55430-1447
FDA Number: n/a   *Fax:* 763-566-8829
E-mail: ppisales@pkgplus.com
Web site: www.pkgplus.com
Medical Products Sales Volume: $300,000
Annual Revenue: $5-$10 Million
Year Founded: 1979
Total Employees: 5   *Marketing Staff:* 1   *Sales Staff:* 5
Ownership: Private
Federal Procurement Eligibility: Small Business
Distribution: Manufacturer Direct, Manufacturer Through Manufacturer Reps, OEM
General Admin.: James Thole/President, Chief Executive Officer
    Vicki Awe/Vice President Human Resources
    Charles Elsberry/Vice President, General Manager
Mktg./Adv.: James Thole/Director Marketing
    Kent Olson/Manager Contract Sales
    Charles Elsberry/Manager National Sales
    James Thole/Manager Sales Training
Production: Jeff Roers/Director Quality Assurance
    Ron Monkman/Manager Materials
  Tray, Custom/Special Procedure   General
  Tray, Sterilization, Instrument   Surgery

PACKAGING PRODUCTS CORP.   800-225-0484
198 Herman Melville Blvd.,   **508-997-5150**
New Bedford, MA 02740
FDA Number: n/a   *Fax:* 508-993-9807
E-mail: sales@pkgprod.com
Web site: www.pkgprod.com
Medical Products Sales Volume: $2,300,000
Annual Revenue: $10-$25 Million
Year Founded: 1961
Total Employees: 19   *Marketing Staff:* 3   *Sales Staff:* 5
Ownership: Private
Produces/Sells CE-marked Devices: N
Federal Procurement Eligibility: Small Business
Distribution: Manufacturer Direct
General Admin.: Ted Heidenreich/President
    Dan Lipcan/Vice President, General Manager
Mktg./Adv.: Robert Heidenreich/Manager Contract Sales
Production: Jody Alty/Manager Customer Services
  Box, Transportation, Container, Specimen   General
  Container, Specimen Mailer And Storage, Temperature Control   Pathology
  Pack, Cold, Chemical   General

PACKAGING SERVICE CORP. (PSC)
  See Olsen Medical

PACON MANUFACTURING CORPORATION   732-357-8020
400 B Pierce Street, Somerset, NJ 08873
FDA Number: 2219905   *Fax:* 732-764-9080
E-mail: info@paconmfg.com
Web site: www.paconmfg.com
Medical Products Sales Volume: $26,000,000
Annual Revenue: $5-$10 Million
Year Founded: 2005
Total Employees: 225   *Marketing Staff:* 3   *Sales Staff:* 3
Ownership: Private
Quality System Registration Information: ISO9002
Produces/Sells CE-marked Devices: N
Federal Procurement Eligibility: Small Business
Distribution: Manufacturer Direct, Manufacturer Through Distributor, OEM
General Admin.: Michael Shannon/President
Mktg./Adv.: Kip Thomas/Manager National Sales

PACON MANUFACTURING CORPORATION 732-357-8020 *(cont'd)*
Robert Lewis/Vice President Sales
Production: Lawrence Shannon/Vice President Manufacturing

Contract Assembly	General
Contract Packaging	General
Cover, Other	General
Drape, Surgical	Surgery
Drape, Surgical, Disposable	Surgery
Dressing, Non-Adherent	General
Packaging Material	General
Packaging, Sterilization	General
Tape, Adhesive	General
Towel, Surgical	Surgery
Wrap, Sterilization	General

PACSGEAR, INC.   **925-846-9600**
7020 Koll Center Parkway, Suite 100, Pleasanton, CA 94566
FDA Number: 3005180827

System, Communication, Image, Digital	Radiology

PACTIV CORPORATION   **888-828-2850**
1900 W. Field Court, Lake Forest, IL 60045   **847-482-2000**
FDA Number: n/a
Web site: www.pactiv.com
Medical Products Sales Volume: $2,921,000,000
Total Employees: 12000
Ownership: TENNECO, INC.
Stock Symbol: PTV
Traded On: NYSE
Produces/Sells CE-marked Devices: Y
Distribution: Manufacturer Direct, Manufacturer Through Manufacturer Reps, Importer, Exporter
General Admin.: Richard L. Wambold/President, Chief Executive Officer
John M. Schwab/Vice President, General Manager
Production: Wade Thomas/Vice President Logistics
Research: Laurie Mester/Vice President Research & Development

Foodservice Product/Equipment	General
Tray, Foodservice	General

PAGE SOUTHERLAND PAGE, LLP   **512-472-6721**
400 West Cesar Chavez Street, Suite 500,
Austin, TX 78701
FDA Number: n/a   *Fax:* 512-477-3211
E-mail: aus@pspaec.com
Web site: www.pspaec.com
Annual Revenue: $25-$50 Million
Year Founded: 1898
Total Employees: 300   *Marketing Staff:* 7
Ownership: Private
Produces/Sells CE-marked Devices: N
Federal Procurement Eligibility: Small Business
General Admin.: James M. Wright, AIA/Principal
John N. Cryer, III, AIA/Principal
Lawrence W. Speck, FAIA/Principal
Matthew Kreisle, III, AIA/Principal
Mattie J. Flabiano, III, AIA/Principal
Mktg./Adv.: Rita Harris/Coord. Marketing

Service, Architectural	General
Service, Engineering/Design	General

PAIN MANAGEMENT TECHNOLOGIES   **888-267-5422**
1340 Home Ave. Building A, Akron, OH 44310   **216-776-1335**
FDA Number: 1528161   *Fax:* 888-304-5454
E-mail: info@paintechnology.com
Web site: www.paintechnology.com
Ownership: Private
Produces/Sells CE-marked Devices: N

Joint, Hip, External Brace	Physical Med
Joint, Knee, External Brace	Physical Med
Pack, Hot Or Cold, Water Circulating	Physical Med
Stimulator, Nerve, Transcutaneous (Pain Relief, TENS)	Cns/Neurology
Stimulator, Nerve, Transcutaneous Elec. (Speech Disorder)	Cns/Neurology

PAINLESS SHOE CO.
See PLS Shoe Co.

PAKO MEDICAL IMAGING
See Afp Imaging Corp.

PAL HEALTH SYSTEMS   **800-223-2957**
1805 Riverway Drive, Pekin, IL 61554
FDA Number: 1423627
Ownership: Private
Produces/Sells CE-marked Devices: N

Orthosis, Limb Brace	Physical Med

PALCO LABS, INC.   **800-346-4488**
8030 Soquel Avenue, Suite 104,   **831-476-3151**
Santa Cruz, CA 95062
FDA Number: n/a   *Fax:* 831-476-1114

PALCO LABS, INC.   **800-346-4488** *(cont'd)*
E-mail: info@palcolabs.com
Web site: www.palcolabs.com
Medical Products Sales Volume: $7,500,000
Annual Revenue: $10-$25 Million
Year Founded: 1979
Total Employees: 30   *Marketing Staff:* 5   *Sales Staff:* 3
Ownership: Private
Produces/Sells CE-marked Devices: Y
Federal Procurement Eligibility: Small Business
Distribution: Manufacturer Direct, Manufacturer Through Distributor, Manufacturer Through Manufacturer Reps, OEM, Exclusive Distributor, Importer, Exporter
General Admin.: David Levin/President, Chief Executive Officer
Mktg./Adv.: Laurie Weeden/Director Marketing
Laurie Weeden/Director Sales
Production: Diane Lane/Director Quality Assurance
Richella Goo/Director Regulatory Affairs
Steve Burnett/Manager Production

Alarm, Enuresis	Gastroenterology/Urology
Injector, Insulin	Gastroenterology/Urology
Lancet, Blood	General
Needle, Blood Collection	General
Syringe, Insulin	General

PALCO MARKETING, INC.   **763-559-5539**
8555 Revere Ln N #600, Maple Grove, MN 55369
FDA Number: 2135149
Ownership: Private
Produces/Sells CE-marked Devices: N

Sunglasses (Including Photosensitive)	Ophthalmology

PALISADES DENTAL, LLC   **201-569-0050**
111 Cedar Lane, Englewood, NJ 07631
FDA Number: 3003963943

Drill, Dental, Intraoral	Dental And Oral
Handpiece, Air-Powered, Dental	Dental And Oral

PALL BIOMEDICAL PRODUCTS CO.
See Pall Corporation

PALL BIOMEDICAL, INC.
See Pall Lifesciences Puerto Rico Llc

PALL CORPORATION   **800-645-6532**
25 Harbor Park Drive,   **516-484-5400**
Port Washington, NY 11050
FDA Number: 2432733
E-mail: info@pall.com   *Fax:* 516-801-9754
Web site: www.pall.com
Annual Revenue: More than $1 Billion
Total Employees: 10828
Ownership: Public
Stock Symbol: PLL
Traded On: NYSE
Produces/Sells CE-marked Devices: N
General Admin.: Mr. Eric Krasnoff/Chief Executive Officer, Chairman
Lisa McDermott/Chief Financial Officer, Treasurer
Donald Stevens/President
Roberto Perez/Vice President
Mktg./Adv.: Ms. Carol Flint/Vice President Corporate Communications

Condenser, Heat And Moisture (Artificial Nose)	Anesthesiology
Filter, Bacterial, Breathing Circuit	Anesthesiology
Filter, Blood, Cardiopulmonary Bypass, Arterial Line	Cardiovascular
Filter, Blood, Cardiotomy Suction Line, Cardiopulmonary	Cardiovascular
Filter, Infusion Line	General
Filter, Pre-Bypass, Cardiopulmonary Bypass	Cardiovascular
Microfilter, Blood Transfusion	Anesthesiology
Mixer, Blood Bank, Donor Blood	Hematology

PALL CORPORATION   **800-521-1520**
600 S. Wagner Road, Ann Arbor, MI 48103   **734-665-0651**
FDA Number: n/a   *Fax:* 734-913-6114
E-mail: info@pall.com
Web site: www.pall.com
Medical Products Sales Volume: $2,000,000,000
Annual Revenue: More than $1 Billion
Year Founded: 1946
Total Employees: 9400
Ownership: Pall Corporation
Stock Symbol: PLL
Traded On: NYSE
Quality System Registration Information: ISO9001
Produces/Sells CE-marked Devices: N
Distribution: Manufacturer Through Distributor, OEM
General Admin.: Eric Krasnoff/Chief Executive Officer
Abbott Hilelson/Vice President Human Resources
Larry O'Connell/Vice President, General Manager
Mktg./Adv.: Carol Flint/Manager Marketing & Communications
Pat Radowitz/Public Relations Specialist

PALL CORPORATION
800-521-1520 *(cont'd)*

Eric Wigner/Senior Director Business Development
Production: Paul Kohn/Vice President Manufacturing
Research: John Miller/Vice President Research & Development

Contract Manufacturing	General
Filter Paper	Chemistry
Filter, Air	General
Filter, Bacterial, Breathing Circuit	Anesthesiology
Filter, Bacteriological, Laboratory	Chemistry
Filter, Blood, Cardiopulmonary Bypass, Arterial Line	Cardiovascular
Filter, Blood, Cardiotomy Suction Line, Cardiopulmonary	Cardiovascular
Filter, Conduction, Anesthesia	Anesthesiology
Filter, Gas	General
Filter, Infusion Line	General
Filter, Intravenous Tubing	General
Filter, Membrane	Chemistry
Filter, Ventilator	Anesthesiology
Media, Filter	General
Microfilter, Blood Transfusion	Anesthesiology
Purification Filter, Water, Particulate	Chemistry
Ultrafiltration Equipment	Chemistry

Medical Product Subsidiaries (Listed Separately)
Pall Corporation

PALL DENTAL
See Pall Medical

PALL LIFESCIENCES PUERTO RICO LLC
516-801-9064
Carr. 194, Km. O.4, Fajardo, PR 00738
FDA Number: 2647898
Web site: www.pall.com
Ownership: Private
Produces/Sells CE-marked Devices: N

Condenser, Heat And Moisture (Artificial Nose)	Anesthesiology
Filter, Bacterial, Breathing Circuit	Anesthesiology
Filter, Blood, Cardiopulmonary Bypass, Arterial Line	Cardiovascular
Filter, Blood, Cardiotomy Suction Line, Cardiopulmonary	Cardiovascular
Filter, Infusion Line	General
Filter, Pre-Bypass, Cardiopulmonary Bypass	Cardiovascular
Microfilter, Blood Transfusion	Anesthesiology

PALL MEDICAL
800-521-1520
600 S. Wagner Rd., Ann Arbor, MI 48103
734-665-0651
FDA Number: n/a
Fax: 734-913-6495
Web site: www.pall.com
Ownership: PALL CORPORATION
Quality System Registration Information: ISO9001
Produces/Sells CE-marked Devices: Y
Distribution: Manufacturer Direct, Manufacturer Through Distributor, OEM

Dental Laboratory Equipment	Dental And Oral

PALL PNEUMATIC PRODUCTS CORPORATION
See Pneumatic Products Corporation

PALL ULTRAFINE HEALTHCARE DIV.
See Pall Corporation

PALMER CAP-CHUR, INC.
770-942-4395
421 Tidwell Rd, Powder Springs, GA 30127
FDA Number: n/a
Fax: 770-874-7339
E-mail: info@palmercap-chur.com
Web site: www.palmercap-chur.com
Annual Revenue: $0-$1 Million
Ownership: Private
Produces/Sells CE-marked Devices: N
Federal Procurement Eligibility: Small Business
Distribution: Manufacturer Direct, Manufacturer Through Distributor, Service Direct, Exclusive Distributor, Exporter

Injector, Medication (Inoculator)	General
Syringe, Hypodermic	General

PALMER CHEMICAL & EQUIPMENT CO., INC.
See Palmer Cap-Chur, Inc.

PALMER INDUSTRIES
800-847-1304
P O Box 5707, Endicott, NY 13763
607-754-2957
FDA Number: 7000685
Fax: 607-754-1954
E-mail: palmer@palmerind.com
Web site: www.palmerind.com
Annual Revenue: $1-$5 Million
Year Founded: 1973
Total Employees: 50   *Marketing Staff:* 3   *Sales Staff:* 5
Ownership: Private
Produces/Sells CE-marked Devices: N
Federal Procurement Eligibility: Small Business
Distribution: Manufacturer Direct
General Admin.: Jack Palmer/President
Mktg./Adv.: Lisa Carter/Manager Advertising
Production: Jack Palmer/Vice President Manufacturing
Research: Mildred Palmer/Vice President Research & Development

Control, Hand Driving, Automobile, Mechanical	Physical Med
Wheelchair, Manual	Physical Med

PALMER INDUSTRIES
800-847-1304 *(cont'd)*

Wheelchair, Powered	Physical Med
Wheelchair, Special Grade	Physical Med

PALMERO HEALTH CARE
800-344-6424
120 Goodwin Pl., Stratford, CT 06615
203-377-6424
FDA Number: 1219113
Fax: 203-377-8988
E-mail: custserv@palmerohealth.com
Web site: www.palmerohealth.com
Total Employees: 25   *Marketing Staff:* 3   *Sales Staff:* 16
Ownership: Private
Quality System Registration Information: ISO9002
Produces/Sells CE-marked Devices: N
Federal Procurement Eligibility: Small Business
Distribution: Manufacturer Through Distributor
General Admin.: Kenneth Palmero/President
        Rhonda Palmero/Vice President
Mktg./Adv.: Chris McDevitt/Director Marketing
        Mary Ann Mure/Manager International & National Sales
Purchasing: Mary Ann Mure/Credit Manager

Accessories, Retractor, Dental	Dental And Oral
Apron, Lead, Radiographic	Radiology
Container, Sterilization (Tray)	General
Cotton, Roll	Dental And Oral
Cover, Other	General
Cup, Prophylaxis	Dental And Oral
Disinfector, Liquid	General
Dispenser, Towel	General
Drape, Surgical, Reusable	Surgery
Kit, First Aid	Surgery
Sanitizer	General
Soap	General
Towel/Towelette, Paper	General
Tray, Surgical Instrument	Surgery
Wipe, Instrument	General

PALMERO SALES/MANUFACTURING CO., INC.
See Palmero Health Care

PALOMAR MEDICAL TECHNOLOGIES
800-725-6627
15 Network Drive, Burlington, MA 01803
781-993-2300
FDA Number: 1223483
Fax: 781-993-2330
E-mail: info@palomarmedical.com
Web site: www.palomarmedical.com
Medical Products Sales Volume: $126,540,000
Annual Revenue: $100-$500 Million
Year Founded: 1991
Total Employees: 78   *Marketing Staff:* 5   *Sales Staff:* 19
Ownership: Public
Stock Symbol: PMTI
Traded On: NASDAQ
Produces/Sells CE-marked Devices: Y
Federal Procurement Eligibility: Small Business
Distribution: Manufacturer Direct, Manufacturer Through Distributor, Manufacturer Through Manufacturer Reps, Exclusive Distributor
General Admin.: Paul Weiner/Chief Financial Officer, Senior Vice President
        Dr. Michael Smotrich/Chief Technology Officer
        Joseph Caruso/President, Chief Executive Officer
Mktg./Adv.: Paul Wiener/Senior Vice President Marketing & Sales
Production: Steve Armstrong/Vice President Operations
Research: Gregory Altshuler/Vice President Research & Development

Lamp, Infrared	Physical Med
Laser, Surgical	Surgery

PALUMBO ORTHOPAEDICS
800-292-7223
8206 Leesburg Pike, Ste. 402,
703-790-0200
Vienna, VA 22182
FDA Number: n/a
Fax: 703-790-0854
E-mail: Mark@palumbobraces.com
Web site: www.palumbobrace.com
Medical Products Sales Volume: $1,500,000
Annual Revenue: $1-$5 Million
Total Employees: 19   *Marketing Staff:* 1   *Sales Staff:* 4
Ownership: Private
Produces/Sells CE-marked Devices: N
Federal Procurement Eligibility: Small Business
Distribution: Manufacturer Direct, Manufacturer Through Distributor, Manufacturer Through Manufacturer Reps, Importer, Exporter
General Admin.: P. M. Palumbo/Chief Executive Officer
Mktg./Adv.: Michael P. Horinko/Manager National Sales

Anklet	Physical Med
Immobilizer, Ankle	Orthopedics
Immobilizer, Knee	Orthopedics
Joint, Knee, External Brace	Physical Med
Support, Ankle	Orthopedics
Support, Back	Orthopedics
Support, Elbow	Orthopedics
Support, Knee	Physical Med

PALUMBO ORTHOPAEDICS   800-292-7223 (cont'd)
Support, Wrist   Physical Med

PAN PROBE BIOTECH, INC.   858-689-9936
7396 Trade St., San Diego, CA 92121
FDA Number: 2031779

Enzyme Immunoassay, Amphetamine	Toxicology
Enzyme Immunoassay, Barbiturate	Toxicology
Enzyme Immunoassay, Benzodiazepine	Toxicology
Enzyme Immunoassay, Cannabinoids	Toxicology
Enzyme Immunoassay, Methadone	Toxicology
Enzyme Immunoassay, Opiates	Toxicology
Enzyme Immunoassay, Phencyclidine	Toxicology
Gas Chromatography, Methamphetamine	Toxicology
High Pressure Liquid Chromatography, Tricyclic Drug	Toxicology
System, Test, Drugs of Abuse	Chemistry
Test, Human Chorionic Gonadotropin, Serum	Immunology

PAN-AMERICAN   404-966-4230
1480-f Terrill Mill Rd., Suite 662, Marietta, GA 30067
FDA Number: 3006385441
Ownership: Private
Produces/Sells CE-marked Devices: N
Pack, Hot Or Cold, Reusable   Physical Med

PAN-OPTICS INC.
See Marcolin Usa

PANADENT CORP.   800-368-9777
22573 Barton Road, Grand Terrace, CA 92313   909-783-1841
FDA Number: 2031961   Fax: 909-783-1896
E-mail: info@panadent.com
Web site: www.panadent.com
Medical Products Sales Volume: $1,500,000
Year Founded: 1974
Total Employees: 8   Marketing Staff: 6   Sales Staff: 7
Ownership: Private
Quality System Registration Information: ISO9001
Produces/Sells CE-marked Devices: Y
Federal Procurement Eligibility: Small Business, Female Owned
Distribution: Manufacturer Direct, Manufacturer Through Distributor, Exporter
General Admin.: Thomas Lee/Executive Vice President, General Manager
    Arlene Lee/President
Mktg./Adv.: Thomas Lee/Vice President Marketing
    Thomas Lee/Vice President Services & Sales

Articulators	Dental And Oral
Face Bow	Dental And Oral
Gauge, Depth, Instrument, Dental	Dental And Oral
Implant, Fixation Device, Condylar Plate	Orthopedics

PANAMAX
See Panamax, Inc.

PANAMAX, INC.   800-472-5555
1690 Corporate Circle, Petaluma, CA 94954   707-283-5900
FDA Number: n/a   Fax: 707-283-5901
E-mail: custrelations@panamax.com
Web site: www.panamax.com/
Medical Products Sales Volume: $20,900,000
Annual Revenue: $25-$50 Million
Year Founded: 1975
Total Employees: 93   Marketing Staff: 11   Sales Staff: 14
Ownership: Private
Quality System Registration Information: ISO9001
Produces/Sells CE-marked Devices: N
Federal Procurement Eligibility: Small Business
Distribution: Manufacturer Through Distributor, Manufacturer Through
Manufacturer Reps, OEM, Exporter
General Admin.: Henry F. Moody/Owner
    Bill Pollock/President
    Donna Oates/Program Manager
    Bob Smith/Vice President
Mktg./Adv.: John Maloney/Vice President Sales
Power Systems, Uninterruptible (UPS)   General

PANATREX, INC.   714-630-5582
1648 Sierra Madre Cir., Placentia, CA 92870-6626
FDA Number: 2031929
Ownership: Private
Produces/Sells CE-marked Devices: N

Delivery System, Allergen And Vaccine	General
Speculum, Vaginal, Non-Metal	Obstetrics/Gynecology

PANCRETEC, INC
See Hospira, Inc

PANEX CORP.   800-662-4499
12300 Highway A1A Alt, Suite 103,
Palm Beach Gardens, FL 33410
FDA Number: 1052733
E-mail: jcjahn@worldnet.att.net   Fax: 800-662-4499

PANEX CORP.   800-662-4499 (cont'd)
Annual Revenue: $1-$5 Million
Total Employees: 5   Marketing Staff: 10   Sales Staff: 12
Ownership: Private
Produces/Sells CE-marked Devices: N
Federal Procurement Eligibility: Small Business
Distribution: Manufacturer Direct, Manufacturer Through Distributor, Manufacturer
Through Manufacturer Reps
General Admin.: Robert W. Jahn/President, Chief Executive Officer
Mktg./Adv.: John C. Jahn/Vice President Marketing & Sales
Finance: John C. Jahn/Controller
Otoscope   Ear/Nose/Throat

PANORAMIC CORPORATION   800-654-2027
4321 Goshen Road, Fort Wayne, IN 46818   260-489-2291
FDA Number: 1832462   Fax: 260-489-5683
E-mail: Sales@pancorp.com
Web site: www.pancorp.com
Annual Revenue: $10-$25 Million
Year Founded: 1986
Total Employees: 50   Marketing Staff: 6   Sales Staff: 4
Ownership: Young Innovations, Inc.
Stock Symbol: YDNT
Traded On: NASDAQ
Produces/Sells CE-marked Devices: Y
Distribution: Manufacturer Direct, Exporter
General Admin.: Steve Yaggy/General Manager
Production: Doug Pack/Director Operations
Finance: Carey Sipe/Controller

Film, X-Ray, Dental, Extraoral	Dental And Oral
Pantograph	Dental And Oral
Radiographic Unit, Diagnostic, Dental (X-Ray)	Dental And Oral

PAOLI CHAIR COMPANY
See Paoli, Inc.

PAOLI, INC.   800-457-7415
PO Box 30, Paoli, IN 47454-0030   812-865-1525
FDA Number: 9310052   Fax: 812-865-1516
E-mail: paoli@paoli.com
Web site: www.paoli.com
Medical Products Sales Volume: $2,500,000
Year Founded: 1926
Total Employees: 625
Ownership: Private
Produces/Sells CE-marked Devices: N
Federal Procurement Eligibility: GSA Contract
General Admin.: Mike McCracken/Chief Executive Officer
    Tom Tolone/President
Mktg./Adv.: Steve Smith/Coord. Sales
    Mike Heazlift/Manager Advertising
    Steve Smith/Manager Market Research
    Mike Heazlitt/Vice President Marketing & Sales

Chair, Geriatric	General
Chair, Other	General
Chair, Rehabilitation	General

PAPER CONVERTING OF AMERICA CORP.   718-385-9100
633 Marlborough Rd., Brooklyn, NY 11226
FDA Number: 2436772
Ownership: Private
Produces/Sells CE-marked Devices: N
Pad, Menstrual, Unscented   Obstetrics/Gynecology

PAPER MANUFACTURERS CO.
See Perfecseal

PAPER PAK INDUSTRIES   909-392-1764
One Paper Pak Way, Washington, GA 30673
FDA Number: 3004578592
Linen, Bed   General

PAPER SYSTEMS INC.   800-950-8590
185 S. Pioneer Blvd., P.O. Box 150,   513-746-6841
Springboro, OH 45066
FDA Number: n/a   Fax: 513-746-6959
E-mail: marketing@papersystems.com
Web site: www.papersystems.com
Annual Revenue: $25-$50 Million
Total Employees: 200   Marketing Staff: 4   Sales Staff: 9
Ownership: Private
Produces/Sells CE-marked Devices: N
Federal Procurement Eligibility: Small Business
Distribution: Manufacturer Direct, Manufacturer Through Distributor
General Admin.: Pat Barnes/Manager Human Resources
    Larry Curk/President
Mktg./Adv.: Lee Wagoner/Director Marketing & Sales
Production: Byron Cates/Manager Materials
Paper, Chart, Record, Medical   General

PAPER SYSTEMS INC. 800-950-8590 *(cont'd)*
Paper, Recording, Data General

PAPERPAK 800-428-8363
545 West Terrace Drive, San Dimas, CA 91773 909-971-5000
FDA Number: 7000686 Fax: 909-971-5627
E-mail: info@paperpak.com
Web site: www.paperpak.com
Total Employees: 1000 *Marketing Staff:* 7 *Sales Staff:* 50
Ownership: Private
Produces/Sells CE-marked Devices: N
Federal Procurement Eligibility: Small Business, VA Contract
Distribution: Manufacturer Direct, Manufacturer Through Distributor, Manufacturer Through Manufacturer Reps, Exporter
Mktg./Adv.: Diane Whitmer/Director Marketing
  Rick Finlayson/Vice President Marketing
  Mike Fagan/Vice President Sales
  Diaper, Adult General
  Facial Tissue General
  Linen, Bed General
  Pad, Incontinence (Underpad) General
  Pad, Menstrual, Unscented Obstetrics/Gynecology

PAPPAS SURGICAL INSTRUMENTS, LLC 508-429-1049
7 October Hill Rd., Holliston, MA 01746
FDA Number: 3005038091
Ownership: Private
Produces/Sells CE-marked Devices: N
  Curette Orthopedics
  Osteotome (Orthopedic) Surgery
  Rasp, Bone Orthopedics

PARA SCIENTIFIC, INC. 503-636-4121
17170 Wall St., Lake Oswego, OR 97034
FDA Number: 3022881 Fax: 503-636-4046
E-mail: ericvc@msn.com
Medical Products Sales Volume: $300,000
Year Founded: 1985
Total Employees: 2
Ownership: Private
Produces/Sells CE-marked Devices: N
Federal Procurement Eligibility: Small Business
  Analyzer, Parasite Concentration Microbiology

PARA TECH COATING, INC. 800-999-4942
35 Argonaut, Aliso Viejo, CA 92656 949-855-8010
FDA Number: n/a Fax: 949-855-8993
E-mail: info@parylene.com
Web site: www.parylene.com
Medical Products Sales Volume: $3,100,000
Annual Revenue: $1-$5 Million
Total Employees: 25 *Marketing Staff:* 2 *Sales Staff:* 2
Ownership: Private
Quality System Registration Information: ISO9002
Produces/Sells CE-marked Devices: Y
Federal Procurement Eligibility: Small Business
Distribution: Manufacturer Direct, Manufacturer Through Manufacturer Reps, Exclusive Distributor, Importer, Exporter
General Admin.: Jeffrey Stewart/President, Chief Executive Officer
Mktg./Adv.: Bruce Allen/Director National Accounts
  Maury Swoveland/Manager National Sales
Production: George Glasgow/Director Quality Assurance
  Paul Stewart/Vice President Manufacturing
  Equipment, Device Coating, Protective General
  Material, Raw, Production General
  Service, Device Coating, Protective General

PARADIGM BIODEVICES, INC. 781-982-9950
800 Hingham St. Suite 102n, Suite 207S, Rockland, MA 02370
FDA Number: 1226153 Fax: 781-982-9008
E-mail: info@paradigmbiodevices.com
Web site: http://www.paradigmbiodevices.com
Year Founded: 1997
Ownership: Private
Produces/Sells CE-marked Devices: N
  Orthopedic Manual Surgical Instrument Orthopedics

PARADIGM LASERS, INC. 509-232-2040
3718 S. Union Ct., Spokane Valley, WA 99206
FDA Number: 1319821 Fax: 509-232-1947
Ownership: Private
Produces/Sells CE-marked Devices: N
  Laser, Surgical Surgery

PARADIGM MEDICAL INC. 800-931-2739
116 Spadina Ave., Ste. 407, 416-362-0844
Toronto, ONT M5V-2 Canada
FDA Number: n/a Fax: 416-362-0729

PARADIGM MEDICAL INC. 800-931-2739 *(cont'd)*
E-mail: info@paradigmmed.com
Web site: www.paradigmmed.com
Year Founded: 1994
Total Employees: 10
Ownership: Private
Produces/Sells CE-marked Devices: N
Distribution: Exclusive Distributor, Importer

PARADIGM MEDICAL INDUSTRIES, INC. 801-977-8970
2355 South 1070 West, Salt Lake City, UT 84119
FDA Number: 1722205
Ownership: Public
Stock Symbol: OMED
Traded On: OTC Bulletin
Produces/Sells CE-marked Devices: N
  Lamp, Slit, Biomicroscope, AC-Powered Ophthalmology
  Laser, System, Phacolysis Ophthalmology
  Perimeter, AC-Powered Ophthalmology
  Perimeter, Automatic, AC-Powered Ophthalmology
  Phacofragmentation Unit Ophthalmology
  Scanner, Ultrasonic (Pulsed Echo) Radiology
  Tonometer, AC-Powered Ophthalmology
  Topographer, Corneal Ophthalmology

PARADIGM-TREX, LLC 858-646-5756
10455 Pacific Center Ct., San Diego, CA 92121
FDA Number: 2032507
Ownership: Private
Produces/Sells CE-marked Devices: N
  Laser, Surgical Surgery

PARAGON FOOT ORTHOTIC LABORATORY LTD. 250-721-1112
1650 Cedar Hill Cross Rd., Victoria, BC V8P-2P6 Canada
FDA Number: n/a Fax: 250-721-1160
Year Founded: 1976
Total Employees: 10
Ownership: Private
Produces/Sells CE-marked Devices: N
Distribution: Manufacturer Direct, Exclusive Distributor

PARAGON GROUP OF PLASTICS COMPANIES, IN.
See Paragon Medical, Inc.

PARAGON MANUFACTURING CORP 425-438-0800
2615 W. Casino Rd., Suite 4c, Everett, WA 98204
FDA Number: 3006434078 Fax: 425-438-0400
Ownership: Private
Produces/Sells CE-marked Devices: N
  Regulator, Thermal, Cardiopulmonary Bypass Cardiovascular

PARAGON MEDICAL, INC. 800-225-6975
8 Matchett Industrial Park Dr., 574-594-2140
Pierceton, IN 46562
FDA Number: 1834331 Fax: 574-594-2154
E-mail: info@paragonmedical.com
Web site: www.paragonmedical.com
Year Founded: 1991
Total Employees: 600 *Marketing Staff:* 2 *Sales Staff:* 20
Ownership: Private
Quality System Registration Information: ISO9001
Produces/Sells CE-marked Devices: N
Federal Procurement Eligibility: Small Business
Distribution: Manufacturer Direct
General Admin.: Tobias Buck/Chief Executive Officer, Chairman
  Gary McGill/President, Chief Operating Officer
Mktg./Adv.: Greg Hall/Director International & National Sales
  Cory Colman/Vice President Business Development
Production: Rick Stetler/Director Operations
Finance: Debbie Yingling/Chief Financial Officer, Vice President Finance
  Awl Orthopedics
  Container, Surgical Instrument Surgery
  Instrument, Manual, General Surgical Surgery
  Instrument, Surgical, Powered, Pneumatic Orthopedics
  Probe Orthopedics
  Tray, Surgical Instrument Surgery
Medical Product Subsidiaries (Listed Separately)
  Mark Machine
  Ortho-Craft, Incorporated

PARAGON MEDSYSTEMS, LLC. 858-613-1200
15920 Bernardo Center Dr., San Diego, CA 92127
FDA Number: 2032077
  Stimulator, Nerve, ENT Ear/Nose/Throat

PARAGON VISION SCIENCES, INC. 800-528-8279
947 E. Impala Avenue, Mesa, AZ 85204 480-892-7602
FDA Number: 2022012 Fax: 480-926-7369
E-mail: info@paragonvision.com

PARAGON VISION SCIENCES, INC. 800-528-8279 (cont'd)
Web site: www.paragonvision.com
Medical Products Sales Volume: $2,400,000
Annual Revenue: $10-$25 Million
Year Founded: 2000
Total Employees: 40 Marketing Staff: 8 Sales Staff: 7
Ownership: Private
Stock Symbol: UVICF
Quality System Registration Information: ISO9002
Produces/Sells CE-marked Devices: Y
Federal Procurement Eligibility: Small Business
Distribution: Manufacturer Through Distributor, Manufacturer Through Manufacturer Reps
General Admin.: Joe Sicari/President, Chief Executive Officer
  Paul Michael Hawkins/Vice President
  Larry Warhus/Vice President, General Manager
Medical Admin.: Tim Koch/Director Clinical Affairs
Mktg./Adv.: Jeanne Bear/Vice President International Sales
  Kathleen Shafer/Vice President Marketing
  Greg Kline/Vice President Sales
Production: Henry Maya/Manager Manufacturing
  Hank Stute/Vice President Manufacturing
Research: Herman Neidlinger/Director Research & Development
  Bill Meyers/Vice President Research & Development
  Lens, Contact, Gas-Permeable Ophthalmology

PARAGONDX, LLC 919-653-4748
133 Southcenter Ct., Suite 200, Bay 2, Morrisville, NC 27560
FDA Number: 3004949858

PARAMARK CORPORATION 443-436-9400
2605 Lord Baltimore Dr., Suite H, Baltimore, MD 21244
FDA Number: 3004517009 Fax: 443-436-9409
E-mail: sales@paramarkcorp.com
Web site: www.paramarkcorp.com
Ownership: Private
Produces/Sells CE-marked Devices: N
  Dispenser, Medication, Liquid General

PARAMEDIC INC. 1 800 465-1255
3535, boul. St. Francis, 418-542-1255
Saguenay, QUE G7X 2 Canada
FDA Number: n/a Fax: 418-542-5959
E-mail: info@paramedic-canada.com
Web site: http://paramedic-canada.com
Year Founded: 1985
Total Employees: 25
Ownership: Private
Produces/Sells CE-marked Devices: N
Distribution: Exclusive Distributor

PARAMEDIC INSTRUMENTATION LTD. 604-266-1354
2835 Oliver Cres, Vancouver, BC V6L 1T1 Canada
FDA Number: n/a Fax: 604-263-3203
E-mail: paramedicinstrumentatio@gmail.com
Web site: http://www.paramedicinstrumentation.com
Year Founded: 1969
Total Employees: 10
Ownership: Private
Produces/Sells CE-marked Devices: N
Distribution: Manufacturer Direct, Importer

PARAMEDICAL DISTRIBUTORS 800-245-3278
2020 Grand Ave., Kansas City, MO 64141-9777 816-421-6203
FDA Number: n/a Fax: 800-462-4707
Medical Products Sales Volume: $15,000,000
Annual Revenue: $10-$25 Million
Total Employees: 160 Marketing Staff: 4 Sales Staff: 3
Ownership: Knit-Rite, Inc.
Produces/Sells CE-marked Devices: Y
Federal Procurement Eligibility: Small Business
Distribution: Manufacturer Direct, Manufacturer Through Distributor, Manufacturer Through Manufacturer Reps, OEM, Importer, Exporter
General Admin.: Perry H. Bacon/President, Chief Executive Officer
  Chris Yering/Vice President Human Resources
  Chris Vering/Vice President, General Manager
Mktg./Adv.: Perry H. Bacon/Director National Accounts
  Jeff Dalbey/Director Product Development
  Les Chubick/Manager Advertising
  Bruce Coffin/Manager Contract Sales
  Perry H. Bacon/Manager International & National Sales
  Jeff Dalbey/Manager Product Development
  Chris Vering/Vice President Business Development
  Matt Steigenga/Vice President Marketing
Production: Terry L. Tate/Manager Customer Services
  Leo Hawkins/Manager Materials
  Ron Hercules/Senior Vice President Production

PARAMEDICAL DISTRIBUTORS 800-245-3278 (cont'd)
  Ron Hercules/Vice President Manufacturing
Research: Jeff Dalbey/Vice President Research & Development

Anklet	Physical Med
Bandage, Cast	Physical Med
Bandage, Elastic	General
Bandage, Tubular	General
Bars, Spreader	Orthopedics
Belt, Lumbosacral	Orthopedics
Belt, Rib (Support)	Orthopedics
Belt, Traction, Pelvic, Orthopedic	Orthopedics
Binder, Ankle	Orthopedics
Cane	Physical Med
Cast	Orthopedics
Collar, Cervical Neck	Orthopedics
Corset	Orthopedics
Crutch	Physical Med
Cushion, Foot	Orthopedics
Cutter, Cast	Orthopedics
Goniometer, Orthopedic	Orthopedics
Halter, Head, Traction, Orthopedic	Orthopedics
Insoles, Medical	General
Legging, Compression, Non-Inflatable	General
Nail, Fixation, Bone	Orthopedics
Orthosis, Other	Physical Med
Oven	Chemistry
Pad, Pressure, Foam (Elbow, Heel)	General
Pad, Pressure, Gel	General
Prosthesis, Foot	Orthopedics
Prosthesis, Joint, Other	Orthopedics
Protector, Finger	Orthopedics
Reacher (Handicapped)	General
Shoe, Cast	Physical Med
Sling, Arm	Physical Med
Sling, Leg	Orthopedics
Sock, Fracture	Orthopedics
Sock, Non-Compression	General
Splint, Molded, Plastic	Orthopedics
Splint, Traction	Orthopedics
Stockinette	Orthopedics
Stockinette, Cast	Orthopedics
Stocking, Support (Anti-Embolic)	General
Strap, Clavicle	Orthopedics
Support, Abdominal	Physical Med
Support, Ankle	Orthopedics
Support, Arch	Physical Med
Support, Arm	Physical Med
Support, Back	Orthopedics
Support, Clavicle	Orthopedics
Support, Elbow	Orthopedics
Support, Foot	Orthopedics
Support, Hand	Orthopedics
Support, Knee	Physical Med
Support, Leg	Physical Med
Support, Wrist	Physical Med
Tips And Pads, Cane, Crutch And Walker	Physical Med
Traction Unit, Static, Bed	Orthopedics
Traction Unit, Static, Chair	Orthopedics
Traction Unit, Static, Other	Orthopedics
Utensil, Food	Physical Med
Walker, Mechanical	Physical Med

PARAMIT CORP. 408-782-5600
18735 Madrone Pkwy., Morgan Hill, CA 95037
FDA Number: 3003537036 Fax: 408-782-9991
Web site: www.paramit.com
Ownership: Private
Produces/Sells CE-marked Devices: N
General Admin.: Mr. Billoo Rataul/President, Chief Executive Officer
Mktg./Adv.: Ms. Jim Creel/Vice President Marketing & Sales
Research: Mr. Carl Chun/Vice President Engineering
Finance: Ms. Tom La Rose/Chief Financial Officer
  Device, Storage, Image, Digital Radiology

PARAMOUNT MANUFACTURING 503-612-8442
10360 Sw Spokane Court, Tualatin, OR 97062
FDA Number: 3019856
Ownership: Private
Produces/Sells CE-marked Devices: N
  Cushion, Flotation Physical Med

PARAMOUNT PRODUCTS USA 800-881-9003
150 N.W. 176 Street, Suite E, Miami, FL 33169 305-651-2126
FDA Number: n/a Fax: 305-651-4589
Web site: www.paramountproductsusa.com
Annual Revenue: $0-$1 Million
Ownership: Private
Produces/Sells CE-marked Devices: N
Federal Procurement Eligibility: Small Business
Distribution: Manufacturer Direct, Manufacturer Through Distributor, Manufacturer Through Manufacturer Reps, Importer, Exporter

PARAMOUNT PRODUCTS USA
800-881-9003 *(cont'd)*

Apron, Surgical	Surgery
Cap, Surgical	Surgery
Cover, Head, Surgical	Surgery
Glove, Patient Examination	General

PARAMOUNT SURGICALS, INC.
877-486-4629
3475 West Alton Gloor Blvd.,
956-541-1220
Brownsville, TX 78520
FDA Number: 3006404019   *Fax:* 956-544-6090
E-mail: info@paramountsurgicals.com
Web site: www.paramountsurgicals.com
Ownership: Private
Produces/Sells CE-marked Devices: N

Appliance, Fixation, Spinal Intervertebral Body	Orthopedics
Orthosis, Fixation, Pedicle, Spinal	Orthopedics

PARASCRIPT LLC
888-772-7478
6273 Monarch Park Place, Longmont, CO 80503
303-381-3100
FDA Number: n/a   *Fax:* 303-381-3101
Web site: http://www.parascript.com
Ownership: Private
Produces/Sells CE-marked Devices: N
General Admin.: Mr. Bill Pearlman/Chief Executive Officer
       Dr. Alexander Filatov/Chief Technology Officer
Mktg./Adv.: Mr. Mike Fenton/Vice President Sales
Research: Dr. Illa Losev/Chief Scientist

PARASITIC DISEASE CONSULTANTS
770-496-1370
2177-J Flintstone Dr., P.O. Box 616, Tucker, GA 30085
FDA Number: n/a   *Fax:* 770-938-7189
E-mail: info@Parasitic.com
Web site: www.parasitic.com
Medical Products Sales Volume: $300,000
Annual Revenue: $0-$1 Million
Year Founded: 1983
Ownership: Private
Produces/Sells CE-marked Devices: N
Federal Procurement Eligibility: Small Business
Distribution: Service Direct
General Admin.: Irving G. Kagan/Chief Executive Officer

Service, Consulting	General

PARATECH, INC.
800-435-9358
PO BOX 1000, Frankfort, IL 60423-7748
815-469-3911
FDA Number: n/a   *Fax:* 815-469-7748
E-mail: paratech@paratech.us
Web site: www.paratech.com
Annual Revenue: $0-$1 Million
Total Employees: 30   *Marketing Staff:* 5   *Sales Staff:* 5
Ownership: Private
Produces/Sells CE-marked Devices: N
Federal Procurement Eligibility: Small Business
Distribution: Manufacturer Through Distributor
General Admin.: Howard Leibovitz/President
Mktg./Adv.: Peter Nielsen/Vice President Marketing

Extrication Equipment	General
Rescue Equipment	General

PARCO SCIENTIFIC CO.
877-592-5837
P.O. Box 851559, Westland, MI 48185
FDA Number: n/a   *Fax:* 519-737-9133
E-mail: info@parcoscientific.com
Web site: www.parcoscientific.com
Medical Products Sales Volume: $2,500,000
Annual Revenue: $1-$5 Million
Year Founded: 1959
Ownership: Private
Produces/Sells CE-marked Devices: N
Federal Procurement Eligibility: Small Business, Female Owned
Distribution: Manufacturer Direct, Service Direct, Importer, Exporter

Camera, Other	General
Microscope	Hematology
Monitor, Utilization, Equipment	General

PARCO SCIENTIFIC CO., INSTRUMENT GROUP
See Parco Scientific Co.

PARE SURGICAL, INC.
303-689-0187
7332 South Alton Way, Unit H, Centennial, CO 80112
FDA Number: 1723265   *Fax:* 303-689-0579
E-mail: quikstitch@pare.net
Web site: www.paresurgical.com
Annual Revenue: $0-$1 Million
Year Founded: 1994
Total Employees: 5
Ownership: Private
Quality System Registration Information: ISO9002
Produces/Sells CE-marked Devices: Y

PARE SURGICAL, INC.
303-689-0187 *(cont'd)*
Federal Procurement Eligibility: Small Business
Distribution: Manufacturer Through Manufacturer Reps

Bag, Specimen, Laparoscopic	Surgery
Endoscope	Gastroenterology/Urology
Forceps	Orthopedics
Laparoscope, General & Plastic Surgery	Surgery
Retractor, Fiberoptic	Gastroenterology/Urology
Suture Apparatus, Stomach And Intestinal	Gastroenterology/Urology

PAREXEL INTERNATIONAL CORP.
781-487-9900
195 West St., Waltham, MA 02451
FDA Number: n/a   *Fax:* 781-487-0525
E-mail: clientmaster@parexel.com
Web site: www.parexel.com
Medical Products Sales Volume: $285,000,000
Total Employees: 3900   *Marketing Staff:* 15   *Sales Staff:* 35
Ownership: Public
Stock Symbol: PRXL
Traded On: NASDAQ
Produces/Sells CE-marked Devices: N
Distribution: Service Direct
General Admin.: Josef H. von Rickenbach/Chairman, Chief Executive Officer
       Dr. Ulf Schneider/Chief Administrative Officer
       James Winschel/Chief Financial Officer, Senior Vice President
       Dr. Mark Goldberg/Chief Operating Officer
Mktg./Adv.: Ms. Jennifer Baird/Director Public Relations
Finance: Mr. James Winschel/Chief Financial Officer

Service, Consulting	General
Service, Publication Acquisition	General

PARI RESPIRATORY EQUIPMENT, INC.
800-327-8632
2943 Oak lake Boulevard, Midlothian, VA 23112
804-253-7274
FDA Number: 1123526   *Fax:* 804-253-0260
E-mail: productinfo@pari.com
Web site: www.pari.com
Medical Products Sales Volume: $25,100,000
Annual Revenue: $25-$50 Million
Year Founded: 1906
Total Employees: 33   *Marketing Staff:* 4   *Sales Staff:* 12
Ownership: Pari Gmbh
Quality System Registration Information: ISO9000
Produces/Sells CE-marked Devices: N
Federal Procurement Eligibility: Small Business
Distribution: Manufacturer Direct, Manufacturer Through Distributor, Manufacturer Through Manufacturer Reps, Service Direct
General Admin.: Werner Gutmann/President
Mktg./Adv.: Rob Lee/Director Marketing & Sales
       Susan Verille/Director National Accounts

Nebulizer, Non-Heated	Anesthesiology

PARIMIST FUNDING CORP.
800-645-6598
40 Commerce Place, Hicksville, NY 11801-5210
516-931-7500
FDA Number: n/a   *Fax:* 516-937-3777
E-mail: info@parimist.com
Web site: http://parimist.com/
Medical Products Sales Volume: $9,500,000
Annual Revenue: $5-$10 Million
Total Employees: 9
Ownership: Private
Produces/Sells CE-marked Devices: N
Federal Procurement Eligibility: Small Business
Distribution: Service Direct
General Admin.: Paul Eidelkind/President
Mktg./Adv.: Howard Lebowitz/Vice President Sales
Finance: Richard Smith/Chief Financial Officer

Service, Equipment Leasing	General

PARIS MIKI, INC.
425-883-2464
2863 152nd Ne, Redmond, WA 98052
FDA Number: 3031026
Ownership: Private
Produces/Sells CE-marked Devices: N

Frame, Spectacle (Eyeglasses)	Ophthalmology
Lens, Spectacle/Eyeglasses, Non-Custom	Ophthalmology

PARK DENTAL RESEARCH CORP./IMPLANT CENTER
800-243-7372
19 West 34th St., Ste. 301,
212-736-3765
New York, NY 10001
FDA Number: 2431337   *Fax:* 212-268-6845
E-mail: parkdental@aol.com
Web site: www.parkdentalresearch.com
Annual Revenue: $0-$1 Million
Ownership: Private
Quality System Registration Information: ISO9001
Produces/Sells CE-marked Devices: N

PARK DENTAL RESEARCH 800-243-7372 *(cont'd)*

Federal Procurement Eligibility: Small Business
Distribution: Manufacturer Direct

Bone Grafting Material, Dental, With Biologic Component	Dental And Oral
Implant, Endosseous	Dental And Oral
Instrument, Manual, General Surgical	Surgery

PARK SURGICAL CO., INC. 800-633-7878
5001 New Utrecht Avenue, **718-436-9200**
Brooklyn, NY 11219

FDA Number: 7000874
E-mail: parksurgic@aol.com *Fax:* 718-854-2431
Web site: www.parksurgical.com
Medical Products Sales Volume: $4,600,000
Year Founded: 1925
Total Employees: 24
Ownership: Private
Produces/Sells CE-marked Devices: N
Federal Procurement Eligibility: Small Business
Distribution: Manufacturer Direct
General Admin.: Daniel Dube/President
    James Dube/Secretary
Mktg./Adv.: Peter Dube/Vice President Sales

Amplifier, Voice	Ear/Nose/Throat
Bandage, Other	General
Device, Incontinence, Mechanical/Hydraulic	Gastroenterology/Urology
Hearing-Aid	Ear/Nose/Throat
Larynx, Artificial Battery-Powered	Ear/Nose/Throat

PARKELL, INC. 800-243-7446
300 Executive Dr., Edgewood, NY 11717-9816 **631-249-1134**

FDA Number: 2411797 *Fax:* 631-249-1242
E-mail: info@parkell.com
Web site: www.parkell.com
Ownership: Private
Quality System Registration Information: ISO9001
Produces/Sells CE-marked Devices: Y
Federal Procurement Eligibility: Small Business
Distribution: Manufacturer Direct, Manufacturer Through Distributor
General Admin.: Karen Mitchell/Chief Executive Officer
    Robert Burke/Vice President
Mktg./Adv.: Dave Selander/Director Communications
    Michael Bellew/Manager Sales Training
    Charles Cassar/Vice President Business Development
Production: Matt Amaturo/Director Quality Assurance
    Dan Schechter/Director Regulatory Affairs
Research: Nelson Gendusa/Director Research
IS: Mike Sharp/Vice President Technology

Activator, Ultraviolet, Polymerization	Dental And Oral
Adhesive, Dental	Dental And Oral
Cement, Dental	Dental And Oral
Crown And Bridge, Temporary, Resin	Dental And Oral
Electrosurgical Unit, General Purpose (ESU)	Surgery
Endodontic Instrument	Dental And Oral
Locator, Apex, Root	Dental And Oral
Material, Impression	Dental And Oral
Mirror, Mouth	Dental And Oral
Paper, Articulation	Dental And Oral
Post, Root Canal	Dental And Oral
Scaler, Ultrasonic	Dental And Oral
Syringe, Restorative And Impression Material	Dental And Oral
Tester, Pulp	Dental And Oral
Tooth Bonding Agent, Resin Restoration	Dental And Oral

PARKER ANDERSON LLC 888-799-4289
5030 Paradise Road, Suite A-214, Las Vegas, NV 89119

FDA Number: 3006072740
Ownership: Private
Produces/Sells CE-marked Devices: N

Bandage, Adhesive	Surgery
Gauze, Non-Absorbable, X-Ray Detectable (Internal Sponge)	Surgery
Gauze/sponge, Nonresorbable For External Use	Surgery
Sponge, Gauze	Dental And Oral

PARKER ATHLETIC PRODUCTS, LLC
See Parker Medical Associates, Llc

PARKER HANNIFIN CORPORATION. 805-658-2984
3007 Bunsen Avenue, Units K And L, Ventura, CA 93003

FDA Number: 2029412

Monitor, Uterine Contraction, External	Obstetrics/Gynecology
Oximeter, Intracardiac	Cardiovascular
Probe, Uptake, Nuclear	Radiology

PARKER LABORATORIES, INC. 800-631-8888
286 Eldridge Rd., Fairfield, NJ 07004 **973-276-9500**

FDA Number: 2212018 *Fax:* 973-276-9510
E-mail: parker@parkerlabs.com
Year Founded: 1958
Total Employees: 60

PARKER LABORATORIES, INC. 800-631-8888 *(cont'd)*

Ownership: Private
Quality System Registration Information: ISO9001
Produces/Sells CE-marked Devices: Y
Distribution: Manufacturer Through Distributor, OEM, Exporter
General Admin.: Neal Buchalter/President
Mktg./Adv.: Martin King/Director International Sales
    Joan Bartello/Manager Advertising
    Tom Rodenberg/Manager National Sales
Production: Mary Ann Hohensee/Director Quality Assurance
    Nick Economou/Manager Operations

Cover, Other	General
Electrode, Gel	Cardiovascular
Gel, Electrode, Electrocardiograph	Cardiovascular
Gel, Electrode, TENS	Physical Med
Gel, Ultrasonic Coupling	Physical Med
Gel, Ultrasonic Transmission	General
Lubricant, Patient	General
Solution, Instrument Cleaner	General
Warmer, Gel	General

PARKER MEDICAL 303-799-1990
7275 S. Revere Pkwy, Suite 804, Englewood, CO 80112-5105

FDA Number: 1724737 *Fax:* 303-799-1996
E-mail: writeme@parkermedical.com
Web site: www.parkermedical.com
Medical Products Sales Volume: $1,200,000
Year Founded: 1994
Total Employees: 8
Ownership: Private
Quality System Registration Information: ISO9001
Produces/Sells CE-marked Devices: Y
Federal Procurement Eligibility: Small Business
Distribution: Exclusive Distributor
Mktg./Adv.: Ms. Joyce Hersh/Communications Director

Laryngoscope, Flexible	Anesthesiology
Stylet, Tracheal Tube	Anesthesiology
Tube, Tracheal (Endotracheal)	Anesthesiology

PARKER MEDICAL ASSOCIATES, LLC 704-370-0400
2401 Distribution St., Charlotte, NC 28203

FDA Number: 3003010533
Ownership: Private
Produces/Sells CE-marked Devices: N

Splint, Extremity, Non-inflatable, External, Non-sterile	Surgery
Stethoscope, Manual	Cardiovascular

PARKES SCIENTIFIC CANADA INC. 780-484-1849
108 Ave. #17360, Edmonton, ALB T5S-1E8 Canada

FDA Number: n/a *Fax:* 780-484-0601
E-mail: parkesci@msn.com
Year Founded: 1985
Total Employees: 10
Ownership: Private
Produces/Sells CE-marked Devices: N
Distribution: Manufacturer Direct, Exclusive Distributor

PARKS MEDICAL ELECTRONICS, INC. 503-649-7007
PO Box 5669, Aloha, OR 97007

FDA Number: 9200844 *Fax:* 503-591-9753
E-mail: info@parksmed.com
Web site: www.parksmed.com
Year Founded: 1961
Total Employees: 55
Ownership: Private
Produces/Sells CE-marked Devices: Y
Federal Procurement Eligibility: Small Business
Distribution: Manufacturer Direct, Manufacturer Through Distributor, Manufacturer Through Manufacturer Reps, Service Direct, Exporter
General Admin.: Gary Parks/General Manager
    Debbie Scotter/Managing Director
    Loren E. Parks/President, Chief Executive Officer

Detector, Air Bubble	Gastroenterology/Urology
Detector, Blood Flow, Ultrasonic (Doppler)	Cardiovascular
Flowmeter, Blood, Ultrasonic	Gastroenterology/Urology
Monitor, Blood Flow, Ultrasonic	Obstetrics/Gynecology
Monitor, Fetal Doppler Ultrasound	Obstetrics/Gynecology
Plethysmograph, Ocular	Cns/Neurology

PARMATECH CORPORATION 800-709-1555
2221 Pine View Way, Petaluma, CA 94954 **707-778-2266**

FDA Number: n/a *Fax:* 707-778-2262
E-mail: dlauck@parmatech.com
Web site: www.parmatech.com
Year Founded: 1973
Ownership: Private
Produces/Sells CE-marked Devices: N
General Admin.: Mr. Brian McBride/General Manager
Mktg./Adv.: Mr. Dan Lauck/Sales Manager

PARMATECH CORPORATION   800-709-1555 *(cont'd)*
Production: Mr. Rob Hall/Manager Operations
       Ms. Suzanne Stites/Manager Quality Assurance

PARMELEE INDUSTRIES, INC.   800-821-5218
8101 Lenexa Drive, Lenexa, KS 66214   **913-599-5555**
FDA Number: 1923298   *Fax:* 913-894-5234
E-mail: info@ussafety.com
Web site: http://ussafety.com/
Medical Products Sales Volume: $18,600,000
Annual Revenue: $25-$50 Million
Year Founded: 1935
Total Employees: 70
Ownership: Private
Produces/Sells CE-marked Devices: N
Federal Procurement Eligibility: Small Business, GSA Contract
Distribution: Manufacturer Direct, Manufacturer Through Distributor, Manufacturer Through Manufacturer Reps, OEM, Service Direct, Importer, Exporter
    Frame, Spectacle (Eyeglasses)   Ophthalmology

PARNELL PHARMACEUTICALS, INC.   415-256-1800
1525 Francisco Blvd., Ste. 15, San Rafael, CA 94901
FDA Number: 2936950
    Saliva, Artificial   Dental And Oral

PARR EMERGENCY PRODUCT SALES, INC.
See Bound Tree Medical, Llc

PARR INSTRUMENT CO.   800-872-7720
211 Fifty-Third Street, Moline, IL 61265   **309-762-7716**
FDA Number: 7000286   *Fax:* 309-762-9453
E-mail: parr@parrinst.com
Web site: www.parrinst.com
Medical Products Sales Volume: $20,400,000
Annual Revenue: $10-$25 Million
Year Founded: 1899
Total Employees: 90   *Marketing Staff:* 10   *Sales Staff:* 10
Ownership: Private
Stock Symbol: SRT
Traded On: NYSE
Quality System Registration Information: ISO9001; ISO9002
Produces/Sells CE-marked Devices: Y
Federal Procurement Eligibility: Small Business
Distribution: Manufacturer Direct, Manufacturer Through Distributor
General Admin.: M. R. Steffenson/President
Mktg./Adv.: Sherman Hamel/Vice President Marketing & Sales
    Calorimeter   Chemistry
    Disintegrator, Biological Cell   Microbiology
    Reaction Apparatus   Microbiology

PARSONS A.D.L. INC.   800-263-1281
R.R. #2, 1986 Sideroad 15,   **905-936-3580**
Tottenham, ONT L0G 1 Canada
FDA Number: 9049908   *Fax:* 905-936-3585
E-mail: custserv@parsonsadl.com
Web site: www.parsonsadl.com
Year Founded: 1982
Total Employees: 24   *Marketing Staff:* 1   *Sales Staff:* 2
Ownership: Private
Produces/Sells CE-marked Devices: Y
Federal Procurement Eligibility: Small Business
Distribution: Manufacturer Through Distributor, OEM, Exclusive Distributor, Importer, Exporter

PARTER MEDICAL PRODUCTS   800-666-8282
17015 Kingsview Ave., Carson, CA 90746-1220   **310-327-4417**
FDA Number: 2024311   *Fax:* 310-327-8601
E-mail: info@partermedical.com
Web site: partermedical.com
Medical Products Sales Volume: $6,500,000
Annual Revenue: $5-$10 Million
Year Founded: 1984
Total Employees: 135   *Marketing Staff:* 1   *Sales Staff:* 4
Ownership: Private
Quality System Registration Information: ISO9002
Produces/Sells CE-marked Devices: N
Federal Procurement Eligibility: Small Business
Distribution: Manufacturer Through Distributor, OEM, Service Direct, Exporter
General Admin.: Parviz Hassanzadeh/President, Chief Executive Officer
       Hengameh Hassanzadeh/Vice President
Mktg./Adv.: Parviz Hassanzadeh/Director Marketing & Product Development
    Container, Specimen, All Types   General
    Contract Sterilization   General
    Dish, Petri   Chemistry
    Pipette   Chemistry

PARTERRE VINYL FLOORING SYSTEMS   888-338-1029
Brooklyn Navy Yard, Bldg. 292, Ste. 402,   **718-858-4001**
Brooklyn, NY 11205
FDA Number: n/a   *Fax:* 718-858-0330
E-mail: info@parterreflooring.com
Web site: www.parterreflooring.com
Annual Revenue: $5-$10 Million
Total Employees: 10   *Sales Staff:* 43
Ownership: Private
Produces/Sells CE-marked Devices: N
Federal Procurement Eligibility: Small Business
Distribution: Manufacturer Direct, Service Direct, Importer
General Admin.: Wally Ruttgeizer/Chief Executive Officer
Mktg./Adv.: T. Fred Roche/Director Marketing
       T. Fred Roche/Executive Vice President Marketing & Sales
    Flooring   General

PARVO MEDICS, INC.   801-942-7796
6526 S. State St. Ste. 202, Murray, UT 84107
FDA Number: 1725061
    Computer, Pulmonary Function Data   Anesthesiology

PASADENA SCIENTIFIC INDUSTRIES   717-227-1220
5125 Pine View Dr., Glen Rock, PA 17327
FDA Number: 1123760
Ownership: Private
Produces/Sells CE-marked Devices: N
    Reading System, Closed-Circuit Television   Ophthalmology

PASCAL CO., INC.   425-602-3633
2929 N.e. Northup Way, Bellevue, WA 98004
FDA Number: 3011632
    Accessories, Retractor, Dental   Dental And Oral
    Agent, Polishing, Abrasive, Oral Cavity   Dental And Oral
    Cord, Retraction   Dental And Oral
    Evacuator, Oral Cavity   Dental And Oral
    Forceps, Articulation Paper   Dental And Oral
    Handle, Instrument, Dental   Dental And Oral
    Material, Impression Tray, Resin   Dental And Oral
    Matrix, Dental   Dental And Oral
    Paper, Articulation   Dental And Oral
    Solution, Sterilizing, Cold   Dental And Oral
    Sterilant, Medical Device   General
    Varnish, Cavity   Dental And Oral

PASCAL COMPANY, INC.   800-426-8051
PO Box 1478, Bellevue, WA 98009-1478   **425-827-4694**
FDA Number: 3011632   *Fax:* 425-827-6893
Medical Products Sales Volume: $7,000,000
Annual Revenue: $5-$10 Million
Total Employees: 30   *Marketing Staff:* 2   *Sales Staff:* 16
Ownership: Private
Quality System Registration Information: ISO9002
Produces/Sells CE-marked Devices: Y
Federal Procurement Eligibility: Small Business
Distribution: Manufacturer Through Distributor
General Admin.: Ben Paschall/Chief Executive Officer
Mktg./Adv.: Janet Siwinski/Manager International Marketing & Sales
       Janice Lewsky/Vice President National Marketing & Sales
Production: Vince Pentarelli/Director Regulatory Affairs
       Joe Pellicano/Plant Manager
       David Watton/Vice President Operations
    Accessories, Retractor, Dental   Dental And Oral
    Agent, Polishing, Abrasive, Oral Cavity   Dental And Oral
    Applicator, Tipped, Absorbent, Non-Sterile   General
    Cleaner, Medical Device   General
    Cord, Retraction   Dental And Oral
    Cup, Prophylaxis   Dental And Oral
    Evacuator, Oral Cavity   Dental And Oral
    Forceps, Articulation Paper   Dental And Oral
    Handle, Instrument, Dental   Dental And Oral
    Instrument, Dental, Manual   Dental And Oral
    Kit, Dental Prophylaxis   Dental And Oral
    Matrix, Dental   Dental And Oral
    Medical Disinfectants/Cleaners for Instruments   General
    Nebulizer, Medicinal   Ear/Nose/Throat
    Paper, Articulation   Dental And Oral
    Tray, Fluoride   Dental And Oral
    Varnish, Cavity   Dental And Oral

PASMAN MEDEQ, INC.   574-252-5690
3296 Cambridge Ct., Mishawaka, IN 46545
FDA Number: 105956
Ownership: Private
Produces/Sells CE-marked Devices: N
    Orthosis, Lumbosacral   Physical Med

PASSY & PASSY
See Passy-Muir Inc.

MANUFACTURER PROFILES

PASSY-MUIR INC.
800-634-5397
PMB 273, 4521 Campus Dr., Irvine, CA 92612 — **949-833-8255**
FDA Number: 2024841 — Fax: 949-833-8299
E-mail: info@passy-muir.com
Web site: www.passy-muir.com
Year Founded: 1985
Total Employees: 25
Ownership: Private
Produces/Sells CE-marked Devices: Y
Federal Procurement Eligibility: Small Business, Minority Owned, Female Owned
Distribution: Manufacturer Direct, Manufacturer Through Distributor
General Admin.: Patricia E. Passy/Chief Executive Officer, Chairman
    Melissa S. Fontes/President

Adapter, Tube, Tracheal	Anesthesiology
Anatomical Training Model	General
Catheter, Oxygen, Tracheal	Anesthesiology
Communication Equipment	General
Mask, Oxygen, Other	General
Material, Training, Audiovisual	General
Moist Therapy Pack Conditioner	Physical Med
Tube, Tracheal/Bronchial, Differential Ventilation	Anesthesiology
Tube, Tracheostomy (Breathing Tube), ENT	Ear/Nose/Throat
Tube, Tracheostomy (W/Wo Connector)	Anesthesiology
Valve, Breathing	Anesthesiology
Valve, Non-Rebreathing	Anesthesiology
Valve, Prosthesis	Physical Med
Valve, Speaking, Tracheal	Ear/Nose/Throat

PATA ENTERPRISES, INC.
603-883-4534
1120 North Mesquite St., San Antonio, TX 78202
FDA Number: 3003644608
Ownership: Private
Produces/Sells CE-marked Devices: N

Mattress, Non-Powered Flotation Therapy	Physical Med

PATCRAFT COMMERCIAL
800-241-4014
PO BOX 2128, Dalton, GA 30722-2128 — **706-279-4000**
FDA Number: n/a — Fax: 706-517-7760
E-mail: info@patcraft.com
Web site: www.patcraft.com
Annual Revenue: $0-$1 Million
Total Employees: 660
Ownership: Private
Produces/Sells CE-marked Devices: N
Federal Procurement Eligibility: Small Business
Distribution: Manufacturer Through Distributor, Manufacturer Through Manufacturer Reps, Importer, Exporter
General Admin.: Julian Saul/Chief Executive Officer
    Bob Chandler/Vice President
Mktg./Adv.: Doug Enck/Vice President Sales
IS: Bill Richards/Director Tech. Services
    Gene Autry/Manager Tech. Services

Carpeting	General
Floor Mat	General

PATHFINDER THERAPEUTICS, INC.
615-783-0094
2969 Armory Drive, Suite 100a, Nashville, TN 37204
FDA Number: 3006587863 — Fax: 615) 783-0554
E-mail: sales@2pti.com
Web site: www.pathsurg.com
Ownership: Private
Produces/Sells CE-marked Devices: N

Tracking, Soft Tissue, Intraoperative	Cns/Neurology

PATHLIGHTER, INC.
877-728-4544
105 Riverside Dr., Ormond Beach, FL 32176
FDA Number: 3003527627
E-mail: wippco@aol.com
Web site: www.pathlighter.com
Ownership: Private
Produces/Sells CE-marked Devices: N

Cane	Physical Med

PATHWAY MEDICAL TECHNOLOGIES
(425) 636-4000
10801 120th Ave NE, Kirkland, WA 98033
FDA Number: 3003603429 — Fax: (425) 636-4001
E-mail: customerservice@pathwaymedical.com
Web site: www.pathwaymedical.com
Ownership: Private
Produces/Sells CE-marked Devices: N
General Admin.: Mr. Paul Buckman/President, Chief Executive Officer
Mktg./Adv.: Mr. Tonm Douthitt/Senior Vice President Marketing
    Mr. Mike Napack/Vice President U.S. Sales
Research: Mr. Scott Youmans/Vice President Engineering
Finance: Mr. Michael Behlke/Executive Vice President Finance

Catheter, Peripheral, Atherectomy	Cardiovascular

PATHWORK DIAGNOSTICS INC.
1-877-808-0006
595 Penobscot Drive, — **650-366-1003**
Redwood City, CA 94063
FDA Number: n/a — Fax: 650-599-9083
E-mail: webmaster@pathworkdx.com
Web site: www.pathworkdx.com
Year Founded: 2003
Ownership: Private
Produces/Sells CE-marked Devices: N
General Admin.: W. David Henner/Chief Medical Officer, Vice President
    Deborah Neff/President, Chief Executive Officer
Mktg./Adv.: David Craford/Vice President Commercial Operations
    Shawn Becker/Vice President Marketing
    Mr. Mark McDonough/Vice President Sales

PATIENT CARE DIVISION
See Zimmer Orthopaedic Surgical Products

PATIENT HANDLING TECHNOLOGIES
See Hovertech International

PATIENT INSTRUMENTATION CORP.
610-799-4436
4117 Rte. 309, Schnecksville, PA 18078-2509
FDA Number: n/a — Fax: 610-799-4466
E-mail: patientins@juno.com
Medical Products Sales Volume: $400,000
Annual Revenue: $0-$1 Million
Total Employees: 6 — *Marketing Staff:* 4 — *Sales Staff:* 4
Ownership: Private
Produces/Sells CE-marked Devices: N
Federal Procurement Eligibility: Small Business
Distribution: Service Direct
General Admin.: Peter Esherick/President
    Helen K. Esherick/Secretary
Research: David Esherick/Director Tech. Development

Component, Metal, Other	General
Detector, Leakage, Medical Gas	General
Equipment, Cleaning, Air	General
Service, Consulting	General
Service, Maintenance/Repair	General

PATIENT TRANSFER SYSTEMS, INC.
800-633-4725
5456 Northwood Dr., Center Valley, PA 18034
FDA Number: 2523170

Stretcher, Hand-Carried	General
Transfer Device, Patient, Manual	General

PATIENT TRANSFER SYSTEMS, INC.
See Airpal Patient Transfer Systems Inc.

PATIENT'S PRIDE, INC.
866-607-7433
395 Del Monte Ctr.,, Ste. 182, — **831-626-3344**
Monterey, CA 93940
FDA Number: 3004158994 — Fax: 831-855-0107
Web site: www.patientspride.com
Ownership: Private
Produces/Sells CE-marked Devices: N

Binder, Perineal	General

PATRIOT PRODUCTS
909-988-6578
12460 N. Park Ave., Chino, CA 91710
FDA Number: 3005449993
Ownership: Private
Produces/Sells CE-marked Devices: N

Tourniquet, Non-Pneumatic, Surgical	Surgery

PATTERSON COMPANIES, INC.
800-328-5536
1031 Mendota Heights Road, St. Paul, MN 55120 — **651-686-1600**
FDA Number: n/a — Fax: 651-686-9331
Web site: www.pattersoncompanies.com
Ownership: Private
Stock Symbol: PDCO
Traded On: NASDAQ
Produces/Sells CE-marked Devices: N
General Admin.: Peter L. Frechette/Chairman
    R. Stephen Armstrong/Chief Financial Officer, Executive Vice President
    Mr. Scott Anderson/President, Chief Executive Officer
    Jerome E. Thygesen/Vice President Human Resources
Production: Daniel H. Peckskamp/Vice President Operations

PATTERSON MEDICAL HOLDINGS, INC.
800-323-5547
1000 Remington Blvd., Suite 210, — **630-378-6000**
Bolingbrook, IL 60440
FDA Number: 1418324 — Fax: 630-378-6010
E-mail: sp@patterson-medical.com
Web site: www.sammonspreston.com
Annual Revenue: $50-$100 Million
Ownership: BISSELL HEALTHCARE, INC.

PATTERSON MEDICAL HOLDINGS, INC.   800-323-5547 *(cont'd)*

Produces/Sells CE-marked Devices: N
Federal Procurement Eligibility: Small Business
Distribution: Manufacturer Direct, Manufacturer Through Distributor

Accessories, Cart, Multipurpose	General
Accessories, Traction	Physical Med
Accessories, Wheelchair	Physical Med
Adapter, Hygiene	Physical Med
Adaptor, Grooming	Physical Med
Armboard, Wheelchair	Physical Med
Armrest, Wheelchair	Physical Med
Attachment, Bag (Crutch, Walker, Wheelchair)	Physical Med
Attachment, Commode, Wheelchair	Physical Med
Band, Support, Pelvic	Physical Med
Bandage, Cast	Physical Med
Bars, Parallel, Exercise	Physical Med
Bars, Parallel, Powered	Physical Med
Bars, Parallel, Walking	Physical Med
Bath, Hydro-Massage (Whirlpool)	Physical Med
Bath, Paraffin	Physical Med
Bath, Portable	General
Bath, Sitz, Physical Medicine	Physical Med
Bedpan	General
Belt, Lumbosacral	Orthopedics
Belt, Traction, Pelvic, Orthopedic	Orthopedics
Belt, Wheelchair	Physical Med
Bib	General
Biofeedback Device	Cns/Neurology
Brace, Joint, Ankle (External)	Physical Med
Brake, Extension, Wheelchair	Physical Med
Caliper, Skinfold	General
Cane	Physical Med
Cast	Orthopedics
Chair, Adjustable, Mechanical	Physical Med
Chair, Bath	General
Chair, Geriatric, Wheeled	General
Chair, Pediatric	General
Chair, Rehabilitation	General
Chair, Seat Lifting (Standing Aid)	General
Chair, Shower	General
Collar, Cervical Neck	Orthopedics
Collar, Ice	General
Commode (Toilet)	General
Commode Seat	General
Communication System, Non-Powered	Physical Med
Compression Unit, Intermittent (Anti-Embolism Pump)	Cardiovascular
Cover, Cast	General
Crutch	Physical Med
Cuff, Pusher, Wheelchair	Physical Med
Cup, Geriatric Feeding	General
Cushion, Foot	Orthopedics
Cushion, Wheelchair (Pad)	Physical Med
Cutter, Pill	General
Diathermy, Shortwave	Physical Med
Dynamometer, Grip-Strength (Squeeze)	Anesthesiology
Dynamometer, Other	Cns/Neurology
Elastomer, Other	General
Electrode, Diathermy	Physical Med
Equipment, Therapy, Handicapped/Physical	Physical Med
Ergometer, Bicycle	Cardiovascular
Ergometer, Other	Anesthesiology
Exercise Stair	Physical Med
Exerciser, Arm	Physical Med
Exerciser, Bicycle	Physical Med
Exerciser, Chest	Physical Med
Exerciser, Hand	Physical Med
Exerciser, Leg And Ankle	Physical Med
Exerciser, Measuring	Physical Med
Exerciser, Non-Measuring	Physical Med
Exerciser, Other	Physical Med
Exerciser, Shoulder	Physical Med
Exerciser, Trapeze	Physical Med
Exerciser, Wrist	Physical Med
Floor Mat	General
Footrest, Wheelchair	Physical Med
Goniometer, Mechanical	Physical Med
Halter, Head, Traction	Physical Med
Heater, Hot Pack	Physical Med
Holder, Infant Position	General
Immobilizer, Ankle	Orthopedics
Immobilizer, Arm	Orthopedics
Immobilizer, Elbow	Orthopedics
Immobilizer, Knee	Orthopedics
Immobilizer, Shoulder	Orthopedics
Immobilizer, Wrist/Hand	Orthopedics
Lamp, Infrared	Physical Med
Legging, Compression, Non-Inflatable	General
Lift, Bath, Non-AC-Powered	General
Lift, Patient	General
Mattress, Alternating Pressure (Or Pads)	Physical Med
Mattress, Reduction, Pressure	General
Mirror, Laryngeal	Ear/Nose/Throat

PATTERSON MEDICAL HOLDINGS, INC.   800-323-5547 *(cont'd)*

Mirror, Posture	Physical Med
Mirror, Speech	Ear/Nose/Throat
Moist Therapy Pack	Physical Med
Monitor, Blood Pressure, Indirect, Automatic	Cardiovascular
Orthosis, Cervical	Physical Med
Orthosis, Limb Brace	Physical Med
Orthosis, Other	Physical Med
Pack, Cold	General
Pack, Hot Or Cold, Disposable	Physical Med
Pack, Hot Or Cold, Reusable	Physical Med
Pack, Moist Heat	Physical Med
Pad, Incontinence (Underpad)	General
Pad, Pressure, Air	General
Pad, Pressure, Animal Skin	General
Pad, Pressure, Foam (Elbow, Heel)	General
Pad, Pressure, Foam Convoluted	General
Pad, Pressure, Gel	General
Padding, Cast/Splint	General
Pillow, Bath	General
Pillow, Cervical	Orthopedics
Pressure Pad, Alternating, Reusable	General
Protector, Heel	General
Rail, Bath	General
Rail, Commode	General
Ramp, Wheelchair	General
Reacher (Handicapped)	General
Restraint, Wheelchair	General
Scale, Platform, Wheelchair	Physical Med
Scale, Stand-On	General
Scissors, Bandage/Gauze/Plaster	General
Scooter (Motorized 3-Wheeled Vehicle)	Physical Med
Sling, Arm	Physical Med
Sling, Arm, Overhead Supported	Physical Med
Sling, Overhead Suspension, Wheelchair	Physical Med
Sphygmomanometer, Aneroid (Arterial Pressure)	General
Sphygmomanometer, Mercury (Arterial Pressure)	General
Splint, Abduction, Congenital Hip Dislocation	Physical Med
Splint, Abduction, Shoulder	Orthopedics
Splint, Extremity, Inflatable, External	Surgery
Splint, Extremity, Non-Inflatable, External	Surgery
Splint, Hand, And Component	Physical Med
Splint, Molded, Plastic	Orthopedics
Splint, Other	Orthopedics
Splint, Traction	Orthopedics
Spreader, Plaster (Cast)	Orthopedics
Stethoscope, Manual	Cardiovascular
Stimulator, Muscle, Electrical-Powered (EMS)	Physical Med
Stimulator, Muscle, Low Intensity	Physical Med
Stimulator, Nerve, Transcutaneous (Pain Relief, TENS)	Cns/Neurology
Stimulator, Ultrasound, Muscle	Physical Med
Stockinette, Cast	Orthopedics
Stocking, Elastic	General
Stocking, Elastic, Physical Medicine	Physical Med
Stroller, Adaptive	Physical Med
Support, Abdominal	Physical Med
Support, Ankle	Orthopedics
Support, Arch	Physical Med
Support, Arm	Physical Med
Support, Back	Orthopedics
Support, Clavicle	Orthopedics
Support, Elbow	Orthopedics
Support, Foot	Orthopedics
Support, Hand	Orthopedics
Support, Head And Trunk, Wheelchair	Physical Med
Support, Knee	Physical Med
Support, Leg	Physical Med
Support, Patient Position	Anesthesiology
Support, Wrist	Physical Med
Table, Examination/Treatment	General
Table, Mechanical	Physical Med
Table, Overbed	General
Table, Physical Medicine, Powered	Physical Med
Table, Physical Therapy	Physical Med
Table, Traction	Orthopedics
Tips And Pads, Cane, Crutch And Walker	Physical Med
Traction Unit, Static, Chair	Orthopedics
Transfer Aid	Physical Med
Transfer Device, Patient, Manual	General
Tray, Walker	General
Tray, Wheelchair	Physical Med
Treadmill, Mechanical	Physical Med
Treadmill, Powered	Physical Med
Utensil, Food	Physical Med
Utensil, Handicapped Aid	Physical Med
Walker, Mechanical	Physical Med
Wheelchair, Manual	Physical Med

Medical Product Subsidiaries (Listed Separately)
  Midland Manufacturing Co., Inc.

PATTERSON MEDICAL SUPPLY, INC. 262-387-8720
W68 N158 Evergreen Blvd., Cedarburg, WI 53012
FDA Number: 2128677

Accessories, Wheelchair	Physical Med
Adapter, Hygiene	Physical Med
Adaptor, Dressing	Physical Med
Adaptor, Grooming	Physical Med
Adaptor, Recreational	Physical Med
Alarm, Overload, External Limb, Powered	Physical Med
Armrest, Wheelchair	Physical Med
Attachment, Narrowing, Wheelchair	Physical Med
Band, Support, Pelvic	Physical Med
Bandage, Elastic	General
Brace, Joint, Ankle (External)	Physical Med
Cane	Physical Med
Climber, Curb, Wheelchair	Physical Med
Cover, Cast	General
Crutch	Physical Med
Cushion, Wheelchair (Pad)	Physical Med
Discriminator, Two-point	Cns/Neurology
Dressing, Other	General
Elastomer, Silicone (Scar Management)	Surgery
Electrode, Cutaneous	Cns/Neurology
Esthesiometer	Cns/Neurology
Exerciser, Non-Measuring	Physical Med
Goniometer, Non-Powered	Orthopedics
Joint, Knee, External Brace	Physical Med
Joint, Wrist, External Limb Component, Mechanical	Physical Med
Massager, Therapeutic	Physical Med
Massager, Therapeutic, Manual	Physical Med
Material, Impression Tray, Resin	Dental And Oral
Medical Disinfectants/Cleaners for Instruments	General
Orthosis, Abdominal	Physical Med
Orthosis, Cervical	Physical Med
Orthosis, Corrective Shoe	Physical Med
Orthosis, Limb Brace	Physical Med
Orthosis, Lumbosacral	Physical Med
Pack, Hot Or Cold, Reusable	Physical Med
Pack, Moist Heat	Physical Med
Protector, Skin Pressure	General
Scissors, Orthopedic	Orthopedics
Sling, Arm	Physical Med
Splint, Extremity, Non-Inflatable, External	Surgery
Splint, Hand, And Component	Physical Med
Splint, Traction	Orthopedics
Sponge, Gauze	Dental And Oral
Support, Arm	Physical Med
Support, Head And Trunk, Wheelchair	Physical Med
Table, Mechanical	Physical Med
Tape, Orthopedic	Orthopedics
Teletherapy System, Radionuclide	Radiology
Tips And Pads, Cane, Crutch And Walker	Physical Med
Toothbrush, Manual	Dental And Oral
Tourniquet, Pneumatic	Surgery
Transfer Aid	Physical Med
Tray, Wheelchair	Physical Med
Utensil, Food	Physical Med
Utensil, Handicapped Aid	Physical Med
Walker, Mechanical	Physical Med

PATTERSON PRECISION, INC. 956-943-6119
561 Industrial Way, PORT ISABEL, TX 78578
FDA Number: 2028841 *Fax:* 956-943-6529
E-mail: info@pattersonprecision.com
Web site: http://pattersonprecision.com/
Medical Products Sales Volume: $100,000
Annual Revenue: $1-$5 Million
Year Founded: 1991
Total Employees: 2
Ownership: Private
Produces/Sells CE-marked Devices: N
Federal Procurement Eligibility: Small Business

PATTERSON TECHNOLOGY CENTER, INC 800-475-5036
2202 Althoff Drive, Effingham, IL 62401-1267 217-347-5964
FDA Number: 1424139 *Fax:* 217-342-6950
E-mail: craig.kabbes@pattersondental.com
Web site: www.pattersoncompanies.com
Annual Revenue: $50-$100 Million
Year Founded: 1983
Total Employees: 230
Ownership: PATTERSON COMPANIES, INC.
Produces/Sells CE-marked Devices: N

Powder, Porcelain	Dental And Oral
Radiographic Unit, Diagnostic, Intraoral	Dental And Oral

PATTON MEDICAL DEVICES 877-763-7678
31058 N. Lamar Blvd., Austin, TX 78705 512-279-4545
FDA Number: 3006035654
Year Founded: 2004

PATTON MEDICAL DEVICES 877-763-7678 *(cont'd)*
Total Employees: 30
Ownership: Private
Produces/Sells CE-marked Devices: N
General Admin.: Chris C. Donnelly/Chief Financial Officer, Executive Vice President
Terrance Gregg/Executive Chairman
John S. Burns/President
Mktg./Adv.: Liz Walker/Vice President Marketing
Rick E. Wittenbraker/Vice President Sales
Research: William J. Ambruzs/Vice President Research & Development

Catheter, Intravascular, Therapeutic, Short-term Less Than 30 Days	General

PATTON SURGICAL CORP. 1.877.641.0469
6300 Bridgepoint Pkwy. 512-329-0469
Building Two, Ste. 420
Austin, TX 78730
FDA Number: 1651380 *Fax:* 512-328-9113
E-mail: info@pattonsurgical.com
Web site: www.pattonsurgical.com
Ownership: Private
Produces/Sells CE-marked Devices: Y
Distribution: Manufacturer Direct, Manufacturer Through Distributor, Manufacturer Through Manufacturer Reps
General Admin.: Dr. Michael Patton/Chief Medical Officer, Vice President
Ms. Rebecca Foletta/Manager
Mr. Ron Baker/President, Chief Executive Officer
Finance: Ms. Christine Mallory/Vice President Finance & Operations

Electrosurgical Unit, Cutting & Coagulation Device	Surgery
Laparoscope, General & Plastic Surgery	Surgery
Speculum, Vaginal, Non-Metal	Obstetrics/Gynecology
Trocar, Laparoscopic	Surgery

PAUL ARPIN MFG. 408-263-4974
1347 Highland Ct., Milpitas, CA 95035
FDA Number: 2953183
Ownership: Private
Produces/Sells CE-marked Devices: N

Mirror, General & Plastic Surgery	Surgery

PAUSCH LLC 732-747-6110
808 Shrewsbury Ave., Tinton Falls, NJ 07724
FDA Number: 2243057 *Fax:* 732-747-6882
E-mail: info@pauschusa.com
Web site: www.pausch.de
Year Founded: 1930
Ownership: HANS PAUSCH GMBH & CO. KG
Quality System Registration Information: ISO9001
Produces/Sells CE-marked Devices: N
Federal Procurement Eligibility: Small Business

Device, Limiting, Beam, Diagnostic, X-Ray	Radiology
Holder, Radiographic Cassette, Wall-Mounted	Radiology
Mount, X-Ray Tube, Diagnostic	Radiology
Spot Film Device	Radiology
Table, Radiographic, Non-Tilting, Powered	Radiology
Table, Radiographic, Tilting	Radiology

PAWLING CORP., ARCHITECTURAL PROD. DIV. 800-431-3456
32 Nelson Hill Road, PO Box 200, 845-373-9300
Wassaic, NY 12592
FDA Number: 9330093 *Fax:* 845-373-7827
E-mail: sales@pawling.com
Web site: www.pawling.com
Medical Products Sales Volume: $5,000,000
Annual Revenue: $50-$100 Million
Year Founded: 1945
Total Employees: 65 *Marketing Staff:* 1
Ownership: Private
Quality System Registration Information: ISO9001
Produces/Sells CE-marked Devices: N
Federal Procurement Eligibility: Small Business, GSA Contract
Distribution: Manufacturer Through Distributor, Manufacturer Through Manufacturer Reps, OEM
General Admin.: Rick Raible/Vice President
Mktg./Adv.: Greg Holen/Director National Sales

Bumper Guard, Corner	General
Floor Mat	General
Rail, Wall Side	General

PAYTON ASSOCIATES INC.
See Payton Scientific Inc.

PAYTON SCIENTIFIC INC. 716-876-1813
964 Kenmore Avenue, Buffalo, NY 14216
FDA Number: 1317363 *Fax:* 716-876-8957
E-mail: paytonscientific@att.net
Web site: www.paytonscientific.com
Medical Products Sales Volume: $400,000

PAYTON SCIENTIFIC INC.
716-876-1813 *(cont'd)*
Annual Revenue: $0-$1 Million
Year Founded: 1968
Total Employees: 5   Sales Staff: 3
Ownership: Private
Produces/Sells CE-marked Devices: N
Federal Procurement Eligibility: Small Business
Distribution: Manufacturer Direct, Manufacturer Through Manufacturer Reps
General Admin.: R. W. Baker/President, Chief Executive Officer
   Paul Baker/Vice President, General Manager
Mktg./Adv.: Paul Baker/Director Marketing
   Allene Baker/Director National Accounts
   Robert Baker/Manager International & National Sales
   Paul Baker/Manager International Marketing & Sales
   G. Chadwick/Manager Marketing
Research: A. Baker/Manager Research

Aggregometer, Platelet	Hematology
Analyzer, Platelet Aggregation	Hematology
Analyzer, Platelet Aggregation, Automated	Hematology
Recorder, Paper Chart	Cardiovascular

PBS BIOTECH, INC
1 (805) 482-727
4023 Camino Ranchero AõÉ,™É_o Suite I, Camarillo, CA 93012
FDA Number: n/a   Fax: 1 (805) 383-772
E-mail: info@pbsbiotech.com
Web site: www.pbsbiotech.com
Year Founded: 2007
Ownership: Private
Produces/Sells CE-marked Devices: N
General Admin.: Mr. Brian Less/President, Chief Executive Officer
Mktg./Adv.: Mr. James Schultz/Vice President Marketing & Sales
Production: Mr. Oscar Garza/Vice President Manufacturing & Operations
Research: Mr. Randy Ray/Vice President Engineering
   Mr. Dainel Giroux/Vice President Research & Development

PCA INDUSTRIES, INC.
See Sports Play Equipment, Inc.

PCI
800-309-8935
12201 Magnolia Avenue, Riverside, CA 92503
FDA Number: n/a
Web site: http://pci-intl.com
Year Founded: 1984
Ownership: Private
Produces/Sells CE-marked Devices: N
General Admin.: Mr. Bob Eng/Chief Executive Officer
Research: Mr. Tarik Naheiri/Vice President Engineering
Finance: Mr. Jeff Cartwright/Chief Financial Officer

Generator, Oxygen	Anesthesiology

PCI TECHNOLOGY
See Brady Precision Converting, Llc

PCI TRANSAID
See Artromick

PCL-RIA INC.
See Oxis International, Inc.

PCN, INC.
508-880-7140
125 John Hancock Road, Taunton, MA 02780
FDA Number: 88163
Ownership: Private
Produces/Sells CE-marked Devices: N

Electrosurgical Unit, Cutting & Coagulation Device	Surgery

PCP CHAMPION
800-888-0867
300 Congress St., Ripley, OH 45167-1411
FDA Number: n/a   Fax: 800-667-5984
Web site: www.surgicalappliance.com
Annual Revenue: $0-$1 Million
Ownership: Truform Orthotics & Prosthetics
Produces/Sells CE-marked Devices: N
Federal Procurement Eligibility: Small Business
Distribution: Manufacturer Direct

Cane	Physical Med
Walker, Mechanical	Physical Med

PDG PRODUCT DESIGN GROUP, INC.
888-858-4422
Unit 102, 366 East Kent Ave. South,
604-323-9220
Vancouver, BC V5X 4 Canada
FDA Number: 9681827   Fax: 604-323-9097
E-mail: info@prodgroup.com
Web site: www.prodgroup.com
Year Founded: 1996
Total Employees: 25   Marketing Staff: 3   Sales Staff: 50
Ownership: Private
Produces/Sells CE-marked Devices: Y
Distribution: Manufacturer Through Distributor, Manufacturer Through Manufacturer Reps, Exporter

PDI COMMUNICATION SYSTEMS
800-992-7734
40 Greenwood Lane, Springboro, OH 45066
800-628-9870
FDA Number: n/a   Fax: 937-743-5664
E-mail: cfocht@pdiarm.com
Web site: www.pdiarm.com
Medical Products Sales Volume: $10,000,000
Annual Revenue: $10-$25 Million
Year Founded: 1976
Ownership: Private
Produces/Sells CE-marked Devices: N
Federal Procurement Eligibility: Small Business
Distribution: Manufacturer Through Distributor

Computer Equipment	General
Mount, Monitor (Support)	General
Mount, Television Set	General
Recorder, Videotape/Videodisc	General
Television, Patient Room	General

PDI, A DIVISION OF DEROYAL INDUSTRIES, INC
800-251-9864
720 Northern Rd., Mount Juliet, TN 37122
865-362-6022
FDA Number: 1055080
E-mail: customerservice@deroyal.com
Web site: www.deroyal.com
Year Founded: 1973
Ownership: DEROYAL INDUSTRIES, INC.
Produces/Sells CE-marked Devices: N

Basin, Emesis	General
Bedpan	General
Container, Medication, Graduated Liquid	General
Container, Specimen, Non-sterile	General
Tray, Surgical	Surgery

PDS HEALTH, INC.
800-440-2417
112 Intracoastal Pointe Drive, Jupiter, FL 33477
FDA Number: 3006306378
Ownership: Private
Produces/Sells CE-marked Devices: N

Computer, Chemistry Analyzer	Chemistry

PDS MANUFACTURING, INC.
817-329-2701
577 Commerce St., Suite A, Southlake, TX 76092
FDA Number: 3005832736

Cryosurgical Unit	Surgery

PDT, INC.
406-626-4153
12201 Moccasin Ct., Missoula, MT 59808
FDA Number: 3003963832

Curette, Periodontic	Dental And Oral
Explorer, Operative	Dental And Oral
Handle, Instrument, Dental	Dental And Oral
Probe, Periodontic	Dental And Oral
Scaler, Periodontic	Dental And Oral

PEACE MEDICAL
800-537-9564
50 S. Center St., Unit 11, Orange, NJ 07050-3587
973-672-2120
FDA Number: 2243990   Fax: 973-672-3404
E-mail: info@peacemedical.com
Web site: www.peacemedical.com
Annual Revenue: $1-$5 Million
Total Employees: 10
Ownership: Private
Quality System Registration Information: ISO9000
Produces/Sells CE-marked Devices: N
Federal Procurement Eligibility: Small Business, Female Owned
Distribution: Manufacturer Direct
General Admin.: Tim Fegan/President, Chief Executive Officer
   Diane L. Sellitto/Vice President, General Manager
Mktg./Adv.: Tim Fegan/Vice President Marketing & Sales
Production: Jen Masson/Director Quality Assurance

Alarm, Oxygen Depletion	Anesthesiology
Chamber, Isolation, Patient Care	General
Chamber, Isolation, Patient Transport	General
Evacuator, Fume	Chemistry
Filter, Air	General
Holder, Gas Cylinder	Anesthesiology
Hood, Oxygen, Infant	General
Isolation Unit, Surgical	General
Rack, Bedpan	General
Tent, Mist	General
Tent, Oxygen (Canopy)	Anesthesiology
Tent, Pediatric Aerosol	General

PEACE MEDICAL, INC.
800-537-9564
50 South Center St., Unit 11, Orange, NJ 07050
973-672-2120
FDA Number: 2243990   Fax: 973-672-3404
E-mail: info@peacemedical.com
Web site: www.peacemedical.com
Ownership: Private
Produces/Sells CE-marked Devices: N

PEACE MEDICAL, INC.   800-537-9564 (cont'd)
Chamber, Isolation, Patient Care	General
Tent, Pediatric Aerosol	General

PEAK ENTERPRISES INC   941-373-0046
635 South Orange Avenue, Suite 8, Sarasota, FL 34236
FDA Number: 1063242   Fax: 941-373-0048
E-mail: contact@peak21.com
Web site: www.peak21.com
Medical Products Sales Volume: $300,000
Year Founded: 1996
Total Employees: 2
Ownership: Private
Produces/Sells CE-marked Devices: N
Federal Procurement Eligibility: Small Business
General Admin.: Thomas Oechslin/President

Toothbrush, Manual	Dental And Oral

PEAK SURGICAL INC.   888-792-7325
2464 Embarcadero Way, Palo Alto, CA 94303   650-331-3020
FDA Number: n/a   Fax: 650-331-3293
E-mail: info@peaksurgical.com
Web site: www.peaksurgical.com
Ownership: Private
Produces/Sells CE-marked Devices: N
General Admin.: John Tighe/President, Chief Executive Officer
Mktg./Adv.: Andre Bessette/Vice President Marketing
       John Cifarelli/Vice President Sales
Production: Jeff Heer/Vice President Operations
       Grace Carlson/Vice President Regulatory & Clinical Affairs
Research: Paul Davison/Vice President Research & Development
Finance: Lori Munoz/Vice President Finance

PEARCE-TURK DENTAL LAB   800-835-2776
201 North Emporia, Wichita, KS 67202   316-263-0284
FDA Number: 3004133908   Fax: 316-263-5869
E-mail: tphillips@dentalservices.net
Web site: www.dentalservices.net
Ownership: Private
Produces/Sells CE-marked Devices: N

Crown, Preformed	Dental And Oral
Device, Anti-Snoring	Ear/Nose/Throat
Device, Repositioning, Jaw	Dental And Oral
Mouthguard	Dental And Oral

PEARL BATHS, INC.   800-328-2531
9224 73rd Avenue North, Minneapolis, MN 55428
FDA Number: n/a   Fax: 763-424-9808
Web site: www.pearlbaths.com
Ownership: Private
Produces/Sells CE-marked Devices: N
Distribution: Manufacturer Through Distributor

Bath, Hydro-Massage (Whirlpool)	Physical Med

PEARLE VISION   800-937-3937
4000 Luxottica Place, Mason, OH 45040   877-486-6486
FDA Number: n/a
Web site: www.pearlevision.com
Ownership: Private
Produces/Sells CE-marked Devices: N
Federal Procurement Eligibility: Small Business
Distribution: Manufacturer Direct

Eyeglasses	Ophthalmology

PECHINEY PLASTIC PKG., AN ALCAN COMPANY   323-721-6777
5416 Union Pacific Ave., Commerce, CA 90022
FDA Number: 2023811
Web site: www.pechineyplasticpackaging.com
Ownership: Private
Produces/Sells CE-marked Devices: N

Pack, Sterilization Wrapper (Bag And Accessories)	Surgery

PECTUS SERVICES   757-224-0177
549 Pompton Ave., Suite 210, Cedar Grove, NJ 07009
FDA Number: 3005737684

Orthosis, Thoracic	Physical Med

PEDIA PALS, LLC   888-733-4272
965 Highway 169 N., Plymouth, MN 55441   763-546-4161
FDA Number: 1528482   Fax: 763-546-4501
E-mail: akochsiek@pediapals.com
Web site: www.pediapals.com
Medical Products Sales Volume: $1,200,000
Annual Revenue: $1-$5 Million
Year Founded: 1998
Total Employees: 4   Marketing Staff: 2   Sales Staff: 2
Ownership: Health and Technology
Produces/Sells CE-marked Devices: Y

PEDIA PALS, LLC   888-733-4272 (cont'd)
Federal Procurement Eligibility: Small Business, Female Owned, GSA Contract
Distribution: Manufacturer Direct, Manufacturer Through Manufacturer Reps, OEM, Exclusive Distributor, Exporter
General Admin.: Mr. Ed Powell/Chief Executive Officer, General Manager
Mktg./Adv.: Ms. Brenda Dupont/Admin. Marketing & Sales
       Ms. Ann Kochsiek/Vice President, Director Marketing

Accessories, Speculum	Surgery
Cuff, Blood Pressure	Cardiovascular
Holder, Intravascular Catheter	General
Otoscope	Ear/Nose/Throat
Percussor	Cns/Neurology
Speculum, Ophthalmic	Ophthalmology
Stethoscope, Manual	Cardiovascular
Syringe, Irrigating	General
Table, Examination/Treatment	General
Table, Mechanical	Physical Med

PEDIATRIC INTENSIVE THERAPY, INC.   786-543-8165
18639 S.w. 107th Ave., Miami, FL 33157
FDA Number: 3004518475
Ownership: Private
Produces/Sells CE-marked Devices: N

Component, Exercise	Physical Med

PEDIATRIC SEATING DIST., INC.   416-604-9219
2833 Dundas St W, Toronto M6P 1Y6 Canada
FDA Number: 9680551

Accessories, Wheelchair	Physical Med

PEDICRAFT, INC.   800-223-7649
4134 St. Augustine Road,   904-396-9627
Jacksonville, FL 32247
FDA Number: 1043568   Fax: 904-346-3947
E-mail: info@pedicraft.com
Web site: www.pedicraft.com
Medical Products Sales Volume: $3,000,000
Annual Revenue: $1-$5 Million
Year Founded: 1966
Total Employees: 13   Marketing Staff: 3   Sales Staff: 5
Ownership: Private
Produces/Sells CE-marked Devices: N
Federal Procurement Eligibility: Small Business
Distribution: Manufacturer Direct
General Admin.: Eric A. Nord/Chief Executive Officer
       Doug Maynard/President
Production: Bobbie Nord/Manager Regulatory Affairs

Bassinet (Infant Bed)	General
Bed, Pediatric (Crib)	General
Board, Arm	Anesthesiology
Furniture, Patient Room	General
Mattress, Bed	General
Restraint, Crib	General
Restraint, Protective (Body)	General

PEDIFIX, INC.   800-424-5561
310 Guinea Road, Brewster, NY 10509   845-277-2850
FDA Number: 2431499   Fax: 845-277-2851
E-mail: info@pedifix.com
Web site: www.pedifix.com
Medical Products Sales Volume: $1,100,000
Annual Revenue: $10-$25 Million
Year Founded: 1885
Total Employees: 25   Marketing Staff: 5   Sales Staff: 5
Ownership: Private
Produces/Sells CE-marked Devices: N
Federal Procurement Eligibility: Small Business
Distribution: Manufacturer Direct, Manufacturer Through Distributor, Manufacturer Through Manufacturer Reps, Exclusive Distributor
General Admin.: Dennis Case/Chief Financial Officer, Treasurer
       Dennis Case/President, Chief Executive Officer
Mktg./Adv.: Caroline Bochnia/Director Marketing & Advertising
       Richard Ovadek/Director Product Development
       Jon Case/Vice President Sales

Analyzer, Gait	Orthopedics
Bandage, Elastic	General
Bandage, Other	General
Cushion, Foot	Orthopedics
Immobilizer, Ankle	Orthopedics
Orthosis, Limb Brace	Physical Med
Pad, Pressure, Soft Rubber	General
Production Equipment	General
Separator, Toe	Orthopedics
Shield, Bunion	Orthopedics
Splint, Molded, Plastic	Orthopedics
Splint, Temporary Training	Physical Med
Support, Ankle	Orthopedics
Support, Arch	Physical Med

PEDIFIX, INC.
800-424-5561 *(cont'd)*
Support, Foot — Orthopedics

PEDIGO PRODUCTS
360-695-3500
4000 S.E. Columbia Way, Vancouver, WA 98661
FDA Number: n/a — *Fax:* 360-696-1700
E-mail: custserv@pedigo.usa.com
Web site: www.pedigo-usa.com
Medical Products Sales Volume: $8,000,000
Annual Revenue: $5-$10 Million
Year Founded: 1947
Total Employees: 100 — *Marketing Staff:* 2 — *Sales Staff:* 5
Ownership: Private
Produces/Sells CE-marked Devices: N
Federal Procurement Eligibility: Small Business, GSA Contract, VA Contract
Distribution: Manufacturer Direct, Manufacturer Through Distributor, OEM
General Admin.: Rick Pedigo/President, Chief Operating Officer
Mktg./Adv.: Tom Hillebrand/Vice President Marketing & Sales
Production: Bill Byer/Manager Customer Services
Larry White/Manager Materials

Bassinet (Infant Bed)	General
Cabinet Casework, General Purpose	General
Cabinet, Warming	General
Cart, Instrument	Surgery
Cart, Laundry	General
Cart, Supply, Operating Room	Surgery
Footstool	General
Infusion Stand	General
Laundry Hamper	General
Stand, Basin	General
Stand, Operating Room Instrument (Mayo)	Surgery
Stool, Operating Room, Adjustable	Surgery
Stretcher, Transfer	Surgery
Table, Instrument, Surgical	Surgery
Table, Operating Room, Mechanical	Surgery
Waste Receptacle, Kick Bucket	General

PEDINOL PHARMACAL, INC.
800-733-4665
631-293-9500
30 Banfi Plaza, Farmingdale, NY 11735-1528
FDA Number: 2425128 — *Fax:* 631-293-7359
E-mail: info@pedinol.com
Medical Products Sales Volume: $25,000,000
Annual Revenue: $25-$50 Million
Year Founded: 1971
Total Employees: 56 — *Marketing Staff:* 3 — *Sales Staff:* 37
Ownership: Private
Produces/Sells CE-marked Devices: N
Federal Procurement Eligibility: Small Business
Distribution: Manufacturer Through Distributor
General Admin.: Richard Strauss/President, Chief Executive Officer
Gary Strauss/Vice President, General Manager
Mktg./Adv.: Jim Prendergast/Manager National Sales
William Thomas/Vice President Business Development
A. T. Buatti/Vice President Marketing

Bandage, Elastic	General
Component, Cast	Orthopedics
Culture Media, Antibiotic Assay	Microbiology
Drying Unit	Chemistry
Lotion, Skin Care	General
Shoe, Cast	Physical Med
Solution, Antibacterial Cleaner	General
Swabs, Cotton	General
Tape, Gauze, Adhesive	General

PEDORS SHOES
800-750-6729
770-218-7414
1349 Old 41 Hwy. #130, Marietta, GA 30060
FDA Number: n/a — *Fax:* 800-446-3101
E-mail: info@pedors.com
Web site: www.pedors.com
Medical Products Sales Volume: $700,000
Annual Revenue: $1-$5 Million
Year Founded: 1995
Total Employees: 10 — *Marketing Staff:* 5 — *Sales Staff:* 5
Ownership: Private
Produces/Sells CE-marked Devices: N
Federal Procurement Eligibility: Small Business
Distribution: Manufacturer Direct, Manufacturer Through Distributor, Importer, Exporter
General Admin.: Mr. John O'Hare/Chief Executive Officer, Chief Financial Officer
Ms. Lindsay Chisholm/General Manager
Stephen O'Hare/President
Mktg./Adv.: Russell McMillan/Director Marketing

Insoles, Medical	General
Orthosis, Corrective Shoe	Physical Med
Shoe, Orthopedic	Orthopedics

PEEL-A-WAY CO.
See Polysciences, Inc.

PEERLESS INJECTION MOLDING, LLC.
310-768-8023
14600 S. Main Street, Gardena, CA 90248
FDA Number: 3004601221
Ownership: Private
Produces/Sells CE-marked Devices: N
Laser, Surgical — Surgery

PEGASUS BIOLOGICS, INC.
949-585-9430
10 Pasteur, Suite 150, Irvine, CA 92618
FDA Number: 3005147058

Dressing, Burn, Porcine	Surgery
Dura-Substitute	Cns/Neurology
Mesh, Surgical (Steel Gauze)	Surgery

PEGASUS IMAGING CORP.
800-875-7009
813-875-7575
4001 N. Riverside Drive, Tampa, FL 33603
FDA Number: 1063288 — *Fax:* 813-875-7705
E-mail: support@jpg.com
Web site: www.pegasusimaging.com
Medical Products Sales Volume: $4,300,000
Year Founded: 1991
Total Employees: 46
Ownership: Private
Produces/Sells CE-marked Devices: N
Distribution: Manufacturer Direct, OEM
Mktg./Adv.: Ms. Jaime Cornelison/Director Marketing & Advertising
Image Processing System — Radiology

PEGASUS PRODUCTS INC.
800-865-6767
204-483-3151
1 Paisley Rd., Carroll, MAN R0K-0K0 Canada
FDA Number: n/a — *Fax:* 204-483-3141
E-mail: pegasus@pegasuswalkers.com
Web site: www.pegasusproducts.com
Year Founded: 1991
Total Employees: 10
Ownership: Private
Produces/Sells CE-marked Devices: N
Distribution: Manufacturer Direct, Exporter

PEGASUS RESEARCH CORP.
877-632-0255
714-241-7077
**3505 Cadillac Avenue Suite G-5,
Costa Mesa, CA 92626**
FDA Number: 2026969 — *Fax:* 714-241-7177
E-mail: ken.m@pegasusontheweb.com
Web site: www.pegasusontheweb.com
Medical Products Sales Volume: $500,000
Annual Revenue: $1-$5 Million
Year Founded: 1981
Total Employees: 11 — *Marketing Staff:* 1 — *Sales Staff:* 10
Ownership: Private
Produces/Sells CE-marked Devices: N
Federal Procurement Eligibility: Small Business
Distribution: Manufacturer Through Distributor, Manufacturer Through Manufacturer Reps, OEM, Importer, Exporter
General Admin.: Kenneth G. Miller/President
Michael Henigman/Vice President, General Manager
Mktg./Adv.: Michael Henigman/Manager National Sales
Rose Henigman/Sales Specialist
Production: Mina Carrasco/Customer Service Representative
Sara Perez/Director Quality Assurance
Keith Miller/Vice President Manufacturing

Compressor, Air, Portable	Anesthesiology
Humidifier, Heated	Anesthesiology
Humidifier, Respiratory Gas, (Direct Patient Interface)	Anesthesiology
Mask, Oxygen, Low Concentration, Venturi	Anesthesiology
Nebulizer, Heated	Anesthesiology
Service, Engineering/Design	General

PEKNAMED
See Microtek Medical, Inc

PELICAN PRODUCTS, LLC
864-699-4181
209 Jones Rd., Spartanburg, SC 29307
FDA Number: 3004088989
Case, Contact Lens — Ophthalmology

PELIKAN TECHNOLOGIES, INC
757-224-0177
1072 East Meadow Circle, Palo Alto, CA 94303
FDA Number: 3005310882
Ownership: Private
Produces/Sells CE-marked Devices: N

PELLERIN MILNOR CORP.
800-469-8780
504-467-9591
PO Box 400, Kenner, LA 70063-0400
FDA Number: 9310054 — *Fax:* 504-468-3094
E-mail: mktg@milnor.com
Web site: www.milnor.com
Medical Products Sales Volume: $46,700,000
Year Founded: 1987

PELLERIN MILNOR CORP.   800-469-8780 *(cont'd)*
Total Employees: 600   Marketing Staff: 8   Sales Staff: 10
Ownership: Private
Produces/Sells CE-marked Devices: Y
Federal Procurement Eligibility: Small Business
Distribution: Manufacturer Through Distributor
General Admin.: James W. Pellerin/President, Chief Executive Officer
Mktg./Adv.: Gary Gauthier/Manager Advertising
     Rick Kelly/Vice President Marketing
Research: Russ Poy/Vice President Engineering
Finance: Peter T. Youngblood/Vice President Finance
Laundry Equipment	General
Washer, Laundry	General

PELSTAR LLC (HEALTH O METER PROFESSIONAL)   800-815-6615
7400 West 100th Place, Bridgeview, IL 60455   **708-598-9100**
FDA Number: 1420128   Fax: 708-233-5472
E-mail: HomProCS@pelstarllc.com
Web site: www.healthometermedical.com
Medical Products Sales Volume: $1,700,000
Year Founded: 2001
Total Employees: 20
Ownership: Private
Quality System Registration Information: ISO9001
Produces/Sells CE-marked Devices: N
Federal Procurement Eligibility: Small Business
Distribution: Manufacturer Through Distributor, Exporter
Mktg./Adv.: Joe Giglio/Director Sales
Scale, Chair	General
Scale, Infant	General
Scale, Platform, Wheelchair	Physical Med
Scale, Stand-On	General

PELTON & CRANE   704-588-2126
11727 Fruehauf Dr., Charlotte, NC 28273
FDA Number: 1017522
Ownership: Danaher Corporation
Amalgamator, Dental, AC-Powered	Dental And Oral
Chair, Dental (With Unit)	Dental And Oral
Illuminator, Radiographic Film	Radiology
Light, Surgical Operating, Dental	Dental And Oral
Operative Dental Treatment Unit	Dental And Oral
Sterilizer, Steam (Autoclave)	General

PELTON & CRANE CO.,   800-659-6560
11727 Fruehauf Dr., Charlotte, NC 28241-7800   **704-588-2126**
FDA Number: n/a   Fax: 704-587-7237
E-mail: customerservice@pelton.net
Web site: www.pelton.net
Medical Products Sales Volume: $65,000,000
Annual Revenue: $50-$100 Million
Total Employees: 225
Ownership: Private
Quality System Registration Information: ISO9002
Produces/Sells CE-marked Devices: N
Distribution: Manufacturer Through Distributor
General Admin.: John Spencer/Chief Executive Officer
     Darrell Mc Givern/Vice President, General Manager
Mktg./Adv.: George Szalony/Sales Specialist
     Jason Spencer/Vice President Sales
Production: Bob Mc Nelis/Manager Regulatory Affairs
Chair, Dental	Dental And Oral
Chair, Dental (With Unit)	Dental And Oral
Ejector, Saliva	Ear/Nose/Throat
Evacuator, Oral Cavity	Dental And Oral
Light, Dental	Dental And Oral
Light, Dental, Intraoral	Dental And Oral
Sterilizer, Dry Heat, Dental	Dental And Oral
Sterilizer, Steam (Autoclave)	General
Sterilizer, Steam (Autoclave), Surgical	Surgery
Stool, Dental	Dental And Oral
Tester, Pulp	Dental And Oral
Tip, Suction	Anesthesiology
Tip, Suction Tube (Yankauer, Poole, Etc.)	Surgery

PELTON SHEPHERD INDUSTRIES   800-258-3423
812b Luce St., Stockton, CA 95203   **209-460-0893**
FDA Number: 2938257   Fax: 209-460-1003
E-mail: sales@peltonshepherd.com
Medical Products Sales Volume: $1,500,000
Annual Revenue: $1-$5 Million
Total Employees: 25   Marketing Staff: 2   Sales Staff: 2
Ownership: Private
Produces/Sells CE-marked Devices: N
Federal Procurement Eligibility: Small Business, Minority Owned, Female Owned
Distribution: Manufacturer Through Distributor, OEM
General Admin.: Alicia M. Shepherd/President

PELTON SHEPHERD INDUSTRIES   800-258-3423 *(cont'd)*
Mktg./Adv.: Pat Shepherd/Manager Marketing
     Susan Stanger/Manager Marketing
Production: William Zulim/Vice President Manufacturing
Linen	General
Moist Therapy Pack	Physical Med
Pack, Hot Or Cold, Reusable	Physical Med
Pack, Moist Heat	Physical Med
Probe, Other	General
Wrap, Sterilization	General

PELTOR, INC.   800-444-4774
90 Mechanic St., Southbridge, MA 01550   **508-764-5500**
FDA Number: n/a
E-mail: peltor.comms@mmm.com
Web site: www.peltor.com
Annual Revenue: $1-$5 Million
Ownership: Private
Produces/Sells CE-marked Devices: N
Distribution: Manufacturer Through Distributor
Eyeglasses, Safety	Ophthalmology
Protector, Hearing (Circumaural)	Ear/Nose/Throat
Ventilator, Other	Anesthesiology

PELVIC BINDER, INC.   877-451-3000
3982 Fm 2653 South, Cumby, TX 75433
FDA Number: 3003887052
Orthosis, Truncal/Limb	Physical Med
Splint, Clavicle	Physical Med

PEMACO, INC.   1-800-435-6487
2030 S. 3rd St., St. Louis, MO 63104   **314-231-3399**
FDA Number: 1938146   Fax: 314-231-4484
E-mail: pemaco@pemaco.us
Web site: /www.pemaco.us
Annual Revenue: $0-$1 Million
Total Employees: 21   Marketing Staff: 1   Sales Staff: 2
Ownership: Private
Produces/Sells CE-marked Devices: N
Distribution: Manufacturer Through Distributor, Exporter
General Admin.: Richard L. Perkowski/President
     Kenneth F.Perkowski/Vice President
Production: Desiree Koss/Customer Service Representative
     Rosemary Acosta/Director Quality Assurance
     Stephanie Sullens/Manager Customer Services
     Kathleen Perkowski/Manager Materials
Purchasing: Gail Riggs/Credit Manager
Cement, Dental	Dental And Oral
Cleaner, Ultrasonic, Medical Instrument	General
Dental Laboratory Equipment	Dental And Oral
Foil, Dental	Dental And Oral
Wax, Dental	Dental And Oral

PEMACO, INC.   314-231-3399
2030 South 3rd St., Saint Louis, MO 63104
FDA Number: 1938146
Cleaner, Ultrasonic, Medical Instrument	General
Wax, Dental	Dental And Oral

PEMCO, INC. - MEDICAL DIV.   216-524-2990
5663 Brecksville Road, Cleveland, OH 44131-1510
FDA Number: 1519227   Fax: 216-642-8646
E-mail: pemco@pemcomed.com
Web site: www.pemcomed.com
Medical Products Sales Volume: $1,200,000
Annual Revenue: $1-$5 Million
Year Founded: 1955
Total Employees: 15   Marketing Staff: 1   Sales Staff: 2
Ownership: Rultract, Inc.
Produces/Sells CE-marked Devices: Y
Federal Procurement Eligibility: Small Business
Distribution: Manufacturer Direct, Manufacturer Through Distributor, Exporter
General Admin.: William J. Koteles/President, Chief Executive Officer
Mktg./Adv.: Bilas Hazra/Manager International Marketing & Sales
     William J. Koteles/Vice President Marketing & Sales
Production: William J. Koteles/Manager Regulatory Affairs
     Ivan Kovacs/Vice President Manufacturing
Catheter, Vascular, Cardiopulmonary Bypass	Cardiovascular
Retractor, Surgical	Surgery

PENBERTHY, INC.
See Tyco Valves and Controls

PENCO PRODUCTS INC.   800-562-1000
2024 Cressman Road, P O Box 158, Skippack, PA 19474   **610-666-0500**
FDA Number: n/a   Fax: 610-666-7561
E-mail: customerservice@pencoproducts.com
Web site: www.pencoproducts.com

PENCO PRODUCTS INC.
800-562-1000 (cont'd)
Annual Revenue: $50-$100 Million
Year Founded: 1869
Total Employees: 500   Sales Staff: 32
Ownership: Private
Produces/Sells CE-marked Devices: N
Distribution: Manufacturer Through Distributor
General Admin.: Mark Horita/President
Mktg./Adv.: Philip Krugler/Manager Marketing
        Don Travis/Vice President Marketing & Sales
Production: Kirit Patel/Vice President Manufacturing
Finance: Michael P. Boniello/Vice President Finance
   Cabinet Casework, General Purpose   General
   Cabinet, Instrument   General
   Cart, Multipurpose   General
   Furniture, General   General

PENDRAGON MEDICAL INC.
800-667-5941
20 Devlin Place, Aurora, ONT L4G 5W6 Canada
FDA Number: n/a   Fax: 905-727-3806
E-mail: sales@pendragonmedicalinc.com
Web site: http://pendragonmedicalinc.com/
Year Founded: 1992
Total Employees: 10
Ownership: Private
Produces/Sells CE-marked Devices: N
Distribution: Exclusive Distributor, Importer

PENETRATING INNOVATIONS, INC.
608-845-3270
415 Venture Court, Verona, WI 53593
FDA Number: 3004183698
Ownership: Private
Produces/Sells CE-marked Devices: N
   Accessory, Assisted Reproduction   Obstetrics/Gynecology

PENFLEX
800-232-3539
610-367-2260
105-B Industrial Drive, Gilbertsville, PA 19525
FDA Number: n/a   Fax: 610-367-2248
E-mail: Sales@Penflex.com
Web site: www.penflex.com
Annual Revenue: $0-$1 Million
Year Founded: 1902
Ownership: Private
Produces/Sells CE-marked Devices: N
Federal Procurement Eligibility: Small Business
Distribution: Manufacturer Direct, Manufacturer Through Distributor
Mktg./Adv.: Claire Thompson/Sales Manager
Production: Alex Kouzine/Product Engineer
        Janet R. Ellison/Quality Control, Product Engineer
   Blanket, Infant   General
   Component, Metal, Other   General

PENINSULA LABORATORIES, INC.
800-650-4442
650-592-5392
305 Old County Road,
San Carlos, CA 94070
FDA Number: 7000290   Fax: 650-595-4071
E-mail: info@penlabs.com
Web site: www.bachem.com
Medical Products Sales Volume: $2,200,000
Annual Revenue: $5-$10 Million
Year Founded: 1999
Total Employees: 20   Marketing Staff: 7   Sales Staff: 7
Ownership: Private
Stock Symbol: BANB
Traded On: Switzerland
Produces/Sells CE-marked Devices: N
Federal Procurement Eligibility: Small Business
Distribution: Manufacturer Direct
General Admin.: Hiroshi Morihara/Chief Executive Officer
        Ben Lim/Manager Human Resources
        Bosco Fong/President
Mktg./Adv.: Jim Hampton/Vice President Business Development
Production: Mohammed Anwer/Vice President Manufacturing
   Media, Supporting   Chemistry
   Reagent, Protein, Total   Chemistry

PENINSULA MEDICAL, INC.
831-430-9066
108 Whispering Pines Drive, Suite 115, Santa Cruz, CA 95066
FDA Number: 2954307
   Binder, Medical, Therapeutic   General

PENN CARE MEDICAL PRODUCTS
800-392-7233
330-544-0777
1317 North Rd., Niles, OH 44446
FDA Number: n/a   Fax: 330-544-0022
Web site: www.penncare.net
Annual Revenue: $0-$1 Million
Year Founded: 1984
Ownership: Private

PENN CARE MEDICAL PRODUCTS
800-392-7233 (cont'd)
Produces/Sells CE-marked Devices: N
Federal Procurement Eligibility: Small Business
Distribution: Exclusive Distributor
General Admin.: Stephanie Clemens/Administrator
        John Hanysh/Information Technology Administrator
        Shawn Bryant/President
        Don Bloom/Vice President, General Manager
Mktg./Adv.: Taylor Pease/Sales Manager
   Computer Software, Home Healthcare   General
   Rescue Equipment   General

PENN DIAGNOSTICS
301-279-5958
14 Clemson Court, Rockville, MD 20850
FDA Number: 3005662876
Ownership: Private
Produces/Sells CE-marked Devices: N
   Image Processing System   Radiology
   Nuclear Magnetic Resonance Imaging System   Radiology

PENN UNITED TECHNOLOGY, INC.
724-352-1507
799 N. Pike Rd., Cabot, PA 16023
FDA Number: 3002942776   Fax: 724-352-4970
E-mail: customer_service@pennunited.com
Web site: www.pennunited.com
Annual Revenue: $50-$100 Million
Total Employees: 700   Marketing Staff: 2   Sales Staff: 15
Ownership: Private
Quality System Registration Information: ISO9002
Produces/Sells CE-marked Devices: N
Distribution: Manufacturer Direct, Manufacturer Through Distributor, Manufacturer Through Manufacturer Reps
General Admin.: Mr. William Jones/President
Mktg./Adv.: Mr. Dennis Muir/Manager Sales
Production: Dave Jones/Vice President Manufacturing
        Jerry Purcell/Vice President Operations
   Component, Metal, Other   General
   Service, Engineering/Design   General
   Stapler, Surgical   Surgery

PENNER MANUFACTURING INC
800-732-0717
402-694-5003
102 Grant Street, PO Box 523, Aurora, NE 68818
FDA Number: 1922538   Fax: 402-694-5319
E-mail: sales@pennercareinc.com
Web site: www.pennerpatientcare.com
Ownership: Private
Produces/Sells CE-marked Devices: N
   Bath, Hydro-Massage (Whirlpool)   Physical Med
   Bath, Sitz, Physical Medicine   Physical Med
   Chair, With Casters   Physical Med
   Lift, Bath, Non-AC-Powered   General
   Lift, Patient   General
   Scale, Infant   General
   Table, Obstetrical, AC-Powered   Obstetrics/Gynecology

PENNSYLVANIA GLASS PRODUCTS CO.
412-621-2853
430 N. Craig St., Pittsburgh, PA 15213-1105
FDA Number: 7000689   Fax: 412-621-2854
E-mail: dykema@ibm.net
Web site: www.dykemarubberband.com
Annual Revenue: $1-$5 Million
Total Employees: 25
Ownership: Private
Produces/Sells CE-marked Devices: N
Federal Procurement Eligibility: Small Business
Distribution: Manufacturer Direct
General Admin.: L. C. Dykema/President
Mktg./Adv.: Alice Oehlschlager/Manager Sales
Production: Mr. Samuel McKibben/Associate Product Manager
   Bottle, Sterile Solution   General
   Dropper, Nose   Ear/Nose/Throat

PENNSYLVANIA SCALE CO.
800-233-0473
717-295-6935
1042 New Holland Ave, Burle Business Center,
Lancaster, PA 17601
FDA Number: n/a   Fax: 717-295-6941
E-mail: rsw@pascale.com
Web site: pennsylvaniascalecompany.net
Annual Revenue: $1-$5 Million
Year Founded: 1908
Ownership: Private
Produces/Sells CE-marked Devices: N
Federal Procurement Eligibility: Small Business
Distribution: Manufacturer Direct, Manufacturer Through Distributor, OEM, Importer, Exporter
General Admin.: Rob Woodward/Vice President, General Manager
IS: Alex Shirk/Tech. Specialist
   Scale, Infant   General

PENNSYLVANIA SCALE CO. — 800-233-0473 (cont'd)
Scale, Laboratory	Chemistry
Scale, Platform, Wheelchair	Physical Med

PENNWALT CORP., S. S. WHITE DIV.
See S.S. White Burs Inc.

PENRAD TECHNOLOGIES, INC. — 763-475-3388
10580 Wayzata Blvd, Suite 200, Minnetonka, MN 55305
FDA Number: 3004174244   Fax: 763-475-2815
E-mail: penrad@penrad.com
Web site: http://penrad.com
Year Founded: 1995
Ownership: Private
Produces/Sells CE-marked Devices: N
Mktg./Adv.: Mr. Dan Bickford/Executive Vice President Marketing & Sales
Device, Storage, Image, Digital	Radiology

PENTAGON CO., THE — 800-414-8888 / 818-785-5112
15500 Erwin Street, Suite 1122, Van Nuys, CA 91411
FDA Number: n/a   Fax: 818-785-5814
E-mail: donnam@pentagonco.com
Web site: www.pentagonco.com
Medical Products Sales Volume: $3,000,000
Annual Revenue: $1-$5 Million
Year Founded: 1960
Total Employees: 7   Marketing Staff: 2   Sales Staff: 7
Ownership: PENTAGON TECHNOLOGY, INC.
Produces/Sells CE-marked Devices: N
Federal Procurement Eligibility: Small Business
Distribution: Manufacturer Through Manufacturer Reps
General Admin.: Donna Materna/President
Contract Manufacturing	General

PENTAX MEDICAL COMPANY — 800-431-5880 / 201-571-2300
102 Chestnut Ridge Road, Montvale, NJ 07645
FDA Number: 2518897   Fax: 201-391-4189
E-mail: BEnerson@pentaxmedical.com
Web site: www.pentaxmedical.com
Medical Products Sales Volume: $257,000,000
Year Founded: 1979
Total Employees: 258
Ownership: Private
Produces/Sells CE-marked Devices: Y
Federal Procurement Eligibility: Small Business
Distribution: Manufacturer Through Manufacturer Reps
General Admin.: David Woods/President
Mktg./Adv.: Mac Tonegawa/Director Product Management
          Cindy Corsaro/Manager Marketing
Production: Paul Silva/Director Regulatory Affairs
          Rick Stribley/Vice President Operations
Finance: Thomas McFarland/Controller
Accessories, Cleaning, Endoscopic	Gastroenterology/Urology
Adapter, Bulb, Endoscope, Miscellaneous	Gastroenterology/Urology
Bronchoscope, Non-Rigid	Ear/Nose/Throat
Camera, Video, Endoscopic	General
Camera, Video, Multi-Image	General
Cart, Equipment, Video	General
Cart, Instrument	Surgery
Cart, Monitor	General
Cart, Multipurpose	General
Choledochoscope, Flexible Or Rigid	Gastroenterology/Urology
Cleaner, Ultrasonic, Medical Instrument	General
Colonoscope, Gastro-Urology	Gastroenterology/Urology
Computer Software	General
Computer Software, Hospital/Nursing Management	General
Computer, Image, Endoscopic	General
Computer, Patient Data Management	General
Cystoscope	Gastroenterology/Urology
Duodenoscope, Esophago/Gastro	Gastroenterology/Urology
Endoscope, Fiberoptic	Surgery
Enteroscope	Gastroenterology/Urology
Forceps, Endoscopic	Gastroenterology/Urology
Gastroscope, Flexible	Gastroenterology/Urology
Laparoscope, General & Plastic Surgery	Surgery
Laryngoscope	Ear/Nose/Throat
Light Source, Endoscope, Xenon Arc	Surgery
Light Source, Fiberoptic, Routine	Gastroenterology/Urology
Nasopharyngoscope (Flexible Or Rigid)	Ear/Nose/Throat
Nephroscope, Flexible	Gastroenterology/Urology
Observerscope	General
Printer, Image, Video	General
Pump, Aspiration, Portable	Anesthesiology
Scope, Fiberoptic Intubation	Anesthesiology
Sigmoidoscope, Flexible	Gastroenterology/Urology
Snare, Endoscopic	Surgery
Teaching Attachment, Endoscopic	Gastroenterology/Urology
Transducer, Ultrasonic, Diagnostic	Radiology

PENTAX MEDICAL COMPANY — 800-431-5880 (cont'd)
Ureteroscope	Gastroenterology/Urology

Medical Product Subsidiaries (Listed Separately)
Kaypentax

PENTAX SOUTHERN REGION SERVICE CENTER — 201-571-2300
8934 Kirby Dr., Houston, TX 77054
FDA Number: 3006035604
Bronchoscope, Rigid	Ear/Nose/Throat
Camera, Television, Endoscopic (Without Audio)	Surgery
Choledochoscope, Flexible Or Rigid	Gastroenterology/Urology
Colonoscope, Gastro-Urology	Gastroenterology/Urology
Cystoscope	Gastroenterology/Urology
Device, Storage, Image, Digital	Radiology
Duodenoscope, Esophago/Gastro	Gastroenterology/Urology
Endoscope	Gastroenterology/Urology
Esophagoscope, General & Plastic Surgery	Gastroenterology/Urology
Gastroscope, Gastro-Urology	Gastroenterology/Urology
Laparoscope, General & Plastic Surgery	Surgery
Laryngoscope, Flexible	Anesthesiology
Laryngostroboscope	Ear/Nose/Throat
Light Source, Endoscope, Xenon Arc	Surgery
Light Source, Fiberoptic, Routine	Gastroenterology/Urology
Nasopharyngoscope (Flexible Or Rigid)	Ear/Nose/Throat
Nephroscope Set	Gastroenterology/Urology
Scanner, Ultrasonic (Pulsed Doppler)	Radiology
Sigmoidoscope, Flexible	Gastroenterology/Urology
Teaching Attachment, Endoscopic	Gastroenterology/Urology
Transducer, Ultrasonic, Diagnostic	Radiology
Ureteroscope	Gastroenterology/Urology

PENTAX WEST COAST SERVICE CENTER — 800-431-5880
10410 Pioneer Blvd., Unit 2, Santa Fe Springs, CA 90670
FDA Number: 3005930542
Ownership: Private
Produces/Sells CE-marked Devices: N
Bronchoscope, Rigid	Ear/Nose/Throat
Camera, Television, Endoscopic (Without Audio)	Surgery
Choledochoscope, Flexible Or Rigid	Gastroenterology/Urology
Colonoscope, Gastro-Urology	Gastroenterology/Urology
Cystoscope	Gastroenterology/Urology
Device, Storage, Image, Digital	Radiology
Duodenoscope, Esophago/Gastro	Gastroenterology/Urology
Endoscope	Gastroenterology/Urology
Esophagoscope, General & Plastic Surgery	Gastroenterology/Urology
Gastroscope, Gastro-Urology	Gastroenterology/Urology
Laparoscope, General & Plastic Surgery	Surgery
Laryngoscope, Flexible	Anesthesiology
Laryngostroboscope	Ear/Nose/Throat
Light Source, Endoscope, Xenon Arc	Surgery
Light Source, Fiberoptic, Routine	Gastroenterology/Urology
Nasopharyngoscope (Flexible Or Rigid)	Ear/Nose/Throat
Nephroscope Set	Gastroenterology/Urology
Scanner, Ultrasonic (Pulsed Doppler)	Radiology
Sigmoidoscope, Flexible	Gastroenterology/Urology
Teaching Attachment, Endoscopic	Gastroenterology/Urology
Transducer, Ultrasonic, Diagnostic	Radiology
Ureteroscope	Gastroenterology/Urology

PENTRON CLINICAL TECHNOLOGIES — 203-265-7397
68-70 North Plains Industrial, Road, Wallingford, CT 06492
FDA Number: 3003690896
Activator, Ultraviolet, Polymerization	Dental And Oral
Applicator, Resin	Dental And Oral
Base, Denture, Relining, Repairing, Rebasing, Resin	Dental And Oral
Burr, Dental	Dental And Oral
Cement, Dental	Dental And Oral
Crown And Bridge, Temporary, Resin	Dental And Oral
Crown, Preformed	Dental And Oral
Dam, Rubber	Dental And Oral
Disk, Abrasive	Dental And Oral
Gutta Percha	Dental And Oral
Instrument, Diamond, Dental	Dental And Oral
Material, Impression	Dental And Oral
Material, Tooth Shade, Resin	Dental And Oral
Post, Root Canal	Dental And Oral
Resin, Root Canal Filling	Dental And Oral
Sealant, Pit And Fissure, And Conditioner, Resin	Dental And Oral
Splint, Endodontic Stabilizer	Dental And Oral
Tooth Bonding Agent, Resin Restoration	Dental And Oral
Tray, Impression	Dental And Oral
Varnish, Cavity	Dental And Oral

PENTRON LABORATORY TECHNOLOGIES — 800-551-0283 / 203-265-7397
53 N. Plains Industrial Rd., Wallingford, CT 06492
FDA Number: 1219277   Fax: 877-677-8844
Web site: www.pentron.com
Annual Revenue: $50-$100 Million
Year Founded: 1967
Ownership: Private

PENTRON LABORATORY TECHNOLOGIES 800-551-0283 (cont'd)
Quality System Registration Information: ISO9001
Produces/Sells CE-marked Devices: Y
Federal Procurement Eligibility: Small Business
Distribution: Manufacturer Direct, Manufacturer Through Distributor, Manufacturer Through Manufacturer Reps, OEM, Service Direct, Exclusive Distributor

Adhesive, Bracket And Conditioner, Resin	Dental And Oral
Agent, Polishing, Abrasive, Oral Cavity	Dental And Oral
Alloy, Amalgam	Dental And Oral
Alloy, Gold Based, For Clinical Use	Dental And Oral
Alloy, Precious Metal, For Clinical Use	Dental And Oral
Antigen, Antiserum, Control, IGE, Peroxidase	Immunology
Disk, Abrasive	Dental And Oral
Material, Impression	Dental And Oral
Material, Tooth Shade, Resin	Dental And Oral
Metal, Base	Dental And Oral
Point, Abrasive	Dental And Oral
Teeth, Porcelain	Dental And Oral
Tooth Bonding Agent, Resin Restoration	Dental And Oral
Toothbrush, Powered	Dental And Oral

PENTRON LABORATORY TECHNOLOGIES 203-265-7397
53 North Plains Industrial Rd., Wallingford, CT 06492
FDA Number: 1219277

Adhesive, Bracket And Conditioner, Resin	Dental And Oral
Alloy, Gold Based, For Clinical Use	Dental And Oral
Alloy, Precious Metal, For Clinical Use	Dental And Oral
Base, Denture, Relining, Repairing, Rebasing, Resin	Dental And Oral
Cement, Dental	Dental And Oral
Crown And Bridge, Temporary, Resin	Dental And Oral
Crown, Preformed	Dental And Oral
Implant, Subperiosteal	Dental And Oral
Instrument, Diamond, Dental	Dental And Oral
Material, Impression	Dental And Oral
Material, Tooth Shade, Resin	Dental And Oral
Metal, Base	Dental And Oral
Post, Root Canal	Dental And Oral
Powder, Porcelain	Dental And Oral
Remover, Crown	Dental And Oral
Resin, Root Canal Filling	Dental And Oral
Sealant, Pit And Fissure, And Conditioner, Resin	Dental And Oral
Splint, Endodontic Stabilizer	Dental And Oral
Teeth, Porcelain	Dental And Oral
Tooth Bonding Agent, Resin Restoration	Dental And Oral

PENUMBRA, INC. 1.888.272.4606
1351 Harbor Bay Parkway, Alameda, CA 94502 510.748.3200
FDA Number: 3005168196 Fax: 510.748.3232
E-mail: info@penumbrainc.com
Web site: www.penumbrainc.com
Ownership: Private
Produces/Sells CE-marked Devices: N

Catheter, Angioplasty, Transluminal, Peripheral	Cardiovascular
Catheter, Percutaneous	Cardiovascular
Pump, Aspiration, Portable	Anesthesiology
Suction Apparatus, Ward Use, Portable, AC-Powered	Surgery

PEPCO
See Frederick Tool Corp.

PEPEX BIOMEDICAL INC. 314-633-5053
4041 Forest Park, St. Louis, MO 63108
FDA Number: n/a
E-mail: information@pepex.com
Web site: http://www.pepex.com
Ownership: Private
Produces/Sells CE-marked Devices: N
General Admin.: Mr. Steven Collins/President, Chief Executive Officer
Research: Dr. Mark Vreeke/Vice President Research & Development
Finance: Mr. Joseph Driver/Chief Financial Officer

PEPIN MANUFACTURING, INC. 800-291-6505
1875 Hwy. 61 South, Lake City, MN 55041 651-345-5655
FDA Number: n/a Fax: 651-345-5656
E-mail: info@pepinmfg.com
Web site: www.pepinmfg.com
Medical Products Sales Volume: $2,500,000
Annual Revenue: $5-$10 Million
Year Founded: 1993
Total Employees: 35   Marketing Staff: 2   Sales Staff: 5
Ownership: Private
Quality System Registration Information: ISO9002
Produces/Sells CE-marked Devices: Y
Federal Procurement Eligibility: Small Business
Distribution: Manufacturer Through Distributor, Manufacturer Through Manufacturer Reps, OEM, Exclusive Distributor
General Admin.: Jeff Solberg/President, Chief Executive Officer
Mktg./Adv.: Paul Lusic/Vice President Marketing & Sales
Production: Daniel Denn/Plant Manager
            Jeff Solberg/Vice President Manufacturing & Development

PEPIN MANUFACTURING, INC. 800-291-6505 (cont'd)

Bandage, Other	General
Contract Assembly	General
Contract Manufacturing	General
Electrode, TENS	Cns/Neurology
Material, Raw, Production	General
Service, Printing	General
Tape, Adhesive	General

PER-SE TECHNOLOGIES 877-737-3773
1145 sanctuary prkwy sutit 200, 770-444-5300
Alpharetta, GA 30004
FDA Number: n/a Fax: 770-444-5243
E-mail: askus@per-se.com
Web site: www.per-se.com
Medical Products Sales Volume: $372,700,000
Annual Revenue: $100-$500 Million
Total Employees: 500
Ownership: Public
Stock Symbol: PSTI
Traded On: NASDAQ
Produces/Sells CE-marked Devices: N
Federal Procurement Eligibility: Small Business
Distribution: Manufacturer Direct
General Admin.: Philip Pead/Chief Executive Officer
            Philip Jordan/President
            Karl Straub/Senior Vice President
Mktg./Adv.: Deborah Sunday/Director Marketing
Research: Tim Aligheri/Vice President Product Development
Finance: Chris Perkins/Chief Financial Officer
            Michele Howard/Vice President Corporate & Investor Relations

Computer, Patient Data Management	General

PER4MAX MEDICAL, LLC 866-648-6891
1000 Post & Paddock, Ste. 302, 972-641-6773
Grand Prairie, TX 75050
FDA Number: 3004013215 Fax: 972-782-9011
E-mail: sales@per4max.com
Web site: www.per4max.com
Ownership: Private
Produces/Sells CE-marked Devices: N

Wheelchair, Special Grade	Physical Med

PERCEPTICS CORPORATION 800-448-8544
9737 Cogdill Rd., Suite 200N, 865-966-9200
Knoxville, TN 37932
FDA Number: n/a Fax: 865-966-9330
E-mail: sales@perceptics.com
Web site: www.perceptics.com
Annual Revenue: $10-$25 Million
Ownership: Private
Quality System Registration Information: ISO9001
Produces/Sells CE-marked Devices: Y
Distribution: Manufacturer Direct

Unit, Examination, Lens, Contact	Ophthalmology

PERCEPTIVE SCIENTIFIC INSTRUMENTS, INC.
See Leica Microsystems (San Jose) Corporation

PERCEPTIVE SYSTEMS, INC.
See Leica Microsystems (San Jose) Corporation

PERCIVAL SCIENTIFIC INC. 800-695-2743
505 Research Drive, Perry, IA 50220 515-465-9363
FDA Number: 7000291 Fax: 515-465-9464
E-mail: sales@percival-scientific.com
Web site: www.percival-scientific.com
Medical Products Sales Volume: $5,300,000
Annual Revenue: $1-$5 Million
Year Founded: 1886
Total Employees: 70   Marketing Staff: 1   Sales Staff: 2
Ownership: Private
Produces/Sells CE-marked Devices: Y
Federal Procurement Eligibility: Small Business, GSA Contract
Distribution: Manufacturer Direct, Manufacturer Through Manufacturer Reps
Mktg./Adv.: H. Donald Fronc/Vice President Marketing & Sales
Production: Karl Lundy/Customer Service Representative
            Mitch Yates/Manager Materials
            Henry Imberti/Vice President, Engineer
Finance: Gary Wheelock/Chief Financial Officer

Chamber, Constant Temperature (Environmental)	Microbiology
Incubator, Aerobic	Microbiology

PERCUSSIONAIRE CORPORATION 208-263-2549
1655 Glengary Bay Rd., Sagle, ID 83860
FDA Number: 3029845 Fax: 208-263-0577
E-mail: sales@percussionaire.com
Web site: www.percussionaire.com
Annual Revenue: $0-$1 Million

PERCUSSIONAIRE CORPORATION   208-263-2549 *(cont'd)*
Year Founded: 1954
Ownership: Percussionaire Corporation
Quality System Registration Information: ISO9002
Produces/Sells CE-marked Devices: Y
Federal Procurement Eligibility: Small Business
Distribution: Manufacturer Direct, Manufacturer Through Distributor, Manufacturer Through Manufacturer Reps, Importer, Exporter
General Admin.: Forrest Bird/President, Chief Executive Officer

Ventilator, Continuous (Respirator)	Anesthesiology
Ventilator, Neonatal Respirator	General
Ventilator, Non-Continuous (Respirator)	Anesthesiology

Medical Product Subsidiaries (Listed Separately)
  Percussionaire Corporation

PERCUSSIONAIRE CORPORATION BIRD AIRLODGE
  See Percussionaire Corporation

PERCUTANEOUS SYSTEMS, INCORPORATED   650-493-4200
3260 Hillview Avenue, Suite 100, Palo Alto, CA 94304
FDA Number: 3004786058
Web site: http://www.percsys.com
Ownership: Private
Produces/Sells CE-marked Devices: N
General Admin.: Robert Behl/Chief Executive Officer

Accessories, Catheter, G-U	Gastroenterology/Urology
Catheter, Straight	Gastroenterology/Urology
Dislodger, Stone, Basket, Ureteral, Metal	Gastroenterology/Urology

PEREGRINE PHARMACEUTICALS, INC.   714-508-6000
14282 Franklin Ave., Tustin, CA 92780
FDA Number: n/a   Fax: 714-838-5817
Web site: www.peregrineinc.com
Annual Revenue: $0-$1 Million
Year Founded: 1981
Total Employees: 133
Ownership: Public
Stock Symbol: PPHM
Traded On: NASDAQ
Produces/Sells CE-marked Devices: N
Federal Procurement Eligibility: Small Business
Distribution: Service Direct
General Admin.: Steven W King/President, Chief Executive Officer

Antibody, Monoclonal	Microbiology

PEREGRINE SURGICAL, LTD.   215-348-0456
51 Britain Drive, Doylestown, PA 18901
FDA Number: 2529392

Cannula, Ophthalmic	Ophthalmology
Cutter, Vitreous Aspiration, AC-Powered	Ophthalmology
Endoilluminator	Ophthalmology
Fiberoptic Light Source & Carrier	Ear/Nose/Throat
Fluid, Intraocular	Ophthalmology
Laser, Ophthalmic	Ophthalmology
Marker, Sclera (Ocular)	Ophthalmology
Needle, Aspiration And Injection, Disposable	Surgery
Speculum, Ophthalmic	Ophthalmology
Therapeutic Deep Heat Vitrectomy	Ophthalmology
Tubing, Non-Invasive	Surgery

PERENY EQUIPMENT CO., GI DIV.
  See Unique/Pereny

PERFECSEAL   877-828-7501
PO Box 2968, 3500 North Main St.,   920-303-7000
Oshkosh, WI 54903
FDA Number: 1467001   Fax: 920-303-7002
E-mail: perfecseal@bemis.com
Web site: www.perfecseal.com
Medical Products Sales Volume: $102,500,000
Year Founded: 1996
Total Employees: 820
Ownership: BEMIS CO.
Quality System Registration Information: ISO9000; ISO9001; ISO9002
Produces/Sells CE-marked Devices: N
Federal Procurement Eligibility: Small Business
Distribution: Manufacturer Direct
General Admin.: Jeffrey Curler/Chief Executive Officer
           Paul Verbeten/President
Mktg./Adv.: Thomas R. Pech, Jr./Manager Marketing & Communications
           Ed Haedt/Vice President Marketing
           Sandra Mathison/Vice President Sales
Production: Jeff Caldwell/Director Quality Assurance
Research: Bruce Hergert/Vice President Research & Development

Component, Paper	General
Packaging Material	General

PERFECT CARE   718-805-7800
8927 126 St., Richmond Hill, NY 11418
FDA Number: 2438848

PERFECT CARE   718-805-7800 *(cont'd)*
Ownership: Private
Produces/Sells CE-marked Devices: N

Attachment, Commode, Wheelchair	Physical Med
Cane	Physical Med
Crutch	Physical Med
Tips And Pads, Cane, Crutch And Walker	Physical Med
Transfer Aid	Physical Med
Transfer Device, Patient, Manual	General
Walker, Mechanical	Physical Med

PERFECT FIT GLOVE   800-245-6837
85 Innsbruck Drive, Buffalo, NY 14227   716-668-2000
FDA Number: 9001569   Fax: 716-668-1264
E-mail: gloveinfo@sperianprotection.com
Web site: www.perfectfitglove.com
Medical Products Sales Volume: $9,400,000
Annual Revenue: $25-$50 Million
Year Founded: 1973
Total Employees: 210   Marketing Staff: 3   Sales Staff: 22
Ownership: SPERIAN PROTECTION
Quality System Registration Information: ISO9001
Produces/Sells CE-marked Devices: N
Federal Procurement Eligibility: Small Business
Distribution: Manufacturer Through Distributor
General Admin.: Joseph Hoerner/President
Mktg./Adv.: Bill Alico/Vice President Marketing & Sales
Production: Ed Mesanovic/Vice President Manufacturing

Glove, Other	General

PERFECT FIT, L.P.   972-955-6836
6315 Riverview Lane, Dallas, TX 75248
FDA Number: 3003550188
Ownership: Private
Produces/Sells CE-marked Devices: N

Articulators	Dental And Oral

PERFECT OPTICS, INC.
  See General Scientific Corp.

PERFECT SMILE CORPORATION   800-520-1906
29313 Clemens Road, #2E, Westlake, OH 44145   440-617-2200
FDA Number: 1530874   Fax: 440-617-8330
E-mail: info@4theperfectsmile.com
Web site: www.theperfectsmile.org
Medical Products Sales Volume: $800,000
Annual Revenue: $1-$5 Million
Year Founded: 2002
Total Employees: 9   Marketing Staff: 1   Sales Staff: 2
Ownership: Private
Produces/Sells CE-marked Devices: N
Federal Procurement Eligibility: Small Business

Carboxymethylcellulose Sodium (40-100%)	Dental And Oral

PERFECTION ENTERPRISES   818-764-3447
7250 Hinds Ave., North Hollywood, CA 91605
FDA Number: 2032671
Ownership: Private
Produces/Sells CE-marked Devices: N

Table, Radiographic, Tilting	Radiology

PERFECTO PRODUCTS MFG., INC.   404-352-3863
1800 Marietta Blvd., Atlanta, GA 30318
FDA Number: 1039259
Ownership: Private
Produces/Sells CE-marked Devices: N

Medical Disinfectants/Cleaners for Instruments	General

PERFEX CORP.   800-848-8483
32 Case St., Poland, NY 13431   315-826-3600
FDA Number: n/a   Fax: 315-826-7471
E-mail: perfex@ntcnet.com
Web site: www.perfexonline.com
Medical Products Sales Volume: $800,000
Annual Revenue: $1-$5 Million
Year Founded: 1976
Total Employees: 13   Marketing Staff: 3   Sales Staff: 3
Ownership: Private
Quality System Registration Information: ISO9000; ISO9001
Produces/Sells CE-marked Devices: N
Federal Procurement Eligibility: Small Business
Distribution: Manufacturer Direct, Manufacturer Through Distributor
General Admin.: Michael Kubick/President, Chief Executive Officer
Mktg./Adv.: Jon Skaly/Director Marketing
           Johann Skaly/Manager Marketing

Housekeeping Equipment	General

PERFORM MANUFACTURING INCORPORATED 913-722-1557
1624 South 45th St., Kansas City, KS 66106
FDA Number: 3003677528
Ownership: Private
Produces/Sells CE-marked Devices: N
  Medical Disinfectants/Cleaners for Instruments   General

PERFORMANCE ATTAINMENT ASSOCIATES 800-835-2766
12805 Lake Blvd, #3, PO Box 528, 651-257-3040
Lindstrom, MN 55045
FDA Number: n/a   Fax: 651-257-7210
E-mail: info@spineproducts.com
Web site: www.spineproducts.com
Annual Revenue: $0-$1 Million
Ownership: Private
Produces/Sells CE-marked Devices: Y
Distribution: Manufacturer Direct, Exporter
  Analyzer, Motion   General

PERFORMANCE HEALTH, INC.
  See Biofreeze Performance Health, Inc.

PERFORMANCE MACHINE TECHNOLOGIES 661-294-8617
25141 W. Avenue Stanford, Valencia, CA 91355-1227
FDA Number: n/a   Fax: 661-294-1290
E-mail: pmtinc1@sbcglobal.net
Web site: www.pmtinc.org
Annual Revenue: $1-$5 Million
Year Founded: 1995
Total Employees: 20
Ownership: Private
Quality System Registration Information: ISO9002
Produces/Sells CE-marked Devices: N
Federal Procurement Eligibility: Small Business
Distribution: Manufacturer Through Distributor
General Admin.: Dennis E. Moran/President, Chief Executive Officer
  Orthopedic Manual Surgical Instrument   Orthopedics

PERFORMANCE ORTHOPEDICS 804-288-2717
6716 Patterson Ave., #B, Richmond, VA 23226-3433
FDA Number: n/a   Fax: 804-270-0169
Ownership: Private
Produces/Sells CE-marked Devices: N
Federal Procurement Eligibility: Small Business
Distribution: Manufacturer Direct
General Admin.: Richard B. Caspari/President
  Equipment, Traction, Powered   Physical Med
  Holder, Leg, Arthroscopy   Orthopedics
  Pliers, Surgical   Orthopedics
  Tray, Custom/Special Procedure   General

PERFORMANCE SYSTEMATIX INC 616-949-9090
5569 33RD Street S.E., Grand Rapids, MI 49512
FDA Number: 1832535   Fax: 616-949-5154
E-mail: info@psix.com
Web site: www.psix.com
Medical Products Sales Volume: $1,200,000
Annual Revenue: $5-$10 Million
Year Founded: 1984
Total Employees: 20
Ownership: Private
Produces/Sells CE-marked Devices: N
Federal Procurement Eligibility: Small Business
Distribution: OEM
General Admin.: Karlis Vizulis/President
  Karlis Mateus/Vice President, General Manager
Mktg./Adv.: John W. Grover/Manager International & National Sales
  Karwyn Bursma/Manager Marketing
  Contract Manufacturing   General
  Filter, Air   General
  Media, Filter   General

PERFORMANCE WATER SYSTEMS, LLC 708-396-0136
13601 S. Kenton Avenue, Crestwood, IL 60445
FDA Number: 3004168891
  Purification System, Water   Gastroenterology/Urology

PERGRINE PHARM
  See Peregrine Pharmaceuticals, Inc.

PERIMED, INC. 877-374-3589
6785 Wallings Rd., Ste. 2C-2D, 440-877-0537
North Royalton, OH 44133
FDA Number: 2246823   Fax: 440-877-0534
E-mail: USAinfo@perimed-instruments.com
Web site: www.perimed.se
Medical Products Sales Volume: $2,000,000
Annual Revenue: $1-$5 Million
Total Employees: 6

PERIMED, INC. 877-374-3589 *(cont'd)*
Ownership: Private
Stock Symbol: N/A
Quality System Registration Information: ISO9000
Produces/Sells CE-marked Devices: Y
Distribution: Manufacturer Direct
General Admin.: Sue Sidhu/Office Manager
  Avtar Sidhu/President
Mktg./Adv.: Samuel Pakvis/Sales Specialist
  Mr. Robert Kostelny/Sales Specialist
  Peter Delaney/Vice President Marketing & Sales
  Analyzer, Doppler Spectrum   General
  Computer Software   General
  Doppler, Blood Flow, Transcranial   Cardiovascular
  Laser, Combination   General
  Monitor, Oxygen   General

PERIMMUNE
  See Intracel Corporation

PERIO PRODUCTS, INC. 800-841-3221
6156 Wilcox Rd., Dublin, OH 43016 614-791-1207
FDA Number: n/a   Fax: 614-792-0484
E-mail: questions@perio-inc.com
Web site: www.perio-inc.com
Medical Products Sales Volume: $900,000
Annual Revenue: $0-$1 Million
Year Founded: 1903
Ownership: Private
Produces/Sells CE-marked Devices: N
Federal Procurement Eligibility: Small Business
Distribution: Manufacturer Direct, Manufacturer Through Manufacturer Reps
  Dentifrice   Dental And Oral
  Electrolysis Equipment, Other   General

PERIO PROTECT LLC 202-672-5430
3929 Bayless Ave., St. Louis, MO 63125
FDA Number: 3005167547
  Tray, Fluoride, Disposable   Dental And Oral

PERIOPTIX, INC. 949-366-3333
1001 Avenida Pico, #C62, San Clemente, CA 92763
FDA Number: 3004951219
E-mail: customerservice@perioptix.com
Web site: http://www.perioptix.com
Ownership: Private
Produces/Sells CE-marked Devices: N
  Light, Examination, Battery-Powered   General
  Loupe, Binocular, Low Power   Ophthalmology
  Shield, Eye, Ophthalmic   Ophthalmology

PERIPHERAL DYNAMICS INC. 800-253-0253
5150 Campus Drive, 610-825-7090
Plymouth Meeting, PA 19462
FDA Number: n/a   Fax: 610-834-7708
E-mail: sales@pdiscan.com
Web site: www.pdiscan.com
Annual Revenue: $5-$10 Million
Year Founded: 1969
Total Employees: 100   *Marketing Staff:* 2   *Sales Staff:* 5
Ownership: INDUCTOTHERM INDUSTRIES, INC.
Produces/Sells CE-marked Devices: Y
Distribution: Manufacturer Direct, Manufacturer Through Distributor, Manufacturer Through Manufacturer Reps, Service Direct
Mktg./Adv.: RON DEMARCO/Director Marketing
  Mr. Ron DeMarco/Manager Marketing & Public Relations
Finance: Mr. Graham L. Gross/Vice President Admin., Chief Financial Officer
  Camera, Video   General
  Component, Electronic   General
  Stainer, Slide, Automated   Pathology

PERKIN ELMER WALLAC, INC. 800-638-6692
9238 Gaither Rd., Gaithersburg, MD 20877-1486 301-963-3200
FDA Number: 9200621   Fax: 301-963-7780
E-mail: lifescienesusa@perkinelmer.com
Web site: www.perkinelmer.com/lifesciences
Medical Products Sales Volume: $23,000,000
Annual Revenue: $25-$50 Million
Total Employees: 91   *Marketing Staff:* 7   *Sales Staff:* 25
Ownership: Eg & G, Inc.
Quality System Registration Information: ISO9001; ISO9002; ISO9003
Produces/Sells CE-marked Devices: N
Distribution: Manufacturer Direct, Service Direct
General Admin.: Jerry Ronner/President
  Craig Rine/Vice President
Mktg./Adv.: Chanda Breakiron/Director Marketing
  Chanda Breakiron/Manager Marketing
Production: Paul Davis/Director Quality Assurance
  Paul Davis/Manager Regulatory Affairs

MANUFACTURER PROFILES

PERKIN ELMER WALLAC, INC. 800-638-6692 *(cont'd)*
Frey Lindquist/Product Manager

Analyzer, Chemistry, Radioimmunoassay, Automated	Chemistry
Counter, Gamma, General Use	Toxicology
Counter, Scintillation	Chemistry
Counter, Scintillation, Liquid, Toxicology	Toxicology
Detector, Beta/Gamma	Chemistry
Fluorometer	Immunology
Fluorometric, Cortisol	Chemistry
Harvester, Cell	Microbiology
Luminometer	Chemistry
Microplate	General
Monitor, Radiation	Radiology
Photometer	Chemistry
Pipette	Chemistry
Pipetting And Diluting System, Automated	Chemistry
Reader, Microplate	General
Washer, Microplate	General

PERKIN-ELMER CORP.
See Perkinelmer Life And Analytical Sciences

PERKINELMER 800-762-4000
940 Winter Street, Waltham, MA 02451 **203-925-4602**
FDA Number: 3006159931 *Fax:* 203-944-4904
E-mail: CustomerCareUS@perkinelmer.com
Web site: www.perkinelmer.com
Annual Revenue: More than $1 Billion
Total Employees: 7900
Ownership: E G & G WALLAC
Stock Symbol: PKI
Traded On: NYSE
Quality System Registration Information: ISO9001
Produces/Sells CE-marked Devices: N
Federal Procurement Eligibility: Small Business
Distribution: Service Direct
General Admin.: Dr. Daniel Marshak/Chief Scientific Officer
Robert F. Friel/President, Chief Executive Officer
Finance: Mr. Frank Wilson/Chief Financial Officer

Antibody, Other	General
Column, Chromatography	Chemistry
Control, Hemoglobin	Hematology
Control, Hemoglobin, Abnormal	Hematology
Densitometer/Scanner (Integrating, Reflectance, TLC, Radio)	Chemistry
Electrofocusing Equipment	Chemistry
Electrophoresis Equipment, Gel	Chemistry
Electrophoretic Separation, Alkaline Phosphatase Isoenzymes	Chemistry
Hemoglobin S	Hematology
Hemoglobinometer, Electrophoretic Analysis System	Hematology
Infrared Spectroscopy Measurement, Urinary Calculi (Stone)	Chemistry
Monitor, Neonatal	Obstetrics/Gynecology
Quantitation, Hemoglobin, Abnormal	Hematology
Standard/Control, Hemoglobin, Normal/Abnormal	Hematology
System, Test, Amino Acids, Free Carnitines And Acylcarnitines Tandem Mass Spectrometry	Chemistry
Test, Glycosylated Hemoglobin Assay	Hematology
Test, Hemoglobin Bart's	Hematology

Medical Product Subsidiaries (Listed Separately)
Perkinelmer Life And Analytical Sciences

PERKINELMER LIFE AND ANALYTICAL SCIENCES 800-323-5891
2200 Warrenville Rd., Downers Grove, IL 60515 **630-969-6000**
FDA Number: 1419712 *Fax:* 630-322-5511
Web site: http://las.perkinelmer.com
Total Employees: 9100
Ownership: PerkinElmer
Stock Symbol: PKI
Traded On: NYSE
Produces/Sells CE-marked Devices: N

Pipetting And Diluting System, Automated	Chemistry
Station Pipetting	Chemistry

PERKINELMER LIFE AND ANALYTICAL SCIENCES 800-446-0035
549 Albany St., Boston, MA 02118 **617-482-9595**
FDA Number: 1224609 *Fax:* 617-482-1380
E-mail: CustomerCareUS@perkinelmer.com
Web site: www.perkinelmer.com
Annual Revenue: $25-$50 Million
Ownership: PERKINELMER
Quality System Registration Information: ISO9002
Produces/Sells CE-marked Devices: Y

PERKINELMER LIFE AND ANALYTICAL SCIENCES 800-762-4000
940 Winter Street, Waltham, MA 02451 **203-925-4602**
FDA Number: 300615993 *Fax:* 203-944-4904
E-mail: CustomerCareUS@perkinelmer.com

PERKINELMER LIFE AND ANALYTICAL 800-762-4000 *(cont'd)*
Web site: www.perkinelmer.com
Medical Products Sales Volume: $1,000,000,000
Ownership: PERKINELMER LIFE SCIENCES, INC.
Quality System Registration Information: ISO9001
Produces/Sells CE-marked Devices: N
Distribution: Manufacturer Direct

Absorption, Atomic, Mercury	Toxicology
Analyzer, Carbon	Chemistry
Analyzer, Carbon Hydrogen	Chemistry
Analyzer, Carbon Hydrogen Nitrogen	Chemistry
Analyzer, Gas, Hydrogen	Anesthesiology
Atomizer, Flameless	Chemistry
Balance, Electronic	Chemistry
Balance, Ultramicro (0.0001 mg Accuracy)	Chemistry
Calorimeter	Chemistry
Cell, Spectrophotometer	Chemistry
Chromatography Equipment, Gas	Chemistry
Chromatography Equipment, Liquid	Chemistry
Chromatography, Liquid, Performance, High	Toxicology
Computer, Clinical Laboratory	Chemistry
Injector, Sample	Chemistry
Photometer, Flame, General Use	Toxicology
Sampler, Particulate	General
Spectrometer, Infrared	Chemistry
Spectrophotometer, Atomic Absorption, General Use	Toxicology
Spectrophotometer, Fluorescence	Chemistry
Spectrophotometer, Infrared	Chemistry
Spectrophotometer, U.V./Visible	Chemistry
Spectrophotometer, Ultraviolet	Chemistry

PERKINELMER OPTOELECTRONICS 800-775-6786
44370 Christy Street, Fremont, CA 94538-3180 **510-979-6500**
FDA Number: n/a *Fax:* 510-687-1140
E-mail: opto@perkinelmer.com
Web site: optoelectronics.perkinelmer.com
Annual Revenue: $0-$1 Million
Ownership: Private
Quality System Registration Information: ISO9000
Produces/Sells CE-marked Devices: Y
Distribution: Importer, Exporter

Component, Electrical	General
Light, Other	General

PERKINELMER WALLACE INC.
See Perkinelmer Life And Analytical Sciences

PERKINS ELECTRONICS 877-923-4545
700 International Parkway, Suite 100, **214-828-4545**
Richardson, TX 75081
FDA Number: 1642869 *Fax:* 214-827-6319
E-mail: sales@perkinselectronics.com
Web site: www.perkinselectronics.com
Annual Revenue: $1-$5 Million
Year Founded: 1987
Total Employees: 33 *Marketing Staff:* 2 *Sales Staff:* 3
Ownership: Private
Quality System Registration Information: ISO9001
Produces/Sells CE-marked Devices: Y
Federal Procurement Eligibility: Small Business
Distribution: Manufacturer Through Distributor, OEM
Mktg./Adv.: Mr. Joe Cox/Director Sales

Device, Storage, Image, Digital	Radiology
Display, Cathode-Ray Tube	Cardiovascular
Image Intensification System	Radiology
Image Processing System	Radiology
Recorder, Videotape/Videodisc	General

PERKINS MANUFACTURING COMPANY
See Perkins Electronics

PERLINK CORPORATION
See PI Medical Co., Llc.

PERMA PURE LLC 800-337-3762
8 Executive Drive, Toms River, NJ 08755 **732-244-0010**
FDA Number: 2244684 *Fax:* 732-244-8140
E-mail: info@permapure.com
Web site: www.permapure.com
Medical Products Sales Volume: $4,000,000
Annual Revenue: $10-$25 Million
Year Founded: 1972
Total Employees: 75 *Marketing Staff:* 1 *Sales Staff:* 8
Ownership: HALMA plc
Stock Symbol: HLMA
Traded On: London
Quality System Registration Information: ISO9001
Produces/Sells CE-marked Devices: Y
Distribution: Manufacturer Direct, Manufacturer Through Distributor, OEM, Exporter
General Admin.: David A. Leighty/President

PERMA PURE LLC   800-337-3762 (cont'd)

Mktg./Adv.: Desmond Morrissey/Vice President Sales
Production: Robert Rozek/Manager Regulatory Affairs
     Scott Rush/Vice President Operations
Finance: Michael Zemble/Vice President Finance

Dryer, Respiratory/Anesthesia Equipment	General
Filter, Ventilator	Anesthesiology
Humidifier, Respiratory Gas, (Direct Patient Interface)	Anesthesiology
Kit, Anesthesia, Conduction	Anesthesiology
Tubing, Flexible, Medical Gas, Low-Pressure	Anesthesiology

PERMA TYPE COMPANY, INC.   860-747-9999
83 Northwest Dr., Plainville, CT 06062
FDA Number: 1215296

Appliance, Incontinence, Urosheath Type	Gastroenterology/Urology
Bag, Drainage, Ostomy (With Adhesive)	General

PERMABOND INTERNATIONAL   800-653-6523
10 Feinder Ave., Bridgewater, NJ 08807   908-575-7200
FDA Number: n/a   *Fax:* 860-379-9173
E-mail: info.americas@permabond.com
Web site: www.permabond.com
Annual Revenue: $10-$25 Million
Ownership: National Starch And Chemical Co.
Produces/Sells CE-marked Devices: N
Distribution: Manufacturer Direct

Adhesive, Liquid	General

PERMATRON CORP.   800-882-8012
1180 Pratt Avenue, Elk Grove Village, IL 60007   847-434-1421
FDA Number: n/a   *Fax:* 847-434-1429
E-mail: sales@permatron.com
Web site: www.permatron.com
Medical Products Sales Volume: $1,700,000
Annual Revenue: $1-$5 Million
Year Founded: 1957
Total Employees: 20
Ownership: Private
Produces/Sells CE-marked Devices: N
Federal Procurement Eligibility: Small Business, Female Owned
Distribution: Manufacturer Direct, Manufacturer Through Distributor, Manufacturer Through Manufacturer Reps, OEM, Exporter
General Admin.: Leslye Sandberg/President
Mktg./Adv.: Shelly Lynn/Manager Contract Sales
     Shelly Lynn/Manager International & National Sales
     Gayle Matthies/Vice President Marketing & Communications

Filter, Air	General

PERMEABLE CONTACT LENSES, INC.
See The Lifestyle Co. Inc.

PERMEABLE TECHNOLOGIES
See The Lifestyle Co. Inc.

PERMEDICS, INC.   (877) 473-7633
1475 South Victoria Ct.,   909-478-5000
San Bernardino, CA 92408
FDA Number: 2032139   *Fax:* 909-478-5016
E-mail: webmaster@permedics.com
Web site: www.permedics.com
Ownership: Private
Produces/Sells CE-marked Devices: N

System, Planning, Radiation Therapy Treatment	Radiology

PERMOBIL, INC.   800-736-0925
6961 Eastgate Blvd., Lebanon, TN 37090   615-547-1889
FDA Number: 1221084   *Fax:* 800-231-3256
E-mail: info@permobilusa.com
Web site: www.permobil.com
Medical Products Sales Volume: $40,000,000
Year Founded: 1963
Total Employees: 100   *Marketing Staff:* 4   *Sales Staff:* 30
Ownership: PERMOBIL AB
Produces/Sells CE-marked Devices: N
Federal Procurement Eligibility: Small Business, VA Contract
Distribution: Manufacturer Through Distributor
General Admin.: Goran Udden/Chief Executive Officer
     Larry Jackson/President
Mktg./Adv.: Barry Steelman/Director Marketing
     John Coffay/Manager National Sales
     John Richards/Manager National Sales
     Tom Rolick/Vice President Business Development
Production: Darin Lowery/Director Customer Services

Wheelchair, Powered	Physical Med
Wheelchair, Special Grade	Physical Med

PERRIGO NEW YORK, INC.   269-686-2916
1700 Bathgate Ave., Bronx, NY 10457
FDA Number: 2434221

PERRIGO NEW YORK, INC.   269-686-2916 (cont'd)

Lubricant, Patient	General
Polyvinyl Methylether Maleic Acid-Calcium-Sodium Dbl. Salt	Dental And Oral

PERRY BAROMEDICAL CORP.   800-741-4376
3660 Interstate Parkway,   561-840-0395
Riviera Beach, FL 33404
FDA Number: 1036464   *Fax:* 561-840-0398
E-mail: baromed@aol.com
Web site: www.perrybaromedical.com
Medical Products Sales Volume: $8,000,000
Annual Revenue: $1-$5 Million
Year Founded: 1992
Total Employees: 4   *Marketing Staff:* 2   *Sales Staff:* 4
Ownership: ADATIF MEDICAL
Quality System Registration Information: ISO9002
Produces/Sells CE-marked Devices: N
Federal Procurement Eligibility: Small Business
Distribution: Manufacturer Direct
General Admin.: W. Robert Bryant/Director
     Wayne Mc Cullough/President, Chief Operating Officer
Production: Glen Norris/Director Quality Assurance
     Ray Weiss/Vice President, Director Operations
Finance: John Pierrard/Chief Financial Officer

Chamber, Hyperbaric	Anesthesiology

PERRY CHEMICAL & MFG. CO., INC.   800-592-6614
2335 South 30th Street (47909), PO Box 6419,   317-474-3404
Lafayette, IN 47903
FDA Number: 2954345   *Fax:* 317-474-3423
E-mail: perry@perryfoam.com
Web site: www.perrychemical.com
Medical Products Sales Volume: $100,000
Annual Revenue: $10-$25 Million
Year Founded: 1960
Ownership: Private
Produces/Sells CE-marked Devices: N
Federal Procurement Eligibility: Small Business
Distribution: Manufacturer Direct, Manufacturer Through Distributor, Manufacturer Through Manufacturer Reps, OEM

Pillow, Cervical(for Mild Sleep Apnea)	Ear/Nose/Throat

PERRY DIVISION
See Ansell Healthcare Products, Inc.

PERSONAL DIAGNOSTICS, INC.
See Ebi, Llc

PERSONAL MOBILITY PRODUCTS LTD.   604-576-1323
17780 56th Ave., Ste. 102, Surrey, BC V3S-4T7 Canada
FDA Number: n/a   *Fax:* 604-576-1400
Year Founded: 1996
Total Employees: 10
Ownership: Private
Produces/Sells CE-marked Devices: N
Distribution: Exclusive Distributor, Importer

PERSONAL PERFORMANCE MEDICAL CORP.   801-364-3100
50 South 900 East, Suite 1, Salt Lake City, UT 84102
FDA Number: 3003603920
Ownership: Private
Produces/Sells CE-marked Devices: N

Orthosis, Cranial	Cns/Neurology

PERSONAL PRODUCTS CO, DIV MCNEIL-PPC, INC.
See Mcneil-Ppc, Inc.

PERSONNA MEDICAL/DIV. OF AMERICAN SAFETY RAZOR CO.   800-457-2222
One Razor Blade Ln., Verona, VA 24482   540-248-8000
FDA Number: 9911010   *Fax:* 540-248-1648
E-mail: medical@asrco.com
Web site: www.asrco.com/medical/
Medical Products Sales Volume: $297,500,000
Annual Revenue: $100-$500 Million
Year Founded: 1875
Total Employees: 450   *Marketing Staff:* 4   *Sales Staff:* 35
Ownership: American Safety Razor Co.
Stock Symbol: RAZR
Quality System Registration Information: ISO9001
Produces/Sells CE-marked Devices: Y
Federal Procurement Eligibility: Small Business, GSA Contract, VA Contract
Distribution: Manufacturer Through Distributor, Manufacturer Through Manufacturer Reps, OEM, Exporter
General Admin.: John Paterson/Vice President, General Manager
Mktg./Adv.: Bill Thomas/Manager Regional Sales
     Jim Boe/Manager Regional Sales
Production: Debra Eckard/Product Manager

Biopsy Instrument	Gastroenterology/Urology

PERSONNA MEDICAL/DIV. OF AMERICAN 800-457-2222 *(cont'd)*

Blade, Scalpel	Surgery
Handle, Scalpel	Surgery
Instrument, Manual, General Surgical	Surgery
Knife, Microtome	Pathology
Scalpel, One-Piece (Knife)	Surgery
Surgical, Razor	Surgery

PERSYST DEVELOPMENT CORP. 928-708-0705
1060 Sandretto Drive, Suite E2, Prescott, AZ 86305
FDA Number: 2031720   *Fax:* 928-771-1209
E-mail: sales@eeg-persyst.com
Web site: www.eeg-persyst.com
Medical Products Sales Volume: $1,000,000
Annual Revenue: $1-$5 Million
Year Founded: 1988
Total Employees: 6
Ownership: Private
Produces/Sells CE-marked Devices: N
Federal Procurement Eligibility: Small Business
Distribution: Manufacturer Through Distributor

Analyzer, Spectrum, EEG Signal	Cns/Neurology

PETER PEPPER PRODUCTS, INC. 800-496-0204
17929 S. Susana Road, PO Box 5769,   310-639-0390
Compton, CA 90224
FDA Number: n/a   *Fax:* 310-639-6013
E-mail: customerservice@peterpepper.com
Web site: www.peterpepper.com
Annual Revenue: $10-$25 Million
Year Founded: 1952
Total Employees: 30   *Sales Staff:* 60
Ownership: Private
Produces/Sells CE-marked Devices: N
Federal Procurement Eligibility: Small Business, Female Owned, GSA Contract
Distribution: Manufacturer Through Distributor, Manufacturer Through Manufacturer Reps, OEM, Importer, Exporter
General Admin.: Sigi Pepper/President, Chief Executive Officer
          Kip Pepper/Vice President, General Manager
Mktg./Adv.: Kip Pepper/Vice President Marketing & Sales
Production: Michael Pepper/Director Operations
          Bob Caseres/Vice President Manufacturing

Cart, Equipment, Video	General
Cart, Other	General
Holder, Medical Chart	General
Holder, X-Ray Film	Dental And Oral
Rack, Medical Chart	General
Table, Other	General
Waste Receptacle, General Purpose	General

PETER SCHIFF ENTERPRISE 931-537-6505
4900 Forrest Hill Rd., Cookeville, TN 38506
FDA Number: 1044143

Balloon, Intra-Aortic (With Control System)	Cardiovascular
Cable, Electrode	Physical Med
Circulatory Assist Unit, Left Ventricular	Cardiovascular
Fibrillator, AC-Powered	Cardiovascular

PETERSON AIR PURIFIERS, LLC 952-703-8962
9555 James Avenue South, Suite 220, Bloomington, MN 55431
FDA Number: 3004039224
Ownership: Private
Produces/Sells CE-marked Devices: N

Purifier, Air, Ultraviolet	General

PETRA MANUFACTURING CO. 800-888-7387
6600 W. Armitage Ave., Chicago, IL 60707   773-622-1475
FDA Number: 9200858   *Fax:* 773-622-9448
E-mail: sales@petramanufacturing.com
Web site: www.petramanufacturing.com
Annual Revenue: $5-$10 Million
Total Employees: 80   *Marketing Staff:* 6   *Sales Staff:* 8
Ownership: Private
Quality System Registration Information: ISO9002
Produces/Sells CE-marked Devices: N
Federal Procurement Eligibility: Small Business
Distribution: Manufacturer Direct
General Admin.: Norman Hofberg/Chairman
          Norman Hoffberg/President, Chief Executive Officer
          Don India/Vice President, General Manager
Production: Susan Doherty/Vice President Operations

Apron, Laboratory	Chemistry
Bib	General
Boot, Bath	General
Cover, Mattress, Waterproof	General
Cover, Microscope	Microbiology

PETRARCH SYSTEMS, INC.
See United Chemical Technologies, Inc.

PETROLAB COMPANY 518-783-5133
874 Albany Shaker Road, Latham, NY 12110-1416
FDA Number: n/a   *Fax:* 518-783-5185
E-mail: info@petrolab.com
Web site: www.petrolab.com
Year Founded: 1984
Total Employees: 11   *Marketing Staff:* 1   *Sales Staff:* 4
Ownership: Ametek
Stock Symbol: AME
Traded On: NYSE
Quality System Registration Information: ISO9000
Produces/Sells CE-marked Devices: Y
Federal Procurement Eligibility: Small Business
Distribution: Exclusive Distributor
General Admin.: Michael Palmer/Vice President, General Manager
Mktg./Adv.: Angel Schell/Director Marketing
          Michael Palmer/Manager Contract Sales
          Richard Palmer/Manager International & National Sales
          Michael Palmer/Vice President Sales

Bath, Kinematic Viscosity	Chemistry
Densitometer	Cardiovascular
Viscometer	Chemistry

PFB INTER-APPAREL CORP. 800-828-7629
1930 Harrison Street, Suite 304,   954-342-0800
Hollywood, FL 33020
FDA Number: n/a   *Fax:* 954-342-0806
E-mail: Sales@pfbia.com
Web site: www.pfbia.com
Medical Products Sales Volume: $400,000
Annual Revenue: $1-$5 Million
Year Founded: 1991
Total Employees: 8
Ownership: Private
Produces/Sells CE-marked Devices: N
Federal Procurement Eligibility: Small Business, Minority Owned
Distribution: Manufacturer Direct, Manufacturer Through Manufacturer Reps, Exporter
General Admin.: Frantz Pilorge/President
Mktg./Adv.: Arlene Mcfarlane/Vice President Marketing & Sales

Cap, Surgical	Surgery
Coat, Laboratory	General
Cover, Shoe, Operating Room	Surgery
Gown, Isolation, Surgical	Surgery
Gown, Patient, Disposable	General
Suit, Scrub, Disposable	Surgery
Suit, Surgical	Surgery

PFG PRECISION OPTICS, INC. 228-875-0165
733 Bienville Blvd., Ocean Springs, MS 39564
FDA Number: n/a   *Fax:* 228-875-9354
E-mail: sales@pfgoptics.com
Web site: www.pfgoptics.com
Annual Revenue: $10-$25 Million
Total Employees: 60   *Marketing Staff:* 1   *Sales Staff:* 2
Ownership: Private
Quality System Registration Information: ISO9001
Produces/Sells CE-marked Devices: N
Federal Procurement Eligibility: Small Business
Distribution: Manufacturer Direct, OEM, Importer, Exporter

Component, Optical	General
Gonioscope (Prism)	Ophthalmology

PFINGST & COMPANY, INC. 908-561-6400
105 Snyder, South Plainfield, NJ 07080-1915
FDA Number: 2410005   *Fax:* 908-561-3213
E-mail: CustomerService@PfingstCo.com
Web site: www.pfingstco.com
Annual Revenue: $0-$1 Million
Year Founded: 1905
Total Employees: 20   *Marketing Staff:* 2   *Sales Staff:* 4
Ownership: Private
Produces/Sells CE-marked Devices: N
Federal Procurement Eligibility: Small Business
Distribution: Manufacturer Through Distributor
General Admin.: Greg Pfingst/Chief Executive Officer
          Valire Harding/Managing Director
          Karl Ptingst/Vice President

Burr, Dental Excavating	Dental And Oral

PFIZER / WYETH CONSUMER HEALTHCARE INC. 212-733-2323
235 East 42nd Street, New York, NY 10017
FDA Number: n/a
Web site: www.wyeth.com
Annual Revenue: More than $1 Billion
Total Employees: 50527
Ownership: Public
Stock Symbol: WYE

PFIZER / WYETH CONSUMER HEALTHCARE INC. 212-733-2323
(cont'd)
- Traded On: NYSE
- Produces/Sells CE-marked Devices: N
- Distribution: Manufacturer Direct
- General Admin.: Robert Essner/Chairman
  - Bernard Poussot/President, Chief Executive Officer
  - Contract Manufacturing, Pharmaceuticals/Chemicals — General
- Medical Product Subsidiaries (Listed Separately)
  - Covidien Lp

PFIZER, INC. 212-573-2323
235 East 42nd St., New York, NY 10017-5755
- FDA Number: n/a
- Web site: www.pfizer.com
- Annual Revenue: More than $1 Billion
- Year Founded: 1849
- Total Employees: 81800
- Ownership: Public
- Stock Symbol: PFE
- Traded On: NYSE
- Produces/Sells CE-marked Devices: N
- Distribution: Manufacturer Direct
- General Admin.: Jeffrey Kindler/Chief Executive Officer, Chairman
  - Corey Goodman/President
  - Natale Ricciardi/President
  - Mary McLeod/Senior Vice President Human Resources
  - Amy Schulman/Senior Vice President, General Counsel
- Medical Admin.: Joe Feczko/Chief Medical Officer
- Mktg./Adv.: William Ringo/Senior Vice President Business Development
  - Sally Susman/Senior Vice President Customer Relations
- Production: Ian Read/President Operations
- Research: Martin Mackay/President Research
- Finance: Frank D'Amelio/Chief Financial Officer
  - Contract Manufacturing, Pharmaceuticals/Chemicals — General
- Medical Product Subsidiaries (Listed Separately)
  - Howmedica France

PFS MED, INC. 541-349-9646
3295 Cross St., Eugene, OR 97402
- FDA Number: 3031035

Brace, Joint, Ankle (External)	Physical Med
Joint, Hip, External Brace	Physical Med
Joint, Knee, External Brace	Physical Med
Orthosis, Limb Brace	Physical Med

PGM 585-458-4300
1305 Emerson St., Rochester, NY 14606-3098
- FDA Number: n/a — Fax: 585-458-7281
- E-mail: thockenberger@pgmcorp.com
- Web site: www.pgmcorp.com
- Medical Products Sales Volume: $20,800,000
- Annual Revenue: $25-$50 Million
- Year Founded: 1967
- Total Employees: 112 — Marketing Staff: 1 — Sales Staff: 3
- Ownership: Private
- Quality System Registration Information: ISO9001; ISO9002
- Produces/Sells CE-marked Devices: N
- Federal Procurement Eligibility: Small Business
- Distribution: Manufacturer Direct, Service Direct
- General Admin.: Mr. William Hockenberger/Chairman
  - Mr. Mike Hockenberger/President, Chief Executive Officer
  - Michelle Fre/Vice President Human Resources
- Mktg./Adv.: Mr. Todd Hockenberger/Director Business Development
- Production: Matt O'Connor/Director Quality Assurance
  - Mr. Jerry Gebhard/Manager Materials
  - Mr. Jeff Hockenberger/Manager Production
  - Mr. Robert Flanagan/Managing Engineer
- Finance: Doug Cauwels/Chief Financial Officer

Contract Manufacturing	General
Service, Engineering/Design	General

PHACO SOLUTIONS, INC. 209-536-9707
19395 Village Dr., Sonora, CA 95370
- FDA Number: 3004142717 — Fax: 209-536-9708
- E-mail: info@phacosolutions.com
- Web site: www.phacosolutions.com
- Ownership: Private
- Produces/Sells CE-marked Devices: N

Fluidic, Phacoemulsification/fragmentation	Ophthalmology

PHAKOSYSTEMS, INC. 416-503-4200
14 Plastics Ave, Toronto M8Z 4B7 Canada
- FDA Number: 8020411

Stand, Instrument, AC-Powered, Ophthalmic	Ophthalmology

PHAMATECH INC. 858-643-5555
10151 Barnes Canyon Rd, San Diego, CA 92121
- FDA Number: 2031229

Container, Specimen, Urine, Drugs Of Abuse, Over The Counter	Chemistry
Enzyme Immunoassay, Barbiturate	Toxicology
Enzyme Immunoassay, Benzodiazepine	Toxicology
Enzyme Immunoassay, Cannabinoids	Toxicology
Enzyme Immunoassay, Methadone	Toxicology
Enzyme Immunoassay, Opiates	Toxicology
Enzyme Immunoassay, Phencyclidine	Toxicology
Gas Chromatography, Methamphetamine	Toxicology
Kit, Pregnancy Test, Over The Counter, HCG	Chemistry
Kit, Test, Multiple, Drugs Of Abuse, Over The Counter	Toxicology
Radioimmunoassay, Follicle Stimulating Hormone	Chemistry
Radioimmunoassay, Human Chorionic Gonadotropin	Chemistry
Radioimmunoassay, Luteinizing Hormone	Chemistry

PHARAOH TRADING COMPANY 866-929-4913 / 216-749-6070
Knollwood Plaza, Suite 241
9701 Brookpark Road
Cleveland, OH 44129
- FDA Number: 1528184 — Fax: 216-749-7327
- E-mail: pharaohtrading@earthlink.net
- Medical Products Sales Volume: $990,000
- Annual Revenue: $0-$1 Million
- Total Employees: 5 — Marketing Staff: 2 — Sales Staff: 3
- Ownership: Private
- Produces/Sells CE-marked Devices: N
- Federal Procurement Eligibility: Small Business, Minority Owned, GSA Contract
- Distribution: Exclusive Distributor, Importer, Exporter
- General Admin.: Bill M. Bebawi/Chief Executive Officer

Apron, Laboratory	Chemistry
Bib	General
Blade, Surgical, Saw, General & Plastic Surgery	Surgery
Cover, Shoe, Conductive	General
Depressor, Tongue	General
Glove, Other	General
Glove, Patient Examination, Latex	General
Glove, Patient Examination, Vinyl	General
Gown, Isolation, Surgical	Surgery
Linen	General
Mask, Surgical	Surgery
Service, Import/Export	General
Sponge, Gauze	Dental And Oral
Thermometer, Electronic	General

PHARMA PAC, LLC 601-743-9771
14124 Hwy 16 West, De Kalb, MS 39328
- FDA Number: 3003982004 — Fax: 601-743-9772
- E-mail: jhiggins@pharmapacllc.com
- Ownership: Private
- Produces/Sells CE-marked Devices: N

Lubricant, Vaginal, Patient	General

PHARMA-PLAST USA, INC.
See Unomedical, Inc.

PHARMA-TURM, INC.
See Vetter Pharma-Turm, Inc.

PHARMACAL RESEARCH LABS. INC. 800-243-5350 / 203-755-4908
P.O. Box 369, Naugatuck, CT 06770
- FDA Number: n/a — Fax: 203-755-4309
- Web site: www.pharmacal.com
- Annual Revenue: $0-$1 Million
- Ownership: Private
- Produces/Sells CE-marked Devices: N
- Federal Procurement Eligibility: Small Business
- Distribution: Manufacturer Direct, Service Direct
- General Admin.: Ken Shapiro/President
- Finance: Jerry Shapiro/Chief Financial Officer

Disinfector, Liquid	General
Solution, Antibacterial Cleaner	General

PHARMACEUTICAL CONSULTANTS, INC.
See Artromick

PHARMACEUTICAL INNOVATIONS, INC. 973-242-2900
897 Frelinghuysen Ave., Newark, NJ 07114-2122
- FDA Number: 9200860 — Fax: 973-242-0578
- E-mail: info@pharminnovations.com
- Web site: www.pharminnovations.com
- Year Founded: 1971
- Total Employees: 60
- Ownership: Private
- Quality System Registration Information: ISO9001
- Produces/Sells CE-marked Devices: Y
- Federal Procurement Eligibility: Small Business
- Distribution: Manufacturer Through Distributor, Exporter
- General Admin.: Gilbert Buchalter/President
- Mktg./Adv.: B S/Sales Representative

PHARMACEUTICAL INNOVATIONS, INC. 973-242-2900 *(cont'd)*

Production: Nelson Carvalho/Plant Manager

Accessories, Laser	General
Disinfector, Liquid	General
Disinfector, Medical Device	General
Dressing, Gel	General
Electrode, TENS	Cns/Neurology
Equipment, Device Coating, Protective	General
Gel, Electrode, Electrocardiograph	Cardiovascular
Gel, Electrode, Electrosurgical	Surgery
Gel, Electrode, Stimulator	Cns/Neurology
Gel, Electrode, TENS	Physical Med
Gel, Support	Immunology
Gel, Ultrasonic Coupling	Physical Med
Gel, Ultrasonic Transmission	General
Guide, Device, Ultrasonic	General
Holder, Electrosurgical Electrode	Surgery
Lubricant, Patient	General
Monitor, Eye Movement, Diagnostic	Ophthalmology
Pad, Breast	Obstetrics/Gynecology
Soap	General
Tips And Pads, Cane, Crutch And Walker	Physical Med
Warmer, Anesthesia Tube	Dental And Oral

PHARMACIA & UPJOHN CO. 212-573-1000
7000 Portage Rd., Kalamazoo, MI 49001
FDA Number: 1810189
Ownership: Private
Produces/Sells CE-marked Devices: N

Agent, Hemostatic, Non-Absorbable, Collagen-Based	Surgery
Pipetting And Diluting System, Automated	Chemistry
Punch, Gelfoam	Ear/Nose/Throat

PHARMACIA DELTEC, INC.
See Smiths Medical Asd, Inc.

PHARMACIA LKB NUCLEAR, INC.
See Perkin Elmer Wallac, Inc.

PHARMAFFAIR INC. 416-444-8090
52 Sanfield Road, Toronto, ONT M3B-2B7 Canada
FDA Number: n/a   Fax: 416-444-4246
E-mail: maha@pharmaffair.ca
Web site: http://www.pharmaffair.ca
Year Founded: 1991
Total Employees: 10
Ownership: Private
Produces/Sells CE-marked Devices: N

PHARMAJET 303-526-4278
24797 Foothills Drive North, Golden, CO 80401
FDA Number: 3004977013   Fax: 303-526-4052
E-mail: Callender@pharmajet.com
Web site: www.pharmajet.com
Medical Products Sales Volume: $200,000
Annual Revenue: $1-$5 Million
Total Employees: 3
Ownership: Private
Produces/Sells CE-marked Devices: N
Federal Procurement Eligibility: Small Business

Injector, Syringe	General

PHARMALUCENCE, INC. 781.275.7120
54 Loomis Street, Bedford, MA 01730
FDA Number: 1219718   Fax: 781.275.5191
Ownership: Private
Produces/Sells CE-marked Devices: N

PHARMASCIENCE MEDICAL DIVISION 800-340-9735
6111 Royalmount Ave., 514-340-1114
Montreal, QUE H4T-2 Canada
FDA Number: n/a   Fax: 514-737-5673
E-mail: service@pharmascience.com
Web site: www.pharmascience.com
Year Founded: 1983
Total Employees: 25
Ownership: Private
Produces/Sells CE-marked Devices: N
Distribution: Manufacturer Direct, Exclusive Distributor

PHARMASYSTEMS INC. 888-475-2500
361 Steelcase Rd. W, Unit 10, 905-475-2500
Markham, ONT L3R-3 Canada
FDA Number: n/a   Fax: 905-475-7155
Web site: http://www.pharmasystems.com
Year Founded: 1962
Ownership: Private
Produces/Sells CE-marked Devices: N
Distribution: Manufacturer Direct, Exclusive Distributor

PHARMAX CANADA LIMITED 800-269-7898
80 Galaxy Blvd., Unit 4, 416-675-3333
Toronto, ONT M9W-4 Canada
FDA Number: n/a   Fax: 416-675-9176
E-mail: hodgins@istar.ca
Web site: www.pharmax.ca
Year Founded: 1976
Total Employees: 10
Ownership: Private
Produces/Sells CE-marked Devices: N
Distribution: Manufacturer Direct, Exclusive Distributor

PHASE II MEDICAL MFG., INC. 603-332-8900
88 Airport Drive, Suite 100, Rocheseter, NH 03867
FDA Number: 1225492   Fax: 603-332-3766
E-mail: info@phaseiimed.com
Web site: www.phaseiimed.com
Annual Revenue: $1-$5 Million
Year Founded: 1995
Total Employees: 38
Ownership: Private
Quality System Registration Information: ISO9000
Produces/Sells CE-marked Devices: Y
Federal Procurement Eligibility: Small Business

Connector, Airway (Extension)	Anesthesiology

PHELAN MANUFACTURING CORP. 800-328-2358
2523 Minnehaha Ave., 612-724-3677
Minneapolis, MN 55404
FDA Number: 2126376   Fax: 612-724-3678
Web site: www.phelanmfgcorp.com
Annual Revenue: $0-$1 Million
Total Employees: 7
Ownership: Private
Produces/Sells CE-marked Devices: N
Federal Procurement Eligibility: Small Business
Distribution: Manufacturer Direct
General Admin.: W. Buelow/Executive Vice President
           Tom Farr/Office Manager
             L. Phelan/President
Production: D. Pederson/Vice President Manufacturing

Accessories, Operating Room, Table	Surgery
Cart, Other	General
Container, Sterilization (Tray)	General
Footstool, Conductive	General
Hanger, Intravenous	General
Hanger, Urologic	Gastroenterology/Urology
Hook, Other	Surgery
Infusion Stand	General
Mount, Monitor (Support)	General
Punch, Biopsy, Surgical	Dental And Oral
Rack, Surgical Instrument	Surgery
Screen, Anesthesia	Anesthesiology
Stand, Basin	General
Stirrup	Gastroenterology/Urology
Stripper, Vein, Reusable	Surgery
Suction Apparatus, Single Patient, Portable, Non-Powered	Surgery
Support, Arm	Physical Med
Table, Instrument, Surgical	Surgery
Tubing, Non-Invasive	Surgery

PHENOMENEX, INC. 310-212-0555
2320 W. 205th St., Torrance, CA 90501-1456
FDA Number: 7000163   Fax: 310-328-7768
Medical Products Sales Volume: $5,000,000
Annual Revenue: $10-$25 Million
Total Employees: 150
Ownership: Private
Produces/Sells CE-marked Devices: N
Federal Procurement Eligibility: Small Business
Distribution: Manufacturer Direct, Importer, Exporter
General Admin.: Fasha Mahjoor/President
            Nader Ghaemmagami/Vice President Human Resources
Mktg./Adv.: Sid Doshi/Director Marketing
            Dave Townsend/Director National Accounts
            Steve Suh/Manager International Sales
            Tom Cleveland/Manager Product Development
            Sue Bielinski/Manager Sales Training
            Doug McCrory/Vice President Sales
Production: Steve Cohen/Vice President Operations
Research: Faizy Ahmed/Vice President Research & Development

Accessories, Chromatography (Gas, Gel, Liquid, Thin Layer)	Chemistry
Chromatography, Liquid, Performance, High	Toxicology
Column, Liquid Chromatography	Toxicology

PHEROMONE SCIENCE CORP. 416-861-9854
443 King St. E, Toronto, ONT M5A-1L5 Canada
FDA Number: n/a   Fax: 416-861-9950

PHEROMONE SCIENCE CORP.   416-861-9854 *(cont'd)*
E-mail: cneuman@pheromonesciences.com
Web site: www.pheromonesciences.com
Year Founded: 1997
Total Employees: 7
Ownership: Public
Stock Symbol: TSX:
Traded On: Vancouver
Quality System Registration Information: ISO9002
Produces/Sells CE-marked Devices: Y
Distribution: Manufacturer Direct

PHILADELPHIA BIOLOGICS CENTER
See Churchill Medical Systems, Inc.

PHILADELPHIA BIOLOGICS CENTER
See Medical Specialties, Inc.

PHILADELPHIA VISION CENTER   215-568-0700
1100 Market St., Philadelphia, PA 19107
FDA Number: 2531444   *Fax:* 215-568-1063
Ownership: Private
Produces/Sells CE-marked Devices: N
  Frame, Spectacle (Eyeglasses)   Ophthalmology

PHILIPS AVENT   800-542-8368
475 Supreme Dr., Bensenville, IL 60106-1161   630-350-2600
FDA Number: n/a
Web site: www.avent.com
Medical Products Sales Volume: $50,000,000
Annual Revenue: $50-$100 Million
Year Founded: 1984
Ownership: PHILIPS GMBH
Produces/Sells CE-marked Devices: N
Federal Procurement Eligibility: Small Business
Distribution: Manufacturer Direct, Importer, Exporter
  Bottle, Nursing   Obstetrics/Gynecology
  Nipple, Feeding   General
  Pacifier   General
  Pad, Breast   Obstetrics/Gynecology
  Pump, Breast, Powered   Obstetrics/Gynecology
  Shield, Nipple   Obstetrics/Gynecology

PHILIPS COMPONENTS
See Narragansett Imaging

PHILIPS DENTAL
See Del Medical Systems

PHILIPS DOMESTIC APPLIANCES AND PERSONAL CARE
See Philips Electronics North America

PHILIPS ELECTRONICS NORTH AMERICA   800-682-7664
2820 B. St. NW, Suite 101, Auburn, WA 98001
FDA Number: 3003418460
Web site: www.medical.philips.com
Annual Revenue: More than $1 Billion
Total Employees: 17346
Ownership: PHILIPS MEDICAL SYSTEMS INTERNATIONAL B.V.
Stock Symbol: PHG
Traded On: NYSE
Produces/Sells CE-marked Devices: N
  Toothbrush, Powered   Dental And Oral
  Unit, Ultraviolet Sanitation/sterilization (for Toothbrushes), Non-sterile   Dental And Oral

PHILIPS HEALTHCARE   614-865-8956
836 North St, Bld 500, Tewksbury, MA 01876
FDA Number: 3007182075
Web site: www.medical.philips.com
Total Employees: 35551
Ownership: KONINKLIJKE PHILIPS ELECTRONICS NV
Stock Symbol: PHG
Traded On: NYSE
Produces/Sells CE-marked Devices: N
  Analyzer, Gas, Oxygen, Gaseous Phase   Anesthesiology
  Attachment, Breathing, Positive End Expiratory Pressure   Anesthesiology
  Mask, Gas, Anesthesia   Anesthesiology
  Oximeter, Whole Blood   Hematology
  Ventilator, Non-Continuous (Respirator)   Anesthesiology

PHILIPS HEALTHCARE INFORMATICS, INC   800-934-7372
4100 East Third Ave, Suite 101,   650-293-2300
Foster City, CA 94404
FDA Number: 2954704
Web site: www.healthcare.philips.com
Annual Revenue: More than $1 Billion
Total Employees: 35551
Ownership: Public
Stock Symbol: PHG
Traded On: NYSE
Produces/Sells CE-marked Devices: N
  Image Processing System   Radiology

PHILIPS HEALTHCARE INFORMATICS, INC 800-934-7372 *(cont'd)*
  System, Communication, Image, Digital   Radiology

PHILIPS LIGHTING CO.   800-555-0050
200 Franklin Square Drive, Somerset, NJ 08875-6800
FDA Number: 2247247
Web site: www.lighting.philips.com
Medical Products Sales Volume: $100,000,000
Annual Revenue: More than $1 Billion
Year Founded: 1891
Total Employees: 57166
Ownership: PHILLIPS ELECTRONICS NORTH AMERICA
Stock Symbol: PHG
Traded On: NYSE
Quality System Registration Information: ISO9001
Produces/Sells CE-marked Devices: N
Federal Procurement Eligibility: Small Business
Distribution: Manufacturer Through Distributor, Manufacturer Through Manufacturer Reps, Exclusive Distributor
  Lamp, Other   General
  Phototherapy Unit (Bilirubin Lamp)   General

PHILIPS LIGHTING CO.   800-555-0050
505 Hoult Rd., Fairmont, WV 26554
FDA Number: 1120644
Web site: www.lighting.philips.com
Annual Revenue: More than $1 Billion
Total Employees: 57166
Ownership: KONINKLIJKE PHILIPS ELECTRONICS NV
Stock Symbol: PHG
Traded On: NYSE
Produces/Sells CE-marked Devices: N
  Booth, Sun Tan   Physical Med
  Control, Drug Mixture   Toxicology
  Light, Ultraviolet, Dermatologic   Surgery
  Phototherapy Unit, Neonatal   General

PHILIPS MEDICAL SYSTEMS   978-659-4252
1525 Ranchero Conejo Blvd, Thousand Oaks, CA 91320
FDA Number: 2023339
Web site: www.medical.philips.com
Total Employees: 35551
Ownership: Public
Stock Symbol: PHG
Traded On: NYSE
Produces/Sells CE-marked Devices: N
  Adapter, Lead Switching, Electrocardiograph   Cardiovascular
  Electrocardiograph, Ambulatory (With Analysis Algorithm)   Cardiovascular
  Electrocardiograph, Ambulatory(without Analysis)   Cardiovascular
  Recorder, Magnetic Tape/Disc   Cardiovascular
  Transmitter/Receiver System, ECG, Telephone Multi-Channel   Cardiovascular
  Transmitter/Receiver System, ECG, Telephone Single-Channel   Cardiovascular

PHILIPS MEDICAL SYSTEMS
See Philips Medical Systems North America Co.

PHILIPS MEDICAL SYSTEMS   978-659-3000
3000 Minuteman Rd, Andover, MA 01810
FDA Number: 1218950
Web site: www.medical.philips.com
Annual Revenue: More than $1 Billion
Total Employees: 35551
Ownership: Public
Stock Symbol: PHG
Traded On: NYSE
Produces/Sells CE-marked Devices: N
  Aid, Resuscitation, Cardiopulmonary   Cardiovascular
  Analyzer, Gas, Carbon-Dioxide, Gaseous Phase (Capnograph)   Anesthesiology
  Attachment, Breathing, Positive End Expiratory Pressure   Anesthesiology
  Connector, Airway (Extension)   Anesthesiology
  Detector, Arrhythmia Alarm   Cardiovascular
  Gas Machine, Analgesia   Anesthesiology
  Gas, Calibrated (Specified Concentration)   Anesthesiology
  Image Processing System   Radiology
  Monitor, Blood Pressure, Indirect (Arterial)   Cardiovascular
  Monitor, Cardiac (Cardiotachometer & Rate Alarm)   Cardiovascular
  Monitor, Physiological, Patient   Cardiovascular
  Monitor, Physiological, Patient(without Arrhythmia Detection Or Alarms)   Cardiovascular
  Oximeter, Intracardiac   Cardiovascular
  Transducer, Ultrasonic   Cardiovascular

PHILIPS MEDICAL SYSTEMS   1-800-722-9377
3000 Minuteman Road,   -
Andover,, MA 01810
FDA Number: 1218950
Annual Revenue: $0-$1 Million
Total Employees: 10
Ownership: Philips Medical Systems North America
Traded On: NYSE
Quality System Registration Information: ISO9000

PHILIPS MEDICAL SYSTEMS
1-800-722-9377 *(cont'd)*

Produces/Sells CE-marked Devices: Y
Distribution: Service Direct
General Admin.: Richard Porte/Chief Executive Officer, General Manager
Donna Haire/Director
Mktg./Adv.: Ross Heaton/Director Marketing
R. Heaton/Manager Advertising

Aid, Resuscitation, Cardiopulmonary	Cardiovascular
Analyzer, Gas, Carbon-Dioxide, Gaseous Phase (Capnograph)	Anesthesiology
Auxiliary Power Supply, Low Energy Defibrillator (AC or DC)	Cardiovascular
Cable, Electrode	Physical Med
Connector, Airway (Extension)	Anesthesiology
Cuff, Blood Pressure	Cardiovascular
Defibrillator, External, Automatic	Cardiovascular
Detector, Arrhythmia Alarm	Cardiovascular
Display, Cathode-Ray Tube	Cardiovascular
Electroencephalograph	Cns/Neurology
Gas Machine, Analgesia	Anesthesiology
Image Processing System	Radiology
Monitor, Cardiac (Cardiotachometer & Rate Alarm)	Cardiovascular
Monitor, Fetal Doppler Ultrasound	Obstetrics/Gynecology
Monitor, Physiological, Patient	Cardiovascular
Monitor, Physiological, Patient(without Arrhythmia Detection Or Alarms)	Cardiovascular
Pacemaker, Cardiac, External Transcutaneous (Non-Invasive)	Cardiovascular
Probe, Ultrasonic	Radiology
Recorder, Magnetic Tape/Disc	Cardiovascular
Recorder, Paper Chart	Cardiovascular
Scanner, Ultrasonic (Pulsed Echo)	Radiology
Scanner, Ultrasonic, Abdominal	Radiology
Scanner, Ultrasonic, General Purpose	Radiology
Scanner, Ultrasonic, Obstetrical/Gynecological, Mobile	Obstetrics/Gynecology
Scanner, Ultrasonic, Other	Radiology
Scanner, Ultrasonic, Pediatric	Radiology
Scanner, Ultrasonic, Small Parts	Radiology
Scanner, Ultrasonic, Vascular	Radiology
Stethoscope, Manual	Cardiovascular
System, Communication, Image, Digital	Radiology
Transducer, Ultrasonic	Cardiovascular
Transducer, Ultrasonic, Obstetrical	Obstetrics/Gynecology
Urinometer, Electrical	Gastroenterology/Urology

PHILIPS MEDICAL SYSTEMS (CLEVELAND), INC. 978-659-4663
5520 Nobel Drive, Fitchburg, WI 53711
FDA Number: 3004022368
Web site: www.medical.philips.com
Annual Revenue: More than $1 Billion
Total Employees: 35551
Ownership: Public
Stock Symbol: PHG
Traded On: NYSE
Produces/Sells CE-marked Devices: N

Nuclear Magnetic Resonance Imaging System	Radiology
System, Planning, Radiation Therapy Treatment	Radiology

PHILIPS MEDICAL SYSTEMS (PMMS PUERTO RICO), INC
978-659-4663

**200 Winston Churchill Ave. Suite
302 Mercurio St. Apolo Shopping Center
Est De San Geraldo, PR 00926**
FDA Number: 2649965
Web site: www.medical.philips.com
Annual Revenue: More than $1 Billion
Total Employees: 35551
Ownership: Public
Stock Symbol: PHG
Traded On: NYSE
Produces/Sells CE-marked Devices: N

PHILIPS MEDICAL SYSTEMS NORTH AMERICA 800-934-7372
2301 Fifth Ave.,, Ste. 200, Seattle, WA 98121
FDA Number: 3030677
Web site: www.medical.philips.com
Annual Revenue: More than $1 Billion
Total Employees: 35551
Ownership: Public
Stock Symbol: PHG
Traded On: NYSE
Quality System Registration Information: ISO9000; ISO9001
Produces/Sells CE-marked Devices: N
Distribution: Manufacturer Direct

Aperture, Radiographic	Radiology
Block, Beam Shaping, Radionuclide	Radiology
Board, Arm	Anesthesiology
Camera, Focal Spot, Radiographic	Radiology
Camera, X-Ray, Fluorographic, Cine Or Spot	Radiology
Cart, Patient (Stretcher)	Anesthesiology
Changer, Film, Radiographic	Radiology
Collimator, Radiographic, Automatic	Radiology
Collimator, Radiographic, Manual	Radiology

PHILIPS MEDICAL SYSTEMS NORTH AMERICA 800-934-7372
(cont'd)

Collimator, Therapeutic X-Ray, Dermatological	Radiology
Collimator, Therapeutic X-Ray, High Voltage	Radiology
Collimator, Therapeutic X-Ray, Low Voltage	Radiology
Collimator, Therapeutic X-Ray, Orthovoltage	Radiology
Computer, Cardiac Catheterization Laboratory	Cardiovascular
Cone, Radiographic	Radiology
Couch, Radiation Therapy, Powered	Radiology
Device, Limiting, Beam, Teletherapy, Radionuclide	Radiology
Display, Cathode-Ray Tube	Cardiovascular
Generator, Diagnostic X-Ray, High Voltage, 3-Phase	Radiology
Generator, Diagnostic X-Ray, High Voltage, Single Phase	Radiology
Generator, Radiographic, Capacitor Discharge	Radiology
Generator, Therapeutic X-Ray, Dermatological (Grenz Ray)	Radiology
Generator, Therapeutic X-Ray, High Voltage	Radiology
Generator, Therapeutic X-Ray, Low Voltage	Radiology
Grid, Radiographic	Radiology
Hanger, X-Ray Tube	Radiology
Holder, Head, Radiographic	Radiology
Holder, Radiographic Cassette, Wall-Mounted	Radiology
Housing, X-Ray Tube, Diagnostic	Radiology
Housing, X-Ray Tube, Therapeutic	Radiology
Monitor, Patient Position, Light Beam	Radiology
Mount, X-Ray Tube, Diagnostic	Radiology
Radiographic Picture Archiving/Communication System (PACS)	Radiology
Radiographic Unit, Diagnostic, Tomographic	Radiology
Radiographic Unit, Digital Subtraction Angiographic (DSA)	Radiology
Radiographic/Fluoroscopic Unit, Angiographic	Radiology
Radiographic/Fluoroscopic Unit, Image-Intensified	Radiology
Radiographic/Fluoroscopic Unit, Mobile C-Arm	Radiology
Scanner, Computed Tomography, X-Ray (CAT, CT)	Cns/Neurology
Scanner, Computed Tomography, X-Ray, Full Body	Radiology
Scanner, Computed Tomography, X-Ray, Special Procedure	Radiology
Scanner, Magnetic Resonance (NMR/MRI)	Radiology
Scanner, Ultrasonic, Other	Radiology
Source, Teletherapy, Radionuclide	Radiology
Spot Film Device	Radiology
Stand, Cardiovascular	Radiology
Stand, Vascular	Radiology
Support, Patient Position	Anesthesiology
System, X-Ray, Mobile	Radiology
Table, Radiographic, Non-Tilting, Powered	Radiology
Table, Radiographic, Stationary Top	Radiology
Table, Radiographic, Tilting	Radiology
Table, Urological, Radiographic	Gastroenterology/Urology
Teletherapy System, Radionuclide	Radiology
Test Pattern, Radiographic	Radiology
Transducer, Ultrasonic	Cardiovascular
Tube, Image Amplifier, X-Ray	Radiology
Tube, X-Ray	Radiology

Medical Product Subsidiaries (Listed Separately)
Philips Medical Systems
Respironics, Inc

PHILIPS MEDICAL SYSTEMS NORTH AMERICA CO.
800-934-7372

**22100 Bothell Everett Highway,
Bothell, WA 98021**
425-487-7000
FDA Number: 1217116
Web site: www.medical.philips.com
Annual Revenue: More than $1 Billion
Total Employees: 35551
Ownership: Public
Stock Symbol: PHG
Traded On: NYSE
Produces/Sells CE-marked Devices: N

Defibrillator, External, Automatic	Cardiovascular
System, Network And Communication, Physiological Monitors	Cardiovascular

PHILIPS MEDICAL SYSTEMS(CLEVELAND), INC. 440-483-3765
595 Miner Rd., Cleveland, OH 44143
FDA Number: 1525965
Web site: www.medical.philips.com
Annual Revenue: More than $1 Billion
Total Employees: 35551
Ownership: Public
Stock Symbol: PHG
Traded On: NYSE
Produces/Sells CE-marked Devices: N

Camera, Gamma (Nuclear/Scintillation)	Radiology
Image Processing System	Radiology
Nuclear Magnetic Resonance Imaging System	Radiology
Scanner, Computed Tomography, X-Ray, Special Procedure	Radiology
Scanner, Emission Computed Tomography	Radiology

PHILIPS MEDICAL SYSTEMS, NEW CLINICAL VENTURES   408-321-9100
3860 North First Street, San Jose, CA 95134
FDA Number: 2916556
Web site: www.medical.philips.com
Annual Revenue: More than $1 Billion
Total Employees: 35551
Ownership: Public
Stock Symbol: PHG
Traded On: NYSE
Produces/Sells CE-marked Devices: N

Accelerator, Linear, Medical	Radiology
Camera, Gamma (Nuclear/Scintillation)	Radiology
Connector, Airway (Extension)	Anesthesiology
Gas, Calibrated (Specified Concentration)	Anesthesiology
Scale, Stand-On	General
Scanner, Emission Computed Tomography	Radiology
Stethoscope, Esophageal	Anesthesiology
Transmitter/Receiver, Physiological Signal, Infrared	Cardiovascular

PHILIPS ORAL HEALTHCARE, INC.   425-396-2000
22100 Bothell Everett Highway, Bothell, WA 98021
FDA Number: 3026630
Web site: www.medical.philips.com
Annual Revenue: More than $1 Billion
Total Employees: 35551
Ownership: Public
Stock Symbol: PHG
Traded On: NYSE
Produces/Sells CE-marked Devices: N

Irrigator, Oral	Dental And Oral
Toothbrush, Powered	Dental And Oral
Unit, Ultraviolet Sanitation/sterilization (for Toothbrushes), Non-sterile	Dental And Oral

PHILIPS REMOTE CARDIAC SERVICES   800-367-1095
7 Waterside Crossing, Windsor, CT 06095
FDA Number: n/a   *Fax:* 860-298-6125
Web site: www.remotecardiacservices.com
Medical Products Sales Volume: $100,000
Annual Revenue: $0-$1 Million
Ownership: Public
Stock Symbol: AEX
Traded On: NYSE
Produces/Sells CE-marked Devices: N
Federal Procurement Eligibility: Small Business

Computer, ECG Interpretation (Arrhythmia)	Cardiovascular
Telemetry Unit, Physiological, ECG	Cardiovascular
Transmitter/Receiver System, ECG, Telephone Multi-Channel	Cardiovascular

PHILIPS ROXANE LABORATORIES
See Roxane Laboratories

PHILIPS ULTRASOUND INTERNATIONAL
See Philips Medical Systems

PHILIPS ULTRASOUND, INC.   425-487-7000
1 Echo Dr., Reedsville, PA 17084-8603
FDA Number: 2518586
Web site: www.medical.philips.com
Annual Revenue: More than $1 Billion
Total Employees: 35551
Ownership: Public
Stock Symbol: PHG
Traded On: NYSE
Produces/Sells CE-marked Devices: N

Phonocardiograph	Cardiovascular
Scanner, Ultrasonic (Pulsed Doppler)	Radiology
Scanner, Ultrasonic (Pulsed Echo)	Radiology
Transducer, Ultrasonic	Cardiovascular

PHILLIPS ENVIRONMENTAL PRODUCTS, INC.   406-388-5999
290 Arden Dr., Belgrade, MT 59714
FDA Number: 3005027352
Ownership: Private
Produces/Sells CE-marked Devices: N

Bedpan	General

PHILLIPS PLASTICS CORP.   877-508-0252
1201 Hanley Road, Hudson, WI 54016
FDA Number: 2183833   *Fax:* 715-381-3291
E-mail: info@phillipsplastics.com
Web site: www.phillipsplastics.com
Medical Products Sales Volume: $250,000,000
Annual Revenue: $100-$500 Million
Year Founded: 1964
Total Employees: 1500
Ownership: Private
Stock Symbol: QCOM
Traded On: NASDAQ
Quality System Registration Information: ISO9000; ISO9001; ISO9002

PHILLIPS PLASTICS CORP.   877-508-0252 *(cont'd)*
Produces/Sells CE-marked Devices: Y
Distribution: Manufacturer Direct, Manufacturer Through Distributor, Manufacturer Through Manufacturer Reps

Component, Metal, Other	General
Component, Other	General
Contract Assembly	General
Contract Manufacturing	General
Molding, Custom	General
Molding, Injection	General

PHILLIPS PLASTICS CORPORATION, PHILLIPS MEDICAL   715-232-4608
415 Red Cedar St., Menomonie, WI 54751
FDA Number: 2134945
Ownership: Private
Produces/Sells CE-marked Devices: N

PHILLIPS PLASTICS CORPORATION, PHILLIPS MEDICAL NEW RICHMOND   877.508.0252
705 Wisconsin Dr., New Richmond, WI 54017   715-246-7070
FDA Number: 2134944
Ownership: Private
Produces/Sells CE-marked Devices: N

Hyperthermia Unit, Microwave	Radiology
Laparoscope, General & Plastic Surgery	Surgery

PHILLIPS SAFETY PRODUCTS   516-482-9001
123 Lincoln Blvd., Middlesex, NJ 08846
FDA Number: 3004183518
Ownership: Private
Produces/Sells CE-marked Devices: N

Barrier, Control Panel, X-Ray, Moveable	Radiology

PHILLIPS ULTRASOUND   800-982-2011
22100 Bothell Everett Hwy., P.O. Box 3003,   425-487-7000
Bothell, WA 98021
FDA Number: 3019216   *Fax:* 425-482-8834
E-mail: linda.likkel@philips.com
Web site: www.medical.philips.com
Total Employees: 2600
Ownership: Public
Stock Symbol: PGH
Traded On: NYSE
Quality System Registration Information: ISO9001
Produces/Sells CE-marked Devices: Y
Distribution: Manufacturer Direct, Manufacturer Through Distributor, Manufacturer Through Manufacturer Reps, Service Direct, Exclusive Distributor

Guide, Device, Ultrasonic	General
Probe, Ultrasonic	Radiology
Scanner, Ultrasonic (Pulsed Doppler)	Radiology
Scanner, Ultrasonic (Pulsed Echo)	Radiology
Scanner, Ultrasonic, Abdominal	Radiology
Scanner, Ultrasonic, General Purpose	Radiology
Scanner, Ultrasonic, Obstetrical/Gynecological	Obstetrics/Gynecology
Scanner, Ultrasonic, Obstetrical/Gynecological, Mobile	Obstetrics/Gynecology
Scanner, Ultrasonic, Other	Radiology
Scanner, Ultrasonic, Pediatric	Radiology
Scanner, Ultrasonic, Small Parts	Radiology
Scanner, Ultrasonic, Vascular	Radiology
System, Communication, Image, Digital	Radiology
Transducer, Ultrasonic	Cardiovascular
Transducer, Ultrasonic, Diagnostic	Radiology
Transducer, Ultrasonic, Obstetrical	Obstetrics/Gynecology

PHIPPS & BIRD, INC.   800-955-7621
1519 Summit Avenue, Richmond, VA 23230   804-254-2737
FDA Number: 1121097   *Fax:* 804-254-2955
E-mail: mail@phippsbird.com
Web site: www.phippsbird.com
Medical Products Sales Volume: $1,700,000
Annual Revenue: $1-$5 Million
Year Founded: 1925
Total Employees: 15
Ownership: Private
Stock Symbol: PHMD
Traded On: NASDAQ
Quality System Registration Information: ISO9001
Produces/Sells CE-marked Devices: Y
Federal Procurement Eligibility: Small Business, Female Owned
Distribution: Manufacturer Through Distributor, OEM, Exporter
General Admin.: Wes Skaperdas/General Manager
    Wes Skaperdas/President, Chief Executive Officer
    Pat Skaperdas/Vice President, General Manager
Mktg./Adv.: Wes Skaperdas/Director National Accounts
    Kevin Byrd/Director Product Development
Production: Rick Marshall/Director Quality Assurance
    Jeannette Wescott/Manager Operations

PHIPPS & BIRD, INC. — 800-955-7621 (cont'd)

George Catlin/Manager Production

Analyzer, Metabolism	Anesthesiology
Aspirator, Emergency Suction	General
Bath, Tissue Flotation	Microbiology
Compressor, Air, Portable	Anesthesiology
Device, Measurement, Velocity, Conduction, Nerve	Cns/Neurology
Fork, Tuning	Cns/Neurology
Oscilloscope	General
Plethysmograph, Volume	Anesthesiology
Pneumograph	Anesthesiology
Simulator, ECG	Cardiovascular
Sphygmomanometer, Mercury (Arterial Pressure)	General
Stirrer	Chemistry
Warmer, Solution	Chemistry

PHOENIX BIO-TECH CORP. — 800-701-7450 / 905-826-6330

6810 Kitimat Rd., Unit 1,
Mississauga, ONT L5N-5 Canada

FDA Number: 9615918
Fax: 905-826-3288
E-mail: info@phoenixbiotech.com
Web site: www.phoenixbiotech.com
Year Founded: 1992
Total Employees: 10
Ownership: Private
Produces/Sells CE-marked Devices: N
Distribution: Manufacturer Direct, Exclusive Distributor

PHOENIX BIOMEDICAL PRODUCTS, INC. — 9056708299

7085 Tomken Rd., Mississauga, ONT L5S-1R7 Canada

FDA Number: n/a
Fax: 9056700195
E-mail: stardish@phoenix-biomed.com
Web site: www.phoenix-biomed.com
Medical Products Sales Volume: $5,000,000
Year Founded: 1980
Total Employees: 45   Marketing Staff: 2   Sales Staff: 2
Ownership: Private
Quality System Registration Information: ISO9002
Produces/Sells CE-marked Devices: N
Federal Procurement Eligibility: Small Business
Distribution: Manufacturer Direct, Manufacturer Through Distributor, Exporter

PHOENIX DENTAL, INC. — 877-463-9905 / 810-750-2328

3452 West Thompson Rd., Fenton, MI 48430

FDA Number: 1836322
Fax: 810-750-7495
E-mail: info@phoenixdental.com
Web site: www.phoenixdental.com
Ownership: Private
Produces/Sells CE-marked Devices: N
Distribution: Exclusive Distributor

Liner, Cavity, Calcium Hydroxide	Dental And Oral

PHOENIX DIAGNOSTICS, INC. — 800-688-2595 / 508-655-8310

8 Tech Circle, Natick, MA 01760

FDA Number: 1222035
Fax: 508-655-8273
Web site: www.phoenixdiagnostics.com
Annual Revenue: $0-$1 Million
Year Founded: 1989
Ownership: Private
Produces/Sells CE-marked Devices: N
Federal Procurement Eligibility: Small Business
Distribution: Manufacturer Direct, Manufacturer Through Distributor, Service Direct, Exporter
General Admin.: Ram Nunna/President, Chief Executive Officer
Mktg./Adv.: John MacPhee/Vice President Business Development
Al Jordan/Vice President Marketing & Sales
Production: Robert Welch/Vice President Manufacturing

Contract Manufacturing	General
Control, Blood Gas	Chemistry
Control, Electrolyte (Assayed And Unassayed)	Chemistry
Control, Enzyme (Assayed And Unassayed)	Chemistry
Control, Multi Analyte, All Kinds (Assayed And Unassayed)	Chemistry
Electrode, Ion Specific, Chloride	Chemistry
Electrode, Ion Specific, Potassium	Chemistry
Electrode, Ion Specific, Sodium	Chemistry
Reagent, Calibration	General
Reagent, Other	General

PHOENIX GROUP, THE — 800-370-6808 / 303-287-6808

4965 Kingston St., Denver, CO 80239

FDA Number: 1718371
Web site: www.falconrehab.com
Ownership: Private
Produces/Sells CE-marked Devices: N

Component, Wheelchair	Physical Med

PHOENIX MEDICAL DEVICES, LLC — 800-689-9892

2458 Alton Parkway, Irvine, CA 92606

FDA Number: 3004620982
Fax: 949-724-1191

PHOENIX MEDICAL DEVICES, LLC — 800-689-9892 (cont'd)

E-mail: support@pmddirect.com
Web site: www.pmddirect.com
Ownership: Private
Quality System Registration Information: ISO9001
Produces/Sells CE-marked Devices: N

Stimulator, Muscle, Electrical-Powered (EMS)	Physical Med

PHOENIX METAL PRODUCTS, INC. — 516-546-4200

100 Bennington Avenue, Freeport, NY 11520-4601

FDA Number: n/a
Fax: 516-546-2594
E-mail: contactus@phoenixmetalproducts.com
Web site: www.phoenixmetalproducts.com
Year Founded: 1991
Ownership: Private
Produces/Sells CE-marked Devices: N
Federal Procurement Eligibility: Small Business
Distribution: Manufacturer Direct
General Admin.: Robert E. Wolf/Chief Executive Officer

Box, Transportation, Container, Specimen	General
Cabinet, Storage, Slide	General

PHOENIX ORTHODONTICS, INC. — 800-642-3009

2401 S.W. Stonecreek Ct., Blue Springs, MO 64015

FDA Number: 1933314
Fax: 816-228-4872
E-mail: sales@phoenixorthodontics.com
Web site: www.phoenixorthodontics.com
Year Founded: 1990
Ownership: Private
Produces/Sells CE-marked Devices: N

Bracket, Metal, Orthodontic	Dental And Oral

PHOENIX POWER SYSTEMS INC.
See Maxwell Technologies Power Systems

PHOENIX PRECISION INST./VIRIS
See Virtis, An Sp Industries Company

PHOENIX SEATING SYSTEMS, LLC
See Phoenix Group, The

PHONE ALERT CORP.
See Actall Corp.

PHONIC EAR, INC. — 800-227-0735 / 707-769-1110

3880 Cypress Drive, Petaluma, CA 94954-7600

FDA Number: 2918633
Fax: 707-769-9624
E-mail: marketing@phonicear.com
Web site: www.phonicear.com
Medical Products Sales Volume: $21,300,000
Year Founded: 1963
Total Employees: 80
Ownership: Public
Traded On: Copenhagen
Quality System Registration Information: ISO9001
Produces/Sells CE-marked Devices: Y
Federal Procurement Eligibility: Small Business
Distribution: Manufacturer Direct, Manufacturer Through Distributor, OEM, Exporter
General Admin.: Rick Pimentel/President, Chief Operating Officer
Mktg./Adv.: Paul Hickey/Director Sales
John Merline/Manager Marketing Communications

Hearing-Aid	Ear/Nose/Throat
Speech Therapy Unit (Trainer)	Ear/Nose/Throat
Trainer, Auditory	Ear/Nose/Throat

PHONIC EAR, LTD. — 800-263-8700 / 905-677-3231

7475 Kimbel St,
Mississauga, ON L5S 1 Canada

FDA Number: n/a
Fax: 905-677-7760
E-mail: jm@oticon.ca
Web site: www.oticon.com
Year Founded: 1904
Total Employees: 100   Marketing Staff: 2   Sales Staff: 5
Ownership: Private
Produces/Sells CE-marked Devices: N
Federal Procurement Eligibility: Small Business
Distribution: Manufacturer Direct, Exclusive Distributor, Importer

PHOTO RESEARCH, INC. — 818-341-5151

9731 Topanga Canyon Place, Chatsworth, CA 91311-4135

FDA Number: 9200866
Fax: 818-341-7070
E-mail: sales@photoresearch.com
Web site: www.photoresearch.com
Medical Products Sales Volume: $2,900,000
Annual Revenue: $5-$10 Million
Year Founded: 1941
Total Employees: 40   Marketing Staff: 10   Sales Staff: 37
Ownership: Excel Technology, Inc.
Stock Symbol: XLTC

PHOTO RESEARCH, INC.   818-341-5151 (cont'd)
Traded On: NASDAQ
Produces/Sells CE-marked Devices: Y
Federal Procurement Eligibility: Small Business
Distribution: Manufacturer Direct, Manufacturer Through Distributor, Manufacturer Through Manufacturer Reps
General Admin.: Ms. Paulette Sark/Office Manager
       Mr. Francis Dominic/President
Mktg./Adv.: Mrs. Corey Albertson/Admin. Marketing & Sales
       Mr. Mike Klein/Director Marketing & Sales

Colorimeter, General Use	Chemistry
Computer Software	General
Equipment/Service, Quality Control	General
Meter, Light, Photomicrographic	Microbiology
Photometer	Chemistry
Radiometer, Phototherapy	General

PHOTOACTIF   480-827-1212
7211 E. Southern Avenue, Suite C-110, Mesa, AZ 85209
FDA Number: 3005823576

Lamp, Infrared	Physical Med
Laser, Surgical	Surgery

PHOTOMEDEX, INC.   215-619-3600
147 Keystone Dr., Mongomeryville, PA 18936
FDA Number: 2523356   Fax: 215-619-3208
E-mail: info@photomedex.com
Web site: www.photomedex.com
Ownership: Public
Stock Symbol: PHMD
Traded On: NASDAQ
Produces/Sells CE-marked Devices: N
General Admin.: Mr. Jeffery Levatter/Chief Technology Officer
       Mr. Michael Stewart/Executive Vice President
       Mr. Dennis McGrath/President, Chief Executive Officer, Chairman
Finance: Ms. Christina Allgeier/Chief Financial Officer

Dressing, Wound and Burn, Hydrogel	Surgery
Drill, Surgical, ENT (Electric Or Pneumatic)	Ear/Nose/Throat
Electrosurgical, Cutting & Coagulation Accessories, Laparoscopic & Endoscopic, Reprocessed	Surgery
Irrigator, Sinus	Ear/Nose/Throat
Laser, Neodymium:YAG, Surgical, Pulmonary	Anesthesiology
Laser, Surgical	Surgery
Tubing, Non-Invasive	Surgery

PHOTOMEDEX, INC.   760-602-3300
2375 Camino Vida Roble, Suite B, Carlsbad, CA 92011
FDA Number: 2031934
Ownership: PhotoMedex, Inc.
Produces/Sells CE-marked Devices: N

Laser, Surgical	Surgery

PHOTOMETRICS LTD.
See Roper Scientific, Inc.

PHOTON TECHNOLOGY INTERNATIONAL, INC.   609-894-4420
300 Birmingham Road, Birmingham, NJ 08011-0272
FDA Number: n/a   Fax: 609-894-1579
E-mail: marketing@pti-nj.com
Web site: www.pti-nj.com
Medical Products Sales Volume: $9,000,000
Annual Revenue: $5-$10 Million
Year Founded: 1983
Total Employees: 50   *Marketing Staff:* 1   *Sales Staff:* 11
Ownership: Private
Stock Symbol: PHTO
Traded On: OTC Bulletin
Produces/Sells CE-marked Devices: Y
Federal Procurement Eligibility: Small Business
Distribution: Manufacturer Direct, Manufacturer Through Distributor, Manufacturer Through Manufacturer Reps
General Admin.: Mr. Charles G. Marianik/President, Chief Executive Officer
       Mr. Ira Saltiel/Vice President
       Mr. Ronald Kovach/Vice President, Corporate Secretary
Production: Mr. Chuck J. Marianik/Vice President Operations
Research: Mr. Richard Wiggins/Senior Director Research & Development
Finance: Mr. Alan Meltzer/Controller

Camera, Video	General
Component, Optical	General
Spectrophotometer, Fluorescence	Chemistry
Spectrophotometer, U.V./Visible	Chemistry

PHOTOPROTECTIVE TECHNOLOGIES   800-219-9993
6610 Topper Ridge, San Antonio, TX 78233   210-493-6353
FDA Number: n/a   Fax: 210-493-7043
E-mail: info@pptworldwide.com
Web site: www.pptworldwide.com
Medical Products Sales Volume: $100,000
Annual Revenue: $0-$1 Million

PHOTOPROTECTIVE TECHNOLOGIES   800-219-9993 (cont'd)
Total Employees: 8   *Sales Staff:* 2
Ownership: Private
Produces/Sells CE-marked Devices: N
Federal Procurement Eligibility: Small Business
Distribution: Manufacturer Direct
General Admin.: Jim Gallas/President

Lens, Spectacle/Eyeglasses, Non-Custom	Ophthalmology
Light, Other	General

PHOTOVAC LASER CORP., INC.   614-875-3300
3513 Farm Bank Way, Grove City, OH 43123
FDA Number: n/a   Fax: 614-875-3311
E-mail: info@photovaclaser.com
Web site: www.photovaclaser.com
Medical Products Sales Volume: $350,000
Annual Revenue: $0-$1 Million
Year Founded: 1994
Total Employees: 6   *Marketing Staff:* 1   *Sales Staff:* 1
Ownership: Private
Quality System Registration Information: ISO9000
Federal Procurement Eligibility: Small Business, Female Owned
Distribution: Service Direct
General Admin.: Christopher Zelich/President

Cable, Laser, Fiberoptic	Surgery
Laser, Surgical	Surgery
Service, Consulting	General
Service, Engineering/Design	General
Service, Maintenance/Repair	General
Service, Used Equipment	General

PHOTOVOLT CORP.
See Spectrum Laboratories, Inc.

PHOXXOR   251-408-0208
5600 Commerce Blvd. East A, Mobile, AL 36619-0037
FDA Number: 3004112822   Fax: 251-408-0201
E-mail: doris.kohler@phoxxor.com
Web site: www.phoxxor.com
Year Founded: 2003
Total Employees: 15   *Marketing Staff:* 2   *Sales Staff:* 4
Ownership: Private
Produces/Sells CE-marked Devices: N
Federal Procurement Eligibility: Small Business
Distribution: Manufacturer Through Distributor, Service Direct, Exporter
General Admin.: Doris Kohler/Admin. Human Resources
       Martin Von Sury/President, Chief Executive Officer
       Jeff Browning/Production and Sales Support
Mktg./Adv.: John Rhim/Director International Sales
       Dennis Brown/Director Marketing
Production: Heinz Camenzind/Director Manufacturing
       Ron Bowman/Director Quality Control & Regulatory Affairs
Research: Alan Kim/Director Research & Development
       Perry Choi/Director Technology
IS: Harshana Nakandala/Computer Engineer
       Harshana Nakandala/Web Master

Imager, X-Ray, Solid State (Flat Panel/Digital)	Radiology
Mount, X-Ray Tube, Diagnostic	Radiology

PHYGEN, LLC   800-939-7008
2301 Dupont Drive, Suite 510, Irvine, CA 92612   949-752-7885
FDA Number: 3005032381   Fax: 949-752-7886
E-mail: info@phyginespine.com
Web site: www.phygenspine.com
Ownership: Private
Produces/Sells CE-marked Devices: N

Appliance, Fixation, Spinal Interlaminal	Orthopedics
Appliance, Fixation, Spinal Intervertebral Body	Orthopedics
Orthosis, Fixation, Pedicle, Spinal	Orthopedics
Orthosis, Fixation, Spinal, Spondylolisthesis	Orthopedics
Orthosis, Spinal Pedicle Fixation, For Degenerative Disc Disease	Orthopedics

PHYSICAL FITNESS, INC.
See Team America Health & Fitness, Inc

PHYSICAL SUPPORT SYSTEMS, INC.
See Boston Brace International, Inc.

PHYSICIAN ENGINEERED PRODUCTS, INC.   800-622-6240
103 Smith Street, Fryeburg, ME 04037   207-935-1256
FDA Number: 2183604   Fax: 207-935-1257
E-mail: sales@peponline.com
Web site: http://peponline.com
Year Founded: 1984
Ownership: Private
Produces/Sells CE-marked Devices: N
Federal Procurement Eligibility: Small Business
Distribution: Manufacturer Direct, Service Direct, Exclusive Distributor
Mktg./Adv.: Mr. Tony Martineau/Director Marketing & Sales

Light, Other	General

PHYSICIAN ENGINEERED PRODUCTS, INC.   800-622-6240
(cont'd)

Pad, Neonatal Eye	General
Phototherapy Unit, Neonatal	General

PHYSICIAN INDUSTRIES, INC.
See Integra Lifesciences Corp.

PHYSICIANS PRACTICE MANAGEMENT   800-252-6635
320 W. 8th St, Suite 218, Bloomington, IN 47404
FDA Number: n/a   Fax: 800-331-4604
E-mail: contact@ppminc.biz
Web site: www.ppminc.biz
Annual Revenue: $0-$1 Million
Year Founded: 1978
Total Employees: 18   Marketing Staff: 2   Sales Staff: 6
Ownership: Private
Produces/Sells CE-marked Devices: N
Distribution: Manufacturer Direct, Manufacturer Through Distributor
General Admin.: Fred Schmucker/President
    Mary Beth Schmucker/Vice President, Secretary
Mktg./Adv.: Becky Fase/Manager Marketing & Sales
Finance: Kristen Brynestad/Director Finance
IS: Cory Myers/Manager Tech. Support

Computer Software	General

PHYSIO-CONTROL CORPORATION
See Physio-Control, Inc.

PHYSIO-CONTROL, INC.   800-442-1142
11811 Willows Road NE, Redmond, WA 98052   425-867-4000
FDA Number: 3015876   Fax: 425-867-4121
E-mail: shiggins@physio-control.com
Web site: www.physiocontrol.com
Total Employees: 925   Marketing Staff: 20   Sales Staff: 200
Ownership: Medtronic, Inc.
Quality System Registration Information: ISO9001
Produces/Sells CE-marked Devices: Y
Distribution: Manufacturer Direct, Manufacturer Through Distributor, Exporter
General Admin.: Jon Tremmel/President
Mktg./Adv.: Sandra Higgins/Manager Corporate Affairs
    Harry Norris/Vice President Strategic Marketing & Communications
Production: Michael Willingham/Vice President Regulatory Affairs
Research: Randy L. Merry/Vice President Research & Development
Finance: Jerry Ng/Vice President Finance

Analyzer, Gas, Carbon-Dioxide, Gaseous Phase (Capnograph)	Anesthesiology
Battery	General
Cart, Other	General
Defibrillator, Battery-Powered, Low Energy	Cardiovascular
Defibrillator, External, Automatic	Cardiovascular
Defibrillator/Monitor, Battery-Powered	Cardiovascular
Electrode, Defibrillator	Cardiovascular
Electrode, Electrocardiograph	Cardiovascular
Gel, Electrode, Electrocardiograph	Cardiovascular
Monitor, Cardiac (Cardiotachometer & Rate Alarm)	Cardiovascular
Monitor, Physiological, Acute Care	Anesthesiology
Pacemaker, Cardiac, External Transcutaneous (Non-Invasive)	Cardiovascular

PHYSIODYNAMICS, INC.   303-713-0605
7200 East Dry Creek Rd.,, Suite A-202, Centennial, CO 80112
FDA Number: n/a
Ownership: Private
Produces/Sells CE-marked Devices: N

Stimulator, Muscle, Electrical-Powered (EMS)	Physical Med

PHYSIOLOGICAL TRAINING CO.
See Pinnacle Technology Group, Inc.

PHYSIOMEDICS MANUFACTURING, LLC   952-201-1463
15320 Minnetonka Blvd., Suite 104, Minnetonka, MN 55345
FDA Number: 3005521729
Ownership: Private
Produces/Sells CE-marked Devices: N

Chair, Adjustable, Mechanical	Physical Med

PHYSIOSONICS, INC   425-732-2814
2002 156th Avenue Ne # 150, Bellevue, WA 98007-3828
FDA Number: n/a
Ownership: Private
Produces/Sells CE-marked Devices: N
General Admin.: Mr. Michael Weitz/Secretary
    Mr. Randy Serroels/Vice President

PHYSIPRO INC.   800-668-2252
10 Ave. Sud, #370,   819-823-2252
Sherbrooke, QUE J1G-2 Canada
FDA Number: n/a   Fax: 819-565-3337
E-mail: physipro@abacon.com
Web site: www.physipro.com
Year Founded: 1987
Ownership: Private

PHYSIPRO INC.   800-668-2252 *(cont'd)*
Produces/Sells CE-marked Devices: N
Distribution: Manufacturer Direct, Exclusive Distributor

PHYSITEMP INSTRUMENTS, INC.   800-452-8510
154 Huron Avenue, Clifton, NJ 07013-2949   973-779-5577
FDA Number: 2242483   Fax: 973-779-5954
E-mail: physitemp@aol.com
Web site: www.physitemp.com
Medical Products Sales Volume: $1,900,000
Annual Revenue: $0-$1 Million
Year Founded: 1969
Total Employees: 7
Ownership: Private
Produces/Sells CE-marked Devices: Y
Federal Procurement Eligibility: Small Business
Distribution: Manufacturer Direct, OEM
General Admin.: Ronald Feller/Manager Personnel
    Ronald R. Feller/President, Chief Executive Officer
    Chris Proffitt/Vice President, General Manager
Mktg./Adv.: Michele Cantwell/Director Marketing & Advertising
    Lawrence Lee/Director Product Development
    Wilda Sabater/Manager International & National Sales
Production: Chris Proffitt/Director Quality Assurance
    Ronald Feller/Manager Regulatory Affairs

Monitor, Temperature (Self-Contained)	General
Probe, Temperature	General
Stage, Microscope	Pathology
Thermometer, Electronic	General
Thermometer, Electronic, Continuous	General
Thermometer, Laboratory	Chemistry
Vibration Threshold Measurement Device	Cns/Neurology

PHYTRON, INC.   800-96P-HYTR
600 Blair Park Road, Suite 220,   802-872-1600
Williston, VT 05495
FDA Number: n/a   Fax: 802-872-0311
E-mail: info@phytron.com
Web site: www.phytron.com
Medical Products Sales Volume: $1,400,000
Annual Revenue: $1-$5 Million
Year Founded: 1947
Total Employees: 106
Ownership: Private
Quality System Registration Information: ISO9001
Produces/Sells CE-marked Devices: Y
Federal Procurement Eligibility: Small Business
Distribution: OEM
General Admin.: Wahid Lahmadi/President
Mktg./Adv.: Wahid Lahmadi/Manager National Sales
Production: Heri Schmid/Vice President Manufacturing
Research: Heri Schmid/Vice President Research & Development

Contract Manufacturing	General
System, Robot	General

PI PROFESSIONAL THERAPY PRODUCTS   888-818-9632
PO Box 1067, Athens, TN 37371-1067   423-744-8000
FDA Number: n/a   Fax: 423-746-1327
E-mail: sroy@pi-inc.com
Web site: www.pi-ptp.com
Annual Revenue: $1-$5 Million
Year Founded: 1991
Total Employees: 75   Marketing Staff: 1   Sales Staff: 5
Ownership: Sealtech, Inc.
Quality System Registration Information: ISO9002
Produces/Sells CE-marked Devices: N
Federal Procurement Eligibility: Small Business
Distribution: Manufacturer Direct, Manufacturer Through Manufacturer Reps, Exporter
General Admin.: Gary Hosack/President
    Gary Hosack/Vice President, General Manager
Mktg./Adv.: Sonya Roy/Director Marketing & Sales
    Gary Hosack/Director Product Development
Production: Mary Gray/Director Quality Assurance
    David Key/Manager Materials

Pack, Cold	General
Pack, Hot Or Cold, Reusable	Physical Med

PI-PTP   888-818-9632
215 Rocky Mount Road, PO Box 1067,   423-745-6213
Athens, TN 37371
FDA Number: 1054296   Fax: 423-744-1364
E-mail: jmurray@pi-inc.com
Web site: www.pi-ptp.com
Year Founded: 1991
Ownership: P.I., INC.
Quality System Registration Information: ISO9001

PI-PTP
888-818-9632 *(cont'd)*

Produces/Sells CE-marked Devices: N
Distribution: Manufacturer Direct, Manufacturer Through Distributor, Manufacturer Through Manufacturer Reps, OEM
Mktg./Adv.: Mr. Jay Murray/Manager Sales

Pack, Hot Or Cold, Disposable	Physical Med
Pack, Hot Or Cold, Reusable	Physical Med
Regulator, Thermal, Cardiopulmonary Bypass	Cardiovascular

PIBBS INC., P.S.
718-445-8046

133-15 32nd Ave., Flushing, NY 11354-4008
FDA Number: 2433167   *Fax:* 718-461-3910
E-mail: info@pibbs.com
Web site: /www.pibbs.com
Annual Revenue: $1-$5 Million
Total Employees: 80   *Marketing Staff:* 5   *Sales Staff:* 10
Ownership: Private
Produces/Sells CE-marked Devices: N
Federal Procurement Eligibility: Small Business
Distribution: Manufacturer Through Distributor, Importer, Exporter
General Admin.: Damiano Petruccelli/President, Chief Executive Officer
Mktg./Adv.: Gianna Petruccelli/Manager Advertising
        Armando Petruccelli/Vice President Sales
Production: Giulio Petruccelli/Vice President Manufacturing

Chair, Examination And Treatment	General
Lamp, Examination (Light)	General

PICIS INC.
781-557-3000

100 Quannapowitt Parkway, Suite 405, Wakefield, MA 01880
FDA Number: 3005244943

PICIS, INC.
781-557-3000

9500 W. Higgins,, Suite 1100, Rosemont, IL 60018
FDA Number: 3006076247

PICO-TESLA INC.
303-795-3222

7852 South Elati, Suite 202, Littleton, CO 80120
FDA Number: n/a
E-mail: info@pico-tesla.com
Web site: http://www.pico-tesla.com
Ownership: Private
Produces/Sells CE-marked Devices: N
General Admin.: Mr. Allen Braswell, Jr./Chief Executive Officer
        Dr. Jerry Jacobson/Chief Scientific Officer

PIERCE BAC-T, INC.
651-636-5901

367-a West County Rd., D, New Brighton, MN 55112
FDA Number: 2182981
Ownership: Private
Produces/Sells CE-marked Devices: N

Culture Media, Non-Selective And Non-Differential	Microbiology

PIERCE BIOTECHNOLOGY
800-487-4885

30 Commerce Way, Woburn, MA 01801-1059
781-937-0890
FDA Number: n/a   *Fax:* 815-968-7316
E-mail: webmaster@endogen.com
Web site: www.endogen.com
Medical Products Sales Volume: $9,000,000,000
Total Employees: 21   *Marketing Staff:* 7   *Sales Staff:* 8
Ownership: Private
Produces/Sells CE-marked Devices: N
Federal Procurement Eligibility: Small Business
Distribution: Manufacturer Direct, Manufacturer Through Distributor, Manufacturer Through Manufacturer Reps, Service Direct, Exporter
General Admin.: Owen A. Dempsey/President, Chief Executive Officer
Mktg./Adv.: Alan Kotik/Director Marketing
        Lee Anne Beausang/Director Product Development
        Dennis Walczewski/Manager International & National Sales
        Uli Schmidt/Vice President Business Development
Production: Monique Morimoto/Director Quality Assurance
        Judy Andrews/Vice President Manufacturing
Finance: Chip Catlin/Chief Financial Officer
        Chip Catlin/Vice President Finance

Antibody, Monoclonal	Microbiology
Antibody, Other	General
Antibody, Polyclonal	Microbiology
Enzyme Immunoassay, Other	Chemistry

PIERCE CHEMICAL COMPANY
800-874-3723

P.O. Box 117, Rockford, IL 61105-0117
815-968-0747
FDA Number: 1416690   *Fax:* 815-968-7316
E-mail: pierce.cs@thermofisher.com
Web site: www.piercenet.com
Total Employees: 160
Ownership: PERBIO SCIENCE
Traded On: Stockholm
Quality System Registration Information: ISO9001
Produces/Sells CE-marked Devices: N

PIERCE CHEMICAL COMPANY
800-874-3723 *(cont'd)*

Federal Procurement Eligibility: Small Business
Distribution: Manufacturer Direct, Manufacturer Through Distributor, Manufacturer Through Manufacturer Reps, OEM, Exporter
General Admin.: Robb Anderson/President, Chief Executive Officer
        Theodore Frank/Vice President, General Manager
Mktg./Adv.: Jeremy Wright/Manager International Sales
Production: Robert Knop/Manager Regulatory Affairs

Dialyzer, Laboratory	Chemistry
Electrophoresis Equipment, Cellulose Acetate Membrane	Chemistry
Electrophoresis Equipment, Gel	Chemistry
Electrophoresis Equipment, Liquid	Chemistry
Electrophoresis Equipment, Paper	Chemistry
Electrophoresis Equipment, Starch Block	Chemistry
Electrophoresis Equipment, Thin-Layer	Chemistry
Electrophoresis Instrumentation	Immunology
Equipment, Immunoelectrophoresis, Rocket	Immunology
Labware, Basic, Reusable	Chemistry
Plate, Hot	Chemistry
Reagent, Analyzer, Amino Acid	Microbiology
Solvent	Chemistry
Standard, Amino Acid	Chemistry
Standard/Control, Hemoglobin, Normal/Abnormal	Hematology
Stationary Liquid Phase	Chemistry

PIKO HEALTHCARE PRODUCTS, INC.
888-737-5656

908 Main St., Louisville, CO 80027
303-666-6340
FDA Number: n/a   *Fax:* 303-666-6380
E-mail: marketing@pikohealth.com
Web site: www.pikohealth.com
Year Founded: 2000
Total Employees: 25
Ownership: Private
Quality System Registration Information: ISO9000; ISO9001
Produces/Sells CE-marked Devices: Y
Federal Procurement Eligibility: Small Business
Distribution: Manufacturer Direct, Manufacturer Through Manufacturer Reps, OEM
General Admin.: Mr. Lee Paul/Managing Director
        Mr. Tom McKevitt/President, Chief Executive Officer

Meter, Peak Flow, Spirometry	Anesthesiology
Spirometer, Monitoring (Volumeter)	Anesthesiology

PILLAR SURGICAL, INC.
800-367-0445

PO Box 8141, La Jolla, CA 92038-8141
619-645-8401
FDA Number: 2030657   *Fax:* 619-758-1431
E-mail: sales@silmaximplants.com
Web site: www.silmaximplants.com
Annual Revenue: $0-$1 Million
Ownership: Dow Corning Corp.
Quality System Registration Information: ISO9001
Produces/Sells CE-marked Devices: N
Federal Procurement Eligibility: Small Business
Distribution: Manufacturer Direct

Elastomer, Silicone (Scar Management)	Surgery
Elastomer, Silicone Block	Surgery
Malar Implant	Surgery
Polymer, ENT Synthetic-PIFE, Silicon Elastomer	Ear/Nose/Throat
Prosthesis, Chin, Internal	Surgery
Prosthesis, Nose, Internal	Surgery

PILLING COMPANY
See Teleflex Medical

PILLING WECK (CANADA) INC.
800-387-9699

165 Gibson Dr., Ste. 1,
905-943-9000
Markham, ONT L3R-3 Canada
FDA Number: n/a   *Fax:* 905-943-9001
E-mail: pwsales@pillingweck.com
Web site: www.pillingweck.com
Year Founded: 1982
Total Employees: 25
Ownership: Private
Produces/Sells CE-marked Devices: N
Distribution: Exclusive Distributor, Importer

PILOT PERFORMANCE RESOURCE MANAGEMENT
905-792-3130

25 Great Lakes Drive, P.O. Box 68584,
Brampton, ONT L6R 0 Canada
FDA Number: n/a   *Fax:* 905-792-3047
E-mail: info@pilotims.com
Web site: www.pilotiso.com
Year Founded: 1994
Total Employees: 10
Ownership: Private
Produces/Sells CE-marked Devices: N

MANUFACTURER PROFILES

PINE TREE ORTHOPEDIC LAB L.L.C.   207-897-5558
175 Park Street, Livermore Falls, ME 04254
FDA Number: 3006196605
E-mail: info@pinetreeorthopedic.com
Ownership: Private
Produces/Sells CE-marked Devices: N
  Brace, Joint, Ankle (External)   Physical Med
  Orthosis, Corrective Shoe   Physical Med

PINMED, INC   412-687-6964
245 Melwood Ave., #501, Pittsburgh, PA 15213
FDA Number: 3005970337
  Transmitter/Receiver System, Physiological, Telephone   Cardiovascular

PINNACLE TECHNOLOGY GROUP, INC.   800-345-5123
7076 Schnipke Drive, Ottawa Lake, MI 49267   734-568-6600
FDA Number: 2020256   *Fax:* 734-568-6601
E-mail: service@pinnacletec.com
Web site: www.pinnacletec.com
Annual Revenue: $1-$5 Million
Year Founded: 1964
Total Employees: 41   *Marketing Staff:* 2   *Sales Staff:* 4
Ownership: Private
Quality System Registration Information: ISO9000
Produces/Sells CE-marked Devices: Y
Federal Procurement Eligibility: Small Business
Distribution: Manufacturer Direct, Manufacturer Through Distributor, OEM, Service Direct, Exporter
General Admin.: Rick Wasserman/President, Chief Executive Officer
Mktg./Adv.: Hope Aguirre/Manager Admin. & Sales
        Mr. Nick Fasciana/Marketing & Sales Representative
Purchasing: Mr. Dennis Neiger/Purchasing Agent
  Anatomical Training Model   General
  Monitor, ECG, Arrhythmia   Cardiovascular
  Simulator, Arrhythmia   Cardiovascular

PIONEER CENTER FOR HUMAN SERVICES   815-344-1230
4001 West Dayton St., Mchenry, IL 60050
FDA Number: 1419534   *Fax:* 815-344-3815
E-mail: sryndak@pioneercenter.org
Web site: http://www.pioneercenter.org
Ownership: Private
Produces/Sells CE-marked Devices: N
  Cuff, Blood Pressure   Cardiovascular
  General Purpose Hematology Device   Hematology
  Tray, Blood Collection   Hematology

PIONEER LABORATORIES, INC.
See Pioneer Surgical Technology

PIONEER MEDICAL SYSTEMS   800-234-0683
3408 Howell Street, Suite D, Duluth, GA 30096   770-476-0837
FDA Number: 3005191230   *Fax:* 770-497-8224
E-mail: jrj@pioneermed.com
Web site: www.pioneermed.com
Medical Products Sales Volume: $150,000
Annual Revenue: $5-$10 Million
Year Founded: 1985
Total Employees: 6
Ownership: Private
Produces/Sells CE-marked Devices: N
Federal Procurement Eligibility: Small Business
Distribution: Manufacturer Direct, Manufacturer Through Manufacturer Reps
General Admin.: George McKay/President
Mktg./Adv.: James R. Johnson/Manager International & National Sales
        James R. Johnson/Vice President Marketing & Sales
Finance: Mr. Peter Abate/Vice President, Corporate Controller
  Communication System, Emergency Alert, Personal   General
  Container, Medication, Home-Use   General
  Nurse Call System   General

PIONEER MICROFILMING, INC.
See Pioneer Micrographix

PIONEER MICROGRAPHIX   800-551-6436
228 South Mill Street, South Lyon, MI 48178
FDA Number: n/a   *Fax:* 248-437-7940
E-mail: BHAAS@PioneerImagingSolutions.com
Web site: www.pioneerimagingsolutions.com
Annual Revenue: $0-$1 Million
Ownership: Private
Produces/Sells CE-marked Devices: N
Federal Procurement Eligibility: Small Business
Distribution: Service Direct
  Microfilm/Microfiche Equipment   General

PIONEER OPTICS CO.   860-286-0071
35 Griffin Road South, Bloomfield, CT 06002
FDA Number: n/a   *Fax:* 860-286-0171
E-mail: info@pioneeroptics.com

PIONEER OPTICS CO.   860-286-0071 *(cont'd)*
Web site: www.pioneeroptics.com
Annual Revenue: $0-$1 Million
Year Founded: 1991
Ownership: Private
Quality System Registration Information: ISO9002
Produces/Sells CE-marked Devices: N
Federal Procurement Eligibility: Small Business
Distribution: Manufacturer Direct, OEM
  Accessories, Laser   General

PIONEER SURGICAL TECHNOLOGY   800-557-9909
375 River Park Circle, Marquette, MI 49855   906-226-9909
FDA Number: 1833824   *Fax:* 906-226-4443
E-mail: sales@pioneersurgical.com
Web site: www.pioneersurgical.com
Medical Products Sales Volume: $26,800,000
Annual Revenue: $25-$50 Million
Year Founded: 1992
Total Employees: 140   *Marketing Staff:* 5   *Sales Staff:* 5
Ownership: Private
Quality System Registration Information: ISO9001
Produces/Sells CE-marked Devices: Y
Federal Procurement Eligibility: Small Business
Distribution: Manufacturer Direct, Manufacturer Through Distributor, Manufacturer Through Manufacturer Reps, OEM, Service Direct, Exclusive Distributor, Exporter
General Admin.: Mr. Eric Baldwin/General Manager
        Mr. Jeff Millin/President, Chief Executive Officer
Mktg./Adv.: Mr. Fred Taccolini/Director Communications
  Cerclage, Fixation   Orthopedics
  Implant, Fixation Device, Spinal   Orthopedics
  Plate, Fixation, Bone   Orthopedics
  Rod, Fixation, Intramedullary   Orthopedics
  Screw, Fixation, Bone   Orthopedics
  Suture, Non-Absorbable, Steel, Monofilament & Multifilament   Surgery

PIPER MEDICAL PRODUCTS   916-834-3283
4007 Seaport Blvd., West Sacramento, CA 95691
FDA Number: n/a
E-mail: sdpiper@pipermedical.com
Web site: www.pipermedical.com
Annual Revenue: $0-$1 Million
Total Employees: 4   *Marketing Staff:* 1   *Sales Staff:* 1
Ownership: Private
Produces/Sells CE-marked Devices: N
Distribution: Manufacturer Through Distributor
General Admin.: S. David Piper/President
Production: Mat Stewart/Vice President Manufacturing
  Nebulizer, Medicinal   Ear/Nose/Throat

PIPER PRODUCTS, INC.   800-492-3431
300 South 84th Ave., Wausau, WI 54401   715-842-2724
FDA Number: n/a   *Fax:* 715-842-3125
E-mail: info@piperonline.net
Web site: www.piperonline.net
Annual Revenue: $5-$10 Million
Total Employees: 60   *Marketing Staff:* 1   *Sales Staff:* 4
Ownership: Private
Produces/Sells CE-marked Devices: N
Federal Procurement Eligibility: Small Business
Distribution: Manufacturer Through Distributor, Manufacturer Through Manufacturer Reps, OEM, Exporter
General Admin.: Roger Sweeney/President, Chief Executive Officer
        Jennifer Sweeney/Vice President Human Resources
        Tony Sweeney/Vice President, General Manager
Mktg./Adv.: Kelly Kubisiak/Coord. Marketing
        Tony Sweeney/Manager National Sales
  Cart, Foodservice   General
  Foodservice Product/Equipment   General
  Station, Nourishment   General

PIRANHA PLASTICS, LLC.   408-855-9650
3531 Thomas Rd., Santa Clara, CA 95054
FDA Number: 3003914021
Ownership: Private
Produces/Sells CE-marked Devices: N
  Computer, Oxygen-Uptake   Anesthesiology

PISCES PRODUCTIONS, INC.   800-822 - 5333
380-a Morris St., Sebastopol, CA 95472   707-829-1496
FDA Number: 3004159020
E-mail: info@piscespro.com
Web site: www.piscespro.com
Ownership: Private
Produces/Sells CE-marked Devices: N
  Chair, Blood Donor   General

PISHARODI SURGICALS, INC.   956-541-6725
3475 W. Alton Gloor Blvd, Brownsville, TX 78520
FDA Number: 3003909293
Appliance, Fixation, Spinal Intervertebral Body	Orthopedics
Orthosis, Fixation, Pedicle, Spinal	Orthopedics

PL CUSTOM BODY & EQUIPMENT CO. INC.   800-752-8786
2201 Atlantic Ave., Manasquan, NJ 08736-1010
FDA Number: n/a   Fax: 732-223-8456
Web site: www.plcustom.com
Year Founded: 1946
Ownership: Private
Produces/Sells CE-marked Devices: N
Distribution: Manufacturer Direct
General Admin.: Jean S. Smock/Chief Executive Officer
Ambulance	General

PL MEDICAL CO., LLC.   800-874-0120
321 Ellis St., New Britain, CT 06051   860-223-8882
FDA Number: 2435343   Fax: 860-223-5941
E-mail: info@plmedical.com
Web site: www.plmedical.com
Medical Products Sales Volume: $1,000,000
Annual Revenue: $1-$5 Million
Year Founded: 1988
Total Employees: 8   Marketing Staff: 4   Sales Staff: 4
Ownership: Private
Quality System Registration Information: ISO9002
Produces/Sells CE-marked Devices: N
Federal Procurement Eligibility: Small Business, Female Owned
Distribution: Manufacturer Through Distributor, Importer
General Admin.: Sushil K. Kanwar/Chief Executive Officer
Mktg./Adv.: Puja Vij/Director National Accounts
    Sushil K. Kanwar/Director National Accounts
    Albert Monet/Manager Contract Sales
    Rajiv Prasad/Vice President Marketing
Production: Sushil K. Kanwar/Manager Regulatory Affairs
Blade, Scalpel	Surgery
Cassette, Radiographic Film	Radiology
Contract Packaging	General
Envelope, Film, X-Ray	Radiology
Film, X-Ray	Radiology
Sanitizer	General
Screen, Intensifying, Radiographic	Radiology

PLACON CORPORATION   800-541-1535
6096 McKee Road, Madison, WI 53719-5114   608-271-5634
FDA Number: n/a   Fax: 608-271-3162
E-mail: package@placon.com
Web site: www.placon.com
Medical Products Sales Volume: $1,300,000
Annual Revenue: $50-$100 Million
Year Founded: 1966
Total Employees: 300   Marketing Staff: 2   Sales Staff: 13
Ownership: Private
Quality System Registration Information: ISO9001
Produces/Sells CE-marked Devices: N
Federal Procurement Eligibility: Small Business
Distribution: Manufacturer Direct
Mktg./Adv.: Lauren Foos/National Sales Representative
    Jennifer Lauderback/Sales Representative
Container, Sterilization (Tray)	General
Foam, Plastic	General

PLAINVIEW BATTERIES, INC.   800-642-2354
23 Newtown Rd., Plainview, NY 11803   516-249-2873
FDA Number: n/a   Fax: 516-249-2876
E-mail: info@energexbatteries.com
Web site: www.energexbatteries.com
Medical Products Sales Volume: $1,500,000
Annual Revenue: $1-$5 Million
Year Founded: 1986
Total Employees: 10   Marketing Staff: 1   Sales Staff: 3
Ownership: Private
Produces/Sells CE-marked Devices: N
Federal Procurement Eligibility: Small Business, Female Owned
Distribution: Manufacturer Direct
General Admin.: Bernard Erde/Chief Executive Officer
    Lynn Erde/President
Mktg./Adv.: Larry Rubin/Manager National Sales
    Bernard Erde/Vice President Marketing
Battery	General
Battery, Hearing-Aid	Ear/Nose/Throat

PLANET LLC   800-338-2010
1212 Fourier Drive, Madison, WI 53717   608-827-5555
FDA Number: 2133431   Fax: 608-827-5050
E-mail: planet@orbitec.com

PLANET LLC   800-338-2010 (cont'd)
Web site: www.planet-llc.com
Year Founded: 1995
Ownership: Private
Quality System Registration Information: ISO9000
Produces/Sells CE-marked Devices: N
Federal Procurement Eligibility: Small Business
Distribution: Manufacturer Direct, Manufacturer Through Distributor
Mktg./Adv.: Mrs. Marty Gustafson/Admin. Marketing & Sales
Alarm, Overload, External Limb, Powered	Physical Med

PLANMECA U.S.A. INC   630-529-2300
100 N. Gary, Suite A, Roselle, IL 60172
FDA Number: 8030876   Fax: 630-529-1929
E-mail: sales@planmeca.com
Web site: www.planmeca.com
Medical Products Sales Volume: $9,400,000
Annual Revenue: $25-$50 Million
Year Founded: 1988
Total Employees: 60   Marketing Staff: 17   Sales Staff: 16
Ownership: Planmeca Oy
Quality System Registration Information: ISO9000; ISO9001
Produces/Sells CE-marked Devices: Y
Federal Procurement Eligibility: Small Business, GSA Contract
Distribution: Manufacturer Through Distributor, Importer
General Admin.: Robert Pienkowski/President
    Heikki Kyostila/President, Chief Executive Officer
Mktg./Adv.: Jim Fritz/Sales Specialist
Production: Ari Kontkanen/Manager Product Support
Chair, Dental	Dental And Oral
Chair, Dental (With Unit)	Dental And Oral
Light, Surgical Operating, Dental	Dental And Oral
Radiographic Unit, Diagnostic, Dental (X-Ray)	Dental And Oral
Radiographic Unit, Diagnostic, Intraoral	Dental And Oral
Stool, Dental	Dental And Oral

PLANMED, INC.
See Fischer Medical Technologies Inc.

PLANO MOLDING CO.
See Plano Molding Co.

PLASCO, INC.   847-662-4400
Carretera Presta La Amistad, Km.19, Acuna, Coahila Mexico
FDA Number: 9616564
Container, IV	General
Device, Assist, CPR	Anesthesiology
Mask, Oxygen, Non-Rebreathing	Anesthesiology
Orthosis, Limb Brace	Physical Med
Valve, Non-Rebreathing	Anesthesiology
Ventilator, Emergency, Manual (Resuscitator)	Anesthesiology

PLASDENT CORP.   909-620-0289
1290 Price St., Pomona, CA 91767
FDA Number: 2029234
Ownership: Private
Produces/Sells CE-marked Devices: N
Absorber, Saliva, Paper	Dental And Oral
Chair, Examination And Treatment	General
Evacuator, Oral Cavity	Dental And Oral
Gauze/sponge, Nonresorbable For External Use	Surgery
Material, Impression Tray, Resin	Dental And Oral
Mirror, Mouth	Dental And Oral
Mouthpiece, Saliva Ejector	Dental And Oral
Retainer, Surgical	Surgery
Syringe Unit, Air And/Or Water	Dental And Oral
Syringe, Restorative And Impression Material	Dental And Oral
Toothbrush, Manual	Dental And Oral
Tray, Surgical Instrument	Surgery
Unit, Operative Dental, Accessories	Dental And Oral

PLASKOLITE WEST INC.   800-562-8883
2225 E. Del Amo Blvd., Compton, CA 90220-6303   310-637-2103
FDA Number: n/a   Fax: 310-637-2450
E-mail: jason@plaskolitecontinental.com
Web site: www.plaskolitecontinental.com
Annual Revenue: $25-$50 Million
Year Founded: 1950
Total Employees: 38   Marketing Staff: 1   Sales Staff: 4
Ownership: Henkel
Quality System Registration Information: ISO9002
Produces/Sells CE-marked Devices: N
Federal Procurement Eligibility: Small Business, GSA Contract
Distribution: Manufacturer Direct, Manufacturer Through Manufacturer Reps,
Service Direct, Exclusive Distributor, Exporter
General Admin.: Jason Shen/General Manager
    Jim Dunn/President
Production: Dean Coassin/Manager Regulatory Affairs
Material, Acrylic, Dental	Dental And Oral

PLASTEK INDUSTRIES, INC.   **336-271-3210**
880 Huffman St., Greensboro, NC 27405
FDA Number: 1017320
Evacuator, Oral Cavity   Dental And Oral

PLASTI PRODUCTS, INC.   **800-527-5396**
14315 C-Circle, Omaha, NE 68144
FDA Number: n/a   *Fax:* 402-330-1120
E-mail: info@plastiproducts.com
Web site: www.plastiproducts.com
Ownership: Private
Produces/Sells CE-marked Devices: N
Federal Procurement Eligibility: Small Business
Distribution: Exclusive Distributor
General Admin.: Rodney Laible/President
    Dan Brown/Vice President, General Manager
Mktg./Adv.: Jim Ciurej/Vice President Marketing
Container, Medication, Graduated Liquid   General
Container, Sharpes   General
Container, Specimen, All Types   General
Dispenser, Other   General

PLASTIC AND METAL CENTER, INC.   **949-770-8230**
23162 La Cadena Drive, Laguna Hills, CA 92653
FDA Number: n/a   *Fax:* 949-770-8478
E-mail: sales@plastic-metal.com
Web site: www.plastic-metal.com
Annual Revenue: $1-$5 Million
Year Founded: 1993
Total Employees: 20   *Marketing Staff:* 1   *Sales Staff:* 2
Ownership: Private
Produces/Sells CE-marked Devices: N
Federal Procurement Eligibility: Small Business
Distribution: Manufacturer Direct, OEM, Service Direct
General Admin.: Fred Carr/Vice President
Accessories, Arthroscope   Orthopedics
Accessories, Cardiopulmonary Bypass   Cardiovascular
Bag, Polymeric Mesh, Pacemaker   Cardiovascular
Cleanroom Equipment   General
Contract Packaging   General
Ring, Teething, Fluid-Filled   Dental And Oral
Tray, Walker   General
Valve, Heart, Mechanical   Cardiovascular

PLASTIC ENDO, LLC   **866-752-3636**
318 Half Day Rd., #247, Buffalo Grove, IL 60089
FDA Number: 3005897690
Web site: www.plasticendo.com
Ownership: Private
Produces/Sells CE-marked Devices: N
File, Pulp Canal, Endodontic   Dental And Oral

PLASTIC PRODUCTS COMPANY
See Plastics One, Inc.

PLASTICARDS, INC. DBA RAINBOW PRINTING CO.   **800-536-9705**
3711 Boettler Oaks Dr.,   **330-896-5555**
Uniontown, OH 44685
FDA Number: 1531157   *Fax:* 330-896-5556
E-mail: info@rainbow-printing.com
Web site: www.rainbow-printing.com
Ownership: Private
Produces/Sells CE-marked Devices: Y
Goniometer, Non-Powered   Orthopedics

PLASTICOID CO., THE   **410-398-2800**
249 W. High St., Elkton, MD 21921-5235
FDA Number: n/a   *Fax:* 410-398-2803
E-mail: info@plasticoid.com
Web site: www.plasticoid.com
Annual Revenue: $1-$5 Million
Total Employees: 80
Ownership: Private
Produces/Sells CE-marked Devices: N
Federal Procurement Eligibility: Small Business
Distribution: Manufacturer Direct, Manufacturer Through Manufacturer Reps, OEM
General Admin.: Harry Thompson/Manager Admin. Services
    James Palinras/President
Mktg./Adv.: Monty Bose/Manager Sales
Production: Bernard Puszcz/Manager Quality Control
    Ray W. Jones/Vice President Manufacturing
Research: William Maes/Supervisor Product Development
Component, Rubber   General
Component, Silicone   General
Dropper, Medicine   General
Molding, Custom   General
Stopper   General

PLASTICS ONE, INC.   **540-772-7950**
6591 Merriman Road S.W., Roanoke, VA 24018-6664
FDA Number: 1118193   *Fax:* 540-989-7519
E-mail: info@plastics1.com
Web site: www.plastics1.com
Annual Revenue: $10-$25 Million
Year Founded: 1949
Total Employees: 250   *Marketing Staff:* 1   *Sales Staff:* 6
Ownership: Private
Quality System Registration Information: ISO9001
Produces/Sells CE-marked Devices: N
Federal Procurement Eligibility: Small Business
Distribution: Manufacturer Direct, OEM
General Admin.: David Wallenborn/President
Mktg./Adv.: John Richardson/Vice President Marketing & Sales
Production: Ted Lineberry/Vice President Manufacturing
    Palmer Bland/Vice President Operations
Cable, Electrode   Physical Med
Cable/Lead, ECG   Cardiovascular
Cable/Lead, EEG   Cns/Neurology
Cable/Lead, EMG   Cns/Neurology
Cable/Lead, TENS   Cns/Neurology
Cannula, Other   General
Molding, Custom   General

PLASTOCON, INC.   **800-966-0103**
1200 W. Second St.,   **262-569-3131**
Oconomowoc, WI 53066
FDA Number: 2183047   *Fax:* 262-569-3135
E-mail: Jerry.Marks@plastocon.com
Web site: www.plastoconinc.com
Annual Revenue: $1-$5 Million
Total Employees: 75   *Marketing Staff:* 5   *Sales Staff:* 3
Ownership: Private
Produces/Sells CE-marked Devices: N
Federal Procurement Eligibility: Small Business
Distribution: Manufacturer Direct, Manufacturer Through Manufacturer Reps, OEM, Exporter
General Admin.: Jim Nurmi/President, Chief Executive Officer
    Joe Chmielewski/Vice President Admin.
    Joe Chmielewski/Vice President Human Resources
    Jim Nurmi/Vice President, General Manager
Mktg./Adv.: Bob Ayer/Director National Accounts
    Dave Ozminkowski/Director Product Development
    Andy Shawholtz/Manager Contract Sales
    Andy Shawholtz/Manager Sales
    Joe Chmielewski/Vice President Business Development
    Bob Ayer/Vice President Marketing & Sales
Production: Barb Edwards/Director Quality Assurance
    Shirley Piepen/Manager Materials
    Joe Chmielewski/Manager Regulatory Affairs
    Joe Chmielewski/Vice President Manufacturing
Research: Dave Ozminkowski/Vice President Engineering
    Dave Ozminkowski/Vice President Research & Development
Basin, Emesis   General
Basin, Wash   General
Cart, Foodservice   General
Container, Specimen, All Types   General
Dispenser, Soap   General
Foodservice Product/Equipment   General
Holder, Thermometer   General
Molding, Custom   General
Tray, Foodservice   General
Tray, Medicine   General

PLATINUM SURGICAL INSTRUMENTS, INC.   **262-798-8540**
2325 Parklawn Dr., Suite F, Waukesha, WI 53186
FDA Number: 3006369878
Ownership: Private
Produces/Sells CE-marked Devices: N
Orthopedic Manual Surgical Instrument   Orthopedics

PLATT LUGGAGE, INC.   **800-222-1555**
4051 W. 51st St., Chicago, IL 60632   **773-838-2000**
FDA Number: n/a   *Fax:* 773-838-2010
E-mail: info@plattcases.com
Web site: www.plattluggage.com
Medical Products Sales Volume: $1,000,000
Annual Revenue: $5-$10 Million
Year Founded: 1921
Total Employees: 75   *Marketing Staff:* 2   *Sales Staff:* 20
Ownership: Private
Produces/Sells CE-marked Devices: N
Federal Procurement Eligibility: Small Business
Distribution: Manufacturer Direct, Manufacturer Through Distributor, Manufacturer Through Manufacturer Reps, OEM, Importer, Exporter
General Admin.: Allan Evavold/Executive Vice President
    Marc Platt/President

2013 MEDICAL DEVICE REGISTER

PLATT LUGGAGE, INC. 800-222-1555 *(cont'd)*
Mktg./Adv.: Allan Evavold/Director Marketing
Kathy Anweiler/Manager National Sales
Purchasing: Steve Pyrka/Purchasing Agent
Case, Protection, Equipment General

PLAYTEX PRODUCTS INC.
See Energizer Personal Care Division

PLAZA MEDICAL, INC. 877-695-4441
9780 E. Girard, Denver, CO 80231 303-695-4441
FDA Number: 1718118 Fax: 303-695-4442
E-mail: plazamedi@aol.com
Web site: www.plazamedical.net
Medical Products Sales Volume: $950,000
Annual Revenue: $0-$1 Million
Year Founded: 1970
Total Employees: 5 *Marketing Staff:* 2 *Sales Staff:* 3
Ownership: Private
Produces/Sells CE-marked Devices: N
Federal Procurement Eligibility: Small Business
Distribution: Manufacturer Direct, Exporter
General Admin.: Rick Rice/President
Centrifuge, Hematocrit Hematology

PLAZA TOWEL HOLDER, INC. 877-874-8394
P.O. Box 4737, Wichita, KS 67204 316-267-4233
FDA Number: 9330097 Fax: 316-264-3515
E-mail: lenox@southwind.net
Medical Products Sales Volume: $300,000
Annual Revenue: $0-$1 Million
Total Employees: 6 *Marketing Staff:* 1 *Sales Staff:* 1
Ownership: LENNOX MANUFACTURING
Produces/Sells CE-marked Devices: N
Federal Procurement Eligibility: Small Business, Female Owned
Distribution: Manufacturer Through Distributor, Exporter
General Admin.: Arlene Lenox/President, Chief Executive Officer
Mktg./Adv.: Robert Shingler/Director Product Development
Arlene Lenox/Manager Contract Sales
Clip, Towel Surgery

PLC MEDICAL SYSTEMS 800-232-8422
10 Forge Pk., Franklin, MA 02038 508-541-8800
FDA Number: 1287243 Fax: 508-541-7980
Medical Products Sales Volume: $6,000,000
Total Employees: 70
Ownership: Public
Stock Symbol: PLC
Traded On: AMEX
Produces/Sells CE-marked Devices: Y
Distribution: Manufacturer Direct, Exclusive Distributor
General Admin.: Robert Rudko/Chairman
Medical Admin.: Ms. Susan Papalia/Vice President Clinical Affairs
Mktg./Adv.: Jack Serino/Vice President Marketing & Sales
Research: Steve Linhares/Vice President Research & Development
Finance: Pat Murphy/Chief Financial Officer
Purchasing: Robert Dion/Buyer
Laser, Surgical Surgery
System, Laser, Transmyocardial Revascularization Cardiovascular

PLC MEDICAL SYSTEMS
See Plc Systems Inc.

PLC SYSTEMS INC. 508-541-8800
459 Fortune Boulevard, Milford, MA 01757
FDA Number: 1287243 Fax: 508-541-7980
E-mail: info@plcmed.com
Web site: www.plcmed.com
Medical Products Sales Volume: $6,500,000
Annual Revenue: $5-$10 Million
Year Founded: 1987
Total Employees: 30
Ownership: Public
Stock Symbol: PLCSF
Traded On: OTC Bulletin
Quality System Registration Information: ISO9000
Produces/Sells CE-marked Devices: Y
Federal Procurement Eligibility: Small Business
Distribution: Manufacturer Direct
General Admin.: Dr. Robert Rudko/Chief Scientific Officer
Mr. Mark R. Tauscher/President, Chief Executive Officer
Production: Mr. Kenneth Luppi/Vice President Operations
Finance: Mr. James Thomasch/Chief Financial Officer, Senior Vice President Finance
Laser, Surgical Surgery
System, Laser, Transmyocardial Revascularization Cardiovascular

PLC SYSTEMS, LASER ENGINEERING, INC.DIV.
See Plc Medical Systems

PLEXAR ASSOCIATES, INC. 216-932-2069
3722 Meadowbrook Blvd., University Heights, OH 44118
FDA Number: 1531231 Fax: 216-932-7047
E-mail: dprohler@plexar.com
Web site: www.plexar.com
Medical Products Sales Volume: $700,000
Year Founded: 1986
Total Employees: 25
Ownership: Private
Produces/Sells CE-marked Devices: N
Federal Procurement Eligibility: Small Business
Distribution: Manufacturer Direct, Manufacturer Through Distributor
System, Communication, Image, Digital Radiology

PLEXUS BIOMEDICAL INC. 901-763-2900
7495 Hwy 64, Oakland, TN 38060
FDA Number: 3005550381
Applier, Pressure, Physical Medicine Physical Med

PLEXUS CORP 425-482-1300
20001 N. Creek Pkwy, Bothell, WA 98011
FDA Number: 9200252 Fax: 425-482-1401
E-mail: info@plexus.com
Web site: www.plexus.com
Medical Products Sales Volume: $1,460,000,000
Annual Revenue: More than $1 Billion
Year Founded: 1980
Total Employees: 250
Ownership: Plexus Corp.
Stock Symbol: PLXS
Traded On: NASDAQ
Quality System Registration Information: ISO9001
Produces/Sells CE-marked Devices: Y
Federal Procurement Eligibility: Small Business
Distribution: Manufacturer Direct, Service Direct
General Admin.: Mr. Dean Foate/Chief Executive Officer
Mr. Paul Ehlers/President
Production: Mr. Mike Abbey/Manager Quality Assurance & Regulatory Affairs
Mr. David Rhoden/Plant General Manager
Contract Manufacturing General
Contract Manufacturing, Product, Durable General
Contract R&D, Equipment General
Service, Engineering/Design General

PLEXUS CORP. 877-733-5919
55 Jewelers Park Drive, PO Box 156, 920-722-3451
Neenah, WI 54956
FDA Number: 2183715 Fax: 920-751-5395
E-mail: plexus_marketing@plexus.com
Web site: www.plexus.com
Medical Products Sales Volume: $1,460,000,000
Annual Revenue: More than $1 Billion
Year Founded: 1980
Total Employees: 7800
Ownership: Public
Stock Symbol: PLXS
Traded On: NASDAQ
Quality System Registration Information: ISO9001; ISO9002
Produces/Sells CE-marked Devices: Y
Distribution: Manufacturer Direct, Service Direct, Exporter
General Admin.: Dean Foate/Chief Executive Officer
Dave Rust/Vice President Human Resources
Mktg./Adv.: Joe Nussbaum/Director Business Development
IS: Bob Kronser/Executive Vice President, Chief Technology Services
Contract Manufacturing General
Service, Engineering/Design General
Medical Product Subsidiaries (Listed Separately)
Plexus Corp

PLEXUS ELECTRONIC ASSEMBLY 847 793 4400
2400 Millbrook Dr., Buffalo Grove, IL 60089
FDA Number: 3004105270 Fax: 847 793 4481
Ownership: Private
Produces/Sells CE-marked Devices: N
Catheter, Intravascular, Diagnostic Cardiovascular
Locator, Vein, Liquid Crystal General
Scanner, Ultrasonic (Pulsed Doppler) Radiology
Scanner, Ultrasonic (Pulsed Echo) Radiology
Suction Apparatus, Ward Use, Portable, AC-Powered Surgery
Transducer, Ultrasonic, Diagnostic Radiology

PLITEK, L.L.C 800-966-1250
69 Rawls Road, Des Plaines, IL 60018 847-827-6680
FDA Number: 1423628 Fax: 847-827-6733
E-mail: info@plitek.com
Web site: www.plitek.com
Medical Products Sales Volume: $4,600,000
Annual Revenue: $10-$25 Million

PLITEK, L.L.C   800-966-1250 *(cont'd)*
Year Founded: 1962
Total Employees: 62   *Marketing Staff: 2*   *Sales Staff: 9*
Ownership: Private
Quality System Registration Information: ISO9001
Produces/Sells CE-marked Devices: N
Federal Procurement Eligibility: Small Business
Distribution: Manufacturer Direct, Manufacturer Through Distributor, Manufacturer Through Manufacturer Reps, OEM, Importer, Exporter
General Admin.: Karl Hoffman/Chief Executive Officer
            Joe Weber/Vice President, General Manager
Mktg./Adv.: Jay Kelley/Director Marketing
            Roger Engel/Director Product Development
Production: Jeff Gilchrist/Product Manager
            Sid Patterson/Vice President Manufacturing

Component, Other	General
Component, Plastic	General
Contract Manufacturing	General
Service, Engineering/Design	General

PLITRON MANUFACTURING, INC.   (1-800-754-8766
8-601 Magnetic Dr,   **416-667-9914**
Toronto, ON M3J 3 Canada
FDA Number: n/a   Fax: 416-667-8928
E-mail: sales@plitron.com
Web site: www.plitron.com
Medical Products Sales Volume: $2,000,000
Total Employees: 75   *Marketing Staff: 1*   *Sales Staff: 3*
Ownership: Private
Quality System Registration Information: ISO9000
Produces/Sells CE-marked Devices: Y
Distribution: Manufacturer Direct, Exporter

PLOMERIA ESPECIALIZADA DE BAJA   626-336-4561
CALIFORNIA, S.A. DE
Calle Maquiladoras No. 322, Seccion Dorada,
Nueva Tijuana, Baja California Mexico
FDA Number: 9616607

Bath, Paraffin	Physical Med
System, Water, Reproduction, Assisted, And Purification	Obstetrics/Gynecology

PLS SHOE CO.   866 712 7463
21500 Osborne St., Canoga Park, CA 91304   **818-734-7080**
FDA Number: 3004574391   Fax: 818 734 9040
E-mail: PAINLESSSHOE@SBCGLOBAL.NET
Web site: WWW.PAINLESSSHOE.COM
Ownership: Private
Produces/Sells CE-marked Devices: N

Orthosis, Corrective Shoe	Physical Med
Orthosis, Limb Brace	Physical Med

PLUROMED, INC   781-932-0574
175-F New Boston Street, Woburn, MA 01801
FDA Number: 3008867907   Fax: 419-828-6350
E-mail: info@pluromed.com
Web site: http://www.pluromed.com
Ownership: Private
Produces/Sells CE-marked Devices: N
General Admin.: Jean-Marie Vogel/Chief Executive Officer
            James Wilkie/Chief Operating Officer
            James Rolke/Chief Technology Officer
Mktg./Adv.: John Merhige/Vice President Market Development
Production: John Nagle/Director Quality Control

Catheter, Urological	Gastroenterology/Urology

PLYMOLD   800-533-0480
615 Centennial Drive, Kenyon, MN 55946   **507-789-5111**
FDA Number: n/a   Fax: 507-789-8315
E-mail: seating@plymold.com
Web site: www.foldcraft.com
Medical Products Sales Volume: $51,000,000
Annual Revenue: $1-$5 Million
Year Founded: 1948
Total Employees: 250
Ownership: Private
Federal Procurement Eligibility: Small Business, GSA Contract
Distribution: Manufacturer Through Manufacturer Reps
General Admin.: Steve Sheppard/Chief Executive Officer
            Chuck Mayhew/President
Mktg./Adv.: Ray Leaf/Supervisor Advertising
            Larry DeBoer/Vice President Marketing & Sales
Production: John Melburg/Vice President Manufacturing

Table, Other	General

PM COMPANY   800-327-4359
1500 Kemper Meadow Drive,   **513-825-7626**
Cincinnati, OH 45240
FDA Number: n/a   Fax: 513-825-2877
E-mail: info@pmcompany.com
Web site: www.pmcompany.com
Medical Products Sales Volume: $38,000,000
Year Founded: 1905
Total Employees: 50   *Marketing Staff: 4*   *Sales Staff: 20*
Ownership: Private
Produces/Sells CE-marked Devices: N
Federal Procurement Eligibility: Small Business
Distribution: Manufacturer Through Distributor
General Admin.: Cheryl Fritz/Manager Human Resources
            Deirdre O'Neill/Owner, Chief Executive Officer
            Mike Webster/President
Mktg./Adv.: Jim Feight/Manager National Sales
            Sharon Bliss/Marketing Communications Specialist
Production: Mike Roberts/Director Operations
            Jean Ann Sisk/Manager Customer Services
            Darlene Walsh/Product Manager
            Davis Mark/Product Manager

Component, Paper	General
Office Product	General

PM COMPANY HEALTHCARE GROUP
See Perfecseal

PM GLOVES, INC.   800-788-9486
13808 Magnolia Avenue, Chino, CA 91710-7027   **909-465-9188**
FDA Number: 2083656   Fax: 909-465-0028
E-mail: pmgloves@pmgloves.com
Medical Products Sales Volume: $3,000,000
Annual Revenue: $1-$5 Million
Total Employees: 7   *Marketing Staff: 1*   *Sales Staff: 3*
Ownership: Private
Quality System Registration Information: ISO9002; ISO9003
Produces/Sells CE-marked Devices: Y
Distribution: Manufacturer Through Distributor
General Admin.: Wei-Teng Lin/Chief Executive Officer
Mktg./Adv.: Andy K. Lin/Manager Marketing
            Gloria Ling/Manager Marketing

Box, Glove	Microbiology
Glove, Autopsy	Pathology
Glove, Other	General
Glove, Patient Examination	General
Glove, Patient Examination, Latex	General
Glove, Patient Examination, Vinyl	General
Glove, Utility	General
Mask, Face	General

PMD
See Paramedical Distributors

PML MICROBIOLOGICALS   800-628-7014
27120 S.W. 95th Avenue,   **503-570-2500**
Wilsonville, OR 97070
FDA Number: 3017344   Fax: 800-765-4415
E-mail: orders@pmlmicro.com
Web site: www.pmlmicro.com
Medical Products Sales Volume: $15,000,000
Annual Revenue: $10-$25 Million
Year Founded: 1969
Total Employees: 91   *Marketing Staff: 2*   *Sales Staff: 5*
Ownership: Public
Stock Symbol: PMLi
Quality System Registration Information: ISO9001
Produces/Sells CE-marked Devices: N
Federal Procurement Eligibility: Small Business, VA Contract
Distribution: Manufacturer Direct, Manufacturer Through Distributor, OEM
General Admin.: Ron Torland/Chairman
            Ken Minton/Chief Executive Officer
            Anita Webb/Vice President Human Resources & Personnel
Mktg./Adv.: Nally Reutov/Coord. Marketing & Sales
            Bill Smutny/Vice President Marketing & Sales
Production: Ruth Martin/Manager Customer Services
            Chris Pagella/Manager Materials
            Tim Schroeder/Vice President Operations
            Minda Evalle/Vice President Tech. Affairs
Finance: Ron Horne/Controller

Concentrator, Clinical Sample	Chemistry
Culture Media, For Isolation Of Pathogenic Neisseria	Microbiology
Culture Media, General Nutrient Broth	Microbiology
Culture Media, Mueller Hinton Agar Broth	Microbiology
Culture Media, Multiple Biochemical Test	Microbiology
Culture Media, Non-Propagating Transport	Microbiology
Culture Media, Non-Selective And Differential	Microbiology
Culture Media, Non-Selective And Non-Differential	Microbiology
Culture Media, Selective And Differential	Microbiology

PML MICROBIOLOGICALS 800-628-7014 (cont'd)

Culture Media, Selective And Non-Differential	Microbiology
Culture Media, Selective Broth	Microbiology
Culture Media, Single Biochemical Test	Microbiology
Culture Media, Supplements	Microbiology
Disc, Strip And Reagent, Microorganism Differentiation	Microbiology
Loop, Inoculating	Microbiology
Stain, Acridine Orange	Pathology
Stain, Microbiological	Microbiology
Test, Agar Plate	Microbiology
Test, Agar Tube	Microbiology
Transport System, Aerobic	Microbiology
Transport System, Anaerobic	Microbiology

PMT CORP. 800-626-5463
1500 Park Rd., Chanhassen, MN 55317-9593 952-470-0866
FDA Number: 2182979 Fax: 952-470-0865
E-mail: info@pmtcorp.com
Web site: www.pmtcorp.com
Annual Revenue: $10-$25 Million
Year Founded: 1979
Total Employees: 100 *Marketing Staff:* 3 *Sales Staff:* 32
Ownership: Private
Quality System Registration Information: ISO9001
Produces/Sells CE-marked Devices: Y
Federal Procurement Eligibility: Small Business
Distribution: Manufacturer Direct
General Admin.: Eric Caille/General Manager
　　　　Alfred A. Iversen/President

Biopsy Instrument, Suction	Gastroenterology/Urology
Cable/Lead, EEG	Cns/Neurology
Catheter, Epidural	Obstetrics/Gynecology
Catheter, Suction, With Tip	General
Electrode, Cortical	Cns/Neurology
Electrode, Depth	Cns/Neurology
Electrode, Electroencephalographic	Cns/Neurology
Electrode, Electrosurgical, Return (Ground, Dispersive)	Surgery
Expander, Skin, Inflatable	Surgery
Expander, Surgical, Skin Graft	Surgery
Flowmeter, Blood, Other	Cardiovascular
Instrument, Microsurgical	Cns/Neurology
Monitor, Temperature (With Probe)	Anesthesiology
Monitor, Temperature, Surgery	Surgery
Orthosis, Cervical	Physical Med
Orthosis, Lumbosacral	Physical Med
Orthosis, Thoracic	Physical Med
Probe, Temperature	General
Tip, Suction Tube (Yankauer, Poole, Etc.)	Surgery

PNAVEL SYSTEMS, INC. 718-645-6304
1502 East 14th Street, Suite 2, Brooklyn, NY 11230
FDA Number: 3006358051

Instrument, Manual, General Surgical	Surgery

PNEMOSIM
See Cardionics, Inc.

PNEU-MOBILITY, INC. 610-266-8500
944 Marcon Blvd, Ste. 110, Allentown, PA 18109-9312
FDA Number: n/a Fax: 610-266-8230
Ownership: Private
Produces/Sells CE-marked Devices: N

Massager, Therapeutic	Physical Med

PNEUMATIC PRODUCTS CORPORATION 352-873-5793
4647 S.W. 40th Ave., Ocala, FL 34474-5799
FDA Number: n/a Fax: 352-873-5770
E-mail: pneumatic.products.sales@spx.com
Web site: www.pneumaticproducts-spx.com
Annual Revenue: $50-$100 Million
Total Employees: 200 *Marketing Staff:* 2 *Sales Staff:* 15
Ownership: UNITED DOMINION INDUSTRIES
Quality System Registration Information: ISO9000
Produces/Sells CE-marked Devices: N
Distribution: Manufacturer Through Manufacturer Reps
Mktg./Adv.: Doug Blocksom/Vice President Marketing & Sales

Desiccator	Chemistry
Equipment, Cleaning, Air	General
Filter, Air	General

PNEUMEX, INC. 800-447-5792
2605 North Boyer Ave., Sandpoint, ID 83864 208-265-4105
FDA Number: 3032760 Fax: 208-265-9651
E-mail: pneumex@pneumex.com
Web site: www.pneumex.com
Year Founded: 1987
Total Employees: 22
Ownership: Private
Produces/Sells CE-marked Devices: Y
Federal Procurement Eligibility: Female Owned

PNEUMEX, INC. 800-447-5792 (cont'd)
Distribution: Manufacturer Direct, Manufacturer Through Distributor, Manufacturer Through Manufacturer Reps, Service Direct, Exporter

Component, Exercise	Physical Med
Exerciser, Powered	Anesthesiology
Isokinetic Testing And Evaluation System	Physical Med
Pressure Measurement, System, Intermittent	Physical Med

PNEUMRX INC 650-625-8910
530 Logue Ave, Mountain View, CA 94043
FDA Number: 3005823838 Fax: 650-625-8915
E-mail: info@pneumrx.com
Web site: http://www.pneumrx.com/
Year Founded: 2004
Ownership: Private
Produces/Sells CE-marked Devices: N

Biopsy Instrument	Gastroenterology/Urology
Kit, Biopsy Needle	Gastroenterology/Urology
Needle, Aspiration And Injection, Disposable	Surgery
Needle, Aspiration And Injection, Reusable	Surgery
Needle, Biopsy, Cardiovascular	Cardiovascular

POCHEMCO, INC. 413-536-2900
724 Main Street, Holyoke, MA 01040
FDA Number: 1219469 Fax: 413-536-4956
E-mail: pochemcoinc@msn.com
Medical Products Sales Volume: $100,000
Year Founded: 1969
Total Employees: 2
Ownership: Private
Produces/Sells CE-marked Devices: N
Federal Procurement Eligibility: Small Business
Distribution: Manufacturer Direct, Manufacturer Through Distributor, Manufacturer Through Manufacturer Reps, Service Direct

Buffer, pH	Hematology
Chromatographic Barbiturate Identification (Thin Layer)	Toxicology
Counter, Platelet, Manual	Hematology
Fluid, White Cell Diluting	Hematology
Formaldehyde (Formalin, Formol)	Pathology
Formalin, Neutral Buffered	Pathology
Formalin-Saline	Pathology
Indicator Method, Protein Or Albumin (Urinary, Non-Quant.)	Chemistry
Reagent, General Purpose	Pathology
Solution, Isotonic	Hematology
Solution, Pathology, Lugol's	Pathology
Stain, Aldehyde Fuchsin	Pathology
Stain, Crystal Violet, Histology	Pathology
Stain, Eosin Y	Pathology
Stain, Giemsa	Pathology
Stain, Grams Iodine	Pathology
Stain, Microbiological	Microbiology
Stain, Reticulocyte	Hematology
Stain, Safranin	Pathology
Stain, Wright's	Pathology

POCKET NURSE ENTERPRISES, INC. 800-225-1600
200 1st Street, Ambridge, PA 15003 412-630-2950
FDA Number: n/a Fax: 412-630-2951
E-mail: info@pocketnurse.com
Web site: www.pocketnurse.com
Medical Products Sales Volume: $18,000,000
Annual Revenue: $10-$25 Million
Year Founded: 1992
Total Employees: 36 *Marketing Staff:* 3 *Sales Staff:* 7
Ownership: Private
Produces/Sells CE-marked Devices: Y
Federal Procurement Eligibility: Small Business
Distribution: Exclusive Distributor
General Admin.: Mr. Anthony Battaglia/President
　　　　　Mr. John Fullum/Vice President
Mktg./Adv.: Ms. Deborah Coltrane/Director Marketing & Strategic Planning
Finance: Mr. Timothy Taylor/Chief Financial Officer

Anatomical Training Model	General
Hemostat	Orthopedics
Light Source, Flash	Chemistry
Penlight, Battery-Powered	Ophthalmology
Scissors, Bandage/Gauze/Plaster	General
Simulator, Blood Pressure	Cardiovascular
Simulator, Heart Sound	Cardiovascular
Simulator, Lung	Anesthesiology
Stethoscope, Mechanical	General
Training Manikin, CPR (Resuscitation)	General
Training Manikin, Intravenous Arm	General
Training Manikin, Other	General
Training Manikin, Wound Moulage	General

PODO TECHNOLOGY, INC 770-353-0723
5 Concourse Parkway, Ste 3000, Atlanta, GA 30328
FDA Number: 3003855545
E-mail: info@podotechnology.com

PODO TECHNOLOGY, INC — 770-353-0723 (cont'd)
Web site: www.podotechnology.com
Ownership: Private
Produces/Sells CE-marked Devices: N
Platform, Force-Measuring — Physical Med

POERSCH METAL MFG. CO. — 773-722-0890
4027 West Kinzie St., Chicago, IL 60624-1807
FDA Number: 1450233 — Fax: 773-722-4122
E-mail: rckruse@poerschmetal.com
Web site: www.poerschmetal.com
Ownership: Private
Produces/Sells CE-marked Devices: N
Holder, Radiographic Cassette, Wall-Mounted — Radiology

POGO, INC. — 507-280-8868
410 1st. Ave. N.w., Rochester, MN 55901
FDA Number: 2133720
Ownership: Private
Produces/Sells CE-marked Devices: N
Laryngoscope, Rigid — Anesthesiology

POINT MEDICAL CORP. — 219-663-1775
891 E. Summit St., Crown Point, IN 46307-2700
FDA Number: 9002237 — Fax: 219-663-2877
E-mail: khanlon@pointmedical.com
Web site: www.pointmedical.com
Medical Products Sales Volume: $13,500,000
Annual Revenue: $10-$25 Million
Year Founded: 1990
Total Employees: 160 — Marketing Staff: 4 — Sales Staff: 8
Ownership: Private
Quality System Registration Information: ISO9001
Produces/Sells CE-marked Devices: N
Federal Procurement Eligibility: Small Business
Distribution: OEM
General Admin.: Rick Ferraro/President
Mktg./Adv.: Mike Basta/Director International Sales
Frank DeBartola/Director National Marketing & Sales
Production: Dan Winter/Director Engineering
Tom Hanlon/Director Operations
Joe Farag/Manager Production
Contract Manufacturing — General
Equipment, Extruding/Molding — General
Molding, Custom — General

POINT PLASTICS, INC.
See Quality Scientific Plastics

POINT SOURCE INC. — 937-855-6020
1864 Dayton Pike, Germantown, OH 45327
FDA Number: n/a — Fax: 937-855-6025
E-mail: Info@PointSource-Inc.com
Web site: www.pointsource-inc.com
Annual Revenue: $0-$1 Million
Year Founded: 1992
Ownership: Private
Produces/Sells CE-marked Devices: N
Federal Procurement Eligibility: Small Business, Female Owned
Distribution: Manufacturer Direct, OEM
Laser, Surgical — Surgery
Light Source, Endoscopic — Obstetrics/Gynecology
Light, Surgical Headlight — Dental And Oral

POINTCARE TECHNOLOGIES INC. — 508-281-6925
181 Cedar Hill St., Marlboro, MA 01752
FDA Number: 3004086182
Counter, Cell, Differential Classifier, Automated — Hematology

POINTE CONCEPTION MEDICAL, INCORPORATED — 805-964-8104
749 Ward Drive, Goleta, CA 93111
FDA Number: 3006990600
Ownership: Private
Produces/Sells CE-marked Devices: N

POINTE SCIENTIFIC, INC. — 800-445-9853 / 734-487-8300
5449 Research Drive, Canton, MI 48188
FDA Number: 1827821 — Fax: 734-483-1592
E-mail: sales@pointescientific.com
Web site: www.pointescientific.com/
Medical Products Sales Volume: $5,000,000
Annual Revenue: $5-$10 Million
Year Founded: 1981
Total Employees: 30 — Marketing Staff: 4 — Sales Staff: 3
Ownership: Private
Produces/Sells CE-marked Devices: Y
Federal Procurement Eligibility: Small Business, GSA Contract, VA Contract

POINTE SCIENTIFIC, INC. — 800-445-9853 (cont'd)
Distribution: Manufacturer Direct, Manufacturer Through Distributor, OEM, Importer, Exporter
General Admin.: Janusz M. Szyszko/President, Chief Executive Officer
Kay Newel/Vice President, General Manager
Mktg./Adv.: Bill Walters/Director Marketing
Larry Noel/Manager National Sales
Production: Mr. Timothy F. Sheehan/Director Quality Assurance & Regulatory Affairs
Bill Walters/Director Tech. Operations
IS: Ron Jamison/Manager Tech. Support
Contract Manufacturing, Reagent — General
NAD Reduction/NADH Oxidation, Lactate Dehydrogenase — Chemistry
NADH Oxidation/NAD Reduction, AST/SGOT — Chemistry
Reagent, Cholesterol (Total Test System) — Chemistry
Test, Glycosylated Hemoglobin Assay — Hematology
Urease And Glutamic Dehydrogenase, Urea Nitrogen — Chemistry

POLAR CRYOGENICS, INC. — 503-239-5252
2734 S.e. Raymond, Portland, OR 97202
FDA Number: 3019317
Box, Glove — Microbiology
Electrode, Blood pH — Chemistry
Gas, Calibrated (Specified Concentration) — Anesthesiology
Laser, Surgical — Surgery

POLAR ELECTRO INC. — 1-800-227-1314
1111 Marcus Ave., Ste. M15, Lake Success, NY 11042-1034
FDA Number: n/a — Fax: 516-364-5454
E-mail: customer.service.usa@polar.fi
Web site: www.polarusa.com
Total Employees: 82
Ownership: Polar Electro Oy
Produces/Sells CE-marked Devices: N
Federal Procurement Eligibility: Small Business
Distribution: Manufacturer Direct, Manufacturer Through Distributor, Manufacturer Through Manufacturer Reps, OEM
General Admin.: Philippe Duleyrie/President
Mktg./Adv.: Stephen C. Cooper/Director Marketing
Greg Wagner/Director Sales
Allison Herrforth/Marketing Representative
Greg Varro/Marketing Representative
Computer Equipment — General
Monitor, ECG — Cardiovascular
Monitor, Heart Rate, Other — Cardiovascular
Monitor, Pulse Rate — Anesthesiology

POLAR PLASTIC LTD. — 514-331-0207
4210 Thimens Blvd., St. Laurent, QUE H4R 2B9 Canada
FDA Number: 9200541 — Fax: 514-331-7604
E-mail: polar@polarplastic.com
Web site: www.polarplastic.com
Year Founded: 1972
Total Employees: 250 — Marketing Staff: 3 — Sales Staff: 10
Ownership: Private
Produces/Sells CE-marked Devices: N
Federal Procurement Eligibility: Small Business
Distribution: Manufacturer Through Distributor, Exporter

POLAR PRODUCTS, INC. — 800-763-8423 / 330-253-9973
3380 Cavalier Trail, Stow, OH 44224
FDA Number: n/a — Fax: 330-253-4233
E-mail: jake@polarsoftice.com
Web site: www.polarsoftice.com
Medical Products Sales Volume: $2,500,000
Annual Revenue: $1-$5 Million
Year Founded: 1983
Ownership: Private
Stock Symbol: N/A
Produces/Sells CE-marked Devices: N
Federal Procurement Eligibility: Small Business
Distribution: Manufacturer Direct, Manufacturer Through Distributor, Manufacturer Through Manufacturer Reps, OEM
Mktg./Adv.: Mr. Jacob Graessle/Sales Associate
Chilling Unit — Physical Med
Compress, Moist Heat — Physical Med
Massager, Therapeutic, Manual — Physical Med
Pack, Cold — General
Pack, Hot Or Cold, Reusable — Physical Med
Pack, Hot Or Cold, Water Circulating — Physical Med
Pack, Moist Heat — Physical Med

POLAR USA, INC.
See Polar Electro Inc.

POLAR WARE CO. — 800-237-3655 / 920-458-3561
2806 N. 15th St., Sheboygan, WI 53083
FDA Number: 2183714 — Fax: 920-458-2205
E-mail: customerservice@polarware.com

POLAR WARE CO. 800-237-3655 *(cont'd)*

Web site: www.polarware.com
Annual Revenue: $1-$5 Million
Year Founded: 1907
Total Employees: 250   Marketing Staff: 1   Sales Staff: 4
Ownership: Private
Produces/Sells CE-marked Devices: N
Federal Procurement Eligibility: Small Business, GSA Contract
Distribution: Manufacturer Through Distributor, Manufacturer Through
Manufacturer Reps, OEM, Exporter
General Admin.: Walt Vollrath/President, Chief Executive Officer
Mktg./Adv.: Jim Stephani/Manager International Marketing & Sales
          Stephanie Wittmus/Manager Market Development
          Jim Stephani/Manager Sales
          Rick Carr/Vice President Marketing & Sales
Production: Lee Wolf/Vice President Manufacturing

Basin, Emesis	General
Basin, Sponge	General
Basin, Wash	General
Bath, Sitz, Physical Medicine	Physical Med
Bedpan	General
Bedpan, Fracture	General
Bowl, Solution	General
Bowl, Sponge	General
Container, Sterilization (Tray)	General
Cup, Medicine	General
Holder, Thermometer	General
Jar, Applicator	Surgery
Jar, Dressing	Surgery
Jar, Forceps	Surgery
Tray, Surgical Instrument	Surgery
Urinal	General

POLARIS CONTRACT SERVICES, A DIVISION OF 508-748-1160
SIPPICON, INC.

7 Barnabas Rd., Marion, MA 02738-1421
FDA Number: n/a   Fax: 508-748-3626
E-mail: randall.l.goode@lmco.com
Web site: www.polariscs.com
Annual Revenue: $5-$10 Million
Total Employees: 120   Sales Staff: 2
Ownership: SIPPICAN, INC.
Quality System Registration Information: ISO9001
Produces/Sells CE-marked Devices: N
Federal Procurement Eligibility: Small Business
General Admin.: William E. Walsh/Chief Executive Officer
          Donna O'Connor/Vice President Human Resources
          Howard Mott/Vice President, General Manager
Mktg./Adv.: Richard Wicker/Director Marketing
          Richard Wicker/Director National Accounts
Production: William Inman/Director Quality Assurance

Contract Manufacturing	General

POLDER, INC. 800-431-2133
  914-937-8200

8 Slater St., Port Chester, NY 10573
FDA Number: n/a   Fax: 914-937-8297
E-mail: info@polder.com
Web site: www.polder.com/
Total Employees: 35   Marketing Staff: 1   Sales Staff: 4
Ownership: Private
Quality System Registration Information: ISO9001
Produces/Sells CE-marked Devices: N
Distribution: Exclusive Distributor
General Admin.: Calvin Scott/President
Mktg./Adv.: Joan Scire/Sales Representative

Foodservice Product/Equipment	General

POLIVKA LOGAN DESIGN

See Logic Product Development

POLY SCIENTIFIC R&D CORP. 800-645-5825
  631-586-0400

70 Cleveland Ave., Bay Shore, NY 11706-1224
FDA Number: 2429783   Fax: 631-254-0618
E-mail: polyrnd@polyrnd.com
Web site: www.polyrnd.com
Year Founded: 1969
Total Employees: 40   Marketing Staff: 4   Sales Staff: 8
Ownership: Private
Produces/Sells CE-marked Devices: N
Federal Procurement Eligibility: Small Business
Distribution: Manufacturer Direct
General Admin.: John J. Caggiano/President
          Joseph C. Caggiano/Vice President
Mktg./Adv.: Joseph Carl/Manager Sales
Finance: Denise M. Caggiano/Controller

Acetone	Chemistry
Adhesive, Albumin Based	Pathology
Cup, Medicine	General

POLY SCIENTIFIC R&D CORP. 800-645-5825 *(cont'd)*

Fluid, Bouin's	Pathology
Formaldehyde (Formalin, Formol)	Pathology
Formalin, Neutral Buffered	Pathology
Glutaraldehyde (Fixative)	Pathology
Media, Mounting	Pathology
Mercuric Chloride Formulations For Tissue	Pathology
Reagent, Other	General
Silver Nitrate	Pathology
Sirius Red	Pathology
Solution, Isotonic	Hematology
Solution, Pathology, Carnoy's	Pathology
Solution, Pathology, Decalcifier, Acid Containing	Pathology
Solution, Pathology, Fontanna Silver	Pathology
Solution, Pathology, Formalin-Alcohol-Acetic Acid	Pathology
Solution, Pathology, Lugol's	Pathology
Solution, Pathology, Zenker's	Pathology
Stain, Acid Fuchsin	Pathology
Stain, Alcian Blue	Pathology
Stain, Ammoniacal Silver Hydroxide Silver Nitrate	Pathology
Stain, Aniline Blue	Pathology
Stain, Biebrich Scarlet	Pathology
Stain, Carbol Fuchsin	Pathology
Stain, Congo Red	Pathology
Stain, Crystal Violet, Histology	Pathology
Stain, Eosin Y	Pathology
Stain, Giemsa, Hematology	Hematology
Stain, Gold Chloride	Pathology
Stain, Grams Iodine	Pathology
Stain, Hematology	Pathology
Stain, Hematoxylin	Pathology
Stain, Hematoxylin, Mayer's	Pathology
Stain, Light Green	Pathology
Stain, Luxol Fast Blue	Pathology
Stain, Mallory's Trichrome	Pathology
Stain, Metanil Yellow	Pathology
Stain, Methenamine Silver	Pathology
Stain, Methyl Green	Pathology
Stain, Methylene Blue	Pathology
Stain, Methylene Blue, New	Hematology
Stain, Microbiological	Microbiology
Stain, Mucicarmine	Pathology
Stain, Nuclear Fast Red	Pathology
Stain, Oil Red O	Pathology
Stain, Other	Pathology
Stain, Papanicolau	Pathology
Stain, Phosphotungstic Acid Hematoxylin	Pathology
Stain, Reagent, Schiff	Pathology
Stain, Safranin	Pathology
Stain, Sudan Black B	Pathology
Stain, Van Gieson's	Pathology
Stain, Weigert's Iron Hematoxylin	Pathology
Stain, Wright's, Hematology	Hematology
Test, Ethyl Alcohol	Toxicology

POLY-OPTICAL PRODUCTS INC.

See Trimedyne, Inc.

POLYCHROME MEDICAL 763-585-9328

2700 Freeway Blvd., Suite 750, Brooklyn Center, MN 55430
FDA Number: 2134435   Fax: 763-585-9329
E-mail: info@polychromemedical.com
Web site: www.polychromemedical.com
Medical Products Sales Volume: $1,200,000
Year Founded: 1995
Total Employees: 15   Marketing Staff: 1   Sales Staff: 1
Ownership: Private
Produces/Sells CE-marked Devices: N
Federal Procurement Eligibility: Small Business, Female Owned
Distribution: Manufacturer Direct, OEM

Iontophoresis Unit, Physical Medicine	Physical Med
Test, Cystic Fibrosis	Chemistry

POLYCOM INC. 978-924-6000

100 Minuteman Rd., Andover, MA 01810
FDA Number: 3003702744   Fax: 978-292-5900
Ownership: Private
Produces/Sells CE-marked Devices: N

System, Communication, Image, Digital	Radiology

POLYCONVERSIONS, INC. 888-893-3330
  217-893-3330

505 Condit Dr., Rantoul, IL 61866
FDA Number: 1423205   Fax: 217-893-3003
E-mail: info@polyconversions.com
Web site: www.polyconversions.com
Medical Products Sales Volume: $2,000,000
Annual Revenue: $1-$5 Million
Year Founded: 1994
Total Employees: 50   Marketing Staff: 3   Sales Staff: 7
Ownership: Private
Produces/Sells CE-marked Devices: Y

POLYCONVERSIONS, INC.   888-893-3330 *(cont'd)*
Federal Procurement Eligibility: Small Business
Distribution: Manufacturer Direct, Manufacturer Through Distributor, Manufacturer Through Manufacturer Reps, OEM, Exporter
Accessories, Apparel, Surgical   Surgery

POLYFOAM PACKERS CORP.
See Thermosafe Brands

POLYGELL LLC.   973-884-8995
30 Leslie Ct., Whippany, NJ 07981
FDA Number: 3005621376   *Fax:* 973-884-1331
Web site: http://www.polygel.com
Ownership: Private
Produces/Sells CE-marked Devices: N

Bandage, Cast	Physical Med
Bandage, Elastic	General
Dressing, Wound, Occlusive	Surgery
Elastomer, Silicone (Scar Management)	Surgery
Orthosis, Limb Brace	Physical Med
Protector, Skin Pressure	General
Splint, Temporary Training	Physical Med

POLYGENEX INTERNATIONAL, INC.
See Polyzen, Inc.

POLYLC INC.   410-992-5400
9151 Rumsey Rd., Ste. 180, Columbia, MD 21045
FDA Number: n/a   *Fax:* 410-730-8340
E-mail: polylc@aol.com
Web site: www.polylc.com
Annual Revenue: $1-$5 Million
Total Employees: 5   *Sales Staff:* 1
Ownership: Private
Produces/Sells CE-marked Devices: N
Federal Procurement Eligibility: Small Business
Distribution: Manufacturer Direct, Manufacturer Through Distributor, Service Direct, Exclusive Distributor, Importer
General Admin.: Andrew Alpert/Chief Executive Officer
Column, Liquid Chromatography   Toxicology

POLYMED SURGICAL INC.   800-361-9840
387, avenue Sainte-Croix,   514-737-2524
Saint-Laurent, QUE H4N 2 Canada
FDA Number: n/a   *Fax:* 514-737-9135
E-mail: contact@polymed.ca
Web site: www.polymed.ca
Year Founded: 1976
Total Employees: 25
Ownership: Private
Produces/Sells CE-marked Devices: N
Distribution: Exclusive Distributor, Importer

POLYMEDCO, INC.   800-431-2123
510 Furnace Dock Rd.,   914-739-5400
Cortlandt Manor, NY 10567
FDA Number: 3022762   *Fax:* 914-739-5890
E-mail: info@polymedco.com
Web site: www.polymedco.com
Annual Revenue: $10-$25 Million
Year Founded: 1980
Total Employees: 50
Ownership: Private
Produces/Sells CE-marked Devices: N
Federal Procurement Eligibility: Small Business
Distribution: Manufacturer Direct, Manufacturer Through Distributor, Manufacturer Through Manufacturer Reps, Exclusive Distributor, Exporter

Antigen, Tumor Marker, Bladder (Basement Membrane Complexes)	Immunology
Kit, Breast Cancer Detection	Obstetrics/Gynecology

Medical Product Subsidiaries (Listed Separately)
Bion Diagnostic Sciences, Inc.

POLYMER CONCEPTS, INC.   877-820-3163
7561-8 Tyler Blvd., Mentor, OH 44060-4867   440-953-9605
FDA Number: 1527181   *Fax:* 440-953-9602
E-mail: PCI1999@aol.com
Web site: www.polymerconcept.com
Medical Products Sales Volume: $400,000
Annual Revenue: $0-$1 Million
Year Founded: 1998
Total Employees: 5
Ownership: Private
Produces/Sells CE-marked Devices: N
Federal Procurement Eligibility: Small Business
Distribution: Manufacturer Direct, Manufacturer Through Distributor, OEM
General Admin.: Mr. Chris Callsen/President, Chief Executive Officer
Mktg./Adv.: Mr. Kevin Callsen/Director Marketing

Cushion, Table, Surgical	Surgery
Cushion, Wheelchair (Pad)	Physical Med

POLYMER CONCEPTS, INC.   877-820-3163 *(cont'd)*
Protector, Skin Pressure   General

POLYMER LABORATORIES, NOW A PART OF VARIAN, INC.   800-767-3963
Amherst Fields Research Park   413-253-9554
160 Old Farm Road
Amherst, MA 01002
FDA Number: n/a   *Fax:* 413-253-2476
E-mail: Online@polymerlabs.com
Web site: www.polymerlabs.com
Year Founded: 1976
Ownership: Varian Inc
Quality System Registration Information: ISO9001
Produces/Sells CE-marked Devices: Y
Distribution: Manufacturer Direct, Importer, Exporter
Mktg./Adv.: Laura Watson/Vice President Marketing
     John McConville/Vice President Sales

Accessories, Chromatography (Gas, Gel, Liquid, Thin Layer)	Chemistry
Chromatography Equipment, Ion Exchange	Toxicology
Chromatography Equipment, Liquid	Chemistry
Chromatography, Liquid, Performance, High	Toxicology
Column, Chromatography	Chemistry
Column, Liquid Chromatography	Toxicology
Contract Manufacturing, Reagent	General
High Pressure Liquid Chromatography, Tricyclic Drug	Toxicology
Instrumentation, High Pressure Liquid Chromatography	Toxicology
Molecular Weight Equipment	Chemistry
Polymer, Synthetic, Other	General
Reagent, Other	General
Resin, Other	General
Resins, Ion Exchange, Liquid Chromatography	Toxicology
Test, Direct Agglutination, Toxoplasma Gondii	Microbiology
Viscometer	Chemistry

POLYMER TECHNOLOGY SYSTEMS, INC.   317-870-5610
7736 Zionsville Rd., Indianapolis, IN 46268
FDA Number: 1836135
Web site: www.cardiochek.com
Year Founded: 1992
Ownership: Private
Produces/Sells CE-marked Devices: N

Alpha-Ketobutyric Acid And NADH (U.V.), Hydroxybutyric	Chemistry
Colorimetric Method, Triglycerides	Chemistry
Control, Multi Analyte, All Kinds (Assayed And Unassayed)	Chemistry
Enzymatic Esterase-Oxidase, Cholesterol	Chemistry
Enzymatic Method, Creatinine	Chemistry
LDL & VLDL Precipitation, HDL	Chemistry
Lipoprotein, High Density, HDL, Over-The-Counter	Chemistry
Reagent, Glucose (Test System)	Chemistry
System, Test, Blood Glucose, Over-The-Counter	Chemistry
System, Test, Low-Density, Lipoprotein	Chemistry

POLYONE   866-765-9663
10 Ruckle Ave., Farmingdale, NJ 07727   (732) 938-5980
FDA Number: n/a   *Fax:* 705-324-9284
Web site: www.polyone.com
Ownership: GEON/SYNERGISTICS
Stock Symbol: C:SGX-A
Traded On: NYSE
Quality System Registration Information: ISO9002
Produces/Sells CE-marked Devices: N
Distribution: Manufacturer Direct
General Admin.: Allen Jones/General Manager
Mktg./Adv.: Frank Tomachi/Director Marketing
     Jerry O'Grady/Manager National Sales
Production: Phil Donataccio/Vice President Manufacturing
Component, Plastic   General

POLYSCIENCE, DIVISION OF PRESTON INDUSTRIES INC.   800-229-7569
6600 W. Touhy Ave., Niles, IL 60714   847-647-0611
FDA Number: n/a   *Fax:* 847-647-1155
E-mail: sales@polyscience.com
Web site: www.polyscience.com
Annual Revenue: $10-$25 Million
Year Founded: 1963
Total Employees: 140
Ownership: Private
Quality System Registration Information: ISO9001
Produces/Sells CE-marked Devices: Y
Federal Procurement Eligibility: Small Business
Distribution: Manufacturer Direct, OEM, Exporter
General Admin.: Wayne Walter/Director, General Manager
     Philip Preston/President
Mktg./Adv.: Sue Gibbons/Manager Customer Services & Sales

Chilling Unit	Physical Med
Circulator, Water Bath	Chemistry

POLYSCIENCE, DIVISION OF PRESTON 800-229-7569 *(cont'd)*

Heater, Immersion	Microbiology
Shaker, Waterbath	Chemistry

POLYSCIENCES, INC. 800-523-2575

400 Valley Rd., Warrington, PA 18976-2522 215-343-6484

FDA Number: 2518071 *Fax:* (800) 343-3291
E-mail: info@polysciences.com
Web site: www.polysciences.com
Annual Revenue: $10-$25 Million
Year Founded: 1961
Total Employees: 85 *Marketing Staff:* 1
Ownership: Private
Produces/Sells CE-marked Devices: Y
Federal Procurement Eligibility: Small Business
Distribution: Manufacturer Direct, OEM, Importer, Exporter
General Admin.: Michael H. Ott/President, Chief Executive Officer
  Walter Baker/Vice President
Mktg./Adv.: Debra A. Sesholtz/Director Marketing
Production: Walter Baker/Vice President Operations
IS: David A. Templer/Vice President Technology

2nd Antibody (Species Specific Anti-Animal Gamma Globulin)	Immunology
Acetone	Chemistry
Cassette, Tissue	Pathology
Celloidin	Pathology
Chemical, Heparin Coating	Cardiovascular
Container, Embedding	Pathology
Fluid, Bouin's	Pathology
Formaldehyde (Formalin, Formol)	Pathology
Formalin, Neutral Buffered	Pathology
Gelatin	Pathology
Kit, Mycobacteria Identification	Microbiology
Media, Mounting	Pathology
Media, Mounting, Water Soluble	Pathology
Mounting Media, Oil Soluble	Pathology
Oil, Immersion	Hematology
Osmium Tetroxide	Pathology
Paraffin, All Formulations	Pathology
Paraformaldehyde	Pathology
Polyethylene Glycol (Carbowax)	Pathology
Protargol S	Pathology
Radioautographic Equipment	Chemistry
Silver Nitrate	Pathology
Slide, Microscope	Pathology
Stain, Acridine Orange	Pathology
Stain, Aldehyde Fuchsin	Pathology
Stain, Ammoniacal Silver Hydroxide Silver Nitrate	Pathology
Stain, Aniline Blue	Pathology
Stain, Auramine O	Pathology
Stain, Biebrich Scarlet	Pathology
Stain, Brilliant Yellow	Pathology
Stain, Carbol Fuchsin	Pathology
Stain, Carmine	Pathology
Stain, Chlorazol Black E	Pathology
Stain, Dye Solution	Pathology
Stain, Eosin Y	Pathology
Stain, Giemsa	Pathology
Stain, Giemsa, Hematology	Hematology
Stain, Hematoxylin	Pathology
Stain, Hematoxylin, Harris's	Pathology
Stain, Indigocarmine	Pathology
Stain, Light Green	Pathology
Stain, Luxol Fast Blue	Pathology
Stain, Metanil Yellow	Pathology
Stain, Methyl Green	Pathology
Stain, Microbiological	Microbiology
Stain, Neutral Red	Pathology
Stain, Oil Red O	Pathology
Stain, Orange G	Pathology
Stain, Other	Pathology
Stain, Papanicolau	Pathology
Stain, Periodic Acid Schiff (PAS)	Pathology
Stain, Pyronin	Pathology
Stain, Safranin	Pathology
Stain, Toluidine Blue	Pathology
Stain, Trypan Blue	Pathology
Stain, Wright's	Pathology
Tissue Embedding Equipment/Reagent	Pathology
Tweezers	General

Medical Product Subsidiaries (Listed Separately):
Bangs Laboratories, Inc.

POLYSORT 330-665-5918

4000 Embassy Pkwy., Suite 400, Akron, OH 44333
FDA Number: n/a *Fax:* 330-665-5152
E-mail: jbraver@polysort.com
Web site: www.polysort.com
Total Employees: 20
Ownership: Private
Produces/Sells CE-marked Devices: N

POLYSORT 330-665-5918 *(cont'd)*

Mktg./Adv.: John Braver/Director Business Development
Computer Software General

POLYVISION INC. 888-645-7788

875 East Patriot Blvd, Suite 201, Reno, NV 89511 775-850-2050

FDA Number: 2953748 *Fax:* 775-850-2060
E-mail: customerservice@polycore-usa.com
Web site: www.polycore.com
Medical Products Sales Volume: $14,000,000
Total Employees: 45
Ownership: Polycore Optical Pte. Ltd.
Produces/Sells CE-marked Devices: Y
Federal Procurement Eligibility: Small Business

Lens, Spectacle/Eyeglasses, Non-Custom	Ophthalmology

POLYZEN, INC. 919-319-9599

1041 Classic Road, Apex, NC 27539
FDA Number: 1064859 *Fax:* 919-319-8428
E-mail: info@polyzen.com
Web site: www.polyzen.com
Year Founded: 1991
Total Employees: 60 *Marketing Staff:* 1 *Sales Staff:* 2
Ownership: Private
Produces/Sells CE-marked Devices: N
Federal Procurement Eligibility: Small Business, Minority Owned
Distribution: Manufacturer Direct, Manufacturer Through Manufacturer Reps, OEM, Service Direct, Exporter
General Admin.: Tilak M. Shah/President, Chief Executive Officer

Bag, Plastic	General
Catheter, Cardiovascular, Balloon Type	Cardiovascular
Cover, Other	General
Film, X-Ray	Radiology
Glove, Other	General
Polymer, Synthetic, Other	General
Prophylactic (Condom)	General
Sheath, Endoscopic	Gastroenterology/Urology
Tubing, Radiopaque	General

POMDEVICES LLC 866-514-0325

5302 NC Highway 55, Suite 102, 919-200-6538
Durham, NC 27713
FDA Number: n/a *Fax:* 866-209-3941
E-mail: bizdev@pomdevices.com
Web site: http://sonamba.com
Year Founded: 2009
Ownership: Private
Produces/Sells CE-marked Devices: N
General Admin.: Mr. Adjit Pense/Chief Executive Officer
  Mr. Trey Weaver/Chief Technology Officer
Mktg./Adv.: Mr. John Riester/Director Business Development
  Mr. Robert Burke/Vice President Marketing

POMPANO PRECISION PRODUCTS, INC. 800-628-8333

1100 S.w. 12th Avenue, 954-946-6059
Deerfield Beach, FL 33069
FDA Number: 3003413730 *Fax:* 954-782-0910
E-mail: george@pompanoprecision.com
Web site: www.pompanoprecision.com
Ownership: Private
Produces/Sells CE-marked Devices: N

Rasp, Bone	Orthopedics

PONDUS MEDICAL, INC. 215-219-9152

5044 Davis Drive, PO Box 2079, Doylestown, PA 18901
FDA Number: 3006791380 *Fax:* (267) 224-4482
Ownership: Private
Produces/Sells CE-marked Devices: N

Scale, Sponge, Surgical, Electrically-powered	General

POP OLIGOS, LLC 301-461-0457

9430 Key West Ave., Rockville, MD 20850
FDA Number: 3005800650
Ownership: Private
Produces/Sells CE-marked Devices: N

Reagents, Specific, Analyte	Hematology

POPPER & SONS, INC.
See Cadence Science Inc.

POREX CORPORATION 800-241-0195

500 Bohannon Rd., Fairburn, GA 30213-2828 770-964-1421
FDA Number: 1043678
Web site: www.porex.com
Ownership: Hlth Corporation
Stock Symbol: SNTC
Traded On: NASDAQ
Produces/Sells CE-marked Devices: N
Distribution: OEM, Importer, Exporter

POREX CORPORATION 800-241-0195 *(cont'd)*
General Admin.: Kim A. Davis/President, Chief Executive Officer
Phil White/Vice President Human Resources
Finance: Don Jackson/Vice President Finance

Applicator, Sample	Chemistry
Equipment, Laboratory, Gen. Purpose (Specific Medical Use)	Chemistry
Filter, Blood, Dialysis	Gastroenterology/Urology
Foam, Plastic	General
Kit, Sampling, Blood	General
Molding, Custom	General
Serum Separation System	Hematology
Swabs, Specimen Collection	General

Medical Product Subsidiaries (Listed Separately)
Medegen
Porex Surgical, Inc.

POREX SURGICAL, INC. 800-521-7321
15 Dart Rd., Newnan, GA 30265 1-770-254-4400
FDA Number: 1057129 Fax: 1-678-423-1435
E-mail: surgical.info@porexsurgical.com
Web site: www.porexsurgical.com
Annual Revenue: $5-$10 Million
Total Employees: 50 *Marketing Staff:* 4 *Sales Staff:* 7
Ownership: Public
Produces/Sells CE-marked Devices: Y
Distribution: Manufacturer Direct, Manufacturer Through Distributor, Manufacturer Through Manufacturer Reps
General Admin.: William Midgette/President, Chief Executive Officer
Mktg./Adv.: John O'Shaughnessy/Manager International & National Sales
Darlene Robinson/Manager Marketing & Communications
Jeff Williams/Vice President Marketing & Sales
Production: Kent Iverson/Manager Manufacturing
Jerri Davis/Manager Regulatory Affairs
Research: Sebastien Henry/Vice President Research & Development

Kit, Surgical (General)	Surgery
Marker, Skin	Surgery
Mesh, Surgical, Polymeric	Surgery
Prosthesis, Chin, Internal	Surgery
Prosthesis, Soft Tissue	Surgery
Suction Apparatus, Single Patient, Portable, Non-Powered	Surgery

PORI & ROWE ASSOC., INC. 650-359-5175
1825 Palmetto Ave., Pacifica, CA 94044
FDA Number: 2916631
Ownership: Private
Produces/Sells CE-marked Devices: N

Transmitter/Receiver System, Physiological, Telephone	Cardiovascular

POROUS MEDIA CORP. 651-653-2000
1350 Hammond Rd., Saint Paul, MN 55110
FDA Number: 2132517

Filter, Bacterial, Breathing Circuit	Anesthesiology
Filter, Pre-Bypass, Cardiopulmonary Bypass	Cardiovascular
Humidifier, Respiratory Gas, (Direct Patient Interface)	Anesthesiology

PORTA-LUNG INC. 303-288-7575
747 Sheridan Blvd, Unit 6 D, Lakewood, CO 80214
FDA Number: 1720621 Fax: 303-288-7577
E-mail: portalung@comcast.net
Web site: www.porta-lung.com
Medical Products Sales Volume: $160,000
Annual Revenue: $0-$1 Million
Total Employees: 3 *Marketing Staff:* 1 *Sales Staff:* 1
Ownership: Private
Quality System Registration Information: ISO9001
Produces/Sells CE-marked Devices: Y
Federal Procurement Eligibility: Small Business
Distribution: Manufacturer Direct, Manufacturer Through Distributor, Manufacturer Through Manufacturer Reps, Exporter
General Admin.: Dano S. Carbone/President, Chief Executive Officer
Bryan L. Weingarten/Vice President

Ventilator, External Body, Negative Pressure, (Cuirass)	Anesthesiology

PORTABLE MEDICAL LABORATORIES, INC. 858-755-7385
544 S. Nardo Avenue, Solana Beach, CA 92075-0667
FDA Number: 2024663 Fax: 858-259-6022
E-mail: info@portable-medical-lab.com
Web site: www.portable-medical-lab.com
Medical Products Sales Volume: $200,000
Annual Revenue: $0-$1 Million
Year Founded: 1984
Total Employees: 2 *Marketing Staff:* 3 *Sales Staff:* 3
Ownership: Private
Produces/Sells CE-marked Devices: N
Federal Procurement Eligibility: Small Business
Distribution: Manufacturer Direct, Manufacturer Through Distributor, OEM, Exclusive Distributor, Importer, Exporter
General Admin.: Claude D. Jones/Chairman

PORTABLE MEDICAL LABORATORIES, INC. 858-755-7385
(cont'd)
Warren R. Sanborn/President, Chief Executive Officer
Mktg./Adv.: Warren R. Sanborn/Manager International & National Sales

Equipment, Laboratory, Gen. Purpose (Specific Medical Use)	Chemistry
Microscope	Hematology
Microscope, Fluorescence/U.V.	Pathology

PORTABLE POWER SYSTEMS, INC. 303-460-8261
405 West 115th Ave., Suite 3, Denver, CO 80234
FDA Number: 1722325
Ownership: Private
Produces/Sells CE-marked Devices: N

System, X-Ray, Mobile	Radiology

PORTACARE LLC 509-928-0650
13023 Tall Tree Rd., Spokane, WA 99216
FDA Number: 3034543 Fax: 509-928-4427
E-mail: jakuntz@portacare.com
Web site: www.portacare.com
Ownership: Private
Produces/Sells CE-marked Devices: N

Bath, Hydro-Massage (Whirlpool)	Physical Med
Walker, Mechanical	Physical Med
Wheelchair, Manual	Physical Med

PORTAL, INC. 435-753-3598
1350 N 200 W., Suite 6, Logan, UT 84341
FDA Number: 3003799782

Holder, Head, Radiographic	Radiology
Nuclear Magnetic Resonance Imaging System	Radiology
Scanner, Computed Tomography, X-Ray, Special Procedure	Radiology

PORTER INSTRUMENT DIVISION PARKER HANNIFIN CORP 800-457-2001
245 Township Line Rd., Hatfield, PA 19440-0907 215-723-4000
FDA Number: 2518157 Fax: 215-723-5106
E-mail: dental@parker.com
Web site: www.porterinstrument.com
Annual Revenue: $25-$50 Million
Year Founded: 1968
Total Employees: 170
Ownership: Public
Traded On: Paris
Produces/Sells CE-marked Devices: Y
Federal Procurement Eligibility: Small Business
Distribution: Manufacturer Through Distributor
General Admin.: Mike Howard/General Manager
Mktg./Adv.: Michael J. Lynam/Manager Marketing & Sales
Production: Steve Loeffler/Manager Quality Assurance & Engineering
Amy L. Englebert/Manager Regulatory Affairs
Joe Cotellese/Managing Director Production

Flowmeter, Back-Pressure Compensated, Thorpe Tube	Anesthesiology
Gas-Machine, Analgesia	Anesthesiology
Gas-Machine, Anesthesia	Anesthesiology
Resuscitator, Pulmonary, Manual (Demand Valve)	General
Scavenger, Gas	Anesthesiology

PORTIONPAC CHEMICAL CORP. 312-226-0400
400 N. Ashland Ave., Chicago, IL 60622
FDA Number: n/a Fax: 312-226-5400
E-mail: info@portionpaccorp.com
Web site: www.portionpaccorp.com
Annual Revenue: $1-$5 Million
Ownership: Private
Produces/Sells CE-marked Devices: N
Federal Procurement Eligibility: Small Business
Distribution: Manufacturer Direct

Solution, Antibacterial Cleaner	General

PORTLAND HEARING AID SPECIALISTS, INC. 503-261-9309
8505 SE Stark St, Portland, OR 97216
FDA Number: 3026265
Ownership: Private
Produces/Sells CE-marked Devices: N

Hearing-Aid	Ear/Nose/Throat

PORTLAND WELDING SUPPLY 207-772-3036
40 Madison St., South Portland, ME 04106
FDA Number: 1221338
Ownership: Private
Produces/Sells CE-marked Devices: N

Gas, Calibrated (Specified Concentration)	Anesthesiology

PORTO-LIFT CORP. 800-321-1454
PO Box 5, Higgins Lake, MI 48627 989-821-6688
FDA Number: 1824365 Fax: 989-821-8084
E-mail: www.portolift@voyager.net
Medical Products Sales Volume: $900,000

PORTO-LIFT CORP.   800-321-1454 (cont'd)
Annual Revenue: $0-$1 Million
Year Founded: 1942
Total Employees: 8   *Marketing Staff:* 1   *Sales Staff:* 1
Ownership: Private
Produces/Sells CE-marked Devices: N
Federal Procurement Eligibility: Small Business
Distribution: Manufacturer Through Distributor, Manufacturer Through Manufacturer Reps
General Admin.: Wayne H. Teeter/President

Lift, Bath, Non-AC-Powered	General
Lift, Patient	General
Scale, Chair, Transfer	General
Unit, Evaluation, Height, Lift	Orthopedics

PORVAIR FILTRATION GROUP INC   803-327-5008
454 South Anderson Road, BTC 514, Rock Hill, SC 29730
FDA Number: n/a   *Fax:* 803-327-1052
E-mail: info@porvairfiltration.com
Web site: www.porvairfiltration.com
Medical Products Sales Volume: $76,800,000
Ownership: Private
Stock Symbol: PRV
Traded On: London
Quality System Registration Information: ISO9001
Produces/Sells CE-marked Devices: N
Federal Procurement Eligibility: Small Business
Distribution: Manufacturer Direct, Manufacturer Through Distributor, Manufacturer Through Manufacturer Reps
Mktg./Adv.: Helen Heiford/Market Manager
         Mr. Roy Rigby/Sales Specialist

Filter, Air	General
Filter, Gas	Anesthesiology
Filter, Membrane	Chemistry
Filter, Syringe	General
Media, Filter	General
Purification Filter, Water, Particulate	Chemistry

POS-T-VAC, INC.   800-279-7434
1701 North 14th Ave., P.O. Box 1436, Dodge City, KS 67801
FDA Number: 1931563
E-mail: postvac@pld.com
Web site: www.postvac.com
Ownership: Private
Produces/Sells CE-marked Devices: N

Clamp, Bone	Orthopedics
Clamp, Other	Surgery
Prosthesis, Penis, Rigid Rod, External	Gastroenterology/Urology

POSEY CO., J.T.
See J. T. Posey Co.

POSITECNA
See Alimed, Inc.

POSITIVE ELECTRICAL PRODUCTS, INC.
See Frederick Tool Corp.

POSITIVEID CORPORATION   561-805-8000
1690 South Congress Avenue, Suite 200, Delray Beach, FL 33445
FDA Number: n/a   *Fax:* 561-805-8001
Web site: http://positiveidcorp.com
Year Founded: 2009
Total Employees: 20
Ownership: Public
Stock Symbol: PSID
Traded On: NASDAQ
Produces/Sells CE-marked Devices: N
General Admin.: Mr. Scott Silverman/Chairman, Chief Executive Officer
         Mr. William Caragol/President, Chief Financial Officer

POSITRON CORPORATION   866-613-7587
9715 Kincaid Blvd., Suite 1000, Fishers, IN 46038   317-576-0183
FDA Number: 3007219383   *Fax:* 317-576-0358
E-mail: contact@positron.com
Web site: www.positron.com
Medical Products Sales Volume: $2,200,000
Total Employees: 10   *Marketing Staff:* 2   *Sales Staff:* 3
Ownership: Public
Stock Symbol: POSC
Traded On: OTC Bulletin
Produces/Sells CE-marked Devices: N
Distribution: Manufacturer Direct
General Admin.: Mr. Patrick Rooney/Chief Executive Officer
         Mr. Joseph Oliverio/Chief Technology Officer
Mktg./Adv.: Mr. Peter Webner/Director Business Development
Production: Mr. Ron Hinton/Director Quality Assurance & Regulatory Affairs
Research: Mr. Timothy Gabel/Vice President Engineering

POSITRON CORPORATION   866-613-7587 (cont'd)
Finance: Mr. Corey Conn/Chief Financial Officer

Camera, Positron	Radiology
Scanner, Emission Computed Tomography	Radiology
Shield, Protective, Personnel	Radiology

POSITRON INDUSTRIES INC.   1-888-577-5254
5101 rue Buchan, Suite 220, Montreal, QC H4P 2 Canada   514-345-2200
FDA Number: 8020357   *Fax:* 514-345-2271
E-mail: info@positronpower.com
Web site: www.positroninc.com
Total Employees: 300   *Marketing Staff:* 15   *Sales Staff:* 15
Ownership: Private
Quality System Registration Information: ISO9002
Produces/Sells CE-marked Devices: N
Distribution: OEM

POSSIS MEDICAL, INC.   800-633-7231
100 Global View Drive, Warrendale, PA 15086   1 724-940-6800
FDA Number: 2183460   *Fax:* 1 412-767-4120
E-mail: info@medrad.com
Web site: www.possis.com
Medical Products Sales Volume: $66,654,592
Annual Revenue: $50-$100 Million
Year Founded: 1956
Total Employees: 269   *Marketing Staff:* 11   *Sales Staff:* 80
Ownership: Medrad, Inc.
Quality System Registration Information: ISO9001
Produces/Sells CE-marked Devices: Y
Distribution: Manufacturer Direct, Exporter
General Admin.: Robert G. Dutcher/President, Chief Executive Officer
         Irving R. Colacci/Vice President Legal Affairs, Corporate Counsel
Mktg./Adv.: John C. Riles/Director Marketing
         Bonnie Carney/Manager National Accounts
         Mr. Shawn McCarrey/Vice President Marketing & Sales
Production: Tim Anderson/Director Quality Assurance
         Pete Vaillant/Manager Materials
         Mark D. Stenoien/Manager Regulatory Affairs
         Robert J. Scott/Vice President Manufacturing Operations & Information Technology
Research: Eric Thor/Director Research
         James D. Gustafson/Senior Vice President Research & Development
Finance: Jules L. Fisher/Chief Financial Officer, Vice President Finance

Catheter, Continuous Flush	Cardiovascular
Catheter, Embolectomy (Fogarty Type)	Cardiovascular
Catheter, Intravascular Occluding, Temporary	Cardiovascular
Catheter, Peripheral, Atherectomy	Cardiovascular
Catheter, Thrombectomy	Cardiovascular

POST GLOVER LIFELINK   800-287-4123
167 Gap Way., Erlanger, KY 41018   859-283-5900
FDA Number: n/a   *Fax:* 859-372-6272
E-mail: judyk@pglifelink.com
Web site: www.pglifelink.com
Medical Products Sales Volume: $5,000,000
Annual Revenue: $5-$10 Million
Year Founded: 1957
Total Employees: 35   *Marketing Staff:* 2   *Sales Staff:* 4
Ownership: Private
Stock Symbol: halma
Traded On: London
Quality System Registration Information: ISO9000
Produces/Sells CE-marked Devices: N
Federal Procurement Eligibility: Small Business
Distribution: Manufacturer Direct, Manufacturer Through Distributor, Manufacturer Through Manufacturer Reps, Exporter
General Admin.: Ms. Judith Kathman/President
Production: Mr. Keith Van Kerckhove/Manager Engineering
         Mrs. Caroll Roden/Manager Quality Systems
         Mr. Glenn Coyle/Plant & Production Manager
Finance: Mr. Joseph Tanner/Vice President Finance

Headwall System (Patient Room)	General
Illuminator, Radiographic Film	Radiology
Isolation Unit, Surgical	General
Monitor, Line Isolation	Cardiovascular

POST MEDICAL, INC.   800-876-8678
226 Creekstone Ridge, Woodstock, GA 30188   770-928-4100
FDA Number: 1034525   *Fax:* 770-928-4949
E-mail: sales@postmedical.com
Web site: www.postmedical.com
Medical Products Sales Volume: $1,000,000
Annual Revenue: $1-$5 Million
Total Employees: 10   *Marketing Staff:* 3   *Sales Staff:* 3
Ownership: Private
Produces/Sells CE-marked Devices: N

POST MEDICAL, INC.
800-876-8678 *(cont'd)*
Federal Procurement Eligibility: Small Business
Distribution: Manufacturer Direct, Manufacturer Through Distributor, Exporter
General Admin.: Rip Thead/General Manager
   William Thead/President, Chief Executive Officer
Mktg./Adv.: Rip Thead/Director National Accounts
   Rip Thead/Director Product Development
   William Thead/Manager Advertising
   Rip Thead/Manager Contract Sales
   Bill Thead/Manager Market Research
   W. H. Thead/Vice President Business Development
   Rip Thead/Vice President Marketing & Sales
Production: Rip Thead/Director Quality Assurance
   Bill Thead/Manager Regulatory Affairs
   Rip Thead/Vice President Manufacturing
Research: Rip Thead/Vice President Research & Development

Needle, Hypodermic, Single Lumen With Syringe	General
Rack, Test Tube	Chemistry
Tray, Custom/Special Procedure	General
Waste Disposal Unit, Sharps	General
Waste Disposal Unit, Syringe	General

POSTCRAFT CO.
800-528-4844
625 W. Rillito St., Tucson, AZ 85705-5441 **520-624-2531**
FDA Number: n/a *Fax:* 520-884-0013
Web site: www.postcraft.com
Annual Revenue: $1-$5 Million
Total Employees: 23 *Marketing Staff:* 2 *Sales Staff:* 2
Ownership: Private
Produces/Sells CE-marked Devices: N
Federal Procurement Eligibility: Small Business
Distribution: Manufacturer Direct, Manufacturer Through Distributor, Exporter
General Admin.: Bruce S. Beyer/President, Chief Executive Officer
Mktg./Adv.: Andi L. Cross/Manager International & National Sales
   Donna M. Beyer/Vice President Marketing

Apron, Laboratory	Chemistry
Bib	General
Cover, Mattress	General
Cover, Mattress, Waterproof	General
Curtain, Cubicle	General
Curtain, Shower	General
Glove, Other	General
Glove, Utility	General

POSTURE DYNAMICS, INC.
732-278-2081
415 Jarob Court, Point Pleasant, NJ 08742
FDA Number: 2249161 *Fax:* 732-295-3304
E-mail: AJVB43@aol.com
Ownership: Private
Produces/Sells CE-marked Devices: N
Federal Procurement Eligibility: Small Business
General Admin.: Dr. Anthony Barone/President

Chair, Position, Electric	Physical Med
Orthosis, Lumbar	Physical Med

POSTURE PRO, INC.
714-847-8607
18584 Main Street, Beach Center, CA 92648
FDA Number: 3006990604
E-mail: sales@posturepro.com
Web site: www.posturepro.com
Ownership: Private
Produces/Sells CE-marked Devices: N

Traction Unit, Non-Powered	Orthopedics

POSTURIZER, INC.
631-399-4385
89 Lincoln Avenue, Mastic Beach, NY 11951-1619
FDA Number: 3004198501
Ownership: Private
Produces/Sells CE-marked Devices: N

Exerciser, Non-Measuring	Physical Med

POTTY MD, LLC
865-584-6700
6512 Baum Dr. Suite 14, Knoxville, TN 37919
FDA Number: 3005739654

Alarm, Enuresis	Gastroenterology/Urology

POWELL LABS
800-210-6549
480 Roe Avenue, Elmira, NY 14901 **607-732-1901**
FDA Number: 2438397 *Fax:* 607-732-1901
E-mail: jimpowell@infoblvd.net
Web site: www.powi.com
Ownership: Private
Produces/Sells CE-marked Devices: N
Distribution: Manufacturer Direct

Irrigator, Oral	Dental And Oral

POWELL PRODUCTS, INC.
800-840-9205
4940 Northpark Drive, **719-260-7887**
Colorado Springs, CO 80918
FDA Number: 1722647 *Fax:* 719-260-7885
E-mail: stephen@powellproducts.com
Web site: www.powellproducts.com
Medical Products Sales Volume: $5,700,000
Year Founded: 1959
Total Employees: 80 *Marketing Staff:* 2 *Sales Staff:* 3
Ownership: Private
Quality System Registration Information: ISO9001
Produces/Sells CE-marked Devices: N
Federal Procurement Eligibility: Small Business
Distribution: Manufacturer Direct, Manufacturer Through Distributor, OEM

Cultured Animal And Human Cells	Pathology
Swabs, Alcohol	General
Swabs, Antiseptic	General
Swabs, Oral Care	General
Swabs, Specimen Collection	General
Tip, Rubber, Oral-Hygiene	Dental And Oral

POWER MEDICAL INTERVENTIONS, INC.
267-775-8154
2021 Cabot Blvd., Langhorne, PA 19047
FDA Number: 2532140
Ownership: Public
Stock Symbol: PMII
Traded On: NASDAQ
Produces/Sells CE-marked Devices: N

Probe, Gastrointestinal	Gastroenterology/Urology
Staple, Implantable	Surgery

POWER PRODUCTS, INC.-SPLINTEK
816-531-1900
3325 Wyoming St., Kansas City, MO 64111
FDA Number: 3003460151

Mouthguard	Dental And Oral

POWER SWITCH CORPORATION
See Martek Power

POWERLUNG, INC.
713-465-1180
10690 Shadow Wood Dr., Suite 100, Houston, TX 77043
FDA Number: 3006084514

Exerciser, Non-Measuring	Physical Med

POWERS SCIENTIFIC, INC.
800-998-0500
PO Box 268, Pipersville, PA 18947 **215-230-7100**
FDA Number: 2531478
E-mail: info@powersscientific.com
Web site: www.powersscientific.com
Medical Products Sales Volume: $300,000
Annual Revenue: $1-$5 Million
Year Founded: 1984
Total Employees: 2
Ownership: Private
Federal Procurement Eligibility: Small Business
Distribution: Manufacturer Through Distributor
General Admin.: Gail Bartholomeow/Chief Executive Officer
Mktg./Adv.: Gail Bartholomeow/Manager Advertising
   Wendy Pappas/Marketing Officer
   Gail Bartholomeow/Vice President Marketing & Sales

Chamber, Constant Temperature (Environmental)	Microbiology
Incubator, Aerobic	Microbiology
Refrigerator, Laboratory	General

POWERVAR, INC.
800-369-7179
1450 Lakeside Drive, Waukegan, IL 60085 **847-596-7000**
FDA Number: n/a *Fax:* 847-596-7100
E-mail: info@powervar.com
Web site: www.powervar.com
Medical Products Sales Volume: $15,000,000
Annual Revenue: $25-$50 Million
Total Employees: 52 *Marketing Staff:* 2 *Sales Staff:* 5
Ownership: Private
Quality System Registration Information: ISO9001
Produces/Sells CE-marked Devices: Y
Federal Procurement Eligibility: Small Business
Distribution: Manufacturer Direct, Manufacturer Through Manufacturer Reps, OEM
General Admin.: Scot Moeller/Chief Operating Officer
   George Lannert/President, Chief Executive Officer
Mktg./Adv.: Tom Gornick/Manager National Sales
   Tom Gornick/Vice President International & National Sales
   Dennis Ver Mulm/Vice President Marketing

Power System, Isolated	General
Power Systems, Uninterruptible (UPS)	General

POWERWAY, INC.
800-964-9004
317-624-4000
429 N. Pennsylvania Street, Suite 400,
Indianapolis, IN 46204
FDA Number: n/a   Fax: 317-624-4040
E-mail: info@powerwayinc.com
Web site: www.powerwayinc.com
Medical Products Sales Volume: $25,900,000
Annual Revenue: $10-$25 Million
Year Founded: 1987
Total Employees: 300   *Marketing Staff:* 4   *Sales Staff:* 25
Ownership: Private
Quality System Registration Information: ISO9000; ISO9001
Produces/Sells CE-marked Devices: N
Federal Procurement Eligibility: Small Business
Distribution: Manufacturer Direct, Manufacturer Through Manufacturer Reps
General Admin.: Ted Wozniak/Chief Executive Officer
    Steve Scott/Chief Technology Officer
Mktg./Adv.: Jenna Martin/Director Marketing
    Jerry Abbott/Vice President International Sales
    Jerry Abbott/Vice President Sales
Production: Jodi Martz/Manager Materials
   Computer Software   General

PPDI/BUNTING DIV.
See Pdi Communication Systems

PPI-TIME ZERO INC.
973-278-6500
262 Buffalo Ave., Paterson, NJ 07503
FDA Number: 2244698
   Goniometer, AC-powered   Orthopedics
   Transmitter/Receiver System, Physiological, Telephone   Cardiovascular

PPR DIRECT, INC.
800-526-3668
718-965-8600
74 20th St., Brooklyn, NY 11232-1100
FDA Number: 7000706   Fax: 718-965-9729
Annual Revenue: $10-$25 Million
Total Employees: 48
Ownership: Private
Produces/Sells CE-marked Devices: N
Federal Procurement Eligibility: Small Business
Distribution: Manufacturer Direct
General Admin.: Leonard Feldman/President
Mktg./Adv.: Margaret Hickey/Manager Sales
    Larry Brown/Vice President Sales
   Disinfector, Liquid   General
   Exerciser, Other   Physical Med
   Pillow, Cervical   Orthopedics
   Stool, Bedside   General
   Support, Back   Orthopedics

PRACTICAL SYSTEMS, INC.
800-237-8154
727-376-7900
11617 Prospect Rd., Odessa, FL 33556
FDA Number: n/a   Fax: 800-330-3800
E-mail: gphpsi1@gate.net
Web site: www.practicalsystems.com
Annual Revenue: $5-$10 Million
Total Employees: 45   *Marketing Staff:* 1   *Sales Staff:* 7
Ownership: Private
Produces/Sells CE-marked Devices: N
Distribution: Manufacturer Direct
General Admin.: Patrick Hernandez/President
    Tom Smith/Vice President, General Manager
Production: Matthew Hernandez/Manager Operations
   Production Equipment   General

PRACTICAL THINGS, LLC.
310-951-6906
3267 East 3300 South,, Suite 105, Salt Lake City, UT 84109
FDA Number: 3004584997
Ownership: Private
Produces/Sells CE-marked Devices: N
   Head Rest, Neurosurgical   Cns/Neurology

PRACTICEWORKS SYSTEMS, LLC.
See Carestream Dental LLC

PRAIRIE LABS
952-908-7654
637 12th Ave., South, Hopkins, MN 55343
FDA Number: 2184059
   Hearing-Aid   Ear/Nose/Throat

PRAIRIE PRODUCTS, INC.
717-292-1089
4660 Raycom Rd.,, Industrial Park, Dover, PA 17315
FDA Number: 2522949
   Sunglasses (Including Photosensitive)   Ophthalmology

PRAXAIR DISTRIBUTION INC., SOUTHEAST LLC
440-234-1075
403 Zell Dr., Orlando, FL 32824
FDA Number: 1038820
   Gas, Calibrated (Specified Concentration)   Anesthesiology

PRAXAIR DISTRIBUTION INC., SOUTHEAST LLC
440-234-1075
(cont'd)
   Laser, Surgical   Surgery

PRAXAIR DISTRIBUTION MID-ATLANTIC LLC
610-695-7628
One Steel Rd. East, U.S. Industrial Park, Morrisville, PA 19067
FDA Number: 2523408
Annual Revenue: $5-$10 Million
Year Founded: 1973
Total Employees: 900   *Marketing Staff:* 15   *Sales Staff:* 90
Ownership: Private
Quality System Registration Information: ISO9001
Produces/Sells CE-marked Devices: N
Federal Procurement Eligibility: Small Business
Distribution: Manufacturer Direct
   Gas, Calibrated (Specified Concentration)   Anesthesiology
   Gas, GLC   Toxicology
   Gauge, Gas Pressure, Cylinder/Pipeline   Anesthesiology
   Laser, Surgical   Surgery
   Regulator, Pressure, Gas Cylinder   Anesthesiology
   Sterilizer, Ethylene-Oxide Gas   General

PRAXAIR DISTRIBUTION, INC.
(925) 439-1508
1930 Loveridge Rd., Pittsburg, CA 94565
FDA Number: 2911183
Ownership: Private
Produces/Sells CE-marked Devices: N
   Gas, Calibrated (Specified Concentration)   Anesthesiology

PRAXAIR DISTRIBUTION, INC.
1.800.PRAXAIR
1-716.879.4077
39 Old Ridgebury Road,
Danbury, CT 06810
FDA Number: 1648589   Fax: 1-716.879.2040
E-mail: info@praxair.com
Web site: www.praxair.com
Ownership: Private
Produces/Sells CE-marked Devices: N
   Gas, Calibrated (Specified Concentration)   Anesthesiology

PRAXAIR, INC.
800-PRAXAIR
716-879-4077
39 Old Ridgebury Rd., Danbury, CT 06810
FDA Number: n/a   Fax: 716-879-2040
Web site: www.praxair.com
Total Employees: 17000
Ownership: Private
Produces/Sells CE-marked Devices: N
Distribution: Manufacturer Direct, Manufacturer Through Distributor, OEM, Service Direct, Exclusive Distributor, Importer, Exporter
General Admin.: E. G. Hotard/President
   Medical Admin.: Bharat Kohli/Director Health Care
Mktg./Adv.: Paul Bilek/Vice President Marketing & Sales
Production: Bill Therrien/Vice President Manufacturing
   Sampler, Gas   Chemistry
   Stand, Gas Cylinder   Anesthesiology

PRAXAIR-PUERTO RICO
440-234-1075
Rt. 931 & 189, Gurabo, PR 00778
FDA Number: 2648972
   Gas, Calibrated (Specified Concentration)   Anesthesiology
   Incubator/Water Bath, Microbiology   Microbiology
   Laser, Surgical   Surgery

PRAXIS, LLC.
508-400-3969
1110 Washington St., Holliston, MA 01746
FDA Number: 1226596
Ownership: Private
Produces/Sells CE-marked Devices: N
   Adhesive, Soft Tissue Approximation   Surgery
   Device, Incontinence, Occlusion, Urethral   Gastroenterology/Urology

PRD, INC.
812-279-8885
747 Washboard Road, Springville, IN 47462
FDA Number: 3006365154   Fax: 812-279-3867
E-mail: PRD.Sales@prd-inc.com
Web site: www.spcmfg.com
Ownership: Private
Produces/Sells CE-marked Devices: N
   Speculum, Vaginal, Non-Metal   Obstetrics/Gynecology

PRE PAK PRODUCTS, INC.
800-544-7257
760-643-0390
4055 Oceanside Blvd., Suite L,
Oceanside, CA 92056
FDA Number: 2028658   Fax: 800-577-3725
E-mail: info@prepakproducts.com
Web site: www.prepakproducts.com
Medical Products Sales Volume: $1,800,000
Annual Revenue: $1-$5 Million
Year Founded: 1987
Total Employees: 11   *Marketing Staff:* 2   *Sales Staff:* 2

PRE PAK PRODUCTS, INC. 800-544-7257 *(cont'd)*

Ownership: Private
Produces/Sells CE-marked Devices: N
Federal Procurement Eligibility: Small Business
Distribution: Manufacturer Direct, Manufacturer Through Distributor, Service Direct
General Admin.: Jim Ray/Chief Executive Officer, Vice President Marketing
    Judy Ray/President
Mktg./Adv.: Jim Ray/Director Product Development
    Rebecca Myer/Manager International & National Sales
Production: Sheila Moore/Manager Customer Services
Finance: Carrie Gabel/Chief Financial Officer

Equipment, Therapy, Handicapped/Physical	Physical Med
Exerciser, Leg And Ankle	Physical Med
Exerciser, Non-Measuring	Physical Med
Exerciser, Other	Physical Med
Lotion, Skin Care	General
Support, Arm	Physical Med
Tubing, Other	General

PREAT CORP. 800-232-7732
2976 Long Valley Rd., P.O. Box 1030, 805-693-8666
Santa Ynez, CA 93460

FDA Number: 2918719 *Fax:* 805-693-8106
E-mail: info@preat.com
Web site: www.preat.com
Year Founded: 1980
Ownership: Private
Quality System Registration Information: ISO9001
Produces/Sells CE-marked Devices: N
Federal Procurement Eligibility: Small Business
Distribution: Manufacturer Direct, Manufacturer Through Distributor, Exclusive Distributor, Importer, Exporter

Attachment, Precision	Dental And Oral
Base, Denture, Relining, Repairing, Rebasing, Resin	Dental And Oral
Material, Impression	Dental And Oral

PRECEPT MEDICAL PRODUCTS, INC. 800-438-5827
370 Airport Road, PO Box 2400, 828-681-0209
Arden, NC 28704

FDA Number: 903882 *Fax:* 828-687-3605
E-mail: info@preceptmed.com
Web site: www.preceptmed.com
Annual Revenue: $25-$50 Million
Total Employees: 400
Ownership: Private
Produces/Sells CE-marked Devices: N
Federal Procurement Eligibility: Small Business
Distribution: Manufacturer Direct, Manufacturer Through Distributor, Manufacturer Through Manufacturer Reps, OEM, Exporter
General Admin.: John Sopcisak/Chief Executive Officer, Chief Financial Officer
    Michael Boyd/President
Mktg./Adv.: Vicki Careccia/Marketing Coordinator

Cap, Surgical	Surgery
Clothing, Protective	General
Coat, Laboratory	General
Cover, Shoe, Conductive	General
Drape, Surgical, Disposable	Surgery
Dress, Scrub, Disposable	Surgery
Gown, Isolation, Surgical	Surgery
Gown, Operating Room, Disposable	Surgery
Gown, Patient, Disposable	General
Mask, Surgical	Surgery
Pack, Surgical (Drape)	Surgery
Sheeting, Stretcher	General

PRECIMED
See GREATBATCH MEDICAL

PRECIOUS LIFE SAVING PRODUCTS, INC. 416-644-0011
101-200 Ronson Dr, Toronto M9W 5Z9 Canada

FDA Number: 9680958

Anti-Choke Device, Suction	Ear/Nose/Throat

PRECISA BALANCES USA INC. 877-PRE-CISA
540 Powder Springs St., Suite 8, 770-794-4450
Marietta, GA 30064

FDA Number: n/a *Fax:* 770-794-4639
E-mail: sales@precisausa.com
Web site: www.precisausa.com
Medical Products Sales Volume: $375,000
Annual Revenue: $0-$1 Million
Total Employees: 2
Ownership: Private
Quality System Registration Information: ISO9001
Produces/Sells CE-marked Devices: Y
Federal Procurement Eligibility: Small Business
Distribution: Manufacturer Direct, Manufacturer Through Manufacturer Reps, Service Direct
General Admin.: Victor Valles/President, Chief Executive Officer

PRECISA BALANCES USA INC. 877-PRE-CISA *(cont'd)*

Balance (General Use)	Chemistry
Balance, Analytical	Chemistry
Balance, Electronic	Chemistry
Balance, Semimicro (0.01 mg Accuracy)	Chemistry
Meter, pH, Portable	Chemistry

PRECISE DENTAL INTERNACIONAL S.A.C.V. 818-992-5333
925 Parque Cuzin Belenes Norte, Zapopan, Jalisoo Mexico

FDA Number: 9680728

Gutta Percha	Dental And Oral
Point, Paper, Endodontic	Dental And Oral

PRECISE OPTICS/PME, INC. 800-242-6604
239 S. Fehr Way, Bay Shore, NY 11706-1207 631-242-6600

FDA Number: 2429479 *Fax:* 631-242-4421
E-mail: info@preciseoptics.com
Year Founded: 1953
Total Employees: 30
Ownership: Private
Produces/Sells CE-marked Devices: N
Federal Procurement Eligibility: Small Business
Distribution: OEM
Mktg./Adv.: Robert Corso/Manager Marketing
Production: Glenn Corso/Manager Manufacturing

Camera, X-Ray, Fluorographic, Cine Or Spot	Radiology
Photofluoroscope (Cardiac Catheterization)	Radiology
Radiographic Unit, Digital	Radiology
Radiographic/Fluoroscopic Unit, Fixed	Radiology
Radiographic/Fluoroscopic Unit, Image-Intensified	Radiology
Radiographic/Fluoroscopic Unit, Special Procedure	Radiology
System, X-Ray, Mobile	Radiology
Tube, Image Amplifier, X-Ray	Radiology

PRECISE PLASTICS 814-474-5504
7700 Middle Rd., Fairview, PA 16415

FDA Number: 3001748889

Device, Anti-Snoring	Ear/Nose/Throat

PRECISION ACOUSTICS INDUSTRIES, INC. 212-986-6470
501 5th Ave., New York, NY 10017-6103

FDA Number: 2432246
Annual Revenue: $0-$1 Million
Total Employees: 6
Ownership: Private
Produces/Sells CE-marked Devices: N
Distribution: Manufacturer Direct
General Admin.: Michael Davis/President
Mktg./Adv.: Mark Davis/Vice President Marketing & Sales

Audiometer	Ear/Nose/Throat

PRECISION ASSEMBLY CORPORATION 973-664-9889
198 Green Pond Road, Rockaway, NJ 07866

FDA Number: 2248636 *Fax:* 973-538-5421
E-mail: sales@pac-adm.com
Web site: www.pac-adm.com
Annual Revenue: $1-$5 Million
Total Employees: 11
Ownership: Public
Stock Symbol: ADMT
Traded On: NASDAQ
Quality System Registration Information: ISO9001
Produces/Sells CE-marked Devices: Y
Federal Procurement Eligibility: Small Business
Distribution: Manufacturer Direct, Manufacturer Through Manufacturer Reps, Importer, Exporter
General Admin.: Thomas R. Petrie/President, Chief Executive Officer
Mktg./Adv.: Andre' Dimino/Vice President Business Development
Production: Randall Vlasak/Manager Regulatory Affairs

Column, Life Support (Electrical/Gas)	General
Computer, Patient Monitor	Anesthesiology
Contract R&D, Diagnostics	General

PRECISION BIOLOGIC, INC. 800-267-2796
140 Eileen Stubbs Avenue, 902-468-6422
Dartmouth, NS B3B 0 Canada

FDA Number: 8043599 *Fax:* 902-468-6421
E-mail: info@precisionbiologic.com
Web site: www.precisionbiologic.com
Year Founded: 1983
Total Employees: 28 *Marketing Staff:* 3 *Sales Staff:* 5
Ownership: Private
Quality System Registration Information: ISO9001
Produces/Sells CE-marked Devices: Y
Federal Procurement Eligibility: Small Business
Distribution: Manufacturer Direct, Manufacturer Through Manufacturer Reps, Exporter

PRECISION BIOMETRICS, INC.   650-508-2600
981-a Industrial Rd., San Carlos, CA 94070
FDA Number: 2950325
  Biofeedback Device   Cns/Neurology

PRECISION CAST PLASTIC PARTS, LLC.   530-241-5189
2278 Crescent Moon Dr., Redding, CA 96001
FDA Number: 3032870
  Audiometer   Ear/Nose/Throat

PRECISION CHARTS, INC.   800-645-5410
130 Wilbur Place, Dept. P.C., Bohemia, NY 11716   631-567-6100
FDA Number: 2433063   *Fax:* 631-567-6224
E-mail: info@pcicharts.com
Web site: www.pcicharts.com
Ownership: Private
Quality System Registration Information: ISO9001
Produces/Sells CE-marked Devices: N
Federal Procurement Eligibility: Small Business
Distribution: OEM
  Office Product   General
  Paper, Chart, Record, Medical   General
  Paper, Recording, Data   General
  Paper, Recording, ECG/EEG   General
  Recorder, Paper Chart   Cardiovascular

PRECISION CONVERTERS
See Brady Precision Converting, Llc

PRECISION DENTAL INT, INC.   818-992-1888
21361 Deering Ct., Canoga Park, CA 91304
FDA Number: 2022845
Ownership: Private
Produces/Sells CE-marked Devices: N
  Drill, Dental, Intraoral   Dental And Oral
  Holder, X-Ray Film   Dental And Oral
  Mirror, Mouth   Dental And Oral
  Post, Root Canal   Dental And Oral

PRECISION DENTAL LABORATORIES, INC.   701-280-9089
6 Broadway Suite 200, Fargo, ND 58102
FDA Number: 3003616146
  Device, Anti-Snoring   Ear/Nose/Throat

PRECISION DYNAMICS CORP.   800-772-1122
13880 Del Sur St., San Fernando, CA 91340-3440   818-897-1111
FDA Number: 2020282   *Fax:* 818-899-4045
E-mail: info@pdcorp.com
Web site: www.pdcorp.com
Medical Products Sales Volume: $50,000,000
Annual Revenue: $50-$100 Million
Year Founded: 1956
Total Employees: 550   *Marketing Staff:* 50
Ownership: Private
Quality System Registration Information: ISO9001
Produces/Sells CE-marked Devices: Y
Federal Procurement Eligibility: Small Business
Distribution: Manufacturer Through Distributor
General Admin.: Gary Hutchinson/President, Chief Executive Officer
Mktg./Adv.: Scott Hirst/Director Marketing
          Daniel Hobin/Director Marketing & Communications
          Chuck Hugues/Director Sales
          Nick Curtin/Vice President Marketing & Sales
          Robin Barber/Vice President Sales
Production: Hosmel Galan/Vice President Operations
  Amniotome   Obstetrics/Gynecology
  Bag, Body   General
  Bag, Collection, Urine, Newborn   General
  Bag, Drainage (Incontinence)   Gastroenterology/Urology
  Bag, Leg   Gastroenterology/Urology
  Bracelet, Identification   General
  Clamp, Umbilical   Obstetrics/Gynecology
  Collector, Urine, Disposable   Gastroenterology/Urology
  Cover, Arm Board   General
  Cover, Mattress, Waterproof   General
  Cover, Other   General
  Labware, Basic, Disposable   Chemistry
  Marker, Skin   Surgery
  Perforator, Amniotic Membrane   Obstetrics/Gynecology
  Splint, Other   Orthopedics
  Splint, Pneumatic   Orthopedics
  Tray, Impression, Foot   Orthopedics

PRECISION ELECTROLYSIS NEEDLES, INC.   800-206-7771
166 Bay Spring Ave., Barrington, RI 02806   401-246-1155
FDA Number: 1221892
E-mail: uniprobeorders@aol.com
Web site: www.uniprobe.com
Ownership: Private
Produces/Sells CE-marked Devices: N

PRECISION ELECTROLYSIS NEEDLES, INC.   800-206-7771
(cont'd)
  Epilator, High-Frequency, Needle-Type   Surgery

PRECISION FABRICS GROUP, INC.   888-733-5759
301 E. Meadowview Rd., Forest Oaks, NC 27406
FDA Number: 1066748
Ownership: Private
Produces/Sells CE-marked Devices: N
  Cover, Mattress   General
  Fiber, Absorbent   General

PRECISION FABRICS GROUP, INC.   888-733-5759
323 Virginia Ave., Vinton, VA 24179
FDA Number: 1126193
Ownership: Private
Produces/Sells CE-marked Devices: N
  Cover, Mattress   General

PRECISION INSTRUMENTS, INC.
See Performance Orthopedics

PRECISION LABORATORIES, INC.   800-327-4792
830 Sunshine Ln., Altamonte Springs, FL 32714   407-774-8022
FDA Number: 1043599   *Fax:* 407-774-8133
E-mail: info@precisionweb.com
Web site: www.precisionweb.com
Medical Products Sales Volume: $1,900,000
Total Employees: 25
Federal Procurement Eligibility: Small Business
  Hearing-Aid   Ear/Nose/Throat

PRECISION MEDICAL DEVICES, INC.   717-795-9480
5020 Ritter Rd., Ste. #211, Mechanicsburg, PA 17055
FDA Number: 2523013   *Fax:* 717-795-9468
E-mail: weverhart@precisionmd.com
Annual Revenue: $1-$5 Million
Year Founded: 1983
Total Employees: 10
Ownership: Private
Quality System Registration Information: ISO9001
Produces/Sells CE-marked Devices: N
Federal Procurement Eligibility: Small Business
Distribution: Manufacturer Through Manufacturer Reps, OEM
General Admin.: Harvey Muskat/Chief Financial Officer, Treasurer
          Peter Sayet/President, Chief Executive Officer
          Francisco Tejada/Vice President
Production: Lloyd Sutherland/Chief Engineer
  Component, Traction, Invasive   Orthopedics
  Dispenser, Cement   Orthopedics
  Mixing Equipment, Cement   Orthopedics
  Syringe, Piston   General

PRECISION MEDICAL MANUFACTURING CORPORATION   866-633-4626
852 SETON CT., WHEELING, IL 60090   847-229-1551
FDA Number: 1416666   *Fax:* 847-229-1511
E-mail: kris@precisionmm.com
Web site: www.precisionmm.com
Year Founded: 1914
Total Employees: 15   *Marketing Staff:* 2   *Sales Staff:* 1
Ownership: Private
Produces/Sells CE-marked Devices: N
Federal Procurement Eligibility: Small Business
Distribution: Manufacturer Through Distributor
General Admin.: Mrs. Janice Polites/Chief Executive Officer
  Adenotome   Ear/Nose/Throat
  Anoscope, Non-Powered   Gastroenterology/Urology
  Curette   Orthopedics
  Dilator, Esophageal (Metal Olive) Gastro-Urology   Gastroenterology/Urology
  Holder, Head, Neurosurgical (Skull Clamp)   Cns/Neurology
  Mallet, Bone   Orthopedics
  Osteotome, Manual (Plastic Surgery)   Surgery
  Rack, Surgical Instrument   Surgery
  Retractor, Abdominal   Surgery
  Retractor, Manual   Cns/Neurology
  Retractor, Other   Surgery
  Retractor, Surgical   Surgery
  Retractor, Vaginal   Obstetrics/Gynecology
  Ring, Laparotomy   Gastroenterology/Urology
  Snare, Tonsil   Ear/Nose/Throat
  Speculum, Vaginal, Metal   Obstetrics/Gynecology
  Surgical Instrument, Cardiovascular   Cardiovascular

PRECISION MEDICAL PRODUCTS, INC.   717-335-3700
44 Denver Road, PO Box 300, Denver, PA 17517
FDA Number: 2531321   *Fax:* 717-335-0007
E-mail: contactpmp@precmed.net
Web site: www.pmp.net

PRECISION MEDICAL PRODUCTS, INC.　717-335-3700 *(cont'd)*
　Medical Products Sales Volume: $13,400,000
　Annual Revenue: $10-$25 Million
　Year Founded: 1997
　Total Employees: 140
　Ownership: Private
　Quality System Registration Information: ISO9002
　Produces/Sells CE-marked Devices: N
　Federal Procurement Eligibility: Small Business
　Distribution: Manufacturer Direct, OEM
　General Admin.: Douglas N. Yocom/President, Chief Executive Officer
　Production: Mr. Robert Rhoads Jr./Vice President Manufacturing

Component, Metal, Other	General
Component, Plastic	General
Contract Assembly	General
Contract Manufacturing	General
Contract Manufacturing, Product, Disposable	General
Contract Manufacturing, Product, Durable	General
Contract Packaging	General
Molding, Custom	General
Needle, Hypodermic	General
Packaging, Sterilization	General
Service, Engineering/Design	General
Tray, Custom/Special Procedure	General

PRECISION MEDICAL TECHNOLOGIES　574-267-6385
2059 N. Pound Dr., Warsaw, IN 46582
　FDA Number: 1835296　Fax: (574) 268-9240
　E-mail: info@premedtec.com
　Ownership: Private
　Produces/Sells CE-marked Devices: N

Orthopedic Manual Surgical Instrument	Orthopedics

PRECISION MEDICAL, INC.　800-272-7285
300 Held Drive, Northampton, PA 18067　610-262-6090
　FDA Number: 2523148　Fax: 610-262-6080
　E-mail: info@precisionmedical.com
　Web site: www.precisionmedical.com
　Medical Products Sales Volume: $9,800,000
　Annual Revenue: $10-$25 Million
　Year Founded: 1981
　Total Employees: 104　*Marketing Staff:* 2　*Sales Staff:* 8
　Ownership: Private
　Quality System Registration Information: ISO9001
　Produces/Sells CE-marked Devices: Y
　Federal Procurement Eligibility: Small Business, GSA Contract, VA Contract
　Distribution: Manufacturer Direct, Manufacturer Through Distributor, Manufacturer Through Manufacturer Reps, OEM, Exporter
　General Admin.: Mike Krupa/President
　　　　　Clyde Shuman/Vice President
　Mktg./Adv.: Tim Clark/Executive Director Marketing & Sales
　　　　　Tim Clark/Manager International Sales
　　　　　Tim Clark/Manager National Sales
　　　　　Tim Clark/Vice President Sales
　Production: Jim Parker/Director Quality Assurance
　　　　　John Ondush/Manager Materials

Alarm, Breathing Circuit	Anesthesiology
Compressor, Air, Portable	Anesthesiology
Fitting, Quick Connect (Gas Connector)	General
Fixation Device, Tracheal Tube	Anesthesiology
Flowmeter, Back-Pressure Compensated, Thorpe Tube	Anesthesiology
Gauge, Gas Pressure, Cylinder/Pipeline	Anesthesiology
Humidifier, Non-Heated	Anesthesiology
Humidifier, Respiratory Gas, (Direct Patient Interface)	Anesthesiology
Pump, Aspiration, Portable	Anesthesiology
Pump, Nebulizer, Electric	Ear/Nose/Throat
Regulator, Pressure, Gas Cylinder	Anesthesiology
Regulator, Vacuum	General
Support, Breathing Tube	Anesthesiology
Valve, Switching (Ploss)	Anesthesiology

PRECISION METAL PRODUCTS INC.　619-448-2711
850 West Bradley Ave., El Cajon, CA 92020
　FDA Number: n/a　Fax: 619-448-2005
　E-mail: sales@pmp-elcajon.com
　Web site: www.pmp-elcajon.com/
　Year Founded: 1963
　Ownership: Private
　Produces/Sells CE-marked Devices: N

PRECISION METAL SERVICES, INC.　800-635-4885
418 Stump Road, Montgomeryville, PA 18936　215-661-0225
　FDA Number: n/a　Fax: 215-661-0366
　E-mail: pms@precisionmetalservices.com
　Web site: www.precisionmetalservices.com
　Year Founded: 1975
　Total Employees: 5
　Ownership: Private
　Quality System Registration Information: ISO9001

PRECISION METAL SERVICES, INC.　800-635-4885 *(cont'd)*
　Produces/Sells CE-marked Devices: N
　Distribution: OEM, Importer, Exporter
　General Admin.: James J. Noonan/Executive Vice President
　　　　　Mark L. Payton/Import Manager
　　　　　Martin J. Payton/President
　　　　　Martin J. Payton/Vice President
　　　　　Rick Robie/Warehouse Manager
　Mktg./Adv.: Arlene King/Account Executive
　　　　　Sergey V. Gorbachev/Marketing Coordinator
　　　　　Bill King/Sales Manager
　　　　　Cesar Martinez/Sales Manager
　　　　　Don Payton/Sales Specialist
　Production: Richard C. Robie/Quality Control Manager/Traffic Manager
　　　　　Ray Coniglio/Vice President Operations
　Finance: Kathryn H. Rogers/Controller
　Purchasing: Sharon A. McElwee/Purchasing Manager/Sales Coordinator

Component, Metal, Other	General

PRECISION MICROCURRENT, INC.　503-443-6100
705 S.springbrook Rd., Bld.a-135, Newberg, OR 97132
　FDA Number: 2028697

Stimulator, Nerve, Transcutaneous (Pain Relief, TENS)	Cns/Neurology

PRECISION OPTICAL CO. INC.
　See H.L. Bouton Co., Inc.

PRECISION OPTICAL PRODUCTS　866-472-4436
4950 Waring Rd., Suite 2a, San Diego, CA 92120
　FDA Number: 2021370　Fax: 888-951-5627
　E-mail: info@popsandiego.com
　Web site: www.popsandiego.com
　Ownership: Private
　Produces/Sells CE-marked Devices: N

Lens, Spectacle/Eyeglasses, Non-Custom	Ophthalmology

PRECISION OPTICS CORP.　800-447-2812 Ex
22 E. Broadway, Gardner, MA 01440-3338　978-630-1800
　FDA Number: 1222616　Fax: 978-630-1487
　E-mail: info@poci.com
　Web site: www.poci.com
　Total Employees: 30　*Marketing Staff:* 2　*Sales Staff:* 2
　Ownership: Public
　Stock Symbol: POCI
　Traded On: OTC Bulletin
　Quality System Registration Information: ISO9001
　Produces/Sells CE-marked Devices: N
　Federal Procurement Eligibility: Small Business
　Distribution: Manufacturer Through Distributor, OEM
　General Admin.: Richard E. Forkey/President
　Mktg./Adv.: Chuck Gerlowski/Director Business Development

Accessories, Photographic, Endoscopic	Gastroenterology/Urology
Arthroscope	Orthopedics
Contract Manufacturing	General
Coupler, Optical, Laparoscopic	General
Endoscope	Gastroenterology/Urology
Endoscope, Fiberoptic	Surgery
Laparoscope, General & Plastic Surgery	Surgery
Laryngoscope	Ear/Nose/Throat
Mirror, Mouth	Dental And Oral
Nasopharyngoscope (Flexible Or Rigid)	Ear/Nose/Throat
Ophthalmoscope, Battery-Powered	Ophthalmology
Otoscope	Ear/Nose/Throat
Service, Engineering/Design	General
Speculum, Illuminated	Surgery

PRECISION PLASTIC MOLDING, INC.　865-982-5552
28035 Hwy. 31 North, Jemison, AL 35085
　FDA Number: 3004775225

Booth, Sun Tan	Physical Med

PRECISION POLYMER PRODUCTS　610-326-0921
815 South St., Pottstown, PA 19464
　FDA Number: n/a　Fax: 610-327-6267
　E-mail: contact@precisionpolymer.com
　Web site: www.precisionpolymer.com
　Ownership: Private
　Quality System Registration Information: ISO9001
　Produces/Sells CE-marked Devices: N
　Federal Procurement Eligibility: Small Business
　Distribution: OEM
　General Admin.: Joe Voytilla/Chief Executive Officer
　　　　　Susan J. Rufibach/General Manager

Component, Rubber	General
Component, Silicone	General
Contract Manufacturing	General
Molding, Custom	General

PRECISION PRODUCTION, INC.   216-252-0372
15215 Chatfield Ave., Cleveland, OH 44111
FDA Number: n/a   *Fax:* 216-252-6056
E-mail: sales@precisionproduction.com
Web site: www.precisionproduction.com
Ownership: Private
Produces/Sells CE-marked Devices: N
  Contract Manufacturing   General

PRECISION PRODUCTS, INC.   800-220-9221
681 North Varnell Rd., Tunnel Hill, GA 30755   **706-673-6900**
FDA Number: 3004824912   *Fax:* 706-673-9304
E-mail: sales@ppiparts.com
Web site: www.ppiparts.com
Ownership: Private
Produces/Sells CE-marked Devices: N
  Retractor, Surgical   Surgery

PRECISION PROSTHETICS & ORTHOTICS, INC.   314-843-3339
11102 S.lindbergh Business Ct., St. Louis, MO 63123
FDA Number: 3003460137
Ownership: Private
Produces/Sells CE-marked Devices: N
  Orthosis, Cranial   Cns/Neurology

PRECISION QUINCY CORP.   800-338-0079
1625 W. Lake Shore Drive, Woodstock, IL 60098   **815-338-2675**
FDA Number: n/a   *Fax:* 815-338-2960
E-mail: pqsales@precisionquincy.com
Web site: www.precisionquincy.com
Medical Products Sales Volume: $19,100,000
Annual Revenue: $10-$25 Million
Year Founded: 1960
Total Employees: 85   *Marketing Staff:* 2   *Sales Staff:* 7
Ownership: Private
Produces/Sells CE-marked Devices: N
Federal Procurement Eligibility: Small Business
Distribution: Manufacturer Direct, Manufacturer Through Manufacturer Reps, OEM, Service Direct, Exporter
General Admin.: John Guanci/President, Chief Executive Officer
Mktg./Adv.: Jami Switzer/Manager Advertising & Public Relations
        Wayne Stanek/Vice President Sales
  Oven   Chemistry
  Waste Receptacle, Contaminated   General

PRECISION REHABILITATION INC.   800-895-5891
4 Cataraqui St., Ste. 316, Suite 316,   **613-541-7838**
Kingston, ONT K7K-1 Canada
FDA Number: n/a   *Fax:* 613-541-7838
Year Founded: 1990
Total Employees: 10
Ownership: Private
Produces/Sells CE-marked Devices: N
Distribution: Exclusive Distributor

PRECISION SCLERO   727-517-0729
12408 Chickasaw Trail, Largo, FL 33774
FDA Number: 3004471697
  Adapter, Holder, Syringe   Physical Med

PRECISION SURGICAL INTL., INC.   800-776-8493
PO Box 726, Noblesville, IN 46061   **317-776-3843**
FDA Number: 1834268   *Fax:* 317-776-3826
E-mail: sales@psint.net
Web site: www.psint.net
Medical Products Sales Volume: $500,000
Annual Revenue: $0-$1 Million
Year Founded: 1993
Total Employees: 3
Ownership: Private
Produces/Sells CE-marked Devices: N
Federal Procurement Eligibility: Small Business
General Admin.: Mr. Mike Kseniak/President, Owner
  Cutter, Surgical   Surgery
  Forceps, General & Plastic Surgery   Surgery
  General Use Surgical Scissors   Surgery
  Handle, Scalpel   Surgery
  Hemostat   Orthopedics
  Holder, Needle   Gastroenterology/Urology
  Retractor, Surgical   Surgery
  Scissors, Ophthalmic   Ophthalmology
  Scissors, Wire Cutting, ENT   Ear/Nose/Throat

PRECISION SYSTEMS, INC.   508-655-7010
16 Tech Circle, Natick, MA 01760-1029
FDA Number: 1250003   *Fax:* 508-653-6999
E-mail: precisionsystems@msn.com
Web site: www.nbizz.com/precisionsystemsinc

PRECISION SYSTEMS, INC.   508-655-7010 *(cont'd)*
Medical Products Sales Volume: $2,000,000
Year Founded: 1964
Total Employees: 25   *Marketing Staff:* 4   *Sales Staff:* 4
Ownership: Private
Produces/Sells CE-marked Devices: N
Federal Procurement Eligibility: Small Business
Distribution: Manufacturer Direct, Manufacturer Through Distributor, OEM, Exporter
General Admin.: Charles A. Bell/President, Chief Executive Officer
Production: Robert Atwood/Vice President Manufacturing
  Computer, Chemistry Analyzer   Chemistry
  Dialysis Unit Test Equipment   Gastroenterology/Urology
  Osmometer   Chemistry
  Standard/Control, All Types   Chemistry

PREDICTIVE BIOSCIENCES   781-402-1780
128 Spring Street, 400 Level, B Annex, Lexington,, MA 02421
FDA Number: n/a   *Fax:* 781-402-1785
E-mail: info@predictivebiosci.com
Web site: http://www.predictivebiosci.com
Year Founded: 2006
Ownership: Private
Produces/Sells CE-marked Devices: N
General Admin.: Mr. Anthony Shuber/Chief Technology Officer
      Dr. Peter Klemm/President, Chief Executive Officer
Mktg./Adv.: Mr. Eugene Chiu/Vice President Commercial Operations
      Dr. Andy Hu/Vice President Strategic Planning
Finance: Mr. Vikram Lamba/Chief Financial Officer

PREEMINENT, LLC   925989-0977
1440 Maria Ln., Suite 250, Walnut Creek, CA 94596
FDA Number: 3004361489
Ownership: Private
Produces/Sells CE-marked Devices: N
  Traction Unit, Non-Powered   Orthopedics

PREFERRED MEDICAL PRODUCTS   800-441-1161
PO Box 100, Ducktown, TN 37326   **423-496-3738**
FDA Number: 1038913   *Fax:* 423-496-3758
E-mail: wandas@preferred-medical.com
Web site: www.preferred-medical.com
Medical Products Sales Volume: $2,600,000
Year Founded: 1991
Total Employees: 45
Ownership: Private
Produces/Sells CE-marked Devices: N
Federal Procurement Eligibility: Small Business
Distribution: Manufacturer Direct
General Admin.: Mrs. J. Randall Pittman/Chief Executive Officer
      Mr. J. Ryan Pittman/General Manager
  Cover, Camera   Surgery
  Cover, Other   General
  Cover, Probe, Transducer   Surgery
  Drape, Surgical, Disposable   Surgery

PREFERRED SOLUTIONS, LLC   757-224-0177
467 Swan Ave., Hohenwald, TN 38462
FDA Number: 3006396266
  Adaptor, Dressing   Physical Med

PREISER SCIENTIFIC, INC.   800-624-8285
94 Oliver St., P.O. Box 1330,   **304-727-2902**
St. Albans, WV 25177
FDA Number: n/a   *Fax:* 304-727-2932
E-mail: preiser@preiser.com
Web site: www.preiser.com
Medical Products Sales Volume: $250,000
Annual Revenue: $5-$10 Million
Year Founded: 1924
Total Employees: 42   *Marketing Staff:* 10   *Sales Staff:* 10
Ownership: Private
Quality System Registration Information: ISO9001
Produces/Sells CE-marked Devices: N
Federal Procurement Eligibility: Small Business
Distribution: Manufacturer Direct, Manufacturer Through Distributor, Manufacturer Through Manufacturer Reps, Service Direct, Exclusive Distributor, Importer, Exporter
General Admin.: G. Preiser/Chief Executive Officer
      A. E. Preiser/President
      J. Gatens/Vice President, General Manager
Mktg./Adv.: J. Gatens/Director National Accounts
      K. Westfall/Director Product Development
      A. E. Preiser/Manager Advertising & Market Research
      C. Cline/Manager International & National Sales
      John Gatens/Manager National Sales
      S. Lette/Manager Sales Training
      J. Gatens/Vice President Business Development

MANUFACTURER PROFILES

PREISER SCIENTIFIC, INC.   800-624-8285 *(cont'd)*
Production: D. Meddings/Director Quality Assurance & Regulatory Affairs
K. Westfall/Manager Materials

Balance, Analytical	Chemistry
Calorimeter	Chemistry
Forceps, Biopsy, Electric	Gastroenterology/Urology
Furnace, Porcelain	Dental And Oral

Medical Product Subsidiaries (Listed Separately)
Standard Instrumentation, Div. Preiser Scientific

PREMIER BRANDS OF AMERICA, INC.   914-667-6200
31 South Street, Mount Vernon, NY 10550
FDA Number: 2434554   *Fax:* 914-662-3610
Ownership: Private
Produces/Sells CE-marked Devices: N

Bandage, Adhesive	Surgery
Dusting Powder, Surgical	Surgery
Protector, Skin Pressure	General

PREMIER DENTAL PRODUCTS CO.   888-670-6100
1710 Romano Dr., Plymouth Meeting, PA 19462   **610-239-6000**
FDA Number: 2511556   *Fax:* 610-239-6100
E-mail: dentalinfo@premusa.com
Web site: www.premusa.com
Year Founded: 1913
Total Employees: 110   *Sales Staff:* 35
Ownership: Private
Produces/Sells CE-marked Devices: N
Federal Procurement Eligibility: Small Business
Distribution: Manufacturer Through Manufacturer Reps
General Admin.: Gary Charlestein/Chief Executive Officer
Jack Ruppel/President

Agent, Polishing, Abrasive, Oral Cavity	Dental And Oral
Brush, Dermabrasion	Surgery
Burnisher, Operative, Dental	Dental And Oral
Carrier, Amalgam, Operative	Dental And Oral
Carver, Dental Amalgam, Operative	Dental And Oral
Carver, Wax, Dental	Dental And Oral
Cement, Dental	Dental And Oral
Chisel, Bone, Surgical	Dental And Oral
Condenser, Amalgam And Foil, Operative	Dental And Oral
Cord, Retraction	Dental And Oral
Cotton, Roll	Dental And Oral
Cryosurgical Unit	Surgery
Cup, Prophylaxis	Dental And Oral
Curette, Endodontic	Dental And Oral
Curette, Operative	Dental And Oral
Curette, Periodontic	Dental And Oral
Curette, Surgical, Dental	Dental And Oral
Cutter, Operative	Dental And Oral
Driver, Band, Orthodontic	Dental And Oral
Electrosurgical Unit, Cutting & Coagulation Device	Surgery
Elevator, Surgical, Dental	Dental And Oral
Excavator, Dental, Operative	Dental And Oral
Explorer, Operative	Dental And Oral
File, Bone, Surgical	Dental And Oral
File, Margin Finishing, Operative	Dental And Oral
Filling, Instrument Plastic, Dental	Dental And Oral
Forceps, Articulation Paper	Dental And Oral
Forceps, Rongeur, Surgical	Dental And Oral
Forceps, Rubber Dam Clamp	Dental And Oral
Forceps, Tooth Extractor, Surgical	Dental And Oral
Hand Instrument, Calculus Removal	Dental And Oral
Handle, Instrument, Dental	Dental And Oral
Hemostat, Surgical	Dental And Oral
Hoe, Periodontic	Dental And Oral
Holder, Needle, Other	Surgery
Instrument, Diamond, Dental	Dental And Oral
Knife, Margin Finishing, Operative	Dental And Oral
Knife, Periodontic	Dental And Oral
Mallet, Surgical, General & Plastic Surgery	Surgery
Marker, Periodontic	Dental And Oral
Material, Tooth Shade, Resin	Dental And Oral
Pessary, Vaginal	Obstetrics/Gynecology
Pliers, Operative	Dental And Oral
Plugger, Root Canal, Endodontic	Dental And Oral
Probe, Periodontic	Dental And Oral
Pusher, Band, Orthodontic	Dental And Oral
Remover, Crown	Dental And Oral
Retainer, Matrix	Dental And Oral
Retractor, All Types	Dental And Oral
Scaler, Periodontic	Dental And Oral
Scissors, Collar And Crown	Dental And Oral
Scissors, Surgical Tissue, Dental (Oral)	Dental And Oral
Sealant, Pit And Fissure, And Conditioner, Resin	Dental And Oral
Setter, Band, Orthodontic	Dental And Oral
Spreader, Pulp Canal Filling Material, Endodontic	Dental And Oral
Teeth, Porcelain	Dental And Oral
Tooth Bonding Agent, Resin Restoration	Dental And Oral
Tray, Impression	Dental And Oral
Varnish, Cavity	Dental And Oral

PREMIER DENTAL PRODUCTS CO.   888-670-6100 *(cont'd)*
Warmer, Anesthesia Tube	Dental And Oral

Medical Product Subsidiaries (Listed Separately)
Premier Medical Products

PREMIER HEART, LLC.   888-380-8338
110 Main Street, Suite 201-88,   **516-883-3383**
Port Washington, NY 11050
FDA Number: n/a   *Fax:* 516-883-5812
E-mail: info@premierheart.com
Web site: http://www.premierheart.com
Ownership: Private
Produces/Sells CE-marked Devices: N

Computer, Diagnostic, Programmable	Cardiovascular

PREMIER MEDICAL PRODUCTS   888-PREMUSA
1710 Romano Dr., Plymouth Meeting, PA 19462   **610-239-6000**
FDA Number: 2521453   *Fax:* 610-239-6171
E-mail: medinfo@premusa.com
Web site: www.premusa.com
Year Founded: 1980
Ownership: Private
Quality System Registration Information: ISO9001
Produces/Sells CE-marked Devices: Y
Federal Procurement Eligibility: Small Business
Distribution: Manufacturer Through Distributor
General Admin.: Gary Charlestein/Chief Executive Officer
Jack Ruppel/President
Kevin Brown/Vice President
Mktg./Adv.: Toni Banet/Admin. Marketing

Adapter, Needle	Cardiovascular
Cannula, Insufflation, Uterine	Obstetrics/Gynecology
Cannula, Suction, Uterine	Obstetrics/Gynecology
Clipper, Nail	General
Container, Liquid Nitrogen	Anesthesiology
Cryosurgical Unit	Surgery
Curette, Ear	Ear/Nose/Throat
Curette, Suction, Endometrial	Obstetrics/Gynecology
Curette, Uterine	Obstetrics/Gynecology
Dilator, Uterine	Obstetrics/Gynecology
Electrode, Other	General
Electrosurgical Equipment, General Purpose	Surgery
Electrosurgical Unit, Cutting & Coagulation Device	Surgery
Equipment, Cleaning, Air	General
Forceps, Biopsy, Gynecological	Obstetrics/Gynecology
Hook, IUD Removal	Obstetrics/Gynecology
Instrument, Diamond, Dental	Dental And Oral
Instrument, Electrosurgery, Laparoscopic	Surgery
Pessary, Vaginal	Obstetrics/Gynecology
Punch, Biopsy	Gastroenterology/Urology
Retractor, Vaginal	Obstetrics/Gynecology
Scissors, Suture	Surgery
Sound, Uterine	Obstetrics/Gynecology
Speculum, Vaginal, Metal	Obstetrics/Gynecology
System, Evacuation, Smoke, Laser	Surgery
Tenaculum, Uterine	Obstetrics/Gynecology

PREMIER RESEARCH   215-282-5500
1500 Market Street, Suite 3500, Philadelphia, PA 19102
FDA Number: n/a   *Fax:* 215-282-5528
E-mail: info@premier-research.com
Ownership: Private
Produces/Sells CE-marked Devices: N

PREMIERE BIOMEDICAL, INC.
See Toray International America Inc.

PREMIUM LATEX PRODUCTS, INC.
See Bio-Flex International, Inc.

PRENATAL CRADLE, INC.   800-383-3068
P O BOX 443, Hamburg, MI 48139-0443   **989-386-6038**
FDA Number: 1834182   *Fax:* 989-386-6020
E-mail: prenatal@prenatalcradle.com
Web site: www.aboutbabiesinc.com
Ownership: Private
Produces/Sells CE-marked Devices: N
Federal Procurement Eligibility: Small Business
Distribution: Manufacturer Direct

Orthosis, Thoracic	Physical Med

PRENTKE ROMICH COMPANY   800-262-1984
1022 Heyl Road, Wooster, OH 44691   **800-262-1933**
FDA Number: 1526550   *Fax:* 330-263-4829
E-mail: info@prentrom.com
Web site: www.prentrom.com
Medical Products Sales Volume: $17,500,000
Annual Revenue: $10-$25 Million
Year Founded: 1966
Total Employees: 90   *Marketing Staff:* 8   *Sales Staff:* 24

PRENTKE ROMICH COMPANY   800-262-1984 (cont'd)
Ownership: Private
Produces/Sells CE-marked Devices: Y
Federal Procurement Eligibility: Small Business
Distribution: Manufacturer Direct
General Admin.: Heidi McCullough/Admin. Human Resources
    Barry Romich/Chief Executive Officer
    Dave Moffatt/President, Chief Operating Officer
Mktg./Adv.: Lisa Fannin/Manager Advertising
    Rod McMichael/Manager Contracts
    Cherie Weaver/Manager Market Research
    Lisa Maynard/Manager Sales Training
Production: Dan Widmer/Director Manufacturing
    Steve Bucher/Director Quality Assurance
    Mark Dodez/Manager Materials
Research: Marvin Indermuhle/Vice President Research & Development & Production
Finance: Jan Hughes/Director Finance

Aid, Control, Environmental, Controlled, Breath	Physical Med
Amplifier, Voice	Ear/Nose/Throat
Communication Equipment	General
Computer Software	General

PREPARED MEDIA LABORATORY INC
See Pml Microbiologicals

PRESCIENT MEDICAL INC.   866-376-0500
2005 S. Easton Rd., Suite 204,   **205-933-1150**
Doylestown, PA 18901
FDA Number: n/a   *Fax:* 205-933-1149
E-mail: info@prescientmedical.com
Web site: www.prescientmedical.com
Year Founded: 2004
Ownership: Private
Produces/Sells CE-marked Devices: N
General Admin.: Patricia Scheller/Chief Executive Officer
    James Brennan III/Chief Scientific Officer
    Michele Frank/General Counsel
    Ilana Odess/General Manager
Production: Dennis Genito/Vice President Regulatory Affairs
Finance: Scott Durbin/Chief Financial Officer

PRESCO-WEBBER CORPORATION   336-722-1067
440 Cotton St., Winston Salem, NC 27101-5071
FDA Number: 7000701   *Fax:* 336-748-8546
E-mail: batomlinson@earthlink.net
Web site: www.presco-webber.com
Medical Products Sales Volume: $300,000
Annual Revenue: $0-$1 Million
Total Employees: 8
Ownership: Private
Federal Procurement Eligibility: Small Business
Distribution: Manufacturer Through Distributor
General Admin.: Vicki Tomlinson/Chairman
    Brent A. Tomlinson/President, Chief Executive Officer
Mktg./Adv.: Brent Tomlinson/Manager Contract Sales

Screen, Bedside	General

PRESCOTT IDEAS, LLC   520-886-4399
8960 E. Anna Place, Tucson, AZ 85710
FDA Number: 3005932408

Software, Blood Bank (Stand-Alone Products)	Hematology

PRESCRIPTION OPTICAL, INC.   800-284-8886
P.O.Box 1088, St. Cloud, MN 56302
FDA Number: n/a   *Fax:* 800-284-4449
E-mail: info@prescriptionoptical.com
Web site: www.prescriptionoptical.com
Medical Products Sales Volume: $3,000,000
Annual Revenue: $1-$5 Million
Ownership: Private
Produces/Sells CE-marked Devices: N
Federal Procurement Eligibility: Small Business
Distribution: Manufacturer Direct

Lens, Spectacle/Eyeglasses, Custom (Prescription)	Ophthalmology

PRESERVATION SOLUTIONS, INC.   262-723-6715
980 Proctor Dr., Elkhorn, WI 53121
FDA Number: 2132588   *Fax:* 262-723-4013
E-mail: brader@preservationsolutions.com
Web site: www.preservationsolutions.com
Annual Revenue: $1-$5 Million
Year Founded: 1994
Total Employees: 11   *Marketing Staff:* 1   *Sales Staff:* 2
Ownership: Private
Produces/Sells CE-marked Devices: N
Federal Procurement Eligibility: Small Business

PRESERVATION SOLUTIONS, INC.   262-723-6715 (cont'd)
Distribution: Manufacturer Direct, Manufacturer Through Distributor, Manufacturer Through Manufacturer Reps, OEM
Mktg./Adv.: Laura Torhorst/Manager Customer Services & Sales

Accessories, Cleaning, Endoscopic	Gastroenterology/Urology
Dressing, Wound and Burn, Occlusive	Surgery
Media, Transport/Storage, Organ/Tissue	Cardiovascular
Perfusion System, Kidney	Gastroenterology/Urology

PRESERVE INTERNATIONAL   800-995-1607
P.O. Box 17003, Reno, NV 89511
FDA Number: n/a   *Fax:* 209-664-1728
Web site: www.preserveinternational.com
Annual Revenue: $1-$5 Million
Total Employees: 9   *Marketing Staff:* 2   *Sales Staff:* 2
Ownership: Private
Produces/Sells CE-marked Devices: N
Federal Procurement Eligibility: Small Business, Female Owned
Distribution: Manufacturer Direct

Disinfector, Liquid	General

PRESSURE-TECH, INC.   760-470-2831
102 Woodcleft Ave., Freeport, NY 11520
FDA Number: 3006788920
Ownership: Private
Produces/Sells CE-marked Devices: N

Chamber, Hyperbaric	Anesthesiology

PRESTIGE AMERITECH   817-595-1131
7426 Tower St., Ft. Worth, TX 76118
FDA Number: 3005022483
Ownership: Merit Medical Systems, Inc.

Mask, Surgical	Surgery

PRESTIGE MEDICAL CORPORATION   800-762-3333
8600 Wilbur Ave., Northridge, CA 91324-4499   **818-993-3030**
FDA Number: 7000702   *Fax:* 818-993-4151
E-mail: prestige@prestigemed.com
Web site: www.prestigemed.com
Medical Products Sales Volume: $10,000,000
Annual Revenue: $5-$10 Million
Total Employees: 50   *Marketing Staff:* 3   *Sales Staff:* 7
Ownership: Private
Produces/Sells CE-marked Devices: Y
Federal Procurement Eligibility: Small Business
Distribution: Exclusive Distributor, Importer
General Admin.: Richard Rashman/Chief Executive Officer
    Dennis Shick/General Manager
    Richard Rashman/President
    Dennis Shick/Vice President, General Manager
Mktg./Adv.: Rick Love/Director Marketing
    Jacquie Dunder/Director National Accounts
    Dennis Shick/Director Product Development
    Dennis Shick/Manager International & National Sales
    Brian Spangerberg/Manager National Sales
    Brian Spangenberg/Manager Sales Training
Production: Robert Albious/Director Quality Assurance
    Dennis Shick/Manager Regulatory Affairs
    Dennis Shick/Vice President Manufacturing
Research: Dennis Shick/Vice President Research & Development

Forceps, Hemostatic	Surgery
Otoscope	Ear/Nose/Throat
Scissors, Bandage/Gauze/Plaster	General
Sphygmomanometer, Aneroid (Arterial Pressure)	General
Stethoscope, Mechanical	General
Thermometer, Electronic	General

PRESTO ABSORBENT PRODUCTS, INC.   715-839-2085
3925 N. Hastings Way, Eau Claire, WI 54703
FDA Number: 3004789162

Garment, Protective, For Incontinence	Gastroenterology/Urology

PRESTO ABSORBENT PRODUCTS-ATLANTA   715-839-2085
1070 Atlanta Industrial Drive, Marietta, GA 30066
FDA Number: 3004789162
Ownership: Private
Produces/Sells CE-marked Devices: N

Garment, Protective, For Incontinence	Gastroenterology/Urology

PRETIKA CORPORATION, NORTH AMERICA MARKET HEADQUAR   949-481-8818
16 Salermo, Laguna Niguel, CA 92677
FDA Number: 2032852
E-mail: customerservice@pretika.com
Web site: www.pretikafacebodyspa.com
Ownership: Private
Produces/Sells CE-marked Devices: N

Brush, Dermabrasion	Surgery

MANUFACTURER PROFILES

PRETIKA CORPORATION, NORTH AMERICA   949-481-8818
(cont'd)
| Motor, Surgical Instrument, Pneumatic-Powered | Surgery |
| Vibrator, Therapeutic | Physical Med |

PREVENTIVE DENTISTRY PRODUCTS, INC.   714-979-4191
3197-F Airport Loop Dr., Costa Mesa, CA 92626-3424
FDA Number: n/a   Fax: 714.557.1505
Ownership: Private
Produces/Sells CE-marked Devices: N
Federal Procurement Eligibility: Small Business, Female Owned
Distribution: Manufacturer Direct, Manufacturer Through Manufacturer Reps
| Floss, Dental | Dental And Oral |
| Mirror, Mouth | Dental And Oral |

PREVENTIVE TECHNOLOGIES, INC.   704-849-2416
1150 Crews Rd., Suite H, Matthews, NC 28105
FDA Number: 1061053
Web site: preventech.comÉ_Z
Ownership: Private
Produces/Sells CE-marked Devices: N
Agent, Polishing, Abrasive, Oral Cavity	Dental And Oral
Cup, Prophylaxis	Dental And Oral
Handpiece, Contra- And Right-Angle Attachment, Dental	Dental And Oral

PREXION INC.   650-212-0300
411 Borel Avenue, Suite 550, San Mateo, CA 94402
FDA Number: 3007038334
E-mail: info@prexion.com   Fax: 650-212-0310
Web site: http://www.prexion.com
Year Founded: 2007
Ownership: Private
Produces/Sells CE-marked Devices: N
General Admin.: Mr. Kazuo Takahashi/Chief Executive Officer
   Mr. Robert Meier/President, Chief Operating Officer
| X-ray, Tomography, Computed, Dental | Radiology |

PRIDE INDUSTRIES   800-550-6005
10030 Foothills Blvd., Roseville, CA 95747-7102   916-788-2100
FDA Number: n/a   Fax: 916-788-2552
Web site: www.prideindustries.com
Medical Products Sales Volume: $145,000,000
Year Founded: 1966
Total Employees: 4100
Ownership: Private
Produces/Sells CE-marked Devices: N
General Admin.: Michael Ziegler/Chief Executive Officer

PRIDE MOBILITY PRODUCTS CORP.   800-800-8586
182 Susquehanna Avenue, Exeter, PA 18643   570-655-5574
FDA Number: 2523375   Fax: 570-655-4305
E-mail: etempleton@pridemobility.com
Web site: www.pridemobility.com
Year Founded: 1986
Total Employees: 700
Ownership: Private
Produces/Sells CE-marked Devices: N
Distribution: Manufacturer Through Distributor
General Admin.: Scott Meuser/President, Chief Executive Officer
Mktg./Adv.: Dan Meuser/Director National Accounts
   Craig Otto/Vice President International Sales
   Mark A. Miller/Vice President Marketing
   Dan Meuser/Vice President Sales
Chair, Seat Lifting (Standing Aid)	General
Scooter (Motorized 3-Wheeled Vehicle)	Physical Med
Wheelchair, Powered	Physical Med

PRIDE MOBILITY PRODUCTS CORP.   800-800-8586
182 Susquehanna Avenue, Exeter, PA 18643
FDA Number: 2531465
Ownership: Private
Produces/Sells CE-marked Devices: N
Chair, Position, Electric	Physical Med
Cushion, Wheelchair (Pad)	Physical Med
Scooter (Motorized 3-Wheeled Vehicle)	Physical Med
Wheelchair, Powered	Physical Med

PRIDENT INTERNATIONAL INC.   717-849-4229
570 West College Ave., York, PA 17404
FDA Number: 3005652240
Web site: www.dentsply.com
Ownership: Dentsply International, Inc.
Produces/Sells CE-marked Devices: N

PRIMAPHARM, INC.   (949) 278-1597
3443 Tripp Court, San Diego, CA 92121
FDA Number: 1000135880
E-mail: tony@primapharm.net
Ownership: Private

PRIMAPHARM, INC.   (949) 278-1597 *(cont'd)*
Produces/Sells CE-marked Devices: N
| Fluid, Intraocular | Ophthalmology |

PRIMARY CARE SOLUTIONS, INC.   888-212-5336
40420 Free Fall Avenue, Zephyrhills, FL 33540   813-779-7226
FDA Number: 1066336   Fax: 813-715-4084
E-mail: rmaddix@primarycaresolutionsinc.com
Web site: www.primarycaresolutionsinc.com
Ownership: Private
Produces/Sells CE-marked Devices: N
Distribution: Manufacturer Through Distributor, OEM
| Catheter, Suction, With Tip | General |

PRIMARY MEDICAL CO., INC.   727-520-1920
6541 44TH STREET N / SUITE 6003, PINELLAS PARK, FL 33781
FDA Number: 1058755   Fax: 727-520-1922
E-mail: info@primedco.com
Year Founded: 1992
Total Employees: 3
Ownership: Private
Produces/Sells CE-marked Devices: N
Federal Procurement Eligibility: Female Owned
Airway, Oropharyngeal, Anesthesia	Anesthesiology
Connector, Airway (Extension)	Anesthesiology
Cuff, Blood Pressure	Cardiovascular
Forceps, Tube Introduction	Anesthesiology
Laryngoscope	Ear/Nose/Throat
Stylet, Tracheal Tube	Anesthesiology
Support, Breathing Tube	Anesthesiology
Transducer, Stethoscope	Anesthesiology

PRIME DENTAL MANUFACTURING, INC.   773-539-5927
3735 West Belmont Avenue, Chicago, IL 60618
FDA Number: 1424442   Fax: 773-539-6919
E-mail: primedental@hotmail.com
Web site: www.primedentalmfg.com
Medical Products Sales Volume: $2,100,000
Year Founded: 1999
Total Employees: 30
Ownership: Private
Quality System Registration Information: ISO9001
Produces/Sells CE-marked Devices: Y
Federal Procurement Eligibility: Small Business
Distribution: Manufacturer Through Distributor, OEM, Exporter
General Admin.: Mr. Pedro Segura/President, Chief Executive Officer
Production: Dr. Chah Shen/Vice President Quality Assurance & Regulatory Affairs
| Material, Tooth Shade, Resin | Dental And Oral |

PRIME ENGINEERING   800-827-8263
4202 W Sierra Madre Avenue, Fresno, CA 93722   559-276-0991
FDA Number: n/a   Fax: 559-276-3544
E-mail: info@primeengineering.com
Web site: www.primeengineering.com
Annual Revenue: $1-$5 Million
Year Founded: 1984
Total Employees: 15   Marketing Staff: 2   Sales Staff: 2
Ownership: Private
Produces/Sells CE-marked Devices: Y
Federal Procurement Eligibility: Small Business, Female Owned
Distribution: Manufacturer Through Distributor, Manufacturer Through Manufacturer Reps, Exporter
General Admin.: Ms. Mary Wilson Boegel/President
   Mr. Mark Allen/Vice President
Mktg./Adv.: Mr. Mark Allen/Manager Contract Sales
Production: Peggy Woodward/Customer Service Representative
Finance: Mr. Bruce Boegel/Chief Financial Officer
Bars, Parallel, Walking	Physical Med
Equipment, Therapy, Handicapped/Physical	Physical Med
Support, Patient Position	Anesthesiology
Table, Physical Therapy	Physical Med

PRIME MATERIALS CORP.   877-755-1649
6 Treadeasy Avenue, PO Box 71,   585-815-0400
Batavia, NY 14021
FDA Number: 3003409616   Fax: 585-815-0401
E-mail: treadeasy@primematerialscorp.com
Web site: www.treadeasy.com
Medical Products Sales Volume: $3,000,000
Year Founded: 2001
Total Employees: 30   Sales Staff: 16
Ownership: Private
Produces/Sells CE-marked Devices: N
Federal Procurement Eligibility: Small Business
Distribution: Manufacturer Through Distributor, Manufacturer Through Manufacturer Reps
| Orthosis, Corrective Shoe | Physical Med |

PRIME SOLUTIONS
510-490-2299
4261 Business Center Drive, Fremont, CA 94538
FDA Number: n/a
Fax: 510-490-2177
E-mail: Sales@primesol.com
Web site: www.primesol.com
Medical Products Sales Volume: $1,700,000
Year Founded: 1988
Total Employees: 17
Ownership: Private
Produces/Sells CE-marked Devices: N
Federal Procurement Eligibility: Small Business
Distribution: Service Direct
Mktg./Adv.: Mr. Alex Sagatelian/Sales Representative
  Service, Modification, Product
General

PRIMED INSTRUMENTS, INC.
877-565-0565
905-565-0565
1080 Tristar Dr., Unit 14,
Mississauga, ONTAR L5T 1 Canada
FDA Number: 9680488
Fax: 877-565-0566
E-mail: info@primedinstruments.com
Web site: www.primedinstruments.com
Year Founded: 1993
Total Employees: 4
Ownership: Private
Produces/Sells CE-marked Devices: Y
Federal Procurement Eligibility: Small Business
Distribution: Manufacturer Direct, Manufacturer Through Distributor, Manufacturer Through Manufacturer Reps, OEM, Exporter

PRIMELINE MEDICAL PRODUCTS INC.
780-497-7600
3rd Floor, 1259-91 Street SW, Edmonton, ALB T6X 1E9 Canada
FDA Number: n/a
Fax: 780-497-7670
E-mail: info@primed.ca
Web site: http://www.primed.ca
Year Founded: 1995
Total Employees: 25
Ownership: Private
Produces/Sells CE-marked Devices: N
Distribution: Exclusive Distributor, Exporter

PRIMERADX
508-618-2300
171 Forbes Blvd, Suite 2000, Mansfield, MA 02048
FDA Number: n/a
Fax: 508-339-0452
E-mail: Info@PrimeraDx.com
Web site: www.primeradx.com
Ownership: Private
Produces/Sells CE-marked Devices: N
General Admin.: Ms. Lilly Kong/Chief Scientific Officer
  Dr. Matthew McManus/President, Chief Executive Officer
Mktg./Adv.: Mr. David Jackson/Vice President Business Development
  Mr. Jeff Liter/Vice President Corporate Development
  Mr. Daniel Bowman/Vice President Marketing & Sales
Production: Mr. Gary Riordan/Vice President Regulatory Affairs
Finance: Mr. Ted Myles/Chief Financial Officer
IS: Mr. Louise Hlousek/Vice President Systems

PRIMESOURCE HEALTHCARE, INC.
800-317-0711
2100 East Lake Cook Road, Suite 1100, Buffalo Grove, IL 60089
FDA Number: n/a
Fax: 800-434-7113
Web site: www.pshcs.com
Annual Revenue: $50-$100 Million
Year Founded: 1996
Total Employees: 150
Marketing Staff: 4
Sales Staff: 85
Ownership: Private
Produces/Sells CE-marked Devices: N
Distribution: Manufacturer Through Distributor, Manufacturer Through Manufacturer Reps, OEM, Exclusive Distributor, Importer
General Admin.: Shaun McMeans/Chief Operating Officer, Chief Financial Officer
  Joe Potenza/Chief Operating Officer, Senior Vice President
  Brad Walker/President, Chief Executive Officer
  Bruce Hoadley/Regional Vice President
  Mark Jungers/Regional Vice President
  Scott Billman/Regional Vice President
  Sam Stein/Vice President, General Manager
Mktg./Adv.: Ron Flora/Director Product Development
  Craig Stevens/Manager International & National Sales
  Gary Gregory/Senior Vice President Marketing & Sales
  Jason Fowler/Vice President Business Development
Bowl, Solution
General
Kit, Cholecystectomy
Gastroenterology/Urology
Tray, Custom/Special Procedure
General

PRIMESOURCE SURGICAL
See Primesource Healthcare, Inc.

PRIMO, INC.
770-486-7394
417A Dividend Dr., Peachtree City, GA 30269
FDA Number: 1064818
Fax: 770-486-6298

PRIMO, INC.
770-486-7394 (cont'd)
Web site: www.primoinc.net
Ownership: Private
Produces/Sells CE-marked Devices: N
Accessories, Traction | Physical Med
Attachment, Narrowing, Wheelchair | Physical Med
Brace, Joint, Ankle (External) | Physical Med
Cover, Mattress | General
Joint, Knee, External Brace | Physical Med
Protector, Skin Pressure | General
Restraint, Patient, Conductive | Anesthesiology
Restraint, Protective (Body) | General
Shoe, Cast | Physical Med
Shoe, Operating Room | Surgery
Sling, Arm | Physical Med
Wheelchair, Special Grade | Physical Med

PRIMROSE MEDICAL, INC.
508-660-8688
478 High Plain St., Walpole, MA 02081
FDA Number: 1220905
Fax: 508-660-8699
E-mail: fletcher@primrosemedical.com
Web site: www.primrosemedical.com
Annual Revenue: $0-$1 Million
Ownership: Private
Produces/Sells CE-marked Devices: N
Federal Procurement Eligibility: Small Business
Distribution: Manufacturer Through Distributor, Manufacturer Through Manufacturer Reps, OEM
General Admin.: Fletcher Longley/President, Chief Executive Officer
Production: Thomas Koteles/Manager Operations
Kit, Administration, Intravenous | General
Lock, Catheter | General
Molding, Injection | General
Needle, Other | General
Scalpel, One-Piece (Knife) | Surgery
Tube, Feeding | General
Tube, Gastro-Enterostomy | Gastroenterology/Urology
Tubing, Urethane | General

PRIMUS DIAGNOSTICS
800-377-4752
816-523-7491
4231 E. 75th Terrace, Kansas City, MO 64132
FDA Number: 1931251
Fax: 816-361-1974
E-mail: sales@primusdiagnostics.com
Web site: www.primusdiagnostics.com
Medical Products Sales Volume: $10,000,000
Annual Revenue: $10-$25 Million
Total Employees: 40
Ownership: Trinity Biotech Plc
Produces/Sells CE-marked Devices: Y
Distribution: OEM, Exporter
General Admin.: Thomas Reidy/President
Production: Richard Bethay/General Manager Operations
Analyzer, Chemistry, Photometric, Discrete | Chemistry
Hemoglobin S | Hematology
Quantitation, Hemoglobin, Abnormal | Hematology
Test, Glycosylated Hemoglobin Assay | Hematology

PRIMUS STERILIZER COMPANY, LLC.
620-793-7900
5520 10th Street, Great Bend, KS 67530
FDA Number: 1954304
Sterilizer, Steam (Autoclave)
General

PRINCE & IZANT NUTEC METAL JOINING
216-362-7000
12999 Plaza Drive, Cleveland, OH 44130
FDA Number: 3005634790
Alloy, Gold Based, For Clinical Use | Dental And Oral
Alloy, Precious Metal, For Clinical Use | Dental And Oral

PRINCESS UNIFORMS ACCESSORIES
800-845-5455
72 Agan Road, Abbeville, SC 29620
FDA Number: n/a
Fax: 864-366-9719
Web site: princessuniforms.net
Annual Revenue: $1-$5 Million
Ownership: Private
Produces/Sells CE-marked Devices: N
Federal Procurement Eligibility: Small Business
Distribution: Manufacturer Through Distributor
Gown, Other
General

PRINCETON BIOMEDITECH CORP.
732-274-1000
4242 U.S. Hwy 1, Monmouth Junction, NJ 08852-1905
FDA Number: 2246703
Fax: 732-274-1010
E-mail: info@pbmc.com
Web site: www.pbmc.com
Medical Products Sales Volume: $13,000,000
Annual Revenue: $25-$50 Million
Year Founded: 1988
Total Employees: 100
Marketing Staff: 5
Sales Staff: 5
Ownership: Private

PRINCETON BIOMEDITECH CORP. 732-274-1000 *(cont'd)*

Quality System Registration Information: ISO9001
Produces/Sells CE-marked Devices: Y
Federal Procurement Eligibility: Small Business, Minority Owned
Distribution: Manufacturer Direct, Manufacturer Through Distributor, OEM, Importer, Exporter
General Admin.: Jemo Kang/President, Chief Executive Officer
Mktg./Adv.: Roger Kang/Director Business Development
    Walter Kang/Director Marketing
    Brian Lee/Manager International Marketing & Sales
Production: W. Yoon/Director Operations
    G. S. Han/Manager Production
    Y. W. Kim/Manager Quality Assurance & Regulatory Affairs
Research: K. Kim/Manager Research
IS: SH Kim/Manager Systems

Alpha-Fetoprotein RIA Test System	Immunology
Antigen, Streptococcus SPP.	Microbiology
Antiserum, CF, Rubella	Microbiology
Enzyme Linked Immunoabsorbent Assay, Chlamydia Group	Microbiology
Kit, Pregnancy Test	Obstetrics/Gynecology
Radioimmunoassay, Other	Chemistry
System, Test, Drugs of Abuse	Chemistry
Test, Bacterial Diagnostic	Microbiology
Test, Cancer Detection, Other	Hematology
Test, Disease, Lyme	Immunology
Test, Fertility Monitoring	Obstetrics/Gynecology
Test, Infectious Mononucleosis	Immunology
Test, Influenza	Microbiology
Test, Myocardial Infarction (Heart Attack)	Chemistry

Medical Product Subsidiaries (Listed Separately)
Lifesign

PRINCETON CASE CO., INC. 908-687-1750

667 Lehigh Ave., Union, NJ 07083
FDA Number: n/a   Fax: 908-687-1755
Web site: www.princetoncase.com
Annual Revenue: $1-$5 Million
Year Founded: 1964
Ownership: Private
Produces/Sells CE-marked Devices: N
Federal Procurement Eligibility: Small Business
Distribution: Manufacturer Direct, Manufacturer Through Manufacturer Reps, OEM

Case, Protection, Equipment	General
Contract Manufacturing	General

PRINCETON INSTRUMENTS - ACTON 978-263-3584

15 Discovery Way, Acton, MA 01720
FDA Number: n/a   Fax: 978-263-5086
E-mail: moreinfo@piacton.com
Web site: www.acton-research.com
Medical Products Sales Volume: $4,700,000
Annual Revenue: $10-$25 Million
Year Founded: 1961
Total Employees: 50   *Marketing Staff:* 2   *Sales Staff:* 10
Ownership: ROPER INDUSTRIES
Stock Symbol: ROP
Traded On: NYSE
Produces/Sells CE-marked Devices: Y
Federal Procurement Eligibility: Small Business
Distribution: Manufacturer Direct, Manufacturer Through Manufacturer Reps, Exporter
General Admin.: Mr. Eugene Yazbak/President
Mktg./Adv.: Ms. Debby Flint-Baum/Manager Advertising
    Mr. Richard Merk/Vice President Marketing & Sales
Production: Mr. William Keating/Vice President Manufacturing
Research: Mr. Michael Case/Vice President Research & Development
Finance: Mr. Joseph McCadden/Vice President Finance, Human Resources

Filter, Lens	Ophthalmology
Laser, Combination	General
Monochromator, for Clinical Use	Chemistry
Spectrophotometer, U.V./Visible	Chemistry
System, Laser, Excimer, Ophthalmic	Ophthalmology

PRINCETON LABORATORY SERVICES, LLC 732-738-8108

340 Mac Lane, Keasbey, NJ 08832
FDA Number: 3005244717

Crown, Preformed	Dental And Oral

PRINCETON MEDICAL GROUP, INC. 800-875-0869

1189 Royal Links Dr., Mt. Pleasant, SC 29466   **843-849-0869**
FDA Number: 1055890   Fax: 843-971-1600
E-mail: prnceton@bellsouth.net
Medical Products Sales Volume: $2,500,000
Annual Revenue: $1-$5 Million
Year Founded: 1990
Total Employees: 21   *Marketing Staff:* 2   *Sales Staff:* 18
Ownership: Private
Quality System Registration Information: ISO9001; ISO9002

PRINCETON MEDICAL GROUP, INC. 800-875-0869 *(cont'd)*

Produces/Sells CE-marked Devices: Y
Federal Procurement Eligibility: Small Business, Female Owned
Distribution: Manufacturer Through Manufacturer Reps, Importer, Exporter
General Admin.: Mr. Joseph G. Frick/Chief Operating Officer
    Ms. Francesca M. Frick/President, Chief Executive Officer
Mktg./Adv.: Mr. Joseph G. Frick/Vice President Marketing & Sales

Anoscope, Non-Powered	Gastroenterology/Urology
Brace, Drill	Orthopedics
Chisel, Osteotome, Surgical	Dental And Oral
Clamp, Aorta	Cardiovascular
Clamp, Circumcision	Obstetrics/Gynecology
Clamp, Fixation, Cholangiography	Surgery
Clamp, Intestinal	Gastroenterology/Urology
Clamp, Muscle, Ophthalmic	Ophthalmology
Clamp, Surgical, General & Plastic Surgery	Surgery
Clamp, Vascular	Cardiovascular
Curette, Ear	Ear/Nose/Throat
Curette, Surgical	Surgery
Curette, Uterine	Obstetrics/Gynecology
Dilator, Uterine	Obstetrics/Gynecology
Dilator, Vascular	Cardiovascular
Endoscope, Rigid	Surgery
Forceps	Orthopedics
Forceps, Biopsy, Gynecological	Obstetrics/Gynecology
Forceps, Biopsy, Non-Electric	Gastroenterology/Urology
Forceps, Dressing	Surgery
Forceps, Gallbladder (Biliary Duct)	Gastroenterology/Urology
Forceps, General & Plastic Surgery	Surgery
Forceps, Grasping, Atraumatic	Surgery
Forceps, Hemostatic	Surgery
Forceps, Sponge	Surgery
Forceps, Surgical, Gynecological	Obstetrics/Gynecology
Fork, Tuning, ENT	Ear/Nose/Throat
Goniometer, Non-Powered	Orthopedics
Guide, Gigli Saw	Orthopedics
Hammer, Percussion	Cns/Neurology
Handle, Instrument, Laparoscopic (Electrocautery)	Surgery
Handle, Scalpel	Surgery
Holder, Needle, Laparoscopic	Surgery
Instrument, Knot Tying, Suture, Laparoscopic	Surgery
Laryngoscope	Ear/Nose/Throat
Mallet, Other	Surgery
Mirror, ENT	Ear/Nose/Throat
Needle, Aspiration And Injection, Disposable	Surgery
Needle, Aspiration And Injection, Reusable	Surgery
Probe, Lacrimal	Ophthalmology
Probe, Other	General
Punch, Biopsy	Gastroenterology/Urology
Punch, Dermal	Surgery
Rasp, Ear	Ear/Nose/Throat
Rasp, Nasal	Ear/Nose/Throat
Resectoscope	Gastroenterology/Urology
Retractor, ENT (Thoracic)	Ear/Nose/Throat
Retractor, Vaginal	Obstetrics/Gynecology
Rongeur, Intervertebral Disk	Orthopedics
Rongeur, Nasal	Ear/Nose/Throat
Scissors, General Dissecting	General
Scissors, Iris	Ophthalmology
Scissors, Laparoscopy, Bipolar, Electrosurgical	Surgery
Scissors, Orthopedic	Orthopedics
Scissors, Plastic Surgery (Dissecting)	Surgery
Sound, Uterine	Obstetrics/Gynecology
Speculum, Ear	Ear/Nose/Throat
Speculum, Ophthalmic	Ophthalmology
Speculum, Vaginal, Metal	Obstetrics/Gynecology
Spreader, Rib	Orthopedics
Sterilization Indicator	Surgery
Stripper, Tendon	Surgery
Surgical Instrument, Obstetric/Gynecologic	Obstetrics/Gynecology
Telescope, Laryngeal-Bronchial	Ear/Nose/Throat
Tenaculum, Uterine	Obstetrics/Gynecology
Tray, Sterilization, Instrument	Surgery
Tray, Surgical Instrument	Surgery
Trocar, Cardiovascular	Cardiovascular
Trocar, Gastro-Urology	Gastroenterology/Urology
Trocar, Laparoscopic	Surgery
Tube, Aspirating, Flexible, Connecting	Anesthesiology

PRINCETON SEPARATIONS, INC. 732-431-3338

100 Commerce Drive, East Freehold, NJ 07728
FDA Number: 2245624

Electrophoresis Equipment, Liquid	Chemistry
Electrophoretic, Protein Fractionation	Chemistry

PRINCIPLE BUSINESS ENT. 1-800-467-3224

Pine Lake Industrial Pk.,   **419-352-1551**
Dunbridge, OH 43414
FDA Number: 1525567   Fax: 419-352-8340
E-mail: consumerinfo@tranquilityproducts.com
Ownership: Private

PRINCIPLE BUSINESS ENT. 1-800-467-3224 (cont'd)
Produces/Sells CE-marked Devices: N
Garment, Protective, For Incontinence Gastroenterology/Urology

PRINCIPLE BUSINESS ENTERPRISES, INC. 800-467-3224
Pine Lake Industrial Park, P.O. Box 129, **419-352-1551**
Dunbridge, OH 43414
FDA Number: 9310057 Fax: 419-352-8340
E-mail: info@tranquilityproducts.com
Web site: www.tranquilityproducts.com
Annual Revenue: $1-$5 Million
Total Employees: 175 *Marketing Staff:* 5 *Sales Staff:* 5
Ownership: Private
Produces/Sells CE-marked Devices: Y
Federal Procurement Eligibility: Female Owned
Distribution: Manufacturer Through Distributor
Cover, Heel Stirrup Orthopedics
Diaper, Adult General
Garment, Protective, For Incontinence Gastroenterology/Urology
Mitt/Washcloth, Patient General
Pad, Incontinence (Underpad) General
Pant, Incontinence General
Slippers General

PRINCO INSTRUMENTS, INC. 800-221-9237
1020 Industrial Blvd., **215-355-1500**
Southampton, PA 18966
FDA Number: n/a Fax: 215-355-7766
Web site: www.princoinstruments.com
Year Founded: 1910
Ownership: Private
Produces/Sells CE-marked Devices: N
Federal Procurement Eligibility: Small Business
Distribution: Manufacturer Direct
Thermometer, Laboratory Chemistry

PRINT MEDIA, INC. 800-994-3318
9002 NW 105th Way, Miami, FL 33178 **305-884-0700**
FDA Number: 3005133883 Fax: 305-884-0702
E-mail: service@printmedia-inc.com
Web site: www.printmedia-inc.com
Annual Revenue: $5-$10 Million
Ownership: Private
Quality System Registration Information: ISO9002
Produces/Sells CE-marked Devices: Y
Federal Procurement Eligibility: Small Business, Minority Owned, GSA Contract,
VA Contract
Distribution: Manufacturer Through Distributor, OEM
General Admin.: Robert Gonzalez/President, Chief Executive Officer
Mktg./Adv.: Adrian Mandreanu/Director Marketing & Sales
Cassette, Audio Tape Cardiovascular
Paper, Chart, Record, Medical General
Paper, Recording, Data General
Paper, Recording, ECG/EEG General
Tape, Television & Video, Endoscopic Gastroenterology/Urology
Unit, Imaging, Thermal Radiology

PRISM CLINICAL IMAGING, INC. 414-727-1930
851 S 70th St., Suite 103, Milwaukee, WI 53214
FDA Number: 3005517190
Image Processing System Radiology
Nuclear Magnetic Resonance Imaging System Radiology

PRISM TECHNOLOGIES, INC.
See Pristech Products, Inc

PRISMATIK DENTALCRAFT, INC. 949-440-2683
2181 Dupont Drive, Irvine, CA 92612
FDA Number: 3005477956
Powder, Porcelain Dental And Oral

PRISTECH PRODUCTS, INC 800-432-8722
6952 Fairgrounds Pkwy., PO Box 680728, **210-520-8051**
San Antonio, TX 78238
FDA Number: 1450530 Fax: 210-509-7463
E-mail: webinfo@pristech.com
Web site: www.pristech.com
Medical Products Sales Volume: $3,000,000
Year Founded: 1992
Total Employees: 35
Ownership: Private
Quality System Registration Information: ISO9002
Produces/Sells CE-marked Devices: Y
Federal Procurement Eligibility: Small Business
Distribution: Manufacturer Direct, Manufacturer Through Distributor, Manufacturer
Through Manufacturer Reps
General Admin.: Grant Haussman/President
Mktg./Adv.: Michelle Hernandez/Coord. Marketing
Barb Wells/Director Marketing Admin. & Sales

PRISTECH PRODUCTS, INC 800-432-8722 (cont'd)
Extractor, Vacuum, Fetal Obstetrics/Gynecology
Pack, Cold General
Pack, Hot Or Cold, Disposable Physical Med
Pack, Hot Or Cold, Reusable Physical Med
Pack, Hot, Chemical General

PRISTINE GLOVES
See World Medical Supply Usa., Inc.

PRITCHETT & HULL ASSOCIATES INC. 800-241-4925
3440 Oakcliff Rd. N.E., Ste. 110, **770-451-0602**
Atlanta, GA 30340
FDA Number: n/a Fax: 800-752-0510
E-mail: phsales@p-h.com
Web site: www.p-h.com
Ownership: Private
Produces/Sells CE-marked Devices: N
Federal Procurement Eligibility: Small Business, Female Owned
Distribution: Manufacturer Direct
Material, Training, Audiovisual General

PRIVA (USA), INC. 516-255-1736
96 Atlantic Ave., Lynbrook, NY 11563
FDA Number: 3005357548
Ownership: Private
Produces/Sells CE-marked Devices: N
Cover, Mattress General

PRIZM MEDICAL, INC. 770-622-0933
P. O. Box 40, Oakwood, GA 30566
FDA Number: 1055808 Fax: 678-714-7243
E-mail: webmaster@prizm-medical.com
Year Founded: 1992
Ownership: Private
Quality System Registration Information: ISO9003
Produces/Sells CE-marked Devices: Y
Federal Procurement Eligibility: Small Business
Distribution: Manufacturer Direct, Manufacturer Through Distributor, Exporter
Electrode, Cutaneous Cns/Neurology
Electrode, Other General
Electrotherapeutic Unit General
Stimulator, Muscle, Powered, Invasive Physical Med
Stimulator, Nerve, Transcutaneous (Pain Relief, TENS) Cns/Neurology
Thermometer, Electronic, Continuous General

PRIZM MEDICAL, INC. 800-447-4422
P.O.Box 40, Oakwood, GA 30566 **770-622-0933**
FDA Number: 1055808 Fax: 678-714-7243
Ownership: Private
Produces/Sells CE-marked Devices: N
General Admin.: Jim Johnson/President, Chief Executive Officer
Electrode, Cutaneous Cns/Neurology
Kit, Administration, Intravenous General
Stimulator, Muscle, Powered, Invasive Physical Med
Stimulator, Nerve, Transcutaneous (Pain Relief, TENS) Cns/Neurology

PRO BED MEDICAL TECHONOGIES, INC. 800-816-8243
602-30930 Wheel Ave., **604-852-3096**
Abbotsford, BC V2T 6 Canada
FDA Number: 8044130 Fax: 604-852-3097
E-mail: splummer@pro-bed.com
Web site: www.pro-bed.com
Year Founded: 1989
Total Employees: 5 *Marketing Staff:* 1 *Sales Staff:* 2
Ownership: Private
Produces/Sells CE-marked Devices: N
Distribution: Manufacturer Direct, Manufacturer Through Distributor, Manufacturer
Through Manufacturer Reps

PRO CUSTOM LABS 866-776-5227
190 Resolute Ln., Port Ludlow, WA 98365
FDA Number: 3005226856
Brace, Joint, Ankle (External) Physical Med

PRO MED PHARMACIES, INC. 806-379-7311
3615 Sw 45th Avenue, Amarillo, TX 79109-5662
FDA Number: n/a Fax: 806-371-0447
E-mail: dgadry@cmc-nhhc.com
Web site: www.promedpharmacies.com/
Medical Products Sales Volume: $2,500,000
Annual Revenue: $1-$5 Million
Year Founded: 1986
Total Employees: 31 *Marketing Staff:* 3
Ownership: Private
Produces/Sells CE-marked Devices: N
Federal Procurement Eligibility: Small Business
Distribution: Service Direct
General Admin.: Don B. Chrysler/Chief Executive Officer

MANUFACTURER PROFILES

PRO MED PHARMACIES, INC.
806-379-7311 (cont'd)

Mktg./Adv.: Keely O'Neal/Director Services & Sales
Finance: David Gadry/Chief Financial Officer
System, Delivery, Drug, Unit-Dose

General

PRO ORTHOPEDIC DEVICES, INC.
800-523-5611
2884 E. Ganley Road, Tucson, AZ 85706
520-294-4401

FDA Number: n/a
Fax: 520-294-6116
E-mail: info@proorthopedic.com
Web site: www.proorthopedic.com
Medical Products Sales Volume: $1,000,000
Annual Revenue: $5-$10 Million
Year Founded: 1994
Total Employees: 35   *Marketing Staff:* 4   *Sales Staff:* 25
Ownership: Private
Produces/Sells CE-marked Devices: Y
Federal Procurement Eligibility: Small Business
Distribution: Manufacturer Through Distributor, Manufacturer Through Manufacturer Reps, Exporter
General Admin.: Jerry Detty/President, Chief Executive Officer
Mktg./Adv.: Jerry Detty/Manager International Marketing & Sales

Belt, Support, Pelvic	Physical Med
Brace, Joint, Ankle (External)	Physical Med
Joint, Hip, External Brace	Physical Med
Joint, Hip, External Limb Component	Physical Med
Joint, Knee, External Brace	Physical Med
Support, Ankle	Orthopedics
Support, Arch	Physical Med
Support, Arm	Physical Med
Support, Back	Orthopedics
Support, Elbow	Orthopedics
Support, Foot	Orthopedics
Support, Hand	Orthopedics
Support, Knee	Physical Med
Support, Leg	Physical Med
Support, Thigh	Physical Med
Support, Wrist	Physical Med

PRO PRODUCTS CORPORATION, INC.
See Ardus Medical, Inc.

PRO SCIENTIFIC INC.
800-584-3776
99 Willenbrock Road, Oxford, CT 06478
203-267-4600

FDA Number: 1225070
Fax: 203-267-4606
E-mail: sales@proscientific.com
Web site: www.proscientific.com
Medical Products Sales Volume: $1,000,000
Year Founded: 1992
Total Employees: 10   *Marketing Staff:* 2   *Sales Staff:* 3
Ownership: Private
Produces/Sells CE-marked Devices: Y
Federal Procurement Eligibility: Small Business, Female Owned
Distribution: Manufacturer Direct, Manufacturer Through Distributor, Manufacturer Through Manufacturer Reps, OEM, Exclusive Distributor, Importer, Exporter
General Admin.: Richard M. Yacko/President
Mktg./Adv.: Patricia A. Yacko/Vice President Marketing & Sales

Bath, Water (Constant Temperature)	Chemistry
Blender/Mixer	Chemistry
Centrifuge, Blood Bank, Diagnostic	Hematology
Centrifuge, Floor	Pathology
Centrifuge, General (Over 5,000 rpm)	Toxicology
Centrifuge, General (Up to 5,000 rpm)	Pathology
Centrifuge, Hematocrit	Hematology
Centrifuge, Microhematocrit	Hematology
Centrifuge, Refrigerated	Pathology
Centrifuge, Tabletop	Pathology
Circulator, Water Bath	Chemistry
Cytocentrifuge	Pathology
Homogenizer, Tissue	Microbiology
Incubator, Aerobic	Microbiology
Incubator, Anaerobic	Microbiology
Oven	Chemistry
Shaker, Waterbath	Chemistry
Shaker/Stirrer	Chemistry
Sterilizer, Dry Heat	General

PRO TRAINERS' CHOICE COMPANY
801-375-6600
Po Box 3953, 5803 Nw Newberry Hill Rd., Silverdale, WA 98383

FDA Number: 3004733525
Pack, Hot Or Cold, Water Circulating   Physical Med

PRO-COMM, INC.
800-920-1476
1105 Industrial Pkwy., Brick, NJ 08724
732-206-0660

FDA Number: 2248206
Fax: 732-458-1919
E-mail: pro-comm222@aol.com
Web site: www.procomm222.com
Annual Revenue: $1-$5 Million
Total Employees: 13   *Marketing Staff:* 2   *Sales Staff:* 2
Ownership: Private
Produces/Sells CE-marked Devices: N

PRO-COMM, INC.
800-920-1476 (cont'd)

Federal Procurement Eligibility: Small Business
Distribution: Manufacturer Direct, Manufacturer Through Distributor, Manufacturer Through Manufacturer Reps
General Admin.: Robert Sepulveda/President
Mktg./Adv.: Robert Sepulveda/Manager National Sales
   Sheryl J. Visone/Vice President Marketing

Accelerator, Linear, Medical	Radiology
Accessories, Radiotherapy	Radiology

PRO-DEX, INC
800-562-6204
2361 McGaw Ave., Irvine, CA 92614
949-769-3200

FDA Number: 2081135
Fax: 949-769-3281
E-mail: SalesCA@pro-dex.com
Web site: www.pro-dex.com
Ownership: Private
Produces/Sells CE-marked Devices: N

Handpiece, Air-Powered, Dental	Dental And Oral
Implant, Endosseous	Dental And Oral
Injector, Jet, Mechanical-Powered	Dental And Oral
Motor, Surgical Instrument, AC-Powered	Surgery
Motor, Surgical Instrument, Pneumatic-Powered	Surgery
Scaler, Ultrasonic	Dental And Oral

PRO-DEX, INC.
800-562-6204
2361 McGaw Ave., Irvine, CA 92614
714-546-4045

FDA Number: 2081135
Ownership: Public
Stock Symbol: PDEX
Traded On: NASDAQ
Produces/Sells CE-marked Devices: N
General Admin.: Mr. Mark Murphy/President, Chief Executive Officer
   Mr. Phillip Brown/Vice President, General Manager
Mktg./Adv.: Mr. Paul Rudzinski/Vice President Sales
Production: Mr. Richard Van Kirk/Vice President Manufacturing
   Mr. Joseph Rotino/Vice President Quality Assurance
Finance: Mr. Harold Hurwitz/Chief Financial Officer

Handpiece, Air-Powered, Dental	Dental And Oral
Implant, Endosseous	Dental And Oral
Injector, Jet, Mechanical-Powered	Dental And Oral
Motor, Surgical Instrument, AC-Powered	Surgery
Motor, Surgical Instrument, Pneumatic-Powered	Surgery
Scaler, Ultrasonic	Dental And Oral

PRO-OPTICS, INC.
800-323-3846
317 Woodwork Lane, Palatine, IL 60067-4993

FDA Number: 1419844
Fax: 847-991-9696
E-mail: jb@proopticsinc.com
Web site: www.proopticsinc.com
Annual Revenue: $1-$5 Million
Total Employees: 75   *Marketing Staff:* 1   *Sales Staff:* 2
Ownership: Private
Produces/Sells CE-marked Devices: N
Federal Procurement Eligibility: Small Business
Distribution: Manufacturer Direct, Manufacturer Through Distributor, Manufacturer Through Manufacturer Reps, Exporter
General Admin.: Jay L. Blomquist/President, Chief Executive Officer
   Richard A. Dimberg/Vice President
Mktg./Adv.: Jay L. Blomquist/Director National Accounts
   Donald Gill/Director Product Development
   Richard A. Dimberg/Manager Contract Sales
   Jay L. Blomquist/Manager International & National Sales
   Jay L. Blomquist/Manager National Sales
   Richard A. Dimberg/Vice President Marketing
Production: Donald Gill/Director Quality Assurance
   Donald Gill/Manager Materials
   Richard A. Dimberg/Manager Regulatory Affairs
Shield, Eye, Ophthalmic   Ophthalmology

PRO-TECH SERVICES, INC.
800-350-5511
4338 Harbour Pointe Blvd SW,
425-322-0300
Mukilteo, WA 98275

FDA Number: 3026456
Fax: 425-322-0397
E-mail: sales@pro-tech.com
Web site: www.pro-tech.com
Medical Products Sales Volume: $4,700,000
Year Founded: 1987
Total Employees: 50
Ownership: Private
Quality System Registration Information: ISO9001
Produces/Sells CE-marked Devices: Y
Federal Procurement Eligibility: Small Business
Distribution: Manufacturer Direct, Manufacturer Through Distributor, OEM, Exclusive Distributor, Exporter
General Admin.: Robert Hezlep/Business Manager
   Jim Johnson/President, Chief Executive Officer
Mktg./Adv.: Mr. William Goodwin/Director International Sales
   Scott Cole RPSGT/Director Regional Sales

PRO-TECH SERVICES, INC.   800-350-5511 (cont'd)
Todd Ramsey RRT/Director Regional Sales
Production: Kim Morrow/Manager Customer Services

Monitor, Apnea	General
Monitor, Ventilatory Frequency	Anesthesiology
Recorder, Ventilatory Effort	Anesthesiology

PRO-TEX INTERNATIONAL, INC.   800-680-9361
5038 Salida Blvd., PO Box 1038, Salida, CA 95368   **209-545-1691**
FDA Number: 2954935   Fax: 209-545-3533
E-mail: info@protexfaceshields.com
Web site: www.protexfaceshields.com
Ownership: Private
Produces/Sells CE-marked Devices: N

Accessories, Apparel, Surgical	Surgery
Device, Anti-Snoring	Ear/Nose/Throat
Device, Repositioning, Jaw	Dental And Oral
Mouthguard	Dental And Oral

PRO-WESTERN PLASTICS LTD.   800-661-9835
30 Riel Dr., P.O. Box 261,   **780-459-4491**
St. Albert, ALBER T8N-1 Canada
FDA Number: n/a   Fax: 800-428-4756
E-mail: wayne.hunt@pro-westernplastics.com
Web site: www.pro-westernplastics.com
Medical Products Sales Volume: $2,000,000
Year Founded: 1969
Total Employees: 240
Ownership: Private
Produces/Sells CE-marked Devices: N
Distribution: Manufacturer Direct, Manufacturer Through Distributor, Exporter

PRO-ZOOICS RESEARCH ASSOCIATES   650-322-2455
711 Central Ave., Menlo Park, CA 94025
FDA Number: 3005002464
Ownership: Private
Produces/Sells CE-marked Devices: N

Traction Unit, Non-Powered	Orthopedics

PROACT, LTD.   814-231-2158
112 W. Foster Ave., 202 C, State College, PA 16801
FDA Number: 2183839   Fax: 814-234-7215
E-mail: adarr@proactltd.com
Annual Revenue: $1-$5 Million
Year Founded: 1989
Ownership: Private
Produces/Sells CE-marked Devices: Y
Federal Procurement Eligibility: Small Business
Distribution: Exclusive Distributor
General Admin.: Allan Darr/President

Biopsy Instrument	Gastroenterology/Urology
Clamp, Surgical, General & Plastic Surgery	Surgery
Kit, Biopsy Needle	Gastroenterology/Urology

PROBED MEDICAL TECHNOLOGIES INC.   800-816-8243
30930 Wheel Ave. #602,   **604-852-3096**
Abbotsford, BC V2T-6 Canada
FDA Number: n/a   Fax: 604-852-3097
E-mail: info@pro-bed.com
Web site: www.pro-bed.com
Year Founded: 1989
Total Employees: 10
Ownership: Private
Produces/Sells CE-marked Devices: N
Distribution: Manufacturer Direct, Exclusive Distributor, Exporter

PROBLEM SOLVING CONCEPTS, INC.   800-755-2150
8021 Knue Rd., Suite 100, Indianapolis, IN 46250
FDA Number: 1836517

Image Processing System	Radiology

PROCEDURE PRODUCTS, INC.   360-693-1832
6622 SE Oakridge Drive, Gladstone, OR 97027
FDA Number: 3020778   Fax: 360-690-4473
E-mail: ppr@pacifier.com
Web site: www.procedureproducts.com
Medical Products Sales Volume: $1,900,000
Annual Revenue: $1-$5 Million
Year Founded: 1985
Total Employees: 2
Ownership: Private
Produces/Sells CE-marked Devices: N
Federal Procurement Eligibility: Small Business, Female Owned
Distribution: Manufacturer Direct

Introducer, Syringe Needle	General
Needle, Hypodermic, Single Lumen With Syringe	General
Syringe, Other	General

PROCESS METRIX   800-995-9902
6622 Owens Drive, Pleasanton, CA 94588-3334   **(925) 460-0385**
FDA Number: n/a   Fax: (925) 460-0728
E-mail: jhoog@processmetrix.com
Web site: www.processmetrix.com
Annual Revenue: $25-$50 Million
Total Employees: 9
Ownership: Private
Produces/Sells CE-marked Devices: Small Business
Federal Procurement Eligibility: Small Business
Distribution: Manufacturer Direct, Manufacturer Through Distributor, Manufacturer Through Manufacturer Reps
General Admin.: Donald Holve/President
Mktg./Adv.: Janice Holve/Vice President Marketing
Production: Tom Harvill/Vice President Manufacturing
Research: Mike Bonin/Vice President Research & Development

Analyzer, Particle	Chemistry
Equipment, Control, Pollution	General

PROCTER & GAMBLE   800-764-7483
1 Procter and Gamble Plaza,   **513-983-1100**
Cincinnati, OH 45201
FDA Number: 1523399
Web site: www.pg.com
Annual Revenue: More than $1 Billion
Year Founded: 1837
Total Employees: 138000
Ownership: Public
Stock Symbol: PG
Traded On: NYSE
Produces/Sells CE-marked Devices: N
Distribution: Manufacturer Direct
General Admin.: A. G. Lafley/Chief Executive Officer, Chairman
Clayton C. Daley/Chief Financial Officer, Chairman
Steven W. Jemison/Chief Legal Officer
Robert A. McDonald/Chief Operating Officer
Bruce Brown/Chief Technology Officer
Charlotte R. Otto/External Relations Officer
Moheet Nagrath/Human Resources Associate
Susan E. Arnold/President
Filippo Passerini/President, CTO
Mktg./Adv.: Marc S. Pritchard/Marketing Officer
Finance: Mariano Martin/Business Development Officer
Valarie L. Sheppard/Vice President, Corporate Controller
Jon R. Moeller/Vice President, Treasurer
Purchasing: R. Keith Harrison/Product Supply Officer

Adhesive, Denture, Polymer, Polyacrylamide	Dental And Oral
Diaper, Pediatric	General
Enzyme Immunoassay, Methadone	Toxicology
Enzyme Immunoassay, Phenobarbital	Toxicology
Floss, Dental	Dental And Oral
Freezer, Laboratory, General Purpose	Chemistry
Labware, Basic, Disposable	Chemistry
Labware, Basic, Reusable	Chemistry
Mitt/Washcloth, Patient	General
Pad, Incontinence (Underpad)	General
Pad, Menstrual, Unscented	Obstetrics/Gynecology
Pant, Incontinence	General
Tampon, Menstrual, Scented	Obstetrics/Gynecology
Tampon, Menstrual, Unscented	Obstetrics/Gynecology

Medical Product Subsidiaries (Listed Separately)
Blendax Gmbh
Tambrands Manufacturing, Inc.

PROCTER & GAMBLE CO.   513-622-4851
6200 Bryan Park Rd., Brown Summit, NC 27214
FDA Number: 1062366
Ownership: Private
Produces/Sells CE-marked Devices: N

Polyvinyl Methylether Maleic Acid-Calcium-Sodium Dbl. Salt	Dental And Oral

PROCTER & GAMBLE PAPER PRODUCT CO.   229-430-8260
512 Liberty Expressway -se, Albany, GA 31705
FDA Number: 1066015

Pack, Hot Or Cold, Disposable	Physical Med

PRODESSE, INC.   888-589-6974
n15w22180 watertown road #8,   **262-446-0700**
Waukesha, WI 53186
FDA Number: 2135145   Fax: 262-446-0600
E-mail: info@prodesse.com
Web site: www.prodesse.com
Year Founded: 1995
Total Employees: 25   *Sales Staff:* 3
Ownership: Private
Produces/Sells CE-marked Devices: Y
Federal Procurement Eligibility: Small Business
Distribution: Manufacturer Direct, Manufacturer Through Distributor, OEM

MANUFACTURER PROFILES

PRODESSE, INC. — 888-589-6974 (cont'd)
General Admin.: Tom Shannon/Chief Executive Officer
Steven Visuri/Chief Scientific Officer
Mktg./Adv.: Mr. Andy Shrago/Vice President Marketing & Sales

Antiserum, Fluorescent, Adenovirus 1-33	Microbiology
Chlamydia, DNA Reagents	Microbiology
Cytomegalovirus, DNA Reagents	Microbiology
Epstein-Barr Virus, DNA Reagents	Microbiology
Legionella DNA Reagents	Microbiology
Mycoplasma SPP. DNA Reagents	Microbiology
Reagent, Clostridium Difficile Toxin	Microbiology
Reagent, Virus, General	Pathology
Test, Influenza	Microbiology

PRODRIVE SYSTEMS, INC. — 866-937-8882
812a Commerce Dr., Ogdensburg, NY 13669
FDA Number: 3006067907
Ownership: Private
Produces/Sells CE-marked Devices: N
General Admin.: Jean Castonguay/President, Chief Executive Officer

Burr, Dental	Dental And Oral
Handpiece, Air-Powered, Dental	Dental And Oral
Handpiece, Belt and/or Gear Driven, Dental	Dental And Oral

PRODUCT DESIGN GROUP — 888-858-4422 / 604-323-9220
103-366 Kent Ave South East, Vancouver, BC V5X-4 Canada
Fax: 604-323-9097
FDA Number: 9681827
E-mail: info@prodgroup.com
Web site: www.prodgroup.com
Year Founded: 1995
Total Employees: 15
Ownership: Private
Produces/Sells CE-marked Devices: Y
Distribution: Manufacturer Direct, Manufacturer Through Distributor, Exporter

PRODUCT DEVELOPMENT INDUSTRIES, INC. — 520-881-2556
4500 East Speedway Blvd., #50, Tucson, AZ 85712
FDA Number: 2032107
Ownership: Private
Produces/Sells CE-marked Devices: N

Alloy, Gold Based, For Clinical Use	Dental And Oral

PRODUCT INVESTIGATIONS, INC. — 610-825-5855
151 E. 10th Avenue, Conshohocken, PA 19428
FDA Number: n/a
Fax: 610-825-7288
E-mail: info@productinvestigations.com
Web site: www.productinvestigations.com
Medical Products Sales Volume: $610,000
Annual Revenue: $0-$1 Million
Year Founded: 1975
Total Employees: 12
Ownership: Private
Produces/Sells CE-marked Devices: N
Federal Procurement Eligibility: Small Business
Distribution: Service Direct
General Admin.: Joseph Shelanski/Chief Executive Officer
Samuel Shelanski/President

Contract R&D, Diagnostics	General

PRODUCTION RESEARCH CORP.
See The After Market Group

PRODUCTOS RUBBERMAID, SOCIEDAD ANONIMA DE CAPITAL — 540-542-8363
Kmi-Ote, Carretera Cadereyta-Allende, Cadereyta Jimenez 67450 Mexico
FDA Number: 9616719

Cane	Physical Med
Cane, Safety Walk	Physical Med
Crutch	Physical Med
Tips And Pads, Cane, Crutch And Walker	Physical Med
Walker, Mechanical	Physical Med

PRODUCTS FOR MEDICINE — 800-333-3087 / 714-991-8222
1201 East Ball Road, Suite H, Anaheim, CA 92805
Fax: 714-991-8200
FDA Number: 2028833
E-mail: custserv@productsformedicine.com
Web site: www.productsformedicine.com
Medical Products Sales Volume: $800,000
Year Founded: 1989
Total Employees: 5
Ownership: Private
Produces/Sells CE-marked Devices: N
Federal Procurement Eligibility: Small Business
Distribution: Manufacturer Direct, Manufacturer Through Distributor, OEM, Service Direct

Accessories, Apparel, Surgical	Surgery
Light Source, Endoscope, Xenon Arc	Surgery

PRODUCTS FOR MEDICINE — 800-333-3087 (cont'd)

Microscope, Surgical	Ear/Nose/Throat
Sterilization Process Indicator, Physical/Chemical	General
Wrap, Sterilization	General

PRODUCTS GROUP INTERNATIONAL, INC. — 800-336-5299 / 303-823-6330
447 Main St., Lyons, CO 80540
Fax: 303-823-6339
FDA Number: n/a
E-mail: grant@productsgroup.com
Web site: www.productsgroup.com
Annual Revenue: $1-$5 Million
Ownership: Private
Produces/Sells CE-marked Devices: Y
Federal Procurement Eligibility: Small Business
Distribution: Manufacturer Direct, Manufacturer Through Manufacturer Reps, Exporter
General Admin.: Grant Gillig/President, Chief Executive Officer

Gel, Ultrasonic Transmission	General
Scanner, Ultrasonic, Other	Radiology
Service, Used Equipment	General
Transducer, Ultrasonic	Cardiovascular

PRODUCTS INTERNATIONAL CO. — 800-521-5123 / 602-257-0141
2320 W. Holly St., Phoenix, AZ 85009-2703
Fax: 602-253-7148
FDA Number: 9200894
E-mail: information@tabband.com
Web site: www.tabband.com
Medical Products Sales Volume: $300,000
Year Founded: 1962
Total Employees: 7
Ownership: Private
Produces/Sells CE-marked Devices: Y
Federal Procurement Eligibility: Small Business
Distribution: Manufacturer Direct, Manufacturer Through Distributor, Manufacturer Through Manufacturer Reps, Exporter
General Admin.: Carl Twentier/President, Chief Executive Officer
Mktg./Adv.: Mike Ferring/Vice President Marketing

Bracelet, Identification	General
Label, Bar Code	General
Splint, Molded, Plastic	Orthopedics

PROFESSIONAL CONVALESCENT PRODUCTS
See Pcp Champion

PROFESSIONAL DENTAL LABORATORY CORPORATION — 574-294-3631
1400 West Indiana Avenue, P.o. Box 877, Elkhart, IN 46515
FDA Number: 3004974484
E-mail: prodentalab@frontier.com
Ownership: Private
Produces/Sells CE-marked Devices: N

Device, Anti-Snoring	Ear/Nose/Throat

PROFESSIONAL DISPOSABLES INTERNATIONAL, INC. — 800-999-6423 / 845-365-1700
Two Nice Pak Park, Orangeburg, NY 10962-1318
Fax: 845-365-1729
FDA Number: 2411192
E-mail: bnewman@pdipdi.com
Web site: www.pdipdi.com
Medical Products Sales Volume: $35,000,000
Annual Revenue: $25-$50 Million
Year Founded: 1977
Total Employees: 25   *Marketing Staff:* 4   *Sales Staff:* 22
Ownership: Private
Quality System Registration Information: ISO9001
Produces/Sells CE-marked Devices: Y
Distribution: Manufacturer Through Distributor, Manufacturer Through Manufacturer Reps, OEM, Exporter
General Admin.: Robert P. Julius/Chief Executive Officer
Zachary Julius/President
Dennis Brody/Vice President Human Resources & Personnel
Mktg./Adv.: Joann Reilly/Director Marketing
Jennifer Rhoda Marsh/Director National Accounts
Anna Cepeda-Mays/Market Manager
Bryan Nye/Marketing Coordinator
Beth Newman/Senior Mktg Manager
Terry Hunt/Vice President National Accounts
Frank Mascaro/Vice President Sales
Production: Dwayne Calek/Director Quality Assurance
Doreen Conoscenti/Manager Materials
Dave Jones/Manager Regulatory Affairs
Mike Sarno/Vice President Manufacturing
Research: Gary Vance/Vice President Research & Development

Brush, Scrub, Operating Room	Surgery
Disinfector, Liquid	General
Jelly, Lubricating	General
Kit, Surgical (General)	Surgery
Lubricant, Patient	General

PROFESSIONAL DISPOSABLES   800-999-6423 (cont'd)

Sanitizer	General
Soap	General
Solution, Patient Preparation	General
Swabs, Alcohol	General
Towel/Towelette, Paper	General

PROFESSIONAL HEARING AID SERVICE   724-548-4801
141 South Jefferson St., Kittanning, PA 16201
FDA Number: 2530181
Web site: www.beltone.com
Ownership: Private
Produces/Sells CE-marked Devices: N

Hearing-Aid	Ear/Nose/Throat

PROFESSIONAL HEARING AID SERVICE   316-942-4992
851 North West St., Wichita, KS 67203
FDA Number: 1933440

Hearing-Aid	Ear/Nose/Throat

PROFESSIONAL PRODUCT CO.   619-231-1951
4250 4th Ave., San Diego, CA 92112-1628
FDA Number: n/a
Medical Products Sales Volume: $350,000
Annual Revenue: $0-$1 Million
Ownership: Private
Produces/Sells CE-marked Devices: N
Federal Procurement Eligibility: Small Business
Distribution: Manufacturer Direct, Importer, Exporter

Agent, Polishing, Abrasive, Oral Cavity	Dental And Oral
Alloy, Amalgam	Dental And Oral
Applicator, Cotton	Dental And Oral
Band, Elastic, Orthodontic	Dental And Oral
Base, Denture, Relining, Repairing, Rebasing, Resin	Dental And Oral
Burr, Dental	Dental And Oral
Cement, Dental	Dental And Oral
Crown And Bridge, Temporary, Resin	Dental And Oral
Crown, Preformed	Dental And Oral
Disinfector, Liquid	General
Evacuator, Oral Cavity	Dental And Oral
Floss, Dental	Dental And Oral
Glove, Other	General
Glove, Patient Examination, Latex	General
Handle, Instrument, Dental	Dental And Oral
Handpiece, Contra- And Right-Angle Attachment, Dental	Dental And Oral
Instrument, Diamond, Dental	Dental And Oral
Liner, Cavity, Calcium Hydroxide	Dental And Oral
Material, Dental Filling	Dental And Oral
Material, Impression	Dental And Oral
Material, Impression Tray, Resin	Dental And Oral
Material, Investment	Dental And Oral
Mercury	Dental And Oral
Needle, Acupuncture	Anesthesiology
Needle, Dental	Dental And Oral
Reliner, Denture, OTC	Dental And Oral
Retainer, Matrix	Dental And Oral
Solution, Antibacterial Cleaner	General
Wax, Dental	Dental And Oral

PROFESSIONAL PRODUCT RESEARCH CO., INC.
See Ppr Direct, Inc.

PROFESSIONAL PRODUCTS, INC.   800-234-9004
54 Hugh Adams Dr., De Funiak Springs, FL 32435
FDA Number: 1026765
Web site: www.ezywrap.com
Year Founded: 1958
Ownership: Private
Produces/Sells CE-marked Devices: Y
Federal Procurement Eligibility: Small Business
Distribution: Manufacturer Direct

Belt, Traction, Pelvic, Orthopedic	Orthopedics
Binder, Abdominal	General
Brace, Joint, Ankle (External)	Physical Med
Joint, Knee, External Brace	Physical Med
Orthosis, Cervical-Thoracic, Rigid	Physical Med
Orthosis, Lumbosacral	Physical Med
Orthosis, Rib Fracture, Soft	Physical Med
Protector, Skin Pressure	General
Sling, Arm	Physical Med
Splint, Clavicle	Physical Med
Splint, Hand, And Component	Physical Med

PROFESSIONAL SPECIALTIES CO. INC.
See Profex Medical Products

PROFESSIONAL TAPE CO. INC.
See Timemed Labeling Systems, Inc.

PROFESSIONAL'S CHOICE SPORTS MEDICINE   800-331-9421
PRODUCTS, INC.
2025 Gillestie way suite #106,
El Cajon, CA 92020
FDA Number: n/a   *Fax:* 800-670-7180
E-mail: info@profchoice.com
Web site: www.profchoice.com
Medical Products Sales Volume: $7,100,000
Annual Revenue: $10-$25 Million
Year Founded: 1976
Total Employees: 80   *Marketing Staff:* 5   *Sales Staff:* 5
Ownership: Private
Produces/Sells CE-marked Devices: Y
Federal Procurement Eligibility: Small Business, Female Owned
Distribution: Manufacturer Direct, Manufacturer Through Distributor, Manufacturer Through Manufacturer Reps
General Admin.: Dal Scott/President
    Nina Scott/Vice President, General Manager
Mktg./Adv.: Barbara Gallagher/Director Marketing
    Cindy Lang/Sales Associate
    Monty Crist/Vice President Marketing & Sales
Production: Tony Lang/Vice President Manufacturing

Orthosis, Other	Physical Med
Orthosis, Rib Fracture, Soft	Physical Med
Shoe, Orthopedic	Orthopedics
Splint, Abduction, Shoulder	Orthopedics
Support, Ankle	Orthopedics
Support, Back	Orthopedics
Support, Elbow	Orthopedics
Support, Knee	Physical Med
Support, Thigh	Physical Med
Support, Wrist	Physical Med

PROFEX MEDICAL PRODUCTS   800-325-0196
2224 E. Person Ave., Memphis, TN 38114   901-452-7485
FDA Number: 1043615   *Fax:* 901-454-9850
E-mail: wallace@profexmed.com
Web site: www.profexmedical.com
Year Founded: 1938
Ownership: Private
Produces/Sells CE-marked Devices: N
Federal Procurement Eligibility: Small Business
Distribution: Manufacturer Through Distributor
General Admin.: Stephen E. Zwick/Chief Executive Officer

Attachment, Bag (Crutch, Walker, Wheelchair)	Physical Med
Board, Spine	Orthopedics
Chair, Examination And Treatment	General
Component, Exercise	Physical Med
Container, Specimen, All Types	General
Container, Urine Specimen	General
Cover, Arm Board	General
Cover, Bedrail	General
Cover, Cart	General
Cover, Mattress, Conductive	General
Cover, Mattress, Waterproof	General
Cover, Stool	General
Crutch	Physical Med
Cup, Medicine	General
Cushion, Other	General
Cushion, Stool	General
Cushion, Wheelchair (Pad)	Physical Med
Dropper, Eye	Ophthalmology
Dropper, Medicine	General
Finger Cot	General
Holder, Medical Chart	General
Holder, Thermometer	General
Jar, Applicator	Surgery
Jar, Blade	Surgery
Labware, Basic, Reusable	Chemistry
Liner, Kick Bucket	General
Liner, Laundry Hamper	General
Mattress, Air Flotation	General
Mattress, Operating Table	General
Pad, Dressing	General
Pad, Pressure, Foam (Elbow, Heel)	General
Pad, Pressure, Foam Convoluted	General
Restraint, Ankle/Foot	General
Restraint, Arm	General
Restraint, Patient, Conductive	Anesthesiology
Restraint, Protective (Body)	General
Restraint, Vest	General
Restraint, Wheelchair	General
Restraint, Wrist/Hand	General
Sand Bag	Radiology
Stirrup	Gastroenterology/Urology
Strap, Restraining	General
Support, Patient Position	Anesthesiology
Support, Patient Position, Radiographic	Radiology
Table, Blood Donor	Hematology

PROFEX MEDICAL PRODUCTS   800-325-0196 (cont'd)

Table, Examination/Treatment	General
Table, Physical Therapy	Physical Med
Tips And Pads, Cane, Crutch And Walker	Physical Med
Transfer Device, Patient, Manual	General
Tray, Wheelchair	Physical Med
Unit, Examining/Treatment, ENT	Ear/Nose/Throat
Urinometer, Non-Electrical	Gastroenterology/Urology

PROFILES, INC.   800-959-3171

7 First St., Palmer Industrial Park,   **413-283-7790**
Palmer, MA 01069
FDA Number: n/a   Fax: 413-283-6372
E-mail: ldalton@profiles-inc.com
Web site: www.profiles-inc.com
Year Founded: 1965
Total Employees: 28
Ownership: Private
Quality System Registration Information: ISO9001
Produces/Sells CE-marked Devices: N
Federal Procurement Eligibility: Small Business
Distribution: Manufacturer Direct
Mktg./Adv.: Mr. Derek Brock/Sales Engineer

Metal, Medical	General

PROGENY DENTAL   888-924-3800

1407 Barclay Blvd, Buffalo Grove, IL 60089   **847-850-3800**
FDA Number: 2027890   Fax: 847-850-3801
E-mail: info@progeny-inc.com
Web site: www.progenydental.com
Medical Products Sales Volume: $15,000,000
Year Founded: 2004
Total Employees: 40
Ownership: McDonough Medical Products Corporation
Quality System Registration Information: ISO9001
Produces/Sells CE-marked Devices: Y
Federal Procurement Eligibility: Small Business
Distribution: Manufacturer Through Manufacturer Reps, OEM, Exporter
General Admin.: Ed McDonough/Chief Executive Officer
Mktg./Adv.: Carole Howard-Lee/Director Marketing & Sales
     John MacLennan/Vice President, Director Marketing

Camera, Video	General
Radiographic Unit, Diagnostic, Dental (X-Ray)	Dental And Oral

Medical Product Subsidiaries (Listed Separately)
    3M Company

PROGENY, INC.   847-415-9800

675 Heathrow Dr., Lincolnshire, IL 60069
FDA Number: 1423380

Cable	Physical Med
Camera, Television, Surgical (Without Audio)	Surgery
Collimator, Radiographic, Automatic	Radiology
Collimator, Radiographic, Manual	Radiology
Grid, Radiographic	Radiology
Radiographic Unit, Diagnostic, Dental, Extraoral	Dental And Oral
System, X-ray, Extraoral Source, Digital	Radiology

PROGNOSTIX, INC.   216-445-1380

10265 Carnegie Avenue, Cleveland, OH 44106
FDA Number: 3004860239

Myeloperoxidase, Immunoassay, System, Test	Immunology

PROGRESSIVE APPLIANCE CORP.   978-649-9334

9 Gloria Ave., Tyngsboro, MA 01879
FDA Number: 1225708

Orthosis, Lumbosacral	Physical Med

PROGRESSIVE DENTAL SERVICES LAB   800-516-0789

21006 No. 22nd Street, Suite B-1,   **602-993-5250**
Phoenix, AZ 85024
FDA Number: 2032828   Fax: 602-993-7739
E-mail: pcochran@dentalservices.net
Web site: www.dentalservices.net
Ownership: Private
Produces/Sells CE-marked Devices: N

Mouthguard	Dental And Oral

PROGRESSIVE DENTAL   800-443-3106
SUPPLY/PROGRESSIVE ORTHODONTICS SEMINARS

1701 E. Edinger Avenue, Suite C-1,   **714-973-2266**
Santa Ana, CA 92705
FDA Number: 9001022   Fax: 714-973-0145
E-mail: info@posortho.com
Web site: www.posortho.com
Medical Products Sales Volume: $8,000,000
Year Founded: 1980
Total Employees: 25   Marketing Staff: 1   Sales Staff: 3
Ownership: Private

PROGRESSIVE DENTAL   800-443-3106 (cont'd)

Quality System Registration Information: ISO9001
Produces/Sells CE-marked Devices: Y
Federal Procurement Eligibility: Small Business
Distribution: OEM, Exporter
General Admin.: B. D. McGann/President

Aligner, Bracket, Orthodontic	Dental And Oral
Contract Manufacturing, Product, Durable	General
Refractor, Ophthalmic	Ophthalmology

PROGRESSIVE DYNAMICS MEDICAL, INC.   269-781-4241

507 Industrial Rd., Marshall, MI 49068-1758
FDA Number: 1831160   Fax: 269-781-7802
E-mail: sales@progressivedyn.com
Web site: www.progressivedynamicsmedical.com
Medical Products Sales Volume: $5,000,000
Annual Revenue: $10-$25 Million
Year Founded: 1964
Total Employees: 110   Marketing Staff: 2   Sales Staff: 5
Ownership: Private
Quality System Registration Information: ISO9001
Produces/Sells CE-marked Devices: Y
Federal Procurement Eligibility: Small Business
Distribution: Manufacturer Direct, Manufacturer Through Distributor, Manufacturer Through Manufacturer Reps, OEM
General Admin.: David Gregory/Director Human Resources
     Ralph McGee/President, Chief Executive Officer
     Thomas Phlipot/Vice President, General Manager
Mktg./Adv.: Kellie Kinsey/Director National Accounts
     David Dykehouse/Manager Sales
Production: Thomas Phlipot/Director Engineering
     Dennis Madison/Manager Materials
     Robert Bauer/Manager Regulatory Affairs

Contract Manufacturing	General
Cover, Other	General
Fiberoptic Light Source & Carrier	Ear/Nose/Throat
Hypothermia Unit	General
Hypothermia Unit (Blanket, Plumbing & Heat Exchanger)	Anesthesiology
Illuminator, Fiberoptic (For Endoscope)	Gastroenterology/Urology
Light Source, Endoscopic	Obstetrics/Gynecology
Light Source, Fiberoptic, Routine	Gastroenterology/Urology
Light, Surgical, Fiberoptic	Surgery

PROGRESSIVE IV'S, INC.

See I.V. House, Inc.

PROGRESSIVE MEDICAL INTERNATIONAL   800-764-0636

2460 Ash Street, Vista, CA 92081   **760-597-5500**
FDA Number: 2087166   Fax: 760-597-5501
E-mail: pmi@progressivemed.com
Web site: www.progressivemed.com
Medical Products Sales Volume: $600,000
Annual Revenue: $1-$5 Million
Year Founded: 1992
Total Employees: 9   Marketing Staff: 2   Sales Staff: 6
Ownership: Private
Produces/Sells CE-marked Devices: N
Federal Procurement Eligibility: Small Business
Distribution: Exclusive Distributor, Importer, Exporter
General Admin.: Marc D. Lawrence/President, Chief Executive Officer
Mktg./Adv.: Mark A. Cervenka/Director Product Development
     Jenny Hansen/Manager Advertising
     Mark Cervenka/Manager International & National Sales
     Mark Cervenka/Vice President International Marketing & Sales
     Mark Cervenka/Vice President Sales

Facility, Equipment, Medical, Mobile	General
Service, Used Equipment	General

PROGRESSIVE MEDICAL SYSTEMS, INC.   602-421-2484

1221 West Warner Rd.,suite 103, Tempe, AZ 85284
FDA Number: 2032842
Ownership: Private
Produces/Sells CE-marked Devices: N

Irrigator, Colonic	Gastroenterology/Urology

PROGRESSIVE OPERATIONS, INC.   314-570-5153

8455 Wabash Avenue, St. Louis, MO 63134
FDA Number: 3006031865
Ownership: Private
Produces/Sells CE-marked Devices: N

Collector, Urine, Powered, Non Indwelling Catheter	Gastroenterology/Urology

PROGRESSIVE TECHNOLOGY, INC.   916-632-6715

4130 Citrus Ave #17, Rocklin, CA 95677
FDA Number: 2939457

Aligner, Bracket, Orthodontic	Dental And Oral

PROGROUP INSTRUMENT CORP.
800-471-1916
4947 Fosterburg Road, Alton, IL 62002
618-258-7393
FDA Number: n/a
Fax: 618-259-4582
E-mail: shovey@wellpro.us
Web site: www.wellpro.us
Medical Products Sales Volume: $300,000
Annual Revenue: $1-$5 Million
Year Founded: 1991
Total Employees: 4
Ownership: Private
Stock Symbol: HAR.
Traded On: NYSE
Produces/Sells CE-marked Devices: Y
Federal Procurement Eligibility: Small Business
Distribution: Manufacturer Direct, Manufacturer Through Distributor, Manufacturer Through Manufacturer Reps, OEM, Service Direct, Exporter
General Admin.: Scott A. Hovey/President
  Microtiter Diluting/Dispensing Device — Microbiology

PROLAB SCIENTIFIC
800-556-5226
2213 le Chatelier St.,
450-682-5118
Laval, QUE H7L-5 Canada
FDA Number: n/a
Fax: 450-682-6468
E-mail: info@prolabscientific.com
Web site: http://www.prolabscientific.com
Year Founded: 1974
Total Employees: 25
Ownership: Private
Produces/Sells CE-marked Devices: N
Distribution: Exclusive Distributor

PROMA, INC.
310-327-0035
730 East Kingshill Pl., Carson, CA 90746
FDA Number: 2020475
  Light, Surgical Operating, Dental — Dental And Oral
  Operative Dental Treatment Unit — Dental And Oral

PROMATURA GROUP, LLC
800-201-1483
19 County Road 168, Oxford, MS 38655
662-234-0158
FDA Number: n/a
Fax: 662-234-0288
E-mail: info@promatura.com
Web site: www.promatura.com
Medical Products Sales Volume: $900,000
Annual Revenue: $1-$5 Million
Year Founded: 1985
Total Employees: 17 — *Marketing Staff:* 2 — *Sales Staff:* 2
Ownership: Private
Federal Procurement Eligibility: Small Business, Female Owned
Distribution: Service Direct
General Admin.: Margaret A. Wylde/President, Chief Executive Officer
  Bernie Smith/Vice President, General Manager
Mktg./Adv.: Edie Smith/Vice President Market Research
  Service, Consulting — General

PROMEDIC, INC.
239-498-2155
24301 woodsage drive, Bonita Springs, FL 34134-2015
FDA Number: 1834325
Fax: 239-236-0354
E-mail: info@promedic.cc
Web site: www.promedic.cc
Year Founded: 1992
Total Employees: 1 — *Marketing Staff:* 1
Ownership: Private
Produces/Sells CE-marked Devices: Y
Federal Procurement Eligibility: Small Business
Distribution: Manufacturer Through Distributor
  Analyzer, Gas, Carbon-Dioxide, Gaseous Phase (Capnograph) — Anesthesiology
  Circuit, Breathing (W Connector, Adapter, Y Piece) — Anesthesiology
  Filter, Bacterial, Breathing Circuit — Anesthesiology
  Laryngoscope, Rigid — Anesthesiology
  Light, Examination, Battery-Powered — General

PROMEDICA, INC.
  See Promedica, Inc.

PROMEGA CORP.
800-356-9526
2800 Woods Hollow Rd., Madison, WI 53711
608-274-4330
FDA Number: 2134567
Fax: 608-277-2516
E-mail: custserv@promega.com
Web site: www.promega.com
Annual Revenue: $100-$500 Million
Year Founded: 1978
Total Employees: 920
Ownership: Private
Quality System Registration Information: ISO9001
Produces/Sells CE-marked Devices: N
Federal Procurement Eligibility: Small Business
Distribution: Manufacturer Direct, Manufacturer Through Manufacturer Reps, Exporter

PROMEGA CORP.
800-356-9526 *(cont'd)*
  Antibody, Monoclonal — Microbiology
  Antibody, Other — General
  Device, Semen Analysis — Obstetrics/Gynecology
  Enzyme, Cell (Erythrocytic And Leukocytic) — Hematology
  Equipment, Laboratory, Gen. Purpose (Specific Medical Use) — Chemistry
  Reagent, General Purpose — Pathology
  Test, DNA-Probe, Other — Microbiology

PROMETHEAN MEDICAL TECHNOLOGIES, INC.
763-259-0559
105 Old Highway #8, Suite 1, New Brighton, MN 55112
FDA Number: 2134713
  Washer, Receptacle, Waste, Body — General

PROMETHEUS LABORATORIES INC
888-423-5227
9410 Carroll Park Drive, San Diego, CA 92121
FDA Number: n/a
Fax: 877-816-4019
E-mail: exus@prometheuslabs.com
Web site: www.prometheuslabs.com
Ownership: Private
Produces/Sells CE-marked Devices: N
General Admin.: Mr. Joseph Limber/President, Chief Executive Officer
  Ms. Toni Wayne/Vice President Human Resources
  Mr. William Franzblau/Vice President Legal Affairs, Corporate
Counsel
Production: Mr. Frederick Fletcher/Vice President Operations
Research: Dr. Sharat Singh/Vice President Research & Development
Finance: Mr. Peter Westlake/Vice President Finance

PROMETIC BIOTHERAPEUTICS, INC.
301-917-6320
9800 Medical Center Dr., Suite C-110, Rockville, MD 20850
FDA Number: n/a
Fax: 301-838-9023
E-mail: info@prometic.us
Web site: www.prometic.com
Medical Products Sales Volume: $3,200,000
Annual Revenue: $1-$5 Million
Year Founded: 1994
Ownership: Public
Stock Symbol: PLI
Traded On: Toronto
Quality System Registration Information: ISO9001; ISO9002
Produces/Sells CE-marked Devices: N
Federal Procurement Eligibility: Small Business
Distribution: Manufacturer Direct
General Admin.: Pierre Laurin/President, Chairman, Chief Executive Officer
Finance: Bruce Pritchard/Chief Financial Officer
  Contract R&D, Diagnostics — General

PROMEX TECHNOLOGIES, LLC
317-736-0128
3049 Hudson St., Franklin, IN 46131
FDA Number: 1833550
  Applicator, Radionuclide, Manual — Radiology
  Biopsy Instrument — Gastroenterology/Urology
  Cutter, Vitreous Aspiration, AC-Powered — Ophthalmology
  Drill, Surgical, ENT (Electric Or Pneumatic) — Ear/Nose/Throat
  Guide, Surgical, Needle — Surgery
  Introducer, Catheter — Cardiovascular
  Kit, Biopsy Needle — Gastroenterology/Urology
  Motor, Surgical Instrument, AC-Powered — Surgery
  Needle, Spinal, Short-Term — General
  Pin, Fixation, Threaded — Orthopedics

PROMIDENT LLC
845-634-3997
242 North Main St., Clarkstown, NY 10956
FDA Number: 2433005
Ownership: Private
Produces/Sells CE-marked Devices: N
  Burr, Dental — Dental And Oral
  Handpiece, Air-Powered, Dental — Dental And Oral
  Handpiece, Contra- And Right-Angle Attachment, Dental — Dental And Oral
  Post, Root Canal — Dental And Oral

PROPORTIONAL TECHNOLOGIES, INC.
800-759-7325
8022 El Rio St., Houston, TX 77054
713-747-7324
FDA Number: 1648536
Fax: 713-747-7325
Web site: www.proportionaltech.com
Ownership: Private
Produces/Sells CE-marked Devices: N
  Camera, Gamma (Nuclear/Scintillation) — Radiology

PROPPER MANUFACTURING CO., INC.
800-832-4300
36-04 Skillman Ave.,
718-392-6650
Long Island City, NY 11101
FDA Number: 2410251
Fax: 718-482-8909
E-mail: marketing@proppermfg.com
Web site: www.proppermfg.com
Annual Revenue: $25-$50 Million
Year Founded: 1935
Total Employees: 160 — *Marketing Staff:* 3 — *Sales Staff:* 20

PROPPER MANUFACTURING CO., INC.   800-832-4300 (cont'd)

Ownership: Private
Quality System Registration Information: ISO9001
Produces/Sells CE-marked Devices: Y
Federal Procurement Eligibility: Small Business
Distribution: Manufacturer Through Distributor, Importer, Exporter
General Admin.: B. Schuman/Chief Executive Officer
         Graeme Silbert/Chief Operating Officer
         M. Tozzi/Manager Human Resources
         Georgina Deloatch/Program Manager
         Marian Schuman/Vice Chairman
Mktg./Adv.: Andrew Sharavara/Director Corporate Marketing
         Bill Hull/Director National Accounts
         Dene Bourne/Director National Accounts
         J. Raber/Manager Contract Sales
         Kevin Davis/Vice President National Sales
Production: Arvid Rodin/Director Quality Assurance & Regulatory Affairs
         Alston Jones/Manager Materials
         Lionel Florus/Vice President Operations
         Joseph Nussenbaum/Vice President Technology & Product Development
Research: Mahesh Patel/Vice President Research & Development

Blade, Scalpel	Surgery
Clip, Removable (Skin)	Surgery
Coverslip, Microscope Slide	Pathology
Cuff, Blood Pressure	Cardiovascular
Handle, Knife Blade	Surgery
Handle, Scalpel	Surgery
Hemacytometer	Hematology
Hemocytometer	Hematology
Lancet, Blood	General
Laryngoscope, Surgical	Surgery
Ophthalmoscope, AC-Powered	Ophthalmology
Ophthalmoscope, Battery-Powered	Ophthalmology
Oscillometer	Cardiovascular
Otoscope	Ear/Nose/Throat
Pack, Sterilization Wrapper (Bag And Accessories)	Surgery
Packaging, Sterilization	General
Pipette, Sahli	Hematology
Reagent, Occult Blood	Hematology
Scalpel, One-Piece (Knife)	Surgery
Slide, Microscope	Pathology
Speculum, Ear	Ear/Nose/Throat
Speculum, Nasal	Ear/Nose/Throat
Sphygmomanometer, Aneroid (Arterial Pressure)	General
Sphygmomanometer, Electronic, Automatic	General
Sphygmomanometer, Electronic, Manual	General
Sphygmomanometer, Mercury (Arterial Pressure)	General
Spirometer, Diagnostic (Respirometer)	Anesthesiology
Sterilization Process Indicator, Biological	General
Sterilization Process Indicator, Chemical	General
Sterilization Process Indicator, Physical/Chemical	General
Tourniquet, Non-Pneumatic, Surgical	Surgery
Tube, Capillary Blood Collection	Hematology
Wrap, Sterilization	General

PROQUEST CANADA INC.   905-607-7190
4167 Treetop Crescent, Mississauga, ONT L5L-2L7 Canada
FDA Number: n/a   Fax: 905-607-3590
E-mail: sylviak@interlog.com
Year Founded: 1999
Total Employees: 10
Ownership: Private
Produces/Sells CE-marked Devices: N
Distribution: Manufacturer Direct, Exclusive Distributor, Exporter

PRORHYTHM, INC.   631-981-3907
105 Comac St., Ronkonkoma, NY 11779
FDA Number: 3005741810

Catheter, Electrode Recording, Or Probe	Cardiovascular

PROSCIENCE INC., GLASS SHOP DIVISION   1-888-335-9113
770 Birchmount Rd., Unit 25,   416-699-5555
Scarborough, ONT M1K-5 Canada
FDA Number: n/a   Fax: 416-751-4224
E-mail: proscience@bellnet.ca
Web site: www.proscience.com
Year Founded: 1912
Total Employees: 25
Ownership: Private
Produces/Sells CE-marked Devices: N
Distribution: Manufacturer Direct

PROSEC PROTECTION SYSTEMS, INC.   732-886-0990
1985 Swarthmore Ave., Suite 7, Lakewood, NJ 08701
FDA Number: 2249805

Occluder, Umbilical	General

PROSTHETICS BY NELSON, INC.
See Nelson Prosthetic & Orthotic Laboratory

PROSUN TANNING INTERNATIONAL, LLC.   800-874-2776
2442 23rd Street North,   727-825-0400
St. Petersburg, FL 33713
FDA Number: 1058796   Fax: 727-825-0700
E-mail: sales@prosun.com
Web site: www.prosun.com
Medical Products Sales Volume: $2,700,000
Annual Revenue: $5-$10 Million
Year Founded: 1972
Total Employees: 30   Marketing Staff: 2   Sales Staff: 10
Ownership: Private
Quality System Registration Information: ISO9001
Produces/Sells CE-marked Devices: Y
Federal Procurement Eligibility: Small Business
Distribution: Manufacturer Direct, Exclusive Distributor

Booth, Sun Tan	Physical Med

PROSURGE INSTRUMENTS, INC.   866-832-7874
199 Laidlaw Avenue, Jersey City, NJ 07306-2511   201-714-7003
FDA Number: 2249443   Fax: 201-714-9550
E-mail: sales@prosurge.com
Web site: www.prosurge.com
Medical Products Sales Volume: $500,000
Annual Revenue: $0-$1 Million
Year Founded: 1999
Total Employees: 2   Marketing Staff: 1   Sales Staff: 1
Ownership: Private
Produces/Sells CE-marked Devices: N
Federal Procurement Eligibility: Small Business
Distribution: Exclusive Distributor, Importer, Exporter
General Admin.: Muhammad Razi/President
Mktg./Adv.: Arshan Mughal/Manager Marketing & Sales

Accessories, Retractor, Dental	Dental And Oral
Applicator, Clip (Forceps)	General
Clamp, Vascular	Cardiovascular
Cleaner, Forceps, Biopsy	Cardiovascular
Cover, Biopsy Forceps	Gastroenterology/Urology
Dissector, Tonsil	Ear/Nose/Throat
Forceps	Orthopedics
Forceps, Articulation Paper	Dental And Oral
Forceps, Biopsy	Surgery
Forceps, Biopsy, Bronchoscope (Rigid)	Anesthesiology
Forceps, Biopsy, Gynecological	Obstetrics/Gynecology
Forceps, Biopsy, Non-Electric	Gastroenterology/Urology
Forceps, Dressing	Surgery
Forceps, Dressing, Dental	Dental And Oral
Forceps, ENT	Ear/Nose/Throat
Forceps, Endoscopic	Gastroenterology/Urology
Forceps, General & Plastic Surgery	Surgery
Forceps, Grasping, Atraumatic	Surgery
Forceps, Grasping, Traumatic	Surgery
Forceps, Hemostatic	Surgery
Forceps, Intestinal (Clamps)	Gastroenterology/Urology
Forceps, Obstetrical	Obstetrics/Gynecology
Forceps, Ophthalmic	Ophthalmology
Forceps, Rongeur, Surgical	Dental And Oral
Forceps, Rubber Dam Clamp	Dental And Oral
Forceps, Sponge	Surgery
Forceps, Surgical, Gynecological	Obstetrics/Gynecology
Forceps, Tissue	Surgery
Forceps, Tooth Extractor, Surgical	Dental And Oral
Forceps, Utility	Surgery
Forceps, Wire Closure, ENT	Ear/Nose/Throat
Forceps, Wire Holding	Orthopedics
General Use Surgical Scissors	Surgery
Handle, Knife, Laparoscopic	Surgery
Hemostat	Orthopedics
Hemostat, Surgical	Dental And Oral
Holder, Needle	Gastroenterology/Urology
Holder, Speculum, ENT	Ear/Nose/Throat
Holder/Scissors, Needle, Laparoscopic	Surgery
Instrument, Dental, Manual	Dental And Oral
Instrument, Dissecting, Laparoscopic	Surgery
Instrument, Microsurgical	Cns/Neurology
Pliers, Surgical	Orthopedics
Remover, Foreign Body, Bronchoscope (Non-Rigid)	Anesthesiology
Scissors, Bandage/Gauze/Plaster	General
Scissors, Cardiovascular	Cardiovascular
Scissors, Ear	Ear/Nose/Throat
Scissors, General Dissecting	General
Scissors, Gynecological	Obstetrics/Gynecology
Scissors, Iris	Ophthalmology
Scissors, Nasal	Ear/Nose/Throat
Scissors, Neurosurgical (Dura)	Cns/Neurology
Scissors, Orthopedic	Orthopedics
Scissors, Plastic Surgery (Dissecting)	Surgery
Scissors, Rectal	Gastroenterology/Urology

PROSURGE INSTRUMENTS, INC.   866-832-7874 (cont'd)

Scissors, Surgical Tissue, Dental (Oral)	Dental And Oral
Scissors, Tenotomy	Ophthalmology
Scissors, Umbilical	Obstetrics/Gynecology
Scissors, Wire Cutting, ENT	Ear/Nose/Throat
Sharpener, Instrument, Surgical	Surgery
Speculum, Ear	Ear/Nose/Throat
Speculum, Nasal	Ear/Nose/Throat
Speculum, Ophthalmic	Ophthalmology
Speculum, Rectal	Gastroenterology/Urology
Speculum, Vaginal, Metal	Obstetrics/Gynecology
Speculum, Vaginal, Metal, Fiberoptic	Obstetrics/Gynecology
Surgical Instrument, Manual (General Use)	Surgery
Tenaculum, Other (Forceps)	Surgery
Tray, Surgical	Surgery
Urinal	General
Wire, Orthodontic	Dental And Oral

PROTATEK REFERENCE LABORATORY   480-545-8499
574 East Alamo Dr., Suite 90, Chandler, AZ 85225
FDA Number: 2029179   Fax: 480-545-8409
Web site: www.protatek.com
Ownership: Private
Produces/Sells CE-marked Devices: N

Antigen, CF, Typhus Fever Group	Microbiology

PROTECH LEADED EYEWEAR   561-627-9769
10415 riverside drive, Palm Beach Gardens, FL 33410
FDA Number: 1063300   Fax: 561-627-0923
E-mail: info@protecheyewear.com
Web site: www.protecheyewear.com
Ownership: Protech,Leaded Eyewear, Inc.
Quality System Registration Information: ISO9001
Produces/Sells CE-marked Devices: Y
Production: Ms. Ingrid Bergman/Manager Quality Assurance & Regulatory Affairs

Apron, Lead, Radiographic	Radiology
Barrier, Control Panel, X-Ray, Moveable	Radiology
Glove, Protective, Radiographic	Radiology
Shield, Eye, Ophthalmic	Ophthalmology
Shield, Gonadal	Radiology
Shield, Protective, Personnel	Radiology
Shield, X-Ray	Radiology
Shield, X-Ray, Lead-Plastic	Radiology
Shield, X-Ray, Portable	Radiology
Shield, X-Ray, Transparent	Radiology

PROTECH PROFESSIONAL PRODUCTS, INC.   561-493-9818
2900 Nw Commerce Park Dr., #10, Boynton Beach, FL 33426
FDA Number: 2435952

Base, Denture, Relining, Repairing, Rebasing, Resin	Dental And Oral
Cleaner, Denture	Dental And Oral
Material, Tooth Shade, Resin	Dental And Oral
Sealant, Pit And Fissure, And Conditioner, Resin	Dental And Oral

PROTECTAIR INC.   800-235-7932
59 Eisenhower Ln., Lombard, IL 60148   800-235-7932
FDA Number: n/a   Fax: 630-916-9115
E-mail: protectair@msn.com
Web site: www.protectairinc.com
Medical Products Sales Volume: $3,000,000
Total Employees: 12   Marketing Staff: 2   Sales Staff: 4
Ownership: Private
Produces/Sells CE-marked Devices: N
Federal Procurement Eligibility: Small Business
Distribution: Manufacturer Direct, Manufacturer Through Manufacturer Reps
General Admin.: Larry Montgomery/President, Chief Executive Officer
Mktg./Adv.: Diane Michaelis/Manager Contract Sales

Blade, Saw, Cast Cutting	Orthopedics
Component, Cast	Orthopedics
Immobilizer, Ankle	Orthopedics
Immobilizer, Shoulder	Orthopedics
Joint, Knee, External Brace	Physical Med
Support, Ankle	Orthopedics
Surgical Instrument, Manual (General Use)	Surgery

PROTECTION PRODUCTS, INC.   800-869-6818
PO Box 59367, Homewood, AL 35259-9367   205-271-3131
FDA Number: 1053198   Fax: 205-271-3111
E-mail: al@p-p-i.com
Web site: www.p-p-i.com
Annual Revenue: $1-$5 Million
Total Employees: 10   Marketing Staff: 2   Sales Staff: 2
Ownership: Private
Federal Procurement Eligibility: Small Business
Distribution: OEM
General Admin.: Albert E. Ritchey/Chief Executive Officer
    Thomas C. Reeves/President
Mktg./Adv.: Don Barrington/Vice President Marketing & Sales
Production: Michelle Waite/Manager Customer Services
    Sue Coalson/Manager Operations

PROTECTION PRODUCTS, INC.   800-869-6818 (cont'd)
Contract Packaging   General

PROTECTIVE LINING CO.   800-221-9712
601 39th St., Brooklyn, NY 11232   718-854-3838
FDA Number: n/a   Fax: 718-854-4658
Web site: www.prolining.com
Annual Revenue: $10-$25 Million
Year Founded: 1951
Ownership: Private
Produces/Sells CE-marked Devices: N
Distribution: Manufacturer Direct, Manufacturer Through Distributor, Manufacturer Through Manufacturer Reps, OEM, Service Direct, Exclusive Distributor

Cover, Mattress, Conductive	General
Liner, Kick Bucket	General
Packaging, Sterilization	General

PROTECTIVE MEDICAL PRODUCTS (PMP) INC.   888-669-9470
95 chemin Du Lac,   819-669-9470
Gatineau, QUE J8P-4 Canada
FDA Number: n/a   Fax: 888-669-8995
E-mail: information@pmpint.com
Web site: http://www.pmpint.com
Year Founded: 1992
Total Employees: 10
Ownership: Private
Produces/Sells CE-marked Devices: N
Distribution: Manufacturer Direct, Exclusive Distributor

PROTECTOR CANADA INC.   800-268-6594
1111 Flint Rd., Unit 23,   416-665-7766
Toronto, ON M3J 3 Canada
FDA Number: n/a   Fax: 416-665-6923
E-mail: shield@protectorcanada.com
Web site: www.protectorcanada.com
Medical Products Sales Volume: $3,000,000
Year Founded: 1983
Total Employees: 25   Marketing Staff: 2   Sales Staff: 4
Ownership: Private
Produces/Sells CE-marked Devices: N
Distribution: Manufacturer Through Distributor, OEM, Importer, Exporter

PROTECTOSEAL CO.   800-323-2268
225 W. Foster Avenue,   630-595-0800
Bensenville, IL 60106
FDA Number: 7000881   Fax: 630-595-8059
E-mail: info@protectoseal.com
Web site: www.protectoseal.com
Annual Revenue: $0-$1 Million
Year Founded: 1970
Total Employees: 50   Marketing Staff: 2   Sales Staff: 12
Ownership: Private
Quality System Registration Information: ISO9001
Produces/Sells CE-marked Devices: Y
Federal Procurement Eligibility: Small Business, GSA Contract
Distribution: Manufacturer Through Distributor
General Admin.: Larry Borowczyk/President
Mktg./Adv.: Carol Beem/Executive Advertising
    Carol Beem/Vice President Marketing
    Ross Giordano/Vice President Sales
Production: J. Roche/Vice President Manufacturing

Cabinet, Medicine	General
Cabinet, Narcotic Control	General
Waste Receptacle, General Purpose	General

PROTECTUS MEDICAL DEVICES INC.   800-778-8438
110 First Ave., NE, Suite 1006, Minneapolis, MN 55413
FDA Number: n/a
E-mail: moreinfo@protectusmedical.com
Web site: www.protectusmedical.com
Ownership: Private
Produces/Sells CE-marked Devices: N
General Admin.: Mr. Jack Dillard/Chief Operating Officer, Executive Vice President
    Mr. John Ollinger/Director
    Dr. John Salstrom/President, Chief Executive Officer, Director
Medical Admin.: Dr. Dan Hartley/Medical Director
Mktg./Adv.: Mr. Ronald Ginn/Executive Vice President Marketing & Sales

PROTEIN SCIENCES CORP.   800-488-7099
1000 Research Pkwy., Meriden, CT 06450-7149   203-686-0800
FDA Number: n/a   Fax: 203-686-0268
E-mail: psc@proteinsciences.com
Web site: www.proteinsciences.com
Annual Revenue: $5-$10 Million
Total Employees: 15   Marketing Staff: 2
Ownership: Private
Produces/Sells CE-marked Devices: N

MANUFACTURER PROFILES

PROTEIN SCIENCES CORP. — 800-488-7099 (cont'd)
Federal Procurement Eligibility: Small Business
General Admin.: Daniel Adams/President, Chief Executive Officer
 Manon Cox/Vice President, General Manager
Production: Monica Rogers/Director Quality Assurance
Research: Gale Smith/Chief Scientist
 Separator, Protein — Chemistry
 Service, Design, Implant, Custom — Orthopedics

PROTEK MEDICAL PRODUCTS, INC. — 319-545-7100
4125 Westcor Court, Coralville, IA 52241
FDA Number: 1934029
 Cover, Barrier, Protective — General
 Drape, Surgical — Surgery
 Transducer, Ultrasonic, Diagnostic — Radiology

PROTEUS BIOMEDICAL, INC. — 650-632-4031
2600 Bridge Parkway, Suite 101, Redwood City, CA 94065
FDA Number: n/a   *Fax:* 650-632-4071
E-mail: info@proteusbiomed.com
Web site: www.proteusbiomed.com
Ownership: Private
Produces/Sells CE-marked Devices: N
General Admin.: Andrew M. Thompson/Chief Executive Officer
 Dr. Mark J. Zdeblick/Chief Technology Officer
Medical Admin.: Dr. George M. Savage/Chief Medical Officer
Finance: Joy Berberich/Vice President Finance
 Monitor, Cardiac (Cardiotachometer & Rate Alarm) — Cardiovascular

PROTEX CENTRAL INC. — 800-274-0888 / 402-463-0666
1239 N. Minnesota Avenue, PO Box 1467, Hastings, NE 68902
FDA Number: n/a   *Fax:* 402-463-6057
E-mail: info@protexcentral.com
Web site: www.protexcentral.com/
Medical Products Sales Volume: $3,000,000
Annual Revenue: $0-$1 Million
Year Founded: 1966
Total Employees: 47
Ownership: Private
Federal Procurement Eligibility: Small Business
Distribution: Service Direct
General Admin.: Denny Mullen/President
 Nurse Call System — General

PROTEX MEDICAL PRODUCTS, INC. — 877-776-8395 / 318-324-1155
913 Wood St., P.O. Box 2172, West Monroe, LA 71291
FDA Number: 3004112799   *Fax:* 318-324-0363
E-mail: protexmedical@yahoo.com
Web site: www.protexmedical.com
Ownership: Private
Produces/Sells CE-marked Devices: N
 Cover, Limb — Physical Med

PROTOCOL SYSTEMS, INC.
See Welch Allyn Protocol Inc.

PROTOMED — 303-422-2207
1329 West 121st Avenue, Westminster, CO 80234
FDA Number: 3004830697
 Template — Orthopedics

PROTOTYPE & PLASTIC MOLD CO., INC. — 203-632-2800
35 Industrial Park Pl., Middletown, CT 06457
FDA Number: n/a   *Fax:* 203-632-2249
E-mail: prototypeand.plastic@snet.net
Web site: www.prototypeplastic.com
Medical Products Sales Volume: $6,000,000
Annual Revenue: $5-$10 Million
Total Employees: 80   *Marketing Staff:* 1   *Sales Staff:* 2
Ownership: Private
Produces/Sells CE-marked Devices: N
Federal Procurement Eligibility: Small Business
Distribution: Manufacturer Direct
General Admin.: Victor de Jong/President
Mktg./Adv.: John Rose/Vice President Marketing & Sales
Production: Paul Testa/Director Operations
 Jeryl Greenawalt/Director Quality Assurance
 Contract Manufacturing — General
 Molding, Injection — General

PROTRON TECHNOLOGIES — 201-297-7377
PO Box 234, Alpine, NJ 07620
FDA Number: n/a
E-mail: info@Stethotron.com
Web site: www.Stethotron.com
Ownership: Private
Produces/Sells CE-marked Devices: N

PROTRON TECHNOLOGIES — 201-297-7377 (cont'd)
 Stethoscope, Electronic-Amplified — Surgery

PROUDFOOT COMPANY, INC. — 800-445-0034 / 203-459-0031
588 Pepper St., Monroe, CT 06468-0276
FDA Number: 9330100   *Fax:* 203-459-0033
E-mail: info@theproudfootcompany.com
Web site: www.noisemaster.com
Annual Revenue: $0-$1 Million
Total Employees: 13   *Marketing Staff:* 3   *Sales Staff:* 3
Ownership: Private
Produces/Sells CE-marked Devices: N
Federal Procurement Eligibility: Small Business
Distribution: Manufacturer Direct, Manufacturer Through Distributor, Importer, Exporter
General Admin.: Jim Loseth/General Manager
 David Proudfoot/President
 Room, Acoustical — Ear/Nose/Throat

PROUROCARE MEDICAL INC. — 925-476-9093
6440 Flying Cloud Dr., Suite 101, Eden Prairie, MN 55344
FDA Number: n/a   *Fax:* 952-843-7031
Web site: www.prourocare.com
Year Founded: 2006
Ownership: Public
Stock Symbol: PUMD
Traded On: OTC Bulletin
Produces/Sells CE-marked Devices: N
General Admin.: Richard Carlson/Chief Executive Officer
Finance: Richard Thon/Chief Financial Officer

PROVATION MEDICAL, INC. — 888-952-6673 / 612-313-1500
800 Washington Ave North, Suite 400, Minneapolis, MN 55401
FDA Number: 3006561961
Web site: www.provationmedical.com
Ownership: Private
Produces/Sells CE-marked Devices: N
 Accessories, Surgical Camera — Surgery
 Device, Storage, Image, Digital — Radiology
 System, Communication, Image, Digital — Radiology

PROVEN PROCESS MEDICAL DEVICES, INC. — 508-261-0806
110 Forbes Blvd., Mansfield, MA 02048
FDA Number: 3003174284
 Analyzer, Medical Image — Radiology
 Pump, Infusion, Implantable, General — General
 Pump, Infusion, Implantable, Non-Programmable — General

PROVON MEDICAL GROUP
See Gojo Industries, Inc

PROWESS, INC. — 925-356-0360
1370 Ridgewood Dr., #20, Chico, CA 95973
FDA Number: 2939248
 Simulator, Radiotherapy, Special Purpose — Radiology
 System, Planning, Radiation Therapy Treatment — Radiology
 Tester, Radiology — Radiology

PRU-DENT MANUFACTURING CO. — 800-631-2339
1929 S Wright Blvd, Schaumburg, IL 60193
FDA Number: 1419247
E-mail: retip@pru-dent.us
Web site: www.pru-dent.us
Medical Products Sales Volume: $300,000
Annual Revenue: $0-$1 Million
Total Employees: 14
Ownership: Private
Produces/Sells CE-marked Devices: N
Federal Procurement Eligibility: Small Business
Distribution: Manufacturer Direct, Manufacturer Through Distributor
General Admin.: John H. Prusaitis/Chief Executive Officer
 Curette — Orthopedics
 Explorer, Operative — Dental And Oral
 File, Periodontic — Dental And Oral
 Handle, Instrument, Dental — Dental And Oral
 Probe — Orthopedics
 Scaler, Rotary — Dental And Oral
 Service, Maintenance/Repair — General

PRU-DENT MFG. INC. — 847-301-1170
1929 S. Wright Blvd., Schaumburg, IL 60193
FDA Number: 1419247
 Handle, Instrument, Dental — Dental And Oral

PRYOR PRODUCTS — 800-854-2280 / 619-724-8244
1819 Peacock Blvd., Oceanside, CA 92056-3578
FDA Number: 9200899   *Fax:* 619-724-0944
E-mail: pryorproducts@pryorproducts.com

PRYOR PRODUCTS
800-854-2280 *(cont'd)*
Web site: www.pryorproducts.com
Year Founded: 1972
Total Employees: 100   *Marketing Staff:* 1   *Sales Staff:* 1
Ownership: Private
Produces/Sells CE-marked Devices: Y
Federal Procurement Eligibility: Small Business
Distribution: Manufacturer Direct, OEM
General Admin.: Jeff W. Pryor/Chief Executive Officer, Chief Financial Officer
          Paul Pryor/Chief Operating Officer
          Jon Willmschen/President

Attachment, Oxygen Canister/IV Pole, Wheelchair	General
Cabinet, Other	General
Clamp, Other	Surgery
Hanger, Intravenous	General
Infusion Stand	General
Stand, Instrument, Ophthalmic	Ophthalmology
Track And Carrier, Intravenous	General
Walker, Mechanical	Physical Med

PRZYBYLA & ASSOCIATES INC.
See Wisap America

PS PRODUCTS, LLC
215-661-9595
329 Bradford Lane, Lansdale, PA 19446
FDA Number: 98937
Ownership: Private
Produces/Sells CE-marked Devices: N

Orthosis, Abdominal	Physical Med

PS SOLUTIONS, INC.
972-548-8080
411 Interchange St., Mckinney, TX 75071
FDA Number: 3001623253

Device, Positive Pressure Breathing, Intermittent	Anesthesiology

PSC CORP.
See Olsen Medical

PSC MEDICAL, INC.
888-986-4276
813-287-0810
4930 W. Nassau Street, #284, Tampa, FL 33607
FDA Number: n/a   *Fax:* 603-258-4770
E-mail: info@pscmedical.com
Web site: www.pscmedical.com
Medical Products Sales Volume: $500,000
Year Founded: 2001
Total Employees: 4
Ownership: Private
Quality System Registration Information: ISO9002
Produces/Sells CE-marked Devices: Y
Federal Procurement Eligibility: Small Business
Distribution: Manufacturer Direct, Manufacturer Through Distributor, Manufacturer Through Manufacturer Reps
General Admin.: Mr. Arie Koren/President, Owner
          Mr. Gil Adler/Principal
          Mr. David Cohen/Vice President, General Manager

Drape, Surgical, Disposable	Surgery

PSG CONTROLS, INC.
800-523-2558
215-257-3621
1225 Tunnel Road, Perkasie, PA 18944
FDA Number: 9200836   *Fax:* 215-257-4288
E-mail: sales@psgcontrols.com
Web site: www.psgcontrols.com
Medical Products Sales Volume: $5,200,000
Year Founded: 1978
Total Employees: 60
Ownership: Private
Produces/Sells CE-marked Devices: N
Federal Procurement Eligibility: Small Business, GSA Contract
Distribution: Manufacturer Through Distributor, Manufacturer Through Manufacturer Reps, OEM
General Admin.: Mr. Thane Tagg/President
Production: Mr. Jack Turner/Chief Engineer

Controller, Temperature, Other	General
Monitor, Temperature (With Probe)	Anesthesiology
Thermometer, Electronic, Continuous	General

PSI
See Welch Allyn Protocol Inc.

PSI INFUSION INC.
See Medtronic Minimed

PSI/EYE-KO, INC.
636-447-1010
804 Corporate Centre Dr., O'fallon, MO 63368
FDA Number: 1929756

Cannula, Ophthalmic	Ophthalmology
Hook, Ophthalmic	Ophthalmology
Knife, Ophthalmic	Ophthalmology
Needle, Aspiration And Injection, Disposable	Surgery
Needle, Aspiration And Injection, Reusable	Surgery
Probe, Lacrimal	Ophthalmology

PSI/EYE-KO, INC.
636-447-1010 *(cont'd)*

Retractor, Ophthalmic	Ophthalmology
Spatula, Ophthalmic	Ophthalmology
Speculum, Ophthalmic	Ophthalmology

PSS BIO INSTRUMENTS, INC.
925-960-9182
6052 Industrial Way, Suite H, Livermore, CA 94551
FDA Number: 3005684145
Ownership: Private
Produces/Sells CE-marked Devices: N

Pipetting And Diluting System, Automated	Chemistry

PST
413-447-8051
1520 East St., Pittsfield, MA 01201
FDA Number: n/a   *Fax:* 413-447-8052
E-mail: info@pst-corp.com
Web site: www.pst-corp.com
Medical Products Sales Volume: $2,000,000
Annual Revenue: $1-$5 Million
Year Founded: 1993
Total Employees: 8   *Marketing Staff:* 1   *Sales Staff:* 2
Ownership: Private
Produces/Sells CE-marked Devices: Y
Federal Procurement Eligibility: Small Business, Female Owned
Distribution: OEM, Service Direct, Exclusive Distributor
General Admin.: Sandra Kristensen/President, Chief Executive Officer
Mktg./Adv.: Dean P. Barbalias/Director Marketing & Advertising
          Joan Couture/Manager Contract Sales
          Dean P. Barbalias/Manager International & National Sales
Production: Sandra Kristensen/Director Quality Assurance

Container, Sterilization (Tray)	General

PSYCHE SYSTEMS
800-345-1514
508-473-1500
321 Fortune Blvd., Milford, MA 01757
FDA Number: 1221871   *Fax:* 508-478-4717
E-mail: sales@psychesystems.com
Web site: www.psychesystems.com
Annual Revenue: $1-$5 Million
Total Employees: 40   *Marketing Staff:* 5   *Sales Staff:* 8
Ownership: Private
Produces/Sells CE-marked Devices: N
Federal Procurement Eligibility: Small Business
Distribution: Manufacturer Direct
General Admin.: Robert Sage/President, Chief Executive Officer
Mktg./Adv.: Suzanne Caron/Director Product Development
          Debbie Drennan/Manager Advertising
          Patricia Salem/Manager Marketing
          Patricia Salem/Marketing Representative
          Richard DeSimone/Vice President Marketing & Sales
Production: Suzanne Caron/Director Quality Assurance

Computer Software	General
Computer, Clinical Laboratory	Chemistry
Service, Computer	General
Software, Blood Bank (Stand-Alone Products)	Hematology

PSYCHEMEDICS CORP.
800-628-8073
978-206-8220
125 Nagog Park, Suite 200, Acton, MA 01720
FDA Number: n/a   *Fax:* 978-264-9236
E-mail: info@psychemedics.com
Web site: www.psychemedics.com
Medical Products Sales Volume: $23,400,000
Annual Revenue: $10-$25 Million
Year Founded: 1989
Total Employees: 97   *Marketing Staff:* 3   *Sales Staff:* 8
Ownership: Public
Stock Symbol: PMD
Traded On: AMEX
Produces/Sells CE-marked Devices: Y
Federal Procurement Eligibility: Small Business
Distribution: Manufacturer Direct
General Admin.: Ray Kubacki/President, Chief Executive Officer
          Mr. William Thistle/Senior Vice President, General Counsel
          Mr. Ray Ruddy/Vice President
Mktg./Adv.: Mr. Jim Dyke/Vice President Sales
Research: Dr. Michael Schaffer/Vice President Lab. Operations

Contract Laboratory	General
Enzyme Immunoassay, Opiates	Toxicology
Radioimmunoassay, Cannabinoid (S)	Toxicology
Radioimmunoassay, Cocaine Metabolite	Toxicology
Radioimmunoassay, Phencyclidine	Toxicology
Thin Layer Chromatography, Metamphetamine	Toxicology

PSYCHMEDICS CORP.
978-206-8220
125 Nagog Park, Action, MA 01720
FDA Number: 3005115810   *Fax:* 800-628-8073
Web site: http://www.psychemedics.com
Ownership: Public
Stock Symbol: PMD

PSYCHMEDICS CORP.   978-206-8220 *(cont'd)*

Traded On: NASDAQ
Produces/Sells CE-marked Devices: N
General Admin.: Mr. Raymond Kubacki/President, Chief Executive Officer
    Mr. William Thistle/Senior Vice President, General Counsel
Research: Dr. Michael Schaffer, Ph.D/Vice President Lab. Operations
Finance: Mr. Raymond Ruddy/Vice President, Controller

Enzyme Immunoassay, Opiates	Toxicology
Radioimmunoassay, Cannabinoid (S)	Toxicology
Radioimmunoassay, Cocaine Metabolite	Toxicology
Radioimmunoassay, Phencyclidine	Toxicology
Thin Layer Chromatography, Metamphetamine	Toxicology

PTR OPTICS

See Optometrics Llc

PULLEY-KELLAM CO., INC.   260-356-6326

245 Erie St., Huntington, IN 46750
FDA Number: 1832125
                Fax: 260-356-1928
E-mail: info@pulleykellam.com
Medical Products Sales Volume: $7,000,000
Year Founded: 1961
Total Employees: 22   *Marketing Staff:* 1   *Sales Staff:* 1
Ownership: Private
Quality System Registration Information: ISO9001
Produces/Sells CE-marked Devices: N
Federal Procurement Eligibility: Small Business, Female Owned
Distribution: OEM
General Admin.: Ms. Marla Foster/Chief Executive Officer, Vice President
Marketing
               Mr. James Foster/President
               Mr. Charles Kellam/Secretary, Treasurer
Production: Mr. Maury Pulley/Vice President Manufacturing, General Manager

Powered Medical Examination Table	General
Table, Examination/Treatment	General
Table, Mechanical	Physical Med
Table, Obstetrical, AC-Powered	Obstetrics/Gynecology
Table, Obstetrical, Manual	Obstetrics/Gynecology

PULMONARY DIAGNOSTICS

See Telediagnostic Systems

PULMONOX MEDICAL CORPORATION   888-464-8742

5243-53 Ave, Tofield, ALB T0B 4J0 Canada   **780-662-3968**
FDA Number: 9680537   *Fax:* 780-662-4255
E-mail: sales@pulmonox.com
Web site: www.pulmonox.com
Year Founded: 1993
Total Employees: 50
Ownership: Private
Produces/Sells CE-marked Devices: N
Distribution: Manufacturer Direct

PULMONX   650-364-0400

700 Chesapeake Drive, Redwood City, CA 94063
FDA Number: 3007797756   *Fax:* 650-364-0403
E-mail: customerservice@pulmonx.com
Web site: www.pulmonx.com
Ownership: Private
Produces/Sells CE-marked Devices: N

Spirometer, Diagnostic (Respirometer)	Anesthesiology
Tube, Tracheal (Endotracheal)	Anesthesiology

PULNIX AMERICA INC.   800-445-5444

1330 Orleans Drive, Sunnyvale, CA 94089   **408-747-0300**
FDA Number: n/a   *Fax:* 408-747-0660
E-mail: camerasales.americas@jai.com
Web site: www.pulnix.com
Annual Revenue: $5-$10 Million
Year Founded: 1963
Total Employees: 100
Ownership: TAKENAKA GROUP CENTER
Quality System Registration Information: ISO9001
Produces/Sells CE-marked Devices: Y
Federal Procurement Eligibility: Small Business
Distribution: Manufacturer Direct, Manufacturer Through Distributor, OEM,
Importer, Exporter
General Admin.: Joegreen Amdersem/President, Chief Executive Officer
Mktg./Adv.: Ken Zinsin/Director Marketing & Sales
          Toshi Hori/Director Product Development
          Vicki Stuart/Manager Customer Services & Sales
Production: Howard Myers/Director Quality Assurance
          Cecelia Cordoncillo/Manager Materials

Camera, Other	General

PULPDENT CORP.   800-343-4342

80 Oakland St., Watertown, MA 02471-0780   **617-926-6666**
FDA Number: 1215305   *Fax:* 617-926-6262
E-mail: pulpdent@pulpdent.com

PULPDENT CORP.   800-343-4342 *(cont'd)*

Web site: www.pulpdent.com
Annual Revenue: $10-$25 Million
Year Founded: 1947
Ownership: Private
Quality System Registration Information: ISO9001
Produces/Sells CE-marked Devices: Y
Distribution: Manufacturer Through Distributor, OEM, Exporter

Accessories, Retractor, Dental	Dental And Oral
Adhesive, Bracket And Conditioner, Resin	Dental And Oral
Agent, Polishing, Abrasive, Oral Cavity	Dental And Oral
Alloy, Amalgam	Dental And Oral
Band, Material, Orthodontic	Dental And Oral
Broach, Endodontic	Dental And Oral
Burnisher, Operative, Dental	Dental And Oral
Carrier, Amalgam, Operative	Dental And Oral
Carver, Wax, Dental	Dental And Oral
Cement, Dental	Dental And Oral
Dam, Rubber	Dental And Oral
File, Pulp Canal, Endodontic	Dental And Oral
Forceps, Articulation Paper	Dental And Oral
Forceps, Tooth Extractor, Surgical	Dental And Oral
Frame, Rubber Dam	Dental And Oral
Handle, Scalpel	Surgery
Hemostat, Surgical	Dental And Oral
Holder, Needle	Gastroenterology/Urology
Holder, X-Ray Film	Dental And Oral
Liner, Cavity, Calcium Hydroxide	Dental And Oral
Material, Impression	Dental And Oral
Matrix, Dental	Dental And Oral
Mouthpiece, Saliva Ejector	Dental And Oral
Needle, Dental	Dental And Oral
Paper, Articulation	Dental And Oral
Pliers, Operative	Dental And Oral
Plugger, Root Canal, Endodontic	Dental And Oral
Point, Paper, Endodontic	Dental And Oral
Point, Silver, Endodontic	Dental And Oral
Preparer, Root Canal, Endodontic	Dental And Oral
Pusher, Band, Orthodontic	Dental And Oral
Reamer, Pulp Canal, Endodontic	Dental And Oral
Remover, Crown	Dental And Oral
Resin, Root Canal Filling	Dental And Oral
Retainer, Matrix	Dental And Oral
Scaler, Periodontic	Dental And Oral
Scissors, Disposable	General
Sealant, Pit And Fissure, And Conditioner, Resin	Dental And Oral
Splint, Endodontic Stabilizer	Dental And Oral
Spreader, Pulp Canal Filling Material, Endodontic	Dental And Oral
Sterilizer, Glass Bead	Dental And Oral
Tester, Pulp	Dental And Oral
Tooth Bonding Agent, Resin Restoration	Dental And Oral
Tray, Impression	Dental And Oral
Zinc Oxide Eugenol	Dental And Oral

PULSE BIOMEDICAL INC.   610-666-5510

1305 catfish lane, Norristown, PA 19403
FDA Number: 2529508   *Fax:* 610-666-5630
E-mail: info@qrscard.com
Web site: www.qrscard.com
Medical Products Sales Volume: $700,000
Year Founded: 1990
Total Employees: 7
Ownership: Private
Quality System Registration Information: ISO9001
Produces/Sells CE-marked Devices: N
Federal Procurement Eligibility: Small Business
Distribution: Manufacturer Direct, Manufacturer Through Distributor, Manufacturer
Through Manufacturer Reps, OEM
General Admin.: Mrs. Rosemarie DeLucia/Director Admin.

Cable/Lead, ECG	Cardiovascular
Electrocardiograph, Multi-Channel	Cardiovascular
Recorder, Long-Term, ECG, Portable (Holter Monitor)	Cardiovascular

PULSE MEDICAL INC.   800-342-5973

4131 S.W. 47th Avenue, Suite 1404,   **954-587-8867**
Davie, FL 33314
FDA Number: 3001238025   *Fax:* 954-587-8853
E-mail: info@rci-pulsemed.com
Web site: www.rci-pulsemed.com
Medical Products Sales Volume: $1,800,000
Annual Revenue: $5-$10 Million
Year Founded: 1982
Total Employees: 25   *Marketing Staff:* 15   *Sales Staff:* 15
Ownership: Private
Produces/Sells CE-marked Devices: N
Federal Procurement Eligibility: Small Business, Minority Owned, Female Owned
Distribution: Manufacturer Direct, Manufacturer Through Distributor, Manufacturer
Through Manufacturer Reps, OEM, Exporter
General Admin.: Gordon Boyce/Chief Executive Officer

PULSE MEDICAL INC.　　800-342-5973 *(cont'd)*
Barb Boyce/President

Apron, Lead, Radiographic	Radiology
Eyeglasses, Safety	Ophthalmology
Illuminator, Radiographic Film	Radiology
Shield, X-Ray, Portable	Radiology
System, Marking, Film, Radiographic	Radiology

PULSE MEDICAL INSTRUMENTS, INC.　　301-816-9212 ex
5951 Halpine Rd., Rockville, MD 20851-2452
FDA Number: 1126084　　　　　　Fax: 703-816-0042
E-mail: ehotchkiss@pmifit.com
Web site: www.pmifit.com
Ownership: Private
Produces/Sells CE-marked Devices: N

Pupillometer, AC-Powered	Ophthalmology

PULSE SCIENTIFIC, INC.　　800-363-7907
**5100 S. Service Rd., Unit 18,　　9053338188
Burlington, ONT L7L-6 Canada**
FDA Number: 8044007　　　　　　Fax: 9053330500
E-mail: info@pulsescientific.com
Web site: www.pulsescientific.com
Medical Products Sales Volume: $1,200,000
Year Founded: 1992
Total Employees: 10
Ownership: Private
Produces/Sells CE-marked Devices: N
Distribution: Manufacturer Direct, Manufacturer Through Distributor, Manufacturer Through Manufacturer Reps, OEM, Exclusive Distributor, Exporter

PULSE SYSTEMS, INC.　　505-662-7599
422 Connie Ave., Los Alamos, NM 87544
FDA Number: n/a　　　　　　Fax: 505-662-7748
E-mail: pulsesystems@psilasers.com
Web site: www.psilasers.com
Year Founded: 1979
Ownership: Private
Produces/Sells CE-marked Devices: N
Federal Procurement Eligibility: Small Business
Distribution: OEM
General Admin.: Edward J. McLellan/President, Chief Executive Officer
Mktg./Adv.: Linda L. McLellan/Vice President, General Manager Marketing

Laser, Carbon-Dioxide, Surgical	Surgery
Service, Engineering/Design	General

PURDUE FREDERICK COMPANY　　800-877-5666
One Stamford Forum, Stamford, CT 06901　　203-588-8000
FDA Number: 9310059　　　　　　Fax: 203-588-8850
E-mail: customer.service@pharma.com
Web site: www.purduepharma.com
Medical Products Sales Volume: $43,600,000
Year Founded: 1955
Total Employees: 310　　Marketing Staff: 45　　Sales Staff: 922
Ownership: Private
Produces/Sells CE-marked Devices: N
Federal Procurement Eligibility: Small Business
Distribution: Manufacturer Through Manufacturer Reps
General Admin.: Irwin Block/Executive Director
　　　　　　Michael Friedman/President
Mktg./Adv.: Mark Alfonso/Vice President Marketing
　　　　　　Russ Gasdia/Vice President Sales

Brush, Scrub, Operating Room	Surgery
Pad, Medicated	General
Solution, Patient Preparation	General
Solution, Surgical Scrub	General
Swabs, Antiseptic	General

PURDY ELECTRONICS CORP.　　408-523-8225
755 North Pastoria Avenue, Sunnyvale, CA 94085
FDA Number: n/a　　　　　　Fax: 408-733-1287
E-mail: sales@purdyelectronics.com
Web site: www.purdyelectronics.com
Annual Revenue: $5-$10 Million
Year Founded: 1930
Total Employees: 15　　Marketing Staff: 5　　Sales Staff: 5
Ownership: Private
Produces/Sells CE-marked Devices: N
Distribution: Manufacturer Direct, Manufacturer Through Distributor, Manufacturer Through Manufacturer Reps, Importer, Exporter
General Admin.: Bruce Bastl/Chief Executive Officer
Mktg./Adv.: Linda Wooliever/Director Marketing
　　　　　　Joel Lee/Manager International & National Sales

Cart, Monitor	General
Component, Electronic	General
Vision Aid, Electronic, Battery-Powered	Ophthalmology

PURE WATER SOLUTIONS, INC.　　877-202-5871
520 D Topeka Way, Castle Rock, CO 80109　　303-660-9093
FDA Number: 1724740　　　　　　Fax: 303-663-9779
E-mail: PUREWATER@PUREWATERSOLUTIONS.US
Web site: WWW.PUREWATERSOLUTIONS.US
Year Founded: 1990
Total Employees: 11
Ownership: Private
Produces/Sells CE-marked Devices: N

Purification System, Water	Gastroenterology/Urology

PURE WATER, INC.　　864-375-0105
311 W. Market St., Anderson, SC 29624
FDA Number: 1066681
Ownership: Private
Produces/Sells CE-marked Devices: N

Purification System, Water	Gastroenterology/Urology
Tank, Holding, Dialysis	Gastroenterology/Urology

PUREGAS　　800-521-5351
226A Commerce Street, Broomfield, CO 80020　　303-427-3700
FDA Number: n/a　　　　　　Fax: 303-657-2205
E-mail: info@puregas.com
Web site: www.puregas.com
Medical Products Sales Volume: $2,600,000
Annual Revenue: $5-$10 Million
Year Founded: 1954
Total Employees: 30
Ownership: Private
Produces/Sells CE-marked Devices: Y
Federal Procurement Eligibility: Small Business
Distribution: Manufacturer Direct, Manufacturer Through Distributor, OEM, Exporter
Mktg./Adv.: Thomas Mandl/Director Business Development

Chromatography (Gas), Clinical Use	Toxicology
Chromatography Equipment, Gas	Chemistry

PURELINE ORALCARE, INC.　　831-662-9500
804 Estates Dr., Aptos, CA 95003
FDA Number: 3004957169

Dilator, Nasal	Ear/Nose/Throat

PURETEC INDUSTRIAL WATER　　805-652-0552
3151 Sturgis Rd., Oxnard, CA 93030
FDA Number: 2028755

Purifier, Water	Chemistry

PURICORE INC.　　484-321-2700
508 Lapp Rd., Malvern, PA 19355
FDA Number: 3005856705　　　　Fax: 1 484.321.2725
Ownership: Private
Produces/Sells CE-marked Devices: N

Cleanser, Root Canal	Dental And Oral
Medical Disinfectants/Cleaners for Instruments	General
Sterilant, Medical Device	General

PURIFIED PROTEIN, INC.　　866-339-6589
3443 Tripp Court, San Diego, CA 92121-1009　　(949) 278-1597
FDA Number: n/a　　　　　　Fax: 858-259-8268
E-mail: tony@primapharm.net
Web site: www.primapharm.net
Annual Revenue: $1-$5 Million
Year Founded: 1989
Total Employees: 31　　Marketing Staff: 1　　Sales Staff: 1
Ownership: Private
Produces/Sells CE-marked Devices: N
Federal Procurement Eligibility: Small Business
Distribution: Manufacturer Direct
General Admin.: Zakaria Hassanein/President, Chief Executive Officer
Production: Arshad Chaudry/Director Quality Assurance & Quality Control
　　　　　　Tony Dzaibo/Manager Regulatory Affairs

Compound, Resinous, Composite	Dental And Oral

PURITAN BENNETT CORP.　　925-463-4371
2800 Airwest Blvd., Plainfield, IN 46168
FDA Number: 1825511
Web site: www.puritanbennett.com
Ownership: Covidien Ltd.
Produces/Sells CE-marked Devices: N

Canister, Liquid Oxygen, Portable	Anesthesiology
Lung, Membrane (For Long-Term Respiratory Support)	Anesthesiology
Regulator, Pressure, Gas Cylinder	Anesthesiology

PURITAN BENNETT CORP.
See Mallinckrodt, Inc.

PURITAN MEDICAL PRODUCTS COMPANY LLC　　800-321-2313
31 School St., Guilford, ME 04443-0149　　207-876-3311
FDA Number: 1216735　　　　　　Fax: 800-323-4153

MANUFACTURER PROFILES

PURITAN MEDICAL PRODUCTS COMPANY LLC   800-321-2313
(cont'd)
E-mail: info@hwppuritan.com
Web site: www.puritanmedproducts.com
Annual Revenue: $25-$50 Million
Year Founded: 1919
Total Employees: 320   *Marketing Staff:* 4   *Sales Staff:* 35
Ownership: Private
Quality System Registration Information: ISO9000; ISO9001
Produces/Sells CE-marked Devices: Y
Federal Procurement Eligibility: Small Business
Distribution: Manufacturer Direct, Manufacturer Through Distributor, Manufacturer Through Manufacturer Reps, OEM, Exporter
General Admin.: Terry Young/Chief Executive Officer
Mktg./Adv.: Timothy Templet/Director Marketing
     Timothy Templet/Director National Accounts
     Timothy Templet/Director Product Development
     Timothy Templet/Manager International & National Sales
     Timothy Templet/Manager Sales
Production: William Young/Manager Regulatory Affairs

Applicator, Cotton	Dental And Oral
Applicator, ENT	Ear/Nose/Throat
Applicator, Other	General
Applicator, Proctoscopic	Gastroenterology/Urology
Applicator, Tipped, Absorbent	General
Applicator, Tipped, Absorbent, Non-Sterile	General
Applicator, Tipped, Absorbent, Sterile	General
Applicator, Vaginal	Obstetrics/Gynecology
Blade, Tongue	Surgery
Brush, Cytology	General
Brush, Other	General
Depressor, Tongue	General
Depressor, Tongue, Dental	Dental And Oral
Depressor, Tongue, ENT, Wood	Ear/Nose/Throat
Scraper, Cytology (Cervical)	Obstetrics/Gynecology
Spatula, Cervical, Cytology	Obstetrics/Gynecology
Swabs, Antiseptic	General
Swabs, Cotton	General
Swabs, Oral Care	General
Swabs, Specimen Collection	General

PUTNAM PRECISION PRODUCTS   845-278-2141
3859 Danbury Road, Brewster, NY 10509-9806
FDA Number: 1318997   *Fax:* 845-278-6808
E-mail: shamilton@putnamprecision.com
Total Employees: 200
Ownership: Private
Quality System Registration Information: ISO9001
Produces/Sells CE-marked Devices: Y
Production: Sean Hamilton/Director Operations

Applier, Surgical Staple	Surgery
Applier, Surgical, Clip	Surgery
Cannula, Surgical, General & Plastic Surgery	Surgery
Chisel, Surgical, Manual	Surgery
Clip, Instrument	Surgery
Component, Metal, Other	General
Component, Plastic	General
Contract Manufacturing	General
Handle, Instrument, Laparoscopic (Electrocautery)	Surgery
Scissors, Laparoscopy	Surgery
Sleeve, Trocar	Surgery
Stapler, Laparoscopic	Surgery
Surgical Instrument, Disposable	Surgery
Surgical Instrument, Orthopedic, Battery-Powered	Surgery
Trocar, Laparoscopic	Surgery
Trocar, Short	Surgery

PVA   518-371-2684
15 Solar Drive, Halfmoon, NY 12065
FDA Number: n/a   *Fax:* 518-371-2688
E-mail: info@pva.net
Web site: www.pva.net
Medical Products Sales Volume: $2,500,000
Year Founded: 1992
Total Employees: 65   *Marketing Staff:* 2   *Sales Staff:* 4
Ownership: Private
Produces/Sells CE-marked Devices: Y
Federal Procurement Eligibility: Small Business
Distribution: Manufacturer Through Manufacturer Reps, OEM
General Admin.: Anthony J. Hynes/Chief Executive Officer
Mktg./Adv.: Frank R. Hart/Director Marketing
     John A. Bova/Director National Accounts
     Karah Anderson/Sales Associate

Production Equipment	General

PYNE CORP.
See Fujifilm Medical Systems Usa, Inc.

PYNG MEDICAL CORP.   1-800-349-7964
13511 Crestwood Pl. #7,   604-303-7964
Richmond, BC V6V-2 Canada
FDA Number: n/a
E-mail: pyngmed@axionet.com   *Fax:* 604-303-7987
Web site: www.pyng.com
Year Founded: 1992
Total Employees: 10
Ownership: Private
Produces/Sells CE-marked Devices: N
Distribution: Manufacturer Direct, Exporter

PYRABACK.COM   713-859-7568
10339 Belfast Rd., La Porte, TX 77571
FDA Number: 3005098698
Ownership: Private
Produces/Sells CE-marked Devices: N

Component, Exercise	Physical Med

PYRAMID INDUSTRIES, LLC   888-343-3352
3911 Schaad Rd., Unit 102, Knoxville, TN 37921   865-769-0299
FDA Number: 1055932   *Fax:* 865-769-0398
E-mail: info@pyramidindllc.com
Web site: www.pyramidindllc.com
Medical Products Sales Volume: $2,000,000
Annual Revenue: $1-$5 Million
Year Founded: 2001
Total Employees: 14   *Marketing Staff:* 2   *Sales Staff:* 3
Ownership: Private
Produces/Sells CE-marked Devices: N
Federal Procurement Eligibility: Small Business
Distribution: Manufacturer Through Distributor, Manufacturer Through Manufacturer Reps, Service Direct, Importer
General Admin.: Joe Petringa/President
Mktg./Adv.: Jim Britton/Senior Mktg Manager
     Chuck Brewer/Senior Sales Manager

Back Rest	General
Chair, Flotation Therapy	General
Cushion, Wheelchair (Pad)	Physical Med
Mattress, Air Flotation	General
Mattress, Reduction, Pressure	General
Transfer Device, Patient, Manual	General

PYRAMID MEDICAL LLC   800-764-1154
10940 Portal Drive, Los Alamitos, CA 90720   714-826-2777
FDA Number: n/a   *Fax:* 714-826-3875
E-mail: ultrasound@pyramidmedical.com
Web site: www.pyramidmed.com
Medical Products Sales Volume: $2,400,000
Annual Revenue: $5-$10 Million
Year Founded: 1978
Total Employees: 14   *Marketing Staff:* 2   *Sales Staff:* 6
Ownership: Private
Produces/Sells CE-marked Devices: Y
Federal Procurement Eligibility: Small Business
Distribution: Service Direct, Exclusive Distributor, Importer, Exporter
General Admin.: Hap Burnett/President
     Don Kennebeck/Vice President
Mktg./Adv.: DAN HENRY/Managing Director, General Manager Marketing
Production: KRISTEN KENNEBECK/Customer Service Representative
IS: DON WAUCHOPE/Manager Information Systems

Echocardiograph (Ultrasonic Scanner)	Cardiovascular
Equipment, Ultrasound, Doppler, Evaluation, Fetal	Obstetrics/Gynecology
Service, Parts, Repair	General
Service, Used Equipment	General

PYRAMID MEDICAL, INC.
See Pyramid Medical Llc

PYRAMID ORTHODONTICS   800-752-8884
4328 Redwood Hwy., Ste. 100,   415-479-6400
San Rafael, CA 94903
FDA Number: 2950152   *Fax:* 415-479-2745
E-mail: pyramid@pyramidorthodontics.com
Web site: www.pyramidorthodontics.com
Medical Products Sales Volume: $2,000,000
Annual Revenue: $1-$5 Million
Year Founded: 1989
Total Employees: 5   *Marketing Staff:* 3   *Sales Staff:* 3
Ownership: Private
Quality System Registration Information: ISO9001
Produces/Sells CE-marked Devices: Y
Federal Procurement Eligibility: Small Business
Distribution: Manufacturer Direct, Exporter
General Admin.: Rodney Schmitt/Chief Executive Officer
Mktg./Adv.: Rodney Schmitt/Manager Advertising
     Rodney Schmitt/Vice President Marketing & Sales
Production: Rodney Schmitt/Vice President Manufacturing

PYRAMID ORTHODONTICS · 800-752-8884 (cont'd)
Research: Rodney Schmitt/Vice President Research & Development

Band, Elastic, Orthodontic	Dental And Oral
Bracket, Metal, Orthodontic	Dental And Oral
Bracket, Plastic, Orthodontic	Dental And Oral
Clamp, Wire, Orthodontic	Dental And Oral
Pliers, Orthodontic	Dental And Oral
Wire, Orthodontic	Dental And Oral

PYROMETER INSTRUMENT CO. · 800-468-7976
92 North Main Street Bldg 18D, · **609-443-5522**
Windsor, NJ 08561
FDA Number: 7000303 · *Fax:* 609-443-5590
E-mail: sales@pyrometer.com
Web site: www.pyrometer.com
Annual Revenue: $0-$1 Million
Year Founded: 1928
Total Employees: 15
Ownership: Private
Quality System Registration Information: ISO9001
Produces/Sells CE-marked Devices: N
Federal Procurement Eligibility: Small Business
Distribution: Manufacturer Direct
General Admin.: D. Crozier/Chief Executive Officer
　　　　　Judd Parrish/President
Mktg./Adv.: Amy Larison/Manager International & National Sales
Production: A. Dmitriyev/Plant Manager

Pyrometer	General
Thermometer, Laboratory	Chemistry

Q'STRAINT · 800-987-9987
100 Sheldon Dr., Unit 18, Cambridge, ONT N1R-7S7 Canada
FDA Number: n/a · *Fax:* 519-622-0021
E-mail: sales@qstraint.com
Web site: www.qstraint.com
Year Founded: 1980
Total Employees: 25
Ownership: Private
Produces/Sells CE-marked Devices: N
Distribution: Manufacturer Direct, Exporter

Q-MED, INC. · 732-544-5544
100 Metro Park S., 3rd Fl., South Amboy, NJ 08878
FDA Number: n/a · *Fax:* 732-544-5404
Medical Products Sales Volume: $3,300,000
Annual Revenue: $1-$5 Million
Total Employees: 45
Ownership: Private
Produces/Sells CE-marked Devices: N
Federal Procurement Eligibility: Small Business
Distribution: Manufacturer Direct
General Admin.: Michael W. Cox/President
　　　　　Teri Kraf/Vice President
Mktg./Adv.: Jane Murray/Director Marketing
　　　　　John Siegel/Manager National Sales
Production: Amy Woodruff/Project Coord.

Electrocardiograph, Single Channel	Cardiovascular
Monitor, Blood Pressure, Venous	Cardiovascular
Monitor, ECG, Ambulatory, Real-Time	Cardiovascular
Recorder, Long-Term, ECG, Portable (Holter Monitor)	Cardiovascular

Q-TEKNOLOGIES, INC. · 321-631-3915
391 Brookcrest Circle, Rockledge, FL 32955
FDA Number: 1061816
Ownership: Private
Produces/Sells CE-marked Devices: N

Tourniquet, Non-Pneumatic, Surgical	Surgery

Q.I. MEDICAL, INC. · 800-837-8361
440-C Lower Grass Valley Road, · **530-265-4820**
Nevada City, CA 95959
FDA Number: 2950467 · *Fax:* 530-265-9416
E-mail: info@qimedical.com
Web site: www.qimedical.com
Annual Revenue: $1-$5 Million
Year Founded: 1992
Total Employees: 5 · *Marketing Staff:* 1 · *Sales Staff:* 1
Ownership: Private
Produces/Sells CE-marked Devices: N
Federal Procurement Eligibility: Small Business
Distribution: Manufacturer Through Distributor
General Admin.: Hilary R. Hedman/President
Production: Sheila Campbell/Director Quality Assurance & Regulatory Affairs

Culture Media, General Nutrient Broth	Microbiology
Dispenser, Fluid	General
Filter, Bacteriological, Laboratory	Chemistry
Incubator, Aerobic	Microbiology
Plate, Culture	Microbiology

Q.I. MEDICAL, INC. · 800-837-8361 (cont'd)

Syringe, Piston	General
Transfer Unit, IV Fluid	General

Q.T.I. CORP. · 760-723-9825
879 Del Valle Drive, Fallbrook, CA 92028
FDA Number: 2032792
Ownership: Private
Produces/Sells CE-marked Devices: N

Delivery System, Allergen And Vaccine	General

QBC DIAGNOSTICS, INC. · 814-342-6205
168 Bradford Drive, Port Matilda, PA 16870
FDA Number: 3005599574 · *Fax:* 814-692-7662
Web site: http://www.qbcdiagnostics.com
Year Founded: 2005
Total Employees: 50
Ownership: Private
Produces/Sells CE-marked Devices: N

Counter, Cell, Differential Classifier, Automated	Hematology
Kit, Mycobacteria Identification	Microbiology
Labware, Blood Collection	Chemistry
Serum Separation System	Hematology

QC SCIENCES · 866-709-0523
4851 Lake Brook Dr, Glen Allen, VA 23060
FDA Number: 1125806

Cultured Animal And Human Cells	Pathology
Preservative, Cytological	Pathology
Reagent, General Purpose	Pathology

QED BIOSCIENCE, INC. · 800-929-2114
10919 Technology Place, Suite C, · **858-675-2405**
San Diego, CA 92127
FDA Number: n/a · *Fax:* 858-592-1509
E-mail: info@qedbio.com
Web site: www.qedbio.com
Medical Products Sales Volume: $700,000
Annual Revenue: $1-$5 Million
Year Founded: 1995
Total Employees: 10 · *Marketing Staff:* 2 · *Sales Staff:* 2
Ownership: Private
Produces/Sells CE-marked Devices: N
Federal Procurement Eligibility: Small Business
Distribution: Manufacturer Direct, Manufacturer Through Distributor, Manufacturer Through Manufacturer Reps, OEM, Service Direct, Exclusive Distributor, Importer, Exporter
General Admin.: Dr. Eileen Skaletsky/President, Chief Executive Officer
Production: Ms. Jennifer Johnson/Manager Operations

2nd Antibody (Species Specific Anti-Animal Gamma Globulin)	Immunology
Antibody, Monoclonal	Microbiology
Antigen, Enzyme Linked Immunoabsorbent Assay, Cryptococcus	Microbiology
Gel, Support	Immunology
Kit, Serological, Positive Control	Microbiology

QED, INC. · 859-231-0338
750 Enterprise Dr., Lexington, KY 40510
FDA Number: 1037039

Box, Battery, Rechargeable (Endoscopic)	Gastroenterology/Urology
Camera, Television, Surgical (Without Audio)	Surgery
Headlamp, Operating, AC-Powered	Ophthalmology
Headlamp, Operating, Battery-Operated	Ophthalmology
Headlight, Fiberoptic Focusing	Gastroenterology/Urology
Lamp, Surgical	Surgery
Light Source, Fiberoptic, Routine	Gastroenterology/Urology
Light, Fiberoptic, Dental	Dental And Oral
Light, Surgical Headlight	Dental And Oral
Mirror, Mouth	Dental And Oral

QED/ADVANCED RESEARCH TECHNOLOGIES
See Qed Bioscience, Inc.

QFC PLASTICS, INC. · 817-649-7400
728 111th St., Arlington, TX 76011
FDA Number: 1648571

Applicator, Tipped, Absorbent, Non-Sterile	General
Clamp, Bone	Orthopedics
Clamp, Surgical, General & Plastic Surgery	Surgery
Container, Specimen, Non-sterile	General
Forceps	Orthopedics
Gauze/sponge, Nonresorbable For External Use	Surgery
Tray, Surgical	Surgery

QIAGEN GAITHERSBURG, INC. · 800-344-3631
1201 Clopper Rd., Gaithersburg, MD 20878 · **301-944-7090**
FDA Number: 1122376 · *Fax:* 240-632-7121
Web site: www.qiagen.com
Year Founded: 1987
Ownership: Private
Produces/Sells CE-marked Devices: N

QIAGEN GAITHERSBURG, INC.   800-344-3631 *(cont'd)*

Applicator, Tipped, Absorbent, Sterile	General
Chlamydia, DNA Reagents	Microbiology
Colorimeter, General Use	Chemistry
Culture Media, General Nutrient Broth	Microbiology
Cytomegalovirus, DNA Reagents	Microbiology
DNA Device, Hepatitis B, Viral	Microbiology
DNA-Probe, Reagent	Microbiology
Dish, Tissue Culture	Pathology
Kit, DNA Detection, Human Papillomavirus	Microbiology
Neisseria, DNA Reagents	Microbiology
Pipetting And Diluting System, Automated	Chemistry
Plate, Culture	Microbiology
Reagents, Specific, Analyte	Hematology
Spatula, Cervical, Cytology	Obstetrics/Gynecology
Test, DNA-Probe, Other	Microbiology

QIAGEN SCIENCES, INC.   301-944-7090
19300 Germantown Rd., Germantown, MD 20874
FDA Number: 3003572099
Web site: http://www.qiagen.com
Ownership: Private
Produces/Sells CE-marked Devices: N
General Admin.: Mr. Peer Schatz/Chief Executive Officer
Mktg./Adv.: Mr. Bernd Uder/Senior Vice President Sales
       Mr. Ulrich Shriek/Vice President Corporate Development
       Dr. Thomas Schweinz/Vice President Marketing
Production: Mr. Douglas Liu/Vice President Operations
Research: Dr. Joachimm Schorr/Senior Vice President Research & Development
Finance: Mr. Roland Sackers/Chief Financial Officer

Concentrator, Clinical Sample	Chemistry
Reagent, General Purpose	Pathology
Reagents, Specific, Analyte	Hematology

QINETIQ NORTH AMERICA   703-752-9595
7918 Jones Branch Drive, Suite 350, McLean, VA 22102
FDA Number: n/a
E-mail: info@analex.com
Web site: www.analex.com
Annual Revenue: $10-$25 Million
Total Employees: 200
Ownership: Private
Quality System Registration Information: ISO9001
Produces/Sells CE-marked Devices: N
Federal Procurement Eligibility: Small Business, Female Owned

Service, Consulting	General

QLT INC.   800-663-5486
887 Great Northern Way,   **604-872-7881**
Vancouver, BC V5T-4 Canada
FDA Number: n/a   *Fax:* 604-875-0001
E-mail: CorpDev@qltinc.com
Web site: www.qltinc.com
Year Founded: 1986
Ownership: Private
Produces/Sells CE-marked Devices: N
Distribution: Manufacturer Direct, Exclusive Distributor

QMD MEDICAL   800-665-9950
9800 Clark St., Montreal, QUE H3L 2R3 Canada   **514-381-9955**
FDA Number: n/a   *Fax:* 514-381-8751
E-mail: jayoub@qel.ca
Web site: www.qmdmedical.com
Medical Products Sales Volume: $2,500,000
Total Employees: 80   *Marketing Staff:* 5   *Sales Staff:* 5
Ownership: QUALITY ELASTICS LTD.
Produces/Sells CE-marked Devices: N
Distribution: Manufacturer Through Distributor, OEM

QPSI MASS, LLC   413-789-6500
609 Silver St., Agawam, MA 01001-2986
FDA Number: 1226389
Ownership: Private
Produces/Sells CE-marked Devices: N

Tampon, Menstrual, Unscented	Obstetrics/Gynecology

QRP, INC.   800-832-3882
3925 N. Runway Drive, PO Box 28802,   **520-790-3533**
Tucson, AZ 85726
FDA Number: 2031472   *Fax:* 520-790-3530
E-mail: info@qrpgloves.com
Web site: www.qrpgloves.com
Medical Products Sales Volume: $1,400,000
Annual Revenue: $5-$10 Million
Year Founded: 1974
Total Employees: 24   *Marketing Staff:* 2   *Sales Staff:* 4
Ownership: Private
Quality System Registration Information: ISO9000

QRP, INC.   800-832-3882 *(cont'd)*
Produces/Sells CE-marked Devices: Y
Federal Procurement Eligibility: Small Business
Distribution: Manufacturer Through Distributor
General Admin.: William Casselman/Chief Executive Officer
       Duncan Casselman/President
Mktg./Adv.: Fred Buchanan/Director Sales
       Laurie Casselman/Vice President Export Sales
Finance: Tom Stash/Controller

Cleanroom Equipment	General

QRS DIAGNOSTIC, LLC   800-465-8408
14755 27th Avenue N., Plymouth, MN 55447   **763-559-8492**
FDA Number: n/a   *Fax:* 763-559-2961
E-mail: info@QRSdiagnostic.com
Web site: www.QRSdiagnostic.com
Year Founded: 1995
Total Employees: 30   *Marketing Staff:* 3   *Sales Staff:* 8
Ownership: Private
Quality System Registration Information: ISO9001
Produces/Sells CE-marked Devices: Y
Federal Procurement Eligibility: Small Business
Distribution: Manufacturer Direct, Manufacturer Through Distributor, OEM
General Admin.: Spencer Lien/Chief Executive Officer
       Amy Ptak/General Manager

Electrocardiograph, Interpretive	Cardiovascular
Oximeter, Pulse	General
Spirometer, Monitoring (Volumeter)	Anesthesiology

QS/1 DATA SYSTEMS   800-845-7558
201 West Saint John Street,   **(864) 253-8600**
Spartanburg, SC 29306
FDA Number: n/a
E-mail: success@qs1.com
Web site: www.qs/.com
Annual Revenue: $10-$25 Million
Total Employees: 560
Ownership: Private
Produces/Sells CE-marked Devices: Y
Federal Procurement Eligibility: Small Business
Distribution: Manufacturer Direct

Computer Software, Hospital/Nursing Management	General

QSA-GLOBAL INC.   781-272-2000
40 North Ave., Burlington, MA 01803
FDA Number: 1226007
Ownership: Private
Produces/Sells CE-marked Devices: N

Applicator, Radionuclide, Remote-Controlled	Radiology
Calibrator Source, Nuclear Sealed	Radiology
Calibrator, Dose, Radionuclide	Radiology
Holder, Radiographic Cassette, Wall-Mounted	Radiology
Phantom, Flood Source, Nuclear	Radiology
Source, Brachytherapy, Radionuclide	Radiology

QSUM BIOPSY DISPOSABLES LLC   720-304-2135
6539 Stearns Ave., Boulder, CO 80303
FDA Number: 3005675811

Drape, Surgical	Surgery
Kit, Surgical Instrument, Disposable	Surgery

QUAD MED   800-933-7334
11210 Philips Ind. Blvd. E., Suite 10   **904-880-2323**
PO Box 550773
Jacksonville, FL 32255
FDA Number: n/a   *Fax:* 877-367-7759
E-mail: quadmed@bellsouth.net
Web site: www.quadmed.com
Medical Products Sales Volume: $900,000
Year Founded: 1992
Total Employees: 6
Ownership: Private
Produces/Sells CE-marked Devices: Y
Federal Procurement Eligibility: Small Business, Female Owned
Distribution: Exclusive Distributor
General Admin.: Lisa M. Price/President

Facility, Equipment, Medical, Mobile	General

QUADRICISER CORPORATION   865-689-5003
6624 Central Ave. Pike, Knoxville, TN 37912
FDA Number: 3004930646

Exerciser, Non-Measuring	Physical Med

QUADRIS MEDICAL   507-389-4319
2030 Lookout Dr., North Mankato, MN 56003
FDA Number: 3005521856
Ownership: Private
Produces/Sells CE-marked Devices: N

QUADRIS MEDICAL
507-389-4319 *(cont'd)*
Bandage, Adhesive — Surgery
Kit, Wound Dressing — Surgery

QUADROMED INC.
800-363-0192
514-332-3287
2365 Rue Guenette,
St-Laurent, QC H4R 2 Canada
FDA Number: n/a — Fax: 514-332-477
E-mail: info@quadromed.com
Year Founded: 1986
Total Employees: 14 — Marketing Staff: 1 — Sales Staff: 5
Ownership: Private
Produces/Sells CE-marked Devices: N
Distribution: Exclusive Distributor, Importer

QUALICON
800-863-6842
302-695-8754
Route 141 and Henry Clay Rd.,
Wilmington, DE 19880
FDA Number: n/a — Fax: 302-695-5301
E-mail: info@qualicon.com
Web site: www.qualicon.com
Ownership: DU PONT DE NEMOURS AND COMPANY
Produces/Sells CE-marked Devices: N
Mktg./Adv.: Lisa Mulliror/Manager Media
Test, Bacteria Characterization — General
Test, DNA-Probe, Other — Microbiology

QUALIGEN, INC.
760-918-9165
2042 Corte Del Nogal, Carlsbad, CA 92011
FDA Number: 2032087
Antigen, Prostate-Specific (PSA), Management, Cancer — Immunology
Calibrator, Secondary, Clinical Chemistry — Chemistry
Colorimeter, General Use — Chemistry
Control, Analyte (Assayed And Unassayed) — Chemistry
Radioimmunoassay, Free Thyroxine — Chemistry
Radioimmunoassay, Testosterones And Dihydrotestosterone — Chemistry
Radioimmunoassay, Thyroid Stimulating Hormone — Chemistry
Test, Prostate Specific Antigen, Free, (noncomplexed) To Distinguish Prostate Cancer From Benign Conditions — Immunology

QUALIS GROUP LLC
515-243-3000
4600 Park Ave., Des Moines, IA 50321
FDA Number: 1927596
Ownership: Private
Produces/Sells CE-marked Devices: N
Detector/Remover, Lice — General
Lubricant, Patient — General
Lubricant, Vaginal, Patient — General
Radioimmunoassay, Human Chorionic Gonadotropin — Chemistry

QUALISYS DIAGNOSTICS INC.
877-825-4797
514-636-6898
522 Meloche Ave., Dorval, QUE H9P-2T2 Canada
FDA Number: n/a — Fax: 514-636-1380
E-mail: customer@qualisyscanada.com
Web site: www.qualisyscanada.com
Year Founded: 1997
Total Employees: 10
Ownership: Private
Produces/Sells CE-marked Devices: N
Distribution: Exclusive Distributor

QUALITEL CORPORATION
425-423-8388
4608 150th Avenue Ne, Redmond, WA 98052
FDA Number: 3024673
Catheter, Intravascular, Therapeutic, Long-term Greater Than 30 Days — General
Shunt, Central Nerve, With Component — Cns/Neurology

QUALITICO DIST'S, INC.
813-264-4788
14025 Clubhouse Cr. #2503, Tampa, FL 33624
FDA Number: 1066302
Ownership: Private
Produces/Sells CE-marked Devices: N
Lancet, Blood — General

QUALITY ASPIRATORS
800-858-2121
972-298-2669
1419 Goodwin Lane, Duncanville, TX 75116
FDA Number: 161260 — Fax: 972-298-6592
E-mail: support@qualityaspirators.com
Web site: www.q-optics.com
Medical Products Sales Volume: $1,500,000
Annual Revenue: $1-$5 Million
Year Founded: 1979
Total Employees: 12
Ownership: Private
Quality System Registration Information: ISO9001
Produces/Sells CE-marked Devices: Y
Federal Procurement Eligibility: Small Business
Distribution: Manufacturer Direct, Manufacturer Through Distributor, OEM, Exporter

QUALITY ASPIRATORS
800-858-2121 *(cont'd)*
General Admin.: Corless Wiley/President
Mktg./Adv.: Keith Wiley/Manager International Marketing & Sales
Aspirator, Surgical — Surgery
Loupe, Diagnostic/Surgical — Surgery
Surgical Instrument, Disposable — Surgery
Tip, Suction, Fiberoptic Illuminated — Anesthesiology

QUALITY ASSURED SERVICES DBA ALERE HOME MONITORING PRODUCTS
800-298-4515
407-563-2860
70 S. Keller Rd., Orlando, FL 32810
FDA Number: 3004469004 — Fax: 407-563-2861
Ownership: Alere, Inc.
Produces/Sells CE-marked Devices: N

QUALITY ASSURED SERVICES INC.
See QUALITY ASSURED SERVICES DBA ALERE HOME MONITORING PRODUCTS

QUALITY BIORESOURCES, INC.
888-674-7224
830-372-4797
1015 North Austin St., Seguin, TX 78155
FDA Number: 1645368 — Fax: 830-372-4799
E-mail: cbriell@qualbio.com
Web site: www.qualbio.com
Medical Products Sales Volume: $1,800,000
Annual Revenue: $1-$5 Million
Year Founded: 1992
Total Employees: 24
Ownership: Private
Produces/Sells CE-marked Devices: N
Federal Procurement Eligibility: Small Business
Distribution: OEM
General Admin.: Ms. Claudia Briell/President, Chief Executive Officer
Production: Mr. Marc Henriquez/Director Facility & Manufacturing
Ms. Cara Vela/Quality Control, Product Engineer
2nd Antibody (Species Specific Anti-Animal Gamma Globulin) — Immunology
ATP Release (Luminescence) — Hematology
Antibody, Polyclonal — Microbiology
Contract Assembly — General
Contract Manufacturing, Reagent — General
Contract Packaging — General
Contract R&D, Diagnostics — General
Reagent, Quality Control — General

QUALITY CABLE ASSEMBLY, LLC
248-236-9915
3204 Adventure Lane, Oxford, MI 48371-1638
FDA Number: 3004198730 — Fax: 248-236-9931
Web site: www.qcallc.com
Ownership: Private
Produces/Sells CE-marked Devices: N
Cable/Lead, ECG, With Transducer And Electrode — Cardiovascular

QUALITY CONTRACT MANUFACTURING, LLC
770-965-3300
4362 Thurmond Tanner Rd., Flowery Branch, GA 30542
FDA Number: 3004546535
Laser, Surgical — Surgery

QUALITY CONTROL CORP.
708-887-5400
7315 W. Wilson Ave., Harwood Heights, IL 60706
FDA Number: 3005566540
Infusion Stand — General

QUALITY ELECTRODYNAMICS
440-484-2228
777 Beta Drive, Cleveland, OH 44143
FDA Number: 3005686103
Ownership: Private
Produces/Sells CE-marked Devices: N
Coil, Magnetic Resonance, Specialty — Radiology

QUALITY HEARING
651-770-5282
2115 County Rd., D East, Suite A100, Maplewood, MN 55109
FDA Number: 2132278
Hearing-Aid — Ear/Nose/Throat

QUALITY MONITOR SYSTEMS, INC.
800-743-5747
719-596-2187
1950 Victor Pl., Colorado Springs, CO 80915
FDA Number: n/a — Fax: 719-596-0322
E-mail: sales@qualmonsys.com
Web site: www.qualmonsys.com
Medical Products Sales Volume: $800,000
Annual Revenue: $1-$5 Million
Year Founded: 1978
Total Employees: 6 — Sales Staff: 2
Ownership: Private
Produces/Sells CE-marked Devices: N
Federal Procurement Eligibility: Small Business, GSA Contract, VA Contract
Distribution: Service Direct
General Admin.: Dennis Heath/Chairman
Stanley Helm/President

QUALITY MONITOR SYSTEMS, INC. 800-743-5747 *(cont'd)*
Monitor, Bed Patient

General

QUALITY PACKAGING INDUSTRIES LLC 573-334-6700
5830 State Highway V, Jackson, MO 63755
FDA Number: 1932082

Fax: 573-334-8032
E-mail: lstewart@wahlco-dwtool.com
Web site: qualitypackagingind.com
Medical Products Sales Volume: $2,900,000
Annual Revenue: $5-$10 Million
Year Founded: 2002
Total Employees: 50
Ownership: Private
Produces/Sells CE-marked Devices: N
Federal Procurement Eligibility: Small Business, Female Owned
Distribution: Service Direct
General Admin.: Mrs. Linda Stewart/President, Owner
Mktg./Adv.: Mrs. Tonya Russo/Vice President, Director Marketing
Production: Ms. Rebecca Powell/Director Quality Control
    Mr. Donnie McCarty/Product Manager
Garment, Protective, For Incontinence

Gastroenterology/Urology

QUALITY PRODUCTS OF MONTANA 406-544-0305
4022 Timberlane, Missoula, MT 59802
FDA Number: 3003650767
Ownership: Private
Produces/Sells CE-marked Devices: N
Pack, Sterilization Wrapper (Bag And Accessories)

Surgery
Wrap, Sterilization

General

QUALITY RAPID SERVICE MOUNTS, INC. 800-418-8342
8617 Eagle Point Blvd., Lake Elmo, MN 55042 715-248-7049
FDA Number: n/a

Fax: 651-738-7617
E-mail: sales@qrsmounts.com
Web site: www.qrsmounts.com
Medical Products Sales Volume: $100,000
Year Founded: 1995
Ownership: Private
Produces/Sells CE-marked Devices: N
Federal Procurement Eligibility: Small Business
Distribution: Manufacturer Direct, Manufacturer Through Distributor
Electrode, Electrocardiograph

Cardiovascular
Mount, Equipment

General
Paper, Recording, ECG/EEG

General

QUALITY SCIENTIFIC PLASTICS 800-426-9595
1260 Holm Road, Petaluma, CA 94954-1182 707-762-6689
FDA Number: n/a

Fax: 707-762-7198
E-mail: corinne_christenson@porex.com
Medical Products Sales Volume: $9,100,000
Annual Revenue: $25-$50 Million
Year Founded: 1998
Total Employees: 110
Ownership: POINT PLASTICS, INC.
Quality System Registration Information: ISO9001
Federal Procurement Eligibility: Small Business
Distribution: Manufacturer Through Distributor, OEM, Exporter
Production: Corinne Christenson/Vice President Customer Service
Labware, Basic, Disposable

Chemistry
Pipette Tip

Chemistry
Tube, Centrifuge

Chemistry
Tube, Culture

Microbiology
Tube, Test

Chemistry

QUALITY SOFTWARE SYSTEMS 800-777-3020
210 B East Spring Valley Rd., Dayton, OH 45458 937-885-2255
FDA Number: n/a

Fax: 937-885-2252
E-mail: sales@pqsystems.com
Web site: http://www.pqsystems.com/
Medical Products Sales Volume: $1,000,000
Annual Revenue: $0-$1 Million
Total Employees: 6 *Marketing Staff:* 2 *Sales Staff:* 2
Ownership: Private
Produces/Sells CE-marked Devices: N
Federal Procurement Eligibility: Small Business
Distribution: Manufacturer Direct
General Admin.: Jeffrey Caspari/President, Chief Executive Officer
Mktg./Adv.: Jeff Caspari/Vice President Marketing & Sales
Computer Software

General

QUALITY SYSTEMS, INC. 800-888-7955
18111 Von Karman Ave., Suite 600, 949-255-2600
Irvine, CA 92612
FDA Number: n/a

Fax: 949-255-2605
E-mail: qsi@qsii.com
Web site: www.qsii.com
Annual Revenue: $25-$50 Million
Year Founded: 1974

QUALITY SYSTEMS, INC. 800-888-7955 *(cont'd)*
Total Employees: 237
Ownership: Public
Stock Symbol: QSII
Traded On: NASDAQ
Produces/Sells CE-marked Devices: N
Federal Procurement Eligibility: Small Business
Distribution: Manufacturer Through Manufacturer Reps
General Admin.: Mr. Steve Plochocki/Chief Executive Officer
    Mr. Donn Neufield/Executive Vice President
    Mr. Patrick Cline/President
Finance: Mr. Paul Holt/Chief Financial Officer
Computer Equipment

General
Computer Software

General

QUALITYWORX, INC. 877-825-4379
11 Valley Road, Kinnelon, NJ 07405-2313 973-492-0015
FDA Number: n/a

Fax: 973-406-4706
E-mail: info@qualityworxinc.com
Web site: www.qualityworxinc.com
Total Employees: 9
Ownership: Private
Produces/Sells CE-marked Devices: N
Federal Procurement Eligibility: Small Business, Female Owned
General Admin.: Ilene Butka/President
    Elizabeth Fretz/Vice President, General Manager
Computer Software

General
Service, Computer

General

QUANTACHROME 800-989-2476
1900 Corporate Drive, Boynton Beach, FL 33426 561-731-4999
FDA Number: n/a

Fax: 561-732-9888
E-mail: qc.sales@quantachrome.com
Web site: www.quantachrome.com
Medical Products Sales Volume: $8,500,000
Annual Revenue: $1-$5 Million
Year Founded: 1968
Total Employees: 85 *Marketing Staff:* 15 *Sales Staff:* 15
Ownership: Private
Produces/Sells CE-marked Devices: Y
Federal Procurement Eligibility: Small Business
Distribution: Manufacturer Direct, Service Direct
General Admin.: Scott Lowell/President
Mktg./Adv.: Robert Swinson/Director Marketing
    Thomas O'Connor/Director Marketing & Sales
Analyzer, Particle

Chemistry
Analyzer, Water Vapor

Anesthesiology
Contract Laboratory

General
Medical Product Subsidiaries (Listed Separately)
Quantachrome Gmbh

QUANTEL-USA, INC. 406-586-0131
601 Haggerty Ln., Bozeman, MT 59715
FDA Number: 3031037
Ownership: Private
Produces/Sells CE-marked Devices: N
Laser, Surgical

Surgery

QUANTERIX CORPORATION 617-301-9400
One Kendall Square, Suite B14201, Cambridge, MA 02139
FDA Number: n/a

Fax: 617-301-9401
E-mail: info@quanterix.com
Web site: www.quanterix.com
Ownership: Private
Produces/Sells CE-marked Devices: N
General Admin.: Dr. Martin Madaus/Executive Chairman
Mktg./Adv.: Dr. David Hanlon/Director Marketing
Production: Mr. David Fournier/Director Engineering
Research: Dr. David Duffy/Senior Director Research & Development

QUANTERRON, INC.
See Apothecary Products, Inc.

QUANTIMETRIX CORPORATION 800-624-8380
2005 Manhattan Beach Blvd., 310-536-0006
Redondo Beach, CA 90278
FDA Number: 7000640

Fax: 310-297-3639
E-mail: info@4qc.com
Web site: www.4qc.com
Ownership: Private
Produces/Sells CE-marked Devices: Y
Federal Procurement Eligibility: Small Business
Distribution: Manufacturer Direct, Manufacturer Through Distributor, OEM, Exporter
General Admin.: Mr. Robert Ban/President, Chief Executive Officer, Chairman
Mktg./Adv.: Ms. Monica Jacobs/Manager Marketing Communications
    Ms. Yolanda Louis/Manager Sales
Research: Mrs. Jennifer Morais/Manager Research & Development

QUANTIMETRIX CORPORATION   800-624-8380 *(cont'd)*
Finance: Mr. Edward Cleek/Chief Financial Officer
Control, Enzyme (Assayed And Unassayed) — Chemistry
Control, Multi Analyte, All Kinds (Assayed And Unassayed) — Chemistry
Control, Urinalysis (Assayed And Unassayed) — Chemistry
Electrophoretic Separation, Alkaline Phosphatase Isoenzymes — Chemistry
Electrophoretic Separation, Lipoproteins — Chemistry
Reagent, Protein, Total — Chemistry

QUANTRONIX CORP.
See Quantronix Lasers

QUANTRONIX LASERS   1-800-289-7707
41 Research Way, East Setauket, NY 11733   631-784-6100
FDA Number: n/a   *Fax:* 631-784-6101
E-mail: www.quantronixlasers.com
Web site: www.quantronixlasers.com
Annual Revenue: $25-$50 Million
Year Founded: 1967
Ownership: Private
Produces/Sells CE-marked Devices: N
Federal Procurement Eligibility: Small Business
Distribution: Manufacturer Direct
Accessories, Laser — General
Laser, Dental — Dental And Oral
Laser, Laboratory — Chemistry
Laser, Nd:YAG, Surgical — Surgery
Laser, Ophthalmic — Ophthalmology
Laser, Surgical — Surgery
Medical Product Subsidiaries (Listed Separately)
Quatronix

QUANTRX BIOMEDICAL CORP.   503-252-9565
5920 NE 112th Avenue, Portland, OR 97220
FDA Number: 3005981667   *Fax:* 503-252-9732
Web site: http://www.quantrx.com
Ownership: Private
Stock Symbol: QTXB
Traded On: OTC Bulletin
Produces/Sells CE-marked Devices: N
General Admin.: Mr. Walter Witoshkin/Chairman, Chief Executive Officer
     Dr. William Flemming/Chief Scientific Officer
Finance: Mr. Sasha Affanasiev/Chief Financial Officer, Senior Vice President Finance
Enzyme Immunoassay, Amphetamine — Toxicology
Enzyme Immunoassay, Barbiturate — Toxicology
Enzyme Immunoassay, Benzodiazepine — Toxicology
Enzyme Immunoassay, Cannabinoids — Toxicology
Enzyme Immunoassay, Cocaine And Cocaine Metabolites — Toxicology
Enzyme Immunoassay, Methadone — Toxicology
Enzyme Immunoassay, Phencyclidine — Toxicology
Gas Chromatography, Methamphetamine — Toxicology
Radioimmunoassay, Tricyclic Antidepressant Drugs — Toxicology
Tampon, Menstrual, Unscented — Obstetrics/Gynecology
Test, Follicle Stimulating Hormone (fsh), Over The Counter — Toxicology
Thin Layer Chromatography, Metamphetamine — Toxicology
Thin Layer Chromatography, Morphine — Toxicology

QUANTUM BIOENGINEERING, LTD.   954-474-4707
7951 S.w. 6th St., Plantation, FL 33324
FDA Number: 3002851558
Accessories, Implant, Dental, Endosseous — Dental And Oral
Implant, Endosseous — Dental And Oral

QUANTUM DEVICES, INC.   608-924-3000
112 Orbison Street, Barneveld, WI 53507
FDA Number: 3004181270
Lamp, Infrared — Physical Med

QUANTUM INTERCONNECT, INC.   817-231-1400
3400 Northern Cross Blvd., Fort Worth, TX 76137
FDA Number: 3004087736
Ownership: Private
Produces/Sells CE-marked Devices: N
Electrosurgical Unit, Cutting & Coagulation Device — Surgery

QUANTUM LABS, INC.   800-328-8213
452 Northco Dr., Suite 180,   763-545-1984
Minneapolis, MN 55432
FDA Number: 2183760   *Fax:* 800-485-9565
E-mail: gloves@quantumlabs.com
Web site: www.quantumlabs.com
Medical Products Sales Volume: $2,500,000
Annual Revenue: $1-$5 Million
Total Employees: 7
Ownership: Private
Produces/Sells CE-marked Devices: N
Federal Procurement Eligibility: Small Business
Distribution: Manufacturer Direct, Manufacturer Through Manufacturer Reps
General Admin.: Michael Stefanson/Chief Executive Officer

QUANTUM LABS, INC.   800-328-8213 *(cont'd)*
Glove, Patient Examination — General

QUANTUM MEDICAL CONCEPTS, LLC.   503-708-0702
3518 Se 21st Ave., Portland, OR 97202
FDA Number: 3004517245
Tray, Surgical — Surgery

QUANTUM MEDICAL IMAGING, LLC   631-567-5800
2002 Orville Dr N Suite B, Ronkonkoma, NY 11779
FDA Number: 2438474   *Fax:* 631-567-5074
E-mail: info@qmiteam.com
Web site: www.quantummedical.net
Medical Products Sales Volume: $70,000,000
Year Founded: 1999
Total Employees: 100
Ownership: Private
Federal Procurement Eligibility: Small Business, Female Owned
Distribution: Manufacturer Through Distributor
Chair, Adjustable, Mechanical — Physical Med
Generator, Diagnostic X-Ray, High Voltage, Single Phase — Radiology
Holder, Radiographic Cassette, Wall-Mounted — Radiology
Mount, X-Ray Tube, Diagnostic — Radiology
Radiographic Unit, Diagnostic — Radiology
Table, Radiographic, Non-Tilting, Powered — Radiology
Table, Radiographic, Stationary Top — Radiology

QUANTUM MEDICAL SYSTEMS
See Siemens Medical Systems, Inc., Ultrasound Group

QUARTET TECHNOLOGY, INC.   978-649-4328
87 Progress Avenue, Tyngsboro, MA 01879
FDA Number: 1221664   *Fax:* 978-649-8363
E-mail: info@qtiusa.com
Web site: www.qtiusa.com
Medical Products Sales Volume: $900,000
Year Founded: 1994
Total Employees: 5
Ownership: Private
Produces/Sells CE-marked Devices: N
Federal Procurement Eligibility: Small Business
Distribution: Manufacturer Direct, Manufacturer Through Distributor
General Admin.: Mr. Michael Rourke/President, Chief Executive Officer
Mktg./Adv.: Mr. Aaron Breen/Vice President Marketing & Sales
Environmental Control System, Powered — Physical Med
Environmental Control System, Powered, Remote — Physical Med

QUARTZ SCIENTIFIC, INC.   800-229-2186
819 East St., Fairport Harbor, OH 44077-5564   440-354-2186
FDA Number: n/a   *Fax:* 440-354-6381
E-mail: sales@qsiquartz.com
Web site: www.qsiquartz.com
Medical Products Sales Volume: $4,900,000
Annual Revenue: $5-$10 Million
Year Founded: 1963
Total Employees: 30   *Marketing Staff:* 1   *Sales Staff:* 3
Ownership: Private
Quality System Registration Information: ISO9002
Produces/Sells CE-marked Devices: N
Federal Procurement Eligibility: Small Business, Female Owned
Distribution: Manufacturer Direct, Service Direct, Exporter
General Admin.: Paula Weber/Director Human Resources
     James R. Atwell/President, Chief Executive Officer
Mktg./Adv.: David North/Manager Marketing & Sales
     David North/Manager National Sales
     Ms. Jessica Snyder/Sales Associate
Beaker (Laboratory) — Chemistry
Labware, Basic, Reusable — Chemistry
Tube, Test — Chemistry

QUATRO COMPOSITES   858-513-4300
13250 Gregg St. Suite A-1, Poway, CA 92064
FDA Number: n/a   *Fax:* 858-513-3628
E-mail: molly.sitzmann@quatrocomposites.com
Web site: www.quatrocomposites.com
Year Founded: 2004
Total Employees: 70
Ownership: Private
Produces/Sells CE-marked Devices: N
Federal Procurement Eligibility: Small Business
Distribution: Manufacturer Direct, OEM
Mktg./Adv.: MOLLY SITZMANN/Manager Marketing & Sales
     DOUG ROBERTS/Vice President Sales
Accessories, Fixation, Orthopedic — Orthopedics
Accessories, Operating Room, Table — Surgery
Fixation Device, Extra-Cranial (Head Frame) — Orthopedics
Table, Radiographic — Radiology

MANUFACTURER PROFILES

QUATRO COMPOSITES   858-513-4300 *(cont'd)*
Table, Surgical, Orthopedic   Orthopedics

QUATRONIX
41 Research Way, East Setauket, NY 11733   **800-289-7707**
FDA Number: n/a   **631-784-6100**
E-mail: lasers@quantron.com   *Fax:* 631-784-6101
Web site: www.quantron.com
Annual Revenue: $25-$50 Million
Year Founded: 1967
Total Employees: 80   *Marketing Staff:* 2   *Sales Staff:* 15
Ownership: Quantronix Lasers
Quality System Registration Information: ISO9002
Produces/Sells CE-marked Devices: Y
Distribution: Manufacturer Direct, OEM
General Admin.: Qiang Fu/President
Mktg./Adv.: Prithvi Virasinghe/Director Marketing
              David Heck/Vice President Sales
Research: James Zhang/Vice President Research & Development
Accessories, Laser   General
Laser, Dental   Dental And Oral
Laser, Laboratory   Chemistry
Laser, Nd:YAG, Surgical   Surgery
Laser, Ophthalmic   Ophthalmology
Laser, Surgical   Surgery

QUDEN INC.
8 Maple, Cp 510, Knowlton J0E 1V0 Canada   **450-243-6101**
FDA Number: 9615394
Floss, Dental   Dental And Oral
Probe, Periodontic   Dental And Oral
Toothbrush, Manual   Dental And Oral

QUEEN SCREW & MANUFACTURING INC.   781-894-8110
60 Farwell St., Boston, MA 02154
FDA Number: n/a   *Fax:* 617-894-0907
E-mail: queenscrew@queenscrew.com
Web site: www.queenscrew.com
Medical Products Sales Volume: $3,000,000
Annual Revenue: $5-$10 Million
Total Employees: 50   *Marketing Staff:* 1   *Sales Staff:* 1
Ownership: Private
Quality System Registration Information: ISO9002
Produces/Sells CE-marked Devices: N
Federal Procurement Eligibility: Small Business
Distribution: OEM
General Admin.: Dominic A. DeJulio/President
Mktg./Adv.: Peter G. Babigian/Director Marketing
              Peter G. Babigian/Manager Advertising
Production: Michael DeJulio/Vice President Manufacturing
Component, Plastic   General
Contract Assembly   General
General Medical Device   General

QUELAB LABORATORIES INC.
5615 Fullum, Montreal, QUE H2G 2H6 Canada   **800-361-1434**
FDA Number: n/a   **514-277-2558**
E-mail: info@quelab.qc.ca   *Fax:* 514-277-4714
Web site: www.quelab.com
Year Founded: 1974
Total Employees: 100
Ownership: Private
Produces/Sells CE-marked Devices: N
Distribution: Manufacturer Direct, Exporter

QUEST
See Quest Diagnostics, Inc.

QUEST DIAGNOSTICS, INC.
3 Giralda Farms, Madison, NJ 07940   **800-222-0446**
FDA Number: n/a   **973-520-2700**
E-mail: media@questdiagnostics.com   *Fax:* 973-520-2900
Web site: www.questdiagnostics.com
Medical Products Sales Volume: $6,200,000,000
Annual Revenue: More than $1 Billion
Year Founded: 1967
Total Employees: 43000
Ownership: Public
Stock Symbol: DGX
Traded On: NYSE
Produces/Sells CE-marked Devices: N
Distribution: Service Direct
General Admin.: Mr. Surya N. Mohapatara/Chairman, Chief Executive Officer
Medical Admin.: Dr. Jon Cohen/Chief Medical Officer
Mktg./Adv.: Ms. Laure Park/Vice President Communications
Production: Mr. Wayne Simmons/Vice President Operations
Finance: Robert A. Hagemann/Chief Financial Officer
Contract Laboratory   General

QUEST INC.
704 Metro Dr., Lebanon, PA 17042-9138   **717-273-8118**
FDA Number: n/a   *Fax:* 717-273-2580
E-mail: Info@paquest.com
Web site: www.paquest.com
Annual Revenue: $1-$5 Million
Year Founded: 1950
Ownership: Private
Produces/Sells CE-marked Devices: N
Federal Procurement Eligibility: Small Business
Distribution: Service Direct
General Admin.: Art J. Mack/Executive Director
Mktg./Adv.: Cathy Edward/Manager Advertising
              Cathy Edward/Vice President Marketing
Production: Cathy Edward/Vice President Manufacturing
Finance: Holly Manwiller/Financial Executive
Contract Packaging   General

QUEST INTL., INC.
8127 Nw 29th Street, Doral, FL 33122   **305-592-6991**
FDA Number: 1061839
Anti-DNA Antibody, Antigen and Control   Immunology
Anti-RNP-Antibody, Antigen And Control   Immunology
Anti-SM-Antibody, Antigen And Control   Immunology
Antibody IGM, IF, Epstein-Barr Virus   Microbiology
Antinuclear Antibody (Enzyme-Labeled), Antigen, Controls   Immunology
Campylobacter Pylori   Microbiology
Enzyme Linked Immunoabsorbent Assay, Cytomegalovirus   Microbiology
Enzyme Linked Immunoabsorbent Assay, Herpes Simplex Virus   Microbiology
Enzyme Linked Immunoabsorbent Assay, Mumps Virus   Microbiology
Enzyme Linked Immunoabsorbent Assay, Rubella   Microbiology
Enzyme Linked Immunoabsorbent Assay, Rubeola   Microbiology
Enzyme Linked Immunoabsorbent Assay, Toxoplasma Gondii   Microbiology
Enzyme Linked Immunoabsorbent Assay, Treponema Pallidum   Microbiology
Enzyme Linked Immunoabsorbent Assay, Varicella-Zoster   Microbiology
Epstein-Barr Virus, Other   Microbiology
Extractable Antinuclear Antibody (Rnp/Sm), Antigen/Control   Immunology
Kit, Earmold Impression   Ear/Nose/Throat
System, Test, Anticardiolipin, Immunological   Immunology
Test, Thyroid Autoantibody   Immunology
Thyroglobulin, Antigen, Antiserum, Control   Immunology

QUEST MEDICAL, INC.
1 Allentown Pkwy., Allen, TX 75002-4211   **800-627-0226**
FDA Number: 1649914   **972-390-9800**
E-mail: custserveweb@questmedical.com   *Fax:* 972-390-7173
Web site: www.questmedical.com
Medical Products Sales Volume: $23,000,000
Annual Revenue: $25-$50 Million
Year Founded: 1994
Total Employees: 150
Ownership: Atrion Medical Products, Inc.
Stock Symbol: QMED
Traded On: NASDAQ
Quality System Registration Information: ISO9001
Produces/Sells CE-marked Devices: Y
Federal Procurement Eligibility: Small Business
Distribution: Manufacturer Direct, Manufacturer Through Distributor, Exporter
General Admin.: Ken Jones/President
Mktg./Adv.: Ken Jones/Manager National Sales
Production: Doug Bryan/Director Quality Assurance
              Michael Witkowski/Manager Materials
              Doug Bryan/Manager Regulatory Affairs
Activated Whole Blood Clotting Time   Hematology
Adapter, Stopcock, Manifold, Cardiopulmonary Bypass   Cardiovascular
Catheter, Perfusion   Cardiovascular
Detector, Bubble, Cardiopulmonary Bypass   Cardiovascular
Gauge, Pressure, Coronary, Cardiopulmonary Bypass   Cardiovascular
Heat Exchanger, Heart-Lung Bypass   Cardiovascular
Infusion Stand   General
Probe, Lacrimal   Ophthalmology
Set, Administration, Intravenous, Needle-Free   General
Snare, Surgical   Surgery
Transducer, Blood Pressure, Extravascular   Cardiovascular
Tubing, Fluid Delivery   General
Valve, CPB Check, Retrograde, In-Line   Anesthesiology

QUEST MEDICAL, INC.
See St. Jude Medical Neuromodulation Division

QUEST STAR MEDICAL, INC.
10180 Viking Drive, Eden Prairie, MN 55344-7222   **800-525-6718**
FDA Number: 2183836   **952-941-7345**
E-mail: info@queststarmedical.com   *Fax:* 952-941-7019
Web site: www.queststarmedical.com
Medical Products Sales Volume: $800,000
Year Founded: 2001
Total Employees: 10
Ownership: Private

QUEST STAR MEDICAL, INC.   800-525-6718 *(cont'd)*
Produces/Sells CE-marked Devices: Y
Federal Procurement Eligibility: Small Business
Distribution: Manufacturer Direct, Manufacturer Through Distributor, Exporter
General Admin.: George Joseph/President, Chief Executive Officer, Chief Financial Officer
Mktg./Adv.: E Jackson/Manager International Marketing
  Monitor, Blood Glucose (Test)   Gastroenterology/Urology
  Reagent, Glucose (Test System)   Chemistry

QUESTAR CORP.   215-862-5277
6204 Ingham Rd., New Hope, PA 18938
FDA Number: n/a   *Fax:* 215-862-0512
Web site: www.questarcorporation.com
Total Employees: 35
Ownership: Private
Produces/Sells CE-marked Devices: N
Federal Procurement Eligibility: Small Business
Distribution: Manufacturer Direct, Manufacturer Through Distributor, Manufacturer Through Manufacturer Reps
General Admin.: Donald J. Bandurick/Chief Executive Officer
    Earlene J. Austin/President
Research: Douglas Knight/Research Consultant
  Microscope, Operating, AC-Powered, Ophthalmic   Ophthalmology

QUESTECH INTERNATIONAL, INC.   800-966-5367
3810 Gunn Highway, Tampa, FL 33624   **813-960-7000**
FDA Number: 1038611   *Fax:* 813-960-2700
E-mail: echurch@questec.biz
Web site: www.questechproducts.com
Medical Products Sales Volume: $700,000
Annual Revenue: $5-$10 Million
Year Founded: 1988
Total Employees: 7   *Sales Staff:* 3
Ownership: Private
Produces/Sells CE-marked Devices: N
Federal Procurement Eligibility: Small Business, Female Owned
Distribution: Manufacturer Through Distributor, Manufacturer Through Manufacturer Reps, Exclusive Distributor, Importer, Exporter
General Admin.: Randall Krafft/Chief Executive Officer
    Sam Chan/Director International Operations
Mktg./Adv.: Daniel Morton/Manager Market Research
    Wayne Albright/Vice President Sales
Production: Edward Church/Director Quality Assurance
Research: Edward Church/Vice President Research & Development
  Cleaner, Lens, Contact   Ophthalmology
  Dispenser, Soap   General
  Pad, Heating, Electrical   Physical Med
  Pad, Heating, Powered   Physical Med
  Service, Consulting   General
  Service, Engineering/Design   General
  Service, Import/Export   General
  Thermometer, Electronic, Continuous   General

QUESTRON TECHNOLOGIES CORPORATION   905-363-1223
6725 Millcreek Drive, Unit 7,
Mississauga, ONT L5N 5 Canada
FDA Number: n/a   *Fax:* 905-363-1227
E-mail: info@qtechcorp.com
Web site: www.qtechcorp.com
Year Founded: 1989
Total Employees: 25
Ownership: Private
Produces/Sells CE-marked Devices: N
Distribution: Manufacturer Direct, Exclusive Distributor, Importer, Exporter

QUEUE SYSTEMS
See Kendro Laboratory Products

QUICARE, LTD.   208-676-8015
P.O. Box 3667, Coeur d'Alene, ID 83816
FDA Number: n/a   *Fax:* (208) 676 8034
E-mail: info@quicare.com
Web site: www.quicare.com
Year Founded: 2003
Ownership: Private
Produces/Sells CE-marked Devices: N
General Admin.: Eyal Wachtenberg/Chairman
    Nissim Greisas/Chief Operating Officer
Research: Dan Eylon/Vice President Research & Development

QUICK POINT INC.   636-343-9400
1717 Fenpark Drive, Fenton, MO 63026
FDA Number: 3001177326
E-mail: sales@quickpoint.com
Web site: www.quickpoint.com
Ownership: Private
Produces/Sells CE-marked Devices: N

QUICK POINT INC.   636-343-9400 *(cont'd)*
  Kit, First Aid
    Surgery

QUIDEL CORP.   (800) 874-1517
10165 McKellar Court, San Diego, CA 92121   **858-552-1100**
FDA Number: 2024674
E-mail: ir@quidel.com
Web site: www.quidel.com
Year Founded: 1979
Ownership: QUIDEL CORPORATION
Stock Symbol: QDEL
Traded On: NASDAQ
Produces/Sells CE-marked Devices: N
  Antigen, Antiserum, Complement C1 Inhibitor (Inactivator)   Immunology
  Antigen, Antiserum, Control, Complement C1q   Immunology
  Antinuclear Antibody (Enzyme-Labeled), Antigen, Controls   Immunology
  Column, Chromatography, Hydroxyproline   Chemistry
  DNA-Probe, Gardnerella Vaginalis   Microbiology
  Indicator, pH, Dye (Urinary, Non-Quantitative)   Chemistry
  Phenylphosphate, Alkaline Phosphatase Or Isoenzymes   Chemistry
  Reagent, Immunoassay, Activator, C3, Complement   Immunology

QUIDEL CORPORATION   800-874-1517
10165 McKellar Ct., San Diego, CA 92121-4299   **619-552-1100**
FDA Number: 2024674   *Fax:* 858-455-4960
E-mail: ir@quidel.com
Web site: www.quidel.com
Medical Products Sales Volume: $106,000,000
Annual Revenue: More than $1 Billion
Year Founded: 1979
Ownership: Public
Stock Symbol: QDEL
Traded On: NASDAQ
Quality System Registration Information: ISO9001
Produces/Sells CE-marked Devices: N
Federal Procurement Eligibility: Small Business
Distribution: Manufacturer Direct, Manufacturer Through Distributor, Manufacturer Through Manufacturer Reps, Exclusive Distributor, Exporter
General Admin.: Dr. Timothy Stenzel/Chief Scientific Officer
    Mr. Douglas Bryant/President, Chief Executive Officer
Mktg./Adv.: Mr. Robert Bujarski/Senior Vice President Business Development
Production: Mr. Scott McCloud/Senior Vice President Operations
    Dr. John Tamerious/Senior Vice President Regulatory Affairs
Finance: Mr. John Radak/Chief Financial Officer
  Antibody, Monoclonal   Microbiology
  Antigen, Antiserum, Control, Luteinizing Hormone   Immunology
  Antigen, CF (Including CF Control), Influenza Virus   Microbiology
  Antigen, Streptococcus SPP.   Microbiology
  Antisera, Fluorescent, All Types, Staphylococcus SPP.   Microbiology
  Antiserum, Streptococcus SPP.   Microbiology
  Campylobacter Pylori   Microbiology
  Chlamydia Trachomatis   Microbiology
  Enzyme Linked Immunoabsorbent Assay, Chlamydia Group   Microbiology
  Kit, Pregnancy Test   Obstetrics/Gynecology
  Radioimmunoassay, Human Chorionic Gonadotropin   Chemistry
  Reagent, Occult Blood   Hematology
  Test, Allergy   Immunology
  Test, Antibiotic Susceptibility   Microbiology
  Test, Disease, Lyme   Immunology
  Test, Fertility Monitoring   Obstetrics/Gynecology
  Test, Human Chorionic Gonadotropin   Immunology
  Test, Infectious Mononucleosis   Immunology
Medical Product Subsidiaries (Listed Separately)
  Quidel

QUINCY SPECIALTIES CO.   217-222-4057
631 Vermont St., Quincy, IL 62306
FDA Number: 9200906   *Fax:* 217-222-4065
E-mail: qcyspec@quincyspecialtiesco.com
Web site: www.quincyspecialtiesco.com
Medical Products Sales Volume: $900,000
Annual Revenue: $0-$1 Million
Year Founded: 1935
Total Employees: 9
Ownership: Private
Produces/Sells CE-marked Devices: N
Federal Procurement Eligibility: Small Business
Distribution: Manufacturer Direct, Manufacturer Through Distributor
General Admin.: Dwight C. Seeley/President, Chief Executive Officer
    Doris Timpe/Vice President, Secretary
  Apron, Laboratory   Chemistry

QUINT COMPANY   215-533-1988
3725 Castor Ave., Philadelphia, PA 19124
FDA Number: n/a   *Fax:* 215-533-7784
E-mail: sales@quintco.com
Web site: www.quintco.com
Annual Revenue: $5-$10 Million
Year Founded: 1849

QUINT COMPANY — 215-533-1988 (cont'd)

Total Employees: 40   Marketing Staff: 2   Sales Staff: 2
Ownership: Private
Produces/Sells CE-marked Devices: N
Federal Procurement Eligibility: Small Business
Distribution: Manufacturer Direct
General Admin.: Harry Feby Jr./General Manager
    Edward Howell/President

Labeling Equipment	General
Pen, Marking, Surgical	Ophthalmology

QUINTRON INSTRUMENT COMPANY — 800-542-4448
3712 W. Pierce St., Milwaukee, WI 53215-1032   **414-645-4222**
FDA Number: 2124914   Fax: 414-645-3484
E-mail: sales@quintron-usa.com
Web site: www.quintron-usa.com
Year Founded: 1962
Ownership: Private
Quality System Registration Information: ISO9000; ISO9001
Produces/Sells CE-marked Devices: Y
Federal Procurement Eligibility: Small Business
Distribution: Manufacturer Direct, Manufacturer Through Distributor, Manufacturer Through Manufacturer Reps, OEM, Exporter
General Admin.: Steve Hamilton/President, Chief Executive Officer

Analyzer, Trace Gas, Breath	Anesthesiology
Container, Specimen, All Types	General
Gas, Collecting Vessel	Anesthesiology
Recorder, Chart, Laboratory	Chemistry

R & D BATTERIES, INC. — 800-950-1945
3300 Corporate Center Drive,   **952-890-0629**
Burnsville, MN 55306
FDA Number: n/a   Fax: 952-890-7912
E-mail: info@rdbatteries.net
Web site: www.rdbatteries.net
Medical Products Sales Volume: $12,000
Annual Revenue: $10-$25 Million
Year Founded: 1989
Total Employees: 42   Marketing Staff: 12   Sales Staff: 14
Ownership: Private
Produces/Sells CE-marked Devices: N
Federal Procurement Eligibility: Small Business
Distribution: Manufacturer Direct
General Admin.: Randall C. Noddings/President, Chief Executive Officer
    Barbara J. Noddings/Vice President Human Resources
    Barbara J. Noddings/Vice President, General Manager
Mktg./Adv.: Jake Kaluza/Admin. Contract Sales
    Jake Kaluza/Manager International & National Sales
Production: Julie Maldenhauer/Admin. Production
    James Brooks/Director Quality Assurance
    James Brooks/Manager Regulatory Affairs

Box, Battery, Rechargeable (Endoscopic)	Gastroenterology/Urology
Communication System, Powered	Physical Med
Exerciser, Powered	Anesthesiology

R & D MEDICAL PRODUCTS, INC. — 949-472-9346
20492 Crescent Bay Drive #106, Lake Forest, CA 92630
FDA Number: 9031339   Fax: 949-472-9347
E-mail: admin@rdmedicalproducts.com
Web site: www.medicalelectrodes.com
Medical Products Sales Volume: $1,300,000
Annual Revenue: $1-$5 Million
Year Founded: 1997
Total Employees: 17   Marketing Staff: 1   Sales Staff: 1
Ownership: Private
Quality System Registration Information: ISO9001
Produces/Sells CE-marked Devices: N
Federal Procurement Eligibility: Small Business, Minority Owned
Distribution: Manufacturer Through Distributor, OEM
General Admin.: David Sheraton/Chief Executive
    Ms. Joana Prunean/Vice President Corporate Operations

Electrode, Electrocardiograph	Cardiovascular
Stimulator, Nerve, Transcutaneous (Pain Relief, TENS)	Cns/Neurology
Suction Apparatus, Single Patient, Portable, Non-Powered	Surgery

R & D SYSTEMS, INC. — 612-656-4533
614 McKinley Place N.E., Minneapolis, MN 55413-2647
FDA Number: 2182501
Web site: www.rndsystems.com
Medical Products Sales Volume: $104,000
Annual Revenue: $50-$100 Million
Total Employees: 450   Marketing Staff: 30   Sales Staff: 30
Ownership: Public
Stock Symbol: TECH
Traded On: NASDAQ
Produces/Sells CE-marked Devices: N
Federal Procurement Eligibility: Small Business
Distribution: Manufacturer Direct, Manufacturer Through Distributor, OEM

R & D SYSTEMS, INC. — 612-656-4533 (cont'd)

General Admin.: Thomas E. Oland/President, Chief Executive Officer
    Lea Simone/Vice President Human Resources
Mktg./Adv.: John Syverud/Director National Accounts
    Johanna LaBresh/Manager Advertising
    Marty Kissel/Vice President Business Development
Production: Ralph Hogancamp/Manager Regulatory Affairs
    Mary Poole/Product Manager
Research: Lisa Jarvis/Vice President Research & Development

Calibrator, Cell Indices	Hematology
Calibrator, Hemoglobin And Hematocrit Measurement	Hematology
Calibrator, Platelet Counting	Hematology
Calibrator, Red Cell And White Cell Counting	Hematology
Control, Cell Counter, Normal And Abnormal	Hematology
Control, Hemoglobin	Hematology
Control, Platelet	Hematology
Hematology Quality Control Mixture	Hematology

Medical Product Subsidiaries (Listed Separately)
R&D System Europe Ltd.

R & R INDUSTRIES, INC. — 800-234-5611
1000 Calle Cordillera, San Clemente, CA 92673   **949-361-9238**
FDA Number: 2029336   Fax: 949-361-9360
E-mail: service@rrind.com
Web site: www.rrind.com
Ownership: Private
Produces/Sells CE-marked Devices: N

Glove, Protective, Radiographic	Radiology
Orthosis, Abdominal	Physical Med
Orthosis, Limb Brace	Physical Med
Orthosis, Lumbar	Physical Med
Support, Arm	Physical Med

R AND L HEARING SERVICES — 800-444-8920
3005 Niagara Lane   Ste. 2,   **763-383-1429**
Minneapolis, MN 55447
FDA Number: 2183866   Fax: 763-383-1437
E-mail: billl@rllabs.net
Web site: www.rllabs.net
Annual Revenue: $1-$5 Million
Year Founded: 1988
Total Employees: 28   Sales Staff: 1
Ownership: Private
Produces/Sells CE-marked Devices: Y
Federal Procurement Eligibility: Small Business
Distribution: Manufacturer Through Distributor, Service Direct, Importer
General Admin.: Frederick W. Lewis/President, Chief Executive Officer

Hearing-Aid	Ear/Nose/Throat
Service, Maintenance/Repair	General

R MEDICAL SUPPLY — 800-882-7578
620 Valley Forge Rd, #F, Hillsborough, NC 27278   **919-245-3600**
FDA Number: 2950523   Fax: 919-245-3606
E-mail: rmed3@earthlink.net
Annual Revenue: $1-$5 Million
Year Founded: 1991
Ownership: Private
Produces/Sells CE-marked Devices: N
Federal Procurement Eligibility: Small Business
Distribution: Manufacturer Through Distributor, Exclusive Distributor, Importer
General Admin.: Rick Crafts/President

Belt, Sanitary	Obstetrics/Gynecology
Cannula, Suction, Uterine	Obstetrics/Gynecology
Catheter, Bartholin Gland	Gastroenterology/Urology
Colposcope	Obstetrics/Gynecology
Cryosurgical Unit, Gynecologic	Obstetrics/Gynecology
Curette, Suction, Endometrial	Obstetrics/Gynecology
Curette, Uterine	Obstetrics/Gynecology
Dilator, Cervical, Expandable	Obstetrics/Gynecology
Dilator, Cervical, Hygroscopic-Laminaria	Obstetrics/Gynecology
Dilator, Uterine	Obstetrics/Gynecology
Dilator, Vaginal	Obstetrics/Gynecology
Electrosurgical Equipment, Special Purpose	Surgery
Forceps, Biopsy, Gynecological	Obstetrics/Gynecology
Hook, IUD Removal	Obstetrics/Gynecology
Kit, Pregnancy Test	Obstetrics/Gynecology
Monitor, Fetal Doppler Ultrasound	Obstetrics/Gynecology
Pessary, Vaginal	Obstetrics/Gynecology
Radioimmunoassay, Human Chorionic Gonadotropin	Chemistry
Speculum, Vaginal, Metal	Obstetrics/Gynecology
Warmer, Gel	General

R&B WIRE PRODUCTS, INC. — 800-634-0555
2902 West Garry Street, Santa Ana, CA 92704   **714-549-3355**
FDA Number: n/a   Fax: 714-549-0625
E-mail: sales@rbwire.com
Web site: www.rbwire.com
Medical Products Sales Volume: $4,000,000
Annual Revenue: $5-$10 Million

R&B WIRE PRODUCTS, INC. 800-634-0555 (cont'd)
Year Founded: 1946
Total Employees: 35
Ownership: Private
Produces/Sells CE-marked Devices: N
Federal Procurement Eligibility: Small Business, GSA Contract
Distribution: Manufacturer Through Distributor
General Admin.: Richard Rawlins/President, Chief Executive Officer
Mktg./Adv.: Santiago Meza/Manager Planning
Frank Rowe/Vice President Marketing & Sales
Finance: Christine Arakaki/Vice President Admin., Finance

Cart, Laundry	General
Cart, Multipurpose	General
Cart, Other	General
Housekeeping Equipment	General
Laundry Equipment	General
Laundry Hamper	General
Stand, Laundry Hamper	General

R&DA CO. 508-747-5803
37 Dwight Avenue, Plymouth, MA 02360-2159
FDA Number: n/a
Fax: 508-747-5803
E-mail: fencing_SaEF@comcast.net
Medical Products Sales Volume: $100,000
Annual Revenue: $0-$1 Million
Total Employees: 1
Ownership: Private
Produces/Sells CE-marked Devices: Y
Federal Procurement Eligibility: Small Business
Distribution: Manufacturer Direct, Manufacturer Through Manufacturer Reps
General Admin.: Harry A. Shamir/President, Chief Executive Officer

Card, Identification	General
Equipment, Cleaning, Air	General
Equipment, Control, Pollution	General
Equipment, Marking, Electrochemical	General
Identification, Alert, Medical	General
Service, Engineering/Design	General

R&R MEDICAL, INC. 877-776-9972
2225 Park Place Dr., Slatington, PA 18080
FDA Number: 3005215751
Ownership: Private
Produces/Sells CE-marked Devices: N

Fixation Appliance, Multiple Component	Orthopedics
Pin, Fixation, Threaded	Orthopedics

R. A. FISCHER CO. 800-525-3467
8751 White Oak Ave., Northridge, CA 91325 818-407-0855
FDA Number: n/a
Fax: 818-775-2941
E-mail: orders@rafischer.com
Web site: http://www.rafischer.com/
Ownership: A.R. Hinkel Co., Inc.
Produces/Sells CE-marked Devices: N

Epilator, High-Frequency, Needle-Type	Surgery
Iontophoresis Unit, Physical Medicine	Physical Med

R. A. JONES & CO., INC. 859-341-0400
2701 Crescent Springs Rd., Covington, KY 41017
FDA Number: n/a
Fax: 859-341-0519
E-mail: sales@oystar.rajones.com
Web site: www.rajones.com
Annual Revenue: $50-$100 Million
Year Founded: 1905
Total Employees: 500
Ownership: Public
Produces/Sells CE-marked Devices: N
Distribution: Manufacturer Direct
General Admin.: Jack C. Collins/Chief Operating Officer
Ralph J. Olson/President, Chief Executive Officer
John Tamashasky/Vice President Human Resources
Mktg./Adv.: Paula E. Holmes/Director Marketing
Mark A. Logan/Vice President Marketing & Sales
Production: John Finck/Vice President Manufacturing

Packaging Equipment	General

R. B. ANNIS INSTRUMENTS, INC. 317-637-9282
1101 N. Delaware St., Indianapolis, IN 46202-2529
FDA Number: 9200072
Fax: 317-637-9282
E-mail: info@rbannis.com
Web site: www.rbannis.com
Medical Products Sales Volume: $800,000
Annual Revenue: $0-$1 Million
Year Founded: 1928
Total Employees: 8
Ownership: Private
Produces/Sells CE-marked Devices: N
Federal Procurement Eligibility: Small Business
Distribution: Manufacturer Direct, OEM, Exporter

R. B. ANNIS INSTRUMENTS, INC. 317-637-9282 (cont'd)
General Admin.: M.E. Scott/President, Chief Executive Officer
Production: M. Scott/Manager Materials

Component, Electrical	General
Component, Metal, Other	General
Demagnetizer	General
Detector, Metal, Magnetic	Ophthalmology
Fluxmeter	General
Gaussmeter	General
Magnetic Unit, Therapeutic	Physical Med
Magnetometer	General

R. B. WILLIAMS CO., INC. 800-843-7346
2616 First Avenue North, St. Petersburg, FL 33713
FDA Number: n/a
Fax: 727-821-7927
E-mail: info@rbwillamsco.com
Web site: www.rbwilliamsco.com
Ownership: Private
Produces/Sells CE-marked Devices: N

Dressing, Other	General

R. D. EQUIPMENT, INC. 508-362-7498
230 Percival Dr., West Barnstable, MA 02668
FDA Number: 2975127
Fax: 508-362-7498
E-mail: info@rdequipment.com
Web site: www.rdequipment.com
Total Employees: 5 Marketing Staff: 5 Sales Staff: 5
Ownership: Private
Produces/Sells CE-marked Devices: N
Federal Procurement Eligibility: Small Business
Distribution: Manufacturer Direct, Manufacturer Through Distributor, OEM, Service Direct
General Admin.: Richard Dagostino/President
Diana Pontieri/Vice President, General Manager
Mktg./Adv.: Diana Pontieri/Manager National Sales

Bag, Leg	Gastroenterology/Urology
Chair, Shower	General
Fork	Orthopedics
Telephone Equipment	General

R. SABEE COMPANY 920-882-7350
1718 W. 8th St., Appleton, WI 54914-4957
FDA Number: 2123423
Fax: 920-882-7351
E-mail: info@rsabeecompany.com
Web site: www.rsabeecompany.com
Medical Products Sales Volume: $30,000,000
Annual Revenue: $25-$50 Million
Total Employees: 220 Marketing Staff: 2 Sales Staff: 3
Ownership: Private
Produces/Sells CE-marked Devices: N
Federal Procurement Eligibility: Small Business
Distribution: Manufacturer Direct, Manufacturer Through Distributor, Manufacturer Through Manufacturer Reps, Exclusive Distributor
General Admin.: Anthony Sabee/President
Mktg./Adv.: Sherry Ahlman/Director Marketing
Sherry Ahlman/Director National Accounts
Sherry Ahlman/Manager Contract Sales
Sherry Ahlman/Manager International & National Sales
Lois Sabee/Vice President Marketing
Production: Nancy Pingel/Director Quality Assurance
Joe M. Donovan/Manager Materials

Cap, Surgical	Surgery
Diaper, Pediatric	General
Drape, Surgical	Surgery
Gown, Examination	General
Pad, Incontinence (Underpad)	General
Sheeting, Examination Table	General
Towel, Surgical	Surgery
Wrap, Sterilization	General

R.A. FISCHER COMPANY 800-525-3467
8751 White Oak Avenue, Northridge, CA 91325 818-407-0855
FDA Number: 2011113
Fax: 818-775-2941
E-mail: orders@rafischer.com
Web site: www.rafischer.com
Medical Products Sales Volume: $400,000
Year Founded: 1948
Total Employees: 5
Ownership: A.R. Hinkel Co., Inc.
Produces/Sells CE-marked Devices: N
Federal Procurement Eligibility: Small Business
Distribution: Manufacturer Through Distributor
General Admin.: William Schuler/President, Chief Executive Officer
Production: Jerry Van Orden/Vice President Manufacturing

Epilator, High-Frequency, Needle-Type	Surgery
Iontophoresis Equipment	Chemistry

R.A.E. TECHNOLOGIES INC.
905-428-6384
48 Barbour Crescent, Ajax, ONT L1S-6Z6 Canada
FDA Number: n/a
E-mail: raydel@home.com   Fax: 905-427-2685
Year Founded: 1985
Total Employees: 10
Ownership: Private
Produces/Sells CE-marked Devices: N
Distribution: Manufacturer Direct

R.C. SMITH COMPANY
800-747-7648
952-854-0711
14200 Southcross Drive W.,
Burnsville, MN 55306
FDA Number: n/a
E-mail: info@rcsmith.com   Fax: 952-854-8160
Web site: www.rcsmith.com
Medical Products Sales Volume: $8,800,000
Annual Revenue: $5-$10 Million
Year Founded: 1965
Total Employees: 38
Ownership: Private
Produces/Sells CE-marked Devices: N
Federal Procurement Eligibility: Small Business, GSA Contract, VA Contract
Distribution: Manufacturer Through Manufacturer Reps
General Admin.: Peter J. Smith/President
Mktg./Adv.: Peter J. Smith/Manager Sales

Cabinet Casework, Laboratory	Chemistry
Cabinet Casework, Modular	General
Cabinet Casework, Pharmacy	General
Station, Nursing	General

R.C.A. RUBBER COMPANY, THE
800-321-2340
330-784-1291
1833 E. Market St., P.O. Box 9240,
Akron, OH 44305
FDA Number: 9330102
E-mail: info@rcarubber.com   Fax: 330-784-2899
Web site: www.rcarubber.com
Year Founded: 1931
Total Employees: 240   Marketing Staff: 4   Sales Staff: 6
Ownership: Private
Produces/Sells CE-marked Devices: N
Federal Procurement Eligibility: Small Business, Female Owned
Distribution: Manufacturer Through Distributor
Mktg./Adv.: D. Harris/Manager Advertising

Bumper Guard, Corner	General
Component, Plastic	General
Component, Rubber	General
Floor Mat	General
Flooring	General

R.J. LINDQUIST CO.
213-382-1268
2419 James M. Wood Blvd., Los Angeles, CA 90006
FDA Number: 2011548

Chronaximeter, Physical Medicine	Physical Med
Diathermy, Shortwave	Physical Med
Massager, Therapeutic	Physical Med
Stimulator, Neuromuscular, External Functional	Cns/Neurology
Stimulator, Ultrasound, Muscle	Physical Med

R.J.S. ACOUSTIC SERVICES, INC.
800-826-3180
11919 Ne Glisan, Portland, OR 97220-2144
FDA Number: 3004136292
Ownership: Private
Produces/Sells CE-marked Devices: N

Hearing-Aid	Ear/Nose/Throat

R2 DIAGNOSTICS, INC.
574-288-4377
1801 Commerce Dr., South Bend, IN 46628
FDA Number: 1835316

Fibrin Split Products	Hematology
Partial Thromboplastin Time	Hematology
Plasma, Coagulase, Human/Horse/Rabbit	Microbiology
Plasma, Deficient, Factor, Coagulation	Hematology
Prothrombin Time	Hematology
Reagent, General Purpose	Pathology
Test, Antithrombin III, Two Stage Clotting Time	Hematology
Test, Fibrinogen	Hematology
Test, Qualitative And Quantitative Factor Deficiency	Hematology
Test, Systemic Lupus Erythematosus	Immunology
Test, Thrombin Time	Hematology
Thromboplastin, Activated Partial	Hematology

R4 VASCULAR, INC.
612-770-4038
Meridian Business Center, Suite 150, 7550 Meridian Cir N,
Osseo, MN 55369
FDA Number: 3006242715

Holder, Intravascular Catheter	General

RA MEDICAL SYSTEMS, INC.
760-804-1648
2270 Camino Vida Roble, Suite L, Carlsbad, CA 92011
FDA Number: 2032864

Laser, Surgical	Surgery
System, Laser, Photodynamic Therapy	Surgery

RACER-MATE, INC.
800-522-3610
206-524-6625
3016 N.E. Blakeley St., Seattle, WA 98105-4012
FDA Number: n/a
E-mail: sales@racermateinc.com   Fax: 206-523-4961
Web site: www.racermateinc.com
Annual Revenue: $0-$1 Million
Total Employees: 10   Marketing Staff: 4   Sales Staff: 4
Ownership: Private
Produces/Sells CE-marked Devices: N
Federal Procurement Eligibility: Small Business
Distribution: Manufacturer Direct
General Admin.: Wilfried Baatz/President
     Chuck Wurster/Vice President, General Manager
Mktg./Adv.: Charles Wurster/Vice President Marketing
Production: Gary Walters/Vice President Manufacturing

Computer, Stress Exercise	Cardiovascular
Exerciser, Bicycle	Physical Med
Monitor, Physiological, Stress Exercise	Cardiovascular

RACINE & CO. INC.
See Smith Time, Inc.

RADCAL CORP.
800-423-7169
626-357-7921
426 W. Duarte Rd., Monrovia, CA 91016-4544
FDA Number: 7000889
E-mail: sales@radcal.com   Fax: 626-357-8863
Web site: www.radcal.com
Annual Revenue: $5-$10 Million
Year Founded: 1973
Total Employees: 50   Marketing Staff: 4   Sales Staff: 7
Ownership: Private
Quality System Registration Information: ISO9001
Produces/Sells CE-marked Devices: Y
Federal Procurement Eligibility: Small Business
Distribution: Manufacturer Direct, Manufacturer Through Distributor, Manufacturer Through Manufacturer Reps, OEM, Exporter
General Admin.: Ken Mettler/President
Mktg./Adv.: Ken Mettler/Manager International Sales
     John Gilmor/Manager Sales
     Ken Mettler/Vice President Marketing & Sales

Computer Software	General
Device, Limiting, Beam, Diagnostic, X-Ray	Radiology
Monitor, Radiation	Radiology
Phantom, Computed Axial Tomography (CAT, CT)	Radiology
Tester, Radiology Quality Assurance	Radiology

RADD PRECISION INC.
905-760-1045
60 Citation Dr., Concord, ONT L4K-2W9 Canada
FDA Number: n/a   Fax: 905-760-1046
Year Founded: 1984
Total Employees: 10
Ownership: Private
Produces/Sells CE-marked Devices: N
Distribution: Manufacturer Direct

RADELIN SCREENS
See Mci Optonix, Div. Of Usr Optonix Inc.

RADIANCE MEDICAL SYSTEMS
See Endologix, Inc.

RADIANT ELECTRIC HEAT INC.
262-502-1282
Radiant Electric HeatÉ_Z N112W14600 Mequ,
Germantown, WI 53022
FDA Number: 3006369657
Ownership: Private
Produces/Sells CE-marked Devices: N

Heating Unit, Powered	Physical Med

RADIATION MANAGEMENT CONSULTANTS
See Rmc Medical

RADIATION MONITORING DEVICES, INC.
800-532-3763
617-668-6800
44 Hunt St., Watertown, MA 02472
FDA Number: 1219248
E-mail: info@rmdinc.com   Fax: 617-926-9980
Web site: www.rmdinc.com
Medical Products Sales Volume: $9,800,000
Year Founded: 1974
Ownership: Private
Quality System Registration Information: ISO9000; ISO9003
Produces/Sells CE-marked Devices: Y
Federal Procurement Eligibility: Small Business
Distribution: Manufacturer Direct, OEM, Exporter

RADIATION MONITORING DEVICES, INC. 800-532-3763 (cont'd)
General Admin.: Gerald Entine/President
Jack Paster/Vice President
Research: Michael Squillante/Vice President Research

Analyzer, Lead	General
Counter, Radiation	Radiology
Monitor, Radiation	Radiology
Probe, Other	General
Probe, Uptake, Nuclear	Radiology

RADIATION PRODUCTS DESIGN, INC. 800-497-2071
5218 Barthel Industrial Dr., 763-497-2071
Albertville, MN 55301
FDA Number: 2182762 Fax: 763-497-2295
E-mail: sales@rpdinc.com
Web site: www.rpdinc.com
Medical Products Sales Volume: $2,000,000
Annual Revenue: $1-$5 Million
Ownership: Private
Produces/Sells CE-marked Devices: N
Federal Procurement Eligibility: Small Business
Distribution: Manufacturer Direct, Manufacturer Through Distributor, Exporter

Accessories, Radiotherapy	Radiology
Applicator, Radionuclide, Manual	Radiology
Block, Beam Shaping, Radionuclide	Radiology
Caliper	Orthopedics
Contract Manufacturing	General
Dispenser, Mercury And/Or Alloy	Dental And Oral
Holder, Head, Radiographic	Radiology
Holder, Syringe, Leaded	Radiology
Infusion Stand	General
Lift, Patient	General
Phantom, Anthropomorphic, Radiographic	Radiology
Phantom, Computed Axial Tomography (CAT, CT)	Radiology
Protractor	Orthopedics
Shield, Gonadal	Radiology
Shield, Protective, Personnel	Radiology
Shield, X-Ray, Brick	Radiology
Stain, Dye Solution	Pathology
Support, Patient Position, Radiographic	Radiology
Table, Radiographic, Stationary Top	Radiology
Test Pattern, Radiographic	Radiology

RADIATION SHIELD TECHNOLOGIES, INC. 866-733-6766
1825 Ponce De Leon Blvd, Suite 456, Coral Gables, FL 33134
FDA Number: 3003794732 Fax: 866-533-6766
E-mail: info@radshield.com
Web site: www.radshield.com
Ownership: Private
Produces/Sells CE-marked Devices: N

Apron, Lead, Radiographic	Radiology

RADIENT PHARMACEUTICALS 714-505-4460
2492 Walnut Avenue Suite 100, Tustin, CA 92780-6953
FDA Number: 2030936 Fax: 714-505-4464
E-mail: Info@amdl.com
Web site: www.amdl.com
Medical Products Sales Volume: $60,000
Year Founded: 1987
Total Employees: 320
Ownership: Public
Stock Symbol: ADL
Traded On: AMEX
Quality System Registration Information: ISO9001
Produces/Sells CE-marked Devices: N
Federal Procurement Eligibility: Small Business
Distribution: Manufacturer Direct, Manufacturer Through Distributor, Exclusive Distributor, Importer, Exporter
General Admin.: Linda McKenzie/Office Manager
Gary Dreher/President, Chief Executive Officer
Research: Andrea Small-Howard/Manager Research & Development
Finance: Akio Ariura/Chief Financial Officer

Campylobacter Pylori	Microbiology

RADIO SHACK 800-843-7422
300 Radioshack Circle, Mail Stop Wf4-136, 817-415-3700
Fort Worth, TX 76102
FDA Number: 1641033
E-mail: RadioShack.Customer.Care@RadioShack.com
Web site: http://www.radioshackcorporation.com/
Annual Revenue: More than $1 Billion
Total Employees: 36800
Ownership: Private
Stock Symbol: RSH
Traded On: NYSE
Produces/Sells CE-marked Devices: N
Distribution: Service Direct, Exclusive Distributor
General Admin.: Julian C. Day/Chief Executive Officer, Chairman

RADIO SHACK 800-843-7422 (cont'd)
James F. Gooch/Chief Financial Officer, Executive Vice President
Lee D. Applbaum/Executive Vice President
Peter J. Whitsett/Executive Vice President
John G. Ripperton/Senior Vice President
Production: Bryan Bevin/Executive Vice President Operations
Finance: Martin O. Moad/Vice President, Controller

Communication System, Room Status	General
Cuff, Blood Pressure	Cardiovascular
Monitor, Blood Pressure, Finger	Cardiovascular
Telephone Equipment	General
Thermometer, Electronic	General

RADIOGRAPHIC AND DATA SOLUTIONS, INC. 612-379-7152
2101 Kennedy St. Ne, Suite 190, Minneapolis, MN 55413
FDA Number: 3003873056
Ownership: Private
Produces/Sells CE-marked Devices: N

Camera, X-Ray, Fluorographic, Cine Or Spot	Radiology

RADIOGRAPHIC DIGITAL IMAGING, INC. 310-921-9559
2580 West 237th St., Torrance, CA 90505
FDA Number: n/a Fax: 310-921-2559
E-mail: info@cobrascan.com
Web site: www.icrcompany.com
Annual Revenue: $1-$5 Million
Year Founded: 1991
Total Employees: 15 Marketing Staff: 2 Sales Staff: 30
Ownership: Private
Produces/Sells CE-marked Devices: Y
Distribution: Manufacturer Direct, Manufacturer Through Distributor
General Admin.: Stephen Neushul/President, Chief Executive Officer
Peter Neushul/Vice President, General Manager
Mktg./Adv.: Hunter Adler/Director Marketing

Computer Software	General
Image Digitizer	Radiology
Imager, X-Ray, Electrostatic	Radiology
Scanner, Computed Tomography, X-Ray, Full Body	Radiology
Transmitter, Image & Data, Radiographic	Radiology

RADIOLOGICAL IMAGING TECHNOLOGY, INC. 719-590-1077
5065 List Drive, Colorado Springs, CO 80919-3321
FDA Number: 1722661 Fax: 719-590-1071
Web site: www.radimage.com
Year Founded: 1993
Ownership: Private
Produces/Sells CE-marked Devices: N
Distribution: Manufacturer Direct
General Admin.: Daniel Ritt/President, Chief Executive Officer
Mktg./Adv.: Ellen Ritt/Vice President Marketing

Accelerator, Linear, Medical	Radiology

RADIOLOGY INFORMATION SYSTEMS, INC. 877-722-6747
43676 Trade Center Place, Suite 100, 703-713-3313
Dulles, VA 20166
FDA Number: 1125622 Fax: 703-713-3343
Web site: www.radinfosystems.com
Ownership: Private
Produces/Sells CE-marked Devices: N

Computer and Software, Medical	General

RADIOLOGY SUPPORT DEVICES 800-221-0527
1904 E. Dominguez St., 310-518-0527
Long Beach, CA 90810
FDA Number: 9003310 Fax: 310-518-0806
E-mail: Information@RSDPhantoms.com
Web site: www.rsdphantoms.com
Medical Products Sales Volume: $2,500,000
Annual Revenue: $0-$1 Million
Year Founded: 1988
Total Employees: 26 Marketing Staff: 1 Sales Staff: 2
Ownership: Private
Federal Procurement Eligibility: Small Business
Distribution: Manufacturer Direct, Manufacturer Through Distributor, Manufacturer Through Manufacturer Reps, Importer, Exporter
General Admin.: Samuel W. Alderson/President
Research: Samuel W. Alderson/Director Research

Anatomical Training Model	General
Calibrator, Radioisotope	Radiology
Phantom, Anthropomorphic, Nuclear	Radiology
Phantom, Anthropomorphic, Radiographic	Radiology
Phantom, Mammographic	Radiology
Phantom, Radiotherapy	Radiology
Simulator, Lung	Anesthesiology

RADIOMED CORPORATION 866-649-0300
One Industrial Way, Tyngsboro, MA 01879-1400 978-649-0300
FDA Number: 3004047528 Fax: 978-649-0333

RADIOMED CORPORATION 866-649-0300 (cont'd)
E-mail: info@radiomed.com
Web site: www.radiomed.com
Total Employees: 20   Sales Staff: 3
Ownership: Iba
Stock Symbol: IBAB
Traded On: Brussels
Produces/Sells CE-marked Devices: Y
Distribution: Manufacturer Direct
Mktg./Adv.: Mr. Bruce Taylor/Manager National Sales
Production: Mr. Matt Blum/Manager Medical Products

Accelerator, Linear, Medical	Radiology
Scanner, Computed Tomography, Cine	Radiology
Scanner, Computed Tomography, X-Ray, Special Procedure	Radiology

RADIOMETER AMERICA, INC. 800-736-0600
810 Sharon Drive, Westlake, OH 44145 **440-871-8900**
FDA Number: 8020503   Fax: 440-871-2633
E-mail: support@radiometeramerica.com
Web site: www.radiometeramerica.com
Medical Products Sales Volume: $30,400,000
Annual Revenue: $50-$100 Million
Year Founded: 1935
Total Employees: 67   Marketing Staff: 18   Sales Staff: 50
Ownership: Private
Quality System Registration Information: ISO9001; ISO9002
Produces/Sells CE-marked Devices: Y
Federal Procurement Eligibility: Small Business, GSA Contract, VA Contract
Distribution: Manufacturer Through Distributor
General Admin.: Carolyn Paris/Manager Human Resources
    Russell Christian/President
Mktg./Adv.: Ed Grover/Director Corporate Accounts
    Rob Guerin/Director Marketing & Business Development
    Jan Weaver/Manager Marketing Services
Production: Vince Sigmund/Director Regulatory Affairs
Finance: Judith A. Dobbins/Controller

Analyzer, Blood Gas pH	Anesthesiology
Analyzer, Chemistry, Electrolyte	Chemistry
Analyzer, Concentration, Oxyhemoglobin, Blood Phase	Toxicology
Analyzer, Gas, Carbon-Dioxide, Partial Pressure, Blood	Anesthesiology
Analyzer, Gas, Carboxyhemoglobin, Blood Phase, Non-Indw.	Toxicology
Analyzer, Gas, Oxygen, Partial Pressure, Blood Phase	Anesthesiology
Analyzer, Ion, Hydrogen-Ion pH, Blood Phase, Non-Indwelling	Anesthesiology
Computer Software	General
Computer, Patient Data Management	General
Control, Blood Gas	Chemistry
Control, Electrolyte (Assayed And Unassayed)	Chemistry
Electrode, Blood Gas, Carbon-Dioxide	Anesthesiology
Electrode, Blood Gas, Oxygen	Anesthesiology
Electrode, Blood pH	Chemistry
Electrode, Transcutaneous, Carbon-Dioxide	Anesthesiology
Electrode, Transcutaneous, Oxygen	Anesthesiology
Hemoglobinometer	Hematology
Hemoglobinometer, Automated	Hematology
Kit, Sampling, Arterial Blood	Anesthesiology
Kit, Sampling, Blood Gas	General
Meter, pH, Blood	Chemistry
Monitor, Blood Gas, Transcutaneous Carbon-Dioxide	Anesthesiology
Monitor, Blood Gas, Transcutaneous Oxygen	Anesthesiology
Monitor, Transcutaneous, Carbon-Dioxide	Anesthesiology
Monitor, Transcutaneous, Oxygen	Anesthesiology
Oximeter, Whole Blood	Hematology
Oxyhemoglobin/Carboxyhemoglobin Curve, Carbon-Monoxide	Toxicology
Tube, Capillary	Chemistry

RADIOMETRIC, DIV. LASER PRECISION CORP.
See Laser Probe, Inc.

RADIONICS, INC.
See Integra Radionics

RADIUM ACCESSORIES SERVICE, INC. 305-289-1361
34 Coco Plum Dr., Marathon, FL 33050
FDA Number: 2431373   Fax: 305-743-8312
E-mail: radaccess@earthlink.net
Web site: www.radiumaccessories.com
Ownership: Private
Produces/Sells CE-marked Devices: N
General Admin.: Marie Golly/President

Applicator, Vaginal	Obstetrics/Gynecology

RADIUS CORP. 800-626-6223
207 Railroad St., Kutztown, PA 19530
FDA Number: 2531570

Toothbrush, Manual	Dental And Oral

RADIUS MEDICAL TECHNOLOGIES, INC. 978-263-4466
15 Craig Road, Acton, MA 01720
FDA Number: 1225894
Web site: http://www.radiusmed.com
Year Founded: 1991

RADIUS MEDICAL TECHNOLOGIES, INC. 978-263-4466 (cont'd)
Ownership: Private
Produces/Sells CE-marked Devices: N

Catheter, Angioplasty, Transluminal, Peripheral	Cardiovascular
Catheter, Embolectomy (Fogarty Type)	Cardiovascular
Guidewire, Catheter	Cardiovascular

RADIUS MEDICAL, LLC
See Biostructures, Llc

RADIX CORP. 204-697-2349
#2-572 South Fifth St., Pembina, ND 58271
FDA Number: n/a   Fax: 204-694-1422
E-mail: info@radix-online.com
Web site: www.radix-online.com
Medical Products Sales Volume: $3,500,000
Annual Revenue: $1-$5 Million
Year Founded: 1957
Total Employees: 2   Marketing Staff: 2   Sales Staff: 24
Ownership: NORTH AMERICAN CASELINE, INC.
Produces/Sells CE-marked Devices: N
Federal Procurement Eligibility: Small Business, Female Owned
Distribution: Manufacturer Direct, Manufacturer Through Manufacturer Reps
General Admin.: Andy Kraljevic/President
Mktg./Adv.: David Spearman/Vice President Marketing & Sales

Cabinet, Bedside	General
Chair, Geriatric	General
Chair, Other	General
Contract Manufacturing	General
Furniture, Patient Room	General
Table, Other	General

RADLINK, INC. 310-643-6900
2400 Marine Ave, Redondo Beach, CA 90278
FDA Number: 2032516   Fax: 310-643-6906
Web site: www.radlink.com
Ownership: Private
Produces/Sells CE-marked Devices: N

Image Digitizer	Radiology
Imager, X-Ray, Solid State (Flat Panel/Digital)	Radiology

RADNOTI GLASS TECHNOLOGY, INC. 800-428-1416
227 W. Maple Ave., Monrovia, CA 91016 **626-357-8827**
FDA Number: n/a   Fax: 626-303-2998
E-mail: sales@radnoti.com
Web site: www.radnoti.com
Annual Revenue: $0-$1 Million
Ownership: Private
Produces/Sells CE-marked Devices: N
Federal Procurement Eligibility: Small Business
Distribution: Manufacturer Through Distributor, Exclusive Distributor
General Admin.: Desmond L. Radnoti/President
Production: Alex Radnoti/Vice President Operations

Bath, Tissue Flotation	Microbiology
Electrode, pH	Gastroenterology/Urology
Homogenizer, Tissue	Microbiology
Molecular Weight Equipment	Chemistry
Pipette, Diluting	Hematology

RADQUAL LLC 508-833-1005
PO Box 82, Weare, NH 03281
FDA Number: 3003227308   Fax: 603-415-0160
Web site: http://www.radqual.com
Year Founded: 2001
Ownership: Private
Produces/Sells CE-marked Devices: N
Production: Mr. Keith Allberg/Director Manufacturing & Quality Assurance

Calibrator Source, Nuclear Sealed	Radiology
Marker, X-Ray	Radiology
Phantom, Flood Source, Nuclear	Radiology

RADSCAN MEDICAL EQUIPMENT, INC. 623-580-0556
23620 N. 20th Dr., Suite 16, Phoenix, AZ 85085
FDA Number: 2032841
Ownership: Private
Produces/Sells CE-marked Devices: N

Bed, Scanning, Nuclear/Fluoroscopic	Radiology
Cradle, Patient, Radiographic	Radiology
Table, Radiographic	Radiology

RAF TABTRONICS LLC 386-736-1698
200 Lexington Ave., Deland, FL 32724
FDA Number: n/a   Fax: 386-736-7338
E-mail: info@tabtronics.com
Web site: www.raftabtronics.com
Medical Products Sales Volume: $150,000
Annual Revenue: $0-$1 Million
Ownership: Private
Produces/Sells CE-marked Devices: N
Federal Procurement Eligibility: Small Business, Minority Owned

RAF TABTRONICS LLC — 386-736-1698 (cont'd)

Distribution: Manufacturer Direct, Manufacturer Through Manufacturer Reps, OEM
General Admin.: Barbara Radcliffe/Admin., General Manager
Robert Malkani/Chief Executive Officer, Chairman
Victor Quinn/Chief Technology Officer
James Tabbi/President, Chief Operating Officer
Production: John Belna/Managing Engineer
Bruce Pratt/Vice President Operations

Component, Electronic	General

RAF TECHNOLOGIES

See Raf Tabtronics Llc

RAHD ONCOLOGY PRODUCTS — 800-844-0103

10762 Indian Head Industrial Blvd, — 314-524-0103
St. Louis, MO 63132
FDA Number: n/a — Fax: 314-890-0866
E-mail: rtp@rahd.com
Web site: www.rahd.com
Medical Products Sales Volume: $1,400,000
Annual Revenue: $1-$5 Million
Year Founded: 1990
Total Employees: 12 — *Marketing Staff:* 2 — *Sales Staff:* 4
Ownership: Private
Produces/Sells CE-marked Devices: Y
Federal Procurement Eligibility: Small Business, VA Contract
Distribution: Manufacturer Direct
General Admin.: J. Michael Cantrell/General Manager
Mark Russell/President, Chief Executive Officer
Mktg./Adv.: Michael Zeleznik/Director Product Development
Mike Cantrell/Manager Contract Sales
Mark Russell/Sales Representative
Alex Sabo/Vice President Marketing
Production: Laura Earley/Director Quality Assurance
Mike Cantrell/Manager Materials

Contract Assembly	General
Radiotherapy Treatment Planning Unit	Radiology

RAHNS SPECIALTY METALS — 800-523-1777

140 Bridge Street, Collegeville, PA 19426 — 610-489-7211
FDA Number: 7000735 — Fax: 610-489-2996
E-mail: mselya@rsmusinor.com
Web site: www.rahnsspecialtymetals.com
Annual Revenue: $10-$25 Million
Total Employees: 70 — *Marketing Staff:* 5 — *Sales Staff:* 5
Ownership: ARCELOR
Quality System Registration Information: ISO9002
Produces/Sells CE-marked Devices: N
Federal Procurement Eligibility: Small Business
Distribution: Manufacturer Through Distributor, Manufacturer Through
Manufacturer Reps, OEM, Exclusive Distributor
General Admin.: Daniel P. Rico/President, Chief Executive Officer
Mktg./Adv.: Michael Selya/Vice President Marketing
Production: Scott Hubler/Manager Production

Suture, Stainless Steel	Surgery

RAICHEM, DIVISION OF HEMAGEN DIAGNOSTICS, INC. — 800-438-6100

8225 Mercury Ct., San Diego, CA 92111-1203 — 858-569-8009
FDA Number: 2022395 — Fax: 858-569-6208
E-mail: info@raichem.com
Web site: www.hemagen.com
Medical Products Sales Volume: $7,300,000
Annual Revenue: $10-$25 Million
Year Founded: 1985
Total Employees: 46 — *Marketing Staff:* 3 — *Sales Staff:* 3
Ownership: Hemagen Diagnostics, Inc.
Stock Symbol: HMGN
Traded On: OTC Bulletin
Produces/Sells CE-marked Devices: Y
Federal Procurement Eligibility: Small Business, GSA Contract, VA Contract
Distribution: Manufacturer Direct, Manufacturer Through Distributor, OEM,
Exclusive Distributor, Exporter
General Admin.: William Hales/President
Mktg./Adv.: Ms. Michelle Egyed/Sales Specialist
Finance: Deborah Ricci/Chief Financial Officer
IS: Nina Catibayan/Manager Tech. Services

2, 4-dinitrophenylhydrazine, Lactate Dehydrogenase	Chemistry
ATP and CK (Enzymatic), Creatine	Chemistry
Alpha-1-Lipoprotein, Antigen, Antiserum, Control	Immunology
Antigen, Antiserum, Control, Lipoprotein, Low Density	Immunology
Azo-Dyes, Colorimetric, Bilirubin And Conjugates	Chemistry
Colorimetric Method, Gamma-Glutamyl Transpeptidase	Chemistry
Colorimetric Method, Triglycerides	Chemistry
Control, Analyte (Assayed And Unassayed)	Chemistry
Enzymatic Method, Ammonia	Chemistry
Enzymatic, Carbon-Dioxide	Chemistry
Hexokinase, Glucose	Chemistry

RAICHEM, DIVISION OF HEMAGEN — 800-438-6100 (cont'd)

Immunoassay, Other	Toxicology
LDL & VLDL Precipitation, Cholesterol Via Esterase-Oxidase	Chemistry
LDL & VLDL Precipitation, HDL	Chemistry
Lipase Hydrolysis/Glycerol Kinase Enzyme, Triglycerides	Chemistry
NAD Reduction/NADH Oxidation, Lactate Dehydrogenase	Chemistry
NADH Oxidation/NAD Reduction, AST/SGOT	Chemistry
Nephelometric Method, Immunoglobulins (G, A, M)	Chemistry
Phosphatase, Acid	Hematology
Phosphatase, Alkaline	Hematology
Phosphorus Reagent (Test System)	Chemistry
Photometric Method, Magnesium	Chemistry
Reagent, Acetylcholine Chloride	Toxicology
Reagent, Albumin, Colorimetric	Chemistry
Reagent, Amylase, Colorimetric	Chemistry
Reagent, Blood Urea Nitrogen (BUN)	Chemistry
Reagent, Calcium (Test System)	Chemistry
Reagent, Chloride (Test System)	Chemistry
Reagent, Cholesterol (Total Test System)	Chemistry
Reagent, Creatinine (Test System)	Chemistry
Reagent, Glucose (Test System)	Chemistry
Reagent, Iron (Test System)	Chemistry
Reagent, NAD-NADH, Alcohol Enzyme Method	Toxicology
Reagent, Other	General
Reagent, Protein, Total	Chemistry
SGPT, Ultraviolet	Chemistry
Standard, Lipid	Chemistry
Standard/Control, All Types	Chemistry
Test, C-Reactive Protein	Immunology
Test, C-Reactive Protein, FITC	Immunology
U.V. Method, CPK Isoenzymes	Chemistry
Urease And Glutamic Dehydrogenase, Urea Nitrogen	Chemistry
Uricase (Colorimetric), Uric Acid	Chemistry

RAINBOW ELECTRO-TECHNOLOGIES, INC. — 516-933-0327

41 Moss Ln., Jericho, NY 11753-1816
FDA Number: 2438697
Ownership: Private
Produces/Sells CE-marked Devices: N

Laser, Surgical	Surgery

RAINDANCE TECHNOLOGIES, INC. — 888-724-6440

44 Hartwell Avenue, Lexington, MA 02421 — 781-861-6300
FDA Number: n/a — Fax: 781-861-1233
E-mail: info@raindancetech.com
Web site: www.raindancetech.com
Ownership: Private
Produces/Sells CE-marked Devices: N
General Admin.: Mr. S. Roopom Banerjee/President, Chief Executive Officer
Mktg./Adv.: Mr. Christopher McNary/Commercial Director
Production: Mr. Roch Kelly/Senior Vice President Operations
Research: Dr. Darren Link, Ph.D./Vice President Research & Development
IS: Mr. Michael Olex/Vice President Systems

RALEIGH LIONS CLINIC FOR THE BLIND, INC. — 919-256-4220

3200 Bush St., Raleigh, NC 27609
FDA Number: 1058533 — Fax: 919-850-3442
Web site: www.rlcb.net
Ownership: Private
Produces/Sells CE-marked Devices: N

Bandage, Adhesive	Surgery

RALSTON GROUP — 334-875-2298

656 Lake Lanier Rd., Selma, AL 36701
FDA Number: 1065408

Component, Exercise	Physical Med

RAM PLUS, LLC — 435-781-1646

983 N. 2175 W., Vernal, UT 84078
FDA Number: 3004511389
Ownership: Private
Produces/Sells CE-marked Devices: N

Exerciser, Non-Measuring	Physical Med

RAM SCIENTIFIC, INC. — 800-535-6734

7 odell plaza, Yonkers, NY 10703 — 914-969-7900
FDA Number: 2246954 — Fax: 914-969-7022
E-mail: info@ramsci.com
Web site: www.ramsci.com
Annual Revenue: $1-$5 Million
Year Founded: 1990
Total Employees: 8
Ownership: Private
Quality System Registration Information: ISO9001
Produces/Sells CE-marked Devices: N
Federal Procurement Eligibility: Small Business, Female Owned
Distribution: Exclusive Distributor, Importer
General Admin.: Monique Muri/President, Chief Executive Officer

Hematocrit Tube, Rack, Sealer, Holder	Hematology
Tube, Blood Microcollection	Chemistry

RAM SCIENTIFIC, INC. 800-535-6734 (cont'd)
Tube, Capillary Blood Collection Hematology

RAMCO INNOVATIONS/ SUNX SENSORS 800-280-6933
PO Box 65310, 1207 Maple Street, 515-225-6933
West Des Moines, IA 50265
FDA Number: n/a
E-mail: sales@ramcoinnovations.com Fax: 515-225-0063
Web site: www.sunx-ramco.com
Year Founded: 1962
Total Employees: 5
Ownership: Private
Produces/Sells CE-marked Devices: Y
Federal Procurement Eligibility: Small Business
Distribution: Importer
General Admin.: Joe Fitzgerald/President, Chief Executive Officer
Mktg./Adv.: Mike Reelitz/Manager Advertising
Production: Mike Reelitz/Manager Materials
Computer Equipment General

RAMCO LABORATORIES, INC. 281-313-1200
4100 Greenbriar Drive, Suite 200, Stafford, TX 77477
FDA Number: 1650223
E-mail: Ramco@ramcolab.com Fax: 281-313-1251
Web site: www.ramcolab.com
Medical Products Sales Volume: $540,000
Annual Revenue: $1-$5 Million
Year Founded: 1976
Total Employees: 7 Marketing Staff: 1 Sales Staff: 1
Ownership: Private
Produces/Sells CE-marked Devices: Y
Federal Procurement Eligibility: Small Business
Distribution: Manufacturer Direct, OEM, Exclusive Distributor, Exporter
General Admin.: Clarence P. Alfrey/Chief Executive Officer
Lani Wheeler/Office Manager
Jeffrey Grubb/President
Mktg./Adv.: Lorah Horn/Manager International Marketing
Billy J. Ryals/Manager Sales
Production: Candice L. Gorin/Director Quality Assurance
Tami A. Grubb/Manager Regulatory Affairs
Antigen, ID, Candida Albicans Microbiology
Antiserum, Latex Agglutination, Cryptococcus Neoformans Microbiology
Enzyme Immunoassay, Other Chemistry
Immunochemical, Transferrin Immunology
Radioimmunoassay, Ferritin Microbiology
Radioimmunoassay, Other Chemistry
Test, Qualitative And Quantitative Factor Deficiency Hematology

RAMPIT, INC.
See Tj Rampit, Inc.

RAMPMASTER DIVISION OF THORWELD 416-741-2501
174 Milvan Dr., Weston, ONT M9L 1Z9 Canada
FDA Number: 9201078
E-mail: info@rampmaster.com Fax: 416-741-7223
Web site: www.rampmaster.com
Total Employees: 10
Ownership: Private
Produces/Sells CE-marked Devices: Y
Distribution: Manufacturer Direct, Manufacturer Through Distributor, Exporter

RAMPUS, INC.
See Tj Rampit, Inc.

RAMSEY - A THERMO SENTRON CO.
See Thermo Fisher Scientific (Sales And Service)

RAMSEY ANALYTICAL
See Applied Biosystems

RAMSEY MACHINE 724-787-3059
1392 Darlington Rd., Ligonier, PA 15658
FDA Number: 3003159877
Accessories, Wheelchair Physical Med

RAMSEY TECHNOLOGY, INC.
See Thermo Fisher Scientific (Sales And Service)

RAMSOFT, INC. 416-674-1347
37 Bankview Cir, Etobicoke M9W 6S6 Canada
FDA Number: 9680028
Scanner, Ultrasonic (Pulsed Echo) Radiology
System, Communication, Image, Digital Radiology
Tester, Radiology Radiology

RAMVAC DENTAL PRODUCTS INC 800-572-6822
3100 First Avenue, Spearfish, SD 57783 605-642-4614
FDA Number: 2183905 Fax: 605-642-3776
E-mail: ramvac@ramvac.com
Web site: www.ramvac.com
Medical Products Sales Volume: $1,900,000
Annual Revenue: $5-$10 Million

RAMVAC DENTAL PRODUCTS INC 800-572-6822 (cont'd)
Year Founded: 2002
Total Employees: 30
Ownership: Dentalez Group
Quality System Registration Information: ISO9001
Produces/Sells CE-marked Devices: N
Federal Procurement Eligibility: Small Business, VA Contract
Distribution: Manufacturer Through Distributor
General Admin.: Mr. Matt Olson/General Manager
Evacuator, Oral Cavity Dental And Oral
Pump, Suction Operatory Dental And Oral

RAMÇ-HART, INC. 973-448-0305
95 Allen Street, PO Box 400, Netcong, NJ 07857-0400
FDA Number: n/a Fax: 973-448-0315
E-mail: carl@ramehart.com
Web site: www.ramehart.com
Medical Products Sales Volume: $5,000,000
Annual Revenue: $1-$5 Million
Year Founded: 1962
Total Employees: 15 Marketing Staff: 1 Sales Staff: 2
Ownership: Private
Produces/Sells CE-marked Devices: N
Federal Procurement Eligibility: Small Business, GSA Contract
Distribution: Manufacturer Direct
General Admin.: Ken Christiansen/President
Adapter, Syringe General
Goniometer, AC-powered Orthopedics
Goniometer, Orthopedic Orthopedics
Stopper General

RANA MEDICAL 888-297-7889
205 Stephen St., 204-822-6595
Morden, MAN R6M-1 Canada
FDA Number: n/a Fax: 204-822-3852
E-mail: rana@ranamedical.com
Web site: www.ranamedical.com
Year Founded: 1988
Total Employees: 50
Ownership: Private
Produces/Sells CE-marked Devices: N
Distribution: Manufacturer Direct

RAND SPECIALTY CO. INC., J.R.
See J.R. Rand Corp.

RAND-SCOT INC. 800-467-7967
401 Linden Center Drive, Fort Collins, CO 80524 970-484-7967
FDA Number: n/a Fax: 970-484-3800
E-mail: info@randscot.com
Web site: www.randscot.com
Medical Products Sales Volume: $1,300,000
Annual Revenue: $1-$5 Million
Year Founded: 1980
Total Employees: 17 Marketing Staff: 2 Sales Staff: 5
Ownership: Private
Produces/Sells CE-marked Devices: N
Federal Procurement Eligibility: Small Business, GSA Contract, VA Contract
Distribution: Manufacturer Through Manufacturer Reps
General Admin.: Ms. Erin Thames/Administrator
Joel Lerich/President, Chief Executive Officer
Mktg./Adv.: Fred Ekstam/Director National Accounts
Kate Stephens/Manager Sales
Chair, Other General
Chair, Seat Lifting (Standing Aid) General
Exerciser, Leg And Ankle Physical Med
Patient Transfer Unit General

RANDAL MINOR OCULAR PROSTHETICS INC. 813-949-2500
1628 Dale Mabry Hwy., Ste. 110, Lutz, FL 33548
FDA Number: 3005133837
E-mail: Randalminor@tampabay.rr.com
Web site: www.remeyes.com
Ownership: Private
Produces/Sells CE-marked Devices: N
Button, Iris, Eye, Artificial Ophthalmology
Conformer, Ophthalmic Ophthalmology
Shell, Scleral Ophthalmology

RANDALL FAICHNEY CORP.
See Ranfac Corp.

RANDALL L. SULHOFF LIFE PLUS INTERNATIONAL
See Life Plus International

RANDOLPH ENGINEERING, INC. 781-961-6070
26 Thomas Patten Dr., Randolph, MA 02368
FDA Number: 1293762
Frame, Spectacle (Eyeglasses) Ophthalmology

RANDOLPH ENGINEERING, INC. 781-961-6070 *(cont'd)*
Sunglasses (Including Photosensitive) — Ophthalmology

RANFAC CORP. 800-2RANFAC
Avon Industrial Park, 30 Doherty Ave., **508-588-4400**
Avon, MA 02322
FDA Number: 1211566 Fax: 508-584-8588
E-mail: info@ranfac.com
Web site: www.ranfac.com
Annual Revenue: $10-$25 Million
Year Founded: 1888
Total Employees: 50 *Marketing Staff:* 1 *Sales Staff:* 1
Ownership: Private
Produces/Sells CE-marked Devices: Y
Distribution: Manufacturer Direct, OEM, Exclusive Distributor, Exporter
General Admin.: Robert M. Adler/President
Chris Whelan/Senior Vice President
Barry Zimble/Vice President, General Manager
Production: Brad Horton/Vice President Manufacturing

Cannula, Epidural	Obstetrics/Gynecology
Cannula, Ophthalmic	Ophthalmology
Cannula, Other	General
Catheter, Cholangiography	Surgery
Catheter, Infusion	Surgery
Catheter, Other	Gastroenterology/Urology
Catheter, Sialoglycoprotein	Gastroenterology/Urology
Device, Closure, Puncture, Hemostatic	Cardiovascular
Instrument, Knot Tying, Suture, Laparoscopic	Surgery
Instrument, Passing, Ligature, Knot Tying	Cns/Neurology
Introducer, Spinal Needle	Anesthesiology
Laparoscope, Gynecologic	Obstetrics/Gynecology
Needle, Aspiration And Injection, Reusable	Surgery
Needle, Aspiration, Cyst, Laparoscopic	Surgery
Needle, Biopsy, Cardiovascular	Cardiovascular
Needle, Biopsy, Mammary	Obstetrics/Gynecology
Needle, Blunt	General
Needle, Bone Marrow	Surgery
Needle, Endoscopic	Gastroenterology/Urology
Needle, Hypodermic	General
Needle, Insufflation, Laparoscopic	Surgery
Needle, Intra-Arterial	Cardiovascular
Needle, Ophthalmic	Ophthalmology
Needle, Pneumoperitoneum, Simple	Gastroenterology/Urology
Needle, Pneumoperitoneum, Spring Loaded	Gastroenterology/Urology
Needle, Radiographic	Radiology
Needle, Spinal, Short-Term	General
Retractor, Laparoscopy, Other	Surgery
Stylet, Catheter	Cardiovascular

RANGER ALL SEASON CORP. 800-225-3811
2002 Kingbird Ave., George, IA 51237 **712-475-2811**
FDA Number: 1933703 Fax: 712-475-3320
E-mail: sales@rangerallseason.com
Web site: www.rangerallseason.com
Ownership: Private
Produces/Sells CE-marked Devices: N
Federal Procurement Eligibility: Small Business
Distribution: Manufacturer Through Manufacturer Reps, Exclusive Distributor
General Admin.: Larry Kruse/Chief Executive Officer
Mktg./Adv.: Randy Riecks/Vice President Marketing
Scooter (Motorized 3-Wheeled Vehicle) — Physical Med

RANGER WHEELCHAIRS LTD. 888.745.7888
14722 64th Ave., Unit 16, **604-590-4333**
Surrey, BC V3S-1 Canada
FDA Number: n/a Fax: 604-590-4337
E-mail: sales@rangerwheelchairs.com
Web site: http://www.rangerwheelchairs.com
Year Founded: 1982
Total Employees: 10
Ownership: Private
Produces/Sells CE-marked Devices: N
Distribution: Manufacturer Direct

RANIR CORP. 800-253-0906
4701 E. Paris Ave. S.E., **616-698-8880**
Grand Rapids, MI 49512
FDA Number: 1825660 Fax: 616-222-0710
E-mail: contact@ranir.com
Web site: www.ranir.com
Medical Products Sales Volume: $29,000,000
Annual Revenue: $25-$50 Million
Total Employees: 400 *Marketing Staff:* 5 *Sales Staff:* 5
Ownership: Private
Produces/Sells CE-marked Devices: N
Federal Procurement Eligibility: Small Business
Distribution: Manufacturer Direct
General Admin.: Richard Peck/Chairman

RANIR CORP. 800-253-0906 *(cont'd)*
Richard Peck/Chief Executive Officer
Mktg./Adv.: Ken Hank/President Marketing
Production: Garry M. Hammerlund/Executive Vice President Operations

Device, Anti-Snoring	Ear/Nose/Throat
Eraser, Dental Stain	Dental And Oral
Floss, Dental	Dental And Oral
Mirror, Mouth	Dental And Oral
Mouthguard	Dental And Oral
Scaler, Periodontic	Dental And Oral
Scraper, Tongue	Dental And Oral
Toothbrush, Manual	Dental And Oral
Toothbrush, Powered	Dental And Oral

RANIR, LLC 616-698-8880
4701 East Paris Avenue SE, Grand Rapids, MI 49512
FDA Number: n/a Fax: 616-222-0710
E-mail: contact@ranir.com
Web site: www.ranir.com
Year Founded: 1979
Total Employees: 400 *Marketing Staff:* 6 *Sales Staff:* 8
Ownership: Private
Quality System Registration Information: ISO9001
Produces/Sells CE-marked Devices: N
Federal Procurement Eligibility: Small Business
Distribution: Manufacturer Direct, Manufacturer Through Manufacturer Reps
General Admin.: Christine Henisee/President
Mktg./Adv.: Michael Young/Senior Vice President Sales
Research: Jeff Fisher/Senior Vice President Research & Development

Floss, Dental	Dental And Oral
Protector, Mouth Guard	Dental And Oral
Toothbrush, Ionic, Battery-Powered	Dental And Oral
Toothbrush, Manual	Dental And Oral
Toothbrush, Powered	Dental And Oral

RAPID AID LTD. 800-265-3468
4120A Sladeview Crescent, Units 1-4, **905-820-4788**
Mississauga, ONT L5L-5 Canada
FDA Number: n/a Fax: 905-820-9226
E-mail: sales@rapidaid.com
Web site: www.rapidaid.com
Year Founded: 1975
Total Employees: 100
Ownership: Private
Produces/Sells CE-marked Devices: N
Distribution: Manufacturer Direct, Exporter

RAPID DEPLOYMENT PRODUCTS 877-433-7569
157 Railroad Avenue, Ivyland, PA 18974 **215-953-9190**
FDA Number: n/a Fax: 215-354-1413
E-mail: feedback@prolitespineboards.com
Web site: www.prolitespineboards.com
Medical Products Sales Volume: $3,000,000
Annual Revenue: $1-$5 Million
Year Founded: 1999
Total Employees: 16 *Marketing Staff:* 5 *Sales Staff:* 5
Ownership: Private
Produces/Sells CE-marked Devices: Y
Federal Procurement Eligibility: Small Business
Distribution: Manufacturer Through Distributor
General Admin.: Thomas Richmond/Vice President, General Manager
Mktg./Adv.: Rae Lehman/National Director Marketing

Extrication Equipment	General
Mask, Face	General
Pack, Hot Or Cold, Disposable	Physical Med
Rescue Equipment	General
Strap, Restraining	General
Stretcher, Emergency, Other	General
Stretcher, Hand-Carried	General
Transfer Aid	Physical Med

RAPID DIAGNOSTIC TECHNOLOGIES
See Quidel Corporation

RAPID DIAGNOSTICS, DIV. OF MP 800-888-7008
BIOMEDICALS, LLC
1429 Rollins Road, Burlingame, CA 94010 **650-558-0395**
FDA Number: 2954282 Fax: 650-558-0397
E-mail: rapidtest@rapiddiag.com
Web site: www.mpbio.com
Medical Products Sales Volume: $2,300,000
Year Founded: 2003
Total Employees: 26
Ownership: Mp Biomedicals Diagnostics Division
Produces/Sells CE-marked Devices: N
Federal Procurement Eligibility: Small Business
Distribution: Manufacturer Direct, Manufacturer Through Distributor, Manufacturer Through Manufacturer Reps, OEM, Service Direct, Exclusive Distributor, Exporter

RAPID DIAGNOSTICS, DIV. OF MP   800-888-7008 (cont'd)

Enzyme Immunoassay, Amphetamine	Toxicology
Enzyme Immunoassay, Barbiturate	Toxicology
Enzyme Immunoassay, Benzodiazepine	Toxicology
Enzyme Immunoassay, Cannabinoids	Toxicology
Enzyme Immunoassay, Cocaine And Cocaine Metabolites	Toxicology
Enzyme Immunoassay, Methadone	Toxicology
Enzyme Immunoassay, Opiates	Toxicology
Enzyme Immunoassay, Phencyclidine	Toxicology
Enzyme Immunoassay, Propoxyphene	Toxicology
Gas Chromatography, Methamphetamine	Toxicology
Kit, Pregnancy Test, Over The Counter, HCG	Chemistry
Radioimmunoassay, Human Chorionic Gonadotropin	Chemistry
Radioimmunoassay, Luteinizing Hormone	Chemistry
Thin Layer Chromatography, Metamphetamine	Toxicology

RAPID DIAGNOSTICS, DIVISION OF ICN BIOMEDICALS, INC.

See Rapid Diagnostics, Div. Of Mp Biomedicals, Llc

RAPID MICRO BIOSYSTEMS INC.   781-271-1444

One Oak Park Drive, 2nd Floor, Bedford, MA 01730
FDA Number: n/a   Fax: 781-271-9905
E-mail: info@rapidmicrobio.com
Ownership: Private
Produces/Sells CE-marked Devices: N
General Admin.: Mr. Steve Delity/President, Chief Executive Officer
Mktg./Adv.: Ms. Julie Sperry/Commercial Director
Research: Mr. Sarath Krishnaswamy/Vice President Research & Development
Finance: Mr. Michael Ellis/Chief Financial Officer
IS: Mr. David Jones/Director Tech. Services

RAPID PATHOGEN SCREENING   877-921-0080

7227 Delainey Court,   941-556-1850
Lakewood Ranch, FL 34240
FDA Number: 3006602209
E-mail: info@RPSdetectors.com   Fax: 941-556-1851
Ownership: Private
Produces/Sells CE-marked Devices: N

Antigen, CF (Including CF Control), Adenovirus 1-33	Microbiology

RAPID PATHOGEN SCREENING, INC.   941-556-1850

101 Philips Park Dr., S Williamsport, PA 17702
FDA Number: 3006036259

Antigen, CF (Including CF Control), Adenovirus 1-33	Microbiology

RAPID POWER TECHNOLOGIES, INC.   800-332-1111

18 Graysbridge Rd., Brookfield, CT 06804-0291   203-775-0411
FDA Number: n/a   Fax: 203-775-0666
E-mail: marketing@rapidpower.com
Annual Revenue: $1-$5 Million
Total Employees: 175   Marketing Staff: 2   Sales Staff: 6
Ownership: Private
Produces/Sells CE-marked Devices: N
Federal Procurement Eligibility: Small Business
Distribution: Manufacturer Direct, Manufacturer Through Manufacturer Reps, Service Direct
General Admin.: Ronald Viola/President
Mktg./Adv.: Pam Kromer/Manager Advertising
    Pete Cambria/Manager Sales
Research: Bill Shaughnessy/Vice President Research & Development

Power System, Isolated	General
Regulator, Line Voltage	General
Transformer, Endoscope	Surgery

RARE EARTH MEDICAL, INC.

See Cardiofocus, Inc.

RAULAND-BORG CORP.   800-752-7725

3450 W. Oakton St., Skokie, IL 60076-2951   847-679-0900
FDA Number: 9200919   Fax: 847-679-4106
E-mail: info@rauland.com
Web site: www.rauland.com
Annual Revenue: $50-$100 Million
Total Employees: 250
Ownership: Private
Produces/Sells CE-marked Devices: N
Federal Procurement Eligibility: Small Business
Distribution: Manufacturer Through Distributor
General Admin.: Norman Kidder/President, Chief Executive Officer
    Karen York/Vice President Human Resources
Mktg./Adv.: Robert Barthi/Director National Accounts
    Larry Ball/Manager Marketing
    Maureen Pajerski/Vice President Marketing
Production: Ed O'Connor/Manager Publications
    John Gutknecht/Vice President Manufacturing

Clock, Elapsed Time	General
Communication Equipment	General
Computer Software, Hospital/Nursing Management	General
Nurse Call System	General

RAULAND-BORG CORP.   800-752-7725 (cont'd)

Pager, Non-Radio	General

RAVEN BIOLOGICAL LABORATORIES, INC.   800-728-5702

8607 Park Drive, PO Box 27261, Omaha, NE 68127   402-593-0781
FDA Number: 1921058
E-mail: info@ravenlabs.com   Fax: 402-593-0921
Web site: www.ravenlabs.com
Medical Products Sales Volume: $3,600,000
Annual Revenue: $1-$5 Million
Year Founded: 1949
Total Employees: 42   Marketing Staff: 2   Sales Staff: 3
Ownership: Private
Produces/Sells CE-marked Devices: Y
Federal Procurement Eligibility: Small Business, GSA Contract, VA Contract
Distribution: Manufacturer Direct, Manufacturer Through Distributor, Manufacturer Through Manufacturer Reps, OEM, Exporter
General Admin.: Robert V. Dwyer/President, Chief Executive Officer
Mktg./Adv.: Chris R. Dwyer/Director Marketing & Product Development
    Dan Dwyer/Manager National Sales
Production: Wendy Royalty-Hahn/Director Quality Assurance
    Deb Dwyer/Vice President Manufacturing
Research: Russ Nyberg/Vice President Research & Development

Indicator, Biological, Liquid Chemical Steril. Process	General
Sterilization Process Indicator, Biological	General
Test, Agar Tube	Microbiology

RAYLABCON, INC.

See Rayson Co. Inc., W.R.

RAYMAX MEDICAL CORP.   905-791-3020

20 Strathearn Ave, Unit 3, Brampton, ONT L6T 4P7 Canada
FDA Number: 8022203   Fax: 905-791-3375
E-mail: sales@raymaxmedical.com
Web site: www.raymaxmedical.com
Year Founded: 1978
Total Employees: 10
Ownership: Private
Quality System Registration Information: ISO9001
Produces/Sells CE-marked Devices: N
Federal Procurement Eligibility: Minority Owned
Distribution: Manufacturer Through Distributor, OEM, Exporter

RAYONIX INC.   800-463-2262

5685 boul. De l'Ormiere,   418-871-1026
Quebec, QUE G1P-1 Canada
FDA Number: n/a   Fax: 418-871-2438
Year Founded: 1980
Total Employees: 10
Ownership: Private
Produces/Sells CE-marked Devices: N
Distribution: Exclusive Distributor, Importer

RAYOVAC   800-331-4522

601 Rayovac Drive, Madison, WI 53744-4960   608-275-4694
FDA Number: n/a   Fax: 608-275-4973
E-mail: pilarzyk@rayovac.com
Web site: www.rayovac.com
Medical Products Sales Volume: $50,000
Year Founded: 1906
Ownership: LEE CO., THOMAS
Stock Symbol: ROV
Traded On: NYSE
Quality System Registration Information: ISO9001
Produces/Sells CE-marked Devices: Y
Federal Procurement Eligibility: Small Business, GSA Contract, VA Contract
Distribution: Manufacturer Direct, Manufacturer Through Distributor, Manufacturer Through Manufacturer Reps, OEM
General Admin.: David A. Jones/Chief Executive Officer
    Kent Hussey/President
    Mark Joslyn/Vice President Human Resources
Mktg./Adv.: Janna Rose/Director Product Development
    Jim Pilarzyk/Division Manager
    Steve Shanesy/Executive Vice President Marketing
    Jerry Albright/Vice President Marketing
    Randy Raymond/Vice President Sales
Production: Tom Quick/Director Quality Assurance
    Ken Biller/Executive Vice President Manufacturing
Research: Dr. Paul Cheeseman/Senior Vice President Tech. Research & Development

Battery	General
Battery, Hearing-Aid	Ear/Nose/Throat
Charger, Battery	General
Light, Other	General

RAYOVAC CANADA, INC.
800-268-0425
9056244448
5448 Timberlea Blvd.,
Mississauga, ONT L4W-2 Canada
FDA Number: n/a
Fax: 9056292571
Web site: www.rayovac.com
Year Founded: 1906
Total Employees: 25
Ownership: Private
Produces/Sells CE-marked Devices: N
Distribution: Exclusive Distributor

RAYOVAC CORP.
See Rayovac

RAYSON CO. INC., W.R.
800-526-1526
910-259-8100
720 S. Dickerson St., Burgaw, NC 28425
FDA Number: 2431400
Fax: 910-259-8110
E-mail: info@wrrayson.com
Web site: www.wrrayson.com
Medical Products Sales Volume: $4,200,000
Annual Revenue: $1-$5 Million
Year Founded: 1969
Total Employees: 35   *Marketing Staff:* 3   *Sales Staff:* 4
Ownership: Private
Produces/Sells CE-marked Devices: N
Federal Procurement Eligibility: Small Business
Distribution: Manufacturer Through Distributor, Exporter
General Admin.: Michael Dimartino/President, Chief Executive Officer
    Jean Swanson/Vice President
Mktg./Adv.: Wendy Watts/Market Manager
   Container, Specimen Mailer And Storage   Pathology
   Coverslip, Microscope Slide   Pathology
   Slide, Microscope   Pathology

RAYTEL MEDICAL CORP.
See Philips Remote Cardiac Services

RAYTHEON APPLIANCES, COMMERCIAL LAUNDRY
See Unimac

RAZEL SCIENTIFIC INSTRUMENTS, INC.
877-324-9914
203-324-9914
PO Box 111, St. Albans, VT 05478
FDA Number: 1280565
Fax: 802-527-5095
E-mail: info@razelscientific.com
Web site: www.razelscientific.com
Medical Products Sales Volume: $820,000
Annual Revenue: $0-$1 Million
Year Founded: 1968
Total Employees: 10
Ownership: Private
Produces/Sells CE-marked Devices: Y
Federal Procurement Eligibility: Small Business
Distribution: Manufacturer Direct, Manufacturer Through Distributor, OEM, Exporter
General Admin.: M. Nesin/President
   Pump, Infusion   General
   Pump, Infusion, Laboratory   Chemistry
   Pump, Infusion, Syringe   General

RAZORAID INCORPORATED
410-585-1395
7301 Park Heights Ave., Suite 207, Baltimore, MD 21208-5407
FDA Number: 3003652857
Ownership: Private
Produces/Sells CE-marked Devices: N
   Forceps   Orthopedics

RBM SERVICES, LLC.
865-483-0067
101-b Valley Court, Oak Ridge, TN 37830
FDA Number: 2320968
E-mail: Contact@rbm-services.com
Ownership: Private
Produces/Sells CE-marked Devices: N
   Light, Surgical, Fiberoptic   Surgery
   Pump, Infusion   General

RCD COMPONENTS, INC.
877-723-2667
603-669-0054
520 E. Industrial Park,
Manchester, NH 03109
FDA Number: n/a
Fax: 603-669-5455
E-mail: Sales@rcdcomponents.com
Web site: www.rcdcomponents.com
Annual Revenue: $50-$100 Million
Total Employees: 500   *Marketing Staff:* 2   *Sales Staff:* 15
Ownership: Private
Quality System Registration Information: ISO9001
Produces/Sells CE-marked Devices: N
General Admin.: Louis J. Arcidy/President
    Maria Grisanzio/Vice President Human Resources
Mktg./Adv.: Chris Monroe/Manager Sales Training

RCD COMPONENTS, INC.
877-723-2667 *(cont'd)*
   Al Arcidy/Vice President Marketing
   Louis M. Arcidy/Vice President Sales
Production: Mark Arcidy/Vice President Manufacturing
Research: Michael Arcidy/Vice President Research & Development
   Contract Manufacturing   General

RCMEX, S.A. DE C.V.
915-598-4072
Av. Profr. Ramon Rivera Lara, Juarez 31857 Mexico
FDA Number: 9680256
   Gown, Surgical   Surgery

RD INDUSTRIES, INC.
800-759-7090
402-453-9070
11811 Calhoun Road, Omaha, NE 68152-1346
FDA Number: 1931237
Fax: 402-455-8242
E-mail: rlaible@rdindustries.com
Web site: rdindustries.com
Medical Products Sales Volume: $4,900,000
Year Founded: 1982
Total Employees: 68
Ownership: Private
Quality System Registration Information: ISO9000
Produces/Sells CE-marked Devices: N
Federal Procurement Eligibility: Small Business
Distribution: Manufacturer Through Distributor
   Container, Sharpes   General

RD MEDICAL MFG. INC.
787-716-6363
Road 183, Km 21.6, Las Piedras Industrial Park,
Las Piedras, PR 00771
FDA Number: 96933
Fax: 787-716-6372
E-mail: rdm@rdmedical.com
Web site: www.rdmedical.com
Ownership: Private
Produces/Sells CE-marked Devices: N
   IV Start Kit   Surgery
   Kit, Administration, Intravenous   General
   Kit, Sampling, Arterial Blood   Anesthesiology
   Kit, Surgical Instrument, Disposable   Surgery
   Kit, Suture Removal   Surgery
   Laparoscope, Gynecologic   Obstetrics/Gynecology
   Set, Administration, Intravenous, Needle-Free   General
   Tube, Aspirating, Flexible, Connecting   Anesthesiology

RD PLASTICS COMPANY, INC.
800-795-7007
615-781-0007
P.O. Box 111300, Nashville, TN 37222
FDA Number: 2320740
Fax: 615-781-2828
E-mail: plastics@rdplastics.com
Web site: www.rdplastics.com
Ownership: Private
Produces/Sells CE-marked Devices: N
   Container, Specimen, All Types   General
   Container, Specimen, Non-sterile   General

RD SERVICE, DIVISION OF NICRAM ENVIRO INC.
800-667-0127
514-331-2007
2760 Paulus St.,
Saint-Laurent, QUE H4S-1 Canada
FDA Number: n/a
Fax: 514-331-8147
E-mail: sales@nicram.com
Web site: www.rdservice.com
Year Founded: 1985
Total Employees: 25
Ownership: Private
Produces/Sells CE-marked Devices: N
Distribution: Exclusive Distributor

RDF CORP.
800-445-8367
603-882-5195
23 Elm Avenue, Hudson, NH 03051
FDA Number: 7000306
Fax: 603-882-6925
E-mail: sensor@rdfcorp.com
Web site: www.rdfcorp.com
Medical Products Sales Volume: $6,100,000
Annual Revenue: $5-$10 Million
Year Founded: 1955
Total Employees: 69
Ownership: Private
Quality System Registration Information: ISO9001
Produces/Sells CE-marked Devices: N
Federal Procurement Eligibility: Small Business, Minority Owned, Female Owned
Distribution: Manufacturer Direct, Manufacturer Through Distributor, Manufacturer Through Manufacturer Reps, OEM, Service Direct, Importer
General Admin.: Naresh Puri/Chief Executive Officer
    Dennis Wilkinson/Vice President Human Resources
Mktg./Adv.: Randy A. Gauthier/Vice President Marketing & Sales
Production: Paul Siemiesz/Director Quality Assurance
   Thermometer, Laboratory   Chemistry
   Thermometer, Laboratory, Recording   General

RDL SUPPLY
214-630-3965
11240 Gemini Lane, Dallas, TX 75229
FDA Number: n/a
Fax: 214-560-0326
E-mail: sales@rdlsupply.com
Web site: www.rdlsupply.com
Annual Revenue: $0-$1 Million
Year Founded: 1981
Ownership: Private
Quality System Registration Information: ISO9000
Produces/Sells CE-marked Devices: N
Federal Procurement Eligibility: Female Owned
Distribution: Manufacturer Direct
   Equipment, Therapy, Handicapped/Physical — Physical Med
   Rail, Bath — General

REA INCORPORATED
330-666-7414
4808 Pin Oak Road, Akron, OH 44333
FDA Number: 9042955
Fax: 330-666-7414
E-mail: info@medicalmilestones.com
Web site: www.medicalmilestones.com
Annual Revenue: $0-$1 Million
Ownership: Private
Quality System Registration Information: ISO9002
Produces/Sells CE-marked Devices: N
Distribution: Manufacturer Through Distributor, Manufacturer Through Manufacturer Reps, OEM, Exclusive Distributor, Importer, Exporter
General Admin.: Robert E. Anthony/President

REACH GLOBAL INDUSTRIES, INC. (REACHGOOD)
888-518-8389
8 Corporate Park, Suite 300, Irvine, CA 92606
949-309-2958
FDA Number: 2031343
Fax: 949-203-8787
E-mail: info@rgihq.com
Web site: www.rgihq.com
Medical Products Sales Volume: $2,000,000
Annual Revenue: $1-$5 Million
Year Founded: 1997
Total Employees: 15   *Marketing Staff:* 2   *Sales Staff:* 2
Ownership: Private
Quality System Registration Information: ISO9000; ISO9001; ISO9002
Produces/Sells CE-marked Devices: Y
Federal Procurement Eligibility: Small Business, Minority Owned
Distribution: Manufacturer Direct, Manufacturer Through Distributor, Manufacturer Through Manufacturer Reps, OEM, Exclusive Distributor, Importer
   Appliance, Incontinence, Urosheath Type — Gastroenterology/Urology
   Catheter, Ureteral, Gastro-Urology — Gastroenterology/Urology
   Catheter, Urethral — Gastroenterology/Urology
   Collector, Urine — Gastroenterology/Urology
   Drainage System, Urine, Closed — Gastroenterology/Urology
   Lubricant, Patient — General
   Urinal — General
   Uroflowmeter — Gastroenterology/Urology

READ DENTAL LAB
337-496-3706
1508 Ford St., Lake Charles, LA 70601
FDA Number: 3004967957
   Alloy, Precious Metal, For Clinical Use — Dental And Oral
   Teeth, Porcelain — Dental And Oral

READE ADVANCED MATERIALS
401-433-7000
PO Box 15039, East Providence, RI 02915-0039
FDA Number: n/a
Fax: 401-433-7001
E-mail: rcg@reade.com
Web site: www.reade.com
Annual Revenue: $10-$25 Million
Year Founded: 1773
Ownership: Private
Quality System Registration Information: ISO9001; ISO9002
Produces/Sells CE-marked Devices: Y
Distribution: Manufacturer Direct, Importer, Exporter
General Admin.: E. S. Reade/Vice President, General Manager
Mktg./Adv.: Charles Reade/Manager International & National Sales
        Bethany Cochran/Manager Sales
        Karen Ramos/Manager Sales
Production: Steve Munson/Manager Materials
   Electrode, Biopotential, Surface, Composite — Physical Med
   Foil, Ophthalmic — Ophthalmology
   Solvent — Chemistry

READE METALS & MINERALS CORP.
See Reade Advanced Materials

REAGENTS APPLICATIONS, INC.
See Raichem, Division Of Hemagen Diagnostics, Inc.

REAL IDEAS REHABILITATION DIV. INC.
604-820-8916
34142 York Ave, Mission V2V 6Y5 Canada
FDA Number: 9613812

REAL IDEAS REHABILITATION DIV. INC.
604-820-8916 *(cont'd)*
   Table, Mechanical — Physical Med

RECIGNO LABORATORIES INC.
215-659-7755
509 Davisville Rd., Willow Grove, PA 19090
FDA Number: 3006059066
   Alloy, Gold Based, For Clinical Use — Dental And Oral
   Alloy, Precious Metal, For Clinical Use — Dental And Oral
   Metal, Base — Dental And Oral

RECOGNITION EXPRESS
800-573-6444
502 Sunnyside Avenue, Wheaton, IL 60187
630-668-6540
FDA Number: n/a
Fax: 630-668-1396
E-mail: recogexprs@aol.com
Web site: www.recognitionexpress.com
Annual Revenue: $0-$1 Million
Total Employees: 6   *Sales Staff:* 2
Ownership: Private
Produces/Sells CE-marked Devices: N
Federal Procurement Eligibility: Small Business
Distribution: Manufacturer Direct
General Admin.: Tom Denson/Chief Executive Officer
Mktg./Adv.: Mary Sue Wysocki/Vice President Sales
Production: Jackie Cummings/Vice President Manufacturing
   Sign, Hospital — General

RECREATION EQUIPMENT UNLIMITED, INC.
412-731-3000
P.O. Box 4700, Pittsburgh, PA 15206
FDA Number: n/a
Fax: 412-731-3052
E-mail: nobsbb@aol.com
Web site: www.sportmasterinc.com
Medical Products Sales Volume: $50,000
Annual Revenue: $0-$1 Million
Year Founded: 1967
Total Employees: 10   *Sales Staff:* 3
Ownership: Private
Produces/Sells CE-marked Devices: N
Federal Procurement Eligibility: Small Business
Distribution: Manufacturer Direct
Mktg./Adv.: Mary Fullen/Manager Contract Sales
        Jean McCue/Manager Sales Training
   Table, Examination/Treatment — General
   Wheelchair, Manual — Physical Med

RECREATIONAL INNOVATIONS CO.
See Noir Manufacturing

RECTO MOLDED PRODUCTS INC., QUINN HEALTHCARE PRODU
513-871-5544
4425 Appleton St., Cincinnati, OH 45209
FDA Number: 1527461
Ownership: Private
Produces/Sells CE-marked Devices: N
   Exhaust System, Surgical — Surgery

REDFIELD CORP.
800-678-4472
336 West Passaic St, Rochelle Park, NJ 07662
201-845-3990
FDA Number: 2246437
Fax: 201-845-3993
E-mail: info@redfieldcorp.com
Web site: www.redfieldcorp.com
Medical Products Sales Volume: $550,000
Annual Revenue: $1-$5 Million
Year Founded: 1987
Total Employees: 4   *Sales Staff:* 9
Ownership: Private
Produces/Sells CE-marked Devices: N
Federal Procurement Eligibility: Small Business
Distribution: Service Direct
General Admin.: Mr. Andrew Gould/Chief Executive
        Mr. Donald Osur/President
   Ligator, Hemorrhoidal — Gastroenterology/Urology

REDI-TECH MEDICAL PRODUCTS,LLC
800-824-1793
529 Front Street, Suite 125, Cleveland, OH 44017
FDA Number: 3005137477
Fax: 440-234-5801
E-mail: info@redi-tech.com
Web site: www.redi-tech.com
Medical Products Sales Volume: $800,000
Annual Revenue: $0-$1 Million
Year Founded: 2003
Total Employees: 4   *Marketing Staff:* 1   *Sales Staff:* 2
Ownership: Private
Produces/Sells CE-marked Devices: N
Federal Procurement Eligibility: Small Business
Distribution: Exclusive Distributor
General Admin.: Frank T. Costanzo/Chairman, Chief Executive Officer
        Edmond L. Lonergan/President

REDI-TECH MEDICAL PRODUCTS,LLC   800-824-1793 (cont'd)
Finance: Curt B. Westrom/Chief Financial Officer

Bag, Bile Collection	Gastroenterology/Urology
Cannula, Intrauterine Insemination	Obstetrics/Gynecology
Catheter, Imaging, Ultrasonic	Radiology
Catheter, Salpingography	Obstetrics/Gynecology
Catheter, Tenckhoff	Gastroenterology/Urology
Drain, Nasobiliary	Gastroenterology/Urology
Kit, Tubing, Dialysis, Peritoneal	Gastroenterology/Urology
Stent, Ureteral	Gastroenterology/Urology

REDITAC MEDICAL USA, LLC   225-923-3592
1555 Cottondale Drive, Suite 4, Baton Rouge, LA 70815-4162
FDA Number: 3003952528
Ownership: Private
Produces/Sells CE-marked Devices: N

Bed, Air Fluidized	Physical Med

REDMAN POWERCHAIRS   800-727-6684
1601 S Pantano Parkway #107, Tucson, AZ 85710
FDA Number: n/a   Fax: 520-546-5530
E-mail: info@RedmanPowerChair.com
Web site: www.redmanpowerchair.com
Medical Products Sales Volume: $2,000,000
Annual Revenue: $1-$5 Million
Year Founded: 1989
Ownership: Private
Produces/Sells CE-marked Devices: N
Federal Procurement Eligibility: Small Business
Distribution: Exclusive Distributor

Wheelchair, Powered	Physical Med

REDMAN WHEELCHAIRS
See Redman Powerchairs

REDWOOD TOXICOLOGY LABORATORIES, INC.   800-255-2159
3650 Westwind Blvd., Santa Rosa, CA 95403   707-577-7959
FDA Number: 3004145089   Fax: 707-577-8102
E-mail: sales@redwoodtoxicology.com
Web site: www.redwoodtoxicology.com
Ownership: Alere, Inc.
Stock Symbol: IMA
Traded On: AMEX
Produces/Sells CE-marked Devices: N
General Admin.: Albert Berger/President

Enzyme Immunoassay, Amphetamine	Toxicology
Enzyme Immunoassay, Barbiturate	Toxicology
Enzyme Immunoassay, Cannabinoids	Toxicology
Enzyme Immunoassay, Cocaine And Cocaine Metabolites	Toxicology
Enzyme Immunoassay, Opiates	Toxicology
Enzyme Immunoassay, Phencyclidine	Toxicology
Radioimmunoassay, Tricyclic Antidepressant Drugs	Toxicology
Thin Layer Chromatography, Metamphetamine	Toxicology

REDYREF A DIVISION OF DAWNEX INDUSTRIES   800-628-3603
38-61 11th Street, Long Island City, NY 11101   718-784-3690
FDA Number: n/a   Fax: 718-784-3696
E-mail: sales@redyref.com
Web site: www.redyref.com
Medical Products Sales Volume: $3,400,000
Annual Revenue: $1-$5 Million
Year Founded: 1913
Total Employees: 40
Ownership: Private
Federal Procurement Eligibility: Small Business
Distribution: Manufacturer Through Distributor, Exclusive Distributor

Speculum, Vaginal, Non-Metal	Obstetrics/Gynecology

REEDSPECTRUM
See Clariant

REEL R&D, INC.   800-348-7335
9533 Sunnyside Ave.,   831-336-3960
Ben Lomond, CA 95005
FDA Number: 2939597   Fax: 831-336-3532
E-mail: info@spiints.com
Web site: www.spiimts.com
Medical Products Sales Volume: $5,000,000
Annual Revenue: $1-$5 Million
Total Employees: 18   Marketing Staff: 2   Sales Staff: 12
Ownership: Private
Quality System Registration Information: ISO9000
Produces/Sells CE-marked Devices: Y
Federal Procurement Eligibility: Small Business
Distribution: Manufacturer Direct, Manufacturer Through Manufacturer Reps, Exporter
General Admin.: Roger Lee/President, Chief Executive Officer
Mktg./Adv.: Paul Martin/Vice President Sales
Production: Paul Martin/Vice President Manufacturing
Research: Roger Lee/Vice President Research & Development

REEL R&D, INC.   800-348-7335 (cont'd)

Splint, Other	Orthopedics
Splint, Traction	Orthopedics

REEVES EMERGENCY MANAGEMENT SYSTEMS, LLC.   301-698-1596
1704 W. 7th Street, Frederick, MD 21702
FDA Number: 3004157808
Web site: www.reevesems.com
Ownership: Private
Produces/Sells CE-marked Devices: N

Stretcher, Hand-Carried	General
Transfer Device, Patient, Manual	General

REFLEX INDUSTRIES, INC.   619-562-1821
9530 Pathway St., Suite 105, Santee, CA 92071
FDA Number: 2020651

Adsorbents, Ion Exchange	Toxicology
Detector, Beta/Gamma	Chemistry

REFLEX TECHNOLOGIES, INC.   305-892-0584
12565 Palm Rd., Suite B, North Miami, FL 33181-2611
FDA Number: 1059007
Ownership: Private
Produces/Sells CE-marked Devices: N

Monitor, Muscle, Dental	Dental And Oral
Stimulator, Nerve, Transcutaneous (Pain Relief, TENS)	Cns/Neurology
Stimulator, Neuromuscular, External Functional	Cns/Neurology
Unit, Anesthesia, Dental, Electric	Dental And Oral

REFRACTEC, INC.   949-784-2600
5 Jenner, Suite 150, Irvine, CA 92618
FDA Number: 2032402
Ownership: Private
Produces/Sells CE-marked Devices: N

Cautery, Radiofrequency, AC-Powered	Ophthalmology
Electrosurgical, Radio Frequency, Refractive Correction	Ophthalmology
Marker, Ocular	Ophthalmology

REGAL MEDI-SPA CO., INC.   905-477-7689
166 Torbay Rd, Markham L3R 1G6 Canada
FDA Number: 9680644

Transfer Device, Patient, Manual	General

REGAL PLASTICS PRODUCTS, INC.
See Team Vantage Molding Llc.

REGANES, INC.
See Avid Medical

REGEN BIOLOGICS, INC.   415-562-0800
411 Hackensack Ave., Hackensack, NJ 07601
FDA Number: 2956141
E-mail: info@regenbio.com
Web site: www.regenbio.com
Year Founded: 1990
Ownership: Public
Stock Symbol: RGBI
Traded On: OTC Bulletin
Produces/Sells CE-marked Devices: Y
General Admin.: Gerald Bisbee/President, Chief Executive Officer, Chairman
Production: John Dichiara/Senior Vice President Medical & Regulatory Affairs
Research: William Rodkey/Vice President Scientific Affairs
Finance: Brion Umidi/Senior Vice President Finance

Arthroscope	Orthopedics
Suture, Non-Absorbable, Synthetic, Polyester	Surgery

REGENCY MEDICAL SUPPLIES   800-663-1012
4437 Canada Way, Burnaby, BC V5G-1J3 Canada   604-434-1383
FDA Number: n/a   Fax: 604-435-8150
E-mail: regmed@axionet.com
Web site: www.regencymed.com
Year Founded: 1966
Total Employees: 25
Ownership: Private
Produces/Sells CE-marked Devices: N
Distribution: Exclusive Distributor

REGENCY PRODUCT INTERNATIONAL   800-845-7931
4732 E 26TH STREET, VERNON, CA 90040-2002   323-266-2500
FDA Number: 9002285   Fax: 323-266-7958
E-mail: info@regencyproducts.com
Web site: www.regencyproducts.com
Annual Revenue: $0-$1 Million
Year Founded: 1990
Total Employees: 6
Ownership: Private
Produces/Sells CE-marked Devices: Y
Federal Procurement Eligibility: Small Business, Minority Owned

REGENCY PRODUCT INTERNATIONAL 800-845-7931 *(cont'd)*

Distribution: Manufacturer Direct, Manufacturer Through Distributor, Manufacturer Through Manufacturer Reps, OEM, Exclusive Distributor, Importer, Exporter
General Admin.: Mr. David Soomekh/President, Chief Executive Officer

Cushion, Other	General
Cushion, Wheelchair (Pad)	Physical Med
Pack, Hot Or Cold, Reusable	Physical Med
Pack, Hot Or Cold, Water Circulating	Physical Med
Pillow, Cervical	Orthopedics
Support, Hot/Cold Pack	Physical Med

REGENERATION TECHNOLOGIES, INC.

See RTI Biologics Inc.

REGENERON PHARMACEUTICALS, INC. 914-345-7400

777 Old Saw Mill River Road, Tarrytown, NY 10591
FDA Number: n/a   *Fax:* 914-347-2847
E-mail: info@regeneron.com
Web site: www.regeneron.com
Medical Products Sales Volume: $63,400,000
Annual Revenue: $10-$25 Million
Year Founded: 1988
Total Employees: 588
Ownership: Public
Stock Symbol: REGN
Traded On: NASDAQ
Produces/Sells CE-marked Devices: N
General Admin.: Dr. George D. Yancopoulos/Chief Scientific Officer & Executive Vice President
          Dr. Leonard S. Schleifer/President, Chief Executive Officer
Medical Admin.: Dr. Hans-Peter Guler/Vice President Clinical Services
Mktg./Adv.: Ms. Suzanne Blaug/Vice President Marketing & Sales
Production: Dr. Randall Rupp/Senior Vice President Manufacturing
          Mr. Stephen L. Holst/Vice President Quality Assurance & Regulatory Affairs
Finance: Mr. Murray A. Goldberg/Chief Financial Officer, Senior Vice President Finance
          Mr. Charles Poole/Vice President Public Communications & Investor Relations

Contract Manufacturing, Pharmaceuticals/Chemicals	General

REGENT HOSPITAL PRODUCTS LTD.

See Molnlycke Health Care Inc.

REGENT LABS, INC. 954-426-4403

700 West Hillsboro Blvd., Bldg. #2-206, Deerfield Bch, FL 33441
FDA Number: 1058743

Adhesive, Denture, Karaya	Dental And Oral
Cleaner, Denture	Dental And Oral

REGIONAL MEDIA LABORATORIES, INC.

See Remel

REGIONAL ORGAN BANK OF ILLINOIS, INC.

See Allosource

REGIS TECHNOLOGIES, INC. 800-323-8144
                                          847-967-6000

8210 N. Austin Avenue,
Morton Grove, IL 60053
FDA Number: 7000312   *Fax:* 847-967-1214
E-mail: sales@registech.com
Web site: www.registech.com
Medical Products Sales Volume: $4,300,000
Annual Revenue: $10-$25 Million
Year Founded: 1956
Total Employees: 53
Ownership: Private
Produces/Sells CE-marked Devices: N
Federal Procurement Eligibility: Small Business
Distribution: Manufacturer Direct, Exporter
General Admin.: Dr. Louis Glunz/Chief Executive Officer
          Susan E. Lye/General Manager
          Louis Glunz/President
Mktg./Adv.: David McCleary/Manager Business Development
          Lori A. Hoffman/Senior Project Manager
Production: Steve Jerger/Director Quality Assurance

Chromatography, Liquid, Performance, High	Toxicology
Contract Manufacturing, Pharmaceuticals/Chemicals	General
Labware, Basic, Reusable	Chemistry

REGUPOL AMERICA 800-537-8737

33 Keystone Drive, Lebanon, PA 17042
FDA Number: n/a   *Fax:* 717-675-2199
Web site: www.regupol.com
Ownership: Bsw Berleburger Schaumstoffwerk Gmbh
Produces/Sells CE-marked Devices: Y

Flooring	General
Foam, Plastic	General

REHAB INNOVATIONS, INC. 402-445-4335

8727 Ames Ave., Omaha, NE 68134
FDA Number: 3004099452

Exerciser, Non-Measuring	Physical Med
Wheelchair, Manual	Physical Med

REHABILITATION CENTER FOR CHILDREN INC. 204-452-4311

633 Wellington Cres, Winnipeg R3M 0A8 Canada
FDA Number: 9615318

Walker, Mechanical	Physical Med

REHABILITATION SERVICES, INC. 888-300-4548
9841 SW 100 Ave., Miami, FL 33176 305-271-0012
FDA Number: n/a   *Fax:* 305-273-1221
E-mail: rehabsvcs @ gmail.com
Web site: www.rehabserv.com
Medical Products Sales Volume: $200,000
Annual Revenue: $0-$1 Million
Year Founded: 1974
Ownership: Private
Quality System Registration Information: ISO9002
Produces/Sells CE-marked Devices: Y
Federal Procurement Eligibility: Small Business
Distribution: Service Direct
General Admin.: Dr. Robert Lessne/President, Chief Executive Officer

Contract Manufacturing	General
Service, Engineering/Design	General

REHABILITATION TECHNICAL 919-732-1705
COMPONENTS, CORP.

3913 Devonwood Road, Hillsborough, NC 27278
FDA Number: n/a
Annual Revenue: $0-$1 Million
Year Founded: 1971
Ownership: Private
Produces/Sells CE-marked Devices: N
Federal Procurement Eligibility: Small Business
Distribution: Manufacturer Through Distributor, Importer

Belt, Traction, Pelvic	Physical Med
Exerciser, Non-Measuring	Physical Med
Insoles, Medical	General
Joint, Knee, External Brace	Physical Med
Sling, Arm	Physical Med
Splint, Hand, And Component	Physical Med

REHABTEK LLC 847-853-8380

2510 Wilmette Ave., Wilmette, IL 60091
FDA Number: 2000019555

Exerciser, Powered	Anesthesiology

REHAMED INTL. LLC. 800-577-4424
522 West Mowry Drive, Homestead, FL 33030 305-247-8300
FDA Number: 1063923   *Fax:* 305-247-8304
E-mail: steve@grouprmt.com
Web site: www.grouprmt.com
Medical Products Sales Volume: $600,000
Year Founded: 1996
Total Employees: 5
Ownership: Private
Produces/Sells CE-marked Devices: N
Federal Procurement Eligibility: Small Business
Distribution: Manufacturer Through Distributor
Mktg./Adv.: Mr. Stephen Roche/Director Marketing & Business Development

Ergometer, Treadmill	Cardiovascular
Lift, Bath, Non-AC-Powered	General

REHEAT CO., INC. 800-373-4328
10 School St., Danvers, MA 01923 978-777-4441
FDA Number: n/a   *Fax:* 978-777-7958
E-mail: reheatco@reheat.com
Web site: www.reheat.com
Medical Products Sales Volume: $1,200,000
Annual Revenue: $1-$5 Million
Year Founded: 1986
Total Employees: 10   *Marketing Staff:* 3   *Sales Staff:* 15
Ownership: Private
Produces/Sells CE-marked Devices: N
Federal Procurement Eligibility: Small Business
Distribution: Manufacturer Direct, Manufacturer Through Distributor, Manufacturer Through Manufacturer Reps
General Admin.: Paul Meinerth/President, Chief Executive Officer
Mktg./Adv.: Wayne Reutter/Manager Product Marketing
Production: Janet Fitzgerald/Customer Service Representative
          Nick Childs/Industrial Engineer
Purchasing: Bill Deorio/Vice President Purchasing

Component, Electrical	General
Controller, Temperature, Programmable	Chemistry
Dryer, Labware	Chemistry

REHEAT CO., INC.   800-373-4328 *(cont'd)*
Plate, Hot   Chemistry

REICHERT OPHTHALMIC INSTR., DIV. LEICA, INC./NY
See Reichert, Inc.

REICHERT SCIENTIFIC INSTRUMENTS
See Leica Microsystems, Inc., Educational & Analytical Division

REICHERT, INC.   888-849-8955
3362 Walden Avenue, Depew, NY 14043   **716-686-4500**
FDA Number: 1319721   *Fax:* 716-686-4545
E-mail: info@reichert.com
Web site: www.reichert.com
Medical Products Sales Volume: $14,100,000
Annual Revenue: $25-$50 Million
Total Employees: 147
Ownership: Private
Quality System Registration Information: ISO9000; ISO9001
Produces/Sells CE-marked Devices: Y
Federal Procurement Eligibility: Small Business, GSA Contract
Distribution: Manufacturer Through Distributor
General Admin.: Tim Levindofske/Chief Operating Officer
     John Burgess/President
Mktg./Adv.: Graham Hodge/Director Marketing & Sales
     David Biggins/Manager Product Development
Research: Bruce Siskowski/Director Research & Development
Frame, Trial, Ophthalmic	Ophthalmology
Lamp, Slit, Biomicroscope, AC-Powered	Ophthalmology
Lens, Set, Trial, Ophthalmic	Ophthalmology
Measurer, Lens, AC-Powered	Ophthalmology
Projector, Ophthalmic	Ophthalmology
Refractor, Ophthalmic	Ophthalmology
Tonometer, AC-Powered	Ophthalmology
Topographer, Corneal	Ophthalmology

REICHERT-JUNG
See Leica Microsystems, Inc., Educational & Analytical Division

REICHERT-JUNG SCIENTIFIC INSTRUMENTS
See Leica Microsystems, Inc., Educational & Analytical Division

REID OPTICAL LABORATORY, INC.
See Southern Reid Optical Laboratory, Inc.

REID ROWELL
See Solvay Pharmaceuticals

REIMERS SYSTEMS, INC.   877-734-6377
8210-D Cinder Bed Road, Lorton, VA 22079   **703-952-0240**
FDA Number: 1122095   *Fax:* 703-952-0244
E-mail: info@ReimersSystems.com
Web site: www.ReimersSystems.com
Medical Products Sales Volume: $700,000
Year Founded: 1994
Total Employees: 9   *Marketing Staff:* 1   *Sales Staff:* 2
Ownership: Private
Produces/Sells CE-marked Devices: N
Federal Procurement Eligibility: Small Business
Distribution: Manufacturer Direct
General Admin.: Stephen D. Reimers/President, Owner
Mktg./Adv.: Regina Sonnenrein/Manager International & National Sales
     Ishtiaque Alam/Manager International Marketing Operations
Production: Ramesh Kumar/Manager Engineering
Chamber, Hyperbaric	Anesthesiology
System, Pipeline, Gas	General

REINA IMAGING   800-752-4918
6107 West Lou Ave., Crystal Lake, IL 60014   **815-356-8181**
FDA Number: 1450835
Ownership: Private
Produces/Sells CE-marked Devices: N
Grid, Radiographic	Radiology
Holder, Radiographic Cassette, Wall-Mounted	Radiology

REJUVENESS PHARAMCEUTICALS, INC.   518-584-5017
125 High Rock Ave., Saratoga Springs, NY 12866
FDA Number: 1320762
Ownership: Private
Produces/Sells CE-marked Devices: N
Elastomer, Silicone (Scar Management)	Surgery

RELAXOBAK, INC   866-369-6914
4956 W 300 N., P.O. Box 2613, Anderson, IN 46018-2613
FDA Number: 1616728
Web site: www.relaxobak.com
Medical Products Sales Volume: $50,000
Annual Revenue: $0-$1 Million
Year Founded: 1963
Ownership: Private
Produces/Sells CE-marked Devices: N
Federal Procurement Eligibility: Small Business

RELAXOBAK, INC   866-369-6914 *(cont'd)*
Distribution: Manufacturer Direct
Orthosis, Lumbosacral	Physical Med

RELIA DIAGNOSTIC SYSTEMS, LLC   415-344-0844
One Market, suite 1475, Steuart Tower,
San Francisco, CA 94105
FDA Number: 2954941
Ownership: Private
Produces/Sells CE-marked Devices: N
Radioimmunoassay, Thyroid Stimulating Hormone	Chemistry

RELIABLE BIOPHARMECEUTICAL   314-429-7700
1945 Walton Rd., St. Louis, MO 63114
FDA Number: 059605   *Fax:* 314-429-0937
E-mail: info@reliablebiopharm.com
Web site: www.reliablebiopharm.com
Annual Revenue: $10-$25 Million
Year Founded: 1968
Total Employees: 62   *Marketing Staff:* 2   *Sales Staff:* 1
Ownership: Private
Produces/Sells CE-marked Devices: N
Distribution: Manufacturer Direct
Mktg./Adv.: Dwayne Sharpe/Director Marketing
Contract Manufacturing, Pharmaceuticals/Chemicals	General
Contract Manufacturing, Reagent	General

RELIABLE CHEMICAL CO.
See Reliable Biopharmeceutical

RELIANCE DENTAL MFG., CO.   708-597-6694
5805 West 117th Place, Alsip, IL 60803
FDA Number: 1415367
Base, Denture, Relining, Repairing, Rebasing, Resin	Dental And Oral
Crown And Bridge, Temporary, Resin	Dental And Oral
Material, Impression Tray, Resin	Dental And Oral
Tray, Impression	Dental And Oral

RELIANCE MEDICAL CORP.   800-633-8423
5981 Graham Ct, Livermore, CA 94550   **510-732-9950**
FDA Number: 1523545   *Fax:* 510-785-8182
E-mail: mel@mdresource.com
Web site: www.mdresource.com
Annual Revenue: $0-$1 Million
Ownership: Medical Device Resource Corporation
Produces/Sells CE-marked Devices: Y
Federal Procurement Eligibility: Small Business
Distribution: Manufacturer Through Manufacturer Reps
Accessories, Operating Room, Table	Surgery
Aspirator, Liposuction	Surgery
Chair, Ophthalmic, AC-Powered	Ophthalmology
Chair, Ophthalmic, Manual	Ophthalmology
Stand, Instrument, AC-Powered, Ophthalmic	Ophthalmology
Stool, Anesthetist's	Anesthesiology
Unit, Examining/Treatment, ENT	Ear/Nose/Throat

RELIANCE MEDICAL PRODUCTS, INC.
See HAAG-STREIT USA, INC.

RELIEF WRAP LTD.   519-442-5071
15a Oak Ave, Paris N3L 3C6 Canada
FDA Number: 9680641
Pack, Moist Heat	Physical Med

RELIEVANT MEDSYSTEMS INC.   650-368-1000
2688 Middlefield Road Suite A, Redwood City, CA 94063
FDA Number: 3006789852
E-mail: info@Relievant.com
Web site: www.relievant.com
Ownership: Private
Produces/Sells CE-marked Devices: N
General Admin.: Mr. Alex DiNello/President, Chief Executive Officer
Electrosurgical Unit, Cutting & Coagulation Device	Surgery

REM SYSTEMS   305-499-4800
625 East 10 Ave., Hialeah, FL 33010-1660
FDA Number: n/a   *Fax:* 305-885-8677
E-mail: info@remsystems.com
Web site: www.remsystems.com
Medical Products Sales Volume: $1,000,000
Annual Revenue: $5-$10 Million
Total Employees: 20   *Marketing Staff:* 2   *Sales Staff:* 4
Ownership: Private
Produces/Sells CE-marked Devices: N
Federal Procurement Eligibility: Small Business
Distribution: Exclusive Distributor, Exporter
Mktg./Adv.: Joe Carignan/Director National Accounts
Cabinet Casework, General Purpose	General
Cabinet, X-Ray Transfer	Radiology
Cart, Multipurpose	General

REM SYSTEMS
305-499-4800 *(cont'd)*

Cart, Other	General
Cart, Supply	General
Office Equipment	General
Stand/Holder, Equipment, Laboratory	Chemistry
Storage Unit, X-Ray Film	Radiology

Medical Product Subsidiaries (Listed Separately)
Kardex Systems, Inc.

REMED SCIENTIFIC LTD.
604-899-8985
238 Alvin Narod Mews, Ste. 238,
Vancouver, BC V6B-5 Canada
FDA Number: n/a
E-mail: info@remed.bc.ca   *Fax:* 604-899-8986
Web site: www.remed.bc.ca
Year Founded: 1998
Total Employees: 10
Ownership: Private
Produces/Sells CE-marked Devices: N
Distribution: Exclusive Distributor, Exporter

REMEDPAR
800-624-3994
615-859-1303
101 Old Stone Bridge Road,
Goodlettsville, TN 37072
FDA Number: 1051467
E-mail: RMPInfo@ReMedPar.com   *Fax:* 615-859-4165
Web site: www.remedpar.com
Medical Products Sales Volume: $30,000,000
Annual Revenue: $10-$25 Million
Year Founded: 1980
Total Employees: 43   *Marketing Staff:* 4   *Sales Staff:* 8
Produces/Sells CE-marked Devices: N
Federal Procurement Eligibility: Small Business
Distribution: Service Direct, Exclusive Distributor
General Admin.: Mr. Edward A. Sloan/President, Chief Executive Officer
     Mr. Mark A. Suffridge/Senior Vice President
Mktg./Adv.: Mrs. Wanda Legate/Vice President Marketing & Sales
Finance: Ms. Kim Ames/Chief Financial Officer

Service, Parts, Repair	General
Service, Used Equipment	General

REMEDY HEARING AIDS
760-754-8151
2420 Vista Way, Ste. 112, Oceanside, CA 92054-6190
FDA Number: 2031348
E-mail: wgobitas@cox.net   *Fax:* 760-754-8150
Web site: www.4hearingaids.com
Year Founded: 1993
Ownership: Private
Produces/Sells CE-marked Devices: N

Hearing-Aid	Ear/Nose/Throat

REMEL
800-255-6730
913-888-0939
12076 Santa Fe Drive, Lenexa, KS 66215-3519
FDA Number: 1924669   *Fax:* 800-621-8251
E-mail: remel@remel.com
Web site: www.remel.com
Year Founded: 1972
Total Employees: 50   *Marketing Staff:* 10   *Sales Staff:* 40
Ownership: Fisher Scientific Co., Llc.
Produces/Sells CE-marked Devices: N
Federal Procurement Eligibility: Small Business
Distribution: Manufacturer Direct, Manufacturer Through Manufacturer Reps, OEM, Importer, Exporter
General Admin.: Susanne Garay/President
     Lyndon Davis/Vice President Human Resources
Mktg./Adv.: Mary Ann Silvius/Director Business Development
     Sean O'Connor/Director Marketing
     Scott Puyear/Manager International Sales
     Jeff Papi/Vice President Marketing & Sales
     Nancy Cote/Vice President National Accounts
Production: Dee Ann Berry/Director Customer Services
     Bill Leverich/Manager Quality Assurance
     Gerald Lillian/Vice President Operations
     Bob Booth/Vice President Quality Assurance & Regulatory Affairs
Finance: Rob Chestnut/Chief Financial Officer
IS: LaNae Druen/Manager Tech. Services

Culture Media, Anaerobic Transport	Microbiology
Culture Media, For Isolation Of Pathogenic Neisseria	Microbiology
Culture Media, General Nutrient Broth	Microbiology
Culture Media, Mueller Hinton Agar Broth	Microbiology
Culture Media, Multiple Biochemical Test	Microbiology
Culture Media, Non-Propagating Transport	Microbiology
Culture Media, Non-Selective And Differential	Microbiology
Culture Media, Non-Selective And Non-Differential	Microbiology
Culture Media, Selective And Differential	Microbiology
Culture Media, Selective And Non-Differential	Microbiology
Culture Media, Selective Broth	Microbiology
Culture Media, Single Biochemical Test	Microbiology

REMEL
800-255-6730 *(cont'd)*

Culture Media, Supplements	Microbiology
Disc, Strip And Reagent, Microorganism Differentiation	Microbiology
Kit, Screening, Staphylococcus Aureus	Microbiology

Medical Product Subsidiaries (Listed Separately)
Chrisope Technologies, Inc.
Remel Atlanta, Div. Of Remel, Inc.
Separation Technology Inc

REMEL ATLANTA, DIV. OF REMEL, INC.
800-255-6730
770-409-0713
2797 Peterson Pl., Norcross, GA 30071
FDA Number: 1031428
E-mail: remel@remel.com   *Fax:* 770-409-0789
Web site: www.remelinc.com
Year Founded: 1973
Total Employees: 25
Ownership: Remel
Produces/Sells CE-marked Devices: N
Distribution: Manufacturer Direct, OEM, Exporter
General Admin.: Suzanne gary/President
Mktg./Adv.: Gerald Lillian/Vice President Marketing
Production: Jim Belei/Director Operations
     Bob Booth/Director Quality Assurance
     Scott Kendall/Manager Regulatory Affairs
     Gary Pearson/Vice President Safety

Culture Media, General Nutrient Broth	Microbiology
Disc, Strip And Reagent, Microorganism Differentiation	Microbiology
Kit, Identification, Anaerobic	Microbiology
Kit, Identification, Enterobacteriaceae	Microbiology
Kit, Identification, Glucose (Non-Ferment)	Microbiology
Kit, Identification, Neisseria Gonorrhoeae	Microbiology
Kit, Identification, Yeast	Microbiology
Kit, Screening, Staphylococcus Aureus	Microbiology
Test, Bacterial Diagnostic	Microbiology

REMEL-LAKE CHARLES, DIVISION OF REMEL INC.
800-256-4376
3941 Ryan St., Lake Charles, LA 70605
FDA Number: 1625984

Kit, Quality Control	Microbiology

REMINGTON MEDICAL EQUIPMENT LTD.
800-267-5822
905-470-7790
401 Bently St. #9,
Markham, ONT L3R-9 Canada
FDA Number: n/a
E-mail: mail@remingtonmedical.com   *Fax:* 905-470-7787
Web site: www.remingtonmedical.com
Year Founded: 1983
Total Employees: 10
Ownership: Private
Produces/Sells CE-marked Devices: N
Distribution: Exclusive Distributor, Importer

REMINGTON PRODUCTS CO.
See Remington Products Company Llc

REMINGTON PRODUCTS COMPANY LLC
800-491-1571
330-335-1571
961 Seville Rd., Wadsworth, OH 44281-0506
FDA Number: 1523560
E-mail: jwert@remprod.com   *Fax:* 330-336-9462
Web site: www.remprod.com
Annual Revenue: $10-$25 Million
Year Founded: 1932
Total Employees: 140   *Marketing Staff:* 2   *Sales Staff:* 6
Ownership: Private
Quality System Registration Information: ISO9001
Produces/Sells CE-marked Devices: N
Distribution: Manufacturer Direct, Exporter
General Admin.: Timothy Remington/President
Mktg./Adv.: Gerry Gross/Director Product Development
     Jeff Wert/Vice President Marketing & Sales

Board, Foot	Orthopedics
Orthosis, Corrective Shoe	Physical Med

REMOTE TECHNOLOGIES, INC.
800-733-9729
914-937-3293
P.O. Box 1185, Greenwich, CT 06836
FDA Number: 1222777
E-mail: questions@remotetechnologies.com   *Fax:* 914-939-3460
Web site: www.remotetechnologies.net
Annual Revenue: $1-$5 Million
Year Founded: 1991
Total Employees: 6   *Marketing Staff:* 1   *Sales Staff:* 2
Ownership: Private
Produces/Sells CE-marked Devices: Y
Federal Procurement Eligibility: Female Owned
Distribution: OEM
General Admin.: Cheryl Makrinos/Chief Executive Officer

REMOTE TECHNOLOGIES, INC.   800-733-9729 *(cont'd)*
  System, X-Ray, Mobile   Radiology

RENAISSANCE PLASTICS CO., THE   716-426-2078
155 Pineview Dr., Amherst, NY 14228
FDA Number: n/a   Fax: 716-426-5493
Web site: www.ultratool.com
Medical Products Sales Volume: $15,000,000
Annual Revenue: $50-$100 Million
Total Employees: 600   *Marketing Staff:* 2   *Sales Staff:* 15
Ownership: Private
Quality System Registration Information: ISO9002
Produces/Sells CE-marked Devices: N
Federal Procurement Eligibility: Small Business
General Admin.: Joe Betro/President
Mktg./Adv.: Dan Hanlon/Vice President Sales
Production: Dave Leaderer/Director Quality Assurance
  Cleanroom Equipment   General
  Component, Plastic   General
  Contract Manufacturing   General
  Contract R&D, Diagnostics   General

RENAL SOLUTIONS INC.   (866) 466-3436
770 Commonwealth Drive, Suite 101,   724-772-6900
Warrendale, PA 15086
FDA Number: 3005778453
Web site: www.renalsolutionsinc.com   Fax: (724) 772-6925
Ownership: Private
Produces/Sells CE-marked Devices: N
  Dialysate Delivery System, Sorbent Regenerated   Gastroenterology/Urology
  Dialyzer, High Permeability   Gastroenterology/Urology

RENAL SYSTEMS INCORPORATED
  See Minntech Corporation

RENEW BIOCARE CORP.   415-367-3646
1001 Bayhill Dr., 2nd Fl, San Bruno, CA 94066
FDA Number: 2954717
  Implant, Endosseous   Dental And Oral

RENFRO CORPORATION   336-719-8345
661 Linville Road, Mount Airy, NC 27030
FDA Number: 3002854239
  Stocking, Elastic   General

RENICK ENT., INC.   561-863-4183
1211 West 13th St., Riviera Beach, FL 33404
FDA Number: 1056829   Fax: 561-863-4185
E-mail: mike@rei-usa.com
Web site: www.rei-usa.com
Medical Products Sales Volume: $1,000,000
Annual Revenue: $0-$1 Million
Year Founded: 1990
Total Employees: 25   *Marketing Staff:* 1   *Sales Staff:* 3
Ownership: Private
Quality System Registration Information: ISO9001; ISO9002
Produces/Sells CE-marked Devices: N
Federal Procurement Eligibility: Small Business
Distribution: Manufacturer Direct, Manufacturer Through Distributor, Importer, Exporter
  Barrier, Control Panel, X-Ray, Moveable   Radiology
  Cannula, Surgical, General & Plastic Surgery   Surgery
  Chisel, Osteotome, Surgical   Dental And Oral
  Contract Manufacturing   General
  Drill, Dental, Intraoral   Dental And Oral
  Implant, Endosseous   Dental And Oral
  Screw, Fixation, Intraosseous   Dental And Oral

RENO MICRO PRECISION LTEE.   514-728-4785
8422 10th Ave., Montreal, QUE H1Z-3B5 Canada
FDA Number: n/a   Fax: 514-728-3973
Year Founded: 1969
Total Employees: 10
Ownership: Private
Produces/Sells CE-marked Devices: N
Distribution: Manufacturer Direct, Exporter

RENOX INC.
  See Boc Gases

RENU MEDICAL INC.   877-252-1110
9800 Evergreen Way, Everett, WA 98204
FDA Number: 3034520   Fax: 425-353-9116
E-mail: sales@renumedical.com
Web site: http://www.renumedical.com
Year Founded: 2000
Ownership: Private
Produces/Sells CE-marked Devices: N
  Circuit, Breathing (W Connector, Adapter, Y Piece)   Anesthesiology
  Mask, Gas, Anesthesia   Anesthesiology

RENU MEDICAL INC.   877-252-1110 *(cont'd)*
  Mask, Oxygen, Aerosol Administration   Anesthesiology
  Mask, Oxygen, Low Concentration, Venturi   Anesthesiology
  Mask, Scavenging   Anesthesiology
  Nebulizer, Medicinal, Non-Ventilatory (Atomizer)   Anesthesiology
  Oximeter, Tissue Saturation, Reprocessed   Cardiovascular
  Pressure Infusor, IV Container   General
  Sleeve, Compressible Limb   Cardiovascular
  Stethoscope, Manual   Cardiovascular
  Tourniquet   General
  Trocar, Laryngeal   Ear/Nose/Throat

REPAK SURGICAL CO.
  See Standard Textile

REPCO   800-726-1852
1227 W. Magnolia Avenue, Suite 310,   713-467-3085
Fort Worth, TX 76104
FDA Number: 1626406   Fax: 817-927-0559
E-mail: none@aol.com
Medical Products Sales Volume: $150,000
Annual Revenue: $0-$1 Million
Total Employees: 3
Ownership: Private
Produces/Sells CE-marked Devices: N
Federal Procurement Eligibility: Small Business, GSA Contract
Distribution: Manufacturer Direct, Exclusive Distributor
General Admin.: Les G. Coleman/President, Chief Executive Officer
  Instrument, Diamond, Dental   Dental And Oral
  Kit, Instruments and Accessories, Surgical   Surgery

REPEX MEDICAL PRODUCTS, INC.   305-740-0133
5240 SW 64th Avenue, Miami, FL 33155-6431
FDA Number: n/a   Fax: 305-740-0134
E-mail: repexmed@aol.com
Web site: www.repexmedical.com
Medical Products Sales Volume: $400,000
Year Founded: 1993
Total Employees: 4   *Marketing Staff:* 1   *Sales Staff:* 1
Ownership: Private
Produces/Sells CE-marked Devices: Y
Federal Procurement Eligibility: Small Business, Minority Owned, Female Owned
Distribution: Manufacturer Direct, Manufacturer Through Distributor, Manufacturer Through Manufacturer Reps, OEM, Exclusive Distributor, Exporter
General Admin.: Suely P. Argianas/President
  Circuit, Breathing, Ventilator   Anesthesiology
  Compressor, Air, Portable   Anesthesiology
  Humidifier, Heat/Moisture Exchange   Anesthesiology
  Service, Import/Export   General
  Ventilator, Other   Anesthesiology
  Ventilator, Volume (Critical Care)   Anesthesiology

REPLACEMENT PARTS INDUSTRIES, INC.   800-221-9723
20338 Corisco St., Chatsworth, CA 91313-5019   818-882-8611 ex
FDA Number: 100061766   Fax: 818-882-7028
E-mail: order@rpiparts.com
Web site: www.rpiparts.com
Medical Products Sales Volume: $4,000,000
Annual Revenue: $1-$5 Million
Year Founded: 1972
Total Employees: 26   *Marketing Staff:* 1
Ownership: Private
Quality System Registration Information: ISO9001
Produces/Sells CE-marked Devices: N
Federal Procurement Eligibility: Small Business
Distribution: Manufacturer Direct
General Admin.: Ira F. Lapides/President, Chief Executive Officer
Mktg./Adv.: Jim Wisniewski/Director Product Development
        Sherry Lapides/Vice President Customer Relations
        Joan D. Woodlock/Vice President Marketing
Production: Ray Martinez/Manager Quality Control
  Phototherapy Unit, Neonatal   General
  Service, Parts, Repair   General
  Warmer, Radiant, Infant   General

REPRO-MED SYSTEMS, INC.   800-624-9600
24 Carpenter Rd., Chester, NY 10918   845-469-2042
FDA Number: 1318360   Fax: 845-469-5518
E-mail: info@rmsmedicalproducts.com
Ownership: Public
Stock Symbol: REPR
Traded On: OTC Bulletin
Produces/Sells CE-marked Devices: N
  Catheter, Suction (Tracheal Aspirating Tube)   Anesthesiology
  Electrocautery Unit, Endoscopic   Obstetrics/Gynecology
  Prosthesis, Penis, Rigid Rod, External   Gastroenterology/Urology
  Stirrup   Gastroenterology/Urology

RES-Q PRODUCTS INC. 250-285-2890
P.O. Box 661, Quathiaski Cove, BC V0P-1N0 Canada
FDA Number: n/a   *Fax:* 250-285-2898
E-mail: resq@connected.bc.ca
Web site: www.hypothermia-ca.com
Year Founded: 1983
Total Employees: 10
Ownership: Private
Produces/Sells CE-marked Devices: N
Distribution: Manufacturer Direct, Exclusive Distributor, Importer

RESEARCH APPLIANCE CO.
See Thermo Fisher Scientific

RESEARCH INSTRUMENTATION 440-729-1649
ASSOCIATES, INC.
8753 Mayfield Rd., Chesterland, OH 44026
FDA Number: 1523880
Plethysmograph, Volume   Anesthesiology

RESEARCH ORGANICS, INC. 800-321-0570
4353 East 49th Street, Cleveland, OH 44125-1083   216-883-8025
FDA Number: n/a   *Fax:* 216-883-1576
E-mail: info@resorg.com
Web site: www.resorg.com
Medical Products Sales Volume: $14,000,000
Year Founded: 1953
Total Employees: 85   *Marketing Staff:* 7   *Sales Staff:* 7
Ownership: Private
Quality System Registration Information: ISO9001
Produces/Sells CE-marked Devices: N
Federal Procurement Eligibility: Small Business
Distribution: Manufacturer Direct, Manufacturer Through Distributor, Service Direct, Exporter
General Admin.: Annie Harlan-Gray/Director Human Resources
     Rob Sternfeld/President, Chief Executive Officer
Mktg./Adv.: Mr. Boaz Parran/Director Marketing
     Alan Miller/Manager National Sales
     Teri Durdella/Sales Assistant
Production: Amy Mutere/Director Quality Assurance & Quality Control
     Kim Johnson/Manager Customer Services
     Stan Biel/Plant Engineer
Research: Dan Flowers/Director Research & Development
Finance: John Mazzarella/Controller
Purchasing: Glenn Miller/Manager Materials, Director Purchasing
Peptides   Chemistry

RESEARCH PRODUCTS INTERNATIONAL CORP. 800-323-9814
410 N. Business Center Dr.,   847-635-7330
Mount Prospect, IL 60056
FDA Number: n/a   *Fax:* 847-635-1177
E-mail: service@rpicorp.com
Web site: www.rpicorp.com
Annual Revenue: $0-$1 Million
Total Employees: 15
Ownership: Private
Produces/Sells CE-marked Devices: N
Federal Procurement Eligibility: Small Business
Distribution: Manufacturer Direct
General Admin.: Robert Schudie/President
Mktg./Adv.: Al Eccker/Vice President Marketing
Beaker (Laboratory)   Chemistry
Stand/Holder, Equipment, Laboratory   Chemistry

RESEARCH TRIANGLE INSTITUTE 866-RTI-1958
3040 Cornwallis Rd., PO Box 12194,   919-485-2666
Research Triangle Park, NC 27709
FDA Number: 1046518
E-mail: listen@rti.org
Web site: www.rti.org
Ownership: Private
Produces/Sells CE-marked Devices: N
Control, Analyte (Assayed And Unassayed)   Chemistry
Control, Urinalysis (Assayed And Unassayed)   Chemistry

RESEARCH, INC. 952-941-3300
7128 Shady Oak Road, Eden Prairie, MN 55344
FDA Number: n/a   *Fax:* 952-949-9559
E-mail: knouis@researchinc.com
Web site: www.researchinc.com
Annual Revenue: $5-$10 Million
Year Founded: 1952
Total Employees: 25   *Marketing Staff:* 3   *Sales Staff:* 7
Ownership: Private
Produces/Sells CE-marked Devices: Y
Federal Procurement Eligibility: Small Business
Distribution: Manufacturer Through Manufacturer Reps

RESEARCH, INC. 952-941-3300 *(cont'd)*
General Admin.: Brad Yopp/Chief Financial Officer, Chairman
     Bill Hayland/President
Mktg./Adv.: Chad Carney/Director Marketing
Production: Bruce Bailey/Director Engineering
Heater, Electrical Instrument   General
Lamp, Infrared   Physical Med

RESMED CORP. 800-424-0737
9001 Spectrum Center Blvd.,   1 (858) 836-500
San Diego, CA 92123
FDA Number: 2183969   *Fax:* 1 (858) 836-550
E-mail: reception@resmed.com
Web site: www.resmed.com
Annual Revenue: $500 Million-$1 Billion
Ownership: RESMED INC.
Produces/Sells CE-marked Devices: N
General Admin.: Mr. Peter C Farrell/Chairman
     Mr. Lasse Beijer/Chief Operating Officer
     Mr. Kieran T. Gallahue/President, Chief Executive Officer
     Mr. David Pendarvis/Senior Vice President
Finance: Mr. Brett Sandercock/Chief Financial Officer
Humidifier, Respiratory Gas, (Direct Patient Interface)   Anesthesiology

RESMED INC. 800-424-0737
9001 Spectrum Center Blvd.,   858-836-5000
San Diego, CA 92123
FDA Number: 3007573469   *Fax:* 858-836-5501
E-mail: reception@resmed.com
Web site: http://www.resmed.com
Year Founded: 1989
Ownership: Public
Stock Symbol: RMD
Traded On: NYSE
Produces/Sells CE-marked Devices: N
General Admin.: Peter C. Farrell/Chairman
     Mr. Robert Douglas/Chief Operating Officer
Finance: Brett Sandercock/Chief Financial Officer
Humidifier, Respiratory Gas, (Direct Patient Interface)   Anesthesiology
Ventilator, Non-Continuous (Respirator)   Anesthesiology

RESMED WEST COAST WAREHOUSE 858-746-2576
23650 Brodiaea, Moreno valley, CA 92553
FDA Number: 3007009701
Ownership: RESMED CORP.
Stock Symbol: RMD
Traded On: NYSE
Produces/Sells CE-marked Devices: N
Humidifier, Respiratory Gas, (Direct Patient Interface)   Anesthesiology
Ventilator, Non-Continuous (Respirator)   Anesthesiology

RESONANCE INNOVATIONS LLC 402-934-2650
10957 Lake Ridge Drive, Omaha, NE 68136
FDA Number: 1932898
Image Processing System   Radiology
Nuclear Magnetic Resonance Imaging System   Radiology

RESONANCE TECHNOLOGY, INC. 818-882-1997
18121 Parthenia St., Northridge, CA 91325
FDA Number: 2029299
Nuclear Magnetic Resonance Imaging System   Radiology

RESONANT MEDICAL 877-985-2442
2050 Bleury Street, Suite 200,   514-985-2442
Montreal, QUEBE H3A 2 Canada
FDA Number: 3004747535   *Fax:* 514-985-2662
E-mail: info@resonantmedical.com
Web site: http://www.resonantmedical.com
Ownership: Private
Produces/Sells CE-marked Devices: N

RESOUND CORPORATION
See Gn Resound Corporation

RESPAN PROD. INC. 800-267-4063
8 Erinville Dr., Erin, ONT N0B 1T0 Canada   519-833-9774
FDA Number: 8022007   *Fax:* 519-833-7453
E-mail: info@respan.com
Web site: www.respan.com
Year Founded: 1981
Total Employees: 23   *Marketing Staff:* 3   *Sales Staff:* 3
Ownership: Private
Quality System Registration Information: ISO9002
Produces/Sells CE-marked Devices: Y
Federal Procurement Eligibility: Small Business, Female Owned
Distribution: Manufacturer Through Distributor, Manufacturer Through Manufacturer Reps, OEM, Service Direct, Exclusive Distributor, Importer

RESPIRATORY DIAGNOSTICS, INC.　425-881-8300
47987 Fremont Blvd., Fremont, CA 94538
FDA Number: n/a
Ownership: Private
Produces/Sells CE-marked Devices: N

Cable, Electrode	Physical Med
Cable/Lead, ECG, With Transducer And Electrode	Cardiovascular
Electrode, Electrosurgical, Return (Ground, Dispersive)	Surgery
Electrosurgical Unit, Cutting & Coagulation Device	Surgery
Generator, Radiofrequency Lesion	Cns/Neurology

RESPIRATORY SCIENCE INDUSTRIES LTD　516-561-6161
1325 M St., Elmont, NY 11003
FDA Number: 2434898
Medical Products Sales Volume: $4,600,000
Year Founded: 1977
Total Employees: 25
Federal Procurement Eligibility: Small Business

Cylinder, Gas (Empty)	Anesthesiology
Wheelchair, Manual	Physical Med

RESPIRATORY SERVICES, INC.
See Fuller Medical Co.

RESPIRATORY SUPPORT PRODUCTS, INC.
See Smiths Medical Asd, Inc.

RESPIRATORY TECHNOLOGIES, INC.　651-379-8999
1380 Energy Lane, Suite 113, St. Paul, MN 55108
FDA Number: 3004961434

Percussor, Powered	Anesthesiology

RESPIRCARE　800-267-6352
1000 Thomas Spratt Pl.,　613-737-7711
Ottawa, ONT K1G-5 Canada
FDA Number: n/a　Fax: 613-737-7144
E-mail: info@respircare.com
Web site: www.respircare.com
Year Founded: 1980
Total Employees: 100
Ownership: Private
Produces/Sells CE-marked Devices: N
Distribution: Exclusive Distributor

RESPIRONICS CALIFORNIA, INC.　724-387-4559
2271 Cosmos Ct., Carlsbad, CA 92011
FDA Number: 2031642
Web site: www.respironics.com
Ownership: Public
Stock Symbol: RESP
Traded On: NASDAQ
Produces/Sells CE-marked Devices: N

Adapter, Y	Gastroenterology/Urology
Analyzer, Gas, Carbon-Dioxide, Gaseous Phase (Capnograph)	Anesthesiology
Analyzer, Gas, Oxygen, Partial Pr., Blood Phase, Indwelling	Anesthesiology
Computer, Pulmonary Function Data	Anesthesiology
Continuous, Ventilator, Home Use	Anesthesiology
Electrode, Blood pH	Chemistry
Electrode, Cutaneous	Cns/Neurology
Flowmeter, Gas (Oxygen), Calibrated	Anesthesiology
Mask, Oxygen, Aerosol Administration	Anesthesiology
Mixer, Breathing Gases, Anesthesia Inhalation	Anesthesiology
Monitor, Carbon-Dioxide, Cutaneous	Anesthesiology
Monitor, Oxygen, Cutaneous	Anesthesiology
Oximeter, Ear	Cardiovascular
Oximeter, Intracardiac	Cardiovascular
Rebreathing Unit	Anesthesiology
Spirometer, Diagnostic (Respirometer)	Anesthesiology
Spirometer, Monitoring (Volumeter)	Anesthesiology
Tube, Tracheostomy (W/Wo Connector)	Anesthesiology
Ventilator, Continuous (Respirator)	Anesthesiology
Ventilator, Continuous, Non-Life Supporting	Anesthesiology

RESPIRONICS COLORADO　800-345-6443
12301 N Grant St #190, Thornton, CO 80241　800-345-6443
FDA Number: 1718784　Fax: 303-255-9000
Web site: www.respironics.com
Medical Products Sales Volume: $2,000,000
Annual Revenue: $1-$5 Million
Total Employees: 285　Marketing Staff: 5　Sales Staff: 5
Ownership: RESPIRONICS PENNSYLVANIA
Stock Symbol: RESP
Traded On: NASDAQ
Quality System Registration Information: ISO9000; ISO9001
Produces/Sells CE-marked Devices: Y
Federal Procurement Eligibility: Small Business
Distribution: Manufacturer Direct
General Admin.: Dennis Metney/President, Chief Executive Officer
　Geoffrey Waters/Vice President, General Manager
Mktg./Adv.: Derek Glinsman/Manager Marketing

RESPIRONICS COLORADO　800-345-6443 *(cont'd)*
Robert Fary/Manager Sales

Attachment, Breathing, Positive End Expiratory Pressure	Anesthesiology
Circuit, Breathing (W Connector, Adapter, Y Piece)	Anesthesiology
Concentrator, Oxygen	Anesthesiology
Continuous Positive Airway Pressure Unit (CPAP, CPPB)	Anesthesiology
Monitor, Airway Pressure (Gauge/Alarm)	Anesthesiology
Monitor, Oxygen (Ventilatory) W/Wo Alarm	Anesthesiology
Oximeter, Finger	General
Ventilator, External Body, Negative Pressure, (Cuirass)	Anesthesiology
Ventilator, Other	Anesthesiology
Ventilator, Time Cycled (Iron Lung)	Anesthesiology
Ventilator, Volume (Critical Care)	Anesthesiology

RESPIRONICS GEORGIA, INC.　724-387-4559
175 Chastain Meadows Ct., Kennesaw, GA 30144-3724
FDA Number: 1040777
Web site: www.respironics.com
Medical Products Sales Volume: $494,000,000
Total Employees: 2600　Marketing Staff: 31　Sales Staff: 108
Ownership: Public
Stock Symbol: RESP
Traded On: NASDAQ
Quality System Registration Information: ISO9000; ISO9001; ISO9002; ISO9003
Produces/Sells CE-marked Devices: Y
Distribution: Manufacturer Direct, Manufacturer Through Distributor, OEM, Exporter
General Admin.: John Miclot/Chief Executive Officer
　Criag Reynolds/Chief Operating Officer
Mktg./Adv.: Geoff Waters/Vice President International Sales
　John Frank/Vice President Marketing
Research: Doug Mechlenburg/Vice President Research & Development

Analyzer, Gas, Oxygen, Continuous Monitor	Anesthesiology
Computer Software	General
Concentrator, Oxygen	Anesthesiology
Continuous Positive Airway Pressure Unit (CPAP, CPPB)	Anesthesiology
Meter, Peak Flow, Spirometry	Anesthesiology
Monitor, Apnea	General
Monitor, Neonatal, Heart Rate	General
Nebulizer, Medicinal	Ear/Nose/Throat
Oximeter, Pulse	General
Recorder, Long-Term, Trend	General
Recorder, Paper Chart	Cardiovascular
Simulator, ECG	Cardiovascular
Simulator, Respiration	Anesthesiology
Sleep Assessment Equipment	Cns/Neurology
Ventilator, Other	Anesthesiology

RESPIRONICS MISSOURI　978-659-4252
2039 Concourse Dr., St. Louis, MO 63146
FDA Number: 1937850
Web site: www.respironnics.com
Medical Products Sales Volume: $2,500,000
Annual Revenue: $1-$5 Million
Total Employees: 10　Marketing Staff: 2　Sales Staff: 2
Ownership: Public
Stock Symbol: RESP
Traded On: NASDAQ
Produces/Sells CE-marked Devices: N
Federal Procurement Eligibility: Small Business, Female Owned
Distribution: Manufacturer Direct, OEM, Service Direct
General Admin.: Dale E. Walters/Chief Executive Officer
　Matt Walters/President
Mktg./Adv.: Brian Guerra/Director Marketing
　Brian Guerra/Manager National Sales
Production: Brian Guerra/Manager Materials

Bilirubin (Total and Unbound) Neonate Test System	Chemistry
Pack, Hot Or Cold, Disposable	Physical Med
Phototherapy Unit, Neonatal	General
Temperature Strip, Forehead, Liquid Crystal	General
Thermometer, Chemical Color Change	General
Thermometer, Liquid Crystals	Surgery
Warmer, Heel, Infant	Physical Med

RESPIRONICS NEW JERSEY, INC.　800-804-3443
5 Wood Hollow Road,　973-571-2600
Parsippany, NJ 07054
FDA Number: 2243193　Fax: 973-857-9521
E-mail: Info@respironics.com
Web site: www.respironics.com
Year Founded: 1976
Total Employees: 25　Marketing Staff: 10　Sales Staff: 10
Ownership: Public
Stock Symbol: RESP
Traded On: NASDAQ
Quality System Registration Information: ISO9002
Produces/Sells CE-marked Devices: Y
Distribution: Manufacturer Direct, Manufacturer Through Distributor
General Admin.: Susan Lloyd/Vice President

RESPIRONICS NEW JERSEY, INC.   800-804-3443 *(cont'd)*

Mktg./Adv.: Dirk Von Hollen/Director Product Development
Mia Mischuk-O'Brien/Manager Advertising
Matt Conlon/Manager National Sales
Production: Lauren Ziegler/Director Quality Assurance

Compressor, Air, Portable	Anesthesiology
Exerciser, Respiratory	Anesthesiology
Meter, Peak Flow, Spirometry	Anesthesiology
Mouthpiece, Breathing	Anesthesiology
Nebulizer, Medicinal	Ear/Nose/Throat
Nebulizer, Medicinal, Non-Ventilatory (Atomizer)	Anesthesiology
Spirometer, Therapeutic (Incentive)	Anesthesiology

RESPIRONICS NOVAMETRIX, LLC.   724-387-4559
5 Technology Dr., Wallingford, CT 06492-1942

FDA Number: 1219324
Web site: www.respironics.com
Ownership: Public
Stock Symbol: RESP
Traded On: NASDAQ
Produces/Sells CE-marked Devices: N

Adapter, Y	Gastroenterology/Urology
Analyzer, Gas, Carbon-Dioxide, Gaseous Phase (Capnograph)	Anesthesiology
Analyzer, Gas, Oxygen, Gaseous Phase	Anesthesiology
Analyzer, Gas, Oxygen, Partial Pr., Blood Phase, Indwelling	Anesthesiology
Attachment, Breathing, Positive End Expiratory Pressure	Anesthesiology
Computer, Pulmonary Function Data	Anesthesiology
Electrode, Blood pH	Chemistry
Electrode, Cutaneous	Cns/Neurology
Flowmeter, Gas (Oxygen), Calibrated	Anesthesiology
Mask, Oxygen, Aerosol Administration	Anesthesiology
Monitor, Airway Pressure (Gauge/Alarm)	Anesthesiology
Monitor, Carbon-Dioxide, Cutaneous	Anesthesiology
Monitor, Oxygen, Cutaneous	Anesthesiology
Oximeter, Ear	Cardiovascular
Oximeter, Intracardiac	Cardiovascular
Rebreathing Unit	Anesthesiology
Spirometer, Monitoring (Volumeter)	Anesthesiology

RESPIRONICS, INC   800-345-6443   724-387-5200
1010 Murry Ridge Ln.,
Murrysville, PA 15668

FDA Number: 2518422   *Fax:* 724-387-5010
Web site: www.respironics.com
Annual Revenue: $25-$50 Million
Year Founded: 1976
Total Employees: 4200   *Marketing Staff:* 15   *Sales Staff:* 25
Ownership: Public
Stock Symbol: RESP
Traded On: NASDAQ
Quality System Registration Information: ISO9001
Produces/Sells CE-marked Devices: Y
Federal Procurement Eligibility: Small Business
Distribution: Manufacturer Direct, OEM
General Admin.: Gerald E. McGinnis/Chairman
Daniel J. Bevevino/Chief Financial Officer, Vice President
John L. Miclot/President, Chief Executive Officer
William Lacourciere/President, Chief Executive Officer
Steven P. Fulton/Vice President, General Counsel
Joseph Vincent/Vice President, General Manager
Mktg./Adv.: Phil Nuzzo/Director Marketing
Russell Hayden/Director National Accounts
Craig B. Reynolds/Executive Vice President, Chief Operating Officer Marketing
Patrick Shannon/Manager International Marketing & Sales
Production: Les Mace/Director Engineering
Robert Schiffman/Director Quality Assurance
Joel Maynard/Vice President Operations

Analyzer, Gas, Carbon-Dioxide, Partial Pressure, Blood	Anesthesiology
Analyzer, Gas, Oxygen, Partial Pressure, Blood Phase	Anesthesiology
Attachment, Breathing, Positive End Expiratory Pressure	Anesthesiology
Drain, Tee (Water Trap)	Anesthesiology
Electrode, Transcutaneous, Carbon-Dioxide	Anesthesiology
Electrode, Transcutaneous, Oxygen	Anesthesiology
Humidifier, Respiratory Gas, (Direct Patient Interface)	Anesthesiology
Mask, Gas, Anesthesia	Anesthesiology
Monitor, Airway Pressure (Gauge/Alarm)	Anesthesiology
Monitor, Cardiac Output, Flowmeter	Cardiovascular
Oximeter, Finger	General
Oximeter, Pulse	General
Spirometer, Diagnostic (Respirometer)	Anesthesiology
Ventilator, Emergency, Manual (Resuscitator)	Anesthesiology
Ventilator, External Body, Negative Pressure, (Cuirass)	Anesthesiology
Ventilator, Non-Continuous (Respirator)	Anesthesiology

RESPIRONICS, INC. SLEEP THERAPY   724-387-4559
312 Alvin Dr., New Kensington, PA 15068

FDA Number: 300722052
Ownership: Public

RESPIRONICS, INC. SLEEP THERAPY   724-387-4559 *(cont'd)*

Stock Symbol: RESP
Traded On: NASDAQ
Produces/Sells CE-marked Devices: N

Ventilator, Non-Continuous (Respirator)	Anesthesiology

RESPOND INDUSTRIES, INC.   1-800-523-8999   303-463-3200
9500 Woodend Rd., Edwardsville, KS 66111

FDA Number: n/a   *Fax:* 303-940-0867
E-mail: info@respondindustries.com
Web site: www.respondindustries.com
Total Employees: 4   *Marketing Staff:* 2   *Sales Staff:* 1
Ownership: Private
Produces/Sells CE-marked Devices: N
Distribution: Manufacturer Through Distributor

Bandage, Adhesive	Surgery
Bandage, Elastic	General
Canister, Liquid Oxygen, Portable	Anesthesiology
Fiber, Absorbent	General
Kit, First Aid	Surgery
Mouthpiece, Breathing	Anesthesiology
Pack, Hot Or Cold, Disposable	Physical Med
Pad, Alcohol	General
Sheet, Burn	General
Sling, Arm	Physical Med
Splint, Extremity, Non-Inflatable, External	Surgery

RESPONSE BIOMEDICAL CORP.   888-591-5577   604-456-6010
1781 75th Ave. W.,
Vancouver, BC V6P 6 Canada

FDA Number: 3004205692   *Fax:* 604-456-6066
E-mail: info@responsebio.com
Web site: www.responsebio.com
Year Founded: 1991
Total Employees: 50
Ownership: Public
Stock Symbol: RBM
Traded On: TSX Venture Exchange
Produces/Sells CE-marked Devices: Y

RESPONSE GENETICS INC.   323-224-3900
1640 Marengo St., Los Angeles, CA 90033

FDA Number: n/a   *Fax:* 323-224-3096
Web site: http://www.responsegenetics.com
Year Founded: 1999
Ownership: Private
Produces/Sells CE-marked Devices: N
General Admin.: Ms. Kathleen Danenberg/President, Chief Executive Officer
Ms. Denise Mcnairn/Vice President, General Counsel
Production: Ms. Janine Cooc/Vice President Regulatory Affairs
Finance: Mr. David O'Toole/Chief Financial Officer

REST ASSURED INC.   800-852-7378   602-437-9201
4006 S. 21st Street, PO Box 163,
Phoenix, AZ 85040

FDA Number: n/a   *Fax:* 602-437-8857
E-mail: racustomserve2@qwest.net
Web site: www.restassuredinc.com
Medical Products Sales Volume: $1,800,000
Annual Revenue: $0-$1 Million
Year Founded: 1978
Total Employees: 22   *Marketing Staff:* 1   *Sales Staff:* 1
Ownership: Private
Produces/Sells CE-marked Devices: N
Federal Procurement Eligibility: Small Business, Minority Owned, Female Owned
Distribution: Manufacturer Direct, Service Direct, Exclusive Distributor, Exporter
General Admin.: Ms. Shirleen D. Fossum/President
Mr. Kenneth A. Rohde/Vice President
Mktg./Adv.: Mr. Gary L. Monson/Director Marketing & Sales
Production: Mr. Gary L. Monson/Director Quality Assurance & Regulatory Affairs
Research: Mr. Gary L. Monson/General Manager Research
Finance: Ms. Janel C. Rohde/Vice President, Treasurer

Commode (Toilet)	General

RESTORATION ROBOTICS, INC   (650) 965-3612
1383 Shorebird Way, Mountain View, CA 94043

FDA Number: n/a   *Fax:* (650) 965-3624
E-mail: contactus@restorationrobotics.com
Web site: www.restorationrobotics.com
Year Founded: 2007
Ownership: Private
Produces/Sells CE-marked Devices: N
General Admin.: Mr. Mohan Bodduluri/Chief Technology Officer
Mr. James McCollum/President, Chief Executive Officer
Mr. Miguel Canales/Vice President
Ms. Lena Vinitskaya/Vice President Legal Affairs, Corporate Counsel

RESTORATION ROBOTICS, INC
(650) 965-3612 *(cont'd)*
Production: Mr. Kevin O'Brien/Vice President Manufacturing & Engineering

RESTORATIVE CARE OF AMERICA INC
800-627-1595
727-573-1595
12221 33rd Street N.,
Saint Petersburg, FL 33716
FDA Number: 1051118   Fax: 727-573-1886
E-mail: inquire@rcai.com
Web site: www.rcai.com
Medical Products Sales Volume: $10,000,000
Annual Revenue: $5-$10 Million
Year Founded: 1975
Total Employees: 91   Marketing Staff: 3   Sales Staff: 30
Ownership: Private
Quality System Registration Information: ISO9001
Produces/Sells CE-marked Devices: Y
Federal Procurement Eligibility: Small Business, VA Contract
Distribution: Manufacturer Direct, Manufacturer Through Distributor, Exporter
General Admin.: Bud Hess/President, Chief Executive Officer
Mktg./Adv.: Connie Wassermann/Manager Advertising
   Nancy Tiller/Manager Contract Sales
   Nancy Tiller/Manager International Sales
Production: Jerry Kelly/Director Quality Assurance
   Fred Kenefsky/Manager Materials
Research: Steve Sensabaugh/Manager Research & Development

Immobilizer, Elbow	Orthopedics
Immobilizer, Knee	Orthopedics
Orthosis, Limb Brace	Physical Med
Orthosis, Thoracic	Physical Med
Splint, Abduction, Congenital Hip Dislocation	Physical Med
Splint, Hand, And Component	Physical Med
Splint, Molded, Plastic	Orthopedics
Splint, Other	Orthopedics
Support, Elbow	Orthopedics
Support, Foot	Orthopedics
Support, Knee	Physical Med
Support, Wrist	Physical Med

RESTORATIVE HEALTH SERVICES
615-225-6090
800 Nw Broad Street, Suite 126, Mboro, TN 37129
FDA Number: 3003897775

Orthosis, Cranial	Cns/Neurology

RESTORATIVE MEDICAL, INC.
270-422-5454
332 E Broadway, Brandenburg, KY 40108
FDA Number: 1528759

Joint, Hip, External Brace	Physical Med
Joint, Knee, External Brace	Physical Med
Orthosis, Limb Brace	Physical Med
Orthosis, Lumbosacral	Physical Med
Splint, Temporary Training	Physical Med
Support, Arm	Physical Med

RESTORATIVE THERAPIES INC.
(800) 609-9166
443 552-0401
907 South Lakewood Ave.,
Baltimore, MD 21224
FDA Number: 3004733458   Fax: (410) 878-2466
E-mail: support@restorative-therapies.com
Web site: www.restorative-therapies.com
Ownership: Private
Produces/Sells CE-marked Devices: N

Biofeedback Device	Cns/Neurology
Exerciser, Powered	Anesthesiology
Stimulator, Neuromuscular, External Functional	Cns/Neurology

RESTORE MEDICAL INC.
904-296-9600
6743 Southpoint Drive, North, Jacksonville, FL 32216
FDA Number: 3003968839   Fax: 904-296-6457
E-mail: rsjaxwebmaster@medtronic.com
Web site: www.restoremedical.com
Year Founded: 1999
Ownership: Medtronic, Inc.
Produces/Sells CE-marked Devices: N

Device, Anti-Snoring	Ear/Nose/Throat

RETIGO INC, T.C.
   See Statcorp, Inc.

RETONE, INC.
866-864-3271
4280 Sunrise Rd., Eagan, MN 55122
FDA Number: 2134242
Ownership: Private
Produces/Sells CE-marked Devices: N

Hearing-Aid	Ear/Nose/Throat

RETRACTABLE TECHNOLOGIES, INC.
888-806-2626
972-294-1010
511 Lobo Lane, Little Elm, TX 75068
FDA Number: 1647137   Fax: 972-292-3600
E-mail: rti@vanishpoint.com
Web site: www.vanishpoint.com

RETRACTABLE TECHNOLOGIES, INC.
888-806-2626 *(cont'd)*
Medical Products Sales Volume: $11,000,000
Annual Revenue: $10-$25 Million
Year Founded: 1994
Total Employees: 90
Ownership: Public
Stock Symbol: RVP
Traded On: AMEX
Quality System Registration Information: ISO9001
Produces/Sells CE-marked Devices: Y
Federal Procurement Eligibility: Small Business
Distribution: Manufacturer Through Distributor
General Admin.: Mr. Douglas Cowen/Chief Financial Officer, Vice President
   Steve Wisner/Executive Vice President
   Thomas J. Shaw/President, Chief Executive Officer
Mktg./Adv.: Mr. Shayne Blythe/Director Marketing & Sales
   Judy Zhu/Director Product Development
   Kathryn Duesman/Manager Sales Training
   Russell Kuhlman/Vice President Sales
Production: Mr. Lawrence Salerno/Director Operations

Catheter, Intravascular, Therapeutic, Short-term Less Than 30 Days	General
Needle, Hypodermic, Single Lumen, Reprocessed	General
Set, Administration, Intravenous, Needle-Free	General
Syringe, Antistick	General
Syringe, Other	General
Syringe, Piston	General

RETROACTIVE BIOSCIENCE
859-431-4660
One Moock Road, Suite 3, Wilder, KY 41071
FDA Number: 3004363278   Fax: 859-392-2750
E-mail: cust_service@retroactivebioscience.com
Web site: www.retroactivebioscience.com
Medical Products Sales Volume: $2,300,000
Year Founded: 1999
Total Employees: 5
Ownership: Private
Quality System Registration Information: ISO9000
Produces/Sells CE-marked Devices: Y
Federal Procurement Eligibility: Small Business
Distribution: Manufacturer Direct, Manufacturer Through Distributor, OEM, Exclusive Distributor, Exporter
Medical Admin.: Dr. Ronald Thompson/Medical Director
Mktg./Adv.: Mr. Justin Thompson/Director Business Development
   Mr. Robert Williams/Vice President Global Marketing
Production: Mr. James Thompson/Vice President, General Manager Regulatory Affairs
Research: Mr. Robert Hassman/Managing Partner

Lubricant, Patient	General

REU
   See Recreation Equipment Unlimited, Inc.

REVALESIO CORPORATION
253-922-2600
5102 20th Street East, Building 100, Tacoma, WA 98424
FDA Number: 3006282168

Bandage, Liquid	Surgery
Solution, Saline(wound Dressing)	Surgery

REVELATION ENGINEERING
   See Revelation Industries

REVELATION INDUSTRIES
800-833-2139
406-587-5978
101 East Oak Street, Bozeman, MT 59715
FDA Number: n/a   Fax: 406-587-5930
E-mail: info@revelationindustries.com
Web site: www.revelationindustries.com
Medical Products Sales Volume: $2,300,000
Annual Revenue: $0-$1 Million
Year Founded: 1987
Total Employees: 125   Sales Staff: 1
Ownership: Private
Produces/Sells CE-marked Devices: N
Federal Procurement Eligibility: Small Business
Distribution: Manufacturer Direct, Manufacturer Through Distributor
General Admin.: Steve Nettik/President
   Ben Lindeman/Vice President

Labeler, X-Ray Film	Radiology

REVERE HEALTHCARE LTD.
800-826-4900
847-516-4900
10 Spring St., Cary, IL 60013
FDA Number: n/a   Fax: 847-516-9941
E-mail: information@reverehc.com
Web site: www.reverehc.com
Medical Products Sales Volume: $700,000
Annual Revenue: $0-$1 Million
Year Founded: 1985
Total Employees: 10   Marketing Staff: 1   Sales Staff: 1
Ownership: Private
Produces/Sells CE-marked Devices: N

MANUFACTURER PROFILES

REVERE HEALTHCARE LTD.   800-826-4900 *(cont'd)*
Federal Procurement Eligibility: Small Business
Distribution: Service Direct
General Admin.: Grant Shumway/President
  Service, Consulting   General

REVERSE MEDICAL CORPORATION   877.639.0081
13700 Alton Parkway, Suite 167,   949.215.0660
Irvine, CA 92618
FDA Number: 3007170829   *Fax:* 949.215.0661
E-mail: info@reversemed.com
Web site: www.reversemed.com
Ownership: Private
Produces/Sells CE-marked Devices: N
General Admin.: Mr. Michael Henson/Chairman
         Mr. Brian Strauss/Chief Technology Officer
         Mr. Gerard Harper/Director
         Mr. Jeffery Valko/President, Chief Executive Officer
Mktg./Adv.: Mr. Joe Glab/National Sales Manager
Research: Ms. Lynn Shimada/Vice President Engineering
  Device, Retrieval, Percutaneous   Cardiovascular

REVISION OPTICS   949-707-2740
25651 Atlantic Ocean Drive, Suite A1, Lake Forest, CA 92630
FDA Number: n/a   *Fax:* 949-707-2744
E-mail: info@revisionoptics.com
Web site: http://www.revisionoptics.com
Ownership: Private
Produces/Sells CE-marked Devices: N
General Admin.: Mr. Randy Alexander/Chairman
         Mr. John Kilcoyne/President, Chief Executive Officer
Medical Admin.: Ms. Lynne Archer/Vice President Clinical Affairs
Production: Mr. Ali Dahi/Vice President Process Development
         Ms. Audrey Munnerlyn/Vice President Regulatory Affairs
Research: Mr. Keith Holliday/Vice President Research & Development
Finance: Mr. Louis Bunn/Chief Financial Officer
  Implant, Corneal   Ophthalmology

REVOLUTION EYEWEAR, INC.   310-777-8399
997 Flower Glen Rd., Simi Valley, CA 93065
FDA Number: 2087485
  Frame, Spectacle (Eyeglasses)   Ophthalmology
  Sunglasses (Including Photosensitive)   Ophthalmology

REVOLUTIONS MEDICAL CORP.   843-971-6917
2073 Shell Ring Circle, Mount Pleasant, SC 29466
FDA Number: n/a   *Fax:* 843-971-6917
E-mail: sales@revolutionsmedical.com
Web site: www.revolutionsmedical.com
Ownership: Public
Stock Symbol: RMCP
Traded On: OTC Bulletin
Produces/Sells CE-marked Devices: N
General Admin.: Rondald Wheet/Chief Executive Officer, Chairman
         Thomas O'Brien/President
  Syringe, Antistick   General
  Syringe, Piston   General

REVTEK INDUSTRIES, LLC   503-659-1650
4288 S.E. International Way, Portland, OR 97222
FDA Number: n/a   *Fax:* 503-659-2931
E-mail: sales@revtek.com
Web site: www.revtek.com
Medical Products Sales Volume: $9,000,000
Annual Revenue: $5-$10 Million
Year Founded: 2000
Total Employees: 97   *Marketing Staff:* 1   *Sales Staff:* 4
Ownership: Private
Quality System Registration Information: ISO9002
Federal Procurement Eligibility: Small Business
Distribution: Manufacturer Direct, Manufacturer Through Manufacturer Reps
General Admin.: Ralph Carter/President, Chief Executive Officer
Mktg./Adv.: Rhodes Gustafson/Manager Advertising
         Rhodes Gustafson/Vice President Marketing & Sales
Production: Dennis Reinking/Director Quality Assurance
  Component, Metal, Other   General

REXAM CARTONS
See Keller Crescent

REXHAM CORP.
See Keller Crescent

REXHAM INDUSTRIAL
See Keller Crescent

REXHAM PACKAGING
See Keller Crescent

REXTON, A DIVISION OF SIEMENS HEARING   763-553-0787
INSTRUMENTS, IN.
5010 Cheshire Lane North, Suite 2, Plymouth, MN 55446
FDA Number: 1419512   *Fax:* 763-553-9129
Web site: www.rexton.com
Ownership: Siemens Ag
Stock Symbol: SI
Traded On: NYSE
Produces/Sells CE-marked Devices: N
  Audiometer   Ear/Nose/Throat
  Hearing-Aid   Ear/Nose/Throat

REXTON, INC.
See REXTON, A DIVISION OF SIEMENS HEARING INSTRUMENTS, IN.

REZNIK INSTRUMENT, INC.   847-673-3444
7337 North Lawndale, Skokie, IL 60076
FDA Number: 1419997
Ownership: Private
Produces/Sells CE-marked Devices: N
  Accessories, Photographic, Endoscopic   Gastroenterology/Urology
  Cannula, Suprapubic, With Trocar   Gastroenterology/Urology
  Electrosurgical Unit, Anesthesiology Accessories   Surgery
  Forceps, Surgical, Gynecological   Obstetrics/Gynecology
  Illuminator, Fiberoptic (For Endoscope)   Gastroenterology/Urology
  Insufflator, Laparoscopic   Obstetrics/Gynecology
  Laparoscope, Gynecologic   Obstetrics/Gynecology
  Needle, Endoscopic   Gastroenterology/Urology
  Sound, Uterine   Obstetrics/Gynecology

RF DESIGN, INC.   810-632-6000
10143 Bergin Rd., Howell, MI 48843
FDA Number: 1834183
  Apron, Lead, Dental   Dental And Oral

RF INDUSTRIES, INC.   800-233-1728
7610 Miramar Road, San Diego, CA 92126-4202   858-549-6340
FDA Number: 2032351   *Fax:* 858-549-6345
E-mail: rfi@rfindustries.com
Web site: www.rfindustries.com
Medical Products Sales Volume: $15,200,000
Annual Revenue: $5-$10 Million
Year Founded: 1979
Total Employees: 87   *Marketing Staff:* 3   *Sales Staff:* 6
Ownership: Public
Stock Symbol: RFIL
Traded On: NASDAQ
Quality System Registration Information: ISO9000; ISO9001
Produces/Sells CE-marked Devices: N
Federal Procurement Eligibility: Small Business
Distribution: Manufacturer Through Distributor, OEM
General Admin.: Howard Hill/President, Chief Executive Officer
         Terri Gross/Vice President Human Resources
         Joe La Fay/Vice President, General Manager
Mktg./Adv.: Linda Heida/Manager Advertising
         Manny Gutsche/Vice President Marketing & Sales
Production: Ronnie Rice/Director Quality Assurance
         Diane Nelson/Manager Materials
         Conrad Neri/Vice President Manufacturing
         Bob Macias/Vice President Product Assurance & Regulatory Affairs
Research: J. David McReynolds/Research & Development Associate
  Component, Electronic   General
  Current Limiter, Patient Leads   Cardiovascular
  Monitor, ECG   Cardiovascular

RF SURGICAL INC.
See RF Surgical Systems, Inc.

RF SURGICAL SYSTEMS INC. TECHNICAL CENTER
See RF Surgical Systems, Inc.

RF SURGICAL SYSTEMS INC.   760-994-8198
TECHNICAL CENTER
9740 Appaloosa Road, Suite 150, San Diego, CA 92131
FDA Number: 3005883396
Web site: http://www.rfsurg.com/
Medical Products Sales Volume: $12,000,000
Annual Revenue: $10-$25 Million
Ownership: Private
Produces/Sells CE-marked Devices: N
  Counter, Sponge, Surgical   Surgery
  Sponge, Gauze   Dental And Oral

RF SURGICAL SYSTEMS, INC.   425-283-0678
3326 160th Avenue SE, Suite 220, Bellevue, WA 98008
FDA Number: n/a   *Fax:* 425-283-0677
E-mail: info@rfsurg.com
Web site: http://www.rfsurg.com
Ownership: Private
Produces/Sells CE-marked Devices: N

RF SURGICAL SYSTEMS, INC.   425-283-0678 (cont'd)
General Admin.: Dr. Jeffery Scott/Chairman
Mktg./Adv.: Mr. Matt DePiero/Sales Manager

RF TECHNOLOGIES   800-669-9946
3125 N. 126th St., Brookfield, WI 53005   **262-790-1771**
FDA Number: n/a   Fax: 262-790-1784
E-mail: info@rft.com
Web site: www.rft.com
Annual Revenue: $10-$25 Million
Year Founded: 1987
Total Employees: 150   Marketing Staff: 1   Sales Staff: 30
Ownership: Private
Produces/Sells CE-marked Devices: Y
Federal Procurement Eligibility: Small Business, GSA Contract
Distribution: Manufacturer Direct, Manufacturer Through Manufacturer Reps, OEM, Exporter
General Admin.: Mr. Mark Harwood/President
   Glenn Jonas/President, Chief Executive Officer
Mktg./Adv.: Mr. Greg Wingrove/Vice President Corporate Accounts
Research: Mr. Wyndham Gary/Vice President Engineering
Finance: Mr. Joseph Siekierski/Chief Financial Officer
Communication Equipment	General
Communication System, Emergency Alert, Personal	General
Communication System, Room Status	General
Elevator, Other	General
Monitor, Bed Occupancy	General
Nurse Call System	General
Pager, Non-Radio	General
Security Equipment/Supplies	General

RF TECHNOLOGIES, INC.
See Rf Technologies

RG ELECTRONICS, INC.   888-877-5682
100 Spring Creek Dr., Liberty Hill, TX 78642
FDA Number: 1651164
Ownership: Private
Produces/Sells CE-marked Devices: N
Monitor, Bed Patient	General

RGI MEDICAL MANUFACTURING INC.   352-378-3633
2321 N.w. 66th Ct., Ste. W4, Gainesville, FL 32653
FDA Number: 3004994611
Connector, Catheter	Surgery
Twister, Wire	Orthopedics

RHAMDEC INC.   800-4-MYDESC
P.O. Box 4296, Santa Clara, CA 95056   **408-495-5590**
FDA Number: n/a   Fax: 408-496-5593
E-mail: sales@mydesc.com
Web site: www.mydesc.com
Total Employees: 4   Marketing Staff: 1
Ownership: Private
Produces/Sells CE-marked Devices: N
Federal Procurement Eligibility: Small Business, Minority Owned
Distribution: Manufacturer Direct
General Admin.: Ronald H. Arima/President
Mktg./Adv.: Si Arima/Director Marketing & Sales
Accessories, Wheelchair	Physical Med

RHEIN MEDICAL, INC.   800-637-4346
5460 Beaumont Center Blvd., Suite 500   **813-885-5050**
Suite 500
Tampa, FL 33634
FDA Number: 1051791   Fax: 813-885-9346
E-mail: info@rheinmedical.com
Web site: www.rheinmedical.com
Medical Products Sales Volume: $4,300,000
Year Founded: 1988
Total Employees: 18
Ownership: Private
Quality System Registration Information: ISO9000; ISO9001; ISO9002; ISO9003
Produces/Sells CE-marked Devices: Y
Federal Procurement Eligibility: Small Business, VA Contract
Distribution: Manufacturer Direct, Manufacturer Through Distributor, Manufacturer Through Manufacturer Reps, OEM, Service Direct, Exclusive Distributor, Importer, Exporter
General Admin.: John A. Bee/President, Chief Executive Officer
Production: Carl E. Wortham/Vice President Operations
Aspirator, Ophthalmic	Ophthalmology
Clamp, Surgical, General & Plastic Surgery	Surgery
Container, Sterilization (Tray)	General
Curette, Ophthalmic	Ophthalmology
Cystotome, Ophthalmic	Ophthalmology
Forceps, General & Plastic Surgery	Surgery
Forceps, Ophthalmic	Ophthalmology
Forceps, Tissue	Surgery
Hook, Ophthalmic	Ophthalmology

RHEIN MEDICAL, INC.   800-637-4346 (cont'd)
Knife, Keratome	Ophthalmology
Knife, Ophthalmic	Ophthalmology
Knife, Scalpel	Surgery
Needle, Ophthalmic	Ophthalmology
Retractor, Ophthalmic	Ophthalmology
Scissors, Iris	Ophthalmology
Scissors, Ophthalmic	Ophthalmology
Scissors, Plastic Surgery (Dissecting)	Surgery
Medical Product Subsidiaries (Listed Separately)
Rhein Mfg., Inc.

RHEIN MFG., INC.   314-997-1775
2269 Grissom Dr., St. Louis, MO 63146
FDA Number: 1932214
Blade, Scalpel	Surgery
Forceps, Ophthalmic	Ophthalmology
Needle, Aspiration And Injection, Disposable	Surgery
Retractor, Ophthalmic	Ophthalmology

RHEOLOGICS, INC.   610-524-5427
15 East Uwchlan Avenue, Suite 414, Exton, PA 19341
FDA Number: 2531989   Fax: 610-524-9440
E-mail: info@rheologics.com
Web site: www.rheologics.com
Medical Products Sales Volume: $300,000
Year Founded: 1997
Total Employees: 5   Marketing Staff: 1   Sales Staff: 1
Ownership: Private
Produces/Sells CE-marked Devices: N
Federal Procurement Eligibility: Small Business
General Admin.: Mr. Ray Mannion/President, Chief Operating Officer
   Dr. Anders H. Boss/Vice President
   Mr. Dick Johnson/Vice President
Production: Mr. Nathan Krieger/Product Engineer
   Mr. Bill Hogenauer/Vice President Tech. Development
Viscometer, Plasma	Chemistry

RHEONIX   607-257-1242
22 Thornwood Drive, Ithaca, NY 14850
FDA Number: n/a   Fax: 607-257-0979
E-mail: info@rheonix.com
Web site: http://www.rheonix.com
Ownership: Private
Produces/Sells CE-marked Devices: N
General Admin.: Mr. Gregory Galvin/Chief Executive Officer, Chairman
   Mr. Peng Zhou/Chief Scientific Officer, Senior Vice President
   Mr. Tony Eisenhunt/President
Mktg./Adv.: Mr. Richard Montagna/Senior Vice President Corporate Development
Production: Mr. Lincoln Young/Director Engineering
Finance: Mr. Christopher Smith/Chief Financial Officer

RHODES INC., M.H.   800-548-4637
105 Nutmeg Rd. S., South Windsor, CT 06074   **860-673-3281**
FDA Number: n/a   Fax: 860-673-8633
E-mail: customer-service@mhrhodes.com
Web site: www.mhrhodes.com
Medical Products Sales Volume: $15,000,000
Annual Revenue: $10-$25 Million
Total Employees: 200   Sales Staff: 9
Ownership: OWOSSO CORP.
Stock Symbol: RHMH
Traded On: NASDAQ
Produces/Sells CE-marked Devices: N
Federal Procurement Eligibility: Small Business
Distribution: Manufacturer Direct, Manufacturer Through Manufacturer Reps, OEM
General Admin.: J. Morelli/President
Mktg./Adv.: H. Matles/Vice President Marketing & Sales
Timer, General Laboratory	Hematology

RHODES MEDICAL PRODUCTS INC.   904-233-0928
1116 Celebrant Dr., Jacksonville, FL 32225
FDA Number: 3004031664
Ownership: Private
Produces/Sells CE-marked Devices: N
Holder, Head, Radiographic	Radiology

RHYTEC INCORPORATED   781-474-9832
130 Turner Street, Building 2, South Waltham, MA 02453
FDA Number: 3004948955
Electrosurgical Unit, Cutting & Coagulation Device	Surgery

RHYTHMLINK INTERNATIONAL, LLC   866-633-3754
1140 First St. South, Columbia, SC 29209   **803-252-1222**
FDA Number: 1067162   Fax: 803-252-1111
E-mail: sales@rhythmlink.com
Web site: www.rhythmlink.com
Ownership: Private
Produces/Sells CE-marked Devices: N

RHYTHMLINK INTERNATIONAL, LLC 866-633-3754 (cont'd)

Distribution: Manufacturer Direct
General Admin.: Shawn Regan/Chief Executive Officer
          Michael O'Leary/Chief Operating Officer
Mktg./Adv.: Lori Melton/Director Marketing & Communications

Electrode, Cutaneous	Cns/Neurology
Electrode, Electroencephalographic	Cns/Neurology
Electrode, Needle	Cns/Neurology
Electrode, Needle, Diagnostic Electromyograph	Physical Med
Instrument, Manual, General Surgical	Surgery
Stimulator, Nerve, ENT	Ear/Nose/Throat
Syringe, Piston	General

RICCA CHEMICAL COMPANY LLC 817-461-5601
1490 Lammers Pike, Batesville, IN 47006

FDA Number: 3006365273
Ownership: Private
Produces/Sells CE-marked Devices: N

Counter, Platelet, Manual	Hematology
Diazonium Colorimetry, Urobilinogen (Urinary, Non-Quant.)	Chemistry
Fixative, Acid Containing	Pathology
Fixative, Alcohol Containing	Pathology
Fixative, Metallic Containing	Pathology
Fluid, Bouin's	Pathology
Fluid, Red Cell Diluting	Hematology
Fluid, White Cell Diluting	Hematology
Formaldehyde (Formalin, Formol)	Pathology
Formalin, Neutral Buffered	Pathology
Reagent, General Purpose	Pathology
Solution, Copper Sulfate, For Specific Gravity Test	Hematology
Solution, Isotonic	Hematology
Solution, Pathology, Carnoy's	Pathology
Solution, Pathology, Decalcifier, Acid Containing	Pathology
Solution, Pathology, Formalin-Alcohol-Acetic Acid	Pathology
Solution, Pathology, Lugol's	Pathology
Solution, Pathology, Orth's	Pathology
Solution, Pathology, Zenker's	Pathology
Stain, Brilliant Cresyl Blue	Pathology
Stain, Carbol Fuchsin	Pathology
Stain, Crystal Violet, Histology	Pathology
Stain, Dye Solution	Pathology
Stain, Eosin Y	Pathology
Stain, Giemsa	Pathology
Stain, Gold Chloride	Pathology
Stain, Grams Iodine	Pathology
Stain, Hematoxylin	Pathology
Stain, Hematoxylin, Harris's	Pathology
Stain, Metanil Yellow	Pathology
Stain, Methylene Blue	Pathology
Stain, Papanicolau	Pathology
Stain, Reagent, Schiff	Pathology
Stain, Reticulocyte	Hematology
Stain, Safranin	Pathology
Stain, Toluidine Blue	Pathology
Stain, Wright's	Pathology
Sudan III	Pathology
Turbidimetric Method, Protein Or Albumin (Urinary)	Chemistry

RICCA CHEMICAL COMPANY LLC 888-467-4222
1841 Broad St., Pocomoke City, MD 21851 817-461-5601

Fax: 817-795-8848

FDA Number: 1125908
E-mail: llowy@riccachemical.com
Web site: riccachemical.com
Year Founded: 2000
Ownership: Private
Quality System Registration Information: ISO9001
Produces/Sells CE-marked Devices: N
Federal Procurement Eligibility: Small Business
Distribution: Manufacturer Through Distributor

Brilliant Cresyl Blue	Hematology
Counter, Platelet, Manual	Hematology
Crystal Violet	Hematology
Diazonium Colorimetry, Urobilinogen (Urinary, Non-Quant.)	Chemistry
Fixative, Acid Containing	Pathology
Fixative, Alcohol Containing	Pathology
Fixative, Metallic Containing	Pathology
Fluid, Bouin's	Pathology
Fluid, White Cell Diluting	Hematology
Formaldehyde (Formalin, Formol)	Pathology
Formalin, Neutral Buffered	Pathology
Gold Chloride (Colorimetric), Bromide	Toxicology
Reagent, General Purpose	Pathology
Solution, Copper Sulfate, For Specific Gravity Test	Hematology
Solution, Isotonic	Hematology
Solution, Pathology, Carnoy's	Pathology
Solution, Pathology, Decalcifier, Acid Containing	Pathology
Solution, Pathology, Formalin-Alcohol-Acetic Acid	Pathology
Solution, Pathology, Lugol's	Pathology
Solution, Pathology, Orth's	Pathology
Solution, Pathology, Zenker's	Pathology
Stain, Carbol Fuchsin	Pathology

RICCA CHEMICAL COMPANY LLC 888-467-4222 (cont'd)

Stain, Crystal Violet, Histology	Pathology
Stain, Dye Solution	Pathology
Stain, Eosin Y	Pathology
Stain, Giemsa	Pathology
Stain, Grams Iodine	Pathology
Stain, Hematoxylin	Pathology
Stain, Hematoxylin, Harris's	Pathology
Stain, Metanil Yellow	Pathology
Stain, Methylene Blue	Pathology
Stain, Papanicolau	Pathology
Stain, Reagent, Schiff	Pathology
Stain, Reticulocyte	Hematology
Stain, Safranin	Pathology
Stain, Toluidine Blue	Pathology
Stain, Wright's	Pathology
Turbidimetric Method, Protein Or Albumin (Urinary)	Chemistry

RICCA CHEMICAL COMPANY, LLC 817-461-5601
448 West Fork Dr., Arlington, TX 76012

FDA Number: 1625587   Fax: 817-795-8848
E-mail: customerservice@riccachemical.com
Web site: www.riccachemical.com
Year Founded: 1975
Ownership: Private
Produces/Sells CE-marked Devices: N

Counter, Platelet, Manual	Hematology
Diazonium Colorimetry, Urobilinogen (Urinary, Non-Quant.)	Chemistry
Fixative, Acid Containing	Pathology
Fixative, Alcohol Containing	Pathology
Fixative, Metallic Containing	Pathology
Fluid, Bouin's	Pathology
Fluid, Red Cell Diluting	Hematology
Fluid, White Cell Diluting	Hematology
Formaldehyde (Formalin, Formol)	Pathology
Formalin, Neutral Buffered	Pathology
Reagent, General Purpose	Pathology
Reagent, Protein, Total	Chemistry
Solution, Copper Sulfate, For Specific Gravity Test	Hematology
Solution, Isotonic	Hematology
Solution, Pathology, Carnoy's	Pathology
Solution, Pathology, Decalcifier, Acid Containing	Pathology
Solution, Pathology, Formalin-Alcohol-Acetic Acid	Pathology
Solution, Pathology, Lugol's	Pathology
Solution, Pathology, Orth's	Pathology
Solution, Pathology, Zenker's	Pathology
Stain, Brilliant Cresyl Blue	Pathology
Stain, Carbol Fuchsin	Pathology
Stain, Crystal Violet, Histology	Pathology
Stain, Dye Solution	Pathology
Stain, Eosin Y	Pathology
Stain, Giemsa	Pathology
Stain, Gold Chloride	Pathology
Stain, Grams Iodine	Pathology
Stain, Hematoxylin	Pathology
Stain, Hematoxylin, Harris's	Pathology
Stain, Metanil Yellow	Pathology
Stain, Methylene Blue	Pathology
Stain, Papanicolau	Pathology
Stain, Safranin	Pathology
Stain, Toluidine Blue	Pathology
Stain, Wright's	Pathology
Sudan III	Pathology
Turbidimetric Method, Protein Or Albumin (Urinary)	Chemistry

RICE LAKE WEIGHING SYSTEMS 800-472-6703
230 W. Coleman St., Rice Lake, WI 54868-9902 715-234-9171

FDA Number: n/a   Fax: 715-234-6967
E-mail: prodinfo@rlws.com
Web site: www.rlws.com
Medical Products Sales Volume: $60,000,000
Year Founded: 1945
Total Employees: 300   Marketing Staff: 15   Sales Staff: 40
Ownership: Private
Quality System Registration Information: ISO9001
Produces/Sells CE-marked Devices: N
Federal Procurement Eligibility: Small Business, GSA Contract
Distribution: Manufacturer Through Distributor
General Admin.: Mark Johnson/President, Chief Executive Officer
Mktg./Adv.: Jim Sexton/Vice President Marketing
          Frank Page/Vice President Sales

Balance, Analytical	Chemistry
Balance, Electronic	Chemistry
Balance, Mechanical	Chemistry
Computer Software	General
Scale, Chair, Transfer	General
Scale, Infant	General
Scale, Stand-On	General

RICH-MAR CORPORATION
800-762-4665
PO Box 879, 15499 E 590 Rd, Inola, OK 74036-9802 **918-543-2222**
FDA Number: 1623423 *Fax:* 918-543-3334
E-mail: info@richmarweb.com
Web site: www.richmarweb.com
Medical Products Sales Volume: $2,300,000
Annual Revenue: $5-$10 Million
Year Founded: 1972
Total Employees: 32
Ownership: Private
Quality System Registration Information: ISO9001
Produces/Sells CE-marked Devices: N
Federal Procurement Eligibility: Small Business, GSA Contract
Distribution: OEM, Exclusive Distributor
General Admin.: Ken Coffey/President
Mktg./Adv.: Greg Dorholt/Director Marketing
Production: David Richards/Manager Regulatory Affairs

Diathermy, Ultrasonic (Physical Therapy)	Physical Med
Electrode, Other	General
Gel, Ultrasonic Transmission	General
Lamp, Infrared	Physical Med
Stimulator, Muscle, Electrical-Powered (EMS)	Physical Med
Stimulator, Ultrasound, Muscle	Physical Med

RICHARD DANZ AND SONS, INC.
212-697-5722
104 East 40th St., New York, NY 10016
FDA Number: 2428741
Medical Products Sales Volume: $2,000,000
Year Founded: 1938
Total Employees: 50
Ownership: Private
Federal Procurement Eligibility: Small Business

Conformer, Ophthalmic	Ophthalmology
Prosthesis, Eye, Internal (Sphere)	Surgery

RICHARD SCIENTIFIC, INC.
800-840-3030
285 Bel Marin Keys Blvd, Suite M, **415-883-2888**
Novato, CA 94949
FDA Number: n/a *Fax:* 415-382-1922
E-mail: info@richardscientific.com
Web site: www.richardscientific.com
Annual Revenue: $1-$5 Million
Year Founded: 1985
Total Employees: 14 *Marketing Staff:* 2 *Sales Staff:* 9
Ownership: Private
Quality System Registration Information: ISO9000
Federal Procurement Eligibility: Small Business
Distribution: Exclusive Distributor
General Admin.: Richard Devereaux/Chief Executive Officer
Mktg./Adv.: Jim Powers/Vice President Sales

Chromatography, Liquid, Performance, High	Toxicology

RICHARD WESCHLER/VPR&D
See Cdc Products Corp.

RICHARD WOLF MEDICAL INSTRUMENTS CORP.
800-323-9653

353 Corporate Woods Pkwy., **847-913-1113**
Vernon Hills, IL 60061
FDA Number: 1418749 *Fax:* 847-913-1488
E-mail: marketing@richardwolfusa.com
Web site: www.richardwolfusa.com
Medical Products Sales Volume: $21,900,000
Year Founded: 1972
Total Employees: 175 *Marketing Staff:* 25 *Sales Staff:* 87
Ownership: Private
Quality System Registration Information: ISO9000
Produces/Sells CE-marked Devices: Y
Federal Procurement Eligibility: Small Business, GSA Contract
Distribution: Manufacturer Through Manufacturer Reps, Importer, Exporter
General Admin.: Mr. Alfons Notheis/Chief Executive Officer
Mktg./Adv.: Mr. Kevin Gallagher/Director Marketing & Sales

Accessories, Arthroscope	Orthopedics
Accessories, Cleaning, Endoscopic	Gastroenterology/Urology
Accessories, Photographic, Endoscopic	Gastroenterology/Urology
Applicator, Clip (Forceps)	General
Arthroscope	Orthopedics
Aspirator, Surgical	Surgery
Aspirator, Thoracic (Suction Unit)	Cardiovascular
Atomizer And Tip, ENT	Ear/Nose/Throat
Biopsy Instrument, Mechanical, Gastrointestinal	Gastroenterology/Urology
Biopsy Instrument, Suction	Gastroenterology/Urology
Bit, Drill	Orthopedics
Bronchoscope, Non-Rigid	Ear/Nose/Throat
Bronchoscope, Rigid	Ear/Nose/Throat
Bronchoscope, Rigid, Non-Ventilating	Anesthesiology
Bronchoscope, Rigid, Ventilating	Anesthesiology
Brush, Cytology, Endoscopic	Gastroenterology/Urology

RICHARD WOLF MEDICAL
800-323-9653 *(cont'd)*

Bulb, Inflation (Endoscope)	Gastroenterology/Urology
Cable, Electrosurgical Unit	Surgery
Camera, Still, Endoscopic	Surgery
Camera, Still, Surgical	Surgery
Camera, Television, Endoscopic (Without Audio)	Surgery
Camera, Video, Endoscopic	General
Cannula, Drainage, Arthroscopy	Orthopedics
Cannula, Extraction, Appendix	Surgery
Cannula, Suction, Uterine	Obstetrics/Gynecology
Cannula, Suprapubic, With Trocar	Gastroenterology/Urology
Carrier, Sponge, Endoscopic	Gastroenterology/Urology
Cart, Equipment, Video	General
Catheter, Suction (Tracheal Aspirating Tube)	Anesthesiology
Choledochoscope, Flexible Or Rigid	Gastroenterology/Urology
Clamp, Penile	Gastroenterology/Urology
Clip, Tubal Occlusion	Obstetrics/Gynecology
Coagulator, Hysteroscopic (With Accessories)	Obstetrics/Gynecology
Coagulator, Laparoscopic, Unipolar	Obstetrics/Gynecology
Coagulator/Cutter, Endoscopic, Bipolar	Obstetrics/Gynecology
Coagulator/Cutter, Endoscopic, Unipolar	Obstetrics/Gynecology
Colposcope	Obstetrics/Gynecology
Container, Sterilization (Tray)	General
Culdoscope	Obstetrics/Gynecology
Cystometer, Electrical Recording	Gastroenterology/Urology
Cystoscope	Gastroenterology/Urology
Cystourethroscope	Gastroenterology/Urology
Dilator, Blunt	Surgery
Dilator, Fascia, Umbilical	Surgery
Dilator, Urethral, Mechanical	Gastroenterology/Urology
Electrocautery Unit, Endoscopic	Obstetrics/Gynecology
Electrode, Electrosurgical, Active (Blade)	Surgery
Electrode, Electrosurgical, Active, Foot Controlled	Surgery
Electrosurgical Equipment, General Purpose	Surgery
Electrosurgical Unit, General Purpose (ESU)	Surgery
Endoscope, Direct Vision	Surgery
Endoscope, Electronic (Videoendoscope)	Surgery
Endoscope, Flexible	Gastroenterology/Urology
Endoscope, Neurological	Cns/Neurology
Endoscope, Rigid	Surgery
Endoscope, Transcervical (Amnioscope)	Obstetrics/Gynecology
Equipment, Suction/Irrigation, Laparoscopic	Surgery
Esophagoscope (Flexible Or Rigid)	Ear/Nose/Throat
Fitting, Luer	General
Forceps, Biopsy, Gynecological	Obstetrics/Gynecology
Forceps, Electrosurgical	Surgery
Forceps, Endoscopic	Gastroenterology/Urology
Forceps, Grasping, Atraumatic	Surgery
Forceps, Grasping, Flexible Endoscopic	Gastroenterology/Urology
Forceps, Grasping, Traumatic	Surgery
Forceps, Lung	Surgery
Forceps, Specimen	Gastroenterology/Urology
Forceps, Sponge	Surgery
Forceps, Stone Manipulation	Gastroenterology/Urology
Gastroscope, General & Plastic Surgery	Gastroenterology/Urology
Gastroscope, Rigid	Gastroenterology/Urology
Generator, Power, Electrosurgical	Surgery
Headlight, ENT	Ear/Nose/Throat
Heater, Perineal, Radiant, Non-Contact	Obstetrics/Gynecology
Holder, Guide, Catheter	Cardiovascular
Holder, Laparoscope	Obstetrics/Gynecology
Holder, Leg, Arthroscopy	Orthopedics
Holder/Scissors, Needle, Laparoscopic	Surgery
Hysteroscope	Obstetrics/Gynecology
Illuminator, Fiberoptic (For Endoscope)	Gastroenterology/Urology
Insert, Tubal Occlusion	Obstetrics/Gynecology
Instrument, Dissecting, Laparoscopic	Surgery
Instrument, Dissecting, Myoma, Laparoscopic	Surgery
Instrument, Knot Tying, Suture, Laparoscopic	Surgery
Instrument, Needle Holder/Knot Tying	Surgery
Instrument, Passing, Suture, Laparoscopic	Surgery
Instrument, Surgical, Powered, Pneumatic	Orthopedics
Insufflator, Carbon-Dioxide, Automatic (For Endoscope)	Gastroenterology/Urology
Insufflator, Hysteroscopic	Obstetrics/Gynecology
Insufflator, Laparoscopic	Obstetrics/Gynecology
Insufflator, Other	Surgery
Lamp, Endoscopic, Incandescent	Surgery
Laparoscope, General & Plastic Surgery	Surgery
Laparoscope, Gynecologic	Obstetrics/Gynecology
Laryngoscope, Rigid	Anesthesiology
Laryngostroboscope	Ear/Nose/Throat
Light Source, Endoscope, Xenon Arc	Surgery
Light Source, Endoscopic	Obstetrics/Gynecology
Light Source, Fiberoptic, Routine	Gastroenterology/Urology
Light, Surgical, Endoscopic	Surgery
Lithotriptor, Electro-Hydraulic, Percutaneous	Gastroenterology/Urology
Lithotriptor, Extracorporeal Shock-wave, Urological	Gastroenterology/Urology
Lithotriptor, Ultrasonic	Gastroenterology/Urology
Mediastinoscope	Surgery
Mediastinoscope, ENT	Ear/Nose/Throat
Microscope, Surgical	Ear/Nose/Throat
Microscope, Surgical, General & Plastic Surgery	Surgery

MANUFACTURER PROFILES

RICHARD WOLF MEDICAL   800-323-9653 *(cont'd)*

Monitor, Video, Endoscope	General
Nasopharyngoscope (Flexible Or Rigid)	Ear/Nose/Throat
Needle, Aspiration, Cyst, Laparoscopic	Surgery
Needle, Endoscopic	Gastroenterology/Urology
Needle, Insufflation, Laparoscopic	Surgery
Needle, Pneumoperitoneum, Simple	Gastroenterology/Urology
Nephroscope, Flexible	Gastroenterology/Urology
Nephroscope, Rigid	Gastroenterology/Urology
Obturator, Endoscopic	Gastroenterology/Urology
Otoscope	Ear/Nose/Throat
Printer, Image, Video	General
Probe, Electrocauterization, Multi-Use	Surgery
Probe, Suction, Irrigator/Aspirator, Laparoscopic	Surgery
Proctoscope	Surgery
Punch, Biopsy	Gastroenterology/Urology
Rasp, Surgical, General & Plastic Surgery	Surgery
Recorder, Paper Chart	Cardiovascular
Recorder, Videotape/Videodisc	General
Resectoscope	Gastroenterology/Urology
Resectoscope Working Element	Gastroenterology/Urology
Retractor, Abdominal	Surgery
Retractor, Bladder	Gastroenterology/Urology
Sampler, Blood, Fetal	Obstetrics/Gynecology
Sheath, Endoscopic	Gastroenterology/Urology
Sigmoidoscope, Rigid, Non-Electrical	Gastroenterology/Urology
Snare, Endoscopic	Surgery
Solution, Instrument, Laparoscopic, Anti-Fog	General
Speculum, Vaginal, Metal	Obstetrics/Gynecology
Stripper, Vein, Reusable	Surgery
System, Camera, 3-Dimensional	Surgery
Tape, Television & Video, Endoscopic	Gastroenterology/Urology
Teaching Attachment, Endoscopic	Gastroenterology/Urology
Telescope, Rigid, Endoscopic	Gastroenterology/Urology
Tenaculum, Uterine	Obstetrics/Gynecology
Thoracoscope	Cardiovascular
Trainer, Laparoscopy	Surgery
Transilluminator, AC-Powered, Other	Ophthalmology
Transilluminator, Battery-Powered	Ophthalmology
Trocar, Abdominal	Gastroenterology/Urology
Trocar, Amniotic	Obstetrics/Gynecology
Trocar, Antrum	Ear/Nose/Throat
Trocar, Gallbladder	Gastroenterology/Urology
Trocar, Gastro-Urology	Gastroenterology/Urology
Trocar, Laryngeal	Ear/Nose/Throat
Trocar, Other	General
Trocar, Short	Surgery
Trocar, Thoracic	Cardiovascular
Tubal Occlusive Device	Obstetrics/Gynecology
Tube, Bronchial (W/Wo Connector)	Anesthesiology
Tube, Smoke Removal, Endoscopic	Gastroenterology/Urology
Ureteroscope	Gastroenterology/Urology
Ureterotome	Gastroenterology/Urology
Urethrometer	Gastroenterology/Urology
Urethroscope	Gastroenterology/Urology
Urethrotome	Gastroenterology/Urology
Urodynamic Measurement System	Gastroenterology/Urology
Uroflowmeter	Gastroenterology/Urology
Vaginoscope	Obstetrics/Gynecology
Ventilator, Pressure Cycled (IPPB Machine)	Anesthesiology
Warmer, Endoscope	Surgery
Yoke, Medical Gas	Anesthesiology

RICHARD-ALLAN SCIENTIFIC   269-544-5628
4481 Campus Dr., Kalamazoo, MI 49008
FDA Number: 1831638

Accessories, Microtome	Pathology
Buffer, pH	Hematology
Cassette, Tissue	Pathology
Container, Embedding	Pathology
Container, Specimen Mailer And Storage	Pathology
Container, Specimen, Non-sterile	General
Fixative, Acid Containing	Pathology
Fixative, Alcohol Containing	Pathology
Fixative, Formalin Containing	Pathology
Formalin, Neutral Buffered	Pathology
Fuchsin, Basic	Pathology
Hematoxylin Weigert's	Pathology
Immunohistochemistry Reagents And Kits	Pathology
Microscope, Light	Pathology
Periodic Acid	Pathology
Reagent, General Purpose	Pathology
Solution, Copper Sulfate, For Specific Gravity Test	Hematology
Solution, Pathology, Decalcifier, Acid Containing	Pathology
Solution, Pathology, Lugol's	Pathology
Solution, Pathology, Zenker's	Pathology
Stain, Aniline Blue	Pathology
Stain, Biebrich Scarlet	Pathology
Stain, Carbol Fuchsin	Pathology
Stain, Chemical Solution	Pathology
Stain, Congo Red	Pathology
Stain, Crystal Violet, Histology	Pathology

RICHARD-ALLAN SCIENTIFIC   269-544-5628 *(cont'd)*

Stain, Dye Powder	Pathology
Stain, Dye Solution	Pathology
Stain, Eosin Y	Pathology
Stain, Fast Green	Pathology
Stain, Giemsa	Pathology
Stain, Gold Chloride	Pathology
Stain, Grams Iodine	Pathology
Stain, Hematoxylin	Pathology
Stain, Hematoxylin, Harris's	Pathology
Stain, Hematoxylin, Mayer's	Pathology
Stain, Iron	Pathology
Stain, Jenner Stain	Pathology
Stain, Light Green	Pathology
Stain, Mallory's Trichrome	Pathology
Stain, Methenamine Silver	Pathology
Stain, Methyl Green	Pathology
Stain, Methylene Blue	Pathology
Stain, Microbiological	Microbiology
Stain, Mucicarmine	Pathology
Stain, Nuclear Fast Red	Pathology
Stain, Papanicolau	Pathology
Stain, Pyronin	Pathology
Stain, Reagent, Schiff	Pathology
Stain, Reticulocyte	Hematology
Stain, Safranin	Pathology
Stain, Van Gieson's	Pathology
Stain, Weigert's Iron Hematoxylin	Pathology
Stain, Wright's	Pathology
Tourniquet, Non-Pneumatic, Surgical	Surgery

RICHARD-JAMES, INC.   978-532-0666
2 Centennial Dr., Peabody, MA 01960
FDA Number: 1221628   *Fax:* 978-532-0034
E-mail: drichard@richard-james.com
Total Employees: 9   *Marketing Staff:* 1
Ownership: Private
Quality System Registration Information: ISO9001
Produces/Sells CE-marked Devices: Y
Federal Procurement Eligibility: Small Business
Distribution: OEM
General Admin.: Wayne Richard/President

Fluid, Intraocular	Ophthalmology

RICHARDS LABORATORIES, INC.   800-453-1210
55 E. Center, Pleasant Grove, UT 84062-2233   801-785-2500
FDA Number: n/a
Web site: richardslabs.infogenix.com
Annual Revenue: $0-$1 Million
Ownership: Private
Produces/Sells CE-marked Devices: N
Federal Procurement Eligibility: Small Business
Distribution: Service Direct

Service, Consulting	General

RICHARDS MEDICAL COMPANY
See Smith & Nephew Inc.- Orthopaedics Division

RICHARDS MICRO-TOOL, INC.   508-746-6900
250 Nicks Road,, Plymouth, MA 02360-2800
FDA Number: 122211   *Fax:* 508-747-4339
E-mail: sales@richardsmicrotool.com
Web site: www.richardsmicrotool.com
Medical Products Sales Volume: $2,900,000
Annual Revenue: $5-$10 Million
Year Founded: 1961
Total Employees: 40   *Marketing Staff:* 1   *Sales Staff:* 3
Ownership: Private
Quality System Registration Information: ISO9002
Produces/Sells CE-marked Devices: N
Federal Procurement Eligibility: Small Business, GSA Contract
Distribution: Manufacturer Direct, OEM, Service Direct, Importer
General Admin.: Michael Fucillo/General Manager
Mktg./Adv.: Phil Samuels/Director Marketing
        Dave Paquette/Manager National Sales
        Mike Fucillo/Vice President Business Development
Production: Ron Harris/Manager Materials

Contract Manufacturing	General
Drill, Bone	Orthopedics
Drill, Cranial	Cns/Neurology
Osteotome (Orthopedic)	Surgery
Reamer	Orthopedics

RICHARDS SURGICAL MANUFACTURING CO.
See Smith & Nephew Inc.- Orthopaedics Division

RICHARDS-WILCOX, INC.   800-253-5668
600 S. Lake St., Aurora, IL 60506   630-897-6951
FDA Number: n/a   *Fax:* 630-897-6994
E-mail: mail@richardswilcox.com

RICHARDS-WILCOX, INC.   800-253-5668 (cont'd)
Web site: www.richardswilcox.com
Medical Products Sales Volume: $40,000,000
Annual Revenue: $50-$100 Million
Year Founded: 1880
Total Employees: 210   *Sales Staff:* 30
Ownership: Private
Produces/Sells CE-marked Devices: N
Federal Procurement Eligibility: Small Business, GSA Contract, VA Contract
Distribution: Manufacturer Through Distributor, Manufacturer Through Manufacturer Reps
General Admin.: Manfred Haiderer/President
  Cabinet Casework, General Purpose   General
  Office Equipment   General
  Office Product   General

RICHARDSON ACCESS ELEVATOR INC.   800-268-7745
1244 Trafalgar St.,   **519-455-0906**
London, ONT N5Z-1 Canada
FDA Number: n/a   *Fax:* 519-453-6993
E-mail: sales@richardsonaccess.com
Web site: www.richardsonaccess.com
Year Founded: 1987
Ownership: Private
Produces/Sells CE-marked Devices: N
Distribution: Exclusive Distributor, Importer

RICHARDSON ELECTRONICS CANADA LTD.   800-348-5580
4 Paget Rd., Unit 1,   **905-789-3000**
Brampton, ONT L6T-5 Canada
FDA Number: n/a   *Fax:* 905-789-3050
E-mail: jfenn@rell.com
Web site: www.rell.com
Year Founded: 1947
Total Employees: 250
Ownership: Private
Produces/Sells CE-marked Devices: N
Distribution: Exclusive Distributor

RICHARDSON LIMITED   602-843-6365
11633 N. 38th Avenue, Phoenix, AZ 85029
FDA Number: 3005722915
Ownership: Private
Produces/Sells CE-marked Devices: N
  Lens, Contact (Other Material)   Ophthalmology

RICHARDSON PRODUCTS, INC.   888-928-7297
9408 Gulfstream Road, Frankfort, IL 60423   **815-464-3575**
FDA Number: 3004526603   *Fax:* 815-464-3576
E-mail: RPI@RICHARDSONPRODUCTS.COM
Web site: www.richardsonproducts.com
Year Founded: 1989
Ownership: Private
Produces/Sells CE-marked Devices: N
  Accessories, Wheelchair   Physical Med
  Adapter, Hygiene   Physical Med
  Adaptor, Dressing   Physical Med
  Adaptor, Grooming   Physical Med
  Adaptor, Recreational   Physical Med
  Armrest, Wheelchair   Physical Med
  Bandage, Elastic   General
  Component, Exercise   Physical Med
  Compression Instrument   Orthopedics
  Cover, Mattress   General
  Depressor, Tongue   General
  Dynamometer, Non-Powered   Orthopedics
  Exerciser, Non-Measuring   Physical Med
  Gauge, Measuring   Ear/Nose/Throat
  Goniometer, Non-Powered   Orthopedics
  Helmet, Cranial, For Protective Use   Physical Med
  Joint, Knee, External Brace   Physical Med
  Mirror, General & Plastic Surgery   Surgery
  Mirror, Mouth   Dental And Oral
  Scale, Platform, Wheelchair   Physical Med
  Splint, Hand, And Component   Physical Med
  Tips And Pads, Cane, Crutch And Walker   Physical Med
  Transfer Aid   Physical Med
  Tray, Wheelchair   Physical Med
  Utensil, Food   Physical Med
  Utensil, Handicapped Aid   Physical Med

RICHARDSON-VICKS
  See Procter & Gamble

RICHLYN LABORATORIES
  See Global Pharmaeuticals: A Division Of Impax Labs Inc.

RICHMOND DIAGNOSTICS, INC.   732-246-2429
100 Jersey Ave., Suite 202-a,, Bldg. B,
New Brunswick, NJ 08901
FDA Number: 2248933
  Hematocrit Control   Hematology

RICHMOND PRODUCTS, INC.   505-275-2406
4400 Silver Se, Albuquerque, NM 87108
FDA Number: 1035253
  Chart, Visual Acuity   Ophthalmology
  Illuminator, Color Vision Plate   Ophthalmology
  Lens, Set, Trial, Ophthalmic   Ophthalmology
  Screen, Tangent, Felt (Campimeter)   Ophthalmology
  Screen, Tangent, Target   Ophthalmology
  Shield, Eye, Ophthalmic   Ophthalmology
  Tester, Color Vision   Ophthalmology

RICKMAN TOOL, INC.
  See Rochester Medical Implants

RICO SUCTION LABS, INC.   800-845-8490
326 MacArthur Ln., Burlington, NC 27217   **336-585-0313**
FDA Number: 1034117   *Fax:* 336-584-3661
E-mail: info@ricosuction.com
Web site: www.ricosuction.com
Medical Products Sales Volume: $300,000
Annual Revenue: $0-$1 Million
Year Founded: 1952
Total Employees: 2   *Marketing Staff:* 2   *Sales Staff:* 2
Ownership: Private
Quality System Registration Information: ISO9001
Produces/Sells CE-marked Devices: N
Federal Procurement Eligibility: Small Business, Female Owned, GSA Contract
Distribution: Manufacturer Direct, Manufacturer Through Distributor, OEM, Exporter
General Admin.: JOE MICHAEL/President, Chief Executive Officer
  Aspirator, Tracheal   Ear/Nose/Throat
  Bottle, Collection, Vacuum (Aspirator)   General
  Catheter, Suction (Tracheal Aspirating Tube)   Anesthesiology

RICON CORP.   800-322-2884
7900 Nelson Road,   **818-267-3000**
Panorama City, CA 91402
FDA Number: n/a   *Fax:* 818-267-3001
E-mail: sales@riconcorp.com
Web site: www.riconcorp.com
Medical Products Sales Volume: $17,000,000
Annual Revenue: $50-$100 Million
Year Founded: 1971
Total Employees: 300   *Marketing Staff:* 3   *Sales Staff:* 12
Ownership: Private
Quality System Registration Information: ISO9001
Produces/Sells CE-marked Devices: N
Distribution: Manufacturer Through Distributor, Manufacturer Through Manufacturer Reps, OEM, Exclusive Distributor, Exporter
General Admin.: William Baldwin/President
Mktg./Adv.: Oscar Pardinas/Vice President Marketing & Sales
          Jerry Dann/Vice President National Sales
Production: Stan Saucier/Vice President Engineering & Operations
Finance: Dave Chaimowitz/Chief Financial Officer
  Lift, Wheelchair   General

RIDALCO INDUSTRIES INC.   613-745-9161
1551 Michael St., Ottawa, ONT K1B-3T4 Canada
FDA Number: n/a   *Fax:* 613-745-6452
E-mail: info@ridalco.com
Web site: www.ridalco.com
Year Founded: 1946
Total Employees: 50
Ownership: Private
Produces/Sells CE-marked Devices: N
Distribution: Manufacturer Direct, Exporter

RIDEAU ORTHODONTIC MFG., LTD.   613-283-6841
69 Beckwith St N, Smiths Falls K7A 2B6 Canada
FDA Number: 9681560
  Retainer, Screw Expansion, Orthodontic   Dental And Oral

RIDGE DIAGNOSTICS INC.   877-743-4301
12390 El Camino Real, Suite 170, San Diego, CA 92130
FDA Number: n/a   *Fax:* 877-743-4301
Web site: http://www.ridgedx.com
Ownership: Private
Produces/Sells CE-marked Devices: N
General Admin.: Ms. Lonna Williams/Chief Executive Officer
          Dr. John Bilello/Chief Scientific Officer
          Dr. Bo Pi/Chief Technology Officer
Medical Admin.: Dr. Perry Renshaw/Chief Medical Officer

RIDGE DIAGNOSTICS INC.   877-743-4301 *(cont'd)*
Finance: Mr. David Vandertie/Chief Financial Officer

RIEGEL CONSUMER PRODUCTS DIV.   800-845-2232
P.O. Box E, 51 Riegel Road,   **803-275-2541**
Johnston, SC 29832
FDA Number: 9310060   Fax: 803-275-2219
E-mail: rbailey2@midsouth.rr.com
Web site: www.riegellinen.com
Total Employees: 600   *Marketing Staff:* 3   *Sales Staff:* 8
Ownership: Mount Vernon Mills Inc.
Produces/Sells CE-marked Devices: N
Distribution: Manufacturer Direct, Manufacturer Through Distributor, Importer
General Admin.: Bill Josey/President
Mktg./Adv.: Theresa Thornburg/Director Product Development
     Bob Bailey/Vice President Sales

Blanket, Infant	General
Cover, Mattress	General
Linen	General
Linen, Bed	General
Towel, Surgical	Surgery

RIEGEL TEXTILE
See Riegel Consumer Products Div.

RIESE ENTERPRISES, INC.
See Biosure, Inc.

RIFTON EQUIPMENT   800-571-8198
PO Box 260, Rifton, NY 12471-0260   **800-571-8198**
FDA Number: 6028514   Fax: 800-336-5948
E-mail: sales@rifton.com
Web site: www.rifton.com
Medical Products Sales Volume: $8,000,000
Annual Revenue: $5-$10 Million
Total Employees: 50   *Marketing Staff:* 6   *Sales Staff:* 30
Ownership: Private
Produces/Sells CE-marked Devices: Y
Federal Procurement Eligibility: Small Business
Distribution: Manufacturer Direct
General Admin.: John Rhodes/Chief Executive Officer
Mktg./Adv.: Clare Stober/Manager Advertising
     Jeff Kipphut/Vice President Marketing & Sales
Production: Hans Boller/Manager Regulatory Affairs
Research: Kirk Wareham/Vice President Research & Development

Aid, Living, Handicapped	General
Chair, Adjustable, Mechanical	Physical Med
Chair, Bath	General
Chair, Pediatric	General
Chair, Shower	General
Commode (Toilet)	General
Commode Seat	General
Equipment, Therapy, Handicapped/Physical	Physical Med
Lift, Patient	General
Patient Transfer Unit	General
Transfer Aid	Physical Med
Walker, Mechanical	Physical Med

RIGEL MEDICAL ELECTRONICS
See Marcal Medical, Inc.

RIGID FX ORTHOPEDICS, INCORPORATED   877-707-1404
9230 Neils Thompson Dr, Suite 111,   **512-443-7770**
Austin, TX 78758
FDA Number: 3003599693
Web site: www.rigidfx.com
Ownership: Private
Produces/Sells CE-marked Devices: N

Fixation Appliance, Multiple Component	Orthopedics

RILEY MEDICAL, INC.   800-245-3300
27 Wrights Landing, Auburn, ME 04210   **207-786-2775**
FDA Number: 1220906   Fax: 207-786-5553
E-mail: info@rileymedical.com
Web site: www.rileymed.com
Medical Products Sales Volume: $10,000,000
Annual Revenue: $5-$10 Million
Total Employees: 100   *Marketing Staff:* 2   *Sales Staff:* 6
Ownership: Symmetry Medical, Inc.
Stock Symbol: SMA
Traded On: NYSE
Quality System Registration Information: ISO9001
Produces/Sells CE-marked Devices: Y
Federal Procurement Eligibility: Small Business
Distribution: Manufacturer Direct, Manufacturer Through Distributor, OEM, Exclusive Distributor, Exporter
General Admin.: Edward Riley/Chief Executive Officer
     Edward Riley/President
Mktg./Adv.: Chris Melino/Director Marketing & Sales
Production: Richard Campbell/Manager Materials

RILEY MEDICAL, INC.   800-245-3300 *(cont'd)*

Container, Sterilization (Tray)	General
Packaging, Sterilization	General
Tray, Custom/Special Procedure	General
Tray, Sterilization, Instrument	Surgery
Tray, Surgical	Surgery

RIM MEDICAL, LLC.   828-859-2000
2160 Highway 292, PO Box 880, Inman, SC 29349
FDA Number: 3005853078   Fax: 858-777-3588
E-mail: info@rimmedical.com
Web site: www.rimdirect.com
Ownership: Private
Produces/Sells CE-marked Devices: N

RING COMMUNICATIONS, INC.   516-585-7464
57 Trade Zone Dr., Ronkonkoma, NY 11779-7343
FDA Number: n/a   Fax: 516-585-7410
E-mail: mail@ringcomm.com
Web site: www.ringcomm.com
Annual Revenue: $1-$5 Million
Total Employees: 9   *Marketing Staff:* 1   *Sales Staff:* 2
Ownership: Private
Produces/Sells CE-marked Devices: N
Federal Procurement Eligibility: Small Business
Distribution: Manufacturer Through Distributor
General Admin.: Peter R. McLean/President
Mktg./Adv.: Craig Krsanac/Vice President Sales
Production: Kjell Solem/Vice President Manufacturing

Communication System, Emergency Alert, Personal	General
Telephone Equipment	General

RINZ-L-O   248-548-3993
340 West Maplehurst, Ferndale, MI 48220
FDA Number: 1833589
Ownership: Private
Produces/Sells CE-marked Devices: N

Orthosis, Cervical	Physical Med
Pack, Hot Or Cold, Disposable	Physical Med
Support, Patient Position	Anesthesiology

RIPP RESTRAINTS, INC.   800-544-8344
1220 East Industrial Dr., PO Box 740071,   **386-775-2812**
Orange City, FL 32763
FDA Number: 1052735   Fax: 386-775-2912
E-mail: info@ripprestraints.com
Web site: www.ripprest.com
Ownership: Private
Produces/Sells CE-marked Devices: N

Restraint, Patient, Conductive	Anesthesiology

RISMED ONCOLOGY SYSTEMS   256-534-6993
2494 Washington Street, Huntsville, AL 35811-1663
FDA Number: 3003835335   Fax: 256-534-6996
E-mail: info@rismed.com
Web site: www.rismed.com
Medical Products Sales Volume: $500,000
Annual Revenue: $10-$25 Million
Year Founded: 1977
Total Employees: 6   *Marketing Staff:* 1   *Sales Staff:* 3
Ownership: Private
Produces/Sells CE-marked Devices: N
Federal Procurement Eligibility: Small Business, Minority Owned
Distribution: Manufacturer Direct
General Admin.: Jose A. Rodriguez/Chief Executive Officer, Chairman
     Liliana Di Nardo/President, General Manager
Mktg./Adv.: Daniel Alberto Rangel/Director Marketing
     Monica Machado/Manager International & National Sales

Accessories, Blood Circuit, Hemodialysis	Gastroenterology/Urology
Cannula, Hemodialysis	Gastroenterology/Urology
Concentrate, Dialysis, Hemodialysis (Liquid or Powder)	Gastroenterology/Urology
Dialysate Delivery System, Central Multiple Patient	Gastroenterology/Urology
Dialyzer, Capillary, Hollow Fiber (Hemodialysis)	Gastroenterology/Urology
Hemodialysis Unit (Kidney Machine)	Gastroenterology/Urology
Purification System, Water, Reverse Osmosis	Chemistry

RITA MEDICAL SYSTEMS
See Angiodynamics, Inc.

RITE TIME CORPORATION   800-266-2924
2950 East Dover St., Mesa, AZ 85213-6952   **480-832-1592**
FDA Number: 2030765   Fax: 480-641-6368
E-mail: sandra@RiteTime.com
Web site: www.FaceDownRecovery.com
Annual Revenue: $0-$1 Million
Ownership: Private
Produces/Sells CE-marked Devices: N
Federal Procurement Eligibility: Small Business, Female Owned
Distribution: Manufacturer Direct

RITE TIME CORPORATION   800-266-2924 (cont'd)

General Admin.: Mr. Alfred Heitz/President
Ms. Sandra Heitz Willwater/Vice President

Bed, Manual	General
Plinth	Physical Med

RITE-DENT MANUFACTURING CORP.   305-693-8626
3750 East 10th Court, Hialeah, FL 33013

FDA Number: 1064592   Fax: 305-693-8630
E-mail: info@ritedent.com
Web site: www.ritedent.com
Annual Revenue: $1-$5 Million
Year Founded: 1981
Total Employees: 10   *Marketing Staff:* 2   *Sales Staff:* 3
Ownership: Private
Produces/Sells CE-marked Devices: N
Federal Procurement Eligibility: Small Business, Minority Owned
Distribution: Manufacturer Direct, Manufacturer Through Distributor, Manufacturer Through Manufacturer Reps, Exclusive Distributor, Importer, Exporter
General Admin.: Dr. Oscar Lopez/Chief Executive Officer
Mr. Cesar Veliz/Chief Financial Officer, Vice President
Mktg./Adv.: Mr. Juan Carlos Cabello/Manager Accounts
Mrs. Maria Alvarado/Vice President Sales

Amalgamator, Dental, AC-Powered	Dental And Oral
Base, Denture, Relining, Repairing, Rebasing, Resin	Dental And Oral
Burr, Dental	Dental And Oral
Cement, Dental	Dental And Oral
Crown, Preformed	Dental And Oral
Dam, Rubber	Dental And Oral
Dental Cement w/out Zinc-Oxide Eugenol as an Ulcer Covering for Pain Relief	Dental And Oral
Dress, Surgical	Surgery
Gutta Percha	Dental And Oral
Liner, Cavity, Calcium Hydroxide	Dental And Oral
Material, Impression	Dental And Oral
Material, Impression Tray, Resin	Dental And Oral
Material, Tooth Shade, Resin	Dental And Oral
Matrix, Dental	Dental And Oral
Paper, Articulation	Dental And Oral
Point, Paper, Endodontic	Dental And Oral
Resin, Root Canal Filling	Dental And Oral
Sealant, Pit And Fissure, And Conditioner, Resin	Dental And Oral
Strip, Polishing Agent	Dental And Oral
Tooth Bonding Agent, Resin Restoration	Dental And Oral
Tray, Impression	Dental And Oral
Varnish, Cavity	Dental And Oral
Zinc Oxide Eugenol	Dental And Oral

RITTER MEDICAL PRODUCTS
See Midmark Corporation

RIVER MEDICAL, INC.
See Alaris Medical Systems, Inc

RIVERAIN MEDICAL GROUP   800-990-3387
3020 South Tech Blvd., Miamisburg, OH 45342   937-425-6811

FDA Number: 3005156333   Fax: 937-425-6493
E-mail: info@riverainmedical.com
Web site: http://www.riverainmedical.com
Year Founded: 2004
Ownership: Private
Produces/Sells CE-marked Devices: N
General Admin.: Dr. Diane Hirakawa/Chairman, Chief Executive Officer
Mr. Steve Worrell/Chief Technology Officer
Medical Admin.: Dr. David Fryd/Vice President Clinical Affairs
Mktg./Adv.: Mr. Rich Bares/Executive Vice President Marketing & Sales
Production: Mr. Kendall Cobb/Director Operations
Finance: Mr. David House/Chief Financial Officer

Analyzer, Medical Image	Radiology

RIVERBANK LABORATORIES   630-232-2207
2613 kaneville ct., PO Box 110, Geneva, IL 60134

FDA Number: 1416612   Fax: 630-232-7606
E-mail: riverbanklabs@aol.com
Web site: www.riverbanklabs.com
Medical Products Sales Volume: $500,000
Annual Revenue: $1-$5 Million
Year Founded: 1921
Total Employees: 12
Ownership: Private
Produces/Sells CE-marked Devices: N
Distribution: Manufacturer Through Distributor, Exporter
General Admin.: Robert Swanson/President, General Manager
Mktg./Adv.: Mary Robinson/Vice President Sales

Fork, Tuning, ENT	Ear/Nose/Throat
Hammer, Percussion	Cns/Neurology
Pinwheel	Cns/Neurology

RIVERPOINT MEDICAL   503-517-8001
809 Ne 25th Ave, Portland, OR 97232

FDA Number: 3006981798
Ownership: Private
Produces/Sells CE-marked Devices: N

Biopsy Instrument	Gastroenterology/Urology
Headlamp, Operating, Battery-Operated	Ophthalmology
Suture, Non-Absorbable, Silk	Surgery
Suture, Non-Absorbable, Synthetic, Polyamide	Surgery
Suture, Non-Absorbable, Synthetic, Polyester	Surgery
Suture, Non-Absorbable, Synthetic, Polyethylene	Surgery
Suture, Non-Absorbable, Synthetic, Polypropylene	Surgery

RIVERTRAIL MOBILITY   501-745-6790
369 Factory Road, Clinton, AR 72031

FDA Number: 3004433931
Ownership: Private
Produces/Sells CE-marked Devices: N

Wheelchair, Powered	Physical Med

RJL SYSTEMS, INC.   586-790-0200
33939 Harper Ave., Clinton Township, MI 48035

FDA Number: 1831675

Plethysmograph, Impedance	Cardiovascular

RK FROOM & CO., INC.   310-327-5125
903 Cunningham Lane, Salem, OR 97302

FDA Number: 3004198659

Armboard, Wheelchair	Physical Med
Component, Exercise	Physical Med
Splint, Traction	Orthopedics

RKL TECHNOLOGIES, INC.   800-738-8007
245 Citation Circle, Corona, CA 92880-2523   951-738-8000

FDA Number: 2031692   Fax: 951-738-8008
Web site: www.rkltech.com
Ownership: Private
Produces/Sells CE-marked Devices: N

Device, Spinal Vertebral Body Replacement	Orthopedics
Orthopedic Manual Surgical Instrument	Orthopedics

RLI PROFESSIONAL TECHNOLOGIES
See Rlisys Practice Solutions, Inc.

RLISYS PRACTICE SOLUTIONS, INC.   800-447-2205
One Aloha Lane, Peoria, IL 61615-1431   309-691-3700

FDA Number: n/a   Fax: 309-683-2203
E-mail: Mkane@rlisys.com
Web site: http://rlisys.com/
Annual Revenue: $5-$10 Million
Year Founded: 1984
Total Employees: 30   *Marketing Staff:* 2   *Sales Staff:* 3
Ownership: Division of THE SWATCH GROUP (U.S.) Inc.
Produces/Sells CE-marked Devices: N
Distribution: Manufacturer Direct
General Admin.: Martin Kane/President

Computer Software, Hospital/Nursing Management	General

RMC MEDICAL   800-332-0672
6940 State Road Bldg C,   215-824-4100
Philadelphia, PA 19154

FDA Number: n/a   Fax: 215-824-1371
E-mail: info@rmcmedical.com
Web site: www.rmcmedical.com
Annual Revenue: $0-$1 Million
Total Employees: 7   *Marketing Staff:* 1   *Sales Staff:* 1
Ownership: Private
Produces/Sells CE-marked Devices: N
Federal Procurement Eligibility: Small Business
Distribution: Manufacturer Through Distributor
General Admin.: Roger Linnemann/President
Mktg./Adv.: Lois White/Manager Sales
Gil Cosnett/Manager Sales Training

Service, Waste Management	General

RMED INTERNATIONAL   866-624-1403
675 Industrial Blvd., Delta, CO 81416-2811

FDA Number: n/a   Fax: 708-345-8290
Web site: www.tushies.com
Medical Products Sales Volume: $1,000,000
Annual Revenue: $0-$1 Million
Ownership: Public
Produces/Sells CE-marked Devices: N
Federal Procurement Eligibility: Small Business
Distribution: Manufacturer Direct, Importer, Exporter
General Admin.: Edward Reiss/Chairman
Brenda Schenk/President, Chief Executive Officer

Diaper, Pediatric	General

RMO, INC.
800-525-6375
650 West Colfax Avenue, Denver, CO 80204
303-592-8200
FDA Number: 1718476
Fax: 303-592-8209
E-mail: rmosales@rmortho.com
Web site: www.rmortho.com
Medical Products Sales Volume: $22,000,000
Annual Revenue: $25-$50 Million
Year Founded: 1933
Ownership: Private
Quality System Registration Information: ISO9001
Produces/Sells CE-marked Devices: Y
Distribution: Manufacturer Direct, Manufacturer Through Distributor, Exporter
General Admin.: Jody Hardy/President
Tony Zakhem/Vice Chairman

Adhesive, Bracket And Conditioner, Resin	Dental And Oral
Band, Elastic, Orthodontic	Dental And Oral
Band, Material, Orthodontic	Dental And Oral
Band, Preformed, Orthodontic	Dental And Oral
Bracket, Metal, Orthodontic	Dental And Oral
Bracket, Plastic, Orthodontic	Dental And Oral
Clasp, Preformed	Dental And Oral
Crown, Preformed	Dental And Oral
Cutter, Operative	Dental And Oral
Driver, Band, Orthodontic	Dental And Oral
Face Bow	Dental And Oral
Headgear, Extraoral, Orthodontic	Dental And Oral
Lock, Wire, And Ligature, Intraoral	Dental And Oral
Maintainer, Space Preformed, Orthodontic	Dental And Oral
Material, Impression	Dental And Oral
Mesh, Metal	Gastroenterology/Urology
Pliers, Orthodontic	Dental And Oral
Pusher, Band, Orthodontic	Dental And Oral
Retainer, Screw Expansion, Orthodontic	Dental And Oral
Spring, Orthodontic	Dental And Oral
Tray, Impression	Dental And Oral
Tube, Orthodontic	Dental And Oral
Tucker, Ligature, Orthodontic	Dental And Oral
Wire, Orthodontic	Dental And Oral

RMS COMPANY
763-783-5074
8600 Evergreen Blvd., Minneapolis, MN 55433-6036
FDA Number: 2183946
Fax: 763-786-1305
E-mail: bjohnson@machine.com
Web site: www.rmsmachining.com
Medical Products Sales Volume: $27,000,000
Annual Revenue: $50-$100 Million
Year Founded: 1967
Total Employees: 320   *Marketing Staff:* 6   *Sales Staff:* 16
Ownership: Cretex, Inc.
Quality System Registration Information: ISO9001
Produces/Sells CE-marked Devices: N
Federal Procurement Eligibility: Small Business
Distribution: Manufacturer Through Manufacturer Reps
General Admin.: Sue Osbakken/Manager Human Resources
Lee Zachman/President
Mktg./Adv.: Bruce Johnson/Director Marketing & Sales
Production: Patrick Biggins/Director Quality Assurance
Finance: Vicki Bentz/Director Finance

Component, Metal, Other	General
Component, Other	General
Contract Assembly	General
Contract Manufacturing	General

RMS INSTRUMENTS
905-677-5533
6877-1 Goreway Dr., Mississauga, ONT L4V 1L9 Canada
FDA Number: n/a
Fax: 905-677-5030
E-mail: rms@rmsinst.com
Web site: www.rmsinst.com
Total Employees: 15
Ownership: Private
Produces/Sells CE-marked Devices: N
Federal Procurement Eligibility: Small Business
Distribution: Manufacturer Direct, Manufacturer Through Manufacturer Reps, OEM

RMS MEDICAL PRODUCTS
800-624-9600
24 Carpenter Road, Chester, NY 10918
845-469-2042
FDA Number: n/a
Fax: 845-469-5518
E-mail: info@rmsmedicalproducts.com
Web site: www.repro-med.com
Medical Products Sales Volume: $3,000,000
Annual Revenue: $1-$5 Million
Year Founded: 1980
Total Employees: 20   *Marketing Staff:* 5   *Sales Staff:* 15
Ownership: Rms Medical Products
Produces/Sells CE-marked Devices: Y
Federal Procurement Eligibility: Small Business
Distribution: Manufacturer Direct, Manufacturer Through Distributor, Manufacturer Through Manufacturer Reps, Exporter

RMS MEDICAL PRODUCTS
800-624-9600 *(cont'd)*
General Admin.: Andy Selfon/Chief Executive Officer
Andrew Seafon/President
Mktg./Adv.: Manal Habib/Director Marketing
Ron Tortorella/Director Product Development
Keith Perlmutter/Vice President Marketing & Sales
Production: William Jablesnik/Manager Regulatory Affairs
Ron Tortorella/Vice President Manufacturing
Research: Andy Sealfon/Vice President Research & Development

Brush, Endometrial	Obstetrics/Gynecology
Curette, Uterine	Obstetrics/Gynecology
Electrocautery Unit, Gynecologic	Obstetrics/Gynecology
Kit, Biopsy	General
Stirrup	Gastroenterology/Urology

RNA MEDICAL, A DIVISION OF BIONOSTICS, INC.
800-533-6162
7 Jackson Road, Devens, MA 01434
978-772-9070
FDA Number: n/a
Fax: 978-772-9071
E-mail: info@rnamedical.com
Web site: www.rnamedical.com
Annual Revenue: $1-$5 Million
Total Employees: 100   *Marketing Staff:* 1   *Sales Staff:* 5
Ownership: Bionostics, Inc.
Quality System Registration Information: ISO9000
Produces/Sells CE-marked Devices: Y
Federal Procurement Eligibility: Small Business
Distribution: Manufacturer Through Manufacturer Reps, Exclusive Distributor
Mktg./Adv.: Paul Shea/Director Business Development
Dan Massucco/Director Sales
Patricia Gowdy/Marketing & Advertising Assistant
Michael J. Melville/Vice President Business Development
Production: Tara Simpson/Product Manager

Calibrator, Blood Gas	General
Control, Blood Gas	Chemistry
Control, Electrolyte (Assayed And Unassayed)	Chemistry
Control, Hemoglobin	Hematology
Tonometer (Calibration And Q.C. Of Blood Gas Instruments)	Chemistry

RND SIGNS
800-328-4009
7605 Equitable Drive, Eden Prairie, MN 55344
952-926-1315
FDA Number: n/a
Fax: 952-926-3840
E-mail: info@rndsigns.com
Web site: www.rndsigns.com
Medical Products Sales Volume: $270,000
Annual Revenue: $0-$1 Million
Year Founded: 1985
Total Employees: 5   *Sales Staff:* 2
Ownership: Private
Produces/Sells CE-marked Devices: N
Federal Procurement Eligibility: Small Business
Distribution: Manufacturer Direct
General Admin.: Deb Bielefeld/Office Manager
Richard Rendahl/President

Pouch, Telemetry	General

RNK PRODUCTS, INC.
612-414-0289
12700 Diamond Drive, Burnsville, MN 55337
FDA Number: 3004595287

Stethoscope, Electronic (Auscultoscope)	Cardiovascular

ROBELL RESEARCH, INC.
212-755-6577
635 Madison Ave., New York, NY 10022
FDA Number: 2437696
Fax: 212-755-3263
E-mail: info@supersmile.com
Web site: www.supersmile.com
Ownership: Private
Produces/Sells CE-marked Devices: N
Distribution: Manufacturer Direct, Manufacturer Through Distributor, Manufacturer Through Manufacturer Reps, Exclusive Distributor

Toothbrush, Manual	Dental And Oral

ROBERT B. SCOTT OCULARISTS OF FLORIDA, INC.
See KUBLY OCULAR PROSTHETICS INC.

ROBERT JOSEPH CRAIG SA DE CV
905-5600803
Blvd De Santa Monica 106-204, Jardines De, Tlalnepantla Mexico
FDA Number: 8030624

Electrode, Electrosurgical, Return (Ground, Dispersive)	Surgery

ROBERTS & GORDON CANADA, INC.
905-945-5403
76 Main St. West, Unit 10, Grimsby, ON L3M-1R6 Canada
FDA Number: n/a
Fax: 905-945-0511
Year Founded: 1923
Total Employees: 6
Ownership: Private
Produces/Sells CE-marked Devices: N

ROBERTS & GORDON CANADA, INC.   905-945-5403 *(cont'd)*
Distribution: Manufacturer Through Distributor, Manufacturer Through Manufacturer Reps

ROBERTS LABORATORY
See Conmed Corporation

ROBERTS OXYGEN CO., INC.   301-315-9090
17011 Railroad St., Gaithersburg, MD 20877
FDA Number: 1150053
  Gas, Calibrated (Specified Concentration)   Anesthesiology

ROBERTSON HARNESS   702-564-4286
261 West Cyress Dr., A, PO Box 90086, Henderson, NV 89009
FDA Number: 86703
E-mail: RobertsonHarness@cox.net
Web site: www.robertsonharness.com
Ownership: Private
Produces/Sells CE-marked Devices: N
  Treadmill, Powered   Physical Med

ROBI
See Allosource

ROBIN INSTRUMENTS INC.
See General Devices

ROBINS, A.H.
See Pfizer / Wyeth Consumer Healthcare Inc.

ROBINSON AUDIOLOGY LABORATORIES   810-754-3511
8033 East 10 Mile Rd., #104, Centerline, MI 48015
FDA Number: 1828921
Ownership: Private
Produces/Sells CE-marked Devices: N
  Hearing-Aid   Ear/Nose/Throat

ROBOMEDICA, INC.   877-762-6633
One Technology Drive, Bldg. C, Suite C-511, Irvine, CA 92618
FDA Number: 2032560
  Lift, Bath, Non-AC-Powered   General
  Lift, Patient   General

ROBOT COUPE USA, INC.,   815-722-8400
SCIENTIFIC-INDUSTRIAL DIV.
1101 Buell Avenue, Joliet, IL 60435
FDA Number: n/a   Fax: 815-722-3125
E-mail: robotcoupesi@comcast.net
Web site: www.robotcoupe-si.com
Annual Revenue: $0-$1 Million
Year Founded: 1992
Ownership: Private
Produces/Sells CE-marked Devices: N
Federal Procurement Eligibility: Small Business
Distribution: Manufacturer Through Distributor
General Admin.: Jay Williams/President
Mktg./Adv.: Tom McPeck/Vice President Marketing
  Mixer, Clinical Laboratory   Chemistry

ROBOT RESEARCH, INC., SENSOMATICS DIV.   858-642-2400
6795 Flanders Dr., San Diego, CA 92121
FDA Number: n/a
Ownership: Fischer Medical Technologies Inc.
Quality System Registration Information: ISO9000
Produces/Sells CE-marked Devices: Y
Distribution: Manufacturer Direct, Manufacturer Through Manufacturer Reps
  Monitor, Bed Patient   General

ROBOZ SURGICAL INSTRUMENT CO., INC.   800-424-2984
PO Box 10710, Gaithersburg, MD 20898-0710   301-590-0055
FDA Number: 1180552   Fax: 301-590-1290
E-mail: info@roboz.com
Web site: www.roboz.com
Medical Products Sales Volume: $3,400,000
Annual Revenue: $5-$10 Million
Year Founded: 1953
Total Employees: 20
Ownership: Private
Produces/Sells CE-marked Devices: Y
Federal Procurement Eligibility: Small Business
Distribution: Manufacturer Direct
Mktg./Adv.: Raymond Hodgson/General Manager, Manager International Marketing and Sales
  Applier, Surgical Staple   Surgery
  Applier, Surgical, Clip   Surgery
  Blade, Scalpel   Surgery
  Cannula, Other   General
  Clamp, Bulldog   Surgery
  Clip, Suture   Surgery
  Clip, Wound   Surgery
  Curette, Surgical   Surgery

ROBOZ SURGICAL INSTRUMENT CO., INC.   800-424-2984 *(cont'd)*
  Forceps, Dressing   Surgery
  Forceps, Hemostatic   Surgery
  Handle, Scalpel   Surgery
  Holder, Needle, Other   Surgery
  Instrument, Microsurgical   Cns/Neurology
  Needle, Suture, Disposable   Surgery
  Remover, Clip   Surgery
  Remover, Staple, Surgical   Surgery
  Rongeur, Other   Surgery
  Sterilizer, Dry Heat   General

ROCHE BIOMEDICAL LABORATORIES, INC.
See Lab Corp.

ROCHE DIAGNOSTICS   800-361-2070
201 Armand-Frappier Blvd.,   514-686-7050
Laval, QUE H7V 4 Canada
FDA Number: 8020003   Fax: 514-686-7009
E-mail: luc.lavigne@roche.com
Web site: www.roche.com/diagnostics/
Medical Products Sales Volume: $40,000,000
Year Founded: 1971
Total Employees: 250   Marketing Staff: 56   Sales Staff: 125
Ownership: F. HOFFMANN - LA ROCHE LTD.
Traded On: NYSE
Produces/Sells CE-marked Devices: Y
Distribution: Service Direct, Exclusive Distributor

ROCHE DIAGNOSTICS CORP.   317-521-2834
Marginal Rd., Punto Oro, Industrial Development,
Ponce, PR 00731
FDA Number: 2627723
  Glucose Dehydrogenase, Glucose   Chemistry

ROCHE DIAGNOSTICS OPERATIONS   317-521-2000
9115 Hague Rd., PO Box 50457, Indianapolis, IN 46250
FDA Number: 1823260
E-mail: indianapolis.mediarelations@roche.com
Web site: www.roche-diagnostics.us
Annual Revenue: $0-$1 Million
Year Founded: 1986
Total Employees: 3900
Ownership: Boehringer Mannheim Gmbh
Quality System Registration Information: ISO9001
Produces/Sells CE-marked Devices: N
Distribution: Manufacturer Through Distributor, Manufacturer Through Manufacturer Reps
General Admin.: Jean Luc Belingard/President
                 Steven Glow/Vice President Human Resources
Mktg./Adv.: James Johnson/Vice President Sales
Production: Edward Kimmelman/Manager Regulatory Affairs
  Alpha-Ketobutyric Acid And NADH (U.V.), Hydroxybutyric   Chemistry
  Analyzer, Chemistry, ELISA   Chemistry
  Analyzer, Chemistry, Enzyme   Chemistry
  Analyzer, Chemistry, Multi-Channel, Programmable   Chemistry
  Analyzer, Chemistry, Photometric, Discrete   Chemistry
  Analyzer, Chemistry, Sequential Multiple, Continuous Flow   Chemistry
  Analyzer, Chemistry, Therapeutic Drug Monitor (TDM)   Chemistry
  Analyzer, Chemistry, Urinalysis   Chemistry
  Analyzer, Chemistry, Urine   Chemistry
  Analyzer, Coagulation, Automated   Hematology
  Antigen, Antiserum, Control, Albumin   Immunology
  Calibrator, Primary, Clinical Chemistry   Chemistry
  Calibrator, Secondary, Clinical Chemistry   Chemistry
  Catalytic Method, AST/SGOT   Chemistry
  Catalytic Method, Amylase   Chemistry
  Catalytic Method, Creatine Phosphokinase   Chemistry
  Chromatographic Separation, CPK Isoenzymes   Chemistry
  Complexone, Cresolphthalein, Calcium   Chemistry
  Control, Coagulation, Plasma   Hematology
  Control, Enzyme (Assayed And Unassayed)   Chemistry
  Control, Multi Analyte, All Kinds (Assayed And Unassayed)   Chemistry
  Densitometer/Scanner (Integrating, Reflectance, TLC, Radio)   Chemistry
  Dispenser, Brush   Surgery
  Electrode, Ion Specific, Urea Nitrogen   Chemistry
  Electrophoresis Equipment, Thin-Layer   Chemistry
  Enzymatic (U.V.), Pyruvic Acid   Chemistry
  Enzymatic Esterase-Oxidase, Cholesterol   Chemistry
  Enzymatic Method, Alcohol Dehydrogenase, Ultraviolet   Toxicology
  Enzymatic Method, Ammonia   Chemistry
  Fructose-1, 6-Diphosphate And NADH (U.V.), Aldolase   Chemistry
  Genetic Engineering   Microbiology
  Hexokinase, Glucose   Chemistry
  Indophenol, Berthelot, Urea Nitrogen   Chemistry
  Kinetic Method, Gamma-Glutamyl Transpeptidase   Chemistry
  Kit, Screening, Urine   Microbiology
  L-Isocitrate And NADP (U.V.), Isocitric Dehydrogenase   Chemistry
  L-Leucine-4-Nitroanilide (Colorimetric), Leucine   Chemistry
  Lancet, Blood   General

ROCHE DIAGNOSTICS OPERATIONS   317-521-2000 *(cont'd)*

Lipase Hydrolysis/Glycerol Kinase Enzyme, Triglycerides	Chemistry
Monitor, Blood Glucose (Test)	Gastroenterology/Urology
NAD Reduction/NADH Oxidation, Lactate Dehydrogenase	Chemistry
NADP Reduction (U.V.), Glucose-6-Phosphate Dehydrogenase	Hematology
Nitrophenylphosphate, Acid Phosphatase	Chemistry
Nitrophenylphosphate, Alkaline Phosphatase Or Isoenzymes	Chemistry
Photometer, Reflectance	Chemistry
Pinwheel	Cns/Neurology
Pipette, Diluting	Hematology
Prothrombin Time	Hematology
Reagent, Acetylcholine Chloride	Toxicology
Reagent, Bilirubin (Total Or Direct Test System)	Chemistry
Reagent, Creatinine (Test System)	Chemistry
Reagent, Glucose (Test System)	Chemistry
Reagent, Kinase, Phosphate, Creatine	Chemistry
Reagent, Protein, Total	Chemistry
SGPT, Ultraviolet	Chemistry
Stain, Fetal Hemoglobin	Hematology
Standard/Control, All Types	Chemistry
Stethoscope, Direct (Acoustic), Ultrasonic	Surgery
Thromboplastin, Activated Partial	Hematology

ROCHE DIAGNOSTICS/BOEHRINGER MANNHEIM CORP.
See Roche Diagnostics Operations

ROCHE INSULIN DELIVERY SYSTEMS INC.   800-280-7801
11800 Exit 5 Parkway, Fishers, IN 46037   763-795-5200
FDA Number: 2183996   *Fax:* 763-795-5300
E-mail: info.insulindelivery@roche.com
Web site: www.disetronic-usa.com
Medical Products Sales Volume: $26,800,000
Annual Revenue: $50-$100 Million
Year Founded: 1984
Total Employees: 180   *Marketing Staff:* 5   *Sales Staff:* 80
Ownership: Disetronic Medical Systems Ag
Produces/Sells CE-marked Devices: Y
Federal Procurement Eligibility: Small Business
Distribution: Manufacturer Direct, Manufacturer Through Distributor, OEM, Importer
General Admin.: Patrik DeHaes/Chief Executive Officer
Mktg./Adv.: Rem Laan/Director Marketing
     Zoe Myers/Director National Accounts
     Randall Cole/Manager National Sales

Infusion Pump, Insulin	General

ROCHE MOLECULAR SYSTEMS, INC.   925-730-8110
4300 Hacienda Drive, Pleasanton, CA 94588
FDA Number: 3004141078

Analyzer, Chemistry, Micro	Chemistry
Assay, Hybridization And/or Nucleic Acid Amplification For Detection Of Hepatitis C Rna, Hepatitis C Virus	Microbiology
Concentrator, Clinical Sample	Chemistry
DNA-Probe, Nucleic Acid Amplification, Chlamydia	Microbiology
Drug Metabolizing Enzyme Genotyping Systems	Toxicology
Monitor, Test, Hiv-1	Hematology
Neisseria, DNA Reagents	Microbiology
Reagents, Specific, Analyte	Hematology
Software, Blood Bank (Stand-Alone Products)	Hematology
System, Nucleic Acid Amplification, Mycobacterium Tuberculosis Complex	Microbiology

ROCHESTER ELECTRO MEDICAL, INC.   813-963-2933
4212 Cypress Gulch Drive, Lutz, FL 33559
FDA Number: 2126558

Cable, Electrode	Physical Med
Electrode, Cutaneous	Cns/Neurology
Electrode, Nasopharyngeal	Cns/Neurology
Electrode, Needle	Cns/Neurology
Electrode, Needle, Diagnostic Electromyograph	Physical Med
Gel, Electrode, Stimulator	Cns/Neurology
Monitor, Ventilatory Frequency	Anesthesiology
Stimulator, Muscle, Diagnostic	Physical Med
Tester, Electrode/Lead, Electroencephalograph	Cns/Neurology
Thermometer, Electronic, Continuous	General

ROCHESTER MEDICAL CORP.   800-615-2364
One Rochester Medical Dr.,   507-533-9600
Stewartville, MN 55976
FDA Number: 2130787   *Fax:* 507-533-9725
E-mail: info@rocm.com
Web site: http://www.rocm.com
Ownership: Private
Stock Symbol: ROCM
Traded On: NASDAQ
Produces/Sells CE-marked Devices: N
General Admin.: Mr. Anthony Conway/President, Chief Executive Officer, Chairman
Mktg./Adv.: Mr. Jim Carper/Vice President Marketing
Production: Mr. Rob Anglin/Vice President Quality Assurance & Regulatory Affairs
Finance: Mr. David Jonas/Chief Financial Officer

Appliance, Incontinence, Urosheath Type	Gastroenterology/Urology

ROCHESTER MEDICAL CORP.   800-615-2364 *(cont'd)*

Catheter and Accessories, Urological	Gastroenterology/Urology
Catheter, Retention Type, Balloon	Gastroenterology/Urology
Catheter, Urethral	Gastroenterology/Urology
Collector, Urine	Gastroenterology/Urology
Device, Transurethral, For Controlled Urination	Gastroenterology/Urology
Kit, Catheterization, Sterile Urethral	Gastroenterology/Urology

ROCHESTER MEDICAL IMPLANTS   574-223-8198
1202 E. 4th Street, Rochester, IN 46975-0547
FDA Number: 1836249
E-mail: info@rmi.us.com
Web site: www.rickmantool.com
Year Founded: 1992
Total Employees: 26   *Marketing Staff:* 1   *Sales Staff:* 1
Ownership: Private
Produces/Sells CE-marked Devices: N
Distribution: Manufacturer Direct
General Admin.: Edward Rickman/President
     Eddie Rickman Jr./Vice President
Mktg./Adv.: Roy Shepard/Manager Contract Sales

Implant, Fixation Device, Spinal	Orthopedics

ROCHESTER MEDICAL IMPLANTS   800- 371-6851
1202 East 4th Street, Noblesville, IN 46975-9104   317- 214-7076
FDA Number: 1836249   *Fax:* 317- 214-7081
E-mail: info@rmi.us.com
Ownership: Private
Produces/Sells CE-marked Devices: N

Appliance, Fixation, Spinal Intervertebral Body	Orthopedics
Orthosis, Fixation, Pedicle, Spinal	Orthopedics
Orthosis, Fixation, Spinal, Spondylolisthesis	Orthopedics
Prosthesis, Hip, Cement Restrictor	Orthopedics

ROCHESTER MIDLAND, CORP.   800-836-1627
333 Hollenbeck St, Rochester, NY 14621   585-336-2200
FDA Number: 1314897
Web site: www.rochestermidland.com
Annual Revenue: $25-$50 Million
Year Founded: 1888
Total Employees: 600
Ownership: Private
Produces/Sells CE-marked Devices: N
Distribution: Manufacturer Direct, Manufacturer Through Distributor, Exporter
General Admin.: H.D. Calkins/Chief Executive Officer, Chairman
     Bradley Calkins/President
     Katherine Calkins/Senior Vice President, General Manager
Mktg./Adv.: Jim Bruno/Market Manager

Cleaner, Medical Device	General
Disinfector, Liquid	General
Pad, Menstrual, Unscented	Obstetrics/Gynecology
Solution, Antibacterial Cleaner	General
Tampon, Menstrual, Unscented	Obstetrics/Gynecology

ROCHESTER OPTICAL MFG. COMPANY   585-254-0022
1260 Lyell Avenue, Rochester, NY 14606-2040
FDA Number: 1317695   *Fax:* 585-254-0066
E-mail: info@rochesteroptical.com
Web site: www.rochesteroptical.com
Medical Products Sales Volume: $3,100,000
Annual Revenue: $1-$5 Million
Year Founded: 1989
Total Employees: 15   *Marketing Staff:* 1   *Sales Staff:* 6
Ownership: Private
Produces/Sells CE-marked Devices: N
Federal Procurement Eligibility: Small Business, Minority Owned, VA Contract
Distribution: Manufacturer Direct
General Admin.: Mr. Patrick Ho/Chief Executive Officer

Eyeglasses, Safety	Ophthalmology
Frame, Spectacle (Eyeglasses)	Ophthalmology
Goggles, Protective, Eye	Ophthalmology
Lens, Contact(rigid Gas Permeable)-extended Wear	Ophthalmology
Lens, Spectacle/Eyeglasses, Custom (Prescription)	Ophthalmology
Lens, Spectacle/Eyeglasses, Non-Custom	Ophthalmology
Sunglasses (Including Photosensitive)	Ophthalmology

ROCHESTER SCIENTIFIC CO. INC.
See Fisher Scientific Co., Llc.

ROCK VALLEY TEXTILES   608-752-6866
111 Avon St., Janesville, WI 53545
FDA Number: 3006067515
Ownership: Private
Produces/Sells CE-marked Devices: N

Linen, Bed	General

ROCKET MEDICAL PLC.

800-707-7625
781-749-6223

150 Recreation Park Drive, Unit 3,
Hingham, MA 02043

FDA Number: 3004056053
E-mail: usa@rocketmedical.com
Web site: www.rocketmedical.com
Medical Products Sales Volume: $400,000
Annual Revenue: $10-$25 Million
Year Founded: 1964
Total Employees: 3
Ownership: Private
Quality System Registration Information: ISO9001
Produces/Sells CE-marked Devices: Y
Federal Procurement Eligibility: Small Business
Distribution: Manufacturer Direct, Manufacturer Through Distributor, Importer, Exporter
General Admin.: Robi Bernberg/Chief Executive Officer
Mktg./Adv.: Bruce Carmell/Vice President Marketing & Sales
Production: Jackie Irwin/Manager Regulatory Affairs
Les Todd/Vice President Manufacturing

Amniotome	Obstetrics/Gynecology
Applicator, Electrode, Scalp, Fetal	Obstetrics/Gynecology
Aspirator, Endocervical	Obstetrics/Gynecology
Aspirator, Endometrial	Obstetrics/Gynecology
Brush, Cytology	General
Cannula With Inflatable Balloon (Distal Tip)	Surgery
Cannula, Aortic	Cardiovascular
Cannula, Insufflation, Uterine	Obstetrics/Gynecology
Cannula, Intrauterine Insemination	Obstetrics/Gynecology
Cannula, Manipulator/Injector, Uterine	Obstetrics/Gynecology
Cannula, Suction, Uterine	Obstetrics/Gynecology
Cannula, Venous	Cardiovascular
Catheter, Assisted Reproduction	Obstetrics/Gynecology
Catheter, Biliary, General & Plastic Surgery	Surgery
Catheter, Imaging, Ultrasonic	Radiology
Catheter, Intrauterine, With Introducer	Obstetrics/Gynecology
Catheter, Nephrostomy, General & Plastic Surgery	Surgery
Catheter, Perfusion	Cardiovascular
Catheter, Salpingography	Obstetrics/Gynecology
Catheter, Sampling, Chorionic Villus	Obstetrics/Gynecology
Catheter, Transfer, Intrafallopian	Obstetrics/Gynecology
Collector, Urine, Disposable	Gastroenterology/Urology
Curette, Suction, Endometrial	Obstetrics/Gynecology
Curette, Uterine	Obstetrics/Gynecology
Dilator, Cervical, Fixed Size	Obstetrics/Gynecology
Dosimeter, Radiation	Radiology
Drain, Thoracic (Chest)	Anesthesiology
Electrode, Clip, Fetal Scalp (And Applicator)	Obstetrics/Gynecology
Endoscope, Fetal Blood Sampling	Obstetrics/Gynecology
Equipment, In Vitro Fertilization/Embryo Transfer	Obstetrics/Gynecology
Forceps, Biopsy	Surgery
Forceps, Biopsy, Gynecological	Obstetrics/Gynecology
Forceps, Dressing	Surgery
Forceps, Hemostatic	Surgery
Forceps, Obstetrical	Obstetrics/Gynecology
Forceps, Sponge	Surgery
Forceps, Surgical, Gynecological	Obstetrics/Gynecology
Forceps, Tissue	Surgery
General Use Surgical Scissors	Surgery
Guide, Needle	Surgery
Hook, Surgical, General & Plastic Surgery	Surgery
Instrument, Microsurgical	Cns/Neurology
Irrigator, Suction	General
Kit, Mid-Stream Collection	General
Kit, Sampling, Endometrial	Obstetrics/Gynecology
Light Source, Fiberoptic, Routine	Gastroenterology/Urology
Loop, Inoculating	Microbiology
Manometer, Spinal Fluid	General
Needle, Aspiration And Injection, Disposable	Surgery
Needle, Bone Marrow	Surgery
Needle, Dental	Dental And Oral
Pelvimeter	Obstetrics/Gynecology
Pelvimeter, External	Obstetrics/Gynecology
Probe, Suction, Irrigator/Aspirator, Laparoscopic	Surgery
Pump, Abortion Unit, Vacuum	Obstetrics/Gynecology
Punch, Biopsy	Gastroenterology/Urology
Retractor, Surgical	Surgery
Scissors, Disposable	General
Speculum, Vaginal, Metal	Obstetrics/Gynecology
Surgical Instrument, Obstetric/Gynecologic, General	Obstetrics/Gynecology

ROCKFORD MEDICAL & SAFETY CO.

800-435-9451
815-394-4809

2420 Harrison Avenue, PO Box 5646,
Rockford, IL 61125

FDA Number: 1419164
E-mail: firensafety@msn.com
Web site: www.r-m-s-c.com
Medical Products Sales Volume: $1,160,000
Annual Revenue: $1-$5 Million
Year Founded: 1976

ROCKFORD MEDICAL & SAFETY CO.

800-435-9451 *(cont'd)*

Total Employees: 18   *Marketing Staff:* 3   *Sales Staff:* 6
Ownership: FIRE & SAFETY EQUIPMENT OF ROCKFORD, INC.
Produces/Sells CE-marked Devices: N
Federal Procurement Eligibility: Small Business
Distribution: Manufacturer Direct
General Admin.: Steve Long/President, Chief Executive Officer
Mktg./Adv.: Mrs. Diana Bliss/Admin. Marketing & Sales

Airway, Esophageal (Obturator)	Anesthesiology
Apron, Laboratory	Chemistry
Aspirator, Emergency Suction	General
Blanket, Rescue	General
Board, Cardiac Compression	Cardiovascular
Board, Spine	Orthopedics
Cannula, Nasal, Oxygen	Anesthesiology
Catheter, Suction (Tracheal Aspirating Tube)	Anesthesiology
Cutter, Ring	General
Dressing, Universal	General
Eyeglasses, Safety	Ophthalmology
Fountain, Eye Wash	Chemistry
Kit, Burn	General
Kit, First Aid	Surgery
Kit, Labor and Delivery	Obstetrics/Gynecology
Mask, Oxygen, Partial Rebreathing	General
Monitor, Blood Pressure, Indirect (Arterial)	Cardiovascular
Pack, Cold	General
Pack, Hot Or Cold, Reusable	Physical Med
Resuscitator, Pulmonary, Gas	General
Sand Bag	Radiology
Scissors, Bandage/Gauze/Plaster	General
Sign, Hospital	General
Sphygmomanometer, Electronic, Manual	General
Splint, Pneumatic	Orthopedics
Stretcher, Hand-Carried	General
Stretcher, Transfer	Surgery
Strip, Adhesive	Surgery
Suit, Pneumatic Counterpressure (Anti-Shock)	Cardiovascular
Training Manikin, CPR (Resuscitation)	General
Training Manikin, Intravenous Arm	General
Training Manikin, Other	General
Tubing, Oxygen Connecting	General

ROCKLAND IMMUNOCHEMICALS, INC.

800-656-ROCK
610-369-1008

PO Box 326, Gilbertsville, PA 19525

FDA Number: 2517886
E-mail: fendrick@rockland-inc.com
Web site: www.rockland-inc.com
Medical Products Sales Volume: $9,000,000
Total Employees: 35
Ownership: Private
Produces/Sells CE-marked Devices: N
Federal Procurement Eligibility: Small Business, Minority Owned, Female Owned, VA Contract
Distribution: Manufacturer Direct, OEM, Exporter
General Admin.: Natalie Joy Cappel/Chairman
James Fendrick/Vice President

Anti-Human Serum, Manual	Hematology
Antibody, Polyclonal	Microbiology
Antigen, Antiserum, Control, Ferritin	Immunology
Antigen, Antiserum, Control, IGG	Immunology
Antigen, Antiserum, Control, IGG, FITC	Immunology
Antigen, Antiserum, Control, IGG, Peroxidase	Immunology
Antigen, Antiserum, Control, IGG, Rhodamine	Immunology
Column, Chromatography, Hydroxyproline	Chemistry
Complement	Immunology
Enzyme Immunoassay, Other	Chemistry
IGG (FD Fragment Specific), Antigen, Antiserum, Control	Immunology
IGG, Ferritin, Antigen, Antiserum, Control	Immunology
Reagent, Glucose (Test System)	Chemistry
Reagent, Other	General
Serum, Animal	Pathology
Serum, Biological, General	Toxicology
Serum, Human	Pathology

ROCKLAND INDUSTRIES, INC.

800-876-2566
410-522-2505

1601 Edison Hwy., Baltimore, MD 21213

FDA Number: n/a
E-mail: mail@roc-lon.com
Web site: www.roc-lon.com
Medical Products Sales Volume: $10,000,000
Annual Revenue: $50-$100 Million
Total Employees: 1000
Ownership: Private
Federal Procurement Eligibility: GSA Contract
Distribution: Manufacturer Direct, Exporter
General Admin.: Mark R. Berman/Chief Executive Officer
Mktg./Adv.: Darlene Sanders/Director Marketing
Mark Kresel/Vice President Sales

ROCKLAND INDUSTRIES, INC.   800-876-2566 *(cont'd)*
Sheet, Drape   Surgery

ROCKLAND TECHNIMED LIMITED RTL   845-426-1136
3 Larissa Court, Airmont, NY 10952-3833
FDA Number: n/a   *Fax:* 845-426-1109
E-mail: info@technimed.com
Web site: www.technimed.com
Medical Products Sales Volume: $4,900,000
Annual Revenue: $0-$1 Million
Year Founded: 1999
Total Employees: 10   *Marketing Staff:* 2   *Sales Staff:* 4
Ownership: Private
Produces/Sells CE-marked Devices: N
Federal Procurement Eligibility: Small Business, Minority Owned
Distribution: Manufacturer Through Distributor
General Admin.: Mr. Pradeep M. Gupte/Chief Executive Officer, Chairman
     Dr. Robert DeLaPaz/Director
     Mr. Elliot Cole, Esq./Director
     Mr. George E Heinze/President, General Director
Mktg./Adv.: Gary Mascitis/Vice President Marketing & Sales
Research: Dr. John Pile-Spellman/Vice President Clinical Research
Computer Software   General
Computer, Radiographic Image Analysis   Radiology
Media, Radiographic Injectable Contrast   Radiology
Service, Consulting   General

ROCKLAND, INC.
See Rockland Immunochemicals, Inc.

ROCKWELL MEDICAL TECHNOLOGIES   248-960-9009
308 N. Iowa Street, Washington, IA 52353
FDA Number: 1954315
Ownership: Private
Produces/Sells CE-marked Devices: N

ROCKWELL MEDICAL TECHNOLOGIES, INC.   800-449-3353
30142 S. Wixom Rd., Wixom, MI 48393-3440   248-960-9009
FDA Number: 1835498   *Fax:* 248-960-9119
E-mail: sales@rockwellmed.com
Web site: www.rockwellmed.com
Medical Products Sales Volume: $28,000,000
Annual Revenue: $25-$50 Million
Year Founded: 1995
Total Employees: 150
Ownership: Public
Stock Symbol: RMTI
Traded On: NASDAQ
Produces/Sells CE-marked Devices: N
Distribution: Manufacturer Direct, Exporter
General Admin.: Mr. Robert L. Chioini/Chief Executive Officer, Chairman
Finance: Mr. Thomas Klema/Chief Financial Officer, Vice President Finance
Concentrate, Dialysis, Hemodialysis (Liquid or Powder)   Gastroenterology/Urology
Medical Product Subsidiaries (Listed Separately)
Rockwell Medical Technologies, Inc.

ROCKWELL MEDICAL TECHNOLOGIES, INC.   248-960-9009
30142 Wixom Road, Wixom, MI 48393
FDA Number: 1652176   *Fax:* 248 960-9119
E-mail: invest@rockwellmed.com
Web site: www.rockwellmed.com
Ownership: Private
Produces/Sells CE-marked Devices: N

ROCKWELL MEDICAL TECHNOLOGIES, INC.   248-960-9009
604 High Tech Ct., Greer, SC 29650
FDA Number: 1065847
Ownership: Rockwell Medical Technologies, Inc.
Produces/Sells CE-marked Devices: N
Concentrate, Dialysis, Hemodialysis (Liquid or Powder)   Gastroenterology/Urology

ROCKY MOUNTAIN ANAPLASTOLOGY, INC.   303-973-8482
3405 South Yarrow St., Suite C, Denver, CO 80227
FDA Number: 1721657
Eye, Artificial, Non-Custom   Ophthalmology
Prosthesis, Ear, Internal   Surgery
Prosthesis, Finger, Polymer   Orthopedics
Prosthesis, Nose, Internal   Surgery

ROCKY MOUNTAIN MEDICAL CORP.
See Rmed International

ROCKY MOUNTAIN REAGENTS,INC.   303-762-0800
3207 W. Hampden Avenue, Englewood, CO 80110-3261
FDA Number: 1711690   *Fax:* 303-762-1240
E-mail: info@rmreagents.com
Web site: www.rmreagents.com
Medical Products Sales Volume: $1,400,000
Annual Revenue: $0-$1 Million
Total Employees: 13

ROCKY MOUNTAIN REAGENTS,INC.   303-762-0800 *(cont'd)*
Ownership: Private
Produces/Sells CE-marked Devices: N
Federal Procurement Eligibility: Small Business, Female Owned
Distribution: Manufacturer Direct
General Admin.: Phyllis Sordelet/Chief Executive Officer
Brilliant Cresyl Blue   Hematology
Crystal Violet   Hematology
Diluent, Blood Cell   Hematology
Ferric Chloride, Phenylketones (Urinary, Non-Quantitative)   Chemistry
Fluid, Red Cell Diluting   Hematology
Fluid, White Cell Diluting   Hematology
Formaldehyde (Formalin, Formol)   Pathology
Formalin, Neutral Buffered   Pathology
Formalin-Saline   Pathology
Mercuric Chloride Formulations For Tissue   Pathology
Silver Nitrate   Pathology
Solution, Pathology, Formalin-Alcohol-Acetic Acid   Pathology
Solution, Pathology, Lugol's   Pathology
Stain, Alizarin Red   Pathology
Stain, Aniline Blue   Pathology
Stain, Carbol Fuchsin   Pathology
Stain, Congo Red   Pathology
Stain, Crystal Violet, Histology   Pathology
Stain, Eosin Y   Pathology
Stain, Fast Green   Pathology
Stain, Giemsa, Hematology   Hematology
Stain, Grams Iodine   Pathology
Stain, Light Green   Pathology
Stain, Methyl Green   Pathology
Stain, Methylene Blue   Pathology
Stain, Methylene Blue, New   Hematology
Stain, Microbiological   Microbiology
Stain, Mucicarmine   Pathology
Stain, Neutral Red   Pathology
Stain, Oil Red O   Pathology
Stain, Phloxine B   Pathology
Stain, Ponceau   Pathology
Stain, Ponceau, Hematology   Hematology
Stain, Reticulocyte   Hematology
Stain, Safranin   Pathology
Stain, Toluidine Blue   Pathology
Stain, Toluidine Blue, Hematology   Hematology
Stain, Wright's   Pathology
Stain, Wright's, Hematology   Hematology
Titrimetric With EDTA And Indicator, Calcium   Chemistry
Turbidimetric Method, Protein Or Albumin (Urinary)   Chemistry

ROCKY MOUNTAIN RESEARCH, INC.   801-359-6060
825 North 300 West, Suite 410, Salt Lake City, UT 84103
FDA Number: 1721220   *Fax:* 801-359-6073
Ownership: Private
Quality System Registration Information: ISO9001
Produces/Sells CE-marked Devices: Y
Clamp, Tubing, Blood, Automatic   Gastroenterology/Urology
Detector, Bubble, Cardiopulmonary Bypass   Cardiovascular
Monitor, Cardiopulmonary Level Sensing   Cardiovascular

ROCKY MOUNTAIN/ORTHODONTICS
See Rmo, Inc.

RODALE ELECTRONICS, INC.   631-231-0044 x1
20 Oser Ave., Hauppauge, NY 11788
FDA Number: 2429649   *Fax:* 631-231-1345
E-mail: ljust@rodaleelectronics.com
Web site: www.rodaleelectronics.com
Ownership: Private
Produces/Sells CE-marked Devices: N
Device, Peripheral Electromag. Field to Aid Wound Healing   Surgery

RODENSTOCK NORTH AMERICA, INC.   614-409-2820
2150 Bixby Rd., Lockbourne, OH 43137-9273
FDA Number: 3003367235
Ownership: Private
Produces/Sells CE-marked Devices: N
Lens, Spectacle/Eyeglasses, Non-Custom   Ophthalmology

ROERIG INC.
See Pfizer, Inc.

ROGER L. GOODMAN, D.D.S., P.C.   517-676-5200
200 Temple St., Mason, MI 48854-1837
FDA Number: 1834299
Ownership: Private
Produces/Sells CE-marked Devices: N
Sterilant, Medical Device   General
Sterilizer, Chemical   General

ROGERS FOAM CORP.   714-538-3033
808 West Nicholas Avenue, Orange, CA 92868-1320
FDA Number: 2032301   *Fax:* 714-538-3013
E-mail: rfcca@aol.com

ROGERS FOAM CORP.   714-538-3033 *(cont'd)*
Web site: www.rogersfoam.com
Medical Products Sales Volume: $30,000,000
Year Founded: 1947
Total Employees: 40
Ownership: Private
Stock Symbol: SEE
Traded On: NYSE
Produces/Sells CE-marked Devices: N
Federal Procurement Eligibility: Small Business
  Accessories, Fixation, Orthopedic   Orthopedics
  Collar, Cervical Neck   Orthopedics
  Sponge, Other   General

ROGERS FOAM CORPORATION   859-497-0702
120 Clarence Dr., Woodland Industrial Park,
Mt. Sterling, KY 40353
FDA Number: 3004082002
  Tray, Surgical   Surgery

ROGERS FOAM CORPORATION   617-623-3010
609 Boone Trail Road, Clinchport, VA 24244
FDA Number: 3006784172
Ownership: Private
Produces/Sells CE-marked Devices: N
  Cover, Mattress   General
  Mattress, Air Flotation   General

ROHE SCIENTIFIC CORPORATION
See Philips Medical Systems

ROHO GROUP, THE   800-851-3449
100 N. Florida Avenue, Belleville, IL 62221-5429   **618-277-9173**
FDA Number: 1419507   *Fax:* 618-277-9561
E-mail: intl@therohogroup.com
Web site: www.therohogroup.com
Medical Products Sales Volume: $13,000,000
Year Founded: 1973
Total Employees: 165   *Marketing Staff:* 4   *Sales Staff:* 24
Ownership: Private
Quality System Registration Information: ISO9002
Produces/Sells CE-marked Devices: Y
Federal Procurement Eligibility: Small Business, VA Contract
Distribution: Manufacturer Through Distributor, Exclusive Distributor
General Admin.: Tom Oleksy/President, Chief Executive Officer
Mktg./Adv.: Scott Fiss/Director National Accounts
       Dennis Clapper/Director Product Development
       Tom Borcherding/Manager International & National Sales
       Tom Hartmann/Manager National Sales
       Jackie Wiegart/Marketing Specialist
       Melissa Keim/Vice President Marketing
       Tom Borcherding/Vice President Sales
Production: John Schwartz/Director Quality Assurance
       Chris Hall/Vice President Manufacturing
Research: David Parsons/Vice President Research & Development
  Cover, Mattress   General
  Cushion, Flotation   Physical Med
  Cushion, Other   General
  Mattress, Bed   General

ROLDAN PRODUCTS CORP.   866-922-6800
448 Sovereign Court, Ballwin, MO 63021   **636-527-6800**
FDA Number: 9200933   *Fax:* 636-527-4770
E-mail: roldanexport@aol.com
Web site: www.roldanexport.com
Medical Products Sales Volume: $1,000,000
Annual Revenue: $1-$5 Million
Year Founded: 1926
Total Employees: 6
Ownership: Private
Produces/Sells CE-marked Devices: Y
Federal Procurement Eligibility: Small Business
Distribution: Manufacturer Direct, Manufacturer Through Distributor, OEM, Exporter
General Admin.: J. G. Roldan/President, Chief Executive Officer
       A. J. Roldan/Vice President
Mktg./Adv.: Tony Roldan/Manager Marketing
Finance: Linda Roldan/Treasurer
  Lamp, Examination (Light)   General
  Lamp, Other   General
  Lamp, Ultraviolet, Physical Medicine   Physical Med
  Light, High Intensity   Radiology
  Light, Other   General
  Light, Overbed   General
  Loupe, Diagnostic/Surgical   Surgery
  Viewer/Magnifier   Hematology

ROLL A BOUT CORP.   888-736-6151
3240 Barratts Chapel Rd., Frederica, DE 19946   **302-335-5057**
FDA Number: 2531619   *Fax:* 302-335-5484
E-mail: customerservice@roll-a-bout.com
Web site: www.roll-a-bout.com
Ownership: Private
Produces/Sells CE-marked Devices: N
  Tips And Pads, Cane, Crutch And Walker   Physical Med
  Walker, Mechanical   Physical Med

ROLLENS PROFESSIONAL PRODUCTS, INC.   800-898-7474
16610 Amberstone Way, Parker, CO 80134   **303-840-2238**
FDA Number: 1725059   *Fax:* 303-840-8015
E-mail: dlw526@indra.com
Medical Products Sales Volume: $1,500,000
Year Founded: 1989
Total Employees: 7   *Marketing Staff:* 1   *Sales Staff:* 2
Ownership: Private
Produces/Sells CE-marked Devices: N
General Admin.: Donald Wilson/President
  Sunglasses (Including Photosensitive)   Ophthalmology

ROLLITURE CORP.   650-652-5675
665 Clearfield Dr., Millbrae, CA 94030
FDA Number: 2939952
Web site: www.rollens.com
Ownership: Private
Produces/Sells CE-marked Devices: N
  Orthosis, Lumbosacral   Physical Med

ROLLS EQUIPMENT
See Invacare Corporation

ROLOKE   800-533-8212
127 W. Hazel Street, Inglewood, CA 90302   **310-674-7500**
FDA Number: n/a   *Fax:* 310-673-7773
E-mail: info@roloke.com
Web site: www.roloke.com
Medical Products Sales Volume: $1,200,000
Year Founded: 1968
Total Employees: 13   *Marketing Staff:* 2
Ownership: Private
Produces/Sells CE-marked Devices: N
Federal Procurement Eligibility: Small Business
Distribution: Manufacturer Direct, Manufacturer Through Distributor, Exporter
  Collar, Cervical Neck   Orthopedics
  Pillow, Cervical   Orthopedics

ROMAINE, INC.
See Romaine, Inc. D.B.A. Koldcare

ROMAINE, INC. D.B.A. KOLDCARE   800-294-7101
2026 Sterling Ave., Elkhart, IN 46516-4220   **574-294-7101**
FDA Number: n/a   *Fax:* 574-294-4961
E-mail: info@koldcare.com
Web site: www.koldcare.com
Medical Products Sales Volume: $1,000,000
Annual Revenue: $0-$1 Million
Year Founded: 1980
Total Employees: 9   *Marketing Staff:* 1   *Sales Staff:* 1
Ownership: Private
Quality System Registration Information: ISO9002
Produces/Sells CE-marked Devices: Y
Federal Procurement Eligibility: Small Business
Distribution: Manufacturer Through Distributor, Exclusive Distributor, Exporter
General Admin.: Meg Patton/President, Chief Executive Officer
Mktg./Adv.: Michele Yoder/Supervisor Marketing & Sales
Production: Andrea Cramer/Manager Process Control
       Andrea Cramer/Manager Regulatory Affairs
  Bandage, Other   General
  Blanket, Fire   General
  Compress, Cold   General
  Dressing, Wound and Burn, Occlusive   Surgery
  Electrode, Gel   Cardiovascular
  Kit, Burn   General

ROMAN RESEARCH, INC.   800-451-5700
800 Franklin St, Hanson, MA 02341   **781-447-3411**
FDA Number: 1217996   *Fax:* 781-447-0995
E-mail: custserv@romanresearch.com
Web site: www.romanresearch.com
Medical Products Sales Volume: $20,100,000
Annual Revenue: $1-$5 Million
Year Founded: 1970
Total Employees: 110   *Marketing Staff:* 1   *Sales Staff:* 1
Ownership: Private
Produces/Sells CE-marked Devices: N
Federal Procurement Eligibility: Small Business

ROMAN RESEARCH, INC. 800-451-5700 *(cont'd)*
Distribution: Manufacturer Direct, Manufacturer Through Distributor, Manufacturer Through Manufacturer Reps, Service Direct, Exporter
General Admin.: Dale Southworth/President
Gerry Finn/Vice President
Mktg./Adv.: Bill Russell/Director Marketing

Perforator, Ear	Ear/Nose/Throat
Perforator, Ear-Lobe	Ear/Nose/Throat

ROMC, INC. 508-829-4602
37 Kris Allen Drive, Holden, MA 01520
FDA Number: 3004562778 Fax: 508-829-5123
E-mail: dmcnally@microendoscope.com
Web site: www.microendoscope.com
Medical Products Sales Volume: $200,000
Annual Revenue: $1-$5 Million
Year Founded: 2003
Total Employees: 3 *Marketing Staff:* 1 *Sales Staff:* 1
Ownership: Private
Produces/Sells CE-marked Devices: N
Federal Procurement Eligibility: Small Business
Distribution: Manufacturer Through Distributor
General Admin.: Mr. David McNally/President
Production: Mr. Jim Bomnneville/Director Manufacturing

Arthroscope	Orthopedics
Endoilluminator	Ophthalmology
Endoscope	Gastroenterology/Urology
Endoscope, Fetal Blood Sampling	Obstetrics/Gynecology
Endoscope, Fiberoptic	Surgery
Endoscope, Neurological	Cns/Neurology

ROMED, LLC 562-438-8904
4224 Massachusetts St., Long Beach, CA 90814-2939
FDA Number: 2032681 Fax: 562-438-8904
E-mail: RoMedLLC@aol.com
Web site: www.nursefriendly.com/Comfeeze
Medical Products Sales Volume: $14,000
Annual Revenue: $0-$1 Million
Year Founded: 2001
Total Employees: 2 *Marketing Staff:* 1 *Sales Staff:* 1
Ownership: Private
Produces/Sells CE-marked Devices: N
Federal Procurement Eligibility: Small Business, Female Owned
Distribution: Manufacturer Direct, Manufacturer Through Manufacturer Reps

Circuit, Breathing (W Connector, Adapter, Y Piece)	Anesthesiology

RONDEX PRODUCTS, INC. 815-226-0452
P.O. Box 1829, Rockford, IL 61110-0329
FDA Number: 1419464 Fax: 815-216-0458
E-mail: request@rondex.com
Web site: www.rondex.com
Annual Revenue: $5-$10 Million
Year Founded: 1978
Ownership: Private
Produces/Sells CE-marked Devices: Y
Federal Procurement Eligibility: Small Business
Distribution: Manufacturer Direct, Manufacturer Through Distributor, OEM
Mktg./Adv.: G. Baldwin/Manager Marketing

Device, Assist, CPR	Anesthesiology
Mask, Oxygen, Other	General
Valve, Non-Rebreathing	Anesthesiology

RONPAK, INC. 732-968-8000
4301 New Brunswick Avenue, South Plainfield, NJ 07080-1291
FDA Number: 2247897 Fax: 310-445-4277
E-mail: dmorris@ronpak.com
Web site: www.ronpak.com
Medical Products Sales Volume: $14,000,000
Year Founded: 1942
Total Employees: 80
Ownership: Private
Produces/Sells CE-marked Devices: N
Federal Procurement Eligibility: Small Business

Sterilization Indicator	Surgery

RONTRON ENGINEERING, INC. 203-488-5020
131 Commercial Pkwy., Branford, CT 06405
FDA Number: 1225083 Fax: 203-315-4994
E-mail: sales@rontroneng.com
Web site: rontroneng.com
Medical Products Sales Volume: $400,000
Annual Revenue: $0-$1 Million
Year Founded: 1978
Total Employees: 16 *Marketing Staff:* 1 *Sales Staff:* 2
Ownership: Privately held
Produces/Sells CE-marked Devices: Y
Federal Procurement Eligibility: Small Business
Distribution: OEM, Exporter

RONTRON ENGINEERING, INC. 203-488-5020 *(cont'd)*

Electrosurgical Unit, Cutting & Coagulation Device	Surgery
Electrosurgical Unit, General Purpose (ESU)	Surgery

ROPER SCIENTIFIC
See Princeton Instruments - Acton

ROPER SCIENTIFIC, INC. 800-874-9789
3440 E. Britannia Drive, Tucson, AZ 85706-5006 520-889-9933
FDA Number: n/a Fax: 520-573-1944
E-mail: info@roperscientific.com
Web site: www.roperscientific.com
Annual Revenue: $25-$50 Million
Total Employees: 90 *Marketing Staff:* 10 *Sales Staff:* 15
Ownership: ROPER INDUSTRIES
Traded On: NYSE
Quality System Registration Information: ISO9002
Produces/Sells CE-marked Devices: Y
Federal Procurement Eligibility: Small Business
Distribution: Manufacturer Direct, OEM
General Admin.: Thomas Connelly/President
Lucy Rumney/Vice President Human Resources
Mktg./Adv.: Rachel Belleci/Admin. National Sales
Jim Schumacher/Director Sales
Mike Meade/Manager National Sales
Tracey Eddy/Marketing Communications Assistant
Mark Christenson/Vice President Business Development
Scott Sternberg/Vice President Business Development
Patrick Lordi/Vice President Marketing & Sales
Research: Jim Pisa/Vice President Research & Development

Computer Software	General
Contract R&D, Diagnostics	General

ROQUETTE AMERICA 319-524-5757
1417 Exchange St., PO Box 6647, Keokuk, IA 52632-6647
FDA Number: 1910565 Fax: 319-526-2345
E-mail: rai.sales@roquette.com
Web site: www.roquette.com
Medical Products Sales Volume: $94,000,000
Year Founded: 1991
Total Employees: 470
Ownership: ROQUETTE FRERE
Produces/Sells CE-marked Devices: Y
Federal Procurement Eligibility: Small Business
Distribution: Manufacturer Direct
General Admin.: Mike Jorgenson/President, Chief Executive Officer
Mktg./Adv.: Don Wiggins/Manager National Sales
Production: Clark McGrew/Manager Quality Assurance

Sensitivity Test Powder, Antimicrobial	Microbiology

RORKE DATA, INCORPORATED 757-224-0177
7626 Golden Triangle Drive, Eden Prairie, MN 55344
FDA Number: 3004413161

Device, Storage, Image, Digital	Radiology

ROSE TECHNOLOGIES 425-637-2344
13400 NE 20th Street, STE 32, Bellevue, WA 98005
FDA Number: 3033514 Fax: 425-637-8655
E-mail: chade@rosestudios.com
Web site: www.rosetechnologies.com
Ownership: Private
Produces/Sells CE-marked Devices: N
Federal Procurement Eligibility: Small Business

Reagent, Glucose (Test System)	Chemistry

ROSE TECHNOLOGIES COMPANY 616-233-3000
1440 Front Ave, Grand Rapids, MI 49504
FDA Number: 1836324 Fax: 616-233-3099
E-mail: vroege1@rose-technologies.com
Web site: www.rose-technologies.com
Medical Products Sales Volume: $1,500,000
Annual Revenue: $1-$5 Million
Year Founded: 1998
Total Employees: 20
Ownership: Private
Produces/Sells CE-marked Devices: N
Distribution: OEM
General Admin.: Mr. Todd Grimm/President
Mr. Eric Vroegop/Vice President

Accessories, Catheter	Surgery
Cannula, Catheter	Cardiovascular
Cannula, Venous	Cardiovascular
Catheter, Arterial	Cardiovascular
Contract Manufacturing	General
Tube, Tracheal (Endotracheal)	Anesthesiology
Tubing, Silicone	General

ROSKAMP CHAMPION
800-366-2563
2975 Airline Circle, Waterloo, IA 50703
319-232-8444
FDA Number: n/a
E-mail: sales@cpmroskamp.com
Web site: www.cpmroskamp.com
Ownership: Private
Quality System Registration Information: ISO9000
Produces/Sells CE-marked Devices: Y
Federal Procurement Eligibility: Small Business
Distribution: Manufacturer Direct, Manufacturer Through Distributor, Manufacturer Through Manufacturer Reps, Service Direct, Exclusive Distributor
  Contract Manufacturing   General

ROSKAMP MANUFACTURING, INC.
See Roskamp Champion

ROSS DISPOSABLE PRODUCTS
800-649-6526
411 Bradwick Drive, Unit 12,
(905) 660-4799
Concord, ON L4K 2 Canada
FDA Number: 9200934   *Fax:* (905) 660-7885
E-mail: RossDisposable@aol.com
Web site: www.rossdisposable.bizland.com
Medical Products Sales Volume: $985,000
Year Founded: 1960
Total Employees: 5
Ownership: Private
Produces/Sells CE-marked Devices: N
Federal Procurement Eligibility: Small Business
Distribution: Manufacturer Direct, Exclusive Distributor, Importer

ROSS LABORATORIES
See Abbott Laboratories

ROSS PRODUCTS DIVISION
See Abbott Laboratories

ROSYS, INC.
See Xiril

ROTBURG INSTRUMENTS OF AMERICA INC.
954-331-8046
1560 Sawgrass Corporate Pkwy., 4th Floor, Sunrise, FL 33323
FDA Number: 3004632084   *Fax:* 954-331-4601
E-mail: info@rotburg.com
Web site: www.rotburg.com
Ownership: Private
Produces/Sells CE-marked Devices: N
  Cystoscope   Gastroenterology/Urology
  Electrocautery Unit, Gynecologic   Obstetrics/Gynecology
  Electrode, Electrosurgical, Return (Ground, Dispersive)   Surgery
  Electrosurgical Unit, Cutting & Coagulation Device   Surgery
  Forceps, Biopsy, Non-Electric   Gastroenterology/Urology
  Laparoscope, Gynecologic   Obstetrics/Gynecology
  Retractor   Orthopedics
  Ureteroscope   Gastroenterology/Urology

ROTH DRUG CO.
312-733-1478
669 West Ohio St., --, Chestnut Street, IL 60610
FDA Number: 1419646
  Cement, Dental   Dental And Oral
  Preparer, Root Canal, Endodontic   Dental And Oral

ROTOFLEX INTERNATIONAL INC.
800-387-3825
420 Ambassador Dr.,
905-670-8700
Mississauga, ONT L5T 1 Canada
FDA Number: n/a   *Fax:* 905-670-3402
Web site: www.rotoflex.com
Medical Products Sales Volume: $25,000,000
Total Employees: 200   *Marketing Staff:* 10   *Sales Staff:* 20
Ownership: Private
Quality System Registration Information: ISO9000
Produces/Sells CE-marked Devices: Y
Federal Procurement Eligibility: Small Business
Distribution: Manufacturer Direct, Exporter

ROWLEY BIOCHEMICAL INSTITUTE
978-739-4883
10 Electronics Avenue, Danvers Industrial Park,
Danvers, MA 01923
FDA Number: 1219125   *Fax:* 978-739-5640
E-mail: info@rowleybio.com
Web site: www.rowleybio.com
Annual Revenue: $0-$1 Million
Total Employees: 5
Ownership: Private
Produces/Sells CE-marked Devices: N
Federal Procurement Eligibility: Small Business
Distribution: Manufacturer Direct
General Admin.: Martin E. Hecht/Chief Executive Officer
Mktg./Adv.: Debbie Monahan/Manager Advertising
Production: Anne E. Parsons/Manager Production
  Fluid, Bouin's   Pathology

ROWLEY BIOCHEMICAL INSTITUTE
978-739-4883 *(cont'd)*
  Hematoxylin Weigert's   Pathology
  Resorcin Fuchsin   Pathology
  Stain, Alcian Blue   Pathology
  Stain, Congo Red   Pathology
  Stain, Eosin Y   Pathology
  Stain, Giemsa   Pathology
  Stain, Hematoxylin, Harris's   Pathology
  Stain, Hematoxylin, Mayer's   Pathology
  Stain, Iron   Pathology
  Stain, Methylene Blue   Pathology
  Stain, Microbiological   Microbiology
  Stain, Mucicarmine   Pathology
  Stain, Nuclear Fast Red   Pathology
  Stain, Phosphotungstic Acid Hematoxylin   Pathology
  Stain, Reagent, Schiff   Pathology
  Stain, Romanowsky   Hematology
  Stain, Van Gieson's   Pathology

ROX MEDICAL
949-361-8899
150 Calle Iglesia, Suite A, San Clemente, CA 92672
FDA Number: 3004614328   *Fax:* 949-361-8833
E-mail: info@roxmedical.com
Web site: www.roxmedical.com/
Ownership: Private
Produces/Sells CE-marked Devices: N
General Admin.: Mr. Rodney Brenneman/President, Chief Executive Officer
Mktg./Adv.: Mr. Trent Reutiman/Vice President Marketing
         Mr. Martin Chambers/Vice President Sales
Production: Ms. Helene Lamielle/Vice President Quality Assurance & Regulatory Affairs
  Clip, Implantable   Surgery

ROXANE LABORATORIES
800-962-8364
P.O. Box 16532, Columbus, OH 43216-6532
FDA Number: n/a   *Fax:* 614-308-3540
Web site: www.roxane.com
Medical Products Sales Volume: $75,000,000
Annual Revenue: $50-$100 Million
Ownership: Boehringer Ingelheim Pharmacueticals Inc.
Produces/Sells CE-marked Devices: N
Distribution: Manufacturer Through Distributor
  Saliva, Artificial   Dental And Oral
  System, Delivery, Drug, Unit-Dose   General

ROXON MEDI-TECH LTD.
800-361-6991
9400 Pascal Gagnon,
514-326-7780
St-Leonard, QUE H1P 1 Canada
FDA Number: n/a   *Fax:* 514-326-8420
E-mail: montreal@roxon.ca
Web site: www.roxon.ca
Year Founded: 1975
Total Employees: 50
Ownership: Private
Produces/Sells CE-marked Devices: N
Distribution: Exclusive Distributor, Importer

ROXON--UNIVERSAL MEDICAL LTD.
(800) 667-7408
#144, 15501 - 89A Avenue,
(604) 420-7743
Surrey, BC V3R 0 Canada
FDA Number: n/a   *Fax:* (800) 861-7780
E-mail: vancouver@roxon.ca
Web site: www.roxon.ca
Year Founded: 1995
Total Employees: 10
Ownership: Private
Produces/Sells CE-marked Devices: N
Distribution: Exclusive Distributor

ROYAL CONVERTING, INC.
-800-251-9864
200 DeBusk Lane, Powell, TN 37849
865-938-7828
FDA Number: 1060681
E-mail: customerservice@deroyal.com
Ownership: Private
Produces/Sells CE-marked Devices: N
  Cushion, Table, Surgical   Surgery
  Cushion, Wheelchair (Pad)   Physical Med
  Dressing, Wound, Hydrogel W/out Drug And/or Biologic   Surgery
  Dressing, Wound, Hydrophilic   Surgery
  Dressing, Wound, Occlusive   Surgery
  Protector, Skin Pressure   General
  Support, Patient Position   Anesthesiology

ROYAL DENTAL MANUFACTURING, INC.
425-743-0988
12414 Highway 99, Everett, WA 98204
FDA Number: 3022707   *Fax:* 425-743-3588
E-mail: apeterson@royaldental.com
Web site: www.royaldental.com/
Medical Products Sales Volume: $6,800,000

ROYAL DENTAL MANUFACTURING, INC. 425-743-0988 *(cont'd)*
Annual Revenue: $10-$25 Million
Year Founded: 1976
Total Employees: 70
Ownership: Private
Produces/Sells CE-marked Devices: N
Federal Procurement Eligibility: Small Business, Minority Owned
Distribution: Manufacturer Through Distributor, Exporter
General Admin.: Harold Tai/President, Chief Executive Officer
 Carl Grinolds/Vice President, Secretary
Mktg./Adv.: Anita Peterson/Manager Exports
 Raymond Tai/Manager Product Development
 Chuck DePree/Vice President Marketing
 Howard Sorenson/Vice President Sales
Production: Daryl Glassey/Manager Customer Services

Chair, Dental	Dental And Oral
Stool, Dental	Dental And Oral

Medical Product Subsidiaries (Listed Separately)
Biotec, Inc.
Proma, Inc.

ROYAL PAPER PRODUCTS, INC. 800-666-6655
PO Box 151, Coatesville, PA 19320 610-384-3400
FDA Number: 2523490 *Fax:* 610-384-5106
E-mail: sales@royalpaper.com
Web site: www.royalpaper.com
Medical Products Sales Volume: $4,700,000
Annual Revenue: $25-$50 Million
Year Founded: 1949
Total Employees: 37 Marketing Staff: 3 Sales Staff: 167
Ownership: Private
Produces/Sells CE-marked Devices: N
Federal Procurement Eligibility: Small Business
Distribution: Manufacturer Direct, Importer
General Admin.: David Milberg/President
 Fred B. Leibowitz/Vice President, General Manager
Mktg./Adv.: Todd J. Strauss/Manager Advertising

Foodservice Product/Equipment	General
Glove, Patient Examination, Latex	General
Glove, Patient Examination, Vinyl	General
Towel/Towelette, Paper	General

ROYCE MEDICAL 800-521-0601
742 Pancho Road, Camarillo, CA 93012 805-484-2600
FDA Number: n/a *Fax:* 800-889-5722
E-mail: info@roycemedical.com
Web site: www.roycemedical.com
Medical Products Sales Volume: $9,000,000
Year Founded: 1972
Total Employees: 109 Sales Staff: 40
Ownership: Private
Federal Procurement Eligibility: Small Business, GSA Contract
Distribution: Manufacturer Direct, Exporter
General Admin.: Jeff Haines/President, Chief Executive Officer
Mktg./Adv.: Dwane Lindberg/Manager International Marketing & Sales
Production: Carlos Ballina/Vice President Manufacturing

Immobilizer, Knee	Orthopedics
Material, Casting	Dental And Oral
Orthosis, Limb Brace	Physical Med
Support, Ankle	Orthopedics
Support, Back	Orthopedics
Support, Knee	Physical Med
Support, Leg	Physical Med
Support, Wrist	Physical Med

ROYCE ROLLS RINGER CO. 800-253-9638
PO Box 1831, 16 Riverview Terrace, 616-361-9266
Grand Rapids, MI 49501
FDA Number: 9310062 *Fax:* 616-361-5976
E-mail: roycerol@msn.com
Web site: www.RoyceRolls.net
Medical Products Sales Volume: $4,000,000
Annual Revenue: $1-$5 Million
Year Founded: 1925
Total Employees: 26
Ownership: Private
Produces/Sells CE-marked Devices: N
Federal Procurement Eligibility: Small Business
Distribution: Manufacturer Direct
General Admin.: Matthew Royce/Chief Executive Officer
 Charles Royce/President
 S. A. Royce/Secretary, Treasurer
 Charles Royce/Vice President
Mktg./Adv.: Bill Swartz/Director Marketing

Cart, Housekeeping	General
Cart, Laundry	General
Cart, Other	General
Dispenser, Tissue, Toilet	General

ROYCE ROLLS RINGER CO. 800-253-9638 *(cont'd)*
Housekeeping Equipment General

ROYCO APPARATUS LTD. 905-893-1972
P.O. Box 277, Kleinburg, ONT L0J-1C0 Canada
FDA Number: n/a *Fax:* 905-893-0968
E-mail: 7983royce@rogers.com
Year Founded: 1970
Total Employees: 10
Ownership: Private
Produces/Sells CE-marked Devices: N
Distribution: Manufacturer Direct, Exclusive Distributor

ROYDENT DENTAL PRODUCTS 800.992.7767
608 Rolling Hills Drive, Johnson City, TN 37604 717-845-7511
FDA Number: 3004146638 *Fax:* 888.769.3368
E-mail: information@roydent.com
Web site: www.roydent.com
Ownership: Dentsply International, Inc.
Stock Symbol: XRAY
Traded On: NASDAQ
Produces/Sells CE-marked Devices: N

Base, Denture, Relining, Repairing, Rebasing, Resin	Dental And Oral
Broach, Endodontic	Dental And Oral
Crown And Bridge, Temporary, Resin	Dental And Oral
Drill, Dental, Intraoral	Dental And Oral
File, Pulp Canal, Endodontic	Dental And Oral
Gauge, Depth, Instrument, Dental	Dental And Oral
Gutta Percha	Dental And Oral
Material, Impression	Dental And Oral
Paper, Articulation	Dental And Oral
Point, Paper, Endodontic	Dental And Oral
Post, Root Canal	Dental And Oral
Reamer, Pulp Canal, Endodontic	Dental And Oral

ROZINN BY SCOTTCARE CORPORATION 800-243-9412
4791 West 150th Street, Cleveland, OH 44135 216-361-0550
FDA Number: 2435544 *Fax:* 216-267-6129
E-mail: info@scottcare.com
Web site: www.rozinn.com
Annual Revenue: $10-$25 Million
Year Founded: 1979
Total Employees: 60 Marketing Staff: 6 Sales Staff: 30
Ownership: Scottcare Corporation
Stock Symbol: brk.a
Traded On: NYSE
Produces/Sells CE-marked Devices: Y
Distribution: Manufacturer Direct, Manufacturer Through Distributor, Manufacturer Through Manufacturer Reps, OEM
General Admin.: Mark Rosoff/President
Mktg./Adv.: Roland Bates/Director Marketing & Advertising
 Snehraj Merchant/Director Product Development
 Karl Ziemann/Manager International Sales
 George Falcone/Manager Sales
 Nicusor Ilie/Product & Services Manager
Production: Richard Gordon/Director Quality Assurance
 Mark Rosoff/Manager Regulatory Affairs
Purchasing: Christina Ferrante/Manager Purchasing

Battery	General
Circulatory Assist Unit, Cardiac	Cardiovascular
Electrocardiograph, Ambulatory (With Analysis Algorithm)	Cardiovascular
Recorder, Long-Term, Blood Pressure, Portable	Cardiovascular
Recorder, Long-Term, ECG	Cardiovascular
Recorder, Long-Term, ECG, Portable (Holter Monitor)	Cardiovascular
Service, Maintenance/Repair	General
Service, Used Equipment	General
Telemetry Unit, Physiological, ECG	Cardiovascular

ROZYNSKI & ASSOCIATES 202-974-6222
2120 L Street, NW, Suite 245, Washington, DC 20037
FDA Number: n/a *Fax:* 202-974-6262
E-mail: ed@rozynski-associates.com
Web site: www.rozynski-associates.com
Medical Products Sales Volume: $400,000
Annual Revenue: $0-$1 Million
Year Founded: 2003
Total Employees: 4 Marketing Staff: 2 Sales Staff: 2
Ownership: Private
Produces/Sells CE-marked Devices: N
Federal Procurement Eligibility: Small Business
Distribution: Service Direct
General Admin.: Mr. William Merkin/Co-Managing Director
 Mr. Edward Rozynski/President, Owner
Mktg./Adv.: Ms. Raelyn Campbell/Director International Business Development
 Ms. Kristin Pomeroy/Manager Advertising & Market Research
IS: Ms. Elaine Bayliff/Web Master

Service, Consulting	General

ROZYNSKI & ASSOCIATES
202-974-6222 *(cont'd)*
Service, Licensing, Device, Medical
General

RPC
800-647-3873
PO Box 35849, Tucson, AZ 85740
520-888-5551
FDA Number: 2028411
Fax: 520-888-5557
E-mail: mhonstein@compuserve.com
Web site: www.rpc-rabrenco.com
Annual Revenue: $5-$10 Million
Year Founded: 1991
Ownership: Private
Produces/Sells CE-marked Devices: N
Distribution: Manufacturer Direct, Manufacturer Through Distributor, OEM, Exclusive Distributor, Importer, Exporter
General Admin.: Mr. Michael Honstein/Chief Operating Officer
Mr. Vern Taaffe/President, Chief Executive Officer
Mktg./Adv.: Ms. Brenda Johnson/Admin. Marketing & Sales
Strip, Test, Reagent, Residuals For Dialysate, Disinfectant | Gastroenterology/Urology
Tube, Capillary Blood Collection | Hematology

RPI OF ATLANTA
800-554-1501
120 Interstate N. Pkwy. E., Ste. 440,
770-850-1126
Atlanta,, GA 30339
FDA Number: n/a
Fax: 770-952-7492
E-mail: stickdoc@intracell.net
Web site: www.intracell.net
Annual Revenue: $0-$1 Million
Total Employees: 6 | *Marketing Staff:* 2 | *Sales Staff:* 4
Ownership: Private
Produces/Sells CE-marked Devices: Y
Federal Procurement Eligibility: Small Business
Distribution: Manufacturer Direct, Manufacturer Through Distributor
General Admin.: Pat E. Belcher/President
Mktg./Adv.: Ginger McClure/Coord. Marketing
Pat Belcher/Manager Sales
Stimulator, Muscle, Low Intensity | Physical Med

RS MEDICAL
800-683-0353
14001 S.E. First St., Vancouver, WA 98684
FDA Number: 1644243
Fax: 800-929-6476
Web site: www.rsmedical.com
Medical Products Sales Volume: $50,000,000
Year Founded: 1990
Total Employees: 500
Ownership: Private
Produces/Sells CE-marked Devices: Y
Federal Procurement Eligibility: Small Business
Distribution: Manufacturer Direct
General Admin.: Rick Terrell/President
Mktg./Adv.: Randy Murphy/Vice President Marketing
Bruce Hatch/Vice President Sales
Production: Mike Rodeman/Vice President Operations
Research: Mike McGraw/Vice President Product Development
Bill Carroll/Vice President Research
Finance: Tom Pierce/Vice President Finance
Electrode, Cutaneous | Cns/Neurology
Joint, Knee, External Brace | Physical Med
Orthosis, Lumbar | Physical Med
Stimulator, Electro-Analgesic | Cns/Neurology
Stimulator, Muscle, Electrical-Powered (EMS) | Physical Med
Stimulator, Neuromuscular, External Functional | Cns/Neurology
Traction Unit, Non-Powered | Orthopedics
Unit, Therapy, Current, Interferential | Cns/Neurology

RSB SPINE LLC.
866-241-2104
2530 Superior Ave., Suite 703, Cleveland, OH 44114
FDA Number: 3003597504
Fax: 216-241-2820
E-mail: aturchek@rbsurgical.com
Web site: www.rsbspine.com
Ownership: Private
Produces/Sells CE-marked Devices: N
General Admin.: Mr. John Redmond/Chief Executive Officer
Production: Ms. Lisa Hower/Manager Operations
Mr. William Parsons/Manager Quality Assurance
Research: Mr. James Moran/Vice President Engineering
Appliance, Fixation, Spinal Intervertebral Body | Orthopedics
Device, Spinal Vertebral Body Replacement | Orthopedics
Drill, Manual (With Burr, Trephine & Accessories) | Cns/Neurology

RSTI (RADIOLOGICAL SERVICE TRAINING INSTITUTE)
800-229-7784
30745 Solon Road, Solon, OH 44139
440-349-4700
FDA Number: 1528026
Fax: 440-349-2053
E-mail: rsti@infinet.com
Web site: www.rsti-training.com
Medical Products Sales Volume: $1,000,000
Annual Revenue: $5-$10 Million

RSTI (RADIOLOGICAL SERVICE TRAINING 800-229-7784 *(cont'd)*
Year Founded: 1985
Total Employees: 10 | *Marketing Staff:* 5 | *Sales Staff:* 10
Ownership: Private
Produces/Sells CE-marked Devices: N
Federal Procurement Eligibility: Small Business
Distribution: Manufacturer Direct
General Admin.: Terry Speth/President
Kathy Speth/Vice President Personnel
Mktg./Adv.: Terry Speth/Director Sales Training
Anna Morrison/Manager Marketing
Jim Monro/Vice President Marketing & Sales
IS: Dale Cover/Manager Tech. Training
Service, Maintenance/Repair | General
Training Aid | Orthopedics
Medical Product Subsidiaries (Listed Separately)
Jannx Medical Systems Inc.

RTC INC.-MEMCATH TECHNOLOGIES LLC
651-450-7400
1777 Oakdale Ave.,, West St. Paul, MN 55118
FDA Number: 2184110
Ownership: Private
Produces/Sells CE-marked Devices: N
Accessories, Catheter, G-U | Gastroenterology/Urology
Nasopharyngoscope (Flexible Or Rigid) | Ear/Nose/Throat
Sheath, Endoscopic | Gastroenterology/Urology

RTECH, INC.
877-783-2446
739 Brandywine Drive, Moorestown, NJ 08057
856-222-0604
FDA Number: 2248593
Fax: 856-222-1204
E-mail: service@rtechmedical.com
Web site: www.rtech medical.com
Ownership: Private
Produces/Sells CE-marked Devices: N
Airway, Nasopharyngeal (Breathing Tube) | Anesthesiology
Laryngoscope, Rigid | Anesthesiology

RTF MFG. CO. LLC.
800-836-0744
793 Rt. 66, Hudson, NY 12534-9801
FDA Number: 1320893
Fax: 518-828-2257
E-mail: info@rtfmanufacturing.com
Web site: www.rtfmanufacturing.com
Ownership: Private
Produces/Sells CE-marked Devices: N
Freezer, Blood Storage | Hematology

RTI BIOLOGICS INC.
877-343-6832
11621 Research Circle, Alachua, FL 32615
386-418-8888
FDA Number: 3002719998
Fax: 386-418-0342
E-mail: webmanager@rtix.com
Web site: www.rtix.com
Year Founded: 1998
Ownership: Public
Stock Symbol: RTIX
Traded On: NASDAQ
Produces/Sells CE-marked Devices: N
General Admin.: Mr. Dean Bergy/Chairman, Director
Brian K. Hutchison/Chief Executive Officer, Chairman
Thomas F. Rose/Chief Operating Officer, Vice President
Ms. Caroline Harthill/Chief Scientific Officer
Dr. Karl Koschatzky/Vice President International Affairs
Mktg./Adv.: Mr. Roger Rose/Commercial Director
Finance: Mr. Robert Jordheim/Chief Financial Officer
Filler, Calcium Sulfate Preformed Pellets | Orthopedics
Passer, Wire, Orthopedic | Orthopedics
Screw, Fixation, Bone | Orthopedics
Screwdriver | Orthopedics
Tap, Bone | Orthopedics
Tray, Surgical Instrument | Surgery
Valve, Heart, Tissue | Cardiovascular
Medical Product Subsidiaries (Listed Separately)
Tutogen Medical Gmbh

RTI ELECTRONICS, INC.
800-222-7537
1275 Bloomfield Avenue, Building 5, Unit 29A,
973-439-0242
Fairfield, NJ 07004
FDA Number: n/a
Fax: 973-439-0248
E-mail: info@rtielectronics.com
Web site: www.rtielectronics.com
Medical Products Sales Volume: $1,000,000
Annual Revenue: $1-$5 Million
Year Founded: 1981
Total Employees: 3
Ownership: Private
Produces/Sells CE-marked Devices: Y
Federal Procurement Eligibility: Small Business
Distribution: Exclusive Distributor
Mktg./Adv.: Mr. Robert Morrison/Admin. National Sales

RTI ELECTRONICS, INC.
800-222-7537 *(cont'd)*

Camera, Focal Spot, Radiographic — Radiology
Tester, Radiology Quality Assurance — Radiology

RTI ELECTRONICS, INC.
(714) 765-8200
1800 E. Via Burton, Anaheim, CA 92806-1213
FDA Number: n/a
Fax: (714) 765-8201
Web site: www.rtie-corp.com
Medical Products Sales Volume: $250,000
Annual Revenue: $10-$25 Million
Total Employees: 110   *Marketing Staff:* 1   *Sales Staff:* 7
Ownership: SELAS CORPORATION OF AMERICA
Stock Symbol: SLS
Traded On: AMEX
Produces/Sells CE-marked Devices: N
Distribution: Manufacturer Through Distributor, OEM
General Admin.: Carle Bryant/Vice President Human Resources
       Steve M. Binnix/Vice President, General Manager
Mktg./Adv.: Bill Wentzel/Director Product Development
       Steve M. Binnix/Vice President Business Development
       Jeanne Kurth/Vice President Sales
Production: Brue Wilson/Director Quality Assurance
       Linda Ogg/Manager Materials
       Jonathan Smith/Vice President Manufacturing
Component, Electronic — General

RTR INDUSTRIES, INC.
519-438-3691
700 York St, London N5W 2S8 Canada
FDA Number: 9681282
Pack, Hot Or Cold, Reusable — Physical Med

RUBBERMAID COMMERCIAL PRODUCTS LLC
800-347-9800
3124 Valley Ave., Winchester, VA 22601-2636
540-667-8700
FDA Number: 9320110
Fax: 540-542-8309
Web site: www.rubbermaidcommercial.com
Ownership: Public
Stock Symbol: NWL
Traded On: NYSE
Quality System Registration Information: ISO9002
Produces/Sells CE-marked Devices: N
Distribution: Manufacturer Through Distributor
General Admin.: W. Michael Moorefield/President, General Manager
Mktg./Adv.: Judy Cline/Director Marketing & Sales
Cart, Housekeeping — General
Cart, Multipurpose — General
Housekeeping Equipment — General
Waste Receptacle, General Purpose — General

RUBICOR MEDICAL, INC.
650-587-3446
600 Chesapeake Drive, Redwood City, CA 94063
FDA Number: 3004014191
Binder, Elastic — General
Biopsy Instrument — Gastroenterology/Urology
Electrosurgical Unit, Cutting & Coagulation Device — Surgery

RUBIN & POOR, INC.
973-762-9009
155 Maplewood Ave, #5, Maplewood, NJ 07040
FDA Number: 2438963
Software, Blood Bank (Stand-Alone Products) — Hematology

RUDOLPH ALBERT CO., THE
See Albert International, Inc.

RUDOLPH RESEARCH ANALYTICAL
973-584-1558
55 Newburgh Road, Hackettstown, NJ 07840
FDA Number: n/a
Fax: 973-584-5440
E-mail: info@rudolphresearch.com
Web site: www.rudolphresearch.com
Medical Products Sales Volume: $5,700,000
Annual Revenue: $1-$5 Million
Total Employees: 34
Ownership: Private
Produces/Sells CE-marked Devices: N
Federal Procurement Eligibility: Small Business
Distribution: Manufacturer Direct, Manufacturer Through Manufacturer Reps
General Admin.: Richard C. Spanier/President, Chief Executive Officer
Polarimeter — Chemistry
Refractometer — Chemistry

RUGGLES CORPORATION
See Elekta Inc.

RUHLING ENTERPRISES, INC.
616-364-0090
4598 Plainfield Ne, Grand Rapids, MI 49525
FDA Number: 1832733
Hearing-Aid — Ear/Nose/Throat

RUPERT INDUSTRIES, DIV C&J ASSOC. INC
See E-Z-On Products Inc. Of Florida

RUPP + BOWMAN CO.
See Global Focus (G.F.M.D. Ltd.)

RUSH MEDICAL
401-461-9132
18 Gallup Ave., Cranston, RI 02910
FDA Number: 3004649027
Ownership: Private
Produces/Sells CE-marked Devices: N
Bandage, Elastic — General
Clamp, Line — Gastroenterology/Urology

RUSH-BERIVON, INC.
800-251-7874
1010 19th St., P.O. Box 1851, Meridian, MS 39302
601-693-6344
FDA Number: 1018798
Fax: 601-693-6348
E-mail: sales@rushpin.com
Web site: www.netdoor.com/com/berivon
Medical Products Sales Volume: $700,000
Annual Revenue: $0-$1 Million
Total Employees: 5   *Marketing Staff:* 1   *Sales Staff:* 1
Ownership: Private
Produces/Sells CE-marked Devices: N
Distribution: Manufacturer Direct
General Admin.: Leslie Rush/President
       Beryl R. Webb/Vice President
Mktg./Adv.: Vi Stinnette/Director Advertising
Bender — Orthopedics
Driver, Surgical, Pin — Surgery
Extractor, Nail — Orthopedics
Holder, Leg — Surgery
Mallet, Bone — Orthopedics
Passer, Wire, Orthopedic — Orthopedics
Pin, Fixation, Smooth — Orthopedics
Rack, Surgical Instrument — Surgery
Reamer — Orthopedics

RUSHABH INSTRUMENTS, LLC
215-491-0081
1750a Costner Dr., Warrington, PA 18976
FDA Number: 3003639866
Stainer, Slide, Automated — Pathology

RUSHMORE LABORATORIES
See Abbott Laboratories

RX HONING MACHINE CORPORATION
800-346-6464
1301 E. Fifth St., Mishawaka, IN 46544-2827
574-259-1606
FDA Number: n/a
Fax: 574-259-9163
E-mail: info@rxhoning.com.
Web site: www.rxhoning.com
Medical Products Sales Volume: $500,000
Annual Revenue: $0-$1 Million
Total Employees: 7   *Marketing Staff:* 2   *Sales Staff:* 2
Ownership: Private
Produces/Sells CE-marked Devices: Y
Federal Procurement Eligibility: Small Business
Distribution: Manufacturer Direct
General Admin.: R. J . Watson/President
Mktg./Adv.: Marvin Yocum/Director Product Development
Research: Marvin Yocum/Vice President Research & Development
Arthroscope — Orthopedics
Instrument, Dental, Manual — Dental And Oral
Instrument, Manual, General Surgical — Surgery
Instrument, Microsurgical — Cns/Neurology
Kit, Instruments and Accessories, Surgical — Surgery
Service, Maintenance/Repair — General
Sharpener, Dental — Dental And Oral
Sharpener, Instrument, Surgical — Surgery
Sharpener, Knife — Surgery
Surgical Instrument, Manual (General Use) — Surgery
Surgical Instrument, Orthopedic, AC-Powered Motor — Orthopedics
Training Aid — Orthopedics

RX TEXTILES, INC.
704-283-9787
3107 Chamber Dr., Monroe, NC 28110
FDA Number: 1061153
Bandage, Cast — Physical Med
Bandage, Elastic — General
Cover, Limb — Physical Med
Drape, Surgical — Surgery
Protector, Skin Pressure — General

RYCOR MEDICAL, INC.
800-227-9267
2053 Atwater Drive, North Port, FL 34288
216-226-4900
FDA Number: 1529287
Fax: 941-240-5839
E-mail: info@rycormedical.com
Web site: www.rycormedical.com
Medical Products Sales Volume: $200,000
Annual Revenue: $0-$1 Million
Year Founded: 1980
Total Employees: 3
Ownership: Private

RYCOR MEDICAL, INC.   800-227-9267 *(cont'd)*
Produces/Sells CE-marked Devices: N
Federal Procurement Eligibility: Small Business
Distribution: Manufacturer Direct
General Admin.: Clifford Limpert/President
Mktg./Adv.: Ryan Limpert/Manager National Sales

Bin, Storage	General
Component, Traction, Non-Invasive	Orthopedics
Contract Manufacturing, Product, Durable	General
Stirrup	Gastroenterology/Urology
Table, Surgical, Manual	General

RYDER INTERNATIONAL CORP.
See Atrion Medical Products, Inc.

RYMED TECHNOLOGIES, INC.   615-790-8093
137 Third Avenue North, Franklin, TN 37064
FDA Number: 3005951712   *Fax:* 615-790-8984
E-mail: info@rymedtech.com
Web site: http://www.rymedtech.com
Ownership: Private
Produces/Sells CE-marked Devices: N
General Admin.: Ms. Dana Ryan/President, Chief Executive Officer
Production: Mr. James Kaiser/Vice President Operations

Kit, Administration, Intravenous	General

RYNEL, INC.   207-882-0200
11 Twin Rivers Dr, Wiscasset, ME 04578
FDA Number: 1225263

Bandage, Liquid	Surgery
Dressing, Wound, Hydrophilic	Surgery

S & S ORTHOPEDIC LTD.   336-626-5167
701 Westmont Drive, Asheboro, NC 27205-4263
FDA Number: 1063482   *Fax:* 336-626-2822
E-mail: sefcik@asheboro.com
Year Founded: 1992
Ownership: Private
Produces/Sells CE-marked Devices: N
Federal Procurement Eligibility: Small Business
Distribution: Manufacturer Through Distributor, OEM, Exporter
Production: Frank Sefcik/Vice President, Engineer

Surgical Instrument, Orthopedic, Battery-Powered	Surgery

S & S X-RAY PRODUCTS, INC.   800-231-1747
10625 Telge Road, Houston, TX 77095   281-815-1300
FDA Number: 3003848601   *Fax:* 281-815-1444
E-mail: info@ssxray.com
Web site: www.ssxray.com
Year Founded: 1947
Ownership: Private
Quality System Registration Information: ISO9001
Produces/Sells CE-marked Devices: N
Federal Procurement Eligibility: Small Business
Distribution: Manufacturer Through Distributor
General Admin.: Dr. Norman Shoenfeld/President, Chief Executive Officer
    Mr. Fred Sopenoff/Vice President
Mktg./Adv.: Mr. Donald Thurston/Manager National Sales
    Mr. Jim Beegle/Manager National Sales

Accelerator, Linear, Medical	Radiology

Medical Product Subsidiaries (Listed Separately)
    S&S Medcart

S & T MICROLAB AG
See Eriem Surgical

S & T MICROSURGICAL AG
See Eriem Surgical

S JACKSON INC.   800-368-5225
PO Box 4487, Alexandria, VA 22303   703-370-4900
FDA Number: 1111225   *Fax:* 703-370-1679
E-mail: supramid@mindspring.com
Web site: www.supramid.com
Medical Products Sales Volume: $900,000
Annual Revenue: $0-$1 Million
Total Employees: 10   *Marketing Staff:* 5   *Sales Staff:* 5
Ownership: Private
Produces/Sells CE-marked Devices: N
Federal Procurement Eligibility: Small Business
Distribution: Manufacturer Direct, Manufacturer Through Distributor, OEM, Exporter
General Admin.: J. Jackson/President, Chief Executive Officer
    S. S. Jackson/Secretary, Treasurer
Mktg./Adv.: M. Dawson/Manager National Sales
Production: Sallie Jackson/Manager Materials
    C. Boutwell/Manager Regulatory Affairs

Mesh, Surgical, Polymeric	Surgery
Prosthesis, Chin, Internal	Surgery
Prosthesis, Eye, Internal (Sphere)	Surgery

S JACKSON INC.   800-368-5225 *(cont'd)*

Prosthesis, Rhinoplasty	Surgery
Suture, Non-Absorbable, Synthetic, Polyamide	Surgery

S&B BIOMEDICS, INC.   972-288-3278
844 Dalworth Drive, Suite 6, Mesquite, TX 75149-4162
FDA Number: 9320163   *Fax:* 972-288-3279
Annual Revenue: $0-$1 Million
Total Employees: 5   *Marketing Staff:* 1   *Sales Staff:* 1
Ownership: Private
Produces/Sells CE-marked Devices: N
Federal Procurement Eligibility: Small Business
Distribution: Manufacturer Direct, Importer, Exporter
General Admin.: A. J. Segars/President
Mktg./Adv.: Jack E. Burroughs/Vice President Marketing

Prosthesis, Ankle, Semi-Constrained, Metal/Polymer	Orthopedics
Prosthesis, Foot	Orthopedics

S&G ENTERPRISES, INC.   800-233-3721
N115 W19000 Edison Drive,   262-251-8300
Germantown, WI 53022
FDA Number: 9330109   *Fax:* 262-251-1616
E-mail: info@ramflat.com
Web site: www.ramflat.com
Medical Products Sales Volume: $1,000,000
Annual Revenue: $0-$1 Million
Year Founded: 1961
Total Employees: 3
Ownership: Private
Produces/Sells CE-marked Devices: N
Federal Procurement Eligibility: Small Business, GSA Contract
Distribution: Manufacturer Direct, OEM
General Admin.: Ola Tyshynsky/Office Manager
    Mark J. Griffith/President
Production: Mark J. Griffith/Product Engineer

Compactor, Fixed	General
Component, Other	General
Crusher, Vial, Laboratory	General

S&K REAGENTS, INC.
See Rocky Mountain Reagents, Inc.

S&S INFICON, INC.
See Infimed, Inc.

S&S MEDCART   800-231-1747
10625 Telge Road, Houston, TX 77095   281-815-1300
FDA Number: n/a   *Fax:* 281-815-1444
E-mail: information@medcart.com
Web site: www.medcart.com
Total Employees: 25   *Marketing Staff:* 3   *Sales Staff:* 12
Ownership: S & S X-Ray Products, Inc.
Produces/Sells CE-marked Devices: N
Federal Procurement Eligibility: VA Contract
Distribution: Manufacturer Direct, Manufacturer Through Manufacturer Reps
General Admin.: Dr. Norman Shoenfeld/President, Chief Executive Officer
Mktg./Adv.: Mr. Kenny Jones/Manager Sales

Cart, Medicine	General

S&S TECHNOLOGY   281-815-1300
10625 Telge Road, Houston, TX 77095
FDA Number: ÿ1650045   *Fax:* 281-815-1444
E-mail: info@ss-technology.com
Web site: www.ss-technology.com
Medical Products Sales Volume: $13,900,000
Annual Revenue: $10-$25 Million
Year Founded: 1999
Total Employees: 115   *Marketing Staff:* 2   *Sales Staff:* 9
Ownership: Private
Produces/Sells CE-marked Devices: N
Federal Procurement Eligibility: Small Business
Distribution: Manufacturer Through Distributor, OEM, Exporter
General Admin.: Tom Chando/Chief Operating Officer
    Dr. Norman Shoenfeld/President
Mktg./Adv.: Jennifer Williams/Coord. Marketing & Trade Show
    Donald Thurston/Manager International & National Sales
Production: Kevin Bradley/Director Engineering

Apron, Lead, Radiographic	Radiology
Block, Therapy, Radiation	Radiology
Cabinet, Other	General
Cabinet, Storage, Catheter	General
Cabinet, X-Ray Transfer	Radiology
Cart, Anesthetist's	Anesthesiology
Cart, Dressing	General
Cart, Emergency, Cardiopulmonary Resuscitation (Crash)	Anesthesiology
Cart, Equipment, Video	General
Cart, Instrument	Surgery
Cart, Isolation	General
Cart, Medicine	General
Cart, Monitor	General

S&S TECHNOLOGY
281-815-1300 (cont'd)

Cart, Multipurpose	General
Cart, Other	General
Cart, Supply, Operating Room	Surgery
Densitometer, Radiographic	Radiology
Dryer, Film, Radiographic	Dental And Oral
Holder, Radiographic Cassette, Wall-Mounted	Radiology
Holder, X-Ray Film	Dental And Oral
Illuminator, Radiographic Film	Radiology
Labeler, X-Ray Film	Radiology
Safelight, X-Ray	Radiology
Sensor, Optical Contour, Physical Medicine	Physical Med
Shield, Gonadal	Radiology
Shield, X-Ray	Radiology
Storage Unit, X-Ray Film	Radiology
Support, Patient Position, Radiographic	Radiology
Tape, Measuring, Ruler And Caliper	Surgery
Viewer, Radiographic Film, Motorized	Radiology

S&S X-RAY PRODUCTS, INC.
See S&S Technology

S&W BY HAUSMANN
888-428-7626
130 Union Street, Northvale, NJ 07647
201-767-0255
FDA Number: 7000718
Fax: 201-767-1369
E-mail: info@hausmann.com
Web site: www.s-wenterprises.com
Medical Products Sales Volume: $6,800,000
Annual Revenue: $1-$5 Million
Year Founded: 1971
Total Employees: 95   *Marketing Staff:* 1   *Sales Staff:* 3
Ownership: Aaron Carlson Corporation
Produces/Sells CE-marked Devices: N
Federal Procurement Eligibility: Small Business
Distribution: Manufacturer Direct, Manufacturer Through Distributor
General Admin.: Jason Horner/President
Mktg./Adv.: Mr. Brian Buhl/Director Sales

Bars, Parallel, Exercise	Physical Med
Cabinet Casework, Patient Room	General
Cabinet, Bedside	General
Cabinet, Medicine	General
Cart, Instrument	Surgery
Chair, Blood Donor	General
Furniture, Patient Room	General
Mirror, Posture	Physical Med
Table, Examination/Treatment	General
Table, Physical Therapy	Physical Med

S. RONCI CO., INC.
See Allen Medical Systems, Inc.

S.A.T. INC.
See Spirig Advanced Technologies, Inc.

S.C.I. SCIENCE CENTER, INC.
800-345-0774
PO Box 994, Santa Fe, NM 87505
505-982-8029
FDA Number: n/a
Fax: 505-983-2851
E-mail: info@sciloops.com
Web site: www.sciloops.com
Medical Products Sales Volume: $400,000
Annual Revenue: $0-$1 Million
Year Founded: 1962
Total Employees: 3   *Marketing Staff:* 2   *Sales Staff:* 1
Ownership: Private
Produces/Sells CE-marked Devices: N
Federal Procurement Eligibility: Small Business, Minority Owned
Distribution: Manufacturer Direct, OEM, Exporter
General Admin.: Patrick O. Aranda/President
Production: Paul Marquez/Manufacturing Technician
    Joe Chavez/Vice President Manufacturing

Loop, Inoculating	Microbiology

S.E. INTERNATIONAL, INC.
800-293-5759
436 Farm Road, PO Box 39,
931-964-3561
Summertown, TN 38483
FDA Number: n/a
Fax: 931-964-3564
E-mail: radiationinfo@seintl.com
Web site: www.seintl.com
Medical Products Sales Volume: $2,500,000
Annual Revenue: $1-$5 Million
Year Founded: 1979
Total Employees: 19   *Marketing Staff:* 2   *Sales Staff:* 3
Ownership: Private
Produces/Sells CE-marked Devices: Y
Federal Procurement Eligibility: Small Business, Female Owned
Distribution: Manufacturer Direct, Manufacturer Through Distributor, OEM
General Admin.: Susan Skinner/President, Chief Executive Officer
Mktg./Adv.: Corey Walker/Director Marketing
Production: Beth Cramer/Customer Service Representative

Counter, Radiation	Radiology
Dosimeter, Radiation	Radiology

S.E. INTERNATIONAL, INC.
800-293-5759 (cont'd)

Monitor, Radiation	Radiology

S.P. ARTIFICIAL EYE CO.
270-665-5515
374 Broadway, La Center, KY 42056
FDA Number: 1032906
Ownership: Private
Produces/Sells CE-marked Devices: N

Eye, Artificial, Non-Custom	Ophthalmology

S.S. WHITE BURS INC.
800-535-2877
1145 Towbin Ave., Lakewood, NJ 08701-5932
732-905-1100
FDA Number: 2245654
Fax: 732-905-0987
E-mail: staff@sswhiteburs.com
Web site: www.sswhiteburs.com
Annual Revenue: $10-$25 Million
Total Employees: 390   *Marketing Staff:* 8   *Sales Staff:* 20
Ownership: Private
Quality System Registration Information: ISO9001
Produces/Sells CE-marked Devices: N
Distribution: Manufacturer Through Distributor
General Admin.: Tom Gallop/Chief Executive Officer
    William N. Babcock/President
Mktg./Adv.: Brian Reichert/Director National Accounts
    Ron Doan/Director Product Development
Production: Wayne Boylan/Vice President Manufacturing

Agent, Polishing, Abrasive, Oral Cavity	Dental And Oral
Burr, Dental	Dental And Oral
Burr, Dental Excavating	Dental And Oral
Glove, Patient Examination, Latex	General
Instrument, Diamond, Dental	Dental And Oral
Point, Abrasive	Dental And Oral

S.W. FLORIDA PROSTHETIC CLINIC
239-936-0033
13691 Metro Pkwy., Suite 100, Ft Myers, FL 33912-4348
FDA Number: 1058004
Ownership: Private
Produces/Sells CE-marked Devices: N

Eye, Artificial, Non-Custom	Ophthalmology

S4 TECH INC
703-467-9034
22831 Silverbrook Center Dr. #135, Sterling, VA 20166
FDA Number: 3005024421
Web site: www.s4-tech.com
Ownership: Private
Produces/Sells CE-marked Devices: N

Pack, Hot Or Cold, Water Circulating	Physical Med

S4J MANUFACTURING SERVICES, INC.
888-S4J-LUER
2685 N.E. 9th Avenue, Cape Coral, FL 33909
239-574-9400
FDA Number: n/a
Fax: 239-574-9567
E-mail: sales@s4jluer.com
Web site: www.s4jluer.com
Medical Products Sales Volume: $1,500,000
Annual Revenue: $1-$5 Million
Year Founded: 1964
Total Employees: 15
Ownership: Private
Quality System Registration Information: ISO9001
Produces/Sells CE-marked Devices: N
Federal Procurement Eligibility: Small Business
Distribution: Manufacturer Direct, OEM, Service Direct, Exporter
General Admin.: Steven E. Gyure/President, Chief Executive Officer
Mktg./Adv.: Phillip G. Mullas/Manager Marketing
Production: Douglas S. Gyure/Vice President Production

Contract Manufacturing	General
Contract Manufacturing, Product, Durable	General
Fitting, Luer	General
Fitting, Quick Connect (Gas Connector)	General
Manifold, Gas	Chemistry
Manifold, Liquid	Chemistry
Stopcock	General

SA SCIENTIFIC, INC.
800-272-2710
4919 Golden Quail, San Antonio, TX 78240
210-699-8800
FDA Number: 1645225
Fax: 210-699-6545
E-mail: info@sascientific.com
Web site: www.sascientific.com
Annual Revenue: $5-$10 Million
Year Founded: 1984
Total Employees: 50
Ownership: Private
Produces/Sells CE-marked Devices: N
Distribution: Manufacturer Through Distributor, OEM
General Admin.: Harbi Shadfan/President

Antigen, (Febrile), Agglutination, Brucella SPP.	Microbiology
Antigen, All Types, Escherichia Coli	Microbiology
Antigen, Febrile	Microbiology
Antigen, IHA, Toxoplasma Gondii	Microbiology

SA SCIENTIFIC, INC. 800-272-2710 *(cont'd)*

Antigen, Salmonella SPP.	Microbiology
Antigen, Slide And Tube, Francisella Tularensis	Microbiology
Antigen, Streptococcus SPP.	Microbiology
Antisera, Fluorescent, All Globulins, Proteus SPP.	Microbiology
Antiserum, Escherichia Coli	Microbiology
Antiserum, H. Influenzae	Microbiology
Antiserum, Listeria Monocytogenes	Microbiology
Antiserum, N. Meningitidis	Microbiology
Antiserum, Positive And Negative Febrile Antigen Control	Microbiology
Antiserum, Salmonella SPP.	Microbiology
Antiserum, Shigella SPP.	Microbiology
Antiserum, Streptococcus SPP.	Microbiology
Antiserum, Vibrio Cholerae	Microbiology
Candida Species, Antibody Detection	Microbiology
Kit, Pregnancy Test	Obstetrics/Gynecology
Kit, Pregnancy Test, Over The Counter, HCG	Chemistry
Streptolysin O	Pathology
Test, C-Reactive Protein	Immunology
Test, Human Chorionic Gonadotropin	Immunology
Test, Infectious Mononucleosis	Immunology
Test, Rheumatoid Factor	Immunology
Test, Rotavirus	Microbiology
Test, Sickle Cell	Hematology
Test, Syphilis (RPR or VDRL)	Microbiology
Test, Systemic Lupus Erythematosus	Immunology

SABHI, INC. 601-956-3169
1303 Riverwood Dr., Jackson, MS 39211
FDA Number: 1050855
Ownership: Private
Produces/Sells CE-marked Devices: N
Culture Media, Selective And Differential — Microbiology

SABIN CORPORATION 800-264-4510
3800 Constitution Avenue, PO Box 788 812-323-4500
PO Box 788
Bloomington, IN 47402
FDA Number: 1836564 *Fax:* 812-339-3395
E-mail: sabin@sabincorp.com
Web site: www.sabincorp.com
Medical Products Sales Volume: $7,700,000
Annual Revenue: $10-$25 Million
Year Founded: 1969
Total Employees: 140
Ownership: COOK GROUP
Quality System Registration Information: ISO9002
Produces/Sells CE-marked Devices: N
Federal Procurement Eligibility: Small Business
Distribution: Manufacturer Direct
General Admin.: Dan Peterson/General Manager
Bob Lendman/President, Chief Executive Officer
Mktg./Adv.: Bruce DeMars/Director Product Development
Production: Mike Davis/Director Quality Assurance
Jim Boltinghouse/Manager Materials
Scott Lewis/Plant Manager
Component, Plastic — General

SABLE INDUSTRIES 800-890-0251
4751 Oceanside Blvd., Unit G, 760-758-4553
Oceanside, CA 92056
FDA Number: n/a *Fax:* 760-758-8085
E-mail: sableind@ix.netcom.com
Annual Revenue: $0-$1 Million
Total Employees: 11 *Sales Staff:* 3
Ownership: Private
Produces/Sells CE-marked Devices: N
Federal Procurement Eligibility: Small Business, Female Owned, VA Contract
Distribution: Manufacturer Direct, Manufacturer Through Distributor, Manufacturer Through Manufacturer Reps, OEM
General Admin.: Alexandra Mondiadis/Owner
Julie Butler/President

Blade, Knife, Laparoscopic	Surgery
Blade, Scalpel	Surgery
Instrument, Microsurgical	Cns/Neurology
Knife, Cataract	Ophthalmology
Knife, Myringotomy	Ear/Nose/Throat

SABOLICH PROSTHETIC & RESEARCH CENTER
See Hanger Orthopedic Group, Inc.

SACOR INC. 800-263-3557
12 - 300 Steelcase Rd. W., 905-752-0146
Markham, ONT L3R 2 Canada
FDA Number: n/a *Fax:* 905-752-0185
E-mail: info@sacor.com
Web site: www.sacor.com
Year Founded: 1995
Total Employees: 25

SACOR INC. 800-263-3557 *(cont'd)*
Ownership: Private
Produces/Sells CE-marked Devices: N
Distribution: Exclusive Distributor, Importer, Exporter

SAEBO, INC. 888-284-5433
2725 Water Ridge Parkway, Suite 320, Charlotte, NC 28217
FDA Number: 3005539258
Orthosis, Limb Brace — Physical Med

SAES MEMRY 203-739-1100
3 Berkshire Blvd., Bethel, CT 06801
FDA Number: n/a *Fax:* 203-798-6606
E-mail: info@memry.com
Web site: www.memry.com
Annual Revenue: $25-$50 Million
Ownership: SAES GETTERS SPA
Quality System Registration Information: ISO9001
Produces/Sells CE-marked Devices: Y
Federal Procurement Eligibility: Small Business
Distribution: Manufacturer Direct, OEM, Service Direct
General Admin.: James Binch/Chairman, Chief Executive Officer
Robert Belcher/Chief Financial Officer, Vice President
James Binch/President
Mktg./Adv.: Krishine Carroll/Manager Marketing
Phillipe Poncet/Vice President Business Development
Vikki Hazelwood/Vice President Sales
IS: Ming Wu/Vice President Technology
Contract Manufacturing — General
Contract R&D, Equipment — General

SAFARI DENTAL INC. 800-567-0013
94D boul. Des Enterprises, 450-433-5754
Boisbriand, QUE J7E-2 Canada
FDA Number: n/a *Fax:* 450-433-5987
E-mail: info@dental-safari.com
Web site: www.dental-safari.com
Year Founded: 1994
Total Employees: 10
Ownership: Private
Produces/Sells CE-marked Devices: N
Distribution: Manufacturer Direct

SAFC BIOSCIENCES, INC. 1 800-255-6032
13804 West 107th St., Lenexa, KS 66215 913-469-5580
FDA Number: 1924540 *Fax:* 913-469-5584
Ownership: Private
Produces/Sells CE-marked Devices: N

Culture Media, Synthetic Cell And Tissue	Pathology
Serum, Animal	Pathology
Trypsin	Pathology

SAFC BIOSCIENCES, INC. 913-469-5580
320 Swampbridge Rd., Denver, PA 17517
FDA Number: 2550030

Culture Media, Synthetic Cell And Tissue	Pathology
Trypsin	Pathology

SAFCO PRODUCTS COMPANY 800-328-3020
9300 W. Research Center Rd., 763-536-6700
New Hope, MN 55428
FDA Number: 9201147 *Fax:* 763-536-6777
E-mail: info@safcoproducts.com
Web site: www.safcoproducts.com
Annual Revenue: $5-$10 Million
Total Employees: 150 *Marketing Staff:* 2 *Sales Staff:* 15
Ownership: Private
Produces/Sells CE-marked Devices: N
Distribution: Manufacturer Through Distributor, Manufacturer Through Manufacturer Reps
Mktg./Adv.: Nat Porter/Director Marketing & Sales
Steve Greseth/Director Product Development
Sandy Edstrom/Manager Advertising
Tom Hosinski/Manager National Sales
Waste Receptacle, General Purpose — General

SAFE SOLUTIONS, INC. 616-677-2850
2530 Hayes St., Marne, MI 49435
FDA Number: 3003723243
Detector/Remover, Lice — General

SAFE-GUARD TECHNOLOGIES CORP. 800-220-1245
1111 Hector St., Conshohocken, PA 19428-2311 610-834-1903
FDA Number: n/a *Fax:* 610-834-0769
E-mail: safegdpack@aol.com
Web site: www.safe-guardtech.com
Annual Revenue: $1-$5 Million
Total Employees: 35

SAFE-GUARD TECHNOLOGIES CORP. 800-220-1245 (cont'd)
Ownership: Private
Produces/Sells CE-marked Devices: N
Federal Procurement Eligibility: Small Business
Distribution: Manufacturer Direct, OEM, Exclusive Distributor
General Admin.: Bernard J. Dillon/President
Mktg./Adv.: Linda Barnett/Manager Contracts
        Stephen Phillips/Manager Marketing
        John McGee/Vice President Sales
Production: Larry Conroy/Manager Production
        Ted Barnett/Vice President Manufacturing
Finance: George Rule/Chief Financial Officer

Container, Frozen Donor Tissue Storage	General
Container, Slide Mailer	Microbiology
Container, Specimen Mailer And Storage	Pathology
Container, Specimen Mailer And Storage, Temperature Control	Pathology
Container, Specimen, All Types	General
Contract Manufacturing, Product, Disposable	General
Contract Packaging	General
Foam, Plastic	General

SAFE-T-RACK SYSTEMS, INC. 800-344-0619
4325 Dominguez Road, Suite A, 916-632-1121
Rocklin, CA 95677
FDA Number: n/a   Fax: 916-632-1173
E-mail: info@safe-t-racksystems.com
Web site: www.safe-t-racksystems.com
Medical Products Sales Volume: $1,000,000
Annual Revenue: $0-$1 Million
Year Founded: 1982
Total Employees: 25   *Marketing Staff:* 3   *Sales Staff:* 6
Ownership: Private
Produces/Sells CE-marked Devices: Y
Federal Procurement Eligibility: Small Business, GSA Contract
Distribution: Manufacturer Direct, Manufacturer Through Distributor, Manufacturer Through Manufacturer Reps
General Admin.: Don Despy/President
        Becky Evans/Vice President Personnel
Mktg./Adv.: Becky Evans/Manager International & National Sales

Component, Metal, Other	General
Cylinder, Compressed Gas, With Valve	Anesthesiology
Safety Equipment, Laboratory	Chemistry

SAFE-TEC CLINICAL PRODUCTS, INC. 800-356-6033
142 Railroad Drive, Ivyland, PA 18974 215-364-5582
FDA Number: 2528905   Fax: 215-364-7335
E-mail: sales@safe-tecinc.com
Web site: www.safe-tecinc.com
Medical Products Sales Volume: $500,000
Annual Revenue: $1-$5 Million
Year Founded: 1988
Total Employees: 5   *Marketing Staff:* 2   *Sales Staff:* 2
Ownership: Private
Federal Procurement Eligibility: Small Business
Distribution: Manufacturer Direct, OEM, Service Direct, Exclusive Distributor
General Admin.: Andy Ring/Chief Operating Officer

Dispenser, Fluid	General
Labware, Blood Collection	Chemistry
Tube, Capillary Blood Collection	Hematology

SAFECARE CORPORATION 225-753-4664
6352 Quinn Drive Suite A, Baton Rouge, LA 70817
FDA Number: 3003897809   Fax: 225-753-4664
E-mail: evan@safecaremedical.com
Ownership: Private
Produces/Sells CE-marked Devices: N

Syringe, Antistick	General
Syringe, Piston	General

SAFECROSS FIRST AID LTD. 416-665-0050
1111 Alness St, Toronto M3J 2J1 Canada
FDA Number: 9680884

Kit, First Aid	Surgery

SAFEGARD MEDICAL PRODUCTS, INC. 800-389-7173
52 Dragon Ct., Woburn, MA 01801 781-935-2275
FDA Number: 1226314   Fax: 781-935-8424
E-mail: sales@safegardmedical.com
Web site: www.safegardmedical.com
Total Employees: 1   *Marketing Staff:* 1   *Sales Staff:* 1
Ownership: Preco Industries
Produces/Sells CE-marked Devices: N
Federal Procurement Eligibility: Small Business

Syringe, Piston	General

SAFEGUARD MEDICAL TECHNOLOGIES, LLC 330-547-2166
14200 Ellsworth Rd., Berlin Center, OH 44401
FDA Number: 3003227527

SAFEGUARD MEDICAL TECHNOLOGIES, LLC 330-547-2166
(cont'd)
Ownership: Private
Produces/Sells CE-marked Devices: N

Device, Needle Destruction	General

SAFEPRO USA INC. 904-880-1958
11497 Columbia Park Dr., West Suite 9, Jacksonville, FL 32258
FDA Number: 3003641035
Ownership: Private
Produces/Sells CE-marked Devices: N

Syringe, Antistick	General

SAFER SLEEP LLC 425-861-8262
3322 West End Avenue, Suite 705, Nashville, TN 37203
FDA Number: 3005551612

Gas-Machine, Anesthesia	Anesthesiology

SAFERAIL INC.
See Cweco, Inc.

SAFESLIDEBOARD.COM 770-675-2978
56 Strickland Drive S.w., Mableton, GA 30126
FDA Number: 3004361326
Ownership: Private
Produces/Sells CE-marked Devices: N

Accessories, Wheelchair	Physical Med

SAFESTITCH MEDICAL INC. 305-575-4145
4400 Biscayne Blvd, Suite 760, Miami, FL 33137
FDA Number: 3007802906
Web site: http://www.safestitch.com/
Year Founded: 2005
Ownership: Public
Stock Symbol: SFES
Traded On: OTC Bulletin
Produces/Sells CE-marked Devices: N
General Admin.: Dr. Stewart Davis/Chief Operating Officer
        Mr. Jeffrey Spragens/President, Chief Executive Officer
Medical Admin.: Dr. Charles Filipi/Medical Director
Finance: Mr. Adam Jackson/Chief Financial Officer, Vice President Finance

Dilator, Esophageal	Gastroenterology/Urology
Staple, Implantable	Surgery
Stapler, Surgical	Surgery

SAFETEC OF AMERICA, INC. 800-456-7077
887 Kensington Avenue, Buffalo, NY 14215 716-895-1822
FDA Number: 1319744   Fax: 716-895-2969
E-mail: sales@safetec.com
Web site: www.safetec.com
Medical Products Sales Volume: $10,000,000
Annual Revenue: $5-$10 Million
Total Employees: 50   *Marketing Staff:* 3   *Sales Staff:* 6
Ownership: Private
Produces/Sells CE-marked Devices: N
Federal Procurement Eligibility: Small Business, GSA Contract
Distribution: Manufacturer Through Distributor, OEM
General Admin.: Scott A. Weinstein/President, Chief Executive Officer
Mktg./Adv.: Mrs. Clarice Otminski/Director Marketing
        Mr. Rick Merlino/Director National Accounts
        Ms. Kelly Ticco/Manager Market Research
Production: Ms. Denise Kruszka/Manager Regulatory Affairs

Bottle, Medicine Spray	General
Container, Sharpes	General
Disinfector, Liquid	General
Dispenser, Liquid, Unit-Dose	General
Dispenser, Other	General
Dispenser, Soap	General
Dispenser, Towel	General
Dressing, Gel	General
Encapsulator, Fluid	General
Fiber, Absorbent	General
Kit, Emergency, Cardiopulmonary Resuscitation	General
Pad, Medicated	General
Sanitizer	General
Solution, Antibacterial Cleaner	General
Towel/Towelette, Paper	General

SAFETY 1ST MEDICAL, INC. 800-997-2331
1740 E. Garry Avenue #109, Santa Ana, CA 92705 949-476-5555
FDA Number: 2029274   Fax: 949-476-5559
E-mail: cwilhelm@safety1stmedical.com
Web site: www.safety1stmedical.com
Medical Products Sales Volume: $900,000
Annual Revenue: $1-$5 Million
Total Employees: 10   *Marketing Staff:* 1   *Sales Staff:* 3
Ownership: Private
Produces/Sells CE-marked Devices: N
Federal Procurement Eligibility: Small Business, GSA Contract

SAFETY 1ST MEDICAL, INC.   800-997-2331 *(cont'd)*
Distribution: Manufacturer Direct, Manufacturer Through Distributor, Manufacturer Through Manufacturer Reps, OEM, Importer, Exporter
General Admin.: E. Craig Wilhelm/President, Chief Executive Officer
Mktg./Adv.: Ronda K. Wilhelm/Director Advertising
     Lee Connerton/Director Market Research
     Dan Daley/Director National Accounts
     Robert Gremel/Director Product Development
     Robert J. Mohan/Vice President Sales
Production: Carroll Councilman/Director Quality Assurance
     Richard Eichler/Manager Materials

Syringe, Antistick	General
Syringe, Other	General
Syringe, Piston	General

SAFETY SYRINGE CORPORATION OF AMERICA, INC.   415-454-8054
58 Oakdale Avenue, San Rafael, CA 94901
FDA Number: 2954909   Fax: 415-457-5983
E-mail: itgllc@worldnet.att.net
Web site: www.itg-llc.biz
Annual Revenue: $50-$100 Million
Year Founded: 1979
Total Employees: 12   *Marketing Staff:* 6   *Sales Staff:* 50
Ownership: Private
Produces/Sells CE-marked Devices: N
Federal Procurement Eligibility: Small Business
Distribution: Manufacturer Direct

Syringe, Antistick	General

SAFETY SYRINGES, INC.   760-918-9908
2875 Loker Avenue East, Carlsbad, CA 92010
FDA Number: 2029163

Syringe, Antistick	General
Syringe, Piston	General

SAFETY TEK INSTRUMENTS GROUP
    See Linear Laboratories Corporation

SAFETY TODAY INC.   800-263-1251
90 Morton Ave E,   519-752-9035
Brantford, ONT N3R 7 Canada
FDA Number: n/a   Fax: 519-752-5258
E-mail: infocanada@safetytoday.com
Web site: http://www.safetytoday.com
Year Founded: 1984
Total Employees: 10
Ownership: Private
Produces/Sells CE-marked Devices: N
Distribution: Manufacturer Direct, Exclusive Distributor, Importer

SAFILO USA   973-952-2800
801 Jefferson Rd., Parsippany, NJ 07054
FDA Number: 2241997   Fax: 1-973-5601598
E-mail: 2241997
Web site: www.safilo.com
Year Founded: 1934
Total Employees: 350   *Marketing Staff:* 14
Ownership: Public
Produces/Sells CE-marked Devices: N
Distribution: Manufacturer Direct
General Admin.: Claudio Gottardi/President
Mktg./Adv.: Jaimie LaFrano/Director Marketing
     Bill Harrison/Director National Accounts
     Francesco DeGrossi/Director Product Development
     Flora Maltessieh/Manager Advertising
     Tom Carberry/Manager National Sales
     Deborah Kelly/Vice President Marketing
     Dick Russo/Vice President Sales
Production: Lorenzo Bugin/Vice President Manufacturing

Eyeglasses	Ophthalmology

SAGAX INTERNATIONAL
    See Thermo Biostar, Inc.

SAGE IN-VITRO FERTILIZATION INC.   203-601-5200
1979 East Locust St., Pasadena, CA 91107
FDA Number: 2031459

Media, Reproductive	Obstetrics/Gynecology
Microtools, Assisted Reproduction	Obstetrics/Gynecology
System, Water, Reproduction, Assisted, And Purification	Obstetrics/Gynecology

SAGE INSTRUMENTS
    See Orion Research, Inc.

SAGE LABORATORIES, INC.   800-960-0599
8 Executive Drive, Hudson, NH 03051   (603) 459 1600
FDA Number: n/a   Fax: (603) 459 1605
E-mail: info@sagelabs.com
Web site: www.sage-labs.com

SAGE LABORATORIES, INC.   800-960-0599 *(cont'd)*
Annual Revenue: $0-$1 Million
Total Employees: 28
Ownership: Private
Produces/Sells CE-marked Devices: N
Federal Procurement Eligibility: Small Business, Minority Owned
Distribution: Manufacturer Through Distributor, Manufacturer Through Manufacturer Reps
General Admin.: J. R. Chen/President
Mktg./Adv.: B. Earl Raborn/Vice President Marketing & Sales

Dressing, Wound and Burn, Hydrogel	Surgery
Kit, Wound Dressing	Surgery
Pad, Electrode	Cardiovascular
Pad, Incontinence (Underpad)	General
Stimulator, Wound Healing	Physical Med

SAGE PHARMACEUTICALS, INC.   318-635-1594
5408 Interstate Dr., Shreveport, LA 71109
FDA Number: 2319121   Fax: 318-635-1595
E-mail: sagepharma@sagepharm.com
Web site: www.sagepharmonline.com
Ownership: Private
Produces/Sells CE-marked Devices: N

Dressing, Wound and Burn, Hydrogel	Surgery

SAGE PRODUCTS, INC.   800-323-2220
3909 Three Oaks Road, Cary, IL 60013   815-455-4700
FDA Number: 1419181
Web site: www.sageproducts.com
Year Founded: 1971
Ownership: Private
Produces/Sells CE-marked Devices: N
Federal Procurement Eligibility: Small Business
Distribution: Manufacturer Through Distributor
General Admin.: Vince Foglia/Chairman, Chief Executive Officer
     D. Scott Brown/Chief Operating Officer
     Paul Hills/Director
Mktg./Adv.: Paul Hanifl/Vice President Business Development

Accessories, Apparel, Surgical	Surgery
Applicator, Tipped, Absorbent, Non-Sterile	General
Block, Bite	Cns/Neurology
Catheter, Suction, With Tip	General
Gown, Isolation, Surgical	Surgery
Kit, Admission (Patient Utensil)	General
Kit, Blood Collection, Phlebotomy	Cardiovascular
Needle, Hypodermic, Single Lumen With Syringe	General
Operative Dental Treatment Unit	Dental And Oral
Patient Personal Hygiene Kit	Dental And Oral
Patient Transfer Unit	General
Protector, Skin Pressure	General
Toothbrush, Manual	Dental And Oral
Waste Disposal Unit, Sharps	General
Waste Receptacle, Contaminated	General

SAGE SCIENCE INC.   888-744-2244
500 Cummings Center, Suite 3150,   978-922-1832
Beverly, MA 01915
FDA Number: n/a   Fax: 617-812-0540
E-mail: info@sagescience.com
Web site: http://www.sagescience.com
Ownership: Private
Produces/Sells CE-marked Devices: N
General Admin.: Mr. Gary Paul Magnant/Chief Executive Officer
     Mr. Todd Barbera/Chief Operating Officer
     Dr. T. Chris Boles/Chief Scientific Officer

SAGE SYSTEM, INC.
    See T&S Brass And Bronze Works, Inc.

SAGENTIA INC   410-654-0090
11403 Cronhill Drive, Suite B, Owings Mills, MD 21117
FDA Number: n/a   Fax: 410-654-0138
E-mail: USmedical@sagentia.com
Web site: www.genesismedical.com
Medical Products Sales Volume: $138,000,000
Annual Revenue: $25-$50 Million
Year Founded: 1986
Total Employees: 230   *Marketing Staff:* 1   *Sales Staff:* 3
Ownership: Summit Haus Communication, Ltd.
Stock Symbol: SGA
Traded On: London
Quality System Registration Information: ISO9001
Produces/Sells CE-marked Devices: N
Federal Procurement Eligibility: Small Business
Distribution: Service Direct
General Admin.: Mr. PAUL CARON/President
     Mr. Paul Caron/Vice President
Mktg./Adv.: Mr. Paul Fearis/Vice President Sales

MANUFACTURER PROFILES

SAGENTIA INC   410-654-0090 *(cont'd)*
Contract R&D, Equipment   General

SAGIAN
See Beckman Coulter Inc. (Sagian Operation)

SAGINAW MEDICAL SERVICE, INC.   989-793-4444
3960 Tittabawassee Rd., Saginaw, MI 48604
FDA Number: 1831953   *Fax:* 989-921-0971
E-mail: info@saginawmedical.com
Web site: www.saginawmedical.com
Ownership: Private
Produces/Sells CE-marked Devices: N
   Cushion, Wheelchair (Pad)   Physical Med

SAINT-AMAND MANUFACTURING CO., INC.
See Samco Scientific Corporation

SAINT-GOBAIN PERFORMANCE   800-798-1554
PLASTICS--AKRON
2664 Gilchrist Rd., Akron, OH 44305   330-798-9240
FDA Number: 1519258   *Fax:* 330-798-6968
E-mail: bradley.e.hanson@saint-gobain.com
Web site: www.medical.saint-gobain.com
Ownership: Saint-Gobain Performance Plastics
Stock Symbol: 12500
Traded On: Paris
Quality System Registration Information: ISO9001
Produces/Sells CE-marked Devices: Y
Distribution: Manufacturer Direct, Manufacturer Through Distributor, OEM, Exporter
Mktg./Adv.: Anthony Pagliaro, Jr./Manager Business Development
     Christopher McDonald/Manager National Sales
     Brad Hanson/Market Manager
Production: Nicola Roberts/Supervisor Customer Service
   Fitting, Other   General
   Polymer, Synthetic, Other   General
   Sealer, Packaging   General
   Tubing, Fluid Delivery   General
   Tubing, Non-Conductive   General
   Tubing, Other   General
   Tubing, Plastic   General
   Tubing, Polyethylene   General
   Tubing, Polyvinyl Chloride   General
   Tubing, Silicone   General
   Tubing, Urethane   General
   Tubing, Vinyl   General

SAINT-GOBAIN PERFORMANCE   800-541-6880
PLASTICS/CLEARWATER
4451 110th Ave, North, Clearwater, FL 33762   727-531-4191
FDA Number: 1035360   *Fax:* 727-530-5603
Medical Products Sales Volume: $4,000,000
Annual Revenue: $5-$10 Million
Year Founded: 1982
Total Employees: 50   *Marketing Staff:* 2   *Sales Staff:* 5
Ownership: Private
Produces/Sells CE-marked Devices: N
Federal Procurement Eligibility: Small Business
Distribution: Manufacturer Direct, Manufacturer Through Manufacturer Reps, OEM
General Admin.: Larry Carpenter/President, Chief Executive Officer
     Linda Carpenter/Vice President Human Resources
Mktg./Adv.: Jerry Stadt/Vice President Marketing & Sales
Production: Richard Burger/Vice President Operations
   Component, Plastic   General
   Elastomer, Other   General
   Molding, Custom   General
   Polymer, Synthetic, Other   General
   Stent, Ureteral   Gastroenterology/Urology
   Tube, Drainage   Gastroenterology/Urology
   Tube, Myringotomy   Ear/Nose/Throat
   Tubing, Other   General
   Tubing, Plastic   General

SAJAN, INC.   877-426-9505
625 Whitetail Blvd, River Falls, WI 54022   715-426-9505
FDA Number: n/a   *Fax:* 715-426-0105
E-mail: solutions@sajan.com
Web site: www.sajan.com
Medical Products Sales Volume: $1,400,000
Year Founded: 1997
Total Employees: 41
Ownership: Private
Quality System Registration Information: ISO9000
Produces/Sells CE-marked Devices: N
Federal Procurement Eligibility: Small Business
Distribution: Service Direct
   Service, Consulting   General

SAKURA FINETEK U.S.A., INC.   800-725-8723
1750 West 214th Street, Torrance, CA 90501   310-972-7800
FDA Number: 2083544   *Fax:* 310-972-7888
E-mail: mail@sakuraus.com
Web site: www.sakuraus.com
Annual Revenue: $50-$100 Million
Total Employees: 150   *Marketing Staff:* 7   *Sales Staff:* 25
Ownership: Private
Quality System Registration Information: ISO9001
Produces/Sells CE-marked Devices: Y
Federal Procurement Eligibility: Small Business, Minority Owned
Distribution: Manufacturer Direct, Manufacturer Through Distributor, Importer, Exporter
General Admin.: Kenichi Matsumoto/Chairman, Chief Executive Officer
     Anthony C. Marotti/President
     Takashi Tsuzuki/President, Chief Executive Officer
Mktg./Adv.: Robert Weingard/Manager National Sales
     Gilles Lefebvre/Vice President Marketing & Sales
Production: Hisa Kimura/Manager Materials
     Wolfgang Mueller/Senior Vice President Production
Finance: Kam Patel/Controller
   Cassette, Tissue   Pathology
   Centrifuge, Cell Washing   Hematology
   Microtome, Cryostat   Pathology
   Microtome, Rotary   Pathology
   Slide And Coverslip   Hematology
   Stainer, Slide, Hematology, Automated   Hematology
   Tissue Embedding Equipment/Reagent   Pathology
   Tissue Processor, Automated   Pathology

SAKURA MEDICAL CORPORATION
See Konica Minolta Medical Imaging Usa, Inc.

SALADAX BIOMEDICAL, INC.   610-419-6731
116 Research Dr., Bethlehem, PA 18015
FDA Number: 3005567065   *Fax:* 610-849-5001
E-mail: info@saladax.com
Web site: www.saladax.com
Ownership: Private
Produces/Sells CE-marked Devices: N
General Admin.: Dr. Salvatore Salamone/Chief Executive Officer
     Ms. Adrienne Choma/Chief Operating Officer
     Mr. Toni Klich/Director Admin. & Finance
Mktg./Adv.: Mr. Keith Galloway/Vice President Marketing & Sales
Production: Mr. Gary Feiss/Vice President Regulatory & Clinical Affairs
Research: Ms. Jodi Courtney/Director Research & Development
   Calibrator, Drug Specific   Toxicology
   Control, Drug Specific   Toxicology
   Reagents, Specific, Analyte   Hematology

SALIENT SURGICAL TECHNOLOGIES INC.   800-354-2808
180 International Drive, Portsmouth, NH 03801
FDA Number: 1226420   *Fax:* 603-742-1488
Web site: http://salientsurgical.com
Year Founded: 1999
Ownership: Private
Produces/Sells CE-marked Devices: N
General Admin.: Mr. Joseph Army/President, Chief Executive Officer
Finance: Mr. Richard Altieri/Chief Financial Officer, Vice President Finance
   Electrosurgical Unit, Cutting & Coagulation Device   Surgery

SALIMETRICS, LLC   800-790-2258
101 Innovation Blvd., Suite 302,   814-234-7748
State College, PA 16803
FDA Number: 3003760091   *Fax:* 814-234-1608
E-mail: sales@salimetrics.com
Web site: www.salimetrics.com
Year Founded: 1998
Ownership: Private
Produces/Sells CE-marked Devices: Y
Federal Procurement Eligibility: Small Business
Distribution: Manufacturer Direct, Manufacturer Through Distributor
   Calibrator, Secondary, Clinical Chemistry   Chemistry
   Container, Specimen Mailer And Storage   Pathology
   Control, Multi Analyte, All Kinds (Assayed And Unassayed)   Chemistry
   Enzyme Immunoassay, Other   Chemistry
   Radioimmunoassay, Progesterone   Chemistry
   Syringe, Irrigating   General

SALK INC.   800-343-4497
119 Braintree St. #701, 4th Floor,   617-232-4030
Boston, MA 02134
FDA Number: 9320166   *Fax:* 617-735-9402
E-mail: info@salkinc.com
Web site: www.salkinc.com
Medical Products Sales Volume: $2,500,000
Annual Revenue: $1-$5 Million
Year Founded: 1945

SALK INC.   800-343-4497 (cont'd)

Total Employees: 35
Ownership: Private
Produces/Sells CE-marked Devices: N
Federal Procurement Eligibility: Small Business
Distribution: Manufacturer Direct
General Admin.: Mr. Lawrence Salk/President

Bib	General
Garment, Protective, For Incontinence	Gastroenterology/Urology
Gown, Patient, Reusable	General
Pad, Incontinence (Underpad)	General
Pant, Incontinence	General
Slippers	General

SALMON MEDICAL INNOVATIONS, LLC   866-268-3376
5017 Worthington Drive, Bethesda, MD 20816   301-320-3514

FDA Number: 3005783148   Fax: 240-396-6174
E-mail: info@salmonmedical.com
Web site: www.salmonmedical.com
Ownership: Private
Produces/Sells CE-marked Devices: N

Protector, Dental	Anesthesiology

SALSBURY INDUSTRIES   800-640-4341
1010 E. 62nd St., Los Angeles, CA 90001-1510   323-846-6700

FDA Number: n/a   Fax: 323-846-6800
E-mail: salsbury@hospitalhardware.com
Web site: www.hospitalhardware.com
Medical Products Sales Volume: $5,000,000
Annual Revenue: $10-$25 Million
Total Employees: 60
Ownership: Private
Produces/Sells CE-marked Devices: N
Federal Procurement Eligibility: Small Business
Distribution: Manufacturer Direct
General Admin.: Dennis Fraher/President
Mktg./Adv.: Brian Fraher/Director Marketing
     Ricardo Alva/Manager International & National Sales
     Brian Fraher/Vice President Sales

Curtain, Cubicle	General
Hanger, Intravenous	General
Track And Carrier, Cubicle Curtain	General
Track And Carrier, Intravenous	General

SALTER LABS   800-235-4203
100 W. Sycamore Rd., Arvin, CA 93203-0608   661-854-3166

FDA Number: 2921601   Fax: 661-854-3850
E-mail: salterlabs@us.salterlabs.com
Web site: www.salterlabs.com
Total Employees: 400   Marketing Staff: 7   Sales Staff: 16
Ownership: Private
Quality System Registration Information: ISO9001
Produces/Sells CE-marked Devices: Y
Federal Procurement Eligibility: Small Business
Distribution: Manufacturer Through Distributor, Manufacturer Through
Manufacturer Reps, OEM, Exporter
General Admin.: Peter W. Salter/President, Chief Executive Officer
     Jerry Berkstresser/Vice President, General Manager
Mktg./Adv.: Rod Tabor/Director Marketing
     Al Piraino/Director National Accounts
     Bill Leonard/Manager National Sales
Production: Ray Johnson/Manager Materials
     Jim Curti/Manager Regulatory Affairs
Research: Jim Chua/Director Research & Development

Analyzer, Gas, Carbon-Dioxide, Gaseous Phase (Capnograph)	Anesthesiology
Analyzer, Gas, Oxygen, Gaseous Phase	Anesthesiology
Cannula, Nasal	General
Cannula, Nasal, Oxygen	Anesthesiology
Conserver, Oxygen	Anesthesiology
Drain, Tee (Water Trap)	Anesthesiology
Fixation Device, Tracheal Tube	Anesthesiology
Humidifier, Non-Heated	Anesthesiology
Mask, Oxygen, Low Concentration, Venturi	Anesthesiology
Mask, Oxygen, Non-Rebreathing	Anesthesiology
Nebulizer, Direct Patient Interface	Anesthesiology
Nebulizer, Medicinal	Ear/Nose/Throat
Nebulizer, Medicinal, Non-Ventilatory (Atomizer)	Anesthesiology
Oxygen	Anesthesiology
Recorder, Ventilatory Effort	Anesthesiology
Regulator, Pressure, Gas Cylinder	Anesthesiology
Spirometer, Diagnostic (Respirometer)	Anesthesiology
Tubing, Flexible, Medical Gas, Low-Pressure	Anesthesiology
Tubing, Oxygen Connecting	General

Medical Product Subsidiaries (Listed Separately)
     Salter Labs

SALTER LABS   800-421-0024
100 W. Sycamore Road, Arvin, CA 93203   805-854-3166

FDA Number: 2921601   Fax: 661-854-3850

SALTER LABS   800-421-0024 (cont'd)

E-mail: salterlabs@us.salterlabs.com
Ownership: Salter Labs
Produces/Sells CE-marked Devices: N

Analyzer, Carbon	Chemistry
Analyzer, Gas, Carbon-Monoxide, Gaseous Phase	Anesthesiology
Analyzer, Gas, Oxygen, Gaseous Phase	Anesthesiology
Cannula, Nasal, Oxygen	Anesthesiology
Drain, Tee (Water Trap)	Anesthesiology
Mask, Oxygen, Low Concentration, Venturi	Anesthesiology
Mask, Oxygen, Non-Rebreathing	Anesthesiology
Nebulizer, Direct Patient Interface	Anesthesiology
Regulator, Pressure, Gas Cylinder	Anesthesiology
Spirometer, Diagnostic (Respirometer)	Anesthesiology

SALTIME, INC.
See Boston Rheology, L.L.C.

SALTON, INC.   202-408-9213
1955 Field Court, Lake Forest, IL 60045

FDA Number: 1421727

Massager, Therapeutic	Physical Med
Stimulator, Transcutaneous Electrical, For Cosmetic Use	Cns/Neurology
Toothbrush, Powered	Dental And Oral

SALUMEDICA, L.L.C.   404-589-1727
4451 Atlanta Rd. Se, Suite 138, Smyrna, GA 30080

FDA Number: 1067104

Bit, Drill	Orthopedics
Cuff, Nerve	Cns/Neurology
Orthopedic Manual Surgical Instrument	Orthopedics
Prosthesis, Knee, Hemi-, Tibial Resurfacing, Uncemented	Orthopedics
Tray, Surgical	Surgery

SALVATORI OPHTHALMICS MANUFACTURING CORPORATION
See Unilens Corp., Usa

SALVIN DENTAL SPECIALTIES, INC.   800-535-6566
3450 Latrobe Drive, Charlotte, NC 28211   704-442-5400

FDA Number: 1066741   Fax: 704-442-5424
E-mail: orders@salvin.com
Web site: www.salvin.com
Medical Products Sales Volume: $3,200,000
Year Founded: 1981
Total Employees: 20
Ownership: Private
Federal Procurement Eligibility: Small Business

Blade, Scalpel	Surgery
Burr, Dental	Dental And Oral
Caliper	Orthopedics
Chisel, Osteotome, Surgical	Dental And Oral
Curette, Periodontic	Dental And Oral
Curette, Surgical, Dental	Dental And Oral
Elevator, Surgical, General & Plastic Surgery	Surgery
Evacuator, Oral Cavity	Dental And Oral
File, Bone, Surgical	Dental And Oral
Forceps	Orthopedics
Forceps, Rongeur, Surgical	Dental And Oral
Forceps, Tooth Extractor, Surgical	Dental And Oral
Gauge, Depth, Instrument, Dental	Dental And Oral
Handle, Scalpel	Surgery
Hemostat, Surgical	Dental And Oral
Holder, Needle, Orthopedic	Orthopedics
Instrument, Diamond, Dental	Dental And Oral
Light, Fiberoptic, Dental	Dental And Oral
Light, Surgical Headlight	Dental And Oral
Mallet, Bone	Orthopedics
Mirror, Mouth	Dental And Oral
Remover, Crown	Dental And Oral
Retractor, All Types	Dental And Oral
Scissors, Surgical Tissue, Dental (Oral)	Dental And Oral
Screwdriver	Orthopedics
Tray, Surgical	Surgery
Trephine, Bone	Orthopedics

SAM MEDICAL PRODUCTS   503-639-5474
4909 South Coast Hwy., #245, Newport, OR 97365

FDA Number: 3023316

Component, Traction, Non-Invasive	Orthopedics
Orthosis, Sacroiliac, Soft	Physical Med
Splint, Extremity, Non-Inflatable, External	Surgery
Splint, Hand, And Component	Physical Med

SAMADHI TANK CO.   888-755-7700
PO Box 2119, Nevada City, CA 95959-1942   530-477-1319

FDA Number: n/a   Fax: 530-477-1953
E-mail: float@samadhitank.com
Web site: www.samadhitank.com
Medical Products Sales Volume: $200,000
Annual Revenue: $0-$1 Million
Year Founded: 1972
Total Employees: 3   Marketing Staff: 1   Sales Staff: 3

SAMADHI TANK CO.
888-755-7700 *(cont'd)*
Ownership: Private
Federal Procurement Eligibility: Small Business, Female Owned
Distribution: Manufacturer Direct, Manufacturer Through Distributor, Exclusive Distributor, Importer, Exporter
General Admin.: Lee Perry/Chief Executive Officer
Mktg./Adv.: Glenn Perry/Director Product Development
Production: Glenn Perry/Manager Production
  Tank, Full Body (Bath) .... General

SAMCO SCIENTIFIC CORPORATION
800-522-3359
1050 Arroyo Avenue,
818-838-2400
San Fernando, CA 91340
FDA Number: 3003750373
Fax: 818-838-2488
E-mail: customerservice@samcosci.com
Web site: www.samcosci.com
Medical Products Sales Volume: $34,200,000
Year Founded: 1971
Total Employees: 300   *Sales Staff:* 1
Ownership: FISHER SCIENTIFIC CO.
Traded On: NYSE
Quality System Registration Information: ISO9001
Produces/Sells CE-marked Devices: N
Federal Procurement Eligibility: Small Business, GSA Contract
Distribution: Manufacturer Through Distributor, OEM, Exporter
General Admin.: Tuyen Nguyen/General Manager
Mktg./Adv.: Valerie Buschey/Vice President Sales
Production: Sandy McKenzie/Manager Customer Services
  Martha Gonzalez/Manager Materials
  Theresa Modugno/Manager Regulatory Affairs
  Block, Therapy, Radiation .... Radiology
  Container, Specimen, All Types .... General
  Container, Urine Specimen .... General
  Pipette, Micro .... Chemistry
  Pipette, Pasteur .... Hematology

SAMMANN CO., SEE AIDS DIV.
800-348-2508
9935 E. U.S. 12, Michigan City, IN 46360-1282
219-872-4413
FDA Number: 1831687
Fax: 219-872-4695
E-mail: glasses@peeperspecs.com
Web site: www.sammann.com
Medical Products Sales Volume: $2,000,000
Annual Revenue: $1-$5 Million
Total Employees: 14   *Marketing Staff:* 2   *Sales Staff:* 10
Ownership: Private
Produces/Sells CE-marked Devices: N
Federal Procurement Eligibility: Small Business
Distribution: Manufacturer Direct, OEM, Importer, Exporter
General Admin.: P. N. Sammann/Chief Executive Officer
Mktg./Adv.: Diane Reed/Manager Marketing
Production: Mike Glossinger/Manager Production
  Eyeglasses .... Ophthalmology
  Lens, Spectacle/Eyeglasses, Custom (Prescription) ...... Ophthalmology
  Scissors, Bandage/Gauze/Plaster .... General
  Scissors, Disposable .... General
  Spectacle, Magnifier .... Ophthalmology
  Sunglasses (Including Photosensitive) .... Ophthalmology

SAMMONS INC., FRED
See Patterson Medical Holdings, Inc.

SAMMONS PRESTON ROLYAN
See Patterson Medical Holdings, Inc.

SAMPLE SOLUTIONS, LLC
970-323-5440
540 Highway 50 Business Loop, Olathe, CO 81425
FDA Number: 3004198972
Ownership: Private
Produces/Sells CE-marked Devices: N

SAMPLIFY SYSTEMS INC.
408-249-1500
160 Saratoga Avenue, Suite 150, Santa Clara, CA 95051
FDA Number: n/a
Web site: http://www.samplify.com
Ownership: Private
Produces/Sells CE-marked Devices: N
Distribution: OEM
General Admin.: Mr. Al Wegener/Chief Technology Officer
  Mr. Tom Sparkman/President, Chief Executive Officer
Mktg./Adv.: Mr. Allan Evans/Vice President Marketing
Research: Mr. Richard Tobias/Vice President Engineering

SAN DIEGO SWISS MACHINING, INC.
858-571-6636
9177 Aero Dr., Suite A, San Diego, CA 92123
FDA Number: 2029155
  Mirror, Endoscopic .... Surgery
  Mirror, Mouth .... Dental And Oral
  Plugger, Root Canal, Endodontic .... Dental And Oral

SAN DIEGO SWISS MACHINING, INC.
858-571-6636 *(cont'd)*
  Spreader, Pulp Canal Filling Material, Endodontic .... Dental And Oral

SAN-I-PAK,PACIFIC INC.
800-875-7264
23535 South Bird Road, Tracy, CA 95304
209-836-2310
FDA Number: n/a
Fax: 209-836-2336
E-mail: info@sanipak.com
Web site: www.sanipak.com
Medical Products Sales Volume: $4,600,000
Year Founded: 1978
Total Employees: 50   *Marketing Staff:* 4   *Sales Staff:* 7
Ownership: Private
Federal Procurement Eligibility: Small Business
Distribution: Manufacturer Direct
General Admin.: John Hall/President
Production: Julie Longpre/Director Medical Products
  Clothing, Protective .... General
  Container, Sterilization (Tray) .... General
  Equipment, Control, Pollution .... General
  Generator, Aerosol .... Ear/Nose/Throat
  Sterilizer, Steam (Autoclave) .... General
  Sterilizer/Compactor .... General

SAN-MAR LABORATORIES, INC.
914-592-3130
4 Warehouse Ln., Elmsford, NY 10523
FDA Number: 2431229
  Condom .... Obstetrics/Gynecology

SAN-TEK - SANTAIR
See Santek, Div. Tjernlund Products, Inc.

SANARUS MEDICAL, INC.
925-460-5730
4696 Willow Rd., Pleasanton, CA 94588
FDA Number: 3003515897
  Biopsy Instrument .... Gastroenterology/Urology
  Cannula, Surgical, General & Plastic Surgery .... Surgery
  Cryosurgical Unit .... Surgery
  Guide, Surgical, Needle .... Surgery

SANAX PROTECTIVE PRODUCTS, INC.
800-379-9929
236 Upland Avenue,
617-964-1365
Newton Highlands, MA 02461
FDA Number: 123519
Fax: 617-965-7316
E-mail: sanax@comcast.net
Web site: www.sanaxinc.com
Annual Revenue: $1-$5 Million
Total Employees: 18172   *Marketing Staff:* 1   *Sales Staff:* 4
Ownership: Private
Quality System Registration Information: ISO9000
Produces/Sells CE-marked Devices: Y
Federal Procurement Eligibility: Small Business
Distribution: Manufacturer Through Distributor
General Admin.: Alex Freedman/President
Production: Donna Medin/Vice President Operations
  Bandage, Elastic .... General
  Cap, Surgical .... Surgery
  Cover, Barrier, Protective .... General
  Cover, Head, Surgical .... Surgery
  Cover, Shoe, Operating Room .... Surgery
  Glove, Patient Examination .... General
  Goggles, Protective, Eye .... Ophthalmology
  Gown, Other .... General
  Mask, Face .... General

SANDARE INTL., INC.
972-293-7440
910 K.c.k. Way, Cedar Hill, TX 75104
FDA Number: 1627187
  Complexone, Cresolphthalein, Calcium .... Chemistry
  Control, Hemoglobin .... Hematology
  Ferrozine (Colorimetric) Iron Binding Capacity .... Chemistry
  Phosphorus Reagent (Test System) .... Chemistry
  Photometric Method, Iron (Non-Heme) .... Chemistry
  Reagent, Bilirubin (Total Or Direct Test System) .... Chemistry
  Reagent, Chloride (Test System) .... Chemistry
  Reagent, Cyanomethemoglobin, With Standard .... Hematology
  Reagent, Protein, Total .... Chemistry
  Test, Glycosylated Hemoglobin Assay .... Hematology
  Thymolphthalein Monophosphate, Acid Phosphatase ... Chemistry
  Thymolphthalein Monophosphate, Alkaline Phosphatase .. Chemistry

SANDERS DATA SYSTEMS, LLC
650-857-0455
3980 Bibbits Dr., Palo Alto, CA 94303
FDA Number: 2950426
Fax: 650-856-0455
E-mail: bill@sandersdata.com
Web site: www.sandersdata.com
Year Founded: 1991
Ownership: Private
Produces/Sells CE-marked Devices: N
Federal Procurement Eligibility: Small Business
Distribution: Manufacturer Direct, OEM

SANDERS DATA SYSTEMS, LLC 650-857-0455 *(cont'd)*
General Admin.: William Sanders/President, Owner
Computer, Cardiac Catheterization Laboratory   Cardiovascular

SANDERS MEDICAL PRODUCTS, INC. 865-588-8998
520 Bearden Park Circle, Knoxville, TN 37919
FDA Number: 1062620
Calibrator Source, Nuclear Sealed   Radiology
Phantom, Flood Source, Nuclear   Radiology

SANDERSON PLUMBING PRODUCTS, SANI-MED DIV.
See Sani-Med, A Division Of Sanderson Plumbing Products, Inc.

SANDERSON-MACLEOD, INC. 866-522-3481
1199 S. Main St., Palmer, MA 01069-0050   413-283-3481
FDA Number: 1220744   Fax: 413-289-1919
E-mail: tsnyder@sandersonmacleod.com
Web site: www.sandersonmacleod.com
Annual Revenue: $5-$10 Million
Year Founded: 1958
Total Employees: 100   Marketing Staff: 2   Sales Staff: 2
Ownership: Private
Produces/Sells CE-marked Devices: N
Federal Procurement Eligibility: Small Business
Distribution: OEM
General Admin.: Eric Sanderson/President
   Linda Mitchell/Vice President Human Resources
   Jim Pascale/Vice President, General Manager
Mktg./Adv.: Ted Snyder/Manager Sales
Accessories, Cleaning Brushes (For Endoscope)   Gastroenterology/Urology
Brush, Biopsy, Bronchoscope (Non-Rigid)   Anesthesiology
Brush, Burr Cleaning   Dental And Oral
Brush, Cleaning, Tracheal Tube   Ear/Nose/Throat
Brush, Cytology, Endoscopic   Gastroenterology/Urology
Brush, Other   General
Collector, Specimen   Microbiology
Contract Manufacturing   General
Labware, Basic, Disposable   Chemistry
Stylet, Catheter   Cardiovascular

SANDFIRE SCIENTIFIC LTD. 604-886-9003
1019 Venture Way, Gibsons, BC V0N-1V7 Canada
FDA Number: n/a   Fax: 604-886-6709
E-mail: info@sandfire.com
Web site: www.sandfire.com
Year Founded: 1975
Total Employees: 10
Ownership: Private
Produces/Sells CE-marked Devices: N
Distribution: Manufacturer Direct

SANDHILL SCIENTIFIC, INC. 800-468-4556
9150 Commerce Center Circle, #500,   303-470-7020
Highlands Ranch, CO 80129
FDA Number: 2023374   Fax: 303-470-2975
E-mail: sales@sandhillsci.com
Web site: www.sandhillsci.com
Medical Products Sales Volume: $2,700,000
Annual Revenue: $10-$25 Million
Year Founded: 1981
Total Employees: 35   Marketing Staff: 3   Sales Staff: 25
Ownership: Private
Quality System Registration Information: ISO9001
Produces/Sells CE-marked Devices: Y
Federal Procurement Eligibility: Small Business, GSA Contract, VA Contract
Distribution: Manufacturer Through Manufacturer Reps, Importer, Exporter
General Admin.: Mr. Rick F. Jory/President, Chief Executive Officer
Mktg./Adv.: Ms. Becky Jones/Manager National Sales
   Mr. Stu Wildhorn/Vice President Sales
Production: Mr. Guy B. Harris/Director Quality Assurance
   Ms. Sandi McDonald/Manager Materials
   Mr. Thomas D. Stuebe/Vice President, Director Engineering
IS: Mr. Jerry E. Mabary/Vice President, Tech. Director
Analyzer, Motility, Gastrointestinal, Electrical   Gastroenterology/Urology
Electrode, pH   Gastroenterology/Urology
Monitor, Esophageal Motility, And Tube   Gastroenterology/Urology
Monitor, pH   Anesthesiology
Probe, Gastrointestinal   Gastroenterology/Urology
Probe, Rectal, Non-Powered   Gastroenterology/Urology

SANDOZ NUTRITION
See Novartis Nutrition

SANDS CANADA INC. 800-563-0911
P.O. Box 1752, Brockville, ONT K6V-6K8 Canada   613-345-2687
FDA Number: n/a   Fax: 613-345-2455
E-mail: sands@cybertap.com
Web site: www.sands.ca
Year Founded: 1987
Total Employees: 25

SANDS CANADA INC. 800-563-0911 *(cont'd)*
Ownership: Private
Produces/Sells CE-marked Devices: N
Distribution: Manufacturer Direct, Exclusive Distributor, Importer

SANDSPUR ENTERPRISES INC.
See Encompas Unlimited, Inc.

SANDSTONE MEDICAL TECHNOLOGIES, LLC 205-290-8251
102 Oxmoor Rd., Suite 130, Birmingham, AL 35209-5964
FDA Number: 3003991952   Fax: 205-290-4269
Web site: www.sandstonemedicaltechnologies.com
Ownership: Private
Produces/Sells CE-marked Devices: N
Laser, Surgical   Surgery

SANDSTROM TRADE & TECHNOLOGY, INC. 800-699-0745
610 Niagara St., P.O. Box 850,   905-732-1307
Welland, ONT L3C 1 Canada
FDA Number: 8022207   Fax: 905-735-6948
E-mail: stx@sandstrom.on.ca
Web site: www.sandstrom.on.ca
Year Founded: 1987
Total Employees: 3
Ownership: Private
Quality System Registration Information: ISO9001
Produces/Sells CE-marked Devices: Y
Federal Procurement Eligibility: Small Business, Female Owned
Distribution: Manufacturer Direct, Manufacturer Through Distributor, OEM, Exporter

SANDT PRODUCTS, INC. 800-441-8764 ex
1275 Loop Rd., Lancaster, PA 17601   717-299-4900
FDA Number: n/a   Fax: 717-299-2468
E-mail: info@sandtproducts.com
Web site: www.sandtproducts.com
Annual Revenue: $5-$10 Million
Total Employees: 40   Marketing Staff: 1   Sales Staff: 6
Ownership: Private
Produces/Sells CE-marked Devices: N
Distribution: Manufacturer Direct, Manufacturer Through Distributor, OEM
General Admin.: Roger W. Sandt/President
Production: Paul J. Xander/Vice President Manufacturing
Component, Paper   General

SANDVIK MEDTECH 901-384-5907
4477 Getwell Rd., P.O. Box 1990, Memphis, TN 38118
FDA Number: n/a
E-mail: medical@sandvik.com
Web site: www.sandvik.com/medical
Year Founded: 1862
Ownership: Sandvik Materials Technology
Produces/Sells CE-marked Devices: N
Distribution: Manufacturer Direct, Manufacturer Through Distributor, Exporter

SANFORD, L.P. 800-323-0749
1 Pencil St., Shelbyville, TN 37160
FDA Number: n/a
Ownership: Private
Produces/Sells CE-marked Devices: N
Marker, Skin   Surgery

SANI-MED, A DIVISION OF SANDERSON 800-647-1042
PLUMBING PRODUCTS, INC.
PO Box 1367, Columbus, MS 39703   601-328-4000
FDA Number: 9200114   Fax: 601-329-4362
E-mail: jtrip@sppi.com
Web site: www.benekeseats.com
Medical Products Sales Volume: $50,000,000
Annual Revenue: $50-$100 Million
Year Founded: 1893
Total Employees: 810   Marketing Staff: 2   Sales Staff: 5
Ownership: Private
Produces/Sells CE-marked Devices: N
Federal Procurement Eligibility: Female Owned
Distribution: Manufacturer Direct, Manufacturer Through Distributor, Manufacturer Through Manufacturer Reps, OEM
General Admin.: Sandra Sanderson/President, Chief Executive Officer
   Gayle Booker/Vice President Personnel
Mktg./Adv.: Penny Sansing/Manager Advertising
   Johnny Triplett/Manager Sales
Production: Allen Bennett/Manager Materials
Commode Seat   General
Lift, Patient   General

SANIJET CORP. 877-934-0477
6200 Maple Avenue, Dallas, TX 75235   972-745-2283
FDA Number: 3002984272   Fax: 214-352-0348

SANIJET CORP. 877-934-0477 *(cont'd)*
E-mail: info@sanijet.com
Web site: www.sanijet.com
Ownership: Private
Produces/Sells CE-marked Devices: N
Bath, Hydro-Massage (Whirlpool) — Physical Med

SANITARIUM EQUIPMENT CO.
See Battle Creek Equipment Co.

SANITOR MANUFACTURING CO. 800-379-5314
1221 W. Centre Avenue, Portage, MI 49024 269-327-3001
FDA Number: 9310063 — Fax: 269-327-4562
E-mail: customerservice@sanitorusa.com
Web site: www.sanitorusa.com
Medical Products Sales Volume: $500,000
Annual Revenue: $5-$10 Million
Year Founded: 1931
Total Employees: 10 — Marketing Staff: 4 — Sales Staff: 4
Ownership: Private
Produces/Sells CE-marked Devices: N
Federal Procurement Eligibility: Small Business
Distribution: Manufacturer Direct, Manufacturer Through Distributor, Manufacturer Through Manufacturer Reps, Exporter
Mktg./Adv.: Mike Fawley/Director Marketing
Production: Bill Gilman/Manager Production
Commode Seat — General
Cover, Seat, Toilet, Sanitary — General
Housekeeping Equipment — General

SANKER INTL., INC. 817-645-8015
3516 County Road 801, Cleburne, TX 76031
FDA Number: 2951210
E-mail: DrSanker@hydrotsii.com
Ownership: Private
Produces/Sells CE-marked Devices: N
Pack, Hot Or Cold, Water Circulating — Physical Med

SANMINA-SCI CORP. 408-964-3555
2700 North First Street, San Jose, CA 95134
FDA Number: n/a — Fax: 408-964-3636
E-mail: info@sanmina-sci.com
Web site: www.sanmina-sci.com
Annual Revenue: $50-$100 Million
Total Employees: 250
Ownership: Public
Quality System Registration Information: ISO9000
Produces/Sells CE-marked Devices: N
Distribution: Manufacturer Through Distributor
Monitor, Cardiopulmonary Level Sensing — Cardiovascular

SANMINA-SCI ENCLOSURES
See Sanmina-Sci Corp.

SANMINA-SCI USA, INC. 256-882-4800
13000 South Memorial Pkwy., Huntsville, AL 35803
FDA Number: 1037998
Glucose Dehydrogenase, Glucose — Chemistry
Reagent, Glucose (Test System) — Chemistry
System, Hyperthermia, Rf/microwave (benign Prostatic Hyperplasia), Thermotherapy Gastroenterology/Urology
System, Test, Blood Glucose, Over-The-Counter — Chemistry

SANMINA-SCI USA, INC. 408-904-2117
2700 North First Street, San Jose, CA 95134
FDA Number: 2954951 — Fax: 1 408 964 3636
Ownership: Private
Produces/Sells CE-marked Devices: N
Monitor, Cardiac (Cardiotachometer & Rate Alarm) — Cardiovascular

SANOFI DIAGNOSTICS PASTEUR, INC.
See Biorad Laboratories

SANOMEDICS DEVELOPMENT CORP. 305-433-7814
80 SW 8th Street, Suite 2180, Miami, FL 33130
FDA Number: 3008029837 — Fax: 305-433-5129
Web site: http://www.sanomedics.com
Ownership: Private
Produces/Sells CE-marked Devices: N
General Admin.: Mr. Craig Sizer/Chairman
Mr. Gary O'Hara/Chief Technology Officer
Mr. Keith Houlihan/President
Production: Mr. Dom Gatto/Vice President Operations
Finance: Mr. Steve Relis/Chief Financial Officer
Thermometer, Electronic — General

SANTA BARBARA MEDCO, INC. 651-452-1977
1270 Eagan Industrial Road, Eagan, MN 55121
FDA Number: 2022602
Dilator, Nasal — Ear/Nose/Throat
Kit, Earmold Impression — Ear/Nose/Throat

SANTA BARBARA MEDCO, INC. 651-452-1977 *(cont'd)*
Protector, Hearing (Insert) — Ear/Nose/Throat
Tube, Tympanostomy — Ear/Nose/Throat

SANTA FE RUBBER PRODUCTS, INC. 562-693-2776
12306 East Washington Blvd., Whittier, CA 90606
FDA Number: 2020752 — Fax: 562-693-4936
E-mail: Lterrones@santaferubber.com
Web site: www.santaferubber.com
Ownership: Private
Produces/Sells CE-marked Devices: N
General Admin.: Mr. William Krames/President, Chief Executive Officer
Mr. Michael Peterman/Vice President
Production: Mr. David Steen/Vice President Tech. Development
Humidifier, Respiratory Gas, (Direct Patient Interface) — Anesthesiology

SANTE FEMININE LIMITED 678-314-1649
1649 Sands Place,, Suite C, Marietta, GA 30067
FDA Number: 3004824921
Ownership: Private
Produces/Sells CE-marked Devices: N
Radiographic Unit, Diagnostic, Mammographic — Radiology
Scanner, Ultrasonic (Pulsed Echo) — Radiology

SANTEK, DIV. TJERNLUND PRODUCTS, INC. 800-255-4208
1601 9th St., St. Paul, MN 55110-6794 651-426-2993
FDA Number: 9200946 — Fax: 651-426-9547
E-mail: fanmail@tjfans.com
Web site: www.tjernlund.com
Medical Products Sales Volume: $10,000,000
Annual Revenue: $10-$25 Million
Total Employees: 60 — Marketing Staff: 4 — Sales Staff: 10
Ownership: Private
Produces/Sells CE-marked Devices: N
Federal Procurement Eligibility: Small Business
Distribution: Manufacturer Through Distributor, OEM
General Admin.: Bob Tjernlund/Chief Executive Officer
Mktg./Adv.: Rick Wagner/Manager Contract Sales
Tom Tjernlund/Vice President Marketing & Sales
Production: Tom Tjernlund/Manager Product Distribution
Equipment, Cleaning, Air — General
Filter, Air — General

SANUWAVE INC. 866-581-6843
11680 Great Oaks Way, Suite 350, 770-419-7525
Alpharetta, GA 30022
FDA Number: 1062240
E-mail: marketing@sanuwave.com.
Web site: www.sanuwave.com
Ownership: Private
Produces/Sells CE-marked Devices: N
General Admin.: Mr. Christopher Cashman/President, Chief Executive Officer
Mktg./Adv.: Mr. Bernie Laurel/Vice President Marketing & Sales
Production: Mr. Pete Stegagno/Vice President Operations
Research: Dr. Iulian Cioanta/Vice President Research & Development
Finance: Mr. Barry Jenkins/Chief Financial Officer
Massager, Therapeutic — Physical Med

SAPHEON INC 707-703-4371
3579 Westwind Blvd., Santa Rosa, CA 95403
FDA Number: n/a
E-mail: info@sapheoninc.com
Web site: http://www.sapheoninc.com
Ownership: Private
Produces/Sells CE-marked Devices: N
General Admin.: Mr. Don Crawford/Chief Executive Officer
Medical Admin.: Dr. Rod Raabe/Chief Medical Officer
Mktg./Adv.: Mr. Gary McCord/Vice President New Business
Production: Mr. Bruce Choi/Vice President Quality Systems
Ms. Elsa Chi Abruzzo/Vice President Regulatory Affairs
Research: Mr. Jack Chu/Vice President Research
Finance: Mr. Harry Phillips/Vice President Finance

SARNS, 3M HEALTH CARE
See Terumo Cardiovascular Systems, Corp

SARSTEDT, INC. 800-257-5101
PO Box 468, 1025, St. James Church Road, 828-465-4000
Newton, NC 28658
FDA Number: 2242368 — Fax: 828-465-0718
E-mail: info@sarstedt.com
Web site: www.sarstedt.com
Medical Products Sales Volume: $29,500,000
Year Founded: 1961
Total Employees: 200
Ownership: Private
Quality System Registration Information: ISO9001
Produces/Sells CE-marked Devices: Y

SARSTEDT, INC.   800-257-5101 *(cont'd)*

Federal Procurement Eligibility: Small Business, GSA Contract
Distribution: Manufacturer Direct, OEM
General Admin.: Peter Rumswinkel/Vice President, General Manager

Analyzer, Chemistry, Centrifuge	Chemistry
Analyzer, Sedimentation Rate, Automated	Hematology
Analyzer, Sedimentation Rate, Erythrocyte	Hematology
Blender/Mixer	Chemistry
Bottle, Tissue Culture, Roller	Pathology
Centrifuge, Cell Washing	Hematology
Container, Specimen Mailer And Storage	Pathology
Container, Specimen Mailer And Storage, Temperature Control	Pathology
Dish, Tissue Culture	Pathology
Equipment, Laboratory, Gen. Purpose (Specific Medical Use)	Chemistry
Flask, Tissue Culture	Pathology
Heat-Sealing Device	Hematology
Labware, Blood Collection	Chemistry
Lancet, Blood	General
Mixer, Blood Tube	Hematology
Mixer/Scale, Blood	Hematology
Pipette, Micro	Chemistry

SARTORIUS OMNIMARK INSTRUMENT CORP   480-784-2200
1320 South Priest Drive, Tempe, AZ 85281

FDA Number: n/a   Fax: 480-784-4738
E-mail: info@omniwww.com
Web site: http://www.sartorius-omnimark.com
Medical Products Sales Volume: $3,100,000
Annual Revenue: $100-$500 Million
Year Founded: 1991
Total Employees: 796
Ownership: Private
Quality System Registration Information: ISO9000; ISO9001; ISO9002
Produces/Sells CE-marked Devices: N
Federal Procurement Eligibility: Small Business, Female Owned
Distribution: Manufacturer Direct, Exclusive Distributor

Sensor, Moisture	General

SARTORIUS STEDIM SUS INC.   925-689-6650
1910 Mark Court, Concord, CA 94520

FDA Number: 3003914055   Fax: 925-689-6988
E-mail: techsupport@sartorius-stedim.com
Web site: www.sartorius.com
Annual Revenue: $100-$500 Million
Total Employees: 796
Ownership: Private
Produces/Sells CE-marked Devices: Y
Federal Procurement Eligibility: Small Business
Distribution: Manufacturer Direct, Manufacturer Through Distributor, Manufacturer Through Manufacturer Reps, OEM, Exclusive Distributor

Dish, Tissue Culture	Pathology
Tissue Culture, Accessories, Dental	Hematology

SAS SHOEMAKERS   877-782-7463
101 New Laredo HWY,   **210-924-6507**
San Antonio, TX 78224

FDA Number: n/a   Fax: 210-921-7896
Web site: www.sasshoes.com
Year Founded: 1976
Ownership: Private
Produces/Sells CE-marked Devices: N
Federal Procurement Eligibility: Small Business
Distribution: Manufacturer Direct

Shoe, Conductive	Surgery
Shoe, Operating Room	Surgery

SATIETY, INC.   877-728-7288
2470 Embarcadero Way, Palo Alto, CA 94303   **650-320-2100**

FDA Number: n/a   Fax: 650-320-2150
E-mail: info@satietyinc.com
Web site: www.satietyinc.com
Year Founded: 2001
Ownership: Private
Produces/Sells CE-marked Devices: N
General Admin.: Eric Reuter/President, Chief Executive Officer, Director
Mktg./Adv.: Rachel Croft/Vice President Marketing
Production: Robert Gaffney/Vice President Operations
     Dr. Allan Abati/Vice President Quality Assurance & Regulatory Affairs
Research: John Gaiser/Vice President Research & Development

SAUDER MANUFACTURING CO.   800-537-1530
930 W. Barre Rd., Archbold, OH 43502   **419-445-7670**

FDA Number: n/a   Fax: 419-446-3697
E-mail: sales@saudercontract.com
Web site: www.saudercontract.com
Annual Revenue: $25-$50 Million
Year Founded: 1946
Total Employees: 310   *Marketing Staff:* 4   *Sales Staff:* 15

SAUDER MANUFACTURING CO.   800-537-1530 *(cont'd)*

Ownership: SAUDER WOODWORKING CO.
Produces/Sells CE-marked Devices: N
Distribution: Manufacturer Direct, Manufacturer Through Distributor, Manufacturer Through Manufacturer Reps, OEM, Importer, Exporter
General Admin.: Virgil Miller/President, Chief Executive Officer
Mktg./Adv.: Bob Borcherdt/Manager Contract Sales
     Kelvin Friesen/Vice President Marketing & Sales

Chair, Other	General

SAVAGE LABORATORIES
See Altana, Inc.

SAVANT INSTRUMENTS, INC.
See Thermo Savant

SAVARIA CORPORATION   800-661-5112
107 Alfred Kuehne Blvd.,   **905-791-5555**
Brampton, ONT L6T-4 Canada

FDA Number: n/a   Fax: 905-791-2222
E-mail: info@concordelevator.com
Web site: www.savaria.com
Year Founded: 1978
Total Employees: 100
Ownership: Private
Produces/Sells CE-marked Devices: N
Distribution: Manufacturer Direct

SAVE THE GONADS, LTD.   513-385-8147
P.O. Box 53111, Cincinnati, OH 45253

FDA Number: 3003917267   Fax: 513-385-8148
E-mail: pam@savethegonads.com
Web site: www.savethegonads.com
Ownership: Private
Produces/Sells CE-marked Devices: N

Shield, Gonadal	Radiology

SAVE-A-LIFE LLC   585-624-3732
62 Buggywhip Trail, Honeoye Falls, NY 14472

FDA Number: 3005776067
Ownership: Young Innovations, Inc.
Produces/Sells CE-marked Devices: N

Anti-Choke Device, Suction	Ear/Nose/Throat

SAVILLE 1300, INC.   888-824-9929
200 Culver Blvd., Suite D,   **909-338-8360**
Playa del Rey, CA 90293

FDA Number: 2030307   Fax: 909-338-8370
E-mail: David@saville1300inc.com
Web site: www.saville1300inc.com
Medical Products Sales Volume: $1,200,000
Annual Revenue: $1-$5 Million
Year Founded: 1986
Total Employees: 5
Ownership: Private
Produces/Sells CE-marked Devices: N
Federal Procurement Eligibility: Small Business
Distribution: Manufacturer Through Manufacturer Reps, Exclusive Distributor
General Admin.: David M. Mindel/Chief Executive Officer
     Robert Harvey/Vice President, General Manager
Mktg./Adv.: Sherry Mindel/Vice President Sales

Prosthesis, Breast, External	Surgery

SAVOY MEDICAL SUPPLY   631-234-7003
745 Calebs Pass, Hauppauge, NY 11788

FDA Number: 2429623   Fax: 631-234-7004
E-mail: don@savoymed.com
Web site: www.savoymed.com
Medical Products Sales Volume: $6,400,000
Year Founded: 1960
Total Employees: 40
Ownership: Private
Federal Procurement Eligibility: Small Business
Distribution: Manufacturer Through Distributor
Production: Joe Galante/Manager Operations

Drape, Surgical	Surgery
Kit, Surgical (General)	Surgery
Surgical Instrument, Manual (General Use)	Surgery
Tray, Surgical	Surgery

SAW INSTRUMENTS   866-459-2774
Schwertberger Str. 16, Bonn D-53177   **+49 228 8128760**

FDA Number: n/a
E-mail: info@saw-instruments.de
Web site: www.saw-instruments.de
Ownership: Private
Produces/Sells CE-marked Devices: N

MANUFACTURER PROFILES

SBW MEDICAL
See Medical Action Industries, Inc

SBW MEDICAL PRODUCTS, INC.
See Medical Action Industries, Inc

SC/OIS ORTHODONTICS   1-(800) 448-732
3300 University Drive, Suite 250, Coral Springs, FL 33065
FDA Number: n/a
Web site: www.oisortho.com
Ownership: DARBY GROUP COMPANY
Quality System Registration Information: ISO9002
Produces/Sells CE-marked Devices: N
Federal Procurement Eligibility: Small Business
Distribution: Manufacturer Direct, Exclusive Distributor
Mktg./Adv.: Marti Fauber/Manager Sales

Activator, Ultraviolet, Polymerization	Dental And Oral
Compound, Resinous, Composite	Dental And Oral
Dental Laboratory Equipment	Dental And Oral
Elastomer, Silicone Rubber	General
Handpiece, Belt and/or Gear Driven, Dental	Dental And Oral
Instrument, Dental, Manual	Dental And Oral
Wax, Dental	Dental And Oral

SCA HYGIENE PRODUCTS
See Sca Personal Care, North America

SCA HYGIENE PRODUCTS INC.   800-361-6944
2010 Winston Park Dr., Ste. 300,   905-339-3539
Oakville, ONT L6H-5 Canada
FDA Number: n/a   *Fax:* 905-339-1792
E-mail: rick.foltz@hygiene.sca.se
Web site: www.sca.se
Year Founded: 1979
Total Employees: 100
Ownership: Private
Produces/Sells CE-marked Devices: N
Distribution: Manufacturer Direct, Exclusive Distributor

SCA PERSONAL CARE, NORTH AMERICA   270-796-9300
7030 Louisville Rd., Bowling Green, KY 42103
FDA Number: 1039577

Cover, Mattress	General
Dressing, Other	General
Forceps	Orthopedics
Garment, Protective, For Incontinence	Gastroenterology/Urology

SCA PERSONAL CARE, NORTH AMERICA   270-796-9300
7030 Louisville Road, Bowling Green, KY 42101
FDA Number: 1039577   *Fax:* 270-796-3181
E-mail: info@sca.com
Web site: www.sca.com
Annual Revenue: More than $1 Billion
Total Employees: 51999
Ownership: Private
Produces/Sells CE-marked Devices: Y
Distribution: Manufacturer Through Distributor
General Admin.: Lennart Persson/Chief Financial Officer, Executive Vice President
    Kenneth Eriksson/Chief Operating Officer
    Jan Johansson/President, Chief Executive Officer

Cover, Mattress	General
Garment, Protective, For Incontinence	Gastroenterology/Urology
Pad, Incontinence (Underpad)	General
Pant, Incontinence	General

SCALE ELECTRONIC DEVELOPMENT INC.
See Algen Scale Corp.

SCALE-TRONIX, INC.   800-873-2001
200 E. Post Rd., White Plains, NY 10601-4903   914-948-8117
FDA Number: 1419590   *Fax:* 914-948-0581
E-mail: sales@scale-tronix.com
Web site: www.scale-tronix.com
Year Founded: 1975
Total Employees: 38
Ownership: Private
Produces/Sells CE-marked Devices: Y
Federal Procurement Eligibility: Small Business, Female Owned
Distribution: Manufacturer Direct, Manufacturer Through Manufacturer Reps
General Admin.: Carolyn Lepler/Chief Executive Officer
    Dave Hale/President
Mktg./Adv.: Joe Drago/Vice President Sales
Production: Don Winkleman/Plant Manager

Chair, Dialysis (With Scale)	Gastroenterology/Urology
Scale, Bed	General
Scale, Chair	General
Scale, Infant	General
Scale, Platform, Wheelchair	Physical Med
Scale, Stand-On	General
Scale, Surgical Sponge	General

SCANDINAVIAN FORMULAS, INC.   215-453-2507
140 East Church St., Sellersville, PA 18960
FDA Number: 2528972
Stain, Chemical Solution   Pathology

SCANDITRONIX - WELLHOFER NORTH AMERICA   901-386-2242
3150 Stage Post Drive, Suite 110, Bartlett, TN 38113
FDA Number: 2246563   *Fax:* 901-382-9453
E-mail: info@scanditronix-wellhofer.com
Web site: www.scanditronix-wellhofer.com
Medical Products Sales Volume: $7,000,000
Annual Revenue: $5-$10 Million
Year Founded: 1996
Total Employees: 10   *Sales Staff:* 3
Ownership: Public
Traded On: Brussels
Quality System Registration Information: ISO9001
Produces/Sells CE-marked Devices: Y
Federal Procurement Eligibility: Small Business, GSA Contract, VA Contract
Distribution: Manufacturer Direct, Service Direct, Importer
Mktg./Adv.: Mark Marsico/Manager Advertising & Sales
    Sandra Wilson/Manager Business Development

Monitor, Radiation	Radiology
Phantom, Anthropomorphic, Radiographic	Radiology
Tester, Radiology	Radiology

SCANDIUS BIOMEDICAL, INC.   978-486-4088
11a Beaver Brook Road, Littleton, MA 01460
FDA Number: 3004824670   *Fax:* 978-486-4108
Web site: www.covidien.com
Ownership: Covidien Ltd.
Stock Symbol: COV
Traded On: NYSE
Produces/Sells CE-marked Devices: N

Fastener, Fixation, Biodegradable, Soft Tissue	Orthopedics
Fastener, Fixation, Non-Biodegradable, Soft Tissue	Orthopedics

SCANLAN INTERNATIONAL, INC.   800-328-9458
One Scanlan Plaza, St. Paul, MN 55107-1629   651-298-0997
FDA Number: 2126670   *Fax:* 651-298-0018
E-mail: info@scanlangroup.com
Web site: www.scanlaninternational.com
Medical Products Sales Volume: $2,200,000
Year Founded: 1921
Total Employees: 34
Ownership: Private
Quality System Registration Information: ISO9001
Produces/Sells CE-marked Devices: Y
Federal Procurement Eligibility: Small Business, GSA Contract
Distribution: Manufacturer Through Distributor
General Admin.: Julie Reilly/Executive Vice President
    Timothy M. Scanlan/President, Chief Executive Officer
Mktg./Adv.: Mark J. Anderson/Manager Marketing & Communications
    Walter Olson/Vice President Business Development
    Frank Coolong/Vice President Sales
Research: Kenneth R. Blake/Vice President Research & Development

Bottle, Collection, Vacuum (Aspirator)	General
Clamp, Bulldog	Surgery
Clamp, Peripheral Vascular	Cardiovascular
Clamp, Surgical, General & Plastic Surgery	Surgery
Clamp, Vascular	Cardiovascular
Clip, Aneurysm (Intracranial)	Cns/Neurology
Container, Sterilization (Tray)	General
Cover, Clamp	Surgery
Dilator, Vascular	Cardiovascular
Dissector, Surgical, General & Plastic Surgery	Surgery
Forceps	Orthopedics
Forceps, Hemostatic	Surgery
Forceps, Suction	Surgery
Forceps, Tissue	Surgery
Hemostat, Surgical	Dental And Oral
Holder, Needle	Gastroenterology/Urology
Instrument, Manual, General Surgical	Surgery
Instrument, Microsurgical	Cns/Neurology
Instrument, Passing, Ligature, Knot Tying	Cns/Neurology
Kit, Instruments and Accessories, Surgical	Surgery
Kit, Surgical Instrument, Disposable	Surgery
Label, Device	General
Ligator, Hemorrhoidal	Gastroenterology/Urology
Loop, Vascular	Cardiovascular
Loupe, Binocular, Low Power	Ophthalmology
Marker, Ostia, Aorto-Saphenous Vein	Surgery
Marker, Skin	Surgery
Protector, Surgical Instrument	Surgery
Punch, Aortic	Cardiovascular
Rack, Surgical Instrument	Surgery
Retractor, Abdominal	Surgery
Retractor, Cardiac	Cardiovascular

SCANLAN INTERNATIONAL, INC.   800-328-9458 (cont'd)

Retractor, Mammary	Obstetrics/Gynecology
Retractor, Other	Surgery
Retractor, Surgical	Surgery
Rongeur, Rib	Orthopedics
Scissors, Bandage/Gauze/Plaster	General
Scissors, Cardiovascular	Cardiovascular
Scissors, Neurosurgical (Dura)	Cns/Neurology
Scissors, Orthopedic	Orthopedics
Scissors, Pediatric	General
Scissors, Plastic Surgery (Dissecting)	Surgery
Scissors, Tenotomy	Ophthalmology
Scissors, Thoracic	Cardiovascular
Surgical Instrument, Cardiovascular	Cardiovascular
Surgical Instrument, Manual (General Use)	Surgery
System, Coding, Color, Instrument	Dental And Oral
Valvulotome	Cardiovascular

SCANNEX, INC.   954-974-2000
5100 W. Copans Rd, Bldg 1000, Margate, FL 33063
FDA Number: 1047190
Ownership: Private
Produces/Sells CE-marked Devices: N

Scanner, Ultrasonic (Pulsed Echo)	Radiology

SCANTEK MEDICAL, INC.   973-527-7100
1705 Route 46 West, Unit 5, Ledgewood, NJ 07852
FDA Number: 2247290

Thermographic Device, Liquid Crystal, Non-Powered	Radiology

SCANTIBODIES LABORATORY, INC.   619-258-9300
9336 Abraham Way, Santee, CA 92071
FDA Number: 2020808

Calibrator, Primary, Clinical Chemistry	Chemistry
Control, Multi Analyte, All Kinds (Assayed And Unassayed)	Chemistry
Kit, Pregnancy Test, Over The Counter, HCG	Chemistry
Radioimmunoassay, ACTH	Chemistry
Radioimmunoassay, Calcitonin	Chemistry
Radioimmunoassay, Luteinizing Hormone	Chemistry
Radioimmunoassay, Parathyroid Hormone	Chemistry
Radioimmunoassay, Thyroid Stimulating Hormone	Chemistry
Test, Immunity, Cell-Mediated, Mycobacterium Tuberculosis	Microbiology
Test, Luteinizing Hormone (lh), Over The Counter	Chemistry

SCAPA MEDICAL   310-419-0567
540 N. Oak St., Inglewood, CA 90302-2942
FDA Number: 2024442   *Fax:* 310-419-4150
E-mail: appsupport@scapamedical.com
Web site: www.scapamedical.com
Medical Products Sales Volume: $22,000,000
Annual Revenue: $100-$500 Million
Total Employees: 90   *Marketing Staff:* 2   *Sales Staff:* 19
Ownership: Public
Traded On: London
Quality System Registration Information: ISO9001
Produces/Sells CE-marked Devices: N
Distribution: OEM
General Admin.: Mr. Steve Lennon/President, Chief Operating Officer
Mktg./Adv.: Mr. Rich Malaspina/Executive Vice President Marketing & Sales
    Mr. Tony Ieraci/Manager Marketing Communications
    Mr. Mark McDonough/Manager Sales
    Ms. Andrea Gross/Marketing Coordinator
    Mr. Christian Touey/Sales Representative
    Mr. Jim Shauck/Sales Representative
    Mr. Neil Muchin/Sales Representative
    Ms. Melinda Plumlee/Sales Representative
Production: Mr. Stephen Sloat/Applications Specialist
    Mr. Tony Kibler/Applications Specialist
Research: Ms. Laura Yao/Chemist

Dressing, Permeable, Moisture	General
Dressing, Wound and Burn, Occlusive	Surgery
Strip, Adhesive	Surgery

SCC SOFT COMPUTER   800-763-8352
5400 Tech Data Drive, Clearwater, FL 33760   **727-789-0100**
FDA Number: 1058332   *Fax:* 727-789-0124
E-mail: sales@softcomputer.com
Web site: www.softcomputer.com
Medical Products Sales Volume: $62,500,000
Annual Revenue: $50-$100 Million
Year Founded: 1979
Total Employees: 500   *Marketing Staff:* 6   *Sales Staff:* 15
Ownership: Private
Produces/Sells CE-marked Devices: N
Federal Procurement Eligibility: Small Business
Distribution: Manufacturer Direct, Exclusive Distributor
General Admin.: Gilbert Hakim/Chief Executive Officer
    Jean Hakim/President
    Armin Hakim/Vice President Human Resources

SCC SOFT COMPUTER   800-763-8352 (cont'd)
Mktg./Adv.: Ellie Vahman/Director Marketing & Sales
    Donna Kopotic/Manager Marketing
Production: Elizabeth Paul/Director Quality Assurance
    Magdy Ebeid/Vice President Operations
Finance: Iraj Gheysari/Chief Financial Officer

Computer Equipment	General
Computer Software	General
Computer Software, Hospital/Nursing Management	General
Computer, Clinical Laboratory	Chemistry
Computer, Patient Data Management	General
Service, Consulting	General
Software, Blood Bank (Stand-Alone Products)	Hematology

SCENAR TRAINING CENTER   248-318-2001
12222 Merit Dr., Suite 955, Dallas, TX 75251
FDA Number: n/a
Ownership: Private
Produces/Sells CE-marked Devices: N

Biofeedback Device	Cns/Neurology

SCEPTER MEDICAL, INC.
See Promedica, Inc.

SCHAAN HEALTHCARE PRODUCTS INC.   800-667-3786
820 45th St. W., Saskatoon, SK S7K-4E4 Canada   **306-664-1188**
FDA Number: n/a   *Fax:* 306-664-6676
E-mail: cschaan@schaanhealthcareproducts.ca
Web site: http://www.schaanhealthcareproducts.ca
Year Founded: 1980
Total Employees: 25
Ownership: Private
Produces/Sells CE-marked Devices: N
Distribution: Exclusive Distributor, Importer

SCHAERER MAYFIELD USA   800-755-6381
4900 Charlemar Drive, Cincinnati, OH 45227   **513-561-2241**
FDA Number: 1525725   *Fax:* 513-561-0195
E-mail: info@schaerermayfieldusa.com
Web site: www.schaerermayfieldusa.com
Medical Products Sales Volume: $1,500,000
Year Founded: 1978
Total Employees: 20   *Marketing Staff:* 6   *Sales Staff:* 3
Ownership: Schaerer Ag, M.
Quality System Registration Information: ISO9001
Produces/Sells CE-marked Devices: Y
Federal Procurement Eligibility: Small Business
Distribution: Manufacturer Direct
General Admin.: Jerry Harvey/President, Chief Executive Officer
Mktg./Adv.: James McCafferty/Vice President Marketing
    James F. McCafferty/Vice President Marketing & Sales
Production: Carol Wolfram/Manager Customer Services
    Michael C. Molloy/Product Director
    David Deye/Vice President Manufacturing
Purchasing: Jeff Wylds/Purchasing Agent

Bed, Pediatric (Crib)	General
Clamp, Skull	Cns/Neurology
Head Rest, Neurosurgical	Cns/Neurology
Holder, Head, Neurosurgical (Skull Clamp)	Cns/Neurology
Retractor, Brain	Cns/Neurology
Retractor, Self-Retaining	Gastroenterology/Urology
Retractor, Self-Retaining, Neurology	Cns/Neurology
Rongeur, Manual, Neurosurgical	Cns/Neurology
Scanner, Computed Tomography, X-Ray (CAT, CT)	Cns/Neurology
Stereotaxy Equipment	Cns/Neurology
Stretcher, Wheeled (Mobile)	General
Table, Instrument, Surgical	Surgery
Table, Mechanical	Physical Med
Table, Surgical, Electrical	Surgery
Table, Surgical, Orthopedic	Orthopedics

SCHEIN DENTAL EQUIPMENT CORP., THE
See Henry Schein, Inc.

SCHELL, INC.   800-821-5001
P.O. Box 12689, St. Petersburg, FL 33733-2689   **727-821-5000**
FDA Number: 9320168   *Fax:* 727-822-8800
E-mail: actionusa@hotmail.com
Medical Products Sales Volume: $2,500,000
Annual Revenue: $1-$5 Million
Total Employees: 75   *Marketing Staff:* 2   *Sales Staff:* 4
Ownership: ACTION U.S.A.
Produces/Sells CE-marked Devices: N
Federal Procurement Eligibility: Small Business, Female Owned
Distribution: Manufacturer Direct, Manufacturer Through Distributor, Manufacturer Through Manufacturer Reps, OEM, Importer, Exporter
General Admin.: Ranya Hahn/President, Chief Executive Officer
    Matt Laura/Vice President, General Manager
Mktg./Adv.: James Weiss/Director Product Development
    Stephen Hahn/Manager Sales

SCHELL, INC. 800-821-5001 (cont'd)
S. H. Wallace/Vice President Marketing & Sales

Bag, Medical, Physician	General
Case, Protection, Equipment	General

SCHERING-PLOUGH CORP., CONTACT LENS DIV.
See Ciba Vision

SCHERING-PLOUGH CORP., SCHOLL FOOTCARE
See Schering-Plough Health Care Products

SCHERING-PLOUGH HEALTH CARE PRODUCTS 901-320-2011
3030 Jackson Ave., Memphis, TN 38151
FDA Number: 1020060
Web site: www.schering-plough.com
Medical Products Sales Volume: $300,000,000
Ownership: Schering-Plough Corp.
Produces/Sells CE-marked Devices: N
Distribution: Manufacturer Direct

Cushion, Foot	Orthopedics
Exerciser, Non-Measuring	Physical Med
Tape, Adhesive	General

SCHERING-PLOUGH HEALTHCARE PRODUCTS, INC. 862-245-5115
4207 Michigan Avenue Rd. N.e., Cleveland, TN 37311
FDA Number: 1031623

Bandage, Adhesive	Surgery
Cryosurgical Unit	Surgery
Dilator, Nasal	Ear/Nose/Throat
Insoles, Medical	General
Orthosis, Corrective Shoe	Physical Med

SCHIAPPARELLI BIOSYSTEMS
See Alfa Wassermann, Inc.

SCHICK TECHNOLOGIES, INC. 718-937-5765
30-30 47th Ave., Long Island City, NY 11101
FDA Number: 2436911 Fax: 718-937-5962
Web site: www.schicktech.com
Annual Revenue: $50-$100 Million
Year Founded: 1992
Total Employees: 2388
Ownership: Public
Stock Symbol: SCHK
Traded On: NASDAQ
Quality System Registration Information: ISO9001
Produces/Sells CE-marked Devices: Y
Federal Procurement Eligibility: Small Business
Distribution: Manufacturer Direct, Manufacturer Through Distributor, Manufacturer Through Manufacturer Reps, OEM, Service Direct, Exporter
General Admin.: Simone Blank/Chief Financial Officer, Executive Vice President
Jeffrey T. Solvin/Chief Operating Officer, Executive Vice President
Jost C. Fischer/President, Chief Executive Officer, Chairman

Computer Software	General
Densitometer, Bone, Single Photon	Radiology
Imager, X-Ray, Solid State (Flat Panel/Digital)	Radiology
Operative Dental Treatment Unit	Dental And Oral
Radiographic Unit, Diagnostic, Dental (X-Ray)	Dental And Oral
Radiographic Unit, Diagnostic, Dental, Extraoral	Dental And Oral
Radiographic Unit, Diagnostic, Intraoral	Dental And Oral
Radiographic Unit, Digital	Radiology
System, X-ray, Extraoral Source, Digital	Radiology

SCHIFFMAYER PLASTICS CORPORATION 800-621-1092
1201 Armstrong St., Algonquin, IL 60102-3599 847-658-8140
FDA Number: n/a Fax: 847-658-0863
E-mail: sales@schiffmayerplastics.com
Web site: www.schiffmayerplastics.com
Ownership: Private
Produces/Sells CE-marked Devices: N

Waste Disposal Unit, Surgical Instrument (Sharps)	Surgery

SCHILLER AMERICA, INC. 786-845-0620
2131 N.w. 79th Ave., Doral, FL 33122
FDA Number: 2084041 Fax: 1-786-845-0602
E-mail: sales@schilleramerica.com
Web site: www.schilleramerica.com
Ownership: Private
Produces/Sells CE-marked Devices: N

Analyzer, ECG	Cardiovascular
Monitor, Physiological, Patient	Cardiovascular
Spirometer, Diagnostic (Respirometer)	Anesthesiology

SCHLEICHER & SCHUELL, INC. 800-245-4024
10 Optical Avenue, PO Box 2012, 603-352-3810
Keene, NH 03431
FDA Number: 9200954 Fax: 603-357-3627
E-mail: techserv@s-and-s.com
Web site: www.s-and-s.com
Total Employees: 115 Marketing Staff: 5 Sales Staff: 6

SCHLEICHER & SCHUELL, INC. 800-245-4024 (cont'd)
Ownership: Schleicher & Schuell Gmbh
Distribution: Manufacturer Direct, Manufacturer Through Distributor, OEM
General Admin.: Gary Henricken/Chief Executive Officer
Rick Watkins/Director Human Resources
Dr. Werner Specht/President
Mktg./Adv.: Miles Kirk/Director Marketing & Sales
Judith Peter/Manager International & National Sales
Matt Andrus/Manager Marketing Communications
Bernie Kosmoski/Manager National Sales
Production: Janet LaRoche/Applications Specialist
Daniel O'Leary/Director Manufacturing
Michael Harvey/Manager Regulatory Affairs
Research: Michael Harvey/Director Research & Development
David Reilly/Director Scientific Affairs
Finance: Sergei Galeano/Director Finance

Chromatography Equipment, Paper	Chemistry
Filter Paper	Chemistry
Filter, Air	General
Filter, Bacteriological, Laboratory	Chemistry
Filter, Membrane	Chemistry
Filter, Syringe	General
Labware, Basic, Disposable	Chemistry
Labware, Basic, Reusable	Chemistry
Swabs, Specimen Collection	General
Unit, Filter, Membrane	Chemistry

SCHLEUNIGER, INC. 877-902-1470
87 Colin Drive, Manchester, NH 03103 603-668-8117
FDA Number: n/a Fax: 603-668-8119
E-mail: sales@schleuniger.com
Web site: www.schleuniger-na.com
Medical Products Sales Volume: $6,700,000
Year Founded: 1988
Total Employees: 40 Marketing Staff: 2 Sales Staff: 9
Ownership: SCHLEUNIGER AG
Produces/Sells CE-marked Devices: N
Federal Procurement Eligibility: Small Business, GSA Contract
Distribution: Manufacturer Through Manufacturer Reps
General Admin.: Mike Rizzo/President
Peter Doyon/Vice President, General Manager
Mktg./Adv.: Karen Brown/Communication Specialist
Christine Wheeler/Manager Marketing Communications
Karyn Fearon/Manager Sales

Cutter, Wire And Pin	Orthopedics

SCHNEIDER (USA), INC.
See Boston Scientific Corp.

SCHNEIDER INTERNATIONAL LTD. 201-568-5166
600 Sylvan Avenue, East Wing - First Floor,
Englewood, NJ 07632
FDA Number: n/a Fax: 201-568-1312
E-mail: info@silimports.com
Web site: www.silimports.com
Medical Products Sales Volume: $800,000
Annual Revenue: $0-$1 Million
Year Founded: 1962
Total Employees: 7
Ownership: Private
Produces/Sells CE-marked Devices: N
Federal Procurement Eligibility: Small Business
Distribution: Importer, Exporter
General Admin.: Elliot J. Porwich/President

Service, Import/Export	General

SCHNEIDER PLASTIC ENTERPRISES, INC.
See Packaging Plus Llc

SCHOELLY IMAGING, INC. 1 (508) 926 885
722 Plantation Street, Worcester, MA 01605
FDA Number: 3005305991 Fax: 1 (508) 852 111
Ownership: Private
Produces/Sells CE-marked Devices: N

Accessories, Laser, Endoscopic	Surgery
Arthroscope	Orthopedics
Camera, Television, Endoscopic (Without Audio)	Surgery
Cystoscope	Gastroenterology/Urology
Fiberoptic Light Source & Carrier	Ear/Nose/Throat
Laparoscope, General & Plastic Surgery	Surgery
Nasopharyngoscope (Flexible Or Rigid)	Ear/Nose/Throat
Operative Dental Treatment Unit	Dental And Oral
Ureteroscope	Gastroenterology/Urology

SCHOLL INC. FOOTCARE DIV.
See Schering-Plough Health Care Products

SCHOLLE CHEMICAL CORP. 404-761-0604
2300 West Point Ave., Atl, GA 30337
FDA Number: 1413547

SCHOLLE CHEMICAL CORP.   404-761-0604 *(cont'd)*
Collodion   Pathology

SCHOLTEN SURGICAL INSTRUMENTS, INC.   209-365-1393
170 Commerce St. #101, Lodi, CA 95240-0722
FDA Number: 2936330
E-mail: info@bioptome.com   *Fax:* 209-365-1437
Web site: www.bioptome.com
Medical Products Sales Volume: $200,000
Annual Revenue: $0-$1 Million
Year Founded: 1979
Total Employees: 7
Ownership: Private
Quality System Registration Information: ISO9001
Produces/Sells CE-marked Devices: N
Federal Procurement Eligibility: Small Business
Distribution: Manufacturer Direct, Service Direct
General Admin.: Arie Scholten/Chief Executive Officer
     Jim Van Andel/Chief Operating Officer

Biopsy Device, Endomyocardial	Cardiovascular
Cleaner, Forceps, Biopsy	Cardiovascular
Lead, Pacemaker, Temporary Myocardial	Cardiovascular
Retractor, Rib	Orthopedics

SCHOLZ X-RAY CORP., FRANK
See Frank Scholz X-Ray Corp.

SCHOTT GLASS TECHNOLOGIES, INC.   570-457-7485
400 York Ave., Duryea, PA 18642-2026
FDA Number: n/a
E-mail: sgt@schottglasstech.com   *Fax:* 570-457-6960
Web site: www.us.schott.com
Annual Revenue: $50-$100 Million
Total Employees: 475   *Marketing Staff:* 4   *Sales Staff:* 21
Ownership: Schott Corporation
Quality System Registration Information: ISO9001
Produces/Sells CE-marked Devices: N
Distribution: Manufacturer Direct
Mktg./Adv.: Stephen J. Sokach/Manager Marketing
     Josephy Rudy/Manager National Sales
Production: Philip Kolatis/Director Quality Assurance
     Steven P. Krenitsky/Vice President Operations

Cable, Laser, Fiberoptic	Surgery
Eyeglasses	Ophthalmology
Eyeglasses, Safety	Ophthalmology
Sunglasses (Including Photosensitive)	Ophthalmology

SCHOTT NORTH AMERICA, INC.   315-255-2791
62 Columbus Street, Auburn, NY 13021-3137
FDA Number: n/a
E-mail: fiberoptics.auburn@us.schott.com   *Fax:* 315-255-2695
Web site: www.us.schott.com/fiberoptics
Annual Revenue: $50-$100 Million
Year Founded: 1999
Total Employees: 90   *Marketing Staff:* 2   *Sales Staff:* 13
Ownership: Schott Corporation
Produces/Sells CE-marked Devices: Y
Federal Procurement Eligibility: Small Business
Distribution: Manufacturer Direct, Manufacturer Through Distributor, Manufacturer Through Manufacturer Reps, OEM, Service Direct, Exporter
Mktg./Adv.: Domenic Bucci/Director Marketing
     Anthony Cappabianca/Director National Sales
     Tom Bender/Director Product Development
     John Harrington/Manager Contract Sales
     Michelle Cottrell/Manager Marketing & Advertising
Production: Karen Walter/Director Quality Assurance
     Anthony Cappabianca/Product Manager

Component, Optical	General
Fiberoptic Light Source & Carrier	Ear/Nose/Throat
Light, Other	General

SCHOTT-FOSTEC, LLC
See Schott North America, Inc.

SCHROEDER AMERICAN, INC.   210 662 8200
5620 Business Park, San Antonio, TX 78218
FDA Number: 3006786400
E-mail: INFO@SCHROEDERAMERICA.COM   *Fax:* 210 667 2600
Web site: www.schroederamerica.com
Ownership: Private
Produces/Sells CE-marked Devices: N

SCHUELER & COMPANY, INC.   516-487-1500
PO BOX 528, Stratford, CT 06615-0528
FDA Number: n/a
E-mail: rburchman@shc123.com   *Fax:* 516-487-5494
Web site: www.schuelerinc.com
Annual Revenue: $1-$5 Million
Ownership: Private
Quality System Registration Information: ISO9000

SCHUELER & COMPANY, INC.   516-487-1500 *(cont'd)*
Produces/Sells CE-marked Devices: Y
Federal Procurement Eligibility: Small Business
Distribution: Exclusive Distributor, Exporter
General Admin.: Martin Wolf/Chief Executive Officer
     Robyn A. Burchman/Managing Director
Mktg./Adv.: Peter McCann/Director Marketing

Accessories, Bite Blocks (For Endoscope)	Gastroenterology/Urology
Accessories, Laser, Endoscopic	Surgery
Apron, Lead, Radiographic	Radiology
Aspirator, Tracheal	Ear/Nose/Throat
Balance, Electronic	Chemistry
Balance, Mechanical	Chemistry
Bandage, Gauze	General
Bed, Electric	General
Bed, Manual	General
Blade, Scalpel	Surgery
Board, Spine	Orthopedics
Bulb, Inflation	General
Cabinet, Medicine	General
Cassette, Radiographic Film	Radiology
Chair, Blood Drawing	General
Chair, Dental	Dental And Oral
Container, Sterilization (Tray)	General
Cuff, Blood Pressure	Cardiovascular
Cuff, Tracheal Tube, Inflatable	Anesthesiology
Cutter, X-Ray Film	Radiology
Depressor, Tongue	General
Depressor, Tongue, Dental	Dental And Oral
Dosimeter, Radiation	Radiology
Dryer, Film, Radiographic	Dental And Oral
Duplicator, X-Ray Film	Radiology
Eyeglasses, Safety	Ophthalmology
Film, X-Ray	Radiology
Film, X-Ray, Dental, Extraoral	Dental And Oral
Film, X-Ray, Dental, Intraoral	Dental And Oral
Filter, Aspirator	Surgery
Footstool, Non-Conductive	General
Forceps, General & Plastic Surgery	Surgery
Gel, Ultrasonic Transmission	General
General Use Surgical Scissors	Surgery
Glove, Protective, Radiographic	Radiology
Holder, X-Ray Film	Dental And Oral
Illuminator, Radiographic Film	Radiology
Immobilizer, Infant (Circumcision Board)	Orthopedics
Instrument, Manual, General Surgical	Surgery
Jelly, Lubricating, Transurethral Surgical Instrument	Gastroenterology/Urology
Lamp, Examination (Light)	General
Lamp, Examination, Ceiling Mounted (Light)	General
Patient Transfer Unit	General
Penlight, Battery-Powered	Ophthalmology
Positioner, Tooth, Preformed	Dental And Oral
Processor, Radiographic Film, Automatic	Radiology
Processor, Radiographic Film, Automatic, Dental	Dental And Oral
Processor, Radiographic Film, Manual	Radiology
Restraint, Vest	General
Safelight, X-Ray	Radiology
Scale, Infant	General
Scale, Stand-On	General
Scissors, Bandage/Gauze/Plaster	General
Sheeting, Stretcher	General
Speculum, Vaginal, Metal	Obstetrics/Gynecology
Sphygmomanometer, Aneroid (Arterial Pressure)	General
Splint, Extremity, Inflatable, External	Surgery
Splint, Wire Board	Orthopedics
Stand, Basin	General
Sterilizer, Dry Heat	General
Sterilizer, Steam (Autoclave)	General
Stethoscope, Manual	Cardiovascular
Storage Unit, X-Ray Film	Radiology
Stretcher, Emergency, Other	General
Stretcher, Hydraulic	General
Stretcher, Transfer	Surgery
Stretcher, Wheeled (Mobile)	General
Strip, Test	Chemistry
Surgical Instrument, Obstetric/Gynecologic, General	Obstetrics/Gynecology
Table, Blood Donor	Hematology
Table, Examination/Treatment	General
Tank, Developing, TLC	Toxicology
Toothbrush, Manual	Dental And Oral
Tourniquet	General
Tourniquet, Pneumatic	Surgery
Viewer, Radiographic Film, Motorized	Radiology

SCHUERCH CORP.   617-773-0927
48 Oval Road, Quincy, MA 02169
FDA Number: 1223962
E-mail: info@schuredmed.com   *Fax:* 617-328-5012
Web site: www.schuredmed.com
Medical Products Sales Volume: $500,000
Annual Revenue: $1-$5 Million

SCHUERCH CORP.   617-773-0927 *(cont'd)*
Year Founded: 1994
Total Employees: 5   Marketing Staff: 5   Sales Staff: 30
Ownership: Private
Produces/Sells CE-marked Devices: N
Federal Procurement Eligibility: Small Business
Distribution: Manufacturer Direct, Manufacturer Through Distributor, Manufacturer Through Manufacturer Reps, OEM

Accessories, Operating Room, Table	Surgery
Table, Surgical, Manual	General
Transfer Device, Patient, Manual	General

SCHUKRA MANUFACTURING INC.   800-663-7248
310 Carlingview Dr.,   **416-213-1074**
Toronto, ON M9W 5 Canada
FDA Number: n/a   Fax: 416-213-1085
E-mail: info@schukra.net
Web site: www.schukra.net
Medical Products Sales Volume: $10,000,000
Year Founded: 1995
Total Employees: 60   Marketing Staff: 4   Sales Staff: 4
Ownership: SCHUKRA OF NORTH AMERICA, LTD.
Produces/Sells CE-marked Devices: N
Distribution: Manufacturer Through Distributor, Manufacturer Through Manufacturer Reps, Exporter

SCHULLER CORP.
See Johns Manville

SCHUMANN INC., A.   978-369-6782
167 Hayward Mill Road, Concord, MA 01742-3919
FDA Number: 1219134
Annual Revenue: $0-$1 Million
Total Employees: 2
Ownership: Private
Produces/Sells CE-marked Devices: N
Federal Procurement Eligibility: Small Business
Distribution: Exclusive Distributor
General Admin.: R. Schumann/President

Analyzer, Visual Function	Ophthalmology
Dermabrasion Unit	Surgery
Magnet, AC-Powered	Ophthalmology
Magnet, Permanent	Ophthalmology

SCI GEN, INC.   310-324-6576
333 E. Gardena Blvd., Gardena, CA 90248
FDA Number: 2028815   Fax: 310-324-7993
E-mail: Scigen@Scigen.peachhost.com
Web site: www.ScigenUS.com
Medical Products Sales Volume: $1,200,000
Year Founded: 1992
Total Employees: 10
Ownership: Private
Produces/Sells CE-marked Devices: Y
Federal Procurement Eligibility: Small Business, Minority Owned
Distribution: Manufacturer Direct, Manufacturer Through Distributor, Manufacturer Through Manufacturer Reps, OEM, Service Direct, Exclusive Distributor

Acid, Hematein	Pathology
Agent, Chelating, Decalcification	Pathology
Chrome Alum Hematoxylin	Pathology
Clearing Agent	Pathology
Clearing Oil	Pathology
Container, Embedding	Pathology
Container, Specimen Mailer And Storage, Temperature Control	Pathology
Decalcifier Solution, Electrolytic	Pathology
Dispenser, Paraffin	Pathology
Fixative, Acid Containing	Pathology
Fixative, Alcohol Containing	Pathology
Fixative, Formalin Containing	Pathology
Fixative, Metallic Containing	Pathology
Fluid, Bouin's	Pathology
Formaldehyde (Formalin, Formol)	Pathology
Formalin, Neutral Buffered	Pathology
Glutaraldehyde (Fixative)	Pathology
Media, Mounting	Pathology
Media, Mounting, Water Soluble	Pathology
Mounting Media, Oil Soluble	Pathology
Paraffin, All Formulations	Pathology
Paraformaldehyde	Pathology
Polyethylene Glycol (Carbowax)	Pathology
Reagent, General Purpose	Pathology
Solution, Formalin/Sodium Acetate	Pathology
Solution, Pathology, Decalcifier, Acid Containing	Pathology
Solution, Pathology, Formalin-Alcohol-Acetic Acid	Pathology
Stain, Crystal Violet, Histology	Pathology
Stain, Dye Powder	Pathology
Stain, Eosin B	Pathology
Stain, Eosin Y	Pathology
Stain, Hematoxylin	Pathology
Stain, Hematoxylin, Mayer's	Pathology

SCI GEN, INC.   310-324-6576 *(cont'd)*

Stain, Phloxine B	Pathology

SCI INTERNATIONAL INC.   301-696-8879
5902 Enterprise Court, Frederick, MD 21703
FDA Number: 3003791481

Kit, Pregnancy Test, Over The Counter, HCG	Chemistry
Test, Luteinizing Hormone (lh), Over The Counter	Chemistry

SCI TECHNOLOGIES INC.
See Questech International, Inc.

SCI-DENT, INC.   800-323-4145
210 Dowdle St. #2, Algonquin, IL 60102   **847-658-3111**
FDA Number: 1419493   Fax: 847-658-0115
Medical Products Sales Volume: $1,000,000
Annual Revenue: $0-$1 Million
Total Employees: 10   Marketing Staff: 1   Sales Staff: 2
Ownership: Private
Produces/Sells CE-marked Devices: N
Federal Procurement Eligibility: Small Business
Distribution: Manufacturer Direct, Manufacturer Through Distributor, Service Direct, Exporter
General Admin.: Robert O'Connor/President

Burnisher, Operative, Dental	Dental And Oral
Carver, Dental Amalgam, Operative	Dental And Oral
Condenser, Amalgam And Foil, Operative	Dental And Oral
Curette, Periodontic	Dental And Oral
Curette, Surgical, Dental	Dental And Oral
Excavator, Dental, Operative	Dental And Oral
Explorer, Operative	Dental And Oral
Filling, Instrument Plastic, Dental	Dental And Oral
Knife, Periodontic	Dental And Oral
Plugger, Root Canal, Endodontic	Dental And Oral
Probe, Periodontic	Dental And Oral
Pusher, Band, Orthodontic	Dental And Oral
Scaler, Periodontic	Dental And Oral
Spreader, Pulp Canal Filling Material, Endodontic	Dental And Oral
Tucker, Ligature, Orthodontic	Dental And Oral

SCIARRA LABORATORIES, INC   516-933-7853
485-09 South Broadway, Hicksville, NY 11801-5071
FDA Number: 2436227   Fax: 516-933-7807
E-mail: sciarralabs@att.net
Web site: www.sciarralabs.com
Medical Products Sales Volume: $700,000
Annual Revenue: $1-$5 Million
Year Founded: 1993
Total Employees: 7   Marketing Staff: 1   Sales Staff: 2
Ownership: Private
Produces/Sells CE-marked Devices: N
Federal Procurement Eligibility: Small Business
Distribution: Manufacturer Through Distributor
General Admin.: John Sciarra/President, Chief Executive Officer
    Carolyn LaRegina/Vice President Human Resources & Personnel
    Christopher Sciarra/Vice President, General Manager
Mktg./Adv.: John Sciarra/Director National Accounts & Sales
Production: Christopher Sciarra/Director Quality Assurance
    Carolyn LaRegina/Manager Materials

Accessory, Barium Sulfate, Methyl Methacrylate For Cranioplasty	Cns/Neurology

SCICAN   800-667-7733
1440 Don Mills Rd.,   **416-445-1600**
Toronto, ON M3B 3 Canada
FDA Number: n/a   Fax: 416-445-2727
E-mail: CustService.ca@scican.com
Web site: www.scican.com
Year Founded: 1957
Total Employees: 180
Ownership: SciCan, Division of Lux & Zwingenberger Ltd.
Quality System Registration Information: ISO9001
Produces/Sells CE-marked Devices: Y
Distribution: Manufacturer Direct, Manufacturer Through Distributor, Exclusive Distributor, Exporter

SCICAN INC.   800-572-1211
701 Technology Drive, Canonsburg, PA 15317   **724-820-1600**
FDA Number: 2529090   Fax: 724-820-1479
Web site: www.scican.com
Year Founded: 1957
Ownership: Scican
Produces/Sells CE-marked Devices: N
Federal Procurement Eligibility: Small Business
Distribution: Manufacturer Through Distributor

Packaging, Sterilization	General
Sterilization Indicator	Surgery
Sterilizer, Steam (Autoclave)	General
Test, Equipment, Sterilization	General

SCICON TECHNOLOGIES CORP.
888-295-8630
661-295-8630
27525 Newhall Ranch Road, Suite 2,
Valencia, CA 91355
FDA Number: n/a
Fax: 661-295-6611
E-mail: rfq@scicontech.com
Web site: www.scicontech.com
Medical Products Sales Volume: $5,100,000
Annual Revenue: $0-$1 Million
Year Founded: 1989
Total Employees: 50   Marketing Staff: 2   Sales Staff: 10
Ownership: Private
Quality System Registration Information: ISO9001
Produces/Sells CE-marked Devices: N
Federal Procurement Eligibility: Small Business
Distribution: OEM, Service Direct
General Admin.: Scott Turner/President
Mktg./Adv.: Brad Bulger/Vice President Marketing
   Service, Engineering/Design   General

SCIENCARE CORP.
   See Respironics Colorado

SCIENCE 20/20, INC.
760-753-7928
681 Encinitas Blvd, Suite 302, Encinitas, CA 92024
FDA Number: 2032221
Fax: 760-753-6127
E-mail: science2020@abac.com
Web site: www.science2020.com
Medical Products Sales Volume: $400,000
Year Founded: 1998
Total Employees: 3
Ownership: Private
Produces/Sells CE-marked Devices: N
Federal Procurement Eligibility: Small Business
   Chart, Visual Acuity   Ophthalmology

SCIENCE APPLICATIONS
INTERNATIONAL CORP.
800-430-7629

10260 Campus Point Drive, San Diego, CA 92121
858-826-6000
FDA Number: n/a
Fax: 858-826-7191
E-mail: info@saic.com
Web site: www.saic.com
Medical Products Sales Volume: $8,200,000,000
Year Founded: 1969
Total Employees: 4300
Ownership: Public
Federal Procurement Eligibility: VA Contract
Distribution: Service Direct
General Admin.: Larry Kull/President
    Dr. J.R. Beyster/Senior Vice President
Mktg./Adv.: Joan Moore/Director Communications
    Gloria Kosman/Vice President Sales
    Jeff Anderson/Vice President Sales
   Service, Consulting   General

SCIENCETECH INC.
519-644-0135
1450 Global Drive, London, ONT N6N 1R3 Canada
FDA Number: n/a
Fax: 519-644-0136
E-mail: sales@sciencetech-inc.com
Web site: www.sciencetech-inc.com
Year Founded: 1985
Total Employees: 25
Ownership: Private
Produces/Sells CE-marked Devices: N
Distribution: Manufacturer Direct, Exclusive Distributor

SCIENT'X USA, INC.
407-571-2550
1015 Maitland Center Commons, Suite 106A,
Maitland, FL 32751
FDA Number: 3003807094
Fax: 407-571-2551
E-mail: info@scientxusa.com
Web site: www.scientxusa.com
Medical Products Sales Volume: $1,900,000
Year Founded: 2002
Total Employees: 25
Ownership: Private
Produces/Sells CE-marked Devices: Y
Federal Procurement Eligibility: Small Business
   Appliance, Fixation, Spinal Interlaminal   Orthopedics
   Appliance, Fixation, Spinal Intervertebral Body   Orthopedics
   Orthosis, Fixation, Pedicle, Spinal   Orthopedics

SCIENTECH, INC.
303-444-1361
5649 Arapahoe Avenue, Boulder, CO 80303-1399
FDA Number: 9200960
Fax: 303-444-9229
E-mail: inst@scientech-inc.com
Web site: www.scientech-inc.com
Medical Products Sales Volume: $2,200,000
Annual Revenue: $1-$5 Million

SCIENTECH, INC.
303-444-1361 (cont'd)
Year Founded: 1968
Total Employees: 15   Marketing Staff: 1   Sales Staff: 1
Ownership: Private
Quality System Registration Information: ISO9001
Produces/Sells CE-marked Devices: Y
Federal Procurement Eligibility: Small Business
Distribution: Manufacturer Direct, Manufacturer Through Distributor, Manufacturer Through Manufacturer Reps, OEM, Service Direct, Exporter
General Admin.: Thomas O'Rourke/President
Mktg./Adv.: Tom Campbell/Vice President Marketing
   Accessories, Laser   General
   Balance, Electronic   Chemistry
   Balance, Macro (0.1 mg Accuracy)   Chemistry
   Balance, Semimicro (0.01 mg Accuracy)   Chemistry
   Calorimeter   Chemistry
   Scale, Laboratory   Chemistry

SCIENTEK HOSPITAL AND LABORATORY
EQUIPMENT
866-321-3828

7943A Progress Way,
604-940-8084
Delta, BC V4G 1 Canada
FDA Number: n/a
Fax: 604-940-8085
E-mail: sales@scientek.net
Web site: http://www.scientek.net
Year Founded: 1982
Total Employees: 100
Ownership: Private
Produces/Sells CE-marked Devices: N
Distribution: Manufacturer Direct, Exporter

SCIENTEK MEDICAL EQUIPMENT
604-273-9094
11151 Bridgeport Rd., Richmond, BC V6X 1T3 Canada
FDA Number: n/a
Fax: 604-273-1262
E-mail: sales@scientek.net
Medical Products Sales Volume: $10,000,000
Total Employees: 50   Marketing Staff: 7   Sales Staff: 7
Ownership: CHALMERS
Stock Symbol: CYL
Traded On: Montreal
Quality System Registration Information: ISO9003
Produces/Sells CE-marked Devices: N
Federal Procurement Eligibility: Small Business
Distribution: Manufacturer Through Distributor

SCIENTIFIC DEVICE LABORATORY INC.
847-803-9495
411 E. Jarvis Ave., Des Plaines, IL 60018
FDA Number: 1420513
   Reagent, General Purpose   Pathology
   Slide, Control, Quality   Microbiology

SCIENTIFIC GAS PROD./ASHLAND CHEM.
   See Scott Medical Products

SCIENTIFIC GLASS & INSTRUMENTS, INC.
877-682-1481
PO Box 6, Houston, TX 77001-0006
FDA Number: 7000325
Fax: 713-682-3054
E-mail: glasscom@aol.com
Web site: www.sginstr.com
Medical Products Sales Volume: $300,000
Annual Revenue: $0-$1 Million
Year Founded: 1945
Total Employees: 7   Marketing Staff: 2   Sales Staff: 2
Ownership: Private
Quality System Registration Information: ISO9000
Produces/Sells CE-marked Devices: N
Federal Procurement Eligibility: Small Business
Distribution: Manufacturer Direct, OEM, Exporter
General Admin.: James A. Muller/Chief Executive Officer
Mktg./Adv.: Robert D. Muller/Manager Advertising
    Robert D. Muller/Vice President Marketing & Sales
Production: Robert F. Muller/Vice President Manufacturing
   Distilling Unit, Molecular   Chemistry
   Manometer, Laboratory   Chemistry
   Molecular Weight Equipment   Chemistry

SCIENTIFIC GROWTH
   See Meritech, Inc.

SCIENTIFIC IMAGING, INC.
303-681-9402
97 Slate Lane, Mt. Crested Butte, CO 81225
FDA Number: 1722077
   Computer and Software, Medical   General

SCIENTIFIC IMAGING, LLC
770-926-3060
9878 Main Street, Suite 125, Woodstock, GA 30188
FDA Number: 3006157994
Ownership: Private
Produces/Sells CE-marked Devices: N

SCIENTIFIC IMAGING, LLC

770-926-3060 *(cont'd)*
Device, Measurement, Velocity, Conduction, Nerve — Cns/Neurology

SCIENTIFIC INDUSTRIES, INC.

888-850-6208
70 Orville Drive, Bohemia, NY 11716-2512 — **631-567-4700**
FDA Number: 9200963 — Fax: 631-567-5896
E-mail: info@scientificindustries.com
Web site: www.scientificindustries.com
Medical Products Sales Volume: $3,400,000
Annual Revenue: $1-$5 Million
Year Founded: 1954
Total Employees: 15
Ownership: Public
Stock Symbol: SCND
Traded On: OTC Bulletin
Produces/Sells CE-marked Devices: Y
Federal Procurement Eligibility: Small Business
Distribution: Manufacturer Direct, Manufacturer Through Distributor, Manufacturer Through Manufacturer Reps, Exclusive Distributor, Exporter
General Admin.: Helena Santos/President, Chief Executive Officer
    Robert Nichols/Vice President, Secretary
Mktg./Adv.: Chere Griffin/Director Marketing

Blender/Mixer	Chemistry
Disrupter, Cell	Microbiology
Homogenizer, Tissue	Microbiology
Incubator, Test Tube, Stationary	Microbiology
Mixer, Clinical Laboratory	Chemistry
Refrigerator, Biological	Microbiology
Shaker/Stirrer	Chemistry
Stirrer	Chemistry
Tissue Culture Apparatus	Microbiology

SCIENTIFIC INSTRUMENT SERVICES, INC.

908-788-5550
1027 Old York Road, Ringoes, NJ 08551
FDA Number: n/a — Fax: 908-806-6631
E-mail: sisexp@sisweb.com
Web site: www.sisweb.com
Annual Revenue: $1-$5 Million
Total Employees: 25 — *Marketing Staff:* 1 — *Sales Staff:* 5
Ownership: Private
Produces/Sells CE-marked Devices: Y
Federal Procurement Eligibility: Small Business
Distribution: Manufacturer Direct, Service Direct
General Admin.: John Manura/President, Chief Executive Officer
    Christopher Baker/Vice President, General Manager

Accessories, Chromatography (Gas, Gel, Liquid, Thin Layer)	Chemistry

SCIENTIFIC PHARMACEUTICALS, INC.

800-634-3047
3221 Producer Way, Pomona, CA 91768-3916 — **909-595-9922**
FDA Number: 2022039 — Fax: 909-595-0331
E-mail: scipharm@msn.com
Web site: www.scipharm.com
Annual Revenue: $1-$5 Million
Year Founded: 1979
Total Employees: 35 — *Marketing Staff:* 3 — *Sales Staff:* 3
Ownership: Private
Quality System Registration Information: ISO9001
Produces/Sells CE-marked Devices: Y
Federal Procurement Eligibility: Small Business
Distribution: Manufacturer Direct, Manufacturer Through Distributor, Manufacturer Through Manufacturer Reps, OEM, Exporter
General Admin.: Jan. A. Orlowski/President
Production: David V. Butler/Vice President Manufacturing

Adhesive, Bracket And Conditioner, Resin	Dental And Oral
Agent, Polishing, Abrasive, Oral Cavity	Dental And Oral
Cement, Dental	Dental And Oral
Coating, Filling Material, Resin	Dental And Oral
Glove, Patient Examination	General
Material, Impression Tray, Resin	Dental And Oral
Material, Tooth Shade, Resin	Dental And Oral
Sealant, Pit And Fissure, And Conditioner, Resin	Dental And Oral
Syringe, Restorative And Impression Material	Dental And Oral
Varnish	Dental And Oral
Varnish, Cavity	Dental And Oral
Veneer, Dental	Dental And Oral
Zinc Oxide Eugenol	Dental And Oral

SCIENTIFIC PLASTICS, INC.

212-967-1199
243 West 30th St., New York, NY 10001
FDA Number: 2434220

Hearing-Aid	Ear/Nose/Throat

SCIENTIFIC PRODUCTS & EQUIPMENT LTD.

800-268-1956
(S.P.E.)
95 Barber Greene Road, Suite 303,
North York, ONT M3C 3 Canada
FDA Number: n/a — Fax: 416-443-2570
E-mail: info@scipro.com

SCIENTIFIC PRODUCTS & EQUIPMENT LTD.

800-268-1956
(cont'd)
Web site: www.scipro.com
Year Founded: 1983
Total Employees: 10
Ownership: Private
Produces/Sells CE-marked Devices: N
Distribution: Exclusive Distributor

SCIENTIMED CORP.

510-763-5405
4109 Balfour Ave., Oakland, CA 94610
FDA Number: 2939021
Ownership: Private
Produces/Sells CE-marked Devices: N

Condom	Obstetrics/Gynecology
Cover, Shoe, Operating Room	Surgery
Glove, Patient Examination	General
Glove, Surgical, Plastic Surgery	Surgery
Gown, Isolation, Surgical	Surgery
Gown, Patient	Surgery
Gown, Surgical	Surgery
Shoe And Shoe Cover, Conductive	Anesthesiology

SCIFIT

800-278-3933
5151 S. 110th E. Avenue, Tulsa, OK 74146 — **918-359-2000**
FDA Number: 3002114262 — Fax: 918-359-2012
E-mail: info@scifit.com
Web site: www.scifit.com
Medical Products Sales Volume: $2,500,000
Year Founded: 1987
Total Employees: 32 — *Sales Staff:* 5
Ownership: Private
Produces/Sells CE-marked Devices: N
Federal Procurement Eligibility: Small Business, GSA Contract, VA Contract
Distribution: Manufacturer Direct, Manufacturer Through Distributor, Manufacturer Through Manufacturer Reps
General Admin.: Larry Born/Chief Executive Officer
    Denton Smith/President

Equipment, Therapy, Handicapped/Physical	Physical Med

SCIMAGE, INC.

866-724-6243
4916 El Camino Real, Suite 200, — **650-694-4858**
Los Altos, CA 94022
FDA Number: 2952596 — Fax: 650-694-4861
E-mail: chris_carr@scimage.com
Year Founded: 1993
Total Employees: 48 — *Marketing Staff:* 3 — *Sales Staff:* 16
Ownership: Private
Produces/Sells CE-marked Devices: N
Federal Procurement Eligibility: Small Business, Minority Owned
Distribution: Manufacturer Direct, OEM, Service Direct
General Admin.: Mr. Sai Raya/Chief Executive Officer
Mktg./Adv.: Mr. Rob Tinker/Manager National Operations
    Mr. Richard Taylor/Manager National Sales
Production: Mr. Skip Strasser/Director Tech. Operations
Finance: Mrs. Mahadvi Raya/Chief Financial Officer

Computer, Cardiac Catheterization Laboratory	Cardiovascular
Computer, Radiographic Image Analysis	Radiology
Image Processing System	Radiology
System, Communication, Image, Digital	Radiology

SCIMED/BOSTON SCIENTIFIC CORPORATION
See Boston Scientific - Maple Grove

SCIMEDX CORPORATION

800-221-5598
100 Ford Road, Suite 100-08, — **973-625-8822**
Denville, NJ 07834
FDA Number: 2247139 — Fax: 973-625-8796
E-mail: info@scimedx.com
Web site: www.scimedx.com
Medical Products Sales Volume: $4,200,000
Annual Revenue: $5-$10 Million
Year Founded: 1986
Total Employees: 38 — *Marketing Staff:* 1 — *Sales Staff:* 3
Ownership: Private
Quality System Registration Information: ISO9001
Produces/Sells CE-marked Devices: Y
Federal Procurement Eligibility: Small Business
Distribution: Manufacturer Direct, Manufacturer Through Distributor, Manufacturer Through Manufacturer Reps, OEM, Importer, Exporter
General Admin.: Thomas L. Britten/President, Chief Executive Officer

Antibody, Anti-Smooth Muscle, Indirect Immunofluorescent	Immunology
Antibody, Antimitochondrial, Indirect Immunofluorescent	Immunology
Antibody, Antinuclear, Indirect Immunofluorescent, Antigen	Immunology
Antibody, Multiple Auto, Indirect Immunofluorescent	Immunology
Antibody, Other	General
Reagent, Legionella Detection	Microbiology
Test, DNA-Probe, Other	Microbiology

SCIMEDX CORPORATION 800-221-5598 *(cont'd)*
Test, Thyroid Autoantibody Immunology

SCION CARDIO-VASCULAR, INC. 305-259-8880
14256 SW 119 Ave., Miami, FL 33186
FDA Number: 1055965
E-mail: ggolik@scioncv.com Fax: 305-259-8878
Web site: www.scioncv.com
Annual Revenue: $1-$5 Million
Year Founded: 1999
Total Employees: 6 Marketing Staff: 2 Sales Staff: 20
Ownership: Private
Quality System Registration Information: ISO9001; ISO9003
Produces/Sells CE-marked Devices: Y
Federal Procurement Eligibility: Small Business
Distribution: Manufacturer Direct, Manufacturer Through Manufacturer Reps,
Service Direct, Exporter
General Admin.: Mr. Ernie Manzano/General Manager
Mktg./Adv.: Lorraine OToole/Director Sales
Device, Hemostasis, Vascular Cardiovascular
Dislodger, Stone, Flexible Gastroenterology/Urology
Dressing, Wound, Hydrophilic Surgery

SCIREQ INC. 514-286-1429
6600 St-Urbain, Suite 300, Montreal, QUE H2S 3G8 Canada
FDA Number: n/a Fax: 514-286-1627
E-mail: sales@scireq.com
Web site: www.scireq.com
Year Founded: 1997
Total Employees: 10
Ownership: Private
Produces/Sells CE-marked Devices: N
Distribution: Manufacturer Direct, Exclusive Distributor, Exporter

SCITON, INC. 888-646-6999
9255 Commercial St., Palo Alto, CA 94303 650-493-9155
FDA Number: 2953696 Fax: 650-493-9146
E-mail: marketing@sciton.com
Year Founded: 1997
Ownership: Private
Quality System Registration Information: ISO9001
Produces/Sells CE-marked Devices: N
Laser, Surgical Surgery

SCIVOLUTIONS, INC. 704-853-0100
2260 Raeford Court, Gastonia, NC 28052
FDA Number: 1225475 Fax: 704-853-0400
E-mail: orders@granuderm.com
Web site: www.scivolutions.com
Ownership: Private
Produces/Sells CE-marked Devices: N
Bandage, Adhesive Surgery

SCJ ENTERPRISES, INC. 516-797-8903
3 riviera drive east, Massapequa, NY 11758-8509
FDA Number: 2437412 Fax: 516-797-8906
E-mail: JParis@Technologist.com
Web site: www.scjenterprises.com
Medical Products Sales Volume: $100,000
Annual Revenue: $0-$1 Million
Year Founded: 1995
Total Employees: 2
Ownership: Private
Produces/Sells CE-marked Devices: N
Federal Procurement Eligibility: Small Business
Distribution: Manufacturer Direct
Monitor, Bed Patient General

SCODENCO, INC. 918-627-6795
7405 East 31st Pl., Tulsa, OK 74145
FDA Number: 1646667
Ownership: Private
Produces/Sells CE-marked Devices: N
Handpiece, Contra- And Right-Angle Attachment, Dental Dental And Oral
Teeth, Artificial, Posterior With Metal Insert Dental And Oral

SCOOTER-TOTE 604-517-3990
739 Princess Rd., New Westminster, BC V3M-6V6 Canada
FDA Number: n/a Fax: 604-517-3926
E-mail: henrid@bc.sympatico.ca
Web site: www.infostuff.com/ScooterTote/index.html
Year Founded: 1987
Ownership: Private
Produces/Sells CE-marked Devices: N
Distribution: Manufacturer Direct

SCOPE TECHNOLOGY, INC. 860-963-1141
28 Quassett Road, Pompfret, CT 06258
FDA Number: 81534 Fax: 860-928-7036

SCOPE TECHNOLOGY, INC. 860-963-1141 *(cont'd)*
E-mail: rgreene@scopetech.com
Annual Revenue: $1-$5 Million
Ownership: Private
Produces/Sells CE-marked Devices: N
Fiberoptic Light Source & Carrier Ear/Nose/Throat

SCOTFOAM
See Foamex Innovations

SCOTSMAN ICE SYSTEMS
See Scotsman Industries

SCOTSMAN INDUSTRIES 800-SCOTSMAN
775 Corporate Woods Pkwy., 847-215-4500
Vernon Hills, IL 60061
FDA Number: n/a Fax: 847-913-9844
E-mail: customer.service@scotman/ice.com
Web site: www.scotsmanindustries.com
Annual Revenue: $1-$5 Million
Total Employees: 100
Ownership: SCOTTSMAN INDUSTRIES
Quality System Registration Information: ISO9000
Produces/Sells CE-marked Devices: N
Distribution: Manufacturer Direct, Manufacturer Through Distributor, Manufacturer
Through Manufacturer Reps, OEM, Exclusive Distributor
General Admin.: Randy Rossi/President
Mktg./Adv.: Jospeh Clark/Director Marketing
Mike Dowell/Director Sales
Charles Janousky/Manager Advertising & Promotions
Dispenser, Ice General

SCOTT AVIATION
See Avox Systems

SCOTT CO., DAVID, MEDICAL SALES DIV.
See David Scott Company

SCOTT HEALTH CARE
See Sca Personal Care, North America

SCOTT LABORATORIES, LEXINGTON DIV.
See Gibson Laboratories

SCOTT MEDICAL PRODUCTS 800-233-4334
6097 Easton Road, Building 3, 215-766-8861
Plumsteadville, PA 18949
FDA Number: n/a Fax: 215-766-7250
Web site: www.scottecatalog.com
Medical Products Sales Volume: $6,500,000
Annual Revenue: $5-$10 Million
Ownership: Scott Medical Products
Quality System Registration Information: ISO9002
Produces/Sells CE-marked Devices: Y
Distribution: Manufacturer Direct, OEM
Electrode, Blood pH Chemistry
Gas Mixtures, Medical General
Medical Product Subsidiaries (Listed Separately)
Scott Medical Products

SCOTT ORTHOTIC LABS, INC. 866-648-9148
1709 Heath Parkway, 970-484-5017
Fort Collins, CO 80524
FDA Number: 3003684341 Fax: 970-498-9529
E-mail: info@scottorthotic.com
Web site: www.scottorthotic.com
Ownership: Private
Produces/Sells CE-marked Devices: N
Brace, Joint, Ankle (External) Physical Med
Joint, Hip, External Brace Physical Med
Joint, Knee, External Brace Physical Med
Orthosis, Limb Brace Physical Med
Stirrup, External Brace Component Physical Med
Walker, Mechanical Physical Med

SCOTT SPECIALTIES, INC. 785-527-5627
1820 East 7th St., Concordia, KS 66901
FDA Number: 1933909
Ownership: Private
Produces/Sells CE-marked Devices: N
Ankle/Foot, External Limb Component Physical Med
Belt, Traction, Pelvic, Orthopedic Orthopedics
Binder, Abdominal General
Binder, Breast Obstetrics/Gynecology
Binder, Elastic General
Cushion, Wheelchair (Pad) Physical Med
Halter, Head, Traction, Orthopedic Orthopedics
Joint, Knee, External Brace Physical Med
Orthosis, Cervical Physical Med
Orthosis, Lumbosacral Physical Med
Orthosis, Rib Fracture, Soft Physical Med
Orthosis, Sacroiliac, Soft Physical Med

SCOTT SPECIALTIES, INC. — 785-527-5627 (cont'd)

Protector, Skin Pressure	General
Shoe, Cast	Physical Med
Sling, Arm	Physical Med
Splint, Clavicle	Physical Med
Splint, Hand, And Component	Physical Med

SCOTT SPECIALTIES, INC. — 785-527-5627
1827 Meadowlark Rd., Clay Center, KS 67432
FDA Number: 1933910

Ankle/Foot, External Limb Component	Physical Med
Belt, Traction, Pelvic, Orthopedic	Orthopedic
Binder, Abdominal	General
Binder, Breast	Obstetrics/Gynecology
Binder, Elastic	General
Cushion, Wheelchair (Pad)	Physical Med
Halter, Head, Traction, Orthopedic	Orthopedics
Joint, Knee, External Brace	Physical Med
Orthosis, Cervical	Physical Med
Orthosis, Lumbosacral	Physical Med
Orthosis, Rib Fracture, Soft	Physical Med
Orthosis, Sacroiliac, Soft	Physical Med
Protector, Skin Pressure	General
Shoe, Cast	Physical Med
Sling, Arm	Physical Med
Splint, Clavicle	Physical Med
Splint, Hand, And Component	Physical Med

SCOTT SPECIALTIES, INC./CMO INC./GINNY INC. — 800-255-7136
512 M St., Belleville, KS 66935-1546 — 785-527-5627
FDA Number: 1917910 — *Fax:* 785-527-5713
E-mail: linda.ashton@scottspecialties.com
Web site: www.scottspecialties.com
Medical Products Sales Volume: $16,300,000
Annual Revenue: $10-$25 Million
Year Founded: 1962
Total Employees: 150 — *Marketing Staff:* 1 — *Sales Staff:* 1
Ownership: Private
Produces/Sells CE-marked Devices: Y
Federal Procurement Eligibility: Small Business, GSA Contract
Distribution: Manufacturer Through Distributor, Manufacturer Through Manufacturer Reps, OEM, Exporter
General Admin.: Wilson Scott/Chief Executive Officer
　Jim McDonald/President
Mktg./Adv.: Linda Ashton/Vice President Marketing & Sales
Production: Tim Wellendorf/Vice President Manufacturing
Research: Lanie Engle/Vice President Product Development

Belt, Lumbosacral	Orthopedics
Belt, Rib (Support)	Orthopedics
Belt, Traction, Pelvic	Physical Med
Belt, Traction, Pelvic, Orthopedic	Orthopedics
Binder, Abdominal	General
Collar, Cervical Neck	Orthopedics
Immobilizer, Arm	Orthopedics
Immobilizer, Knee	Orthopedics
Immobilizer, Shoulder	Orthopedics
Joint, Knee, External Brace	Physical Med
Orthosis, Cervical	Physical Med
Orthosis, Lumbosacral	Physical Med
Orthosis, Rib Fracture, Soft	Physical Med
Orthosis, Sacroiliac, Soft	Physical Med
Pad, Pressure, Animal Skin	General
Shoe, Cast	Physical Med
Sling, Arm	Physical Med
Splint, Clavicle	Physical Med
Splint, Hand, And Component	Physical Med
Support, Abdominal	Physical Med
Support, Ankle	Orthopedics
Support, Back	Orthopedics
Support, Clavicle	Orthopedics
Support, Elbow	Orthopedics
Support, Knee	Physical Med
Support, Leg	Physical Med
Support, Wrist	Physical Med

SCOTT SPECIALTY GASES
See Scott Medical Products

SCOTT SPECIALTY GASES — 215-766-8861
6141 Easton Road Box 310, Plumsteadville, PA 18949
FDA Number: 2518435 — *Fax:* 215-766-2476
E-mail: solutions.center@airliquide.com
Web site: www.scottecatalog.com
Year Founded: 1960
Total Employees: 500
Ownership: Private
Produces/Sells CE-marked Devices: N
Distribution: Manufacturer Direct, Exporter

Gas, Calibrated (Specified Concentration)	Anesthesiology
Gas, Reattachment Procedure, Retinal	Ophthalmology

SCOTT SPECIALTY GASES — 215-766-8861 (cont'd)

Regulator, Pressure, Gas Cylinder	Anesthesiology

SCOTT TECHNOLOGY LLC — 203-888-2783
1 Jacks Hill Rd., Oxford, CT 06478
FDA Number: 3003617315

Bed, Electric	General
Bed, Flotation Therapy, Powered	Physical Med
Mattress, Air Flotation	General
Mattress, Non-Powered Flotation Therapy	Physical Med

SCOTT THERAPEUTIC DESIGNS, INC.
See Freedom Designs, Inc.

SCOTT-GROSS CO., INC. — 800-967-6874
664 Magnolia Ave., Lexington, KY 40505-3706 — 859-737-5452
FDA Number: n/a
Web site: www.scottgross.com
Ownership: Private
Produces/Sells CE-marked Devices: N

Cryosurgical Unit	Surgery

SCOTTCARE CORPORATION — 800-243-9412
4791 W. 150th St., Cleveland, OH 44135 — 216-362-0550
FDA Number: 1527715 — *Fax:* 216-267-6129
E-mail: info@scottcare.com
Web site: www.scottcare.com
Medical Products Sales Volume: $1,025
Annual Revenue: $10-$25 Million
Year Founded: 1987
Total Employees: 45 — *Marketing Staff:* 3 — *Sales Staff:* 25
Ownership: BERKSHIRE HATHWAY - SCOTT FETZER DIV.
Stock Symbol: BRK-A
Traded On: NYSE
Produces/Sells CE-marked Devices: Y
Distribution: Manufacturer Direct, Manufacturer Through Manufacturer Reps
General Admin.: Mr. Kenneth M. Zajaczkowski/President, General Manager
Mktg./Adv.: Mr. William Kulp/Director Marketing & Business Development
　Mr. Robert Ody/Manager Sales
Purchasing: Mr. David Shipe/Purchasing Agent

Circulatory Assist Unit, Cardiac	Cardiovascular
Detector, Arrhythmia Alarm	Cardiovascular
Monitor, ECG	Cardiovascular
Transmitter/Receiver System, Physiological, Radiofrequency	Cardiovascular

Medical Product Subsidiaries (Listed Separately)
Nicore Equipment & Leasing, Inc.
Rozinn By Scottcare Corporation

SCOTTCARE CORPORATION — 813-901-0019
4897 W. Waters Ave., Suite J, Tampa, FL 33634
FDA Number: 1063268
E-mail: billw@nicore.com
Web site: www.nicore.com
Year Founded: 1997
Ownership: Private
Produces/Sells CE-marked Devices: N
Distribution: Manufacturer Direct
General Admin.: Bill V. Wooley/President, Chief Executive Officer
　Garrett R. Bates/Vice President
Production: Jeff Mogiliewicz/Director Quality Assurance

Pump, Counterpulsating, External	Cardiovascular

SCOTTY TECHNOLOGY OF THE AMERICAS, INC. — 910-395-6100
6714 Netherlands Drive, Wilmington, NC 28405
FDA Number: 3003415616
Ownership: Private
Produces/Sells CE-marked Devices: N

Communication System, Powered	Physical Med

SCP SCIENCE — 800-361-6820
21800 Clark Graham Ave., — 514-457-0701
Baie D'Urfe, QUE H9X-4 Canada
FDA Number: n/a — *Fax:* 514-457-4499
E-mail: sales@scpscience.com
Web site: www.scpscience.com
Year Founded: 1980
Total Employees: 25
Ownership: Private
Produces/Sells CE-marked Devices: N
Distribution: Manufacturer Direct, Exclusive Distributor

SCS CORPORATION — 630-797-7300
1901 Powis Court, West Chicago, IL 60185
FDA Number: 1424527 — *Fax:* 630-797-7305
E-mail: cja@scscorp.com
Web site: www.scscorp.com
Year Founded: 1996
Total Employees: 8 — *Marketing Staff:* 1 — *Sales Staff:* 1
Ownership: Private

SCS CORPORATION   630-797-7300 (cont'd)
Produces/Sells CE-marked Devices: N
Federal Procurement Eligibility: Small Business
Distribution: Manufacturer Through Distributor
Needle, Hypodermic, Single Lumen With Syringe   General

SCULPTEC DENTAL DESIGN INC.   801-942-1874
6841 South 1300 East, Cottonwood Heights, UT 84121
FDA Number: 3004590946
Ownership: Private
Produces/Sells CE-marked Devices: N
System, Optical Impression, Computer Assisted Design And Manufacturing (cad/cam)
Of Dental Restorations   Dental And Oral

SCYTEK LABORATORIES, INC.   435-755-9848
205 South 600 West, Logan, UT 84321
FDA Number: 3004074729

Buffer, pH	Hematology
Culture Media, Synthetic Cell And Tissue	Pathology
Fixative, Formalin Containing	Pathology
Formalin, Neutral Buffered	Pathology
Immunohistochemistry Reagents And Kits	Pathology
Media, Mounting, Water Soluble	Pathology
Reagent, General Purpose	Pathology
Reagents, Specific, Analyte	Hematology
Stain, Eosin Y	Pathology
Stain, Hematoxylin	Pathology
Stain, Hematoxylin, Mayer's	Pathology
Stain, Methyl Green	Pathology
Stain, Nuclear Fast Red	Pathology
Trypsin	Pathology

SDI DIAGNOSTICS, INC.   800-678-5782
10 Hampden Drive, Easton, MA 02375   508-238-7033
FDA Number: 1220253   Fax: 508-230-2752
E-mail: sales@sdidiagnostics.com
Web site: www.sdidiagnostics.com
Annual Revenue: $1-$5 Million
Total Employees: 50   Marketing Staff: 2   Sales Staff: 8
Ownership: Private
Produces/Sells CE-marked Devices: Y
Federal Procurement Eligibility: Small Business, GSA Contract
Distribution: Manufacturer Through Distributor
General Admin.: Michael J. Boyle/President
Mktg./Adv.: Mr. Cosimo Cariolo/Director Marketing
    Ms. Dianne MacAdam/Manager Market Research
    Ms. Cynthia Minkle/Sales Associate
Production: Pat DeStoop/Manager Materials

Clip, Nose	Anesthesiology
Filter, Bacteriological, Laboratory	Chemistry
Filter, Conduction, Anesthesia	Anesthesiology
Monitor, Ventilation	Anesthesiology
Mouthpiece, Breathing	Anesthesiology
Pneumotachometer	Anesthesiology

SDI MEDICAL CONSULTANTS   619-267-1391
4190 Bonita Road, Suite # 211, Bonita, CA 91902
FDA Number: n/a   Fax: 619-267-1389
E-mail: sdimedical@sbcglobal.net
Web site: http://sdimedical.com/
Medical Products Sales Volume: $100,000
Annual Revenue: $0-$1 Million
Year Founded: 2002
Total Employees: 2   Marketing Staff: 1   Sales Staff: 2
Ownership: Private
Produces/Sells CE-marked Devices: N
Federal Procurement Eligibility: Small Business
Distribution: Service Direct, Exclusive Distributor, Importer, Exporter
General Admin.: Robert Rizo/President

Scanner, Ultrasonic, Obstetrical/Gynecological	Obstetrics/Gynecology
Service, Import/Export	General
Sink, Hospital	General

SDS (SUMMIT DENTAL SYSTEMS)   800-275-3368
3560 NW 53rd Court, Fort Lauderdale, FL 33309   954-730-3636
FDA Number: 1121867   Fax: 954-730-3602
E-mail: sds@summitdental.com
Web site: www.summitdental.com
Medical Products Sales Volume: $1,700,000
Annual Revenue: $1-$5 Million
Year Founded: 1986
Total Employees: 24   Marketing Staff: 2   Sales Staff: 5
Ownership: Private
Stock Symbol: SYD
Traded On: NYSE
Produces/Sells CE-marked Devices: N
Federal Procurement Eligibility: Small Business
Distribution: Manufacturer Through Distributor, Manufacturer Through Manufacturer Reps, OEM, Exporter

SDS (SUMMIT DENTAL SYSTEMS)   800-275-3368 (cont'd)
General Admin.: Cesar Coral/President, Chief Executive Officer
Mktg./Adv.: Veronica Coral/Vice President Exports
    Robert Billoni/Vice President U.S. Sales
Production: Tony Bock/Manager Customer Services
    Willie Pettis/Manager Production
Research: Leo Batista/Manager Research & Development

Chair, Dental	Dental And Oral
Chair, Dental (With Unit)	Dental And Oral
Cuspidor	Dental And Oral
Evacuator, Oral Cavity	Dental And Oral
Holder, X-Ray Film	Dental And Oral
Light, Dental	Dental And Oral
Light, Fiberoptic, Dental	Dental And Oral
Pump, Suction Operatory	Dental And Oral
Stool, Dental	Dental And Oral
Syringe Unit, Air And/Or Water	Dental And Oral

SDS DE MEXICO, S.A. DE C.V.   714-516-7484
Circuito Sur 31, Parque Industrial Nelson, Mexicali 21395 Mexico
FDA Number: 9680845

Cutter, Operative	Dental And Oral
Pliers, Orthodontic	Dental And Oral

SDS-SURGICAL ACUITY   888-822-8489
3225 Deming Way, Suite 120,   608-831-2404
Middleton, WI 53562
FDA Number: n/a   Fax: 608-831-2004
E-mail: carol@focus100.com
Web site: www.surgicalacuity.com
Medical Products Sales Volume: $150,000,000
Total Employees: 75   Marketing Staff: 5   Sales Staff: 30
Ownership: Kerr Corporation
Stock Symbol: SYD
Produces/Sells CE-marked Devices: Y
Federal Procurement Eligibility: Small Business, VA Contract
Distribution: Manufacturer Direct, Exporter
General Admin.: Brian Wilt/Chief Operating Officer
Mktg./Adv.: Brian McManus/Vice President International Sales
    Garrett Sato/Vice President International Sales
Production: Carol Naab/Product Manager

Light, Surgical, Fiberoptic	Surgery
Telescope, Spectacle, Low-Vision	Ophthalmology

SEA HORSE BIO SCIENCE   800-671-0633
16 Esquire Road, North Billerica, MA 01862   978-671-1600
FDA Number: n/a   Fax: 978-671-1611
E-mail: sales@seahorsebio.com
Web site: www.thermogenicimaging.com
Medical Products Sales Volume: $2,500,000
Year Founded: 2000
Total Employees: 60   Marketing Staff: 2   Sales Staff: 6
Ownership: Private
Stock Symbol: BDX
Traded On: NYSE
Produces/Sells CE-marked Devices: N
Federal Procurement Eligibility: Small Business
Distribution: Manufacturer Direct
General Admin.: Jay Teich/Chief Executive Officer
Mktg./Adv.: Steve Chomicz/Vice President Marketing & Sales
Research: Andy Neilson/Vice President Engineering & Development
IS: Jim Orrell/Vice President Software
Analyzer, Chemistry, Fluorescence Immunoassay   Chemistry

SEA-LONG MEDICAL SYSTEMS, INC.   502-969-4949
1983 South Park Rd., Louisville, KY 40219
FDA Number: 1037230
Tent, Oxygen (Canopy)   Anesthesiology

SEA-VIEW OPTICAL, INC.   561-276-5099
1715 S. Federal Hwy., Delray Beach, FL 33483-3329
FDA Number: n/a   Fax: 561-274-9697
E-mail: EYECARE@SEAVIEWOPTICAL.NET
Web site: www.seaviewoptical.net
Medical Products Sales Volume: $500,000
Annual Revenue: $0-$1 Million
Total Employees: 8   Marketing Staff: 1   Sales Staff: 7
Ownership: Private
Produces/Sells CE-marked Devices: N
Federal Procurement Eligibility: Small Business
Distribution: Manufacturer Direct
General Admin.: Richard Bergida/President

Eyeglasses	Ophthalmology
Spectacle, Magnifier	Ophthalmology

MANUFACTURER PROFILES

SEABERG COMPANY INC., THE
27350 SW 95th Ave, Suite 3038,
Wilsonville, OR 97070
     800-818-4726
     503.639.5474

FDA Number: n/a
E-mail: info@sammedical.com
    Fax: 503-639-5425
Web site: www.sammedical.com
Medical Products Sales Volume: $500,000
Annual Revenue: $1-$5 Million
Total Employees: 7   *Marketing Staff:* 1   *Sales Staff:* 1
Ownership: Private
Quality System Registration Information: ISO9001
Produces/Sells CE-marked Devices: Y
Federal Procurement Eligibility: Small Business, Female Owned
Distribution: Manufacturer Through Distributor
General Admin.: Dr. Sam Scheinberg/Chief Executive Officer
        Cheryl Scheinberg/President
  Splint, Other   Orthopedics

SEAHORSE BIOSCIENCE INC.
16 Esquire Road, North Billerica, MA 01862
     978-671-1600

FDA Number: 3006774903
E-mail: sales@seahorsebio.com
Web site: http://www.seahorsebio.com
Year Founded: 2001
Ownership: Private
Produces/Sells CE-marked Devices: N
General Admin.: Mr. Jay Teich/President, Chief Executive Officer
Mktg./Adv.: Mr. Steve Chomicz/Vice President Marketing & Sales
Research: Mr. Andy Neilson/Vice President Product Development
Finance: Mr. Jim Orrell/Vice President Admin., Finance
  Equipment, Laboratory, Gen. Purpose (Specific Medical Use)   Chemistry

SEALY INC.
One Office Parkway, Trinity, NC 27370
     800-697-3259
     336-861-3500

FDA Number: n/a
E-mail: david.mullen@mullen.com
    Fax: 336-861-3501
Web site: www.sealyinc.com
Medical Products Sales Volume: $74,000,000
Annual Revenue: $0-$1 Million
Total Employees: 130
Ownership: Public
Stock Symbol: ZZ
Traded On: NYSE
Federal Procurement Eligibility: Small Business
Distribution: Manufacturer Through Distributor
General Admin.: Ronald Jones/President
Mktg./Adv.: David McIlquham/Vice President Marketing
        Gary Fazio/Vice President Sales
  Mattress, Bed   General

SEALY MATTRESS CO.
See Sealy Inc.

SEAMED CORP.
See Plexus Corp

SEASPINE
2302 La Mirada Drive, Vista, CA 92081-7862
     760-727-8399

FDA Number: 2032593
E-mail: info@seaspine.com
    Fax: 760-727-8809
Web site: www.seaspine.com
Medical Products Sales Volume: $2,800,000
Annual Revenue: $10-$25 Million
Year Founded: 2002
Total Employees: 16
Ownership: Private
Stock Symbol: ATEC
Traded On: NYSE
Produces/Sells CE-marked Devices: N
Federal Procurement Eligibility: Small Business
  Orthosis, Fixation, Pedicle, Spinal   Orthopedics

SEATTLE SYSTEMS
See Lumedx Corp.

SEATTLE SYSTEMS
26296 Twelve Trees Lane N.W., Bldg. 1, Poulsbo, WA 98370
     360-697-5656

FDA Number: n/a
E-mail: customerservice@seattle-systems.com
    Fax: 800-568-6463
Web site: www.seattle-systems.com
Medical Products Sales Volume: $19,000,000
Annual Revenue: $25-$50 Million
Total Employees: 250   *Marketing Staff:* 7   *Sales Staff:* 11
Ownership: HANGER ORTHOPEDIC GROUP, INC.
Stock Symbol: CCASX
Traded On: NYSE
Quality System Registration Information: ISO9001
Produces/Sells CE-marked Devices: Y
Federal Procurement Eligibility: Small Business

SEATTLE SYSTEMS
     360-697-5656 *(cont'd)*

Distribution: Manufacturer Direct, Manufacturer Through Distributor, Manufacturer Through Manufacturer Reps
General Admin.: J.G. Cairns/Chief Executive Officer, Chairman
        Kelly Kschinka/Director Human Resources
Mktg./Adv.: David Adams/Director Marketing
        Christopher Welch/Director Sales
        Hans Schaepper/Manager International Sales
        Michael Douglas/Manager National Sales
Production: Scott Sloaum/Director Manufacturing
        Anna Reyes-Potts/Director Operations
        Anna Reyes-Potts/Manager Regulatory Affairs
Research: Stewart Atkinson/Director Research & Development
Finance: Laurence Leslie/Chief Financial Officer
  Collar, Cervical Neck   Orthopedics
  Immobilizer, Elbow   Orthopedics
  Immobilizer, Knee   Orthopedics
  Shoe, Cast   Physical Med
Medical Product Subsidiaries (Listed Separately)
  Lenox Hill Brace / Seattle Systems

SEBIA ELECTROPHORESIS
400-1705 Corporate Drive, Norcross, GA 30093
     800-835-6497
     770-446-3707

FDA Number: 9032488
E-mail: info@sebia-usa.com
    Fax: 770-446-8511
Web site: www.sebia-usa.com
Annual Revenue: $10-$25 Million
Year Founded: 1997
Ownership: Private
Quality System Registration Information: ISO9001
Produces/Sells CE-marked Devices: Y
Federal Procurement Eligibility: VA Contract
Distribution: Manufacturer Direct
General Admin.: Mr. Steve Thorne/President
Mktg./Adv.: Mr. Robert Liedke/Director Sales
        Ms. Diane Reik/Market Manager
Finance: Mr. Gary Mahoski/Controller
IS: Ms. Karen Anderson/Technical Manager
  Densitometer, Laboratory   Chemistry
  Densitometer/Scanner (Integrating, Reflectance, TLC, Radio)   Chemistry
  Electrophoresis Equipment, Gel   Chemistry
  Electrophoresis Instrumentation   Immunology
  Electrophoretic Separation, Alkaline Phosphatase Isoenzymes   Chemistry
  Electrophoretic Separation, Lipoproteins   Chemistry
  Electrophoretic, Lactate Dehydrogenase Isoenzymes   Chemistry
  Electrophoretic, Protein Fractionation   Chemistry
  Equipment, Immunoelectrophoresis, Rocket   Immunology
  Hemoglobin A2 Quantitation   Hematology
  Hemoglobin C (Abnormal Hemoglobin Variant)   Hematology
  Hemoglobin F Quantitation   Hematology
  Hemoglobin S   Hematology

SEBOTEK HEARING SYSTEMS, LLC
See SEBOTEK HEARING SYSTEMS, LLC

SECA CORP.
1352 Charwood Road, Suite E,
Hanover, MD 21076
     800-542-7322
     410-694-9330

FDA Number: 1120986
E-mail: info.NLIII@seca.com
    Fax: 410-694-9680
Web site: www.seca-online.com
Medical Products Sales Volume: $8,200,000
Year Founded: 1840
Total Employees: 16   *Marketing Staff:* 5   *Sales Staff:* 36
Ownership: VOGEL AND HALKE GMBH
Quality System Registration Information: ISO9002
Produces/Sells CE-marked Devices: Y
Federal Procurement Eligibility: Small Business, GSA Contract
Distribution: Manufacturer Through Distributor, Importer, Exporter
General Admin.: Sonke Vogel/President
        Jeff Mayes/Vice President, General Manager
Mktg./Adv.: Jeff Mayes/Director Marketing
        David Vasquez/Manager Regional Sales
        Michael Peck/Manager Regional Sales
  Exerciser, Powered   Anesthesiology
  Meter, Patient Height   General
  Scale, Chair   General
  Scale, Infant   General
  Scale, Stand-On   General

SECHRIST INDUSTRIES, INC.
4225 E. La Palma Avenue, Anaheim, CA 92807
     800-732-4747
     714-579-8400

FDA Number: 2020676
E-mail: info@sechristusa.com
    Fax: 714-579-0814
Web site: www.sechristusa.com
Medical Products Sales Volume: $21,900,000
Year Founded: 1973
Total Employees: 90
Ownership: Private

SECHRIST INDUSTRIES, INC.   800-732-4747 (cont'd)
Produces/Sells CE-marked Devices: Y
Federal Procurement Eligibility: Small Business
Distribution: Manufacturer Direct, Exporter
General Admin.: James R. Sechrist/President, Chief Executive Officer
Mktg./Adv.: Craig T. Townsend/Director National Accounts
      Craig T. Townsend/Vice President Marketing & Sales
Production: Greg Godfrey/Director Quality Assurance
      Steve Smith/Manager Materials

Chamber, Hyperbaric	Anesthesiology
Mixer, Breathing Gases, Anesthesia Inhalation	Anesthesiology
Ventilator, Continuous (Respirator)	Anesthesiology

SECO PRODUCTS CORPORATION
See Piper Products, Inc.

SECOND EXPOSURE, INC.   985-845-0933
P.O. Box 609, Madisonville, LA 70447
FDA Number: n/a   Fax: 985-845-0955
E-mail: bruce@secondexposure.com
Web site: www.secondexposure.com
Medical Products Sales Volume: $1,500,000
Annual Revenue: $1-$5 Million
Year Founded: 1987
Total Employees: 10   Marketing Staff: 1   Sales Staff: 5
Ownership: Private
Produces/Sells CE-marked Devices: N
Federal Procurement Eligibility: Small Business
Distribution: Exporter
General Admin.: Bruce Crawford/President

Service, Used Equipment	General

SECOND SKIN RUBBER PRODUCTS   1-888-565-SKIN
5484 Royalmount Ave.,   514-344-3333
Mont-Royal, QUE H4P-1 Canada
FDA Number: n/a   Fax: 514-344-3253
E-mail: info@secondskinrubber.com
Web site: http://secondskinrubber.com
Year Founded: 1995
Total Employees: 10
Ownership: Private
Produces/Sells CE-marked Devices: N
Distribution: Exclusive Distributor, Importer

SECOND SOURCE, THE   800-776-3924
1480 N. Claremont Blvd., Claremont, CA 91711   909-399-3691
FDA Number: n/a   Fax: 909-399-3643
E-mail: info@thesecondsource.com
Web site: www.thesecondsource.com
Medical Products Sales Volume: $4,700,000
Annual Revenue: $1-$5 Million
Year Founded: 1980
Total Employees: 668   Sales Staff: 2
Ownership: Private
Produces/Sells CE-marked Devices: N
Distribution: Exclusive Distributor, Importer, Exporter
General Admin.: Steve Boland/Chief Executive Officer
Mktg./Adv.: Becky Young/Sales Associate

Lamp, Other	General

SECTOR MEDICAL CORP.   770-975-1384
320 Northpoint Pkwy., Suite Q, Acworth, GA 30102
FDA Number: 3004355310
Ownership: Private
Produces/Sells CE-marked Devices: N

Recorder, Ventilatory Effort	Anesthesiology

SECURE CARE PRODUCTS, INC.   800-451-7917
39 Chenell Dr., Concord, NH 03301-8501   603-223-0745
FDA Number: n/a   Fax: 603-227-0200
E-mail: jmcauly@securecare.com
Web site: www.securecare.com
Year Founded: 1979
Total Employees: 52
Ownership: Private
Quality System Registration Information: ISO9001
Produces/Sells CE-marked Devices: Y
Federal Procurement Eligibility: Small Business
Distribution: Manufacturer Through Distributor, OEM
General Admin.: Forrest McKerley/Chief Executive Officer
      Harold Baldwin/President
Mktg./Adv.: Michael McKerley/Manager National Accounts
      John McAuley/Vice President Marketing & Sales

Bracelet, Identification	General
Cart, Laundry	General
Equipment, Building Security	General
Monitor, Bed Patient	General
Security Equipment/Supplies	General

SECURE CARE PRODUCTS, INC.   800-451-7917 (cont'd)
Wristlet, Patient Return	Gastroenterology/Urology

SECURE PRODUCTS   469-233-0385
914 Thistle Green Lane, Duncanville, TX 75137
FDA Number: 3005112471
Ownership: Private
Produces/Sells CE-marked Devices: N

Cane	Physical Med

SECURITY ENGINEERED MACHINERY   800-225-9293
5 Walkup Drive, Westborough, MA 01581   508-366-1488
FDA Number: n/a   Fax: 508-366-6814
E-mail: info@semshred.com
Web site: www.semshred.com
Medical Products Sales Volume: $19,700,000
Annual Revenue: $10-$25 Million
Year Founded: 1967
Total Employees: 31   Marketing Staff: 2
Ownership: Private
Stock Symbol: SPW
Traded On: AMEX
Produces/Sells CE-marked Devices: N
Federal Procurement Eligibility: Small Business, GSA Contract
Distribution: Manufacturer Direct, Exporter
General Admin.: Leonard Rosen/Chief Executive Officer
      Peter Dempsey/President
      David Lefrancois/Vice President, General Manager
Mktg./Adv.: Leonard Rosen/Director Marketing
      David Lefrancois/Director Product Development
      Mr. Michael Paciello/Manager Commercial Sales
      Steve Sarja/Manager International Sales
      Peter Dempsey/Manager National Sales
Production: Larry Parker/Director Quality Assurance
      Ray Tift/Manager Materials
Finance: Michael Byrne/Chief Financial Officer

Service, Waste Management	General
Waste Disposal Unit, Syringe	General

SEECOR, INC.   972-288-3278
844 Dalworth Drive, Suite 6, Mesquite, TX 75149-4162
FDA Number: 9200967   Fax: 972-288-3279
E-mail: jeb8afwwii@ev1.net
Web site: www.seecor.com
Medical Products Sales Volume: $200,000
Annual Revenue: $0-$1 Million
Year Founded: 1975
Total Employees: 3   Marketing Staff: 2   Sales Staff: 2
Ownership: Private
Produces/Sells CE-marked Devices: N
Federal Procurement Eligibility: Small Business
Distribution: Manufacturer Direct, Manufacturer Through Distributor, Manufacturer Through Manufacturer Reps, OEM, Importer, Exporter
General Admin.: Jack E. Burroughs, Sr/President, Chairman, Chief Executive Officer
Medical Admin.: L. Siegel/Vice President, Medical Director

Catheter, Other	Gastroenterology/Urology
Detector, His Bundle	Cardiovascular
Fibrillator	Cardiovascular
Fibrillator, AC-Powered	Cardiovascular
Pacemaker, Heart, External	Cardiovascular

SEGAMI CORPORATION   410-381-2311
8325 Guilford Rd., Suite B, Columbia, MD 21046
FDA Number: 3003370689

Image Processing System	Radiology
System, Communication, Image, Digital	Radiology

SEGUFIX SYSTEMS LTD.   1-877-734-8349
110 Queen St.,   506-328-8636
Woodstock, NB E7M-2 Canada
FDA Number: 8022046   Fax: 506-328-4742
E-mail: segufix-canada@segufix.com
Web site: www.segufix.com
Year Founded: 1980
Total Employees: 5   Marketing Staff: 5
Ownership: Private
Produces/Sells CE-marked Devices: N
Distribution: Manufacturer Direct, Exclusive Distributor, Importer

SEIICHI MANUFACTURING
See Ultrascope

SEIKO OPTICAL PRODUCTS   201-529-9099
575 Corporate Dr., Mahwah, NJ 07430-2330
FDA Number: 2434293
E-mail: csmail@seikoeyewear.com
Web site: www.seikoeyewear.com
Annual Revenue: $1-$5 Million

SEIKO OPTICAL PRODUCTS — 201-529-9099 (cont'd)

Year Founded: 1881
Ownership: Seiko Optical Products Co.,Ltd
Produces/Sells CE-marked Devices: N
Distribution: Manufacturer Through Distributor, Manufacturer Through Manufacturer Reps

Lens, Spectacle/Eyeglasses, Non-Custom	Ophthalmology

SEILER PRECISION MICROSCOPES, DIV. OF SEILER INSTRUMENT CO. — 800-489-2282

3433 Tree Court Industrial Blvd., — 314-968-2282
St. Louis, MO 63122
FDA Number: 1927430 — Fax: 314-968-3601
E-mail: micro@seilerinst.com
Web site: www.seilerinst.com
Annual Revenue: $0-$1 Million
Year Founded: 1945
Total Employees: 145 — Marketing Staff: 1 — Sales Staff: 2
Ownership: Private
Quality System Registration Information: ISO9001
Produces/Sells CE-marked Devices: Y
Federal Procurement Eligibility: Small Business
Distribution: Manufacturer Direct, Manufacturer Through Distributor, Exclusive Distributor, Importer, Exporter
General Admin.: Eric P. Seiler/President
Mktg./Adv.: Dane Carlson/Manager Sales

Colposcope	Obstetrics/Gynecology
Lamp, Microscope	Pathology
Loupe, Diagnostic/Surgical	Surgery
Microscope, Light	Pathology
Microscope, Surgical	Ear/Nose/Throat

SEIRIN-AMERICA, INC. — 800-337-9338

230 Libbey Pkwy., Weymouth, MA 02189 — 781-340-1827
FDA Number: 1222113 — Fax: 781-340-1637
E-mail: info@seirinamerica.com
Web site: www.seirinamerica.com
Medical Products Sales Volume: $500,000
Annual Revenue: $0-$1 Million
Year Founded: 1990
Total Employees: 5
Ownership: Private
Quality System Registration Information: ISO9000; ISO9002
Produces/Sells CE-marked Devices: Y
Federal Procurement Eligibility: Small Business
Distribution: Exclusive Distributor, Importer
General Admin.: Thomas Riihimaki/Chief Executive Officer

Needle, Acupuncture, Single Use	General

SEITZ TECHNICAL PRODUCTS, INC. — 610-268-2228

729 Newark Road, Avondale, PA 19311-0338
FDA Number: n/a — Fax: 610-268-2229
E-mail: sales@seitz.com
Web site: www.seitz.com
Medical Products Sales Volume: $1,800,000
Year Founded: 1982
Total Employees: 18 — Marketing Staff: 1 — Sales Staff: 1
Ownership: Private
Produces/Sells CE-marked Devices: Y
Federal Procurement Eligibility: Small Business
Distribution: Manufacturer Direct, OEM
General Admin.: John R. Seitz/President

Camera, Television, Endoscopic (Without Audio)	Surgery
Camera, Television, Microsurgical (Without Audio)	Surgery
Camera, Video	General
Cart, Instrument/Equipment, Laparoscopy	Surgery

SEKISUI DIAGNOSTICS, LLC — 800-999-6578

115 Summit Dr., Exton, PA 19341 — 800-999-6578
FDA Number: 2523813 — Fax: 610-594-8585
E-mail: info@equaldiagnostics.com
Web site: www.equaldiagnostics.com
Medical Products Sales Volume: $7,000,000
Annual Revenue: $5-$10 Million
Total Employees: 26 — Marketing Staff: 2 — Sales Staff: 14
Ownership: Genzyme
Quality System Registration Information: ISO9001
Produces/Sells CE-marked Devices: N
Federal Procurement Eligibility: Small Business
Distribution: Exclusive Distributor, Importer
General Admin.: Allan Murphy/Chief Executive Officer
Mktg./Adv.: Allan Murphy/Vice President Marketing & Sales

Contract Manufacturing, Reagent	General

SELCO PRODUCTS COMPANY — 800-257-3526

605 S. East St., Anaheim, CA 92805-4842 — 714-917-1333
FDA Number: n/a — Fax: 714-917-1355

SELCO PRODUCTS COMPANY — 800-257-3526 (cont'd)

E-mail: sales@selcoproducts.com
Web site: www.selcoproducts.com
Medical Products Sales Volume: $5,000,000
Annual Revenue: $10-$25 Million
Year Founded: 1958
Total Employees: 32 — Marketing Staff: 2 — Sales Staff: 30
Ownership: Private
Produces/Sells CE-marked Devices: N
Federal Procurement Eligibility: Small Business
Distribution: Exclusive Distributor
General Admin.: Tim Wilkinson/President
Mktg./Adv.: Michelle Blakeslee/Coord. Marketing

Component, Other	General

SELECT ENGINEERING, INC. — 800-971-4500

260 Lunenburg St., Fitchburg, MA 01420 — 978-345-4400
FDA Number: n/a — Fax: 978-345-6030
E-mail: info@selectengineering.com
Web site: www.selectengineering.com
Medical Products Sales Volume: $12,000,000
Annual Revenue: $10-$25 Million
Total Employees: 45 — Marketing Staff: 2 — Sales Staff: 2
Ownership: Private
Quality System Registration Information: ISO9001
Produces/Sells CE-marked Devices: N
Federal Procurement Eligibility: Small Business
Distribution: Manufacturer Direct, OEM
General Admin.: Steven R. Aho/Chief Executive Officer
Mktg./Adv.: David Rainville/Director Marketing
David Rainville/Manager International & National Sales

Electrode, Electrocardiograph	Cardiovascular

SELECT FABRICATORS, INC. — 585-393-0650

5310 North Street, Building 5, Canandaigua, NY 14424
FDA Number: 3003595697

Dressing, Other	General

SELECT MEDICAL PRODUCTS, INC. — 800-276-7237

6531 47th St. N., Pinellas Park, FL 33781 — 727-527-7801
FDA Number: n/a — Fax: 888-276-7237
E-mail: abieling@hotmail.com
Web site: www.selectmedicalproducts.com
Medical Products Sales Volume: $2,100,000
Annual Revenue: $1-$5 Million
Year Founded: 1993
Total Employees: 28 — Marketing Staff: 3 — Sales Staff: 3
Ownership: Private
Produces/Sells CE-marked Devices: N
Federal Procurement Eligibility: Small Business, GSA Contract, VA Contract
Distribution: Manufacturer Direct, Manufacturer Through Distributor
General Admin.: Ross P. Bieling/President, Chief Executive Officer
Mktg./Adv.: Alan C. Bieling/Director National Accounts
Alan C. Bieling/Manager National Sales

Exerciser, Passive, Non-Measuring (CPM Machine)	Physical Med
Pad, Pressure, Animal Skin	General
Padding, Cast/Splint	General
Splint, Extremity, Non-Inflatable, External	Surgery

SELECT MEDICAL SYSTEMS — 800-441-1973

30 Winter Sport Lane, PO Box 966, — 802-862-1017
Williston, VT 05495
FDA Number: 1222636 — Fax: 802-862-3767
E-mail: info@selectmedical.com
Web site: www.selectmedical.com
Medical Products Sales Volume: $1,000,000
Year Founded: 1986
Total Employees: 3
Ownership: Private
Produces/Sells CE-marked Devices: N
Federal Procurement Eligibility: Small Business
Distribution: Manufacturer Direct, Manufacturer Through Distributor, Exporter
General Admin.: Michel Lajeunesse/President, Chief Executive Officer
Mktg./Adv.: Michel Lajeunesse/Director Product Development
Production: Monique Girard/Manager Materials
Monique Girard/Vice President Manufacturing

Aspirator, Endocervical	Obstetrics/Gynecology
Cannula, Intrauterine Insemination	Obstetrics/Gynecology
Curette, Suction, Endometrial	Obstetrics/Gynecology
Device, Semen Analysis	Obstetrics/Gynecology

SELECTIVE MED COMPONENTS, INC. — 740-397-7838

564 Harcourt Rd., Mount Vernon, OH 43050
FDA Number: 1528764

Electrode, Cutaneous	Cns/Neurology
Iontophoresis Device, Dental	Dental And Oral
Stimulator, Nerve, Transcutaneous (Pain Relief, TENS)	Cns/Neurology

SELF CARE SYSTEMS
See Biomerica, Inc.

SELF REGULATION SYSTEMS, INC.　800-345-5642
8672 154th Avenue NE,, Bldg. F,　425-882-1101
Redmond, WA 98052
FDA Number: 3021815　*Fax:* 425-882-1935
E-mail: info@srsmedical.com
Web site: www.srsmedical.com
Medical Products Sales Volume: $1,100,000
Year Founded: 1979
Total Employees: 12
Ownership: SRS MEDICAL SYSTEMS, INC.
Produces/Sells CE-marked Devices: Y
Federal Procurement Eligibility: Small Business
Distribution: Manufacturer Direct, Manufacturer Through Manufacturer Reps, OEM, Exporter
General Admin.: Kevin Connolly/Chief Executive Officer
Mktg./Adv.: Jane Stansbury/Vice President Marketing
Biofeedback Device	Cns/Neurology
Perineometer	Obstetrics/Gynecology
Valve, Other	Chemistry

SELF-PROGRAMMED CONTROL CENTER　800-782-2256
11949 Jefferson Blvd., #104,　310-301-3317
Culver City, CA 90230
FDA Number: 2025188　*Fax:* 310-306-3917
E-mail: stresscard@aol.com
Web site: www.stresscards.com
Medical Products Sales Volume: $200,000
Annual Revenue: $0-$1 Million
Year Founded: 1985
Total Employees: 2　*Marketing Staff:* 1
Ownership: Private
Produces/Sells CE-marked Devices: N
Federal Procurement Eligibility: Small Business, Minority Owned
Distribution: Manufacturer Through Distributor
General Admin.: Dr. Alfred A. Barrios/President, Chief Executive Officer
Biofeedback Device	Cns/Neurology

SELFCARE, INC.
See Inverness Medical Inc.

SELLSTROM MANUFACTURING CO.　800-323-7402
1 Sellstrom Drive, Palatine, IL 60067　847-358-2000
FDA Number: 1419319　*Fax:* 847-358-8564
E-mail: sellstrom@sellstrom.com
Web site: www.sellstrom.com
Medical Products Sales Volume: $7,100,000
Annual Revenue: $10-$25 Million
Year Founded: 1923
Total Employees: 100　*Marketing Staff:* 3　*Sales Staff:* 47
Ownership: Private
Quality System Registration Information: ISO9002
Produces/Sells CE-marked Devices: N
Federal Procurement Eligibility: Small Business
Distribution: Manufacturer Direct
General Admin.: Barbara Sellstrom/Chairman
　　　　David Peters/President
Mktg./Adv.: Thomas E. Barr/Director Marketing
　　　Richard Ondra/Director National Accounts
　　　J. R. Franklin/Vice President Marketing & Sales
Production: Garry Adams/Director Quality Assurance
Eyeglasses	Ophthalmology
Goggles, Protective, Eye	Ophthalmology
Mask, Face	General
Protector, Hearing (Insert)	Ear/Nose/Throat
Safety Equipment, Laboratory	Chemistry

SEM
See Security Engineered Machinery

SEMPRUS BIOSCIENCES　617-577-7755
One Kendall Square, Building 1400W, 1st Floor,
Cambridge, MA 02139
FDA Number: n/a　*Fax:* 617-577-7756
E-mail: info@semprusbio.com
Web site: http://www.semprusbio.com
Ownership: Private
Produces/Sells CE-marked Devices: N
General Admin.: Mr. David Luchino/Chief Executive Officer
　　　　Dr. Christopher Loose/Chief Technology Officer
Mktg./Adv.: Mr. Donald Anderson/Vice President Business Development
Research: Mr. Laurence Roth/Vice President Product Development

SENDX MED, INC.　760-930-6300
1945 Palomar Oaks Way, Carlsbad, CA 92009
FDA Number: 2027541　*Fax:* 760-930-6310
E-mail: admin@sendx.com

SENDX MED, INC.　760-930-6300 *(cont'd)*
Annual Revenue: $0-$1 Million
Ownership: Private
Produces/Sells CE-marked Devices: N
Federal Procurement Eligibility: Small Business
Distribution: Manufacturer Direct
Electrode, Ion Specific, Calcium	Chemistry
Electrode, Ion Specific, Chloride	Chemistry
Electrode, Ion Specific, Potassium	Chemistry
Electrode, Ion Specific, Sodium	Chemistry
Electrode, pH	Gastroenterology/Urology
Meter, pH, General Use	Toxicology
Multi Analyte Mixture, Calibrator	Chemistry
Radioimmunoassay, Human Chorionic Gonadotropin	Chemistry

SENECARE ENTERPRISES, INC.　800-442-4577
350 A Central Ave., Bohemia, NY 11716　631-567-9375
FDA Number: n/a　*Fax:* 631-567-9105
E-mail: seneskin@aol.com
Web site: www.senecare.com
Annual Revenue: $1-$5 Million
Total Employees: 12　*Marketing Staff:* 2　*Sales Staff:* 8
Ownership: Private
Quality System Registration Information: ISO9000
Produces/Sells CE-marked Devices: N
Federal Procurement Eligibility: Small Business
Distribution: Manufacturer Direct, Manufacturer Through Distributor, Exporter
General Admin.: Dr. Karl Eilender/President, Chief Executive Officer
　　　　Holly Lidowsky/Vice President Human Resources
Mktg./Adv.: Leslie Strauss/Director Marketing
　　　Leslie Strauss/Director National Accounts
　　　Arnold Bruckner/Director Product Development
　　　Holly Lidowski/Manager Advertising
　　　Holly Lidowski/Manager Market Research
　　　Leslie Strauss/Vice President International Marketing & Sales
Production: Ed Lidowski/Manager Materials
IS: Arnold Bruckner/Manager Tech. Development
Leg Rest	General
Pad, Medicated	General
Protector, Heel	General
Protector, Skin Pressure	General

SENIOR TECHNOLOGIES　800-824-2996
PO Box 80238, 1620 N 20th Circle,　402-475-4002
Lincoln, NE 68503
FDA Number: 1929691　*Fax:* 402-475-4281
E-mail: sales@seniortech.com
Web site: www.seniortechnologies.com
Medical Products Sales Volume: $30,000,000
Annual Revenue: $25-$50 Million
Total Employees: 150
Ownership: STANLEY WORKS
Stock Symbol: SWK
Traded On: NYSE
Quality System Registration Information: ISO9000
Produces/Sells CE-marked Devices: Y
Federal Procurement Eligibility: Small Business
Distribution: Manufacturer Direct, Manufacturer Through Distributor, Manufacturer Through Manufacturer Reps, OEM, Service Direct, Exclusive Distributor, Exporter
General Admin.: Kelly White/Manager Human Resources
　　　　Kevin Pope/President, Chief Executive Officer
Mktg./Adv.: Mr. Ted Algaier/Vice President National Accounts
　　　Eric Perry/Vice President Sales
Production: Don Kringel/Director Quality Assurance
　　　Mike Selting/Vice President Manufacturing
Research: Marvin Jacques/Vice President Engineering
Finance: Mike Balters/Chief Financial Officer
Communication System, Emergency Alert, Personal	General
Monitor, Bed Occupancy	General
Monitor, Bed Patient	General
Nurse Call System	General

SENITECH MEDICAL INSTRUMENTS　760-918-1904
6351 Corte Del Abeto, #a105, Carlsbad, CA 92009
FDA Number: n/a
Ownership: Private
Produces/Sells CE-marked Devices: N
Pliers, Orthodontic	Dental And Oral

SENMED, SUTURES DIVISION
See Ethicon, Inc.

SENNHEISER ELECTRONIC CORP.　877-736-6434
One Enterprise Drive, Old Lyme, CT 06371　860-434-9190
FDA Number: n/a　*Fax:* 860-434-1759
E-mail: info@sennheiserusa.com
Web site: www.sennheiserusa.com
Medical Products Sales Volume: $24,100,000

SENNHEISER ELECTRONIC CORP. 877-736-6434 (cont'd)
Annual Revenue: $25-$50 Million
Year Founded: 1991
Total Employees: 100
Ownership: Sennheiser Electronic Kg
Stock Symbol: SECI
Traded On: NASDAQ
Produces/Sells CE-marked Devices: Y
Federal Procurement Eligibility: Small Business, GSA Contract
Distribution: Manufacturer Direct, Manufacturer Through Distributor
General Admin.: John C. Falcone/President, Chief Executive Officer
Mktg./Adv.: Denise Lavoie/Manager Product Sales
Stefanie Reichert/Vice President International Marketing
Amplifier, Voice — Ear/Nose/Throat
Device, Assistive Listening — Ear/Nose/Throat

SENORX, INC. 949-362-4800
11 Columbia, Aliso Viejo, CA 92656
FDA Number: 2032230
Ownership: C. R. Bard, Inc.
Stock Symbol: SENO
Traded On: NASDAQ
Produces/Sells CE-marked Devices: N
Biopsy Instrument — Gastroenterology/Urology
Clip, Implantable — Surgery
Electrosurgical Unit, Cutting & Coagulation Device — Surgery
Staple, Implantable — Surgery

SENSABLE TECHNOLOGIES, INC. 781-937-8315
181 Ballardvale Street, Wilmington, MA 01887
FDA Number: 1000580006 — *Fax:* 781-937-8325
Web site: http://www.sensable.com
Year Founded: 1993
Ownership: Private
Produces/Sells CE-marked Devices: N
General Admin.: Mr. Curt Rawley/Chairman, Chief Executive Officer
Mr. David Chen/Chief Technology Officer
Mr. Bob Steingart/President, Chief Operating Officer
Mktg./Adv.: Mr. Mark Tatkow/Vice President Business Development
Ms. Joan Lockhart/Vice President Marketing & Sales
Research: Mr. Joe Wisnewski/Vice President Engineering
Finance: Mr. Bob Kittler/Chief Financial Officer
System, Optical Impression, Computer Assisted Design And Manufacturing (cad/cam) Of Dental Restorations — Dental And Oral

SENSE TECHNOLOGY, INC. 800-628-9416
4241 William Penn Highway, 1st Floor, 724-733-2277
Murrysville, PA 15668
FDA Number: 2530787 — *Fax:* 724-733-1531
E-mail: info@pulstarfras.com
Web site: www.pulstarfras.com
Medical Products Sales Volume: $400,000
Year Founded: 1989
Total Employees: 5
Ownership: Private
Produces/Sells CE-marked Devices: N
Federal Procurement Eligibility: Small Business
Distribution: Manufacturer Direct, Manufacturer Through Distributor, OEM
General Admin.: Joseph M. Evans/President
Plunger-Like Joint Manipulator — Physical Med

SENSIDYNE, INC. 800-451-9444
16333 Bay Vista Drive, Clearwater, FL 33760 727-530-3602
FDA Number: 1064593 — *Fax:* 727-539-0550
E-mail: info@sensidyne.com
Web site: www.sensidyne.com
Medical Products Sales Volume: $15,000,000
Annual Revenue: $10-$25 Million
Year Founded: 1983
Total Employees: 100 — *Marketing Staff:* 3 — *Sales Staff:* 9
Ownership: SIEGEL-ROBERT, INC.
Quality System Registration Information: ISO9000; ISO9001
Produces/Sells CE-marked Devices: Y
Federal Procurement Eligibility: Small Business
Distribution: Manufacturer Direct, Manufacturer Through Distributor, Manufacturer Through Manufacturer Reps, OEM, Exclusive Distributor
General Admin.: Bretta Day/Human Resources Associate
Gordon Dore/President
Howard Mills/Vice President, General Manager
Mktg./Adv.: Joe Troy/Manager Marketing & Advertising
Bob Horton/Marketing Associate
Production: George Mason/Director Quality Assurance & Regulatory Affairs
Glenn Warr/Vice President Manufacturing
Calibrator, Respiratory Therapy Unit — Anesthesiology
Component, Other — General
Detector, Leakage, Medical Gas — General
Monitor, Blood Gas, Oxygen — Anesthesiology
Monitor, Contamination, Environmental, Personal — General

SENSIDYNE, INC. 800-451-9444 (cont'd)
Pump, Air, Non-Manual, Endoscopic — Gastroenterology/Urology
Sensor, Oxygen — Anesthesiology
Medical Product Subsidiaries (Listed Separately)
Ventrex, Inc.

SENSITECH, INC. 800-843-8367
800 Cummings Ctr. #258, 978-927-7033
Beverly, MA 01915
FDA Number: n/a — *Fax:* 978-921-2112
E-mail: info@sensitech.com
Web site: www.sensitech.com
Annual Revenue: $5-$10 Million
Ownership: Private
Produces/Sells CE-marked Devices: Y
Distribution: Manufacturer Through Manufacturer Reps
General Admin.: Eric Schultz/Chief Executive Officer
Mktg./Adv.: John Carr/Vice President Marketing
Computer Equipment — General

SENSOMOTORIC INSTRUMENTS, INC. 888-SMI-USA1
97 Chapel St., Needham, MA 02492 781-453-1377
FDA Number: 3002674187 — *Fax:* 781-453-1378
E-mail: info@smiusa.com
Web site: www.smi.de
Medical Products Sales Volume: $600,000
Annual Revenue: $1-$5 Million
Year Founded: 1991
Total Employees: 6
Ownership: Private
Produces/Sells CE-marked Devices: Y
Federal Procurement Eligibility: Small Business, VA Contract
Distribution: Manufacturer Direct
Monitor, Eye Movement — Ophthalmology

SENSOR DYNAMICS, INC. 510-623-1459
4568 Enterprise St., Fremont, CA 94538
FDA Number: 2951564 — *Fax:* 510-623-9827
E-mail: lseng@sensordynamics.com
Web site: www.sensordynamics.com
Medical Products Sales Volume: $1,600,000
Year Founded: 1992
Total Employees: 15
Federal Procurement Eligibility: Small Business
Monitor, Cardiac (Cardiotachometer & Rate Alarm) — Cardiovascular

SENSOR SCIENTIFIC, INC. 800-524-1610
6 Kings Bridge Road, Fairfield, NJ 07004 973-227-7790
FDA Number: 2248573 — *Fax:* 973-227-8063
E-mail: sales@sensorsci.com
Web site: www.sensorsci.com
Medical Products Sales Volume: $1,800,000
Annual Revenue: $5-$10 Million
Year Founded: 1983
Total Employees: 20 — *Marketing Staff:* 3 — *Sales Staff:* 6
Ownership: Private
Quality System Registration Information: ISO9001
Produces/Sells CE-marked Devices: Y
Federal Procurement Eligibility: Small Business
Distribution: Manufacturer Direct
General Admin.: G. Robert Brinley/President
Mktg./Adv.: Alana Svab/Director Sales
Production: Ralph Espenshade/Director Quality Assurance
Research: Dr. Russell Bolton/Vice President Engineering
Monitor, Skin Resistance/skin Temperature, For Insulin Reactions — General
Probe, Temperature — General
Thermistor — General
Thermometer, Electronic — General

SENSOREX CORP. 714-895-4344
11751 Markon Drive, Garden Grove, CA 92841
FDA Number: n/a — *Fax:* 714-894-4839
E-mail: info@sensorex.com
Web site: www.sensorex.com
Annual Revenue: $5-$10 Million
Year Founded: 1972
Total Employees: 45 — *Marketing Staff:* 4
Ownership: Private
Produces/Sells CE-marked Devices: N
Federal Procurement Eligibility: Small Business
Distribution: Manufacturer Direct, OEM
Mktg./Adv.: Mike Ross/Manager International Marketing & Sales
IS: Scott Edwards/Manager Tech. Services
Electrode, Laboratory pH — Chemistry

SENSORMATIC ELECTRONICS 800-241-6678
6600 Congress Ave, Boca Raton, FL 33487 561-912-6000
FDA Number: n/a

SENSORMATIC ELECTRONICS   800-241-6678 *(cont'd)*
E-mail: www.adt.com@adt.com
Web site: www.sensormatic.com
Medical Products Sales Volume: $1,017,500,000
Total Employees: 5700
Ownership: Allied Signal, Inc.
Stock Symbol: SRM
Traded On: NYSE
Produces/Sells CE-marked Devices: Y
Distribution: Manufacturer Through Distributor, Manufacturer Through Manufacturer Reps

Bracelet, Identification	General
Camera, Other	General
Equipment, Building Security	General
Identification, Alert, Medical	General

SENSORMEDICS CORP.
See CAREFUSION 211, INC..

SENSORS, INC.   734-429-2100
6812 S. State Road, Saline, MI 48176-9274
FDA Number: 9918031   *Fax:* 734-429-4080
E-mail: rwilson@sensors-inc.com
Web site: www.sensors-inc.com
Year Founded: 1976
Total Employees: 100   *Marketing Staff:* 2
Ownership: Private
Federal Procurement Eligibility: Small Business
Distribution: OEM
General Admin.: Donald M. Soenen/Chief Executive Officer
        Andrew R. Realing/President
Mktg./Adv.: Robert L. Wilson/Vice President Marketing & Sales
Production: Allen Dryer/Vice President Manufacturing
Research: Atul Shah/Vice President Engineering
        Gideva Eden/Vice President Research & Development

Component, Electronic	General
Monitor, Gas, Atmospheric, Environmental	General

SENSORTEK
See Physitemp Instruments, Inc.

SENSORY AIDS CORP.
See Humanware

SENSYM ICT   800-573-6796
1804 McCarthy Blvd., Milpitas, CA 95035   **408-954-6700**
FDA Number: n/a   *Fax:* 408-954-9458
E-mail: kris.lafko@invensys.com
Web site: www.sensym-ict.com
Medical Products Sales Volume: $19,200,000
Annual Revenue: $25-$50 Million
Year Founded: 1999
Total Employees: 248   *Sales Staff:* 4
Ownership: INVENSYS PLC
Stock Symbol: BTR
Traded On: London
Quality System Registration Information: ISO9001
Produces/Sells CE-marked Devices: Y
Federal Procurement Eligibility: Small Business
Distribution: Manufacturer Through Distributor, Manufacturer Through Manufacturer Reps
Mktg./Adv.: Kris Lafko/Director Marketing & Sales
        David Kertes/Manager International Marketing & Sales

Component, Electronic	General
Transducer, Blood Pressure	General

SENTARA HEALTH MANAGEMENT   800-736-8272
6015 Poplar Hall Dr., Norfolk, VA 23502-3800   **757-455-7976**
FDA Number: n/a   *Fax:* 757-552-7176
Web site: www.sentara.com
Annual Revenue: $1-$5 Million
Year Founded: 1888
Ownership: Private
Produces/Sells CE-marked Devices: N
Distribution: Service Direct
General Admin.: John F. Malbon/Chairman
        David Bernd/President, Chief Executive Officer

Mass Screening System	Chemistry

SENTECH MEDICAL SYSTEMS, INC.   954-340-0500
4200 N.w. 120th Ave., Coral Springs, FL 33065
FDA Number: 1058219

Bed, Flotation Therapy, Powered	Physical Med
Bed, Patient Rotation, Powered	Physical Med
Mattress, Air Flotation	General

SENTECH SYSTEMS INC.   800-263-8534
1445 Bonhill Rd. #10,   **905-564-7411**
Mississauga, ONT L5T-1 Canada
FDA Number: n/a   *Fax:* 905-567-7413

SENTECH SYSTEMS INC.   800-263-8534 *(cont'd)*
E-mail: sentech@on.aibn.com
Web site: www.sentech.ca
Year Founded: 1992
Total Employees: 25
Ownership: Private
Produces/Sells CE-marked Devices: N
Distribution: Manufacturer Direct

SENTIENT SYSTEMS TECHNOLOGY INC.
See Dynavox Systems Inc.

SENTREHEART INC.   650-354-1200
300 Saginaw Drive, Redwood City, CA 94063
FDA Number: 3005802238   *Fax:* 650-354-1204
E-mail: info@sentreheart.com
Web site: www.sentreheart.com
Ownership: Private
Produces/Sells CE-marked Devices: N

Catheter, Percutaneous	Cardiovascular
Cutter, Surgical	Surgery
Guidewire, Catheter	Cardiovascular
Instrument, Manual, General Surgical	Surgery
Suture, Non-Absorbable, Synthetic, Polyamide	Surgery

SENTRON, INC.   253-851-7881
7117 Stinson Avenue, Suite C, Gig Harbor, WA 98335
FDA Number: n/a   *Fax:* 253-851-7899
E-mail: info@sentronph.com
Web site: www.sentronph.com
Annual Revenue: $1-$5 Million
Total Employees: 10
Ownership: Private
Quality System Registration Information: ISO9001
Produces/Sells CE-marked Devices: Y
Federal Procurement Eligibility: Small Business
Distribution: Manufacturer Direct, Manufacturer Through Distributor, OEM
Mktg./Adv.: Eric Amundson/Director Marketing
        Paul Richer/Manager National Sales

Meter, pH, Portable	Chemistry

SENTRY BATTERY CORP.   800-747-0199
62 Colin Drive, Manchester, NH 03103   **603-624-9090**
FDA Number: n/a   *Fax:* 603-606-6295
E-mail: sales@sentrybattery.com
Web site: www.sentrybattery.com
Medical Products Sales Volume: $1,200,000
Annual Revenue: $1-$5 Million
Year Founded: 1992
Total Employees: 3   *Marketing Staff:* 1   *Sales Staff:* 1
Ownership: Private
Produces/Sells CE-marked Devices: N
Federal Procurement Eligibility: Small Business
Distribution: Manufacturer Direct, Manufacturer Through Distributor
General Admin.: Raymond Ege/Chief Executive Officer
        Russell Ege/President
Mktg./Adv.: Raymond Ege/Manager International & National Sales

Battery	General

SENTRY TECHNOLOGY CORP.   800-645-7217
1881 Lakeland Avenue, Ronkonkoma, NY 11779   **800-645-4224**
FDA Number: n/a   *Fax:* 631-739-2117
E-mail: sentry@sentrytechnology.com
Web site: www.sentrytechnology.com
Medical Products Sales Volume: $10,000,000
Annual Revenue: $10-$25 Million
Year Founded: 1966
Total Employees: 65   *Sales Staff:* 15
Ownership: Public
Stock Symbol: SKVY
Traded On: OTC Bulletin
Produces/Sells CE-marked Devices: N
Distribution: Manufacturer Direct
General Admin.: Peter L. Murdoch/President, Chief Executive Officer
Research: Jonathan G. Granoff/Director Technology
        Robert D. Furst/Director Technology

Bracelet, Identification	General
Security Equipment/Supplies	General

SEPARATION TECHNOLOGY INC   800-777-6668
582 Monroe Road, Suite 1424, Sanford, FL 32771   **407-788-8791**
FDA Number: 1721649   *Fax:* 407-788-3677
E-mail: custserv@separationtechnology.com
Web site: www.separationtechnology.com
Year Founded: 1988
Ownership: Thermo Fisher Scientific
Produces/Sells CE-marked Devices: Y
Distribution: Manufacturer Direct, Manufacturer Through Distributor, OEM

SEPARATION TECHNOLOGY INC 800-777-6668 *(cont'd)*

General Admin.: Jami Meeks/President

Centrifuge, General (Over 5,000 rpm)	Toxicology
Centrifuge, Hematocrit	Hematology
Centrifuge, Microhematocrit	Hematology
Centrifuge, Tabletop	Pathology
Cytocentrifuge	Pathology
Hematocrit Control	Hematology
Hematocrit, Automated	Hematology
Hematocrit, Manual	Hematology
Tube, Capillary Blood Collection	Hematology

SEPOR, INC. 800-753-6463
718 N. Fries Ave., P.O. Box 578, 310-830-6601
Wilmington, CA 90748

FDA Number: n/a

Fax: 310-830-9336

E-mail: info@sepor.com
Web site: www.sepor.com
Annual Revenue: $1-$5 Million
Year Founded: 1953
Ownership: Private
Produces/Sells CE-marked Devices: N
Federal Procurement Eligibility: Small Business
Distribution: Manufacturer Direct, Service Direct

Balance, Analytical	Chemistry

SEPTRX INC 510-225-9170
47533 Westinghouse Drive, Suite C, Fremont, CA 94539

FDA Number: n/a

Fax: 510-952-4446

E-mail: info@septrx.com
Web site: www.septrx.com
Ownership: Private
Produces/Sells CE-marked Devices: N

SEQUAL TECHNOLOGIES INC. 800-826-4610
11436 Sorrento Valley Rd., 858-202-3100
San Diego, CA 92121

FDA Number: 2030505

Fax: 858-558-1915

E-mail: medicalsales@sequal.com
Web site: www.sequal.com
Ownership: Private
Produces/Sells CE-marked Devices: Y
Federal Procurement Eligibility: Small Business
Distribution: Manufacturer Direct, Manufacturer Through Distributor, Manufacturer Through Manufacturer Reps, Importer

Generator, Oxygen, Portable	Anesthesiology

SEQUENOM, INC 1-877-443-6663
3595 John Hopkins Court, 858-202-9000
San Diego, CA 92121

FDA Number: n/a

Fax: 858-202-9001

E-mail: sales-us@sequenom.com
Web site: www.sequenom.com
Ownership: Private
Produces/Sells CE-marked Devices: N
General Admin.: Dr. Harry Hixson/Chairman, Chief Executive Officer
　　　　　Dr. Charles Cantor/Chief Scientific Officer
Medical Admin.: Dr. Alan Bombard/Chief Medical Officer
Mktg./Adv.: Mr. Michael Monko/Senior Vice President Marketing & Sales
Production: Mr. Larry Myres/Vice President Operations
Research: Mr. William Welch/Vice President Diagnostics
　　　　　Dr. Ronald Lindsay/Vice President Research & Development
Finance: Mr. Paul Maier/Chief Financial Officer

SEQUENT MEDICAL INC. 949-830-9600
11A Columbia, Aliso Viejo, CA 92656

FDA Number: n/a

Fax: 949-830-9658

E-mail: info@sequentmedical.com
Web site: http://www.sequentmedical.com/
Year Founded: 2007
Ownership: Private
Produces/Sells CE-marked Devices: N
General Admin.: Dr. Robert Rosenbluth/Chairman
　　　　　Mr. Brian Cox/Chief Technology Officer, Vice President
　　　　　Mr. Thomas Wilder III/President, Chief Executive Officer
Research: Mr. Philippe Marchand/Director Research & Development
　　　　　Dr. William Patterson/Vice President Research & Development

SEQUOIA-TURNER CORP.
See Abbott Hematology, Diagnostics Div.

SEQWRIGHT INC. 800-720-4363
2575 West Bellfort, Suite 2001, 713-528-4363
Houston, TX 77054

FDA Number: n/a
E-mail: seq@seqwright.com
Web site: http://www.seqwright.com
Year Founded: 1994

SEQWRIGHT INC. 800-720-4363 *(cont'd)*

Ownership: Private
Produces/Sells CE-marked Devices: N
General Admin.: Dr. Fei Lu/Chief Executive Officer
Production: Dr. Meredith Berry/Director Quality Assurance

SERACARE LIFE SCIENCES 800-676-1881
37 Birch St., Milford, MA 01757 508-244-6400

FDA Number: 3007088335

Fax: 508.634.3334

E-mail: info@seracarewebsite.com
Web site: www.seracare.com
Medical Products Sales Volume: $8,300,000
Annual Revenue: $25-$50 Million
Year Founded: 1984
Total Employees: 50　　　　Marketing Staff: 1　　　　Sales Staff: 13
Ownership: Public
Stock Symbol: SRLS
Traded On: OTC Bulletin
Produces/Sells CE-marked Devices: N
Federal Procurement Eligibility: Small Business
Distribution: Manufacturer Direct
General Admin.: Ms. Susan Vogt/President, Chief Executive Officer
Mktg./Adv.: Mr. Michael Steele/Vice President Business Development
　　　　　Mr. David Olsen/Vice President Corporate Affairs
　　　　　Mr. Bill Smutny/Vice President Marketing & Sales
Production: Mr. Ronald Dilling/Vice President Operations
Finance: Mr. Gregory Gould/Chief Financial Officer

Antibodies, Gliadin	Immunology
Antibody Igm, If, Cytomegalovirus Virus	Microbiology
Antisera, IF, Toxoplasma Gondii	Microbiology
Control, Multi Analyte, All Kinds (Assayed And Unassayed)	Chemistry
Kit, Quality Control, Blood Banking	Hematology
Kit, Serological, Positive Control	Microbiology
Serum, Animal	Pathology
Serum, Human	Pathology

SERADYN, INC. 800-428-4072
7998 Georgetown Road, Suite 1000, 317-610-3800
Indianapolis, IN 46268

FDA Number: 1836010

Fax: 317-610-3888

E-mail: info@seradyn.com
Web site: www.seradyn.com
Medical Products Sales Volume: $7,300,000
Year Founded: 1984
Total Employees: 90　　　　Sales Staff: 4
Ownership: Liberty Industries, Inc
Stock Symbol: APO
Traded On: NASDAQ
Quality System Registration Information: ISO9001
Produces/Sells CE-marked Devices: N
Federal Procurement Eligibility: Small Business
Distribution: Manufacturer Direct, OEM
Mktg./Adv.: Rick Galloway/Director Marketing
Production: Jim Kircher/Director Operations

Antibody, Monoclonal	Microbiology
Immunoassay, Other	Toxicology
Reagent, Other	General
Test, Infectious Mononucleosis	Immunology
Test, Rheumatoid Factor	Immunology

SERAGEN DIAGNOSTICS
See Seradyn, Inc.

SERATRONICS INC.
See Fresenius Usa, Inc.

SERFILCO LTD.
See Filterspun

SERIM RESEARCH CORP. 574-264-3440
3506 Reedy Dr, Elkhart, IN 46514

FDA Number: 1833387

Campylobacter Pylori	Microbiology
Detector, Blood Leakage	Gastroenterology/Urology
Dialyzer Reprocessing System	Gastroenterology/Urology
Filter, Blood, Dialysis	Gastroenterology/Urology
Purification System, Water	Gastroenterology/Urology
Sterilant, Medical Device	General
Sterilization Process Indicator, Physical/Chemical	General
Strip, Indicator, pH, Dialysate	Gastroenterology/Urology
Test, Urine Leukocyte	Hematology

SERITEX INC. 973-472-4200
1 Madison St., East Rutherford, NJ 07073

FDA Number: 2246775

Fax: 973-472-0222

E-mail: instruments@seritex.com
Web site: www.seritex.com
Medical Products Sales Volume: $1,400,000
Annual Revenue: $0-$1 Million
Year Founded: 1986

SERITEX INC. 973-472-4200 (cont'd)
Total Employees: 5   Marketing Staff: 1   Sales Staff: 1
Ownership: Private
Produces/Sells CE-marked Devices: N
Federal Procurement Eligibility: Small Business
Distribution: Exclusive Distributor
General Admin.: William Kattermann/President, Chief Executive Officer
Mktg./Adv.: Emil Kattermann/Vice President Marketing
Caliper, Skinfold   General
Orchidometer   General

SEROLA BIOMECHANICS, INC. 815-636-2780
5281 Zenith Parkway, Loves Park, IL 61111
FDA Number: 3006563279   Fax: -815-636-2781
E-mail: julie@serola.net
Web site: www.serola.net
Ownership: Private
Produces/Sells CE-marked Devices: N
Band, Support, Pelvic   Physical Med
Support, Arm   Physical Med
Traction Unit, Non-Powered   Orthopedics

SEROLOGICALS CORP 678-728-2000
5655 Spalding Dr, Norcross, GA 30092
FDA Number: n/a   Fax: 678-728-2247
Ownership: Private
Quality System Registration Information: ISO9001; ISO9002
Produces/Sells CE-marked Devices: Y
Federal Procurement Eligibility: Small Business
Distribution: Manufacturer Direct, Manufacturer Through Manufacturer Reps
Analyzer, Chemistry, Enzyme Immunoassay   Chemistry
Analyzer, Chemistry, Fluorescence Immunoassay   Chemistry
Contract Manufacturing, Reagent   General
Culture Media, Supplements   Microbiology
Heparin   Pathology
Immunochemical, Transferrin   Immunology
Plasma, Control, Normal   Hematology
Serum, Biological, General   Toxicology
Standard, Lipid   Chemistry
Thrombin   Hematology
Trypsin   Pathology

SERRANO INTERNATIONAL 760-773-5140
45-175 Panorama Drive, Suite G, Palm Desert, CA 92260
FDA Number: 2082000   Fax: 760-773-1790
E-mail: esqualitat@aol.com
Medical Products Sales Volume: $1,000,000
Annual Revenue: $0-$1 Million
Total Employees: 4   Marketing Staff: 2   Sales Staff: 2
Ownership: Private
Produces/Sells CE-marked Devices: N
Federal Procurement Eligibility: Small Business, Minority Owned
Distribution: Manufacturer Through Distributor, Exclusive Distributor, Importer, Exporter
General Admin.: Jose Luis Serrano/President, Chief Executive Officer
Mktg./Adv.: Kenneth Massey/Manager International & National Sales
Margot Fagan/Vice President Marketing
Service, Import/Export   General

SERUM INTERNATIONAL INC. 800-361-7726
4400 Autoroute Chomeoey, 450-625-8511
Laval, QUEBE H7R-6 Canada
FDA Number: n/a   Fax: 450-625-7172
E-mail: serum@serum.ca
Web site: www.serum.ca
Year Founded: 1962
Total Employees: 25
Ownership: Private
Produces/Sells CE-marked Devices: N
Distribution: Importer

SERV-A-PURE COMPANY 800-338-4905
1101 Columbus Ave., Bay City, MI 48708
FDA Number: 1836317
Purification System, Water   Gastroenterology/Urology

SERVICE FILTRATION CORP.
See Filterspun

SERVICIOS PARACLINICLOS S.A. 01800 581 9157
Ave Madero 3330 Pte, Mitras Sur,
Monterrey N.L. 64020 Mexico
FDA Number: n/a   Fax: 0181-8333 8400
E-mail: serviclinicos@serviclinicos.com
Web site: www.serviclinicos.com
Medical Products Sales Volume: $1,578,947
Total Employees: 14   Marketing Staff: 2   Sales Staff: 8
Ownership: Private
Produces/Sells CE-marked Devices: N

SERVICIOS PARACLINICLOS S.A. 01800 581 9157 (cont'd)
Distribution: Manufacturer Through Distributor, Exclusive Distributor, Importer

SERVOLIFT/EASTERN CORP. 800-727-3786
266 Hancock St., Boston, MA 02125-2155 617-825-9000
FDA Number: 9310024   Fax: 617-825-1292
E-mail: servolift@servolift.com
Web site: www.servolift.com
Medical Products Sales Volume: $20,300,000
Annual Revenue: $10-$25 Million
Year Founded: 1926
Total Employees: 200   Marketing Staff: 2   Sales Staff: 7
Ownership: Private
Federal Procurement Eligibility: Small Business
Distribution: Manufacturer Through Distributor, Manufacturer Through Manufacturer Reps
General Admin.: Ira Kaplan/Chief Executive Officer
Ira Kaplan/President
Arthur Vershlow/Vice President Human Resources
Mktg./Adv.: Stephanie Kaplan Hamilton/Director Marketing
Jonathon Vershow/Director National Accounts
Flavian Iovanel/Director Product Development
Stephanie Kaplan Hamilton/Manager Advertising
Ira Kaplan/Manager International & National Sales
Shari Kaplan/Manager National Sales
Shari Kaplan/Manager Sales Training
John Frishman/Vice President Marketing & Sales
Production: Bo Manic/Vice President Manufacturing
Research: Flavian Iovanel/Vice President Research & Development
Cart, Foodservice   General
Cart, Other   General
Conveyor, Tray   General

SERVOMEX 800-862-0200
525 Julie Rivers Drive, Suite 185, 281-295-5800
Sugar Land, TX 77478
FDA Number: n/a   Fax: 281-295-5899
E-mail: info@servomex.com
Web site: www.servomex.com
Annual Revenue: $1-$5 Million
Year Founded: 1952
Total Employees: 41   Marketing Staff: 1   Sales Staff: 25
Ownership: Public
Stock Symbol: SXS
Traded On: London
Quality System Registration Information: ISO9000
Produces/Sells CE-marked Devices: N
Distribution: Manufacturer Through Manufacturer Reps, OEM
Mktg./Adv.: Jane Hammond/Manager Marketing Services
Sensor, Oxygen   Anesthesiology

SETHCO DIV.
See Met-Pro Corporation

SETON IDENTIFICATION PRODUCTS
See Champion America

SETON NAME PLATE CORP.
See Champion America

SETTLER MEDICAL ELECTRONICS INC.
723 Queenston St, Winnipeg R3N 0X8 Canada
FDA Number: 8022045
Meter, pH, Portable   Chemistry

SEVEN CONTINENTS INC.
See Questech International, Inc.

SEVEN HARVEST INTL. IMPORT & EXPORT 765-456-3584
108 North Dixon Rd., Kokomo, IN 46901
FDA Number: 1120797
Airway, Oropharyngeal, Anesthesia   Anesthesiology
Circuit, Breathing (W Connector, Adapter, Y Piece)   Anesthesiology
Clip, Nose   Anesthesiology
Mouthpiece, Breathing   Anesthesiology
Wrench   Orthopedics

SGARLATO LABORATORIES, INC. 800-421-5303
2315 S. Bascom Ave, Suite#200, 408-626-9600
Campbell, CA 95008
FDA Number: 2939320   Fax: 408-626-9629
E-mail: Sales@sgarlatolabs.com
Web site: www.sgarlatolabs.com
Medical Products Sales Volume: $300,000
Annual Revenue: $1-$5 Million
Year Founded: 1986
Total Employees: 4   Marketing Staff: 5   Sales Staff: 5
Ownership: Private
Quality System Registration Information: ISO9001
Produces/Sells CE-marked Devices: Y

MANUFACTURER PROFILES

SGARLATO LABORATORIES, INC.   800-421-5303 (cont'd)
Federal Procurement Eligibility: Small Business
Distribution: Manufacturer Direct, Manufacturer Through Distributor, Manufacturer Through Manufacturer Reps
General Admin.: Dr. Thomas E. Sgarlato/President, Chief Executive Officer
     Mr. Sean Cervantes/Vice President
Production: Lucinda Rodriquez/Director Operations
     Michael McDougall/Director Quality Assurance & Regulatory Affairs
     Jen Millen/Manager Customer Services
     Erik Lupercio/Manager Warehouse

Prosthesis, Foot	Orthopedics
Prosthesis, Toe	Orthopedics
System, Delivery, Drug, Non-invasive	General

SHADOW SHIELD   866-838-8400
42 Shandelin Ct, Alamo, CA 94507   **925-743-0569**
FDA Number: n/a   *Fax:* 530-272-7248
E-mail: rwestcpa@sbcglobal.net
Annual Revenue: $0-$1 Million
Ownership: Private
Produces/Sells CE-marked Devices: N
Federal Procurement Eligibility: Minority Owned
Distribution: Manufacturer Direct, Manufacturer Through Distributor

Shield, Gonadal	Radiology

SHAMIR INSIGHT, INC.   877-514-833
9938 Via Pasar, San Diego, CA 92126
FDA Number: 2086480   *Fax:* 877-285-4863
E-mail: information@shamirlens.com
Web site: www.shamirlens.com
Year Founded: 1972
Total Employees: 845
Ownership: SHAMIR OPTICAL INDUSTRY
Stock Symbol: SHMR
Traded On: NASDAQ
Produces/Sells CE-marked Devices: N
General Admin.: Mr. Raanan Naftalovich/Chief Executive Officer

Case, Contact Lens	Ophthalmology

SHAMIR USA, INC.   818-889-6292
30077 Agoura Rd, Suite 220, Agoura Hills, CA 91301
FDA Number: 2028425
E-mail: michael@shamirusa.com
Web site: www.shamir.co.il
Year Founded: 1972
Total Employees: 845
Ownership: SHAMIR OPTICAL INDUSTRY
Stock Symbol: SHMR
Traded On: NASDAQ
Produces/Sells CE-marked Devices: N
General Admin.: Mr. Dagan Avishai/Business Manager
     Mr. Giora Ben-Zeev/Chairman
     Mr. Eyal Hayardeny/President, Chief Executive Officer
Finance: Mr. Yagen Moshe/Chief Financial Officer

Cleaner, Lens, Contact	Ophthalmology

SHAMROCK MEDICAL, INC.   503-233-5055
3620 S.E. Powell Blvd., Portland, OR 97202
FDA Number: 3022169   *Fax:* 503-234-6974
E-mail: info@shamrockmedical.com
Web site: www.shamrockmedical.com
Medical Products Sales Volume: $100,000
Annual Revenue: $0-$1 Million
Year Founded: 1980
Total Employees: 5   *Marketing Staff:* 2   *Sales Staff:* 2
Ownership: Private
Produces/Sells CE-marked Devices: N
Federal Procurement Eligibility: Small Business, Female Owned
Distribution: Manufacturer Direct
General Admin.: Arlene Henley/President

Belt, Traction, Pelvic, Orthopedic	Orthopedics
Cushion, Stool	General
Halter, Head, Traction	Physical Med
Pillow, Cervical	Orthopedics
Support, Back	Orthopedics
Traction Unit, Non-Powered	Orthopedics

SHANTEL MEDICAL SUPPLY   888-577-5688
5600 Peck Road, Arcadia, CA 91006   **626-358-7530**
FDA Number: 2087188   *Fax:* 626-599-8171
E-mail: info@shantel.com
Web site: www.shantel.com
Medical Products Sales Volume: $1,500,000
Year Founded: 1990
Total Employees: 10
Ownership: Private
Produces/Sells CE-marked Devices: N
Federal Procurement Eligibility: Small Business

SHANTEL MEDICAL SUPPLY   888-577-5688 (cont'd)
Diathermy, Ultrasonic (Physical Therapy)   Physical Med

SHAPEMASTER USA, INC.   866-531-3586
7633 E. 63rd Place, Suite 300, Tulsa, OK 74133   **918-392-3475**
FDA Number: 3006214320   *Fax:* 918-392-3471
E-mail: karent@shapemasterusa.com
Web site: www.shapemasterusa.com
Ownership: Private
Produces/Sells CE-marked Devices: N

Exerciser, Powered	Anesthesiology

SHARED P.E.T. IMAGING, LLC   330-491-0480
4912 Higbee Ave, Nw Suite 100, Canton, OH 44718
FDA Number: 3004082056

Image Processing System	Radiology

SHARED SYSTEMS, INC.   888-474-2733
PO Box 211587, 3961 Columbia Rd,   **706-868-0408**
Augusta, GA 30917
FDA Number: 1055356   *Fax:* 706-855-6588
E-mail: sharinc@bellsouth.net
Web site: www.sharedsystems.com
Medical Products Sales Volume: $300,000
Annual Revenue: $0-$1 Million
Year Founded: 1991
Total Employees: 5
Ownership: Private
Quality System Registration Information: ISO9001
Produces/Sells CE-marked Devices: N
Federal Procurement Eligibility: Small Business
Distribution: OEM
General Admin.: Robert C. Hicks/President, Chief Executive Officer
Production: Gregory Oblak/Manager Production
Research: T. S. Enriquez/Vice President Research & Development

Component, Other	General
Contract Manufacturing, Reagent	General
Kit, Quality Control	Microbiology
Kit, Serological, Negative Control	Microbiology
Kit, Serological, Positive Control	Microbiology
Reagent, Cholesterol (Total Test System)	Chemistry
Test, Bacterial Diagnostic	Microbiology

SHARN, INC.   800-325-3671
4517 George Road Suite 200,   **813-889-9614**
Tampa, FL 33634
FDA Number: 1035845   *Fax:* 813-886-2701
E-mail: mailbox@sharn.com
Web site: www.sharn.com
Medical Products Sales Volume: $6,100,000
Year Founded: 1983
Total Employees: 38
Ownership: Private
Stock Symbol: BPK.L
Traded On: London
Produces/Sells CE-marked Devices: Y
Federal Procurement Eligibility: Small Business, GSA Contract
Distribution: Manufacturer Direct, Importer, Exporter
General Admin.: Judy Tomlinson/Managing Director
     Bruce A. Tomlinson/President, Chief Executive Officer
Mktg./Adv.: Julie Anderson/Director Product Development
     Judy Tomlinson/Manager International & National Sales

Airway, Nasopharyngeal (Breathing Tube)	Anesthesiology
Airway, Oropharyngeal, Anesthesia	Anesthesiology
Biofeedback Device	Cns/Neurology
Brush, Other	General
Cuff, Blood Pressure	Cardiovascular
Dispenser, Medication, Liquid	General
Monitor, Temperature, Surgery	Surgery
Oximeter, Pulse	General
Sensor, Oxygen	Anesthesiology
Shield, Eye, Ophthalmic	Ophthalmology
Stethoscope, Esophageal, With Electrical Conductors	Anesthesiology
Strap, Head, Gas Mask	Anesthesiology
Stylet, Tracheal Tube	Anesthesiology
Temperature Strip, Forehead, Liquid Crystal	General
Thermometer, Liquid Crystals	Surgery
Vaporizer, Anesthesia, Non-Heated	Anesthesiology

SHARP CORPORATION   800-892-6197
23 Carland Road,   **610-279-3550**
Conshohocken, PA 19428
FDA Number: 2210051   *Fax:* 610-279-4712
E-mail: info@sharpcorporation.com
Web site: www.sharpcorporation.com
Medical Products Sales Volume: $102,600,000
Year Founded: 1952
Total Employees: 500   *Marketing Staff:* 2   *Sales Staff:* 10

SHARP CORPORATION 800-892-6197 *(cont'd)*
Ownership: SUPERIOR GROUP, INC.
Produces/Sells CE-marked Devices: N
Federal Procurement Eligibility: Small Business
Distribution: Service Direct
General Admin.: George Burke/President, Chief Executive Officer
        Ray Renza/Vice President Human Resources
Mktg./Adv.: William J. Walker/Vice President Marketing & Sales
Production: Doug Hill/Vice President Manufacturing & Operations
        Marc Feinberg/Vice President Quality Systems
Research: Steve Verespy/Vice President Engineering
  Contract Packaging   General

SHARP IVERS-LEE
  See Sharp Corporation

SHARPS COMPLIANCE CORP. 713-432-0300
9220 Kirby Drive, Suite 500, Houston, TX 77054
FDA Number: 1651383   *Fax:* 713-838-0508
E-mail: sharps@sharpsinc.com
Web site: www.sharpsinc.com
Medical Products Sales Volume: $10,500,000
Annual Revenue: $5-$10 Million
Year Founded: 1992
Total Employees: 29   *Marketing Staff:* 3   *Sales Staff:* 8
Ownership: Public
Stock Symbol: SCOM
Traded On: OTC Bulletin
Produces/Sells CE-marked Devices: N
Federal Procurement Eligibility: Small Business
Distribution: Manufacturer Direct, Manufacturer Through Distributor, Manufacturer Through Manufacturer Reps, OEM, Exclusive Distributor, Importer
Mktg./Adv.: Mr. Bill Turpin/Vice President Marketing & Business Development
Production: Mr. Mark Iske/Vice President Operations
  Infusion Stand   General
  Waste Disposal Unit, Sharps   General

SHAW THERAPEUTICS, INC.
  See Circaid Medical Products, Inc.

SHAW-WALKER
  See Knoll, Inc.

SHEATHING TECHNOLOGIES, INC. 408-782-2720
18431 Technology Dr., Morgan Hill, CA 95037
FDA Number: 2950776
  Transducer, Ultrasonic, Diagnostic   Radiology

SHEEPSKIN RANCH, INC. 800-366-9950
3408 Indale Road, Fort Worth, TX 76116 817-738-2485
FDA Number: 1947926   *Fax:* 817-738-1970
E-mail: info@sheepskinranch.com
Web site: www.sheepskinranch.com
Medical Products Sales Volume: $600,000
Annual Revenue: $0-$1 Million
Year Founded: 1982
Total Employees: 10   *Marketing Staff:* 1   *Sales Staff:* 2
Ownership: COMPU-TTY, INC.
Produces/Sells CE-marked Devices: N
Federal Procurement Eligibility: Small Business, Minority Owned, Female Owned, VA Contract
Distribution: Manufacturer Through Distributor, Manufacturer Through Manufacturer Reps, Exporter
General Admin.: Sidney Ander/Chief Executive Officer
        Barbara Ander/President
Mktg./Adv.: Bryan Davis/Vice President Marketing
  Armrest, Wheelchair   Physical Med
  Cushion, Wheelchair (Pad)   Physical Med
  Pad, Pressure, Animal Skin   General

SHEFFIELD PHARMACEUTICALS 800-222-1087
170 Broad St., New London, CT 06320 860-442-4451
FDA Number: 1210513   *Fax:* 860-442-0356
E-mail: general@sheffield-labs.com
Web site: www.sheffield-labs.com
Medical Products Sales Volume: $22,600,000
Annual Revenue: $10-$25 Million
Year Founded: 1850
Total Employees: 150
Ownership: Private
Federal Procurement Eligibility: Small Business, Minority Owned
  Homopolymer, Karaya and Ethylene-Oxide   Dental And Oral
  Lubricant, Vaginal, Patient   General

SHELBY ELASTICS, LLC OF NORTH CAROLINA 800-562-4507
639 North Post Rd., Shelby, NC 28150
FDA Number: 1067005
  Bandage, Elastic   General

SHELBY-WILLIAMS INDUSTRIES 800-873-3252
5303 East Morris Blvd., Morristown, TN 37813 423-586-7000
FDA Number: 9330144   *Fax:* 423-586-2260
E-mail: swisales@shelbywilliams.com
Web site: www.shelbywilliams.com
Annual Revenue: $50-$100 Million
Year Founded: 1959
Total Employees: 1000
Ownership: Falcon Products, Inc.
Stock Symbol: FCP
Traded On: NYSE
Federal Procurement Eligibility: GSA Contract
Distribution: Manufacturer Through Manufacturer Reps, Importer, Exporter
General Admin.: Franklin Jacobs/Chief Executive Officer
        Robert Coulter/President, Chief Operating Officer
Mktg./Adv.: Mike Sandlock/Director Advertising
        Linda Crews/Director National Accounts
        Mike Sandlock/Manager Advertising
        Bob Harmon/Manager Sales
Production: Dennis Gurley/Vice President Manufacturing
  Chair, Geriatric   General
  Chair, Other   General
  Furniture, General   General
  Furniture, Patient Room   General

SHELDON ENTERPRISES, INC. 727-443-1677
609 Richards Ave # 102, P.O. Box 996, Clearwater, FL 33765
FDA Number: n/a   *Fax:* 800-497-2892
E-mail: sheldonentinc@yahoo.com
Web site: http://sheldonentinc.com
Medical Products Sales Volume: $599,000
Annual Revenue: $0-$1 Million
Year Founded: 1971
Ownership: Private
Produces/Sells CE-marked Devices: N
Federal Procurement Eligibility: Small Business, Female Owned
Distribution: Manufacturer Direct, Exclusive Distributor
  Cart, Other   General
  Chamber, Isolation, Patient Transport   General
  Grid, Radiographic   Radiology
  Holder, X-Ray Film   Dental And Oral
  Marker, X-Ray   Radiology
  Stool, Bedside   General
  Storage Unit, X-Ray Film   Radiology

SHELDON MFG., INC. 503-640-3000
300 North 26th Ave., Cornelius, OR 97113
FDA Number: 3024716
  Incubator/Water Bath, Microbiology   Microbiology

SHELHIGH, INC. 908-206-8706
650 Liberty Ave., Union, NJ 07083
FDA Number: 2247123
Web site: www.shelhigh.com
Ownership: Private
Produces/Sells CE-marked Devices: N
  Catheter, Vascular, Cardiopulmonary Bypass   Cardiovascular
  Dura-Substitute   Cns/Neurology
  Mesh, Surgical (Steel Gauze)   Surgery
  Mesh, Surgical, Polymeric   Surgery
  Pledget And Intracardiac Patch, PETP, PTFE, Polypropylene   Cardiovascular
  Ring, Annuloplasty   Cardiovascular

SHEPARD MEDICAL PRODUCTS 800-354-5683
260 E Lies Road, Carol Stream, IL 60188-9418 630-462-6720
FDA Number: 1422291   *Fax:* 708-447-9879
E-mail: chriswright@eagle-gloves.com
Web site: www.eagle-gloves.com
Medical Products Sales Volume: $2,100,000
Annual Revenue: $10-$25 Million
Total Employees: 12   *Marketing Staff:* 4   *Sales Staff:* 4
Ownership: Private
Quality System Registration Information: ISO9002
Distribution: Manufacturer Direct, Manufacturer Through Distributor
General Admin.: Christopher Wright/President, Chief Executive Officer
        Catherine Constontino/Vice President, General Manager
Mktg./Adv.: Steve Buschardt/Director Marketing
        Tim Sheehorn/Director National Accounts
        Kyle B. Pearce/Vice President Marketing & Sales
Production: William Lavencamp/Director Quality Assurance
        William Lavencamp/Manager Regulatory Affairs
  Glove, Patient Examination   General

SHEPHERD CASTER CORPORATION 800-253-0868
203 Kerth St., St. Joseph, MI 49085-2623 269-983-7351
FDA Number: n/a   *Fax:* 269-983-3091
E-mail: info@shepherdscasters.com
Web site: www.shepherdcasters.com

SHEPHERD CASTER CORPORATION 800-253-0868 (cont'd)
Annual Revenue: $10-$25 Million
Total Employees: 125   *Marketing Staff:* 2   *Sales Staff:* 8
Ownership: MARMON GROUP, INC., THE
Produces/Sells CE-marked Devices: N
Distribution: Manufacturer Direct, Manufacturer Through Distributor, OEM
General Admin.: Dennis Jones/President
Mktg./Adv.: Brian Hakeem/Director Marketing
Production: Melba Little/Director Quality Assurance
Casters, Hospital Equipment   General
Chair, Other   General

SHEPHERD PRODUCTS U.S., INC.
See Shepherd Caster Corporation

SHERCON INC. 800-228-3218
6262 Katella Ave, Cypress, CA 90630 **714-548-3999**
FDA Number: n/a   *Fax:* 714-548-3991
E-mail: hans.nilarp@shercon.com
Web site: www.shercon.com
Annual Revenue: $0-$1 Million
Year Founded: 1946
Ownership: Private
Produces/Sells CE-marked Devices: N
Federal Procurement Eligibility: Small Business
Distribution: Manufacturer Direct
Biofeedback Device   Cns/Neurology
Component, Silicone   General
Tape, Adhesive   General

SHERIDAN CATHETER CORP.
See Covidien Lp, Formerly Registered As Kendall

SHERMAN OPHTHALMIC SUPPLIES, INC. 714-738-0209
428 South Brea Blvd., Suite #B, Brea, CA 92821
FDA Number: 2028370   *Fax:* 714-529-8384
E-mail: drkirschen@sbcglobal.net
Ownership: Private
Produces/Sells CE-marked Devices: N
Nuclear Magnetic Resonance Imaging System   Radiology

SHERWOOD - DAVIS & GECK
See Covidien Lp

SHERWOOD MEDICAL COMPANY
See Covidien Lp

SHERWOOD, HARSCO CORP. 716-505-4831
2111 Liberty Dr., Niagara Falls, NY 14304
FDA Number: 3004550118
Ownership: Private
Produces/Sells CE-marked Devices: N
Regulator, Pressure, Gas Cylinder   Anesthesiology

SHIELDING INTERNATIONAL, INC. 800-292-2247
2150 NW Andrews Drive, P.O. Box Z, **541-475-7211**
Madras, OR 97741
FDA Number: 3014842   *Fax:* 541-475-6628
E-mail: info@shieldingintl.com
Web site: www.shieldingintl.com
Medical Products Sales Volume: $3,000,000
Annual Revenue: $1-$5 Million
Year Founded: 1958
Total Employees: 22   *Marketing Staff:* 4   *Sales Staff:* 4
Ownership: Private
Produces/Sells CE-marked Devices: Y
Federal Procurement Eligibility: Small Business, Female Owned
Distribution: Manufacturer Through Distributor, Exporter
General Admin.: Susan Kovari/Chief Executive Officer
     Brent Moschetti/President
     Doug Lofting/Vice President, General Manager
Apron, Lead, Radiographic   Radiology
Curtain, Protective, Radiographic   Radiology
Glove, Protective, Radiographic   Radiology
Shield, Gonadal   Radiology
Shield, Protective, Personnel   Radiology
Shield, X-Ray, Lead-Plastic   Radiology

SHIELDING INTL., INC. 541-475-7211
2150 N.w. Andrews Dr., Madras, OR 97741
FDA Number: 3020118
Apron, Lead, Dental   Dental And Oral
Apron, Lead, Radiographic   Radiology
Glove, Protective, Radiographic   Radiology
Shield, Gonadal   Radiology
Shield, Protective, Personnel   Radiology

SHIMADZU MEDICAL SYSTEMS 800-228-1429
20101 S. Vermont Avenue, Torrance, CA 90502 **310-217-8855**
FDA Number: n/a   *Fax:* 310-217-0661
E-mail: info@shimadzumed.com

SHIMADZU MEDICAL SYSTEMS 800-228-1429 (cont'd)
Web site: http://www.shimadzu.com
Total Employees: 40
Ownership: SHIMADZU CORP.
Quality System Registration Information: ISO9000; ISO9001; ISO9002
Produces/Sells CE-marked Devices: Y
Federal Procurement Eligibility: Small Business, VA Contract
Distribution: Manufacturer Through Distributor, Importer
General Admin.: Akinori Yamaguchi/Assistant General Manager
     Ryuichi Ban/Vice President, General Manager
Mktg./Adv.: Frank Serrao/Director Marketing & Sales
     James Mekker/Manager Business Development
     Vickie L. Standridge/Manager Communications
     Donald Karle/Manager National Operations
     Tom Kloetzly/Manager National Sales
     Burl Taylor/Manager Regional Sales
     Wendy De Castro/Manager Regional Sales
     Randy Walker/Services Manager
Finance: Tepsuya Kiyozumi/Controller
Gel, Ultrasonic Transmission   General
Generator, Diagnostic X-Ray, High Voltage, 3-Phase   Radiology
Generator, Diagnostic X-Ray, High Voltage, Single Phase   Radiology
Radiographic Unit, Diagnostic, Fixed (X-Ray)   Radiology
Radiographic Unit, Digital Subtraction Angiographic (DSA)   Radiology
Radiographic/Fluoroscopic Unit, Angiographic   Radiology
Radiographic/Fluoroscopic Unit, Mobile C-Arm   Radiology
Radiographic/Fluoroscopic Unit, Special Procedure   Radiology
Scanner, Computed Tomography, X-Ray, Full Body   Radiology
Scanner, Ultrasonic, Abdominal   Radiology
Scanner, Ultrasonic, Other   Radiology
System, X-Ray, Mobile   Radiology
Table, Radiographic, Tilting   Radiology
Transducer, Ultrasonic   Cardiovascular

SHINAMERICA, INC. 651-291-7909
710 Fourth St., Desmet, SD 57231
FDA Number: 2135402
Syringe, Piston   General

SHINEMOUND ENTERPRISE, INC. 978-436-9980
17a Sterling Road, North Billerica, MA 01862
FDA Number: 1221921   *Fax:* 978-436-9983
E-mail: shinemound@earthlink.net
Web site: www.shinemound.com
Medical Products Sales Volume: $16,000,000
Year Founded: 1988
Total Employees: 6
Ownership: Private
Quality System Registration Information: ISO9002
Produces/Sells CE-marked Devices: Y
Federal Procurement Eligibility: Small Business, Minority Owned
Distribution: Manufacturer Through Distributor, OEM, Importer
Glove, Patient Examination, Latex   General
Glove, Patient Examination, Poly   General
Glove, Patient Examination, Vinyl   General
Gown, Patient, Disposable   General
Mask, Face   General

SHIPPERT MEDICAL TECHNOLOGIES CORP. 800-888-8663
6248 South Troy Circle, Unit A, **303-754-0044**
Centennial, CO 80111
FDA Number: 1718903   *Fax:* 800-284-0864
E-mail: info@shippertmedical.com
Web site: www.shippertmedical.com
Medical Products Sales Volume: $900,000
Annual Revenue: $1-$5 Million
Year Founded: 1978
Total Employees: 13   *Marketing Staff:* 2   *Sales Staff:* 5
Ownership: Private
Quality System Registration Information: ISO9001
Produces/Sells CE-marked Devices: Y
Federal Procurement Eligibility: Small Business
Distribution: Manufacturer Direct, Manufacturer Through Distributor, OEM, Exporter
General Admin.: Ron Shippert/Chief Executive Officer
     Sarah Shippert/President
Mktg./Adv.: Angela Mediger/Director Marketing
Production: Sarah M. Lake/Manager Regulatory Affairs
Research: Mark Gabrielson/Vice President Research & Development
Finance: Allison Therwhanger/Chief Financial Officer
Button, Nasal Septal   Ear/Nose/Throat
Cannula, Surgical, General & Plastic Surgery   Surgery
Contract Manufacturing   General
Dressing, Non-Adherent   General
Dressing, Other   General
Electrocautery Unit, Battery-Powered   Surgery
Electrosurgical Equipment, General Purpose   Surgery
Laryngoscope   Ear/Nose/Throat

SHIPPERT MEDICAL TECHNOLOGIES CORP.   800-888-8663
(cont'd)

Legging, Compression, Non-Inflatable	General
Otoscope	Ear/Nose/Throat
Packing, Surgical	Surgery
Splint, Nasal	Ear/Nose/Throat
Tray, Custom/Special Procedure	General
Tube, Myringotomy	Ear/Nose/Throat

SHOFU DENTAL CORPORATION   800-827-4638
1225 Stone Drive, San Marcos, CA 92069   760-736-3277
FDA Number: 2916735   *Fax:* 760-736-3276
E-mail: customer-service@shofu.com
Web site: www.shofu.com
Year Founded: 1971
Total Employees: 36   *Marketing Staff:* 3   *Sales Staff:* 15
Ownership: Shofu Inc.
Quality System Registration Information: ISO9001
Produces/Sells CE-marked Devices: Y
Distribution: Manufacturer Direct, Manufacturer Through Distributor, Manufacturer Through Manufacturer Reps, Importer
General Admin.: Brian Melonakos/President
Mktg./Adv.: Randy Bailey/Manager National Sales
      Lynne Calliott/Market Manager
Production: David Morais/Manager Operations

Accessories, Retractor, Dental	Dental And Oral
Agent, Polishing, Abrasive, Oral Cavity	Dental And Oral
Articulators	Dental And Oral
Burr, Dental	Dental And Oral
Cement, Dental	Dental And Oral
Dam, Rubber	Dental And Oral
Disk, Abrasive	Dental And Oral
Handpiece, Air-Powered, Dental	Dental And Oral
Instrument, Diamond, Dental	Dental And Oral
Point, Abrasive	Dental And Oral
Source, Heat, Bleaching, Teeth, Dental	Dental And Oral
Syringe, Restorative And Impression Material	Dental And Oral
Wheel, Polishing Agent	Dental And Oral

SHONEY SCIENTIFIC, INC.   262-970-0170
West 223 North 720 Saratoga Drive,, Suite 120, Waukesha, WI 53186
FDA Number: 2183650   *Fax:* 253-650-6972
Web site: www.shoney.com
Medical Products Sales Volume: $100,000
Year Founded: 1986
Total Employees: 3
Ownership: Public

Cannula, Surgical, General & Plastic Surgery	Surgery
Catheter, Suction (Tracheal Aspirating Tube)	Anesthesiology
Curette, Ear	Ear/Nose/Throat
Dilator, Cervical, Fixed Size	Obstetrics/Gynecology
Orthosis, Limb Brace	Physical Med
Punch, Biopsy, Surgical	Dental And Oral
Sound, Uterine	Obstetrics/Gynecology
Speculum, Ear	Ear/Nose/Throat
Syringe Unit, Air And/Or Water	Dental And Oral

SHOPPERS HOME HEALTH CARE DONCASTER   800-363-1020
243 Consumers Rd.,   416-493-1220
North York, ONT M2J-4 Canada
FDA Number: n/a   *Fax:* 416-490-7316
E-mail: customerservice@shoppersdrugmart.ca
Web site: www.shoppersdrugmart.ca
Year Founded: 1980
Total Employees: 100
Ownership: Private
Produces/Sells CE-marked Devices: N

SHOPRIDER CANADA MOBILITY PRODUCTS   888-999-0895
1360 Cliveden Ave, Delta, BC V3M 6K2 Canada   604-273-5173
FDA Number: n/a   *Fax:* 604-273-9312
Year Founded: 1989
Total Employees: 10
Ownership: Private
Produces/Sells CE-marked Devices: N
Distribution: Exclusive Distributor, Importer

SHORE MEDICAL, INC.
See Truer Medical, Inc.

SHORELINE HEALTHCO INC.   888-233-7038
23 Victoria St., P.O. Box 628,   519-482-3046
Clinton, ONT N0M-1 Canada
FDA Number: n/a   *Fax:* 519-482-7306
E-mail: mpenner@odyssey.on.ca
Web site: www.shorelinehealthco.com
Year Founded: 1990
Total Employees: 10

SHORELINE HEALTHCO INC.   888-233-7038 *(cont'd)*
Ownership: Private
Produces/Sells CE-marked Devices: N

SHOWERFLOSS, INC.   800-723-2300
20930 Persimmon Pl., Estero, FL 33928   239-992-8686
FDA Number: 1056603   *Fax:* 941-729-1470
E-mail: info@showerfloss.com
Web site: www.showerfloss.com
Medical Products Sales Volume: $500,000
Annual Revenue: $0-$1 Million
Year Founded: 1986
Total Employees: 12
Ownership: Private
Produces/Sells CE-marked Devices: N
Federal Procurement Eligibility: Small Business
Distribution: Manufacturer Direct, Manufacturer Through Distributor, Service Direct

Irrigator, Oral	Dental And Oral

SHRINK NANOTECHNOLOGIES, INC.   760-804-8844
2038 Corte Del Nogal, Suite 110, Carlsbad, CA 92011
FDA Number: n/a   *Fax:* 760-804-8845
E-mail: info@shrinknano.com
Web site: http://www.shrinknano.com
Ownership: Public
Stock Symbol: INKN
Traded On: NASDAQ
Produces/Sells CE-marked Devices: N
General Admin.: Mark Baum/President, Chief Executive Officer

SHUKLA MEDICAL   888-474-8552)
151 Old New Brunswick Rd,   732-474-1769
Piscataway, NJ 08854
FDA Number: 2183899   *Fax:* 732-474-1869
E-mail: customer.service@shuklamedical.com
Web site: www.shuklamedical.com
Ownership: Private
Produces/Sells CE-marked Devices: N

Extractor, Nail	Orthopedics
Orthopedic Manual Surgical Instrument	Orthopedics

SHUMSKY POST-OP PILLOWS
See Shumsky Therapeutic Products

SHUMSKY THERAPEUTIC PRODUCTS   888-333-3677
811 E 4th St, Dayton, OH 45402   937-223-2203
FDA Number: n/a   *Fax:* 800-414-8943
E-mail: pillows@shumsky.com
Web site: www.therapeuticpillows.com
Annual Revenue: $5-$10 Million
Total Employees: 94
Ownership: Private
Produces/Sells CE-marked Devices: N
Federal Procurement Eligibility: Small Business, Female Owned
Distribution: Exclusive Distributor
General Admin.: Jayne Miller/Chief Executive Officer
      Mike Emoff/President
Mktg./Adv.: Lynne Booher/Director Marketing & Sales
      Kisten Phillips/Manager National Sales

Support, Abdominal	Physical Med

SHURE MANUFACTURING CORP.   800-227-4873
1901 W. Main St., Washington, MO 63090   636-390-7100
FDA Number: n/a   *Fax:* 636-390-7171
E-mail: sales@shureusa.com
Web site: www.shureusa.com
Year Founded: 1945
Total Employees: 25
Ownership: Private
Produces/Sells CE-marked Devices: N
Federal Procurement Eligibility: Small Business
Distribution: Manufacturer Direct, Manufacturer Through Distributor, Manufacturer Through Manufacturer Reps, OEM, Importer, Exporter
General Admin.: Daniel Richardson/Chief Executive Officer
      Andrew Richardson/President
Mktg./Adv.: Peter Richardson/Vice President Sales

Furniture, General	General
Security Equipment/Supplies	General

SHUTTLE SYSTEMS BY CONTEMPORARY DESIGN CO.   800-334-5633
10005 Mt. Baker Hwy., Glacier, WA 98244-5089   360-599-2833
FDA Number: 3032322   *Fax:* 360-599-2171
E-mail: gary@shuttlesystems.com
Web site: www.shuttlesystems.com
Year Founded: 1962
Total Employees: 10
Ownership: Private

SHUTTLE SYSTEMS BY CONTEMPORARY 800-334-5633 (cont'd)
Traded On: NYSE
Produces/Sells CE-marked Devices: N
Federal Procurement Eligibility: Small Business
Distribution: Manufacturer Through Manufacturer Reps, Exporter
General Admin.: Gary Graham/President, Chief Executive Officer
   Exerciser, Non-Measuring   Physical Med

SI-BONE INC.   408-207-0700
550 South Winchester Blvd., Suite 620, San Jose, CA 95128
FDA Number: 3007700286   Fax: 408-557-8312
E-mail: info@SI-BONE.com
Web site: http://www.si-bone.com/
Ownership: Private
Produces/Sells CE-marked Devices: N
General Admin.: Mr. Jeffrey Dunn/President, Chief Executive Officer
  Medical Admin.: Dr. Mark Reiley/Chief Medical Officer
Mktg./Adv.: Mr. Jeffrey Polack/Vice President Marketing
          Mr. Kevin Shaw/Vice President Sales
Research: Mr. Garret Mauldin/Vice President Engineering
Finance: Mr. Dan Murray/Chief Financial Officer
   Screw, Fixation, Bone   Orthopedics

SI-BONE INC.   408-207-0700
550 South Winchester Blvd., Suite 620, San Jose, CA 95128
FDA Number: 3007700286   Fax: 408-557-8312
E-mail: info@SI-BONE.com
Web site: www.si-bone.com
Ownership: Private
Produces/Sells CE-marked Devices: N
General Admin.: Mr. Dan Murray/Chief Financial Officer, Vice President Operations
         Mr. Jeffery Dunn/President, Chief Executive Officer
  Medical Admin.: Mr. Mark Reiley/Chief Medical Officer
Mktg./Adv.: Mr. Jeff Polack/Vice President Marketing
          Mr. Kevin Shaw/Vice President Sales

Bit, Drill	Orthopedics
Guide, Surgical, Instrument	Surgery
Hammer, Surgical	Surgery
Knife, Orthopedic	Orthopedics
Orthopedic Manual Surgical Instrument	Orthopedics
Screw, Fixation, Bone	Orthopedics

SICEL TECHNOLOGIES, INC.   919-465-2236
3800 Gateway Centre Blvd., Suite 308, Morrisville, NC 27560
FDA Number: 3004725397

Accelerator, Linear, Medical	Radiology
Radiotherapy Unit, Charged-Particle	Radiology

SICHEL SLEEP PRODUCTS   610-292-8700
1210 Stanbridge St., Norristown, PA 19401
FDA Number: n/a   Fax: 610-292-9096
E-mail: sichelbed@aol.com
Web site: www.sichelbed.com
Annual Revenue: $0-$1 Million
Total Employees: 15
Ownership: Private
Produces/Sells CE-marked Devices: N
Federal Procurement Eligibility: Small Business
Distribution: Manufacturer Direct, Manufacturer Through Distributor, Manufacturer Through Manufacturer Reps
General Admin.: Robert Burwinkle/President
Mktg./Adv.: Ellen Burnwinkle/Manager Advertising
         Ellen Burnwinkle/Vice President Marketing & Sales

Cushion, Other	General
Mattress, Bed	General

SICK OPTIC-ELECTRONIC, INC.
See Sick, Inc.

SICK, INC.   800-325-7425
                     952-941-6780
6900 West 110th Street, Minneapolis, MN 55438
FDA Number: n/a   Fax: 952-941-9287
E-mail: info@sick.com
Web site: www.sickusa.com
Total Employees: 250   Sales Staff: 40
Ownership: SICK AG
Quality System Registration Information: ISO9000
Produces/Sells CE-marked Devices: Y
Federal Procurement Eligibility: Female Owned

Production Equipment	General
Reader, Bar Code	General

SIDMAR MFG., INC.   800-330-7260
                     763-389-9594
31530 - 125th St. NW, Princeton, MN 55371
FDA Number: 2134295   Fax: 763-389-9385
E-mail: Joe@sidmar.com
Web site: www.sidmar.com
Medical Products Sales Volume: $1,000,000
Annual Revenue: $1-$5 Million

SIDMAR MFG., INC.   800-330-7260 (cont'd)
Year Founded: 1992
Total Employees: 11
Ownership: Private
Produces/Sells CE-marked Devices: N
Distribution: Manufacturer Direct, Manufacturer Through Manufacturer Reps, Exporter
General Admin.: Mr. Joseph Holland/President
   Massager, Therapeutic   Physical Med

SIEBE NORTH, INC.
See North Safety Products

SIEMANS QUANTUM INC.
See Siemens Medical Systems, Inc., Ultrasound Group

SIEMENS CORP.
See Siemens Medical

SIEMENS CREDIT CORP.   800-327-4443
                     800-798-7721
170 Wood Avenue, South Iselin, NJ 08830
FDA Number: n/a   Fax: 908-429-6075
E-mail: info.usa.sfs@siemens.com
Web site: www.usa.siemens.com/finance
Medical Products Sales Volume: $200,000,000
Annual Revenue: $100-$500 Million
Total Employees: 1933
Ownership: Siemens Medical
Produces/Sells CE-marked Devices: Y
Distribution: Service Direct
General Admin.: Dominik Asam/Chief Executive Officer
Finance: Dr. Peter Moritz/Chief Financial Officer
   Service, Equipment Leasing   General

SIEMENS ELEMA PACEMAKER SYSTEMS
See St. Jude Medical Cardiac Rhythm Management Div.

SIEMENS ELEMA VENTILATOR SYSTEMS
See Siemens Medical Systems, Inc.

SIEMENS GAMMASONICS, INC.
See Siemens Medical Systems, Inc., Nuclear Med. Group

SIEMENS HEALTH SERVICES
See Delta Health Technologies, Llc

SIEMENS HEALTHCARE DIAGNOSTICS INC   866-637-4448
101 Silvermine Rd, Brookfield, CT 06804
FDA Number: 1226181
Web site: http://diagnostics.siemens.com
Ownership: Siemens Ag
Stock Symbol: SI
Traded On: NYSE
Produces/Sells CE-marked Devices: N

Electrode, Ion Specific, Chloride	Chemistry
Electrode, Ion Specific, Potassium	Chemistry
Equipment, Laboratory, Gen. Purpose (Specific Medical Use)	Chemistry
Hexokinase, Glucose	Chemistry
Lipase Hydrolysis/Glycerol Kinase Enzyme, Triglycerides	Chemistry
NAD Reduction/NADH Oxidation, CPK Or Isoenzymes	Chemistry
NAD Reduction/NADH Oxidation, Lactate Dehydrogenase	Chemistry
Radioimmunoassay, Free Thyroxine	Chemistry
Radioimmunoassay, Immunoglobulins (G, A, M)	Chemistry
Urease And Glutamic Dehydrogenase, Urea Nitrogen	Chemistry

SIEMENS HEALTHCARE DIAGNOSTICS INC   800-255-3232
2 Edgewater Drive, Norwood, MA 02062
FDA Number: 1217157   Fax: 888-242-1997
Web site: http://diagnostics.siemens.com
Ownership: Siemens Ag
Stock Symbol: SI
Traded On: NYSE
Produces/Sells CE-marked Devices: N
Distribution: Manufacturer Direct, Manufacturer Through Distributor, Manufacturer Through Manufacturer Reps, Importer, Exporter

Analyzer, Blood Gas pH	Anesthesiology
Analyzer, Chemistry, Electrolyte	Chemistry
Analyzer, Chemistry, Micro	Chemistry
Analyzer, Chemistry, Radioimmunoassay, Automated	Chemistry
Analyzer, Chemistry, Therapeutic Drug Monitor (TDM)	Chemistry
Analyzer, Coagulation, Automated	Hematology
Analyzer, Gas, Carbon-Dioxide, Partial Pressure, Blood	Anesthesiology
Analyzer, Gas, Oxygen, Partial Pressure, Blood Phase	Anesthesiology
Analyzer, Ion, Hydrogen-Ion pH, Blood Phase, Non-Indwelling	Anesthesiology
Bilirubin (Total and Unbound) Neonate Test System	Chemistry
Co-Oximeter	Hematology
Electrode, Ion Specific, Calcium	Chemistry
Electrode, Ion Specific, Chloride	Chemistry
Electrode, Ion Specific, Potassium	Chemistry
Electrode, Laboratory pH	Chemistry
Electrophoresis Equipment, Gel	Chemistry
Electrophoresis Instrumentation	Immunology
Electrophoretic Separation, Lipoproteins	Chemistry
Electrophoretic, Lactate Dehydrogenase Isoenzymes	Chemistry

SIEMENS HEALTHCARE DIAGNOSTICS INC   800-255-3232
(cont'd)

Electrophoretic, Protein Fractionation	Chemistry
Fluorometric Method, CPK Or Isoenzymes	Chemistry
Instrument, Coagulation, Automated	Hematology
Photometer, Flame Emission	Chemistry
Photometer, Flame, General Use	Toxicology
Photometer, Flame, Potassium	Chemistry
Prothrombin Time	Hematology
Radioimmunoassay, Cortisol	Chemistry
Radioimmunoassay, Digoxin (125-I), Rabbit, Solid Phase	Toxicology
Radioimmunoassay, Ferritin	Microbiology
Radioimmunoassay, Free Thyroxine	Chemistry
Radioimmunoassay, Immunoreactive Insulin	Chemistry
Radioimmunoassay, Prolactin (Lactogen)	Chemistry
Radioimmunoassay, T3 Uptake	Chemistry
Radioimmunoassay, T4	Chemistry
Radioimmunoassay, Thyroid Stimulating Hormone	Chemistry
Radioimmunoassay, Thyroxine Binding Globulin	Chemistry
Radioimmunoassay, Total Thyroxine	Chemistry
Radioimmunoassay, Total Triiodothyronine	Chemistry
Radioimmunoassay, Vitamin B12	Chemistry
Reagent, Calibration	General
Reagent, General Purpose	Pathology
Solution, pH Buffer	Chemistry
Standard/Control, All Types	Chemistry
Thromboplastin, Activated Partial	Hematology

SIEMENS HEALTHCARE DIAGNOSTICS INC   866-637-4448
333 Coney Street, E Walpole, MA 02032
FDA Number: 1219913
Web site: http://diagnostics.siemens.com
Ownership: Siemens Ag
Stock Symbol: SI
Traded On: NYSE
Produces/Sells CE-marked Devices: N

Acid, Ascorbic, 2, 4-dinitrophenylhydrazine (spectrophotometric)	Chemistry
Container, Specimen Mailer And Storage	Pathology
Cuvette, Thermostated	Chemistry
Fluorometric, Cortisol	Chemistry
Radioimmunoassay, Follicle Stimulating Hormone	Chemistry
Radioimmunoassay, Progesterone	Chemistry
Radioimmunoassay, Prolactin (Lactogen)	Chemistry
Radioimmunoassay, Total Triiodothyronine	Chemistry

SIEMENS HEALTHCARE DIAGNOSTICS INC   574-295-7516
3400 Middlebury St, Elkhart, IN 46515
FDA Number: 1824828
Web site: http://diagnostics.siemens.com
Ownership: Siemens Ag
Stock Symbol: SI
Traded On: NYSE
Produces/Sells CE-marked Devices: N

Control, Urinalysis (Assayed And Unassayed)	Chemistry

SIEMENS HEALTHCARE DIAGNOSTICS INC   973-584-4649
62 Flanders-Barley Road, Flanders, NJ 07836
FDA Number: 2247117
Web site: http://diagnostics.siemens.com
Ownership: Siemens Ag
Stock Symbol: SI
Traded On: NYSE
Produces/Sells CE-marked Devices: Y
Distribution: Manufacturer Direct

Analyzer, Chemistry, Enzyme Immunoassay	Chemistry

SIEMENS HEALTHCARE DIAGNOSTICS INC   800-434-2447
725 Potter St, Berkeley, CA 94710
FDA Number: 3003932969   *Fax:* 510-705-5902
Web site: http://diagnostics.siemens.com
Ownership: Siemens Ag
Stock Symbol: SI
Traded On: NYSE
Produces/Sells CE-marked Devices: N

Assay, Hybridization And/or Nucleic Acid Amplification For Detection Of Hepatitis C Rna, Hepatitis C Virus	Microbiology
Reagent, General Purpose	Pathology
Test, Hiv Detection	Immunology

SIEMENS HEALTHCARE DIAGNOSTICS INC   317-240-0012
7750 West Morris St., Indianapolis, IN 46231
FDA Number: 1835506
Web site: http://diagnostics.siemens.com
Ownership: Siemens Ag
Stock Symbol: SI
Traded On: NYSE
Produces/Sells CE-marked Devices: N

SIEMENS HEALTHCARE DIAGNOSTICS INC
   See WILEX, Inc.

SIEMENS HEALTHCARE DIAGNOSTICS INC.   302-631-6311
500 Gbc Dr., Mailstop 514, Newark, DE 19702
FDA Number: 2517506
Web site: http://diagnostics.siemens.com
Ownership: Siemens Ag
Stock Symbol: SI
Traded On: NYSE
Produces/Sells CE-marked Devices: N

Antigen, Antiserum, Control, Prealbumin, FITC	Immunology
Calibrator, Drug Mixture	Toxicology
Calibrator, Drug Specific	Toxicology
Colorimetry, Acetaminophen	Toxicology
Enzyme Immunoassay, Barbiturate	Toxicology
Enzyme Immunoassay, Benzodiazepine	Toxicology
Enzyme Immunoassay, Cannabinoids	Toxicology
Enzyme Immunoassay, Cocaine And Cocaine Metabolites	Toxicology
Enzyme Immunoassay, Methadone	Toxicology
Enzyme Immunoassay, Other	Chemistry
Enzyme Immunoassay, Phencyclidine	Toxicology
Enzyme Immunoassay, Valproic Acid	Toxicology
Lipase Hydrolysis/Glycerol Kinase Enzyme, Triglycerides	Chemistry
Lipase-Esterase, Enzymatic, Photometric, Lipase	Chemistry
Radioimmunoassay, Methaqualone	Toxicology
Test, C-Reactive Protein	Immunology

SIEMENS HEALTHCARE DIAGNOSTICS INC.   914-631-8000
511 Benedict Avenue, Tarrytown, NY 10591
FDA Number: 2432235   *Fax:* 914-524-2132
Web site: http://diagnostics.siemens.com
Annual Revenue: More than $1 Billion
Ownership: Siemens Ag
Stock Symbol: SI
Traded On: NYSE
Quality System Registration Information: ISO9001
Produces/Sells CE-marked Devices: Y
Distribution: Manufacturer Direct, Manufacturer Through Distributor
General Admin.: Mr. Donal Quinn/Chief Executive Officer
     Mr. Jim Reid Anderson/President, Chief Executive Officer
     Mr. Arnd Kaldowski/Senior Vice President
     Mr. Joe Bernardo/Senior Vice President
Mktg./Adv.: Ms. Linda Langendonk/Manager Communications
Finance: Mr. Jochen Schmitz/Chief Financial Officer

Acetone	Chemistry
Analyzer, Amino Acid	Microbiology
Analyzer, BUN (Blood Urea Nitrogen)	Chemistry
Analyzer, Carbon	Chemistry
Analyzer, Chemistry, Electrolyte	Chemistry
Analyzer, Chemistry, Enzyme	Chemistry
Analyzer, Chemistry, Enzyme Immunoassay	Chemistry
Analyzer, Chemistry, Micro	Chemistry
Analyzer, Chemistry, Multi-Channel, Fixed	Chemistry
Analyzer, Chemistry, Radioimmunoassay, Automated	Chemistry
Analyzer, Chemistry, Sequential Multiple, Continuous Flow	Chemistry
Analyzer, Chemistry, Single Channel, Programmable	Chemistry
Analyzer, Chemistry, Urinalysis	Chemistry
Analyzer, Chemistry, Urinalysis, Automated	Chemistry
Analyzer, Platelet Aggregation	Hematology
Analyzer, Protein	Chemistry
Analyzer, Pulmonary Function	Anesthesiology
Chromatography Equipment, Liquid	Chemistry
Chromatography, Liquid, Performance, High	Toxicology
Computer, Clinical Laboratory	Chemistry
Computer, Hematology Analyzer	Hematology
Computer, Pulmonary Function Laboratory	Anesthesiology
Counter, Cell	Microbiology
Counter, Cell Or Particle, Automated	Hematology
Counter, Cell, Differential Classifier, Automated	Hematology
Counter, Platelet, Automated	Hematology
Cytocentrifuge	Pathology
Dialyzer, Laboratory	Chemistry
Diazo (Colorimetric), Nitrite (Urinary, Non-Quantitative)	Chemistry
Diazonium Colorimetry, Urobilinogen (Urinary, Non-Quant.)	Chemistry
Electrode, Blood pH	Chemistry
Electrode, Specific Ion	Chemistry
Enzymatic Method, Blood, Occult, Fecal	Chemistry
Enzymatic Method, Blood, Occult, Urinary	Chemistry
Enzyme Immunoassay, Valproic Acid	Toxicology
Ferric Chloride, Phenylketones (Urinary, Non-Quantitative)	Chemistry
Fluorometer, Toxicology	Toxicology
Fluorometric Method, Triglycerides	Chemistry
Hexokinase, Glucose	Chemistry
High Pressure Liquid Chromatography, Tricyclic Drug	Toxicology
Indicator Method, Protein Or Albumin (Urinary, Non-Quant.)	Chemistry
Kit, Identification, Neisseria Gonorrhoeae	Microbiology
Lipase Hydrolysis/Glycerol Kinase Enzyme, Triglycerides	Chemistry
Metallic Reduction Method, Glucose (Urinary, Non-Quant.)	Chemistry
Microtome, Cryostat	Pathology
Monitor, Blood Glucose (Test)	Gastroenterology/Urology
Nephelometer	Chemistry
Nitroprusside, Ketones (Urinary, Non-Quantitative)	Chemistry

SIEMENS HEALTHCARE DIAGNOSTICS INC.   914-631-8000
(cont'd)

Phosphatase, Acid	Hematology
Photometer, Flame, General Use	Toxicology
Photometer, Reflectance	Chemistry
Radioimmunoassay, Estradiol	Chemistry
Radioimmunoassay, Prostate-Specific Antigen (PSA)	Immunology
Radioimmunoassay, Sisomicin	Toxicology
Radioimmunoassay, Testosterones And Dihydrotestosterone	Chemistry
Radioimmunoassay, Total Triiodothyronine	Chemistry
Radioimmunoassay, Vitamin B12	Chemistry
Reagent, Albumin, Colorimetric	Chemistry
Reagent, Analyzer, Amino Acid	Microbiology
Reagent, Bilirubin (Total Or Direct Test System)	Chemistry
Reagent, Calcium (Test System)	Chemistry
Reagent, Chloride (Test System)	Chemistry
Reagent, Cholesterol (Total Test System)	Chemistry
Reagent, Glucose (Test System)	Chemistry
Reagent, Kinase, Phosphate, Creatine	Chemistry
Reagent, Protein, Total	Chemistry
SGOT, Ultraviolet	Chemistry
SGPT, Ultraviolet	Chemistry
Serum Separation System	Hematology
Serum, Biological, General	Toxicology
Solution, Pathology, Newcomer's	Pathology
Spectrophotometer, Ultraviolet	Chemistry
Spectrophotometer, Visible	Chemistry
Stain, Biological, General	Pathology
Stainer, Slide, Hematology	Hematology
Stainer, Slide, Hematology, Automated	Hematology
Stainer, Tissue, Automated	Pathology
Standard, Amino Acid	Chemistry
Standard, Carbohydrate	Chemistry
Standard/Control, All Types	Chemistry
Stick, Urinalysis Test	Chemistry
System, Test, Acid, Methylmalonic, Urinary	Chemistry
Tissue Processor (Infiltrator)	Pathology
Titrator	Chemistry
Turbidimetric Method, Protein Or Albumin (Urinary)	Chemistry
Urease, Photometric, Urea Nitrogen	Chemistry
Uricase (Coulometric), Uric Acid	Chemistry

SIEMENS HEALTHCARE DIAGNOSTICS INC.   310-645-8200
5210 Pacific Concourse Drive, Los Angeles, CA 90045
FDA Number: 3005250747   *Fax:* 310-645-9999
E-mail: usa.med@siemens.com
Web site: http://diagnostics.siemens.com
Medical Products Sales Volume: $198,700,000
Annual Revenue: $100-$500 Million
Ownership: Siemens Ag
Stock Symbol: SI
Traded On: NYSE
Quality System Registration Information: ISO9001
Produces/Sells CE-marked Devices: Y
Federal Procurement Eligibility: Small Business
Distribution: Manufacturer Direct, Manufacturer Through Distributor

Antigen, Antiserum, Control, IGE	Immunology
Antigen, Prostate-Specific (PSA), Management, Cancer	Immunology
Control, Multi Analyte, All Kinds (Assayed And Unassayed)	Chemistry
Enzyme Immunoassay, Digitoxin	Toxicology
Enzyme Linked Immunoabsorbent Assay, Cytomegalovirus	Microbiology
Enzyme Linked Immunoabsorbent Assay, Rubella	Microbiology
Enzyme Linked Immunoabsorbent Assay, Toxoplasma Gondii	Microbiology
Fluorescent Immunoassay, Tobramycin	Toxicology
Hepatitis B Test (B Core, BE Antigen & Antibody, B Core IGM)	Microbiology
Immunoassay, Other	Toxicology
Radioimmunoassay, ACTH	Chemistry
Radioimmunoassay, Aldosterone	Chemistry
Radioimmunoassay, Amikacin	Toxicology
Radioimmunoassay, Amphetamine	Toxicology
Radioimmunoassay, Androstenedione	Chemistry
Radioimmunoassay, Barbiturate	Toxicology
Radioimmunoassay, C Peptides Of Proinsulin	Chemistry
Radioimmunoassay, Calcitonin	Chemistry
Radioimmunoassay, Cannabinoid (S)	Toxicology
Radioimmunoassay, Cocaine Metabolite	Toxicology
Radioimmunoassay, Cortisol	Chemistry
Radioimmunoassay, Cyclic AMP	Chemistry
Radioimmunoassay, Dehydroepiandrosterone (Free And Sulfate)	Chemistry
Radioimmunoassay, Digitoxin (3-H)	Toxicology
Radioimmunoassay, Digoxin (125-I), Rabbit, 2nd Antibody	Toxicology
Radioimmunoassay, Estradiol	Chemistry
Radioimmunoassay, Estriol	Chemistry
Radioimmunoassay, Ferritin	Microbiology
Radioimmunoassay, Folic Acid	Chemistry
Radioimmunoassay, Follicle Stimulating Hormone	Chemistry
Radioimmunoassay, Free Thyroxine	Chemistry
Radioimmunoassay, Gastrin	Chemistry
Radioimmunoassay, Gentamicin (125-I), Second Antibody	Toxicology
Radioimmunoassay, Glucagon	Chemistry
Radioimmunoassay, Human Chorionic Gonadotropin	Chemistry

SIEMENS HEALTHCARE DIAGNOSTICS INC.   310-645-8200
(cont'd)

Radioimmunoassay, Human Growth Hormone	Chemistry
Radioimmunoassay, Human Placental Lactogen	Chemistry
Radioimmunoassay, Immunoreactive Insulin	Chemistry
Radioimmunoassay, LSD (125-I)	Toxicology
Radioimmunoassay, Luteinizing Hormone	Chemistry
Radioimmunoassay, Morphine (125-I), Goat Antibody	Toxicology
Radioimmunoassay, Parathyroid Hormone	Chemistry
Radioimmunoassay, Progesterone	Chemistry
Radioimmunoassay, Prolactin (Lactogen)	Chemistry
Radioimmunoassay, T3 Uptake	Chemistry
Radioimmunoassay, T4	Chemistry
Radioimmunoassay, Testosterones And Dihydrotestosterone	Chemistry
Radioimmunoassay, Theophylline	Toxicology
Radioimmunoassay, Thyroid Stimulating Hormone	Chemistry
Radioimmunoassay, Thyroxine Binding Globulin	Chemistry
Radioimmunoassay, Tobramycin	Toxicology
Radioimmunoassay, Total Thyroxine	Chemistry
Radioimmunoassay, Total Triiodothyronine	Chemistry
Radioimmunoassay, Vitamin B12	Chemistry
System, Test, Drugs of Abuse	Chemistry
Tartrate Inhibited, Acid Phosphatase (Prostatic)	Chemistry
Test, Allergy	Immunology
Test, Alpha-Fetoprotein	Pathology

SIEMENS HEALTHCARE DIAGNOSTICS INC.   800-242-3233
600 Tradeport Blvd, Suite 601, Atlanta, GA 30354
FDA Number: 1058613
Web site: http://diagnostics.siemens.com
Ownership: Siemens Ag
Stock Symbol: SI
Traded On: NYSE
Produces/Sells CE-marked Devices: N

SIEMENS HEALTHCARE DIAGNOSTICS, INC   800-242-3233
2040 Enterprise Blvd., West Sacramento, CA 95691
FDA Number: 2919016   *Fax:* 888-242-1997
Web site: http://diagnostics.siemens.com
Ownership: Siemens Ag
Stock Symbol: SI
Traded On: NYSE
Produces/Sells CE-marked Devices: N

Disc, Strip And Reagent, Microorganism Differentiation	Microbiology
Kit, Identification, Anaerobic	Microbiology
Kit, Yeast Screening	Microbiology
Panel, Identification, Gram Negative	Microbiology
Panel, Identification, Gram Positive	Microbiology
Test System, Antimicrobial Susceptibility, Automated	Microbiology

SIEMENS HEARING INSTRUMENTS, INC.   800-766-4500
10 Constitution Avenue, P.O. Box 1397,   **732-568-6600**
Piscataway, NJ 08855
FDA Number: 2217809   *Fax:* 732-562-6640
E-mail: customerservice@siemens-hearing.com
Web site: www.siemens-hearing.com
Medical Products Sales Volume: $63,700,000
Year Founded: 1882
Total Employees: 357
Ownership: Siemens Ag
Stock Symbol: SI
Traded On: NYSE
Quality System Registration Information: ISO9001
Produces/Sells CE-marked Devices: Y
Federal Procurement Eligibility: Small Business
Distribution: Manufacturer Through Distributor
General Admin.: Christi M. Pedra/President, Chief Executive Officer

Audiometer	Ear/Nose/Throat
Battery, Hearing-Aid	Ear/Nose/Throat
Computer Software	General
Hearing-Aid	Ear/Nose/Throat
System, Analysis, Hearing-Aid	Ear/Nose/Throat

SIEMENS KWU INC.
See Siemens Medical

SIEMENS MED. LABS., INC.
See Siemens Medical Solutions Usa, Inc

SIEMENS MEDICAL   732-590-5441
186 Wood Ave. S., 2nd Floor, Iselin, NJ 08830
FDA Number: n/a   *Fax:* 732-590-5475
Web site: www.medical.siemens.com
Total Employees: 27000
Ownership: Public
Produces/Sells CE-marked Devices: Y
Distribution: Manufacturer Direct
General Admin.: Horst Langer/Chairman, Chief Executive Officer
     Aldert Hoser/President

Hearing-Aid	Ear/Nose/Throat

Medical Product Subsidiaries (Listed Separately)

SIEMENS MEDICAL   732-590-5441 *(cont'd)*
Nokia Siemens Networks
Siemens Credit Corp.
Siemens Medical Systems, Inc., Nuclear Med. Group

SIEMENS MEDICAL CORP.
See Siemens Medical Solutions Usa, Inc.

SIEMENS MEDICAL SOLUTIONS HEALTH   800-888-7436
SERVICES CORP.

215 N. Admiral Byrd Road,   801-539-4600
Salt Lake City, UT 84116
FDA Number: n/a
E-mail: medseriesfour@smed.com
Web site: www.smed.com
Medical Products Sales Volume: $7,600,000
Year Founded: 1989
Ownership: Public
Stock Symbol: SI
Traded On: NASDAQ
Produces/Sells CE-marked Devices: N
Federal Procurement Eligibility: Small Business
Distribution: Manufacturer Direct

Computer Software	General
Computer Software, Hospital/Nursing Management	General
Computer, Bar Code	General
Computer, Clinical Laboratory	Chemistry
Computer, Patient Data Management	General
Service, Computer	General

SIEMENS MEDICAL SOLUTIONS HEALTH   888-321-1777
SERVICES DIVISION

51 Valley Stream Pkwy, Malvern, PA 19355   888-826-9702
FDA Number: 2530132   Fax: 610-448-1534
E-mail: usa.med@siemens.com
Web site: www.medical.siemens.com
Ownership: Siemens Ag
Stock Symbol: SI
Traded On: NYSE
Produces/Sells CE-marked Devices: N

Monitor, Physiological, Patient(without Arrhythmia Detection Or Alarms)	Cardiovascular
Software, Blood Bank (Stand-Alone Products)	Hematology

SIEMENS MEDICAL SOLUTIONS USA, INC   888-826-9702
2500 Millbrook Dr., Suite B, Buffalo Grove, IL 60089
FDA Number: 3006814109
E-mail: usa.med@siemens.com
Web site: www.medical.siemens.com
Ownership: Siemens Ag
Stock Symbol: SI
Traded On: NYSE
Produces/Sells CE-marked Devices: N

Scanner, Ultrasonic (Pulsed Doppler)	Radiology
Scanner, Ultrasonic (Pulsed Echo)	Radiology
System, Imaging, Laparoscopy, Ultrasonic	Radiology
Transducer, Ultrasonic, Diagnostic	Radiology

SIEMENS MEDICAL SOLUTIONS USA, INC   888-826-9702
400 W. Morgan Road, Suite 100, Ann Arbor, MI 48108
FDA Number: 1836549
E-mail: usa.med@siemens.com
Web site: www.medical.siemens.com
Ownership: Siemens Ag
Stock Symbol: SI
Traded On: NYSE
Produces/Sells CE-marked Devices: N

Image Processing System	Radiology

SIEMENS MEDICAL SOLUTIONS USA, INC   888-826-9702
51 Valley Stream Parkway, Malvern, PA 19355   610-448-4153
FDA Number: 2910081
Web site: www.medical.siemens.com
Total Employees: 150
Ownership: Siemens Ag
Stock Symbol: SI
Traded On: NYSE
Quality System Registration Information: ISO9001
Produces/Sells CE-marked Devices: Y
Distribution: Manufacturer Direct, Importer
General Admin.: Mr. Donald Rucker/Chief Medical Officer, Vice President
    Mr. Robert H. Bea/Chief Operating Officer, Vice President
    Holger Schmidt/President
    Mr. Heinrich Kolem/President
    Mr. Erich R. Reinhardt/President, Chief Executive Officer
    Mr. Marc Lauterbach/Senior Chairman
    Mr. Kulin Hemani/Vice President
    Laura Timmons/Vice President Human Resources
Mktg./Adv.: Colleen Smith/Manager Advertising

SIEMENS MEDICAL SOLUTIONS USA, INC   888-826-9702 *(cont'd)*
   Ingrid Padilla/Manager Media
   Mr. Jeff Kloss/Manager National Sales
   Mr. Guillaume Grousset/Senior Mktg Manager
   Mr. Gordon M. Rice/Senior Vice President Sales
   Terry Moore/Vice President Business Development
   Ms. Ursula Sieberg/Vice President Market Development
   Mr. Martin Forbes/Vice President Sales
Production: Roland Betz/Director Quality Assurance
Research: Joerg Stein/Vice President Product Development
Finance: Ms. Julie Bourgeois/Controller

Accelerator, Linear, Medical	Radiology
Block, Beam Shaping, Radionuclide	Radiology
Couch, Radiation Therapy, Powered	Radiology
Facility, Equipment, Medical, Mobile	General
Simulator, Radiotherapy, Special Purpose	Radiology
System, Planning, Radiation Therapy Treatment	Radiology
Table, Examination/Treatment	General

SIEMENS MEDICAL SOLUTIONS USA, INC   888-826-9702
Pony Farm Industrial Park, 139 Commerce Rd,
Oneonta, NY 13820
FDA Number: n/a
E-mail: usa.med@siemens.com
Web site: www.medical.siemens.com
Ownership: Siemens Ag
Stock Symbol: SI
Traded On: NYSE
Produces/Sells CE-marked Devices: N

Nuclear Magnetic Resonance Imaging System	Radiology

SIEMENS MEDICAL SOLUTIONS USA, INC.   610-448-3184
20 Valley Stream Pkwy, Malvern, PA 19355
FDA Number: 3002329443
Web site: www.medical.siemens.com
Ownership: Siemens Ag
Stock Symbol: SI
Traded On: NYSE
Produces/Sells CE-marked Devices: N

SIEMENS MEDICAL SOLUTIONS USA, INC.   865-218-2534
203 Dunavant Drive, Rockford, TN 37853
FDA Number: 3006365753
Web site: www.medical.siemens.com
Ownership: Siemens Ag
Stock Symbol: SI
Traded On: NYSE
Produces/Sells CE-marked Devices: N

SIEMENS MEDICAL SOLUTIONS USA, INC.   847-304-7700
2501 North Barrington Road, Hoffman Estates, IL 60192
FDA Number: 1423253   Fax: 847-304-7701
E-mail: usa.med@siemens.com
Web site: www.medical.siemens.com
Ownership: Siemens Ag
Stock Symbol: SI
Traded On: NYSE
Produces/Sells CE-marked Devices: N
General Admin.: Dr. Heinrich Kolem/Chief Executive Officer
    Mr. Donald Rucker/Chief Medical Officer, Vice President
    Ms. Janet Dillione/Chief Operating Officer
    Mr. Heinrich Kolem/President, Chief Executive Officer
Finance: Mr. Klaus P Stegemann/Chief Financial Officer

Camera, Gamma (Nuclear/Scintillation)	Radiology
Collimator, Radiographic, Manual	Radiology
Image Processing System	Radiology
Nuclear Magnetic Resonance Spectroscopic System	Radiology
Radiographic/Fluoroscopic Unit, Angiographic	Radiology
Scanner, Computed Tomography, X-Ray, Special Procedure	Radiology
Scanner, Emission Computed Tomography	Radiology
Scanner, Nuclear, Tomographic	Radiology

SIEMENS MEDICAL SOLUTIONS USA, INC.   865-218-2534
3100 Stockcreek Blvd, Rockford, TN 37853
FDA Number: 3006365759
Web site: www.medical.siemens.com
Ownership: Siemens Ag
Stock Symbol: SI
Traded On: NYSE
Produces/Sells CE-marked Devices: N

Scanner, Computed Tomography, X-Ray (CAT, CT)	Cns/Neurology
Scanner, Emission Computed Tomography	Radiology

SIEMENS MEDICAL SOLUTIONS USA, INC.   888-826-9702
51 Valley Stream Parkway,   610-448-4500
Malvern, PA 19355
FDA Number: 3002329443
E-mail: usa.med@siemens.com   Fax: 610-448-2554

MANUFACTURER PROFILES

Web site: www.medical.siemens.com
Medical Products Sales Volume: $1,400,000
Total Employees: 5000
Ownership: Siemens Ag
Stock Symbol: SI
Traded On: NYSE
Quality System Registration Information: ISO9000; ISO9001; ISO9002
Produces/Sells CE-marked Devices: N
Distribution: Manufacturer Direct, Importer
General Admin.: Mr. Donald Rucker/Chief Medical Officer, Vice President
Mr. Robert H. Bea/Chief Operating Officer, Vice President
Dr. Heinrich Kolem/President
Dr. Erich R Reinhardt/President, Chief Executive Officer
Mktg./Adv.: Mr. Rick Legleiter/Senior Vice President Customer Relations
Mr. Gordon M. Rice/Senior Vice President Sales

Accelerator, Linear, Medical	Radiology
Aligner, Beam, X-Ray (Collimator)	Dental And Oral
Aperture, Radiographic	Radiology
Aspirator, Ultrasonic	Obstetrics/Gynecology
Battery, Mobile Radiographic Unit	Radiology
Calibrator Source, Nuclear Sealed	Radiology
Camera, Gamma (Nuclear/Scintillation)	Radiology
Camera, Television, Microsurgical (With Audio)	Surgery
Camera, Television, Microsurgical (Without Audio)	Surgery
Camera, Videotape, Surgical	Surgery
Camera, X-Ray, Fluorographic, Cine Or Spot	Radiology
Cart, Multipurpose	General
Changer Programmer, Radiographic Film/Cassette	Radiology
Changer, Cassette, Radiographic	Radiology
Changer, Film, Radiographic	Radiology
Changer, Radiographic Film/Cassette	Radiology
Cineangiograph (Cardiac Catheterization)	Radiology
Collimator, Radiographic, Automatic	Radiology
Collimator, Radiographic, Manual	Radiology
Collimator, Therapeutic X-Ray, Orthovoltage	Radiology
Collimator, X-Ray	Dental And Oral
Component, Electronic	General
Computer, Cardiac Catheterization Laboratory	Cardiovascular
Computer, ECG Interpretation (Arrhythmia)	Cardiovascular
Computer, Nuclear Medicine	Radiology
Computer, Patient Data Management	General
Computer, Patient Monitor	Anesthesiology
Computer, Radiographic Data	Radiology
Computer, Radiographic Image Analysis	Radiology
Computer, Stress Exercise	Cardiovascular
Computer, Ultrasound	Radiology
Cradle, Patient, Radiographic	Radiology
Cradle, Radiographic, Powered	Radiology
Cyclotron	Radiology
Defibrillator, Line-Powered	Cardiovascular
Defibrillator/Monitor, Line-Powered	Cardiovascular
Dental Laboratory Equipment	Dental And Oral
Detector, Arrhythmia Alarm	Cardiovascular
Detector, Blood Flow, Ultrasonic (Doppler)	Cardiovascular
Device, Limiting, Beam, Diagnostic, X-Ray	Radiology
Device, Limiting, Beam, Teletherapy	Radiology
Device, Limiting, Beam, Teletherapy, Radionuclide	Radiology
Doppler, Blood Flow, Transcranial	Cardiovascular
Echocardiograph (Ultrasonic Scanner)	Cardiovascular
Electrocardiograph, Interpretive	Cardiovascular
Electrocardiograph, Multi-Channel	Cardiovascular
Electrocardiograph, Single Channel	Cardiovascular
Electrosurgical Unit, Anesthesiology Accessories	Surgery
Electrosurgical Unit, Dental	Dental And Oral
Electrosurgical Unit, General Purpose (ESU)	Surgery
Exerciser, Nuclear Diagnostic (Cardiac Stress Table)	Radiology
Filter, Radiographic	Radiology
Gantry, Nuclear Imaging	Radiology
Generator, Diagnostic X-Ray, High Voltage, 3-Phase	Radiology
Generator, Diagnostic X-Ray, High Voltage, Single Phase	Radiology
Generator, High Voltage, X-Ray, Therapeutic	Radiology
Generator, Therapeutic X-Ray, Orthovoltage	Radiology
Grid, Radiographic	Radiology
Hanger, X-Ray Tube	Radiology
Holder, Head, Radiographic	Radiology
Holder, Radiographic Cassette, Wall-Mounted	Radiology
Holder, X-Ray Film	Dental And Oral
Holder, X-Ray Film Cassette, Vertical	Radiology
Housing, X-Ray Tube, Diagnostic	Radiology
Housing, X-Ray Tube, Therapeutic	Radiology
Image Intensification System	Radiology
Instrument, Microsurgical	Cns/Neurology
Kit, Biopsy, Ultrasonic Aspiration	General
Lamp, Operating Room	General
Lamp, Surgical	Surgery
Light, Surgical, Ceiling Mounted	Surgery
Lithotriptor, Extracorporeal Shock-wave, Urological	Gastroenterology/Urology
Lithotriptor, Extracorporeal, Gallstone	Gastroenterology/Urology
Lithotriptor, Ultrasonic	Gastroenterology/Urology
Microscope, Operating, AC-Powered, Ophthalmic	Ophthalmology

Microscope, Surgical	Ear/Nose/Throat
Microscope, Surgical, General & Plastic Surgery	Surgery
Microscope, Surgical, Neurosurgical	Cns/Neurology
Monitor, Blood Pressure, Indirect (Arterial)	Cardiovascular
Monitor, Blood Pressure, Indirect, Anesthesiology	Anesthesiology
Monitor, Blood Pressure, Indirect, Automatic	Cardiovascular
Monitor, Blood Pressure, Indirect, Semi-Automatic	Cardiovascular
Monitor, Blood Pressure, Indirect, Surgery	Surgery
Monitor, Blood Pressure, Indirect, Surgery, Powered	Surgery
Monitor, Blood Pressure, Indirect, Transducer	Anesthesiology
Monitor, Blood Pressure, Invasive (Arterial)	Cardiovascular
Monitor, Blood Pressure, Invasive (Arterial), Anesthesia	Anesthesiology
Monitor, Blood Pressure, Venous	Cardiovascular
Monitor, Cardiac (Cardiotachometer & Rate Alarm)	Cardiovascular
Monitor, Cardiac Output, Dye (Central Venous & Arterial)	Surgery
Monitor, Cardiac Output, Thermal (Balloon Type Catheter)	Surgery
Monitor, Cardiac Output, Trend (Arterial Pressure Pulse)	Surgery
Monitor, ECG	Cardiovascular
Monitor, ECG, Ambulatory, Real-Time	Cardiovascular
Monitor, ECG, Anesthesia	Anesthesiology
Monitor, ECG, Arrhythmia	Cardiovascular
Monitor, ECG, Surgery	Surgery
Monitor, EEG	Cns/Neurology
Monitor, Fetal Doppler Ultrasound	Obstetrics/Gynecology
Monitor, Heart Rate, R-Wave (ECG)	Cardiovascular
Monitor, Neonatal, Physiological	Obstetrics/Gynecology
Monitor, Physiological, Acute Care	Anesthesiology
Monitor, Physiological, Cardiac Catheterization	Cardiovascular
Monitor, Physiological, Stress Exercise	Cardiovascular
Monitor, Pressure, Cardiac, Ventricular	Cardiovascular
Monitor, Pulse Rate	Anesthesiology
Monitor, X-Ray Tube	Radiology
Mount, Surgical Microscope	Surgery
Mount, X-Ray Tube, Diagnostic	Radiology
Nuclear Magnetic Resonance Imaging System	Radiology
Phantom, Flood Source, Nuclear	Radiology
Phonocardiograph	Cardiovascular
Phototimer, Radiographic Mobile	Radiology
Probe, Transesophageal	Cardiovascular
Probe, Ultrasonic	Radiology
Probe, Uptake, Nuclear	Radiology
Radiographic Picture Archiving/Communication System (PACS)	Radiology
Radiographic Unit, Diagnostic	Radiology
Radiographic Unit, Diagnostic, Chest	Radiology
Radiographic Unit, Diagnostic, Dental (X-Ray)	Dental And Oral
Radiographic Unit, Diagnostic, Dental, Extraoral	Dental And Oral
Radiographic Unit, Diagnostic, Fixed (X-Ray)	Radiology
Radiographic Unit, Diagnostic, Head	Radiology
Radiographic Unit, Diagnostic, Intraoral	Dental And Oral
Radiographic Unit, Diagnostic, Mammographic	Radiology
Radiographic Unit, Diagnostic, Mobile, Explosion-Safe	Radiology
Radiographic Unit, Diagnostic, Photofluorographic	Radiology
Radiographic Unit, Diagnostic, Polytomographic	Radiology
Radiographic Unit, Diagnostic, Portable (X-Ray)	Radiology
Radiographic Unit, Diagnostic, Skeletal	Radiology
Radiographic Unit, Diagnostic, Tomographic	Radiology
Radiographic Unit, Digital	Radiology
Radiographic Unit, Digital Subtraction Angiographic (DSA)	Radiology
Radiographic/Fluoroscopic Unit, Angiographic	Radiology
Radiographic/Fluoroscopic Unit, Angiographic, Digital	Radiology
Radiographic/Fluoroscopic Unit, Fixed	Radiology
Radiographic/Fluoroscopic Unit, Image-Intensified	Radiology
Radiographic/Fluoroscopic Unit, Mobile C-Arm	Radiology
Radiographic/Fluoroscopic Unit, Special Procedure	Radiology
Radiotherapy Treatment Planning Unit	Radiology
Recorder, Radiographic Video Tape	Radiology
Recorder, X-Ray Image	Radiology
Scanner, Computed Tomography, X-Ray (CAT, CT)	Cns/Neurology
Scanner, Computed Tomography, X-Ray, Full Body	Radiology
Scanner, Computed Tomography, X-Ray, Head	Radiology
Scanner, Computed Tomography, X-Ray, Special Procedure	Radiology
Scanner, Emission Computed Tomography	Radiology
Scanner, Magnetic Resonance (NMR/MRI)	Radiology
Scanner, Nuclear Emission Computed Tomography (ECT)	Radiology
Scanner, Nuclear, Rectilinear	Radiology
Scanner, Nuclear, Tomographic	Radiology
Scanner, Positron Emission Tomography (PET)	Radiology
Scanner, Ultrasonic (Pulsed Doppler)	Radiology
Scanner, Ultrasonic (Pulsed Echo)	Radiology
Scanner, Ultrasonic, Abdominal	Radiology
Scanner, Ultrasonic, Breast (Mammographic)	Obstetrics/Gynecology
Scanner, Ultrasonic, General Purpose	Radiology
Scanner, Ultrasonic, Obstetrical/Gynecological	Obstetrics/Gynecology
Scanner, Ultrasonic, Obstetrical/Gynecological, Mobile	Obstetrics/Gynecology
Scanner, Ultrasonic, Other	Radiology
Scanner, Ultrasonic, Pediatric	Radiology
Scanner, Ultrasonic, Small Parts	Radiology
Scanner, Ultrasonic, Vascular	Radiology
Screen, Intensifying, Radiographic	Radiology
Simulator, Radiotherapy	Radiology
Spot Film Device	Radiology

SIEMENS MEDICAL SOLUTIONS USA, INC. 888-826-9702 *(cont'd)*

Stretcher, Radiographic	Radiology
Support, Patient Position, Radiographic	Radiology
Synchronizer, Nuclear Camera	Radiology
System, Recording, Data, Anesthesiology	Anesthesiology
System, X-Ray, Mobile	Radiology
Table, Operating Room, AC-Powered	Surgery
Table, Operating Room, Mechanical	Surgery
Table, Radiographic	Radiology
Table, Radiographic, Non-Tilting, Powered	Radiology
Table, Radiographic, Tilting	Radiology
Table, Surgical With Orthopedic Accessories, AC-Powered	Surgery
Table, Surgical, Electrical	Surgery
Table, Surgical, Orthopedic	Orthopedics
Table, Urological (Cystological)	Gastroenterology/Urology
Table, Urological, Radiographic	Gastroenterology/Urology
Telemetry Unit, Physiological, ECG	Cardiovascular
Television Monitor, Microscope	General
Television Monitor, Operating Room	General
Therapeutic X-Ray System	Radiology
Transducer, Ultrasonic	Cardiovascular
Transducer, Ultrasonic, Diagnostic	Radiology
Transducer, Ultrasonic, Intravaginal	Obstetrics/Gynecology
Transducer, Ultrasonic, Obstetrical	Obstetrics/Gynecology
Transmitter/Receiver System, Physiological, Radiofrequency	Cardiovascular
Tube, Image Amplifier, X-Ray	Radiology
Tube, X-Ray	Radiology
Ventilator, Anesthesia Unit	Anesthesiology
Ventilator, Continuous (Respirator)	Anesthesiology
Ventilator, High-Frequency	Anesthesiology
Ventilator, Neonatal Respirator	General
Ventilator, Volume (Critical Care)	Anesthesiology

SIEMENS MEDICAL SOLUTIONS USA, INC. 650-969-9112
ULTRASOUND DIVISION

1230 Shorebird Way, Mountain View, CA 94039-7393
FDA Number: 2936884   *Fax:* 650 968 1833
E-mail: usa.med@siemens.com
Web site: www.medical.siemens.com
Ownership: Siemens Ag
Stock Symbol: SI
Traded On: NYSE
Produces/Sells CE-marked Devices: N
General Admin.: Mr. Robert H. Bea/Chief Operating Officer, Vice President
          Mr. Klaus Hambuechen/President
Mktg./Adv.: Mr. Rick Legleiter/Senior Vice President Customer Relations
          Mr. Gordon M. Rice/Supervisor Sales
          Mr. Arnd Kaldowski/Vice President Marketing & Sales

Catheter, Intravascular, Diagnostic	Cardiovascular
Scanner, Ultrasonic (Pulsed Doppler)	Radiology
Scanner, Ultrasonic (Pulsed Echo)	Radiology
Transducer, Ultrasonic, Diagnostic	Radiology

SIEMENS MEDICAL SOLUTIONS USA, 888-826-9702
MOLECULAR IMAGING

810 Innovation Dr, Knoxville, TN 37932-2571
FDA Number: 1034973   *Fax:* 865-218-3000
Web site: www.medical.siemens.com
Ownership: SIEMENS AG
Stock Symbol: SI
Traded On: NYSE
Produces/Sells CE-marked Devices: N

Calibrator Source, Nuclear Sealed	Radiology
Image Processing System	Radiology
Scanner, Emission Computed Tomography	Radiology

SIEMENS MEDICAL SYSTEMS, INC. 800-437-2437

16 Electronics Ave., Danvers, MA 01923
FDA Number: n/a
E-mail: usa.med@siemens.com
Web site: www.medical.siemens.com
Ownership: Public
Stock Symbol: SI
Traded On: NYSE
Quality System Registration Information: ISO9001
Produces/Sells CE-marked Devices: N
Distribution: Manufacturer Direct

Analyzer, Gas, Oxygen, Continuous Monitor	Anesthesiology
Circuit, Breathing, Ventilator	Anesthesiology
Computer Equipment	General
Monitor, Bed Patient	General
Ventilator, Other	Anesthesiology

SIEMENS MEDICAL SYSTEMS, INC., NUCLEAR 847-304-7700
MED. GROUP

2501 N. Barrington Road, Hoffman Estates, IL 60195
FDA Number: 1423253   *Fax:* 847-304-7701
E-mail: usa.med@siemens.com
Web site: www.medical.siemens.com

SIEMENS MEDICAL SYSTEMS, INC., NUCLEAR 847-304-7700
(cont'd)
Medical Products Sales Volume: $1,400,000
Year Founded: 1861
Ownership: Siemens Medical
Stock Symbol: SI
Traded On: NYSE
Quality System Registration Information: ISO9000; ISO9001
Produces/Sells CE-marked Devices: Y
Federal Procurement Eligibility: Small Business
Distribution: Manufacturer Direct, OEM, Exporter

Camera, Gamma (Nuclear/Scintillation)	Radiology
Computer, Nuclear Medicine	Radiology
Scanner, Positron Emission Tomography (PET)	Radiology

SIEMENS MEDICAL SYSTEMS, INC., 800-964-4114
ULTRASOUND GROUP

22010 S.E. 51st St., Issaquah, WA 98029
FDA Number: 3023245
E-mail: usa.med@siemens.com
Web site: www.medical.siemens.com
Ownership: Siemens Ag
Stock Symbol: SI
Traded On: NYSE
Quality System Registration Information: ISO9001
Produces/Sells CE-marked Devices: Y
Distribution: Manufacturer Direct, Manufacturer Through Distributor, Manufacturer Through Manufacturer Reps, Importer, Exporter

Analyzer, Ultrasonic Unit	General
Scanner, Ultrasonic (Pulsed Doppler)	Radiology
Scanner, Ultrasonic (Pulsed Echo)	Radiology
Scanner, Ultrasonic, General Purpose	Radiology
Scanner, Ultrasonic, Other	Radiology
Scanner, Ultrasonic, Pediatric	Radiology
Scanner, Ultrasonic, Small Parts	Radiology
Scanner, Ultrasonic, Vascular	Radiology
Stimulator, Growth, Bone, Electromagnetic, Dental	Dental And Oral

SIEMENS MEDICAL SYSTEMS, ONCOLOGY CARE SYSTEMS
See Siemens Medical Solutions Usa, Inc

SIEMENS WATER TECHNOLOGIES 978-614-7359

10875 Kempwood, Houston, TX 77043
FDA Number: 1648705
E-mail: information.water@siemens.com
Web site: www.water.siemens.com
Ownership: Public
Stock Symbol: SI
Traded On: NYSE
Produces/Sells CE-marked Devices: N

System, Water Purification, General Medical Use	Gastroenterology/Urology

SIEMENS WATER TECHNOLOGIES 866-926-8420
1335 Ford St., Colorado Springs, CO 80915 978-614-7359
FDA Number: 1723687
E-mail: information.water@siemens.com
Web site: www.water.siemens.com
Ownership: Public
Stock Symbol: SI
Traded On: NYSE
Produces/Sells CE-marked Devices: N

System, Water Purification, General Medical Use	Gastroenterology/Urology

SIEMENS WATER TECHNOLOGIES 866.926.8420

1700 East 28th St., Signal Hill, CA 90807
FDA Number: 2029022
E-mail: information.water@siemens.com
Web site: www.water.siemens.com
Ownership: Public
Stock Symbol: SI
Traded On: NYSE
Produces/Sells CE-marked Devices: N

System, Water Purification, General Medical Use	Gastroenterology/Urology

SIEMENS WATER TECHNOLOGIES 866-926-8420

6125 Guion Rd., Indianapolis, IN 46254
FDA Number: 3004057358
E-mail: information.water@siemens.com
Web site: www.water.siemens.com
Ownership: Public
Stock Symbol: SI
Traded On: NYSE
Produces/Sells CE-marked Devices: N

System, Water Purification, General Medical Use	Gastroenterology/Urology

SIEMENS WATER TECHNOLOGIES 866-926-8420

6550 Trade Center Dr., Jacksonville, FL 32254
FDA Number: 1064564
E-mail: information.water@siemens.com

SIEMENS WATER TECHNOLOGIES — 866-926-8420 (cont'd)

Web site: www.water.siemens.com
Ownership: Public
Stock Symbol: SI
Traded On: NYSE
Produces/Sells CE-marked Devices: N
  System, Water Purification, General Medical Use   Gastroenterology/Urology

SIEMENS WATER TECHNOLOGIES — 866-926-8420

960 Ames Avenue, Milpitas, CA 95035   **408-946-1520**
FDA Number: 3004158969
E-mail: information.water@siemens.com
Web site: www.water.siemens.com
Ownership: Public
Stock Symbol: SI
Traded On: NYSE
Produces/Sells CE-marked Devices: N
  System, Water Purification, General Medical Use   Gastroenterology/Urology

SIEMENS, STROMBERG - CARLSON

See Nokia Siemens Networks

SIEMENS-PACESETTER INC.

See St. Jude Medical Cardiac Rhythm Management Div.

SIENCO, INC. — 800-432-1624

7985 Vance Drive, Suite 104, Arvada, CO 80003   **303-420-1148**
FDA Number: 9200981   *Fax:* 303-379-4403
E-mail: sienco@sienco.com
Web site: www.sienco.com
Annual Revenue: $0-$1 Million
Total Employees: 5   *Marketing Staff:* 1   *Sales Staff:* 2
Ownership: Private
Produces/Sells CE-marked Devices: Y
Federal Procurement Eligibility: Small Business
Distribution: Manufacturer Direct, Manufacturer Through Distributor, Exporter
General Admin.: Barbara DeBiase/Director
    Jon Henderson/President
Production: John Feicht/Director Manufacturing
  Activated Whole Blood Clotting Time   Hematology
  Analyzer, Coagulation, Automated   Hematology
  Stirrer   Chemistry

SIENTRA, INC — 888-423-7600

11220 Grader St., Suite 100, Dallas, TX 75238   **214-348-1571**
FDA Number: 1651189   *Fax:* 214-348-1855
E-mail: info@sientra
Web site: www.sientra.com
Medical Products Sales Volume: $400,000
Year Founded: 1997
Ownership: Private
Stock Symbol: CVD
Traded On: NYSE
Quality System Registration Information: ISO9000; ISO9001; ISO9002
Produces/Sells CE-marked Devices: N
Federal Procurement Eligibility: Small Business
Distribution: Manufacturer Through Distributor, Manufacturer Through
Manufacturer Reps, Exclusive Distributor
  Splint, Nasal   Ear/Nose/Throat

SIERRA MOLECULAR INC. — 209-536-0886

21109 Longeway Rd. # C, Sonora, CA 95370
FDA Number: 2953142
  Kit, Identification, Neisseria Gonorrhoeae   Microbiology
  Reagent, General Purpose   Pathology
  Transport System, Aerobic   Microbiology

SIERRA SCIENTIFIC INSTRUMENTS, INC. — 310-641-8492

5757 Century Blvd., Suite 660, Los Angeles, CA 90045
FDA Number: 3005344223
  Analyzer, Motility, Gastrointestinal, Electrical   Gastroenterology/Urology

SIGMA INSTRUMENTS, INC. — 724-776-9500

506 Thomson Park Dr., Cranberry Township, PA 16066
FDA Number: 2531782
  Plunger-Like Joint Manipulator   Physical Med

SIGMA INTERNATIONAL, LLC. — 800-356-3454

711 Park Avenue, Medina, NY 14103-0756   **585-798-3901**
FDA Number: 1314492   *Fax:* 585-798-3909
E-mail: customersupport@sigmapumps.com
Web site: www.sigmapumps.com
Medical Products Sales Volume: $6,600,000
Annual Revenue: $5-$10 Million
Year Founded: 1992
Total Employees: 75   *Marketing Staff:* 2   *Sales Staff:* 8
Ownership: Private
Produces/Sells CE-marked Devices: N
Federal Procurement Eligibility: Small Business, GSA Contract, VA Contract

SIGMA INTERNATIONAL, LLC. — 800-356-3454 (cont'd)

Distribution: Manufacturer Direct, Manufacturer Through Distributor, Manufacturer
Through Manufacturer Reps, OEM, Exporter
General Admin.: Roger Hungerford/President, Chief Executive Officer
    Michelle Klotzbach/Vice President Human Resources
Mktg./Adv.: Bill Fithian/Director National Accounts
    Kathy Wolski/Manager Sales Training
    David Wolski/Vice President Marketing & Sales
Production: Gary Lawton/Director Quality Assurance & Regulatory Affairs
    David Feltz/Manager Materials
    Gary Lawton/Manager Regulatory Affairs
    Matt Rich/Vice President Manufacturing
  Pump, Infusion   General

SIGMA PRODUCTS LTD. — 845-778-4200

2274 Albany Post Road, Walden, NY 12586
FDA Number: n/a   *Fax:* 845-778-4199
E-mail: sigmanet@frontiernet.net
Web site: www.conefor.com
Medical Products Sales Volume: $400,000
Year Founded: 1983
Total Employees: 2
Ownership: Public
Federal Procurement Eligibility: Small Business
Distribution: Manufacturer Through Distributor, OEM, Importer
General Admin.: Steven Fodor/President
  Electrode, Electrosurgical, Active, Foot Controlled   Surgery
  Electrode, Electrosurgical, Return (Ground, Dispersive)   Surgery

SIGMA-ALDRICH CORP. — 800-521-8956

3050 Spruce St., St. Louis, MO 63103   **314-771-5765**
FDA Number: 1938173   *Fax:* 314-771-5757
E-mail: sig-ald@sial.com
Web site: www.sigmaaldrich.com
Annual Revenue: $50-$100 Million
Ownership: Public
Stock Symbol: SIAL
Traded On: NASDAQ
Quality System Registration Information: ISO9000; ISO9001
Produces/Sells CE-marked Devices: N
Distribution: Manufacturer Direct
General Admin.: Rakesh Sachdev/Chief Financial Officer, Senior Vice President
    Jai Nagarkatti/President, Chief Executive Officer, Chairman
    Doug Rau/Vice President Human Resources
Mktg./Adv.: Mr. Gerrit J.C. van den Dool/Vice President Sales
Finance: Kirk Richter/Vice President, Treasurer
  Contract Manufacturing   General
  Lipase-Esterase, Enzymatic, Photometric, Lipase   Chemistry
  Sterilizer, Loop, Inoculating   Microbiology
  Vial, Liquid Scintillation Counting   Chemistry
Medical Product Subsidiaries (Listed Separately)
  Fluka Chemie Ag
  Sigma-Aldrich Chemie Steinheim/Albuch Gmbh

SIGMA-ALDRICH MANUFACTURING, LLC — 314-286-6600

3500 Dekalb St., St. Louis, MO 63118
FDA Number: 1943967
  Phosphatase, Acid   Hematology

SIGMA-ALDRICH MANUFACTURING, LLC. — 913-469-5580

3506 South Broadway, St. Louis, MO 63118
FDA Number: 1937991
  Culture Media, Synthetic Cell And Tissue   Pathology
  Solution, Balanced Salt   Pathology

SIGMACON HEALTH PRODUCTS CORP. — 800-898-7455

436 Limestone Crescent,   **416-665-6616**
North York, ON M3J 2 Canada
FDA Number: n/a   *Fax:* 416-665-8395
E-mail: info@sigmacon.com
Web site: www.sigmacon.com
Total Employees: 25   *Marketing Staff:* 3   *Sales Staff:* 3
Ownership: Private
Produces/Sells CE-marked Devices: Y
Federal Procurement Eligibility: Small Business
Distribution: Exclusive Distributor

SIGMAMOTOR INC.

See Sigma International, Llc.

SIGNAL MEDICAL CORP. — 810-364-7070

400 Pyramid Dr., Marysville, MI 48040
FDA Number: 1836001
Ownership: Private
Produces/Sells CE-marked Devices: N
  Prosthesis, Hip, Semi-Const., Metal/Ceramic/Ceramic, Cem.   Orthopedics
  Prosthesis, Hip, Semi-Const., Metal/Poly., Porous Uncemented   Orthopedics
  Prosthesis, Toe, Hemi-, Phalangeal   Orthopedics

SIGNAL MEDICAL CORPORATION
800-246-6324
314-775-0518
1000 Des Peres Road, Suite 140,
St. Louis, MO 63131
FDA Number: 1932213
Fax: 314-775-0524
E-mail: whiteside@whitesidebio.com
Web site: www.whitesidebio.com
Annual Revenue: $1-$5 Million
Year Founded: 1992
Total Employees: 4
Ownership: Private
Quality System Registration Information: ISO9001
Produces/Sells CE-marked Devices: Y
Federal Procurement Eligibility: Small Business
Distribution: Manufacturer Direct, Manufacturer Through Manufacturer Reps
General Admin.: Leo Whiteside/Chief Executive Officer
　　Debbie Latorre/Office Manager
Production: Ms. Michelle Himmelmann/Customer Service Representative
　　Mr. Brian Katerberg/Engineer

Blade, Surgical, Saw, General & Plastic Surgery	Surgery
Cable	Physical Med
Immobilizer, Knee	Orthopedics
Joint, Hip, External Limb Component	Physical Med
Prosthesis, Femoral Head	Orthopedics
Prosthesis, Hip (Metal Stem/Ceramic Self-Locking Ball)	Orthopedics
Retractor	Orthopedics
Screw, Fixation, Bone	Orthopedics
Support, Knee	Physical Med

SIGNET ARMORLITE, INC.
760-744-4000
1001 Armorlite Dr., San Marcos, CA 92069
FDA Number: 2022060

Lens, Spectacle (prescription), For Reading Discomfort	Ophthalmology
Lens, Spectacle/Eyeglasses, Non-Custom	Ophthalmology

SIGNET PATHOLOGY SYSTEMS, INC.
See Covance Research Products Inc.

SIGVARIS CORPORATION
800-363-4999
514-336-2362
4535 Dobrin,
Ville St-Laurent, QUE H4R 2 Canada
FDA Number: n/a
Fax: 514-336-8736
Web site: www.sigvaris.com
Year Founded: 1988
Ownership: Private
Produces/Sells CE-marked Devices: N
Distribution: Exclusive Distributor

SIGVARIS INC.
800-322-7744
770-631-1778
1119 Hwy. 74 S., Peachtree City, GA 30269
FDA Number: n/a
Fax: 800-481-5488
E-mail: clair.ford@ganzoni.com
Web site: www.sigvarisusa.com
Ownership: Ganzoni Gmbh
Produces/Sells CE-marked Devices: N
Distribution: Manufacturer Through Distributor
General Admin.: Charles E. Handschin/President, Chief Executive Officer
Mktg./Adv.: Michael Leonard/Director Product Development
　　Ms. Clair Ford/Marketing Communications Specialist

Stocking, Elastic	General

SIHI PUMPS INC.
See Sterling Fluid Systems (Usa)

SILICON KINETICS
858-646-5444
10455 Pacific Center Court, San Diego, CA 92121
FDA Number: n/a
Fax: 858-646-5401
E-mail: infosk@siliconkinetics.com
Web site: http://www.siliconkinetics.com
Year Founded: 2002
Ownership: Private
Produces/Sells CE-marked Devices: N
General Admin.: Mr. Hus Tigli/Chief Executive Officer
Research: Dr. John Ervin/Director Research & Engineering

SILIPOS INC.
800-229-4404
716-283-0700
704 Williams Road, Niagara Falls, NY 14304
FDA Number: 2435506
Fax: 716-283-0600
E-mail: saksmarketing@silipos.com
Web site: www.silipos.com
Medical Products Sales Volume: $38,000,000
Annual Revenue: $25-$50 Million
Year Founded: 1989
Total Employees: 75
Sales Staff: 20
Ownership: Private
Quality System Registration Information: ISO9001
Produces/Sells CE-marked Devices: Y
Federal Procurement Eligibility: Small Business
Distribution: Manufacturer Through Distributor, Manufacturer Through Manufacturer Reps, OEM

SILIPOS INC.
800-229-4404 *(cont'd)*
General Admin.: Joel E. Bickel/Chief Executive Officer
　　Richard Greco/President
　　Eileen Burkett/Vice President Human Resources
　　Marcy Zasucha/Vice President, General Manager
Mktg./Adv.: Alf Steinbach/Director Marketing
　　Peter Bickel/Director National Accounts
　　Robert Govid/Director Product Development
　　Francine Fishman/Manager Advertising
　　Brian Sinder/Manager Contract Sales
　　Robert Mogel/Manager International & National Sales
　　Peter Sciacca/Manager Market Research
　　Lewis Freeman/Manager National Sales
　　David Arnoio/Manager Sales Training
　　Richard Melchner/Vice President Business Development
　　Allison Jennings/Vice President Marketing
　　Gisela Pena/Vice President Sales
Production: Pam Netal/Director Quality Assurance
　　Tom Roman/Manager Materials
　　Claire France/Manager Regulatory Affairs
　　Robert Kalinek/Vice President Manufacturing
Research: Robert Corbett/Vice President Research & Development

Cushion, Wheelchair (Pad)	Physical Med
Dressing, Other	General

Medical Product Subsidiaries (Listed Separately)
Geligne Medical

SILMED, INC.
435-753-7307
97 West 300 South, Millville, UT 84326-0438
FDA Number: 3003603914
Ownership: Private
Produces/Sells CE-marked Devices: N

Button, Nasal Septal	Ear/Nose/Throat

SILOR OPTICAL OF FLORIDA, INC.
See Essilor Of America, Inc.

SILTRON EMERGENCY SYSTEMS
800-874-3392
815-459-7142
290 E. Prairie, Crystal Lake, IL 60014
FDA Number: n/a
Fax: 815-459-6126
E-mail: info@siltron.com
Annual Revenue: $1-$5 Million
Total Employees: 50
Marketing Staff: 4
Sales Staff: 4
Ownership: Private
Produces/Sells CE-marked Devices: N
Distribution: Manufacturer Through Manufacturer Reps, Exporter
General Admin.: Nick Shaw/President

Light, Other	General

SILTRON ILLUMINATION, INC.
See Siltron Emergency Systems

SILVER BAY, LLC
941-306-5812
1431 Tallevast Rd., Sarasota, FL 34243
FDA Number: 3006182559

Lamp, Infrared	Physical Med

SILVER EAGLE LABS INC.
650-522-9700
204 W. Spear Street, Carson City, NV 89703
FDA Number: 3005940466

Dilator, Nasal	Ear/Nose/Throat

SILVER RING SPLINT CO.
434-971-4052
1140 East Market St., Charlottesville, VA 22902
FDA Number: 1122273

Splint, Hand, And Component	Physical Med

SILVER STAR MOBILITY
800-555-4385
541-857-5012
578 Mason Way, Medford, OR 97501
FDA Number: n/a
Fax: 541-857-5160
E-mail: info@silverstarmobility.com
Web site: www.silverstarmobility.com
Medical Products Sales Volume: $100,000
Annual Revenue: $1-$5 Million
Year Founded: 1989
Total Employees: 3
Marketing Staff: 2
Sales Staff: 4
Ownership: Silver Star Mobility
Quality System Registration Information: ISO9001
Produces/Sells CE-marked Devices: N
Federal Procurement Eligibility: Small Business
Distribution: Manufacturer Through Distributor
General Admin.: Dennis Mortimore/President, Chief Executive Officer
Mktg./Adv.: David Mortimore/Vice President Marketing & Sales
Production: Sara Davis/Customer Service Representative
　　Scotty Butler/Customer Service Representative
　　Yvette Crume/Customer Service Representative
　　Steve Herzog/Vice President Manufacturing
　　Jeff Phebus/Vice President Quality Assurance & Quality Control
IS: Lance Griffen/Tech. Specialist

SILVER STAR MOBILITY   800-555-4385 *(cont'd)*
    Lift, Wheelchair   General
    Medical Product Subsidiaries (Listed Separately)
    Silver Star Mobility

SILVERGLIDE SURGICAL TECHNOLOGIES   303-444-1970
    5398 Manhattan Circle, Suite 120, Boulder, CO 80303
    FDA Number: 1724439   *Fax:* 303-444-6273
    Year Founded: 1997
    Electrosurgical Unit, Cutting & Coagulation Device   Surgery
    Tray, Surgical Instrument   Surgery

SILVERPLATTER EDUCATION, INC.
    See Healthstream, Inc.

SILVERSTONE PACKAGING, INC.-YOUR ONE   800-413-1108
STOP SUPPLIER
    1401 Lakeland Avenue, Bohemia, NY 11716   **631-244-2630**
    FDA Number: n/a   *Fax:* 631-244-2638
    E-mail: info@silverstonepackaging.com
    Web site: www.silverstonepackaging.com
    Annual Revenue: $1-$5 Million
    Year Founded: 2002
    Total Employees: 5   *Marketing Staff:* 1   *Sales Staff:* 4
    Ownership: Private
    Produces/Sells CE-marked Devices: N
    Federal Procurement Eligibility: Small Business
    Distribution: Manufacturer Through Distributor
    Bag, Garbage   General
    Ball, Cotton   General
    Dispenser, Soap   General
    Glove, Other   General
    Glove, Patient Examination, Vinyl   General
    Mask, Face   General
    Packaging Material   General
    Tape, Adhesive   General
    Towel/Towelette, Paper   General

SIM INC.
    See Surgical Instrument Manufacturers, Inc.

SIM MEDICAL SALES   574-268-0341
    PO BOX 0895, Warsaw, IN 46581
    FDA Number: n/a
    E-mail: info@simmedicalsales.com
    Web site: www.simmedicalsales.com
    Medical Products Sales Volume: $1,000,000
    Annual Revenue: $0-$1 Million
    Ownership: Private
    Produces/Sells CE-marked Devices: N
    Federal Procurement Eligibility: Small Business
    Distribution: Manufacturer Through Manufacturer Reps
    Bit, Drill   Orthopedics
    Blade, Bone Cutting   Orthopedics
    Blade, Surgical, Saw, General & Plastic Surgery   Surgery
    Burr   Ear/Nose/Throat
    Burr, Cranial   Cns/Neurology
    Burr, Orthopedic   Orthopedics
    Burr, Other   Surgery
    Burr, Podiatric   Orthopedics

SIM NET, INC.   804-752-2776
    10471 Cobbs Rd., Glen Allen, VA 23059
    FDA Number: n/a   *Fax:* 804-752-2864
    E-mail: simnetinc3@aol.com
    Web site: www.simnetinc.com
    Ownership: Private
    Produces/Sells CE-marked Devices: N
    Radiographic Unit, Diagnostic   Radiology
    Radiographic Unit, Diagnostic, Tomographic   Radiology
    Simulator, Radiotherapy, Special Purpose   Radiology

SIM-KAR LIGHTING FIXTURE
    See Simkar Corporation

SIMBEX, LLC   603-448-2367
    10 Water Street, Room 410, Lebanon, NH 03766
    FDA Number: 3003647304
    Prosthesis Alignment Device   Physical Med
    Treadmill, Powered   Physical Med

SIMKAR CORPORATION   800-523-3602
    700 Ramona, Philadelphia, PA 19120-4691   **215-831-7700**
    FDA Number: 9200984   *Fax:* 215-831-7703
    E-mail: lighting@simkar.com
    Web site: www.simkar.com
    Annual Revenue: $1-$5 Million
    Total Employees: 550   *Marketing Staff:* 2   *Sales Staff:* 7
    Ownership: Private
    Produces/Sells CE-marked Devices: N
    Distribution: Manufacturer Through Distributor

SIMKAR CORPORATION   800-523-3602 *(cont'd)*
    General Admin.: Bill Eagle/President
    Mktg./Adv.: Ken Bopf/Director National Accounts
         Bud Drago/Manager Advertising
         Anne Young/Manager Exports
         Bart Lawrence/Manager Marketing
    Production: Joe Mroz/Director Quality Assurance
    Lamp, Other   General
    Light, Other   General
    Light, Overbed   General

SIMMLER, INC.   800-325-0786
    4564 North Square Dr., P.O. Box 350,   **636-376-8347**
    High Ridge, MO 63049
    FDA Number: 1950226   *Fax:* 636-376-8324
    E-mail: simmler@primary.net
    Web site: www.simmler.com
    Medical Products Sales Volume: $1,000,000
    Annual Revenue: $0-$1 Million
    Total Employees: 4   *Marketing Staff:* 1   *Sales Staff:* 1
    Ownership: Private
    Produces/Sells CE-marked Devices: N
    Federal Procurement Eligibility: Small Business, Female Owned
    Distribution: Manufacturer Direct
    General Admin.: T. Joyce Erb/President, Chief Executive Officer
         Dave Kremer/Vice President
    Mktg./Adv.: Dave Kremer/Director Product Development
    Stain, Fetal Hemoglobin   Hematology

SIMMONS HEALTHCARE, INC.
    See Gf Health Products, Inc

SIMON & COMPANY INC., H.R.   800-638-9460
    3515 Marmenco Ct., Baltimore, MD 21230-3411   **410-636-5555**
    FDA Number: n/a   *Fax:* 410-636-4415
    E-mail: sales@hrsimon.com
    Web site: www.hrsimon.com
    Medical Products Sales Volume: $8,000,000
    Total Employees: 45   *Marketing Staff:* 3   *Sales Staff:* 7
    Ownership: Private
    Produces/Sells CE-marked Devices: N
    Federal Procurement Eligibility: Small Business
    Distribution: Manufacturer Through Distributor, Importer, Exporter
    General Admin.: H. R. Simon/President
    Mktg./Adv.: Jason M. Simon/Vice President Marketing
    Chemical, Film Processor   Radiology
    Film, X-Ray   Radiology
    Mixer, Chemical, Film, X-Ray   Radiology
    Processor, Cine Film   Radiology
    Processor, Radiographic Film, Automatic   Radiology
    Processor, Radiographic Film, Automatic, Dental   Dental And Oral

SIMON & SIMON MOBILITY SERVICES   210-614-1414
    9207 Huebner Rd., San Antonio, TX 78240
    FDA Number: 3003106692
    Cushion, Wheelchair (Pad)   Physical Med

SIMON DECHATLET LABS   952-541-9622
    4484 North Dixie Drive, Dayton, OH 45414
    FDA Number: n/a
    Ownership: Private
    Produces/Sells CE-marked Devices: N
    Mouthguard   Dental And Oral

SIMPEX MEDICAL, INC.   800-851-9753
    401 E. Prospect Ave., Mount Prospect, IL 60056
    FDA Number: 3025266   *Fax:* 800-705-8443
    E-mail: info@simpexmedical.com
    Web site: www.simpexmedical.com
    Year Founded: 1991
    Ownership: Private
    Produces/Sells CE-marked Devices: N
    Federal Procurement Eligibility: Small Business
    Distribution: Manufacturer Direct, Manufacturer Through Distributor, Exporter
    Mktg./Adv.: Richard Gorski/Manager International & National Sales
         Sue V. Magee/Manager National Sales
    Bit, Drill   Orthopedics
    Container, Sterilization (Tray)   General
    Cutter, Wire And Pin   Orthopedics
    Drill, Bone   Orthopedics
    Pin, Fixation, Smooth   Orthopedics
    Pin, Fixation, Threaded   Orthopedics
    Wire, Bone   Orthopedics

SIMPLE ORTHOPAEDIC SOLUTIONS, LLC   317-414-1558
    9337 North 700 East, Darlington, IN 47940
    FDA Number: 3005047044
    Ownership: Private
    Produces/Sells CE-marked Devices: N

SIMPLE ORTHOPAEDIC SOLUTIONS, LLC 317-414-1558 (cont'd)
Accessories, Operating Room, Table — Surgery

SIMPLE SLANT 828-245-8962
1218 Spooky Hollow Rd., Marion, NC 28752
FDA Number: 3004822523
Ownership: Private
Produces/Sells CE-marked Devices: N
Table, Mechanical — Physical Med

SIMPLER IMPLANTS INC. 800-565-3559
Suite 404-1023 Wolfe Ave., (604) 736-9890
Vancouver, BC V6H 1 Canada
FDA Number: n/a
E-mail: simpler@simplerimplants.com Fax: (606) 736-9747
Web site: www.simplerimplants.com
Year Founded: 1987
Total Employees: 10
Ownership: Private
Produces/Sells CE-marked Devices: N
Distribution: Manufacturer Direct, Exclusive Distributor

SIMPLEXGRINNELL LP 800-746-7539
50 Technology Dr, 978-731-2500
Westminster, MA 01441
FDA Number: n/a
Web site: www.simplexgrinnell.com Fax: 978-731-7856
Ownership: Private
Produces/Sells CE-marked Devices: N
Distribution: Manufacturer Direct
Clock, Elapsed Time — General
Physician Registry — General
Recorder, Transient — General

SIMPLICITY ORTHOPEDIC SOLUTIONS, LLC 866-623-0033
77 Main St., Second Floor, Andover, MA 01810
FDA Number: n/a
E-mail: info@simplicityortho.com
Web site: www.simplicityortho.com
Ownership: Private
Produces/Sells CE-marked Devices: N
Screw, Fixation, Bone — Orthopedics

SIMPLIFIED SYSTEMS, INC. 305-672-7676
4014 Chase Ave., Ste. P.H., Miami, FL 33140-3421
FDA Number: n/a
Web site: http://thecommunicatorfl.com
Medical Products Sales Volume: $1,000,000
Annual Revenue: $0-$1 Million
Ownership: Private
Produces/Sells CE-marked Devices: N
Federal Procurement Eligibility: Small Business
Distribution: Manufacturer Through Distributor
Communication Equipment — General
Scaler, Ultrasonic — Dental And Oral

SIMPLOMATIC MANUFACTURING CO. 773-342-7757
816 N. Kostner Ave., Chicago, IL 60651-3423
FDA Number: n/a Fax: 773-342-8329
E-mail: info@simplomatic.com
Web site: www.simplomatic.com
Annual Revenue: $0-$1 Million
Total Employees: 70 Marketing Staff: 4 Sales Staff: 4
Ownership: Private
Produces/Sells CE-marked Devices: N
Federal Procurement Eligibility: Female Owned
Distribution: Manufacturer Direct
General Admin.: Pat V. DiBenedetto/General Manager
Jo Anne Cippola/President
Mktg./Adv.: David Hahn/Vice President Marketing & Sales
Equipment, Extruding/Molding — General
Production Equipment — General

SIMPLY CLEAN AIR & WATER, INC. 860-231-0687
28 Shepard Drive, Newington, CT 06131
FDA Number: 3004114902
Purification System, Water — Gastroenterology/Urology

SIMPORT PLASTICS LTD. 450-464-1723
2588 Bernard-Pilon, Beloeil, QUE J3G 4S5 Canada
FDA Number: 8020301 Fax: 450-464-3394
E-mail: info@simport.com
Web site: www.simport.com
Year Founded: 1975
Total Employees: 200 Marketing Staff: 3 Sales Staff: 7
Ownership: Private
Produces/Sells CE-marked Devices: Y
Federal Procurement Eligibility: Small Business

SIMPORT PLASTICS LTD. 450-464-1723 (cont'd)
Distribution: Manufacturer Through Distributor, Exporter

SIMPSON ELECTRIC CO. 715-588-3311
520 Simpson Avenue, PO Box 99,
Lac du Flambeau, WI 54538
FDA Number: 9200988 Fax: 715-588-3326
E-mail: rbarma@simpsonelectric.com
Web site: www.simpsonelectric.com
Medical Products Sales Volume: $10,000,000
Year Founded: 1934
Total Employees: 130 Marketing Staff: 6 Sales Staff: 15
Ownership: Private
Federal Procurement Eligibility: Minority Owned, GSA Contract
Distribution: Manufacturer Through Distributor, OEM, Exporter
General Admin.: Edward Herter/President
Mktg./Adv.: Ron Barma/Manager Advertising
Saul Mariasis/Manager International Marketing & Sales
Jack Femmel/Manager National Sales
Production: Libby Schulz/Manager Production
Detector, Microwave Leakage — General
Dosimeter, Radiation — Radiology
Generator, Electronic Noise (For Audiometric Testing) — Ear/Nose/Throat
Meter, Leakage Current (Ammeter) — General
Monitor, Temperature (With Probe) — Anesthesiology
Pyrometer — General
Recorder, Long-Term, Trend — General
Thermometer, Electronic — General
Voltmeter — Chemistry

SIMS DELTEC, INC.
See Smiths Medical Asd, Inc.

SIMULAIDS, INC. 800-431-4310
16 Simulaids Drive, PO Box 1289, 845-679-2475
Saugerties, NY 12477
FDA Number: 1317199
E-mail: info@simulaids.com Fax: 845-679-8996
Web site: www.simulaids.com
Medical Products Sales Volume: $1,000,000
Annual Revenue: $10-$25 Million
Year Founded: 1999
Total Employees: 93 Marketing Staff: 2 Sales Staff: 2
Ownership: Public
Stock Symbol: ARTL
Traded On: NASDAQ
Produces/Sells CE-marked Devices: Y
Federal Procurement Eligibility: Small Business, GSA Contract
Distribution: Manufacturer Through Distributor
Mktg./Adv.: Greg Zindulka/Manager Product Development
Production: Jane Boice/Manager Materials
Jack McNeff/Vice President Operations
Stretcher, Hand-Carried — General
Training Manikin, CPR (Resuscitation) — General
Training Manikin, Intravenous Arm — General
Training Manikin, Other — General
Training Manikin, Wound Moulage — General

SINGER MEDICAL PRODUCTS INC., MD SYSTEMS DIV. 630-860-6500
3800 Buckner, El Paso, TX 79925
FDA Number: 1419974
Ownership: Private
Produces/Sells CE-marked Devices: N
Audiometer — Ear/Nose/Throat
Electrode, Needle — Cns/Neurology
Stimulator, Nerve, ENT — Ear/Nose/Throat
Tester, Auditory Impedance — Ear/Nose/Throat

SINGER MEDICAL PRODUCTS, INC. 800-222-2572
790 Maple Lane, Bensenville, IL 60106-1513 630-860-6500
FDA Number: n/a Fax: 630-860-3672
Annual Revenue: $5-$10 Million
Year Founded: 1986
Total Employees: 6 Sales Staff: 2
Ownership: Private
Produces/Sells CE-marked Devices: N
Federal Procurement Eligibility: Small Business
Distribution: Manufacturer Direct, Manufacturer Through Manufacturer Reps
General Admin.: Theodore Singer/President, Chief Executive Officer
Mktg./Adv.: Deborah Singer/Director Marketing
Production: Bob Brown/Manager Materials
Audiometer — Ear/Nose/Throat
Stimulator, Nerve Locating — Cns/Neurology
Tester, Auditory Impedance — Ear/Nose/Throat

SINGLETON CORP.
888-456-0643
3280 W. 67th Place, Cleveland, OH 44102
216-651-7800
FDA Number: n/a
Fax: 216-651-4247
Web site: www.singletoncorp.com
Annual Revenue: $0-$1 Million
Ownership: Private
Produces/Sells CE-marked Devices: N
Federal Procurement Eligibility: Small Business, Female Owned
Distribution: Manufacturer Direct, Manufacturer Through Manufacturer Reps, Exporter

Chamber, Constant Temperature (Environmental)	Microbiology

SINOVUS BIOTECH, INC.
631-924-1135
3661 Horseblock Road, Medford, NY 11763
FDA Number: n/a
Fax: 631-924-6033
E-mail: info@sinovus.com
Web site: www.sinovus.com
Total Employees: 70
Ownership: Chembio Diagnostic Systems, Inc.
Federal Procurement Eligibility: Small Business
Distribution: Manufacturer Direct, Manufacturer Through Distributor
General Admin.: Lawrence Siebert/Chairman
Tomas Haendler/President
Mktg./Adv.: Avi Pelossof/Director Marketing
Javan Esfandiari/Director Product Development
Production: Karen Keskinen/Director Quality Assurance

SINTIES SCIENTIFIC, INC.
See Scifit

SIPPICAN, INC.
See Polaris Contract Services, A Division Of Sippicon, Inc.

SIRCHIE FINGER PRINT LABORATORIES
800-356-7311
100 Hunter Place, Youngsville, NC 27596
919-554-2244
FDA Number: 1055300
Fax: 919-554-2266
E-mail: sirchieinfo@sirchie.com
Web site: www.sirchie.com
Annual Revenue: $5-$10 Million
Year Founded: 1927
Ownership: Private
Produces/Sells CE-marked Devices: N
Federal Procurement Eligibility: Small Business
Distribution: Manufacturer Direct, Manufacturer Through Distributor, Manufacturer Through Manufacturer Reps, Importer, Exporter

Alcohol Breath Trapping Device	Toxicology
Kit, Forensic Evidence	Pathology
Kit, Forensic Evidence, Sexual Assault	Obstetrics/Gynecology
Kit, Screening, Urine	Microbiology
System, Test, Drugs of Abuse	Chemistry

SIRIUS GENOMICS INC.
604-484-7195
1125 Howe Street, Suite 603, Vancouver, BC V6Z 2K8 Canada
FDA Number: n/a
Fax: 604-484-7190
E-mail: cwagner@siriusgenomics.com
Web site: http://www.siriusgenomics.com
Year Founded: 2001
Ownership: Private
Produces/Sells CE-marked Devices: N

SIRONA DENTAL SYSTEMS INC.
718-482-2011
30-30 47th Avenue, Suite 500, Long Island City, NY 11101
FDA Number: n/a
Fax: 718-937-5962
E-mail: contact@sirona.com
Web site: www.sirona.com
Year Founded: 1877
Ownership: Public
Stock Symbol: SIRO
Traded On: NASDAQ
Produces/Sells CE-marked Devices: N
General Admin.: Simone Blank/Chief Financial Officer, Executive Vice President
Jeffrey T. Slovin/Chief Operating Officer, Executive Vice President
Mr. Theo Haar/Executive Vice President
Jost Fischer/President, Chief Executive Officer, Chairman

SIRONA DENTAL SYSTEMS LLC
800-659-5977
4835 Sirona Drive, Suite 100,
704-587-0453
Charlotte, NC 28273
FDA Number: 1064812
Fax: 704-587-9394
E-mail: marketing@sirona.com
Web site: www.sirona.com
Annual Revenue: $500 Million-$1 Billion
Total Employees: 2280
Ownership: Private
Stock Symbol: SIRO
Traded On: NASDAQ
Produces/Sells CE-marked Devices: N
Distribution: Manufacturer Through Distributor

SIRONA DENTAL SYSTEMS LLC
800-659-5977 *(cont'd)*
General Admin.: Ms. Simone Blank/Chief Financial Officer, Executive Vice President
Mr. Jeffrey T. Slovin/Chief Operating Officer, Executive Vice President
Theo Haar/Executive Vice President
Mr. Jost Fischer/President, Chief Executive Officer, Chairman
Finance: Mr. Nicholas W. Alexos/Director Finance

Film, X-Ray, Dental, Extraoral	Dental And Oral

SIRONA USA, LLC
See Sirona Dental Systems Llc

SISBRO INTERNATIONAL TECHNOLOGY, INC.
See Spi Sports/Science Inc.

SISTEMAS MEDICOS ALARIS
858-458-7000
Ave. Ferrocarril No. 16y17y18, Km. 14 1/2 Centro Ind. Limon,
Tijuana, Bc. - Mexico
FDA Number: 9616066
Ownership: Private
Produces/Sells CE-marked Devices: N

SITA ASSOCIATES
630-968-3727
720 Williamsburg Court, Oak Brook, IL 60523
FDA Number: 1419306
Ownership: Private
Produces/Sells CE-marked Devices: N

Chromatographic Separation, Lecithin-Sphingomyelin Ratio	Chemistry
Lowry (Colorimetric), Total Protein	Chemistry
Reagent, Creatinine (Test System)	Chemistry

SKEDCO, INC.
503-639-2119
16420 S.W. 72nd Avenue, PO Box 230487, Portland, OR 97281
FDA Number: n/a
Fax: 503-639-4538
E-mail: skedco@skedco.com
Web site: www.skedco.com
Annual Revenue: $1-$5 Million
Year Founded: 1981
Ownership: Private
Produces/Sells CE-marked Devices: Y
Federal Procurement Eligibility: Small Business, Minority Owned, Female Owned, GSA Contract
Distribution: Manufacturer Direct, Manufacturer Through Distributor, OEM, Exporter
General Admin.: Hang Lee Calkin/Chief Executive Officer
Bud Calkin/Vice President, General Manager

Board, Spine	Orthopedics
Cushion, Flotation	Physical Med
Rescue Equipment	General
Stretcher, Emergency, Other	General
Stretcher, Hand-Carried	General

SKELETAL KINETICS, LLC
408-366-5000
10201 Bubb Rd., Cupertino, CA 95014
FDA Number: 3003890476

Dispenser, Cement	Orthopedics
Filler, Calcium Sulfate Preformed Pellets	Orthopedics
Metacrylate, Methyl, Cranioplasty	Cns/Neurology

SKIL-CARE CORP.
800-431-2972
29 Wells Avenue, Yonkers, NY 10701-6605
914-963-2040
FDA Number: 2431497
Fax: 914-963-2567
E-mail: customerservice@skil-care.com
Web site: www.skil-care.com
Medical Products Sales Volume: $10,200,000
Annual Revenue: $10-$25 Million
Year Founded: 1978
Total Employees: 125 *Marketing Staff:* 4 *Sales Staff:* 34
Ownership: Private
Produces/Sells CE-marked Devices: Y
Federal Procurement Eligibility: Small Business, GSA Contract
Distribution: Manufacturer Direct, Manufacturer Through Distributor, Exporter
General Admin.: Arnold Silverman/President
Martin Prenske/Vice President
Mktg./Adv.: Dan Jungwirth/Manager National Sales
Production: Stephen Warren/Vice President Production

Accessories, Wheelchair	Physical Med
Bag, Drainage (Incontinence)	Gastroenterology/Urology
Clothing, Protective	General
Cover, Bedrail	General
Cushion, Wheelchair (Pad)	Physical Med
Holder, Catheter	Gastroenterology/Urology
Protector, Skin Pressure	General
Restraint, Protective (Body)	General

SKIN DEEP, INC.
215-728-1035
1926 Cottman Ave., Philadelphia, PA 19111
FDA Number: 2523747
Ownership: Private

SKIN DEEP, INC.   215-728-1035 *(cont'd)*
Produces/Sells CE-marked Devices: N
  Epilator, High-Frequency, Needle-Type   Surgery

SKINNER INC., J.J.
See Merit Medical Systems Inc.

SKINSCIENCE LABS, INC.   212-265-4600
330 West 58th St., Suite 211, New York, NY 10019
FDA Number: 3004427935
Ownership: Private
Produces/Sells CE-marked Devices: N
  Brush, Dermabrasion   Surgery

SKYNDEX BIO-MEDICAL SYSTEMS INC.
See Caldwell, Justiss & Co., Inc.

SKYTRON   800-759-8766
5085 Corporate Exchange Blvd. S.E.,   616-656-2900
Grand Rapids, MI 49512
FDA Number: 1825014   *Fax:* 616-656-1563
E-mail: sales@skytron.us
Web site: www.skytron.us
Year Founded: 1972
Total Employees: 100
Ownership: Private
Produces/Sells CE-marked Devices: N
Federal Procurement Eligibility: Small Business
Distribution: Manufacturer Through Distributor, OEM
General Admin.: Dave Mehney/President
Mktg./Adv.: Mike Breslin/Director National Accounts
       Randy Tomaszewski/Vice President Marketing
       Tom Maher/Vice President, Manager Sales
  Cabinet, Table And Tray, Anesthesia   Anesthesiology
  Cabinet, Warming   General
  Examination Device, AC-Powered   General
  Lamp, Examination (Light)   General
  Lamp, Examination, Ceiling Mounted (Light)   General
  Lamp, Surgical   Surgery
  Light, Surgical, Ceiling Mounted   Surgery
  Radiographic Picture Archiving/Communication System (PACS)   Radiology
  Sink, Hospital   General
  System, Evacuation, Smoke, Laser   Surgery
  Table, Surgical, Electrical   Surgery
  Table, Surgical, Hydraulic   Surgery
  Washer/Disinfector   General

SKYWAY MACHINE, INC   530-243-5151
4451 Caterpillar Road, Redding, CA 96003
FDA Number: n/a   *Fax:* 530-243-5104
E-mail: sales@skywaytuffwheels.com
Web site: www.skywaytuffwheels.com
Annual Revenue: $1-$5 Million
Year Founded: 1963
Total Employees: 15   *Marketing Staff:* 2   *Sales Staff:* 3
Ownership: Private
Produces/Sells CE-marked Devices: N
Federal Procurement Eligibility: Small Business, GSA Contract
Distribution: Manufacturer Direct, Manufacturer Through Distributor, OEM, Service Direct, Exporter
General Admin.: Mrs. Lynne Cross/Admin. Human Resources
       Mr. Kenneth Coster/President, Chief Executive Officer
Mktg./Adv.: Mr. Parrey Cremeans/Manager Sales
       Mr. Bart Weems/Sales Associate
  Accessories, Wheelchair   Physical Med

SLAWNER LTD., J.   514-731-3378
5713, ch. de la CA'te-des-Neiges,
Montreal, QUE H3S 1 Canada
FDA Number: n/a   *Fax:* 514-731-4571
E-mail: info@slawner.com
Medical Products Sales Volume: $2,900,000
Total Employees: 35   *Marketing Staff:* 3   *Sales Staff:* 10
Ownership: Private
Produces/Sells CE-marked Devices: N
Federal Procurement Eligibility: Small Business
Distribution: Manufacturer Direct, Service Direct

SLEEP DEVICES, INC.   866-935-9166
506 West Cherry Street, Kissimmee, FL 34741   407-935-1008
FDA Number: 3004639925   *Fax:* 407-935-9750
E-mail: customerservice@sonapillow.com
Web site: http://sonapillow.com/
Medical Products Sales Volume: $100,000
Annual Revenue: $0-$1 Million
Year Founded: 2004
Total Employees: 6   *Marketing Staff:* 1   *Sales Staff:* 2
Ownership: Private
Produces/Sells CE-marked Devices: N

SLEEP DEVICES, INC.   866-935-9166 *(cont'd)*
Federal Procurement Eligibility: Small Business, Minority Owned
Distribution: OEM, Exclusive Distributor
Mktg./Adv.: Ms. Carol Sommers/Vice President Sales
  Pillow   General

SLEEP GROUP SOLUTIONS   305-830-0327
1875 Ne 168th Street, North Miami, FL 33162
FDA Number: 3007075845
Ownership: Private
Produces/Sells CE-marked Devices: N
  Rhinoanemometer (Measurement Of Nasal Decongestion)   Anesthesiology

SLEEP SAUNA
See Sleep Sauna, Inc.

SLEEP SAUNA, INC.   800-229-5210
608 13th Avenue, Council Bluffs, IA 51501   712-323-3269
FDA Number: n/a   *Fax:* 800-320-9612
E-mail: questions@delasco.com
Web site: www.sleepsauna.com
Ownership: Dermatologic Lab & Supply, Inc.
Produces/Sells CE-marked Devices: N
Federal Procurement Eligibility: Small Business, Female Owned
Distribution: Exclusive Distributor, Exporter
General Admin.: Eugene Friedman/President
Mktg./Adv.: Polly Friedman/Director Marketing & Sales
  Clothing, Protective   General

SLEEP SOLUTIONS, INC.
See NovaSom, Inc.

SLEEPMED INCORPORATED   800-334-5085
200 Corporate Place, Ste. 5-B,   978-536-7400
Peabody, MA 01960
FDA Number: n/a   *Fax:* 978-535-9778
E-mail: eegservices@sleepmed.md
Web site: www.sleepmed.md
Annual Revenue: $100-$500 Million
Total Employees: 650   *Marketing Staff:* 3   *Sales Staff:* 25
Ownership: Private
Produces/Sells CE-marked Devices: N
Distribution: Service Direct
General Admin.: David Lewis/President, Chief Executive Officer
Mktg./Adv.: Mary Safko/Vice President Corporate Marketing
       Mary Safko/Vice President Market Development
       Stuart Tuthill/Vice President Marketing & Product Development
       Dan Moore/Vice President National Marketing & Sales
Production: Nancy Foote/Director Quality Assurance
       Troy Roberts/Vice President Engineering & Product Development
Finance: Carl Iberger/Chief Financial Officer
       Joe Rose/Vice President Finance & Operations
  Camera, Video   General
  Monitor, EEG   Cns/Neurology
  Sleep Assessment Equipment   Cns/Neurology
Medical Product Subsidiaries (Listed Separately)
  Digitrace Care Services, Inc.

SLEEPNET CORPORATION   800-742-3646
5 Merrill Industrial Drive, Hampton, NH 03842   603-758-6600
FDA Number: 1222088   *Fax:* 603-758-6699
E-mail: sleepnet@sleep-net.com
Web site: www.sleep-net.com
Year Founded: 1989
Total Employees: 25   *Marketing Staff:* 1   *Sales Staff:* 5
Ownership: Private
Produces/Sells CE-marked Devices: Y
Federal Procurement Eligibility: Small Business
Distribution: Manufacturer Direct, Manufacturer Through Distributor, Manufacturer Through Manufacturer Reps
General Admin.: Tom Moulton/President, Chief Executive Officer
Mktg./Adv.: Mr. Frank Petruno/Director Sales
       Richard Kerry/Manager International & National Sales
       Deidre Christiansen/Marketing & Sales Representative
Production: Jennifer Kennedy/Director Quality Assurance
  Continuous Positive Airway Pressure Unit (CPAP, CPPB)   Anesthesiology
  Ventilator, Continuous (Respirator), Accessory   Anesthesiology
  Ventilator, Non-Continuous (Respirator)   Anesthesiology

SLIDE FREE LLC   601-213-3758
22 Lake Eddins 163815, Pachuta, MS 39347
FDA Number: 3006162801
  Cushion, Wheelchair (Pad)   Physical Med

SLM INSTRUMENTS, INC.
See Thermo Spectronic

SLOAN CORP.   800-782-3742
13316 A St., Omaha, NE 68144   402-597-5700
FDA Number: 1932271   *Fax:* 888-323-8565

SLOAN CORP.   800-782-3742 *(cont'd)*

E-mail: info@sloanco.com
Web site: www.sloanco.com
Ownership: Private
Produces/Sells CE-marked Devices: N

Accessories, Apparel, Surgical	Surgery
Cover, Shoe, Operating Room	Surgery
Gown, Surgical	Surgery
Suit, Surgical	Surgery

SLOAN VALVE CO.   800-9VA-LVE9
10500 Seymour Ave.,   **847-671-4300**
Franklin Park, IL 60131

FDA Number: n/a   *Fax:* 847-671-6944
E-mail: customer.service@sloanvalve.com
Web site: www.sloanvalve.com
Year Founded: 1906
Total Employees: 750
Ownership: Private
Produces/Sells CE-marked Devices: N
Distribution: Manufacturer Through Distributor, Manufacturer Through Manufacturer Reps
General Admin.: C. S. Allen/President, Chief Executive Officer
Mktg./Adv.: Susan Kennedy/Director Marketing
       Christine Nicosia/Director National Accounts
       Fred Hawley/Manager International Sales
       Ben Owen/Manager National Sales
Production: Bob Bednarz/Director Manufacturing

Building Material	General
Cleaner, Bedpan (Sterilizer)	General
Housekeeping Equipment	General
Scrub Machine, Surgical	Surgery

SM CO., SEIICHI MANUFACTURING
See Ultrascope

SMALL BEGINNINGS INC.   760-949-7707
17525 Alder Street, Suite 28, Hesperia, CA 92345

FDA Number: 2032476

Evacuator, Oral Cavity	Dental And Oral
Linen, Bed	General
Pad, Neonatal Eye	General

SMALL BONE INNOVATIONS, INC.   215-428-1791
1380 S. Pennsylvania Ave., Morrisville, PA 19067

FDA Number: 3003640913   *Fax:* 215-428-1795
E-mail: customerservice@totalsmallbone.com
Ownership: Private
Produces/Sells CE-marked Devices: N
General Admin.: Mr. Anthony Viscogliosi/Chief Executive Officer, Chairman
       Mr. Steve Ward/Chief Operating Officer, Chief Financial Officer
       Mr. Thomas Crowley/President
Mktg./Adv.: Mr. James Hook/Senior Vice President Sales

Bit, Drill	Orthopedics
Brace, Drill	Orthopedics
Broach	Orthopedics
Brush, Scrub, Operating Room	Surgery
Burr, Orthopedic	Orthopedics
Countersink	Orthopedics
Cutter, Wire And Pin	Orthopedics
Elevator, Surgical, General & Plastic Surgery	Surgery
Fixation Appliance, Multiple Component	Orthopedics
Forceps	Orthopedics
Forceps, General & Plastic Surgery	Surgery
Gauge, Depth	Orthopedics
Guide, Surgical, Instrument	Surgery
Impactor	Orthopedics
Orthopedic Manual Surgical Instrument	Orthopedics
Osteotome (Orthopedic)	Surgery
Pin, Fixation, Smooth	Orthopedics
Plate, Fixation, Bone	Orthopedics
Pliers, Orthodontic	Dental And Oral
Pliers, Surgical	Orthopedics
Prosthesis, Elbow, Hemi-, Radial, Polymer	Orthopedics
Prosthesis, Elbow, Semi-Constrained	Orthopedics
Prosthesis, Finger, Constrained, Metal/Polymer	Orthopedics
Prosthesis, Finger, Constrained, Polymer	Orthopedics
Prosthesis, Toe, Hemi-, Phalangeal	Orthopedics
Prosthesis, Wrist, 3 Part Metal-Plastic-Metal Articulation	Orthopedics
Prosthesis, Wrist, Carpal Trapezium	Orthopedics
Prosthesis, Wrist, Hemi-, Ulnar	Orthopedics
Rod, Fixation, Intramedullary	Orthopedics
Scaler, Periodontic	Dental And Oral
Screw, Fixation, Bone	Orthopedics
Screwdriver	Orthopedics
Surgical Instrument, Orthopedic, AC-Powered Motor	Orthopedics
Template	Orthopedics
Tray, Surgical	Surgery
Tray, Surgical Instrument	Surgery

SMALL BONE INNOVATIONS, INC.   (866) SBi-TIPS
1380 S. Pennsylvania Avenue,   **(215) 428-1791**
Morrisville, PA 19067

FDA Number: 3003640913   *Fax:* (215) 428-1795
E-mail: customerservice@totalsmallbone.com
Web site: www.totalsmallbone.com
Medical Products Sales Volume: $417,100
Annual Revenue: $0-$1 Million
Total Employees: 22   *Marketing Staff:* 4   *Sales Staff:* 4
Ownership: Private
Quality System Registration Information: ISO9001
Produces/Sells CE-marked Devices: Y
Distribution: Manufacturer Direct, Importer
General Admin.: J. J. Martin/Chief Executive Officer
       J. J. Martin/President
Mktg./Adv.: J. J. Martin/Director Marketing
       J. J. Martin/Manager International & National Sales
Production: J. P. Lescuyer/Vice President Manufacturing

Brace, Drill	Orthopedics
Broach	Orthopedics
Brush, Scrub, Operating Room	Surgery
Burr, Orthopedic	Orthopedics
Countersink	Orthopedics
Cutter, Wire And Pin	Orthopedics
Elevator, Surgical, General & Plastic Surgery	Surgery
Fixation Appliance, Multiple Component	Orthopedics
Forceps	Orthopedics
Gauge, Depth	Orthopedics
Guide, Surgical, Instrument	Surgery
Hammer, Surgical	Surgery
Impactor	Orthopedics
Joint, Shoulder, External Limb Component	Physical Med
Osteotome, Manual (Plastic Surgery)	Surgery
Pin, Fixation, Smooth	Orthopedics
Plate, Fixation, Bone	Orthopedics
Pliers, Orthodontic	Dental And Oral
Prosthesis, Elbow, Hemi-, Radial, Polymer	Orthopedics
Prosthesis, Elbow, Semi-Constrained	Orthopedics
Prosthesis, Finger	Orthopedics
Prosthesis, Toe, Hemi-, Phalangeal	Orthopedics
Prosthesis, Wrist, 3 Part Metal-Plastic-Metal Articulation	Orthopedics
Prosthesis, Wrist, Carpal Trapezium	Orthopedics
Prosthesis, Wrist, Hemi-, Ulnar	Orthopedics
Rasp, Bone	Orthopedics
Scaler, Periodontic	Dental And Oral
Screw, Fixation, Bone	Orthopedics
Screwdriver	Orthopedics
Staple, Fixation, Bone	Orthopedics
Template	Orthopedics
Tray, Surgical	Surgery

SMART MEDICAL TECHNOLOGY, INC   630-964-1689
8404 S. Wilmette Ave, Suite B, Darien, IL 60561

FDA Number: 3005643982

Lift, Patient	General

SMC LTD.   715-247-3500
360 Reed Street, Somerset, WI 54025

FDA Number: 3004595311
E-mail: inquiry@smcltd.com
Web site: http://www.smcltd.com
Year Founded: 1988
Ownership: Private
Produces/Sells CE-marked Devices: N

Exerciser, Non-Measuring	Physical Med
Perfusion System, Kidney	Gastroenterology/Urology

SMC MEDICAL MANUFACTURING DIVISION
See SMC Ltd.

SMC MEDICAL-TECH CORP.
See Venes Technology Corp.

SMEAD MANUFACTURING CO.   1-88-USE-SMEAD
600 Smead Blvd., Hastings, MN 55033-2219   **651-437-4111**

FDA Number: n/a   *Fax:* 800-959-9134
Web site: www.smead.com
Medical Products Sales Volume: $497,000,000
Year Founded: 1906
Total Employees: 2900   *Marketing Staff:* 21   *Sales Staff:* 53
Ownership: Private
Produces/Sells CE-marked Devices: N
Federal Procurement Eligibility: Female Owned
Distribution: Manufacturer Through Distributor
General Admin.: Sharon Avent/President
       Dean Schwanke/Vice President Human Resources
Mktg./Adv.: David Fasbender/Senior Vice President Sales
       Albert Arends/Vice President Marketing
       Thomas Sullivan/Vice President Sales
Production: Wally Glashan/Vice President Manufacturing

SMEAD MANUFACTURING CO.   1-88-USE-SMEAD *(cont'd)*

Computer Equipment	General
Office Product	General
Storage Unit, X-Ray Film	Radiology

SMI   920-876-3361

Industrial Park, 544 Sohn Drive, Elkhart Lake, WI 53020
FDA Number: 2183576   Fax: 920-876-2289
E-mail: sohn@excel.net
Web site: www.smi-div.com
Medical Products Sales Volume: $7,100,000
Year Founded: 1971
Total Employees: 85
Ownership: Private
Quality System Registration Information: ISO9001
Produces/Sells CE-marked Devices: N
Federal Procurement Eligibility: Small Business
Distribution: Manufacturer Direct
General Admin.: W. J. Beaudry/President
    Walter A. Daum/Vice President
Production: Paula Allen/Director Quality Assurance
    Timothy Leon/Manager Materials

Bandage, Adhesive	Surgery
Bandage, Butterfly	General
Contract Manufacturing	General
Cuff, Blood Pressure	Cardiovascular
Electrode, Electrosurgical, Return (Ground, Dispersive)	Surgery
Electrode, Gel	Cardiovascular
Electrode, TENS	Cns/Neurology
Patch, Transdermal	General
Strip, Test	Chemistry
Tape, Adhesive	General

SMILE BRITE DISTRIBUTING LLC   585-248-9260

5 Boughton Avenue, Pittsford, NY 14534
FDA Number: 3004553132

Cleaner, Denture	Dental And Oral
Cleaner, Denture, Mechanical	Dental And Oral

SMISSON-CARTLEDGE BIOMEDICAL   1-866-944-9992

487 Cherry St, Third Street Tower, Macon, GA 31201
FDA Number: 3006158088   Fax: 478-744-9996
E-mail: billy@t3med.com
Ownership: Private
Produces/Sells CE-marked Devices: N
Mktg./Adv.: Mr. Billy Williams/Vice President Sales

Pump, Infusion	General

SMITH & NEPHEW

See Smith & Nephew, Inc., Endoscopy Division

SMITH & NEPHEW CASTING & BANDAGING SA. DE CV   012-82-61774

Ave.de Los Encinos S/n Esq.ave, Del Parque,parque Ind. Villa, Florida, Reynosa Tamaulipas Mexico
FDA Number: 9612388

Bandage, Cast	Physical Med

SMITH & NEPHEW INC., ENDOSCOPY DIV.   978-749-1000

76 S. Meridian Ave., Oklahoma City, OK 73107-6512
FDA Number: 1643264
Web site: www.endo.smith-nephew.com
Ownership: SMITH & NEPHEW PLC.
Stock Symbol: SN
Traded On: London
Produces/Sells CE-marked Devices: N

Accessories, Surgical Camera	Surgery
Arthroscope	Orthopedics
Camera, Television, Endoscopic (Without Audio)	Surgery
Component, Traction, Non-Invasive	Orthopedics
Device, Communications, Images, Ophthalmic	Ophthalmology
Device, Storage, Image, Digital	Radiology
Electrosurgical Unit, Cutting & Coagulation Device	Surgery
Endoscope	Gastroenterology/Urology
Image Processing System	Radiology
Insufflator, Laparoscopic	Obstetrics/Gynecology
Laparoscope, General & Plastic Surgery	Surgery
Laparoscope, Gynecologic	Obstetrics/Gynecology
Light Source, Endoscope, Xenon Arc	Surgery
Monitor, Infusion, Gravity Flow	General
Pump, Infusion	General
Radiographic/Fluoroscopic Unit, Image-Intensified	Radiology
Surgical Instrument, Orthopedic, Battery-Powered	Surgery
Traction Unit, Non-Powered	Orthopedics

SMITH & NEPHEW INC.- ORTHOPAEDICS DIVISION   800-238-7538

1450 Brooks Rd., Memphis, TN 38116   **901-399-5081**
FDA Number: 1020279   Fax: 901-332-7289
Web site: global.smith-nephew.com

SMITH & NEPHEW INC.- ORTHOPAEDICS   800-238-7538 *(cont'd)*

Medical Products Sales Volume: $1,598,000,000
Annual Revenue: More than $1 Billion
Total Employees: 9190
Ownership: Smith & Nephew, Inc.
Stock Symbol: SN
Traded On: London
Quality System Registration Information: ISO9000; ISO9001; ISO9002
Produces/Sells CE-marked Devices: N
Distribution: Manufacturer Direct, Manufacturer Through Distributor, Manufacturer Through Manufacturer Reps
General Admin.: David J. Illingworth/Chief Executive
    James A. Ralston/Chief Legal Officer
    Elizabeth Bolgiano/Director Human Resources
    R. Gordon Howe/Senior Vice President Planning and Development
Medical Admin.: Joe Woody/President of Advanced Wound Management
    Michael Frazzette/President of Endoscopy
    Joseph DeVivo/President of Orthopaedic Reconstruction
    Mark Augusti/President of Orthopaedic Trauma
Finance: Adrian Hennah/Chief Financial Officer

Accessories, Light, Surgical	Surgery
Acid, Hyaluronic, Intraarticular	Physical Med
Adapter, Electrosurgical Unit, Cable	Surgery
Adapter, Unit, Electrosurgical, Hand-Controlled	Surgery
Appliance, Fix., Nail/Blade/Plate Comb., Multiple Component	Orthopedics
Applier, Surgical Staple	Surgery
Awl	Orthopedics
Bender	Orthopedics
Bit, Drill	Orthopedics
Blade, Bone Cutting	Orthopedics
Blade, Scalpel	Surgery
Blade, Surgical, Saw, General & Plastic Surgery	Surgery
Bolt, Nut, Washer	Orthopedics
Brace, Drill	Orthopedics
Broach	Orthopedics
Burr, Other	Surgery
Caliper, Orthopedic	Orthopedics
Camera, Video, Endoscopic	General
Cart, Equipment, Video	General
Cart, Traction	Orthopedics
Cement, Orthopedic (Bone)	Orthopedics
Cerclage, Fixation	Orthopedics
Chisel (Osteotome)	Surgery
Chisel, Orthopedic	Orthopedics
Chisel, Surgical, Manual	Surgery
Clamp, Surgical, General & Plastic Surgery	Surgery
Compression Instrument	Orthopedics
Container, Sterilization (Tray)	General
Corkscrew	Orthopedics
Countersink	Orthopedics
Curette	Orthopedics
Curette, Surgical	Surgery
Cutter, Wire And Pin	Orthopedics
Driver, Prosthesis	Orthopedics
Extractor, Nail	Orthopedics
Filler, Calcium Sulfate Preformed Pellets	Orthopedics
Forceps	Orthopedics
Forceps, Fixation	Surgery
Forceps, General & Plastic Surgery	Surgery
Forceps, Hemostatic	Surgery
Forceps, Sponge	Surgery
Forceps, Tissue	Surgery
Forceps, Wire Holding	Orthopedics
Gauge, Depth	Orthopedics
Goniometer, Orthopedic	Orthopedics
Gouge, Surgical, General & Plastic Surgery	Surgery
Halter, Head, Traction, Orthopedic	Orthopedics
Hammer, Surgical	Surgery
Handle, Knife Blade	Surgery
Handle, Scalpel	Surgery
Hemostat	Orthopedics
Holder, Electrosurgical Electrode	Surgery
Holder, Needle	Gastroenterology/Urology
Holder, Needle, Laparoscopic	Surgery
Holder, Needle, Other	Surgery
Holder/Scissors, Needle, Laparoscopic	Surgery
Hollow Mill Set	Orthopedics
Hook, Skin	Surgery
Hook, Surgical, General & Plastic Surgery	Surgery
Implant, Fixation Device, Condylar Plate	Orthopedics
Implant, Fixation Device, Proximal Femoral	Orthopedics
Instrument, Bending (Contouring)	Orthopedics
Instrument, Surgical, Powered, Pneumatic	Orthopedics
Jig, Piston Cutting, ENT	Ear/Nose/Throat
Kit, Instruments and Accessories, Surgical	Surgery
Kit, Surgical Instrument, Disposable	Surgery
Knife, Orthopedic	Orthopedics
Knife, Scalpel	Surgery
Lavage Unit, Water Jet	General
Light Source, Fiberoptic, Routine	Gastroenterology/Urology

SMITH & NEPHEW INC.- ORTHOPAEDICS   800-238-7538 *(cont'd)*

Lubricant, Instrument	General
Mirror, Laryngeal	Ear/Nose/Throat
Mixing Equipment, Cement	Orthopedics
Motor, Surgical Instrument, AC-Powered	Surgery
Nail, Fixation, Bone	Orthopedics
Needle, Conduction, Anesthesia (W/Wo Introducer)	Anesthesiology
Osteotome (Orthopedic)	Surgery
Osteotome, Manual (Plastic Surgery)	Surgery
Passer	Orthopedics
Pin, Fixation, Smooth	Orthopedics
Pin, Fixation, Threaded	Orthopedics
Pinwheel	Cns/Neurology
Plate, Fixation, Bone	Orthopedics
Pliers, Surgical	Orthopedics
Probe	Orthopedics
Prosthesis, Elbow, Semi-Constrained	Orthopedics
Prosthesis, Femoral	Orthopedics
Prosthesis, Hip (Metal Stem/Ceramic Self-Locking Ball)	Orthopedics
Prosthesis, Hip, Acetabular Mesh	Orthopedics
Prosthesis, Hip, Cement Restrictor	Orthopedics
Prosthesis, Hip, Femoral Component, Cemented, Metal	Orthopedics
Prosthesis, Hip, Hemi-, Femoral, Metal/Polymer	Orthopedics
Prosthesis, Hip, Semi-Const., Metal/Poly., Porous Uncemented	Orthopedics
Prosthesis, Hip, Semi-Constr., Metal/Ceramic, Cemented/NC	Orthopedics
Prosthesis, Hip, Semi-Constrained, Metal/Polymer	Orthopedics
Prosthesis, Knee, Femorotibial, Non-Constrained	Orthopedics
Prosthesis, Knee, Femorotibial, Semi-Constrained	Orthopedics
Prosthesis, Knee, Patellofemoral, Semi-Constrained	Orthopedics
Prosthesis, Knee, Patellofemorotibial, Semi-Constrained	Orthopedics
Prosthesis, Shoulder	Orthopedics
Prosthesis, Shoulder, Constr., Metal/Metal or Polymer/Cem.	Orthopedics
Prosthesis, Shoulder, Hemi-, Humeral	Orthopedics
Prosthesis, Toe, Constrained, Polymer	Orthopedics
Prosthesis, Upper Femoral	Orthopedics
Protector, Skin Pressure	General
Rack, Surgical Instrument	Surgery
Rasp, Bone	Orthopedics
Rasp, Surgical, General & Plastic Surgery	Surgery
Reamer	Orthopedics
Retractor, Surgical	Surgery
Rod, Fixation, Intramedullary	Orthopedics
Rongeur, Other	Surgery
Rongeur, Rib	Orthopedics
Saw, Manual, And Accessories	Surgery
Scalpel, One-Piece (Knife)	Surgery
Scissors, Orthopedic	Orthopedics
Scissors, Suture	Surgery
Screw, Fixation, Bone	Orthopedics
Screwdriver	Orthopedics
Skid, Bone	Orthopedics
Spatula, Orthopedic	Orthopedics
Staple, Fixation, Bone	Orthopedics
Stereotaxy Equipment	Cns/Neurology
Stimulator, Growth, Bone, Non-Invasive	Orthopedics
Stripper, Surgical	Orthopedics
Stripper, Tendon	Surgery
Suture, Stainless Steel	Surgery
Syringe, Piston	General
Table, Surgical, Orthopedic	Orthopedics
Tap, Bone	Orthopedics
Tape, Measuring, Ruler And Caliper	Surgery
Tape, Television & Video, Endoscopic	Gastroenterology/Urology
Tip, Suction, Electrosurgical	Surgery
Traction Unit, Non-Powered	Orthopedics
Tray, Surgical	Surgery
Trephine, Bone	Orthopedics
Twister, Wire	Orthopedics

SMITH & NEPHEW ORTHOPAEDICS, INC.
See Smith & Nephew Inc.- Orthopaedics Division

SMITH & NEPHEW PERRY
See Ansell Healthcare Products, Inc.

SMITH & NEPHEW RICHARDS
See Smith & Nephew Inc.- Orthopaedics Division

SMITH & NEPHEW SIGMA, INC
See Sigma International, Llc.

SMITH & NEPHEW, INC.   800-876-1261
970 lake carillon dr., suite 110,   **727-392-1261**
saint petersburg, FL 33716
FDA Number: 3006760724
Web site: www.smith-nephew.com   *Fax:* 727-392-6914
Annual Revenue: $1-$5 Million
Year Founded: 1856
Total Employees: 320
Ownership: Smith & Nephew Plc.
Stock Symbol: SN
Traded On: London
Produces/Sells CE-marked Devices: N

SMITH & NEPHEW, INC.   800-876-1261 *(cont'd)*
Distribution: Manufacturer Direct
General Admin.: Mr. Joe Woody/President
　　　　　　　Barbara Rohan/Vice President Government Affairs
Mktg./Adv.: Peter Metcalfe/Senior Vice President Marketing
Production: Charlie Hoac/Vice President Operations
Research: Tanya Rhodes/Vice President Research & Development
Finance: Mr. Adrian Hennah/Chief Financial Officer

Accessories, Catheter	Surgery
Adhesive Strip, Waterproof	General
Adhesive, Liquid	General
Bag, Drainage (Incontinence)	Gastroenterology/Urology
Bag, Drainage, Ostomy (With Adhesive)	General
Bag, Urinary Collection	General
Bag, Urinary, Ileostomy	Gastroenterology/Urology
Bandage, Adhesive	Surgery
Bandage, Liquid	Surgery
Catheter, Irrigation	Surgery
Catheter, Urinary, Condom	Gastroenterology/Urology
Cement, Stomal Appliance, Ostomy	Gastroenterology/Urology
Colostomy Appliance, Disposable	Gastroenterology/Urology
Device, Incontinence, Fecal	Gastroenterology/Urology
Drainage Unit, Urinary	General
Dressing, Foam	General
Dressing, Gel	General
Dressing, Layer, Charcoal	General
Dressing, Non-Adherent	General
Dressing, Other	General
Dressing, Permeable, Moisture	General
Kit, Wound Drainage	General
Lavage Unit, Water Jet	General
Lotion, Skin Care	General
Ostomy Appliance (Ileostomy, Colostomy)	Gastroenterology/Urology
Solution, Ostomy, Odor Control	Gastroenterology/Urology
Solvent, Adhesive Tape	Surgery
Strip, Adhesive	Surgery
Tape, Gauze, Adhesive	General

Medical Product Subsidiaries (Listed Separately)
Smith & Nephew Inc.- Orthopaedics Division

SMITH & NEPHEW, INC.   901-396-2121
6409 E. Holmes Rd., Mem, TN 38141
FDA Number: 3005551626
Ownership: SMITH & NEPHEW PLC.
Stock Symbol: SN
Traded On: London
Produces/Sells CE-marked Devices: Y

Prosthesis, Hip, Semi-Const., Metal/Poly., Porous Uncemented	Orthopedics
Prosthesis, Knee, Femorotibial, Non-Constrained	Orthopedics

SMITH & NEPHEW, INC.   800-876-1261
970 Lake Carillon Dr., Suite 110,   **727-392-1261**
Saint Petersburg, FL 33716
FDA Number: 3006760724
Web site: http://global.smith-nephew.com   *Fax:* 727-392-6914
Ownership: Private
Produces/Sells CE-marked Devices: N

Accessories, Catheter	Surgery
Bag, Drainage (Incontinence)	Gastroenterology/Urology
Bandage, Other	General
Drain, Tee (Water Trap)	Anesthesiology
Dressing, Other	General
Dressing, Universal	General
Lavage Unit, Water Jet	General
Pump, Alternating Pressure Pad	General
Solvent, Adhesive Tape	Surgery

SMITH & NEPHEW, INC.   800-343-5717
University Business Park   **978-749-1000**
12500 Network, Suite 112
San Antonio, TX 78249
FDA Number: 1651491
E-mail: Endo.Inquiry@smith-nephew.com   *Fax:* 978-749-1599
Web site: www.obi.com
Medical Products Sales Volume: $2,000,000
Year Founded: 1856
Total Employees: 20
Ownership: SMITH & NEPHEW PLC.
Stock Symbol: SN
Traded On: London
Quality System Registration Information: ISO9001
Produces/Sells CE-marked Devices: N
Production: Mark Niederauer/Director Operations

Implant, Endosseous (Bone Filling and/or Augmentation)	Dental And Oral

SMITH & NEPHEW, INC., EDOSCOPY DIVISION
See Smith & Nephew, Inc., Endoscopy Division

SMITH & NEPHEW, INC., ENDOSCOPY DIVISION   800-343-8386
130 Forbes Blvd., Mansfield, MA 02048   **978-749-1000**
FDA Number: 1219602   Fax: 978-748-1599
Web site: www.endo.smith-nephew.com
Total Employees: 1300
Ownership: Smith & Nephew Plc.
Stock Symbol: SN
Traded On: London
Quality System Registration Information: ISO9001
Produces/Sells CE-marked Devices: Y
Distribution: Manufacturer Direct, Manufacturer Through Manufacturer Reps, Exporter
General Admin.: Ron Sparks/President
    Tom Finnerty/Vice President Human Resources
Mktg./Adv.: Eric Halvorson/Director Product Marketing
    Ruth Kane/Manager Marketing Communications
    Philip Hasskarl/Manager Sales Training
    Ruben Rosales/Senior Vice President International & National Sales
    John Konsin/Vice President Marketing
    Jerry Goodman/Vice President National Sales
Production: Sally Maher/Director Regulatory Affairs
    Hooks Johnston/Senior Vice President Operations
Research: Bryant Moore/Vice President Research & Development

Accessories, Arthroscope	Orthopedics
Accessories, Operating Room, Table	Surgery
Arthroscope	Orthopedics
Blade, Bone Cutting	Orthopedics
Camera, Other	General
Cannula, Surgical, General & Plastic Surgery	Surgery
Chisel, Surgical, Manual	Surgery
Container, Sterilization (Tray)	General
Cover, Shoe, Operating Room	Surgery
Cutter, Orthopedic	Orthopedics
Forceps	Orthopedics
Forceps, Wire Holding	Orthopedics
Gauge, Depth	Orthopedics
Gouge, Surgical, General & Plastic Surgery	Surgery
Guide, Surgical, Instrument	Surgery
Guide, Surgical, Needle	Surgery
Instrument, Microsurgical	Cns/Neurology
Knife, Surgical	Dental And Oral
Laparoscope, General & Plastic Surgery	Surgery
Needle, Spinal, Short-Term	General
Needle, Suture, Disposable	Surgery
Pump, Infusion	General
Scalpel, One-Piece (Knife)	Surgery
Snare, Surgical	Surgery
Staple, Fixation, Bone	Orthopedics
Stylet, Surgical	Surgery
Suture, Non-Absorbable	Surgery
Syringe, Piston	General
Tape, Measuring, Ruler And Caliper	Surgery
Tray, Surgical Instrument	Surgery

SMITH & NEPHEW, INC., ENDOSCOPY DIVISION   800-343-8386
150 Minuteman Road, Andover, MA 01810-1031   **978-749-1000**
FDA Number: 3003604053   Fax: 978-749-1599
E-mail: endo.inquiry@smith-nephew.com
Web site: www.endo.smith-nephew.com
Total Employees: 1300
Ownership: SMITH & NEPHEW PLC.
Stock Symbol: SN
Traded On: London
Produces/Sells CE-marked Devices: Y
Distribution: Manufacturer Direct, Manufacturer Through Manufacturer Reps, Exporter
General Admin.: Mike Frazzette/President
    Tom Finnerty/Vice President Human Resources
    Jerry Goodman/Vice President, General Manager
    Joe Darling/Vice President, General Manager
Mktg./Adv.: Mark Cole/Director Education
    Tom May/Director Marketing
    Travis Lee/Director Marketing
    Ruth Kane/Director Marketing & Communications
    Ruben Rosales/Senior Vice President International Sales
    Sally Maher/Vice President Business Development
    Joe Metzger/Vice President Corporate Communications
Production: Diane Minear/Director Regulatory Affairs
    Nigel Wilkinson/Vice President Quality Assurance & Regulatory Affairs
Finance: Ian Ashton/Vice President Finance

Accessories, Arthroscope	Orthopedics
Arthroscope	Orthopedics
Blade, Surgical, Saw, General & Plastic Surgery	Surgery
Cable, Fiberoptic	General
Camera, Cine, Endoscopic (With Audio)	Surgery
Camera, Cine, Endoscopic (Without Audio)	Surgery
Camera, Still, Endoscopic	Surgery
Camera, Television, Endoscopic (With Audio)	Surgery

SMITH & NEPHEW, INC., ENDOSCOPY DIVISION   800-343-8386
(cont'd)

Camera, Television, Endoscopic (Without Audio)	Surgery
Camera, Video	General
Camera, Video, Endoscopic	General
Camera, Video, Multi-Image	General
Cannula, Drainage, Arthroscopy	Orthopedics
Cannula, Other	General
Cart, Emergency, Cardiopulmonary Resuscitation (Crash)	Anesthesiology
Cart, Equipment, Video	General
Coagulator, Laparoscopic, Unipolar	Obstetrics/Gynecology
Coagulator/Cutter, Endoscopic, Unipolar	Obstetrics/Gynecology
Cutter, Orthopedic	Orthopedics
Dissector, Surgical, General & Plastic Surgery	Surgery
Drill, Bone	Orthopedics
Electrosurgical Unit, Cutting & Coagulation Device	Surgery
Endoscope, Direct Vision	Surgery
Endoscope, Electronic (Videoendoscope)	Surgery
Endoscope, Rigid	Surgery
Fastener, Fixation, Non-Biodegradable, Soft Tissue	Orthopedics
Fiber, Absorbent	General
Forceps	Orthopedics
Forceps, Endoscopic	Gastroenterology/Urology
Forceps, Grasping, Atraumatic	Surgery
Forceps, Grasping, Traumatic	Surgery
Holder, Leg, Arthroscopy	Orthopedics
Holder, Needle, Curved, Laparoscopic	Surgery
Holder, Needle, Laparoscopic	Surgery
Holder, Shoulder, Arthroscopy	Surgery
Holder/Scissors, Needle, Laparoscopic	Surgery
Hysteroscope	Obstetrics/Gynecology
Illuminator, Fiberoptic (For Endoscope)	Gastroenterology/Urology
Instrument, Dissecting, Laparoscopic	Surgery
Instrument, Microsurgical	Cns/Neurology
Instrument, Needle Holder/Knot Tying	Surgery
Insufflator, Carbon-Dioxide, Automatic (For Endoscope)	Gastroenterology/Urology
Insufflator, Laparoscopic	Obstetrics/Gynecology
Insufflator, Other	Surgery
Irrigator, Suction	General
Knife, Meniscus	Surgery
Knife, Orthopedic	Orthopedics
Laparoscope, General & Plastic Surgery	Surgery
Laparoscope, Gynecologic	Obstetrics/Gynecology
Light Source, Endoscope, Xenon Arc	Surgery
Light Source, Endoscopic	Obstetrics/Gynecology
Light Source, Fiberoptic, Routine	Gastroenterology/Urology
Monitor, Video, Endoscope	General
Nasopharyngoscope (Flexible Or Rigid)	Ear/Nose/Throat
Needle, Insufflation, Laparoscopic	Surgery
Obturator, Endoscopic	Gastroenterology/Urology
Printer, Image, Video	General
Probe, Electrocauterization, Single-Use	Surgery
Probe, Radiofrequency Lesion	Cns/Neurology
Prosthesis, Hip, Semi-Const., Metal/Ceramic/Ceramic, Cem.	Orthopedics
Prosthesis, Hip, Semi-Const., Metal/Poly., Porous Uncemented	Orthopedics
Pump, Infusion	General
Regulator, Vacuum	General
Saw, Powered, And Accessories	Cns/Neurology
Scissors with Removable Tips, Laparoscopy	Surgery
Scissors, Orthopedic	Orthopedics
Screw, Fixation, Bone	Orthopedics
Stripper, Vein, External	Cardiovascular
Surgical Instrument, Orthopedic, Battery-Powered	Surgery
Tape, Television & Video, Endoscopic	Gastroenterology/Urology
Tray, Surgical Instrument	Surgery
Trocar, Abdominal	Gastroenterology/Urology
Trocar, Gallbladder	Gastroenterology/Urology
Trocar, Gastro-Urology	Gastroenterology/Urology

SMITH & NEPHEW, INC., ENDOSCOPY DIVISION   978-749-1073
737 North Detroit St., Warsaw, IN 46580
FDA Number: 3004503399
Web site: www.smith-nephew.com
Ownership: SMITH & NEPHEW PLC.
Stock Symbol: SN
Traded On: London
Produces/Sells CE-marked Devices: N

SMITH & NEPHEW, MEXICO INC.   901-396-2121
San Francisco Cuautlalpan #101, Naucalpan, Edo. De Mexico Mexico
FDA Number: 9616082

Component, Cast	Orthopedics

SMITH & UNDERWOOD LABORATORIES
See Thorn Smith Laboratories

SMITH COMPANIES DENTAL PRODUCTS   800-336-3263
4368 Enterprise St., Fremont, CA 94538-6305   **510-490-8999**
FDA Number: 2952490   Fax: 510-659-1855
E-mail: info@smithdental.com
Web site: www.smithdental.com

SMITH COMPANIES DENTAL PRODUCTS 800-336-3263 *(cont'd)*
Medical Products Sales Volume: $1,600,000
Year Founded: 1987
Total Employees: 15
Ownership: Private
Produces/Sells CE-marked Devices: Y
Federal Procurement Eligibility: Small Business, Female Owned
Distribution: Manufacturer Direct, Manufacturer Through Distributor, Exporter
General Admin.: Mr. Barry Walter/General Manager

Device, Storage, Image, Digital	Radiology
Printer, Radiographic Duplicator	Radiology
Processor, Radiographic Film, Automatic, Dental	Dental And Oral

SMITH GROUP 800-227-3008
301 Battery Street, 7th Floor, 415-227-0100
San Francisco, CA 94111
FDA Number: n/a Fax: 734.780.8346
E-mail: ken.lerch@smithgroup.com
Web site: www.smithgroup.com
Annual Revenue: $10-$25 Million
Total Employees: 130 *Marketing Staff:* 3 *Sales Staff:* 3
Ownership: Private
Produces/Sells CE-marked Devices: N
Distribution: Service Direct
General Admin.: Steven J. Isaacs/President, Chief Executive Officer
Production: James T. Hannon/Senior Vice President Production

Contract R&D, Equipment	General
Service, Architectural	General

Medical Product Subsidiaries (Listed Separately)
Trelleborg Sealing Solutions

SMITH METAL PRODUCTS 651-248-9650
30625 Olinda Trail, Lindstrom, MN 55045
FDA Number: n/a Fax: 651-257-2767
E-mail: mikebrown@smithmetals.com
Web site: www.mimparts.com
Annual Revenue: $5-$10 Million
Ownership: Private
Quality System Registration Information: ISO9002
Produces/Sells CE-marked Devices: N
Federal Procurement Eligibility: Female Owned
Distribution: Manufacturer Direct
General Admin.: Ron Carlson/Vice President, General Manager
Mktg./Adv.: Michael Brown/Director Marketing

Component, Metal, Other	General
Contract Manufacturing	General

SMITH RIVER BIOLOGICALS 276-930-2369
9388 Charity Hwy., Ferrum, VA 24088
FDA Number: 1120889

Culture Media, For Isolation Of Pathogenic Neisseria	Microbiology
Culture Media, General Nutrient Broth	Microbiology
Culture Media, Mueller Hinton Agar Broth	Microbiology
Culture Media, Multiple Biochemical Test	Microbiology
Culture Media, Non-Propagating Transport	Microbiology
Culture Media, Non-Selective And Differential	Microbiology
Culture Media, Non-Selective And Non-Differential	Microbiology
Culture Media, Propagating Transport	Microbiology
Culture Media, Selective And Differential	Microbiology
Culture Media, Selective And Non-Differential	Microbiology
Culture Media, Selective Broth	Microbiology
Culture Media, Single Biochemical Test	Microbiology

SMITH SPORTS OPTICS, INC. 208-726-4477
280 Northwood Way, P.o. Box 2999, Ketchum, ID 83340
FDA Number: 3022808

Sunglasses (Including Photosensitive)	Ophthalmology

SMITH TIME, INC. 804-977-7440
P.O. Box 496, Ivy, VA 22945-0496
FDA Number: 9200914 Fax: 804-977-7456
E-mail: chipshoi@minospring.com
Medical Products Sales Volume: $1,000,000
Total Employees: 10
Ownership: Private
Produces/Sells CE-marked Devices: N
Federal Procurement Eligibility: Small Business
Distribution: Manufacturer Through Distributor, Importer
General Admin.: Roger B. Smith/President
Mktg./Adv.: Jeffrey Smith/Vice President Marketing

Timer, General Laboratory	Hematology

SMITHERS MEDICAL PRODUCTS, INC. 330-497-0690
4850 Shuffel Dr., N.w., North Canton, OH 44720-5436
FDA Number: 1527616 Fax: 330-497-0392
E-mail: smpjeffrey@sbcglobal.net
Web site: www.alphacradle.com
Annual Revenue: $1-$5 Million
Year Founded: 1981

SMITHERS MEDICAL PRODUCTS, INC. 330-497-0690 *(cont'd)*
Ownership: Private
Produces/Sells CE-marked Devices: N
Federal Procurement Eligibility: Female Owned
Distribution: Manufacturer Direct

Immobilizer, Therapy, Radiation	Radiology
Support, Patient Position	Anesthesiology

SMITHKLINE BEECHAM CONSUMER HEALTHCARE
See Gsk Consumer Healthcare

SMITHLINE BEECHAM CONSUMER HEALTHCARE
See Gsk Consumer Healthcare

SMITHS MEDICAL ASD 800-424-8662
5700 W. 23rd Avenue, Gary, IN 46406-2617 219-989-9150
FDA Number: 1824231 Fax: 219-844-9031
E-mail: info@smiths-medical.com
Web site: www.smiths-medical.com
Medical Products Sales Volume: $25,000,000
Annual Revenue: $25-$50 Million
Year Founded: 1978
Total Employees: 285
Ownership: Smiths Medical Asd, Inc.
Stock Symbol: SMIN
Traded On: London
Quality System Registration Information: ISO9001
Produces/Sells CE-marked Devices: Y
Federal Procurement Eligibility: Small Business
Distribution: Manufacturer Direct, Manufacturer Through Distributor, OEM, Exporter
General Admin.: Mark Stuart/General Manager
Production: John Sandie/Manager Engineering
  Mark Stuart/Manager Facilities
  Julie Bradley/Manager Quality Systems

Adhesive, Liquid	General
Airway, Bi-Nasopharyngeal (With Connector)	Anesthesiology
Airway, Nasopharyngeal (Breathing Tube)	Anesthesiology
Aspirator, Thoracic (Suction Unit)	Cardiovascular
Balloon, Epistaxis (Nasal)	Ear/Nose/Throat
Button, Tracheostomy Tube	Anesthesiology
Cannula, Tracheostomy	Ear/Nose/Throat
Component, Silicone	General
Connector, Airway (Extension)	Anesthesiology
Contract Manufacturing	General
Cuff, Tracheostomy Tube	Ear/Nose/Throat
Device, Incontinence, Occlusion, Urethral	Gastroenterology/Urology
Drain, Tee (Water Trap)	Anesthesiology
Drain, Thoracic (Chest)	Anesthesiology
Implant, Female Incontinence	Obstetrics/Gynecology
Kit, Cricothyrotomy	Anesthesiology
Kit, Tracheotomy	Anesthesiology
Larynx, Artificial Battery-Powered	Ear/Nose/Throat
Needle, Emergency Airway	Anesthesiology
Needle, Other	General
Prosthesis, Larynx	Ear/Nose/Throat
Tube, Laryngectomy	Ear/Nose/Throat
Tube, Tracheal (Endotracheal)	Anesthesiology
Tube, Tracheal/Bronchial, Differential Ventilation	Anesthesiology
Tube, Tracheostomy (Breathing Tube), ENT	Ear/Nose/Throat
Tube, Tracheostomy (W/Wo Connector)	Anesthesiology
Tubing, Other	General
Tubing, Silicone	General
Valve, Speaking, Tracheal	Ear/Nose/Throat
Ventilator, Pressure Cycled (IPPB Machine)	Anesthesiology

SMITHS MEDICAL ASD INC. 800-258-5361
10 Bowman Drive, Keene, NH 03431 603-352-3812
FDA Number: 1217052 Fax: 603-352-3703
E-mail: info@smiths-medical.com
Web site: www.smiths-medical.com
Annual Revenue: $100-$500 Million
Total Employees: 20
Ownership: Public
Stock Symbol: SMIN
Traded On: London
Quality System Registration Information: ISO9001
Produces/Sells CE-marked Devices: N
Federal Procurement Eligibility: Small Business
Distribution: Manufacturer Direct, Manufacturer Through Distributor, OEM
General Admin.: Stuart Beesley/Chief Information Officer
  Pennie Boyko/Director Human Resources
  Srini Seshadri/Managing Director
Mktg./Adv.: Paul Harris/Director Communications
Finance: Chris Taft/Director Finance

Airway, Nasopharyngeal (Breathing Tube)	Anesthesiology
Airway, Oropharyngeal, Anesthesia	Anesthesiology
Attachment, Breathing, Positive End Expiratory Pressure	Anesthesiology
Attachment, Intermittent Mandatory Ventilation (IMV)	Anesthesiology
Bag, Reservoir (Blood)	Anesthesiology

SMITHS MEDICAL ASD INC. 800-258-5361 *(cont'd)*

Cannula, Nasal, Oxygen	Anesthesiology
Catheter, Conduction, Anesthesia	Anesthesiology
Catheter, Suction (Tracheal Aspirating Tube)	Anesthesiology
Circuit, Breathing (W Connector, Adapter, Y Piece)	Anesthesiology
Condenser, Heat And Moisture (Artificial Nose)	Anesthesiology
Connector, Airway (Extension)	Anesthesiology
Drain, Tee (Water Trap)	Anesthesiology
Filter, Bacterial, Breathing Circuit	Anesthesiology
Filter, Conduction, Anesthesia	Anesthesiology
Gas, Collecting Vessel	Anesthesiology
Heater, Breathing System W/Wo Controller	Anesthesiology
Humidifier, Respiratory Gas, (Direct Patient Interface)	Anesthesiology
Laryngoscope, Rigid	Anesthesiology
Mask, Gas, Anesthesia	Anesthesiology
Mask, Oxygen, Aerosol Administration	Anesthesiology
Mask, Oxygen, Low Concentration, Venturi	Anesthesiology
Monitor, Airway Pressure (Inspiratory Force)	Anesthesiology
Mouthpiece, Breathing	Anesthesiology
Nebulizer, Direct Patient Interface	Anesthesiology
Needle, Conduction, Anesthesia (W/Wo Introducer)	Anesthesiology
Percussor, Powered	Anesthesiology
Spirometer, Therapeutic (Incentive)	Anesthesiology
Strap, Head, Gas Mask	Anesthesiology
Stylet, Tracheal Tube	Anesthesiology
Tube, Tracheostomy (W/Wo Connector)	Anesthesiology
Tubing, Flexible, Medical Gas, Low-Pressure	Anesthesiology
Tubing, Ventilator	Anesthesiology
Valve, Non-Rebreathing	Anesthesiology
Ventilator, Emergency, Manual (Resuscitator)	Anesthesiology

SMITHS MEDICAL ASD, INC. 800-433-5832
1265 Grey Fox Road, St. Paul, MN 55112 651-633-2556

FDA Number: 2183502 *Fax:* 651-628-7459
E-mail: info.md@smiths-medical.com
Web site: www.smiths-medical.com
Medical Products Sales Volume: $34,300,000
Year Founded: 1983
Total Employees: 500 *Marketing Staff:* 13 *Sales Staff:* 120
Ownership: Smiths Medical Asd, Inc.
Stock Symbol: SMIN
Traded On: London
Quality System Registration Information: ISO9001
Produces/Sells CE-marked Devices: Y
Federal Procurement Eligibility: Small Business
Distribution: Manufacturer Direct, Manufacturer Through Distributor, Manufacturer Through Manufacturer Reps, Exporter
General Admin.: James Stitt/President
Mktg./Adv.: Brian Johnson/Director Marketing
　　　　　Martha Sewall/Vice President Marketing
　　　　　Jeanette Bousquet/Vice President Sales
Production: Tom Rasmussen/Vice President Manufacturing
　　　　　Russ Davies/Vice President Quality Assurance & Regulatory Affairs
Research: Rhall Pope/Vice President Research & Development
Finance: Karen Linnard/Vice President Finance
IS: Ron Johnston/Director Information Services

Analyzer, Gas, Carbon-Dioxide, Gaseous Phase (Capnograph)	Anesthesiology
Catheter, Arterial	Cardiovascular
Catheter, Hemodialysis	Gastroenterology/Urology
Catheter, Intraspinal, Subcutaneous, Implantable	General
Catheter, Multiple Lumen	Surgery
Catheter, Pediatric, General & Plastic Surgery	Surgery
Catheter, Percutaneous	Cardiovascular
Catheter, Peripheral, Atherectomy	Cardiovascular
Catheter, Peritoneal	Surgery
Catheter, Vascular, Cardiopulmonary Bypass	Cardiovascular
Needle, Other	General
Oximeter, Ear	Cardiovascular
Port, Vascular Access	Cardiovascular
Pump, Infusion, Ambulatory	General
Pump, Infusion, Patient Controlled Analgesia (PCA)	General
Set, Administration, Intravenous, Needle-Free	General

SMITHS MEDICAL ASD, INC. 614-791-5568
201 West Queen St., Southington, CT 06489

FDA Number: 1219611
Ownership: Private
Produces/Sells CE-marked Devices: N

Catheter, Intravascular, Therapeutic, Short-term Less Than 30 Days	General

SMITHS MEDICAL ASD, INC. 847-793-0135
330 Corporate Woods Dr., Vernon Hills, IL 60061

FDA Number: 1417519
Ownership: Private
Produces/Sells CE-marked Devices: N

Cannula, Nasal, Oxygen	Anesthesiology
Circulator, Breathing Circuit	Anesthesiology
Drain, Tee (Water Trap)	Anesthesiology
Filter, Bacterial, Breathing Circuit	Anesthesiology
Humidifier, Non-Direct Patient Interface (Home-Use)	Anesthesiology

SMITHS MEDICAL ASD, INC. 847-793-0135 *(cont'd)*

Humidifier, Respiratory Gas, (Direct Patient Interface)	Anesthesiology
Mask, Oxygen, Aerosol Administration	Anesthesiology
Mask, Oxygen, Non-Rebreathing	Anesthesiology
Mouthpiece, Breathing	Anesthesiology
Nebulizer, Direct Patient Interface	Anesthesiology
Sterilant, Medical Device	General
Thermometer, Mercury	General
Tubing, Ventilator	Anesthesiology

SMITHS MEDICAL ASD, INC. 1 800 258 5361
5200 Upper Metro Place, Suite 200, 1 214 618 0218
Dublin, OH 43017

FDA Number: 1221261 *Fax:* 1 614 734 0254
E-mail: info.asd@smiths-medical.com
Web site: www.smiths-medical.com
Medical Products Sales Volume: $84,600,000
Annual Revenue: $50-$100 Million
Total Employees: 576
Ownership: Smiths Medical Asd, Inc.
Stock Symbol: SMIN
Traded On: London
Quality System Registration Information: ISO9001
Produces/Sells CE-marked Devices: Y
Distribution: Manufacturer Direct, Exporter
General Admin.: Stuart Beesley/Chief Information Officer
　　　　　Pennie Boyko/Director Human Resources
　　　　　Srini Seshadri/Managing Director
　　　　　Mark Nevens/Vice President Human Resources
Mktg./Adv.: Paul Harris/Director Communications
　　　　　Peter Healy/Manager Contract Sales
　　　　　Deniss Dutson/Vice President Business Development
　　　　　Mark Beran/Vice President Marketing & Sales
Production: Mark Sheehan/Director Materials
　　　　　Rich Norton/Vice President Manufacturing
Finance: Chris Taft/Director Finance

Bag, Reservoir (Blood)	Anesthesiology
Equipment, Suction/Irrigation, Laparoscopic	Surgery
Humidifier, Respiratory Gas, (Direct Patient Interface)	Anesthesiology
Infuser, Pressure (Blood Pump)	General
Nebulizer, Direct Patient Interface	Anesthesiology
Pressure Infusor, IV Container	General
Spirometer, Therapeutic (Incentive)	Anesthesiology
Warmer, Blanket	General
Warmer, Blood and Plasma	Hematology
Warmer, Blood, Non-Electromagnetic Radiation	Anesthesiology
Warmer, Blood, Water Bath	Hematology
Warmer, Infusion Fluid, Thermal	General
Warmer, Irrigation Solution	General

SMITHS MEDICAL ASD, INC.
See Smiths Medical OEM

SMITHS MEDICAL ASD, INC. 610-578-9600
9255 Customhouse Plaza, Suite N, San Diego, CA 92154

FDA Number: 2020364
Ownership: Private
Produces/Sells CE-marked Devices: N

Analyzer, Gas, Carbon-Dioxide, Gaseous Phase (Capnograph)	Anesthesiology
Catheter, Conduction, Anesthesia	Anesthesiology
Connector, Airway (Extension)	Anesthesiology
Electrode, Cutaneous	Cns/Neurology
Humidifier, Respiratory Gas, (Direct Patient Interface)	Anesthesiology
Monitor, Airway Pressure (Gauge/Alarm)	Anesthesiology
Oximeter, Ear	Cardiovascular
Regulator, Thermal, Cardiopulmonary Bypass	Cardiovascular
Thermometer, Electronic, Continuous	General
Tube, Aspirating, Flexible, Connecting	Anesthesiology
Tube, Tracheal (Endotracheal)	Anesthesiology

SMITHS MEDICAL MD, INC.
See Smiths Medical Asd, Inc.

SMITHS MEDICAL OEM 800-258-5361
5200 Upper Metro Place, Suite 200, 614-210-7300
Dublin, OH 43017

FDA Number: n/a *Fax:* 614-889-2651
E-mail: OEM.Inquiries@smiths-medical.com
Web site: http://www.smiths-medical.com
Medical Products Sales Volume: $95,000,000
Total Employees: 1300 *Marketing Staff:* 13 *Sales Staff:* 46
Ownership: Public
Stock Symbol: MDEX
Traded On: NYSE
Quality System Registration Information: ISO9001
Produces/Sells CE-marked Devices: N
Distribution: Manufacturer Through Distributor, Manufacturer Through Manufacturer Reps, OEM, Exporter
General Admin.: Mr. Srini Seshadri/President
Mktg./Adv.: Mr. Stuart Morris-Hopkins/Vice President Marketing & Sales

SMITHS MEDICAL OEM 800-258-5361 (cont'd)

Production: Mr. Ron Frisbie/Vice President Operations
Mr. Russ Davies/Vice President Quality Assurance & Regulatory Affairs
Finance: Mr. Rob White/Vice President Finance

Adapter, Stopcock, Manifold, Cardiopulmonary Bypass	Cardiovascular
Catheter, Continuous Flush	Cardiovascular
Catheter, Other	Gastroenterology/Urology
Clamp, Tubing	General
Dome, Pressure Transducer	General
Filter, Air	General
Filter, Bacterial, Breathing Circuit	Anesthesiology
Filter, Intravenous Tubing	General
Fitting, Luer	General
Flushing Device, Automatic	Anesthesiology
Kit, Administration, Intravenous	General
Kit, Intravenous Extension Tubing	General
Kit, Pressure Monitoring (Air/Gas)	General
Lock, Catheter	General
Manifold, Liquid	Chemistry
Monitor, Blood Pressure, Invasive (Arterial)	Cardiovascular
Monitor, Blood Pressure, Venous, Central	Surgery
Plug, Catheter	Gastroenterology/Urology
Pump, Industrial	General
Pump, Infusion, Ambulatory	General
Pump, Infusion, Syringe	General
Stopcock	General
Transducer, Blood Pressure	General
Transfer Unit, IV Fluid	General
Valve, Catheter Flush	Cardiovascular
Valve, Catheter Flush, Continuous	Cardiovascular

SMITHS MEDICAL PM, INC. 800-558-2345

N7 W22025 Johnson Drive, Waukesha, WI 53186 262-542-3100
FDA Number: 2182466 Fax: 262-542-0718
E-mail: info.pm@smiths-medical.com
Web site: www.smiths-medical.com
Medical Products Sales Volume: $13,000,000
Annual Revenue: $25-$50 Million
Year Founded: 1999
Total Employees: 140 Marketing Staff: 7 Sales Staff: 18
Ownership: SMITHS MEDICAL
Stock Symbol: SMIN
Traded On: London
Quality System Registration Information: ISO9001
Produces/Sells CE-marked Devices: Y
Federal Procurement Eligibility: Small Business
Distribution: Manufacturer Direct, Manufacturer Through Distributor, OEM, Exporter
General Admin.: Stuart Beesley/Chief Information Officer
Pennie Boyko/Director Human Resources
Srini Seshadri/Managing Director
Mktg./Adv.: Paul Harris/Director Communications
Maria Cartier/Director Product Marketing
Rob Sweitzer/Director Sales
Marilyn Lemsky/Manager Advertising & Communications
Production: Guy Smith/Manager Engineering
Linda Korn/Manager Materials
Don Alexander/Vice President Regulatory Affairs
Finance: Chris Taft/Director Finance
Mary Hamkins/Vice President Finance

Analyzer, Gas, Carbon-Dioxide, Gaseous Phase (Capnograph)	Anesthesiology
Monitor, Bed Patient	General
Monitor, Blood Pressure, Indirect, Surgery	Surgery
Monitor, ECG	Cardiovascular
Oximeter, Pulse	General

SMOKEMASTER INC.

See Air Quality Engineering, Inc.

SMP TECHNOLOGY 408-778-4777

15940 Concord Circle, Morgan Hill, CA 95037-5461
FDA Number: n/a Fax: 408-778-4646
E-mail: Design@smptech.com
Web site: www.smptech.com
Annual Revenue: $1-$5 Million
Year Founded: 1990
Total Employees: 50 Marketing Staff: 1 Sales Staff: 1
Ownership: Private
Produces/Sells CE-marked Devices: N
Federal Procurement Eligibility: Small Business, Female Owned
Distribution: OEM
General Admin.: Ann Brannon/President
Thomas A. Roberts/Vice President Corporate Operations

Service, Engineering/Design	General

SMS MEDSERIES4 DIVISION

See Siemens Medical Solutions Health Services Corp.

SMS TECHNOLOGIES, INC. 858-587-6900

9877 Waples St., San Diego, CA 92121
FDA Number: 3002779318 Fax: 858-457-2069
E-mail: info@smstech.com
Web site: www.smstech.com
Ownership: Private
Produces/Sells CE-marked Devices: N

Counter, Sponge, Surgical	Surgery

SNAP LABORATORIES, L.L.C. 847-777-0000

5210 Capitol Drive, Wheeling, IL 60025
FDA Number: 1423640 Fax: 847-465-3404
E-mail: don@snaplab.com
Web site: www.snaplab.com
Ownership: Private
Produces/Sells CE-marked Devices: N
Distribution: Manufacturer Through Manufacturer Reps

Recorder, Ventilatory Effort	Anesthesiology

SNG PROSTHETIC EYE INSTITUTE 561-391-7099

6018 S.w.18th St., #c-2, Boca Raton, FL 33433
FDA Number: 1058740
Ownership: Private
Produces/Sells CE-marked Devices: N

Eye, Artificial, Non-Custom	Ophthalmology

SNOW PRODUCTS, INC. 847-381-5222

27w996 Industrial Ave. #6, Barrington, IL 60010
FDA Number: 1450936
Ownership: Private
Produces/Sells CE-marked Devices: N

Clamp, Dialysis Arm	Gastroenterology/Urology

SNS BIOSYSTEMS 805-925-1616

527-B East Oak St., Santa Maria, CA 93454
FDA Number: 2029076
Ownership: Private
Stock Symbol: ABI
Traded On: NYSE
Produces/Sells CE-marked Devices: N

Cup, Prophylaxis	Dental And Oral
Sterilization Process Indicator, Biological	General

SNUG SEAT, INC. 800-336-7684

12801 E. Independence Blvd., PO Box 1739, 704-882-0668
Matthews, NC 28106
FDA Number: 1053060 Fax: 704-882-0751
E-mail: sales@snugseat.com
Web site: www.snugseat.com
Medical Products Sales Volume: $1,700,000
Annual Revenue: $5-$10 Million
Year Founded: 1988
Total Employees: 23 Marketing Staff: 2 Sales Staff: 4
Ownership: Private
Produces/Sells CE-marked Devices: Y
Federal Procurement Eligibility: Small Business
Distribution: Manufacturer Through Distributor, Manufacturer Through Manufacturer Reps, OEM, Exclusive Distributor, Importer, Exporter
Mktg./Adv.: Steve Scribner/Vice President Sales

Chair, Pediatric	General
Stand/Holder, Equipment, Laboratory	Chemistry
Wheelchair, Manual	Physical Med

SNUGFLEECE INTERNATIONAL INC. 800-824-1177

2740 Poleline Rd., Pocatello, ID 83201-6112 208-233-9622
FDA Number: 3032664 Fax: 208-234-0936
E-mail: sales@snugfleece.com
Web site: www.snugfleece.com
Annual Revenue: $0-$1 Million
Year Founded: 1988
Total Employees: 6
Ownership: Private
Produces/Sells CE-marked Devices: N
Federal Procurement Eligibility: Small Business
Distribution: Manufacturer Direct

Protector, Skin Pressure	General

SNYDER GENERAL CORPORATION

See Aaf International

SNYDER LABORATORIES INC.

See Zimmer Orthopaedic Surgical Products

SO-LOW ENVIRONMENTAL EQUIPMENT 513-772-9410

10310 Spartan Dr., Cincinnati, OH 45215-1277
FDA Number: 1526542 Fax: 513-772-0570
E-mail: solow@ixnetcom.com
Web site: www.so-low.com
Medical Products Sales Volume: $7,000,000
Annual Revenue: $5-$10 Million

SO-LOW ENVIRONMENTAL EQUIPMENT   513-772-9410 (cont'd)

Year Founded: 1960
Total Employees: 48
Ownership: Public
Produces/Sells CE-marked Devices: Y
Federal Procurement Eligibility: Small Business
Distribution: Manufacturer Direct, Manufacturer Through Distributor, Manufacturer Through Manufacturer Reps
Mktg./Adv.: Dave Collins/Manager Contract Sales
    Jim Leidenbor/Manager International Marketing & Sales
    Dan Hensler/Manager National Sales
    James Schum/Vice President Sales

Chamber, Constant Temperature (Environmental)	Microbiology
Freezer, Blood Storage	Hematology
Freezer, Laboratory, Biological	Chemistry
Freezer, Laboratory, General Purpose	Chemistry
Freezer, Laboratory, Ultra-Low Temperature	Chemistry
Refrigerator, Biological	Microbiology
Refrigerator, Explosion-Proof	Chemistry
Refrigerator, Laboratory	General
Refrigerator, Pharmacy	General

SODERBERG OPTICAL, INC.   800-755-5655
230 Eva St., St. Paul, MN 55107-1605   651-291-1400

FDA Number: 2183437   Fax: 651-291-7764
E-mail: info@soseyes.com
Web site: www.soseyes.com
Medical Products Sales Volume: $35,000,000
Annual Revenue: $25-$50 Million
Total Employees: 475   Marketing Staff: 3   Sales Staff: 23
Ownership: Private
Quality System Registration Information: ISO9001
Produces/Sells CE-marked Devices: N
Distribution: Manufacturer Direct, Manufacturer Through Distributor
Mktg./Adv.: Dan Henderson/Manager Sales Training
    Craig Giles/Vice President Marketing & Sales
Production: Ed Schmidt/Manager Materials
Finance: Robert Grundtner/Treasurer

Eyeglasses	Ophthalmology
Lens, Contact (Other Material)	Ophthalmology

SOFFER & SONS CO., M.
See Geri-Care Products

SOFIE BIOSCIENCES   310-242-6794
6162 Bristol Parkway, Culver City, CA 90230

FDA Number: n/a
E-mail: inquiry@sofiebio.com
Web site: http://www.sofiebio.com
Ownership: Private
Produces/Sells CE-marked Devices: N
General Admin.: Mr. Patrick Phelps/President, Chief Executive Officer
Mktg./Adv.: Dr. Jennifer Cho/Director Business Development
Finance: Mr. Philip Czernin/Director Finance

SOFT COMPUTER CONSULTANTS, INC.
See Scc Soft Computer

SOFT INNOVATIONS, INC.   909-678-3540
22300 Baxter Rd., Wildomar, CA 92595

FDA Number: n/a
Ownership: Private
Produces/Sells CE-marked Devices: N

Prosthesis, Breast, External, No Adhesive	Surgery

SOFT-FLEX
See Progressive Dynamics Medical, Inc.

SOFTCARE INNOVATIONS INC.   1-800-663-1509
541 Mill Street., Suite 2,   (519) 744-1228
Kitchener, ONT N2G 2 Canada

FDA Number: n/a   Fax: (519) 744-9630
E-mail: ingenuity@mayhew.ca
Web site: www.softcarein.com
Year Founded: 1995
Total Employees: 10
Ownership: Private
Produces/Sells CE-marked Devices: N
Distribution: Manufacturer Direct, Exclusive Distributor, Exporter

SOFTCHROME, INC.   925-743-1285
2551 San Ramon Valley Blvd.,, Suite 101,
San Ramon, CA 94583

FDA Number: 2950245   Fax: 925-743-9821
E-mail: eyetint@aol.com
Web site: www.softchrometinting.com
Medical Products Sales Volume: $400,000
Year Founded: 1986
Total Employees: 4
Ownership: Private

SOFTCHROME, INC.   925-743-1285 (cont'd)

Produces/Sells CE-marked Devices: N
Federal Procurement Eligibility: Small Business
Distribution: Manufacturer Direct, Manufacturer Through Distributor

System, Identification, Lens, Contact	Ophthalmology

SOFTSERT, INC.   516-887-2056
19 Reunion Road, Rye Brook, NY 10573

FDA Number: 2431502   Fax: 516-887-5070
E-mail: lensdoc@optonline.net
Web site: www.Softsert.com
Annual Revenue: $0-$1 Million
Year Founded: 1977
Total Employees: 10   Marketing Staff: 2   Sales Staff: 2
Ownership: Private
Produces/Sells CE-marked Devices: N
Federal Procurement Eligibility: Small Business
Distribution: Manufacturer Direct, Manufacturer Through Distributor
General Admin.: Dr. Michael Feldman/Chief Executive Officer
Mktg./Adv.: William Smith/Manager Marketing

Inserter/Remover, Lens, Contact	Ophthalmology

SOHN MANUFACTURING, INC.
See Smi

SOHNIKS ENDOSCOPY, INC.   800-495-0297
325 Armour Avenue, St. Paul, MN 55075   651-452-4059

FDA Number: 2134298   Fax: 451-452-4056
E-mail: sales@sohniks.com
Web site: www.sohniks.com
Ownership: Private
Produces/Sells CE-marked Devices: N

Accessories, Arthroscopic	Orthopedics
Endoscope, Rigid	Surgery
Mirror, Endoscopic	Surgery

SOKEN PRODUCTS, INC.   972-939-8072
1906 Robin Meadow Dr., Carrollton, TX 75007

FDA Number: 1629773

Stimulator, Muscle, Electrical-Powered (EMS)	Physical Med

SOL ENTERPRISES, INC.   800-510-8267
3101 Northside Ave., Richmond, VA 23228

FDA Number: 1125259

Booth, Sun Tan	Physical Med

SOLA CUSTOM COATINGS, INC.   858-509-9899
9117 South East Saint Helens, Street, Clackamas, OR 97015

FDA Number: 81338
Ownership: Private
Produces/Sells CE-marked Devices: N

Lens, Spectacle/Eyeglasses, Non-Custom	Ophthalmology

SOLA OPTICAL USA INC.
See Paragon Vision Sciences, Inc.

SOLA-SYNTEX OPHTHALMICS
See Paragon Vision Sciences, Inc.

SOLACE THERAPEUTICS, INC   760-431-0153
5865 Avenida Encinas, Suite 142b, Carlsbad, CA 92008

FDA Number: 2032663
Ownership: Private
Produces/Sells CE-marked Devices: N

Device, Incontinence, Occlusion, Urethral	Gastroenterology/Urology

SOLAR LIGHT CO.   215-517-8700
100 E. Glenside Avenue, Glenside, PA 19038

FDA Number: 2520713   Fax: 215-517-8747
E-mail: info@solarlight.com
Web site: www.solar.com
Medical Products Sales Volume: $1,300,000
Year Founded: 1966
Total Employees: 15
Ownership: Private
Produces/Sells CE-marked Devices: N
Federal Procurement Eligibility: Small Business
Distribution: Manufacturer Direct, Manufacturer Through Distributor
General Admin.: Ms. Deserie Bayron/Office Manager
Mktg./Adv.: Mr. John Forrest/Sales Representative

Detector, Ultraviolet	Dental And Oral
Radiometer, Ultraviolet	General

SOLARCARE TECHNOLOGIES CORPORATION
See Orasure Technologies, Inc.

SOLARCHROMIC, INC.   719-591-9264
2103 Essex Lane, Colorado Springs, CO 80909

FDA Number: n/a
E-mail: solaz@solarchromic.com
Web site: www.solarchromic.com
Ownership: Private

SOLARCHROMIC, INC.
719-591-9264 *(cont'd)*
Produces/Sells CE-marked Devices: N
Federal Procurement Eligibility: Small Business
Distribution: Manufacturer Direct
Sunglasses (Including Photosensitive) — Ophthalmology

SOLARIS, INC.
414-918-9180
6737 West Washington St., Suite 3260, West Allis, WI 53214
FDA Number: 2135152
Binder, Medical, Therapeutic — General
Orthosis, Limb Brace — Physical Med
Prosthesis Alignment Device — Physical Med
Stocking, Elastic — General

SOLARIUS DEVELOPMENT INC.
800-731-1220
550 Weddell Drive #3, Sunnyvale, CA 94089
408-541-0151
FDA Number: n/a
Fax: 408-541-0153
E-mail: inquiry@solarius-inc.com
Web site: www.solarius-inc.com
Medical Products Sales Volume: $800,000
Annual Revenue: $1-$5 Million
Year Founded: 1998
Total Employees: 10
Ownership: Private
Produces/Sells CE-marked Devices: N
Federal Procurement Eligibility: Small Business
Distribution: Manufacturer Direct, Manufacturer Through Manufacturer Reps, Importer
General Admin.: Peter Joshua/President
Mktg./Adv.: Eva Weppner/Manager Marketing
    Adam Donoghue/Manager Sales
    Randy Leifheit/Manager Sales
Device, Measurement, Potential, Skin — Cns/Neurology
Gauge, Measuring — Ear/Nose/Throat

SOLDER ABSORBING TECH., INC.
See Spirig Advanced Technologies, Inc.

SOLID STATE CONTROLS
See Ametek Solidstate Controls

SOLID STATE SONICS & ELECTRONICS, INC.
785-232-0497
4137 Lower Silver Lake Rd, Topeka, KS 66618
FDA Number: n/a
Fax: 785-232-0498
E-mail: info@solidstatesonics.com
Web site: www.solidstatesonics.com
Ownership: Private
Produces/Sells CE-marked Devices: N
Federal Procurement Eligibility: Small Business
Distribution: Manufacturer Direct, Service Direct, Importer, Exporter
Tester, Defibrillator — Cardiovascular

SOLIDPHASE, INC.
207-797-0211
1039 Riverside Street Suite 3, Portland, ME 04103
FDA Number: 1223963
Fax: 207-797-0227
E-mail: solidphase@msn.com
Ownership: Private
Produces/Sells CE-marked Devices: N
Federal Procurement Eligibility: Small Business
Distribution: Manufacturer Direct
Radioimmunoassay, Follicle Stimulating Hormone — Chemistry
Radioimmunoassay, Luteinizing Hormone — Chemistry
Radioimmunoassay, Total Thyroxine — Chemistry

SOLO BAMBINI
650-340-1773
729 Occidental Ave., San Mateo, CA 94402
FDA Number: 2951585
Frame, Spectacle (Eyeglasses) — Ophthalmology

SOLO STEP, INC.
866-631-1117
2522 W. 41st St. #318, Sioux Falls, SD 57105
605-271-2014
FDA Number: 3004183707
Fax: 866-453-9442
E-mail: info@solostep.com
Web site: www.solostep.com
Ownership: Private
Produces/Sells CE-marked Devices: N
Transfer Aid — Physical Med

SOLOMON TECHNOLOGY LABS
520-568-8007
22374 N. Dietz Dr., Maricopa, AZ 85239
FDA Number: 2030432
E-mail: sales@solomontechnologylabs.com
Web site: www.solomontechnologylabs.com
Ownership: Private
Produces/Sells CE-marked Devices: N
Scanner, Ultrasonic, Obstetrical/Gynecological — Obstetrics/Gynecology

SOLON MANUFACTURING CO.
800-341-6640
338 Madison Avenue, Suite 7,
207-474-6213
Skowhegan, ME 04976
FDA Number: 1220081
Fax: 207-474-7320
E-mail: cgiguere@solonme.com
Web site: www.solonme.com
Medical Products Sales Volume: $7,300,000
Year Founded: 1936
Total Employees: 85   *Marketing Staff:* 1   *Sales Staff:* 7
Ownership: Private
Quality System Registration Information: ISO9001
Produces/Sells CE-marked Devices: N
Federal Procurement Eligibility: Small Business, GSA Contract, VA Contract
Distribution: Manufacturer Direct, Manufacturer Through Distributor, Manufacturer Through Manufacturer Reps, OEM, Importer, Exporter
General Admin.: Iver Mossberg/Chief Executive Officer
    Steve Clark/General Manager
Mktg./Adv.: Don Petersen/Director National Marketing & Sales
    Joseph Rini/Director National Sales
    Coreen A. Giguere/Manager Sales
Production: Peter Martell/Engineer
    Ken Downey/Manager Quality Assurance
Finance: Gary Bulmer/Controller, Credit Manager
Applicator, Cotton — Dental And Oral
Applicator, ENT — Ear/Nose/Throat
Applicator, Proctoscopic — Gastroenterology/Urology
Applicator, Tipped, Absorbent — General
Applicator, Vaginal — Obstetrics/Gynecology
Brush, Cytology — General
Depressor, Tongue — General
Depressor, Tongue, ENT, Wood — Ear/Nose/Throat
Scraper, Cytology (Cervical) — Obstetrics/Gynecology
Spatula, Cervical, Cytology — Obstetrics/Gynecology
Speculum, Vaginal, Non-Metal — Obstetrics/Gynecology
Spoon, Medicine — General
Swabs, Cotton — General

SOLOS ENDOSCOPY
800-388-6445
65 Sprague Street, West B
617-360-9700
Boston/Dedham Commerce Park
Boston, MA 02136
FDA Number: n/a
Fax: 617-360-9740
Web site: http://www.solosendoscopy.com
Ownership: Private
Stock Symbol: SNDY
Traded On: OTC Bulletin
Produces/Sells CE-marked Devices: N
Finance: Mr. Fred Schieman/Chief Financial Officer
Accessories, Light, Surgical — Surgery
Accessories, Surgical Camera — Surgery
Arthroscope — Orthopedics
Camera, Television, Endoscopic (Without Audio) — Surgery
Cannula, Ophthalmic — Ophthalmology
Cannula, Suprapubic, With Trocar — Gastroenterology/Urology
Carrier, Ligature — Surgery
Clamp, Surgical, General & Plastic Surgery — Surgery
Coagulator, Culdoscopic — Obstetrics/Gynecology
Drape, Patient, Ophthalmic — Ophthalmology
ENT Manual Surgical Instrument — Ear/Nose/Throat
Electrosurgical Unit, Cutting & Coagulation Device — Surgery
Endoscope — Gastroenterology/Urology
Forceps, ENT — Ear/Nose/Throat
Forceps, General & Plastic Surgery — Surgery
Forceps, Obstetrical — Obstetrics/Gynecology
General Use Surgical Scissors — Surgery
Image Processing System — Radiology
Instrument, Manual, General Surgical — Surgery
Insufflator, Hysteroscopic — Obstetrics/Gynecology
Insufflator, Laparoscopic — Obstetrics/Gynecology
Laparoscope, General & Plastic Surgery — Surgery
Laparoscope, Gynecologic — Obstetrics/Gynecology
Light Source, Endoscope, Xenon Arc — Surgery
Light, Surgical, Endoscopic — Surgery
Light, Surgical, Fiberoptic — Surgery
Phacofragmentation Unit — Ophthalmology
Punch, ENT — Ear/Nose/Throat
Sponge, Ophthalmic — Ophthalmology
Tubing, Non-Invasive — Surgery

SOLOS ENDOSCOPY, INC.
See Conmed Corporation

SOLSTICE CORP.
207-874-7922
68 Marginal Way, 4th Floor, Portland, ME 04101
FDA Number: 1221946
Applicator, Tipped, Absorbent, Non-Sterile — General
System, Marking, Film, Radiographic — Radiology

SOLTA MEDICAL, INC.
877-782-2286
25881 Industrial Boulevard, Hayward, CA 94545
FDA Number: 2954746   *Fax:* 510-782-2287
Web site: www.solta.com
Year Founded: 2008
Ownership: Public
Stock Symbol: SLTM
Traded On: NASDAQ
Produces/Sells CE-marked Devices: N
General Admin.: Mr. Clint Carnell/Chief Operating Officer
     Mr. Len Debenedictis/Chief Technology Officer
     Mr. Stephen Fanning/President, Chairman, Chief Executive
Officer
Mktg./Adv.: Mr. Jeff Nardoci/Vice President Global Marketing
     Mr. William Brodie/Vice President International Sales
Production: Mr. Doug Heigel/Vice President Operations
     Ms. Kristine Foss/Vice President Regulatory & Clinical Affairs
Finance: Mr. Jack Glenn/Chief Financial Officer
     Mr. H. Daniel Ferrari/Vice President Finance

Electrosurgical Equipment, General Purpose	Surgery
Electrosurgical Unit, Cutting & Coagulation Device	Surgery
Laser, Surgical	Surgery
Massager, Therapeutic	Physical Med

SOLTEC CORP.
800-423-2344
12977 Arroyo St., San Fernando, CA 91340-1548
818-365-0800
FDA Number: 9200997   *Fax:* 818-365-7839
E-mail: Sales@SoltecCorp.com
Web site: www.solteccorp.com
Medical Products Sales Volume: $3,600,000
Annual Revenue: $5-$10 Million
Year Founded: 1968
Total Employees: 22   *Marketing Staff:* 2   *Sales Staff:* 9
Ownership: Private
Quality System Registration Information: ISO9000; ISO9001; ISO9002
Produces/Sells CE-marked Devices: Y
Federal Procurement Eligibility: Small Business
Distribution: Manufacturer Direct, Exclusive Distributor, Importer, Exporter
General Admin.: Marvin Solomon/Chief Executive Officer
     Byron McIntire/President
Mktg./Adv.: Polly Dodson/Manager Advertising
     Byron McIntire/Manager International & National Sales
     Byron McIntire/Manager Market Research
     Paul Nelson/Vice President Business Development
     Byron McIntire/Vice President Sales

Amplifier, Transducer Signal (W Signal Conditioner)	Cardiovascular
Analyzer, Signal Isolation	Cardiovascular
Analyzer, Spectrum, EEG Signal	Cns/Neurology
Computer Software	General
Conditioner, Signal, Physiological	Cns/Neurology
Counter, Scintillation	Chemistry
Gauge, Measuring	Ear/Nose/Throat
Gauge, Pressure	General
Gauge, Strain	General
Oscilloscope	General
Recorder, Chart, Laboratory	Chemistry
Recorder, Paper Chart	Cardiovascular
Recorder, Videotape/Videodisc	General
System, Robot	General
Thermometer, Laboratory	Chemistry
Voltmeter	Chemistry

SOLUBLE SYSTEMS, LLC
877) 222-2681
11830 Canon Blvd, Suite A,
757-877-8899
Newport News, VA 23606
FDA Number: 3006784174
E-mail: info@solublesystems.com   *Fax:* (757) 877-8870
Web site: www.solublesystems.com
Ownership: Private
Produces/Sells CE-marked Devices: N

Dressing, Wound, Hydrogel W/out Drug And/or Biologic	Surgery

SOLUTEK CORP.
800-403-0770
94 Shirley St., Boston, MA 02119-3036
617-445-5335
FDA Number: n/a   *Fax:* 617-445-9623
Total Employees: 40
Ownership: Private
Produces/Sells CE-marked Devices: N
Federal Procurement Eligibility: Small Business
Distribution: Manufacturer Through Distributor, OEM, Exporter
General Admin.: Marlowe A. Sigal/Chief Executive Officer
Mktg./Adv.: John McMahon/Manager National Sales
Production: Tom Colletti/Manager Production

Blender/Mixer	Chemistry
Chemical, Film Processor	Radiology

SOLVAY PHARMACEUTICALS
800-241-1643
901 Sawyer Rd., Marietta, GA 30062
770-578-9000
FDA Number: n/a   *Fax:* 770-578-5597
Web site: www.solvaypharmaceuticals-us.com
Annual Revenue: $0-$1 Million
Year Founded: 1863
Total Employees: 9000
Ownership: Solvay Pharma US Holdings, Inc.
Produces/Sells CE-marked Devices: N
Distribution: Manufacturer Through Manufacturer Reps
General Admin.: Stephen Hill/President
     Contract Manufacturing, Pharmaceuticals/Chemicals   General

SOMAGEN DIAGNOSTICS INC.
800-661-9993
9220 - 25 Avenue,
780.702.9500
Edmonton, ALB T6N 1 Canada
FDA Number: n/a   *Fax:* 780.438.6595
E-mail: info@somagen.com
Web site: www.somagen.com
Year Founded: 1988
Total Employees: 50
Ownership: Private
Produces/Sells CE-marked Devices: N
Distribution: Exclusive Distributor

SOMANETICS CORP.
800-359-7662
2600 Troy Center Drive, Troy, MI 48084
248-244-1400
FDA Number: 1831181   *Fax:* 248-244-0978
E-mail: customerservice@somanetics.com
Web site: www.somanetics.com
Annual Revenue: $25-$50 Million
Total Employees: 75   *Marketing Staff:* 4   *Sales Staff:* 40
Ownership: Covidien Lp
Stock Symbol: SMTS
Traded On: NASDAQ
Quality System Registration Information: ISO9001
Produces/Sells CE-marked Devices: Y
Federal Procurement Eligibility: Small Business
Distribution: Manufacturer Direct, Manufacturer Through Distributor, Manufacturer
Through Manufacturer Reps
General Admin.: Mary Ann Victor/Chief Administrative Officer
     Bruce Barrett/President, Chief Executive Officer
Mktg./Adv.: Dominic Spadafore/Vice President Marketing & Sales
Production: Pam Winters/Vice President Manufacturing
     Pamela Winters/Vice President Quality Assurance
Research: Mr. Arik Anderson/Senior Vice President Research & Development
Finance: Mr. William Iacona/Chief Financial Officer

Oximeter, Tissue Saturation	Cardiovascular
Pledget And Intracardiac Patch, PETP, PTFE, Polypropylene	Cardiovascular

SOMATICS, LLC
847-234-6761
910 Sherwood Drive , #23, Green Oaks, IL 60044
FDA Number: 1420295

Block, Bite	Cns/Neurology
Electroconvulsive Therapy Unit (Electroshock)	Cns/Neurology

SOMERVELL LABORATORIES
254-897-4085
1102a Bluebonnet St., Glen Rose, TX 76043
FDA Number: 1651664
Ownership: Private
Produces/Sells CE-marked Devices: N

Gel, Support	Immunology

SOMNOMED INC.
940-381-5200
3537 Teasley Lane, Denton, TX 76210
FDA Number: 3005598536
Ownership: Private
Produces/Sells CE-marked Devices: N

Device, Anti-Snoring	Ear/Nose/Throat

SONARMED, INC.
317-489-3161
5513 West 74th St., Indianapolis, IN 46268
FDA Number: n/a   *Fax:* 866-853-3684
Web site: http://www.sonarmed.com
Year Founded: 2005
Ownership: Private
Produces/Sells CE-marked Devices: N
General Admin.: Mr. Jeff Mansfield/Chief Technology Officer
     Mr. David Wortman/Executive Chairman
     Mr. Andy Cothrel/President
Production: Ms. Laura Lyons/Vice President Quality Control & Regulatory Affairs

SONGBIRD HEARING, INC.
732-828-8300
303 George St., Suite 307, New Brunswick, NJ 08901
FDA Number: 2249293

Hearing-Aid	Ear/Nose/Throat

SONIC INNOVATIONS
4246 Riverboat Road, Suite 300,
Salt Lake City, UT 84123
(888) 678-4327
801-365-2800

FDA Number: 1724310
Fax: 801-365-3000
E-mail: info@sonici.com
Web site: www.sonici.com
Medical Products Sales Volume: $105,490,000
Annual Revenue: $100-$500 Million
Year Founded: 1991
Total Employees: 664 *Marketing Staff:* 7 *Sales Staff:* 17
Ownership: Otix Global Inc.
Quality System Registration Information: ISO9001
Produces/Sells CE-marked Devices: Y
Distribution: Manufacturer Direct, Manufacturer Through Distributor, OEM
General Admin.: Samuel Westover/Chief Executive Officer, Chairman
Michael Halloran/Chief Financial Officer, Vice President
Vicky Johnson/Manager Human Resources
Paul Wennerholm/President, Chief Operating Officer
Michael Nilsson/Vice President
Brent Shimada/Vice President General Counsel & Secretary
Mktg./Adv.: Merritt Johns/Manager Marketing
Merritt Johns/Market Manager
Rob Wolf/Vice President Marketing & Sales
Production: Christie Mitchell/Vice President Manufacturing & Operations
Mike Monahan/Vice President National Operations
David Whittle/Vice President Quality Assurance & Quality Control
Research: Victor Bray/Vice President Research
Jerry DaBell/Vice President Research & Development

Hearing-Aid	Ear/Nose/Throat
Hearing-Aid, Plate, Face	Ear/Nose/Throat

SONIC NEEDLE CORP.
See Misonix, Inc.

SONIC SYSTEMS, INC.
See Sonicwall, Inc.

SONICOR INSTRUMENT CORP.
50 Capital Drive, Wallingford, CT 06492
800-864-5022
203-265-6048

FDA Number: n/a
Fax: 203-793-1668
E-mail: customerservice@sonicor.com
Web site: www.sonicor.com
Medical Products Sales Volume: $4,500,000
Annual Revenue: $5-$10 Million
Ownership: Private
Produces/Sells CE-marked Devices: Y
Federal Procurement Eligibility: Small Business
Distribution: Manufacturer Direct, Manufacturer Through Manufacturer Reps, Exporter

Cleaner, Denture, Mechanical	Dental And Oral
Cleaner, Lens, Contact	Ophthalmology
Cleaner, Ultrasonic, Medical Instrument	General

SONICWALL, INC.
2001 Logic Drive, San Jose, CA 95124-3452
888-557-6642
408-745-9600

FDA Number: n/a
Fax: 408-745-9300
Web site: www.sonicwall.com
Medical Products Sales Volume: $1,000,000
Annual Revenue: $1-$5 Million
Total Employees: 20
Ownership: Private
Produces/Sells CE-marked Devices: N
Federal Procurement Eligibility: Small Business
Distribution: Manufacturer Direct
General Admin.: Mr. Matt Medeiros/President, Chief Executive Officer
Mktg./Adv.: Mr. Steve Franzese/Vice President International Marketing
Mr. Marvin Blough/Vice President Worldwide sales and service
Finance: Mr. Robert D. Selvi/Chief Financial Officer

Cleaner, Ultrasonic, Medical Instrument	General
Disintegrator, Biological Cell	Microbiology
Drill, Cannulated	Orthopedics
Probe, Ultrasonic	Radiology
Solution, Instrument Cleaner	General
Washer, Pipette	Chemistry

SONITUS MEDICAL INC.
1825 S. Grant Street, Suite 350, San Mateo, CA 94402
650-838-0325

FDA Number: n/a
Fax: 650-838-0326
Web site: http://www.sonitusmedical.com
Ownership: Private
Produces/Sells CE-marked Devices: N
General Admin.: Mr. Amir Abolfathi/Chief Executive Officer
Mktg./Adv.: Mr. Kurt Carlson/Vice President Corporate Development
Mr. Jason Shelton/Vice President Marketing
Production: Mr. Sam Mostafavi/Vice President Quality Assurance
Dr. Robert Chin/Vice President Regulatory Affairs
Research: Mr. Tim Proulx/Director Research & Development

SONITUS MEDICAL INC.
650-838-0325 *(cont'd)*
Finance: Mr. Richard Vicenti/Chief Financial Officer

SONO DIAGNOSTICS, INC.
See Ideal Medical Source, Inc.

SONOCO
4633 Dues Drive, Cincinnati, OH 45246-1008
513-874-7655

FDA Number: 9200207
Fax: 513-870-3983
E-mail: maryalice@cin-made.com
Web site: www.sonoco.com.
Medical Products Sales Volume: $3,700,000,000
Annual Revenue: $1-$5 Million
Year Founded: 1899
Total Employees: 17700 *Marketing Staff:* 1 *Sales Staff:* 3
Ownership: Private
Stock Symbol: SON
Traded On: NYSE
Produces/Sells CE-marked Devices: N
Distribution: Manufacturer Direct, Manufacturer Through Distributor, Manufacturer Through Manufacturer Reps
General Admin.: Bob Frey/Chief Executive Officer
Hartmut Geisselbrecht/General Manager
Mktg./Adv.: Mary Royse/Manager Sales
Production: Erik Frey/Vice President Manufacturing

Box, Transportation, Container, Specimen	General
Container, Specimen Mailer And Storage	Pathology
Container, Specimen, All Types	General

SONOCO CRELLIN, INC.
87 Center St., Chatham, NY 12037
518-392-2000

FDA Number: n/a
Fax: 518-392-2022
E-mail: scott.peterson@sonoco.com
Web site: www.sonococrellin.com
Annual Revenue: $50-$100 Million
Year Founded: 1946
Total Employees: 250 *Marketing Staff:* 5 *Sales Staff:* 5
Ownership: SONOCO PRODUCTS
Stock Symbol: SON
Traded On: NYSE
Quality System Registration Information: ISO9000; ISO9002
Produces/Sells CE-marked Devices: Y
Federal Procurement Eligibility: Small Business
Distribution: Manufacturer Direct
General Admin.: Mike Tucker/Executive Vice President
Bob Puechl/Vice President
Production: Eric Pearson/Director Quality Assurance
Research: Vic Des Rosiers/Vice President Research & Development

Equipment/Service, Quality Control	General
Molding, Injection	General
Polymer, Synthetic, Other	General
Service, Engineering/Design	General

SONOCO-STANCAP DIVISION
3150 Clinton Ct., Norcross, GA 30071
(800) 264-7494
(770) 476-9088

FDA Number: n/a
Fax: 770-476-0765
E-mail: david.murphy@sonoco.com
Web site: www.sonoco.com
Annual Revenue: $0-$1 Million
Total Employees: 50 *Marketing Staff:* 4 *Sales Staff:* 6
Ownership: SONOCO CORPORATION
Stock Symbol: SON
Traded On: NYSE
Produces/Sells CE-marked Devices: N
Distribution: Manufacturer Direct, Manufacturer Through Distributor, Manufacturer Through Manufacturer Reps, Exporter
General Admin.: Diana Simmons/Manager Admin.
Howard Ward/President
Mktg./Adv.: John McGeady/Manager National Sales
Smitty Thomas/Vice President Marketing & Sales
Production: Tom Johnson/Vice President Manufacturing

Cover, Other	General
Dentifrice	Dental And Oral
Foodservice Product/Equipment	General
Labware, Basic, Disposable	Chemistry

SONOGAGE, INC.
26650 Renaissance Pkwy., Cleveland, OH 44128
216-464-1119

FDA Number: 1526843

Scanner, Ultrasonic (Pulsed Echo)	Radiology

SONOMA ORTHOPEDIC PRODUCTS, INC.
3589 Westwind Boulevard, Santa Rosa, CA 95403
707-526-1335

FDA Number: 3007038372
Fax: 707-526-2022
Web site: http://www.sonomaorthopedics.com/
Year Founded: 2005
Ownership: Private
Produces/Sells CE-marked Devices: N

Plate, Fixation, Bone	Orthopedics

SONOMA ORTHOPEDIC PRODUCTS, INC. 707-526-1335 (cont'd)

Rod, Fixation, Intramedullary	Orthopedics
Screw, Fixation, Bone	Orthopedics

SONOMED, INC. 800-227-1285
1979 Marcus Ave., Suite C105, 516-354-0900
Lake Success, NY 11042
FDA Number: 2433682 Fax: 516-354-5902
E-mail: info@sonomedescalon.com
Web site: www.sonomedinc.com
Medical Products Sales Volume: $9,500,000
Annual Revenue: $5-$10 Million
Year Founded: 1983
Total Employees: 30
Ownership: Escalon Medical Corp.
Stock Symbol: ESMC
Traded On: NASDAQ
Produces/Sells CE-marked Devices: Y
Federal Procurement Eligibility: Small Business
Distribution: Manufacturer Direct, Manufacturer Through Distributor, Manufacturer Through Manufacturer Reps, Service Direct, Exclusive Distributor
General Admin.: Mr. Richard Depiano/Chief Executive Officer
　　　　　Mr. Barry Durante/Executive Vice President
Production: Mr. Mark Wallace/Manager Regulatory Affairs
Purchasing: Mrs. Judi Herman/Director Purchasing

Camera, Gamma (Nuclear/Scintillation)	Radiology
Pachometer	Ophthalmology
Scanner, Ultrasonic (Pulsed Echo)	Radiology
Scanner, Ultrasonic, Ophthalmic	Radiology
Transducer, Ultrasonic, Diagnostic	Radiology

SONOMETRICS CORPORATION 519-474-6464
500 Nottinghill Road, London, ONT N6K 3P1 Canada
FDA Number: n/a Fax: 519-474-6426
E-mail: sales@sonometrics.com
Web site: www.sonometrics.com
Year Founded: 1993
Total Employees: 25
Ownership: Private
Produces/Sells CE-marked Devices: N
Distribution: Manufacturer Direct, Exporter

SONOSITE, INC. 888-482-9449
21919 30th Drive SE, Bothell, WA 98021-3904 425-951-1200
FDA Number: 3032367
Web site: www.sonosite.com
Medical Products Sales Volume: $171,000,000
Year Founded: 1998
Total Employees: 600 *Marketing Staff:* 10 *Sales Staff:* 51
Ownership: Public
Stock Symbol: SONO
Traded On: NASDAQ
Quality System Registration Information: ISO9002
Produces/Sells CE-marked Devices: Y
Federal Procurement Eligibility: Small Business
Distribution: Manufacturer Direct, Manufacturer Through Distributor, Manufacturer Through Manufacturer Reps
General Admin.: Michael J. Schuh/Chief Financial Officer, Vice President
　　　　　Mr. Marcus Smith/Chief Financial Officer, Vice President
　　　　　Dr. Juin-Jet Hwang/Chief Technology Officer
　　　　　Kevin M. Goodwin/President, Chief Executive Officer
　　　　　Mr. Graham Cox/Senior Vice President International Marketing Operations
Medical Admin.: Dr. Diku Mandavia/Chief Medical Officer
Mktg./Adv.: Mr. brian Noyes/Vice President Marketing
Production: Ms. Mary Moore/Vice President Regulatory Affairs
Research: John S. Bowers/Senior Vice President Development

Equipment, Ultrasound, Doppler, Evaluation, Fetal	Obstetrics/Gynecology
Guidewire, Catheter	Cardiovascular
Image Processing System	Radiology
Plethysmograph, Impedance	Cardiovascular
Scanner, Ultrasonic (Pulsed Doppler)	Radiology
Scanner, Ultrasonic (Pulsed Echo)	Radiology
System, Communication, Image, Digital	Radiology
System, Imaging, Laparoscopy, Ultrasonic	Radiology
Transducer, Ultrasonic, Diagnostic	Radiology

SONOTECH INC. 800-458-4254
774 Marine Dr., Bellingham, WA 98225 360-671-9121
FDA Number: 2523891 Fax: 360-671-9024
E-mail: sonotech@sonotech-inc.com
Web site: www.sonotech-inc.com
Medical Products Sales Volume: $500,000
Annual Revenue: $1-$5 Million
Year Founded: 1988
Total Employees: 15 *Marketing Staff:* 1 *Sales Staff:* 1
Ownership: Private
Quality System Registration Information: ISO9001

SONOTECH INC. 800-458-4254 (cont'd)
Produces/Sells CE-marked Devices: N
Federal Procurement Eligibility: Small Business, Female Owned
Distribution: Manufacturer Direct, Exporter
General Admin.: Margaret J. Larson/President, Chief Executive Officer
Mktg./Adv.: Marian Larson/Marketing & Sales Specialist
Production: Delilah Bragg/Director Operations
　　　　　Roger St. Claire/Manager Quality Assurance

Gel, Ultrasonic Transmission	General
Scanner, Ultrasonic (Pulsed Echo)	Radiology

SONTEC INSTRUMENTS INC. 303-790-9411
7248 S. Tuscon Way, Englewood, CO 80112-6415
FDA Number: 1720747 Fax: 303-792-2606
E-mail: sales@sontecinstruments.com
Web site: www.sontecinstruments.com
Total Employees: 15 *Sales Staff:* 4
Ownership: Private
Produces/Sells CE-marked Devices: N
Federal Procurement Eligibility: Small Business
Distribution: Manufacturer Direct, OEM, Importer, Exporter
General Admin.: Dennis Scanlan/President, Chief Executive Officer
　　　　　Caron Scanlan/Vice President, General Manager

Contract Manufacturing, Product, Disposable	General
Instrument, Manual, General Surgical	Surgery

SONTRA MEDICAL CORPORATION
See Echo Therapeutics, Inc.

SONY CORPORATION OF AMERICA, MEDICAL SYS
See Sony Electronics, Inc., Medical Systems Div.

SONY ELECTRONICS, INC., MEDICAL 800-686-7669
SYSTEMS DIV.
One Sony Drive, Park Ridge, NJ 07656 201-358-4261
FDA Number: 2246606 Fax: 201-358-4977
E-mail: medical@am.sony.com
Web site: www.sony.com/medical
Medical Products Sales Volume: $110,000
Annual Revenue: More than $100 Million
Total Employees: 2 *Marketing Staff:* 9 *Sales Staff:* 16
Quality System Registration Information: ISO9000; ISO9001; ISO9002
Federal Procurement Eligibility: Small Business, GSA Contract, VA Contract
Distribution: Manufacturer Direct, Manufacturer Through Manufacturer Reps, OEM, Service Direct
General Admin.: Gordon Marzano/Manager Human Resources
　　　　　Steve Blum/Vice President
Mktg./Adv.: Tom Danisiewicz/Director Marketing
　　　　　Louise Nardone/Manager Advertising
　　　　　George Santanello/Manager Marketing
　　　　　Jim Ng/Manager Marketing
　　　　　Mark Wagner/Manager Marketing
Production: Erwin Ishmael/Director Customer Services
　　　　　John Kefalos/Manager Regulatory Affairs
Finance: Kristen Moloney/Controller

Accessories, Surgical Camera	Surgery
Camera, Microscope	Microbiology
Camera, Video	General
Camera, Video, Endoscopic	General
Camera, Video, Multi-Image	General
Camera, Videotape, Surgical	Surgery
Cart, Equipment, Video	General
Computer Software	General
Endoscope And Accessories, AC-Powered	Surgery
Monitor, Video, Endoscope	General
Printer, Image, Video	General
Projector, X-Ray Film	Radiology
Radiographic Picture Archiving/Communication System (PACS)	Radiology
Recorder, Videotape/Videodisc	General
Tape, Television & Video, Endoscopic	Gastroenterology/Urology
Television Monitor, Microscope	General
Television Monitor, Operating Room	General
Television System, Slow Scan	Radiology
Unit, Imaging, Thermal	Radiology

SONY OF CANADA LTD., MEDICAL SYSTEMS 800-361-5535
115 Gordon Baker Rd., 416-499-1414
Toronto, ONT M2H-3 Canada
FDA Number: n/a Fax: 416-499-8290
E-mail: general_enquiries@sony.ca
Web site: www.sony.ca
Year Founded: 1986
Ownership: SONY CORPORATION, JAPAN
Produces/Sells CE-marked Devices: N
Distribution: Exclusive Distributor, Importer

SOPER BROTHERS & ASSOCIATES 713-521-1263
1213 Hermann Dr., Suite 320, Houston, TX 77004
FDA Number: 1000220575

SOPER BROTHERS & ASSOCIATES 713-521-1263 (cont'd)

Conformer, Ophthalmic	Ophthalmology
Eye, Artificial, Non-Custom	Ophthalmology
Shell, Scleral	Ophthalmology

SOQUELEC LIMITED 514-482-6427
5757 Cavendish Blvd., Ste. 101,
Montreal, QUE H4W-2 Canada
FDA Number: n/a *Fax:* 514-482-1929
E-mail: sales@soquelec.com
Web site: www.soquelec.com
Year Founded: 1974
Total Employees: 10
Ownership: Private
Produces/Sells CE-marked Devices: N
Distribution: Exclusive Distributor

SORB TECHNOLOGY, INC. 405-682-1993
3631 S.w. 54th St., Oklahoma City, OK 73119
FDA Number: 1647143

Accessories, Blood Circuit, Hemodialysis	Gastroenterology/Urology
Concentrate, Dialysis, Hemodialysis (Liquid or Powder)	Gastroenterology/Urology
Dialysate Delivery System, Sorbent Regenerated	Gastroenterology/Urology
Purification System, Water	Gastroenterology/Urology

SORBA MEDICAL SYSTEMS, INC. 800-SOR-BA13
165 Bishops Way, Suite 152, 262-827-2740
Brookfield, WI 53005
FDA Number: 2183850 *Fax:* 262-827-2759
E-mail: jbarney@sorba.com
Web site: www.sorba.com
Medical Products Sales Volume: $1,000,000
Annual Revenue: $0-$1 Million
Total Employees: 10 *Marketing Staff:* 2 *Sales Staff:* 2
Ownership: Private
Produces/Sells CE-marked Devices: N
Federal Procurement Eligibility: Small Business, VA Contract
Distribution: Manufacturer Direct, Exporter
General Admin.: Jill Barney/President, General Manager
  John Allen/Secretary
  William Rose/Vice President
Mktg./Adv.: R. J. Collins/Manager International & National Sales
Production: Jill Barney/Executive Vice President Production
Finance: Kathy Moeschberger/Treasurer

Monitor, Cardiac Output, Impedance Plethysmography	Surgery

SORBOTHANE, INC. 800-838-3906
2144 State Rte. 59, Kent, OH 44240-7142 330-678-9444
FDA Number: 1525878 *Fax:* 330-678-1303
E-mail: sales@sorbothane.com
Web site: www.sorbothane.com
Medical Products Sales Volume: $1,900,000
Year Founded: 1982
Total Employees: 20
Ownership: Private
Produces/Sells CE-marked Devices: N
Federal Procurement Eligibility: Small Business
Distribution: Manufacturer Direct, Manufacturer Through Distributor
General Admin.: Robert E. Boyd/President
Mktg./Adv.: James Forsyth/Manager Market Research
Production: Nate Adair/Director Quality Assurance
  James Forsyth/Vice President Manufacturing
Research: Michael Zanin/Vice President Research & Development

Orthosis, Corrective Shoe	Physical Med

SORIN GROUP USA 800-289-5759
14401 W. 65th Way, Arvada, CO 80004-3599 303-425-5508
FDA Number: 1718850 *Fax:* 303-467-6584
E-mail: customerservice@sorin.com
Web site: www.soringroup-usa.com
Medical Products Sales Volume: $139,050,000
Annual Revenue: $100-$500 Million
Year Founded: 1999
Total Employees: 675 *Marketing Staff:* 10 *Sales Staff:* 45
Ownership: Sorin S.p.A.
Produces/Sells CE-marked Devices: N
Distribution: Manufacturer Direct, OEM
General Admin.: Rodger Stewart/President
Mktg./Adv.: Don Todd/Vice President Marketing
  Don Todd/Vice President Sales
Research: Steve Hunley/Research & Development Associate

Accessories, Cardiopulmonary Bypass	Cardiovascular
Adapter, Stopcock, Manifold, Cardiopulmonary Bypass	Cardiovascular
Autotransfusion Unit (Blood)	Anesthesiology
Cannula, Catheter	Cardiovascular
Clamp, Cannula	Gastroenterology/Urology
Clamp, Line	Gastroenterology/Urology
Clamp, Tubing, Blood, Automatic	Gastroenterology/Urology

SORIN GROUP USA 800-289-5759 (cont'd)

Computer, Patient Data Management	General
Connector, Tubing, Blood	Cardiovascular
Console, Heart-Lung Machine, Cardiopulmonary Bypass	Cardiovascular
Filter, Blood, Cardiopulmonary Bypass, Arterial Line	Cardiovascular
Filter, Blood, Cardiotomy Suction Line, Cardiopulmonary	Cardiovascular
Hematocrit, Automated	Hematology
Holder, Transducer	Anesthesiology
Kit, Blood, Transfusion	General
Kit, Tubing, Blood, Anti-Regurgitation	Gastroenterology/Urology
Monitor, Blood Pressure, Invasive (Arterial)	Cardiovascular
Monitor, Physiological, Cardiac Catheterization	Cardiovascular
Oxygenator, Cardiopulmonary Bypass	Cardiovascular
Oxygenator, Extracorporeal Perfusion	Anesthesiology
Oxygenator, Organ Preservation	Surgery
Pump, Blood, Cardiopulmonary Bypass, Roller Type	Cardiovascular
Pump, Extracorporeal Perfusion	Cardiovascular
Reservoir, Blood, Cardiopulmonary Bypass	Cardiovascular
Stopcock	General
Tie Gun, Dialysis	Gastroenterology/Urology
Transducer, Blood Pressure, Extravascular	Cardiovascular
Tube, Pump, Cardiopulmonary Bypass	Cardiovascular
Valve, CPB Check, Retrograde, In-Line	Anesthesiology

Medical Product Subsidiaries (Listed Separately)
  Ela Medical, Inc.

SORNA CORPORATION 651-406-9900
2020 Silver Bell Road, Suite 17, Eagan, MN 55122
FDA Number: 2135398

Device, Storage, Image, Digital	Radiology

SORRENTO BIOCHEMICAL, INC. 858-259-0717
3443 Tripp Ct., San Diego, CA 92121
FDA Number: 2031382
Ownership: Private
Produces/Sells CE-marked Devices: N

Control, Analyte (Assayed And Unassayed)	Chemistry

SOS REHABILITATION PRODUCTS INC. 800-667-3422
3359 RUE GRIFFITH, 514-737-3422
St-Laurent, QUE H4T 1 Canada
FDA Number: n/a *Fax:* 514-731-5086
E-mail: info@sosrehab.com
Web site: www.sosrehab.com
Year Founded: 1988
Total Employees: 10
Ownership: Private
Produces/Sells CE-marked Devices: N
Distribution: Exclusive Distributor, Importer

SOTA PRECISION OPTICS, INC. 714-532-6100
1073 North Batavia St., Orange, CA 92867
FDA Number: 3000190675

Operative Dental Treatment Unit	Dental And Oral

SOUND FEELINGS 818-757-0600
18375 Ventura Blvd. #8000, Tarzana, CA 91356-4218
FDA Number: n/a *Fax:* 818-999-3518
E-mail: information@soundfeelings.com
Web site: www.soundfeelings.com
Annual Revenue: $0-$1 Million
Year Founded: 1984
Total Employees: 4
Ownership: Private
Produces/Sells CE-marked Devices: N
Federal Procurement Eligibility: Small Business
Distribution: Manufacturer Direct, Manufacturer Through Manufacturer Reps,
  Service Direct, Exclusive Distributor, Exporter
General Admin.: Howard Richman/President
Mktg./Adv.: Jackie Adair/Director Marketing

Card, Identification	General
Chart, Anatomical Training	General
Material, Training, Audiovisual	General

SOUND SURGICAL TECHNOLOGIES LLC 888-471-4777
357 So. McCaslin, Suite 100, 303-384-9133
Louisville, CO 80027
FDA Number: 1725012 *Fax:* 720-294-2948
E-mail: info@vaser.com
Web site: www.LipoSelection.com
Medical Products Sales Volume: $4,500,000
Year Founded: 1998
Total Employees: 49
Ownership: Private
Stock Symbol: LSV
Traded On: NASDAQ
Quality System Registration Information: ISO9003
Produces/Sells CE-marked Devices: Y
Federal Procurement Eligibility: Small Business, VA Contract

SOUND SURGICAL TECHNOLOGIES LLC 888-471-4777 *(cont'd)*
Distribution: Manufacturer Direct, Manufacturer Through Distributor, Exporter
General Admin.: Dan Goldberger/Chief Executive Officer
Douglas Foote/General Counsel
Mktg./Adv.: Kristy Matteson/Director Marketing
Carter Morgan/Vice President Sales
Production: Steve Smith/Director Quality Assurance & Quality Control
Finance: John Sullivan/Chief Financial Officer
IS: William W. Cimino/Chief Technologist
Aspirator, Liposuction	Surgery
Cannula, Surgical, General & Plastic Surgery	Surgery
Surgical Instrument, Ultrasonic	Surgery

SOUND TECHNIQUES SYSTEMS, LLC 201-271-0700
710 Denbish Blvd., Newport News, VA 23608
FDA Number: 3003991862
Ownership: Private
Produces/Sells CE-marked Devices: N
Masker, Tinnitus	Ear/Nose/Throat

SOUNDCURE 617-419-1800
33 Arch Street, Boston, MA 02110
FDA Number: n/a   *Fax:* 617-226-4590
Web site: http://www.alliedminds.com/Portfolio/SoundCure/Overview
Year Founded: 2009
Ownership: Allied Minds
Produces/Sells CE-marked Devices: N
General Admin.: Mr. Bill Perry/General Manager

SOUNDTEC, INC. 405-842-5045
2601 Northwest Expressway, Suite 400w,
Oklahoma City, OK 73112
FDA Number: 1651971
Ownership: Private
Produces/Sells CE-marked Devices: N
Hearing Aid, Direct Drive, Partially Implanted	Ear/Nose/Throat

SOURCE MEDICAL CORPORATION 888-871-5945
60 International Blvd., 416-213-5000
Toronto, ON M9W 6 Canada
FDA Number: n/a   *Fax:* 416-213-5199
E-mail: ebusiness@sourcemedical.com
Web site: www.sourcemedical.com
Medical Products Sales Volume: $300,000,000
Year Founded: 1997
Total Employees: 600   *Marketing Staff:* 8   *Sales Staff:* 55
Ownership: ALLEGIANCE HEALTHCARE/MDS, INC.
Produces/Sells CE-marked Devices: N
Federal Procurement Eligibility: Small Business
Distribution: Exclusive Distributor, Importer

SOURCE ONE TECHNOLOGIES 408-376-3400
120 Knowles Dr., Los Gatos, CA 95032
FDA Number: 2954796
Electrosurgical Unit, Cutting & Coagulation Device	Surgery

SOURCE PRODUCTION & EQUIPMENT CO., INC. 504-464-9471
113 Teal St., Saint Rose, LA 70087
FDA Number: 1000437833   *Fax:* 504-467-7685
E-mail: spec@spec150.com
Ownership: Private
Produces/Sells CE-marked Devices: N

SOURCE-RAY, INC. 631-244-8200
167 Keyland Ct., Bohemia, NY 11716
FDA Number: 3004606964   *Fax:* 631-244-7464
E-mail: sales@sourceray.com
Web site: www.sourceray.com
Ownership: Private
Produces/Sells CE-marked Devices: N
Federal Procurement Eligibility: Small Business
Distribution: Manufacturer Direct, OEM, Exclusive Distributor
System, X-Ray, Mobile	Radiology

SOURCEMEDICAL 866-245-8093
100 Grandview Place, Suite 400, Birmingham, AL 35243
FDA Number: n/a   *Fax:* 205-278-1416
E-mail: therapy@sourcemed.net
Web site: www.sourcemed.net
Annual Revenue: $0-$1 Million
Ownership: Private
Produces/Sells CE-marked Devices: N
Federal Procurement Eligibility: Small Business
Distribution: Manufacturer Direct
Computer Software	General

SOUTH AMERICAN DENTAL EXPORT CORP. 305-512-4705
8205 West 20th Avenue, Hialeah, FL 33014
FDA Number: 1051788   *Fax:* 305-693-8630

SOUTH AMERICAN DENTAL EXPORT CORP. 305-512-4705
(cont'd)
E-mail: sadec@rite-dent.com
Web site: www.rite-dent.com
Medical Products Sales Volume: $1,500,000
Annual Revenue: $1-$5 Million
Year Founded: 1981
Total Employees: 9   *Marketing Staff:* 3   *Sales Staff:* 4
Ownership: Private
Quality System Registration Information: ISO9001
Produces/Sells CE-marked Devices: N
Federal Procurement Eligibility: Small Business, Minority Owned
Distribution: Manufacturer Direct, Manufacturer Through Distributor, Exclusive Distributor, Importer, Exporter
General Admin.: Maria Alvarado/President, Chief Executive Officer
Dr. Oscar Lopez/President, Chief Executive Officer
Cesar E. Veliz/Vice President, General Manager
Mktg./Adv.: Dr. Oscar Lopez/Director Marketing
Ulisses Lopez/Manager Advertising
Maria Alvarado/Manager International & National Sales
Juan Carlos Cabello/Manager Sales Training
William Lopez/Vice President Marketing & Business Development
Production: Cesar E. Veliz/Director Quality Assurance
Dr. Oscar Lopez/Manager Materials
Cesar E. Veliz/Vice President Manufacturing & Development
Service, Import/Export	General

SOUTH EAST INSTRUMENTS CORP. 352-332-0125
3706 N.w. 97th. Blvd., Gainesville, FL 32606
FDA Number: 1052939
Scaler, Ultrasonic	Dental And Oral

SOUTHERN CATS, INC.
See Atlas Medical Technologies

SOUTHERN ILLINOIS X-RAY MARKERS 618-253-7375
513 East Locust, Harrisburg, IL 62946
FDA Number: 3005099236
Ownership: Private
Produces/Sells CE-marked Devices: N
System, Marking, Film, Radiographic	Radiology

SOUTHERN OPTICAL LABORATORY, INC. 800-333-8498
501 Merritt Ave, Nashville, TN 37203 615-259-2303
FDA Number: n/a   *Fax:* 615-256-6631
Web site: www.southern-optical.com
Annual Revenue: $0-$1 Million
Year Founded: 1975
Ownership: Private
Produces/Sells CE-marked Devices: N
Federal Procurement Eligibility: Small Business
Distribution: Manufacturer Direct
Lens, Spectacle/Eyeglasses, Custom (Prescription)	Ophthalmology

SOUTHERN PACIFIC COAST CORP.
See Life Guard

SOUTHERN REID OPTICAL LABORATORY, INC. 800-765-7343
1856 Corporate Dr. Suite 150, 678-380-7425
Norcross, GA 30093
FDA Number: n/a   *Fax:* 678-380-7437
Web site: www.southern-optical.com
Annual Revenue: $0-$1 Million
Ownership: Private
Produces/Sells CE-marked Devices: N
Federal Procurement Eligibility: Small Business
Distribution: Manufacturer Through Distributor
Lens, Spectacle/Eyeglasses, Non-Custom	Ophthalmology

SOUTHERN TIER PLASTICS, INC. 607-723-2601
94 Industrial Park, P.O. Box 2015, Binghamton, NY 13902
FDA Number: n/a   *Fax:* 607-772-9881
E-mail: info@southerntierplastics.com
Web site: www.southerntierplastics.com
Annual Revenue: $0-$1 Million
Year Founded: 1967
Ownership: Private
Produces/Sells CE-marked Devices: N
Federal Procurement Eligibility: Small Business
Distribution: Manufacturer Direct
General Admin.: Jack Gwyn/Chief Executive Officer
Joyce Gray/President
Speculum, Vaginal, Non-Metal	Obstetrics/Gynecology

SOUTHLAND CRYOGENICS, INC. 800-872-2796
8350 Mosley Rd., Houston, TX 77075-1112 972-243-1311
FDA Number: n/a   *Fax:* 972-243-1370
E-mail: kgrimes@aeriform.com
Annual Revenue: $0-$1 Million

SOUTHLAND CRYOGENICS, INC.
800-872-2796 *(cont'd)*

Total Employees: 2   Marketing Staff: 2   Sales Staff: 1
Ownership: AERIFORM COMPANY
Produces/Sells CE-marked Devices: N
Federal Procurement Eligibility: Small Business
Distribution: Manufacturer Through Distributor
Mktg./Adv.: Keith Grimes/Manager Sales

Cryosurgical Unit	Surgery
Flask, Dewar	Chemistry
Regulator, Pressure, Gas Cylinder	Anesthesiology
Resuscitator, Emergency Oxygen	Dental And Oral

SOUTHMEDIC INC.
800-463-7146
50 Alliance Blvd., Barrie, ONT L4M-5K3 Canada   **705-726-9383**
FDA Number: 8022032   Fax: 705-728-9537
E-mail: contactus@southmedic.com
Web site: www.southmedic.com
Year Founded: 1983
Total Employees: 50   Marketing Staff: 2   Sales Staff: 9
Ownership: Private
Quality System Registration Information: ISO9001
Produces/Sells CE-marked Devices: Y
Federal Procurement Eligibility: Small Business, Female Owned
Distribution: Manufacturer Through Distributor, OEM, Exclusive Distributor, Importer, Exporter

SOUTHPAW ENTERPRISES, INC.
800-228-1698
PO Box 1047, Dayton, OH 45401   **937-252-7676**
FDA Number: n/a   Fax: 937-252-8502
E-mail: therapy@southpawenterprises.com
Web site: www.southpawenterprises.com
Medical Products Sales Volume: $3,100,000
Annual Revenue: $5-$10 Million
Year Founded: 1976
Total Employees: 34   Marketing Staff: 1   Sales Staff: 4
Ownership: Private
Produces/Sells CE-marked Devices: N
Federal Procurement Eligibility: Small Business
Distribution: Manufacturer Direct, Service Direct
General Admin.: Franklin D. Howard/President, Chief Executive Officer
Mktg./Adv.: Anna Wenning/Director Marketing & Advertising
     Priscilla Gillman/Manager Sales Training
Production: Kris Gant/Manager Regulatory Affairs
     Andy Roussey/Vice President Manufacturing & Development

Massager, Therapeutic	Physical Med
Scissors, Pediatric	General

SOUTHSIDE BIOTECHNOLOGY
440-974-4074
8780 Tyler Blvd., Mentor, OH 44060
FDA Number: 1527827   Fax: 440-974-4074
E-mail: sside8780@aol.com
Year Founded: 1988
Ownership: Private
Produces/Sells CE-marked Devices: N
Federal Procurement Eligibility: Small Business
Distribution: Manufacturer Direct

Accessories, Catheter, G-U	Gastroenterology/Urology
Tube, Gastro-Enterostomy	Gastroenterology/Urology

SOUTHWEST ARTIFICIAL EYES, INC.
210-737-3937
6323 Sovereign St # 159, San Antonio, TX 78201
FDA Number: 1648192   Fax: 210-737-2112
Ownership: Private
Produces/Sells CE-marked Devices: N

Conformer, Ophthalmic	Ophthalmology
Eye, Artificial, Non-Custom	Ophthalmology
Shell, Scleral	Ophthalmology

SOUTHWEST TECHNOLOGIES, INC.
800-247-9951
1746 Levee Road, North Kansas City, MO 64030   **816-221-2442**
FDA Number: 1929833   Fax: 816-221-3995
E-mail: info@elastogel.com
Web site: www.elastogel.com
Medical Products Sales Volume: $2,500,000
Annual Revenue: $1-$5 Million
Year Founded: 1981
Total Employees: 37   Marketing Staff: 3   Sales Staff: 5
Ownership: Private
Quality System Registration Information: ISO9000
Produces/Sells CE-marked Devices: Y
Federal Procurement Eligibility: Small Business, GSA Contract, VA Contract
Distribution: Manufacturer Through Distributor, OEM, Exporter
General Admin.: Cathy Moyer/Human Resources Representative
     Ed Stout/President, Chief Executive Officer
     John Phillips/Vice President, General Manager
Mktg./Adv.: Mr. James Ford/Director International Marketing & Sales
     Angela McKessor/Manager Contract Sales
     Robert Lange/National Accounts Representative

SOUTHWEST TECHNOLOGIES, INC.
800-247-9951 *(cont'd)*

     Angela McKessor/Vice President Medical Marketing
Production: Bob Scott/Director Quality Assurance
     Matt Mayes/Engineer
     Kurt Shouse/Manager Materials
     Bob Scott/Manager Regulatory Affairs
Research: Edward I. Stout/Director Research
     Ed Stout/Vice President Research & Development
Finance: Cathy Phillips/Controller

Collar, Cervical Neck	Orthopedics
Cushion, Flotation	Physical Med
Cushion, Other	General
Cushion, Wheelchair (Pad)	Physical Med
Dressing, Gel	General
Dressing, Other	General
Dressing, Wound and Burn, Occlusive	Surgery
Exerciser, Hand	Physical Med
Pack, Hot Or Cold, Reusable	Physical Med
Padding, Cast/Splint	General

SOYEE PRODUCTS, INC.
800-574-4743
459 Thompson Road, Thompson, CT 06277   **860-923-3400**
FDA Number: 2435881   Fax: 877-397-6933
E-mail: sales@soyeeproductsny.com
Web site: www.soyeeproductsny.com
Medical Products Sales Volume: $280,000
Annual Revenue: $1-$5 Million
Total Employees: 2   Marketing Staff: 6   Sales Staff: 6
Ownership: Private
Quality System Registration Information: ISO9002
Produces/Sells CE-marked Devices: Y
Federal Procurement Eligibility: Small Business
Distribution: Importer
General Admin.: Fred Spring/Chief Executive Officer
     Maureen Lee/Vice President, General Manager
Mktg./Adv.: Fred Spring/Vice President Marketing & Sales
Production: Maureen Lee/Manager Materials

Cassette, Radiographic Film	Radiology
Grid, Radiographic	Radiology
Holder, X-Ray Film	Dental And Oral
Screen, Intensifying, Radiographic	Radiology

Medical Product Subsidiaries (Listed Separately)
   X-Ray Accessory Corp.

SPACE MAINTAINERS LAB
(800) 423-3270
9129 Lurline Ave., Chatsworth, CA 91311   **818-998-7460**
FDA Number: 2082148   Fax: 818.341.4684
Ownership: Private
Produces/Sells CE-marked Devices: N

Device, Anti-Snoring	Ear/Nose/Throat
Device, Repositioning, Jaw	Dental And Oral
Dilator, Nasal	Ear/Nose/Throat
Retainer, Screw Expansion, Orthodontic	Dental And Oral
Tray, Fluoride, Disposable	Dental And Oral
Ventilator, Non-Continuous (Respirator)	Anesthesiology

SPACE TABLES, INC.
800-328-2580
11511 95th Avenue N., Maple Grove, MN 55369   **763-494-6969**
FDA Number: n/a   Fax: 763-494-6979
E-mail: info@spacetables.com
Web site: www.spacetables.com
Medical Products Sales Volume: $2,500,000
Annual Revenue: $1-$5 Million
Total Employees: 10   Marketing Staff: 30   Sales Staff: 30
Produces/Sells CE-marked Devices: N
Federal Procurement Eligibility: Small Business, GSA Contract, VA Contract
Distribution: Manufacturer Direct, Manufacturer Through Manufacturer Reps, OEM
General Admin.: Cheryl Erickson/President

Furniture, General	General

SPACEAGE CONTROL, INC.
661-273-3000
38850 20th Street East, Palmdale, CA 93550
FDA Number: n/a   Fax: 661-273-4240
E-mail: email@spaceagecontrol.com
Web site: http://spaceagecontrol.com/
Medical Products Sales Volume: $2,100,000
Annual Revenue: $1-$5 Million
Year Founded: 1968
Total Employees: 25
Ownership: Private
Quality System Registration Information: ISO9001
Produces/Sells CE-marked Devices: N
Federal Procurement Eligibility: Small Business
Distribution: Manufacturer Direct, Manufacturer Through Manufacturer Reps, OEM, Exclusive Distributor

Probe, Other	General
Prosthesis, Sensory	Cns/Neurology

SPACELABS BURDICK, INC.
See Cardiac Science Corp.

SPACELABS HEALTHCARE
5150 220th Avenue SE, Issaquah, WA 98029
800-522-7025
425-657-7200
FDA Number: 3023361
Fax: 425-657-7212
Web site: www.spacelabshealthcare.com
Ownership: Private
Produces/Sells CE-marked Devices: N
General Admin.: Deepak Chopra/Chief Executive Officer
Finance: Alan Edrick/Chief Financial Officer

Analyzer, Gas, Carbon-Dioxide, Gaseous Phase (Capnograph)	Anesthesiology
Analyzer, Gas, Nitrous-Oxide, Gaseous Phase	Anesthesiology
Analyzer, Gas, Oxygen, Gaseous Phase	Anesthesiology
Computer, Diagnostic, Pre-Programmed, Single-Function	Cardiovascular
Detector, Arrhythmia Alarm	Cardiovascular
Display, Cathode-Ray Tube	Cardiovascular
Electrorheograph	General
Gas-Machine, Anesthesia	Anesthesiology
Monitor, Physiological, Patient	Cardiovascular
Oximeter, Ear	Cardiovascular
System, Network And Communication, Physiological Monitors	Cardiovascular
Transmitter/Receiver System, ECG, Telephone Multi-Channel	Cardiovascular
Ventilator, Continuous (Respirator)	Anesthesiology

SPACELABS MEDICAL INC.
5150 220th Ave Se, Issaquah, WA 98029
(800) 522-7025
425-657-7200
FDA Number: 3023361
Fax: 425-657-7212
Web site: www.spacelabshealthcare.com
Year Founded: 1958
Ownership: Private
Produces/Sells CE-marked Devices: N
General Admin.: Deepak Chopra/Chief Executive Officer
David Tilley/Chief Operating Officer
Roy Hays/Chief Technology Officer
Jim Roop/President
Victor Sze/Secretary, General Counsel
Finance: Alan Edrick/Chief Financial Officer

Analyzer, Gas, Carbon-Dioxide, Gaseous Phase (Capnograph)	Anesthesiology
Analyzer, Gas, Nitrous-Oxide, Gaseous Phase	Anesthesiology
Analyzer, Gas, Oxygen, Gaseous Phase	Anesthesiology
Computer and Software, Medical	General
Computer, Blood Pressure	Cardiovascular
Computer, Diagnostic, Pre-Programmed, Single-Function	Cardiovascular
Computer, Diagnostic, Programmable	Cardiovascular
Detector, Arrhythmia Alarm	Cardiovascular
Display, Cathode-Ray Tube	Cardiovascular
Electrocardiograph, Ambulatory(without Analysis)	Cardiovascular
Electroencephalograph	Cns/Neurology
Gas Machine, Analgesia	Anesthesiology
Monitor, Blood Pressure, Indirect, Semi-Automatic	Cardiovascular
Monitor, Cardiac (Cardiotachometer & Rate Alarm)	Cardiovascular
Monitor, Perinatal	Obstetrics/Gynecology
Monitor, Physiological, Patient	Cardiovascular
Oximeter, Ear	Cardiovascular
Oximeter, Intracardiac	Cardiovascular
Recorder, Magnetic Tape/Disc	Cardiovascular
System, Network And Communication, Physiological Monitors	Cardiovascular
Thermometer, Electronic	General
Transmitter/Receiver System, ECG, Telephone Multi-Channel	Cardiovascular
Transmitter/Receiver System, Physiological, Radiofrequency	Cardiovascular

SPACESAVER CORPORATION
1450 Janesville Avenue,
Fort Atkinson, WI 53538
800-492-3434
920-563-6362
FDA Number: 9201004
Fax: 920-563-2702
E-mail: ssc@spacesaver.com
Web site: www.spacesaver.com
Medical Products Sales Volume: $30,900,000
Annual Revenue: $50-$100 Million
Year Founded: 1972
Total Employees: 400
Ownership: Ki
Quality System Registration Information: ISO9001
Produces/Sells CE-marked Devices: N
Federal Procurement Eligibility: Small Business, GSA Contract
Distribution: Manufacturer Through Distributor, Exclusive Distributor
General Admin.: Paul Olsen/Executive Vice President
Mktg./Adv.: David Klumb/Director Marketing
Mark Haubenshield/Vice President Sales
Production: Brian Patterman/Director Quality Assurance
James Muth/Vice President Operations

Bin, Storage	General
Cabinet Casework, General Purpose	General
Cabinet, Other	General
Storage Unit, X-Ray Film	Radiology

SPADINA INDUSTRIES INC.
110 Apex St., Saskatoon, SK S7R-1C8 Canada
800-665-2337
306-652-7344
FDA Number: n/a
Fax: 306-384-6311
E-mail: spadina@sasktel.net
Web site: www.spadina.com
Year Founded: 1988
Total Employees: 10
Ownership: Private
Produces/Sells CE-marked Devices: N
Distribution: Manufacturer Direct

SPAN PACKAGING SERVICES LLC.
4611-a Dairy Dr., Greenville, SC 29607
864-627-4155
FDA Number: 1063707
Fax: 864-627-0233
Web site: www.spanps.com
Ownership: Private
Produces/Sells CE-marked Devices: N

Agent, Polishing, Abrasive, Oral Cavity	Dental And Oral
Bandage, Adhesive	Surgery
Cover, Barrier, Protective	General
Disinfector, Medical Device	General
Lubricant, Patient	General
Medical Disinfectants/Cleaners for Instruments	General
Saliva, Artificial	Dental And Oral
Solvent, Adhesive Tape	Surgery

SPAN-AMERICA MEDICAL SYSTEMS, INC.
70 Commerce Center, Greenville, SC 29615
800-888-6752
864-288-8877
FDA Number: 1041130
Web site: www.spanamerica.com
Medical Products Sales Volume: $43
Annual Revenue: $25-$50 Million
Year Founded: 1970
Total Employees: 319   *Sales Staff:* 30
Ownership: Public
Stock Symbol: SPAN
Traded On: NASDAQ
Produces/Sells CE-marked Devices: N
Federal Procurement Eligibility: Small Business
Distribution: Manufacturer Through Distributor, OEM
General Admin.: Thomas D. Henrion/Chairman
Richard C. Coggins/Chief Financial Officer, Treasurer
James D. Ferguson/President, Chief Executive Officer
Mktg./Adv.: Clyde A. Shew/Vice President Marketing & Sales
Production: Robert E. Ackley/Vice President Operations
Wanda J. Totton/Vice President Quality Control

Cushion, Foot	Orthopedics
Cushion, Wheelchair (Pad)	Physical Med
Mattress, Air Flotation	General
Mattress, Bed	General
Pad, Pressure, Foam Convoluted	General
Pillow, Cervical	Orthopedics
Restraint, Patient, Conductive	Anesthesiology
Support, Head, Surgical, ENT	Ear/Nose/Throat
Support, Patient Position	Anesthesiology

SPARCO, INC.
2605 Oceanside Blvd., Ste. F,
Oceanside, CA 92054
800-783-8309
760-727-8309
FDA Number: 2937454
Fax: 760-734-4299
E-mail: sparco@flash-guard.com
Web site: www.sparcoinc.com
Annual Revenue: $0-$1 Million
Ownership: Private
Produces/Sells CE-marked Devices: N
Federal Procurement Eligibility: Small Business
Distribution: Manufacturer Direct, Manufacturer Through Distributor, Manufacturer Through Manufacturer Reps, Service Direct
General Admin.: Mr. Jonathan Searle/President, Chief Executive Officer

Sterilizer, Steam (Autoclave)	General
Table, Surgical With Orthopedic Accessories, AC-Powered	Surgery

SPARTAN BIOSCIENCES
6 Gurdwara Road, Suite 204q,
Ottawa, ONTAR K2E 8 Canada
877-228-7756
613-228-7756
FDA Number: n/a
Fax: 613-228-8636
E-mail: info@spartanbio.com
Web site: http://www.spartanbio.com
Year Founded: 2005
Ownership: Private
Produces/Sells CE-marked Devices: N

SPARTAN CHEMICAL COMPANY, INC.
1110 Spartan Dr., Maumee, OH 43537-0110
800-537-8990
419-897-5551
FDA Number: n/a
Fax: 419-536-8423
E-mail: customerservice@spartanchemical.com
Web site: www.spartanchemical.com
Year Founded: 1956

SPARTAN CHEMICAL COMPANY, INC.   800-537-8990 (cont'd)

Total Employees: 170	*Marketing Staff:* 4	*Sales Staff:* 68

Ownership: Private
Produces/Sells CE-marked Devices: N
Distribution: Manufacturer Through Distributor
General Admin.: Gordon Hufford/Corporate Vice President
    Stephen H. Swigart/President
    J. B. Waters/Secretary Treasurer
Mktg./Adv.: Sharon Elfring/International Sales Representative
    Mary Grace Miller/Manager Market Research
    R. C. LeMasters/Manager Sales Training
    Greg Ford/Vice President Sales
Production: Ron Cook/Manager Regulatory Affairs
    Jim Lenardson/Vice President Operations
Research: William J. Schalitz/Director Research & Development

Disinfector, Liquid	General
Dispenser, Soap	General
Encapsulator, Fluid	General
Solution, Antibacterial Cleaner	General
Washer/Disinfector	General
Washer/Sterilizer	General

SPARTAN USA, INC.

See Obtura Spartan

SPARTON CORPORATION   440-878-4630

22740 Lunn Road, Strongsville, OH 44149
FDA Number: 3003144120
Web site: http://sparton.com
Ownership: Private
Produces/Sells CE-marked Devices: N
General Admin.: Ms. Cary Wood/President, Chief Executive Officer
Mktg./Adv.: Mr. Mike Osborne/Senior Vice President Business Development
Production: Mr. Gordon Madlock/Senior Vice President Operations
    Mr. Steve Korwin/Senior Vice President Quality Assurance
Finance: Mr. Greg Slome/Chief Financial Officer

Analyzer, Chemistry, Urinalysis, Automated	Chemistry
Centrifuge, Cell Washing, Automated, Immuno-Hematology	Hematology
Chamber, Oxygen, Topical, Extremity	Surgery
Dialyzer Reprocessing System	Gastroenterology/Urology
Diluter, Blood Cell, Automated	Hematology
Pump, Infusion	General
Sensor, Pressure, Aneurysm, Implantable	Cardiovascular
System, Immunomagnetic, Circulating Cancer Cell, Enumeration	Immunology
Warmer, Infusion Fluid, Thermal	General

SPARTON ELECTRONICS   800.772.7866

425 N. Martingale Road, Suite 2050,
Schaumburg, IL 60173
FDA Number: 1834311
E-mail: mhammouri@sparton.com
Web site: http://www.sparton.com
Annual Revenue: $100-$500 Million
Year Founded: 1900
Ownership: Public
Stock Symbol: SPA
Traded On: NYSE
Quality System Registration Information: ISO9001
Produces/Sells CE-marked Devices: Y
Mktg./Adv.: Mr. Al Houghtaling/Vice President Business Development
Production: Mr. Monte Hammouri/Director Quality Assurance & Regulatory Affairs

Contract Manufacturing	General
Contract R&D, Equipment	General

Medical Product Subsidiaries (Listed Separately)
Sparton Electronics Florida, Inc.

SPARTON ELECTRONICS FLORIDA, INC.   800-824-0682

5612 Johnson Lake Rd.,   386-985-4631
De Leon Springs, FL 32130
FDA Number: 1058092   *Fax:* 386-985-5036
E-mail: medical@sparton.com
Web site: www.sparton.com
Medical Products Sales Volume: $1,500,000
Year Founded: 1900

Total Employees: 750	*Marketing Staff:* 4	*Sales Staff:* 10

Ownership: Sparton Corporation
Stock Symbol: SPA
Traded On: NYSE
Quality System Registration Information: ISO9001
Produces/Sells CE-marked Devices: Y
Distribution: Manufacturer Direct, Manufacturer Through Distributor, OEM
General Admin.: Douglas E. Johnson/Chief Operating Officer, Senior Executive Vice President
Mktg./Adv.: Robert Kundinger/Director Business Development
Production: Mrs. Annette Sobolewski/Director Operations
    Michael Lodge/Director Quality Assurance
    Mr. Michael Sobolewski/Senior Vice President Medical Products

Contract Manufacturing	General

SPARTON ELECTRONICS FLORIDA, INC.   800-824-0682 (cont'd)

Contract Manufacturing, Product, Durable	General
Contract R&D, Equipment	General
Service, Engineering/Design	General

SPARTON ELECTRONICS, INC.   800-443-4132

30167 Power Line Rd., Brooksville, FL 34602   352-799-6520
FDA Number: 1055575
Ownership: Private
Produces/Sells CE-marked Devices: N

SPARTON MEDICAL SYSTEMS   440-878-4630

22740 Lunn Rd., Strongsville, OH 44149
FDA Number: 3003144120
Web site: http://www.sparton.com
Year Founded: 1900
Ownership: Public
Stock Symbol: SPA
Traded On: NYSE
Produces/Sells CE-marked Devices: N

Analyzer, Chemistry, Photometric, Discrete	Chemistry
Analyzer, Chemistry, Urinalysis	Chemistry
Chamber, Oxygen, Topical, Extremity	Surgery
Dialyzer Reprocessing System	Gastroenterology/Urology
Diluter, Blood Cell, Automated	Hematology
Generator, Oxygen, Portable	Anesthesiology

SPARTON MEDICAL SYSTEMS

See Sparton Electronics Florida, Inc.

SPATIAL DATA SYSTEMS INC.

See Titan Corporation/Systems & Imagery Division

SPAULDING CLINICAL RESEARCH   262-334-6020

525 S Silverbrook Dr, West Bend, WI 53095
FDA Number: n/a   *Fax:* 262-334-6067
E-mail: info@spauldingclinical.com
Web site: http://www.spauldingclinical.com
Ownership: Private
Produces/Sells CE-marked Devices: N
General Admin.: Mr. Randol Spaulding/Chief Executive Officer
Medical Admin.: Dr. Jay Mason/Chief Medical Officer
Mktg./Adv.: Mr. Kevin Geno/Vice President International Sales
Production: Mr. Daniel Selness/Senior Vice President Operations
    Mr. Paul Schultz/Vice President Quality Assurance

SPEC CONNECTION INTL INC.   813-618-0400

37325 Sr 54, Zephyrhills, FL 33542
FDA Number: 1063155
Ownership: Private
Produces/Sells CE-marked Devices: N

Analyzer, Gas, Carbon-Dioxide, Blood Phase, Indwelling	Anesthesiology
Gas, Calibrated (Specified Concentration)	Anesthesiology
Laser, Surgical	Surgery
Tonometer (Calibration And Q.C. Of Blood Gas Instruments)	Chemistry
Transport System, Anaerobic	Microbiology

SPECIAL GAS SERVICES INC   919-621-0980

PO Box 727, Mount Laurel, NJ 08054
FDA Number: n/a   *Fax:* 609-784-0964
E-mail: specialgas@aol.com
Web site: www.specialgas.com
Medical Products Sales Volume: $1,500,000
Year Founded: 1985
Total Employees: 3
Ownership: Private
Produces/Sells CE-marked Devices: N
Federal Procurement Eligibility: Small Business
Distribution: Manufacturer Through Distributor

Cylinder, Gas (Empty)	Anesthesiology
Holder, Gas Cylinder	Anesthesiology

SPECIAL PRODUCTS, INC.   800-538-6836

2540 Greenwood Drive,   407-344-0550
Kissimmee, FL 34744
FDA Number: 2919265   *Fax:* 407-344-3674
E-mail: drjack@betterendo.com
Web site: www.BetterEndo.com/SPI
Medical Products Sales Volume: $400,000
Year Founded: 1978
Total Employees: 5
Ownership: Private
Produces/Sells CE-marked Devices: N
Federal Procurement Eligibility: Small Business
Distribution: Manufacturer Direct, Manufacturer Through Distributor, Manufacturer Through Manufacturer Reps
General Admin.: Dr. JOHN JACKLICH/President
Finance: Mrs. M. JACKLICH, C.P.A./Treasurer

File, Pulp Canal, Endodontic	Dental And Oral

SPECIAL PRODUCTS, INC. 800-538-6836 (cont'd)
Syringe, Periodontic, Endodontic — Dental And Oral

SPECIALEYES LLC 813-645-2855
6447 Parkland Dr., Suite 2020, Sarasota, FL 34243
FDA Number: 3004927493
Lenses, Soft Contact, Daily Wear — Ophthalmology

SPECIALITIES ELECTRONICS CO., INC. 609-267-5593
43 Washington St., Mt. Holly, NJ 08060
FDA Number: 2523869
Ownership: Private
Produces/Sells CE-marked Devices: N
Probe, Uptake, Nuclear — Radiology
Test, Thyroid Autoantibody — Immunology

SPECIALIZED HEALTH PRODUCTS INTERNATIONAL, INC. 800-306-3360
585 W. 500 S., Bountiful, UT 84010 — 801-298-3360
FDA Number: 1723684 — Fax: 801-298-1759
E-mail: pevans@shpi.com
Web site: www.shpi.com
Medical Products Sales Volume: $16,500,000
Annual Revenue: $1-$5 Million
Year Founded: 1993
Total Employees: 31 — Marketing Staff: 1 — Sales Staff: 6
Ownership: Public
Stock Symbol: SHPI
Traded On: OTC Bulletin
Produces/Sells CE-marked Devices: Y
Federal Procurement Eligibility: Small Business
Distribution: Manufacturer Through Distributor, OEM, Exclusive Distributor, Exporter
General Admin.: Jeff Soinski/President, Chief Executive Officer
Donald Solomon/Vice President, General Manager
Mktg./Adv.: Mary Jo Benak/Director Marketing & Sales
Ross Davis/Director Marketing & Sales
Mark Ferguson/Director Product Development
Paul Evans/Vice President Business Development
Production: Mark Nelson/Director Quality Assurance
Introducer, Catheter — Cardiovascular
Kit, Administration, Intravenous — General
Needle, Blood Collection — General
Needle, Hypodermic — General
Port, Vascular Access — Cardiovascular
Syringe, Other — General

SPECIALIZED MEDICAL DEVICES, LLC 800-463-1874
300 Running Pump Rd, Lancaster, PA 17603 — 717-392-8570
FDA Number: 2530180 — Fax: 717-392-8578
E-mail: sales@specializedmedical.com
Web site: www.specializedmedical.com
Total Employees: 130 — Marketing Staff: 3 — Sales Staff: 5
Ownership: Teleflex Medical
Stock Symbol: TFX
Traded On: NYSE
Quality System Registration Information: ISO9001
Produces/Sells CE-marked Devices: Y
Distribution: Manufacturer Direct, OEM
General Admin.: Edward Burton/General Manager
Margie Helig/Human Resources Representative
Mary Burton/Vice President
Mktg./Adv.: Jack Fulton/Director Sales
Steve Bergstrom/Manager Sales
Production: Greg Myers/Director Manufacturing & Tech. Services
Terry Corl/Manager Quality Assurance
Component, Metal, Other — General
Contract Manufacturing — General
Punch, Surgical — Surgery
Service, Engineering/Design — General

SPECIALTEAM MEDICAL SERVICES, INC. 714-694-0348
22445 E. La Palma Ave., Ste F, Yorba Linda, CA 92887
FDA Number: 9041455 — Fax: 714-694-0171
E-mail: billy@specialteam.com
Web site: www.specialteam.com
Medical Products Sales Volume: $1,750,000
Annual Revenue: $1-$5 Million
Year Founded: 1996
Total Employees: 21 — Sales Staff: 1
Ownership: Private
Quality System Registration Information: ISO9002
Produces/Sells CE-marked Devices: Y
Federal Procurement Eligibility: Small Business
Distribution: Manufacturer Direct, Service Direct, Exporter
General Admin.: Billy Teeple/Chief Operating Officer, Vice President
Terry Bagwell/President, Chief Executive Officer
Contract Assembly — General

SPECIALTEAM MEDICAL SERVICES, INC. 714-694-0348 (cont'd)
Contract Manufacturing — General
Contract Manufacturing, Product, Disposable — General
Contract Packaging — General
Contract Sterilization — General

SPECIALTY CARE 800-349-4374
One American Center — (615) 345-5400
3100 West End Avenue, Suite 800
Nashville, TN 37203
FDA Number: 2433882 — Fax: (615) 345-5405
E-mail: info@specialtycare.net
Web site: www.surgicalservices.com
Annual Revenue: $25-$50 Million
Total Employees: 215
Ownership: TELEFLEX, INC.
Stock Symbol: SGSI
Traded On: OTC Bulletin
Produces/Sells CE-marked Devices: N
Distribution: Service Direct
General Admin.: Kevin Gordon/Chairman
Paul D'Alesio/Chief Financial Officer, Treasurer
Todd Riddell/President, Chief Executive Officer
Mktg./Adv.: Craig Little/Senior Vice President Corporate Development
Production: Arlene Campbell/Vice President Operations
Service, Equipment Leasing — General
Service, Repair, Endoscopic — General
Tray, Surgical Instrument — Surgery

SPECIALTY COATING SYSTEMS, INC. 800-356-8260
7645 Woodland Dr., Indianapolis, IN 46278 — 317-244-1200
FDA Number: n/a — Fax: 317-240-2092
E-mail: lwolgemuth@scscoatings.com
Web site: www.scscoatings.com
Year Founded: 1971
Total Employees: 300
Ownership: Private
Quality System Registration Information: ISO9001
Produces/Sells CE-marked Devices: N
Federal Procurement Eligibility: Small Business
Distribution: Manufacturer Direct, Manufacturer Through Distributor, Service Direct, Exporter
General Admin.: Wendy Walters/Director Human Resources
Terry Bush/President, Chief Executive Officer
Mktg./Adv.: Timothy Bender/Vice President Marketing & Sales
IS: Dr. Rakesh Kumar/Vice President Technology
Equipment, Device Coating, Protective — General
Service, Device Coating, Protective — General

SPECIALTY GASES OF AMERICA, INC. 419-729-7732
6055 Brent Dr., Toledo, OH 43611
FDA Number: 3003326978
Gas, Calibrated (Specified Concentration) — Anesthesiology

SPECIALTY HEALTH PRODUCTS, INC. 623-582-4950
21636 North 14th Ave.,, Suite A-1, Phoenix, AZ 85027
FDA Number: 2027347
Irrigator, Colonic — Gastroenterology/Urology

SPECIALTY LABORATORIES, INC. 800-421-7110
27027 Tourney Rd., Valencia, CA 91355 — 661-799-6543
FDA Number: n/a — Fax: 661-799-6634
E-mail: specialty@specialtylabs.com
Web site: www.specialtylabs.com
Year Founded: 1975
Ownership: QUEST DIAGNOSTICS, INC.
Produces/Sells CE-marked Devices: N
Federal Procurement Eligibility: Small Business
Contract Laboratory — General

SPECIALTY LENS CORP. 800-366-1382
3955 South 210 West, Salt Lake City, UT 84107
FDA Number: 1724601
Ownership: Private
Produces/Sells CE-marked Devices: N
Lens, Spectacle/Eyeglasses, Non-Custom — Ophthalmology

SPECIALTY MANUFACTURERS, MEDICAL PRODUCTS DIVISION 317-241-2457
2410 Executive Drive, Indianapolis, IN 46241
FDA Number: 3006039198 — Fax: 317-241-4420
E-mail: dlucas@spcmfg.com
Web site: www.spcmfg.com
Ownership: Private
Produces/Sells CE-marked Devices: N
Speculum, Vaginal, Non-Metal — Obstetrics/Gynecology

SPECIALTY MANUFACTURING CO., THE   651-653-0599
5858 Centerville Rd., St. Paul, MN 55127-6804
FDA Number: n/a   Fax: 651-653-0989
E-mail: info@specialtymfg.com
Web site: www.specialtymfg.com
Medical Products Sales Volume: $5,000,000
Annual Revenue: $25-$50 Million
Year Founded: 1901
Total Employees: 250   Marketing Staff: 1   Sales Staff: 5
Ownership: Private
Produces/Sells CE-marked Devices: N
Federal Procurement Eligibility: Small Business, Female Owned
Distribution: Manufacturer Direct, OEM, Exclusive Distributor
General Admin.: Dan McKeown/President, Chief Executive Officer
     Mark Nosbush/Vice President, General Manager
Mktg./Adv.: Dave Furth/Director Marketing
     Dave Furth/Director National Accounts & Sales
     Robert Pfegler/Director Product Development
     Dave Furth/Manager Advertising
     Kevin Carlson/Manager Contract Sales
     David Furth/Manager Sales Training

Pump, Infusion	General
Valve, Other	Chemistry

SPECIALTY MANUFACTURING, INC.   800-269-6204
2210 Midland Road, Saginaw, MI 48603-3440   989-790-9011
FDA Number: 1831948   Fax: 989-790-9106
E-mail: kwiechmann@smimfg.com
Web site: www.smimfg.com
Medical Products Sales Volume: $1,600,000
Year Founded: 1979
Total Employees: 25   Marketing Staff: 3   Sales Staff: 3
Ownership: Private
Quality System Registration Information: ISO9002
Produces/Sells CE-marked Devices: N
Federal Procurement Eligibility: Small Business, Female Owned
Distribution: OEM
General Admin.: Kristi Wiechmann/Chief Financial Officer, Vice President
     Kathy Thompson/President
     Kristi Wiechmann/Vice President
Mktg./Adv.: Dennis Vowell/Manager Marketing
     Mr. Steve Smith/Manager Sales

Catheter, Other	Gastroenterology/Urology
Component, Silicone	General
Silicone Sheeting	General
Tubing, Silicone	General

SPECIALTY MEDICAL PRODUCTS CO.   801-295-6023
3063 South Davis Blvd., Bountiful, UT 84010
FDA Number: 1721432

Clamp, Umbilical	Obstetrics/Gynecology
Tubing, Non-Invasive	Surgery

SPECIALTY MEDICAL SUPPLIES, INC.   954-752-5603
3882 NW 124th Avenue,, Coral Springs, FL 33065
FDA Number: n/a   Fax: 954-757-8074
E-mail: info@specialtyms.com
Web site: www.specialtymedicalsupplies.com
Medical Products Sales Volume: $1,600,000
Annual Revenue: $5-$10 Million
Year Founded: 1999
Total Employees: 10
Ownership: Private
Quality System Registration Information: ISO9001
Produces/Sells CE-marked Devices: Y
Federal Procurement Eligibility: Small Business
Distribution: Manufacturer Direct

Pad, Alcohol	General

SPECIALTY SURGICAL INSTRUMENTATION, INC.   800-251-3000
3034 Owen Drive, Antioch, TN 37013   615-883-9090
FDA Number: n/a   Fax: 615-883-9107
E-mail: louwallace@specialty-surgical.com
Web site: www.ssiultra.com
Annual Revenue: $25-$50 Million
Year Founded: 1976
Total Employees: 74   Marketing Staff: 1   Sales Staff: 30
Ownership: Private
Produces/Sells CE-marked Devices: N
Federal Procurement Eligibility: Small Business
Distribution: Manufacturer Direct, Exclusive Distributor
General Admin.: Charles O. Mann/Executive Vice President
     Louis C. Wallace/President, Chief Executive Officer
Mktg./Adv.: Mickey Wormsley/Manager Contract Sales
     Aaron Priest/Manager Sales
     Les McClimans/Manager Sales
     Mickey Wormsley/Vice President Business Development

SPECIALTY SURGICAL INSTRUMENTATION, INC.   800-251-3000
(cont'd)
     Les McClimans/Vice President Sales
Production: Steve Tanner/Manager Regulatory Affairs
     Dale Reese/Product Specialist

Instrument, Microsurgical	Cns/Neurology
Laser, Combination	General
Laser, Surgical	Surgery
Surgical Instrument, Disposable	Surgery

SPECIALTY SURGICAL PRODUCTS, INC.   406-961-0102
1131 North U.S. Hwy. 93, Victor, MT 59875
FDA Number: 3031984   Fax: 406-961-0103
E-mail: info@ssp-inc.com
Web site: www.ssp-inc.com
Year Founded: 1997
Ownership: Private
Quality System Registration Information: ISO9001
Produces/Sells CE-marked Devices: Y
Federal Procurement Eligibility: Small Business
Distribution: Manufacturer Direct, Manufacturer Through Manufacturer Reps
Production: Customer Service/Customer Service Representative

Catheter, Biliary	Gastroenterology/Urology
Dilator, Rectal	Gastroenterology/Urology
Expander, Skin, Inflatable	Surgery
Mesh, Surgical, Polymeric	Surgery
Protector, Skin Pressure	General
Sizer, Mammary, Breast Implant Volume	Surgery

SPECLINC   800-468-9276
361 Haynes Rd., Dyersburg, TN 38024   731-286-4211
FDA Number: 1034771   Fax: 731-286-0213
E-mail: speclinc@gmail.com
Web site: www.speclinc.com
Ownership: Private
Produces/Sells CE-marked Devices: N

Speculum, Ear	Ear/Nose/Throat

SPECMAT TECHNOLOGIES INC.   011-441-5687
215 Dunavant Dr., Rockford, TN 37853
FDA Number: 3004709721
Ownership: Private
Produces/Sells CE-marked Devices: N

Wheelchair, Manual	Physical Med

SPECTRA GASES, INC.   800-932-0624
3434 Rt. 22 W., Branchburg, NJ 08876   908-252-9300
FDA Number: n/a   Fax: 908-252-0811
E-mail: info@spectragases.com
Web site: www.spectragases.com
Medical Products Sales Volume: $34,900,000
Annual Revenue: $50-$100 Million
Year Founded: 1980
Total Employees: 143   Marketing Staff: 2   Sales Staff: 25
Ownership: Private
Quality System Registration Information: ISO9000; ISO9001
Produces/Sells CE-marked Devices: N
Federal Procurement Eligibility: Small Business
Distribution: Manufacturer Direct, Exporter
General Admin.: Andrew Dietz/President
Mktg./Adv.: Mr. Michael Baselice/Manager Marketing

Laser, Excimer, Surgical	Surgery

SPECTRA INDUSTRIES CORP.   800-220-7050
322 W. Oak Lane, Manor, PA 19036   610-622-6700
FDA Number: n/a   Fax: 610-259-9040
E-mail: sales@spectracor.com
Web site: www.spectracor.com
Medical Products Sales Volume: $500,000
Annual Revenue: $0-$1 Million
Total Employees: 10   Marketing Staff: 1   Sales Staff: 2
Ownership: Private
Produces/Sells CE-marked Devices: N
Federal Procurement Eligibility: Small Business
Distribution: Manufacturer Direct, Manufacturer Through Distributor, OEM, Exporter
General Admin.: Mario DiGiulio/Chief Executive Officer
     Mario DiGiulio/President
Mktg./Adv.: Barbara Hoffert/Manager Advertising
     Marian N. Gabriele/Sales Representative
     Margaret Redding/Vice President Marketing
Production: George R. Harper/Vice President Manufacturing

Orthosis, Corrective Shoe	Physical Med

SPECTRA MEDICAL DEVICES, INC.   978-657-0889
260-H Fordham Road, Wilmington, MA 01887
FDA Number: 1224960   Fax: 978-657-4339
E-mail: arthur@spectramedical.com

SPECTRA MEDICAL DEVICES, INC.   978-657-0889 *(cont'd)*
Web site: www.spectramedical.com
Medical Products Sales Volume: $2,200,000
Annual Revenue: $5-$10 Million
Year Founded: 1995
Total Employees: 12   *Marketing Staff:* 2   *Sales Staff:* 2
Ownership: Private
Produces/Sells CE-marked Devices: N
Federal Procurement Eligibility: Small Business
Distribution: OEM
General Admin.: anthony arrigo/President
Mktg./Adv.: joe harms/National Sales Representative
Production: scott henderson/Director Manufacturing & Engineering
robert duffett/Director Operations

Applicator, Other	General
Bag, Laundry, Infection Control	General
Blade, Scalpel	Surgery
Introducer, Spinal Needle	Anesthesiology
Needle, Conduction, Anesthesia (W/Wo Introducer)	Anesthesiology
Needle, Radiographic	Radiology
Needle, Spinal, Short-Term	General
Stylet, Needle	General
Syringe, Anesthesia	Anesthesiology
Syringe, Other	General
Trocar, Other	General

SPECTRA MEDICAL DEVICES, INC.   866-938-8649
4C Henshaw St., Woburn, MA 01801   **781-938-8649**
FDA Number: 9012618   Fax: 781-938-0357
E-mail: rduffett95@aol.com
Annual Revenue: $5-$10 Million
Year Founded: 1995
Total Employees: 15   *Marketing Staff:* 4   *Sales Staff:* 5
Ownership: Private
Produces/Sells CE-marked Devices: N
Federal Procurement Eligibility: Small Business, Female Owned
Distribution: Manufacturer Direct, OEM, Exclusive Distributor
General Admin.: Tony Arrigo/President, Chief Executive Officer
Mktg./Adv.: Phylis Dias/Manager Marketing & Sales
Production: Robert Duffett/Manager Regulatory Affairs

Applicator, Other	General
Bag, Garbage	General
Blade, Scalpel	Surgery
Catheter, Epidural	Obstetrics/Gynecology
Contract Manufacturing	General
Drape, Surgical	Surgery
Fitting, Luer	General
Glove, Surgical	General
Kit, Administration, Intra-Arterial	General
Kit, Intravenous Extension Tubing	General
Kit, Pressure Monitoring (Air/Gas)	General
Pipette, Quantitative, Hematology	Hematology
Slide, Microscope	Pathology
Syringe, Laboratory	Chemistry
Syringe, Other	General
Tube, Capillary	Chemistry
Tubing, Fluid Delivery	General
Tubing, Hypodermic	General
Tubing, Other	General
Tubing, Oxygen Connecting	General
Tubing, Plastic	General
Tubing, Polyethylene	General
Tubing, Polypropylene	General
Tubing, Polyvinyl Chloride	General
Tubing, Radiopaque	General
Tubing, Silicone	General
Tubing, Urethane	General
Tubing, Vinyl	General
Valve, Other	Chemistry

SPECTRA-PHYSICS LAZORS   877-835-9620
3635 Peterson Way, Santa Clara, CA 95054   **408-980-4300**
FDA Number: n/a   Fax: 408-980-6921
E-mail: sales@spectra-physics.com
Web site: www.newport.com/spectra-physics
Medical Products Sales Volume: $3,000,000
Annual Revenue: $1-$5 Million
Total Employees: 970
Ownership: Public
Produces/Sells CE-marked Devices: N
Distribution: Manufacturer Direct, Exporter
General Admin.: Patrick L. Edsell/President
Mktg./Adv.: Leif Alexandersson/Vice President Sales
Research: Norm Hodgson/Manager Research & Development

Accessories, Laser	General
Ophthalmoscope, Laser	Ophthalmology

SPECTRA-PHYSICS, INC.
See Spectra-Physics Lazors

SPECTRA-TECH
See Thermo Spectra-Tech

SPECTRA-TINT   585-546-8050
250 Cumberland Street, Suite 228, Rochester, NY 14605
FDA Number: 1317783

Fixative, Alcohol Containing	Pathology
Fixative, Formalin Containing	Pathology
Formalin, Neutral Buffered	Pathology
Gelatin For Specimen Adhesion	Pathology
Solution, Pathology, Decalcifier, Acid Containing	Pathology
Solution, Pathology, Formalin-Alcohol-Acetic Acid	Pathology
Stain, Eosin Y	Pathology

SPECTRACELL LABORATIES   800.227.5227
10401 Town Park Drive, Houston, TX 77072   **713.621.3101**
FDA Number: n/a   Fax: 713.621.3234
E-mail: spec1@spectracell.com
Web site: http://www.spectracell.com
Year Founded: 1993
Ownership: Private
Produces/Sells CE-marked Devices: N
General Admin.: Mr. William Stanber/Chief Executive Officer
Mktg./Adv.: Mr. Otto Schaefer/Vice President Sales
Production: Dr. John Crawford/Senior Vice President Operations
Finance: Mr. William Preece/Chief Financial Officer

SPECTRAL DIAGNOSTICS INC.   888-426-4264
135-2 The West Mall,   **416-626-3233**
Toronto, ON M9C 1 Canada
FDA Number: 9617857   Fax: 416-626-7383
E-mail: info@spectraldx.com
Web site: www.spectraldx.com
Year Founded: 1991
Total Employees: 100   *Marketing Staff:* 8   *Sales Staff:* 35
Ownership: Public
Stock Symbol: SDI
Traded On: Toronto
Quality System Registration Information: ISO9001
Produces/Sells CE-marked Devices: N
Distribution: Manufacturer Direct, Manufacturer Through Manufacturer Reps, Exporter

SPECTRAL INSTRUMENTS, INC.   520-884-8821
420 North Bonita Ave, Tucson, AZ 85745
FDA Number: n/a   Fax: 520-884-8803
E-mail: info@specinst.com
Web site: www.specinst.com
Annual Revenue: $1-$5 Million
Ownership: Private
Produces/Sells CE-marked Devices: N
Federal Procurement Eligibility: Small Business
Distribution: Manufacturer Direct, Manufacturer Through Distributor, Manufacturer Through Manufacturer Reps, OEM

Camera, Other	General
Spectrophotometer, U.V./Visible	Chemistry

SPECTRAL MOLECULAR IMAGING INC.   310-858-1670
250 N. Robertson Blvd., Suite 427, Beverly Hills, CA 90211
FDA Number: n/a   Fax: 310-858-1699
E-mail: info@opmol.com
Web site: http://www.spectralmi.com
Ownership: Private
Produces/Sells CE-marked Devices: N
General Admin.: Dr. Erik Lindsley/President
Mktg./Adv.: Dr. Sam Raz/Vice President Business Development

SPECTRALINK CORPORATION   800-676-5465
5755 Central Avenue, Boulder, CO 80301   **303-440-5330**
FDA Number: n/a   Fax: 303-440-5331
E-mail: info@spectralink.com
Web site: www.spectralink.com
Medical Products Sales Volume: $144,800,000
Annual Revenue: $50-$100 Million
Year Founded: 1990
Total Employees: 650
Ownership: Public
Stock Symbol: SLNK
Traded On: NASDAQ
Quality System Registration Information: ISO9001
Produces/Sells CE-marked Devices: N
Federal Procurement Eligibility: GSA Contract
Distribution: Manufacturer Direct, Manufacturer Through Distributor, OEM
General Admin.: John Elms/President, Chief Executive Officer
Mktg./Adv.: Mark Mitton/Manager Advertising & Public Relations
Jill Kenney/Vice President Marketing & Sales
Ben Guderian/Vice President Strategic Development
Production: John Kelley/Vice President Manufacturing

SPECTRALINK CORPORATION
800-676-5465 *(cont'd)*
Communication Equipment — General
Telephone Equipment — General

SPECTRALYTICS
800-543-0163
145 3rd St. South, PO Box L, Dassel, MN 55325
320-275-2118
FDA Number: n/a
Fax: 320-275-2993
E-mail: sales@spectralytics.com
Web site: www.spectralytics.com
Medical Products Sales Volume: $1,700,000
Annual Revenue: $5-$10 Million
Year Founded: 1990
Total Employees: 30 — *Marketing Staff:* 1 — *Sales Staff:* 2
Ownership: Private
Quality System Registration Information: ISO9002
Produces/Sells CE-marked Devices: N
Federal Procurement Eligibility: Small Business
Distribution: Manufacturer Direct, Manufacturer Through Manufacturer Reps
General Admin.: Gary Oberg/President, Chief Executive Officer
Joanne Kotila/Vice President Human Resources
Mktg./Adv.: Kurt Krueger/Director Marketing
Kurt Krueger/Manager National Sales
Production: Bob Deitz/Director Quality Assurance
Service, Engineering/Design — General

SPECTRAMED INC., CARDIOPULMONARY DIV.
See CAREFUSION 211, INC..

SPECTRAN SPECIALTY OPTICS CO.
See Ofs, Specialty Photonics Division

SPECTRANETICS CORP.
800-633-0960
9965 Federal Drive, Colorado Springs, CO 80921
719-447-2000
FDA Number: 1721279
Fax: 877-447-2022
E-mail: info@bv.spectranetics.com
Web site: www.spectranetics.com
Medical Products Sales Volume: $71,600,000
Year Founded: 1984
Total Employees: 311
Ownership: Public
Stock Symbol: SPNC
Traded On: NASDAQ
Quality System Registration Information: ISO9000; ISO9001
Produces/Sells CE-marked Devices: Y
Federal Procurement Eligibility: Small Business
Distribution: Manufacturer Direct, Manufacturer Through Manufacturer Reps, Importer, Exporter
General Admin.: Mr. Scott Drake/Chief Executive Officer
Mr. Roger Wertheimer/Senior Vice President Human Resources
Mr. Frank Rivas/Vice President
Mr. Roger Wertheimer/Vice President General Counsel & Secretary
Mktg./Adv.: Mr. Jason Hein/Senior Vice President Marketing & Sales
Mr. Shar Matin/Senior Vice President Product Development
Ms. Renee Boehme/Vice President Sales
Finance: Guy Childs/Chief Financial Officer, Senior Vice President Finance
Catheter, Myoplasty, Laser, Coronary — Cardiovascular
Device, Removal, Pacemaker Electrode, Percutaneous — Cardiovascular
Laser, Excimer, Surgical — Surgery

SPECTRASCIENCE, INC.
858-847-0200
11568-11 Sorrento Valley Rd., San Diego, CA 92121
FDA Number: 2183611
Fax: 858-847-0880
E-mail: info@spectrascience.com
Web site: www.spectrascience.com
Ownership: Public
Stock Symbol: SCIE
Traded On: OTC Bulletin
Produces/Sells CE-marked Devices: N
Finance: Jim Hitchin/Chief Financial Officer
Jim Dorst/Chief Financial Officer, Vice President Finance
Analyzer, Diagnostic, Fiberoptic (Colon) — Gastroenterology/Urology
Catheter, Percutaneous — Cardiovascular
Forceps, Biopsy, Non-Electric — Gastroenterology/Urology
Laser, Angioplasty, Peripheral — Cardiovascular
Sensor, Electro-optical(for Cervical Cancer) — Obstetrics/Gynecology

SPECTREX CORP.
800-822-3940
3580 Haven Avenue,
650-365-6567
Redwood City, CA 94063
FDA Number: 7000904
E-mail: info@spectrex.com
Fax: 650-365-5845
Web site: www.spectrex.com
Medical Products Sales Volume: $1,000,000
Annual Revenue: $0-$1 Million
Year Founded: 1966
Total Employees: 4 — *Marketing Staff:* 1 — *Sales Staff:* 1
Ownership: Private
Produces/Sells CE-marked Devices: Y

SPECTREX CORP.
800-822-3940 *(cont'd)*
Federal Procurement Eligibility: Small Business
Distribution: Manufacturer Direct, Manufacturer Through Distributor, Service Direct, Exporter
General Admin.: John M. Hoyte/President
Stan Figone/Vice President
Production: Steve Figone/Vice President Production
Counter, Cell — Microbiology
Sampler, Gas — Chemistry
Spectrophotometer, U.V./Visible — Chemistry

SPECTRO ANALYTICAL INSTRUMENTS INC.
800-548-5809
160 Authority Drive, Fitchburg, MA 01420
978-342-3400
FDA Number: n/a
Fax: 978-342-8695
E-mail: info@spectro-usa.com
Web site: www.spectro-usa.com
Annual Revenue: $10-$25 Million
Year Founded: 1979
Total Employees: 15 — *Marketing Staff:* 4 — *Sales Staff:* 15
Ownership: Private
Produces/Sells CE-marked Devices: N
Federal Procurement Eligibility: Small Business
Distribution: Manufacturer Direct, Importer, Exporter
General Admin.: Tom Bloomer/President
Mktg./Adv.: Thomas Bloamer/Vice President Marketing
Analyzer, Carbon Hydrogen Nitrogen — Chemistry
Mass Spectrometer, Clinical Use — Toxicology

SPECTRO INDUSTRIES INC.
See Mckesson Drug Co.

SPECTROCELL, INC.
215-572-7605
143 Montgomery Ave., Oreland, PA 19075
FDA Number: n/a
Fax: 215-885-2792
E-mail: spectrocell@comcast.net
Web site: www.spectrocell.com
Annual Revenue: $1-$5 Million
Year Founded: 1955
Ownership: Private
Produces/Sells CE-marked Devices: N
Federal Procurement Eligibility: Small Business
Distribution: Manufacturer Direct
General Admin.: Michael J. Serianni/President
Production: Gerald Serianni/Vice President Manufacturing
Cuvette, Spectrophotometer — Chemistry
Cuvette, Thermostated — Chemistry
Spectrophotometer, U.V./Visible — Chemistry
Stirrer — Chemistry
Viscometer — Chemistry

SPECTRON CORP.
425-827-9317
934 S. Burlington Blvd # 603, Burlington, WA 98233
FDA Number: n/a
Fax: 425-458-4412
E-mail: jim@spectroncorp.com
Web site: www.spectroncorp.com
Medical Products Sales Volume: $2,000,000
Annual Revenue: $1-$5 Million
Year Founded: 1973
Total Employees: 10 — *Marketing Staff:* 4 — *Sales Staff:* 4
Ownership: Private
Produces/Sells CE-marked Devices: N
Federal Procurement Eligibility: Small Business
Distribution: Exclusive Distributor
General Admin.: James R. Tompkins/President
Mktg./Adv.: Julie Reid/Manager Clinical Sales
Gene Hulsey/Manager International Marketing & Sales
Analyzer, Blood Gas pH — Anesthesiology
Analyzer, Chemistry, Multi-Channel, Fixed — Chemistry
Analyzer, Chemistry, Single Channel, Programmable — Chemistry
Analyzer, Gas, Oxygen, Sampling — Anesthesiology
Camera, Gamma (Nuclear/Scintillation) — Radiology
Chromatography, Liquid, Performance, High — Toxicology
Counter, Cell — Microbiology
Counter, Gamma, General Use — Toxicology
Diffractometer, X-Ray — Chemistry
Fluorometer — Immunology
Mass Spectrometer, Clinical Use — Toxicology
Microscope, Laboratory, Electron — Microbiology
Microtome, Cryostat — Pathology
Nuclear Magnetic Resonance Imaging System — Radiology
Osmometer — Chemistry
Photometer, Flame, General Use — Toxicology
Scanner, Computed Tomography, X-Ray (CAT, CT) — Cns/Neurology
Service, Used Equipment — General
Spectrograph, Mass — Chemistry
Spectrophotometer, U.V./Visible — Chemistry
Sterilizer, Steam (Autoclave) — General
Tissue Processor, Automated — Pathology

SPECTRON ENGINEERING, INC.   303-733-1060
255 Yuma Ct., Denver, CO 80223
FDA Number: n/a   Fax: 303-733-2432
E-mail: sales@spectronengineering.com
Web site: www.spectronengineering.com
Annual Revenue: $0-$1 Million
Total Employees: 10
Ownership: Private
Produces/Sells CE-marked Devices: N
Federal Procurement Eligibility: Small Business
Distribution: Manufacturer Through Distributor

Densitometer, Laboratory	Chemistry
Image Processing System	Radiology
Spectrophotometer, Ultraviolet	Chemistry
Spectrophotometer, Visible	Chemistry

SPECTRONIC INSTRUMENTS, INC.
See Thermo Spectronic

SPECTRONIC UNICAM
See Thermo Spectronic

SPECTRONICS CORPORATION   800-274-8888
956 Brush Hollow Road,   516-333-4840
Westbury, NY 11590
FDA Number: 2419818   Fax: 516-333-4840
E-mail: info@spectroline.com
Web site: www.spectroline.com
Medical Products Sales Volume: $20,000,000
Annual Revenue: $10-$25 Million
Year Founded: 1955
Total Employees: 190   *Marketing Staff:* 2   *Sales Staff:* 5
Ownership: Private
Quality System Registration Information: ISO9001
Produces/Sells CE-marked Devices: N
Federal Procurement Eligibility: Small Business
Distribution: Manufacturer Direct, Manufacturer Through Distributor, OEM, Importer, Exporter
General Admin.: B. William Cooper/Chief Executive Officer
      Barbara Heslin/Manager Personnel
      Jonathan D. Cooper/President
Mktg./Adv.: Betty Cheng/Director National Accounts
      Gary D. Fixel/Director Sales
      Alice McKeown/Manager Corporate Communications
      Gerri Curry/Manager International Accounts
      Michael Newmark/Manager Sales
Production: Gloria Blusk/Manager Customer Services
      John Duerr/Vice President Manufacturing

Bilirubinometer	Chemistry
Cabinet, Chromatography (U.V.) Viewing	Chemistry
Cabinet, Other	General
Cassette, Radiographic Film	Radiology
Duplicator, X-Ray Film	Radiology
Grid, Radiographic	Radiology
Lamp, Examination (Light)	General
Lamp, Other	General
Lamp, Ultraviolet, Germicidal	General
Lamp, Ultraviolet, Physical Medicine	Physical Med
Photometer	Chemistry
Radiometer, Phototherapy	General
Radiometer, Ultraviolet	General
Screen, Intensifying, Radiographic	Radiology

SPECTROS CORPORATION   650-851-4040
808 Portola Rd, Portola Valley, CA 94028
FDA Number: 3004957206   Fax: 650-851-4099
E-mail: info@spectros.com
Web site: http://www.spectros.com
Ownership: Private
Produces/Sells CE-marked Devices: N
General Admin.: Mr. David Benaron/Chief Executive Officer

Oximeter, Tissue Saturation	Cardiovascular

SPECTRUM AQUATICS   800-791-8056
7100 Spectrum Ln., Missoula, MT 59808   406-542-9781
FDA Number: n/a   Fax: 406-728-7143
E-mail: info@spectrumaquatics.com
Web site: www.spectrumaquatics.com
Year Founded: 1975
Total Employees: 50   *Marketing Staff:* 2   *Sales Staff:* 8
Ownership: Private
Produces/Sells CE-marked Devices: N
Distribution: Manufacturer Direct, Manufacturer Through Distributor
General Admin.: Dave Murray/President
Mktg./Adv.: George Bowman/Vice President Marketing & Sales
Production: Joe Weimer/Vice President Manufacturing

Bath, Hydro-Massage (Whirlpool)	Physical Med
Unit, Evaluation, Height, Lift	Orthopedics

SPECTRUM ASSEMBLY INC.   760-752-7008
970 Los Vallecitos Blvd., Suite 140, San Marcos, CA 92069
FDA Number: 3002672225

Unit, Therapy, Current, Interferential	Cns/Neurology

SPECTRUM DENTAL LLC.   310-845-8345
8554 Hayden Place, Culver City, CA 90232
FDA Number: 3003840077

Dam, Rubber	Dental And Oral

SPECTRUM DESIGNS MEDICAL, INC.   800-239-6399
6387-B Rose Lane, Carpinteria, CA 93013   805-684-7678
FDA Number: 2028306   Fax: 805-684-0497
E-mail: service@spectrumdesignsmedical.com
Web site: www.spectrumdesignsmedical.com
Annual Revenue: $1-$5 Million
Year Founded: 1987
Total Employees: 10   *Marketing Staff:* 4   *Sales Staff:* 2
Ownership: Private
Quality System Registration Information: ISO9001
Produces/Sells CE-marked Devices: Y
Federal Procurement Eligibility: Small Business
Distribution: Manufacturer Direct, Manufacturer Through Distributor, OEM
General Admin.: Jim Dishman/President, Chief Executive Officer
      Donna Dishman/Vice President, General Manager
Mktg./Adv.: Donna Dishman/Director Marketing
      Donna Dishman/Director National Accounts

Elastomer, Silicone (Scar Management)	Surgery
Elastomer, Silicone Block	Surgery
Implant, Muscle, Pectoralis	Surgery
Malar Implant	Surgery
Prosthesis, Chin, Internal	Surgery
Prosthesis, Nose, Internal	Surgery

SPECTRUM HEARING SYSTEMS, INC.   704-237-9100
18636 Starcreek Drive, Suite E, Cornelius, NC 28031
FDA Number: 3004743369

Hearing-Aid	Ear/Nose/Throat

SPECTRUM INTERNATIONAL, INC.   925-768-1122
1130 Burnett Avenue, Suite J, Clyde, CA 94520
FDA Number: 3006015832

Laser, Surgical	Surgery

SPECTRUM LABORATORIES, INC.   800-634-3300
18617 Broadwick St.,   310-885-4600
Rancho Dominguez, CA 90220
FDA Number: 2025136   Fax: 310-885-4666
E-mail: customerservice@spectrapor.com
Web site: www.spectrumlabs.com
Annual Revenue: $10-$25 Million
Year Founded: 1970
Total Employees: 125   *Marketing Staff:* 3   *Sales Staff:* 4
Ownership: Spectrum Laboratories, Inc.
Stock Symbol: SPTM
Traded On: NASDAQ
Quality System Registration Information: ISO9000
Federal Procurement Eligibility: Small Business
Distribution: Manufacturer Direct, Manufacturer Through Distributor, OEM
General Admin.: Roy T. Eddleman/Chief Executive Officer
      Laura Sarconi/Manager Human Resources
      F. Jesus Martinez/President
      Malcolm Morrison/Vice President, General Manager
Mktg./Adv.: Bob Sodul/Director National Accounts
      Leanna Levine/Director Product Development
      Bob Sodul/Vice President Marketing & Sales
Production: Malcolm Morrison/Director Quality Assurance
      Cheryl Lomonaco/Manager Materials
      Malcolm Morrison/Vice President Manufacturing
Research: Leanna Levine/Vice President Research & Development
Finance: Larry Womack/Chief Financial Officer

Accessories, Chromatography (Gas, Gel, Liquid, Thin Layer)	Chemistry
Concentrator, Clinical Sample	Chemistry
Contract R&D, Equipment	General
Dialyzer, Capillary, Hollow Fiber (Hemodialysis)	Gastroenterology/Urology
Dialyzer, Laboratory	Chemistry
Drape, Surgical, Disposable	Surgery
Filter, Gas	Anesthesiology
Filter, Membrane	Chemistry
Filter, Syringe	General
Injector, Sample	Chemistry
Kit, Tubing, Dialysis, Peritoneal	Gastroenterology/Urology
Office Product	General
Pump, Infusion	General
Sterilizer, Steam (Autoclave)	General
Syringe, Bulb	General
System, Peritoneal Dialysis, Automatic	Gastroenterology/Urology
Ultrafiltration Equipment	Chemistry

SPECTRUM LABORATORIES, INC.
800-634-3300 *(cont'd)*
Unit, Filter, Membrane
Chemistry

SPECTRUM LABORATORY PRODUCTS, INC.
800-813-1514
14422 S. San Pedro St., Gardena, CA 90248-2027
310-516-8000
FDA Number: n/a
E-mail: sales@spectrumchemical.com
Web site: www.spectrumchemical.com
Year Founded: 1971
Ownership: Private
Quality System Registration Information: ISO9000; ISO9001
Produces/Sells CE-marked Devices: N
Federal Procurement Eligibility: Small Business, Female Owned
Distribution: Manufacturer Direct, Manufacturer Through Distributor
General Admin.: Marc Hayem/Chief Executive Officer

Contract Manufacturing	General
Contract Manufacturing, Pharmaceuticals/Chemicals	General
Eyeglasses, Safety	Ophthalmology
Fountain, Eye Wash	Chemistry
Plug, Electrical	General
Safety Equipment, Laboratory	Chemistry
Shower, Emergency	Chemistry
Stain, Chemical Solution	Pathology

SPECTRUM LASER & TECHNOLOGIES, INC
719-264-7632
2270 Garden of the Gods Road, Suite 103,
Colorado Springs, CO 80907
FDA Number: 1724675
Fax: 719-548-8289
E-mail: inform@spectrumlaser.com
Web site: www.spectrumlaser.com
Medical Products Sales Volume: $2,000,000
Annual Revenue: $1-$5 Million
Year Founded: 1997
Total Employees: 20   *Marketing Staff:* 2   *Sales Staff:* 2
Ownership: Private
Quality System Registration Information: ISO9001
Produces/Sells CE-marked Devices: N
Federal Procurement Eligibility: Small Business
Distribution: Manufacturer Direct, Manufacturer Through Distributor

Laser, Healing, Wound	Surgery
Laser, Therapy, Pain	Cns/Neurology

SPECTRUM MEDICAL INDUSTRIES, INC.
See Spectrum Laboratories, Inc.

SPECTRUM MEDICAL MARKET CONSULTANTS
514-696-0303
475 Westminster Ave.,
Dollard-des-Ormeaux, QUE H9G-2 Canada
FDA Number: n/a
Fax: 514-696-0373
E-mail: spectrum@SprintUS.com
Year Founded: 1986
Total Employees: 25
Ownership: Private
Produces/Sells CE-marked Devices: N

SPECTRUM MICROGON
See Spectrum Laboratories, Inc.

SPECTRUM OPTICAL
323-931-4349
6154 West 6th. Street, Los Angeles, CA 90048
FDA Number: 2085342
Fax: 323-931-5667
E-mail: spctrmopt@aol.com
Medical Products Sales Volume: $300,000
Year Founded: 2000
Ownership: Private
Produces/Sells CE-marked Devices: N
Federal Procurement Eligibility: Small Business

Frame, Spectacle (Eyeglasses)	Ophthalmology
Sunglasses (Including Photosensitive)	Ophthalmology

SPECTRUM PRODUCTS USA
800-338-7581
3701 West Roanoke, Phoenix, AZ 85009
FDA Number: 2032008

Stretcher, Hand-Carried	General

SPECTRUM QUALITY PRODUCTS, INC.
See Spectrum Laboratory Products, Inc.

SPECTRUM SYSTEMS, LLC
717-845-5339
465 Ogontz St., --, York, PA 17403
FDA Number: 3006791424
Ownership: Private
Produces/Sells CE-marked Devices: N

Instrument, Diamond, Dental	Dental And Oral

SPECTRUM TECHNOLOGY
513-471-8770
3120 Warsaw Avenue, Cincinnati 45205
FDA Number: 3004363288
Ownership: Private
Produces/Sells CE-marked Devices: N

SPECTRUM TECHNOLOGY
513-471-8770 *(cont'd)*
Pouch, Colostomy
Gastroenterology/Urology

SPECTRUM TECHNOLOGY, INC.
See Vectron International

SPECTRUM-BRANDS
800-237-6541
601 Rayovac Drive, Madison, WI 53711-2497
608-275-3340
FDA Number: 1280159
Fax: 800-275-4973
E-mail: germano@rayovac.com
Web site: www.spectrumbrands.com
Annual Revenue: $1-$5 Million
Year Founded: 1900
Total Employees: 1000   *Marketing Staff:* 3   *Sales Staff:* 2
Ownership: Rayovac Corporation
Quality System Registration Information: ISO9002
Produces/Sells CE-marked Devices: N
Federal Procurement Eligibility: Small Business, GSA Contract, VA Contract
Distribution: Manufacturer Direct, Manufacturer Through Distributor, Exclusive Distributor, Importer, Exporter
Mktg./Adv.: Jennifer Clark/Director Marketing

Battery, Hearing-Aid	Ear/Nose/Throat

SPEECHEASY INTERNATIONAL, LLC
252-551-9042
112 Staton Rd., Greenville, NC 27834
FDA Number: 3004522031
Fax: (252) 413-0950
E-mail: info@speecheasy.com
Ownership: Private
Produces/Sells CE-marked Devices: N

Anti-Stammering Device	Ear/Nose/Throat

SPEED QUEEN CO.
See Unimac

SPEEDENT DENTAL SUPPLIES
800-706-0644
9591 Central Ave., Montclair, CA 91763
FDA Number: 3004672853
Ownership: Private
Produces/Sells CE-marked Devices: N

Implant, Endosseous	Dental And Oral

SPEEDLINE TECHNOLOGIES, INC.
508-520-0083
16 Forge Park, Franklin, MA 02038
FDA Number: n/a
Fax: 508-520-2288
E-mail: ctsc@speedlinetech.com
Web site: www.speedlinetechnologies.com
Annual Revenue: $25-$50 Million
Ownership: COOKSON ELECTRONICS
Stock Symbol: CKSN
Traded On: London
Produces/Sells CE-marked Devices: Y
Distribution: Manufacturer Direct, Manufacturer Through Manufacturer Reps
General Admin.: Ken Cavallaro/Chief Executive Officer
Mktg./Adv.: Craig Lazinsky/Director Marketing Services
         Allen Duck/Manager International & National Sales
Production: Chip Hosey/Manager Regulatory Affairs

Dispenser, Liquid, Laboratory	Chemistry

Medical Product Subsidiaries (Listed Separately)
Specialty Coating Systems, Inc.

SPEEDY PRODUCTS CO.
800-388-2001
225 Cash St., Jacksonville, TX 75766
903-586-2531
FDA Number: n/a
E-mail: info@SpeedyProducts.com
Web site: www.speedyproducts.com
Annual Revenue: $0-$1 Million
Ownership: Private
Produces/Sells CE-marked Devices: N
Federal Procurement Eligibility: Small Business
Distribution: Manufacturer Direct

Clamp, Tubing	General

SPEGAS INDUSTRIES LTD.
See Oridion Medical Inc.

SPELLMAN HIGH VOLTAGE ELECTRONICS CORP.
631-630-3000
475 Wireless Blvd., Hauppauge, NY 11788
FDA Number: 2429877
Fax: 631-435-1620
E-mail: service@spellmanhv.com
Web site: www.spellmanhv.com
Medical Products Sales Volume: $33,000,000
Annual Revenue: $25-$50 Million
Total Employees: 400   *Marketing Staff:* 2   *Sales Staff:* 7
Ownership: Private
Quality System Registration Information: ISO9000; ISO9001; ISO9002
Produces/Sells CE-marked Devices: Y
Distribution: Manufacturer Direct
General Admin.: S. M. Skeist/Chief Executive Officer
         Richard Projain/Managing Director

SPELLMAN HIGH VOLTAGE   631-630-3000 (cont'd)
Dr. Loren Skeist/President
Mktg./Adv.: Jim Donley/Manager Marketing
    Dennis Bay/Vice President Sales
    Eric Marko/Vice President Sales
Production: Bill Hartman/Director Quality Assurance
    Robert Barone/Vice President Manufacturing
Research: Cliff Scapellati/Vice President Engineering
Finance: Rosalie Casarona/Controller

Generator, Diagnostic X-Ray, High Voltage, 3-Phase	Radiology
Generator, Diagnostic X-Ray, High Voltage, Single Phase	Radiology
Generator, High Voltage, X-Ray, Therapeutic	Radiology
Tube, Image Amplifier, X-Ray	Radiology

SPENCER TECHNOLOGIES   800-684-0586
701 16th Avenue, Seattle, WA 98122-4525   206-329-7220
FDA Number: 3033518   Fax: 206-329-7230
E-mail: info@spencertechnologies.com
Web site: www.spencertechnologies.com
Annual Revenue: $1-$5 Million
Year Founded: 1987
Total Employees: 125   Marketing Staff: 2   Sales Staff: 3
Ownership: Private
Produces/Sells CE-marked Devices: N
Federal Procurement Eligibility: Small Business
Distribution: Manufacturer Through Distributor, OEM
General Admin.: Scott M. Seidel/President, Chief Executive Officer
Medical Admin.: David T. Dobson/Vice President Clinical Services
    Merrill P. Spencer/Vice President, Medical Director
Mktg./Adv.: Gail Ingram Kinner/Coord. Marketing
    Joe Farnsworth/Director Sales
    David T. Dobson/Vice President Marketing & Sales
Production: Tony Williams/Director Quality Assurance & Regulatory Affairs
    Grant Mattson/Vice President Manufacturing & Engineering
Research: Mark A. Moehring/Manager Research & Development

Doppler, Blood Flow, Transcranial	Cardiovascular
Fixation Device, Extra-Cranial (Head Frame)	Orthopedics

SPENCO MEDICAL   800-387-9538
6905 Millcreek Dr., Unit 12,   905-858-3565
Mississauga, ONT L5N-6 Canada
FDA Number: n/a   Fax: 905-858-3570
E-mail: spenco@spenco.ca
Web site: www.spenco.ca
Year Founded: 1995
Total Employees: 10
Ownership: Private
Produces/Sells CE-marked Devices: N
Distribution: Exclusive Distributor

SPENCO MEDICAL CORP.   254-772-6000
PO Box 2501, Waco, TX 76702-2501
FDA Number: 1619779   Fax: 254-751-3372
E-mail: spenco@spenco.com
Web site: www.spenco.com
Annual Revenue: $25-$50 Million
Year Founded: 1967
Total Employees: 500   Marketing Staff: 4   Sales Staff: 50
Ownership: Private
Quality System Registration Information: ISO9001
Produces/Sells CE-marked Devices: Y
Federal Procurement Eligibility: VA Contract
Distribution: Manufacturer Through Distributor, Manufacturer Through Manufacturer Reps, Exporter
General Admin.: Steven B. Smith/Chief Executive Officer
    Euneta Jones/Vice President Human Resources
Mktg./Adv.: Gwen Sumner/Admin. International Sales
    Mr. Blake Boulden/Marketing Product Specialist

Cushion, Foot	Orthopedics
Cushion, Wheelchair (Pad)	Physical Med
Dressing, Wound and Burn, Occlusive	Surgery
Pad, Pressure, Foam (Elbow, Heel)	General
Pad, Pressure, Gel	General
Support, Ankle	Orthopedics
Support, Arch	Physical Med
Support, Foot	Orthopedics

SPERIAN EYE & FACE PROTECTION INC.   401-232-1200
10 Thurber Blvd., Smithfield, RI 02917
FDA Number: 3005664148
Ownership: Sperian Protection
Produces/Sells CE-marked Devices: N

Frame, Spectacle (Eyeglasses)	Ophthalmology
Shield, Eye, Ophthalmic	Ophthalmology

SPERIAN PROTECTION   800-343-3411
900 Douglas Pike, Smithfield, RI 02917
FDA Number: n/a

SPERIAN PROTECTION   800-343-3411 (cont'd)
E-mail: information@sperianprotection.com
Web site: www.sperianprotection.com
Total Employees: 200   Sales Staff: 40
Ownership: Public
Stock Symbol: SPR
Traded On: Paris
Quality System Registration Information: ISO9001
Produces/Sells CE-marked Devices: Y
Federal Procurement Eligibility: Small Business
Distribution: Manufacturer Through Distributor, Manufacturer Through Manufacturer Reps, Importer, Exporter
General Admin.: Brice de La Morandiere/Chief Executive Officer
Mktg./Adv.: Tracy Benevides/Marketing Coordinator
Finance: Jerome Ronze/Chief Financial Officer

Lift, Patient	General

Medical Product Subsidiaries (Listed Separately)
  Sperian Eye & Face Protection Inc.

SPERIAN PROTECTION OPTICAL-TITMUS
See Sperian Eye & Face Protection Inc.

SPERTI DRUG PRODUCTS, INC.
See Kbd, Inc.

SPERTI SUNLAMP COMPANY
See Kbd, Inc.

SPEX GROUP, INC.
See Horiba Jobin Yvon Inc

SPEX INDUSTRIES, INC.
See Horiba Jobin Yvon Inc

SPI SPORTS/SCIENCE INC.   800-322-0688
3506 Cedar Springs, Suite 1400,   214-740-9797
Dallas, TX 75201
FDA Number: 902932   Fax: 214-740-0605
E-mail: spi@spiinc-tx.com
Web site: www.spiinc-tx.com
Ownership: Private
Produces/Sells CE-marked Devices: N
Federal Procurement Eligibility: Small Business, Female Owned
General Admin.: Suzanne Harper/President

Analyzer, Composition, Weight, Patient	General
Orthosis, Limb Brace	Physical Med

SPI, INC.
See Spi Sports/Science Inc.

SPIN-CAST PLASTICS, INC.   800-422-3625
3300 N. Kenmore St., South Bend, IN 46628   219-232-8066
FDA Number: n/a   Fax: 219-232-6036
E-mail: inquire@spincast.com
Web site: www.spincast.com
Medical Products Sales Volume: $5,900,000
Total Employees: 90   Marketing Staff: 1   Sales Staff: 2
Ownership: QUIXOTE CORPORATION
Produces/Sells CE-marked Devices: N
Federal Procurement Eligibility: Small Business
Distribution: Manufacturer Direct, OEM
General Admin.: Eric Strom/Vice President, General Manager
Mktg./Adv.: Rick Szymanowski/Manager National Sales
Production: David Eggleston/Product Manager
    Ken Clark/Vice President Manufacturing

Cabinet, Other	General
Service, Engineering/Design	General
Waste Receptacle, General Purpose	General

SPINAL DESIGNS INTL.   701-265-4927
708 Division Ave S., Cavalier, ND 58220
FDA Number: 2184146
Ownership: Private
Produces/Sells CE-marked Devices: N

Traction Unit, Non-Powered	Orthopedics

SPINAL ELEMENTS, INC.   760-607-0121
2744 Loker Ave. W. Suite 100, Carlsbad, CA 92008
FDA Number: 3004893332

Appliance, Fixation, Spinal Intervertebral Body	Orthopedics
Device, Spinal Vertebral Body Replacement	Orthopedics
Orthopedic Manual Surgical Instrument	Orthopedics
Prosthesis, Hip, Cement Restrictor	Orthopedics

SPINAL KINETICS, INC.   609-254-3999
595 N Pastoria Avenue, Sunnyvale, CA 94085
FDA Number: 3004987282

Orthopedic Manual Surgical Instrument	Orthopedics
Prosthesis, Spine, Intervertebral Disc	Orthopedics

SPINAL MODULATION INC.   650-543-6800
1135 O'Brien Drive, Menlo Park, CA 94025
FDA Number: n/a   Fax: 650-327-2336

SPINAL MODULATION INC.   650-543-6800 *(cont'd)*
E-mail: info@spinalmodulation.com
Web site: http://www.spinalmodulation.com
Year Founded: 2004
Ownership: Private
Produces/Sells CE-marked Devices: N
General Admin.: Mr. Lynn Elliott/Chief Technology Officer
     Mr. David Wood/President, Chief Executive Officer
Medical Admin.: Dr. Jeff Kramer/Director Clinical Affairs
Mktg./Adv.: Mr. Dan Brounstein/Director Marketing
Production: Mr. Timothy Placek/Vice President Quality Assurance & Regulatory
Affairs

SPINAL SOLUTIONS, INC.   800-922-5155
1971 Old Covington Rd., Suite 103,   **770-922-2434**
Conyers, GA 30013
FDA Number: n/a   Fax: 770-922-2076
E-mail: spinalsolution@mindspring.com
Web site: www.spinalsolution.net
Ownership: Private
Produces/Sells CE-marked Devices: N

Brace, Joint, Ankle (External)	Physical Med
Joint, Hip, External Brace	Physical Med
Orthosis, Cervical-Thoracic, Rigid	Physical Med
Orthosis, Lumbosacral	Physical Med
Orthosis, Thoracic	Physical Med
Orthosis, Truncal/Limb	Physical Med

SPINAL SPECIALTIES, INC.
See Integra Lifesciences Corp.

SPINAL TRACTION PRODUCTS, LLC.   636-947-9086
5 Lake Forest Ct. East, St. Charles, MO 63301
FDA Number: 1954387
Ownership: Private
Produces/Sells CE-marked Devices: N

Traction Unit, Non-Powered	Orthopedics

SPINDLER & HOYER, INC
See Linos Photonics, Inc

SPINE SMITH PARTNERS L.P.   512-206-0770
8140 N. Mopac, Bldg Ii, Suite 120, Austin, TX 78759
FDA Number: 3006404071

Brace, Drill	Orthopedics
Orthopedic Manual Surgical Instrument	Orthopedics
Retractor, Surgical	Surgery
Suction Apparatus, Single Patient, Portable, Non-Powered	Surgery

SPINE WAVE, INC.   203-944-9494
Two Enterprise Dr., Suite 302, Shelton, CT 06484
FDA Number: 3004638600

Accessories, Arthroscopic	Orthopedics
Awl	Orthopedics
Bender	Orthopedics
Curette	Orthopedics
Device, Spinal Vertebral Body Replacement	Orthopedics
Dispenser, Cement	Orthopedics
Extractor, Nail	Orthopedics
Forceps	Orthopedics
Impactor	Orthopedics
Instrument, Manual, General Surgical	Surgery
Orthopedic Manual Surgical Instrument	Orthopedics
Orthosis, Fixation, Pedicle, Spinal	Orthopedics
Orthosis, Fixation, Spinal, Spondylolisthesis	Orthopedics
Osteotome, Manual (Plastic Surgery)	Surgery
Passer, Wire, Orthopedic	Orthopedics
Plate, Fixation, Bone	Orthopedics
Probe	Orthopedics
Rasp, Bone	Orthopedics
Retractor, Surgical	Surgery
Rongeur, Rib	Orthopedics
Screwdriver	Orthopedics
Tamp	Orthopedics
Tap, Bone	Orthopedics
Template	Orthopedics
Tray, Surgical Instrument	Surgery
Wrench	Orthopedics

SPINE360   512.327.6400
5000 Plaza On The Lake, Suite 175, Austin, TX 78746
FDA Number: 3005841736
E-mail: info@spine360.c
Web site: www.spine360.com
Ownership: Private
Produces/Sells CE-marked Devices: N

Appliance, Fixation, Spinal Intervertebral Body	Orthopedics
Orthosis, Fixation, Spinal, Spondylolisthesis	Orthopedics

SPINEALIGN MEDICAL, INC.   925.227.9800
5880 W. Las Positas Blvd.,, Suite 52, Pleasanton, CA 94588
FDA Number: 3006794240   Fax: 925.892.9808
E-mail: info@spinealignmedical.com
Web site: www.spinealignmedical.com
Ownership: Private
Produces/Sells CE-marked Devices: N

Bit, Drill	Orthopedics
Device, Spinal Vertebral Body Replacement	Orthopedics
Dispenser, Cement	Orthopedics
Orthopedic Manual Surgical Instrument	Orthopedics
Spinal Channeling Instrument, Vertebroplasty	Orthopedics

SPINECRAFT LLC   708-531-9700
2215 Entreprise Dr., Westchester, IL 60154
FDA Number: 3004717358

Appliance, Fixation, Spinal Interlaminal	Orthopedics
Filler, Calcium Sulfate Preformed Pellets	Orthopedics
Orthosis, Fixation, Pedicle, Spinal	Orthopedics
Orthosis, Fixation, Spinal, Spondylolisthesis	Orthopedics

SPINEDOK, DIVISION OF ALTRUEON LLC.   650-755-7750
235 Westlake Center, #212, Daly City, CA 94015
FDA Number: n/a   Fax: 650-648-0447
E-mail: service@spinedok.com
Web site: http://www.spinedok.com
Ownership: Private
Produces/Sells CE-marked Devices: N
General Admin.: Mr. John Rambo/Chief Executive Officer
     Mr. Vincent Chang/Chief Operating Officer

SPINEMATRIX, INC.   330-665-6780
202 Montrose West Ave., Suite 360, Akron, OH 44321
FDA Number: 1531144

Electromyograph, Diagnostic	Physical Med

SPINEOLOGY GROUP, LLC   888-377-4633
7800 3rd Street N., Suite 600,   **651-256-8500**
St. Paul, MN 55128
FDA Number: 2135156   Fax: 651-256-8505
E-mail: webinfo@spineology.com
Web site: http://www.spineology.com
Ownership: Private
Produces/Sells CE-marked Devices: N
General Admin.: Mr. James Rybicki/Chairman
     Mr. John Booth/Chief Executive Officer
Mktg./Adv.: Mr. Daniel McPhillips/Vice President Marketing
     Mr. Timothy Walnofer/Vice President Sales
IS: Ms. Karen Roche/Vice President Technology

Appliance, Fixation, Spinal Intervertebral Body	Orthopedics
Catheter, Balloon (Foley Type)	Surgery
Electrode, Needle	Cns/Neurology
Instrument, Manual, General Surgical	Surgery
Mesh, Orthopedic (Metallic)	Orthopedics
Mesh, Surgical (Steel Gauze)	Surgery
Orthopedic Manual Surgical Instrument	Orthopedics
Prosthesis, Hip, Cement Restrictor	Orthopedics
Surgical Instrument, Disposable	Surgery
System, Facet Screw Spinal Device	Orthopedics

SPINEOVATIONS   858-812-3003
4445 Eastgate Mall, Suite 200, San Diego, CA 92121
FDA Number: n/a   Fax: 858-812-2001
E-mail: info@spineovations.com
Web site: www.spineovations.com
Ownership: Private
Produces/Sells CE-marked Devices: N
General Admin.: Dr. Neville Alleyne/Chairman
     Mr. M. Ross Simmonds/Chief Executive Officer
     Dr. William Taylor/Chief Scientific Officer
     Mr. Stuart Young/President

SPINERX TECHNOLOGY   713-983-9979
6100 Brittmoore Rd., Suite S, Houston, TX 77041
FDA Number: 3004096438
Ownership: Private
Produces/Sells CE-marked Devices: N

Equipment, Traction, Powered	Physical Med
Isokinetic Testing And Evaluation System	Physical Med

SPINEWORKS MEDICAL INC.
See SPINEALIGN MEDICAL, INC.

SPINUS, LLC   603-758-1444
8 Merrill Industrial Dr., Hampton, NH 03842
FDA Number: 3005279854

Electrosurgical Unit, Cutting & Coagulation Device	Surgery
Knife, Orthopedic	Orthopedics
Tape, Measuring, Ruler And Caliper	Surgery
Tube, Ear Suction	Ear/Nose/Throat

SPINUS, LLC 603-758-1444 (cont'd)
Tube, Tonsil Suction   Ear/Nose/Throat

SPIO INC. 253-893-0390
25826 108th Ave. Se, Kent, WA 98030
FDA Number: 3005979000
Orthosis, Abdominal	Physical Med
Orthosis, Limb Brace	Physical Med
Orthosis, Lumbar	Physical Med
Orthosis, Lumbosacral	Physical Med
Orthosis, Thoracic	Physical Med
Orthosis, Truncal/Limb	Physical Med

SPIRACLE TECHNOLOGY 714-418-1091
16520 Harbor Blvd., Unit D, Fountain Valley, CA 92708
FDA Number: 2030745   *Fax:* 741-418-1095
E-mail: info@spiracle.com
Web site: www.spiracle.com
Ownership: Private
Produces/Sells CE-marked Devices: N
Flowmeter, Gas (Oxygen), Calibrated	Anesthesiology
Monitor, Airway Pressure (Gauge/Alarm)	Anesthesiology
Regulator, Pressure, Gas Cylinder	Anesthesiology
Valve, Non-Rebreathing	Anesthesiology
Ventilator, Emergency, Powered (Resuscitator)	Anesthesiology

SPIRATION INC. 866-497-1700
6675 185th Ave. N.E., Redmond, WA 98052 425-497-1700
FDA Number: 3004450998   *Fax:* 425-497-1912
E-mail: info@spiration.com
Web site: www.spiration.com
Year Founded: 1999
Ownership: Private
Produces/Sells CE-marked Devices: Y
General Admin.: Mr. Gregory Sessler/Chief Operating Officer
    Xavier Gonzalez/Chief Scientific Officer, Vice President
    Richard Shea/President, Chief Executive Officer
Medical Admin.: Steven Springmeyer/Vice President, Medical Director
Mktg./Adv.: Nancy Hill/Vice President Marketing
Valve, Breathing	Anesthesiology

SPIRAX SARCO, INC. 800-575-0394
1150 Nortpoint Blvd., Blythewood, SC 29016 803-714-2000
FDA Number: n/a   *Fax:* 803-714-2222
E-mail: InsideSalesLeads@Spirax.com
Web site: www.spiraxsarco.com/us
Medical Products Sales Volume: $94,000,000
Annual Revenue: $50-$100 Million
Year Founded: 1983
Total Employees: 330
Ownership: Spirax Sarco Limited
Stock Symbol: LON
Traded On: London
Quality System Registration Information: ISO9001
Produces/Sells CE-marked Devices: N
Federal Procurement Eligibility: Small Business
Distribution: Manufacturer Direct, Manufacturer Through Manufacturer Reps,
Service Direct, Exporter
General Admin.: Anthony Scrivin/President
Mktg./Adv.: Dawn Cartwright/Manager Marketing Communications
    Justin C. O'Dowd/Vice President Marketing & Sales
Production: Peter Moreton/Vice President Manufacturing
Check Valve, Retrograde Flow (In-Line)	General
Filter, Steam	General

SPIRE CORP. 800-510-4815
One Patriots Park, Bedford, MA 01730-2396 781-275-6000
FDA Number: 1223643   *Fax:* 781-275-7470
E-mail: info@spirecorp.com
Web site: www.spirecorp.com
Medical Products Sales Volume: $21,700,000
Annual Revenue: $10-$25 Million
Year Founded: 1969
Total Employees: 113   *Marketing Staff:* 3   *Sales Staff:* 3
Ownership: Public
Stock Symbol: SPIR
Traded On: NASDAQ
Quality System Registration Information: ISO9001
Produces/Sells CE-marked Devices: Y
Federal Procurement Eligibility: Small Business
Distribution: Manufacturer Through Distributor, Service Direct
General Admin.: Roger Little/President, Chief Executive Officer
    Mark Little/Vice President, General Manager
Mktg./Adv.: Nader Kalkhoran/Manager Marketing & Sales
Production: Rick Oliver/Applications Engineer
    Rick Oliver/Manager Operations
    Don Fickett/Manager Regulatory Affairs

SPIRE CORP. 800-510-4815 (cont'd)
Finance: Gregory Towle/Controller
Equipment, Device Coating, Protective	General
Service, Device Coating, Protective	General
Service, Engineering/Design	General
Service, Modification, Product	General

SPIRIG ADVANCED TECHNOLOGIES, INC. 413-788-6191
144 Oakland St., Springfield, MA 01108-1787
FDA Number: n/a   *Fax:* 413-788-0490
E-mail: sat@spirig.com
Web site: www.spirig.org
Medical Products Sales Volume: $350,000
Year Founded: 1978
Total Employees: 3   *Marketing Staff:* 2   *Sales Staff:* 2
Ownership: Private
Produces/Sells CE-marked Devices: Y
Federal Procurement Eligibility: Small Business
Distribution: Manufacturer Direct, OEM, Importer
General Admin.: Ernst Spirig/Chief Executive Officer
    Laurie Topjian/General Manager
Cleanroom Equipment	General
Label, Device	General
Microscope	Hematology
Timeclock	General

SPIROMETRICS MEDICAL EQUIPMENT CO., LLC 207-657-6700
22 Shaker Road, Gray, ME 04039
FDA Number: 1720605   *Fax:* 207-657-4123
E-mail: Wcyr@spirometrics.com
Web site: www.spirometrics.com
Ownership: Private
Quality System Registration Information: ISO9001
Produces/Sells CE-marked Devices: Y
Distribution: Manufacturer Direct, OEM
Filter, Bacterial, Breathing Circuit	Anesthesiology
Meter, Peak Flow, Spirometry	Anesthesiology

SPIROTECH
See Thermo Fisher Scientific

SPIRUS MEDICAL, INC. 781-297-7220
1063 Turnpike Street, PO Box 258, Stoughton, MA 02072
FDA Number: 3005814162   *Fax:* 781-297-5059
E-mail: info@spirusmed.com
Web site: www.spirusmed.com
Year Founded: 2005
Ownership: Private
Quality System Registration Information: ISO9001
Produces/Sells CE-marked Devices: N
Colonoscope, Gastro-Urology	Gastroenterology/Urology
Endoscope	Gastroenterology/Urology
Lubricant, Patient	General
Sheath, Endoscopic	Gastroenterology/Urology

SPIVEY INTERNATIONAL INC. 415-333-6800
58 Genebern Way, San Francisco, CA 94112
FDA Number: n/a   *Fax:* 415-333-6888
E-mail: gloves@spiveyinternational.com
Web site: www.spiveyinternational.com
Annual Revenue: $1-$5 Million
Year Founded: 1989
Total Employees: 15   *Marketing Staff:* 3   *Sales Staff:* 3
Ownership: Private
Produces/Sells CE-marked Devices: N
Federal Procurement Eligibility: Small Business, Female Owned
Distribution: Exclusive Distributor
General Admin.: Lisa Spivey/President
Glove, Other	General
Glove, Patient Examination, Latex	General
Service, Consulting	General

SPLASH SHIELD, INC. 800-536-6686
52 Dragon Ct., Woburn, MA 01801 781-935-9060
FDA Number: 1223404   *Fax:* 888-697-4435
E-mail: splashield@aol.com
Web site: www.splashshield.org
Medical Products Sales Volume: $490,000
Annual Revenue: $1-$5 Million
Year Founded: 1990
Total Employees: 5
Ownership: Private
Produces/Sells CE-marked Devices: N
Federal Procurement Eligibility: Small Business
Distribution: Manufacturer Through Distributor, OEM
General Admin.: Patrick Grant/President
Mktg./Adv.: Neil Simmons/Vice President Marketing & Sales
Production: John W. Burke, Jr./Vice President Manufacturing
Research: Peter Gazzara/Vice President Research & Development

MANUFACTURER PROFILES

SPLASH SHIELD, INC.   800-536-6686 *(cont'd)*
Mask, Face   General

SPLENODEX CANADA INC.   514-224-1080
109 Ch Des Ormes Rr 121,
Sainte-Anne-Des-Lacs J0R 1 Canada
FDA Number: 8022300
Medical Disinfectants/Cleaners for Instruments   General

SPORT TECH, INC.   434-982-5752
391 Ridge Lee Drive, Charlottesville, VA 22903
FDA Number: 3003651467
Goniometer, Non-Powered   Orthopedics

SPORTIME
See Abilitations

SPORTKAT, LLC   800.743.0575
1497 Poinsettia Avenue, Suite 157,   760-599-8600
Vista, CA 92081
FDA Number: 2031091
E-mail: info@sportkat.com   *Fax:* 760.599.8610
Web site: www.sportkat.com
Ownership: Private
Produces/Sells CE-marked Devices: N
Stimulator, Vestibular Acceleration, Therapeutic   Cns/Neurology

SPORTS PLAY EQUIPMENT, INC.   800-727-8180
5642 Natural Bridge, St. Louis, MO 63120-1628   314-389-4140
FDA Number: n/a   *Fax:* 314-389-9034
E-mail: awilhelm@primary.net
Web site: www.sportsplayinc.com
Annual Revenue: $1-$5 Million
Total Employees: 60
Ownership: Private
Produces/Sells CE-marked Devices: N
Federal Procurement Eligibility: Small Business
Distribution: Manufacturer Through Distributor, OEM
General Admin.: Brain Kearns/President
    Keith Panchot/Vice President, General Manager
Mktg./Adv.: Jay E. Blanke/Director Marketing
    Arthur Wilhelm/Director Sales
    Angela Williams/Manager National Sales
Adaptor, Recreational   Physical Med
Component, Exercise   Physical Med

SPORTSBANDS, INC.   302-322-1148
181 South Dupont Hwy., New Castle, DE 19720
FDA Number: 3006791455
Ownership: Private
Produces/Sells CE-marked Devices: N
Bandage, Elastic   General

SPORTSGUARD LABORATORIES, INC.   800-401-1776
267 Martinel Dr, Kent, OH 44240   330-673-6932
FDA Number: 3003587221
E-mail: sales@sportsguard.com
Web site: www.sportsguard.com
Ownership: Private
Produces/Sells CE-marked Devices: N
Mouthguard   Dental And Oral

SPRAYWAY, INC.   800-332-9000
484 Vista Avenue, Addison, IL 60101-4468   630-628-3000
FDA Number: n/a   *Fax:* 630-543-7797
E-mail: linda@spraywayinc.com
Web site: www.spraywayinc.com
Year Founded: 1947
Total Employees: 15   *Marketing Staff:* 10   *Sales Staff:* 5
Ownership: Private
Produces/Sells CE-marked Devices: N
Federal Procurement Eligibility: Small Business
Distribution: Manufacturer Through Distributor, Exporter
General Admin.: Tony Schwab/President
Mktg./Adv.: Bob Potvin/Vice President Sales
Production: Steve Engler/Manager Regulatory Affairs
Carpeting   General
Housekeeping Equipment   General
Office Product   General

SPRING BIOSCIENCE   510-979-9460
46755 Fremont Blvd, Fremont, CA 94538
FDA Number: 3007038395
Web site: www.springbio.com
Ownership: Private
Produces/Sells CE-marked Devices: N
Immunohistochemical Reagent, Antibody (monoclonal Or Polyclonal) To P63 Protein In
Nucleus Of Prostatic Basal Cells   Hematology

SPRING HEALTH PRODUCTS, INC.   800-800-1680
705 General Washington Ave., Ste. 701,   610-630-9171
Norristown, PA 19403
FDA Number: n/a
E-mail: springhealth@atxmail.com   *Fax:* 610-630-9730
Web site: www.springhealthproducts.com
Annual Revenue: $1-$5 Million
Total Employees: 15
Ownership: Private
Produces/Sells CE-marked Devices: N
Federal Procurement Eligibility: Small Business
Distribution: Manufacturer Through Distributor
General Admin.: Alex Lieb/Vice President
Burr, Dental   Dental And Oral
Drill, Dental, Intraoral   Dental And Oral
Glove, Surgical   General
Instrument, Diamond, Dental   Dental And Oral
Light, Dental   Dental And Oral

SPRINGER-PENGUIN, INC.   800-835-8500
11 Brookdale Place, PO Box 310,   914-699-3200
Mount Vernon, NY 10551
FDA Number: n/a
E-mail: jspringer21@juno.com   *Fax:* 914-699-3231
Web site: www.springerpenguin.com
Medical Products Sales Volume: $1,000,000
Annual Revenue: $1-$5 Million
Total Employees: 25   *Marketing Staff:* 4   *Sales Staff:* 4
Ownership: Private
Produces/Sells CE-marked Devices: N
Federal Procurement Eligibility: Small Business, VA Contract
Distribution: Manufacturer Through Distributor
General Admin.: Gerard K. Springer/President
Mktg./Adv.: Gerard K. Springer/Director Marketing
    Vicki Matos/Manager Sales Training
Production: Gerard K. Springer/Vice President Manufacturing
Refrigerator, Pharmacy   General

SPS MEDICAL
See Sps Medical Supply Corp.

SPS MEDICAL SUPPLY CORP.   800-722-1529
6789 W. Hennetta Road, Rush, NY 14543   585-359-0130
FDA Number: 1319130   *Fax:* 585-359-0167
E-mail: info@spsmedical.com
Web site: www.spsmedical.com
Medical Products Sales Volume: $4,100,000
Annual Revenue: $5-$10 Million
Year Founded: 1987
Total Employees: 48   *Marketing Staff:* 5   *Sales Staff:* 26
Ownership: Private
Produces/Sells CE-marked Devices: N
Federal Procurement Eligibility: Small Business, Female Owned
Distribution: Manufacturer Through Distributor, OEM
General Admin.: Charles Hughes/General Manager
    Nancy Hughes/President
Mktg./Adv.: Jackie Nale/Director Marketing
    Georgi Jossifov/Manager International & National Sales
    Mariann Burke/Manager Marketing
    Ray Averill/Manager Sales Training
Production: Rex Norton/Manager Materials
    Gary Socola/Manager Quality Assurance & Regulatory Affairs
Packaging Material   General
Packaging, Sterilization   General
Sterilization Process Indicator, Biological   General
Sterilization Process Indicator, Chemical   General

SQI DIAGNOSTICS   416-674-9500
36 Meteor Dr., Toronto, ONT M9W-1A4 Canada
FDA Number: 3008564556
E-mail: Sales@sqidiagnostics.com   *Fax:* 416-674-9300
Web site: www.sqidiagnostics.com
Year Founded: 1999
Total Employees: 25
Ownership: Public
Stock Symbol: SQD
Traded On: TSX Venture Exchange
Produces/Sells CE-marked Devices: N

SQUARE D COMPANY   1 847 397 2600
1415 Roselle Road, Palatine, IL 60067
FDA Number: 9201012
Web site: www.squared.com   *Fax:* 1 847 925 7500
Total Employees: 350   *Marketing Staff:* 20
Ownership: GROUPE SCHNEIDER
Quality System Registration Information: ISO9000
Produces/Sells CE-marked Devices: Y
Distribution: Manufacturer Through Distributor

SQUARE D COMPANY — 1 847 397 2600 (cont'd)

General Admin.: Charlie Denny/Chief Executive Officer
Mktg./Adv.: Frank Sullivan/Vice President Marketing & Sales
Production: Hal Grant/Vice President Manufacturing

Clock, Elapsed Time	General
Meter, Leakage Current (Ammeter)	General
Monitor, Line Isolation	Cardiovascular
Power System, Isolated	General
Tester, Grounding System	General
Tester, Isolated Power System	General
Timer, General Laboratory	Hematology

SQUAREONE MEDICAL, INC. — 805-987-2457
1640 Pierside Ln., Camarillo, CA 93010
FDA Number: 2028171
Ownership: Private
Produces/Sells CE-marked Devices: N

Syringe, Piston	General

SQUIBB CORP.
See Bristol-Myers Group Company

SQUIBB-NOVO INC.
See Novo Nordisk Pharmaceuticals, Inc.

SQUIRE-COGSWELL AEROS INSTRUMENTS INC
See Ohio Medical Corp.

SR INSTRUMENTS, INC. — 800-654-6360 / 716-693-5977
600 Young St., Tonawanda, NY 14150-4105
FDA Number: 1317256 *Fax:* 716-693-5854
E-mail: sri@srinstruments.com
Web site: www.srscales.com
Year Founded: 1973
Total Employees: 48   *Marketing Staff:* 1   *Sales Staff:* 1
Ownership: Private
Quality System Registration Information: ISO9002
Produces/Sells CE-marked Devices: Y
Federal Procurement Eligibility: Small Business, GSA Contract
Distribution: Manufacturer Direct, Manufacturer Through Distributor, Manufacturer Through Manufacturer Reps, OEM
General Admin.: Todd Drachenburg/General Manager
John Siegel/President
Mktg./Adv.: Teresa Eyring/Market Manager
Gerald Petrotto/Project Manager
David Low/Senior Sales Manager
Production: June Drachenburg/Manager Regulatory Affairs

Component, Electronic	General
Component, Other	General
Contract Manufacturing	General
Contract R&D, Equipment	General
Lift, Patient	General
Scale, Bed	General
Scale, Chair	General
Scale, Infant	General
Scale, Laboratory	Chemistry
Scale, Platform, Wheelchair	Physical Med
Scale, Stand-On	General
Service, Engineering/Design	General

SRC MEDICAL, INC. — 781-826-9100
263 Winter Street, Assinippi, MA 02339
FDA Number: 1218347

Applicator, Vaginal	Obstetrics/Gynecology
Dropper, Ear	Ear/Nose/Throat

SRI SURGICAL — 813-891-9550
12425 Race Track Roa, Tampa, FL 33626
FDA Number: 1527607 *Fax:* (813) 818-9076
E-mail: info@srisurgical.com
Ownership: Private
Produces/Sells CE-marked Devices: N

Cover, Shoe, Operating Room	Surgery
Instrument, Manual, General Surgical	Surgery
Tray, Surgical Instrument	Surgery

SRI SURGICAL — 813-891-9550
6801 Longe St., Stockton, CA 95206
FDA Number: 2954327

Cover, Shoe, Operating Room	Surgery
Drape, Surgical	Surgery
Gown, Surgical	Surgery
Instrument, Manual, General Surgical	Surgery
Kit, Surgical (General)	Surgery
Table, Obstetrical	Obstetrics/Gynecology
Tray, Surgical Instrument	Surgery
Wrap, Sterilization	General

SRI/SURGICAL EXPRESS — 813-818-9550
12425 Race Track Road, Tampa, FL 33626
FDA Number: 1056591 *Fax:* 813-818-9076
Ownership: Private

SRI/SURGICAL EXPRESS — 813-818-9550 (cont'd)

Produces/Sells CE-marked Devices: N

Applicator, ENT	Ear/Nose/Throat
Cover, Shoe, Operating Room	Surgery
Drape, Surgical	Surgery
Gown, Isolation, Surgical	Surgery
Gown, Surgical	Surgery
Instrument, Manual, General Surgical	Surgery
Kit, Surgical (General)	Surgery
Kit, Wound Dressing	Surgery
Surgical Instrument, Manual (General Use)	Surgery
Table, Obstetrical	Obstetrics/Gynecology
Tray, Surgical Instrument	Surgery
Wrap, Sterilization	General

SRL MEDICAL
See CAREFUSION 211, INC..

SROUFE HEALTHCARE PRODUCTS LLC — 888-894-4171 / 260-894-4171
PO Box 347, 601 Sroufe St., Ligonier, IN 46767
FDA Number: 1832148 *Fax:* 260-894-4092
E-mail: sales@sroufe.com
Web site: www.sroufe.com
Medical Products Sales Volume: $8,000,000
Annual Revenue: $5-$10 Million
Year Founded: 1975
Total Employees: 125
Ownership: Private
Produces/Sells CE-marked Devices: Y
Federal Procurement Eligibility: Small Business, GSA Contract, VA Contract
Distribution: Manufacturer Direct, Manufacturer Through Distributor, Manufacturer Through Manufacturer Reps, OEM, Service Direct, Exclusive Distributor, Exporter
General Admin.: Jon Sroufe/Chief Executive Officer
Jeff Wells/President
Mktg./Adv.: Jeff Wells/Manager Advertising
Jeff Wells/Vice President Marketing & Sales
Production: Roger Niles/Manager Quality Assurance
Research: Jon Sroufe/Vice President Research & Development

Belt, Rib (Support)	Orthopedics
Immobilizer, Knee	Orthopedics
Shoe, Cast	Physical Med
Sling, Arm	Physical Med
Slippers	General
Splint, Pneumatic	Orthopedics
Support, Wrist	Physical Med
Walker, Mechanical	Physical Med

SRS MEDICAL SYSTEMS
See Fasstech

SRS MEDICAL SYSTEMS, INC. — 800-345-5642 / 425-882-1101
8672 N.E. 154th Ave., Redmond, WA 98052
FDA Number: 3021815 *Fax:* 1-425-882-1935
E-mail: info@srsmedical.com
Web site: www.srsmedical.com
Ownership: Private
Produces/Sells CE-marked Devices: N

Biofeedback Device	Cns/Neurology
Clamp, Penile	Gastroenterology/Urology
Perineometer	Obstetrics/Gynecology
Pessary, Vaginal	Obstetrics/Gynecology

SSCOR — 800-434-5211 / 818-504-4054
11064 Randall St., Sun Valley, CA 91352
FDA Number: 2022724 *Fax:* 818-504-6032
E-mail: marketing@sscor.com
Web site: www.sscor.com
Medical Products Sales Volume: $1,400,000
Year Founded: 1980
Total Employees: 16   *Marketing Staff:* 1   *Sales Staff:* 1
Ownership: Private
Quality System Registration Information: ISO9001
Produces/Sells CE-marked Devices: N
Federal Procurement Eligibility: Small Business
Distribution: Manufacturer Through Distributor, OEM
General Admin.: Jonathan H. Kim Kim/Administrator
Sam D. Say/President, Chief Executive Officer
Production: William Marinero/Manager Materials
Jesus Gasaway/Vice President Tech. Affairs

Aspirator, Emergency Suction	General

SSI MEDICAL TECHNOLOGIES, LLC — 860-621-3223
24b Robert Porter Rd., Southington, CT 06489
FDA Number: 3005110411
Ownership: Private
Produces/Sells CE-marked Devices: N

Electrosurgical Unit, Cutting & Coagulation Device	Surgery
Laparoscope, General & Plastic Surgery	Surgery

MANUFACTURER PROFILES

SSI SURGICAL SERVICES, INC   **407-249-1946**
5776 Hoffner Ave, Ste 200, Orlando, FL 32822
FDA Number: 3005736025
E-mail: info@surgicalservices.com
Web site: www.surgicalservices.com
Ownership: Teleflex Medical
Stock Symbol: TFX
Traded On: NYSE
Produces/Sells CE-marked Devices: N
General Admin.: Mr. Todd Riddell/President, Chief Executive Officer
Mktg./Adv.: Mr. Craig Little/Senior Vice President Marketing & Sales
Finance: Mr. Paul D'Alesio/Chief Financial Officer

SST
See Dynavox Systems Inc.

ST. FRANCIS MEDICAL TECHNOLOGIES, INC.   **408-548-6500**
1201 Marina Village Parkway, Suite 200, Alameda, CA 94501
FDA Number: 2953720
Ownership: Private
Produces/Sells CE-marked Devices: N

Orthosis, Lumbar	Physical Med

ST. JOHN COMPANIES   **800-435-4242**
25167 Anza Drive, PO Box 800460,   **805-257-0233**
Santa Clarita, CA 91380
FDA Number: n/a   *Fax:* 805-257-1017
E-mail: cs@stjohninc.com
Web site: www.stjohninc.com
Year Founded: 1956
Total Employees: 15
Ownership: Private
Produces/Sells CE-marked Devices: N
Federal Procurement Eligibility: Small Business
Distribution: Manufacturer Direct, Manufacturer Through Distributor, OEM, Exporter
General Admin.: A. F. Press/Chief Executive Officer, Chairman
Mktg./Adv.: Donna Brooks/Director Marketing & Communications
    Tracey Carpentier/President Marketing & Sales

Collar, Cervical Neck	Orthopedics
Cover, Film, X-Ray	Radiology
Envelope, Film, X-Ray	Radiology
Film, X-Ray	Radiology
Filter, Radiographic	Radiology
Forms, Medical And Patient	General
Gel, Ultrasonic Transmission	General
Labeler, X-Ray Film	Radiology
Marker, Skin	Surgery
Monitor, X-Ray Film Processor Quality Control	Radiology
Office Product	General
Shield, X-Ray	Radiology

ST. JUDE MEDICAL ATRIAL FIBRILLATION   **800-328-3873**
14901 DeVeau Pl., Minnetonka, MN 55345-2126   **612-933-4700**
FDA Number: 2182269   *Fax:* 952-933-7131
Web site: www.sjm.com
Ownership: St. Jude Medical, Inc.
Stock Symbol: STJ
Traded On: NYSE
Produces/Sells CE-marked Devices: N
Distribution: Manufacturer Direct, OEM, Exclusive Distributor
General Admin.: Jane Song/President

Accessories, Catheter	Surgery
Cable, Pacemaker	Cardiovascular
Cable/Lead, ECG, With Transducer And Electrode	Cardiovascular
Catheter, Electrode Recording, Or Probe	Cardiovascular
Catheter, Other	Gastroenterology/Urology
Catheter, Percutaneous	Cardiovascular
Device, Hemostasis, Vascular	Cardiovascular
Dilator, Vessel, Percutaneous Catheterization	Cardiovascular
Electrode, Pacemaker, Temporary	Cardiovascular
Guide, Catheter	Cardiovascular
Guidewire	Cardiovascular
Introducer, Catheter	Cardiovascular
Lead, Pacemaker, Temporary Endocardial	Cardiovascular
Surgical Instrument, Disposable	Surgery

ST. JUDE MEDICAL ATRIAL FIBRILLATION   **800-748-7335**
6500 Wedgwood Rd., Maple Grove, MN 55311   **763-383-0900**
FDA Number: 3004028841   *Fax:* 763-383-2600
E-mail: epicor@sjm.com
Web site: www.sjm.com
Ownership: St. Jude Medical, Inc.
Stock Symbol: STJ
Traded On: NYSE
Produces/Sells CE-marked Devices: N
General Admin.: Mr. John C. Heinmiller/Chief Financial Officer, Executive Vice President
    Mr. Frank J. Callaghan/President

ST. JUDE MEDICAL ATRIAL FIBRILLATION 800.748.7335 *(cont'd)*
    Mr. Daniel J. Starks/President, Chief Executive Officer, Chairman

Clip, Implantable	Surgery
Device, Retrieval, Percutaneous	Cardiovascular
Introducer, Catheter	Cardiovascular

ST. JUDE MEDICAL ATRIAL FIBRILLATION (ENDOCARDIAL SOLUTIONS)
See St. Jude Medical Atrial Fibrillation (Endocardial Solutions)

ST. JUDE MEDICAL CARDIAC RHYTHM   **800-777-2237**
MANAGEMENT DIV.
15900 Valley View Ct., Sylmar, CA 91342-3577   **818-362-6822**
FDA Number: 2017865   *Fax:* 818-364-5814
Web site: www.sjm.com
Ownership: ST. JUDE MEDICAL, INC.
Stock Symbol: STJ
Traded On: NYSE
Quality System Registration Information: ISO9001; ISO9002
Produces/Sells CE-marked Devices: Y
Distribution: Manufacturer Direct, OEM, Importer, Exporter
General Admin.: Mr. John C. Heinmiller/Chief Financial Officer, Executive Vice President
    Mr. Daniel J. Starks/President, Chief Executive Officer, Chairman
    Mr. Paul Bae/Vice President Human Resources

Adapter, Lead, Pacemaker	Cardiovascular
Catheter, Percutaneous	Cardiovascular
Catheter, Steerable	Cardiovascular
Dual Chamber, Anti-Tachycardia, Pulse Generator	Cardiovascular
Introducer, Catheter	Cardiovascular
Kit, Repair, Pacemaker	Cardiovascular
Lead, Pacemaker, Implantable Endocardial	Cardiovascular
Lead, Pacemaker, Implantable Myocardial	Cardiovascular
Pacemaker, Heart, External	Cardiovascular
Pacemaker, Heart, Implantable, Dual Chamber	Cardiovascular
Pacemaker, Heart, Implantable, Programmable	Cardiovascular
Pacemaker, Heart, Implantable, Rate Responsive	Cardiovascular

ST. JUDE MEDICAL NEUROMODULATION   **800-727-7846**
DIVISION
6901 Preston Rd., Plano, TX 75024   **972-309-8000**
FDA Number: 1627487   *Fax:* 972-309-8150
E-mail: info@ans-medical.com
Web site: www.ans-medical.com
Annual Revenue: $100-$500 Million
Year Founded: 1981
Total Employees: 950   *Marketing Staff:* 41   *Sales Staff:* 235
Ownership: St. Jude Medical, Inc.
Stock Symbol: STJ
Traded On: NYSE
Quality System Registration Information: ISO9001
Produces/Sells CE-marked Devices: Y
Federal Procurement Eligibility: Small Business
Distribution: Manufacturer Direct, Manufacturer Through Distributor, Manufacturer Through Manufacturer Reps
General Admin.: RJ Steines/Chief Financial Officer, Vice President
    Mr. Christopher Chavez/President, Chief Executive Officer
    Kimberley Elting/Vice President General Counsel & Secretary
    Jason Whitehair/Vice President Human Resources
Mktg./Adv.: Linda Thomas/Director Corporate Communications
    Alan Mock/Vice President Marketing
    Paul Hanchin/Vice President Sales
    Ray Dougan/Vice President Special Projects
    Rohan Hoare/Vice President Strategic Development
Production: Dennis Alexander/Vice President Manufacturing
    Bruce Horowitz/Vice President Production
    Drew Johnson/Vice President Regulatory & Clinical Affairs
Research: John Erickson/Vice President Research & Development

Stimulator, Nerve, Battery-Powered	Anesthesiology
Stimulator, Peripheral Nerve, Implantable (Pain Relief)	Cns/Neurology
Stimulator, Spinal Cord, Implantable (Pain Relief)	Cns/Neurology

ST. JUDE MEDICAL, INC.   **800-328-9634**
One St. Jude Medical Drive,   **651-483-2000**
St. Paul, MN 55117
FDA Number: 2126673   *Fax:* 651-482-8318
E-mail: afcustomerservice@sjm.com
Web site: www.sjm.com
Medical Products Sales Volume: $1,528,000,000
Annual Revenue: More than $1 Billion
Year Founded: 1976
Total Employees: 12000
Ownership: Public
Stock Symbol: STJ
Traded On: NYSE
Quality System Registration Information: ISO9001
Produces/Sells CE-marked Devices: Y

ST. JUDE MEDICAL, INC. 800-328-9634 *(cont'd)*
Distribution: Manufacturer Through Distributor, Manufacturer Through Manufacturer Reps
General Admin.: Dr. Mark D. Carlson/Chief Medical Officer, Vice President
Dr. Eric S. Fain/President
Mr. Christopher G. Chavez/President
Ms. Jane J. Song/President
Mr. Denis M. Gestin/President International Operations
Mr. Daniel Starks/President, Chief Executive Officer, Chairman
Ms. Pamela S. Krop/Vice President, General Counsel
Mktg./Adv.: Ms. Angela D. Craig/Vice President Customer Relations

Accessories, Catheter	Surgery
Catheter, Other	Gastroenterology/Urology
Catheter, Vascular, Long-Term	Cardiovascular
Defibrillator, Battery-Powered	Cardiovascular
Lead, Pacemaker (Catheter)	Cardiovascular
Prosthesis, Cardiac Valve	Cardiovascular
Prosthesis, Cardiac Valve, Biological	Cardiovascular
Ring, Annuloplasty	Cardiovascular
Sizer, Heart Valve Prosthesis	Cardiovascular
Valve, Heart, Mechanical	Cardiovascular
Valve, Heart, Tissue	Cardiovascular

Medical Product Subsidiaries (Listed Separately)
Irvine Biomedical, Inc.
St. Jude Medical
St. Jude Medical Atrial Fibrillation
St. Jude Medical Atrial Fibrillation (Endocardial Solutions)
St. Jude Medical Atrial Fibrillation (Epicor Medical)
St. Jude Medical Cardiac Rhythm Management Div.
St. Jude Medical Neuromodulation Division
St. Jude Medical, Puerto Rico, B.V.

ST. JUDE MEDICAL, PUERTO RICO, B.V. 787-746-1111
Lot 20, Caguas West Industrial Park, Caguas, PR 00726-0998
FDA Number: 2648612   Fax: 787-746-5272
Web site: www.sjm.com
Ownership: St. Jude Medical, Inc.
Stock Symbol: STJ
Traded On: NYSE
Produces/Sells CE-marked Devices: N
General Admin.: Mr. John C. Heinmiller/Chief Financial Officer, Executive Vice President
Mr. Daniel J. Starks/President, Chief Executive Officer, Chairman
Mr. Paul Bae/Vice President Human Resources

Device, Hemostasis, Vascular	Cardiovascular
Ring, Annuloplasty	Cardiovascular

ST. JUDE MEDICAL. PUERTO RICO, LLC 787-746-1111
Lot A Interior - #2 St Km 67.5, Santana Industrial Park, Arecibo, PR 00612
FDA Number: 3006705815
Ownership: Private
Produces/Sells CE-marked Devices: N

Dual Chamber, Implantable Pulse Generator	Cardiovascular
Programmer, Pacemaker	Cardiovascular

ST. PAUL BIOTECH 714-903-1000
11555 Monarch St., Garden Grove, CA 92841
FDA Number: 3004581865
Ownership: Private
Produces/Sells CE-marked Devices: N

Antigen, Prostate-Specific (PSA), Management, Cancer	Immunology
Antiserum, Fluorescent, Mycobacterium Tuberculosis	Microbiology
Assay, Enzyme Linked Immunosorbent, Hepatitis C Virus	Microbiology
Campylobacter Pylori	Microbiology
Enzymatic Esterase-Oxidase, Cholesterol	Chemistry
Enzyme Immunoassay, Amphetamine	Toxicology
Enzyme Immunoassay, Barbiturate	Toxicology
Enzyme Immunoassay, Cannabinoids	Toxicology
Enzyme Immunoassay, Cocaine And Cocaine Metabolites	Toxicology
Enzyme Immunoassay, Methadone	Toxicology
Enzyme Linked Immunoabsorbent Assay, Chlamydia Group	Microbiology
Enzyme Linked Immunoabsorbent Assay, Neisseria Gonorrhoeae	Microbiology
Hepatitis B Test (B Core, BE Antigen & Antibody, B Core IGM)	Microbiology
Kit, Pregnancy Test, Over The Counter, HCG	Chemistry
Kit, Test, Malaria	Toxicology
Liquid Chromatography, Morphine	Toxicology
Radioimmunoassay, Luteinizing Hormone	Chemistry
System, Test, Blood Glucose, Over-The-Counter	Chemistry
Test, Follicle Stimulating Hormone (fsh), Over The Counter	Toxicology
Test, Methamphetamine, Over The Counter	Toxicology
Test, Rheumatoid Factor	Immunology
Test, Syphilis, Treponemal	Hematology
Thin Layer Chromatography, Metamphetamine	Toxicology

STA-SOF BREAST COMPRESSOR-CLAMP 310-470-8798
10571 Wyton Dr., Los Angeles, CA 90024
FDA Number: 2025413

STA-SOF BREAST COMPRESSOR-CLAMP 310-470-8798 *(cont'd)*
Clamp, Bone	Orthopedics

STAAR SURGICAL CO. 800-292-7902
1911 Walker Ave., Monrovia, CA 91016-4846   626-303-7902
FDA Number: 2023826   Fax: 626-303-2962
E-mail: info@staar.com
Web site: www.staar.com
Annual Revenue: $1-$5 Million
Year Founded: 1982
Total Employees: 230
Ownership: Public
Stock Symbol: STAA
Traded On: NASDAQ
Produces/Sells CE-marked Devices: Y
Federal Procurement Eligibility: Small Business
Distribution: Manufacturer Through Manufacturer Reps
General Admin.: Mr. Barry Caldwell/Chief Executive Officer
Deborah Andrews/Chief Executive Officer, Vice President
David Bailey/President International Operations
Mktg./Adv.: Ms. Robin Hughes/Vice President Marketing
Production: Mr. Paul Hambrick/Vice President Operations
Mr. John Santos/Vice President Quality Assurance & Regulatory Affairs
Research: Mr. Craig Felberg/Vice President Research & Development

Folders and Injectors, Intraocular Lens (IOL)	Ophthalmology
Guide, Intraocular Lens	Ophthalmology
Kit, Surgical Instrument, Disposable	Surgery
Lens, Contact (Other Material)	Ophthalmology
Lens, Intraocular	Ophthalmology
Phacofragmentation Unit	Ophthalmology

Medical Product Subsidiaries (Listed Separately)
Circuit Tree Medical, Inc.

STACKBIN CORPORATION 800-333-1603
29 Powder Hill Rd., Lincoln, RI 02865-4424   401-333-1600
FDA Number: n/a   Fax: 401-333-1952
E-mail: info@stackbin.com
Web site: www.stackbin.com
Medical Products Sales Volume: $5,000,000
Annual Revenue: $1-$5 Million
Total Employees: 22   *Marketing Staff:* 2   *Sales Staff:* 3
Ownership: Private
Produces/Sells CE-marked Devices: N
Federal Procurement Eligibility: Small Business
Distribution: Manufacturer Direct
General Admin.: William Shaw/Chief Executive Officer
Scott Shaw/Vice President
Mktg./Adv.: Scott Shaw/Director Marketing
Joe Laginhas/Manager Sales

Accessories, Cart, Multipurpose	General
Bin, Storage	General
Cabinet Casework, General Purpose	General
Cart, Multipurpose	General
Furniture, General	General
Storage Unit, X-Ray Film	Radiology

STACO, INC.
See Kimble Chase Life Science And Research Products Llc

STAINO, LLC 845-887-5746
11617 State Route 97, Long Eddy, NY 12760
FDA Number: 3005744794   Fax: 845-231-6036
E-mail: service@staino.com
Web site: www.staino.com
Ownership: Private
Produces/Sells CE-marked Devices: N

Floss, Dental	Dental And Oral
Toothbrush, Manual	Dental And Oral

STAIR SYSTEMS, INC. 336-852-9122
3723-a West Market Street, Greensboro, NC 27403
FDA Number: 3004361320
Ownership: Private
Produces/Sells CE-marked Devices: N

System, Communication, Image, Digital	Radiology

STAIRMASTER HEALTH AND FITNESS PRODUCTS 800-628-8458
1886 Prarie Way, Louisville, CO 80027
FDA Number: n/a
E-mail: customerservice@nautilus.com
Web site: www.nautilus.com
Ownership: Stairmaster Health And Fitness Products
Produces/Sells CE-marked Devices: N
Federal Procurement Eligibility: Small Business
Distribution: Manufacturer Direct

Equipment, Therapy, Handicapped/Physical	Physical Med

Medical Product Subsidiaries (Listed Separately)
Stairmaster Health And Fitness Products

MANUFACTURER PROFILES

STAIRMASTER HEALTH AND FITNESS   800-628-8458 *(cont'd)*
Stairmaster Sports/Medical Products Gmbh

STAIRMASTER SPORTS/MEDICAL PRODUCTS
See Stairmaster Health And Fitness Products

STALLION TECHNOLOGIES INC.   315-476-4330
1201 East Fayette St., Syracuse, NY 13210
FDA Number: 1320938
E-mail: sti@stalliontech.com   *Fax:* 253-399-4256
Web site: www.stalliontech.com
Medical Products Sales Volume: $800,000
Year Founded: 1992
Total Employees: 8
Ownership: Private
Produces/Sells CE-marked Devices: N
Federal Procurement Eligibility: Small Business
Distribution: Manufacturer Through Distributor, Manufacturer Through
Manufacturer Reps, OEM, Exclusive Distributor, Exporter
General Admin.: Marshall Ma/President
   Image Processing System   Radiology

STALLION TECHNOLOGIES, INC.   315-476-4330
1201 East Fayette Street, Syracuse, NY 13210
FDA Number: n/a
E-mail: sti@stalliontech.com   *Fax:* 253-399-4256
Web site: www.stalliontech.com
Year Founded: 1992
Ownership: Private
Produces/Sells CE-marked Devices: Y
Federal Procurement Eligibility: Small Business
Distribution: Manufacturer Through Distributor, Manufacturer Through
Manufacturer Reps, OEM, Exclusive Distributor
   Camera, X-Ray, Fluorographic, Cine Or Spot   Radiology
   Cineangiograph (Cardiac Catheterization)   Radiology
   Computer, Radiographic Image Analysis   Radiology
   Image Processing System   Radiology
   Imager, X-Ray, Solid State (Flat Panel/Digital)   Radiology
   Radiographic Unit, Digital   Radiology
   Radiographic Unit, Digital Subtraction Angiographic (DSA)   Radiology
   Radiographic/Fluoroscopic Unit, Angiographic   Radiology
   Radiographic/Fluoroscopic Unit, Angiographic, Digital   Radiology
   Radiographic/Fluoroscopic Unit, Fixed   Radiology
   Radiographic/Fluoroscopic Unit, Image-Intensified   Radiology
   Radiographic/Fluoroscopic Unit, Mobile C-Arm   Radiology
   Radiographic/Fluoroscopic Unit, Non-Image-Intensified   Radiology
   Radiographic/Fluoroscopic Unit, Special Procedure   Radiology
   Storage Device, Fluoroscopic Image   Radiology

STAN-PAK
See St. Jude Medical Neuromodulation Division

STANBIO LABORATORY, INC.   830-249-0772
1261 N. Main St., Boerne, TX 78006-3014
FDA Number: 1616487
E-mail: stanbio@stanbio.com   *Fax:* 830-249-0851
Web site: www.stanbio.com
Medical Products Sales Volume: $4,000,000
Annual Revenue: $5-$10 Million
Year Founded: 1960
Total Employees: 50   *Marketing Staff:* 4   *Sales Staff:* 14
Ownership: Private
Quality System Registration Information: ISO9001
Produces/Sells CE-marked Devices: N
Federal Procurement Eligibility: Small Business, GSA Contract
Distribution: Manufacturer Through Distributor, OEM, Importer, Exporter
General Admin.: William R. Pippin/President, Chief Executive Officer
Mktg./Adv.: Albert E. Blanco/Vice President Marketing
   Colorimetry, Acetaminophen   Toxicology
   Control, Hemoglobin   Hematology
   Detergent   Hematology
   Diacetyl-Monoxime, Urea Nitrogen   Chemistry
   Dye-Binding, Albumin, Bromcresol, Green   Chemistry
   Enzymatic Method, Glucose (Urinary, Non-Quantitative)   Chemistry
   Kit, Pregnancy Test   Obstetrics/Gynecology
   Phosphatase, Alkaline   Hematology
   Phosphorus Reagent (Test System)   Chemistry
   Radiometric, Fe59, Iron Binding Capacity   Chemistry
   Reagent, Amylase, Colorimetric   Chemistry
   Reagent, Bilirubin (Total Or Direct Test System)   Chemistry
   Reagent, Blood Urea Nitrogen (BUN)   Chemistry
   Reagent, Calcium (Test System)   Chemistry
   Reagent, Chloride (Test System)   Chemistry
   Reagent, Cholesterol (Total Test System)   Chemistry
   Reagent, Creatinine (Test System)   Chemistry
   Reagent, Cyanomethemoglobin, With Standard   Hematology
   Reagent, Iron (Test System)   Chemistry
   Reagent, Kinase, Phosphate, Creatine   Chemistry
   Reagent, Other   General
   Reagent, Protein, Total   Chemistry
   Reagent, Streptolysin O/Antistreptolysin-Titer   Microbiology

STANBIO LABORATORY, INC.   830-249-0772 *(cont'd)*
   Solution, pH Buffer   Chemistry
   Stain, Giemsa   Pathology
   Standard/Control, All Types   Chemistry
   Test, C-Reactive Protein   Immunology
   Test, Glycosylated Hemoglobin Assay   Hematology
   Test, Human Chorionic Gonadotropin   Immunology
   Test, Rheumatoid Factor   Immunology
   Test, Syphilis (RPR or VDRL)   Microbiology
   Uricase (Colorimetric), Uric Acid   Chemistry

STANBIO LIFE SCIENCES, DIVISION OF   (800) 545-4437
STANBIO LABORATORY
25235 Leer Dr., Elkhart, IN 46514   **(574) 264-7384**
FDA Number: 1832837   *Fax:* 574) 266-0062
Ownership: Private
Produces/Sells CE-marked Devices: N
   Enzymatic Esterase-Oxidase, Cholesterol   Chemistry
   Nitroprusside, Ketones (Urinary, Non-Quantitative)   Chemistry

STAND-RITE MANUFACTURING CO.   562-782-6346
16655 Grand Ave., Bellflower, CA 90706-5037
FDA Number: 2032885
Ownership: Private
Produces/Sells CE-marked Devices: N
   Table, Mechanical   Physical Med
   Wheelchair, Standup   Physical Med

STANDARD CAP & SEAL
See Sonoco-Stancap Division

STANDARD DENTAL LAB   952-541-9622
431 Clark Street, Clarksburg, WV 26301
FDA Number: 3004136305
Ownership: Private
Produces/Sells CE-marked Devices: N
   Mouthguard   Dental And Oral

STANDARD IMAGING, INC.   608-831-0025
3120 Deming Way, Middleton, WI 53562
FDA Number: 2184007
   Accelerator, Linear, Medical   Radiology
   Calibrator, Dose, Radionuclide   Radiology
   Monitor, Patient Position, Light Beam   Radiology
   Phantom, Anthropomorphic, Radiographic   Radiology
   Pliers, Surgical   Orthopedics
   Radiotherapy Unit, Charged-Particle   Radiology
   Shield, Protective, Personnel   Radiology
   Tester, Radiology   Radiology

STANDARD INSTRUMENTATION, DIV. PREISER   800-624-8285
SCIENTIFIC
94 Oliver St., St. Albans, WV 25177   **304-727-2902**
FDA Number: n/a   *Fax:* 304-727-2932
E-mail: preiser@preiser.com
Web site: www.preiser.com
Medical Products Sales Volume: $1,000,000
Annual Revenue: $5-$10 Million
Year Founded: 1924
Total Employees: 42   *Marketing Staff:* 10   *Sales Staff:* 10
Ownership: Preiser Scientific, Inc.
Quality System Registration Information: ISO9001
Produces/Sells CE-marked Devices: N
Federal Procurement Eligibility: Female Owned
General Admin.: G. Preiser/Chief Executive Officer
       A. E. Preiser/President
       J. Gatens/Vice President, General Manager
Mktg./Adv.: C. Cline/Director Marketing
       K. Westfall/Director Product Development
       S. Gatens/Manager Advertising
       D. Meddings/Manager Contract Sales
       C. Cline/Manager International & National Sales
       J. Gatens/Manager Market Research
       J. Gatens/Manager National Sales
       D. Meddings/Manager Sales Training
       J. Gatens/Vice President Business Development
Production: C. Parrish/Director Quality Assurance
       J. Gatens/Manager Regulatory Affairs
   Calorimeter   Chemistry
   Dispenser, Pipette   Chemistry
   Fluorometer   Immunology
   Forceps   Orthopedics
   Freezer, Laboratory, General Purpose   Chemistry
   Microscope, Fluorescence/U.V.   Pathology
   Microscope, Inverted Stage, Tissue Culture   Pathology
   Microscope, Phase Contrast   Pathology
   Pipette Tip   Chemistry
   Sterilizer, Steam (Autoclave)   General
   Vial, Liquid Scintillation Counting   Chemistry

STANDARD INSTRUMENTATION, DIV. PREISER   800-624-8285
(cont'd)
Viscometer	Chemistry
Washer, Pipette	Chemistry

STANDARD SUPPLY CO.   800-453-7036
3424 S. Main St., Salt Lake City, UT 84165-0009   801-486-3371
FDA Number: n/a   Fax: 801-466-2362
E-mail: swalker@standardsupply.com
Web site: www.standardsupply.com
Annual Revenue: $5-$10 Million
Total Employees: 38   *Marketing Staff:* 2   *Sales Staff:* 10
Ownership: Private
Produces/Sells CE-marked Devices: N
Federal Procurement Eligibility: Small Business
Distribution: Exclusive Distributor
General Admin.: C. R. Stillman/President, Chief Executive Officer
          Loyd Steffensen/Vice President, General Manager
Mktg./Adv.: Steve Walker/Manager Sales
Battery	General
Service, Maintenance/Repair	General

STANDARD TEXTILE   800-999-0400
One Knollcrest Drive, Cincinnati, OH 45237   513-761-9255
FDA Number: 1527185   Fax: 513-761-0467
E-mail: info@standardtextile.com
Web site: www.standardtextile.com
Medical Products Sales Volume: $111,200,000
Year Founded: 1940
Total Employees: 2000   *Marketing Staff:* 10   *Sales Staff:* 101
Ownership: Private
Produces/Sells CE-marked Devices: Y
Federal Procurement Eligibility: GSA Contract, VA Contract
Distribution: Manufacturer Direct
General Admin.: Amanda Poitra/Director Human Resources
          Gary Heiman/President, Chief Executive Officer
Mktg./Adv.: Richard Stewart/Director Product Development
          Norman A. Frankel/Vice President Marketing & Sales
          Kim Heiman/Vice President, Manager Sales
Production: Brad Bushman/Director Quality Assurance
          Brad Bushman/Manager Regulatory Affairs
          Steve Tracey/Senior Vice President Manufacturing
          Steve Tracey/Vice President Manufacturing
Accessories, Apparel, Surgical	Surgery
Clothing, Protective	General
Curtain, Cubicle	General
Drape, Surgical	Surgery
Gown, Operating Room, Reusable	Surgery
Gown, Surgical	Surgery
Mattress, Bed	General
Pad, Incontinence (Underpad)	General
Wrapper, Surgical Instrument (Sterile)	General

STANDARD TEXTILE AUGUSTA, INC.   513-761-9255
1701 Goodrich St., Augusta, GA 30904
FDA Number: 3003714402
Fiber, Absorbent	General

STANDARD TEXTILE CO., INC.   888-999-0400
PO Box 371805, Cincinnati, OH 45222   513-761-9255
FDA Number: 1039147   Fax: 513-761-0467
E-mail: info@standardtextile.com
Web site: www.standardtextile.com
Year Founded: 1940
Total Employees: 1200   *Marketing Staff:* 10   *Sales Staff:* 75
Ownership: Private
Produces/Sells CE-marked Devices: Y
Distribution: Manufacturer Direct
Bag, Laundry, Operating Room	General
Blanket, Infant	General
Drape, Surgical	Surgery
Gown, Examination	General
Gown, Patient	Surgery
Gown, Surgical	Surgery
Linen	General
Linen, Bed	General
Pad, Incontinence (Underpad)	General
Wrap, Sterilization	General
Medical Product Subsidiaries (Listed Separately)
Standard Textile Co., Inc.

STANDING STONE, INC.   203-227-8710
49 Richmondville Ave, Westport, CT 06880
FDA Number: 3005643424
Computer, Chemistry Analyzer	Chemistry

STANLEY STORAGE SYSTEMS
See Stanley Vidmar

STANLEY SUPPLY & SERVICES, INC   800-225-5370
335 Willow Street,   978-682-2000
North Andover, MA 01845
FDA Number: n/a   Fax: 800-366-9662
E-mail: sales@stanleyworks.com
Web site: www.stanleysupplyservices.com
Medical Products Sales Volume: $33,000,000
Year Founded: 1963
Total Employees: 110   *Marketing Staff:* 3   *Sales Staff:* 29
Ownership: STANLEY WORKS
Stock Symbol: SWK
Traded On: NYSE
Produces/Sells CE-marked Devices: N
Federal Procurement Eligibility: Small Business, GSA Contract
Distribution: Exclusive Distributor
Mktg./Adv.: Steve Mitchell/Director Business Development
          Tom Seratti/Director Sales
          Erin Walsh/Media Planner
          Ron Broussard/National Sales Representative
Case, Protection, Equipment	General

STANLEY VIDMAR   800-523-9462
11 Grammes Road, Allentown, PA 18103
FDA Number: n/a   Fax: 800-523-9934
E-mail: custserv3@stanleyworks.com
Web site: www.stanleyvidmar.com
Annual Revenue: $25-$50 Million
Total Employees: 500   *Marketing Staff:* 2   *Sales Staff:* 40
Ownership: STANLEY WORKS
Stock Symbol: SWK
Traded On: NYSE
Quality System Registration Information: ISO9002
Produces/Sells CE-marked Devices: N
Federal Procurement Eligibility: GSA Contract
Distribution: Manufacturer Direct, Manufacturer Through Distributor, Manufacturer Through Manufacturer Reps, Exporter
General Admin.: Dave Fabris/President
Mktg./Adv.: Mark Weigel/Director Marketing
          Joe Micek/Director National Accounts
          Mark Weigel/Manager Advertising
          Dave Fabris/Vice President Sales
Production: Stephanie Heffelfinger/Director Customer Services
          John Flamisch/Director Engineering
          Mark Weigel/Product Manager
Cabinet, Instrument	General
Cabinet, Laboratory	Chemistry
Cabinet, Medicine	General
Cabinet, Narcotic Control	General
Cabinet, Other	General
Cabinet, Storage, Catheter	General
Cabinet, Table And Tray, Anesthesia	Anesthesiology
Cart, Emergency, Cardiopulmonary Resuscitation (Crash)	Anesthesiology
Cart, Instrument	Surgery

STAR CASE MANUFACTURING CO., INC.   800-822-7827
648 Superior Avenue, Munster, IN 46321   219-922-4440
FDA Number: n/a   Fax: 219-922-4442
E-mail: star@starcase.com
Web site: www.starcase.com
Medical Products Sales Volume: $1,800,000
Annual Revenue: $1-$5 Million
Year Founded: 1975
Total Employees: 50   *Marketing Staff:* 6   *Sales Staff:* 12
Ownership: Private
Produces/Sells CE-marked Devices: N
Federal Procurement Eligibility: Small Business, GSA Contract
Distribution: Manufacturer Direct
General Admin.: Mr. Dennis Toma/President, Chief Executive Officer
Mktg./Adv.: Ralph Hoopes/Manager Advertising
          Ralph Hoopes/Vice President Business Development
          Ralph G. Hoopes/Vice President Marketing & Sales
Production: Darren Eason/Director Quality Assurance
Case, Protection, Equipment	General
Component, Electrical	General
Container, Surgical Instrument	Surgery

STAR CUSHION PRODUCTS, INC.   618-539-7070
5 Commerce Dr., Freeburg, IL 62243
FDA Number: 1423735
Cushion, Wheelchair (Pad)	Physical Med
Mattress, Non-Powered Flotation Therapy	Physical Med

STAR DENTAL MANUFACTURING
See Dentalez Group

STAR INDUSTRIES   323-588-4141
2426 E. Washington Blvd., Los Angeles, CA 90021-2939
FDA Number: n/a   Fax: 323-588-1937

STAR INDUSTRIES
323-588-4141 *(cont'd)*

Web site: www.starind.com
Annual Revenue: $1-$5 Million
Total Employees: 14   Marketing Staff: 6   Sales Staff: 6
Ownership: Private
Produces/Sells CE-marked Devices: N
Distribution: Manufacturer Direct
General Admin.: Kermit Hillseth/President
     Damian Hillseth/Vice President
Mktg./Adv.: Mary Coffey/Vice President Sales

Service, Used Equipment	General

STAR MEDICAL SYSTEMS
800-626-3006
8301 Torresdale Avenue, Suite 13,
215-333-9518
Philadelphia, PA 19136

FDA Number: n/a   Fax: 215-333-9211
E-mail: info1@starmedsys.com
Web site: www.starmedsys.com
Annual Revenue: $1-$5 Million
Year Founded: 1991
Total Employees: 50   Marketing Staff: 2   Sales Staff: 2
Ownership: Private
Produces/Sells CE-marked Devices: N
Federal Procurement Eligibility: Small Business
Distribution: Manufacturer Direct, Manufacturer Through Distributor, Manufacturer Through Manufacturer Reps, Exporter
General Admin.: Alec Palmer/President

Brace, Joint, Ankle (External)	Physical Med
Collar, Cervical Neck	Orthopedics
Support, Wrist	Physical Med

STAR TECH HEALTH SERVICES, LLC.
801-229-1114
1219 South 1840 West, Bonnie, UT 84058

FDA Number: 1724621

Biofeedback Device	Cns/Neurology

STAR X-RAY CO., INC.
800-374-2163
63 Ranick Dr., Amityville, NY 11701-2821
631-842-3010

FDA Number: 9310066   Fax: 631-842-5901
E-mail: erosen@starxray.com
Web site: www.starxray.com
Annual Revenue: $1-$5 Million
Total Employees: 33
Ownership: Private
Quality System Registration Information: ISO9001
Produces/Sells CE-marked Devices: Y
Federal Procurement Eligibility: Small Business
Distribution: Manufacturer Through Distributor
General Admin.: Eric Rosen/President, Chief Executive Officer

Apron, Lead, Dental	Dental And Oral
Apron, Lead, Radiographic	Radiology
Holder, X-Ray Film	Dental And Oral
Illuminator, Radiographic Film	Radiology
Light, Other	General
Processor, Radiographic Film, Automatic, Dental	Dental And Oral
Safelight, X-Ray	Radiology

STARCHILD LABS
805-564-7194
57 Tierra Cielo Lane, Santa Barbara, CA 93105

FDA Number: 2938638

Alarm, Enuresis	Gastroenterology/Urology

STARGATE INTERNATIONAL, INC.
303-840-8206
10235 South Progress Way, #7, Parker, CO 80134

FDA Number: 3004160935

Lamp, Non-heating, For Adjunctive Use In Pain Therapy	Physical Med

STARION INSTRUMENTS
800-782-7466
1227 innsbruck dr, Sunnyvale, CA 94089
408-522-5200 EX

FDA Number: 2954339
E-mail: customerservice@Starioninstruments.com
Web site: www.starioninstruments.com
Year Founded: 2003
Ownership: Private
Produces/Sells CE-marked Devices: N
Mktg./Adv.: Charles Gilbride/Director Business Development
     Charles Gilbride/Director Marketing

Cautery, Radiofrequency, AC-Powered	Ophthalmology
Cautery, Thermal, AC-Powered	Ophthalmology
Cautery, Thermal, Battery-Powered	Ophthalmology
Electrosurgical Unit, Cutting & Coagulation Device	Surgery

STARKEY CALIFORNIA
952-947-4734
2536 Woodland Dr., Anaheim, CA 92801

FDA Number: 2026166
Ownership: Starkey Laboratories, Inc.

Hearing-Aid	Ear/Nose/Throat

STARKEY EAST
952-947-4734
535 Route 38 East, Suite 230, Cherry Hill, NJ 08002

FDA Number: 2246475
Ownership: Starkey Laboratories, Inc.

Hearing-Aid	Ear/Nose/Throat
Masker, Tinnitus	Ear/Nose/Throat

STARKEY FLORIDA
952-947-4734
2200 North Commerce Parkway, Weston, FL 33326

FDA Number: 1049183
Ownership: Starkey Laboratories, Inc.

Hearing-Aid	Ear/Nose/Throat

STARKEY GLENCOE
952-947-4734
2915 10th St. East, Glencoe, MN 55336

FDA Number: 2183732
Ownership: Starkey Laboratories, Inc.

Cotton, Roll	Dental And Oral
Kit, Earmold Impression	Ear/Nose/Throat

STARKEY LABORATORIES, INC.
800-328-8602
6700 Washington Ave. South,
952-941-6401
Eden Prairie, MN 55344

FDA Number: 2125608
E-mail: sales@starkey.com
Web site: http://www.starkey.com
Annual Revenue: $0-$1 Million
Year Founded: 1967
Total Employees: 4000   Marketing Staff: 17
Ownership: Private
Produces/Sells CE-marked Devices: N
Distribution: Manufacturer Direct, Manufacturer Through Manufacturer Reps
General Admin.: Mr. Jerry Ruzicka/President
     Mr. William Austin/President, Chief Executive Officer
     Mr. Rob Duchscher/Vice President Information Technology
Medical Admin.: Mr. Scott Nelson/Chief Medical Officer
Mktg./Adv.: Mr. Brandon Sawalich/Senior Vice President Sales
Production: Mr. Keith Guggenberger/Senior Vice President Operations
Research: Dr. Brent Edwardsd/Vice President Research
IS: Dr. Timothy Trine/Technical Director

Audiometer	Ear/Nose/Throat
Battery, Hearing-Aid	Ear/Nose/Throat
Calibrator, Hearing-Aid/Earphone And Analysis Systems	Ear/Nose/Throat
Chamber, Acoustic, Testing	Ear/Nose/Throat
Hearing-Aid	Ear/Nose/Throat
Holder, Speculum, ENT	Ear/Nose/Throat
Masker, Tinnitus	Ear/Nose/Throat
Meter, Leakage Current (Ammeter)	General
Mold, Middle Ear	Ear/Nose/Throat
Otoscope	Ear/Nose/Throat
Stethoscope, Electronic-Amplified	Surgery
System, Analysis, Hearing-Aid	Ear/Nose/Throat
Tester, Auditory Impedance	Ear/Nose/Throat
Unit, Therapy, Tinnitus	Ear/Nose/Throat

Medical Product Subsidiaries (Listed Separately)
Nu-Ear Electronics
Starkey California
Starkey East
Starkey Florida
Starkey Glencoe
Starkey Northwest
Starkey Southeast
Starkey Southwest

STARKEY NORTHWEST
800-537-5300
2255 N.E. 194th Ave., Portland, OR 97230-7437
612-941-6401

FDA Number: n/a   Fax: 503-667-9017
Web site: www.starkey.com
Total Employees: 92   Marketing Staff: 3   Sales Staff: 3
Ownership: Starkey Laboratories, Inc.
Produces/Sells CE-marked Devices: Y
Distribution: Manufacturer Direct
General Admin.: William Austin/Chief Executive Officer
     Jerry Ruzicka/President
Mktg./Adv.: Brandon Sawalich/Vice President Sales
Production: Keith Guggenberger/Senior Vice President Operations
Research: Dr. Brent Edwards/Vice President Research

Hearing-Aid	Ear/Nose/Throat

STARKEY SOUTHEAST
952-947-4734
5300 Oakbrook Pkwy.,, Bldg. 100, Suite 130,
Norcross, GA 30093

FDA Number: 1039190
Ownership: Starkey Laboratories, Inc.

Hearing-Aid	Ear/Nose/Throat

STARKEY SOUTHWEST
3100 Alvin Devane Blvd., Austin, TX 78741
952-947-4734
FDA Number: 1625545
Ownership: Starkey Laboratories, Inc.
Hearing-Aid
Ear/Nose/Throat

STARKMAN SURGICAL SUPPLY LTD.
1243 Bathurst St.,
Toronto, ONT M5R-3 Canada
800-387-0330
416-534-8411
FDA Number: n/a
Fax: 416-534-0203
Year Founded: 1931
Total Employees: 50
Ownership: Private
Produces/Sells CE-marked Devices: N
Distribution: Exclusive Distributor

STARMET CORPORATION
2229 Main St., Concord, MA 01742-3813
978-369-5410
FDA Number: n/a
Fax: 978-369-4045
E-mail: sales@starmet.com
Web site: www.starmet.com
Annual Revenue: $25-$50 Million
Total Employees: 213   *Marketing Staff:* 1   *Sales Staff:* 12
Ownership: Public
Stock Symbol: NUCM
Traded On: NASDAQ
Quality System Registration Information: ISO9002
Federal Procurement Eligibility: Small Business
Distribution: Manufacturer Direct
General Admin.: Robert E. Quinn/President
Mktg./Adv.: John D. Nicholson/Manager Advertising
     John D. Nicholson/Manager Business
     John D. Nicholson/Manager International Marketing & Sales
     Donald T. King/Manager Sales
Production: John D. Nicholson/Product Manager
     Bruce Zukauskas/Vice President Manufacturing
Research: William Nachtrab/Vice President Research & Development
Amalgam, Dental, Powder
Dental And Oral
Source, Wire, Radioactive Iridium
Radiology

STARPLEX SCIENTIFIC CORP.
705 Industrial Drive Sw, Cleveld, TN 37311
423-479-4108
FDA Number: 3006623380
Ownership: Private
Produces/Sells CE-marked Devices: N
Container, Specimen, All Types
General
Container, Specimen, Non-sterile
General
Culture Media, Non-Propagating Transport
Microbiology

STARPLEX SCIENTIFIC INC.
50A Steinway Blvd.,
Etobicoke, ONT M9W 6 Canada
800-665-0954
416-674-7474
FDA Number: n/a
Fax: 416-674-6067
E-mail: info@starplexscientific.com
Web site: www.starplexscientific.com
Year Founded: 1975
Total Employees: 150   *Marketing Staff:* 1   *Sales Staff:* 4
Ownership: Apotex Scientific, Inc.
Quality System Registration Information: ISO9001
Produces/Sells CE-marked Devices: Y
Federal Procurement Eligibility: Small Business
Distribution: Manufacturer Through Distributor, Exclusive Distributor

STARR INDUSTRIES/PORTABLE ENTRY SYSTEMS
87 Taylor St, Quincy, MI 49082
800-677-8377
517-639-7401
FDA Number: 1836411
Fax: 517-639-3098
E-mail: starindustries@chartermi.net
Medical Products Sales Volume: $5,000,000
Annual Revenue: $10-$25 Million
Year Founded: 1989
Total Employees: 60   *Marketing Staff:* 4   *Sales Staff:* 4
Ownership: Private
Produces/Sells CE-marked Devices: N
Distribution: Manufacturer Direct, Manufacturer Through Distributor
General Admin.: Mr. Jim Starr/Co-Owner, Vice President
Ramp, Wheelchair
General

STARS
6630 Exchequer Drive, Baton Rouge, LA 70809
225-752-4912
FDA Number: 2320553
Fax: 225-752-8523
E-mail: BradC@scoliosis.com
Web site: www.scoliosis.com
Ownership: Private
Distribution: Manufacturer Direct
Orthosis, Lumbosacral
Physical Med

STARS
225-752-4912 *(cont'd)*
Stimulator, Scoliosis, Neuromuscular, Functional
Orthopedics

STARSURGICAL, INC.
7781 Lakeview Dr., Burlington, WI 53105-8119
888-609-2470
FDA Number: 2135151
Fax: 262-539-2096
E-mail: osteo@tds.net
Year Founded: 2000
Ownership: Private
Quality System Registration Information: ISO9000
Produces/Sells CE-marked Devices: N
Federal Procurement Eligibility: Small Business
Distribution: Manufacturer Direct
Adhesive, Wound Closure
Surgery
Mesh, Surgical, Polymeric
Surgery

STAT HEALTHCARE CORPORATION
6215 3rd St. SE, Unit C12,
Calgary, ALB T2H-2 Canada
800-567-6001
403-297-0700
FDA Number: n/a
Fax: 403-297-0709
E-mail: stat@cadvision.com
Year Founded: 1989
Total Employees: 25
Ownership: Private
Produces/Sells CE-marked Devices: N
Distribution: Exclusive Distributor

STAT-CHEK COMPANY
P.O. Box 9636, Bend, OR 97708
800-248-6618
541-322-2870
FDA Number: n/a
Fax: 541-322-1890
E-mail: statchek@clearwire.net
Web site: http://stat-chek.com
Medical Products Sales Volume: $200,000
Annual Revenue: $0-$1 Million
Year Founded: 1962
Total Employees: 6
Ownership: Private
Produces/Sells CE-marked Devices: N
Federal Procurement Eligibility: Small Business, Female Owned
Distribution: Manufacturer Direct, Manufacturer Through Distributor
Communication System, Powered
Physical Med
Holder, Medical Chart
General
Label, Device
General
Physician Registry
General

STAT-CHEK COMPANY (THE)
See Stat-Chek Company

STATCO HEARING AID LABORATORY
4000 Mccain Blvd., North Little Rock, AR 72116
501-771-2444
FDA Number: 2318075
Ownership: Private
Produces/Sells CE-marked Devices: N
Hearing-Aid, Master
Ear/Nose/Throat

STATCORP, INC.
14476 Duval Place West #303,
Jacksonville, FL 32218
800-992-0014
904-786-5113
FDA Number: 1051575
Fax: 904-786-6101
E-mail: RHALL@statcorp.net
Web site: www.statcorp.net
Medical Products Sales Volume: $2,300,000
Annual Revenue: $5-$10 Million
Year Founded: 1989
Total Employees: 28   *Marketing Staff:* 2   *Sales Staff:* 4
Ownership: Private
Quality System Registration Information: ISO9002
Produces/Sells CE-marked Devices: Y
Federal Procurement Eligibility: Small Business
Distribution: Manufacturer Direct, Manufacturer Through Distributor, Manufacturer Through Manufacturer Reps, OEM, Service Direct
General Admin.: James M. Shepherd/President, Chief Executive Officer
     Andy Woods/Vice Chairman
Mktg./Adv.: Roger Hall/Vice President Marketing
Production: Wayne Emmert/Manager Regulatory Affairs
Cuff, Blood Pressure
Cardiovascular
Inflator, Cuff
General
Microfilter, Blood Transfusion
Anesthesiology

STATE CHEMICAL MANUFACTURING CO.
3100 Hamilton Ave., Cleveland, OH 44114
800-321-8180
216-861-7114
FDA Number: n/a
Fax: 888-771-9670
E-mail: customerservice@statechemical.com
Web site: http://www.stateindustrial.com
Annual Revenue: $0-$1 Million
Total Employees: 300   *Marketing Staff:* 6   *Sales Staff:* 400
Ownership: Private
Produces/Sells CE-marked Devices: N

STATE CHEMICAL MANUFACTURING CO. 800-321-8180 *(cont'd)*
Distribution: Manufacturer Direct

Disinfector, Liquid	General
Solution, Antibacterial Cleaner	General

STATE TRADING CORP. OF AMERICA, THE
See State Trading Corporation Of India, Ltd.

STATE TRADING CORPORATION OF INDIA, LTD. 212-244-3317
350 5th Ave., Ste. 1124, 11th Fl., New York, NY 10118
FDA Number: n/a   *Fax:* 212-244-3319
E-mail: stcnewyork@aol.com
Medical Products Sales Volume: $600,000,000
Total Employees: 2000
Ownership: State Trading Corporation Of India, Ltd., The
Stock Symbol: STTC-BO
Traded On: Bombay
Produces/Sells CE-marked Devices: N
Distribution: Exporter

Accessories, Apparel, Surgical	Surgery
Bag, Blood	Hematology
Blade, Surgical, Saw, General & Plastic Surgery	Surgery
Cannula, Injection	Gastroenterology/Urology
Cap, Surgical	Surgery
Catheter, Suction (Tracheal Aspirating Tube)	Anesthesiology
Catheter, Urethral	Gastroenterology/Urology
Cover, Other	General
Cover, Shoe, Operating Room	Surgery
Glove, Patient Examination, Latex	General
Glove, Surgical	General
Gown, Isolation, Surgical	Surgery
Kit, Administration, Blood	General
Kit, Administration, Intravenous	General
Kit, Blood Donor	Hematology
Kit, Maternity	Obstetrics/Gynecology
Linen, Bed	General
Sheet, Drape	Surgery
Suit, Surgical	Surgery
Suture, Catgut	Surgery
Suture, Non-Absorbable, Steel, Monofilament & Multifilament	Surgery
Suture, Non-Absorbable, Synthetic, Polyamide	Surgery
Suture, Non-Absorbable, Synthetic, Polyester	Surgery
Suture, Silk	Surgery
Syringe, Other	General
Thermometer, Mercury	General
Tube, Feeding	General
Tube, X-Ray	Radiology

STATLAB MEDICAL PRODUCTS, INC. 800-442-3573
106 Hillside Drive, Lewisville, TX 75057 972-436-1010
FDA Number: 1640981   *Fax:* 972-436-1369
E-mail: mlduke@statlab.com
Web site: www.statlab.com
Medical Products Sales Volume: $4,900,000
Annual Revenue: $10-$25 Million
Year Founded: 1977
Total Employees: 30   *Marketing Staff:* 3   *Sales Staff:* 9
Ownership: Private
Produces/Sells CE-marked Devices: N
Federal Procurement Eligibility: Small Business
Distribution: Manufacturer Direct, Manufacturer Through Distributor, Exporter
General Admin.: John Bickel/President, Chief Executive Officer
          David Bickel/Vice President
Mktg./Adv.: Daniel Bickel/Vice President Marketing & Sales

Blade, Scalpel	Surgery
Brush, Cytology	General
Cassette, Tissue	Pathology
Container, Specimen Mailer And Storage	Pathology
Container, Specimen, All Types	General
Coverslip, Microscope Slide	Pathology
Dressing, Aerosol	General
Fixative, Formalin Containing	Pathology
Formalin, Neutral Buffered	Pathology
Mounting Media, Oil Soluble	Pathology
Preservative, Cytological	Pathology
Reagent, General Purpose	Pathology
Slide, Microscope	Pathology
Solution, Pathology, Decalcifier, Acid Containing	Pathology
Spatula, Cervical, Cytology	Obstetrics/Gynecology
Stain, Hematoxylin	Pathology
Stain, Papanicolau	Pathology

STATLABS, INC.
See Statcorp, Inc.

STATRAD 800-835-3723
13915 Danielson St, Suite 200, Poway,, CA 92064
FDA Number: 3008008144
Web site: www.statrad.com
Ownership: Private

STATRAD 800-835-3723 *(cont'd)*
Produces/Sells CE-marked Devices: N

STATSPIN, INC. 800-782-8774
60 Glacier Drive, Westwood, MA 02090-1825 781-551-0100
FDA Number: n/a   *Fax:* 781-551-0036
E-mail: info1@statspin.com
Web site: www.statspinvet.com
Medical Products Sales Volume: $16,800,000
Annual Revenue: $5-$10 Million
Year Founded: 1986
Total Employees: 151   *Marketing Staff:* 5   *Sales Staff:* 2
Ownership: Iris International, Inc.
Stock Symbol: IRIS
Traded On: NASDAQ
Quality System Registration Information: ISO9001
Produces/Sells CE-marked Devices: Y
Federal Procurement Eligibility: Small Business
Distribution: Manufacturer Through Distributor, OEM
General Admin.: Robert Mello/President
Mktg./Adv.: Pam Pasakarnis/Vice President Marketing & Sales
Production: John Forte/Director Operations
          Richard Vincins/Director Quality Assurance & Regulatory Affairs
Research: Kevin Sullivan/Director Research & Development
IS: Jessica Thibeault/Tech. Specialist

Analyzer, Sedimentation Rate, Erythrocyte	Hematology
Block, Heating	Chemistry
Centrifuge, General (Over 5,000 rpm)	Toxicology
Centrifuge, General (Up to 5,000 rpm)	Pathology
Centrifuge, Microhematocrit	Hematology
Clearing Agent	Pathology
Cytocentrifuge	Pathology
Hematocrit Tube, Rack, Sealer, Holder	Hematology
Spinner, Slide, Automated	Hematology
Tube, Capillary Blood Collection	Hematology

STATSURE DIAGNOSTIC SYSTEMS, INC. 508-872-2625
1881 Worcester Road, Framingham, MA 01701
FDA Number: 3026209
Ownership: Public
Stock Symbol: SSUR
Traded On: OTC Bulletin
Produces/Sells CE-marked Devices: N

Absorber, Saliva, Paper	Dental And Oral
Applicator, Tipped, Absorbent, Non-Sterile	General
Container, Specimen, Non-sterile	General

STAXI CORPORATION LTD. 877-677-8294
201 Millway Ave., Unit 5, 905-760-8103
Concord, ONT L4K-5 Canada
FDA Number: n/a   *Fax:* 905-760-8106
E-mail: info@staxi.com
Web site: www.staxi.com
Year Founded: 1999
Total Employees: 25
Ownership: Private
Produces/Sells CE-marked Devices: N
Distribution: Manufacturer Direct, Exclusive Distributor

STC COMPANIES
See Sunrise Medical, Inc.

STC MEDICAL CORP.
See Orasure Technologies, Inc.

STC TECHNOLOGIES, INC.
See Orasure Technologies, Inc.

STD MED, INC. 781-828-4400
75 Mill Street, PO Box 420, Stoughton, MA 02072
FDA Number: 1222928   *Fax:* 781-344-5895
E-mail: sales@stdmed.com
Web site: www.stdmed.com
Medical Products Sales Volume: $13,900,000
Annual Revenue: $10-$25 Million
Year Founded: 1953
Total Employees: 140   *Marketing Staff:* 2   *Sales Staff:* 4
Ownership: Private
Quality System Registration Information: ISO9001
Produces/Sells CE-marked Devices: N
Federal Procurement Eligibility: Small Business
Distribution: OEM
Mktg./Adv.: Andrea Patisteas/Vice President Sales

Electrosurgical Unit, Cutting & Coagulation Device	Surgery
Scissors, Disposable	General
Suction Apparatus, Single Patient, Portable, Non-Powered	Surgery

STEALTH PRODUCTS 800-965-9229
103 John Kelly Dr, Burnet, TX 78611
FDA Number: 3004473024

STEALTH PRODUCTS
800-965-9229 *(cont'd)*
Accessories, Wheelchair — Physical Med

STEALTH THERAPEUTICS INC
608-577-4484
5520 Nobel Dr Suite 150, Fitchburg, WI 53711
FDA Number: n/a
Web site: www.stealththerapeutics.com
Ownership: Private
Produces/Sells CE-marked Devices: N
General Admin.: Mr. Peter Drumm/Chief Executive Officer
Mr. Bradley Glenn/Chief Technology Officer

STEDIM BIOSYSTEMS, INC.
800-914-6644
925-689-6650
1910 Mark Ct., Concord, CA 94520
Fax: 925-689-6988
FDA Number: 3003914055
E-mail: info@stedim.com
Web site: www.stedim.com
Medical Products Sales Volume: $11,900,000
Annual Revenue: $25-$50 Million
Year Founded: 1978
Total Employees: 65 — *Marketing Staff:* 2 — *Sales Staff:* 12
Ownership: Public
Stock Symbol: DIM
Traded On: Paris
Quality System Registration Information: ISO9001; ISO9002
Produces/Sells CE-marked Devices: N
Federal Procurement Eligibility: Small Business
Distribution: Manufacturer Direct, Exporter
General Admin.: Chris Rombach/President
Mktg./Adv.: Dave Belomy/Director Marketing & Sales
Production: Felicia Adler/Manager Quality Assurance & Regulatory Affairs
Finance: Jeff Mitchell/Financial Executive
IS: Maxime Lok/Manager Tech. Services
Container, Specimen, All Types — General
Dispenser, Fluid — General

STEEGER USA, LLC
800-554-2082
864-472-7000
2353 Highway 292, Inman, SC 29349
Fax: 864-472-7073
FDA Number: n/a
E-mail: info@steegerusa.com
Web site: www.steegerusa.com
Medical Products Sales Volume: $4,000,000
Annual Revenue: $1-$5 Million
Total Employees: 10 — *Marketing Staff:* 3 — *Sales Staff:* 3
Ownership: Private
Produces/Sells CE-marked Devices: Y
Federal Procurement Eligibility: Small Business
Distribution: Manufacturer Direct, OEM, Exclusive Distributor, Importer, Exporter
General Admin.: Dan Hargett/Chief Executive Officer
Myra Lambert/Executive Assistant
Susan Sonnleitner/Executive Assistant
Mktg./Adv.: Ray Owens/Representative Tech. Sales
Tim Stillwell/Vice President Sales
Research: Kenneth Stenstrom/Director Technology
Twister, Wire — Orthopedics

STEELCRAFT, INC.
800-225-7710
508-865-4445
115 W. Main St., Millbury, MA 01527
Fax: 508-865-4600
FDA Number: 1219107
E-mail: djb@steelcraft-inc.com
Medical Products Sales Volume: $1,000,000
Annual Revenue: $10-$25 Million
Total Employees: 50 — *Marketing Staff:* 2 — *Sales Staff:* 3
Ownership: Private
Produces/Sells CE-marked Devices: Y
Federal Procurement Eligibility: Small Business
Distribution: Manufacturer Direct, Manufacturer Through Distributor, OEM, Exporter
General Admin.: Douglas Backman/President, Chief Executive Officer
Production: Don Small/Vice President Manufacturing
Accessories, Cart, Multipurpose — General
Cart, Other — General
Casters, Hospital Equipment — General
Infusion Stand — General
Mount, Equipment — General
Mount, Monitor (Support) — General

STEELE CANVAS BASKET CO., INC.
800-541-8929
617-889-0202
201 Williams St., P.O. Box 6267 IMCN, Chelsea, MA 02150
Fax: 617-889-0524
FDA Number: n/a
E-mail: steele-canvas@msn.com
Medical Products Sales Volume: $400,000
Annual Revenue: $0-$1 Million
Total Employees: 40
Ownership: Private
Produces/Sells CE-marked Devices: N

STEELE CANVAS BASKET CO., INC.
800-541-8929 *(cont'd)*
Federal Procurement Eligibility: Small Business
Distribution: Manufacturer Through Distributor
General Admin.: John J. Lordan/President
Cart, Laundry — General
Cover, Laundry Hamper — General
Laundry Hamper — General
Liner, Laundry Hamper — General
Stand, Laundry Hamper — General

STEINER LABORATORIES
866-317-1348
714-783-7827
590 Farrington Hwy., #524 Suite 132, Kapolei, HI 96707
FDA Number: 3005138409
E-mail: staff@steinerlabs.com
Web site: www.steinerlabs.com
Ownership: Private
Produces/Sells CE-marked Devices: N
Accessories, Implant, Dental, Endosseous — Dental And Oral
Graft, Bone — Orthopedics
Implant, Endosseous (Bone Filling and/or Augmentation) — Dental And Oral
Tricalcium Phosphate Granules for Dental Bone Repair — Dental And Oral

STELKAST COMPANY
888-273-1583
724-941-6368
200 Hidden Valley Rd., Mcmurray, PA 15317
Fax: 724-941-5987
FDA Number: 2530191
E-mail: info@stelkast.com
Web site: http://www.stelkast.com
Year Founded: 1992
Ownership: Private
Produces/Sells CE-marked Devices: N
Prosthesis, Hip, Femoral Component, Cemented, Metal — Orthopedics
Prosthesis, Hip, Semi-Constr., Metal/Ceramic, Cemented/NC — Orthopedics
Prosthesis, Hip, Semi-Constrained Acetabular — Orthopedics
Prosthesis, Hip, Semi-Constrained, Metal/Polymer — Orthopedics
Prosthesis, Hip, Semi-Constrained, Metal/Polymer, Uncemented — Orthopedics
Prosthesis, Knee, Femorotibial, Non-Constrained — Orthopedics
Prosthesis, Knee, Patellofemorotibial, Semi-Constrained — Orthopedics
Prosthesis, Shoulder, Non-Constrained, Metal/Polymer Cem. — Orthopedics

STELLAR TECHNOLOGIES, INC.
888-566-9094
763-493-8556
9200 Xylon Avenue North, Suite 100, Brooklyn Park, MN 55445
Fax: 763-493-8507
FDA Number: 2135130
E-mail: dforcelle@stellar-technologies.com
Web site: www.stellar-technologies.com
Medical Products Sales Volume: $8,300,000
Annual Revenue: $10-$25 Million
Year Founded: 1995
Total Employees: 115 — *Marketing Staff:* 2 — *Sales Staff:* 20
Ownership: Private
Quality System Registration Information: ISO9001
Produces/Sells CE-marked Devices: N
Federal Procurement Eligibility: Small Business, Female Owned
Distribution: Manufacturer Through Manufacturer Reps
General Admin.: Estelle Forcelle/Chief Executive Officer
Mktg./Adv.: Dennis Forcelle/Director Marketing & Sales
Production: Tom Warren/Director Quality Assurance
Equipment/Service, Quality Control — General

STELLARTECH RESEARCH CORP.
408-331-3000
1346 Bordeaux Dr., Sunnyvale, CA 94089
FDA Number: 2952366
Electrosurgical Unit, Cutting & Coagulation Device — Surgery

STELLATE SYSTEMS
514-486-1306
300-345 Av Victoria, Westmount H3Z 2N2 Canada
FDA Number: 9680936
Analyzer, Spectrum, EEG Signal — Cns/Neurology

STELRAY PLASTIC PRODUCTS, INC
203-735-2331
50 Westfield Ave., Ansonia, CT 06401
FDA Number: 3003283852
Mouthguard — Dental And Oral

STELREMA CORP.
814-422-8892
4055 East 250 North, Knox, IN 46534
FDA Number: 1828935
Ownership: Private
Produces/Sells CE-marked Devices: N
Bracket, Plastic, Orthodontic — Dental And Oral

STENTOR INC., A PHILIPS MEDICAL SYSTEMS CO.
See Philips Healthcare Informatics, Inc

STENTYS INC.
609-853-0100
103 Carnegie Center, Princeton, NJ 08540
FDA Number: n/a
Fax: 609-275 6155
Web site: http://www.stentys.com
Ownership: Public

MANUFACTURER PROFILES

STENTYS INC.   609-853-0100 *(cont'd)*
Stock Symbol: STNT
Traded On: Paris
Produces/Sells CE-marked Devices: N
General Admin.: Mr. Gonzague Issenmann/Chief Executive Officer
         Mr. Hikmat Hojeibane/Chief Technology Officer
Medical Admin.: Dr. RenAc Spaargaren/Chief Medical Officer
Mktg./Adv.: Mr. Paul Geudens/Vice President Marketing & Sales
Production: Mr. Benoit Vandenbossche/Director Operations
         Mr. Luc Morisset/Director Quality Control & Regulatory Affairs
Finance: Mr. Stanislas Piot/Chief Financial Officer

STEP FORWARD CO.   253-631-0683
11109 Se Kent-kangley Road, Kent, WA 98030
FDA Number: 3021074

Insoles, Medical	General

STEPAN CO.   800-745-7837
22 W. Frontage Road, Northfield, IL 60093   847-446-7500
FDA Number: n/a   *Fax:* 847-501-2100
E-mail: order.placement@stepan.com
Web site: www.stepan.com
Medical Products Sales Volume: $1,172,600,000
Annual Revenue: More than $100 Million
Year Founded: 1932
Total Employees: 363
Ownership: Public
Stock Symbol: SCL
Traded On: NYSE
Federal Procurement Eligibility: Small Business
Distribution: Manufacturer Direct, Manufacturer Through Distributor, OEM, Exporter
General Admin.: F. Quinn Stepan/Chief Executive Officer
         Michael Gumkowski/Director Human Resources
         James Hartlage/Senior Vice President Admin.
         John Venegoni/Vice President, General Manager
         Ronald Siemon/Vice President, General Manager
Mktg./Adv.: Gilbert Eshoo/Vice President Sales
Production: David Milner/Director Regulatory Affairs
         M. Mirghanbari/Vice President Manufacturing
Research: Earl Wagener/Vice President Research & Development
Finance: Walter Klein/Vice President Finance
IS: James Hartlage/Senior Vice President Technology

Disinfector, Liquid	General
Solution, Antibacterial Cleaner	General

STEPHAN WOOD PRODUCTS, INC.   989-348-5496
605 Huron, P.O. Box 669, Grayling, MI 49738-0669
FDA Number: 1828689   *Fax:* 989-348-2427
Ownership: Private
Produces/Sells CE-marked Devices: N

Splint, Temporary Training	Physical Med

STEPHEN TOBIAS HEARING CENTER   617-770-3395
382 Quincy Avenue, Quincy, MA 02169
FDA Number: 3006176517

Hearing-Aid, Plate, Face	Ear/Nose/Throat

STEPHENS INSTRUMENTS, INC.   800-354-7848
2500 Sandersville Rd, Lexington, KY 40511   859-259-4924
FDA Number: 1045379   *Fax:* 859-259-4926
E-mail: stephensinst@aol.com
Web site: www.stephensinst.com
Medical Products Sales Volume: $1,000,000
Ownership: Private
Produces/Sells CE-marked Devices: N
Federal Procurement Eligibility: Small Business, Minority Owned
Distribution: Manufacturer Through Distributor, Manufacturer Through Manufacturer Reps, OEM, Exporter

Blade, Scalpel	Surgery
Caliper, Ophthalmic	Ophthalmology
Cannula, Cyclodialysis (Eye)	Ophthalmology
Cannula, Lacrimal (Eye)	Ophthalmology
Cannula, Ophthalmic	Ophthalmology
Container, Sterilization (Tray)	General
Depressor, Orbital	Ophthalmology
Dilator, Lacrimal	Ophthalmology
Forceps, Ophthalmic	Ophthalmology
Holder, Needle, Other	Surgery
Hook, Ophthalmic	Ophthalmology
Hook, Scleral Fixation	Ophthalmology
Hook, Strabismus	Ophthalmology
Kit, Irrigation, Eye	Ophthalmology
Knife, Cataract	Ophthalmology
Knife, Keratome	Ophthalmology
Knife, Ophthalmic	Ophthalmology
Needle, Ophthalmic	Ophthalmology
Probe, Lacrimal	Ophthalmology
Probe, Ophthalmic	Ophthalmology

STEPHENS INSTRUMENTS, INC.   800-354-7848 *(cont'd)*

Probe, Trabeculotomy	Ophthalmology
Retractor, Ophthalmic	Ophthalmology
Scissors, Corneal	Ophthalmology
Scissors, Enucleation	Ophthalmology
Scissors, Iris	Ophthalmology
Scissors, Ophthalmic	Ophthalmology
Scissors, Tenotomy	Ophthalmology
Spatula, Ophthalmic	Ophthalmology
Speculum, Ophthalmic	Ophthalmology
Spoon, Ophthalmic	Ophthalmology
Spud, Ophthalmic	Ophthalmology

STEREO OPTICAL CO., INC.   800-344-9500
8623 W. Bryn Mawr Ave.,, Suite 502,   1.773.867.0380
Chicago, IL 60631
FDA Number: 1419226   *Fax:* 773-777-4985
E-mail: sales@stereoooptical.com
Web site: www.stereooptical.com
Medical Products Sales Volume: $4,300,000
Annual Revenue: $1-$5 Million
Total Employees: 20   *Marketing Staff:* 1   *Sales Staff:* 3
Ownership: Public
Produces/Sells CE-marked Devices: Y
Distribution: Manufacturer Direct, Manufacturer Through Manufacturer Reps, OEM
General Admin.: Mr. William Baker/Vice President
Mktg./Adv.: Mr. Chris Albu/Manager International Sales
         Ms. Mackenzie Rakers/Manager National Sales

Analyzer, Peripheral Vision	Ophthalmology
Analyzer, Visual Function	Ophthalmology
Chart, Visual Acuity	Ophthalmology
Refractometer, Ophthalmic	Ophthalmology
Retinoscope, Battery-Powered	Ophthalmology
Stereoscope, AC-Powered	Ophthalmology
Target, Fusion/Stereoscopic	Ophthalmology
Tester, Color Vision	Ophthalmology

STEREOIMAGING CORPORATION   978-649-8592
164 Westford Rd. Suite 17, Tyngsboro, MA 01879
FDA Number: 3003850172
Ownership: Private
Produces/Sells CE-marked Devices: N

Microscope, Surgical	Ear/Nose/Throat

STEREOTACTIC MEDICAL SYSTEMS, INC.
See Compass International, Inc.

STEREOTAXIS, INC.   866-646-2346
4320 Forest Park Ave., Suite 100,   314-615-6940
St. Louis, MO 63108
FDA Number: 3003084417   *Fax:* 314-678-6159
E-mail: kim.wright@stereotaxis.com
Web site: www.stereotaxis.com
Ownership: Public
Stock Symbol: STSX
Traded On: NASDAQ
Produces/Sells CE-marked Devices: N
General Admin.: Mr. Michael Kaminski/President, Chief Executive Officer
         Ms. Karen Duros/Senior Vice President, General Counsel, Secretary
         Mr. Pierre Rivaux/Vice President
Mktg./Adv.: Mr. Frank Cheng/Senior Vice President Marketing & Business Development
Finance: Mr. Daniel Johnston/Chief Financial Officer

Control System, Catheter, Steerable	Cardiovascular
Guidewire, Catheter	Cardiovascular
Imager, X-Ray, Solid State (Flat Panel/Digital)	Radiology

STEREX CORP.   800-603-5045
4501 126th Avenue, North,   727-573-5045
Clearwater, FL 33762
FDA Number: 1214368   *Fax:* 727-573-3058
Medical Products Sales Volume: $100,000
Year Founded: 1986
Total Employees: 5
Ownership: Private
Produces/Sells CE-marked Devices: N
Federal Procurement Eligibility: Small Business

Holder, Syringe, Leaded	Radiology
Needle, Aspiration And Injection, Disposable	Surgery
Syringe, Cartridge	Dental And Oral

STERI-DENT CORP.
See Cpac Equipment, Inc.

STERI-SHIELD PRODUCTS   805-692-4972
336 S. Fairview Ave, Goleta, CA 93117
FDA Number: 2954770

Holder, X-Ray Film	Dental And Oral

STERICON, INC.   708-865-8790
2315 Gardner Road, Broadview, IL 60153
FDA Number: 1419421   Fax: 708-865-2094
E-mail: stericon@stericon.com
Web site: www.stericon.com
Medical Products Sales Volume: $2,700,000
Year Founded: 1975
Total Employees: 37
Ownership: Private
Quality System Registration Information: ISO9001
Produces/Sells CE-marked Devices: N
Federal Procurement Eligibility: Small Business
Distribution: Manufacturer Direct, Manufacturer Through Distributor
General Admin.: Clifford Faust/Chief Executive Officer
Mktg./Adv.: Gregory Faust/Director Marketing
         John McDowell/Director Product Development
Production: Dan Bernier/Director Quality Assurance

Bag, Blood	Hematology
Bag, Plastic	General
Bag, Reservoir (Blood)	Anesthesiology
Container, Frozen Donor Tissue Storage	General

STERICYCLE   847-367-5910
28161 N. Keith Dr., Lake Forest, IL 60045
FDA Number: 3007097064   Fax: 847-367-9493
E-mail: investor@stericycle.com
Web site: http://www.stericycle.com
Year Founded: 1989
Ownership: Public
Stock Symbol: SRCL
Traded On: NASDAQ
Produces/Sells CE-marked Devices: N
General Admin.: Mr. Mark Miller/Chief Executive Officer
         Mr. Richard Kogler/Chief Operating Officer
Finance: Mr. Frank ten Brink/Chief Financial Officer

Container, Sharpes	General
Needle, Hypodermic, Single Lumen With Syringe	General
Needle, Hypodermic, Single Lumen, Reprocessed	General

STERIGENICS INTERNATIONAL, INC.   800-472-4508
                                                     630-928-1700
2015 Spring Road, Suite 650,
Oak Brook, IL 60523
FDA Number: 1450293   Fax: 630-928-1701
E-mail: info@sterigenics.com
Web site: www.sterigenics.com
Medical Products Sales Volume: $11,300,000
Annual Revenue: $100-$500 Million
Year Founded: 2004
Total Employees: 14
Ownership: Private
Quality System Registration Information: ISO9002
Produces/Sells CE-marked Devices: N
Federal Procurement Eligibility: Small Business
Distribution: Manufacturer Direct, Manufacturer Through Distributor, OEM, Service Direct
General Admin.: David Meyer/President, Chief Executive Officer
Mktg./Adv.: Patrick Hughes/Vice President Marketing & Sales
Production: Kathy Hoffman/Vice President Quality Assurance & Regulatory Affairs
         John Gilbert/Vice President, Engineer
Research: Lisa Foster/Vice President Laboratories
Finance: Fred Ruegsegger/Chief Financial Officer

Contract Laboratory	General
Contract Sterilization	General
Forceps, Sterilizer Transfer	General
Sterilizer, Ethylene-Oxide Gas	General
Sterilizer, Radiation	General

STERILATOR COMPANY, INC.   585-968-2377
30 Water Street, Cuba, NY 14727-1023
FDA Number: 1317154   Fax: 585-968-4847
Medical Products Sales Volume: $600,000
Annual Revenue: $0-$1 Million
Year Founded: 1999
Total Employees: 10
Federal Procurement Eligibility: Small Business
Distribution: Manufacturer Direct, Exporter
General Admin.: Shawn A. Doyle/President

Sterilization Process Indicator, Biological	General

STERILE RESOURCES, INC.   800-317-6472
                                                   804-897-4061
1565 Oakbridge Terrace, Powhatan, VA 23139
FDA Number: 3004121310   Fax: 804-897-4064
Web site: www.sterileresources.com
Ownership: Private
Produces/Sells CE-marked Devices: N

Sterilizer, Steam (Autoclave)	General

STERILE SYSTEMS, DIVISION OF MEDTRONIC, INC.
See Medtronic Dlp

STERILE TECHNOLOGIES, INC.   518-793-7077
63 Park Rd., Queensbury, NY 12804
FDA Number: n/a   Fax: 518-793-8357
E-mail: voman-sti@adelphea.net
Web site: www.steriletech.com
Annual Revenue: $1-$5 Million
Year Founded: 1987
Total Employees: 8   Marketing Staff: 1   Sales Staff: 1
Ownership: Private
Produces/Sells CE-marked Devices: Y
Federal Procurement Eligibility: Small Business
Distribution: Manufacturer Direct, OEM, Service Direct, Exporter
General Admin.: Roman M. Stienss/President, Chief Executive Officer

Service, Equipment Leasing	General
Test, Equipment, Sterilization	General

STERILEX CORP.   800-511-1659
                                                   410-581-8860
11409 Cronhill Drive Suite L,
Owings Mills, MD 21117
FDA Number: 1125516   Fax: 410-581-8864
E-mail: faith@sterilex.com
Web site: www.sterilex.com
Medical Products Sales Volume: $2,700,000
Year Founded: 1995
Total Employees: 15
Ownership: Private
Produces/Sells CE-marked Devices: Y
Federal Procurement Eligibility: Small Business

Operative Dental Treatment Unit	Dental And Oral

STERILIS INC.   714-437-9801
17092 Newhope St., Fountain Valley, CA 92708
FDA Number: 2032220   Fax: 714-437-9806
E-mail: dkochmanski@suturainc.com
Ownership: Private
Produces/Sells CE-marked Devices: N

Surgical Instrument, Obstetric/Gynecologic	Obstetrics/Gynecology

STERILIZATION SERVICES   404-344-8423
6005 Boatrock Blvd., Atlanta, GA 30336-2703
FDA Number: 1048735   Fax: 404-344-8665
E-mail: tfisher@sterilization-services.com
Web site: www.sterilization-services.com
Medical Products Sales Volume: $790,000
Annual Revenue: $5-$10 Million
Year Founded: 1976
Total Employees: 6   Marketing Staff: 1   Sales Staff: 1
Ownership: Private
Quality System Registration Information: ISO9002
Produces/Sells CE-marked Devices: N
Federal Procurement Eligibility: Small Business
General Admin.: Tom Fisher/General Manager
Production: Jonathan Wallace/Manager Quality Assurance & Regulatory Affairs
         David Connor/Plant Manager
         Jodie Jefferson/Plant Manager

Contract Sterilization	General

STERILIZATION SERVICES OF TENNESSEE, INC.   901-947-2217
2396 Florida St., Memphis, TN 38109-2563
FDA Number: 1048014   Fax: 901-774-0879
E-mail: tfisher@sterilization-services.com
Web site: www.sterilization-services.com
Medical Products Sales Volume: $600,000
Annual Revenue: $0-$1 Million
Year Founded: 1976
Total Employees: 8   Marketing Staff: 1   Sales Staff: 1
Ownership: Private
Federal Procurement Eligibility: Small Business
Distribution: Service Direct
General Admin.: Tom Fisher/General Manager
Mktg./Adv.: Dan Eberdt/Manager National Sales
Production: Jonathan Wallace/Manager Quality Assurance & Regulatory Affairs
         Jodie Jefferson/Plant Manager

Contract Sterilization	General

STERILIZATION SERVICES OF VIRGINIA, INC.   804-236-1652
5674 Eastport Blvd., Richmond, VA 23231-4443
FDA Number: 1123137   Fax: 804-236-1655
E-mail: tfisher@sterilization-services.com
Web site: www.sterilization-services.com
Medical Products Sales Volume: $1,000,000
Annual Revenue: $0-$1 Million
Year Founded: 1990
Total Employees: 10   Marketing Staff: 1   Sales Staff: 1
Produces/Sells CE-marked Devices: N

MANUFACTURER PROFILES

STERILIZATION SERVICES OF VIRGINIA, INC. 804-236-1652
(cont'd)
Federal Procurement Eligibility: Small Business
Distribution: Service Direct
General Admin.: Tom Fisher/General Manager
Mktg./Adv.: Dan Eberdt/Manager National Sales
Production: Jonathan Wallace/Manager Quality Assurance & Regulatory Affairs
      David Connor/Plant Manager
Contract Sterilization   General

STERILMED, INC. 763-488-3400
11400 73rd Ave. North, #100, Maple Grove, MN 55369
FDA Number: 2134070
Ownership: Ethicon Endo-Surgery, Inc.
Produces/Sells CE-marked Devices: N
Finance: Mr. Mike Gustafson/President

Accessories, Arthroscopic	Orthopedics
Airway, Oropharyngeal, Anesthesia	Anesthesiology
Applier, Hemostatic Clip	Cns/Neurology
Arthroscope	Orthopedics
Bit, Drill	Orthopedics
Blade, Surgical, Saw, General & Plastic Surgery	Surgery
Burr, Surgical, General & Plastic Surgery	Surgery
Cable, Electrode	Physical Med
Catheter, Angiography, Reprocessed	Cardiovascular
Catheter, Biliary, Reprocessed	Gastroenterology/Urology
Catheter, Recording, Electrode, Reprocessed	Cardiovascular
Chisel, Surgical, Manual	Surgery
Clamp, Vascular, Reprocessed	Cardiovascular
Dislodger, Stone, Basket, Ureteral, Metal	Gastroenterology/Urology
Dislodger, Stone, Basket, Ureteral, Metal, Reprocessed	Gastroenterology/Urology
Dissector, Surgical, General & Plastic Surgery	Surgery
Drape, Surgical	Surgery
Electrode, Ablation, Tissue, Conduction, Percutaneous	Cardiovascular
Electrode, Electrosurgical, Active, Urological, Reprocessed	Gastroenterology/Urology
Electrode, Electrosurgical, Return (Ground, Dispersive)	Surgery
Electrosurgical Unit, Cutting & Coagulation Device	Surgery
Endoilluminator, Reprocessed	Ophthalmology
Endoscope	Gastroenterology/Urology
Fixation Appliance, Multiple Component	Orthopedics
Forceps, Biopsy, Electric, Reprocessed	Gastroenterology/Urology
Forceps, Biopsy, Non-Electric	Gastroenterology/Urology
Gown, Surgical	Surgery
Injector And Syringe, Angiographic, Balloon Inflation, Reprocessed	Cardiovascular
Laparoscope, General & Plastic Surgery, Reprocessed	Gastroenterology/Urology
Laser, Ophthalmic	Ophthalmology
Laser, Surgical	Surgery
Mask, Oxygen, Aerosol Administration	Anesthesiology
Monitor, Bed Patient	General
Needle, Phacoemulsification, Reprocessed	Ophthalmology
Orthopedic Manual Surgical Instrument	Orthopedics
Oximeter, Reprocessed	Anesthesiology
Oximeter, Tissue Saturation, Reprocessed	Cardiovascular
Retractor, Fiberoptic	Gastroenterology/Urology
Retractor, Surgical	Surgery
Scalpel, Ultrasonic, Reprocessed	Surgery
Sleeve, Compressible Limb	Cardiovascular
Snare, Flexible, Reprocessed	Gastroenterology/Urology
Stabilizer, Heart, Non-compression, Reprocessed	Cardiovascular
Staple, Implantable, Reprocessed	Surgery
Stapler, Surgical	Surgery
Tap, Bone	Orthopedics
Tourniquet, Pneumatic	Surgery
Unit, Electrosurgical, Endoscopic (with Or Without Accessories), Reprocessed Gastroenterology/Urology	

STERILOGIC WASTE SYSTEMS, INC. 315-455-5600
6691 Pickard Dr., Syracuse, NY 13211
FDA Number: 2531812
Ownership: Private
Produces/Sells CE-marked Devices: N

Container, Sharpes	General
Needle, Hypodermic, Single Lumen With Syringe	General

STERIMARK/ETIGAM 419-868-1800
1031 Calle Trepadora #D, Toledo, OH 43635-2796
FDA Number: n/a   Fax: 419-868-1837
E-mail: info@etigam.nl
Web site: www.etigam.nl
Annual Revenue: $25-$50 Million
Ownership: Private
Quality System Registration Information: ISO9002
Produces/Sells CE-marked Devices: N
Distribution: Manufacturer Direct
General Admin.: Leo Tak/Chief Executive Officer
Production: Frank Reynolds/Vice President Operations
Research: Eddie McCoy/Director Technology
Contract Sterilization   General

STERIMED, INC. 770-387-0771
10 River Ct., Cartersville, GA 30120
FDA Number: 1037978   Fax: 111-111-1111
E-mail: sterimed@bellsouth.net
Web site: www.sterion.net
Year Founded: 1984
Ownership: Private
Produces/Sells CE-marked Devices: N
Federal Procurement Eligibility: Small Business
Distribution: Manufacturer Through Manufacturer Reps

Drape, Surgical	Surgery
Radiographic/Fluoroscopic Unit, Angiographic	Radiology

STERION, INCORPORATED 800-328-7958
13828 Lincoln St. N.E., Ham Lake, MN 55304 763-755-9516
FDA Number: 2183160   Fax: 763-755-9466
E-mail: info@sterion.com
Web site: www.aspensurgical.com
Medical Products Sales Volume: $7,000,000
Annual Revenue: $5-$10 Million
Year Founded: 1982
Total Employees: 70   *Marketing Staff:* 3   *Sales Staff:* 30
Ownership: Public
Stock Symbol: STEN
Traded On: NASDAQ
Quality System Registration Information: ISO9002
Produces/Sells CE-marked Devices: Y
Federal Procurement Eligibility: Small Business, GSA Contract, VA Contract
Distribution: Manufacturer Direct, Manufacturer Through Distributor, Manufacturer Through Manufacturer Reps, OEM, Exporter
Mktg./Adv.: Kevin Dey/Director International Business Development
      Bill Maass/Vice President Marketing
      Jess Carsello/Vice President Sales
Production: Jim Lannan/Director Quality Assurance

Accessories, Light, Surgical	Surgery
Cap, Tip, Syringe	General
Clamp, Bulldog	Surgery
Container, Evacuated	General
Cover, Clamp	Surgery
Cover, Other	General
Holder, Intravascular Catheter	General
Label, Device	General
Loop, Vascular	Cardiovascular
Marker, Identification, Suture	Surgery
Protector, Surgical Instrument	Surgery
Solvent, Adhesive Tape	Surgery
Sterilization Process Indicator, Chemical	General
Syringe, Antistick	General
Tape, Adhesive	General

STERIPLEX CORP.
See Multisorb Technologies, Inc.

STERIS BIOLOGICAL OPERATIONS FACILITY 440-354-2600
9325 Pinecone Dr., Mentor, OH 44060
FDA Number: 3004080920
Ownership: Steris Corporation
Stock Symbol: STE
Traded On: NYSE
Produces/Sells CE-marked Devices: N
General Admin.: Mr. Peter A. Burke/Chief Technology Officer, Senior Vice President
      Mr. Les C. Vinney/President, Chief Executive Officer
      Mr. Timothy L. Chapman/Senior Vice President
      Mr. Mark D. McGinley/Senior Vice President, General Counsel
Finance: Mr. William L. Aamoth/Vice President, Treasurer

Culture Media, General Nutrient Broth	Microbiology
Indicator, Biological, Liquid Chemical Steril. Process	General
Sterilization Process Indicator, Biological	General
Sterilization Process Indicator, Physical/Chemical	General
Wrap, Sterilization	General

STERIS CORPORATION 814-452-3100
2424 West 23rd Street, Erie, PA 16506
FDA Number: 2515984
Web site: www.steris.com
Ownership: Steris Corporation
Stock Symbol: STE
Traded On: NYSE
Produces/Sells CE-marked Devices: N
General Admin.: Mr. Peter A. Burke/Chief Technology Officer, Senior Vice President
      Mr. Les C. Vinney/President, Chief Executive Officer
      Mr. Timothy L. Chapman/Senior Vice President
      Mr. Mark D. McGinley/Senior Vice President, General Counsel
Finance: Mr. William L. Aamoth/Vice President, Treasurer

Disinfector, Medical Device	General
Kit, Irrigation, Sterile	Gastroenterology/Urology
Purification System, Water	Gastroenterology/Urology

STERIS CORPORATION   814-452-3100 *(cont'd)*
Sterilizer, Ethylene-Oxide Gas   General
Sterilizer, Steam (Autoclave)   General

STERIS CORPORATION   334-277-6660
2720 Gunter Park Drive, Montgomery, AL 36109
FDA Number: 1043572   *Fax:* 334-271-3579
Web site: www.steris.com
Ownership: Steris Corporation
Stock Symbol: STE
Traded On: NYSE
Produces/Sells CE-marked Devices: N
General Admin.: Mr. Peter A. Burke/Chief Technology Officer, Senior Vice President
   Mr. Les C. Vinney/President, Chief Executive Officer
   Mr. Timothy L. Chapman/Senior Vice President
   Mr. Mark D. McGinley/Senior Vice President, General Counsel
Finance: Mr. William L. Aamoth/Vice President, Treasurer
Accessories, Operating Room, Table   Surgery
Accessories, Surgical Camera
Holder, Head, Neurosurgical (Skull Clamp)   Cns/Neurology
Lamp, Surgical   Surgery
Light, Surgical, Ceiling Mounted   Surgery
Light, Surgical, Fiberoptic   Surgery
Table, Obstetrical   Obstetrics/Gynecology
Table, Operating Room, AC-Powered   Surgery
Table, Surgical, Orthopedic   Orthopedics
Unit, Examining/Treatment, ENT   Ear/Nose/Throat
Warmer, Irrigation Solution   General

STERIS CORPORATION   800-884-9550
5960 Heisley Road, Mentor, OH 44060-1834   440-354-2600
FDA Number: 1527821
Web site: http://www.steris.com
Medical Products Sales Volume: $846,000,000
Annual Revenue: More than $1 Billion
Year Founded: 1987
Total Employees: 5100
Ownership: Public
Stock Symbol: STE
Traded On: NYSE
Quality System Registration Information: ISO9001
Produces/Sells CE-marked Devices: Y
Distribution: Manufacturer Direct, Manufacturer Through Distributor
General Admin.: Mr. Michael J. Tokich/Chief Financial Officer, Senior Vice President
   Mr. Peter A. Burke/Chief Technology Officer, Senior Vice President
   Mr. Walter M. Rosebrough/President, Chief Executive Officer
   Mr. Mark D. McGinley/Senior Vice President, General Counsel
Finance: Mr. William L. Aamoth/Vice President Treasury
Accessories, Cleaning, Endoscopic   Gastroenterology/Urology
Disinfector, Liquid   General
Lamp, Surgical   Surgery
Light, Surgical, Ceiling Mounted   Surgery
Sterilant, Medical Device   General
Sterilization Process Indicator, Biological   General
Sterilization Process Indicator, Physical/Chemical   General
Sterilizer, Chemical   General
Table, Instrument, Surgical   Surgery
Washer/Sterilizer   General
Medical Product Subsidiaries (Listed Separately)
Steris Biological Operations Facility
Steris Corporation
Steris Isomedix Services

STERIS CORPORATION   440-354-2600
6100 Heisley Road, Mentor, OH 44060
FDA Number: 3003950207   *Fax:* 440-350-7078
Web site: www.steris.com
Ownership: Steris Corporation
Stock Symbol: STE
Traded On: NYSE
Produces/Sells CE-marked Devices: N
General Admin.: Mr. Peter A. Burke/Chief Technology Officer, Senior Vice President
   Mr. Les C. Vinney/President, Chief Executive Officer
   Mr. Timothy L. Chapman/Senior Vice President
   Mr. Mark D. McGinley/Senior Vice President, General Counsel
Finance: Mr. William L. Aamoth/Vice President, Treasurer

STERIS CORPORATION   440-354-2600
6515 Hopkins Road, Mentor, OH 44060
FDA Number: 3000251274
Web site: www.steris.com
Ownership: Steris Corporation
Stock Symbol: STE
Traded On: NYSE

STERIS CORPORATION   440-354-2600 *(cont'd)*
Produces/Sells CE-marked Devices: N
General Admin.: Mr. Peter A. Burke/Chief Technology Officer, Senior Vice President
   Mr. Les C. Vinney/President, Chief Executive Officer
   Mr. Timothy L. Chapman/Senior Vice President
   Mr. Mark D. McGinley/Senior Vice President, General Counsel
Finance: Mr. William L. Aamoth/Vice President, Treasurer
Accessories, Germicide, Cleaning, For Endoscopes   Gastroenterology/Urology
Sterilant, Medical Device   General
Sterilization Process Indicator, Physical/Chemical   General
Sterilizer, Chemical   General
Suction Apparatus, Operating Room, Wall Vacuum-Powered   Surgery
Wrap, Sterilization   General

STERIS CORPORATION   314-290-4600
7501 Page Avenue, St. Louis, MO 63133
FDA Number: 1937531   *Fax:* 314-290-4605
Web site: www.steris.com
Ownership: Steris Corporation
Stock Symbol: STE
Traded On: NYSE
Produces/Sells CE-marked Devices: N
General Admin.: Mr. Peter A. Burke/Chief Technology Officer, Senior Vice President
   Mr. Les C. Vinney/President, Chief Executive Officer
   Mr. Timothy L. Chapman/Senior Vice President
   Mr. Mark D. McGinley/Senior Vice President, General Counsel
Finance: Mr. William L. Aamoth/Vice President, Treasurer
Brush, Scrub, Operating Room   Surgery
Cleaner, Ultrasonic, Medical Instrument   General
Disinfector, Medical Device   General
Sterilant, Medical Device   General

STERIS CORPORATION   314-290-4703
8525 Page Boulevard, St. Louis, MO 63114
FDA Number: 1933443   *Fax:* 314-290-4605
Web site: www.steris.com
Ownership: Steris Corporation
Stock Symbol: STE
Traded On: NYSE
Produces/Sells CE-marked Devices: N
General Admin.: Mr. Peter A. Burke/Chief Technology Officer, Senior Vice President
   Mr. Les C. Vinney/President, Chief Executive Officer
   Mr. Timothy L. Chapman/Senior Vice President
   Mr. Mark D. McGinley/Senior Vice President, General Counsel
Finance: Mr. William L. Aamoth/Vice President, Treasurer
Brush, Scrub, Operating Room   Surgery
Cleaner, Ultrasonic, Medical Instrument   General
Disinfector, Medical Device   General

STERIS CORPORATION-DISTRIBUTION CENTER
See Steris Corporation

STERIS ISOMEDIX SERVICES   973-887-2754
9 Apollo Drive, Whippany, NJ 07981-1423
FDA Number: 9320097   *Fax:* 973-887-6591
E-mail: Larry_Winters@steris.com
Web site: www.isomedix.com
Medical Products Sales Volume: $50,000,000
Annual Revenue: $50-$100 Million
Total Employees: 25   *Marketing Staff:* 2   *Sales Staff:* 10
Ownership: Steris Corporation
Stock Symbol: ISO
Traded On: OTC Bulletin
Quality System Registration Information: ISO9001; ISO9002
Produces/Sells CE-marked Devices: Y
Federal Procurement Eligibility: Small Business
Distribution: Service Direct
General Admin.: John Masefield/Chief Executive Officer
   Tom DeAngelo/President
   George R. Dietz/Senior Vice President
   Susan Johnson/Vice President Human Resources
   Peter Baker/Vice President, General Manager
Mktg./Adv.: Glenn Parton/Coord. Sales
   Grace Masefield/Director Marketing
Production: Charles Tuoby/Director Quality Assurance
   Jon Young/Manager Regulatory Affairs
Contract Sterilization   General

STERISIL, INC.   719-481-0937
835 S. Highway 105, Suite D, Palmer Lake, CO 80133
FDA Number: 3005844469
Operative Dental Treatment Unit   Dental And Oral

STERITEC PRODUCTS, INC.   303-660-4201
599 Topeka Way, Suite 400, Castle Rock, CO 80109
FDA Number: 2028456

STERITEC PRODUCTS, INC. 303-660-4201 *(cont'd)*
Sterilization Process Indicator, Physical/Chemical — General

STERLING DIAGNOSTIC IMAGING, INC.
See Agfa Corporation

STERLING DIAGNOSTICS, INC. 800-637-2661
36645 Metro Court, Sterling Heights, MI 48312 586-979-2141
FDA Number: 1831796 *Fax:* 586-979-4971
E-mail: info@sterlingdiagnostics.com
Web site: www.sterlingdiagnostics.com
Medical Products Sales Volume: $1,500,000
Year Founded: 1984
Total Employees: 14
Ownership: Private
Produces/Sells CE-marked Devices: N
Federal Procurement Eligibility: Small Business
Distribution: Manufacturer Direct, Manufacturer Through Distributor, Manufacturer Through Manufacturer Reps, OEM, Exporter

Colorimetric Method, Gamma-Glutamyl Transpeptidase	Chemistry
Colorimetric Method, Lipoproteins	Chemistry
Colorimetry, Salicylate	Toxicology
Complexone, Cresolphthalein, Calcium	Chemistry
Differential Rate Kinetic Method, CPK Or Isoenzymes	Chemistry
Diluent, Blood Cell	Hematology
Dye-Binding, Albumin, Bromcresol, Green	Chemistry
Emulsion, Oil, (Titrimetric), Lipase	Chemistry
Enzymatic Esterase-Oxidase, Cholesterol	Chemistry
Ferrozine (Colorimetric) Iron Binding Capacity	Chemistry
Fluid, Red Cell Lysing	Hematology
Hexokinase, Glucose	Chemistry
Indophenol, Berthelot, Urea Nitrogen	Chemistry
Lipase Hydrolysis/Glycerol Kinase Enzyme, Triglycerides	Chemistry
NAD Reduction/NADH Oxidation, CPK Or Isoenzymes	Chemistry
NAD Reduction/NADH Oxidation, Lactate Dehydrogenase	Chemistry
NADH Oxidation/NAD Reduction, AST/SGOT	Chemistry
Nitrophenylphosphate, Alkaline Phosphatase Or Isoenzymes	Chemistry
Phosphorus Reagent (Test System)	Chemistry
Photometric Method, Magnesium	Chemistry
Reagent, Acetylcholine Chloride	Toxicology
Reagent, Amylase, Colorimetric	Chemistry
Reagent, Bilirubin (Total Or Direct Test System)	Chemistry
Reagent, Chloride (Test System)	Chemistry
Reagent, Creatinine (Test System)	Chemistry
Reagent, Cyanomethemoglobin, With Standard	Hematology
Reagent, Glucose (Test System)	Chemistry
Reagent, Streptolysin O/Antistreptolysin-Titer	Microbiology
SGOT, Ultraviolet	Chemistry
SGPT, Colorimetric	Chemistry
SGPT, Ultraviolet	Chemistry
Test, C-Reactive Protein	Immunology
Test, Rheumatoid Factor	Immunology
Test, Sickle Cell	Hematology
Test, Systemic Lupus Erythematosus	Immunology
Tetraphenyl Borate, Colorimetry, Potassium	Chemistry
Thymolphthalein Monophosphate, Alkaline Phosphatase	Chemistry
Urease And Glutamic Dehydrogenase, Urea Nitrogen	Chemistry

STERLING DRUG INC.
See Bayer Healthcare Llc, Consumer Care

STERLING FLUID SYSTEMS (USA) 716-773-6450
303 Industrial Blvd., Grand Island, NY 14072
FDA Number: n/a *Fax:* 716-773-2330
E-mail: mail@sihi.com
Web site: www.sterlingamericas.com
Year Founded: 1960
Ownership: STERLING FLUID SYSTEMS GROUP
Quality System Registration Information: ISO9001
Produces/Sells CE-marked Devices: N
Federal Procurement Eligibility: GSA Contract, VA Contract
Distribution: Manufacturer Through Distributor
General Admin.: George Grasso/President
Mktg./Adv.: R. McIntosh/Manager Sales
Production: Ronald Machens/Manager Engineering

Equipment, Cleaning, Air	General
Pump, Vacuum, Central	Anesthesiology

STERLING MEDICAL PRODUCTS 800-537-5320
401 Market St., Prophetstown, IL 61277 815-537-5303
FDA Number: 1422598 *Fax:* 815-537-5119
Total Employees: 25 *Marketing Staff:* 1 *Sales Staff:* 1
Ownership: Private
Produces/Sells CE-marked Devices: N
Federal Procurement Eligibility: Small Business
Distribution: Manufacturer Direct, Manufacturer Through Manufacturer Reps, OEM
Mktg./Adv.: Mel Snitchler/Director Marketing
Mel Snitchler/General Manager Marketing

Kit, Circumcision, Disposable Tray	Obstetrics/Gynecology
Kit, Disposable Procedure	Cardiovascular
Kit, Incision And Drainage	Surgery

STERLING MEDICAL PRODUCTS 800-537-5320 *(cont'd)*

Kit, Surgical Instrument, Disposable	Surgery
Kit, Suture	Surgery
Kit, Suture Removal	Surgery
Kit, Wound Dressing	Surgery
Scissors, Disposable	General
Surgical Instrument, Disposable	Surgery

STERLING MEDICAL-PRODUCTS INTL., INC. 815-537-5303
401 Market St., Prophetstown, IL 61277
FDA Number: 1422598

Kit, Surgical Instrument, Disposable	Surgery

STERLING MULTI-PRODUCTS, INC. 815-537-2381
326 West 5th St., Prophetstown, IL 61277
FDA Number: 1419591

Kit, Surgical Instrument, Disposable	Surgery
Surgical Instrument, Disposable	Surgery

STERLING MULTI-PRODUCTS, INC.
See Sterling Medical Products

STERLING OPTICAL KAHN CONSULT INC.
See Sterling Vision, Inc.

STERLING VISION, INC. 800-332-6302
520 Eighth Avenue, New York, NY 10018 516-390-2100
FDA Number: n/a *Fax:* 516-390-2111
Web site: www.sterlingoptical.net
Total Employees: 300
Ownership: Public
Produces/Sells CE-marked Devices: N
Distribution: Manufacturer Through Manufacturer Reps, Exclusive Distributor
General Admin.: Dr. Alan Cohen/Chief Executive Officer
Joseph Silver/Executive Vice President
Joseph Silver/General Counsel
Robert Greenberg/President
Mktg./Adv.: Jerry Darnell/Vice President Sales
Finance: Sabastian Giordano/Chief Financial Officer

Eyeglasses	Ophthalmology
Frame, Spectacle (Eyeglasses)	Ophthalmology
Lenses, Soft Contact, Daily Wear	Ophthalmology

STERN INC., WALTER 516-883-9100
68 Sintsink Drive East, P.O. Box 571,
Port Washington, NY 11050
FDA Number: n/a
Medical Products Sales Volume: $2,000,000
Ownership: Private
Produces/Sells CE-marked Devices: N
Federal Procurement Eligibility: Small Business
Distribution: Importer

Forceps	Orthopedics
Labware, Basic, Reusable	Chemistry

STERNE EQUIPMENT CO., LTD. 905-457-2524
20 Strathearn Avenue Unit #4,
Brampton, ONTAR L6T 4 Canada
FDA Number: 9681201 *Fax:* 905-457-3396
E-mail: info@sternemedical.com
Web site: www.sternemedical.com
Year Founded: 1986
Total Employees: 25
Ownership: Private
Produces/Sells CE-marked Devices: N
Distribution: Manufacturer Direct, Exclusive Distributor

STERNGOLD 800-243-9942
23 Frank Mossberg Drive, PO Box 2967, 508-226-5660
Attleboro, MA 02703
FDA Number: 2921595 *Fax:* 800-531-2685
E-mail: info@sterngold.com
Web site: www.sterngold.com
Medical Products Sales Volume: $11,000,000
Year Founded: 1897
Total Employees: 30 *Marketing Staff:* 4 *Sales Staff:* 11
Ownership: Private
Produces/Sells CE-marked Devices: Y
Federal Procurement Eligibility: Small Business, GSA Contract
Distribution: Manufacturer Direct, Exporter
General Admin.: Rev. Laura Greige/Human Resources Representative
David M. Sklarski/President
Mktg./Adv.: Dulcina Jorge/Director International Sales
Victoria Savino/Director Marketing
James Ellison CDT/Director Product Development
Joanne Santos/Director Sales
Gordon Craig/Vice President Business Development
Production: Lee Clermont/Director Quality Assurance
Purchasing: Vidya Pai/Director Purchasing

STERNGOLD
800-243-9942 (cont'd)

Adhesive, Dental Impression	Dental And Oral
Alloy, Gold Based, For Clinical Use	Dental And Oral
Alloy, Precious Metal, For Clinical Use	Dental And Oral
Attachment, Precision	Dental And Oral
Base, Denture, Relining, Repairing, Rebasing, Resin	Dental And Oral
Burr, Dental	Dental And Oral
Cement, Dental	Dental And Oral
Crown And Bridge, Temporary, Resin	Dental And Oral
Curing Unit, Acrylic	Dental And Oral
Dental Laboratory Equipment	Dental And Oral
Implant, Endosseous	Dental And Oral
Instrument, Diamond, Dental	Dental And Oral
Material, Casting	Dental And Oral
Post, Root Canal	Dental And Oral
Varnish	Dental And Oral

STEROGENE BIOSEPARATIONS, INC.
800-535-2284
5922 Farnsworth Ct., Carlsbad, CA 92008
760-929-0455
FDA Number: n/a
Fax: 760-929-8720
E-mail: info@sterogene.com
Web site: www.sterogene.com
Annual Revenue: $1-$5 Million
Total Employees: 20   *Marketing Staff:* 2   *Sales Staff:* 2
Ownership: Private
Produces/Sells CE-marked Devices: N
Federal Procurement Eligibility: Small Business
Distribution: Manufacturer Direct
General Admin.: Susan Szathmary/Executive Vice President
     Peter Grandics/President
Mktg./Adv.: Darren Whitley/Director Sales
Research: Peter Grandics/Director Research

Monitor, EEG	Cns/Neurology
Resins, Ion Exchange, Liquid Chromatography	Toxicology

STERYLAB USA, LLC
317-736-8306
2916 Graham Rd., Suite C, Franklin, IN 46131
FDA Number: 3005561465
Fax: 317-736-8443
E-mail: sterylab-USA@sterylab.it
Web site: www.sterylab.it
Ownership: Private
Produces/Sells CE-marked Devices: N

Biopsy Instrument	Gastroenterology/Urology
Kit, Biopsy Needle	Gastroenterology/Urology

STETHOCAP, INC.
866-691-4181
1520 Industrial Dr, Unit F, Lake In The Hills, IL 60156
FDA Number: 3006187138
Fax: 847-574-7641
Ownership: Private
Produces/Sells CE-marked Devices: N

Stethoscope, Manual	Cardiovascular

STETHOGRAPHICS, INC.
508-320-2841
1153 Centre St., Suite 40, Boston, MA 02130
FDA Number: 3004047676
E-mail: support@stethographics.com
Web site: www.stethographics.com
Ownership: Private
Produces/Sells CE-marked Devices: N

Computer, Pulmonary Function Interpretator (Diagnostic)	Anesthesiology
Phonocardiograph	Cardiovascular

STEUART LABORATORIES
877-210-9664
142 South Main St., Mabel, MN 55954
507-493-5516
FDA Number: n/a
E-mail: order@steuartlabs.com
Web site: www.steuartlaboratories.com
Annual Revenue: $0-$1 Million
Ownership: Private
Produces/Sells CE-marked Devices: N
Federal Procurement Eligibility: Small Business
Distribution: Manufacturer Direct

Lotion, Skin Care	General

STEVEN R. YOUNG OCULARIST, INC.
510-836-2123
411 30th Street, Suite 512, Oakland, CA 94609
FDA Number: 2935668

Eye, Artificial, Non-Custom	Ophthalmology

STEVENS METALLURGICAL CORP.
800-794-7887
239 E. 78th St., New York, NY 10021-0817
212-861-2645
FDA Number: n/a
Fax: 212-706-7410
E-mail: info@stevensmetallurgical.com
Web site: www.stevensmetallurgical.com
Medical Products Sales Volume: $200,000
Annual Revenue: $0-$1 Million
Year Founded: 1967
Total Employees: 1   *Marketing Staff:* 1   *Sales Staff:* 1
Ownership: Private

STEVENS METALLURGICAL CORP.
800-794-7887 (cont'd)
Produces/Sells CE-marked Devices: N
Federal Procurement Eligibility: Small Business
Distribution: Service Direct
General Admin.: Larry Stevens/Chief Executive Officer, Vice President Marketing

Alloy, Precious Metal, For Clinical Use	Dental And Oral
Osmium Tetroxide	Pathology

STEVENSON INDUSTRIES, INC.
310-459-9393
881 Alma Real Dr., Suite 310, Pacific Palisades, CA 90272
FDA Number: 2032500
Ownership: Private
Produces/Sells CE-marked Devices: N

Ventilator, Non-Continuous (Respirator)	Anesthesiology

STEWART EFI, LCC
800-678-7931
630 Central Park Avenue, Yonkers, NY 10704
914-965-0816
FDA Number: n/a
Fax: 914-992-7835
E-mail: sales@stewartefi.com
Web site: www.stewartefi.com
Medical Products Sales Volume: $28,000,000
Annual Revenue: $50-$100 Million
Year Founded: 1936
Total Employees: 185   *Marketing Staff:* 2   *Sales Staff:* 7
Ownership: Private
Quality System Registration Information: ISO9001
Federal Procurement Eligibility: Small Business
General Admin.: Dan Stokes/Chief Executive Officer
     Bernie Rosselli/President
     Anna Cicio/Vice President Human Resources
Mktg./Adv.: John Labas/Director Marketing
     Christine Fox/Manager Marketing
     John Labas/Vice President Marketing & Sales
Production: Edward Rish/Director Quality Assurance
     Mary Knapp/Manager Materials

Component, Metal, Other	General
Contract Manufacturing	General

STEWART STAMPING CORP.
See Stewart Efi, Lcc

STEWART STAMPING/EFI, INC.
See Stewart Efi, Lcc

STI
See Surgical Technologies, Inc.

STI OPTRONICS, INC.
425-827-0460
2755 Northrup Way, Bellevue, WA 98004-1495
FDA Number: n/a
Fax: 425-828-3517
Web site: www.stioptronics.com
Annual Revenue: $0-$1 Million
Ownership: Private
Produces/Sells CE-marked Devices: N
Federal Procurement Eligibility: Small Business, Minority Owned
Distribution: Manufacturer Direct

Contract R&D, Diagnostics	General

STICHT INC., HERMAN H.
800-221-3203
45 Main Street, Brooklyn, NY 11201
718-852-7602
FDA Number: 9201025
Fax: 718-852-7915
E-mail: stichtco@aol.com
Web site: www.stichtco.com/
Medical Products Sales Volume: $2,000,000
Annual Revenue: $1-$5 Million
Total Employees: 17
Ownership: Private
Produces/Sells CE-marked Devices: N
Federal Procurement Eligibility: Small Business, Female Owned
Distribution: Manufacturer Direct
General Admin.: Paul H. Plotkin/President
Production: Allen Butterfield/Vice President Production

Tester, Conductivity, Floor And Equipment	General

STIEFEL
888-784-3335
20 T.W. Alexander Drive, Research Triangle Park, NC 27709
FDA Number: n/a
E-mail: customerservice@glades.com
Web site: www.stiefel-us.com
Annual Revenue: $0-$1 Million
Year Founded: 1991
Ownership: Stiefel Laboratories, Inc.
Produces/Sells CE-marked Devices: N
Federal Procurement Eligibility: Small Business
Distribution: Manufacturer Through Distributor
General Admin.: Bob Cunard/President
Production: Chris Schneider/Vice President Operations

Lotion, Skin Care	General

STIEFEL LABORATORIES, INC.   **800-724-1565**
255 Alhambra Circle,   **305-443-3800**
Coral Gables, FL 33134
FDA Number: n/a
E-mail: medicalaffairs@stiefel.com
Web site: www.stiefel.com
Ownership: Private
Produces/Sells CE-marked Devices: Y
Federal Procurement Eligibility: Small Business
Distribution: Manufacturer Direct, Manufacturer Through Manufacturer Reps, Exporter
  Lotion, Skin Care   General
Medical Product Subsidiaries (Listed Separately)
Stiefel

STIEFEL LABORATORIES, INC.   **518-239-6901**
6290 Route 145, Oak Hill, NY 12460
FDA Number: 1314819
E-mail: medicalaffairs@stiefel.com   *Fax:* 518-239-6341
Web site: www.stiefel.com
Ownership: STIEFEL LABORATORIES, INC.
Produces/Sells CE-marked Devices: N
  Dressing, Wound and Burn, Hydrogel   Surgery
  Polyvinyl Methylether Maleic Acid-Calcium-Sodium Dbl. Salt   Dental And Oral
  Punch, Biopsy   Gastroenterology/Urology

STIK STOPPERS, INC.   **541-726-7869**
3777 Douglas Dr., Springfield, OR 97478
FDA Number: 3032878
Ownership: Private
Produces/Sells CE-marked Devices: N
  Container, Sharpes   General

STILL RIVER SYSTEMS, INC.
See Mevion Medical Systems

STILLE BETA, INC.
See Surgical Table Services Co.

STILLE-SONESTA, INC.   **800-665-1614**
1610 I35 North, Suite 203, Carrolton, TX 75006   **214-741-2464**
FDA Number: 1648279   *Fax:* 214-741-2605
E-mail: info@stille-usa.com
Web site: www.stille.se
Medical Products Sales Volume: $600,000
Year Founded: 1841
Total Employees: 5   *Marketing Staff:* 2   *Sales Staff:* 50
Ownership: Stille AB
Traded On: Stockholm
Quality System Registration Information: ISO9002
Produces/Sells CE-marked Devices: Y
Federal Procurement Eligibility: Small Business
Distribution: Manufacturer Direct, Exclusive Distributor
General Admin.: Tara Woodruff/President
  Chair, Examination And Treatment   General
  Chair, Other   General
  Chair, Position, Electric   Physical Med
  Chair, Posture, For Cardiac And Pulmonary Treatment   Anesthesiology
  Chair, Surgical, AC-Powered   Surgery
  Chair/Table, Medical   General
  Table, Examination/Treatment   General
  Table, Other   General
  Table, Radiographic   Radiology
  Table, Radiographic, Tilting   Radiology
  Table, Surgical, Electrical   Surgery
  Table, Ultrasound   General
  Table, Urological (Cystological)   Gastroenterology/Urology
  Table, Urological, Radiographic   Gastroenterology/Urology

STINGER INDUSTRIES   **615-896-1652**
1152 Park Ave., Murfreesboro, TN 37129
FDA Number: 3003348395
  Monitor, Physiological, Patient(without Arrhythmia Detection Or Alarms)   Cardiovascular

STINSON MANUFACTURING   **800-932-2885**
N. 414 Sycamore, PO Box 3644,   **509-534-1509**
Spokane, WA 99202
FDA Number: n/a   *Fax:* 509-534-1424
E-mail: customerservice@stinsonmfg.com
Web site: www.stinsonmfg.com
Medical Products Sales Volume: $1,300,000
Annual Revenue: $1-$5 Million
Year Founded: 1945
Total Employees: 14
Ownership: Private
Produces/Sells CE-marked Devices: N
Federal Procurement Eligibility: Small Business
Distribution: Manufacturer Through Distributor
General Admin.: S. L. Boots/President

STINSON MANUFACTURING   **800-932-2885** *(cont'd)*
Mktg./Adv.: Gary Bugbey/Manager Sales
  Ramp, Wheelchair   General

STL INTERNATIONAL, INC. / TEETER HANG UPS   **253-840-5252**
9902 162nd St. Ct. E, Puyallup, WA 98375
FDA Number: 3022192
E-mail: sales@teeterhangups.com   *Fax:* 253-840-5757
Web site: www.teeterhangups.com
Medical Products Sales Volume: $4,100,000
Year Founded: 1981
Total Employees: 22   *Marketing Staff:* 2   *Sales Staff:* 2
Ownership: Private
Produces/Sells CE-marked Devices: Y
Federal Procurement Eligibility: Small Business
Distribution: Manufacturer Direct, Manufacturer Through Distributor, Manufacturer Through Manufacturer Reps, Exporter
General Admin.: Randall Hill/Chief Executive Officer
        Jill Holmly/Chief Operating Officer
        Roger Teeter/President
Mktg./Adv.: Kim Grotzke/Director Marketing
Purchasing: Brandon Johnson/Purchasing Agent
  Inversion Unit   Orthopedics

STOCKERYALE   **800-814-9552**
275 Kesmark, Montreal, QUEBE H9B 3J1 Canada   **514-685-1005**
FDA Number: n/a   *Fax:* 514-685-3307
E-mail: lasers@stockeryale.com
Web site: www.stockeryale.com
Total Employees: 200
Ownership: Public
Stock Symbol: STKR
Traded On: NASDAQ
Produces/Sells CE-marked Devices: N
Federal Procurement Eligibility: Small Business
Distribution: Manufacturer Direct, Manufacturer Through Distributor

STOELTING   **800-558-5807**
502 Hwy. 67, Kiel, WI 53042   **920-894-2293**
FDA Number: 7000233   *Fax:* 920-894-7029
E-mail: cleaning@stoelting.com
Web site: www.stoelting.com
Annual Revenue: $5-$10 Million
Year Founded: 1905
Total Employees: 15   *Marketing Staff:* 1   *Sales Staff:* 3
Ownership: STOELTING LLC
Quality System Registration Information: ISO9001
Produces/Sells CE-marked Devices: N
Federal Procurement Eligibility: Small Business, GSA Contract
Distribution: Manufacturer Direct, Manufacturer Through Manufacturer Reps, OEM, Service Direct, Exporter
Mktg./Adv.: Chris Swainbank/Director Product Development
        Claudette Barbino/Manager Advertising
Production: Hugh Swainbank/Director Quality Assurance
  Cleaner, Ultrasonic, Medical Instrument   General

STOELTING CO.   **630-860-9700**
620 Wheat Ln., Wood Dale, IL 60191
FDA Number: 1417837
Ownership: Private
Produces/Sells CE-marked Devices: N
  Biofeedback Device   Cns/Neurology

STONE MARRACCINI & PATTERSON
See Smith Group

STONESTREET ONE   **502-708-3500**
9960 Corporate Campus Drive, Louisville, KY 40223
FDA Number: n/a   *Fax:* 502-708-3520
Web site: http://stonestreetone.com
Year Founded: 2000
Ownership: Private
Produces/Sells CE-marked Devices: N

STONHOUSE MANUFACTURING   **231-548-5630**
7693 Barney Rd, Alanson, MI 49706-9214
FDA Number: 3005971162
Ownership: Private
Produces/Sells CE-marked Devices: N
  Instrument, Manual, General Surgical   Surgery

STONY BROOK, INC.   **563-388-0588**
12047 70th Avenue, Blue Grass, IA 52726
FDA Number: 1932994
E-mail: F0511@aol.com   *Fax:* 563-381-1160
Year Founded: 1960
Total Employees: 1
Ownership: Private
Produces/Sells CE-marked Devices: N

STONY BROOK, INC.　563-388-0588 *(cont'd)*
Lubricant, Patient　　　　　　　　　　　　　　General

STORAGE BATTERY SYSTEMS, INC.　800-554-2243
N. 56 W. 16665 Ridgewood Drive,　262-703-5800
Menomonee Falls, WI 53051
FDA Number: n/a　　　　　　　　　Fax: 262-703-3073
E-mail: sbs@sbsbattery.com
Web site: www.sbsbattery.com
Medical Products Sales Volume: $22,900,000
Annual Revenue: $10-$25 Million
Year Founded: 1915
Total Employees: 40　　*Marketing Staff:* 6　　*Sales Staff:* 12
Ownership: Private
Federal Procurement Eligibility: Small Business
Distribution: Manufacturer Direct, OEM
General Admin.: Scott Rubenzer/President
Mktg./Adv.: Michael K. Jackson/Director Marketing & Sales
　　　　Bob Rubenzer/Vice President Marketing
　　　　Glen Wilder/Vice President Marketing
Research: Bill Rubenzer/Vice President Research
Battery　　　　　　　　　　　　　　　General
Power Systems, Uninterruptible (UPS)　　　General

STORTZ CO.
See Psg Controls, Inc.

STORZ INSTRUMENT COMPANY
See Bausch & Lomb Surgical

STORZ LITHOTRIPSY-AMERICA-ATLANTA, KARL
See Karl Storz Lithotripsy-America, Inc.

STORZ OPHTHALMICS, INC.
See Bausch & Lomb, Inc.

STRATAGENE　　800-424-5444
11011 N. Torrey Pines Road,　858-373-6300
La Jolla, CA 92037
FDA Number: n/a　　　　　　　　Fax: 858-535-0034
E-mail: Diane_Haines@stratagene.com
Web site: www.stratagene.com
Medical Products Sales Volume: $128,000,000
Annual Revenue: $50-$100 Million
Year Founded: 1984
Total Employees: 459
Ownership: Agilent Technologies, Inc.
Stock Symbol: STGN
Traded On: NASDAQ
Produces/Sells CE-marked Devices: N
Federal Procurement Eligibility: Small Business, GSA Contract
Distribution: Manufacturer Direct, OEM, Exporter
General Admin.: Joseph A. Sorge/Chief Executive Officer
Mktg./Adv.: Nicolas H. Roelofs/Senior Vice President Marketing & Sales
　　　　John R. Pouk/Vice President Sales
Contract R&D, Equipment　　　　　　　General
Incubator, Aerobic　　　　　　　　Microbiology

STRATCOM　　514-421-2705
1743 Sunnybrooke,
Dollard-des-Ormeaux, QUE H9B-1 Canada
FDA Number: n/a　　　　　　　　Fax: 514-421-2705
E-mail: stratcom@pagebleu.com
Web site: www.pagebleu.com/stratcom/
Year Founded: 1988
Total Employees: 10
Ownership: Private
Produces/Sells CE-marked Devices: N

STRATEGIC DIAGNOSTICS INC.　800-544-8881
111 Pendacar Dr., Newark, DE 19702　302-456-6789
FDA Number: n/a　　　　　　　　Fax: 302-456-6770
Web site: www.sdix.com
Ownership: Public
Stock Symbol: SDIX
Traded On: NASDAQ
Produces/Sells CE-marked Devices: N
Federal Procurement Eligibility: Small Business
Distribution: Manufacturer Direct, Manufacturer Through Distributor
General Admin.: Francis M. DiNuzzo/President, Chief Executive Officer
　　　　Darlene Pence/Vice President Human Resources
Mktg./Adv.: Deborah Day Barbara/Vice President Business Development
　　　　Monette Greenway/Vice President Marketing & Sales
Research: James W. Stave/Vice President Research & Development
Finance: Kevin J. Bratton/Chief Financial Officer, Vice President Finance
Photometer　　　　　　　　　　　Chemistry

STRATEGIC DIAGNOSTICS, INC.　800-544-8881
111 Pencader Dr., Newark, DE 19702　302-456-6785
FDA Number: 3005462533　　　　　Fax: 302-456-6782

STRATEGIC DIAGNOSTICS, INC.　800-544-8881 *(cont'd)*
E-mail: sales@sdix.com
Web site: www.sdix.com
Ownership: Private
Produces/Sells CE-marked Devices: N
General Admin.: Mr. Fran DiNuzzo/President, Chief Executive Officer
Research: Dr. Klaus Lindpainter/Vice President Research & Development, Chief Scientific Officer
Finance: Mr. Kevin Bratton/Chief Financial Officer, Vice President Finance
Antigen, Antiserum, Control, Lipoprotein, Low Density　Immunology

STRATEGIC POLYMER SCIENCES INC.　814-238-7400
200 Innovation Blvd., Suite 237, State College, PA 16803
FDA Number: n/a　　　　　　　　Fax: 814-238-7401
E-mail: info@strategicpolymers.com
Web site: http://www.strategicpolymers.com
Year Founded: 2006
Ownership: Private
Produces/Sells CE-marked Devices: N
General Admin.: Dr. Qiming Zhang/Chief Technology Officer, Vice President
　　　　Mr. Ralph Russo/President, Chief Executive Officer
　　　　Mr. Paul Rehrig/Program Director
Production: Dr. Shihai Zhang/Director Engineering
　　　　Dr. Dean Anderson/Director Operations

STRATFORD-COOKSON COMPANY
See Darby Dental Supply Co.

STRAUMANN MANUFACTURING, INC.　978-747-2575
60 Minuteman Rd., Andover, MA 01810
FDA Number: 1222315
Ownership: Private
Produces/Sells CE-marked Devices: N
Abutment, Implant, Dental, Endosseous　　Dental And Oral
Accessories, Implant, Dental, Endosseous　Dental And Oral
Implant, Endosseous　　　　　　　Dental And Oral
Screw, Fixation, Intraosseous　　　　Dental And Oral

STRAUMANN MANUFACTURING, INC.　978-747-2575
916a 113th St., Arlington, TX 76011
FDA Number: 3005106405
Ownership: Private
Produces/Sells CE-marked Devices: N
Accessories, Implant, Dental, Endosseous　Dental And Oral
Alloy, Precious Metal, For Clinical Use　Dental And Oral
Crown And Bridge, Temporary, Resin　　Dental And Oral
Implant, Endosseous　　　　　　　Dental And Oral
Material, Tooth Shade, Resin　　　　Dental And Oral
Metal, Base　　　　　　　　　Dental And Oral
Powder, Porcelain　　　　　　　Dental And Oral

STRECK LABORATORIES, INC.　800-843-0912
7002 South 109th Street, Omaha, NE 68128　402-333-1982
FDA Number: 1950302　　　　　　Fax: 402-333-4094
E-mail: custserv@streck.com
Web site: www.streck.com
Medical Products Sales Volume: $45,000,000
Annual Revenue: $25-$50 Million
Year Founded: 1971
Total Employees: 290　　*Marketing Staff:* 8　　*Sales Staff:* 9
Ownership: Private
Quality System Registration Information: ISO9001
Produces/Sells CE-marked Devices: N
Federal Procurement Eligibility: Small Business, GSA Contract
Distribution: Manufacturer Direct, Manufacturer Through Distributor, Manufacturer Through Manufacturer Reps, OEM, Exporter
General Admin.: Wayne Ryan/Chief Executive Officer
　　　　Connie Ryan/President
　　　　Lori Briggs/Vice President Human Resources
Mktg./Adv.: Teri Thiele/Manager Advertising
　　　　Jodi Gnader/Manager Contract Sales
　　　　Kerstin Zedrosser/Manager International & National Sales
　　　　Jodi Gnader/Vice President Sales
Production: Carol Thompson/Director Quality Assurance
　　　　Carol Thompson/Manager Regulatory Affairs
Research: Hal Sornson/Vice President Research & Development
Finance: Bob Stonacek/Controller
Analyzer, Sedimentation Rate, Automated　Hematology
Bath, Ice　　　　　　　　　　Microbiology
Calibrator, Primary, Clinical Chemistry　Chemistry

STRENUMED, INC.　805-477-1000
1833 Portola Road,, Suite K, Ventura, CA 93003
FDA Number: 2030425　　　　　　Fax: 805-477-1367
E-mail: doug@strenumed.com
Web site: www.strenumed.com
Annual Revenue: $1-$5 Million
Year Founded: 1995
Total Employees: 20　　*Marketing Staff:* 4　　*Sales Staff:* 4

STRENUMED, INC.   805-477-1000 *(cont'd)*
Ownership: Private
Produces/Sells CE-marked Devices: Y
Federal Procurement Eligibility: Small Business, Minority Owned, Female Owned
Distribution: Manufacturer Direct, Manufacturer Through Distributor, Exporter
General Admin.: Mr. Douglas Walker/President
Mktg./Adv.: Ms. Brenda Acosta/Vice President Marketing

Accessories, Powered Drill	Cns/Neurology
Instrument, Surgical, Powered, Pneumatic	Orthopedics

STRETCHAIR PATIENT TRANSFER SYSTEMS   800-237-1162
8110 Ulmerton Rd., Largo, FL 33771   **352-854-2929**
FDA Number: 1043565   *Fax:* 727-536-0666
E-mail: horn@stretchair.com
Web site: http://www.stretchair.com
Ownership: Private
Produces/Sells CE-marked Devices: N

STRETCHAIR PATIENT TRANSFER SYSTEMS, INC,   800-237-1162
8110 Ulmerton Road, Largo, FL 33771   **727-531-2444**
FDA Number: 2424022   *Fax:* 727-536-0666
E-mail: lbauman@stretchair.com
Web site: www.stretchair.com
Medical Products Sales Volume: $1,700,000
Annual Revenue: $1-$5 Million
Year Founded: 1973
Total Employees: 23   *Marketing Staff:* 2   *Sales Staff:* 2
Ownership: MLA SYSTEMS, INC.
Produces/Sells CE-marked Devices: N
Federal Procurement Eligibility: Small Business
Distribution: Manufacturer Direct, Manufacturer Through Distributor, OEM, Service Direct, Exclusive Distributor, Exporter
General Admin.: E. A . Scordato/Chairman, Chief Executive Officer
    Kathy Marro/Human Resources Representative
Mktg./Adv.: Pia Johansson/Director Marketing
    Lawrence Bauman/Vice President Marketing & Sales
Production: Wayne Mauney/Customer Service Representative
    Robert Novack/Director Facility & Manufacturing
Research: George Assoian/Director Research & Engineering

Chair, Examination And Treatment	General
Scale, Chair, Transfer	General
Wheelchair, Special Grade	Physical Med

STRIKER CORP.   800 253 3210
4100 East Milham Avenue, Kalamazoo, MI 49001   **269 323 7700**
FDA Number: n/a   *Fax:* 800 999 3811
Web site: www.stryker.com
Annual Revenue: More than $1 Billion
Total Employees: 17594   *Sales Staff:* 6664
Ownership: STRYKER CORPORATION
Stock Symbol: SYK
Traded On: NYSE
Quality System Registration Information: ISO9001
Produces/Sells CE-marked Devices: Y
Federal Procurement Eligibility: Small Business
Distribution: Service Direct
General Admin.: John W. Brown/Chairman
    Stephen P. MacMillan/President, Chief Executive Officer
Finance: Dean H. Bergy/Vice President Admin., Chief Financial Officer
    Curt R. Hartman/Vice President Finance
    Tony M. McKinney/Vice President, Chief Administrative Officer

Accessories, Arthroscope	Orthopedics
Bone Mill	Orthopedics
Chisel (Osteotome)	Surgery
Chisel, Bone, Surgical	Dental And Oral
Chisel, Nasal	Ear/Nose/Throat
Chisel, Osteotome, Surgical	Dental And Oral
Chisel, Surgical, Manual	Surgery
Clamp, Cannula	Gastroenterology/Urology
Clamp, Surgical, General & Plastic Surgery	Surgery
Cover, Biopsy Forceps	Gastroenterology/Urology
Cutter, Wire And Pin	Orthopedics
Electrosurgical Equipment, General Purpose	Surgery
Instrument, Bending (Contouring)	Orthopedics
Mesh, Orthopedic (Metallic)	Orthopedics
Osteotome, Manual (Plastic Surgery)	Surgery
Plate, Fixation, Bone	Orthopedics
Prosthesis, Craniofacial	Ear/Nose/Throat
Rasp, Nasal	Ear/Nose/Throat
Rasp, Surgical, General & Plastic Surgery	Surgery
Retractor, All Types	Dental And Oral
Retractor, Manual	Cns/Neurology
Retractor, Non-Self-Retaining	Gastroenterology/Urology
Retractor, Surgical	Surgery
Scissors, Nasal	Ear/Nose/Throat
Scissors, Surgical Tissue, Dental (Oral)	Dental And Oral
Scissors, Wire Cutting, ENT	Ear/Nose/Throat

STRIKER CORP.   800 253 3210 *(cont'd)*

Screw, Cranioplasty Plate	Cns/Neurology
Screw, Fixation, Bone	Orthopedics
Stereotaxy Equipment	Cns/Neurology

STRIKER LEIBINGER
See Striker Corp.

STRITE INDUSTRIES LTD.   800-267-7333
298 Shepherd Ave.,   **519-658-9361**
Cambridge, ON N3C 1 Canada
FDA Number: n/a   *Fax:* 519-658-6925
E-mail: sales@strite.com
Web site: www.speedsystem.com
Medical Products Sales Volume: $2,500,000
Year Founded: 1964
Total Employees: 40   *Marketing Staff:* 1   *Sales Staff:* 3
Ownership: Private
Produces/Sells CE-marked Devices: N
Federal Procurement Eligibility: Small Business
Distribution: Manufacturer Direct, Manufacturer Through Manufacturer Reps, OEM

STRUBLE AND MOFFITT CO.
See White Knight Engineered Products

STRUCTURE PROBE, INC., SPI SUPPLIES   800-2424-SPI
569 East Gay St., PO Box 656,   **610-436-5400**
West Chester, PA 19380
FDA Number: n/a   *Fax:* 610-436-5755
E-mail: spi3spi@2spi.com
Web site: www.2spi.com/
Medical Products Sales Volume: $2,000,000
Annual Revenue: $1-$5 Million
Year Founded: 1970
Total Employees: 30
Ownership: Private
Produces/Sells CE-marked Devices: N
Federal Procurement Eligibility: Small Business, GSA Contract
Distribution: Manufacturer Through Distributor, Importer, Exporter
General Admin.: Kim Murray/Corporate Secretary
    Dr. Charles A. Garber/President, Chief Executive Officer
Mktg./Adv.: Eugene Rodek/Vice President Sales
IS: Dr. Andrew W. Blackwood/Vice President Technology

Desiccator	Chemistry

STRYKER BIOTECH   508-416-5200
35 South St., Hopkinton, MA 01748
FDA Number: 1224732   *Fax:* 508 416 5395
Web site: www.stryker.com
Ownership: Stryker Corp.
Stock Symbol: SYK
Traded On: NYSE
Produces/Sells CE-marked Devices: N
General Admin.: Mark A. Philip/President

Filler, Bovine Protein Mixture, Bone Morphogenetic Proteins, Collagen Scaffold, Osteoinduction	Physical Med

STRYKER BIOTECH
See OLYMPUS BIOTECH CORPORATION

STRYKER COMMUNICATIONS CORP.   866-726-3705
1410 Lakeside Parkway,   **972-410-7100**
Flower Mound, TX 75028
FDA Number: 2031963   *Fax:* 408-754-2969
E-mail: cansari@strykercom.com
Web site: www.strykercom.com
Medical Products Sales Volume: $12,000,000
Year Founded: 1999
Total Employees: 150
Ownership: Stryker Corp.
Stock Symbol: SYK
Traded On: NYSE
Produces/Sells CE-marked Devices: N
Federal Procurement Eligibility: Small Business
Mktg./Adv.: Chad Croasdale/National Director Marketing

Cabinet, Table And Tray, Anesthesia	Anesthesiology
Endoscope And Accessories, AC-Powered	Surgery
Laparoscope, General & Plastic Surgery	Surgery
Light, Surgical, Ceiling Mounted	Surgery
Suction Apparatus, Operating Room, Wall Vacuum-Powered	Surgery
System, Communication, Image, Digital	Radiology
Table, Operating Room, AC-Powered	Surgery

STRYKER CORP.   800-726-2725
2825 Airview Boulevard, Kalamazoo, MI 49002   **269-385-2600**
FDA Number: 300885397   *Fax:* 269-385-1062
Web site: www.stryker.com
Medical Products Sales Volume: $6,000,500,000
Annual Revenue: More than $1 Billion
Year Founded: 1941

STRYKER CORP.   800-726-2725 (cont'd)

Total Employees: 16026   Sales Staff: 3500
Ownership: Public
Stock Symbol: SYK
Traded On: NYSE
Quality System Registration Information: ISO9000
Produces/Sells CE-marked Devices: N
Distribution: Manufacturer Direct, Exporter
General Admin.: Michael P. Mogul/President
   William R. Enquist/President
   Mr. Andrew Fox-Smith/President International Operations
   Mr. Stephen P. MacMillan/President, Chief Executive Officer
   Ms. Bronwen R. Taylor/Vice President
   Mr. Curtis E. Hall/Vice President, General Counsel
Mktg./Adv.: Ms. Katherine A. Owen/Vice President Strategic Planning
Production: Ms. Elizabeth A. Staub/Vice President Quality Assurance & Regulatory Affairs
Finance: Ms. Jeanne M. Blondia/Vice President, Treasurer

Arthroscope	Orthopedics
Catheter, Percutaneous	Cardiovascular
Cutter, Cast	Orthopedics
Cutter, Wire And Pin	Orthopedics
Drill, Bone	Orthopedics
Driver, Wire	Orthopedics
Embolization Device	Cardiovascular
Handpiece, Belt and/or Gear Driven, Dental	Dental And Oral
Handpiece, Contra- And Right-Angle Attachment, Dental	Dental And Oral
Irrigator, Suction	General
Lavage Unit, Surgical	Surgery
Lavage Unit, Water Jet	General
Light Source, Fiberoptic, Routine	Gastroenterology/Urology
Mixing Equipment, Cement	Orthopedics
Monitor, Video, Endoscope	General
Osteotome, Roto With Blade	Dental And Oral
Rack, Surgical Instrument	Surgery
Reamer	Orthopedics
Regulator, Pressure, Gas Cylinder	Anesthesiology
Retractor	Orthopedics
Retractor, All Types	Dental And Oral
Retractor, Fiberoptic	Gastroenterology/Urology
Saw, Bone Cutting	Orthopedics
Saw, Bone Cutting, Micro	Orthopedics
Saw, Bone, Pneumatic	Orthopedics
Saw, Electric	Cardiovascular
Saw, Other	Surgery
Screwdriver	Orthopedics
Shoe, Cast	Physical Med
Splint, Clavicle	Physical Med
Television Monitor, Microscope	General
Television Monitor, Operating Room	General
Tip, Suction	Anesthesiology
Tip, Suction Tube (Yankauer, Poole, Etc.)	Surgery
Trephine, Bone	Orthopedics
Vacuum, Cast Cutter	Orthopedics

Medical Product Subsidiaries (Listed Separately)
Boston Scientific-Neurovascular
Everest Biomedical Instruments Co.
Gaymar Industries, Inc.
Howmedica Osteonics Corp.
Link Technology, Inc.
OLYMPUS BIOTECH CORPORATION
Stryker Biotech
Stryker Communications Corp.
Stryker Endoscopy

STRYKER CORP., SURGICAL DIV.

See Stryker Corp.

STRYKER ENDOSCOPY   800-435-0220

5900 Optical Ct, San Jose, CA 95138   408-754-2000
FDA Number: 2936485   Fax: 800-754-2505
Web site: www.strykerendo.com
Medical Products Sales Volume: $200,000,000
Total Employees: 500   Marketing Staff: 22   Sales Staff: 130
Ownership: Stryker Corp.
Stock Symbol: SYK
Traded On: NYSE
Quality System Registration Information: ISO9001
Produces/Sells CE-marked Devices: Y
Distribution: Manufacturer Direct, Manufacturer Through Manufacturer Reps, OEM, Exporter
General Admin.: John Brown/Chief Executive Officer
   Lee Lovely/Director Human Resources
   Bill Enquist/President
   Si Johnson/President
Mktg./Adv.: Brady Shirley/Director Marketing
   Keric De Chant/Director National Accounts
   Mike Pierce/Vice President Business Development
   Tim Scannell/Vice President Marketing & Sales

STRYKER ENDOSCOPY   800-435-0220 (cont'd)

Production: John Haller/Director Operations
   Margaret Cox/Manager Materials
   Carlos Gonzalez/Vice President Quality Assurance & Regulatory Affairs
Research: William Change/Vice President Research & Development
Finance: Doug Smith/Vice President Finance

Arthroscope	Orthopedics
Camera, Television, Surgical (With Audio)	Surgery
Camera, Videotape, Surgical	Surgery
Insufflator, Laparoscopic	Obstetrics/Gynecology
Laparoscope, General & Plastic Surgery	Surgery
Light, Surgical Headlight	Dental And Oral
Monitor, Video, Endoscope	General
Orthopedic Manual Surgical Instrument	Orthopedics
Surgical Instrument, Orthopedic, AC-Powered Motor	Orthopedics
Tape, Television & Video, Endoscopic	Gastroenterology/Urology
Television Monitor, Microscope	General
Television Monitor, Operating Room	General
Trocar, Laparoscopic	Surgery

STRYKER GI   866-672-5757

1420 Lakeside Parkway, Suite 110,   877-795-3539
Flower Mound, TX 75028
FDA Number: 3006370937
Web site: www.stryker.com   Fax: 866-519-2598
Ownership: STRYKER CORPORATION
Stock Symbol: SYK
Traded On: NYSE
Produces/Sells CE-marked Devices: N
General Admin.: Mr. Stephen P. MacMillan/President, Chief Executive Officer

Colonoscope, Gastro-Urology	Gastroenterology/Urology
Cover, Biopsy Forceps	Gastroenterology/Urology
Endoscope	Gastroenterology/Urology
Garment, Protective, For Incontinence	Gastroenterology/Urology
Laparoscope, General & Plastic Surgery	Surgery

STRYKER HOWMEDICA OSTEONICS   201-831-5000

325 Corporate Drive, Mahwah, NJ 07430
FDA Number: 2249697
Web site: www.stryker.com
Ownership: STRYKER CORPORATION
Stock Symbol: SYK
Traded On: NYSE
Produces/Sells CE-marked Devices: N

Prosthesis, Hip, Semi-Const., Metal/Poly., Porous Uncemented	Orthopedics
Prosthesis, Hip, Semi-Constrained, Metal/Polymer	Orthopedics
Prosthesis, Knee, Femorotibial, Non-Constrained	Orthopedics
Prosthesis, Knee, Femorotibial, Semi-Constrained	Orthopedics
Prosthesis, Knee, Patellofemorotibial, Semi-Constrained	Orthopedics

STRYKER IMAGING   888-795-4624

1410 Lakeside Pkwy., Ste. 600,   972-410-5000
Flower Mound, TX 75028
FDA Number: 1064427   Fax: 972-410-5010
E-mail: Imaging-Support@stryker.com
Web site: http://imaging.stryker.com
Ownership: STRYKER CORPORATION
Stock Symbol: SYK
Traded On: NYSE
Produces/Sells CE-marked Devices: N
General Admin.: Mark B. Lipscomb/General Manager
   Mr. Andrew Fox-Smith/President International Operations
   Mr. Stephen P. MacMillan/President, Chief Executive Officer

Device, Storage, Image, Digital	Radiology
Image Processing System	Radiology
System, Communication, Image, Digital	Radiology

STRYKER INSTRUMENTS, INSTRUMENTS DIV.   800-253-3210

4100 East Milham Ave., Kalamazoo, MI 49001   269 323 7700
FDA Number: 1811755   Fax: 800-999-3811
E-mail: Custsvc@Strykerinc.com
Web site: www.instrumedinc.com
Ownership: STRYKER CORPORATION
Stock Symbol: SYK
Traded On: NYSE
Produces/Sells CE-marked Devices: N
General Admin.: Mr. Stephan MacMillian/President, Chief Executive Officer, Chairman
Finance: Mr. Tony McKinney/Vice President Accounting
   Ms. Jeanne Blondia/Vice President Treasury

Accessories, Apparel, Surgical	Surgery
Accessories, Powered Drill	Cns/Neurology
Applier, Cast	Orthopedics
Arthroscope	Orthopedics
Autotransfusion Unit (Blood)	Anesthesiology
Bandage, Adhesive	Surgery
Bit, Surgical	Surgery
Blade, Saw, Surgical, Cardiovascular	Cardiovascular

STRYKER INSTRUMENTS, INSTRUMENTS DIV.   800-253-3210
(cont'd)

Blade, Surgical, Saw, General & Plastic Surgery	Surgery
Bone Cement	Orthopedics
Bottle, Collection, Breathing System (Uncalibrated)	Anesthesiology
Bottle, Collection, Vacuum (Aspirator)	General
Brush, Dermabrasion	Surgery
Burr	Ear/Nose/Throat
Burr, Dental	Dental And Oral
Burr, Surgical, General & Plastic Surgery	Surgery
Canister, Suction	Cardiovascular
Cannula, Sinus	Ear/Nose/Throat
Catheter, Conduction, Anesthesia	Anesthesiology
Catheter, Intravascular, Therapeutic, Short-term Less Than 30 Days	General
Chisel, Bone, Surgical	Dental And Oral
Component, Cast	Orthopedics
Controller, Foot, Handpiece And Cord	Dental And Oral
Cover, Cast	General
Cover, Shoe, Operating Room	Surgery
Curette	Orthopedics
Cutter, Cast, AC-Powered	Orthopedics
Dermatome	Surgery
Dispenser, Cement	Orthopedics
Drill, Bone, Powered	Dental And Oral
Drill, Dental, Intraoral	Dental And Oral
Drill, Surgical, ENT (Electric Or Pneumatic)	Ear/Nose/Throat
Driver, Wire, And Bone Drill, Manual	Dental And Oral
EIA, Blastomyces Dermatitidis	Microbiology
Electrosurgical Unit, Cutting & Coagulation Device	Surgery
Evacuator, Vapor, Cement Monomer	Orthopedics
Exhaust System, Surgical	Surgery
Fastener, Fixation, Biodegradable, Soft Tissue	Orthopedics
File, Bone, Surgical	Dental And Oral
File, Margin Finishing, Operative	Dental And Oral
Filler, Bone Cement (for Vertebroplasty)	Orthopedics
Gauze, Non-Absorbable, X-Ray Detectable (Internal Sponge)	Surgery
Gown, Surgical	Surgery
Guard, Disk	Dental And Oral
Guide, Surgical, Instrument	Surgery
Guide, Surgical, Needle	Surgery
Handpiece, Contra- And Right-Angle Attachment, Dental	Dental And Oral
Handpiece, Rotary Bone Cutting	Dental And Oral
Helmet, Surgical	Surgery
Hood, Surgical	Surgery
Instrument, Manual, General Surgical	Surgery
Instrument, Surgical, Powered, Pneumatic	Orthopedics
Introducer, Catheter	Cardiovascular
Irrigator, Oral	Dental And Oral
Knife, Surgical	Dental And Oral
Lamp, Surgical	Surgery
Lavage Unit, Water Jet	General
Light, Surgical, Instrument	Surgery
Mask, Surgical	Surgery
Metacrylate, Methyl, Cranioplasty	Cns/Neurology
Mixing Equipment, Cement	Orthopedics
Monitor, Pressure, Intracompartmental	Orthopedics
Motor, Drill, Electric	Cns/Neurology
Motor, Drill, Pneumatic	Cns/Neurology
Motor, Surgical Instrument, AC-Powered	Surgery
Motor, Surgical Instrument, Pneumatic-Powered	Surgery
Obturator, Cement	Orthopedics
Operative Dental Treatment Unit	Dental And Oral
Orthopedic Manual Surgical Instrument	Orthopedics
Orthosis, Cervical	Physical Med
Pack, Sterilization Wrapper (Bag And Accessories)	Surgery
Probe	Orthopedics
Prosthesis, Hip, Cement Restrictor	Orthopedics
Pump, Infusion	General
Pump, Infusion, Elastomeric	General
Pump, Infusion, Patient Controlled Analgesia (PCA)	General
Regulator, Pressure, Gas Cylinder	Anesthesiology
Saw, Electric	Cardiovascular
Saw, Electric Bone	Dental And Oral
Saw, Pneumatically Powered	Surgery
Saw, Powered, And Accessories	Cns/Neurology
Saw, Surgical, ENT (Electric Or Pneumatic)	Ear/Nose/Throat
Sponge, Gauze	Dental And Oral
Stereotaxy Equipment	Cns/Neurology
Suction Apparatus, Operating Room, Wall Vacuum-Powered	Surgery
Suction Apparatus, Single Patient, Portable, Non-Powered	Surgery
Suit, Surgical	Surgery
Surgical Instrument, Orthopedic, AC-Powered Motor	Orthopedics
Surgical Instrument, Orthopedic, Battery-Powered	Surgery
Syringe, Piston	General
Tourniquet, Pneumatic	Surgery
Trap, Sterile Specimen	Anesthesiology
Tray, Surgical Instrument	Surgery
Tubing, Non-Invasive	Surgery
Wire, Fixation, Intraosseous	Dental And Oral

STRYKER MEDICAL   800-869-0770
2825 Airview Boulevard, Kalamazoo, MI 49002   269 389 2600
FDA Number: 1831750   *Fax:* 269 389 1062
E-mail: jo.johnson@stryker.com
Web site: www.stryker.com
Medical Products Sales Volume: $400,000
Year Founded: 1941
Total Employees: 15   *Marketing Staff:* 12   *Sales Staff:* 126
Ownership: STRYKER CORPORATION
Stock Symbol: SYK
Traded On: NYSE
Quality System Registration Information: ISO9001
Produces/Sells CE-marked Devices: Y
Federal Procurement Eligibility: Small Business
Distribution: Manufacturer Direct
General Admin.: Mr. John Brown/Chief Executive Officer
      Mr. John Ferrell/Director Human Resources
      Mr. Stephen Johnson/President
      Mr. Jim Cunniff/Vice President, General Manager
Mktg./Adv.: Mr. Fred Taccolini/Director National Accounts
      Mr. Jeff Gerlach/Vice President Marketing
      Mr. Jim Heath/Vice President Sales
Production: Mr. Larry Carpenter/Director Engineering
      Mr. Wilf Ruiz/Director Quality Assurance
      Mr. Wilf Ruiz/Director Regulatory Affairs
      Mr. Jon Crawford/Vice President Operations

Accessories, Traction (Cart, Frame, Cord, Weight)	Orthopedics
Bassinet (Infant Bed)	General
Bed, Birthing	General
Bed, Electric	General
Bed, Hydraulic	General
Bed, Patient Rotation, Manual	Physical Med
Bed, Patient Rotation, Powered	Physical Med
Cabinet, Bedside	General
Cart, Patient (Stretcher)	Anesthesiology
Chair, Examination And Treatment	General
Cover, Mattress	General
Frame, Turning	Orthopedics
Furniture, Patient Room	General
Headwall System (Patient Room)	General
Mattress, Bed	General
Mattress, Silicone, And Chair Cushion	General
Pad, Pressure, Gel, Operating Table	General
Stool, Operating Room, Adjustable	Surgery
Stretcher, Hydraulic	General
Stretcher, Radiographic	Radiology
Stretcher, Transfer	Surgery
Stretcher, Wheeled (Mobile)	General
Stretcher, Wheeled, Mechanical	Physical Med
Table, Obstetrical, Manual	Obstetrics/Gynecology
Table, Radiographic, Tilting	Radiology
Table, Surgical, Manual	General
Table, Surgical, Orthopedic	Orthopedics
Transfer Device, Patient, Manual	General
Unit, Examining/Treatment, ENT	Ear/Nose/Throat
Wheelchair, Manual	Physical Med

STRYKER MEDICAL/MEDIQUIP DIVISION
See Medical Technologies Co.

STRYKER PUERTO RICO, LTD.   939-307-2500
Hwy. 3, Km. 131.2, Las Guasimas Ind. Park, Arroyo, PR 00714
FDA Number: 2648666   *Fax:* 939-307-2501
Ownership: STRYKER CORPORATION
Stock Symbol: SYK
Traded On: NYSE
Produces/Sells CE-marked Devices: N

Analyzer, Chemistry, Radioimmunoassay	Chemistry
Arthroscope	Orthopedics
Autotransfusion Unit (Blood)	Anesthesiology
Basin, Emesis	General
Biopsy Instrument	Gastroenterology/Urology
Bottle, Collection, Vacuum (Aspirator)	General
Burr, Surgical, General & Plastic Surgery	Surgery
Canister, Suction	Cardiovascular
Cannula, Sinus	Ear/Nose/Throat
Catheter, Conduction, Anesthesia	Anesthesiology
Catheter, Irrigation	Surgery
Catheter, Suction (Tracheal Aspirating Tube)	Anesthesiology
Catheter, Suction, With Tip	General
Connector, Tubing, Blood, Infusion, T-Type	Gastroenterology/Urology
Cutter, Surgical	Surgery
Dispenser, Cement	Orthopedics
Electrosurgical Unit, Cutting & Coagulation Device	Surgery
Endoscope	Gastroenterology/Urology
Evacuator, Vapor, Cement Monomer	Orthopedics
Expander, Skin, Inflatable	Surgery
Filler, Bone Cement (for Vertebroplasty)	Orthopedics
Gauze, Non-Absorbable, X-Ray Detectable (Internal Sponge)	Surgery
Instrument, Manual, General Surgical	Surgery

STRYKER PUERTO RICO, LTD.   939-307-2500 *(cont'd)*

Insufflator, Laparoscopic	Obstetrics/Gynecology
Irrigator, Oral	Dental And Oral
Kit, Irrigation, Sterile	Gastroenterology/Urology
Knife, Surgical	Dental And Oral
Lamp, Surgical	Surgery
Lavage Unit, Water Jet	General
Light, Surgical, Instrument	Surgery
Mixing Equipment, Cement	Orthopedics
Monitor, Pressure, Intracompartmental	Orthopedics
Obturator, Cement	Orthopedics
Orthopedic Manual Surgical Instrument	Orthopedics
Prosthesis, Hip, Cement Restrictor	Orthopedics
Pump, Infusion	General
Sponge, Gauze	Dental And Oral
Suction Apparatus, Operating Room, Wall Vacuum-Powered	Surgery
Suction Apparatus, Single Patient, Portable, Non-Powered	Surgery
Syringe, Piston	General
Tube, Drainage	Gastroenterology/Urology
Tubing, Fluid Delivery	General
Tubing, Non-Invasive	Surgery

STRYKER SCOPES

See Stryker Endoscopy

STRYKER SPINE   866-457-7463

2 Pearl Ct, Allendale, NJ 07401   **201-760-8000**

FDA Number: 3004024955   *Fax:* 201-760-8108
Web site: http://www.stryker.com
Total Employees: 3800
Ownership: STRYKER CORPORATION
Stock Symbol: SYK
Traded On: NYSE
Quality System Registration Information: ISO9001
Produces/Sells CE-marked Devices: Y
Distribution: Manufacturer Direct, Manufacturer Through Manufacturer Reps

Appliance, Fixation, Spinal Interlaminal	Orthopedics
Bit, Drill	Orthopedics
Cement, Orthopedic (Bone)	Orthopedics
Cerclage, Fixation	Orthopedics
Container, Sterilization (Tray)	General
Cutter, Wire And Pin	Orthopedics
Device, Spinal Vertebral Body Replacement	Orthopedics
Drill, Bone	Orthopedics
Drill, Cannulated	Orthopedics
Drill, Cranial	Cns/Neurology
Driver, Bone Staple	Orthopedics
Driver, Prosthesis	Orthopedics
Driver, Surgical, Pin	Surgery
Driver/Extractor, Bone Nail/Pin	Orthopedics
Extractor, Nail	Orthopedics
Fixation Appliance, Multiple Component	Orthopedics
Forceps	Orthopedics
Forceps, Wire Holding	Orthopedics
Gauge, Depth	Orthopedics
Guide	Orthopedics
Guide, Drill	Orthopedics
Guide, Gigli Saw	Orthopedics
Impactor	Orthopedics
Implant, Fixation Device, Proximal Femoral	Orthopedics
Mallet, Bone	Orthopedics
Mesh, Surgical (Steel Gauze)	Surgery
Mixing Equipment, Cement	Orthopedics
Nail, Fixation, Bone	Orthopedics
Orthosis, Fixation, Spinal, Spondylolisthesis	Orthopedics
Osteotome (Orthopedic)	Surgery
Passer, Wire, Orthopedic	Orthopedics
Pin, Fixation, Smooth	Orthopedics
Pin, Fixation, Threaded	Orthopedics
Plate, Bone, Skull, Preformed, Non-Alterable	Cns/Neurology
Plate, Fixation, Bone	Orthopedics
Prosthesis Implantation Instrument, Orthopedic	Orthopedics
Prosthesis, Ankle, Semi-Constrained, Metal/Polymer	Orthopedics
Prosthesis, Ankle, Talar Component	Orthopedics
Prosthesis, Ankle, Tibial Component	Orthopedics
Prosthesis, Diaphysis, Custom	Orthopedics
Prosthesis, Elbow, Semi-Constrained	Orthopedics
Prosthesis, Femoral	Orthopedics
Prosthesis, Hip, Acetabular Component, Metal, Non-Cemented	Orthopedics
Prosthesis, Hip, Acetabular Mesh	Orthopedics
Prosthesis, Hip, Cement Restrictor	Orthopedics
Prosthesis, Hip, Hemi-, Femoral, Metal/Polymer	Orthopedics
Prosthesis, Hip, Semi-Const., Metal/Poly., Porous Uncemented	Orthopedics
Prosthesis, Hip, Semi-Constr., Metal/Ceramic, Cemented/NC	Orthopedics
Prosthesis, Hip, Semi-Constrained (Cemented Acetabular)	Orthopedics
Prosthesis, Hip, Semi-Constrained, Metal/Polymer	Orthopedics
Prosthesis, Hip, Semi-Constrained, Metal/Polymer, Uncemented	Orthopedics
Prosthesis, Joint, Other	Orthopedics
Prosthesis, Knee, Femorotibial, Constrained, Metal/Polymer	Orthopedics
Prosthesis, Knee, Femorotibial, Non-Constrained	Orthopedics
Prosthesis, Knee, Femorotibial, Semi-Constrained	Orthopedics
Prosthesis, Knee, Femorotibial, Semi-Constrained, Trunnion	Orthopedics

STRYKER SPINE   866-457-7463 *(cont'd)*

Prosthesis, Knee, Hemi-, Femoral	Orthopedics
Prosthesis, Knee, Hemi-, Patellar Resurfacing, Uncemented	Orthopedics
Prosthesis, Knee, Hemi-, Tibial Resurfacing, Uncemented	Orthopedics
Prosthesis, Knee, Hinged (Metal-Metal)	Orthopedics
Prosthesis, Knee, Patellar	Orthopedics
Prosthesis, Knee, Patellofemoral, Semi-Constrained	Orthopedics
Prosthesis, Knee, Patellofemorotibial, Semi-Constrained	Orthopedics
Prosthesis, Knee, Total	Orthopedics
Prosthesis, Shoulder	Orthopedics
Prosthesis, Shoulder, Hemi-, Humeral	Orthopedics
Prosthesis, Upper Femoral	Orthopedics
Prosthesis, Wrist, 3 Part Metal-Plastic-Metal Articulation	Orthopedics
Punch, Bone	Orthopedics
Punch, Femoral Neck	Orthopedics
Pusher, Socket	Orthopedics
Rasp, Bone	Orthopedics
Reamer	Orthopedics
Retractor	Orthopedics
Rod, Fixation, Intramedullary	Orthopedics
Saw, Bone Cutting	Orthopedics
Screw, Fixation, Bone	Orthopedics
Screwdriver	Orthopedics
Staple, Fixation, Bone	Orthopedics
Tap, Bone	Orthopedics
Template	Orthopedics
Tray, Surgical Instrument	Surgery
Wire, Bone	Orthopedics
Wrench	Orthopedics

Medical Product Subsidiaries (Listed Separately)
Striker Corp.

STS DIVISION OF ETHOX INTERNATIONAL   800.836.4850

7500 West Henrietta Rd., Rush, NY 14543   **585.533.1672**

FDA Number: 1314417   *Fax:* 585.533.1796
E-mail: info@ethoxsts.com
Web site: www.ethoxsts.com
Ownership: Ethox International
Produces/Sells CE-marked Devices: N

Block, Bite	Cns/Neurology
Catheter, Irrigation	Surgery
Container, Sterilization (Tray)	General
Cuff, Blood Pressure	Cardiovascular
Pressure Infusor, IV Container	General
Pump, Infusion	General
Sterilization Process Indicator, Biological	General
Tube, Gastrointestinal	Gastroenterology/Urology

STS DUOTEK, INC   800-836-4850

370 Summit Point Drive, Henrietta, NY 14467   **585-321-5000**

FDA Number: 1316257   *Fax:* 585-321-3058
E-mail: info@stsduotek.com
Web site: www.stsduotek.com
Medical Products Sales Volume: $4,500,000
Annual Revenue: $10-$25 Million
Year Founded: 1978
Total Employees: 75   *Marketing Staff:* 4   *Sales Staff:* 4
Ownership: Ethox Sts Life Sciences Div
Quality System Registration Information: ISO9002
Produces/Sells CE-marked Devices: N
Federal Procurement Eligibility: Small Business
Distribution: Manufacturer Direct
General Admin.: Annette Borrelli/Executive Assistant
          Lynn Martin/Executive Vice President
          James Whitbourne/President
Mktg./Adv.: Gerard F. Whitbourne/Vice President Marketing & Sales
Production: Carolyn Eastman/Vice President Regulatory Affairs

Contract Laboratory	General
Contract Packaging	General
Contract R&D, Diagnostics	General
Contract Sterilization	General
Packaging, Sterilization	General
Sterilization Process Indicator, Biological	General

STUART ALLYN CO., INC.   413-443-7306

17 Taconic Park Dr., Pittsfield, MA 01202

FDA Number: 1222688   *Fax:* 413-443-7672
E-mail: info@stuartallyn.com
Web site: www.stuartallyn.com
Ownership: Private
Produces/Sells CE-marked Devices: N
General Admin.: Mr. Allyn Scace/Vice President
Finance: Mr. Stuart Scace/President

Probe, Periodontic	Dental And Oral

STUDEBAKER-WORTHINGTON LEASING CORP.   800-645-7242

100 Jericho Quadrangle, Jericho, NY 11753

FDA Number: n/a   *Fax:* 516-938-5604
E-mail: webmaster@studebaker.com
Web site: www.studebaker.com

STUDEBAKER-WORTHINGTON LEASING CORP. 800-645-7242
(cont'd)
   Ownership: Private
   Produces/Sells CE-marked Devices: N
   Distribution: Service Direct
     Service, Equipment Leasing   General

STURGES MANUFACTURING COMPANY, INC. 315-732-6159
2030 Sunset Ave., Utica, NY 13503
   FDA Number: 3002786781
   E-mail: info@sturgesstraps.com   *Fax:* 315.732.2314
   Web site: www.sturgesstraps.com
   Ownership: Private
   Produces/Sells CE-marked Devices: N
     Bandage, Cast   Physical Med

STYLOPTIC INTL., S.A. DE C.V. 301-242-2330
274 Playa Villa Del Mar, Mexico City Mexico
   FDA Number: 9616076
     Frame, Spectacle (Eyeglasses)   Ophthalmology

SUAREZ CORPORATION INDUSTRIES 330-494-5504
7800 Whipple Avenue N.w., North Canton, OH 44720
   FDA Number: 1528424
     Pad, Heating, Powered   Physical Med

SUBURBAN ADULT SERVICES, INC. 716-496-5551
441 Indian Church Rd., West Seneca, NY 14224
   FDA Number: 3003735309
     Fiber, Absorbent   General

SUBURBAN ADULT SERVICES, INC. (888)496-5551
960 West Maple Court, Elma, NY 14059 (716)805-1555
   FDA Number: 3003480567   *Fax:* (716)805-1444
   Web site: www.sasinc.org
   Ownership: Private
   Produces/Sells CE-marked Devices: N
     Fiber, Absorbent   General

SUBURBAN OSTOMY SUPPLY CO., INC.
   See Invacare Supply Group, An Invacare Co.

SUBURBAN OSTOMY, AN INVACARE COMPANY
   See Invacare Supply Group, An Invacare Co.

SUBURBAN SURGICAL CO., INC. 800-323-7366
275 Twelfth St., Wheeling, IL 60090 847-537-9320
   FDA Number: 7000350   *Fax:* 847-537-9061
   E-mail: ssurgical@aol.com
   Web site: www.suburban-surgical.com
   Medical Products Sales Volume: $13,700,000
   Year Founded: 1943
   Total Employees: 200
   Ownership: Private
   Produces/Sells CE-marked Devices: N
   Federal Procurement Eligibility: Small Business, GSA Contract, VA Contract
   Distribution: Manufacturer Direct, Manufacturer Through Distributor
   General Admin.: James M. Pinkerman/President
   Mktg./Adv.: Todd Pinkerman/Manager National Sales
   Production: Jimmy Pinkerman/Manager Production
     Cabinet Casework, General Purpose   General
     Cabinet Casework, Laboratory   Chemistry
     Cabinet Casework, Modular   General
     Cabinet, Bedside   General
     Cabinet, Medicine   General
     Cabinet, Table And Tray, Anesthesia   Anesthesiology
     Cage, Animal   Microbiology
     Cart, Emergency, Cardiopulmonary Resuscitation (Crash)   Anesthesiology
     Cart, Foodservice   General
     Cart, Instrument   Surgery
     Cart, Laundry   General
     Cart, Multipurpose   General
     Cart, Orthopedic Supply (Cast)   Orthopedics
     Cart, Supply   General
     Cart, Supply, Operating Room   Surgery
     Isolation Unit, Surgical   General
     Sink, Laboratory   Chemistry
     Table, Examination/Treatment   General
     Table, Surgical, Manual   General

SUDBURY SYSTEMS 800-876-8888
490 Boston Post Rd., Sudbury, MA 01776 508-443-1100
   FDA Number: n/a   *Fax:* 978-218-1129
   Annual Revenue: $1-$5 Million
   Total Employees: 30
   Ownership: Private
   Produces/Sells CE-marked Devices: N
   Federal Procurement Eligibility: Small Business
   Distribution: Manufacturer Direct, Manufacturer Through Manufacturer Reps, Service Direct
   General Admin.: Gerald Delaney/President

SUDBURY SYSTEMS 800-876-8888 (cont'd)
   Mktg./Adv.: William Cudina/Vice President Marketing & Sales
     Computer Software   General

SUDOR INC. 705-445-0606
P.O. Box 383, Collingwood, ONT L9Y-3Z7 Canada
   FDA Number: n/a   *Fax:* 705-445-8383
   E-mail: sudor@lynx.org
   Web site: www.groundhealth.com
   Year Founded: 1986
   Total Employees: 10
   Ownership: Private
   Produces/Sells CE-marked Devices: N
   Distribution: Manufacturer Direct, Exclusive Distributor

SUGAR BEET PRODUCTS COMPANY
   See Deb Sbs, Inc.

SUKOL SCIENTIFIC, INC. 305-885-0045
10100 NW 116th Way # 18, Miami, FL 33178
   FDA Number: n/a   *Fax:* 305-885-0046
   E-mail: info@sukol.us
   Web site: www.sukol.us
   Ownership: Private
   Produces/Sells CE-marked Devices: N
     Component, Cast   Orthopedics

SULLIVAN-SCHEIN DENTAL EQUIPMENT
   See Henry Schein, Inc.

SULTAN HEALTHCARE, INC.
   See Dshealthcare Inc.

SULZER CALCITEK, INC.
   See Zimmer Dental, Inc.

SULZER DENTAL, INC.
   See Zimmer Dental, Inc.

SULZER MITROFLOW CORP. 604-270-7751
11220 Voyageur Way #1, Richmond, BC V6X-3E1 Canada
   FDA Number: n/a   *Fax:* 604-270-6308
   E-mail: sales@mitroflow.com
   Web site: www.mitroflow.com
   Year Founded: 1982
   Total Employees: 100
   Ownership: Private
   Produces/Sells CE-marked Devices: N
   Distribution: Manufacturer Direct, Exporter

SULZER OSCOR, INC.
   See Oscor, Inc.

SUMITCON INC.
   See Caire, Inc.

SUMMER INFANT, INC. 800-268-6237
1275 Park East Drive, Woonsocket, RI 02895 401-671-6550
   FDA Number: 3003657928
   E-mail: customerservice@summerinfant.com
   Web site: www.summerinfant.com
   Ownership: Public
   Stock Symbol: SUMR
   Traded On: NASDAQ
   Produces/Sells CE-marked Devices: N
   General Admin.: Jason P. Macari/President, Chief Executive Officer

SUMMERS LABORATORIES
   See Electron Microscopy Sciences

SUMMIT BUSINESS PRODUCTS, INC. 260-244-1820
995 E. Business 30, Columbia City, IN 46725
   FDA Number: 1836590
   Web site: www.summit-bp.com
   Ownership: Private
   Produces/Sells CE-marked Devices: N
     Template   Orthopedics

SUMMIT DOPPLER SYSTEMS, INC. 800-554-5090
4620 Technology Drive, Unit 100, 303-423-7572
Golden, CO 80403
   FDA Number: 3003892563   *Fax:* 303-940-7165
   E-mail: info@summitdoppler.com
   Web site: www.summitdoppler.com
   Medical Products Sales Volume: $2,000,000
   Year Founded: 2003
   Total Employees: 10
   Ownership: Private
   Produces/Sells CE-marked Devices: Y
   Federal Procurement Eligibility: Small Business
   Distribution: Manufacturer Direct, Manufacturer Through Distributor, Manufacturer Through Manufacturer Reps, OEM

SUMMIT DOPPLER SYSTEMS, INC.   800-554-5090 (cont'd)
Monitor, Fetal, Ultrasonic   Obstetrics/Gynecology

SUMMIT HILL LABORATORIES   800-922-0722
1 Sheila Dr, Tinton Falls, NJ 07724   **732-933-0800**
FDA Number: n/a   Fax: 732-933-0055
E-mail: sales@summithilllaboratories.com
Web site: www.summithilllaboratories.com
Year Founded: 1964
Ownership: Private
Produces/Sells CE-marked Devices: N
Federal Procurement Eligibility: Small Business
Distribution: Manufacturer Through Distributor
Purifier, Air, Ultraviolet   General

SUMMIT INDUSTRIES, INC.   800-729-9729
2901 W. Lawrence Avenue,   **773-588-2444**
Chicago, IL 60625
FDA Number: 1450503   Fax: 773-588-3424
E-mail: summitinfo@summitindustries.net
Web site: www.summitindustries.net
Medical Products Sales Volume: $9,900,000
Annual Revenue: $10-$25 Million
Year Founded: 1984
Total Employees: 72   Marketing Staff: 5   Sales Staff: 5
Ownership: Private
Produces/Sells CE-marked Devices: N
Federal Procurement Eligibility: Small Business
Distribution: Manufacturer Through Distributor
General Admin.: Ken Petrella/Chief Operating Officer, General Manager
     Jim Walsh/President, Chief Executive Officer
Mktg./Adv.: Greg Oravec/Manager Contract Sales
     Greg Oravec/Manager International Sales
     Gail Orzechowski/Manager Sales
     Tom Sterne/Manager Sales
Production: Don Matson/Manager Regulatory Affairs
     Greg Oravec/Senior Product Manager
     Lori Adams/Senior Product Manager
Processor, Radiographic Film, Automatic   Radiology
Radiographic Unit, Diagnostic   Radiology
Medical Product Subsidiaries (Listed Separately)
Lantiseptic Division, Summit Industries, Inc.

SUMMIT LIFTS, INC.   866-378-6648
18505 E. 163rd Street, Lake Winnebago, MO 64034
FDA Number: 3004153586
Transport, Patient, Powered   Physical Med

SUMMIT TECHNOLOGIES INC.   800-268-7916
2333 Wyecroft Rd., Unit 1,   **905-847-7300**
Oakville, ONT L6L-6 Canada
FDA Number: n/a   Fax: 905-847-7308
E-mail: cservice@summittech.on.ca
Web site: www.summittech.on.ca
Year Founded: 1982
Ownership: Private
Produces/Sells CE-marked Devices: N
Distribution: Exclusive Distributor

SUN BIOMEDICAL LABORATORIES, INC.   888-440-8388
604 Vpr Center, 1001 Lower Landing Road,   **856-401-1080**
Blackwood, NJ 08012
FDA Number: 2248645   Fax: 856-401-1090
E-mail: sales@sunbiomed.com
Web site: www.sunbiomed.com
Medical Products Sales Volume: $1,000,000
Annual Revenue: $5-$10 Million
Year Founded: 1993
Total Employees: 24
Ownership: Private
Stock Symbol: HGRLF
Traded On: Sydney
Quality System Registration Information: ISO9002
Produces/Sells CE-marked Devices: N
Federal Procurement Eligibility: Small Business
Distribution: Manufacturer Direct, Manufacturer Through Distributor, Manufacturer
Through Manufacturer Reps, OEM, Service Direct, Importer, Exporter
Mktg./Adv.: Ms. Tracey Natoli/Account Specialist
     Mrs. Kim McNally/Admin. Marketing & Sales
Production: Mrs. Alice Sun/Vice President Operations
Enzyme Immunoassay, Benzodiazepine   Toxicology
Enzyme Immunoassay, Cannabinoids   Toxicology
Immunoassay, Other   Toxicology
Kit, Pregnancy Test, Over The Counter, HCG   Chemistry
Kit, Test, Multiple, Drugs Of Abuse, Over The Counter   Toxicology
Test, Human Chorionic Gonadotropin, Serum   Immunology

SUN FABRICATIONS   916-635-3583
2660 Mercantile Dr., Suite A, Rancho Cordova, CA 95742
FDA Number: n/a
Ownership: Private
Produces/Sells CE-marked Devices: N
Booth, Sun Tan   Physical Med

SUN GLITZ CORP.   800-287-0911
111 S. McVicker Drive, Energy, IL 62933   **618-942-5915**
FDA Number: 1421974   Fax: 618-942-2168
E-mail: foambandage@yahoo.com
Web site: www.foambandage.com
Medical Products Sales Volume: $300,000
Year Founded: 1980
Total Employees: 1
Ownership: Private
Produces/Sells CE-marked Devices: N
Federal Procurement Eligibility: Small Business, Female Owned
Distribution: Manufacturer Direct, Manufacturer Through Distributor, Manufacturer
Through Manufacturer Reps, Exporter
General Admin.: Nola Janene McVicker/President
Bandage, Adhesive   Surgery

SUN MEDICAL, INC.   800-678-6633
2607 Aero Drive, Grand Prairie, TX 72052   **817-633-1373**
FDA Number: 1627662   Fax: 817-640-1840
E-mail: sunmed@sunmedicalinc.com
Web site: www.sunmedicalinc.com
Annual Revenue: $1-$5 Million
Year Founded: 1978
Total Employees: 8   Marketing Staff: 5   Sales Staff: 3
Ownership: Private
Produces/Sells CE-marked Devices: N
Federal Procurement Eligibility: Small Business
Distribution: Manufacturer Direct, Manufacturer Through Distributor, Manufacturer
Through Manufacturer Reps, Exporter
General Admin.: Stephen Polk/President
     Larry Adair/Vice President
Production: Stephen Polk/Manager Regulatory Affairs
Cannula, Suction, Uterine   Obstetrics/Gynecology
Extractor, Vacuum, Fetal   Obstetrics/Gynecology
Laser, Carbon-Dioxide, Surgical   Surgery
Service, Maintenance/Repair   General
System, Evacuation, Smoke, Laser   Surgery

SUN METAL PRODUCTS, INC.   219-267-3281
P.O. Box 1508, Warsaw, IN 46581-1508
FDA Number: n/a   Fax: 219-267-2446
E-mail: info@rims.com
Web site: www.sunmetal.com
Medical Products Sales Volume: $1,500,000
Annual Revenue: $10-$25 Million
Total Employees: 180   Marketing Staff: 1   Sales Staff: 4
Ownership: Private
Quality System Registration Information: ISO9001
Produces/Sells CE-marked Devices: N
Federal Procurement Eligibility: Small Business
Distribution: OEM
General Admin.: Robert M. Piecuch/President
Mktg./Adv.: J. Steven Music/Manager Marketing & Sales
Accessories, Wheelchair   Physical Med

SUN NUCLEAR CORP.   321-259-6862
425-a Pineda Court, Melbourne, FL 32940
FDA Number: 1038814
Accelerator, Linear, Medical   Radiology
Calibrator, Dose, Radionuclide   Radiology
Collimator, Therapeutic X-Ray, Orthovoltage   Radiology
Nuclear Magnetic Resonance Imaging System   Radiology
Probe, Uptake, Nuclear   Radiology
Source, Brachytherapy, Radionuclide   Radiology
Teletherapy System, Radionuclide   Radiology
Tester, Radiology   Radiology

SUN TECHNOLOGIES, INC.   (770) 643-0622
3700 Mansell Road,, Suite# 125, Alpharetta,, GA 30022
FDA Number: 3005831223   Fax: 770) 643-0623
Ownership: Private
Produces/Sells CE-marked Devices: N
Booth, Sun Tan   Physical Med

SUN-MED   800-433-2797
12393 Belcher Road, Suite #450, Largo, FL 33773   **727-530-7099**
FDA Number: 1036445   Fax: 727-531-3991
E-mail: info@sun-med.com
Web site: www.sunmedusa.com
Medical Products Sales Volume: $8,000,000
Annual Revenue: $5-$10 Million

SUN-MED
800-433-2797 *(cont'd)*

Total Employees: 22   Marketing Staff: 6   Sales Staff: 6
Ownership: Siemens Medical Solutions USA, Inc.
Produces/Sells CE-marked Devices: N
Federal Procurement Eligibility: Small Business
Distribution: Manufacturer Through Distributor
General Admin.: John King/General Manager
Sue Delaney/Manager
Sue Delaney/Office Manager
Barry L. Wall/President, Chief Executive Officer
Mktg./Adv.: Michael Mullinax/Director Advertising
Barry L. Wall/Director Marketing & Sales
Neal Meyers/Director New Product Development
Roger Hall/Vice President, Manager Sales
Production: Barry L. Wall/Manager Regulatory Affairs
Purchasing: Angel Dixon/Director Purchasing

Airway, Nasopharyngeal (Breathing Tube)	Anesthesiology
Airway, Oropharyngeal, Anesthesia	Anesthesiology
Bag, Breathing	Anesthesiology
Bandage, Adhesive	Surgery
Clip, Nose	Anesthesiology
Connector, Airway (Extension)	Anesthesiology
Flowmeter, Back-Pressure Compensated, Thorpe Tube	Anesthesiology
Flowmeter, Gas (Oxygen), Calibrated	Anesthesiology
Forceps	Orthopedics
Laryngoscope	Ear/Nose/Throat
Laryngoscope, Rigid	Anesthesiology
Mask, Gas, Anesthesia	Anesthesiology
Protector, Dental	Anesthesiology
Shield, Eye, Ophthalmic	Ophthalmology
Stethoscope, Esophageal	Anesthesiology
Stethoscope, Manual	Cardiovascular
Stethoscope, Mechanical	General
Stylet, Tracheal Tube	Anesthesiology
Transducer, Stethoscope	Anesthesiology
Tube, Tracheal (Endotracheal)	Anesthesiology

SUNBEAM PRODUCTS, INC.
601-671-2277
224 Russell Dr., Waynesboro, MS 39367

FDA Number: 3006162833
Ownership: Private
Produces/Sells CE-marked Devices: N

Pad, Heating, Powered	Physical Med

SUNBEAM PRODUCTS, INC.
561-912-4100
2381 Executive Center Dr., Boca Raton, FL 33431

FDA Number: 1043899
Web site: www.sunbeam.com
Ownership: Private
Produces/Sells CE-marked Devices: N

Analyzer, Body Composition	Cardiovascular
Bag, Ice	General
Bottle, Hot/Cold Water	General
Cuff, Blood Pressure	Cardiovascular
Humidifier, Non-Direct Patient Interface (Home-Use)	Anesthesiology
Monitor, Blood Pressure, Indirect, Semi-Automatic	Cardiovascular
Pack, Hot Or Cold, Disposable	Physical Med
Pack, Hot Or Cold, Reusable	Physical Med
Pad, Heating, Powered	Physical Med
Scale, Stand-On	General
Toothbrush, Powered	Dental And Oral

SUNBOX COMPANY
800-548-3968
19217 Orbit Dr., Gaithersburg, MD 20879
301-869-5980
Fax: 301-977-2281

FDA Number: n/a
E-mail: sunbox@aol.com
Web site: www.sunbox.com
Annual Revenue: $1-$5 Million
Year Founded: 1985
Total Employees: 12   Sales Staff: 3
Ownership: Private
Produces/Sells CE-marked Devices: N
Federal Procurement Eligibility: Small Business
Distribution: Manufacturer Direct, Manufacturer Through Distributor, Exclusive Distributor, Importer
General Admin.: Neal Owens/Chief Executive Officer
Frank Kall/General Manager

Light, Other	General

SUNCO LLC
901-412-7589
4187 Senator St., Memphis, TN 38118

FDA Number: 3005940264
Ownership: Private
Produces/Sells CE-marked Devices: N

Mattress, Non-Powered Flotation Therapy	Physical Med

SUNCOAST HEARING AIDS & REPAIR SERVICES
See Suncoast Laboratories

SUNCOAST LABORATORIES
714-229-9178
6888 Lincoln Ave. # G, Buena Park, CA 90620
Fax: 714-229-9187

FDA Number: 3004615749
Ownership: Private
Produces/Sells CE-marked Devices: N

Hearing Aid, Air Conduction, Transcutaneous System	Ear/Nose/Throat

SUNCOAST MEDICAL MANUFACTURING INC.
See Bovie Medical Corp.

SUNDANCE ENTERPRISES, INC.
317-831-6447
236 E. Washington St., Po. Box 146, Mooresville, IN 46158

FDA Number: 1836394

Cushion, Flotation	Physical Med

SUNDANCE SPAS, INC.
800-883-7727
14525 Monte Vista Avenue, Chino, CA 91710
909-606-7733
Fax: 909-606-0195

FDA Number: n/a
E-mail: info@sundancespas.com
Web site: www.sundancespas.com
Medical Products Sales Volume: $54,500,000
Annual Revenue: $50-$100 Million
Year Founded: 1998
Total Employees: 950   Marketing Staff: 5   Sales Staff: 5
Ownership: JACUZZI, INC.
Quality System Registration Information: ISO9001
Distribution: OEM
General Admin.: Jonathan Clark/President, Chief Executive Officer
Mktg./Adv.: Jerry Greer/Director Marketing & Sales
Rob Olney/Director Product Development
Patrick Kenny/Manager International & National Sales
Aim'ee Caudle/Manager Sales Training
Production: Steve Purcell/Vice President Manufacturing

Bath, Portable	General

SUNEVA MEDICAL, INC.
858-550-9999
5870 Pacific Center Blvd., San Diego, CA 92121

FDA Number: 3003707320
E-mail: info@sunevamedical.com
Web site: http://www.sunevamedical.com
Year Founded: 2009
Ownership: Private
Produces/Sells CE-marked Devices: N
General Admin.: Mr. Philip Ranker/Chief Financial Officer, Vice President
Mr. Niv Caviar/President, Chief Executive Officer
Medical Admin.: Dr. Lisa Misell/Director Clinical Affairs
Mktg./Adv.: Mr. Joseph Rudman/Vice President Sales
Production: Ms. Karon Morrell/Senior Vice President Regulatory Affairs

Cystoscope	Gastroenterology/Urology
Implant, Collagen, Dermal (Aesthetic Use)	Surgery

SUNFLOWER MEDICAL L.L.C.
888-321-3382
206 Jerrerson, Ellis, KS 67637
785-726-2486
Fax: 785-726-4131

FDA Number: 1954156
E-mail: sales@sunflowermedical.com
Web site: www.sunflowermedical.com
Medical Products Sales Volume: $3,040,000
Year Founded: 1998
Total Employees: 17
Ownership: Private
Produces/Sells CE-marked Devices: N
Federal Procurement Eligibility: Small Business, VA Contract
Distribution: Manufacturer Through Distributor

Mattress, Air Flotation	General

SUNGLASS INTERNATIONAL LLC
888-478-6764
71 Cypress St., Warwick, RI 02888

FDA Number: 3005042764
Ownership: Private
Produces/Sells CE-marked Devices: N

Lens, Spectacle/Eyeglasses, Non-Custom	Ophthalmology
Sunglasses (Including Photosensitive)	Ophthalmology

SUNI MEDICAL IMAGING, INC.
408-227-6698
6840 Via Del Oro, San Jose, CA 95119

FDA Number: 3003952803

System, X-ray, Extraoral Source, Digital	Radiology

SUNLITE PLASTICS, INC.
262-253-0600
W194 N11340 McCormick Dr., Germantown, WI 53022
Fax: 262-253-0601

FDA Number: 2128508
E-mail: info@sunliteplastics.com
Web site: www.sunliteplastics.com
Year Founded: 1946
Total Employees: 55   Marketing Staff: 1   Sales Staff: 6
Ownership: Private
Quality System Registration Information: ISO9001
Produces/Sells CE-marked Devices: N
Distribution: Manufacturer Direct

SUNLITE PLASTICS, INC.   262-253-0600 *(cont'd)*
General Admin.: Brant Stanford/President
Mktg./Adv.: Barbara Stanford/Vice President Business Development
Production: Julie Skowronski/Director Operations
    William Elesh/Manager Regulatory Affairs
Finance: John Feistel/Chief Financial Officer

Catheter, Multiple Lumen	Surgery
Contract Manufacturing	General
Polymer, Synthetic, Other	General
Tube, Blood Collection	Chemistry
Tube, Double Lumen For Intestinal Decompression	Gastroenterology/Urology
Tube, Drainage	Gastroenterology/Urology
Tube, Enema	Gastroenterology/Urology
Tube, Feeding	General
Tubing, Connecting	General
Tubing, Fluid Delivery	General
Tubing, Multi-Lumen	General
Tubing, Non-Conductive	General
Tubing, Non-Invasive	Surgery
Tubing, Other	General
Tubing, Plastic	General
Tubing, Polyethylene	General
Tubing, Polypropylene	General
Tubing, Polyvinyl Chloride	General
Tubing, Radiopaque	General
Tubing, Urethane	General
Tubing, Vinyl	General

SUNMED HEALTHCARE   727-531-7266
12393 Belcher Road, Suite 460, Largo, FL 33773
FDA Number: n/a   Fax: 727-489-5914
E-mail: info@sun-med.com
Web site: www.sunmedhealthcare.com
Annual Revenue: $5-$10 Million
Year Founded: 1980
Total Employees: 22
Ownership: Siemens Medical Solutions USA, Inc.
Produces/Sells CE-marked Devices: N
Federal Procurement Eligibility: Small Business
Distribution: Manufacturer Through Distributor
General Admin.: Mr. Randall Green/President
Mktg./Adv.: Mrs. Stella Lampl/International Marketing, Sales Associate

Adapter, Anesthesia	Anesthesiology
Airway, Nasopharyngeal (Breathing Tube)	Anesthesiology
Bag, Breathing	Anesthesiology
Block, Bite, Intubation	Anesthesiology
Bougie, Esophageal, ENT	Ear/Nose/Throat
Clip, Nose	Anesthesiology
Lamp, Laryngoscope	Ear/Nose/Throat
Laryngoscope	Ear/Nose/Throat
Laryngoscope, Flexible	Anesthesiology
Laryngoscope, Rigid	Anesthesiology
Mask, Gas, Anesthesia	Anesthesiology
Protector, Dental	Anesthesiology
Stimulator, Nerve, Anesthesia	Anesthesiology
Stimulator, Peripheral Nerve, Blockade Monitor	Anesthesiology
Strap, Head, Gas Mask	Anesthesiology
Stylet, Tracheal Tube	Anesthesiology
Support, Breathing Tube	Anesthesiology

SUNMED USA LLC.   310-531-8222
841 Apollo Street, Suite 334, El Segundo, CA 90245
FDA Number: 3005837148
Ownership: Private
Produces/Sells CE-marked Devices: N

Bandage, Adhesive	Surgery
Condenser, Heat And Moisture (Artificial Nose)	Anesthesiology
Gauze/sponge, Nonresorbable For External Use	Surgery
Mask, Oxygen, Non-Rebreathing	Anesthesiology

SUNMED, INC.
See Sunmedica

SUNMEDICA   530-229-1600
1661 Zachi Way, Redding, CA 96003
FDA Number: 1721819   Fax: 530-229-9457
E-mail: kathy@sunmedica.com
Web site: www.sunmedica.com
Medical Products Sales Volume: $400,000
Annual Revenue: $0-$1 Million
Year Founded: 1986
Total Employees: 6   Marketing Staff: 2   Sales Staff: 2
Ownership: Private
Quality System Registration Information: ISO9001
Produces/Sells CE-marked Devices: Y
Federal Procurement Eligibility: Small Business
Distribution: Manufacturer Direct, Manufacturer Through Distributor, Manufacturer Through Manufacturer Reps
General Admin.: Ronald M. Carn/President
    Pat Kinyon/Vice President, General Manager

SUNMEDICA   530-229-1600 *(cont'd)*

Contract Manufacturing	General
Splint, Extremity, Non-Inflatable, External	Surgery

SUNNEX BIOTECHNOLOGIES   877-778-6639
167 Lombard Ave., Suite 657,   204-956-2476
Winnipeg, MB R3B-0 Canada
FDA Number: n/a   Fax: 204-949-0627
E-mail: mwaldman@sunnexbiotech.com
Web site: www.sunnexbiotech.com
Year Founded: 1990
Total Employees: 5
Ownership: Private
Produces/Sells CE-marked Devices: N
Distribution: Manufacturer Direct, Manufacturer Through Distributor, Exporter

SUNNEX, INC.   800-445-7869
3 Huron Drive, Natick, MA 01760-1314   508-651-0009
FDA Number: 1226709   Fax: 508-651-0099
E-mail: sunnex@sunnex.com
Web site: www.sunnexonline.com
Medical Products Sales Volume: $5,600,000
Annual Revenue: $5-$10 Million
Year Founded: 2001
Total Employees: 24
Ownership: Private
Quality System Registration Information: ISO9002; ISO9003
Produces/Sells CE-marked Devices: Y
Federal Procurement Eligibility: Small Business
Distribution: Manufacturer Direct, Manufacturer Through Distributor, Manufacturer Through Manufacturer Reps
General Admin.: Lars-Arne. Lundholm/Chief Executive Officer
Mktg./Adv.: Jennifer Butler/Manager Marketing

Lamp, Examination (Light)	General
Lamp, Examination, Ceiling Mounted (Light)	General
Lamp, Other	General
Light, Surgical, Floor Standing	Surgery

SUNNYDALE INDUSTRIES, INC.   800-346-3515
6859 Audrain Road 9139,   573-682-2128
Centralia, MO 65240
FDA Number: 1419451   Fax: 573-682-2121
E-mail: sdale@socket.net
Web site: www.sunnydalegoss.com
Medical Products Sales Volume: $500,000
Annual Revenue: $0-$1 Million
Year Founded: 1980
Total Employees: 30   Marketing Staff: 1   Sales Staff: 1
Ownership: Private
Produces/Sells CE-marked Devices: N
Federal Procurement Eligibility: Small Business
Distribution: Manufacturer Through Distributor
General Admin.: Larry Stark/General Manager
Production: Andy Prevo/Manager Production

Tent, Mist	General
Tent, Oxygen (Canopy)	Anesthesiology
Tent, Pediatric Aerosol	General

SUNNYREC CORP.   310-638-4368
20505 Belshaw Ave., Carson, CA 90746
FDA Number: 2032280
Ownership: Private
Produces/Sells CE-marked Devices: N

Cushion, Wheelchair (Pad)	Physical Med

SUNOPTIC TECHNOLOGIES   877-677-2832
6018 Bowdendale Ave., Jacksonville, FL 32216   904-737-7611
FDA Number: 1035968   Fax: 904-733-4832
E-mail: sales.dept@sunoptictech.com
Web site: www.sunoptictech.com
Medical Products Sales Volume: $8,000,000
Annual Revenue: $5-$10 Million
Total Employees: 60   Marketing Staff: 1   Sales Staff: 3
Ownership: Private
Quality System Registration Information: ISO9001
Produces/Sells CE-marked Devices: Y
Federal Procurement Eligibility: Small Business
Distribution: Manufacturer Through Distributor, OEM, Service Direct, Exporter
General Admin.: Christopher Black/President, Chief Executive Officer
Mktg./Adv.: David Naylor/Director International Sales
    David Mutch/Vice President, Director Marketing
Production: Jose Galarza/Applications Engineer
    Janice Lee/Director Quality Assurance
    Eric VanDenhende/Managing Engineer

Accessories, Surgical Camera	Surgery
Cable, Fiberoptic	General
Camera, Television, Endoscopic (Without Audio)	Surgery
Fiberoptic Light Source & Carrier	Ear/Nose/Throat

SUNOPTIC TECHNOLOGIES 877-677-2832 *(cont'd)*

Handpiece, Fiberoptic	Dental And Oral
Headlight, ENT	Ear/Nose/Throat
Headlight, Fiberoptic Focusing	Gastroenterology/Urology
Illuminator, Fiberoptic (For Endoscope)	Gastroenterology/Urology
Illuminator, Fiberoptic, Surgical Field	Cns/Neurology
Lamp, Surgical, Xenon	Surgery
Light Source, Endoscope, Xenon Arc	Surgery
Light Source, Endoscopic	Obstetrics/Gynecology
Light Source, Fiberoptic, Routine	Gastroenterology/Urology
Light Source, Photographic, Fiberoptic	Gastroenterology/Urology
Light, Dental	Dental And Oral
Light, Fiberoptic, Dental	Dental And Oral
Light, Headband, Surgical	Surgery
Light, High Intensity	Radiology
Light, Surgical Headlight	Dental And Oral
Light, Surgical, Connector	Surgery
Light, Surgical, Endoscopic	Surgery
Light, Surgical, Fiberoptic	Surgery
Light, Surgical, Floor Standing	Surgery
Light, Surgical, Instrument	Surgery

SUNQUEST INFORMATION SYSTEMS, INC 520-570-2347
250 S. Williams Blvd, Tucson, AZ 85711
FDA Number: 2029302
E-mail: proposal@sunquestinfo.com
Ownership: Private
Produces/Sells CE-marked Devices: N

Computer, Chemistry Analyzer	Chemistry
Digital Image, Storage And Communications, Non-diagnostic, Laboratory Information System	Chemistry
System, Communication, Image, Digital	Radiology

SUNRIDGE INTERNATIONAL INC. 480-837-6165
16857 Saguaro Blvd, Fountain Hills, AZ 85268
FDA Number: n/a Fax: 480-837-6870
E-mail: info@sunridgeint.com
Ownership: Public
Stock Symbol: SNDZ
Traded On: OTC Bulletin
Produces/Sells CE-marked Devices: N

SUNRISE LABS, INC. 888-420-9600
5 Dartmouth Drive, Auburn, NH 03032 603-644-4500
FDA Number: n/a Fax: 603-622-9797
E-mail: info@sunriselabs.com
Web site: www.SunriseLabs.com
Medical Products Sales Volume: $2,300,000
Annual Revenue: $1-$5 Million
Year Founded: 1992
Total Employees: 27 *Marketing Staff:* 1 *Sales Staff:* 3
Ownership: Private
Produces/Sells CE-marked Devices: N
Federal Procurement Eligibility: Small Business
Distribution: Service Direct
General Admin.: Bruce Pierson/Chief Operating Officer
  Drew Sunstein/President

Service, Engineering/Design	General

SUNRISE MACHINE AND TOOL, INC. 218-847-3386
1380 Legion Rd., Detroit Lakes, MN 56501
FDA Number: 2132280

Chair, With Casters	Physical Med
Lift, Bath, Non-AC-Powered	General

SUNRISE MEDICAL 800-333-4000
7477 E. Dry Creek Pkwy., Longmont, CO 80503 303-218-4500
FDA Number: 9019832 Fax: 303-218-4590
E-mail: webmaster@sunmed.com
Web site: www.sunrisemedical.com
Medical Products Sales Volume: $267,400,000
Year Founded: 1983
Total Employees: 400 *Marketing Staff:* 20 *Sales Staff:* 100
Ownership: Private
Traded On: NASDAQ
Quality System Registration Information: ISO9001
Produces/Sells CE-marked Devices: N
Federal Procurement Eligibility: Small Business
Distribution: Manufacturer Through Distributor
General Admin.: Mr. Mike Hammes/Chief Executive Officer
Mktg./Adv.: Mrs. Kristin Mastin/Director Marketing
  Mr. Pieter Leenhouts/Vice President Marketing

Accessories, Walker	General
Accessories, Wheelchair	Physical Med
Aid, Living, Handicapped	General
Attachment, Oxygen Canister/IV Pole, Wheelchair	General
Bed, Adjustable Hospital	General
Bed, Electric, Home-Use	General
Bed, Manual	General

SUNRISE MEDICAL 800-333-4000 *(cont'd)*

Bedpan	General
Bedrail	General
Cannula, Nasal	General
Carrier, Container, Oxygen, Portable	General
Chair, Bath	General
Commode (Toilet)	General
Commode Seat	General
Communication Equipment	General
Computer, Patient Data Management	General
Concentrator, Oxygen	Anesthesiology
Continuous Positive Airway Pressure Unit (CPAP, CPPB)	Anesthesiology
Cushion, Ring, Foam Rubber	General
Cushion, Wheelchair (Pad)	Physical Med
Furniture, Patient Room	General
Humidifier, Heated	Anesthesiology
Humidifier, Non-Heated	Anesthesiology
Lift, Patient	General
Mask, Other	General
Mattress, Air Flotation	General
Mattress, Bed	General
Mattress, Reduction, Pressure	General
Nebulizer, Ultrasonic	Anesthesiology
Pad, Pressure, Foam (Elbow, Heel)	General
Pad, Pressure, Foam Convoluted	General
Rail, Bath	General
Rail, Commode	General
Table, Overbed	General
Transfer Device, Patient, Manual	General
Tray, Walker	General
Tube, Suction	General
Tubing, Oxygen Connecting	General
Unit, Control, Bed, Patient, Powered	General
Urinal	General

Medical Product Subsidiaries (Listed Separately)
Dynavox Systems Inc.

SUNRISE MEDICAL HHG INC 303-218-4505
2010 E Spruce Cir, Olathe, KS 66062
FDA Number: 3003460145

Accessories, Wheelchair	Physical Med
Belt, Wheelchair	Physical Med
Cushion, Wheelchair (Pad)	Physical Med
Support, Head And Trunk, Wheelchair	Physical Med
Tray, Wheelchair	Physical Med

SUNRISE MEDICAL HHG INC (800) 333-4000
2842 Business Park Avenue,
Fresno, CA 93727
FDA Number: 2937137
Ownership: Private
Produces/Sells CE-marked Devices: N

Accessories, Wheelchair	Physical Med
Belt, Wheelchair	Physical Med
Component, Wheelchair	Physical Med
Cushion, Flotation	Physical Med
Cushion, Wheelchair (Pad)	Physical Med
Protector, Skin Pressure	General
Support, Head And Trunk, Wheelchair	Physical Med
Tray, Wheelchair	Physical Med

SUNRISE MEDICAL HHG INC 303-218-4505
7128 Ambassasor Rd., Baltimore, MD 21244
FDA Number: 1123832 Fax: 303-218-4590
E-mail: Webmaster@Sunmed.com
Web site: www.sunrisemedical.com
Ownership: Private
Produces/Sells CE-marked Devices: N

Accessories, Wheelchair	Physical Med
Belt, Wheelchair	Physical Med
Chair, With Casters	Physical Med
Cushion, Wheelchair (Pad)	Physical Med
Support, Head And Trunk, Wheelchair	Physical Med
Transfer Device, Patient, Manual	General
Tray, Wheelchair	Physical Med

SUNRISE MEDICAL LTC.
See Joerns Healthcare, Inc

SUNRISE MEDICAL, INC. 800-333-4000
7477 E. Dry Creek Pkwy., Longmont, CO 80503
FDA Number: 1720745 Fax: 303-218-4590
Web site: www.sunrisemedical.com
Total Employees: 4000
Ownership: Private
Stock Symbol: SMD
Traded On: NYSE
Quality System Registration Information: ISO9000
Produces/Sells CE-marked Devices: N
Distribution: Manufacturer Direct, Manufacturer Through Distributor

Accessories, Wheelchair	Physical Med

SUNRISE MEDICAL, INC.　800-333-4000 *(cont'd)*

Bed, Electric	General
Bed, Manual	General
Cane	Physical Med
Commode (Toilet)	General
Component, Wheelchair	Physical Med
Concentrator, Oxygen	Anesthesiology
Continuous Positive Airway Pressure Unit (CPAP, CPPB)	Anesthesiology
Crutch	Physical Med
Cushion, Flotation	Physical Med
Cushion, Wheelchair (Pad)	Physical Med
Lift, Bath, Non-AC-Powered	General
Lift, Patient	General
Nebulizer, Direct Patient Interface	Anesthesiology
Oxygen	Anesthesiology
Protector, Skin Pressure	General
Rail, Bath	General
Scooter (Motorized 3-Wheeled Vehicle)	Physical Med
Walker, Mechanical	Physical Med
Wheelchair, Manual	Physical Med
Wheelchair, Powered	Physical Med

Medical Product Subsidiaries (Listed Separately)
Dynavox Systems Inc.
Joerns Healthcare, Inc
Norsk Hydro ASA
Norsk Medisinaldepot
Sopur Gmbh

SUNROC / TELKEE, INC.　800-478-6762
60 Starlifter Avenue, Kent County Aero Park,　302-678-7800
Dover, DE 19901
FDA Number: 7000737　　　　*Fax:* 302-678-7811
E-mail: lhorrocks@telkee.com
Web site: www.telkee.com
Medical Products Sales Volume: $500,000
Total Employees: 6
Ownership: Private
Produces/Sells CE-marked Devices: N
Federal Procurement Eligibility: Small Business
Distribution: Manufacturer Through Distributor
General Admin.: Anthony Salamone/President
Production: Mark Wood/Manager Production

Cabinet, Narcotic Control	General

SUNSCOPE INTL., INC.
See Biosensors International - Usa

SUNSHINE HEART, INC.　1 952 345 4200
7651 Anagram Dr, Eden Prairie, MN 55344
FDA Number: n/a
Web site: www.sunshineheart.com
Ownership: Private
Produces/Sells CE-marked Devices: N

SUNSTAR BUTLER　800-J BUTLER
4635 W. Foster Ave., Chicago, IL 60630-1709　773-777-4000
FDA Number: 1413787　　　　*Fax:* 773-777-5101
E-mail: web_support@jbutler.com
Web site: www.jbutler.com
Total Employees: 300
Ownership: Private
Quality System Registration Information: ISO9000
Produces/Sells CE-marked Devices: Y
Distribution: Manufacturer Direct, Manufacturer Through Distributor, Importer, Exporter
General Admin.: Mike Bava/President, Chief Operating Officer
Mktg./Adv.: Dennis Roy/Director Marketing
　　　　Lisa Smith/Director Marketing
　　　　Dan Descary/Vice President International Sales
　　　　John Hennessy/Vice President Marketing & Sales
　　　　Denny Eatherton/Vice President New Business
　　　　Mandy Chia/Vice President New Product Development
　　　　James Doyle/Vice President Sales
Production: John Shimkus/Vice President Operations
Finance: Richard McMahon/Chief Financial Officer, Vice President Finance

Brush, Scrub, Operating Room	Surgery
Cup, Prophylaxis	Dental And Oral
Dressing, Wound, Hydrogel W/out Drug And/or Biologic	Surgery
Floss, Dental	Dental And Oral
Kit, Plaque Disclosing	Dental And Oral
Mirror, Mouth	Dental And Oral
Pick, Massaging	Dental And Oral
Rinse, Oral, Antibacterial (by Physical Means)	Dental And Oral
Scraper, Tongue	Dental And Oral
Toothbrush, Manual	Dental And Oral
Toothbrush, Powered	Dental And Oral
Tray, Impression	Dental And Oral
Varnish, Cavity	Dental And Oral

SUNSTAR BUTLER　800-J BUTLER *(cont'd)*

Wax, Dental	Dental And Oral

SUNTECH MEDICAL, INC.　800-421-8626
507 Airport Boulevard, Suite 117,　919-654-2300
Morrisville, NC 27560
FDA Number: 1036863　　　　*Fax:* 919-654-2301
E-mail: Sales@SunTechMed.com
Web site: www.SunTechMed.com
Medical Products Sales Volume: $15,000,000
Annual Revenue: $10-$25 Million
Year Founded: 1980
Total Employees: 80
Ownership: SunTech Medical Group, Ltd.　UK
Quality System Registration Information: ISO9001
Produces/Sells CE-marked Devices: Y
Distribution: Manufacturer Direct, Manufacturer Through Distributor, Manufacturer Through Manufacturer Reps, OEM, Exporter
General Admin.: Dayn McBee/Chief Executive Officer
Mktg./Adv.: Mr. Kenneth Anderson/Director Marketing
　　　　Don WIldmon/Vice President Sales
Production: Mr. Keith Robinson/Vice President Customer Service
Research: David Gallick/Vice President Engineering

Monitor, Blood Pressure, Indirect, Automatic	Cardiovascular
Monitor, Physiological, Stress Exercise	Cardiovascular

SUPERDIMENSION INC.　800-387-9016
161 Cheshire Lane North, Suite 100,　763-210-4015
Minneapolis, MN 55441
FDA Number: 3004962788　　　　*Fax:* 866-706-9639
E-mail: info.us@superdimension.com
Web site: http://www.superdimension.com
Ownership: Private
Produces/Sells CE-marked Devices: N
General Admin.: Mr. Rick Buchholz/Chief Financial Officer, Vice President
　　　　Mr. Daniel Sullivan/President, Chief Executive Officer
Mktg./Adv.: Mr. Thomas Borillo/Vice President Sales
Production: Mr. Daniel Bulver/Vice President Operations
　　　　Mr. Jonathan Kuvach/Vice President Quality Control & Regulatory Affairs
Research: Mr. Jay Johnson/Vice President Research & Development

Forceps, Biopsy, Non-Electric	Gastroenterology/Urology
Needle, Aspiration And Injection, Disposable	Surgery
Scanner, Computed Tomography, X-Ray, Special Procedure	Radiology

SUPERIOR AUTOCATHETER ENTERPRISES　800-243-1467
2137 Vermillion Street, Suite 250,　651-437-7704
Hastings, MN 55033
FDA Number: 9310070　　　　*Fax:* 651-437-3277
E-mail: sac@webblake.net
Web site: http://sacguards.com/
Medical Products Sales Volume: $200,000
Year Founded: 1971
Total Employees: 2　　*Marketing Staff:* 2　　*Sales Staff:* 2
Ownership: Private
Produces/Sells CE-marked Devices: N
Federal Procurement Eligibility: Small Business, Female Owned, VA Contract
Distribution: Manufacturer Direct
General Admin.: Donald Eddy/Chief Executive Officer
Research: Barbara Eddy/Manager Research

Protector, Dental	Anesthesiology

SUPERIOR DENTAL
See Superior Dental & Test

SUPERIOR DENTAL & TEST
See Superior Dental & Test

SUPERIOR DENTAL / TT &
See Superior Dental & Test

SUPERIOR MEDICAL LIMITED　800-268-7944
520 Champagne Dr.,　416-635-9797
Toronto, ONT M3J 2 Canada
FDA Number: n/a　　　　*Fax:* 416-635-8931
E-mail: info@superiormedical.com
Web site: www.superiormedical.com
Year Founded: 1978
Total Employees: 20　　*Marketing Staff:* 3　　*Sales Staff:* 6
Ownership: Private
Produces/Sells CE-marked Devices: N
Distribution: Exclusive Distributor

SUPERIOR PRODUCTS, INC.　216-651-9400
3786 Ridge Rd., Cleveland, OH 44144
FDA Number: 1529989

Cannula, Nasal, Oxygen	Anesthesiology
Conserver, Oxygen	Anesthesiology
Flowmeter, Back-Pressure Compensated, Thorpe Tube	Anesthesiology

SUPERIOR PRODUCTS, INC.   216-651-9400 *(cont'd)*

Humidifier, Respiratory Gas, (Direct Patient Interface)	Anesthesiology
Nebulizer, Direct Patient Interface	Anesthesiology
Regulator, Pressure, Gas Cylinder	Anesthesiology
Regulator, Vacuum	General
Tubing, Flexible, Medical Gas, Low-Pressure	Anesthesiology
Unit, Filter, Membrane	Chemistry
Yoke, Medical Gas	Anesthesiology

SUPERIOR SURGICAL SUPPLY   610-622-0740
28 N. Lansdowne Ave., Lansdowne, PA 19050
FDA Number: n/a
Medical Products Sales Volume: $100,000
Annual Revenue: $0-$1 Million
Ownership: Private
Produces/Sells CE-marked Devices: N
Federal Procurement Eligibility: Small Business
Distribution: Manufacturer Through Distributor, OEM
General Admin.: Michael Thaete/President
Mktg./Adv.: Michael Thaete/Manager Advertising
            Michael Thaete/Vice President Marketing & Sales
Production: Michael Thaete/Vice President Manufacturing

Belt, Rib (Support)	Orthopedics
Bib	General
Strap, Restraining	General
Strap, Tracheostomy Tube	Anesthesiology
Support, Abdominal	Physical Med
Support, Hernia	Gastroenterology/Urology

SUPERIOR UNIFORM GROUP   727-397-9611
10055 Seminole Blvd., Seminole, FL 33772
FDA Number: 2431345
E-mail: info@superioruniformgroup.com
Web site: www.superioruniformgroup.com
Annual Revenue: $100-$500 Million
Year Founded: 1920
Total Employees: 525
Ownership: Public
Stock Symbol: SGC
Traded On: NASDAQ
Produces/Sells CE-marked Devices: N
General Admin.: Gerald M. Benstock/Chairman
            Michael Benstock/Chief Executive Officer
            Andrew D. Demott/Chief Financial Officer, Treasurer

Clothing, Protective	General

SUPERNOVA DIAGNOSTICS, INC   301-792-4345
20271 Goldenrod Lane, Suite 2028, Germantown, MD 20876
FDA Number: n/a
E-mail: ncampbell@supernovadiagnostics.com
Web site: www.supernovadiagnostics.com
Ownership: Private
Produces/Sells CE-marked Devices: N
General Admin.: Mr. Neil Campbell/President, Chief Executive Officer

SUPERQUAD, LLC   800-659-4548
8265 Sierra College Blvd, Suite 316,   916-791-0505
Roseville, CA 95661
FDA Number: 2951244   *Fax:* 916-791-0585
E-mail: sales@superquad.com
Web site: www.wijit.com
Medical Products Sales Volume: $600,000
Annual Revenue: $0-$1 Million
Year Founded: 1996
Total Employees: 7
Ownership: Private
Federal Procurement Eligibility: Small Business
Distribution: Manufacturer Direct

Accessories, Wheelchair	Physical Med

SUPERSCREW-SUPERSPRING CO.   800-494-7594
135 Stables Way, Highwood, IL 60040   1-847-266-8023
FDA Number: 1424160   *Fax:* 847-266-8024
E-mail: ssss@superscrewsuperspring.com
Web site: www.superscewsuperspring.com
Annual Revenue: $0-$1 Million
Year Founded: 1997
Total Employees: 2   *Marketing Staff:* 2   *Sales Staff:* 2
Ownership: Private
Produces/Sells CE-marked Devices: Y
Distribution: Manufacturer Direct, Manufacturer Through Distributor

Retainer, Screw Expansion, Orthodontic	Dental And Oral

SUPERSTAT CORP.   800-487-3786
2015 University Dr.,   310-605-1655
Rancho Dominguez, CA 90220
FDA Number: 2031101
E-mail: info@superstat.biz   *Fax:* 310-537-6141

SUPERSTAT CORP.   800-487-3786 *(cont'd)*
Web site: www.superstat.biz
Ownership: Private
Produces/Sells CE-marked Devices: N

Agent, Hemostatic, Non-Absorbable, Collagen-Based	Surgery

SUPERTECH, INC.   800-654-1054
P.O. Box 186, Elkhart, IN 46515-0186   574-264-4310
FDA Number: 9046422   *Fax:* 574-264-9551
E-mail: sales@supertechx-ray.com
Web site: www.supertechx-ray.com
Annual Revenue: $1-$5 Million
Year Founded: 1973
Total Employees: 5   *Marketing Staff:* 1   *Sales Staff:* 3
Ownership: Private
Produces/Sells CE-marked Devices: Y
Federal Procurement Eligibility: Small Business
Distribution: Manufacturer Direct, Manufacturer Through Distributor, Exporter
General Admin.: Mr. David B. McNitt/President, Chief Executive Officer
Mktg./Adv.: Ms. Judy McNitt-Mell/Vice President Marketing & Sales

Barrier, Control Panel, X-Ray, Moveable	Radiology
Calculator, Technique, Radiographic	Radiology
Computer Software	General
Computer, Radiographic Data	Radiology
Densitometer, Radiographic	Radiology
Filter, Radiographic	Radiology
Glove, Protective, Radiographic	Radiology
Magnet, Permanent, MRI (Magnetic Resonance Imaging)	Radiology
Phantom, Anthropomorphic, Radiographic	Radiology
Phantom, Mammographic	Radiology
Phantom, Radiotherapy	Radiology
Sensitometer, Radiographic	Radiology
Shield, Gonadal	Radiology
Shield, Magnetic Field	Radiology
Shield, Ophthalmic, Radiological	Radiology
Shield, Protective, Personnel	Radiology
Shield, X-Ray, Transparent	Radiology
Table, Surgical, Manual	General
Table, Ultrasound	General
Test Pattern, Radiographic	Radiology
Tester, Radiology Quality Assurance	Radiology

SUPERTECHS, INC.   301-309-6695
9610 Medical Center Dr., Suite 101, Rockville, MD 20850
FDA Number: 1124976

Reagents, Specific, Analyte	Hematology

SUPERTEX INDUSTRIAL, S.A. DE C.V.   656-65-57
Carretera a Bosques De San, Isidro # 1136,
Zapopan, Jalisco Mexico
FDA Number: 8030666

Glove, Patient Examination	General

SUPERTEX, INC.   800-222-9883
1235 Bordeaux Drive, Sunnyvale, CA 94089   408-222-8888
FDA Number: n/a   *Fax:* 408-222-4800
E-mail: prodinfo@supertex.com
Web site: www.supertex.com
Medical Products Sales Volume: $98,020,000
Annual Revenue: $50-$100 Million
Year Founded: 1976
Total Employees: 290   *Marketing Staff:* 11   *Sales Staff:* 7
Ownership: Public
Stock Symbol: SUPX
Traded On: NASDAQ
Quality System Registration Information: ISO9001
Produces/Sells CE-marked Devices: N
Federal Procurement Eligibility: Small Business
Distribution: Manufacturer Through Distributor, Manufacturer Through Manufacturer Reps, OEM, Exporter
General Admin.: Richard Siegel/Executive Vice President
            Carol Klemstein/Manager Human Resources
            Henry Pao/President, Chief Executive Officer
Mktg./Adv.: Brian Hedayati/Director Marketing
            Jim Adams/Manager Advertising
            Mr. Michael Lee/Vice President Design
            Mr. Dilip Kapur/Vice President Products
            Pete Petersen/Vice President Sales
Production: Mr. William Ingram/Vice President Production
Research: Ben Choy/Vice President Research & Development
IS: Mr. Franklin Gonzales/Vice President Technology

Component, Electrical	General

SUPPLEYES, INC.   800-727-3725
4890 Hammond Industrial Drive, Suite A,   678-455-0486
Cumming, GA 30041
FDA Number: n/a   *Fax:* 678-455-0491
E-mail: suppleyes@bellsouth.com

SUPPLEYES, INC.   800-727-3725 *(cont'd)*
Web site: www.suppleyes.net
Medical Products Sales Volume: $300,000
Annual Revenue: $0-$1 Million
Year Founded: 1999
Total Employees: 4
Ownership: Private
Produces/Sells CE-marked Devices: N
Federal Procurement Eligibility: Small Business
Distribution: Manufacturer Direct
General Admin.: Tom Hixon/Chief Executive Officer
    Darryl Archer/Office Manager
    Steve Richardson/President

Component, Paper	General
Light, Other	General

SUPPLIES INC.
See Suppleyes, Inc.

SUPPORO CANADA INC.   800-361-6857
9675 Papineau #175,   **514-384-4424**
Montreal, QUE H2B-3 Canada
FDA Number: n/a   Fax: 514-382-4868
E-mail: order@supporo.com
Web site: www.supporo.com
Year Founded: 1994
Total Employees: 25
Ownership: Private
Produces/Sells CE-marked Devices: N
Distribution: Manufacturer Direct

SUPPORT SYSTEMS INTERNATIONAL, INC.
See Hill-Rom Manufacturing, Inc.

SUPRACOR, INC.   800-787-7226
2050 Corporate Ct., San Jose, CA 95131   **408-432-1616**
FDA Number: 2951293   Fax: 408-432-1975
E-mail: bstern@supracor.com
Web site: www.supracor.com
Year Founded: 1982
Ownership: Private
Produces/Sells CE-marked Devices: Y
Distribution: Manufacturer Through Manufacturer Reps

Cover, Mattress	General
Cushion, Wheelchair (Pad)	Physical Med

SUPREME SCREW PRODUCTS, INC.   718-293-6600
1368 Cromwell Avenue, Bronx, NY 10452
FDA Number: 2435714   Fax: 718-293-6602
E-mail: sspnet@msn.com
Medical Products Sales Volume: $800,000
Annual Revenue: $0-$1 Million
Year Founded: 1963
Total Employees: 15
Ownership: Private
Produces/Sells CE-marked Devices: N
Federal Procurement Eligibility: Small Business, Minority Owned
Distribution: Manufacturer Direct

Screw, Fixation, Bone	Orthopedics

SURCO PRODUCTS   800-556-0111
RIDC Industrial Park, 292 Alpha Drive,   **412-252-7000**
Pittsburgh, PA 15238
FDA Number: n/a   Fax: 412-252-1005
E-mail: info@SURCO.com
Web site: www.surco.com
Annual Revenue: $0-$1 Million
Year Founded: 1948
Total Employees: 15   Marketing Staff: 4   Sales Staff: 4
Ownership: Private
Produces/Sells CE-marked Devices: N
Federal Procurement Eligibility: Small Business
Distribution: Manufacturer Through Distributor, Manufacturer Through Manufacturer Reps, OEM
General Admin.: Arnold Zlotnik/President
Mktg./Adv.: A. Howard/Director Marketing

Disinfector, Liquid	General
Solution, Ostomy, Odor Control	Gastroenterology/Urology

SURCO PRODUCTS, INC.
See Surco Products

SURE-LOK, INC.   866-787-3565
2501 Baglyos Circle, Bethlehem, PA 18020   **610-814-0300**
FDA Number: n/a   Fax: 610-814-0644
E-mail: info@sure-lok.com
Web site: www.sure-lok.com
Medical Products Sales Volume: $2,000,000
Annual Revenue: $10-$25 Million

SURE-LOK, INC.   866-787-3565 *(cont'd)*
Year Founded: 2005
Total Employees: 30
Ownership: Private
Quality System Registration Information: ISO9002
Produces/Sells CE-marked Devices: N
Federal Procurement Eligibility: Small Business
Distribution: Manufacturer Through Distributor
General Admin.: Robert Joseph/President
Mktg./Adv.: Ed Cardona/Director Product Development
    Jerry Crunk/Director Sales
    Sabrina Burdge/Marketing Associate
Production: Christine Roe/Manager Customer Services

Restraint	Physical Med
Restraint, Protective (Body)	General

SURE-TECH DIAGNOSTIC ASSOCIATES, INC.   314-894-8933
11040 Lin Valle Dr., Suite D, St. Louis, MO 63123
FDA Number: 1938095

Stain, Fetal Hemoglobin	Hematology

SUREFIRE MEDICAL, INC   888-321-5212
8601 Turnpike Drive, Suite 206,   **303-426-1222**
Westminster, CO 80031
FDA Number: n/a   Fax: 303-426-1223
Ownership: Private
Produces/Sells CE-marked Devices: N
General Admin.: Dr. James Chomas/Chief Executive Officer
Medical Admin.: Dr. Aravind Arepally/Chief Medical Officer
Mktg./Adv.: Mr. Stephen Cambridge/Vice President Sales

SUREHANDS LIFT & CARE SYSTEMS   800-724-5305
982 Rte. 1, Pine Island, NY 10969   **845-258-6500**
FDA Number: n/a   Fax: 845-258-6634
E-mail: info@surehands.com
Web site: www.surehands.com
Medical Products Sales Volume: $2,000,000
Annual Revenue: $1-$5 Million
Year Founded: 1976
Total Employees: 13   Marketing Staff: 1   Sales Staff: 38
Ownership: Private
Quality System Registration Information: ISO9000
Produces/Sells CE-marked Devices: N
Federal Procurement Eligibility: Small Business, GSA Contract, VA Contract
Distribution: Exclusive Distributor
General Admin.: Thomas F. Herceg/President, Chief Executive Officer
Mktg./Adv.: Joyce Moraczewski/Coord. Marketing
    Carol Colegrove/Coord. Sales
Production: Ellen Karnas/Customer Service Representative
IS: Ray Stramka/Tech. Specialist

Lift, Patient	General

SURGE MEDICAL SOLUTIONS, LLC.   616-977-2516
3710 Sysco Ct. S.e., Grand Rapids, MI 49512
FDA Number: 3003964340

Catheter, Vascular, Cardiopulmonary Bypass	Cardiovascular
Clamp, Surgical, General & Plastic Surgery	Surgery
Stool, Operating Room, Adjustable	Surgery
Stretcher, Hand-Carried	General
Suction Apparatus, Operating Room, Wall Vacuum-Powered	Surgery
Surgical Instrument, Cardiovascular	Cardiovascular

SURGI-AID ENDOSCOPICS, INC.   480-988-0916
3553 E. Wildhorse Dr., Gilbert, AZ 85297
FDA Number: 2025880
Ownership: Private
Produces/Sells CE-marked Devices: N

Biopsy Instrument, Mechanical, Gastrointestinal	Gastroenterology/Urology
Forceps, Biopsy, Bronchoscope (Non-Rigid)	Anesthesiology
Forceps, Biopsy, Bronchoscope (Rigid)	Anesthesiology
Forceps, Biopsy, Non-Electric	Gastroenterology/Urology

SURGI-VISION, INC.   949-900-6833
5 Musick, Irvine, CA 92618
FDA Number: 1125732   Fax: 949-900-6834
Year Founded: 1998
Ownership: Private
Produces/Sells CE-marked Devices: N
General Admin.: Steve Gorlin/Chief Executive Officer, Chairman
Finance: John Thomas/Chief Financial Officer

Coil, Magnetic Resonance, Specialty	Radiology
Drape, Surgical	Surgery
Holder, Head, Neurosurgical (Skull Clamp)	Cns/Neurology
Nuclear Magnetic Resonance Imaging System	Radiology
Sterotaxic Unit	Cns/Neurology

SURGIC AID, INC.   800-338-5213
37 Crystal Avenue, #287, Derry, NH 03038-1714   **603-437-6280**
FDA Number: 1219308

SURGIC AID, INC.   800-338-5213 (cont'd)

E-mail: mdsolutions@cs.com
Medical Products Sales Volume: $500,000
Annual Revenue: $0-$1 Million
Total Employees: 5   Marketing Staff: 1   Sales Staff: 2
Ownership: Private
Produces/Sells CE-marked Devices: N
Federal Procurement Eligibility: Small Business
Distribution: Manufacturer Through Distributor
General Admin.: Paul W. O'Reilly/President
Mktg./Adv.: Paul O' Reilly/Director National Accounts
        Paul O' Reilly/Manager International Marketing & Sales
        Paul O' Reilly/Manager National Sales
        Diana O'Reilly/Vice President Marketing
Production: Paul O' Reilly/Manager Regulatory Affairs

Dressing, Tracheostomy Tube	Ear/Nose/Throat
Dressing, Wound and Burn, Occlusive	Surgery
Gauze, Non-Absorbable, X-Ray Detectable (Internal Sponge)	Surgery
Sponge, Dissector	Pathology
Sponge, External, Neurological	Cns/Neurology
Sponge, Gauze	Dental And Oral
Sponge, Internal	Cns/Neurology
Sponge, Neuro	Cns/Neurology
Sponge, X-Ray Detectable	Surgery

SURGICA CORPORATION   800-979-5090

PO Box 723, #4, Pollock Pines, CA 95726   916-933-5056
FDA Number: 2953190   Fax: 916-933-5260
E-mail: surgica@surgica.com
Web site: www.surgica.com
Medical Products Sales Volume: $400,000
Year Founded: 1997
Total Employees: 5
Ownership: Private
Produces/Sells CE-marked Devices: N
Federal Procurement Eligibility: Small Business
Distribution: Manufacturer Through Manufacturer Reps, Exclusive Distributor

Device, Embolization, Artificial	Cns/Neurology

SURGICAL ACCESSORIES, INC.
See Signal Medical Corporation

SURGICAL APPLIANCE INDUSTRIES   800-888-0458

3960 Rosslyn Dr., Cincinnati, OH 45209-1195   513-271-4594
FDA Number: n/a   Fax: 800-309-9055
Web site: www.surgicalappliance.com
Annual Revenue: $25-$50 Million
Total Employees: 800
Ownership: Private
Produces/Sells CE-marked Devices: N
Federal Procurement Eligibility: Small Business
Distribution: Manufacturer Direct, Manufacturer Through Distributor
General Admin.: L. Thomas Applegate/Chief Executive Officer
Mktg./Adv.: Tim Faust/Manager International & National Sales
        Tim Pennington/Manager National Marketing & Sales
        Patrick Stinwell/Vice President Marketing

Bars, Spreader	Orthopedics
Belt, Rib (Support)	Orthopedics
Belt, Traction, Pelvic	Physical Med
Brace, Joint, Ankle (External)	Physical Med
Collar, Cervical Neck	Orthopedics
Halter, Head, Traction	Physical Med
Orthosis, Lumbosacral	Physical Med
Orthosis, Sacroiliac, Soft	Physical Med
Splint, Abduction, Shoulder	Orthopedics
Splint, Clavicle	Physical Med
Support, Ankle	Orthopedics
Support, Back	Orthopedics
Support, Hand	Orthopedics
Support, Knee	Physical Med
Support, Wrist	Physical Med
Truss, Hernia (Belt)	Gastroenterology/Urology

Medical Product Subsidiaries (Listed Separately)
Airway Division Of Surgical Appliance Industries, Inc.

SURGICAL APPLIANCE INDUSTRIES INC.
See Pcp Champion

SURGICAL APPLIANCES
See Surgical Appliance Industries

SURGICAL DESIGN CORP.   914-273-2445

3 Macdonald Ave., Armonk, NY 10504
FDA Number: 2428191   Fax: 914-273-2691
E-mail: info@surgical.com
Web site: www.surgicaldesign.com
Ownership: Private
Produces/Sells CE-marked Devices: N

Phacofragmentation Unit	Ophthalmology

SURGICAL EYE ENTERPRISE   636-282-2800

1763 Engle Dr., Arnold, MO 63010
FDA Number: 1933756
Ownership: Private
Produces/Sells CE-marked Devices: N

Forceps, Ophthalmic	Ophthalmology

SURGICAL IMPLANT GENERATION NETWORK (SIGN)   509-371-1107

451 Hills St., Richland, WA 99354
FDA Number: 3034525   Fax: 509-371-1316
E-mail: info@sign-post.org
Web site: www.sign-post.org
Ownership: Private
Produces/Sells CE-marked Devices: N

Awl	Orthopedics
Bit, Drill	Orthopedics
Cannula, Surgical, General & Plastic Surgery	Surgery
Clamp, Circumcision	Obstetrics/Gynecology
Extractor, Nail	Orthopedics
Gauge, Depth	Orthopedics
Guide, Surgical, Instrument	Surgery
Orthopedic Manual Surgical Instrument	Orthopedics
Probe	Orthopedics
Reamer	Orthopedics
Rod, Fixation, Intramedullary	Orthopedics
Screw, Fixation, Bone, Non-Spinal, Metallic	Orthopedics
Screwdriver	Orthopedics
Starter, Bone Screw	Orthopedics
Template	Orthopedics

SURGICAL IMPLANTS, INC.   941-366-1882

962 S. Tamiami Trail, Suite 203, Sarasota, FL 34236
FDA Number: 1833498   Fax: 941-366-1734
E-mail: surgicalimplants@aol.com
Annual Revenue: $0-$1 Million
Total Employees: 2
Ownership: Private
Produces/Sells CE-marked Devices: N
Federal Procurement Eligibility: Small Business
Distribution: Manufacturer Direct, Service Direct
General Admin.: Douglas W. Stuart/Chief Executive Officer

Service, Consulting	General

SURGICAL INFORMATION SYSTEMS, INC.   800-930-0895

**11605 Haynes Bridge Rd., Suite 200,   678-507-1610
Alpharetta, GA 30004**
FDA Number: 1057202   Fax: 678-507-1616
E-mail: sales@sisfirst.com
Web site: www.sisfirst.com
Ownership: Private
Produces/Sells CE-marked Devices: N
General Admin.: Mr. Edward Daih;/Chief Executive Officer
        Mr. Eric Nilsson/Chief Technology Officer
Mktg./Adv.: Mr. Kermit Randa/Senior Vice President Marketing & Sales
Production: Mr. Doug Rempfer/Senior Vice President Operations
Research: Mr. Bobby Roberts/Vice President Development
Finance: Mr. Bruce Duner/Chief Financial Officer
        Ms. Deborah Zumbado/Controller

Computer and Software, Medical	General

SURGICAL INSTRUMENT MANUFACTURERS, INC.   800-521-2985

1650 Headland Drive, St. Louis, MO 63026-2915   636-349-4960
FDA Number: 1935627   Fax: 636-326-2417
E-mail: info@surinst.com
Web site: www.simsurgical.com
Medical Products Sales Volume: $3,500,000
Annual Revenue: $0-$1 Million
Year Founded: 2001
Total Employees: 38   Marketing Staff: 1   Sales Staff: 2
Ownership: Private
Quality System Registration Information: ISO9000
Produces/Sells CE-marked Devices: N
Federal Procurement Eligibility: Small Business
Distribution: Manufacturer Direct
General Admin.: William Bartling/President

Cannula, Ophthalmic	Ophthalmology
Clip, Iris Retractor	Ophthalmology
Coagulator/Cutter, Endoscopic, Bipolar	Obstetrics/Gynecology
Curette, Ear	Ear/Nose/Throat
Curette, Nasal	Ear/Nose/Throat
Dilator, Lacrimal	Ophthalmology
Elevator, Surgical, General & Plastic Surgery	Surgery
Forceps, Ophthalmic	Ophthalmology
Hook, Ophthalmic	Ophthalmology
Hook, Surgical, General & Plastic Surgery	Surgery
Instrument, Microsurgical	Cns/Neurology

SURGICAL INSTRUMENT   800-521-2985 *(cont'd)*

Kit, Surgical Instrument, Disposable	Surgery
Knife, Ear	Ear/Nose/Throat
Knife, Ophthalmic	Ophthalmology
Needle, Suture, Ophthalmic	Ophthalmology
Retractor, Surgical	Surgery
Scissors, Ophthalmic	Ophthalmology
Spatula, Ophthalmic	Ophthalmology
Speculum, Ophthalmic	Ophthalmology
Surgical Instrument, Cardiovascular	Cardiovascular
Suture, Absorbable, Ophthalmic	Ophthalmology
Tube, Ear Suction	Ear/Nose/Throat

SURGICAL LASER TECHNOLOGIES, INC.   800-366-4758
147 Keystone Drive,   **215-619-3600**
Montgomeryville, PA 18936

FDA Number: n/a   *Fax:* 215-619-3208
E-mail: info@photomedex.com
Web site: www.photomedex.com
Medical Products Sales Volume: $16,000,000
Annual Revenue: $10-$25 Million
Year Founded: 1984
Total Employees: 100   *Marketing Staff:* 2   *Sales Staff:* 15
Ownership: Public
Stock Symbol: PHMD
Traded On: NASDAQ
Quality System Registration Information: ISO9001
Produces/Sells CE-marked Devices: Y
Federal Procurement Eligibility: GSA Contract, VA Contract
Distribution: Manufacturer Direct, Manufacturer Through Distributor, Manufacturer Through Manufacturer Reps, OEM, Service Direct, Exporter
General Admin.: Michael R. Stewart/President, Chief Executive Officer
Mktg./Adv.: Stewart Jaffe/Director Marketing
　　　　　Al Intintoli/Director Product Development
　　　　　E. Kevin Scanlon/Manager National Sales

Accessories, Laser	General
Accessories, Laser, Endoscopic	Surgery
ENT Manual Surgical Instrument	Ear/Nose/Throat
Instrument, Microsurgical	Cns/Neurology
Laser, Carbon-Dioxide, Surgical	Surgery
Laser, Diode, Laparoscopy	Surgery
Laser, Excimer, Surgical	Surgery
Laser, Nd:YAG, Laparoscopy	Surgery
Laser, Nd:YAG, Surgical	Surgery
Laser, Neodymium:YAG, Surgical, Gynecologic	Obstetrics/Gynecology
Laser, Surgical	Surgery
Laser, Surgical, Holmium	Surgery
Lithotriptor, Laser	Gastroenterology/Urology
Tip, Suction, Electrosurgical	Surgery

SURGICAL PRODUCTS SPECIALTIES   604-536-4000
1908 168th St., Surrey, BC V4P-2W7 Canada

FDA Number: n/a   *Fax:* 604-536-4032
E-mail: info@surgicalproducts.ca
Web site: http://surgicalproducts.ca
Year Founded: 1994
Total Employees: 10
Ownership: Private
Produces/Sells CE-marked Devices: N
Distribution: Exclusive Distributor, Importer

SURGICAL SAFETY PRODUCTS, INC.   800-953-7889
2018 Oak Terrace, Suite 400, Sarasota, FL 34231   **941-927-7874**

FDA Number: n/a   *Fax:* 941-925-0515
E-mail: donl@ssp-inc.com
Web site: www.ssp-inc.com
Annual Revenue: $0-$1 Million
Total Employees: 7   *Marketing Staff:* 3   *Sales Staff:* 2
Ownership: Public
Stock Symbol: SURG
Traded On: OTC Bulletin
Produces/Sells CE-marked Devices: N
Federal Procurement Eligibility: Small Business
Distribution: Manufacturer Direct, Manufacturer Through Distributor
General Admin.: Don Lawrence/Chief Operating Officer, Vice President
　　　　　Frank M. Clark/President, Chief Executive Officer
Mktg./Adv.: Leann Spofford/Director Marketing
　　　　　Mike Williams/Vice President Sales

Computer Software, Hospital/Nursing Management	General
Eyeglasses, Safety	Ophthalmology
Surgical Instrument, Disposable	Surgery

SURGICAL SERVICES
See Specialty Care

SURGICAL SPECIALTIES CORPORATION   800-523-3332
100 Dennis Drive, Reading, PA 19606   **610-404-1000**

FDA Number: 2522801   *Fax:* 610-404-4010
E-mail: info@surgicalspecialties.com

SURGICAL SPECIALTIES CORPORATION   800-523-3332 *(cont'd)*

Web site: www.surgicalspecialties.com
Medical Products Sales Volume: $25,100,000
Year Founded: 2003
Total Employees: 200
Ownership: Private
Quality System Registration Information: ISO9001
Produces/Sells CE-marked Devices: Y
Federal Procurement Eligibility: Small Business
Distribution: Manufacturer Through Distributor, Manufacturer Through Manufacturer Reps
General Admin.: Pete Molinaro/President
Mktg./Adv.: Steve Bryant/Vice President Sales

Suture, Absorbable	Surgery
Suture, Absorbable, Synthetic	Surgery
Suture, Non-Absorbable	Surgery
Suture, Non-Absorbable, Silk	Surgery
Suture, Non-Absorbable, Steel, Monofilament & Multifilament	Surgery
Suture, Non-Absorbable, Synthetic, Polyamide	Surgery
Suture, Non-Absorbable, Synthetic, Polyester	Surgery
Suture, Non-Absorbable, Synthetic, Polypropylene	Surgery
Wax, Bone	Surgery

SURGICAL SUPPLY SERVICE
See Medco Supply Company

SURGICAL TABLE SERVICES CO.   800-248-2382
526 South Main St., Akron, OH 44311   **330-253-7766**

FDA Number: n/a   *Fax:* 330-253-4374
E-mail: sts-co@lek.net
Web site: www.sts-co.net
Annual Revenue: $1-$5 Million
Ownership: STILLE
Produces/Sells CE-marked Devices: N
Federal Procurement Eligibility: Small Business
Distribution: Manufacturer Through Distributor, Manufacturer Through Manufacturer Reps, OEM, Importer

Table, Other	General

SURGICAL TABLE SERVICES COMPANY   330-253-7766
526 South Main St., Suite 701e, Akron, OH 44311

FDA Number: 3003917495

Table, Surgical, Electrical	Surgery

SURGICAL TABLES INCORPORATED   888-737-5044
2 Debush Avenue, Building A Unit 2, Middleton, MA 01949

FDA Number: 3004957.147

Table, Radiographic	Radiology

SURGICAL TECHNOLOGIES, INC.   800-777-9987
292 E. Lafayette Frontage Road,   **651-227-9953**
St. Paul, MN 55107

FDA Number: 2183319   *Fax:* 651-227-7859
E-mail: scanlanjoe@surgicaltechnologies.com
Web site: www.surgicaltechnologies.com
Medical Products Sales Volume: $400,000
Year Founded: 1981
Total Employees: 7
Ownership: Private
Produces/Sells CE-marked Devices: N
Federal Procurement Eligibility: Small Business
Distribution: OEM
General Admin.: Kenneth R. Blake/Vice President, General Manager
Mktg./Adv.: Mark J. Anderson/Manager Marketing Communications
　　　　　Joseph Scanlan/Vice President Business Development

Cleanroom Equipment	General
Contract Assembly	General
Contract Manufacturing	General
Contract Sterilization	General
Packaging Material	General
Service, Consulting	General
Service, Engineering/Design	General
Test, Equipment, Sterilization	General
Thermoforming, Extrusion, Custom	General

SURGICAL TECHNOLOGY LABORATORIES INC.   803-462-1714
610 Clemson Rd., Columbia, SC 29229

FDA Number: 1825527

Airway, Oropharyngeal, Anesthesia	Anesthesiology
Prosthesis, Chin, Internal	Surgery
Prosthesis, Nose, Internal	Surgery
Splint, Nasal	Ear/Nose/Throat

SURGICAL TOOLS, INC.   800-774-2040
1106 Monroe St., Bedford, VA 24523   **540-587-7193**

FDA Number: 1219153   *Fax:* 540-587-7197
E-mail: info@surgicaltools.com
Web site: www.surgicaltools.com
Annual Revenue: $1-$5 Million

SURGICAL TOOLS, INC.   800-774-2040 (cont'd)

Year Founded: 1995
Ownership: Private
Produces/Sells CE-marked Devices: N
Federal Procurement Eligibility: Small Business
Distribution: Manufacturer Direct, Manufacturer Through Manufacturer Reps, Service Direct, Exclusive Distributor, Importer

Accessories, Apparel, Surgical	Surgery
Blade, Scalpel	Surgery
Camera, Other	General
Container, Surgical Instrument	Surgery
General Medical Device	General
Headlight, Fiberoptic Focusing	Gastroenterology/Urology
Sponge, Other	General
System, Evacuation, Smoke, Laser	Surgery
Tray, Medicine	General

SURGICHIP, INC.   561-694-7776

4398 Hickory Dr., Palm Beach Gardens, FL 33418
FDA Number: 3004892065

Marker, Skin	Surgery

SURGICOUNT MEDICAL, INC.   951-587-6201

43460 Ridge Park Drive Suite 140, Temecula, CA 92590
FDA Number: 3005868511
Ownership: Private
Produces/Sells CE-marked Devices: N

Counter, Sponge, Surgical	Surgery

SURGIDEV CORP.

See Advanced Vision Science

SURGIDYNE, INC.

See Aspen Surgical

SURGIKOS, INC.

See Johnson & Johnson Medical Division Of Ethicon, Inc.

SURGILIGHT, INC.   407-482-4555

23 Alafaya Woods Blvd., Box 170, Oviedo, FL 32765
FDA Number: 1061914   Fax: 407-482-0505
E-mail: surgilightsales@aol.com
Web site: www.surgilight.com
Annual Revenue: $1-$5 Million
Total Employees: 10
Ownership: Public
Stock Symbol: SLGT
Traded On: OTC Bulletin
Produces/Sells CE-marked Devices: Y
General Admin.: Dr. Colette Cozean/Chief Executive Officer, Chairman
            Mr. Timothy Shea/President, Chief Operating Officer

Laser, Surgical	Surgery

SURGIMARK, INC.   800-228-1186

2516 W Washington Avenue, Yakima, WA 98903   509-965-1911
FDA Number: 3023415   Fax: 509-965-4852
Web site: www.surgimark.com
Medical Products Sales Volume: $600,000
Year Founded: 1983
Total Employees: 4
Ownership: Private
Federal Procurement Eligibility: Small Business, Female Owned
Distribution: Manufacturer Direct
General Admin.: Barbara Yarger/President

Aspirator, Surgical	Surgery
Kit, Incision And Drainage	Surgery

SURGIMEDICS   800-840-9906

2950 Mechanic St., Lake City, PA 16423
FDA Number: 3003640911   Fax: 814-774-0778
Web site: www.surgimedics.com
Ownership: Private
Produces/Sells CE-marked Devices: N

Bottle, Collection, Vacuum (Aspirator)	General
Exhaust System, Surgical	Surgery
Mask, Surgical	Surgery
Regulator, Vacuum	General
Tube, Smoke Removal, Endoscopic	Gastroenterology/Urology
Tubing, Non-Invasive	Surgery

SURGIMEDICS/TMP

See Novosci Corp.

SURGIN SURGICAL INSTRUMENTATION, INC.   800-753-7400
(SURGIN INC.)

37 Shield, Irvine, CA 92618   714-832-6300
FDA Number: 2023739   Fax: 714-832-0300
E-mail: surgin@surgin.com
Web site: www.surgin.com
Medical Products Sales Volume: $4,900,000
Year Founded: 1981

SURGIN SURGICAL INSTRUMENTATION, INC.   800-753-7400
(cont'd)

Total Employees: 55
Ownership: Private
Quality System Registration Information: ISO9001
Produces/Sells CE-marked Devices: Y
Federal Procurement Eligibility: Small Business
Distribution: Manufacturer Direct, Manufacturer Through Distributor, Manufacturer Through Manufacturer Reps, OEM, Exclusive Distributor, Exporter
General Admin.: Mr. Armand Maaskamp/President

Frame, Spectacle (Eyeglasses)	Ophthalmology
Keratome, AC-Powered	Ophthalmology
Staple, Implantable	Surgery
Stopcock	General
Tubing, Irrigation	Surgery
Tubing, Non-Invasive	Surgery

SURGIQUEST, INC.   203-799-2400

12 Cascade Blvd., Suite 2b, Orange, CT 06477
FDA Number: 3006217371   Fax: 203-799-2401
E-mail: information@surqiquest.com
Web site: http://www.surqiquest.com
Year Founded: 2006
Ownership: Private
Produces/Sells CE-marked Devices: N
General Admin.: Mr. Kurt Azarbarzin/Chief Executive Officer
Mktg./Adv.: Mr. Carlos Babini/Executive Vice President Marketing & Sales
            Ms. Jane Ann Zavalishin/Manager Business
Production: Mr. Dan Donovan/Director Operations
Finance: Mr. David Hildenbrand/Vice President Finance, Controller

Laparoscope, General & Plastic Surgery	Surgery
Laparoscope, General & Plastic Surgery, Reprocessed	Gastroenterology/Urology

SURGISTAR INC.   800-995-7086

2310 La Mirada Dr., Vista, CA 92081   760-598-2480
FDA Number: 2028661   Fax: 760-598-2481
E-mail: info@surgistar.com
Web site: www.surgistar.com
Medical Products Sales Volume: $8,000,000
Annual Revenue: $5-$10 Million
Year Founded: 1992
Ownership: Private
Quality System Registration Information: ISO9001
Produces/Sells CE-marked Devices: N
Distribution: Manufacturer Direct, Manufacturer Through Distributor, OEM, Exclusive Distributor

Cannula, Suprapubic, With Trocar	Gastroenterology/Urology
Drum, Eye Knife Test	Ophthalmology
Knife, Ophthalmic	Ophthalmology
Knife, Surgical	Dental And Oral
Trocar, Cardiovascular	Cardiovascular
Trocar, ENT	Ear/Nose/Throat
Trocar, Gastro-Urology	Gastroenterology/Urology
Trocar, Laryngeal	Ear/Nose/Throat
Trocar, Other	General
Trocar, Sinus	Ear/Nose/Throat
Trocar, Tracheal	Ear/Nose/Throat

Medical Product Subsidiaries (Listed Separately)
Sterilab Inc.

SURGITECH INC.   800-443-7563

1211 West Vista Way, Vista, CA 92083   760-477-8191
FDA Number: 2032723   Fax: 760-758-9587
E-mail: Admin@SurgiTechinc.com
Web site: www.surgitechinc.com
Ownership: Private
Produces/Sells CE-marked Devices: N

Orthosis, Cervical-Thoracic, Rigid	Physical Med
Orthosis, Limb Brace	Physical Med
Orthosis, Lumbar	Physical Med
Unit, Therapy, Current, Interferential	Cns/Neurology

SURGITREND LTD.

See Shippert Medical Technologies Corp.

SURMET CORP.   800-262-8783

31 B St., Burlington, MA 01803   781-272-8250
FDA Number: n/a   Fax: 781-272-9185
E-mail: lmgoldman@surmet.com
Web site: www.surmet.com
Annual Revenue: $1-$5 Million
Total Employees: 15   Sales Staff: 3
Ownership: Private
Produces/Sells CE-marked Devices: N
Federal Procurement Eligibility: Small Business, Minority Owned
Distribution: Manufacturer Direct, OEM, Service Direct
General Admin.: Suri A. Sastri/President, Chief Executive Officer
            Richard Cooke/Vice President
Research: Richard Cooke/Vice President Research & Development

SURMET CORP.
800-262-8783 (cont'd)
Service, Device Coating, Protective | General

SURMODICS, INC.
866-787-6639
9924 W. 74th St., Eden Prairie, MN 55344-3523 | 952-500-7000
FDA Number: 3001374820 | Fax: 952-500-7001
E-mail: info@surmodics.com
Web site: www.surmodics.com
Annual Revenue: $50-$100 Million
Year Founded: 1979
Total Employees: 225   Marketing Staff: 3   Sales Staff: 4
Ownership: Public
Stock Symbol: SRDX
Traded On: NASDAQ
Quality System Registration Information: ISO9001
Produces/Sells CE-marked Devices: Y
Federal Procurement Eligibility: Small Business
Distribution: Manufacturer Direct, Manufacturer Through Distributor, Manufacturer Through Manufacturer Reps, OEM
General Admin.: Mr. Gary Maharaj/Chief Executive Officer
    Mr. Phil Ankeny/Chief Financial Officer, Vice President
    Dr. Arthur Tipton/Chief Scientific Officer, Senior Vice President
    Jan Webster/Vice President Human Resources
Mktg./Adv.: Mr. Charlie Olson/Senior Vice President Business Development
    Mr. Brian Robey/Senior Vice President Product Development
    Mr. Joseph Stitch/Vice President Corporate Development

Enzyme Immunoassay, Other	Chemistry
Equipment, Device Coating, Protective	General
Reagent, Other	General
Service, Device Coating, Protective	General

SUROS SURGICAL SYSTEMS, INC
877-887-8767
6100,6110,6120 Technology Center Drive, Indianapolis, IN 46278
FDA Number: 3003862400
E-mail: info@hologic.com
Web site: www.hologic.com
Ownership: Hologic, Inc.
Stock Symbol: HOLX
Traded On: NASDAQ
Produces/Sells CE-marked Devices: N

Biopsy Instrument	Gastroenterology/Urology
Guide, Surgical, Needle	Surgery
Marker, Radiographic, Implantable	Surgery
Radiographic Unit, Diagnostic, Mammographic	Radiology

SURVIVAL TECHNOLOGY, INC.
See Meridian Medical Technologies

SUTER DENTAL MANUFACTURING COMPANY, INC.
800-368-8376
632 Cedar St., Chico, CA 95928-5015 | 530-893-8376
FDA Number: 2923282 | Fax: 530-893-0473
E-mail: info@suterdental.com
Web site: www.suterdental.com
Year Founded: 1929
Total Employees: 12
Ownership: Private
Produces/Sells CE-marked Devices: Y
Federal Procurement Eligibility: Small Business
Distribution: Manufacturer Direct, Manufacturer Through Distributor, Exporter
Mktg./Adv.: Mark O. Ziemkowski/Director Marketing

Burnisher, Operative, Dental	Dental And Oral
Carver, Dental Amalgam, Operative	Dental And Oral
Carver, Wax, Dental	Dental And Oral
Chisel, Bone, Surgical	Dental And Oral
Condenser, Amalgam And Foil, Operative	Dental And Oral
Curette, Periodontic	Dental And Oral
Cutter, Operative	Dental And Oral
Excavator, Dental, Operative	Dental And Oral
Explorer, Operative	Dental And Oral
File, Margin Finishing, Operative	Dental And Oral
File, Periodontic	Dental And Oral
Filling, Instrument Plastic, Dental	Dental And Oral
Gauge, Depth, Instrument, Dental	Dental And Oral
Handle, Instrument, Dental	Dental And Oral
Hoe, Periodontic	Dental And Oral
Instrument, Dental, Manual	Dental And Oral
Knife, Margin Finishing, Operative	Dental And Oral
Probe, Periodontic	Dental And Oral
Scaler, Periodontic	Dental And Oral
Sharpener, Dental	Dental And Oral

SUTURA, INC.
714-437-9801
17080 Newhope St., Fountain Valley, CA 92708
FDA Number: 2031768
Ownership: Public
Stock Symbol: SUTU
Traded On: OTC Bulletin

SUTURA, INC.
714-437-9801 (cont'd)
Produces/Sells CE-marked Devices: N

Instrument, Passing, Ligature, Knot Tying	Cns/Neurology
Laparoscope, General & Plastic Surgery	Surgery
Suture, Non-Absorbable, Synthetic, Polyethylene	Surgery
Unit, Sanitation/Sterilization, Toothbrush, Ultraviolet	Dental And Oral

SUTURTEK INCORPORATED
978-251-8088
51 Middlesex St., N. Chelmsford, MA 01863
FDA Number: 3003683512 | Fax: 978-251-8585
E-mail: info@SuturTek.com
Web site: www.suturtek.com
Ownership: Private
Produces/Sells CE-marked Devices: N

Guide, Surgical, Needle	Surgery
Instrument, Passing, Ligature, Knot Tying	Cns/Neurology
Needle, Suture, Disposable	Surgery
Suture, Absorbable, Natural	Surgery
Suture, Non-Absorbable, Steel, Monofilament & Multifilament	Surgery
Tray, Surgical Instrument	Surgery

SV LIFE SCIENCES
617-367-8100
60 State Street, Suite 3650, Boston, MA 02109
FDA Number: n/a | Fax: 617-367-1590
E-mail: info@svlsa.com
Web site: http://www.svlsa.com
Year Founded: 1993
Ownership: Private
Produces/Sells CE-marked Devices: N
General Admin.: Mr. James Garvey/Chairman, Chief Executive Officer
    Ms. Denise Marks/Chairman, Chief Financial Officer
    Mr. Paul Wallace/Partner

SVELTE MEDICAL SYSTEMS INC.
908-264-2194
675 Central Avenue, Suite 2, New Providence, NJ 07974
FDA Number: n/a | Fax: 908-728-9981
E-mail: info@sveltemedical.com
Web site: www.sveltemedical.com
Year Founded: 2007
Ownership: Private
Produces/Sells CE-marked Devices: N
General Admin.: Mr. Mark Pomeranz/President, Chief Executive Officer
   Medical Admin.: Ms. Michele Snyder/Director Clinical Affairs
Mktg./Adv.: Mr. William Easterbrook/Director Product Development
    Mr. Tim Shannon/Vice President Marketing & Sales
Production: Mr. Mark Kielek/Vice President Quality Assurance
Finance: Mr. Michael Johnson/Chief Financial Officer

Stent, Cardiovascular	Cardiovascular

SWANK OPTICAL CO.
See Marcolin Usa

SWB ELBOW BRACE, LTD.
760-564-9853
56059 Winged Foot, La Quinta, CA 92253
FDA Number: n/a | Fax: 760-564-9981
E-mail: swbelbow@dc.rr.com
Web site: www.swbelbow.com
Year Founded: 1987
Ownership: Private
Produces/Sells CE-marked Devices: N
Federal Procurement Eligibility: Small Business, Female Owned
Distribution: Manufacturer Direct
General Admin.: Shirley W. Hays/Owner, General Manager

Immobilizer, Elbow	Orthopedics
Support, Elbow	Orthopedics

SWEAT CHIROPRACTIC CLINIC
770-457-4430
3288 Chamblee Tucker Road, Atlanta, GA 30341
FDA Number: 1039671 | Fax: 770-454-8328
E-mail: drmattsweat@sweatinstitute.com
Web site: www.sweatinstitute.com
Ownership: Private
Produces/Sells CE-marked Devices: N
General Admin.: Dr. Roy Sweat/Chief Executive Officer
    Ms. Tina Shotts/Office Manager
Finance: Ms. Tecla Sweat/Chief Financial Officer

Percussor	Cns/Neurology

SWEDE-O, INC.
651-674-8301
6459 Ash St., Branch, MN 55056
FDA Number: 3000138370

Brace, Joint, Ankle (External)	Physical Med

SWEET COMPUTER SERVICES, INC.
See Ortivus

SWEN SONIC CORP.
See Blue Wave Ultrasonics

SWENSON CANADA INC.   800-561-2863
80 Orfus Rd., Toronto, ONT M6A-1M1 Canada   416-787-4500
FDA Number: n/a   Fax: 416-787-0551
E-mail: sales@swenson-ca.com
Web site: www.swenson-ca.com
Year Founded: 1922
Total Employees: 50
Ownership: Private
Produces/Sells CE-marked Devices: N
Distribution: Manufacturer Direct

SWISS AMERICAN PRODUCTS, INC.   800-633-8872
2055 Luna Rd., Ste. 126, Carrollton, TX 75006
FDA Number: 1649690
   Dressing, Other   General
   Dressing, Wound and Burn, Hydrogel   Surgery

SWISS IMPLANTS, INC.   805-781-8700
3046 South Higuera Street, Suite E, San Luis Obispo, CA 93401
FDA Number: 2032531
Ownership: Private
Produces/Sells CE-marked Devices: N
   Abutment, Implant, Dental, Endosseous   Dental And Oral

SWISS NF METALS INC.   800-387-5031
461 Alden Road, Unit 26 & 27,   416-510-2220
Markham, ONT M3B-3 Canada
FDA Number: n/a   Fax: 416-510-2207
E-mail: info@swissnf.com
Web site: www.swissnf.com
Year Founded: 1979
Total Employees: 10
Ownership: Private
Produces/Sells CE-marked Devices: N
Distribution: Exclusive Distributor

SWISSLOG TRANSLOGIC CORPORATION   800-525-1841
10825 E. 47th Ave., Denver, CO 80239-2913   303-371-7770
FDA Number: n/a   Fax: 303-373-7932
E-mail: healthcare@swisslog.com
Web site: www.translogic-corp.com
Medical Products Sales Volume: $50,000,000
Total Employees: 291   *Marketing Staff:* 4   *Sales Staff:* 17
Ownership: Private
Produces/Sells CE-marked Devices: N
Federal Procurement Eligibility: Small Business
Distribution: Manufacturer Direct
General Admin.: Charles Kegley/Chief Executive Officer
Mktg./Adv.: Craig Swank/Manager Marketing
     Nancy Warehime/Marketing Associate
     Bjorn Berg/Vice President Business Development
     Paul Collings/Vice President International Sales
     Jim Patrician/Vice President Marketing & Sales
Production: Dennis McWherter/Manager Production
   Bag, Plastic   General
   Computer Equipment   General
   Computer Software   General
   Conveyor, Guided Vehicle   General
   Delivery System, Pneumatic Tube   General
   Elevator, Other   General

SWISSRAY AMERICA, INC.   908 353 0971
One Tower Center Blvd., East Brunswick, NJ 08816
FDA Number: n/a   Fax: 908 353 1237
E-mail: info@swissray.com
Web site: www.swissray.com
Medical Products Sales Volume: $18,000,000
Annual Revenue: $10-$25 Million
Total Employees: 60   *Marketing Staff:* 6   *Sales Staff:* 18
Ownership: Swissray International, Inc.
Quality System Registration Information: ISO9001; ISO9002
Produces/Sells CE-marked Devices: Y
Federal Procurement Eligibility: Small Business
Distribution: Manufacturer Direct, Manufacturer Through Distributor, Manufacturer Through Manufacturer Reps, OEM
General Admin.: Ueli Laupper/Chief Executive Officer
     Mike Baker/Vice President, General Manager
Mktg./Adv.: Steve Barrlaski/Manager Contract Sales
     Andreas C. Keller/Vice President Business Development
   Radiographic Unit, Diagnostic   Radiology
   Radiographic Unit, Digital   Radiology

SWISSRAY CORPORATION
See Swissray America, Inc.

SWISSRAY EMPOWER, INC.
See Medimaging Tecnology, Inc.

SWISSRAY INTERNATIONAL (HQ) INC.   908-353-0971
One Tower Center Blvd., East Brunswick, NJ 08816
FDA Number: 3031197   Fax: 908-353-1237
E-mail: info@swissray.com
Web site: www.swissray.com
Year Founded: 1968
Total Employees: 126
Ownership: Private
Produces/Sells CE-marked Devices: Y
General Admin.: Terry Ross/Chief Executive Officer, Chairman
     Ruedi Laupper/President, Director
     Josef Laupper/Secretary
     Ueli Laupper/Vice President
Finance: Michael Laupper/Chief Financial Officer
Medical Product Subsidiaries (Listed Separately)
Swissray International, Inc.

SWISSRAY MEDICAL SYSTEMS INC.
See Swissray America, Inc.

SWISSTECH
See Nypro Inc.

SWIVELIER CO., INC.   845-353-1455
600 Bradley Hill Rd., Blauvelt, NY 10913-1187
FDA Number: 9201037   Fax: 845-353-1512
E-mail: info@swivelier.com
Web site: www.swivelier.com
Year Founded: 1947
Total Employees: 100
Ownership: Private
Produces/Sells CE-marked Devices: N
Federal Procurement Eligibility: Small Business
Distribution: Manufacturer Through Distributor
General Admin.: Michael Schwartz/President
Mktg./Adv.: Michael Schwartz/Manager Sales
Production: Gerry Phelan/Vice President Manufacturing
   Lamp, Examination (Light)   General
   Light, Overbed   General
   Light, Surgical, Ceiling Mounted   Surgery

SYBRON CORP., ANALYTICAL PRODUCTS DIV.
See Servomex

SYBRON CORP./MEDIATECH DIV.
See Mediatech, Inc.

SYBRON DENTAL SPECIALTIES, INC.   800-537-7824
1717 W. Collins Ave, Orange, CA 92867   714-516-7400
FDA Number: n/a
E-mail: frances.zee@sybrondental.com
Web site: http://www.sybrondental.com
Ownership: Public
Produces/Sells CE-marked Devices: Y
Distribution: Manufacturer Through Distributor, Manufacturer Through Manufacturer Reps, OEM, Importer, Exporter
   Aligner, Bracket, Orthodontic   Dental And Oral
   Band, Elastic, Orthodontic   Dental And Oral
   Band, Material, Orthodontic   Dental And Oral
   Band, Preformed, Orthodontic   Dental And Oral
   Bracket, Metal, Orthodontic   Dental And Oral
   Cement, Dental   Dental And Oral
   Clamp, Wire, Orthodontic   Dental And Oral
   Headgear, Extraoral, Orthodontic   Dental And Oral
   Hemostat, Surgical   Dental And Oral
   Material, Impression   Dental And Oral
   Pliers, Orthodontic   Dental And Oral
   Pusher, Band, Orthodontic   Dental And Oral
   Retainer, Screw Expansion, Orthodontic   Dental And Oral
   Scissors, Collar And Crown   Dental And Oral
   Setter, Band, Orthodontic   Dental And Oral
   Toothbrush, Manual   Dental And Oral
   Tube, Orthodontic   Dental And Oral
   Tucker, Ligature, Orthodontic   Dental And Oral
   Wax, Dental   Dental And Oral
   Wire, Orthodontic   Dental And Oral
Medical Product Subsidiaries (Listed Separately)
Allesee Orthodontic Appliances
Allesee Orthodontic Appliances (Calexico)
Allesee Orthodontic Appliances, Inc. - Connecticut
Attachments International, Inc.
Kerr Corp.
Kerrhawe Sa
Metrex Research Corp.
Ormco Corp.

SYBRONENDO   800-346-3636
1717 W. Collins Ave., Orange, CA 92867
FDA Number: n/a   Fax: 714-516-7911
Web site: www.sybronendo.com
Medical Products Sales Volume: $10,000,000

SYBRONENDO
800-346-3636 *(cont'd)*
Annual Revenue: $10-$25 Million
Ownership: Public
Stock Symbol: DHR
Traded On: NYSE
Quality System Registration Information: ISO9000
Produces/Sells CE-marked Devices: N
Federal Procurement Eligibility: Small Business
Distribution: Manufacturer Direct, Exclusive Distributor, Exporter

Electrocautery Unit, Line-Powered	Surgery
Gutta Percha	Dental And Oral
Reamer, Pulp Canal, Endodontic	Dental And Oral
Tester, Pulp	Dental And Oral
Wax, Dental	Dental And Oral

SYLVAN CORP.
800-628-3836
32 Billot Avenue, N. Huntingdon, PA 15642
724-864-9350
FDA Number: 9000618
Fax: 724-864-7138
E-mail: sylmed@capslock.net
Web site: WWW.SYLVANMEDICAL.COM
Annual Revenue: $0-$1 Million
Year Founded: 1984
Ownership: Private
Produces/Sells CE-marked Devices: N
Distribution: Manufacturer Direct

Light Source, Fiberoptic, Routine	Gastroenterology/Urology

SYLVAN CORP.
See Sylvan Fiberoptics

SYLVAN FIBEROPTICS
800-628-3836
P.O. Box 501, Irwin, PA 15642
724-864-9350
FDA Number: n/a
Fax: 724-864-7138
E-mail: sylmed@capslock.net
Web site: http://www.sylvanmed.com
Medical Products Sales Volume: $500,000
Annual Revenue: $0-$1 Million
Year Founded: 1984
Total Employees: 6   *Marketing Staff:* 1   *Sales Staff:* 2
Ownership: Private
Produces/Sells CE-marked Devices: N
Federal Procurement Eligibility: Small Business
Distribution: Manufacturer Direct
General Admin.: James G. Fedorka/President, Chief Executive Officer

Transilluminator, Battery-Powered	Ophthalmology

SYLVANIA
See Osram Sylvania Inc.

SYMBIOS MEDICAL PRODUCTS, LLC
317-225-4447
7301 Georgetown Rd, Suite 150, Indianapolis, IN 46268
FDA Number: 3005203102
Ownership: Private
Produces/Sells CE-marked Devices: N
General Admin.: W. Herbert Senft II/Executive Vice President
Mktg./Adv.: Carolyn Rae/Market Manager
Production: Jen Ramo/Product Director

Accessories, Catheter	Surgery
Catheter, Conduction, Anesthesia	Anesthesiology
Pump, Infusion, Elastomeric	General

SYMMETRIC DESIGNS, LTD.
800-537-1724
125 Knott Place,
250-537-2177
Salt Spring Island, BC V8K 2 Canada
FDA Number: 9680670
Fax: 250-537-1998
E-mail: sales@symmetric-designs.com
Web site: www.symmetric-designs.com
Year Founded: 1986
Total Employees: 10
Ownership: Private
Produces/Sells CE-marked Devices: N
Distribution: Manufacturer Direct, Exporter

SYMMETRICOM TIMING, TEST & MEASUREMENT
800-544-0233
34 Tozer Road, Beverly, MA 01915
978-927-8220
FDA Number: n/a
Fax: 978-927-4099
E-mail: us-info@symmetricom.com
Web site: www.symmetricom.com
Annual Revenue: $25-$50 Million
Total Employees: 200   *Marketing Staff:* 3   *Sales Staff:* 11
Ownership: Symmetricom, Inc.
Stock Symbol: SYMM
Traded On: NASDAQ
Quality System Registration Information: ISO9001
Produces/Sells CE-marked Devices: Y
Federal Procurement Eligibility: Small Business, GSA Contract
Distribution: Manufacturer Direct, Manufacturer Through Distributor, Manufacturer Through Manufacturer Reps, OEM, Service Direct, Exporter

SYMMETRICOM TIMING, TEST &
800-544-0233 *(cont'd)*
General Admin.: Michele Shindleman/Vice President Human Resources
Mktg./Adv.: Dr. Bruce Bromage/Executive Vice President Sales
     John Hirsekorn/Vice President Marketing & Sales
Production: Edward Anemoduris/Vice President Manufacturing
Research: Scott Davis/Manager Development
     R. Michael Garvey/Vice President Research & Development

Clock, Elapsed Time	General

SYMMETRY MEDICAL INC.
See Symmetry Medical, Inc.

SYMMETRY MEDICAL NEW BEDFORD
508-998-4493
New Bedford Industrial Park, New Bedford, MA 02745
FDA Number: 1218840
Web site: www.symmetrymedical.com
Ownership: Symmetry Medical, Inc.
Stock Symbol: SMA
Traded On: NYSE
Produces/Sells CE-marked Devices: N

Curette, Nasal	Ear/Nose/Throat
Curette, Surgical	Surgery
ENT Manual Surgical Instrument	Ear/Nose/Throat
Electrosurgical Unit, Cutting & Coagulation Device	Surgery
Instrument, Manual, General Surgical	Surgery
Orthopedic Manual Surgical Instrument	Orthopedics
Punch, Nasal	Ear/Nose/Throat
Scissors, General Dissecting	General
Scissors, Orthopedic	Orthopedics
Surgical Instrument, G-U, Manual	Gastroenterology/Urology

SYMMETRY MEDICAL USA, INC
207-786-2775
111 N. Clay, Claypool, IN 46510
FDA Number: 3005061536
Web site: www.symmetrymedical.com
Ownership: Symmetry Medical, Inc.
Stock Symbol: SMA
Traded On: NYSE
Produces/Sells CE-marked Devices: N

Instrument, Manual, General Surgical	Surgery
Orthopedic Manual Surgical Instrument	Orthopedics

SYMMETRY MEDICAL USA, INC.
574-267-8700
486 West 350 North, Warsaw, IN 46582
FDA Number: 1828464
Fax: 574-267-7306
Web site: www.symmetrymedical.com
Total Employees: 1795
Ownership: Symmetry Medical, Inc.
Stock Symbol: SMA
Traded On: NYSE
Produces/Sells CE-marked Devices: N
General Admin.: Reese Myers/Director
Mktg./Adv.: Dean Trippiedi/Senior Vice President Sales
Production: Michele Schlichtenmyer/Quality Control, Product Engineer
Research: Barry Parker/Senior Vice President Development
Finance: James Norris/Accountant

Awl	Orthopedics
Bender	Orthopedics
Bit, Surgical	Surgery
Blade, Scalpel	Surgery
Blade, Surgical, Saw, General & Plastic Surgery	Surgery
Bone Mill	Orthopedics
Cannula, Surgical, General & Plastic Surgery	Surgery
Clamp, Bone	Orthopedics
Curette	Orthopedics
Cutter, Surgical	Surgery
Cutter, Wire And Pin	Orthopedics
Driver, Surgical, Pin	Surgery
Elevator, Surgical, Dental	Dental And Oral
Elevator, Surgical, General & Plastic Surgery	Surgery
File, Bone, Surgical	Dental And Oral
File, Surgical, General & Plastic Surgery	Surgery
Forceps	Orthopedics
Forceps, Rongeur, Surgical	Dental And Oral
Gauge, Depth	Orthopedics
Gauge, Depth, Instrument, Dental	Dental And Oral
General Use Surgical Scissors	Surgery
Guide, Surgical, Instrument	Surgery
Handle, Instrument, Dental	Dental And Oral
Handle, Scalpel	Surgery
Hemostat	Orthopedics
Holder, Needle	Gastroenterology/Urology
Holder, Needle, Orthopedic	Orthopedics
Hook, Surgical, General & Plastic Surgery	Surgery
Instrument, Manual, General Surgical	Surgery
Instrument, Surgical, Powered, Pneumatic	Orthopedics
Knife, Nasal	Ear/Nose/Throat
Knife, Orthopedic	Orthopedics
Mallet, Surgical, General & Plastic Surgery	Surgery
Motor, Surgical Instrument, Pneumatic-Powered	Surgery
Orthopedic Manual Surgical Instrument	Orthopedics

SYMMETRY MEDICAL USA, INC.   574-267-8700 *(cont'd)*

Osteotome, Manual (Plastic Surgery)	Surgery
Pliers, Surgical	Orthopedics
Probe	Orthopedics
Punch, Antrum	Ear/Nose/Throat
Punch, Surgical	Surgery
Rasp, Bone	Orthopedics
Retractor, All Types	Dental And Oral
Retractor, Surgical	Surgery
Rongeur, Rib	Orthopedics
Scissors, Nasal	Ear/Nose/Throat
Scissors, Ophthalmic	Ophthalmology
Scissors, Surgical Tissue, Dental (Oral)	Dental And Oral
Surgical Instrument, Orthopedic, AC-Powered Motor	Orthopedics
Surgical Instrument, Orthopedic, Battery-Powered	Surgery
Tamp	Orthopedics
Tape, Measuring, Ruler And Caliper	Surgery
Tray, Impression	Dental And Oral
Trephine, Bone	Orthopedics
Tube, Ear Suction	Ear/Nose/Throat
Tube, Tonsil Suction	Ear/Nose/Throat
Wrench	Orthopedics

SYMMETRY MEDICAL, INC.   574-268-2252
3724 N. State Rd. 15, Warsaw, IN 46582
FDA Number: 3004776227
Web site: www.symmetrymedical.com
Year Founded: 1976
Total Employees: 2449
Ownership: Public
Stock Symbol: SMA
Traded On: NYSE
Quality System Registration Information: ISO9001
Produces/Sells CE-marked Devices: Y
Federal Procurement Eligibility: Small Business
Distribution: Manufacturer Through Distributor, OEM, Importer, Exporter
General Admin.: Mr. Thomas Sullivan/Chief Executive Officer
    Mr. Fred L. Hite/Chief Financial Officer, Senior Vice President
    Mr. Michael Curtis/Chief Operating Officer
    Mr. Michael W. Curtis/Chief Operating Officer, Senior Vice President
Mktg./Adv.: Mr. Brian S. Moore/Executive Vice President Business Development
    Mr. Jose Fernandez/Senior Vice President Product Development
Production: Mr. D. Darin Martin/Senior Vice President Quality Assurance
Finance: Ms. Ronda Harris/Chief Accountant

Contract Manufacturing	General
Orthopedic Manual Surgical Instrument	Orthopedics

Medical Product Subsidiaries (Listed Separately)
Riley Medical, Inc.
Symmetry Medical New Bedford
Symmetry Medical Usa, Inc
Symmetry Medical Usa, Inc.
Symmetry Medical, Inc. - Polyvac
Symmetry Medical/Ssi
Symmetry Tnco

SYMMETRY MEDICAL, INC. - POLYVAC   207-786-2775
253 Abby Rd., Manchester, NH 03103
FDA Number: 1221053
Web site: www.symmetrymedical.com
Ownership: Symmetry Medical, Inc.
Stock Symbol: SMA
Traded On: NYSE
Produces/Sells CE-marked Devices: N

Tray, Surgical	Surgery
Tray, Surgical Instrument	Surgery
Wrap, Sterilization	General

SYMMETRY MEDICAL/SSI   615-883-9090
200 River Hills Drive, Nashville, TN 37210
FDA Number: 3007208013
Web site: www.symmetrymedical.com
Ownership: Symmetry Medical, Inc.
Stock Symbol: SMA
Traded On: NYSE
Produces/Sells CE-marked Devices: N

SYMMETRY TNCO   888-447-6661
15 Colebrook Blvd., Whitman, MA 02382   781-447-6661
                                 Fax: 781-447-2132
FDA Number: 1219597
E-mail: info@tnco-inc.com
Web site: www.tnco-inc.com
Medical Products Sales Volume: $7,600,000
Annual Revenue: $5-$10 Million
Year Founded: 1964
Total Employees: 60   *Marketing Staff:* 1   *Sales Staff:* 2
Ownership: Symmetry Medical, Inc.
Stock Symbol: SMA
Traded On: NYSE

SYMMETRY TNCO   888-447-6661 *(cont'd)*
Produces/Sells CE-marked Devices: Y
Federal Procurement Eligibility: Small Business
Distribution: Manufacturer Direct, Manufacturer Through Distributor, OEM
General Admin.: Mr. Win Sargent/Chief Financial Officer, Controller
    Karin B. Dolan/President, Chief Executive Officer
Mktg./Adv.: Mr. Nicholas Burke/Manager Sales
Production: Mr. Joseph Talkowski/Director Operations
Research: Frank DiFrancesco/Vice President Research & Development
Purchasing: Mr. Brian Braasch/Buyer

Accessories, Arthroscope	Orthopedics
Arthroscope	Orthopedics
Curette	Orthopedics
Cutter, Orthopedic	Orthopedics
ENT Manual Surgical Instrument	Ear/Nose/Throat
Forceps	Orthopedics
Instrument, Microsurgical	Cns/Neurology
Knife, Meniscus	Surgery
Knife, Orthopedic	Orthopedics
Probe	Orthopedics
Punch, Other	Surgery
Scissors, Orthopedic	Orthopedics
Service, Maintenance/Repair	General

SYMPHONY MEDICAL PRODUCTS   877-470-9995
6320 N.w. 84th Avenue, Miami, FL 33166   305-470-9994
                                 Fax: 305-470-9962
FDA Number: 9055896
E-mail: Info@symxcorp.com
Web site: www.symphonymedical.com
Medical Products Sales Volume: $32,000,000
Annual Revenue: $50-$100 Million
Year Founded: 1999
Total Employees: 40
Ownership: Private
Produces/Sells CE-marked Devices: N
Federal Procurement Eligibility: Small Business, Minority Owned
Distribution: Manufacturer Direct

Bed, Electric	General
Bed, Hydraulic	General
Bed, Manual	General
Bed, Pediatric (Crib)	General
Mattress, Non-Powered Flotation Therapy	Physical Med
Stretcher, Hand-Carried	General
Stretcher, Wheeled (Mobile)	General
Stretcher, Wheeled, Powered	Physical Med
Transfer Device, Patient, Manual	General

SYMYX TECHNOLOGIES, INC.   408-764-2000
1263 East Arques Avenue, Sunnyvale, CA 94085
FDA Number: n/a
Web site: www.symyx.com
Annual Revenue: $50-$100 Million
Year Founded: 1994
Total Employees: 540
Ownership: Private
Stock Symbol: SMMX
Traded On: NASDAQ
Produces/Sells CE-marked Devices: N
Distribution: Manufacturer Direct, Manufacturer Through Manufacturer Reps, Service Direct, Exclusive Distributor, Importer, Exporter
General Admin.: Isy Goldwasser/Chief Executive Officer
    Rex S. Jackson/Chief Financial Officer, Executive Vice President
    Trevor Heritage/President

Computer Software	General

SYN-OPTICS
See Stryker Endoscopy

SYNAPSE BIOMEDICAL INC.   440-774-2488
300 Artino St., Oberlin, OH 44074
FDA Number: 3005868392
                                 Fax: 440-774-2572
E-mail: info@synapsebiomedical.com
Web site: www.synapsebiomedical.com
Year Founded: 2002
Ownership: Private
Produces/Sells CE-marked Devices: N
General Admin.: Mr. Moustapha Diop/Chief Operating Officer
    Mr. Anthony Ignagni/President, Chief Executive Officer
Mktg./Adv.: Mr. Timothy Crish/Director Product Development
    Steven Annunziato/Senior Vice President Marketing & Sales
Production: Mr. James Gelbke/Director Manufacturing

Stimulator, Diaphragmatic/Phrenic Nerve, Implantable	Cns/Neurology

SYNCARDIA SYSTEMS, INC.   866-771-9437
1992 E. Silverlake Rd., Tucson, AZ 85713   520-545-1234
                                 Fax: 520-903-1783
FDA Number: 3003761017
E-mail: info@syncardia.com
Web site: www.syncardia.com
Year Founded: 2001

SYNCARDIA SYSTEMS, INC. 866-771-9437 (cont'd)
Ownership: Private
Produces/Sells CE-marked Devices: Y
General Admin.: Mike Gaul/Chief Operating Officer
    Marvin Slepian/Chief Scientific Officer
    Richard Smith/Chief Technology Officer
    Rodger Ford/President, Chief Executive Officer
Mktg./Adv.: Donald Isaacs/Director Communications
    J. David Mackstaller/Vice President Corporate Development
Production: Carole Marcot/Vice President Quality Assurance & Regulatory Affairs
Finance: Dena Richter/Chief Financial Officer
    Circulatory Assist Unit, Left Ventricular — Cardiovascular

SYNCHROTECH MEDICAL CORPORATION
See Cardio Command, Inc.

SYNCOR INT'L CORP./NUCLEAR PHARMACY DIV.
See Nuclear Pharmacy Services

SYNECTIC MEDICAL PRODUCT DEVELOPMENT 203-877-8488
60 Commerce Park, Milford, CT 06460
FDA Number: 9045002   Fax: 203-874-4290
E-mail: jstein@synectic.net
Web site: www.synectic.com
Medical Products Sales Volume: $620,000
Annual Revenue: $1-$5 Million
Year Founded: 1981
Total Employees: 10   *Marketing Staff:* 2   *Sales Staff:* 1
Ownership: Private
Produces/Sells CE-marked Devices: N
Federal Procurement Eligibility: Small Business
Distribution: Service Direct
General Admin.: Jeffrey Stein/President
Mktg./Adv.: Robert Kundinger/Director Sales
    Cynthia Rubin/Marketing Coordinator
Cannula, Suprapubic, With Trocar	Gastroenterology/Urology
Coagulator, Laparoscopic, Unipolar	Obstetrics/Gynecology
Coagulator/Cutter, Endoscopic, Bipolar	Obstetrics/Gynecology
Coagulator/Cutter, Endoscopic, Unipolar	Obstetrics/Gynecology
Contract R&D, Diagnostics	General
Equipment, Suction/Irrigation, Laparoscopic	Surgery
Forceps, Endoscopic	Gastroenterology/Urology
Forceps, Grasping, Atraumatic	Surgery
Forceps, Grasping, Flexible Endoscopic	Gastroenterology/Urology
Forceps, Grasping, Traumatic	Surgery
Holder, Needle, Laparoscopic	Surgery
Holder/Scissors, Needle, Laparoscopic	Surgery
Instrument, Dissecting, Laparoscopic	Surgery
Instrument, Needle Holder/Knot Tying	Surgery
Insufflator, Laparoscopic	Obstetrics/Gynecology
Irrigator, Suction	General
Needle, Insufflation, Laparoscopic	Surgery
Probe, Electrocauterization, Multi-Use	Surgery
Probe, Electrocauterization, Single-Use	Surgery
Probe, Suction, Irrigator/Aspirator, Laparoscopic	Surgery
Scissors with Removable Tips, Laparoscopy	Surgery
Scissors, Disposable	General
Service, Attorney, Patent	General
Service, Engineering/Design	General
Stapler, Surgical	Surgery
Trocar, Abdominal	Gastroenterology/Urology
Trocar, Gastro-Urology	Gastroenterology/Urology

SYNERGENT BIOCHEM, INC. 562-809-3389
12026 Centralia Ave., Unit G & H, Hawaiian Gardens, CA 90716
FDA Number: 2032335   Fax: 562-809-6191
E-mail: info@synergentbiochem.com
Web site: www.synergentbiochem.com
Year Founded: 2000
Ownership: Private
Produces/Sells CE-marked Devices: N
Control, Analyte (Assayed And Unassayed)	Chemistry
Control, Drug Mixture	Toxicology
Control, Multi Analyte, All Kinds (Assayed And Unassayed)	Chemistry
Multi Analyte Mixture, Calibrator	Chemistry

SYNERGETICS USA, INC. 800-600-0565
3845 Corporate Centre Dr., 636-939-5100
O'Fallon, MO 63368
FDA Number: 1932402   Fax: 636-939-6885
E-mail: customerservice@synergeticsusa.com
Web site: www.synergeticsusa.com
Year Founded: 1991
Total Employees: 350
Ownership: Public
Stock Symbol: SURG
Traded On: NASDAQ
Produces/Sells CE-marked Devices: N
General Admin.: Mr. David Hable/Chief Executive Officer
    Jerry Malis/Chief Scientific Officer & Executive Vice President

SYNERGETICS USA, INC. 800-600-0565 (cont'd)
Mktg./Adv.: Kurt Gampp/Executive Vice President, Chief Operating Officer Marketing
Finance: Pamela Boone/Chief Financial Officer
Cannula, Ophthalmic	Ophthalmology
Cautery, Radiofrequency, AC-Powered	Ophthalmology
Condenser, Heat And Moisture (Artificial Nose)	Anesthesiology
Cutter, Vitreous Aspiration, AC-Powered	Ophthalmology
Electrosurgical Unit, Cutting & Coagulation Device	Surgery
Endoilluminator	Ophthalmology
Forceps, Ophthalmic	Ophthalmology
General Use Surgical Scissors	Surgery
Instrument, Manual, General Surgical	Surgery
Instrument, Microsurgical	Cns/Neurology
Laser, Surgical	Surgery
Magnet, Permanent	Ophthalmology
Photocoagulator	Ophthalmology
Plate, Bone, Skull (Cranioplasty)	Cns/Neurology
Pump, Infusion	General
Scissors, Ophthalmic	Ophthalmology
Transilluminator, AC-Powered, Ophthalmic	Ophthalmology

SYNERGETICS, INC.
See Synergetics Usa, Inc.

SYNERGISTIC CONCEPTS, LTD. 419-448-4868
1660 W. Market St., Suite D, Tiffin, OH 44883
FDA Number: 3006194522
| Table, Physical Medicine, Powered | Physical Med |

SYNERGY REHAB TECHNOLOGIES, INC. 407-344-8440
2701 Wortham Lane, Kissimmee, FL 34744
FDA Number: 3004181143   Fax: 407-344-8449
E-mail: lauras@synergyrehab.net
Web site: www.synergyrehab.net
Ownership: Private
Produces/Sells CE-marked Devices: N
Production: Ms. Laura Shantz/Vice President Manufacturing
Finance: Mr. Paul Barattiero/President
| Cushion, Wheelchair (Pad) | Physical Med |

SYNERGY TECHNOLOGIES, INC. 218-879-4610
240 Erkkila Road, Esko, MN 55733
FDA Number: 9038179   Fax: 218-879-4610
E-mail: mkrohn@syntechinc.com
Web site: www.syntechinc.com
Ownership: Private
Produces/Sells CE-marked Devices: N
Federal Procurement Eligibility: Small Business, Female Owned
Distribution: Manufacturer Direct
General Admin.: Mr. Jeff Fisher/Chief Executive Officer
    Ms. Mary Krohn/President, Chief Financial Officer
| Basin, Emesis | General |

SYNERGY USA 786-222-1710
13899 Biscayne Blvd, Suite 101, Nmb, FL 33181
FDA Number: 3006002539
Ownership: Private
Produces/Sells CE-marked Devices: N
Diazo (Colorimetric), Nitrite (Urinary, Non-Quantitative)	Chemistry
Disc, Strip And Reagent, Microorganism Differentiation	Microbiology
Test, Urine Leukocyte	Hematology
Thermometer, Electronic	General
Unit, Ultraviolet Sanitation/sterilization (for Toothbrushes), Non-sterile	Dental And Oral
pH Paper, Obstetric	Obstetrics/Gynecology

SYNERMED INTERNATIONAL INC. 800-361-3552
1688 50th Ave., Lachine, QUE H8T-2V5 Canada 514-633-1112
FDA Number: n/a   Fax: 514-633-8039
E-mail: synermed@synermed.ca
Year Founded: 1989
Total Employees: 50
Ownership: Private
Produces/Sells CE-marked Devices: N
Distribution: Manufacturer Direct, Exclusive Distributor

SYNERMED INTL., INC. 317-896-1565
17408 Tiller Court, Ste. 1900, Westfield, IN 46074
FDA Number: 3003593973
Analyzer, Chemistry, Micro	Chemistry
Azo-Dye, Calcium	Chemistry
Catalytic Method, Amylase	Chemistry
Electrode, Ion Specific, Chloride	Chemistry
Electrode, Ion Specific, Potassium	Chemistry
Electrode, Ion Specific, Sodium	Chemistry
Enzymatic Esterase-Oxidase, Cholesterol	Chemistry
Enzymatic, Carbon-Dioxide	Chemistry
Ferrozine (Colorimetric) Iron Binding Capacity	Chemistry
Indicator Method, Protein Or Albumin (Urinary, Non-Quant.)	Chemistry
Kinetic Method, Gamma-Glutamyl Transpeptidase	Chemistry
Lipase Hydrolysis/Glycerol Kinase Enzyme, Triglycerides	Chemistry

SYNERMED INTL., INC.   317-896-1565 *(cont'd)*

Multi Analyte Mixture, Calibrator	Chemistry
NAD Reduction/NADH Oxidation, CPK Or Isoenzymes	Chemistry
NAD Reduction/NADH Oxidation, Lactate Dehydrogenase	Chemistry
NADH Oxidation/NAD Reduction, AST/SGOT	Chemistry
Nitrophenylphosphate, Alkaline Phosphatase Or Isoenzymes	Chemistry
Phosphoric-Tungstic Acid (Spectrophotometric), Chloride	Chemistry
Phosphorus Reagent (Test System)	Chemistry
Photometric Method, Magnesium	Chemistry
Reagent, Bilirubin (Total Or Direct Test System)	Chemistry
Reagent, Creatinine (Test System)	Chemistry
Reagent, Glucose (Test System)	Chemistry
Reagent, Protein, Total	Chemistry
SGPT, Ultraviolet	Chemistry
Urease And Glutamic Dehydrogenase, Urea Nitrogen	Chemistry
Uricase (Colorimetric), Uric Acid	Chemistry

SYNERON, INC.   949-716-6670
3 Goodyear Unit A, Irvine, CA 92618
FDA Number: 3004772125   *Fax:* 949-716-8287
E-mail: info@syneron.com
Web site: www.syneron.com
Year Founded: 2000
Ownership: SYNERON MEDICAL LTD.
Stock Symbol: ELOS
Traded On: NASDAQ
Produces/Sells CE-marked Devices: N
Finance: Fabian Tenenbaum/Business Specialist
      David Seligman/Chief Financial Officer
      Judith Kleinman/Vice President Public Communications & Investor
Relations

SYNOVIS LIFE TECHNOLOGIES, INC   800-255-4018
2575 University Ave. W, St. Paul, MN 55114   **651-796-7300**
FDA Number: 2183620   *Fax:* 651-642-9018
Web site: http://www.synovislife.com
Total Employees: 390
Ownership: Public
Stock Symbol: SYNO
Traded On: NASDAQ
Produces/Sells CE-marked Devices: N
General Admin.: Mr. Richard W. Kramp/President, Chief Executive Officer
Mktg./Adv.: Mr. Tim Floeder/Vice President Corporate Development
      Ms. Jodi Brendel/Vice President Marketing & Sales
Production: Mr. Mary L. Frick/Vice President Quality Assurance & Regulatory
Affairs
Research: Dr. Daniel Mooradian/Vice President Research & Development
Finance: Mr. Brett Reynolds/Chief Financial Officer

Clamp, Vascular	Cardiovascular
Dilator, Vessel, Surgical	Cardiovascular
Dura-Substitute	Cns/Neurology
Mesh, Surgical (Steel Gauze)	Surgery
Pledget And Intracardiac Patch, PETP, PTFE, Polypropylene	Cardiovascular

SYNOVIS MICRO COMPANIES ALLIANCE, INC.   800-510-3318
439 Industrial Ln., Birmingham, AL 35211-4464   **205-941-0111**
FDA Number: 1062741   *Fax:* 205-941-1522
E-mail: info@synovismicro.com
Web site: www.synovismicro.com
Ownership: SYNOVIS LIFE TECHNOLOGIES, INC
Stock Symbol: SYNO
Traded On: NASDAQ
Produces/Sells CE-marked Devices: N
Mktg./Adv.: Terry Harrell/Director Sales

Cuff, Nerve	Cns/Neurology
Device, Anastomotic, Microvascular	Cardiovascular
Flowmeter, Blood, Other	Cardiovascular
Forceps	Orthopedics
Instrument, Manual, General Surgical	Surgery
Tray, Surgical Instrument	Surgery
Wrap, Sterilization	General

SYNOVIS SURGICAL INNOVATIONS   800-255-4018
2575 University Avenue W., St. Paul, MN 55114   **651-796-7300**
FDA Number: 2183620   *Fax:* 651-642-9018
E-mail: hr@synovislife.com
Web site: www.synovissurgical.com
Medical Products Sales Volume: $55,830,000
Year Founded: 1985
Ownership: Ferraris Group, Plc
Stock Symbol: SYNO
Traded On: NASDAQ
Quality System Registration Information: ISO9001
Produces/Sells CE-marked Devices: Y
Distribution: Manufacturer Direct, Manufacturer Through Distributor, Manufacturer
Through Manufacturer Reps
General Admin.: Tim Scanlan/Chairman
      David Buche/Chief Operating Officer, Vice President

SYNOVIS SURGICAL INNOVATIONS   800-255-4018 *(cont'd)*
      Richard Kramp/President, Chief Executive Officer
Medical Admin.: Mary Frick/Vice President Clinical Affairs
Research: Dr. Daniel Mooradian/Vice President Research & Development
Finance: Brett Reynolds/Chief Financial Officer, Vice President Finance

Clamp, Vascular	Cardiovascular
Dilator, Vessel, Surgical	Cardiovascular
Dura-Substitute	Cns/Neurology
Graft, Bovine	Surgery
Mesh, Surgical, Polymeric	Surgery

SYNOVIS SURGICAL INNOVATIONS, A DIVISION OF SYNOVIS LIFE TECHNOLOGIES, INC.
See Synovis Surgical Innovations

SYNTEC, INC.   636-566-6500
733 Mansion Rd., Winfield, MO 63389
FDA Number: 1933422

Cutter, Vitreous Aspiration, AC-Powered	Ophthalmology

SYNTEC, INC.   636-566-6500
812 Truman Blvd., Crystal City, MO 63019
FDA Number: 1933597
Ownership: Private
Produces/Sells CE-marked Devices: N

Irrigator, Ocular Surgery	Ophthalmology

SYNTECH INTERNATIONAL   949-752-9642
17171 Daimler Ave., Irvine, CA 92614
FDA Number: 3005142514

Oximeter, Intracardiac	Cardiovascular
Sleeve, Compressible Limb	Cardiovascular

SYNTERMED, INC.   404-814-5277
Tower Place Ctr., Suite 1800, 3340 Peachtree Rd.,
Atlanta, GA 30326
FDA Number: 1066019   *Fax:* 404-303-1197
E-mail: info@syntermed.com
Web site: www.syntermed.com
Medical Products Sales Volume: $150,000
Year Founded: 1999
Total Employees: 2
Ownership: Private
Quality System Registration Information: ISO9000
Produces/Sells CE-marked Devices: N
Federal Procurement Eligibility: Small Business
Distribution: Manufacturer Direct, OEM
General Admin.: Mr. Michael Lee/Chief Executive Officer, Chairman

Computer and Software, Medical	General

SYNTEX DENTAL PRODUCTS INC.
See Dentalez Group

SYNTHES (USA)   719 481 5300
1051 Synthes Avenue, P.O. Box 366, Monument, CO 80132
FDA Number: 1719045
Web site: www.synthes.com
Ownership: Synthes Inc.
Stock Symbol: SYST
Traded On: Switzerland
Produces/Sells CE-marked Devices: N

Appliance, Fixation, Spinal Intervertebral Body	Orthopedics
Cannula, Surgical, General & Plastic Surgery	Surgery
Cerclage, Fixation	Orthopedics
Chisel, Bone, Surgical	Dental And Oral
Chisel, Surgical, Manual	Surgery
Drill, Bone, Powered	Dental And Oral
Filter, Bacterial, Breathing Circuit	Anesthesiology
Forceps, General & Plastic Surgery	Surgery
Guide, Surgical, Instrument	Surgery
Hammer, Surgical	Surgery
Hook, Surgical, General & Plastic Surgery	Surgery
Lock, Wire, And Ligature, Intraoral	Dental And Oral
Nail, Fixation, Bone	Orthopedics
Needle, Aspiration And Injection, Disposable	Surgery
Pin, Fixation, Threaded	Orthopedics
Plate, Fixation, Bone	Orthopedics
Regulator, Pressure, Gas Cylinder	Anesthesiology
Retractor	Surgery
Retractor, Fiberoptic	Gastroenterology/Urology
Rod, Fixation, Intramedullary	Orthopedics
Scalpel, One-Piece (Knife)	Surgery
Screw, Fixation, Bone	Orthopedics
Screw, Fixation, Intraosseous	Dental And Oral
Suture, Non-Absorbable, Steel, Monofilament & Multifilament	Surgery
Tape, Measuring, Ruler And Caliper	Surgery
Tray, Surgical Instrument	Surgery

SYNTHES (USA)   610-719-5000
35 Airport Road, Horseheads, NY 14845
FDA Number: 3003506883

SYNTHES (USA)   610-719-5000 *(cont'd)*

E-mail: info@synthes.com
Web site: http://us.synthes.com
Annual Revenue: More than $1 Billion
Year Founded: 1974
Total Employees: 9000
Ownership: Synthes Inc.
Stock Symbol: SYST
Traded On: Switzerland
Produces/Sells CE-marked Devices: N

Accessories, Fixation, Orthopedic	Orthopedics
Appliance, Fix., Nail/Blade/Plate Comb., Multiple Component	Orthopedics
Appliance, Fixation, Spinal Interlaminal	Orthopedics
Bit, Drill	Orthopedics
Blade, Surgical, Saw, General & Plastic Surgery	Surgery
Bolt, Nut, Washer	Orthopedics
Burr, Surgical, General & Plastic Surgery	Surgery
Cerclage, Fixation	Orthopedics
Component, Traction, Invasive	Orthopedics
Cover, Burr Hole (Cranial)	Cns/Neurology
Fixation Appliance, Multiple Component	Orthopedics
Fixation Appliance, Single Component	Orthopedics
Guide, Surgical, Instrument	Surgery
Implant, Endosseous	Dental And Oral
Implant, Fixation Device, Condylar Plate	Orthopedics
Implant, Fixation Device, Proximal Femoral	Orthopedics
Mesh, Surgical (Steel Gauze)	Surgery
Orthosis, Fixation, Pedicle, Spinal	Orthopedics
Orthosis, Fixation, Spinal, Spondylolisthesis	Orthopedics
Orthosis, Fusion, Intervertebral, Spinal	Orthopedics
Pin, Fixation, Smooth	Orthopedics
Pin, Fixation, Threaded	Orthopedics
Plate, Bone, Orthodontic	Dental And Oral
Plate, Fixation, Bone	Orthopedics
Reamer	Orthopedics
Rod, Fixation, Intramedullary	Orthopedics
Screw, Fixation, Bone	Orthopedics
Screw, Fixation, Intraosseous	Dental And Oral
Tap, Bone	Orthopedics
Traction Unit, Non-Powered	Orthopedics
Wire, Fixation, Intraosseous	Dental And Oral
Wire, Surgical	Orthopedics

SYNTHES (USA) - BRANDYWINE TECHNICAL CENTER   800-523-0322

1302 Wrights Lane East,
West Chester, PA 19380   610-719-5000
FDA Number: 2530088   *Fax:* 800-796-8437
E-mail: info@synthes.com
Web site: http://us.synthes.com
Year Founded: 1974
Total Employees: 9000
Ownership: Synthes Inc.
Stock Symbol: SYST
Traded On: NYSE
Produces/Sells CE-marked Devices: N
Distribution: Manufacturer Through Manufacturer Reps
General Admin.: Charles Hedgepath/Chief Executive Officer

Bit, Drill	Orthopedics
Bit, Surgical	Surgery
Broach	Orthopedics
Chisel, Surgical, Manual	Surgery
Curette	Orthopedics
Cutter, Surgical	Surgery
Dissector, Surgical, General & Plastic Surgery	Surgery
Forceps	Orthopedics
Gauge, Depth	Orthopedics
Guide, Surgical, Instrument	Surgery
Hammer, Surgical	Surgery
Hook, Surgical, General & Plastic Surgery	Surgery
Laser, Surgical	Surgery
Lock, Wire, And Ligature, Intraoral	Dental And Oral
Plate, Bone, Skull, Preformed, Alterable	Cns/Neurology
Plate, Fixation, Bone	Orthopedics
Pliers, Surgical	Orthopedics
Protractor	Orthopedics
Rasp, Other	Surgery
Reamer	Orthopedics
Retractor	Orthopedics
Screw, Fixation, Bone	Orthopedics
Suture, Non-Absorbable, Steel, Monofilament & Multifilament	Surgery

SYNTHES (USA) - DEVELOPMENT CENTER   719-481-5300

1230 Wilson Dr., West Chester, PA 19380
FDA Number: 2939274
Web site: www.synthes.com
Ownership: Synthes Inc.
Stock Symbol: SYST
Traded On: Switzerland

SYNTHES (USA) - DEVELOPMENT CENTER   719-481-5300 *(cont'd)*

Produces/Sells CE-marked Devices: N

Cement, Hydroxyapatite	Surgery
Dispenser, Cement	Orthopedics
Filler, Calcium Sulfate Preformed Pellets	Orthopedics
Mesh, Surgical (Steel Gauze)	Surgery
Mesh, Surgical, Polymeric	Surgery
Metacrylate, Methyl, Cranioplasty	Cns/Neurology
Mixing Equipment, Cement	Orthopedics
Needle, Aspiration And Injection, Disposable	Surgery
Plate, Bone, Skull, Preformed, Alterable	Cns/Neurology
Spatula, Surgical, General & Plastic Surgery	Surgery
Stylet, Surgical	Surgery
Syringe, Piston	General

SYNTHES INC.   800-523-0322

1302 Wrights Ln. E., West Chester, PA 19380   610-719-5000
FDA Number: n/a
E-mail: info@synthes.com
Web site: www.synthes.com
Medical Products Sales Volume: $2,759,700,000
Annual Revenue: More than $1 Billion
Year Founded: 1974
Total Employees: 9070
Ownership: Public
Stock Symbol: SYST
Traded On: Switzerland
Produces/Sells CE-marked Devices: Y
Medical Product Subsidiaries (Listed Separately)
Synthes (Usa)
Synthes (Usa) - Brandywine Technical Center
Synthes (Usa) - Development Center
Synthes Gmbh
Synthes Jennersville
Synthes San Diego

SYNTHES JENNERSVILLE   484-356-9728

108 Willowbrook Lane, West Chester, PA 19382
FDA Number: 3003787298
Web site: www.synthes.com
Ownership: Synthes Inc.
Stock Symbol: SYST
Traded On: Switzerland
Produces/Sells CE-marked Devices: N

Drill, Bone, Powered	Dental And Oral
Screw, Fixation, Intraosseous	Dental And Oral

SYNTHES SAN DIEGO   858-452-1266

6244 Ferris Square, Suite B, San Diego, CA 92121-3239
FDA Number: 3004699960
Ownership: Synthes Inc.
Produces/Sells CE-marked Devices: N

Accessories, Arthroscopic	Orthopedics
Awl	Orthopedics
Orthopedic Manual Surgical Instrument	Orthopedics
Orthosis, Fixation, Spinal, Spondylolisthesis	Orthopedics
Posterior Metal/polymer Spinal System, Fusion	Orthopedics

SYNTRON BIORESEARCH, INC.   800-854-6226

2774 Loker Avenue W., Carlsbad, CA 92008   760-930-2200
FDA Number: 2025760   *Fax:* 760-930-2212
E-mail: marketing@syntron.net
Web site: www.syntron.net
Medical Products Sales Volume: $23,000,000
Annual Revenue: $10-$25 Million
Year Founded: 1986
Total Employees: 140   *Marketing Staff:* 9   *Sales Staff:* 9
Ownership: Private
Quality System Registration Information: ISO9001
Produces/Sells CE-marked Devices: N
Federal Procurement Eligibility: Small Business, Minority Owned
Distribution: Manufacturer Direct, Manufacturer Through Distributor, Manufacturer Through Manufacturer Reps, OEM, Service Direct, Exporter
General Admin.: Charles Yu/General Manager
       James Lee/President

Kit, Pregnancy Test	Obstetrics/Gynecology
System, Test, Drugs of Abuse	Chemistry
Test, Bacteria Characterization	General
Test, Fertility Monitoring	Obstetrics/Gynecology

SYNVASIVE TECHNOLOGY, INC.   800-925-2337

4925 Robert J. Mathews Pkwy.,   916-939-3913
El Dorado Hills, CA 95762
FDA Number: 2950261   *Fax:* 916-939-3919
Web site: www.synvasive.com
Annual Revenue: $5-$10 Million
Total Employees: 32   *Marketing Staff:* 2   *Sales Staff:* 2

SYNVASIVE TECHNOLOGY, INC.   800-925-2337 *(cont'd)*
Ownership: Private
Quality System Registration Information: ISO9001
Produces/Sells CE-marked Devices: Y
Federal Procurement Eligibility: Small Business
Distribution: Manufacturer Direct, Manufacturer Through Distributor, Manufacturer Through Manufacturer Reps, OEM, Service Direct, Exclusive Distributor, Exporter
General Admin.: Michael G. Fisher/President, Chief Executive Officer
Mktg./Adv.: Tony Pasciuto/Director Sales

Blade, Bone Cutting	Orthopedics
Guide, Drill, Ligament	Orthopedics
Guide, Surgical, Instrument	Surgery
Orthopedic Manual Surgical Instrument	Orthopedics

SYRACUSE MEDICAL DEVICES, INC.   315-449-0657
214 Hurlburt Road, Syracuse, NY 13224-1821
FDA Number: n/a   *Fax:* 315-449-0756
E-mail: syrmed@twcny.rr.com
Medical Products Sales Volume: $230,000
Annual Revenue: $0-$1 Million
Year Founded: 1958
Total Employees: 2   *Sales Staff:* 2
Ownership: Private
Produces/Sells CE-marked Devices: N
Federal Procurement Eligibility: Small Business
Distribution: Manufacturer Direct
General Admin.: Geoffrey Guisbond/President, Chief Executive Officer

Dilator, Vaginal	Obstetrics/Gynecology

SYRACUSE PLASTICS OF NORTH CAROLINA, INC.   919-467-5151
100 Falcone Pkwy., Po Box 1067, Cary, NC 27511-6712
FDA Number: n/a   *Fax:* 919-460-1013
E-mail: sales@syrplas.com
Web site: www.Syracuseplastics.com
Annual Revenue: $5-$10 Million
Total Employees: 72   *Marketing Staff:* 2   *Sales Staff:* 2
Ownership: Private
Produces/Sells CE-marked Devices: N
Federal Procurement Eligibility: Small Business
Distribution: Manufacturer Direct
General Admin.: Rich Harvey/General Manager
     Tom Falcone/President
Production: Eric Donati/Manager Manufacturing
     Irvin Glasgow/Manager Quality Assurance

Molding, Custom	General

SYRIS SCIENTIFIC   800-714-1374 / 207-657-7050
22 Shaker Road, Gray, ME 04039
FDA Number: 3003864773   *Fax:* 207-657-7051
E-mail: pwilkinson@syrisscientific.com
Web site: www.syrisscientific.com
Medical Products Sales Volume: $570,000
Year Founded: 1997
Total Employees: 4
Ownership: ZELLWEGER LUWA
Produces/Sells CE-marked Devices: Y
Federal Procurement Eligibility: Small Business
Distribution: Manufacturer Direct, Service Direct
General Admin.: Ms. Pam Wilkinson/Executive Managing Director

Accessories, Light, Surgical	Surgery

SYSMED   214-820-2176
2625 Elm St., Ste. 102, Dallas, TX 75226-1453
FDA Number: 9916060
Web site: www.sysmed.org/
Total Employees: 14   *Marketing Staff:* 1   *Sales Staff:* 5
Ownership: Medco
Produces/Sells CE-marked Devices: N
General Admin.: Jeff Butler/Chief Operating Officer
Mktg./Adv.: Chad Johnson/Manager Sales
Production: Rex Moses/Manager Production Services

Communication System, Powered	Physical Med
Environmental Control System,, Powered, Remote	Physical Med

SYSMEX AMERICA INC.   1-800-462-1262
One Nelson C. White Parkway, Mundelein, IL 60060
FDA Number: 1422681
E-mail: communications@sysmex.com
Web site: http://www.sysmex.com/us
Ownership: Sysmex Corp.
Produces/Sells CE-marked Devices: N
General Admin.: Mr. Andre Ezers/Executive Vice President
     Mr. John Kershaw/President, Chief Executive Officer
Production: Mr. John Neal/Vice President Operations
IS: Ms. Judy Bosko/Vice President Tech. Services

SYSMEX REAGENTS AMERICA, INC.   847-996-4512
10716 Reagan St., Los Alamitos, CA 90720
FDA Number: 2916738

Diluent, Blood Cell	Hematology
Fluid, Red Cell Lysing	Hematology

SYSTEC COMPUTER ASSOCIATES, INC.   631-473-5620
28 N. County Road, Mount Sinai, NY 11766-1518
FDA Number: 2435501   *Fax:* 631-476-0732
E-mail: lifetec@systec.com
Web site: www.systec.com
Medical Products Sales Volume: $1,200,000
Year Founded: 1980
Total Employees: 15   *Marketing Staff:* 1   *Sales Staff:* 1
Ownership: Private
Produces/Sells CE-marked Devices: N
Federal Procurement Eligibility: Small Business
Distribution: Manufacturer Direct, Exclusive Distributor
General Admin.: William Bongiorno/President, Chief Executive Officer

Computer Software	General

SYSTEM ANALYSIS CORP.
See Psyche Systems

SYSTEM ONE
See Physicians Practice Management

SYSTEM SENSOR   800-736-7672, 630-377-6580
3825 Ohio Ave., Saint Charles, IL 60174
FDA Number: 3004529690   *Fax:* 630-377-6495
E-mail: info@systemsensor.com
Web site: www.systemsensor.com
Year Founded: 1984
Ownership: Private
Produces/Sells CE-marked Devices: N

Scale, Stand-On	General
Transmitter/Receiver System, Physiological, Radiofrequency	Cardiovascular

SYSTEMEDICS/DYATRON
See Medical Systems Support, Inc.

SYSTEMS PLUS, INC.
See Medical Manager Health Systems, Inc.

T & L SHARPENING, INC.   574-583-3868
2663 S. Freeman Rd., P.o. Box 338, Monticello, IN 47960
FDA Number: 3003541440
Ownership: Private
Produces/Sells CE-marked Devices: N

Orthopedic Manual Surgical Instrument	Orthopedics

T&S BRASS AND BRONZE WORKS, INC.   800-476-4103
2 Saddleback Cove, P.O. Box 1088, Travelers Rest, SC 29690
FDA Number: n/a   *Fax:* 800-868-0084
Web site: www.tsbrass.com
Annual Revenue: $0-$1 Million
Year Founded: 1947
Ownership: Private
Produces/Sells CE-marked Devices: Y
Federal Procurement Eligibility: Small Business
Distribution: Manufacturer Through Distributor

Kit, Irrigation, Eye	Ophthalmology
Washer, Cart	General

T+D METAL PRODUCTS   757-224-0177
602 E. Walnut, Watseka, IL 60970
FDA Number: 3004068465

Cart, Emergency, Cardiopulmonary Resuscitation (Crash)	Anesthesiology

T.B. CLIFT LIMITED   800-563-7205, 709-753-6850
34 O'Leary Ave., P.O. Box 8870, St. John's, MAN A1B-3 Canada
FDA Number: n/a   *Fax:* 709-753-7654
E-mail: tbclift@nfld.net
Web site: www.tbclift.com
Year Founded: 1929
Total Employees: 25
Ownership: Private
Produces/Sells CE-marked Devices: N
Distribution: Exclusive Distributor

T.C. DYNAMICS, INC.   248-706-2021
5235 Greer Rd., West Bloomfield, MI 48234
FDA Number: 3004059463
Ownership: Private
Produces/Sells CE-marked Devices: N

Exerciser, Powered	Anesthesiology

T2 BIOSYSTEMS   781-457-1200
101 Hartwell Avenue, Lexington, MA 02421
FDA Number: n/a   *Fax:* 781-351-3080

T2 BIOSYSTEMS   781-457-1200 (cont'd)

E-mail: info@t2biosystems.com
Web site: http://www.t2biosystems.com
Ownership: Private
Produces/Sells CE-marked Devices: N
General Admin.: Mr. John McDonough/Chief Executive Officer
Mktg./Adv.: Mr. Kirtland Poss/Senior Vice President Corporate Development
         Mr. Rahul Dhanda/Vice President Marketing
Research: Dr. Parris Wellman/Vice President Product Development
         Dr. Tom Lowery/Vice President Research & Development

TA INSTRUMENTS   302-427-4000

109 Lukens Drive, New Castle, DE 19720
FDA Number: n/a   Fax: 302-427-4001
E-mail: info@tainstruments.com
Web site: www.tainst.com
Medical Products Sales Volume: $26,400,000
Annual Revenue: More than $100 Million
Year Founded: 1996
Total Employees: 170   Marketing Staff: 15   Sales Staff: 20
Ownership: Waters Corp.
Stock Symbol: WAT
Traded On: NYSE
Quality System Registration Information: ISO9002
Produces/Sells CE-marked Devices: Y
Federal Procurement Eligibility: Small Business
Distribution: Manufacturer Direct, Manufacturer Through Distributor, Manufacturer Through Manufacturer Reps, Exporter
General Admin.: Patrick Y. Howard/President, Chief Executive Officer
Mktg./Adv.: Robert Hassel/Director Product Development
         George Dallas/Manager Marketing
         Terry Kelly/Vice President Marketing & Sales
Purchasing: Ed Butcher/Manager Purchasing

Calorimeter	Chemistry
Mass Spectrometer, Clinical Use	Toxicology

TABBIES, DIV. OF XERTREX INTERNATIONAL, INC.   800-822-2437

1530 W. Glenlake Ave., Itasca, IL 60143-1171   630-773-4160
FDA Number: n/a   Fax: 630-773-4696
E-mail: sales@tabbies.com
Web site: www.tabbies.com
Annual Revenue: $5-$10 Million
Year Founded: 1955
Total Employees: 60
Ownership: Private
Produces/Sells CE-marked Devices: N
Distribution: Manufacturer Through Distributor
General Admin.: Dennis W. Cunningham/President

Labeler, X-Ray Film	Radiology
Marker, X-Ray	Radiology

TABTRONICS, INC.   937-222-9969

2153 Winners Circle, Dayton, OH 45404
FDA Number: 1529102
E-mail: sales@Tabtronics.net
Web site: www.tabtronics.net
Ownership: Private
Produces/Sells CE-marked Devices: N

TACTILE SYSTEMS TECHNOLOGY INC   866-435-3948

1331 Tyler St. N.E., Ste. 200,   952-224-4060
Minneapolis, MN 55413
FDA Number: 3004183730   Fax: 866-435-3949
E-mail: info@tactilesystems.com
Web site: www.flexitouch.com
Year Founded: 1995
Ownership: Private
Produces/Sells CE-marked Devices: N
Federal Procurement Eligibility: Small Business, Female Owned
Distribution: Manufacturer Direct
General Admin.: Gerald R. Mattys/Chief Executive Officer
Mktg./Adv.: Mary Rausch/Director Marketing

Massager, Powered Inflatable Tube	Physical Med

TACTX MEDICAL/PRODUXX, INC.

See Creganna-Tactx Medical

TAGA MEDICAL TECHNOLOGIES   800-651-9490

34675 Vokes Drive, Suite 105,   440-602-8242
Eastlake, OH 44095
FDA Number: 3003499865
E-mail: tima@tagamed.com   Fax: 440-602-6989
Web site: www.tagamed.com
Medical Products Sales Volume: $110,000
Annual Revenue: $1-$5 Million
Year Founded: 1999

TAGA MEDICAL TECHNOLOGIES   800-651-9490 (cont'd)

Ownership: Private
Produces/Sells CE-marked Devices: N
Federal Procurement Eligibility: Small Business
Distribution: Manufacturer Through Distributor
General Admin.: Tim Austin/President, Chief Executive Officer, Chairman
Mktg./Adv.: Tim Austin/President Marketing & Sales
         Tim Austin/President New Product Development
Research: Gary Austin/Vice President Research & Development

Controller, Temperature, Humidifier	General
Dryer, Respiratory/Anesthesia Equipment	General
General Medical Device	General

TAGG INDUSTRIES L.L.C.   800-548-3514

23210 Del Lago, Laguna Hills, CA 92653   949-770-9029
FDA Number: 2083412   Fax: 949-770-3016
E-mail: info@taggmed.com
Web site: www.taggmed.com
Medical Products Sales Volume: $2,800,000
Annual Revenue: $1-$5 Million
Year Founded: 1984
Total Employees: 10   Marketing Staff: 2   Sales Staff: 15
Ownership: Private
Produces/Sells CE-marked Devices: Y
Federal Procurement Eligibility: Small Business, GSA Contract, VA Contract
Distribution: Manufacturer Direct, Manufacturer Through Distributor, Manufacturer Through Manufacturer Reps, OEM, Importer, Exporter
General Admin.: Terry Shirley/President, Chief Executive Officer
Mktg./Adv.: Consuelo Habal/Director National Accounts
         Frank Erlet/Manager Marketing

Attachment, Oxygen Canister/IV Pole, Wheelchair	General
Box, Transportation, Container, Specimen	General
Container, Specimen, All Types	General
Dressing, Other	General
Equipment, Therapy, Handicapped/Physical	Physical Med
Joint, Knee, External Brace	Physical Med
Mask, Oxygen, Aerosol Administration	Anesthesiology
Resuscitator, Cardiopulmonary	Cardiovascular
Valve, Non-Rebreathing	Anesthesiology

TAIHSIN ENTERPRISES INC.

See Life Guard

TAILORED LABEL PRODUCTS, INC.   800-727-1344

W165 N5731 Ridgewood Drive,   262-703-5000
Menomonee Falls, WI 53051
FDA Number: 2184127   Fax: 262-703-5010
E-mail: sales@tailoredlabel.com
Web site: www.tailoredlabel.com
Medical Products Sales Volume: $1,700,000
Annual Revenue: $5-$10 Million
Year Founded: 1984
Total Employees: 30   Marketing Staff: 3   Sales Staff: 9
Ownership: Private
Produces/Sells CE-marked Devices: N
Federal Procurement Eligibility: Small Business
Distribution: Manufacturer Direct, Manufacturer Through Distributor, Manufacturer Through Manufacturer Reps, Exporter
General Admin.: Michael Erwin/President
Mktg./Adv.: Kevin Machan/Director Marketing
         Brock Klaus/Manager National Sales
Production: Jim Brown/Managing Engineer

Adhesive Strip, Hypoallergenic	General
Adhesive Strip, Waterproof	General
Adhesive, Wound Closure	Surgery
Bandage, Adhesive	Surgery
Bandage, Butterfly	General
Component, Other	General
Component, Paper	General
Computer, Bar Code	General
Contract Assembly	General
Contract Manufacturing	General
Contract Manufacturing, Product, Disposable	General
Cushion, Ring, Foam Rubber	General
Dressing, Foam	General
Electrode, TENS	Cns/Neurology
Foam, Plastic	General
Gel, Electrode, TENS	Physical Med
Label, Bar Code	General
Label, Device	General
Label/Tag, Sterile	Surgery
Labeling Equipment	General
Marker, X-Ray	Radiology
Pad, Eye	Ophthalmology
Printer, Bar Code	General
Service, Printing	General
Strip, Adhesive	Surgery
Tag, Device Status	General
Tape, Adhesive	General
Tape, Adhesive, Hypoallergenic	General

TAILORED LABEL PRODUCTS, INC.   800-727-1344 *(cont'd)*
Tape, Adhesive, Waterproof   General

TAIYO TECH. OF AMERICA   847-466-7905
1355 Remington Road, Suite F, Schaumburg, IL 60173
FDA Number: n/a   *Fax:* 847-806-0758
Total Employees: 2   *Marketing Staff:* 2   *Sales Staff:* 2
Ownership: Private
Produces/Sells CE-marked Devices: N
Federal Procurement Eligibility: Small Business
Distribution: Service Direct
General Admin.: H. Tsuji/President
   Contract Manufacturing   General

TAK SYSTEMS   800-333-9631
14 Kendricks Road, Suite 5,   508-295-9630
Wareham, MA 02571
FDA Number: 1222665
E-mail: Cheryl@taksystems.com   *Fax:* 508-291-3240
Web site: www.taksystems.com
Medical Products Sales Volume: $1,700,000
Annual Revenue: $1-$5 Million
Year Founded: 1987
Total Employees: 21   *Marketing Staff:* 2   *Sales Staff:* 2
Ownership: Private
Produces/Sells CE-marked Devices: N
Federal Procurement Eligibility: Small Business, Minority Owned, GSA Contract, VA Contract
Distribution: Manufacturer Direct
General Admin.: Michael Diesso/President
Mktg./Adv.: C. A. Cavacas/Manager International Marketing & Sales
   Component, Plastic   General
   Material, Impression   Dental And Oral

TAKARA BELMONT USA, INC.   800-223-1192
101 Belmont Dr., Somerset, NJ 08873
FDA Number: 2243976   *Fax:* (732)356-1035
E-mail: gstern@belmontequip.com
Web site: www.belmontequip.com
Medical Products Sales Volume: $25,000,000
Annual Revenue: $25-$50 Million
Ownership: Takara Belmont Usa, Inc.
Produces/Sells CE-marked Devices: N
Distribution: Manufacturer Through Distributor
General Admin.: Hidetaka Yoshikawa/Chairman
      Masa Ando/Chief Operating Officer, General Manager
Mktg./Adv.: Fred Robinson/Vice President Marketing & Sales
   Chair, Dental   Dental And Oral
   Light, Dental   Dental And Oral
   Radiographic Unit, Diagnostic, Dental (X-Ray)   Dental And Oral
   Radiographic Unit, Diagnostic, Dental, Extraoral   Dental And Oral
   Stool, Dental   Dental And Oral

TAKARA COMPANY NY. INC.
See Takara Belmont Usa, Inc.

TAKE ONE LLC   602-997-2888
10807 North Cave Creek Rd., Phoenix, AZ 85020
FDA Number: 2032651
Ownership: Private
Produces/Sells CE-marked Devices: N
   Sunglasses (Including Photosensitive)   Ophthalmology

TAKE-ALONG LIFTS, LLC   877-667-6515
125 Pumpkin Hill Rd.,   877-667-6515
New Milford, CT 06776
FDA Number: 300697408   *Fax:* 877-667-6515
E-mail: TakeAlongLifts@UReach.com
Web site: www.TakeAlongLifts.com
Year Founded: 1999
Ownership: Private
Produces/Sells CE-marked Devices: N
Federal Procurement Eligibility: Small Business, Minority Owned
Distribution: Manufacturer Direct, Manufacturer Through Distributor
General Admin.: Mr. Alexander Brandorff/President
   Lift, Bath, Non-AC-Powered   General
   Lift, Patient   General

TALISMAN LIMITED   703-242-4200
421 F Church St., N.e., Vienna, VA 22180
FDA Number: 3004585612
   Software, Blood Bank (Stand-Alone Products)   Hematology

TALK-A-PHONE CO.   773-539-1100
5013 N. Kedzie Avenue, Chicago, IL 60625-4988
FDA Number: 9330119   *Fax:* 773-539-1241
E-mail: info@talkaphone.com
Web site: www.talkaphone.com
Ownership: Private

TALK-A-PHONE CO.   773-539-1100 *(cont'd)*
Produces/Sells CE-marked Devices: N
Federal Procurement Eligibility: Small Business
Distribution: Manufacturer Through Distributor
General Admin.: C. Z. Lieberman/Chief Executive Officer
Mktg./Adv.: Bob Shanes/Vice President Marketing & Sales
   Communication Equipment   General
   Pager, Non-Radio   General
   Physician Registry   General
   Telephone Equipment   General

TALLADIUM, INC.   661-295-0900
27360 West Muirfield Ln., Valencia, CA 91355
FDA Number: 2023129
   Alloy, Precious Metal, For Clinical Use   Dental And Oral
   Metal, Base   Dental And Oral

TALON ACRYLICS, INC.   888-433-2551
710 Strauss Ave, Winchester, OR 97495-8930   503-262-9307
FDA Number: 3032727   *Fax:* 503-253-0550
E-mail: talon@talonacrylics.com
Web site: www.talonacrylics.com
Ownership: Private
Produces/Sells CE-marked Devices: N
Federal Procurement Eligibility: Small Business
Distribution: Manufacturer Direct, Exporter
General Admin.: Mr. SHERMAN WATSON/President, Chief Executive Officer
   Base, Denture, Relining, Repairing, Rebasing, Resin   Dental And Oral
   Device, Repositioning, Jaw   Dental And Oral
   Material, Acrylic, Dental   Dental And Oral
   Prosthesis, Dental   Dental And Oral

TAMARAC SYSTEMS CORP.
See Cardiac Science Corp.

TAMARACK HABILITATION   763-795-0057
TECHNOLOGIES, INC.
1670 94th Lane NE, Blaine, MN 55449
FDA Number: 2133465   *Fax:* 763-795-0058
E-mail: tamarack@oandp.com
Web site: www.oandp.com/tamarack
Medical Products Sales Volume: $1,000,000
Year Founded: 1990
Total Employees: 12
Ownership: Private
Produces/Sells CE-marked Devices: N
Federal Procurement Eligibility: Small Business
   Accessories, Wheelchair   Physical Med
   Brace, Joint, Ankle (External)   Physical Med
   Cover, Limb   Physical Med

TAMBRANDS MANUFACTURING, INC.   513-634-2466
2879 Hotel Rd., Auburn, ME 04210
FDA Number: 1219109
   Tampon, Menstrual, Scented   Obstetrics/Gynecology
   Tampon, Menstrual, Unscented   Obstetrics/Gynecology

TAMCENAN CORP.   800-950-0113
1703 S. Minnesota Ave.,   605-334-0113
Sioux Falls, SD 57105
FDA Number: 1721624   *Fax:* 605-334-8247
E-mail: erlkoenig@sio.midco.net
Year Founded: 1988
Total Employees: 10   *Marketing Staff:* 2   *Sales Staff:* 5
Ownership: Private
Produces/Sells CE-marked Devices: N
Federal Procurement Eligibility: Small Business
Distribution: Manufacturer Direct
General Admin.: Thomas C. White/Chief Executive Officer
   Implant, Eye Valve   Ophthalmology
   Marker, Sclera (Ocular)   Ophthalmology
   Probe, Lacrimal   Ophthalmology
   Shunt, Intraocular   Ophthalmology

TAMPA HYPERBARIC ENTERPRISE   813-391-9473
10104 Lake Cove Lane, Tampa, FL 33618
FDA Number: 1059249   *Fax:* 813-931-0441
E-mail: oxyman@oxytank.com
Web site: www.oxytank.com
Total Employees: 2
Ownership: Private
Produces/Sells CE-marked Devices: N
Distribution: Manufacturer Direct
General Admin.: Michael Capria/President
   Chamber, Hyperbaric Oxygen   Physical Med

TAMPA WORK SERVICES   813-663-9555
5602 East Columbus Dr., Tampa, FL 33619
FDA Number: 3006227305

TAMPA WORK SERVICES   813-663-9555 *(cont'd)*
Ownership: Private
Produces/Sells CE-marked Devices: N
  Bandage, Adhesive   Surgery

TAMSCO TOOLS
  See Trans American Medical / Tamsco Instruments

TAN AMERICA-INDOOR SUNSYSTEM   800-350-2826
11151 Trade Center Dr.,   **916-503-7281**
Rancho Cordova, CA 95670
FDA Number: n/a   Fax: 916-638-0685
E-mail: salesca@heartlandtan.com
Web site: www.tanamerica.com
Medical Products Sales Volume: $15,000,000
Annual Revenue: $10-$25 Million
Ownership: Private
Produces/Sells CE-marked Devices: N
Distribution: Manufacturer Direct, Exporter
  Booth, Sun Tan   Physical Med

TAN SOURCE SUPPLY, INC.   913-451-7000
12142a State Line Rd., Leawood, KS 66209
FDA Number: 3003168809
Ownership: Private
Produces/Sells CE-marked Devices: N
  Booth, Sun Tan   Physical Med

TANDD CORPORATION   518-669-9227
PO Box 321, Saratoga Springs, FL 12866
FDA Number: n/a
E-mail: inquiries@tandd.com
Web site: www.tandd.com
Ownership: Private
Produces/Sells CE-marked Devices: N

TANDEM MEDICAL, INC.   760-943-0100
535 Encinitas Blvd, Suite 109, Encinitas, CA 92024
FDA Number: 2031881   Fax: 760-943-0143
E-mail: jdhaldeman@tanmed.com
Web site: www.autodose.com
Medical Products Sales Volume: $2,800,000
Annual Revenue: $1-$5 Million
Year Founded: 1997
Total Employees: 30   Marketing Staff: 2   Sales Staff: 4
Ownership: Private
Quality System Registration Information: ISO9001
Produces/Sells CE-marked Devices: Y
Federal Procurement Eligibility: Small Business
Distribution: Manufacturer Direct
General Admin.: Mr. Marc Lieberman/President, Chief Executive Officer
Mktg./Adv.: Ms. JD Haldeman/Vice President Marketing & Business Development
Production: Mr. Dave Brengle/Vice President Engineering & Operations
    Mr. Albert Misajon/Vice President Quality Assurance & Regulatory
Affairs
Finance: Mr. Greg Simmons/Chief Financial Officer
  Pump, Infusion, Elastomeric   General

TANGENT MEDICAL TECHNOLOGIES INC.   734-330-2668
58 Parkland Plaza, Suite 300, Ann Arbor, MI 48103
FDA Number: n/a   Fax: 734-213-0600
Web site: http://www.tangentmedical.com
Year Founded: 2009
Ownership: Private
Produces/Sells CE-marked Devices: N
General Admin.: Mr. Jeff Williams/Chief Executive Officer
Production: Mr. Jamie Olson/Vice President Operations
    Ms. Kay Fuller/Vice President Regulatory & Clinical Affairs

TANGLE, INC.   650-616-7900
439c Eccles Ave., South San Francisco, CA 94080
FDA Number: 3004511013
  Exerciser, Non-Measuring   Physical Med

TANITA CORPORATION OF AMERICA, INC.   877-682-6482
2625 S. Clearbrook Drive,   **847-640-9241**
Arlington Heights, IL 60005
FDA Number: 1423937   Fax: 847-640-9261
E-mail: PROSALES@tanita.com
Web site: www.tanita.com
Annual Revenue: $25-$50 Million
Ownership: Private
Quality System Registration Information: ISO9001
Produces/Sells CE-marked Devices: Y
Federal Procurement Eligibility: Small Business
Distribution: Manufacturer Through Distributor
General Admin.: Kiyoshi Izumisawa/Executive Vice President, General Manager
    Zentaro Yamazaki/President

TANITA CORPORATION OF AMERICA, INC. 877-682-6482 *(cont'd)*
Mktg./Adv.: John Skaggs/Director Marketing
    Dan McNulty/Vice President Sales
Production: Rhoda Lynn Valera/Manager Regulatory Affairs
    Jim Montagnino/Vice President Technology & Product Development
  Analyzer, Body Composition   Cardiovascular
  Scale, Infant   General
  Scale, Stand-On   General

TANOX BIOSYSTEMS, INC.   713-664-2288
10301 Stella Link Road, Suite 110, Houston, TX 77025-5497
FDA Number: n/a   Fax: 713-664-8914
E-mail: info@tanox.com
Annual Revenue: $0-$1 Million
Year Founded: 1986
Total Employees: 130
Ownership: Public
Stock Symbol: TNOX
Traded On: NASDAQ
Produces/Sells CE-marked Devices: N
Federal Procurement Eligibility: Minority Owned, Female Owned
Distribution: Manufacturer Direct
General Admin.: Mr. Jeff Organ/Chief Operating Officer
    Ms. Michelle DeSantis/Coordinator
    Dr. Ashraf Hanna/Director
    Nancy T. Chang/President, Chief Executive Officer
Mktg./Adv.: Mr. Joe Welch/Vice President Marketing & Business Development
  Antibody, Monoclonal   Microbiology

TAP EXPRESS, INC.   305-468-0038
8424 Nw 61 St., Miami, FL 33166
FDA Number: 1058192
Ownership: Private
Produces/Sells CE-marked Devices: N
  Band, Elastic, Orthodontic   Dental And Oral

TAPCO MEDICAL, INC.   818-225-5376
23981 Craftsman Road, Calabasas, CA 91302
FDA Number: n/a   Fax: 818-222-1276
E-mail: kimm@mundymed.com
Medical Products Sales Volume: $400,000
Year Founded: 1994
Total Employees: 3
Ownership: Private
Produces/Sells CE-marked Devices: Y
Federal Procurement Eligibility: Small Business
  Cart, Instrument/Equipment, Laparoscopy   Surgery
  Cover, Camera   Surgery
  Glove, Protective, Radiographic   Radiology
  Staple, Fixation, Bone   Orthopedics
  Sterilization Indicator   Surgery

TAPCON, INC.   800-247-3587
521 Sheperd Street, Garland, TX 75042   **972-276-0178**
FDA Number: 1717926   Fax: 972-494-5332
E-mail: tapcon@gte.net
Web site: www.tapconinc.com
Medical Products Sales Volume: $800,000
Annual Revenue: $1-$5 Million
Year Founded: 1975
Total Employees: 4
Ownership: Private
Produces/Sells CE-marked Devices: N
Federal Procurement Eligibility: Small Business
Distribution: Manufacturer Direct, Manufacturer Through Distributor, Service Direct
Mktg./Adv.: Jim Reynolds/Director Sales
Production: Tim Boyle/Vice President Manufacturing
  Equipment, Cleaning, Air   General

TAPE-O-CORPORATION   800-752-4944
35 Crosby Road, Dover, NH 03820-4340   **603-743-6636**
FDA Number: 3003640109   Fax: 603-743-6645
E-mail: info@tape-o.com
Web site: www.tape-o.com
Medical Products Sales Volume: $2,500,000
Annual Revenue: $5-$10 Million
Year Founded: 1952
Total Employees: 30   Marketing Staff: 2   Sales Staff: 5
Ownership: Private
Produces/Sells CE-marked Devices: Y
Federal Procurement Eligibility: Small Business
Distribution: Manufacturer Direct, Manufacturer Through Distributor, Manufacturer
Through Manufacturer Reps, Service Direct, Importer, Exporter
General Admin.: Stuart Bauder/President
    Debra Miesfeldt/Vice President
Mktg./Adv.: Ernie Goulet/Vice President Sales
Production: Thomas Hand/Plant & Production Manager
  Bandage, Adhesive   Surgery

MANUFACTURER PROFILES

TAPE-O-CORPORATION   800-752-4944 *(cont'd)*
- Bandage, Elastic   General
- Solvent, Adhesive Tape   Surgery

TAPELESS WOUND CARE PRODUCTS, LLC.   866-714-9199
PO Box 4515, ENGLEWOOD, CO 80155   303-881-9355
- FDA Number: 1723835
- E-mail: tapefree@aol.com   *Fax: 303-699-8880*
- Web site: www.tapelesswoundcare.com
- Medical Products Sales Volume: $190,000
- Annual Revenue: $0-$1 Million
- Year Founded: 2003
- Total Employees: 3
- Ownership: Private
- Produces/Sells CE-marked Devices: N
- Federal Procurement Eligibility: Small Business
- Distribution: Manufacturer Direct, Manufacturer Through Distributor, OEM, Exclusive Distributor
- General Admin.: Mr. John Finamore/Chief Executive Officer, Chief Financial Officer
  - Dr. Barry Shesol/President, Chief Operating Officer
- Accessories, Apparel, Surgical   Surgery
- Bag, Ice   General
- Bandage, Elastic   General
- Bandage, Other   General

TAPEMARK   800-535-1998
1685 Marthaler Lane,   651-455-1611
West St. Paul, MN 55118
- FDA Number: 2182681
- E-mail: tmsales@tapemark.com   *Fax: 651-450-8403*
- Web site: www.tapemark.com
- Annual Revenue: $50-$100 Million
- Year Founded: 1952
- Total Employees: 200
- Ownership: Private
- Quality System Registration Information: ISO9001
- Produces/Sells CE-marked Devices: N
- Distribution: OEM
- General Admin.: Robert Klas/Chief Executive Officer
  - Ms. Pat Mork/Director Human Resources
  - Andy Rensink/President, Chief Operating Officer
- Mktg./Adv.: Steve Larsen/Manager Sales
  - Julie Karlson/Market Manager
  - Kim Mueller/Vice President Marketing & Sales
- Production: Steve Rau/Director Engineering
  - Matt Bilbo/Director Operations
  - Marilyn Tucker/Vice President Quality Assurance & Regulatory Affairs
- Research: Tom Yetter/Vice President Research & Development
- Contract Manufacturing   General
- Contract Manufacturing, Pharmaceuticals/Chemicals   General
- Contract Manufacturing, Product, Disposable   General
- Contract Manufacturing, Reagent   General
- Contract Packaging   General
- Dilator, Nasal   Ear/Nose/Throat
- Holder, X-Ray Film   Dental And Oral
- Iontophoresis Unit, Physical Medicine   Physical Med

TAPESWITCH CORPORATION   800-234-8273
100 Schmitt Blvd., Farmingdale, NY 11735   631-630-0442
- FDA Number: n/a   *Fax: 631-630-0454*
- E-mail: sales@tapeswitch.com
- Web site: www.tapeswitch.com
- Medical Products Sales Volume: $1,000,000
- Annual Revenue: $10-$25 Million
- Total Employees: 90
- Ownership: CTS
- Produces/Sells CE-marked Devices: Y
- Distribution: Manufacturer Direct, Manufacturer Through Distributor, Manufacturer Through Manufacturer Reps
- General Admin.: Mike Steele/President
- Mktg./Adv.: Bob Espinosa/Supervisor Sales Support
- Floor Mat   General
- Monitor, Bed Occupancy   General
- Monitor, Bed Patient   General

TARGESON INC.   877-290-4043
3550 General Atomics Court, MS 02-444,   858-427-3675
San Diego, CA 92121
- FDA Number: n/a   *Fax: 877-859-0981*
- Web site: http://www.targeson.com
- Ownership: Private
- Produces/Sells CE-marked Devices: N
- General Admin.: Mr. Jack DeFranco/President, Chief Executive Officer
- Research: Dr. Joshua Rychak/Vice President Research & Development

TARGET COMPACTION, INC.   315-363-3077
510 Lake Rd., Oneida, NY 13421
- FDA Number: 2438463

TARGET COMPACTION, INC.   315-363-3077 *(cont'd)*
- Ownership: Private
- Produces/Sells CE-marked Devices: N
- Lift, Bath, Non-AC-Powered   General

TARO PHARMACEUTICALS, INC.   905-791-8276
130 East Dr, Brampton L6T 1C1 Canada
- FDA Number: 8022154
- Jelly, Lubricating, Transurethral Surgical Instrument   Gastroenterology/Urology

TARRY MANUFACTURING   800-688-2779
22 Shelter Rock Lane, Danbury, CT 06810-8156   203-794-1438
- FDA Number: 1226711
- E-mail: customerservice@tarrymfg.com   *Fax: 203-792-5581*
- Web site: www.tarrymfg.com
- Annual Revenue: $1-$5 Million
- Year Founded: 1982
- Ownership: Private
- Produces/Sells CE-marked Devices: Y
- Federal Procurement Eligibility: Small Business
- Distribution: Manufacturer Direct, Manufacturer Through Distributor, Manufacturer Through Manufacturer Reps, Exporter
- Armboard, Wheelchair   Physical Med
- Bandage, Adhesive   Surgery
- Board, Arm   Anesthesiology
- Cover, Mattress   General
- Incubator, Neonatal   General
- Protector, Skin Pressure   General
- Support, Breathing Tube   Anesthesiology
- Warmer, Radiant, Infant   General

TARTAN ORTHOPEDICS, LTD.   888-287-1456
10651 Irma Drive, Unit C, Northglenn, CO 80233   303-287-1456
- FDA Number: 1718669
- E-mail: dsanders@tartanortho.com   *Fax: 303-287-4739*
- Web site: www.tartanortho.com
- Medical Products Sales Volume: $500,000
- Annual Revenue: $0-$1 Million
- Year Founded: 1974
- Total Employees: 10   *Sales Staff: 20*
- Ownership: Private
- Produces/Sells CE-marked Devices: N
- Federal Procurement Eligibility: Small Business
- Distribution: Manufacturer Direct, Manufacturer Through Distributor, Exporter
- General Admin.: David G. Sanders/President
- Mktg./Adv.: Russ Blanden/Vice President Marketing
- Production: Dan Durbin/Vice President Manufacturing
- Research: Sandy Covey/Manager Research
- Apron, Surgical   Surgery
- Belt, Abdominal   Gastroenterology/Urology
- Belt, Support, Pelvic   Physical Med
- Belt, Traction, Pelvic, Orthopedic   Orthopedics
- Binder, Abdominal   General
- Binder, Breast   Obstetrics/Gynecology
- Binder, Wrist   Orthopedics
- Brace, Joint, Ankle (External)   Physical Med
- Cage, Knee   Physical Med
- Immobilizer, Ankle   Orthopedics
- Immobilizer, Elbow   Orthopedics
- Immobilizer, Knee   Orthopedics
- Immobilizer, Shoulder   Orthopedics
- Immobilizer, Wrist/Hand   Orthopedics
- Joint, Knee, External Brace   Physical Med
- Orthosis, Cervical   Physical Med
- Orthosis, Cervical-Thoracic, Rigid   Physical Med
- Orthosis, Lumbosacral   Physical Med
- Orthosis, Rib Fracture, Soft   Physical Med
- Orthosis, Sacroiliac, Soft   Physical Med
- Pad, Pressure, Foam (Elbow, Heel)   General
- Restraint, Ankle/Foot   General
- Restraint, Protective (Body)   General
- Restraint, Wrist/Hand   General
- Shoe, Cast   Physical Med
- Sling, Arm   Physical Med
- Sling, Arm, Overhead Supported   Physical Med
- Sling, Knee   Orthopedics
- Splint, Abduction, Congenital Hip Dislocation   Physical Med
- Splint, Clavicle   Physical Med
- Splint, Extremity, Non-Inflatable, External   Surgery
- Support, Ankle   Orthopedics
- Support, Arm   Physical Med
- Support, Clavicle   Orthopedics

TASK MICRO-ELECTRONICS INC.   514-697-6616
16700 TransCanada Hwy, Montreal, QUE H9H-4M7 Canada
- FDA Number: n/a   *Fax: 514-697-6466*
- E-mail: info@taskmicro.com
- Web site: www.taskmicro.com
- Year Founded: 1987
- Total Employees: 100

TASK MICRO-ELECTRONICS INC.   514-697-6616 *(cont'd)*
Ownership: Private
Produces/Sells CE-marked Devices: N
Distribution: Manufacturer Direct, Exporter

TATUM SURGICAL   888-360-5550 / 727-536-4880
14010 Roosevelt Blvd, Suite # 705,
Clearwater, FL 33762
FDA Number: 1054986   Fax: 727-531-6005
E-mail: tatumsurgical@tampabay.rr.com
Web site: www.tatumsurgical.com
Medical Products Sales Volume: $200,000
Year Founded: 1981
Total Employees: 5
Ownership: Suncoast Dental, Inc.
Quality System Registration Information: ISO9001
Produces/Sells CE-marked Devices: Y
Federal Procurement Eligibility: Small Business
Distribution: Exclusive Distributor
General Admin.: Ms. Norma Woods/President

System, Implant, Tooth	Dental And Oral

TAUB PRODUCTS & FUSION CO., INC.
See George Taub Products & Fusion Co., Inc.

TAUT, INC.   800-231-8288 / 630-232-2507
2571 Kaneville Ct., Geneva, IL 60134
FDA Number: n/a   Fax: 630-232-8005
E-mail: info@taut.com
Web site: www.taut.com
Medical Products Sales Volume: $3,600,000
Total Employees: 45
Ownership: Private
Quality System Registration Information: ISO9002
Produces/Sells CE-marked Devices: Y
Federal Procurement Eligibility: Small Business
Distribution: Manufacturer Direct, Manufacturer Through Distributor, OEM, Exporter
General Admin.: G. G. McFarlane/Executive Vice President
     R. H. McFarlane/President
Mktg./Adv.: Matthew McFarlane/Vice President Corporate Development
     Raul Brizuela/Vice President Marketing & Sales
Production: Max Cloat/Director Quality Assurance
     R. D. Kenseth/Vice President Operations

Cart, Instrument/Equipment, Laparoscopy	Surgery
Catheter, Cholangiography	Surgery
Catheter, Intravenous	Cardiovascular
Catheter, Peritoneal	Surgery
Clip, Other	Surgery
Drain, Penrose	Gastroenterology/Urology
Introducer, Catheter	Cardiovascular
Kit, Cholecystectomy	Gastroenterology/Urology
Kit, Laparoscopy	Gastroenterology/Urology
Kit, Wound Drainage	General
Trocar, Laparoscopic	Surgery
Tube, Drainage	Gastroenterology/Urology

TAVA SURGICAL INSTRUMENTS   800 569-6738 / 912-921-7575
4837 McGrath St., Ste. J, Ventura, CA 93003
FDA Number: 2025102   Fax: 805-560-5260
E-mail: customerservice@brasselerusa.com
Web site: http://www.tavasurgical.com
Year Founded: 1977
Ownership: Private
Produces/Sells CE-marked Devices: Y
Distribution: Manufacturer Through Manufacturer Reps
Production: Mr. Christopher Feitel/Manager Quality Assurance & Regulatory Affairs

Accessories, Powered Drill	Cns/Neurology
Blade, Surgical, Saw, General & Plastic Surgery	Surgery
Burr	Ear/Nose/Throat
Burr, Dental	Dental And Oral
Burr, Surgical, General & Plastic Surgery	Surgery
Instrument, Surgical, Powered, Pneumatic	Orthopedics
Lavage Unit, Water Jet	General
Motor, Drill, Pneumatic	Cns/Neurology
Pin, Fixation, Smooth	Orthopedics
Pin, Fixation, Threaded	Orthopedics
Saw, Powered, And Accessories	Cns/Neurology
Suction Apparatus, Operating Room, Wall Vacuum-Powered	Surgery
Surgical Instrument, Orthopedic, AC-Powered Motor	Orthopedics
Wrap, Sterilization	General

TAYLOR   800-255-0626 / 815-624-8333
750 N. Blackhawk Blvd., P.O. Box 410,
Rockton, IL 61072
FDA Number: 1420149   Fax: 815-624-8000
E-mail: info@taylor-company.com
Web site: www.taylor-company.com
Year Founded: 1926

TAYLOR   800-255-0626 *(cont'd)*
Total Employees: 375
Ownership: Carrier Commercial Refrigeration
Stock Symbol: UTX
Traded On: NYSE
Quality System Registration Information: ISO9001
Produces/Sells CE-marked Devices: Y
Distribution: Exclusive Distributor
General Admin.: Marguerite Stuck/Director Human Resources
Mktg./Adv.: Tricia Bennett/Manager Marketing Services
     Stephen Neas/Vice President Marketing & Sales
Production: Debra Magee/Vice President Operations

Dispenser, Fluid	General
Foodservice Product/Equipment	General

TAYLOR FREEZER COMPANY
See Taylor

TAYLOR INDUSTRIES, INC.   800-339-1361 / 573-893-5412
2706 Industrial Drive, Jefferson City, MO 65109
FDA Number: 2133585   Fax: 573-893-3647
E-mail: taylor@taylor-ind.com
Web site: www.taylor-ind.com
Medical Products Sales Volume: $600,000
Annual Revenue: $0-$1 Million
Year Founded: 1994
Total Employees: 5   Marketing Staff: 2   Sales Staff: 10
Ownership: Private
Produces/Sells CE-marked Devices: N
Federal Procurement Eligibility: Small Business, VA Contract
Distribution: Manufacturer Direct, Manufacturer Through Distributor, Manufacturer Through Manufacturer Reps, OEM, Exporter
General Admin.: Mr. Kevin Holtmeyer/Admin., General Manager
Mktg./Adv.: Mr. Michael Ballard/President, Chief Executive Officer, Marketing Manager
Production: Mr. Otis Jessee/Chief Engineer

Electrode, ECG, Radiolucent	Cardiovascular
Electrode, Electrocardiograph	Cardiovascular
Electrode, Electrocardiograph, Long-Term	Cardiovascular
Electrode, Electrocardiograph, Multi-Function	Cardiovascular
Electrode, Gel	Cardiovascular
Electrode, Holter	Cardiovascular
Gel, Electrode, Electrocardiograph	Cardiovascular
Pad, Electrode	Cardiovascular
Recorder, Paper Chart	Cardiovascular
Stimulator, Muscle, Electrical-Powered (EMS)	Physical Med
Stimulator, Muscle, Low Intensity	Physical Med
Stimulator, Muscle, Powered, Invasive	Physical Med
Stimulator, Neuromuscular, Functional Walking, Non-Invasive	Physical Med
Tape, Adhesive, Hypoallergenic	General

TAYLOR LTD., EDWARD
See Western Medical, Ltd.

TAYLOR WHARTON   800-898-2657 / 251-443-8680
4075 Hamilton Blvd., Theodore, AL 36582
FDA Number: n/a   Fax: 251-443-2209
E-mail: twsales@harsco.com
Web site: www.taylorwharton.com
Medical Products Sales Volume: $3,000,000
Annual Revenue: More than $100 Million
Total Employees: 45   Marketing Staff: 3   Sales Staff: 12
Ownership: HARSCO CORP.
Stock Symbol: HSC
Traded On: NYSE
Quality System Registration Information: ISO9001
Federal Procurement Eligibility: Small Business
Distribution: Manufacturer Direct, Manufacturer Through Distributor, OEM, Service Direct, Importer, Exporter
General Admin.: Ronald W. Kaplan/President

Cleanroom Equipment	General
Refrigerator, Biological	Microbiology

TAYLOR'S MFG.   336-886-4192
524 Barker Ave, High Point, NC 27262
FDA Number: 1067142
Ownership: Private
Produces/Sells CE-marked Devices: N

Bed, Manual	General

TAYLORCRAFT, INC.   877-376-4756
313 Harbor Watch Dr., Chesapeake, VA 23320
FDA Number: 3005403332

Shoe, Cast	Physical Med

TBL, INC.   816-233-5487
751 South 4th St., St. Joseph, MO 64507
FDA Number: 3002265489

Preservative, Cytological	Pathology

TC IMAGING SOLUTIONS
757-224-0177
2432 Cheyenne Trail, Traverse City, MI 49684
FDA Number: 3005916116
Device, Communications, Images, Ophthalmic — Ophthalmology

TCP RELIABLE, INC.
888-TCP-3393
551 Raritan Center Pkwy., Edison, NJ 08837 **732-346-9200**
FDA Number: n/a
Fax: 732-346-0295
E-mail: Sales@TCPreliable.com
Web site: www.tcpreliable.com
Medical Products Sales Volume: $9,600,000
Annual Revenue: $5-$10 Million
Year Founded: 1990
Total Employees: 45 *Marketing Staff:* 2 *Sales Staff:* 5
Ownership: Public
Produces/Sells CE-marked Devices: N
Federal Procurement Eligibility: Small Business
Distribution: Manufacturer Direct, Service Direct
General Admin.: Mr. Frank Hajduk/Chief Operating Officer
   Mr. Maurice Barakat/President, Chief Executive Officer
Mktg./Adv.: Ms. Donna Swisher/Coord. Sales
   Mr. Michael Paterno/Sales Representative
Case, Protection, Equipment — General
Controller, Temperature, Other — General
Pack, Cold — General
Service, Engineering/Design — General

TCS SCIENTIFIC CORP.
215-862-3910
6467 StoneyHill Road, New Hope, PA 18938
FDA Number: 9201044
Fax: 215-862-4710
E-mail: mail@tcssci.com
Web site: www.tcssci.com
Medical Products Sales Volume: $1,000,000
Annual Revenue: $0-$1 Million
Total Employees: 3 *Marketing Staff:* 1 *Sales Staff:* 1
Ownership: Private
Produces/Sells CE-marked Devices: N
Federal Procurement Eligibility: Small Business
Distribution: Manufacturer Direct, Manufacturer Through Manufacturer Reps, OEM
General Admin.: Wayne Albert/Owner, Chief Executive Officer
Analyzer, Gas, Oxygen, Partial Pressure, Blood Phase — Anesthesiology
Computer Software — General

TDM/TDX LAB., INC.
See Specialty Laboratories, Inc.

TDS HEALTHCARE SYSTEMS CORPORATION
See Eclipsys Corporation

TDS U-BEST DENTAL TECHNOLOGY
866-686-1899
2941 E. Miraloma Ave. #6 & 7,
714-666-2288
Anaheim, CA 92806
FDA Number: 3006301978
Fax: 714-666-2388
E-mail: ubestdental@yahoo.com
Web site: www.ubestdental.com
Ownership: Private
Produces/Sells CE-marked Devices: N
Teeth, Artificial, Backing And Facing — Dental And Oral

TEAM AMERICA HEALTH & FITNESS, INC
800-642-5419
675 Racquet Club Ln,
805-777-0168
Thousand Oaks, CA 91360
FDA Number: 2014789
Fax: 805-499-4861
E-mail: exergenie@earthlink.net
Web site: www.exergenie.com
Medical Products Sales Volume: $700,000
Annual Revenue: $0-$1 Million
Year Founded: 1975
Total Employees: 4
Ownership: TEAM AMERICA HEALTH & FITNESS, INC.
Produces/Sells CE-marked Devices: N
Federal Procurement Eligibility: Small Business
Distribution: Manufacturer Direct, Manufacturer Through Distributor
Production: Jim Warren/Manager Production
Exerciser, Non-Measuring — Physical Med

TEAM TECHNOLOGIES MOLDING
630-937-0380
1300 Nagel Blvd., Batavia, IL 60510
FDA Number: 3006187135
Evacuator, Oral Cavity — Dental And Oral

TEAM TECHNOLOGIES, INC.
423-587-2199
5949 Commerce Blvd., Morristown, TN 37814
FDA Number: 1051594
Brush, Scrub, Operating Room — Surgery
Catheter, Suction (Tracheal Aspirating Tube) — Anesthesiology
Floss, Dental — Dental And Oral
Handpiece, Contra- And Right-Angle Attachment, Dental — Dental And Oral
Mirror, Mouth — Dental And Oral

TEAM TECHNOLOGIES, INC.
423-587-2199 *(cont'd)*
Mouthpiece, Saliva Ejector — Dental And Oral
Polyvinyl Methylether Maleic Acid/Carboxymethylcellulose — Dental And Oral
Scraper, Tongue — Dental And Oral
Spatula, Cervical, Cytology — Obstetrics/Gynecology
Toothbrush, Manual — Dental And Oral

TEAM VANTAGE MOLDING LLC.
651-464-3900
22455 Everton Avenue N., Forest Lake, MN 55025-0370
FDA Number: 2183970
Fax: 651-982-1299
E-mail: sales@teamvantage.com
Web site: www.teamvantage.com
Medical Products Sales Volume: $4,300,000
Annual Revenue: $10-$25 Million
Year Founded: 1996
Total Employees: 65 *Marketing Staff:* 2 *Sales Staff:* 2
Ownership: Private
Quality System Registration Information: ISO9001
Produces/Sells CE-marked Devices: N
Federal Procurement Eligibility: Small Business
Distribution: Manufacturer Direct, Service Direct
General Admin.: Ray Newkirk/President, Chief Executive Officer
Mktg./Adv.: Randy Kvalheim/Manager National Sales
Production: Lester Jones/Director Quality Assurance
   Phil Hage/Plant Manager
Molding, Custom — General

TEARSCIENCE INC.
919-467-4007
5151 McCrimmon Parkway, Ste 250, Morrisville, NC 27560
FDA Number: 3008169506
E-mail: info@tearscience.com
Web site: http://www.lipiflow.com
Year Founded: 2005
Ownership: Private
Produces/Sells CE-marked Devices: N
Caliper, Ophthalmic — Ophthalmology
Camera, Ophthalmic, AC-Powered (Fundus) — Ophthalmology
Lamp, Slit, Biomicroscope, AC-Powered — Ophthalmology

TEARTEC
816-518-8626
7400 N.w. Whipple Ln., Kansas City, MO 64152
FDA Number: 1932161
Ownership: Private
Produces/Sells CE-marked Devices: N
Applicator, Tipped, Absorbent, Non-Sterile — General

TEC COACH CO.
See Medtec Ambulance Corp.

TECA CORP.
See Oxford Instruments

TECAN SYSTEMS
800-231-0711
2450 Zanker Rd., San Jose, CA 95131 **408-953-3100**
FDA Number: 2916719
Fax: 408-953-3101
E-mail: helpdesk-sy@tecan.com
Web site: www.tecan.com
Annual Revenue: $100-$500 Million
Total Employees: 1116
Ownership: Tecan Group Ag, Ltd.
Quality System Registration Information: ISO9001
Produces/Sells CE-marked Devices: Y
Federal Procurement Eligibility: Small Business
Distribution: OEM
General Admin.: Mike Baronian/Chairman
   Thomas P. Bachmann/Chief Executive Officer
Diluter — Chemistry
Dispenser, Fluid — General
Microtiter Diluting/Dispensing Device — Microbiology
Pipette, Diluting — Hematology
Pipetting And Diluting System, Automated — Chemistry
Pump, Infusion — General
Pump, Laboratory — Chemistry
System, Robot — General
Valve, Other — Chemistry

TECAN U.S., INC.
1 800 352 5128
4022 Stirrup Creek Rd., Ste. 310,
919-361-5200
Durham, NC 27709
FDA Number: 1037985
Fax: 919-361-5201
E-mail: Sales-Americas@Tecan.com
Web site: www.tecan.com
Annual Revenue: $100-$500 Million
Ownership: Tecan Group Ag, Ltd.
Traded On: Switzerland
Quality System Registration Information: ISO9001
Produces/Sells CE-marked Devices: Y
Federal Procurement Eligibility: Small Business
Distribution: Manufacturer Direct, Manufacturer Through Distributor
General Admin.: Dr. Emile C. Sutcliffe/Chief Executive Officer

TECAN U.S., INC. 1 800 352 5128 (cont'd)

Diane Bell/Manager Human Resources
Carl Severinghaus/President
Jaye McDermott/Vice President, General Manager
Mktg./Adv.: Elaine Carraher/Director Marketing
Peter Siesel/Vice President Sales
Production: Ron Wheeler/Manager Quality Assurance

Computer Software	General
Container, Medication, Graduated Liquid	General
Equipment, Test, Western Blot	Microbiology
Fluorometer	Immunology
Reader, Microplate	General
System, Robot	General
Washer, Microplate	General

TECH SPRAY, L.P. 800-858-4043
P.O. Box 949, Amarillo, TX 79105-0949 806-372-8523
FDA Number: n/a *Fax:* 806-372-8750
E-mail: tsales@techspray.com
Web site: www.techspray.com
Annual Revenue: $25-$50 Million
Total Employees: 230 *Marketing Staff:* 6 *Sales Staff:* 20
Ownership: Private
Produces/Sells CE-marked Devices: N
Federal Procurement Eligibility: Small Business
Distribution: Manufacturer Through Distributor
General Admin.: Richard Russell/Chief Executive Officer
Jimmy Witcher/President
Mktg./Adv.: Bo Maurer/Director Marketing & Sales
Kevin Pawlowaki/Manager Advertising
Bill Butler/Manager Sales
Research: Steve Cook/Director Technology
Finance: Sam Spadlin/Chief Financial Officer

Production Equipment	General

TECH MEDICAL, INC.
See The Tech Group

TECH PROTOTYPE
See Technh, Inc

TECH/OPS
See Landauer, Inc.

TECHALLOY CO., INC.
See Rahns Specialty Metals

TECHDEVICE CORPORATION 888-TECHDEV
650 Pleasant St., Watertown, MA 02472 617-972-5800
FDA Number: 3003712030 *Fax:* 617-972-5815
E-mail: info@techdevice.com
Web site: www.techdevice.com
Ownership: Private
Produces/Sells CE-marked Devices: N

Guidewire	Cardiovascular

TECHLAB, INC. 800-832-4522
2001 Kraft Drive, Blacksburg, VA 24060-6364 540-953-1664
FDA Number: 1122855 *Fax:* 540-953-1665
E-mail: techlab@techlab.com
Web site: www.techlab.com
Medical Products Sales Volume: $3,100,000
Annual Revenue: $1-$5 Million
Year Founded: 1989
Total Employees: 40 *Marketing Staff:* 1 *Sales Staff:* 1
Ownership: Private
Produces/Sells CE-marked Devices: N
Federal Procurement Eligibility: Small Business
Distribution: Manufacturer Direct, Manufacturer Through Distributor, Manufacturer Through Manufacturer Reps, OEM, Importer, Exporter
General Admin.: Dr. Tracy Wilkins/President, Chief Executive Officer
Dr. David Lyerly/Vice President
Mktg./Adv.: Ms. Pauline Hahn/Director Marketing
Ms. Pauline Hahn/Manager International Sales
Ms. Betty Polk/Manager National Sales
Production: Ms. Donna Evans/Director Quality Assurance
Ms. Donna Evans/Manager Regulatory Affairs
Mr. David Wall/Vice President Operations
Research: Dr. David Lyerly/Manager Research & Development

Antigen, Antiserum, Control, Lactoferrin	Immunology
Test, Bacterial Diagnostic	Microbiology

TECHMAN INT'L CORP. 508-248-2900
242 Sturbridge Rd., Charlton, MA 01507
FDA Number: 1225807
Ownership: Private
Produces/Sells CE-marked Devices: N

Colposcope	Obstetrics/Gynecology
Fiberoptic Light Source & Carrier	Ear/Nose/Throat
Headlight, Fiberoptic Focusing	Gastroenterology/Urology
Light Source, Fiberoptic, Routine	Gastroenterology/Urology

TECHMAN INT'L CORP. 508-248-2900 (cont'd)

Microscope, Surgical	Ear/Nose/Throat
Retractor, Fiberoptic	Gastroenterology/Urology

TECHMED CORP.
See Empi, Inc.

TECHMIRE LTD. 514-694-4110
185 Voyageur, Pointe Claire,, QC H9R 6B2 Canada
FDA Number: n/a *Fax:* 514-694-2634
E-mail: info@techmire.com
Total Employees: 80 *Marketing Staff:* 5 *Sales Staff:* 2
Ownership: Public
Produces/Sells CE-marked Devices: N
Distribution: Manufacturer Direct, Exporter

TECHNE CORPORATION 612-379-8854
614 McKinley Place N.E., Minneapolis, MN 55413
FDA Number: n/a *Fax:* 612-379-6580
Web site: http://www.techne-corp.com
Year Founded: 1981
Ownership: Public
Stock Symbol: TECH
Traded On: NASDAQ
Produces/Sells CE-marked Devices: N

TECHNH, INC 603-424-4404
8 Continental Blvd., PO Box 476, Merrimack, NH 03054
FDA Number: 1223651 *Fax:* 603-424-5820
E-mail: sales@technh.com
Web site: www.technh.com
Medical Products Sales Volume: $9,000,000
Annual Revenue: $5-$10 Million
Year Founded: 1982
Total Employees: 100 *Marketing Staff:* 2 *Sales Staff:* 3
Ownership: Private
Quality System Registration Information: ISO9001
Produces/Sells CE-marked Devices: N
Federal Procurement Eligibility: Small Business
Distribution: Manufacturer Direct, Manufacturer Through Manufacturer Reps
General Admin.: Richard Grosky/President, Chief Executive Officer
Deborah Cochran/Vice President Human Resources
Mktg./Adv.: Roger Somers/Director Marketing
Doug Waterman/Director Product Development
Roger Somers/Manager Advertising
Production: Kim Rice/Director Quality Assurance
Craig Stern/Manager Materials
Kim Rice/Manager Regulatory Affairs
Gregory Gardner/Vice President Manufacturing
Purchasing: Craig Stern/Manager Purchasing

Germ-Free Apparatus	Microbiology
Molding, Custom	General
Molding, Injection	General

TECHNICAL INSTRUMENTS (TI) 650-651-3000
1826 Rollins Road, Burlingame, CA 94010-2215
FDA Number: 7000354 *Fax:* 650-651-3001
E-mail: info@techinst.com
Web site: www.techinst.com
Medical Products Sales Volume: $4,800,000
Annual Revenue: $10-$25 Million
Total Employees: 29 *Marketing Staff:* 2 *Sales Staff:* 12
Ownership: Private
Produces/Sells CE-marked Devices: N
Federal Procurement Eligibility: Small Business
Distribution: Manufacturer Through Distributor
General Admin.: F. E. Lundy/President, Chief Executive Officer
Brian Lundy/Vice President, General Manager
Mktg./Adv.: Mr. Eric Wishan/Senior Sales Manager
Production: David Blevins/Manager Materials
Finance: Dennis Milosky/Chief Financial Officer

Micromanipulator, Laboratory	Microbiology
Microscope	Hematology
Microscope, Laboratory, Optical	Microbiology
Microscope, Laser, Scanning, Acoustic	Microbiology
Microscope, Surgical, General & Plastic Surgery	Surgery

TECHNICAL MARKETING, INC. 954-370-0855
1776 N. Pine Island Road, Suite 306, Plantation, FL 33322-5253
FDA Number: 1039746 *Fax:* 954-474-3866
E-mail: tmusa@bellsouth.net
Medical Products Sales Volume: $1,500,000
Annual Revenue: $1-$5 Million
Total Employees: 12
Ownership: Private
Federal Procurement Eligibility: Small Business, GSA Contract, VA Contract
Distribution: Exclusive Distributor, Importer, Exporter
General Admin.: William Leibstone/President
Jean Claude Kappler/Vice President

TECHNICAL MARKETING, INC.
954-370-0855 *(cont'd)*

Contract Manufacturing, Pharmaceuticals/Chemicals	General
Glove, Patient Examination	General
Glove, Surgical	General
Service, Import/Export	General

TECHNICAL MOLDED PRODUCTS, INC.
970-484-9111

3713 Canal Dr., Fort Collins, CO 80524
FDA Number: n/a
E-mail: info@techmolded.com *Fax:* 970-484-4242
Web site: www.techmolded.com
Medical Products Sales Volume: $250,000
Annual Revenue: $0-$1 Million
Year Founded: 1977
Ownership: Private
Produces/Sells CE-marked Devices: N
Federal Procurement Eligibility: Small Business
Distribution: Manufacturer Through Distributor, Exporter

Splint, Molded, Plastic	Orthopedics
Splint, Other	Orthopedics

TECHNICAL PRODUCTS INTERNATIONAL, INC.
800-729-4421

5918 Evergreen Blvd, St. Louis, MO 63134-2302
314-522-8671
FDA Number: n/a
E-mail: information@vibratome.com *Fax:* 314-522-6360
Web site: www.vibratome.com
Medical Products Sales Volume: $400,000
Annual Revenue: $1-$5 Million
Year Founded: 1984
Total Employees: 2   *Marketing Staff:* 2   *Sales Staff:* 4
Ownership: Private
Quality System Registration Information: ISO9000
Produces/Sells CE-marked Devices: Y
Federal Procurement Eligibility: Small Business
Distribution: Manufacturer Direct, Manufacturer Through Distributor
General Admin.: Douglas Martin/Chief Executive Officer
James Unnerstall/Vice President, General Manager
Mktg./Adv.: Drew Mehta/Manager Sales Support
Sophie Montgomery/Marketing & Sales Specialist
Production: Ms. Robyn Davis/Customer Service Representative

Microtome, Cryostat	Pathology
Microtome, Sliding	Pathology
Remover, Tissue	Surgery
Stainer, Tissue, Automated	Pathology

TECHNICAL PRODUCTS, INC.
800-226-8434

805 Marathon Parkway, Suite 150,
770-236-8452
Lawrenceville, GA 30045
FDA Number: 1061771
E-mail: techprodincgausa@mindspring.com *Fax:* 770-236-8453
Web site: www.tpi-ga.com
Year Founded: 1967
Total Employees: 16   *Sales Staff:* 4
Ownership: Private
Quality System Registration Information: ISO9001
Produces/Sells CE-marked Devices: N
Federal Procurement Eligibility: Small Business, Female Owned
Distribution: Manufacturer Direct
Mktg./Adv.: Ms. Kristin Counts/Admin. Marketing
Mr. Eric Thompson/Vice President, Manager Sales

Catheter, Irrigation	Surgery
Catheter, Malecot (Gastrostomy Tube)	Gastroenterology/Urology
Catheter, Multiple Lumen	Surgery
Conformer, Ophthalmic	Ophthalmology
Connector, Catheter	Surgery
Elastomer, Silicone Block	Surgery
Instrument, Manual, General Surgical	Surgery
Kit, Incision And Drainage	Surgery
Mesh, Surgical, Polymeric	Surgery
Plug, Punctum	Ophthalmology
Polymer, ENT Synthetic-PIFE, Silicon Elastomer	Ear/Nose/Throat
Prosthesis, Tendon, Passive	Orthopedics
Silastic Elastomer (Angular Deformity Prevention)	Orthopedics
Spacer, Tendon	Orthopedics
Suction Apparatus, Single Patient, Portable, Non-Powered	Surgery
Valve, Speaking, Tracheal	Ear/Nose/Throat

TECHNICARE ULTRASOUND
See Johnson & Johnson

TECHNICLONE INTERNATIONAL CORP.
See Peregrine Pharmaceuticals, Inc.

TECHNICON
See Siemens Healthcare Diagnostics Inc.

TECHNICON DATA SYSTEMS CORP.
See Eclipsys Corporation

TECHNICUFF CORP.
800-276-2833
2525 Industrial, Leesburg, FL 34748
352-326-2833
FDA Number: 1058002 *Fax:* 352-326-2027
E-mail: sales@technicuff.com
Web site: www.technicuff.com
Medical Products Sales Volume: $500,000
Year Founded: 1992
Total Employees: 6
Ownership: Private
Produces/Sells CE-marked Devices: N
Federal Procurement Eligibility: Small Business, Female Owned
Distribution: Manufacturer Direct, Manufacturer Through Distributor, Manufacturer Through Manufacturer Reps, OEM
General Admin.: Mr. Bill Yandell/Chief Executive Officer, Chairman
Mrs. Julie Yandell/Chief Information Officer

Cuff, Blood Pressure	Cardiovascular

TECHNIPOWER (A POWER DESIGNS CO.)
800-682-8235
14 Commerce Dr., Danbury, CT 06810
203-748-7001
FDA Number: n/a *Fax:* 203-797-9285
E-mail: sales@technipowersystems.com
Annual Revenue: $1-$5 Million
Total Employees: 24   *Marketing Staff:* 2   *Sales Staff:* 2
Ownership: Private
Produces/Sells CE-marked Devices: N
Federal Procurement Eligibility: Small Business
Distribution: Manufacturer Direct, Manufacturer Through Distributor, Manufacturer Through Manufacturer Reps, OEM
General Admin.: Anthony Intino/President
Mktg./Adv.: Rick Diachenko/Vice President Marketing & Sales

Power System, Isolated	General

TECHNISCAN, INC.
888-268-3030
13216 South Highland Dr., Suite 200,
801-521-0444
Salt Lake City, UT 84106
FDA Number: n/a *Fax:* 801-747-1099
E-mail: wdunn@techniscanmedical.com
Web site: www.techniscanmedicalsystems.com
Annual Revenue: $50-$100 Million
Year Founded: 1984
Total Employees: 19
Ownership: Private
Produces/Sells CE-marked Devices: N
Federal Procurement Eligibility: Small Business
General Admin.: Mr. Barry Hanover/Chief Operating Officer
Mr. Dave Robinson/President, Chief Executive Officer
Medical Admin.: Mrs. Karleen Callahan/Director Clinical Affairs
Research: Mr. Steven A. Johnson/Chief Scientist

Scanner, Ultrasonic (Pulsed Echo)	Radiology

TECHNO SCIENTIFIC INC.
905-760-1745
259 Edgeley Blvd., Unit 11-12, Concord, ONT L4K 3Y5 Canada
FDA Number: n/a *Fax:* 905-760-1746
E-mail: technoscientific@bellnet.ca
Web site: www.technoscientific.com
Year Founded: 1980
Total Employees: 25
Ownership: Private
Produces/Sells CE-marked Devices: N
Distribution: Manufacturer Direct, Exporter

TECHNO-AIDE MANUFACTURING CO. INC.
See Techno-Aide, Inc.

TECHNO-AIDE, INC.
800-251-2629
7117 Centennial Blvd., Nashville, TN 37209-1018
615-350-7030
FDA Number: n/a *Fax:* 615-350-7879
E-mail: davidm@techno-aide.com
Web site: www.techno-aide.com
Medical Products Sales Volume: $6,000,000
Annual Revenue: $5-$10 Million
Total Employees: 50   *Marketing Staff:* 2   *Sales Staff:* 5
Ownership: Private
Produces/Sells CE-marked Devices: N
Federal Procurement Eligibility: Small Business
Distribution: Manufacturer Through Distributor, Exporter
Mktg./Adv.: David McCall/Vice President Sales

Apron, Lead, Radiographic	Radiology
Duplicator, X-Ray Film	Radiology
Furniture, General	General
Holder, X-Ray Film Cassette, Vertical	Radiology
Labeler, X-Ray Film	Radiology
Marker, X-Ray	Radiology
Sand Bag, X-Ray	Radiology
Support, Patient Position, Radiographic	Radiology

TECHNOFROLICS 617-441-8870
11 Miller Street, Somerville, MA 02143
FDA Number: 3005260990
Device, Storage, Image, Digital   Radiology

TECHNOLOGIES OF STERILIZATION WITH 1-866-715-0003
OZONE (TSO3) INC.
2505 Dalton Ave.,   418-653-4389
Ste-Foy, QUE G1P-3 Canada
FDA Number: n/a   *Fax:* 418-653-5726
E-mail: info@tso3.com
Web site: http://www.tso3.com
Year Founded: 1998
Total Employees: 25
Ownership: Private
Produces/Sells CE-marked Devices: N
Distribution: Manufacturer Direct

TECHNOLOGY DELIVERY SYSTEMS, INC. 866-629-4359
Lsu-emtc Bldg, 340, East Parker St., Suite 240,
Baton Rouge, LA 70808
FDA Number: 3004088999
Laser, Surgical   Surgery
Ureteroscope   Gastroenterology/Urology

TECHNOLOGY FOR IMAGING, INC.
See Conmed Linvatec

TECHNOLOGY PRODUCTS INC.
See Caridianbct Inc.

TECHNOMEDIC INC. 416-743-0009
4 Racine Road, Unit 7, Etobicoke, ONT M9W 5W7 Canada
FDA Number: n/a   *Fax:* 416-745-8901
E-mail: technomedic@bellnet.ca
Web site: http://www.technomedic.ca
Year Founded: 1997
Total Employees: 10
Ownership: Private
Produces/Sells CE-marked Devices: N
Distribution: Exclusive Distributor, Importer

TECHNY INDUSTRIES INC.
See Del Medical Systems

TECHSTYLES MANUFACTURING DIVISION 800-826-4490
16415 Addison Road, Suite 660,   972-732-7694
Addison, TX 75001
FDA Number: 1650928   *Fax:* 972-732-7842
E-mail: info@encompassmed.net
Web site: www.encompassgroup.net/encompassmed
Year Founded: 1982
Total Employees: 15
Ownership: Encompass Group, Llc
Quality System Registration Information: ISO9001
Produces/Sells CE-marked Devices: Y
Federal Procurement Eligibility: Small Business
Distribution: Manufacturer Through Distributor, OEM, Importer, Exporter
Accessories, Apparel, Surgical   Surgery
Surgical Instrument, Disposable   Surgery

TECHSTYLES, INC.
See Encompass Medical

TECHULON INC. 540-443-9254
2200 Kraft Drive, Suite 2475, Blacksburg, VA 24060
FDA Number: n/a   *Fax:* 206-202-0418
Web site: http://www.techulon.com
Ownership: Private
Produces/Sells CE-marked Devices: N
General Admin.: Mr. Frank Akers/President
Research: Dr. Joshua Bryson/Chief Scientist

TECHWORLD CORPORATION, INC. 1-888-658-8108
721 E Lancaster Avenue, Twc-01,   484-237-8059
Downingtown, PA 19335
FDA Number: 3005151526
E-mail: info@techworldcorp.com
Web site: www.techworldcorp.com
Ownership: Private
Produces/Sells CE-marked Devices: N
Douche, Vaginal   Obstetrics/Gynecology
Irrigator, Powered Nasal   Ear/Nose/Throat

TECNI-QUIP 800-826-1245
960 Crossroads Blvd., PO Box 2050,   830-401-4400
Seguin, TX 78155
FDA Number: 9310072   *Fax:* 830-401-0600
E-mail: tqcarts@tqind.com
Web site: www.tqind.com

TECNI-QUIP 800-826-1245 *(cont'd)*
Medical Products Sales Volume: $2,200,000
Annual Revenue: $1-$5 Million
Year Founded: 1961
Total Employees: 27   *Marketing Staff:* 2   *Sales Staff:* 3
Ownership: Private
Produces/Sells CE-marked Devices: N
Federal Procurement Eligibility: Small Business, Female Owned, GSA Contract
Distribution: Manufacturer Direct, Manufacturer Through Distributor
General Admin.: Charles R. Clement/Chief Executive Officer, Vice President
    Mike Reilly/President, Chief Financial Officer
Mktg./Adv.: Jo Beth Reilly/Director National Accounts
    Lon Ray/Manager National Sales
    Jo Beth Reilly/Vice President Marketing
Cabinet Casework, General Purpose   General
Cart, Foodservice   General
Cart, Housekeeping   General
Cart, Laundry   General
Cart, Multipurpose   General
Cart, Supply   General
Cart, Waste   General
Cover, Cart   General
Laundry Equipment   General

TECNOMED INTERNATIONAL S.A. DE C.V. 01 55 5519 7234
Andalucia 25, Colonia Alamos,
Ciudad De Mexico, DF CP 03 Mexico
FDA Number: n/a   *Fax:* 01 55 5519 5810
E-mail: informes@grupotecnomed.com
Web site: www.grupotecnomed.com
Medical Products Sales Volume: $2,100,000
Year Founded: 1993
Total Employees: 26   *Marketing Staff:* 1   *Sales Staff:* 6
Ownership: Private
Produces/Sells CE-marked Devices: Y
Federal Procurement Eligibility: Small Business
Distribution: Manufacturer Through Manufacturer Reps, Exclusive Distributor, Importer

TECO DIAGNOSTICS 800-222-9880
1268 N. Lakeview Ave., Anaheim, CA 92807   1-714-463-1111
FDA Number: 1832216   *Fax:* 1-714-463-1169
E-mail: tecodiag@pacbell.net
Web site: www.tecodiag.com
Annual Revenue: $5-$10 Million
Total Employees: 44   *Marketing Staff:* 4   *Sales Staff:* 4
Ownership: Private
Produces/Sells CE-marked Devices: Y
Federal Procurement Eligibility: Minority Owned, Female Owned
Distribution: Manufacturer Through Distributor, OEM, Exclusive Distributor, Exporter
General Admin.: Dr. K. C. Chen/Chief Executive Officer
    K. C. Chen/President, Chief Executive Officer
Mktg./Adv.: Happy Chen/Vice President Marketing & Sales
2, 4-dinitrophenylhydrazine, Lactate Dehydrogenase   Chemistry
Analyzer, Chemistry, Photometric, Discrete   Chemistry
Azo-Dyes, Colorimetric, Bilirubin And Conjugates   Chemistry
Catalytic Method, Amylase   Chemistry
Colorimetric Method, Gamma-Glutamyl Transpeptidase   Chemistry
Hexokinase, Glucose   Chemistry
Kinetic Method, Gamma-Glutamyl Transpeptidase   Chemistry
Kit, Pregnancy Test   Obstetrics/Gynecology
Kit, Pregnancy Test, Over The Counter, HCG   Chemistry
Nephelometric Method, Immunoglobulins (G, A, M)   Chemistry
Phosphatase, Acid   Hematology
Phosphatase, Alkaline   Hematology
Phosphorus Reagent (Test System)   Chemistry
Pipette   Chemistry
Radioimmunoassay, Thyroid Stimulating Hormone   Chemistry
Reagent, Amylase, Colorimetric   Chemistry
Reagent, Bilirubin (Total Or Direct Test System)   Chemistry
Reagent, Blood Urea Nitrogen (BUN)   Chemistry
Reagent, Calcium (Test System)   Chemistry
Reagent, Chloride (Test System)   Chemistry
Reagent, Cholesterol (Total Test System)   Chemistry
Reagent, Creatinine (Test System)   Chemistry
Reagent, Kinase, Phosphate, Creatine   Chemistry
Reagent, Protein, Total   Chemistry
Reagent, Streptolysin O/Antistreptolysin-Titer   Microbiology
Reagent, Test, Fluoride   Toxicology
Strip, Test   Chemistry
Test, Rheumatoid Factor   Immunology

TECO DIAGNOSTICS 714-693-7788
1268 North Lakeview Ave., Anaheim, CA 92807
FDA Number: 1832216
Agglutination Method, Human Chorionic Gonadotropin   Chemistry
Analyzer, Chemistry, Photometric, Discrete   Chemistry
Analyzer, Chemistry, Urinalysis   Chemistry

TECO DIAGNOSTICS   714-693-7788 *(cont'd)*

Calibrator, Primary, Clinical Chemistry	Chemistry
Catalytic Method, Amylase	Chemistry
Colorimeter, General Use	Chemistry
Colorimetry, Cholinesterase	Toxicology
Complexone, Cresolphthalein, Calcium	Chemistry
Control, Multi Analyte, All Kinds (Assayed And Unassayed)	Chemistry
Differential Rate Kinetic Method, CPK Or Isoenzymes	Chemistry
Dye-Binding, Albumin, Bromcresol, Green	Chemistry
Electrode, Ion Specific, Sodium	Chemistry
Emulsion, Olive Oil (Turbidimetric), Lipase	Chemistry
Enzymatic Esterase-Oxidase, Cholesterol	Chemistry
Enzymatic Method, Ammonia	Chemistry
Enzymatic Method, Glucose (Urinary, Non-Quantitative)	Chemistry
Enzymatic, Carbon-Dioxide	Chemistry
Enzyme Immunoassay, Amphetamine	Toxicology
Enzyme Immunoassay, Cannabinoids	Toxicology
Enzyme Immunoassay, Cocaine	Toxicology
Enzyme Immunoassay, Non-Radiolabeled, Total Thyroxine	Chemistry
Equipment, Laboratory, Gen. Purpose (Specific Medical Use)	Chemistry
Ferrozine (Colorimetric) Iron Binding Capacity	Chemistry
Fluorometry, Morphine	Toxicology
Gas Chromatography, Methamphetamine	Toxicology
Hexokinase, Glucose	Chemistry
Indicator Method, Protein Or Albumin (Urinary, Non-Quant.)	Chemistry
Kinetic Method, Gamma-Glutamyl Transpeptidase	Chemistry
Kit, Pregnancy Test, Over The Counter, HCG	Chemistry
Kit, Screening, Urine	Microbiology
LDL & VLDL Precipitation, HDL	Chemistry
Labware, Blood Collection	Chemistry
Lipase Hydrolysis/Glycerol Kinase Enzyme, Triglycerides	Chemistry
NAD Reduction/NADH Oxidation, Lactate Dehydrogenase	Chemistry
NADH Oxidation/NAD Reduction, AST/SGOT	Chemistry
Naphthyl Phosphate, Acid Phosphatase	Chemistry
Nitrophenylphosphate, Alkaline Phosphatase Or Isoenzymes	Chemistry
Nitroprusside, Ketones (Urinary, Non-Quantitative)	Chemistry
Nitrosalicylate Reduction, Amylase	Chemistry
Phosphorus Reagent (Test System)	Chemistry
Photometric Method, Magnesium	Chemistry
Qualitative Chemical Reactions, Urinary Calculi (Stone)	Chemistry
Quantitation, Antithrombin III	Hematology
Radioimmunoassay, Cholyglycine, Bile Acids	Chemistry
Radioimmunoassay, Thyroid Stimulating Hormone	Chemistry
Reagent, Bilirubin (Total Or Direct Test System)	Chemistry
Reagent, Chloride (Test System)	Chemistry
Reagent, Creatinine (Test System)	Chemistry
Reagent, Glucose (Test System)	Chemistry
Reagent, Occult Blood	Hematology
Reagent, Protein, Total	Chemistry
SGOT, Ultraviolet	Chemistry
SGPT, Colorimetric	Chemistry
SGPT, Ultraviolet	Chemistry
Starch-Dye Bound Polymer, Amylase	Chemistry
System, Test, Low-Density, Lipoprotein	Chemistry
Test, C-Reactive Protein	Immunology
Test, Glycosylated Hemoglobin Assay	Hematology
Test, Human Chorionic Gonadotropin, Serum	Immunology
Test, Rheumatoid Factor	Immunology
Test, Urine Leukocyte	Hematology
Tetraphenyl Borate, Colorimetry, Potassium	Chemistry
Tetrazolium Int Dye-Diaphorase, Lactate Dehydrogenase	Chemistry
Thymolphthalein Monophosphate, Acid Phosphatase	Chemistry
Thymolphthalein Monophosphate, Alkaline Phosphatase	Chemistry
Uranyl Acetate/Zinc Acetate, Sodium	Chemistry
Urease And Glutamic Dehydrogenase, Urea Nitrogen	Chemistry
Urease, Photometric, Urea Nitrogen	Chemistry
Uricase (Colorimetric), Uric Acid	Chemistry
Whole Blood Hemoglobin Determination	Hematology

TECOGICS SCIENTIFIC LTD.   1-888-298-9922
2430 Magnus Avenue,   **613-238-8403**
Ottawa, ONT K1G 1 Canada
FDA Number: n/a   *Fax:* 613-238-8789
E-mail: info@exnflex.com
Web site: www.exnflex.com
Year Founded: 1990
Total Employees: 10
Ownership: Private
Produces/Sells CE-marked Devices: N
Distribution: Manufacturer Direct, Exclusive Distributor

TECOMET, A SUBSIDIARY OF VIASYS HEALTHCARE INC.   978-658-3379
115 Eames St., Wilmington, MA 01887
FDA Number: 1225675   *Fax:* 978-658-4334
E-mail: sales.tecomet@viasyshc.com
Web site: www.tecomet.com
Medical Products Sales Volume: $21,100,000
Year Founded: 1995
Total Employees: 180

TECOMET, A SUBSIDIARY OF VIASYS   978-658-3379 *(cont'd)*
Ownership: Jencons (Scientific) Ltd.
Stock Symbol: VAS
Traded On: NYSE
Quality System Registration Information: ISO9002
Produces/Sells CE-marked Devices: N
Federal Procurement Eligibility: Small Business
Distribution: OEM
General Admin.: Giulio Perillo/President
Mktg./Adv.: Jean-Paul Burtin/Vice President Marketing & International Sales

Contract Manufacturing	General

TECSTAR MFG. COMPANY   262-255-5790
W190 N11701 Moldmakers Way, Germantown, WI 53022
FDA Number: 2134846

Floss, Dental	Dental And Oral

TECTRIX
See CYBEX INTERNATIONAL, INC.

TED PELLA, INC.   800-237-3526
4595 Mountain Lakes Blvd.,   **530-243-2200**
Redding, CA 96003
FDA Number: 2954792   *Fax:* 530-243-3761
E-mail: sales@tedpella.com
Web site: http://www.tedpella.com
Year Founded: 1968
Ownership: Private
Quality System Registration Information: ISO9001; ISO9002
Produces/Sells CE-marked Devices: Y
Federal Procurement Eligibility: Small Business
Distribution: Manufacturer Direct, Manufacturer Through Manufacturer Reps, OEM, Exporter
Mktg./Adv.: Mr. Jack Vermeulen/Director Sales

Decalcifier Device, Electrolytic	Pathology
Microscope, Laboratory, Optical	Microbiology
Microscope, Light	Pathology
Stainer, Tissue, Automated	Pathology
Tissue Processor, Automated	Pathology

TED PELLA, INC.   800-237-3526
750 Pierce Road, Suite 2,   **530-243-2200**
Clifton Park, NY 12065
FDA Number: n/a   *Fax:* 530-243-3761
E-mail: sales@tedpella.com
Web site: http://www.tedpella.com
Annual Revenue: $0-$1 Million
Ownership: Private
Produces/Sells CE-marked Devices: N
Federal Procurement Eligibility: Small Business
Distribution: Manufacturer Direct, Importer, Exporter
General Admin.: Peter W. Fullam/President, Chief Executive Officer
         Dianne B. Fullam/Secretary, Treasurer

Cabinet Casework, General Purpose	General
Evaporator	Chemistry
Micromanipulator, Laboratory	Microbiology
Microscope, Laboratory, Electron	Microbiology
Monitor, Bed Patient	General
Scissors, General Dissecting	General
Stage, Microscope	Pathology
Stand/Holder, Equipment, Laboratory	Chemistry
Tweezers	General
Wipe, Instrument	General

TEFTEC CORP.   210-477-0330
12450 Network Blvd., San Antonio, TX 78249
FDA Number: 1650371
Ownership: Private
Produces/Sells CE-marked Devices: N

Wheelchair, Powered	Physical Med

TEGAL SCIENTIFIC, INC.   707-763-5600
140 2nd Street, Ste 318, Petaluma, CA 94952
FDA Number: n/a   *Fax:* 707-765-9311
E-mail: submission@tegal.com
Web site: www.tegal.com
Annual Revenue: $0-$1 Million
Total Employees: 10
Ownership: Private
Produces/Sells CE-marked Devices: N
Federal Procurement Eligibility: Small Business
Distribution: Manufacturer Through Manufacturer Reps
General Admin.: L. Rigali/Chief Executive Officer

Hood, Fume	Toxicology
Viscometer	Chemistry

Medical Product Subsidiaries (Listed Separately)
    Berghof/America

TEGRA MEDICAL INC.
508-541-4200
9 Forge Park, Franklin, MA 02038
FDA Number: n/a   *Fax:* 508-553-4100
E-mail: info@tegramedical.com
Web site: http://www.tegramedical.com
Medical Products Sales Volume: $10,000,000
Year Founded: 2007
Total Employees: 140   *Marketing Staff:* 3   *Sales Staff:* 3
Ownership: Private
Quality System Registration Information: ISO9002
Produces/Sells CE-marked Devices: N
Federal Procurement Eligibility: Small Business
Distribution: OEM
General Admin.: Mr. Jerry Mazzenga/Chief Technology Officer
     Mr. Bob Roche/President, Chief Executive Officer
Mktg./Adv.: Mr. Tom Burns/Vice President Business Development
Production: Mr. Jean Mattar/Vice President Quality Assurance & Regulatory Affairs
Finance: Mr. Joe Kajano/Chief Financial Officer, Vice President Finance

Cannula, Epidural	Obstetrics/Gynecology
Cannula, Injection	Gastroenterology/Urology
Cannula, Ophthalmic	Ophthalmology
Cannula, Other	General
Cannula, Suprapubic, With Trocar	Gastroenterology/Urology
Cannula, Venous	Cardiovascular
Cannula, Ventricular	Cns/Neurology
Component, Metal, Other	General
Contract Manufacturing	General
Contract Manufacturing, Product, Disposable	General
Contract R&D, Diagnostics	General
Drill, Bone	Orthopedics
Introducer, Spinal Needle	Anesthesiology
Needle, Angiographic	Cns/Neurology
Needle, Aspiration And Injection, Disposable	Surgery
Needle, Aspiration And Injection, Reusable	Surgery
Needle, Biopsy, Cardiovascular	Cardiovascular
Needle, Biopsy, Mammary	Obstetrics/Gynecology
Needle, Blunt	General
Needle, Bone Marrow	Surgery
Needle, Cardiac	Cardiovascular
Needle, Cholangiography	Cardiovascular
Needle, Dental	Dental And Oral
Needle, Endoscopic	Gastroenterology/Urology
Needle, Hypodermic	General
Needle, Insufflation, Laparoscopic	Surgery
Needle, Intra-Arterial	Cardiovascular
Needle, Intravenous	General
Needle, Ophthalmic	Ophthalmology
Needle, Other	General
Needle, Radiographic	Radiology
Needle, Spinal, Short-Term	General
Pin, Fixation, Smooth	Orthopedics
Pin, Fixation, Threaded	Orthopedics
Stimulator, Neurological	Surgery
Stylet, Needle	General
Trocar, Laparoscopic	Surgery
Trocar, Other	General
Trocar, Short	Surgery
Tubing, Hypodermic	General
Tubing, Other	General
Tunneler, Surgical	Surgery

TEGRANT CORPORATION, PROTEXIC BRANDS
800-289-9966
724-843-8200
800 5th Ave., P.O. Box 448,
New Brighton, PA 15066
FDA Number: n/a   *Fax:* 724-843-4845
E-mail: packagingna@tegrant.com
Web site: www.protexic.com
Medical Products Sales Volume: $198,000,000
Annual Revenue: $100-$500 Million
Year Founded: 1962
Total Employees: 1500   *Marketing Staff:* 2   *Sales Staff:* 50
Ownership: Tegrant Corporation
Quality System Registration Information: ISO9002
Produces/Sells CE-marked Devices: N
Distribution: Manufacturer Direct, Manufacturer Through Distributor, Manufacturer Through Manufacturer Reps
General Admin.: Ron Leach/President, Chief Executive Officer
     Bill Kelly/Senior Vice President
     Rick Foltz/Vice President
Mktg./Adv.: Ron Tankus/Director Business Development

Case, Protection, Equipment	General
Computer Equipment	General
Molding, Custom	General
Packaging Material	General

Medical Product Subsidiaries (Listed Separately)
Thermosafe Brands

TEGRANT CORPORATION, THERMOSAFE BRANDS
1 800 323 7442
3930 Ventura Drive Suite 450, Arlington Heights, IL 60084
FDA Number: n/a   *Fax:* 847-398-0653
E-mail: customer.support@tegrant.com
Web site: www.thermosafe.com
Annual Revenue: $100-$500 Million
Year Founded: 1962
Total Employees: 300   *Marketing Staff:* 9   *Sales Staff:* 35
Ownership: Tegrant Corporation
Quality System Registration Information: ISO9002
Produces/Sells CE-marked Devices: N
Distribution: Manufacturer Direct, Manufacturer Through Distributor, Manufacturer Through Manufacturer Reps
General Admin.: Dan Filippini/Vice President
Mktg./Adv.: Rich Ellinger/Director Marketing
     Kevin Grogan/Vice President, Director Marketing

Case, Protection, Equipment	General
Chest, Dry Ice	General
Container, Frozen Donor Tissue Storage	General
Container, Specimen Mailer And Storage	Pathology
Container, Specimen, All Types	General

TEI BIOSCIENCES INC.
617-268-1616
7 Elkins St., Boston, MA 02127
FDA Number: 3004170064   *Fax:* (617) 268-3906
E-mail: info@teibio.com
Web site: www.teibio.com
Ownership: Private
Produces/Sells CE-marked Devices: N

Dressing, Burn, Porcine	Surgery
Mesh, Surgical (Steel Gauze)	Surgery
Mesh, Surgical, Polymeric	Surgery

TEK MARKETING, INC.
215-364-4941
98 Railroad Dr., Warminster, PA 18974-1454
FDA Number: 2531990
Ownership: Private
Produces/Sells CE-marked Devices: N

Processor, Radiographic Film, Automatic	Radiology

TEKIA, INC.
949-699-1300
17 Hammond Street, Suite 414, Irvine, CA 92718
FDA Number: 2031474   *Fax:* 949-699-1302
E-mail: AIOL@tekia.com
Web site: http://www.tekia.com
Medical Products Sales Volume: $3,000,000
Year Founded: 1995
Total Employees: 20   *Marketing Staff:* 2   *Sales Staff:* 2
Ownership: Private
Quality System Registration Information: ISO9001
Produces/Sells CE-marked Devices: Y
Federal Procurement Eligibility: Small Business
Distribution: Manufacturer Through Distributor, OEM, Exporter
General Admin.: Gene Currie/President, Chief Executive Officer
Production: Pascale David/Vice President Quality Assurance & Regulatory Affairs
Research: Larry W. Blake/Vice President Research & Development

Folders and Injectors, Intraocular Lens (IOL)	Ophthalmology
Lens, Intraocular	Ophthalmology

TEKNA SOLUTIONS, INC.
269-978-3500
3400 Tech Circle, Kalamazoo, MI 49008
FDA Number: 3005694091

Cart, Emergency, Cardiopulmonary Resuscitation (Crash)	Anesthesiology
Powered Medical Examination Table	General
Table, Operating Room, AC-Powered	Surgery

TEKQUEST INDUSTRIES
800-327-7175
403-324-5887
4200 St. John's Parkway, Sanford, FL 32771
FDA Number: 1036037   *Fax:* 407-324-3991
E-mail: customerservice@rushhampton.com
Web site: http://tekquestindustries.com/
Medical Products Sales Volume: $800,000
Annual Revenue: $5-$10 Million
Year Founded: 1999
Total Employees: 10
Ownership: Private
Produces/Sells CE-marked Devices: N
Federal Procurement Eligibility: Small Business
Mktg./Adv.: Mr. Kent Arblaster/Director Marketing & Sales

Accessories, Operating Room, Table	Surgery
Table, Anesthetist's	Anesthesiology

TEKSCAN, INC.
800-248-3669
617-464-4500
307 West First St.,
South Boston, MA 02127
FDA Number: 1221639   *Fax:* 617-464-4266
E-mail: marketing@tekscan.com

TEKSCAN, INC.   800-248-3669 *(cont'd)*

Web site: www.tekscan.com
Medical Products Sales Volume: $3,000,000
Annual Revenue: $5-$10 Million
Total Employees: 60   *Marketing Staff:* 6   *Sales Staff:* 8
Ownership: Private
Quality System Registration Information: ISO9001
Produces/Sells CE-marked Devices: N
Federal Procurement Eligibility: Small Business
Distribution: Manufacturer Direct, Manufacturer Through Distributor, Manufacturer Through Manufacturer Reps
General Admin.: Steve Jacobs/President
Mktg./Adv.: Norman Murphy/Manager Market Research
     Kerry Sullivan/Manager Marketing & Communications
     Amy Robinson/Marketing Assistant
     Charles Malacaria/Vice President Business Development
Research: Thomas Papakostas/Director Research & Development

Analyzer, Gait	Orthopedics
Computer Equipment	General
Dental Laboratory Equipment	Dental And Oral
Paper, Articulation	Dental And Oral
Pressure Measurement, System, Intermittent	Physical Med

TEKTONE SOUND & SIGNAL MANUFACTURING, INC.   828-524-9967

277 Industrial Park Rd., Franklin, NC 28734
FDA Number: 3001757821

Environmental Control System, Powered	Physical Med

TEL-TRON TECHNOLOGIES CORPORATION   904-255-1921

220 Fentress Blvd., Daytona Beach, FL 32114-1228
FDA Number: n/a   *Fax:* 904-258-3782
E-mail: info@tel-tron.com
Web site: www.tel-tron.com
Medical Products Sales Volume: $1,300,000
Annual Revenue: $1-$5 Million
Year Founded: 1945
Total Employees: 20   *Marketing Staff:* 1   *Sales Staff:* 5
Ownership: Private
Produces/Sells CE-marked Devices: N
Federal Procurement Eligibility: Small Business
Distribution: Manufacturer Direct, Manufacturer Through Distributor
General Admin.: Rick Dawson/Chief Executive Officer
     Brian Dawson/Vice President, General Manager
Mktg./Adv.: Meg Dawson/Director Marketing
     Rick Taylor/Vice President Sales

Communication System, Emergency Alert, Personal	General

TELE-MADE DISPOSABLES, INC.   888-822-4299

3215 Huffman Eastgate Rd., Huffman, TX 77336
FDA Number: 1644196

Bed, Electric	General
Cushion, Flotation	Physical Med
Cushion, Wheelchair (Pad)	Physical Med
Mattress, Air Flotation	General

TELECATION   800-584-9964 / 800-677-0067

7112 W. Jefferson Avenue, Suite 307, Lakewood, CO 80235
FDA Number: n/a   *Fax:* 505-994-3574
E-mail: sales@telecation.com
Web site: www.telecation.com
Medical Products Sales Volume: $400,000
Annual Revenue: $0-$1 Million
Year Founded: 1984
Total Employees: 6   *Marketing Staff:* 2   *Sales Staff:* 5
Ownership: OPS SYSTEMS INC
Produces/Sells CE-marked Devices: N
Federal Procurement Eligibility: Small Business
Distribution: Manufacturer Direct, Manufacturer Through Manufacturer Reps, OEM, Exporter
General Admin.: John Dorner/President, Chief Executive Officer
Mktg./Adv.: Melanie Hazlett/Manager Marketing & Sales
Production: Linda Vautrin-Hale/Product Manager

Computer Software	General

TELEDIAGNOSTIC SYSTEMS   800-227-3224 / 650-625-9001

2483 Old Middlefield Way, Suite 202, Mountain View, CA 94043
FDA Number: 2917957   *Fax:* 650-625-9004
E-mail: tb@telediagnostic.com
Web site: www.telediagnostic.com
Medical Products Sales Volume: $600,000
Annual Revenue: $1-$5 Million
Year Founded: 1972
Total Employees: 6
Ownership: Private

TELEDIAGNOSTIC SYSTEMS   800-227-3224 *(cont'd)*

Produces/Sells CE-marked Devices: N
Federal Procurement Eligibility: Small Business, VA Contract
Distribution: Manufacturer Direct, OEM
General Admin.: Larry Woodard/President, Chief Executive Officer
     Tom Buescher/Vice President, General Manager
Mktg./Adv.: Tom Buescher/Vice President Business Development

Sleep Assessment Equipment	Cns/Neurology
Transmitter/Receiver, EEG, Telephone	Cns/Neurology

TELEDYNE ANALYTICAL INSTRUMENTS   888-789-8168 / 626-934-1500

16830 Chestnut St., City of Industry, CA 91749
FDA Number: 2026424   *Fax:* 626-961-2538
E-mail: ask_tai@teledyne.com
Web site: www.teledyne-ai.com
Medical Products Sales Volume: $2,500,000
Annual Revenue: $25-$50 Million
Total Employees: 140   *Marketing Staff:* 2   *Sales Staff:* 7
Ownership: Altair Corporation
Stock Symbol: TDY
Traded On: NYSE
Quality System Registration Information: ISO9001
Produces/Sells CE-marked Devices: Y
Distribution: Manufacturer Direct, Manufacturer Through Distributor, Manufacturer Through Manufacturer Reps, OEM
General Admin.: Tom Compas/General Manager
     April Hancock/Manager Human Resources
Mktg./Adv.: Vasu Narasimhan/Director Business Development
     Kunal Kothari/Director Marketing & Sales
Production: Steve Broy/Director Engineering
     Roger Starlin/Manager Quality Assurance

Analyzer, Gas, Oxygen, Gaseous Phase	Anesthesiology
Monitor, Oxygen (Ventilatory) W/Wo Alarm	Anesthesiology

TELEDYNE ELECTRONIC DEVICES

See Teledyne Analytical Instruments

TELEFELX MEDICAL   610-948-5100

155 South Limerick Road, Limerick, PA 19468-1699
FDA Number: 1417411   *Fax:* 610-948-5101
Web site: www.teleflexmedical.com
Ownership: Teleflex Medical
Stock Symbol: TFX
Traded On: NYSE
Produces/Sells CE-marked Devices: N

Computer, Pulmonary Function Data	Anesthesiology
Humidifier, Respiratory Gas, (Direct Patient Interface)	Anesthesiology
Thermometer, Electronic, Continuous	General

TELEFLEX INC.   610-948-5100

155 South Limerick Road, Limerick, PA 19468-1699
FDA Number: n/a   *Fax:* 610-948-5101
Web site: www.teleflex.com
Year Founded: 1979
Ownership: Public
Stock Symbol: TFX
Traded On: NYSE
Produces/Sells CE-marked Devices: N
General Admin.: Jeffrey P. Black/Chief Executive Officer, Chairman
     Mr. Richard Meier/Chief Financial Officer, Executive Vice President
     Mr. Laurence Miller/Executive Vice President
     Mr. John Suddarth/President
Production: Mr. Vince Northfield/Executive Vice President Operations

TELEFLEX MEDICAL   919-433-4829

1805 A Tw Alexander Drive, Durham, NC 27703
FDA Number: 3004943382
Web site: www.teleflexmedical.com
Ownership: Teleflex Medical
Stock Symbol: TFX
Traded On: NYSE
Produces/Sells CE-marked Devices: Y
General Admin.: Mr. R. Ernest Waaser/President

Chisel (Osteotome)	Surgery
Clamp, Vascular	Cardiovascular
Curette, Surgical, Dental	Dental And Oral
Dilator, Vessel, Surgical	Cardiovascular
File, Bone, Surgical	Dental And Oral
Forceps, Tooth Extractor, Surgical	Dental And Oral
Hemostat	Orthopedics
Holder, Speculum, ENT	Ear/Nose/Throat
Knife, Surgical	Dental And Oral
Laryngoscope, Rigid	Anesthesiology
Mirror, Mouth	Dental And Oral
Needle, Biopsy, Cardiovascular	Cardiovascular
Retractor, All Types	Dental And Oral
Stylet, Tracheal Tube	Anesthesiology
Surgical Instrument, Cardiovascular	Cardiovascular

TELEFLEX MEDICAL 919-433-4829 *(cont'd)*
Tube, Aspirating, Flexible, Connecting — Anesthesiology

TELEFLEX MEDICAL 800-334-9751
2917 Weck Drive, — 919-544-8000
Research Triangle Park, NC 27709
FDA Number: 1044475 — *Fax:* 919-433-4989
Web site: www.teleflexmedical.com
Annual Revenue: $50-$100 Million
Total Employees: 375 — *Marketing Staff:* 4 — *Sales Staff:* 62
Ownership: Teleflex Medical
Stock Symbol: TFX
Traded On: NYSE
Quality System Registration Information: ISO9001
Produces/Sells CE-marked Devices: Y
Distribution: Manufacturer Direct, Manufacturer Through Distributor, Manufacturer Through Manufacturer Reps, Importer, Exporter
General Admin.: Mr. Jeffrey Black/Chairman, Chief Executive Officer
    Mr. Richard Meier/Chief Financial Officer, Executive Vice President
Production: Mr. Vince Northfield/Executive Vice President Operations

Applier, Surgical, Clip	Surgery
Catheter, Intravascular, Diagnostic	Cardiovascular
Clip, Ligature	Surgery
Clip, Scalp	Cns/Neurology
Electrode, Electrosurgical, Return (Ground, Dispersive)	Surgery
Electrode, Pacemaker, Temporary	Cardiovascular
Electrosurgical Unit, Cutting & Coagulation Device	Surgery
Instrument, Clip Removal	Cns/Neurology
Retractor, Self-Retaining, Neurology	Cns/Neurology
Retractor, Surgical	Surgery
Staple, Removable (Skin)	Surgery
Surgical Instrument, Cardiovascular	Cardiovascular
Tray, Surgical Instrument	Surgery

TELEFLEX MEDICAL 866-246-6990
4024 Stirrup Creek, — 919-544-8000
Research Triangle Park, NC 27703
FDA Number: 3005747797 — *Fax:* 919-433-4989
E-mail: askteleflexmedical@teleflexmedical.com
Web site: www.teleflexmedical.com
Medical Products Sales Volume: $1,021,885,000
Annual Revenue: More than $1 Billion
Year Founded: 1938
Total Employees: 1939
Ownership: Private
Stock Symbol: TFX
Traded On: NYSE
Produces/Sells CE-marked Devices: Y
General Admin.: Mr. R. Ernest Waaser/President
    Ms. Julie McDowell/Senior Vice President
    Mr. Jens Boy/Vice President, General Manager
Mktg./Adv.: Mr. Renee Bryan/Senior Director Strategic Business Development
    Mr. Tim Hopper/Vice President Marketing

Protector, Dental	Anesthesiology

Medical Product Subsidiaries (Listed Separately)
Arrow International, Inc.
Pilling Surgical, Teleflex Medical
Specialized Medical Devices, Llc
Ssi Surgical Services, Inc
Teleflex Medical
Teleflex Medical
Teleflex Medical Oem
Tfx Medical Oem

TELEFLEX MEDICAL
See Tfx Medical Oem

TELEFLEX MEDICAL 866-246-6990
920 Westport Parkway, Fort Worth, TX 76177
FDA Number: 3005428244
Web site: www.teleflexmedical.com
Ownership: Teleflex Medical
Stock Symbol: TFX
Traded On: NYSE
Produces/Sells CE-marked Devices: Y
General Admin.: Mr. R. Ernest Waaser/President
Mktg./Adv.: Mr. Jeffrey D. Brown/Senior Vice President International Sales

Ventilator, Emergency, Manual (Resuscitator)	Anesthesiology

TELEFLEX MEDICAL OEM 800-458-2553
375 Forbes Boulevard, — 508-964-6021
Mansfield, MA 02048
FDA Number: 1221601 — *Fax:* 508-964-6078
Web site: www.deknatel.com
Ownership: Teleflex Medical
Stock Symbol: TFX
Traded On: NYSE

TELEFLEX MEDICAL OEM 800-458-2553 *(cont'd)*
Produces/Sells CE-marked Devices: Y
General Admin.: Mr. R. Ernest Waaser/President

Suture, Non-Absorbable, Synthetic, Polyamide	Surgery
Suture, Non-Absorbable, Synthetic, Polyester	Surgery

TELEMED SYSTEMS INC. 800-481-6718
8 Kane Industrial Drive, Hudson, MA 01749 — 978-567-9033
FDA Number: 1222168 — *Fax:* 978-567-8904
E-mail: info@telemedsystems.com
Web site: www.telemedsystems.com
Medical Products Sales Volume: $2,400,000
Year Founded: 1988
Total Employees: 24 — *Marketing Staff:* 3
Ownership: Private
Quality System Registration Information: ISO9001
Produces/Sells CE-marked Devices: Y
Federal Procurement Eligibility: Small Business
Distribution: Manufacturer Direct, Importer, Exporter
General Admin.: Michael J. Carroll/President, Chief Executive Officer
Mktg./Adv.: Cathy Kelly/Manager Business
    Michael J. Carroll/Vice President Marketing & Sales
Production: Ernest Hartland/Director Quality Assurance & Regulatory Affairs
    Patrica Arntzen/Manager Materials
    D. Mason/Vice President Manufacturing
Research: Gil Wilcox/Vice President Research & Development

Balloon, Occlusion, Cerebrovascular	Cns/Neurology
Basket, Biliary Stone Retrieval	Gastroenterology/Urology
Bottle, Hot/Cold Water	General
Brush, Cytology	General
Cannula, Other	General
Catheter, Balloon, Dilatation, Vessel	Gastroenterology/Urology
Catheter, Occlusion	Cardiovascular
Cleanroom Equipment	General
Forceps, Biopsy	Surgery
Guidewire	Cardiovascular
Needle, Other	General
Papillotome	Surgery
Stent, Other	Obstetrics/Gynecology

TELEMEDX CORP. 800-231-1009
2550 S Sam Houston Pkwy W, — 713-655-7600
Houston, TX 77047
FDA Number: 1641703 — *Fax:* 713-655-7799
E-mail: ray@telemedx.com
Web site: www.telemedx.com
Annual Revenue: $1-$5 Million
Year Founded: 1976
Ownership: Private
Produces/Sells CE-marked Devices: N
Federal Procurement Eligibility: Small Business
Distribution: Manufacturer Direct, Service Direct
General Admin.: Ray Mitchell/President, Chief Executive Officer, Chairman
Mktg./Adv.: Matthew Mitchell/Vice President Business Admin.

Transmitter/Receiver, EEG, Telephone	Cns/Neurology

TELESCAN MEDICAL SYSTEMS 800-388-4324
26424 Table Meadow Road, — 530-269-0461
Auburn, CA 95602
FDA Number: 2020393 — *Fax:* 530-269-0464
E-mail: telscan@quiknet.com
Web site: www.globalcard.com
Annual Revenue: $0-$1 Million
Year Founded: 1976
Total Employees: 6
Ownership: Private
Produces/Sells CE-marked Devices: N
Federal Procurement Eligibility: Small Business
Distribution: Manufacturer Direct
General Admin.: Stanley Wegner/President

Scanner, Long-Term, ECG, Recording	Cardiovascular

TELESTO MEDTECH LLC 831-621-8011
635 E. Rockwell St., Arlington Heights, IL 60005
FDA Number: 3006084892

Bandage, Compression	General

TELETRONICS
See Instrumentarium Imaging, Inc.

TELEVERE SYSTEMS 800-385-9593
1611 Center Avenue, Janesville, WI 53545
FDA Number: 2954358

Device, Storage, Image, Digital	Radiology
Image Processing System	Radiology

TELEVIDEO SYSTEMS, INC. 408-954-8333
2562 Seaboard Ave, San Jose, CA 95131
FDA Number: n/a — *Fax:* 408-954-0622

MANUFACTURER PROFILES

TELEVIDEO SYSTEMS, INC. 408-954-8333 *(cont'd)*
E-mail: info@televideo.com
Web site: www.televideo.com
Medical Products Sales Volume: $21,000,000
Annual Revenue: $25-$50 Million
Year Founded: 1975
Ownership: Private
Produces/Sells CE-marked Devices: N
Federal Procurement Eligibility: Small Business, Minority Owned
Distribution: Manufacturer Through Distributor, Importer, Exporter
Computer Equipment | General

TELEVITAL, INC. 408-441-1199
1309 Harefield Ct., San Jose, CA 95131
FDA Number: 3005596982
E-mail: info@televital.com
Web site: www.televital.com
Ownership: Private
Produces/Sells CE-marked Devices: N
Transmitter/Receiver System, Physiological, Radiofrequency | Cardiovascular

TELEVOX SOFTWARE, INC. 800-644-4266
1110 Montlimar Drive, Suite 700, 251-633-9252
Mobile, AL 36609
FDA Number: n/a Fax: 251-633-2420
E-mail: info@televox.com
Web site: www.televox.com
Medical Products Sales Volume: $45,000,000
Annual Revenue: $25-$50 Million
Year Founded: 1992
Total Employees: 250 Marketing Staff: 14 Sales Staff: 23
Ownership: Private
Produces/Sells CE-marked Devices: N
Federal Procurement Eligibility: Small Business
Distribution: Manufacturer Direct, Manufacturer Through Manufacturer Reps
General Admin.: Neil Armentrout/President
Fran Smith/Vice President, General Manager
Medical Admin.: Larry Thompson/Manager Medical Div.
Mktg./Adv.: Jackie Pietri/Manager Marketing
Computer Software, Hospital/Nursing Management | General

TELEX COMMUNICATIONS, INC.-HEARING 800-328-8212
INSTRUMENT GRP.
1200 Portland Avenue S, Burnsville, MN 55357 952-884-4051
FDA Number: J211339 Fax: 952-884-0043
E-mail: hig@telex.com
Web site: www.telex.com
Medical Products Sales Volume: $308,000,000
Annual Revenue: More than $100 Million
Year Founded: 1932
Total Employees: 210 Marketing Staff: 1 Sales Staff: 13
Ownership: Private
Quality System Registration Information: ISO9002
Federal Procurement Eligibility: Small Business, Minority Owned, GSA Contract, VA Contract
Distribution: Manufacturer Through Manufacturer Reps
General Admin.: Ned Jackson/Chief Executive Officer
Edward P. Bravn/President
Edward P. Bravin/Vice President, General Manager
Mktg./Adv.: John Wesenberg/Director National Accounts
Patrick Henry/Director Sales
Greg Hovland/Manager Contract Sales
Glen Mazzone/Manager International Sales
Production: Radu Serbu/Chief Engineering Officer
Karen Wolfe/Manager Materials
Dan LaForge/Manager Quality Assurance
Hearing-Aid | Ear/Nose/Throat
Trainer, Auditory | Ear/Nose/Throat
Medical Product Subsidiaries (Listed Separately)
Topcon Omni Systems, Inc.

TELIOS PHARMACEUTICALS
See INTEGRA LIFE

TELKEE, INC.
See Sunroc / Telkee, Inc.

TELLUS MEDICAL PRODUCTS, INC. 760-200-9772
77-971 Wildcat Drive, Suite C, Palm Desert, CA 92211
FDA Number: 1649697
Bandage, Adhesive | Surgery
Bandage, Elastic | General
Pack, Hot Or Cold, Disposable | Physical Med

TELOS MEDICAL EQUIPMENT (AUSTIN & 800-934-3029
ASSOC., INC.)
1109 Sturbridge Road, Fallston, MD 21047-1905 410-877-3029
FDA Number: 1121721 Fax: 410-877-0544

TELOS MEDICAL EQUIPMENT (AUSTIN & 800-934-3029 *(cont'd)*
E-mail: telosusa@aol.com
Web site: www.telosmedical.com
Medical Products Sales Volume: $495,000
Annual Revenue: $0-$1 Million
Total Employees: 10
Ownership: Private
Produces/Sells CE-marked Devices: Y
Federal Procurement Eligibility: Small Business, GSA Contract, VA Contract
Distribution: Exclusive Distributor
General Admin.: Al G. Austin/President
Mktg./Adv.: Al E. Austin/Manager International Marketing & Sales
Finance: Joyce C. Austin/Treasurer
Accessories, Fixation, Orthopedic | Orthopedics
Board, Arm | Anesthesiology
Densitometer, Radiography, Digital, Quantitative | Radiology
Driver, Bone Staple | Orthopedics
Holder, Leg, Arthroscopy | Orthopedics
Laparoscope, General & Plastic Surgery | Surgery
Pressure Measurement, System, Intermittent | Physical Med
Support, Patient Position | Anesthesiology
Table, Surgical, Orthopedic | Orthopedics

TELSAR LABORATORIES INC 800-255-9938
1 Enviroway, Suite 100, Wood River, IL 62095 618-254-5555
FDA Number: n/a Fax: 618-254-5554
E-mail: telsar@telsar.com
Web site: www.telsar.com
Medical Products Sales Volume: $1,000,000
Annual Revenue: $1-$5 Million
Year Founded: 1984
Total Employees: 10 Marketing Staff: 3 Sales Staff: 3
Ownership: Private
Produces/Sells CE-marked Devices: N
Federal Procurement Eligibility: Small Business
Distribution: Manufacturer Direct, Manufacturer Through Distributor, Manufacturer Through Manufacturer Reps, OEM, Service Direct, Exclusive Distributor, Importer, Exporter
General Admin.: J. Peter Zimmer/President, Chief Executive Officer
Accessories, Laser | General
Arm Rest | Physical Med
Laser, Nd:YAG, Surgical | Surgery
Laser, Surgical | Surgery
Service, Maintenance/Repair | General
System, Cooling, Laser | Surgery

TELSAR LABORATORIES, INC. 800-255-9938
319 Ridge Street, Alton, IL 62002 618-254-0555
FDA Number: 1423368 Fax: 618-462-0531
E-mail: info@telsar.com
Web site: www.telsar.com
Ownership: Private
Produces/Sells CE-marked Devices: N
Laser, Surgical | Surgery

TEMEDCO, LTD. 210-798-0978
1141 N. Loop 1604 E #105, Box 418, San Antonio, TX 78232
FDA Number: 3004028536
Applier, Surgical Staple | Surgery

TEMP-TRONIX 800-223-8367
7350-B Trade St., San Diego, CA 92121 858-578-4530
FDA Number: 2020598 Fax: 858-578-4532
E-mail: tempeuro@inetmail.att.net
Year Founded: 1967
Total Employees: 5
Ownership: Private
Produces/Sells CE-marked Devices: N
Federal Procurement Eligibility: Small Business, Minority Owned, Female Owned, VA Contract
Distribution: Manufacturer Direct, Manufacturer Through Distributor
General Admin.: Charlie Mize/President
Thermometer, Electronic, Continuous | General

TEMPTEK INC.
See Thermotek Inc.

TEMPTIME CORPORATION 973-984-6000
116 American Rd., Greystone Park, NJ 07950
FDA Number: 3004437723 Fax: (973) 984-1520
Ownership: Private
Produces/Sells CE-marked Devices: N

TEMPUR CANADA 519-660-4154
1807 Wonderland Road N., London, ONT N6G 5C2 Canada
FDA Number: n/a Fax: 519-679-4793
E-mail: inquiries@tempurpedic.com
Web site: www.tempurcanada.com
Year Founded: 1990

TEMPUR CANADA   519-660-4154 *(cont'd)*
Total Employees: 10
Ownership: Private
Produces/Sells CE-marked Devices: N
Distribution: Exclusive Distributor

TEMPUR PRODUCTION USA, INC.   276-431-7174
12907 Tempurpedic Parkway, Albuquerque, NM 87121
FDA Number: 3006429287
Ownership: Private
Produces/Sells CE-marked Devices: N
  Mattress, Non-Powered Flotation Therapy   Physical Med

TEMPUR PRODUCTION USA, INC.   276-431-7174
203 Tempur Pedic Drive,, Suite 102, Duffield, VA 24244
FDA Number: 3003256125
  Accessories, Wheelchair   Physical Med
  Bed, Patient Rotation, Powered   Physical Med
  Mattress, Air Flotation   General
  Mattress, Non-Powered Flotation Therapy   Physical Med

TEMPUR-MED INC.
See Tempur-Medical, Inc.

TEMPUR-MEDICAL, INC.   888-255-3302
1713 Jaggie Fox Way, Lexington, KY 40511   859-259-0754
FDA Number: 1528236   *Fax:* 859-514-4423
E-mail: customerservice@tempurmed.com
Web site: www.tempurmed.com
Medical Products Sales Volume: $1,700,000
Year Founded: 2000
Total Employees: 11
Ownership: TEMPUR-PEDIC, INC.
Produces/Sells CE-marked Devices: N
Federal Procurement Eligibility: Small Business, GSA Contract, VA Contract
Distribution: Manufacturer Direct, Manufacturer Through Distributor, OEM
General Admin.: Joel Guerin/President
Production: Rick Fontaine/Director Regulatory Affairs
  Accessories, Operating Room, Table   Surgery
  Bed, Patient Rotation, Powered   Physical Med
  Cover, Mattress   General
  Cushion, Wheelchair (Pad)   Physical Med
  Mattress, Air Flotation   General
  Mattress, Non-Powered Flotation Therapy   Physical Med
  Pillow, Cervical   Orthopedics

TEMPUR-PEDID
See Tempur-Medical, Inc.

TEMREX CORP.   516-868-6221
112 Albany Ave., P.o. Box 182, Freeport, NY 11520
FDA Number: 2429849
  Alloy, Precious Metal, For Clinical Use   Dental And Oral
  Block, Bite   Cns/Neurology
  Cement, Dental   Dental And Oral
  Crown And Bridge, Temporary, Resin   Dental And Oral
  Holder, X-Ray Film   Dental And Oral
  Liner, Cavity, Calcium Hydroxide   Dental And Oral
  Spatula, Surgical, General & Plastic Surgery   Surgery
  Tooth Bonding Agent, Resin Restoration   Dental And Oral
  Tray, Impression   Dental And Oral
  Zinc Oxide Eugenol   Dental And Oral

TEMREX CORPORATION   800-645-1226
112 Albany Ave., Freeport, NY 11520-4702   516-868-6221
FDA Number: 2429849   *Fax:* 516-868-5700
E-mail: temrex@centurytel.net
Web site: www.temrex.com
Annual Revenue: $0-$1 Million
Total Employees: 15   *Marketing Staff:* 3   *Sales Staff:* 4
Ownership: Private
Quality System Registration Information: ISO9001
Produces/Sells CE-marked Devices: Y
Federal Procurement Eligibility: Small Business
Distribution: Manufacturer Through Distributor, Exporter
General Admin.: Ethan A. Levander/President
Production: Joseph W. Jones/Manager Production
         Jackie Prather/Product Manager
  Accessories, Retractor, Dental   Dental And Oral
  Agent, Polishing, Abrasive, Oral Cavity   Dental And Oral
  Block, Bite, ENT   Ear/Nose/Throat
  Cement, Dental   Dental And Oral
  Crown And Bridge, Temporary, Resin   Dental And Oral
  Holder, X-Ray Film   Dental And Oral
  Liner, Cavity, Calcium Hydroxide   Dental And Oral
  Material, Dental Filling   Dental And Oral
  Material, Tooth Shade, Resin   Dental And Oral
  Sharpener, Dental   Dental And Oral
  Source, Heat, Bleaching, Teeth, Dental   Dental And Oral
  Tooth Bonding Agent, Resin Restoration   Dental And Oral
  Tray, Impression   Dental And Oral

TEMREX CORPORATION   800-645-1226 *(cont'd)*
  Zinc Oxide Eugenol   Dental And Oral

TEMTEK/THERMOTEK INC.
See Thermotek Inc.

TENET MEDICAL ENGINEERING, INC.   888-836-3863
5540 1A St. SW, Calgary, ALB T2H 0E7 Canada   403-571-0750
FDA Number: 9681741   *Fax:* 403-571-0752
E-mail: kwmoore@tenetmedical.com
Web site: www.tenetmedical.com
Annual Revenue: $0-$1 Million
Year Founded: 1994
Total Employees: 10
Distribution: Manufacturer Direct, Exclusive Distributor
General Admin.: Ken Moore/President
Production: Brent King/Director Engineering
  Accessories, Operating Room, Table   Surgery

TENGION INC   610-292-8364
2900 Potshop Ln 100, East Norriton, PA 19403
FDA Number: n/a
Web site: www.tengion.com
Ownership: Private
Produces/Sells CE-marked Devices: N
General Admin.: Dr. Deepak Jain/Chief Technology Officer
         Dr. Tim Bertram/President
         Mr. Mark Stejbach/Vice President
Finance: Mr. A. Brian Davis/Chief Financial Officer, Vice President Finance

TENNECO PACKAGING
See Pactiv Corporation

TENNESSEE MEDICAL EQUIPMENT, INC.   800-200-4808
4637 Hwy 19 East, Ripley, TN 38063   731-635-2119
FDA Number: 1057435   *Fax:* 731-635-5887
E-mail: tnmed@aeneas.net
Web site: www.tnmedicalequipment.com
Ownership: Private
Produces/Sells CE-marked Devices: N
  Generator, Oxygen, Portable   Anesthesiology
  Humidifier, Respiratory Gas, (Direct Patient Interface)   Anesthesiology
  Nebulizer, Medicinal, Non-Ventilatory (Atomizer)   Anesthesiology
  Pump, Aspiration, Portable   Anesthesiology
  Regulator, Pressure, Gas Cylinder   Anesthesiology

TENNEY ENGINEERING, INC.
See Thermal Product Solutions

TENSYS MEDICAL, INC.   888-722-7800
5825 Oberlin Drive, Suite 100,   858-552-1941
San Diego, CA 92121
FDA Number: 2032673   *Fax:* 858-552-2094
E-mail: support@tensysmedical.com
Web site: www.tensysmedical.com
Medical Products Sales Volume: $1,000,000
Year Founded: 1995
Total Employees: 35
Ownership: Private
Produces/Sells CE-marked Devices: N
Federal Procurement Eligibility: Small Business
Distribution: Manufacturer Direct
General Admin.: Mr. Michael Martin/Chief Executive Officer
Mktg./Adv.: Mr. Bill Markle/Vice President, Manager Business
         Mr. Scott Schlesner/Vice President, Manager Sales
  Monitor, Blood Pressure, Indirect, Semi-Automatic   Cardiovascular

TENTE CASTERS, INC.   800-783-2470
2266 Southpark Drive, Hebron, KY 41048   859-586-5558
FDA Number: n/a   *Fax:* 859-586-5859
E-mail: info@tente-us.com
Web site: www.tente.com
Medical Products Sales Volume: $19,600,000
Year Founded: 1979
Total Employees: 81   *Marketing Staff:* 1   *Sales Staff:* 10
Ownership: Tente Rollen Gmbh & Co.
Quality System Registration Information: ISO9001
Produces/Sells CE-marked Devices: N
Federal Procurement Eligibility: Small Business
Distribution: Manufacturer Through Distributor, OEM, Importer, Exporter
General Admin.: Mr. Bradford M. Hood/Managing Director
Mktg./Adv.: Mrs. Sabine Batsche/Manager Marketing
         Mr. Aaron Romer/Manager Sales
Production: Mrs. Sue Dinkel/Manager Materials
  Casters, Hospital Equipment   General

TEPCO, INC.
See Tapcon, Inc.

MANUFACTURER PROFILES

TEPHA, INCORPORATED — 781-357-1709
99 Hayden Avenue, Suite 360, Lexington, MA 02421
FDA Number: 3005670760
E-mail: contact@tepha.com
Fax: (781) 357-1701
Ownership: Private
Produces/Sells CE-marked Devices: N
Mesh, Surgical, Polymeric — Surgery

TEPNEL LIFECODES CORPORATION — 203-328-9500
550 West Ave., Stamford, CT 06902
FDA Number: 1226100
Ownership: Private
Produces/Sells CE-marked Devices: N
Reagents, Specific, Analyte — Hematology
Test, Qualitative, For Hla, Non-diagnostic — Hematology

TEPROMARK INTERNATIONAL, INC. — 800-645-2622
7518 N. St. Louis #1047, Skokie, IL 60076
FDA Number: n/a
E-mail: customerservice@tepromark.com
Web site: www.tepromark.com
Annual Revenue: $0-$1 Million
Year Founded: 1971
Ownership: Private
Federal Procurement Eligibility: Small Business
Distribution: Manufacturer Direct, Manufacturer Through Distributor, Manufacturer Through Manufacturer Reps, OEM, Service Direct, Exclusive Distributor
Bumper Guard, Corner — General
Carpeting — General
Cover, Other — General
Floor Mat — General
Floor Mat, Antibacterial — General
Rail, Wall Side — General
Rails, Equipment — General

TERAMEDICA, INC. — 414-908-7713
10400 Innovation, Suite 200, Milwaukee, WI 53226
FDA Number: 3003856807
Device, Storage, Image, Digital — Radiology

TERARECON, INC. — 877-354-1100 / 650-372-1100
4000 East 3rd Avenue, Suite 200, Foster City,, CA 94404
FDA Number: 2954793
E-mail: info@terarecon.com
Fax: 650-372-1101
Web site: www.terarecon.com
Year Founded: 1997
Ownership: Private
Produces/Sells CE-marked Devices: N
General Admin.: Motoaki Saito/Chief Executive Officer
Robert Taylor/President, Chief Operating Officer
Production: Toshiaki Sakaguchi/Senior Vice President Operations
Finance: Lakshmi Lakshminarayan/Senior Vice President Finance
IS: Vikram Simha/Senior Vice President Technology
Image Processing System — Radiology
Scanner, Emission Computed Tomography — Radiology
Scanner, Ultrasonic (Pulsed Doppler) — Radiology
System, Communication, Image, Digital — Radiology

TERASON REVOLUTIONIZING ULTRASOUND
See Terason Revolutionizing Ultrasound

TERATECH CORP. — 781-270-4143
77-79 Terrace Hall Ave., Burlington, MA 01803
FDA Number: 3002315840
Scanner, Ultrasonic (Pulsed Echo) — Radiology

TERRA NOVA BIOTECHNOLOGY CO. LTD. — 800-851-1677 / 709-737-4026
P.O. Box 13340, St. John's, NF A1B-4 Canada
FDA Number: n/a
E-mail: tnb@morgan.ucs.mun.ca
Fax: 709-737-2101
Web site: www.mun.ca/seabright/tnb/
Year Founded: 1988
Total Employees: 25
Ownership: Private
Produces/Sells CE-marked Devices: N
Distribution: Manufacturer Direct, Exporter

TERRISS-CONSOLIDATED INDUSTRIES — 800-342-1611 / 732-988-0909
807 Summerfield Ave., Asbury Park, NJ 07712
FDA Number: n/a
E-mail: terriss@terriss.com
Fax: 732-502-0526
Web site: www.terriss.com
Year Founded: 1895
Total Employees: 13
Ownership: Private

TERRISS-CONSOLIDATED INDUSTRIES — 800-342-1611 *(cont'd)*
Produces/Sells CE-marked Devices: N
Federal Procurement Eligibility: Small Business, Female Owned
Distribution: Manufacturer Direct
General Admin.: Zipporah Epstein/Chief Executive Officer
Mktg./Adv.: Marc J. Epstein/Director Marketing & Product Development
Edward Della Zanna/Manager International & National Sales
Ed Della Zanna/Vice President Marketing & Sales
Production: Stephen Bodnovich/Vice President Production
Bowl, Solution — General
Cabinet, Laboratory — Chemistry
Container, Specimen, All Types — General
Filter Paper — Chemistry
Jar, Applicator — Surgery
Jar, Forceps — Surgery
Sink, Laboratory — Chemistry

TERUMO CARDIOVASCULAR SYSTEMS
See Terumo Cardiovascular Systems, Corp

TERUMO CARDIOVASCULAR SYSTEMS (TCVS) — 800-283-7866 / 410-398-8500
125 Blue Ball Road, Elkton, MD 21921
FDA Number: 1124841
Fax: 410-392-7171
Web site: www.terumo-cvs.com
Year Founded: 1921
Total Employees: 500
Ownership: Terumo Corporation
Stock Symbol: 4543
Traded On: Tokyo
Produces/Sells CE-marked Devices: N
General Admin.: Mark Sutter/Chief Executive Officer
Shukri F.Khuri/Vice President
Adapter, Stopcock, Manifold, Cardiopulmonary Bypass — Cardiovascular
Blade, Saw, Surgical, Cardiovascular — Cardiovascular
Cannula, Catheter — Cardiovascular
Catheter, Suction (Tracheal Aspirating Tube) — Anesthesiology
Catheter, Vascular, Cardiopulmonary Bypass — Cardiovascular
Filter, Blood, Cardiopulmonary Bypass, Arterial Line — Cardiovascular
Heat Exchanger, Heart-Lung Bypass — Cardiovascular
Heat Exchanger, Heart-Lung Bypass, AC-Powered — Cardiovascular
Monitor, Blood Gas, On-Line, Cardiopulmonary Bypass — Cardiovascular
Oxygenator, Cardiopulmonary Bypass — Cardiovascular
Pump, Blood, Cardiopulmonary Bypass, Non-Roller Type — Cardiovascular
Reservoir, Blood, Cardiopulmonary Bypass — Cardiovascular
Supplies, Blood Bank — Hematology
Transducer, Blood Pressure, Extravascular — Cardiovascular
Trap, Sterile Specimen — Anesthesiology
Tube, Pump, Cardiopulmonary Bypass — Cardiovascular

TERUMO CARDIOVASCULAR SYSTEMS (TCVS) — 714-258-8001
1311 Valencia Ave., Tustin, CA 92780
FDA Number: 2023117
Fax: 714-258-1230
Web site: www.terumo-cvs.com
Annual Revenue: More than $1 Billion
Year Founded: 1921
Total Employees: 500
Ownership: Terumo Corporation
Stock Symbol: 4543
Traded On: Tokyo
Produces/Sells CE-marked Devices: N
General Admin.: Mark Sutter/Chief Executive Officer
Shukri F.Khuri/Vice President
Adapter, Stopcock, Manifold, Cardiopulmonary Bypass — Cardiovascular
Analyzer, Gas, Oxygen, Partial Pr., Blood Phase, Indwelling — Anesthesiology
Analyzer, Ion, Hydrogen-Ion (pH), Blood Phase, Indwelling — Anesthesiology
Catheter, Suction (Tracheal Aspirating Tube) — Anesthesiology
Filter, Blood, Cardiopulmonary Bypass, Arterial Line — Cardiovascular
Monitor, Blood Gas, On-Line, Cardiopulmonary Bypass — Cardiovascular
Oxygenator, Cardiopulmonary Bypass — Cardiovascular
Reservoir, Blood, Cardiopulmonary Bypass — Cardiovascular
Transducer, Blood Pressure, Extravascular — Cardiovascular
Trap, Sterile Specimen — Anesthesiology

TERUMO CARDIOVASCULAR SYSTEMS (TCVS) — 800-283-7866 / 508-881-4858
28 Howe St., Ashland, MA 01721
FDA Number: 1212122
Fax: 508-231-5210
Web site: www.terumo-cvs.com
Annual Revenue: More than $1 Billion
Year Founded: 1921
Total Employees: 500
Ownership: Terumo Corporation
Stock Symbol: 4543
Traded On: Tokyo
Produces/Sells CE-marked Devices: N
General Admin.: Mark Sutter/Chief Executive Officer
Shukri F.Khuri/Vice President
Accessories, Blood Circuit, Hemodialysis — Gastroenterology/Urology
Accessories, Cardiopulmonary Bypass — Cardiovascular
Adapter, Stopcock, Manifold, Cardiopulmonary Bypass — Cardiovascular
Autotransfusion Unit (Blood) — Anesthesiology

TERUMO CARDIOVASCULAR SYSTEMS (TCVS) 800-283-7866
(cont'd)

Bag, Blood, Collection	Hematology
Blade, Saw, Surgical, Cardiovascular	Cardiovascular
Bottle, Collection, Vacuum (Aspirator)	General
Catheter, Suction (Tracheal Aspirating Tube)	Anesthesiology
Catheter, Suction, With Tip	General
Catheter, Vascular, Cardiopulmonary Bypass	Cardiovascular
Clamp, Bone	Orthopedics
Clamp, Surgical, General & Plastic Surgery	Surgery
Collector, Urine	Gastroenterology/Urology
Container, Specimen Mailer And Storage	Pathology
Controller, Suction, Intracardiac, Cardiopulmonary Bypass	Cardiovascular
Detector, Bubble, Cardiopulmonary Bypass	Cardiovascular
Dialyzer, High Permeability	Gastroenterology/Urology
Dilator, Vessel, Surgical	Cardiovascular
Drape, Surgical	Surgery
Filter, Bacterial, Breathing Circuit	Anesthesiology
Filter, Blood, Cardiopulmonary Bypass, Arterial Line	Cardiovascular
Filter, Blood, Cardiotomy Suction Line, Cardiopulmonary	Cardiovascular
Filter, Pre-Bypass, Cardiopulmonary Bypass	Cardiovascular
Heat Exchanger, Heart-Lung Bypass	Cardiovascular
Kit, Administration, Intravenous	General
Kit, Irrigation, Sterile	Gastroenterology/Urology
Microfilter, Blood Transfusion	Anesthesiology
Monitor, Blood Gas, On-Line, Cardiopulmonary Bypass	Cardiovascular
Needle, Hypodermic, Single Lumen With Syringe	General
Oxygenator, Cardiopulmonary Bypass	Cardiovascular
Probe, Blood Flow, Extravascular	Cardiovascular
Protector, Transducer, Dialysis	Gastroenterology/Urology
Pump, Blood, Cardiopulmonary Bypass, Non-Roller Type	Cardiovascular
Regulator, Vacuum	General
Reservoir, Blood, Cardiopulmonary Bypass	Cardiovascular
Sensor, Blood Gas, In-Line, Cardiopulmonary Bypass	Cardiovascular
Sucker, Cardiotomy Return, Cardiopulmonary Bypass	Cardiovascular
Suction Apparatus, Operating Room, Wall Vacuum-Powered	Surgery
Supplies, Blood Bank	Hematology
Surgical Instrument, Cardiovascular	Cardiovascular
Surgical Instrument, Disposable	Surgery
Syringe, Irrigating	General
Syringe, Piston	General
Thermometer, Electronic, Continuous	General
Transducer, Blood Pressure, Extravascular	Cardiovascular
Transfer Unit, Blood	Hematology
Trap, Sterile Specimen	Anesthesiology
Tube, Double Lumen For Intestinal Decompression	Gastroenterology/Urology
Tube, Pump, Cardiopulmonary Bypass	Cardiovascular
Tubing, Non-Invasive	Surgery
Valve, CPB Check, Retrograde, In-Line	Anesthesiology
Valve, Pressure Relief, Cardiopulmonary Bypass	Cardiovascular
Wrap, Sterilization	General

TERUMO CARDIOVASCULAR SYSTEMS CORP.
See Terumo Cardiovascular Systems (Tcvs)

TERUMO CARDIOVASCULAR SYSTEMS CORP.
See Terumo Cardiovascular Systems (Tcvs)

TERUMO CARDIOVASCULAR SYSTEMS CORPORATION
See Terumo Cardiovascular Systems (Tcvs)

TERUMO CARDIOVASCULAR SYSTEMS, CORP 800-521-2818
6200 Jackson Rd., Ann Arbor, MI 48103-9300 734-663-4145
FDA Number: 1828100   *Fax:* 734-741-6079
Web site: www.terumo-cvs.com
Annual Revenue: More than $1 Billion
Year Founded: 1921
Total Employees: 500
Ownership: Terumo Corporation
Stock Symbol: 4543
Traded On: Tokyo
Quality System Registration Information: ISO9001
Produces/Sells CE-marked Devices: Y
Distribution: Manufacturer Direct, Manufacturer Through Distributor, Manufacturer Through Manufacturer Reps
General Admin.: Mark Sutter/Chief Executive Officer
    Gael Tisack/General Counsel
    Mac Ritchie/Vice President
    Matt GrayBill/Vice President Human Resources
Mktg./Adv.: Mark DiLemente/Director National Accounts
    Dana Currier/Manager International Sales
    Barbara Schmid/Manager Marketing Communications
    Mark DiClemente/Manager National Sales
    Pat Elliot/Vice President Global Marketing
Production: Paul Western/Manager Manufacturing
    Steve Arick/Manager Regulatory Affairs

Accessories, Cardiopulmonary Bypass	Cardiovascular
Adapter, Stopcock, Manifold, Cardiopulmonary Bypass	Cardiovascular
Blade, Saw, Surgical, Cardiovascular	Cardiovascular
Catheter, Vascular, Cardiopulmonary Bypass	Cardiovascular
Console, Heart-Lung Machine, Cardiopulmonary Bypass	Cardiovascular
Controller, Gas, Cardiopulmonary Bypass	Cardiovascular

TERUMO CARDIOVASCULAR SYSTEMS, CORP 800-521-2818
(cont'd)

Controller, Pump Speed, Cardiopulmonary Bypass	Cardiovascular
Controller, Temperature, Cardiopulmonary Bypass	Cardiovascular
Defoamer, Cardiopulmonary Bypass	Cardiovascular
Detector, Bubble, Cardiopulmonary Bypass	Cardiovascular
Dilator, Vessel, Surgical	Cardiovascular
Filter, Blood, Cardiotomy Suction Line, Cardiopulmonary	Cardiovascular
Flowmeter, Blood, Intravenous	Cardiovascular
Flowmeter, Gas (Oxygen), Calibrated	Anesthesiology
Gauge, Pressure, Coronary, Cardiopulmonary Bypass	Cardiovascular
Generator, Pulsatile Flow, Cardiopulmonary Bypass	Cardiovascular
Heart-Lung Bypass Unit (Cardiopulmonary)	Cardiovascular
Heat Exchanger, Heart-Lung Bypass	Cardiovascular
Hypo/Hyperthermia Unit, Mobile	General
Kit, Administration, Cardioplegia Solution	Cardiovascular
Monitor, Blood Flow, Ultrasonic	Obstetrics/Gynecology
Monitor, Blood Gas, On-Line, Cardiopulmonary Bypass	Cardiovascular
Monitor, Cardiopulmonary Level Sensing	Cardiovascular
Monitor, Pressure, Venous, Central, Powered	Cardiovascular
Monitor, Temperature (With Probe)	Anesthesiology
Motor, Surgical Instrument, AC-Powered	Surgery
Oxygenator, Cardiopulmonary Bypass	Cardiovascular
Perfusion Unit	General
Pump, Blood, Cardiopulmonary Bypass, Non-Roller Type	Cardiovascular
Pump, Blood, Cardiopulmonary Bypass, Roller Type	Cardiovascular
Pump, Blood, Hemodialysis Unit	Gastroenterology/Urology
Pump, Extracorporeal Perfusion	Cardiovascular
Pump, Infusion	General
Reservoir, Blood, Cardiopulmonary Bypass	Cardiovascular
Saw, Electric	Cardiovascular
Sphygmomanometer, Aneroid (Arterial Pressure)	General
Sucker, Cardiotomy Return, Cardiopulmonary Bypass	Cardiovascular
Support, Arm	Physical Med
Thermometer, Chemical Color Change	General
Thermometer, Electronic, Continuous	General
Trap, Bubble	Cardiovascular
Tube, Pump, Cardiopulmonary Bypass	Cardiovascular
Tubing, Flexible, Medical Gas, Low-Pressure	Anesthesiology

TERUMO HEART INC. (THI) 800-803-8385
6180 Jackson Road, Ann Arbor, MI 48103 800-262-3304
FDA Number: 3005228872   *Fax:* 734-741-6456
E-mail: thi.customerservice@terumomedical.com
Web site: www.terumoheart.com
Year Founded: 1921
Ownership: Terumo Corporation
Stock Symbol: 4543
Traded On: Tokyo
Produces/Sells CE-marked Devices: N
General Admin.: Chisato Nojiri/Chief Executive Officer
    Dr. David Munjal/Vice President

TERUMO HEART, INC
See Terumo Heart Inc. (Thi)

TERUMO MEDICAL CORP. 800-283-7866
2101 Cottontail Lane, Somerset, NJ 08873 908-302-4900
FDA Number: 2243441   *Fax:* 908-302-3083
Web site: http://www.terumomedical.com
Medical Products Sales Volume: $180,000,000
Annual Revenue: More than $1 Billion
Year Founded: 1921
Total Employees: 7500   *Marketing Staff:* 62   *Sales Staff:* 120
Ownership: Terumo Corporation
Stock Symbol: 4543
Traded On: Tokyo
Quality System Registration Information: ISO9001
Produces/Sells CE-marked Devices: Y
Federal Procurement Eligibility: Minority Owned
Distribution: Manufacturer Through Distributor, Manufacturer Through Manufacturer Reps, Importer, Exporter
General Admin.: Wataru Umemura/Chief Operating Officer, Vice President Operations
    Bruce Van Klompenberg/Manager Personnel
    Ron Devore/President
Production: Maryann Kehoe/Manager Regulatory Affairs
    Rusty Pierce/Plant Manager

Kit, Sampling, Blood	General
Kit, Sampling, Blood Gas	General
Needle, Blood Collection	General
Spectrophotometer, U.V./Visible	Chemistry
Syringe, Insulin	General
Tube, Blood Collection	Chemistry

TERUMO MEDICAL CORP. 800-283-7866
302 North 45th Ave., Suite 1, Phoenix, AZ 85043 602-484-7842
FDA Number: 2080985   *Fax:* 602-484-7951
Web site: www.terumomedical.com
Ownership: Terumo Corporation

TERUMO MEDICAL CORP. 800-283-7866 *(cont'd)*
Stock Symbol: 4543
Traded On: Tokyo
Produces/Sells CE-marked Devices: N

TERUMO MEDICAL CORP. 800-283-7866
State Line Business Park 662-280-2643
8655 Commerce Drive, Suite 101
Southaven, MS 38671
FDA Number: 3006119144 *Fax:* 662-393-8208
Web site: www.terumomedical.com
Ownership: Terumo Corporation
Stock Symbol: 4543
Traded On: Tokyo
Produces/Sells CE-marked Devices: N

TERUMO MEDICAL CORPORATION 800-283-7866
8750 NW 36th Street, Suite 600, Miami, FL 33178 305-477-4822
FDA Number: 3003706012 *Fax:* 305-477-4872
Web site: www.terumomedical.com
Ownership: Terumo Corporation
Stock Symbol: 4543
Traded On: Tokyo
Produces/Sells CE-marked Devices: N

TERUMO MEDICAL CORPORATION 800-283-7866
950 Elkton Blvd., P.O.Box 605, Elkton, MD 21921 410-392-8500
FDA Number: 1118880 *Fax:* 410-392-7218
Web site: www.terumomedical.com
Year Founded: 1921
Total Employees: 7500
Ownership: Terumo Corporation
Stock Symbol: 4543
Traded On: Tokyo
Produces/Sells CE-marked Devices: N
General Admin.: Mr. Takashi Wachi/Chairman

Catheter, Intravascular, Therapeutic, Short-term Less Than 30 Days	General
Catheter, Percutaneous	Cardiovascular
Colorimeter, General Use	Chemistry
Culture Media, Synthetic Cell And Tissue	Pathology
Guidewire, Catheter	Cardiovascular
Holder, Needle	Gastroenterology/Urology
Introducer, Catheter	Cardiovascular
Kit, Administration, Intravenous	General
Labware, Blood Collection	Chemistry
Needle, Fistula	Gastroenterology/Urology
Needle, Hypodermic	General
Needle, Hypodermic, Single Lumen With Syringe	General
Radioimmunoassay, Estradiol	Chemistry
Radioimmunoassay, Progesterone	Chemistry
Serum Separation System	Hematology
Set, Administration, Intravenous, Needle-Free	General
Stopcock	General
Supplies, Blood Bank	Hematology
Surgical Instrument, Cardiovascular	Cardiovascular
Syringe, Antistick	General
Syringe, Piston	General
System, Peritoneal Dialysis, Automatic	Gastroenterology/Urology

TERUMO MEDICAL PRODUCTS (HANGZHOU) CO., LTD.
See Terumo Medical Corp.

TESA MEASUREMENT SYSTEMS
See Brown & Sharpe Inc.

TESCOM CORP. 800-447-9635
12616 Industrial Blvd., Elk River, MN 55330-2491 763-441-6330
FDA Number: 2126665 *Fax:* 763-241-3224
E-mail: icd@tescom.com
Web site: www.tescom.com
Medical Products Sales Volume: $33,000,000
Annual Revenue: $25-$50 Million
Year Founded: 1916
Total Employees: 150
Ownership: Private
Quality System Registration Information: ISO9001
Produces/Sells CE-marked Devices: N
Federal Procurement Eligibility: Small Business
Distribution: Manufacturer Direct, Manufacturer Through Distributor, OEM
General Admin.: Don Glesmann/Chief Executive Officer
Ed Cunnington/Chief Operating Officer
Mktg./Adv.: Vikki Nehring/Account Specialist
Steve Horner/Director Marketing

Regulator, Pressure, Gas Cylinder	Anesthesiology

TESSEK CHROMATOGRAPHY
See Melcor Technologies, Inc.

TESTO, INC. 800-227-0729
40 White Lake Road, Sparta, NJ 07871
FDA Number: n/a
E-mail: Info@testo.com
Web site: www.testo.com
Medical Products Sales Volume: $1,300,000
Annual Revenue: $1-$5 Million
Ownership: Testo Gmbh & Co.
Quality System Registration Information: ISO9001
Produces/Sells CE-marked Devices: N
Federal Procurement Eligibility: Small Business
Distribution: Manufacturer Through Distributor, Manufacturer Through Manufacturer Reps

Foodservice Product/Equipment	General
Thermometer, Laboratory	Chemistry

TESTOTERM, INC.
See Testo, Inc.

TETHYS BIOSCIENCE INC. 888-697-7339
5858 Horton Street, Suite 550, 510-420-6700
Emeryville, CA 94608
FDA Number: n/a *Fax:* 510-601-0371
E-mail: clientservices@tethysbio.com
Web site: http://tethysbio.com
Ownership: Private
Produces/Sells CE-marked Devices: N
General Admin.: Mr. Mickey Urdea/Chairman, Chief Executive Officer
Mr. David Hodgson/Chief Information Officer
Mr. Michael McKenna/Chief Scientific Officer
Dr. Steven Watkins/Chief Technology Officer
Mr. R. Michael Richey/President
Finance: Mr. Mohan Iyer/Business Development Officer
Ms. Matthew Ferguson/Chief Financial Officer

TETRA CO., THE
See Tetra Medical Supply Corp.

TETRA COMPUTER SYSTEMS, LLC 856-728-6835
328 Bryn Mawr Drive, Williamstown, NJ 08094
FDA Number: 3005983065
Ownership: Private
Produces/Sells CE-marked Devices: N

Adaptor, Recreational	Physical Med

TETRA MEDICAL SUPPLY CORP. 800-621-4041
6364 W. Gross Point Road, Niles, IL 60714-3916 847-647-0590
FDA Number: 1418270 *Fax:* 847-647-9034
E-mail: sales@tetramed.com
Web site: www.tetramed.com
Medical Products Sales Volume: $700,000
Annual Revenue: $1-$5 Million
Year Founded: 1913
Total Employees: 12 *Marketing Staff:* 2 *Sales Staff:* 4
Ownership: Private
Produces/Sells CE-marked Devices: Y
Federal Procurement Eligibility: Small Business, Female Owned, GSA Contract
Distribution: Manufacturer Direct, Manufacturer Through Distributor, Exporter
General Admin.: Constance A. Shier/Chairman, Chief Financial Officer
James A. Shier/President, General Manager
Mktg./Adv.: Sandy Ketteman/Director Marketing & Sales
Constance A. Shier/Manager Advertising

Bag, Ice	General
Bandage, Elastic	General
Bandage, Tubular	General
Belt, Lumbosacral	Orthopedics
Belt, Rib (Support)	Orthopedics
Belt, Traction, Pelvic, Orthopedic	Orthopedics
Binder, Abdominal	General
Binder, Ankle	Orthopedics
Binder, Wrist	Orthopedics
Collar, Cervical Neck	Orthopedics
Collar, Ice	General
Cushion, Other	General
Electrode, Metallic With Soft Pad Covering	Physical Med
Gel, Electrode, TENS	Physical Med
Halter, Head, Traction, Orthopedic	Orthopedics
Heating Unit, Powered	Physical Med
Immobilizer, Ankle	Orthopedics
Immobilizer, Arm	Orthopedics
Immobilizer, Cervical	Orthopedics
Immobilizer, Elbow	Orthopedics
Immobilizer, Infant (Circumcision Board)	Orthopedics
Immobilizer, Knee	Orthopedics
Immobilizer, Shoulder	Orthopedics
Immobilizer, Wrist/Hand	Orthopedics
Mattress, Water	General
Moist Therapy Pack	Physical Med
Orthosis, Other	Physical Med
Pack, Cold	General

TETRA MEDICAL SUPPLY CORP.   800-621-4041 *(cont'd)*

Pack, Cold, Chemical	General
Pack, Hot Or Cold, Reusable	Physical Med
Pack, Hot, Chemical	General
Pad, Pressure, Foam (Elbow, Heel)	General
Pad, Pressure, Water Cushion	General
Pillow, Cervical	Orthopedics
Shoe, Cast	Physical Med
Shoe, Orthopedic	Orthopedics
Sling, Arm	Physical Med
Sling, Knee	Orthopedics
Sling, Leg	Orthopedics
Splint, Molded, Aluminum	Orthopedics
Splint, Padded Stays	Orthopedics
Splint, Traction	Orthopedics
Stimulator, External, Neuromuscular, Functional	Physical Med
Stockinette	Orthopedics
Stocking, Support (Anti-Embolic)	General
Support, Abdominal	Physical Med
Support, Ankle	Orthopedics
Support, Arm	Physical Med
Support, Back	Orthopedics
Support, Clavicle	Orthopedics
Support, Elbow	Orthopedics
Support, Foot	Orthopedics
Support, Hand	Orthopedics
Support, Hot/Cold Pack	Physical Med
Support, Knee	Physical Med
Support, Leg	Physical Med
Support, Thigh	Physical Med
Support, Wrist	Physical Med
Traction Unit, Static, Bed	Orthopedics

TETRACORE, INC   240-268-5400
9901 Belward Campus Dr., Suite 300, Rockville, MD 20850
FDA Number: 3003517954

TEX-CARE MEDICAL   800-441-8510
2908 Alamance Road, Burlington, NC 27215   336-570-5870
FDA Number: 1063411   *Fax:* 336-226-7220
E-mail: russd@texcaremedical.com
Web site: www.texcaremedical.com
Medical Products Sales Volume: $12,000,000
Ownership: FLYNT AMTEX, INC.
Produces/Sells CE-marked Devices: N
Federal Procurement Eligibility: Small Business
Distribution: Manufacturer Direct, Manufacturer Through Distributor, Manufacturer Through Manufacturer Reps, OEM, Exclusive Distributor, Exporter

Accessories, Apparel, Surgical	Surgery
Bandage, Cast	Physical Med
Component, Cast	Orthopedics
Drape, Surgical	Surgery
Mask, Surgical	Surgery
Shield, Heat, Infant	General
Sock, Non-Compression	General
Stockinette	Orthopedics

TEX-CARE MEDICAL, DIV. FLYNT AMTEX INC.
See Tex-Care Medical

TEX-PRO WESTERN LIMITED   800-663-9266
828 Powell St., Vancouver, BC V6A-1H8 Canada   604-254-9551
FDA Number: n/a   *Fax:* 604-254-2550
E-mail: sales@texpro.net
Web site: www.texpro.net
Year Founded: 1967
Total Employees: 50
Ownership: Private
Produces/Sells CE-marked Devices: N
Distribution: Manufacturer Direct, Exclusive Distributor, Importer

TEX-TENN CORP.   800-251-3027
108-118 Kwick Way Lane, PO Box 8219,   423-477-2611
Gray, TN 37615
FDA Number: 6211212   *Fax:* 423-477-4154
E-mail: smiller@textenn.com
Web site: www.textenn.com
Medical Products Sales Volume: $3,000,000
Annual Revenue: $10-$25 Million
Year Founded: 1981
Total Employees: 150   *Marketing Staff:* 4   *Sales Staff:* 9
Ownership: Private
Produces/Sells CE-marked Devices: N
Federal Procurement Eligibility: Small Business, Female Owned
Distribution: Manufacturer Direct, Manufacturer Through Manufacturer Reps, Service Direct, Exporter
General Admin.: C. John Seifert/President, Chief Executive Officer
Mktg./Adv.: Jeff Dahill/Director Product Development
          Susan Miller/Manager Sales
          Katy Seifert/Vice President, Director Marketing

TEX-TENN CORP.   800-251-3027 *(cont'd)*

Cushion, Wheelchair (Pad)	Physical Med
Mattress, Alternating Pressure (Or Pads)	Physical Med
Pad, Pressure, Foam (Elbow, Heel)	General

TEXAS EYE PROSTHETICS LLC   713-524-1001
4203 Montrose Blvd., Suite 380, Houston, TX 77006
FDA Number: 3006419344   *Fax:* 713-524-1004
E-mail: TexasEyePros@aol.com
Web site: www.texaseyeprosthetics.com
Ownership: Private
Produces/Sells CE-marked Devices: N

Button, Iris, Eye, Artificial	Ophthalmology
Conformer, Ophthalmic	Ophthalmology
Eye, Artificial, Non-Custom	Ophthalmology
Shell, Scleral	Ophthalmology

TEXAS FIBERS
See Leggett & Platt Inc.

TEXAS MEDICAL INDUSTRIES, INC.   800-332-9556
1409 Industrial Drive, Royse City, TX 75189-9559   972-636-9556
FDA Number: 1625408   *Fax:* 972-635-9539
E-mail: danielle@tmiunited.com
Web site: www.tmiunited.com
Medical Products Sales Volume: $1,000,000
Annual Revenue: $1-$5 Million
Year Founded: 1968
Ownership: Private
Produces/Sells CE-marked Devices: N
Federal Procurement Eligibility: Small Business
Distribution: Manufacturer Direct, Manufacturer Through Manufacturer Reps, OEM, Exporter

Accessories, Traction	Physical Med
Accessories, Traction (Cart, Frame, Cord, Weight)	Orthopedics
Bandage, Elastic	General
Belt, Traction, Pelvic, Orthopedic	Orthopedics
Binder, Abdominal	General
Crutch	Physical Med
Equipment, Laboratory, Gen. Purpose (Specific Medical Use)	Chemistry
Halter, Head, Traction	Physical Med
Orthosis, Cervical	Physical Med
Orthosis, Limb Brace	Physical Med
Orthosis, Lumbosacral	Physical Med
Orthosis, Rib Fracture, Soft	Physical Med
Prosthesis, Splint, Nasal, External	Surgery
Protector, Skin Pressure	General
Restraint, Protective (Body)	General
Shoe, Cast	Physical Med
Sling, Arm	Physical Med
Sling, Arm, Overhead Supported	Physical Med
Splint, Abduction, Congenital Hip Dislocation	Physical Med
Splint, Clavicle	Physical Med
Splint, Extremity, Non-Inflatable, External	Surgery
Splint, Hand, And Component	Physical Med
Splint, Traction	Orthopedics
Sponge, External, Rubber	Surgery
Support, Patient Position	Anesthesiology
Tips And Pads, Cane, Crutch And Walker	Physical Med

TEXAS MEDICAL PRODUCTS, INC.
See Novosci Corp.

TEXAS ORTHOPAEDIC PRODUCTS &   888-373-4009
SERVICES, L.L.C.
805 Riding Club Road, Rockwall, TX 75087-2193   972-772-8776
FDA Number: n/a   *Fax:* 972-772-1930
Web site: topsproducts.com
Annual Revenue: $0-$1 Million
Total Employees: 10
Ownership: Private
Produces/Sells CE-marked Devices: N
Distribution: Manufacturer Direct, Manufacturer Through Distributor, Manufacturer Through Manufacturer Reps, OEM

Band, Support, Pelvic	Physical Med
Bandage, Elastic	General
Belt, Traction, Pelvic, Orthopedic	Orthopedics
Binder, Abdominal	General
Brace, Joint, Ankle (External)	Physical Med
Cane	Physical Med
Component, Exercise	Physical Med
Crutch	Physical Med
Joint, Knee, External Brace	Physical Med
Orthosis, Abdominal	Physical Med
Orthosis, Cervical	Physical Med
Orthosis, Cervical-Thoracic, Rigid	Physical Med
Orthosis, Limb Brace	Physical Med
Orthosis, Lumbar	Physical Med
Orthosis, Lumbosacral	Physical Med
Orthosis, Rib Fracture, Soft	Physical Med
Shoe, Cast	Physical Med

TEXAS ORTHOPAEDIC PRODUCTS & 888-373-4009 (cont'd)

Sling, Arm	Physical Med
Splint, Abduction, Congenital Hip Dislocation	Physical Med
Splint, Clavicle	Physical Med
Stimulator, Muscle, Diagnostic	Physical Med
Support, Arm	Physical Med
Tips And Pads, Cane, Crutch And Walker	Physical Med

TEXAS PHOTONICS, INC. 972-412-7111
3213 Main Street, Rowlett, TX 75088
FDA Number: n/a   Fax: 972-412-5440
E-mail: texasop@earthlink.net
Web site: www.texas-photonics.com
Medical Products Sales Volume: $100,000
Annual Revenue: $1-$5 Million
Year Founded: 2003
Total Employees: 9   Marketing Staff: 1   Sales Staff: 1
Ownership: Private
Produces/Sells CE-marked Devices: N
Federal Procurement Eligibility: Small Business
Distribution: Manufacturer Direct, Manufacturer Through Manufacturer Reps, OEM, Exporter
General Admin.: Mr. John Spor/President

Detector, Electrochemical, Chromatography, Liquid	Toxicology
Detector, Ultraviolet	Dental And Oral
Laser, Diode, Laparoscopy	Surgery
Oximeter, Whole Blood	Hematology

TEXFI INDUSTRIES
See Asheboro Elastics Corp.

TEXSTAR TECHNOLOGY INC. 806-748-1184
2306-d 120th St., Lubbock, TX 79423
FDA Number: 3004770593
Ownership: Private
Produces/Sells CE-marked Devices: N

Tray, Impression	Dental And Oral

TFI HEALTHCARE 800-526-0178
600 W. Wythe St., Petersburg, VA 23803
FDA Number: n/a   Fax: 804-861-6664
Web site: www.tfihealthcare.com
Year Founded: 1979
Total Employees: 60
Ownership: Private
Produces/Sells CE-marked Devices: N
Federal Procurement Eligibility: Small Business
Distribution: Manufacturer Through Distributor, Manufacturer Through Manufacturer Reps
General Admin.: Joseph Battiston/President
David Battiston/Vice President

Chair, Bath	General
Commode (Toilet)	General
Commode Seat	General
Rail, Bath	General
Walker, Mechanical	Physical Med

TFX MEDICAL OEM 800-548-6600
50 Plantation Drive, Jaffrey, NH 03452 603-532-7706
FDA Number: 1221019   Fax: 603-532-6108
E-mail: sales@tfx.com
Web site: www.tfx.com
Year Founded: 1981
Ownership: Teleflex Medical
Stock Symbol: TFX
Traded On: NYSE
Quality System Registration Information: ISO9001
Produces/Sells CE-marked Devices: Y
Federal Procurement Eligibility: Small Business
Distribution: OEM
General Admin.: Emily Tinkham/Manager Human Resources
Production: Sue Geikie/Manager Customer Services
Mr. Bob Ginn/Manager Quality Assurance
Lori Connolly/Plant Manager
Finance: Neil Tansey/Chief Financial Officer

Catheter, Angiographic	Cns/Neurology
Catheter, Conduction, Anesthesia	Anesthesiology
Catheter, Epidural	Obstetrics/Gynecology
Catheter, Intravascular, Therapeutic, Short-term Less Than 30 Days	General
Catheter, Other	Gastroenterology/Urology
Catheter, Percutaneous	Cardiovascular
Component, Metal, Other	General
Component, Plastic	General
Dilator, Catheter	Surgery
Dilator, Other	Surgery
Dilator, Vessel, Percutaneous Catheterization	Cardiovascular
Endoscope	Gastroenterology/Urology
Guidewire	Cardiovascular
Guidewire, Catheter	Cardiovascular
Guidewire, Catheter, Radiological	Radiology

TFX MEDICAL OEM 800-548-6600 (cont'd)

Introducer, Catheter	Cardiovascular
Introducer, Syringe Needle	General
Needle, Catheter	Surgery
Needle, Other	General
Surgical Instrument, Cardiovascular	Cardiovascular
Tube, Gastrointestinal	Gastroenterology/Urology
Tubing, Braided	General
Tubing, Conductive	General
Tubing, Flexible, Medical Gas, Low-Pressure	Anesthesiology
Tubing, Fluid Delivery	General
Tubing, Multi-Lumen	General
Tubing, Non-Conductive	General
Tubing, Nylon	General
Tubing, Other	General
Tubing, Plastic	General
Tubing, Polyethylene	General
Tubing, Polypropylene	General
Tubing, Polytetrafluoroethylene	General
Tubing, Radiopaque	General

TG MEDICAL USA INC. 626-969-7838
TG Medical USA Inc., 165 North Aspan Avenue, Azusa, CA 91702
FDA Number: 8043848   Fax: 626-969-7823
E-mail: davidlim@topgloveusa.com
Web site: www.topglove.com.my
Annual Revenue: $10-$25 Million
Year Founded: 1992
Ownership: Private
Quality System Registration Information: ISO9001
Produces/Sells CE-marked Devices: Y
Distribution: Manufacturer Direct, Manufacturer Through Distributor, OEM, Importer
General Admin.: Wilson Lim/Manager
Edwyn Poon/Office Manager
David Lim/President

Glove, Patient Examination	General
Glove, Patient Examination, Latex	General
Glove, Patient Examination, Poly	General
Glove, Surgical	General

TG MEDICAL USA, INC.
See Tg Medical Usa Inc.

THALES / THOMSON COMPONENTS AND TUBES CORP.
See Thales Components Corporation

THALES COMPONENTS CORPORATION 973-812-9000
40G Commerce Way, PO Box 540, Totowa, NJ 07511-0540
FDA Number: 2244774   Fax: 973-812-9050
E-mail: information@thalescomponents-us.com
Web site: www.thalescomponents-us.com
Medical Products Sales Volume: $9,100,000
Year Founded: 1973
Total Employees: 46   Sales Staff: 41
Ownership: Thales Electron Devices
Stock Symbol: TCSFY
Traded On: NASDAQ
Quality System Registration Information: ISO9002; ISO9003
Produces/Sells CE-marked Devices: Y
Federal Procurement Eligibility: Small Business
Distribution: OEM
General Admin.: Stephen Shpock/President, Chief Executive Officer
Mktg./Adv.: Jeff Ohstrom/Manager Contract Sales

Camera, Television, Endoscopic (Without Audio)	Surgery
Camera, X-Ray, Fluorographic, Cine Or Spot	Radiology
Component, Electronic	General
Image Intensification System	Radiology
Imager, X-Ray, Solid State (Flat Panel/Digital)	Radiology
Radiographic Unit, Digital	Radiology
Tube, Image Amplifier, X-Ray	Radiology

THAYER MEDICAL CORP. 520-790-5393
4575 South Palo Verde Rd.,, Suite 337, Tucson, AZ 85714
FDA Number: 2026894

Drain, Tee (Water Trap)	Anesthesiology
Mask, Gas, Anesthesia	Anesthesiology
Mouthpiece, Breathing	Anesthesiology
Nebulizer, Direct Patient Interface	Anesthesiology
Nebulizer, Medicinal	Ear/Nose/Throat
Percussor, Powered	Anesthesiology

THE 50 DEGREE COMPANY 321-956-0050
315 Stan Drive, W. Melbourne, FL 32904
FDA Number: 3006424674

Pack, Hot Or Cold, Reusable	Physical Med

THE AFTER MARKET GROUP 888-824-8200
39400 Taylor Parkway, N. Ridgeville, OH 44039
FDA Number: n/a   Fax: 800-468-0033
Web site: www.aftermarketgroup.com

THE AFTER MARKET GROUP 888-824-8200 *(cont'd)*
Annual Revenue: $1-$5 Million
Ownership: Public
Traded On: NYSE
Produces/Sells CE-marked Devices: N
Federal Procurement Eligibility: Small Business

Accessories, Wheelchair	Physical Med
Attachment, Commode, Wheelchair	Physical Med
Belt, Wheelchair	Physical Med
Board, Foot	Orthopedics
Component, Wheelchair	Physical Med
Cushion, Wheelchair (Pad)	Physical Med
Device, Anti-Tip, Wheelchair	Physical Med
Footrest, Wheelchair	Physical Med
Handrim, Wheelchair	Physical Med
Holder, Crutch and Cane, Wheelchair	Physical Med
Infusion Stand	General
Leg Rest	General
Restraint, Wheelchair	General
Support, Back	Orthopedics
Support, Foot	Orthopedics
Support, Head And Trunk, Wheelchair	Physical Med
Tips And Pads, Cane, Crutch And Walker	Physical Med
Tray, Wheelchair	Physical Med

THE AFTERMARKET GROUP 888-TAG-8200
10173 Croyden Way, Sacramento, CA 95827 440-329-6000
FDA Number: 2950340 Fax: 800-468-0033
Web site: www.aftermarketgroup.com
Year Founded: 1996
Ownership: Invacare Corporation
Stock Symbol: IVC
Traded On: NYSE
Produces/Sells CE-marked Devices: N

Accessories, Wheelchair	Physical Med

THE ALGER COMPANY, INC. 800-320-1043
320 Flightline Rd., Lago Vista, TX 78645
FDA Number: 1625407

Spud, Ophthalmic	Ophthalmology

THE ALIGN-RIGHT PILLOW CO. LTD. 800-331-0907
881 Guelph Street, 519-742-9873
Kitchener, ONTAR N2H 1 Canada
FDA Number: 9616712 Fax: 519-578-7409
E-mail: info@alignright.com
Web site: www.alignright.com
Ownership: Private
Produces/Sells CE-marked Devices: N

THE ALOE INSTITUTE 941-727-0042
5808 42nd Street East, Bradenton, FL 34203
FDA Number: n/a Fax: 941-753-5232
E-mail: catalogjfc@aol.com
Web site: www.thealoeinstitute.org
Medical Products Sales Volume: $3,000,000
Annual Revenue: $1-$5 Million
Year Founded: 1986
Total Employees: 2 *Marketing Staff:* 2
Ownership: Private
Produces/Sells CE-marked Devices: N
Federal Procurement Eligibility: Small Business
Distribution: Manufacturer Direct, Manufacturer Through Distributor, Manufacturer Through Manufacturer Reps, Exporter
General Admin.: Jess F. Clarke/President, Chief Executive Officer
Mktg./Adv.: Chris Sykes/Manager Advertising
      Curtis Clarke/Manager International & National Sales
      Jess F. Clarke/Vice President Marketing

Lotion, Skin Care	General
Lubricant, Patient	General

Medical Product Subsidiaries (Listed Separately)
  Winning Solutions, Inc.

THE AMCOR GROUP LTD. 800-584-6484
685A Gotham Parkway, Carlstadt, NJ 07072-2403
FDA Number: n/a Fax: 201-460-9481
E-mail: management@amcorgroupusa.com
Web site: www.amcorgroupusa.com
Total Employees: 10
Ownership: Amcor Ltd.
Quality System Registration Information: ISO9002
Produces/Sells CE-marked Devices: N
Distribution: Manufacturer Through Distributor, Importer

Counter, Air Ion	General
Generator, Ionized Air	Anesthesiology

THE ANSAR GROUP, INC. 888-883-7804
240 South Eighth St., Philadelphia, PA 19107 215-922-6088
FDA Number: 3000210032 Fax: 215-922-6463

THE ANSAR GROUP, INC. 888-883-7804 *(cont'd)*
E-mail: info@ans-hrv.com
Web site: www.ans-hrv.com
Ownership: Private
Produces/Sells CE-marked Devices: N

Monitor, Cardiac (Cardiotachometer & Rate Alarm)	Cardiovascular

THE ANTHROS MEDICAL GROUP 785-544-6592
807 East Spring, Highland, KS 66035
FDA Number: 1932356

Bed, Manual	General
Cart, Emergency, Cardiopulmonary Resuscitation (Crash)	Anesthesiology
Chair, Adjustable, Mechanical	Physical Med
Walker, Mechanical	Physical Med

THE ARC OTSEGO
See Arc/Otsego

THE ART OF LIVING INSTITUTE 713-621-0366
7815 Fondren Rd., Houston, TX 77074
FDA Number: 3004159419
Ownership: Private
Produces/Sells CE-marked Devices: N

Kit, Enema (For Cleaning Purposes)	Gastroenterology/Urology

THE BIOFEEDBACK INSTITUTE OF LOS 800-246-3526
ANGELES
6542 Hayes Dr., Los Angeles, CA 90048-5320 323-930-8500
FDA Number: 2024687
Web site: www.biocompresearch.org
Year Founded: 1970
Ownership: Private
Produces/Sells CE-marked Devices: N

Biofeedback Device	Cns/Neurology

THE BREMER GROUP CO. 800-428-2304
11243-5 St. Johns Industrial, Pkwy. South, 904-645-0004
Jacksonville, FL 32246
FDA Number: 1062838 Fax: 904-645-0990
E-mail: bremergroup@bremer.net
Web site: www.bremergroup.com
Medical Products Sales Volume: $3,500,000
Year Founded: 1994
Total Employees: 14
Ownership: Private
Produces/Sells CE-marked Devices: N
Federal Procurement Eligibility: Small Business

Orthosis, Thoracic	Physical Med

THE BURROWS CO. 847-537-7300
230 West Palatine Road, Wheeling, IL 60090-0747
FDA Number: n/a Fax: 847-537-7786
Web site: www.burrowsco.com
Medical Products Sales Volume: $100,000,000
Year Founded: 1932
Ownership: Private
Produces/Sells CE-marked Devices: N
Distribution: Exclusive Distributor

Glove, Surgical	General

THE C. D. SPARLING COMPANY 734-455-3121
498 Farmer St, Plymouth, MI 48170-1206
FDA Number: 7000725 Fax: 734-455-7322
E-mail: info@cdsparling.com
Web site: www.cdsparling.com
Medical Products Sales Volume: $600,000
Annual Revenue: $1-$5 Million
Year Founded: 1946
Total Employees: 10 *Sales Staff:* 3
Ownership: Private
Produces/Sells CE-marked Devices: N
Federal Procurement Eligibility: Small Business
Distribution: Manufacturer Through Distributor, Manufacturer Through Manufacturer Reps, OEM
General Admin.: Torb Guenther/President

Rail, Bath	General

THE CARNEGIE TEXTILE CO. 800-633-4136
31100 Solon Road, P.O. Box 14, Solon, OH 44139 440-542-1180
FDA Number: n/a Fax: 440-542-1188
E-mail: info@carnegietextile.com
Web site: www.carnegietextile.com
Medical Products Sales Volume: $1,000,000
Annual Revenue: $1-$5 Million
Year Founded: 1939
Ownership: Private
Produces/Sells CE-marked Devices: N
Federal Procurement Eligibility: Small Business

MANUFACTURER PROFILES

THE CARNEGIE TEXTILE CO.   800-633-4136 *(cont'd)*
Distribution: Exclusive Distributor

Diaper, Pediatric	General
Drape, Surgical	Surgery
Drape, Surgical, Reusable	Surgery
Housekeeping Equipment	General
Legging, Compression, Non-Inflatable	General
Linen	General
Mitt/Washcloth, Patient	General
Service, Engraving	General
Sheet, Drape	Surgery
Towel/Towelette, Paper	General

THE COOPER COMPANIES, INC   925-460-3600
6140 Stoneridge Mall Road, Suite 590, Pleasanton, CA 94588
FDA Number: n/a
Web site: www.coopercos.com
Ownership: Public
Stock Symbol: COO
Traded On: NYSE
Produces/Sells CE-marked Devices: N
General Admin.: Ms. Carol R Kaufman/Chief Administrative Officer
     Mr. Eugene J Midlock/Chief Financial Officer, Senior Vice President
     Mr. Robert S Weiss/President, Chief Executive Officer
     Mr. Albert G White/Vice President
     Mr. Daniel G McBride/Vice President, General Counsel

THE DAAVLIN COMPANY   800-322-8546
205 West Bement Street, PO Box 626,   419-636-6304
Bryan, OH 43506
FDA Number: 1526255
E-mail: sales@daavlin.com   *Fax:* 419-636-1739
Web site: www.daavlin.com
Medical Products Sales Volume: $4,500,000
Annual Revenue: $1-$5 Million
Year Founded: 1981
Total Employees: 29   *Sales Staff:* 3
Ownership: Private
Produces/Sells CE-marked Devices: Y
Federal Procurement Eligibility: Small Business, VA Contract
Distribution: Manufacturer Direct
General Admin.: David Swanson/President, Chief Executive Officer
Mktg./Adv.: Cris McNeal/Director National Accounts
     David Swanson/Manager International & National Sales
Production: Lissa Whitman/Manager Materials
     Mrs. Tracy McKelvey/Manager Operations
     Chad Reynolds/Manager Regulatory Affairs

Lamp, Ultraviolet, Physical Medicine	Physical Med

THE DIAL CORPORATION, A HENKEL COMPANY   480-754-3425
15501 North Dial Boulevard, Scottsdale, AZ 85260
FDA Number: 2085936
Web site: www.henkel.com
Medical Products Sales Volume: $1,500,000,000
Ownership: HENKEL GMBH & CO. KG, CARL
Produces/Sells CE-marked Devices: N
Distribution: Manufacturer Direct, Manufacturer Through Distributor, OEM, Service Direct, Importer, Exporter

Soap	General

THE EARMOLD CO., LTD.   800-798-2198
814 Eighth St., Salem, VA 24153   540-389-1642
FDA Number: 1123452
Ownership: Private
Produces/Sells CE-marked Devices: N

Hearing-Aid	Ear/Nose/Throat

THE ELECTRODE STORE   360-829-0400
Post Office Box 188, Enumclaw, WA 98022
FDA Number: 2022388
E-mail: info@electrodestore.com   *Fax:* 360-829-0402
Web site: www.electrodestore.com
Medical Products Sales Volume: $1,700,000
Annual Revenue: $1-$5 Million
Total Employees: 18
Ownership: Private
Quality System Registration Information: ISO9001
Produces/Sells CE-marked Devices: Y
Federal Procurement Eligibility: Small Business
Distribution: Manufacturer Direct, Manufacturer Through Distributor, OEM, Importer, Exporter
General Admin.: Tim Cooke/Chief Executive Officer
Production: Camille Cooke/Director Operations

Cable/Lead, EMG	Cns/Neurology
Collodion	Pathology
Compressor, Air, Portable	Anesthesiology
Electrode, Biopotential, Surface, Metallic	Physical Med

THE ELECTRODE STORE   360-829-0400 *(cont'd)*

Electrode, Electroencephalographic	Cns/Neurology
Electrode, Electromyographic	Cns/Neurology
Electrode, Needle	Cns/Neurology
Electrode, Needle, Diagnostic Electromyograph	Physical Med
Electrode, Neurological	Cns/Neurology
Needle, Blunt	General
Solvent	Chemistry

THE EVERCARE COMPANY   800-435-6223
3440 Preston Ridge Road, Suite 650,   770-570-5000
Alpharetta, GA 30005
FDA Number: 9200530   *Fax:* 770-570-5001
E-mail: customerservice@evercare.com
Web site: www.evercare.com
Medical Products Sales Volume: $15,600,000
Annual Revenue: $25-$50 Million
Year Founded: 1956
Total Employees: 310   *Marketing Staff:* 10   *Sales Staff:* 7
Ownership: Private
Produces/Sells CE-marked Devices: Y
Federal Procurement Eligibility: Small Business, GSA Contract
Distribution: Manufacturer Direct, Manufacturer Through Distributor, Manufacturer Through Manufacturer Reps, Importer, Exporter
General Admin.: N. D. McKay/Chairman
     Nick Mc Kay/Chief Executive Officer
     Douglas Taeckens/President
Mktg./Adv.: Larry McKay/Manager National Sales
     Larry Moore/Manager National Sales
     Nicholas McKay/Vice President Marketing & Sales
Production: Bryan Bennett/Director Manufacturing

Cleanroom Equipment	General
Kit, Prep	General
Remover, Particulate	Surgery
Strip, Adhesive	Surgery

THE EYE CONCERN, INC.   480-962-5841
1450 S. Dobson Rd., Suite #a-206, Mesa, AZ 85202
FDA Number: 3005147029

Eye, Artificial, Non-Custom	Ophthalmology

THE FEMALE HEALTH CO.   312-595-9123
515 N. State, St. #2225, Chicago, IL 60611
FDA Number: n/a   *Fax:* 312-595-9122
E-mail: info@femalehealth.com
Web site: www.femalehealth.com
Ownership: Public
Stock Symbol: FHCO
Traded On: OTC Bulletin
Quality System Registration Information: ISO9001
Produces/Sells CE-marked Devices: Y
Distribution: Manufacturer Through Distributor
General Admin.: Michael Pope/Vice President, General Manager
Production: Nicholas Twitchen/Manager Quality Assurance

Condom	Obstetrics/Gynecology

THE FOREDOM ELECTRIC CO.   203-792-8622
16 Stony Hill Rd., Bethel, CT 06801
FDA Number: 1217202   *Fax:* 203-796-7861
Web site: www.foredom.net
Ownership: Private
Produces/Sells CE-marked Devices: N

Percussor, Powered	Anesthesiology

THE FREDERICKS COMPANY   215-947-2500
2400 Philmont Ave., Huntingdon Valley, PA 19006-0067
FDA Number: n/a   *Fax:* 215-947-7464
E-mail: sjablonski@frederickscom.com
Web site: www.fredericks.com
Medical Products Sales Volume: $1,000,000
Annual Revenue: $0-$1 Million
Year Founded: 1938
Total Employees: 115   *Sales Staff:* 10
Ownership: Private
Quality System Registration Information: ISO9001
Produces/Sells CE-marked Devices: N
Distribution: Manufacturer Direct

Ampule	Gastroenterology/Urology
Transducer, Force	General

THE GILLETTE COMPANY   617-421-7000
800 Boylston St., Prudential Tower Bldg. Fl.45,
Boston, MA 02199
FDA Number: 1216894
Ownership: Private
Produces/Sells CE-marked Devices: N

Irrigator, Oral	Dental And Oral

THE GILLETTE COMPANY   617-421-7000 *(cont'd)*
Toothbrush, Powered   Dental And Oral

THE GOTZEN GROUP, INC.   905-607-1494
7-3505 Laird Rd, Mississauga L5L 5Y7 Canada
FDA Number: 9615032
Radiographic Unit, Diagnostic, Intraoral   Dental And Oral

THE HEARING AID FACTORY, INC.   407-649-9696
710 West Colonial Dr., #101, Orlando, FL 32804
FDA Number: 1058001
Ownership: Private
Produces/Sells CE-marked Devices: N
    Hearing-Aid   Ear/Nose/Throat

THE HILLIARD CORPORATION   607-733-7121
100 West. 4th Street, Elmira, NY 14902
FDA Number: n/a   *Fax:* 607-737-1108
E-mail: hilliard@hilliardcorp.com
Web site: www.hilliardcorp.com
Medical Products Sales Volume: $63,700,000
Year Founded: 1905
Total Employees: 372   *Marketing Staff:* 3
Ownership: Private
Produces/Sells CE-marked Devices: N
Federal Procurement Eligibility: Small Business
Distribution: Manufacturer Through Distributor, Manufacturer Through
Manufacturer Reps
Mktg./Adv.: Greg Bickham/Manager Regional Sales
    Filter Paper   Chemistry
    Filter, Bacteriological, Laboratory   Chemistry

THE HORIZON PHOENIX GROUP LIMITED   800-718-8218
3219 Yonge St., Ste. 248,   416-347-2565
Toronto, ONT M4N-3 Canada
FDA Number: n/a   *Fax:* 416-347-4313
E-mail: timd@horizonphoenix.com
Web site: www.horizonphoenix.biz
Year Founded: 1994
Total Employees: 50
Ownership: Private
Produces/Sells CE-marked Devices: N

THE HORTON CO.
See Horton Emergency Vehicles

THE HYGENIC CORP.   800-321-2135
1245 Home Avenue, Akron, OH 44310-2575
FDA Number: 1519375   *Fax:* 330-633-9359
E-mail: feedback@hygenic.com
Web site: www.hygenic.com
Medical Products Sales Volume: $20,300,000
Year Founded: 1930
Total Employees: 125
Ownership: Private
Quality System Registration Information: ISO9001
Produces/Sells CE-marked Devices: Y
Federal Procurement Eligibility: Small Business
Distribution: Manufacturer Direct, Manufacturer Through Distributor, Manufacturer
Through Manufacturer Reps, OEM, Importer
General Admin.: Mr. Stewart Lorenzen/President, Chief Executive Officer
Mktg./Adv.: Mr. Herm Rottinghaus/Vice President Marketing & Sales
    Mr. John Vatalaro/Vice President Sales
Production: Mr. Ralph Buster/Director Quality Assurance & Regulatory Affairs
    Mr. Earl DeCarli/Executive Vice President, Chief Operating Officer
Production
Research: Mr. Jeff Sullivan/Vice President Research & Development
Finance: Mr. Kurt Marhoefer/Chief Financial Officer
    Mr. Niels Lichti/Vice President Finance, Controller
    Bag, Leg   Gastroenterology/Urology
    Band, Elastic, Orthodontic   Dental And Oral
    Bath, Paraffin   Physical Med
    Component, Exercise   Physical Med
    Dam, Rubber   Dental And Oral
    Exerciser, Non-Measuring   Physical Med
    Tourniquet, Non-Pneumatic, Surgical   Surgery
    Tubing, Non-Invasive   Surgery
    Wax, Dental   Dental And Oral
    Wrap, Sterilization   General

THE HYMED GROUP CORP.   610-865-9876
1890 Bucknell Dr., Bethlehem, PA 18015
FDA Number: 2530949   *Fax:* 610-691-5930
E-mail: hymed@hymed.com
Web site: www.hymed.com
Year Founded: 1995
Ownership: Private
Quality System Registration Information: ISO9001
Produces/Sells CE-marked Devices: N

THE HYMED GROUP CORP.   610-865-9876 *(cont'd)*
Federal Procurement Eligibility: Small Business
Distribution: Manufacturer Through Distributor
Mktg./Adv.: Anita M. Petito/Vice President Business Development
    Bottle, Medicine Spray   General
    Dressing, Other   General
    Dressing, Periodontal   Dental And Oral
    Dressing, Wound and Burn, Hydrogel   Surgery
    Dressing, Wound and Burn, Occlusive   Surgery
    Dropper, Eye   Ophthalmology
    Solution, Antibacterial Cleaner   General

THE JUDGE ROTENBERG EDUCATIONAL   781-828-2202
CENTER, INC.
240 Turnpike St., Canton, MA 02021-2341
FDA Number: 1222743   *Fax:* 781-828-2804
E-mail: j.gomes@judgerc.org
Web site: www.judgerc.org
Medical Products Sales Volume: $56,900,000
Year Founded: 1971
Total Employees: 300
Ownership: Private
Produces/Sells CE-marked Devices: N
Federal Procurement Eligibility: Small Business
Distribution: Manufacturer Direct
    Device, Conditioning, Aversion   Cns/Neurology

THE KAHN COMPANIES   860-529-8643
885 Wells Road, Wethersfield, CT 06109
FDA Number: 7000566   *Fax:* 860-529-1895
E-mail: info@kahn.com
Web site: www.kahn.com
Medical Products Sales Volume: $700,000
Annual Revenue: $5-$10 Million
Year Founded: 1945
Total Employees: 26
Ownership: Private
Quality System Registration Information: ISO9001
Produces/Sells CE-marked Devices: Y
Federal Procurement Eligibility: Small Business
Distribution: Manufacturer Direct, Manufacturer Through Manufacturer Reps, OEM,
Importer, Exporter
General Admin.: Jeffrey Kahn/President, Chief Executive Officer
    David Kahn/Vice President
Mktg./Adv.: David A. Kahn/Director Marketing
Production: Baldwin Levy/Manager Production
    John W. Sutcliffe, III/Manager Quality Control
    Robert T. Bailey/Product Manager
    Equipment, Filtering, Air, ETO   General
    Hygrometer (Humidity Indicator)   Anesthesiology

THE KENDAL CO.
See Covidien Lp, Formerly Registered As Kendall

THE KENDALL COMPANY
See Covidien Lp, Formerly Registered As Kendall

THE KENDRICK CO., INC.   800-523-0178
6139 Germantown Ave., Philadelphia, PA 19144   215-438-1122
FDA Number: 2515123   *Fax:* 215-438-8065
Web site: www.thekendrickcompany.com
Ownership: Private
Produces/Sells CE-marked Devices: N
    Stocking, Elastic   General
    Truss, Umbilical   Gastroenterology/Urology

THE KIPPGROUP
See Medegen

THE LAGADO CORP.   303-789-0933
2890 South Tejon St., Englewood, CO 80110
FDA Number: 1719531
    Lens, Contact (Other Material)   Ophthalmology
    Lens, Contact, Polymethylmethacrylate   Ophthalmology

THE LIFESTYLE CO. INC.   800-622-0777
1800 Route 34 North, Suite 401,   732-972-8585
Wall Township, NJ 07719
FDA Number: 2249258   *Fax:* 732-972-9205
E-mail: lenses@lifestylecompany.com
Web site: www.lifestylecompany.com
Medical Products Sales Volume: $1,200,000
Annual Revenue: $1-$5 Million
Year Founded: 1995
Total Employees: 4
Ownership: Private
Produces/Sells CE-marked Devices: N
Federal Procurement Eligibility: Small Business
Distribution: Manufacturer Direct, Manufacturer Through Distributor, Exporter
General Admin.: Tom Seidner/President, Chief Executive Officer

THE LIFESTYLE CO. INC.
800-622-0777 *(cont'd)*

Production: Emma Hudson/Director Services
Dan Cyriacks/Product Manager
Research: Dr. Martin R. Riehm/Director Research

Accessories, Solution, Lens, Contact	Ophthalmology
Cleaner, Lens, Contact	Ophthalmology
Lens, Other	Ophthalmology
Resin, Plastic	General

THE LIFESTYLE GP COMPANY, L.L.C.
888-379-6645

2530 Trailmate Dr., Sarasota, FL 34243
FDA Number: 3004719382
Ownership: Private
Produces/Sells CE-marked Devices: N

Lens, Contact (Other Material)	Ophthalmology

THE LUDLOW COMPANY LP

See Covidien Lp, Formerly Registered As Ludlow

THE LYONS COMPANIES
502-267-0087

11401 Electron Dr., Louisville, KY 40299-3857
FDA Number: n/a   *Fax:* 502-267-8464
Web site: www.lyons-companies.com
Annual Revenue: $5-$10 Million
Year Founded: 1952
Ownership: Private
Produces/Sells CE-marked Devices: N
Federal Procurement Eligibility: Small Business
Distribution: Manufacturer Through Distributor, Manufacturer Through Manufacturer Reps, OEM

Mount, Monitor (Support)	General
Radiographic Unit, Diagnostic, Chest	Radiology
Shield, X-Ray	Radiology

THE MASON BOX COMPANY
800-225-2708
508-695-9381

521 Mt. Hope St., PO Box 129,
N. Attleboro, MA 02761
FDA Number: n/a   *Fax:* 508-695-3210
E-mail: sales@masonbox.com
Web site: www.masonbox.com
Medical Products Sales Volume: $7,100,000
Year Founded: 1891
Total Employees: 100
Ownership: Private
Quality System Registration Information: ISO9002
Produces/Sells CE-marked Devices: N
Federal Procurement Eligibility: Small Business
Distribution: Manufacturer Direct, Service Direct

Box, Transportation, Container, Specimen	General

THE MEDIPATTERN CORPORATION
416-744-0009

3080 Yonge St., Suite 4070, Toronto, ON M4N 3N1 Canada
FDA Number: 3005311473   *Fax:* 416-744-6899
E-mail: sales@medipattern.com
Web site: www.medipattern.com
Year Founded: 1999
Ownership: Public
Stock Symbol: MKI
Traded On: TSX Venture Exchange
Produces/Sells CE-marked Devices: N

THE METRIX CO.
800-752-3148
563-556-8800

4400 Chavenelle Road, Dubuque, IA 52002-2655
FDA Number: 1937141   *Fax:* 563-556-4704
E-mail: info@metrixco.com
Web site: www.metrixco.com
Medical Products Sales Volume: $9,200,000
Annual Revenue: $10-$25 Million
Year Founded: 1964
Total Employees: 100   *Marketing Staff:* 1   *Sales Staff:* 3
Ownership: Private
Quality System Registration Information: ISO9001
Produces/Sells CE-marked Devices: N
Federal Procurement Eligibility: Small Business
Distribution: Manufacturer Through Distributor, OEM
General Admin.: John Schoen/Chief Executive Officer
Karen Smith/Manager Human Resources
Donnelle Fuerste/President
Mktg./Adv.: Dave Wagner/Manager Sales
Mike FitzPatrick/Manager Sales
Production: Shari Johnson/Manager Materials
Jeff Gensler/Manager Quality Control
Dave Jacobs/Project Engineer
Jim Oldham/Project Engineer
Purchasing: Mr. Dan Schoen/Purchasing Agent

Bag, Blood	Hematology
Bag, Blood, Collection	Hematology
Bottle, Collection, Vacuum (Aspirator)	General
Bottle, Evacuated	General

THE METRIX CO.
800-752-3148 *(cont'd)*

Container, Evacuated	General
Container, IV	General
Contract Manufacturing	General
Filter, Intravenous Tubing	General
Kit, Administration, Blood	General
Kit, Blood Donor	Hematology
Serum, Animal	Pathology
Serum, Biological, General	Toxicology
Transfer Unit, Blood	Hematology
Tubing, Fluid Delivery	General

THE MICROOPTICAL CORPORATION
781-326-8111

33 Southwest Park, Westwood, MA 02090
FDA Number: 3003066842
Ownership: Private
Produces/Sells CE-marked Devices: N

Laparoscope, General & Plastic Surgery	Surgery

THE MYO TOOL CO.
530-272-7306

1020-d Mccourtney Road, Grass Valley, CA 95949
FDA Number: 3005738169
E-mail: info@myotool.com
Web site: www.myotool.com
Ownership: Private
Produces/Sells CE-marked Devices: N

Massager, Therapeutic, Manual	Physical Med

THE NATIONAL IMPLANT REGISTRY

See Medicalert Foundation International

THE NATIONAL WHEEL-O-VATOR CO., INC.
800-551-9095
309-923-2611

509 W. Front St., Roanoke, IL 61561-0348
FDA Number: 1422384   *Fax:* 309-923-5091
E-mail: sales@wheelovator.com
Web site: www.wheelovator.com
Medical Products Sales Volume: $25,000,000
Annual Revenue: $5-$10 Million
Year Founded: 1982
Total Employees: 125
Ownership: Private
Produces/Sells CE-marked Devices: N
Federal Procurement Eligibility: Small Business, GSA Contract, VA Contract
Distribution: Manufacturer Through Distributor, Importer, Exporter
General Admin.: Gregory L. Harmon/President
Mktg./Adv.: Kevin Brinkman/Director Product Development

Elevator, Wheelchair	Physical Med
Lift, Patient	General
Lift, Wheelchair	General

THE NEUROLOGICAL RESEARCH AND DEVELOPMENT GROUP
800-327-6759

115 Rotary Drive, West Hazleton, PA 18202
570-501-7713
FDA Number: 7000672   *Fax:* 570-501-3734
E-mail: sales@neuropedic.com
Web site: www.neuropedic.com
Medical Products Sales Volume: $2,700,000
Annual Revenue: $1-$5 Million
Year Founded: 1972
Total Employees: 19   *Marketing Staff:* 2   *Sales Staff:* 6
Ownership: Private
Produces/Sells CE-marked Devices: N
Federal Procurement Eligibility: Small Business, GSA Contract
Distribution: Manufacturer Direct, Manufacturer Through Distributor, Manufacturer Through Manufacturer Reps
General Admin.: Antonio Nunez/President
Mktg./Adv.: Douglas B Phillips/Manager National Sales
Douglas B Phillips/Vice President Marketing & Sales

Bed, Electric	General
Cover, Mattress, Waterproof	General
Mattress, Bed	General
Mattress, Reduction, Pressure	General
Pillow	General

THE NEWMAN GROUP, LLC
847-283-9177

42 Sherwood Terrace, Suite 2, Lake Bluff, IL 60044
FDA Number: 3006265099

Monitor, Fetal, Ultrasonic	Obstetrics/Gynecology
Transducer, Ultrasonic, Diagnostic	Radiology

THE OPTICAL SHOP
405-514-0903

1111 S. Eastern Ave., Oklahoma City, OK 73129
FDA Number: 3004080824
Ownership: Private
Produces/Sells CE-marked Devices: N

Frame, Spectacle (Eyeglasses)	Ophthalmology
Lens, Spectacle/Eyeglasses, Non-Custom	Ophthalmology

THE ORTHOTIC GROUP, INC.
800-551-3008
905-477-8511
160 Markland Street,
Markham, ONT L6C 0 Canada
FDA Number: n/a
Fax: 905-946-8100
Year Founded: 1985
Total Employees: 10
Ownership: Private
Produces/Sells CE-marked Devices: N
Distribution: Manufacturer Direct, Exporter

THE ORVIS CO., INC.
802-362-3622
P. O. Box 798, Manchester, VT 05254
FDA Number: 1291645
E-mail: customerservice@orvis.com
Ownership: Private
Produces/Sells CE-marked Devices: N
Sunglasses (Including Photosensitive) — Ophthalmology

THE PANDAH CO.
336-993-4579
408 Drayton Park, Kernersville, NC 27284
FDA Number: 1061026
Electrode, Electrocardiograph — Cardiovascular

THE PERISTAT GROUP, INC.
714-928-8507
3721 Fillmore St, San Francisco, CA 94123
FDA Number: 2032872
Ownership: Private
Produces/Sells CE-marked Devices: N
Grid, Amsler — Ophthalmology
Perimeter, Automatic, AC-Powered — Ophthalmology

THE PETTIBON SYSTEM
888-774-6258
(888) 774-6258
3214 50th St CT, Suite 102C,
Gig Harbor, WA 98335
FDA Number: 3005033444
Fax: 800-738-4266
Web site: www.pettibonsystem.com
Year Founded: 1987
Ownership: Private
Produces/Sells CE-marked Devices: N
Component, Exercise — Physical Med
Exerciser, Non-Measuring — Physical Med
Massager, Therapeutic — Physical Med
Traction Unit, Non-Powered — Orthopedics
Vibrator, Therapeutic — Physical Med

THE PHANTOM LABORATORY, INC.
800-525-1190
518-692-1190
PO Box 511, Salem, NY 12865-0511
FDA Number: 1320150
Fax: 518-692-3329
E-mail: info@phantomlab.com
Web site: www.phantomlab.com
Medical Products Sales Volume: $750,000
Year Founded: 1989
Total Employees: 9
Ownership: Private
Quality System Registration Information: ISO9001
Produces/Sells CE-marked Devices: Y
Federal Procurement Eligibility: Small Business
General Admin.: Joshua Levy/President
Accelerator, Linear, Medical — Radiology
Phantom, Anthropomorphic, Radiographic — Radiology
Test Pattern, Radiographic — Radiology

THE PROMETHEUS GROUP
603-749-0733
1 Washington St., Suite 303, Dover, NH 03820
FDA Number: 1224842
Biofeedback Device — Cns/Neurology
Perineometer — Obstetrics/Gynecology
Stimulator, Incontinence (Non-Implantable), Electrical — Gastroenterology/Urology
Uroflowmeter — Gastroenterology/Urology

THE QUALITY ASSURANCE SERVICE CORP.
706-863-6536
310 Commerce Dr., Martinez, GA 30907
FDA Number: 1032263
Control, Drug Mixture — Toxicology

THE REESE PHARMACEUTICAL CO.
800-321-7178
216-231-6441
10617 Frank Ave., Cleveland, OH 44106
FDA Number: 1518939
Fax: 216-231-6444
E-mail: reese@apk.net
Web site: www.reesechemical.com
Year Founded: 1907
Ownership: Private
Produces/Sells CE-marked Devices: N
Bandage, Elastic — General
Kit, Pregnancy Test, Over The Counter, HCG — General Chemistry

THE REGENTS OF THE UNIVERSITY OF MICHIGAN
734-615-8433
3003 S. State, Rm 1072, Ann Arbor, MI 48109-1274
FDA Number: 1836318
Ownership: Private
Produces/Sells CE-marked Devices: N
Scanner, Emission Computed Tomography — Radiology

THE RENAISSANCE CO.
480-969-1731
708 South Drew St., Mesa, AZ 85201
FDA Number: 2032837
Ownership: Private
Produces/Sells CE-marked Devices: N
Orthosis, Lumbosacral — Physical Med

THE RESPIRATORY GROUP
314-659-4311
4150 Carr Lane, St. Louis, MO 63119
FDA Number: 1937613
Conserver, Oxygen — Anesthesiology
Nebulizer, Direct Patient Interface — Anesthesiology
Regulator, Pressure, Gas Cylinder — Anesthesiology

THE RICHMOND LIGHT CO.
888-276-0559
804-276-0559
2301 Falkirk Drive, Richmond, VA 23236
FDA Number: 1120522
Fax: 804-276-5378
E-mail: trlc@trlc.com
Web site: www.trlc.com
Medical Products Sales Volume: $400,000
Year Founded: 1979
Total Employees: 5
Ownership: Private
Produces/Sells CE-marked Devices: N
Federal Procurement Eligibility: Small Business, VA Contract
Distribution: Manufacturer Direct
Light, Ultraviolet, Dermatologic — Surgery

THE ROHO GROUP
See Roho Group, The

THE SAUNDERS GROUP
800-445-9836
952-368-9214
4250 Norex Drive, Chaska, MN 55318-3047
FDA Number: 2184030
Fax: 952-368-9249
E-mail: sales1@thesaundersgroup.com
Web site: www.thesaundersgroup.com
Medical Products Sales Volume: $16,200,000
Year Founded: 1982
Total Employees: 30
Ownership: Private
Produces/Sells CE-marked Devices: Y
Federal Procurement Eligibility: Small Business
Distribution: Manufacturer Through Distributor
Accessories, Traction — Physical Med
Band, Support, Pelvic — Physical Med
Component, Traction, Non-Invasive — Orthopedics
Exerciser, Non-Measuring — Physical Med
Goniometer, Non-Powered — Orthopedics
Halter, Head, Traction, Orthopedic — Orthopedics
Orthosis, Cervical — Physical Med
Orthosis, Cervical-Thoracic, Rigid — Physical Med
Orthosis, Limb Brace — Physical Med
Orthosis, Lumbar — Physical Med
Orthosis, Lumbosacral — Physical Med
Orthosis, Thoracic — Physical Med
Pack, Hot Or Cold, Reusable — Physical Med
Strap, Head, Gas Mask — Anesthesiology
Support, Patient Position — Anesthesiology
Traction Unit, Non-Powered — Orthopedics

THE SCALE SHOP LTD.
888-844-2031
709-747-2031
86 Clyde Ave., Mount Peal, NF A1N-4S2 Canada
FDA Number: n/a
Fax: 709-747-1338
E-mail: wayne@scaleshop.nf.net
Year Founded: 1985
Total Employees: 10
Ownership: Private
Produces/Sells CE-marked Devices: N
Distribution: Manufacturer Direct

THE SEWING SOURCE, INC.
800-849-6945
252-478-3900
802 East Nash St., Spring Hope, NC 27882
FDA Number: 1038209
Fax: 252-478-4728
Ownership: Private
Produces/Sells CE-marked Devices: N
Drape, Surgical, ENT — Ear/Nose/Throat
Dress, Surgical — Surgery
Gown, Examination — General
Gown, Isolation, Surgical — Surgery
Gown, Patient — Surgery
Gown, Surgical — Surgery

THE SEWING SOURCE, INC. 800-849-6945 *(cont'd)*
Pack, Sterilization Wrapper (Bag And Accessories) Surgery
Sudan IV Pathology
Suit, Surgical Surgery

THE SMARTPILL CORPORATION 800-644-4162
847 Main Street, Buffalo, NY 14203-1109 716-882-0701
FDA Number: 1320877 *Fax:* 716-882-0706
E-mail: info@smartpillcorp.com
Web site: www.smartpillcorp.com
Medical Products Sales Volume: $3,000,000
Annual Revenue: $0-$1 Million
Year Founded: 2005
Total Employees: 27 *Marketing Staff:* 2
Ownership: Private
Stock Symbol: NGNM
Traded On: NASDAQ
Produces/Sells CE-marked Devices: N
Federal Procurement Eligibility: Small Business
Distribution: Exclusive Distributor
General Admin.: David Barthel/President, Chief Executive Officer
Mktg./Adv.: Jack Semler/Director Product Development
Production: Chuck Currie/Product Manager
Research: Jack Semler/Vice President Research & Development
Controller, Infusion, Intravenous Cardiovascular

THE SOULE CO., INC. 813-907-6000
4322 Pet Ln., Lutz, FL 33559
FDA Number: 1059079
Accelerator, Linear, Medical Radiology

THE STEADY-ARM COMPANY, INC. 570-358-3632
Rr 1 Box 353, Ulster, PA 18850-9513
FDA Number: 2532058
Ownership: Private
Produces/Sells CE-marked Devices: N
Adaptor, Recreational Physical Med

THE STEVENS COMPANY LTD. 800-268-0184
425 Railside Drive, 905-791-8600
Brampton, ONT L7A 0 Canada
FDA Number: n/a *Fax:* 905-791-6143
E-mail: rachadala@stevens.ca
Web site: www.stevens.ca
Year Founded: 1874
Total Employees: 250
Ownership: Private
Produces/Sells CE-marked Devices: N
Distribution: Exclusive Distributor

THE SYNAPTIC CORP. 800-685-7246
3176 S. Peoria St., Ste. 110, Aurora, CO 80014 303-696-6325
FDA Number: 1722014 *Fax:* 303-696-7396
E-mail: info@synapticusa.com
Web site: www.synapticusa.com
Ownership: Private
Produces/Sells CE-marked Devices: N
Stimulator, Nerve, Transcutaneous (Pain Relief, TENS) Cns/Neurology

THE TECH GROUP
See The Tech Group

THE TECH GROUP TEMPE 480-281-4400
640 South Rockford Dr., Tempe, AZ 85281
FDA Number: n/a *Fax:* 480-281-4401
E-mail: www.techgroup.com
Web site: www.techgroup.com
Ownership: West Pharmaceutical Services, Inc.
Stock Symbol: WST
Traded On: NYSE
Produces/Sells CE-marked Devices: N
General Admin.: David Moffitt/Managing Director
Robert S. Hargesheimer/President
Mktg./Adv.: Shari Krusniak/Market Manager
Production: Mike Treadaway/Vice President Operations
Autotransfusion Unit (Blood) Anesthesiology
Inhaler, Nasal Ear/Nose/Throat

THE TRI W-G GROUP
See Tri W-G Group

THE UNIVERSAL HANDICYCLE WHEELCHAIR 604-595-8632
2214 Belmont Ave, Victoria V8R 3Z8 Canada
FDA Number: 9681500
Wheelchair, Manual Physical Med

THEKEN ORTHOPEDIC LLC 330-753-9923
1100 Nola Avenue, Barberton, OH 44203
FDA Number: n/a *Fax:* 330-753-9925
E-mail: info@thekenorthopaedic.com

THEKEN ORTHOPEDIC LLC 330-753-9923 *(cont'd)*
Web site: www.thekenortho.com
Year Founded: 1992
Ownership: Private
Produces/Sells CE-marked Devices: N
Fixation Device, Spinal (External) Orthopedics

THEKEN SPINE LLC 1-866-942-8698
1153 Medina Road, Medina, OH 44256
FDA Number: 3008657535 *Fax:* 1-877-558-6227
E-mail: spine.info@integralife.com
Web site: www.thekenspine.com
Year Founded: 1998
Ownership: Private
Produces/Sells CE-marked Devices: N
Appliance, Fixation, Spinal Interlaminal Orthopedics
Appliance, Fixation, Spinal Intervertebral Body Orthopedics
Device, Spinal Vertebral Body Replacement Orthopedics
Orthosis, Fixation, Pedicle, Spinal Orthopedics
Orthosis, Fixation, Spinal, Spondylolisthesis Orthopedics
Orthosis, Fusion, Intervertebral, Spinal Orthopedics
Prosthesis, Hip, Cement Restrictor Orthopedics
Screw, Fixation, Bone Orthopedics

THEKEN SPINE, LLC 1-866-942-8698
1153 Medina Road, Medina, OH 44256
FDA Number: 1530901 *Fax:* 877-558-6227
E-mail: info@thekenspine.com
Web site: www.thekenspine.com
Ownership: THEKEN SPINE LLC
Produces/Sells CE-marked Devices: N
Appliance, Fixation, Spinal Intervertebral Body Orthopedics
Device, Spinal Vertebral Body Replacement Orthopedics
Intervertebral Fusion Device With Bone Graft, Cervical Orthopedics
Orthosis, Fixation, Pedicle, Spinal Orthopedics
Prosthesis, Hip, Cement Restrictor Orthopedics

THEKEN SURGICAL,LLC
See Theken Spine, Llc

THER OX, INC. 949-757-1999
17500 Cartwright Rd.,, Suite 100, Irvine, CA 92612
FDA Number: n/a *Fax:* 949-757-1989
E-mail: info@therox.com
Web site: www.therox.com
Annual Revenue: $0-$1 Million
Total Employees: 380 *Marketing Staff:* 2 *Sales Staff:* 3
Ownership: Private
Quality System Registration Information: ISO9000; ISO9001; ISO9002
Produces/Sells CE-marked Devices: Y
Distribution: Exclusive Distributor
General Admin.: Paul Zalesky/Chief Operating Officer
Production: Greg Watson/Vice President Manufacturing
Linda D'abatz/Vice President Regulatory Affairs
Research: Bill Peterson/Senior Director Research & Development
Regulator, Oxygen, Mechanical General

THERA-KINETICS
See JACE SYSTEMS, INC

THERA-P-CUSHION 800-567-9926
46 Dufflaw Road, 9056607431
Toronto, ONT M6A 2 Canada
FDA Number: n/a *Fax:* 416-782-7993
E-mail: info@therapyproducts.com
Web site: www.therapyproducts.com
Year Founded: 1987
Total Employees: 10
Ownership: Private
Produces/Sells CE-marked Devices: N
Distribution: Manufacturer Direct, Exporter

THERA-TRONICS, INC. 800-267-6211
623 Mamaroneck Avenue, 613-592-3400
Mamaroneck, NY 10543
FDA Number: 2436016 *Fax:* 914-698-1790
E-mail: TheraTronics@aol.com
Web site: www.theratronics.com
Medical Products Sales Volume: $900,000
Annual Revenue: $1-$5 Million
Year Founded: 1946
Total Employees: 10 *Marketing Staff:* 1 *Sales Staff:* 4
Ownership: Private
Produces/Sells CE-marked Devices: N
Federal Procurement Eligibility: Small Business, Female Owned
Distribution: Service Direct, Exclusive Distributor
General Admin.: Neil H. Dublet/Chief Executive Officer
Mktg./Adv.: Lorraine Dublet/Manager Marketing
Bath, Hydro-Massage (Whirlpool) Physical Med

THERA-TRONICS, INC.   800-267-6211 *(cont'd)*

Component, Exercise	Physical Med
Diathermy, Ultrasonic (Physical Therapy)	Physical Med
Equipment, Therapy, Handicapped/Physical	Physical Med
Exercise Stair	Physical Med
Exerciser, Bicycle	Physical Med
Pack, Hot Or Cold, Reusable	Physical Med
Stimulator, Muscle, Electrical-Powered (EMS)	Physical Med
Stimulator, Nerve, Transcutaneous (Pain Relief, TENS)	Cns/Neurology
Table, Mechanical	Physical Med
Table, Other	General
Traction Unit, Static, Other	Orthopedics
Treadmill, Powered	Physical Med

THERADYNE PRODUCTS DIVISION   800-328-4014
395 Ervin Industrial Drive,   763-502-6190
Jordan, MN 55352
FDA Number: 2126669
E-mail: tonyp@kurt.com   *Fax:* 952-492-3443
Web site: www.theradyne.com
Annual Revenue: $1-$5 Million
Year Founded: 1963
Total Employees: 450
Ownership: KURT MANUFACTURING CO.
Produces/Sells CE-marked Devices: N
Federal Procurement Eligibility: Small Business
Distribution: Manufacturer Direct, Manufacturer Through Distributor, Importer, Exporter
General Admin.: Bill Kuban/President, Chief Executive Officer
        Kern Walker/Vice President Human Resources
        Roger DeLacey/Vice President, General Manager
Mktg./Adv.: Jeff Thaves/Division Manager

Accessories, Wheelchair	Physical Med
Wheelchair, Manual	Physical Med
Wheelchair, Powered	Physical Med
Wheelchair, Standup	Physical Med

THERAFIN CORPORATION   800-843-7234
19747 Wolf Rd., Mokena, IL 60448-0848   708-479-7300
FDA Number: n/a   *Fax:* 708-479-1515
Medical Products Sales Volume: $1,400,000
Annual Revenue: $1-$5 Million
Total Employees: 16   *Marketing Staff:* 2   *Sales Staff:* 2
Ownership: Private
Produces/Sells CE-marked Devices: N
Federal Procurement Eligibility: Small Business
Distribution: Manufacturer Direct, Manufacturer Through Distributor, OEM, Exclusive Distributor
General Admin.: Julie Fink/General Manager
        Gilbert L. Fink/President
Mktg./Adv.: Jim Dyes/Manager Sales
IS: Todd Fink/Systems Engineer

Accessories, Wheelchair	Physical Med
Adapter, Hygiene	Physical Med
Adaptor, Dressing	Physical Med
Adaptor, Grooming	Physical Med
Adaptor, Recreational	Physical Med
Armboard, Wheelchair	Physical Med
Armrest, Wheelchair	Physical Med
Band, Support, Pelvic	Physical Med
Board, Scooter, Prone	Physical Med
Chair, Seat Lifting (Standing Aid)	General
Communication System, Non-Powered	Physical Med
Component, Exercise	Physical Med
Cushion, Wheelchair (Pad)	Physical Med
Exerciser, Non-Measuring	Physical Med
Holder, Crutch and Cane, Wheelchair	Physical Med
Reacher (Handicapped)	General
Service, Parts, Repair	General
Telephone, Handicapped Use	Physical Med
Transfer Aid	Physical Med
Transfer Device, Patient, Manual	General
Tray, Wheelchair	Physical Med
Utensil, Food	Physical Med
Utensil, Handicapped Aid	Physical Med
Walker, Mechanical	Physical Med
Wheelchair, Powered	Physical Med

THERAFIN CORPORATION   800-843-7234
19747 Wolf Rd., Mokena, IL 60448
FDA Number: 3003760853

Accessories, Wheelchair	Physical Med
Adapter, Hygiene	Physical Med
Adaptor, Dressing	Physical Med
Adaptor, Grooming	Physical Med
Adaptor, Recreational	Physical Med
Applier, Pressure, Physical Medicine	Physical Med
Armboard, Wheelchair	Physical Med
Band, Support, Pelvic	Physical Med
Board, Scooter, Prone	Physical Med

THERAFIN CORPORATION   800-843-7234 *(cont'd)*

Component, Exercise	Physical Med
Cushion, Wheelchair (Pad)	Physical Med
Exerciser, Non-Measuring	Physical Med
Holder, Crutch and Cane, Wheelchair	Physical Med
Support, Head And Trunk, Wheelchair	Physical Med
Transfer Aid	Physical Med
Tray, Wheelchair	Physical Med
Utensil, Food	Physical Med
Utensil, Handicapped Aid	Physical Med
Walker, Mechanical	Physical Med

THERAFIRM, A KNIT RITE COMPANY   800-562-2701
120 Osage Avenue, Kansas City, KS 66105   913-281-4600
FDA Number: 1064876   *Fax:* 913-281-5455
E-mail: customerservice@knitrite.com
Web site: www.therafirm.com
Annual Revenue: $5-$10 Million
Year Founded: 1950
Total Employees: 55   *Marketing Staff:* 3   *Sales Staff:* 21
Ownership: KNIT RITE, INC.
Produces/Sells CE-marked Devices: Y
Federal Procurement Eligibility: Small Business, VA Contract
Distribution: Manufacturer Direct, Manufacturer Through Distributor, Manufacturer Through Manufacturer Reps, OEM, Exporter
General Admin.: Ron Hercules/Chief Operating Officer, Vice President
        Ms. Lisa Trussell/Manager Human Resources
        Perry Bacon/President, Chief Executive Officer
Mktg./Adv.: Ron Hercules/Manager International & National Sales
Production: Judy Saunders/Director Quality Assurance
        James Ray/Vice President Manufacturing
Research: Robert Ward/Director Research & Development

Brace, Joint, Ankle (External)	Physical Med
Joint, Knee, External Brace	Physical Med
Stocking, Support (Anti-Embolic)	General
Support, Wrist	Physical Med

THERAGENICS CORP.   770-271-0233
5203 Bristol Industrial Way, Buford, GA 30518
FDA Number: 1037598   *Fax:* 770-831-4369
Web site: www.theragenics.com
Medical Products Sales Volume: $38,000,000
Annual Revenue: $25-$50 Million
Year Founded: 1981
Total Employees: 161   *Marketing Staff:* 2   *Sales Staff:* 1
Ownership: Public
Stock Symbol: TGX
Traded On: NYSE
Produces/Sells CE-marked Devices: Y
Federal Procurement Eligibility: Small Business
Distribution: Manufacturer Direct, Manufacturer Through Distributor, Exclusive Distributor
General Admin.: Frank Tarallo/Chief Financial Officer, Treasurer
        M. Christine Jacobs/President, Chief Executive Officer
        Mr. Joseph Plante/Vice President
Mktg./Adv.: Bruce W. Smith/Executive Vice President Business Development
        Mr. C. Russell Small/Executive Vice President Marketing & Sales

Component, Electrical	General
Source, Brachytherapy, Radionuclide	Radiology

Medical Product Subsidiaries (Listed Separately)
Cp Medical Corporation
Galt Medical Corp.

THERAKOS, INC., A JOHNSON & JOHNSON COMPANY   877-865-6850

1001 US Route 202, Raritan, NJ 08869-0606   610-280-1000
FDA Number: 2523595   *Fax:* 610-280-1087
E-mail: bskillman@tksus.jnj.com
Web site: www.therakos.com
Total Employees: 50
Ownership: Public
Stock Symbol: JNJ
Traded On: NYSE
Quality System Registration Information: ISO9001
Produces/Sells CE-marked Devices: Y
Distribution: Manufacturer Direct
General Admin.: Ray Davis/President
        Tatia Troy/Vice President Human Resources
Mktg./Adv.: William Skillman/Vice President Marketing & Sales
Research: Harold Walder/Vice President Research & Development

Bottle, Sterile Solution	General
Extracorporeal Photopheresis System	Gastroenterology/Urology

THERALASE INC.   866-843-5273
102-29 Gervais Dr.,   416-447-8455
Toronto, ON M3C 1 Canada
FDA Number: 3003614490   *Fax:* 416-447-3020

MANUFACTURER PROFILES

THERALASE INC.   866-843-5273 *(cont'd)*
Web site: www.theralase.com
Year Founded: 1995
Total Employees: 10
Ownership: Public
Stock Symbol: TLT
Traded On: TSX Venture Exchange
Produces/Sells CE-marked Devices: N
Distribution: Manufacturer Direct

THERALIGHT, INC.   760-930-8000
2794 Loker Ave. West,suite 105, Carlsbad, CA 92010
FDA Number: 2032580

Laser, Surgical	Surgery
Light, Ultraviolet, Dermatologic	Surgery

THERAMED CORPORATION   800-305-4441
6891 Edwards Blvd.,   905-564-5009
Mississauga, ONT L5T 2 Canada
FDA Number: n/a   *Fax:* 905-564-4776
E-mail: theramed@theramed.com
Year Founded: 1995
Total Employees: 10
Ownership: Private
Produces/Sells CE-marked Devices: N
Distribution: Exclusive Distributor, Importer

THERAPEASE INNOVATION, LLC   435-671-0886
32 North 1025 East, Lindon, UT 84042
FDA Number: 3004828695

Exerciser, Powered	Anesthesiology

THERAPEUTIC ALLIANCES, INC.   937-879-0734
333 North Broad St., Fairborn, OH 45324
FDA Number: 1529150   *Fax:* 937-879-5211
E-mail: info@ergys.com
Web site: www.musclepower.com
Ownership: Private
Produces/Sells CE-marked Devices: N

Biofeedback Device	Cns/Neurology
Stimulator, Muscle, Electrical-Powered (EMS)	Physical Med

THERAPEUTIC DIMENSIONS, INC.   509-323-9275
319 W Hastings Rd., Po Box 28307, Spokane, WA 99218
FDA Number: 3031209

Exerciser, Non-Measuring	Physical Med
Transfer Aid	Physical Med

THERAPEUTIC SILICONE TECHNOLOGIES, INC.   212-606-0830
909 Fifth Avenue, New York, NY 10021
FDA Number: 1221628
Ownership: Private
Produces/Sells CE-marked Devices: N

Needle, Hypodermic, Single Lumen With Syringe	General
Silicone, Liquid, Injectable	Surgery
Syringe, Piston	General

THERAPIST'S CHOICE MEDICAL SUPPLIES   800-263-6618
944 Lawrence Ave. West,   416-781-7210
Toronto, ONT M6A-1 Canada
FDA Number: n/a   *Fax:* 416-781-8406
E-mail: tfox@therapistschoice.com
Web site: http://www.therapistschoice.com
Year Founded: 1991
Total Employees: 25
Ownership: Private
Produces/Sells CE-marked Devices: N

THERAPY INNOVATIONS LLC   541-550-7347
840 Se Woodland Blvd, Suite 185, Bend, OR 97702
FDA Number: 3006227146

Pack, Hot Or Cold, Reusable	Physical Med

THERASONICS MEDICAL SYSTEMS INC.
See Exogen, Inc.

THERATECH, INC.   800-788-1705
1109 Myatt Blvd., Madison, TN 37115
FDA Number: 2320963   *Fax:* 800-485-2626
E-mail: customerservice@stimsupply.com
Web site: www.stimsupply.com
Medical Products Sales Volume: $3,000,000
Annual Revenue: $1-$5 Million
Year Founded: 1980
Ownership: Private
Produces/Sells CE-marked Devices: N
Federal Procurement Eligibility: Small Business
Distribution: Manufacturer Direct, Manufacturer Through Distributor, Manufacturer Through Manufacturer Reps, Importer

THERATECH, INC.   800-788-1705 *(cont'd)*

Stimulator, Nerve, Transcutaneous (Pain Relief, TENS)	Cns/Neurology
Unit, Therapy, Current, Interferential	Cns/Neurology

THERATECHNOLOGIES INC.   514-336-7800
2310 Alfred-Nobel Blvd., St-Laurent, QUE H4S-2A4 Canada
FDA Number: n/a   *Fax:* 514-336-7242
E-mail: thera@theratech.com
Web site: www.theratech.com
Year Founded: 1993
Total Employees: 100
Ownership: Private
Produces/Sells CE-marked Devices: N
Distribution: Manufacturer Direct, Exporter

THERATEST LABORATORIES, INC.   800-441-0771
1111 N. Main St., Lombard, IL 60148   630-627-6069
FDA Number: 1421346   *Fax:* 630-627-4231
E-mail: tony@theratest.com
Web site: www.Theratest.com
Medical Products Sales Volume: $1,500,000
Annual Revenue: $1-$5 Million
Year Founded: 1988
Total Employees: 6
Ownership: Private
Produces/Sells CE-marked Devices: N
Federal Procurement Eligibility: Small Business
Distribution: Manufacturer Direct, OEM, Service Direct, Importer, Exporter

Anti-DNA Antibody (Enzyme-Labeled), Antigen, Control	Immunology
Antigen, Antiserum, Control, Whole Human Serum	Immunology
Antinuclear Antibody (Enzyme-Labeled), Antigen, Controls	Immunology
System, Test, Antibodies, B2 - Glycoprotein I (b2 - Gpi)	Immunology
System, Test, Anticardiolipin, Immunological	Immunology
Test, Rheumatoid Factor	Immunology

THERICS, LLC
See Integra Spine

THERMADYNE HOLDINGS, CORP.   940-381-1388
800 Henrietta Creek Rd., Roanoke, TX 76262
FDA Number: 1625393

Regulator, Pressure, Gas Cylinder	Anesthesiology
Ventilator, Non-Continuous (Respirator)	Anesthesiology

THERMAGE, INC.   1-888-437-2935
25881 Industrial Blvd., Hayward, CA 94545   510-782-2286
FDA Number: 2954746   *Fax:* 510-782-2287
E-mail: info@thermage.com
Web site: www.thermage.com
Year Founded: 1995
Ownership: Public
Stock Symbol: THRM
Traded On: NASDAQ
Produces/Sells CE-marked Devices: N
General Admin.: Clint Carnell/Chief Operating Officer
    Stephen Fanning/President, Chief Executive Officer
Finance: Jack Glenn/Chief Financial Officer

Electrosurgical Unit, Cutting & Coagulation Device	Surgery

THERMAL LOGIC, INC.   318-345-5603
204 Timber Lane, Monroe, LA 71203
FDA Number: 2320555
Ownership: Private
Produces/Sells CE-marked Devices: N

Pack, Hot Or Cold, Reusable	Physical Med

THERMAL PRODUCT SOLUTIONS   800-586-2473
2121 Reach Road, Williamsport, PA 17701   570-326-7304
FDA Number: n/a   *Fax:* 570-326-7304
E-mail: TPSinfo@tps.spx.com
Web site: www.tenney.com
Medical Products Sales Volume: $12,000,000
Annual Revenue: $10-$25 Million
Total Employees: 100
Ownership: Public
Stock Symbol: TNNYB
Traded On: OTC Bulletin
Quality System Registration Information: ISO9001
Federal Procurement Eligibility: Small Business
Distribution: Manufacturer Direct, Manufacturer Through Manufacturer Reps, OEM, Service Direct, Exporter
General Admin.: Michael Grausam/President, Chairman, Chief Executive Officer
    Stuart Lunick/Vice President, General Manager
Mktg./Adv.: Tara Kechane/Director Marketing
    Tara Kechane/Manager Advertising

Chamber, Constant Temperature (Environmental)	Microbiology

THERMAL PRODUCT SOLUTIONS   800-216-7725
2121 Reach Road, Williamsport, PA 17701   570-326-1770
FDA Number: 9200144   *Fax:* 570-326-7304
E-mail: TPSinfo@tps.spx.com
Web site: www.blue-m.com
Annual Revenue: $50-$100 Million
Total Employees: 100
Ownership: SPX
Stock Symbol: BMEC
Traded On: NASDAQ
Quality System Registration Information: ISO9001
Produces/Sells CE-marked Devices: N
Federal Procurement Eligibility: Small Business
Distribution: Manufacturer Direct, Manufacturer Through Distributor, Manufacturer Through Manufacturer Reps, OEM, Service Direct, Exporter
General Admin.: Ed Osborn/President
Mktg./Adv.: Erin Hall/Coord. Marketing
     Keith Itsell/Manager International & National Sales

Bath, Viscosity	Chemistry
Bath, Water (Constant Temperature)	Chemistry
Chamber, Constant Temperature (Environmental)	Microbiology
Incubator, Aerobic	Microbiology
Oven	Chemistry
Oven, Paraffin	Pathology
Shaker, Waterbath	Chemistry

THERMASOLUTIONS, INC.   651-209-3900
1889 Buerkle Road, Birchwood, MN 55110
FDA Number: 3005699784

Warmer, Dialysate, Peritoneal	Gastroenterology/Urology

THERMCRAFT, INC   336-784-4800
3950 Overdale Road, PO Box 12037,
Winston Salem, NC 27117
FDA Number: n/a   *Fax:* 336-784-0634
E-mail: info@thermcraftinc.com
Web site: www.thermcraftinc.com
Medical Products Sales Volume: $6,500,000
Annual Revenue: $5-$10 Million
Year Founded: 1971
Total Employees: 49   *Marketing Staff:* 2   *Sales Staff:* 5
Ownership: Private
Produces/Sells CE-marked Devices: N
Federal Procurement Eligibility: Small Business
Distribution: Manufacturer Through Manufacturer Reps, OEM
General Admin.: Morris L. Crafton/Chief Executive Officer, General Manager
Mktg./Adv.: Thomas Crafton/Director Business Development
     James Miller/Manager International & National Sales
     Thomas Crafton/Vice President Sales

Oven	Chemistry

THERMIONICS CORP.   800-800-5728
1214 Bunn Avenue, Suite 5,   217-529-4280
Springfield, IL 62703
FDA Number: 1055265   *Fax:* 800-200-5728
E-mail: sales@thermipaq.com
Web site: www.thermipaq.com
Medical Products Sales Volume: $2,500,000
Annual Revenue: $1-$5 Million
Year Founded: 1990
Total Employees: 14   *Marketing Staff:* 1   *Sales Staff:* 2
Ownership: Private
Produces/Sells CE-marked Devices: N
Federal Procurement Eligibility: Small Business
Distribution: Manufacturer Direct, Manufacturer Through Distributor, Manufacturer Through Manufacturer Reps, OEM
General Admin.: Gregg Harwood/Chief Executive Officer
Mktg./Adv.: Jay Bush/Vice President Sales
Production: Neil Puhse/General Manager Operations

Bottle, Hot/Cold Water	General
Pack, Hot Or Cold, Reusable	Physical Med
Pad, Heating, Powered	Physical Med

THERMO - INDUSTRIAL HYGIENE DIVISION   508-520-0430
27 Forge Pkwy., Franklin, MA 02038
FDA Number: n/a   *Fax:* 508-520-2800
E-mail: info.eid@thermo.com
Web site: www.thermo.comrmp
Annual Revenue: $0-$1 Million
Year Founded: 1956
Total Employees: 300   *Marketing Staff:* 15   *Sales Staff:* 20
Ownership: Thermo Electron Corporation
Stock Symbol: TMO
Traded On: NYSE
Distribution: Manufacturer Through Distributor, Manufacturer Through Manufacturer Reps, Exporter
General Admin.: Gerard Abraham/General Manager

THERMO - INDUSTRIAL HYGIENE DIVISION   508-520-0430
(cont'd)
Mktg./Adv.: Bob Foster/Vice President Marketing & Sales

Analyzer, Mercury	Chemistry
Computer, Chemistry Analyzer	Chemistry
Spectrograph, Mass	Chemistry

THERMO ALKO
See Thermo Fisher Scientific Inc.

THERMO BIOSTAR, INC.   800-637-3717
331 S. 104th St, Louisville, CO 80027   303-530-3888
FDA Number: 1720655   *Fax:* 303-530-6601
E-mail: info@thermobiostar.com
Web site: www.thermobiostar.com
Medical Products Sales Volume: $13,400,000
Annual Revenue: $25-$50 Million
Year Founded: 2005
Total Employees: 180   *Marketing Staff:* 12   *Sales Staff:* 100
Ownership: Thermo Electron Corporation
Federal Procurement Eligibility: Small Business
Distribution: Manufacturer Direct
General Admin.: George Stebbings/Director Human Resources
     Noel Doheny/President, Chief Executive Officer
Mktg./Adv.: Chris Lynn/Vice President Marketing
     Bob Bush/Vice President Sales
Production: John Adams/Director Regulatory Affairs
     Craig Reinhardt/Vice President Manufacturing
Research: Barry Polisky/Vice President Research
     John Dorson/Vice President Research & Development

Antigen, Streptococcus SPP.	Microbiology
Chlamydia, DNA Reagents	Microbiology
Test, Influenza	Microbiology

THERMO CARDIOSYSTEMS, INC.
See Thoratec Corporation

THERMO ELECTRIC COMPANY   800-523-2002
1193 McDermott Drive, West Chester, PA 19380   610-692-7990
FDA Number: n/a   *Fax:* 610-430-1325
E-mail: info@te-direct.com
Web site: tepasales@te-direct.com
Ownership: Private
Produces/Sells CE-marked Devices: N

Bath, Paraffin	Physical Med
Bed, Air Fluidized	Physical Med
Fluidotherapy Unit	Physical Med

THERMO FISHER SCIENTIFIC   800-345-0206
22 Friars Drive, Hudson, NH 03051   603-595-0505
FDA Number: 9002630   *Fax:* 603-595-0106
E-mail: info@matrixtechcorp.com
Web site: www.matrixtechcorp.com
Medical Products Sales Volume: $35,100,000
Annual Revenue: $25-$50 Million
Total Employees: 400   *Marketing Staff:* 10   *Sales Staff:* 50
Ownership: Fisher Scientific Co., Llc.
Stock Symbol: TMO
Traded On: NYSE
Produces/Sells CE-marked Devices: Y
Federal Procurement Eligibility: Small Business, GSA Contract
Distribution: Manufacturer Direct
General Admin.: William Henderson/Chief Executive Officer
     Verner Anderson/President
Mktg./Adv.: Victor Torti/Director Product Development
     Raymond Mercier/Manager National Sales
     Marc Hamel/Senior Vice President Marketing
     Marc Hamel/Vice President Sales
Production: Jeffrey Johns/Director Quality Assurance
     Nick Cakounes/Manager Materials
     Brad Hogg/Senior Vice President Operations
Research: Victor Torti/Vice President Research & Development

Diluter	Chemistry
Dispenser, Other	General
Pipette Tip	Chemistry
Pipetter	Hematology
Stand/Holder, Equipment, Laboratory	Chemistry

THERMO FISHER SCIENTIFIC   800-241-6898
500 Technology Ct., Smyrna, GA 30082   770-319-9999
FDA Number: 7000314   *Fax:* 770-319-0336
E-mail: sales@thermoandersen.com
Web site: www.thermo.com
Medical Products Sales Volume: $3,000,000
Annual Revenue: $10-$25 Million
Year Founded: 1956
Total Employees: 100   *Marketing Staff:* 2   *Sales Staff:* 6
Ownership: Thermo Electron Corporation
Stock Symbol: TMO

MANUFACTURER PROFILES

THERMO FISHER SCIENTIFIC   800-241-6898 *(cont'd)*
Traded On: NYSE
Quality System Registration Information: ISO9001
Produces/Sells CE-marked Devices: Y
Federal Procurement Eligibility: Small Business
Distribution: Manufacturer Direct, Manufacturer Through Distributor, Manufacturer Through Manufacturer Reps
General Admin.: Herbert Schloesser/President
Mktg./Adv.: Wes Davis/Director Product Development
     James R. Morton/Division Manager
     Rob Ford/Manager International Sales
     Jim Morton/Manager National Sales
     Sam Lanasa/Vice President Business Development
     Sam Lanasa/Vice President Marketing & Sales
Production: Larry Kline/Manager Materials
     Ray White/Vice President Manufacturing

Sampler, Air	General
Sampler, Particulate	General

THERMO FISHER SCIENTIFIC   877-843-7668
81 Wyman Street, Waltham, MA 02454-9046   781-622-1000
FDA Number: n/a   *Fax:* 781-622-1207
E-mail: info@thermo.com
Web site: www.thermo.com
Annual Revenue: More than $1 Billion
Year Founded: 1956
Total Employees: 11000
Ownership: Public
Stock Symbol: TMO
Traded On: NYSE
Quality System Registration Information: ISO9001
Produces/Sells CE-marked Devices: Y
Distribution: Manufacturer Direct
General Admin.: Marijn Dekkers/Chief Executive Officer
Mktg./Adv.: Keith Bisogno/Director Corporate Marketing

Bath, Kinematic Viscosity	Chemistry
Bath, Tissue Flotation	Microbiology
Bath, Viscosity	Chemistry
Circulator, Water Bath	Chemistry
Incubator/Water Bath, Microbiology	Microbiology
Regulator, Temperature	Chemistry
Shaker, Waterbath	Chemistry

Medical Product Subsidiaries (Listed Separately)
Thermo Uscs

THERMO FISHER SCIENTIFIC   800-437-2999
PO Box 712099, Cincinnati, OH 45271   814-353-2300
FDA Number: n/a   *Fax:* 814-353-2305
E-mail: tech@thermohypersil.com
Web site: www.thermo.com
Year Founded: 1956
Ownership: Public
Stock Symbol: TMO
Traded On: NYSE
Produces/Sells CE-marked Devices: N
Distribution: Manufacturer Direct, Manufacturer Through Distributor, OEM
General Admin.: Paul Ross/General Manager
Mktg./Adv.: Eric Stover/Manager Product Development
     Steve Kozel/Manager Sales
Production: Fred Heiss/Manager Engineering
     Richard Leathers/Manager Production

Chromatography, Liquid, Performance, High	Toxicology
Column, Liquid Chromatography	Toxicology

THERMO FISHER SCIENTIFIC (ASHEVILLE) LLC   828-658-4400
275 Aiken Road, Asheville, NC 28804
FDA Number: 1036832
Ownership: Private
Produces/Sells CE-marked Devices: N

Centrifuge, Blood Bank, Diagnostic	Hematology
Centrifuge, Cell Washing	Hematology
Freezer, Blood Storage	Hematology

THERMO FISHER SCIENTIFIC (ASHEVILLE) LLC   740-373-4763
Millcreek Rd., Marietta, OH 45750
FDA Number: 1523845

Accessory, Assisted Reproduction	Obstetrics/Gynecology
Box, Glove	Microbiology
Chamber, Environmental, Platelet Storage	Hematology
Freezer, Blood Cell	Hematology
Freezer, Blood Storage	Hematology
Incubator/Water Bath, Microbiology	Microbiology
Shaker/Stirrer	Chemistry
Warmer, Blood and Plasma	Hematology
Warmer, Blood, Non-Electromagnetic Radiation	Anesthesiology

THERMO FISHER SCIENTIFIC (ROCHESTER)   585-899-7600
75 Panorama Creek Dr., Panorama, NY 14625
FDA Number: 1314344

THERMO FISHER SCIENTIFIC (ROCHESTER)   585-899-7600
(cont'd)

Bottle, Tissue Culture, Roller	Pathology
Chamber, Slide Culture	Pathology
Coverslip, Microscope Slide	Pathology
Dish, Tissue Culture	Pathology
Equipment, Laboratory, Gen. Purpose (Specific Medical Use)	Chemistry
Flask, Tissue Culture	Pathology
Plate, Radial Immunodiffusion	Immunology
Suspension System, Cell Culture	Pathology

THERMO FISHER SCIENTIFIC (SALES AND SERVICE)   800-227-8891

PROCESS INSTRUMENTS DIVISION   763-783-2500
501 90th Avenue N.W.
Minneapolis, MN 55433
FDA Number: n/a   *Fax:* 763-783-2525
E-mail: sales.pharmaceutical.us@thermo.com
Web site: www.thermo.com
Year Founded: 1956
Total Employees: 600
Ownership: Public
Stock Symbol: TMO
Traded On: NYSE
Quality System Registration Information: ISO9001
Produces/Sells CE-marked Devices: Y
Distribution: Manufacturer Through Manufacturer Reps
Mktg./Adv.: Joergen Olsson/Vice President Sales

Production Equipment	General

THERMO FISHER SCIENTIFIC -   800-227-8891
CHECKWEIGHING, METAL AND X-RAY DETECTION

501 90th Avenue NW, Minneapolis, MN 55433   763-783-2500
FDA Number: n/a   *Fax:* 763-783-2525
E-mail: barb.jurek@thermoallencoding.com
Web site: www.thermo.com
Medical Products Sales Volume: $5,000,000
Annual Revenue: $1-$5 Million
Year Founded: 1956
Total Employees: 4
Ownership: Private
Stock Symbol: TMO
Traded On: NYSE
Quality System Registration Information: ISO9001
Distribution: Manufacturer Through Distributor, OEM
Mktg./Adv.: Barbara Jurek/Coord. Sales

Service, Printing	General

THERMO FISHER SCIENTIFIC - FAIRPORT   585-899-7600
236 Perinton Parkway, Fairport, NY 14450
FDA Number: 3004548426

Suspension System, Cell Culture	Pathology

THERMO FISHER SCIENTIFIC - LABORATORY   800-662-7477
EQUIPMENT DIVISION HEADQUARTERS

450 Fortune Boulevard, Milford, MA 01757   866-984-3766
FDA Number: n/a   *Fax:* 740-373-6770
E-mail: info.sampleprep@thermo.com
Web site: www.thermo.com
Year Founded: 1956
Ownership: Jouan, Inc.
Stock Symbol: TMO
Traded On: NYSE
Quality System Registration Information: ISO9001
Produces/Sells CE-marked Devices: Y
Federal Procurement Eligibility: GSA Contract
Distribution: Manufacturer Direct, Manufacturer Through Distributor, Manufacturer Through Manufacturer Reps, Exporter
General Admin.: Susan Jezierny/Director Human Resources
Mktg./Adv.: R. Barrow/Manager National Sales
     J. Perkins/Manager Sales Training
Production: Bob Thornton/Vice President Manufacturing

Centrifuge, Blood Bank, Diagnostic	Hematology
Centrifuge, Cell Washing	Hematology
Centrifuge, Cell Washing, Automated, Immuno-Hematology	Hematology
Centrifuge, Continuous Flow	Chemistry
Centrifuge, Explosion-Proof	Chemistry
Centrifuge, Floor	Pathology
Centrifuge, General (Over 5,000 rpm)	Toxicology
Centrifuge, General (Up to 5,000 rpm)	Pathology
Centrifuge, Hematocrit	Hematology
Centrifuge, Microhematocrit	Hematology
Centrifuge, Microsedimentation	Hematology
Centrifuge, Refrigerated	Pathology
Centrifuge, Tabletop	Pathology
Cytocentrifuge	Pathology

THERMO FISHER SCIENTIFIC - LABORATORY   800-662-7477
(cont'd)

Hematocrit, Manual	Hematology

THERMO FISHER SCIENTIFIC INC.   563-556-2241
2555 Kerper Blvd., Dubuque, IA 52001
FDA Number: n/a
Web site: www.thermofisher.com
Annual Revenue: $0-$1 Million
Total Employees: 30000
Ownership: Thermo Fisher Scientific
Quality System Registration Information: ISO9001
Produces/Sells CE-marked Devices: Y
Distribution: Manufacturer Direct, Manufacturer Through Distributor, Exporter
General Admin.: David Ross/Manager Human Resources
　　　　　Ken Townsend/President, Chief Executive Officer
Mktg./Adv.: Kathy Regan/Manager Marketing Communications
　　　　　Rick Haber/Manager National Sales
　　　　　John Stork/Vice President Marketing & Sales
Production: Michael Regan/Director Quality Assurance & Regulatory Affairs
　　　　　Nicholas White/Vice President Manufacturing
Research: Dennis Smith/Vice President Engineering & Development
Finance: Brenda Hoefler/Vice President Finance

Bath, Dry (Constant Temperature)	Chemistry
Block, Heating	Chemistry
Demineralizer	Chemistry
Dispenser, Other	General
Distilling Unit	Chemistry
Filter, Bacteriological, Laboratory	Chemistry
Filter, Membrane	Chemistry
Furnace, Porcelain	Dental And Oral
Incubator/Water Bath, Microbiology	Microbiology
Meter, Dialysate Conductivity	Gastroenterology/Urology
Oven	Chemistry
Packaging, Sterilization	General
Plate, Hot	Chemistry
Purification System, Water, Deionization	Chemistry
Purification System, Water, Reverse Osmosis	Chemistry
Reverse Osmosis Membrane Equipment	Chemistry
Shaker/Stirrer	Chemistry
Sterilization Process Indicator, Biological	General
Sterilization Process Indicator, Chemical	General
Sterilizer, Laboratory	Microbiology
Sterilizer, Steam (Autoclave)	General
Sterilizer, Vapor	General
Still, Water	Chemistry
Stirrer	Chemistry
Tissue Culture Apparatus	Microbiology

THERMO FISHER SCIENTIFIC INC.   781-622-1000
81 Wyman Street, Waltham, MA 02454
FDA Number: n/a　　　　　　　　*Fax:* 781-622-1207
Web site: www.thermo.com
Medical Products Sales Volume: $2,000,000
Annual Revenue: $5-$10 Million
Year Founded: 1975
Total Employees: 34500
Ownership: Public
Stock Symbol: TMO
Traded On: NYSE
Produces/Sells CE-marked Devices: N
Distribution: Manufacturer Direct, Manufacturer Through Distributor, OEM
General Admin.: Peter M. Wilver/Chief Financial Officer, Senior Vice President
　　　　　Marc N. Casper/President, Chief Executive Officer
　　　　　Alan J. Malus/Senior Vice President
　　　　　Edward A. Pesicka/Senior Vice President
　　　　　Gregory J. Herrema/Senior Vice President

Calibrator, Blood Gas	General
Calibrator, Gas, Pressure	Anesthesiology
Calibrator, Secondary, Clinical Chemistry	Chemistry
Co-Oximeter	Hematology
Control, Blood Gas	Chemistry
Control, Electrolyte (Assayed And Unassayed)	Chemistry
Control, Hemoglobin	Hematology
Electrode, Blood Gas, Carbon-Dioxide	Anesthesiology
Electrode, Blood Gas, Oxygen	Anesthesiology
Electrode, Blood pH	Chemistry
Electrode, Ion Selective (Non-Specified)	Chemistry
Electrode, Ion Specific, Calcium	Chemistry
Electrode, Ion Specific, Chloride	Chemistry
Electrode, Ion Specific, Potassium	Chemistry
Electrode, Ion Specific, Sodium	Chemistry
Electrode, Other	General
Gas, Calibrated (Specified Concentration)	Anesthesiology
Lamp, Other	General
Mass Spectrometer, Clinical Use	Toxicology
Multi Analyte Mixture, Calibrator	Chemistry
Photometer, Flame, Lithium	Chemistry
Photometer, Flame, Potassium	Chemistry
Photometer, Flame, Sodium	Chemistry

THERMO FISHER SCIENTIFIC INC.   781-622-1000 *(cont'd)*

Reaction Apparatus	Microbiology
Reagent, Blood Gas/pH	General
Reagent, Calibration	General
Reagent, Other	General
Solution, Instrument Cleaner	General
Solution, pH Buffer	Chemistry
Standard/Control, All Types	Chemistry

Medical Product Subsidiaries (Listed Separately)
Dionex Corp.

THERMO NESLAB
See Thermo Fisher Scientific

THERMO NUTECH
See Eberline Services

THERMO NUTECH / EBERLINE SERVICES
See Eberline Services

THERMO ORIEL   203-377-8282
150 Long Beach Blvd., Stratford, CT 06615
FDA Number: 7000281　　　　　*Fax:* 203-378-2457
E-mail: oriel.sales@newport.com
Web site: www.oriel.com
Annual Revenue: $1-$5 Million
Total Employees: 110
Ownership: Thermo Electron Corporation
Produces/Sells CE-marked Devices: Y
Distribution: Manufacturer Direct, OEM, Exporter
General Admin.: Allen Smith/President
　　　　　Debbie Berggren/Vice President Human Resources
Mktg./Adv.: William K. Anderson/Manager International Marketing & Sales
Research: Z. Drozdowicz/Vice President Research & Development

Filter, Membrane	Chemistry
Instrument, Manual, General Surgical	Surgery
Lamp, Microscope	Pathology
Monochromator, for Clinical Use	Chemistry
Radiometer, Phototherapy	General
Spectrograph, Mass	Chemistry

THERMO PRODUCTS, LLC   (877) 903-5600
7767 S.valentia St, Centennial, CO 80112   (303) 985-9134
FDA Number: 3007057211　　　*Fax:* (303) 479-9705
Web site: http://thermo-products.com
Ownership: Private
Produces/Sells CE-marked Devices: N

Temperature Strip, Forehead, Liquid Crystal	General

THERMO SAVANT   800-634-8886
100 Colin Drive, Holbrook, NY 11741-4306   631-244-2929
FDA Number: 9320167　　　　*Fax:* 631-244-0606
E-mail: savantec@savec.com
Web site: www.thermosavant.com
Medical Products Sales Volume: $20,000,000
Total Employees: 95　　*Marketing Staff:* 5　　*Sales Staff:* 6
Ownership: Thermo Electron Corporation
Quality System Registration Information: ISO9001
Federal Procurement Eligibility: Small Business, GSA Contract
Distribution: Manufacturer Direct, Exporter
General Admin.: Mark Shon/President
Mktg./Adv.: Craig Chin/Director Marketing
Production: Michael Mattern/Manager Production
Research: Bob Evans/Vice President Engineering
Finance: Gary Berg/Controller

Centrifuge, Tabletop	Pathology
Drying Unit	Chemistry
Evaporator	Chemistry
Pump, Laboratory	Chemistry

THERMO SCIENTIFIC HAMILTON   920-794-6800
1316 18th St., Two Rivers, WI 54241
FDA Number: n/a　　　　　　*Fax:* 920-794-6409
Web site: www.hamiltonlab.com
Ownership: Thermo Fisher Scientific
Produces/Sells CE-marked Devices: N
Distribution: Exclusive Distributor

Cabinet Casework, General Purpose	General
Cabinet Casework, Laboratory	Chemistry
Cabinet Casework, Modular	General
Cabinet, Laboratory	Chemistry
Furniture, General	General
Hood, Fume	Toxicology

THERMO SPECTRA-TECH   800-243-9186
2 Research Drive, PO Box 869,   203-926-8998
Shelton, CT 06484
FDA Number: n/a　　　　　　*Fax:* 203-926-8909
E-mail: info@spectra-tech.com
Web site: www.spectra-tech.com
Medical Products Sales Volume: $2,200,000

THERMO SPECTRA-TECH
800-243-9186 *(cont'd)*
Annual Revenue: $0-$1 Million
Total Employees: 49　　*Marketing Staff:* 3　　*Sales Staff:* 5
Ownership: THERMAL OPTEK CORPORATION
Federal Procurement Eligibility: Small Business
Distribution: Manufacturer Direct, OEM, Service Direct, Importer
General Admin.: Gregg Ressler/President
Mktg./Adv.: Ed Manke/Director Marketing
　　Peter Troost/Director Product Development
　　Ed Manke/Manager Advertising
　　Debbie Esposito/Manager National Sales

Computer Software	General
System, Automated, Microbiological	Microbiology

THERMO SPECTRONIC
820 Linden Avenue, Rochester, NY 14625-2710　**800-654-9955**
585-248-4000
FDA Number: 7000320　　*Fax:* 585-248-4200
E-mail: info@thermospectronic.com
Web site: www.thermo.com/spectronic
Medical Products Sales Volume: $20,000,000
Annual Revenue: $10-$25 Million
Year Founded: 1967
Total Employees: 499　　*Marketing Staff:* 5　　*Sales Staff:* 12
Ownership: Thermo Electron Corporation
Quality System Registration Information: ISO9001
Produces/Sells CE-marked Devices: Y
Federal Procurement Eligibility: Small Business, GSA Contract
Distribution: Manufacturer Direct, Manufacturer Through Distributor, Manufacturer Through Manufacturer Reps, OEM, Exporter
General Admin.: Mark Whiteman/Chief Executive Officer
　　Mike Whiteman/President
Mktg./Adv.: Zbigniew Stanek/Director Market Research & Planning
　　Guy Lachance/Director National Accounts
　　Prabhakar Rao/Director Product Development
　　John Deluca/Manager International & National Sales
　　Ms. Kati Chenot/Marketing Communications Specialist
Production: George Gudz/Director Quality Assurance
　　Cathy Dayton/Product Manager
Finance: Brian Davis/Vice President Finance

Cell, Spectrophotometer	Chemistry
Disintegrator, Biological Cell	Microbiology
Fluorometer	Immunology
Fluorometer, Toxicology	Toxicology
Spectrophotometer, Fluorescence	Chemistry
Spectrophotometer, U.V./Visible	Chemistry

THERMO SPECTRONIC [UNICAM]
See Thermo Spectronic

THERMO USCS
120 Bishops Way, Suite 100, Box 0951,　**800-558-6377**
Brookfield, WI 53008
FDA Number: n/a　　*Fax:* 262-784-5779
E-mail: info@us-cs.com
Web site: www.us-cs.com
Year Founded: 1969
Total Employees: 160　　*Marketing Staff:* 4　　*Sales Staff:* 25
Ownership: Thermo Fisher Scientific
Stock Symbol: TMO
Traded On: NYSE
Produces/Sells CE-marked Devices: N
Distribution: Service Direct
General Admin.: Christine A. Miller/Executive Vice President
　　Scott D. McFadden/Vice President, General Manager
Mktg./Adv.: Dick Sandretti/Manager Marketing

Service, Consulting	General

THERMO-SONICS INC.
See Ts Scientific

THERMOGENESIS CORP.
2711 Citrus Road, Rancho Cordova, CA 95742　**800-783-8357**
916-858-5100
FDA Number: 2950374　　*Fax:* 916-858-5199
E-mail: sales@thermogenesis.com
Web site: www.thermogenesis.com
Medical Products Sales Volume: $16,800,000
Annual Revenue: $10-$25 Million
Year Founded: 1986
Total Employees: 60　　*Marketing Staff:* 3　　*Sales Staff:* 5
Ownership: Public
Stock Symbol: KOOL
Traded On: NASDAQ
Quality System Registration Information: ISO9001
Produces/Sells CE-marked Devices: Y
Federal Procurement Eligibility: Small Business
Distribution: Manufacturer Direct, Manufacturer Through Distributor, OEM, Exporter
General Admin.: Mr. J. Melville Engle/Chief Executive Officer

THERMOGENESIS CORP.
800-783-8357 *(cont'd)*
Mr. Matthew Plaven/Chief Operating Officer, Chief Financial Officer
Mktg./Adv.: Mr. Hal Baker/Vice President Commercial Operations
Production: Mr. Jorge Artiles/Vice President Quality Control & Regulatory Affairs
Research: Mr. Menachem Shavit/Vice President Engineering

Autotransfusion Unit (Blood)	Anesthesiology
Bag, Blood, Collection	Hematology
Centrifuge, Refrigerated	Pathology
Cord Blood Processing System And Storage Container	Hematology
Freezer, Blood Storage	Hematology
Refrigerator, Blood Bank	Hematology
Syringe, Piston	General
Warmer, Blood and Plasma	Hematology
Warmer, Infusion Fluid, Thermal	General

THERMOMETRICS
See Ge Industrial, Sensing

THERMOPEUTIX INC.
9925b Business Park Ave., San Diego, CA 92131　**858-549-1760**
FDA Number: 3005034471

Stent, Cardiovascular	Cardiovascular
System, Hypothermia, Intravenous, Cooling	Cns/Neurology

THERMOPLASTIC COMFORT SYSTEMS, INC.
2619 Lime Avenue, Signal Hill, CA 90755　**562-426-2970**
FDA Number: 2032807

Base, Denture, Relining, Repairing, Rebasing, Resin	Dental And Oral

THERMOSAFE BRANDS
3930 Ventura Drive, Suite 450,　**847-398-0110**
Arlington Heights, IL 60004　**800-323-7442**
FDA Number: 9200881　　*Fax:* 847-398-0653
E-mail: info@thermosafe.com
Web site: www.thermosafe.com
Annual Revenue: $50-$100 Million
Year Founded: 1946
Total Employees: 499
Ownership: Tegrant Corporation, Protexic Brands
Quality System Registration Information: ISO9001
Produces/Sells CE-marked Devices: N
Federal Procurement Eligibility: Small Business
Distribution: Manufacturer Direct
General Admin.: Ken Harris/Director, General Manager
Mktg./Adv.: Kevin Grogan/Director Marketing
Production: Ken Sears/Vice President Manufacturing

Chest, Dry Ice	General
Container, Slide Mailer	Microbiology
Container, Specimen Mailer And Storage	Pathology
Container, Specimen Mailer And Storage, Temperature Control	Pathology
Container, Specimen, All Types	General
Container, Transport, Kidney	Gastroenterology/Urology
Container, Urine Specimen	General
Foodservice Product/Equipment	General
Labware, Basic, Disposable	Chemistry
Labware, Basic, Reusable	Chemistry
Pack, Cold	General
Rack, Test Tube	Chemistry

THERMOSURGERY TECHNOLOGIES, INC.
2901 W. Indian School Road, Phoenix, AZ 85017-4162　**602-264-7300**
FDA Number: 2027460　　*Fax:* 602-248-3809
E-mail: corporate@thermosurgery.com
Web site: www.thermosurgery.com
Medical Products Sales Volume: $2,100,000
Annual Revenue: $0-$1 Million
Year Founded: 1990
Total Employees: 6　　*Sales Staff:* 1
Ownership: Private
Produces/Sells CE-marked Devices: Y
Federal Procurement Eligibility: Small Business, VA Contract
Distribution: Manufacturer Through Distributor
General Admin.: Mr. Gene Hedin/Chief Executive Officer, Chairman

Electrosurgical Unit, Cutting & Coagulation Device	Surgery

THERMOTEK INC.
1454 Halsey Way, Carrollton, TX 75007-4409　**877-242-3232**
972-242-3232
FDA Number: 1648700　　*Fax:* 972-446-1195
E-mail: info@thermotekusa.com
Web site: www.thermotekusa.com
Medical Products Sales Volume: $1,000,000
Annual Revenue: $10-$25 Million
Year Founded: 1993
Total Employees: 18　　*Marketing Staff:* 2　　*Sales Staff:* 6
Ownership: Private
Stock Symbol: AAON
Traded On: NASDAQ
Quality System Registration Information: ISO9001

THERMOTEK INC.   877-242-3232 *(cont'd)*

Produces/Sells CE-marked Devices: Y
Federal Procurement Eligibility: Small Business
Distribution: Manufacturer Direct, OEM, Exporter
General Admin.: Jim Hartman/Chief Operating Officer
     Tony Quisenberry/President
Mktg./Adv.: Tony Quisenberry/Director Marketing
     Tony Quisenberry/Vice President Sales
Production: Debra Thomas/Director Customer Services
     Sara Lee/Director Quality Assurance
     Niran Bolachandra/Manager Engineering

Binder, Medical, Therapeutic	General
Hypo/Hyperthermia Unit, Mobile	General
Pack, Hot Or Cold, Water Circulating	Physical Med

THERMOTEX THERAPY SYSTEMS LTD.   800-975-0253
6115 4th St. SE #15,   **403-252-5335**
Calgary, ALB T2H-2 Canada
FDA Number: n/a   *Fax:* 403-252-9772
E-mail: info@thermotex.com
Web site: www.thermotex.com
Year Founded: 1996
Total Employees: 10
Ownership: Private
Produces/Sells CE-marked Devices: N
Distribution: Manufacturer Direct, Exporter

THEROKENETICS, INC.
    See JACE SYSTEMS, INC

THEROX, INC.   949-757-1999
17500 Cartwright Rd Suite 100, Irvine, CA 92614
FDA Number: 2030964

Catheter, Intravascular, Diagnostic	Cardiovascular
System, Oxygen, Aqueous	Cardiovascular

THINKING SYSTEMS CORPORATION   727-217-0909
750 94th Avenue North, Suite 211, Saint Petersburg, FL 33702
FDA Number: 1066247   *Fax:* 727-217-0938
E-mail: sales@thinkingsystems.com
Web site: www.thinkingsystems.com
Medical Products Sales Volume: $1,000,000
Year Founded: 1996
Total Employees: 12
Ownership: Private
Stock Symbol: PACS
Produces/Sells CE-marked Devices: N
Federal Procurement Eligibility: Small Business
General Admin.: Xiaoyi Wang/President

Device, Storage, Image, Digital	Radiology
Image Processing System	Radiology
System, Communication, Image, Digital	Radiology

THINOPTX, INC.   276-623-2258
15856 Porterfield Highway, Abingdon, VA 24211-0784
FDA Number: 3003670444
Ownership: Private
Produces/Sells CE-marked Devices: N

Lens, Intraocular	Ophthalmology

THIRD WAVE TECHNOLOGIES, INC.   888-898-2357
502 South Rosa Rd., Madison, WI 53719-1256   **608-273-8933**
FDA Number: 2134294
Web site: www.twt.com
Year Founded: 1993
Total Employees: 179
Ownership: Hologic
Stock Symbol: TWTI
Traded On: NASDAQ
Produces/Sells CE-marked Devices: N

Concentrator, Clinical Sample	Chemistry
Control, Analyte (Assayed And Unassayed)	Chemistry
Cystic Fibrosis System	Gastroenterology/Urology
Drug Metabolizing Enzyme Genotyping Systems	Toxicology
Kit, DNA Detection, Human Papillomavirus	Microbiology
Reagent, General Purpose	Pathology
Reagents, Specific, Analyte	Hematology

THOMAS MEDICAL INC.   800-556-0349
5610 WEST 82 2ND STREET,   **770-360-7778**
INDIANPOLIS, IN 46278
FDA Number: 9006852   *Fax:* 770-360-7779
E-mail: info@thomasmedical.com
Web site: www.thomasmedical.com
Medical Products Sales Volume: $1,900,000
Annual Revenue: $1-$5 Million
Total Employees: 12   *Marketing Staff:* 5   *Sales Staff:* 150
Ownership: Private
Stock Symbol: TSMA

THOMAS MEDICAL INC.   800-556-0349 *(cont'd)*

Quality System Registration Information: ISO9001
Produces/Sells CE-marked Devices: Y
Federal Procurement Eligibility: Small Business
Distribution: Manufacturer Direct, Manufacturer Through Distributor, Manufacturer Through Manufacturer Reps, OEM, Service Direct, Exclusive Distributor, Importer, Exporter
General Admin.: Thomas J. Zinnanti/President, Chief Executive Officer
Mktg./Adv.: Andre Keeve/Director National Accounts
     Aaron Ingram/Director Product Development
     Emmanuel Kuehn/Manager International & National Sales
     Scott Marcus/Manager National Marketing & Sales

Accessories, Laser, Endoscopic	Surgery
Aspirator, Endocervical	Obstetrics/Gynecology
Aspirator, Endometrial	Obstetrics/Gynecology
Curette, Uterine	Obstetrics/Gynecology
Electrode, Other	General
Electrosurgical Equipment, General Purpose	Surgery
Elevator, Uterine	Obstetrics/Gynecology
Hook, IUD Removal	Obstetrics/Gynecology
Injector & Accessories, Manipulator, Uterine	Obstetrics/Gynecology
Scissors, Umbilical	Obstetrics/Gynecology
Tenaculum, Uterine	Obstetrics/Gynecology

THOMAS MEDICAL PRODUCTS, INC.   866-446-3003
65 Great Valley Pkwy., Malvern, PA 19355   **610-296-3000**
FDA Number: 2529252   *Fax:* 610-296-4591
E-mail: tmpinfo@ge.com
Web site: http://www.thomas-medical.com
Total Employees: 70
Ownership: Public
Stock Symbol: VITL
Traded On: NASDAQ
Quality System Registration Information: ISO9000
Produces/Sells CE-marked Devices: Y
Distribution: Manufacturer Direct, OEM
General Admin.: Joseph Thomas/Chief Executive Officer
     Joseph Thomas/President
Research: David Catlin/Vice President Research & Development

Adapter, Stopcock, Manifold, Cardiopulmonary Bypass	Cardiovascular
Catheter, Angioplasty, Transluminal, Peripheral	Cardiovascular
Catheter, Percutaneous	Cardiovascular
Introducer, Catheter	Cardiovascular

THOMAS MEDICAL PRODUCTS, INC.   866-446-3003
65 Great Valley Pkwy., Malvern, PA 19355   **610-296-3000**
FDA Number: 2529252   *Fax:* 610-296-4591
E-mail: info@thomas-medical.com
Year Founded: 1990
Ownership: Vital Signs, Inc.
Stock Symbol: VITL
Traded On: NASDAQ
Produces/Sells CE-marked Devices: N
Mktg./Adv.: Mark Kesti/Vice President Marketing & Sales

Accessories, Catheter	Surgery
Adapter, Stopcock, Manifold, Cardiopulmonary Bypass	Cardiovascular
Catheter, Angioplasty, Transluminal, Peripheral	Cardiovascular
Catheter, Intravascular, Therapeutic, Short-term Less Than 30 Days	General
Catheter, Percutaneous	Cardiovascular
Dilator, Vessel, Percutaneous Catheterization	Cardiovascular
Introducer, Catheter	Cardiovascular
Kit, Anesthesia, Conduction	Anesthesiology
Needle, Hypodermic, Single Lumen With Syringe	General
Surgical Instrument, Cardiovascular	Cardiovascular
Trocar, Cardiovascular	Cardiovascular
Tubing, Fluid Delivery	General

THOMAS OCULAR PROSTHETICS LABS, INC.   901-753-4724
1900 Kirby Parkway, Suite 102, Germantown, TN 38138
FDA Number: 1057440

Eye, Artificial, Non-Custom	Ophthalmology

THOMAS PRODUCTS DIVISION   920-457-4891
3524 Washington Avenue, Sheboygan, WI 53082
FDA Number: n/a   *Fax:* 920-451-4238
E-mail: leads@rtpumps.com
Web site: www.thomaspumps.com
Annual Revenue: $100-$500 Million
Year Founded: 1953
Total Employees: 460   *Marketing Staff:* 20   *Sales Staff:* 25
Ownership: Public
Quality System Registration Information: ISO9001
Produces/Sells CE-marked Devices: Y
Distribution: Manufacturer Direct, Manufacturer Through Distributor, OEM, Exporter
General Admin.: Mr. James Kregel/General Manager
Mktg./Adv.: Scott Johnston/Director Marketing
     David Droege/Manager Advertising
     James Gartman/Manager National Sales

THOMAS PRODUCTS DIVISION 920-457-4891 (cont'd)

Production: Paul Healy/Director Quality Assurance
Dan Pfister/Manager Regulatory Affairs
David Endsley/Vice President Manufacturing
Finance: Don Helf/Controller

Compressor, Air, Portable	Anesthesiology
Pump, Aspiration, Portable	Anesthesiology
Pump, Vacuum, Central	Anesthesiology

THOMPSON CONTRACT INC. 631-589-7337

41 Keyland Court, Bohemia, NY 11716
FDA Number: n/a Fax: 631-589-7339
E-mail: mthompson@kusch-usa.com
Web site: www.kusch.com
Medical Products Sales Volume: $1,200,000
Annual Revenue: $50-$100 Million
Year Founded: 1991
Total Employees: 10 Marketing Staff: 9 Sales Staff: 25
Ownership: Private
Federal Procurement Eligibility: Small Business
Distribution: Manufacturer Through Distributor
General Admin.: Dieter Kusch/Chief Executive Officer
Mktg./Adv.: Hanns Jorg Aderhold/Director Marketing
Justin Thompson/Manager National Sales

Chair, Geriatric	General
Chair, Other	General
Chair, Pediatric	General
Furniture, General	General
Table, Other	General

THOMPSON ENGINEERING 858-748-5677

11472 Tree Hollow Lane, San Diego, CA 92128
FDA Number: 3004620767

Circuit, Breathing (W Connector, Adapter, Y Piece)	Anesthesiology

THOMPSON MEDICAL SPECIALTIES 800-777-4949
952-285-4186

3404 Library Ln., St. Louis Park, MN 55426
FDA Number: n/a Fax: 952-285-4188
Web site: www.thompsonmedical.com
Medical Products Sales Volume: $800,000
Annual Revenue: $0-$1 Million
Ownership: Private
Produces/Sells CE-marked Devices: N
Federal Procurement Eligibility: Small Business
Distribution: Manufacturer Direct

Accessories, Wheelchair	Physical Med
Attachment, Bag (Crutch, Walker, Wheelchair)	Physical Med
Belt, Wheelchair	Physical Med
Component, Exercise	Physical Med
Cushion, Wheelchair (Pad)	Physical Med
Protector, Skin Pressure	General
Restraint, Protective (Body)	General
Support, Head And Trunk, Wheelchair	Physical Med

THOMPSON OCULAR PROSTHETICS, INC. 210-223-3754

4118 Mccullough Ave., Suite 16, San Antonio, TX 78212
FDA Number: 1646945

Conformer, Ophthalmic	Ophthalmology
Eye, Artificial, Non-Custom	Ophthalmology
Shell, Scleral	Ophthalmology

THOMPSON RETRACTOR

See Thompson Surgical Instruments, Inc.

THOMPSON SURGICAL INSTRUMENTS, INC. 800-227-7543
231-922-0177

10170 E. Cherry Bend Road,
Traverse City, MI 49684
FDA Number: 9201077 Fax: 231-922-0174
E-mail: danf@thompsonsurgical.com
Web site: www.thompsonsurgical.com
Medical Products Sales Volume: $1,400,000
Annual Revenue: $1-$5 Million
Year Founded: 1983
Total Employees: 20 Marketing Staff: 3 Sales Staff: 3
Ownership: Private
Stock Symbol: IART
Quality System Registration Information: ISO9000
Produces/Sells CE-marked Devices: Y
Federal Procurement Eligibility: Small Business
Distribution: Manufacturer Direct, Exporter
General Admin.: Daniel K. Farley/President
Mktg./Adv.: Rhonda White/Director Marketing
Johnnie Lynch/Manager Advertising
Bill Dawson/Manager International & National Sales

Holder, Instrument, Laparoscopic	Surgery
Holder, Laparoscope	Obstetrics/Gynecology
Holder, Retractor	Surgery
Instrument, Manual, General Surgical	Surgery
Retractor, Abdominal	Surgery

THOMPSON SURGICAL INSTRUMENTS, INC. 800-227-7543
(cont'd)

Retractor, Bladder	Gastroenterology/Urology
Retractor, Other	Surgery
Retractor, Self-Retaining, Neurology	Cns/Neurology
Retractor, Surgical	Surgery
Retractor, Vaginal	Obstetrics/Gynecology
Surgical Instrument, Orthopedic, AC-Powered Motor	Orthopedics

THOMSON COMPONENTS AND TUBES CORP.

See Thales Components Corporation

THOMSON INDUSTRIES, INC. 540-633-3549

203A West Rock Road, Radford, VA 24141
FDA Number: n/a Fax: 540-633-0294
E-mail: : thomson@thomsonlinear.com
Web site: http://literature.thomsonlinear.com
Total Employees: 600
Ownership: Private
Quality System Registration Information: ISO9001; ISO9002
Produces/Sells CE-marked Devices: N
Distribution: Manufacturer Direct
General Admin.: Dr. Alex N. Beavers/Chief Executive Officer
Jodi Baldassin/Vice President Human Resources
Mktg./Adv.: Sam Sher/Director Marketing
Production: Paul Cadmus/Vice President Manufacturing

Contract Assembly	General

THONET INDUSTRIES, INC.

See Gf Health Products, Inc

THORATEC CORPORATION 800-456-1477
925-847-8600

6101 Stoneridge Drive, Pleasanton, CA 94588
FDA Number: 2916596 Fax: 925-847-8571
E-mail: customer.service@thoratec.com
Web site: http://www.thoratec.com
Annual Revenue: $100-$500 Million
Total Employees: 1209
Ownership: Private
Stock Symbol: THOR
Traded On: NASDAQ
Produces/Sells CE-marked Devices: Y
Distribution: Manufacturer Direct
General Admin.: David V. Smith/Chief Financial Officer, Executive Vice President
Mr. Lawrence Cohen/President
Gerhard F. Burbach/President, Chief Executive Officer

Introducer, Catheter	Cardiovascular
Prosthesis, Heart	Cardiovascular
Prosthesis, Vascular Graft, Less Than 6mm Diameter	Cardiovascular
Prosthesis, Vascular Graft, Of 6mm And Greater Diameter	Cardiovascular

THORN EMI ELECTRON TUBES, INC.

See Adit/Electron Tubes

THORN SMITH LABORATORIES 231-882-7251

7755 Narrow Gauge Rd., Beulah, MI 49617
FDA Number: 1824234 Fax: 231-882-4804
E-mail: auric@thornsmithlabs.com
Web site: www.thornsmithlabs.com
Annual Revenue: $0-$1 Million
Total Employees: 6
Ownership: Private
Produces/Sells CE-marked Devices: N
Federal Procurement Eligibility: Small Business
Distribution: Manufacturer Direct, Manufacturer Through Distributor, Exporter
General Admin.: Robert M. Brown/President
Production: Melanie S. Cederholm/Plant Manager

Sterilization Process Indicator, Chemical	General
Sterilization Process Indicator, Physical/Chemical	General

THOUGHT TECHNOLOGY LTD. 800-361-3651
514-489-8251

2180 Belgrave Avenue,
Montreal, QUEBE H4A 2 Canada
FDA Number: n/a Fax: 514-489-8255
E-mail: mail@thoughttechnology.com
Web site: www.thoughttechnology.com
Year Founded: 1974
Total Employees: 45 Marketing Staff: 4 Sales Staff: 10
Ownership: Private
Produces/Sells CE-marked Devices: Y
Federal Procurement Eligibility: Small Business
Distribution: Manufacturer Direct, Manufacturer Through Distributor, Manufacturer Through Manufacturer Reps, Exporter

THOUGHT TECHNOLOGY LTD. 800-361-3651
514-489-8251

8205 Montreal / Toronto Boulevard, Suite 223,
Montreal West, QUE H4X 1 Canada
FDA Number: 9201079 Fax: 514-489-8255
E-mail: mail@thoughttechnology.com
Web site: www.thoughttechnology.com

THOUGHT TECHNOLOGY LTD.   800-361-3651 *(cont'd)*
Year Founded: 1974
Total Employees: 45   *Marketing Staff:* 4   *Sales Staff:* 6
Ownership: Private
Quality System Registration Information: ISO9001
Produces/Sells CE-marked Devices: Y
Federal Procurement Eligibility: Small Business
Distribution: Manufacturer Direct, Manufacturer Through Distributor, OEM

THREE M COMPANY
See 3m Co.

THREE PALM SOFTWARE   408-356-3240
367 Penn Way, Los Gatos, CA 95032
FDA Number: 3007038409   Fax: (650) 898-3219
E-mail: info@threepalmsoft.com
Web site: http://threepalmsoft.com
Ownership: Private
Produces/Sells CE-marked Devices: N

Image Processing System	Radiology

THREE RIVERS HOLDINGS, LLC   480-833-1829
1826 West Broadway Rd., Suite 43, Mesa, AZ 85202
FDA Number: 2032827

Accessories, Wheelchair	Physical Med
Platform, Force-Measuring	Physical Med
Pressure Measurement, System, Intermittent	Physical Med

THREE-D ORTHOPEDIC, DIV. DEROYAL INDUSTRIES, INC.   800-251-9864
101 Rose Hill Industrial Park,   865-362-6022
Rose Hill, VA 24281
FDA Number: 1122762
E-mail: customerservice@deroyal.com
Web site: www.deroyal.com
Year Founded: 1973
Ownership: DEROYAL INDUSTRIES, INC.
Produces/Sells CE-marked Devices: N

Ankle/Foot, External Limb Component	Physical Med
Bandage, Elastic	General
Belt, Traction, Pelvic, Orthopedic	Orthopedics
Belt, Wheelchair	Physical Med
Brace, Joint, Ankle (External)	Physical Med
Cover, Cast	General
Cushion, Table, Surgical	Surgery
Halter, Head, Traction, Orthopedic	Orthopedics
Joint, Knee, External Brace	Physical Med
Orthosis, Limb Brace	Physical Med
Orthosis, Lumbosacral	Physical Med
Pack, Hot Or Cold, Disposable	Physical Med
Protector, Skin Pressure	General
Restraint, Protective (Body)	General
Shoe, Cast	Physical Med
Sling, Arm	Physical Med
Splint, Clavicle	Physical Med
Splint, Hand, And Component	Physical Med

THYSSENKRUPP ACCESS CORP.   1-800-829-9760
4001 E. 138th St., Grandview, MO 64030   816-767-5453
FDA Number: 1925312   Fax: 816-763-4467
E-mail: michael.bolton@tkaccess.com
Web site: www.tkaccess.com
Annual Revenue: $50-$100 Million
Year Founded: 1947
Total Employees: 350   *Marketing Staff:* 4   *Sales Staff:* 50
Ownership: ThyssenKrupp AG
Produces/Sells CE-marked Devices: N
Distribution: Manufacturer Through Distributor, Manufacturer Through Manufacturer Reps
Mktg./Adv.: Michael Bolton/Manager Marketing

Chair, Geriatric	General
Elevator, Other	General
Elevator, Wheelchair	Physical Med
Lift, Stair Climbing	General
Lift, Wheelchair	General
Transport, Patient, Powered	Physical Med

TI-BA ENTERPRISES, INC.   585-247-1212
25 Hytec Circle, Rochester, NY 14606
FDA Number: 2438931   Fax: 585-247-1395
E-mail: info@ti-ba.com
Web site: www.ti-ba.com
Annual Revenue: $5-$10 Million
Year Founded: 1979
Total Employees: 10   *Marketing Staff:* 1   *Sales Staff:* 2
Ownership: Private
Quality System Registration Information: ISO9000
Produces/Sells CE-marked Devices: N
Federal Procurement Eligibility: Small Business

TI-BA ENTERPRISES, INC.   585-247-1212 *(cont'd)*
Distribution: Manufacturer Through Distributor, Manufacturer Through Manufacturer Reps, OEM, Service Direct, Exclusive Distributor, Importer, Exporter
General Admin.: Don Titus/Chief Executive Officer
    Bill Titus/President
    Marianne Pastecki/Vice President, General Manager

Camera, Radiographic Photospot	Radiology
Chemical, Film Processor	Radiology
Computer, Radiographic Data	Radiology
Film, X-Ray	Radiology
Image Digitizer	Radiology
Image Processing System	Radiology
Processor, Cine Film	Radiology
Processor, Radiographic Film, Automatic	Radiology
Projector, X-Ray Film	Radiology
Radiographic Unit, Diagnostic, Dental (X-Ray)	Dental And Oral
Safelight, X-Ray	Radiology
Shield, X-Ray	Radiology

TIARA MEDICAL SYSTEMS, INC.
See Care Fusion 205, Inc.

TIBA MEDICAL, INC.   503-222-1500
2701 Nw Vaughn St., Suite 470, Portland, OR 97210
FDA Number: 3004006751
Ownership: Private
Produces/Sells CE-marked Devices: N

TIBURON MEDICAL ENTERPRISES   909-654-2333
915 Industrial Way, San Jacinto, CA 92582
FDA Number: 2031918   Fax: 951-654-2331
E-mail: tiburon@linkline.net
Medical Products Sales Volume: $1,800,000
Total Employees: 30
Ownership: Private
Produces/Sells CE-marked Devices: N
Federal Procurement Eligibility: Small Business
General Admin.: Mr. Juan Ordaz/Vice President

Brace, Joint, Ankle (External)	Physical Med
Joint, Hip, External Brace	Physical Med
Joint, Knee, External Brace	Physical Med
Orthosis, Lumbar	Physical Med
Splint, Hand, And Component	Physical Med

TICONIUM CO.   800-833-2343
413 North Pearl Street, Albany, NY 12201   518-434-3147
FDA Number: n/a   Fax: 518-434-1288
E-mail: ticonium@cmpindustries.com
Web site: www.cmpindustry.com
Ownership: Private
Quality System Registration Information: ISO9002
Produces/Sells CE-marked Devices: N
Federal Procurement Eligibility: Small Business
Distribution: Manufacturer Direct, Exporter

Alloy, Gold Based, For Clinical Use	Dental And Oral
Alloy, Precious Metal, For Clinical Use	Dental And Oral
Base, Denture, Relining, Repairing, Rebasing, Resin	Dental And Oral
Casting Unit, Dental	Dental And Oral
Disk, Abrasive	Dental And Oral
Metal, Base	Dental And Oral
Point, Abrasive	Dental And Oral

TIDI PRODUCTS, LLC   800-521-1314
570 Enterprise Dr., Neenah, WI 54956-4865
FDA Number: n/a   Fax: 800-837-7770
Web site: www.tidiproducts.com
Ownership: Private
Quality System Registration Information: ISO9001
Produces/Sells CE-marked Devices: Y
Distribution: Manufacturer Through Distributor

Cover, Thermometer	General
Sponge, Other	General
Thermometer, Electronic, Continuous	General
Tray, Fluoride	Dental And Oral

TIDI PRODUCTS, LLC   920-751-4380
570 Enterprise Dr., Neenah, WI 54956
FDA Number: 2182318

Absorber, Saliva, Paper	Dental And Oral
Accessories, Surgical Camera	Surgery
Bedpan	General
Cotton, Roll	Dental And Oral
Cover, Shoe, Operating Room	Surgery
Fiber, Absorbent	General
Garment, Protective, For Incontinence	Gastroenterology/Urology
Gauze/sponge, Nonresorbable For External Use	Surgery
Gown, Examination	General
Gown, Isolation, Surgical	Surgery
Linen, Bed	General
Microscope, Surgical	Ear/Nose/Throat
Mouthpiece, Saliva Ejector	Dental And Oral

MANUFACTURER PROFILES

TIDI PRODUCTS, LLC   920-751-4380 *(cont'd)*
- Operative Dental Treatment Unit — Dental And Oral
- Radiographic/Fluoroscopic Unit, Image-Intensified — Radiology
- Sheet, Burn — General
- Sponge, Gauze — Dental And Oral
- System, X-Ray, Mobile — Radiology
- Thermometer, Electronic, Continuous — General
- Wrap, Sterilization — General

TILLER MIND BODY, INC.   210-308-8888
10911 West Ave., San Antonio, TX 78213
FDA Number: 1648139
- Irrigator, Colonic — Gastroenterology/Urology

TILLOTSON HEALTHCARE CORP.   888-335-7500
10 Glenshaw St., Orangeburg, NY 10962   845-365-8200
FDA Number: n/a   *Fax:* 845-365-8201
E-mail: info@dynarex.com
Web site: www.thcnet.com
Annual Revenue: $50-$100 Million
Total Employees: 270   *Marketing Staff:* 2   *Sales Staff:* 4
Ownership: Private
Produces/Sells CE-marked Devices: Y
Distribution: Manufacturer Through Distributor, Manufacturer Through Manufacturer Reps, OEM, Exporter
General Admin.: Thomas N. Tillotson/Chairman
    Thomas N. Tillotson/Chief Executive Officer
    Thomas N. Tillotson/President
Mktg./Adv.: Denise Caron/Coord. Marketing
    Debi Moline/Manager Contract Sales
    Larry D. Sheldon/Manager International & National Sales
    Larry D. Sheldon/Senior Vice President Marketing & Sales
Production: Pauline Grader/Manager Materials
    Judith Genzale/Manager Regulatory Affairs
Research: Frank W. Perrella, PhD/Vice President Research & Development
Finance: Mark C. Olsen/Chief Financial Officer
- Bandage, Elastic — General
- Fiber, Absorbent — General
- Glove, Patient Examination, Latex — General
- Glove, Patient Examination, Poly — General
- Glove, Surgical, Plastic Surgery — Surgery
- Sling, Arm — Physical Med
- Sponge, External — Surgery
- Sponge, External, Synthetic — Surgery
- Sponge, Gauze — Dental And Oral
- Sponge, Internal — Cns/Neurology
Medical Product Subsidiaries (Listed Separately)
Best Glove Manufacturing Ltd.

TILLOTSON RUBBER CO., INC.   781-402-1731
59 Waters Ave., Everett, MA 02149
FDA Number: 1280080
Ownership: Private
Produces/Sells CE-marked Devices: N
- Glove, Patient Examination, Latex — General
- Rotator, Transverse — Physical Med

TIMEKEEPING SYSTEMS, INC.   216-595-0890
30700 Bainbridge Road, Solon, OH 44128
FDA Number: n/a   *Fax:* 216-595-0991
E-mail: sales@guard1.com
Web site: www.guardl.com
Total Employees: 30   *Marketing Staff:* 1   *Sales Staff:* 2
Ownership: Private
Produces/Sells CE-marked Devices: N
Distribution: Manufacturer Direct
General Admin.: Barry Markwitz/Chief Executive Officer
Mktg./Adv.: Neil Sheehan/Director Marketing
    Heather Meens/Director Product Development
    David Buck/Manager International & National Sales
- Computer Equipment — General
- Security Equipment/Supplies — General

TIMELY NEUROPATHY TESTING, LLC   225-638-5343
9553 Island Rd, Ventress, LA 70783
FDA Number: 3006305783
- Esthesiometer — Cns/Neurology

TIMEMED LABELING SYSTEMS, INC.   800-323-4840
144 Tower Drive, Burr Ridge, IL 60527   630-986-1800
FDA Number: 1419467   *Fax:* 630-986-0016
E-mail: PhilKashuba@TimeMed.com
Web site: www.timemed.com
Medical Products Sales Volume: $40,000,000
Year Founded: 1950
Total Employees: 100   *Marketing Staff:* 5   *Sales Staff:* 32
Ownership: Private
Produces/Sells CE-marked Devices: N
Federal Procurement Eligibility: Small Business, GSA Contract

TIMEMED LABELING SYSTEMS, INC.   800-323-4840 *(cont'd)*
Distribution: Manufacturer Direct, Manufacturer Through Distributor, OEM
General Admin.: Mike Casale/Chief Operating Officer, Vice President
    Jerry Nerad/President
Mktg./Adv.: Phil Kashuba/Director Marketing
    Kevin Muldowney/Manager Advertising
    Mark Bouchard/Manager National Sales
Finance: Marilyn Opelka/Controller
- Computer, Patient Data Management — General
- Label, Bar Code — General
- Label, Device — General
- Tape, Adhesive — General

TIMM MEDICAL TECHNOLOGIES, INC.   800-966-2796
6585 City West Pkwy., Eden Prairie, MN 55344   952-947-9410
FDA Number: 2134022   *Fax:* 952-947-9411
E-mail: CustomerService@TimmMedical.com
Web site: www.timmmedical.com
Medical Products Sales Volume: $10,500,000
Annual Revenue: $10-$25 Million
Total Employees: 50   *Marketing Staff:* 6   *Sales Staff:* 36
Ownership: Private
Stock Symbol: VVUS
Quality System Registration Information: ISO9001
Produces/Sells CE-marked Devices: Y
Federal Procurement Eligibility: Small Business
Distribution: Manufacturer Direct
General Admin.: Jerry Mattys/Chief Executive Officer
Mktg./Adv.: Robert Pilon/Director Marketing
    Stevan Bastrow/Vice President Sales
Production: John Antil/Manager Materials
    Dave Johnson/Vice President Manufacturing
    Mark McKoskey/Vice President Manufacturing
    Mark McKoskey/Vice President Operations
Research: David Anderson/Vice President Research & Development
- Catheter, Urethral, Diagnostic — Gastroenterology/Urology
- Device, Dysfunction, Erectile — Gastroenterology/Urology
- General Medical Device — General
- Monitor, Penile Tumescence — Gastroenterology/Urology
- Prosthesis, Penile — Gastroenterology/Urology
- Urodynamic Measurement System — Gastroenterology/Urology

TIN WORLDWIDE, INC.
See Bsn Medical, Inc

TINCHER/BUTLER DENTAL LABS   800-225-4699
525 First Avenue, South Charleston, WV 25303   304-744-4671
FDA Number: 1118096   *Fax:* 304-744-8452
E-mail: dwithrow@dentalservices.net
Ownership: Private
Produces/Sells CE-marked Devices: N
- Base, Denture, Relining, Repairing, Rebasing, Resin — Dental And Oral
- Crown, Preformed — Dental And Oral
- Device, Anti-Snoring — Ear/Nose/Throat
- Device, Repositioning, Jaw — Dental And Oral
- Mouthguard — Dental And Oral

TINGLE X-RAY LLC   349-162-8905
5481 Skyland Blvd. East, Coaling, AL 35453
FDA Number: 1033419
- Radiographic Unit, Diagnostic, Tomographic — Radiology
- Table, Radiographic, Stationary Top — Radiology

TINNITUS CARE INC.   888-535-6160
66 East 80th Street, Suite 1a,   212-535-6160
Manhattan, NY 10021
FDA Number: 3005494827
Ownership: Private
Produces/Sells CE-marked Devices: N

TINO, S.A. DE C.V.   800-024-77-55
Hospital #631, Guadalajara, JALIS 44200 Mexico   33-36-142-110
FDA Number: n/a   *Fax:* 33-36-142-687
E-mail: info@tino.com.mx
Web site: www.tino.com.mx
Medical Products Sales Volume: $2,352,941
Year Founded: 1975
Total Employees: 26   *Marketing Staff:* 4   *Sales Staff:* 8
Ownership: Private
Produces/Sells CE-marked Devices: N
Federal Procurement Eligibility: Small Business
Distribution: Exclusive Distributor, Importer

TIP, INC.   314-729-2969
2 Muirfield Ln., PO Box 410208, St. Louis, MO 63141
FDA Number: 1931878   *Fax:* 314-576-2678
E-mail: tipinc86@earthlink.net
Annual Revenue: $0-$1 Million
Year Founded: 1986

TIP, INC.　314-729-2969 (cont'd)

Total Employees: 2
Ownership: Private
Produces/Sells CE-marked Devices: N
Federal Procurement Eligibility: Female Owned
Distribution: Service Direct
General Admin.: Dr. Chanatip Rujanavech/President
　　　Dr. Naris Rujanavech/Vice President, General Manager
　Container, Specimen Mailer And Storage　Pathology

TIPAL INSTRUMENTS LTD.　514-484-9741

128 Prom Ronald, Montreal-Ouest H4X 1M8 Canada
FDA Number: 8022200
　Stereotaxy Equipment　Cns/Neurology

TIPP MACHINE & TOOL, INC.　937-387-0880

4201 Little York Road, Dayton, OH 45414
FDA Number: 1530966　Fax: 937-387-0881
E-mail: tmti@tippmachine.com
Web site: www.tippmachine.com
Medical Products Sales Volume: $13,000,000
Year Founded: 1947
Total Employees: 125　Sales Staff: 5
Ownership: Private
Quality System Registration Information: ISO9002
Produces/Sells CE-marked Devices: N
Federal Procurement Eligibility: Small Business
Distribution: Manufacturer Direct
Mktg./Adv.: Mr. Jerry Webb/Vice President Sales
　Implant, Collagen (Non-Aesthetic Use)　Surgery

TISPORT, LLC　800-545-2266　509-586-6117

1426 East Third Ave.,
Kennewick, WA 99337
FDA Number: 3032618　Fax: 866-586-2413
E-mail: customerservice@tilite.com
Web site: www.tilite.com
Total Employees: 100　Marketing Staff: 3　Sales Staff: 4
Ownership: Private
Produces/Sells CE-marked Devices: Y
Distribution: Manufacturer Through Manufacturer Reps
　Wheelchair, Manual　Physical Med

TISSUE BANKS INTERNATIONAL　800-756-4824　(415) 455-9000

2597 Kerner Blvd., San Rafael, CA 94901
FDA Number: 3007215572　Fax: (415) 455-5801
E-mail: nctb@tbionline.org
Web site: www.tbionline.org
Medical Products Sales Volume: $2,000,000
Annual Revenue: $1-$5 Million
Ownership: TISSUE BANKS INTERNATIONAL
Produces/Sells CE-marked Devices: N
Federal Procurement Eligibility: Small Business
Distribution: Service Direct
General Admin.: James H. Forsell/Senior Vice President
　Medical Admin.: Robert I. Branick/Medical Director
　Filler, Bone Void, Osteoinduction　Physical Med
　Graft, Bone　Orthopedics
　Orthopedic Manual Surgical Instrument　Orthopedics

TISSUE CULTURE BIOLOGICALS　800-845-1445　559-688-9391

19766 S Highway 99 Unit A, Suite 300,
Tulare, CA 93274
FDA Number: 2919166　Fax: 559-688-2377
E-mail: sales@tcbio.com
Web site: www.tcbio.com
Medical Products Sales Volume: $400,000
Year Founded: 1977
Total Employees: 6
Ownership: Private
Produces/Sells CE-marked Devices: N
Federal Procurement Eligibility: Small Business
Distribution: Manufacturer Direct, Manufacturer Through Distributor, OEM, Importer, Exporter
　Serum, Animal　Pathology

TITAN CORPORATION/SYSTEMS & IMAGERY DIVISION　800-622-8554

1200 S. Woody Burke Road, PO Box 550,
Melbourne, FL 32901　321-727-0660
FDA Number: 7000237　Fax: 321-952-1689
E-mail: sales@dba.titan.com
Web site: www.titan.com/dbasystems/
Medical Products Sales Volume: $2,000,000
Annual Revenue: $1-$5 Million
Total Employees: 250　Marketing Staff: 5　Sales Staff: 5
Ownership: Public

TITAN CORPORATION/SYSTEMS & IMAGERY　800-622-8554
(cont'd)

Stock Symbol: TTN
Traded On: NASDAQ
Produces/Sells CE-marked Devices: N
Federal Procurement Eligibility: Small Business
Distribution: Manufacturer Direct, Manufacturer Through Manufacturer Reps
General Admin.: James Shaw/President
Mktg./Adv.: Richard Reynolds/Director Marketing
　　　Andre Lachance/Vice President Business Development
Research: Glenn Turner/Director Research & Development
　Image Digitizer　Radiology
　Image Processing System　Radiology

TITAN IMPLANTS, INC.　1-866-439-0470　201-439-0026

18 Columbia Ave., Bergenfield, NJ 07621
FDA Number: 2249649　Fax: 201-439-1145
E-mail: support@titanimplants.com
Web site: www.titanimplants.com
Annual Revenue: $0-$1 Million
Year Founded: 2000
Total Employees: 5　Marketing Staff: 1　Sales Staff: 2
Ownership: Private
Quality System Registration Information: ISO9000
Produces/Sells CE-marked Devices: N
Federal Procurement Eligibility: Small Business, Minority Owned
Distribution: Manufacturer Direct, Service Direct
General Admin.: Cyril Chen/President, Chief Executive Officer
Mktg./Adv.: Dr. Alvin Charles Jacobs/Director Marketing
　　　S. Emmanuel/Manager International & National Sales
Production: Lynn Howard/Manager Regulatory Affairs
　Implant, Endosseous　Dental And Oral

TITAN SPINE LLC.　1-866-822-7800　262-242-7801

6140 W. Executive Drive, Suite A,
Mequon, WI 53092
FDA Number: 3006340236　Fax: 262-242-7802
E-mail: tsinfo@titanspine.com
Web site: http://www.titanspine.com
Ownership: Private
Produces/Sells CE-marked Devices: N
General Admin.: Dr. Peter Ulrrich/Chief Executive Officer
　　　Mr. Kevin Gemas/President
Mktg./Adv.: Mr. Chad Patterson/Director Product Development
　　　Mr. Steve Cichy/Vice President Marketing & Sales
Production: Mr. Scott Van Ellis/Director Quality Assurance & Regulatory Affairs
　　　Mr. Mark Berg/Vice President Operations
　　　Mr. Mike Berg/Vice President Operations
Research: Ms. Jennifer Schneider/Senior Vice President Research & Development
　Device, Spinal Vertebral Body Replacement　Orthopedics

TITERTEK INSTRUMENTS, INC.　256-859-8600

330 Wynn Drive, Huntsville, AL 35805-1961
FDA Number: 1028229　Fax: 256-859-8671
E-mail: inquiry@titertek.com
Web site: www.titertek.com
Medical Products Sales Volume: $5,100,000
Annual Revenue: $5-$10 Million
Total Employees: 44
Ownership: Private
Produces/Sells CE-marked Devices: N
Federal Procurement Eligibility: Small Business
Distribution: Manufacturer Direct
General Admin.: James Haines/President
　Adhesive, Liquid　General
　Counter, Gamma, General Use　Toxicology
　Microplate　General
　Microtiter Diluting/Dispensing Device　Microbiology
　Station Pipetting　Chemistry

TITMUS OPTICAL INC.　800-446-1802　804-452-5200

690 HP Way, 3811 CorPOrate Drive,
Chester, VA 23836
FDA Number: 1118530　Fax: 804-862-3734
E-mail: info@titmus.com
Web site: www.titmus.com
Medical Products Sales Volume: $15,900,000
Annual Revenue: $25-$50 Million
Year Founded: 1908
Total Employees: 253　Marketing Staff: 7　Sales Staff: 12
Ownership: SPERIAN PROTECTION
Quality System Registration Information: ISO9001; ISO9002
Produces/Sells CE-marked Devices: Y
Federal Procurement Eligibility: Small Business
Distribution: Manufacturer Through Distributor, Manufacturer Through Manufacturer Reps
General Admin.: Tom Goeltz/President

TITMUS OPTICAL INC. 800-446-1802 *(cont'd)*

Mktg./Adv.: Joe Parsons/Director Sales
Donna Martin/Manager Advertising
Sameet Rajguru/Manager Product Marketing
Richard Masters/Vice President Marketing
Production: David Devine/Director Quality Assurance
Jim Troy/Manager Materials
Jeffery Pughe/Vice President Operations

Analyzer, Visual Function	Ophthalmology
Lens, Spectacle/Eyeglasses, Custom (Prescription)	Ophthalmology
Tester, Color Vision	Ophthalmology

TITRONICS RESEARCH & DEVELOPMENT CO. 800-705-2307

400 Stephans Street, PO Box 470, 319-545-7377
Tiffin, IA 52340
FDA Number: 1933956 *Fax:* 319-545-7380
E-mail: info@titronics.com
Web site: www.titronics.com
Medical Products Sales Volume: $1,000,000
Annual Revenue: $1-$5 Million
Year Founded: 1972
Total Employees: 10 *Marketing Staff:* 1 *Sales Staff:* 3
Ownership: Private
Quality System Registration Information: ISO9001
Produces/Sells CE-marked Devices: N
Federal Procurement Eligibility: Small Business
Distribution: Manufacturer Direct, Manufacturer Through Distributor, Exporter
General Admin.: Mr. Roger Titone/President, Chief Executive Officer, Director

Monitor, Temperature, Neurosurgery, Direct Contact, Powered	Cns/Neurology

TJ RAMPIT, INC. 800-876-9498

338 Bidwell Road, Coldwater, MI 49036
FDA Number: n/a *Fax:* 517-278-9023
E-mail: Information@tjrampitusa.com
Web site: tjrampitusa.com
Annual Revenue: $0-$1 Million
Ownership: Private
Produces/Sells CE-marked Devices: N
Federal Procurement Eligibility: Small Business
Distribution: Manufacturer Direct

Ramp, Wheelchair	General

TJN MANUFACTURING,INC. 563-322-2162

416 Perry St., Davenport, IA 52801
FDA Number: 1931814

Table, Physical Therapy	Physical Med

TKI MEDCON INC. 800-854-0166

1066 Somerset St. W, Unit 100, 613-798-1411
Ottawa, ONT K1Y-4 Canada
FDA Number: n/a *Fax:* 613-798-8106
E-mail: tki@comnet.ca
Year Founded: 1994
Total Employees: 10
Ownership: Private
Produces/Sells CE-marked Devices: N
Distribution: Manufacturer Direct, Exporter

TL TATE MFG, INC. 765-452-8283

1500 N Webster Street, Kokomo, IN 46901
FDA Number: 1833757 *Fax:* 765-452-0769
E-mail: sales@tltate.com
Web site: www.tltate.com
Medical Products Sales Volume: $700,000
Annual Revenue: $0-$1 Million
Ownership: Private
Produces/Sells CE-marked Devices: Y
Federal Procurement Eligibility: Small Business
Distribution: Manufacturer Direct
General Admin.: Chuck Simon/General Manager
Timothy Tate/President

Cannula, Surgical, General & Plastic Surgery	Surgery
Cutter, Skin Graft, Expanded Mesh	Surgery
Guide, Surgical, Instrument	Surgery

TMA EBERLINE
See Eberline Services

TMI
See Technical Marketing, Inc.

TMJ APPLIANCE 800 865-7246

130 Black Ferry Court, Littleton, NC 27850 434-636-2537
FDA Number: 1122655 *Fax:* 208-988-4834
E-mail: sellam003@yahoo.com
Web site: N/A
Medical Products Sales Volume: $65,000
Annual Revenue: $1-$5 Million
Year Founded: 1980

TMJ APPLIANCE 800 865-7246 *(cont'd)*

Total Employees: 7 *Sales Staff:* 4
Ownership: Private
Produces/Sells CE-marked Devices: Y
Federal Procurement Eligibility: Small Business
Distribution: Importer
General Admin.: John Lenkey/President

Prosthesis, Facial, Mandibular Implant	Ear/Nose/Throat

TMJ SOLUTION, INC 805-650-3391

1793 Eastman Ave, Ventura, CA 93003
FDA Number: 2031049

Implant, Joint, Temporomandibular	Dental And Oral
Orthopedic Manual Surgical Instrument	Orthopedics

TMP TECHNOLOGIES, INC. 716-895-6100

1200 Northland Avenue, Buffalo, NY 14215
FDA Number: 1381802 *Fax:* 716-895-6396
E-mail: info@tmptech.com
Web site: www.tmptech.com
Medical Products Sales Volume: $8,900,000
Annual Revenue: $10-$25 Million
Year Founded: 1945
Total Employees: 65 *Marketing Staff:* 1 *Sales Staff:* 4
Ownership: Private
Quality System Registration Information: ISO9001
Produces/Sells CE-marked Devices: N
Federal Procurement Eligibility: Small Business
Distribution: Manufacturer Direct, Manufacturer Through Manufacturer Reps, OEM
General Admin.: Jeffrey Dorn/Chief Executive Officer
Robert Flowers/Vice President, General Manager
Mktg./Adv.: Jim Peczonczyk/Sales Specialist
Gary Ashe/Vice President Sales
Production: Ed Purizhansky/Chief Engineer
Wayne Fabiszewski/Manager Quality Assurance
Don Pfister/Vice President Manufacturing

Applicator, Other	General
Catheter, Retention Type	Gastroenterology/Urology
Component, Other	General
Contract Assembly	General
Contract Manufacturing	General
Contract Manufacturing, Product, Disposable	General
Contract R&D, Equipment	General
Elastomer, Other	General
Kit, Wound Dressing	Surgery
Service, Engineering/Design	General
Splint, Temporary Training	Physical Med
Sponge, External, Synthetic	Surgery

TMX ENGINEERING & MANUFACTURING, INC. 714-641-5884

2141 S. Standard Ave., Santa Ana, CA 92707
FDA Number: 3005185555

Guide, Surgical, Needle	Surgery

TNA (TAMI NORTH AMERICA) 514.334.7417

2865 Sabourin Street, St-Laurent, QUE H4S 1M9 Canada
FDA Number: n/a *Fax:* 514.334.3409
E-mail: nfo@tami-america.com
Web site: http://www.tami-na.com
Year Founded: 1999
Ownership: TAMI INDUSTRIES (France)
Produces/Sells CE-marked Devices: N
Distribution: Manufacturer Direct, Exclusive Distributor

TNC DEVICES, INC. 504-286-7794

50 Mcdonald Blvd., Aston, PA 19013
FDA Number: 3006199673
Ownership: Private
Produces/Sells CE-marked Devices: N

Catheter, Suction (Tracheal Aspirating Tube)	Anesthesiology

TNCO, INC.
See Symmetry Tnco

TOEFCO ENGINEERING COATING SYSTEMS 800-555-6495

1220 N. 14th St., Niles, MI 49120 269-683-0188
FDA Number: n/a *Fax:* 269-683-8408
Web site: www.toefco.com
Annual Revenue: $5-$10 Million
Total Employees: 75
Ownership: Private
Quality System Registration Information: ISO9002
Produces/Sells CE-marked Devices: N
Distribution: Manufacturer Direct
General Admin.: Arthur McEwee/President, Chief Executive Officer

Service, Device Coating, Protective	General
Service, Printing	General

TOEFCO ENGINEERING, INC.
See Toefco Engineering Coating Systems

TOLMAR INC.
(1-877-986-5627
970-212-4931
701 Centre Ave., Fort Collins, CO 80526
FDA Number: 3006218434
E-mail: info@tolmar.com
Ownership: Private
Produces/Sells CE-marked Devices: N

TOMAS L. ORTEGA
956-630-2887
San Borja 1361, Mexico City Mexico
FDA Number: 8030655
  Eye, Artificial, Non-Custom   Ophthalmology
  Prosthesis, Eye, Internal (Sphere)   Surgery

TOMOPHASE CORPORATION
781-229-5700
One North Avenue, Burlington, MA 01803
FDA Number: n/a   *Fax:* 781-229-5737
E-mail: info@tomophase.com
Web site: http://www.tomophase.com
Year Founded: 2003
Ownership: Private
Produces/Sells CE-marked Devices: N
General Admin.: Dr. Peter Norris/Chief Executive Officer
          Mr. Ralph Johnston/President, Chief Operating Officer

TOMOTHERAPY INCORPORATED
608-824-2800
1209 Deming Way, Madison, WI 53717
FDA Number: 3003873069   *Fax:* 608-824-2996
Web site: www.tomotherapy.com
Year Founded: 1997
Total Employees: 665   *Sales Staff:* 63
Ownership: Public
Stock Symbol: TOMO
Traded On: NASDAQ
Produces/Sells CE-marked Devices: Y
General Admin.: Dr. Frederick Robinson/Chief Executive Officer
          Mr. Steven Brooks/Chief Operating Officer
          Mr. Paul Reckwerdt/President
Mktg./Adv.: Mr. Delwin Coufal/Vice President Marketing
Production: Mr. Kenneth Buroker/Vice President Quality Assurance & Regulatory Affairs
  Accelerator, Linear, Medical   Radiology
  System, Planning, Radiation Therapy Treatment   Radiology

TOMTEC
877-866-8323
203-281-6790
1000 Sherman Avenue, Hamden, CT 06514
FDA Number: n/a   *Fax:* 203-248-5724
E-mail: info@tomtec.com
Web site: www.tomtec.com/
Medical Products Sales Volume: $6,500,000
Annual Revenue: $10-$25 Million
Year Founded: 1967
Total Employees: 68   *Marketing Staff:* 6   *Sales Staff:* 16
Ownership: Private
Produces/Sells CE-marked Devices: Y
Federal Procurement Eligibility: Small Business
Distribution: Manufacturer Direct, OEM, Exporter
General Admin.: William Harris/Chief Information Officer
          Thomas W. Astle/President
          James Hass/Vice President, General Manager
Mktg./Adv.: Jay Zebora/Manager Contract Sales
          Robert Speziale/Vice President Marketing & Sales
Production: Howard Tomlin/Director Quality Assurance
          Ronald Schyed/Vice President Manufacturing
          Russell House/Vice President Operations
Finance: James Hass/Controller
IS: Eichi Sengoku/Manager Tech. Development
          Michael Randi/Manager Tech. Services
  Equipment, Laboratory, Gen. Purpose (Specific Medical Use)   Chemistry
  Harvester, Cell   Microbiology
  Microplate   General
  Pipetting And Diluting System, Automated   Chemistry
  Stainer, Slide, Automated   Pathology

TOMY TECH U.S.A., INC.
800-545-8669
510-440-1976
40479 Encyclopedia Circle,
Fremont, CA 94538
FDA Number: n/a   *Fax:* 510-440-1975
E-mail: info@tomytech.com
Web site: http://www.tomytech.com
Total Employees: 3   *Marketing Staff:* 1   *Sales Staff:* 2
Ownership: Tomy Seiko Co. Ltd.
Produces/Sells CE-marked Devices: N
Federal Procurement Eligibility: Small Business
Distribution: Manufacturer Direct
Mktg./Adv.: Leanne Goyn/Account Executive
          Bernadette Holtz/Manager Advertising
          Bernadette Holtz/Vice President Marketing & Sales

TOMY TECH U.S.A., INC.
800-545-8669 *(cont'd)*
  Sterilizer, Steam (Autoclave)   General

TOOLMEX CORPORATION
800-992-4766
508-653-8897
1075 Worchester Road, Natick, MA 01760-1510
FDA Number: 1220429   *Fax:* 508-653-5110
E-mail: tools@toolmex.com
Web site: www.toolmex.com
Medical Products Sales Volume: $31,100,000
Year Founded: 1973
Total Employees: 65   *Marketing Staff:* 6   *Sales Staff:* 6
Ownership: Private
Quality System Registration Information: ISO9001
Produces/Sells CE-marked Devices: N
Federal Procurement Eligibility: Small Business
Distribution: Manufacturer Through Distributor, Exclusive Distributor
General Admin.: Arkadiusz Kielb/President
Mktg./Adv.: George Pytko/Manager Sales
  Clip, Towel   Surgery
  Cover, Shoe, Operating Room   Surgery
  Curette, Adenoid   Ear/Nose/Throat
  Curette, Surgical, Dental   Dental And Oral
  Curette, Uterine   Obstetrics/Gynecology
  Cutter, Wire And Pin   Orthopedics
  Forceps, Dressing   Surgery
  Forceps, Hemostatic   Surgery
  Forceps, Obstetrical   Obstetrics/Gynecology
  Forceps, Surgical, Gynecological   Obstetrics/Gynecology
  Forceps, Tissue   Surgery
  Forceps, Wire Holding   Orthopedics
  Gag, Mouth   Ear/Nose/Throat
  Handle, Knife Blade   Surgery
  Handle, Scalpel   Surgery
  Holder, Needle   Gastroenterology/Urology
  Holder, Needle, Other   Surgery
  Instrument, Dental, Manual   Dental And Oral
  Instrument, Microsurgical   Cns/Neurology
  Knife, Scalpel   Surgery
  Nipper, Malleus   Ear/Nose/Throat
  Pliers, Orthodontic   Dental And Oral
  Retractor, Manual   Cns/Neurology
  Scissors, Collar And Crown   Dental And Oral
  Scissors, Surgical Tissue, Dental (Oral)   Dental And Oral
  Scissors, Suture   Surgery
  Scissors, Umbilical   Obstetrics/Gynecology

TOOLS FOR SURGERY, LLC
631-444-4448
1339 Stony Brook Rd., Stony Brook, NY 11790
FDA Number: 3004550973
  Bulb, Inflation (Endoscope)   Gastroenterology/Urology
  Catheter, Multiple Lumen   Surgery
  Clamp, Surgical, General & Plastic Surgery   Surgery
  Dilator, Rectal   Gastroenterology/Urology
  Rod, Colostomy   Gastroenterology/Urology
  Staple, Implantable   Surgery
  Surgical Instrument, G-U, Manual   Gastroenterology/Urology

TOOTHTICKLER ENTERPRISES, INC.
651-429-5187
5222 E. Bald Eagle Blvd., White Bear Lake, MN 55110
FDA Number: 2135347
Ownership: Private
Produces/Sells CE-marked Devices: N
  Toothbrush, Powered   Dental And Oral

TOP TERUMO CARDIOVASCULAR SYSTEMS (TCVS)
See Terumo Cardiovascular Systems (Tcvs)

TOP END WHEELCHAIR SPORTS, INC.
See Invacare Top End Sports And Recreation Products

TOP SHELF MANUFACTURING, LLC
209-834-8185
1851 E. Paradise Road, Suite B, Tracy, CA 95304
FDA Number: 3003890514
  Brace, Joint, Ankle (External)   Physical Med
  Component, Exercise   Physical Med
  Joint, Knee, External Brace   Physical Med
  Orthosis, Limb Brace   Physical Med
  Orthosis, Lumbosacral   Physical Med
  Shoe, Cast   Physical Med
  Sling, Arm   Physical Med
  Splint, Hand, And Component   Physical Med
  Traction Unit, Non-Powered   Orthopedics

TOPCON CANADA INC.
800-361-3515
450-430-7771
110 Provencher Ave.,
Boisbriand, QUE J7G-1 Canada
FDA Number: n/a   *Fax:* 450-430-6457
E-mail: info@topcon.ca
Web site: www.topcon.ca
Year Founded: 1963
Total Employees: 50

TOPCON CANADA INC.   800-361-3515 (cont'd)
Ownership: Topcon Medical Systems, Inc.
Produces/Sells CE-marked Devices: N
Distribution: Exclusive Distributor

TOPCON MEDICAL SYSTEMS, INC.   800-223-1130
37 West Century Road, Paramus, NJ 07652-1408   **201-261-9450**
FDA Number: 2242863   *Fax:* 201-599-5250
E-mail: tmsinfo@topcon.com
Web site: www.TopconMedical.com
Medical Products Sales Volume: $14,800,000
Annual Revenue: $50-$100 Million
Year Founded: 1970
Total Employees: 86
Ownership: UTI/Star Guide
Quality System Registration Information: ISO9001
Produces/Sells CE-marked Devices: Y
Federal Procurement Eligibility: Small Business
Distribution: Manufacturer Direct, Manufacturer Through Distributor
General Admin.: Mr. Dave Mudrick/Chief Financial Officer, Executive Vice President
     Mr. Paul Iwasaki/President
     Mr. Randy Samuels/Vice President, General Counsel
Mktg./Adv.: Mr. Robert Gibson/Director Marketing
     Mr. James Jarmusch/Director Sales
     Mr. Ray Wright/Director Sales
     Mr. Stephen Hamilton/Director Sales
     Mr. Tom Koike/Vice President International Marketing & Sales
     Mr. Donald Winfield/Vice President Marketing
Production: Mr. Jim Bashant/Product Manager
     Mr. Mark Iguchi/Product Manager
     Mr. Ricardo Almiron/Product Manager
Research: Dr. Eugene Huang/Managing Director Research & Development

Camera, Ophthalmic, AC-Powered (Fundus)	Ophthalmology
Chair, Examination And Treatment	General
Chair, Ophthalmic, AC-Powered	Ophthalmology
Chair, Ophthalmic, Manual	Ophthalmology
Computer and Software, Medical, Ophthalmic Use	Ophthalmology
Frame, Trial, Ophthalmic	Ophthalmology
Illuminator, Radiographic Film	Radiology
Keratometer	Ophthalmology
Keratoscope, AC-Powered	Ophthalmology
Laboratory Equipment, Ophthalmic	Ophthalmology
Lamp, Slit, Biomicroscope, AC-Powered	Ophthalmology
Lens, Set, Trial, Ophthalmic	Ophthalmology
Measurer, Lens, AC-Powered	Ophthalmology
Microscope, Operating, AC-Powered, Ophthalmic	Ophthalmology
Ophthalmoscope, AC-Powered	Ophthalmology
Projector, Ophthalmic	Ophthalmology
Pupillometer, AC-Powered	Ophthalmology
Refractometer, Ophthalmic	Ophthalmology
Refractor, Ophthalmic	Ophthalmology
Stand, Instrument, AC-Powered, Ophthalmic	Ophthalmology
Stereoscope, AC-Powered	Ophthalmology
Table, Ophthalmic, Instrument, Powered	Ophthalmology
Tonometer, AC-Powered	Ophthalmology
Topographer, Corneal	Ophthalmology

Medical Product Subsidiaries (Listed Separately)
Topcon Canada Inc.

TOPERA MEDICAL   617-453-8001
6190 Cornerstone Court, Suite 220, San Diego, CA 92121
FDA Number: n/a
E-mail: info@toperamedical.com
Web site: www.toperamedical.com
Ownership: Private
Produces/Sells CE-marked Devices: N
General Admin.: Dr. Edward Kerslake/Chief Executive Officer
     Dr. Sanjiv Narayan/Chief Scientific Officer
Mktg./Adv.: Ms. Amy Siegel/Vice President Marketing
Finance: Ms. Diane Marcou/Chief Financial Officer

TOPEX, INC   203-748-5918
10 Precision Road, Danbury, CT 06810
FDA Number: 3006110296

Therapeutic X-Ray System	Radiology

TOPEZ ORTHOPEDICS, INC   303-865-5105
4820 N. 63 Rd., #104, Boulder, CO 80301
FDA Number: 3005663955
Ownership: Private
Produces/Sells CE-marked Devices: N

Prosthesis, Ankle, Semi-Constrained, Metal/Polymer	Orthopedics

TORAX MEDICAL, INC.   651-361-8900
4188 Lexington Avenue North, Shoreview, MN 55126
FDA Number: n/a   *Fax:* 651-361-8910
E-mail: info@toraxmedical.com
Web site: www.toraxmedical.com

TORAX MEDICAL, INC.   651-361-8900 (cont'd)
Ownership: Private
Produces/Sells CE-marked Devices: N
General Admin.: Mr. Todd Berg/President, Chief Executive Officer
Mktg./Adv.: Mr. Brent Collins/Vice President Market Development
Research: Mr. Jon St. Germain/Vice President Research & Development
Finance: Mr. Brian Mower/Vice President Finance

TORAY INTERNATIONAL AMERICA INC.   800-662-1777
140 Cypress Station Dr., Ste. 210,   **281-587-2299**
Houston, TX 77090
FDA Number: 2435106   *Fax:* 281-587-9933
E-mail: s.lewis@toray-intl.com
Web site: www.torayusa.com/medical
Year Founded: 1988
Ownership: Private
Stock Symbol: N/A
Produces/Sells CE-marked Devices: Y
Distribution: Manufacturer Direct, Exclusive Distributor, Importer, Exporter
General Admin.: Ms. Karen Newbolt/Assistant Manager
     Susan Lewis/Manager Admin.
Production: Dennis M. Metcalf/Director Medical Products

Catheter, Percutaneous (Valvuloplasty)	Cardiovascular
Guidewire, Catheter	Cardiovascular

TORBOT GROUP INC., JOBSKIN DIVISION   800-207-1074
653 Miami Street, Toledo, OH 43605   **419-724-1475**
FDA Number: 3004083786   *Fax:* 419-724-1476
E-mail: Jobskincs@torbot.com
Web site: www.torbotgarments.com
Total Employees: 28
Ownership: Torbot Group, Inc.
Produces/Sells CE-marked Devices: N
Federal Procurement Eligibility: Small Business
Distribution: Manufacturer Direct, Manufacturer Through Distributor
General Admin.: Greg Johnson/General Manager

Binder, Medical, Therapeutic	General
Elastomer, Silicone (Scar Management)	Surgery

TORBOT GROUP, INC.   800-545-4254
1367 Elmwood Ave., Cranston, RI 02910   **401-780-8737**
FDA Number: 2417346   *Fax:* 401-780-8740
E-mail: contactus@torbot.com
Web site: www.torbot.com
Medical Products Sales Volume: $5,000,000
Annual Revenue: $1-$5 Million
Year Founded: 1999
Total Employees: 20   *Marketing Staff:* 1   *Sales Staff:* 2
Ownership: Private
Produces/Sells CE-marked Devices: Y
Federal Procurement Eligibility: Small Business, Female Owned
Distribution: Manufacturer Direct, Manufacturer Through Distributor, Exporter
General Admin.: David Nathanson/Chief Operating Officer
     Mr. Gregory Johnson/General Manager
Mktg./Adv.: Ms. Lisa Blanchette/Manager Sales
     Mr. Lawrence Sadwin/Vice President Business Development
Production: Claire Hebert/Supervisor Customer Service

Adhesive, Liquid	General
Bag, Drainage (Incontinence)	Gastroenterology/Urology
Bag, Drainage, Ostomy (With Adhesive)	General
Bag, Urinary Collection	General
Bag, Urinary, Ileostomy	Gastroenterology/Urology
Cement, Stomal Appliance, Ostomy	Gastroenterology/Urology
Collector, Ostomy	Gastroenterology/Urology
Colostomy Appliance, Disposable	Gastroenterology/Urology
Irrigator, Ostomy	Gastroenterology/Urology
Ostomy Appliance (Ileostomy, Colostomy)	Gastroenterology/Urology

Medical Product Subsidiaries (Listed Separately)
Torbot Group Inc., Jobskin Division

TORK   914-664-3542
1 Grove St., Mount Vernon, NY 10550-2401
FDA Number: n/a   *Fax:* 914-664-5052
E-mail: emintzer@tork.com
Web site: www.tork.com
Annual Revenue: $10-$25 Million
Year Founded: 1922
Total Employees: 200
Ownership: Private
Produces/Sells CE-marked Devices: N
Federal Procurement Eligibility: Small Business
Distribution: Manufacturer Through Distributor, Manufacturer Through Manufacturer Reps, OEM, Exporter
General Admin.: Sam Shanker/Chief Executive Officer
Mktg./Adv.: Tony Collins/Director Marketing & Sales
     Elliot Mintzer/Manager Marketing
Production: Len Caponigro/Manager Production

TORK   914-664-3542 *(cont'd)*
Security Equipment/Supplies   General

TORNADO INDUSTRIES   800-822-8867
7401 W. Lawrence Ave., Chicago, IL 60706   708-867-5100
FDA Number: n/a   Fax: 708-867-6968
E-mail: marketing@tornadovac.com
Web site: www.tornadovac.com
Annual Revenue: $1-$5 Million
Total Employees: 110   *Sales Staff:* 31
Ownership: Private
Produces/Sells CE-marked Devices: N
Federal Procurement Eligibility: Small Business, Female Owned
Distribution: Manufacturer Through Distributor
General Admin.: Linda Breuer/President
Mktg./Adv.: Michael Schaffer/Vice President Sales
Production: Tom Bogusevic/Vice President Manufacturing
Finance: Gary Cirone/Vice President Finance
Housekeeping Equipment   General

TORNIER INC.   800-611-2992
100 Cummings Center, Suite 444c,   978-232-9997
Beverly, MA 01915
FDA Number: 1226487
Ownership: Private
Produces/Sells CE-marked Devices: N
Cutter, Wire And Pin   Orthopedics
Fastener, Fixation, Biodegradable, Soft Tissue   Orthopedics
Fastener, Fixation, Non-Biodegradable, Soft Tissue   Orthopedics
Guide, Surgical, Instrument   Surgery
Instrument, Manual, General Surgical   Surgery
Mallet, Surgical, General & Plastic Surgery   Surgery
Mesh, Surgical, Polymeric   Surgery
Needle, Suture, Disposable   Surgery
Orthopedic Manual Surgical Instrument   Orthopedics
Pin, Fixation, Threaded   Orthopedics
Plate, Fixation, Bone   Orthopedics
Prosthesis, Wrist, Carpal Trapezium   Orthopedics
Punch, Surgical   Surgery
Rasp, Other   Surgery
Screw, Fixation, Bone   Orthopedics
Staple, Fixation, Bone   Orthopedics
Suture, Non-Absorbable, Synthetic, Polyethylene   Surgery
Suture, Non-Absorbable, Synthetic, Polypropylene   Surgery
Tray, Surgical Instrument   Surgery

TORONTO RESEARCH CHEMICALS INC.   800-727-9240
2 Brisbane Rd., Toronto, ONT M3J-2J8 Canada   416-665-9696
FDA Number: n/a   Fax: 416-665-4439
E-mail: torresch@interlog.com
Web site: www.trc-canada.com
Year Founded: 1982
Ownership: Private
Produces/Sells CE-marked Devices: N
Distribution: Manufacturer Direct

TOSHIBA AMERICA MEDICAL SYSTEMS   800-421-1968
2441 Michelle Dr., Tustin, CA 92780-7014   714-730-5000
FDA Number: 2020563   Fax: 714-832-2570
E-mail: mktgcomm@tams.com
Web site: www.medical.toshiba.com
Medical Products Sales Volume: $400,000,000
Year Founded: 1969
Total Employees: 920
Ownership: Private
Quality System Registration Information: ISO9000; ISO9001
Produces/Sells CE-marked Devices: Y
Distribution: Manufacturer Direct, Exclusive Distributor
General Admin.: Mr. Toshiya Miyaguchi/President
    Frederic J. Friedberg/Senior Vice President, General Counsel
    Lawrence Dentice/Senior Vice President, General Manager
    Mr. Donald Fowler/Senior Vice President, General Manager
Mktg./Adv.: Cathy Wolfe/Director Corporate Communications
    Mr. Aaron Hudy/Vice President Sales
Production: Mr. Doug Ryan/Vice President Manufacturing & Development
Finance: Mr. Kevin Abbott/Chief Financial Officer
Image Processing System   Radiology
Nuclear Magnetic Resonance Imaging System   Radiology
Radiographic Unit, Diagnostic   Radiology
Radiographic/Fluoroscopic Unit, Angiographic   Radiology
Radiographic/Fluoroscopic Unit, Image-Intensified   Radiology
Scanner, Computed Tomography, X-Ray, Special Procedure   Radiology
Scanner, Emission Computed Tomography   Radiology
Scanner, Nuclear, Tomographic   Radiology
Scanner, Ultrasonic (Pulsed Doppler)   Radiology
Scanner, Ultrasonic (Pulsed Echo)   Radiology
Scanner, Ultrasonic, Pediatric   Radiology
Scanner, Ultrasonic, Small Parts   Radiology
Simulator, Radiotherapy   Radiology

TOSHIBA AMERICA MEDICAL SYSTEMS   800-421-1968 *(cont'd)*
System, Communication, Image, Digital   Radiology
System, X-Ray, Mobile   Radiology
Table, Radiographic, Non-Tilting, Powered   Radiology
Table, Radiographic, Tilting   Radiology
Transducer, Ultrasonic, Diagnostic   Radiology

TOSHIBA AMERICA MEDICAL SYSTEMS, INC.   800-421-1968
280 Utah Ave., South San Francisco, CA 94080-6883
FDA Number: 2020563
Ownership: Private
Produces/Sells CE-marked Devices: N
Nuclear Magnetic Resonance Imaging System   Radiology

TOSHIBA AMERICA MRI, INC.
See Toshiba America Medical Systems, Inc.

TOSOH BIOSCIENCE LLC   800-366-4875
156 Keystone Drive,   215-283-5000
Montgomeryville, PA 18936
FDA Number: n/a   Fax: 215-283-5035
E-mail: techservice.tbl@tosoh.com
Web site: www.tosohbioscience.com
Annual Revenue: $10-$25 Million
Year Founded: 1987
Total Employees: 25
Ownership: TOSOH CORP.
Quality System Registration Information: ISO9002
Produces/Sells CE-marked Devices: N
Distribution: Manufacturer Direct, Manufacturer Through Distributor, OEM,
Importer, Exporter
General Admin.: Shigeru Nakatani/Executive Vice President
    Hiroyuki Uchida/President, Chief Executive Officer
Mktg./Adv.: Dr. Roy Eksteen/Director Marketing
    Thomas Higley/Manager New Product Development
High Performance Liquid Chromatography, Cyclosporine   Chemistry

TOSOH BIOSCIENCE, INC.   614-317-1909
3600 Gantz Road, Grove City, OH 43123
FDA Number: 3005529799
E-mail: info.diag.am@tosoh.com
Web site: www.diagnostics.us.tosohbioscience.com
Year Founded: 1989
Ownership: TOSOH CORP.
Produces/Sells CE-marked Devices: N
Radioimmunoassay, Dehydroepiandrosterone (Free And Sulfate)   Chemistry
Radioimmunoassay, Follicle Stimulating Hormone   Chemistry
Radioimmunoassay, Luteinizing Hormone   Chemistry
Radioimmunoassay, Prolactin (Lactogen)   Chemistry
Radioimmunoassay, Testosterones And Dihydrotestosterone   Chemistry
Radioimmunoassay, Total Triiodothyronine   Chemistry

TOSOH BIOSCIENCE, INC.   800-248-6764
6000 Shoreline Court, Suite 101,   614-317-1909
South San Francisco, CA 94080
FDA Number: 2950409
E-mail: info.diag.am@tosoh.com
Web site: www.diagnostics.us.tosohbioscience.com
Year Founded: 1989
Ownership: TOSOH CORP.
Produces/Sells CE-marked Devices: N
Antigen, Antiserum, Control, Carcinoembryonic Antigen   Immunology
Antigen, Antiserum, Control, Myoglobin   Immunology
Antigen, Prostate-Specific (PSA), Management, Cancer   Immunology
Enzymatic Method, Troponin Subunit   Chemistry
Fluorometer, Chemistry   Chemistry
Fluorometric Method, CPK Or Isoenzymes   Chemistry
Fluorometric, Cortisol   Chemistry
Hemoglobin A2 Quantitation   Hematology
Kit, Test, Alpha-fetoprotein For Testicular Cancer   Immunology
Radioassay, Triiodothyronine Uptake   Chemistry
Radioimmunoassay, C Peptides Of Proinsulin   Chemistry
Radioimmunoassay, Estradiol   Chemistry
Radioimmunoassay, Ferritin   Microbiology
Radioimmunoassay, Folic Acid   Chemistry
Radioimmunoassay, Follicle Stimulating Hormone   Chemistry
Radioimmunoassay, Free Thyroxine   Chemistry
Radioimmunoassay, Human Growth Hormone   Chemistry
Radioimmunoassay, Immunoglobulins (D, E)   Immunology
Radioimmunoassay, Immunoreactive Insulin   Chemistry
Radioimmunoassay, Luteinizing Hormone   Chemistry
Radioimmunoassay, Progesterone   Chemistry
Radioimmunoassay, Prolactin (Lactogen)   Chemistry
Radioimmunoassay, Testosterones And Dihydrotestosterone   Chemistry
Radioimmunoassay, Thyroid Stimulating Hormone   Chemistry
Radioimmunoassay, Total Thyroxine   Chemistry
Radioimmunoassay, Total Triiodothyronine   Chemistry
Radioimmunoassay, Vitamin B12   Chemistry
System, Test, Carbohydrate Antigen (ca19-9), For Monitoring And Management Of
Pancreatic Cancer   Immunology

TOSOH BIOSCIENCE, INC.   800-248-6764 *(cont'd)*

System, Test, Immunological, Antigen, Tumor	Immunology
Tartrate Inhibited, Acid Phosphatase (Prostatic)	Chemistry
Test, Antigen (CA125), Tumor-Associated, Ovarian, Epithelial	Immunology
Test, Beta 2 - Microglobulin	Immunology
Test, Glycosylated Hemoglobin Assay	Hematology
Test, Thyroid Autoantibody	Immunology

TOSOHAAS
See Tosoh Bioscience Llc

TOTAL CARE
See Total Care

TOTAL HEALTH PRODUCTS/EAST ATLANTIC TRD.
See East Atlantic Trading/Triangle Healthcare Inc.

TOTAL HEALTHCARE EQUIPMENT (T.H.E.) MEDICAL   800-565-7075

75 Dyment Rd., Barrie, ONT L4N 3H6 Canada   **705-733-0022**
FDA Number: n/a   *Fax:* 705-733-3432
E-mail: theadmin@themedical.com
Web site: www.themedical.com
Year Founded: 1992
Total Employees: 10
Ownership: Private
Produces/Sells CE-marked Devices: N
Distribution: Manufacturer Direct, Exclusive Distributor, Importer

TOTAL INNOVATIVE MANUFACTURING   616-738-8299
12688 New Holland St., Holland, MI 49424
FDA Number: 3004598639
Ownership: Private
Produces/Sells CE-marked Devices: N

Transfer Device, Patient, Manual	General

TOTAL MOLDING SERVICES, INC.   215-538-9613
354 East Broad St., Trumbauersville, PA 18970
FDA Number: 2529596   *Fax:* 215-538-2519
E-mail: info@totalmoldingservices.com
Web site: www.totalmoldingservices.com
Year Founded: 1985
Total Employees: 40   *Sales Staff:* 2
Ownership: Private
Produces/Sells CE-marked Devices: Y
Distribution: Exclusive Distributor
General Admin.: Ms. Elizabeth Hrycko/Admin. Human Resources
   Mr. Thomas McNutt, Jr./President
Production: Mrs. Cynthia Dise/Customer Service Representative
   Mr. Nathan Scherff/Designer

Adapter, Stopcock, Manifold, Cardiopulmonary Bypass	Cardiovascular
Adapter, Y	Gastroenterology/Urology
Applier, Surgical Staple	Surgery
Bag, Blood, Collection	Hematology
Cap, Surgical	Surgery
Cap, Tip, Syringe	General
Conformer, Ophthalmic	Ophthalmology
Detector, Air Bubble	Gastroenterology/Urology
Electrocautery Unit, Endoscopic	Obstetrics/Gynecology
Exerciser, Non-Measuring	Physical Med
Guard, Disk	Dental And Oral
Mouthguard	Dental And Oral
Occluder, Ophthalmic	Ophthalmology
Shield, Eye, Ophthalmic	Ophthalmology
Spatula, Surgical, General & Plastic Surgery	Surgery
Syringe, Angioplasty	Cardiovascular
Syringe, Other	General
Tube, Gastrointestinal	Gastroenterology/Urology

TOTAL MOTION RESTORATION, LLC   678-910-0156
9990 Devonshire St., Douglasville, GA 30135
FDA Number: 3005418721

Traction Unit, Non-Powered	Orthopedics

TOTAL MOTION, INC.   281-386-8747
19606 Piney Place Court, Houston, TX 77094
FDA Number: 3005257745
E-mail: Sales@Total-Motion.com
Web site: www.total-motion.com
Ownership: Private
Produces/Sells CE-marked Devices: N

Exerciser, Non-Measuring	Physical Med

TOTAL ORTHOPEDIC
See Total Care

TOTAL TITANIUM   618-473-2429
140 E. Monroe St., Hecker, IL 62248
FDA Number: n/a   *Fax:* 618-473-2156
Medical Products Sales Volume: $250,000
Annual Revenue: $0-$1 Million
Total Employees: 12   *Sales Staff:* 2

TOTAL TITANIUM   618-473-2429 *(cont'd)*
Ownership: Private
Produces/Sells CE-marked Devices: N
Federal Procurement Eligibility: Small Business
Distribution: Manufacturer Direct
General Admin.: Brian Casey/President, Chief Executive Officer
   Ron Casey/Vice President

Cannula, Ophthalmic	Ophthalmology
Hook, Ophthalmic	Ophthalmology
Knife, Ear	Ear/Nose/Throat
Knife, Ophthalmic	Ophthalmology
Molding, Injection	General
Retractor, Ophthalmic	Ophthalmology
Ring, Ophthalmic (Flieringa)	Ophthalmology
Spatula, Ophthalmic	Ophthalmology
Tube, Ear Suction	Ear/Nose/Throat

TOTAL TITANIUM, INC.   618-473-2429
140 East Monroe St., Hecker, IL 62248
FDA Number: 1424658

Caliper, Ophthalmic	Ophthalmology
Cannula, Ophthalmic	Ophthalmology
Curette, Ophthalmic	Ophthalmology
Dilator, Lacrimal	Ophthalmology
Forceps, Ophthalmic	Ophthalmology
Hook, Ophthalmic	Ophthalmology
Knife, Ophthalmic	Ophthalmology
Marker, Ocular	Ophthalmology
Probe, Lacrimal	Ophthalmology
Retractor, Ophthalmic	Ophthalmology
Ring, Ophthalmic (Flieringa)	Ophthalmology
Scissors, Ophthalmic	Ophthalmology
Spatula, Ophthalmic	Ophthalmology
Speculum, Ophthalmic	Ophthalmology

TOTER, INC.   800-772-0071   704-872-8171
841 Meacham Road, PO Box 5338, Statesville, NC 28677
FDA Number: n/a   *Fax:* 704-878-0734
E-mail: info@toter.com
Web site: www.toter.com
Medical Products Sales Volume: $38,100,000
Annual Revenue: $25-$50 Million
Year Founded: 1962
Total Employees: 150
Ownership: Private
Produces/Sells CE-marked Devices: N
Federal Procurement Eligibility: Small Business, GSA Contract
Distribution: Manufacturer Through Distributor, Manufacturer Through Manufacturer Reps
Mktg./Adv.: John Ford/Manager Advertising
   Brian Park/Manager International & National Sales
   Sherwyn Beaver/Manager Sales Training
Production: Ira Bradley/Director Quality Assurance
   Don Sexton/Manager Manufacturing

Cart, Waste	General

TOTO KIKI USA, INC.   888-295-8134   770-282-8686
1155 Southern Road, Morrow, GA 30260
FDA Number: n/a   *Fax:* 770-282-8698
E-mail: custservice@totousa.com
Web site: www.totousa.com
Medical Products Sales Volume: $100,000
Annual Revenue: $1-$5 Million
Year Founded: 1917
Total Employees: 400   *Marketing Staff:* 6   *Sales Staff:* 24
Ownership: Private
Traded On: Tokyo
Federal Procurement Eligibility: Small Business
Distribution: Exclusive Distributor
General Admin.: Yasuji Moriyana/Chief Executive Officer
   Toshio Kitano/President
Mktg./Adv.: Kazuo Watanabe/Director Marketing
   Newbold Warden/Manager Marketing & Advertising

Commode Seat	General

TOUCH BIONICS   614-388-8075
3455 Mill Run Drive, Hilliard, OH 43026
FDA Number: 3008018840   *Fax:* 614-388-8079
E-mail: info@touchbionics.com
Web site: www.livingskin.com
Ownership: Private
Produces/Sells CE-marked Devices: N

Prosthesis, Finger	Orthopedics
Prosthesis, Finger, Total	Orthopedics
Prosthesis, Hand	Orthopedics

TOUCH TURNER COMPANY
888-811-1962
360-651-1962
13621 103rd Avenue NE,
Arlington, WA 98223
FDA Number: n/a
Fax: 360-658-9380
E-mail: sales@touchturner.com
Web site: www.touchturner.com
Medical Products Sales Volume: $200,000
Annual Revenue: $0-$1 Million
Year Founded: 1950
Total Employees: 3   *Marketing Staff:* 1   *Sales Staff:* 1
Ownership: Private
Produces/Sells CE-marked Devices: N
Federal Procurement Eligibility: Small Business, Female Owned
Distribution: Manufacturer Direct, Manufacturer Through Manufacturer Reps, OEM, Importer, Exporter
Mktg./Adv.: Karen Rieger/Director Marketing
     Karen Rieger/Manager Sales Training
     Karen Rieger/President, Director Marketing
Production: Dennis Rieger/Vice President Manufacturing

Page Turner (Handicapped)	General

TOWER MANUFACTURING CO.
See Premier Medical Products

TOWER MEDICAL SYSTEM, LTD.
631-699-3200
917-11 Lincoln Ave., Holbrook, NY 11741
FDA Number: 3003747574
Fax: 631-699-3201
E-mail: info@towermedicalsystems.com
Web site: www.towermedicalsystems.com
Medical Products Sales Volume: $90,000
Annual Revenue: $1-$5 Million
Year Founded: 1989
Total Employees: 10   *Marketing Staff:* 5   *Sales Staff:* 3
Ownership: Private
Produces/Sells CE-marked Devices: N
Federal Procurement Eligibility: Small Business, Female Owned
Distribution: Manufacturer Direct, Manufacturer Through Distributor, Manufacturer Through Manufacturer Reps, Exporter
General Admin.: Josephine Chillemi/President
     Anthony Chillemi/Vice President
Mktg./Adv.: Vivian Chillemi/Manager National Marketing & Sales

Cabinet, Other	General
Radiographic/Fluoroscopic Unit, Mobile C-Arm	Radiology
Table, Examination/Treatment	General
Table, Radiographic, Non-Tilting, Powered	Radiology
Table, Radiographic, Stationary Top	Radiology
Table, Radiographic, Tilting	Radiology

TOWIC MEDICAL, INC.
847-823-2215
303 S Clifton, PO Box 883, Park Ridge, IL 60068-0883
FDA Number: 1450221
Fax: 847-823-2230
E-mail: towicimi@attbi.com
Medical Products Sales Volume: $440,000
Year Founded: 1986
Total Employees: 4
Ownership: Private
Produces/Sells CE-marked Devices: N
Federal Procurement Eligibility: Small Business, Female Owned
Distribution: Manufacturer Direct, Manufacturer Through Manufacturer Reps
General Admin.: J. Mrowiec/Chief Executive Officer
     K. Toter/President
Mktg./Adv.: J. Reinthaler/Manager Advertising
     M. Lenz/Manager Market Research
     W. Toter/Manager Product Development

Bag, Drainage, Nasogastric	General

TOWN & COUNTRY DENTAL STUDIOS
516-868-8641
275 South Main St., Freeport, NY 11520
FDA Number: 3005193491

Device, Anti-Snoring	Ear/Nose/Throat

TOYAD CORP.
See Chestnut Ridge Foam, Inc.

TP LABORATORIES INC.
See Tp Orthodontics, Inc.

TP ORTHODONTICS, INC.
800-348-8856
219-785-2591
100 Center Plaza, La Porte, IN 46350-9672
FDA Number: 1815540
Fax: 219-324-3029
E-mail: info@tportho.com
Web site: www.tportho.com
Year Founded: 1940
Total Employees: 400   *Marketing Staff:* 6   *Sales Staff:* 20
Ownership: Private
Quality System Registration Information: ISO9001
Produces/Sells CE-marked Devices: Y
Federal Procurement Eligibility: Small Business

TP ORTHODONTICS, INC.
800-348-8856 *(cont'd)*
Distribution: Manufacturer Direct, Manufacturer Through Distributor, Exclusive Distributor, Exporter
General Admin.: Mr. Andrew Kesling/Chief Executive Officer
     Mr. John Skierkowski/Manager Personnel
     Mr. Andrew Kesling/President
Mktg./Adv.: Mrs. Mary Knaup/Director Advertising
     Mrs. Cassia Coelho/Manager Sales
     Ms. Sandra Hoefer/Vice President Marketing & Sales
Production: Mr. Douglas Biege/Manager Regulatory Affairs
     Mr. William Beesley/Vice President Manufacturing
Purchasing: Mrs. Norma Szczepaniak/Manager Purchasing

Adhesive, Dental	Dental And Oral
Band, Material, Orthodontic	Dental And Oral
Bracket, Metal, Orthodontic	Dental And Oral
Component, Ceramic	General
Headgear, Extraoral, Orthodontic	Dental And Oral
Orthodontic Instrument	Dental And Oral
Pliers, Orthodontic	Dental And Oral
Positioner, Tooth, Preformed	Dental And Oral
Protector, Mouth Guard	Dental And Oral
Retainer, Screw Expansion, Orthodontic	Dental And Oral
Splint, Other	Orthopedics
Tray, Impression	Dental And Oral
Tube, Orthodontic	Dental And Oral
Wire, Orthodontic	Dental And Oral

TPC ADVANCED TECHNOLOGY, INC.
800-560-8222
626-810-4337
18525 East Gale Ave., City of Industry, CA 91748
FDA Number: 2031508
E-mail: danny@kingstwodental.com
Annual Revenue: $1-$5 Million
Total Employees: 3   *Marketing Staff:* 2   *Sales Staff:* 2
Ownership: Private
Produces/Sells CE-marked Devices: N
Distribution: OEM
Mktg./Adv.: Scott Beckley/Vice President Sales

Activator, Ultraviolet, Polymerization	Dental And Oral
Amalgamator, Dental, AC-Powered	Dental And Oral
Applicator, Tipped, Absorbent, Non-Sterile	General
Carboxymethylcellulose Sodium (40-100%)	Dental And Oral
Chair, Dental	Dental And Oral
Cup, Prophylaxis	Dental And Oral
Drill, Dental, Intraoral	Dental And Oral
Handpiece, Air-Powered, Dental	Dental And Oral
Holder, X-Ray Film	Dental And Oral
Illuminator, Radiographic Film	Radiology
Light, Fiberoptic, Dental	Dental And Oral
Scaler, Periodontic	Dental And Oral
Scaler, Ultrasonic	Dental And Oral
Syringe, Restorative And Impression Material	Dental And Oral

TPV MANUFACTURINGü
978-425-8940
2 Shaker Road, Unit A101, Shirley, MA 01464
FDA Number: n/a
Fax: 978-425-8924
E-mail: sales@trstpe.com
Web site: www.trstpe.com
Annual Revenue: $1-$5 Million
Total Employees: 9   *Marketing Staff:* 1   *Sales Staff:* 1
Ownership: Private
Produces/Sells CE-marked Devices: N
Federal Procurement Eligibility: Small Business, Minority Owned
Distribution: Manufacturer Direct
General Admin.: Jonas Angus/President

Elastomer, Other	General

TR GROUP, INC.
800-752-6900
847-724-6600
903 Wedel Lane, Glenview, IL 60025
FDA Number: 1422399
Fax: 847-724-8566
E-mail: information@trequipment.com
Web site: www.trequipment.com
Ownership: Private
Produces/Sells CE-marked Devices: N
Mktg./Adv.: Sharon Grason/Director Marketing

Bath, Hydro-Massage (Whirlpool)	Physical Med
Bath, Sitz, Non-Powered	Physical Med
Lift, Bath, Non-AC-Powered	General
Lift, Patient	General
Pack, Hot Or Cold, Disposable	Physical Med
Patient Transfer Unit, Powered	General
Stretcher, Wheeled (Mobile)	General
Transfer Device, Patient, Manual	General
Walker, Mechanical	Physical Med

TRA & ACCESSORIES
909-305-1944
449 West Allen Ave. Suite 107, San Dimas, CA 91773
FDA Number: 2028947
Ownership: Private
Produces/Sells CE-marked Devices: N

TRA & ACCESSORIES 909-305-1944 *(cont'd)*
Tonometer, Manual   Ophthalmology

TRAC ABOUT, INC. 800-458-8616
PO Box 502, 1801 SE 9th St.,   316-283-5660
Newton, KS 67114
FDA Number: 1954330   *Fax: 316-283-0693*
E-mail: info@tracabout.com
Web site: www.tracabout.com
Medical Products Sales Volume: $200,000
Year Founded: 1985
Total Employees: 3
Ownership: Private
Produces/Sells CE-marked Devices: Y
Federal Procurement Eligibility: Small Business
Distribution: Manufacturer Direct, Manufacturer Through Distributor, Manufacturer Through Manufacturer Reps, OEM
General Admin.: Mr. Darren Wells/President
            Mr. Steve Wells/Vice President
Production: Mr. Lloyd Wolf/Vice President Operations
Wheelchair, Powered   Physical Med

TRAC ELECTRONICS 919-876-8088
1100 West Chatham St., Cary, NC 27511
FDA Number: 1058550
Ownership: Private
Produces/Sells CE-marked Devices: N
System, X-Ray, Mobile   Radiology

TRACE LABORATORIES-EAST 410-584-9099
5 N. Park Drive, Hunt Valley, MD 21030
FDA Number: n/a   *Fax: 410-584-9117*
E-mail: traceeast@tracelabs.com
Web site: www.tracelabs.com
Annual Revenue: $1-$5 Million
Year Founded: 1980
Total Employees: 20   Marketing Staff: 1   Sales Staff: 5
Ownership: Private
Quality System Registration Information: ISO9001
Produces/Sells CE-marked Devices: N
Federal Procurement Eligibility: Small Business
Distribution: Service Direct
General Admin.: Scott Opperhauser/Vice President, General Manager
Mktg./Adv.: Mary T. Opperhauser/Director Marketing
Production: Renee Michalkiewicz/Director Manufacturing
Research: John Radman/Director Research & Development
Contract Laboratory   General
Monitor, Radiation   Radiology
Spectrometer, Infrared   Chemistry
Tube, X-Ray   Radiology
Vehicle/Equipment, Recreational (Handicapped)   General

TRACE MEDICAL EQUIPMENT, INC. 800-323-3786
5000 Varsity Drive, Lisle, IL 60532   630-963-9696
FDA Number: 1422281   *Fax: 630-963-1611*
E-mail: tracemed@aol.com
Medical Products Sales Volume: $920,000
Year Founded: 1981
Total Employees: 7
Ownership: Private
Produces/Sells CE-marked Devices: N
Federal Procurement Eligibility: Small Business
Bed, Pediatric (Crib)   General
Lift, Bath, Non-AC-Powered   General

TRACER DESIGNS, INC. 805-933-2616
333 South 11th St., Santa Paula, CA 93060
FDA Number: 2024944
Bone Mill   Orthopedics

TRACERLAB
See Mirion Technologies

TRACEY TECHNOLOGIES CORP. 281-445-1666
16720 Hedgecroft Dr., Suite 208, Houston, TX 77060
FDA Number: 1651254
Aberrometer, Ophthalmic   Ophthalmology
Refractometer, Ophthalmic   Ophthalmology

TRACK CORPORATION 616-850-9444
17024 Taft Road, Spring Lake, MI 49456
FDA Number: 3004976290
Table, Physical Medicine, Powered   Physical Med

TRACO MEDICAL EQUIPMENT 605-339-9339
3505 S. Norton Ave, Sioux Falls, SD 57105
FDA Number: n/a   *Fax: 605-334-3025*
Web site: www.tracomedical.com
Year Founded: 1983

TRACO MEDICAL EQUIPMENT 605-339-9339 *(cont'd)*
Ownership: Private
Produces/Sells CE-marked Devices: N
Federal Procurement Eligibility: Small Business
Distribution: Manufacturer Direct, Service Direct, Exporter
General Admin.: Ken Smith/President
Service, Used Equipment   General

TRACOR HOLDINGS
See Tremetrics

TRACOR INC.
See Tremetrics

TRACOR INSTRUMENTS AUSTIN, INC.
See Tremetrics

TRACOUSTICS INC.
See Starkey Laboratories, Inc.

TRADEMARK MEDICAL
See Trademark Medical Llc

TRADEMARK MEDICAL LLC 800-325-9044
449 Soverign Ct, St. Louis, MO 63011   636-527-2288
FDA Number: 1937137   *Fax: 636-527-0255*
E-mail: info@trademarkmedical.com
Web site: www.trademarkmedical.com
Medical Products Sales Volume: $1,200,000
Year Founded: 1976
Total Employees: 8   Marketing Staff: 2   Sales Staff: 5
Ownership: Private
Produces/Sells CE-marked Devices: Y
Federal Procurement Eligibility: Small Business, VA Contract
Distribution: Manufacturer Direct, Manufacturer Through Distributor, Manufacturer Through Manufacturer Reps, Exclusive Distributor
Mktg./Adv.: Robert Egan/President, Director Sales
            Peter Digasbarro/Vice President National Sales
Finance: J. M. Peckham/Manager Acctg.
Analyzer, Composition, Weight, Patient   General
Aspirator, Emergency Suction   General
Box, Glove   Microbiology
Communication Equipment   General
Cover, Cast   General
Cover, Other   General
Crusher, Pill   General
Cutter, Pill   General
Eyeglasses, Safety   Ophthalmology
Goggles, Protective, Eye   Ophthalmology
Monitor, Temperature, Surgery   Surgery
Pad, Pressure, Foam (Elbow, Heel)   General
Remover, Blade, Scalpel   General
Shield, Protective, Personnel   Radiology
Stand/Holder, Equipment, Laboratory   Chemistry
Temperature Strip, Forehead, Liquid Crystal   General
Thermometer, Chemical Color Change   General
Thermometer, Liquid Crystals   Surgery
Toothbrush, Powered   Dental And Oral
Tube, Connecting   General
Tube, Nasogastric   Anesthesiology

TRADEWINDS REHABILITATION CENTER, INC. 219-949-4000
5901 West 7th Ave., Gary, IN 46406
FDA Number: 1833484   *Fax: 219-944-8134*
E-mail: cskozen@tradewindservices.org
Web site: www.tradewindservices.org
Ownership: Private
Produces/Sells CE-marked Devices: N
Accessories, Apparel, Surgical   Surgery
Gown, Isolation, Surgical   Surgery

TRADEX INTERNATIONAL 800-456-8370
5300 Tradex Pkwy, Cleveland, OH 44102
FDA Number: 1527823   *Fax: 216-651-4770*
Web site: www.tradexgloves.com
Medical Products Sales Volume: $5,000,000
Annual Revenue: $1-$5 Million
Year Founded: 1988
Ownership: Private
Produces/Sells CE-marked Devices: N
Federal Procurement Eligibility: Small Business, Minority Owned
Distribution: Manufacturer Through Distributor
General Admin.: Saji Daniels/President, Chief Executive Officer
Glove, Patient Examination, Latex   General
Glove, Patient Examination, Vinyl   General

TRADEX MEDICAL PRODUCTS, INC.
See Tradex International

TRADIS INC.
See Comfort Touch

TRAINER'S CHOICE INC.
800-706-9834
705-721-5138
205-480 Huronia Road,
Barrie, ONT L4N 6 Canada
FDA Number: n/a   *Fax:* 705-733-8057
E-mail: info@trainerschoice.on.ca
Web site: www.trainerschoice.on.ca
Year Founded: 1989
Total Employees: 10
Ownership: Private
Produces/Sells CE-marked Devices: N
Distribution: Manufacturer Direct, Exclusive Distributor

TRAINEX CORPORATION
See Medcom, Inc.

TRAN PA-C, INC.
321-276-5407
3348 Herringridge Dr., Orlando, FL 32812
FDA Number: 3005761465
Ownership: Private
Produces/Sells CE-marked Devices: N

Scalpel, One-Piece (Knife)	Surgery

TRANS AMERICAN MEDICAL
800-626-9232
708-430-7777
7633 W. 100th Pl., Bridgeview, IL 60455
FDA Number: n/a   *Fax:* 708-430-7873
E-mail: info@tamsco.biz
Web site: www.tamsco.biz
Medical Products Sales Volume: $600,000
Annual Revenue: $0-$1 Million
Year Founded: 1992
Total Employees: 5   *Marketing Staff:* 1   *Sales Staff:* 1
Ownership: Trans American Medical / Tamsco Instruments
Produces/Sells CE-marked Devices: N
Federal Procurement Eligibility: Small Business
Distribution: Manufacturer Through Distributor, Manufacturer Through Manufacturer Reps, OEM, Exporter
General Admin.: Jay Younis/President, Chief Executive Officer

Forceps, Hemostatic	Surgery
General Use Surgical Scissors	Surgery
Holder, Needle	Gastroenterology/Urology
Scissors, Bandage/Gauze/Plaster	General
Scissors, Iris	Ophthalmology

TRANS AMERICAN MEDICAL / TAMSCO INSTRUMENTS
708-430-7777
7633 W. 100th Pl, Bridgeview, IL 60455-2433
FDA Number: 7000740   *Fax:* 708-430-7873
E-mail: info@tamsco.biz
Web site: www.tamsco.biz
Medical Products Sales Volume: $600,000
Annual Revenue: $1-$5 Million
Year Founded: 1979
Total Employees: 5   *Marketing Staff:* 1   *Sales Staff:* 3
Ownership: Private
Produces/Sells CE-marked Devices: Y
Federal Procurement Eligibility: Small Business, Minority Owned
Distribution: Manufacturer Through Distributor, Manufacturer Through Manufacturer Reps, OEM
General Admin.: M. Younis/President
Mktg./Adv.: Jay Younis/Manager International & National Sales
     Jay Younis/Vice President Marketing & Sales
Production: M. Younis/Vice President Manufacturing
Research: Peter Ryan/Vice President Research & Development

Curette	Orthopedics
Curette, Ear	Ear/Nose/Throat
Cutter, Ring	General
Elevator, Surgical, Dental	Dental And Oral
Filling, Instrument Plastic, Dental	Dental And Oral
Forceps	Orthopedics
Gag, Mouth	Ear/Nose/Throat
General Use Surgical Scissors	Surgery
Hammer, Percussion	Cns/Neurology
Hemostat	Orthopedics
Holder, Needle	Gastroenterology/Urology
Instrument, Clip Removal	Cns/Neurology
Kit, Dissecting	Pathology
Knife, Scalpel	Surgery
Laryngoscope	Ear/Nose/Throat
Mirror, Mouth	Dental And Oral
Otoscope	Ear/Nose/Throat
Pliers, Surgical	Orthopedics
Retractor, All Types	Dental And Oral
Scissors, Bandage/Gauze/Plaster	General
Scissors, Collar And Crown	Dental And Oral
Scissors, Disposable	General
Scissors, Ear	Ear/Nose/Throat
Scissors, Iris	Ophthalmology
Scissors, Plastic Surgery (Dissecting)	Surgery
Scissors, Surgical Tissue, Dental (Oral)	Dental And Oral

TRANS AMERICAN MEDICAL / TAMSCO
708-430-7777 *(cont'd)*

Scissors, Umbilical	Obstetrics/Gynecology
Spatula, Surgical, General & Plastic Surgery	Surgery
Speculum, Ear	Ear/Nose/Throat
Speculum, Nasal	Ear/Nose/Throat
Speculum, Vaginal, Metal	Obstetrics/Gynecology

Medical Product Subsidiaries (Listed Separately)
Trans American Medical

TRANS AMERICAN MEDICAL, INC.
801-796-7335
965 West 325 North, Lindon, UT 84042
FDA Number: 1058541   *Fax:* 801.796.7363
E-mail: info@transamericanmedical.com
Web site: www.transamericanmedical.com
Ownership: Private
Stock Symbol: AMMD
Traded On: NASDAQ
Produces/Sells CE-marked Devices: N

Brush, Dermabrasion	Surgery
Curtain, Protective, Radiographic	Radiology

TRANS MED USA, INC.
978-670-6000
77 Alexander Road, #9, Billerica, MA 01821-5043
FDA Number: n/a   *Fax:* 978-670-6020
E-mail: paul@transmed-usa.com
Web site: www.transmed-usa.com
Annual Revenue: $10-$25 Million
Total Employees: 39379   *Marketing Staff:* 2   *Sales Staff:* 4
Ownership: Private
Federal Procurement Eligibility: Small Business
Distribution: Exclusive Distributor, Exporter
General Admin.: Ebi Masalehdan/President, Treasurer
Mktg./Adv.: David Kelly/Manager Contract Sales
     Helen Silveira/Manager Market Research

Service, Import/Export	General

TRANS-ATLANTIC DENTAL
609-695-0168
46 Arctic Pkwy., Trenton, NJ 08638-3041
FDA Number: 2249320   *Fax:* 609-695-0168
E-mail: UniFlexTAD@msn.com
Web site: www.uniflex.bizhosting.comuniflextad.htm
Ownership: Private
Produces/Sells CE-marked Devices: N
Federal Procurement Eligibility: Small Business, Female Owned
Distribution: Manufacturer Direct, Manufacturer Through Manufacturer Reps

Base, Denture, Relining, Repairing, Rebasing, Resin	Dental And Oral

TRANS-GENOMIC
888-233-9283
408-894-9200
12325 Emmet Street, Omaha, NE 68164
FDA Number: n/a   *Fax:* 402-452-5453
E-mail: info@transgenomic.com
Web site: www.transgenomic.com
Medical Products Sales Volume: $4,000,000
Annual Revenue: $1-$5 Million
Year Founded: 1997
Total Employees: 60   *Marketing Staff:* 1   *Sales Staff:* 2
Ownership: TRANS-GENOMIC
Stock Symbol: TBIO
Traded On: OTC Bulletin
Federal Procurement Eligibility: Small Business
Distribution: Manufacturer Direct, Importer, Exporter
General Admin.: Collin De'Silva/Chief Executive Officer
     Dough G. Jerde/Chief Scientific Officer
Production: Bart Poulsen/Vice President Manufacturing

Column, Liquid Chromatography	Toxicology

TRANS-TYPE OF MARYLAND, INC.
301-695-7087
108 Byte Drive, Suite 101, Frederick, MD 21702
FDA Number: 1122530

Test, Leukocyte Typing	Hematology

TRANS1 INCORPORATED
910-332-1700
411 Landmark Dr., Wilmington, NC 28412
FDA Number: 3004578806
Ownership: Public
Stock Symbol: TSON
Traded On: NASDAQ
Produces/Sells CE-marked Devices: N

Appliance, Fixation, Spinal Intervertebral Body	Orthopedics
Arthroscope	Orthopedics
System, Facet Screw Spinal Device	Orthopedics

TRANSAMERICAN TECHNOLOGIES INTERNATIONAL
800-322-7373
925-355-0750
2246 Camino Ramon, San Ramon, CA 94583
FDA Number: 2938071   *Fax:* 925-355-0777
E-mail: ussales@ttimedical.com
Web site: www.ttimedical.com

TRANSAMERICAN TECHNOLOGIES 800-322-7373 *(cont'd)*

Medical Products Sales Volume: $600,000
Annual Revenue: $1-$5 Million
Year Founded: 1984
Total Employees: 6
Ownership: Private
Quality System Registration Information: ISO9001
Produces/Sells CE-marked Devices: Y
Federal Procurement Eligibility: Small Business
Distribution: Manufacturer Direct, Manufacturer Through Distributor, Manufacturer Through Manufacturer Reps, OEM, Service Direct, Importer, Exporter
General Admin.: Allen R. Howes/President, Chief Executive Officer
Mktg./Adv.: Jason Botting/Director Sales
Production: Steve Freer/Vice President Operations
Finance: Andrea Wong/Controller

Accessories, Laser	General
Accessories, Light, Surgical	Surgery
Accessories, Photographic, Endoscopic	Gastroenterology/Urology
Accessories, Surgical Camera	Surgery
Cannula, Suction, Pool-Tip	Surgery
Cannula, Suction/Irrigation, Laparoscopic	Surgery
Coagulator, Laparoscopic, Unipolar	Obstetrics/Gynecology
Coagulator/Cutter, Endoscopic, Unipolar	Obstetrics/Gynecology
Component, Other	General
Electrode, Electrosurgery, Laparoscopic	Surgery
Electrode, Electrosurgical, Return (Ground, Dispersive)	Surgery
Endoscope	Gastroenterology/Urology
Kit, Instruments and Accessories, Surgical	Surgery
Lamp, Surgical, Xenon	Surgery
Laser, Neodymium:YAG, Surgical, Gynecologic	Obstetrics/Gynecology
Laser, Surgical	Surgery
Light Source, Fiberoptic, Routine	Gastroenterology/Urology
Micromanipulator	General
Monitor, Video, Endoscope	General
Photocoagulator	Ophthalmology

TRANSATLANTIC ENGINEERING 818-716-0663
21637 Dumetz Road, Woodland Hills, CA 91364
FDA Number: n/a
E-mail: Reggie@mirthless.com   *Fax:* 818-716-0663
Total Employees: 1
Ownership: Private
Produces/Sells CE-marked Devices: N
Federal Procurement Eligibility: Female Owned
Distribution: Service Direct
Mktg./Adv.: Willy Bruyns/Account Executive
                    yvonne williams/Director Public Relations

Utensil, Food	Physical Med

TRANSFUSION TECHNOLOGIES
See Haemonetics Corp.

TRANSGENOMIC, INC. 888-233-9283
12325 Emmet Street, Omaha, NE 68164
FDA Number: n/a   *Fax:* 402-452-5453
Web site: www.transgenomic.com
Ownership: Private
Produces/Sells CE-marked Devices: N
General Admin.: Dr. Rodney Markin/Chairman
                    Mr. Craig Tuttle/President, Chief Executive Officer
Mktg./Adv.: Mr. Chad Richards/Commercial Director
Production: Ms. Katrina Fahlin/Vice President Quality Assurance
Research: Ms. Katherine Richardson/Vice President Research & Development
Finance: Mr. Brett Frevert/Chief Financial Officer

TRANSILWRAP CO., INC. 800-972-8858
9201 W. Belmont Avenue, 909-944-9981
Franklin Park, IL 60131
FDA Number: 1929456   *Fax:* 909-944-7270
Web site: www.transilwrap.com
Ownership: Private
Produces/Sells CE-marked Devices: N

Accessories, Wheelchair	Physical Med
Monitor, Bed Patient	General

TRANSITIONS OPTICAL, INC. 727-545-0400
9251 Belcher Rd., Pinellas Park, FL 33782
FDA Number: 1052967

Lens, Spectacle/Eyeglasses, Non-Custom	Ophthalmology
Sunglasses (Including Photosensitive)	Ophthalmology

TRANSLITE 281-240-3111
8410 Highway 90 A, Sugar Land, TX 77478
FDA Number: 1648557

Computer and Software, Medical	General
Light, Examination, Battery-Powered	General
Microscope, Light	Pathology
Transilluminator, AC-Powered, Ophthalmic	Ophthalmology

TRANSLOGIC CORP.
See Swisslog Translogic Corporation

TRANSMED
See Metro Medical Supply Wholesale

TRANSMED SCIENTIFIC
See U.F.I.

TRANSMOTION MEDICAL INC. 866-860-8447
1441 Wolf Creek Trail, Sharon Center, OH 44274
FDA Number: 3004082462

Chair, Surgical, AC-Powered	Surgery

TRANSONIC SYSTEMS INC. 800-353-3569
34 Dutch Mill Road 607-257-5300
Warren Road Business Park
Ithaca, NY 14850
FDA Number: 1319030   *Fax:* 607-257-7256
E-mail: support@transonic.com
Web site: www.transonic.com
Medical Products Sales Volume: $14,000,000
Annual Revenue: $10-$25 Million
Year Founded: 1983
Total Employees: 110   *Marketing Staff:* 6   *Sales Staff:* 19
Ownership: Valley Capital Corporation
Quality System Registration Information: ISO9000; ISO9001
Produces/Sells CE-marked Devices: Y
Federal Procurement Eligibility: Small Business
Distribution: Manufacturer Direct, Manufacturer Through Distributor, Manufacturer Through Manufacturer Reps, OEM
General Admin.: Bruce Kilmartin/Chief Operating Officer
                    Cornelis J. Drost/President, Chief Executive Officer
Medical Admin.: Mark Alsberge/Vice President Medical Affairs
Mktg./Adv.: Susan Eymann/Manager Advertising
Production: Bruce Kilmartin/Vice President Manufacturing
Finance: Howard Phipps/Vice President Finance

Flowmeter, Blood, Other	Cardiovascular
Monitor, Hemodialysis Unit Conductivity	Gastroenterology/Urology
Perfusion Apparatus	Pathology

TRANSPHOTON CORPORATION 305-234-0836
14350 S.w. 142nd Ave., Miami, FL 33186
FDA Number: 3003380231

Camera, Gamma (Nuclear/Scintillation)	Radiology
Scanner, Emission Computed Tomography	Radiology

TRANSTRACHEAL SYSTEMS, INC. 800-527-2667
109 Inverness Dr. E., Ste. C, 303-790-4766
Englewood, CO 80112
FDA Number: 1721097   *Fax:* 303-790-4588
E-mail: cservice@tto2.com
Web site: www.TTO2.com
Annual Revenue: $1-$5 Million
Year Founded: 1984
Total Employees: 9   *Marketing Staff:* 2   *Sales Staff:* 2
Ownership: Private
Quality System Registration Information: ISO9002
Produces/Sells CE-marked Devices: Y
Distribution: Manufacturer Through Distributor, Exporter
General Admin.: Shawn Gillespie/Chief Operating Officer
                    Les Peterson/President, Chief Executive Officer
Mktg./Adv.: Dan Baird/Director National Accounts
                    John Goodman/Manager International & National Sales
Production: Scott Durkop/Director Quality Assurance
IS: John Goodman/Vice President Tech. Services

Cannula, Nasal, Oxygen	Anesthesiology
Catheter, Oxygen, Tracheal	Anesthesiology
ENT Manual Surgical Instrument	Ear/Nose/Throat
Eyeglasses	Ophthalmology
Tray, Surgical	Surgery
Tube, Tracheostomy (W/Wo Connector)	Anesthesiology

TRANSYLVANIA VOCATIONAL SERVICES 828-884-3195
11 Mountain Industrial Drive, PO Box 1115, Brevard, NC 28712
FDA Number: n/a   *Fax:* 828-884-3102
E-mail: info@tvsinc.org
Web site: www.tvsinc.org
Medical Products Sales Volume: $5,800,000
Annual Revenue: $0-$1 Million
Year Founded: 1967
Total Employees: 129
Ownership: Private
Produces/Sells CE-marked Devices: N
Federal Procurement Eligibility: Small Business
Distribution: Manufacturer Through Distributor
General Admin.: Nancy Stricker/Chief Executive Officer
                    Becky Alderman/Chief Operating Officer

TRANSYLVANIA VOCATIONAL SERVICES 828-884-3195 *(cont'd)*
Contract Manufacturing .... General

TRAV-L-FILE, INC.
See Leeco Industries, Inc.

TRAVANTI PHARMA INCORPORATED 651-730-1008
2520 Pilot Knob Rd., Suite 100, Mendota Heights, MN 55120
FDA Number: 2135154
Iontophoresis Device, Dental .... Dental And Oral

TRAVEL RAMP, INC. (888) 661-7267
13900 NW 126th Ter, P.O. Box 2015, 386-462-5267
Alachua, FL 32615
FDA Number: n/a .... Fax: (386) 462-7744
E-mail: info@travelrampinc.com
Web site: http://www.travelrampinc.com
Annual Revenue: $0-$1 Million
Year Founded: 1985
Ownership: Private
Produces/Sells CE-marked Devices: N
Federal Procurement Eligibility: Small Business, Female Owned
Distribution: Manufacturer Through Distributor, Exporter
Ramp, Wheelchair .... General

TRAVENOL-GENENTECH DIAGNOSTICS
See Genentech, Inc.

TRAVERSE MEDICAL MONITORS DIV.
See Sensors, Inc.

TRAX CLEANROOM PRODUCTS 800-520-8729
3352 Swetzer Rd., P.O. Box 2089, 916-652-1080
Loomis, CA 95650
FDA Number: n/a .... Fax: 916-652-1083
E-mail: traxcorp@traxindprod.com
Web site: www.traxindprod.com
Medical Products Sales Volume: $100,000
Annual Revenue: $1-$5 Million
Year Founded: 1978
Total Employees: 9   *Marketing Staff:* 1   *Sales Staff:* 3
Ownership: Private
Produces/Sells CE-marked Devices: N
Federal Procurement Eligibility: Small Business
Distribution: Manufacturer Direct, Manufacturer Through Distributor, Manufacturer Through Manufacturer Reps, OEM
General Admin.: Fred Vodicka/Chief Executive Officer
          Mr. Peter Gort/President
          Ms. Kathy Gort/Vice President
Mktg./Adv.: Don Fries/Director Marketing
          Mr. Del Marks/Manager National Sales
Production: Jeremy Jensen/Manager Production
Component, Plastic .... General
Cover, Cart .... General
Cover, Mattress, Conductive .... General
Cover, Other .... General
Curtain, Cubicle .... General

TRAX INDUSTRIAL PRODUCTS CORP.
See Trax Cleanroom Products

TRAXYZ MEDICAL, INC. 781-249-6254
24 Lido Lane, Bedford, MA 01730
FDA Number: 3005044893
Ownership: Private
Produces/Sells CE-marked Devices: N
Radiographic Unit, Diagnostic, Mammographic .... Radiology

TRAY-PAK CORPORATION 888-926-1777
Tuckerton Road & Reading Crest Avenue 610-926-5800
PO Box 14804
Reading, PA 19612
FDA Number: n/a .... Fax: 610-926-9140
E-mail: sales@traypak.com
Web site: www.traypak.com
Medical Products Sales Volume: $22,200,000
Annual Revenue: $25-$50 Million
Year Founded: 1975
Total Employees: 300   *Marketing Staff:* 2   *Sales Staff:* 10
Ownership: Private
Quality System Registration Information: ISO9001
Produces/Sells CE-marked Devices: N
Federal Procurement Eligibility: Small Business
Distribution: Manufacturer Direct, Manufacturer Through Distributor, Manufacturer Through Manufacturer Reps, Service Direct
General Admin.: Tom Hessen/Chief Operating Officer
          David Bestwick/President, Chief Executive Officer
          John Carl/Vice President Human Resources
Mktg./Adv.: Steve Maguire/Director Product Development
          John Carl/Manager Sales Training

TRAY-PAK CORPORATION 888-926-1777 *(cont'd)*
          Randy Simcox/Vice President Marketing & Sales
Production: Paul Chen/Director Quality Assurance
          Tom Ruffing/Manager Materials
Container, Surgical Instrument .... Surgery
Contract Packaging .... General
Labeling Equipment .... General
Thermoforming, Extrusion, Custom .... General
Tray, Foodservice .... General

TRAYCO 512-341-3709
1101 West Pecan St., Pflugerville, TX 78660
FDA Number: 1649265 .... Fax: 512-251-6017
E-mail: traycomfg@aol.com
Ownership: Private
Produces/Sells CE-marked Devices: N
Accessories, Wheelchair .... Physical Med
Tray, Wheelchair .... Physical Med

TREASURE DENTAL LABORATORY 800-325-5244
3735 Washington Parkway, Idaho Falls, ID 83404 208-524-1888
FDA Number: n/a .... Fax: 208-528-5443
E-mail: info@treasuredental.com
Web site: www.treasuredental.com
Year Founded: 1968
Ownership: Private
Produces/Sells CE-marked Devices: N
Federal Procurement Eligibility: Small Business
Distribution: Manufacturer Direct
Crown And Bridge, Temporary, Resin .... Dental And Oral
Crown, Preformed .... Dental And Oral

TREK DIAGNOSTIC SYSTEMS 800-871-8909
982 Keynote Circle, Ste. 6, Cleveland, OH 44131 216-351-8735
FDA Number: 1530126 .... Fax: 216-351-5456
E-mail: info@trekds.com
Web site: www.trekds.com
Year Founded: 1999
Total Employees: 150
Ownership: Private
Quality System Registration Information: ISO9001
Produces/Sells CE-marked Devices: Y
Federal Procurement Eligibility: Small Business
Distribution: Manufacturer Direct, Manufacturer Through Distributor, Service Direct, Exclusive Distributor, Importer, Exporter
General Admin.: Michael D. Burke/Chief Executive Officer
Mktg./Adv.: Ms. Jenny Lorbach/Director Marketing
          Tim Seekely/Director National Accounts
          Paul Daga/Manager International & National Sales
          Ms. Liz Lloyd/Market Manager
Production: Teri Anacker/Director Quality Assurance
Research: Nadine Sullivan/Chief Scientist
Finance: Pamela Gornall/Chief Financial Officer
Analyzer, Overnight Suscept. System, Automated .... Microbiology
Susceptibility Test Panels, Antimicrobial .... Microbiology
System, Automated, Microbiological .... Microbiology
System, Blood Culturing .... Microbiology
Test System, Antimicrobial Susceptibility, Automated .... Microbiology
Test, Antimicrobial Susceptibility .... Microbiology
Medical Product Subsidiaries (Listed Separately)
Trek Diagnostic Systems, Inc.

TREK DIAGNOSTIC SYSTEMS, INC. 608-8373788
210 Business Park Dr., Sun Prairie, WI 53590
FDA Number: 2183729
Ownership: Trek Diagnostic Systems
Produces/Sells CE-marked Devices: N
Culture Media, Antimicrobial Susceptibility Test .... Microbiology
Culture Media, Mueller Hinton Agar Broth .... Microbiology
Culture Media, Non-Selective And Non-Differential .... Microbiology
Monitor, Microbial Growth .... Microbiology
Powders, Antimycobacterial Susceptibility Test .... Microbiology
System, Blood Culturing .... Microbiology

TRELLEBORG SEALING SOLUTIONS 800-466-1727
510 Burbank St., Broomfield, CO 80020 303-465-1727
FDA Number: n/a .... Fax: 303-469-4874
E-mail: variseal@ix.netcom.com
Web site: www.tss.trelleborg.com
Medical Products Sales Volume: $2,000,000
Annual Revenue: $10-$25 Million
Year Founded: 1978
Total Employees: 150   *Marketing Staff:* 2   *Sales Staff:* 4
Ownership: Private
Quality System Registration Information: ISO9000
Produces/Sells CE-marked Devices: N
Distribution: Manufacturer Direct, Manufacturer Through Distributor, Manufacturer Through Manufacturer Reps

TRELLEBORG SEALING SOLUTIONS   800-466-1727 *(cont'd)*
General Admin.: Tom Potosky/General Manager
Production: Don Collins/Manager Quality Assurance
    Tim Miller/Product Manager

Component, Other	General
Component, Plastic	General

TREMETRICS   800-825-0121
7625 Golden Triangle Drive,   **952-278-4423**
Eden Prairie, MN 55344
FDA Number: 1625391
E-mail: info@tremetrics.com   *Fax:* 952-903-4100
Web site: www.tremetrics.com
Medical Products Sales Volume: $2,100,000
Annual Revenue: $5-$10 Million
Total Employees: 27   Marketing Staff: 1   Sales Staff: 1
Ownership: WILLIAM DEMANT HOLDING A/S
Traded On: Copenhagen
Produces/Sells CE-marked Devices: N
Federal Procurement Eligibility: Small Business, VA Contract
Distribution: Manufacturer Through Distributor, Manufacturer Through
Manufacturer Reps
General Admin.: Ron Perlt/Vice President
Mktg./Adv.: Jack Foreman/Manager Product Development & Sales

Audiometer	Ear/Nose/Throat
Calibrator, Audiometer	Ear/Nose/Throat
Chamber, Acoustic, Testing	Ear/Nose/Throat
Chromatography Equipment, Gas	Chemistry
Computer Software	General

TRESTLE CORP.   949-673-1907
199 Technology Dr., Suite 105, Irvine, CA 92618-2446
FDA Number: 2032160
Ownership: Private
Produces/Sells CE-marked Devices: N

Micrometer, Microscope	Pathology

TREVOR OWEN LIMITED   866-487-2224
80 Barbados Blvd., Unit 5,   **416-267-8231**
Scarborough, ONT M1J-1 Canada
FDA Number: n/a
E-mail: Sales@TrevorOwenLtd.com   *Fax:* 416-267-1035
Web site: http://www.trevorowenltd.com
Year Founded: 1952
Total Employees: 25
Ownership: Private
Produces/Sells CE-marked Devices: N
Distribution: Manufacturer Direct

TREX ENTERPRISES CORP.   808-442 -7000
427 Ala Makani Street, Kahului, HI 96732
FDA Number: 2956505   *Fax:* 808-442-7001
E-mail: info@trexenterprises.com
Web site: www.trexenterprises.com
Ownership: Private
Produces/Sells CE-marked Devices: N

System, X-Ray, Mobile	Radiology

TREYMED, INC.   262-820-1294
N56 W 24790 N. Corporate Cir., #c, Sussex, WI 53089
FDA Number: 2134715

Analyzer, Gas, Carbon-Dioxide, Gaseous Phase (Capnograph)	Anesthesiology
Computer, Pulmonary Function Data	Anesthesiology

TRI HAWK CORPORATION   866-874-4295
150 Highland Rd., Massena, NY 13662-421550   **315-764-7664**
FDA Number: n/a   *Fax:* 315-764-8128
Web site: www.trihawk.com
Medical Products Sales Volume: $2,500,000
Annual Revenue: $1-$5 Million
Year Founded: 1969
Ownership: Private
Quality System Registration Information: ISO9002
Produces/Sells CE-marked Devices: Y
Federal Procurement Eligibility: Small Business
Distribution: Manufacturer Direct, Exporter

Burr, Dental	Dental And Oral
Burr, Surgical, General & Plastic Surgery	Surgery
Orthosis, Other	Physical Med
Support, Arch	Physical Med

TRI HAWK INC.   877-874-4295
P.O. Box 619,
Morrisburg, ONTAR K0C 1 Canada
FDA Number: n/a   *Fax:* 1-613-543-4501
Web site: www.trihawk.com
Year Founded: 1969
Total Employees: 50

TRI HAWK INC.   877-874-4295 *(cont'd)*
Ownership: Private
Produces/Sells CE-marked Devices: N
Distribution: Manufacturer Direct, Exporter

TRI W-G GROUP   800-437-8011
215 12th Avenue NE, PO Box 905,   **701-845-3984**
Valley City, ND 58072
FDA Number: 1717548   *Fax:* 701-845-2023
E-mail: triwg@triwg.com
Web site: www.triwg.com
Total Employees: 40
Ownership: Private
Produces/Sells CE-marked Devices: N
Federal Procurement Eligibility: Small Business, GSA Contract
Distribution: Manufacturer Direct, Manufacturer Through Distributor, Exporter
General Admin.: George Gaukler/Chief Executive Officer
Mktg./Adv.: Duane Fast/Vice President Marketing

Bars, Parallel, Exercise	Physical Med
Bars, Parallel, Powered	Physical Med
Exerciser, Non-Measuring	Physical Med
Table, Examination/Treatment	General
Table, Other	General
Table, Physical Medicine, Powered	Physical Med
Table, Physical Therapy	Physical Med

TRI-CITY OPTICAL   727-528-8873
5600 115th Ave. North, Suite B, Clearwater, FL 33760
FDA Number: 3003768944
Ownership: Private
Produces/Sells CE-marked Devices: N

Lens, Spectacle/Eyeglasses, Non-Custom	Ophthalmology

TRI-CLOVER, INC., ALPHA-LAVAL GROUP
See Alfa Laval Inc.

TRI-CONTINENT SCIENTIFIC, INC.   530-274-4240
12555 Loma Rica Dr., #2, Grass Valley, CA 95945
FDA Number: 2937957

Microtiter Diluting/Dispensing Device	Microbiology
Pipetting And Diluting System, Automated	Chemistry

TRI-D CORP.
19625 62nd Ave. S.,, Ste. B101, Kent, WA 98032
FDA Number: 3003650644

Binder, Medical, Therapeutic	General

TRI-FI KNITTING, LLC   423-855-0501
4641 Shallowford Rd., Chattanooga, TN 37411
FDA Number: 3005423373

Bandage, Elastic	General

TRI-MAG, INC.   559-651-2222
1601 Clancy Ct., Visalia, CA 93291-9253
FDA Number: n/a   *Fax:* 559-651-0188
E-mail: sales@tri-mag.com
Web site: www.tri-mag.com
Annual Revenue: $5-$10 Million
Total Employees: 80
Ownership: Private
Quality System Registration Information: ISO9000
Produces/Sells CE-marked Devices: Y
Federal Procurement Eligibility: Small Business, Minority Owned
Distribution: Manufacturer Direct, Manufacturer Through Distributor, Manufacturer
Through Manufacturer Reps, OEM

Component, Electronic	General

TRI-MED INC.
See Smiths Medical Pm, Inc.

TRI-MEDICS, INC.   401-490-5321
10 Pine Tree Lane, Lincoln, RI 02865
FDA Number: 3003644992
Ownership: Private
Produces/Sells CE-marked Devices: N

Positioner, Socket	Orthopedics

TRI-POINT MEDICAL CORPORATION
See Closure Medical

TRI-STAR INDUSTRIES LTD.   902-742-9254
88 Forest Street, Yarmouth, NS B5A 4B4 Canada
FDA Number: n/a   *Fax:* 902-742-7632
E-mail: info@tri-star.ca
Web site: www.tri-star.ca
Total Employees: 60   Marketing Staff: 5   Sales Staff: 3
Ownership: Private
Quality System Registration Information: ISO9000
Produces/Sells CE-marked Devices: N
Federal Procurement Eligibility: Small Business

TRI-STAR INDUSTRIES LTD.   902-742-9254 (cont'd)
Distribution: Manufacturer Direct, OEM, Exclusive Distributor, Importer, Exporter

TRI-STAR MEDICAL, INC.   708-645-1107
14227 Winchester Court, Orland Park, IL 60467
FDA Number: 71279
Ownership: Private
Produces/Sells CE-marked Devices: N
  Therapeutic X-Ray System   Radiology

TRI-STATE HOSPITAL SUPPLY CORP.   800-248-4058
301 Catrell Drive, PO Box 170,   517-546-5400
Howell, MI 48843
FDA Number: 1824619   Fax: 517-546-9388
E-mail: info@tshsc.com
Web site: www.tshsc.com
Year Founded: 1961
Total Employees: 723   *Marketing Staff:* 5   *Sales Staff:* 100
Ownership: Private
Quality System Registration Information: ISO9000; ISO9001
Produces/Sells CE-marked Devices: Y
Federal Procurement Eligibility: GSA Contract
Distribution: Manufacturer Direct, Manufacturer Through Distributor, Exclusive Distributor
General Admin.: Mr. Tom Archipley/President, Chief Executive Officer
       Mr. Mike Obsitnik/Vice President
       Mr. Ron Dooley/Vice President
Mktg./Adv.: Jerry Roberts/Director Product Development
       Marie Parmer/Manager Advertising
       Mr. Tom Archipley II/Manager Market Research
       Mr. Tom Barrett/Manager National Sales
       Cynthia Obsitnik/Manager Sales
       Mr. Richard Schild/Manager Sales Training
       Mr. Mike Goro/Vice President Marketing & Sales
Production: Karen Kowalczyk/Director Quality Assurance & Regulatory Affairs
       Nate Chapman/Manager Materials
Research: Don Propp/Director Research & Development

Bag, Body	General
Clamp, Circumcision	Obstetrics/Gynecology
Cushion, Other	General
Dressing, Other	General
Kit, Maternity	Obstetrics/Gynecology
Kit, Pelvic Exam	Obstetrics/Gynecology
Kit, Shroud	Pathology
Kit, Surgical Instrument, Disposable	Surgery
Pad, Menstrual, Unscented	Obstetrics/Gynecology
Surgical Instrument, Disposable	Surgery
Trap, Mucus	Anesthesiology
Tray, Circumcision, Reusable	Obstetrics/Gynecology

TRI-STATE HOSPITAL SUPPLY CORP.
See Centurion Medical Products Corporation

TRI-STATE HOSPITAL SUPPLY CORP.
See Centurion Medical Products Corp.

TRI-STATE SURGICAL SUPPLY & EQUIPMENT   800-424-5227
409 Hoyt St., Brooklyn, NY 11231-4858   718-624-1000
FDA Number: 2434110   Fax: 718-624-0666
E-mail: tristateequip@aol.com
Medical Products Sales Volume: $13,800,000
Annual Revenue: $0-$1 Million
Year Founded: 1976
Total Employees: 66   *Marketing Staff:* 12   *Sales Staff:* 6
Ownership: Private
Produces/Sells CE-marked Devices: N
Federal Procurement Eligibility: Small Business
Distribution: Service Direct, Exclusive Distributor, Importer
General Admin.: Jacob Hoffman/Chief Executive Officer
       Ben Zelman/General Manager
Production: Eli Steinberg/Manager Operations
Research: Jacob Schwartz/Manager Research
Purchasing: Moshe M. Spira/Director Purchasing

Furniture, General	General
Lotion, Skin Care	General
Solution, Antibacterial Cleaner	General

TRI-TECH MEDICAL, INC.   800-253-8692
35401 Avon Commerce Parkway,   440-937-6244
Avon, OH 44011
FDA Number: 1530881   Fax: 440-937-5060
E-mail: internationalsales@tri-techmedical.com
Web site: www.tri-techmedical.com
Medical Products Sales Volume: $1,200,000
Year Founded: 1989
Total Employees: 15
Ownership: Private
Produces/Sells CE-marked Devices: N
Federal Procurement Eligibility: Small Business

TRI-TECH MEDICAL, INC.   800-253-8692 (cont'd)
  Flowmeter, Gas (Oxygen), Calibrated   Anesthesiology
  Gauge, Gas Pressure, Cylinder/Pipeline   Anesthesiology

TRI-TRONICS CO., INC.   800-237-0946
7705 Cheri Court, Tampa, FL 33634-2419   813-886-4000
FDA Number: n/a   Fax: 813-884-8818
E-mail: info@ttco.com
Web site: www.ttco.com
Year Founded: 1954
Ownership: Private
Produces/Sells CE-marked Devices: N
Distribution: Manufacturer Through Distributor
  Transilluminator, Fiber Optic   Ear/Nose/Throat

TRIA BEAUTY, INC.   925-701-2540
5880 W. Las Positas Blvd, Suite 52, Pleasanton, CA 94588
FDA Number: 3005572989
  Laser, Surgical   Surgery

TRIAD DISPOSABLES   800-288-1288
19355 Janacek Court, Brookfield, WI 53045   262-641-1500
FDA Number: 2128643   Fax: 262-641-1452
E-mail: info@triad-group.net
Web site: www.triad-group.net
Medical Products Sales Volume: $4,000,000
Year Founded: 1988
Total Employees: 50
Ownership: Private
Produces/Sells CE-marked Devices: N
Federal Procurement Eligibility: Small Business
Distribution: Manufacturer Through Distributor, OEM
  Gel, Electrode, Electrosurgical   Surgery
  Jelly, Lubricating, Transurethral Surgical Instrument   Gastroenterology/Urology

TRIAID, INC.   301-759-3525
637 North Centre St., Cumberland, MD 21502
FDA Number: 1124832
  Attachment, Commode, Wheelchair   Physical Med
  Chair, With Casters   Physical Med
  Walker, Mechanical   Physical Med
  Wheelchair, Special Grade   Physical Med

TRIANGLE BIOMEDICAL SCIENCES, INC.   919-384-9393
3014 Croasdaile Drive, Durham, NC 27705-2507
FDA Number: 1055757   Fax: 919-384-9595
E-mail: sales@trianglebiomedical.com
Web site: www.trianglebiomedical.com
Medical Products Sales Volume: $2,200,000
Annual Revenue: $1-$5 Million
Year Founded: 1984
Total Employees: 20   *Marketing Staff:* 4   *Sales Staff:* 4
Ownership: Private
Produces/Sells CE-marked Devices: N
Federal Procurement Eligibility: Small Business
Distribution: Manufacturer Direct, Manufacturer Through Distributor, OEM, Importer
General Admin.: Jack E. Hunnell/Chief Executive Officer
Mktg./Adv.: Greg Geyer/Manager International & National Sales
       Valerie Abbott/Marketing & Communications Officer
Production: Lisa Veasey/Manager Operations
  Contract R&D, Equipment   General

TRIANGLE RESEARCH AND DEVELOPMENT CORP.
See Triangle Biomedical Sciences, Inc.

TRIBORO SUPPLIES INC   800-369-7546
994 Grand Blvd., Deer Park, NY 11729   631-595-2221
FDA Number: n/a   Fax: 631-595-9845
E-mail: triboro1@msn.com
Web site: www.luckyseven.com.pk
Medical Products Sales Volume: $1,000,000
Annual Revenue: $1-$5 Million
Year Founded: 1980
Total Employees: 5   *Marketing Staff:* 2   *Sales Staff:* 1
Ownership: Private
Quality System Registration Information: ISO9002
Produces/Sells CE-marked Devices: N
Federal Procurement Eligibility: Small Business
Distribution: Manufacturer Direct
General Admin.: Zafar Iqbal/President
Mktg./Adv.: Mr. M. Saeed/Manager Contract Sales
Production: Azhar Iqbal/Director Quality Assurance
       Mr. M. Iqbal/Vice President Manufacturing

Cutter, Ring	General
Forceps	Orthopedics
Forceps, Surgical, Gynecological	Obstetrics/Gynecology
General Use Surgical Scissors	Surgery
Laryngoscope	Ear/Nose/Throat

TRICO METAL PRODUCTS, INC.   800-457-1376
2309 Wyandotte Rd., Willow Grove, PA 19090   **215-659-2673**
FDA Number: n/a
Web site: www.tricometal.com
Annual Revenue: $1-$5 Million
Ownership: Private
Produces/Sells CE-marked Devices: N
Federal Procurement Eligibility: Small Business
Distribution: Manufacturer Direct, OEM, Service Direct, Exporter
  Accessories, Wheelchair   Physical Med
  Head Rest, Neurosurgical   Cns/Neurology

TRICONTINENT   800-937-4738
12555 Loma Rica Drive, Grass Valley, CA 95945   **530-273-8888**
FDA Number: 7000364   *Fax:* 530-273-2586
E-mail: liquidhandling@tricontinent.com
Web site: www.tricontinent.com
Medical Products Sales Volume: $6,500,000
Year Founded: 1975
Total Employees: 85   *Marketing Staff:* 1   *Sales Staff:* 4
Ownership: HITACHI CHEMICAL LTD.
Stock Symbol: 4217
Traded On: Tokyo
Quality System Registration Information: ISO9001
Produces/Sells CE-marked Devices: Y
Federal Procurement Eligibility: Small Business
Distribution: Manufacturer Direct, Manufacturer Through Distributor, Manufacturer Through Manufacturer Reps, OEM
General Admin.: Randy Dismukes/Manager Personnel
    Brenton Hanlon/President
Mktg./Adv.: Mik Bajka/Director Product Development
    Arthur McGeown/Manager National Sales
    Thomas Hecker/Manager National Sales
    Scott Snyder/Manager Product Development
    Steve Walters/Manager Product Development
    Aimee Driggs/Marketing Communications Specialist
Production: Amy Drake/Manager Customer Services
    Tammie Hamilton/Manager Manufacturing
    John McDaniels/Manager Materials
    Jerry Mitchell/Manager Regulatory Affairs
  Dispenser, Fluid   General
  Microtiter Diluting/Dispensing Device   Microbiology
  Pipette Tip   Chemistry
  Pipetter   Hematology
  Pump, Infusion, Syringe   General
  Washer, Microplate   General

TRIDENT MEDICAL PRODUCTS   800-647-4448
1201 Summit Avenue, Fort Worth, TX 76102   **817-335-4031**
FDA Number: 1643569   *Fax:* 817-820-0241
E-mail: trident@flash.net
Medical Products Sales Volume: $400,000
Year Founded: 1986
Ownership: Private
Produces/Sells CE-marked Devices: N
Federal Procurement Eligibility: Small Business
Distribution: Manufacturer Direct, Manufacturer Through Distributor, OEM, Exporter
General Admin.: Tim Tatom/Vice President, General Manager
  Drape, Patient, Ophthalmic   Ophthalmology
  Shield, Eye, Ophthalmic   Ophthalmology

TRIDIEN MEDICAL   800-474-4225
1691 North Delilah St., Corona, CA 92879   **951-549-6800**
FDA Number: 2032518   *Fax:* 954-340-0511
E-mail: jedwards@tridien.com
Web site: www.tridien.com
Ownership: Private
Produces/Sells CE-marked Devices: N
  Bed, Patient Rotation, Powered   Physical Med
  Cushion, Flotation   Physical Med
  Mattress, Air Flotation   General
  Mattress, Non-Powered Flotation Therapy   Physical Med
  Protector, Skin Pressure   General
  Table, Surgical With Orthopedic Accessories, AC-Powered   Surgery

TRIDIEN MEDICAL   954-340-0500
4200 NW 120th Avenue, Coral Springs, FL 33065
FDA Number: 1055581
Ownership: Private
Produces/Sells CE-marked Devices: N
Mktg./Adv.: Ms. Jackie Edwards/Vice President Sales
  Lamp, Infrared   Physical Med
  Pad, Heating, Powered   Physical Med

TRIFORMATION SYSTEMS, INC.
See Enabling Technologies Company

TRIGG LABORATORIES, INC.   757-224-0177
28650 Braxton Avenue, Valencia, CA 91355
FDA Number: 3003963141
  Condom   Obstetrics/Gynecology

TRIGON TECHNOLOGY, INC.   269-699-7182
23126 South Shore Dr., Edwardsburg, MI 49112
FDA Number: 1835047
Ownership: Private
Produces/Sells CE-marked Devices: N
  Stain, Dye Solution   Pathology

TRIGROUP TECHNOLOGIES, LTD.   972-226-4600
200 Adell Blvd., Sunnyvale, TX 75182
FDA Number: 1645179
Ownership: Private
Produces/Sells CE-marked Devices: N
  Mouthguard   Dental And Oral
  Mouthpiece, Saliva Ejector   Dental And Oral
  Wax, Dental   Dental And Oral

TRILLING MEDICAL TECHNOLOGIES INC.
See Water-Jel Technologies

TRILLING RESOURCES LTD.
See Water-Jel Technologies

TRILLIUM DIAGNOSTICS, LLC.   866-364-0028
246 Sylvan Rd., Bangor, ME 04401   **207-945-0900**
FDA Number: 1226556   *Fax:* 207-942-0346
E-mail: info@trilliumdx.com
Web site: trilliumdx.com
Ownership: Private
Produces/Sells CE-marked Devices: Y
Federal Procurement Eligibility: Small Business
Distribution: Manufacturer Direct, Manufacturer Through Distributor
General Admin.: Bruce H Davis/President
    Kathleen Thompson Davis/Vice President
  Hematology Quality Control Mixture   Hematology
  Reagents, Specific, Analyte   Hematology

TRILLIUM HEARING TECHNOLOGIES, INC.   813-864-2292
13803 W. Hillsborough Ave., Tampa, FL 33635
FDA Number: 1066373
  Hearing-Aid   Ear/Nose/Throat

TRIMEDYNE, INC.   800-733-5273
15091 Bake Parkway, Irvine, CA 92618-2501   **949-951-3800**
FDA Number: 1419951   *Fax:* 949-855-8206
E-mail: info@trimedyne.com
Web site: www.trimedyne.com
Medical Products Sales Volume: $6,200,000
Annual Revenue: $5-$10 Million
Year Founded: 1980
Total Employees: 26   *Marketing Staff:* 1   *Sales Staff:* 3
Ownership: Public
Stock Symbol: TMED
Traded On: OTC Bulletin
Quality System Registration Information: ISO9000
Produces/Sells CE-marked Devices: Y
Federal Procurement Eligibility: Small Business
Distribution: Manufacturer Through Distributor, Manufacturer Through Manufacturer Reps, OEM, Service Direct, Exporter
General Admin.: Marvin P. Loeb/Chairman, Chief Executive Officer
    Sudele Seron/Director Human Resources
    Glenn Yeik/President, Chief Operating Officer
Mktg./Adv.: Craig Smith/Director Marketing
    Brian Kenney/Vice President Marketing & Sales
Production: Laurie Cartwright/Manager Regulatory Affairs
  Accessories, Laser   General
  Laser, Surgical, Holmium   Surgery
  Prosthesis, Spine, Intervertebral Disc   Orthopedics

TRINITY BIOTECH, INC.   1.800.325.3424
2823 Girts Road, Jamestown, NY 14701   **716-483-3851**
FDA Number: 1318354   *Fax:* 716-488-1990
E-mail: customerservice@trinityusa.com
Web site: www.trinitybiotech.com
Medical Products Sales Volume: $15,400,000
Annual Revenue: $25-$50 Million
Year Founded: 1992
Total Employees: 80
Ownership: Public
Stock Symbol: TRIBY
Traded On: NASDAQ
Quality System Registration Information: ISO9000; ISO9001
Produces/Sells CE-marked Devices: N
Federal Procurement Eligibility: Small Business
Distribution: Manufacturer Through Distributor, OEM

TRINITY BIOTECH, INC.   1.800.325.3424 *(cont'd)*

General Admin.: Brendan Farrell/President
            Ian Woodward/Vice President, General Manager
Mktg./Adv.: Mark Smith/Director Marketing & Sales
Production: Bonnie DeJoy/Director Quality Assurance
Finance: Bill Reese/Controller

Antibody, Antimitochondrial, Indirect Immunofluorescent	Immunology
Antisera, Cf, Herpesvirus Hominis 1, 2	Microbiology
Antiserum, CF, Cytomegalovirus	Microbiology
Antiserum, CF, Epstein-Barr Virus	Microbiology
Antiserum, CF, Varicella-Zoster	Microbiology
Calibrator, Primary, Clinical Chemistry	Chemistry
Contract R&D, Diagnostics	General
Culture Media, Non-Propagating Transport	Microbiology
Electrophoretic Separation, Lipoproteins	Chemistry
Immunochemical, Thyroglobulin Autoantibody	Immunology
Instrument, Coagulation, Automated	Hematology
Lipase-Esterase, Enzymatic, Photometric, Lipase	Chemistry
Lipoprotein, Low Density, Removal	Gastroenterology/Urology
Radioimmunoassay, Free Thyroxine	Chemistry
Radioimmunoassay, Thyroid Stimulating Hormone	Chemistry
Radioimmunoassay, Thyroxine Binding Globulin	Chemistry
Radioimmunoassay, Total Thyroxine	Chemistry
Radioimmunoassay, Total Triiodothyronine	Chemistry

TRINITY ORTHOPEDICS, LLC   858. 689. 4113

8817 Production Ave., San Diego, CA 92121
FDA Number: 3006700424   Fax: 858. 689. 4115
E-mail: info@trinity-ortho.com
Web site: www.trinity-ortho.com
Ownership: Private
Produces/Sells CE-marked Devices: N

Orthopedic Manual Surgical Instrument	Orthopedics
Orthosis, Spinal Pedicle Fixation, For Degenerative Disc Disease	Orthopedics

TRINITY STERILE, INC.   410-860-5123

201 Kiley Dr., Salisbury, MD 21802
FDA Number: 1123010   Fax: 410.860.2913
E-mail: an34@aol.com
Ownership: Private
Produces/Sells CE-marked Devices: N

Catheter, Suction (Tracheal Aspirating Tube)	Anesthesiology
Catheter, Suction, With Tip	General
Kit, Urinary Drainage Collection	Gastroenterology/Urology
Syringe, Irrigating	General
Tray, Surgical Instrument	Surgery

TRION, INC.   800-884-0002
                           919-775-2201

101 McNeil Road, Sanford, NC 27330
FDA Number: 7000919   Fax: 919-777-6399
E-mail: sales@trioninc.com
Web site: www.trioninc.com
Medical Products Sales Volume: $34,568,000
Annual Revenue: $25-$50 Million
Year Founded: 1947
Total Employees: 130
Ownership: Public
Stock Symbol: FJC
Traded On: NYSE
Federal Procurement Eligibility: Small Business, GSA Contract
Distribution: Manufacturer Through Distributor, Manufacturer Through
Manufacturer Reps, OEM, Exporter
General Admin.: Steven Schneider/Chief Executive Officer
            Gary Waters/Vice President Human Resources
Mktg./Adv.: Brian H. Boender/Vice President Marketing & Sales
Production: Jerry Stephens/Vice President Manufacturing

Filter, Air	General

TRIONIX RESEARCH LABORATORY, INC.   330-425-9055

8037 Bavaria Rd., Twinsburg, OH 44087
FDA Number: 1527587

Scanner, Emission Computed Tomography	Radiology
Scanner, Nuclear, Tomographic	Radiology

TRIPATH IMAGING   800-636-7284

8271 154th Ave. N.E., Redmond, WA 98052-3878   425-869-7284
FDA Number: n/a   Fax: 425-556-3064
E-mail: rbromfield@neopath.com
Annual Revenue: $10-$25 Million
Total Employees: 175
Ownership: Public
Stock Symbol: NPTH
Traded On: NASDAQ
Produces/Sells CE-marked Devices: N
Distribution: Manufacturer Direct
General Admin.: Alan C. Nelson/Chairman
            Ronald R. Bromfield/President, Chief Executive Officer
Production: Mary Norton/Vice President Regulatory Affairs
Research: James Lee/Vice President Research & Development

TRIPATH IMAGING   800-636-7284 *(cont'd)*

Analyzer, Chemistry, Micro	Chemistry
Locator, Cell, Automated	Hematology

TRIPATH IMAGING, INC.   919-206-7140

780 Plantation Dr., Burlington, NC 27215
FDA Number: 1062336

Antinuclear Antibody (Enzyme-Labeled), Antigen, Controls	Immunology
Buffer, pH	Hematology
Control, Multi Analyte, All Kinds (Assayed And Unassayed)	Chemistry
Cultured Animal And Human Cells	Pathology
Cytocentrifuge	Pathology
Filter, Cell Collection, Tissue Processing	Pathology
Fixative, Alcohol Containing	Pathology
Immunohistochemistry Reagents And Kits	Pathology
Microscope, Automated, Image Analysis, Immunohistochemistry, Operator Intervention, Nuclear Intensity & Percent Positivity	Hematology
Microscope, Automated, Image Analysis, Operator Intervention	Hematology
Preservative, Cytological	Pathology
Processor, Slide, Cytology, Automated	Pathology
Reagent, General Purpose	Pathology
Reagents, Specific, Analyte	Hematology
Slide, Microscope	Pathology
Stain, Dye Solution	Pathology
Stainer, Slide, Automated	Pathology
Tissue Processor, Automated	Pathology

TRIPATH IMAGING, INC.   919-206-7140

8271 154th Ave., N.e., Redmond, WA 98052
FDA Number: 3026575

Reader, Slide, Cytology, Cervical, Automated	Pathology

TRIPLE G SYSTEMS GROUP, INC.   905-305-0041

600-3100 Steeles Ave E, Markham L3R 8T3 Canada
FDA Number: 9615148

Computer and Software, Medical	General

TRIREME MEDICAL INC.   925-931-1300

7060 Koll Center Parkway, Suite 300, Pleasanton, CA 94566
FDA Number: 3008089360   Fax: 925-931-1361
Web site: http://trirememedical.com
Year Founded: 2005
Ownership: Private
Produces/Sells CE-marked Devices: N
General Admin.: Dr. Eitan Konstantino/President, Chief Executive Officer
   Medical Admin.: Dr. Lian Cunningham/Vice President Clinical Affairs
Mktg./Adv.: Mr. Christopher Haig/Vice President Marketing & Business
Development
Production: Mr. Tanhum Feld/Designer
            Ms. Shiva Ardakani/Vice President Quality Control & Regulatory Affairs
Research: Ms. Maria Pizarro/Vice President Research & Development

Catheter, Percutaneous	Cardiovascular
Stent, Coronary, Drug-eluting	Cardiovascular

TRIVASCULAR INC.   707-543-8800

3910 Brickway Blvd., Santa Rosa, CA 95403
FDA Number: n/a   Fax: 707-543-8700
E-mail: info@trivascular.com
Web site: http://trivascular.com
Ownership: Private
Produces/Sells CE-marked Devices: N
General Admin.: Mr. Steven Harrison/Chief Financial Officer, Vice President
            Dr. Michael Chobotov/President, Chief Executive Officer
Mktg./Adv.: Mr. Vivek Jayaraman/Vice President Commercial Operations
Production: Dr. Joseph Humphrey/Vice President Manufacturing
            Mr. Lou Molinari/Vice President Manufacturing
            Ms. Shari Allen/Vice President Regulatory & Clinical Affairs
Research: Dr. Robert Whirley/Vice President Research & Development

TRIVIRIX INTERNATIONAL INC.   320-982-8000

925 6th Avenue NE, Milaca, MN 56353
FDA Number: 2183613   Fax: 320-982-8001
E-mail: sales@trivirix.com
Web site: www.trivirix.com
Medical Products Sales Volume: $23,000,000
Year Founded: 1998
Total Employees: 90
Ownership: Private
Produces/Sells CE-marked Devices: Y
Federal Procurement Eligibility: Small Business

Magnet, Test, Pacemaker	Cardiovascular
Probe, Radiofrequency Lesion	Cns/Neurology
Programmer, Pacemaker	Cardiovascular
Pump, Infusion, Implantable, General	General
Stimulator, Electrical, Implanted (Parkinsonian Tremor)	Cns/Neurology
Stimulator, Peripheral Nerve, Implantable (Pain Relief)	Cns/Neurology
Stimulator, Sacral Nerve, Implanted	Cns/Neurology
Stimulator, Spinal Cord, Implantable (Pain Relief)	Cns/Neurology
Transmitter/Receiver System, Physiological, Telephone	Cardiovascular

TRIVIRIX MINNEAPOLIS, INC.
See Trivirix International Inc.

TRLBY INNOVATIVE L.L.C.   860-482-6848
65 New Litchfield St., Torrington, CT 06790
FDA Number: 1225917
E-mail: info@trlby.com
Web site: www.trlby.com
Ownership: Private
Produces/Sells CE-marked Devices: N

Mattress, Air Flotation	General

TROEMNER LLC   800-352-7705
201 Wolf Drive, PO Box 87,   856-686-1600
Thorofare, NJ 08086
FDA Number: 7000920
E-mail: troemner@troemner.com   *Fax:* 856-686-1601
Web site: www.troemner.com
Medical Products Sales Volume: $15,000,000
Year Founded: 1838
Total Employees: 150   *Marketing Staff:* 4   *Sales Staff:* 4
Ownership: Private
Quality System Registration Information: ISO9001
Produces/Sells CE-marked Devices: Y
Federal Procurement Eligibility: Small Business
Distribution: Manufacturer Direct, Manufacturer Through Distributor, Exporter
General Admin.: Will Abele/President
       Mark Kline/Vice President, General Manager
Production: Steve Butler/Vice President Operations

Balance, Mechanical	Chemistry
Block, Heating	Chemistry
Cart, Gas Cylinder (Carrier)	Anesthesiology
Clamp, Other	Surgery
Equipment, Laboratory, Gen. Purpose (Specific Medical Use)	Chemistry
Homogenizer, Tissue	Microbiology
Mixer, Clinical Laboratory	Chemistry
Plate, Hot	Chemistry
Safety Equipment, Laboratory	Chemistry
Scale, Laboratory	Chemistry
Shaker/Stirrer	Chemistry
Stirrer	Chemistry

TRONEX HEALTHCARE INDUSTRIES   800-833-1181
One Tronex Centre, 2 Cranberry Road,   973-627-3800
Parsippany, NJ 07054
FDA Number: 2435161
E-mail: marketing@tronex.healthcare.com   *Fax:* 973-625-7630
Web site: www.tronexcompany.com
Medical Products Sales Volume: $4,600,000
Year Founded: 1989
Total Employees: 35   *Marketing Staff:* 10   *Sales Staff:* 13
Ownership: Private
Quality System Registration Information: ISO9001; ISO9002
Produces/Sells CE-marked Devices: N
Federal Procurement Eligibility: Small Business, Minority Owned, GSA Contract
Distribution: Manufacturer Direct, Manufacturer Through Distributor, Manufacturer Through Manufacturer Reps, OEM, Service Direct, Exclusive Distributor
General Admin.: Poyee L. Tai/Executive Vice President
       Donald C. L. Chu/President, Chief Executive Officer
Mktg./Adv.: Poyee Tai/Director National Accounts
       Daphne Mon/Director Product Development
       Rick Wright/Director Sales
       Bob Larsen/Manager Contract Sales
       Bianca Cenac/Manager Marketing
       Kit Cheung/Manager Sales
       Bob Larsen/Vice President Marketing & Sales
Research: Tom Chen/Vice President Engineering
       P. Pan/Vice President Research & Development
Finance: Dennis McNany/Vice President Finance

Coat, Laboratory	General
Cover, Head, Surgical	Surgery
Cover, Shoe, Conductive	General
Glove, Patient Examination	General
Glove, Patient Examination, Latex	General
Glove, Patient Examination, Specialty	General
Glove, Patient Examination, Vinyl	General
Gown, Examination	General
Gown, Isolation, Surgical	Surgery
Gown, Patient, Disposable	General
Mask, Face	General
Suit, Surgical	Surgery

TROVAGENE, INC   [+1] 858 217 4
11055 Flintkote Ave, Suite B, San Diego, CA 92121
FDA Number: n/a
E-mail: info@trovagene.com   *Fax:* [+1] 858 217 47
Web site: www.trovagene.com
Ownership: Private
Produces/Sells CE-marked Devices: N

TROVAGENE, INC   [+1] 858 217 4 *(cont'd)*
General Admin.: Mr. Kerry Segal/Business Manager
       Mr. Thomas Adams/Chairman
       Dr. Antonius Schuh/Chief Executive Officer
Research: Mr. David Robbins/Vice President Research & Development

TROY MANUFACTURING CO.   440-834-8262
17090 Rapids Road, PO Box 448, Burton, OH 44021
FDA Number: n/a   *Fax:* 440-834-1137
E-mail: troymfg@myepath.com
Medical Products Sales Volume: $1,300,000
Year Founded: 1951
Total Employees: 30
Ownership: Private
Produces/Sells CE-marked Devices: N
Federal Procurement Eligibility: Small Business
Distribution: OEM
General Admin.: Robert Gittings/Chief Financial Officer, Controller
       David S. Cseplo/President
       Charles Fath/Vice President
       Richard Taylor/Vice President
       Wynne Bogert/Vice President

Component, Metal, Other	General
Metal, Medical	General
Surgical Instrument, Disposable	Surgery
Surgical Instrument, Manual (General Use)	Surgery
Trocar, Abdominal	Gastroenterology/Urology
Trocar, Cardiovascular	Cardiovascular
Trocar, ENT	Ear/Nose/Throat
Trocar, Gastro-Urology	Gastroenterology/Urology
Trocar, Laparoscopic	Surgery
Trocar, Other	General

TRU-MOLD SHOES, INC.   800-843-6653
42 Breckenridge Street, Buffalo, NY 14213   716-881-4484
FDA Number: 3004548409
E-mail: info@trumold.com   *Fax:* 716-881-0406
Web site: www.trumold.com
Medical Products Sales Volume: $1,900,000
Annual Revenue: $1-$5 Million
Year Founded: 1950
Total Employees: 35
Ownership: Private
Produces/Sells CE-marked Devices: N
Federal Procurement Eligibility: Small Business, Minority Owned, VA Contract
Distribution: Manufacturer Direct, Manufacturer Through Distributor, Exporter

Shoe, Orthopedic	Orthopedics

TRUARCH, INC.   618-592-6468
6062 E. 800th Ave., Robinson, IL 62454
FDA Number: 3005771134
Ownership: Private
Produces/Sells CE-marked Devices: N

Insoles, Medical	General

TRUDELL MEDICAL MARKETING LTD.   800-265-5494
758 Third Street, London, ON N5V 5J7 Canada   519-685-8800
FDA Number: n/a
E-mail: tmml@tmml.com   *Fax:* 519-685-8993
Web site: www.tmml.com
Year Founded: 1922
Total Employees: 210
Ownership: Private
Produces/Sells CE-marked Devices: N
Distribution: Exclusive Distributor

TRUE FITNESS   800-426-6570
865 Hoff Road, St. Louis, MO 63366   636-272-7100
FDA Number: 1937824
E-mail: info@truefitness.com   *Fax:* 636-272-7148
Web site: www.truefitness.com
Medical Products Sales Volume: $24,100,000
Year Founded: 1981
Total Employees: 240
Ownership: Private
Produces/Sells CE-marked Devices: N
Federal Procurement Eligibility: Small Business, GSA Contract
Distribution: Manufacturer Direct, Manufacturer Through Distributor
General Admin.: Frank Trulaske/President, Chief Executive Officer
Mktg./Adv.: Tom Birkenmeier/Director Marketing
       Steve Ward/Director Product Development
       Keith Hankins/Manager Contract Sales
       Michael Brennan/Manager International Sales
       Keith Hankins/Manager National Sales
       Scott Eyler/Vice President Marketing & Sales
Production: Joe Piccolli/Manager Materials
       Stan Goldfader/Vice President Manufacturing

Exerciser, Other	Physical Med

TRUE FITNESS   800-426-6570 *(cont'd)*
Treadmill, Powered   Physical Med

TRUER MEDICAL, INC.   714-628-9785
1050 North Batavia, Unit C, Orange, CA 92867
FDA Number: 2032273   *Fax:* 714 633-3822
E-mail: sales@truermedical.com
Web site: www.truermedical.com
Ownership: Private
Produces/Sells CE-marked Devices: N
General Admin.: Douglas Mongeon/Chief Executive Officer
Production: Jeff Hunter/Manager Materials
Bougie, Esophageal, ENT	Ear/Nose/Throat
Contract Manufacturing	General
Contract R&D, Diagnostics	General
Stethoscope, Esophageal, With Electrical Conductors	Anesthesiology
Stylet, Tracheal Tube	Anesthesiology
Thermometer, Electronic, Continuous	General
Tubing, Flexible, Medical Gas, Low-Pressure	Anesthesiology

TRUETT LABS   626-334-5106
798 North Coney Ave., Azusa, CA 91702
FDA Number: 2018612   *Fax:* 626-969-3026
Web site: www.truettlabs.com
Total Employees: 40
Ownership: Private
Produces/Sells CE-marked Devices: N
Distribution: Service Direct
Contract Laboratory	General
Media, Coupling, Ultrasound	Radiology

TRUEVISION SYSTEMS, INCORPORATED   805-963-9700
114 East Haley Street, Santa Barbara, CA 93101
FDA Number: 3006140455
Microscope, Surgical	Ear/Nose/Throat

TRUFORM ORTHOTICS & PROSTHETICS   800-888-0458
3960 Rosslyn Drive, Cincinnati, OH 45209-1110   513-271-4594
FDA Number: 9201091   *Fax:* 800-309-9055
E-mail: truform-otc@surgicalappliance.com
Web site: www.truform-otc.com
Annual Revenue: $25-$50 Million
Year Founded: 1893
Total Employees: 350
Ownership: Otto Bock HealthCare Gmbh
Produces/Sells CE-marked Devices: N
Distribution: Manufacturer Through Manufacturer Reps
General Admin.: Tom Applegate/President, Chief Executive Officer
Mktg./Adv.: Patrick Spenlau/Director Marketing
     Tim Pennington/Director National Accounts
     Gary Parsons/Director Product Development
     Thomas Faust/Vice President Business Development
Production: Ginny Faught/Vice President Safety
Accessories, Fixation, Orthopedic	Orthopedics
Accessories, Traction	Physical Med
Bars, Spreader	Orthopedics
Belt, Lumbosacral	Orthopedics
Belt, Rib (Support)	Orthopedics
Belt, Traction, Pelvic, Orthopedic	Orthopedics
Binder, Abdominal	General
Brassiere, Surgical	Surgery
Cage, Knee	Physical Med
Cane	Physical Med
Collar, Cervical Neck	Orthopedics
Component, Exercise	Physical Med
Corset	Orthopedics
Cover, Mattress	General
Crutch	Physical Med
Fixation Appliance, Multiple Component	Orthopedics
Fixation Appliance, Single Component	Orthopedics
Garment, Protective, For Incontinence	Gastroenterology/Urology
Legging, Compression, Non-Inflatable	General
Nail/Blade/Plate Appliance	Orthopedics
Orthosis, Cervical	Physical Med
Orthosis, Cervical-Thoracic, Rigid	Physical Med
Orthosis, Limb Brace	Physical Med
Orthosis, Lumbar	Physical Med
Orthosis, Lumbosacral	Physical Med
Orthosis, Other	Physical Med
Orthosis, Rib Fracture, Soft	Physical Med
Orthosis, Sacroiliac, Soft	Physical Med
Orthosis, Thoracic	Physical Med
Pad, Pressure, Foam (Elbow, Heel)	General
Prosthesis, Breast, External	Surgery
Prosthesis, Breast, Inflatable, Internal	Surgery
Prosthesis, Breast, Non-Inflatable, Internal	Surgery
Prosthesis, Nipple	Obstetrics/Gynecology
Protector, Skin Pressure	General
Restraint, Protective (Body)	General
Sling, Arm	Physical Med

TRUFORM ORTHOTICS & PROSTHETICS   800-888-0458 *(cont'd)*
Splint, Abduction, Congenital Hip Dislocation	Physical Med
Splint, Clavicle	Physical Med
Splint, Hand, And Component	Physical Med
Splint, Molded, Aluminum	Orthopedics
Splint, Padded Stays	Orthopedics
Splint, Traction	Orthopedics
Stocking, Support (Anti-Embolic)	General
Support, Abdominal	Physical Med
Support, Back	Orthopedics
Support, Hernia	Gastroenterology/Urology
Support, Knee	Physical Med
Support, Scrotal	Gastroenterology/Urology
Support, Scrotal, Therapeutic	General
Traction Unit, Hip, Non-Powered, Non-Penetrating	Orthopedics
Traction Unit, Non-Powered	Orthopedics
Traction Unit, Static, Bed	Orthopedics
Traction Unit, Static, Other	Orthopedics
Truss, Hernia (Belt)	Gastroenterology/Urology
Truss, Umbilical	Gastroenterology/Urology
Urinal	General
Walker, Mechanical	Physical Med
Medical Product Subsidiaries (Listed Separately)
Airway Division Of Surgical Appliance Industries, Inc.
Pcp Champion

TRULIFE, INC.   360-697-5656
26296 Twelve Trees Ln., N.w., Poulsbo, WA 98370
FDA Number: 3022549
Ankle/Foot, External Limb Component	Physical Med
Cover, Limb	Physical Med
Joint, Knee, External Brace	Physical Med
Joint, Knee, External Limb Component	Physical Med
Orthosis, Lumbosacral	Physical Med
Orthosis, Truncal/Limb	Physical Med
Pack, Hot Or Cold, Water Circulating	Physical Med
Prosthesis, Thigh Socket, External Component	Physical Med

TRUPPE HEALTH CARE PRODUCTS AND SERVICES LTD.   800-854-1237
2500 Main St., Lambeth, ONT N6P-1P9 Canada   519-352-2041
FDA Number: n/a   *Fax:* 519-652-0249
E-mail: truppehealthcare@on.aibn.com
Year Founded: 1953
Total Employees: 10
Ownership: Private
Produces/Sells CE-marked Devices: N
Distribution: Manufacturer Direct, Exclusive Distributor

TRUTOUCH TECHNOLOGY INC.   866-721-6221
317 Commercial St NE, Suite 112, Albuquerque, NM 87102
FDA Number: n/a   *Fax:* 505-272-7083
Web site: www.trutouchtechnologies.com
Ownership: Private
Produces/Sells CE-marked Devices: N
General Admin.: Dr. Trent Ridder/Chief Technology Officer
     Dr. Richard Gill/President, Chief Executive Officer
Mktg./Adv.: Mr. Oscar Lazaro/Senior Vice President Sales
Research: Mr. Ben Ver Steeg/Vice President Engineering
Finance: Mr. James Dixon/Chief Financial Officer

TRYTON MEDICAL, INC.   919-226-1490
1000 Park Forty Plaza, Suite 325, Durham, NC 27713
FDA Number: n/a   *Fax:* 919-226-1497
E-mail: info@trytonmedical.com
Web site: www.trytonmedical.com
Year Founded: 2003
Ownership: Private
Produces/Sells CE-marked Devices: N
General Admin.: Mr. H. Richard Davis/Chief Technology Officer
     Mr. J. Greg Davis/President, Chief Executive Officer
Mktg./Adv.: Mr. Olivier Delporte/Vice President Sales
Finance: Mr. Brett Farabaugh/Chief Financial Officer
Stent, Cardiovascular	Cardiovascular

TS SCIENTIFIC   800-258-2796
PO Box 198, Perkasie, PA 18944-0198   215-257-4756
FDA Number: 9320151   *Fax:* 215-257-6046
E-mail: kryots@aol.com
Web site: www.tsscientific.com
Medical Products Sales Volume: $1,800,000
Annual Revenue: $1-$5 Million
Year Founded: 1972
Total Employees: 5   *Marketing Staff:* 1   *Sales Staff:* 1
Ownership: Private
Produces/Sells CE-marked Devices: Y
Federal Procurement Eligibility: Small Business
Distribution: Manufacturer Through Manufacturer Reps, Exclusive Distributor
General Admin.: Dermot O. Dinan/President

TS SCIENTIFIC
800-258-2796 *(cont'd)*
Equipment, Bank, Blood, Cryogenic (Liquid Nitrogen) — Hematology
Refrigerator, Biological — Microbiology

TSI INC.
500 Cardigan Road, Shoreview, MN 55126
800-874-2811
651-490-2811
FDA Number: n/a
Fax: 651-490-3824
E-mail: info@tsi.com
Web site: www.tsi.com
Annual Revenue: $5-$10 Million
Ownership: Private
Quality System Registration Information: ISO9001
Produces/Sells CE-marked Devices: Y
Distribution: Manufacturer Through Distributor, OEM
Cleanroom Equipment — General
Flowmeter, Gas, Non-Back-Pressure Compensated, Bourdon Gauge — Anesthesiology
Regulator, Temperature — Chemistry
Spectrometer, Infrared — Chemistry
Medical Product Subsidiaries (Listed Separately)
Twist2it, Inc.

TSI INC.
See Vasamed

TSI INCORPORATED
500 Cardigan Road, Shoreview, MN 55126
800-874-2811
651-490-2811
FDA Number: n/a
Fax: 651-490-3824
E-mail: info@tsi.com
Web site: www.tsi.com
Medical Products Sales Volume: $150,000,000
Annual Revenue: $100-$500 Million
Year Founded: 1961
Total Employees: 300 — *Marketing Staff:* 45 — *Sales Staff:* 50
Ownership: Private
Quality System Registration Information: ISO9002
Produces/Sells CE-marked Devices: Y
Federal Procurement Eligibility: Small Business, GSA Contract
Distribution: Manufacturer Direct, Manufacturer Through Distributor, Manufacturer Through Manufacturer Reps, OEM
Mktg./Adv.: Ron Grogg/Communication Specialist
Production: Brent Kiser/Product Manager
Analyzer, Particle — Chemistry
Analyzer, Protein — Chemistry
Generator, Aerosol — Ear/Nose/Throat
Pump, Nebulizer, Manual — Ear/Nose/Throat

TSI TECHNOLOGIES INC.
259 Edgeley Blvd, Unit 11-12, Concord, ONT L4K-3W7 Canada
905-760-1745
FDA Number: n/a
Fax: 905-760-1746
E-mail: tscientifi@aol.com
Web site: www.technoscientific.com
Year Founded: 1995
Total Employees: 25
Ownership: Private
Produces/Sells CE-marked Devices: N
Distribution: Manufacturer Direct

TSK LABORATORY CANADA INC.
1660 West 75th Avenue, Vancouver, BC V6P6G2 Canada
-604-269-3490
FDA Number: n/a
Fax: 604-269-9489
E-mail: americas@tsklab.com
Web site: www.tsklab.com
Year Founded: 1999
Total Employees: 10
Ownership: Private
Produces/Sells CE-marked Devices: N
Distribution: Exclusive Distributor, Importer

TSS FOAM INDUSTRIES CORP.
2770 West Main Rd., Caledonia, NY 14423
888-435-1083
585-538-2321
FDA Number: 2439010
Fax: 585-538-2876
E-mail: TSSFOAM@rochester.rr.com
Web site: www.tssfoam.net
Ownership: Private
Produces/Sells CE-marked Devices: N
Cushion, Flotation — Physical Med

TSS HUDSON
19 Brent Dr, Hudson, MA 01749
FDA Number: 1036769
Ownership: Private
Produces/Sells CE-marked Devices: N
Tubing, Fluid Delivery — General

TSUGAMI / REM SALES INC.
910 Day Hill Road, Windsor, CT 06095
860-687-3400
FDA Number: n/a
Fax: 860-687-3401
E-mail: jmacgregor@remsales.com
Web site: www.tsugamiusa.com

TSUGAMI / REM SALES INC.
860-687-3400 *(cont'd)*
Medical Products Sales Volume: $20,000,000
Annual Revenue: $100-$500 Million
Year Founded: 1959
Total Employees: 900 — *Marketing Staff:* 20 — *Sales Staff:* 150
Ownership: Private
Produces/Sells CE-marked Devices: N
Distribution: Manufacturer Through Distributor, Manufacturer Through Manufacturer Reps, OEM, Exclusive Distributor, Importer
General Admin.: Mr. Bradley Morris/President Admin.
Tap, Bone — Orthopedics

TSUMURA MEDICAL
See King Pharmaceuticals, Inc.

TTI MEDICAL
See Transamerican Technologies International

TU-WAY AMERICAN GROUP
191 Pearl St., Rockford, OH 45882-0306
800-537-3750
248-649-8790
FDA Number: n/a
Fax: 800-426-3964
E-mail: cs@tuwayamerican.com
Web site: www.tuwaymops.com
Annual Revenue: $0-$1 Million
Year Founded: 1923
Ownership: Private
Produces/Sells CE-marked Devices: N
Federal Procurement Eligibility: Small Business
Distribution: Manufacturer Through Distributor
Mktg./Adv.: Steven F. Grimes/Manager Sales
Production: Sandy Bettinger/Manager Customer Services
Housekeeping Equipment — General

TU-WAY PRODUCTS CO.
See Tu-Way American Group

TUA SYSTEMS, INC.
3645 North Courtenay Pky., Merritt Island, FL 32953
321-453-3200
FDA Number: 1052321
Fax: 321-453-3294
E-mail: tua111@aol.com
Web site: www.tua-rdc.com
Medical Products Sales Volume: $470,000
Annual Revenue: $0-$1 Million
Year Founded: 1988
Total Employees: 9 — *Marketing Staff:* 3 — *Sales Staff:* 16
Ownership: Private
Quality System Registration Information: ISO9000; ISO9001; ISO9002
Produces/Sells CE-marked Devices: N
Federal Procurement Eligibility: Small Business
Distribution: Manufacturer Through Manufacturer Reps, OEM
General Admin.: Dr. Theodore W. Unkel/Chief Executive Officer
Mktg./Adv.: Theodore L. Unkel/Vice President Business Development
Production: Audrey Unkel/Director Quality Assurance
Accessories, Catheter — Surgery
Accessories, Solution, Lens, Contact — Ophthalmology
Contract Manufacturing — General
Service, Device Coating, Protective — General

TUB MASTER LC
413 Virginia Drive, Orlando, FL 32803
800-833-0260
407-314-2176
FDA Number: n/a
Fax: 407-682-3138
E-mail: info@showersolutionsusa.com
Web site: www.tub-master.com
Annual Revenue: $1-$5 Million
Total Employees: 15 — *Marketing Staff:* 1 — *Sales Staff:* 4
Ownership: TUB-MASTER L.C.
Produces/Sells CE-marked Devices: N
Federal Procurement Eligibility: Small Business
Distribution: Manufacturer Direct, Manufacturer Through Distributor, Manufacturer Through Manufacturer Reps, OEM, Exporter
General Admin.: Chuck Johnson/Chief Executive Officer
David A. Webster/President
Mktg./Adv.: Marisa Winsky/Coord. Communications
Accessories, Wheelchair — Physical Med
Aid, Living, Handicapped — General
Chair, Shower — General
Rail, Bath — General

TUBULAR FABRICATORS INDUSTRY, INC.
See TFI Healthcare

TUBULAR FABRICATORS INDUSTRY, INC.
804-733-4000
600 West Wythe St., Petersburg, VA 23803
FDA Number: 2245337
Attachment, Commode, Wheelchair — Physical Med
Cane — Physical Med
Traction Unit, Non-Powered — Orthopedics
Transfer Aid — Physical Med

TUCKER DESIGNS LIMITED
800-780-7979
PO Box 641117, Kenner, LA 70064   **504-464-7479**
FDA Number: 2319127   Fax: 504-464-7480
E-mail: info@tuckerdesigns.com
Web site: www.tuckersling.com
Ownership: Private
Produces/Sells CE-marked Devices: N
Federal Procurement Eligibility: Small Business, Female Owned
Distribution: Manufacturer Direct, Manufacturer Through Distributor, Manufacturer Through Manufacturer Reps, OEM
General Admin.: Keith A. Jarrett/President
     Terry B. Jarrett/Vice President, General Manager
Mktg./Adv.: Gabriela Jarrett/Manager Marketing
   Holder, Infant Position   General

TUCSON MEDICAL CORP.
See Primesource Healthcare, Inc.

TUDOR SCIENTIFIC GLASS CO., INC.
800-336-4666
555 Edgefield Road, Belvedere, SC 29841   **803-279-4666**
FDA Number: n/a   Fax: 803-279-4690
E-mail: sales@tudorscientific.com
Web site: www.tudorscientific.com
Medical Products Sales Volume: $800,000
Annual Revenue: $0-$1 Million
Year Founded: 1956
Total Employees: 7   *Sales Staff:* 3
Ownership: Private
Produces/Sells CE-marked Devices: N
Federal Procurement Eligibility: Small Business
Distribution: Manufacturer Direct
General Admin.: Tom Tudor/President
     Teresa Crawford/Vice President Human Resources
Mktg./Adv.: Rod Barrie/Manager Marketing Research
   Buret   Chemistry
   Collector, Fraction   Chemistry
   Dispenser, Pipette   Chemistry
   Extraction/Chromatography, Ninhydrin, Hydroxyproline   Chemistry
   Heating Mantle   Microbiology
   Pipette   Chemistry
   Pipette Tip   Chemistry
   Pipette, Micro   Chemistry
   Viscometer   Chemistry

TUFF ORTHOPEDIC PRODUCTS
925-595-7053
776 West Lumsden Rd., Suite 104, Brandon, FL 33511
FDA Number: 3006371986
   Accessories, Traction   Physical Med

TUFFCARE
800-367-6160
3999 E. La Palma, Anaheim, CA 92807   **714-632-3999**
FDA Number: n/a   Fax: 714-632-3998
E-mail: Contact@tuffcare.com
Web site: www.tuffcare.com
Medical Products Sales Volume: $14,500,000
Annual Revenue: $25-$50 Million
Year Founded: 1989
Total Employees: 70   *Marketing Staff:* 7   *Sales Staff:* 14
Ownership: Private
Quality System Registration Information: ISO9000; ISO9001
Produces/Sells CE-marked Devices: Y
Federal Procurement Eligibility: Small Business, Minority Owned, GSA Contract, VA Contract
Distribution: Manufacturer Direct
General Admin.: Joseph Chang/President
Mktg./Adv.: Joseph Chang/Manager Advertising
     Joseph Chang/Vice President Marketing
Research: Joseph Chang/Vice President Research & Development
   Accessories, Walker   General
   Accessories, Wheelchair   Physical Med
   Armrest, Wheelchair   Physical Med
   Attachment, Bag (Crutch, Walker, Wheelchair)   Physical Med
   Attachment, Commode, Wheelchair   Physical Med
   Bed, Adjustable Hospital   General
   Bed, Electric, Home-Use   General
   Bed, Manual   General
   Bed, Obese   General
   Bedrail   General
   Belt, Wheelchair   Physical Med
   Brake, Extension, Wheelchair   Physical Med
   Cane   Physical Med
   Cane, Safety Walk   Physical Med
   Chair, Bath   General
   Chair, Shower   General
   Chair, Sitz Bath   General
   Commode (Toilet)   General
   Commode Seat   General
   Component, Wheelchair   Physical Med
   Crutch   Physical Med

TUFFCARE
800-367-6160 *(cont'd)*
   Cushion, Flotation   Physical Med
   Cushion, Flotation, Therapeutic   Physical Med
   Cushion, Wheelchair (Pad)   Physical Med
   Device, Anti-Tip, Wheelchair   Physical Med
   Footrest, Wheelchair   Physical Med
   Lift, Patient   General
   Mattress, Alternating Pressure (Or Pads)   Physical Med
   Mattress, Non-Powered Flotation Therapy   Physical Med
   Pad, Pressure, Air   General
   Pad, Pressure, Foam Convoluted   General
   Pad, Pressure, Gel   General
   Pressure Pad, Alternating, Reusable   General
   Pump, Alternating Pressure Pad   General
   Rail, Bath   General
   Ramp, Wheelchair   General
   Scooter (Motorized 3-Wheeled Vehicle)   Physical Med
   Table, Overbed   General
   Transfer Device, Patient, Manual   General
   Tray, Wheelchair   Physical Med
   Walker, Mechanical   Physical Med
   Weight, IV Pole   General
   Wheelchair, Manual   Physical Med
   Wheelchair, Powered   Physical Med

TULIP MEDICAL PRODUCTS
800-325-6526
PO Box 7368, San Diego, CA 92167   **619-239-6200**
FDA Number: 2028621   Fax: 619-239-5740
E-mail: tulipco@aol.com
Web site: www.tulipmedical.com
Medical Products Sales Volume: $1,200,000
Annual Revenue: $1-$5 Million
Year Founded: 2000
Total Employees: 3
Ownership: Private
Quality System Registration Information: ISO9000
Produces/Sells CE-marked Devices: N
Federal Procurement Eligibility: Small Business
Distribution: Manufacturer Direct, Manufacturer Through Manufacturer Reps
General Admin.: John Johnson/Chairman
     Marcille Pilkington/President, Chief Executive Officer
   Aspirator, Surgical   Surgery
   Camera, Television, Endoscopic (Without Audio)   Surgery
   Cannula, Other   General
   Cannula, Surgical, General & Plastic Surgery   Surgery
   Laparoscope, General & Plastic Surgery   Surgery
   Surgical Instrument, G-U, Manual   Gastroenterology/Urology
   Syringe, Other   General

TULOX PLASTICS CORP.
800-234-1118
401 S. Miller Ave., P.O. Box 984,   **765-664-5155**
Marion, IN 46952
FDA Number: n/a   Fax: 765-664-0257
E-mail: sales@tulox.com
Web site: www.tulox.com
Medical Products Sales Volume: $3,000,000
Annual Revenue: $5-$10 Million
Year Founded: 1983
Total Employees: 60   *Marketing Staff:* 1   *Sales Staff:* 5
Ownership: Private
Quality System Registration Information: ISO9002
Produces/Sells CE-marked Devices: N
Federal Procurement Eligibility: Small Business
Distribution: Manufacturer Direct, Service Direct
General Admin.: John C. Sciaudone/President
Mktg./Adv.: Christopher Sciaudone/Manager National Sales
Production: William E. Patuzzi/Vice President Manufacturing
Finance: Elizabeth Kachel/Controller
   Cabinet, Storage, Catheter   General
   Container, IV   General

TULSA DENTAL PRODUCTS
See Dentsply Tulsa Dental Specialties

TUMBLE FORMS, INC.
262-387-8720
1013 Barker Rd., Dolgeville, NY 11329
FDA Number: 2435707
   Accessories, Wheelchair   Physical Med
   Adapter, Hygiene   Physical Med
   Board, Scooter, Prone   Physical Med
   Chair, Adjustable, Mechanical   Physical Med
   Chair, With Casters   Physical Med
   Chair/Table, Medical   General
   Exerciser, Non-Measuring   Physical Med
   Table, Mechanical   Physical Med

TUNGSTONE POWER INC
800-232-3557
623 Main St., Woburn, MA 01801   **781-937-0011**
FDA Number: n/a   Fax: 781-937-3499
E-mail: sales@tungstonepower.com

TUNGSTONE POWER INC 800-232-3557 (cont'd)
Web site: www.tungstonepower.com
Medical Products Sales Volume: $2,200,000
Annual Revenue: $1-$5 Million
Total Employees: 3   Marketing Staff: 1   Sales Staff: 3
Ownership: Private
Produces/Sells CE-marked Devices: Y
Federal Procurement Eligibility: Small Business
Distribution: Manufacturer Through Distributor, Manufacturer Through
Manufacturer Reps, Exclusive Distributor
General Admin.: R. Jacobs/President
Production: D. Jacobs/Manager Production

Battery	General
Charger, Battery	General

TUNSTALL CANADA INC. 800-892-2205
7540 Bath Rd., 905-677-1144
Mississauga, ONT L4T-1 Canada
FDA Number: n/a
E-mail: sralbert@bellnet.ca   Fax: 905-677-1121
Web site: www.tunstallamerica.com
Year Founded: 1990
Total Employees: 10
Ownership: Private
Produces/Sells CE-marked Devices: N
Distribution: Exclusive Distributor

TURBO WHEELCHAIR CO., INC. 843-322-0486
45 Laurel Bay Rd., Suite 3 & 15, Beaufort, SC 29906
FDA Number: 3004149089

Wheelchair, Manual	Physical Med

TURBO-DOC EMR 800-977-4868
771 Buschmann Road, Suite G, 530-877-8650
Paradise, CA 95969
FDA Number: n/a
E-mail: turbodoc@turbodoc.com   Fax: 530-877-8621
Web site: www.turbo-doc.com
Annual Revenue: $0-$1 Million
Total Employees: 5   Marketing Staff: 4   Sales Staff: 2
Ownership: Private
Produces/Sells CE-marked Devices: N
Federal Procurement Eligibility: Small Business
Distribution: Manufacturer Direct
General Admin.: Lyle B. Hunt/Chief Executive Officer
Mktg./Adv.: Ward Clark/Director Marketing

Computer, Patient Data Management	General

TURNER BIOSYSTEMS, INC. 408-636-2414
645 North Mary Avenue, Sunnyvale, CA 94085
FDA Number: 101052
Ownership: Private
Produces/Sells CE-marked Devices: N

Colorimeter, General Use	Chemistry
Equipment, Laboratory, Gen. Purpose (Specific Medical Use)	Chemistry

TURNER DESIGNS 877-316-8049
845 W. Maude Avenue, Sunnyvale, CA 94085 408-749-0994
FDA Number: 2919015
E-mail: sales@turnerdesigns.com   Fax: 408-749-0998
Web site: www.turnerdesigns.com
Medical Products Sales Volume: $4,200,000
Annual Revenue: $5-$10 Million
Year Founded: 1972
Total Employees: 45   Marketing Staff: 4   Sales Staff: 4
Ownership: Private
Quality System Registration Information: ISO9001
Produces/Sells CE-marked Devices: Y
Federal Procurement Eligibility: Small Business, GSA Contract
Distribution: Manufacturer Direct, Manufacturer Through Distributor, Manufacturer
Through Manufacturer Reps, OEM, Exporter
General Admin.: Mike Mokelke/President, Chief Executive Officer
Mktg./Adv.: Pam Mayerfeld/Director Marketing & Sales
          Rita Juan/Manager Advertising
          Rita Juan/Manager Marketing Services
Production: Wellson Wong/Vice President Manufacturing

Fluorometer	Immunology
Fluorometer, Chemistry	Chemistry
Luminometer	Chemistry

TURNER INSTRUMENTS
See Abbott Hematology, Diagnostics Div.

TURNTINE OCULAR PROSTHETICS, INC 913-962-6299
6342 Long, Suite H, Lenexa, KS 66216
FDA Number: 3003926353

Conformer, Ophthalmic	Ophthalmology
Eye, Artificial, Non-Custom	Ophthalmology

TURNTINE OCULAR PROSTHETICS, INC 913-962-6299 (cont'd)

Shell, Scleral	Ophthalmology

TUTTNAUER USA CO. LTD. 800-624-5836
25 Power Dr., Hauppauge, NY 11788 631-737-4850
FDA Number: 2435367   Fax: 631-737-0720
E-mail: info@tuttnauerusa.com
Web site: www.tuttnauerusa.com
Medical Products Sales Volume: $30,000,000
Annual Revenue: $25-$50 Million
Total Employees: 80   Marketing Staff: 3   Sales Staff: 40
Ownership: Public
Quality System Registration Information: ISO9001; ISO9002
Produces/Sells CE-marked Devices: Y
Federal Procurement Eligibility: Small Business
Distribution: Manufacturer Through Distributor, Exclusive Distributor
General Admin.: Joshua Tuttnauer/Chief Executive Officer
          Ran Tuttnauer/President
          Robert Basile/Vice President Admin.
Mktg./Adv.: Ted Shlisky/Director Product Development
          Frank Krol/Manager Marketing
          Jake Miller/Manager Marketing
          David Morganstern/Manager National Sales
          Bill Soest/Manager Sales
          Jerry Fabricius/Manager Sales
          Hank Dierschke/Manager Training
          Paul J. McNichol/Vice President Sales
Production: Randy Polansky/Manager Materials
          Robert Basile/Manager Regulatory Affairs

Cleaner, Ultrasonic, Medical Instrument	General
Distilling Unit	Chemistry
Sterilizer, Steam (Autoclave)	General
Sterilizer, Steam, Table Top	General
Sterilizer/Compactor	General

TUZIK BOSTON 800-886-6363
104 Longwater Dr., Assinippi Park, 781-878-6363
Norwell, MA 02061
FDA Number: n/a   Fax: 781-878-6938
E-mail: info@tuzikboston.com
Web site: www.tuzikboston.com
Annual Revenue: $0-$1 Million
Ownership: Private
Produces/Sells CE-marked Devices: N
Federal Procurement Eligibility: Small Business
Distribution: Exclusive Distributor
General Admin.: David Tuzik/General Manager
          Joan E. Tuzik/President
Mktg./Adv.: John Tuzik/Vice President Sales

Applier, Surgical, Clip	Surgery
Blade, Scalpel	Surgery
Blade, Surgical, Saw, General & Plastic Surgery	Surgery
Carrier, Ligature	Surgery
Catheter, Suction, With Tip	General
Chisel (Osteotome)	Surgery
Chisel, Bone, Surgical	Dental And Oral
Chisel, Mastoid	Ear/Nose/Throat
Chisel, Middle Ear	Ear/Nose/Throat
Chisel, Nasal	Ear/Nose/Throat
Chisel, Osteotome, Surgical	Dental And Oral
Chisel, Surgical, Manual	Surgery
Clamp, Bone	Orthopedics
Clamp, Carotid Artery	Cns/Neurology
Clamp, Penile	Gastroenterology/Urology
Clamp, Surgical, General & Plastic Surgery	Surgery
Clamp, Uterine	Obstetrics/Gynecology
Clamp, Vascular	Cardiovascular
Cleaner, Ultrasonic, Medical Instrument	General
Clip, Removable (Skin)	Surgery
Cuff, Blood Pressure	Cardiovascular
Cuff, Inflation	General
Curette	Orthopedics
Curette, Adenoid	Ear/Nose/Throat
Curette, Biopsy, Bronchoscope (Non-Rigid)	Anesthesiology
Curette, Biopsy, Bronchoscope (Rigid)	Anesthesiology
Curette, Ear	Ear/Nose/Throat
Curette, Suction, Endometrial	Obstetrics/Gynecology
Curette, Uterine	Obstetrics/Gynecology
Cutter, Ring	General
Cutter, Wire And Pin	Orthopedics
Device, Locking, Clamp, Instestinal	Gastroenterology/Urology
Dilator, Tracheal	Ear/Nose/Throat
Dilator, Vaginal	Obstetrics/Gynecology
Dynamometer, Non-Powered	Orthopedics
Elevator, ENT	Ear/Nose/Throat
Elevator, Surgical, Dental	Dental And Oral
Elevator, Surgical, General & Plastic Surgery	Surgery
Forceps	Orthopedics
Forceps, Biopsy, Bronchoscope (Non-Rigid)	Anesthesiology

TUZIK BOSTON   800-886-6363 (cont'd)

Forceps, Biopsy, Bronchoscope (Rigid)	Anesthesiology
Forceps, Biopsy, Gynecological	Obstetrics/Gynecology
Forceps, Biopsy, Non-Electric	Gastroenterology/Urology
Forceps, Dressing, Dental	Dental And Oral
Forceps, ENT	Ear/Nose/Throat
Forceps, General & Plastic Surgery	Surgery
Forceps, Obstetrical	Obstetrics/Gynecology
Forceps, Rongeur, Surgical	Dental And Oral
Forceps, Surgical, Gynecological	Obstetrics/Gynecology
Forceps, Tube Introduction	Anesthesiology
Gauge, Mastoid	Ear/Nose/Throat
Gouge, Surgical, General & Plastic Surgery	Surgery
Grid, Radiographic	Radiology
Hammer, Surgical	Surgery
Handle, Scalpel	Surgery
Hemostat	Orthopedics
Hemostat, Surgical	Dental And Oral
Holder, Ear Speculum	Ear/Nose/Throat
Holder, Needle	Gastroenterology/Urology
Holder, Needle, Orthopedic	Orthopedics
Holder, Speculum, ENT	Ear/Nose/Throat
Hook, Surgical, General & Plastic Surgery	Surgery
Hook, Tracheal, ENT	Ear/Nose/Throat
Instrument, Clip Removal	Cns/Neurology
Instrument, Microsurgical	Cns/Neurology
Knife, Amputation	Surgery
Knife, Orthopedic	Orthopedics
Knife, Surgical	Dental And Oral
Knife, Tonsil	Ear/Nose/Throat
Mallet, Bone	Orthopedics
Mallet, Surgical, General & Plastic Surgery	Surgery
Mercury	Dental And Oral
Osteotome (Orthopedic)	Surgery
Osteotome, Manual (Plastic Surgery)	Surgery
Percussor	Cns/Neurology
Pledget And Intracardiac Patch, PETP, PTFE, Polypropylene	Cardiovascular
Pledget, Dacron, Teflon, Polypropylene	Cardiovascular
Probe, Gastrointestinal	Gastroenterology/Urology
Prosthesis, Arterial Graft, Synthetic, Greater Than 6mm	Surgery
Prosthesis, Arterial Graft, Synthetic, Less Than 6mm	Surgery
Prosthesis, Vascular Graft, Less Than 6mm Diameter	Cardiovascular
Prosthesis, Vascular Graft, Of 6mm And Greater Diameter	Cardiovascular
Punch, Adenoid	Ear/Nose/Throat
Punch, Biopsy	Gastroenterology/Urology
Punch, Biopsy, Surgical	Dental And Oral
Rasp, Bone	Orthopedics
Rasp, Surgical, General & Plastic Surgery	Surgery
Remover, Intrauterine Device, Contraceptive (Hook Type)	Obstetrics/Gynecology
Retractor	Orthopedics
Retractor, All Types	Dental And Oral
Retractor, Manual	Cns/Neurology
Retractor, Non-Self-Retaining	Gastroenterology/Urology
Retractor, Self-Retaining	Gastroenterology/Urology
Retractor, Surgical	Surgery
Retractor, Vaginal	Obstetrics/Gynecology
Saw, Bone Cutting	Orthopedics
Saw, Nasal	Ear/Nose/Throat
Scissors, Disposable	General
Scissors, Ear	Ear/Nose/Throat
Scissors, Episiotomy	Obstetrics/Gynecology
Scissors, Nasal	Ear/Nose/Throat
Scissors, Ophthalmic	Ophthalmology
Scissors, Orthopedic	Orthopedics
Scissors, Surgical Tissue, Dental (Oral)	Dental And Oral
Scissors, Umbilical	Obstetrics/Gynecology
Scissors, Wire Cutting, ENT	Ear/Nose/Throat
Skid, Bone	Orthopedics
Sound, Urethral, Metal Or Plastic	Gastroenterology/Urology
Spatula, Surgical, General & Plastic Surgery	Surgery
Speculum, Ear	Ear/Nose/Throat
Speculum, Rectal	Gastroenterology/Urology
Speculum, Vaginal, Metal	Obstetrics/Gynecology
Sphygmomanometer, Aneroid (Arterial Pressure)	General
Sphygmomanometer, Mercury (Arterial Pressure)	General
Stethoscope, Electronic (Auscultoscope)	Cardiovascular
Stethoscope, Fetal	Obstetrics/Gynecology
Stripper, Vein, External	Cardiovascular
Surgical Instrument, Cardiovascular	Cardiovascular
Tenaculum, Uterine	Obstetrics/Gynecology
Tip, Suction	Anesthesiology
Tray, Surgical Instrument	Surgery
Tube, Ear Suction	Ear/Nose/Throat
Tube, Tonsil Suction	Ear/Nose/Throat
Twister, Wire	Orthopedics

TUZIK CORPORATION
See Tuzik Boston

TWIST2IT, INC.   877-PRO-PHYS
39-30A 62nd St., Flushing, NY 11377   718-672-4234
FDA Number: n/a   Fax: 718-396-4500

TWIST2IT, INC.   877-PRO-PHYS (cont'd)
E-mail: twist@twist2it.com
Web site: www.twist2it.com
Total Employees: 20
Ownership: Private
Quality System Registration Information: ISO9000; ISO9002
Produces/Sells CE-marked Devices: Y
Federal Procurement Eligibility: Small Business, VA Contract
Distribution: Manufacturer Direct, Manufacturer Through Distributor, OEM, Service Direct, Exclusive Distributor, Importer, Exporter
General Admin.: Robert J. Achtziger/President, Chief Executive Officer
    Leonard B. Shaoul/Vice President
    Robert T. Postal/Vice President
Mktg./Adv.: Ann Smith/Manager Advertising & Market Research
    Margaret Bruce/Manager International & National Sales
Production: Barbara Decker/Manager Regulatory Affairs

Eraser, Dental Stain	Dental And Oral
Handpiece, Air-Powered, Dental	Dental And Oral
Handpiece, Contra- And Right-Angle Attachment, Dental	Dental And Oral
Operative Dental Treatment Unit	Dental And Oral

TWO RIVERS, LLC   423-626-4990
3199 Hwy. 25 E North, Tazewell, TN 37879
FDA Number: 2320646   Fax: 423-626-4990
E-mail: tworivers@communicomm.com
Medical Products Sales Volume: $600,000
Year Founded: 1999
Total Employees: 13
Ownership: Private
Produces/Sells CE-marked Devices: N
Federal Procurement Eligibility: Small Business

Chair, Position, Electric	Physical Med

TWO TECHNOLOGIES
See Two Technologies Inc.

TWO TECHNOLOGIES INC.   215-441-5305
419 Sargon Way, Horsham, PA 19044
FDA Number: n/a   Fax: 215-441-0423
E-mail: real.rugged@2T.com
Web site: www.2t.com
Medical Products Sales Volume: $7,400,000
Annual Revenue: $5-$10 Million
Year Founded: 1987
Total Employees: 45
Ownership: Private
Quality System Registration Information: ISO9001
Produces/Sells CE-marked Devices: Y
Federal Procurement Eligibility: Small Business
Distribution: OEM
General Admin.: David Young/Chief Executive Officer
Mktg./Adv.: Joan Rickards/Vice President Marketing & Sales

Component, Electronic	General

TWO-SIX INC.
See Ii-Vi, Inc.

TYCO ELECTRONICS/PRECISION   503-673-5027
INTERCONNECT
10025 S.w. Freeman Court, Wilsonville, OR 97070
FDA Number: 3026961

Cable, Electrode	Physical Med
Cable/Lead, ECG, With Transducer And Electrode	Cardiovascular
Electrosurgical Unit, Cutting & Coagulation Device	Surgery

TYCO HEALTHCARE GROUP LP   800-445-5025
Two Ludlow Park Drive, Chicopee, MA 01022   413-593-6400
FDA Number: n/a   Fax: 413-593-1372
E-mail: platka@ludlowhq.com
Web site: www.tycohealthcare.com
Medical Products Sales Volume: $22,000,000
Total Employees: 850   Marketing Staff: 2   Sales Staff: 8
Ownership: Covidien
Quality System Registration Information: ISO9001
Produces/Sells CE-marked Devices: N
Distribution: Manufacturer Direct, Manufacturer Through Distributor
General Admin.: Jim Anderson/President
    Levi Carrier/Vice President, General Manager
Mktg./Adv.: Paul Latka/Director Marketing & Sales
    Jim Anderson/Vice President Marketing & Sales
Research: Nilay Sankalia/Vice President Research & Development

Component, Other	General
Contract Manufacturing	General
Dressing, Gel	General
Electrode, Defibrillator	Cardiovascular
Electrode, ECG, Radiolucent	Cardiovascular
Electrode, Electrocardiograph	Cardiovascular
Electrode, Fetal Scalp	Obstetrics/Gynecology
Electrode, Gel	Cardiovascular

MANUFACTURER PROFILES

TYCO HEALTHCARE GROUP LP 800-445-5025 *(cont'd)*

Electrode, Holter	Cardiovascular
Electrode, Neuromuscular Stimulator	Cns/Neurology
Electrode, Other	General
Electrode, Pacemaker, External	Cardiovascular
Electrode, Sweat Test	Chemistry
Pack, Cold	General
Paper, Chart, Record, Medical	General
Paper, Recording, ECG/EEG	General
Recorder, Paper Chart	Cardiovascular

Medical Product Subsidiaries (Listed Separately)
Total Walther Feuerschutz Loschmittel Gmbh

TYCO VALVES AND CONTROLS 309-946-5205
121 W 1st Street, Suite 200, Geneseo, IL 61254
FDA Number: n/a *Fax:* 309-946-5206
E-mail: penberthysales@tycovalves.com
Annual Revenue: $0-$1 Million
Total Employees: 150
Ownership: Private
Quality System Registration Information: ISO9002
Produces/Sells CE-marked Devices: N
Federal Procurement Eligibility: Small Business
Distribution: Manufacturer Through Distributor, Manufacturer Through Manufacturer Reps
Mktg./Adv.: Len Wright/Manager Sales
  Control System, Energy   General

TYKRIS INC. 905-854-3009
**3272 15th Side Rd., P.O. Box 309,
Campbellville, ONT L0P-1 Canada**
FDA Number: n/a *Fax:* 905-851-3012
E-mail: tykris@aol.com
Year Founded: 1984
Ownership: Private
Produces/Sells CE-marked Devices: N
Distribution: Exclusive Distributor, Importer

TYLER MANUFACTURING CO.
See Bestway Products Co.

TYLER RESEARCH CORPORATION 780-448-1249
10328 73rd Ave., Edmonton, ALB T6E-6N5 Canada
FDA Number: n/a *Fax:* 780-433-0479
E-mail: tyler@tylerresearch.com
Web site: www.tylertech.com
Year Founded: 1986
Total Employees: 10
Ownership: Private
Produces/Sells CE-marked Devices: N
Distribution: Manufacturer Direct

TYRX, INC. 866-908-8979 / 732-246-8676
**1 Deer Park Dr., Suite G,
Monmouth Junction, NJ 08852**
FDA Number: 3005619263 *Fax:* 732-246-8677
Web site: www.tyrx.com
Year Founded: 1998
Ownership: Private
Produces/Sells CE-marked Devices: N
General Admin.: Robert White/President, Chief Executive Officer
Medical Admin.: Dr. Daniel Lerner/Chief Medical Officer
Mktg./Adv.: Mr. George Landau/Vice President Business Development
    Randy Mansfield/Vice President Marketing
Production: Mr. Mark Citron/Vice President Quality Control & Regulatory Affairs
Research: Mr. William McJames/Vice President Product Development
Finance: Ray Imp/Chief Financial Officer
  Mesh, Surgical, Polymeric   Surgery

TYSON CONSULTING GROUP 847-459-9189
612 White Pine Rd., Buffalo Grove, IL 60089-3330
FDA Number: n/a *Fax:* 847-215-6141
Total Employees: 3
Ownership: Private
Produces/Sells CE-marked Devices: N
Federal Procurement Eligibility: Small Business
General Admin.: Ted R. Tyson/President
    Patricia Tyson/Vice President
  Service, Consulting   General

TYTEX, INC. 401-762-4100
**601 Park East Dr.,, Highland Industrial Park,
Woonsocket, RI 02895**
FDA Number: 1225157
Ownership: Private
Produces/Sells CE-marked Devices: N

Garment, Protective, For Incontinence	Gastroenterology/Urology
Orthosis, Lumbar	Physical Med

TYTEX, INC. 401-762-4100 *(cont'd)*

Prosthesis, Hip, Semi-constrained, Metal/Ceramic/Ceramic/Metal, Cemented Or Uncemented	Orthopedics

TZ MEDICAL INC. 800-944-0187 / 503-639-0282
**7272 S.W. Durham Road, #800,
Portland, OR 97224**
FDA Number: 3027815 *Fax:* 503-639-0239
E-mail: info@tzmedical.com
Web site: http://tzmedical.com/
Ownership: Private
Quality System Registration Information: ISO9001
Produces/Sells CE-marked Devices: Y
Federal Procurement Eligibility: Small Business
Distribution: Manufacturer Direct, Manufacturer Through Distributor, Manufacturer Through Manufacturer Reps, OEM, Importer, Exporter

Bandage, Compression	General
Clamp, Vascular	Cardiovascular
Defibrillator, Battery-Powered, Low Energy	Cardiovascular
Pacemaker, Cardiac, External Transcutaneous (Non-Invasive)	Cardiovascular
Transmitter/Receiver System, Physiological, Telephone	Cardiovascular

U O EQUIPMENT CO. 800-231-6372 / 713-686-1869
5863 W. 34th St., Houston, TX 77092
FDA Number: 1642145 *Fax:* 713-688-0001
E-mail: CustomerService@UOEquipment.com
Web site: www.UOEquipment.com
Medical Products Sales Volume: $300,000
Annual Revenue: $0-$1 Million
Year Founded: 1981
Total Employees: 5 *Marketing Staff:* 1
Ownership: Private
Produces/Sells CE-marked Devices: N
Federal Procurement Eligibility: Small Business, VA Contract
Distribution: Manufacturer Direct, Manufacturer Through Distributor, Exporter
General Admin.: Robert R. Wright,/President

Aspirator, Emergency Suction	General
Canister, Oxygen	Anesthesiology
Carrier, Container, Oxygen, Portable	General
Cart, Gas Cylinder (Carrier)	Anesthesiology
Cylinder, Compressed Gas, With Valve	Anesthesiology
Cylinder, Oxygen	Anesthesiology
Flowmeter, Gas (Oxygen), Calibrated	Anesthesiology
Kit, Administration, Oxygen	Anesthesiology
Regulator, Oxygen, Mechanical	General
Regulator, Pressure, Gas Cylinder	Anesthesiology
Resuscitator, Cardiopulmonary	Cardiovascular
Resuscitator, Emergency Oxygen	Dental And Oral
Resuscitator, Emergency, Protective, Infection	Anesthesiology
Resuscitator, Pulmonary, Gas	General
Resuscitator, Pulmonary, Manual (Demand Valve)	General
Valve, Non-Rebreathing	Anesthesiology
Ventilator, Emergency, Powered (Resuscitator)	Anesthesiology

U S BIOTEX CORP. 606-652-4700
Route 1 Box 62, Webbville, KY 41180
FDA Number: 1528557

Clearing Oil	Pathology
Fixative, Formalin Containing	Pathology
Formalin, Neutral Buffered	Pathology
Gelatin For Specimen Adhesion	Pathology
Preservative, Cytological	Pathology
Preservative, Polyethylene Glycol	Pathology
Solution, Pathology, Decalcifier, Acid Containing	Pathology

U-LINE CORPORATION 800-779-2547 / 414-354-0300
**8900 N. 55th St., PO Box 245040,
Milwaukee, WI 53224**
FDA Number: n/a *Fax:* 414-354-0349
E-mail: Sales@U-Line.com
Web site: www.u-line.com
Medical Products Sales Volume: $11,800,000
Year Founded: 1962
Total Employees: 200 *Marketing Staff:* 3 *Sales Staff:* 27
Ownership: Private
Produces/Sells CE-marked Devices: Y
Federal Procurement Eligibility: Small Business, GSA Contract
Distribution: Manufacturer Through Distributor
General Admin.: Philip Uihlein/President, Chief Executive Officer
Mktg./Adv.: Jennifer Strafzewski/Director Marketing
    Marnie Uihlein/Manager Advertising
    Richard Uihlein/Vice President Advertising
    Jennifer Straszewski/Vice President Marketing
    Henry Uihlein/Vice President Sales
Production: Dean Byczynski/Director Quality Assurance
    David Barna/Manager Materials
    Keith Wischer/Plant & Production Manager
  Dispenser, Ice   General

U-LINE CORPORATION   800-779-2547 *(cont'd)*
Refrigerator, Foodservice   General

U-SYSTEM, INC.   408-571-0777
110 Rose Orchard Way, San Jose, CA 95134
FDA Number: 2954903
Scanner, Ultrasonic (Pulsed Echo)   Radiology

U-SYSTEM, INC.   (408) 245-1970
447 Indio Way, Sunnyvale, CA 94085
FDA Number: 2024567
E-mail: inquiries@u-systems.com
Web site: www.u-sys.com
Ownership: Private
Produces/Sells CE-marked Devices: N
Scanner, Ultrasonic (Pulsed Echo)   Radiology
Transducer, Ultrasonic, Diagnostic   Radiology

U-SYSTEMS, INC.   408-245-1970
447 Indio Way, Sunnyvale, CA 94085
FDA Number: 2954903
E-mail: inquiries@u-systems.com
Ownership: Private
Produces/Sells CE-marked Devices: N
General Admin.: Mr. Ronald Ho/President, Chief Executive Officer
Production: Ms. Lisa Scott/Vice President Quality Assurance & Regulatory Affairs
Research: Dr. Jiaya Chen/Vice President Engineering
Finance: Mr. Fred Ong/Chief Financial Officer
Scanner, Ultrasonic (Pulsed Echo)   Radiology
Transducer, Ultrasonic, Diagnostic   Radiology

U-TEN CORPORATION   630-289-8058
1286 Humbracht Cir, Bartlett, IL 60103-2051
FDA Number: 1424634   Fax: 630-289-8718
E-mail: yong@u-ten.com
Web site: www.u-ten.com
Medical Products Sales Volume: $470,000
Year Founded: 1994
Total Employees: 4
Ownership: Private
Quality System Registration Information: ISO9002
Produces/Sells CE-marked Devices: Y
Federal Procurement Eligibility: Small Business, Minority Owned
Distribution: Manufacturer Direct, Manufacturer Through Manufacturer Reps, OEM, Importer, Exporter
Cap, Surgical   Surgery
Cover, Shoe, Operating Room   Surgery
Drape, Surgical, Disposable   Surgery
Fiber, Absorbent   General
Sponge, External   Surgery
Sponge, Gauze   Dental And Oral

U.A. MEDICAL PRODUCTS OF GEORGIA
See Thomas Medical Inc.

U.E. SYSTEMS, INC.   800-223-1325
14 Hayes St., Elmsford, NY 10523-2407   914-592-1220
FDA Number: 9201092   Fax: 914-347-2181
E-mail: info@uesystems.com
Web site: www.uesystems.com
Medical Products Sales Volume: $2,500,000
Annual Revenue: $5-$10 Million
Year Founded: 1973
Total Employees: 30   Marketing Staff: 3   Sales Staff: 50
Ownership: Private
Produces/Sells CE-marked Devices: Y
Federal Procurement Eligibility: Small Business, GSA Contract
Distribution: Manufacturer Direct, Manufacturer Through Manufacturer Reps
General Admin.: Michael Osterer/President, Chief Executive Officer
Mktg./Adv.: Alan S. Bandes/Vice President Marketing
Research: Mark Goodman/Vice President Engineering
Detector, Leakage, Medical Gas   General

U.F.I.   805-772-1203
545 Main St., Ste. C-2, Morro Bay, CA 93442-2522
FDA Number: 9201093   Fax: 805-772-5056
E-mail: mail@ufiservingscience.com
Web site: www.ufiservingscience.com
Annual Revenue: $0-$1 Million
Year Founded: 1978
Total Employees: 10   Marketing Staff: 2   Sales Staff: 2
Ownership: Private
Produces/Sells CE-marked Devices: N
Federal Procurement Eligibility: Small Business, Female Owned
Distribution: Manufacturer Direct, Exporter
General Admin.: S. Woodside/President
    Mr. Brian Scholfield/Secretary
Research: H. Hanish/Vice President Research & Development
Accelerometer   Chemistry

U.F.I.   805-772-1203 *(cont'd)*
Amplifier, Biopotential (W Signal Conditioner)   Cardiovascular
Amplifier, Physiological Signal   Cns/Neurology
Amplifier, Transducer Signal (W Signal Conditioner)   Cardiovascular
Cardiograph, Apex (Vibrocardiograph)   Cardiovascular
Cardiograph, Impedance   Cardiovascular
Computer Equipment   General
Computer Software   General
Device, Measurement, Potential, Skin   Cns/Neurology
Electrode, Biopotential, Surface, Metallic   Physical Med
Electrode, Electrocardiograph   Cardiovascular
Electrode, Electromyographic   Cns/Neurology
Electrode, Surface   Anesthesiology
Electroglottograph   Ear/Nose/Throat
Electrorheograph   General
Meter, Skin Resistance, AC-Powered   Physical Med
Meter, Skin Resistance, Battery-Powered   Physical Med
Monitor, Cardiac Output, Impedance Plethysmography   Surgery
Monitor, Impedance Pneumograph   Anesthesiology
Monitor, Pulse Rate   Anesthesiology
Monitor, Respiratory   Surgery
Monitor, Response, Skin, Galvanic   Cns/Neurology
Phlebograph, Impedance   Cardiovascular
Plethysmograph, Impedance   Cardiovascular
Plethysmograph, Photo-Electric, Pneumatic Or Hydraulic   Cardiovascular
Probe, Temperature   General
Recorder, Chart, Laboratory   Chemistry
Recorder, Long-Term, ECG   Cardiovascular
Recorder, Long-Term, ECG, Portable (Holter Monitor)   Cardiovascular
Recorder, Long-Term, Respiration   Anesthesiology
Recorder, Long-Term, Trend   General
Rheoencephalograph   Cns/Neurology
Simulator, ECG   Cardiovascular
Simulator, EEG Test Signal   Cns/Neurology
Tester, Electrocardiograph Cable   Cardiovascular
Tester, Electrode   General
Tester, Electrode, Surface, Electrocardiograph   Cardiovascular
Tester, Electrode/Lead, Electroencephalograph   Cns/Neurology
Transducer, Blood Pressure   General
Transducer, Force   General
Transducer, Stethoscope   Anesthesiology
Transducer, Tremor   Cns/Neurology

U.M.A., INC.   800-842-5578
260 Main St., Dayton, VA 22821-0100   540-879-2040
FDA Number: 2412254   Fax: 540-879-2738
E-mail: umainc@rica.net
Web site: www.umainstruments.com
Annual Revenue: $1-$5 Million
Total Employees: 20   Marketing Staff: 1   Sales Staff: 2
Ownership: Private
Produces/Sells CE-marked Devices: N
Federal Procurement Eligibility: Small Business
Distribution: Manufacturer Direct, OEM, Exporter
General Admin.: Awad M. Da'Mes/President
Mktg./Adv.: Sharon Rathbun/Manager Marketing & Sales
Production: William S. Ham/Director Quality Assurance
Research: Dr. Dahmane Alem/Vice President Research & Development
Meter, Ultrasonic Power   General
Monitor, Blood Pressure, Indirect (Arterial)   Cardiovascular
Monitor, Blood Pressure, Venous   Cardiovascular
Oscillometer   Cardiovascular
Sphygmomanometer, Electronic, Manual   General

U.M.F. INC.
See United Metal Fabricators, Inc.

U.S. ARMY PINE BLUFF ARSENAL   870-540-3000
10020 Kabrich Circle, Pine Bluff, AR 71602-9500
FDA Number: 1648318
Web site: www.pba.army.mi
Ownership: Private
Produces/Sells CE-marked Devices: N
Decontamination Kit   Surgery

U.S. BIOCHEMICAL CORP.
See Usb Corporation

U.S. CATHETER & INSTRUMENT COMPANY
See Bard Electro Physiology

U.S. COUNSELING SERVICES, INC.
See Thermo Uscs

U.S. IMAGING INC.
See Shimadzu Medical Systems

U.S. IOL, INC.   800-354-7848
2500 Sandersville Rd., Lexington, KY 40583   859-259-4925
FDA Number: 1037089   Fax: 859-259-4926
E-mail: usiol@aol.com
Web site: www.usiol.com
Annual Revenue: $1-$5 Million

U.S. IOL, INC.   800-354-7848 *(cont'd)*
Ownership: Private
Quality System Registration Information: ISO9002
Produces/Sells CE-marked Devices: Y
Federal Procurement Eligibility: Small Business, Minority Owned
Distribution: Manufacturer Direct, Manufacturer Through Distributor, OEM
General Admin.: Kanu M. Shukla/Chief Executive Officer
      Dhaval K. Shukla/President
Production: A. K. Shukla/Vice President Manufacturing
   Folders and Injectors, Intraocular Lens (IOL)   Ophthalmology
   Lens, Intraocular   Ophthalmology

U.S. MEDICAL INSTRUMENTS, INC.   619-661-5500
1490 Air Wing Road, San Diego, CA 92154
FDA Number: 2028562
   Syringe, Antistick   General

U.S. MEDICAL SYSTEMS, INC.   512-347-8800
3160 Bee Cave Road, Suite 300c, Austin, TX 78746
FDA Number: 2950487
   Carboxymethylcellulose Sodium   Dental And Oral
   Cleaner, Ultrasonic, Medical Instrument   General
   Handpiece, Air-Powered, Dental   Dental And Oral

U.S. ORTHOTICS, INC.   800-825-5228
8605 Palm River Road, Tampa, FL 33619-4317   813-621-7797
FDA Number: 1043533   *Fax:* 813-623-1055
E-mail: info@usorthotics.com
Web site: www.usorthotics.com
Annual Revenue: $1-$5 Million
Year Founded: 1979
Total Employees: 50   *Marketing Staff:* 3   *Sales Staff:* 3
Ownership: Private
Produces/Sells CE-marked Devices: N
Federal Procurement Eligibility: Small Business, Minority Owned, GSA Contract, VA Contract
Distribution: Manufacturer Direct, Manufacturer Through Manufacturer Reps, OEM, Exporter
General Admin.: Anthony Velazquez/President
   Collar, Cervical Neck   Orthopedics
   Immobilizer, Knee   Orthopedics
   Immobilizer, Shoulder   Orthopedics
   Joint, Hip, External Brace   Physical Med
   Joint, Knee, External Brace   Physical Med
   Orthosis, Other   Physical Med
   Sling, Arm   Physical Med
   Support, Ankle   Orthopedics
   Support, Back   Orthopedics
   Support, Elbow   Orthopedics
   Support, Knee   Physical Med
   Support, Thigh   Physical Med

U.S. TABLE, INC.   847-741-3650
158 North Edison Ave., Elgin, IL 60123
FDA Number: 1056484
Ownership: Private
Produces/Sells CE-marked Devices: N
   Powered Medical Examination Table   General
   Table, Mechanical   Physical Med
   Table, Physical Medicine, Powered   Physical Med
   Table, Physical Therapy   Physical Med
   Table, Surgical, Manual   General

U.S. TECHNOLOGIES, INC.   800-234-0862
1701 Pollitt Dr., Fair Lawn, NJ 07410   201-475-8700
FDA Number: n/a   *Fax:* 201-475-8710
E-mail: info@ustechnologies.com
Web site: www.ustechnologies.com
Annual Revenue: $5-$10 Million
Year Founded: 1987
Ownership: Private
Produces/Sells CE-marked Devices: N
Federal Procurement Eligibility: Small Business
Distribution: Manufacturer Direct, Service Direct
   Service, Maintenance/Repair   General

U.S. VISION OPTICAL, INC.   866-435-7111
1 Harmon Dr., Glen Oaks Industrial Park, Glendora, NJ 08029
FDA Number: 2249712
E-mail: help@eyewearcare.com
Web site: www.usvision.com
Ownership: Private
Produces/Sells CE-marked Devices: N
   Frame, Spectacle (Eyeglasses)   Ophthalmology
   Sunglasses (Including Photosensitive)   Ophthalmology

U.S. WOMEN INSTITUTE   714-378-5606
9940 Takbert Avenue, Suite 303, Fountain Valley, CA 92708
FDA Number: 79559   *Fax:* 714-378-5621

U.S. WOMEN INSTITUTE   714-378-5606 *(cont'd)*
E-mail: dsamimi19@hotmail.com
Ownership: Private
Produces/Sells CE-marked Devices: N
   Surgical Instrument, G-U, Manual   Gastroenterology/Urology

U.S.A. DELTA.INC   305-557-1435
7830 W. 28th Ave., #213, Hialeah, FL 33018
FDA Number: 1064410
   Explorer, Operative   Dental And Oral

U.V. PROCESS SUPPLY, INC.   800-621-1296
1229 W. Cortland, Chicago, IL 60614-4805   773-248-0099
FDA Number: n/a   *Fax:* 773-880-6647
E-mail: info@uvps.com
Web site: www.uvprocess.com
Medical Products Sales Volume: $800,000
Annual Revenue: $1-$5 Million
Year Founded: 1979
Total Employees: 11   *Marketing Staff:* 3   *Sales Staff:* 5
Ownership: Private
Produces/Sells CE-marked Devices: Y
Federal Procurement Eligibility: Small Business
Distribution: Manufacturer Direct, Manufacturer Through Manufacturer Reps, OEM, Exclusive Distributor, Exporter
General Admin.: Mr. Stephen Siegel/Chief Executive Officer
Mktg./Adv.: Mr. Corey Gunzberg/Director Marketing
   Balance, Micro (0.001 mg Accuracy)   Chemistry

U.V. VISION CORP.   480-948-5350
7702 e. doubletree ranch road, suite 300, Scottsdale, AZ 85258
FDA Number: 3005823798
Ownership: Private
Produces/Sells CE-marked Devices: N
   Shield, Eye, Ophthalmic   Ophthalmology

UAS
   See United Air Specialists, Inc.

UBER LUCAS INTL LLC   410-758-3181
11126 Tuckahoe Rd., Denton, MD 21629
FDA Number: 3007033455
Ownership: Private
Produces/Sells CE-marked Devices: N
   Illuminator, Radiographic Film   Radiology

UBI   631-273-2828
25 Davids Drive, Hauppauge, NY 11788-2037
FDA Number: 1079   *Fax:* 631-273-1717
E-mail: pr@unitedbiomedical.com
Web site: www.unitedbiomedical.com
Medical Products Sales Volume: $13,800,000
Annual Revenue: $10-$25 Million
Year Founded: 1974
Total Employees: 285   *Marketing Staff:* 1
Ownership: Private
Produces/Sells CE-marked Devices: N
Federal Procurement Eligibility: Small Business
Distribution: Manufacturer Direct, OEM, Exporter
General Admin.: Mr. Nean Hu/Chairman
      Dr. Chang Yi Wang/Chief Executive Officer
      Dr. Chang Yi Wang/Chief Scientific Officer
      Mrs. Francine Volz/Manager Human Resources
Mktg./Adv.: Dr. Alan M. Walfield/Director Liscensing
Production: Dr. Chung Ho Hung/Vice President Manufacturing & Operations
Research: Dr. Connie Finstad/Manager Clinical Research
      Dr. Joseph Chang/Senior Scientist
      Dr. Kenneth Sokoll/Vice President Development
Finance: Ms. Amy Lin/Controller
   Serum, Screening, Blood   Hematology
   Test, Antibody, Acquired Immune Deficiency Syndrome (AIDS)   Hematology
   Test, Bacterial Diagnostic   Microbiology

UBIMED   310-556-0624
1180 South Beverly Drive Suite#400, Los Angeles, CA 90035
FDA Number: 3005960055
   Bottle, Collection, Vacuum (Aspirator)   General

UBM CANON   800-442-4200
11444 Olympic Blvd. Suite 900, Los Angeles, CA 90064   310-445-8590
FDA Number: n/a   *Fax:* 310-445-4269
E-mail: Reggie@mirthless.com
Web site: 3
Medical Products Sales Volume: $522,555
Annual Revenue: More than $1 Billion
Year Founded: 1980
Total Employees: 200   *Marketing Staff:* 100   *Sales Staff:* 85

UBM CANON 800-442-4200 *(cont'd)*
Ownership: A & A Orthopedic Appliances, Inc.
Stock Symbol: CAN
Traded On: Sydney
Quality System Registration Information: ISO9000; ISO9003
Produces/Sells CE-marked Devices: N
Federal Procurement Eligibility: Small Business, Minority Owned, Female Owned
Distribution: Manufacturer Direct, Manufacturer Through Distributor, Manufacturer Through Manufacturer Reps, Service Direct, Exclusive Distributor, Importer, Exporter

Absorbent, Carbon-Dioxide	Anesthesiology

Medical Product Subsidiaries (Listed Separately)
American Polarizers, Inc.

UBS INSTRUMENTS CORPORATION 818-710-1195
7745 Alabama Avenue, Suite 7, Canoga Park, CA 91304-6645
FDA Number: n/a Fax: 818-710-1242
E-mail: hklee4@hotmail.com
Medical Products Sales Volume: $300,000
Annual Revenue: $0-$1 Million
Total Employees: 2 *Marketing Staff:* 2
Ownership: Private
Produces/Sells CE-marked Devices: N
Federal Procurement Eligibility: Small Business, Minority Owned
Distribution: Service Direct, Exclusive Distributor
General Admin.: Howard K. Lee/President

Centrifuge, Tabletop	Pathology
Electrocardiograph, Multi-Channel	Cardiovascular
Electrode, Electrocardiograph	Cardiovascular
Monitor, ECG, Ambulatory, Real-Time	Cardiovascular
Sterilizer, Steam (Autoclave)	General
Suction Apparatus, Ward Use, Portable, AC-Powered	Surgery

UCB - PHARMA INC.
See UCB Inc.

UCB - PHARMACEUTICALS
See UCB Inc.

UCB INC. 770-970-7500
1950 Lake Park Dr., Smyrna, GA 30080
FDA Number: n/a Fax: 770-970-8857
E-mail: uscommunications@ucb.com
Web site: www.ucb-usa.com
Annual Revenue: $0-$1 Million
Year Founded: 1994
Total Employees: 500
Ownership: Ucb Bioproducts S.A.
Quality System Registration Information: ISO9000
Produces/Sells CE-marked Devices: N
Distribution: Manufacturer Direct, Manufacturer Through Manufacturer Reps, Importer

Contract Manufacturing, Pharmaceuticals/Chemicals	General
Contract R&D, Diagnostics	General

UCI/COULOMETRICS
See Uic, Inc.

UCP BIOSCIENCES, INC. 408-392-0064
1445 Koll Circle, Ste. 111, San Jose, CA 95112
FDA Number: 3004987297 Fax: 408-392-0163
E-mail: info@ucpbiosciences.com
Web site: www.ucpbiosciences.com
Ownership: Private
Produces/Sells CE-marked Devices: N

Enzyme Immunoassay, Amphetamine	Toxicology
Enzyme Immunoassay, Barbiturate	Toxicology
Enzyme Immunoassay, Benzodiazepine	Toxicology
Enzyme Immunoassay, Cannabinoids	Toxicology
Enzyme Immunoassay, Cocaine And Cocaine Metabolites	Toxicology
Enzyme Immunoassay, Methadone	Toxicology
Enzyme Immunoassay, Opiates	Toxicology
Enzyme Immunoassay, Phencyclidine	Toxicology
Enzyme Immunoassay, Propoxyphene	Toxicology
Radioimmunoassay, Tricyclic Antidepressant Drugs	Toxicology
Test System, Nicotine, Cotinine, Metabolites	Toxicology
Thin Layer Chromatography, Cocaine	Toxicology
Thin Layer Chromatography, Metamphetamine	Toxicology

UDL LABORATORIES, INC. 281-240-1000
12720 Dairy Ashford, Sugar Land, TX 77478
FDA Number: 1610608

Dressing, Other	General

UEI 800-547-5740 / 503-644-8723
8030 SW Mimbus, Beaverton, OR 97008
FDA Number: n/a Fax: 503-643-6322
E-mail: info@ueitest.com
Web site: www.ueitest.com
Medical Products Sales Volume: $8,200,000
Annual Revenue: $25-$50 Million

UEI 800-547-5740 *(cont'd)*
Year Founded: 1967
Total Employees: 44 *Marketing Staff:* 5 *Sales Staff:* 12
Ownership: KANE INTERNATIONAL
Produces/Sells CE-marked Devices: Y
Federal Procurement Eligibility: Small Business, GSA Contract
Distribution: Manufacturer Through Distributor
General Admin.: Michael Kane/President
    Jackie Shannon-Hollis/Vice President Human Resources
Mktg./Adv.: Leonard Ogden/Director Marketing
    Gary Lampasona/Director National Accounts
    Leonard Ogden/Director Product Development
    Tim Kilian/Manager Advertising
    Becky Watt/Manager Contract Sales
    Gary Lampasona/Manager International & National Sales
    Jayant Ingle/Manager International & National Sales
    Tim Kilian/Manager Marketing & Communications
    Tim Kilian/Manager Marketing Communications
Production: Benita Ballard/Director Quality Assurance

Thermometer, Electronic	General
Thermometer, Laboratory	Chemistry
Thermometer, Laboratory, Recording	General

UFP TECHNOLOGIES, INC. 630-543-2855
1235 National Avenue, Addison, IL 60101-3179
FDA Number: 7000513 Fax: 630-543-9820
E-mail: info@ufpt.com
Web site: www.ufpt.com
Medical Products Sales Volume: $4,500,000
Annual Revenue: $25-$50 Million
Year Founded: 1963
Total Employees: 45 *Marketing Staff:* 1 *Sales Staff:* 6
Ownership: Public
Stock Symbol: UFPT
Traded On: NASDAQ
Quality System Registration Information: ISO9001
Produces/Sells CE-marked Devices: N
Federal Procurement Eligibility: Small Business
Distribution: Manufacturer Direct
General Admin.: Philip L. Allen/General Manager
Mktg./Adv.: J. Anthony Bushnell/Manager National Sales
Production: Ellen Tarmichael/Manager Materials
    Ed Charhut/Vice President Manufacturing
Finance: Pam Danikowski/Vice President Finance

Contract Manufacturing	General
Cushion, Wheelchair (Pad)	Physical Med
Pad, Pressure, Foam Convoluted	General
Service, Engineering/Design	General

UGM MEDICAL SYSTEMS, INC. 425-487-7000
3611 Market St., Philadelphia, PA 19104
FDA Number: 2529017
Ownership: Private
Produces/Sells CE-marked Devices: N

Scanner, Emission Computed Tomography	Radiology

UHI CORPORATION
See Hill-Rom Manufacturing, Inc.

UHLMANN PACKAGING SYSTEMS, INC. 973-402-8855
44 Indian Lane E., Towaco, NJ 07082-1032
FDA Number: n/a Fax: 973-316-9330
E-mail: info@uhlmann-usa.com
Web site: www.uhlmann.de
Year Founded: 1948
Total Employees: 84 *Marketing Staff:* 2 *Sales Staff:* 8
Ownership: Private
Quality System Registration Information: ISO9001
Produces/Sells CE-marked Devices: N
Federal Procurement Eligibility: Small Business, Female Owned
Distribution: Manufacturer Direct
Mktg./Adv.: Mr. Walter Berghahn/Director Marketing & Business Development
    Mr. Alexander Mayer/Manager National Sales

Packaging Equipment	General
Packaging System, Unit-Dose	General

UIC, INC. 815-744-4477
1225 Channahon Rd., Joliet, IL 60436
FDA Number: n/a Fax: 815-744-1561
E-mail: jbanasek@uicinc.com
Web site: www.uicinc.com
Medical Products Sales Volume: $50,000
Annual Revenue: $5-$10 Million
Year Founded: 1965
Ownership: Private
Produces/Sells CE-marked Devices: Y
Federal Procurement Eligibility: Small Business
Distribution: Manufacturer Direct, Manufacturer Through Distributor

Analyzer, Carbon	Chemistry

UIC, INC.   815-744-4477 *(cont'd)*
Osmometer   Chemistry

ULBRICH STAINLESS STEELS & SPECIAL METALS   800-243-1676

57 Dodge Avenue, North Haven, CT 06473   **203-239-4481**
FDA Number: n/a   Fax: 203-239-7479
E-mail: info@ulbrich.com
Web site: www.ulbrich.com
Annual Revenue: $25-$50 Million
Ownership: Private
Quality System Registration Information: ISO9002
Produces/Sells CE-marked Devices: Y
Federal Procurement Eligibility: Small Business
Distribution: Manufacturer Direct, Manufacturer Through Distributor
General Admin.: Fred C. Ulbrich/Chairman
       Chris Ulbrich/Vice Chairman, Chief Operating Officer
   Alloy, Precious Metal, For Clinical Use   Dental And Oral

ULMER PHARMACAL CO.   800-848-5637
1614 Industry Ave., P.O. Box 408, Park Rapids, MN 56470
FDA Number: n/a   Fax: 218-732-5300
Web site: www.lobanaproducts.com
Annual Revenue: $0-$1 Million
Year Founded: 1919
Total Employees: 5   *Sales Staff:* 2
Ownership: Private
Produces/Sells CE-marked Devices: N
Federal Procurement Eligibility: Small Business, Female Owned
Distribution: Manufacturer Through Distributor
   Cleaner, Ultrasonic, Medical Instrument   General
   Disinfector, Liquid   General
   Jelly, Lubricating   General
   Lotion, Skin Care   General
   Soap   General
   Solvent   Chemistry
   Solvent, Adhesive Tape   Surgery

ULSTER SCIENTIFIC, INC.   845-255-2200
83 South Putt Corners Road, PO Box 819, New Paltz, NY 12561
FDA Number: 1321249   Fax: 845-255-3299
E-mail: info@americansci.com
Web site: www.americansci.com
Medical Products Sales Volume: $1,800,000
Annual Revenue: $0-$1 Million
Year Founded: 1974
Total Employees: 10   *Marketing Staff:* 1   *Sales Staff:* 2
Ownership: American Scientific Resources, Inc.
Stock Symbol: ASRO
Produces/Sells CE-marked Devices: N
Federal Procurement Eligibility: Small Business
Distribution: Manufacturer Direct, Importer, Exporter
General Admin.: Mr. Kenneth Hubbard/Chief Financial Officer, Vice President Operations
       Mr. Peter F. Lordi/President, Chief Executive Officer
   Meter, Peak Flow, Spirometry   Anesthesiology
   Pacifier   General
   Pipette Tip   Chemistry
   Pipetter   Hematology

ULTHERA INC.   877-858-4372
2150 S. Country Club Drive, Suite 21, Mesa, AZ 85210   **480-619-4069**
FDA Number: 3006560326   Fax: 480-619-4071
E-mail: info@ulthera.com
Web site: www.ulthera.com
Ownership: Private
Produces/Sells CE-marked Devices: N
General Admin.: Mr. Matthew Likens/President, Chief Executive Officer
Mktg./Adv.: Mr. James Atkinson/Vice President Marketing & Sales
Production: Dr. Randall Miller/Vice President Regulatory & Clinical Affairs
Research: Mr. Michael Peterson/Vice President Research & Development
   Electrosurgical Unit, Cutting & Coagulation Device   Surgery

ULTI MED, INC.   877-858-4633
287 E. 6th St., Suite 380, St. Paul, MN 55101   **651-291-7909**
FDA Number: 2183771   Fax: 651-291-7074
E-mail: customerservice@ulti-care.com
Web site: www.ulti-care.com
Medical Products Sales Volume: $7,800,000
Annual Revenue: $1-$5 Million
Year Founded: 1988
Total Employees: 50   *Marketing Staff:* 1   *Sales Staff:* 2
Ownership: ULTIMED, INC.
Quality System Registration Information: ISO9002
Produces/Sells CE-marked Devices: N

ULTI MED, INC.   877-858-4633 *(cont'd)*
Federal Procurement Eligibility: Small Business, GSA Contract
Distribution: Manufacturer Direct, Manufacturer Through Distributor, Manufacturer Through Manufacturer Reps, OEM
General Admin.: Thomas Erickson/Chief Executive Officer
       Jim Erickson/President
Mktg./Adv.: Shawn McGreavey/Director National Accounts
       Fred E. Meyer/Manager Advertising
       Fred E. Meyer/Manager Sales Training
Production: Jim Erickson/Director Quality Assurance
       Fred E. Meyer/Vice President Manufacturing & Sales
   Syringe, Insulin   General
Medical Product Subsidiaries (Listed Separately)
   Shinamerica, Inc.

ULTIMATE CONCEPTS, INC.   801-566-3241
5056 Crimson Patch Way, Riverton, UT 84065
FDA Number: 1724619
   Irrigator, Colonic   Gastroenterology/Urology
   Kit, Enema (For Cleaning Purposes)   Gastroenterology/Urology
   Speculum, Rectal   Gastroenterology/Urology

ULTIMATE SPINE, LLC.   562-598-1753
1220 North Barsten Way, Anaheim, CA 92806
FDA Number: 3005598612
   Orthosis, Fixation, Spinal, Spondylolisthesis   Orthopedics

ULTIMATE TRENDS   800-745-3191
1455 East 8125 So., Sandy, UT 84092   **801-554-8534**
FDA Number: 1723418   Fax: 866-389-4822
E-mail: myhomecolonic@earthlink.net
Web site: www.myhomecolonic.com
Year Founded: 1992
Ownership: Private
Produces/Sells CE-marked Devices: N
Federal Procurement Eligibility: Small Business, Female Owned
Distribution: Manufacturer Through Manufacturer Reps
General Admin.: Ms. Lisa Lowder/Owner
   Kit, Enema (For Cleaning Purposes)   Gastroenterology/Urology

ULTIMATE WIREFORMS, INC.   800-999-6484
200 Central St., Bristol, CT 06010-6716   **860-582-9111**
FDA Number: 1221844   Fax: 860-585-6666
E-mail: info@ultimatewireforms.com
Web site: www.ultimatewireforms.com
Annual Revenue: $5-$10 Million
Year Founded: 1988
Total Employees: 67   *Marketing Staff:* 1
Ownership: Private
Produces/Sells CE-marked Devices: Y
Federal Procurement Eligibility: Small Business
Distribution: Manufacturer Through Distributor, OEM
General Admin.: Paul J. Blanchette/Chief Executive Officer
       Alan Bednaz/President
Mktg./Adv.: Robert Nadeau/Vice President Business Development
Production: Michael Brault/Director Manufacturing
       Doreen Goulet/Manager Customer Services
       Bruce Keevers/Manager Regulatory Affairs
Research: Thomas Cameron/General Manager Research & Development
Finance: Nancy Blanchette/Manager Finance
   Aligner, Bracket, Orthodontic   Dental And Oral
   Band, Material, Orthodontic   Dental And Oral
   Clamp, Wire, Orthodontic   Dental And Oral
   Face Bow   Dental And Oral
   Pliers, Orthodontic   Dental And Oral
   Spring, Orthodontic   Dental And Oral
   Tube, Orthodontic   Dental And Oral
   Wire, Orthodontic   Dental And Oral

ULTIMEX CORP.   727-403-3090
6250 42nd St., Unit #30, Pinellas Park, FL 33781
FDA Number: 3004001813
Ownership: Private
Produces/Sells CE-marked Devices: N
   Cushion, Wheelchair (Pad)   Physical Med

ULTRA CLEAN SYSTEMS, INC.   877-935-6624
12700 Dupont Circle, Tampa, FL 33626   **813-925-1003**
FDA Number: 3002811406   Fax: 813-925-1044
E-mail: info@ultracleansystems.com
Web site: www.ultracleansystems.com
Medical Products Sales Volume: $700,000
Annual Revenue: $0-$1 Million
Year Founded: 1999
Total Employees: 7   *Marketing Staff:* 1   *Sales Staff:* 35
Ownership: Private
Produces/Sells CE-marked Devices: N
Federal Procurement Eligibility: Small Business

ULTRA CLEAN SYSTEMS, INC.   877-935-6624 *(cont'd)*
Distribution: Manufacturer Direct, Manufacturer Through Manufacturer Reps
General Admin.: O'Brien Cale/President
Mktg./Adv.: Lee Watkins/Manager International Marketing & Sales

Cleaner, Ultrasonic, Medical Instrument	General
Detergent	Hematology
Disinfector, Liquid	General
Solution, Instrument Cleaner	General

ULTRA RAY INC.   877-338-6857
760 Pacific Rd Unit 12,   **905-338-6857**
Oakville, ONT L6L 6 Canada
FDA Number: n/a   *Fax:* 905-338-5593
E-mail: ultraray@globalserve.net
Year Founded: 1983
Total Employees: 10
Ownership: Private
Produces/Sells CE-marked Devices: N
Distribution: Manufacturer Direct

ULTRA TEC MANUFACTURING, INC.   877-542-0609
1025 E. Chestnut Avenue, Santa Ana, CA 92701   **714-542-0608**
FDA Number: n/a   *Fax:* 714-542-0627
E-mail: info@ultratecusa.com
Web site: www.ultratecusa.com
Medical Products Sales Volume: $1,300,000
Annual Revenue: $1-$5 Million
Year Founded: 1972
Total Employees: 15   *Marketing Staff:* 3   *Sales Staff:* 4
Ownership: Private
Produces/Sells CE-marked Devices: Y
Federal Procurement Eligibility: Small Business
Distribution: Manufacturer Direct, Manufacturer Through Distributor, Manufacturer Through Manufacturer Reps, Service Direct, Exporter
General Admin.: Joseph Rubin/President
Mktg./Adv.: Tim Hazeldine/Vice President Marketing & Sales
Production: Tim Hazeldine/Product Manager
     Robert Rubin/Vice President Manufacturing

Cleaner, Medical Device	General
Production Equipment	General
Saw, Other	Surgery

ULTRA-CAL, INC.   760-741-7207
3014 Laurashawn Ln, Escondido, CA 92026
FDA Number: 7000922   *Fax:* 760-489-0811
Medical Products Sales Volume: $300,000
Annual Revenue: $0-$1 Million
Year Founded: 1975
Total Employees: 4   *Marketing Staff:* 1   *Sales Staff:* 2
Ownership: Private
Produces/Sells CE-marked Devices: N
Federal Procurement Eligibility: Small Business
Distribution: Manufacturer Direct, OEM, Exclusive Distributor, Exporter
General Admin.: J. R. Penney/President, Chief Executive Officer
Mktg./Adv.: Lori A. Fyfe/Vice President Marketing & Sales
Production: Steve Davenport/Manager Materials

Phantom, Computed Axial Tomography (CAT, CT)	Radiology
Phantom, Digital Subtraction Angiography (DSA)	Radiology
Phantom, NMR/MRI	Radiology
Phantom, Ultrasound	Radiology

ULTRA-DERM SYSTEMS   989-792-6110
2201 South Michigan Ave., Saginaw, MI 48602
FDA Number: 1832799

Booth, Sun Tan	Physical Med

ULTRA-LUM, INC.   800-809-6559
1480 N. Claremont Blvd., Claremont, CA 91711   **909-399-3694**
FDA Number: n/a   *Fax:* 909-482-0527
E-mail: info@ultralum.com
Web site: www.ultralum.com
Medical Products Sales Volume: $1,100,000
Annual Revenue: $1-$5 Million
Year Founded: 1988
Total Employees: 15
Ownership: Private
Produces/Sells CE-marked Devices: Y
Federal Procurement Eligibility: Small Business, GSA Contract
Distribution: Manufacturer Direct, Manufacturer Through Distributor, Manufacturer Through Manufacturer Reps, OEM, Service Direct, Exclusive Distributor, Importer, Exporter
Production: Mr. Steven G. Boland/Vice President Operations, General Manager
IS: Ms. Lucy Lee/Tech. Specialist

Counter, Colony	Microbiology
Device, Germicidal, Ultraviolet	General
Electrophoresis Equipment, Gel	Chemistry
Equipment, Test, Western Blot	Microbiology
Illuminator, Ultraviolet	Dental And Oral

ULTRA-LUM, INC.   800-809-6559 *(cont'd)*

Lamp, Ultraviolet (Spectrum A)	General
Transilluminator, Laboratory	Chemistry

ULTRACELL MEDICAL TECHNOLOGIES, INC.   877-SPO-NGE1
183 Providence New London Tpke.,   **860-599-4883**
North Stonington, CT 06359
FDA Number: 1222976   *Fax:* 860-599-4193
E-mail: sales@ultracell.com
Web site: www.ultracell.com
Medical Products Sales Volume: $4,700,000
Annual Revenue: $1-$5 Million
Year Founded: 1991
Total Employees: 24   *Marketing Staff:* 2   *Sales Staff:* 2
Ownership: Private
Quality System Registration Information: ISO9001
Produces/Sells CE-marked Devices: Y
Federal Procurement Eligibility: Small Business
Distribution: Manufacturer Through Distributor, OEM, Service Direct, Exporter
General Admin.: Wayne Korteweg/President, Chief Executive Officer
     Wayne Korteweg/Vice President, General Manager
Mktg./Adv.: Wayne Korteweg/Director National Accounts
     Wayne Korteweg/Director Product Development
Production: Wayne Korteweg/Director Quality Assurance
     Dan Burton/Manager Manufacturing
     Audrey Vitale/Manager Regulatory Affairs

Accessories, Cleaning, Endoscopic	Gastroenterology/Urology
Applicator, Tipped, Absorbent	General
Applicator, Tipped, Absorbent, Sterile	General
Balloon, Epistaxis (Nasal)	Ear/Nose/Throat
Band, Sweat	General
Collector, Sweat	Chemistry
Device, Ultrasound, Sinus	Ear/Nose/Throat
Gauze, Non-Absorbable, X-Ray Detectable (Internal Sponge)	Surgery
Holder, Retractor	Surgery
Packing, Surgical	Surgery
Paddie, Cottonoid	Cns/Neurology
Shield, Corneal	Ophthalmology
Shield, Eye, Ophthalmic	Ophthalmology
Splint, Septal, Intranasal	Ear/Nose/Throat
Sponge, Dissector	Pathology
Sponge, External	Surgery
Sponge, External, Neurological	Cns/Neurology
Sponge, External, Synthetic	Surgery
Sponge, Internal	Cns/Neurology
Sponge, Ophthalmic	Ophthalmology
Sponge, Other	General
Sponge, Rayon Cellulose	General
Sponge, X-Ray Detectable	Surgery
Syringe, Irrigating	General
Trephine, Manual, Ophthalmic (Corneal)	Ophthalmology
Wick, Ear	Ear/Nose/Throat
Wipe, Instrument	General

ULTRADENT PRODUCTS, INC.   801-553-4586
505 West 10200 South, South Jordan, UT 84095
FDA Number: 1718912

Accessories, Retractor, Dental	Dental And Oral
Activator, Ultraviolet, Polymerization	Dental And Oral
Adhesive, Bracket And Conditioner, Resin	Dental And Oral
Agent, Polishing, Abrasive, Oral Cavity	Dental And Oral
Airbrush	Dental And Oral
Applicator, Resin	Dental And Oral
Bracket, Metal, Orthodontic	Dental And Oral
Bracket, Plastic, Orthodontic	Dental And Oral
Burnisher, Operative, Dental	Dental And Oral
Burr, Dental	Dental And Oral
Carver, Dental Amalgam, Operative	Dental And Oral
Cement, Dental	Dental And Oral
Clamp, Rubber Dam	Dental And Oral
Cleaner, Ultrasonic, Medical Instrument	General
Cleanser, Root Canal	Dental And Oral
Cord, Retraction	Dental And Oral
Cup, Prophylaxis	Dental And Oral
Curette, Operative	Dental And Oral
Dam, Rubber	Dental And Oral
Detector, Caries	Dental And Oral
Disk, Abrasive	Dental And Oral
Excavator, Dental, Operative	Dental And Oral
Explorer, Operative	Dental And Oral
File, Pulp Canal, Endodontic	Dental And Oral
Filling, Instrument Plastic, Dental	Dental And Oral
Floss, Dental	Dental And Oral
Handle, Instrument, Dental	Dental And Oral
Handpiece, Air-Powered, Dental	Dental And Oral
Instrument, Diamond, Dental	Dental And Oral
Liner, Cavity, Calcium Hydroxide	Dental And Oral
Mask, Surgical	Surgery
Material, Impression	Dental And Oral
Material, Impression Tray, Resin	Dental And Oral

ULTRADENT PRODUCTS, INC.   801-553-4586 (cont'd)

Material, Tooth Shade, Resin	Dental And Oral
Matrix, Dental	Dental And Oral
Mirror, Mouth	Dental And Oral
Needle, Dental	Dental And Oral
Paper, Articulation	Dental And Oral
Pick, Massaging	Dental And Oral
Pliers, Orthodontic	Dental And Oral
Point, Abrasive	Dental And Oral
Post, Root Canal	Dental And Oral
Powder, Porcelain	Dental And Oral
Protector, Dental	Anesthesiology
Resin, Root Canal Filling	Dental And Oral
Retainer, Matrix	Dental And Oral
Retractor, All Types	Dental And Oral
Sealant, Pit And Fissure, And Conditioner, Resin	Dental And Oral
Source, Heat, Bleaching, Teeth, Dental	Dental And Oral
Strip, Polishing Agent	Dental And Oral
Syringe Unit, Air And/Or Water	Dental And Oral
Syringe, Cartridge	Dental And Oral
Syringe, Periodontic, Endodontic	Dental And Oral
Syringe, Restorative And Impression Material	Dental And Oral
Tooth Bonding Agent, Resin Restoration	Dental And Oral
Toothbrush, Manual	Dental And Oral
Tray, Impression	Dental And Oral
Tricalcium Phosphate Granules for Dental Bone Repair	Dental And Oral
Varnish, Cavity	Dental And Oral
Wheel, Polishing Agent	Dental And Oral
Wire, Orthodontic	Dental And Oral
Zinc Oxide Eugenol	Dental And Oral

ULTRAFLEX SYSTEMS, INC.   800-220-6670
237 South Street, Ste. 200, Pottstown, PA 19464   610-906-1410
Fax: 610-906-1420
FDA Number: 2529550
E-mail: info@ultraflexsystems.com
Web site: www.ultraflexsystems.com
Ownership: Private
Produces/Sells CE-marked Devices: N

Orthosis, Limb Brace	Physical Med
Splint, Hand, And Component	Physical Med

ULTRALIFE BATTERIES, INC.   800-332-5000
2000 Technology Pkwy., Newark, NY 14513   315-332-7100
Fax: 315-331-7800
FDA Number: n/a
E-mail: sales@ulbi.com
Web site: www.ultralifebatteries.com
Annual Revenue: $100-$500 Million
Year Founded: 1991
Total Employees: 1000
Ownership: Public
Stock Symbol: ULBI
Traded On: NASDAQ
Quality System Registration Information: ISO9001
Produces/Sells CE-marked Devices: N
Distribution: Manufacturer Direct, Manufacturer Through Distributor, Manufacturer Through Manufacturer Reps, OEM, Exporter
General Admin.: Mr. William Schmitz/Chief Operating Officer
  Mr. John Kavazanjian/President, Chief Executive Officer
Mktg./Adv.: Mr. Julius Cirin/Vice President Corporate Marketing
  Mr. Eric Lind/Vice President Sales

Battery	General

ULTRALITE ENTERPRISES, INC.   800-241-7506
390 Farmer Ct., Lawrenceville, GA 30045   770-963-0594
Fax: 770-995-7171
FDA Number: 1045025
E-mail: ultralit@bellsouth.net
Web site: www.ultralite-uv.com
Medical Products Sales Volume: $300,000
Annual Revenue: $1-$5 Million
Year Founded: 1976
Total Employees: 5
Federal Procurement Eligibility: Small Business
Distribution: Manufacturer Direct, Exporter
General Admin.: William C. McMillan/President
Production: William C. McMillan/Manager Production

Cabinet, Phototherapy (PUVA)	Surgery

ULTRAMED CORP.
See Boston Scientific Interventional Technologies

ULTRAMED INC.   800-804-3544
50 Sleeles Ave. E, Ste. 15,   905-878-4400
Milton, ONT L9T-4 Canada
Fax: 905-878-5044
FDA Number: n/a
E-mail: ultramed@interhop.net
Web site: www.ultramedinc.com
Year Founded: 1987
Total Employees: 25
Ownership: Private

ULTRAMED INC.   800-804-3544 (cont'd)
Produces/Sells CE-marked Devices: N
Distribution: Exclusive Distributor

ULTRASCOPE   800-677-2673
2401 Distribution Street, Charlotte, NC 28203   704-344-9998
Fax: 704-344-9733
FDA Number: 2028196
E-mail: sales@ultrascopes.com
Web site: www.ultrascopes.com
Medical Products Sales Volume: $700,000
Annual Revenue: $0-$1 Million
Year Founded: 1981
Total Employees: 7   Marketing Staff: 4   Sales Staff: 10
Ownership: Private
Produces/Sells CE-marked Devices: N
Federal Procurement Eligibility: Small Business, Minority Owned, Female Owned
Distribution: Manufacturer Direct, Manufacturer Through Manufacturer Reps
General Admin.: Shirley Masaoka/President, Chief Executive Officer
Production: Shirley Masaoka/Director Quality Assurance

Communication Equipment	General
Stethoscope, Amplified	General
Stethoscope, Manual	Cardiovascular
Stethoscope, Mechanical	General

ULTRASONIC SERVICES, INC.   713-665-4949
7126 Mullins Dr., Houston, TX 77081
FDA Number: 1000151813

Scaler, Ultrasonic	Dental And Oral

ULTRASONIX MEDICAL CORPORATION   604-279-8550
130 - 4311 Viking Way, Richmond, BC V6V 2K9 Canada
Fax: 604-279-8559
FDA Number: 3004877167
E-mail: info@ultrasonix.com
Web site: http://www.ultrasonix.com
Ownership: Private
Produces/Sells CE-marked Devices: N

ULTRASPECT INC.   972-485-4661
2005 Merrick Rd, Ste 336, Merrick, NY 11566
FDA Number: 3004962759
Ownership: Private
Produces/Sells CE-marked Devices: N

ULTRATEC, INC.   800-482-2424
450 Science Drive, Madison, WI 53711   608-238-5400
Fax: 608-238-3008
FDA Number: n/a
E-mail: service@ultratec.com
Web site: www.ultratec.com
Medical Products Sales Volume: $28,700,000
Year Founded: 1978
Total Employees: 300
Ownership: Private
Produces/Sells CE-marked Devices: Y
Federal Procurement Eligibility: Small Business
Distribution: Manufacturer Direct
General Admin.: Robert Engelke/Chief Executive Officer
Mktg./Adv.: Jackie Morgan/Director Marketing & Advertising
  Barbara Dreyfus/Vice President Marketing
  Jayne Turner/Vice President Sales
Production: Pamela Holmes/Manager Regulatory Affairs
  Mark Turner/Vice President Manufacturing
Research: Kevin Colwell/Vice President Research & Development

Communication Equipment	General
Communication System, Emergency Alert, Personal	General
Component, Electronic	General
Service, Printing	General
Telephone Equipment	General
Telephone, Handicapped Use	Physical Med

ULTRATHERMICS INC.
See Bsd Medical Corporation

ULTRAVIOLET PRODUCTS INC.
See Uvp, Llc

ULTRAVOICE, LTD.   800-985-3000
3612 Chapel Rd., Newtown Square, PA 19073
FDA Number: 2529591

Larynx, Artificial Battery-Powered	Ear/Nose/Throat

ULTREO   877-485-8736
9461 Willows Road N.e., Suite 101, Redmond, WA 98052
FDA Number: 3006096757

Toothbrush, Powered	Dental And Oral

ULTROID, LLC AND ULTROID TECHNOLOGIES,   727-865-1929
INCORPORATED
405 Central Ave., Ste. 100, Saint Petersburg, FL 33701
FDA Number: 3004892080

ULTROID, LLC AND ULTROID TECHNOLOGIES,   727-865-1929
(cont'd)
  Electrosurgical, Unit, Gastroenterology   Gastroenterology/Urology

ULTRON SYSTEMS, INC.   805-529-1485
5105 Maureen Lane, Moorpark, CA 93021
FDA Number: n/a   *Fax:* 805-523-1061
E-mail: sales@ultronsystems.com
Web site: www.ultronsystems.com
Medical Products Sales Volume: $1,600,000
Annual Revenue: $5-$10 Million
Year Founded: 1982
Total Employees: 17   *Marketing Staff:* 1   *Sales Staff:* 3
Ownership: Private
Produces/Sells CE-marked Devices: Y
Federal Procurement Eligibility: Small Business, Minority Owned
Distribution: Manufacturer Direct, Manufacturer Through Distributor, Manufacturer Through Manufacturer Reps, OEM, Exclusive Distributor, Exporter
General Admin.: Aki Egerer/President
     Aaron Chan/Vice President, General Manager
Mktg./Adv.: Alvin Egerer/Director Marketing
     Tiffany Wechsler/Manager International & National Sales
  Facility, Equipment, Medical, Mobile   General
  Traction Unit, Static, Other   Orthopedics

ULURU INC.   214-905-5145
4452 Beltway Drive, 4452 Beltway Drive, TX 75001
FDA Number: 3005692382   *Fax:* 214-905-5130
E-mail: mailto:kgray@uluruinc.com
Web site: www.uluruinc.com
Ownership: Private
Produces/Sells CE-marked Devices: N
General Admin.: Mr. Terrance Wallberg/Chief Financial Officer, Vice President
     Mr. Kerry Gray/President, Chief Executive Officer, Director
  Dressing, Wound and Burn, Hydrogel   Surgery

ULVAC NORTH AMERICA CORP.
  See Ulvac Technologies, Inc.

ULVAC TECHNOLOGIES, INC.   800-998-5822
401 Griffin Brook Dr., Methuen, MA 01844   978-686-7550
FDA Number: n/a   *Fax:* 978-689-6300
E-mail: bbilodeau@ulvac.com
Web site: www.ulvac.com
Medical Products Sales Volume: $39,100,000
Annual Revenue: $25-$50 Million
Year Founded: 1992
Total Employees: 40   *Marketing Staff:* 6   *Sales Staff:* 6
Ownership: ULVAC JAPAN, LTD
Produces/Sells CE-marked Devices: N
Federal Procurement Eligibility: Small Business
Distribution: Manufacturer Direct, Manufacturer Through Manufacturer Reps
General Admin.: Peter Goebel/Chief Operating Officer
     Haru Obinata/President, Chief Executive Officer
Mktg./Adv.: Rob Gardner/Director Marketing & Sales
     Robert Bilodeau/Manager National Sales
Production: Wayne Anderson/Director Production
Purchasing: Susan Zilaro/Director Contracts
  Analyzer, Gas, Helium, Gaseous Phase   Anesthesiology
  Calorimeter   Chemistry
  Mass Spectrometer, Clinical Use   Toxicology
  Pump, Vacuum, Central   Anesthesiology

UMI INTL.   888-511-8655
2 E. Union Avenue, PO Box 170,   201-804-8044
East Rutherford, NJ 07073
FDA Number: 1225677   *Fax:* 201-804-8046
E-mail: umimedical@umimedical.com
Web site: www.umimedical.com
Year Founded: 1983
Ownership: Private
Quality System Registration Information: ISO9002
Produces/Sells CE-marked Devices: Y
Federal Procurement Eligibility: Small Business, Minority Owned
Distribution: Manufacturer Through Manufacturer Reps, OEM, Exclusive Distributor, Importer, Exporter
  Cassette, Radiographic Film   Radiology
  Grid, Radiographic   Radiology
  Screen, Intensifying, Radiographic   Radiology

UNEEK CONCEPTS, LLC   888-686-7988
6435 Alloway Court, Springfield, VA 22152
FDA Number: 3003884598
Ownership: Private
Produces/Sells CE-marked Devices: N
  Utensil, Handicapped Aid   Physical Med

UNETIXS VASCULAR, INC.   800-486-3849
115 Airport Street,, North Kingstown, RI 02852   401-294-7559
FDA Number: 1222117   *Fax:* 401-294-3893
E-mail: sales@unetixs.com
Web site: www.unetixs.com
Medical Products Sales Volume: $5,600,000
Annual Revenue: $1-$5 Million
Year Founded: 1988
Total Employees: 37   *Marketing Staff:* 1   *Sales Staff:* 4
Ownership: Private
Produces/Sells CE-marked Devices: N
Federal Procurement Eligibility: Small Business
Distribution: Manufacturer Through Distributor, Manufacturer Through Manufacturer Reps, OEM, Exclusive Distributor, Exporter
General Admin.: Peter A. Moscovita/President, Chief Executive Officer
Mktg./Adv.: Anthony Castello/Director Product Development
     Peter A. Moscorita/Manager International & National Sales
Production: Dennis Cabral/Manager Materials
     Russell Straight/Manager Regulatory Affairs
     John Haefele/Vice President Manufacturing & Operations
  Computer Software   General
  Doppler, Flow Mapping   Radiology
  Plethysmograph, Photo-Electric, Pneumatic Or Hydraulic   Cardiovascular
  Plethysmograph, Volume   Anesthesiology
  Scanner, Ultrasonic, Vascular   Radiology
  Thermometer, Infrared   General

UNETTE CORPORATION   973-328-6800
88 N. Main St., Wharton, NJ 07885-1600
FDA Number: n/a   *Fax:* 973-537-1010
E-mail: info@unette.com
Web site: www.unette.co.uk
Medical Products Sales Volume: $8,000,000
Annual Revenue: $5-$10 Million
Year Founded: 1955
Ownership: Private
Produces/Sells CE-marked Devices: N
Federal Procurement Eligibility: Small Business
Distribution: Manufacturer Through Manufacturer Reps
  Contract Packaging   General

UNI-FIT CO.   650-363-2000
260-E Main St., Redwood City, CA 94063
FDA Number: n/a   *Fax:* 650-363-2015
E-mail: unifit@aol.com
Web site: www.uni-fit.com
Medical Products Sales Volume: $1,000,000
Annual Revenue: $0-$1 Million
Ownership: Private
Produces/Sells CE-marked Devices: N
Federal Procurement Eligibility: Small Business, Minority Owned
Distribution: Exclusive Distributor, Importer
  Knife, Other   Surgery
  Tweezers   General

UNI-LAC CORPORATION
  See Univac Dental Company

UNI-PATCH OEM DIVISION OF COVIDIEN
  See Covidien Lp, Formerly Registered As Uni-Patch

UNI/USE SYSTEMS DIVISION OF PARKE-DAVIS
  See Lionville Systems, Inc.

UNICARE BIOMEDICAL, INC.   949-643-6707
22971-B Triton Way, Laguna Hills, CA 92653
FDA Number: 2032542   *Fax:* 949-362-0433
E-mail: sales@unicarebiomedical.com
Web site: www.unicarebiomedical.com
Year Founded: 1998
Ownership: Private
Produces/Sells CE-marked Devices: N
Federal Procurement Eligibility: Small Business
Distribution: Manufacturer Direct, Exclusive Distributor
General Admin.: Stan Yang/Vice President
  Graft, Bone   Orthopedics
  Implant, Endosseous (Bone Filling and/or Augmentation)   Dental And Oral
  Plate, Bone, Orthodontic   Dental And Oral

UNICARE BIOMEDICAL, INC.   949-643-6707
22971-b Triton Way, Laguna Hills, CA 92653
FDA Number: 2032542   *Fax:* 949-362-0433
E-mail: info@unicarebiomedical.com
Web site: http://unicarebiomedical.com/
Ownership: Private
Produces/Sells CE-marked Devices: N

MANUFACTURER PROFILES

UNICARE MEDICAL PRODUCTS INC.
800-668-2030
770 Lawrence Ave. W,
416-785-5535
Toronto, ONT M6A-1 Canada
FDA Number: n/a
Year Founded: 1981
Fax: 416-787-8042
Total Employees: 50
Ownership: Private
Produces/Sells CE-marked Devices: N
Distribution: Manufacturer Direct, Exclusive Distributor, Importer

UNICELL INC.
800-718-2347
12160 É_, 103A Avenue, Surre BC V3V 3G8
Canada
FDA Number: N
E-mail: Dixon Freeman/President
Web site: info@unicellinc.com
Ownership: I
Stock Symbol: N
Distribution: Manufacturer Through Manufacturer Reps

UNICLEAN CLEANROOM GARMENT SERVICES
877-544-4432
A UNIFIRST CO., 8 Hixon Pl,
973-313-1173
Maplewood, NJ 07040
FDA Number: n/a
Fax: 973-313-0933
E-mail: jtilton@uniclean.com
Web site: www.uniclean.com
Medical Products Sales Volume: $100,000
Annual Revenue: $5-$10 Million
Total Employees: 3 — *Marketing Staff:* 1 — *Sales Staff:* 4
Ownership: WINDROSE MEDICAL PROPERTIES TRUST
Stock Symbol: UNF
Traded On: NYSE
Quality System Registration Information: ISO9002
Produces/Sells CE-marked Devices: N
Federal Procurement Eligibility: Small Business
Distribution: Service Direct
General Admin.: Mike Bovino/General Manager
Mktg./Adv.: Jim Mara/Manager Sales
Production: Ms. Suneela Mistry/Manager Quality Assurance
  Cleanroom Equipment — General

UNICOM
800-556-2828
6 Blackstone Valley Place, Suite 402,
401-765-3000
Lincoln, RI 02865
FDA Number: n/a
Fax: 401-765-6440
Web site: www.unicom-inc.com
Annual Revenue: $5-$10 Million
Year Founded: 1946
Total Employees: 85
Ownership: Private
Produces/Sells CE-marked Devices: N
Federal Procurement Eligibility: Small Business
Distribution: Exclusive Distributor
  Computer, Diagnostic, Programmable — Cardiovascular

UNICOM MICROAGE
See Unicom

UNICOM UNITED CAMERA
See Unicom

UNIFET, INC.
See Sendx Med, Inc.

UNIFLEX INC., MEDICAL PACKAGING DIVISION
800-223-0564
383 W. John St., Hicksville, NY 11802
516-932-2000
FDA Number: n/a
Fax: 516-932-3129
E-mail: sales@uniflexbags.com
Web site: www.uniflexbags.com
Medical Products Sales Volume: $25,000,000
Annual Revenue: $25-$50 Million
Year Founded: 1963
Total Employees: 20 — *Marketing Staff:* 1 — *Sales Staff:* 20
Ownership: Private
Produces/Sells CE-marked Devices: N
Federal Procurement Eligibility: Small Business
Distribution: Manufacturer Through Distributor
General Admin.: Richard Richer/Chief Executive Officer
Mktg./Adv.: Roy Walther/Director National Marketing & Sales
  Jyll Brink/Director National Sales
  Karen Schwaeber/Manager Sales
  Myra Hyman/Manager Sales
Production: Melissa Cantor/Vice President Operations
  Bag, Laundry, Infection Control — General
  Bag, Medical, Physician — General
  Bag, Plastic — General
  Bag, Specimen, Laparoscopic — Surgery
  Cover, Film, X-Ray — Radiology
  Cover, Other — General

UNIFLEX INC., MEDICAL PACKAGING DIVISION
800-223-0564
(cont'd)
  Security Equipment/Supplies — General

UNIFLOW MFG. CO. INC.
See Kold-Draft

UNIFORMS MANUFACTURING, INC.
800-222-1474
7575 E. Redfield Rd., P.O. Box 12716,
480-368-9316
Scottsdale, AZ 85267
FDA Number: n/a
Fax: 480-368-8556
Web site: www.unifmfg.com
Ownership: Private
Produces/Sells CE-marked Devices: N
Distribution: Service Direct
General Admin.: Larry Tucker/Chief Executive Officer
  Apron, Lead, Radiographic — Radiology
  Dress, Surgical — Surgery
  Gown, Examination — General
  Gown, Isolation, Surgical — Surgery
  Gown, Surgical — Surgery

UNILAB SURGIBONE INC.
905-564-3474
5790 Atlantic Dr., Unit 2, Mississauga, ONT L4W-4N8 Canada
FDA Number: n/a
Fax: 905-564-3475
Year Founded: 1990
Total Employees: 10
Ownership: Private
Produces/Sells CE-marked Devices: N
Distribution: Manufacturer Direct, Exclusive Distributor, Exporter

UNILAB, INC.
9058559093
2355 Royal Windsor Dr., Unit 3,
Mississauga, ON L5M-5 Canada
FDA Number: n/a
Fax: 905-855-3384
E-mail: brenda.kelly@unilabfurniture.com
Web site: www.unilabfurniture.com
Medical Products Sales Volume: $2,000,000
Year Founded: 1974
Total Employees: 10 — *Marketing Staff:* 1 — *Sales Staff:* 2
Ownership: Private
Produces/Sells CE-marked Devices: N
Federal Procurement Eligibility: Small Business
Distribution: Manufacturer Through Manufacturer Reps, Exclusive Distributor, Exporter

UNILENS
See Unilens Corp., Usa

UNILENS CORP., USA
800-446-2020
10431 72nd St. North, Largo, FL 33777
941-753-0383
FDA Number: 1034196
Fax: 800-808-8264
E-mail: information@unilens.com
Web site: www.unilens.com
Medical Products Sales Volume: $4,000,000
Annual Revenue: $5-$10 Million
Total Employees: 35 — *Marketing Staff:* 5 — *Sales Staff:* 5
Ownership: Public
Stock Symbol: EYES
Traded On: OTC Bulletin
Produces/Sells CE-marked Devices: N
Federal Procurement Eligibility: Small Business
Distribution: Manufacturer Direct
General Admin.: Al Vitale/President
Mktg./Adv.: Adrian Lupien/Vice President Marketing & Business Development
  Lenses, Soft Contact, Daily Wear — Ophthalmology
  Lenses, Soft Contact, Extended Wear — Ophthalmology
  Spectacle Microscope, Low-Vision — Ophthalmology

UNILENS CORP., USA
727-544-2531
10431 72nd St. North, Largo, FL 33777
FDA Number: 1034196
  Lens, Contact (Other Material) — Ophthalmology
  Lenses, Soft Contact, Daily Wear — Ophthalmology
  Lenses, Soft Contact, Extended Wear — Ophthalmology

UNILIFE MEDICAL SOLUTIONS
1-800-324-7674
250 Cross Farm Lane, York, PA 17406
717-384-3400
FDA Number: 3007710720
Fax: 717-384-3401
E-mail: info@unilife.com
Web site: www.unilife.com
Ownership: Private
Produces/Sells CE-marked Devices: N
General Admin.: Mr. Alan Shortall/Chief Executive Officer
  Mr. Richar Wieland/Chief Financial Officer, Executive Vice President
  Dr. Ramin Mojdeh/Chief Operating Officer
  Mr. Ian Hanson/Director
Mktg./Adv.: Mr. Eugene Shortall/Senior Vice President Business Development

UNILIFE MEDICAL SOLUTIONS   1-800-324-7674 *(cont'd)*
Mr. Michael Ratigan/Vice President Commercial Operations
Mr. Stephen Allan/Vice President Marketing & Communications
Dr. Jack Kelley/Vice President Strategic Marketing & Communications
Production: Mr. Mark Iampietro/Vice President Quality Control & Regulatory Affairs
Research: Dr. Gerald Verollet/Vice President Scientific Affairs

Syringe, Antistick	General
Syringe, Piston	General

UNIMAC   800-587-5458
PO Box 990 Shepard Street, Ripon, WI 54971   **920-748-3121**
FDA Number: n/a   *Fax:* 920-748-4431
E-mail: sales@alliancels.com
Web site: www.uniwash.com
Medical Products Sales Volume: $366,100,000
Annual Revenue: $25-$50 Million
Year Founded: 2004
Ownership: Private
Quality System Registration Information: ISO9001
Produces/Sells CE-marked Devices: N
Federal Procurement Eligibility: Small Business, GSA Contract
Distribution: Manufacturer Through Distributor
Mktg./Adv.: Mr. Kim Shady/Manager National Sales
     Patti Westpfahl/Media Planner

Laundry Equipment	General

UNIMED SURGICAL PRODUCTS, INC.   727-546-1900
10401 Belcher Rd., Largo, FL 33777
FDA Number: 1058746

Electrode, Electrosurgical, Return (Ground, Dispersive)	Surgery

UNION CARBIDE - OXYGEN CONCENTR. DIV.
See Nidek Medical Products Inc.

UNION CARBIDE CORP.
See Praxair, Inc.

UNION SPRINGS PHARMACEUTICALS   877-462-5967
4157 Olympic Blvd, Suite 200, Erlanger, KY 41018
FDA Number: n/a   *Fax:* 859-384-4083
Web site: http://clynsbrands.com
Year Founded: 2006
Ownership: Private
Produces/Sells CE-marked Devices: N
General Admin.: Mr. Robert Griggs/Chairman
Mktg./Adv.: Mr. Mark Steffen/National Sales Manager
     Mr. Steve Coutoure/Vice President Marketing & Sales

UNIPATH COMPANY
See Abbott Hematology, Diagnostics Div.

UNIPATH COMPANY, OXOID DIV.
See Oxoid, Inc.

UNIPATH, A DIVISION OF UL CANADA INC.
See Oxoid, Inc.

UNIQUE INSTRUMENTS, INC.
See Orchid Unique

UNIQUE SPORTS PRODUCTS, INC.   800-554-3707
840 Mcfarland Road, Alpharetta, GA 30004   **770-442-1977**
FDA Number: 1039647   *Fax:* 770-475-2065
E-mail: sales@uniquesports.us
Web site: www.uniquesports.us
Medical Products Sales Volume: $1,500,000
Annual Revenue: $5-$10 Million
Year Founded: 1972
Total Employees: 42
Ownership: Private
Produces/Sells CE-marked Devices: N
Federal Procurement Eligibility: Small Business
Distribution: Manufacturer Direct, Manufacturer Through Distributor, Manufacturer Through Manufacturer Reps, OEM, Exclusive Distributor, Exporter
General Admin.: Gene Niksich/President, Chief Executive Officer
Mktg./Adv.: Connie Smith/Director National Accounts
     Glinda Powers/Manager Advertising
     Mike Niksich/Manager International & National Sales
Production: John Varveries/Director Manufacturing & Quality Assurance
     Joe Bertolini/Manager Materials

Brace, Joint, Ankle (External)	Physical Med
Joint, Knee, External Brace	Physical Med
Protector, Finger	Orthopedics
Support, Arm	Physical Med

UNIQUE TECHNOLOGIES, INC.   610-775-9191
111 Chestnut St., Mohnton, PA 19540
FDA Number: 2531324

Blade, Scalpel	Surgery

UNIQUE/PERENY   800-HED-KILN
P.O. Box 246, 449 Route 31,   **609-466-1900**
Ringoes, NJ 08551
FDA Number: n/a   *Fax:* 609-466-3608
E-mail: sales@hed.com
Web site: www.hed.com
Total Employees: 60
Ownership: Private
Produces/Sells CE-marked Devices: N
Federal Procurement Eligibility: Small Business
Distribution: Manufacturer Direct, Manufacturer Through Manufacturer Reps, OEM, Importer, Exporter
General Admin.: John S. Dennis/President
     Samuel Tricase/Vice President
     James W. Dennis/Vice President, General Manager
Mktg./Adv.: Kathleen Kriskewic/Manager Product Marketing
     Terrance J. Dennis/Vice President Marketing
Production: Irvin L. Palitz/Executive Vice President Production

Material, Casting	Dental And Oral
Oven	Chemistry

UNISENSOR USA, INC.   603-926-5200
One Park Avenue, Suite #6, Hampton, NH 03842
FDA Number: 1226718   *Fax:* 603-926-5038
E-mail: info@unisensor.ch
Web site: www.unisensor.ch
Medical Products Sales Volume: $600,000
Year Founded: 1992
Total Employees: 5
Ownership: Private
Produces/Sells CE-marked Devices: N
Federal Procurement Eligibility: Small Business
Distribution: Manufacturer Direct, Manufacturer Through Distributor

Analyzer, Motility, Gastrointestinal, Electrical	Gastroenterology/Urology
Device, Cystometric, Hydraulic	Gastroenterology/Urology

UNISPLINT CORP.   770-271-0646
4485 Commerce Dr., Suite 106, Buford, GA 30518
FDA Number: 1046292
Annual Revenue: $0-$1 Million
Ownership: Private
Produces/Sells CE-marked Devices: N
Federal Procurement Eligibility: Small Business
Distribution: Manufacturer Direct, Importer, Exporter

Airway, Obstruction Removal (Choke Saver)	General
Band, Material, Orthodontic	Dental And Oral
Fixation Device, Jaw Fracture	Orthopedics
Lock, Wire, And Ligature, Intraoral	Dental And Oral
Splint, Other	Orthopedics

UNISYN MEDICAL TECHNOLOGIES.   877-386-3246
1150 Catamount Dr., Golden, CO 80403   **303-384-3246**
FDA Number: 1724524
Web site: http://www2.unisynmedical.com
Total Employees: 185
Ownership: Private
Produces/Sells CE-marked Devices: N
Mktg./Adv.: Mr. Troy Williams/Vice President Services & Sales

Tester, Radiology Quality Assurance	Radiology

UNIT CHEMICAL CORP.   800-879-8648
7360 Commercial Way, Henderson, NV 89015   **702-564-6454**
FDA Number: n/a   *Fax:* 702-564-6629
E-mail: info@unitchemical.com
Web site: www.unitchemical.com
Medical Products Sales Volume: $600,000
Annual Revenue: $1-$5 Million
Year Founded: 1949
Total Employees: 8
Ownership: Private
Produces/Sells CE-marked Devices: N
Federal Procurement Eligibility: Small Business, Female Owned
Distribution: Manufacturer Direct
General Admin.: Raymond Chaplar/President
Mktg./Adv.: Mike Chaplar/Director Marketing

Cleaner, Bedpan (Sterilizer)	General
Disinfectant, Liquid	General
Disinfector, Medical Device	General
Medical Disinfectants/Cleaners for Instruments	General
Sanitizer	General
Washer/Disinfector	General

UNITED AD LABEL
See Veriad

UNITED AIR SPECIALISTS, INC.   800-252-4647
4440 Creek Rd., Cincinnati, OH 45242   **513-891-0400**
FDA Number: n/a   *Fax:* 513-891-4171

UNITED AIR SPECIALISTS, INC. 800-252-4647 *(cont'd)*
E-mail: sales@uasinc.com
Web site: www.uasinc.com
Annual Revenue: $10-$25 Million
Year Founded: 1966
Total Employees: 80
Ownership: CLARCOR FILTRATION PRODUCTS GROUP
Stock Symbol: CLC
Traded On: NYSE
Quality System Registration Information: ISO9001
Produces/Sells CE-marked Devices: N
Distribution: Manufacturer Through Distributor, Manufacturer Through Manufacturer Reps
General Admin.: Rich Larson/President
Mktg./Adv.: Steve Trame/Vice President Marketing

Equipment, Cleaning, Air	General
Filter, Air	General

UNITED AMERICAN MEDICAL CO, INC.
See Vilex, Inc.

UNITED BIOMEDICAL
See Ubi

UNITED BIOTECH 866-753-5700
45 W Jefryn Blvd., Suite E, Deer Park, NY 11729
FDA Number: 3004506204
Ownership: Private
Produces/Sells CE-marked Devices: N

Cleaner, Ultrasonic, Medical Instrument	General

UNITED BIOTECH, INC. 650-961-2910
211 S. Whisman Road, Suite E, Mountain View, CA 94041-1517
FDA Number: 2937601   *Fax:* 650-961-0766
E-mail: info@unitedbiotech.com
Web site: www.unitedbiotech.com
Medical Products Sales Volume: $1,000,000
Year Founded: 1984
Total Employees: 7
Ownership: Private
Quality System Registration Information: ISO9001
Produces/Sells CE-marked Devices: Y
Federal Procurement Eligibility: Small Business, Minority Owned
Distribution: Manufacturer Direct, Manufacturer Through Distributor, Manufacturer Through Manufacturer Reps, OEM, Exporter
Mktg./Adv.: Mr. Jack Wan/Director International Marketing

Alpha-1 Microglobulin, Antigen, Antiserum, Control	Immunology
Analyzer, Parasite Concentration	Microbiology
Anti-DNA Antibody (Enzyme-Labeled), Antigen, Control	Immunology
Antibody, Toxoplasma Gondii	Microbiology
Antibody, Treponema Pallidum	Microbiology
Antigen, Antiserum, Control, Albumin	Immunology
Antigen, Antiserum, Control, Beta Globulin	Immunology
Antigen, Antiserum, Control, Ferritin	Immunology
Antigen, Antiserum, Control, IGE	Immunology
Antigen, Antiserum, Control, Other	Immunology
Antigen, CF, T. Cruzi	Microbiology
Antigen, Carbohydrate (CA19-9)	Immunology
Antigen, Tumor Marker, Bladder (Basement Membrane Complexes)	Immunology
Antinuclear Antibody (Enzyme-Labeled), Antigen, Controls	Immunology
Campylobacter Pylori	Microbiology
Cytomegalovirus, DNA Reagents	Microbiology
Enzyme Linked Immunoabsorbent Assay, Coccidioides Immitis	Microbiology
Enzyme Linked Immunoabsorbent Assay, Cytomegalovirus	Microbiology
Enzyme Linked Immunoabsorbent Assay, Toxoplasma Gondii	Microbiology
Enzyme-Linked Immunosorbent Assay, Herpes Simplex Virus, HSV-2	Microbiology
Hepatitis B Test (B Core, BE Antigen & Antibody, B Core IGM)	Microbiology
Immunofluorescent Assay, T. Cruzi	Microbiology
Kit, Test, Alpha-fetoprotein For Testicular Cancer	Immunology
Proteins, Amyloid And Precursor	Immunology
Radioimmunoassay, Cortisol	Chemistry
Radioimmunoassay, Follicle Stimulating Hormone	Chemistry
Radioimmunoassay, Human Chorionic Gonadotropin	Chemistry
Radioimmunoassay, Luteinizing Hormone	Chemistry
Radioimmunoassay, Prolactin (Lactogen)	Chemistry
Radioimmunoassay, Prostate-Specific Antigen (PSA)	Immunology
Radioimmunoassay, Thyroid Stimulating Hormone	Chemistry
Reagent, Cysticercosis	Microbiology
Reagent, Leishmanii Serological	Microbiology
Reagent, Serological, Delta, Hepatitis	Microbiology
Rubella, Other Assays	Microbiology
Strip, HAMA IGG, ELISA, In Vitro Test System	Immunology
System, Test, Immunological, Antigen, Tumor	Immunology
System, Test, Tumor Marker, For Detection Of Bladder Cancer	Immunology
Test, Antigen (CA125), Tumor-Associated, Ovarian, Epithelial	Immunology
Test, Bacterial Diagnostic	Microbiology
Test, Beta 2 - Microglobulin	Immunology
Test, C-Reactive Protein	Immunology
Test, Hepatitis A (Antibody and IGM Antibody)	Microbiology
Test, Hiv Detection	Immunology
Test, Rheumatoid Factor	Immunology

UNITED BIOTECH, INC. 650-961-2910 *(cont'd)*

Test, Syphilis (RPR or VDRL)	Microbiology
Test, Thyroid Autoantibody	Immunology
Thyroglobulin, Antigen, Antiserum, Control	Immunology

UNITED CHEMICAL TECHNOLOGIES, INC. 800-385-3153
2731 Bartram Road, Bristol, PA 19007-6893 215-781-9255
FDA Number: 2523730   *Fax:* 215-785-1226
E-mail: customerservice@unitedchem.com
Web site: www.unitedchem.com
Medical Products Sales Volume: $7,800,000
Annual Revenue: $5-$10 Million
Year Founded: 1986
Total Employees: 53   *Marketing Staff:* 3   *Sales Staff:* 6
Ownership: Private
Produces/Sells CE-marked Devices: N
Federal Procurement Eligibility: Small Business
Distribution: Manufacturer Direct, OEM
General Admin.: Michael J. Telepchak/President, Chief Executive Officer
      William Hiltner/Vice President Human Resources
Mktg./Adv.: Bethany Telepchak/Manager National Sales
Production: Scott Vance/Manager Materials
      Mark Connelly/Manager Regulatory Affairs

Column, Chromatography	Chemistry
Component, Silicone	General
Contract Manufacturing	General
Elastomer, Silicone Rubber	General
Material, Raw, Production	General
Plate, Silica Gel, TLC	Toxicology

UNITED CONTACT LENS, INC. 425-743-7343
19111 61st Ave Ne #5, Arlington, WA 98223
FDA Number: 2918644

Lenses, Soft Contact, Daily Wear	Ophthalmology

UNITED DENTAL MANUFACTURERS, INC. 918-878-0450
PO Box 700874, Tulsa, OK 74135-6560
FDA Number: 7000937   *Fax:* 918-878-0451
E-mail: kurt@udm-endo.com
Annual Revenue: $5-$10 Million
Total Employees: 21
Ownership: Public
Stock Symbol: XRAY
Traded On: NYSE
Quality System Registration Information: ISO9002
Produces/Sells CE-marked Devices: Y
Federal Procurement Eligibility: Small Business
Distribution: Exclusive Distributor, Importer, Exporter
General Admin.: Kurt VanHofwegen/Vice President Human Resources
Mktg./Adv.: Kurt Van Hofwegen/Manager International & National Sales
Production: Kurt Van Hofwegen/General Manager Production

Container, Sterilization (Tray)	General
File, Pulp Canal, Endodontic	Dental And Oral
Filling, Instrument Plastic, Dental	Dental And Oral
Gutta Percha	Dental And Oral
Point, Paper, Endodontic	Dental And Oral
Point, Silver, Endodontic	Dental And Oral
Reamer, Pulp Canal, Endodontic	Dental And Oral

UNITED DENTAL MFG., INC. 717-845-7511
608 Rolling Hills Dr., Johnson City, TN 37604
FDA Number: 1048372
Web site: www.dentsply.com
Ownership: Dentsply International, Inc.
Stock Symbol: XRAY
Traded On: NASDAQ
Produces/Sells CE-marked Devices: N

Broach, Endodontic	Dental And Oral
Drill, Dental, Intraoral	Dental And Oral
File, Pulp Canal, Endodontic	Dental And Oral
Filling, Instrument Plastic, Dental	Dental And Oral
Gauge, Depth, Instrument, Dental	Dental And Oral
Gutta Percha	Dental And Oral
Locator, Apex, Root	Dental And Oral
Plugger, Root Canal, Endodontic	Dental And Oral
Point, Paper, Endodontic	Dental And Oral
Point, Silver, Endodontic	Dental And Oral
Reamer, Pulp Canal, Endodontic	Dental And Oral

UNITED ELECTRIC CONTROLS CO. 617-926-1000
180 Dexter Ave., P.O. Box 9143, Watertown, MA 02472-9143
FDA Number: n/a   *Fax:* 617-926-2568
E-mail: sales@ueonline.com
Web site: www.ueonline.com
Annual Revenue: $25-$50 Million
Year Founded: 1931
Ownership: Private
Quality System Registration Information: ISO9002
Produces/Sells CE-marked Devices: Y

UNITED ELECTRIC CONTROLS CO. 617-926-1000 *(cont'd)*
Federal Procurement Eligibility: Small Business
Distribution: Manufacturer Direct, Exporter

Controller, Temperature, Other	General
Probe, Other	General
Probe, Temperature	General
Recorder, Paper Chart	Cardiovascular

UNITED HEARING SYSTEMS, INC. 800-835-2001
137 Norwich Rd, Central Village, CT 06332   **860-564-4130**
FDA Number: 2125604   *Fax:* 860-564-5724
E-mail: mail@unitedhearing.com
Web site: www.unitedhearing.com
Ownership: Private
Produces/Sells CE-marked Devices: N
Federal Procurement Eligibility: Small Business
Distribution: Manufacturer Direct
General Admin.: Ralph T. Campagna/Chief Executive Officer

Hearing Aid, Air Conduction, Transcutaneous System	Ear/Nose/Throat
Hearing-Aid	Ear/Nose/Throat

UNITED LABORATORIES AND MANUFACTURING, LLC 703-787-9600
45000 Underwood Lane, Unit F, Sterling, VA 20166
FDA Number: 3005931760

Massager, Therapeutic	Physical Med
Toothbrush, Powered	Dental And Oral

UNITED LABORATORY PLASTICS 800-722-2499
1724A Westpark Ctr., PO Box 8585,   **636-343-2202**
Saint Louis, MO 63126
FDA Number: n/a   *Fax:* 636-343-6676
E-mail: ulp@unitedlabplastics.com
Web site: www.unitedlabplastics.com
Medical Products Sales Volume: $570,000
Year Founded: 1982
Total Employees: 5
Ownership: Private
Produces/Sells CE-marked Devices: N
Federal Procurement Eligibility: Small Business, Female Owned
General Admin.: Donna M. Sondag/President
Mktg./Adv.: Norma Parker/Manager National Accounts
     Meg Frederick/Manager Sales Training
     Krissie McGrath/Vice President Sales

Component, Plastic	General
Equipment, Laboratory, Gen. Purpose (Specific Medical Use)	Chemistry

UNITED MARKETING, INC.
See United Receptacle

UNITED MCGILL CORP.
See Mcgill Airpressure Corp.

UNITED MEDICAL
See Smith & Nephew, Inc.

UNITED MEDICAL ENTERPRISES 757-224-0177
4049 Allen Station Rd, Augusta, GA 30906
FDA Number: 1062201

Absorber, Saliva, Paper	Dental And Oral
Chair, Dental, Without Operative Unit	Dental And Oral
Gauze/sponge, Nonresorbable For External Use	Surgery
Mask, Surgical	Surgery

UNITED METAL FABRICATORS, INC. 800-638-5322
1316 Eisenhower Blvd.,   **814-266-8726**
Johnstown, PA 15904
FDA Number: 2518399   *Fax:* 814-266-1870
E-mail: customerservice@umf-exam.com
Web site: http://umf-exam.com/
Medical Products Sales Volume: $9,200,000
Annual Revenue: $5-$10 Million
Year Founded: 1955
Total Employees: 107   *Marketing Staff:* 2   *Sales Staff:* 45
Ownership: Private
Produces/Sells CE-marked Devices: Y
Federal Procurement Eligibility: Small Business, GSA Contract, VA Contract
Distribution: Manufacturer Direct, Manufacturer Through Distributor, Manufacturer Through Manufacturer Reps, OEM, Exporter
General Admin.: Thomas D. Jones/President, Chief Executive Officer
Mktg./Adv.: Greg Long/Manager International & National Sales
Production: Mike Pribish/Manager Production

Bassinet (Infant Bed)	General
Cabinet Casework, Modular	General
Cabinet, Instrument	General
Cabinet, Table And Tray, Anesthesia	Anesthesiology
Cart, Other	General
Chair, Blood Drawing	General
Chair, Examination And Treatment	General
Footstool, Operating Room	Surgery

UNITED METAL FABRICATORS, INC. 800-638-5322 *(cont'd)*

Furniture, General	General
Heater, Perineal, Radiant, Non-Contact	Obstetrics/Gynecology
Laundry Hamper	General
Light Source, Incandescent, Diagnostic	Gastroenterology/Urology
Rack, Glove, Operating Room	Surgery
Scale, Infant	General
Stirrup	Gastroenterology/Urology
Stool, Dental	Dental And Oral
Stool, Operating Room, Adjustable	Surgery
Stretcher, Wheeled, Mechanical	Physical Med
Table, Examination/Treatment	General
Table, Instrument, Surgical	Surgery
Table, Obstetrical, Manual	Obstetrics/Gynecology
Table, Physical Medicine, Powered	Physical Med
Table, Surgical, Manual	General
Waste Receptacle, General Purpose	General

UNITED METAL RECEPTACLE CORP.
See United Receptacle

UNITED OXYGEN EQUIPMENT CO.
See U O Equipment Co.

UNITED PLASTIC MOLDERS, INC.
See United Plastic Molders, Inc.

UNITED PRECISION TECHNOLOGY 716-634-4331
4085 David Rd., Williamsville, NY 14221
FDA Number: 1318740
Ownership: Private
Produces/Sells CE-marked Devices: N

Lock, Wire, And Ligature, Intraoral	Dental And Oral

UNITED PRODUCTS & INSTRUMENTS, INC. 800-588-9776
182 Ridge Road, Suite E, Dayton, NJ 08810   **732-274-1155**
FDA Number: 2249760   *Fax:* 732-274-1151
E-mail: sales@unico1.com
Web site: www.unico1.com
Medical Products Sales Volume: $980,000
Year Founded: 1991
Total Employees: 7
Ownership: Private
Quality System Registration Information: ISO9002
Produces/Sells CE-marked Devices: Y
Federal Procurement Eligibility: Small Business
Distribution: Manufacturer Through Distributor, Manufacturer Through Manufacturer Reps, OEM, Exporter
Mktg./Adv.: Mr. Alex Golberg/Coord. Marketing & Sales

Centrifuge, Microhematocrit	Hematology
Centrifuge, Tabletop	Pathology
Counter, Differential Hand Tally	Hematology
Microscope	Hematology
Microscope, Laboratory, Optical	Microbiology
Microscope, Light	Pathology
Spectrophotometer, U.V./Visible	Chemistry
Spectrophotometer, Visible	Chemistry
Tube, Centrifuge	Chemistry

UNITED RECEPTACLE 800-233-0314
1400 Laurel Blvd, Pottsville, PA 17901   **570-622-7715**
FDA Number: 9201108   *Fax:* 570-622-3817
E-mail: united@unitedrecept.com
Web site: www.unitedrecept.com
Medical Products Sales Volume: $500,000
Annual Revenue: $0-$1 Million
Year Founded: 1970
Total Employees: 200   *Marketing Staff:* 10   *Sales Staff:* 9
Ownership: Private
Produces/Sells CE-marked Devices: N
Federal Procurement Eligibility: Small Business, GSA Contract, VA Contract
Distribution: Manufacturer Through Distributor, Manufacturer Through Manufacturer Reps, Exporter
General Admin.: Richard Weiss/Chief Executive Officer
     Richard Weiss/President
Mktg./Adv.: Amber Misstishin/Coord. Advertising
     Layton Dodson/Director Marketing & Sales
     Terry English/Manager Sales
     Andrew Lesh/Market Manager
     Sheryl Beltz/Marketing Coordinator

Waste Receptacle, General Purpose	General

UNITED RECEPTACLE, INC.
See United Receptacle

UNITED SILICA PRODUCTS, INC. 973-209-8854
3 Park Dr., Franklin, NJ 07416
FDA Number: n/a   *Fax:* 973-209-8864
E-mail: quartzsales@unitedsilica.com
Web site: www.unitedsilica.com
Medical Products Sales Volume: $2,300,000
Annual Revenue: $1-$5 Million

UNITED SILICA PRODUCTS, INC.   973-209-8854 *(cont'd)*
Year Founded: 1988
Ownership: Private
Quality System Registration Information: ISO9001
Produces/Sells CE-marked Devices: N
Federal Procurement Eligibility: Small Business, Female Owned
Distribution: Manufacturer Direct, Manufacturer Through Manufacturer Reps
  Flask, Dewar   Chemistry

UNITED STATES CATHETER & INSTRUMENT CO.
See Bard Electro Physiology

UNITED STATES ENDOSCOPY GROUP   800-769-8226
5976 Heisley Road, Mentor, OH 44060   **440-639-4494**
FDA Number: 1528319   *Fax:* 440-639-4495
E-mail: info@usendoscopy.com
Web site: www.usendoscopy.com
Medical Products Sales Volume: $22,000,000
Year Founded: 1991
Total Employees: 202   *Marketing Staff:* 5   *Sales Staff:* 24
Ownership: Private
Quality System Registration Information: ISO9001
Produces/Sells CE-marked Devices: Y
Federal Procurement Eligibility: Small Business
Distribution: Manufacturer Direct, Manufacturer Through Distributor, Manufacturer Through Manufacturer Reps, OEM
General Admin.: Marlin Younker/Chief Executive Officer
       Gretchen Cohen/Executive Vice President
Mktg./Adv.: Allison Hanson/Director Marketing
       Allison Hanson/Manager Advertising
       Jim Sarosy/Manager International Sales
       Gulam Khan/Vice President Business Development
       John Steenburg/Vice President Sales
Production: Don Terriaco/Director Quality Assurance
       Sherri Wright/Manager Materials
       Gretchen Cohen/Manager Regulatory Affairs
       Robert Stuba/Vice President Manufacturing
Research: Dean Secrest/Vice President Research & Development
  Bag, Specimen, Laparoscopic   Surgery
  Brush, Cytology, Endoscopic   Gastroenterology/Urology
  Cannula, Catheter   Cardiovascular
  Catheter, Cholangiography   Surgery
  Forceps, Biopsy   Surgery
  Needle, Endoscopic   Gastroenterology/Urology
  Snare, Endoscopic   Surgery
  Snare, Other   Surgery

UNITED STATES PUMICE CO.   818-882-0300
20219 Bahama Street, Chatsworth, CA 91311
FDA Number: 2014379
  Brush, Dermabrasion, Manual   Surgery

UNITED STATES SURGICAL CORP.
See Covidien Lp, Formerly Registered As United States Surgical

UNITED SYNTEK CORP.   888-665-2326
3557 Denver Dr., Denver, NC 28037   **704-483-4455**
FDA Number: 300021553   *Fax:* 704-483-9588
E-mail: syntek@bellsouth.net
Medical Products Sales Volume: $2,000,000
Annual Revenue: $1-$5 Million
Year Founded: 1991
Total Employees: 8   *Marketing Staff:* 2   *Sales Staff:* 22
Ownership: Private
Produces/Sells CE-marked Devices: Y
Federal Procurement Eligibility: Small Business
Distribution: Exclusive Distributor, Importer
  Frame, Spectacle (Eyeglasses)   Ophthalmology
  Sunglasses (Including Photosensitive)   Ophthalmology

UNITED UNION WIRE, INC.
See Gillis Associated Industries

UNITED-GUARDIAN, INC.   800-645-5566
230 Marcus Blvd., P.O. Box 18050,   **631-273-0900**
Hauppauge, NY 11788
FDA Number: 2410853   *Fax:* 631-273-0858
E-mail: evp@u-g.com
Web site: www.u-g.com
Medical Products Sales Volume: $3,000,000
Annual Revenue: $10-$25 Million
Year Founded: 1942
Total Employees: 43
Ownership: Public
Stock Symbol: UG
Traded On: AMEX
Quality System Registration Information: ISO9001
Produces/Sells CE-marked Devices: N
Federal Procurement Eligibility: Small Business
Distribution: Manufacturer Direct, Manufacturer Through Distributor, Exporter

UNITED-GUARDIAN, INC.   800-645-5566 *(cont'd)*
  Jelly, Lubricating, Transurethral Surgical Instrument   Gastroenterology/Urology

UNITEDHEALTHCARE   800-368-0707
1001 Winstead Dr., Suite 200, Cary, NC 27513
FDA Number: n/a   *Fax:* 919-677-9012
Web site: www.uhc.com
Annual Revenue: More than $1 Billion
Year Founded: 1974
Total Employees: 75000
Ownership: Public
Stock Symbol: UNH
Traded On: NYSE
Produces/Sells CE-marked Devices: N
General Admin.: George L. Mikan III/Chief Operating Officer, Executive Vice President
       Gail K. Boudreaux/Executive Vice President
       Stephen J. Hemsley/President, Chief Executive Officer
  Transmitter, Image & Data, Radiographic   Radiology

UNITEX PRODUCTS
See Angelica Image Apparel

UNITRON HEARING   763-744-3300
2300 Berkshire Ln. North, Suite A, Plymouth, MN 55441
FDA Number: 1824293
  Hearing-Aid   Ear/Nose/Throat

UNITRON INDUSTRIES LTD.   877-492-6244
20 Beasley Dr., P.O. Box 9017,   **519-895-0100**
Kitchener, ONT N2G 4 Canada
FDA Number: n/a   *Fax:* 519-895-0108
E-mail: info.canada@unitron.com
Web site: www.unitron.com
Year Founded: 1964
Total Employees: 600
Ownership: Private
Quality System Registration Information: ISO9000; ISO9001; ISO9002
Produces/Sells CE-marked Devices: Y
Distribution: Manufacturer Through Distributor, Exporter

UNITRON LTD   631-543-2000
73 Mall Drive, Commack, NY 11725
FDA Number: 9201113   *Fax:* 631-589-6975
E-mail: info@unitronusa.com
Web site: www.unitronusa.com
Medical Products Sales Volume: $5,000,000
Annual Revenue: $1-$5 Million
Year Founded: 1952
Total Employees: 25   *Marketing Staff:* 1   *Sales Staff:* 5
Ownership: Private
Produces/Sells CE-marked Devices: Y
Federal Procurement Eligibility: Small Business
Distribution: Manufacturer Direct
General Admin.: Mr. Brian Taub/Chief Executive
       Mr. Jay Berliner/Chief Executive Officer
Mktg./Adv.: Peter I. Indrigo/Director National Accounts
       John D. Coyle/Vice President Marketing & Sales
  Camera, Microscope   Microbiology
  Lamp, Microscope   Pathology
  Microscope, Laboratory, Optical   Microbiology

UNIVAC DENTAL COMPANY   800-523-2559
113 Park Drive, PO Box 447,   **215-540-0800**
Montgomeryville, PA 18936
FDA Number: 2518428   *Fax:* 800-523-7550
E-mail: jmb@universaldentalco.com
Web site: www.universaldentalco.com
Medical Products Sales Volume: $1,000,000
Annual Revenue: $0-$1 Million
Total Employees: 15
Ownership: Private
Produces/Sells CE-marked Devices: N
Federal Procurement Eligibility: Small Business, VA Contract
Distribution: Exclusive Distributor, Importer, Exporter
  Denture, Plastic, Teeth   Dental And Oral
  Teeth, Porcelain   Dental And Oral

UNIVEC, INC.   410-347-9959
4810 Seton Dr., Baltimore, MD 21215
FDA Number: 2437110
Ownership: Public
Stock Symbol: UNVC
Traded On: OTC Bulletin
Produces/Sells CE-marked Devices: N
  Syringe, Antistick   General
  Syringe, Piston   General

UNIVERSAL DIAGNOSTIC SOLUTIONS — 800-416-7567 / 760-754-3288
101 Copperwood Way, Suite A,
Oceanside, CA 92054
FDA Number: n/a
E-mail: info@u-d-s.com
Web site: www.u-d-s.com
Medical Products Sales Volume: $1,500,000
Annual Revenue: $1-$5 Million
Year Founded: 2004
Ownership: Private
Produces/Sells CE-marked Devices: N
Federal Procurement Eligibility: Small Business
Distribution: Importer, Exporter
Scanner, Ultrasonic, General Purpose — Radiology
Fax: 206-374-6495

UNIVERSAL ENTERPRISES. INC.
See Uei

UNIVERSAL GYM EQUIPMENT — 800-843-3906 / 319-365-7561
PO Box 1296, PO Box 1270,
West Point, MS 39773
FDA Number: n/a
E-mail: customerservice@universalgym.com
Web site: www.universalgymequipment.com
Medical Products Sales Volume: $1,000,000
Annual Revenue: $1-$5 Million
Year Founded: 1957
Total Employees: 10   Marketing Staff: 3   Sales Staff: 3
Ownership: Private
Produces/Sells CE-marked Devices: N
Federal Procurement Eligibility: GSA Contract
Distribution: Manufacturer Direct, Manufacturer Through Distributor
General Admin: Steve Sadler/President
Exerciser, Other — Physical Med
Fax: 319-362-6212

UNIVERSAL IMPLANT SYSTEMS, INC. — 202-244-9200
4400 Jenifer St. N.W., Suite 220, Washington, DC 20015-2113
FDA Number: 1122904
Annual Revenue: $0-$1 Million
Ownership: Private
Produces/Sells CE-marked Devices: N
Federal Procurement Eligibility: Small Business
Distribution: Service Direct, Exclusive Distributor
General Admin.: Gerald Marlin/Chief Executive Officer
Implant, Endosseous — Dental And Oral
Prosthesis, Dental — Dental And Oral

UNIVERSAL MEDICAL DESIGN — 888-227-5948
4488 Mountain Lakes Blvd., Redding, CA 96003
FDA Number: n/a
E-mail: karend@unimeddesign.com
Web site: www.unimeddesign.com
Annual Revenue: $0-$1 Million
Total Employees: 22
Ownership: Private
Produces/Sells CE-marked Devices: N
Federal Procurement Eligibility: Small Business
Distribution: Manufacturer Through Distributor
General Admin.: William Durbin/President
Finance: Karen Durbin/Controller
Carrier, Container, Oxygen, Portable — General
Case, Protection, Equipment — General
Contract Manufacturing — General
Fax: 530-547-4808

UNIVERSAL MEDICAL PRODUCTS — 310-839-9738
9435 Venice Blvd, Culver City, CA 90232
FDA Number: n/a
E-mail: support@universalmedicalinc.com
Web site: http://www.universalmedicalinc.com
Annual Revenue: $0-$1 Million
Year Founded: 1982
Ownership: Private
Produces/Sells CE-marked Devices: N
Federal Procurement Eligibility: Small Business, Minority Owned
Distribution: Manufacturer Direct, Manufacturer Through Distributor, Importer, Exporter
Implant, Retinal — Ophthalmology
Laser, Argon, Surgical — Surgery
Laser, Nd:YAG, Surgical — Surgery
Lens, Contact, Hydrophilic — Ophthalmology
Lens, Intraocular — Ophthalmology
Microscope — Hematology
Phacofragmentation Unit — Ophthalmology
Service, Import/Export — General
Fax: 310-839-5473

UNIVERSAL MEDICAL PRODUCTS, INC. — 800-206-1045
1550 N. 20th Circle, Lincoln, NE 68503
FDA Number: n/a
Fax: 402-475-4023

UNIVERSAL MEDICAL PRODUCTS, INC. — 800-206-1045 (cont'd)
Web site: www.u-m-p.com
Annual Revenue: $1-$5 Million
Year Founded: 1997
Ownership: Private
Produces/Sells CE-marked Devices: N
Federal Procurement Eligibility: Small Business, Female Owned
Distribution: Manufacturer Direct, Manufacturer Through Manufacturer Reps
Monitor, Bed Patient — General

UNIVERSAL MEDICAL SYSTEMS, INC.
See Universal Ultrasound

UNIVERSAL MEDICAL TECHNOLOGIES — 415-924-1133
15720 N. Greenway Hayden Loop, Suite 8,
Scottsdale, AZ 85260
FDA Number: 2951178
Pump, Infusion — General

UNIVERSAL MEDICAL, INC. — 800-423.2767
275 Phillips Blvd, Ewing, NJ 08618
FDA Number: 2248680
E-mail: info@universalmedicalinc.com
Annual Revenue: $1-$5 Million
Ownership: Private
Produces/Sells CE-marked Devices: N
Distribution: Manufacturer Direct, Manufacturer Through Distributor, Manufacturer Through Manufacturer Reps
Transmitter/Receiver System, Physiological, Telephone — Cardiovascular
Fax: 800.535.6229

UNIVERSAL PACS, INC. — 225-766-9381
127 Albert Hart Drive, Baton Rouge, LA 70808-6702
FDA Number: 3003897797
E-mail: contact@unipacs.com
Web site: www.unipacs.com
Year Founded: 2003
Ownership: Private
Produces/Sells CE-marked Devices: N
Federal Procurement Eligibility: Small Business
Distribution: Manufacturer Direct
Image Processing System — Radiology
Fax: 225-766-9381

UNIVERSAL SCIENTIFIC
See Metal Techology, Inc.

UNIVERSAL SERVICE ASSOCIATES, INC. — 800-601-1916 / 570-748-4400
500 Ellis Avenue, Darby, PA 19023-2725
FDA Number: 2529583
E-mail: mshields@usainc.com
Web site: www.medical.usainc.com
Medical Products Sales Volume: $2,600,000
Annual Revenue: $0-$1 Million
Year Founded: 1974
Total Employees: 50   Marketing Staff: 1   Sales Staff: 1
Ownership: Private
Produces/Sells CE-marked Devices: N
Federal Procurement Eligibility: Small Business
Distribution: Manufacturer Direct, Exporter
General Admin.: Ms. Mary Shields/Administrator
Support, Patient Position — Anesthesiology
Fax: 570-748-4422

UNIVERSAL SURGICAL APPLIANCE CO. — 305-652-0810
400 N.E. 191 Street, Miami, FL 33179
FDA Number: 1018371
Ownership: Private
Produces/Sells CE-marked Devices: N
Federal Procurement Eligibility: Small Business
Distribution: Manufacturer Through Distributor, Exporter
Binder, Abdominal — General
Joint, Knee, External Brace — Physical Med
Orthosis, Cervical — Physical Med
Orthosis, Limb Brace — Physical Med
Orthosis, Lumbosacral — Physical Med
Orthosis, Rib Fracture, Soft — Physical Med

UNIVERSAL TECHNOLOGY SYSTEMS, INC. — 904-778-8614
5150-4 Timuquana Rd., Jacksonville, FL 32210
FDA Number: 1052741
Stimulator, Muscle, Electrical-Powered (EMS) — Physical Med

UNIVERSAL ULTRASOUND — 800-842-0607 / 914-666-6200
299 Adams Street, Bedford Hills, NY 10507
FDA Number: n/a
E-mail: sales@UniversalUltrasound.com
Web site: www.universalultrasound.com
Medical Products Sales Volume: $23,000,000
Annual Revenue: $10-$25 Million
Year Founded: 1981
Total Employees: 23   Marketing Staff: 6   Sales Staff: 12
Ownership: Private
Fax: 914-666-2454

UNIVERSAL ULTRASOUND
800-842-0607 *(cont'd)*
Quality System Registration Information: ISO9003
Produces/Sells CE-marked Devices: Y
Federal Procurement Eligibility: Small Business
Distribution: Manufacturer Direct, Manufacturer Through Distributor, OEM, Service Direct, Exclusive Distributor, Importer, Exporter
General Admin.: Mr. Ray Starzman/General Manager
    Mr. Peter Brunelli/President, Chief Executive Officer
Mktg./Adv.: Cory Gabel/Coord. Marketing & Trade Show
    Cathy Carducci/Coord. Training
    Mike Mumaw/National Sales Representative
    Richard Brunelli/Sales Representative
Finance: Peter Capurso/Controller
IS: Gabe Hohner/Technical Manager

Echocardiograph (Ultrasonic Scanner)	Cardiovascular
Gel, Ultrasonic Transmission	General
Printer, Image, Video	General
Scanner, Ultrasonic (Pulsed Doppler)	Radiology
Scanner, Ultrasonic, General Purpose	Radiology
Scanner, Ultrasonic, Other	Radiology
Scanner, Ultrasonic, Surgical	Surgery

UNIVERSAL X-RAY CO. OF CANADA LTD.
514-631-4477
1370-55th Avenue, Lachine, QUE H8T 3J8 Canada
FDA Number: n/a   *Fax:* 514-631-3643
E-mail: info@uxr.ca
Web site: www.uxr.ca
Year Founded: 1949
Ownership: Private
Produces/Sells CE-marked Devices: N
Distribution: Exclusive Distributor, Importer

UNIVERSAL/ALLIED IMAGING INC.
See Del Medical Systems

UNIVERSITY OF MIAMI TISSUE BANK
888-UMTISSUE
1600 N.W. 10th Ave. (R-12), Miami, FL 33136
305-243-6786
FDA Number: 1052998   *Fax:* 305-243-4622
E-mail: umtb@med.miami.edu
Medical Products Sales Volume: $2,800,000
Annual Revenue: $1-$5 Million
Total Employees: 24   *Sales Staff:* 2
Ownership: Private
Produces/Sells CE-marked Devices: N
Distribution: Manufacturer Direct, Exporter
General Admin.: Theodore Malinin/Chief Executive Officer
Production: Alvaro Flores/Manager Production

Graft, Bone	Orthopedics

UNIVERSITY OF UTAH HOSPITALS AND CLINICS
801-581-2742
50 North Medical Dr., Salt Lake City, UT 84132
FDA Number: 3004595606
Web site: healthcare.utah.edu
Ownership: Private
Produces/Sells CE-marked Devices: N

Sleeve, Compressible Limb	Cardiovascular

UNIVERSITY OF WASHINGTON
206-616-5130
T-281 Health Science Bldg., Seattle, WA 98195
FDA Number: 3017697

Clip, Tantalum, Ophthalmic	Ophthalmology
Kit, Collection/Transfusion, Marrow, Bone	General

UNOMEDICAL, INC.
800-634-6003
5701-1 S. Ware Rd., McAllen, TX 78503
956-683-8472
FDA Number: n/a   *Fax:* 956-683-8482
E-mail: usa@unomedical.com
Web site: www.unomedical.net
Annual Revenue: $50-$100 Million
Total Employees: 600   *Marketing Staff:* 3   *Sales Staff:* 10
Ownership: Private
Quality System Registration Information: ISO9001; ISO9002
Produces/Sells CE-marked Devices: Y
Distribution: Manufacturer Through Distributor, OEM, Importer, Exporter
General Admin.: Ernie Escobar/Chief Financial Officer, General Counsel
    Erik Hald Nissen/President, Chief Executive Officer
Mktg./Adv.: Thomas B. Jorgensen/Vice President Sales
Production: Sylvia Rodrigues/Manager Customer Services
    Eloy Cruz/Manager Quality Assurance
    Efrain Carrero/Plant Manager
Finance: Celia Gides/Controller
Purchasing: Thomas Beck/Director Purchasing
IS: Baldo Gallardo/Manager Information Systems

Bag, Leg	Gastroenterology/Urology
Bag, Urinary Collection	General
Button, Tracheostomy Tube	Anesthesiology
Catheter, Balloon (Foley Type)	Surgery
Catheter, Other	Gastroenterology/Urology
Catheter, Suction (Tracheal Aspirating Tube)	Anesthesiology

UNOMEDICAL, INC.
800-634-6003 *(cont'd)*

Mask, Gas, Anesthesia	Anesthesiology
Tube, Tracheal (Endotracheal)	Anesthesiology

UNOTECH DIAGNOSTICS, INC.
510-352-3070
2235 Polvorosa Ave., Suite 220, San Leandro, CA 94577
FDA Number: 2953160

Test, Human Chorionic Gonadotropin, Serum	Immunology

UNSMOKE INTERNATIONAL
See Surco Products

UOP
See Guided Wave Inc.

UPLIFT TECHNOLOGIES, INC.
800-387-0896
125-11 Morris Dr.,
902-422-0804
Dartmouth, NS B3B 1 Canada
FDA Number: 9681423   *Fax:* 902-422-0798
E-mail: info@up-lift.com
Web site: www.up-lift.com
Year Founded: 1993
Total Employees: 25
Ownership: Private
Produces/Sells CE-marked Devices: Y
Distribution: Manufacturer Direct, Exporter

UPTAKE MEDICAL CORP.
206-859-4555
1924 1st Avenue, 3rd Floor, Seattle, WA 98101
FDA Number: n/a   *Fax:* 206-859-4557
E-mail: info@uptakemedical.com
Web site: www.uptakemedical.com
Ownership: Private
Produces/Sells CE-marked Devices: N
General Admin.: Mr. J.C. MacRae/Chief Financial Officer, Vice President
    Dr. Steven Kesten/Chief Medical Officer, Vice President
    Mr. Robert Barry/Chief Technology Officer
    Mr. R. King Nelson/President, Chief Executive Officer
Mktg./Adv.: Mr. Mike Numamoto/Vice President Marketing
Production: Dr. Norman Lowe/Head Quality Assurance
    Mr. Greg Watson/Vice President Manufacturing & Development

URESIL, LLC
800-538-7374
5418 W. Touhy Avenue, Skokie, IL 60077-3232
847-982-0200
FDA Number: 1450032   *Fax:* 847-982-0106
E-mail: jims@uresil.com
Web site: www.uresil.com
Medical Products Sales Volume: $2,600,000
Year Founded: 1986
Total Employees: 39   *Marketing Staff:* 2   *Sales Staff:* 3
Ownership: Private
Quality System Registration Information: ISO9002
Produces/Sells CE-marked Devices: N
Federal Procurement Eligibility: Small Business
Distribution: Manufacturer Through Manufacturer Reps
General Admin.: Lev Melinyshyn/President
Mktg./Adv.: Jim Sarns/Senior Vice President Marketing & Sales

Bag, Drainage (Incontinence)	Gastroenterology/Urology
Bandage, Adhesive	Surgery
Catheter, Biliary	Gastroenterology/Urology
Catheter, Intravascular Occluding	Cns/Neurology
Catheter, Nephrostomy	Gastroenterology/Urology
Catheter, Percutaneous	Cardiovascular
Drain, Thoracic (Chest)	Anesthesiology
Guidewire, Catheter, Radiological	Radiology
Suction Apparatus, Single Patient, Portable, Non-Powered	Surgery
Valvulotome	Cardiovascular

URI THERM-Y INC.
See Labthermics Technologies

URIDYNAMICS, INC.
317-915-7896
6786 Hawthorn Park Dr., Indianapolis, IN 46220
FDA Number: 83697
Ownership: Private
Produces/Sells CE-marked Devices: N

Control, Urinalysis (Assayed And Unassayed)	Chemistry

UROCARE PRODUCTS, INC.
800-423-4441
2735 Melbourne Avenue,
909-621-6013
Pomona, CA 91767
FDA Number: 2023344   *Fax:* 909-621-4436
E-mail: sales@urocare.com
Web site: www.urocare.com
Medical Products Sales Volume: $1,300,000
Year Founded: 1976
Total Employees: 19
Ownership: Private
Quality System Registration Information: ISO9001
Produces/Sells CE-marked Devices: N

UROCARE PRODUCTS, INC.
800-423-4441 *(cont'd)*

Federal Procurement Eligibility: Small Business
Distribution: Manufacturer Direct, Manufacturer Through Distributor, OEM, Exclusive Distributor, Importer, Exporter
Mktg./Adv.: Glenn K. Franke/Vice President Marketing & Sales
Production: Raymond Franke/Director Operations

Adhesive Strip, Waterproof	General
Bag, Drainage, Ostomy (With Adhesive)	General
Bag, Leg	Gastroenterology/Urology
Bag, Urinary Collection	General
Bag, Urinary Collection, Ureterostomy	Gastroenterology/Urology
Bag, Urinary, Ileostomy	Gastroenterology/Urology
Catheter, Urinary, Condom	Gastroenterology/Urology
Drainage Unit, Urinary	General
Solution, Antibacterial Cleaner	General
Tape, Adhesive, Waterproof	General
Tube, Drainage	Gastroenterology/Urology
Urinal	General

UROLOGIX, INC.
800-475-1403
763-475-1400

14405 - 21st Avenue North,
Minneapolis, MN 55447
FDA Number: 2133936   Fax: 763-475-1443
E-mail: customerservice@urologix.com
Web site: www.urologix.com
Medical Products Sales Volume: $18,800,000
Annual Revenue: $10-$25 Million
Year Founded: 1991
Ownership: Public
Stock Symbol: ULGX
Traded On: NASDAQ
Quality System Registration Information: ISO9001
Produces/Sells CE-marked Devices: Y
Distribution: Manufacturer Direct
General Admin.: Stryker Warren/Chief Executive Officer
    Gregory J. Fluet/Chief Operating Officer, Executive Vice President

Device, Ablation, Thermal, Ultrasonic	Gastroenterology/Urology
System, Hyperthermia, Rf/microwave (benign Prostatic Hyperplasia), Thermotherapy	Gastroenterology/Urology

UROLOGY-TECH LLC
800-397-3318
806-798-0214

4503 89th S, Lubbock, TX 79424
FDA Number: 1650358   Fax: 806-798-7102
Web site: www.urologytech.com
Ownership: Private
Produces/Sells CE-marked Devices: N

Surgical Instrument, G-U, Manual	Gastroenterology/Urology

UROMEDICA, INC.
763-694-9880

1840 Berkshire Ln. North, Plymouth, MN 55441-3723
FDA Number: 3003477176   Fax: 763-694-9945
E-mail: info@uromedica-inc.com
Web site: www.uromedica-inc.com
Medical Products Sales Volume: $710,000
Year Founded: 1997
Total Employees: 9
Ownership: Private
Quality System Registration Information: ISO9001
Produces/Sells CE-marked Devices: Y
Federal Procurement Eligibility: Small Business
Distribution: Manufacturer Through Distributor
General Admin.: Dr. Timothy Cook/President, Chief Executive Officer

Device, Incontinence, Mechanical/Hydraulic	Gastroenterology/Urology

UROMEND, LLC
540-980-0886

1321 Hopkins Dr., Pulaski, VA 24301
FDA Number: 3004632101

Device, Incontinence, Occlusion, Urethral	Gastroenterology/Urology

UROPLASTY, INC.
952-426-6140

5420 Feltl Road, Minnetonka, MN 55343
FDA Number: 3002647932   Fax: 952-426-6199
E-mail: info.usa@uroplasty.com
Web site: http://uroplasty.com
Year Founded: 1992
Ownership: Public
Stock Symbol: UPI
Traded On: AMEX
Produces/Sells CE-marked Devices: N
General Admin.: Mr. Mahedi Jiwani/Chief Financial Officer, Vice President
    Ms. Susan Hartjes Holman/Chief Operating Officer
    Mr. David Kaysen/President, Chief Executive Officer
Mktg./Adv.: Ms. Nancy Kolb/Vice President Marketing
    Mr. Larry Heinemann/Vice President Sales
Production: Mr. Marc Herregraven/Vice President Manufacturing

Agent, Bulking, Injectable (Gastro-Urology)	Gastroenterology/Urology
Device, Incontinence, Fecal, Implanted	Gastroenterology/Urology
Holder, Needle	Gastroenterology/Urology

UROPLASTY, INC.
952-426-6140 *(cont'd)*

Implant, Collagen, Dermal (Aesthetic Use)	Surgery
Needle, Aspiration And Injection, Disposable	Surgery
Surgical Instrument, G-U, Manual	Gastroenterology/Urology
System, Vocal Cord Medialization	Ear/Nose/Throat

UROVALVE INC.
973-596-1350

211 Warren St., Newark, NJ 07103
FDA Number: n/a
Web site: http://www.urovalve.com
Ownership: Private
Produces/Sells CE-marked Devices: N
General Admin.: Mr. Harvey Homan/President, Chief Executive Officer
Research: Mr. Tom Winegar/Vice President Engineering & Development

US HIFU LLC
704-332-4308

801 E. Morehead St., Suite 201, Charlotte, NC 28202
FDA Number: n/a   Fax: 1-888-874-4384
Web site: http://www.ushifu.com
Year Founded: 2004
Ownership: Private
Produces/Sells CE-marked Devices: N
General Admin.: Mr. Stephen Pucket, Jr./Chief Executive Officer
    Mr. Naren Sanghvi/Chief Scientific Officer
    Mr. Alex Gonzalez/Vice President International Operations
Medical Admin.: Dr. Mark Schoenberg/Chief Medical Officer
    Dr. George Suarez/Medical Director
Mktg./Adv.: Mr. Jim Bobbit/Vice President Corporate Affairs
Research: Mr. Adam Lowe/Vice President Scientific Affairs
Finance: Mr. John Linn/Vice President Finance

US JVC CORP.
See JVC Americas Corp.

US SPINE INC.
561-367-7463

3600 Fau Blvd., Suite 101, Boca Raton, FL 33431
FDA Number: 3004744230
Ownership: Amedica Corporation

Appliance, Fixation, Spinal Interlaminal	Orthopedics
Appliance, Fixation, Spinal Intervertebral Body	Orthopedics
Device, Spinal Vertebral Body Replacement	Orthopedics
Orthosis, Fixation, Pedicle, Spinal	Orthopedics
Orthosis, Fixation, Spinal, Spondylolisthesis	Orthopedics

USA INSTRUMENTS, INC.
330-562-1000

1515 Danner Dr., Aurora, OH 44202
FDA Number: 1529041   Fax: 330-562-1422
Web site: www.gehealthcare.com
Year Founded: 1993
Ownership: Ge Healthcare
Quality System Registration Information: ISO9001
Produces/Sells CE-marked Devices: Y
Federal Procurement Eligibility: Small Business, Minority Owned
Distribution: Manufacturer Direct, Manufacturer Through Distributor, OEM, Service Direct, Exporter

Coil, Magnetic Resonance, Specialty	Radiology
Nuclear Magnetic Resonance Imaging System	Radiology
Test Pattern, Radiographic	Radiology

USA PHOTONICS, INC.
845-348-4900

169 Main St., 1st Flr., Central Nyack, NY 10960
FDA Number: 3003971434

Laser, Surgical	Surgery

USA SCIENTIFIC, INC.
800-522-8477
352-237-6288

P.O. Box 3565, Ocala, FL 34478-3565
FDA Number: n/a   Fax: 352-351-2057
E-mail: infoline@usascientific.com
Web site: www.usascientific.com
Annual Revenue: $0-$1 Million
Year Founded: 1982
Ownership: Private
Produces/Sells CE-marked Devices: N
Distribution: Manufacturer Direct

Pipette Tip	Chemistry
Tube, Centrifuge	Chemistry
Tube, Culture	Microbiology

USA THINK, INC.
605-787-7717

13030 Homer Smith Rd., Piedmont, SD 57769
FDA Number: 3006369279

Activator, Ultraviolet, Polymerization	Dental And Oral

USAEROTEAM
937-226-1900

1300 Grange Hall Road, Dayton, OH 45430
FDA Number: 3004124372   Fax: 937-458-0331
E-mail: jmaag@USAeroteam.com
Web site: www.USAeroteam.com
Annual Revenue: $5-$10 Million
Year Founded: 1985

USAEROTEAM — 937-226-1900 (cont'd)

Total Employees: 125 *Marketing Staff:* 1 *Sales Staff:* 4
Ownership: Private
Quality System Registration Information: ISO9001
Produces/Sells CE-marked Devices: N
Federal Procurement Eligibility: Small Business, Minority Owned
Distribution: Manufacturer Direct, Manufacturer Through Distributor, Manufacturer Through Manufacturer Reps, OEM
General Admin.: Mr. Jeff Maag/Vice President

Prosthesis, Knee, Hemi-, Femoral	Orthopedics

USB CORPORATION — 1-888-362-2447 / 1-408-731-5000

3420 central expressway, santa clara, CA 95051
FDA Number: 3003314809 *Fax:* 1-408-731-5380
E-mail: sales@affymetrix.com
Web site: www.usbweb.com
Medical Products Sales Volume: $7,800,000
Year Founded: 1999
Total Employees: 70
Ownership: Affymetrix, Inc.
Quality System Registration Information: ISO9001; ISO9002
Produces/Sells CE-marked Devices: N
Federal Procurement Eligibility: Small Business
Distribution: Manufacturer Direct, Manufacturer Through Distributor
General Admin.: Michael Lachman/Chief Executive Officer
Mktg./Adv.: Michele Paris/Director Marketing
E. Fred Leffler/Vice President Marketing & Sales

Culture Media, Multiple Biochemical Test	Microbiology
Instrumentation For Clinical Multiplex Test Systems	Chemistry

USB SPECIALTY BIOCHEMICALS

See Usb Corporation

USGI MEDICAL — 949-369-3890

1140 Calle Cordillera, San Clemente, CA 92673
FDA Number: 3004447686 *Fax:* 949-369-3891
E-mail: info@usgimedical.com
Web site: www.usgimedical.com
Ownership: Private
Produces/Sells CE-marked Devices: N

Endoscope	Gastroenterology/Urology
Laparoscope, Gynecologic	Obstetrics/Gynecology
Suture, Non-Absorbable, Synthetic, Polyethylene	Surgery

USHIO AMERICA, INC. — 800-838-7446 / 714-236-8600

5440 Cerritos Avenue, Cypress, CA 90630-4567
FDA Number: n/a *Fax:* 714-229-3180
E-mail: customerservice@ushio.com
Web site: www.ushio.com
Medical Products Sales Volume: $346,200,000
Annual Revenue: $50-$100 Million
Year Founded: 1967
Total Employees: 75 *Marketing Staff:* 7 *Sales Staff:* 16
Ownership: USHIO INC. - JAPAN
Quality System Registration Information: ISO9001; ISO9002
Produces/Sells CE-marked Devices: N
Federal Procurement Eligibility: Small Business
Distribution: Manufacturer Through Distributor, OEM, Exclusive Distributor
General Admin.: Mr. Kenji Hamashima/President, Chief Executive Officer
Mr. Ray Chikami/Vice President Admin.
Mktg./Adv.: Ms. Vereen Koh/Coord. Marketing Communications
Mrs. Julie Maetani/Manager Marketing Communications
Mr. Dave Olsen/Manager Product Development
Mr. George Baer/Manager Sales
Mr. Todd Young/Manager Sales
Mr. Tom Ciurczak/Vice President Marketing & Sales
IS: Mr. Keith Cordero/Manager Tech. Services

Lamp, Other	General
Lamp, Surgical, Xenon	Surgery

USSC PUERTO RICO, INC. — 203-845-1000

Building 911-67, Sabanetas Industrial Park, Ponce, PR 00731
FDA Number: 2647580
Web site: www.covidien.com
Ownership: Covidien Ltd.
Produces/Sells CE-marked Devices: N

Accessories, Cleaning, Endoscopic	Gastroenterology/Urology
Appliance, Fixation, Spinal Intervertebral Body	Orthopedics
Applier, Surgical, Clip	Surgery
Arthroscope	Orthopedics
Biopsy Instrument	Gastroenterology/Urology
Catheter, Percutaneous	Cardiovascular
Catheter, Subcutaneous Intravascular, Implanted	General
Clamp, Surgical, General & Plastic Surgery	Surgery
Clip, Implantable	Surgery
Container, Specimen Mailer And Storage, Temperature Control	Pathology
Curette	Orthopedics
Cutter, Surgical	Surgery

USSC PUERTO RICO, INC. — 203-845-1000 (cont'd)

Dissector, Surgical, General & Plastic Surgery	Surgery
Electrosurgical Unit, Cutting & Coagulation Device	Surgery
Elevator, Surgical, General & Plastic Surgery	Surgery
Endoscope	Gastroenterology/Urology
Fastener, Fixation, Biodegradable, Soft Tissue	Orthopedics
Instrument, Manual, General Surgical	Surgery
Instrument, Passing, Ligature, Knot Tying	Cns/Neurology
Kit, Surgical (General)	Surgery
Laparoscope, General & Plastic Surgery	Surgery
Laparoscope, Gynecologic	Obstetrics/Gynecology
Mediastinoscope	Surgery
Mesh, Surgical, Polymeric	Surgery
Needle, Pneumoperitoneum, Spring Loaded	Gastroenterology/Urology
Orthopedic Manual Surgical Instrument	Orthopedics
Orthosis, Fusion, Intervertebral, Spinal	Orthopedics
Pledget And Intracardiac Patch, PETP, PTFE, Polypropylene	Cardiovascular
Pump, Aspiration, Portable	Anesthesiology
Retractor	Orthopedics
Retractor, Manual	Cns/Neurology
Rongeur, Rib	Orthopedics
Screw, Fixation, Bone	Orthopedics
Staple, Fixation, Bone	Orthopedics
Staple, Implantable	Surgery
Stapler, Surgical	Surgery
Suture Apparatus, Stomach And Intestinal	Gastroenterology/Urology
Suture, Absorbable, Natural	Surgery
Suture, Absorbable, Synthetic	Surgery
Suture, Non-Absorbable, Silk	Surgery
Suture, Non-Absorbable, Steel, Monofilament & Multifilament	Surgery
Suture, Non-Absorbable, Synthetic, Polyamide	Surgery
Suture, Non-Absorbable, Synthetic, Polyethylene	Surgery
Suture, Non-Absorbable, Synthetic, Polypropylene	Surgery
Tray, Surgical Instrument	Surgery
Trocar, Gastro-Urology	Gastroenterology/Urology

USV PHARMACEUTICAL

See Csl Behring

UTAH MEDICAL PRODUCTS, INC. — 800-533-4984 / 801-566-1200

7043 S. 300 W., Midvale, UT 84047
FDA Number: 1718873 *Fax:* 801-566-2062
E-mail: info@utahmed.com
Web site: www.utahmed.com
Medical Products Sales Volume: $28,800,000
Annual Revenue: $25-$50 Million
Year Founded: 1978
Total Employees: 215 *Marketing Staff:* 5 *Sales Staff:* 23
Ownership: Public
Stock Symbol: UTMD
Traded On: NASDAQ
Quality System Registration Information: ISO9000; ISO9001
Produces/Sells CE-marked Devices: Y
Federal Procurement Eligibility: Small Business, GSA Contract, VA Contract
Distribution: Manufacturer Direct, Manufacturer Through Distributor, Manufacturer Through Manufacturer Reps, OEM, Importer, Exporter
General Admin.: Paul Richins/Chief Administrative Officer
Kevin L. Cornwell/President, Chief Executive Officer
Mktg./Adv.: Kevin L. Cornwell/Director Marketing
Mary Teasdale/Director National Accounts
Bruce Wilson/Manager International Sales
Ted Paulos/Manager Market Research
Production: Marci Clawson/Director Customer Services
Jean Teasdale/Director Engineering
Ben Shirley/Director Quality Assurance & Regulatory Affairs
Jean Teasdale/Manager Manufacturing
Dennis Simonaitis/Manager Materials
Research: Ben Shirley/Director Research & Development
Finance: Mr. Greg LeClaire/Chief Financial Officer

Amniotome	Obstetrics/Gynecology
Aspirator, Infant	General
Catheter, Continuous Irrigation	Surgery
Catheter, Intrauterine, With Introducer	Obstetrics/Gynecology
Catheter, Intravascular, Therapeutic, Long-term Greater Than 30 Days	General
Catheter, Umbilical Artery	General
Catheter, Urological	Gastroenterology/Urology
Drain, Thoracic (Chest)	Anesthesiology
Electrode, Electrosurgical, Active (Blade)	Surgery
Electrode, Other	General
Electrosurgical Equipment, Special Purpose	Surgery
Endoscope And Accessories, Battery-Powered	Surgery
Extractor, Vacuum, Fetal	Obstetrics/Gynecology
Hood, Oxygen, Infant	General
Injector & Accessories, Manipulator, Uterine	Obstetrics/Gynecology
Kit, Labor and Delivery	Obstetrics/Gynecology
Kit, Lumbar Puncture	Cns/Neurology
Kit, Urinary Drainage Collection	Gastroenterology/Urology
Microfilter, Blood Transfusion	Anesthesiology
Tube, Gastrointestinal	Gastroenterology/Urology

UTAH MEDICAL PRODUCTS, INC.   800-533-4984 *(cont'd)*
  Tube, Tracheal (Endotracheal)   Anesthesiology

UTAH PIONEER MEDICAL, INC.   801-280-1053
8173 S. Summit Valley Drive, West Jordan, UT 84088
FDA Number: 1722152   *Fax:* 801-280-1052
E-mail: Utahpioneermed@aol.com
Annual Revenue: $0-$1 Million
Year Founded: 1991
Total Employees: 50
Ownership: Private
Produces/Sells CE-marked Devices: N
Federal Procurement Eligibility: Small Business
Distribution: Manufacturer Direct
General Admin.: William D. J. Wallis/President
  Catheter, Cholangiography   Surgery

UTAH RESEARCH & DEVELOPMENT CO. INC.
  See Diacor, Inc.

UTAK LABORATORIES, INC.   800-235-3442
25020 Ave Tibbitts, Valencia, CA 91355   661-294-3935
FDA Number: 2022375   *Fax:* 661-294-9272
E-mail: info@utak.com
Web site: www.utak.com
Medical Products Sales Volume: $800,000
Annual Revenue: $0-$1 Million
Total Employees: 8
Ownership: Private
Produces/Sells CE-marked Devices: N
Federal Procurement Eligibility: Small Business
Distribution: Manufacturer Direct
General Admin.: Lawrence B. Plutchak/President
Mktg./Adv.: Christina Plutchak/Managing Director Marketing & Sales
Production: James Plutchak/Director Operations
  Control, Heavy Metals   Toxicology
  General Hematology Reagent   Pathology
  System, Test, Drugs of Abuse   Chemistry

UTECH PRODUCTS, INC.   800-828-8324
135 Broadway St, Schenectady, NY 12305   518-489-5705
FDA Number: n/a   *Fax:* 518-489-3772
E-mail: webservice@utechproducts.com
Web site: www.utechproducts.com
Medical Products Sales Volume: $3,000,000
Annual Revenue: $1-$5 Million
Ownership: Private
Produces/Sells CE-marked Devices: Y
Federal Procurement Eligibility: Small Business, Minority Owned
Distribution: Exclusive Distributor, Importer, Exporter
  Balance, Analytical   Chemistry
  Calorimeter   Chemistry
  Sterilizer, Steam (Autoclave)   General

UVP, LLC   800-452-6788
2066 W. 11th St., Upland, CA 91786-3509   909-946-3197
FDA Number: 9201098   *Fax:* 909-946-3597
E-mail: info@uvp.com
Web site: www.uvp.com
Medical Products Sales Volume: $8,000,000
Annual Revenue: $10-$25 Million
Year Founded: 1932
Total Employees: 120   *Marketing Staff:* 4   *Sales Staff:* 9
Ownership: Private
Produces/Sells CE-marked Devices: N
Federal Procurement Eligibility: Small Business
Distribution: Manufacturer Direct, Manufacturer Through Distributor, Manufacturer Through Manufacturer Reps, OEM, Exporter
General Admin.: Leighton Smith/President
Mktg./Adv.: Kathleen Buckman/Manager Marketing Services
      Jeff Pieri/Manager Sales
      Alex Waluszko/Vice President Marketing & Sales
Production: Betty Cambruzzi/Manager Customer Services
  Cabinet, Chromatography (U.V.) Viewing   Chemistry
  Electrophoresis Equipment, Gel   Chemistry
  Electrophoresis Equipment, Thin-Layer   Chemistry
  Image Processing System   Radiology
  Lamp, Ultraviolet, Germicidal   General
  Lamp, Ultraviolet, Physical Medicine   Physical Med
  Radiometer, Phototherapy   General
  Sterilizer, Ultraviolet   General
  Transilluminator, AC-Powered, Other   Ophthalmology

V--OPERATIONS MANAGEMENT CONSULTING,   317-570-5830
7350 E 86th St, Indianapolis, IN 46256
FDA Number: 1835831   *Fax:* 317-570-5831
E-mail: aelsbury@omcprecision.com
Web site: www.OMCPrecision.com
Medical Products Sales Volume: $1,800,000

V--OPERATIONS MANAGEMENT CONSULTING,   317-570-5830 *(cont'd)*
Annual Revenue: $1-$5 Million
Year Founded: 1996
Total Employees: 25
Ownership: Private
Produces/Sells CE-marked Devices: Y
Federal Procurement Eligibility: Small Business
Distribution: OEM
General Admin.: Mr. Andrew Elsbury/President, Chief Executive Officer
Research: Mr. Paul Beckwith/Vice President Research & Development & Engineering
Finance: Mrs. Debbie Rowe/Director Finance
  Implant, Fixation Device, Spinal   Orthopedics
  Mesh, Orthopedic (Metallic)   Orthopedics
  Orthopedic Manual Surgical Instrument   Orthopedics
  Orthosis, Fixation, Pedicle, Spinal   Orthopedics
  Staple, Fixation, Bone   Orthopedics

V.I.E.W. VIDEO   800-843-9843
PO Box 77, Saugerties, NY 12477   845) 246-9955
FDA Number: n/a   *Fax:* (845) 246-9966
E-mail: info@view.com
Web site: www.view.com
Annual Revenue: $1-$5 Million
Total Employees: 20   *Marketing Staff:* 3   *Sales Staff:* 7
Ownership: Private
Produces/Sells CE-marked Devices: N
Federal Procurement Eligibility: Small Business
Distribution: Exclusive Distributor, Exporter
General Admin.: Bob Karcy/President, Chief Executive Officer
      Doris Schultz/Vice President, General Manager
Mktg./Adv.: Stephen Kates/Director Marketing
      Timothy Orr/Manager Marketing Operations
      Joe Knipes/Manager National Sales
  Material, Training, Audiovisual   General

V.I.R. ENGINEERING, INC.   805-964-0553
5951 Encina Road, Suite 209, Goleta, CA 93117
FDA Number: 2025521   *Fax:* 805-964-9588
E-mail: rredmond@vir-eng.com
Web site: www.vir-eng.com
Medical Products Sales Volume: $300,000
Year Founded: 1984
Total Employees: 5
Ownership: Private
Produces/Sells CE-marked Devices: N
Federal Procurement Eligibility: Small Business
Distribution: Manufacturer Direct
  Blade, Scalpel   Surgery

V.T.S.,INC.   620-227-7434
1701 N. 14th Ave., Dodge City, KS 67801
FDA Number: 1650924
  Prosthesis, Penis, Inflatable   Surgery
  Prosthesis, Penis, Rigid Rod, External   Gastroenterology/Urology

VACALON COMPANY, INC.   614-577-1945
12960 Stonecreek Dr., Ste. C, Pickerington, OH 43147
FDA Number: 3003377077
  Paper, Articulation   Dental And Oral

VACUMED   800-235-3333
4538 Westinghouse St., Ventura, CA 93003   805-644-7461
FDA Number: 2023529   *Fax:* 805-654-8759
E-mail: info@vacumed.com
Web site: www.vacumed.com
Medical Products Sales Volume: $1,700,000
Annual Revenue: $1-$5 Million
Year Founded: 1968
Total Employees: 10   *Marketing Staff:* 1   *Sales Staff:* 1
Ownership: VACUMETRICS, INC.
Produces/Sells CE-marked Devices: N
Federal Procurement Eligibility: Small Business
Distribution: Manufacturer Direct, Manufacturer Through Distributor, Manufacturer Through Manufacturer Reps, OEM, Importer, Exporter
General Admin.: John Hoppe/President, Chief Executive Officer
Mktg./Adv.: John Hoppe/Director Marketing
      Andrew Huszczuk/Director Product Development
  Analyzer, Gas, Carbon-Dioxide, Gaseous Phase (Capnograph)   Anesthesiology
  Analyzer, Gas, Oxygen, Gaseous Phase   Anesthesiology
  Analyzer, Metabolism   Anesthesiology
  Analyzer, Pulmonary Function   Anesthesiology
  Bag, Breathing   Anesthesiology
  Clip, Nose   Anesthesiology
  Computer, Pulmonary Function Data   Anesthesiology
  Continuous Positive Airway Pressure Unit (CPAP, CPPB)   Anesthesiology
  Exerciser, Bicycle   Physical Med

VACUMED
800-235-3333 *(cont'd)*

Filter, Bacterial, Breathing Circuit	Anesthesiology
Filter, Conduction, Anesthesia	Anesthesiology
Meter, Peak Flow, Spirometry	Anesthesiology
Mouthpiece, Breathing	Anesthesiology
Nebulizer, Non-Heated	Anesthesiology
Paper, Chart, Record, Medical	General
Pneumotachograph	Anesthesiology
Spectrograph, Mass	Chemistry
Spirometer, Diagnostic (Respirometer)	Anesthesiology
Treadmill, Powered	Physical Med
Tubing, Ventilator	Anesthesiology

VACUMETRICS INC.
See Vacumed

VACUUM ATMOSPHERES CO.
310-644-0255

4652 W. Rosecrans Avenue, Hawthorne, CA 90250-6896
FDA Number: 7000375   *Fax:* 310-970-0980
E-mail: sales@vac-atm.com
Web site: www.vac-atm.com
Medical Products Sales Volume: $8,100,000
Annual Revenue: $5-$10 Million
Year Founded: 1960
Total Employees: 80   *Marketing Staff:* 2   *Sales Staff:* 6
Ownership: WEMS, INC.
Produces/Sells CE-marked Devices: Y
Federal Procurement Eligibility: Small Business
Distribution: Manufacturer Direct, Manufacturer Through Manufacturer Reps, OEM
General Admin.: Robert Hood/Chief Executive Officer
    Terry Sweem/President
Mktg./Adv.: John Hamilton/Manager International Marketing & Sales
    Tom Ashimoto/Manager National Sales
    John Hamilton/Manager Sales
    Terry Sweem/Vice President Marketing
Production: Shawn Udell/Director Quality Assurance
    Terry Whelan/Manager Materials

Box, Glove	Microbiology

VAL MED
800-242-5355
504-276-5111

Ace Bayou Group, 3700 Desire Pkwy.,
New Orleans, LA 70126
FDA Number: 2317942   *Fax:* 504-276-6182
E-mail: info@valmedmedical.com
Web site: www.valmedmedical.com
Annual Revenue: $0-$1 Million
Year Founded: 1986
Total Employees: 120
Ownership: Private
Produces/Sells CE-marked Devices: N
Federal Procurement Eligibility: Small Business
Distribution: Manufacturer Direct
General Admin.: Murray Valene/President
Mktg./Adv.: Mr. Dave Wood/General Manager Marketing & Sales

Accessories, Traction (Cart, Frame, Cord, Weight)	Orthopedics
Belt, Traction, Pelvic, Orthopedic	Orthopedics
Cover, Mattress	General
Mattress, Bed	General

VAL-U-MED INC.
800-668-3168
519-753-0855

673 Colborne St., P.O. Box 1206,
Brantford, ONT N3S-3 Canada
FDA Number: n/a   *Fax:* 519-753-0019
E-mail: valumed@bfree.on.ca
Year Founded: 1991
Total Employees: 25
Ownership: Private
Produces/Sells CE-marked Devices: N
Distribution: Manufacturer Direct, Exclusive Distributor

VALEANT CANADA LTD
1-800-361-1448
514-744-6792

4787 Levy Street,
Montreal, QUEBE H4R 2 Canada
FDA Number: n/a   *Fax:* 514-744-6272
Web site: www.valeantcanada.com
Total Employees: 150
Ownership: Icn Pharmaceuticals, Inc.
Stock Symbol: VRX
Traded On: NYSE
Produces/Sells CE-marked Devices: N
Distribution: Manufacturer Direct, OEM, Exporter

VALEO, INC.
800-634-2704
262-695-4800

W248 N5499 Executive Dr., Sussex, WI 53089
FDA Number: n/a   *Fax:* 800-831-9642
E-mail: valeoinfo@valeoinc.com
Web site: www.valeoinc.com
Year Founded: 1988

VALEO, INC.
800-634-2704 *(cont'd)*

Total Employees: 20
Ownership: Private
Produces/Sells CE-marked Devices: N
Federal Procurement Eligibility: Small Business
Distribution: Manufacturer Through Distributor
General Admin.: Lisa Yewer/President
Mktg./Adv.: Chris O'Donnell/Manager Sales
    Phil Welch/Vice President, Manager Sales
Production: Delores Scharmer/Customer Service Representative

Support, Back	Orthopedics
Support, Knee	Physical Med
Support, Wrist	Physical Med

VALERITAS, LLC
508-845-1177

800 Boston Turnpike, Shrewsbury, MA 01545
FDA Number: 1226572
E-mail: gjenkins@valeritas.com
Web site: www.valeritas.com
Ownership: Private
Produces/Sells CE-marked Devices: N
General Admin.: Ms. Kristine Peterson/Chief Executive Officer
    Mr. John Timberlake/President
Production: Mr. Geoffrey Jenkins/Executive Vice President Operations
Finance: Mr. Jim Dentzer/Chief Financial Officer

Injector, Fluid, Non-Electric	General
Pump, Infusion	General

VALIDYNE ENGINEERING SALES CORP.
800-423-5851
818-886-2057

8626 Wilbur Avenue, Northridge, CA 91324
FDA Number: 2018713   *Fax:* 818-886-6512
E-mail: sales@validyne.com
Web site: www.validyne.com
Annual Revenue: $5-$10 Million
Year Founded: 1968
Total Employees: 45   *Sales Staff:* 10
Ownership: Private
Produces/Sells CE-marked Devices: Y
Federal Procurement Eligibility: Small Business
Distribution: Manufacturer Direct

Flowmeter, Pulmonary Function	Anesthesiology

VALLEY BIOMEDICAL PRODUCTS/SER., INC.
540-868-0800

121 Industrial Dr., Winchester, VA 22602
FDA Number: 1121958

Antigen, Antiserum, Control, Whole Human Serum	Immunology
Control, Urinalysis (Assayed And Unassayed)	Chemistry
Diluent, Blood Cell	Hematology
Whole Human Plasma, Antigen, Antiserum, Control	Immunology

VALLEY CRAFT
800-328-1480
651-345-3386

2001 South Highway 61, Lake City, MN 55041
FDA Number: n/a   *Fax:* 651-345-3606
E-mail: customer@valleycraft.com
Web site: www.valleycraft.com
Annual Revenue: $10-$25 Million
Year Founded: 1953
Total Employees: 146   *Marketing Staff:* 1   *Sales Staff:* 6
Ownership: Private
Produces/Sells CE-marked Devices: N
Federal Procurement Eligibility: Small Business
Distribution: Manufacturer Direct, Manufacturer Through Distributor, Manufacturer Through Manufacturer Reps, Importer, Exporter
General Admin.: Mr. Wayne Morris/Manager Plant
Mktg./Adv.: Mr. Grant DesRoches/Director Marketing & Sales
    Ms. Linda Brackee/Manager Inventory Control
    Mr. Dave Hinck/Manager National Accounts
    Mr. Glenn Dwelle/Manager Regional Sales
    Mr. John Pinderski/Manager Regional Sales
    Mr. Kirt Whitney/Manager Regional Sales
    Mrs. Daria Dalager/Marketing Coordinator
Production: Mrs. Jodi Mueller/Manager Customer Services

Accessories, Cart, Multipurpose	General
Cabinet Casework, General Purpose	General
Cabinet Casework, Modular	General
Cabinet Casework, Pharmacy	General
Cabinet, Instrument	General
Cabinet, Medicine	General
Cabinet, Narcotic Control	General
Cabinet, Other	General
Cart, Equipment, Video	General
Cart, Multipurpose	General
Cart, Other	General
Cart, Supply	General
Office Equipment	General
Security Equipment/Supplies	General

VALLEY FORGE SCIENTIFIC CORP.
610-666-7500
136 Green Tree Road, Suite 100, Oaks, PA 19456
FDA Number: 2521567
Fax: 610-666-7565
E-mail: sales@vlfg.com
Web site: www.vlfg.com
Annual Revenue: $5-$10 Million
Year Founded: 1980
Total Employees: 15   *Marketing Staff:* 1
Ownership: Public
Stock Symbol: VLFG
Traded On: NASDAQ
Quality System Registration Information: ISO9000
Produces/Sells CE-marked Devices: Y
Federal Procurement Eligibility: Small Business
Distribution: Manufacturer Through Distributor, Exclusive Distributor
General Admin.: Jerry L. Malis/President, Chief Executive Officer
　　　　Michael Ritchie/Vice President, General Manager
Mktg./Adv.: Susan Anderson/Director Marketing & Business Development
Production: Mr. Anthony Groch/Manager Engineering
　　　　Robert Conrad/Manager Production
　　　　David Solt/Vice President Manufacturing
　　　　Bonnie Ritchie/Vice President Operations

Electrode, Electrosurgical, Return (Ground, Dispersive)	Surgery
Electrosurgical Equipment, Special Purpose	Surgery
Electrosurgical Unit, Cutting & Coagulation Device	Surgery
Irrigator, Suction	General
Laparoscope, Gynecologic	Obstetrics/Gynecology
Loupe, Binocular, Low Power	Ophthalmology
Tubing, Irrigation	Surgery

VALLEY INSTITUTE OF PROSTHETICS AND ORTHOTICS, INC
661-322-1005
1524 21st St., Suite B, Bakersfield, CA 93301-4002
FDA Number: 3003914036
Ownership: Private
Produces/Sells CE-marked Devices: N

Assembly, Knee/Shank/Ankle/Foot, External	Physical Med

VALLEY NATIONAL GASES WV LLC
724-834-9200
1055 Garden Street, Gbg, PA 15601
FDA Number: 2522976

Gas, Calibrated (Specified Concentration)	Anesthesiology

VALLEY PRODUCTS CO.
800-451-8874
717-792-1010
P.O. Box 187, York New Salem, PA 17371-0187
FDA Number: n/a
Fax: 877-792-4964
E-mail: valpro@clothlabels.com
Web site: www.clothlabels.com
Annual Revenue: $1-$5 Million
Year Founded: 1938
Total Employees: 10   *Sales Staff:* 2
Ownership: Private
Produces/Sells CE-marked Devices: N
Federal Procurement Eligibility: Small Business
Distribution: Manufacturer Direct, Exclusive Distributor
General Admin.: John Eyster/President, Chief Executive Officer
Mktg./Adv.: Betsy Doutrich/Director National Accounts
　　　　Andrew Eyster/Director Product Development
　　　　Betsy Doutrich/Vice President, Director Marketing
Production: Andrew Eyster/Director Quality Assurance

Contract Manufacturing	General
Tape, Cotton	General
Tape, Orthopedic	Orthopedics

VALLEY TECHNOLOGY, INC.
541-434-9180
1025 Conger Street, Suite #2, Eugene, OR 97402
FDA Number: 3034535
Ownership: Private
Produces/Sells CE-marked Devices: N

Table, Surgical With Orthopedic Accessories, AC-Powered	Surgery

VALLEYLAB
800-255-8522
303-530-2300
5920 Longbow Dr., Boulder, CO 80301-3299
FDA Number: 1717344
Fax: 303-530-6285
E-mail: valleylab.customerservice@tycohealthcare.com
Web site: www.valleylab.com
Year Founded: 1967
Total Employees: 850
Ownership: Covidien Ltd.
Stock Symbol: COV
Traded On: NYSE
Quality System Registration Information: ISO9002
Produces/Sells CE-marked Devices: Y
Distribution: Manufacturer Direct, Exporter
General Admin.: Ralph Mills/Director Human Resources
　　　　Sherri Hughes-Smith/Manager
　　　　Scott Drake/President

VALLEYLAB
800-255-8522 *(cont'd)*
　　　　Adrianne Muniz/Secretary
Mktg./Adv.: Kathy Rosser/Manager Communications
　　　　Rodney Marcy/Vice President Sales
Production: Bruce Lamb/Vice President Operations
　　　　Terry Hilkemeier/Vice President Quality Assurance & Regulatory Affairs
Research: Paul Hermes/Vice President Research & Development

Aspirator, Surgical	Surgery
Electrode, Electrosurgery, Laparoscopic	Surgery
Electrode, Electrosurgical, Active (Blade)	Surgery
Electrode, Electrosurgical, Return (Ground, Dispersive)	Surgery
Electrode, Gel	Cardiovascular
Electrosurgical Equipment, General Purpose	Surgery
Electrosurgical Equipment, Special Purpose	Surgery
Electrosurgical Unit, Cardiovascular	Cardiovascular
Electrosurgical Unit, Cutting & Coagulation Device	Surgery
Electrosurgical Unit, Gastroenterology	Gastroenterology/Urology
Electrosurgical Unit, General Purpose (ESU)	Surgery
Equipment, Suction/Irrigation, Laparoscopic	Surgery
Exhaust System, Surgical	Surgery
Forceps, Electrosurgical	Surgery
Generator, Radiofrequency Lesion	Cns/Neurology
Handle, Instrument, Laparoscopic (Electrocautery)	Surgery
Irrigator/Coagulator/Cutter, Suction, Laparoscopic	Surgery
System, Evacuation, Smoke, Laser	Surgery

VALMARK, INC.
613-822-3107
P.O. Box 190, Gloucester, ONT K1X-1A4 Canada
FDA Number: n/a
Fax: 613-822-3109
Ownership: Private
Produces/Sells CE-marked Devices: N
Federal Procurement Eligibility: Small Business, Female Owned
Distribution: Exclusive Distributor, Exporter

VALOR MEDICAL, INC.
858-643-1675
6749 Top Gun Street, Suite 109, San Diego, CA 92121
FDA Number: 3006202040
Fax: 858-750-1454
E-mail: info@valormedical.com
Web site: www.valormedical.com
Ownership: Private
Produces/Sells CE-marked Devices: N
General Admin.: H. Clark Adams/Chairman, Chief Executive Officer
Production: Robert Elms/Director Operations
Finance: Dr. Charles Kerber/President

VALPLAST INTL. CORP.
718-361-7440
34-30 31st St., Long Island City, NY 11106
FDA Number: 2436918

Base, Denture, Relining, Repairing, Rebasing, Resin	Dental And Oral
Denture, Plastic, Teeth	Dental And Oral

VALTRONICS USA INC.
440-349 1239
6168 Cochran Rd., Solon, OH 44139
FDA Number: n/a
Fax: 440-349-1040
E-mail: inquiries@valtronicstechnologies.com
Web site: http://www.valtronictechnologies.com
Ownership: Private
Produces/Sells CE-marked Devices: N
General Admin.: Mr. Peter Ruppersberg/Chief Executive Officer
Mktg./Adv.: Mr. Timothy Kline/Vice President Marketing & Sales
Production: Mr. Gregory Stoeckli/Vice President Operations
　　　　Mr. Bertrand Gabry/Vice President Quality Control
Finance: Mr. Charles Fontannaz/Vice President Finance

VALUE PLASTICS
888-404-5837
970-267-5200
3325 S. Timberline Rd, Ft. Collins, CO 80525
FDA Number: n/a
E-mail: sales@valueplastics.com
Web site: http://www.valueplastics.com
Year Founded: 1968
Ownership: Private
Produces/Sells CE-marked Devices: N
Distribution: OEM

VALUED MEDICAL CARE (VMC) INC.
800-673-0555
506-832-1019
262 Robertson Rd., P.O. Box 1188, Hampton, NB E5N-8 Canada
FDA Number: n/a
Fax: 506-832-3603
E-mail: info@vmc1.net
Web site: www.vmc1.net
Year Founded: 1992
Total Employees: 10
Ownership: Private
Produces/Sells CE-marked Devices: N
Distribution: Exclusive Distributor

VAN-TEC INC.
See Boston Scientific Corporation

MANUFACTURER PROFILES

VANCARE, INC.
    1515 1st St., Aurora, NE 68818
    FDA Number: 1933441
    E-mail: pvancare@hamilton.net
    Web site: www.vancare.com
    Medical Products Sales Volume: $2,300,000
    Annual Revenue: $1-$5 Million
    Year Founded: 1993
    Total Employees: 18   *Sales Staff:* 2
    Ownership: Private
    Produces/Sells CE-marked Devices: N
    Federal Procurement Eligibility: Small Business
    Distribution: Manufacturer Through Distributor
    Mktg./Adv.: James A. Vanderheiden/Manager National Sales
      Lift, Patient   General

800-694-4525
402-694-4525
Fax: 402-694-3994

VANCE PRODUCTS, INC.
    See Cook Urological, Inc.

VANCO INDUSTRIES, INC.
    See Spectrum-Brands

VANDENT DENTAL HANDPIECE SALES & SERVICE   **800-826-3368**
    P.O. Box 1229, Eastville, VA 23347   **757-678-7973**
    FDA Number: n/a   *Fax:* 757-678-7975
    E-mail: vandent@esva.net
    Web site: www.vandent.com
    Annual Revenue: $0-$1 Million
    Total Employees: 2
    Ownership: Private
    Produces/Sells CE-marked Devices: N
    Federal Procurement Eligibility: Small Business
    Distribution: Service Direct
    General Admin.: Nan Leighton/Office Manager
               Michael Arpino/President
      Dentifrice   Dental And Oral
      Floss, Dental   Dental And Oral
      Handpiece, Air-Powered, Dental   Dental And Oral
      Handpiece, Belt and/or Gear Driven, Dental   Dental And Oral
      Service, Maintenance/Repair   General

VANDERBILT UNIVERSITY   **615-343-0068**
    2201 West End Ave., Nashville, TN 37235
    FDA Number: 3004909208
      Camera, Gamma (Nuclear/Scintillation)   Radiology

VANNY CORP.   **310-556-1170**
    10390 Sana Monica Blvd., Suite 270, Los Angeles, CA 90025
    FDA Number: 2029171
    Ownership: Private
    Produces/Sells CE-marked Devices: N
      Cabinet, Moist Steam   Physical Med

VANTAGE DENTAL LAB. CORP.
    See Mastercraft Dental Co. Of Texas

VANTAGE INDUSTRIES, INC.   **800-221-4329**
    5070 Phillip Lee Drive, Atlanta, GA 30336
    FDA Number: n/a
    Web site: www.vantageindustries.com
    Medical Products Sales Volume: $500,000
    Ownership: LEGGETT AND PLATT
    Stock Symbol: LEG
    Traded On: NYSE
    Produces/Sells CE-marked Devices: N
    Distribution: OEM
      Cover, Mattress   General
      Cushion, Wheelchair (Pad)   Physical Med
      Floor Mat   General

VANTAGE ORTHOPEDICS   **513-563-1690**
    41 Techview Dr., Cincinnati, OH 45215
    FDA Number: 3002624207
      Orthosis, Limb Brace   Physical Med

VAPOTHERM, INC.   **866-827-6843**
    198 Log Canoe Circle, Stevensville, MD 21666   **410-604-3977**
    FDA Number: 1125759   *Fax:* 410-604-3978
    E-mail: info@vtherm.com
    Web site: www.vtherm.com
    Ownership: Private
    Produces/Sells CE-marked Devices: N
      Humidifier, Respiratory Gas, (Direct Patient Interface)   Anesthesiology

VAR-LAC-OID CHEMICAL CO., INC.   **201-387-0038**
    13 Foster Street, Bergenfield, NJ 07621-4301
    FDA Number: n/a   *Fax:* 201-387-0291
    E-mail: info@cesium-chloride.com
    Web site: www.cesium-chloride.com

VAR-LAC-OID CHEMICAL CO., INC.   **201-387-0038** *(cont'd)*
    Medical Products Sales Volume: $1,000,000
    Annual Revenue: $0-$1 Million
    Year Founded: 1923
    Total Employees: 10   *Marketing Staff:* 1   *Sales Staff:* 3
    Ownership: Private
    Produces/Sells CE-marked Devices: N
    Federal Procurement Eligibility: Small Business, GSA Contract, VA Contract
    Distribution: Manufacturer Direct
    General Admin.: Alan Kessler/President
    Mktg./Adv.: B. Gerald/Manager Sales
      Genetic Engineering   Microbiology

VARIAN ASSOCIATES, INC.
    See Varian Medical Systems

VARIAN EIMAC DIV.
    See Varian Medical Systems X-Ray Products

VARIAN INC   **650-424-5078**
    25200 Commercentre Dr., Lake Forest, CA 92630-8810
    FDA Number: 2026835
    Web site: www.varian.com
    Ownership: Agilent Technologies, Inc.
    Stock Symbol: VAR
    Traded On: NYSE
    Produces/Sells CE-marked Devices: N
      Chromatography Equipment, Ion Exchange   Toxicology
      Chromatography Equipment, Thin Layer   Toxicology
      Container, Specimen Mailer And Storage, Non-sterile   Pathology
      Enzyme Immunoassay, Amphetamine   Toxicology
      Enzyme Immunoassay, Barbiturate   Toxicology
      Enzyme Immunoassay, Benzodiazepine   Toxicology
      Enzyme Immunoassay, Cannabinoids   Toxicology
      Enzyme Immunoassay, Cocaine And Cocaine Metabolites   Toxicology
      Enzyme Immunoassay, Opiates   Toxicology
      Enzyme Immunoassay, Phencyclidine   Toxicology
      Fluorometry, Morphine   Toxicology
      Gas Chromatography, Methamphetamine   Toxicology
      Instrumentation, High Pressure Liquid Chromatography   Toxicology
      Potassium Dichromate, Alcohol   Toxicology
      Radioimmunoassay, Tricyclic Antidepressant Drugs   Toxicology
      Reagent, NAD-NADH, Alcohol Enzyme Method   Toxicology
      Test, Tetrahydrocannabinol   Toxicology
      Thin Layer Chromatography, Opiates   Toxicology
    Medical Product Subsidiaries (Listed Separately)
      Polymer Laboratories, Now A Part Of Varian, Inc.
      Varian Sample Preparation Products
      Varian Vacuum Products

VARIAN MEDICAL SYSTEMS   **800-544-4636**
    3100 Hansen Way, Palo Alto, CA 94304-1038   **415-493-4000**
    FDA Number: 2916710   *Fax:* 650-424-8617
    E-mail: ca@varian.com
    Web site: www.varian.com
    Medical Products Sales Volume: $1,590,000,000
    Annual Revenue: More than $1 Billion
    Year Founded: 1940
    Total Employees: 4800
    Ownership: Public
    Stock Symbol: VAR
    Traded On: NYSE
    Quality System Registration Information: ISO9000; ISO9001
    Produces/Sells CE-marked Devices: Y
    Distribution: Manufacturer Direct, Manufacturer Through Distributor, Manufacturer Through Manufacturer Reps, Exporter
    General Admin.: Elisha W. Finney/Chief Financial Officer, Senior Vice President
               Mr. George A. Zdasiuk/Chief Technology Officer, Vice President
               Mr. John W. Kuo/Corporate Vice President
               Mr. Robert H. Kluge/Corporate Vice President
               Mr. Timothy E. Guertin/President, Chief Executive Officer
               Wendy S Reitherman/Vice President Human Resources
    Mktg./Adv.: Spencer Sias/Director Corporate Communications
    Finance: Mr. Franco N Palomba/Vice President Finance & Operations
             Tai-Yun Chen/Vice President Finance, Controller
      Accelerator, Linear, Medical   Radiology
      Accessories, Radiotherapy   Radiology
      Afterloader, Radiotherapy   Radiology
      Collimator, Therapeutic X-Ray, High Voltage   Radiology
      Computer, Radiographic Data   Radiology
      Image Processing System   Radiology
      Imager, X-Ray, Solid State (Flat Panel/Digital)   Radiology
      Simulator, Radiotherapy   Radiology
      Stereotaxy Equipment   Cns/Neurology
      Synchronizer, ECG/Respirator, Radiographic   Radiology
      System, Communication, Image, Digital   Radiology
      System, Planning, Radiation Therapy Treatment   Radiology
      Tube, X-Ray   Radiology
    Medical Product Subsidiaries (Listed Separately)
      Varian Medical Systems Brachytheraphy

VARIAN MEDICAL SYSTEMS   800-544-4636 *(cont'd)*
Varian Medical Systems Interay
Varian Medical Systems X-Ray Products
Varian Medical Systems, Oncology Systems

VARIAN MEDICAL SYSTEMS BRACHYTHERAPHY 888.666.7847
700 Harris St, Suite 109,   **434-977-8495**
Charlottesville, VA 22903
FDA Number: 1124791   Fax: 434-244-7181
E-mail: vbtinfo@varian.com
Web site: www.varian.com
Ownership: Varian Medical Systems
Stock Symbol: VAR
Traded On: NYSE
Produces/Sells CE-marked Devices: N
  System, Planning, Radiation Therapy Treatment   Radiology

VARIAN MEDICAL SYSTEMS INTERAY   800-468-3729
3235 Fortune Drive, North Charleston, SC 29418   **843-767-3005**
FDA Number: 1035768   Fax: 843-760-0079
E-mail: interay.sales@varian.com
Web site: www.varian.com
Year Founded: 1983
Total Employees: 35
Ownership: Varian Medical Systems
Stock Symbol: VAR
Traded On: NYSE
Quality System Registration Information: ISO9002
Produces/Sells CE-marked Devices: Y
Distribution: Manufacturer Through Distributor, OEM, Exporter
Mktg./Adv.: Steve Kimmel/Manager International Marketing & Sales
Production: Bill Herring/Manager Manufacturing
  Housing, X-Ray Tube, Diagnostic   Radiology
  Scanner, Computed Tomography, X-Ray, Special Procedure   Radiology

VARIAN MEDICAL SYSTEMS X-RAY PRODUCTS   800-432-4422
1678 S. Pioneer Rd., Salt Lake City, UT 84104   **801-972-5000**
FDA Number: 1717855   Fax: 801-973-5050
E-mail: industrial@varian.com
Web site: www.varian.com
Year Founded: 1940
Total Employees: 560   *Marketing Staff:* 10   *Sales Staff:* 10
Ownership: Varian Medical Systems
Stock Symbol: VAR
Traded On: NYSE
Quality System Registration Information: ISO9000
Produces/Sells CE-marked Devices: N
Federal Procurement Eligibility: Small Business
Distribution: Manufacturer Direct, Importer, Exporter
General Admin.: Bob Kluge/Vice President, General Manager
Mktg./Adv.: Steve Clark/Manager Marketing & Sales
Production: Leonard Aoyagi/Manager Manufacturing
  Housing, X-Ray Tube, Diagnostic   Radiology
  Housing, X-Ray Tube, Therapeutic   Radiology
  Image Intensification System   Radiology
  Tube, Image Amplifier, X-Ray   Radiology
  Tube, X-Ray   Radiology

VARIAN MEDICAL SYSTEMS, ONCOLOGY SYSTEMS   800 278-2747
911 Hansen Way, Bldg.3 M/S C-165,   **650-424-5945**
Palo Alto, CA 94304
FDA Number: 2916710   Fax: 650 424-6252
E-mail: planning@varian.com
Web site: www.varian.com
Ownership: Varian Medical Systems
Stock Symbol: VAR
Traded On: NYSE
Produces/Sells CE-marked Devices: N
Mktg./Adv.: Mike Harral/Project Manager
  Accelerator, Linear, Medical   Radiology
  Image Processing System   Radiology
  Radiotherapy Unit, Charged-Particle   Radiology
  Stereotaxy Equipment   Cns/Neurology
  Synchronizer, ECG/Respirator, Radiographic   Radiology
  System, Communication, Image, Digital   Radiology
  System, Planning, Radiation Therapy Treatment   Radiology

VARIAN SAMPLE PREPARATION PRODUCTS   800-421-2825
24201 Frampton Avenue,
Harbor City, CA 90710
FDA Number: 9200070   Fax: 310-539-4270
E-mail: nigel.simpson@spp.varian.com
Annual Revenue: $10-$25 Million
Total Employees: 80   *Marketing Staff:* 8   *Sales Staff:* 12
Ownership: Varian Inc
Quality System Registration Information: ISO9002; ISO9003

VARIAN SAMPLE PREPARATION PRODUCTS   800-421-2825
(cont'd)
Federal Procurement Eligibility: GSA Contract
Distribution: Manufacturer Direct, Manufacturer Through Distributor, Manufacturer Through Manufacturer Reps, OEM, Exporter
General Admin.: Craig Woods/General Manager
Mktg./Adv.: David Stephens/Director Marketing
     David Nau/Manager Product Development
Production: Nigel Simpson/Product Manager
  Chromatography Equipment, Paper   Chemistry
  Column, Chromatography   Chemistry
  Dispenser, Fluid   General
  Tube, Vacuum Sample, With Anticoagulant   Hematology

VARIAN SCIENTIFIC INSTRUMENTS   925-939-2400
2700 Mitchell Dr., Walnut Creek, CA 94598
FDA Number: n/a   Fax: 925-945-2360
E-mail: custserv@varianinc.com
Web site: www.varianinc.com
Ownership: VARIAN, INC.
Produces/Sells CE-marked Devices: N
General Admin.: Garry W. Rogerson/Chief Executive Officer, Chairman
     G. Edward McClammy/Chief Financial Officer, Senior Vice President
     Martin O'Donoghue/Senior Vice President
  Chromatography (Gas), Clinical Use   Toxicology
  Chromatography (Liquid, Gel), Clinical Use   Toxicology
  Mass Spectrometer, Clinical Use   Toxicology

VARIAN VACUUM PRODUCTS   800-882-7426
121 Hartwell Ave., Lexington, MA 02421-3133   **781-861-7200**
FDA Number: n/a   Fax: 781-860-5437
E-mail: custserv@varianinc.com
Web site: www.varianinc.com
Ownership: Varian Inc
Quality System Registration Information: ISO9001
Produces/Sells CE-marked Devices: Y
Distribution: Manufacturer Direct
General Admin.: Garry W. Rogerson/Chief Executive Officer, Chairman
     G. Edward McClammy/Chief Financial Officer, Senior Vice President
     Sergio Piras/Senior Vice President
  Contract R&D, Diagnostics   General
  Pump, Vacuum, Central   Anesthesiology
  Pump, Vacuum, Electric, Suction-Type Electrode   Orthopedics
  Regulator, Vacuum   General

VARIAN X-RAY TUBE PRODUCTS
See Varian Medical Systems X-Ray Products

VARIAN, INC.
See Varian Scientific Instruments

VARIAN, INC.   800-926-3000
3120 Hansen Way, Palo Alto, CA 94304-1030   **650-213-8000**
FDA Number: n/a
E-mail: custserv@varianinc.com
Web site: www.varianinc.com
Ownership: Private
Stock Symbol: VARI
Traded On: NASDAQ
Produces/Sells CE-marked Devices: Y
Federal Procurement Eligibility: Small Business
Distribution: Manufacturer Direct
General Admin.: Garry W. Rogerson/Chief Executive Officer, Chairman
     G. Edward McClammy/Chief Financial Officer, Senior Vice President
  Column, Liquid Chromatography   Toxicology
Medical Product Subsidiaries (Listed Separately)
Varian Inc

VARIETY ABILITY SYSTEMS INC.   800-891-4514
2 Kelvin Ave., Unit 3,   **416-698-1415**
Toronto, ONT M4C-5 Canada
FDA Number: n/a   Fax: 416-698-5860
E-mail: mmifsud@vasi.on.ca
Web site: www.vasi.on.ca
Medical Products Sales Volume: $1,000,000
Year Founded: 1986
Total Employees: 7   *Marketing Staff:* 1   *Sales Staff:* 1
Ownership: Private
Quality System Registration Information: ISO9000; ISO9002
Produces/Sells CE-marked Devices: Y
Federal Procurement Eligibility: Small Business
Distribution: Manufacturer Direct, Manufacturer Through Distributor, Exclusive Distributor, Exporter

VARIMED   800-426-5496
1121 Pagni Dr., Elk Grove Village, IL 60007-6602   847-956-8900
FDA Number: n/a   *Fax:* 847-956-8909
E-mail: sales@varimed.net
Web site: www.unilabel.com
Annual Revenue: $1-$5 Million
Total Employees: 50
Ownership: UNI-LABEL & TAG, INC.
Produces/Sells CE-marked Devices: N
Federal Procurement Eligibility: Small Business
Distribution: Manufacturer Direct, Manufacturer Through Manufacturer Reps, OEM
General Admin.: Jim Brunner/President
  Labeling Equipment   General
  Packaging Material   General

VARIORAW S.A.
  See Axcan Pharma Inc.

VARITECH MEDICAL DEVICES, INC.   815-624-6785
319 Dicop, South Beloit, IL 61080
FDA Number: 3004995568
Ownership: Private
Produces/Sells CE-marked Devices: N
  Light, Surgical, Instrument   Surgery

VARITRONICS, INC.   800-345-1244
620 Parkway, Broomall, PA 19008   610-356-3995
FDA Number: 2518414   *Fax:* 610-356-5222
E-mail: varimed@varitronics.com
Web site: www.varitronics.com
Annual Revenue: $1-$5 Million
Total Employees: 15   *Marketing Staff:* 1   *Sales Staff:* 6
Ownership: Private
Produces/Sells CE-marked Devices: N
Federal Procurement Eligibility: Small Business
Distribution: Manufacturer Direct, Manufacturer Through Manufacturer Reps
General Admin.: Wilfred Klein/President, Chief Executive Officer
Mktg./Adv.: Mr. Mark Minassian/Manager Tech. Sales
Production: Bill Kleinz/Manager Materials
  Cabinet, Instrument, AC-Powered, Ophthalmic   Ophthalmology
  Communication System, Powered   Physical Med

VARLEY & SONS INC., JAMES
  See Jvs Solutions

VARTA MICROBATTERY INC.   800-468-2782
1311 Mamaroneck Ave., Suite120,   914-345-0488
White Plains, NY 10605
FDA Number: n/a
Web site: www.us.varta-microbattery.com
Medical Products Sales Volume: $30,000,000
Ownership: VARTA BATTERIES, AG GERMANY
Quality System Registration Information: ISO9001
Produces/Sells CE-marked Devices: N
Distribution: OEM
  Battery   General
  Battery, Hearing-Aid   Ear/Nose/Throat
  Hearing-Aid   Ear/Nose/Throat

VARTEC SOLUTIONS, INC.   330-655-7930
7570 Foxdale Circle, Hudson, OH 44236
FDA Number: 3005627267
  Support, Breathing Tube   Anesthesiology

VARTEX INSTRUMENT CORP.   718-486-5050
311 Wallabout St., Brooklyn, NY 11206
FDA Number: 2433709
Ownership: Private
Produces/Sells CE-marked Devices: N
  Hemostat, Surgical   Dental And Oral
  Holder, Needle   Gastroenterology/Urology
  Scissors, Disposable   General

VASAMED   800-695-2737
7615 Golden Triangle Drive, Suite C,   952-947-9543
Eden Prairie, MN 55344
FDA Number: 2183943
E-mail: info@vasamed.com   *Fax:* 952-944-6022
Web site: www.vasamed.com
Medical Products Sales Volume: $1,400,000
Annual Revenue: $1-$5 Million
Year Founded: 1989
Total Employees: 33
Ownership: Optical Sensors Incorporated
Stock Symbol: OPTL
Traded On: OTC Bulletin
Produces/Sells CE-marked Devices: N
Federal Procurement Eligibility: Small Business
Distribution: Manufacturer Through Manufacturer Reps

VASAMED   800-695-2737 *(cont'd)*
General Admin.: Mr. John Borgos/General Manager
     Ms. Paulita LaPlante/President, Chief Executive Officer
Mktg./Adv.: Mr. Ramon Diaz/Manager Sales
     Mr. Victor Kimball/Vice President Business Development
  Cuff, Blood Pressure   Cardiovascular
  Flowmeter, Blood, Other   Cardiovascular
  Plethysmograph, Pressure (Body)   Anesthesiology

VASC-ALERT, INC.   765-775-2525
3000 Kent Ave, West Lafayette, IN 47906
FDA Number: 3003574195
E-mail: info@vasc-alert.com   *Fax:* 765-775-2527
Web site: www.vasc-alert.com
Medical Products Sales Volume: $2,000,000
Annual Revenue: $1-$5 Million
Year Founded: 2002
Total Employees: 6   *Marketing Staff:* 1   *Sales Staff:* 2
Ownership: Private
Produces/Sells CE-marked Devices: N
Federal Procurement Eligibility: Small Business
Distribution: Service Direct
  System, Hemodialysis, Remote Accessories   Gastroenterology/Urology

VASCULAR DESIGNS, INC   408-484-9010
4960 Almaden Expressway, San Jose, CA 95118
FDA Number: n/a
E-mail: dorloff@orloffwilliams.com
Web site: www.vasculardesigns.com
Ownership: Private
Produces/Sells CE-marked Devices: N
  Catheter, Infusion   Surgery

VASCULAR INSIGHTS LLC   203-376-3775
395 Boston Post Rd., Madison, CT 06443
FDA Number: 3005831739
Web site: http://www.vascularinsights.com
Ownership: Private
Produces/Sells CE-marked Devices: N
General Admin.: Mr. John Marano/President, Chief Executive Officer
Medical Admin.: Dr. Michael Tal/Chief Medical Officer
  Catheter, Continuous Flush   Cardiovascular

VASCULAR PERFORMANCE PRODUCTS, LLC.   888-364-7004
6945 Southbelt Dr., Se, Caledonia, MI 49316
FDA Number: 3005225457
  Shield, Protective, Personnel   Radiology

VASCULAR SOLUTIONS, INC.   888-240-6001
6464 Sycamore Court North,   763-656-4300
Minneapolis, MN 55369
FDA Number: 2134812   *Fax:* 763-656-4251
Web site: www.vascularsolutions.com
Ownership: Public
Stock Symbol: VASC
Traded On: NASDAQ
Produces/Sells CE-marked Devices: N
General Admin.: Howard Root/Chief Executive Officer
Mktg./Adv.: Mr. William Rutstein/Senior Vice President Sales
Production: Mr. Charmaine Sutton/Senior Vice President Operations
     Mr. Jon Hammond/Vice President Manufacturing
Finance: James Hennen/Chief Financial Officer, Senior Vice President Finance
  Bandage, Compression   General
  Catheter, Embolectomy (Fogarty Type)   Cardiovascular
  Device, Hemostasis, Vascular   Cardiovascular
  Set, Administration, Intravenous, Needle-Free   General
  Syringe, Piston   General

VASCULAR TECHNOLOGY INCORPORATED   800-550-0856
12 Murphy Drive, Nashua, NH 03062   603-594-9700
FDA Number: 1221072   *Fax:* 603-594-0092
E-mail: info@vti-online.com
Web site: www.vti-online.com
Annual Revenue: $1-$5 Million
Ownership: Private
Produces/Sells CE-marked Devices: Y
Federal Procurement Eligibility: Small Business, Minority Owned
Distribution: Manufacturer Direct, Manufacturer Through Distributor, OEM
Mktg./Adv.: David L. Regan/Vice President Sales
Production: Mr. Tim Dutton/Quality Control, Product Engineer
     Gary Douglas/Vice President Manufacturing
  Adapter, Anesthesia   Anesthesiology
  Alarm, Oxygen Depletion   Anesthesiology
  Analyzer, Gas, Oxygen, Continuous Monitor   Anesthesiology
  Analyzer, Gas, Oxygen, Gaseous Phase   Anesthesiology
  Detector, Blood Flow, Ultrasonic (Doppler)   Cardiovascular
  Monitor, Oxygen (Ventilatory) W/Wo Alarm   Anesthesiology

VASCULAR TECHNOLOGY INCORPORATED   800-550-0856
(cont'd)
  Sensor, Oxygen   Anesthesiology

VASCUTECH, INC.
  See Lemaitre Vascular, Inc.

VASOGEN INC.   905-569-2265
2505 Meadowvale Blvd, Mississauga, ONT L5L-4M1 Canada
FDA Number: n/a   *Fax: 905-569-9231*
E-mail: investor@vasogen.com
Web site: www.vasogen.com
Year Founded: 1992
Total Employees: 25
Ownership: Private
Produces/Sells CE-marked Devices: N
Distribution: Manufacturer Direct

VASOMEDICAL INC.   800-455-3327
                                       516-997-4600
180 Linden Ave., Westbury, NY 11590-3228
FDA Number: 2435300   *Fax: 516-997-2299*
E-mail: customerservice@vasomedical.com
Web site: http://www.vasomedical.com
Medical Products Sales Volume: $6,200,000
Annual Revenue: $5-$10 Million
Total Employees: 24
Ownership: Public
Stock Symbol: VASO
Traded On: OTC Bulletin
Quality System Registration Information: ISO9001
Produces/Sells CE-marked Devices: Y
Distribution: Manufacturer Direct, Manufacturer Through Manufacturer Reps
General Admin.: Dr. John Hui/Chief Technology Officer
                Dr. Jun Ma/President, Chief Executive Officer
Mktg./Adv.: Mr. Larry Liebman/Vice President Marketing & Sales
Finance: Mr. Tarachand Singh/Chief Financial Officer
  Cardiac Output Unit, Other   Cardiovascular
  Pump, Counterpulsating, External   Cardiovascular
  Recorder, Magnetic Tape/Disc   Cardiovascular

VASSOL, INC.   312-601-4431
833 West Jackson Blvd., 8th Floor, Chicago, IL 60607
FDA Number: 3003494057
  Image Processing System   Radiology

VAT-TECH, INC.   705-687-8717
684 Muskoka Rd N, Gravenhurst P1P 1E7 Canada
FDA Number: 8022271
  Equipment, Traction, Powered   Physical Med

VAX-D MEDICAL TECHNOLOGIES LLC   813-343-5000
310 Mears Blvd, Oldsmar, FL 34677
FDA Number: 1058809   *Fax: 813-343-5005*
E-mail: info@vaxd.com
Web site: www.vaxd.com
Year Founded: 1989
Total Employees: 12   *Marketing Staff: 3*   *Sales Staff: 3*
Ownership: Private
Quality System Registration Information: ISO9001
Produces/Sells CE-marked Devices: Y
Federal Procurement Eligibility: Small Business
Distribution: Manufacturer Through Distributor, OEM
  Equipment, Traction, Powered   Physical Med

VEC TECHNOLOGIES, INC.   518-257-2010
1 University Pl., Rensselaer, NY 12144-3456
FDA Number: n/a   *Fax: 518-257-2012*
E-mail: info@vectechnologies.com
Web site: www.vectechnologies.com
Annual Revenue: $0-$1 Million
Total Employees: 2
Ownership: Private
Produces/Sells CE-marked Devices: N
Federal Procurement Eligibility: Small Business, Female Owned
Distribution: Manufacturer Direct
General Admin.: Jolene Clarke/President, Chief Executive Officer
Research: Peter Del Vecchio/Chief Scientist
  Culture Media, Synthetic Cell And Tissue   Pathology

VECO, S.A. DE C.V.   55-688-3566
Pirineos No. 263, Col. General Anaya,
Mexico D.F., BENIT 03100 Mexico
FDA Number: n/a   *Fax: 55-688-0252*
E-mail: vecosacv@prodigy.net.mx
Total Employees: 150   *Marketing Staff: 4*   *Sales Staff: 2*
Ownership: DE VECCHI INGENIEROS S.A DE C.V.
Quality System Registration Information: ISO9001
Produces/Sells CE-marked Devices: N
Federal Procurement Eligibility: Small Business

VECO, S.A. DE C.V.   55-688-3566 *(cont'd)*
Distribution: Manufacturer Direct, Service Direct, Exporter

VECTOR ELECTRONICS & TECHNOLOGY, INC.   800-423-5659
11115 Vanowen St., North Hollywood, CA 91605   **818-985-8208**
FDA Number: 9201118   *Fax: 818-985-7708*
E-mail: inquire@vectorelect.com
Web site: www.vectorelect.com
Annual Revenue: $1-$5 Million
Year Founded: 1959
Total Employees: 50   *Sales Staff: 2*
Ownership: Private
Produces/Sells CE-marked Devices: N
Federal Procurement Eligibility: Small Business, Minority Owned
Distribution: Manufacturer Direct, Manufacturer Through Distributor
General Admin.: Rick Bajaria/Chief Executive Officer
Production: Mr. Jerry Rodriguez/Vice President Operations
  Cabinet, Instrument   General

VECTOR FIRSTAID, INC.   800-999-4423
316 N. Corona Avenue, Ontario, CA 91764   **909-937-6470**
FDA Number: n/a   *Fax: 909-937-6460*
E-mail: Sales@vectorfirstaid.com
Web site: www.vectorfirstaid.com
Medical Products Sales Volume: $1,200,000
Annual Revenue: $1-$5 Million
Total Employees: 12   *Marketing Staff: 1*   *Sales Staff: 7*
Ownership: Public
Produces/Sells CE-marked Devices: N
Federal Procurement Eligibility: Small Business, Female Owned
Distribution: Manufacturer Direct, Manufacturer Through Distributor, Manufacturer Through Manufacturer Reps
General Admin.: Lori Martin/Chief Executive Officer
Production: Gary Martin/Vice President Operations
  Bandage, Adhesive   Surgery
  Device, Assist, CPR   Anesthesiology
  Fountain, Eye Wash   Chemistry
  Kit, Burn   General
Medical Product Subsidiaries (Listed Separately)
Cepp Corp.

VECTOR LABORATORIES, INC.   800-227-6666
30 Ingold Road, Burlingame, CA 94010   **650-697-3600**
FDA Number: n/a   *Fax: 650-697-0339*
E-mail: vector@vectorlabs.com
Web site: www.vectorlabs.com
Medical Products Sales Volume: $6,900,000
Year Founded: 1975
Total Employees: 50
Ownership: Private
Produces/Sells CE-marked Devices: N
Federal Procurement Eligibility: Small Business
Distribution: Manufacturer Direct, Manufacturer Through Distributor, OEM
General Admin.: James Whitehead/President
Mktg./Adv.: Judy Decker/Director Marketing
IS: Craig Pow/Manager Tech. Services
  Antibody, Other   General
  Antigen, Antiserum, Control, IGG   Immunology
  Antigen, Antiserum, Control, IGG, FITC   Immunology
  Antigen, Antiserum, Control, IGG, Peroxidase   Immunology
  Antigen, Antiserum, Control, IGM   Immunology
  Antigen, Antiserum, Control, IGM (Mu Chain Specific)   Immunology
  Antigen, Antiserum, Control, Other   Immunology
  Lectins/Protectins   Hematology
  Reagent, Other   General
  Serum, Animal   Pathology
  Serum, Biological, General   Toxicology

VECTOR RESEARCH & DEVELOPMENT   877-883-7455
6824 19th St. #230, University Place, WA 98466   **253-564-5084**
FDA Number: 3003934980
Web site: www.vectorusa.net
Ownership: Private
Produces/Sells CE-marked Devices: N
  Handpiece, Air-Powered, Dental   Dental And Oral

VECTOR SCIENTIFIC, INC.
  See Zoetek Medical Sales & Service, Inc.

VECTOR VISION   800-526-7703
1850 Livingston Rd, Suite E,   **937-548-7970**
Greenville, OH 45331
FDA Number: 1527853   *Fax: 937-548-2773*
Web site: www.vectorvision.com
Annual Revenue: $0-$1 Million
Ownership: Private
Produces/Sells CE-marked Devices: Y
Federal Procurement Eligibility: Small Business

VECTOR VISION
800-526-7703 *(cont'd)*
Distribution: Manufacturer Direct, Manufacturer Through Manufacturer Reps
General Admin.: David W. Evans/President
Production: Brian E. Wilson/Vice President Operations
Analyzer, Visual Function — Ophthalmology
Chart, Visual Acuity — Ophthalmology

VECTRON INTERNATIONAL
717-486-6060
100 Watts St., Mount Holly Springs, PA 17065
FDA Number: n/a
E-mail: ssles@ofc.com
Fax: 717-486-5920
Web site: www.ofc.com
Annual Revenue: $0-$1 Million
Ownership: DOVER CORPORATION
Quality System Registration Information: ISO9001
Produces/Sells CE-marked Devices: N
Distribution: Manufacturer Direct, Manufacturer Through Manufacturer Reps
Component, Electronic — General
Service, Parts, Repair — General

VEE GEE SCIENTIFIC, INC.
800-423-8842
425-823-4518
13600 N.E. 126th, Suite A,
Kirkland, WA 98034
FDA Number: n/a
Fax: 425-820-9826
E-mail: sales@veegee.net
Web site: www.veegee.com
Medical Products Sales Volume: $1,600,000
Year Founded: 1981
Total Employees: 12 — *Marketing Staff:* 3 — *Sales Staff:* 5
Ownership: Private
Quality System Registration Information: ISO9001
Produces/Sells CE-marked Devices: Y
Federal Procurement Eligibility: Small Business
Distribution: Manufacturer Through Distributor, Exclusive Distributor
General Admin.: Guy McFarland/Chief Executive Officer
Bonnie Brice/President
Mktg./Adv.: Paul Wendling/Vice President Business Development
Paul Wendling/Vice President Marketing & Sales
Component, Ceramic — General
Microscope — Hematology
Refractometer — Chemistry

VEGAMED, INC.
787-807-0392
Edificio Multifabril #5, Ave. Las Flores #39,
Vega Baja, PR 00693
FDA Number: 2640118
Calibrator, Hemoglobin And Hematocrit Measurement — Hematology
Clearing Agent — Pathology
Diluent, Blood Cell — Hematology
Drink, Glucose Tolerance — Chemistry
Fluid, Red Cell Lysing — Hematology
Hematology Quality Control Mixture — Hematology
Reagent, General Purpose — Pathology

VELCO TOOL AND DIE CO.
949-855-6638
20551 Pascal Way, Lake Forest, CA 92692
FDA Number: 2029315
E-mail: velco@packbell.net
Fax: 949-855-0458
Web site: http://velco.net/
Medical Products Sales Volume: $600,000
Annual Revenue: $1-$5 Million
Year Founded: 1984
Total Employees: 10
Ownership: Private
Quality System Registration Information: ISO9001
Produces/Sells CE-marked Devices: N
Federal Procurement Eligibility: Small Business, Minority Owned
Distribution: Manufacturer Through Distributor
Instrument, Manual, General Surgical — Surgery

VELCRO CANADA INC.
800-683-5276
905-791-1630
114 East Dr., Brampton, ONT L6T-1C1 Canada
FDA Number: n/a
Fax: 905-791-5329
E-mail: canada@velcro.com
Web site: www.velcro.com
Year Founded: 1964
Total Employees: 100
Ownership: Private
Produces/Sells CE-marked Devices: N
Distribution: Manufacturer Direct, Exclusive Distributor

VELCRO USA, INC.
603-669-4880
406 Brown Ave., Manchester, NH 03101
FDA Number: 1222748
Ownership: Private
Produces/Sells CE-marked Devices: N
Bag, Ice — General

VELCRO USA, INC.
603-669-4880 *(cont'd)*
Pack, Hot Or Cold, Disposable — Physical Med

VELOPEX INTERNATIONAL.
888-835-6739
407-957-3900
105 East 17th St., Saint Cloud, FL 34769
FDA Number: n/a
E-mail: velopex@earthlink.net
Fax: 407-957-3927
Web site: www.velopexusa.com
Medical Products Sales Volume: $300,000
Annual Revenue: $1-$5 Million
Year Founded: 1996
Total Employees: 7 — *Marketing Staff:* 2 — *Sales Staff:* 22
Ownership: MEDIVANCE INSRUMENTS
Quality System Registration Information: ISO9002
Produces/Sells CE-marked Devices: N
Federal Procurement Eligibility: Small Business
Distribution: Manufacturer Through Distributor
General Admin.: Sidney Grant/President
Mktg./Adv.: Tony Urella/Manager National Sales
Image Processing System — Radiology

VELTEK ASSOCIATES, INC.
888-478-3745
610-644-8335
15 Lee Boulevard, Malvern, PA 19355
FDA Number: n/a
E-mail: sales@sterile.com
Fax: 610-644-8336
Web site: www.sterile.com
Medical Products Sales Volume: $6,100,000
Year Founded: 1981
Total Employees: 50 — *Marketing Staff:* 2 — *Sales Staff:* 10
Ownership: Private
Produces/Sells CE-marked Devices: Y
Federal Procurement Eligibility: Small Business
Distribution: Manufacturer Direct, Manufacturer Through Distributor, Manufacturer Through Manufacturer Reps, Importer, Exporter
General Admin.: Art Vellutato/President
IS: Art Vellutato/Vice President Tech. Services
Solvent — Chemistry
Swabs, Alcohol — General

VENES TECHNOLOGY CORP.
800-777-4974
972-988-1218
6701 Democracy Blvd. Ste # 300.,
Bethesda, MD 20817
FDA Number: n/a
E-mail: info@venusinc.com
Fax: 972-602-0185
Web site: www.venusinc.com
Total Employees: 3 — *Marketing Staff:* 1 — *Sales Staff:* 1
Ownership: Venes Technology Corp.
Produces/Sells CE-marked Devices: N
Federal Procurement Eligibility: Small Business
Distribution: Manufacturer Direct
General Admin.: Simon Yung/Chief Executive Officer
Mktg./Adv.: Ken Meng/Manager Advertising
Ken Meng/Vice President Marketing & Sales
Unit, Examination, Lens, Contact — Ophthalmology
Medical Product Subsidiaries (Listed Separately)
Venes Technology Corp.

VENETEC INTERNATIONAL., INC.
888-685-0565
858-509-2400
12555 High Bluff Drive,, Suite 100,
San Diego, CA 92130
FDA Number: 1722045
E-mail: cservice@venetec.com
Fax: 858-350-7899
Web site: www.venetec.com
Medical Products Sales Volume: $6,800,000
Total Employees: 72
Ownership: C. R. Bard, Inc.
Produces/Sells CE-marked Devices: N
Federal Procurement Eligibility: Small Business
Holder, Intravascular Catheter — General
Kit, Administration, Intravenous — General
Transfer Unit, IV Fluid — General

VENOSAN NORTH AMERICA, INC.
800-432-5347
336-629-7181
300 Industrial Park Avenue, PO Box 1067,
Asheboro, NC 27204
FDA Number: 8030999
E-mail: venosan@venosanonline.com
Fax: 800-849-0946
Web site: www.venosanusa.com
Medical Products Sales Volume: $2,000,000
Total Employees: 9 — *Marketing Staff:* 1 — *Sales Staff:* 30
Ownership: Salzmann Medico
Quality System Registration Information: ISO9001
Produces/Sells CE-marked Devices: Y
Federal Procurement Eligibility: Small Business, VA Contract
Distribution: Exclusive Distributor
General Admin.: Phyllis M. Turner/Director Admin.
Robert C. Spalding/President, Chief Executive Officer

VENOSAN NORTH AMERICA, INC.   800-432-5347 (cont'd)
Mktg./Adv.: Steve Cardoza/Vice President Marketing & Sales
Production: Myra Smith/Manager Customer Services
    Dennis L. Shaw/Manager Materials
Finance: Phyllis M. Turner/Controller

Hook, Surgical, General & Plastic Surgery	Surgery
Instrument, Microsurgical	Cns/Neurology
Stocking, Elastic	General
Stocking, Elastic, Physical Medicine	Physical Med
Stripper, Vein, Reusable	Surgery

VENOSCOPE, LLC
See Venoscope, LLC

VENOSCOPE, LLC   800-284-7655
1018 Harding Street, Suite 104,   337-234-8993
Lafayette, LA 70503
FDA Number: n/a   *Fax:* 337-268-4080
E-mail: info@venoscope.com
Web site: www.venoscope.com
Medical Products Sales Volume: $300,000
Annual Revenue: $0-$1 Million
Year Founded: 1989
Total Employees: 3   *Marketing Staff:* 1   *Sales Staff:* 2
Ownership: Private
Produces/Sells CE-marked Devices: Y
Federal Procurement Eligibility: Small Business, VA Contract
Distribution: Manufacturer Direct, Manufacturer Through Distributor, Manufacturer Through Manufacturer Reps, OEM, Exporter
General Admin.: Frank Creaghan/Chief Executive Officer
Mktg./Adv.: Hille Domingue/Director Marketing

Transilluminator, Battery-Powered	Ophthalmology

VENTANA MEDICAL SYSTEMS, INC.   800-227-2155
1910 Innovation Park Dr., Tucson, AZ 85755   520-887-2155
FDA Number: 2028492   *Fax:* 520-229-6855
E-mail: info@ventanamed.com
Web site: www.ventanamed.com
Year Founded: 1991
Total Employees: 952
Ownership: Private
Produces/Sells CE-marked Devices: N
General Admin.: Libo Yang/Chief Executive Officer
    Ms. Mara Aspinall/President
Mktg./Adv.: Mr. Weidong Shan/Vice President Marketing & Sales
Production: Mr. Zhiming Wang/Vice President Manufacturing
Finance: Dr. Chenming Yu/Chief Financial Officer
    Ms. Junwen Wang/Chief Financial Officer

Antigen, Antiserum, Control, Alpha-1-Antitrypsin	Immunology
Antigen, Antiserum, Control, IGM, Peroxidase	Immunology
Antigen, Antiserum, Control, Lambda	Immunology
Buffer, pH	Hematology
Cultured Animal And Human Cells	Pathology
Diastase	Pathology
Fixative, Acid Containing	Pathology
Immunohistochemistry Antibody Assay, C-kit	Hematology
Immunohistochemistry Assay, Antibody, Estrogen Receptor	Pathology
Immunohistochemistry Assay, Antibody, Progesterone Receptor	Pathology
Immunohistochemistry Reagents And Kits	Pathology
Kappa, Peroxidase, Antigen, Antiserum, Control	Immunology
Paraffin, All Formulations	Pathology
Reagent, General Purpose	Pathology
Reagents, Specific, Analyte	Hematology
Resorcin Fuchsin	Pathology
Solution, Silver Carbonate	Pathology
Stain, Alcian Blue	Pathology
Stain, Ammoniacal Silver Hydroxide Silver Nitrate	Pathology
Stain, Carbol Fuchsin	Pathology
Stain, Congo Red	Pathology
Stain, Dye Solution	Pathology
Stain, Giemsa	Pathology
Stain, Hematoxylin	Pathology
Stain, Hematoxylin, Mayer's	Pathology
Stain, Iron	Pathology
Stain, Light Green	Pathology
Stain, Mallory's Trichrome	Pathology
Stain, Methenamine Silver	Pathology
Stain, Methyl Green	Pathology
Stain, Mucicarmine	Pathology
Stain, Nuclear Fast Red	Pathology
Stain, Reagent, Schiff	Pathology
Stainer, Slide, Automated	Pathology
Stainer, Tissue, Automated	Pathology
System, Test, Her-2/neu, Ihc	Pathology
Trypsin	Pathology

VENTION MEDICAL   908-561-0717
6 Century Road, South Plainfield, NJ 07080
FDA Number: n/a   *Fax:* 908-561-3811
E-mail: info@ventionmedical.com

VENTION MEDICAL   908-561-0717 (cont'd)
Web site: http://www.ventionmedical.com/
Ownership: Private
Produces/Sells CE-marked Devices: N
Medical Product Subsidiaries (Listed Separately)
Atek Medical

VENTLAB CORP.   336-753-5000
155 Boyce Drive, Mocksville, NC 27028
FDA Number: 2246980

Attachment, Breathing, Positive End Expiratory Pressure	Anesthesiology
Bottle, Collection, Breathing System (Uncalibrated)	Anesthesiology
Circuit, Breathing (W Connector, Adapter, Y Piece)	Anesthesiology
Condenser, Heat And Moisture (Artificial Nose)	Anesthesiology
Filter, Bacterial, Breathing Circuit	Anesthesiology
Fixation Device, Tracheal Tube	Anesthesiology
Mask, Gas, Anesthesia	Anesthesiology
Mask, Oxygen, Aerosol Administration	Anesthesiology
Nebulizer, Direct Patient Interface	Anesthesiology
Pressure Infusor, IV Container	General
Resuscitator, Manual, Non Self-inflating	Anesthesiology
Tubing, Flexible, Medical Gas, Low-Pressure	Anesthesiology
Ventilator, Emergency, Manual (Resuscitator)	Anesthesiology
Ventilator, Non-Continuous (Respirator)	Anesthesiology

VENTLAB CORPORATION   800-593-4654
155 Boyce Dr., Mocksville, NC 27028   336-753-5000
FDA Number: 2246980   *Fax:* 336-75-5002
E-mail: CSR@Ventlab.com
Web site: www.ventlab.com
Annual Revenue: $10-$25 Million
Year Founded: 1993
Total Employees: 87
Ownership: Private
Quality System Registration Information: ISO9001
Produces/Sells CE-marked Devices: N
Federal Procurement Eligibility: Small Business, Minority Owned
Distribution: Manufacturer Through Distributor, OEM, Importer, Exporter
General Admin.: Bob Martin/President

Mask, Face	General
Pacemaker, Respiratory	Surgery
Resuscitator, Pulmonary, Manual (Demand Valve)	General
System, Delivery, Drug, Unit-Dose	General

VENTRIPOINT DIAGNOSTICS LTD.   206-283-0221
100 West Harrison St., Suite 410, Seattle, WA 98119
FDA Number: n/a   *Fax:* 206-283-2309
E-mail: info@ventripoint.com
Web site: www.ventripoint.com
Year Founded: 2005
Ownership: Public
Stock Symbol: VPT
Produces/Sells CE-marked Devices: N
General Admin.: Joseph Ashley/Chief Executive Officer
Mktg./Adv.: Mark Levine/Vice President Marketing & Sales
Research: Florence Sheehan/Chief Scientist
    Mary-Pierre Waiss/Vice President Clinical Development
    Scott Ashley/Vice President Research & Development
Finance: Ed Garth/Vice President Finance

VENTURA ENTERPRISES   317-745-2989
35 Lawton Avenue, Danville, IN 46122
FDA Number: 9320199   *Fax:* 317-745-3179
E-mail: mobility@venturaenterprises.com
Web site: www.venturaenterprises.com
Annual Revenue: $0-$1 Million
Total Employees: 3
Ownership: Private
Federal Procurement Eligibility: Female Owned
Distribution: Manufacturer Through Distributor
General Admin.: Linda Plunkett/President
Production: Amy Fowler/Manager Operations

Attachment, Bag (Crutch, Walker, Wheelchair)	Physical Med
Cushion, Wheelchair (Pad)	Physical Med

VENTURA RESEARCH & REHAB.
See Ventura Enterprises

VENTURI, INC.   231-929-7732
2299 Traversefield Dr., Traverse City, MI 49686
FDA Number: 1836688

Toothbrush, Manual	Dental And Oral

VENTUS MEDICAL, INC.   650-632-4199
1301 Shoreway Rd., Suite 425, Belmont, CA 94002
FDA Number: 3007038487   *Fax:* 650-632-4198
E-mail: info@ventusmedical.com
Web site: http://www.ventusmedical.com
Ownership: Private
Produces/Sells CE-marked Devices: N

VENTUS MEDICAL, INC.   650-632-4199 *(cont'd)*
General Admin.: Ms. Sandra Gardiner/Chief Financial Officer, Executive Vice President
     Mr. Peter Wyles/President, Chief Executive Officer
Medical Admin.: Dr. Philip Westbrook/Chief Medical Officer
     Ms. Connie Rey/Director Clinical Affairs
Mktg./Adv.: Mr. Glenn Johnson/Vice President Marketing & Sales
Production: Mr. Michael Lopez/Vice President Operations

Dilator, Nasal	Ear/Nose/Throat
Expiratory Resistance Valve, Intranasal, For Obstructive Sleep Apnea	Dental And Oral
Recorder, Ventilatory Effort	Anesthesiology

VERACYTE INC.   650-243-6300
7000 Shoreline Ct., Suite 250, South San Francisco, CA 94080
FDA Number: 3007808978
Fax: 650-243-6301
E-mail: info@veracyte.com
Web site: http://www.veracyte.com
Ownership: Private
Produces/Sells CE-marked Devices: N
General Admin.: Ms. Bonnie Anderson/Chief Executive Officer
     Dr. Giulia Kennedy/Chief Scientific Officer, Vice President
Medical Admin.: Dr. Richard Lanman/Chief Medical Officer
Mktg./Adv.: Mr. Chris Hall/Commercial Director
Research: Dr. William Seltzer/Vice President Lab. Operations
Finance: Ms. Anne Sissel/Vice President Finance

Container, Specimen Mailer And Storage	Pathology
Container, Specimen Mailer And Storage, Temperature Control	Pathology

VERALIGHT INC   (505) 272-7023
800 Bradbury SE, Suite 217, Albuquerque, NM 87106
FDA Number: n/a
Fax: (505) 272-7112
E-mail: info@VeraLight.com
Web site: www.veralight.com
Year Founded: 2004
Ownership: Private
Produces/Sells CE-marked Devices: N
General Admin.: Mr. David VanAvermaete/Chief Executive Officer
     Dr. M. Ries Robinson/Chief Operating Officer
     Mr. Marwood Ediger/Chief Technology Officer
Production: Mr. Scot Dolin/Vice President Engineering & Operations
IS: Mr. John Maynard/Vice President Technology

VERAN MEDICAL TECHNOLOGIES, INC.   314-659-8500
1908 Innerbelt Business Center Dr., St. Louis, MO 63114
FDA Number: 3007222345
E-mail: info@veranmedical.com
Web site: www.veranmedical.com
Ownership: Private
Produces/Sells CE-marked Devices: N
Distribution: Manufacturer Direct
General Admin.: Mr. Troy Holsing/Chief Technology Officer
     Mr. Jerome Edwards/President, Chief Executive Officer
Mktg./Adv.: Mr. Les Carlson/Director Sales
Production: Mr. Mark Hunter/Senior Vice President Operations

X-ray, Tomography, Computed, Dental	Radiology

VERATHON INC.   800-331-2313
20001 North Creek Parkway, Bothell, WA 98011   425-867-1348
FDA Number: 3022472
Fax: 425-883-2896
E-mail: sales@verathon.com
Web site: http://verathon.com
Medical Products Sales Volume: $61,520,000
Annual Revenue: $50-$100 Million
Year Founded: 1984
Total Employees: 100   Marketing Staff: 10   Sales Staff: 30
Ownership: Private
Quality System Registration Information: ISO9000
Produces/Sells CE-marked Devices: Y
Federal Procurement Eligibility: Small Business, GSA Contract, VA Contract
Distribution: Manufacturer Direct, Service Direct
General Admin.: Maureen Graham/Chief Financial Officer, Vice President
     Muriel Doyle/Manager Human Resources
     Gerald Mc Morrow/President, Chief Executive Officer
     Russ Garrison/Vice President, General Manager
Mktg./Adv.: Karen Fournier/Director Marketing & Sales
     Mike Rothmeyer/Manager International Sales
Production: Russ Garrison/Director Quality Assurance
     Chuck Errico/Manager Materials

Flowmeter, Blood, Ultrasonic	Gastroenterology/Urology
Instrument, Volume, Bladder	Gastroenterology/Urology
Scanner, Ultrasonic (Pulsed Echo)	Radiology
Scanner, Ultrasonic, Other	Radiology
Scanner, Ultrasonic, Pediatric	Radiology
Transducer, Ultrasonic, Diagnostic	Radiology

VEREBURN SUPPLY LTD.   800-263-1055
2235 27th Ave. NE,   403-250-7944
Calgary, ALB T2E-7 Canada
FDA Number: n/a
Fax: 403-250-2947
E-mail: corporate@vereburn.com
Year Founded: 1979
Total Employees: 25
Ownership: Private
Produces/Sells CE-marked Devices: N
Distribution: Exclusive Distributor

VERG, INC.   800-563-7676
55 Henlow Bay, #3,   204-949-7676
Winnipeg, MANIT R3G-1 Canada
FDA Number: 9680095
Fax: 204-949-7650
E-mail: fsa@verg.com
Web site: www.verg.com
Year Founded: 1989
Total Employees: 14
Ownership: Private
Quality System Registration Information: ISO9003
Produces/Sells CE-marked Devices: Y
Federal Procurement Eligibility: Small Business
Distribution: Manufacturer Direct, Manufacturer Through Distributor, Manufacturer Through Manufacturer Reps, OEM

VERGASON TECHNOLOGY, INC.   607-589-4429
166 State Route 224, Van Etten, NY 14889
FDA Number: n/a
Fax: 607-589-6955
E-mail: sales@vergason.com
Web site: www.vergason.com
Annual Revenue: $10-$25 Million
Year Founded: 1986
Total Employees: 500
Ownership: Private
Quality System Registration Information: ISO9001
Produces/Sells CE-marked Devices: Y
Federal Procurement Eligibility: Small Business
Distribution: Manufacturer Direct, Service Direct
Mktg./Adv.: Bruce Deiseroth/Manager Market Development
     Julie Wellington/Manager Market Development
     Ed Ward/Sales Associate

Accessories, Decorative	General
Equipment, Device Coating, Protective	General
Service, Device Coating, Protective	General

VERIAD   800-423-4643
650 Columbia Street, Brea, CA 92821
FDA Number: n/a
Web site: www.unitedadlabel.com
Annual Revenue: $25-$50 Million
Year Founded: 1958
Ownership: Public
Quality System Registration Information: ISO9001
Produces/Sells CE-marked Devices: N
Distribution: Manufacturer Direct, Manufacturer Through Manufacturer Reps

Bag, Plastic	General
Label, Device	General
Office Product	General
Solvent, Adhesive Tape	Surgery
Sterilization Process Indicator, Chemical	General

VERICHEM LABORATORIES, INC.   401-461-0180
90 Narragansett Ave., Providence, RI 02907
FDA Number: 1221645

Calibrator, Drug Mixture	Toxicology
Calibrator, Ethyl Alcohol	Toxicology
Calibrator, Primary, Clinical Chemistry	Chemistry
Calibrator, Secondary, Clinical Chemistry	Chemistry
Control, Enzyme (Assayed And Unassayed)	Chemistry

VERIDEX, LLC   877-837-4339
1001 US Highway Route 202 N., Raritan, NJ 08869   585-453-3240
FDA Number: 3004619490
Fax: 585-453-3344
E-mail: VeridexMedicalAffairs@vrxus.jnj.com
Web site: www.immunicon.com
Ownership: Private
Produces/Sells CE-marked Devices: N

Control Material, Blood Circulating Epithelial Cancer Cell	Hematology
System, Immunomagnetic, Circulating Cancer Cell, Enumeration	Immunology

VERIDEX, LLC   (877-837-4339)
1001 US Highway Route 202 North,   1-585-453-3240
Raritan, NJ 08869
FDA Number: 3004619490
Fax: 1-585-453-3344
E-mail: VeridexMedicalAffairs@vrxus.jnj.com
Web site: www.veridex.com/
Ownership: Private

VERIDEX, LLC   (877-837-4339) *(cont'd)*
Produces/Sells CE-marked Devices: N

VERIDIEN CORP.   800-345-5444
7600 Bryan Dairy Road, Suite F,   727-576-1600
Largo, FL 33777
FDA Number: n/a   *Fax:* 727-576-1611
E-mail: info@veridien.com
Web site: www.vrde.com
Medical Products Sales Volume: $1,900,000
Annual Revenue: $0-$1 Million
Year Founded: 1991
Total Employees: 15   *Marketing Staff:* 4   *Sales Staff:* 4
Ownership: Public
Stock Symbol: VRDE
Traded On: OTC Bulletin
Federal Procurement Eligibility: Small Business, VA Contract
Distribution: Manufacturer Through Distributor, Manufacturer Through Manufacturer Reps
General Admin.: Sheldon C. Fenton/President, Chief Executive Officer
Mktg./Adv.: Ken Chester/Director Marketing
     Paul L. Simmons/Director Product Development
     Terry Seagers/Manager National Sales
     Kathy Grazyk/Manager Sales Training
Production: Dr. Jerry Kern/Director Quality Assurance
     Albine L. Otte/Manager Regulatory Affairs
Finance: Cheryl Ballou/Director Finance

Cleaner, Medical Device	General
Solution, Antimicrobial	Microbiology
Towel/Towelette, Paper	General

VERISTA IMAGING INC.   712-353-6225
201 4th Street, Castana, IA 51010
FDA Number: 3006407518

Scanner, Emission Computed Tomography	Radiology

VERITECH CORPORATION   413-525-3368
168 Denslow Road, East Longmeadow, MA 01028-2812
FDA Number: n/a   *Fax:* 413-525-7449
E-mail: info@veritechmedia.com
Web site: www.veritechmedia.com
Medical Products Sales Volume: $2,200,000
Annual Revenue: $5-$10 Million
Year Founded: 1976
Total Employees: 22   *Marketing Staff:* 7   *Sales Staff:* 10
Ownership: Private
Quality System Registration Information: ISO9002
Produces/Sells CE-marked Devices: N
Federal Procurement Eligibility: Small Business
Distribution: Manufacturer Direct
General Admin.: Michael Feldman/Chief Operating Officer, Chief Financial Officer
     Steven Graziano/President, Chief Executive Officer
Mktg./Adv.: Donald H. Wesson/Vice President Marketing & Sales
Production: Jeremy Cole/Vice President Production

Computer, Patient Data Management	General
Material, Training, Audiovisual	General
Training Aid	Orthopedics

VERMED, INC.   802-463-9976
9 Lovell Dr., Bellows Falls, VT 05101
FDA Number: 1219288

Electrode, Electrocardiograph	Cardiovascular

VERMILLION, INC.   512-519-0400
12117 Bee Caves Rd., Building III, Suite 100, Austin, TX 78738
FDA Number: 3004869564   *Fax:* 512-439-6980
E-mail: info@vermillion.com
Web site: www.vermillion.com
Year Founded: 1993
Total Employees: 19   *Sales Staff:* 5
Ownership: Public
Stock Symbol: VRML
Traded On: NASDAQ
Produces/Sells CE-marked Devices: N
General Admin.: Eric Fung/Chief Scientific Officer, Vice President
     Gail Page/President, Chief Executive Officer
Mktg./Adv.: Simon Shorter/Vice President Corporate Development
Research: Lee Lomas/Senior Director Research & Development

VERMONT COMPOSITES, INC.   802-442-9964
Subsidiary of APC, 25 Performance Drive,
Bennington, VT 05201
FDA Number: n/a   *Fax:* 802-447-3642
E-mail: sales@vtcomposites.com
Web site: www.vtcomposites.com
Annual Revenue: $10-$25 Million
Total Employees: 500   *Marketing Staff:* 6   *Sales Staff:* 6
Ownership: Private

VERMONT COMPOSITES, INC.   802-442-9964 *(cont'd)*
Quality System Registration Information: ISO9001
Produces/Sells CE-marked Devices: N
Federal Procurement Eligibility: Small Business, VA Contract
Distribution: OEM, Exporter
General Admin.: Daniel J. Maneely/President
     Garth Kenyon/Vice President

Cradle, Patient, Radiographic	Radiology
Holder, Head, Radiographic	Radiology
Stretcher, Radiographic	Radiology
Support, Patient Position, Radiographic	Radiology
Table, Nuclear Medicine	Radiology
Table, Radiographic, Non-Tilting, Powered	Radiology
Table, Radiographic, Stationary Top	Radiology
Table, Radiographic, Tilting	Radiology
Table, Urological, Radiographic	Gastroenterology/Urology

VERMONT MEDICAL, INC.   800-245-4025
9 Lovell Drive, Bellows Falls, VT 05101-0556   802-463-9976
FDA Number: 1219288   *Fax:* 802-463-9228
E-mail: info@vermed.com
Web site: www.vermed.com
Annual Revenue: $10-$25 Million
Total Employees: 95   *Marketing Staff:* 2   *Sales Staff:* 8
Ownership: Private
Quality System Registration Information: ISO9000
Produces/Sells CE-marked Devices: N
Federal Procurement Eligibility: Small Business
Distribution: Manufacturer Direct, Manufacturer Through Distributor, Manufacturer Through Manufacturer Reps, OEM, Exporter
General Admin.: Richard Kalich/Chief Operating Officer
     Hurley J. Blakeney/President
Mktg./Adv.: Mark Billeci/Director Marketing & Sales
     Ken Booth/Director Product Development
     Casey Schmackenberg/Manager Advertising
Production: Ken Booth/Director Quality Assurance
     Amy-Beth Carter/Manager Customer Services
     Henry Gauthier/Manager Manufacturing & Engineering
     Susan Normandin/Manager Materials
     Ken Booth/Manager Regulatory Affairs

Electrode, Cutaneous	Cns/Neurology
Electrode, Electrocardiograph	Cardiovascular
Electrode, Gel	Cardiovascular
Electrode, Other	General
Stimulator, Nerve, AC-Powered	Anesthesiology
Warmer, Radiant, Infant	General

VERNACARE   800-268-2422
200 Trowers Rd., Unit 3,   905-851-1300
Woodbridge, ONT L4L-5 Canada
FDA Number: n/a   *Fax:* 905-851-7600
E-mail: marketing@varnacare.com
Web site: www.vernacare.com
Year Founded: 1990
Total Employees: 10
Ownership: Private
Produces/Sells CE-marked Devices: N
Distribution: Manufacturer Direct, Exclusive Distributor, Exporter

VERNAY LABORATORIES, INC.   800-666-5227
120 E. South College Street,   937-767-7261
Yellow Springs, OH 45387
FDA Number: n/a   *Fax:* 937-767-7913
E-mail: sales@vernay.com
Web site: www.vernay.com
Medical Products Sales Volume: $44,800,000
Annual Revenue: $50-$100 Million
Year Founded: 1946
Total Employees: 331   *Marketing Staff:* 1   *Sales Staff:* 10
Ownership: Private
Quality System Registration Information: ISO9001
Produces/Sells CE-marked Devices: N
Distribution: Manufacturer Direct, OEM
General Admin.: Mr. Tom Allen/Chief Executive Officer
Mktg./Adv.: Ms. Debbie Laveck/Coord. National Sales
     Ms. Robin Thompson/Coord. National Sales
     Mr. David Juarez/Director National Sales
     Mr. Douglas Stangle/Manager Medical Market
     Mr. Carl Diem/Vice President Worldwide sales and service
Production: Mr. Joe Herold/Director Engineering
     Mr. John Madewell/Director Manufacturing
     Mr. David Engelbert/Manager Quality Systems
     Mr. Gregory Gearhart/Vice President Operations, General Manager
     Mr. John Martin/Vice President Technology & Product Development
Research: Dr. Steve Glancy/Chief Chemist
Finance: Mr. Frank Welling/Chief Financial Officer

Accessories, Catheter	Surgery

VERNAY LABORATORIES, INC.   800-666-5227 *(cont'd)*

Check Valve, Retrograde Flow (In-Line)	General
Component, Other	General
Component, Plastic	General
Component, Rubber	General
Component, Silicone	General
Contract Manufacturing	General
Elastomer, Other	General
Elastomer, Silicone Rubber	General
Guide, Catheter	Cardiovascular
Introducer, Catheter	Cardiovascular
Molding, Custom	General
Molding, Injection	General
Valve, Other	Chemistry

VERNON-BENSHOFF COMPANY, INC.
See Cmp Industries Llc

VERSAMED MEDICAL SYSTEMS, INC.   800-475-9239
2 Blue Hill Plaza, Pearl River, NY 10965   **845-770-2840**
FDA Number: 2249632   *Fax:* 845-770-2850
E-mail: info@versamed.com
Web site: www.versamed.com
Year Founded: 1999
Ownership: Ge Healthcare
Produces/Sells CE-marked Devices: N
General Admin.: Jerry Korten/Chief Executive Officer
       Moustafa El-Gohary/General Manager
       Eyal Dior/President
Mktg./Adv.: David Hammond/Vice President International Marketing & Sales
       Kevin Plihal/Vice President Market Development

Ventilator, Continuous (Respirator)	Anesthesiology

VERTEBRON, INC.   203-380-9340
400 Long Beach Blvd., Stratford, CT 06615
FDA Number: 3004435519
Ownership: Private
Produces/Sells CE-marked Devices: N

Appliance, Fixation, Spinal Intervertebral Body	Orthopedics
Orthosis, Fixation, Pedicle, Spinal	Orthopedics

VERTEX INTERNATIONAL, INC.   540-989-6945
7429 Fort Mason Dr., Roanoke, VA 24018-5383
FDA Number: 3000224509
Ownership: Private
Produces/Sells CE-marked Devices: N

Computer, Chemistry Analyzer	Chemistry

VERTIFLEX (TM), INCORPORATED   866-268-6486
1351 Calle Avanzado, San Clemente, CA 92673   **949-940-1400**
FDA Number: 3005882106   *Fax:* 949-940-1450
Web site: http://www.vertiflexspine.com/
Year Founded: 2005
Ownership: Private
Produces/Sells CE-marked Devices: N
General Admin.: Mr. Moti Altarac/Chief Technology Officer
       Mr. Earl Fender/President, Chief Executive Officer
Mktg./Adv.: Mr. Scott Lynch/Vice President Marketing
       Mr. Jack Carlson/Vice President Sales
Production: Mr. Steve Reitzler/Vice President Regulatory & Clinical Affairs
Research: Mr. Bill Duffell/Vice President Research
Finance: Mr. Jeff Swieki/Vice President Finance

Device, Spinal Vertebral Body Replacement	Orthopedics
Orthosis, Fixation, Pedicle, Spinal	Orthopedics
Orthosis, Fixation, Spinal, Spondylolisthesis	Orthopedics
Orthosis, Spinal Pedicle Fixation, For Degenerative Disc Disease	Orthopedics

VERTOS MEDICAL INC.   877.958.6227.
11 Columbia, Suite B, Aliso Viejo, CA 92656   **408-437-3148**
FDA Number: 3006450448
E-mail: info@vertosmed.com
Web site: www.vertosmed.com
Ownership: Private
Produces/Sells CE-marked Devices: N

Accessories, Arthroscope	Orthopedics
Arthroscope	Orthopedics

VESPO MARKETING ASSOC., INC.   800-49-VESPO
9 Dogwood Drive, P.O. Box 60,   **845-361-2800**
Bloomingburg, NY 12721
FDA Number: n/a   *Fax:* 845-361-2818
E-mail: controls@vespo.com
Web site: www.vespo.com
Medical Products Sales Volume: $5,000,000
Annual Revenue: $1-$5 Million
Year Founded: 1975
Ownership: Private
Produces/Sells CE-marked Devices: Y
Federal Procurement Eligibility: Small Business, Female Owned

VESPO MARKETING ASSOC., INC.   800-49-VESPO *(cont'd)*
Distribution: Exclusive Distributor

Thermometer, Infrared	General

VESS CHAIRS, INC.   414-476-2488
9036 W. Schlinger, West Allis, WI 53214
FDA Number: 1579597   *Fax:* 414-476-3493
Medical Products Sales Volume: $550,000
Annual Revenue: $0-$1 Million
Total Employees: 2   *Marketing Staff:* 2   *Sales Staff:* 2
Ownership: Private
Produces/Sells CE-marked Devices: N
Federal Procurement Eligibility: Small Business, Female Owned
Distribution: Manufacturer Direct
General Admin.: Judith I. Kulpa/President
       Michael F. Conmy/Secretary, Treasurer

Chair, Adjustable, Mechanical	Physical Med
Chair, Examination And Treatment	General

VESSIX VASCULAR, INC.   858-217-0300
26052 Merit Circle, Suite 106, Laguna Hills, CA 92653
FDA Number: n/a
E-mail: info@minnowmedical.com
Web site: http://www.minnowmedical.com
Ownership: Private
Produces/Sells CE-marked Devices: N
General Admin.: Mr. Raymond Cohen/Chief Executive Officer
Mktg./Adv.: Mr. Prabodh Mathur/Director Product Development
       Ms. Sharon Riddle/Vice President Market Development
Finance: Mr. Dan Dearen/Chief Financial Officer

VESTA   714-993-4100
1941 Petra Lane, Placentia, CA 92870
FDA Number: n/a   *Fax:* 714-993-4141
E-mail: extrumed@aol.com
Web site: www.extrumed.com
Medical Products Sales Volume: $2,000,000
Annual Revenue: $1-$5 Million
Total Employees: 20   *Marketing Staff:* 1   *Sales Staff:* 1
Ownership: Private
Quality System Registration Information: ISO9002
Produces/Sells CE-marked Devices: N
Federal Procurement Eligibility: Small Business, Female Owned
Distribution: Manufacturer Direct, OEM, Service Direct, Exclusive Distributor, Importer
General Admin.: Vraj Lathiya/President
Mktg./Adv.: Apur Lathiya/Director Marketing

Polymer, Synthetic, Other	General
Thermoforming, Extrusion, Custom	General
Tubing, Multi-Lumen	General
Tubing, Nylon	General
Tubing, Polyethylene	General
Tubing, Polyvinyl Chloride	General
Tubing, Urethane	General

VESTAR COMPANY
See Gilead Sciences

VESTIBULAR TECHNOLOGIES, LLC   307-637-5711
205 County Road 128a, Suite 200, Cheyenne, WY 82007-1831
FDA Number: 3003652725   *Fax:* 312-896-5856
Web site: www.vestibtech.com
Year Founded: 1996
Ownership: Private
Produces/Sells CE-marked Devices: N

Audiometer	Ear/Nose/Throat
Chart, Visual Acuity	Ophthalmology
Platform, Force-Measuring	Physical Med
Scale, Stand-On	General

VESTURE CORP.   614-864-6400
120 East Pritchard St., Asheville, NC 27203
FDA Number: 48512
Ownership: Private
Produces/Sells CE-marked Devices: N

Pack, Hot Or Cold, Reusable	Physical Med

VESTURE CORPORATION   800-462-4201
120 E. Pritchard St., Asheboro, NC 27203   **336-629-3000**
FDA Number: n/a   *Fax:* 336-629-3100
E-mail: info@vesture.com
Web site: www.vesture.com
Medical Products Sales Volume: $20,000,000
Annual Revenue: $10-$25 Million
Total Employees: 125   *Marketing Staff:* 3   *Sales Staff:* 35
Ownership: BARRY CORPORATION, R.G.
Stock Symbol: RGB
Traded On: NYSE
Produces/Sells CE-marked Devices: N

VESTURE CORPORATION   800-462-4201 *(cont'd)*

Distribution: Manufacturer Through Distributor, Manufacturer Through Manufacturer Reps
General Admin.: Byron Owens/Chief Executive Officer
        Gary Hyatt/President
Mktg./Adv.: Sharon Caughron/Manager International Marketing & Sales
        Wayne Baldwin/Manager National Sales
        Melanie Buchanan/Vice President Marketing
Production: Anthony Day/Manager Materials
Cushion, Other	General
Pad, Heating, Powered	Physical Med
Slippers	General

VET-CO, INC.
See Augusta Medical Systems, Llc

VETTER PHARMA-TURM, INC.   215-321-6930
Heston Hall/Carriage House, Suite 203
1790 Yardley-Langhorne Rd.
Yardley, PA 19067
FDA Number: 9610900   *Fax:* 215-321-6932
E-mail: info@vetter-pharma.com
Web site: www.vetter-pharma.com
Year Founded: 1983
Total Employees: 500
Ownership: VETTER GROUP
Quality System Registration Information: ISO9001
General Admin.: Udo J. Vetter/President
        Jeffrey K. Turms/Vice President, General Manager
Mktg./Adv.: James C. Rhodes/Vice President Marketing & Sales
Aspirator, Nasal	Ear/Nose/Throat
Injector, Syringe	General
Syringe, Cartridge	Dental And Oral

VIA! FOR TRAVEL   800-339-0628
22885 Savi Ranch Parkway, Suite C,   714-455-2007
Yorba Linda, CA 92887
FDA Number: 2028540   *Fax:* 714-455-2008
E-mail: catalogues@viafortravel.com
Web site: www.viafortravel.com
Medical Products Sales Volume: $360,000
Annual Revenue: $1-$5 Million
Year Founded: 1996
Total Employees: 14   *Marketing Staff:* 1   *Sales Staff:* 2
Ownership: Private
Produces/Sells CE-marked Devices: N
Federal Procurement Eligibility: Small Business, Female Owned
General Admin.: Mrs. Michelle Schlosberg/Chief Executive Officer
Production: Mr. David Abramowitz/Director Operations
Toothbrush, Manual	Dental And Oral

VIACIRQ, INC.
See Viacirq, Inc.

VIASYS HEALTHCARE INC.
See CAREFUSION 211, INC..

VIASYS MEDSYSTEMS
See Corpak Medsystems, Inc.

VIASYS NEUROCARE
See Cardinal Healthcare 209, Inc.

VIASYS SLEEP SYSTEMS, LLC.   847-689-8410
9305 Eton Avenue, Chatsworth, CA 91311
FDA Number: 3005279296
Ownership: Private
Produces/Sells CE-marked Devices: N
Ventilator, Non-Continuous (Respirator)	Anesthesiology

VIATRO CORP.
See Great Lakes Medical

VIATRONIX, INC.   631-444-9700
25 Health Sciences Drive, Suite 203,
Stony Brook, NY 11790
FDA Number: 2438935   *Fax:* 631-444-9701
E-mail: support@viatronix.com
Web site: http://www.viatronix.com
Medical Products Sales Volume: $1,500,000
Annual Revenue: $1-$5 Million
Year Founded: 2004
Total Employees: 15
Ownership: Private
Quality System Registration Information: ISO9001
Produces/Sells CE-marked Devices: Y
Federal Procurement Eligibility: Small Business
Distribution: Manufacturer Direct, Manufacturer Through Distributor
General Admin.: Zaffar Hayat/President, Chief Executive Officer
Image Processing System	Radiology
Scanner, Computed Tomography, X-Ray, Special Procedure	Radiology

VIBE 2000   805-377-2709
511 Iguera Dr., Oxnard, CA 93030
FDA Number: 2032873
Ownership: Private
Produces/Sells CE-marked Devices: N
Ring, Teething, Non-Fluid-Filled	Dental And Oral

VIBGYOR OPTICAL SYSTEMS   800-842-4967
1140 N. Phelps, Arlington Heights, IL 60004   847-818-0788
FDA Number: n/a   *Fax:* 847-818-0799
Annual Revenue: $1-$5 Million
Total Employees: 15   *Marketing Staff:* 2   *Sales Staff:* 5
Ownership: Private
Produces/Sells CE-marked Devices: Y
Federal Procurement Eligibility: Small Business, Minority Owned
Distribution: Manufacturer Direct
General Admin.: Victor Verma/President
Mktg./Adv.: Derek Sellers/Vice President Marketing & Sales
Production: Roger Williams/Vice President Manufacturing
Photocoagulator	Ophthalmology

VIBRADERM, INC.   301-279-2899
2100 North Highway 360, Suite 1502, Grand Prairie, TX 75050
FDA Number: 3005037855
Brush, Dermabrasion	Surgery

VICKS MANUFACTURING DIV.
See Procter & Gamble

VICKS TOILETRY PRODUCTS
See Procter & Gamble

VICON   303-799-8686
7388 South Revere Pkwy., #901, Centennial, CO 80112
FDA Number: 1000377231   *Fax:* 303-799-8690
E-mail: info@peakperform.com
Web site: www.vicon.com
Year Founded: 1984
Ownership: Private
Stock Symbol: OMG
Traded On: London
Produces/Sells CE-marked Devices: N
Federal Procurement Eligibility: Small Business, GSA Contract
Distribution: Manufacturer Direct
Optical Position/Movement Recording System	Physical Med

VICON INDUSTRIES INC.   800-645-9116
89 Arkay Dr., Hauppauge, NY 11788   631-952-2288
FDA Number: n/a   *Fax:* 631-951-2288
E-mail: sales@vicon-security.com
Web site: www.vicon-cctv.com
Annual Revenue: $50-$100 Million
Year Founded: 1967
Total Employees: 175   *Marketing Staff:* 6   *Sales Staff:* 30
Ownership: Public
Stock Symbol: VII
Traded On: AMEX
Produces/Sells CE-marked Devices: Y
Federal Procurement Eligibility: Small Business
Distribution: Manufacturer Direct, Manufacturer Through Distributor, Manufacturer Through Manufacturer Reps, Importer, Exporter
General Admin.: Kenneth Darby/President, Chief Executive Officer
Mktg./Adv.: J. C. Caine/Manager International Sales
        Bret McGowan/Vice President Market Development
        Bret McGowan/Vice President Sales
Production: Ray Kleppan/Manager Materials
        Peter Horn/Vice President Quality Assurance
        Yacov Pshtissky/Vice President Tech. Development
Finance: John Badke/Chief Financial Officer, Vice President Finance
IS: Kenny Rohan/Manager Tech. Support
Camera, Video	General
Control System, Energy	General
Lens, Other	Ophthalmology
Security Equipment/Supplies	General

VICOR TECHNOLOGIES INC.   877.528-PD2i (
2300 Corporate Blvd. NW, Suite 123,   800-998-9964
Boca Raton, FL 33431
FDA Number: n/a   *Fax:* 561-995-2449
E-mail: info@vicortech.com
Web site: www.vicortech.com
Ownership: Public
Stock Symbol: VCRT
Traded On: OTC Bulletin
Produces/Sells CE-marked Devices: N
General Admin.: David Fater/Chief Executive Officer
Research: Dr. James Skinner/Director Research & Development
Finance: Thomas Bohannon/Chief Accountant

VICTOR COMPANY OF JAPAN LTD.
See JVC Americas Corp.

VICTOR O. SCHINNERER & COMPANY, INC. 301-961-9800
2 Wisconsin Circle, Chevy Chase, MD 20815-7003
FDA Number: n/a Fax: 301-951-5444
E-mail: vos.info@Schinnerer.com
Web site: www.schinnerer.com
Annual Revenue: $5-$10 Million
Year Founded: 1938
Ownership: Private
Produces/Sells CE-marked Devices: N
Distribution: Service Direct
General Admin.: Jeff Schlingbaum/Chief Financial Officer, Senior Vice President
Steve Giddens/Information Technology Administrator
Lorna Parsons/President
Richard Altmann/Senior Vice President Human Resources
Mktg./Adv.: Mary Jefferson/Senior Vice President Marketing
Service, Insurance General

VICTOR TUBE CORP
See Ccl Containers

VICTORCH MEDITEK, INC. 858-530-9191
7313 Carroll Rd., Suite A-b, San Diego, CA 92121
FDA Number: 2032364
Enzyme Immunoassay, Barbiturate Toxicology
Kit, Pregnancy Test, Over The Counter, HCG Chemistry
Test, Human Chorionic Gonadotropin, Serum Immunology

VICTORY REFRIGERATION, INC. 800-523-5008
110 Woodcrest Road, Cherry Hill, NJ 08003 856-428-4200
FDA Number: n/a Fax: 856-428-7299
E-mail: info@victoryrefrigeration.com
Web site: www.victory-refrig.com
Medical Products Sales Volume: $200,000
Annual Revenue: $25-$50 Million
Year Founded: 1944
Total Employees: 2
Ownership: Private
Produces/Sells CE-marked Devices: Y
Federal Procurement Eligibility: Small Business, GSA Contract
Distribution: Manufacturer Through Manufacturer Reps
General Admin.: Ian Whyte/President
Mktg./Adv.: Jim Hurston/Vice President, Manager Sales
Refrigerator, Foodservice General

VIDA MEDICA, S.A. DE C.V. 5-557-4346
Calle 6 No. 376, Col. Francisco I. Madero,
Mexico D.F. 11480 Mexico
FDA Number: n/a Fax: 5-395-9829
E-mail: vidamedica@prodigy.net.mx
Medical Products Sales Volume: $450,000
Total Employees: 10 Marketing Staff: 1 Sales Staff: 4
Ownership: Private
Produces/Sells CE-marked Devices: N
Distribution: Exclusive Distributor

VIDACARE CORP. 800-680-4911
4350 Lockhill Selma Rd, Suite 150, 866-479-8500
Shavano Park, TX 78249
FDA Number: 3004526033 Fax: 210-375-8537
Web site: http://www.vidacare.com
Year Founded: 2001
Ownership: Private
Produces/Sells CE-marked Devices: N
General Admin.: Mr. Mark Mellin/Chief Executive Officer, Chief Financial Officer
Mr. Michael Voss/Chief Operating Officer
Mr. Clas Runnberg/Director International Operations
Medical Admin.: Dr. Larry Miller/Chief Medical Officer
Production: Mr. Kevin Johnson/Director Operations
Finance: Mr. Rick Magnum/Vice President Finance, Controller
Battery, Rechargeable, Replacement for Class III Device Cardiovascular
Biopsy Instrument, Mechanical, Gastrointestinal Gastroenterology/Urology
Injector, Vertebroplasty (does Not Contain Cement) Orthopedics
Needle, Hypodermic, Single Lumen With Syringe General
Set, Administration, Intravenous, Needle-Free General

VIDAR SYSTEMS CORP. 703-471-7070
365 Herndon Parkway, Herndon, VA 20170
FDA Number: 2027116
Image Digitizer Radiology
Imager, X-Ray, Solid State (Flat Panel/Digital) Radiology

VIDATAK, LLC 734-477-6942
9080 Santa Monica Blvd., Ste. 103, Los Angeles, CA 90069
FDA Number: 2032857
Communication System, Non-Powered Physical Med

VIDCO, INC. 800-638-4326
6175 SW 112th Avenue, 503-641-1804
Beaverton, OR 97008
FDA Number: 3020646
E-mail: info@vidcoinc.com Fax: 503-641-1806
Web site: www.vidcoinc.com
Medical Products Sales Volume: $500,000
Year Founded: 1972
Ownership: Private
Quality System Registration Information: ISO9001
Produces/Sells CE-marked Devices: Y
Federal Procurement Eligibility: Small Business
Distribution: Manufacturer Direct, Manufacturer Through Distributor, Manufacturer Through Manufacturer Reps, OEM, Exporter
Monitor, Bed Patient General
Monitor, ECG, Ambulatory, Real-Time Cardiovascular
Recorder, Paper Chart Cardiovascular
Television Monitor, Operating Room General

VIDENT 800-828-3839
3150 E. Birch St., Brea, CA 92821 714-961-6200
FDA Number: 2082832 Fax: 714-961-6299
E-mail: info@vident.com
Web site: www.vident.com
Medical Products Sales Volume: $2,500,000
Annual Revenue: $25-$50 Million
Year Founded: 1984
Total Employees: 90 Marketing Staff: 12 Sales Staff: 22
Ownership: Private
Quality System Registration Information: ISO9000
Produces/Sells CE-marked Devices: Y
Federal Procurement Eligibility: Small Business
Distribution: Exclusive Distributor
General Admin.: Wayne Whitehill/Chief Executive Officer
Bill Sundheimer/President
Medical Admin.: Dr. Martin Mendelson/Director Clinical Affairs
Mktg./Adv.: Andy Klein/Manager Marketing
Jerry Feeney/Vice President Market Development
Production: William Baker/Manager Regulatory Affairs
Alloy, Gold Based, For Clinical Use Dental And Oral
Alloy, Precious Metal, For Clinical Use Dental And Oral
Base, Denture, Relining, Repairing, Rebasing, Resin Dental And Oral
Compound, Resinous, Composite Dental And Oral
Denture, Plastic, Teeth Dental And Oral
Denture, Preformed Dental And Oral
Furnace, Porcelain Dental And Oral
Implant, Endosseous Dental And Oral
Material, Impression Dental And Oral
Material, Tooth Shade, Resin Dental And Oral
Metal, Base Dental And Oral
Powder, Porcelain Dental And Oral

VIDMAR INC., STANLEY
See Stanley Vidmar

VIGOR THERAPY SOLUTIONS LLC 269-429-0191
4915 Advance Way, Stevensville, MI 49127
FDA Number: 3003681032
Lift, Bath, Non-AC-Powered General
Lift, Patient General

VIKING SYSTEMS INC. 508-366-3668
134 Flanders Rd., Westborough, MA 01581
FDA Number: 1223925 Fax: 508-366-8858
E-mail: Discover3D@vikingsystems.com
Web site: http://www.vikingsystems.com
Ownership: Private
Produces/Sells CE-marked Devices: N
General Admin.: Mr. John Kennedy/President, Chief Executive Officer
Finance: Mr. Robert Mathews/Chief Financial Officer
Accessories, Photographic, Endoscopic Gastroenterology/Urology
Camera, Still, Endoscopic Surgery
Camera, Television, Endoscopic (Without Audio) Surgery
Device, Storage, Image, Digital Radiology
Endoscope Gastroenterology/Urology
Illuminator, Fiberoptic (For Endoscope) Gastroenterology/Urology
Laparoscope, General & Plastic Surgery Surgery
Light Source, Fiberoptic, Routine Gastroenterology/Urology

VILEX, INC. 931-474-7550
111 Moffitt Street, Mcminnville, TN 37110
FDA Number: 1051526
Ownership: Private
Produces/Sells CE-marked Devices: N
Blade, Surgical, Saw, General & Plastic Surgery Surgery
Brush, Biopsy, General & Plastic Surgery Surgery
Driver, Surgical, Pin Surgery
Rasp, Surgical, General & Plastic Surgery Surgery
Saw, Electric Cardiovascular

VILEX, INC.   931-474-7550 *(cont'd)*
Screwdriver	Orthopedics
Surgical Instrument, Orthopedic, AC-Powered Motor	Orthopedics

VILEX, INC.   800-872-4911
345 Old Curry Hollow Road,   **412-655-7550**
Pittsburgh, PA 15236
FDA Number: 2529556   Fax: 800-619-4911
E-mail: info@vilex.com
Web site: www.vilex.com
Medical Products Sales Volume: $600,000
Annual Revenue: $1-$5 Million
Year Founded: 1996
Total Employees: 7   *Sales Staff:* 20
Ownership: Private
Produces/Sells CE-marked Devices: N
Federal Procurement Eligibility: Small Business
Distribution: Manufacturer Direct, Manufacturer Through Manufacturer Reps, Exporter
General Admin.: Dr. Abrahim Lavi/President, Chief Executive Officer
    Sylvia Southard/Vice President, General Manager
Mktg./Adv.: Sylvia Southard/Director National Accounts
Production: Terry Murray/Director Quality Assurance
    Sylvia Southard/Manager Materials

Blade, Bone Cutting	Orthopedics
Burr, Podiatric	Orthopedics
Drill, Bone	Orthopedics
Driver, Wire	Orthopedics
Pin, Fixation, Threaded	Orthopedics
Rasp, Bone	Orthopedics
Saw, Bone Cutting, Micro	Orthopedics
Wire, Surgical	Orthopedics

Medical Product Subsidiaries (Listed Separately)
    Vilex, Inc.

VINDUM ENGINEERING, INC.   925-275-0633
1 Woodview Court, San Ramon, CA 94582-2307
FDA Number: n/a   Fax: 925-275-9697
E-mail: info@vindum.com
Web site: www.vindum.com
Medical Products Sales Volume: $5,000,000
Annual Revenue: $1-$5 Million
Year Founded: 1987
Total Employees: 4   *Marketing Staff:* 3   *Sales Staff:* 3
Ownership: Private
Produces/Sells CE-marked Devices: N
Federal Procurement Eligibility: Small Business
Distribution: Manufacturer Direct, OEM, Exclusive Distributor, Exporter
General Admin.: Ms. Stayc Feil/General Manager
Mktg./Adv.: Ms. Christa Vindum/Vice President Sales

Pump, Laboratory	Chemistry
Tubing, Plastic	General

VINELAND SYRUP INC.   800-642-9124
PO Box 1326, Vineland, NJ 08360
FDA Number: 2226984
E-mail: info@vinelandsyrup.com
Web site: www.vinelandsyrup.com
Ownership: Private
Produces/Sells CE-marked Devices: N

Drink, Glucose Tolerance	Chemistry

VIOPTIX, INC.   510-360-7506
47224 Mission Falls Court, Fremont, CA 94539
FDA Number: 3003965364

Oximeter, Tissue Saturation	Cardiovascular

VIRAL ANTIGENS, INC.
See Meridian Life Science, Inc.

VIROMED LABORATORIES (LABCORP)   800-582-0077
6101 Blue Circle Dr., Minnetonka, MN 55343   **952-563-4024**
FDA Number: 2183472   Fax: 952-563-3215
E-mail: information@viromed.com
Web site: www.viromed.com
Year Founded: 1982
Ownership: Private
Produces/Sells CE-marked Devices: N

Culture Media, Synthetic Cell And Tissue	Pathology
Cultured Animal And Human Cells	Pathology

VIROTECH INTERNATIONAL, INC.   301-924-8000
12 Meem Ave., Suite C, Gaithersburg, MD 20877
FDA Number: 1125815
Ownership: Private
Produces/Sells CE-marked Devices: N

Antigen, Epstein-Barr Virus, Capsid	Microbiology
Assay, Enzyme Linked Immunosorbent, Hepatitis C Virus	Microbiology
Enzyme Linked Immunoabsorbent Assay, Rubella	Microbiology

VIROTECH INTERNATIONAL, INC.   301-924-8000 *(cont'd)*
Enzyme Linked Immunoabsorbent Assay, Toxoplasma Gondii	Microbiology
Enzyme-Linked Immunosorbent Assay, Herpes Simplex Virus, HSV-1	Microbiology
Enzyme-Linked Immunosorbent Assay, Herpes Simplex Virus, HSV-2	Microbiology
System, Identification, Hepatitis B Antigen	Hematology
Test, Donor, Cmv	Immunology
Test, Hiv Detection	Immunology

VIROTEK, L.L.C.   847-634-4500
900 Asbury Dr., Buffalo Grove, IL 60089
FDA Number: 1424360
Ownership: Private
Produces/Sells CE-marked Devices: N

General Purpose Microbiology Diagnostic Device	Microbiology
Lancet, Blood	General

VIRTEC ENTERPRISES, LLC   440-352-8970
11351 Prouty Road, Painesville, OH 44077-2321
FDA Number: 1531143   Fax: 440-352-6280
E-mail: virtec@virtecenterprises.com
Web site: www.virtecenterprises.com
Medical Products Sales Volume: $300,000
Annual Revenue: $0-$1 Million
Year Founded: 1999
Ownership: Private
Produces/Sells CE-marked Devices: N
Federal Procurement Eligibility: Small Business
Distribution: Manufacturer Through Manufacturer Reps, OEM, Importer
General Admin.: Michael Sturdevant/President

Catheter, Suction (Tracheal Aspirating Tube)	Anesthesiology
Service, Consulting	General

VIRTIS, AN SP INDUSTRIES COMPANY   800-431-8232
815 Route 208, Gardiner, NY 12525   **845-255-5000**
FDA Number: 7000381   Fax: 845-255-5338
E-mail: sales@virtis.com
Web site: www.virtis.com
Annual Revenue: $10-$25 Million
Year Founded: 1953
Total Employees: 100   *Marketing Staff:* 16   *Sales Staff:* 16
Ownership: SP INDUSTRIES, INC.
Quality System Registration Information: ISO9000; ISO9001
Produces/Sells CE-marked Devices: Y
Federal Procurement Eligibility: Small Business, GSA Contract
Distribution: Manufacturer Direct, Manufacturer Through Distributor, Manufacturer Through Manufacturer Reps, Importer, Exporter
General Admin.: S. G. Bart/President
Mktg./Adv.: Ken Tenedini/Vice President Marketing & Sales
    Miriam C. Blednick/Vice President Sales

Disintegrator, Biological Cell	Microbiology
Fermentation Equipment	Microbiology
Freeze Drying Equipment	Chemistry
Freezer, Laboratory, General Purpose	Chemistry
Homogenizer, Tissue	Microbiology
Tissue Culture Apparatus	Microbiology

VIRTUAL IMAGING, INC.   954-428-6191
720 S. Powerline Rd., Ste. E, Deerfield Bch, FL 33442
FDA Number: 1064504

Housing, X-Ray Tube, Diagnostic	Radiology
Imager, X-Ray, Solid State (Flat Panel/Digital)	Radiology
Radiographic Unit, Diagnostic	Radiology
System, X-Ray, Mobile	Radiology
Table, Radiographic, Non-Tilting, Powered	Radiology

VIRTUAL RADIOLOGIC CORPORATION   800-737-0610
11995 Singletree Lane, Suite 500,   **952-595-1100**
Eden Prairie, MN 55344
FDA Number: 3007795813   Fax: 952-942-3361
E-mail: info@vrad.com
Web site: http://www.vrad.com
Ownership: Public
Stock Symbol: VRAD
Traded On: NASDAQ
Produces/Sells CE-marked Devices: N
General Admin.: Mr. Rick Jennings/Chief Technology Officer
    Mr. Mike Kolar/General Counsel
    Mr. Rob Kill/President, Chief Executive Officer
Medical Admin.: Dr. Eduard Michel/Chief Medical Officer
Finance: Mr. Len Purkis/Chief Financial Officer

Image Processing System	Radiology

VIRTUALSCOPICS, INC.   585-249-6231
500 Linden Oaks, Rochester, NY 14625
FDA Number: n/a   Fax: 585-218-7350
Web site: www.virtualscopics.com
Ownership: Public
Stock Symbol: VSCP
Traded On: NASDAQ

VIRTUALSCOPICS, INC.
585-249-6231 *(cont'd)*
Produces/Sells CE-marked Devices: N
General Admin.: Molly Henderson/Chief Financial Officer, Senior Vice President
    Dr. Edward Ashton/Chief Scientific Officer
    Dr. Jonathan Riek/Chief Technology Officer
    Jeff Markin/President, Chief Executive Officer
Medical Admin.: Mr. Mark Tengowski/Vice President Clinical Affairs
Production: Ms. Toni Handzel/Director Quality Assurance & Regulatory Affairs
IS: Mr. Colin Rhodes/Director Software

VISCOLAS, INC.
800-548-2694
8801 Consolidated Drive, Soddy Daisy, TN 37379   423-332-0800
FDA Number: 1062612
Fax: 423-332-0802
E-mail: info@viscolas.com
Web site: www.viscolas.com
Medical Products Sales Volume: $500,000
Year Founded: 1991
Total Employees: 7
Ownership: Private
Produces/Sells CE-marked Devices: Y
Federal Procurement Eligibility: Small Business
Distribution: Manufacturer Through Distributor, OEM

Exerciser, Non-Measuring	Physical Med
Insoles, Medical	General
Orthosis, Corrective Shoe	Physical Med
Protector, Skin Pressure	General

VISCOT MEDICAL, LLC
800-221-0658
32 West Street, PO Box 351,   973-887-9273
East Hanover, NJ 07936
FDA Number: 2242656
Fax: 973-887-3961
E-mail: ideas@viscot.com
Web site: www.viscot.com
Medical Products Sales Volume: $5,000,000
Annual Revenue: $1-$5 Million
Year Founded: 1974
Total Employees: 16   *Marketing Staff:* 1   *Sales Staff:* 3
Ownership: Private
Quality System Registration Information: ISO9002
Produces/Sells CE-marked Devices: Y
Federal Procurement Eligibility: Small Business, GSA Contract, VA Contract
Distribution: Manufacturer Through Distributor, OEM
General Admin.: Vincent J. Muccione/President
    Irene T. Muccione/Secretary Treasurer
Mktg./Adv.: Laura I. Boyd/Manager International & National Sales
    Gary J. Muccione/Vice President Marketing
Production: Martin Thomas/Director Quality Assurance

Bib	General
Container, Specimen, All Types	General
Drape, Surgical, Disposable	Surgery
Marker, Skin	Surgery
Towel, Surgical	Surgery
Urinal	General
Wrapper, Surgical Instrument (Sterile)	General

VISEN MEDICAL
781-932-6875 x3
45-47 Wiggins Ave., Bedford, MA 01730
FDA Number: n/a
Fax: 781-937-4994
E-mail: infor@visenmedical.com
Web site: www.visenmedical.com
Year Founded: 2000
Ownership: Private
Produces/Sells CE-marked Devices: N
General Admin.: Wael Yared/Chief Technology Officer
    Kirtland Poss/President, Chief Executive Officer
Mktg./Adv.: Karen Madden/Senior Vice President Corporate Development
    Mr. Robert Sandler/Senior Vice President Marketing
    John Kleijne/Vice President International Sales
Finance: John Ziolkowski/Chief Financial Officer

VISIBILITE INC.
800-926-2466
1221 Labadie, Local 204,   450-677-1441
Longueuil, QUE J4N-1 Canada
FDA Number: n/a
Fax: 450-677-8769
E-mail: visibi@aei.ca
Web site: http://www.visibilite.ca/
Year Founded: 1991
Total Employees: 10
Ownership: Private
Produces/Sells CE-marked Devices: N
Distribution: Exclusive Distributor, Importer

VISICOMM INDUSTRIES
866-221-3131
911A Milwaukee Ave., Burlington, WI 53105   262-767-9032
FDA Number: n/a
Fax: 262-767-9060
Web site: www.50hz.com
Medical Products Sales Volume: $1,400,000

VISICOMM INDUSTRIES
866-221-3131 *(cont'd)*
Annual Revenue: $1-$5 Million
Ownership: Private
Quality System Registration Information: ISO9001
Produces/Sells CE-marked Devices: N
Federal Procurement Eligibility: Small Business, Minority Owned
Distribution: Manufacturer Direct, Exporter

Communication Equipment	General
Pager, Non-Radio	General
Physician Registry	General

VISICU, INC.
410-276-1960
217 E. Redwood St., Ste. 1900, Baltimore, MD 21202
FDA Number: 1125873

System, Network And Communication, Physiological Monitors	Cardiovascular

VISION ASSESSMENT CORP.
847-239-5889
2675 Coyle Ave., Elk Grove Village, IL 60007
FDA Number: 3006446477

Chart, Visual Acuity	Ophthalmology
Target, Fusion/Stereoscopic	Ophthalmology
Tester, Color Vision	Ophthalmology

VISION CHIPS, INC.
949-362-0565
27671 La Paz Road, Laguna Niguel, CA 92677
FDA Number: 2031081

Image Processing System	Radiology

VISION EASE LENS INC.
See Vision-Ease Lens

VISION LABS INC.
See The Lifestyle Co. Inc.

VISION MEDICAL INC.
877-448-1234
#100, 10479 - 184th Street,   780-448-1234
Edmonton, ALB T5S 2 Canada
FDA Number: n/a
Fax: 780-448-7232
E-mail: alvingrenke@visionmedical.ca
Web site: www.visionmedical.ca
Year Founded: 1998
Total Employees: 10
Ownership: Private
Produces/Sells CE-marked Devices: N
Distribution: Exclusive Distributor

VISION MEDICAL INSTRUMENTS, INC.
440-338-5981
8147 Chagrin Mills Rd., Chagrin Falls, OH 44022
FDA Number: 1530131
Ownership: Private
Produces/Sells CE-marked Devices: N

Measurer, Corneal Radius	Ophthalmology

VISION OPTICS TECHNOLOGIES LTD.
866-671-0735
1816 Production Court, Louisville, KY 40299   502-671-0735
FDA Number: 3005761669
Fax: 502-671-0739
E-mail: info@votechnologies.com
Web site: www.votechnologies.com
Ownership: Private
Produces/Sells CE-marked Devices: N

Lens, Spectacle (prescription), For Reading Discomfort	Ophthalmology
Lens, Spectacle/Eyeglasses, Non-Custom	Ophthalmology

VISION PRO LLC
800-892-3937
4309 I-49 South Service Road, Opelousas, LA 70570
FDA Number: 3004750376

Disinfector, Medical Device	General
Exhaust System, Surgical	Surgery

VISION QUEST INDUSTRIES, INC.
800-266-6969
18011 Mitchell So., Irvine, CA 92614   949-261-3865
FDA Number: 2085494
E-mail: info@vqorthocare.com
Web site: www.vqorthocare.com
Year Founded: 1989
Ownership: Private
Produces/Sells CE-marked Devices: N

Component, Exercise	Physical Med
Electrode, Cutaneous	Cns/Neurology
Exerciser, Powered	Anesthesiology
Orthosis, Limb Brace	Physical Med
Stimulator, Muscle, Electrical-Powered (EMS)	Physical Med
Stimulator, Nerve, Transcutaneous (Pain Relief, TENS)	Cns/Neurology
Stimulator, Neuromuscular, External Functional	Cns/Neurology

VISION RESEARCH CORP.
205-942-8011
211 Summit Pkwy., Suite 105, Birmingham, AL 35209
FDA Number: 1036862

Retinoscope, Battery-Powered	Ophthalmology

VISION SYSTEMS GROUP, A DIVISION OF VIKING SYSTEMS
See Viking Systems Inc.

VISION TRAINING PRODUCTS, INC.   **800-348-2225**
4016 N. Home St., Mishawaka, IN 46545   **574-259-2070**
FDA Number: 1820463   *Fax:* 574-259-2102
Web site: www.bernell.com
Annual Revenue: $1-$5 Million
Year Founded: 1954
Ownership: Private
Produces/Sells CE-marked Devices: Y
Federal Procurement Eligibility: Small Business, Female Owned
Distribution: Manufacturer Direct
Production: Al Martin/Vice President Operations, General Manager
Research: Dr. Charles Shearer/Vice President Research & Development

Bar, Prism, Ophthalmic	Ophthalmology
Brush, Haidinger, With Macular Integrity	Ophthalmology
Clip, Lens, Trial, Ophthalmic	Ophthalmology
Cover, Other	General
Fixation Device, AC-Powered, Ophthalmic	Ophthalmology
Gauge, Lens, Ophthalmic	Ophthalmology
Grid, Amsler	Ophthalmology
Lens, Maddox	Ophthalmology
Lens, Spectacle/Eyeglasses, Non-Custom	Ophthalmology
Measurer, Stereopsis	Ophthalmology
Occluder, Ophthalmic	Ophthalmology
Pupillometer	Ophthalmology
Rack, Skiascopic	Ophthalmology
Screen, Tangent, Felt (Campimeter)	Ophthalmology
Target, Fusion/Stereoscopic	Ophthalmology
Tester, Color Vision	Ophthalmology

VISION WHEELCHAIR SEATING SYSTEMS INC.   **416-665-8428**
24-600 Bowes Road, Concord, ONT L4K 4A3 Canada
FDA Number: n/a   *Fax:* 416-665-8978
E-mail: vision-seating@sympatico.ca
Web site: http://www.vision-seating.com
Year Founded: 1992
Total Employees: 10
Ownership: Private
Produces/Sells CE-marked Devices: N
Distribution: Manufacturer Direct, Exporter

VISION-EASE LENS   **800-328-3449**
7000 Sunwood Drive NW, Ramsey, MN 55303   **320-251-8140**
FDA Number: 2124545   *Fax:* 800-289-5456
E-mail: info@vision-ease.com
Web site: www.vision-ease.com
Annual Revenue: $1-$5 Million
Year Founded: 1930
Ownership: Public
Produces/Sells CE-marked Devices: N
Federal Procurement Eligibility: Small Business
Distribution: Manufacturer Direct
Mktg./Adv.: Rich Montag/Vice President Marketing & Sales

Frame, Spectacle (Eyeglasses)	Ophthalmology
Lens, Set, Trial, Ophthalmic	Ophthalmology

VISION-EASE LENS, INC.   **800-328-3449**
7000 Sunwood Drive NW, Ramsey, MN 55303   **320-251-8140**
FDA Number: 2124545   *Fax:* 952-851-6050
E-mail: info@vision-ease.com
Web site: www.vision-ease.com
Medical Products Sales Volume: $104,730,000
Annual Revenue: $25-$50 Million
Year Founded: 2004
Total Employees: 370   *Marketing Staff:* 6   *Sales Staff:* 12
Ownership: Private
Stock Symbol: VELS
Traded On: NASDAQ
Produces/Sells CE-marked Devices: N
Federal Procurement Eligibility: GSA Contract
Distribution: Manufacturer Direct
General Admin.: Paul Burke/Chief Executive Officer
Mktg./Adv.: Jim Misco/Director Sales
        Scott Schaller/Manager Business Development
        Scott Taylor/Manager International Marketing & Sales

Lens, Spectacle/Eyeglasses, Non-Custom	Ophthalmology

VISION-SCIENCES, INC.   **800-874-9975**
40 Ramland Road South, Suite 1,   **845-365-0600**
Orangeburg, NY 10962
FDA Number: 1223490   *Fax:* 845-365-0620
E-mail: info@visionsciences.com
Web site: www.visionsciences.com
Annual Revenue: $5-$10 Million
Ownership: Public
Stock Symbol: VSCI

VISION-SCIENCES, INC.   **800-874-9975** *(cont'd)*
Traded On: NASDAQ
Quality System Registration Information: ISO9001
Produces/Sells CE-marked Devices: Y
Distribution: Manufacturer Through Distributor, Manufacturer Through Manufacturer Reps
General Admin.: Ron Hadani/President, Chief Executive Officer
Mktg./Adv.: Carlos Babini/Vice President Marketing & Sales
Production: Lillian Quintero/Director Quality Assurance
        Jill Johnson/Manager Materials
        Mark Landman/Vice President Operations
Finance: Yoav Cohen/Vice President Finance

Bronchoscope, Non-Rigid	Ear/Nose/Throat
Cystourethroscope	Gastroenterology/Urology
Laryngoscope, Flexible	Anesthesiology
Light Source, Fiberoptic, Routine	Gastroenterology/Urology
Nasopharyngoscope (Flexible Or Rigid)	Ear/Nose/Throat
Scope, Fiberoptic Intubation	Anesthesiology
Sigmoidoscope, Flexible	Gastroenterology/Urology

VISIONARY CONTACT LENS   **714-237-1900**
2940 East Miraloma Ave., Anaheim, CA 92806
FDA Number: 3002830597

Lens, Contact (Other Material)	Ophthalmology

VISIONCARE DEVICES, INC.   **530-243-5047**
1246 Redwood Blvd., Redding, CA 96003
FDA Number: 2939964

Cutter, Vitreous Aspiration, AC-Powered	Ophthalmology
Drape, Pure Latex Sheet, With Self-Retaining Finger Cot	Gastroenterology/Urology
Therapeutic Deep Heat Vitrectomy	Ophthalmology

VISIONCARE OPHTHALMIC   **408-872-9393**
TECHNOLOGIES INC.
14395 Saratoga Ave, Suite 150, Saratoga, CA 95070
FDA Number: 3005251015   *Fax:* 408-872-9395
E-mail: customercare@visioncareinc.net
Web site: www.visioncareinc.net
Ownership: Private
Produces/Sells CE-marked Devices: N
General Admin.: Mr. Richard Powers/Executive Vice President
        Mr. Allen Hill/President, Chief Executive Officer
Mktg./Adv.: Mr. Joaquin Wolff/Commercial Director
        Mr. Chet Kumar/Vice President Business Development
Production: Mr. Yona Katz/Vice President Manufacturing
        Mr. Boris Aradovsky/Vice President Quality Assurance & Regulatory Affairs
Research: Mr. Eli Aharoni/Vice President Research & Development
Finance: Mr. Doron Raz/Vice President Admin., Finance

VISIOPTIC LTD.   **514-842-4601**
1117 St. Catherine St. W, Ste. 324,
Montreal, QUE H3B-1 Canada
FDA Number: n/a
Year Founded: 1973
Total Employees: 10
Ownership: Private
Produces/Sells CE-marked Devices: N
Distribution: Manufacturer Direct

VISTA LIGHTING   **800-576-2135**
1805 Pittsburg Ave., Erie, PA 16502
FDA Number: n/a   *Fax:* 800-576-2136
Web site: www.vistalighting.com
Annual Revenue: $0-$1 Million
Ownership: Jji Lighting Group
Produces/Sells CE-marked Devices: N
Federal Procurement Eligibility: Small Business
Distribution: Manufacturer Direct, Manufacturer Through Distributor, Manufacturer Through Manufacturer Reps
General Admin.: Steve Day/Vice President, General Manager
Production: Joel Gehley/Production Engineer

Console, Patient Service	General
Lamp, Examination (Light)	General
Lamp, Examination, Ceiling Mounted (Light)	General
Light, Other	General
Light, Overbed	General

VISTA MEDICAL LTD.   **1-800-822-3553**
3 - 55 Henlow Bay.,   **204-949-7676**
Winnipeg, MAN R3Y 1 Canada
FDA Number: n/a   *Fax:* 204-949-7650
E-mail: info@vista-medical.com
Web site: www.vistamedical.org
Year Founded: 1989
Total Employees: 25
Ownership: Private
Produces/Sells CE-marked Devices: N

VISTA MEDICAL LTD.
1-800-822-3553 *(cont'd)*
Distribution: Manufacturer Direct, Exclusive Distributor, Exporter

VISTA RESEARCH GROUP, LLC
419-281-3927
1554 Township Road 805, Ashland, OH 44805
FDA Number: 3004522772
Operative Dental Treatment Unit — Dental And Oral

VISTA TECHNOLOGY, INC.
888-468-0020
8432 45th St. NW,
780-468-0020
Edmonton, ALBER T6B-2 Canada
FDA Number: n/a — *Fax:* 780-465-9732
E-mail: sales@vistatechnology.com
Web site: www.vistatechnology.com
Year Founded: 1976
Total Employees: 10
Ownership: Private
Produces/Sells CE-marked Devices: N
Federal Procurement Eligibility: Small Business
Distribution: Manufacturer Direct, Exclusive Distributor, Exporter

VISTAKON, INC.
800-874-5278
7500 Centurion Pkwy, Jacksonville, FL 32256
904-443-1000
FDA Number: 1024871 — *Fax:* 904-443-1252
Web site: www.acuvue.com
Annual Revenue: $0-$1 Million
Total Employees: 600
Ownership: Public
Produces/Sells CE-marked Devices: N
Federal Procurement Eligibility: Minority Owned, Female Owned
Distribution: Manufacturer Direct
General Admin.: Gary Kunkel/President
John Cummings/Vice President
Mktg./Adv.: Richard DeWilde/Vice President Marketing
Thomas Harkleroad/Vice President Sales
Research: Ganesh Kumar/Vice President Research & Development
Lens, Contact (Other Material) — Ophthalmology
Lens, Contact, Disposable — Ophthalmology
Lens, Contact, Extended-Wear — Ophthalmology
Lens, Contact, Hydrophilic — Ophthalmology

VISUAIDE
888-723-7273
445, rue du Parc-Industriel,
450-463-1717
Longueil, QUE J4H 3 Canada
FDA Number: n/a — *Fax:* 450-463-0120
E-mail: ca.info@humanware.com
Web site: www.visuaide.com
Year Founded: 1988
Total Employees: 50
Ownership: Private
Produces/Sells CE-marked Devices: N
Distribution: Manufacturer Direct, Exclusive Distributor

VISUAL MED, INC.
800-324-4464
11110 West Lake Dr., Charlotte, NC 28273
FDA Number: 3005018279
Ownership: Private
Produces/Sells CE-marked Devices: N
System, Communication, Image, Digital — Radiology

VISUAL TELECOMMUNICATIONS NETWORK, INC
703-448-0999
2108 Beach Grove Place, Utica, NY 13501
FDA Number: 3004686793
Monitor, Blood Pressure, Indirect, Semi-Automatic — Cardiovascular

VISUALSONICS INC.
1-866-416-4636
3080 Yonge Street, Suite 6100,
416-484-5000
Toronto, ON M4N 3 Canada
FDA Number: 3003774756 — *Fax:* 416-484-5001
Web site: http://www.visualsonics.com
Year Founded: 1999
Ownership: Sonosite, Inc.
Produces/Sells CE-marked Devices: N

VISX INCORPORATED, A SUBSIDIARY OF AMO INC.
714-247-8656
1328 Kifer Road, Sunnyvale, CA 94089
FDA Number: 3005573878
Lamp, Slit, Biomicroscope, AC-Powered — Ophthalmology
Phacofragmentation Unit — Ophthalmology
Refractometer, Ophthalmic — Ophthalmology
System, Laser, Excimer, Ophthalmic — Ophthalmology

VITA NEEDLE COMPANY
781-444-1780
919 Great Plain Avenue, Needham, MA 02492
FDA Number: 1213680 — *Fax:* 781-444-3956

VITA NEEDLE COMPANY
781-444-1780 *(cont'd)*
E-mail: sales@vitaneedle.com
Web site: www.vitaneedle.com
Medical Products Sales Volume: $6,700,000
Annual Revenue: $1-$5 Million
Year Founded: 1932
Total Employees: 30 — *Marketing Staff:* 1 — *Sales Staff:* 4
Ownership: Private
Produces/Sells CE-marked Devices: N
Federal Procurement Eligibility: Small Business
Distribution: Manufacturer Direct, Manufacturer Through Distributor, OEM, Exporter
General Admin.: Frederick M. Hartman/President, Chief Executive Officer
Mktg./Adv.: Mr. Lance M. Kumm/Vice President Sales
Production: Daniel Howard/Director Quality Assurance
Richard Baudreau/Manager Engineering
Timothy Provost/Manager Materials
Michael A. Larosa/Manager Production
Finance: Mason N. Hartman/Treasurer
Cannula, Other — General
Component, Metal, Other — General
Fitting, Luer — General
Needle, Biopsy, Cardiovascular — Cardiovascular
Needle, Dental — Dental And Oral
Needle, Hypodermic — General
Needle, Hypodermic, Single Lumen With Syringe — General
Needle, Spinal, Short-Term — General

VITACARE MEDICAL PRODUCTS INC.
800-263-9068
331 Bowes Rd., Concorrd, ONT L4K-1J2 Canada
9056602433
FDA Number: n/a — *Fax:* 9056602427
E-mail: vitacare@vitacanada.ca
Web site: www.vitacare.ca
Year Founded: 1984
Total Employees: 25
Ownership: Private
Produces/Sells CE-marked Devices: N
Distribution: Manufacturer Direct, Exclusive Distributor

VITAID LTD.
800-267-9301
300 International Drive, Williamsville, NY 14221
416-633-3261
FDA Number: 1319310 — *Fax:* 800-655-5304
E-mail: support@vitaid.com
Web site: www.vitaid.com
Annual Revenue: $5-$10 Million
Year Founded: 1977
Total Employees: 10 — *Marketing Staff:* 1 — *Sales Staff:* 3
Ownership: Private
Produces/Sells CE-marked Devices: Y
Federal Procurement Eligibility: Small Business
Distribution: Exclusive Distributor, Importer
General Admin.: Will Stewart/President
Mktg./Adv.: Mr. Jeffrey Syrydiuk/Director Business Development
Catheter, Oxygen, Tracheal — Anesthesiology
Continuous Positive Airway Pressure Unit (CPAP, CPPB) — Anesthesiology
Device, Assist, CPR — Anesthesiology
Tube, Tracheal/Bronchial, Differential Ventilation — Anesthesiology

VITAIRE CORP.
800-447-4344
141 Lanza Ave., Bldg 12, 4th Floor,
-
Garfield, NJ 07026
FDA Number: 2431539 — *Fax:* 973-473-2244
Annual Revenue: $0-$1 Million
Total Employees: 15
Ownership: Private
Produces/Sells CE-marked Devices: N
Federal Procurement Eligibility: Small Business
Distribution: Manufacturer Direct
General Admin.: Peter Vayda/President
Equipment, Cleaning, Air — General
Filter, Air — General

VITAL CONCEPTS, INC.
800-984-2300
4334 Brockton Drive SE, Suite F,
616-871-6520
Grand Rapids, MI 49512
FDA Number: 1833708 — *Fax:* 616-871-6525
E-mail: info@vitcon.com
Web site: www.vitcon.com
Medical Products Sales Volume: $1,200,000
Annual Revenue: $1-$5 Million
Year Founded: 2003
Total Employees: 13 — *Marketing Staff:* 2 — *Sales Staff:* 2
Ownership: Private
Quality System Registration Information: ISO9001
Produces/Sells CE-marked Devices: Y
Federal Procurement Eligibility: Small Business

VITAL CONCEPTS, INC.   800-984-2300 *(cont'd)*

Distribution: Manufacturer Direct, Manufacturer Through Distributor, OEM, Exporter
General Admin.: Bernadette Morgan/Office Manager
    Douglas Sheehan/President, Chief Executive Officer
Production: Deborah Matko/Manager Quality Assurance & Quality Control

Contract Manufacturing	General
Contract Manufacturing, Product, Disposable	General
Filter, Air	General
Instrument, Microsurgical	Cns/Neurology
Knife, Laparoscopic	Surgery
Probe, Electrocauterization, Multi-Use	Surgery
Probe, Electrosurgery, Endoscopy	Surgery
Probe, Suction, Irrigator/Aspirator, Laparoscopic	Surgery
Pump, Aspiration, Portable	Anesthesiology
Service, Consulting	General
Sheet, Drape, Disposable	Surgery
Solution, Instrument, Laparoscopic, Anti-Fog	General
Tip, Suction	Anesthesiology
Tray, Custom/Special Procedure	General
Trocar, Laparoscopic	Surgery
Tube, Feeding	General
Tube, Suction	General
Tubing, Connecting	General
Tubing, Other	General
Valve, Other	Chemistry

VITAL CONNECTIONS, INC.   937-667-3880
955 N. Third St., Phoneton, OH 45371
FDA Number: 1527610

Adapter, Lead Switching, Electrocardiograph	Cardiovascular
Cable/Lead, ECG, With Transducer And Electrode	Cardiovascular

VITAL DIAGNOSTICS INC.   714-672-3553
1075 West Lambert Road, Unit D, Brea, CA 92821
FDA Number: 2032799
Ownership: Private
Produces/Sells CE-marked Devices: N

Azo-Dye, Calcium	Chemistry
Calibrator, Primary, Clinical Chemistry	Chemistry
Calibrator, Secondary, Clinical Chemistry	Chemistry
Catalytic Method, Amylase	Chemistry
Colorimetric Method, Lipoproteins	Chemistry
Complexone, Cresolphthalein, Calcium	Chemistry
Control, Multi Analyte, All Kinds (Assayed And Unassayed)	Chemistry
Dye-Binding, Albumin, Bromcresol, Green	Chemistry
Electrode, Blood pH	Chemistry
Electrode, Ion Specific, Chloride	Chemistry
Electrode, Ion Specific, Potassium	Chemistry
Electrode, Ion Specific, Sodium	Chemistry
Electrode, Ion Specific, Urea Nitrogen	Chemistry
Enzymatic Esterase-Oxidase, Cholesterol	Chemistry
Ferrozine (Colorimetric) Iron Binding Capacity	Chemistry
Hexokinase, Glucose	Chemistry
Kinetic Method, Gamma-Glutamyl Transpeptidase	Chemistry
LDL & VLDL Precipitation, Cholesterol Via Esterase-Oxidase	Chemistry
Lipase Hydrolysis/Glycerol Kinase Enzyme, Triglycerides	Chemistry
Multi Analyte Mixture, Calibrator	Chemistry
NAD Reduction/NADH Oxidation, CPK Or Isoenzymes	Chemistry
NAD Reduction/NADH Oxidation, Lactate Dehydrogenase	Chemistry
NADH Oxidation/NAD Reduction, AST/SGOT	Chemistry
Nitrophenylphosphate, Alkaline Phosphatase Or Isoenzymes	Chemistry
Phosphorus Reagent (Test System)	Chemistry
Photometric Method, Iron (Non-Heme)	Chemistry
Photometric Method, Magnesium	Chemistry
Reagent, Bilirubin (Total Or Direct Test System)	Chemistry
Reagent, Creatinine (Test System)	Chemistry
Reagent, Glucose (Test System)	Chemistry
Reagent, Protein, Total	Chemistry
SGPT, Ultraviolet	Chemistry
System, Test, Low-Density, Lipoprotein	Chemistry
Test, C-Reactive Protein, FITC	Immunology
Test, Glycosylated Hemoglobin Assay	Hematology
Urease And Glutamic Dehydrogenase, Urea Nitrogen	Chemistry
Uricase (Colorimetric), Uric Acid	Chemistry
pH Rate Measurement, Carbon-Dioxide	Chemistry

VITAL DIAGNOSTICS INC.   714-672-3553
27 Wellington Road, Lincoln, RI 02865
FDA Number: 3004088125
Ownership: Private
Produces/Sells CE-marked Devices: N

Analyzer, Sedimentation Rate, Automated	Hematology
Electrode, Ion Specific, Chloride	Chemistry
Electrode, Ion Specific, Potassium	Chemistry

VITAL IMAGES,INC.   800-231-0607
5850 Opus Parkway, Suite 300,   952-487-9500
Minnetonka,, MN 55343
FDA Number: 2134213   *Fax:* 952-487-9510
E-mail: info@vitalimages.com

VITAL IMAGES,INC.   800-231-0607 *(cont'd)*

Web site: www.vitalimages.com
Medical Products Sales Volume: $70,500,000
Annual Revenue: $10-$25 Million
Year Founded: 1988
Total Employees: 105   *Marketing Staff:* 6   *Sales Staff:* 30
Ownership: Public
Stock Symbol: VTAL
Traded On: NASDAQ
Quality System Registration Information: ISO9000
Produces/Sells CE-marked Devices: Y
Federal Procurement Eligibility: Small Business
Distribution: Manufacturer Direct, Manufacturer Through Distributor, OEM
General Admin.: Cindy Edwards/Director Human Resources
    Jay D. Miller/President, Chief Executive Officer
Medical Admin.: Vikas Narula/Director Clinical Affairs
Mktg./Adv.: James Chang/Manager International & National Sales
    Steve Canakes/Manager National Sales
    Nicole Gerszewski/Marketing Communications Specialist
    Phil Smith/Vice President Marketing
    Steven P. Canakes/Vice President Sales
Production: Steve Andersen/Director Quality Assurance & Regulatory Affairs
Research: Steve Anderson/Vice President Engineering
Finance: Greg Furness/Chief Financial Officer, Senior Vice President Finance
IS: Vincent Argiro/Chief Technologist

Computer and Software, Medical	General

VITAL METRICS
    See C. R. Bard, Inc., Bard Urological Div.

VITAL SIGNS COLORADO   1-800-932-0760
11039 E. Lansing Circle,   **(973) 790-1330**
Englewood, CO 80112
FDA Number: 1718887   *Fax:* 973-595-9013
E-mail: Customer Service@Vital-Signs.com
Web site: www.vital-signs.com
Annual Revenue: $1-$5 Million
Ownership: Vital Signs, Inc.
Produces/Sells CE-marked Devices: N
Distribution: Manufacturer Direct

Analyzer, Gas, Carbon-Dioxide, Gaseous Phase (Capnograph)	Anesthesiology
Cannula, Nasal, Oxygen	Anesthesiology
Circuit, Breathing (W Connector, Adapter, Y Piece)	Anesthesiology
Circuit, Breathing, Ventilator	Anesthesiology
Condenser, Heat And Moisture (Artificial Nose)	Anesthesiology
Connector, Airway (Extension)	Anesthesiology
Filter, Bacterial, Breathing Circuit	Anesthesiology
Filter, Gas	Anesthesiology
Head Rest, Neurosurgical	Cns/Neurology
Humidifier, Heated	Anesthesiology
Humidifier, Respiratory Gas, (Direct Patient Interface)	Anesthesiology
Kit, Sampling, Arterial Blood	Anesthesiology
Kit, Sampling, Blood Gas	General
Laryngoscope, Rigid	Anesthesiology
Mask, Other	General
Mask, Oxygen, Aerosol Administration	Anesthesiology
Monitor, Airway Pressure (Gauge/Alarm)	Anesthesiology
Nebulizer, Medicinal, Non-Ventilatory (Atomizer)	Anesthesiology
Nebulizer, Non-Heated	Anesthesiology
Needle, Hypodermic, Single Lumen With Syringe	General
Resuscitator, Pulmonary, Manual (Demand Valve)	General
Stethoscope, Esophageal	Anesthesiology
Stethoscope, Esophageal, With Electrical Conductors	Anesthesiology
Stylet, Tracheal Tube	Anesthesiology
Syringe, Arterial Blood Gas	Orthopedics
Thermometer, Electronic	General
Tube, Tracheal (Endotracheal)	Anesthesiology
Tube, Tracheostomy (W/Wo Connector)	Anesthesiology
Tubing, Oxygen Connecting	General
Tubing, Ventilator	Anesthesiology

VITAL SIGNS MN, INC.   973-790-1330
12250 Nicollet Ave., Burnsville, MN 55337
FDA Number: 2183188
E-mail: Customer Service@Vital-Signs.com
Web site: www.vital-signs.com
Ownership: Vital Signs, Inc.
Produces/Sells CE-marked Devices: N

Catheter, Intravascular, Diagnostic	Cardiovascular
Catheter, Irrigation	Surgery
Cuff, Blood Pressure	Cardiovascular
Head Rest, Neurosurgical	Cns/Neurology
Kit, Administration, Intravenous	General
Laparoscope, Gynecologic	Obstetrics/Gynecology
Pressure Infusor, IV Container	General

VITAL SIGNS, INC.   800-932-0760
20 Campus Road, Totowa, NJ 07512   973-790-1330
FDA Number: 2242551
E-mail: Customer Service@Vital-Signs.com

VITAL SIGNS, INC.   800-932-0760 *(cont'd)*

Web site: www.vital-signs.com
Year Founded: 1972
Ownership: GE HEALTHCARE
Stock Symbol: VITL
Traded On: NASDAQ
Quality System Registration Information: ISO9001; ISO9002; ISO9003
Produces/Sells CE-marked Devices: Y
Federal Procurement Eligibility: Small Business
Distribution: Manufacturer Direct, Manufacturer Through Distributor, Manufacturer Through Manufacturer Reps, OEM, Service Direct, Exclusive Distributor
General Admin.: Alex J. Chanin/Chief Information Officer
    Barry Wicker/Chief Operating Officer, Executive Vice President
    Terry D. Wall/President, Chief Executive Officer
    Jay Sturm/Vice President, General Counsel
Mktg./Adv.: Michael Kavinson/Vice President Global Marketing
    Mark Jefferson/Vice President Marketing & Sales
Production: Richard Gordon/Executive Vice President Operations
    Richard Kennedy/Manager Materials
    Anthony Martino/Vice President Quality Assurance & Regulatory Affairs

Airway, Oropharyngeal, Anesthesia	Anesthesiology
Analyzer, Gas, Carbon-Dioxide, Gaseous Phase (Capnograph)	Anesthesiology
Circuit, Breathing, Ventilator	Anesthesiology
Circulator, Breathing Circuit	Anesthesiology
Condenser, Heat And Moisture (Artificial Nose)	Anesthesiology
Connector, Airway (Extension)	Anesthesiology
Cuff, Blood Pressure	Cardiovascular
Exerciser, Respiratory	Anesthesiology
Infuser, Pressure (Blood Pump)	General
Laryngoscope	Ear/Nose/Throat
Mask, Face	General
Mask, Gas, Anesthesia	Anesthesiology
Mask, Other	General
Pressure Infusor, IV Container	General
Resuscitator, Pulmonary, Manual (Demand Valve)	General
Strap, Head, Gas Mask	Anesthesiology
Stylet, Tracheal Tube	Anesthesiology
Tube, Tracheostomy (W/Wo Connector)	Anesthesiology
Ventilator, Emergency, Manual (Resuscitator)	Anesthesiology

Medical Product Subsidiaries (Listed Separately)
  Enginivity Llc
  Thomas Medical Products, Inc.
  Vital Signs Colorado
  Vital Signs Mn, Inc.

VITAL TECHNOLOGY INC.
See Pace Tech, Inc.

VITALAIRE   800-661-8954
2000 Argentia Rd., Plaza 2, Ste. 200,   905-855-0440
Mississauga, ONT L5N-1 Canada
FDA Number: n/a   *Fax:* 905-855-0742
E-mail: vitalair@compusmart.ab.ca
Web site: www.vitalaire.ab.ca
Year Founded: 1995
Total Employees: 100
Ownership: Private
Produces/Sells CE-marked Devices: N
Distribution: Exclusive Distributor

VITALCALL
See Senior Technologies

VITALCOM, INC.   800-888-0077
15222 Del Amo Avenue, Tustin, CA 92780   714-546-0147
FDA Number: 7000871   *Fax:* 714-571-3945
E-mail: inquiries@vitalcom.com
Web site: www.vitalcom.com
Medical Products Sales Volume: $10,000,000
Annual Revenue: $10-$25 Million
Total Employees: 100   *Marketing Staff:* 5   *Sales Staff:* 21
Ownership: Ge Medical Systems Information Technologies
Stock Symbol: VCOM
Traded On: NASDAQ
Quality System Registration Information: ISO9001
Produces/Sells CE-marked Devices: Y
Federal Procurement Eligibility: Small Business
Distribution: Manufacturer Direct
General Admin.: Patrick Bradley/Associate Vice President
    Frank Sample/President, Chief Executive Officer
    Jack Graham/Vice President
Mktg./Adv.: Rex Cawley/Vice President Marketing
Production: Warren Cawley/Product Manager
Research: Stan Reese/Vice President Product Development
Finance: Shelley Thunen/Chief Financial Officer

Computer, Patient Data Management	General
Monitor, Cardiac (Cardiotachometer & Rate Alarm)	Cardiovascular
Telemetry Unit, Physiological, ECG	Cardiovascular

VITALCOM, INC.   800-888-0077 *(cont'd)*
Telemetry Unit, Physiological, Multiple Channel	General

VITALCOR, INC.   800-874-8358
100 East Chestnut Avenue, Westmont, IL 60559   630-325-5500
FDA Number: 1450019   *Fax:* 630-325-0257
E-mail: ghuck@vitalcor.com
Web site: www.vitalcor.com
Medical Products Sales Volume: $1,800,000
Year Founded: 1975
Total Employees: 5
Ownership: Private
Produces/Sells CE-marked Devices: Y
Federal Procurement Eligibility: Small Business, GSA Contract, VA Contract
Distribution: Manufacturer Direct, Manufacturer Through Distributor, Manufacturer Through Manufacturer Reps, Exclusive Distributor, Exporter
General Admin.: Mr. William Huck/Chief Executive Officer, Chairman
Mktg./Adv.: Mr. Gregory Huck/Vice President National Marketing & Sales
Production: Ms. Melinda Marzigliano/Manager Operations

Cable, Laser, Fiberoptic	Surgery
Cannula, Catheter	Cardiovascular
Catheter, Flow Directed	Cardiovascular
Catheter, Intravascular, Diagnostic	Cardiovascular
Catheter, Vascular, Cardiopulmonary Bypass	Cardiovascular
Filter, Blood, Cardiotomy Suction Line, Cardiopulmonary	Cardiovascular
Light, Headband, Surgical	Surgery
Light, Surgical, Fiberoptic	Surgery
Light, Surgical, Instrument	Surgery
Reservoir, Blood, Cardiopulmonary Bypass	Cardiovascular
Retractor, Surgical	Surgery

VITALOG MONITORING, INC.
See Vitalog, Inc

VITALOG, INC   650-366-8676
643 Bair Island Road #212, Redwood City, CA 94063-2754
FDA Number: 9201121   *Fax:* 650-368-5779
E-mail: info@vitalog-med.com
Web site: www.vitalog-med.comcontact.html
Medical Products Sales Volume: $1,000,000
Annual Revenue: $1-$5 Million
Year Founded: 1988
Total Employees: 11   *Marketing Staff:* 3   *Sales Staff:* 2
Ownership: Private
Produces/Sells CE-marked Devices: N
Federal Procurement Eligibility: Small Business, GSA Contract
Distribution: Manufacturer Direct, Manufacturer Through Manufacturer Reps, Importer
General Admin.: Jason Jianguo Sun/President, Chief Executive Officer

Monitor, ECG, Ambulatory, Real-Time	Cardiovascular
Monitor, Physiological, Acute Care	Anesthesiology

VITALOGRAPH, INC.   800-255-6626
13310 W 99th Street, Lenexa, KS 66215
FDA Number: 1924305   *Fax:* 913-888-4259
E-mail: vitcs@vitalograph.com
Web site: www.vitalograph.com
Year Founded: 1971
Ownership: Private
Produces/Sells CE-marked Devices: Y
Distribution: Manufacturer Direct

Analyzer, Gas, Carbon-Monoxide, Gaseous Phase	Anesthesiology
Aspirator, Emergency Suction	General
Computer, Pulmonary Function Data	Anesthesiology
Filter, Bacterial, Breathing Circuit	Anesthesiology
Kit, Emergency, Cardiopulmonary Resuscitation	General
Mask, Face	General
Meter, Peak Flow, Spirometry	Anesthesiology
Mouthpiece, Breathing	Anesthesiology
Reagent, Test, Carbon Monoxide	Toxicology
Recorder, Long-Term, ECG, Portable (Holter Monitor)	Cardiovascular
Resuscitator, Pulmonary, Manual (Demand Valve)	General
Spirometer, Diagnostic (Respirometer)	Anesthesiology
Spirometer, Monitoring (Volumeter)	Anesthesiology
Spirometer, Therapeutic (Incentive)	Anesthesiology
Syringe, Calibration Testing, Spirometer	Anesthesiology

VITALWORKS   800-278-0037
239 Ethan Allen Pky., Ridgefield, CT 06877
FDA Number: n/a   *Fax:* 203-438-8416
E-mail: info@vitalworks.com
Web site: www.vitalworks.com
Ownership: Public
Stock Symbol: VWKS
Traded On: NASDAQ
Produces/Sells CE-marked Devices: N
Distribution: Exclusive Distributor
General Admin.: Joseph M. Walsh/President, Chief Executive Officer
    C. Darren McCormick/Vice President

Computer Software	General

VITALWORKS 800-278-0037 *(cont'd)*
Computer, Radiographic Data — Radiology

VITAMEDICS CORPORATION 800-216-2724x10
19142 S. Molalla Ave., Oregon City, OR 97045-8975
FDA Number: n/a — Fax: 503-656-2992
E-mail: orders@vitamedics.com
Web site: www.vitamedics.com
Annual Revenue: $0-$1 Million
Ownership: Private
Produces/Sells CE-marked Devices: Y
Federal Procurement Eligibility: Small Business, Female Owned
Distribution: Manufacturer Direct, Manufacturer Through Distributor, Service Direct, Exclusive Distributor, Exporter
General Admin.: Anna Rousett/Shipping Manager
Mktg./Adv.: Russ Johnson/Website Administrator
Analyzer, Composition, Weight, Patient — General
Computer Equipment — General
Recorder, Long-Term, Blood Pressure, Portable — Cardiovascular
Recorder, Long-Term, ECG, Portable (Holter Monitor) — Cardiovascular
Spirometer, Monitoring (Volumeter) — Anesthesiology

VITRO DIAGNOSTICS, INC. 303-999-2130
4621 Technology Drive, Golden, CO 80403
FDA Number: n/a — Fax: 303-762-1240
E-mail: Jim@Vitrodiag.com
Web site: http://www.vitrodiag.com
Ownership: Public
Stock Symbol: VODG
Traded On: OTC Bulletin
Produces/Sells CE-marked Devices: N
General Admin.: Dr. Jim Musick/Chief Executive Officer
Finance: Duane Knight/Financial Executive
Immunochemical, Lysozyme (Muramidase) — Chemistry

VIVATONE HEARING SYSTEMS, LLC 203-341-9100
One Gorham Island, Westport, CT 06880
FDA Number: 3004422401
Hearing-Aid — Ear/Nose/Throat

VIVAX MEDICAL CORP. 866-847-7890 / 860-489-7890
89 Putter Ln., Torrington, CT 06790
FDA Number: 1224873 — Fax: 860-489-7935
E-mail: info@vivaxmedical.com
Web site: www.vivaxmedical.com
Medical Products Sales Volume: $2,000,000
Annual Revenue: $1-$5 Million
Year Founded: 1984
Total Employees: 12 — Marketing Staff: 1 — Sales Staff: 3
Ownership: Vivax Medical Corp.
Produces/Sells CE-marked Devices: Y
Distribution: Manufacturer Direct, Manufacturer Through Distributor, Manufacturer Through Manufacturer Reps, Service Direct
General Admin.: Thomas Ellen/Chief Executive Officer, Chairman; John Gildea/General Manager
Mktg./Adv.: Richard Swanson/Vice President Marketing & Sales
Production: Jack Brown/Manager Manufacturing
Finance: Handel You/Chief Financial Officer
Bed, Adjustable Hospital — General
Patient Transfer Unit, Powered — General
Restraint, Protective (Body) — General
Transfer Device, Patient, Manual — General

VIVERSATRONICS
See Varitronics, Inc.

VIVEVE INC. 650-321-3332
450 Sheridan Ave., Palo Alto, CA 94306
FDA Number: 3008175701 — Fax: 650-326-0114
Web site: http://www.viveve.com
Year Founded: 2005
Ownership: Private
Produces/Sells CE-marked Devices: N
General Admin.: Mr. Kerry Pope/Chief Executive Officer
Mktg./Adv.: Ms. Sherree Lucas/Senior Vice President Marketing
Production: Mr. Steve Lopez/Director Operations; Mr. Alan Curtis/Vice President Quality Control & Regulatory Affairs
Electrosurgical Unit, Cutting & Coagulation Device — Surgery

VIVUS, INC. 650-934-5200
1172 Castro St., Mountain View, CA 94040
FDA Number: n/a — Fax: 650-934-5389
E-mail: ir@vivus.com
Web site: www.vivus.com
Medical Products Sales Volume: $17,240,000
Annual Revenue: $25-$50 Million
Year Founded: 1991
Total Employees: 35 — Marketing Staff: 3 — Sales Staff: 10
Ownership: Public

VIVUS, INC. 650-934-5200 *(cont'd)*
Stock Symbol: VVUS
Traded On: NASDAQ
Quality System Registration Information: ISO9001
Federal Procurement Eligibility: Small Business, Female Owned
Distribution: Manufacturer Through Distributor, Manufacturer Through Manufacturer Reps, Exporter
General Admin.: Leland F. Wilson/President, Chief Executive Officer
Mktg./Adv.: Mike O'Meara/Director National Accounts; Lon Roberts/Manager National Sales; Terry Nida/Vice President International Marketing & Sales
Production: Guy Marsh/Vice President Manufacturing; John Dietrich/Vice President Regulatory Affairs
Finance: Richard Walliser/Chief Financial Officer
Device, Dysfunction, Erectile — Gastroenterology/Urology
System, Delivery, Drug, Non-invasive — General

VIVVID INTERNATIONAL 447-040-4013
800 Fern Creek Ave., Orlando, FL 32803
FDA Number: 3006214514
Ownership: Private
Produces/Sells CE-marked Devices: N
Lens, Spectacle (prescription), For Reading Discomfort — Ophthalmology
Lens, Spectacle/Eyeglasses, Non-Custom — Ophthalmology

VLV ASSOCIATES, INC. 973-428-2884
30-C Ridgedale Ave., East Hanover, NJ 07936
FDA Number: 2245539 — Fax: 973-428-2877
E-mail: mv@vlvassociates.com
Web site: www.vlvassociates.com
Annual Revenue: $1-$5 Million
Year Founded: 1982
Total Employees: 28 — Sales Staff: 2
Ownership: Private
Produces/Sells CE-marked Devices: N
Federal Procurement Eligibility: Small Business
Distribution: Manufacturer Through Distributor
General Admin.: Mr. Michael Vaillancourt/President
Biopsy Device, Endomyocardial — Cardiovascular
Forceps, General & Plastic Surgery — Surgery
Introducer, Catheter — Cardiovascular
Kit, Administration, Intravenous — General
Needle, Aspiration And Injection, Disposable — Surgery
Needle, Biopsy, Cardiovascular — Cardiovascular
Needle, Other — General

VMED TECHNOLOGY, INC. (FORMERLY EMS PRODUCTS, INC.) 425-497-9149
16149 Redmond Way #108, Redmond, WA 98052
FDA Number: 2919127 — Fax: 425-497-0260
E-mail: info@vmedtech.com
Web site: www.vmedtech.com
Medical Products Sales Volume: $1,500,000
Annual Revenue: $0-$1 Million
Year Founded: 1990
Total Employees: 5 — Marketing Staff: 1 — Sales Staff: 1
Ownership: Private
Produces/Sells CE-marked Devices: N
Federal Procurement Eligibility: Small Business, VA Contract
Distribution: Manufacturer Direct
General Admin.: Paul D. Ulbrich/Chief Executive Officer
Detector, Blood Flow, Ultrasonic (Doppler) — Cardiovascular
Equipment, Ultrasound, Doppler, Evaluation, Fetal — Obstetrics/Gynecology
Monitor, Blood Flow, Ultrasonic — Obstetrics/Gynecology

VMG MEDICAL, INC. 540-337-1996
542 Walnut Hills Rd., Staunton, VA 24401
FDA Number: 1123402
Component, Traction, Non-Invasive — Orthopedics
Halter, Head, Traction, Orthopedic — Orthopedics
Orthosis, Cervical — Physical Med
Traction Unit, Non-Powered — Orthopedics

VNA SYSTEMS, INC. 404-264-0160
1414 Epping Forest Dr., Atlanta, GA 30319
FDA Number: 1038328
Ownership: Private
Produces/Sells CE-marked Devices: N
Computer and Software, Medical — General

VNUS MEDICAL TECHNOLOGIES, INC. 888-797-8346 / 408-360-7200
5799 Fontanoso Way, San Jose, CA 95138
FDA Number: 2953189 — Fax: 408-365-8480
E-mail: info@vnus.com
Web site: www.vnus.com
Annual Revenue: $50-$100 Million
Year Founded: 1995
Ownership: Public

VNUS MEDICAL TECHNOLOGIES, INC.   888-797-8346 (cont'd)
Stock Symbol: VNUS
Traded On: NASDAQ
Produces/Sells CE-marked Devices: N
General Admin.: Mr. Brian E. Farley/President, Chief Executive Officer
Production: Mr. Mohan F. Sancheti/Vice President Manufacturing
     Mr. William A. Franklin/Vice President Quality Assurance & Regulatory Affairs
Research: Mr. Kirti Kamdar/Senior Vice President Research
Finance: Mr. Peter Osborne/Chief Financial Officer, Vice President Finance

Catheter, Continuous Flush	Cardiovascular
Dilator, Vessel, Percutaneous Catheterization	Cardiovascular
Drape, Surgical	Surgery
Electrosurgical Unit, Cutting & Coagulation Device	Surgery
Forceps, General & Plastic Surgery	Surgery
Guide, Surgical, Needle	Surgery
Guidewire, Catheter	Cardiovascular
Hook, Surgical, General & Plastic Surgery	Surgery
Introducer, Catheter	Cardiovascular
Kit, Surgical (General)	Surgery

VOCAL LABS   360-736-7123
114 W. Pear St., Centralia, WA 98531
FDA Number: 3025260
E-mail: vocallab@comcast.net   *Fax:* 360-736-3373
Total Employees: 5
Ownership: Private
Produces/Sells CE-marked Devices: N
Federal Procurement Eligibility: Small Business

Hearing-Aid	Ear/Nose/Throat

VOCEL   858-679-1919
13400 Sabre Springs Parkway, Suite 255, Rancho Bernardo, CA 92128
FDA Number: 3005960023

Reminder, Medication	Physical Med

VOLCANO CORPORATION   800-228-4728
3661 Valley Centre Drive, Suite 200,   **916-638-8008**
San Diego, CA 92130
FDA Number: 2939520
E-mail: info@volcanocorp.com   *Fax:* 916-638-8812
Web site: www.volcanocorp.com
Year Founded: 2001
Ownership: Public
Stock Symbol: VOLC
Traded On: NASDAQ
Produces/Sells CE-marked Devices: N
General Admin.: John Dahldorf/Chief Financial Officer, Secretary
     David Sheehan/Executive Vice President
     Junichi Osawa/President
     Michel Lussier/President International Operations
     Scott Huennekens/President, Chief Executive Officer
Mktg./Adv.: Joseph Burnett/Executive Vice President Marketing
     George Quinoy/Vice President International Sales
Research: Geoffrey Vince/Vice President Clinical Research

Catheter, Angioplasty, Coronary, Transluminal, Percut. Oper.	Cardiovascular
Catheter, Intravascular, Diagnostic	Cardiovascular
Flowmeter, Blood, Intravenous	Cardiovascular
Guidewire, Catheter	Cardiovascular
Monitor, Physiological, Patient(without Arrhythmia Detection Or Alarms)	Cardiovascular
Scanner, Ultrasonic (Pulsed Echo)	Radiology
Transducer, Blood Pressure, Catheter Tip	Cardiovascular
Transducer, Ultrasonic	Cardiovascular
Transducer, Ultrasonic, Diagnostic	Radiology

VOLK OPTICAL INC.   800-345-8655
7893 Enterprise Drive, Mentor, OH 44060-5309   **440-942-6161**
FDA Number: 1528142   *Fax:* 440-942-2257
E-mail: volk@volk.com
Web site: www.volk.com
Medical Products Sales Volume: $2,500,000
Year Founded: 1974
Total Employees: 50
Ownership: HALMA, PLC
Quality System Registration Information: ISO9001
Produces/Sells CE-marked Devices: Y
Federal Procurement Eligibility: Small Business
Distribution: Manufacturer Direct, Manufacturer Through Distributor, Manufacturer Through Manufacturer Reps, OEM
General Admin.: Peter L. Mastores/President, Chief Executive Officer
Mktg./Adv.: Stephen E. Spisak/Manager International & National Sales
     Mr. Tim Warrell/Manager Marketing
     John Strobel/Vice President Marketing & Sales
Production: Michaeleen Dom/Manager Regulatory Affairs
     Bernard D. Rykaczewski/Vice President Manufacturing
Research: Steven Cech/Vice President Research & Engineering

VOLK OPTICAL INC.   800-345-8655 (cont'd)
Finance: Gary Webel/Chief Financial Officer, Vice President Finance

Lens, Other	Ophthalmology

VOLPI MANUFACTURING USA CO., INC.   315-255-1737
5 Commerce Way, Auburn, NY 13021-1045
FDA Number: 3000239652
Ownership: Private
Produces/Sells CE-marked Devices: N

Accessories, Photographic, Endoscopic	Gastroenterology/Urology

VOLTARC TECHNOLOGIES, INC.   203-578-4600
400 Captain Neville Drive, Waterbury, CT 06705
FDA Number: 1282759   *Fax:* 203-575-3456
E-mail: customer.service@voltarc.com
Web site: www.voltarc.com
Medical Products Sales Volume: $18,000,000
Annual Revenue: $25-$50 Million
Year Founded: 1927
Total Employees: 270   *Marketing Staff:* 2   *Sales Staff:* 10
Ownership: Private
Quality System Registration Information: ISO9000
Produces/Sells CE-marked Devices: N
Federal Procurement Eligibility: Small Business, Minority Owned
Distribution: Manufacturer Direct, Manufacturer Through Distributor, OEM
General Admin.: John J. Andros/Vice President, General Manager
Mktg./Adv.: Robert Spilatore/National Sales Representative

Lamp, Ultraviolet, Physical Medicine	Physical Med

VOLTARC TECHNOLOGIES, INC.
See Perkinelmer Optoelectronics

VOLU-SOL, INC.   801-974-9474
2100 South 5095 West, Salt Lake City, UT 84121
FDA Number: 3002805583   *Fax:* 801-974-9553
E-mail: manager@shopvolusol.com
Web site: www.shopvolusol.com
Annual Revenue: $1-$5 Million
Ownership: Private
Produces/Sells CE-marked Devices: N
Federal Procurement Eligibility: Small Business
Distribution: Manufacturer Through Distributor, Exporter

Buffer, pH	Hematology
Stain, Giemsa, Hematology	Hematology
Stain, Microbiological	Microbiology
Stain, Other	Pathology
Stain, Wright's	Pathology
Stain, Wright's, Hematology	Hematology

VOMARIS INNOVATIONS INC.   866-4 YOUR HEAL
3100 W. Ray Rd, Suite 148,   **480-921-4948**
Chandler, AZ 85226
FDA Number: 3005803853
E-mail: info@vomaris.com
Web site: www.vomaris.com
Ownership: Private
Produces/Sells CE-marked Devices: N
General Admin.: William J. Miller/Chief Operating Officer
     Jeffry B. Skiba/President, Chief Executive Officer

Dressing, Other	General

VON LONDON PHONIX CO   713-772-6666
6103 Glenmont, Houston, TX 77081-1499
FDA Number: 7000295   *Fax:* 713-772-4671
E-mail: mike@phoenixelectrode.com
Web site: www.vl-pc.com
Annual Revenue: $5-$10 Million
Year Founded: 1981
Total Employees: 100   *Marketing Staff:* 10   *Sales Staff:* 10
Ownership: Private
Produces/Sells CE-marked Devices: N
Federal Procurement Eligibility: Small Business
Distribution: Manufacturer Through Distributor, OEM
General Admin.: Ray Burchette/President
     Mike Reif/Vice President, General Manager
Research: Peter Boyle/Vice President Research & Development

Electrode, Ion Selective (Non-Specified)	Chemistry
Electrode, Laboratory pH	Chemistry
Electrode, pH	Gastroenterology/Urology
Meter, pH, Portable	Chemistry

VON WEISE ENGINEERING
See Elite Mattress Manufacturing

VON ZABERN SURGICAL   951-734-7215
4121 Tigris Way, Riverside, CA 92503
FDA Number: 2030599

Orthopedic Manual Surgical Instrument	Orthopedics

VONCO PRODUCTS, INC.
800-323-9077
201 Park Avenue, Lake Villa, IL 60046-8916
847-356-2323
FDA Number: 1419562
Fax: 847-356-8630
E-mail: sales@vonco.com
Web site: www.vonco.com
Annual Revenue: $0-$1 Million
Year Founded: 1955
Total Employees: 125   Marketing Staff: 5   Sales Staff: 6
Ownership: Private
Produces/Sells CE-marked Devices: N
Federal Procurement Eligibility: Small Business
Distribution: Manufacturer Direct, Manufacturer Through Distributor, Manufacturer Through Manufacturer Reps, Exporter
General Admin.: L. Lawrence Laske/Chief Executive
Mktg./Adv.: Mr. Gary Link/National Sales Representative
        Les Laske/Vice President Sales
Production: John LaRoi/Vice President Manufacturing
Purchasing: Tom Laske/Manager Purchasing
  Bag, Ice   General
  Container, Specimen Mailer And Storage   Pathology
  Contract Manufacturing, Product, Disposable   General
  Packaging Equipment   General
  Packaging Material   General

VONEX MEDICAL SUPPLIES INC.
888-866-3920
29-601 Magnetic Dr., Toronto M3J 3J2 Canada
FDA Number: 9617861
Fax: 416-736-6961
E-mail: yury@vonex-medical.com
Web site: www.vonex-medical.com
Year Founded: 1998
Total Employees: 7   Sales Staff: 1
Ownership: Private
Produces/Sells CE-marked Devices: N
Federal Procurement Eligibility: Small Business
Distribution: Manufacturer Direct

VORTRAN MEDICAL TECHNOLOGY
800-434-4034
21 Golden Land Court, Sacramento, CA 95834
916-648-8460
FDA Number: 2951529
Fax: 916-648-9751
E-mail: office@vortran.com
Web site: www.vortran.com
Medical Products Sales Volume: $1,700,000
Annual Revenue: $0-$1 Million
Year Founded: 1997
Total Employees: 18   Marketing Staff: 2
Ownership: Private
Quality System Registration Information: ISO9003
Produces/Sells CE-marked Devices: N
Federal Procurement Eligibility: Small Business, Minority Owned
Distribution: Manufacturer Direct, Manufacturer Through Distributor, Exclusive Distributor
General Admin.: Gordon A. Wong/President
Mktg./Adv.: Merrily Wong/Director Communications
        Jody McCarthy/Director Marketing & Sales
        James Lee/Vice President Marketing & Engineering
Production: Ray Saied/Director Quality Control & Regulatory Affairs
        Glen Thomson/Vice President, Engineer
  Ventilator, Emergency, Powered (Resuscitator)   Anesthesiology

VORUM RESEARCH CORPORATION
800-461-4353
8765 Ash St., Ste. 6,
604-321-7277
Vancouver, BC V6P-6 Canada
FDA Number: n/a
Fax: 604-321-5345
E-mail: canfit@vorum.com
Web site: www.vorum.com
Year Founded: 1989
Total Employees: 16
Ownership: Private
Produces/Sells CE-marked Devices: Y
Distribution: Manufacturer Direct, OEM, Exporter

VOSS MEDICAL PRODUCTS
210-650-3124
4235 Centergate, San Antonio, TX 78217
FDA Number: 1643116
Fax: 210-650-8032
E-mail: vosstec@aol.com
Web site: www.vosstech.com
Medical Products Sales Volume: $3,000,000
Annual Revenue: $1-$5 Million
Year Founded: 1986
Total Employees: 20   Marketing Staff: 1   Sales Staff: 2
Ownership: Voss Technologies Inc
Produces/Sells CE-marked Devices: N
Federal Procurement Eligibility: Small Business
Distribution: Manufacturer Direct
Production: Brady Bragg/Vice President Manufacturing & Operations
Finance: Sara Voss/Chief Financial Officer
  Catheter, Vascular, Cardiopulmonary Bypass   Cardiovascular

VOSS MEDICAL PRODUCTS
210-650-3124 (cont'd)
  Clamp, Vascular   Cardiovascular
  Marker, Ostia, Aorto-Saphenous Vein   Surgery
  Positioner, Socket   Orthopedics
  Table, Operating Room, AC-Powered   Surgery

VOYAGER MEDICAL CORP.
503-223-3881
5550 S.w. Macadam Ave. #310, Portland, OR 97239
FDA Number: 3030962
Ownership: Private
Produces/Sells CE-marked Devices: N
  Massager, Therapeutic   Physical Med

VPI CORPORATION .
  See Coeur Inc., Sheboygan

VPI EXTRUDED PROFILES DIV.
  See Coeur Inc., Sheboygan

VPI MEDICAL PRODUCTS DIV.
  See Coeur Inc., Sheboygan

VQ ORTHOCARE
1390 Decision Street, Suite A, Vista, CA 92081
FDA Number: 2031823
  Brace, Joint, Ankle (External)   Physical Med
  Cover, Limb   Physical Med
  Joint, Knee, External Brace   Physical Med
  Orthosis, Limb Brace   Physical Med
  Orthosis, Lumbosacral   Physical Med
  Prosthesis Alignment Device   Physical Med
  Support, Arm   Physical Med
  Tape, Measuring, Ruler And Caliper   Surgery

VSM HEALTHCARE PRODUCTS
330-673-8227
15547 Main Market Road, Parkman, OH 44080
FDA Number: 1527496
Fax: 330-673-8227
E-mail: OMG369@aol.com
Medical Products Sales Volume: $1,500,000
Annual Revenue: $1-$5 Million
Year Founded: 1983
Total Employees: 15
Ownership: Private
Produces/Sells CE-marked Devices: N
Distribution: Manufacturer Direct, Manufacturer Through Manufacturer Reps, Importer
General Admin.: Mr. Owen Grant/Chief Executive Officer
  Pack, Hot Or Cold, Reusable   Physical Med

VSM MEDTECH (FORMERLY CTF SYSTEMS)
604-540-6044 ex
Unit 1, 1850 Hartley Avenue, Coquitlam, BC V3K 7A1 Canada
FDA Number: n/a
Fax: 604-540-6099
E-mail: sales@ctfmeg.com
Web site: www.vsmmedtech.com
Year Founded: 1970
Total Employees: 100
Ownership: Public
Stock Symbol: VSM
Traded On: Toronto
Produces/Sells CE-marked Devices: Y
Distribution: Manufacturer Direct, Manufacturer Through Distributor, Manufacturer Through Manufacturer Reps, OEM, Service Direct, Exporter

VSM MEDTECH LTD.
604-738-8763
675 West Hastings St., 15th Floor,
Vancouver, BC V6B-1 Canada
FDA Number: n/a
Fax: 604-738-8762
E-mail: corp@vsmmedtech.com
Web site: www.vsmmedtech.com
Year Founded: 1995
Total Employees: 25
Ownership: Private
Produces/Sells CE-marked Devices: N
Distribution: Manufacturer Direct, Exporter

VTS MEDICAL SYSTEMS, INC.
516-249-1703
40 Melville Park Rd., Melville, NY 11747
FDA Number: 1000404456
  Accessories, Surgical Camera   Surgery
  Camera, Television, Surgical (Without Audio)   Surgery

VULCON TECHNOLOGIES
888-522-7746
718 Main St., Grandview, MO 64030
816-966-1212
FDA Number: 1931439
Fax: 816-966-8879
Web site: www.vulcon.com
Ownership: Private
Produces/Sells CE-marked Devices: N
  Blender/Mixer   Chemistry
  Centrifuge, Cell Washing   Hematology
  Hematocrit, Manual   Hematology

MANUFACTURER PROFILES

VULCON TECHNOLOGIES   888-522-7746 *(cont'd)*
Mixer/Scale, Blood   Hematology

VWR CANLAB   800-932-5000
2360 Argentia Rd.,   905-813-7377
Mississauga, ONT L5N-5 Canada
FDA Number: n/a   *Fax:* 905-813-5244
E-mail: solutions@vwrsp.com
Web site: www.vwrsp.com
Year Founded: 1988
Ownership: Private
Produces/Sells CE-marked Devices: N
Distribution: Exclusive Distributor

VYCOR MEDICAL INC   561-558-2020
3651 FAU Blvd, Suite 300, Boca Raton, FL 33431
FDA Number: 3005880844
Ownership: Private   *Fax:* 631.244.1436
Produces/Sells CE-marked Devices: N
Retractor, Self-Retaining   Gastroenterology/Urology

VYGON CORP.   800-473-5414
103a Park Drive, Montgomeryville, PA 18936
FDA Number: 2245270
E-mail: jleaity@vygonusa.com   *Fax:* 215-672-6740
Web site: www.vygonusa.com
Medical Products Sales Volume: $50,000,000
Year Founded: 1962
Total Employees: 7   *Marketing Staff:* 3   *Sales Staff:* 3
Ownership: Vygon S A
Quality System Registration Information: ISO9001
Produces/Sells CE-marked Devices: Y
Federal Procurement Eligibility: Small Business
Distribution: Manufacturer Through Distributor, Manufacturer Through
Manufacturer Reps, OEM, Importer
General Admin.: Roger M. Severn/President, Chief Executive Officer
      John A. Leaity/Vice President

Accessories, Catheter	Surgery
Adapter, Catheter	Surgery
Adapter, Stopcock, Manifold, Cardiopulmonary Bypass	Cardiovascular
Adapter, Syringe	General
Adapter, Y	Gastroenterology/Urology
Bag, Collection, Urine, Newborn	General
Bag, Leg	Gastroenterology/Urology
Bag, Urinary Collection	General
Brush, Scrub, Operating Room	Surgery
Cannula, Epidural	Obstetrics/Gynecology
Cannula, Nasal, Oxygen	Anesthesiology
Catheter, Epidural	Obstetrics/Gynecology
Catheter, Intraspinal, Subcutaneous, Implantable	General
Catheter, Intravenous	Cardiovascular
Catheter, Intravenous, Central	Cardiovascular
Catheter, Multiple Lumen	Surgery
Catheter, Nasal, Oxygen (Tube)	Anesthesiology
Catheter, Pediatric, General & Plastic Surgery	Surgery
Catheter, Perfusion	Cardiovascular
Catheter, Peritoneal Dialysis, Single-Use	Gastroenterology/Urology
Catheter, Rectal	Surgery
Catheter, Suction (Tracheal Aspirating Tube)	Anesthesiology
Catheter, Suction, With Tip	General
Catheter, Umbilical Artery	General
Collector, Urine	Gastroenterology/Urology
Connector, Catheter	Surgery
Connector, Tubing, Blood, Infusion, T-Type	Gastroenterology/Urology
Dilator, Vessel	Gastroenterology/Urology
Drain, Sump	Gastroenterology/Urology
Drain, Thoracic (Chest)	Anesthesiology
Drainage System, Urine, Closed	Gastroenterology/Urology
Drape, Surgical	Surgery
Dressing, Other	General
Dressing, Permeable, Moisture	General
Fitting, Luer	General
Hanger, Intravenous	General
Introducer, Catheter	Cardiovascular
Kit, Administration, Intravenous	General
Kit, Anesthesia, Epidural	Anesthesiology
Kit, Blood, Transfusion	General
Kit, Catheter Care	General
Kit, Catheterization, Intravenous, Winged	Cardiovascular
Kit, Chest Drainage (Thoracentesis Tray)	General
Kit, Intravenous Extension Tubing	General
Kit, Wound Dressing	Surgery
Needle, Intravenous	General
Needle, Scalp	Cns/Neurology
Needle, Spinal, Short-Term	General
Stopcock	General
Stylet, Catheter	Cardiovascular
Stylet, Needle	General
Syringe, Bulb	General
Trap, Mucus	Anesthesiology

VYGON CORP.   800-473-5414 *(cont'd)*

Tube, Feeding	General
Tube, Gastrointestinal	Gastroenterology/Urology
Tube, Stomach Evacuator (Gastric Lavage)	Gastroenterology/Urology
Tube, Suction	General
Tube, Tracheal (Endotracheal)	Anesthesiology
Tubing, Connecting	General
Tubing, Multi-Lumen	General
Tubing, Oxygen Connecting	General
Tubing, Silicone	General
Tubing, Urethane	General

Medical Product Subsidiaries (Listed Separately)
Churchill Medical Systems, Inc.

VYNACRON DENTAL CO.   800-932-7612
6 Orchard Hill Dr., Englishtown, NJ 07726
FDA Number: 2242866
E-mail: sales@vynacron.com,   *Fax:* (732) 928-0096
Annual Revenue: $0-$1 Million
Total Employees: 2
Ownership: Public
Produces/Sells CE-marked Devices: N
Federal Procurement Eligibility: Small Business
Distribution: Manufacturer Direct
General Admin.: Steven Daidone/President
   Base, Denture, Relining, Repairing, Rebasing, Resin   Dental And Oral

VYNACRON DENTAL RESINS, INC.   732-780-6728
1751 Hwy. 9 N., Howell, NJ 07731
FDA Number: 2242866
   Base, Denture, Relining, Repairing, Rebasing, Resin   Dental And Oral

VYSIS   800-553-7042
3100 Woodcreek Drive,   630-271-7000
Downers Grove, IL 60515
FDA Number: n/a
E-mail: vysis-help@vysis.com   *Fax:* 630-271-7138
Web site: www.vysis.com
Medical Products Sales Volume: $11,400,000
Annual Revenue: $25-$50 Million
Year Founded: 1991
Total Employees: 100
Ownership: ATC DIAGNOSTICS, INC.
Traded On: NASDAQ
Quality System Registration Information: ISO9001
Federal Procurement Eligibility: Small Business
Distribution: Manufacturer Direct
General Admin.: John Bishop/Chief Executive Officer
     Susan Zint/Director Human Resources
Mktg./Adv.: Rob Koska/Manager Marketing
     Jim Naumann/Manager National Sales
     Kent Hertzing/Vice President Business Development
     George Kennedy/Vice President Marketing & Sales
Production: Jim Marcella/Vice President Operations
     Russ Enns/Vice President Regulatory Affairs
     russ Enns/Vice President Regulatory Affairs
Research: Steve Seelig/Vice President Research & Development
Finance: Jim Habschmidt/Vice President Finance

Analyzer, Karyotype	Pathology
Probe, Other	General
Test, Cancer Detection, DNA-Probe	Immunology

VYTERIS, INC.   201-703-2299
13-01 Pollitt Dr., Fair Lawn, NJ 07410
FDA Number: n/a
E-mail: info@vyteris.com   *Fax:* 201-703-2295
Web site: www.vyteris.com
Year Founded: 2000
Total Employees: 53
Ownership: Public
Stock Symbol: VYTR
Traded On: OTC Bulletin
Produces/Sells CE-marked Devices: N
General Admin.: Ashutosh Sharma/Chief Executive Officer
Production: George Baskinger/Vice President Quality Assurance & Regulatory
Affairs
Research: Cormac Lyons/Vice President Development
     Michael Reidy/Vice President Research

W&W ASSOCIATES
   See W&W Manufacturing Co.

W&W MANUFACTURING CO.   800-221-0732
800 S. Broadway, Hicksville, NY 11801-5017   516-942-0011
FDA Number: n/a   *Fax:* 516-942-1944
Web site: www.ww-manufacturing.com
Total Employees: 75
Ownership: Private
Produces/Sells CE-marked Devices: N

W&W MANUFACTURING CO.   800-221-0732 *(cont'd)*
Federal Procurement Eligibility: Small Business
Distribution: Manufacturer Direct, Manufacturer Through Manufacturer Reps, OEM, Exporter
General Admin.: Jeffrey Weitzman/President, Chief Executive Officer
Production: Ronie Rosenbaum/Vice President Operations

Analyzer, Battery	General
Battery	General
Charger, Battery	General

W-P INSTRUMENTS INC.
See World Precision Instruments (W.P.I.), Inc.

W. L. GORE & ASSOCIATES, INC.   800-437-8181
PO Box 2400, Flagstaff, AZ 86003   **928-779-2771**
FDA Number: 2017233   *Fax:* 800-942-5315
Web site: www.goremedical.com
Year Founded: 1958
Total Employees: 9000
Ownership: Private
Produces/Sells CE-marked Devices: N

Cover, Cast	General
Device, Occlusion, Cardiac, Transcatheter	Cardiovascular
Drape, Surgical	Surgery
Guide, Surgical, Instrument	Surgery
Introducer, Catheter	Cardiovascular
Mesh, Cardiovascular (Polymeric)	Cardiovascular
Prosthesis, Tracheal, Expandable, Polymeric	Surgery
Sheet, Burn	General
Surgical Instrument, Cardiovascular	Cardiovascular
System, Treatment, Aortic Aneurysm, Endovascular Graft	Cardiovascular

W. L. GORE AND ASSOCIATES, INC.   888-914-4673
555 Papermill Road, Building A Suite 120,   **410-506-7787**
Newark, DE 19711
FDA Number: 1722606   *Fax:* 303-754-2329
E-mail: tshilling@wlgore.com
Web site: www.gore.com
Medical Products Sales Volume: $1,840,000,000
Year Founded: 1958
Total Employees: 7300
Ownership: Private
Produces/Sells CE-marked Devices: Y
Distribution: OEM

Scanner, Ultrasonic (Pulsed Doppler)	Radiology
Scanner, Ultrasonic (Pulsed Echo)	Radiology
Transducer, Ultrasonic, Diagnostic	Radiology

W. LAFRAMBOISE LTD.   800-363-8549
11450 Albert-Hudon,   **514-352-8228**
Montreal-Nord, QUE H1G 3 Canada
FDA Number: n/a   *Fax:* 514-352-0293
E-mail: info@wlaframboise.com
Web site: http://www.wlaframboise.com
Year Founded: 1922
Total Employees: 100
Ownership: Private
Produces/Sells CE-marked Devices: N
Distribution: Manufacturer Direct, Exporter

W. R. GRACE & CO.-CONN   410-531-4000
7500 Grace Drive, Columbia, MD 21044
FDA Number: 3003185577   *Fax:* 410-531-4367
Web site: www.grace.com
Medical Products Sales Volume: $3,000,000,000
Annual Revenue: More than $1 Billion
Year Founded: 1854
Total Employees: 6300
Ownership: Public
Stock Symbol: GRA
Traded On: NYSE
Produces/Sells CE-marked Devices: N
Distribution: Manufacturer Direct, OEM, Exporter
General Admin.: Hudson La Force/Chief Financial Officer, Senior Vice President
         Gloria L. Keesee/Chief Information Officer
         Fred E. Festa/President, Chief Executive Officer
         W. Brian McGowan/Senior Vice President Admin.
         D. Andrew Bonham/Vice President
         Gregory E. Poling/Vice President
         Mark A. Shelnitz/Vice President General Counsel & Secretary
Mktg./Adv.: William M. Corcoran/Vice President Public Affairs
Production: J. P. Forehand/Vice President Operations

Column, Liquid Chromatography	Toxicology
Support, Column, GLC	Toxicology

W.A. BAUM CO., INC.   888-281-6061
620 Oak St., Copiague, NY 11726   **631-226-3940**
FDA Number: 2412762   *Fax:* 631-226-3969
E-mail: info@wabaum.com

W.A. BAUM CO., INC.   888-281-6061 *(cont'd)*
Web site: www.wabaum.com
Medical Products Sales Volume: $10,000,000
Year Founded: 1916
Total Employees: 125
Ownership: Private
Produces/Sells CE-marked Devices: N
Federal Procurement Eligibility: Small Business

Cuff, Blood Pressure	Cardiovascular

W.A. HAMMOND DRIERITE CO.   937-376-2927
138 DAYTON AVE, P.O. Box 460, Xenia, OH 45385
FDA Number: n/a   *Fax:* 937-376-1977
E-mail: drierite@aol.com
Web site: www.drierite.com
Annual Revenue: $0-$1 Million
Year Founded: 1934
Ownership: Private
Produces/Sells CE-marked Devices: N
Federal Procurement Eligibility: Small Business
Distribution: Manufacturer Direct

Desiccator	Chemistry

W.E. MOWREY CO.   800-544-1550
1435 University Ave., St. Paul, MN 55104-4003   **651-646-1895**
FDA Number: n/a   *Fax:* 651-646-1898
E-mail: mowreygold@comcast.net
Web site: http://www.mowreygold.com
Annual Revenue: $0-$1 Million
Ownership: Private
Produces/Sells CE-marked Devices: N
Federal Procurement Eligibility: Small Business
Distribution: Manufacturer Direct, Manufacturer Through Distributor, Manufacturer Through Manufacturer Reps

Alloy, Gold Based, For Clinical Use	Dental And Oral
Material, Casting	Dental And Oral

W.E. MOWREY CO.   651-646-1895
1435 University Ave., Saint Paul, MN 55104
FDA Number: 2182977

Alloy, Gold Based, For Clinical Use	Dental And Oral

W.H.P.M., INC.   978-927-3808
9662 Telstar Ave., El Monte, CA 91731
FDA Number: 2087033

Enzyme Immunoassay, Amphetamine	Toxicology
Enzyme Immunoassay, Cocaine And Cocaine Metabolites	Toxicology
Enzyme Immunoassay, Opiates	Toxicology
Enzyme Immunoassay, Phencyclidine	Toxicology
Radioimmunoassay, Human Chorionic Gonadotropin	Chemistry
Reagent, Occult Blood	Hematology
Test, Tetrahydrocannabinol	Toxicology
Thin Layer Chromatography, Metamphetamine	Toxicology

W.L. GORE & ASSOCIATES, (UK) LTD.   (410) 506-7787
555 Paper Mill Road, Kirkton South, Newark,, DE 19711
FDA Number: n/a   *Fax:* (888) 914-4673
E-mail: ptait@w.l.gore.com
Total Employees: 185   *Marketing Staff:* 1   *Sales Staff:* 10
Ownership: Private
Quality System Registration Information: ISO9002
Produces/Sells CE-marked Devices: Y
Distribution: Manufacturer Direct, Exporter
General Admin.: Collin Goldie/Chief Executive Officer
         John Kennedy/Managing Director

Cleanroom Equipment	General
Suture, Other	Surgery

W.L. GORE & ASSOCIATES, INC.
See W.L. Gore & Associates, Inc., Sealant Technologies Group

W.L. GORE & ASSOCIATES, INC., SEALANT TECHNOLOGIES GROUP   410-392-3200
301 airport rd., Elkton, MD 21921
FDA Number: 3003910212   *Fax:* 410-392-4817
Web site: www.gore.com
Ownership: Private
Quality System Registration Information: ISO9002
Produces/Sells CE-marked Devices: N
Distribution: OEM

W.L. GORE & ASSOCIATES,INC   928-526-3030
1505 North Fourth St., Flagstaff, AZ 86004
FDA Number: 2017233
Ownership: Private
Produces/Sells CE-marked Devices: N
General Admin.: Don Goffena/Manager

Applier, Cast	Orthopedics
Catheter, Biliary	Gastroenterology/Urology

W.L. GORE & ASSOCIATES,INC   928-526-3030 (cont'd)

Catheter, Percutaneous	Cardiovascular
Catheter, Peritoneal	Surgery
Component, Cast	Orthopedics
Cover, Burr Hole (Cranial)	Cns/Neurology
Cover, Cast	General
Device, Occlusion, Cardiac, Transcatheter	Cardiovascular
Dressing, Wound and Burn, Occlusive	Surgery
Dura-Substitute	Cns/Neurology
Endoscope	Gastroenterology/Urology
Floss, Dental	Dental And Oral
Forceps, General & Plastic Surgery	Surgery
Guide, Surgical, Instrument	Surgery
Implant, Endosseous (Bone Filling and/or Augmentation)	Dental And Oral
Introducer, Catheter	Cardiovascular
Malar Implant	Surgery
Mesh, Surgical (Steel Gauze)	Surgery
Mesh, Surgical, Polymeric	Surgery
Orthopedic Manual Surgical Instrument	Orthopedics
Patch, Pericardial	Cardiovascular
Pledget And Intracardiac Patch, PETP, PTFE, Polypropylene	Cardiovascular
Polymer, ENT Composite Synthetic PTFE With Carbon-Fiber	Ear/Nose/Throat
Prosthesis Alignment Device	Physical Med
Prosthesis, Trachea	Surgery
Prosthesis, Vascular Graft, Less Than 6mm Diameter	Cardiovascular
Prosthesis, Vascular Graft, Of 6mm And Greater Diameter	Cardiovascular
Sheet, Burn	General
Shunt, Portosystemic, Endoprosthesis	Cardiovascular
Sphere, Ophthalmic (Implant)	Ophthalmology
Starter, Bone Screw	Orthopedics
Stent, Superficial Femoral Artery	Cardiovascular
Surgical Instrument, Cardiovascular	Cardiovascular
System, Treatment, Aortic Aneurysm, Endovascular Graft	Cardiovascular
System, Vocal Cord Medialization	Ear/Nose/Throat

W.L. GORE & ASSOCIATES,INC   302-738-4880
345 Inverness Dr. S., Bldg. A, Ste. 120, Englewood, CO 80112
FDA Number: 3003910212
Ownership: Private
Produces/Sells CE-marked Devices: N

Implant, Endosseous (Bone Filling and/or Augmentation)	Dental And Oral
Mesh, Surgical, Polymeric	Surgery
Suture, Non-Absorbable, Synthetic, Polypropylene	Surgery

W.O.M. WORLD OF MEDICINE USA, INC.   888-469-4378
4531 36th street, Orlando, FL 32811-6527   **407-438-8810**
FDA Number: 1063750   *Fax:* 407-859-2425
E-mail: info.orlando@womcorp.com
Web site: www.world-of-medicine.com
Medical Products Sales Volume: $3,000,000
Year Founded: 1974
Total Employees: 18   *Marketing Staff:* 7   *Sales Staff:* 7
Ownership: World Of Medicine Usa, Inc.
Quality System Registration Information: ISO9000; ISO9001
Produces/Sells CE-marked Devices: Y
Federal Procurement Eligibility: Small Business
Distribution: Manufacturer Direct, OEM
Mktg./Adv.: Mr. Roland Strelitzki/Director Sales

Flowmeter, Urine, Disposable	Gastroenterology/Urology

WABASH METAL PRODUCTS
See Carver Inc.

WAFERGEN BIOSYSTEMS INC.   510-651-4450
7400 Paseo Padre Parkway, Fremont, CA 94555
FDA Number: n/a   *Fax:* 510-793-8992
E-mail: info@wafergen.com
Web site: http://wafergen.com
Ownership: Public
Stock Symbol: WGBS
Traded On: OTC Bulletin
Produces/Sells CE-marked Devices: N
General Admin.: Alnoor Shivji/Chairman, Chief Executive Officer
     Ms. Mona Chadha/Chief Operating Officer
     David Gelfand/Chief Scientific Officer
Mktg./Adv.: Ms. Janet Lankard/Vice President International Sales
Research: Mr. Syed Husain/Vice President Engineering
Finance: Mr. Donald Huffman/Chief Financial Officer

WAGNER AWNING & MFG., INC.
See Leisure Time

WAHL CLIPPER CORP.   815-548-8342
2900 North Locust St., Sterling, IL 61081
FDA Number: 1410825

Massager, Therapeutic	Physical Med
Surgical, Razor	Surgery
Toothbrush, Powered	Dental And Oral

WAHL CLIPPER CORP.   815-625-6525
2902 N. Locust St., Sterling, IL 61081-0578
FDA Number: 1410825   *Fax:* 815-625-0091
Annual Revenue: $50-$100 Million
Total Employees: 500   *Marketing Staff:* 15   *Sales Staff:* 15
Ownership: Private
Produces/Sells CE-marked Devices: Y
Distribution: Manufacturer Through Manufacturer Reps
General Admin.: John Wahl/Chairman
     Greg Wahl/President
Mktg./Adv.: Pat Anello/Director Marketing
     Jim McCambridge/Director Product Development

Massager, Battery-Powered	Physical Med
Pack, Hot Or Cold, Reusable	Physical Med
Surgical, Razor	Surgery

WAKO CHEMICALS USA, INC.   877-714-1924
1600 Bellwood Road, Richmond, VA 23237-1326   **804-714-1924**
FDA Number: 1627434   *Fax:* 804-271-7791
E-mail: diagnostics@wakousa.com
Web site: www.wakousa.com
Medical Products Sales Volume: $30,000,000
Annual Revenue: $25-$50 Million
Year Founded: 1981
Total Employees: 60   *Marketing Staff:* 5   *Sales Staff:* 5
Ownership: Private
Quality System Registration Information: ISO9001
Produces/Sells CE-marked Devices: N
Federal Procurement Eligibility: Small Business
Distribution: Manufacturer Through Manufacturer Reps
General Admin.: Tonya Mallory/Executive Manager
     A. Fukishima/President
Mktg./Adv.: Michael Ciucci/Manager International & National Sales

Bilirubinometer	Chemistry
Buret	Chemistry
Calibrator, Primary, Clinical Chemistry	Chemistry
Control, Analyte (Assayed And Unassayed)	Chemistry
Diazonium Colorimetry, Urobilinogen (Urinary, Non-Quant.)	Chemistry
Reagent, Other	General
Turbidimetric Method, Protein Or Albumin (Urinary)	Chemistry

WAL-MED, INC.   877-542-3688
11302 E. 164th St., Puyallup, WA 98374   **253-845-6633**
FDA Number: 3032365   *Fax:* 253-845-6458
E-mail: mike.ofarrell@wallace-ofarrell.com
Web site: www.wallace-medical.com
Ownership: Private
Produces/Sells CE-marked Devices: N
Federal Procurement Eligibility: Small Business, Female Owned
Distribution: Manufacturer Direct, Manufacturer Through Distributor, Manufacturer Through Manufacturer Reps

Lubricant, Vaginal, Patient	General

WAL-STAR, INC.   434-685-1094
696 Inman Rd., Danville, VA 24541
FDA Number: 1123461

Chair/Table, Medical	General

WALDMANN LIGHTING
See Waldmann Lighting

WALKER LDJ SCIENTIFIC, INC.   800-962-4638
10 Rockdale Street, Worcester, MA 01606-1922   **508-852-3674**
FDA Number: n/a   *Fax:* 508-856-9931
E-mail: customerservice@walkerscientific.com
Web site: www.walkerscientific.com
Year Founded: 1980
Total Employees: 35
Ownership: Private
Produces/Sells CE-marked Devices: N
Federal Procurement Eligibility: Small Business
Distribution: Manufacturer Direct
Mktg./Adv.: Nancy Bianchini/Manager Advertising
     Steve Dakel/Vice President Marketing & Sales

Demagnetizer	General
Gaussmeter	General

WALKERS, INC., E. C.   800-494-8589
375 Rexdale Boulevard,   **(416) 744-2011**
Toronto, ONT M9W 1 Canada
FDA Number: n/a   *Fax:* (416) 744-2011
E-mail: rick@ecwalkers.com
Web site: www.ecwalkers.com
Total Employees: 15   *Marketing Staff:* 1   *Sales Staff:* 4
Ownership: Private
Quality System Registration Information: ISO9002
Produces/Sells CE-marked Devices: N

WALKERS, INC., E. C. 800-494-8589 (cont'd)
Distribution: Manufacturer Through Distributor

WALKMED INFUSION LLC 303-420-9569
4080 Youngfield St., Wheat Ridge, CO 80033-3862
FDA Number: 1723533
Fax: 303-420-4545
E-mail: info@mckinleymed.com
Web site: www.mckinleymed.com
Medical Products Sales Volume: $1,600,000
Year Founded: 1995
Total Employees: 20   *Marketing Staff:* 2   *Sales Staff:* 22
Ownership: BROE Companies
Quality System Registration Information: ISO9001
Produces/Sells CE-marked Devices: Y
Federal Procurement Eligibility: Small Business, VA Contract
Distribution: Manufacturer Direct, Manufacturer Through Distributor, Manufacturer Through Manufacturer Reps, Service Direct, Exclusive Distributor, Importer
General Admin.: Dr. Randy Hoffman/President
Mktg./Adv.: Mr. Jim Buck/Director Sales
Production: Mr. Ralph Cooey/Director Operations
Research: Mr. Andy Lamborne/Director Research & Development
Finance: Mr. Brian Graff/Director Finance

Container, IV	General
Kit, Administration, Intravenous	General
Pump, Infusion	General
Pump, Infusion, Elastomeric	General
Pump, Infusion, Patient Controlled Analgesia (PCA)	General

WALL LENK CORP. 252-527-4186
PO Box 3349, Kinston, NC 28502-3349
FDA Number: n/a
Fax: 252-527-4189
E-mail: catalog@wlenk.com
Web site: www.wlenk.com
Annual Revenue: $5-$10 Million
Total Employees: 80   *Marketing Staff:* 1   *Sales Staff:* 1
Ownership: Private
Produces/Sells CE-marked Devices: N
Federal Procurement Eligibility: Small Business
Distribution: Manufacturer Direct
General Admin.: Richard B. Davis/President, Chief Executive Officer
Mktg./Adv.: Pete McCurdy/Director Sales
　　　　　Paul A. Ricciarelli/Vice President Marketing & Sales
Production: Ronnie Whitfield/Vice President Manufacturing

Burner	Chemistry

WALLAC, INC.
See PerkinElmer

WALLACE COMPUTER SERVICES, INC 800-782-4892
2275 Cabot Drive, Lisle, IL 60532 630-588-5000
FDA Number: n/a
Fax: 630-588-5172
E-mail: healthcare@wallace.com
Web site: www.wallace.com
Medical Products Sales Volume: $153,000,000
Annual Revenue: More than $100 Million
Year Founded: 1908
Total Employees: 8464   *Marketing Staff:* 75   *Sales Staff:* 1000
Ownership: Public
Stock Symbol: WCS
Traded On: NYSE
Quality System Registration Information: ISO9002
Distribution: Manufacturer Direct
General Admin.: M. David Jones/Chief Executive Officer
　　　　　Mike Duffield/President
Mktg./Adv.: John Edmundson/Director Marketing
　　　　　Janell Begole/Director Sales
　　　　　Gail Provo/Manager Contracts
　　　　　Doug Fitzgerald/Vice President Marketing
　　　　　Tom Brooker/Vice President Sales
Production: Wayne Richter/Vice President Manufacturing

Computer Software, Hospital/Nursing Management	General
Label, Bar Code	General
Printer, Bar Code	General

WALLACH SURGICAL DEVICES, INC. 800-243-2463
235 Edison Road, Orange, CT 06477 203-799-2000
FDA Number: 1219739
Fax: 203-799-2002
E-mail: wallach@wallachsurgical.com
Web site: www.wallachsurgical.com
Medical Products Sales Volume: $11,100,000
Annual Revenue: $5-$10 Million
Year Founded: 1971
Total Employees: 48   *Marketing Staff:* 4   *Sales Staff:* 35
Ownership: Private
Quality System Registration Information: ISO9002
Produces/Sells CE-marked Devices: Y
Federal Procurement Eligibility: Small Business

WALLACH SURGICAL DEVICES, INC. 800-243-2463 (cont'd)
Distribution: Manufacturer Through Distributor, Manufacturer Through Manufacturer Reps
General Admin.: Ronald Wallach/President
　　　　　Edward Carroll/Regional Manager
Mktg./Adv.: Lynn Wallach/Director Marketing & Communications
　　　　　Craig Citron/Director National Accounts
　　　　　Linda Cella/Manager Marketing & Advertising
　　　　　Craig Citron/Vice President Marketing & Sales
Production: Dan Wallach/Manager Materials
　　　　　John Fornabaio/Manager Regulatory Affairs

Colposcope	Obstetrics/Gynecology
Cryoophthalmic Unit	Ophthalmology
Cryosurgical Unit	Surgery
Cryosurgical Unit, Gynecologic	Obstetrics/Gynecology
Electrosurgical Equipment, General Purpose	Surgery
Electrosurgical Unit, General Purpose (ESU)	Surgery
Kit, Pap Smear	Obstetrics/Gynecology
Microscope	Hematology
Microscope, Operating, AC-Powered, Ophthalmic	Ophthalmology
Microscope, Surgical, General & Plastic Surgery	Surgery
Spatula, Cervical, Cytology	Obstetrics/Gynecology
System, Evacuation, Smoke, Laser	Surgery
Unit, Cooling, Cardiac	Cardiovascular

WALLS PRECISION INSTRUMENTS, LLC. 541-894-2520
38800 Deer Creek Rd., Baker City, OR 97814
FDA Number: 1725041

Knife, ENT	Ear/Nose/Throat

WALTER LORENZ SURGICAL, INC.
See Biomet Microfixation Inc.

WAMPOLE LABORATORIES 800-257-9525
2 Research Way, Princeton, NJ 08540 609-627-8000
FDA Number: 2220285
Fax: 800-532-0295
E-mail: info@wampolelabs.com
Web site: www.wampolelabs.com
Medical Products Sales Volume: $13,700,000
Year Founded: 2002
Total Employees: 75   *Marketing Staff:* 5   *Sales Staff:* 38
Ownership: Private
Produces/Sells CE-marked Devices: N
Federal Procurement Eligibility: Small Business, GSA Contract
Distribution: Manufacturer Direct, Manufacturer Through Distributor, Exclusive Distributor
General Admin.: John Bridgen/President
Mktg./Adv.: Jean Zych/Vice President Marketing
　　　　　Joe Vacante/Vice President Sales

Agglutination Method, Human Chorionic Gonadotropin	Chemistry
Anti-Human Globulin, FTA-ABS Test (Coombs)	Microbiology
Anti-SM-Antibody, Antigen And Control	Immunology
Antibody IGM, IF, Epstein-Barr Virus	Microbiology
Antibody Igm, If, Cytomegalovirus Virus	Microbiology
Antibody, Anti-Smooth Muscle, Indirect Immunofluorescent	Immunology
Antibody, Anti-Thyroid, Indirect Immunofluorescent	Immunology
Antibody, Antinuclear, Indirect Immunofluorescent, Antigen	Immunology
Antibody, Herpes Virus	Microbiology
Antibody, Multiple Auto, Indirect Immunofluorescence	Immunology
Antibody, Toxoplasma Gondii	Microbiology
Antideoxyribonuclease, Streptococcus SPP.	Microbiology
Antigen, C. Difficile	Microbiology
Antigen, HA (Including HA Control), Rubella	Microbiology
Antigen, ID, HA, CEP, Entamoeba Histolytica	Microbiology
Antigen, Positive Control, Cryptococcus Neoformans	Microbiology
Antiserum, Fluorescent Antibody For FTA-ABS Test	Microbiology
Calibrator, Hemoglobin And Hematocrit Measurement	Hematology
Campylobacter Pylori	Microbiology
Enzyme Linked Immunoabsorbent Assay, Chlamydia Group	Microbiology
Enzyme Linked Immunoabsorbent Assay, Herpes Simplex Virus	Microbiology
Enzyme Linked Immunoabsorbent Assay, Mumps Virus	Microbiology
Enzyme Linked Immunoabsorbent Assay, Mycoplasma SPP.	Microbiology
Enzyme Linked Immunoabsorbent Assay, Rubella	Microbiology
Enzyme Linked Immunoabsorbent Assay, Rubeola	Microbiology
Enzyme Linked Immunoabsorbent Assay, Treponema Pallidum	Microbiology
Giardia Spp.	Microbiology
Immunoassay, Other	Toxicology
Kit, Pregnancy Test	Obstetrics/Gynecology
Kit, Screening, Urine	Microbiology
Legionella, Spp., ELISA	Microbiology
Reagent, Streptolysin O/Antistreptolysin-Titer	Microbiology
Standard/Control, All Types	Chemistry
Test, C-Reactive Protein	Immunology
Test, Disease, Lyme	Immunology
Test, Infectious Mononucleosis	Immunology
Test, Rheumatoid Factor	Immunology
Test, Rotavirus	Microbiology
Test, Syphilis (RPR or VDRL)	Microbiology
Thyroglobulin, Antigen, Antiserum, Control	Immunology

WANG NMR INC.   925-443-0212
550 N. Canyons Pkwy., Livermore, CA 94550-7632
FDA Number: n/a   Fax: 925-443-0215
E-mail: sales@wangnmr.com
Web site: www.wangnmr.com/
Medical Products Sales Volume: $4,500,000
Annual Revenue: $1-$5 Million
Year Founded: 1984
Total Employees: 25
Ownership: Private
Produces/Sells CE-marked Devices: N
Federal Procurement Eligibility: Small Business
Distribution: Manufacturer Direct
General Admin.: Bert Wang/President
Mktg./Adv.: Tiki Juang/Manager Business

Magnet, Permanent, MRI (Magnetic Resonance Imaging)	Radiology
Magnet, Superconducting, MRI (Magnetic Resonance Imaging)	Radiology

Medical Product Subsidiaries (Listed Separately)
Wang Nmr Inc., Healthcare Product Div.

WARD'S NATURAL SCIENCE ESTABLISHMENT, INC.   800-962-2660
5100 W. Henrietta Rd., P.O. Box 92912,   585-359-2502
Rochester, NY 14692
FDA Number: n/a   Fax: 585-334-6174
E-mail: customer_service@wardsci.com
Web site: www.wardsci.com
Year Founded: 1962
Ownership: Private
Produces/Sells CE-marked Devices: N
Federal Procurement Eligibility: Small Business
Distribution: Manufacturer Direct

Centrifuge, General (Up to 5,000 rpm)	Pathology
Counter, Colony	Microbiology
Freeze Drying Equipment	Chemistry
Labware, Basic, Reusable	Chemistry
Microscope, Phase Contrast	Pathology
Sterilizer, Steam (Autoclave)	General

WARE MEDICS GLASS WORKS, INC.   845-429-6950
PO Box 368, Garnerville, NY 10923
FDA Number: 2431270   Fax: 845-429-6951
E-mail: sales@waremedics.com
Web site: www.waremedics.com
Medical Products Sales Volume: $700,000
Annual Revenue: $0-$1 Million
Year Founded: 1965
Total Employees: 4
Federal Procurement Eligibility: Small Business
Distribution: Manufacturer Through Distributor, Importer, Exporter
General Admin.: Ann Benitto/President
Production: Louis Benitto/Manager Production

Container, Medication, Graduated Liquid	General
Coverslip, Microscope Slide	Pathology
Crusher, Vial, Laboratory	General
Cup, Eye	Ophthalmology
Cup, Medicine	General
Dilator, Vaginal	Obstetrics/Gynecology
Dish, Petri	Chemistry
Dropper, Medicine	General
Hematocrit Tube, Rack, Sealer, Holder	Hematology
Jar, Dressing	Surgery
Lamp, Other	General
Manometer, Spinal Fluid	General
Pipette	Chemistry
Shield, Nipple	Obstetrics/Gynecology
Slide, Microscope	Pathology
Stopper	General
Syringe, Other	General
Thermometer, Mercury	General
Tube, Centrifuge	Chemistry
Tube, Culture	Microbiology
Tube, Sedimentation Rate	Hematology
Urinometer, Non-Electrical	Gastroenterology/Urology

WARING PRODUCTS, DIV. CONAIR CORP.   203-351-9000
1 Crystal Dr., Mcconnellsburg, PA 17233
FDA Number: 2523711
Ownership: Private
Produces/Sells CE-marked Devices: N

Blender/Mixer	Chemistry

WARNER GRAHAM CO., THE   800-872-2300
160 Church Lane, Cockeysville, MD 21030-4921   410-667-6200
FDA Number: 1110202   Fax: 410-628-0617
E-mail: info@warnergraham.com
Web site: www.warnergraham.com
Medical Products Sales Volume: $3,600,000

WARNER GRAHAM CO., THE   800-872-2300 (cont'd)
Year Founded: 1921
Total Employees: 19   Marketing Staff: 1   Sales Staff: 1
Ownership: Private
Produces/Sells CE-marked Devices: N
Federal Procurement Eligibility: Small Business, Female Owned, VA Contract
Distribution: Service Direct, Exclusive Distributor, Importer, Exporter
General Admin.: Ms. Stephanie Hack/Corporate Secretary
         Mary Riepe McWilliams/President
Mktg./Adv.: Mr. Alec Riepe/Director Sales

Alcohol Dehydrogenase, Spec. Reagent - Ethanol Enzyme	Toxicology
Solvent	Chemistry

WASCOMAT LAUNDRY EQUIPMENT   800-645-2204
461 Doughty Blvd., Inwood, NY 11096-0338   516-371-4400
FDA Number: 9330136   Fax: 516-371-4204
E-mail: sales@wascomat.com
Web site: www.wascomat.net
Medical Products Sales Volume: $52,000,000
Year Founded: 1949
Total Employees: 60
Ownership: Bermil Industries
Produces/Sells CE-marked Devices: N
Federal Procurement Eligibility: Small Business
Distribution: Manufacturer Through Distributor
General Admin.: Bernard Milch/Chairman
         Bernard Milch/President
Mktg./Adv.: Eduard Zilberman/Manager Advertising
         Howard Herman/Vice President Marketing & Sales

Laundry Equipment	General
Washer, Laundry	General

WASHEX, INC.   800-433-0933
5000 Central Freeway N.,   940-855-3990
Wichita Falls, TX 76306
FDA Number: n/a   Fax: 940-855-9349
E-mail: bob.montgomery@washex.com
Web site: www.washex.com
Annual Revenue: $10-$25 Million
Year Founded: 1923
Total Employees: 150   Marketing Staff: 3   Sales Staff: 4
Ownership: Private
Produces/Sells CE-marked Devices: Y
Federal Procurement Eligibility: Small Business
Distribution: Manufacturer Through Distributor
Mktg./Adv.: Mr. Bob Montgomery/Senior Vice President Marketing & Sales
Production: Mr. Robert De Hoyos/Chief Engineer
         Mr. Billy Maxwell/Plant Manager
         Mr. Steve Horwitz/Vice President Operations

Laundry Equipment	General

WASHINGTON BIOTECHNOLOGY, INC.   206-292-9734
562 First AvenueS., 7th Floor, Seattle, WA 98104
FDA Number: 3029998   Fax: 206-260-1326
E-mail: wbinc2@qwest.net
Medical Products Sales Volume: $1,000,000
Annual Revenue: $0-$1 Million
Year Founded: 1987
Total Employees: 12
Ownership: Private
Produces/Sells CE-marked Devices: N
Federal Procurement Eligibility: Small Business
Distribution: Service Direct

Campylobacter Pylori	Microbiology
Kit, Identification, Neisseria Gonorrhoeae	Microbiology

WASHINGTON BIOTECHNOLOGY, INC.   410-633-7449
6200 Seaforth Street, Baltimore, MD 21224-6506
FDA Number: n/a   Fax: 410-633-7478
E-mail: sales@washingtonbiotech.com
Web site: www.washingtonbiotech.com
Annual Revenue: $1-$5 Million
Total Employees: 17   Marketing Staff: 1   Sales Staff: 1
Ownership: Private
Produces/Sells CE-marked Devices: N
Federal Procurement Eligibility: Small Business
Distribution: Manufacturer Direct
General Admin.: Sean O'Neill/President, Chief Executive Officer
Mktg./Adv.: Carmen O'Neill/Director Marketing

Animal, Laboratory	Microbiology
Antibody, Monoclonal	Microbiology
Antibody, Polyclonal	Microbiology
Serum, Animal	Pathology

WASHINGTON TRADE INTERNATIONAL, INC.   800-327-3379
2633 Willamette Dr. NE, Lacey, WA 98516   360-493-6013
FDA Number: n/a   Fax: 360-493-6091
E-mail: csvc@washingtontrade.com

WASHINGTON TRADE INTERNATIONAL, INC.
800-327-3379
(cont'd)
Web site: www.washingtontrade.com
Annual Revenue: $1-$5 Million
Year Founded: 1989
Total Employees: 7   *Marketing Staff:* 1   *Sales Staff:* 1
Ownership: Private
Quality System Registration Information: ISO9002
Produces/Sells CE-marked Devices: N
Federal Procurement Eligibility: Small Business
Distribution: Manufacturer Direct, Importer, Exporter
General Admin.: Laura Akhavan/Chief Financial Officer, Vice President
         Cheryl Dowd/Director, General Manager
         Tooradj Akhavan, MIM./President, Chief Executive Officer
Mktg./Adv.: Tony Akhavan/Director Marketing

Glove, Other	General
Glove, Patient Examination, Latex	General
Glove, Patient Examination, Specialty	General
Gown, Patient, Disposable	General
Mask, Face	General
Tissue, Toilet	General

WASHINGTON UNIVERSITY SCHOOL OF MEDICINE
314-362-8525
4921 Parkview Place, St. Louis, MO 63110
FDA Number: 3006396143
E-mail: mpa@wusm.wustl.edu
Web site: www.medschool.wustl.edu
Ownership: Private
Produces/Sells CE-marked Devices: N

Tester, Radiology	Radiology

WASHINGTON-GREENE COUNTY BRANCH PENNSYLVANIA ASSOC
724-228-0770
566 East Maiden St., Wash, PA 15301
FDA Number: 2521990

Kit, Surgical (General)	Surgery
Kit, Suture Removal	Surgery

WATER & POWER TECHNOLOGIES OF TEXAS, INC.
801-974-5500
1501 St. Andrews Rd., Po Box 21743, Columbia, SC 29221
FDA Number: 1066694
Ownership: Private
Produces/Sells CE-marked Devices: N

Purification System, Water	Gastroenterology/Urology

WATER & POWER TECHNOLOGIES, INC.
817-640-1533
1217 W. Corporate Dr., Arlington, TX 76006
FDA Number: 3003550196   *Fax:* 817-633-2790
E-mail: trema.mckamy@wpt.com
Web site: www.wpt.com
Medical Products Sales Volume: $3,000,000
Annual Revenue: $5-$10 Million
Year Founded: 1960
Total Employees: 28   *Sales Staff:* 5
Ownership: TYCO INTERNATIONAL LTD.
Stock Symbol: TYC
Traded On: NYSE
Produces/Sells CE-marked Devices: N
Distribution: Manufacturer Direct, OEM, Service Direct, Exclusive Distributor
General Admin.: Ms. Trema McKamy/Business Manager
         Mr. Michael Ancy/General Manager
Mktg./Adv.: Mr. Gary Arnold/Manager Regional Sales
         Mr. Raul Rodriguez/Manager Regional Sales
         Mr. Scott Gaston/Sales Specialist
         Mr. Luis Rodriguez/Services Manager
Production: Mr. Billy Miles/Manager Operations

Purification System, Water	Gastroenterology/Urology

WATER PIK, INC.
970-221-6129
1730 East Prospect Rd., Fort Collins, CO 80553
FDA Number: 1712259
Ownership: Private
Produces/Sells CE-marked Devices: N

Adhesive, Bracket And Conditioner, Resin	Dental And Oral
Agent, Polishing, Abrasive, Oral Cavity	Dental And Oral
Aligner, Beam, X-Ray (Collimator)	Dental And Oral
Articulators	Dental And Oral
Cement, Dental	Dental And Oral
Condenser, Amalgam And Foil, Operative	Dental And Oral
Crown And Bridge, Temporary, Resin	Dental And Oral
Cup, Prophylaxis	Dental And Oral
Device, Jaw Tracking, For Diagnosis Of Tmj/mpd Disorders	Dental And Oral
Face Bow	Dental And Oral
Handpiece, Contra- And Right-Angle Attachment, Dental	Dental And Oral
Irrigator, Oral	Dental And Oral
Irrigator, Powered Nasal	Ear/Nose/Throat

WATER PIK, INC.
970-221-6129 *(cont'd)*

Material, Impression	Dental And Oral
Material, Impression Tray, Resin	Dental And Oral
Material, Tooth Shade, Resin	Dental And Oral
Matrix, Dental	Dental And Oral
Pick, Massaging	Dental And Oral
Retainer, Matrix	Dental And Oral
Scraper, Tongue	Dental And Oral
Strip, Polishing Agent	Dental And Oral
Toothbrush, Powered	Dental And Oral
Tray, Impression	Dental And Oral
Varnish, Cavity	Dental And Oral

WATER-JEL TECHNOLOGIES
800-275-3433
50 Broad Street, Carlstadt, NJ 07072-2708
201-507-8300
FDA Number: 1219592   *Fax:* 201-507-8325
E-mail: info@waterjel.com
Web site: www.waterjel.com
Year Founded: 1980
Total Employees: 40   *Marketing Staff:* 1   *Sales Staff:* 3
Ownership: Private
Quality System Registration Information: ISO9001
Produces/Sells CE-marked Devices: N
Federal Procurement Eligibility: Small Business
Distribution: Manufacturer Through Distributor
General Admin.: Howard Hirsch/Chief Executive Officer
         Debbie Kinzley/Director Human Resources
         Michael Pisani/President
Mktg./Adv.: Judith Domanski/Director Marketing
         Lane Card/Vice President Sales
Production: Larry Stanchina/Director Quality Assurance
         Cornelia Damsky/Manager Regulatory Affairs
         Carl Haight/Vice President Manufacturing

Blanket, Fire	General
Dressing, Wound and Burn, Occlusive	Surgery
Kit, Burn	General
Mask, Face	General

WATERCLAVE, L.L.C.
913-312-5860
6731 West 121st St., Overland Park, KS 66209
FDA Number: 1934424   *Fax:* 913-312-5861
Web site: www.waterclave.com
Ownership: Private
Produces/Sells CE-marked Devices: N

Sterilizer, Boiling Water	Dental And Oral

WATERLOO CARI ALL
See Waterloo Healthcare, Llc

WATERLOO HEALTHCARE, LLC
800-833-4419
3730 E. Southern Ave, Phoenix, AZ 85040
602-414-3691
FDA Number: 9201129   *Fax:* 602-437-2270
E-mail: info@waterloohealthcare.com
Web site: www.waterloohealthcare.com
Year Founded: 1969
Total Employees: 14   *Marketing Staff:* 1   *Sales Staff:* 5
Ownership: The Bergmann Group
Produces/Sells CE-marked Devices: Y
Federal Procurement Eligibility: Small Business
Distribution: Manufacturer Direct, Manufacturer Through Distributor, Manufacturer Through Manufacturer Reps, Exporter
General Admin.: John M Bergmann/Director, General Manager
Mktg./Adv.: Christina Masengale/Managing Director Marketing & Sales

Accessories, Cart, Multipurpose	General
Cart, Anesthetist's	Anesthesiology
Cart, Dressing	General
Cart, Emergency, Cardiopulmonary Resuscitation (Crash)	Anesthesiology
Cart, Instrument	Surgery
Cart, Isolation	General
Cart, Medicine	General
Cart, Multipurpose	General
Cart, Supply, Operating Room	Surgery

WATERLOO INDUSTRIES, INC.
See Waterloo Healthcare, Llc

WATERMARK MEDICAL LLC.
877-710-6999
1750 Clint Moore Road, Suite 101, Boca Raton, FL 33487
FDA Number: 3008208119
E-mail: info@watermarkmedical.com
Web site: http://www.watermarkmedical.com
Ownership: Private
Produces/Sells CE-marked Devices: N
General Admin.: Mr. Sean Heyniger/Chief Executive Officer
         Mr. Jack Fiedor/Chief Financial Officer, Vice President
         Mr. Greg Poulos/Chief Information Officer
         Mr. Matt Oefinger/Chief Technology Officer
         Mr. David Hruda/Compliance Officer
         Mr. Charlie Alvarez/President
Mktg./Adv.: Mr. Robbie Siegel/Vice President Sales

WATERMARK MEDICAL LLC. 877-710-6999 *(cont'd)*
Recorder, Ventilatory Effort | Anesthesiology

WATERS CHROMATOGRAPHY
See Waters Corp.

WATERS CORP. 800-252-4752
34 Maple St., Milford, MA 01757-3604 508-478-2000
FDA Number: 1218959 *Fax:* 508-872-1990
Web site: www.waters.com
Medical Products Sales Volume: $1,280,000,000
Year Founded: 1958
Total Employees: 4500
Ownership: Public
Stock Symbol: WAT
Traded On: NYSE
Quality System Registration Information: ISO9002
Produces/Sells CE-marked Devices: N
Distribution: Manufacturer Direct, Importer, Exporter
General Admin.: Douglas Berthianume/President, Chief Executive Officer
Mktg./Adv.: Arthur Caputo/Senior Vice President Marketing & Sales
Production: John Ornell/Vice President Operations

Accessories, Chromatography (Gas, Gel, Liquid, Thin Layer)	Chemistry
Analyzer, Amino Acid	Microbiology
Analyzer, Ion, Hydrogen-Ion pH, Blood Phase, Non-Indwelling	Anesthesiology
Chromatography Equipment, Liquid	Chemistry
Chromatography, Liquid, Performance, High	Toxicology
Column, Chromatography	Chemistry
Column, Liquid Chromatography	Toxicology
Computer, Chemistry Analyzer	Chemistry
Polymer, Synthetic, Other	General
Spectrometer, Infrared	Chemistry
Spectrophotometer, U.V./Visible	Chemistry
Synthesizer, Peptide & Protein	Chemistry

Medical Product Subsidiaries (Listed Separately)
Ta Instruments

WATERS CORPORATION 800-252-4752
34 Maple Street, Milford, MA 01757 508-482-2000
FDA Number: 1218959 *Fax:* 508 482 8532
E-mail: waters_quotes@waters.com
Web site: http://www.waters.com
Year Founded: 1958
Ownership: Private
Produces/Sells CE-marked Devices: N
General Admin.: Mr. Arthur Caputo/Executive Vice President
Mr. Douglas Berthiaume/President, Chairman, Chief Executive
Officer
Finance: Mr. John Ornell/Chief Financial Officer, Vice President Finance

Calibrator, Secondary, Clinical Chemistry	Chemistry
Column, Liquid Chromatography	Toxicology
Control, Analyte (Assayed And Unassayed)	Chemistry
Enzyme Immunoassay, Tacrolimus	Toxicology
High Performance Liquid Chromatography, Cyclosporine	Chemistry

WATERS MEDICAL SYSTEMS 800-426-9877
2112-15th St. NW, Rochester, MN 55901 507-288-7777
FDA Number: 2123774 *Fax:* 507-252-3700
E-mail: info@wtrs.com
Web site: www.wtrs.com
Annual Revenue: $25-$50 Million
Year Founded: 1960
Total Employees: 170
Ownership: Waters Instruments, Inc.
Stock Symbol: WTRS
Traded On: NASDAQ
Quality System Registration Information: ISO9002
Produces/Sells CE-marked Devices: Y
Distribution: Manufacturer Direct, Manufacturer Through Distributor, Manufacturer Through Manufacturer Reps
General Admin.: Jerry Grabowski/Chief Executive Officer
Dave Schollman/Vice President, General Manager
Mktg./Adv.: Kathy Hult/Director Marketing
Production: Don Dalland/Vice President Manufacturing

Organ Preservation System	Gastroenterology/Urology
Oximeter, Whole Blood	Hematology

WATERS MEDICAL SYSTEMS, LLC 205-612-5221
2112 15th St. N.w., Rochester, MN 55901
FDA Number: 2123774

Computer, Oxygen-Uptake	Anesthesiology
Oximeter, Intracardiac	Cardiovascular
Oximeter, Whole Blood	Hematology
Perfusion System, Kidney	Gastroenterology/Urology

WAVE FORM SYSTEMS, INC. 800-332-8749
7737 SW Nimbus Avenue, Beaverton, OR 97008 503-626-2100
FDA Number: 3007881723 *Fax:* 503-643-6314
E-mail: info@waveformsys.com

WAVE FORM SYSTEMS, INC. 800-332-8749 *(cont'd)*
Web site: www.waveformsys.com
Medical Products Sales Volume: $3,000,000
Annual Revenue: $1-$5 Million
Ownership: Private
Produces/Sells CE-marked Devices: Y
Federal Procurement Eligibility: Small Business
Distribution: Manufacturer Through Distributor, Manufacturer Through Manufacturer Reps, OEM, Service Direct, Exclusive Distributor, Importer, Exporter

Drape, Surgical	Surgery
Laser, Gastroenterology/Urology	Gastroenterology/Urology
Laser, Nd:YAG, Surgical	Surgery
Laser, Surgical	Surgery
Solution, Instrument Cleaner	General

WAVERLEY GLEN SYSTEMS 1.877.304.5438
480 University Ave., Ste 100, 416.260.2145
Toronto, ONTAR M5G 1 Canada
FDA Number: 9615386 *Fax:* 416.260.5580
E-mail: info@waverleyglen.com
Total Employees: 37 *Marketing Staff:* 1 *Sales Staff:* 4
Ownership: Private
Quality System Registration Information: ISO9001
Produces/Sells CE-marked Devices: N
Distribution: Manufacturer Through Distributor

WAVETEC VISION 949-273-5970
66 Argonaut, Suite 170, Irvine, CA 92618
FDA Number: 2032579 *Fax:* 949-273-5976
E-mail: info@wavetecvision.com
Web site: www.wavetecvision.com
Ownership: Private
Produces/Sells CE-marked Devices: N
General Admin.: Dr. Tom Padrick/Chief Scientific Officer
Mr. Tom Frinzi/President, Chief Executive Officer
Production: Mr. John Taylor/Vice President Operations
Research: Mr. Craig Bender/Vice President Research & Development
Finance: Mr. Scott Cooper/Chief Financial Officer
Aberrometer, Ophthalmic | Ophthalmology

WAVETEC VISION SYSTEMS, INC. 949-273-5970
66 Argonaunt, Suite 170, Aliso Viejo, CA 92656
FDA Number: 2032579 *Fax:* 949.273.5976
E-mail: info@wavetecvision.com
Web site: www.wavetecvision.com
Ownership: Private
Produces/Sells CE-marked Devices: N
Aberrometer, Ophthalmic | Ophthalmology

WAVETOUCH TECHNOLOGIES, LLC 858-924-9283
15970 Bernardo Center Dr., San Diego, CA 92127
FDA Number: 3006346510

Lenses, Soft Contact, Daily Wear	Ophthalmology
Lenses, Soft Contact, Extended Wear	Ophthalmology

WAY & MEANS, INC.
See Labcon North America

WAYNE INTEGRATED TECHNOLOGIES CORP. 631-242-0213
160 Rodeo Dr., Edgewood, NY 11717-8317
FDA Number: n/a *Fax:* 613-242-3278
E-mail: sales@GoWayne.com
Web site: www.gowayne.com
Annual Revenue: $1-$5 Million
Total Employees: 38 *Marketing Staff:* 2 *Sales Staff:* 2
Ownership: Private
Produces/Sells CE-marked Devices: N
Federal Procurement Eligibility: Small Business, Female Owned
Distribution: Manufacturer Through Manufacturer Reps
Mktg./Adv.: Guy Moks/Manager Contract Sales

Component, Metal, Other	General
Contract Manufacturing	General

WCM WASTE & COMPLIANCE 760-930-9101
MANAGEMENT, INC.
6054 Corte Del Cedro, Carlsbad, CA 92009
FDA Number: 2032810
Ownership: Private
Produces/Sells CE-marked Devices: N
Container, Sharpes | General

WCW,INC 518-686-0725
1 Mechanic Street, Hoosick Falls, NY 12090
FDA Number: 1320918

Cushion, Flotation	Physical Med
Mattress, Air Flotation	General
Mattress, Non-Powered Flotation Therapy	Physical Med

WE CARE DESIGN'S, L.L.C.   504-624-8282
428 Bill Dr., Mandeville, LA 70448
FDA Number: 3003502047
  Transfer Aid   Physical Med

WEARTECH INTL., INC.   562-698-7847
13032 Park Street, Santa Fe Springs, CA 90670
FDA Number: 3000300238
  Metal, Base   Dental And Oral

WEAVER & COMPANY   303-366-1804
565-B Nucla Way, Aurora, CO 80011-9319
FDA Number: 1718791   *Fax:* 303-367-5118
E-mail: distributorinquiries@doweaver.com
Web site: www.doweaver.com
Medical Products Sales Volume: $1,100,000
Annual Revenue: $1-$5 Million
Year Founded: 1978
Total Employees: 11   *Marketing Staff:* 2   *Sales Staff:* 2
Ownership: Private
Produces/Sells CE-marked Devices: Y
Federal Procurement Eligibility: Small Business
Distribution: Manufacturer Direct, Manufacturer Through Distributor
General Admin.: David Weaver/President
       Douglas Cleveland/Vice President
  Dressing, Gel   General

WEB-TEX, INC.   888-633-2723
5425 Casgrain, Suite 300,   514-273-5972
Montreal, QC H2T 1 Canada
FDA Number: 8043782   *Fax:* 514-273-4925
E-mail: webtex@total.net
Year Founded: 1985
Total Employees: 50
Ownership: Private
Produces/Sells CE-marked Devices: Y
Federal Procurement Eligibility: Small Business
Distribution: Manufacturer Direct, Exclusive Distributor, Exporter

WEBB MANUFACTURING CO.   800-932-2634
1241 Carpenter St., Philadelphia, PA 19147-5512   215-336-5570
FDA Number: 9201131   *Fax:* 215-336-4422
E-mail: steve@webbmfg.com
Web site: www.webbmfg.com
Medical Products Sales Volume: $2,300,000
Annual Revenue: $0-$1 Million
Year Founded: 1969
Total Employees: 18
Ownership: Private
Produces/Sells CE-marked Devices: N
Federal Procurement Eligibility: Small Business
Distribution: Manufacturer Direct
General Admin.: Steven Krupnick/President, Chief Executive Officer
Mktg./Adv.: Bill Neuhoff/Vice President Marketing
  Bag, Laundry, Infection Control   General
  Biopsy Instrument   Gastroenterology/Urology
  Curtain, Cubicle   General
  Curtain, Shower   General
  Magnet, Permanent, MRI (Magnetic Resonance Imaging)   Radiology
  Track And Carrier, Cubicle Curtain   General

WEBBMED CORPORATION   678-482-1722
615 Emerald Pkwy., Buford, GA 30518
FDA Number: 77881
Ownership: Private
Produces/Sells CE-marked Devices: N
  Massager, Therapeutic   Physical Med

WEBER GLASS WASHER MFG. CORP.
  See Presco-Webber Corporation

WEBSTER ENTERPRISES OF JACKSON COUNTY, INC.   828-586-8981
140 Little Savannah Rd., Sylva, NC 28779
FDA Number: 1034084
  Drape, Surgical   Surgery

WEBSTER ENTERPRISES, INC.   704-586-8981
P.O. Box 220, Webster, NC 28788-0220
FDA Number: 1034084   *Fax:* 704-586-8125
E-mail: grobinson@websterenterprises.org
Annual Revenue: $1-$5 Million
Total Employees: 130   *Marketing Staff:* 1   *Sales Staff:* 1
Ownership: Private
Produces/Sells CE-marked Devices: N
Federal Procurement Eligibility: Small Business
Distribution: Manufacturer Through Distributor
General Admin.: Arlene C. Stewart/Chief Executive Officer

WEBSTER ENTERPRISES, INC.   704-586-8981 *(cont'd)*
  Arlene C. Stewart/Executive Director
Mktg./Adv.: Alan Warshaw/Director Marketing
       Joe Rigdon/Director Product Development
  Drape, Surgical, Disposable   Surgery

WEBSTER LABS, INC.
  See Biosense Webster, Inc

WEBTEC CONVERTING, LLC.   865-246-4342
5900 Middle View Way, Knoxville, TN 37909
FDA Number: 2320643   *Fax:* 865-584-8216
E-mail: questions@webtecllc.com
Web site: www.webtecllc.com
Year Founded: 1998
Ownership: Private
Produces/Sells CE-marked Devices: N
Finance: Mr. Scott Wheatley/Controller
  Bandage, Adhesive   Surgery

WECK & CO. INC., BANDAGE DIV., EDWARD
  See Convatec Professional Services

WECOM, INC.   800-628-4115
20 Warrick Avenue, Glassboro, NJ 08028-2500   609-863-8400
FDA Number: 2244733   *Fax:* 856-863-8408
E-mail: wecom@wecom.com
Web site: www.wecom.com
Medical Products Sales Volume: $3,300,000
Annual Revenue: $5-$10 Million
Year Founded: 1961
Total Employees: 38   *Marketing Staff:* 2   *Sales Staff:* 3
Ownership: Private
Produces/Sells CE-marked Devices: N
Federal Procurement Eligibility: Small Business
Distribution: Manufacturer Direct
  Burr   Ear/Nose/Throat
  Dental Laboratory Equipment   Dental And Oral

WECT INSTRUMENT
  See Conmed Linvatec

WEEVAC, W. MURPHY ENTERPRISES, INC.   613-584-9473
12 La Salle Dr., P.O. Box 1306, Deep River, ONT K0J 1P0 Canada
FDA Number: 8022270   *Fax:* 613-584-2626
E-mail: weevac@on.aicn.com
Year Founded: 1988
Ownership: Private
Produces/Sells CE-marked Devices: N
Distribution: Manufacturer Direct, Exclusive Distributor, Exporter

WEHMER CORPORATION   800-323-0229
1151 N. Main Street, Lombard, IL 60148   630-424-1877
FDA Number: 1418965   *Fax:* 630-424-1898
Web site: www.wehmer.com
Annual Revenue: $1-$5 Million
Year Founded: 1943
Ownership: Private
Quality System Registration Information: ISO9000
Produces/Sells CE-marked Devices: Y
Federal Procurement Eligibility: Small Business
Distribution: Manufacturer Direct, Manufacturer Through Manufacturer Reps
  Aligner, Beam, X-Ray (Collimator)   Dental And Oral
  Cephalometer   Dental And Oral
  Chair, Other   General
  Collimator, X-Ray   Dental And Oral
  Glove, Patient Examination   General
  Grid, Radiographic   Radiology
  Shield, X-Ray   Radiology
  Spatula, Cement   Dental And Oral
  Spatula, Other   Surgery
  Wheel, Polishing Agent   Dental And Oral

WEILER ENGINEERING, INC.   847-697-4900
1395 Gateway Drive, Elgin, IL 60123
FDA Number: n/a   *Fax:* 847-697-4915
E-mail: solutions@weilerengineering.com
Web site: www.weilerengineering.com
Medical Products Sales Volume: $7,300,000
Annual Revenue: $25-$50 Million
Year Founded: 1959
Total Employees: 100   *Marketing Staff:* 1   *Sales Staff:* 4
Ownership: Private
Quality System Registration Information: ISO9001
Produces/Sells CE-marked Devices: Y
Federal Procurement Eligibility: Small Business
Distribution: Manufacturer Direct, Manufacturer Through Manufacturer Reps, Exporter
General Admin.: Gary Weiler/Chief Executive Officer
Mktg./Adv.: Alan Goodman/Manager International Sales

MANUFACTURER PROFILES

WEILER ENGINEERING, INC.   847-697-4900 *(cont'd)*
Chuck Reed/Manager Sales
Carol Zolp/Vice President Sales
Nebulizer, Direct Patient Interface   Anesthesiology

WEIMAN HEALTHCARE SOLUTIONS   800-837-8140
755 Tri-State Parkway, Gurnee, IL 60031-2400   **847-263-3500**
FDA Number: 1450386   *Fax:* 847-263-3700
E-mail: cdemasi@burnishine.com
Web site: http://www.weimanhealthcare.com
Medical Products Sales Volume: $12,000,000
Annual Revenue: $25-$50 Million
Year Founded: 1887
Total Employees: 75   *Marketing Staff:* 3   *Sales Staff:* 9
Ownership: Private
Produces/Sells CE-marked Devices: Y
Federal Procurement Eligibility: Small Business
Distribution: Manufacturer Through Distributor, OEM, Importer, Exporter
General Admin.: Carl DeMasi/President, Chief Executive Officer
Mktg./Adv.: Ron Nelson/Director Marketing
   Herbert Green/Director Product Development
   Carl Demasi/Vice President Marketing
Production: Sylvia Aldrin/Director Quality Assurance
   Melanie Loomis/Manager Materials
   Laurie Philipps/Vice President Manufacturing
Gel, Electrode, TENS   Physical Med
Sanitizer   General
Solvent, Adhesive Tape   Surgery

WEISS AUG CO., INC.   973-887-7600
220 Merry Lane, PO Box 520, East Hanover, NJ 07936
FDA Number: n/a   *Fax:* 973-887-8109
E-mail: marketing@weiss-aug.com
Web site: www.weiss-aug.com
Medical Products Sales Volume: $16,800,000
Annual Revenue: $25-$50 Million
Year Founded: 1972
Total Employees: 120   *Marketing Staff:* 1   *Sales Staff:* 6
Ownership: Private
Quality System Registration Information: ISO9001
Produces/Sells CE-marked Devices: N
Federal Procurement Eligibility: Small Business
Distribution: Manufacturer Direct
General Admin.: Dieter Weissenrieder/President, Chief Executive Officer
Mktg./Adv.: Elisabeth Weissenrieder/Director Marketing
Production: Tom Trokan/Director Quality Assurance
   Doug Bruce/Manager Materials
   Mr. Jeffrey Cole/Vice President Manufacturing
Finance: Pierre Leonard/Controller
Contract Manufacturing   General

WEITBRECHT COMMUNICATIONS, INC.   800-233-9130
926 Colorado Avenue,   **310-452-8613**
Santa Monica, CA 90401
FDA Number: n/a   *Fax:* 310-450-9918
E-mail: sales@weitbrecht.com
Web site: www.weitbrecht.com
Annual Revenue: $1-$5 Million
Total Employees: 8   *Marketing Staff:* 2   *Sales Staff:* 4
Ownership: Private
Produces/Sells CE-marked Devices: N
Federal Procurement Eligibility: Small Business, Female Owned
Distribution: Manufacturer Direct
General Admin.: Barbara Dreyfus/President
Mktg./Adv.: Shelly Stein/Manager National Sales
Environmental Control System, Powered   Physical Med
Telephone, Handicapped Use   Physical Med

WEL INDUSTRIES, INC.   805-985-2462
5114 Terramar Way, Oxnard, CA 93035-1838
FDA Number: 2022476   *Fax:* 805-339-9414
E-mail: info@welindustries.com
Web site: www.welindustries.com
Medical Products Sales Volume: $600,000
Annual Revenue: $0-$1 Million
Year Founded: 1972
Total Employees: 1
Ownership: Private
Produces/Sells CE-marked Devices: N
Federal Procurement Eligibility: Small Business
Distribution: Manufacturer Direct
Catheter, Suction, With Tip   General

WELCH ALLYN PROTOCOL INC.   800-289-2500
8500 S.W. Creekside Pl.,   **503-526-8500**
Beaverton, OR 97008
FDA Number: n/a

WELCH ALLYN PROTOCOL INC.   800-289-2500 *(cont'd)*
Web site: protocol.com
Annual Revenue: $50-$100 Million
Total Employees: 311   *Marketing Staff:* 7   *Sales Staff:* 53
Ownership: Welch Allyn, Inc.
Stock Symbol: PCOL
Traded On: NASDAQ
Quality System Registration Information: ISO9001; ISO9002
Produces/Sells CE-marked Devices: Y
Distribution: Manufacturer Direct, Manufacturer Through Distributor, OEM, Importer, Exporter
General Admin.: Trudel Weidemann/Director Admin.
   James Welch/Vice President, General Manager
   James P. Fee/Vice President, General Manager
Mktg./Adv.: Will Fox/Director Marketing
   Ben Williams/Director National Accounts
   Chris Randall/Director Sales Training
   Grant S. Gibson/Marketing & Communications Officer
   Chris Tew/Vice President Sales
Production: Don Abbey/Vice President Quality Systems
Research: Richard Roa/Vice President Engineering
Finance: Ed Kolasinski/Vice President Finance
Analyzer, Gas, Carbon-Dioxide, Gaseous Phase (Capnograph)   Anesthesiology
Computer, Diagnostic, Programmable   Cardiovascular
Defibrillator, External, Automatic   Cardiovascular
Detector, Arrhythmia Alarm   Cardiovascular
Monitor, Apnea   General
Monitor, Cardiac (Cardiotachometer & Rate Alarm)   Cardiovascular
Monitor, Heart Rate, Other   Cardiovascular
Monitor, Physiological, Patient(without Arrhythmia Detection Or Alarms)   Cardiovascular
Monitor, Pressure, Venous, Central, Powered   Cardiovascular
Monitor, ST Segment (With Alarm)   General
Oximeter, Intracardiac   Cardiovascular
Oximeter, Pulse   General
Recorder, Paper Chart   Cardiovascular
System, Network And Communication, Physiological Monitors   Cardiovascular
Transmitter/Receiver System, Physiological, Radiofrequency   Cardiovascular
Ventilator, Continuous (Respirator), Accessory   Anesthesiology

WELCH ALLYN PROTOCOL, INC.   503 530 7500
8500 s.w. creekside place, Beaverton, OR 97008
FDA Number: 3023750   *Fax:* 503 526 4200
E-mail: info@mrlinc.com
Web site: www.welchallyn.com
Year Founded: 1968
Total Employees: 80
Ownership: Welch Allyn, Inc.
Quality System Registration Information: ISO9001
Produces/Sells CE-marked Devices: N
Federal Procurement Eligibility: Small Business
Distribution: Manufacturer Direct, OEM, Exporter
General Admin.: Dean Milani/President
   Dilip Mehta/Vice President, General Manager
Mktg./Adv.: Adrian Alvarez/Director Marketing
   Michael Garrett/Director Product Development
   Bill Smirles/Vice President Business Development
   Gerald Perozzi/Vice President Sales
Production: Joel Orlinsky/Manager Regulatory Affairs
Defibrillator, Battery-Powered   Cardiovascular
Defibrillator, Battery-Powered, Low Energy   Cardiovascular
Defibrillator, External, Automatic   Cardiovascular
Defibrillator, Line-Powered   Cardiovascular
Defibrillator/Monitor, Battery-Powered   Cardiovascular
Monitor, Blood Pressure, Indirect, Automatic   Cardiovascular
Monitor, ECG   Cardiovascular
Monitor, Physiological, Patient(without Arrhythmia Detection Or Alarms)   Cardiovascular
Pacemaker, Cardiac, External Transcutaneous (Non-Invasive)   Cardiovascular
Recorder, Paper Chart   Cardiovascular
Tester, Defibrillator   Cardiovascular

WELCH ALLYN, INC.   800-535-6663
4341 State St. Rd.,   **315-685-4100**
Skaneateles Falls, NY 13153
FDA Number: 1316463   *Fax:* 315-685-3361
E-mail: info@mail.welchallyn.com
Web site: www.welchallyn.com
Medical Products Sales Volume: $227,300,000
Annual Revenue: $100-$500 Million
Year Founded: 1915
Total Employees: 2700   *Marketing Staff:* 15   *Sales Staff:* 100
Ownership: Private
Quality System Registration Information: ISO9001
Produces/Sells CE-marked Devices: Y
Distribution: Manufacturer Through Distributor
General Admin.: Doug Linquest/Executive Vice President
   Stephen Meyer/Executive Vice President
   Julie Shimer/President, Chief Executive Officer
   Dan Fisher/Senior Vice President Human Resources

WELCH ALLYN, INC.   800-535-6663 (cont'd)

Mktg./Adv.: Eric R. Allyn/Manager Business
    John Moran/Vice President Sales

Accessories, Cleaning, Endoscopic	Gastroenterology/Urology
Analyzer, Middle Ear	Ear/Nose/Throat
Anoscope, Non-Powered	Gastroenterology/Urology
Audiometer	Ear/Nose/Throat
Camera, Television, Endoscopic (Without Audio)	Surgery
Camera, Television, Surgical (Without Audio)	Surgery
Camera, Video, Endoscopic	General
Camera, Video, Multi-Image	General
Cuff, Blood Pressure	Cardiovascular
Depressor, Tongue	General
Electrocardiograph, Ambulatory (With Analysis Algorithm)	Cardiovascular
Endoscope	Gastroenterology/Urology
Endoscope And Accessories, AC-Powered	Surgery
Endoscope, Electronic (Videoendoscope)	Surgery
Endoscope, Fiberoptic	Surgery
Endoscope, Flexible	Gastroenterology/Urology
Endoscope, Rigid	Surgery
Examination Device, AC-Powered	General
Gown, Operating Room, Reusable	Surgery
Headlight, ENT	Ear/Nose/Throat
Lamp, Examination (Light)	General
Lamp, Fluorescein, AC-Powered	Surgery
Lamp, Surgical	Surgery
Laparoscope, Flexible	Surgery
Laparoscope, General & Plastic Surgery	Surgery
Laparoscope, Gynecologic	Obstetrics/Gynecology
Laryngoscope	Ear/Nose/Throat
Laryngoscope, Rigid	Anesthesiology
Light, Dental	Dental And Oral
Light, Examination, Battery-Powered	General
Light, Surgical Headlight	Dental And Oral
Light, Surgical, Endoscopic	Surgery
Loupe, Binocular, Low Power	Ophthalmology
Micrometer, Microscope	Pathology
Microscope	Hematology
Mirror, ENT	Ear/Nose/Throat
Mirror, Laryngeal	Ear/Nose/Throat
Monitor, Blood Pressure, Indirect, Transducer	Anesthesiology
Monitor, ECG, Surgery	Surgery
Monitor, Video, Endoscope	General
Nasopharyngoscope (Flexible Or Rigid)	Ear/Nose/Throat
Ophthalmoscope, Battery-Powered	Ophthalmology
Ophthalmoscope, Direct	Ophthalmology
Otoscope	Ear/Nose/Throat
Perimeter, AC-Powered	Ophthalmology
Power Supply, Endoscopic, Battery-Operated	General
Power Supply, Endoscopic, Line-Operated	General
Probe, Rectal, Non-Powered	Gastroenterology/Urology
Proctoscope	Surgery
Proctosigmoidoscope	Gastroenterology/Urology
Regulator, Line Voltage	General
Retinoscope, AC-Powered	Ophthalmology
Retinoscope, Battery-Powered	Ophthalmology
Sigmoidoscope, Flexible	Gastroenterology/Urology
Sigmoidoscope, Rigid, Electrical	Gastroenterology/Urology
Sigmoidoscope, Rigid, Non-Electrical	Gastroenterology/Urology
Spectacle Microscope, Low-Vision	Ophthalmology
Speculum, Ear	Ear/Nose/Throat
Speculum, Nasal	Ear/Nose/Throat
Speculum, Rectal	Gastroenterology/Urology
Speculum, Vaginal, Metal	Obstetrics/Gynecology
Speculum, Vaginal, Non-Metal	Obstetrics/Gynecology
Sphygmomanometer, Aneroid (Arterial Pressure)	General
Sphygmomanometer, Electronic, Automatic	General
Stethoscope, Amplified	General
Stethoscope, Manual	Cardiovascular
Stethoscope, Mechanical	General
Synoptophore	Ophthalmology
Thermometer, Electronic, Continuous	General
Thoracoscope	Cardiovascular
Tip, Suction	Anesthesiology
Tip, Suction Tube (Yankauer, Poole, Etc.)	Surgery
Transilluminator, AC-Powered, Other	Ophthalmology
Transilluminator, Battery-Powered	Ophthalmology

Medical Product Subsidiaries (Listed Separately)
  Welch Allyn Gmbh
  Welch Allyn Protocol Inc.
  Welch Allyn Protocol, Inc.
  Welch Allyn, Inc.

WELCH ALLYN, INC.   800-535-6663 / 315-685-2993

4341 State Street Road, Skaneateles Falls, NY 13153
FDA Number: 1313399   Fax: 315-685-4091
E-mail: cogentinfo@mail.welchallyn.com
Web site: www.walamp.com
Year Founded: 1915
Ownership: Welch Allyn, Inc.

WELCH ALLYN, INC.   800-535-6663 (cont'd)

Produces/Sells CE-marked Devices: Y
General Admin.: Ms. Karen Roscher/Chief Financial Officer, Executive Vice President
    Mr. Eric Hunt/Chief Information Officer
    Dr. Julie Shimer/President, Chief Executive Officer
    Mr. Andy Clapper/Senior Vice President International Operations
Mktg./Adv.: Bob Kish/Manager International & National Sales

Accessories, Light, Surgical	Surgery
Headlight, ENT	Ear/Nose/Throat
Light Source, Endoscopic	Obstetrics/Gynecology
Light, Other	General
Light, Surgical Headlight	Dental And Oral
Light, Surgical, Endoscopic	Surgery
Light, Surgical, Fiberoptic	Surgery

WELCO-CGI GAS TECHNOLOGIES   440-234-1075

145 Shimersville Rd., Bethlehem, PA 18015
FDA Number: 2529486

Gas, Calibrated (Specified Concentration)	Anesthesiology
Incubator/Water Bath, Microbiology	Microbiology
Laser, Ophthalmic	Ophthalmology
Laser, Surgical	Surgery
Liquid Chromatography, Salicylate	Toxicology
Suture, Non-Absorbable, Synthetic, Polyester	Surgery
Transport System, Anaerobic	Microbiology

WELCON, INC.   800-877-0923 / 817-877-0923

7409 Pebble Drive, Fort Worth, TX 76118
FDA Number: 1218958   Fax: 817-332-1404
E-mail: gpedersen@welcon.com
Web site: www.welcon.com
Annual Revenue: $10-$25 Million
Total Employees: 50   Marketing Staff: 5   Sales Staff: 7
Ownership: Private
Produces/Sells CE-marked Devices: N
Federal Procurement Eligibility: Small Business, GSA Contract, VA Contract
Distribution: Manufacturer Direct, Manufacturer Through Distributor, Manufacturer Through Manufacturer Reps, OEM
Mktg./Adv.: Mr. Gary Pedersen/Vice President Marketing & Sales
Production: Mr. George Hird/Vice President Operations

Bag, Leg	Gastroenterology/Urology
Dispenser, Medication, Liquid	General
Holder, Tracheostomy Tube	Anesthesiology
Kit, Administration, Enteral	Gastroenterology/Urology
Kit, Administration, Parenteral	Gastroenterology/Urology
Kit, Catheterization, Sterile Urethral	Gastroenterology/Urology
Kit, Catheterization, Urinary	Gastroenterology/Urology
Kit, Irrigation, Perineal	Gastroenterology/Urology
Kit, Irrigation, Sterile	Gastroenterology/Urology
Kit, Irrigation, Wound	General
Kit, Tracheostomy Care	Anesthesiology
Pump, Food (Enteral Feeding)	General
Syringe, Catheter	General
Water, Distilled (Irrigation)	Gastroenterology/Urology

WELLAN MEDICAL, INC.   603-676-8601

10 Water Street, Lebanon, NH 03766
FDA Number: 3006095848

Table, Anesthetist's	Anesthesiology

WELLHOFER NORTH AMERICA
  See Scanditronix - Wellhofer North America

WELLS DENTAL, INC.   800-233-0521 / 707-937-0521

5860 Flynn Creek Road, P.O. Box 106, Comptche, CA 95427
FDA Number: n/a   Fax: 707-937-2809
E-mail: info@wellsdental.com
Web site: www.wellsdental.com
Medical Products Sales Volume: $1,500,000
Annual Revenue: $1-$5 Million
Year Founded: 1936
Ownership: Private
Produces/Sells CE-marked Devices: N
Federal Procurement Eligibility: Small Business
Distribution: Manufacturer Direct, Manufacturer Through Distributor, Manufacturer Through Manufacturer Reps, OEM, Exclusive Distributor

Dental Laboratory Equipment	Dental And Oral

WELLS ENDOSCOPIC COMPANY (WECO)
  See Wells Johnson Co.

WELLS GROUP
  See Wells Johnson Co.

WELLS HOSIERY MILLS, INC.   336-633-4881

1758 South Fayetteville St., Asheboro, NC 27204
FDA Number: 3005108032   Fax: 336-633-4862
E-mail: info@wellshosiery.com
Web site: www.wellshosiery.com

WELLS HOSIERY MILLS, INC.   336-633-4881 *(cont'd)*
Ownership: Private
Produces/Sells CE-marked Devices: N
  Stocking, Support (Anti-Embolic)   General

WELLS JOHNSON CO.   800-528-1597
8000 South Kolb Road, Tucson, AZ 85706   **520-298-6069**
FDA Number: 2024022   *Fax:* 520-885-1189
E-mail: sales@wellsgrp.com
Web site: www.wellsgrp.com
Medical Products Sales Volume: $5,000,000
Annual Revenue: $1-$5 Million
Year Founded: 1980
Total Employees: 14   *Marketing Staff:* 2   *Sales Staff:* 3
Ownership: Private
Produces/Sells CE-marked Devices: Y
Federal Procurement Eligibility: Small Business
Distribution: Manufacturer Direct, Manufacturer Through Distributor, Service Direct, Exclusive Distributor, Exporter
General Admin.: Brad Corneliusen/Chief Operating Officer
          John F. Wells/President, Chief Executive Officer
          Elaine Wells/Vice President
Mktg./Adv.: Jason Clark/Senior Sales Manager
          John F. Wells/Vice President Business Development
Production: Joshua Hitchiner/Director Quality Assurance
          Josh Hitchiner/Manager Regulatory Affairs
Aspirator, Liposuction	Surgery
Binder, Abdominal	General
Cannula, Suction, Pool-Tip	Surgery
Cannula, Suction/Irrigation, Laparoscopic	Surgery
Cannula, Surgical, General & Plastic Surgery	Surgery
Catheter, Suction, With Tip	General
Dissector, Surgical, General & Plastic Surgery	Surgery
Elevator, Surgical, General & Plastic Surgery	Surgery
Garment, Protective, For Incontinence	Gastroenterology/Urology
Infusion Stand	General
Needle, Aspiration And Injection, Reusable	Surgery
Pump, Infusion	General
Trap, Sterile Specimen	Anesthesiology
Tube, Aspirating, Flexible, Connecting	Anesthesiology
Tubing, Non-Invasive	Surgery
Tubing, Other	General

WELLS-ENGBERG COMPANY   800-642-3628
129 S. Phelps Ave., Rockford, IL 61125   **815-227-9765**
FDA Number: n/a   *Fax:* 815-227-9737
E-mail: wellseng@aol.com
Web site: www.wells-engberg.com
Total Employees: 10   *Marketing Staff:* 4   *Sales Staff:* 4
Ownership: Private
Produces/Sells CE-marked Devices: N
Federal Procurement Eligibility: Small Business
Distribution: Manufacturer Direct
General Admin.: Dale Engberg/President
  Control, Hand Driving, Automobile, Mechanical   Physical Med

WENDELL-ALAN LTD.   216-881-8299
1768 East 25th St., Cleveland, OH 44114
FDA Number: 3005100672
  Pack, Hot Or Cold, Reusable   Physical Med

WENZEL SPINE INC.   512-469-0600
206 Wild Basin Road, Building A Suite 203, Austin, TX 78746
FDA Number: 3008009850   *Fax:* 512-469-0604
E-mail: info@wenzelspine.com
Web site: http://www.wenzelspine.com
Ownership: Private
Produces/Sells CE-marked Devices: N
General Admin.: Mr. Ryan Crow/Business Manager
          Mr. Chad Neely/Chief Executive Officer
          Dr. Sourabh Mishra/Chief Technology Officer
          Mr. Jon Luedke/Vice President
Medical Admin.: Dr. Warren Neely/Chief Medical Officer
Production: Mr. Andy Anderson/Director Operations
Finance: Mr. Kevin Brady/Chief Financial Officer
          Mr. William Wilson/Director Finance
Appliance, Fixation, Spinal Interlaminal	Orthopedics
Orthosis, Fixation, Spinal, Spondylolisthesis	Orthopedics
Prosthesis, Hip, Cement Restrictor	Orthopedics

WENZELITE MEDICAL SUPPLIES CORP.
  See Wenzelite Rehab Supplies, Llc

WENZELITE REHAB SUPPLIES, LLC   800-706-9255
220 36th Street, 99 Seaview Blvd,   **516-998-4600**
Brooklyn, NY 11232
FDA Number: 2433051   *Fax:* 516-998-4601
E-mail: info@wenzelite.com
Web site: www.wenzelite.com

WENZELITE REHAB SUPPLIES, LLC   800-706-9255 *(cont'd)*
Medical Products Sales Volume: $1,000,000
Year Founded: 1982
Ownership: Drive Medical Design And Manufacturing
Produces/Sells CE-marked Devices: N
Federal Procurement Eligibility: GSA Contract, VA Contract
Distribution: Manufacturer Through Distributor, Manufacturer Through Manufacturer Reps
General Admin.: Abraham Goldstein/President
Mktg./Adv.: Pearl Goldstein/Vice President, Director Marketing
Accessories, Walker	General
Attachment, Oxygen Canister/IV Pole, Wheelchair	General
Chair, Bath	General
Chair, Pediatric	General
Roller, Patient	General
Stroller, Adaptive	Physical Med
Tips And Pads, Cane, Crutch And Walker	Physical Med
Walker, Mechanical	Physical Med

WEPCO PRODUCTS, INC   775-772-5910
1930 Gilly Ln., Concord, CA 94518
FDA Number: 3023901
Ownership: Private
Produces/Sells CE-marked Devices: N
  Electrophoresis Instrumentation   Immunology

WEPCO, INC.
  See Driving Aids Development Corporation

WES-PAK, INC.   1-800-493-7725
11610 Vimy Ridge Rd., Alexander, AR 72002   **800-282-5769**
FDA Number: n/a
E-mail: sales@wespakinc.com
Web site: www.wespakinc.com
Annual Revenue: $1-$5 Million
Total Employees: 25   *Marketing Staff:* 2   *Sales Staff:* 3
Ownership: Private
Produces/Sells CE-marked Devices: N
Federal Procurement Eligibility: Small Business
Distribution: Manufacturer Direct
General Admin.: Frank E. Westerman/President, Chief Executive Officer
Cart, Other	General
Waste Receptacle, Contaminated	General

WESCOR, INC.   800-453-2725
370 West 1700 South, Logan, UT 84321-5294   **435-752-6011**
FDA Number: 1717966   *Fax:* 435-752-4127
E-mail: biomed@wescor.com
Web site: www.wescor.com/biomedical
Medical Products Sales Volume: $11,500,000
Annual Revenue: $10-$25 Million
Year Founded: 1970
Total Employees: 95   *Marketing Staff:* 3   *Sales Staff:* 3
Ownership: Elitech France
Produces/Sells CE-marked Devices: Y
Federal Procurement Eligibility: Small Business
Distribution: Manufacturer Direct, Manufacturer Through Manufacturer Reps, Exporter
General Admin.: Wayne K. Barlow/President, Chief Executive Officer
Mktg./Adv.: Dennis Briscoe/Director Product Development
          Alan Crockett/Manager Advertising
          Kent S. Thomas/Vice President Sales
Production: Brent Thackeray/Manager Quality Assurance & Quality Control
          Paul R. Holman/Vice President Manufacturing & Production
Finance: Janice Wallentine/Chief Financial Officer
Chamber, Slide Culture	Pathology
Collector, Sweat	Chemistry
Cystic Fibrosis System	Gastroenterology/Urology
Cytocentrifuge	Pathology
Iontophoresis Equipment	Chemistry
Iontophoresis Unit (Sweat Rate)	Gastroenterology/Urology
Kit, Identification, Yeast	Microbiology
Kit, Screening, Staphylococcus Aureus	Microbiology
Mycoplasma SPP. DNA Reagents	Microbiology
Oncometer	Microbiology
Oncometer, Laboratory	Chemistry
Osmometer	Chemistry
Stainer, Slide, Automated	Pathology
Stainer, Slide, Hematology	Hematology
Stainer, Slide, Hematology, Automated	Hematology

WESGO/DURAMIC
  See Morgan Advance Ceramics

WESLEY-JESSEN CORP.
  See Ciba Vision

WESSELS AND ASSOCIATES   248-547-7177
131 Cambridge Blvd., Pleasant Ridge, MI 48069-1005
FDA Number: 1836242
Ownership: Private

WESSELS AND ASSOCIATES   248-547-7177 *(cont'd)*
Produces/Sells CE-marked Devices: N

Formaldehyde (Formalin, Formol)	Pathology
Formalin, Neutral Buffered	Pathology

WEST CHEMICAL PRODUCTS INC.
See West Penetone Corp

WEST CO., THE
See West Pharmaceutical Services, Inc.

WEST COAST AUTOMATION, CORP.   509-773-5055
1600 S. Roosevelt, Goldendale, WA 98620
FDA Number: 3002674527
Ownership: Private
Produces/Sells CE-marked Devices: N

Lift, Bath, Non-AC-Powered	General

WEST COAST CHAIN MANUFACTURING COMPANY
See Key-Bak

WEST COAST SURGICAL LLC.   650-728-8095
141 California Ave, Suite 101, Half Moon Bay, CA 94019
FDA Number: 3005619998

Bath, Sitz, Non-Powered	Physical Med
Caliper	Orthopedics
Instrument, Manual, General Surgical	Surgery
Orthopedic Manual Surgical Instrument	Orthopedics
Surgical Instrument, Non-Powered, Neurosurgical	Cns/Neurology
Tray, Surgical Instrument	Surgery

WEST PENETONE CORP   800-631-1652
700 Gotham Pkwy, Carlstadt, NJ 07072   201-567-3000
FDA Number: n/a   *Fax:* 201-510-3973
Web site: www.west-penetone.com
Ownership: WEST CHEMICAL PRODUCTS
Quality System Registration Information: ISO9001
Produces/Sells CE-marked Devices: N
Distribution: Manufacturer Through Distributor, Manufacturer Through Manufacturer Reps, Importer, Exporter

Disinfector, Liquid	General
Solution, Antibacterial Cleaner	General

WEST PHARMACEUTICAL SERVICES DELAWARE ACQUISTION,   903-677-5017
1704 Enterprise St, Athens, TX 75751
FDA Number: 3005159163
Web site: www.westpharma.com
Ownership: WEST PHARMACEUTICAL SERVICES, INC.
Produces/Sells CE-marked Devices: Y

Introducer, Syringe Needle	General

WEST PHARMACEUTICAL SERVICES, INC.   800-231-3000
101 Gordon Dr., Lionville, PA 19341   610-594-2900
FDA Number: n/a   *Fax:* 610-594-3000
E-mail: webmaster@westpharma.com
Web site: www.westpharma.com
Annual Revenue: $500 Million-$1 Billion
Year Founded: 1923
Total Employees: 6323   *Marketing Staff:* 10   *Sales Staff:* 35
Ownership: Public
Stock Symbol: WST
Traded On: NYSE
Quality System Registration Information: ISO9000; ISO9001; ISO9002
Produces/Sells CE-marked Devices: Y
Distribution: Manufacturer Direct, Manufacturer Through Distributor
General Admin.: Dr. Donald E. Morel/Chief Executive Officer, Chairman
     William J. Federici/Chief Financial Officer, Vice President
     Don McMillam/President
     Robert Hargesheimer/President
     Steven A. Ellers/President
     John R. Gailey/Vice President General Counsel & Secretary
     Richard D. Luzzi/Vice President Human Resources
Mktg./Adv.: Frances L. DeGrazio/Vice President Marketing & Business Development
     Jeff Brown/Vice President Sales
Finance: Joseph E. Abbott/Vice President, Corporate Controller
     Michael A. Anderson/Vice President, Treasurer

Component, Metal, Other	General
Component, Other	General
Component, Plastic	General
Component, Rubber	General
Component, Silicone	General
Container, IV	General
Packaging Material	General
Stopper	General

Medical Product Subsidiaries (Listed Separately)
    The Tech Group Tempe

WEST PHARMACEUTICAL SERVICES, INC.   610-594-3105
6453 US Highway 15, Montgomery, PA 17752
FDA Number: 2515707
Web site: www.westpharma.com
Year Founded: 1923
Total Employees: 232
Ownership: WEST PHARMACEUTICAL SERVICES, INC.
Produces/Sells CE-marked Devices: Y

Transfer Unit, IV Fluid	General

WEST PHARMACEUTICAL SERVICES, INC. - LITITZ, PA   717-560-8460
179 W. Airport Road, brickerville, PA 17543
FDA Number: 3004542260   *Fax:* 717-560-8468
Web site: www.westpharma.com
Total Employees: 22
Ownership: WEST PHARMACEUTICAL SERVICES, INC.
Quality System Registration Information: ISO9001
Produces/Sells CE-marked Devices: Y

Transfer Unit, IV Fluid	General

WESTAR MEDICAL PRODUCTS, INC.   425-290-3945
4470 Chennault Beach Road, Ste 2, Mukilteo, WA 98275
FDA Number: 3004418518

Syringe Unit, Air And/Or Water	Dental And Oral

WESTCO SCIENTIFIC INSTRUMENTS   800-445-0759
Suite 1, 117 Old State Road,   (203) 740-2999
Brookfield, CT 06804
FDA Number: n/a   *Fax:* (203) 740-2955
E-mail: Info@WestcoScientific.com
Web site: www.westcoscientific.com
Annual Revenue: $0-$1 Million
Total Employees: 7   *Marketing Staff:* 2   *Sales Staff:* 2
Ownership: Private
Produces/Sells CE-marked Devices: Y
Federal Procurement Eligibility: Small Business
Distribution: Manufacturer Direct, Service Direct
General Admin.: Joe Platano/President
Mktg./Adv.: Aldo Conetta/Manager Advertising
     Anthony Platano/Vice President Marketing

Analyzer, Chemistry, Multi-Channel, Fixed	Chemistry
Distilling Unit	Chemistry
Fluorometer	Immunology

WESTCOAST BRACE & LIMB   813-985-5000
5311 E. Fletcher Ave., Tampa, FL 33617
FDA Number: n/a   *Fax:* 813-985-4499
Web site: www.wcbl.com
Year Founded: 1981
Ownership: Private
Produces/Sells CE-marked Devices: N
Federal Procurement Eligibility: Small Business
Distribution: Manufacturer Direct

Prosthesis, Arm	Orthopedics

WESTCON CONTACT LENS CO.   770-622-9235
611 Eisenhauer St., Grand Junction, CO 81503
FDA Number: 1721446

Lenses, Soft Contact, Daily Wear	Ophthalmology
Lenses, Soft Contact, Extended Wear	Ophthalmology

WESTCON ORTHOPEDICS, INC.   800-382-4975
4 Craig Rd., Neshanic Station, NJ 08853   908-806-8981
FDA Number: 2246920   *Fax:* 908-806-6664
E-mail: info@westconortho.com
Web site: www.westconortho.com
Medical Products Sales Volume: $250,000
Annual Revenue: $0-$1 Million
Year Founded: 1989
Total Employees: 4   *Marketing Staff:* 2   *Sales Staff:* 1
Ownership: Private
Produces/Sells CE-marked Devices: N
Federal Procurement Eligibility: Small Business
Distribution: Manufacturer Direct
General Admin.: R. Schultz/Chief Executive Officer
     Donn M. Gordon/President

Cutter, Wire And Pin	Orthopedics
Driver, Wire	Orthopedics
Driver/Extractor, Bone Nail/Pin	Orthopedics
Pin, Fixation, Smooth	Orthopedics
Pin, Fixation, Threaded	Orthopedics
Wire, Ligature	Surgery

WESTERN CASE, INC.   877-593-2182
14351 Chambers Road, Tustin, CA 92780-6993   714-838-8460
FDA Number: n/a   *Fax:* 714-838-3039
E-mail: info@westerncase.com

WESTERN CASE, INC. 877-593-2182 (cont'd)
Web site: www.westerncase.com
Medical Products Sales Volume: $4,500,000
Annual Revenue: $1-$5 Million
Year Founded: 1981
Total Employees: 60
Ownership: Private
Produces/Sells CE-marked Devices: N
Federal Procurement Eligibility: Small Business
Distribution: Manufacturer Direct, Manufacturer Through Distributor, Manufacturer Through Manufacturer Reps
General Admin.: Laura Darch/Administrator
Martin Smetter/President

Bag, Medical, Physician	General
Cabinet Casework, General Purpose	General
Container, Surgical Instrument	Surgery

WESTERN DIAGNOSTIC IMAGING SYSTEMS, INC. 951-582-9698
4110 Tigris Way, Riverside, CA 92503
FDA Number: n/a
E-mail: pacs@westerndiagnostic.com
Web site: www.westerndiagnostic.com
Medical Products Sales Volume: $3,000,000
Annual Revenue: $1-$5 Million
Ownership: Private
Produces/Sells CE-marked Devices: N
Federal Procurement Eligibility: Small Business
Distribution: Service Direct

Service, Maintenance/Repair	General

WESTERN ENTERPRISES
See Western Medica

WESTERN INSTRUMENT CO.
See Colorado Serum Company

WESTERN LABORATORIES CORP.
See Mesa Laboratories, Inc.

WESTERN MEDICA 800-783-7890
875 Bassett Road, Westlake, OH 44145 440-871-2160
FDA Number: 1526809 Fax: 440-871-2197
E-mail: medica@westernenterprises.com
Web site: www.westernmedica.com
Year Founded: 1950
Total Employees: 250   Marketing Staff: 2   Sales Staff: 5
Ownership: Scott Fetzer Company
Quality System Registration Information: ISO9001
Produces/Sells CE-marked Devices: N
Federal Procurement Eligibility: Small Business
Distribution: Manufacturer Through Distributor, Manufacturer Through Manufacturer Reps, OEM, Exporter
General Admin.: Gary Schuster/General Manager
Byron Crampton/President
Mktg./Adv.: John Brogan/Director Sales
Lisa M. Szpak/Manager Marketing
Research: Tony Scafaro/Vice President Product Development
Tony Scafaro/Vice President Research & Development

Regulator, Oxygen, Mechanical	General

WESTERN MEDICAL PRODUCTS, INC./KOI
See Dgh Technology, Inc.

WESTERN MEDICAL, LTD. 800-628-8276
214 Carnegie Center Suite 100, 609-514-4744
Princeton, NJ 08540
FDA Number: 9320085 Fax: 609-514-8554
E-mail: bbenchoff@dermasciences.com
Web site: www.westernmedical-ltd.com
Medical Products Sales Volume: $2,100,000
Annual Revenue: $5-$10 Million
Year Founded: 1991
Total Employees: 16   Marketing Staff: 1   Sales Staff: 3
Ownership: Private
Produces/Sells CE-marked Devices: N
Federal Procurement Eligibility: Small Business
Distribution: Manufacturer Through Distributor, Exclusive Distributor, Exporter
General Admin.: Chris Fuhrmann/President, Chief Executive Officer
Kendra Manzi/Vice President Human Resources
Mktg./Adv.: Debbie Jones/Director National Accounts
Ruth Fernandez/Manager Contract Sales
Jennifer Galbo/Manager Marketing & Advertising
Brian T. Fuhrmann/Vice President Business Development
Brian T. Fuhrmann/Vice President Marketing
Production: Christine Mariotti/Manager Materials

Bandage, Adhesive	Surgery
Bandage, Elastic	General
Bandage, Gauze	General
Bandage, Tubular	General

WESTERN MEDICAL, LTD. 800-628-8276 (cont'd)

Clothing, Protective	General
Dressing, Other	General
Dressing, Universal	General
Protector, Heel	General
Retainer, Bandage (Elastic Net)	General
Support, Foot	Orthopedics

WESTERN OPHTHALMICS CORPORATION 800-426-9938
19019 36th Ave W, Suite G, 425-672-9332
Lynnwood, WA 98036
FDA Number: 3004206667
E-mail: Info@Western-Ophthalmics.com Fax: 425-672-3528
Web site: www.west-op.com
Medical Products Sales Volume: $360,000
Annual Revenue: $0-$1 Million
Year Founded: 1998
Total Employees: 4
Ownership: Private
Produces/Sells CE-marked Devices: N
Federal Procurement Eligibility: Small Business
Distribution: Manufacturer Through Distributor
General Admin.: Mr. Jack D'Amico/President
Mktg./Adv.: Pete D'Amico/Manager Advertising
Pete D'Amico/Vice President Marketing & Sales

Aesthesiometer	Ophthalmology
Bar, Prism, Ophthalmic	Ophthalmology
Burr, Corneal, Battery-Powered	Ophthalmology
Cannula, Cyclodialysis (Eye)	Ophthalmology
Cannula, Lacrimal (Eye)	Ophthalmology
Case, Contact Lens	Ophthalmology
Cautery, Thermal, AC-Powered	Ophthalmology
Cautery, Thermal, Battery-Powered	Ophthalmology
Chair, Ophthalmic, AC-Powered	Ophthalmology
Chart, Visual Acuity	Ophthalmology
Conformer, Ophthalmic	Ophthalmology
Dilator, Expansive Iris (Accessory)	Ophthalmology
Dilator, Lacrimal	Ophthalmology
Disk, Pinhole, Ophthalmic	Ophthalmology
Distometer	Ophthalmology
Drum, Opticokinetic	Ophthalmology
Electronystagmograph (ENG)	Ophthalmology
Exophthalmometer	Ophthalmology
Eyeglasses, Safety	Ophthalmology
Fixation Device, AC-Powered, Ophthalmic	Ophthalmology
Fixation Device, Battery-Powered, Ophthalmic	Ophthalmology
Forceps, Ophthalmic	Ophthalmology
Frame, Trial, Ophthalmic	Ophthalmology
Gauge, Lens, Ophthalmic	Ophthalmology
Headlamp, Operating, AC-Powered	Ophthalmology
Illuminator, Color Vision Plate	Ophthalmology
Inserter/Remover, Lens, Contact	Ophthalmology
Keratometer	Ophthalmology

WESTERN OPTICAL CORP.
See Western Ophthalmics Corporation

WESTERN SCIENTIFIC CO., INC. 800-48W-ESCO
2112 West Burbank Blvd., Burbank, CA 91506 818-842-9580
FDA Number: 9201139 Fax: 919-942-9459
E-mail: wesco@wescomicroscopes.com
Web site: www.wescomicroscopes.com
Medical Products Sales Volume: $40,000
Annual Revenue: $1-$5 Million
Year Founded: 1962
Ownership: Private
Federal Procurement Eligibility: Small Business
Distribution: Importer
General Admin.: Jeff Jensen/President
Brad Jensen/Vice President, General Manager
Mktg./Adv.: Gary Jensen/Vice President Sales
Production: Gary Jensen/Manager Materials
Research: Brad Jensen/Vice President Research

Microscope	Hematology
Microscope, Laboratory, Optical	Microbiology
Stereoscope, AC-Powered	Ophthalmology

Medical Product Subsidiaries (Listed Separately)
Western Scientific Co., Inc.

WESTERN SCIENTIFIC CO., INC. 877-489-3726
4104 24th St. #183, San Francisco, CA 94114 415-826-5732
FDA Number: n/a Fax: 415-826-5738
E-mail: sales@wescomicroscopes.com
Web site: www.wescomicroscopes.com
Medical Products Sales Volume: $900,000
Year Founded: 1962
Total Employees: 3
Ownership: Western Scientific Co., Inc.
Produces/Sells CE-marked Devices: Y

WESTERN SCIENTIFIC CO., INC. 877-489-3726 (cont'd)
Federal Procurement Eligibility: Small Business
Distribution: OEM, Exclusive Distributor, Importer
Mktg./Adv.: Mr. Gary Jensen/Vice President Sales

Camera, Microscope	Microbiology
Camera, Video	General
Colposcope	Obstetrics/Gynecology
Condenser, Microscope	Pathology
Contrast Enhancement Unit, Microscope	Microbiology
Cover, Microscope	Microbiology
Lamp, Microscope	Pathology
Micrometer, Microscope	Pathology
Microscope	Hematology
Microscope, Fluorescence/U.V.	Pathology
Microscope, Inverted Stage, Tissue Culture	Pathology
Microscope, Laboratory, Optical	Microbiology
Microscope, Light	Pathology
Microscope, Phase Contrast	Pathology
Microscope, Tissue Culture	Microbiology
Stage, Microscope	Pathology
Television Monitor, Microscope	General

WESTERN SYSTEMS RESEARCH, INC. 626-578-7363
127 N. Madison Avenue, Suite 24, Pasadena, CA 91101
FDA Number: 2025854   *Fax:* 626-578-7364
E-mail: ldoleary@4wsr.com
Web site: www.4wsr.com
Medical Products Sales Volume: $900,000
Year Founded: 1986
Total Employees: 5
Ownership: Private
Produces/Sells CE-marked Devices: N
Federal Procurement Eligibility: Small Business
General Admin.: Mr. Scott Barnes/Chief Executive Officer, Chief Operating Officer

Drum, Opticokinetic	Ophthalmology
Nystagmograph	Cns/Neurology

WESTERN TEXTILE PRODUCTOS DE MEXICO 314-225-9400
S.DE R.L. DEC.
Francisco Murguia #514 Nte., M.muzquiz, Coahuila Mexico
FDA Number: 9616081

Cover, Mattress	General
Garment, Protective, For Incontinence	Gastroenterology/Urology

WESTERN WATER PURIFIER CO. 800-55-WATER
PO Box 688, Woodland Hills, CA 91365-0688 818-703-0444
FDA Number: n/a   *Fax:* 818-992-8170
E-mail: reb-wespurco@att.net
Web site: www.westernpurifier.com
Medical Products Sales Volume: $500,000
Annual Revenue: $1-$5 Million
Year Founded: 1971
Total Employees: 18   *Marketing Staff:* 3   *Sales Staff:* 5
Ownership: Private
Quality System Registration Information: ISO9000
Produces/Sells CE-marked Devices: N
Federal Procurement Eligibility: Small Business
Distribution: Importer, Exporter
General Admin.: Robert Baker/President
Production: D. Richards/Vice President Manufacturing

Purifier, Water	Chemistry
Unit, Filter, Membrane	Chemistry

WESTERN/SCOTT FETZER CO. 440-871-2160
1354 Lear Industrial Park, Avon, OH 44011
FDA Number: 1531260

Regulator, Pressure, Gas Cylinder	Anesthesiology

WESTFALIA SEPARATOR AG
See Gea Westfalia Separator, Inc.

WESTINGHOUSE ELECTRIC CORP., LAMP DIV.
See Philips Lighting Co.

WESTLUND ENGINEERING, INC. 727-572-4343
12400 44th St. N., Clearwater, FL 33762
FDA Number: n/a   *Fax:* 727-572-6811
E-mail: westlund@westlundeng.com
Web site: www.westlundeng.com
Medical Products Sales Volume: $2,000,000
Annual Revenue: $1-$5 Million
Year Founded: 1975
Total Employees: 20   *Marketing Staff:* 2   *Sales Staff:* 2
Ownership: Private
Produces/Sells CE-marked Devices: N
Federal Procurement Eligibility: Small Business, Female Owned
Distribution: Manufacturer Direct, Manufacturer Through Manufacturer Reps
General Admin.: Kelly McGaughey/Partner
                  Paul Wright/Partner
                  Rory Westlund/Partner

WESTLUND ENGINEERING, INC. 727-572-4343 (cont'd)
Mktg./Adv.: Rob Pafford/Sales Engineer

Foodservice Product/Equipment	General
Packaging Equipment	General
Sealer, Packaging	General
Service, Engineering/Design	General

WESTMARK INTERNATIONAL
See Phillips Ultrasound

WESTMED, INC. 800-975-7987
5580 S. Nogales Hwy, Tucson, AZ 85706 520-294-7987
FDA Number: 2028807   *Fax:* 520-294-6061
E-mail: sales@westmedinc.com
Web site: www.westmedinc.com
Medical Products Sales Volume: $5,800,000
Year Founded: 1997
Total Employees: 70   *Marketing Staff:* 1   *Sales Staff:* 30
Ownership: Private
Quality System Registration Information: ISO9001
Produces/Sells CE-marked Devices: Y
Federal Procurement Eligibility: Small Business
Distribution: Manufacturer Direct, Manufacturer Through Distributor, Manufacturer Through Manufacturer Reps, Exporter
General Admin.: Robert J. McKinnon/President, Chief Executive Officer
Mktg./Adv.: Mr. Chris Thomas/Vice President Business Development
              Dian Barker/Vice President International Marketing & Sales
Production: Mr. Gary Conger/Director Quality Assurance & Regulatory Affairs
Finance: Marsha Bishop/Chief Financial Officer
Purchasing: Sandy Smith/Purchasing Agent

Meter, Peak Flow, Spirometry	Anesthesiology
Nebulizer, Direct Patient Interface	Anesthesiology
System, Delivery, Drug, Unit-Dose	General

WESTNOFA OF CANADA LTD.
See Radix Corp.

WESTONE LABORATORIES, INC. 719-540-9333
2235 Executive Circle, Colorado Springs, CO 80906
FDA Number: 2094377

Protector, Hearing (Insert)	Ear/Nose/Throat

WESTONE LABORATORIES, INC. 800-552-7203
6287 American Ave., Portage, MI 49002 269-323-8700
FDA Number: 1835346   *Fax:* 269-323-7770
Web site: www.westone.com
Ownership: Private
Produces/Sells CE-marked Devices: N

Protector, Hearing (Insert)	Ear/Nose/Throat

WESTRIDGE LABORATORI 1-800-646-2096
1671 E. Saint Andrew Place, 714-259-9400 Ex
Santa Ana, CA 92705
FDA Number: 3003169402   *Fax:* 714-259-9401
E-mail: customerservice@westridgelabs.com
Web site: www.westridgelabs.com
Ownership: Private
Produces/Sells CE-marked Devices: N

Lubricant, Vaginal, Patient	General

WESTSALIA SEPERATOR, INC.
See Gea Westfalia Separator, Inc.

WESTSIDE PACKAGING, LLC. 909-570-3508
1700 A South Baker Ave., Ontario, CA 91761
FDA Number: 2031532

Accessories, Retractor, Dental	Dental And Oral
Activator, Ultraviolet, Polymerization	Dental And Oral
Agent, Polishing, Abrasive, Oral Cavity	Dental And Oral
Cement, Dental	Dental And Oral
Crown And Bridge, Temporary, Resin	Dental And Oral
Instrument, Diamond, Dental	Dental And Oral
Material, Impression	Dental And Oral
Material, Tooth Shade, Resin	Dental And Oral
Scaler, Ultrasonic	Dental And Oral
Source, Heat, Bleaching, Teeth, Dental	Dental And Oral
Tray, Impression	Dental And Oral
Varnish, Cavity	Dental And Oral

WETMORE ASSOC., INC. 425-303-9520
2815 Wetmore Ave., Everett, WA 98201
FDA Number: 3027770
Ownership: Private
Produces/Sells CE-marked Devices: N

Clothing, Protective, Sun	Surgery

WEXFORD LABS, INC. 314-966-4134
325 Leffingwell Ave., Kirkwood, MO 63122
FDA Number: 1000147951

Medical Disinfectants/Cleaners for Instruments	General

MANUFACTURER PROFILES

WEXLER SURGICAL SUPPLIES   800-414-1076
11333 Chimney Rock Road, Suite 110,   713-723-6900
Houston, TX 77035
FDA Number: n/a   *Fax:* 713-723-6906
E-mail: sales@wexlersurgical.com
Web site: www.wexlersurgical.com
Medical Products Sales Volume: $1,600,000
Year Founded: 1991
Total Employees: 11
Ownership: Private
Produces/Sells CE-marked Devices: Y
Federal Procurement Eligibility: Small Business
Distribution: Exclusive Distributor
Mktg./Adv.: Anna Golod/Manager Business
   Forceps   Orthopedics
   Holder, Needle   Gastroenterology/Urology
   Kit, Instruments and Accessories, Surgical   Surgery
   Scissors, Suture   Surgery

WFR/AQUAPLAST CORP.   800-526-5247
440 Church Road, Avondale, PA 19311   610-268-0585
FDA Number: 2247992   *Fax:* 610-268-0588
E-mail: Sales@Q-Fix.com
Web site: www.wfr-aquaplast.com
Annual Revenue: $0-$1 Million
Ownership: Private
Produces/Sells CE-marked Devices: Y
Federal Procurement Eligibility: Small Business
Distribution: Manufacturer Direct, Exporter
General Admin.: Damon Kirk/President, Chief Executive Officer
   Accelerator, Linear, Medical   Radiology
   Bath, Water (Constant Temperature)   Chemistry
   Couch, Radiation Therapy, Powered   Radiology
   Guard, Graft, Skin   Surgery
   Scissors, Bandage/Gauze/Plaster   General
   Splint, Nasal   Ear/Nose/Throat
   Support, Patient Position, Radiographic   Radiology
   Table, Radiographic   Radiology

WHALE SCIENTIFIC, INC.
See Image Molding, Inc.

WHALEN BIOMEDICAL INCORPORATED   617-868-4433
11 Miller St., Somerville, MA 02143
FDA Number: n/a   *Fax:* 617-868-4304
E-mail: rlwhalen@wbmd.org
Web site: www.wbmd.org
Medical Products Sales Volume: $500,000
Annual Revenue: $1-$5 Million
Year Founded: 1984
Total Employees: 8
Ownership: Whalen Biomedical Inc.
Quality System Registration Information: ISO9000
Produces/Sells CE-marked Devices: Y
Federal Procurement Eligibility: Small Business
Distribution: Manufacturer Direct, OEM, Service Direct, Exporter
General Admin.: Robert L. Whalen/President, Chief Executive Officer
Mktg./Adv.: Craig W. Sherman/Manager Contract Sales
        Pamela N. Rosengard/Vice President Business Development
Production: Christopher L. Richards/Director Quality Assurance
        John C. Norman/Manager Regulatory Affairs
Research: Criag W. Sherman/Vice President Research & Development
   Analyzer, Transcutaneous Nerve Stimulator   Cns/Neurology
   Circulatory Assist Unit, Left Ventricular   Cardiovascular
   Device, Hemostasis, Vascular   Cardiovascular
   Prosthesis, Breast, Inflatable, Internal   Surgery
   Prosthesis, Finger   Orthopedics
   Prosthesis, Heart   Cardiovascular

WHATMAN INC.   732-885-6529
Building One, 800 Centenial Avenue,   800-942-8626
Piscataway, NJ 08854
FDA Number: 2242726   *Fax:* 973-245-8301
E-mail: whatmaninfo@ge.com
Web site: www.whatman.com
Medical Products Sales Volume: $50,600,000
Annual Revenue: $50-$100 Million
Year Founded: 1971
Total Employees: 50   *Marketing Staff:* 6   *Sales Staff:* 20
Ownership: GE HEALTHCARE
Quality System Registration Information: ISO9001
Produces/Sells CE-marked Devices: N
Federal Procurement Eligibility: Small Business
Distribution: Manufacturer Through Distributor
   Chromatography Equipment, Liquid   Chemistry
   Chromatography Equipment, Paper   Chemistry
   Chromatography Equipment, Thin Layer   Toxicology
   Column, Chromatography   Chemistry

WHATMAN INC.   732-885-6529 *(cont'd)*
   Component, Other   General
   Cover, Other   General
   Filter Paper   Chemistry
   Filter, Bacteriological, Laboratory   Chemistry
   Filter, Membrane   Chemistry
   Filter, Syringe   General
   Microfilter, Blood Transfusion   Anesthesiology
   Paper, Ion   Toxicology
   Sprayer, Thin Layer Chromatography   Chemistry

WHEATON BRACE CO.   800-227-6769
336 E. Gundersen Dr., #100,   630-690-5795
Carol Stream, IL 60188
FDA Number: n/a   *Fax:* 630-690-8448
E-mail: sales@wheatonbrace.com
Web site: www.orthseek.com
Annual Revenue: $0-$1 Million
Ownership: Private
Produces/Sells CE-marked Devices: Y
Federal Procurement Eligibility: Small Business, Minority Owned, Female Owned
Distribution: Manufacturer Direct
Mktg./Adv.: Dean Schoeller/Director Marketing
   Collar, Cervical Neck   Orthopedics
   Immobilizer, Knee   Orthopedics
   Immobilizer, Wrist/Hand   Orthopedics
   Orthosis, Limb Brace   Physical Med
   Sling, Arm   Physical Med
   Sling, Knee   Orthopedics
   Sling, Leg   Orthopedics
   Splint, Abduction, Congenital Hip Dislocation   Physical Med
   Splint, Denis Brown   Physical Med
   Splint, Other   Orthopedics
   Strap, Clavicle   Orthopedics

WHEATON SCIENCE PRODUCTS   800-225-1437
1501 North 10th St., Millville, NJ 08332   856-825-1100
FDA Number: 2247898   *Fax:* 856-825-1368
Web site: www.wheatonsci.com
Medical Products Sales Volume: $35,000,000
Annual Revenue: $25-$50 Million
Year Founded: 1888
Ownership: CYPRO
Quality System Registration Information: ISO9001
Produces/Sells CE-marked Devices: Y
Distribution: Manufacturer Through Distributor, Service Direct
General Admin.: Stephen R. Drozdow/President, Chief Executive Officer
Production: Gregory W. Bianco/Vice President Operations
Finance: Danine S. Freeman/Chief Financial Officer, Vice President Finance
   Ampule   Gastroenterology/Urology
   Column, Chromatography   Chemistry
   Desiccator   Chemistry
   Dispenser, Liquid, Unit-Dose   General
   Distilling Unit   Chemistry
   Fermentation Equipment   Microbiology
   Freeze Drying Equipment   Chemistry
   Homogenizer, Tissue   Microbiology
   Labware, Basic, Disposable   Chemistry
   Labware, Basic, Reusable   Chemistry
   Mixer, Clinical Laboratory   Chemistry
   Packaging System, Unit-Dose   General
   Pipette Tip   Chemistry
   Pipette, Micro   Chemistry
   Pipetter   Hematology
   Plate, Hot   Chemistry
   Pump, Laboratory   Chemistry
   Reaction Apparatus   Microbiology
   Shaker/Stirrer   Chemistry
   Spinner System, Cell Culture   Pathology
   Sprayer, Thin Layer Chromatography   Chemistry
   Still, Water   Chemistry
   Stirrer   Chemistry
   Suspension System, Cell Culture   Pathology
   Tissue Culture Apparatus   Microbiology
   Tube, Culture   Microbiology
   Vial, Medication   General

WHEELCHAIR CARRIER, INC.   800-541-3213
203 Matzinger Road, Toledo, OH 43612   419-478-4423
FDA Number: n/a   *Fax:* 419-478-4425
E-mail: wcc@adelphia.net
Web site: www.wheelchaircarrier.com
Medical Products Sales Volume: $500,000
Annual Revenue: $0-$1 Million
Year Founded: 2005
Total Employees: 5   *Marketing Staff:* 1   *Sales Staff:* 2
Ownership: Private
Produces/Sells CE-marked Devices: N
Federal Procurement Eligibility: Small Business

WHEELCHAIR CARRIER, INC. 800-541-3213 (cont'd)
Distribution: Manufacturer Through Distributor, Exporter
Mktg./Adv.: David Makulinski/Product & Sales Manager

Holder, Crutch and Cane, Wheelchair	Physical Med
Wheelchair, Powered	Physical Med

WHEELCHAIR SALES AND SERVICE CO., INC. 877-736-0376
315 Main St., West Springfield, MA 01089 413-736-0376
FDA Number: n/a Fax: 413-736-0377
E-mail: WheelchairDepot@yahoo.com
Web site: www.wheelchairdepot.pridedealer.com
Medical Products Sales Volume: $200,000
Annual Revenue: $0-$1 Million
Year Founded: 1991
Total Employees: 3   *Marketing Staff:* 2   *Sales Staff:* 3
Ownership: Private
Produces/Sells CE-marked Devices: N
Federal Procurement Eligibility: Small Business
Distribution: Service Direct
General Admin.: Thomas Pittsley/President
Mktg./Adv.: Kathleen Vadnais/Manager Advertising & Public Relations

Bath, Portable	General
Bed, Hydraulic	General
Bed, Manual	General
Chair, Seat Lifting (Standing Aid)	General
Scooter (Motorized 3-Wheeled Vehicle)	Physical Med
Service, Parts, Repair	General
Walker, Mechanical	Physical Med
Wheelchair, Manual	Physical Med
Wheelchair, Powered	Physical Med

WHEELCHAIRS OF KANSAS 800-537-6454
204 W. 2nd St., Ellis, KS 67637 785-726-4885
FDA Number: 1931307 Fax: 800-337-2447
E-mail: wokinfo@go2wok.com
Web site: www.wheelchairsofkansas.com
Annual Revenue: $5-$10 Million
Year Founded: 1988
Total Employees: 70   *Marketing Staff:* 2   *Sales Staff:* 30
Ownership: Private
Produces/Sells CE-marked Devices: N
Distribution: Manufacturer Through Distributor, Manufacturer Through Manufacturer Reps
General Admin.: Lee Frickey/President, Chief Executive Officer
    Nancy Guthrie/Vice President Human Resources
Mktg./Adv.: Michele Eberle/Vice President Marketing
    Bernie Taylor/Vice President Sales
Production: Lee Frickey/Manager Regulatory Affairs
    Eric Boss/Vice President Manufacturing

Bed, Adjustable Hospital	General
Bed, Obese	General
Cane	Physical Med
Chair, Shower	General
Commode (Toilet)	General
Crutch	Physical Med
Lift, Patient	General
Mattress, Air Flotation	General
Transfer Device, Patient, Manual	General
Walker, Mechanical	Physical Med
Wheelchair, Manual	Physical Med
Wheelchair, Powered	Physical Med
Wheelchair, Special Grade	Physical Med

WHEELED COACH INDUSTRIES, INC. 800-422-8206
2737 N. Forsyth Rd., Winter Park, FL 32792 407-677-7777
FDA Number: n/a Fax: 407-679-1337
Web site: www.wheeledcoach.com
Total Employees: 500
Ownership: Public
Produces/Sells CE-marked Devices: Y
Distribution: Manufacturer Through Manufacturer Reps
General Admin.: Robert Collins/President
Mktg./Adv.: Abel Del Rio/Manager International Marketing & Sales
    Kent Tyler/Manager Marketing
    Paul Holzapfel/Manager National Sales
    Stan Mikalonis/Vice President Marketing & Sales

Ambulance	General

WHEELIT, INC. 800-523-7508
440 Arco Drive, Toledo, OH 43607-2909 419-531-4900
FDA Number: n/a Fax: 419-531-6415
E-mail: wheelit@solarstop.net
Web site: www.wheelitinc.com
Medical Products Sales Volume: $490,000
Annual Revenue: $0-$1 Million
Year Founded: 1972
Total Employees: 10   *Marketing Staff:* 1
Ownership: Private

WHEELIT, INC. 800-523-7508 (cont'd)
Produces/Sells CE-marked Devices: N
Federal Procurement Eligibility: Small Business
Distribution: OEM
Mktg./Adv.: Tom Skilliter/Manager Sales

Cabinet Casework, General Purpose	General
Cart, Instrument	Surgery
Cart, Multipurpose	General
Cart, Other	General

WHIP MIX CORP. 502-637-1451
1730 East Prospect, Suite 101, Fort Collins, CO 80525
FDA Number: 3007057241
Ownership: Private
Produces/Sells CE-marked Devices: N

Aligner, Beam, X-Ray (Collimator)	Dental And Oral
Articulators	Dental And Oral
Device, Jaw Tracking, For Monitoring Jaw Positions	Dental And Oral
Face Bow	Dental And Oral
Mouthguard	Dental And Oral

WHIP-MIX CORPORATION 800-626-5651
361 farmington Avenue, PO Box 17183, 502-637-1451
Louisville, KY 40217
FDA Number: 1043617 Fax: 502-634-4512
E-mail: asteinbock@whipmix.com
Web site: www.whipmix.com
Medical Products Sales Volume: $23,000,000
Annual Revenue: $10-$25 Million
Year Founded: 1919
Total Employees: 165   *Marketing Staff:* 7   *Sales Staff:* 5
Ownership: Private
Quality System Registration Information: ISO9001
Produces/Sells CE-marked Devices: Y
Federal Procurement Eligibility: Small Business
Distribution: Manufacturer Through Distributor
General Admin.: Allen F. Steinbock/Chief Executive Officer
    David J. Steinbock/Vice President
Mktg./Adv.: Frank Manfre/Vice President Marketing & Sales

Articulators	Dental And Oral
Blender/Mixer	Chemistry
Face Bow	Dental And Oral
Furnace, Porcelain	Dental And Oral
Material, Investment	Dental And Oral
Mixer, Clinical Laboratory	Chemistry
Oven	Chemistry
Wax, Dental	Dental And Oral

WHITBY RESEARCH, INC.
See UCB Inc.

WHITE BITE, INC. 502-222-2647
5006 Hickory Hill Dr., La Grange, KY 40031
FDA Number: 1000123812
Ownership: Private
Produces/Sells CE-marked Devices: N

Crown, Preformed	Dental And Oral

WHITE BURS INC., S.S.
See S.S. White Burs Inc.

WHITE CAP ENT. 781-925-3705
133 Beach Ave., Hull, MA 02045
FDA Number: 1219676
Ownership: Private
Produces/Sells CE-marked Devices: N

Walker, Mechanical	Physical Med

WHITE CONSOLIDATED INC., GIBSON DIV.
See Electrolux Home Products - North America

WHITE CONSOLIDATED INC., TAPPAN DIV.
See Electrolux Home Products - North America

WHITE CONSOLIDATED INDUSTRIES
See Electrolux Home Products - North America

WHITE CONSOLIDATED INDUSTRIES
See Washex, Inc.

WHITE KNIGHT ENGINEERED PRODUCTS
7422 Carmel Executive Park
FDA Number: n/a
General Admin.: Scott Banks/President
Mktg./Adv.: Angel Trimble/Director Marketing
    Greg Winn/Director National Accounts & Sales
    Troy Ohmes/Director Product Development
Production: LuCinda Hodge/Director Quality Assurance

Accessories, Apparel, Surgical	Surgery

WHITE KNIGHT HEALTHCARE
See Precept Medical Products, Inc.

WHITE KNIGHT HEALTHCARE
800-851-4431
Calle 16, Number 780, Agua Prieta, Sonora Mexico
FDA Number: 8030607

Accessories, Apparel, Surgical	Surgery
Cap, Surgical	Surgery
Clothing, Protective, Sun	Surgery
Cover, Shoe, Operating Room	Surgery
Drape, Surgical	Surgery
Drape, Surgical, ENT	Ear/Nose/Throat
Drape, Urological, Disposable	Gastroenterology/Urology
Dress, Surgical	Surgery
Garment, Protective, For Incontinence	Gastroenterology/Urology
Gown, Examination	General
Gown, Isolation, Surgical	Surgery
Gown, Operating Room, Disposable	Surgery
Gown, Patient	Surgery
Gown, Surgical	Surgery
Hood, Surgical	Surgery
Kit, Surgical (General)	Surgery
Linen, Bed	General
Pack, Sterilization Wrapper (Bag And Accessories)	Surgery
Sponge, Gauze	Dental And Oral
Suit, Surgical	Surgery

WHITE KNIGHT MANUFACTURING CO.
See Precept Medical Products, Inc.

WHITE MOUNTAIN IMAGING
603-648-2124
1617 Battle St., Webster, NH 03303
FDA Number: n/a
Fax: 603-648-2197
E-mail: wmi@wmi-t2.com
Web site: www.wmi-t2.com
Medical Products Sales Volume: $15,000,000
Annual Revenue: $25-$50 Million
Total Employees: 35 *Marketing Staff:* 3 *Sales Staff:* 4
Ownership: Private
Produces/Sells CE-marked Devices: N
Federal Procurement Eligibility: Small Business
Distribution: Manufacturer Through Distributor, Exporter
General Admin.: Gary Donoghue/General Manager
Mktg./Adv.: Richard Donoghue/Director Marketing

Chemical, Film Processor	Radiology
Film, X-Ray	Radiology
Monitor, X-Ray Film Processor Quality Control	Radiology

WHITE POWER FILES INC.
See White Systems, Inc.

WHITE STORAGE & RETRIEVAL SYSTEMS, INC.
See White Systems, Inc.

WHITE SURGICAL, INC.
901-758-8768
1644 Dogwood Creek Road, Germantown, TN 38139
FDA Number: 9027113
Federal Procurement Eligibility: Small Business

Table, Surgical, Orthopedic	Orthopedics

WHITE SYSTEMS, INC.
800-275-1442
30 Boright Avenue, Kenilworth, NJ 07033-1015
908-272-6700
FDA Number: n/a
Fax: 908-272-5920
E-mail: info@whitesystems.com
Web site: www.whitesytems.com
Medical Products Sales Volume: $19,300,000
Year Founded: 1946
Total Employees: 100 *Marketing Staff:* 3 *Sales Staff:* 10
Ownership: FKI INDUSTRIES
Produces/Sells CE-marked Devices: N
Federal Procurement Eligibility: Small Business, GSA Contract
Distribution: Manufacturer Through Distributor, Manufacturer Through Manufacturer Reps
General Admin.: Steve Ackerman/President, Chief Executive Officer
Mktg./Adv.: Jill Raab/Director Marketing

Bin, Storage	General
Cabinet, Other	General
Computer Equipment	General
Microfilm/Microfiche Equipment	General

WHITE WESTINGHOUSE APPLIANCE CO.
See Electrolux Home Products - North America

WHITEHALL MANUFACTURING
800-782-7706
15125 Proctor Avenue,
626-968-6681
City of Industry, CA 91746
FDA Number: 2222003
Fax: 626-855-4862
E-mail: info@whitehallmfg.com
Web site: www.whitehallmfg.com
Total Employees: 500
Ownership: Private
Produces/Sells CE-marked Devices: N
Federal Procurement Eligibility: Small Business

WHITEHALL MANUFACTURING
800-782-7706 *(cont'd)*
Distribution: Manufacturer Through Distributor, Manufacturer Through Manufacturer Reps, Exporter
Mktg./Adv.: Bob McCorquodale/Manager Sales
  Tony Catroppa/Vice President Sales

Bath, Hydro-Massage (Whirlpool)	Physical Med
Bath, Paraffin	Physical Med
Chair, Bath	General
Clip, Towel	Surgery
Commode (Toilet)	General
Freezer, Laboratory, General Purpose	Chemistry
Heater, Hot Pack	Physical Med
Lift, Bath, Non-AC-Powered	General
Processor, Radiographic Film, Manual	Radiology
Pump, Blood, Hemodialysis Unit	Gastroenterology/Urology
Rail, Bath	General
Scrub Machine, Surgical	Surgery
Sink, Hospital	General
Tank, Full Body (Bath)	General
Tank, Holding, Dialysis	Gastroenterology/Urology

WHITEHALL/A DIVISION OF ACORN ENGINEERING CO.
626-336-4561
15125 Proctor Ave., City Of Industry, CA 91744
FDA Number: 2222003

Bath, Hydro-Massage (Whirlpool)	Physical Med
Bath, Paraffin	Physical Med
Regulator, Thermal, Cardiopulmonary Bypass	Cardiovascular
System, Water, Reproduction, Assisted, And Purification	Obstetrics/Gynecology
Thermometer, Electronic, Continuous	General

WHITEHILL MANUFACTURING, INC.
281-240-8782
12701 Executive Dr., Ste. 614, Meadows Place, TX 77477
FDA Number: 1644816

Floss, Dental	Dental And Oral

WHITESTONE ACQUISITION CORP.
See HARTMANN USA, Inc.

WHITING & DAVIS COMPANY, INC.
800-876-6374
200 John Dietsch Blvd.,
508-699-4412
Attleboro Falls, MA 02763
FDA Number: 840396
Fax: 508-695-7606
E-mail: info@whitinganddavis.com
Web site: www.whitinganddavis.com
Medical Products Sales Volume: $8,000,000
Annual Revenue: $1-$5 Million
Year Founded: 1876
Total Employees: 56 *Marketing Staff:* 1 *Sales Staff:* 1
Ownership: Public
Produces/Sells CE-marked Devices: N
Federal Procurement Eligibility: Small Business
Distribution: Manufacturer Direct
Mktg./Adv.: Lelia Teixeira/Sales Specialist

Accessories, Radiotherapy	Radiology

WHITMAN CORP.
888-362-4535
1725 Powers St., Cincinnati, OH 45223-2499
513-541-3223
FDA Number: 3000169155
Fax: 513-541-4082
Web site: www.whitcorp.com
Ownership: Private
Produces/Sells CE-marked Devices: N

Orthosis, Limb Brace	Physical Med

WHITMAN GROUP, THE
215-657-9990
3501 Masons Mill Rd., Bldg. 5,
Huntingdon Valley, PA 19006
FDA Number: n/a
Fax: 631-777-2714
E-mail: whitman@whitmangroup.com
Web site: www.whitmangroup.com
Annual Revenue: $1-$5 Million
Total Employees: 80 *Marketing Staff:* 2 *Sales Staff:* 2
Ownership: Private
Produces/Sells CE-marked Devices: N
Distribution: Service Direct
General Admin.: John Whitman/Chief Executive Officer
  Mary Knapp/President
Mktg./Adv.: Nancy Ross/Director Marketing

Service, Consulting	General

WHITNEY PRODUCTS, INC.
800-338-4237
6153 Mulford Street, Unit. C,
847-470-9300
Niles, IL 60714
FDA Number: 1417513
Fax: 847-966-6168
E-mail: info@whitneyproducts.com
Web site: www.whitneyproducts.com
Medical Products Sales Volume: $500,000
Year Founded: 1984
Total Employees: 18 *Marketing Staff:* 1

WHITNEY PRODUCTS, INC.   800-338-4237 (cont'd)
Ownership: Private
Produces/Sells CE-marked Devices: N
Federal Procurement Eligibility: Small Business, GSA Contract, VA Contract
Distribution: Manufacturer Direct, Manufacturer Through Distributor
General Admin.: Steven Whitney/President
Mktg./Adv.: Ms. Barbara Mott/Marketing Coordinator
Production: Alfredo Cruz/Quality Control, Product Engineer

Bag, Medical, Physician	General
Curette	Orthopedics
Hook, Other	Surgery
Knife, Orthopedic	Orthopedics
Rack, Test Tube	Chemistry
Waste Receptacle, Contaminated	General
Waste Receptacle, General Purpose	General

WHITNEY, W.G. CORP.
See Whitney Products, Inc.

WHITTAKER GENERAL MEDICAL
See Mckesson General Medical

WHITTAKER GENERAL SCIENTIFIC
See Mckesson General Medical

WHITTEMORE ENTERPRISES, INC.   800-999-2452
11149 Arrow Route,   909-980-2452
Rancho Cucamonga, CA 91730
FDA Number: 9006160   *Fax:* 909-989-9976
E-mail: sales@wemed1.com
Web site: www.wemed1.com
Medical Products Sales Volume: $6,300,000
Annual Revenue: $5-$10 Million
Year Founded: 1983
Total Employees: 32   *Marketing Staff:* 3   *Sales Staff:* 16
Ownership: Private
Produces/Sells CE-marked Devices: N
Federal Procurement Eligibility: Small Business
Distribution: Manufacturer Direct, Exclusive Distributor, Importer, Exporter
General Admin.: Bill Whittemore/Chief Executive Officer
  Bill Whittemore/Owner
Mktg./Adv.: Cesar Becerra/Manager International Sales
  David Jann/Manager National Sales

Accessories, Light, Surgical	Surgery
Camera, Video, Endoscopic	General
Electrosurgical Unit, General Purpose (ESU)	Surgery
Endoscope	Gastroenterology/Urology
Gas-Machine, Anesthesia	Anesthesiology
Microscope, Surgical, General & Plastic Surgery	Surgery
Service, Used Equipment	General
Sterilizer, Steam (Autoclave), Surgical	Surgery

WHITTLESTONE, INC.   877-608-6455
840 Eubanks Drive, Vacaville, CA 95688
FDA Number: 3003610552

Pump, Breast, Powered	Obstetrics/Gynecology

WI INC   303-762-1693
96 Inverness Drive East, Suite N, Englewood, CO 80112
FDA Number: n/a   *Fax:* 720-294-9506
E-mail: dwright@wiinc.net
Web site: www.wiinc.net
Annual Revenue: $0-$1 Million
Year Founded: 2001
Total Employees: 10
Ownership: Private
Produces/Sells CE-marked Devices: N
General Admin.: Mr. David Wright/President

Contract R&D, Diagnostics	General
Contract R&D, Equipment	General

WIGHTMAN MEDICAL, INC.
See Myoderm

WILBUR CURTIS COMPANY   800-421-6150
6913 Acco St., Montebello, CA 90640   323-837-2300
FDA Number: n/a   *Fax:* 323-837-2406
E-mail: info@wilburcurtis.com
Web site: www.wilburcurtis.com
Medical Products Sales Volume: $36,900,000
Annual Revenue: $0-$1 Million
Year Founded: 1963
Total Employees: 300   *Marketing Staff:* 2   *Sales Staff:* 7
Ownership: Private
Produces/Sells CE-marked Devices: N
Federal Procurement Eligibility: Small Business
Distribution: Manufacturer Through Distributor
General Admin.: R. A. Curtis/President
Mktg./Adv.: Diane Grossman/Manager International Marketing & Sales
  Kevin Curtis/Vice President Marketing
Production: Michael Curtis/Vice President Operations

WILBUR CURTIS COMPANY   800-421-6150 (cont'd)
Foodservice Product/Equipment   General

WILEX, INC.   800-255-3232
Oncogene Science, 100 Acorn Park Drive,   877-229-3711
Cambridge, MA 02140
FDA Number: 1224685   *Fax:* 888-242-1997
E-mail: tcconcogene.med@siemens.com
Web site: www.oncogene.com
Year Founded: 1983
Ownership: Siemens Ag
Stock Symbol: SI
Traded On: NYSE
Produces/Sells CE-marked Devices: N

Antigen, Prostate-Specific (PSA), Management, Cancer	Immunology
System, Test, HER-2/NEU, Monitoring	Immunology

WILKINSON COMPANY, INC.   208-777-8332
590 Clearwater Loop, Suite C, Post Falls, ID 83854
FDA Number: 2016008   *Fax:* 208-777-8592
E-mail: wilkinsoncompany@verizon.net
Medical Products Sales Volume: $200,000
Annual Revenue: $0-$1 Million
Year Founded: 1919
Total Employees: 2   *Sales Staff:* 1
Ownership: Private
Produces/Sells CE-marked Devices: N
Federal Procurement Eligibility: Small Business
Distribution: Manufacturer Direct
General Admin.: John Teets/President

Alloy, Amalgam	Dental And Oral
Alloy, Gold Based, For Clinical Use	Dental And Oral
Alloy, Precious Metal, For Clinical Use	Dental And Oral
Component, Metal, Other	General
Material, Metallic-Stainless Steel, Tantalum, Platinum	Ear/Nose/Throat
Source, Isotope, Sealed, Gold, Titanium, Platinum	Radiology

WILKINSON DENTAL MANUFACTURING CO.
See Wilkinson Company, Inc.

WILKINSON HI-RISE   800-231-3888
11A Kimball Ave., Mount Vernon, NY 10550   954-342-4400
FDA Number: n/a
E-mail: mbracken@whrise.com
Web site: www.wilkinsonhirise.com
Year Founded: 1923
Ownership: Private
Produces/Sells CE-marked Devices: Y
Federal Procurement Eligibility: Small Business
Distribution: Manufacturer Direct, Manufacturer Through Distributor, Manufacturer Through Manufacturer Reps
Mktg./Adv.: Michael Bracken/Sales Specialist

Compactor, Fixed	General
Equipment, Cleaning, Air	General
Waste Receptacle, Contaminated	General

WILL ROSS, DOVER DIV.
See Covidien Lp

WILLIAM LABORATORIES, INC.   800-767-7643
5 Anngina Drive, Unit B, Enfield, CT 06082   860-749-1350
FDA Number: 2243805   *Fax:* 860-749-1351
E-mail: info@williamlabs.com
Web site: www.williamlabs.com
Medical Products Sales Volume: $800,000
Year Founded: 1976
Ownership: Private
Produces/Sells CE-marked Devices: Y
Federal Procurement Eligibility: Small Business, Female Owned
Distribution: Manufacturer Direct

Supplies, Blood Bank	Hematology

WILLIAM LEMBECK, INC.   718-263-3134
54 Continental Ave., Forest Hills, NY 11375
FDA Number: 92292
Ownership: Private
Produces/Sells CE-marked Devices: N

Chart, Visual Acuity	Ophthalmology

WILLIAMS DENTAL CO.
See Ivoclar Vivadent, Inc.

WILLIAMS HEALTHCARE SYSTEMS, LLC.   800-441-4967
158 North Edison Ave., Elgin, IL 60123   847-741-3650
FDA Number: 1415746   *Fax:* 847-741-3661
Web site: www.williamshealthcare.com
Ownership: Private
Produces/Sells CE-marked Devices: N

Bed, Manual	General
Equipment, Traction, Powered	Physical Med

MANUFACTURER PROFILES

WILLIAMS HEALTHCARE SYSTEMS, LLC.   800-441-4967 *(cont'd)*
Stimulator, Neuromuscular, External Functional	Cns/Neurology
Stimulator, Ultrasound, Muscle	Physical Med
Table, Mechanical	Physical Med
Table, Physical Medicine, Powered	Physical Med
Table, Physical Therapy	Physical Med

WILLIAMS SOUND CORP.   800-328-6190
10300 Valley View Road,   952-943-2252
Eden Prairie, MN 55344
FDA Number: 2183450   *Fax: 952-943-2174*
E-mail: info@williamssound.com
Web site: www.williamssound.com
Medical Products Sales Volume: $5,100,000
Year Founded: 1976
Ownership: Private
Produces/Sells CE-marked Devices: N
Federal Procurement Eligibility: Small Business
Distribution: Manufacturer Direct, Manufacturer Through Distributor, Manufacturer Through Manufacturer Reps, OEM
Device, Assistive Listening	Ear/Nose/Throat
Telephone, Handicapped Use	Physical Med

WILLIAMSON MEDICAL DEVICES, INC.   888-239-7884
1401 Sixth Avenue, PO Box 152,   724-763-2285
Ford City, PA 16226
FDA Number: n/a
E-mail: marsha@williamsonmedical.com
Web site: www.turnstand.com
Medical Products Sales Volume: $270,000
Annual Revenue: $0-$1 Million
Year Founded: 1997
Ownership: Private
Produces/Sells CE-marked Devices: N
Federal Procurement Eligibility: Small Business
Distribution: Manufacturer Direct
Transfer Aid	Physical Med

WILLOW GRAPHICS, INC.   631-454-6565
608 Oak St., Copiague, NY 11726
FDA Number: 2433531
Sterilization Process Indicator, Physical/Chemical	General

WILSON GREATBATCH LTD.
See Greatbatch Inc

WILSON OPTICAL LABORATORIES, INC.   866-216-6225
190 Alpha Park, Cleveland, OH 44143   440-442-9277
FDA Number: 1527283   *Fax: 440-449-7851*
E-mail: info@nacl.com
Web site: www.nacl.com
Medical Products Sales Volume: $2,500,000
Annual Revenue: $1-$5 Million
Year Founded: 1974
Total Employees: 50   *Marketing Staff:* 3   *Sales Staff:* 3
Ownership: Private
Quality System Registration Information: ISO9001
Produces/Sells CE-marked Devices: N
Federal Procurement Eligibility: Small Business
Distribution: Manufacturer Direct
General Admin.: Mr. John Wilson/Chief Executive Officer, Chairman
                   Mr. Brian Wilson/President
Mktg./Adv.: Joe Cirincione/Manager National Sales
Sunglasses (Including Photosensitive)	Ophthalmology

WILSON SPINAL SYSTEMS   863-294-6867
3532 Waterfield Pkwy., Lakeland, FL 33803
FDA Number: 1063201
Orthosis, Lumbosacral	Physical Med
Orthosis, Thoracic	Physical Med

WILSON SPORTING GOODS CO.   773-714-6400
8750 W. Bryn Mawr Avenue, Chicago, IL 60631
FDA Number: 1424406   *Fax: 773-714-4565*
E-mail: askwilson@wilson.com
Web site: www.wilson.com
Medical Products Sales Volume: $556,800,000
Year Founded: 2005
Total Employees: 280
Ownership: Private
Stock Symbol: AGPDY
Produces/Sells CE-marked Devices: N
Federal Procurement Eligibility: Small Business
Sunglasses (Including Photosensitive)	Ophthalmology

WILSON-COOK MEDICAL, INC.   336-744-0157
4900 Bethania Station Rd., Winston Salem, NC 27105
FDA Number: n/a
Web site: www.cookmedical.com

WILSON-COOK MEDICAL, INC.   336-744-0157 *(cont'd)*
Annual Revenue: $0-$1 Million
Year Founded: 1963
Ownership: Cook Inc.
Produces/Sells CE-marked Devices: Y
Federal Procurement Eligibility: Small Business
Distribution: Manufacturer Direct, Importer, Exporter
Analyzer, Motility, Gastrointestinal, Electrical	Gastroenterology/Urology
Biopsy Instrument, Mechanical, Gastrointestinal	Gastroenterology/Urology
Bougie, Esophageal, And Gastrointestinal, Gastro-Urology	Gastroenterology/Urology
Brush, Biopsy, Bronchoscope (Non-Rigid)	Anesthesiology
Brush, Cytology, Endoscopic	Gastroenterology/Urology
Cannula, Injection	Gastroenterology/Urology
Catheter, Aspiration	Surgery
Catheter, Balloon (Foley Type)	Surgery
Catheter, Biliary	Gastroenterology/Urology
Catheter, Cholangiography	Surgery
Catheter, Irrigation	Surgery
Dilator, Catheter	Surgery
Dilator, Esophageal	Gastroenterology/Urology
Dislodger, Stone, Flexible	Gastroenterology/Urology
Electrosurgical Unit, Cutting & Coagulation Device	Surgery
Endoscope And Accessories, AC-Powered	Surgery
Forceps, Biopsy, Bronchoscope (Non-Rigid)	Anesthesiology
Forceps, Biopsy, Electric	Gastroenterology/Urology
Forceps, Biopsy, Non-Electric	Gastroenterology/Urology
Guidewire, Catheter, Radiological	Radiology
Kit, Biopsy Needle	Gastroenterology/Urology
Kit, Gastrostomy, Endoscopic, Percutaneous	Gastroenterology/Urology
Lithotriptor, Mechanical, Biliary	Gastroenterology/Urology
Needle, Aspiration And Injection, Disposable	Surgery
Needle, Endoscopic	Gastroenterology/Urology
Prosthesis, Esophageal	Ear/Nose/Throat
Prosthesis, Urethral Sphincter	Gastroenterology/Urology
Snare, Flexible	Gastroenterology/Urology
Snare, Polyp	Surgery
Stent, Other	Obstetrics/Gynecology
System, Cancer Treatment, Hyperthermia, RF/Microwave	Radiology
Tube, Double Lumen For Intestinal Decompression	Gastroenterology/Urology
Tube, Gastro-Enterostomy	Gastroenterology/Urology
Tube, Gastrointestinal	Gastroenterology/Urology
Tube, Single Lumen, W Mercury Wt Balloon	Gastroenterology/Urology

WINCHESTER LABORATORIES LLC   630-377-7880
11 S. 2nd Avenue, St. Charles, IL 60174
FDA Number: 1424524   *Fax: 630-443-1391*
E-mail: howard@winchesterlabs.com
Web site: www.winchesterlabs.com
Medical Products Sales Volume: $240,000
Annual Revenue: $0-$1 Million
Year Founded: 1999
Total Employees: 2
Ownership: Private
Produces/Sells CE-marked Devices: N
Federal Procurement Eligibility: Small Business
Distribution: Manufacturer Through Distributor, Manufacturer Through Manufacturer Reps
General Admin.: Howard Rose/Chief Executive Officer
Mktg./Adv.: Annette Rose/Vice President Marketing
Production: Philip Totton/Manager Regulatory Affairs
Solution, Saline(wound Dressing)	Surgery

WINCHESTER OPTICAL CO.   607-734-4251
1935 Lake St., Elmira, NY 14901-1290
FDA Number: n/a   *Fax: 607-732-0901*
E-mail: customer.service@winoptical.com
Web site: www.winoptical.com
Annual Revenue: $0-$1 Million
Year Founded: 1889
Ownership: Private
Produces/Sells CE-marked Devices: N
Distribution: OEM
Lens, Spectacle/Eyeglasses, Non-Custom	Ophthalmology

WINCO, INC.   800-237-3377
5516 S.w. First Ln., Ocala, FL 34474   352-854-2929
FDA Number: 1027229   *Fax: 352-854-9544*
E-mail: sales@wincomfg.com
Web site: www.wincomfg.com
Medical Products Sales Volume: $10,000,000
Year Founded: 1947
Total Employees: 85   *Marketing Staff:* 2   *Sales Staff:* 7
Ownership: Private
Quality System Registration Information: ISO9001
Produces/Sells CE-marked Devices: Y
Federal Procurement Eligibility: Small Business
Distribution: Manufacturer Through Distributor
Chair, Blood Donor	General
Chair, Geriatric	General

WINCO, INC.   800-237-3377 *(cont'd)*

Chair, Position, Electric	Physical Med
Chair, Surgical, AC-Powered	Surgery
Chair, With Casters	Physical Med
Massager, Therapeutic	Physical Med
Powered Medical Examination Table	General
Stool, Operating Room, Adjustable	Surgery
Table, Examination/Treatment	General
Table, Operating Room, AC-Powered	Surgery
Table, Physical Medicine, Powered	Physical Med
Unit, Examining/Treatment, ENT	Ear/Nose/Throat

WINDERS DENTAL EQUIPMENT   206-772-1522
10624 Crestwood Dr. South, Seattle, WA 98178
FDA Number: 3026644
Ownership: Private
Produces/Sells CE-marked Devices: N

Unit, Operative Dental, Accessories	Dental And Oral

WINDL DENTAL LAB   952-541-9622
314 Maple Dr., New Castle, PA 16105
FDA Number: 3004142684
Ownership: Private
Produces/Sells CE-marked Devices: N

Mouthguard	Dental And Oral

WINDOWCHEM SOFTWARE
See Chemsw, Inc.

WINDQUEST   800-562-4257
3311 Windquest Drive, Holland, MI 49424-9570   616-994-7620
FDA Number: n/a   *Fax:* 616-399-8784
E-mail: customers@windquestco.com
Web site: www.windquestco.com
Medical Products Sales Volume: $6,700,000
Annual Revenue: $0-$1 Million
Total Employees: 125   *Marketing Staff:* 1   *Sales Staff:* 55
Ownership: Private
Produces/Sells CE-marked Devices: N
Federal Procurement Eligibility: Small Business
Distribution: Manufacturer Direct
General Admin.: Eric Wolff/President

Cart, Multipurpose	General
Cart, Other	General
Cart, Supply	General
Cart, Supply, Operating Room	Surgery
Cover, Cart	General

WINDSTONE MEDICAL PACKAGING, INC.   800-637-7056
1602 4th Ave. N., Billings, MT 59101-1521   406-259-6387
FDA Number: 3025168   *Fax:* 406-256-9875
E-mail: info@windstonemedical.com
Web site: www.windstonemedical.com
Medical Products Sales Volume: $5,800,000
Annual Revenue: $5-$10 Million
Year Founded: 1978
Total Employees: 40   *Marketing Staff:* 2   *Sales Staff:* 2
Ownership: Cardio-Med Associates, Cardio-Pak Div.
Quality System Registration Information: ISO9002
Produces/Sells CE-marked Devices: N
Federal Procurement Eligibility: Small Business
Distribution: Manufacturer Direct, Manufacturer Through Distributor, Importer, Exporter
General Admin.: Sam Finkelstein/Chief Executive Officer
     Jeff Smith/Chief Operating Officer
     Troy Bergquist/General Manager
     Eddie McElvoy/President, Chief Financial Officer
Mktg./Adv.: Krista Schmitt/Sales Associate
     Nick Patton/Vice President Sales
Production: Shari Moran/Customer Service Representative
Purchasing: Mike Roberts/Director Purchasing
IS: Lori Baker/Director Information Systems

Contract Packaging	General
Contract Sterilization	General
Injector, Syringe	General
Kit, Surgical (General)	Surgery
Kit, Surgical Instrument, Disposable	Surgery
Pack, Custom/Special Procedure	General
Tray, Custom/Special Procedure	General

WINDSTONE MEDICAL, INC.
See Windstone Medical Packaging, Inc.

WINFIELD LABORATORIES   800-527-4616
P.O. Box 832297, Richardson, TX 75083-2297   972-234-0940
FDA Number: 1629057   *Fax:* 972-234-1150
E-mail: garyc@winfieldlabs.com
Web site: www.winfieldlabs.com
Annual Revenue: $0-$1 Million
Year Founded: 1982

WINFIELD LABORATORIES   800-527-4616 *(cont'd)*
Total Employees: 23   *Marketing Staff:* 4   *Sales Staff:* 4
Ownership: Private
Produces/Sells CE-marked Devices: N
Federal Procurement Eligibility: Small Business
Distribution: Manufacturer Direct, Manufacturer Through Distributor
General Admin.: Gary Cummings/President, Chief Executive Officer

Bandage, Cast	Physical Med
Dressing, Non-Adherent	General
Dressing, Skin Graft, Donor Site	General
Dressing, Universal	General
Dressing, Wound and Burn, Occlusive	Surgery

WINK LENS TECHNOLOGIES   415-332-6694
200 Gate 5 Rd., Suite 201, Sausalito, CA 94965
FDA Number: 3005738090

Sunglasses (Including Photosensitive)	Ophthalmology

WINLAND ELECTRONICS INC.   800-635-4269
1950 Excel Drive, Mankato, MN 56001   507-625-7231
FDA Number: 3000216213   *Fax:* 507-387-2488
Web site: www.winland.com
Ownership: Private
Produces/Sells CE-marked Devices: N

System/device, Pharmacy Compounding	General

WINN-SOL PRODUCTS   414-231-2031
1853 Delaware St., Oshkosh, WI 54901
FDA Number: 2183024
Ownership: Private
Produces/Sells CE-marked Devices: N

Cleaner, Denture	Dental And Oral

WINNING SOLUTIONS INC.
See The Aloe Institute

WINNING SOLUTIONS, INC.   800-899-2563
P.O. Box 612688, Dallas, TX 75261-2688   970-731-6709
FDA Number: n/a   *Fax:* 970-731-6706
E-mail: LJohnson@miracleofaloe.com
Web site: www.miracleofaloe.com
Medical Products Sales Volume: $4,000,000
Annual Revenue: $1-$5 Million
Year Founded: 1986
Total Employees: 12   *Marketing Staff:* 3   *Sales Staff:* 3
Ownership: The Aloe Institute
Produces/Sells CE-marked Devices: N
Federal Procurement Eligibility: Small Business
Distribution: Manufacturer Through Distributor, Manufacturer Through Manufacturer Reps, Exclusive Distributor
General Admin.: J. C. Clarke/President
Mktg./Adv.: J. C. Clarke/Vice President Marketing & Product Development
Production: Chris Clarke/Vice President Manufacturing

Lotion, Skin Care	General

WINSTED CORP.   800-447-2257
10901 Hampshire Avenue S.,   952-944-9050
Minneapolis, MN 55438
FDA Number: n/a   *Fax:* 952-944-1546
E-mail: info@winsted.com
Web site: www.winsted.com
Medical Products Sales Volume: $12,000,000
Year Founded: 1963
Total Employees: 30   *Marketing Staff:* 5   *Sales Staff:* 10
Ownership: Private
Produces/Sells CE-marked Devices: N
Federal Procurement Eligibility: Small Business
Distribution: Manufacturer Through Distributor, Manufacturer Through Manufacturer Reps
General Admin.: Mr. Randy Smith/President, General Manager
Mktg./Adv.: Mr. Bob Pep/Director Marketing
     Mr. Wayne Cook/Manager International & National Sales
     Mr. Brent Liemer/Senior Sales Manager
     Mr. Steve Hoska/Vice President, Director Marketing
Research: Mr. Kent Lilja/Vice President Research & Development

Cabinet, Other	General

WIRE CLOTH MANUFACTURERS INC.   800-947-3626
110 Iron Mountain Road   973-328-1000
Randolph Industrial Park
Mine Hill, NJ 07803
FDA Number: 2244018   *Fax:* 973-328-0919
E-mail: newjerseysales@wireclothman.com
Web site: www.wireclothman.com
Medical Products Sales Volume: $2,300,000
Year Founded: 1965
Total Employees: 25
Ownership: Private

WIRE CLOTH MANUFACTURERS INC. 800-947-3626 *(cont'd)*
Produces/Sells CE-marked Devices: N
Federal Procurement Eligibility: Small Business, Female Owned
Distribution: Manufacturer Through Distributor, Importer, Exporter
General Admin.: Kathleen Hegarty/President
Mktg./Adv.: Kathy Blaber/Manager Sales
Production: Jim Hegarty/Vice President Operations
Splint, Hand, And Component	Physical Med

WIRE CRAFTERS L.L.C. 800-924-9473
6208 Strawberry Lane, **502-363-6691**
Louisville, KY 40214
FDA Number: n/a   Fax: 502-361-3857
E-mail: info@wirecrafters.com
Web site: www.wirecrafters.com
Medical Products Sales Volume: $5,400,000
Annual Revenue: $10-$25 Million
Year Founded: 1967
Total Employees: 73   *Marketing Staff:* 3   *Sales Staff:* 7
Ownership: Private
Produces/Sells CE-marked Devices: N
Federal Procurement Eligibility: Small Business
Distribution: Manufacturer Direct, Manufacturer Through Distributor
General Admin.: Steve Diebold/President, Chief Executive Officer
Mktg./Adv.: Belinda Sliter/Director Marketing
          Milt Tandy/Manager National Sales
          Charlie Hagan/Vice President Sales
Bin, Storage	General
Cabinet, Other	General

WISAP AMERICA 800-233-8448
8231 Melrose Drive, Lenexa, KS 66214 **913-492-5888**
FDA Number: 1640206   Fax: 913-492-9142
E-mail: info@blueendo.com
Web site: www.blueendo.com
Medical Products Sales Volume: $9,000,000
Annual Revenue: $5-$10 Million
Year Founded: 1984
Ownership: Private
Quality System Registration Information: ISO9002
Produces/Sells CE-marked Devices: Y
Federal Procurement Eligibility: Small Business, Female Owned
Distribution: Manufacturer Through Manufacturer Reps, Exclusive Distributor, Importer
General Admin.: Jay Sullivan/President
          Norma Sullivan/President
Accessories, Light, Surgical	Surgery
Accessories, Surgical Camera	Surgery
Applicator, Clip (Forceps)	General
Applicator, Vaginal	Obstetrics/Gynecology
Arthroscope	Orthopedics
Aspirator, Surgical	Surgery
Blade, Electrosurgery, Laparoscopic	Surgery
Blade, Knife, Laparoscopic	Surgery
Brush, Other	General
Camera, Television, Endoscopic (Without Audio)	Surgery
Camera, Video	General
Cannula, Extraction, Appendix	Surgery
Cannula, Suction/Irrigation, Laparoscopic	Surgery
Cart, Instrument/Equipment, Laparoscopy	Surgery
Coagulator, Hysteroscopic (With Accessories)	Obstetrics/Gynecology
Coagulator/Cutter, Endoscopic, Bipolar	Obstetrics/Gynecology
Coagulator/Cutter, Endoscopic, Unipolar	Obstetrics/Gynecology
Coupler, Optical, Laparoscopic	General
Cover, Camera	Surgery
Device, Suturing, Endoscopic	Surgery
Dilator, Blunt	Surgery
Dilator, Fascia, Umbilical	Surgery
Dilator, Port, Laparoscopic	Surgery
Dressing, Non-Adherent	General
Dressing, Skin Graft, Donor Site	General
Electrode, Electrosurgery, Laparoscopic	Surgery
Endoscope, Direct Vision	Surgery
Equipment, Suction/Irrigation, Laparoscopic	Surgery
Forceps, Biopsy	Surgery
Forceps, Grasping, Flexible Endoscopic	Gastroenterology/Urology
Heater, Electrical Instrument	General
Holder, Needle	Gastroenterology/Urology
Hysteroscope	Obstetrics/Gynecology
Instrument, Dissecting, Myoma, Laparoscopic	Surgery
Instrument, Removal, Myoma, Laparoscopic	Surgery
Insufflator, Carbon-Dioxide, Automatic (For Endoscope)	Gastroenterology/Urology
Insufflator, Hysteroscopic	Obstetrics/Gynecology
Insufflator, Other	Surgery
Laparoscope, General & Plastic Surgery	Surgery
Laparoscope, Microlaparoscopy	Surgery
Light Source, Endoscopic	Obstetrics/Gynecology
Motor, Drill, Electric	Cns/Neurology
Needle, Other	General

WISAP AMERICA 800-233-8448 *(cont'd)*
Probe	Orthopedics
Punch, Other	Surgery
Scissors, Laparoscopy	Surgery
Splint, Abduction, Shoulder	Orthopedics
Support, Arm	Physical Med
Television Monitor, Operating Room	General
Trocar, Other	General
Tubing, Other	General
Warmer, Endoscope	Surgery

WISAP USA
See Wisap America

WISCONSIN ALUMINUM FOUNDRY CO., INC. 920-682-8627
838 S. 16th St., Manitowoc, WI 54220
FDA Number: 2126663   Fax: 920-682-4090
E-mail: customerrelations@wafco.com
Web site: store.wafco.com
Medical Products Sales Volume: $2,500,000
Annual Revenue: $50-$100 Million
Total Employees: 460   *Marketing Staff:* 1   *Sales Staff:* 4
Ownership: Private
Produces/Sells CE-marked Devices: N
Federal Procurement Eligibility: Small Business
Distribution: Manufacturer Direct, Manufacturer Through Distributor, Service Direct, Exporter
General Admin.: Philip Jacobs/Chief Executive Officer
          Jim Hatt/President
          Jim Behnke/Vice President Human Resources
Mktg./Adv.: Philip Jacobs/Manager Advertising
          Philip Jacobs/Marketing & Sales Representative
Production: Don Noworatzky/Director Quality Assurance
          Jim Behnke/Manager Regulatory Affairs
Research: Philip Jacobs/Research & Development Associate
Sterilizer, Steam (Autoclave)	General

WISCONSIN PHARMACAL CO. LLC 800-558-6614 Ex
1 Pharmacal Way,, Jackson, WI 53037 **262-677-4121**
FDA Number: 2124143   Fax: 262-677-9006
E-mail: mwundrock@pharmacalway.com
Web site: www.pharmacalway.com
Medical Products Sales Volume: $2,000,000
Annual Revenue: $10-$25 Million
Year Founded: 1896
Total Employees: 55   *Marketing Staff:* 2   *Sales Staff:* 3
Ownership: Private
Produces/Sells CE-marked Devices: N
Federal Procurement Eligibility: Small Business
Distribution: Manufacturer Through Distributor, Manufacturer Through Manufacturer Reps
General Admin.: John Wundrock/President, Chief Executive Officer
          Ben Lanza/Vice President
Research: Mary Wundrock/Vice President Research & Development
Finance: Jeff Potts/Chief Financial Officer
Device, Semen Analysis	Obstetrics/Gynecology
Kit, First Aid	Surgery
Lubricant, Patient	General
Lubricant, Vaginal, Patient	General

WISCONSIN PHARMACAL CO., INC.
See Female Health Company, The

WITHERS PLASTICS, INC.
See Deka Medical

WITT BIOMEDICAL CORPORATION 800-669-1328
305 North Drive, Melbourne, FL 32934 **321-253-5693**
FDA Number: 1039368   Fax: 321-253-0372
E-mail: sales@wittbiomedical.com
Web site: www.medical.philips.com
Medical Products Sales Volume: $33,920,000
Annual Revenue: $25-$50 Million
Year Founded: 1990
Total Employees: 159   *Marketing Staff:* 3   *Sales Staff:* 19
Ownership: Private
Quality System Registration Information: ISO9001
Produces/Sells CE-marked Devices: Y
Federal Procurement Eligibility: Small Business
Distribution: Manufacturer Direct, Exclusive Distributor, Exporter
General Admin.: Mike Wolfe/President, Chief Executive Officer
Mktg./Adv.: Steve Bunting/Manager International Sales
          Ruth Hurley/Vice President Marketing
          Eric Potts/Vice President Sales
Production: Pat Parker/Manager Manufacturing
          Steve Saretsky/Manager Materials
          Paul Rowden/Manager Regulatory Affairs
Finance: Mike Allen/Vice President Finance
Computer, Diagnostic, Programmable	Cardiovascular
Image Processing System	Radiology

WITT BIOMEDICAL CORPORATION — 800-669-1328 (cont'd)

Monitor, Physiological, Patient	Cardiovascular
Recorder, X-Ray Image	Radiology

WITT COMPANY, THE
See Safco Products Company

WOLF X-RAY CORPORATION — 800-356-9729
100 West Industry Court, Deer Park, NY 11729 — 631-242-XRAY
FDA Number: 2427002 — Fax: 631-242-1001
E-mail: info@wolfxray.com
Web site: www.wolfxray.com
Annual Revenue: $10-$25 Million
Total Employees: 140 — Marketing Staff: 2 — Sales Staff: 10
Ownership: Private
Quality System Registration Information: ISO9001; ISO9002
Produces/Sells CE-marked Devices: Y
Distribution: Manufacturer Through Distributor
General Admin.: Martin Wolf/Chief Executive Officer
　　　　　　Howard Wolf/President
Mktg./Adv.: Willa Moats/Manager National Sales
　　　　　William Winters/Vice President Marketing
Production: Hugo Burbano/Vice President Manufacturing

Apron, Lead, Radiographic	Radiology
Cabinet, X-Ray Transfer	Radiology
Caliper, Orthopedic	Orthopedics
Card, Identification	General
Cassette, Radiographic Film	Radiology
Duplicator, X-Ray Film	Radiology
Film, X-Ray	Radiology
Film, X-Ray, Dental, Intraoral	Dental And Oral
Glove, Protective, Radiographic	Radiology
Grid, Radiographic	Radiology
Holder, X-Ray Film	Dental And Oral
Illuminator, Radiographic Film	Radiology
Light, Other	General
Marker, X-Ray	Radiology
Mount, X-Ray Tube, Diagnostic	Radiology
Sand Bag, X-Ray	Radiology
Screen, Intensifying, Radiographic	Radiology
Shield, Ophthalmic, Radiological	Radiology
Shield, X-Ray	Radiology
Storage Unit, X-Ray Film	Radiology
Support, Patient Position, Radiographic	Radiology
System, Marking, Film, Radiographic	Radiology
Timer, Radiographic	Radiology

WOLFE TORY MEDICAL, INC. — 801-281-3000
79 West 4500 South, Suite 18, Salt Lake City, UT 84107
FDA Number: 1722554

Applicator (Laryngo-Tracheal), Topical Anesthesia	Anesthesiology
Device, Cystometric, Hydraulic	Gastroenterology/Urology
Inhaler, Nasal	Ear/Nose/Throat
Syringe, Irrigating	General
Tube, Tracheal (Endotracheal)	Anesthesiology

WOLFF INDUSTRIES, INC.
See Pinnacle Technology Group, Inc.

WONDERWORKS OF AMERICA
See Parterre Vinyl Flooring Systems

WOOD PRO, INC.
See Century Woodworking Corp.

WOODHEAD INDUSTRIES, INC.
See Woodhead L.P.

WOODHEAD L.P. — 847-272-7990
3411 Woodhead Drive, Northbrook, IL 60062-1812
FDA Number: 9201153 — Fax: 847-272-8133
E-mail: customerservice@molex.com
Web site: www.danielwoodhead.com
Medical Products Sales Volume: $85,010,000
Year Founded: 1987
Total Employees: 150
Ownership: Private
Quality System Registration Information: ISO9000; ISO9001
Produces/Sells CE-marked Devices: N
Federal Procurement Eligibility: Small Business
Distribution: Manufacturer Through Distributor
General Admin.: Philippe LeMaitre/Chief Executive Officer
　　　　　　Mark DeWinter/Chief Executive Officer, Chief Operating Officer
　　　　　　Robert Fisher/Chief Financial Officer, Vice President
　　　　　　John Davlantes/Manager Personnel
　　　　　　Terry Spandet/President
Mktg./Adv.: Mike Gies/Director Marketing
　　　　　Dave Oriatti/Director National Accounts
　　　　　Rob Frei/Director Product Development
　　　　　Kathy Eber/Manager Advertising
　　　　　Paul Eitmart/Manager National Sales
　　　　　Pat Stearns/Vice President Sales

WOODHEAD L.P. — 847-272-7990 (cont'd)
　　　　　Patrick Stearns/Vice President Sales
Production: Tom White/Director Manufacturing
　　　　　Ken Bergman/Director Quality Assurance
Finance: David Janek/Treasurer, Controller

Connector, Airway (Extension)	Anesthesiology
Fitting, Quick Connect (Gas Connector)	General
Lamp, Other	General
Meter, Leakage Current (Ammeter)	General
Plug, Catheter	Gastroenterology/Urology
Power System, Isolated	General
Receptacle, Electrical	General
Tester, Receptacle, Electrical	General
Tester, Receptacle, Mechanical	General

WOODHEAD, DANIEL CO.
See Woodhead L.P.

WOODLEAF CORPORATION — 949-675-2121
1700 W. Oceanfront Ave. #d, Newport Beach, CA 92663
FDA Number: 3004574196
Ownership: Private
Produces/Sells CE-marked Devices: N

Dilator, Nasal	Ear/Nose/Throat

WOODLYN, INC. — 800-331-7389
Ophthalmic Instruments and Equipment — 847-952-8330
2920 Malmo Drive
Arlington Heights, IL 60005
FDA Number: 1420317 — Fax: 847-952-0045
E-mail: woody@woodlynintl.com
Web site: www.woodlynintl.com
Medical Products Sales Volume: $1,300,000
Year Founded: 1977
Total Employees: 11
Ownership: Private
Stock Symbol: HLMA
Traded On: London
Produces/Sells CE-marked Devices: N
Federal Procurement Eligibility: Small Business
Distribution: Exclusive Distributor
General Admin.: W. Witt/President
　　　　　　Eileen Bowen/Vice President
Mktg./Adv.: Kathy Mathews/Director Marketing
　　　　　Paul Blenkle/Director Product Development
　　　　　Deanne Davis/Manager Contract Sales
　　　　　W. Witt/Manager Sales Training

Chair, Ophthalmic, AC-Powered	Ophthalmology
Exophthalmometer	Ophthalmology
Frame, Trial, Ophthalmic	Ophthalmology
Keratometer	Ophthalmology
Lamp, Slit, Biomicroscope, AC-Powered	Ophthalmology
Lens, Set, Trial, Ophthalmic	Ophthalmology
Microscope, Operating, AC-Powered, Ophthalmic	Ophthalmology
Projector, Ophthalmic	Ophthalmology
Refractor, Ophthalmic	Ophthalmology
Stand, Instrument, AC-Powered, Ophthalmic	Ophthalmology
Table, Ophthalmic, Instrument, Powered	Ophthalmology

WOODWARD LABORATORIES, INC. — 800-780-6999
125 B Columbia, Aliso Viejo, CA 92656 — 949-362-4600
FDA Number: n/a — Fax: 949-362-4601
E-mail: Jeanette.Glavinic@woodwardlabs.com
Web site: www.woodwardlabs.com
Medical Products Sales Volume: $5,800,000
Year Founded: 1992
Total Employees: 12
Ownership: Private
Produces/Sells CE-marked Devices: N
Federal Procurement Eligibility: Small Business
Distribution: Manufacturer Direct, Manufacturer Through Distributor, Manufacturer Through Manufacturer Reps, OEM, Exclusive Distributor, Exporter
General Admin.: Dr. Kenneth Gerenraich/President
Mktg./Adv.: Mr. Ted Kovacevich/Vice President, Manager Sales

General Medical Device	General
Sanitizer	General
Solution, Antibacterial Cleaner	General
Solution, Antimicrobial	Microbiology

WOODWAY USA, INC. — 262-548-6235
West 229 North 591 Foster Ct., Waukesha, WI 53186
FDA Number: 2133817

Treadmill, Powered	Physical Med

WORK 'N LEISURE PRODUCTS, INC. — 800-884-9629
330 Hopping Brook Road, Holliston, MA 01746 — 508-893-0939
FDA Number: 3003698793 — Fax: 508-893-0938
Ownership: Private
Produces/Sells CE-marked Devices: N

WORK 'N LEISURE PRODUCTS, INC.   800-884-9629 *(cont'd)*
General Admin.: Ms. Audrey Bennett/Business Manager
Mktg./Adv.: Ms. Rene Gilbreath/Sales Manager
Production: Ms. Laura Thomas/Customer Service Representative
Finance: Mr. Wayne Eddy/President

Kit, First Aid	Surgery
Mask, Oxygen, Other	General
Valve, Non-Rebreathing	Anesthesiology
Ventilator, Emergency, Manual (Resuscitator)	Anesthesiology

WORK, INC.   800-898-0301
3 Arlington St., Quincy, MA 02171   **617-691-1500**
FDA Number: 1219693   *Fax:* 617-691-1595
E-mail: workinc@workinc.org
Web site: www.workinc.org
Medical Products Sales Volume: $1,000,000
Year Founded: 1965
Total Employees: 15
Ownership: Private
Produces/Sells CE-marked Devices: N
Federal Procurement Eligibility: Small Business, VA Contract
Distribution: Manufacturer Direct

Bag, Leg	Gastroenterology/Urology
Tube, Feeding	General

WORKLON
See Superior Uniform Group

WORLD CLASS TECHNOLOGY CORPORATION   503-472-8320
1300 Ne Alpha Dr., Mcminnville, OR 97128
FDA Number: 3003971538

Bracket, Metal, Orthodontic	Dental And Oral
Pliers, Orthodontic	Dental And Oral

WORLD DRYER CORP.   800-323-0701
5700 McDermott Drive, Berkeley, IL 60163   **708-449-6950**
FDA Number: n/a   *Fax:* 708-449-6958
E-mail: sales@worlddryer.com
Web site: www.worlddryer.com
Annual Revenue: $10-$25 Million
Total Employees: 65   *Marketing Staff:* 1
Ownership: United Technologies Corporation
Quality System Registration Information: ISO9002
Produces/Sells CE-marked Devices: Y
Federal Procurement Eligibility: Small Business
Distribution: Manufacturer Through Distributor, Manufacturer Through
Manufacturer Reps, Exporter
General Admin.: Tom Vic/General Manager
Mktg./Adv.: Rick. Steffen/Director National Accounts
    Cathy Sibley/Manager Exports
    Bruce Bohner/Manager National Sales
    Rick Steffen/Vice President Sales
Production: Erin Eddy/Manager Engineering
    John Potts/Plant & Production Manager

Basin, Wash	General
Housekeeping Equipment	General
Table, Other	General

WORLD HEART INC.   888-843-5827
4750 Wiley Post Way, Suite 120,   **801-355-6255**
Salt Lake City, UT 84116
FDA Number: 1724471   *Fax:* 801-355-7622
E-mail: info@worldheart.com
Web site: www.worldheart.com
Medical Products Sales Volume: $8,600,000
Annual Revenue: $1-$5 Million
Year Founded: 1969
Total Employees: 23   *Marketing Staff:* 1
Ownership: Public
Stock Symbol: WHRT
Traded On: NASDAQ
Quality System Registration Information: ISO9001
Produces/Sells CE-marked Devices: N
Federal Procurement Eligibility: Small Business
Distribution: OEM
General Admin.: Zaf Zafirelis/President, Chief Executive Officer
Mktg./Adv.: Tim Walker/Director Marketing
    Scott Miles/Director Product Development
Finance: Barbara Madsen/Controller
    Gill Bearnson/Treasurer

Circulatory Assist Unit, Left Ventricular	Cardiovascular

WORLD HEART INC.   801-355-6255
7799 Pardee Lane, Oakland, CA 94621   **510-563-5000**
FDA Number: 2916284   *Fax:* 510-562-5005
E-mail: info@worldheart.com
Web site: www.worldheart.com
Year Founded: 1996

WORLD HEART INC.   801-355-6255 *(cont'd)*
Ownership: Private
Produces/Sells CE-marked Devices: N
General Admin.: C. Ian Ross/Chairman
    Jal Jassawalla/President, Chief Executive Officer
Medical Admin.: Piet Jansen/Medical Director
Mktg./Adv.: Pratap Khanwilkar/Vice President Business Development
Production: John Vajda/Vice President Manufacturing
Research: Phillip Miller/Vice President Research & Development
Finance: Richard Juelis/Chief Financial Officer, Vice President Finance

Circulatory Assist Unit, Left Ventricular	Cardiovascular

WORLD HEART, INC.
See World Heart Inc.

WORLD HEART, INC. (HQ)
See World Heart Inc.

WORLD MEDICAL EQUIPMENT, INC.   800-827-3747
3915 152nd St. NE, Marysville, WA 98271   **360-657-7900**
FDA Number: n/a   *Fax:* 360-657-7901
E-mail: bob@worldmedicalequip.com
Web site: www.worldmedicalequip.com
Medical Products Sales Volume: $3,000,000
Annual Revenue: $1-$5 Million
Year Founded: 1992
Total Employees: 14   *Marketing Staff:* 2   *Sales Staff:* 4
Ownership: Private
Produces/Sells CE-marked Devices: N
Federal Procurement Eligibility: Small Business
Distribution: Manufacturer Direct, Service Direct
General Admin.: Mr. Robert S. Mighell/President
Mktg./Adv.: Ms. Catherine Mighell/Vice President Marketing
Production: Mr. Don Osborne/Product Specialist
    Mr. John Morin/Product Specialist
    Mr. Keith Armstrong/Product Specialist
    Mr. Rich Cram/Product Specialist
Research: Mr. Jim Gigli/Biomedical Engineer

Defibrillator, Line-Powered	Cardiovascular
Defibrillator/Monitor, Battery-Powered	Cardiovascular
Electrocautery Unit, Line-Powered	Surgery
Gas-Machine, Anesthesia	Anesthesiology
Instrument, Manual, General Surgical	Surgery
Light, Surgical, Ceiling Mounted	Surgery
Microscope, Ear	Ear/Nose/Throat
Microscope, Operating, Non-Electric, Ophthalmic	Ophthalmology
Oximeter, Pulse	General
Service, Equipment Leasing	General
Service, Parts, Repair	General
Service, Used Equipment	General
Sterilizer, Steam (Autoclave)	General
Table, Surgical, Electrical	Surgery
Table, Surgical, Manual	General
Table, Surgical, Orthopedic	Orthopedics

WORLD MEDICAL SUPPLY USA., INC.   1-800-827-3747
WORLD MEDICAL SUPPLY USA., INC.   **360-657-7900**
3915 152nd St. NE
Maumelle, WA 98271
FDA Number: 2937863   *Fax:* 360-657-7901
E-mail: bob@worldmedicalequip.com
Web site: www.pristinegloves.com
Medical Products Sales Volume: $500,000
Annual Revenue: $0-$1 Million
Year Founded: 1986
Total Employees: 3   *Marketing Staff:* 1   *Sales Staff:* 1
Ownership: Private
Produces/Sells CE-marked Devices: N
Federal Procurement Eligibility: Small Business
Distribution: Manufacturer Direct, Manufacturer Through Distributor, Service Direct
General Admin.: Richard A. Pascoe/President, Chief Executive Officer

Glove, Other	General
Glove, Surgical	General
Glove, Surgical, Plastic Surgery	Surgery
Glove, Surgical, Powder-Free	Surgery

WORLD OF MEDICINE USA, INC.   407-438-8810
4531 36th St., Orlando, FL 32811-6527
FDA Number: 3003943523   *Fax:* 407-859-2425
E-mail: info.orlando@womcorp.com
Web site: www.world-of-medicine.com
Medical Products Sales Volume: $43,970,000
Annual Revenue: $25-$50 Million
Year Founded: 1974
Total Employees: 18   *Marketing Staff:* 4   *Sales Staff:* 2
Ownership: Coloplast A/S, Denmark
Quality System Registration Information: ISO9001
Produces/Sells CE-marked Devices: Y
Federal Procurement Eligibility: Small Business

WORLD OF MEDICINE USA, INC. 407-438-8810 *(cont'd)*
Distribution: Manufacturer Direct, Manufacturer Through Distributor, OEM, Importer
General Admin.: Peter P. Wiest/President, Chief Executive Officer
Sandra Wiest/Vice President Human Resources
Mktg./Adv.: Roland Strelitzki/Director Marketing & Sales

Accessories, Laser, Endoscopic	Surgery

Medical Product Subsidiaries (Listed Separately)
W.O.M. World Of Medicine Usa, Inc.

WORLD PRECISION INSTRUMENTS 866-606-1974
(W.P.I.), INC.
175 Sarasota Center Blvd., 941-371-1003
Sarasota, FL 34240
FDA Number: 1221000 *Fax:* 941-377-5428
E-mail: wpi@wpiinc.com
Web site: www.wpiinc.com
Year Founded: 1967
Ownership: Private
Produces/Sells CE-marked Devices: Y
Federal Procurement Eligibility: Small Business
Distribution: Manufacturer Direct, OEM, Exclusive Distributor, Importer, Exporter

Amplifier, Microelectrode	General
Computer Equipment	General
Computer Software	General
Dosimeter, Nitrous-Oxide	Anesthesiology
Electrode, Laboratory pH	Chemistry
Electrode, Other	General
Iontophoresis Unit (Sweat Rate)	Gastroenterology/Urology
Meter, pH, Portable	Chemistry
Microelectrode	General
Micromanipulator	General
Puller, Microelectrode	General
Pump, Infusion	General
Pump, Withdrawal/Infusion	Cardiovascular
Recorder, Paper Chart	Cardiovascular
Stimulator, Electrical, Evoked Response	Cns/Neurology
Stimulator, Neurological	Surgery
Tube, Capillary	Chemistry

WORLD TECHNOLOGIES, INC. 847-949-4948
708-6 Diamond Lake Rd., Mundelein, IL 60060
FDA Number: 1424231
Ownership: Private
Produces/Sells CE-marked Devices: N

Radiographic/Fluoroscopic Unit, Image-Intensified	Radiology

WORLDCARE, INC. 617-374-9001
1 Cambridge Center, 5th Floor, Cambridge, MA 02142
FDA Number: 1224994 *Fax:* 617-374-9991
E-mail: info@worldcare.com
Web site: www.worldcare.com
Medical Products Sales Volume: $6,900,000
Year Founded: 1996
Total Employees: 102
Ownership: Private
Produces/Sells CE-marked Devices: N
Federal Procurement Eligibility: Small Business

System, Communication, Image, Digital	Radiology

WORLDHEART, INC. 801-355-6255
4750 Wiley Post Way, Suite 120, Salt Lake City, UT 84116
FDA Number: n/a *Fax:* 801-355-7622
Web site: http://www.worldheart.com
Year Founded: 1996
Ownership: Private
Produces/Sells CE-marked Devices: N
General Admin.: Mr. Morgan Brown/Chief Financial Officer, Executive Vice President
Mr. Jal Jassawalla/Chief Technology Officer, Executive Vice President
Mr. Alex Martin/President, Chief Executive Officer
Research: Mr. Phillip Miller/Vice President Research & Development

WORLDPAK FLEXIBLE PACKAGING, LLC. 775-359-0733
300 E. Parr Blvd., Reno, NV 89512
FDA Number: 3006104083

Pack, Sterilization Wrapper (Bag And Accessories)	Surgery

WORLDWIDE DENTAL, INC.
See Hager Worldwide, Inc.

WORLDWIDE MEDICAL TECHNOLOGIES
See Biocompatibles Inc.

WORLDWIDE PRODUCTS HEAT PACKS 800-554-6340
7031 N. Via De Paesia, Scottsdale, AZ 85258 480-483-8413
FDA Number: n/a *Fax:* 602-443-4878
E-mail: heatpacks@aol.com
Annual Revenue: $0-$1 Million
Year Founded: 1989

WORLDWIDE PRODUCTS HEAT PACKS 800-554-6340 *(cont'd)*
Total Employees: 5
Ownership: Private
Produces/Sells CE-marked Devices: N
Federal Procurement Eligibility: Small Business, Minority Owned, Female Owned
Distribution: Manufacturer Direct, Manufacturer Through Distributor, Manufacturer Through Manufacturer Reps
General Admin.: Michael Slominski/Owner

Heater, Hot Pack	Physical Med
Support, Abdominal	Physical Med

WORTHAM LABORATORIES INC 423-296-0090
6340 Bonny Oaks Dr., Chattanooga, TN 37416
FDA Number: 3003502045

Agent, Hemostatic, Non-Absorbable, Collagen-Based	Surgery
Control, Coagulation, Plasma	Hematology
Control, Plasma, Abnormal	Hematology
Plasma, Control, Fibrinogen	Hematology
Plasma, Control, Normal	Hematology
Prothrombin Time	Hematology
System, Determination, Fibrinogen	Hematology
Thromboplastin, Activated Partial	Hematology

WORTHINGTON BIOCHEMICAL CORP. 800-445-9603
730 Vasser Avenue, Lakewood, NJ 08701 732-942-1660
FDA Number: n/a *Fax:* 732-942-9270
E-mail: office@worthington-biochem.com
Web site: www.worthington-biochem.com
Medical Products Sales Volume: $6,000,000
Annual Revenue: $5-$10 Million
Year Founded: 1947
Total Employees: 50 *Marketing Staff:* 3 *Sales Staff:* 4
Ownership: Private
Produces/Sells CE-marked Devices: N
Federal Procurement Eligibility: Small Business
Distribution: Manufacturer Direct, Manufacturer Through Distributor, OEM, Exporter
General Admin.: Von Worthington/President
Joseph Berardo/Vice President Human Resources
Joseph Berardo/Vice President, General Manager
Mktg./Adv.: Patrice Smoyer/Director National Accounts
David Skrincosky/Director Product Development
Patricia Lundstrom/Manager International & National Sales
Jim Zacka/Vice President Marketing & Business Development
Production: Russell Ryan/Director Quality Control

Control, Enzyme (Assayed And Unassayed)	Chemistry

WORTHINGTON DIAGNOSTICS
See Biomerieux Inc.

WOUND MANAGEMENT TECHNOLOGIES INC 817-820-7077
777 Main Street, Suite 3100, Fort Worth, TX 76102
FDA Number: n/a
Web site: www.wmgtech.com
Ownership: Private
Produces/Sells CE-marked Devices: N
General Admin.: Mr. Scott Haire/Chief Executive Officer, Chairman
Finance: Ms. Deborah Jenkins Hutchinson/President

WOUNDVISION INC. 888-851-0098
450 East 96th Street, Suite 500, Indianapolis, IN 46240
FDA Number: n/a
Web site: http://www.woundvision.com
Ownership: Private
Produces/Sells CE-marked Devices: N
General Admin.: Dr. James Spahn/Chief Executive Officer
Mr. Ken Turro/Chief Operating Officer
Mktg./Adv.: Mr. J.D. Spahn/Executive Vice President Marketing

WPC BRANDS, INC.
See Wisconsin Pharmacal Co. Llc

WR MEDICAL ELECTRONICS CO. 800-635-1312
123 N. Second St., Stillwater, MN 55082-5002 651-430-1200
FDA Number: 2118418 *Fax:* 651-430-8449
E-mail: info@wrmed.com
Web site: www.wrmed.com
Medical Products Sales Volume: $6,000,000
Annual Revenue: $5-$10 Million
Year Founded: 1962
Total Employees: 25 *Marketing Staff:* 1 *Sales Staff:* 6
Ownership: Private
Quality System Registration Information: ISO9001
Produces/Sells CE-marked Devices: Y
Federal Procurement Eligibility: Small Business
Distribution: Manufacturer Direct, Manufacturer Through Distributor, Manufacturer Through Manufacturer Reps, Exporter
General Admin.: Jack Blais/President, Owner
Mktg./Adv.: James Nelson/Director Sales

MANUFACTURER PROFILES

WR MEDICAL ELECTRONICS CO.   **800-635-1312** *(cont'd)*
Elisabeth Thorn/Manager Advertising & Communications
Tony Dabruzzi/Manager International & National Sales
Production: Virginia Benton/Manager Regulatory Affairs

Bath, Paraffin	Physical Med
Computer and Software, Medical	General
Esthesiometer	Cns/Neurology
Iontophoresis Equipment	Chemistry
Kit, Test, Olfactory	Ear/Nose/Throat
Sensor, Moisture	General
Stimulator, Nerve, ENT	Ear/Nose/Throat
Vibration Threshold Measurement Device	Cns/Neurology

WRAP-ADE MACHINE CO., INC.
See Wrapade Packaging Systems, Llc.

WRAPADE PACKAGING SYSTEMS, LLC.   **888-815-8564**
27 Law Drive, Suite B/C, Fairfield, NJ 07004   **973-773-6150**
FDA Number: n/a   *Fax:* 973-773-6010
E-mail: Sales@Wrapade.com
Web site: www.wrapade.com
Medical Products Sales Volume: $3,000,000
Annual Revenue: $1-$5 Million
Year Founded: 2005
Total Employees: 16   *Sales Staff:* 3
Ownership: Private
Produces/Sells CE-marked Devices: Y
Federal Procurement Eligibility: Small Business
Distribution: Manufacturer Direct, Manufacturer Through Manufacturer Reps
General Admin.: William Beattie/President
Mktg./Adv.: Wallace Noonan/Sales Associate

Packaging Equipment	General

WRAPPED IN COMFORT   **877-205-0901**
15760 Via Sonata, San Lorenzo, CA 94580
FDA Number: 3004554581
Ownership: Private
Produces/Sells CE-marked Devices: N

Cover, Barrier, Protective	General
Incubator, Neonatal	General

WRIGHT LINEAR PUMP, INC.
See Wright Therapy Products

WRIGHT LINEAR PUMP, INC.   **800-631-9535**
103-B International Drive, Oakdale, PA 15071
FDA Number: 2522937   *Fax:* 724-695-0406
E-mail: info@wrighttherapy.com
Web site: www.wrighttherapy.com
Year Founded: 1983
Ownership: Private
Stock Symbol: N/A
Produces/Sells CE-marked Devices: N
Federal Procurement Eligibility: Small Business, Female Owned
Distribution: Manufacturer Direct

Sleeve, Compressible Limb	Cardiovascular

WRIGHT MANUFACTURING CO.
See Wright Medical Group, Inc.

WRIGHT MEDICAL GROUP, INC.   **800-238-7117**
5677 Airline Road, Arlington, TN 38002   **901-867-9971**
FDA Number: 1043534   *Fax:* 901-867-9534
E-mail: sales@wmt.com
Web site: www.wmt.com
Medical Products Sales Volume: $55,300,000
Annual Revenue: $100-$500 Million
Year Founded: 1950
Total Employees: 1000
Ownership: Wright Medical Group, Inc.
Stock Symbol: WMGI
Traded On: NASDAQ
Quality System Registration Information: ISO9002; ISO9003
Produces/Sells CE-marked Devices: Y
Federal Procurement Eligibility: Small Business
Distribution: Manufacturer Through Distributor, Exclusive Distributor, Importer, Exporter
General Admin.: Mr. David Stevens/Chairman
    Mr. Lance Berry/Chief Financial Officer, Senior Vice President
    Mr. Frank Bono/Chief Technology Officer, Senior Vice President
    Ms. Lisa Michels/Compliance Officer
    Mr. Robert Palmisano/President, Chief Executive Officer
    Karen Harris/Vice President International Operations
Mktg./Adv.: Mr. Timothy Davis Jr./Senior Vice President Corporate Development
    Mr. John Treace/Senior Vice President Marketing & Sales
    Ms. Julie Tracy/Vice President Communications
Production: Mr. Kyle Joines/Vice President Manufacturing
Finance: Joyce Jones/Vice President Treasury

Chisel, Bone, Surgical	Dental And Oral
Filler, Calcium Sulfate Preformed Pellets	Orthopedics

WRIGHT MEDICAL GROUP, INC.   **800-238-7117** *(cont'd)*

Graft, Bone	Orthopedics
Knife, Surgical	Dental And Oral
Prosthesis, Hip, Acetabular Component, Metal, Non-Cemented	Orthopedics
Prosthesis, Knee, Hemi-, Femoral	Orthopedics
Prosthesis, Knee, Patellofemoral, Semi-Constrained	Orthopedics
Prosthesis, Knee, Patellofemorotibial, Constrained, Metal	Orthopedics
Prosthesis, Knee, Total	Orthopedics
Prosthesis, Shoulder	Orthopedics
Prosthesis, Wrist, Carpal Trapezium	Orthopedics
Prosthesis, Wrist, Semi-Constrained	Orthopedics
Syringe, Piston	General

WRIGHT MEDICAL TECHNOLOGY, INC.
See Wright Medical Group, Inc.

WRIGHT PRODUCTS, INC.   **800-356-6911**
1909 S. Taylorville Road, Suite 100,   **217-423-6911**
Decatur, IL 62525
FDA Number: n/a   *Fax:* 217-423-7282
E-mail: gwslipp@aol.com
Web site: www.wrightproductsinc.com
Annual Revenue: $0-$1 Million
Year Founded: 2001
Total Employees: 10   *Marketing Staff:* 3   *Sales Staff:* 3
Ownership: Private
Produces/Sells CE-marked Devices: N
Federal Procurement Eligibility: Small Business
Distribution: Manufacturer Direct, Manufacturer Through Distributor
General Admin.: Grant A. Wright/President

Transfer Device, Patient, Manual	General

WRIGHT THERAPY PRODUCTS   **800-631-9535**
103-B International Drive, Oakdale, PA 15071
FDA Number: 2522937   *Fax:* 724-695-0406
Web site: http://www.wrighttherapy.com
Ownership: Private
Produces/Sells CE-marked Devices: N
General Admin.: Mr. Ron Billingsly/Chief Operating Officer
    Ms. Carol Wright/Chief Technology Officer, Executive Vice President
    Mr. Michael Hinson/President, Chief Executive Officer
Finance: Ms. Linda Thier/Chief Financial Officer

Sleeve, Compressible Limb	Cardiovascular

WRIGHT-WAY, INC.   **800-241-8839**
175 E. Interstate 30, Garland, TX 75043   **972-240-8839**
FDA Number: n/a   *Fax:* 972-240-0412
E-mail: mobility@wrightwayinc.com
Web site: www.wrightwayinc.com
Medical Products Sales Volume: $900,000
Annual Revenue: $1-$5 Million
Year Founded: 1967
Total Employees: 15   *Marketing Staff:* 2   *Sales Staff:* 4
Ownership: Private
Federal Procurement Eligibility: Small Business
Distribution: Manufacturer Direct, Manufacturer Through Manufacturer Reps, Service Direct
General Admin.: Thomas B. Wright/President
Mktg./Adv.: Randy Smith/Vice President Sales

Scooter (Motorized 3-Wheeled Vehicle)	Physical Med
Vehicle, Handicapped	Physical Med
Vehicle/Equipment, Recreational (Handicapped)	General

WRS GROUP, LTD.   **800-299-3366**
5045 Franklin Avenue, Waco, TX 76710   **254-776-6461**
FDA Number: n/a   *Fax:* 254-776-0640
E-mail: sales@wrsgroup.com
Web site: www.wrsgroup.com
Medical Products Sales Volume: $18,900,000
Annual Revenue: $0-$1 Million
Year Founded: 1969
Total Employees: 70   *Sales Staff:* 6
Ownership: Private
Produces/Sells CE-marked Devices: N
Federal Procurement Eligibility: Small Business, GSA Contract
Distribution: Manufacturer Direct
General Admin.: Scott Salmans/Chief Executive Officer
    Gary Hutchison/Chief Operating Officer
Mktg./Adv.: Gary Hutchison/Director Marketing
    Robin Brown/Sales Representative

Anatomical Training Model	General
Material, Training, Audiovisual	General

Medical Product Subsidiaries (Listed Separately)
Health Edco

WUNDER TOOL & DIE, INC.   **509-922-6415**
17625 E. Euclid Ave., Spokane, WA 99216
FDA Number: 3003254412

WUNDER TOOL & DIE, INC.   509-922-6415 *(cont'd)*
Massager, Therapeutic   Physical Med

WV IV PRO, INC.   304-366-6151
120 Mound Avenue, Fairmont, WV 26554-3309
FDA Number: 3005098956
Ownership: Private
Produces/Sells CE-marked Devices: N
Holder, Intravascular Catheter   General

WY'EAST MEDICAL CORP.   503-657-3101
16700 SE 120th Avenue, PO Box 1625, Clackamas, OR 97015
FDA Number: 3023859   Fax: 503-657-6901
E-mail: contact@wyeastmed.com
Web site: www.wyeastmed.com
Year Founded: 1989
Total Employees: 18   Marketing Staff: 1
Ownership: Private
Produces/Sells CE-marked Devices: N
Federal Procurement Eligibility: Small Business, VA Contract
Distribution: Manufacturer Direct, Manufacturer Through Manufacturer Reps
General Admin.: Stephen Gould/President
Gary Smith/Vice President
Chair, Examination And Treatment   General
Stretcher, Transfer   Surgery
Transfer Device, Patient, Manual   General

WYETH CONSUMER HEALTHCARE INC.
See Pfizer / Wyeth Consumer Healthcare Inc.

WYKLE RESEARCH, INC.   775-887-7500
2222 East College Parkway, Carson City, NV 89706
FDA Number: 2020703
Alloy, Amalgam   Dental And Oral
Amalgamator, Dental, AC-Powered   Dental And Oral
Applicator, Resin   Dental And Oral
Burnisher, Operative, Dental   Dental And Oral
Capsule, Dental, Amalgam   Dental And Oral
Carver, Dental Amalgam, Operative   Dental And Oral
Condenser, Amalgam And Foil, Operative   Dental And Oral
Curette, Periodontic   Dental And Oral
Dispenser, Mercury And/Or Alloy   Dental And Oral
Explorer, Operative   Dental And Oral
Handle, Instrument, Dental   Dental And Oral
Mirror, Mouth   Dental And Oral
Probe, Periodontic   Dental And Oral
Retainer, Matrix   Dental And Oral
Scaler, Periodontic   Dental And Oral
Tooth Bonding Agent, Resin Restoration   Dental And Oral
Varnish, Cavity   Dental And Oral

WYNDGATE TECHNOLOGIES   800-996-3428
**4925 Robert J. Mathews Pkwy.,, Suite 100,   916-404-8400
El Dorado Hills, CA 95762**
FDA Number: 2951268   Fax: 916-404-8484
E-mail: info@wyndgate.com
Web site: www.wyndgate.com
Medical Products Sales Volume: $5,300,000
Year Founded: 1984
Total Employees: 70
Ownership: Global Med Technologies
Stock Symbol: GLOB
Traded On: OTC Bulletin
Produces/Sells CE-marked Devices: N
Federal Procurement Eligibility: Small Business
Distribution: Manufacturer Direct, Manufacturer Through Distributor, Manufacturer Through Manufacturer Reps, Service Direct
Mktg./Adv.: Ms. Patti Larson/Executive Director Product Development & Marketing
Software, Blood Bank (Stand-Alone Products)   Hematology

WYSONG CORPORATION   989-631-0009
7550 Eastman Avenue, Midland, MI 48640-8838
FDA Number: n/a
E-mail: wysong@wysong.net
Web site: www.wysong.net
Annual Revenue: $1-$5 Million
Total Employees: 25   Marketing Staff: 3   Sales Staff: 3
Ownership: Private
Produces/Sells CE-marked Devices: N
Federal Procurement Eligibility: Small Business
Distribution: Manufacturer Direct
General Admin.: R. L. Wysong/President
General Medical Device   General
Kit, Surgical (General)   Surgery
Soap   General

WYSONG MEDICAL CORPORATION
See Wysong Corporation

WYTECH INDUSTRIES, INC.   732-396-3900
960 E. Hazelwood Ave., Rahway, NJ 07065-5503
FDA Number: n/a   Fax: 732-396-4943
E-mail: info@wytech.com
Web site: www.wytech.com
Year Founded: 1975
Total Employees: 90   Marketing Staff: 5   Sales Staff: 17
Ownership: Private
Quality System Registration Information: ISO9001; ISO9002
Produces/Sells CE-marked Devices: N
Federal Procurement Eligibility: Small Business
Distribution: Manufacturer Through Manufacturer Reps, OEM, Exporter
General Admin.: Mr. Anthony J. Casalino/Chief Executive Officer
Mr. Michael Casalino/President
Mktg./Adv.: Paul H. Dowd/Manager International & National Sales
Mr. Paul H. Dowd/Vice President Sales
Production: Victor Ramos/Manager Quality Assurance
Michael J. Casalino/Vice President Operations
IS: Thomas F. Errington/Director Tech. Services
Guidewire   Cardiovascular
Guidewire, Catheter   Cardiovascular
Lead, Pacemaker (Catheter)   Cardiovascular
Stylet, Catheter   Cardiovascular
Stylet, Needle   General
Stylet, Surgical   Surgery
Trocar, Other   General
Wire, Bone   Orthopedics
Wire, Ligature   Surgery
Wire, Orthodontic   Dental And Oral

X P POWER   978-287-7200
305 Foster Street, Littleton, MA 01460
FDA Number: n/a   Fax: 978-287-7222
E-mail: nasales@xppower.com
Web site: www.xpiq.com
Medical Products Sales Volume: $200,000
Annual Revenue: $25-$50 Million
Year Founded: 1982
Total Employees: 3   Marketing Staff: 3   Sales Staff: 6
Ownership: Public
Stock Symbol: XPP
Traded On: London
Quality System Registration Information: ISO9001
Produces/Sells CE-marked Devices: Y
Federal Procurement Eligibility: Small Business
Distribution: Manufacturer Direct, Manufacturer Through Distributor, OEM
General Admin.: Frank Rene/President
Mktg./Adv.: Duane Darrow/Manager Marketing
Julie Thornton/Manager National Accounts
Paul Christiansen/Vice President Marketing
Production: Linda Comolli/Vice President Operations
Research: Sean Ross/Manager Quality Assurance & Research Analysis
Component, Electronic   General

X-CEL CONTACTS   770-622-9235
1120 Sycamore Ave., Suite D, Vista, CA 92083
FDA Number: 2026149
Lens, Contact (Other Material)   Ophthalmology
Lens, Contact(rigid Gas Permeable)-extended Wear   Ophthalmology
Lens, Contact, Polymethylmethacrylate   Ophthalmology

X-CEL CONTACTS   770-622-9235
2775 Premiere Pkwy, Suite 600, Duluth, GA 30097
FDA Number: 1065845
Lens, Contact (Other Material)   Ophthalmology
Lens, Contact(rigid Gas Permeable)-extended Wear   Ophthalmology
Lens, Contact, Polymethylmethacrylate   Ophthalmology
Lenses, Soft Contact, Daily Wear   Ophthalmology

X-CEL OPTICAL CO.   800-747-9235
**806 South Benton Drive, Box 420,   320-251-8404
Sauk Rapids, MN 56379**
FDA Number: 2124540   Fax: 800-232-9235
E-mail: email@x-celoptical.com
Web site: www.x-celoptical.com
Medical Products Sales Volume: $37,000,000
Year Founded: 1937
Total Employees: 185
Ownership: Private
Federal Procurement Eligibility: Small Business
Lens, Spectacle/Eyeglasses, Non-Custom   Ophthalmology

X-CEL X-RAY CORPORATION   800-441-2470
4220 Waller Dr., Crystal Lake, IL 60012-2848   815-455-2470
FDA Number: 1418484   Fax: 815-455-4732
E-mail: xcelxray@mc.net
Web site: www.xcelxray.com
Medical Products Sales Volume: $1,500,000

X-CEL X-RAY CORPORATION   800-441-2470 *(cont'd)*
Annual Revenue: $1-$5 Million
Year Founded: 1972
Total Employees: 13   *Sales Staff:* 2
Ownership: Private
Produces/Sells CE-marked Devices: N
Federal Procurement Eligibility: Small Business
Distribution: Manufacturer Direct, Manufacturer Through Distributor
General Admin.: William W. Morris/President
   Generator, Therapeutic X-Ray, Dermatological (Grenz Ray)   Radiology
   System, X-Ray, Mobile   Radiology
   Therapeutic X-Ray System   Radiology

X-O CORPORATION   214-388-5590
8311 Eastpoint Drive Ste 100, Dallas, TX 75227
FDA Number: 3004483531
   Collector, Ostomy   Gastroenterology/Urology

X-RAY IMAGING SOLUTIONS INC.   847-878-0867
641 Industrial Dr. Unit D, Cary, IL 60013
FDA Number: 3004998575
Ownership: Private
Produces/Sells CE-marked Devices: N
   Cabinet, X-ray System   Radiology

X-RAY SUPPORT INC.   509-242-1011
3020 N. Sullivan Rd., Suite D, Spokane Valley, WA 99216
FDA Number: 3032881
Ownership: Private
Produces/Sells CE-marked Devices: N
   Processor, Radiographic Film, Automatic, Dental   Dental And Oral

X-RAY SUPPORT, INC   888-230-9500
3020 N. Sullivan Rd., Suite D, Spokane Valley, WA 99216
FDA Number: n/a   *Fax:* 509-242-1012
E-mail: info@imagemax.us
Web site: www.imagemax.us
Ownership: Private
Produces/Sells CE-marked Devices: N
Federal Procurement Eligibility: Small Business
Distribution: Manufacturer Direct
   Holder, X-Ray Film   Dental And Oral
   Microfilm/Microfiche Equipment   General
   Storage Unit, X-Ray Film   Radiology

X-RITE, INC.   888-826-3044
4300 44th Street SE, Grand Rapids, MI 49512   616-803-2100
FDA Number: 1836148   *Fax:* 888-826-3045
E-mail: info@xrite.com
Web site: www.x-rite.com
Medical Products Sales Volume: $179,800,000
Annual Revenue: More than $100 Million
Year Founded: 1958
Total Employees: 659
Ownership: X-Rite, Inc.
Stock Symbol: XRIT
Traded On: NASDAQ
Produces/Sells CE-marked Devices: Y
Distribution: Manufacturer Through Distributor
General Admin.: Richard Cook/Chief Executive Officer
         Tony Sanders/Vice President Human Resources
Mktg./Adv.: Jeff Frazine/Manager National Sales
         David Hazlett/Vice President Business Development
         Joan Andrew/Vice President Marketing
Production: Jeff Frazine/Product Manager
         Jeff Smolinski/Vice President Manufacturing & Operations
   Densitometer   Cardiovascular
   Marker, X-Ray   Radiology
   Monitor, X-Ray Film Processor Quality Control   Radiology
   Sensitometer, Radiographic   Radiology
   Silver Recovery Equipment   Radiology
Medical Product Subsidiaries (Listed Separately)
   Labsphere, Inc.
   X-Rite, Inc.

X-SPINE SYSTEMS, INC.   800-903-0640
452 Alexandersville Rd., Miamisburg, OH 45342   937-847-8400
FDA Number: 3005031160   *Fax:* 937-847-8410
E-mail: info@x-spine.com
Web site: www.x-spine.com
Ownership: Private
Produces/Sells CE-marked Devices: N
General Admin.: Dr. David Kirschman/President, Chief Executive Officer
         Mr. Joseph Ryan/Vice President
Production: Mr. Eric Linder/Director Engineering
         Mr. Christopher Canis/Director Operations
Finance: Mr. Michael Schmitz/Chief Financial Officer
   Appliance, Fixation, Spinal Intervertebral Body   Orthopedics

X-SPINE SYSTEMS, INC.   800-903-0640 *(cont'd)*
   Device, Spinal Vertebral Body Replacement   Orthopedics
   Intervertebral Fusion Device With Bone Graft, Cervical   Orthopedics
   Orthosis, Fixation, Pedicle, Spinal   Orthopedics
   Orthosis, Fixation, Spinal, Spondylolisthesis   Orthopedics
   System, Facet Screw Spinal Device   Orthopedics

X-STRAP SYSTEMS   914-968-3381
81 Pondfield Road #157, Bronxville, NY 10708-0850
FDA Number: 2435901   *Fax:* 914-963-2748
E-mail: mivany@x-strap.com
Web site: www.x-strap.com
Medical Products Sales Volume: $1
Annual Revenue: $0-$1 Million
Year Founded: 1987
Ownership: Private
Produces/Sells CE-marked Devices: N
Federal Procurement Eligibility: Small Business
Distribution: Manufacturer Direct, Manufacturer Through Distributor, Manufacturer Through Manufacturer Reps, Exporter
General Admin.: Michael Ivany/President
   Orthosis, Limb Brace   Physical Med

XAVIER ELECTRONICS, INC.   215-788-7554
421 Magnolia Ave., Croydon, PA 19021
FDA Number: n/a   *Fax:* 215-788-7896
E-mail: sales@xavierelectronics.com
Web site: www.xavierelectronics.com
Medical Products Sales Volume: $1,500,000
Annual Revenue: $1-$5 Million
Year Founded: 1978
Ownership: Private
Produces/Sells CE-marked Devices: N
Federal Procurement Eligibility: Small Business
Distribution: Manufacturer Direct
   Computer Software   General

XBACK BRACING SERVICES, INC.   1.800.494.8680
341a W. Main Street, P.O. Box 100,   610-404-4900
Birdsboro, PA 19508
FDA Number: 3005768063   *Fax:* 1.610.404.4905
E-mail: info@xbackbrace.com
Web site: www.xbackbrace.com
Ownership: Private
Produces/Sells CE-marked Devices: N
   Orthosis, Lumbosacral   Physical Med
   Support, Arm   Physical Med

XDX EXPRESSION DIAGNOSTICS
   See XDx Inc.

XDX INC.   415-287-2300
3260 Bayshore Blvd, Brisbane, CA 94005
FDA Number: 3005225997   *Fax:* 415-287-2456
E-mail: service@xdx.com
Web site: www.xdx.com
Year Founded: 2000
Ownership: Private
Produces/Sells CE-marked Devices: N
General Admin.: Mr. Pierre Cassigneul/President, Chief Executive Officer
   Medical Admin.: Dr. James YEe/Chief Medical Officer
Mktg./Adv.: Mr. Matthew Meyer/Vice President Corporate Development
         Mr. Michael Vicari/Vice President Sales
Finance: Jean Viret/Chief Financial Officer
   Cardiac Allograft Gene Expression Profiling Test System   Cardiovascular
   Reagent, General Purpose   Pathology

XEMAX SURGICAL PRODUCTS, INC.   800-257-9470
712 California Blvd., Napa, CA 94559   707-224-7817
FDA Number: 1421873   *Fax:* 707-226-9362
E-mail: customerservice@xemax.com
Web site: www.xemax.com
Medical Products Sales Volume: $600,000
Year Founded: 1990
Total Employees: 7
Ownership: Private
Produces/Sells CE-marked Devices: N
Federal Procurement Eligibility: Small Business
   Light, Examination, Battery-Powered   General

XENNOVATE MEDICAL LLC   608-298-753
1080 University Blvd., Richmond, IN 47374
FDA Number: 3004089989
Web site: www.xennovate.com
Ownership: Private
Produces/Sells CE-marked Devices: N
   Bandage, Liquid   Surgery
   Cement, Stomal Appliance, Ostomy   Gastroenterology/Urology

XENOPORE CORP.
299 Wagaraw Rd., Hawthorne, NJ 07506
800-356-6296
973-423-2400
FDA Number: n/a
Fax: 973-423-2401
E-mail: xenopore@xenopore.com
Web site: www.xenopore.com
Annual Revenue: $0-$1 Million
Ownership: Private
Produces/Sells CE-marked Devices: N
Federal Procurement Eligibility: Small Business
Distribution: Manufacturer Direct, Manufacturer Through Manufacturer Reps

Enzyme Immunoassay, Other	Chemistry
Slide, Microscope	Pathology
Tray, Micro (Mic Plate)	Microbiology

XENOTEC LTD.
511 Hazel Drive, Corona Del Mar, CA 92625
949-640-4053
FDA Number: n/a
Fax: 949-644-2275
E-mail: xenotec@adelphia.net
Web site: www.xenotec.com
Medical Products Sales Volume: $100,000
Annual Revenue: $0-$1 Million
Year Founded: 1989
Total Employees: 2
Ownership: Private
Produces/Sells CE-marked Devices: N
Federal Procurement Eligibility: Small Business
Distribution: Exclusive Distributor, Exporter
General Admin.: William D. DeMayo/President

Electrosurgical Unit, Cutting & Coagulation Device	Surgery
Identification, Alert, Medical	General
Kit, Pregnancy Test	Obstetrics/Gynecology
Lubricant, Instrument	General
Service, Import/Export	General
Sterilizer, Chemical	General
Strip, Test	Chemistry
Syringe, Hypodermic	General

XENOTRONIX, INC.
1031 Miller Dr.,
Altamonte Springs, FL 32701
800-624-9366
407-331-4793
FDA Number: n/a
Fax: 407-331-4708
E-mail: info@xenotronix.com
Web site: www.xenotronix.com
Ownership: Private
Produces/Sells CE-marked Devices: N
Distribution: Manufacturer Direct, OEM
Mktg./Adv.: Lorra R. Geery/Director Marketing
Production: Eric A. Dils/Director Quality Assurance
    Keith P. Mabey/Vice President Manufacturing

Contract Manufacturing	General

XERO PRODUCTS
349 Military Cutoff Road, Wilmington, NC 28405
888-937-6769
910-791-0009
FDA Number: n/a
Fax: 910-791-4479
E-mail: info@drycorp.com
Web site: www.drycorp.com
Annual Revenue: $1-$5 Million
Total Employees: 20   *Marketing Staff:* 2   *Sales Staff:* 6
Ownership: Private
Produces/Sells CE-marked Devices: Y
Federal Procurement Eligibility: Small Business
Distribution: Manufacturer Direct, Manufacturer Through Distributor, Manufacturer Through Manufacturer Reps, Exclusive Distributor, Exporter
General Admin.: Dr. Roy Archambault/Chief Executive Officer
    Corey Heim/Chief Operating Officer
Production: Wiliam Turnbull/Director Operations

Cast	Orthopedics

XERTREX INTERNATIONAL, INC.
See Tabbies, Div. Of Xertrex International, Inc.

XI TEC, INC.
4 New Park Road, East Windsor, CT 06088-9689
800-243-0084
718-783-2298
FDA Number: 9000947
Fax: 860-903-1439
E-mail: sales@xitec.com
Web site: www.xitec.com
Annual Revenue: $5-$10 Million
Year Founded: 1985
Total Employees: 50   *Marketing Staff:* 2   *Sales Staff:* 20
Ownership: Public
Stock Symbol: XTIC
Traded On: NASDAQ
Produces/Sells CE-marked Devices: N
Federal Procurement Eligibility: Small Business
Distribution: Manufacturer Direct, Exclusive Distributor
General Admin.: Michael J. Sullivan/President, Chief Executive Officer
Mktg./Adv.: John Aucoin - VP Finance/Director Marketing
    John Aucoin - VP Finance/Manager Advertising

XI TEC, INC.
800-243-0084 *(cont'd)*
System, X-Ray, Mobile
Radiology

XILLIX TECHNOLOGIES CORP.
13775 Commerce Pkwy., Ste. 100,
Richmond, BC V6V 2 Canada
800-665-2236
604-278-5000
FDA Number: n/a
Fax: 604-278-3356
E-mail: corporateinfo@xillix.com
Web site: www.xillix.com
Total Employees: 35   *Marketing Staff:* 1   *Sales Staff:* 1
Ownership: Public
Stock Symbol: XLX
Traded On: Toronto
Produces/Sells CE-marked Devices: Y

XIMEDIX, INC.
4829 Northpark Drive,
Colorado Springs, CO 80918
800-999-6349
719-264-0410
FDA Number: 1721646
Fax: 719-264-0415
E-mail: customerservice@ximedix.com
Web site: www.ximedix.com
Medical Products Sales Volume: $250,000
Annual Revenue: $0-$1 Million
Year Founded: 1984
Total Employees: 4   *Marketing Staff:* 1   *Sales Staff:* 1
Ownership: RACK Enterprises Inc.
Produces/Sells CE-marked Devices: Y
Federal Procurement Eligibility: Small Business
Distribution: Manufacturer Through Distributor
General Admin.: Vern D. Kornelsen/Secretary, Treasurer
Production: Dan Mitchell/Vice President Operations, General Manager

Fixation Device, Tracheal Tube	Anesthesiology

XINIX RESEARCH, INC.
5 Pheasant Ln., Portsmouth, NH 03801
603-433-9121
FDA Number: 1319204

Probe, Periodontic	Dental And Oral

XINTEC CORP. / CONVERGENT LASER TECH.
1660 South Loop Road, Alameda, CA 94502
510-832-2130
FDA Number: 2938889
Fax: 510-832-1600
E-mail: service@convergentlaser.com
Web site: www.convergentlaser.com
Medical Products Sales Volume: $2,900,000
Year Founded: 1984
Total Employees: 20
Ownership: Private
Produces/Sells CE-marked Devices: N
Federal Procurement Eligibility: Small Business, Minority Owned, Female Owned, GSA Contract, VA Contract
Distribution: Manufacturer Direct, Manufacturer Through Distributor, Manufacturer Through Manufacturer Reps, OEM, Service Direct, Exporter

Laser, Neodymium:YAG, Surgical, Pulmonary	Anesthesiology
Laser, Surgical	Surgery

XINTEC CORPORATION
See Convergent Laser Technologies

XIRIL
91 Lukens Drive, Suite A, New Castle, DE 19720
302-655-7035
FDA Number: n/a
Fax: 302-655-7286
E-mail: sales@xiril.com
Web site: www.xiril.com
Medical Products Sales Volume: $1,900,000
Annual Revenue: $5-$10 Million
Year Founded: 2001
Total Employees: 15   *Marketing Staff:* 7   *Sales Staff:* 7
Ownership: Private
Quality System Registration Information: ISO9000; ISO9002
Produces/Sells CE-marked Devices: Y
Federal Procurement Eligibility: Small Business
Distribution: Manufacturer Direct, Manufacturer Through Manufacturer Reps, OEM, Exporter
General Admin.: Mr. Lee Carter/President
Production: Mr. Wayne Robinson/Product Specialist
Research: Mr. Lee Carter/Vice President Research & Development
IS: Mr. Steven Abdill/Tech. Consultant

Fluorometer	Immunology
Luminometer	Chemistry
Reader, Microplate	General
System, Robot	General
Washer, Microplate	General

XMA
See Xma (X-Ray Marketing Associates, Inc.)

MANUFACTURER PROFILES

XMA (X-RAY MARKETING ASSOCIATES, INC.)
Windham Lakes Business Park
1205 W. Lakeview Court
Romeoville, IL 60446
FDA Number: 1450923
E-mail: info@xma.com
Web site: www.xma.com
Year Founded: 1979
Total Employees: 6   *Marketing Staff:* 1   *Sales Staff:* 1
Ownership: Private
Produces/Sells CE-marked Devices: Y
Federal Procurement Eligibility: Small Business
Distribution: Manufacturer Direct, Manufacturer Through Distributor, Manufacturer Through Manufacturer Reps, OEM, Exclusive Distributor, Importer, Exporter
General Admin.: Amy Pulido/Executive Assistant
Marco Coladipietro/General Manager
Tony Alvarez/President
Sandi Seeger/Secretary
Dan Walsh/Vice President
Production: Ann Miller/Customer Service Representative
Finance: Tom Walker/Treasurer

800-325-8880
630-378-1992
Fax: 630-378-1048

Apron, Lead, Radiographic	Radiology
Barrier, Control Panel, X-Ray, Moveable	Radiology
Battery, Mobile Radiographic Unit	Radiology
Cabinet, X-Ray Transfer	Radiology
Cassette, Radiographic Film	Radiology
Chemical, Film Processor	Radiology
Collimator, Radiographic, Automatic	Radiology
Collimator, Radiographic, Manual	Radiology
Densitometer, Bone, Dual Photon	Radiology
Densitometer, Bone, Single Photon	Radiology
Densitometer, Radiographic	Radiology
Duplicator, X-Ray Film	Radiology
Entrance, X-Ray Darkrooms	Radiology
Envelope, Film, X-Ray	Radiology
Film, X-Ray	Radiology
Film, X-Ray, Special Purpose	Radiology
Filter, Radiographic	Radiology
Generator, Diagnostic X-Ray, High Voltage, 3-Phase	Radiology
Generator, Diagnostic X-Ray, High Voltage, Single Phase	Radiology
Generator, Radiographic, Capacitor Discharge	Radiology
Glove, Protective, Radiographic	Radiology
Grid, Radiographic	Radiology
Holder, X-Ray Film Cassette, Vertical	Radiology
Illuminator, Radiographic Film	Radiology
Image Digitizer	Radiology
Labeler, X-Ray Film	Radiology
Media, Contrast, Radiologic	Radiology
Probe, Ultrasonic	Radiology
Processor, Radiographic Film, Automatic	Radiology
Radiographic Unit, Diagnostic	Radiology
Safelight, X-Ray	Radiology
Sand Bag	Radiology
Sand Bag, X-Ray	Radiology
Shield, X-Ray	Radiology
Silver Recovery Equipment	Radiology
Support, Patient Position, Radiographic	Radiology
Table, Radiographic	Radiology
Table, Radiographic, Non-Tilting, Powered	Radiology
Table, Radiographic, Stationary Top	Radiology
Tube, X-Ray	Radiology
Viewer, Radiographic Film, Motorized	Radiology

XODUS MEDICAL, INC.
Westmoreland Business & Research Park
702 Prominence Drive
New Kensington, PA 15068
FDA Number: 2530138
E-mail: info@xodusmedical.com
Web site: www.xodusmedical.com
Medical Products Sales Volume: $3,700,000
Year Founded: 1994
Total Employees: 40   *Marketing Staff:* 2   *Sales Staff:* 15
Ownership: Private
Quality System Registration Information: ISO9000
Produces/Sells CE-marked Devices: Y
Federal Procurement Eligibility: Small Business, GSA Contract, VA Contract
Distribution: Manufacturer Direct, Manufacturer Through Distributor, Manufacturer Through Manufacturer Reps, OEM, Exporter
General Admin.: Craig Kaforey/President
Production: Mark Kaforey/Vice President Manufacturing

800-963-8776
724-337-5500
Fax: 800-963-6553

Accessories, Laser, Endoscopic	Surgery
Cleaner, Electrosurgical Tip	Surgery
Counter, Sponge, Surgical	Surgery
Drape, Surgical Instrument, Magnetic	Surgery
Drape, Surgical, Disposable	Surgery
Drape, Surgical, Reusable	Surgery
Holder, Knife	Surgery
Holder, Needle, Other	Surgery

XODUS MEDICAL, INC.
800-963-8776 *(cont'd)*

Kit, Surgical (General)	Surgery
Lamp, Surgical	Surgery
Marker, Skin	Surgery
Monitor, Fetal	Obstetrics/Gynecology
Pad, Pressure, Gel	General
Pressure Pad, Alternating, Disposable	General
Strap, Restraining	General

XOFT, INC.
345 Potrero, Sunnyvale, CA 94085
FDA Number: 3005594788
E-mail: info@xoftinc.com
Web site: http://www.xoftinc.com
Ownership: Private
Produces/Sells CE-marked Devices: N
General Admin.: Dr. Thomas Rusch/Chief Technology Officer
Mr. Michael Klein/President, Chief Executive Officer
Medical Admin.: Ms. Kelly Elliott/Vice President Clinical Affairs
Mktg./Adv.: Mr. Robert Kirby/Vice President Business Development
Ms. Lisa Baird/Vice President Marketing
Mr. Dan Arnoff/Vice President Sales
Research: Mr. Robert Burnside/Vice President Research & Development
Finance: Ms. Mhairi Jones/Vice President Finance

408-419-2300
Fax: 408-419-2301

Therapeutic X-Ray System	Radiology

XOMA LTD.
2910 Seventh Street, Berkeley, CA 94710
FDA Number: n/a
Web site: www.xoma
Annual Revenue: $25-$50 Million
Total Employees: 335
Ownership: Public
Stock Symbol: XOMA
Traded On: NASDAQ
Quality System Registration Information: ISO9001
Produces/Sells CE-marked Devices: Y
Distribution: Manufacturer Direct
General Admin.: Steven B. Engle/Chief Executive Officer, Chairman
Patrick J. Scannon/Executive Vice President
Finance: Fred Kurland/Chief Financial Officer, Vice President Finance

510-204-7200
Fax: 510-644-2011

Antibody, Monoclonal	Microbiology
Contract R&D, Diagnostics	General

XOMED SURGICAL PRODUCTS
See Medtronic Xomed, Inc.

XOMED-TREACE
See Medtronic Xomed, Inc.

XONICS PHOTOCHEMICAL INC.
See Allied Diagnostic Imaging Resources, Inc.

XORAN TECHNOLOGIES, INC.
5210 South State Road,
Ann Arbor, MI 48103
FDA Number: 3004198450
E-mail: info@xorantech.com
Web site: www.xorantech.com
Ownership: Private
Produces/Sells CE-marked Devices: N

800-709-6726
734-663-7194
Fax: 734-663-8500

Head Rest, Neurosurgical	Cns/Neurology
Holder, Head, Radiographic	Radiology
Scanner, Computed Tomography, X-Ray (CAT, CT)	Cns/Neurology
Scanner, Computed Tomography, X-Ray, Special Procedure	Radiology

XRADIA INC.
4385 Hopyard Road, Suite 100, Pleasanton,, CA 94588
FDA Number: n/a
E-mail: info@xradia.com
Web site: www.xradia.com
Year Founded: 2000
Ownership: Private
Produces/Sells CE-marked Devices: N
General Admin.: Thomas Miller/Director Admin. & Finance
Wenbing Yun/President, Chief Executive Officer
Michael Feser/Vice President
Mktg./Adv.: S. H. Lau/Vice President Marketing & Sales

925-701-3600
Fax: 925-730-4952

XTOL PRODUCTS CO.
522 Goucher St., Johnstown, PA 15905
FDA Number: 2521578
Ownership: Private
Produces/Sells CE-marked Devices: N

814-255-2298

Tips And Pads, Cane, Crutch And Walker	Physical Med
Transfer Aid	Physical Med

XTRANA, INC.
800-789-6534
303-466-4424
590 Burbank St., Suite 205,
Broomfield, CO 80020
FDA Number: 1724526   *Fax:* 303-466-3326
E-mail: XtraAmp@xtrana.com
Web site: www.xtrana.com
Medical Products Sales Volume: $1,000,000
Total Employees: 15
Ownership: Public
Stock Symbol: XTRN
Traded On: NASDAQ
Produces/Sells CE-marked Devices: N
Federal Procurement Eligibility: Small Business
Distribution: Manufacturer Through Distributor
General Admin.: Timothy Dahltorp/Chief Executive Officer
        Dr. John Gerdes/Chief Scientific Officer, Vice President
Mktg./Adv.: Melanie Harder/Vice President Marketing & Sales
Production: Michael Lands/Vice President Operations
Finance: Dennis Lineberry/Controller
   Reagent, General Purpose   Pathology

XTTRIUM LABORATORIES, INC.
800-587-3721
773-268-5800
415 W. Pershing Road, Chicago, IL 60609-2727
FDA Number: 1410853   *Fax:* 773-924-6002
E-mail: bcreevy@xttrium.com
Web site: www.xttrium.com
Medical Products Sales Volume: $14,000,000
Annual Revenue: $5-$10 Million
Year Founded: 1932
Total Employees: 72
Ownership: Private
Produces/Sells CE-marked Devices: N
Federal Procurement Eligibility: Small Business, Female Owned, VA Contract
Distribution: Manufacturer Direct
General Admin.: Kevin Creevy/President, Chief Executive Officer
        Vijay Verma/Vice President, General Manager
Mktg./Adv.: Brian Creevy/Vice President Marketing & Sales
Production: Ajay Chawla/Director Quality Assurance
Research: Bettakeri Udayakumar/Vice President Research & Development
   Jelly, Lubricating   General
   Pad, Medicated   General
   Sanitizer   General
   Solution, Antibacterial Cleaner   General
   Solution, Instrument Cleaner   General
   Solution, Surgical Scrub   General

Y.I. VENTURES, LLC
314-344-0010
2260 Wendt Street, Algonquin, IL 60102
FDA Number: 2918576
E-mail: info@ydnt.com
Web site: www.ydnt.com
Total Employees: 28   *Marketing Staff:* 2   *Sales Staff:* 3
Ownership: Young Innovations, Inc.
Stock Symbol: YDNT
Traded On: NASDAQ
Produces/Sells CE-marked Devices: N
Federal Procurement Eligibility: Small Business
Distribution: Manufacturer Through Distributor, Manufacturer Through
Manufacturer Reps, Service Direct, Exclusive Distributor, Importer
General Admin.: Melvin Rouse/Chief Executive Officer
Mktg./Adv.: Rick Mustafa/Director Marketing
        Lynn Stavert/Director National Accounts
        Mel Rouse/Director Product Development
Production: Robert Werner/Director Engineering
        Robert Werner/Director Quality Assurance
Finance: Aase Rouse/Chief Financial Officer
   Cannula, Other   General
   Cleaner, Ultrasonic, Medical Instrument   General
   Glove, Utility   General
   Goggles, Protective, Eye   Ophthalmology
   Solution, Antibacterial Cleaner   General

YAMA, INC.
908-206-8706
650 Liberty Ave., Union, NJ 07083
FDA Number: 2248079
Ownership: Private
Produces/Sells CE-marked Devices: N
   Contraceptive Cervical Cap   Obstetrics/Gynecology
   Diaphragm, Contraceptive   Obstetrics/Gynecology
   Pledget And Intracardiac Patch, PETP, PTFE, Polypropylene   Cardiovascular

YAMATO CORPORATION
800-538-1762
719-591-1500
1775 S. Murray Blvd.,
Colorado Springs, CO 80916
FDA Number: n/a   *Fax:* 719-591-1045
E-mail: scales@yamatocorp.com
Web site: www.yamatocorp.com

YAMATO CORPORATION
800-538-1762 *(cont'd)*
Medical Products Sales Volume: $4,000,000
Annual Revenue: $1-$5 Million
Year Founded: 1922
Ownership: YAMATO SCALE CO. LTD.
Quality System Registration Information: ISO9001; ISO9002
Produces/Sells CE-marked Devices: N
Distribution: Manufacturer Through Distributor, Importer, Exporter
   Analyzer, Composition, Weight, Patient   General
   Scale, Infant   General
   Scale, Laboratory   Chemistry
   Scale, Stand-On   General

YAMATO SCIENTIFIC AMERICA, INC.
800-292-6286
925 Walsh Ave., Santa Clara, CA 95050
FDA Number: n/a
E-mail: customerservice@yamato-usa.com
Web site: www.yamato-usa.com
Annual Revenue: $1-$5 Million
Year Founded: 1889
Ownership: YAMATO SCIENTIFIC COMPANY LTD.
Quality System Registration Information: ISO9000
Produces/Sells CE-marked Devices: N
Distribution: Manufacturer Direct, Manufacturer Through Manufacturer Reps
   Bath, Water (Constant Temperature)   Chemistry
   Dryer, Labware   Chemistry
   Equipment, Cleaning, Air   General
   Evaporator   Chemistry
   Freeze Drying Equipment   Chemistry
   Homogenizer, Tissue   Microbiology
   Incubator, Aerobic   Microbiology
   Laminar Air Flow Unit, Mobile   Chemistry
   Mixer, Clinical Laboratory   Chemistry
   Oven   Chemistry
   Sterilizer, Laboratory   Microbiology
   Stirrer   Chemistry
   Washer, Pipette   Chemistry

YAMATO USA INC.
See Yamato Scientific America, Inc.

YAN RAZDOLSKY LTD
847-215-7554
600 W. Lake Cook Rd., Suite 150, Buffalo Grove, IL 60089
FDA Number: n/a
E-mail: yan@razdolsky.com
Web site: www.razdolsky.com
Ownership: Private
Produces/Sells CE-marked Devices: N
   External Mandibular Fixator And/or Distractor   Dental And Oral

YANKEE MEDICAL, INC.
800-649-4591
802-863-4591
276 North Ave., Burlington, VT 05401
FDA Number: n/a   *Fax:* 802-658-3101
Web site: www.yankeemedical.com
Annual Revenue: $1-$5 Million
Total Employees: 50
Ownership: Private
Produces/Sells CE-marked Devices: N
Federal Procurement Eligibility: Small Business
Distribution: Manufacturer Direct
   Contract Manufacturing, Product, Durable   General
   Custom Prosthesis   Orthopedics

YATES & BIRD AND MOTLOID
800-662-5021
312-226-2412
300 N. Elizabeth St., Chicago, IL 60607
FDA Number: n/a   *Fax:* 312-226-2480
E-mail: sales@yate-motloid.com
Web site: www.yates-motloid.com
Annual Revenue: $1-$5 Million
Total Employees: 28   *Marketing Staff:* 2   *Sales Staff:* 3
Ownership: Private
Quality System Registration Information: ISO9002
Produces/Sells CE-marked Devices: N
Federal Procurement Eligibility: Small Business
Distribution: Manufacturer Direct, Manufacturer Through Distributor
General Admin.: Richard Seid/Chief Executive Officer
Mktg./Adv.: Mona Zemsky/Vice President Marketing & Sales
Production: Ron Schwartz/Vice President Manufacturing
   Material, Acrylic, Dental   Dental And Oral
   Orthodontic Instrument   Dental And Oral
   Solvent   Chemistry
   Tray, Impression   Dental And Oral
   Wax, Dental   Dental And Oral

YESWIN CORP.
213-383-8066
3200 Wilshire Blvd South Tower, Ste 1140,
Los Angeles, CA 90010
FDA Number: 2087356
Ownership: Private

YESWIN CORP. 213-383-8066 *(cont'd)*
Produces/Sells CE-marked Devices: N
Orthosis, Lumbar — Physical Med

YORK BARBELL 800-358-9675
3300 Board Rd., York, PA 17405-1707 717-767-6481
FDA Number: n/a
Web site: www.yorkbarbell.com
Ownership: Private
Produces/Sells CE-marked Devices: N
Federal Procurement Eligibility: Small Business
Distribution: Manufacturer Through Distributor, Manufacturer Through
Manufacturer Reps, Importer, Exporter

Board, Quadriceps (Exerciser)	Physical Med
Exerciser, Arm	Physical Med
Exerciser, Chest	Physical Med
Exerciser, Hand	Physical Med
Exerciser, Leg And Ankle	Physical Med
Exerciser, Non-Measuring	Physical Med
Exerciser, Other	Physical Med
Exerciser, Shoulder	Physical Med

YORK X-RAY AND ORTHOPEDIC SUPPLY, INC. 800-334-6427
PO Box 326, 20 Hampton Rd.,, 864-879-2110
Lyman, SC 29365
FDA Number: n/a
E-mail: yorkxrayinc@charter.net *Fax:* 888-329-9675
Web site: www.yorkxray.com
Medical Products Sales Volume: $1,100,000
Annual Revenue: $1-$5 Million
Year Founded: 1983
Total Employees: 8 *Marketing Staff:* 2 *Sales Staff:* 7
Ownership: Private
Produces/Sells CE-marked Devices: N
Federal Procurement Eligibility: Small Business, Female Owned, GSA Contract
Distribution: Exclusive Distributor
General Admin.: Joye W. Atkinson/President, Owner
Joe Poole/Vice President
Mktg./Adv.: John P. Halsey/Manager International & National Sales

Radiographic Unit, Diagnostic, Dental (X-Ray)	Dental And Oral
Radiographic Unit, Diagnostic, Fixed (X-Ray)	Radiology
System, X-Ray, Mobile	Radiology
Table, Radiographic, Non-Tilting, Powered	Radiology
Table, Radiographic, Stationary Top	Radiology
Table, Radiographic, Tilting	Radiology
Videofluoroscopic Unit	Radiology

YOUNG COLORADO, LLC. 800-325-1881
13705 Shoreline Court East, Earth City, MO 63045
FDA Number: 1721374
Web site: www.ydnt.com
Ownership: Young Innovations, Inc.
Stock Symbol: YDNT
Traded On: NASDAQ
Produces/Sells CE-marked Devices: N
General Admin.: George E. Richmond/Chairman
David W. Frank/Secretary
Daniel J. Tarullo/Vice President
Finance: Julia A. Heap/Vice President Finance

Agent, Polishing, Abrasive, Oral Cavity	Dental And Oral
Cleaner, Ultrasonic, Medical Instrument	General
Cup, Prophylaxis	Dental And Oral
Handpiece, Air-Powered, Dental	Dental And Oral
Handpiece, Contra- And Right-Angle Attachment, Dental	Dental And Oral
Mask, Surgical	Surgery
Medical Disinfectants/Cleaners for Instruments	General
Mirror, Mouth	Dental And Oral
Needle, Dental	Dental And Oral
Protector, Dental	Anesthesiology
Scaler, Ultrasonic	Dental And Oral
Sterilant, Medical Device	General
Tray, Fluoride, Disposable	Dental And Oral

YOUNG DENTAL MANUFACTURING CO 1, LLC (800) 325-1881
13705 Shoreline Court East, (314) 344-0010
Earth City, MO 63045
FDA Number: 1628382
Web site: www.ydnt.com
Ownership: Young Innovations, Inc.
Stock Symbol: YDNT
Traded On: NASDAQ
Produces/Sells CE-marked Devices: N
General Admin.: George E. Richmond/Chairman
Arthur L. Herbst/President, Chief Financial Officer
David W. Frank/Secretary
Daniel J. Tarullo/Vice President
Finance: Julia A. Heap/Vice President Finance

Agent, Polishing, Abrasive, Oral Cavity	Dental And Oral

YOUNG DENTAL MANUFACTURING CO 1, LLC (800) 325-1881
(cont'd)

Handpiece, Air-Powered, Dental	Dental And Oral
Handpiece, Contra- And Right-Angle Attachment, Dental	Dental And Oral
Incubator/Water Bath, Microbiology	Microbiology
Mirror, Mouth	Dental And Oral
Needle, Dental	Dental And Oral
Protector, Silicate	Dental And Oral

YOUNG INNOVATIONS LLC DBA PLAK 800-558-6684
SMACKER
755 Trademark Circle, Corona, CA 92879 951-898-7600
FDA Number: 2024980 *Fax:* 951-898-2792
E-mail: store@plaksmacker.com
Web site: www.plaksmacker.com
Ownership: Young Innovations, Inc.
Stock Symbol: YDNT
Traded On: NASDAQ
Produces/Sells CE-marked Devices: N
General Admin.: George E. Richmond/Chairman
Arthur L. Herbst/President, Chief Financial Officer
David W. Frank/Secretary
Daniel J. Tarullo/Vice President
Finance: Julia A. Heap/Vice President Finance

Floss, Dental	Dental And Oral

YOUNG INNOVATIONS, INC. 800-325-1881
13705 Shoreline Court East, 314-344-0010
Earth City, MO 63045
FDA Number: 1925198 *Fax:* 314-344-0021
E-mail: info@ydnt.com
Web site: www.ydnt.com
Medical Products Sales Volume: $45,623,000
Annual Revenue: $50-$100 Million
Year Founded: 1961
Total Employees: 400 *Marketing Staff:* 8 *Sales Staff:* 22
Ownership: Public
Stock Symbol: YDNT
Traded On: NASDAQ
Quality System Registration Information: ISO9000
Produces/Sells CE-marked Devices: N
Federal Procurement Eligibility: Small Business
Distribution: Manufacturer Through Distributor, OEM, Exporter
General Admin.: Mr. Alfred E. Brennan/Chief Executive Officer, Chairman
Mr. Joshua McKey/Vice President
Mktg./Adv.: Mr. Daniel Tarullo/Vice President Business Development
Finance: Mr. Arthur L. Herbst/President
Ms. Julia Carter/Vice President Finance

Absorber, Saliva, Paper	Dental And Oral
Agent, Polishing, Abrasive, Oral Cavity	Dental And Oral
Brush, Other	General
Component, Other	General
Condenser, Amalgam And Foil, Operative	Dental And Oral
Cup, Prophylaxis	Dental And Oral
Disinfector, Medical Device	General
Frame, Rubber Dam	Dental And Oral
Handpiece, Contra- And Right-Angle Attachment, Dental	Dental And Oral
Kit, Plaque Disclosing	Dental And Oral
Mirror, Mouth	Dental And Oral
Needle, Dental	Dental And Oral
Protector, Silicate	Dental And Oral
Tooth Bonding Agent, Resin Restoration	Dental And Oral
Tubing, Other	General

Medical Product Subsidiaries (Listed Separately)
Athena Technology, Inc.
Denticator International, Inc.
Panoramic Corporation
Save-A-Life Llc
Y.I. Ventures, Llc
Young Colorado, Llc.
Young Dental Manufacturing Co 1, Llc
Young Innovations Llc Dba Plak Smacker
Young O/S Llc

YOUNG MICROBRUSH LLC 262-375-4011
1376 Cheyenne Ave., Grafton, WI 53024
FDA Number: 2134751
Ownership: Private
Produces/Sells CE-marked Devices: N

Applicator, Resin	Dental And Oral
Handle, Instrument, Dental	Dental And Oral
Needle, Dental	Dental And Oral
Syringe, Restorative And Impression Material	Dental And Oral

YOUNG O/S LLC 800-325-1881
1663 Fenton Business Park, Fenton, MO 63026
FDA Number: 1926480
Web site: www.ydnt.com

YOUNG O/S LLC   800-325-1881 *(cont'd)*
Ownership: Young Innovations, Inc.
Stock Symbol: YDNT
Traded On: NASDAQ
Produces/Sells CE-marked Devices: N
General Admin.: George E. Richmond/Chairman
       Brian F. Bremer/Partner
       Arthur L. Herbst/President, Chief Financial Officer
       David W. Frank/Secretary
       Daniel J. Tarullo/Vice President
Finance: Julia A. Heap/Vice President Finance

Burr, Dental	Dental And Oral
Cleaner, Ultrasonic, Medical Instrument	General
Condenser, Amalgam And Foil, Operative	Dental And Oral
Filling, Instrument Plastic, Dental	Dental And Oral
Gauge, Depth, Instrument, Dental	Dental And Oral
Gutta Percha	Dental And Oral
Needle, Dental	Dental And Oral
Operative Dental Treatment Unit	Dental And Oral
Plugger, Root Canal, Endodontic	Dental And Oral
Point, Paper, Endodontic	Dental And Oral
Scaler, Ultrasonic	Dental And Oral

YOUNGER MANUFACTURING CO., INC.   800-877-5367
2925 Calfornia St., Torrance, CA 90503   310-783-1533
FDA Number: 2020853   Fax: 310-783-6477
Web site: www.youngeroptics.com
Annual Revenue: $1-$5 Million
Year Founded: 1955
Ownership: Private
Quality System Registration Information: ISO9000
Produces/Sells CE-marked Devices: N
Distribution: OEM, Importer, Exporter

Lens, Spectacle/Eyeglasses, Non-Custom	Ophthalmology

YOUNGER MFG. CO.   310-783-1649
2925 California St., Torrance, CA 90503
FDA Number: 2020853

Lens, Spectacle/Eyeglasses, Non-Custom	Ophthalmology

YOUNGS, INC.   800-523-5454
55 Cherry Lane, Souderton, PA 18964-1550   215-723-4400
FDA Number: 7000934   Fax: 800-544-3239
E-mail: custrep@youngscatalog.com
Web site: www.youngscatalog.com
Medical Products Sales Volume: $1,000,000
Annual Revenue: $5-$10 Million
Year Founded: 1945
Total Employees: 36   *Marketing Staff:* 3   *Sales Staff:* 2
Ownership: Private
Produces/Sells CE-marked Devices: N
Distribution: Exclusive Distributor
General Admin.: Paul O. Young/President

Accessories, Cart, Multipurpose	General
Cabinet, Storage, Catheter	General
Cart, Emergency, Cardiopulmonary Resuscitation (Crash)	Anesthesiology
Cart, Gas Cylinder (Carrier)	Anesthesiology
Cart, Housekeeping	General
Cart, Laundry	General
Cart, Multipurpose	General
Cart, Other	General
Casters, Hospital Equipment	General
Chair, Geriatric	General
Chair, Pediatric	General
Disinfector, Liquid	General
Foodservice Product/Equipment	General
Glove, Patient Examination, Latex	General
Purifier, Air, Ultraviolet	General
Rail, Bath	General
Shield, Protective, Personnel	Radiology
Tips And Pads, Cane, Crutch And Walker	Physical Med
Tray, Medicine	General
Waste Receptacle, Contaminated	General
Wheelchair, Manual	Physical Med

YUASA, INC.
See Enersys

Z SOUND   847-293-5205
6947 West Birchwood Ave., Niles, IL 60714
FDA Number: 64090
Ownership: Private
Produces/Sells CE-marked Devices: N

Hearing-Aid, Group, Or Auditory Trainer	Ear/Nose/Throat

Z TECHNOLOGIES, LLC   404-248-0159
2615 Woodacres Road, Atlanta, GA 30345
FDA Number: 1062203   Fax: 404-248-0159
E-mail: sales@ztekstim.com
Web site: www.ztekstim.com

Z TECHNOLOGIES, LLC   404-248-0159 *(cont'd)*
Medical Products Sales Volume: $200,000
Year Founded: 1998
Ownership: Private
Produces/Sells CE-marked Devices: N
Federal Procurement Eligibility: Small Business
Distribution: Manufacturer Direct

Stimulator, Nerve, Transcutaneous (Pain Relief, TENS)	Cns/Neurology

Z-KAT, INC.   954-927-2044
2903 Simms St., Hollywood, FL 33020
FDA Number: 1066372
Ownership: Private
Produces/Sells CE-marked Devices: N

Image Processing System	Radiology
Stereotaxy Equipment	Cns/Neurology

Z-MAN CORPORATION   616-281-6108
1359 Pickett, SE, Kentwood, MI 49508
FDA Number: n/a   Fax: 616-281-6108
E-mail: info@zmancorp.com
Web site: www.zmancorp.com
Medical Products Sales Volume: $130,000
Year Founded: 1996
Ownership: Private
Produces/Sells CE-marked Devices: N
Federal Procurement Eligibility: Small Business
Distribution: Manufacturer Direct

Clamp, Tubing	General

Z-MEDICA CORPORATION   203-294-0000
4 Fairfield Blvd., Wallingford, CT 06492
FDA Number: 3004138549   Fax: 203-294-0688
E-mail: info@z-medica.com
Web site: http://www.z-medica.com
Year Founded: 2002
Ownership: Private
Produces/Sells CE-marked Devices: N

Dressing, Other	General

Z-PACK, INC.   818-887-4924
6215 Oakdale Ave., Woodland Hills, CA 91367
FDA Number: 3004574428
Ownership: Private
Produces/Sells CE-marked Devices: N

Alarm, Enuresis	Gastroenterology/Urology

Z. HAYDU MANUFACTURING INC.   954-925-1779
1980 Grant St., Hollywood, FL 33020
FDA Number: n/a   Fax: 954-923-1366
E-mail: zhaydumfg@aol.com
Web site: www.zhaydumfg.com
Annual Revenue: $0-$1 Million
Year Founded: 1933
Ownership: Private
Quality System Registration Information: ISO9000
Produces/Sells CE-marked Devices: N
Federal Procurement Eligibility: Small Business
Distribution: Manufacturer Through Distributor

Burr, Dental	Dental And Oral

ZAHOUREK SYSTEMS, INC.   800-950-5025
2198 W. 15th St., Loveland, CO 80538   970-667-9047
FDA Number: n/a   Fax: 970-667-5025
E-mail: info@anatomyinclay.com
Web site: www.anatomyinclay.com
Year Founded: 1989
Ownership: Private
Produces/Sells CE-marked Devices: N
Federal Procurement Eligibility: Small Business
Distribution: Manufacturer Direct
General Admin.: Jon Zahourek/President
       Renee Zahourek/Vice President

Anatomical Training Model	General
Training Aid	Orthopedics
Training Manikin, Other	General

ZANDER MEDICAL SUPPLIES, INC. / ZANDER IVF, INC.   800-820-3029
755, 8th Court, Suite #4, Vero Beach, FL 32962   772-569-5955
FDA Number: 9007950   Fax: 772-569-4430
E-mail: sales@zanderivf.com
Web site: www.zanderivf.com
Medical Products Sales Volume: $3,400,000
Annual Revenue: $1-$5 Million
Year Founded: 1990
Total Employees: 8   *Marketing Staff:* 4   *Sales Staff:* 6
Ownership: Private

ZANDER MEDICAL SUPPLIES, INC. / ZANDER   800-820-3029
(cont'd)
Produces/Sells CE-marked Devices: Y
Federal Procurement Eligibility: Small Business
Distribution: OEM, Exclusive Distributor, Importer, Exporter
General Admin.: Mr. Fred Zander/Chief Executive Officer
         Mr. Fred Zander/President, Owner

Accessory, Assisted Reproduction	Obstetrics/Gynecology
Device, Semen Analysis	Obstetrics/Gynecology
Laser, Combination	General
Micromanipulator	General
Pipette, Micro	Chemistry

ZAP LASERS, LLC   925-930-6777
2621-b Pleasant Hill Rd., Pleasant Hill, CA 94523
FDA Number: 3005212363

Laser, Surgical	Surgery

ZARGIS MEDICAL CORP.   609-488-4608
One Atlantic Street, 1st Floo, Stamford, CT 06901
FDA Number: 3004857240
Web site: http://zargis.com
Ownership: Private
Produces/Sells CE-marked Devices: N
General Admin.: John A. Kallassy/Chief Executive Officer
  Medical Admin.: Dr. Alan Stein, MD, Ph.D./Chief Medical Officer
Research: Dr. Raymond Watrous/Chief Scientist

Phonocardiograph	Cardiovascular
Stethoscope, Electronic (Auscultoscope)	Cardiovascular

ZASSI MEDICAL EVOLUTIONS, INC.   904-261-2169
1886 S. 14th St., Suite 6, Fernandina Beach, FL 32034
FDA Number: 3003895434   *Fax:* 904-261-2172
E-mail: info@zassimedical.com
Web site: www.zassimedical.com
Medical Products Sales Volume: $4,300,000
Year Founded: 1997
Total Employees: 7   *Marketing Staff:* 4   *Sales Staff:* 5
Ownership: Private
Produces/Sells CE-marked Devices: Y
Federal Procurement Eligibility: Small Business
Distribution: Manufacturer Direct, Manufacturer Through Distributor, Manufacturer Through Manufacturer Reps, Exporter
General Admin.: Mr. Peter von Dyck/President, Chief Executive Officer

Catheter, Rectal, Ileostomy, Continent	Gastroenterology/Urology

ZEBEC DATA SYSTEMS, INC., HEALTHCARE MGMT. DIV.   713-782-3480
2425 Fountain View, Houston, TX 77057
FDA Number: n/a   *Fax:* 713-782-8340
E-mail: sales@zebec.net
Web site: www.zebec.net
Ownership: Private
Produces/Sells CE-marked Devices: N
Distribution: Manufacturer Direct
General Admin.: Stephen C. Guistwite/Chief Operating Officer
     Damon J. Small/Information Technology Administrator
     John R. Feltham/President, Chief Executive Officer
Mktg./Adv.: Dennis Chatagnier/Account Executive
Finance: Lizeth Barrera/Controller

Computer Software	General
Computer, Patient Data Management	General

ZEE MEDICAL PRODUCTS CO., INC.
  See Zee Medical, Inc.

ZEE MEDICAL, INC.   800-841-8417   949-252-9500
22 Corporate Park, Irvine, CA 92606
FDA Number: 1828159   *Fax:* 949-252-9649
E-mail: larry@zeemedicalinc.com
Web site: www.zeemedical.com
Medical Products Sales Volume: $249,700,000
Year Founded: 1987
Total Employees: 60
Ownership: Mckesson Corp.
Federal Procurement Eligibility: Small Business
Distribution: Exclusive Distributor
General Admin.: Gary Skelton/President, Chief Executive Officer
     Linda Cook/Vice President Human Resources
Mktg./Adv.: Larry Boss/Director Marketing
     Craig Peoples/Director National Accounts
     Greg Easter/Director Product Development
     Greg Easter/Manager Marketing
     Fred Browne/Vice President Sales
Production: Kevin Lloyd/Director Quality Assurance
     Cindy Larez/Manager Materials
     Paul Fernane/Vice President Operations
Research: Larry Boss/Vice President Product Development

ZEE MEDICAL, INC.   800-841-8417 *(cont'd)*
Finance: Cara Swank/Vice President Finance

Eyeglasses, Safety	Ophthalmology
Kit, First Aid	Surgery
Plug, Ear	Ear/Nose/Throat

ZEE SERVICE, INC.
  See Zee Medical, Inc.

ZEFON INTERNATIONAL   800-282-0073   352-854-8080
5350 S.W. First Lane, Ocala, FL 34474
FDA Number: 1052798   *Fax:* 352-854-7480
E-mail: customer_service@zefon.com
Web site: www.zefon.com
Medical Products Sales Volume: $7,000,000
Annual Revenue: $1-$5 Million
Year Founded: 1988
Total Employees: 67   *Marketing Staff:* 1   *Sales Staff:* 1
Ownership: Private
Produces/Sells CE-marked Devices: N
Federal Procurement Eligibility: Small Business
Distribution: Manufacturer Direct, Manufacturer Through Distributor, OEM
General Admin.: Russell Mantz/President
     Scott Ryan/Vice President, General Manager
Mktg./Adv.: Jeff Mantz/Vice President Sales

Cuff, Blood Pressure	Cardiovascular
Holder, Intravascular Catheter	General

ZEISS, INC.
  See Carl Zeiss Meditec Inc.

ZELTIQ
  See Zeltiq Aesthetics, Inc.

ZELTIQ AESTHETICS, INC.   925-474-2500
4698 Willow Road, Pleasanton, CA 94588
FDA Number: 3007215625   *Fax:* 925-474-2599
Web site: http://www.coolsculpting.com
Year Founded: 2005
Ownership: Private
Produces/Sells CE-marked Devices: N
General Admin.: Mr. Mitchell Levinson/Chief Scientific Officer
     Mr. Gordie Nye/President, Chief Executive Officer
Mktg./Adv.: Ms. Liz Panzica Newman/Vice President Marketing
Research: Dr. John Allison/Vice President Research & Development & Quality Control
Finance: Mr. John Howe/Chief Financial Officer

Laser, Surgical	Surgery
Massager, Therapeutic	Physical Med
Pack, Hot Or Cold, Water Circulating	Physical Med

ZENECA, INC., LUXTRAK BUSINESS GROUP
  See AstraZeneca Pharmaceuticals LP

ZENEX CORPORATION   847-390-0700
850 Elmhurst Rd., Elk Grove Village, IL 60007-2612
FDA Number: 1419329   *Fax:* 847-390-0706
Medical Products Sales Volume: $350,000
Annual Revenue: $0-$1 Million
Total Employees: 10   *Marketing Staff:* 1   *Sales Staff:* 1
Ownership: Private
Produces/Sells CE-marked Devices: N
Federal Procurement Eligibility: Small Business
Distribution: Manufacturer Through Distributor
General Admin.: Elias R. Zenkich/President
Mktg./Adv.: Lorraine La Lond/Coord. Sales
Production: Ilias Zenkich/Vice President Production

Adapter, Lead Switching, Electrocardiograph	Cardiovascular
Electrode, Electrocardiograph	Cardiovascular
Hood, Oxygen, Infant	General

ZENITH MEDICAL INC.   800-747-0216   858-535-0216
10064 Mesa Ridge Ct., Suite 218, San Diego, CA 92121
FDA Number: 2029159   *Fax:* 858-535-9715
E-mail: sales@zenithmedical.com
Web site: www.zenithmedical.com
Medical Products Sales Volume: $750,000
Annual Revenue: $0-$1 Million
Year Founded: 1993
Total Employees: 5
Ownership: Private
Produces/Sells CE-marked Devices: N
Federal Procurement Eligibility: Small Business
Distribution: Manufacturer Direct, Manufacturer Through Distributor
General Admin.: Mark McGlothlin/President
Production: Loraine McNulty/Manager Quality Assurance & Regulatory Affairs

Bag, Specimen, Laparoscopic	Surgery

ZENITH POINT MANUFACTURING   805-499-6808
3867 Old Conejo Rd., Newbury Park, CA 91320
FDA Number: 2032783
Ownership: Private
Produces/Sells CE-marked Devices: N

Post, Root Canal	Dental And Oral
Reamer, Pulp Canal, Endodontic	Dental And Oral

ZENITH/DMG BRAND   800-662-6383
Division of Foremost Dental LLC   **201-894-5500**
242 S. Dean St.
Englewood, NJ 07631
FDA Number: n/a
E-mail: info@zenithdmg.com   Fax: 201-894-0213
Web site: www.zenithdmg.com
Total Employees: 30   *Marketing Staff:* 5   *Sales Staff:* 20
Ownership: Private
Quality System Registration Information: ISO9002
Produces/Sells CE-marked Devices: Y
Federal Procurement Eligibility: Small Business
Distribution: Manufacturer Through Distributor, Manufacturer Through Manufacturer Reps, Exclusive Distributor
General Admin.: Lawrence Katz/President, Chief Executive Officer
Mktg./Adv.: Christine Corsette/Director Marketing
    Jerry Collins/Manager National Sales
    Georgeq Wolfe/Manager Product Development
Production: Joe Zliceski/Manager Regulatory Affairs
Finance: Diane Akerlind/Controller

Alloy, Amalgam	Dental And Oral
Amalgamator, Dental, AC-Powered	Dental And Oral
Capsule, Dental, Amalgam	Dental And Oral
Coating, Filling Material, Resin	Dental And Oral
Gutta Percha	Dental And Oral
Sealant, Pit And Fissure, And Conditioner, Resin	Dental And Oral

ZENITH/OMNI HEARING INSTRUMENTS, INC.   203-624-9857
111 Park St., Suite K, New Haven, CT 06511
FDA Number: 1222908
Ownership: Private
Produces/Sells CE-marked Devices: N

Hearing-Aid	Ear/Nose/Throat

ZENS MANUFACTURING, INC..   414-372-7060
2435 N. Martin Luther King Drive, PO Drawer 12504,
Milwaukee, WI 53212
FDA Number: 2182750   Fax: 414-372-4445
E-mail: sales@zensmfg.com
Ownership: Private
Produces/Sells CE-marked Devices: Y
Federal Procurement Eligibility: Small Business
Distribution: Manufacturer Direct, Manufacturer Through Distributor, Manufacturer Through Manufacturer Reps, OEM, Exporter

Dressing, Other	General

ZEP MANUFACTURING, INC.
See Zep Superior Solutions

ZEP SUPERIOR SOLUTIONS   877-428-9937
1310 Seaboard Ind. Blvd.,   **404-352-1680**
Atlanta, GA 30318
FDA Number: n/a
Web site: www.zep.com
Annual Revenue: $500 Million-$1 Billion
Year Founded: 1937
Total Employees: 2520
Ownership: Public
Stock Symbol: ZEP
Traded On: NYSE
Quality System Registration Information: ISO9001
Produces/Sells CE-marked Devices: Y
Distribution: Manufacturer Through Manufacturer Reps, Exporter
General Admin.: Mark R. Bachmann/Chief Financial Officer, Executive Vice President
    John K. Morgan/President, Chief Executive Officer, Chairman

Disinfector, Liquid	General
Dispenser, Soap	General
Solution, Antibacterial Cleaner	General
Solution, Skin Degreaser	General

ZEPTOMETRIX CORPORATION   800-274-5487
872 Main St., Buffalo, NY 14202-1499   **716-882-0920**
FDA Number: n/a   Fax: 716-882-0959
E-mail: custserv@ZeptoMetrix.com
Web site: www.zeptometrix.com
Annual Revenue: $1-$5 Million
Total Employees: 12   *Marketing Staff:* 1   *Sales Staff:* 1
Ownership: Private
Produces/Sells CE-marked Devices: N

ZEPTOMETRIX CORPORATION   800-274-5487 *(cont'd)*
Federal Procurement Eligibility: Small Business
Distribution: Manufacturer Direct, Manufacturer Through Distributor, OEM, Service Direct, Exclusive Distributor, Importer, Exporter
General Admin.: Dr. James Hengst/President, Chief Executive Officer
Mktg./Adv.: Cathy Dudnanski/Director Marketing & Sales
    Dr. James Hengst/Director Product Development
Production: David Reinlander/Director Quality Assurance
    David Reinlander/Manager Regulatory Affairs

Antibody, Monoclonal	Microbiology
Genetic Engineering	Microbiology
Medium, Lymphocyte Separation	Hematology
Monitor, Test, Hiv-1	Hematology
Standard, Lipid	Chemistry
Strip, HAMA IGG, ELISA, In Vitro Test System	Immunology
Test, Antibody, Acquired Immune Deficiency Syndrome (AIDS)	Hematology

ZERO CASES
See Zero Manufacturing, Inc.

ZERO CORP.
See Zero Manufacturing, Inc.

ZERO ENCLOSURES
See Zero Manufacturing, Inc.

ZERO HALLIBURTON
See Zero Manufacturing, Inc.

ZERO MANUFACTURING, INC.   800-500-9376
500 West 200 North, North Salt Lake, UT 84054   **801-299-7375**
FDA Number: n/a   Fax: 801-299-7389
E-mail: sales@zerocases.com
Web site: www.zerocases.com
Medical Products Sales Volume: $27,500,000
Annual Revenue: $25-$50 Million
Year Founded: 1952
Total Employees: 150
Ownership: Zero Corporation
Quality System Registration Information: ISO9001
Produces/Sells CE-marked Devices: N
Federal Procurement Eligibility: Small Business
Distribution: Manufacturer Direct, Manufacturer Through Distributor, Manufacturer Through Manufacturer Reps, Exclusive Distributor
Mktg./Adv.: Randy Holdaway/Director Marketing & Public Relations
    Nigel Duncan/Vice President Marketing & Sales

Case, Protection, Equipment	General

ZERO PLASTICS
See Zero Manufacturing, Inc.

ZEROWET, INC.   800-438-0938
PO Box 4375,   **310-544-1600**
Palos Verdes Peninsula, CA 90274
FDA Number: 2084203   Fax: 310-544-4411
E-mail: kstamler-zerowet@cox.net
Web site: www.zerowet.com
Medical Products Sales Volume: $400,000
Annual Revenue: $1-$5 Million
Year Founded: 1990
Total Employees: 4   *Marketing Staff:* 2   *Sales Staff:* 2
Ownership: Private
Produces/Sells CE-marked Devices: Y
Federal Procurement Eligibility: Small Business
Distribution: Manufacturer Direct, Manufacturer Through Distributor, OEM, Exporter
General Admin.: Keith Stamler/Chief Executive Officer

Kit, Irrigation, Wound	General
Shield, Syringe	General

ZEST ANCHORS, INC.   800-262-2310
2061 Wineridge Place #100,   **760-743-7744**
Escondido, CA 92029
FDA Number: 2023950   Fax: 800-487-1357
E-mail: zest@zestanchors.com
Web site: www.zestanchors.com
Medical Products Sales Volume: $1,700,000
Annual Revenue: $1-$5 Million
Year Founded: 1943
Ownership: Private
Quality System Registration Information: ISO9001
Produces/Sells CE-marked Devices: Y
Federal Procurement Eligibility: Small Business
Distribution: Manufacturer Direct, OEM, Exporter

Abutment, Implant, Dental, Endosseous	Dental And Oral
Attachment, Precision	Dental And Oral
Implant, Endosseous	Dental And Oral

ZETEK, INC.   800-367-2837
876 Ventura St., Aurora, CO 80011-7917   **303-343-2122**
FDA Number: 1720934   Fax: 720-579-0310

MANUFACTURER PROFILES

ZETEK, INC.   800-367-2837 *(cont'd)*

E-mail: info@zetek.net
Web site: www.zetek.net
Annual Revenue: $0-$1 Million
Total Employees: 5
Ownership: Public
Produces/Sells CE-marked Devices: N
Federal Procurement Eligibility: Small Business
Distribution: Manufacturer Direct
General Admin.: Philip Regas/Chief Executive Officer
     Janice Tague/Office Manager

Device, Fertility, Contraceptive, Diagnostic	Obstetrics/Gynecology
Monitor, Fertility	Obstetrics/Gynecology
Test, Fertility Monitoring	Obstetrics/Gynecology

ZETTLER SYSTEMS, INC.   949-831-5000
75 Columbia, Aliso Viejo, CA 92656

FDA Number: n/a   *Fax:* 949-831-8642
E-mail: sales@azettler.com
Web site: www.azettler.com
Total Employees: 45
Ownership: TYCO INTERNATIONAL LTD.
Stock Symbol: TYC
Traded On: NYSE
Produces/Sells CE-marked Devices: Y
Distribution: Manufacturer Through Distributor
General Admin.: Don Campbell/President
Mktg./Adv.: Rainer Rahaeuser/Manager National Sales

Nurse Call System	General

ZEUS SCIENTIFIC, INC.   800-286-2111
PO Box 38, Raritan, NJ 08869-0038   908-526-3744

FDA Number: 2242436   *Fax:* 908-526-2058
E-mail: info@zeusscientific.com
Web site: www.zeusscientific.com
Medical Products Sales Volume: $4,400,000
Annual Revenue: $10-$25 Million
Year Founded: 1976
Total Employees: 55
Ownership: Private
Quality System Registration Information: ISO9001
Federal Procurement Eligibility: Small Business, VA Contract
Distribution: Manufacturer Direct, Manufacturer Through Distributor, OEM, Exporter
General Admin.: Donald R. Tourville/Chief Executive Officer
     Scott J. Tourville/President
Mktg./Adv.: Joseph B. Turner/Executive Vice President Marketing & Sales
Production: John P. Tourville/Vice President Operations
Research: Mark Kopnitsky/Vice President Research & Development

Antibody IGM, IF, Epstein-Barr Virus	Microbiology
Antibody Igm, If, Cytomegalovirus Virus	Microbiology
Antibody, Anti-Smooth Muscle, Indirect Immunofluorescent	Immunology
Antibody, Antimitochondrial, Indirect Immunofluorescent	Immunology
Antibody, Antinuclear, Indirect Immunofluorescent, Antigen	Immunology
Antibody, Herpes Virus	Microbiology
Antibody, Mycoplasma SPP.	Microbiology
Antibody, Other	General
Antibody, Toxoplasma Gondii	Microbiology
Antibody, Treponema Pallidum	Microbiology
Antibody, Varicella-Zoster	Microbiology
Antinuclear Antibody (Enzyme-Labeled), Antigen, Controls	Immunology
Antiserum, Fluorescent, Rubeola	Microbiology
Antiserum, Neutralization, Herpes Virus Hominis	Microbiology
Campylobacter Pylori	Microbiology
Culture Media, Antimicrobial Susceptibility Test	Microbiology
Enzyme Linked Immunoabsorbent Assay, Cytomegalovirus	Microbiology
Enzyme Linked Immunoabsorbent Assay, Herpes Simplex Virus	Microbiology
Enzyme Linked Immunoabsorbent Assay, Mumps Virus	Microbiology
Enzyme Linked Immunoabsorbent Assay, Mycoplasma SPP.	Microbiology
Enzyme Linked Immunoabsorbent Assay, Rubella	Microbiology
Enzyme Linked Immunoabsorbent Assay, Rubeola	Microbiology
Enzyme Linked Immunoabsorbent Assay, Toxoplasma Gondii	Microbiology
Enzyme Linked Immunoabsorbent Assay, Varicella-Zoster	Microbiology
Epstein-Barr Virus, Other	Microbiology
Extractable Antinuclear Antibody (Rnp/Sm), Antigen/Control	Immunology
Fixative, Acid Containing	Pathology
Legionella Direct & Indirect Fluorescent Antibody Regents	Microbiology
Legionella, Spp., ELISA	Microbiology
Test System, Antineutrophil Cytoplasmic Antibodies (ANCA)	Immunology
Test, Disease, Lyme	Immunology
Test, Nuclear Antigen, Epstein-Barr Virus	Microbiology
Test, Rheumatoid Factor	Immunology

ZEVEX
See Zevex Incorporated

ZEVEX INCORPORATED   800-970-2337
4314 ZEVEX Park Lane,   801-264-1001
Salt Lake City, UT 84123

FDA Number: 1722139   *Fax:* 801-264-1051

ZEVEX INCORPORATED   800-970-2337 *(cont'd)*

E-mail: sales@zevex.com
Web site: www.zevex.com
Medical Products Sales Volume: $41,000,000
Annual Revenue: $25-$50 Million
Year Founded: 1986
Total Employees: 148   *Marketing Staff:* 3   *Sales Staff:* 21
Ownership: Moog Inc.
Stock Symbol: ZVXI
Traded On: NASDAQ
Quality System Registration Information: ISO9001
Produces/Sells CE-marked Devices: Y
Federal Procurement Eligibility: Small Business
Distribution: Manufacturer Direct, Manufacturer Through Manufacturer Reps, OEM
General Admin.: Mr. David J. McNally/Chief Executive Officer, Chairman
     Mr. Phillip L. McStotts/Chief Financial Officer, Treasurer
     Mrs. Barbara Newbold/Human Resources Representative
Mktg./Adv.: Mr. Shawn Fojtik/Vice President Marketing & Sales
Production: Mr. Tim Govin/Vice President Operations
     Mr. Mike Henderson/Vice President Quality Assurance & Regulatory Affairs
Research: Mr. Phil Eggers/Vice President Research & Engineering
Finance: Mrs. Andrea Kendall/Controller

Contract Manufacturing	General
Contract Manufacturing, Product, Durable	General
Contract R&D, Equipment	General
Detector, Air Bubble	Gastroenterology/Urology
Detector, Air, Heart-Lung Bypass	Cardiovascular
Detector, Blood Level	Gastroenterology/Urology
Detector, Bubble, Cardiopulmonary Bypass	Cardiovascular
Detector, Hemodialysis Unit Air Bubble-Foam	Gastroenterology/Urology
Infusion Pump, Enteral	General
Monitor, Cardiopulmonary Level Sensing	Cardiovascular
Perfusion System, Kidney	Gastroenterology/Urology
Phacofragmentation Unit	Ophthalmology
Pump, Infusion, Elastomeric	General
Service, Engineering/Design	General
Transducer, Ultrasonic	Cardiovascular
Tube, Gastrointestinal	Gastroenterology/Urology

ZHANG ENTERPRISES   972-238-8260
400 N. Greenville Ave., Suite 9, Richardson, TX 75081

FDA Number: 1651436
Ownership: Private
Produces/Sells CE-marked Devices: N

Orthosis, Limb Brace	Physical Med
Orthosis, Truncal/Limb	Physical Med
Pack, Moist Heat	Physical Med

ZIAMATIC CORP.   800-711-FIRE
10 W. College Avenue, Yardley, PA 19067-8337   215-493-3618

FDA Number: n/a   *Fax:* 215-493-1401
E-mail: zservice@ziamatic.com
Web site: www.ziamatic.com
Medical Products Sales Volume: $13,000,000
Annual Revenue: $5-$10 Million
Total Employees: 45   *Marketing Staff:* 2   *Sales Staff:* 3
Ownership: Private
Produces/Sells CE-marked Devices: N
Federal Procurement Eligibility: Small Business
Distribution: Manufacturer Through Distributor, Importer, Exporter
General Admin.: Theodore Ziaylek/Chief Executive Officer
     Michael Ziaylek/President
Mktg./Adv.: Ronald La Rue/Vice President Advertising
     Ronald La Rue/Vice President Marketing
     Michael Adams/Vice President Sales
Production: Richard Ossman/Manager Materials

Cabinet Casework, General Purpose	General
Holder, Gas Cylinder	Anesthesiology
Mount, Equipment	General
Rescue Equipment	General

ZIBRA CORP.   800-758-8773
640 American Legion Hwy.,   508-636-6606
Westport, MA 02790

FDA Number: 1222121   *Fax:* 508-636-2155
E-mail: sales@zibracorp.com
Web site: www.zibracorp.com
Annual Revenue: $1-$5 Million
Year Founded: 1984
Total Employees: 10   *Marketing Staff:* 1   *Sales Staff:* 1
Ownership: Private
Produces/Sells CE-marked Devices: N
Federal Procurement Eligibility: Small Business
Distribution: Manufacturer Direct, OEM
General Admin.: Arthur C. McKinley/Chief Executive Officer

Contract Manufacturing	General

ZIBRA CORP.   800-758-8773 *(cont'd)*
Endoscope   Gastroenterology/Urology

ZIEHM IMAGING, INC.   800-503-4952
6280 Hazeltine National Dr., Orlando, FL 32822   **407-615-8560**
FDA Number: 2027299   *Fax:* 407) 6 15-8561
E-mail: mail@ziehm.com
Web site: http://www.ziehm.com
Medical Products Sales Volume: $22,000,000
Annual Revenue: $10-$25 Million
Year Founded: 1972
Total Employees: 50   *Marketing Staff:* 1   *Sales Staff:* 11
Ownership: ATON, GMBH
Quality System Registration Information: ISO9000; ISO9001
Produces/Sells CE-marked Devices: Y
Federal Procurement Eligibility: Small Business
Distribution: Manufacturer Direct, Manufacturer Through Distributor, Manufacturer Through Manufacturer Reps, OEM, Service Direct, Exporter
Mktg./Adv.: Jose Maria Castellon/International Sales Representative
    Mark Axelson/Manager Marketing
    Jayne Miller/Sales Specialist
    Radiographic/Fluoroscopic Unit, Mobile C-Arm   Radiology

ZIEHM INTERNATIONAL, INC.
    See Ziehm Imaging, Inc.

ZIERING MEDICAL WORLDWIDE   310-360-8860
9201 Sunset Boulevard Suite 305, West Hollywood, CA 90069
FDA Number: n/a
E-mail: zieringmedical.com
Ownership: Private
Produces/Sells CE-marked Devices: N

ZILA DENTAL TECHNOLOGIES, INC.   928-899-1231
2410 Harrison St., Batesville, AR 72501
FDA Number: 1649388
Ownership: PROFESSIONAL DENTAL MFG., INC.
Produces/Sells CE-marked Devices: N

Floss, Dental	Dental And Oral
Handpiece, Air-Powered, Dental	Dental And Oral
Pick, Massaging	Dental And Oral
Probe, Periodontic	Dental And Oral
Scaler, Ultrasonic	Dental And Oral
Scraper, Tongue	Dental And Oral
Toothbrush, Manual	Dental And Oral
Toothbrush, Powered	Dental And Oral

ZILA TECHNICAL, INC.   602-266-6700
3418 South 48th St., Suite 9, Phoenix, AZ 85040-1939
FDA Number: 2030577
Ownership: Private
Produces/Sells CE-marked Devices: N

Light, Surgical Operating, Dental	Dental And Oral
Source, Chemiluminescent Light	Obstetrics/Gynecology

ZILA, INC.   800-228-5595
701 Centre Avenue, Fort Collins, CO 80526   **970-212-4500**
FDA Number: 1646353
E-mail: zilapro@zila.com
Web site: www.zila.com
Ownership: Private
Stock Symbol: ZILA
Traded On: NASDAQ
Produces/Sells CE-marked Devices: N
Distribution: Manufacturer Through Manufacturer Reps
General Admin.: David R. Bethune/Chief Executive Officer, Chairman
Finance: Diane E. Klein/Vice President Finance, Treasurer

Agent, Polishing, Abrasive, Oral Cavity	Dental And Oral
Light, Dental	Dental And Oral
Source, Chemiluminescent Light	Obstetrics/Gynecology
Varnish	Dental And Oral

ZIMCOR CORPORATION   616-813-2699
6414 Skyridge Dr. Ne, Belmont, MI 49306
FDA Number: 1836412
Ownership: Private
Produces/Sells CE-marked Devices: N

Blade, Scalpel	Surgery

ZIMMER DENTAL, INC.   800-854-7019
1900 Aston Ave., Carlsbad, CA 92008   **760-929-4300**
FDA Number: 2023141   *Fax:* 760-431-7811
Web site: www.zimmerdental.com
Medical Products Sales Volume: $221,000,000
Annual Revenue: $100-$500 Million
Year Founded: 1927
Total Employees: 410   *Marketing Staff:* 30   *Sales Staff:* 70
Ownership: Zimmer Holdings, Inc.
Stock Symbol: ZMH

ZIMMER DENTAL, INC.   800-854-7019 *(cont'd)*
Traded On: NYSE
Quality System Registration Information: ISO9001
Produces/Sells CE-marked Devices: Y
Distribution: Manufacturer Direct, Manufacturer Through Distributor, Manufacturer Through Manufacturer Reps, Exclusive Distributor
General Admin.: Mr. Harold Flynn/President
    Debbie Miller/Vice President Human Resources
Mktg./Adv.: Mary Davis/Manager Advertising & Communications
    Jennifer Laird/Manager Customer Support
    Michel Madeira/Manager National Sales
    Russell J. Bonafede/Vice President Marketing
    Mr. Michel Madeira/Vice President Sales
Production: Mr. Steve Albright/Director Operations
    Kerry Foote/Director Regulatory Affairs
    Jeff Monroe/Manager Quality Assurance
Research: Mr. Michael Collins/Vice President Research & Development
Finance: Mr. Quentin Blackford/Director Finance
    Chris Kelford/Vice President, Controller

Agent, Hemostatic, Absorbable, Collagen-Based	Surgery
Allograft, Processed	Surgery
Cement, Hydroxyapatite	Surgery
Component, Ceramic	General
Graft, Bone	Orthopedics
Implant, Endosseous	Dental And Oral
Instrument, Dental, Manual	Dental And Oral

ZIMMER HOLDINGS, INC.   800-613-6131
1800 W. Center St., PO Box 708,   **574-267-6131**
Warsaw, IN 46581
FDA Number: 1822565
Web site: www.zimmer.com
Medical Products Sales Volume: $3,898,000,000
Annual Revenue: More than $1 Billion
Year Founded: 1927
Total Employees: 7600
Ownership: Public
Stock Symbol: ZMH
Traded On: NYSE
Quality System Registration Information: ISO9001
Produces/Sells CE-marked Devices: Y
General Admin.: Mr. James T Crines/Chief Financial Officer, Executive Vice President
    Dr. Cheryl Blanchard/Chief Scientific Officer
    Mr. David C. Dvorak/President, Chief Executive Officer
    Mr. Chad F. Phipps/Senior Vice President, General Counsel, Secretary
Finance: Mr. Derek Davis/Vice President Finance, Controller

Accessories, Traction	Physical Med
Accessories, Traction (Cart, Frame, Cord, Weight)	Orthopedics
Applicator, Clip (Forceps)	General
Applier, Cerclage	Orthopedics
Applier, Surgical Staple	Surgery
Applier, Surgical, Clip	Surgery
Aspirator, Wound Suction Pump	General
Autotransfusion Unit (Blood)	Anesthesiology
Awl	Orthopedics
Bandage, Elastic	General
Bars, Spreader	Orthopedics
Bed Cradle	General
Belt, Abdominal	Gastroenterology/Urology
Belt, Lumbosacral	Orthopedics
Belt, Rib (Support)	Orthopedics
Belt, Traction, Pelvic, Orthopedic	Orthopedics
Bender	Orthopedics
Binder, Abdominal	General
Bit, Drill	Orthopedics
Board, Foot	Orthopedics
Bolt, Nut, Washer	Orthopedics
Brace, Drill	Orthopedics
Brace, Joint, Ankle (External)	Physical Med
Broach	Orthopedics
Caliper, Orthopedic	Orthopedics
Cannula, Other	General
Carrier, Ligature	Surgery
Cart, Orthopedic Supply (Cast)	Orthopedics
Cart, Traction	Orthopedics
Cast Walking Heel	Orthopedics
Cement, Orthopedic (Bone)	Orthopedics
Cerclage, Fixation	Orthopedics
Chisel, Bone, Surgical	Dental And Oral
Chisel, Orthopedic	Orthopedics
Chisel, Surgical, Manual	Surgery
Clamp, Bone	Orthopedics
Clip, Scalp	Cns/Neurology
Collar, Cervical Neck	Orthopedics
Component, Traction, Invasive	Orthopedics
Compression Instrument	Orthopedics
Controller, Foot, Handpiece And Cord	Dental And Oral

ZIMMER HOLDINGS, INC.   800-613-6131 *(cont'd)*

Corkscrew	Orthopedics
Countersink	Orthopedics
Crimper, Pin	Orthopedics
Curette	Orthopedics
Curette, Surgical	Surgery
Cutter, Orthopedic	Orthopedics
Cutter, Wire And Pin	Orthopedics
Dermatome	Surgery
Dissector, Surgical, General & Plastic Surgery	Surgery
Drain, T	Gastroenterology/Urology
Drainage Unit, Urinary	General
Dressing, Wound and Burn, Occlusive	Surgery
Drill, Cannulated	Orthopedics
Drill, Intramedullary	Cns/Neurology
Driver, Bone Staple	Orthopedics
Driver, Prosthesis	Orthopedics
Driver, Surgical, Pin	Surgery
Driver/Extractor, Bone Nail/Pin	Orthopedics
Driver/Extractor, Bone Plate	Orthopedics
Elevator, Neurosurgical	Cns/Neurology
Elevator, Orthopedic	Orthopedics
Elevator, Surgical, General & Plastic Surgery	Surgery
Evacuator, Fume	Chemistry
Evacuator, Vapor, Cement Monomer	Orthopedics
Exerciser, Finger, Powered	Physical Med
Exerciser, Leg And Ankle	Physical Med
Exerciser, Trapeze	Physical Med
Expander, Surgical, Skin Graft	Surgery
Extractor, Nail	Orthopedics
Fastener, Fixation, Non-Biodegradable, Soft Tissue	Orthopedics
Finger Cot	General
Forceps	Orthopedics
Forceps, Dressing	Surgery
Forceps, Hemostatic	Surgery
Forceps, Sponge	Surgery
Forceps, Tissue	Surgery
Forceps, Utility	Surgery
Forceps, Wire Holding	Orthopedics
Frame, Traction	Orthopedics
Gauge, Depth	Orthopedics
Goniometer, Orthopedic	Orthopedics
Gouge, Nasal	Ear/Nose/Throat
Gouge, Surgical, General & Plastic Surgery	Surgery
Guide	Orthopedics
Guide, Drill	Orthopedics
Guide, Gigli Saw	Orthopedics
Halter, Head, Traction, Orthopedic	Orthopedics
Handpiece (Brace), Drill	Cns/Neurology
Hemostat	Orthopedics
Holder, Gas Cylinder	Anesthesiology
Holder, Needle, Orthopedic	Orthopedics
Holder, Needle, Other	Surgery
Hollow Mill Set	Orthopedics
Hook, Other	Surgery
Hook, Skin	Surgery
Hook, Surgical, General & Plastic Surgery	Surgery
Immobilizer, Ankle	Orthopedics
Immobilizer, Arm	Orthopedics
Immobilizer, Elbow	Orthopedics
Immobilizer, Knee	Orthopedics
Immobilizer, Shoulder	Orthopedics
Immobilizer, Wrist/Hand	Orthopedics
Impactor	Orthopedics
Implant, Fixation Device, Condylar Plate	Orthopedics
Instrument, Bending (Contouring)	Orthopedics
Joint, Hip, External Brace	Physical Med
Joint, Knee, External Brace	Physical Med
Kit, Burn	General
Kit, Catheterization, Urinary	Gastroenterology/Urology
Kit, Incision And Drainage	Surgery
Kit, Irrigation, Wound	General
Kit, Suction, Airway (Tracheal)	Anesthesiology
Kit, Wound Drainage	General
Kit, Wound Drainage, Closed	Cns/Neurology
Knife, Orthopedic	Orthopedics
Knife, Plaster	Orthopedics
Mallet, Bone	Orthopedics
Mattress, Bed	General
Mesh, Orthopedic (Metallic)	Orthopedics
Mesh, Surgical (Steel Gauze)	Surgery
Mixing Equipment, Cement	Orthopedics
Nail, Fixation, Bone	Orthopedics
Orthosis, Cervical	Physical Med
Orthosis, Limb Brace	Physical Med
Orthosis, Lumbosacral	Physical Med
Orthosis, Other	Physical Med
Orthosis, Rib Fracture, Soft	Physical Med
Orthosis, Sacroiliac, Soft	Physical Med
Osteotome, Manual (Plastic Surgery)	Surgery
Packaging, Sterilization	General
Pad, Pressure, Foam (Elbow, Heel)	General

ZIMMER HOLDINGS, INC.   800-613-6131 *(cont'd)*

Pad, Pressure, Foam Convoluted	General
Passer	Orthopedics
Passer, Wire, Orthopedic	Orthopedics
Pin, Fixation, Smooth	Orthopedics
Pin, Fixation, Threaded	Orthopedics
Plate, Bone, Orthodontic	Dental And Oral
Plate, Fixation, Bone	Orthopedics
Pliers, Surgical	Orthopedics
Prosthesis Implantation Instrument, Orthopedic	Orthopedics
Prosthesis, Ankle, Semi-Constrained, Metal/Polymer	Orthopedics
Prosthesis, Bone Cerclage	Orthopedics
Prosthesis, Elbow, Constrained	Orthopedics
Prosthesis, Elbow, Non-Constrained, Unipolar	Orthopedics
Prosthesis, Elbow, Semi-Constrained	Orthopedics
Prosthesis, Femoral	Orthopedics
Prosthesis, Hip, Acetabular Mesh	Orthopedics
Prosthesis, Hip, Cement Restrictor	Orthopedics
Prosthesis, Hip, Femoral Component, Cemented, Metal	Orthopedics
Prosthesis, Hip, Hemi-, Acetabular, Metal	Orthopedics
Prosthesis, Hip, Hemi-, Femoral, Metal/Polymer	Orthopedics
Prosthesis, Hip, Semi-Constrained, Metal/Polymer	Orthopedics
Prosthesis, Joint, Other	Orthopedics
Prosthesis, Knee, Femorotibial, Constrained, Metal/Polymer	Orthopedics
Prosthesis, Knee, Femorotibial, Non-Constrained	Orthopedics
Prosthesis, Knee, Femorotibial, Semi-Constrained	Orthopedics
Prosthesis, Knee, Patellofemoral, Semi-Constrained	Orthopedics
Prosthesis, Knee, Patellofemorotibial, Semi-Constrained	Orthopedics
Prosthesis, Shoulder	Orthopedics
Prosthesis, Shoulder, Hemi-, Humeral	Orthopedics
Prosthesis, Tibial	Orthopedics
Prosthesis, Upper Femoral	Orthopedics
Protector, Finger	Orthopedics
Protector, Skin Pressure	General
Protractor	Orthopedics
Punch, Bone	Orthopedics
Punch, Femoral Neck	Orthopedics
Pusher, Socket	Orthopedics
Rack, Surgical Instrument	Surgery
Rasp, Bone	Orthopedics
Rasp, Other	Surgery
Raspatory	Surgery
Reamer	Orthopedics
Regulator, Pressure, Gas Cylinder	Anesthesiology
Restraint, Ankle/Foot	General
Restraint, Protective (Body)	General
Restraint, Vest	General
Restraint, Wheelchair	General
Restraint, Wrist/Hand	General
Retractor	Orthopedics
Retractor, Abdominal	Surgery
Retractor, Brain	Cns/Neurology
Retractor, Brain Decompression	Cns/Neurology
Retractor, Laminectomy	Surgery
Retractor, Manual	Cns/Neurology
Retractor, Other	Surgery
Retractor, Self-Retaining, Neurology	Cns/Neurology
Rod, Fixation, Intramedullary	Orthopedics
Saw, Bone Cutting	Orthopedics
Saw, Bone, Pneumatic	Orthopedics
Saw, Manual, And Accessories	Surgery
Scissors, Bandage/Gauze/Plaster	General
Scissors, Disposable	General
Scissors, General Dissecting	Surgery
Scissors, Iris	Ophthalmology
Scissors, Orthopedic	Orthopedics
Scissors, Tenotomy	Ophthalmology
Screw, Cranioplasty Plate	Cns/Neurology
Screw, Fixation, Bone	Orthopedics
Screwdriver	Orthopedics
Separator, Dural	Cns/Neurology
Sharpener, Knife	Surgery
Sheet, Burn	General
Shoe, Cast	Physical Med
Skid, Bone	Orthopedics
Sling, Arm	Physical Med
Sling, Arm, Overhead Supported	Physical Med
Sling, Knee	Orthopedics
Sling, Leg	Orthopedics
Slippers	General
Sock, Fracture	Orthopedics
Spatula, Brain	Cns/Neurology
Spatula, Surgical, General & Plastic Surgery	Surgery
Splint, Abduction, Congenital Hip Dislocation	Physical Med
Splint, Clavicle	Physical Med
Splint, Denis Brown	Physical Med
Splint, Hand, And Component	Physical Med
Splint, Molded, Aluminum	Orthopedics
Splint, Molded, Plastic	Orthopedics
Splint, Nasal	Ear/Nose/Throat
Splint, Padded Stays	Orthopedics
Splint, Traction	Orthopedics

2013 MEDICAL DEVICE REGISTER

ZIMMER HOLDINGS, INC.   800-613-6131 (cont'd)

Spreader, Other	Surgery
Spreader, Plaster (Cast)	Orthopedics
Staple, Fixation, Bone	Orthopedics
Stocking, Support (Anti-Embolic)	General
Strap, Clavicle	Orthopedics
Stripper, Surgical	Orthopedics
Stripper, Tendon	Surgery
Support, Abdominal	Physical Med
Support, Ankle	Orthopedics
Support, Arm	Physical Med
Support, Back	Orthopedics
Support, Clavicle	Orthopedics
Support, Elbow	Orthopedics
Support, Foot	Orthopedics
Support, Hand	Orthopedics
Support, Knee	Physical Med
Support, Leg	Physical Med
Support, Patient Position, Radiographic	Radiology
Support, Wrist	Physical Med
Suture, Laparoscopy	Surgery
Suture, Non-Absorbable, Steel, Monofilament & Multifilament	Surgery
Tamp	Orthopedics
Tap, Bone	Orthopedics
Tape, Measuring, Ruler And Caliper	Surgery
Template	Orthopedics
Template, Femoral Angle Cutting	Orthopedics
Tongs, Skull	Cns/Neurology
Tongs, Skull, Traction	Cns/Neurology
Tourniquet	General
Tourniquet, Air Pressure	Orthopedics
Tourniquet, Automatic Rotating	Cardiovascular
Tourniquet, Pneumatic	Surgery
Traction Unit, Static, Bed	Orthopedics
Traction Unit, Static, Chair	Orthopedics
Tray, Surgical Instrument	Surgery
Trephine, Bone	Orthopedics
Tube, Drainage	Gastroenterology/Urology
Twister, Wire	Orthopedics
Wire, Fixation, Intraosseous	Dental And Oral
Wire, Ligature	Surgery
Wrap, Sterilization	General
Wrench	Orthopedics

Medical Product Subsidiaries (Listed Separately)
Zimmer Dental, Inc.
Zimmer Manufacturing B.V.
Zimmer Orthopaedic Surgical Products
Zimmer Spine
Zimmer Spine, Inc.
Zimmer Trabecular Metal Technology
Zimmer-Wilson-Phillips, Inc

ZIMMER MANUFACTURING B.V.   800-613-6131
Route 1, Km. 123.4, Bldg. 1, Turpeaux Industrial Park,
Mercedita, PR 00715
FDA Number: 2648920
Web site: www.zimmer.com
Ownership: Zimmer Holdings, Inc.
Stock Symbol: ZMH
Traded On: NYSE
Produces/Sells CE-marked Devices: N

Fixation Appliance, Multiple Component	Orthopedics
Implant, Fixation Device, Proximal Femoral	Orthopedics
Implant, Fixation Device, Spinal	Orthopedics
Nail, Fixation, Bone	Orthopedics
Plate, Fixation, Bone	Orthopedics
Plate, Fixation, Bone, Non-Spinal, Metallic	Orthopedics
Prosthesis, Hip, Acetabular Mesh	Orthopedics
Prosthesis, Hip, Femoral Component, Cemented, Metal	Orthopedics
Prosthesis, Hip, Hemi-, Femoral, Metal/Polymer	Orthopedics
Prosthesis, Hip, Semi-Const., Metal/Poly., Porous Uncemented	Orthopedics
Prosthesis, Hip, Semi-Constrained, Metal/Polymer	Orthopedics
Prosthesis, Hip, Semi-Constrained, Metal/Polymer, Uncemented	Orthopedics
Prosthesis, Knee, Femorotibial, Semi-Constrained	Orthopedics
Prosthesis, Knee, Patellofemorotibial, Semi-Constrained	Orthopedics
Rod, Fixation, Intramedullary	Orthopedics
Rod, Fixation, Intramedullary And Accessories, Metallic And Non-collapsible Orthopedics	
Screw, Fixation, Bone	Orthopedics
Screw, Fixation, Bone, Non-Spinal, Metallic	Orthopedics
Template	Orthopedics
Tray, Surgical Instrument	Surgery

ZIMMER MEDIZINSYSTEMS   800-327-3576
25 Mauchly Ste. 300, Irvine, CA 92618   **949-727-3356**
FDA Number: n/a   *Fax:* 949-727-2154
E-mail: info@zimmerusa.com
Web site: www.zimmerusa.com
Medical Products Sales Volume: $750,000
Annual Revenue: $1-$5 Million

ZIMMER MEDIZINSYSTEMS   800-327-3576 (cont'd)
Total Employees: 17   *Sales Staff:* 12
Ownership: Zimmer Elektromedizin Gmbh
Quality System Registration Information: ISO9001
Produces/Sells CE-marked Devices: N
Distribution: Manufacturer Direct
General Admin.: Sarah Soltani/General Manager
      Armin Zimmer/President, Chief Executive Officer

Analgesia Unit, Cryogenic	General
Diathermy, Shortwave	Physical Med
Diathermy, Ultrasonic (Physical Therapy)	Physical Med
Electrode, Cutaneous	Cns/Neurology
Electrode, Neuromuscular Stimulator	Cns/Neurology
Electrode, Other	General
Electrode, TENS	Cns/Neurology
Electrotherapeutic Unit	General
Equipment, Cryotherapy	Physical Med
Laser, Surgical	Surgery
Pack, Hot Or Cold, Reusable	Physical Med
Stimulator, Nerve, Transcutaneous (Pain Relief, TENS)	Cns/Neurology
Stimulator, Ultrasound, Muscle	Physical Med

ZIMMER ORTHOPAEDIC SURGICAL PRODUCTS   800-321-5533
P.O. Box 10, 200 West Ohio Ave.,   **330-343-8801**
Dover, OH 44622
FDA Number: 1526350   *Fax:* 330-343-0995
Web site: www.zimmer.com
Medical Products Sales Volume: $22,800,000
Year Founded: 1951
Total Employees: 100   *Marketing Staff:* 8   *Sales Staff:* 500
Ownership: Zimmer Holdings, Inc.
Stock Symbol: ZMH
Traded On: NYSE
Quality System Registration Information: ISO9001
Produces/Sells CE-marked Devices: Y
Federal Procurement Eligibility: Small Business
Distribution: Manufacturer Through Distributor, Exclusive Distributor
General Admin.: Robin Waltz/Manager Human Resources
Mktg./Adv.: Ian Dawson/Director Marketing
      Gene Rugh/Director Marketing Services
Production: Tim Donaldson/Director Engineering
      Michael Donovan/Director Manufacturing
      Ken Coonce/Vice President Operations

Aspirator, Wound Suction Pump	General
Autotransfusion Unit (Blood)	Anesthesiology
Bandage, Elastic	General
Bars, Spreader	Orthopedics
Belt, Lumbosacral	Orthopedics
Belt, Rib (Support)	Orthopedics
Belt, Support, Pelvic	Physical Med
Belt, Traction, Pelvic, Orthopedic	Orthopedics
Binder, Ankle	Orthopedics
Binder, Wrist	Orthopedics
Cart, Traction	Orthopedics
Cast	Orthopedics
Clip, Other	Surgery
Collar, Cervical Neck	Orthopedics
Cutter, Cast	Orthopedics
Cutter, Skin Graft	Surgery
Cutter, Skin Graft, Expanded Mesh	Surgery
Dermatome	Surgery
Dispenser, Cement	Orthopedics
Expander, Surgical, Skin Graft	Surgery
Frame, Traction	Orthopedics
Halter, Head, Traction, Orthopedic	Orthopedics
Immobilizer, Arm	Orthopedics
Immobilizer, Cervical	Orthopedics
Immobilizer, Elbow	Orthopedics
Immobilizer, Knee	Orthopedics
Immobilizer, Shoulder	Orthopedics
Immobilizer, Wrist/Hand	Orthopedics
Kit, Wound Drainage	General
Kit, Wound Drainage, Closed	Cns/Neurology
Pack, Hot Or Cold, Reusable	Physical Med
Pad, Pressure, Foam (Elbow, Heel)	General
Pad, Pressure, Foam Convoluted	General
Pillow, Cervical	Orthopedics
Sheet, Burn	General
Shoe, Cast	Physical Med
Sling, Arm	Physical Med
Sling, Knee	Orthopedics
Sling, Leg	Orthopedics
Splint, Hand, And Component	Physical Med
Splint, Molded, Aluminum	Orthopedics
Splint, Molded, Plastic	Orthopedics
Splint, Other	Orthopedics
Splint, Padded Stays	Orthopedics
Splint, Traction	Orthopedics
Spreader, Plaster (Cast)	Orthopedics
Stockinette, Cast	Orthopedics

ZIMMER ORTHOPAEDIC SURGICAL PRODUCTS 800-321-5533
(cont'd)

Suction Apparatus, Single Patient, Portable, Non-Powered	Surgery
Support, Back	Orthopedics
Support, Knee	Physical Med
Support, Leg	Physical Med
Tourniquet, Pneumatic	Surgery
Traction Unit, Static, Other	Orthopedics
Tube, Drainage	Gastroenterology/Urology
Tubing, Silicone	General

ZIMMER ORTHOPAEDIC SURGICAL PRODUCTS 704-873-1001
P.O. Box 1838, 2021 Old Mountain Rd., Statesville, NC 28687
FDA Number: 1035617   *Fax:* 704-873-1084
Web site: www.zimmer.com
Ownership: Zimmer Holdings, Inc.
Stock Symbol: ZMH
Traded On: NYSE
Produces/Sells CE-marked Devices: N

Accessories, Operating Room, Table	Surgery
Accessories, Traction	Physical Med
Bandage, Cast	Physical Med
Bandage, Elastic	General
Belt, Traction, Pelvic	Physical Med
Brace, Joint, Ankle (External)	Physical Med
Glove, Surgical	General
Halter, Head, Traction	Physical Med
Joint, Knee, External Brace	Physical Med
Orthosis, Abdominal	Physical Med
Orthosis, Cervical	Physical Med
Orthosis, Limb Brace	Physical Med
Orthosis, Lumbosacral	Physical Med
Orthosis, Sacroiliac, Soft	Physical Med
Pack, Hot Or Cold, Disposable	Physical Med
Protector, Skin Pressure	General
Sheet, Burn	General
Shoe, Cast	Physical Med
Sling, Arm	Physical Med
Splint, Abduction, Congenital Hip Dislocation	Physical Med
Splint, Clavicle	Physical Med
Splint, Extremity, Non-Inflatable, External	Surgery
Splint, Traction	Orthopedics
Stocking, Anti-Embolic, Pneumatic	Cardiovascular
Support, Arm	Physical Med
Support, Patient Position	Anesthesiology
Tourniquet, Pneumatic	Surgery

ZIMMER SPINE 508-643-0983
23 West Bacon St., North Attleboro, MA 02762
FDA Number: 1057469   *Fax:* 508-695-2501
Web site: www.zimmer.com
Total Employees: 31   *Marketing Staff:* 3   *Sales Staff:* 7
Ownership: Zimmer Holdings, Inc.
Stock Symbol: ZMH
Traded On: NYSE
Quality System Registration Information: ISO9001
Produces/Sells CE-marked Devices: Y
Distribution: Manufacturer Through Distributor
General Admin.: Thomas W. Davison/President, Chief Executive Officer
Mktg./Adv.: David Bohrer/Director Marketing
　　　　John T. Sexton/Manager National Sales
　　　　Patricia A. Tecu/Vice President Marketing & Sales
Production: Mark Bliss/Director Quality Assurance
Research: Gene P. DiPoto/Vice President Engineering

Arthroscope	Orthopedics
Endoscope, Neurological	Cns/Neurology
Equipment, Shaving, Disc, Spinal	Orthopedics
Forceps	Orthopedics

ZIMMER SPINE, INC. 800-655-2614
7375 Bush Lake Road,　952-832-5600
Minneapolis, MN 55439
FDA Number: 2184052   *Fax:* 952-832-5620
Web site: www.zimmer.com
Medical Products Sales Volume: $197,000,000
Annual Revenue: $100-$500 Million
Year Founded: 1991
Ownership: Zimmer Holdings, Inc.
Stock Symbol: ZMH
Traded On: NYSE
Produces/Sells CE-marked Devices: N

Appliance, Fixation, Spinal Interlaminal	Orthopedics
Appliance, Fixation, Spinal Intervertebral Body	Orthopedics
Arthroscope	Orthopedics
Awl	Orthopedics
Blade, Surgical, Saw, General & Plastic Surgery	Surgery
Cannula, Surgical, General & Plastic Surgery	Surgery
Chisel, Surgical, Manual	Surgery
Clamp, Surgical, General & Plastic Surgery	Surgery
Compression Instrument	Orthopedics

ZIMMER SPINE, INC. 800-655-2614 *(cont'd)*

Curette	Orthopedics
Cutter, Orthopedic	Orthopedics
Cutter, Surgical	Surgery
Elevator, Orthopedic	Orthopedics
Extractor, Nail	Orthopedics
Gauge, Depth	Orthopedics
Guide, Surgical, Instrument	Surgery
Hammer, Surgical	Surgery
Impactor	Orthopedics
Instrument, Bending (Contouring)	Orthopedics
Orthopedic Manual Surgical Instrument	Orthopedics
Orthosis, Fixation, Cervical Intervertebral Body, Spinal	Orthopedics
Orthosis, Fixation, Pedicle, Spinal	Orthopedics
Orthosis, Fixation, Spinal, Spondylolisthesis	Orthopedics
Orthosis, Fusion, Intervertebral, Spinal	Orthopedics
Orthosis, Spinal Pedicle Fixation, For Degenerative Disc Disease	Orthopedics
Probe	Orthopedics
Rasp, Bone	Orthopedics
Reamer	Orthopedics
Retractor, Surgical	Surgery
Rongeur, Rib	Orthopedics
Screwdriver	Orthopedics
Surgical Instrument, Orthopedic, AC-Powered Motor	Orthopedics
Tamp	Orthopedics
Tap, Bone	Orthopedics
Tape, Measuring, Ruler And Caliper	Surgery
Template	Orthopedics
Tray, Surgical Instrument	Surgery
Wrench	Orthopedics

ZIMMER TRABECULAR METAL TECHNOLOGY 800-613-6131
10 Pomeroy Road, Parsippany, NJ 07054
FDA Number: 3005751028
Web site: www.zimmer.com
Ownership: Zimmer Holdings, Inc.
Stock Symbol: ZMH
Traded On: NYSE
Produces/Sells CE-marked Devices: N

Awl	Orthopedics
Bit, Drill	Orthopedics
Brace, Drill	Orthopedics
Broach	Orthopedics
Caliper	Orthopedics
Compression Instrument	Orthopedics
Corkscrew	Orthopedics
Countersink	Orthopedics
Curette, Surgical	Surgery
Cutter, Orthopedic	Orthopedics
Cutter, Wire And Pin	Orthopedics
Device, Spinal Vertebral Body Replacement	Orthopedics
Driver, Prosthesis	Orthopedics
Dynamometer, Non-Powered	Orthopedics
Extractor, Nail	Orthopedics
Fastener, Fixation, Non-Biodegradable, Soft Tissue	Orthopedics
File	Orthopedics
Fork	Orthopedics
Gauge, Depth	Orthopedics
Guide, Surgical, Instrument	Surgery
Holder, Needle, Orthopedic	Orthopedics
Impactor	Orthopedics
Instrument, Bending (Contouring)	Orthopedics
Knife, Orthopedic	Orthopedics
Mesh, Metal	Gastroenterology/Urology
Mesh, Surgical (Steel Gauze)	Surgery
Obturator, Cement	Orthopedics
Orthopedic Manual Surgical Instrument	Orthopedics
Osteotome (Orthopedic)	Surgery
Osteotome, Manual (Plastic Surgery)	Surgery
Plate, Fixation, Bone	Orthopedics
Positioner, Socket	Orthopedics
Probe	Orthopedics
Prosthesis, Elbow, Hemi-, Radial, Polymer	Orthopedics
Prosthesis, Hip, Cement Restrictor	Orthopedics
Prosthesis, Hip, Hemi-, Femoral, Metal/Polymer	Orthopedics
Prosthesis, Hip, Semi-Const., Metal/Poly., Porous Uncemented	Orthopedics
Prosthesis, Hip, Semi-Const., Uncem., Non-P., M/P, Ca./Phos.	Orthopedics
Prosthesis, Hip, Semi-Constr., Metal/Ceramic, Cemented/NC	Orthopedics
Prosthesis, Hip, Semi-Constrained (Cemented Acetabular)	Orthopedics
Prosthesis, Hip, Semi-Constrained, Metal/Polymer	Orthopedics
Prosthesis, Hip, Semi-Constrained, Metal/Polymer, Uncemented	Orthopedics
Prosthesis, Knee, Femorotibial, Non-Constrained	Orthopedics
Prosthesis, Knee, Femorotibial, Semi-Constrained	Orthopedics
Prosthesis, Knee, Patellofemorotibial, Semi-Constrained	Orthopedics
Prosthesis, Knee, Patfem., S-C., Unc., Por., Ctd., P/M/P	Orthopedics
Prosthesis, Shoulder, Non-Constrained, Metal/Polymer Cem.	Orthopedics
Prosthesis, Shoulder, Semi-Constrained, Metal/Polymer Cem.	Orthopedics
Protractor	Orthopedics
Punch, Femoral Neck	Orthopedics
Pusher, Socket	Orthopedics
Rasp, Bone	Orthopedics
Reamer	Orthopedics

ZIMMER TRABECULAR METAL TECHNOLOGY
800-613-6131
(cont'd)

Retractor, Surgical	Surgery
Rongeur, Rib	Orthopedics
Screw, Fixation, Bone	Orthopedics
Screwdriver	Orthopedics
Starter, Bone Screw	Orthopedics
Surgical Instrument, Orthopedic, AC-Powered Motor	Orthopedics
Tamp	Orthopedics
Template	Orthopedics
Tray, Surgical Instrument	Surgery
Wrench	Orthopedics

ZIMMER-WILSON-PHILLIPS, INC
800-444-4547
214-774-0501
3301 Matrix Drive, Suite 200,
Richardson, TX 75082
FDA Number: 1645485
Fax: 214-774-0511
E-mail: zwilsonphillips.dallas@zimmer.com
Web site: www.zimmer-wilsonphillips.com
Ownership: Zimmer Holdings, Inc.
Stock Symbol: ZMH
Traded On: NYSE
Produces/Sells CE-marked Devices: N
General Admin.: Cheryl Felderhoff/Director Admin.
Rosemary Holt/Director Human Resources
Mr. Mark Phillips/President
Production: Mr. Sam Lunsford/Director Operations
Mr. James Howard/Vice President Operations

ZINETICS MEDICAL, INC.
800-648-4070
801-350-8131
1050 East South Temple,
Salt Lake City, UT 84102
FDA Number: 1721332
Fax: 801-284-8282
E-mail: info@medtronic.com
Web site: www.medtronic.com
Medical Products Sales Volume: $24,900,000
Annual Revenue: $1-$5 Million
Year Founded: 1976
Total Employees: 49   *Marketing Staff:* 2   *Sales Staff:* 3
Ownership: Private
Produces/Sells CE-marked Devices: N
Federal Procurement Eligibility: Small Business
Distribution: Manufacturer Through Manufacturer Reps, OEM
General Admin.: Steve L. Davis/President
Mktg./Adv.: Vince Poulsen/Manager Sales
Production: Margarita Angelo/Director Operations
Richard Vincine/Manager Regulatory Affairs
Research: Milan Heath/Vice President Research & Development

Bag, Enteral Feeding	General
Catheter, Other	Gastroenterology/Urology
Electrode, pH	Gastroenterology/Urology
Monitor, pH	Anesthesiology
Probe	Orthopedics
Tube, Feeding	General

ZIRA INTERNATIONAL INC
See Wells Johnson Co.

ZIRC COMPANY
800-328-3899
763-682-6636
3918 Hwy. 55 S.E., Buffalo, MN 55313
FDA Number: 2126387
Fax: 763-682-6604
E-mail: zirc@zirc.com
Web site: www.zirc.com
Medical Products Sales Volume: $2,200,000
Annual Revenue: $1-$5 Million
Year Founded: 1967
Total Employees: 40   *Marketing Staff:* 1   *Sales Staff:* 18
Ownership: Private
Quality System Registration Information: ISO9001
Produces/Sells CE-marked Devices: Y
Federal Procurement Eligibility: Small Business
Distribution: Manufacturer Through Distributor, OEM, Exclusive Distributor, Exporter
General Admin.: Linda Robasse/General Manager
Jim Campion/President, Chief Executive Officer
Mktg./Adv.: Linda Robasse/Manager Business
Nicolle Folven/Manager Marketing & Sales
James Ortmann/Manager National Sales

Contract Manufacturing, Product, Disposable	General
Dam, Rubber	Dental And Oral
Mirror, Mouth	Dental And Oral
Service, Modification, Product	General
Sterilizer/Compactor	General
Tray, Surgical	Surgery

ZIRC DENTAL PRODUCTS, INC.
See Zirc Company

ZIVIC LABORATORIES
800-422-5227
724-452-5200
178 Toll Gate School Road,
Zelienople, PA 16063
FDA Number: n/a
Fax: 724-452-4506
E-mail: inquiry@zivic.com
Web site: www.zivic.com
Medical Products Sales Volume: $2,000,000
Annual Revenue: $1-$5 Million
Total Employees: 40   *Marketing Staff:* 2   *Sales Staff:* 2
Ownership: Private
Federal Procurement Eligibility: Small Business
Distribution: Manufacturer Direct
General Admin.: Barb Zivic/General Manager
William J. Zivic/President
Mktg./Adv.: Andrea Keller/Manager Contract Sales
Andrea Keller/Manager International & National Sales
Brett Zivic/Sales Associate
Production: George Fritz/Manager Production
Research: Noah Muha/Research & Development Associate

Animal, Laboratory	Microbiology
Knife, Other	Surgery

ZIVIC-MILLER LABORATORIES, INC.
See Zivic Laboratories

ZLB BEHRING L.L.C.
See Csl Behring

ZMI CORP.
See Zoll Medical Corp.

ZOE MEDICAL, INC.
978-887-1410
460 Boston St., Topsfield, MA 01983
FDA Number: 3003294644

Monitor, Blood Pressure, Indirect, Semi-Automatic	Cardiovascular
Monitor, Cardiac (Cardiotachometer & Rate Alarm)	Cardiovascular

ZOETEK MEDICAL SALES & SERVICE, INC.
800-388-6223
585-924-4730
668 Phillips Rd., Victor, NY 14564
FDA Number: n/a
Fax: 585-924-7564
E-mail: info@zoetekemdical.com
Web site: www.zoetekmedical.com
Annual Revenue: $0-$1 Million
Year Founded: 1983
Total Employees: 20   *Marketing Staff:* 2   *Sales Staff:* 4
Ownership: Private
Produces/Sells CE-marked Devices: N
Federal Procurement Eligibility: Small Business
Distribution: Manufacturer Direct, Service Direct, Exclusive Distributor
General Admin.: C.D. Miller/President
Mktg./Adv.: Ms. Jennifer Mousso/Coord. Marketing & Sales
Leah Friends/Vice President Business Development
IS: Mr. Blaise Midnight/Manager Tech. Support

Monitor, ECG, Ambulatory, Real-Time	Cardiovascular
Service, Maintenance/Repair	General
Sterilizer, Steam, Table Top	General
Wrap, Sterilization	General

ZOLL CIRCULATION
800-321-4277
408-541-2140
650 Almanor Ave., Sunnyvale, CA 94085
FDA Number: 3003793491
Fax: 408-541-1030
E-mail: info@zollcirculation.com
Web site: www.zollcirculation.com
Ownership: Zoll Medical Corp.
Stock Symbol: ZOLL
Traded On: NASDAQ
Produces/Sells CE-marked Devices: Y
Production: Mr. Mark Perkins/Director Quality Assurance & Regulatory Affairs

Compressor, Cardiac, External	Cardiovascular
Hypothermia System, Hyperthermia	Cardiovascular

ZOLL DENTAL
800-239-2904
847-647-1819
7450 N. Natchez Avenue, Niles, IL 60714
FDA Number: 1422507
Fax: 847-647-1549
E-mail: ken@zolldental.com
Web site: www.zolldental.com
Year Founded: 1990
Ownership: Private
Stock Symbol: ZOLL
Traded On: NASDAQ
Produces/Sells CE-marked Devices: Y

Burnisher, Operative, Dental	Dental And Oral
Burr, Dental	Dental And Oral
Carver, Wax, Dental	Dental And Oral
Clamp, Rubber Dam	Dental And Oral
Condenser, Amalgam And Foil, Operative	Dental And Oral
Cup, Prophylaxis	Dental And Oral
Curette, Endodontic	Dental And Oral
Curette, Operative	Dental And Oral
Driver, Band, Orthodontic	Dental And Oral

ZOLL DENTAL 800-239-2904 *(cont'd)*

Evacuator, Oral Cavity	Dental And Oral
Excavator, Dental, Operative	Dental And Oral
Explorer, Operative	Dental And Oral
File, Margin Finishing, Operative	Dental And Oral
File, Periodontic	Dental And Oral
Filling, Instrument Plastic, Dental	Dental And Oral
Forceps, Articulation Paper	Dental And Oral
Forceps, Dressing, Dental	Dental And Oral
Forceps, Rubber Dam Clamp	Dental And Oral
Forceps, Tooth Extractor, Surgical	Dental And Oral
Frame, Rubber Dam	Dental And Oral
Gauge, Depth, Instrument, Dental	Dental And Oral
Hand Instrument, Calculus Removal	Dental And Oral
Handle, Instrument, Dental	Dental And Oral
Hemostat	Orthopedics
Instrument, Diamond, Dental	Dental And Oral
Knife, Margin Finishing, Operative	Dental And Oral
Knife, Surgical	Dental And Oral
Mirror, Mouth	Dental And Oral
Pliers, Operative	Dental And Oral
Plugger, Root Canal, Endodontic	Dental And Oral
Probe, Periodontic	Dental And Oral
Pusher, Band, Orthodontic	Dental And Oral
Remover, Crown	Dental And Oral
Retractor, All Types	Dental And Oral
Scissors, Collar And Crown	Dental And Oral
Spreader, Pulp Canal Filling Material, Endodontic	Dental And Oral
Tray, Impression	Dental And Oral
Tucker, Ligature, Orthodontic	Dental And Oral

ZOLL LIFECOR CORPORATION 800-543-3267
121 Freeport Road, Pittsburgh, PA 15238 412-826-9300
FDA Number: 3002158293
E-mail: info@zoll.lifecor.com
Web site: www.zoll.lifecor.com
Ownership: Zoll Medical Corp.
Stock Symbol: ZOLL
Traded On: NASDAQ
Quality System Registration Information: ISO9001
Produces/Sells CE-marked Devices: Y

Wearable, Defibrillator, Automatic, External	Cardiovascular

ZOLL MEDICAL CORP. 800-348-9011
269 Mill Road, Chelmsford, MA 01824 978-421-9655
FDA Number: 1220908 *Fax:* 978-421-0025
E-mail: info@zoll.com
Web site: www.zoll.com
Medical Products Sales Volume: $248,900,000
Annual Revenue: $100-$500 Million
Year Founded: 1980
Total Employees: 225 *Marketing Staff:* 8 *Sales Staff:* 100
Ownership: Public
Stock Symbol: ZOLL
Traded On: NASDAQ
Quality System Registration Information: ISO9001
Produces/Sells CE-marked Devices: Y
Federal Procurement Eligibility: Small Business
Distribution: Manufacturer Direct, Manufacturer Through Distributor, Manufacturer Through Manufacturer Reps
General Admin.: Richard A. Packer/Chief Executive Officer, Chairman
　　　A.Ernest Whiton/Chief Financial Officer, Vice President
　　　Jonathan Rennert/President
　　　Mr. Alex Moghadam/Vice President International Operations
Mktg./Adv.: Mr. Ward Hamilton/Senior Vice President Marketing
Research: Dr. E. Jane Wilson/Vice President Research & Development

Accessories, Pump, Infusion	General
Computer, Blood Pressure	Cardiovascular
Defibrillator, Battery-Powered	Cardiovascular
Defibrillator, External, Automatic	Cardiovascular
Defibrillator, Line-Powered	Cardiovascular
Defibrillator/Monitor, Battery-Powered	Cardiovascular
Defibrillator/Monitor, Line-Powered	Cardiovascular
Display, Cathode-Ray Tube	Cardiovascular
Electrode, Other	General
Monitor, ECG	Cardiovascular
Oximeter, Pulse	General
Pacemaker, Cardiac, External Transcutaneous (Non-Invasive)	Cardiovascular
Pressure Infusor, IV Container	General

Medical Product Subsidiaries (Listed Separately)
Bio-Detek, Inc.
Zoll Circulation
Zoll Lifecor Corporation

ZONARE MEDICAL SYSTEMS, INC. 877-966-2731
420 North Bernardo Avenue, 650-230-2800
Mountain View, CA 94043
FDA Number: 3004189859
E-mail: info@zonare.com *Fax:* 650-230-2828

ZONARE MEDICAL SYSTEMS, INC. 877-966-2731 *(cont'd)*
Web site: www.zonare.com
Ownership: Private
Produces/Sells CE-marked Devices: N
General Admin.: Mr. Timothy Marcotte/Chief Financial Officer, Vice President
　　　Dr. Glen McLaughlin/Chief Technology Officer
　　　Mr. Jay Miller/President, Chief Executive Officer
　　　Mr. Douglas Tefft/Vice President International Affairs
Mktg./Adv.: Mr. Mark Miller/Vice President Marketing & Sales
Finance: Mr. Timothy Heher/Vice President Finance

Scanner, Ultrasonic (Pulsed Doppler)	Radiology
Scanner, Ultrasonic (Pulsed Echo)	Radiology
Transducer, Ultrasonic, Diagnostic	Radiology

ZONDA INC. 214-438-3706
17304 Preston Rd., Suite 800, Dallas, TX 75248
FDA Number: n/a *Fax:* 972-733-6817
E-mail: info@zondaincusa.com
Web site: www.zondaincusa.com
Year Founded: 1984
Ownership: Private
Produces/Sells CE-marked Devices: N
General Admin.: Vera Leonard/President, Chief Executive Officer
Production: Pavel Holik/Director Operations

ZOOM FOCUS EYEWEAR, LLC 800 900 3700
7065-2 Hayvenhurst Ave., 818-785-7773
Lake Balboa, CA 91406
FDA Number: 3006628072
E-mail: info@superfocus.com *Fax:* 818 785 7774
Web site: www.superfocus.com
Ownership: Private
Produces/Sells CE-marked Devices: N

Telescope, Spectacle, Low-Vision	Ophthalmology

ZOUNDS, INC. 480-813-8400
1910 South Stapley Drive, Suite 202, Mesa, AZ 85204
FDA Number: 3005724187
Ownership: Private
Produces/Sells CE-marked Devices: N

Hearing-Aid	Ear/Nose/Throat

ZOUNDS, INC. (888-596-8637)
4405 East Baseline Road, Suite 114, 480-258-6013
Phoenix, AZ 85042
FDA Number: 3005919227
E-mail: info@ZoundsHearing.com
Ownership: Private
Produces/Sells CE-marked Devices: N

Hearing Aid, Air Conduction, Transcutaneous System	Ear/Nose/Throat
Hearing-Aid	Ear/Nose/Throat

ZUTRON MEDICAL LLC 913-967-5943
2830 Roe Ln, Kansas City, KS 66103
FDA Number: 3005299806
Ownership: Private
Produces/Sells CE-marked Devices: N

Bulb, Inflation (Endoscope)	Gastroenterology/Urology
Endoscope	Gastroenterology/Urology

ZYGA TECHNOLOGY INC. 612-455-1061
700 10th Avenue South, Suite 400, MINNEAPOLIS, MN 55415
FDA Number: n/a
Web site: http://www.zygatech.com
Ownership: Private
Produces/Sells CE-marked Devices: N

ZYGO INDUSTRIES, INC. 800-234-6006
7409 SW Tech Center Drive, Suite 125, 503-684-6006
Tigard, OR 97223
FDA Number: 3022509 *Fax:* 503-684-6011
E-mail: zygo@zygo-usa.com
Web site: www.zygo-usa.com
Annual Revenue: $1-$5 Million
Year Founded: 1974
Ownership: Private
Produces/Sells CE-marked Devices: Y
Federal Procurement Eligibility: Small Business
Distribution: Manufacturer Direct, Manufacturer Through Distributor, Manufacturer Through Manufacturer Reps, OEM, Exclusive Distributor, Importer, Exporter

Communication System, Powered	Physical Med
Page Turner (Handicapped)	General

ZYLOWARE CORPORATION 800-765-3700
11-36 46th Road, 718-392-3900
Long Island City, NY 11101
FDA Number: 2428194 *Fax:* 718-392-3955
E-mail: info@zyloware.com

ZYLOWARE CORPORATION
800-765-3700 (cont'd)
Web site: www.zyloware.com
Medical Products Sales Volume: $4,400,000
Year Founded: 1923
Total Employees: 65   Marketing Staff: 3   Sales Staff: 14
Ownership: Private
Produces/Sells CE-marked Devices: Y
Federal Procurement Eligibility: Small Business
Distribution: Manufacturer Direct, Manufacturer Through Distributor, Importer, Exporter
General Admin.: Chris Shyer/President
          Henry Shyer/Vice Chairman
Mktg./Adv.: James Shyer/Executive Vice President Sales
          Yvonne Greico/Manager Contract Sales
          Jodie Hirsch/Manager Marketing
Production: Yvonne Greico/Manager Production
Finance: Martin Weiss/Controller
  Contract Manufacturing   General
  Frame, Spectacle (Eyeglasses)   Ophthalmology
  Sunglasses (Including Photosensitive)   Ophthalmology

ZYMARK CORPORATION
508-435-9500
68 Elm Street, Hopkinton, MA 01748
FDA Number: 7000398   Fax: 508-435-3439
E-mail: solutions@zymark.com
Web site: www.zymark.com
Medical Products Sales Volume: $107,900,000
Annual Revenue: $25-$50 Million
Year Founded: 1995
Total Employees: 200   Marketing Staff: 10   Sales Staff: 20
Ownership: BERWIND GROUP
Stock Symbol: CALP
Traded On: NASDAQ
Quality System Registration Information: ISO9001
Distribution: Manufacturer Direct, Manufacturer Through Manufacturer Reps, OEM, Exporter
General Admin.: Kevin Hrusovsky/President, Chief Executive Officer
Mktg./Adv.: Sharon Correiz/Director Marketing
          Lynda Thomas/Manager Advertising
          John Jorgensen/Manager International & National Sales
          Bob Houser/Manager Training
          Guy Dechamps/Senior Vice President Marketing & Sales
Production: Jack Pinkerman/Manager Materials
          Bruce Bal/Vice President Manufacturing
Research: Rick Bernal/Vice President Research & Development
  Analyzer, Chemistry, ELISA   Chemistry
  Analyzer, Chemistry, Single Channel, Programmable   Chemistry
  Concentrator, Clinical Sample   Chemistry
  Diluter   Chemistry
  Pipetter   Hematology
  Pipetting And Diluting System, Automated   Chemistry
  Medical Product Subsidiaries (Listed Separately)
  Zymark Gmbh

ZYMOGENETICS
206-442-6600
1201 Eastlake Avenue E., Seattle, WA 98102
FDA Number: 3003928063   Fax: 206-442-6608
E-mail: info@zgi.com
Web site: www.zymogenetics.com
Medical Products Sales Volume: $25,400,000
Annual Revenue: $0-$1 Million
Year Founded: 1981
Total Employees: 275   Sales Staff: 1
Ownership: Novo Nordisk A/S
Stock Symbol: ZGEN
Traded On: NASDAQ
Produces/Sells CE-marked Devices: N
Federal Procurement Eligibility: Small Business
General Admin.: Randy Long/Director Human Resources
          Claus Kuhl/President, Chief Executive Officer
          Patrick O'Hara/Vice President
Medical Admin.: Jan Ohestrom/Vice President, Medical Director
Mktg./Adv.: Charlie Hart/Senior Director Business Development
Production: Lynn Rare/Director Regulatory Affairs
  Contract Manufacturing   General

ZYNEX INC.
800-495-6670
303-703-4906
9990 Park Meadows Drive,
Lone Tree, CO 80124
FDA Number: 1723686   Fax: 800-495-6695
E-mail: info@zynexmed.com
Web site: www.zynexmed.com
Year Founded: 1996
Ownership: Public
Stock Symbol: ZYXI
Traded On: OTC Bulletin
Produces/Sells CE-marked Devices: N

ZYNEX INC.
800-495-6670 (cont'd)
General Admin.: Thomas Sandgaard/President, Chief Executive Officer
Production: Mr. David Empey/Director Regulatory Affairs
Finance: Mr. Anthony Scalese/Chief Financial Officer
          Mr. Keith White/Vice President Reimbursement
  Biofeedback Device   Cns/Neurology
  Stimulator, Muscle, Electrical-Powered (EMS)   Physical Med
  Stimulator, Nerve, Transcutaneous (Pain Relief, TENS)   Cns/Neurology
  Unit, Therapy, Current, Interferential   Cns/Neurology

ZYNEX MEDICAL INC.
See Zynex Inc.

1ST AID FIRST
800-613-6770
1690 Lake Hill Rd., Deer Lodge, MT 59722
406-846-1367
FDA Number: n/a   Fax: 406-846-1384
E-mail: staff@1staidkit.com
Ownership: Private
Produces/Sells CE-marked Devices: N
Federal Procurement Eligibility: Small Business
Distribution: Manufacturer Direct
  Kit, First Aid   Surgery

210 INNOVATIONS, LLC
800-210-2298
210 Leonard Drive, Groton, CT 06340
860-445-0210
FDA Number: 3003672078   Fax: 860-445-9999
E-mail: info@safetmate.com
Web site: www.safetmate.com
Ownership: Private
Produces/Sells CE-marked Devices: N
  Component, Wheelchair   Physical Med
  Monitor, Bed Patient   General

21ST CENTURY SCIENTIFIC, INC.
800-448-3680
4931 N Manufacturing Way,
208-667-8800
Coeur D'Alene, ID 83815
FDA Number: 2027797   Fax: 208-667-6600
E-mail: 21st@wheelchairs.com
Web site: www.wheelchairs.com
Ownership: Private
Produces/Sells CE-marked Devices: N
Federal Procurement Eligibility: Small Business
Distribution: Manufacturer Through Distributor
Mktg./Adv.: Mr. R.D. Davidson/Associate Director Marketing
  Wheelchair, Powered   Physical Med

2D CARDIAC IMAGING, INC.
714-777-9900
4745 E. Wesley Drive, Anaheim,, CA 92807
FDA Number: n/a   Fax: 714-777-6699
E-mail: support@2dimaging.com
Web site: www.2dimaging.com
Medical Products Sales Volume: $1,100,000
Annual Revenue: $1-$5 Million
Total Employees: 8   Marketing Staff: 2   Sales Staff: 1
Ownership: Private
Produces/Sells CE-marked Devices: N
Federal Procurement Eligibility: Small Business
Distribution: Service Direct
General Admin.: Daniel A. Duval/President
  Equipment/Service, Quality Control   General

2D IMAGING, INC.
800-449-1332
4745 East Wesley Drive, Anaheim, CA 92807
714-777-9900
FDA Number: n/a   Fax: 714-777-6699
E-mail: support@2dimaging.com
Web site: www.2dimaging.com
Medical Products Sales Volume: $1,400,000
Year Founded: 1987
Total Employees: 4   Marketing Staff: 1   Sales Staff: 3
Ownership: Private
Produces/Sells CE-marked Devices: N
Federal Procurement Eligibility: Small Business
Distribution: Manufacturer Direct, Manufacturer Through Distributor, Manufacturer Through Manufacturer Reps
General Admin.: Duc Dang/President
  Service, Equipment Leasing   General
  Transducer, Ultrasonic   Cardiovascular

3C PACKAGING
919-553-4113
1000 CCC Dr., Clayton, NC 27520
FDA Number: n/a   Fax: 919-553-2581
E-mail: sales@3cpackaging.com
Web site: www.colonialcarton.com
Annual Revenue: $5-$10 Million
Total Employees: 82   Marketing Staff: 1   Sales Staff: 5
Ownership: Private
Produces/Sells CE-marked Devices: N
Federal Procurement Eligibility: Small Business

3C PACKAGING 919-553-4113 (cont'd)
Distribution: Manufacturer Direct, Exclusive Distributor
General Admin.: Joe Elphick/Chief Executive Officer
Mktg./Adv.: Fred Beaudet/Manager International & National Sales
Production: Gary Purcell/Director Quality Assurance
    Packaging Material   General

3COGNITION LLC 516-458-2905
1 Portico Ct., Apt. 302, Great Neck, NY 11021
FDA Number: 3005695971
Ownership: Private
Produces/Sells CE-marked Devices: N
    Accessory - Film Dosimetry System   Radiology

3D MEDICAL CONCEPTS, LLC 205-987-0935
1061 Morgan Park Rd., Pelham, AL 35124
FDA Number: 3004873730   *Fax:* 205-987-0936
E-mail: bev@3dmedicalconcepts.com
Web site: www.3dmedicalconcepts.com
Ownership: Private
Produces/Sells CE-marked Devices: N
General Admin.: Mr. Harry Lee/President, Chairman, Chief Executive Officer
Mktg./Adv.: Mr. Joshua Reardon/Director Marketing & Sales
    Gauze/sponge, Nonresorbable For External Use   Surgery
    Orthopedic Manual Surgical Instrument   Orthopedics

3D SYSTEMS CORPORATION 803-326-3900
333 Three D Systems Circle, Rock Hill, SC 29730
FDA Number: 1000263603
    System, Optical Impression, Computer Assisted Design And Manufacturing (cad/cam)
    Of Dental Restorations   Dental And Oral

3DISC AMERICAS INC. 800-570-0363
45921 Maries Road, Suite 190, Dulles, VA 20166
FDA Number: n/a   *Fax:* 703-430-8320
E-mail: info@3-disc.com
Web site: http://www.3-disc.com
Ownership: Private
Produces/Sells CE-marked Devices: N
General Admin.: Mr. Sung Woon Lee/Chief Executive Officer
    Mr. Jiin Jung/President

3DSHARP, INC. 412-648-9211
6425 Forward Ave., Pittsburgh, PA 15217
FDA Number: 3003639883
Ownership: Private
Produces/Sells CE-marked Devices: N
    Image Processing System   Radiology

3G ULTRASOUND, INC. 201-825-3116
200 Williams Dr., Ramsey, NJ 07446
FDA Number: 3003788308
Ownership: Private
Produces/Sells CE-marked Devices: N
    Scanner, Ultrasonic (Pulsed Echo)   Radiology

3GEN, LLC. 949-481-6384
31521 Rancho Viejo Rd., Suite 104,
San Juan Capistrano, CA 92675
FDA Number: 3003452144   *Fax:* 949-240-7492
E-mail: info@3genllc.com
Web site: www.dermlite.com
Year Founded: 1999
Ownership: Private
Produces/Sells CE-marked Devices: Y
Federal Procurement Eligibility: Small Business
Distribution: Manufacturer Direct, Manufacturer Through Distributor
    Light, Examination, Battery-Powered   General

3M ABERDEEN 605-229-5002
610 N. Brown County Rd. 19, Aberdeen, SD 57401
FDA Number: 1719330
Web site: www.3M.com
Year Founded: 1974
Total Employees: 600
Ownership: 3m Co.
Produces/Sells CE-marked Devices: N
General Admin.: Mr. Patrick D. Campbell/Chief Financial Officer, Senior Vice President
    Mr. Frederick J. Palensky/Chief Technology Officer, Executive Vice President
    Mr. George W. Buckley/President, Chief Executive Officer, Chairman
    Ms. Angela S. Lalor/Senior Vice President Human Resources
Mktg./Adv.: Mr. Robert D. MacDonald/Senior Vice President Marketing & Sales
    Bandage, Adhesive   Surgery
    Mask, Surgical   Surgery

3M CANADA COMPANY 800-364-3577 / 519-451-2500
1840 Oxford St. E.,
London, ONT N5V 3 Canada
FDA Number: 1000283504   *Fax:* 519-452-6597
E-mail: gjmandziuk@mmm.com
Web site: http://solutions.3m.com/wps/portal/3M/en_CA/WW/Country/
Year Founded: 1952
Total Employees: 100
Ownership: Public
Stock Symbol: MMM
Traded On: NYSE
Quality System Registration Information: ISO9000; ISO9002
Produces/Sells CE-marked Devices: N
Distribution: Manufacturer Through Distributor, Service Direct, Exclusive Distributor, Exporter

3M CO. 888-364-3577 / 612-733-1110
3M Center, St. Paul, MN 55144-1000
FDA Number: 2110898   *Fax:* 612-733-9973
E-mail: innovation@mmm.com
Web site: www.3m.com
Medical Products Sales Volume: $1,210,000,000
Annual Revenue: More than $1 Billion
Year Founded: 1902
Total Employees: 76239
Ownership: Public
Stock Symbol: MMM
Traded On: NYSE
Produces/Sells CE-marked Devices: N
Distribution: Manufacturer Direct
General Admin.: Mr. Patrick D. Campbell/Chief Financial Officer, Senior Vice President
    Mr. Frederick J. Palensky/Chief Technology Officer, Executive Vice President
    Mr. George W. Buckley/President, Chief Executive Officer, Chairman
    Ms. Angela S. Lalor/Senior Vice President Human Resources
Mktg./Adv.: Mr. Robert D. MacDonald/Senior Vice President Marketing & Sales
    Bag, Intestine   Surgery
    Bandage, Liquid   Surgery
    Cement, Dental   Dental And Oral
    Colostomy Appliance, Disposable   Gastroenterology/Urology
    Dressing, Wound and Burn, Hydrogel   Surgery
    Electrode, Electrocardiograph   Cardiovascular
    Electrosurgical Unit, Cutting & Coagulation Device   Surgery
    Indicator, Physical/chemical, Storage Temperature   General
    Kit, Intravenous Extension Tubing   General
    Mask, Surgical   Surgery
    Orthosis, Limb Brace   Physical Med
    Pump, Infusion   General
    Solvent, Adhesive Tape   Surgery
    Stethoscope, Electronic (Auscultoscope)   Cardiovascular
    Varnish, Cavity   Dental And Oral
Medical Product Subsidiaries (Listed Separately)
    3m Aberdeen
    3m Company
    3m Espe Dental Products
    3m Flemington
    3m Midwest Distribution Center
    3m Petaluma
    3m Unitek
    3m Valley
    Imtec, A 3m Company

3M CO.
See 3m Hutchinson

3M COMPANY
See 3m Petaluma

3M COMPANY 507-354-8271
1617 N. Front Street, New Ulm, MN 56073
FDA Number: 2183581   *Fax:* 507-359-0111
Web site: www.3M.com
Year Founded: 1962
Total Employees: 650
Ownership: 3m Co.
Stock Symbol: MMM
Traded On: NYSE
Produces/Sells CE-marked Devices: N
General Admin.: Mr. Patrick D. Campbell/Chief Financial Officer, Executive Vice President
    Mr. Frederick J. Palensky/Chief Technology Officer, Executive Vice President
    Mr. George W. Buckley/President, Chief Executive Officer, Chairman
    Ms. Angela S. Lalor/Senior Vice President Human Resources
Mktg./Adv.: Mr. Robert D. MacDonald/Senior Vice President Marketing & Sales
    Cabinet, Aerator, Ethylene-Oxide Gas   General

3M COMPANY   507-354-8271 *(cont'd)*
Cartridge, Ethylene-Oxide   General
Incubator/Water Bath   Chemistry
Sterilization Process Indicator, Biological   General

3M COMPANY
See 3m Co.

3M COMPANY   513-272-5000
5801 Mariemont Ave., Cincinnati, OH 45227
FDA Number: 1510709   *Fax:* 513-272-5072
E-mail: rtaylor@bdfusa.com
Year Founded: 1930
Total Employees: 180
Ownership: Beiersdorf, Inc.
Quality System Registration Information: ISO9001
Produces/Sells CE-marked Devices: Y
Distribution: Manufacturer Direct
Attachment, Commode, Wheelchair   Physical Med
Bandage, Adhesive   Surgery
Bandage, Elastic   General
Bath, Sitz, Non-Powered   Physical Med
Binder, Abdominal   General
Brace, Joint, Ankle (External)   Physical Med
Cane   Physical Med
Cotton, Roll   Dental And Oral
Crutch   Physical Med
Cushion, Wheelchair (Pad)   Physical Med
Garment, Protective, For Incontinence   Gastroenterology/Urology
Halter, Head, Traction, Orthopedic   Orthopedics
Joint, Knee, External Brace   Physical Med
Legging, Compression, Non-Inflatable   General
Orthosis, Cervical   Physical Med
Orthosis, Limb Brace   Physical Med
Orthosis, Rib Fracture, Soft   Physical Med
Orthosis, Sacroiliac, Soft   Physical Med
Orthosis, Truncal/Limb   Physical Med
Pack, Hot Or Cold, Disposable   Physical Med
Pack, Hot Or Cold, Reusable   Physical Med
Pad, Alcohol   General
Pad, Eye   Ophthalmology
Shield, Nipple   Obstetrics/Gynecology
Sling, Arm   Physical Med
Sling, Arm, Overhead Supported   Physical Med
Splint, Clavicle   Physical Med
Splint, Hand, And Component   Physical Med
Sponge, Gauze   Dental And Oral
Stocking, Elastic   General
Support, Arm   Physical Med
Support, Hernia   Gastroenterology/Urology
Support, Leg   Physical Med
Support, Scrotal, Therapeutic   General
Tips And Pads, Cane, Crutch And Walker   Physical Med
Traction Unit, Non-Powered   Orthopedics
Urinal   General
Walker, Mechanical   Physical Med

3M COMPANY   (605) 692-9433
601 22nd Ave. South, PO Box 5227, Brookings, SD 57006
FDA Number: 1717046   *Fax:* (605) 696-1337
Ownership: 3m Co.
Produces/Sells CE-marked Devices: N
Bandage, Adhesive   Surgery
Bandage, Elastic   General
Colostomy Appliance, Disposable   Gastroenterology/Urology
Drape, Surgical   Surgery
Dressing, Wound, Hydrophilic   Surgery
Dressing, Wound, Occlusive   Surgery
Fiber, Absorbent   General
Gel, Electrode, Stimulator   Cns/Neurology
Holder, Intravascular Catheter   General
Pack, Hot Or Cold, Reusable   Physical Med
Protector, Skin Pressure   General
Stethoscope, Manual   Cardiovascular

3M COMPANY   641-585-2700
806 W. Crystal Lake Rd, Forest City, IA 50436
FDA Number: 1933758   *Fax:* 641-585-5892
Web site: www.3M.com
Ownership: 3m Co.
Stock Symbol: MMM
Traded On: NYSE
Produces/Sells CE-marked Devices: N
General Admin.: Mr. Patrick D. Campbell/Chief Financial Officer, Senior Vice President
    Mr. Frederick J. Palensky/Chief Technology Officer, Executive Vice President
    Mr. George W. Buckley/President, Chief Executive Officer, Chairman
    Ms. Angela S. Lalor/Senior Vice President Human Resources

3M COMPANY   641-585-2700 *(cont'd)*
Mktg./Adv.: Mr. Robert D. MacDonald/Senior Vice President Marketing & Sales

3M DENTAL PRODUCTS
See 3m Espe Dental Products

3M EDUMEX, S.A. DE C.V.   651-733-4365
6620 Oriente, Calle Ramon Rivera Lara, Ciudad de Jaurez, CHIHU 32605 Mexico
FDA Number: 9680284
Ownership: Private
Produces/Sells CE-marked Devices: N

3M ESPE DENTAL PRODUCTS   949-863-1360
2111 McGaw Ave., Irvine, CA 92614
FDA Number: 2020493   *Fax:* 949-863-7023
Web site: www.3MESPE.com
Annual Revenue: $5-$10 Million
Total Employees: 400   *Marketing Staff:* 6   *Sales Staff:* 55
Ownership: 3m Co.
Stock Symbol: MMM
Traded On: NYSE
Quality System Registration Information: ISO9000; ISO9001
Produces/Sells CE-marked Devices: Y
Distribution: Manufacturer Direct, Manufacturer Through Distributor, Manufacturer Through Manufacturer Reps, OEM, Service Direct, Importer
General Admin.: Mr. Patrick D. Campbell/Chief Financial Officer, Senior Vice President
    Mr. Frederick J. Palensky/Chief Technology Officer, Executive Vice President
    C. Reich/Division Vice President
    W. G. Meredith/Executive Vice President
    Mr. George W. Buckley/President, Chief Executive Officer, Chairman
    Mr. Angela S. Lalor/Senior Vice President Human Resources
Mktg./Adv.: M. Perpich/Manager Marketing Communications
    Mr. Robert D. MacDonald/Senior Vice President Marketing & Sales
Production: J. P. Kouri/Director Manufacturing
Adhesive, Bracket And Conditioner, Resin   Dental And Oral
Adhesive, Dental   Dental And Oral
Crown And Bridge, Temporary, Resin   Dental And Oral
Crown, Preformed   Dental And Oral
Disk, Abrasive   Dental And Oral
Drill, Dental, Intraoral   Dental And Oral
Filling, Instrument Plastic, Dental   Dental And Oral
Film, X-Ray, Dental, Extraoral   Dental And Oral
Implant, Endosseous   Dental And Oral
Light, Other   General
Material, Dental Filling   Dental And Oral
Material, Impression   Dental And Oral
Material, Restoration, Aesthetic, External   Surgery
Material, Tooth Shade, Resin   Dental And Oral
Matrix, Dental   Dental And Oral
Resinous Compound   Dental And Oral
Screw, Fixation, Intraosseous   Dental And Oral
Sealant, Pit And Fissure, And Conditioner, Resin   Dental And Oral
Sterilization Process Indicator, Physical/Chemical   General
Strip, Polishing Agent   Dental And Oral
Teeth, Porcelain   Dental And Oral

3M ESPE DENTAL PRODUCTS   651-733-7767
2501 SE Otis Corley Drive, Bentonville, AR 72712
FDA Number: 2314911
Ownership: 3m Co.
Stock Symbol: MMM
Traded On: NYSE
Produces/Sells CE-marked Devices: N
Agent, Polishing, Abrasive, Oral Cavity   Dental And Oral
Cleaner, Denture, Mechanical   Dental And Oral
Cup, Prophylaxis   Dental And Oral
Floss, Dental   Dental And Oral
Varnish, Cavity   Dental And Oral

3M FLEMINGTON   908-788-4000
500 Route 202 North, Flemington, NJ 08822
FDA Number: 2222706
Year Founded: 1969
Total Employees: 130
Ownership: 3m Co.
Stock Symbol: MMM
Traded On: NYSE
Produces/Sells CE-marked Devices: N
General Admin.: Mr. Patrick D. Campbell/Chief Financial Officer, Senior Vice President
    Mr. Frederick J. Palensky/Chief Technology Officer, Executive Vice President
    Mr. George W. Buckley/President, Chief Executive Officer, Chairman
    Ms. Angela S. Lalor/Senior Vice President Human Resources

3M FLEMINGTON   908-788-4000 *(cont'd)*
Mktg./Adv.: Mr. Robert D. MacDonald/Senior Vice President Marketing & Sales

Instrument Guard	Surgery
Sterilization Process Indicator, Biological	General
Sterilization Process Indicator, Physical/Chemical	General
Thermometer, Chemical Color Change	General

3M HEALTH CARE CARDIOVASCULAR SYSTEMS
See Terumo Cardiovascular Systems, Corp

3M HEALTH INFORMATION SYSTEMS   800-367-2447
575 W. Murray Blvd., Murray, UT 84123-0900   **801-265-4400**
FDA Number: n/a   *Fax:* 801-263-3658
Web site: http://solutions.3m.com/wps/portal/3M/en_US/3M_Health_Inform
Annual Revenue: $0-$1 Million
Total Employees: 1000
Ownership: Public
Stock Symbol: MMM
Traded On: NYSE
Produces/Sells CE-marked Devices: N
Distribution: Manufacturer Direct, Manufacturer Through Manufacturer Reps
Mktg./Adv.: Cal Klein/Manager Business Development

Computer Software	General

3M HUTCHINSON   320-234-2000
915 Adams St. SE, Hutchinson, MN 55350-2927
FDA Number: 2122594
Web site: www.3m.com
Year Founded: 1947
Ownership: 3M
Stock Symbol: MMM
Traded On: NYSE
Produces/Sells CE-marked Devices: N
General Admin.: Mr. Patrick D. Campbell/Chief Financial Officer, Senior Vice President
    Mrs. Frederick J. Palensky/Chief Technology Officer, Executive Vice President
    Mr. George W. Buckley/President, Chief Executive Officer, Chairman
    Ms. Angela S. Lalor/Senior Vice President Human Resources
Mktg./Adv.: Mr. Robert D. MacDonald/Senior Vice President Marketing & Sales

Bandage, Adhesive	Surgery
Coverslip, Microscope Slide	Pathology

3M MIDWEST DISTRIBUTION CENTER   815-756-5087
3050 Corporate Dr, DeKalb, IL 60115-9299
FDA Number: 3003561612
Web site: www.3M.com   *Fax:* 815-754-2750
Ownership: 3m Co.
Stock Symbol: MMM
Traded On: NYSE
Produces/Sells CE-marked Devices: N
General Admin.: Mr. Patrick D. Campbell/Chief Financial Officer, Senior Vice President
    Mr. Frederick J. Palensky/Chief Technology Officer, Executive Vice President
    Mr. George W. Buckley/President, Chief Executive Officer, Chairman
    Ms. Angela S. Lalor/Senior Vice President Human Resources
Mktg./Adv.: Mr. Robert D. MacDonald/Senior Vice President Marketing & Sales

3M PETALUMA   707-765-3236
1331 Commerce St., Petaluma, CA 94954
FDA Number: n/a
Web site: www.3m.com
Year Founded: 1982
Ownership: 3m Co.
Stock Symbol: MMM
Traded On: NYSE
Produces/Sells CE-marked Devices: N
General Admin.: Mr. Patrick D. Campbell/Chief Financial Officer, Senior Vice President
    Mr. Frederick J. Palensky/Chief Technology Officer, Executive Vice President
    Mr. George W. Buckley/President, Chief Executive Officer, Chairman
    Ms. Angela S. Lalor/Senior Vice President Human Resources
Mktg./Adv.: Mr. Robert D. MacDonald/Senior Vice President Marketing & Sales

Prism, Fresnel, Ophthalmic	Ophthalmology

3M UNITEK   800-634-5300
2724 S. Peck Rd., Monrovia, CA 91016   **626-574-4000**
FDA Number: 2020467   *Fax:* 800-328-2360
Web site: www.3MUnitek.com
Annual Revenue: $10-$25 Million
Year Founded: 1948
Total Employees: 400
Ownership: 3m Co.

3M UNITEK   800-634-5300 *(cont'd)*
Stock Symbol: MMM
Traded On: NYSE
Quality System Registration Information: ISO9001
Produces/Sells CE-marked Devices: N
Distribution: Manufacturer Direct
General Admin.: Mr. Patrick D. Campbell/Chief Financial Officer, Senior Vice President
    Mr. Frederick J. Palensky/Chief Technology Officer, Executive Vice President
    Mr. George W. Buckley/President, Chief Executive Officer, Chairman
    Ms. Angela S. Lalor/Senior Vice President Human Resources
Mktg./Adv.: Mr. Robert D. MacDonald/Senior Vice President Marketing & Sales

Adhesive, Bracket And Conditioner, Resin	Dental And Oral
Adhesive, Dental	Dental And Oral
Aligner, Bracket, Orthodontic	Dental And Oral
Band, Elastic, Orthodontic	Dental And Oral
Band, Material, Orthodontic	Dental And Oral
Band, Preformed, Orthodontic	Dental And Oral
Bracket, Metal, Orthodontic	Dental And Oral
Chair, Operative	Dental And Oral
Clamp, Wire, Orthodontic	Dental And Oral
Component, Ceramic	General
Face Bow	Dental And Oral
Handpiece, Air-Powered, Dental	Dental And Oral
Handpiece, Contra- And Right-Angle Attachment, Dental	Dental And Oral
Handpiece, Direct Drive, AC-Powered	Dental And Oral
Headgear, Extraoral, Orthodontic	Dental And Oral
Instrument, Diamond, Dental	Dental And Oral
Light, Dental, Intraoral	Dental And Oral
Lock, Wire, And Ligature, Intraoral	Dental And Oral
Maintainer, Space Preformed, Orthodontic	Dental And Oral
Material, Impression	Dental And Oral
Material, Impression Tray, Resin	Dental And Oral
Material, Tooth Shade, Resin	Dental And Oral
Metal, Base	Dental And Oral
Orthodontic Instrument	Dental And Oral
Pin, Retentive And Splinting	Dental And Oral
Pusher, Band, Orthodontic	Dental And Oral
Retainer, Screw Expansion, Orthodontic	Dental And Oral
Retractor, All Types	Dental And Oral
Setter, Band, Orthodontic	Dental And Oral
Spring, Orthodontic	Dental And Oral
Syringe Unit, Air And/Or Water	Dental And Oral
Syringe, Restorative And Impression Material	Dental And Oral
Tray, Impression	Dental And Oral
Tube, Orthodontic	Dental And Oral
Tucker, Ligature, Orthodontic	Dental And Oral
Wire, Orthodontic	Dental And Oral

3M VALLEY   402-359-2131
600 E. Meigs Street, Valley, NE 68064
FDA Number: 1929938
Web site: www.3M.com
Year Founded: 1979
Total Employees: 420
Ownership: 3m Co.
Stock Symbol: MMM
Traded On: NYSE
Produces/Sells CE-marked Devices: N
General Admin.: Mr. Patrick D. Campbell/Chief Financial Officer, Senior Vice President
    Mr. Frederick J. Palensky/Chief Technology Officer, Executive Vice President
    Mr. George W. Buckley/President, Chief Executive Officer, Chairman
    Ms. Angela S. Lalor/Senior Vice President Human Resources
Mktg./Adv.: Mr. Robert D. MacDonald/Senior Vice President Marketing & Sales

Bandage, Adhesive	Surgery
Electrode, Electrocardiograph	Cardiovascular
Electrosurgical Unit, Cutting & Coagulation Device	Surgery
Mask, Surgical	Surgery

3S L.L.C.   866-437-2677
9315 Knightbridge Ct., Tampa, FL 33647   **866-437-2677**
FDA Number: n/a
Ownership: Private
Produces/Sells CE-marked Devices: N

Handpiece, Air-Powered, Dental	Dental And Oral

4-D NEUROIMAGING   858-453-6300
9727 Pacific Heights Blvd., San Diego, CA 92121
FDA Number: 2027486

Electroencephalograph	Cns/Neurology
Stimulator, Mechanical, Evoked Response	Cns/Neurology

4D MEDICAL SYSTEMS, INC. / ORTIZ   865-483-5145
1020 Commerce Park Dr., Suite B, Oak Ridge, TN 37830
FDA Number: 3007024536   *Fax:* (865) 483-5351

4D MEDICAL SYSTEMS, INC. / ORTIZ   **865-483-5145** *(cont'd)*
E-mail: info @ 4d-medical.com
Web site: www.4d-medical.com
Ownership: Private
Produces/Sells CE-marked Devices: N
  Camera, Still, Surgical   Surgery

5 STAR IMAGING, INC.   **727-376-0588**
11515 Prosperous Dr., Odessa, FL 33556
FDA Number: 3005097061
Ownership: Private
Produces/Sells CE-marked Devices: N
  Housing, X-Ray Tube, Diagnostic   Radiology

7N GABRIELA NAYDENOV;, INC.   **973-278-0866**
503 East 40th Street, Paterson, NJ 07504
FDA Number: 2249600
Ownership: Private
Produces/Sells CE-marked Devices: N
  Transmitter/Receiver System, Physiological, Telephone   Cardiovascular

883495 ONTARIO, INC.   **613-384-9550**
2-759 Progress Ave, Kingston K7M 6N6 Canada
FDA Number: 9615260
  Ventilator, Continuous (Respirator)   Anesthesiology

928735 ONTARIO, LTD.   **905-660-1030**
8-24 Viceroy Rd, Concord L4K 2L9 Canada
FDA Number: 9615245
  Cover, Mattress   General

SECTION II

GEOGRAPHICAL INDEX

PURPOSE OF THIS SECTION

Identifies manufacturers by geographic location.

FEATURES

◆ U.S. manufacturers and exclusive distributors from the preceding section are organized alphabetically by state, and then by city or municipality within the state.

◆ Canadian and Mexican manufacturers are listed alphabetically by company name at the end of the section.

Health Resources from Grey House Publishing

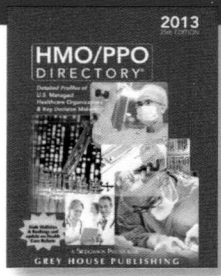

The HMO/PPO Directory

This comprehensive directory details more information about more managed health care organizations than ever before. Over 1,100 HMOs, PPOs and affiliated companies are listed, arranged alphabetically by state. Detailed listings include Key Contact Information, Drug Benefits, Enrollment, Geographical Areas served, Affiliated Physicians & Hospitals, Federal Qualifications, Status, Year Founded, Managed Care Partners, Employer References, Fees & Payment Information and more. *The HMO/PPO Directory* provides the most comprehensive information on the most companies available on the market place today.

600 pages; Softcover ISBN 978-1-59237-876-0, $325.00
Online & Directory Combo: $800.00
Online Database (Single User): $650.00

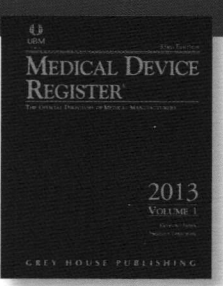

Medical Device Register

Offers fast access to over 13,000 companies - and more than 65,000 products. Volume I: Products, provides the essential information you need when purchasing or specifying medical supplies on every medical device, supply, and diagnostic available in the US. Listings provide FDA codes, Federal Procurement Eligibility, Contact information, Prices and Product Specifications. Volume 2: Suppliers, details the most complete and important data about Suppliers, Manufacturers and Distributors, with Key Executives, Contact Information along with their medical products and specialties. *Medical Device Register* is your only one-stop source for locating suppliers and products; looking for new manufacturers or hard-to-find medical devices; comparing products; know who's selling what and who to buy from cost effectively.

3,000 pages; Two Volumes; Softcover ISBN 978-1-59237-880-7, $350.00
Online Database & Print Combo, $699.00

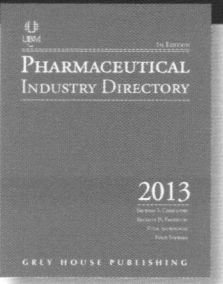

Pharmaceutical Industry Directory

This resource compiles critical information on the multi-billion dollar worldwide Pharmaceutical Industry. Coverage begins with company profiles of 5,000 Pharmaceutical Companies worldwide, with complete contact information, company description, key personnel, areas of clinical development, annual revenue, healthcare revenue, annual research and development expenditure, and number of employees. Each profile also includes a detailed list of the company's prescription drugs in development and brands on the market, over 20,000 in total. An excellent tool for research, portfolio evaluation, new business development, and competitive analyses. This new directory will be a must-have resource for professionals in the pharmaceutical and biotech industries along with public library, university and medical reference collections.

1,000 pages; Softcover ISBN 978-1-61925-174-8, $350.00
Online & Directory Combo: $950.00 | Online Database (Single User): $750.00

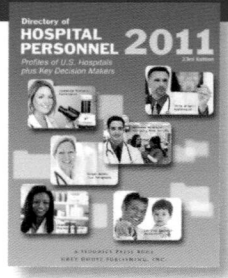

The Directory of Hospital Personnel

The Directory of Hospital Personnel is the best resource you can have at your fingertips when researching or marketing a product or service to the hospital market. A "Who's Who" of the hospital universe, this directory puts you in touch with over 150,000 key decision-makers. Every hospital in the U.S. is profiled, listed alphabetically by city within state. *The Directory of Hospital Personnel* is the only complete source for key hospital decision-makers by name. Whether you want to define or restructure sales territories... locate hospitals with the purchasing power to accept your proposals... or find information on which insurance plans are accepted, *The Directory of Hospital Personnel* gives you the information you need – easily, efficiently, effectively and accurately.

2,500 pages; Softcover ISBN 978-1-59237-856-2, $325.00
Online & Directory Combo: $800.00 | Online Database (Single User): $650.00

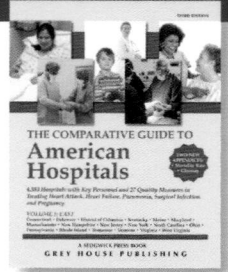

The Comparative Guide to American Hospitals

This new third edition compares and ranks all of the nation's hospitals by 49 measures of quality in the treatment of heart attack, heart failure, pneumonia, surgical procedures, pregnancy care and, new to this edition, children's asthma care, medical imaging and patient satisfaction. Each profile includes the raw percentage for that hospital, the state and US averages and data on the top hospital. Most importantly, The Comparative Guide to American Hospitals provides easy-to-use Regional State by State Statistical Summary Tables for each of the data elements to allow the user to quickly locate hospitals with the best level of service. Plus, a new 30-Day Mortality Chart, Glossary of Terms and Regional Hospital Profile Index make this a must-have source. This new, expanded edition will be a must for the reference collection at all public, medical and academic libraries.

2,000 pages; Four Volume Set; Softcover ISBN 978-1-59237-838-8, $350.00

(800) 562-2139 • www.greyhouse.com

GEOGRAPHICAL INDEX

ALABAMA

Alabaster
Avanti Polar Lipids, Inc. — 800-227-0651
700 Industrial Park Drive, Alabaster, AL 35007

Arab
Atrion Medical Products, Inc. — 800-343-9334
1426 Curt Francis Rd., Arab, AL 35016

Auburn
Capitol Vial — 334-887-8311
2039 Mcmillan Street, Auburn, AL 36832
Health Information Designs, Inc. — 334-502-3262
391 Industry Drive, Auburn, AL 36832

Axis
Lenzing Fibers Inc. — 251-679-2811
12950 US Highway 43 North, Axis, AL 36505

Bay Minette
Dentalez Of Alabama — 251-937-6781
2500 U.s. Highway 31 South, Bay Minette, AL 36507

Birmingham
Alabama Tissue Center, Inc.
500 22nd Street South, Suite 102, Birmingham, AL 35233
Applied Surgical, Llc — 205-259-2050
300 Riverchase Parkway East, Birmingham, AL 35244
Atherotech — 800-719-9807
201 London Parkway, Birmingham, AL 35211
Axcan Pharma Inc. — 800-950-8085
22 Inverness Center Parkway, Birmingham, AL 35242
Bass Medical, Inc — 800-214-9084
2539 John Hawkins Parkway, Suite 101, Birmingham, AL 35244
Biocryst Pharmaceuticals, Inc. — 205-444-4600
2190 Parkway Lake Dr., Birmingham, AL 35244
Biohorizons Implant Systems, Inc. — 888.246.8338
2300 Riverchase Center, Birmingham, AL 35244
Emageon Inc. — 262-369-3379
1200 Corporate Dr, Suite 200, Birmingham, AL 35242
Ergounlimited, Inc. — 205-591-9977
5401 9th Ave. South, Birmingham, AL 35212
Health Science Products, Inc. — 800-237-5794
1489 Hueytown Road, Birmingham, AL 35023-2061
Healthsouth Corporation — 888-476-8849
3660 Grandview Parkway, Suite 200, Birmingham, AL 35243
Intec Industries, Inc. — 205-251-5600
2024 12th Avenue N., Birmingham, AL 35234
Integrated Medical Systems, Inc. — 800-783-9251
1823 27th Ave. S., Birmingham, AL 35209
Klean N Konstant Dental Water Company, Llc — 205-422-3904
2204 Longleaf Blvd., Birmingham, AL 35243
Nidek Medical Products Inc. — 800-822-9255
3949 Valley E. Industrial Dr., Birmingham, AL 35217-1838
Sandstone Medical Technologies, Llc — 205-290-8251
102 Oxmoor Rd., Suite 130, Birmingham, AL 35209-5964
SourceMedical — 866-245-8093
100 Grandview Place, Suite 400, Birmingham, AL 35243
Synovis Micro Companies Alliance, Inc. — 800-510-3318
439 Industrial Ln., Birmingham, AL 35211-4464
Vision Research Corp. — 205-942-8011
211 Summit Pkwy., Suite 105, Birmingham, AL 35209

Citronelle
Citmed — 800-224-8633
18601 South Main St., Citronelle, AL 36522

Cleveland
American Orthopedic Supply Co., Inc. — 205-274-7137
37017 State Hwy. 79, Cleveland, AL 35049

Coaling
Tingle X-Ray Llc — 349-162-8905
5481 Skyland Blvd. East, Coaling, AL 35453

Columbiana
Elastic Corporation Of America — 205-669-3101
455 Highway 70 West, Columbiana, AL 35051

Fayette
Best Manufacturing Co.(Fayette Division) — 706-862-6712
931 Second Ave., S.e., Fayette, AL 35555

Gadsden
Fuller Medical Co. — 256-547-4991
1019 South 4th Street, Gadsden, AL 35901

Georgiana
Nightingale Uniform Co., Inc. — 334-376-2296
210 E. Mill St., P.O. Box 578, Georgiana, AL 36033-0578

Guntersville
Kappler Protective Apparel & Fabrics — 800-600-4019
115 Grimes Drive, Guntersville, AL 35976-9480

Homewood
Protection Products, Inc. — 800-869-6818
PO Box 59367, Homewood, AL 35259-9367

Huntsville
Akribeia, Inc. — 256-564-7450
1251 Washington St., Huntsville, AL 35801
Interact Plus — 800-944-8002
2225 Drake Avenue, Suite 2, Huntsville, AL 35805
Intergraph Corporation — 800-345-4856
P.O. Box 240000, Huntsville, AL 35894-0001
Rismed Oncology Systems — 256-534-6993
2494 Washington Street, Huntsville, AL 35811-1663
Sanmina-Sci Usa, Inc. — 256-882-4800
13000 South Memorial Pkwy., Huntsville, AL 35803
Titertek Instruments, Inc. — 256-859-8600
330 Wynn Drive, Huntsville, AL 35805-1961

Jasper
Beks Incorporated — 630-480-0476
401 14th Avenue N.e., Unit 2, Jasper, AL 35501

Jemison
Precision Plastic Molding, Inc. — 865-982-5552
28035 Hwy. 31 North, Jemison, AL 35085

Madison
Excellance, Inc. — 800-882-9799
453 Lanier Rd., Madison, AL 35758-1896
Intergraph Public Safety — 800-345-4856
19 Interpro Road, Madison, AL 35758

Mobile

Computer Programs And Systems, Inc.   251-639-8100
6600 Wall Street, Mobile, AL 36695
Discovery Hearing Aid Co-Op, Inc.   800-736-9903
4318 Downtowner Loop North,, #k, Mobile, AL 36609
Phoxxor   251-408-0208
5600 Commerce Blvd. East A, Mobile, AL 36619-0037
Televox Software, Inc.   800-644-4266
1110 Montlimar Drive, Suite 700, Mobile, AL 36609

Montgomery

Steris Corporation   334-277-6660
2720 Gunter Park Drive, Montgomery, AL 36109

Moody

Medical Systems Support, Inc.   800-239-2778
2301 Moody Pkwy., Suite 1, Moody, AL 35004

Pelham

Crystal Medical Technology   205-733-0901
153 Cahaba Valley Pkwy., Pelham, AL 35124
Frontier Devices   205-733-0901
153-a Cahaba Valley Parkway, Pelham, AL 35124
3d Medical Concepts, Llc   205-987-0935
1061 Morgan Park Rd., Pelham, AL 35124

Pell City

Bower, Inc.   205-884-7918
830 Pine Harbor Rd., Pell City, AL 35128-6763

Selma

Crown Health Care Laundry Services, Inc.   850-438-7578
3805 Highway 41 North, Selma, AL 36701
Klinger Eye Shields, Inc.   800-848-1244
1108A Singleton Drive, Selma, AL 36701
Ralston Group   334-875-2298
656 Lake Lanier Rd., Selma, AL 36701

Slocomb

Alatech Healthcare, Llc.   334-886-9337
595 E.lawrence Harris Hwy., Slocomb, AL 36375

Talladega

Brecon Knitting Mills, Inc.   800-841-2821
PO BOX 478, Talladega, AL 35161

Theodore

Airgas South, Inc.   251-653-2500
5480 Hamilton Blvd., Theodore, AL 36582
Taylor Wharton   800-898-2657
4075 Hamilton Blvd., Theodore, AL 36582

Tuscaloosa

Howard Instruments, Inc.   205-758-9083
4749 Appletree, Tuscaloosa, AL 35405-5747

Vernon

Marathon Equipment Company   800-269-7237
P.O. Box 1798, Vernon, AL 35592

ALASKA

Anchorage

Alaska Native Tribal Health Consortium   855-882-6842
4000 Ambassador Drive, Anchorage, AK 99508
Marcote, Llc   907-345-1377
1120 E. Huffman Rd. Pmb 348, Anchorage, AK 99516

ARIZONA

Cave Creek

Gri Medical Products, Inc.   800-291-9425
4937 E Red Range Way, Cave Creek, AZ 85331

Cave Creek,

Cardiobeat.Com   480-419-3957
Suite 118, Box 210, 29834 North Cave Creek Road, Cave Creek,, AZ 85331

Chandler

Entech   800-451-0591
7300 West Detroit Street, Chandler, AZ 85226
Magnum Medical   800-336-9710
3265 N. Nevada St., Chandler, AZ 85225
Protatek Reference Laboratory   480-545-8499
574 East Alamo Dr., Suite 90, Chandler, AZ 85225
Vomaris Innovations Inc.   866-4 YOUR HEAL
3100 W. Ray Rd, Suite 148, Chandler, AZ 85226

Corona De Tucson

Action Africa - Artique Refrigeration   520-762-9293
16335 S. Houghton Rd. #115, Corona De Tucson, AZ 85641

Flagstaff

W. L. Gore & Associates, Inc.   800-437-8181
PO Box 2400, Flagstaff, AZ 86003
W.L. Gore & Associates,Inc   928-526-3030
1505 North Fourth St., Flagstaff, AZ 86004

Fountain Hills

Ophthalmic Intl.   480-837-6165
16857 E. Saguaro Blvd, Fountain Hills, AZ 85268
Sunridge International Inc.   480-837-6165
16857 Saguaro Blvd, Fountain Hills, AZ 85268

Gilbert

Hearmore Company Inc.   800-881-4327
75 W Baseline Rd. #9, Gilbert, AZ 85233
Orange-Sol Medical Products, Inc.   800-877-7771
1400 N. Fiesta Blvd. #100, Gilbert, AZ 85233
Surgi-Aid Endoscopics, Inc.   480-988-0916
3553 E. Wildhorse Dr., Gilbert, AZ 85297

Glendale

Emr Tools, Llc   602-579-2694
4814 W. Laurel Ln., Glendale, AZ 85304
Mobile I.V. Systems, Llc   623-434-3136
23630 N. 35th Dr, Glendale, AZ 85310

Kino

Carclo Technical Plastics - Tucson   724-539-1833
1141 W. Grant Road, Kino, AZ 85705

Lake Havasu City

Oto-Med, Inc.   800-433-7703
1090 Empire Dr., Lake Havasu City, AZ 86404

Lakeside

Factor Ii, Inc.   928-537-8387
5642 White Mountain Avenue, Lakeside, AZ 85929-1339

Maricopa

Solomon Technology Labs   520-568-8007
22374 N. Dietz Dr., Maricopa, AZ 85239

Mesa

H & S Technical Services, Inc.   800-923-2486
1833 W. Main St., Suite 119, Mesa, AZ 85201
House Of Hearing   480-649-9609
4020 E. Main St., Mesa, AZ 85205
Image Marketing Corp.   800-466-7032
1636 N. 24th St., PO Box 30935, Mesa, AZ 85275
Paragon Vision Sciences, Inc.   800-528-8279
947 E. Impala Avenue, Mesa, AZ 85204
Photoactif   480-827-1212
7211 E. Southern Avenue, Suite C-110, Mesa, AZ 85209
Rite Time Corporation   800-266-2924
2950 East Dover St., Mesa, AZ 85213-6952
The Eye Concern, Inc.   480-962-5841
1450 S. Dobson Rd., Suite #a-206, Mesa, AZ 85202
The Renaissance Co.   480-969-1731
708 South Drew St., Mesa, AZ 85201
Three Rivers Holdings, Llc   480-833-1829
1826 West Broadway Rd., Suite 43, Mesa, AZ 85202
Ulthera Inc.   877-858-4372
2150 S. Country Club Drive, Suite 21, Mesa, AZ 85210
Zounds, Inc.   480-813-8400
1910 South Stapley Drive, Suite 202, Mesa, AZ 85204

Nogales

Alphaprotech, Inc.   229-242-1931
1287 West Fairway Dr., Nogales, AZ 85621
Denticon International Inc.   952-541-9622
840 North Grand Ave., Suite#13, Nogales, AZ 85621

Paradise Valley

Advanced Dental Systems   480-991-4081
5001 East Desert Jewel Dr., Paradise Valley, AZ 85253

Payson

Health Science Products, Llc   757-224-0177
1010 S. Beeline Hwy, Payson, AZ 85541

Peoria

Medi-Temp Technology Intl., Llc   888-669-0600
14131 N. Rio Vista Blvd. # 8, Peoria, AZ 85381

Phoenix

Accutron, Inc.   800-531-2221
1733 W. Parkside Lane, Phoenix, AZ 85027-2622
Activator Methods International, Ltd   800-598-0224
2950 North 7th St., Suite 200, Phoenix, AZ 85014
Advanced Motion Measurement, Llc   602-263-8657
1202 East Maryland Ave.,, Suite 1j, Phoenix, AZ 85014
Allerderm Laboratories, Inc.   800-365-6868
3400 E. McDowell Rd., Phoenix, AZ 85008

Arizona Industries For The Blind — 602-269-5131
Dept. Economic Security, 3013 W. Linclon St., Phoenix, AZ 85009-5699

Ascent Healthcare Solutions — 480-763-5300
10232 South 51st St., Phoenix, AZ 85044

Avnet, Inc. — 480-643-2000
2211 S. 47th St., Phoenix, AZ 85034

Baxter Healthcare Corporation — 847-473-6141
1606 E. University Dr., Phoenix, AZ 85034

Bio-Concepts, Inc. — 202-772-5333
2424 East University Dr., Phoenix, AZ 85034

Cft, Inc./Life Mask — 800-331-8844
14602 N. Cave Creek Road, Suite B, Phoenix, AZ 85022

Conray, Inc. — 623-465-7881
1950 East Watkins Rd.,, Suite 110, Phoenix, AZ 85034

Custom X-Ray Service, Inc. — (800) 230 - XRA
2120 West Encanto, Phoenix, AZ 85009

Eg & G Amorphous Silicon — 800-528-4225
4250 E. Broadway Rd., Phoenix, AZ 85040

Flowtronics, Inc. — 602-997-1364
10250 N. 19th Ave. Suite B, Phoenix, AZ 85021-1945

Ge Parallel Design, Inc. — 480-222-7000
4313 E Cotton Center Blvd, Suite 100, Phoenix, AZ 85040

Ge Parallel Design, Inc. — 414-721-2584
4313 East Cotton Center Blvd., Suite 100, Phoenix, AZ 85040

I.C. Medical, Inc. — 623-780-0700
2002 W. Quail Ave., Phoenix, AZ 85027

Ir Therapies, Llc — 602-595-3426
19827 North 20th Way, Phoenix, AZ 85024

Knox Company — 800-552-5669
1601 W Deer Valley Road, Phoenix, AZ 85027

Microbiological Specialties — 602-867-7323
3311 East Charter Oak Rd., Phoenix, AZ 85032

Neuromechanical Innovations, Llc — 480-785-8448
11011 South 48th St., Ste. 220, Phoenix, AZ 85044

Products International Co. — 800-521-5123
2320 W. Holly St., Phoenix, AZ 85009-2703

Progressive Dental Services Lab — 800-516-0789
21006 No. 22nd Street, Suite B-1, Phoenix, AZ 85024-5509

Radscan Medical Equipment, Inc. — 623-580-0556
23620 N. 20th Dr., Suite 16, Phoenix, AZ 85085

Rest Assured Inc. — 800-852-7378
4006 S. 21st Street, PO Box 163, Phoenix, AZ 85040-1460

Richardson Limited — 602-843-6365
11633 N. 38th Avenue, Phoenix, AZ 85029

Specialty Health Products, Inc. — 623-582-4950
21636 North 14th Ave.,, Suite A-1, Phoenix, AZ 85027

Spectrum Products Usa — 800-338-7581
3701 West Roanoke, Phoenix, AZ 85009

Take One Llc — 602-997-2888
10807 North Cave Creek Rd., Phoenix, AZ 85020

Terumo Medical Corp. — 800-283-7866
302 North 45th Ave., Suite 1, Phoenix, AZ 85043

Thermosurgery Technologies, Inc. — 602-264-7300
2901 W. Indian School Road, Phoenix, AZ 85017-4162

Waterloo Healthcare, Llc — 800-833-4419
3730 E. Southern Ave, Phoenix, AZ 85040

Zila Technical, Inc. — 602-266-6700
3418 South 48th St., Suite 9, Phoenix, AZ 85040-1939

Zounds, Inc. — (888-596-8637)
4405 East Baseline Road, Suite 114, Phoenix, AZ 85042

Prescott

Jumar Corp. — 928-442-0038
329 N. Alarcon St., Prescott, AZ 86301

Kappa medical, Inc. — 800-634-0880
P.O. Box 11808, Prescott, AZ 86304-1808

Persyst Development Corp. — 928-708-0705
1060 Sandretto Drive, Suite E2, Prescott, AZ 86305

Scottsdale

Arizona Dme--Durable Medical Equipment, Inc. — 888-665-2568
PO BOX 15413, Scottsdale, AZ 85267

Bonovo Orthopedics Inc. — 480-902.3094
7702 East Doubletree Ranch Road, Suite 300, Scottsdale, AZ 85258

Dillon Optics — 480-948-8009
8009 E. Dillon's Way, Scottsdale, AZ 85260

Intelsource Group, Inc — 602-790-8034
15953 N Greenway Hayden Loop Suit I, Scottsdale, AZ 85260

Laboratory Environment Support Systems, Inc. — 800-621-6404
7755 E. Evans, Scottsdale, AZ 85260

Lundy Medical Product, Llc — 480-473-7330
9376 East Bahia, Suite D-101, Scottsdale, AZ 85260

Marcolin Usa — 888-627-2654
7543 E. Tierra Buena Lane, Scottsdale, AZ 85260

Mbf Sales, Llc — 480-422-6742
7025 E Greenway Parkway, #250, Scottsdale, AZ 85254

N-Tech Endoscopy, Inc. — 480-348-7861
14255 N. 79th St., Suite 3, Scottsdale, AZ 85260

Noraxon Usa, Inc. — 800-364-8985
13430 N. Scottsdale Road, Suite #104, Scottsdale, AZ 85254

Orthoscan, Inc. — 866-996-0472
8212 E. Evans Road, Scottsdale, AZ 85260

The Dial Corporation, A Henkel Company — 480-754-3425
15501 North Dial Boulevard, Scottsdale, AZ 85260

The Tech Group — 480-281-4500
14677 N. 74 St., Scottsdale, AZ 85260

U.V. Vision Corp. — 480-948-5350
7702 e. doubletree ranch road, suite 300, Scottsdale, AZ 85258

Uniforms Manufacturing, Inc. — 800-222-1474
7575 E. Redfield Rd., P.O. Box 12716, Scottsdale, AZ 85267-2716

Universal Medical Technologies — 415-924-1133
15720 N. Greenway Hayden Loop, Suite 8, Scottsdale, AZ 85260

Worldwide Products Heat Packs — 800-554-6340
7031 N. Via De Paesia, Scottsdale, AZ 85258

Sedona

Hemo Sapiens, Inc. — 928-202-4453
325 Lookout Dr., Sedona, AZ 86351

Sun Lakes

Micro Hearing Aids — 480-895-2153
10440 East Riggs Rd.,suite 120, Sun Lakes, AZ 85248

Tempe

American Medical Products, Inc. — 800-279-1999
713 South Darrow Drive, Tempe, AZ 85281-3313

Arizona Device Manufacturing — 763-505-0874
2350 West Medtronic Way, Tempe, AZ 85281

Bard Peripheral Vascular, Inc. — 800-321-4254
1625 West Third Street, Tempe, AZ 85281

Capstone Therapeutics — 800-937-5520
1275 W. Washington St., Tempe, AZ 85281

Comtech Efdata — 480-333-2200
2114 West 7th Street, Tempe, AZ 85281

Cranial Technologies, Inc. — 866-362-2263
1395 West Auto Dr., Tempe, AZ 85284

Hanger National Fabrication Facility — 912-691-2030
1119 West Geneva Dr., Tempe, AZ 85282

Innocure, Llc — 480-966-0980
1045 East Sandpiper Dr., Tempe, AZ 85283

Kinetic Muscles, Inc. — 480-557-0448
2103 E Cedar St, #3, Tempe, AZ 85281-7432

Medi-Globe Corporation — 800-966-1431
110 W. Orion St., Suite 136, Tempe, AZ 85283

Mobility Research — 800.332.WALK
P.O. Box 3141, Tempe, AZ 85280

Progressive Medical Systems, Inc. — 602-421-2484
1221 West Warner Rd.,suite 103, Tempe, AZ 85284

Sartorius Omnimark Instrument Corp — 480-784-2200
1320 South Priest Drive, Tempe, AZ 85281

The Tech Group Tempe — 480-281-4400
640 South Rockford Dr., Tempe, AZ 85281

Tolleson

Dotolo Research Western Div. — 623-936-0500
10199 W. Van Buren, Suite 10, Tolleson, AZ 85353

Tucson

Armor Sports Holdings, Llc — 520-623-9800
2030 N. Forbes Blvd., #106, Tucson, AZ 85745

Aztec Orthodontic Laboratory, Inc. — 888-744-1588
7750 N. Redwing Circle, Tucson, AZ 85741

B & H Medical Products, Inc. — 520-296-5544
8925 East Golf Links Rd, Tucson, AZ 85730-1318

Back Solution, The — 800-326-2724
6281 South Park Avenue, Tucson, AZ 85706

Bioptics, Inc. — 800.477.8985
3440 e. britannia dr. suite 150, Tucson, AZ 85714

Boeckeler Instruments, Inc. — 800-552-2262
4650 S. Butterfield Drive, Tucson, AZ 85714

Byron Medical — 800-777-3434
602 W. Rillito, Tucson, AZ 85705

Chief Power Chair, Llc — 520-722-5265
8051 E. Lakeside Pkwy, #113, Tucson, AZ 85730

Competitive Engineering Inc. — 520-746-0270
3371 E. Hemisphere Loop, Tucson, AZ 85706

Cortical Systematics Llc. — 520-444-0666
5324 E. 18th Street, Tucson, AZ 85711

Cybernetic Research Laboratories, Inc. — 520-571-8065
3562 E. 42nd Stravenue, Tucson, AZ 85713

Everest Interscience, Inc. — 800-422-4342
1891 North Oracle Road, Tucson, AZ 85705

Eye Care And Cure — 800-486-6169
4646 S Overland Dr, Tucson, AZ 85714

Hearing Tech, Inc. — 520-297-7555
7225 North Oracle Rd. #111, Tucson, AZ 85704

July Soft — 800-350-7693
610 East Knox Drive, Tucson, AZ 85705

Km Instruments, Llc — 520-529-8455
5941 East Fort Crittendon, Tucson, AZ 85750

Langford Ic Systems, Inc. — 520-745-6201
310 S. Williams Blvd., Suite 270, Tucson, AZ 85711

Lesco Optical — 520-323-1538
4444 East Grant Rd, Tucson, AZ 85712

Lifestyle Medical Mfg — 520-323-0099
6479 E. 22nd St, Tucson, AZ 85710

Lots Corp. — 520-730-6068
10977 E. Tanque Verde Road, Tucson, AZ 85749
Manufacturing & Research, Inc.(Dba Mri Medical) — 520-882-7794
4700 S. Overland Drive, Tucson, AZ 85714
Medfilms, Inc. — 800-535-5593
4910 W. Monte Carlo Drive, Tucson, AZ 85745
Medical Equipment Development, Inc. — 520-743-7874
PO Box 85820, Tucson, AZ 85754-5820
Micro-Vac, Inc. — 800-729-1020
5905 E. 5th St., Tucson, AZ 85711-4522
Mti-Medical Technique, Inc. — 800-426-9053
8060 E. research Court., Tucson, AZ 85710
Oncothyreon Inc. — 520-622-5552
221 East 6th Street, Tucson, AZ 85705
Optical Electronics, Inc. — 520-889-8811
4455 S. Park Ave #106, Tucson, AZ 85714
Postcraft Co. — 800-528-4844
625 W. Rillito St., Tucson, AZ 85705-5441
Prescott Ideas, Llc — 520-886-4399
8960 E. Anna Place, Tucson, AZ 85710
Pro Orthopedic Devices, Inc. — 800-523-5611
2884 E. Ganley Road, Tucson, AZ 85706
Product Development Industries, Inc. — 520-881-2556
4500 East Speedway Blvd., #50, Tucson, AZ 85712
Qrp, Inc. — 800-832-3882
3925 N. Runway Drive, PO Box 28802, Tucson, AZ 85726-8802
Redman Powerchairs — 800-727-6684
1601 S Pantano Parkway #107, Tucson, AZ 85710
Roper Scientific, Inc. — 800-874-9789
3440 E. Britannia Drive, Tucson, AZ 85706-5006
Rpc — 800-647-3873
PO Box 35849, Tucson, AZ 85740
Spectral Instruments, Inc. — 520-884-8821
420 North Bonita Ave, Tucson, AZ 85745
Sunquest Information Systems, Inc — 520-570-2347
250 S. Williams Blvd, Tucson, AZ 85711
Syncardia Systems, Inc. — 866-771-9437
1992 E. Silverlake Rd., Tucson, AZ 85713
Thayer Medical Corp. — 520-790-5393
4575 South Palo Verde Rd.,, Suite 337, Tucson, AZ 85714
Ventana Medical Systems, Inc. — 800-227-2155
1910 Innovation Park Dr., Tucson, AZ 85755
Wells Johnson Co. — 800-528-1597
8000 South Kolb Road, Tucson, AZ 85706
Westmed, Inc. — 800-975-7987
5580 S. Nogales Hwy, Tucson, AZ 85706

Yuma

Centurion Medical Products Corporation — 866-386-0530
3173 East 43rd St., Yuma, AZ 85365

ARKANSAS

Alexander

Wes-Pak, Inc. — 1-800-493-7725
11610 Vimy Ridge Rd., Alexander, AR 72002

Batesville

La Croix Optical Co. — 870-698-1881
PO Box 2556, Batesville, AR 72501
Life Plus International — 800-572-8446
P.O. Box 3749, Batesville, AR 72503
Zila Dental Technologies, Inc. — 928-899-1231
2410 Harrison St., Batesville, AR 72501

Bentonville

Ace Hearing Laboratory, Llc — 877-452-2044
2304 S.E. 14th St., Bentonville, AR 72712
3m Espe Dental Products — 651-733-7767
2501 SE Otis Corley Drive, Bentonville, AR 72712

Clinton

Rivertrail Mobility — 501-745-6790
369 Factory Road, Clinton, AR 72031

Conway

KIMBERLY-CLARK CORP. CONWAY MILL — 501-329-2973
480 Exchange Ave., Conway, AR 72032
Medical Solutions Distribution Group — 501-450-9063
535 Enterprise Ave., Conway, AR 72032

Fayetteville

Caldwell, Justiss & Co., Inc. — 800-643-4343
622 W. Sycamore, Fayetteville, AR 72702

Flippin

Little Shepherd Industries — 870-453-4874
316 River Run Lane, Flippin, AR 72634

Fort Smith

Fox Manufacturing, Inc. — 479-646-1656
5305 Towson Ave., Fort Smith, AR 72901

Greenwood

Armedica Mfg. Corp. — 800-701-5122
212 Bell Rd., PO Box 880, Greenwood, AR 72936

Greers Ferry

H2o Ramps And Lifts, Llc — 501-825-8838
7010 Greers Ferry Rd., Greers Ferry, AR 72067

Hot Springs

Jaeco Orthopedic Specialties, Inc. — 501-623-5944
214 Drexel Street, Hot Springs, AR 71901

Jonesboro

Colson Caster Corporation — 800-643-5515
3700 Airport Road, Jonesboro, AR 72401
Jk Products & Services, Inc. — 870-268-2852
1 Walter Kratz Dr., Jonesboro, AR 72401

Little Rock

Cromwell Architects Engineers — 501-372-2900
101 S. Spring St., Little Rock, AR 72201-2490
Health Care Furnishings, Inc. — 800-648-5744
63 Pebble Beach Drive, Little Rock, AR 72212

Maumelle

Icon Llc — 501-374-2929
8 Ten Tee Circle, Maumelle, AR 72113

Mountain Home

Baxter Healthcare Corporation — 847-473-6141
1900 N. Hwy. 201, Mountain Home, AR 72653

North Little Rock

Statco Hearing Aid Laboratory — 501-771-2444
4000 Mccain Blvd., North Little Rock, AR 72116

Pine Bluff

U.S. Army Pine Bluff Arsenal — 870-540-3000
10020 Kabrich Circle, Pine Bluff, AR 71602-9500

Rogers

Digital Hearing Systems Corp. — 479-925-7700
9679 East High Meadows, Rogers, AR 72756
Du-More, Inc. — 425-489-6088
1751 South First St., Rogers, AR 72756
Northstar Medical. Inc, — 800-457-3217
38 Buckingham Drive, Rogers, AR 72758

Russellville

Grace Manufacturing, Inc. — 479-968-5455
614 SR 247, Russellville, AR 72802

Siloam Springs

Ozark Systems Manufacturing, Llc. — 479-524-9778
501 North Lincoln Street, Siloam Springs, AR 72761

Springdale

Immuno Vision, Inc. — 800-541-0960
1820 Ford Ave., Springdale, AR 72764

Stuttgart

Carter Dental Lab, Llc — 870-673-1568
301 S. Grand St., Stuttgart, AR 72160

Texarkana

Durabuilt Medical Corp. — 800-321-9729
1901 East 50th St., Texarkana, AR 71854

CALIFORNIA

Agoura Hills

Caldera Medical Inc. — 866-422-5337
5171 Clareton Drive, Agoura Hills, CA 91301
Nestor Machine Co Inc — 818-707-1678
5537 Fairview Pl, Agoura Hills, CA 91301
Shamir Usa, Inc. — 818-889-6292
30077 Agoura Rd, Suite 220, Agoura Hills, CA 91301

Alameda

Abbott Diabetes Care Inc. — 510-749-5400
1360 South Loop Rd., Alameda, CA 94502
Berkeley Heartlab, Inc. — 510-747-1740
960 Atlantic Avenue, Suite 100, Alameda, CA 94501
Black Diamond Video, Inc. — 215-348-3896
1151 Harbor Bay Parkway, Suite 208, Alameda, CA 94502
Convergent Laser Technologies — 800-848-8200
1660 S. Loop Road, Alameda, CA 94502
Coolsystems, Inc. — 510-868-5378
1201 Marina Village Parkway, Suite 200, Alameda, CA 94501
Otismed Corporation — 888-684-7633
1600 Harbor Bay Pwy., Alameda, CA 94502
Penumbra, Inc. — 1.888.272.4606
1351 Harbor Bay Parkway, Alameda, CA 94502

St. Francis Medical Technologies, Inc. 408-548-6500
1201 Marina Village Parkway, Suite 200, Alameda, CA 94501
Xintec Corp. / Convergent Laser Tech. 510-832-2130
1660 South Loop Road, Alameda, CA 94502

Alamo
Shadow Shield 866-838-8400
42 Shandelin Ct, Alamo, CA 94507

Alhambra
American Healthcare Products, Inc. 888-784-1888
1068 Westminster Avenue, Alhambra, CA 91803-1231
American Lasers, Inc. 626-300-9330
300 East Main St., Alhambra, CA 91801

Aliso Viejo
Ambry Genetics 866-262-7943
100 Columbia, #200, Aliso Viejo, CA 92656
Cardio-Vascular Sales 888-287-8700
27111 Aliso Creek Rd., Ste. 130, Aliso Viejo, CA 92656
Carl Zeiss Microimaging Ais, Inc 949-425-5700
31 Columbia, Aliso Viejo, CA 92656
Cianna Medical, Inc. 866-920-9444
6 Journey, Suite 125, Aliso Viejo, CA 92656
Clarient, Inc. 888-443-3310
31 Columbia, Aliso Viejo, CA 92656
Global Care Quest 949-330-7450
65 Enterprise, Suite 350, Aliso Viejo, CA 92656
Hampton Research 800-452-3899
34 Journey, Aliso Viejo, CA 92656-3317
Optical Shop Of Aspen 800-647-2345
25 Brookline, Aliso Viejo, CA 92656
Para Tech Coating, Inc. 800-999-4942
35 Argonaut, Aliso Viejo, CA 92656
Senorx, Inc. 949-362-4800
11 Columbia, Aliso Viejo, CA 92656
Sequent Medical Inc. 949-830-9600
11A Columbia, Aliso Viejo, CA 92656
Vertos Medical Inc. 877.958.6227.
11 Columbia, Suite B, Aliso Viejo, CA 92656
Wavetec Vision Systems, Inc. 949-273-5970
66 Argonaut, Suite 170, Aliso Viejo, CA 92656
Woodward Laboratories, Inc. 800-780-6999
125 B Columbia, Aliso Viejo, CA 92656
Zettler Systems, Inc. 949-831-5000
75 Columbia, Aliso Viejo, CA 92656

Alpine
Cornerstone Sensors, Inc. 800-955-1470
2128 ARNOLD WAY, Suite 4, Alpine, CA 91901

Altadena
Dockum Research Lab 626-794-1821
844 East Mariposa St., Altadena, CA 91001

Anaheim
Air Link International 800-388-8237
1189-A, North Grove St., Anaheim, CA 92806
Diamodent 888-281-8850
1577 North Harmony Circle, Anaheim, CA 92806
Discount Dme 714-630-9590
1265 N. Grove St, Suite A, Anaheim, CA 92806
Evermed Corp. 714-777-9997
4999 E. La Palma Ave., Anaheim, CA 92807
Firehouse Medical, Inc. 714-688-1575
1045 Armando St. # D, Anaheim, CA 92806
Hi-Tech Rubber, Inc. 800-924-4832
3191 E. La Palma Avenue, Anaheim, CA 92806
Image Technology, Inc. 800-554-6243
1380 N. Knollwood Circle, Anaheim, CA 92801
Lifemed Of California 800-543-3633
1216 So. Allec St., Anaheim, CA 92805-6301
Lucas Medical, Inc. 714-938-0233
1751 South Douglass Rd., Anaheim, CA 92806
Medivision Endoscopy 800-349-5367
1210 N. Jefferson St, Suite D, Anaheim, CA 92807
Mettler Electronics Corp. 800-854-9305
1333 S. Claudina Street, Anaheim, CA 92805-6235
Mk Battery 800-372-9253
1645 S. Sinclair St., Anaheim, CA 92806
Products For Medicine 800-333-3087
1201 East Ball Road, Suite H, Anaheim, CA 92805
Rti Electronics, Inc. (714) 765-8200
1800 E. Via Burton, Anaheim, CA 92806-1213
Sechrist Industries, Inc. 800-732-4747
4225 E. La Palma Avenue, Anaheim, CA 92807
Selco Products Company 800-257-3526
605 S. East St., Anaheim, CA 92805-4842
Starkey California 952-947-4734
2536 Woodland Dr., Anaheim, CA 92801
Tds U-Best Dental Technology 866-686-1899
2941 E. Miraloma Ave. #6 & 7, Anaheim, CA 92806
Teco Diagnostics 800-222-9880
1268 N. Lakeview Ave., Anaheim, CA 92807

Teco Diagnostics 714-693-7788
1268 North Lakeview Ave., Anaheim, CA 92807
Tuffcare 800-367-6160
3999 E. La Palma, Anaheim, CA 92807
Ultimate Spine, Llc. 562-598-1753
1220 North Barsten Way, Anaheim, CA 92806
Visionary Contact Lens 714-237-1900
2940 East Miraloma Ave., Anaheim, CA 92806
2d Imaging, Inc. 800-449-1332
4745 East Wesley Drive, Anaheim, CA 92807

Anaheim,
2d Cardiac Imaging, Inc. 714-777-9900
4745 E. Wesley Drive, Anaheim,, CA 92807

Apple Valley
Medical Marketplace 760-242-4171
18737 Hwy. 18, Suite 5A, Apple Valley, CA 92307-2311

Aptos
Pureline Oralcare, Inc. 831-662-9500
804 Estates Dr., Aptos, CA 95003

Arcadia
Amrel / American Reliance, Inc. 800-654-9838
11801 Goldring Road, Arcadia, CA 91006-5880
J. T. Posey Co. 800-447-6739
5635 Peck Rd., Arcadia, CA 91006-5851
Shantel Medical Supply 888-577-5688
5600 Peck Road, Arcadia, CA 91006

Artesia
Maxcor Inc (877) ENDO MAX
17517 Fabrica Way, Suite H, Artesia, CA 90703

Arvin
Salter Labs 800-235-4203
100 W. Sycamore Rd., Arvin, CA 93203-0608
Salter Labs 800-421-0024
100 W. Sycamore Road, Arvin, CA 93203

Auburn
Nai Tech Products 866-342-6629
12919 Earhart Avenue, Auburn, CA 95602
Telescan Medical Systems 800-388-4324
26424 Table Meadow Road, Auburn, CA 95602-8959

Azusa
Mortech Manufacturing Company 800) 410-0100
411 N. Aerojet Avenue, Azusa, CA 91702
Tg Medical Usa Inc. 626-969-7838
TG Medical USA Inc., 165 North Aspan Avenue, Azusa, CA 91702
Truett Labs 626-334-5106
798 North Coney Ave., Azusa, CA 91702

Bakersfield
Bioquest Prosthetics 661-325-3338
412 18th St., Bakersfield, CA 93304
Golden Empire Dental Lab Corp. 661-327-1888
929 21st Street, Bakersfield, CA 93301
Kern Surgical Supply, Inc. 800-582-3939
2823 Gibson St., Bakersfield, CA 93308-6105
Valley Institute Of Prosthetics And Orthotics, Inc 661-322-1005
1524 21st St., Suite B, Bakersfield, CA 93301-4002

Baldwin Park
Conrac, Inc. 626-480-0095
5124 Commerce Drive, Baldwin Park, CA 91706
Denovo Dental, Inc. 800-854-7949
5130 Commerce Drive, Baldwin Park, CA 91706
Medi/Nuclear Corp. 800-321-5981
4610 Littlejohn St., Baldwin Park, CA 91706

Beach Center
Posture Pro, Inc. 714-847-8607
18584 Main Street, Beach Center, CA 92648

Bellflower
Alpha-Omega Services, Inc. 800-346-7894
9156 Rose St., Bellflower, CA 90706-6420
Stand-Rite Manufacturing Co. 562-782-6346
16655 Grand Ave., Bellflower, CA 90706-5037

Belmont
Hope Laboratories 650-591-6271
409-a Old County Rd., Belmont, CA 94002
Ventus Medical, Inc. 650-632-4199
1301 Shoreway Rd., Suite 425, Belmont, CA 94002

Ben Lomond
Reel R&D, Inc. 800-348-7335
9533 Sunnyside Ave., Ben Lomond, CA 95005-9345

Benicia

Acrometrix — 707-746-8888
6058 Egret Ct., Benicia, CA 94510
Bio-Rad Laboratories, Diagnostic Group — 800-224-6723
524 Stone Rd, Suite A, Benicia, CA 94510
Bio-Rad Laboratories, Inc — 510-741-6263
5500 East 2nd St, Benicia, CA 94510
Biovir Laboratories, Inc. — 800-442-7342
685 Stone Rd., Unit 6, Benicia, CA 94510
Dusouth Industries — 707-745-5117
651 Stone Rd., Benicia, CA 94510
Medi — 800-947-6334
4814 E. 2nd St., Benicia, CA 94510
Motus Bioengineering Inc. — 707-745-4194
133 Carlisle Way, Benicia, CA 94510

Berkeley

Berkeley Advanced Biomaterials, Inc. — 510-883-0500
901 Grayson Street, Suite 101, Berkeley, CA 94710
Cymed Ostomy Co. — 800-582-0707
1440 4th St # C, Berkeley, CA 94710
Focal Point Opticians — 510-923-0568
2638 Ashby Avenue, Berkeley, CA 94705
Siemens Healthcare Diagnostics Inc — 800-434-2447
725 Potter St, Berkeley, CA 94710
Xoma Ltd. — 510-204-7200
2910 Seventh Street, Berkeley, CA 94710

Beverly Hills

Carole Lewis Stolpe' B.C.O. — 310-271-8801
435 N. Bedford Drive, Suite 411, Beverly Hills, CA 90210
Cyber Medical Imaging, Inc. — 310-859-3802
3054 Franklin Canyon Dr., Beverly Hills, CA 90210
Orthotec, Llc — 800-557-2988
9595 Wilshire Blvd., Suite 502, Beverly Hills, CA 90212-4110
Oxis International, Inc. — 800-547-3686
468 N. Camden Dr., 2nd Floor, Beverly Hills, CA 90210
Spectral Molecular Imaging Inc. — 310-858-1670
250 N. Robertson Blvd., Suite 427, Beverly Hills, CA 90211

Bonita

Pacific Integrated Mfg., Inc. — 619-921-3464
4364 Bonita Rd., #454, Bonita, CA 91902
Sdi Medical Consultants — 619-267-1391
4190 Bonita Road, Suite # 211, Bonita, CA 91902

Box Springs

Cardinal Health 200, Inc — 847-578-6610
1660 Iowa Ave.,, Suite 100/200, Box Springs, CA 92507

Brea

Backstrong International Llc. — 714-671-1150
710 N. Brea Blvd., Suite G, Brea, CA 92821
Beckman Coulter, Inc. — 800-742-2345
250 S. Kraemer Boulevard, PO Box 8000, Brea, CA 92822
Beckman Coulter, Inc. — 800-635-3497
250 South Kraemer Boulevard, Brea, CA 92821-6232
Bio Diagnostic Intl. — 562-691-7850
1300-c- Pioneer Street, Brea, CA 92821
Carolina Liquid Chemistries Corp. — 800-471-7272
510 W. Central Ave., Suite C, Brea, CA 92821
Genchem, Inc. — 714-529-1616
510 W. Central Avenue, Suite D, Brea, CA 92821
Lmi — 714-349-5386
2324 Rain Tree Drive, Brea, CA 92821
Mps Acacia — 800-486-6677
785 Challenger St., Brea, CA 92821
Nurad Medical Solutions Llc — 949-737-7523
396 Cliffwood Park St., Brea, CA 92821
Omnivations — 714-990-0904
445 Capricorn St., Brea, CA 92821
Sherman Ophthalmic Supplies, Inc. — 714-738-0209
428 South Brea Blvd., Suite #B, Brea, CA 92821
Veriad — 800-423-4643
650 Columbia Street, Brea, CA 92821
Vident — 800-828-3839
3150 E. Birch St., Brea, CA 92821
Vital Diagnostics Inc. — 714-672-3553
1075 West Lambert Road, Unit D, Brea, CA 92821

Brentwood

Halt Medical Inc. — 925-634-7943
131 Sand Creek Road, Suite B, Brentwood, CA 94513

Brisbane

Cutera, Inc. — 888-4-CUTERA
3240 Bayshore Blvd, Brisbane, CA 94005
XDx Inc. — 415-287-2300
3260 Bayshore Blvd, Brisbane, CA 94005

Buena Park

Bio-Gate Usa, Inc. — 714-670-2771
6800 Orangethorpe Ave., Unit E, Buena Park, CA 90620

G.E.M. Water Systems, Int'L., Llc — 800-755-1707
6351 Orangethorpe Avenue, Buena Park, CA 90620
Suncoast Laboratories — 714-229-9178
6888 Lincoln Ave. # G, Buena Park, CA 90620

Burbank

Comco, Inc. — 800-796-6626
2151 N. Lincoln St., Burbank, CA 91504
Haskel International, Inc. — 818-843-4000
100 E. Graham Place, Burbank, CA 91502-2027
Imaging3, Inc. — 800-900-9729
3200 W. Valhalla Dr., Burbank, CA 91505
Limerick Incorporate — 818-566-3060
2150 N. Glenoaks Blvd., Burbank, CA 91504
Western Scientific Co., Inc. — 800-48W-ESCO
2112 West Burbank Blvd., Burbank, CA 91506

Burlingame

American Bantex Corp. — 800-633-4839
1815 Rollins Rd., Burlingame, CA 94010
Attachments International, Inc. — 800-999-3003
824 Cowan Rd., Burlingame, CA 94010
G. Hirsch & Co. — 650-692-6435
1815 Rollins Rd., Burlingame, CA 94010
G. Hirsch And Co., Inc. — 650-692-8770
870 Mahler Road, Burlingame, CA 94010
Murdock Laboratories, Inc. — 800 439-2497
123 Primrose Rd., Burlingame, CA 94010
Rapid Diagnostics, Div. Of Mp Biomedicals, Llc — 800-888-7008
1429 Rollins Road, Burlingame, CA 94010
Technical Instruments (Ti) — 650-651-3000
1826 Rollins Road, Burlingame, CA 94010-2215
Vector Laboratories, Inc. — 800-227-6666
30 Ingold Road, Burlingame, CA 94010

Calabasas

Aspyra, Inc. — 800-437-9000
26115-A Mureau Road, Calabasas, CA 91302
Diagnostic Automation/ Cortez Diagnostics Inc,. — 818-591-3030
23961 Craftsman Rd, Suite E/F, Calabasas, CA 91302
Facemaster Of Beverly Hills, Inc. — 818-222-2461
23961 Craftsman Rd.,suite I, Calabasas, CA 92302
Melco Engineering Corp. — 888-635-2688
P.O. Box 8907, Calabasas, CA 91372-8907
Micro Medical Devices, Inc. — 818-874-0000
23945 Calabasas Rd., Suite 110, Calabasas, CA 91302
Tapco Medical, Inc. — 818-225-5376
23981 Craftsman Road, Calabasas, CA 91302

Calabasas Hills

Implant Direct Llc — 818-444-3300
27030 Malibu Hills Rd., Calabasas Hills, CA 91301

Calexico

Allesee Orthodontic Appliances (Calexico) — 714-516-7400
341 E. First St., Calexico, CA 92231
Ortho-Med Intl., Inc. — 760-357-5040
357-a West 2nd St., Calexico, CA 92231-2114
Orthodental Intl., Inc. — 760-357-8070
280 avenida campillo ste m, Calexico, CA 92231

Camarillo

Altair Instruments, Inc. — 805-388-8503
330 North Wood Road, Suite J, Camarillo, CA 93010
Belport Co. Inc., Gingi-Pak Div. — 800-437-1514
4825 Calle Alto, Camarillo, CA 93011-0240
Farley Inc., W.T. — 800-327-5397
931 Via Alondra, Camarillo, CA 93012
Infab Corp. — 805-987-5255
3651 Via Pescador, Camarillo, CA 93012-5050
Kinamed, Inc. — 800-827-5775
820 Flynn Road, Camarillo, CA 93012-8701
Leading Edge Innovations — 805-388-7669
699 Mobil Ave, Camarillo, CA 93010
Medical Packaging Corporation — 800-792-0600
941 Avenida Acaso, Camarillo, CA 93012-8700
Merlin's Medical Supply — 800-639-9322
699 Mobil Avenue, Camarillo, CA 93010
North American Imaging, Inc. — 800-288-8823
924 Via Alondra, Camarillo, CA 93012
Ossur Americas — 800-233-6263
742 Pancho Rd., Camarillo, CA 93012
PBS Biotech, Inc — 1 (805) 482-727
4023 Camino Ranchero AõÉ,™É_o Suite I, Camarillo, CA 93012
Royce Medical — 800-521-0601
742 Pancho Road, Camarillo, CA 93012
Squareone Medical, Inc. — 805-987-2457
1640 Pierside Ln., Camarillo, CA 93010

Cameron Park

Orthogenesis, Inc. — 530-672-8560
4315 Product Drive, #c, Cameron Park, CA 95682

Campbell

Creganna-Tactx Medical — 408-364-7100
1353 Dell Ave., Campbell, CA 95008
Hosmer Dorrance Corp. — 408-379-5151
561 Division St., Campbell, CA 95008
Hosmer-Dorrance Corp. — 800-827-0070
561 Division St., Campbell, CA 95008-6952
Sgarlato Laboratories, Inc. — 800-421-5303
2315 S. Bascom Ave, Suite#200, Campbell, CA 95008

Campbell,

EMKinetics, Inc. — 650-384-0008
583 Division St., Suite A, Campbell,, CA 95008

Canoga Park

Advanced Endoscopy Devices, Inc. — 818-227-2720
22134 Sherman Way, Canoga Park, CA 91303
Cardiac Care Units, Inc. — 818-592-6004
7745 Alabama Avenue, Canoga Park, CA 91304
Neurocybernetics, Inc. — 516-482-9001
21601 Vanowen St., Suite 100, Canoga Park, CA 91303
One Lambda, Inc. — 800-822-8824
21001 Kittridge St., Canoga Park, CA 91303
PLS Shoe Co. — 866 712 7463
21500 Osborne St., Canoga Park, CA 91304
Precision Dental Int, Inc. — 818-992-1888
21361 Deering Ct., Canoga Park, CA 91304
Ubs Instruments Corporation — 818-710-1195
7745 Alabama Avenue, Suite 7, Canoga Park, CA 91304-6645

Capitola

Opap, Inc. — 831-458-5626
3523 Deanes Ln., Capitola, CA 95010

Carlsbad

Aalto Scientific Ltd. — 760-431-7922
1959 Kellogg Ave., Carlsbad, CA 92008
Ablation Frontiers, Inc. — 760-438-4868
6354 Corte Del Abeto, Carlsbad, CA 92011
Alphatec Spine, Inc. — 800-922-1356
5818 El Camino Real, Carlsbad, CA 92008
Beckman Coulter, Inc. — 714-993-8767
2470 Faraday Ave., Carlsbad, CA 92008
Blue Sky Medical Group Incorporated — 727-392-1261
5924 Balfour Ct., Suite 102, Carlsbad, CA 92008
Brendan Technologies Inc. — 760-929-7500
Research Center Plaza, 2236 Rutherford Rd., Ste. 107, Carlsbad, CA 92008
Carlsbad International Export, Inc. — 760-438-5323
1954 Kellogg Ave., Carlsbad, CA 92008
Carol Cole Company — 888-360-9171
3146 Tiger Run Court, Suite 109, Carlsbad, CA 92010
Covidien, Formerly Puritan Bennett Corp — 800-962-9888
2101 Faraday Avenue, Carlsbad, CA 92008
Electro Surface Technologies, Inc. — 760-431-8306
2281 Las Palmas Drive, Suite 101, Carlsbad, CA 92011
GenMark Diagnostics Inc. — 1-800-373-6767
5964 La Place Court, Carlsbad, CA 92008
Hartwell Medical Corp. — 800-633-5900
6352 Corte del Abeto, Suite J, Carlsbad, CA 92011-1408
Intraluminal Therapeutics, Inc. — 800-513-4458
6354 Corte Del Abeto, Suite A, Carlsbad, CA 92009
Ion Vision, Inc. — 760-450-4548
7933 Paseo Membrillo, Carlsbad, CA 92009
Ivd Research, Inc. — 866-794-2126
5909 Sea Lion Place, Suite D, Carlsbad, CA 92010
Kfx Medical — 866-883-8718
5845 Avenida Encinas, Suite 128, Carlsbad, CA 92008
Kinetikos Medical, Inc. — 800-546-3845
6005 Hidden Valley Road, Suite 180, Carlsbad, CA 92009
Life Technologies Corporation — 760-603-7200
5791 Van Allen Way, Carlsbad, CA 92008
Magne Vu — 760-929-8000
1916 Palomar Oaks Way, Suite 150, Carlsbad, CA 92008
Magnevu — 760-929-8000
2225 Faraday Avenue, Suite F, Carlsbad, CA 92008
Mardx Diagnostics, Inc. — 760-929-0500
5919 Farnsworth Ct., Carlsbad, CA 92008
Merlin Labs, Inc. — 760-804-1782
6082 Corte Del Cedro, Carlsbad, CA 92011
Myron L Company — 760-438-2021
2450 Impala Drive, Carlsbad, CA 92010-7226
Ortho Organizers, Inc. — 760-448-8730
1822 Aston Avenue, Carlsbad, CA 92008
Osmetech, Inc. — 800-373-6767
5964 La Place Court, Carlsbad, CA 92008
Photomedex, Inc. — 760-602-3300
2375 Camino Vida Roble, Suite B, Carlsbad, CA 92011
Qualigen, Inc. — 760-918-9165
2042 Corte Del Nogal, Carlsbad, CA 92011
Ra Medical Systems, Inc. — 760-804-1648
2270 Camino Vida Roble, Suite L, Carlsbad, CA 92011
Respironics California, Inc. — 724-387-4559
2271 Cosmos Ct., Carlsbad, CA 92011

Safety Syringes, Inc. — 760-918-9908
2875 Loker Avenue East, Carlsbad, CA 92010
Sendx Med, Inc. — 760-930-6300
1945 Palomar Oaks Way, Carlsbad, CA 92009
Senitech Medical Instruments — 760-918-1904
6351 Corte Del Abeto, #a105, Carlsbad, CA 92009
Shrink Nanotechnologies, Inc. — 760-804-8844
2038 Corte Del Nogal, Suite 110, Carlsbad, CA 92011
Solace Therapeutics, Inc — 760-431-0153
5865 Avenida Encinas, Suite 142b, Carlsbad, CA 92008
Spinal Elements, Inc. — 760-607-0121
2744 Loker Ave. W. Suite 100, Carlsbad, CA 92008
Sterogene Bioseparations, Inc. — 800-535-2284
5922 Farnsworth Ct., Carlsbad, CA 92008
Syntron Bioresearch, Inc. — 800-854-6226
2774 Loker Avenue W., Carlsbad, CA 92008
Theralight, Inc. — 760-930-8000
2794 Loker Ave. West,suite 105, Carlsbad, CA 92010
Wcm Waste & Compliance Management, Inc. — 760-930-9101
6054 Corte Del Cedro, Carlsbad, CA 92009
Zimmer Dental, Inc. — 800-854-7019
1900 Aston Ave., Carlsbad, CA 92008

Carpinteria

Dac International, Inc. — 888-373-3027
6390 Rose Lane, Carpinteria, CA 93013
Dako North America, Inc — 805-566-6655
6392 Via Real, Carpinteria, CA 93013
Ditec Mfg. — 800-332-7083
1019 Mark Avenue, Carpinteria, CA 93013
Helix Medical, Inc. — 800-266-4421
1110 Mark Avenue, Carpinteria, CA 93013-2918
Spectrum Designs Medical, Inc. — 800-239-6399
6387-B Rose Lane, Carpinteria, CA 93013

Carson

Amrex Electrotherapy Equipment — 800-221-9069
641 E. Walnut St., Carson, CA 90746
H.B. Gordon Mfg. Co., Inc. — 310-327-5240
751 East Artesia Blvd., Carson, CA 90746
Jobar Intl., Inc. — 310-222-8682
21022 Figueroa St., Carson, CA 90745-1937
Pacifica Gloves — 800-635-4430
West Coast Distribution, 1709 E. Del Amo Blvd., Carson, CA 90746
Parter Medical Products — 800-666-8282
17015 Kingsview Ave., Carson, CA 90746-1220
Proma, Inc. — 310-327-0035
730 East Kingshill Pl., Carson, CA 90746
Sunnyrec Corp. — 310-638-4368
20505 Belshaw Ave., Carson, CA 90746

CERRITOS

Grand Technology, Inc. — 562-316-7869
12145 Mora Drive, Unit 1, PO Box 4746, CERRITOS, CA 90703
Mediaid Inc. — 714-367-2848
17517 Fabrica Way, Suite H, Cerritos, CA 90703
Millennium Dental Technologies, Inc. — 562-860-2908
10945 South St., Suite 104-A, Cerritos, CA 90703

Chatsworth

Allman Products — 800-223-6889
21101 Itasca St., Chatsworth, CA 91311
American Copak Corp. — 818-576-1000
9175 Eton Ave., Chatsworth, CA 91311
American Medical Mfg., Inc. — 800-426-6476
9410 Desoto Ave., Unit J, Chatsworth, CA 91311
Atlantic Optical Co., Inc. — 800-423-5175
20801 Nordhoff Street, Chatsworth, CA 91311
Burton Medical Products, Inc. — 800-444-9909
21100 Lassen St., Chatsworth, CA 91311
Chad Therapeutics, Inc. — 800-423-8870
21622 Plummer St., Chatsworth, CA 91311
Computrition, Inc. — 800-222-4488
19808 Nordhoff Place, Chatsworth, CA 91311-6607
Cosmetic Laboratories Of America — 818-717-1301
20245 Sunburst Street, Chatsworth, CA 91311-6219
Dolphin Imaging Systems — 800-548-7241
9200 Eton Avenue, Chatsworth, CA 91311-5807
Immunospec Corporation — 818-717-1840
9428 Eton Avenue, Unit O, Chatsworth, CA 91311
Interscan Corp. — 800-458-6153
21700 Nordhoff Street, PO Box 2496, Chatsworth, CA 91313-2496
Iris Diagnostics — 800-776-4747
9172 Eton Ave., Chatsworth, CA 91311
Iris International, Inc. — 800-776-4747
9162 Eton Avenue, Chatsworth, CA 91311-5805
Lasco Diamond Products — 800-621-4726
9950 Canoga Avenue, Unit A-8, PO Box 4657, Chatsworth, CA 91311-6703
Line One Laboratories, Inc. — 800-222-9848
21230 Lassen St., Chatsworth, CA 91311
Natural Wonders Ca Inc. — 818-341-7007
21011 Itasca Street, Suite E, Chatsworth, CA 91311
Pacific Precision Laboratories, Inc. — 800-793-0179
20447 Nordhoff St., Chatsworth, CA 91311

Photo Research, Inc.   818-341-5151
9731 Topanga Canyon Place, Chatsworth, CA 91311-4135
Replacement Parts Industries, Inc.   800-221-9723
20338 Corisco St., Chatsworth, CA 91313-5019
Space Maintainers Lab   (800) 423-3270
9129 Lurline Ave., Chatsworth, CA 91311
United States Pumice Co.   818-882-0300
20219 Bahama Street, Chatsworth, CA 91311
Viasys Sleep Systems, Llc.   847-689-8410
9305 Eton Avenue, Chatsworth, CA 91311

Chatsworth, CA 91311

Advanced Medical Innovations, Inc.   888-367-2641
9410 De Soto Avenue,, Building J, Chatsworth, CA 91311, CA 91311

Chico

Diestco Manufacturing Corp.   800-795-2392
PO Box 6504, Chico, CA 95927
Lares Research   800-347-3289
295 Lockheed Avenue, Chico, CA 95973
Prowess, Inc.   925-356-0360
1370 Ridgewood Dr., #20, Chico, CA 95973
Suter Dental Manufacturing Company, Inc.   800-368-8376
632 Cedar St., Chico, CA 95928-5015

Chino

A Plus International, Inc   909-591-5168
5138 Eucalyptus Ave., Chino, CA 91710
Awi Industries (Usa), Inc.   909-597-0808
14502 Central Avenue, Chino, CA 91710
Bergman Oral Care   877-356-7727
13745 Seminole Dr., Chino, CA 91710
Cw Medical, Inc.   909-591-5220
5595 Daniels St, Suite E, Chino, CA 91710
Genlabs   800-882-5227
5568 Schaefer Ave., Chino, CA 91710
Jacuzzi, Bath Division   800-288-4002
14880 Monte Vista Avenue, Suite 550, Chino, CA 91710
Patriot Products   909-988-6578
12460 N. Park Ave., Chino, CA 91710
Pm Gloves, Inc.   800-788-9486
13808 Magnolia Avenue, Chino, CA 91710-7027
Sundance Spas, Inc.   800-883-7727
14525 Monte Vista Avenue, Chino, CA 91710

Chula Vista

Jt Usa   800-854-2188
515 Otay Valley Rd., Chula Vista, CA 91911-6059

Citrus Heights

Frontier Dental Laboratory   916-965-4471
7916 Alta Sunrise Dr., Ste. 205, Citrus Heights, CA 95610

City of Industry

Brighton Collectibles Inc.   800-628-7687
14022 Nelson Ave., City of Industry, CA 91746
Darnell-Rose Casters   800-327-6355
17915 Railroad St., City of Industry, CA 91748-1113
Dentamerica Inc.   626-912-1388
18688 E. San Jise Ave., City of Industry, CA 91748
Karman Healthcare, Inc.   800-805-2762
19255 San Jose Ave., City of Industry, CA 91748
Life Guard   626-965-1588
18400 San Jose Avenue, City of Industry, CA 91748
Medical & Clinical Consortium (Mcc)   877-622-8378
13740 East Nelson Ave., City of Industry, CA 91746-2048
Omniqur, Inc.   626-336-9737
15342-b East Valley Blvd., City Of Industry, CA 91746
Teledyne Analytical Instruments   888-789-8168
16830 Chestnut St., City of Industry, CA 91749
Tpc Advanced Technology, Inc.   800-560-8222
18525 East Gale Ave., City of Industry, CA 91748
Whitehall Manufacturing   800-782-7706
15125 Proctor Avenue, City of Industry, CA 91746
Whitehall/A Division Of Acorn Engineering Co.   626-336-4561
15125 Proctor Ave., City Of Industry, CA 91744

Claremont

Bhk, Inc.   909-983-2973
1480 N. Claremont Blvd., Claremont, CA 91711-3538
Second Source, The   800-776-3924
1480 N. Claremont Blvd., Claremont, CA 91711
Ultra-Lum, Inc.   800-809-6559
1480 N. Claremont Blvd., Claremont, CA 91711

Clyde

Spectrum International, Inc.   925-768-1122
1130 Burnett Avenue, Suite J, Clyde, CA 94520

Colton

Cardinal Health 203, Inc.   763-398-8305
1016 East Cooley Dr, Suite N, Colton, CA 92324

Commerce

America Green Dent., Mfg.   323-265-7000
3432 E. 14th St., Commerce, CA 90023
Galaxy Medical Manufacturing Co.   800-876-4599
5411 Sheila Street, Commerce, CA 90040-2103
Ideal Brands, Inc.   213-422-8526
1513 Mirasol St., Commerce, CA 90023
Myers-Stevens Group, Inc.   903-566-6696
2931 Vail Ave., Commerce, CA 90040
Pechiney Plastic Pkg., An Alcan Company   323-721-6777
5416 Union Pacific Ave., Commerce, CA 90022

Comptche

Wells Dental, Inc.   800-233-0521
5860 Flynn Creek Road, P.O. Box 106, Comptche, CA 95427

Compton

Hf Pure Water   800-421-5000
203 W. Artesia Blvd., Compton, CA 90220-5550
Peter Pepper Products, Inc.   800-496-0204
17929 S. Susana Road, PO Box 5769, Compton, CA 90224
Plaskolite West Inc.   800-562-8883
2225 E. Del Amo Blvd., Compton, CA 90220-6303

Concord

Acro Associates   800-672-2276
1990 Olivera Rd., Suite A, Concord, CA 94520
Better Hands Glove Products   800-242-2850
P.O. Box 21641, Concord, CA 94521
Biocare Medical, Llc   925-603-8003
4040 Pike Lane, Concord, CA 94520
H.S. International Co., Inc.   800-811-0072
5040 Commercial Circle,, Unit A, Concord, CA 94520
Hartzell & Son, G.   800-950-2206
2372 Stanwell Circle, Concord, CA 94520-4807
Humanware   800-722-3393
175 Mason Circle, Concord, CA 94520
Life Measurement, Inc.   925-676-6002
1850 Bates Ave., Concord, CA 94520
Sartorius Stedim Sus Inc.   925-689-6650
1910 Mark Court, Concord, CA 94520
Stedim Biosystems, Inc.   800-914-6644
1910 Mark Ct., Concord, CA 94520
Wepco Products, Inc   775-772-5910
1930 Gilly Ln., Concord, CA 94518

Corona

Accent Plastics   951-273-7777
1925 Elise Circle, Corona, CA 92879
Alero, Inc.   951-273-7890
1550 Consumer Circle, Corona, CA 92880
Anatomic Concepts, Inc.   951-549-6800
1691 Delilah Street, Corona, CA 92879
Azmec, Inc.   877-862-9632
519 N. Smith Rd, Unit 110, Corona, CA 92880-6911
Colours Wheelchair   800-892-8998
860 E. Parkridge Avenue, Corona, CA 92879
Dansereau Health Products, Inc.   800-423-5657
210 & 250 E. Harrison Street, Corona, CA 92879
Hoosier, Inc.   951-272-3070
1152 California Ave., Corona, CA 92881
Jiffy Mixer Co., Inc.   800-560-2903
1691 California Avenue, Corona, CA 92881
Kap Medical   951-340-4360
1395 Pico St., Corona, CA 92881
Kmi Kolster Methods, Inc.   909-737-5476
3185 Palisades Dr., Corona, CA 92880
Rkl Technologies, Inc.   800-738-8007
245 Citation Circle, Corona, CA 92880-2523
Tridien Medical   800-474-4225
1691 North Delilah St., Corona, CA 92879
Young Innovations Llc Dba Plak Smacker   800-558-6684
755 Trademark Circle, Corona, CA 92879

Corona Del Mar

Xenotec Ltd.   949-640-4053
511 Hazel Drive, Corona Del Mar, CA 92625

Coronado

Dento-Profile Scale Co.   800-936-8610
1010 Eighth Street, Suite A, Coronado, CA 92118

Corte Madera

Alfred Ueda   307-789-2088
145 Uplands Cir., Corte Madera, CA 94925

Costa Mesa

Battery Specialties   800-854-5759
3530 Cadillac Ave., Costa Mesa, CA 92626
C.J.T. Enterprises, Inc.   714-751-6295
PO Box 10028, Costa Mesa, CA 92627
California Medical Laboratories, Inc.   714-556-7365
1570 Sunland Lane, Costa Mesa, CA 92646

Dr. Roth's Footcare Products, Llc.   800-486-0325
261 E. Imperial Hwy, Suite #570, Costa Mesa, CA 92835
E.A. Beck & Co.   949-645-4072
657 West 19th St. Ste. E, P O Box 10857, Costa Mesa, CA 92627
Grams Medical Inc   949-548-7337
2443 Norse Avenue, Costa Mesa, CA 92627-1369
Heart Rate, Inc.   800-237-2271
3190 E Airport Loop, Costa Mesa, CA 92626-6601
Kingsley Mfg. Co.   800-854-3479
1984 Placentia Ave., Costa Mesa, CA 92627
Medic Unique   310-698-0739
2962 Mindanao Dr., Costa Mesa, CA 92626
Medical Cables, Inc.   800-314-51111
1365 Logan Ave., Costa Mesa, CA 92626-4023
Mge Ups Sytems, Inc.   800-523-0142
1660 Scenic Avenue, Costa Mesa, CA 92626-1410
Newport Medical Instruments, Inc.   800-451-3111
1620 Sunflower Ave, Costa Mesa, CA 92626
Packaging Alternatives Corp.   714-662-0277
1685 Toronto Way, Costa Mesa, CA 92626
Pegasus Research Corp.   877-632-0255
3505 Cadillac Avenue Suite G-5, Costa Mesa, CA 92626
Preventive Dentistry Products, Inc.   714-979-4191
3197-F Airport Loop Dr., Costa Mesa, CA 92626-3424

Covina

Arcapco, Inc.   626-966-4556
754 Arrow Grand Circle, Covina, CA 91722
Composites Horizons, Inc.   626-331-0861
1471 Industrial Park St., Covina, CA 91722
Connector Contacts   877-463-9029
714 East Edna Place, Covina, CA 91723
Human Measurement Systems   626-201-2437
1159 N. Conwell Ave. # 311, P.o. Box 2442, Covina, CA 91722
Medsep Corp., A Subsidiary Of Pall Corp.   516-484-5400
1630 Industrial Park St., Covina, CA 91722

Cowan Heights

Ivd Technologies   714-549-5050
2002 S. Grand Ave Ste A, Cowan Heights, CA 92705

Cucamonga

Acro Biotech Llc.   909-466-6892
9500 7th Street Unit M, Cucamonga, CA 91730
Invacare Supply Group   508-429-1000
11231 Jersey Blvd, Suite 101, Cucamonga, CA 91730

Culver City

Allegro Biodiesel Corporation   800-949-4762
6245 Bristol Parkway, Suite 263, Culver City, CA 90230
Inovel Llc   866-546-6835
10111 W. Jefferson Blvd., Culver City, CA 90232
Jason Natural Products Inc., Personal Care Divisio   310-945-4308
8468 Warner Dr., Culver City, CA 90232
Karl Storz Endoscopy-America Inc.   800-421-0837
600 Corporate Pointe, Culver City, CA 90230-7600
Magnet Sales & Manufacturing   800-421-6692
11248 Playa Ct., Culver City, CA 90230
Moldex-Metric, Inc.   800-421-0668
10111 West Jefferson Blvd., Culver City, CA 90232
Mxe, Inc.   800-252-1801
12107 W. Jefferson Blvd., Culver City, CA 90230-6219
Oralgiene Usa, Inc.   800-933-6725
8460 Higuera St., Culver City, CA 90232
Self-Programmed Control Center   800-782-2256
11949 Jefferson Blvd., #104, Culver City, CA 90230
Sofie Biosciences   310-242-6794
6162 Bristol Parkway, Culver City, CA 90230
Spectrum Dental Llc.   310-845-8345
8554 Hayden Place, Culver City, CA 90232
Universal Medical Products   310-839-9738
9435 Venice Blvd, Culver City, CA 90232

Cupertino

Boston Scientific Corp.   408-517-2800
10231 Bubb Rd., Cupertino, CA 95014-4167
Cardeon Corp.   408-253-3319
10600 North Tantau Ave., Cupertino, CA 95014
Cardiovention, Inc.   408-873-3400
19200 Stevens Creek Blvd., #200, Cupertino, CA 95014
Durect Corp.   408.777.1417
2 Results Way, Cupertino, CA 95014
Novare Surgical Systems, Inc.   408-873-3161
10440 Bubb Road, Suite A, Cupertino, CA 95014
Skeletal Kinetics, Llc   408-366-5000
10201 Bubb Rd., Cupertino, CA 95014

Cypress

Creative Medical Technologies   (888) 535-8180
6060 Phyllis Drive, Cypress, CA 90630
Focus Diagnostics, Inc.   800-838-4548
11331 Valley View Street, Cypress, CA 90630
Focus Technologies   800-445-0185
5785 Corporate Avenue, Cypress, CA 90630-4714

Leader Instruments Corp.   800-645-5104
6484 Commerce Dr., Cypress, CA 90630
Medcom, Inc.   800-877-1443
6060 Phyllis Drive, Cypress, CA 90630
Medison America, Inc.   800-829-SONO
11075 Knott Ave, Suite C, Cypress, CA 90630
Neo Pharm Inc.   714-226-0070
10532 Walker St., Suite #b, Cypress, CA 90630
Shercon Inc.   800-228-3218
6262 Katella Ave, Cypress, CA 90630
Ushio America, Inc.   800-838-7446
5440 Cerritos Avenue, Cypress, CA 90630-4567

Daly City

SpineDok, Division of Altrueon LLC.   650-755-7750
235 Westlake Center, #212, Daly City, CA 94015

Danville

BugLab LLC   925-208-1952
310 Freitas Court, Danville, CA 94526
Oridion Medical Inc.   888-674-3466
140 Towne& Country Drive, SuiteB, Danville, CA 94526

Davis

Antibodies, Inc.   800-824-8540
PO Box 1560, Davis, CA 95617-1560
Cedaron Medical, Inc.   800-424-1007
PO Box 2100, Davis, CA 95617
Gold Standard Diagnostics   530-759-8000
2851 Spafford St., Suite A, Davis, CA 95618
Integrated Surgical Systems   530-792-2600
1850 Research Park Drive, Davis, CA 95616

Del Mar

Billups-Rothenberg, Inc.   877-755-3309
PO Box 977, Del Mar, CA 92014-0977
Cbs Scientific Co., Inc.   800-243-4959
po Box 856, Del Mar, CA 92014
Femcap Incorporated   858-792-2624
14058 Mira Montana Drive, Del Mar, CA 92014

Desert Hot Springs

Back Support Systems   800-669-2225
67684 San Andreas, Desert Hot Springs, CA 92240

Diablo

Diablo Sales & Marketing, Inc.   925-648-1611
PO Box 408, Diablo, CA 94526

Diamond Bar

Biosense Webster, Inc   800-729-9010
3333 Diamond Canyon Road, Diamond Bar, CA 91765

Diamond Springs

Adept-Med International, Inc.   800-222-8445
665 Pleasant Valley Rd., Diamond Springs, CA 95619
Co-Oral-Ite Dental Mfg. Co.   530-621-4913
6635 Merchandise Way, Diamond Springs, CA 95619

Dinuba

M.J. Thiesen Co. Inc.   800-443-8773
151 S N ST, Dinuba, CA 93618

Dixon

Complete System Diagnostics, Inc.   800-722-4273
1170 North Lincoln, Suite 108, Dixon, CA 95620

Duarte

Compass Bioscience   626-359-9645
1850 Evergreen St., Duarte, CA 91010-2906
Endodent, Inc.   626-359-5715
851 Meridian St., Duarte, CA 91010

Dublin

Carl Zeiss Meditec Inc.   877-486-7473
5160 Hacienda Drive, Dublin, CA 94568
Dental Technologies, Inc.   800-229-0936
5601 Arnold Rd, Dublin, CA 94568

El Cajon

El Cajon Hearing Aid Center   619-442-5634
761 Arnele Ave., El Cajon, CA 92020
Mit Service, Inc.   800-343-8828
1354 Swallow Drive, Suite 104, El Cajon, CA 92020
Precision Metal Products Inc.   619-448-2711
850 West Bradley Ave., El Cajon, CA 92020
Professional's Choice Sports Medicine Products, Inc.   800-331-9421
2025 Gillestie way suite #106, El Cajon, CA 92020

El Centro

Aisling Industries   760-353-4000
621 East Heil Ave., El Centro, CA 92243

El Dorado Hills

Evans Medical Inc.   916-939-2451
1529 Terracina Drive, El Dorado Hills, CA 95762
Guided Wave Inc.   916-939-4300
5190 Golden Foothill Pkwy., El Dorado Hills, CA 95762-9608
Hayes Medical, Inc.   800-240-0500
1115 Windfield Way, Suite 100, El Dorado Hills, CA 95762
Synvasive Technology, Inc.   800-925-2337
4925 Robert J. Mathews Pkwy., El Dorado Hills, CA 95762
Wyndgate Technologies   800-996-3428
4925 Robert J. Mathews Pkwy.,, Suite 100, El Dorado Hills, CA 95762

El Monte

Lee Pharmaceuticals   626-442-3141
1434 Santa Anita Ave., El Monte, CA 91733
W.H.P.M., Inc.   978-927-3808
9662 Telstar Ave., El Monte, CA 91731

El Segundo

Sunmed Usa Llc.   310-531-8222
841 Apollo Street, Suite 334, El Segundo, CA 90245

Emeryville

Eastman Medical Products Inc.   800-373-4410
2000 Powell St., Suite 1540, Emeryville, CA 94608
Kinemed, Inc.   855-546-3633
5980 Horton Street, Suite 400, Emeryville, CA 94608
Tethys Bioscience Inc.   888-697-7339
5858 Horton Street, Suite 550, Emeryville, CA 94608

Encinitas

Eucardio Laboratory, Inc.   760-632-1824
2216 Silver Peak Place, Encinitas, CA 92024
Hex Laboratory Systems   800-729-2085
1042B El Camino Real, Ste. 308, Encinitas, CA 92024
Medica, Inc.   800-845-6496
336 Encinitas Blvd., Suite 200, Encinitas, CA 92024
Science 20/20, Inc.   760-753-7928
681 Encinitas Blvd, Suite 302, Encinitas, CA 92024
Tandem Medical, Inc.   760-943-0100
535 Encinitas Blvd, Suite 109, Encinitas, CA 92024

Encino

Adelberg Laboratories Inc.   818-784-1141
16821 Oak View Dr., Encino, CA 91436
Jant Pharmacal Corp.   800-676-5565
16255 Ventura Blvd., Suite 505, Encino, CA 91436

Escondido

American Innotek, Inc.   800-366-3941
2320 Meyers Ave., Escondido, CA 92029
Arcmate Mfg. Corp.   888-637-1926
637 S. Vinewood St., Escondido, CA 92029
Datrix   760-480-8874
340 State Place, Escondido, CA 92029
Oralbotic Research, Inc.   760-743-5160
701 South Andreasen Dr., Suite C, Escondido, CA 92029
Ultra-Cal, Inc.   760-741-7207
3014 Laurashawn Ln, Escondido, CA 92026
Zest Anchors, Inc.   800-262-2310
2061 Wineridge Place #100, Escondido, CA 92029

Fairfield

Aalba Dent, Inc.   707-864-3334
400 Watt Dr., Fairfield, CA 94534
Chemsw, Inc.   800-536-0404
4771 Mangels Blvd, Fairfield, CA 94534

Fallbrook

Axelgaard Manufacturing Company, Ltd.   760-728-3430
520 industrial way, Fallbrook, CA 92028-2852
Med-Fit Systems, Inc.   800-831-7665
3553 Rosa Way, Fallbrook, CA 92028
Q.T.I. Corp.   760-723-9825
879 Del Valle Drive, Fallbrook, CA 92028

Ferndale

Notoco Llc.   707-786-4400
660 Berding St., P.o. Box 300, Ferndale, CA 95536

Folsom

Intel Corp. Digital Health Group   916-356-8080
1900 Prairie City Rd., FM7-197, Folsom, CA 95630

Foothill Ranch

Bella Products, Inc.   877-550-5655
27136 Burbank, Foothill Ranch, CA 92610
Nihon Kohden America, Inc.   800-325-0283
90 Icon St., Foothill Ranch, CA 92610
Oakley, Inc.   800-431-1439
One Icon, Foothill Ranch, CA 92610
Ossur Americas, Inc   800-222-4284
19762 Pauling, Foothill Ranch, CA 92610

Fortuna

Barrett Engineering   714-246-4388
606 L Street, Fortuna, CA 95540

Foster City

AB Sciex   1 877-740-2129
110 Marsh Road, Foster City, CA 94404
Applied Biosystems   800-345-5724
850 Lincoln Centre Drive, Foster City, CA 94404
Biocheck, Inc.   650-573-1968
323 Vintage Park Drive, Foster City, CA 94404
Gilead Sciences   650-574-3000
333 Lakeside Dr., Foster City, CA 94404
Invitrogen Corporation   800-955-6288
101 Lincoln Centre Drive, Foster City, CA 94404
Linc Quantum Analytics   800-992-4199
363 Vintage Park Dr., Foster City, CA 94404-1185
Philips Healthcare Informatics, Inc   800-934-7372
4100 East Third Ave, Suite 101, Foster City, CA 94404

Foster City,

Terarecon, Inc.   877-354-1100
4000 East 3rd Avenue, Suite 200, Foster City,, CA 94404

Fountain Valley

Aqua-Cel Corp.   888-254-HEAT
17137 Sparkleberry St, Fountain Valley, CA 92708-3538
Dentalaire Products   800-866-6881
17150 Newhope #407, Fountain Valley, CA 92708
Genie Scientific, Inc.   800-545-8816
17442 Mt. Cliffwood Circle, Fountain Valley, CA 92708
Nobles Medical Technologies, Inc.   714-751-8332
17080 Newhope St., Fountain Valley, CA 92708
Spiracle Technology   714-418-1091
16520 Harbor Blvd., Unit D, Fountain Valley, CA 92708
Sterilis Inc.   714-437-9801
17092 Newhope St., Fountain Valley, CA 92708
Sutura, Inc.   714-437-9801
17080 Newhope St., Fountain Valley, CA 92708
U.S. Women Institute   714-378-5606
9940 Takbert Avenue, Suite 303, Fountain Valley, CA 92708

Fremont

Alara Inc.   800-410-2525
47505 Seabridge Drive, Fremont, CA 94538
Angiodynamics, Inc.   510-771-0400
46421 Landing Parkway, Fremont, CA 94538
Angioscore, Inc.   877-264-4692
5055 Brandin Court, Fremont, CA 94538
Angioscore, Inc.   877-264-4692
5055 Brandin Court, fremont, CA 94538
Boston Scientific-Neurovascular   510-440-7700
47900 Bayside Pkwy., Fremont, CA 94538-6515
Cardima, Inc.   888-354-0300
47266 Benicia St., Fremont, CA 94538-1372
Clean Esd Products, Inc.   510-257-5080
48340 Milmont Drive, Fremont, CA 94538
Cytek Development, Inc.   510-657-0102
4059 Clipper Court, Fremont, CA 94538
Delta Products Corp.   510-668-5100
4405 Cushing Parkway, Fremont, CA 94538
Efotoxpress Inc.   510-979-9100
46560 Fremont Blvd., Unit 115, Fremont, CA 94538
Ems Pacific, Inc.   800-575-5093
4480 Enterprise St., Unit D, Fremont, CA 94538
Encoll Corp.   510-795-8581
4576 Enterprise Street, Fremont, CA 94538
Gentran, Inc.   510-226-9343
42025 Osgood Rd, Fremont, CA 94539
Kyocera Industrial Ceramics Corp.   800-826-0527
472 Kato Terrace, Fremont, CA 94539
Lab Vision Corp.   510-991-2800
47777 Warm Springs Blvd., Fremont, CA 94539
Labo America, Inc.   510-445-1257
920 Auburn Ct., Fremont, CA 94538
Linear Laboratories Corporation   800-536-0262
42025 Osgood Road, Fremont, CA 94539
Medsphere International, Inc   510-656-8232
48531 Warm Springs Blvd., Suite 417, Fremont, CA 94539
Microgenics Corporation   800-232-3342
46360 Fremont Blvd., Fremont, CA 94538
Mission X-Ray   800-676-8718
45459 Industrial Pllace, Suite 1, Fremont, CA 94538-6450
Neo Medical Inc.   888-450-3334
42514 Albrea Street, Fremont, CA 94538
Nidek Inc.   800-223-9044
47651 Westinghouse Drive, Fremont, CA 94539-7474
Nidek, Inc.   510-226-5700
47651 Westinghouse Dr., Fremont, CA 94539
Nitinol Devices & Components, Inc.   510-683-2000
47533 Westinghouse Dr., Fremont, CA 94539
Opnext Inc.   510-580-8828
46429 Landing Parkway, Fremont, CA 94538

Optovue, Inc. — 866-344-8948
45531 Northport Loop West, Fremont, CA 94538
Perkinelmer Optoelectronics — 800-775-6786
44370 Christy Street, Fremont, CA 94538-3180
Prime Solutions — 510-490-2299
4261 Business Center Drive, Fremont, CA 94538
Respiratory Diagnostics, Inc. — 425-881-8300
47987 Fremont Blvd., Fremont, CA 94538
Sensor Dynamics, Inc. — 510-623-1459
4568 Enterprise St., Fremont, CA 94538
SeptRx Inc — 510-225-9170
47533 Westinghouse Drive, Suite C, Fremont, CA 94539
Smith Companies Dental Products — 800-336-3263
4368 Enterprise St., Fremont, CA 94538-6305
Spring Bioscience — 510-979-9460
46755 Fremont Blvd, Fremont, CA 94538
Tomy Tech U.S.A., Inc. — 800-545-8669
40479 Encyclopedia Circle, Fremont, CA 94538-2452
Vioptix, Inc. — 510-360-7506
47224 Mission Falls Court, Fremont, CA 94539
WaferGen Biosystems Inc. — 510-651-4450
7400 Paseo Padre Parkway, Fremont, CA 94555

Fresno

Daniels Sharpsmart, Inc. — 559-351-9593
4144 E. Therese Avenue, Fresno, CA 93727
Minisun, Llc — 559-439-4600
935 Mill Creek Drive, Fresno, CA 93720
Prime Engineering — 800-827-8263
4202 W Sierra Madre Avenue, Fresno, CA 93722
Sunrise Medical Hhg Inc — (800) 333-4000
2842 Business Park Avenue, Fresno, CA 93727

Fullerton

Academy Savant — 800-472-8268
PO Box 3670, Fullerton, CA 92834
Advanced American Biotechnology (Aab) — 714-870-0290
1166 E. Valencia Dr., Unit 6C, Fullerton, CA 92631-5237
Alan's Wheelchairs & Repairs — 800-693-4344
109 South Harbor Blvd.,, Suite B, Fullerton, CA 92832
Aurident, Inc. — 800-422-7373
P.O. Box 7200, 610 South State College Blvd., Fullerton, CA 92631
Covoc Corp. — 800-725-3266
1194 E. Valencia Drive, Fullerton, CA 92831
Elabsupply — 714-446-8740
1001 Starbuck Street, Suite C306, Fullerton, CA 92833
Fastec Medical Systems — 866-463-3633
802 Whitewater Drive, Fullerton, CA 92833
Foam Craft — 714-459-9971
2441 Cypress Way, Fullerton, CA 92831
Fuller Laboratories — 888-826-7660
1135 E. Truslow Avenue, Fullerton, CA 92831

Garden Grove

American Pacific Plastic Fabricators, Inc. — 714-891-3191
7274 Lampson Ave., Garden Grove, CA 92841
Catalina Cylinders — 714-890-0999
7300 Anaconda Avenue, Garden Grove, CA 92841
Genesen Pan America, Inc. — 714-799-1735
7245 Garden Grove Blvd., #d, Garden Grove, CA 92841
Hycor Biomedical, Inc. — 800-382-2527
7272 Chapman Ave., Garden Grove, CA 92841
Sensorex Corp. — 714-895-4344
11751 Markon Drive, Garden Grove, CA 92841
St. Paul Biotech — 714-903-1000
11555 Monarch St., Garden Grove, CA 92841

Gardena

Angelus Medical & Optical Co., Inc. — 310-769-6060
13007 S. Western Avenue, Gardena, CA 90249-1919
Barco Of California — 800-421-1932
350 West Rosecrans Ave., Gardena, CA 90247-0835
Bestway Products Co. — 310-329-0600
16602 S. Broadway St., Gardena, CA 90248
Cweco, Inc. — 800-292-9326
1156 W. 135th St., P.O. Box 2456, Gardena, CA 90247
E-Z Sales & Manufacturing Inc. — 310-324-5980
1432 West 166th Street, Gardena, CA 90247
Lenjoy Medical Engineering, Inc. — 310-353-2481
13112 Crenshaw Blvd., Gardena, CA 90249-2466
Mars Air Doors — 800-421-1266
14716 S. Broadway, Gardena, CA 90248-1814
Midmark Diagnostics Group — 800-643-6275
1125 W 90th Street, Gardena, CA 90248
Mikron Precision, Inc. — 310-515-6221
1558-c West 139th St., Gardena, CA 90249
Onyx Industries, Inc./Quadrtech — 310-851-6161
521 West Rosecrans Avenue, Gardena, CA 90248
Peerless Injection Molding, Llc. — 310-768-8023
14600 S. Main Street, Gardena, CA 90248
Sci Gen, Inc. — 310-324-6576
333 E. Gardena Blvd., Gardena, CA 90248
Spectrum Laboratory Products, Inc. — 800-813-1514
14422 S. San Pedro St., Gardena, CA 90248-2027

Gilroy

Chalgren Enterprises, Inc. — 408-847-3994
380 Tomkins Ct., Gilroy, CA 95020-6315
Jari Electrode Supply — 800-745-1934
380 Tomkins Ct., Gilroy, CA 95020
North Coast Medical, Inc. — 800-821-9319
8100 Camino Arroyo, Gilroy, CA 95020

Glassell

Apc Industries — 323-255-7101
3030 Fletcher Dr., Glassell, CA 90065
Camsight Co., Inc. — 323-259-1900
3380 N. San Fernando Road, Glassell, CA 90065

Glendale

American Dent-All Inc. — 877-864-6294
5140 San Fernando Road, Glendale, CA 91204
Blanchard Ostomy Products — 818-242-6789
1510 Raymond Avenue, Glendale, CA 91201
Crystalmark Dental Systems, Inc. — 818-240-7596
621 Ruberta Ave., Glendale, CA 91201
Edwin Corp. — 1-888-323-3941
425 Hill Dr., Ste. H, Glendale, CA 91206
Imagederm, Inc. — 866-462-4334
632 W Elk Ave, Glendale, CA 91204
Medical Associates Network — 818-500-7711
801 N. Brand Blvd., #690, Glendale, CA 91203

Glendora

Electro-Tech Products Inc. — 909-592-1434
2001 E. Gladstone Street,#a, Glendora, CA 91740
Oasis Medical, Inc. — 800-528-9786
510-528 S. Vermont Ave., Glendora, CA 91741
Ormco Corp. — 800-672-5068
1332 S. Lone Hill Ave., Glendora, CA 91740

Glennville

Hoyle Products, Inc. — 800-345-1950
10675 Highway 155, Glennville, CA 93226

Goleta

Advanced Vision Science — 800-235-5781
5743 Thornwood Drive, Goleta, CA 93117-3801
Allergan — 800-624-4261
71 S. Los Carneros Rd., Goleta, CA 93117
Conmed Linvatec Endoscopy — 800-448-6506
7416 Hollister Avenue, Goleta, CA 93117
Inogen, Inc. — 805-562-0500
326 Bollay Drive, Goleta, CA 93117
La Labs — 805-562-9889
7334 Hollister Ave., Suite H, Goleta, CA 93117
Med Labs Inc. — 800-968-2486
28 Vereda Cordillera, Goleta, CA 93117-5300
Medtronic Neurosurgery — 800-468-9710
125 Cremona Dr., Goleta, CA 93117
Pointe Conception Medical, Incorporated — 805-964-8104
749 Ward Drive, Goleta, CA 93111
Steri-Shield Products — 805-692-4972
336 S. Fairview Ave, Goleta, CA 93117
V.I.R. Engineering, Inc. — 805-964-0553
5951 Encina Road, Suite 209, Goleta, CA 93117

Golita

Karl Storz Imaging — 805-968-5563
175 Cremona Dr., Golita, CA 93117-5502

Granada Hills

Futuremed America, Inc. — 800-222-6780
15700 Devonshire St., Granada Hills, CA 91344-7225

Grand Terrace

Panadent Corp. — 800-368-9777
22573 Barton Road, Grand Terrace, CA 92313

Grass Valley

Applied Science, Inc. — 866-436-6356
983 Golden Gate Terrace, Grass Valley, CA 95945
Biosure, Inc. — 800-345-2267
12301 Loma Rica Drive, Suite G, Grass Valley, CA 95945
Eigen — 888-924-2020
13366 Grass Valley Avenue, Grass Valley, CA 95945
Orthomed Products, Inc. — 800-338-8512
12150 Charles Drive, #5, Grass Valley, CA 95945
The Myo Tool Co. — 530-272-7306
1020-d Mccourtney Road, Grass Valley, CA 95949
Tri-Continent Scientific, Inc. — 530-274-4240
12555 Loma Rica Dr., #2, Grass Valley, CA 95945
Tricontinent — 800-937-4738
12555 Loma Rica Drive, Grass Valley, CA 95945

Half Moon Bay

West Coast Surgical Llc. — 650-728-8095
141 California Ave, Suite 101, Half Moon Bay, CA 94019

Harbor City

Varian Sample Preparation Products   800-421-2825
24201 Frampton Avenue, Harbor City, CA 90710-2105

Hawaiian Gardens

Synergent Biochem, Inc.   562-809-3389
12026 Centralia Ave., Unit G & H, Hawaiian Gardens, CA 90716

Hawthorne

Dolphin Medical Inc.   310-978-0516
12525 Chadron Ave., Hawthorne, CA 90250
Osi Systems, Inc.   310-978-0516
12525 Chadron Avenue, Hawthorne, CA 90250
Osteometer Meditech, Inc.   866-421-7762
12515 Chadron Avenue, Hawthorne, CA 90250
Vacuum Atmospheres Co.   310-644-0255
4652 W. Rosecrans Avenue, Hawthorne, CA 90250-6896

Hayward

GenturaDx   510-725-4767
24590 Clawiter Road, Hayward, CA 94545
Advanced Cell Diagnostics Inc.   510-576-8800
26229 Eden Landing Road, Hayward, CA 94545
Airgas, Northern California And Nevada   916-379-1050
20725 Corsair Blvd., Hayward, CA 94545
Amedica Biotech, Inc.   888-206-9919
28301 Industrial Blvd Suite K, Hayward, CA 94545
Aradigm Corp.   510-265-9000
3929 Point Eden Way, Hayward, CA 94545
Baxter Healthcare Corporation   847-473-6141
21026 Alexander Court, Hayward, CA 94545
Biolog, Inc.   800-284-4949
21124 Cabot Blvd., Hayward, CA 94545-1130
Cholestech Corp.   800-733-0404
3347 Investment Blvd., Hayward, CA 94545-3808
Farallon Medical, Inc.   510-785-0800
3521 Investment Blvd., Suite 1, Hayward, CA 94545
Guava Technologies, Inc.   866-448-2827
25801 Industrial Blvd., Hayward, CA 94545
Hantel Technologies   510-487-1561
721 Sandoval Way, Hayward, CA 94544
Malcomtech International   510-293-0580
26200 Industrial Blvd., Hayward, CA 94545
Maytex Corp.   800-462-9839
23521 Foley Street, Hayward, CA 94545
Mexpo International, Inc.   800-838-8299
2695B McCone Ave., Hayward, CA 94545
Solta Medical, Inc.   877-782-2286
25881 Industrial Boulevard, Hayward, CA 94545
Thermage, Inc.   1-888-437-2935
25881 Industrial Blvd., Hayward, CA 94545

Hayward,

G & K Services   510) 293-5840
3444 Depot Rd., Hayward,, CA 94545

Healdsburg

In Vivo Metric   707-433-2949
PO Box 397, Healdsburg, CA 95448

Hemet

C.A.M. Supply, Inc.   909-851-7114
490 East Menlo Ave., Hemet, CA 92543
Medi-Kid Co.   888-463-3543
P.O. Box 5398, Hemet, CA 92544

Hercules

Bio-Rad Laboratories   800-866-0305
1000 Alfred Nobel Drive, Hercules, CA 94547
Bio-Rad Laboratories Inc., Clinical Systems Div.   800-224-6723
4000 Alfred Nobel Dr., Hercules, CA 94547
Bio-Rad Laboratories, Inc.   800-866-0305
1000 Alfred Nobel Drive, Hercules, CA 94547-1811
Bio-Rad Laboratories, Life Science Group   800-424-6723
2000 Alfred Nobel Dr., Hercules, CA 94547
Biorad Laboratories   800-2BI-ORAD
1000 Alfred Nobel Drive, Hercules, CA 94547
Kontur Kontact Lens Co., Inc.   800-227-1320
642 Alfred Nobel Drive, Hercules, CA 94547-1834

Hesperia

Alltech Associates, Inc.   847-282-2090
17434 Mojave Street, Hesperia, CA 92345
Small Beginnings Inc.   760-949-7707
17525 Alder Street, Suite 28, Hesperia, CA 92345

Hidden Valley Lake

Barrows Company   707-987-0460
18701 Glenwood Road, Hidden Valley Lake, CA 95467

Huntington Beach

Adlib, Inc.   714-895-9529
5142 Bolsa Ave., Suite 106, Huntington Beach, CA 92649

Armm, Inc.   714-848-8190
17744 Sampson Lane, Huntington Beach, CA 92647
Blue White Industries, Inc.   714-893-8529
5300 Business Drive, Huntington Beach, CA 92649
Calmoseptine, Inc.   800-800-3405
16602 Burke Lane, Huntington Beach, CA 92647-4536
Cambro Manufacturing   800-833-3003
5801 Skylab Rd., Huntington Beach, CA 92647
Circular Traction Supply, Inc.   800-247-6535
7602 Talbert Avenue, Unit 9, Huntington Beach, CA 92648
Clinical Pharmacies, Inc.   800-669-6973
21622 Surveyor Circle, #8-C, Huntington Beach, CA 92646
Data Hunter LLC   714-892-5461
5412 Balsa Ave, Unit G, Huntington Beach, CA 92649
Dean Medical Instruments, Inc.   714-893-2772
15502 Commerce Lane, Huntington Beach, CA 92649
Electronic Waveform Laboratory, Inc.   800-874-9283
16168 Beach Blvd., Suite 232, Huntington Beach, CA 92647
Gencosoft Llc.   714-625-8972
17042 Pinehurst Lane, Suite B, Huntington Beach, CA 92647
Hull Anesthesia, Inc.   800-400-4484
7521 Talbert Avenue, Huntington Beach, CA 92648
Medi-Tech Holdings, Inc.   714-841-8603
15209 Springdale Ave., Huntington Beach, CA 92649

Inglewood

Magnetecs   310-670-7700
10524 La Cienega Blvd, Inglewood, CA 90304
Roloke   800-533-8212
127 W. Hazel Street, Inglewood, CA 90302
Scapa Medical   310-419-0567
540 N. Oak St., Inglewood, CA 90302-2942

Irvine

Advanced Sterilization Products   800-595-0200
33 Technology Dr., Irvine, CA 92618
Affinity Medical Technologies Llc   949-477-9495
1732 Reynolds Avenue, Irvine, CA 92614
Agendia Inc.   888-321-2732
22 Morgan, Irvine, CA 92618
Alcon Manufacturing, Ltd.   949-753-1393
15800 Alton Parkway, Irvine, CA 92618
Allergan   800-366-6554
2525 Dupont Dr., Irvine, CA 92623
Alliance Medical Products, Inc.   949-768-4690
9342 Jeronimo Rd., Irvine, CA 92618
Alsius Corp.   949-453-0150
15770 Laguna Canyon, Suite 150, Irvine, CA 92618
American Imex   800-521-8286
16520 Aston St., Irvine, CA 92606
Ampronix, Inc.   800-400-7972
15 Whatney, Irvine, CA 92620
Aspen Medical Products   800-295-2776
6481 Oak Canyon, Irvine, CA 92618
Aubrey Group   949-581-0188
6 Cromwell, Suite 100, Irvine, CA 92618
Baxter Healthcare Corporation, Medication Delivery   949-851-9066
17511 Armstrong Ave, Irvine, CA 92614
Bei Technologies, Inc.   949-341-9500
170 Technology Drive, Irvine, CA 92618
Bien Air Usa, Inc.   800-433-2636
17880 Sky Park Circle, Ste 140, Irvine, CA 92614
Bio-Medical Devices   800-443-3842
17171 Daimler Ave, Irvine, CA 92614
Bio-Rad, Diagnostics Group   800-854-6737
9500 Jeronimo Rd., Irvine, CA 92618-2017
Biolase Technology, Inc.   888-424-6527
4 Cromwell, Irvine, CA 92618
Biomerica, Inc.   800-854-3002
17571 Von Karman Ave, Irvine, CA 92614
Biotemps Dental Laboratory   949-440-2683
2181 Dupont Dr., Irvine, CA 92612
Branan Medical Corp.   866-468-3287
140 Technology, Suite 400, Irvine, CA 92618
Brevet, Inc.   949-474-7000
16661 Jamboree Blvd., Irvine, CA 92606
CANDELIS, INC.   800 800 8600
18821 Bardeen Ave., Irvine, CA 92612
Canon Development Americas, Inc.   949-932-3100
15955 Alton Parkway, Irvine, CA 92618-3731
Cardiomedics, Inc.   888-849-0200
7 Whatney, Suite B, Irvine, CA 92618-2849
Corevalve, Inc.   949-679-2707
2 Jenner, Suite 100, Irvine, CA 92618
Datcard Systems Inc   877-543-3898
7 Goodyear, Irvine, CA 92618
Easi File Corp.   800-800-5563
6 Wrigley St., Irvine, CA 92618
Edwards Lifesciences, Llc.   800-424-3278
One Edwards Way, Irvine, CA 92614
Ellipse Technologies, Inc   949-837-3600
13900 Alton Parkway, Irvine, CA 92618

Endologix, Inc. — 800-983-2284
11 Studebaker, Irvine, CA 92618

Ev3 Neurovascular — 800-716-6700
9775 Toledo Way, Irvine, CA 92618

Freedom Innovations, Inc. — 888-818-6777
30 Fairbanks, Suite 114, Irvine, CA 92618

Hancock/Jaffe Laboratories — 949-261-2900
2807 Mcgaw Ave., Irvine, CA 92614

Healthsonix Inc. — 949-417-8880
14252 Culver Drive, Suite 107, Irvine, CA 92604-0317

Horiba Abx — 888-903-5001
34 Bunsen Drive, Irvine, CA 92618-4210

Indigo Orb, Inc. — 949-784-0303
2454 Alton Parkway, Irvine, CA 92606

Innovative Med Inc. — 877-779-9492
4 Autry, Suite B, Irvine, CA 92618

Interpore Cross International — 800-722-4489
181 Technology Dr., Irvine, CA 92618

Interventional Spine, Inc. — 800-497-0484
13700 Alton Pkwy., Suite 160, Irvine, CA 92618

Intralase Corp. — 714-247-8200
9701 Jeronimo Road, Irvine, CA 92618-1916

Invitrx, Inc. — 877-468-4879
101 Theory, suite 100, Irvine, CA 92617

Irvine Biomedical, Inc. — 888-IBI-9876
2375 Morse Avenue, Irvine, CA 92614-6234

J. Hewitt Incorporated — 800-543-9488
6 Faraday, Unit B, Irvine, CA 92618

J. Morita Usa, Inc. — 888-566-7482
9 Mason, Irvine, CA 92618

Kentec Medical Inc. — 800-825-5996
17871 Fitch, Irvine, CA 92614

Masimo Corp. — 800-326-4890
40, 50 & 60 Parker, Irvine, CA 92618

Medennium, Inc. — 949-789-5385
9 Parker, Suite 150, Irvine, CA 92618

Medical Technical Products — 949-551-4762
14980 Sand Canyon Avenue, Suite 200, Irvine, CA 92618-2102

Meridian America Medicals, Inc. — 800-638-8093
2691 Richter Ave., Suite 104, Irvine, CA 92606

MiCardia Corporation — 949-951-4888
30 Hughes, Suite 206, Irvine, CA 92618

MindFrame Inc — 949-204-0800
12 Goodyear, Suite 125, Irvine, CA 92618

MI Lifesciences — 949-699-3800
17 Hammond, Suite 408, Irvine, CA 92618

Monarch Labs, Llc. — 949-679-3000
17875 Sky Park Circle, Suite K, Irvine, CA 92614

National Medical Products, Inc. — 949-768-1147
57 Parker St., Irvine, CA 92618

Neomatrix, Llc — 877-425-6727
19800 MacArthur Blvd.,, Suite 690, Irvine, CA 92612

Neomend, Inc. — 888-776-4351
60 Technology Drive, Irvine, CA 92618

Newport Corporation — 949-863-3144
1791 Deere Avenue, Irvine, CA 92606

Newport Franklin, Inc. — 800-598-6783
1791 Deere Avenue, Irvine, CA 92606

Nkus Lab — 949-474-9207
2446 Dupont Dr., Irvine, CA 92612-1523

Oct Usa, Inc. — 720-962-5412
17 Hammond, Suite 411, Irvine, CA 92618

Onset Medical Corporation — 949-716-1100
13900 Alton Parkway, Suite 120, Irvine, CA 92618

OvaGene Oncology — 949-748-6415
10 Pasteur, Suite 150, Irvine, CA 92618

PRO-DEX, INC — 800-562-6204
2361 McGaw Ave., Irvine, CA 92614

Passy-Muir Inc. — 800-634-5397
PMB 273, 4521 Campus Dr., Irvine, CA 92612

Pegasus Biologics, Inc. — 949-585-9430
10 Pasteur, Suite 150, Irvine, CA 92618

Phoenix Medical Devices, Llc — 800-689-9892
2458 Alton Parkway, Irvine, CA 92606

Phygen, LLC — 800-939-7008
2301 Dupont Drive, Suite 510, Irvine, CA 92612

Prismatik Dentalcraft, Inc. — 949-440-2683
2181 Dupont Drive, Irvine, CA 92612

Pro-Dex, Inc. — 800-562-6204
2361 McGaw Ave., Irvine, CA 92614

Quality Systems, Inc. — 800-888-7955
18111 Von Karman Ave., Suite 600, Irvine, CA 92612

REVERSE MEDICAL CORPORATION — 877.639.0081
13700 Alton Parkway, Suite 167, Irvine, CA 92618

Reach Global Industries, Inc. (Reachgood) — 888-518-8389
8 Corporate Park, Suite 300, Irvine, CA 92606

Refractec, Inc. — 949-784-2600
5 Jenner, Suite 150, Irvine, CA 92618

Robomedica, Inc. — 877-762-6633
One Technology Drive, Bldg. C, Suite C-511, Irvine, CA 92618

Surgi-Vision, Inc. — 949-900-6833
5 Musick, Irvine, CA 92618

Surgin Surgical Instrumentation, Inc. (Surgin Inc.) — 800-753-7400
37 Shield, Irvine, CA 92618

Syneron, Inc. — 949-716-6670
3 Goodyear Unit A, Irvine, CA 92618

Syntech International — 949-752-9642
17171 Daimler Ave., Irvine, CA 92614

Tekia, Inc. — 949-699-1300
17 Hammond Street, Suite 414, Irvine, CA 92718

Ther Ox, Inc. — 949-757-1999
17500 Cartwright Rd.,, Suite 100, Irvine, CA 92612

Therox, Inc. — 949-757-1999
17500 Cartwright Rd Suite 100, Irvine, CA 92614

Trestle Corp. — 949-673-1907
199 Technology Dr., Suite 105, Irvine, CA 92618-2446

Trimedyne, Inc. — 800-733-5273
15091 Bake Parkway, Irvine, CA 92618-2501

Vision Quest Industries, Inc. — 800-266-6969
18011 Mitchell So., Irvine, CA 92614

Wavetec Vision — 949-273-5970
66 Argonaut, Suite 170, Irvine, CA 92618

Zee Medical, Inc. — 800-841-8417
22 Corporate Park, Irvine, CA 92606

Zimmer Medizinsystems — 800-327-3576
25 Mauchly Ste. 300, Irvine, CA 92618

joimax USA Inc. — 949-859-3472
14 Goodyear, Suite 145, Irvine, CA 92618

3m Espe Dental Products — 949-863-1360
2111 McGaw Ave., Irvine, CA 92614

Irwindale

Biosense Webster — 800-729-9010
15715 Arrow Hwy, Irwindale, CA 91706

La Verne

Bio Cybernetics Intl. — 800-220-4224
1815 Wright Avenue, La Verne, CA 91750

La Jolla

Advanced Biohealing Inc. — 858-754-3863
10933 N. Torrey Pines Road, Suite 200, La Jolla, CA 92037

Bd Diagnostics (Geneohm Sciences, Inc.) — (888) 436-3646
11085 North Torrey Pines Road, Suite 210, La Jolla, CA 92037

Cortechs Labs, Inc. — 858-459-9702
1020 Prospect St., Suite 304, La Jolla, CA 92037

Mobility Inc. — 858-456-8121
5726 La Jolla Blvd., Suite 104, La Jolla, CA 92037

NeuroVigil Inc. — 858-454-5134
7606 Fay Avenue, La Jolla, CA 92037

Osypka Medical, Inc. — 858-454-0021
7855 Ivanhoe Ave., Suite 226, La Jolla, CA 92037

Pillar Surgical, Inc. — 800-367-0445
PO Box 8141, La Jolla, CA 92038-8141

Stratagene — 800-424-5444
11011 N. Torrey Pines Road, La Jolla, CA 92037-1007

La Mirada

Makita Usa Inc. - Drapery Opener Div. — 800-462-5482
14930 Northam St., La Mirada, CA 90638-5753

Packaging Plus Llc — 714-522-5400
14450 Industry Circle, La Mirada, CA 90638

La Puente

Cosmo Health, Inc. — 626-248-7917
15310 Elliot Avenue, Suite 4112, La Puente, CA 91747

La Quinta

Swb Elbow Brace, Ltd. — 760-564-9853
56059 Winged Foot, La Quinta, CA 92253

La Verne

Alpha Scientific Medical, Inc. — 909-802-7000
1751 Yeager Ave., La Verne, CA 91750

Attends Healthcare Products — 252-752-1100
2321 Arrow Highway, La Verne, CA 91750

Edge I-Wear Corp. — 909-598-7679
1775 Curtiss Ct., La Verne, CA 91750

Laguna Beach

Advanced Cardiac Therapeutics Inc. — 877-876-5994
1278 Glenneyre, Suite 139, Laguna Beach, CA 92651

Neuro-Diagnostic Assoc. — 949-497-1207
2514 Temple Hills Drive, Laguna Beach, CA 92651

Laguna Hills

American Diversified Dental Systems — 800-637-2330
22991 La Cadena Drive, Laguna Hills, CA 92653-1314

Applied Cardiac Systems, Inc. — 800-423-2929
22912 El Pacifico Dr., Laguna Hills, CA 92653-1332

Arcoma North America, Inc. — 464-707-0690
23151 Alcalde Drive, Suite C-8, Laguna Hills, CA 92653

Biomedics, Inc. — 949-458-1998
23322 Peralta Drive, Ste. 11, Laguna Hills, CA 92653

Glaukos Corp. — 949-367-9600
26051 Merit Cr #103, Laguna Hills, CA 92653

Mds Products, Inc. — 800-637-2330
22991 La Cadena Drive, Laguna Hills, CA 92653-1314
Med-Logics, Inc. — 800-651-2962
26061 Merit Circle, Suite 102, Laguna Hills, CA 92653
Med-Logics, Inc. — 949-582-3891
26061 Merit Circle, Suite #102, Laguna Hills, CA 92653
Nemoto Medical U.S., Inc. — 949-863-9395
24992 Del Monte St, Laguna Hills, CA 92653-5617
Plastic And Metal Center, Inc. — 949-770-8230
23162 La Cadena Drive, Laguna Hills, CA 92653
Tagg Industries L.L.C. — 800-548-3514
23210 Del Lago, Laguna Hills, CA 92653
Unicare Biomedical, Inc. — 949-643-6707
22971-B Triton Way, Laguna Hills, CA 92653
Unicare Biomedical, Inc. — 949-643-6707
22971-b Triton Way, Laguna Hills, CA 92653
Vessix Vascular, Inc. — 858-217-0300
26052 Merit Circle, Suite 106, Laguna Hills, CA 92653

Laguna Niguel

Pretika Corporation, North America Market Headquar — 949-481-8818
16 Salermo, Laguna Niguel, CA 92677
Vision Chips, Inc. — 949-362-0565
27671 La Paz Road, Laguna Niguel, CA 92677

Lake Balboa

Zoom Focus Eyewear, Llc — 800 900 3700
7065-2 Hayvenhurst Ave., Lake Balboa, CA 91406

Lake Elsinore

Body Therapeutics, Div. Of I-Rep, Inc. — 800-530-3722
508 Chaney Street, Suite 13, Lake Elsinore, CA 92530
I-Rep, Inc. — 800-828-0852
508 Chaney Street #B, Lake Elsinore, CA 92530
N-K Products Company, Div. Of I-Rep,Inc. — 800-462-6509
508 Chaney Street #B, Lake Elsinore, CA 92530

Lake Forest

American Optisurgical Inc. — 800-576-1266
25501 Arctic Ocean Dr., Lake Forest, CA 92630
Ats Medical, Inc. — 949-380-9333
20412 James Bay Circle, Lake Forest, CA 92630
Devax, Inc. — 949-334-2333
20996 Bake Parkway, Suite 106, Lake Forest, CA 92630
I-Flow Corporation — 800-448-3569
20202 Windrow Dr., Lake Forest, CA 92630
R & D Medical Products, Inc. — 949-472-9346
20492 Crescent Bay Drive #106, Lake Forest, CA 92630
Revision Optics — 949-707-2740
25651 Atlantic Ocean Drive, Suite A1, Lake Forest, CA 92630
Varian Inc — 650-424-5078
25200 Commercentre Dr., Lake Forest, CA 92630-8810
Velco Tool And Die Co. — 949-855-6638
20551 Pascal Way, Lake Forest, CA 92692

Lake Forrest

MONOBIND, INC. — 800-854-6265
100 North Pointe Drive, Lake Forrest, CA 92630

Lakeside

Molecular Metallurgy, Inc. — 619-596-7444
11649 Riverside Drive, Suite 139, Lakeside, CA 92040

Lakespur

BioCision LLC — 888-478-2221
12 East Sir Francis Drake Blvd., Suite B, Lakespur, CA 94939

Lancaster

Medi-Tek, Inc. — 661-940-0030
4555 W. Avenue G, Suite # 6, Lancaster, CA 93536

Livermore

Medical Device Resource Corporation — 800-633-8423
5981 Graham Ct, Livermore, CA 94550
Nano-Write Corporation — 925-606-1388
2021 Las Positas Court, Suite 121, Livermore, CA 94551
Pss Bio Instruments, Inc. — 925-960-9182
6052 Industrial Way, Suite H, Livermore, CA 94551
Reliance Medical Corp. — 800-633-8423
5981 Graham Ct, Livermore, CA 94550
Wang Nmr Inc. — 925-443-0212
550 N. Canyons Pkwy., Livermore, CA 94550-7632

Livingston

Fresenius Medical Care North America — 781-699-9068
420 Industrial Dr, Livingston, CA 95334

Lodi

American Mastertech Scientific, Inc. — 209-368-4031
1330 Thurman St., Lodi, CA 95240
Scholten Surgical Instruments, Inc. — 209-365-1393
170 Commerce St. #101, Lodi, CA 95240-0722

Loma Linda

Optivus Proton Therapy, Inc — 888-PROTONS
PO Box 608, Loma Linda, CA 92354

Long Beach

Mac's Lift Gate, Inc. — 800-795-6227
2715 Seaboard Lane, Long Beach, CA 90805-3736
Marine Dynamics Corp. — 951-699-4299
6475 E. Pch, #412, Long Beach, CA 90803
Movincool/Denso Sales California, Inc. — 800-264-9573
3900 Via Oro Avenue, Long Beach, CA 90810
Obagi Medical Products, Inc. — 800-636-7546
3760 Kilroy Airport Way, Suite 500, Long Beach, CA 90806
Radiology Support Devices — 800-221-0527
1904 E. Dominguez St., Long Beach, CA 90810-1002
Romed, Llc — 562-438-8904
4224 Massachusetts St., Long Beach, CA 90814-2939

Loomis

Trax Cleanroom Products — 800-520-8729
3352 Swetzer Rd., P.O. Box 2089, Loomis, CA 95650-2089

Los Alamitos

Pyramid Medical Llc — 800-764-1154
10940 Portal Drive, Los Alamitos, CA 90720
Sysmex Reagents America, Inc. — 847-996-4512
10716 Reagan St., Los Alamitos, CA 90720

Los Altos

Lsvp International, Inc. — 866-969-0100
4692 El Camino Real, Unit 126, Los Altos, CA 94022
Scimage, Inc. — 866-724-6243
4916 El Camino Real, Suite 200, Los Altos, CA 94022

Los Angeles

AMD Technologies Inc. — 800-423-3535
218 Bronwood Avenue, Los Angeles, CA 90049
Airgas West, Inc. — 310-505-9897
11711 South Alameda, Los Angeles, CA 90059
Areeda Assoc., Ltd. — 323-653-5515
1160 Glen Arbor Ave., Los Angeles, CA 90041
Baxter Healthcare Corporation — 847-473-6141
4501 Colorado Blvd., Los Angeles, CA 90039
Biocomp Research Institute — 800-246-3526
6542 Hayes Dr., Los Angeles, CA 90048
Bioplate, Inc. — 310-815-2100
3643 Lenawee Ave., Los Angeles, CA 90016-4310
Camda Corp. — 213-381-0888
3435 Wilshire Blvd.,#990, Los Angeles, CA 90010
Ceremed, Inc. — 310-815-2125
3643 Lenawee Ave., Los Angeles, CA 90016
Compumed, Inc. — 800-421-3395
5777 West Century Blvd.,, Suite 360, Los Angeles, CA 90045
D&M Soomekh International, Inc. — 323-266-2500
1260 South Boyle Ave., Los Angeles, CA 90023
Danbi, Inc. — 310-398-0013
12099 West Washington Blvd., Suite 304, Los Angeles, CA 90066
De Novo Software — 213-384-7000
3250 Wilshire Blvd., Suite 803, Los Angeles, CA 90010
Dent Zar, Inc. — 800-444-1241
6362 Hollywood Blvd., #214, Los Angeles, CA 90028
Dentecon, Inc. — 800-423-6088
1249 S. La Cienega Blvd., Los Angeles, CA 90035
Digitcare Corporation — 888-287-2990
2999 Overland Ave., Ste. 209, Los Angeles, CA 90064
Dio Usa — 213-300-7979
3435 Wilshire Blvd, Suite 2210, Los Angeles, CA 90010
Dreamwrx Dental Laboratory — 949-448-9985
1911 Colorado Blvd., Los Angeles, CA 90041
Equipois Inc. — 866-601-2070
6601 Santa Monica Blvd., Los Angeles, CA 90038
Euro-Frames, Inc. — 800-422-2773
2985 Glendale Blvd., Los Angeles, CA 90039-1801
Exelint International Co. — 800-940-3935
5840 W. Centinela Ave., Los Angeles, CA 90045
Finebrand Co. — 323-588-3228
3720 S. Santa Fe Ave., Los Angeles, CA 90058
General Medical Co. — 800-432-5362
1935 Armacost Ave., Los Angeles, CA 90025-5296
Genesis Digital Imaging, Inc. — (888) 436-3444
12921 W. Washington Blvd, Los Angeles, CA 90066
Gentronics — 800-950-3265
8721 Santa Monica Blvd., Suite 210, Los Angeles, CA 90069
Health Keeper 9000 Usa Inc. — 213-385-3933
680 S. Wilshire Pl., #405, Los Angeles, CA 90005
Health Solutions Medical Products, Corp. — 310-837-9594
9027 Monte Mar Dr., Los Angeles, CA 90035
Intercare Dx, Inc. — 310-242-5634
6080 Center Drive Suite 640, Los Angeles, CA 90045
Intramedical Imaging Llc — 800-519-3959
12340 Santa Monica Blvd., Suite 227, Los Angeles, CA 90025
Irenda Corp. — 323-770-4222
14131 South Avalon Blvd., Los Angeles, CA 90061

Ivory Dental Laboratory — 323-663-6422
4205 Santa Monica Blvd., Los Angeles, CA 90029
Ki-Add Specialized Support Technology, Inc. — 920-468-8100
6500 South Avalon Blvd., Los Angeles, CA 90003-1934
Lazar Research Laboratories, Inc. — 800-824-2066
509 N. Fairfax Avenue, Suite 219, Los Angeles, CA 90036
Medical Systems Ltd. — 310-445-8590
11444 W. Olympic Blvd., Los Angeles, CA 90064
Medical Tactile, Inc. — 310-641-8228
5757 W. Century Blvd #600, Los Angeles, CA 90045
National Cable Molding — 323-225-5611
136 N. San Fernando Rd., Los Angeles, CA 90031
NeuroSigma Inc. — 310-479-3100
10960 Wilshire Boulevard, Suite 1230, Los Angeles, CA 90024
Ocular Prosthetics, Inc. — 323-462-6004
321 N. Larchmont Blvd., Suite # 711, Los Angeles, CA 90004
Online Power, Inc. — 800-227-8899
5701 Smithway St., Los Angeles, CA 90040-9825
Ortho Dermatologics — 310-642-1150
5760 W. 96th St., Los Angeles, CA 90045-5544
Osada, Inc. — 800-426-7232
3000 S. Robertson Blvd., Suite 130, Los Angeles, CA 90034
R.J. Lindquist Co. — 213-382-1268
2419 James M. Wood Blvd., Los Angeles, CA 90006
Response Genetics Inc. — 323-224-3900
1640 Marengo St., Los Angeles, CA 90033
Salsbury Industries — 800-640-4341
1010 E. 62nd St., Los Angeles, CA 90001-1510
Siemens Healthcare Diagnostics Inc. — 310-645-8200
5210 Pacific Concourse Drive, Los Angeles, CA 90045
Sierra Scientific Instruments, Inc. — 310-641-8492
5757 Century Blvd., Suite 660, Los Angeles, CA 90045
Spectrum Optical — 323-931-4349
6154 West 6th. Street, Los Angeles, CA 90048
Sta-Sof Breast Compressor-Clamp — 310-470-8798
10571 Wyton Dr., Los Angeles, CA 90024
Star Industries — 323-588-4141
2426 E. Washington Blvd., Los Angeles, CA 90021-2939
The Biofeedback Institute Of Los Angeles — 800-246-3526
6542 Hayes Dr., Los Angeles, CA 90048-5320
UBM Canon — 800-442-4200
11444 Olympic Blvd. Suite 900, Los Angeles, CA 90064
Ubimed — 310-556-0624
1180 South Beverly Drive Suite#400, Los Angeles, CA 90035
Vanny Corp. — 310-556-1170
10390 Sana Monica Blvd., Suite 270, Los Angeles, CA 90025
Vidatak, Llc — 734-477-6942
9080 Santa Monica Blvd., Ste. 103, Los Angeles, CA 90069
Yeswin Corp. — 213-383-8066
3200 Wilshire Blvd South Tower, Ste 1140, Los Angeles, CA 90010

Los Gatos

Circle Medical Devices — 408-395-0443
101 Cooper Court, Los Gatos, CA 95032
General Cardiac Technology, Inc. — 831-471-2940
15814 Winchester Blvd #105, Los Gatos, CA 95030
Minitool, Inc. — 888-395-1599
634 University Ave., Los Gatos, CA 95032-4416
Source One Technologies — 408-376-3400
120 Knowles Dr., Los Gatos, CA 95032
Three Palm Software — 408-356-3240
367 Penn Way, Los Gatos, CA 95032

Los Osos

Bailey Medical Engineering — 800-413-3216
2216 Sunset Dr., Los Osos, CA 93402
Clinical Controls International — 805-528-4039
2131 10th Street, Los Osos, CA 93402
More Diagnostics, Inc. — 800-758-0978
2020 11th St, PO Box 6714, Los Osos, CA 93412

Lynwood

Backsaver — 310-661-3044
3000 East Imperial Highway, Lynwood, CA 90262

Mcclellan

Bionica, Inc. — 916-643-2222
5112 Bailey Loop, Mcclellan, CA 95652

Menlo Park

Acclarent, Inc. — 877-775-2789
1525-B O'brien Dr., Menlo Park, CA 94025
Corium International, Inc. — 616-656-4563
235 Constitution Drive, Menlo Park, CA 94025
Crux Biomedical Inc. — 650-321-9903
1455 Adams Drive, #1170, Menlo Park, CA 94025
Gynecare — 888-496-3227
235 Constitution Dr., Menlo Park, CA 94025
Immunetech, Inc. — 650-470-7420
888 Oak Grove Ave., Suite 4, Menlo Park, CA 94025
IncellDx Inc. — 650-777-7630
1700 El Camino Real, Menlo Park, CA 94027
Iscience Interventional — 650-421-2700
4055 Campbell Avenue, Menlo Park, CA 94025

Landec Corp. — 650-306-1650
3603 Haven Ave., Menlo Park, CA 94025
Optivia Biotechnology, Inc. — 650-324-3177 ex
115 Constitution Drive, Suite 7, Menlo Park, CA 94025
Pro-Zooics Research Associates — 650-322-2455
711 Central Ave., Menlo Park, CA 94025
Spinal Modulation Inc. — 650-543-6800
1135 O'Brien Drive, Menlo Park, CA 94025

Millbrae

Genlee — 650-697-5831
769 Morningside Drive, Millbrae, CA 94030
L.A.K. Enterprises, Inc. — 800-824-3112
423 Broadway, Suite 501, Millbrae, CA 94030-1905
Rolliture Corp. — 650-652-5675
665 Clearfield Dr., Millbrae, CA 94030

Milpitas

Amo Manufacturing Usa, Llc — 714-247-8656
510 Cottonwood Drive, Milpitas, CA 95035
Fine Pitch Technologies, Inc., A Solectron Subsidi — 408-957-8500
1077 Gibraltar Drive, Milpitas, CA 95035
High Phoenix, Inc. — 886-422-5567
1124 Wrigley Way, Milpitas, CA 95035
Lifescan, Inc. — 800-227-8862
1000 Gibraltar Dr, Milpitas, CA 95035-6314
Nanometrics, Inc. — 408-545-6000
1550 Buckeye Drive, Milpitas, CA 95035
Paul Arpin Mfg. — 408-263-4974
1347 Highland Ct., Milpitas, CA 95035
Sensym Ict — 800-573-6796
1804 McCarthy Blvd., Milpitas, CA 95035
Siemens Water Technologies — 866-926-8420
960 Ames Avenue, Milpitas, CA 95035

Mission Viejo

Alpha Medical Instruments Llc — 949-460-0944
23455 Madero, Suite B, Mission Viejo, CA 92691
Gereonics, Inc. — 949-929-9319
25501 Aria Drive, Mission Viejo, CA 92692
Mobile-Tronics Co., Inc. — 800-368-8181
28570 Marguerite Pkwy. #227, Mission Viejo, CA 92692

Modesto

Medical Vision Industries, Inc. — 800-775-2088
3117 Mchenry Ave., Suite B, Modesto, CA 95350
Nasco — 800-558-9595
4825 Stoddard Road, PO Box 3837, Modesto, CA 95356-9318

Monrovia

Belco Packaging Systems, Inc. — 800-833-1833
910 S. Mountain Avenue, Monrovia, CA 91016
Circuit Tree Medical, Inc. — 626-303-7902
1911 Walker Avenue, Monrovia, CA 91016
Currie Medical Specialties, Inc. — 800-669-3521
730 E. Los Angeles Avenue, Monrovia, CA 91016-4250
Radcal Corp. — 800-423-7169
426 W. Duarte Rd., Monrovia, CA 91016-4544
Radnoti Glass Technology, Inc. — 800-428-1416
227 W. Maple Ave., Monrovia, CA 91016
Staar Surgical Co. — 800-292-7902
1911 Walker Avenue, Monrovia, CA 91016-4846
3m Unitek — 800-634-5300
2724 S. Peck Rd., Monrovia, CA 91016

Montclair

Speedent Dental Supplies — 800-706-0644
9591 Central Ave., Montclair, CA 91763

Montebello

Wilbur Curtis Company — 800-421-6150
6913 Acco St., Montebello, CA 90640

Monterey

Monterey Medical Solutions, Inc. — 831-210-5514
455 Canyon Del Rey Blvd., Suite #411, Monterey, CA 93940
Patient's Pride, Inc. — 866-607-7433
395 Del Monte Ctr.,,, Ste. 182, Monterey, CA 93940

Monterey Park

Kennex Development Inc — 626-458-0598
533 S. Atlantic Blvd, Suite 301, Monterey Park, CA 91754

Moorpark

Koros Usa, Inc. — 805-529-0825
610 Flinn Ave., Moorpark, CA 93021
Ultron Systems, Inc. — 805-529-1485
5105 Maureen Lane, Moorpark, CA 93021

Moraga

Contour Pak, Inc. — 800-926-2228
346 Rheem Blvd., Suite 104, Moraga, CA 94556

Moreno valley

Resmed West Coast Warehouse — 858-746-2576
23650 Brodiaea, Moreno valley, CA 92553

Morgan Hill

Anaerobe Systems — 408-782-7557
15906 Concord Circle, Morgan Hill, CA 95037
Care Wise Medical Products Corp. — 888-462-8725
P.O. Box 1655, Morgan Hill, CA 95037
Hospira, Inc. — 877-946-7747
755 Jarvis Drive, Morgan Hill, CA 95037
John Cudia And Associates, Inc. — 408-782-2628
18440 Technology Dr., #110, Morgan Hill, CA 95037-2844
Paramit Corp. — 408-782-5600
18735 Madrone Pkwy., Morgan Hill, CA 95037
Sheathing Technologies, Inc. — 408-782-2720
18431 Technology Dr., Morgan Hill, CA 95037
Smp Technology — 408-778-4777
15940 Concord Circle, Morgan Hill, CA 95037-5461

Morro Bay

U.F.I. — 805-772-1203
545 Main St., Ste. C-2, Morro Bay, CA 93442-2522

Mountain View

Accessclosure, Inc. — 877-700-6969
645 Clyde Ave., Mountain View, CA 94043
Adinstruments — 888-965-6040
1949 Landings Dr., Mountain View, CA 94043
Ardian Inc. — 650-417-6555
1380 Shorebird Way, Mountain View, CA 94043
Boston Scientific Corporation — 508-652-5578
2011 Stierlin Court, Mountain View, CA 94043
Concentric Medical, Inc. — 650-938-2100
301 East Evelyn Ave., Mountain View, CA 94041
Conceptus, Inc. — 650-962-4000
331 East Evelyn Ave., Mountain View, CA 94041
Depuy Spine, Inc. — 800-227-6633
365 Ravendale Dr., Mountain View, CA 94043
Evolve Manufacturing Technologies Inc. — 650-968-9292
960 Linda Vista Avenue, Mountain View, CA 94043
Hansen Medical, Inc. — 888-404-5801
800 East Middlefield Road, Mountain View, CA 94043
Hitachi Chemical Diagnostics, Inc. — 650-961-5501
630 Clyde Ct., Mountain View, CA 94043
Hotspur Technologies Inc. — 650-969-3150
880 Maude Avenue, Suite A, Mountain View, CA 94043
Huntington Mechanical Laboratories, Inc. — 800-227-8059
1040 La Avenida Street, Mountain View, CA 94043-1422
Impac Medical Systems, Inc. — 888-464-6722
100 W. Evelyn Avenue, Mountain View, CA 94041
IntraPace Inc. — 650-316 4070
967 N. Shoreline Blvd., Mountain View, CA 94043
Iridex Corporation — 800-388-4747
1212 Terra Bella Avenue, Mountain View, CA 94043
Lasercard Systems Corporation — 650-969-4428
1875 N. Shoreline Blvd., Mountain View, CA 94043-1601
Medical Manager Health Systems, Inc. — 800-222-7701
516 Clyde Avenue, Mountain View, CA 94043
Microfit, Inc. — 650-969-7296
1077-b Independence Ave., Mountain View, CA 94043
Ocumetrics, Inc. — 650-960-3955
2224-c Old Middlefield Way, Mountain View, CA 94043
Omnicell — 800-850-6664
1201 Charleston Road, Mountain View, CA 94043
Oxigraf, Inc. — 650-237-0155
1170 Terra Bella Ave., Mountain View, CA 94043
Pneumrx Inc — 650-625-8910
530 Logue Ave, Mountain View, CA 94043
Restoration Robotics, Inc — (650) 965-3612
1383 Shorebird Way, Mountain View, CA 94043
Siemens Medical Solutions Usa, Inc. Ultrasound — 650-969-9112
Division
1230 Shorebird Way, Mountain View, CA 94039-7393
Telediagnostic Systems — 800-227-3224
2483 Old Middlefield Way, Suite 202, Mountain View, CA 94043
United Biotech, Inc. — 650-961-2910
211 S. Whisman Road, Suite E, Mountain View, CA 94041-1517
Vivus, Inc. — 650-934-5200
1172 Castro St., Mountain View, CA 94040
Zonare Medical Systems, Inc. — 877-966-2731
420 North Bernardo Avenue, Mountain View, CA 94043

Murrieta

Abbott Vascular, Cardiac Therapies — 847-937-2388
30590 Cochise Circle, Murrieta, CA 92563
B & C Biotech — 951-894-6650
24910 Washington Ave, Suite 204, Murrieta, CA 92562
Copan Diagnostics, Inc. — 800-216-4016
26055 Jefferson Avenue, Murrieta, CA 92562
Cosmetech — 951-677-5472
26435 John Adams St., Murrieta, CA 92563

Future Dental Technologies, Inc. — 909-894-4203
26398 Deere Ct., Suite 105, Murrieta, CA 92562
International Immunology Corp. — 800-843-2853
PO Box 972, Murrieta, CA 92564-0972
Interventional Technologies, Inc. — 858-268-4488
30590 Cochise Circle, Murrieta, CA 92563
Medical Extrusion Technologies, Inc. — 800-618-4346
26608 Pierce Circle, Murrieta, CA 92562

Napa

Dexta Corporation — 800-733-3982
962 Kaiser Rd., Napa, CA 94558
Dey, L.P. — 800-755-5560
2751 Napa Valley Corporate Drive, Napa, CA 94558-6216
Eldex Laboratories — 800-969-3533
30 Executive Ct., Napa, CA 94558-6278
Marinco Specialty Wiring Devices — 800-767-8541
2655 Napa Valley Corporate Drive, Napa, CA 94558
Xemax Surgical Products, Inc. — 800-257-9470
712 California Blvd., Napa, CA 94559

National City

Friedheim Tool Company — 619-474-3600
1433 Roosevelt Ave., National City, CA 91950
Hyperbaric Technologies, Inc. — 619-336-2022
3224 Hoover Ave., National City, CA 91950

Nevada City

Q.I. Medical, Inc. — 800-837-8361
440-C Lower Grass Valley Road, Nevada City, CA 95959
Samadhi Tank Co. — 888-755-7700
PO Box 2119, Nevada City, CA 95959-1942

Newark

Insound Medical Inc. — 510-792-4000
39660 Eureka Drive, Newark, CA 94560
Mosaic Industries, Inc. — 510-790-8222
5437 Central Avenue, Suite 1, Newark, CA 94560
Novaray, Inc. — 510-619-9200
39655 Eureka Dr., Newark, CA 94560
Novasys Medical, Inc. — 866-784-4777
39684 Eureka Dr., Newark, CA 94560-4805

Newbury Park

Zenith Point Manufacturing — 805-499-6808
3867 Old Conejo Rd., Newbury Park, CA 91320

Newport Beach

Allen Medical Instruments Corp. — 949-646-3215
177 Riverside Avenue, Suite F - 602, Newport Beach, CA 92663-3630
American Medical Bio Care, Inc. — 800-676-1434
1201 Dove St., #520, Newport Beach, CA 92660
Arosurgical Instruments Corp. — 800-776-1751
220 Newport Center Dr., Ste.11101, Newport Beach, CA 92660
Biosensors International - Usa — 949-553-8300
20280 Acacia St., Suite 300, Newport Beach, CA 92660
Biostructures, Llc — 949-553-1743
3700 Campus Dr. Suite 204, Newport Beach, CA 92660
Dentalium Dental Ceramics, Inc. — 949-440-2600
4141 Macarthur Blvd., Newport Beach, CA 92660
Pacifiq Systems Llc — 949-442-2454
5015 Birch St., Newport Beach, CA 92660-2216
Woodleaf Corporation — 949-675-2121
1700 W. Oceanfront Ave. #d, Newport Beach, CA 92663

North Hills

Munchkin, Inc. — 800-247-2223
16689 Schoenborn, North Hills, CA 91343

North Hollywood

Bobrick Washroom Equipment, Inc. — 818-764-1000
11611 Hart St., North Hollywood, CA 91605-5882
Diasol, Inc. — 800-366-0546
1110 Arroyo, North Hollywood, CA 91340
Melrose Mattress, Inc. — 800-500-0233
8241 Lankersheim Blvd., North Hollywood, CA 91605-1614
Perfection Enterprises — 818-764-3447
7250 Hinds Ave., North Hollywood, CA 91605
Vector Electronics & Technology, Inc. — 800-423-5659
11115 Vanowen St., North Hollywood, CA 91605

Northridge

B.G. Industries, Inc. — 800-822-8288
8550 Balboa Blvd., Suite 214, Northridge, CA 91325
Gamma Medica-Ideas, Inc — 877-426-2633
19355 Business Center Dr., Ste. 8, Northridge, CA 91324
Griff Industries, Inc. — 800-709-4743
19761 Bahama St., Northridge, CA 91324
Medtronic Minimed — 800-933-3322
18000 Devonshire, Northridge, CA 91325
Numotech, Inc. — 818-772-1579
9420 Reseda Blvd., Suite 504, Northridge, CA 91324
Prestige Medical Corporation — 800-762-3333
8600 Wilbur Ave., Northridge, CA 91324-4499

R. A. Fischer Co. — 800-525-3467
8751 White Oak Ave., Northridge, CA 91325
R.A. Fischer Company — 800-525-3467
8751 White Oak Avenue, Northridge, CA 91325
Resonance Technology, Inc. — 818-882-1997
18121 Parthenia St., Northridge, CA 91325
Validyne Engineering Sales Corp. — 800-423-5851
8626 Wilbur Avenue, Northridge, CA 91324

Norwalk

Lipomax Mfg., Inc. — 562-623-9364
13055 Tom White Way, Suite G, Norwalk, CA 90650

Novato

Cal Bionics, Inc. — 415-892-1892
1777 Indian Valley Rd., Novato, CA 94947-4223
Diamics, Inc. — 415-883-0414
Six Hamilton Landing Suite 200, Novato, CA 94949
Onyx Medical Inc./Face-It — 800-333-5773
16 Digital Drive, Suite 120, Novato, CA 94949
Richard Scientific, Inc. — 800-840-3030
285 Bel Marin Keys Blvd, Suite M, Novato, CA 94949

Oakland

Adventure Medical Kits — 800-324-3517
7700 Edgewater Drive, Suite 526, Oakland, CA 94624-3021
Cold Ice, Inc. — 800-525-4435
9999 San Leandro St., Oakland, CA 94603
Microworld Medical Instruments, Inc. — 510-534-7401
4640 Malat St., Oakland, CA 94601
Scientimed Corp. — 510-763-5405
4109 Balfour Ave., Oakland, CA 94610
Steven R. Young Ocularist, Inc. — 510-836-2123
411 30th Street, Suite 512, Oakland, CA 94609
World Heart Inc. — 801-355-6255
7799 Pardee Lane, Oakland, CA 94621

Oceanside

Barefoot Medical — 760-967-8225
1902 Calle Buena Ventura, Oceanside, CA 92056
Bd Medical — 760-631-6520
4665 North Ave., Oceanside, CA 92056
Bmw Precision Machining, Inc. — 619-439-6813
2379 Industry St., Oceanside, CA 92054
Clinicon Corp. — 1-800-CLINICON
3025 Industry St., Suite A, Oceanside, CA 92054-4834
Dupaco, Inc. — 800-546-4550
4144 Avenida de la Plata, Oceanside, CA 92056-3512
Pre Pak Products, Inc. — 800-544-7257
4055 Oceanside Blvd., Suite L, Oceanside, CA 92056
Pryor Products — 800-854-2280
1819 Peacock Blvd., Oceanside, CA 92056-3578
Remedy Hearing Aids — 760-754-8151
2420 Vista Way, Ste. 112, Oceanside, CA 92054-6190
Sable Industries — 800-890-0251
4751 Oceanside Blvd., Unit G, Oceanside, CA 92056
Sparco, Inc. — 800-783-8309
2605 Oceanside Blvd., Ste. F, Oceanside, CA 92054
Universal Diagnostic Solutions — 800-416-7567
101 Copperwood Way, Suite A, Oceanside, CA 92054

Ontario

Airgas West, Inc. — 310-505-9897
191 South Kettering Dr., Ontario, CA 91761
Atlas Medical Technologies — 909-923-7887
1137 E. Philadelphia St., Ontario, CA 91761
Azusa Optronics And Manufacturing Inc. — 909-659-3011
2409 S. Vineyard Avenue, Suite B& C, Ontario, CA 91761
Cardinal Health 200, Inc — 847-785-3323
4551 East Philadelphia St, Ontario, CA 91761
Covidien Lp, Formerly Registered As Tyco Healthcare — 800-962-9888
4651 E. Francis Street, Ontario, CA 91761
H & H Co. — 909-390-0373
4435 East Airport Dr., #108, Ontario, CA 91761
Key-Bak — 800-685-2403
4245 Pacific Privado, Ontario, CA 91761-7609
Koaman International — 909-983-4888
656 E. D St., Ontario, CA 91764-4250
Medegen — 800-520-7999
4501 Wall Street, Ontario, CA 91761-8151
Multi Imager Service, Inc — 800-400-4549
990 E. Cedar Street, Ontario, CA 91761
Ophthalmic Innovations Intl., Inc. — 909-937-1033
4290 E. Brickell St., Bldg-a, Ontario, CA 91761
Vector Firstaid, Inc. — 800-999-4423
316 N. Corona Avenue, Ontario, CA 91764
Westside Packaging, Llc. — 909-570-3508
1700 A South Baker Ave., Ontario, CA 91761

Orange

Alpha Medical Products, Inc. — 800-714-2574
1827 E. Chapman Ave., Orange, CA 92867
Denmed Technologies, Inc. — 866-433-6633
1531 West Orangewood Avenue, Orange, CA 92868

Dorex, Inc. — 714-639-0700
954 N. Lemon St., Orange, CA 92867
Eagle Health Supplies, Inc. — 800-755-8999
535 W. Walnut Ave., Orange, CA 92868
Hammill International — 800-228-2129
PO Box 4968, Orange, CA 92613
Handpiece Parts & Products, Inc. — 800-368-3684
707 West Angus Ave., Orange, CA 92868
Kerr Corp. — 949-255-8766
1717 West Collins Ave., Orange, CA 92867
Magnus Mobility Systems — 800-858-7801
1912 W. Business Center Drive, Orange, CA 92867
Rogers Foam Corp. — 714-538-3033
808 West Nicholas Avenue, Orange, CA 92868-1320
Sota Precision Optics, Inc. — 714-532-6100
1073 North Batavia St., Orange, CA 92867
Sybron Dental Specialties, Inc. — 800-537-7824
1717 W. Collins Ave, Orange, CA 92867
Sybronendo — 800-346-3636
1717 W. Collins Ave., Orange, CA 92867
Truer Medical, Inc. — 714-628-9785
1050 North Batavia, Unit C, Orange, CA 92867

Orangevale

Biomagnetics Diagnostics Corp. — 916-987-7078
8864 Greenback Lane, Suite E, Orangevale, CA 95662

Orinda

Athena Feminine Technologies, Inc — 866-308-4436
179 Moraga Way, Orinda, CA 94563
Logovox Systems, Inc. — 925-253-8303
128 Diablo View Dr., Orinda, CA 94563

Oroville

Aztec Heart, Inc. — 530-533-7069
332 Canyon Highlands Dr, Oroville, CA 95966
Nespa Enterprises, Inc. — 888-479-4677
2800 Richter Ave.ste. C, Oroville, CA 95966

Oxnard

American Tooth Industries — 800-235-4639
1200 Stellar Dr., Oxnard, CA 93033-2404
Bright Ideas 4 Therapy, Llc — 805-390-0330
1630 Sophia Dr., PO BOX 7396, Oxnard, CA 93031
Cadco Dental Products — 800-833-8267
600 E. Hueneme Rd., Oxnard, CA 93033-8634
Clive Craig Co. — 800-833-8267
600 East Hueneme Rd., Oxnard, CA 93033
Dux Dental — 800-833-8267
600 E. Hueneme Rd., Oxnard, CA 93033-8600
ERG International — 800-446-1186
361 N. Bernoulli Circle, Oxnard, CA 93030
Frank Stubbs Co., Inc — 800-223-1713
1830 Eastman Avenue, Oxnard, CA 93030
I.V. League Medical — 805-988-1010
460 S. Lombard St., Oxnard, CA 93030
Puretec Industrial Water — 805-652-0552
3151 Sturgis Rd., Oxnard, CA 93030
Vibe 2000 — 805-377-2709
511 Iguera Dr., Oxnard, CA 93030
Wel Industries, Inc. — 805-985-2462
5114 Terramar Way, Oxnard, CA 93035-1838

Pacific Palisades

Orthosource, Inc. — 800-649-5525
17374 Sunset Blvd., Pacific Palisades, CA 90272
Stevenson Industries, Inc. — 310-459-9393
881 Alma Real Dr., Suite 310, Pacific Palisades, CA 90272

Pacifica

Pori & Rowe Assoc., Inc. — 650-359-5175
1825 Palmetto Ave., Pacifica, CA 94044

Pacoima

Nu-Hope Laboratories, Inc. — 800-899-5017
12640 Branford St., Pacoima, CA 91331

Palm Desert

Serrano International — 760-773-5140
45-175 Panorama Drive, Suite G, Palm Desert, CA 92260
Tellus Medical Products, Inc. — 760-200-9772
77-971 Wildcat Drive, Suite C, Palm Desert, CA 92211

Palm Springs

Cardinal Health 207, Inc. — 610-862-0800
1100 Bird Center Dr., Palm Springs, CA 92262
E-Z Floss — 760-325-1888
P.O. BOX 2292, Palm Springs, CA 92263

Palmdale

Elite Medical Products, Inc. — 661-273-6518
38606 Roma Court, Palmdale, CA 93550
Spaceage Control, Inc. — 661-273-3000
38850 20th Street East, Palmdale, CA 93550

Palo Alto

Aesculap, Inc — 650-543-3100
1810 Embarcadero Road, Suite B, Palo Alto, CA 94303
Beckman Coulter Primary Care Diagnostics — 714-961-3712
1050 Page Mill Rd., Bldg. 2-B, Palo Alto, CA 94303-0803
Carbylan Biosurgery, Inc. — 650-855-6777
3181 Porter Drive, Palo Alto, CA 94304
CardioDx — 650-475-2788
2500 Faber Place, Palo Alto, CA 94303
Coapt Systems, Inc. — 650-461-7600
1820 Embarcadero Rd., Palo Alto, CA 94303
Diagnosoft, Inc. — 650-320-9397
3461 Kenneth Drive, Palo Alto, CA 94303
Dpix, Llc — 650-842-9600
3406 Hillview Ave., Palo Alto, CA 94304
Health Hero Network, Inc. — 888-947-8957
2400 Geng Road, Ste. 200, Palo Alto, CA 94303
Nfocus Neuromedical Inc. — 888-483-6287
2191 E. Bayshore Rd., Suite 100, Palo Alto, CA 94303
Peak Surgical Inc. — 888-792-7325
2464 Embarcadero Way, Palo Alto, CA 94303
Pelikan Technologies, Inc — 757-224-0177
1072 East Meadow Circle, Palo Alto, CA 94303
Percutaneous Systems, Incorporated — 650-493-4200
3260 Hillview Avenue, Suite 100, Palo Alto, CA 94304
Sanders Data Systems, Llc — 650-857-0455
3980 Bibbits Dr., Palo Alto, CA 94303
Satiety, Inc. — 877-728-7288
2470 Embarcadero Way, Palo Alto, CA 94303
Sciton, Inc. — 888-646-6999
9255 Commercial St., Palo Alto, CA 94303
Varian Medical Systems — 800-544-4636
3100 Hansen Way, Palo Alto, CA 94304-1038
Varian Medical Systems, Oncology Systems — 800 278-2747
911 Hansen Way, Bldg.3 M/S C-165, Palo Alto, CA 94304-1028
Varian, Inc. — 800-926-3000
3120 Hansen Way, Palo Alto, CA 94304-1030
Viveve Inc. — 650-321-3332
450 Sheridan Ave., Palo Alto, CA 94306

Palos Verdes

Convaid Inc. — 888-266-8243
PO Box 4209, Palos Verdes, CA 90274-9579

Palos Verdes Peninsula

Zerowet, Inc. — 800-438-0938
PO Box 4375, Palos Verdes Peninsula, CA 90274

Panorama City

Ricon Corp. — 800-322-2884
7900 Nelson Road, Panorama City, CA 91402-6090

Paradise

Digital Hearing Aid Center — 530-877-3808
6032 Clark Rd.,suite C, Paradise, CA 95969
Turbo-Doc Emr — 800-977-4868
771 Buschmann Road, Suite G, Paradise, CA 95969

Paramount

Dlc Laboratories, Inc.
7008 Marcelle Street, Paramount, CA 90723

Pasadena

Avery Dennison Corporation — 626-304-2000
150 North Orange Grove Boulevard, Pasadena, CA 91103-3596
Encompass Therapeutic Support Systems — 818-546-2466
100 E. Corson St, Suite 310, Pasadena, CA 91103
Glass Instruments, Inc. — 323-681-0011
2285 E. Foothill Blvd., Pasadena, CA 91107-3687
Konigsberg Instruments, Inc. — 626-449-0016
2000 East Foothill Blvd., Pasadena, CA 91107
Sage In-Vitro Fertilization Inc. — 203-601-5200
1979 East Locust St., Pasadena, CA 91107
Western Systems Research, Inc. — 626-578-7363
127 N. Madison Avenue, Suite 24, Pasadena, CA 91101

Paso Robles

Cornucopia Tool & Plastics, Inc. — 800-235-4144
448 Sherwood Road, P.O. Box 1915, Paso Robles, CA 93447
Hanson Medical, Inc. — 800-771-2215
825 Riverside Avenue, Building #2, Paso Robles, CA 93446

Petaluma

Bibbero Systems, Inc. — 800-242-2376
1300 N. McDowell Blvd., Petaluma, CA 94954
Gcx Corp. — 800-228-2555
3875 Cypress Drive, Petaluma, CA 94954-5635
Helena Plastics — 800-227-1727
3700 Lakeville Highway, Suite 200, Petaluma, CA 94954
Labcon North America — 800-227-1466
3700 Lakeville Highway, Suite 200, Petaluma, CA 94954
Oculus Innovative Sciences, Inc. — 707-283-0550
1135 N. Mc Dowell Blvd, Petaluma, CA 94954

Panamax, Inc. — 800-472-5555
1690 Corporate Circle, Petaluma, CA 94954
Parmatech Corporation — 800-709-1555
2221 Pine View Way, Petaluma, CA 94954
Phonic Ear, Inc. — 800-227-0735
3880 Cypress Drive, Petaluma, CA 94954-7600
Quality Scientific Plastics — 800-426-9595
1260 Holm Road, Petaluma, CA 94954-1182
Tegal Scientific, Inc. — 707-763-5600
140 2nd Street, Ste 318, Petaluma, CA 94952
3m Petaluma — 707-765-3236
1331 Commerce St., Petaluma, CA 94954

Pico Rivera

Cobe Chemical Co. — 562-942-2426
8616 Slauson Ave., Pico Rivera, CA 90660
Deem Precision Products — 562-692-5416
4203 Durfee Avenue, Pico Rivera, CA 90660-0182

Pinole

Ocu-Ease Optical Products, Inc. — 800-521-8984
920 San Pablo Ave, Pinole, CA 94564-1630

Pittsburg

Hospital Systems, Inc. — 925-427-7800
750 Garcia Ave., Pittsburg, CA 94565
Praxair Distribution, Inc. — (925) 439-1508
1930 Loveridge Rd., Pittsburg, CA 94565

Placentia

Bioseal — 800-441-7325
167 W. Orangethorpe Avenue, Placentia, CA 92870
Panatrex, Inc. — 714-630-5582
1648 Sierra Madre Cir., Placentia, CA 92870-6626
Vesta — 714-993-4100
1941 Petra Lane, Placentia, CA 92870

Playa del Rey

Saville 1300, Inc. — 888-824-9929
200 Culver Blvd., Suite D, Playa del Rey, CA 90293

Pleasant Hill

Cirius Group Inc. — 925-685-9300
140 Gregory Lane, Suite 240, Pleasant Hill, CA 94523
Karwoski Dental — 925-938-8977
418 Iron Hill St., Pleasant Hill, CA 94523
Zap Lasers, Llc — 925-930-6777
2621-b Pleasant Hill Rd., Pleasant Hill, CA 94523

Pleasanton

Advanced Stent Technologies — 508-650-8798
6900 Koll Center Pkwy., #415, Pleasanton, CA 94566
Aesthera Corporation — 925-737-2100
6634 Owens Dr., Pleasanton, CA 94588
Assay Technology Inc — 800-833-1258
1252 Quarry Lane, Pleasanton, CA 94566-4756
Christy Manufacturing Corp. — 925-462-7982
1228-f Quarry Ln., Pleasanton, CA 94566
Clarity Medical Systems — 925-463-7984
5775 West Las Positas Blvd., Suite 200, Pleasanton, CA 94588
Coopervision Inc. — 925- 251-6600
5870 Stoneridge Drive # 1, Pleasanton, CA 94588-2733
Covidien — 303-305-2382
5870 Stoneridge Drive, Suite 6, Pleasanton, CA 94588
Deltatrak, Inc. — 800-962-6776
PO Box 398, Pleasanton, CA 94566
Diagnostic Biosystems — 888-896-3350
1020 Serpentine Lane, Suite # 114, Pleasanton, CA 94566
Hitachi High Technologies America — 925-218-2800
5100 Franklin Dr., Pleasanton, CA 94588-3355
Immunoscience, Inc. — 925-460-8111
7066-d Commerce Cir., Pleasanton, CA 94588
NeoTract inc. — 925-401-0700
4473 Willow Road, Suite 100, Pleasanton, CA 94588
Obsidian Medical Technology, Inc. — 832-767-9606
5108 Corona Covet, Pleasanton, CA 94588
Pacsgear, Inc. — 925-846-9600
7020 Koll Center Parkway, Suite 100, Pleasanton, CA 94566
Process Metrix — 800-995-9902
6622 Owens Drive, Pleasanton, CA 94588-3334
Roche Molecular Systems, Inc. — 925-730-8110
4300 Hacienda Drive, Pleasanton, CA 94588
SPINEALIGN MEDICAL, INC. — 925.227.9800
5880 W. Las Positas Blvd.,,, Suite 52, Pleasanton, CA 94588
Sanarus Medical, Inc. — 925-460-5730
4696 Willow Rd., Pleasanton, CA 94588
The Cooper Companies, Inc — 925-460-3600
6140 Stoneridge Mall Road, Suite 590, Pleasanton, CA 94588
Thoratec Corporation — 800-456-1477
6101 Stoneridge Drive, Pleasanton, CA 94588
TriReme Medical Inc. — 925-931-1300
7060 Koll Center Parkway, Suite 300, Pleasanton, CA 94566
Tria Beauty, Inc. — 925-701-2540
5880 W. Las Positas Blvd, Suite 52, Pleasanton, CA 94588

Zeltiq Aesthetics, Inc. — 925-474-2500
4698 Willow Road, Pleasanton, CA 94588

Pleasanton,

Xradia Inc. — 925-701-3600
4385 Hopyard Road, Suite 100, Pleasanton,, CA 94588

Pollock Pines

Surgica Corporation — 800-979-5090
PO Box 723, #4, Pollock Pines, CA 95726

Pomona

Amsino International, Inc. — 800-MD-AMSINO
855 Towne Center Drive, Pomona, CA 91767
Analytical Industries, Inc. — 909-392-6900
2855 Metropolitan Pl., Pomona, CA 91767
Caldon Bioscience, Inc. — 877-CALDON1
2100 South Reservoir St., Pomona, CA 91766
California Medical Innovations — 800-229-5871
873 E. Arrow Highway, Pomona, CA 91767
Immunalysis Corporation — 909-482-0840
829 Towne Center Drive, Pomona, CA 91767
Impact Diagnostic International — 888-628-5118
748 E. Bonita Ave., Unit 211, Pomona, CA 91767
Jay-Y Enterprise Co. — 909-469-4898
632 New York Drive, Pomona, CA 91768
Kc Pharmaceuticals, Inc. — 909-598-9499
3201 Producer Way, Pomona, CA 91768-3915
Mei Beauty Products, Inc. — 909-861-7575
1971 West Holt Ave., Pomona, CA 91768
Oemedic International, Inc. — 886-2-22903959
No. 162, Atlantic Street, Pomona, CA 91768
Plasdent Corp. — 909-620-0289
1290 Price St., Pomona, CA 91767
Scientific Pharmaceuticals, Inc. — 800-634-3047
3221 Producer Way, Pomona, CA 91768-3916
Urocare Products, Inc. — 800-423-4441
2735 Melbourne Avenue, Pomona, CA 91767-1931

Portola Valley

Spectros Corporation — 650-851-4040
808 Portola Rd, Portola Valley, CA 94028

Poway

Alfa Scientific Designs, Inc. — 877-204-5071
13200 Gregg Street, Poway, CA 92064
Caig Laboratories, Inc. — 800-224-4123
12200 Thatcher Court, Poway, CA 92064-6876
Diazyme Laboratories — 858-455-4761
12889 Gregg Court, Poway, CA 92064
Digirad Corp. — 800-947-6134
13950 Stowe Drive, Poway, CA 92064-8803
Mizuho Usa, Inc. — 858-679-0555
12131 Community Road, Poway, CA 92064
Quatro Composites — 858-513-4300
13250 Gregg St. Suite A-1, Poway, CA 92064

Poway,

StatRad — 800-835-3723
13915 Danielson St, Suite 200, Poway,, CA 92064

Rancho Bernardo

Vocel — 858-679-1919
13400 Sabre Springs Parkway, Suite 255, Rancho Bernardo, CA 92128

Rancho California

Griffin Laboratories — 800-330-5969
43391 Business Park Dr., #c5, Rancho California, CA 92590

Rancho Cordova

Biogrip, Inc. — 888-590-4747
P.O. Box 1375, Rancho Cordova, CA 95741
Biomed Products Llc. — 877-424-6633
11300 Sanders Drive, Suite 26, Rancho Cordova, CA 95742
Sun Fabrications — 916-635-3583
2660 Mercantile Dr., Suite A, Rancho Cordova, CA 95742
Tan America-Indoor Sunsystem — 800-350-2826
11151 Trade Center Dr., Rancho Cordova, CA 95670
Thermogenesis Corp. — 800-783-8357
2711 Citrus Road, Rancho Cordova, CA 95742

Rancho Cucamonga

A-1 Engineering — 1 877 929-9920
9450 7th St. Ste. J, Rancho Cucamonga, CA 91730
Air Liquide Healthcare America Corporation — 713-402-2152
12460 Arrow Route, rancho cucamonga, CA 91739
Cardinal Health 207, Inc — 760-778-7255
8822 Flower Road, Suite 140, Rancho Cucamonga, CA 91730
Eagle Laboratories — 800-782-6534
10201-A Trademark Street, Rancho Cucamonga, CA 91730-5850
Eyeonics, Inc. — 949-916-9352
10574 Acacia St., Suite D-1, Rancho Cucamonga, CA 91730
New World Medical, Inc. — 800-832-5327
10763 Edison Ct., Rancho Cucamonga, CA 91730

Whittemore Enterprises, Inc. — 800-999-2452
11149 Arrow Route, Rancho Cucamonga, CA 91730

Rancho Dominguez

Advanced Materials, Inc. — 310-537-5444
20211 South Susana Rd., Rancho Dominguez, CA 90221
Avalon Laboratories, Inc. — 866-938-6613
2610 E Homestead Place, Rancho Dominguez, CA 90220
Biocell Laboratories, Inc. — 800-222-8382
2001 E. University Dr., Rancho Dominguez, CA 90220-6411
Camfil Farr — 800-300-3277
2121 E Paulhan Street, Rancho Dominguez, CA 90220
Caplugs West — 310-537-2300
18704 S. Ferris Place, Rancho Dominguez, CA 90220
Evs Sports Protection — 800-229-4EVS
2146 . Gladwick St, Rancho Dominguez, CA 90220
First Response Solutions — 310-537-3300
2015 University Dr., Rancho Dominguez, CA 90220
Laclede, Inc. — 877-522-5333
2103 E. University Dr., Rancho Dominguez, CA 90220
Spectrum Laboratories, Inc. — 800-634-3300
18617 Broadwick St., Rancho Dominguez, CA 90220
Superstat Corp. — 800-487-3786
2015 University Dr., Rancho Dominguez, CA 90220-6411

Rancho Santa Margarita

Adept Medical Concepts — 949-635-9238
29816 Avenida De Las Banderas, Rancho Santa Margarita, CA 92688
Amest Corp. — 949-766-9692
30394 Esperanza, Rancho Santa Margarita, CA 92688
Applied Medical Resource Corporation — 949-713-8000
22872 Avenida Empresa, Rancho Santa Margarita, CA 92688
Excelladerm Corp. — 877-969-7546
300065 Comercio, Rancho Santa Margarita, CA 92688
Liquidmetal Technologies, Inc. — 949-635-2100
30452 Esperanza, Rancho Santa Margarita, CA 92688
Oncobionic — 518-798-1215
30211 Avenida De Las Banderas, Suite 200, Rancho Santa Margarita, CA 92688

Redding

Biomet Sports Medicine — 530-226-5800
6704 Lockheed Dr., Redding, CA 96002
Cosco — 800-582-6853
1602 Lakeside Drive, Redding, CA 96001
Mallard Medical, Inc. — 530-226-0727
20268 Skypark Dr., Redding, CA 96002
Minto R&D, Inc. — 530-222-2373
20270 Charlanne Drive, Redding, CA 96002
Mobile Designs, Inc. — 530-244-1050
4650 Caterpillar Rd., Redding, CA 96003
Precision Cast Plastic Parts, Llc. — 530-241-5189
2278 Crescent Moon Dr., Redding, CA 96001
Skyway Machine, Inc — 530-243-5151
4451 Caterpillar Road, Redding, CA 96003
Sunmedica — 530-229-1600
1661 Zachi Way, Redding, CA 96003
Ted Pella, Inc. — 800-237-3526
4595 Mountain Lakes Blvd., Redding, CA 96003-1448
Universal Medical Design — 888-227-5948
4488 Mountain Lakes Blvd., Redding, CA 96003
Visioncare Devices, Inc. — 530-243-5047
1246 Redwood Blvd., Redding, CA 96003

Redlands

Climet Instruments Co. — 909-793-2788
1320 W. Colton Ave., Redlands, CA 92374

Redondo Beach

Body Glove — 310-374-3441
201 Herondo Street, Redondo Beach, CA 90277
Quantimetrix Corporation — 800-624-8380
2005 Manhattan Beach Blvd., Redondo Beach, CA 90278-1205
Radlink, Inc. — 310-643-6900
2400 Marine Ave, Redondo Beach, CA 90278

Redwood City

Abbott Vascular Inc. — 800-227-9902
400 Saginaw Drive, Redwood City, CA 94063-4749
Aeroscout — 706-867-0140
1300 Island Drive, Suite 202, Redwood City, CA 94065
Apollo Physical Therapy Products Llc — 650-306-9208
702 Marshall Street, Suite 312, Redwood City, CA 94063
Avinger Inc. — 650-363-2400
400 Chesapeake, Redwood City, CA 94063
Calibra Medical Inc. — 650-298-4710
220 saginaw drive, Redwood City, CA 94063
Cardica, Inc. — 888-544-7194
900 Saginaw Dr., Redwood City, CA 94063
Dream Systems, L.L.C. — 650-369-9227
6 Malory Ct., Redwood City, CA 94061
Electro-Diagnostic Imaging, Inc. — 650-367-9293
200f Twin Dolphin Drive, Redwood City, CA 94065
Genesis Medical Interventional, Inc. — 650-367-7667
652 Bair Island Road, Suite 103, Redwood City, CA 94063

Genomic Health Inc.   866-662-6897
101 Galveston Drive, Redwood City, CA 94063
Gn Resound Corporation   800-582-4327
Seaport Center, 220 Saginaw Drive, Redwood City, CA 94063-4725
Gynesonics Inc.   650-216-3860
604 Fifth Avenue, Redwood City, CA 94063
Heartport   888-478-7678
700 Bay Road, Redwood City, CA 94063
Kelkom Systems   800-985-3556
418 MacArthur Avenue, Redwood City, CA 94063-3414
Modulus Data Systems, Inc.   888-663-8547
386 MAIN STREET, SUITE 200, REDWOOD CITY, CA 94063
Moore Products, A Sale Proprietorship   650-592-1822
596 Teredo Dr., Redwood City, CA 94065
Nor Cal Design   800-525-5402
3600 Haven Ave., #1, Redwood City, CA 94063
Pathwork Diagnostics Inc.   1-877-808-0006
595 Penobscot Drive, Redwood City, CA 94063
Proteus Biomedical, Inc.   650-632-4031
2600 Bridge Parkway, Suite 101, Redwood City, CA 94065
Pulmonx   650-364-0400
700 Chesapeake Drive, Redwood City, CA 94063
Relievant Medsystems Inc.   650-368-1000
2688 Middlefield Road Suite A, Redwood City, CA 94063
Rubicor Medical, Inc.   650-587-3446
600 Chesapeake Drive, Redwood City, CA 94063
Sentreheart Inc.   650-354-1200
300 Saginaw Drive, Redwood City, CA 94063
Spectrex Corp.   800-822-3940
3580 Haven Avenue, Redwood City, CA 94063-4603
Uni-Fit Co.   650-363-2000
260-E Main St., Redwood City, CA 94063
Vitalog, Inc   650-366-8676
643 Bair Island Road #212, Redwood City, CA 94063-2754

Reseda

International Hospital Supply Co.   800-398-9450
6914 Canby Ave., Ste. 105, Reseda, CA 91335-8741

Richmond

Andros, Inc.   510-837-3500
870 Harbour Way South, Richmond, CA 94804-3613
Berkeley Medevices, Inc.   800-227-2388
1330 S. 51st St., Richmond, CA 94804-4628
Digi-Com Electronics   805-522-6223
5327 Jacuzzi Street, Richmond, CA 94804
Incisive, Llc.   510-669-9401
3095 Richmond Pkwy., Suite 213, Richmond, CA 94806
My True Image Mfg.   510-231-5253
999 Marina Way South, Richmond, CA 94804

Rio Dell

Pacific Implant, Inc.   800-336-2282
920 Rio Dell Ave., Rio Dell, CA 95562

Ripon

Medicalibration Physics Consultant Services, Inc.   209-524-6789
558 Van Dyken Way, Ripon, CA 95366

Riverside

Adex Medical, Inc.   800-873-4776
6101 Quail Valley Court, Riverside, CA 92507
Approved Medical Systems   951-353-2453
7101 Jurupa Ave - Unit 4, Riverside, CA 92504
Astro Seal, Inc.   951-787-6670
827-B Palmyrita Avenue, Riverside, CA 92507-1820
Biomed Resource, Inc.   310-323-3888
6646 Doolittle Ave., Riverside, CA 92503
Luxfer Gas Cylinders   800-764-0366
3016 Kansas Avenue, Riverside, CA 92507
PCI   800-309-8935
12201 Magnolia Avenue, Riverside, CA 92503
Pacific Consolidated Industries, Llc   951-479-0872
12201 Magnolia Ave., Riverside, CA 92503
Von Zabern Surgical   951-734-7215
4121 Tigris Way, Riverside, CA 92503
Western Diagnostic Imaging Systems, Inc.   951-582-9698
4110 Tigris Way, Riverside, CA 92503

Rocklin

Cell Marque Corp.   916-746-8977
6600 Sierra College Blvd., Rocklin, CA 95677
Dermasweep, Inc.   916) 632-9134
3715 Atherton Drive,, Suite 2, Rocklin, CA 95765
Progressive Technology, Inc.   916-632-6715
4130 Citrus Ave #17, Rocklin, CA 95677
Safe-T-Rack Systems, Inc.   800-344-0619
4325 Dominguez Road, Suite A, Rocklin, CA 95677-2102

Roseville

Catheffects, Llc.   916-677-1790
1100 Melody Ln., Roseville, CA 95678
New Star Lasers, Inc.   916-677-1900
9085 Foothills Blvd., Roseville, CA 95747

Op-D-Op, Inc.   916-783-5741
8559 Washington Blvd., Roseville, CA 95678-6435
Pride Industries   800-550-6005
10030 Foothills Blvd., Roseville, CA 95747-7102
Superquad, Llc   800-659-4548
8265 Sierra College Blvd, Suite 316, Roseville, CA 95661

Rowland Heights

Al's Merchandise, Inc.   562-690-0139
3652 South Norwich Place, Rowland Heights, CA 91748

S. El Monte

Elite Orthopaedics, Inc.   800-284-1688
1535 Santa Anita Avenue, S. El Monte, CA 91733

Sacramento

Aceme Technologies Int'L.   916-549-2170
278 Howe Avenue, Suite B, Sacramento, CA 95825
Hand Biomechanics Lab, Inc.   800-522-5778
77 Scripps Drive, Suite 104, Sacramento, CA 95825-6209
Immuno Concepts N.A. Ltd.   800-251-5115
9825 Goethe Road, Suite 350, Sacramento, CA 95827-1715
Innovative Imaging, Inc.   800-765-7226
9940 Business Park Drive, Suite 155, Sacramento, CA 95827-1727
Ophthalmic Imaging Systems   800-338-8436
221 Lathrop Way, Ste. I, Sacramento, CA 95815-4215
The Aftermarket Group   888-TAG-8200
10173 Croyden Way, Sacramento, CA 95827
Vortran Medical Technology   800-434-4034
21 Golden Land Court, Sacramento, CA 95834

Salida

Inventive Resources, Inc.   209-545-1663 É_
5038 Salida Blvd., Salida, CA 95368
Pro-Tex International, Inc.   800-680-9361
5038 Salida Blvd., PO Box 1038, Salida, CA 95368

San Anselmo

Go-Mi, Inc.   415-453-3409
740 Fawn Dr., San Anselmo, CA 94960

San Bernardino

Permedics, Inc.   (877) 473-7633
1475 South Victoria Ct., San Bernardino, CA 92408

San Bruno

Renew Biocare Corp.   415-367-3646
1001 Bayhill Dr., 2nd Fl, San Bruno, CA 94066

San Carlos

Biocardia, Inc.   800-624-1179
125 Shoreway Road, SuiteB, San Carlos, CA 94070
L-3 Communications Electron Devices   650-591-8411
960 Industrial Road, San Carlos, CA 94070-4194
Natus Medical Inc.   800-255-3901
1501 Industrial Road, San Carlos, CA 94070
Nektar Therapeutics   650-631-3100
150 Industrial Road, San Carlos, CA 94070
Peninsula Laboratories, Inc.   800-650-4442
305 Old County Road, San Carlos, CA 94070-6241
Precision Biometrics, Inc.   650-508-2600
981-a Industrial Rd., San Carlos, CA 94070

San Clemente

Advanced Refractive Technologies   949-940-1300
1062 Calle Negocio, Suite D, San Clemente, CA 92673
American Qualex, Inc.   800-772-1776
920-A Calle Negocio, San Clemente, CA 92673
C&E Gp Specialists   800-346-2626
1015 Calle Amanecer, San Clemente, CA 92673
Cameron Health Inc   877-742-3411
905 Calle Amanecer, Suite 300, San Clemente, CA 92673
Capistrano Labs, Inc.   949-492-0390
150 Calle Iglesia, Unit B, San Clemente, CA 92672
Composite Manufacturing, Inc.   949-361-7580
970 B Calle Amanecer, San Clemente, CA 92673
Crandall Medical Devices   949-369-9954
2209 Via Gavilan, San Clemente, CA 92673-5643
Creative Biotech Inc.   949-481-5500
814 Calle Negocio, San Clemente, CA 92673
Icu Medical, Inc.   800-824-7890
951 Calle Amanecer, San Clemente, CA 92673-6212
Neuroptics, Inc.   949-250-9792
1001 Avenida Pico, Suite C495, San Clemente, CA 92673
Nichols Institute Diagnostics   949-940-7200
1311 Calle Batido, San Clemente, CA 92673
Perioptix, Inc.   949-366-3333
1001 Avenida Pico, #C62, San Clemente, CA 92763
R & R Industries, Inc.   800-234-5611
1000 Calle Cordillera, San Clemente, CA 92673
ROX Medical   949-361-8899
150 Calle Iglesia, Suite A, San Clemente, CA 92672
Usgi Medical   949-369-3890
1140 Calle Cordillera, San Clemente, CA 92673

Vertiflex (Tm), Incorporated 866-268-6486
1351 Calle Avanzado, San Clemente, CA 92673

San Diego

Prometheus Laboratories Inc 888-423-5227
9410 Carroll Park Drive, San Diego, CA 92121
ARRK Product Development Group 800-735-2775
8880 Rehco Rd., San Diego, CA 92121
Access Scientific Inc. 866-608-8333
12526 High Bluff Drive, Suite 360, San Diego, CA 92130
Accumetrics, Inc. 888-919-9333
3985 Sorrento Valley Blvd., San Diego, CA 92121
Acon Laboratories, Inc. 858-535-2030
10125 Mesa Rim Road., San Diego, CA 92121
Acutus Medical, Inc 858-673-1621
11225 West Bernardo Court, Suite 102, San Diego, CA 92127
Aethlon Medical Inc. 858-459-7800-30
8910 University Center Lane., Suite 660, San Diego, CA 92122
Aim International, Inc. 858-618-2799
16955 Via Del Campo, Suite 260, San Diego, CA 92127
Alaris Medical Systems, Inc 800-854-7128
10221 Wateridge Circle, San Diego, CA 92121-2772
Alliance Pharmaceutical Corp. 858-410-5200
4660 La Jolla Village Drive, Suite 825, San Diego, CA 92122
Ameditech, Inc. 800-635-2452
10340 Camino Santa Fe, Suite F, San Diego, CA 92121
American Contact Lens Inc. 858-487-8684
15970 Bernardo Center Drive, San Diego, CA 92127
American Radiosurgery, Inc. 858-451-6173
16776 Bernardo Center Dr #203, San Diego, CA 92128
Apex Medical Technologies, Inc. 800-345-3208
10064 Mesa Ridge Ct., Suite 202, San Diego, CA 92121-2948
Argen Corp. 800-375-9077
5855 Oberlin Dr., San Diego, CA 92121
Avail Medical Products 858-635-2206
5950 Nancy Ridge Dr, Ste 500, San Diego, CA 92121
Avant Medical Corp. 858-202-1560
10225 Barnes Canyon Rd.,, Suite A113, San Diego, CA 92121
Aviaradx, Inc. 877-886-6739
9640 Towne Centre Dr, Ste. 200, San Diego, CA 92121
Benechill Inc. -
10060 Carroll Canyon Rd., Suite 100, San Diego, CA 92131
Binding Site, Inc., The 800-633-4484
5889 Oberlin Dr., Ste. 101, San Diego, CA 92121-3759
Bioserv Corporation 858-450-3123
5340 Eastgate Mall, San Diego, CA 92121-2804
Biosite Incorporated 888-246-7483
9975 Summers Ridge Rd, San Diego, CA 92121
Biosurplus Inc. 858-550-0800
10805 Vista Sorrento Pkwy, #200, San Diego, CA 92121
Biozyme Laboratories International Ltd. 800-423-8199
9939 Hibert St., Suite 101, San Diego, CA 92131-1029
Boston Scientific Interventional Technologies 858-268-4488
3574 Ruffin Rd., San Diego, CA 92123-2502
Cardinal Health 2200, Inc 847-578-6442
6215 Ferris Square, Suite 100, San Diego, CA 92121
Cardinal Health 303, Inc 800-854-7128
10020 Pacific Mesa Blvd, San Diego, CA 92121
Cardinal Health Manufacturing Llc 858-617-5889
3750 Torrey View Court, San Diego, CA 92130
Cardium Therapeutics Inc. 858-436-1000
12255 El Camino Rea, Suite 250, San Diego, CA 92130
CareFusion MANUFACTURING LLC 800-367-9947
3750 Torrey View Court, San Diego, CA 92130
Carefusion Corporation 888-876-4287
3750 Torrey View Court, San Diego, CA 92130
Carl Zeiss Meditec, Inc. 800-722-6393
10805 Rancho Benardo Road, Suite 210, San Diego, CA 92127
Cdl Technologies Inc. 619-702-1806
645 Front St., Suite 2007, San Diego, CA 92101
Chrontrol Corporation 800-854-1999
PO Box 19537, San Diego, CA 92159
Circaid Medical Products, Inc. 800-247-2243
9323 Chesapeake Dr., Suite B2, San Diego, CA 92123
Clinicomp Intl. 800-350-8202
9655 Towne Centre Drive, San Diego, CA 92121
Conception Technologies 800-995-8081
6835 Flanders Dr. Suite 500, San Diego, CA 92121
Crescent Design, Inc. 858-452-3240
9932 Mesa Rim Rd., Suite B, San Diego, CA 92121
Critical Diagnostics 877-700-1250
3030 Bunker Hill St., Suite 115A, San Diego, CA 92109
Cryocor, Inc. 858-909-2213
9717 Pacific Heights Blvd., San Diego, CA 92121
Cytori Therapeutics, Inc. 877-470-8000
3020 Callan Road, San Diego, CA 92121
Cytori Therapeutics, Inc. 877-470-8000
3020 Callan Road, San Diego, CA 92121-4148
DAW Industries 800-252-2828
5737 Pacific Center Blvd., San Diego, CA 92121
Daniel T Acosta 619-235-8950
635 C Street, Suite 502, San Diego, CA 92101

Dexcom, Inc. 858-200-0200
6340 Sequence Drive, San Diego, CA 92121
Dr Systems, Inc. 800-794-5955
10140 Mesa Rim Rd., San Diego, CA 92121-2914
Enhanced Video Devices, Inc. 858-530-0100
9830 Summers Ridge Road, San Diego, CA 92121
Epitope Diagnostics, Inc. 858-693-7877
8940 Activity Rd., Suite G, San Diego, CA 92126
Ericomp 800-541-8471
10211 Pacific Mesa Blvd., Suite 411, San Diego, CA 92121
Eurogentec North America, Inc. 877-387-6436
11111 Flintkote Avenue, San Diego, CA 92121
Forest Imaging, Inc 619-218-6460
5288 Eastgate Mall, San Diego, CA 92121
Freedom Meditech, Inc. 619-683-3937
10455 Pacific Center Court, San Diego, CA 92121
Gen-Probe, Inc. 800-523-5001
10210 Genetic Center Drive, San Diego, CA 92121-4362
Genzyme Diagnostics 617-252-7500
6659 Top Gun St., San Diego, CA 92121
Habley Medical Technology Corp. 800-729-1994
15721 Bernardo Heights Parkway, Suite B-30, San Diego, CA 92128
Hospira, Inc 877-946-7747
13520 Evening Creek Drive, Suite 200, San Diego, CA 92128
Icd, Inc. 866-791-2503
2232 Verus Street, Suite C, San Diego, CA 92154
Illumina, Inc. 1-800-809-4566
9865 Towne Centre Drive, San Diego, CA 92121
Imak Products Corp. 619-291-9990
2515 Camino Del Rio South,#240, San Diego, CA 92108
Industrial Computer Source 800-523-2320
6260 Sequence Dr., San Diego, CA 92121-4371
Innercool Therapies, Inc.- A Delaware Corporation 858-713-5904
6740 Top Gun Street, San Diego, CA 92121
Innominata dba GENBIO 800-288-4368
15222 Ave. Of Science, Suite A, San Diego, CA 92128
Innovacon, Inc. 858-535-2030
4106 Sorrento Valley Blvd., San Diego, CA 92121
Inova Diagnostics, Inc. 800-545-9495
9900 Old Grove Rd, San Diego, CA 92131-1638
Integra Neurosciences 800-762-1574
5955 Pacific Center Boulevard, San Diego, CA 92121-4309
Integrated Orbital Implants, Inc. 800-424-6537
12625 High Bluff Drive, Suite 314, San Diego, CA 92130-2054
Intergrated Dental Solutions, Inc. 858-643-1143
6195 Cornerstone Court East, Suite 108, San Diego, CA 92121
Inverness Medical Professional Diagnostics-San Die 858-535-2030
4106 Sorrento Valley Boulevard, San Diego, CA 92121
Invivoscribe Technologies, Llc 1 858 224-6601
6330 Nancy Ridge Drive, Suite 106, San Diego, CA 92121
Ivalon, Inc. 800-948-2566
1015 Cordova Street, San Diego, CA 92107
Jaco Medical Equipment Inc. 858-278-7743
4848 Ronson Ct., Suite E, San Diego, CA 92111
Kinetic Diversified Industries, Inc. 858-566-0550
7746 Arjons Dr., San Diego, CA 92126
Kolberg Ocular Products, Inc. 858-695-2021
9663 Tierra Grande St.,, Suite 201, San Diego, CA 92126
Laprostop, Llc 858-705-3838
1845 Newport Avenue, San Diego, CA 92107
Lusys Laboratories Inc. 888-898-3909
10054 Mesa Ridge Court, Suite 118, San Diego, CA 92121
Mast Biosurgery Usa Inc. 858-550-8050
6749 Top Gun St., Suite 108, San Diego, CA 92121
Maxwell Technologies Power Systems 877-511-4324
9244 Balboa Avenue, San Diego, CA 92123
Med Systems 800-345-9061
2631 Ariane Drive, San Diego, CA 92117
Medical Instrumentation & Diagnostics Corp.(Midco) 858-635-2230
7964 Arjons Drive #e, Suite E, San Diego, CA 92126
Medmetric Corp. 800-995-6066
7542 Trade St., San Diego, CA 92121-2412
Medwaves, Incorporated (858) 946-0015
16760 West Bernardo Drive, San Diego, CA 92127
Mfi Medical Equipment Inc 800-633-1558
7929 Silverton Avenue, #610, San Diego, CA 92126
Millenia Diagnostics 858-626-2777
9380 Waples Street Suite 101, San Diego, CA 92121
Millenium Laboratories 877-451-3534
16981 Via Tazon, San Diego, CA 92127
Multiplier Industries Corp. 800-642-2424
2195 Britannia Blvd, Suite 104, San Diego, CA 92154
Nanogen, Inc. 877-626-6436
10398 Pacific Center Ct., San Diego, CA 92121-4340
Naviscan Inc. 858-587-3641
6865 Flanders Dr., Suite B, San Diego, CA 92121
New Laser Science, Inc. 858-487-5880
16776 Bernardo Center Drive, #203, San Diego, CA 92128
Nova Ranger, Inc. 760-274-6344
9885 Mesa Rim Rd., Suite 127, San Diego, CA 92121
Nu-Ear Electronics 800-626-8327
6769 Mesa Ridge Rd., Ste. 100, San Diego, CA 92121

Nu-Ear Electronics 952-947-4734
6769 Mesa Ridge Rd. Suite 100, San Diego, CA 92121
Nuvasive, Inc. 800-475-9131
7475 Lusk Blvd., San Diego, CA 92121
Oncogene Research Products 800-854-3417
10394 Pacific Center Court, San Diego, CA 92121
One Zone Devices 858-350-9284
3525 Del Mar Hts. Road #366, San Diego, CA 92130
Orthorx, Inc. 858-457-3545
8929 University Center Ln.,, Suite 200, San Diego, CA 92122
Pan Probe Biotech, Inc. 858-689-9936
7396 Trade St., San Diego, CA 92121
Paradigm-Trex, Llc 858-646-5756
10455 Pacific Center Ct., San Diego, CA 92121
Paragon Medsystems, Llc. 858-613-1200
15920 Bernardo Center Dr., San Diego, CA 92127
Phamatech Inc. 858-643-5555
10151 Barnes Canyon Rd, San Diego, CA 92121
Precision Optical Products 866-472-4436
4950 Waring Rd., Suite 2a, San Diego, CA 92120
Primapharm, Inc. (949) 278-1597
3443 Tripp Court, San Diego, CA 92121
Professional Product Co. 619-231-1951
4250 4th Ave., San Diego, CA 92112-1628
Purified Protein, Inc. 866-339-6589
3443 Tripp Court, San Diego, CA 92121-1009
Qed Bioscience, Inc. 800-929-2114
10919 Technology Place, Suite C, San Diego, CA 92127-1706
Quidel Corp. (800) 874-1517
10165 McKellar Court, San Diego, CA 92121
Quidel Corporation 800-874-1517
10165 McKellar Ct., San Diego, CA 92121-4299
Raichem, Division Of Hemagen Diagnostics, Inc. 800-438-6100
8225 Mercury Ct., San Diego, CA 92111-1203
Resmed Corp. 800-424-0737
9001 Spectrum Center Blvd., San Diego, CA 92123
Resmed Inc. 800-424-0737
9001 Spectrum Center Blvd., San Diego, CA 92123
Rf Industries, Inc. 800-233-1728
7610 Miramar Road, San Diego, CA 92126-4202
Rf Surgical Systems Inc. Technical Center 760-994-8198
9740 Appaloosa Road, Suite 150, San Diego, CA 92131
Ridge Diagnostics Inc. 877-743-4301
12390 El Camino Real, Suite 170, San Diego, CA 92130
Robot Research, Inc., Sensomatics Div. 858-642-2400
6795 Flanders Dr., San Diego, CA 92121
San Diego Swiss Machining, Inc. 858-571-6636
9177 Aero Dr., Suite A, San Diego, CA 92123
Science Applications International Corp. 800-430-7629
10260 Campus Point Drive, San Diego, CA 92121
Sequal Technologies Inc. 800-826-4610
11436 Sorrento Valley Rd., San Diego, CA 92121-1393
Sequenom, Inc 1-877-443-6663
3595 John Hopkins Court, San Diego, CA 92121
Shamir Insight, Inc. 877-514-833
9938 Via Pasar, San Diego, CA 92126
Silicon Kinetics 858-646-5444
10455 Pacific Center Court, San Diego, CA 92121
Smiths Medical Asd, Inc. 610-578-9600
9255 Customhouse Plaza, Suite N, San Diego, CA 92154
Sms Technologies, Inc. 858-587-6900
9877 Waples St., San Diego, CA 92121
Sorrento Biochemical, Inc. 858-259-0717
3443 Tripp Ct., San Diego, CA 92121
Spectrascience, Inc. 858-847-0200
11568-11 Sorrento Valley Rd., San Diego, CA 92121
SpineOvations 858-812-3003
4445 Eastgate Mall, Suite 200, San Diego, CA 92121
Suneva Medical, Inc. 858-550-9999
5870 Pacific Center Blvd., San Diego, CA 92121
Synthes San Diego 858-452-1266
6244 Ferris Square, Suite B, San Diego, CA 92121-3239
Targeson Inc. 877-290-4043
3550 General Atomics Court, MS 02-444, San Diego, CA 92121
Temp-Tronix 800-223-8367
7350-B Trade St., San Diego, CA 92121
Tensys Medical, Inc. 888-722-7800
5825 Oberlin Drive, Suite 100, San Diego, CA 92121-3709
Thermopeutix Inc. 858-549-1760
9925b Business Park Ave., San Diego, CA 92131
Thompson Engineering 858-748-5677
11472 Tree Hollow Lane, San Diego, CA 92128
Topera Medical 617-453-8001
6190 Cornerstone Court, Suite 220, San Diego, CA 92121
Trinity Orthopedics, Llc 858. 689. 4113
8817 Production Ave., San Diego, CA 92121
TrovaGene, Inc [+1] 858 217 4
11055 Flintkote Ave, Suite B, San Diego, CA 92121
Tulip Medical Products 800-325-6526
PO Box 7368, San Diego, CA 92167
U.S. Medical Instruments, Inc. 619-661-5500
1490 Air Wing Road, San Diego, CA 92154

Valor Medical, Inc. 858-643-1675
6749 Top Gun Street, Suite 109, San Diego, CA 92121
Venetec International., Inc. 888-685-0565
12555 High Bluff Drive, Suite 100, San Diego, CA 92130
Victorch Meditek, Inc. 858-530-9191
7313 Carroll Rd., Suite A-b, San Diego, CA 92121
Volcano Corporation 800-228-4728
3661 Valley Centre Drive, Suite 200, San Diego, CA 92130
Wavetouch Technologies, Llc 858-924-9283
15970 Bernardo Center Dr., San Diego, CA 92127
Zenith Medical Inc. 800-747-0216
10064 Mesa Ridge Ct., Suite 218, San Diego, CA 92121
eBioscience 888-999-1371
10255 Science Center Drive, San Diego, CA 92121
4-D Neuroimaging 858-453-6300
9727 Pacific Heights Blvd., San Diego, CA 92121

San Dimas

Advanced Infusion, Inc. 909-305-9857
466 West Arrow Hwy., Unit H, San Dimas, CA 91773
American Bio-Medical Service Corporation (Abmsc) 800-755-9055
Sales,Service and Refurbishing Center, 631 West Covina Blvd., San Dimas, CA 91773-2913
Anacapa Technologies, Inc. 909-394-7795
301 E. Arrow Hwy, Ste. 106, San Dimas, CA 91773
Labfusions 909-592-8131
437 S. Cataract Ave., Suite 5, San Dimas, CA 91773-2979
Paperpak 800-428-8363
545 West Terrace Drive, San Dimas, CA 91773
Tra & Accessories 909-305-1944
449 West Allen Ave. Suite 107, San Dimas, CA 91773

San Fernando

Charts-Inc. 800-882-9357
12977 Arroyo St., San Fernando, CA 91340
J. L. Shepherd And Assoc. 818-898-2361
1010 Arroyo Ave., San Fernando, CA 91340
Medical Illumination International 800-831-1222
547 Library St., San Fernando, CA 91340
Omnical, Inc. 818-837-7531
557 Jessie St., San Fernando, CA 91340
Precision Dynamics Corp. 800-772-1122
13880 Del Sur St., San Fernando, CA 91340-3440
Samco Scientific Corporation 800-522-3359
1050 Arroyo Avenue, San Fernando, CA 91340-1822
Soltec Corp. 800-423-2344
12977 Arroyo St., San Fernando, CA 91340-1548

San Francisco

Advanced Spine Technology, Inc. 415-241-2400
457 Mariposa St., San Francisco, CA 94107
Aqueduct Medical Incorporated 415-896-0134
665 Third St., Suite 20, San Francisco, CA 94107
Bay Optical Instruments 415-431-8711
2401 15th St., San Francisco, CA 94114
Boost Technology, Llc 415-334-8246
1601 Ocean Ave., San Francisco, CA 94112-1717
Cyprus Personal Care Products, Inc. 415-771-0333
2269 Chestnut Ave., #237, San Francisco, CA 94123
Deka Medical 662-327-9950
665 3rd st ste 20, san francisco, CA 94107
Denart Aesthetic Design, S.F. 415-392-2233
450 Sutter St. Suite 1215, San Francisco, CA 94108
Econnectech Llc. 415-810-9436
2434- 14 Avenue, San Francisco, CA 94116
EmSense Inc. 866-574-7014
150 Spear St., Suite 200, San Francisco, CA 94105
Femsuite, Llc 415-561-2565
16A Funston Ave., San Francisco, CA 94129
Henry's Acupuncture Equipment 415-337-8290
241 Leland Ave., San Francisco, CA 94134
Hong Kong Dental Lab 415-330-9099
9 Silliman Street, Suite C, San Francisco, CA 94134
Invuity, Inc. 866-711-7768
39 Stillman Street, San Francisco, CA 94107
Karetech, Llc 415-824-3769
3573 22nd St., San Francisco, CA 94114
Leemah Electronics, Inc. 415-394-1288
1088 Sansome St., --, San Francisco, CA 94111
Leemah Electronics, Inc. 415-394-1288
1301 Folsom Street, --, San Francisco, CA 94103
Mckesson 800-826-9360
One Post Street, San Francisco, CA 94104
Medical Mfg., Inc. 415-282-5580
1290 Sanchez St., #2, San Francisco, CA 94114
Medweb 800-863-3932
667 Folsom St., San Francisco, CA 94107
Relia Diagnostic Systems, Llc 415-344-0844
One Market,suite 1475, Steuart Tower, San Francisco, CA 94105
Smith Group 800-227-3008
301 Battery Street, 7th Floor, San Francisco, CA 94111
Spivey International Inc. 415-333-6800
58 Genebern Way, San Francisco, CA 94112

The Peristat Group, Inc. — 714-928-8507
3721 Fillmore St, San Francisco, CA 94123
Western Scientific Co., Inc. — 877-489-3726
4104 24th St. #183, San Francisco, CA 94114
iRhythm Technologies, Inc. — 415-632-5700
650 Townsend Street, Suite 350, San Francisco, CA 94103

San Jacinto

Tiburon Medical Enterprises — 909-654-2333
915 Industrial Way, San Jacinto, CA 92582

San Jose

A&D Medical — 800-726-7099
1756 Automation Parkway, San Jose, CA 95131
Airgas, Northern California And Nevada — 916-379-1050
443 Hobson St., San Jose, CA 95110
Align Technology, Inc. — 408-470-1000
2560 orchard parkway, san jose, CA 95131
Ams Innovative Center-San Jose — 800-356-7600
3070 Orchard Drive, San Jose, CA 95134-2011
Baxano, Inc. — 408-514-2200
655 River Oaks Parkway, San Jose, CA 95134
Bd Biosciences — 408-954-6307
2350 Qume Dr., San Jose, CA 95131
Boston Scientific Corp. — 408-935-3400
150 Baytech Dr., San Jose, CA 95134
DFine Inc. — 866-963-3463
3047 Orchard Parkway, San Jose, CA 95134
Ep Technologies, Inc. — 888-272-1001
2710 Orchard Pkwy., San Jose, CA 95134
Flextronics International Ltd. — 408-576-7000
Flextronics International, 2090 Fortune Dr., San Jose, CA 95131
Gdm Electronic And Medical — 408-945-4100
2070 Ringwood Ave., San Jose, CA 95131
Helio Medical Supplies, Inc. — 408-433-3355
606 Charcot Ave., San Jose, CA 95131
Hemosense, Inc. — 877-436-6444
651 River Oaks Parkway, San Jose, CA 95134
Highland Metals, Inc. — 800-368-6484
419 Perrymont Drive, San Jose, CA 95125
Hitachi High Technologies America, Inc. — 800-548-9001
3100 N. First St., San Jose, CA 95134
Intermark (Usa), Inc. — 408-971-2055
1310 Tully Road, Suite 117, San Jose, CA 95122
Laser Dental Innovations — 877-753-5054
745 Dubanski Drive, San Jose, CA 95123
Leica Microsystems (San Jose) Corporation — 800-634-3622
120 Baytech Drive, San Jose, CA 95134-2302
Lobob Laboratories, Inc. — 800-83-LOBOB
1440 Atteberry Lane, San Jose, CA 95131-1410
MOS Plastics Inc. — 408-944-9407
2308 Zanker Rd., San Jose, CA 95131
Magic Walk, Inc. — 408-435-7380
2372 Qume Dr., Suite E, San Jose, CA 95131-1843
Micrus Endovascular Corporation — 888-550-4120
821 Fox Lane, San Jose, CA 95131
Mobilsonic, Inc. — 408-390-4002
19 North 2nd Street, Ste. 206, San Jose, CA 95113
Nds Surgical Imaging, Inc. — 866-637-5237
5750 Hellyer Ave, San Jose, CA 95138
Neoguide Systems, Inc. — 408-321-8844
2712 Orchard Parkway, San Jose, CA 95134
Philips Medical Systems, New Clinical Ventures — 408-321-9100
3860 North First Street, San Jose, CA 95134
SI-Bone INC. — 408-207-0700
550 South Winchester Blvd., Suite 620, San Jose, CA 95128
Sanmina-Sci Corp. — 408-964-3555
2700 North First Street, San Jose, CA 95134
Sanmina-Sci Usa, Inc. — 408-904-2117
2700 North First Street, San Jose, CA 95134
Si-Bone Inc. — 408-207-0700
550 South Winchester Blvd., Suite 620, San Jose, CA 95128
Sonicwall, Inc. — 888-557-6642
2001 Logic Drive, San Jose, CA 95124-3452
Stryker Endoscopy — 800-435-0220
5900 Optical Ct, San Jose, CA 95138
Suni Medical Imaging, Inc. — 408-227-6698
6840 Via Del Oro, San Jose, CA 95119
Supracor, Inc. — 800-787-7226
2050 Corporate Ct., San Jose, CA 95131
Tecan Systems — 800-231-0711
2450 Zanker Rd., San Jose, CA 95131
Televideo Systems, Inc. — 408-954-8333
2562 Seaboard Ave, San Jose, CA 95131
Televital, Inc. — 408-441-1199
1309 Harefield Ct., San Jose, CA 95131
U-System, Inc. — 408-571-0777
110 Rose Orchard Way, San Jose, CA 95134
Ucp Biosciences, Inc. — 408-392-0064
1445 Koll Circle, Ste. 111, San Jose, CA 95112
Vascular Designs, Inc — 408-484-9010
4960 Almaden Expressway, San Jose, CA 95118

Vnus Medical Technologies, Inc. — 888-797-8346
5799 Fontanoso Way, San Jose, CA 95138

San Juan Capistrano

C.E.J. Dental Products Inc. — 949-493-2449
32332 Camino Capistrano #101, San Juan Capistrano, CA 92675
Chi Institute — 949-361-3976
27130a Paseo Espada, Ste 1407, San Juan Capistrano, CA 92675
Imonti And Associates Inc., M. — 949-248-1058
25707 Compass Way, San Juan Capistrano, CA 92675-4003
3gen, Llc. — 949-481-6384
31521 Rancho Viejo Rd., Suite 104, San Juan Capistrano, CA 92675

San Leandro

Ams Industries — 510-667-0673
14680 Doolittel Drive, San Leandro, CA 94577
Con-Cise Contact Lens Co. — 800-772-3911
14450 Doolittle Drive, PO Box 2198, San Leandro, CA 94577-0338
Medical Instrumentation Development Labs — 800-929-5227
557 McCormick Street, San Leandro, CA 94577
Mercator Medsystems, Inc. — 510-614-4550
1670 Alvarado Street, Suite 4, San Leandro, CA 94577
Unotech Diagnostics, Inc. — 510-352-3070
2235 Polvorosa Ave., Suite 220, San Leandro, CA 94577

San Lorenzo

Wrapped In Comfort — 877-205-0901
15760 Via Sonata, San Lorenzo, CA 94580

San Luis Obispo

Alltec Integrated Manufacturing,Inc. — 805-595-3500
4330 Santa Fe Road, San Luis Obispo, CA 93401
Calzyme Laboratories, Inc. — 800-523-9127
3443 Miguelito Court, San Luis Obispo, CA 93401
Deroyal/Lmb, Inc. — 800-251-9864
712 Fiero Lane, No. 37, San Luis Obispo, CA 93401
Dioptics Medical Products, Inc. — 800-959-9040
125 Venture Drive, San Luis Obispo, CA 93401
Fziomed, Inc. — 805-546-0610
231 Bonetti Drive, San Luis Obispo, CA 93401
Swiss Implants, Inc. — 805-781-8700
3046 South Higuera Street, Suite E, San Luis Obispo, CA 93401

San Marcos

Aci Medical, Inc. — 800-667-9451
1857 Diamond St., San Marcos, CA 92078-5129
Anesthesia Associates, Inc. — 760-744-6561
460 Enterprise St., San Marcos, CA 92078-4363
Artventive Medical Group Inc. — 760-471-7700
1797 Playa Vista, San Marcos, CA 92078
Bacton Assay Systems, Inc. — 760-471-4538
772-a Twin Oaks Valley Rd., San Marcos, CA 92069
Cliniqa Corporation — 800-728-9558
774 North Twin Oaks Valley Road, Suite C, San Marcos, CA 92069
Coral Biotechnology — 760-727-8224
110 Bosstick Blvd., San Marcos, CA 92069
International Medical Equipment — 800.543.8496
170 Vallecitos De Oro, San Marcos, CA 92069
Invuity, Inc. — 760-744-4447
334 Via Vera Cruz, Suite 255, San Marcos, CA 92078
Iyia Technologies, Inc. — 760-752-1036
1195 Linda Vista Drive, Suite C, San Marcos, CA 92078
Lancer Orthodontics, Inc. — 760-304-2705
253 Pawnee St., San Marcos, CA 92078
Shofu Dental Corporation — 800-827-4638
1225 Stone Drive, San Marcos, CA 92069
Signet Armorlite, Inc. — 760-744-4000
1001 Armorlite Dr., San Marcos, CA 92069
Spectrum Assembly Inc. — 760-752-7008
970 Los Vallecitos Blvd., Suite 140, San Marcos, CA 92069

San Mateo

Deltagen Inc. — 650-345-7600
1900 S. Norfolk St., Suite 105, San Mateo, CA 94403
E-Y Laboratories, Inc. — 800-821-0044
107 North Amphlett Blvd., San Mateo, CA 94401-1902
Epocrates Inc. — 650-227-1700
1100 Park Place, Suite 300, San Mateo, CA 94403
Halbar North, Inc. — 650-349-4700
#3 West 37th Avenue, San Mateo, CA 94403-4457
PreXion Inc. — 650-212-0300
411 Borel Avenue, Suite 550, San Mateo, CA 94402
Solo Bambini — 650-340-1773
729 Occidental Ave., San Mateo, CA 94402
Sonitus Medical Inc. — 650-838-0325
1825 S. Grant Street, Suite 350, San Mateo, CA 94402

San Pedro

Intusoft — 310-833-0710
P.O. Box 710, San Pedro, CA 90733-9918
Micron Precision Engineering, Inc. — 310-874-4963
939 Evening Shade Dr, San Pedro, CA 90731

San Rafael

Berkeley Nucleonics Corp.   800-234-7858
2955 Kerner Blvd., San Rafael, CA 94901
Bio Plas, Inc.   415-472-3777
4340 Redwood Highway, Suite A15, San Rafael, CA 94903
Marcon Group, Inc.   800-547-5021
655 Du Bois Street, Suite D, San Rafael, CA 94901
Nuprodx, Inc.   888-288-5653
4 Malone Lane, San Rafael, CA 94903
Parnell Pharmaceuticals, Inc.   415-256-1800
1525 Francisco Blvd., Ste. 15, San Rafael, CA 94901
Pyramid Orthodontics   800-752-8884
4328 Redwood Hwy., Ste. 100, San Rafael, CA 94903
Safety Syringe Corporation Of America, Inc.   415-454-8054
58 Oakdale Avenue, San Rafael, CA 94901
Tissue Banks International   800-756-4824
2597 Kerner Blvd., San Rafael, CA 94901

San Ramon

Biogenex Laboratories   800-421-4149
4600 Norris Canyon Road, San Ramon, CA 94583-1320
Bioventrix   925-830-1000
12647 Alcosta Blvd., Suite 400, San Ramon, CA 94583
Breathe Technologies Inc.   925-359-1500
4000 Executive Parkway, Suite 190, San Ramon, CA 94583
Danville Materials   800-827-7940
3420 Fostoria Way, Suite A200, San Ramon, CA 94583
Estech, Inc.   888-378-3240
2603 Camino Ramon, Suite 100, San Ramon, CA 94583
Mirion Technologies   925-543-0800
Bishop Ranch 8, 3000 Executive Parkway Suite 222, San Ramon, CA 94583
Odyssey Thera Inc.   925-242-5000
4550 Norris Canyon Road, Suite 140, San Ramon, CA 94583
Softchrome, Inc.   925-743-1285
2551 San Ramon Valley Blvd.,, Suite 101, San Ramon, CA 94583-1661
Transamerican Technologies International   800-322-7373
2246 Camino Ramon, San Ramon, CA 94583
Vindum Engineering, Inc.   925-275-0633
1 Woodview Court, San Ramon, CA 94582-2307

Santa Ana

Abbott Medical Optics Inc.   866-427-8477
1700 East St. Andrew Pl., Santa Ana, CA 92705
Allez Medical Applications, Inc.   714-641-2098
2141 S. Standard Avenue, Santa Ana, CA 92707
Avail Medical Products, Inc.   858-635-2206
1900 Carnegie Ave., --, Santa Ana, CA 92705
B & L Engineering   714-505-9492
1901 Carnegie Ave., Suite Q, Santa Ana, CA 92705
Choose Manufacturing, Co. Llc   714-327-1698
3310 W. Macarthur Blvd, Santa Ana, CA 92704
Coastal Biocare   714-751-0121
2737 South Croddy Way, Unit D, Santa Ana, CA 92704
Codan Us Corporation   800-332-6326
3511 W. Sunflower Avenue, Santa Ana, CA 92704-6944
Deltronic Corp.   800-451-6922
3900 West Segerstrom Avenue, Santa Ana, CA 92704
Express Manufacturing, Inc.   714-979-2228
3519 West Warner Ave., Santa Ana, CA 92704
Healthcare Service And Supply   714-669-8803
10602 Mira Vista Drive, Santa Ana, CA 92705
Kenlor Industries, Inc.   800-899-9371
1560 East Edinger Ave., Suite A-1, Santa Ana, CA 92705
Kenlor Industries, Inc.   714-647-0770
1560 East Edinger Ave.,, Suite A-1, Santa Ana, CA 92705
Medtronic Cardiovascular Surgery, The Heart Valve Div.   800-328-2518
1851 East Deere Ave., Santa Ana, CA 92705
Merit Cables, Inc.   877-637-4848
830 N. Poinsettia St., Santa Ana, CA 92701
Microtech   714-966-1645
3633 West Macarthur Blvd., Suite 410, Santa Ana, CA 92704
Progressive Dental Supply/Progressive Orthodontics Seminars   800-443-3106
1701 E. Edinger Avenue, Suite C-1, Santa Ana, CA 92705-5011
R&B Wire Products, Inc.   800-634-0555
2902 West Garry Street, Santa Ana, CA 92704
Safety 1st Medical, Inc.   800-997-2331
1740 E. Garry Avenue #109, Santa Ana, CA 92705
Tmx Engineering & Manufacturing, Inc.   714-641-5884
2141 S. Standard Ave., Santa Ana, CA 92707
Ultra Tec Manufacturing, Inc.   877-542-0609
1025 E. Chestnut Avenue, Santa Ana, CA 92701
Westridge Laboratori   1-800-646-2096
1671 E. Saint Andrew Place, Santa Ana, CA 92705-4932

Santa Barbara

Abbeon Cal, Inc.   800-922-0977
123 Gray Avenue, Santa Barbara, CA 93101-1809
Acumed Instruments Corp.   800-234-5045
5662 Calle Real #406, Santa Barbara, CA 91377-2317
Allegiance Group, Inc.   805-569-1694
4025 Lago Dr., Santa Barbara, CA 93110
Channel Industries, Inc.   805-967-0171
839 Ward Drive, Santa Barbara, CA 93111-2920
Cmc Rescue, Inc.   800-235-5741
P.O. Box 6870, Santa Barbara, CA 93160
Giles Scientific, Inc.   800-603-9290
PO Box 4306, Santa Barbara, CA 93140-4306
Greer Medical, Inc.   (800) 424-2155
314 East Carrillo St., Suite 1, Santa Barbara, CA 93101
Intouch Technologies, Inc.   805-562-8686
90 Castilian Dr., Ste. 200, Santa Barbara, CA 93117
Mentor Corp.   800-525-0245
201 Mentor Drive, Santa Barbara, CA 93111
Mentor Ophthalmics, Inc.   800-525-0245
201 Mentor Dr., Santa Barbara, CA 93111
Starchild Labs   805-564-7194
57 Tierra Cielo Lane, Santa Barbara, CA 93105
Truevision Systems, Incorporated   805-963-9700
114 East Haley Street, Santa Barbara, CA 93101

Santa Clara

Abbott Hematology, Diagnostics Div.   800-323-9100
5440 Patrick Henry Dr., Santa Clara, CA 95054
Abbott Vascular, Cardiac Therapies   800-227-9902
3200 Lakeside Dr., Santa Clara, CA 95054-2807
Abbott Vascular, Vascular Solutions   847-937-2388
3200 Lakeside Dr, Santa Clara, CA 95054
Affymetrix, Inc.   888-DNA-CHIP
3420 Central Expy., Santa Clara, CA 95051
Agilent Technologies, Inc.   877-424-4536
5301 Stevens Creek Blvd., Santa Clara, CA 95051
Bacchus Vascular, Inc.   877-622-5082
3110 Coronado Dr., Santa Clara, CA 95054
Benvenue Medical, Inc.   888 717-9333
3052 Bunker Hill Lane, Suite 120, Santa Clara, CA 95054
Cell Biosciences, Inc.   888-607-9692
3040 Oakmead Village Drive, Santa Clara, CA 95051
Coherent, Inc.   800-527-3786
5100 Patrick Henry Drive, Santa Clara, CA 95054
Continuum, Inc.   888-532-1064
3150 Central Expressway, Santa Clara, CA 95051
Eklin Medical Systems   408-492-0057
1605 Wyatt Dr., Santa Clara, CA 95054
Equilasers, Inc   408-588-1212
3350 Scott Blvd., Bldg. 5, Santa Clara, CA 95054
Fiberlite Centrifuge Inc.   408-988-1103
422 Aldo Avenue, Santa Clara, CA 95054
Flossaid Corporation   800-528-3384
3045 Copper Road, Santa Clara, CA 95051-0701
Hologic|r2, Inc.   866-243-2533
2585 Augustine Drive, Santa Clara, CA 95054
Indec Systems, Inc.   408-986-1600
2210 Martin Avenue, Santa Clara, CA 95050
Life Enhancement Technologies, Inc.   408-330-6940
807 Aldo Ave., Suite 101, Santa Clara, CA 95054
Lifescience Plus, Inc.   650-565-8172
473 Sapena Ct., Suite # 7, Santa Clara, CA 95054
LumaSense Technologies Inc.   408-727-1600
3301 Leonard Court, Santa Clara, CA 95054
Medelex, Inc.   800-644-0692
3012 Lawrence Expressway, Santa Clara, CA 95051
Meiji Techno America   800-832-0060
3010 Olcott Street, Santa Clara, CA 95054
Mikron Infrared, Inc.   805-644-9544
3033 Scott Blvd., Santa Clara, CA 95054
NewCardio Inc.   408-516-5000
2350 Mission College Blvd, Suite 1175, Santa Clara, CA 95054
Optimedica Corporation   888-850-1230
3100 Coronado Drive, Santa Clara, CA 95054
Ornim Inc.   866-811-6384
23462 Thornewood Dr, Santa Clara, CA 91321
Piranha Plastics, Llc.   408-855-9650
3531 Thomas Rd., Santa Clara, CA 95054
Rhamdec Inc.   800-4-MYDESC
P.O. Box 4296, Santa Clara, CA 95056
Samplify Systems Inc.   408-249-1500
160 Saratoga Avenue, Suite 150, Santa Clara, CA 95051
Spectra-Physics Lazors   877-835-9620
3635 Peterson Way, Santa Clara, CA 95054
Usb Corporation   1-888-362-2447
3420 central expressway, santa clara, CA 95051
Yamato Scientific America, Inc.   800-292-6286
925 Walsh Ave., Santa Clara, CA 95050

Santa Clarita

Advanced Bionics Corp.   800-678-2575
25129 Rye Canyon Loop, Santa Clarita, CA 91355
Dr.'s Page   888-297-9109
P.O. Box 801764, Santa Clarita, CA 91380-1764
Home-Aid-Healthcare, Inc.   888-297-9109
PO Box 801764, Santa Clarita, CA 91380-1764

St. John Companies
25167 Anza Drive, PO Box 800460, Santa Clarita, CA 91380 — 800-435-4242

Santa Cruz

Beta Technology, Inc.
2841 Mission St., Santa Cruz, CA 95060 — 800-858-2382

Doc's Proplugs, Inc.
719 Swift st, Suite 100, Santa Cruz, CA 95060 — 800-521-2982

Palco Labs, Inc.
8030 Soquel Avenue, Suite 104, Santa Cruz, CA 95062-2032 — 800-346-4488

Peninsula Medical, Inc.
108 Whispering Pines Drive, Suite 115, Santa Cruz, CA 95066 — 831-430-9066

Santa Fe Spgs

Alliance Prosthetics & Orthotics, Inc.
14535 Valley View Ave., Ste U, Santa Fe Spgs, CA 90670 — 562-921-0353

Santa Fe Springs

Adenna Inc.
11932 Baker Place, Santa Fe Springs, CA 90670 — 888-323-3662

Ars Enterprises
12900 Lakeland Road, Santa Fe Springs, CA 90670-4517 — 800-735-9277

Blaine Labs, Inc.
11037 Lockport Place, Santa Fe Springs, CA 90670 — 800-307-8818

Columbia Medical Manufacturing Llc
13577 Larwin Circle, Santa Fe Springs, CA 90670 — 800-454-6612

Crosstex International Ltd., W. Region
14059 Stage Rd., Santa Fe Springs, CA 90670 — 800-707-2737

Jeunique International, Inc.
10528 Pioneer Blvd., Santa Fe Springs, CA 90670 — 800-732-9289

Kodent Inc.
13340 E. Firestone Blvd., Suite J, Santa Fe Springs, CA 90670 — 562-404-8466

Morgan-Gallacher, Inc.
8707 Millergrove Dr., Santa Fe Springs, CA 90670 — 562-695-1232

Pentax West Coast Service Center
10410 Pioneer Blvd., Unit 2, Santa Fe Springs, CA 90670 — 800-431-5880

Weartech Intl., Inc.
13032 Park Street, Santa Fe Springs, CA 90670 — 562-698-7847

Santa Maria

Den-Mat Holdings, Llc
2727 Skyway Dr., Santa Maria, CA 93455 — 800-433-6628

Hardy Diagnostics
1430 West McCoy Lane, Santa Maria, CA 93455 — 800-226-2222

Sns Biosystems
527-B East Oak St., Santa Maria, CA 93454 — 805-925-1616

Santa Monica

Arthronet Medical, Inc.
520 Broadway, Ste. 350, Santa Monica, CA 90401 — 949-254-3343

Bio-Analysis, Inc.
1701 Berkeley St., Santa Monica, CA 90404 — 310-828-7423

Carr Corporation
1547 11th St., Santa Monica, CA 90401 — 800-952-2398

Caspian Designs, Inc.
2632 Lincoln Blvd., Santa Monica, CA 90405 — 310-396-5258

Floss & Go, Inc.
1112 Montana Ave.; Suite D, Santa Monica, CA 90403 — 310-394-6700

Global Healthcheck, Inc.
2417 34th Street, Suite 17, Santa Monica, CA 90405 — 949-757-0639

John Goodman & Associates, Inc.
1734 Colorado Ave., Santa Monica, CA 90404 — 310-828 - 504

Weitbrecht Communications, Inc.
926 Colorado Avenue, Santa Monica, CA 90401-2717 — 800-233-9130

Santa Paula

Hely And Weber
1185 East Main St., Santa Paula, CA 93060 — 800-221-5465

Tracer Designs, Inc.
333 South 11th St., Santa Paula, CA 93060 — 805-933-2616

Santa Rosa

Access Bridges
610 Nason St., Santa Rosa, CA 95404 — 707-546-7671

Macken Instruments, Inc.
3186 Coffee Lane., Santa Rosa, CA 95403 — 707-566-2110

Medtronic Vascular
5345 Skylane Blvd, Santa Rosa, CA 95403 — 707-566-1548

Morgan Medesign, Inc.
947 Piner Place, Santa Rosa, CA 95403 — 888-799-4633

Motion Analysis Corp.
3617 West Wind Blvd., Santa Rosa, CA 95403 — 707-579-6500

Osseon Therapeutics, Inc.
2330 Circadian Way, Santa Rosa, CA 95407 — 877-567-7366

Redwood Toxicology Laboratories, Inc.
3650 Westwind Blvd., Santa Rosa, CA 95403 — 800-255-2159

Sapheon Inc
3579 Westwind Blvd., Santa Rosa, CA 95403 — 707-703-4371

Sonoma Orthopedic Products, Inc.
3589 Westwind Boulevard, Santa Rosa, CA 95403 — 707-526-1335

Trivascular Inc.
3910 Brickway Blvd., Santa Rosa, CA 95403 — 707-543-8800

Santa Ynez

Preat Corp.
2976 Long Valley Rd., P.O. Box 1030, Santa Ynez, CA 93460 — 800-232-7732

Santee

Curapharm, Inc.
10054 Prospect Ave., Suite F, Santee, CA 92071 — 619-449-7388

Reflex Industries, Inc.
9530 Pathway St., Suite 105, Santee, CA 92071 — 619-562-1821

Scantibodies Laboratory, Inc.
9336 Abraham Way, Santee, CA 92071 — 619-258-9300

Saratoga

Meta Fusion, Inc.
15209 Blue Gum Court, Saratoga, CA 95070 — 408-345-0500

VisionCare Ophthalmic Technologies Inc.
14395 Saratoga Ave, Suite 150, Saratoga, CA 95070 — 408-872-9393

Sausalito

Lexicon Branding, Inc.
30 Liberty Ship Way, Suite 3360, Sausalito, CA 94965 — 415-332-1811

Wink Lens Technologies
200 Gate 5 Rd., Suite 201, Sausalito, CA 94965 — 415-332-6694

Scotts Valley

Digital Dynamics, Inc.
5 Victor Square, Scotts Valley, CA 95066 — 800-765-1288

Seal Beach

Orthopedic Sciences, Inc
3020 Old Ranch Parkway, Suite 325, Seal Beach, CA 90740 — 562-799-5550

Sebastopol

Pisces Productions, Inc.
380-a Morris St., Sebastopol, CA 95472 — 800-822 - 5333

Sherman Oaks

Contex, Inc.
4505 Van Nuys Blvd., Sherman Oaks, CA 91403 — 800-626-6839

Signal Hill

Cablestrand Corp.
2660 Signal Pkwy., Signal Hill, CA 90755 — 562-595-4527

Edge Systems Corporation
2277 REDONDO AVENUE, Signal Hill, CA 90755 — 800-603-4996

Integrated Medical Systems, Inc.
1984 Obispo Avenue, Signal Hill, CA 90755 — 562-498-1776

Mellen Air Manufacturing, Inc.
2601 East 28th Street, Suite 307, Signal Hill, CA 90755-2245 — 800-770-6264

Siemens Water Technologies
1700 East 28th St., Signal Hill, CA 90807 — 866.926.8420

Thermoplastic Comfort Systems, Inc.
2619 Lime Avenue, Signal Hill, CA 90755 — 562-426-2970

Simi Valley

Bemco, Inc.
2255 Union Pl., Simi Valley, CA 93065 — 805-583-4970

Eprt Technologies, Inc.
2139 Tapo St., Suite 228, Simi Valley, CA 93063 — 805-522-6223

Freedom Designs, Inc.
2241N. Madera Rd., Simi Valley, CA 93065 — 800-331-8551

Hammer-Plane Inc.
2245 Homewood Avenue, Simi Valley, CA 93063 — 800-398-3017

KnArr Usa Inc.
1890 N. Voyager Avenue, Simi Valley, CA 93063 — 800-465-6877

Revolution Eyewear, Inc.
997 Flower Glen Rd., Simi Valley, CA 93065 — 310-777-8399

Solana Beach

Back Bubble
621 Seabright Ln., Solana Beach, CA 92075 — 858-481-8715

Leasing Innovations Incorporated
437 S. Highway 101, Suite 104, Solana Beach, CA 92075 — 800-532-7388

Metron Optics, Inc.
813 Academy Drive, Solana Beach, CA 92075-0690 — 858-755-4477

Portable Medical Laboratories, Inc.
544 S. Nardo Avenue, Solana Beach, CA 92075-0667 — 858-755-7385

Solvang

Ocularvision, Inc.
687 Alisa Rd, Solvang, CA 93463 — 800-964-9433

Somerset

Astralite Corporation
PO Box 689, Somerset, CA 95684 — 800-345-7703

Sonora

Phaco Solutions, Inc.
19395 Village Dr., Sonora, CA 95370 — 209-536-9707

Sierra Molecular Inc.
21109 Longeway Rd. # C, Sonora, CA 95370 — 209-536-0886

Soquel

Made On Earth   831-475-7352
5044-b Wilder Dr., Soquel, CA 95073

South El Monte

Commerce Atlantic Corp.   626-448-8905
2239 Tyler Ave., Suite B, South El Monte, CA 91733
Gilmore Liquid Air Co., Inc.   626-443-1361
9503 E. Rush St., South El Monte, CA 91733
International Medication Systems, Ltd.   800-423-4136
1886 Santa Anita Ave., South El Monte, CA 91733
Medisol U.S.A., Inc.   626-350-6662
9713 Factorial Way, South El Monte, CA 91733

South Pasadena

Abbott Diagnostics Div.   626-440-0700
820 Mission St., South Pasadena, CA 91030

South San Francisco

Chemux Bioscience, Inc.   650-872-1800
50 South Linden Ave. #7, South San Francisco, CA 94080
Diadexus, Inc.   650-246-6400
343 Oyster Point Blvd., South San Francisco, CA 94080
Ease Labs, Inc.   650-872-7788
338 North Canal St., #9, South San Francisco, CA 94080
Elan   650-877-0900
800 Gateway Boulevard, South San Francisco, CA 94080
Fluidigm Corporation   1-866-358-4354
7000 Shoreline Court, Suite 100, South San Francisco, CA 94080
Fluxion Biosciences Inc.   866-266-8380
384 Oyster Point Blvd. #6, South San Francisco, CA 94080
Genentech, Inc.   888-835-2555
1 DNA Way, South San Francisco, CA 94080-4990
Ita-Med Co.   888-9IT-AMED
310 Littlefield Ave., South San Francisco, CA 94080
Tangle, Inc.   650-616-7900
439c Eccles Ave., South San Francisco, CA 94080
Toshiba America Medical Systems, Inc.   800-421-1968
280 Utah Ave., South San Francisco, CA 94080-6883
Tosoh Bioscience, Inc.   800-248-6764
6000 Shoreline Court, Suite 101, South San Francisco, CA 94080
Veracyte Inc.   650-243-6300
7000 Shoreline Ct., Suite 250, South San Francisco, CA 94080

Spring Valley

Calbiotech, Inc.   866-calbiotech
10461 Austin Dr., #g, Spring Valley, CA 91978
Lumalite, Inc.   800-400-2262
2830 Via Orange Way, Suite B, Spring Valley, CA 91978

Stanton

Newport Glass Works, Ltd.   714-484-8100
PO Box 127, 10564 Fern Avenue, Stanton, CA 90680
Newport Optical Laboratories, Inc.   714-484-3200
10564-C Fern Ave., Stanton, CA 90680

Stockton

Anderson Moulds, Inc.   209-943-1145
3131 E. Anita St., Stockton, CA 95205
Ctronics   800-472-9909
6333 Pacific Avenue, PMB 294, Stockton, CA 95207
Pelton Shepherd Industries   800-258-3423
812b Luce St., Stockton, CA 95203
Sri Surgical   813-891-9550
6801 Longe St., Stockton, CA 95206

Sun Valley

Sscor   800-434-5211
11064 Randall St., Sun Valley, CA 91352

Sunnyvale

EBR Systems, Inc.   1 408 720 1906
686 W. Maude Ave. - Suite 102, Sunnyvale, CA 94085
Accuray Incorporated   888-522-3740
1310 Chesapeake Terrace, Sunnyvale, CA 94089
Accuray, Inc.   888-522-3740
1310 Chesapeake Terrace, Sunnyvale, CA 94089
Acumen Medical, Inc.   408-530-1810
275 Santa Ana Court, Sunnyvale, CA 94085
Addition Technology, Inc.   847-297-8419
155 Moffett Park Drive,, Suite B-1, Sunnyvale, CA 94089
Apherma Corp.   408-524-1634
440 N. Wolfe Road, Sunnyvale, CA 94085
Applied Dental, Inc.   888-841-8481
544 E.Weddell Drive, Suite 9, Sunnyvale, CA 94089-2123
Aptus Endosystems Inc.   877-292-7887
777 N. Pastoria Avenue, Sunnyvale, CA 94085-2918
Arthrocare Corp.   800-797-6520
680 Vaqueros Avenue, Sunnyvale, CA 94085-3523
Asante Solutions Inc.   408-716-5600
1012 Stewart Drive, Sunnyvale, CA 94085
Asthmatx, Inc.   1-877-810-6060
888 Ross Dr., Suite 100, Sunnyvale, CA 94089

Avantec Vascular Corp.   408-329-5425
605 W. W. California Ave, Sunnyvale, CA 94086
Avantis Medical Systems, Inc.   408-733-1901
263 Santa Ana Ct., Sunnyvale, CA 94085
Backproject Corporation   1-888-470-8100
170 N Wolfe Rd, Sunnyvale, CA 94086
Barrx Medical, Incorporated   888-662-2779
540 Oakmead Parkway, Sunnyvale, CA 94085
Bayer Healthcare, Llc   574-256-3430
510 Oakmead Pkwy., Sunnyvale, CA 94085
Cardiva Medical, Inc.   650-964-8900
888 W. Maude Avenue, Sunnyvale, CA 94085
Cepheid   408-541-4191
904 Caribbean Drive, Sunnyvale, CA 94089
Chemdev Instruments, Inc.   408-541-8535
1289 Reamwood Ave., #b, Sunnyvale, CA 94089
CorMatrix Cardiovascular Inc.   877-651-2628
155-a Moffett Park Drive, Suite 240, Sunnyvale, CA 94089
D. Sign Dental Lab, Inc.   757-224-0177
690 W. Fremont Avenue, Suite 9c, Sunnyvale, CA 94087
Diagnostics For The Real World, Ltd.   408-773-1511
840 Del Rey Avenue, Sunnyvale, CA 94085
Dionex Corp.   408-737-0700
1228 Titan Way, P.O. Box 3603, Sunnyvale, CA 94088-3603
Elixir Medical Corporation   408-636-2000
870 Hermosa Ave., Sunnyvale, CA 94085
Ensure Medical, Inc.   408-745-7610
762 San Aleso Ave., Sunnyvale, CA 94085
Equipment Technology Conveyance   408-483-1894
125 Connemara Way #164, Sunnyvale, CA 94087
Flowcardia, Inc.   408-617-0352
745 N. Pastoria Ave., Sunnyvale, CA 94085
Gesturetek Health-Gesturetek Inc   408-216-8087
530 Lakeside Drive,, Suite 280, Sunnyvale, CA 94085
Hayes Manufacturing Services, Inc.   1AŽ408AŽ730AŽ50
1178 Sonora Court, Sunnyvale, CA 94086
Hologic, Inc.   888-773-8376
1240 Elko Drive, Sunnyvale, CA 94089
Imageflow Inc.   408-569-3860
730 Bantry Court, Sunnyvale, CA 94087
Insiphil (Us) Llc   408-616-8700
650 Vaqueros Avenue, Suite F, Sunnyvale, CA 94085-3533
Intella Interventional Systems, Inc.   408-737-7121
870 Hermosa Drive, Sunnyvale, CA 94086
Intraop Medical Corp.   408-636-1020
570 Del Rey Ave, Sunnyvale, CA 94085
Intuitive Surgical, Inc.   888-409-4774
1266 Kifer Road, Sunnyvale, CA 94086-5304
Intuity Medical Inc.   408-530-1700
350 Potrero Avenue, Sunnyvale, CA 94085
Kempf   800-255-6174
1245 Lakeside Dr., #3005, Sunnyvale, CA 94086
Labcyte Inc.   1.408.747.2000
1190 Borregas Avenue, Sunnyvale, CA 94089
Lin-Zhi International, Inc.   408-732-3856
670 Almanor Avenue, Sunnyvale, CA 94085
Med-Surgical Services Inc.   408-617-2000
465 E. Evelyn Ave., Sunnyvale, CA 94086
Meddev Corporation   800-543-2789
730 N. Pastoria Avenue, Sunnyvale, CA 94085
Medtronic Spine Llc   877-690-5353
1221 Crossman Ave., Sunnyvale, CA 94089
Melcor Technologies, Inc.   408-247-0350
1030 E. El Camino Real #435, Sunnyvale, CA 94087
Micrus Corporation   408-830-5900
610 Palomar Avenue, Sunnyvale, CA 94085
Molecular Devices Corp.   800-635-5577
1311 Orleans Drive, Sunnyvale, CA 94089-1136
Onda Corporation   408-745-0383
592 Weddell Drive, Suite 7, Sunnyvale, CA 94089
Pulnix America Inc.   800-445-5444
1330 Orleans Drive, Sunnyvale, CA 94089
Purdy Electronics Corp.   408-523-8225
755 North Pastoria Avenue, Sunnyvale, CA 94085
Solarius Development Inc.   800-731-1220
550 Weddell Drive #3, Sunnyvale, CA 94089
Spinal Kinetics, Inc.   609-254-3999
595 N Pastoria Avenue, Sunnyvale, CA 94085
Starion Instruments   800-782-7466
1227 innsbruck dr, Sunnyvale, CA 94089
Stellartech Research Corp.   408-331-3000
1346 Bordeaux Dr., Sunnyvale, CA 94089
Supertex, Inc.   800-222-9883
1235 Bordeaux Drive, Sunnyvale, CA 94089
Symyx Technologies, Inc.   408-764-2000
1263 East Arques Avenue, Sunnyvale, CA 94085
Turner Biosystems, Inc.   408-636-2414
645 North Mary Avenue, Sunnyvale, CA 94085
Turner Designs   877-316-8049
845 W. Maude Avenue, Sunnyvale, CA 94085
U-System, Inc.   (408) 245-1970
447 Indio Way, Sunnyvale, CA 94085

U-Systems, Inc.   408-245-1970
447 Indio Way, Sunnyvale, CA 94085
Visx Incorporated, A Subsidiary Of Amo Inc.   714-247-8656
1328 Kifer Road, Sunnyvale, CA 94089
Xoft, Inc.   408-419-2300
345 Potrero, Sunnyvale, CA 94085
Zoll Circulation   800-321-4277
650 Almanor Ave., Sunnyvale, CA 94085

Sylmar

Marco Products Company   800-572-USA1
12860 San Fernando Road, Sylmar, CA 91342
Matech, Inc.   818-367-2472
13000 San Fernando Rd., Sylmar, CA 91342
St. Jude Medical Cardiac Rhythm Management Div.   800-777-2237
15900 Valley View Ct., Sylmar, CA 91342-3577

Tarzana

Medic Id's International   800-926-3342
PO Box 571687, Tarzana, CA 91357
Sound Feelings   818-757-0600
18375 Ventura Blvd. #8000, Tarzana, CA 91356-4218

Temecula

Abbott Vascular, Cardiac Therapies   800-227-9902
26531 Ynez Rd., Mailing P.O. Box 9018, Temecula, CA 92589-9018
Abbott Vascular, Vascular Solutions   800-227-9902
26531 Ynez Rd., Temecula, CA 92589
Abbott West Distribution Center   847-937-2388
42301 Zevo Drive, Temecula, CA 92590
Hatch Corporation   800-347-1200
42374 Avenida Alvarado, Suite A, Temecula, CA 92590
Hopkins Imaging   951-302-8416
34721 El Mirador Corte, Temecula, CA 92592
Ims-Ess   951-676-2751
27449 Colt Court, Temecula, CA 92590
Medical Design Concepts, Inc.   951-296-2600
41980 Winchester Rd., Temecula, CA 92590-3666
Next Generation Co.   800-598-4303
41740 Enterprise Cir., North, #108, Temecula, CA 92590-5652
Surgicount Medical, Inc.   951-587-6201
43460 Ridge Park Drive Suite 140, Temecula, CA 92590

Temple City

Micro Bio-Physic Laboratory, Inc.   626-451-6813
5917 Oak Avenue, #357, Temple City, CA 91780

Thousand Oaks

Amgen Inc.   800-28-AMGEN
One Amgen Center Drive, Thousand Oaks, CA 91320-1799
Everybyte, Llc   805-279-3228
3940 Verde Vista Dr., Thousand Oaks, CA 91360-2650
Philips Medical Systems   978-659-4252
1525 Ranchero Conejo Blvd, Thousand Oaks, CA 91320
Team America Health & Fitness, Inc   800-642-5419
675 Racquet Club Ln, Thousand Oaks, CA 91360

Tiburon

Alert Care, Inc.   800-826-7444
98 Main Street, #209, Tiburon, CA 49420

Torrance

Acunetx, Inc.   877-370-0477
2301 W. 205th St., Suite 102, Torrance, CA 90501
Advanced Orthopaedic Solutions, Inc.   866-229-7686
386 Beech Ave., Unit B6, Torrance, CA 90501
Advantage Bag Co.   800-556-6307
22633 Ellinwood Dr., Torrance, CA 90505
Axiom Medical, Inc.   800-221-8569
19320 Van Ness Ave., Torrance, CA 90501
Carley Lamps   310-325-8474
1502 W. 228th St., Torrance, CA 90501
Condex International, Inc.   310-618-8444
2441 W. 205th St. Suite C200e, Torrance, CA 90501
Icrco Inc.   310-921-9559
2580 West 237th Street, Torrance, CA 90505
Intellinetx   877-370-0477
2301 West 205th St., # 102, Torrance, CA 90501
Keller Engineering, Inc.   310-326-6291
3203 Kashiwa St., Torrance, CA 90505
Kenshin Trading Corp.   800-766-1313
22353 South Western Avenue, Suite 201, Torrance, CA 90501
Ledtronics   800-579-4875
23105 Kashiwa Court, Torrance, CA 90505
Life-Like Prosthetics, Llc   310-320-5777
1319 W. Carson St., Torrance, CA 90501
Martek Power   310-202-8820
1111 Knox Street, Torrance, CA 90503
Medical Chemical Corp.   800-424-9394
19430 Van Ness Avenue, Torrance, CA 90501
Medical Electronic Devices, Inc.   310-618-0306
2807 Oregon Ct. #d6, Torrance, CA 90503
Medicool, Inc.   800-426-3227
20460 Gramercy Place, Torrance, CA 90501

Micronova   888-816-4876
3431 W. Lomita Blvd., Torrance, CA 90505-5010
Orthonetx, Inc.   877-370-0477
2301 W. 205th Street #102, Torrance, CA 90501
Phenomenex, Inc.   310-212-0555
2320 W. 205th St., Torrance, CA 90501-1456
Radiographic Digital Imaging, Inc.   310-921-9559
2580 West 237th St., Torrance, CA 90505
Sakura Finetek U.S.A., Inc.   800-725-8723
1750 West 214th Street, Torrance, CA 90501
Shimadzu Medical Systems   800-228-1429
20101 S. Vermont Avenue, Torrance, CA 90502
Younger Manufacturing Co., Inc.   800-877-5367
2925 Calfornia St., Torrance, CA 90503
Younger Mfg. Co.   310-783-1649
2925 California St., Torrance, CA 90503

Tracy

Cct Laser Services   800-808-5273
25421 South Schulte Road, Tracy, CA 95377
San-I-Pak,Pacific Inc.   800-875-7264
23535 South Bird Road, Tracy, CA 95304
Top Shelf Manufacturing, Llc   209-834-8185
1851 E. Paradise Road, Suite B, Tracy, CA 95304

Tulare

Tissue Culture Biologicals   800-845-1445
19766 S Highway 99 Unit A, Suite 300, Tulare, CA 93274

Turlock

Medicalert Foundation International   800-432-5378
2323 Colorado Avenue, Turlock, CA 95382

Tustin

Ambco Electronics   800-345-1079
15052 Redhill Avenue,, Suite D, Tustin, CA 92780
Axiom Analytical, Inc.   949-757-9300
1451 Edinger Ave, Suite A, Tustin, CA 92780
Clinical Resolution Laboratory   213-384-0500
14401 Chambers Road, #200, Tustin, CA 92780
Exiqon Inc.   800-576-6326
15501 Red Hill Avenue, Tustin, CA 92780
Innerspace, Inc.   877.HUM.BIRD
1622 Edinger Avenue, Suite C, Tustin, CA 92780
Innovative Surgical Products, Inc.   714-836-4474
2761 Walnut Avenue, Tustin, CA 92780
Lotus Hygiene Systems Inc.   714-259-8805
15042 Parkway Loop, #b, Tustin, CA 92780
Micro Detect, Inc.   714-832-8234
2852 Walnut Ave., Suite H-1, Tustin, CA 92780
Microvention, Inc.   949-461-3314
1311 valencia avenue, tustin, CA 92780
Neomedix Corp.   949-258-8355
15042 Parkwary Loop, Suite A, Tustin, CA 92780
Peregrine Pharmaceuticals, Inc.   714-508-6000
14282 Franklin Ave., Tustin, CA 92780
Radient Pharmaceuticals   714-505-4460
2492 Walnut Avenue Suite 100, Tustin, CA 92780-6953
Terumo Cardiovascular Systems (Tcvs)   714-258-8001
1311 Valencia Ave., Tustin, CA 92780
Toshiba America Medical Systems   800-421-1968
2441 Michelle Dr., Tustin, CA 92780-7014
Vitalcom, Inc.   800-888-0077
15222 Del Amo Avenue, Tustin, CA 92780
Western Case, Inc.   877-593-2182
14351 Chambers Road, Tustin, CA 92780-6993

Ukiah

Docxs Biomedical Products And Accessories   707-462-2351
564 South Dora, Suite A-1, Ukiah, CA 95482

Union City

Abaxis, Inc.   800-822-2947
3240 Whipple Road, Union City, CA 94587
Aprex, A Division Of Aardex   877-227-3391
2849-B Whipple Road, Union City, CA 94587
Baldur Systems Corporation/ HTI TRADING   800-736-4716
33235 Transit Ave., Union City, CA 94587
K & R Products, Inc.   831-426-6061
33170 Central Avenue, Union City, CA 94587
Mizuho Osi   800-777-4674
30031 Ahern Avenue, Union City, CA 94587-1234

Upland

Accellent Endoscopy   909-982-1025
2052 West 11th St., Upland, CA 91786
Liv International Usa, Inc.   909-931-1719
2335 West Foothill Blvd., Suite 14 And 15, Upland, CA 91784
Mountain Medico, Inc.   909-931-0688
600 North Mountain Ave., #d204, Upland, CA 91786
Uvp, Llc   800-452-6788
2066 W. 11th St., Upland, CA 91786-3509

Vacaville

Whittlestone, Inc.   877-608-6455
840 Eubanks Drive, Vacaville, CA 95688

Valencia

Advanced Bionics Corp.   800-678-2575
28515 Westinghouse Place, Valencia, CA 91355
Bioness Inc.   800-211-9136
25103 Rye Canyon Loop, Valencia, CA 91355
Boston Scientific Neuromodulation Corporation   508-652-5578
25155 Rye Canyon Loop, Valencia, CA 91355
Eckert & Ziegler Isotope Products   661-309-1034
24937 Avenue Tibbitts, Valencia, CA 91355
Isotope Products Laboratories, Inc.   661-309-1010
24937 Ave Tibbitts, Valencia, CA 91355
K-Sera, Inc.   661-775-5988
27525 Newhall Ranch Rd, Unit 8, Valencia, CA 91355
Klm Laboratories, Inc.   800-556-3668
28280 Alta Vista, Valencia, CA 91355
Neotech Products, Inc.   800-966-0500
27822 Fremont Ct, Valencia, CA 91355
Performance Machine Technologies   661-294-8617
25141 W. Avenue Stanford, Valencia, CA 91355-1227
Scicon Technologies Corp.   888-295-8630
27525 Newhall Ranch Road, Suite 2, Valencia, CA 91355
Specialty Laboratories, Inc.   800-421-7110
27027 Tourney Rd., Valencia, CA 91355
Talladium, Inc.   661-295-0900
27360 West Muirfield Ln., Valencia, CA 91355
Trigg Laboratories, Inc.   757-224-0177
28650 Braxton Avenue, Valencia, CA 91355
Utak Laboratories, Inc.   800-235-3442
25020 Ave Tibbitts, Valencia, CA 91355

Valley Springs

Circadian Systems   800-669-7001
8099 Savage Way, Valley Springs, CA 95252

Van Nuys

Garren Scientific, Inc.   800-342-3725
15916 Blythe St., Unit A, Van Nuys, CA 91406
Hemacare Corporation   888-481-1538
15350 Sherman Way,, Suite 350, Van Nuys, CA 91406
Kck Industries   888-800-1967
14941 Calvert St., Van Nuys, CA 91411
Pentagon Co., The   800-414-8888
15500 Erwin Street, Suite 1122, Van Nuys, CA 91411

Ventura

Allied Biomedical   800-276-1322
PO Box 392, Ventura, CA 93003
Biomedical Composites, Ltd.   805-644-4892
4526 Telephone Rd., Suite 204, Ventura, CA 93003
Brasseler Usa - Medical   805-650-5209
4837 McGrath Street, Suite J, Ventura, CA 93003
Implantech Associates, Inc.   800-733-0833
6025 Nicolle Street, Suite B, Ventura, CA 93003
Parker Hannifin Corporation.   805-658-2984
3007 Bunsen Avenue, Units K And L, Ventura, CA 93003
Strenumed, Inc.   805-477-1000
1833 Portola Road,, Suite K, Ventura, CA 93003
Tava Surgical Instruments   800 569-6738
4837 McGrath St., Ste. J, Ventura, CA 93003
Tmj Solution, Inc   805-650-3391
1793 Eastman Ave, Ventura, CA 93003
Vacumed   800-235-3333
4538 Westinghouse St., Ventura, CA 93003

VERNON

Regency Product International   800-845-7931
4732 E 26TH STREET, VERNON, CA 90040-2002

Viats

Living Earth Crafts   800-358-8292
3210 Executive Dr, Viats, CA 92081

Victorville

Bray Corporation   760-345-6689
14149 Calle Contesa, Victorville, CA 92392

Visalia

Tri-Mag, Inc.   559-651-2222
1601 Clancy Ct., Visalia, CA 93291-9253

Vista

Accuech, Llc   800-749-9910
2641 La Mirada Drive, Vista, CA 92081
Aircast Llc   800-321-9549
1430 Decision St., Vista, CA 92081
Almen Laboratories, Inc.   760-806-0040
1672 Gil Way, Vista, CA 92084
Aperio Technologies Inc.   866-478-4111
1360 Park Center Dr., Vista, CA 92081

Autogenomics, Incorporated   760-477-2251
2890 Scott St, Vista, CA 92081
Biner Ellison   800-741-2341
2685 South Melrose Drive, Vista, CA 92081
Biofilm, Inc.   800-848-5900
3225 Executive Ridge, Vista, CA 92081
Biomedical Life Systems, Inc.   800-726-8367
2448 Cades Way, Vista, CA 92085
Breg, Inc., An Orthofix Company   800-897-2734
2611 Commerce Way, Vista, CA 92081
Chattanooga Group   800-321-9549
1430 Decision Street, Vista, CA 37343-0489
Coast Scientific   800-445-1544
1445 Engineer St., Vista, CA 92081
DJO Inc.   800-336-6569
1430 Decision Street, Vista, CA 92081
Davis Medical Electronics, Inc.   800-422-3547
2441 Cades Way, Suite 200, Vista, CA 92081
Integra Biotechnical Llc   760-597-9878
2755 Dos Aarons Way, Suite B, Vista, CA 92081
Medental Intl.   760-727-5889
3008 Palm Hill Dr., Vista, CA 92084
Omni Life Science, Inc.   800-448-OMNI
1390 Decision Street, Vista, CA 92081
Ophthonix Inc.   760-842-5772
1491 Poinsettia Avenue, Vista, CA 92081
Optelec U.S., Inc.   800-828-1056
3030 Enterprise Court, Suite C, Vista, CA 92081
Orthodontic Design And Production, Inc.   760-734-3995
1370 Decision Street, Suite D, Vista, CA 92081
Progressive Medical International   800-764-0636
2460 Ash Street, Vista, CA 92081
Seaspine   760-727-8399
2302 La Mirada Drive, Vista, CA 92081-7862
Sportkat, Llc   800.743.0575
1497 Poinsettia Avenue, Suite 157, Vista, CA 92081
Surgistar Inc.   800-995-7086
2310 La Mirada Dr., Vista, CA 92081
Surgitech Inc.   800-443-7563
1211 West Vista Way, Vista, CA 92083
Vq Orthocare
1390 Decision Street, Suite A, Vista, CA 92081
X-Cel Contacts   770-622-9235
1120 Sycamore Ave., Suite D, Vista, CA 92083

Walnut

Arthrex California, Inc.   800-933-7001
20509 Earlgate St., Walnut, CA 91789
Pac-Dent Intl., Inc.   909-839-0888
21078 Commerce Pointe Dr., Walnut, CA 91789

Walnut Creek

James Consolidated, Inc.   800-884-3317
PO Box 3483, 1867 Ygnacio Valley Rd, Walnut Creek, CA 94598
Kainos Dental Laboratory   925-943-2332
1844 San Miguel Drive, #308b, Walnut Creek, CA 94596
New Deantronics, Ltd.   925-280-8388
1990 N. California Blvd., Suite 1040, Walnut Creek, CA 94596
Preeminent, Llc   925989-0977
1440 Maria Ln., Suite 250, Walnut Creek, CA 94596
Varian Scientific Instruments   925-939-2400
2700 Mitchell Dr., Walnut Creek, CA 94598

Watsonville

Central Welder's Supply, Inc.   800-728-2068
127-d Lee Road, Watsonville, CA 95076

West Covina

Concorde Battery   626-813-1234
2009 San Bernardino Rd., West Covina, CA 91790-1006
Optical Ventures, Inc.   626-915-1533
150 N. Grand Ave., Suite 203, West Covina, CA 91791

West Hollywood

Ziering Medical Worldwide   310-360-8860
9201 Sunset Boulevard Suite 305, West Hollywood, CA 90069

West Sacramento

Affymetrix, Inc.   916-376-1309
890 Embarcadero Dr., West Sacramento, CA 95605
California Scientific   800-284-8112
4005 Seaport, West Sacramento, CA 95691
Crosslink-D, Inc   203-318-8270
3480 Industrial Blvd #105, West Sacramento, CA 95691
Gemini Bio-Products, Inc.   916-273-5215
930 Riverside Parkway, West Sacramento, CA 95605
Piper Medical Products   916-834-3283
4007 Seaport Blvd., West Sacramento, CA 95691
Siemens Healthcare Diagnostics, Inc   800-242-3233
2040 Enterprise Blvd., West Sacramento, CA 95691

Westlake

Matech   818-991-8500
31304 Via Colinas, Suite 102, Westlake, CA 91362

Westlake Village

Dental Innovators, Inc. — 877-921-3919
3016 grandoaks drive, Westlake Village, CA 91361
Medical Resources, Inc. — 800-737-2472
5655 Lindero Cyn. Rd., Suite 104, Westlake Village, CA 91362

Whittier

Collard-Rose Optical Lab — 562-698-2286
12402 Philadelphia St., Whittier, CA 90601
Santa Fe Rubber Products, Inc. — 562-693-2776
12306 East Washington Blvd., Whittier, CA 90606

Wildomar

Soft Innovations, Inc. — 909-678-3540
22300 Baxter Rd., Wildomar, CA 92595

Willits

California Medical Electronics — 707-456-0990
2325 Perch Drive, Willits, CA 95490

Wilmington

Sepor, Inc. — 800-753-6463
718 N. Fries Ave., P.O. Box 578, Wilmington, CA 90748

Winnetka

Energy Prosthetics — 818-675-5083
20438 Acre Street, Winnetka, CA 91306

Woodland

Bentec Medical, Inc. — 757-224-0177
1380 East Beamer St., Woodland, CA 95776
Jr Scientific, Inc. — 530-666-9868
1242-d Commerce Ave., Woodland, CA 95776

Woodland Hills

Andwin Scientific — 800-497-3113
6636 Variel Ave., Woodland Hills, CA 91303
Numask, Inc. — 866-686-2751
6320 Canoga Avenue, Suite#1500, Woodland Hills, CA 91367
Transatlantic Engineering — 818-716-0663
21637 Dumetz Road, Woodland Hills, CA 91364
Western Water Purifier Co. — 800-55-WATER
PO Box 688, Woodland Hills, CA 91365-0688
Z-Pack, Inc. — 818-887-4924
6215 Oakdale Ave., Woodland Hills, CA 91367

Woodside

AeroSurgical Ltd. — 650-530-0032
2995 Woodside Road, Suite 400, Woodside, CA 94062

Yorba Linda

Aaero Swiss, Inc. — 800-394-5808
22347 La Palma Ave, Yorba Linda, CA 92887
CAREFUSION 211, INC.. — 800-231-2466
22745 Savi Ranch Pkwy., Yorba Linda, CA 92887-4645
Nobel Biocare Usa, Llc — 800-579-6515
22715/22725 Savi Ranch Parkway, Yorba Linda, CA 92887
Specialteam Medical Services, Inc. — 714-694-0348
22445 E. La Palma Ave., Ste F, Yorba Linda, CA 92887
Via! For Travel — 800-339-0628
22885 Savi Ranch Parkway, Suite C, Yorba Linda, CA 92887

Yuba City

Andermac, Inc. — 800-824 0214
2626 Live Oak Hwy., Yuba City, CA 95991-8810
Hygiene Specialties, Inc./Andermac, Inc. — 800-824-0214
2626 Live Oak Hwy., Yuba City, CA 95991-8810

Yucaipa

Ingen Technologies, Inc. — 757-224-0177
35193 Avenue A, Suite C, Yucaipa, CA 92399

COLORADO

Adams City

Certol International, Llc — 303-799-9401
6120 E. 58th Ave., Adams City, CO 80022
General Air Service And Supply — 303-892-7003
6330 Colorado Blvd, Adams City, CO 80022

Arvada

Accellent Inc. — 303-424-7300
5000 Independence St., Arvada, CO 80002
Ischemia Technologies, Inc. — 720-540-0200
4600 West 60th Ave., Arvada, CO 80003
Sienco, Inc. — 800-432-1624
7985 Vance Drive, Suite 104, Arvada, CO 80003
Sorin Group Usa — 800-289-5759
14401 W. 65th Way, Arvada, CO 80004-3599

Aurora

A Major Difference, Inc. — 877-315-8638
2950 S. Jamaica Ct., Suite 300, Aurora, CO 80014

Advantage Medical Systems, Inc. — 800-810-1262
2876 South Wheeling Way, Aurora, CO 80014
Alcohol Countermeasure Systems, Inc. — 303-366-5699
1670 Jasper St., Suite G, Aurora, CO 80011
Hosuk America Co. — 303-750-3829
1583 South Tucson Street, Aurora, CO 80012
Marquis Dental Manufacturing Co. — 800-359-3206
15370 Smith Rd., Unit H, Aurora, CO 80011
Marquis Dental Mfg. Co. — 303-344-5222
15370-h Smith Rd., Aurora, CO 80011
Microtech Medical Systems — 303-363-0007
401 Laredo St. - Unit I, Aurora, CO 80011-9207
Natracare, Llc — 303-617-3476
14901 E. Hampden Avenue, Suite 190, Aurora, CO 80014
The Synaptic Corp. — 800-685-7246
3176 S. Peoria St., Ste. 110, Aurora, CO 80014
Weaver & Company — 303-366-1804
565-B Nucla Way, Aurora, CO 80011-9319
Zetek, Inc. — 800-367-2837
876 Ventura St., Aurora, CO 80011-7917

Berthoud

Car-May — 970-532-2816
308 Mountain View Rd, Unit D, Berthoud, CO 80513

Boulder

Analytical Spectral Devices, Inc. — 303-444-6522
2555 55th Street, Suite A, Boulder, CO 80301
Bio-Feedback Systems, Inc. — 303-444-1411
2736 47th St., Boulder, CO 80301-2317
Care Electronics, Inc. — 303-444-2273
4700 Sterling Drive, Suite D, Boulder, CO 80301-2305
Casa Futura Technologies — 303-417-9752
720 31st St, Boulder, CO 80303-2402
Covidien (Formerly Nellcor Puritan Bennett / Tyco Healthcare) — 800-962-9888
6135 Gunbarrel Ave, Boulder, CO 80301
Crosstrees Medical, Inc. — 866-442-2328
4735 Walnut St. Suite E, Boulder, CO 80301
Encision Inc. — 303-444-2600
6797 Winchester Circle, Boulder, CO 80301
Ideas For Living — 303-440-8517
1285 North Cedarbrook Rd., Boulder, CO 80304
Ideatrics, Inc. — 303-417-6353
4845 Pearl East Circle, Suite 101, Boulder, CO 80301
Lexicor Medical Technology, Inc. — 303-443-9944
2840 Wilderness Pl, Suite E, Boulder, CO 80301
Nuclear Cardiology Systems, Inc. — 303-541-0044
5660 Airport Blvd., Suite 101, Boulder, CO 80301
Qsum Biopsy Disposables Llc — 720-304-2135
6539 Stearns Ave., Boulder, CO 80303
Scientech, Inc. — 303-444-1361
5649 Arapahoe Avenue, Boulder, CO 80303-1399
Silverglide Surgical Technologies — 303-444-1970
5398 Manhattan Circle, Suite 120, Boulder, CO 80303
Spectralink Corporation — 800-676-5465
5755 Central Avenue, Boulder, CO 80301
Topez Orthopedics, Inc — 303-865-5105
4820 N. 63 Rd., #104, Boulder, CO 80301
Valleylab — 800-255-8522
5920 Longbow Dr., Boulder, CO 80301-3299

Broomfield

Allpro, Inc. — 800-243-2285
6930 West 116th Ave., Suite 10, P.o. Box 733, Broomfield, CO 80020
Biodesix Inc — 303-417-0500
520 Zang Street, Suite 213, Broomfield, CO 80021
Clinical Reference Systems — 800-237-8401
335 Interlocken Pkway, Broomfield, CO 80021
Colibri Heart Valve, LLC — 303-460-8667
2150 West 6th Avenue, Suite M, Broomfield, CO 80020
Corgenix Medical Corporation — 800-729-5661
11575 Main Street, Broomfield, CO 80020
Fischer Medical Technologies Inc. — 800-777-5345
325 Interlocken Parkway, Building C, Broomfield, CO 80021
Lanx Inc. — 303-443-7500
390 Interlocken Crescent, Broomfield, CO 80021
Puregas — 800-521-5351
226A Commerce Street, Broomfield, CO 80020
Trelleborg Sealing Solutions — 800-466-1727
510 Burbank St., Broomfield, CO 80020
Xtrana, Inc. — 800-789-6534
590 Burbank St., Suite 205, Broomfield, CO 80020

Castle Rock

Pure Water Solutions, Inc. — 877-202-5871
520 D Topeka Way, Castle Rock, CO 80109
Steritec Products, Inc. — 303-660-4201
599 Topeka Way, Suite 400, Castle Rock, CO 80109

Centennial

Allosource — 888-873-8330
6278 South Troy Circle, Centennial, CO 80111

Biomedical Technology Solutions, Inc. 303-653-0100
9800 Mt. Pyramid Court, Ste 350, Centennial, CO 80112
Castle Pines Medical, Inc. 303-442-4514
14883 E Hinsdale Ave, Suite 2, Centennial, CO 80112
Conmed Electrosurgery 800-448-6506
14603 E. Fremont Avenue, Centennial, CO 80112
Dntlworks Equipment Corporation 800-847-0694
7300 South Tucson Way, Centennial, CO 80112
Pare Surgical, Inc. 303-689-0187
7332 South Alton Way, Unit H, Centennial, CO 80112
Physiodynamics, Inc. 303-713-0605
7200 East Dry Creek Rd.,, Suite A-202, Centennial, CO 80112
Shippert Medical Technologies Corp. 800-888-8663
6248 South Troy Circle, Unit A, Centennial, CO 80111
Thermo Products, Llc (877) 903-5600
7767 S.valentia St, Centennial, CO 80112
Vicon 303-799-8686
7388 South Revere Pkwy., #901, Centennial, CO 80112

Co Spgs

Elite Medical Equipment 719-659-7926
5470 Kates Drive, Co Spgs, CO 80919

Colorado Springs

Aspire Biotech, Inc. 719-522-9800
4755 Forge Road Suite 120,, Colorado Springs, CO 80907
Global Sport Technology, Inc 719-574-0584
4745 Signal Rock Rd., Colorado Springs, CO 80922
Harloff Company, Inc. 800-433-4064
650 Ford Street, Colorado Springs, CO 80915-3712
Laser Neurotherapy Development Labs, Inc. 719-264-7632
3855 Interpark Drive, Colorado Springs, CO 80907
Magnisight, Inc. 800-753-4767
3631 N. Stone Avenue, Colorado Springs, CO 80907
Medlogic Global Corporation 800-625-6442
4815 List Dr., Colorado Springs, CO 80919
Mitsui / Mam-A 888-626-3472
10045 Federal Dr., Colorado Springs, CO 80908
Powell Products, Inc. 800-840-9205
4940 Northpark Drive, Colorado Springs, CO 80918
Quality Monitor Systems, Inc. 800-743-5747
1950 Victor Pl., Colorado Springs, CO 80915
Radiological Imaging Technology, Inc. 719-590-1077
5065 List Drive, Colorado Springs, CO 80919-3321
Siemens Water Technologies 866-926-8420
1335 Ford St., Colorado Springs, CO 80915
Solarchromic, Inc. 719-591-9264
2103 Essex Lane, Colorado Springs, CO 80909
Spectranetics Corp. 800-633-0960
9965 Federal Drive, Colorado Springs, CO 80921
Spectrum Laser & Technologies, Inc 719-264-7632
2270 Garden of the Gods Road, Suite 103, Colorado Springs, CO 80907
Westone Laboratories, Inc. 719-540-9333
2235 Executive Circle, Colorado Springs, CO 80906
Ximedix, Inc. 800-999-6349
4829 Northpark Drive, Colorado Springs, CO 80918
Yamato Corporation 800-538-1762
1775 S. Murray Blvd., Colorado Springs, CO 80916-4513

Conifer

Innoventions, Inc. 800-854-6554
9593 Corsair Dr., Conifer, CO 80433-9317

Delta

Rmed International 866-624-1403
675 Industrial Blvd., Delta, CO 81416-2811

Denver

Acceler8 800-810-9897
7000 North Broadway, Building 3-307, Denver, CO 80221
Actall Corp. 800-598-1745
3925 Monaco Parkway, Unit D, Denver, CO 80207
Apdyne Medical Company 800-457-6853
1049 South Vine St., Denver, CO 80209-4622
Colorado Serum Company 303-295-7527
4950 York St., PO Box 16428, Denver, CO 80216-2266
Emerge Medical Inc. 866-553-0376
1530 Blake Street, Suite 204, Denver, CO 80202
Genesee Biomedical, Inc. 800-786-4890
1308 S. Jason St., Denver, CO 80223
Image Molding, Inc. 800-525-1875
4525 Kingston St., Denver, CO 80239-3016
Johns Manville 800-654-3103
P.O. Box 5108, Denver, CO 80217-5108
Labac Systems, Inc. 800-445-4402
4965 Kingston Street, Denver, CO 80239
Medefficiency, Inc. 303-321-7755
8620 Wolff Court, Suite 120, Denver, CO 80031
Optikem International, Inc. 800-525-1752
2172 S. Jason St., Denver, CO 80223
Phoenix Group, The 800-370-6808
4965 Kingston St., Denver, CO 80239
Plaza Medical, Inc. 877-695-4441
9780 E. Girard, Denver, CO 80231

Portable Power Systems, Inc. 303-460-8261
405 West 115th Ave., Suite 3, Denver, CO 80234
Rmo, Inc. 800-525-6375
650 West Colfax Avenue, Denver, CO 80204
Rocky Mountain Anaplastology, Inc. 303-973-8482
3405 South Yarrow St., Suite C, Denver, CO 80227
Spectron Engineering, Inc. 303-733-1060
255 Yuma Ct., Denver, CO 80223
Swisslog Translogic Corporation 800-525-1841
10825 E. 47th Ave., Denver, CO 80239-2913

Denver,

Broadwest Corp. 800-232-2948
304 Elati St, Denver,, CO 80223

Durango

Absolute Air Cleaners & Purifiers, Inc. 888-578-7324
401 Meadow Rd., Durango, CO 81303

Englewood

American Track Roadsters, Inc. 303-986-9300
1500 W. Hampden Ave., Unit 4 - G., Englewood, CO 80110
Asi Medical, Inc. 800-566-9953
14550 East Easter Ave., Suite 700, Englewood, CO 80112
Baxa Corporation 800-567-2292
9540 S Maroon Circle, Suite 400, Englewood, CO 80112
Bell Dental Products, Llc. 800.920.4478
3301 W. Hampden Ave. Unit N, Englewood, CO 80205
Cochlear Americas 303-790-9010
400 Inverness Parkway, Suite 400, Englewood, CO 80112-5128
Confirm Monitoring Systems, Inc. 303-699-3356
109 inverness Drive East, Unit F, Englewood, CO 80112-5105
Crothall 800-447-4476
13111 E. Briarwood Ave. #225, Englewood, CO 80112-3926
Csi International, Inc. 303-795-8273
4301 S. Federal Blvd., Suite 116, Englewood, CO 80110-5310
Denver Optic Company 303-649-9494
14 Inverness Dr. East, Building D, Suite 146, Englewood, CO 80112
Handicaps, Inc. 800-782-4335
4335 S. Santa Fe Drive, Englewood, CO 80110
Helping Hand Trays 303-781-4019
4351 S. Galapago, Englewood, CO 80110-5624
Industrial Specialities Manufacturing, Inc. 800-781-8487
4091 So. Eliot Street, Englewood, CO 80110-4396
Instrumed Oem 800-368-1301
2801 S. Vallejo St., Englewood, CO 80110
Ipax, Inc. 303-975-2444
2700 South Raritan Street, Englewood, CO 80110
Oxy-View, Inc. 877-699-8439
109 Inverness Dr. East, Ste. C, Englewood, CO 80112-5105
Parker Medical 303-799-1990
7275 S. Revere Pkwy, Suite 804, Englewood, CO 80112-5105
Rocky Mountain Reagents,Inc. 303-762-0800
3207 W. Hampden Avenue, Englewood, CO 80110-3261
Sontec Instruments Inc. 303-790-9411
7248 S. Tuscon Way, Englewood, CO 80112-6415
Tapeless Wound Care Products, Llc. 866-714-9199
PO Box 4515, ENGLEWOOD, CO 80155
The Lagado Corp. 303-789-0933
2890 South Tejon St., Englewood, CO 80110
Transtracheal Systems, Inc. 800-527-2667
109 Inverness Dr. E., Ste. C, Englewood, CO 80112-5105
Vital Signs Colorado 1-800-932-0760
11039 E. Lansing Circle, Englewood, CO 80112
W.L. Gore & Associates,Inc 302-738-4880
345 Inverness Dr. S., Bldg. A, Ste. 120, Englewood, CO 80112
Wi Inc 303-762-1693
96 Inverness Drive East, Suite N, Englewood, CO 80112

Erie

Magnum Plastics, Inc. 303-828-3156
425 Bonnell Ave., Erie, CO 80516

Evergreen

Air Lift Unlimited Inc. 800-776-6771
1212 Kerr Gulch, Evergreen, CO 80439-9522

Fort Collins

Dako Colorado, Inc. 454-485-9500
4850 Innovation Dr., Fort Collins, CO 80525-5776
Livengood Engineering Inc. 970-493-2569
1112 Oakridge Dr., #104 Pmb 51, Fort Collins, CO 80525
Rand-Scot Inc. 800-467-7967
401 Linden Center Drive, Fort Collins, CO 80524
Scott Orthotic Labs, Inc. 866-648-9148
1709 Heath Parkway, Fort Collins, CO 80524-3525
Technical Molded Products, Inc. 970-484-9111
3713 Canal Dr., Fort Collins, CO 80524
Tolmar Inc. (1-877-986-5627
701 Centre Ave., Fort Collins, CO 80526
Water Pik, Inc. 970-221-6129
1730 East Prospect Rd., Fort Collins, CO 80553
Whip Mix Corp. 502-637-1451
1730 East Prospect, Suite 101, Fort Collins, CO 80525

Zila, Inc. — 800-228-5595
701 Centre Avenue, Fort Collins, CO 80526

Ft. Collins

Value Plastics — 888-404-5837
3325 S. Timberline Rd, Ft. Collins, CO 80525

Golden

Adventures In Color Technology — 303-271-9644
1800 Jackson St., Suite 214, Golden, CO 80403

Aesthetic Technologies, Inc. — 303-469-0965
14828 West 6th Avenue, Unit B9, Golden, CO 80401

Biovision Technologies, Llc — 303-237-9608
221 Corporate Circle Unit H, Golden, CO 80401

Carsan Engineering, Inc. — 303-237-9608
221 Corporate Circle, Suite H, Golden, CO 80401

Dds Services, Inc. — 720-435-9052
15000 W. 6th Ave., Ste. 150, Golden, CO 80401

Evergreen Research, Inc. — 303-526-7402
433 Park Point Drive, Suite 140, Golden, CO 80401

Lens Dynamics, Inc. — 303-237-6927
14998 W. 6th Ave, #830, Golden, CO 80401

Medical Modeling Inc — 303-273-5344
17301 W. Colfax Ave., Suite 300, Golden, CO 80401

Meinhard Glass Products — 303-277-9776
700 Corporate Circle, Suite A, Golden, CO 80401-5636

Meritech, Inc. — 800-932-7707
600 Corporate Circle, Suite H, Golden, CO 80401

Microlife Medical Home Solutions, Inc. — 1-800-968-1378
2801 Youngfield Street, Suite 241, Golden, CO 80401

Pharmajet — 303-526-4278
24797 Foothills Drive North, Golden, CO 80401

Summit Doppler Systems, Inc. — 800-554-5090
4620 Technology Drive, Unit 100, Golden, CO 80403

Unisyn Medical Technologies — 877-386-3246
1150 Catamount Dr., Golden, CO 80403

Vitro Diagnostics, Inc. — 303-999-2130
4621 Technology Drive, Golden, CO 80403

Grand Junction

Mlw Inc. — 970-434-2222
510 Fruitvale Ct., Suite C, Grand Junction, CO 81504

Westcon Contact Lens Co. — 770-622-9235
611 Eisenhauer St., Grand Junction, CO 81503

Greenwood Village

Accu-Measure, Llc — 800-866-2727
P.O. Box 4411, Greenwood Village, CO 80155-4411

Micromedex, Inc. — 303-486-6400
6200 S. Syracuse Way, Suite 300, Greenwood Village, CO 80111-4740

Hghlnds Ranch

Continental Soft Lens, Inc. — 303-795-2130
9350 Yale Lane, Hghlnds Ranch, CO 80130

Highlands Ranch

Sandhill Scientific, Inc. — 800-468-4556
9150 Commerce Center Circle, #500, Highlands Ranch, CO 80129

Lafayette

Eumedic Incorporated
1369 Forest Park Circle, Ste 100, Lafayette, CO 80026

Lakewood

Archtek, Inc. — 303-763-8916
12105 West Cedar Dr., Lakewood, CO 80228

Caridianbct Inc. — 800-525-2623
10810 W. Collins Ave., Lakewood, CO 80215

Dahlin Laboratory — 952-541-9622
393 South Harlan, Suite 210, Lakewood, CO 80226

Dentsply Friadent Ceramed — 717-849-4229
12860 West Cedar Dr.,suite 110, Lakewood, CO 80228

Elantec Med, Inc. — 303-278-7672
85 S. Union Blvd., Suite M160, Lakewood, CO 80228-2207

Gambro Renal Products — 800-525-2623
14143 Denver West Parkway, Lakewood, CO 80401

Gambro Renal Products, Inc. — 800-525-2623
14143 Denver West Parkway, Lakewood, CO 80401

Gbc, Inc. — (303) 988-6450
190 South Union Blvd., Lakewood, CO 80228

Gnathodontics Ltd. — 800-234-9515
10488 West 6th Place, Lakewood, CO 80215

Long And Rossi Products — 303-233-9581
895 Field St., Lakewood, CO 80215

Mesa Laboratories, Inc. — 800-992-6372
12100 W. 6th Avenue, Lakewood, CO 80228

Porta-Lung Inc. — 303-288-7575
747 Sheridan Blvd, Unit 6 D, Lakewood, CO 80214

Telecation — 800-584-9964
7112 W. Jefferson Avenue, Suite 307, Lakewood, CO 80235

Littleton

Ada Technologies, Inc. — 800-232-0296
8100 Shaffer Parkway, Suite 130, Littleton, CO 80127

Biomed Ink — 720-493-5199
3411 Westhaven Place, Littleton, CO 80126-8036

Multi Marketing & Manufacturing, Inc. — 303-794-5955
PO Box 1070, 5401 Prince Street, Littleton, CO 80160-1070

Pico-Tesla Inc. — 303-795-3222
7852 South Elati, Suite 202, Littleton, CO 80120

Lone Tree

Medical Innovators, Inc. — 888-422-7717
9277 E. Star Hill Lane, Lone Tree, CO 80124

Zynex Inc. — 800-495-6670
9990 Park Meadows Drive, Lone Tree, CO 80124

Longmont

Ball Dynamics International, Llc — 800-752-2255
14215 Mead St., Longmont, CO 80504

MicroPhage Inc. — 303-652-5200
2400 Trade Centre Avenue, Longmont, CO 80503

Nspire Health, Inc — 800-574-7374
1830 Lefthand Circle, Longmont, CO 80501

Parascript LLC — 888-772-7478
6273 Monarch Park Place, Longmont, CO 80503

Sunrise Medical — 800-333-4000
7477 E. Dry Creek Pkwy., Longmont, CO 80503

Sunrise Medical, Inc. — 800-333-4000
7477 E. Dry Creek Pkwy., Longmont, CO 80503

Louisville

Lenox-Maclaren Surgical Corp. — 720-890-9660
657 S. Taylor Avenue, Suite A, Colorado Technology Center, Louisville, CO 80027-3064

Medivance, Inc. — 303-926-1917
1172 Century Dr., Suite 240, Louisville, CO 80027

Medtronic Navigation, Inc. — 888-580-8860
826 Coal Creek Cir., Louisville, CO 80027

Novocol, Inc. — 303-665-7535
416 South Taylor Ave., Louisville, CO 80027

Piko Healthcare Products, Inc. — 888-737-5656
908 Main St., Louisville, CO 80027

Sound Surgical Technologies Llc — 888-471-4777
357 So. McCaslin, Suite 100, Louisville, CO 80027

Stairmaster Health And Fitness Products — 800-628-8458
1886 Prarie Way, Louisville, CO 80027

Thermo Biostar, Inc. — 800-637-3717
331 S. 104th St, Louisville, CO 80027

Loveland

Heska Corporation — 800-GO HESKA
3760 Rocky Mountain Ave, Loveland, CO 80538

Jorgensen Laboratories — 970-669-2500
1450 N. Van Buren Avenue, Loveland, CO 80538-3683

Zahourek Systems, Inc. — 800-950-5025
2198 W. 15th St., Loveland, CO 80538

Lyons

Baseline - Mocon, Inc. — 800-321-4665
19661 Highway 36, P.O. Box 649, Lyons, CO 80540-0649

Products Group International, Inc. — 800-336-5299
447 Main St., Lyons, CO 80540

Monument

Synthes (Usa) — 719 481 5300
1051 Synthes Avenue, P.O. Box 366, Monument, CO 80132

Morrison

Envision Eyes, Llc — 303-880-1031
5368 Wildcat Ct., Morrison, CO 80465

Mt. Crested Butte

Scientific Imaging, Inc. — 303-681-9402
97 Slate Lane, Mt. Crested Butte, CO 81225

Niwot

Crocs, Inc. — 801-455-8558
6328 Monarch Park Place, Niwot, CO 80503

Northglenn

Tartan Orthopedics, Ltd. — 888-287-1456
10651 Irma Drive, Unit C, Northglenn, CO 80233

Olathe

Sample Solutions, Llc — 970-323-5440
540 Highway 50 Business Loop, Olathe, CO 81425

Palmer Lake

Sterisil, Inc. — 719-481-0937
835 S. Highway 105, Suite D, Palmer Lake, CO 80133

Parker

Medtronic Blood Management — 612-514-4000
18501 East Plaza Dr., Parker, CO 80134

Rollens Professional Products, Inc. — 800-898-7474
16610 Amberstone Way, Parker, CO 80134

Stargate International, Inc. — 303-840-8206
10235 South Progress Way, #7, Parker, CO 80134

Sheridan

Aspen Seating, Llc — 866-781-1633
4211 S. Natches Ct., Suite G, Sheridan, CO 80110

Thornton

Respironics Colorado — 800-345-6443
12301 N Grant St #190, Thornton, CO 80241

Westminster

Cerapedics Inc. — 303-974-6275
11025 Dover Street, Suite 1600, Westminster, CO 80021
Linear Medical Corporation — 303-962-5730
1130 West 124th Avenue,, Suite 400, Westminster, CO 80234
Protomed — 303-422-2207
1329 West 121st Avenue, Westminster, CO 80234
Surefire Medical, Inc — 888-321-5212
8601 Turnpike Drive, Suite 206, Westminster, CO 80031

Wheat Ridge

BDC Laboratories — (303) 456-4665
4060 Youngfield Street, Wheat Ridge, CO 80033-3862
Walkmed Infusion Llc — 303-420-9569
4080 Youngfield St., Wheat Ridge, CO 80033-3862

Windsor

Carestream Health, Inc. — 888-777-2072
2000 Howard Smith Avenue West, Windsor, CO 80550

Yardley

Activant Solutions Inc. — 800-776-7438
19 West College Avenue, Yardley, CO 19067

CONNECTICUT

Ansonia

Stelray Plastic Products, Inc — 203-735-2331
50 Westfield Ave., Ansonia, CT 06401

Avon

Ofs, Specialty Photonics Division — 888-438-9936
55 Darling Drive, Avon, CT 06001

Bethel

Duracell Usa — 800-551-2355
8 Research Dr., Berkshire Corporate Park, Bethel, CT 06801
Elvex Corporation — 800-888-6582
13 Trowbridge Dr., Bethel, CT 06801
Focus Medical, Llc. — 866-633-5273
23 Francis J. Clarke Circle, Bethel, CT 06801
Foredom Electric Co. — 203-7304548 EXT
16 Stony Hill Rd., Bethel, CT 06801
Kinetic Instruments, Inc. — 800-233-2346
17 Berkshire Blvd., Bethel, CT 06801
Saes Memry — 203-739-1100
3 Berkshire Blvd., Bethel, CT 06801
The Foredom Electric Co. — 203-792-8622
16 Stony Hill Rd., Bethel, CT 06801

Bloomfield

Degussa - Ney Dental Inc. — 800-221-0168
65 W. Dudley Town Rd., Bloomfield, CT 06002
Deringer-Ney, Inc. — 860-242-2281
Ney Industrial Park, 2 Douglas Street, Bloomfield, CT 06002
Hermell Products, Inc. — 800-233-2342
9 Britton Drive, PO Box 7345, Bloomfield, CT 06002-3616
Pioneer Optics Co. — 860-286-0071
35 Griffin Road South, Bloomfield, CT 06002

Bradford

HistoRx, Inc. — 203-498-7500
35 Northeast Industrial Road, Bradford, CT 06405

Branford

Cas Medical Systems, Inc. — 800-227-4414
44 E. Industrial Rd., Branford, CT 06405
Drm Research Laboratories, Inc. — 203-488-5555
29 Business Park Dr., Branford, CT 06405
HistoRx, Inc. — 877-654-2345
35 Northeast Industrial Road, Branford, CT 06405
Ivy Biomedical Systems, Inc. — 800-247-4614
11 Business Park Drive, Branford, CT 06405
Medical Laser Systems Inc — 203-481-2395
20 Baldwin Dr., Branford, CT 06405
Rontron Engineering, Inc. — 203-488-5020
131 Commercial Pkwy., Branford, CT 06405

Bridgeport

Ats Laboratories, Inc. — 203-579-2700
404 Knowlton St., Bridgeport, CT 06608-1814
Devar Inc. — 800-566-6822
706 Bostwick Avenue, Bridgeport, CT 06605-2396
Lacey Manufacturing Co., LLC — 203-336-0121
1146 Barnum Avenue, PO Box 5156, Bridgeport, CT 06610-0156

Modular Cutting Systems, Inc. — 203-336-3526
650 Clinton Ave., Bridgeport, CT 06605

Bristol

Beekley Corp. — 860-583-4700
One Prestige Lane, Bristol, CT 06010
Colonial/Han-Dee Spring, Llc — 860-589-3231
95 Valley St., PO Box 1079, Bristol, CT 06011
Ultimate Wireforms, Inc. — 800-999-6484
200 Central St., Bristol, CT 06010-6716

Brookfield

Rapid Power Technologies, Inc. — 800-332-1111
18 Graysbridge Rd., Brookfield, CT 06804-0291
Siemens Healthcare Diagnostics Inc — 866-637-4448
101 Silvermine Rd, Brookfield, CT 06804
Westco Scientific Instruments — 800-445-0759
Suite 1, 117 Old State Road, Brookfield, CT 06804

Brookfld Ctr

Feels Good Footwear, Inc — 203-740-8504
1 Whispering Way, Brookfld Ctr, CT 06804

Canaan

Becton Dickinson Medical Systems — 201-847-4570
Grace Way, Canaan, CT 06018
Bicron Electronics — 800-624-2766
50 Barlow St., Canaan, CT 06018

Canton

C.B. Medical L.L.C. — 860-693-2103
26 Center Street, Canton, CT 06019
Kelyniam Global, Inc — 800-280-8192
97 River Road, Canton, CT 60619

Central Village

United Hearing Systems, Inc. — 800-835-2001
137 Norwich Rd, Central Village, CT 06332

Clinton

Bausch & Stroebel Machine Company, Inc. — 866-512-2637
112 Nod Road, Unit 17, Clinton, CT 06413

Danbury

Addent, Inc. — 203-778-0200
43 Miry Brook Road, Danbury, CT 06810
Branson Ultrasonics Corp. — 203-796-2235
41 Eagle Rd., P.o. Box 1961, Danbury, CT 06813
Conoptics, Inc. — 800-748-3349
19 Eagle Rd., Danbury, CT 06810-4127
Kimchuk, Inc. — 203-790-7800
Corporate Drive, Danbury, CT 06810-4130
Lifeline Medical, Inc. — 800-452-4566
22 Shelter Rock Ln., Danbury, CT 06810
Lorad, A Hologic Company — 800-321-4659
36 Apple Ridge Road, Danbury, CT 06810
Miller-Stephenson Chemical Company, Inc. — 800-992-2424
George Washington Highway, Danbury, CT 06810-7378
Praxair Distribution, Inc. — 1.800.PRAXAIR
39 Old Ridgebury Road, Danbury, CT 06810-5113
Praxair, Inc. — 800-PRAXAIR
39 Old Ridgebury Rd., Danbury, CT 06810
Tarry Manufacturing — 800-688-2779
22 Shelter Rock Lane, Danbury, CT 06810-8156
Technipower (A Power Designs Co.) — 800-682-8235
14 Commerce Dr., Danbury, CT 06810
Topex, Inc — 203-748-5918
10 Precision Road, Danbury, CT 06810

Durham

DURHAM MANUFACTURING COMPANY — 800-243-3774
201 Main Street, Durham, CT 06422

East Berlin

Liberty Industries, Inc. — 800-828-5656
133 Commerce St., East Berlin, CT 06023

East Granby

Energy Beam Sciences, Inc. — 800-992-9037
29 B Kripes Road, East Granby, CT 06026-9669

East Hartford

Dur-A-Flex, Inc. — 800-253-3539
95 Goodwin St., East Hartford, CT 06108

East Haven

Micropatent — 800-648-6787
250 Dodge Ave., East Haven, CT 06512

East Norwalk

Buck Scientific, Inc. — 800-562-5566
58 Fort Point St., East Norwalk, CT 06855

East Windsor

Xi Tec, Inc. — 800-243-0084
4 New Park Road, East Windsor, CT 06088-9689

Ellington

Brymill Corporation — 800-777-2796
105 Windermere Ave, Ellington, CT 06029

Enfield

Allesee Orthodontic Appliances, Inc. - Connecticut — 949-255-8766
6 Niblick Rd., Enfield, CT 06082
William Laboratories, Inc. — 800-767-7643
5 Anngina Drive, Unit B, Enfield, CT 06082

Fairfield

Clauss Tools — 800-225-2877
1931 Black Rock Turnpike, Fairfield, CT 06825
General Electric Co. — 800-417-0575
3135 Easton Turnpike, Fairfield, CT 06828
Mcp Systems — 203-367-7761
515 Commerce Drive, Fairfield, CT 06432-5541
Medical Industries Of America Llc. — 203-254-8080
1735 Post Road, Unit 6, Fairfield, CT 06824

Gaylordsville

Intarsia Ltd. — 203-355-1357
14 Martha Ln., Gaylordsville, CT 06755

Glastonbury

Act-Aeromed Copan Technologies Llc. — 951-549-8793
85 Commerce Street, Glastonbury, CT 06033

Greenwich

Mederi Therapeutics Inc — 203-930-9900
8 Sound Shore Drive, Suite 304, Greenwich, CT 06830
Remote Technologies, Inc. — 800-733-9729
P.O. Box 1185, Greenwich, CT 06836

Groton

P.R.I.D.E. Foundation — 800-332-9122
391 Long Hill Road, Groton, CT 06340-1293
210 Innovations, Llc — 800-210-2298
210 Leonard Drive, Groton, CT 06340

Guilford

Bio-Med Devices, Inc. — 800-224-6633
61 Soundview Road, Guilford, CT 06437
Defibtech Llc — 866-333-4248
741Boston Post Rd., Suite 201, Guilford, CT 06437
Genx International — 888-GEN-XNOW
393 Soundview Road, Guilford, CT 06437

Hamden

Brain Tunnelgenix Technologies Corp. — 203-922-0105
375 mather street, Hamden, CT 06514
Mgm Instruments — 800-551-1415
925 Sherman Avenue, Hamden, CT 06514-1117
Tomtec — 877-866-8323
1000 Sherman Avenue, Hamden, CT 06514

Hartford

Aero All Gas Co. — 800-255-4277
3150 Main Street, Hartford, CT 06120
Interex Div. Of Industrial Safety & Supply — 800-671-5080
176 Newington Rd., Hartford, CT 06110-2320

Madison

Vascular Insights LLC — 203-376-3775
395 Boston Post Rd., Madison, CT 06443

Manchester

Lydall, Inc. — 860-646-1233
One Colonial Road, Manchester, CT 06042
Markel Industries, Inc. — 860-646-5303
PO Box 1388, 135A Sheldon Road, Manchester, CT 06040

Meriden

Aplicare, Inc. — 800-760-3236
550 Research Parkway, Meriden, CT 06450
Canberra — 800-255-6370
800 Research Parkway, Meriden, CT 06450
Canberra Industries — 800-243-3955
800 Research Pkwy., Meriden, CT 06450-3215
Cuno Filter Systems — 800-243-6894
400 Research Pkwy., Meriden, CT 06450
Lyons Tool And Die Company — 800-422-9363
185 Research Pkwy., Meriden, CT 06450
Protein Sciences Corp. — 800-488-7099
1000 Research Pkwy., Meriden, CT 06450-7149

Middletown

Bidwell Industrial Group, Inc., Blu-Ray Division — 860-343-5353
2055 S. Main St., Middletown, CT 06457

Contemporary Products, Inc. — 800-424-2444
2055 South Main St., Middletown, CT 04103-1446
Prototype & Plastic Mold Co., Inc. — 203-632-2800
35 Industrial Park Pl., Middletown, CT 06457

Milford

Abbott Associates — 203-878-2370
620 West Avenue, Milford, CT 06461
Accusync Medical Research Corp. — 203-877-1610
132 Research Dr., Milford, CT 06460
Cardiopulmonary Corp. — 203-877-1999
200 Cascade Blvd., Milford, CT 06460
Habilis, Inc. — 203-377-8835
155 Hill St., Milford, CT 06460
Microspecialties, Inc. — 877-874-1933
264 Quarry Road, PO Box 3030, Milford, CT 06460
Synectic Medical Product Development — 203-877-8488
60 Commerce Park, Milford, CT 06460

Monroe

Baltimore Laboratories, Inc. — 203-445-8423
887 Main St., Monroe, CT 06468
Proudfoot Company, Inc. — 800-445-0034
588 Pepper St., Monroe, CT 06468-0276

Mystic

Ami, Inc. — 800-248-4031
1101 Noank Ledyard Road, Mystic, CT 06355
Falck Medical Corporation — 860-536-5162
35 Washington St., Suite 200, Mystic, CT 06355
Medtronic Xomed, Inc. — 800-637-6235
950 Flanders Rd., Mystic, CT 06355

Naugatuck

Custom Bottle/Lerman Container — 800-315-6681
10 Great Hill Road, Naugatuck, CT 06770-0979
Hospital Marketing Svcs. Company, Inc. — 800-786-5094
162 Great Hill Rd., Naugatuck, CT 06770
Made Rite Rocker Inc. — 203-723-5600
44 Gorman St., Naugatuck, CT 06770
Pharmacal Research Labs. Inc. — 800-243-5350
P.O. Box 369, Naugatuck, CT 06770

New Britain

Acme-Monaco Corp. — 860-224-1349
75 Winchell Drive, New Britain, CT 06052-1017
Micro Care Corp. — 800-638-0125
595 John Downey Drive, New Britain, CT 06051
Okay Industries, Inc. — 860-225-8707
200 Ellis St., P.O. Box 2470, New Britain, CT 06050-2470
PI Medical Co., Llc. — 800-874-0120
321 Ellis St., New Britain, CT 06051

New Hartford

Innova Corp. — 860-728-3210
29 Industrial Rd., New Hartford, CT 06057

New Haven

Applied Spine Technologies, Inc. — 203-503-0280
300 George Street, Suite 511, New Haven, CT 06511
Great Age Container — 800.631.7392
220 Frontage Rd., New Haven, CT 06516
Ikonisys, Inc — 203-776-0791
5 Science Park, Suite 1000, New Haven, CT 06511
Zenith/Omni Hearing Instruments, Inc. — 203-624-9857
111 Park St., Suite K, New Haven, CT 06511

New London

Carwild Corp. — 860-442-4914
3 State Pier Road, New London, CT 06320
First Aid Bandage Co., Inc. — 888-813-8214
3 State Pier Road, New London, CT 06320
Sheffield Pharmaceuticals — 800-222-1087
170 Broad St., New London, CT 06320

New Milford

Ispg, Inc. — 860-355-8511
517 Litchfield Road, New Milford, CT 06776-2008
Medical Instill Technologies, Inc. — 860-350-1900
201 Housatonic Avenue, New Milford, CT 06776
Take-Along Lifts, Llc — 877-667-6515
125 Pumpkin Hill Rd., New Milford, CT 06776-4643

Newington

On Site Gas Systems, Inc. — 888-748-3429
35 Budney Road, Newington, CT 06111
Simply Clean Air & Water, Inc. — 860-231-0687
28 Shepard Drive, Newington, CT 06131

Newtown

Dresser Inc., Dresser Measurement Division — 203-426-3115
PO Box 5605, Newtown, CT 06470
Intermed Video Technologies Inc. — 203-270-0677
18 Commerce Road, Newtown, CT 06470

National Video Services, Inc. — 203-270-0677
18 Commerce Road, Newtown, CT 06470-1607

North Haven

Covidien Lp, Formerly Registered As United States — 800-962-9888
Surgical
195 Mcdermott Road, North Haven, CT 06473
Jensen Industries, Inc. — 203-239-2090
50 Stillman Rd., North Haven, CT 06473
Ulbrich Stainless Steels & Special Metals — 800-243-1676
57 Dodge Avenue, North Haven, CT 06473

North Stonington

Ultracell Medical Technologies, Inc. — 877-SPO-NGE1
183 Providence New London Tpke., North Stonington, CT 06359

Norwalk

Aegis Medical — 203-838-9081
10 Wall St., Norwalk, CT 06850
Airpot Corporation — 800-848-7681
35 Lois St., Norwalk, CT 06851
Biowave Corporation — 203-855-8610
16 Knight Street, Norwalk, CT 06851
Cober Electronics, Inc. — 203-855-8755
151 Woodward Avenue, Norwalk, CT 06854-4730
Covidien Lp, Formerly Registered As United States — 800-962-9888
Surgical
150 Glover Ave., Norwalk, CT 06856-5080
Inmark Corporation — 800-899-7947
4 Byington Place, Norwalk, CT 06850-3309
K W Griffen Company — 800-424-5556
100 Pearl St., Norwalk, CT 06850-1629
K. W. Griffen Co. — 203-846-1923
100 Pearl St., Norwalk, CT 06850
Ortholine — 800-243-3351
13 Chapel St., Norwalk, CT 06850-4113

Old Greenwich

Instrumentation For Medicine, Inc. — 203-637-8377
31 Macarthur Dr., Old Greenwich, CT 06870

Old Lyme

Sennheiser Electronic Corp. — 877-736-6434
One Enterprise Drive, Old Lyme, CT 06371

Orange

Light Sources, Inc. — 203-234-7338
37 Robinson Blvd., Orange, CT 06477
Surgiquest, Inc. — 203-799-2400
12 Cascade Blvd., Suite 2b, Orange, CT 06477
Wallach Surgical Devices, Inc. — 800-243-2463
235 Edison Road, Orange, CT 06477

Oxford

Biocompatibles Inc. — 877-783-5463
115 Hurley Road, Bldg. 3, Oxford, CT 06478
Catachem Inc. — 203-262-0330
353 Christian Street, Suite 2, Oxford, CT 06478
Pro Scientific Inc. — 800-584-3776
99 Willenbrock Road, Oxford, CT 06478
Scott Technology Llc — 203-888-2783
1 Jacks Hill Rd., Oxford, CT 06478

Plainville

Edwards Signaling & Security Systems — 800-336-4206
41 Woodford Avenue, Plainville, CT 06062
Innovative Medical Products, Inc. — 800-467-4944
87 Spring Lane, Plainville Industrial Pk, Plainville, CT 06062
Perma Type Company, Inc. — 860-747-9999
83 Northwest Dr., Plainville, CT 06062

Pomfret

Fiberoptics Technology, Inc. — 800-433-5248
1 Fiber Rd., Pomfret, CT 06258

Pompfret

Scope Technology, Inc. — 860-963-1141
28 Quassett Road, Pompfret, CT 06258

Ridgefield

Coactiv Medical Business Solutions — 877-262-2848
900 Ethan Allen Highway, Ridgefield, CT 06877
Dapco Industries — 800-597-2726
241 Ethan Allen Hwy., Ridgefield, CT 06877-6208
Eschenbach Optik Of America, Inc. — 800-487-5389
904 Ethan Allen Hwy., Ridgefield, CT 06877-2826
Js Dental Mfg., Inc. — 800-284-3368
196 North Salem Rd., P.O. Box 904, Ridgefield, CT 06877
Vitalworks — 800-278-0037
239 Ethan Allen Pky., Ridgefield, CT 06877

Shelton

Anton/Bauer - Custom Power Systems — 800-422-3473
14 Progress Drive, Shelton, CT 06484

Centrix, Inc. — 800-235-5862
770 River Rd., Shelton, CT 06484-5458
Dermapac, Inc. — 203-924-7148
33 Hull St., Shelton, CT 06484
Dianon Systems - Labcorp — 800-328-2666
1 Forest Parkway, Shelton, CT 06484
Modern Plastics, Inc. — 800.243.9696
Modern Plastics, Inc., Shelton, CT 06484
Spine Wave, Inc. — 203-944-9494
Two Enterprise Dr., Suite 302, Shelton, CT 06484
Thermo Spectra-Tech — 800-243-9186
2 Research Drive, PO Box 869, Shelton, CT 06484-0869

South Norwalk

Pac Kit Safety Equipment Co. — 800-243-5050
57 Chestnut St., South Norwalk, CT 06854

South Windsor

Enduro Medical Technology, Inc. — 860-289-2299
310 Nutmeg Road South, Unit C-5, South Windsor, CT 06074
Gerber Coburn Optical Inc. — 800-262-8761
55 Gerber Rd., South Windsor, CT 06074
Rhodes Inc., M.H. — 800-548-4637
105 Nutmeg Rd. S., South Windsor, CT 06074

Southington

Northeast Resins & Silicones, Llc. — 860-620-9547
122 Spring St., Unit C-1, Southington, CT 06489
Smiths Medical Asd, Inc. — 614-791-5568
201 West Queen St., Southington, CT 06489
Ssi Medical Technologies, Llc — 860-621-3223
24b Robert Porter Rd., Southington, CT 06489

Stafford Springs

Hobbs Medical, Inc. — 860-684-5875
8 Spring St., Stafford Springs, CT 06076

Stamford

American Diagnostica, Inc. — 888-234-4435
500 West Avenue, Stamford, CT 06902-6360
Aristotle Corp. — 203-358-8000
96 Cummings Point Road, Stamford, CT 06902
Biokinetix Corp. — 203-327-7893
33 Parker Ave., Stamford, CT 06906
Fujifilm Medical Systems Usa, Inc. — 800-431-1850
419 West Avenue, Stamford, CT 06902
Grant Airmass Corporation — 800-243-5237
126 Chestnut Hill Road., PO Box 3456, Stamford, CT 06905
Gyrus Acmi, Inc. — 508-804-2739
300 Stillwater P.o.box 1971, Stamford, CT 06902
Northeastern Sonics — 800-243-2452
130 Lenox Ave., Ste. #23, Stamford, CT 06906
Omega Engineering, Inc. — 800-848-4286
1 Omega Drive, Stamford, CT 06907-0047
Purdue Frederick Company — 800-877-5666
One Stamford Forum, Stamford, CT 06901
Tepnel Lifecodes Corporation — 203-328-9500
550 West Ave., Stamford, CT 06902
Zargis Medical Corp. — 609-488-4608
One Atlantic Street, 1st Floo, Stamford, CT 06901

Stony Creek

Champion America — 800-521-7000
PO Box 3092, Stony Creek, CT 06405

Stratford

Beck-Lee — 800-235-2852
P.O. Box 528, Stratford, CT 06615-0528
In Disposables Inc. — 800-269-4568
P.O.Box 528, Stratford, CT 06615
Kingswood Technology, Inc. — 203-386-1839
44 Rachel Drive, Stratford, CT 06615
Okamoto U.S.A., Inc. — 800-283-7546
18 King St., Stratford, CT 06615-5827
Optima, Inc. — 203-377-8835
111 Research Dr., Stratford, CT 06615
Palmero Health Care — 800-344-6424
120 Goodwin Pl., Stratford, CT 06615
Schueler & Company, Inc. — 516-487-1500
PO BOX 528, Stratford, CT 06615-0528
Thermo Oriel — 203-377-8282
150 Long Beach Blvd., Stratford, CT 06615
Vertebron, Inc. — 203-380-9340
400 Long Beach Blvd., Stratford, CT 06615

Suffield

Agp-Medical, Llc. — 860-416-0590
539 North Main Street, Suffield, CT 06078

Thompson

Soyee Products, Inc. — 800-574-4743
459 Thompson Road, Thompson, CT 06277

Torrington

Bergquist Torrington Company 860-489-0489
89 Commercial Blvd., Torrington, CT 06790
Trlby Innovative L.L.C. 860-482-6848
65 New Litchfield St., Torrington, CT 06790
Vivax Medical Corp. 866-847-7890
89 Putter Ln., Torrington, CT 06790

Trumbull

Coopersurgical, Inc. 800-243-2974
95 Corporate Drive, Trumbull, CT 06611
Jaisons International, Inc. 203-261-1653
22 Bittersweet Lane, Trumbull, CT 06611
Kennedy Center, Inc. 203-365-8522
2440 Reservoir Ave., Trumbull, CT 06611
Korchek Technologies, Llc 203-452-8295
115 Technology Drive, Suite B 206, Trumbull, CT 06611

Vernon

Bio-Plexus, Inc. 800-223-0010
129 Reservoir Road, Vernon, CT 06066

Wallingford

Aloka (Us Headquarters) 800 872-5652
10 Fairfield Blvd., Wallingford, CT 06492-7502
Clinical Dynamics Corp. 800-247-6427
10 Capital Dr., Wallingford, CT 06492
Hitachi Aloka Medical 203-269-5088
10 Fairfield Boulevard, Wallingford, CT 06492
Insite One, Inc. 800-441-0091
135 North Plains Industrial Rd, Wallingford, CT 06492
Lifeline Products, Inc. 203-265-2846
3 Marshall St., Wallingford, CT 06492
Pentron Clinical Technologies 203-265-7397
68-70 North Plains Industrial, Road, Wallingford, CT 06492
Pentron Laboratory Technologies 800-551-0283
53 N. Plains Industrial Rd., Wallingford, CT 06492
Pentron Laboratory Technologies 203-265-7397
53 North Plains Industrial Rd., Wallingford, CT 06492
Respironics Novametrix, Llc. 724-387-4559
5 Technology Dr., Wallingford, CT 06492-1942
Sonicor Instrument Corp. 800-864-5022
50 Capital Drive, Wallingford, CT 06492
Z-Medica Corporation 203-294-0000
4 Fairfield Blvd., Wallingford, CT 06492

Waterbury

Diasys Corporation 800-360-2003
21, West Main Street, Waterbury, CT 06702-2115
Voltarc Technologies, Inc. 203-578-4600
400 Captain Neville Drive, Waterbury, CT 06705

Waterford

Jaypro Corporation 800-243-0533
976 Hartford Tpke., Waterford, CT 06385-4002

West Hartford

El Mar, Inc. 860-729-7232
43 Cody St., West Hartford, CT 06110

West Haven

Marel Corporation 203-934-8187
5 Sawmill Rd., West Haven, CT 06516
Mcneil Healthcare, Inc. 203-932-6263
5 saw mill rd, West Haven, CT 06516

Westport

Energizer Personal Care Division 888-310-4290
300 Nyala Farms Rd., Westport, CT 06880
Interventional Therapies, Llc. 203-291-4893
One Gorham Island, Suite 9, Westport, CT 06880-3217
Standing Stone, Inc. 203-227-8710
49 Richmondville Ave, Westport, CT 06880
Vivatone Hearing Systems, Llc 203-341-9100
One Gorham Island, Westport, CT 06880

Wethersfield

The Kahn Companies 860-529-8643
885 Wells Road, Wethersfield, CT 06109

Willimantic

Hydrofera Llc 866-861-7548
322 Main St., Willimantic, CT 06226

Willington

Mycoscience, Inc. 860-684-0030
25 Village Hill Rd., Willington, CT 06279

Wilton

Beiersdorf, Inc. 800-233-2340
Wilton Corporate Center, 187 Danbury Rd., Wilton, CT 06897
L'Amy, Inc. 800-USA-LAMY
37 Danbury Road, Wilton, CT 06897-4405

Windsor

Arc Home Health Products 800-278-8595
PO Box186, Windsor, CT 06095
Philips Remote Cardiac Services 800-367-1095
7 Waterside Crossing, Windsor, CT 06095
Tsugami / Rem Sales Inc. 860-687-3400
910 Day Hill Road, Windsor, CT 06095

Windsor Locks

Ahlstrom Windsor Locks Llc 860-654-8300
2 Elm St., Windsor Locks, CT 06096-2335

Yalesville

Connecticut Hypodermics, Inc. 203-265-4881
519 Main St., Yalesville, CT 06492-1723

DELAWARE

Clayton

Eagle Mhc 800-637-5100
100 Industrial Blvd., Clayton, DE 19938

Dover

Sunroc / Telkee, Inc. 800-478-6762
60 Starlifter Avenue, Kent County Aero Park, Dover, DE 19901

Frederica

Roll A Bout Corp. 888-736-6151
3240 Barratts Chapel Rd., Frederica, DE 19946

Houston

Country Medical Equipment 302-845-2462
3758 Williamsville Rd., Houston, DE 19954

Middletown

Delstar Technologies, Inc. 800-521-6713
601 Industrial Dr., Middletown, DE 19709

Milford

Dentsply Caulk 800-532-2855
38 West Clarke Avenue, Milford, DE 19963

Milton

Macan Engineering Company 302-645-8068
21 Shay Lane, P.O. BOX 166 Milton, Milton, DE 19968

New Castle

Sportsbands, Inc. 302-322-1148
181 South Dupont Hwy., New Castle, DE 19720
Ta Instruments 302-427-4000
109 Lukens Drive, New Castle, DE 19720
Xiril 302-655-7035
91 Lukens Drive, Suite A, New Castle, DE 19720

Newark

Clinimed, Incorporated 877-CLINIMED
303 Markus Court, Sandy Brae Industrial Park, Newark, DE 19713-1187
Direct Radiography 302-631-2700
600 Technology Drive, Newark, DE 19702
Lightwave Technologies Llc 302-356-2717
121 Continental Drive, Suite 110, Newark, DE 19713
Litecure, Llc 302-709-0408
930 Old Harmony Rd., Suite A, Newark, DE 19713
Midi, Inc. 302-737-4297
125 Sandy Dr., Newark, DE 19713
Siemens Healthcare Diagnostics Inc. 302-631-6311
500 Gbc Dr., Mailstop 514, Newark, DE 19702
Strategic Diagnostics Inc. 800-544-8881
111 Pendacar Dr., Newark, DE 19702
Strategic Diagnostics, Inc. 800-544-8881
111 Pencader Dr., Newark, DE 19702
W. L. Gore And Associates, Inc. 888-914-4673
555 Papermill Road, Building A Suite 120, Newark, DE 19711

Rehoboth

Micron Video International, Inc. 800-564-2766
18585 Coastal Highway,, Suite 149, Rehoboth, DE 19971

Seaford

Fitness Motivation Institute Of America, Inc. 800-538-7790
26685 Sussex Highway Suite A, Seaford, DE 19973

Wilmington

Amelife Llc 302-476-2631
702 West Street, Ste 101, Wilmington, DE 19801
AstraZeneca Pharmaceuticals LP 302-886-3000
1800 Concord Pike, P.O. Box 15437, Wilmington, DE 19850-5437
Delaware Diamond Knives 800-222-5143
3825 Lancaster Pike, Wilmington, DE 19805
Delval Glass, Inc. 302-656-6606
1135 E. 7th St., Wilmington, DE 19801-4501
Jenavalve Technology Inc. 302-295-4897
1000 N. West St., Suite 1200, Wilmington, DE 19801

Qualicon   800-863-6842
Route 141 and Henry Clay Rd., Wilmington, DE 19880-0357

DISTRICT OF COLUMBIA

Washington

American National Red Cross Headquarters   202-303-5640
2025 E Street Nw, Washington, DC 20006
Bioscan, Inc.   800-255-7226
4590 MacArthur Blvd., Washington, DC 20007
Compressus Inc.   202-742-4307
101 Constitution Ave. N.w., Suite 800, Washington, DC 20001
Danaher Corporation   202-828-0850
2000 Pennsylvania Avenue, NW, Suite 800 West, Washington, DC 20006
Rozynski & Associates   202-974-6222
2120 L Street, NW, Suite 245, Washington, DC 20037
Universal Implant Systems, Inc.   202-244-9200
4400 Jenifer St. N.W., Suite 220, Washington, DC 20015-2113

FLORIDA

Alachua

Axogen Inc.   888-296-4361
13859 Progress Blvd., Suite 100, Alachua, FL 32615
Medical Manager Research & Development, Llc   386-462-2148
15151 Nw 99th St., Alachua, FL 32615
Nanotherapeutics, Inc.   386-462-9663
13859 Progress Blvd, Suite 300, Alachua, FL 32615
Novabone Products, Llc   386-462-7660
13631 Progress Blvd, Suite #600, Alachua, FL 32615
Novamin Technology Inc.   386-418-1551
13859 Progress Blvd., #600, Alachua, FL 32615
RTI Biologics Inc.   877-343-6832
11621 Research Circle, Alachua, FL 32615
Travel Ramp, Inc.   (888) 661-7267
13900 NW 126th Ter, P.O. Box 2015, Alachua, FL 32615

Alafaya

Advanced Medical Design International Llc   407-992-6694
1802 N. Alafaya Trail, Suite 132, Alafaya, FL 32826

Altamonte Springs

Precision Laboratories, Inc.   800-327-4792
830 Sunshine Ln., Altamonte Springs, FL 32714
Xenotronix, Inc.   800-624-9366
1031 Miller Dr., Altamonte Springs, FL 32701-2067

Apollo Beach

Lifesaving Systems Corp.   813-645-2748
220 Elsberry Rd., Apollo Beach, FL 33572-2289

Apopka

Custom Medical Products   407-865-7211
3909 East Semoran Blvd., Bldg. 599, Apopka, FL 32703

Boca Raton

Advanced Chemical Sensors Inc.   561-338-3116
3201 N Dixie Hwy Suite 3, Boca Raton, FL 33431-6037
Alrand, Inc./Boca Dental Supply, Inc.   800-5004908
3401 North Federal Hwy., Suite 203, Boca Raton, FL 33431
Beacon Biologicals, Inc.   561-395-1862
5139 pointe alexis Drive, Boca Raton, FL 33433
Binder Biomedical Inc.   561-981-2682
2385 NW Executive Center Drive, Boca Raton, FL 33431
Biotelemetrics, Inc.   561-394-0315
6520 Contempo Ln., Boca Raton, FL 33433-6635
Bsml, Inc.   561-988-4098
7777 Glades Road, Suite 100, Boca Raton, FL 33434
Extra Packaging, Corp.   800-872-7548
631 Golden Harbour Drive, Boca Raton, FL 33432
Health Watch Personal Response Systems   561-994-6699
6400 Park Of Commerce Blvd., Suite 1a, Boca Raton, FL 33487
Intra-Lock International   561-447-8282
6560 West Rogers Circle, Suite 24, Boca Raton, FL 33487
Lexington International, Llc   800-973-4769
777 Yamato Rd., Suite 105, Boca Raton, FL 33431
Mekanika, Inc.   561-417-7244
3998 Fau Blvd., Suite 210, Boca Raton, FL 33431
Nokia Siemens Networks   561-923-9590
900 Broken Sound Pkwy., Boca Raton, FL 33487
Novavision, Inc.   561-558-2040
3651 Fau Blvd., Suite 300, Boca Raton, FL 33431
Ophtec Usa Inc.   561-989-8767
6421 Congress Avenue, Suite 112, Boca Raton, FL 33487
Sensormatic Electronics   800-241-6678
6600 Congress Ave, Boca Raton, FL 33487
Sng Prosthetic Eye Institute   561-391-7099
6018 S.w.18th St., #c-2, Boca Raton, FL 33433
Sunbeam Products, Inc.   561-912-4100
2381 Executive Center Dr., Boca Raton, FL 33431
Us Spine Inc.   561-367-7463
3600 Fau Blvd., Suite 101, Boca Raton, FL 33431

Vicor Technologies Inc.   877.528-PD2i (
2300 Corporate Blvd. NW, Suite 123, Boca Raton, FL 33431
Vycor Medical Inc   561-558-2020
3651 FAU Blvd, Suite 300, Boca Raton, FL 33431
Watermark Medical LLC.   877-710-6999
1750 Clint Moore Road, Suite 101, Boca Raton, FL 33487

Bonita Springs

Bonita Dental Lab   239-495-3368
10915 Bonita Beach Rd., #1152, Bonita Springs, FL 34135
Cejay Engineering, Llc   888-584-3060
24600 South Tamiami Trail, Suite 212-353, Bonita Springs, FL 34134
Promedic, Inc.   239-498-2155
24301 woodsage drive, Bonita Springs, FL 34134-2015

Boynton Beach

Insight Medical Products, Llc   561-742-3650
710 Ne 7th St. Bld# 403, Boynton Beach, FL 33435-3930
Protech Professional Products, Inc.   561-493-9818
2900 Nw Commerce Park Dr., #10, Boynton Beach, FL 33426
Quantachrome   800-989-2476
1900 Corporate Drive, Boynton Beach, FL 33426

Bradenton

Anko Products, Inc., Mityflex Div.   800-446-2656
3007 29th Avenue E., Bradenton, FL 34208
Banco Hearing Centers   941-753-3131
1133 44th Ave W, Bradenton, FL 34207-1439
Dh Biomedical, Inc.   800-600-8791
1712 9th St. W., Bradenton, FL 34205
Ear Tech, Inc.   941-747-8193
3904 9th Ave., West, Bradenton, FL 34205
Glenroe Technologies   800-237-4060
1912 44th Ave., East, Bradenton, FL 34203
Hurricane Medical   941-751-0588
5315 Lena Road, Bradenton, FL 34211
Med X Change, Inc.   941-794-9977
525 8th Street West, Bradenton, FL 34205
The Aloe Institute   941-727-0042
5808 42nd Street East, Bradenton, FL 34203

Brandon

Medical Data Technologies, Inc.   866-643-7424
1421 Oakfield Dr., Brandon, FL 33511
Tuff Orthopedic Products   925-595-7053
776 West Lumsden Rd., Suite 104, Brandon, FL 33511

Brooksville

Sparton Electronics, Inc.   800-443-4132
30167 Power Line Rd., Brooksville, FL 34602

Cape Coral

Greylor Co.   (239) 574-2011
2340 Andalusia Blvd., Cape Coral, FL 33909
S4j Manufacturing Services, Inc.   888-S4J-LUER
2685 N.E. 9th Avenue, Cape Coral, FL 33909

Cape Haze

Harvey Precision Instruments   707-793-2600
217 Fairway Road, Cape Haze, FL 33947

Casselberry

Magnatone Hearing Aid Corp.   800-789-6543
170 N. Cypress Way, Casselberry, FL 32707

Clearwater

Alpha Industries, Inc.   727-443-2673
701 N Martin L King Jr Ave, Clearwater, FL 33757
Bausch & Lomb, Inc.   813-724-6600
21 Park Place Blvd. N., Clearwater, FL 33759
Bovie Medical Corp.   800-537-2790
5115 Ulmerton Road, Clearwater, FL 33760
Boyd Industries, Inc.   800-255-2693
12900 44th St. North, Clearwater, FL 33762
Ellkar Corporation   727-442-8231
1137 Sunnydale Dr., Clearwater, FL 33755
Endo-Therapeutics, Inc.   888-294-2377
15251 Roosevelt Blvd, Suite #204, Clearwater, FL 33760
Exaxol Chemical Corp.   800-739-2965
14325 60th St. North, Clearwater, FL 33760
Eyekon Medical, Inc   800-633-9248
2451 Enterprise Road, Clearwater, FL 33763
Jtl Enterprises   800-699-1008
15395 Roosevelt Blvd, Clearwater, FL 33760
Kree Technologies Usa, Inc.   450-676-9444
11429 53rd Street North, Clearwater, FL 33760
Life Without Pain, Llc   954-786-0007
4600 140th Ave. North, Suite 190, Clearwater, FL 33762
Lincare Holdings, Inc.   727-530-7700
19387 U.S. 19 North, Clearwater, FL 33764
Maverick Technologies, Inc.   727-791-6151
1754 Grove Drive, Clearwater, FL 33759
Mercury Medical   800-237-6418
11300 49th St. N., Clearwater, FL 33762-4800

Pace Tech, Inc. — 800-722-3024
510 Garden Avenue N., Clearwater, FL 33755
Saint-Gobain Performance Plastics/Clearwater — 800-541-6880
4451 110th Ave, North, Clearwater, FL 33762
Scc Soft Computer — 800-763-8352
5400 Tech Data Drive, Clearwater, FL 33760
Sensidyne, Inc. — 800-451-9444
16333 Bay Vista Drive, Clearwater, FL 33760
Sheldon Enterprises, Inc. — 727-443-1677
609 Richards Ave # 102, P.O. Box 996, Clearwater, FL 33765
Sterex Corp. — 800-603-5045
4501 126th Avenue, North, Clearwater, FL 33762-4702
Tatum Surgical — 888-360-5550
14010 Roosevelt Blvd, Suite # 705, Clearwater, FL 33762
Tri-City Optical — 727-528-8873
5600 115th Ave. North, Suite B, Clearwater, FL 33760
Westlund Engineering, Inc. — 727-572-4343
12400 44th St. N., Clearwater, FL 33762
minSURG International, Inc. — 727-466-4550
611 Druid Road Eas, Suite 200, Clearwater, FL 33756

Cocoa

American Quality Mfg., Inc. — 888-999-7577
400 Shearer Blvd, Cocoa, FL 32922
Chamco, Inc. — 888-674-6683
798 Clearlake Rd., Cocoa, FL 32922
GeNO LLC. — 321-785-2645
2941 Oxbow Circle, Cocoa, FL 32926

Coconut Creek

Mergenet Medical Inc. — 888-925-2526
6601 Lyons Road, Suite B1-B4, Coconut Creek, FL 33073

Coral Gables

Crosswell International Corporation — 305-648-0777
101 Madeira Avenue, Coral Gables, FL 33134
Marco-Med U.S.A. — 305-661-7046
1521 Zuleta Ave., Coral Gables, FL 33146
Radiation Shield Technologies, Inc. — 866-733-6766
1825 Ponce De Leon Blvd, Suite 456, Coral Gables, FL 33134
Stiefel Laboratories, Inc. — 800-724-1565
255 Alhambra Circle, Coral Gables, FL 33134-7412

Coral Springs

Abb Concise Optical Group Llc — 800-852-8089
12301 NW 39th Street, Coral Springs, FL 33065
Advantage Medical Electronics, Inc. — 954-345-9800
10630 Wiles Road, Coral Springs, FL 33076
Berghof/America — 800-544-5004
3773 NW 126th Avenue, Building 1, Coral Springs, FL 33065
Inman Orthodontic Laboratories, Inc. — 954-340-8477
9381 W. Sample Rd., Coral Springs, FL 33065
Jason Marine Enterprises, Inc. — 954-346-5240
4311 Northwest 64th Avenue, Coral Springs, FL 33067
New Life Systems, Inc. — 954-972-4600
PO Box 8767, Coral Springs, FL 33075
Sc/Ois Orthodontics — 1-(800) 448-732
3300 University Drive, Suite 250, Coral Springs, FL 33065
Sentech Medical Systems, Inc. — 954-340-0500
4200 N.w. 120th Ave., Coral Springs, FL 33065
Specialty Medical Supplies, Inc. — 954-752-5603
3882 NW 124th Avenue,, Coral Springs, FL 33065
Tridien Medical — 954-340-0500
4200 NW 120th Avenue, Coral Springs, FL 33065

Davie

Pulse Medical Inc. — 800-342-5973
4131 S.W. 47th Avenue, Suite 1404, Davie, FL 33314

Daytona Beach

Amicas, Inc. — 386.253.6222
325 Bill France Blvd., Daytona Beach, FL 32114
Costa Del Mar Sunglasses, Inc. — 800-447-3700
2361 Mason Avenue, Suite 100, Daytona Beach, FL 32117
Florida Manufacturing Corp. — 800-447-2372
501 Beville Road, Daytona Beach, FL 32119
Tel-Tron Technologies Corporation — 904-255-1921
220 Fentress Blvd., Daytona Beach, FL 32114-1228

De Funiak Springs

Professional Products, Inc. — 800-234-9004
54 Hugh Adams Dr., De Funiak Springs, FL 32435

De Leon Springs

Mastercraft Products Corporation — 800-874-6094
5797 Lake Winona Rd, De Leon Springs, FL 32130-0117
Sparton Electronics Florida, Inc. — 800-824-0682
5612 Johnson Lake Rd., De Leon Springs, FL 32130

Debary

audifon USA Inc. — 800-776-0222
403 Chairman Ct, Suite 1, P.O. Box 531700, Debary, FL 32713

Deerfield Bch

Regent Labs, Inc. — 954-426-4403
700 West Hillsboro Blvd., Bldg. #2-206, Deerfield Bch, FL 33441
Virtual Imaging, Inc. — 954-428-6191
720 S. Powerline Rd., Ste. E, Deerfield Bch, FL 33442

Deerfield Beach

Air Dimensions, Inc. — 800-650-3267
1371 W. Newport Center Dr., Deerfield Beach, FL 33442
Cell Science Systems, Ltd. Corp. — 954-426-2304
1239 E. Newport Center Dr., Suite 101, Deerfield Beach, FL 33442
Cte Chem Tec Equipment Co. — 800-222-2177
234 S.W. 12th Avenue, Deerfield Beach, FL 33442
Hygolet Usa — 800-494-6538
349 S.E. 2nd Avenue, Deerfield Beach, FL 33441
Lens Express, Inc. — 800-536-7397
350 S.W. 12th Avenue, Deerfield Beach, FL 33442
Pompano Precision Products, Inc. — 800-628-8333
1100 S.w. 12th Avenue, Deerfield Beach, FL 33069

Deland

Covidien Lp, Formerly Registered As Kendall — 800-962-9888
2010 East International, Speedway Boulevard, Deland, FL 32724
Idm Plastics — 904-734-4740
1813 Patterson Ave., Deland, FL 32724
Norco Medical — 386-734-9080
1501 Lexington Ave., Deland, FL 32724-2117
Raf Tabtronics Llc — 386-736-1698
200 Lexington Ave., Deland, FL 32724

Delray Beach

PositiveID Corporation — 561-805-8000
1690 South Congress Avenue, Suite 200, Delray Beach, FL 33445
Sea-View Optical, Inc. — 561-276-5099
1715 S. Federal Hwy., Delray Beach, FL 33483-3329

doral

Fine & Particular Ey — (914) 834-9227
1723 nw 82nd ave, doral, FL 33126
Quest Intl., Inc. — 305-592-6991
8127 Nw 29th Street, Doral, FL 33122
Schiller America, Inc. — 786-845-0620
2131 N.w. 79th Ave., Doral, FL 33122

Dunedin

Blackhagen Design — 727-736-0582
811-C Douglas Avenue, Dunedin, FL 34698-5071
Microlife Usa, Inc. — 888-314-2599
424 Skinner Blvd.,, Suite C, Dunedin, FL 34698

Dunnellon

Indigenous Peoples Technology And Education Center — 352-465-4545
10575 Sw 147th Circle, Dunnellon, FL 34432

Estero

Showerfloss, Inc. — 800-723-2300
20930 Persimmon Pl., Estero, FL 33928

Fernandina Beach

Leto Medical LLC. — 904-261-8218
1886 S. 14th Street, Suite 6, Fernandina Beach, FL 32034
Zassi Medical Evolutions, Inc. — 904-261-2169
1886 S. 14th St., Suite 6, Fernandina Beach, FL 32034

Fort Lauderdale

Acuderm Inc. — 800-327-0015
5370 NW 35th Terrace, Suite 106, Fort Lauderdale, FL 33309-6335
Cambridge Diagnostic Products, Inc. — 800-525-6262
6880 N.W. 17th Avenue, Fort Lauderdale, FL 33309-1524
Ethicare Products — 800-253-3599
PO Box 5027, Fort Lauderdale, FL 33310-5027
Ideal Medical Source, Inc. — 800-537-0739
2805 East. Oakland Blvd, Suite 352, Fort Lauderdale, FL 33306
Jeremy Ethan Industries, Inc. — 954-772-9779
809 N.w. 57th St., Fort Lauderdale, FL 33309
K Medical — 800-478-5633
PO Box 5224, Fort Lauderdale, FL 33310
Lifesync Corporation — 866-324-3888
One East Broward Blvd,, Suite 1701, Fort Lauderdale, FL 33301
Maguire Enterprises, Inc. — 800-548-9686
10289 NW 46th Street, Fort Lauderdale, FL 33351
Marine Medical Intl., Inc. — 954-523-1404
1414 South Andrews Avenue, Fort Lauderdale, FL 33316
Md Components Inc. — 954-565-5328
3560 NW 53rd Ct., Fort Lauderdale, FL 33309
National Air Ambulance — 800-327-3710
3495 S.W. 9th Avenue, Fort Lauderdale, FL 33315
Nipro Diagnostics, Inc. — 800-342-7226
2400 N.W. 55th Ct., Fort Lauderdale, FL 33309
Originator Corporation — 888-859-5031
832 NW First St., Fort Lauderdale, FL 33311
Sds (Summit Dental Systems) — 800-275-3368
3560 NW 53rd Court, Fort Lauderdale, FL 33309

Fort Myers

Air A Med, Inc. | 800-625-4963
2049 Beacon Manor Dr., Fort Myers, FL 33907
Air Science USA | 800-306-0656
120 6th St., Fort Myers, FL 33907
Cool View, Llc | 865-982-5552
9530 Gladiolus Blossom Ct., Fort Myers, FL 33908
Dawning Technologies, Inc. | 800-332-0499
8140 College Parkway, Suite 202, Fort Myers, FL 33919
Ear-Tronics, Inc. | 239-275-7655
7181 College Pkwy, Suite 14, Fort Myers, FL 33907
Neogemics Laboraties | 866-776-5907
12701 Commonwealth Drive, Suite 5, Fort Myers, FL 33913
Nutra Luxe Md, Llc | 877-241-0459
6835 International Center Blvd, Unit 5, Fort Myers, FL 33912

Fort Pierce

E.M. Adams Co. | 800-225-4788
7496 Commercial Circle, Fort Pierce, FL 34951

Fort Walton Beach

Manufacturing Technology, Inc. | 850-664-6070
70 Ready Ave., N.w., Fort Walton Beach, FL 32548

Ft Myers

S.W. Florida Prosthetic Clinic | 239-936-0033
13691 Metro Pkwy., Suite 100, Ft Myers, FL 33912-4348

Ft. Lauderdale

Ceragroup Industries Inc. | 954-670-0208
6555 N.w. 9th Ave., Suite 211, Ft. Lauderdale, FL 33309
Ethicare | 954-742-3599
P.O. Box 5027, Ft. Lauderdale, FL 33310
Imaging Diagnostic Systems, Inc. | 800-992-9008
5307 NW 35th Terrace, Ft. Lauderdale, FL 33309
J. Pohler | 305-757-7733
8740 Sw 21st Street, Ft. Lauderdale, FL 33324
Mako Surgical Corp. | 954-927-2044
2555 Davie Rd., Suite 110, Ft. Lauderdale, FL 33317
Nutek Orthopaedics, Llc | 954-779-1400
301 SW 7th Street, Ft. Lauderdale, FL 33301
Orbusneich Medical, Inc. | 852-280-2228
5363 N.W. 35th Ave., Ft. Lauderdale, FL 33309-6315

Ft. Myers

Dean B. Scott, Ocularist | 847-965-4455
4101 Evans Ave., Ft. Myers, FL 33901

Gainesville

Exactech, Inc. | 800-392-2832
2320 N.W. 66 Court, Gainesville, FL 32653
Florida Life Systems | 727-321-9554
2632 NW 43rd Street Suite #E-9, Gainesville, FL 32606
Florida Probe Corp. | 352-372-1142
3700 N.w. 91st St., Suite C100, Gainesville, FL 32606
Gator Custom Mobility, Inc. | 352-373-9673
501 NE 23rd Ave., Gainesville, FL 32609
I.M.A. Electronics, Inc. | 352-378-7551
6614 N.w. 26th Terrace, Gainesville, FL 32653
Invivo | 352-336-0010
3650 N.E. 53rd Ave., Gainesville, FL 32608
Mammatech Corp. | 800-626-2273
930 NW 8th Avenue, Gainesville, FL 32601-5071
Medical Device Technologies, Inc. (Md Tech) | 800-338-0440
3600 S.W. 47th Avenue, Gainesville, FL 32608
Moltech Power Systems Inc | 800-677-6937
1908 Nw 67th Pl, Gainesville, FL 32614-7114
Nanoptics, Inc. | 352-378-6620
3014 NE 21st Way, Gainesville, FL 32609-3307
Neurotronics, Inc. | 352-372-9955
912 NE 2nd Street, Suite 5, Gainesville, FL 32601
Noble Anesthesia-Air, Inc. | 772-225-2711
4637Nw 6th Street, Gainesville, FL 32609
Optical Polymer Research, Inc. | 352-378-1027
5921 N.e. 38th St., Gainesville, FL 32609
Rgi Medical Manufacturing Inc. | 352-378-3633
2321 N.w. 66th Ct., Ste. W4, Gainesville, FL 32653
South East Instruments Corp. | 352-332-0125
3706 N.w. 97th. Blvd., Gainesville, FL 32606

Hallandale Beach

Bio-Flex International, Inc. | 800-755-4588
1250 E. Hallandale Beach Blvd., Suite 1, Hallandale Beach, FL 33009

Havana

Freedom Fabrication | 800-304-FREE
815 N. Main St., Suite B, Havana, FL 32333

Hialeah

Arthur Finnieston Clinic | 305-817-1604
2480 W. 82 Street #8, Hialeah, FL 33016
Engler Engineering Corp. | 800-445-8581
1099 E. 47 St., Hialeah, FL 33013-2139

Fen Dental Mfg., Inc. | 305-556-5259
2665 West 81st St., Hialeah, FL 33016
Maramed Orthopedic Systems | 800-327-5830
2480 W. 82nd St., No. 8, Hialeah, FL 33016-2753
Medicore, Inc. | 800-327-8894
2647 West 81 St., Hialeah, FL 33016
Rem Systems | 305-499-4800
625 East 10 Ave., Hialeah, FL 33010-1660
Rite-Dent Manufacturing Corp. | 305-693-8626
3750 East 10th Court, Hialeah, FL 33013
South American Dental Export Corp. | 305-512-4705
8205 West 20th Avenue, Hialeah, FL 33014
U.S.A. Delta.Inc | 305-557-1435
7830 W. 28th Ave., #213, Hialeah, FL 33018

Hollywood

American Bidet Co. | 877-981-1111
1801 Polk St # 1500, P.O. Box - # 1500, Hollywood, FL 33022-1500
Bersa Group, Inc. | 954-920-9991
3430 N. 29th Ave., Hollywood, FL 33020
Critical Care Systems, Inc. | 954-989-4400
5000 Hollywood Blvd., Hollywood, FL 33021
Cryotherapy Pain Relief Products, Inc. | 954-893-9059
3460 Laurel Oaks Lane, Hollywood, FL 33021-8448
Hmb Endoscopy Products | 800-659-5743
3746 SW 30th Avenue, Hollywood, FL 33312
Jodee, Inc. | 800-423-9038
3100 N. 29th Ave., Hollywood, FL 33020
Kollsut Scientific Corporation | 630-290-5746
3286 North 29th Court, Hollywood, FL 33020
Magnivision, Inc. | 954-986-9000
3700 Commerce Parkway, Hollywood, FL 33025
Omiderm Ltd. | 415-753-9989
One Oakwood Blvd., #50, Hollywood, FL 33020
Ortho-Cycle Co., Inc. | 800-82-CYCLE
2026 Scott St., Hollywood, FL 33020
Pfb Inter-Apparel Corp. | 800-828-7629
1930 Harrison Street, Suite 304, Hollywood, FL 33020
Z-Kat, Inc. | 954-927-2044
2903 Simms St., Hollywood, FL 33020
Z. Haydu Manufacturing Inc. | 954-925-1779
1980 Grant St., Hollywood, FL 33020

Homestead

Rehamed Intl. Llc. | 800-577-4424
522 West Mowry Drive, Homestead, FL 33030

Jacksonville

Airgas South, Inc. | 770-590-6200
5837 W. Fifth St., Jacksonville, FL 32254
Alternative Products | 904-378-9081
5351 Ramona Blvd., Suite 7, 8, Jacksonville, FL 32205
Anjon, Llc | 904-730-9373
4801 Dawin Rd., Jacksonville, FL 32207
Aspyra, Inc. | 904-854-2107
8649 Baypine Rd., Jacksonville, FL 32256
Avada Eyewear Inc. | 800-844-2034
5605 Florida Mining Blvd. Bldg. 200, Suite 210, Jacksonville, FL 32257
Avondale Badge Co | 800-874-2551
4114 Herschel St., Suite 101, Jacksonville, FL 32210
Biomet Microfixation Inc. | 800-874-7711
1520 Tradeport Dr., Jacksonville, FL 32218
Bodyline Comfort Systems | 800-874-7715
3730 Kori Rd., Jacksonville, FL 32257
C.E. Tech | 800-333-7477
800 Prudential Dr., Jacksonville, FL 32207
Centennial Products Inc. | 888-604-1004
6900 Philips Hwyd, Suite 45, Jacksonville, FL 32216
Gyrx, Llc | 904-641-2599
10302 Deerwood Park Blvd., Ste. 209, Jacksonville, FL 32256
HealthLink | 800-288-6580
3611 St Johns Bluff Rd. South, Suite 1, Jacksonville, FL 32224
Healthlink | 904-996-7758
3611 St. Johns Bluff Rd. South, Suite 1, Jacksonville, FL 32224
Invotec Intl. | 800-998-8580
6833 Phillips Industrial Blvd., Jacksonville, FL 32256
Johnson & Johnson Vision Care, Inc. | 800-843-2020
7500 Centurion Pkwy, Suite 100, Jacksonville, FL 32256
Kls Martin Lp | 800-625-1557
11239-1 st. johns ind. pkwy. 5, Jacksonville, FL 32246
Kls-Martin L.P. | 800-625-1557
11239-1 St. John`s Industrial, Parkway South, Jacksonville, FL 32250-0249
Marco Ophthalmic, Inc. | 800-874-5274
11825 Central Pkwy., Jacksonville, FL 32224
Medtronic Xomed, Inc. | 800-874-5797
6743 Southpoint Drive North, Jacksonville, FL 32216-0980
National Medical Products | 800-940-6262
9775 Mining Drive, #104, Jacksonville, FL 32257
Pedicraft, Inc. | 800-223-7649
4134 St. Augustine Road, Jacksonville, FL 32247
Quad Med | 800-933-7334
11210 Philips Ind. Blvd. E., Suite 10, PO Box 550773, Jacksonville, FL 32255
Restore Medical Inc. | 904-296-9600
6743 Southpoint Drive, North, Jacksonville, FL 32216

Rhodes Medical Products Inc. — 904-233-0928
1116 Celebrant Dr., Jacksonville, FL 32225
Safepro Usa Inc. — 904-880-1958
11497 Columbia Park Dr., West Suite 9, Jacksonville, FL 32258
Siemens Water Technologies — 866-926-8420
6550 Trade Center Dr., Jacksonville, FL 32254
Statcorp, Inc. — 800-992-0014
14476 Duval Place West #303, Jacksonville, FL 32218
Sunoptic Technologies — 877-677-2832
6018 Bowdendale Ave., Jacksonville, FL 32216
The Bremer Group Co. — 800-428-2304
11243-5 St. Johns Industrial, Pkwy. South, Jacksonville, FL 32246
Universal Technology Systems, Inc. — 904-778-8614
5150-4 Timuquana Rd., Jacksonville, FL 32210
Vistakon, Inc. — 800-874-5278
7500 Centurion Pkwy, Jacksonville, FL 32256

Jacksonville Beach

Dwyer Precision Products, Inc. — 800-422-3894
266 N. 20th St., Jacksonville Beach, FL 32250-2727

Jensen Beach

Enabling Technologies Company — 800-7773687
1601 N.E. Braille Pl., Jensen Beach, FL 34957
Microstim Technology, Inc. — 772-283-0235
3879 NE Skyline Drive, Jensen Beach, FL 34957

Jupiter

Atlas Spine Inc. — 561-741-1108
1555 Jupiter Park Dr., Ste. 4, Jupiter, FL 33458
E-Z-On Products Inc. Of Florida — 800-323-6598
605 Commerce Way W., Jupiter, FL 33458-8893
Ge Medical Systems Information Technologies, Inc. — 414-721-2584
100 Marquette Drive, Jupiter, FL 33468
Nobile Consulting Usa Llc — 866-500-7463
1555 Jupiter Park Dr., Ste. 11, Jupiter, FL 33468
Pds Health, Inc. — 800-440-2417
112 Intracoastal Pointe Drive, Jupiter, FL 33477

Kendall

Beckman Coulter, Inc. — 800-526-3821
11800 Sw 147th Ave., Kendall, FL 33196

Key Largo

Cardiocontrol, Inc. — 973-340-8000
101425 Overseas Hwy, P.O. Box 615, Key Largo, FL 33037

Keystone Heights

Diomedics, Inc. — 888-972-4699
342 S.E. 35th St., Keystone Heights, FL 32656

Kissimmee

Index Instruments U.S. Inc. — 407-932-3688
3305 Commerce Blvd., Kissimmee, FL 34741
Sleep Devices, Inc. — 866-935-9166
506 West Cherry Street, Kissimmee, FL 34741
Special Products, Inc. — 800-538-6836
2540 Greenwood Drive, Kissimmee, FL 34744-3825
Synergy Rehab Technologies, Inc. — 407-344-8440
2701 Wortham Lane, Kissimmee, FL 34744

Lake Park

Barrier Eyewear — 561-317-5324
840 13th St. #31, Lake Park, FL 33403
Emergency Vehicles, Inc. — 800-848-6652
705 13th street, Lake Park, FL 33403-2303

Lake Worth

Intermed Group, Inc. — 561-586-3667
3550 23rd Ave. South, Suite #1, Lake Worth, FL 33461
Mavidon Medical Products — 800-654-0385
1820 2nd Ave N, Lake Worth, FL 33461

Lakeland

Advanced Chemical Technology, Inc. — 863-687-9603
1706 South Combee Rd., Lakeland, FL 33803
Advanced Concept Innovations Llc — 863-577-8055
4100 S. Frontage Rd., Lakeland, FL 33815
Bloodnetusa, Inc. — 863-687-8925
3200 Lakeland Hills Blvd., Lakeland, FL 33805
Independent Brace, Inc. — 863-647-5559
3633 Century Blvd, Ste 1, Lakeland, FL 33811
Maxpak, Llc — 863-682-0123
2808 New Tampa Hwy., Lakeland, FL 33815
Omnia, Inc. — 863-619-8100
3125 Drane Field Rd.,suite 29, Lakeland, FL 33811
Wilson Spinal Systems — 863-294-6867
3532 Waterfield Pkwy., Lakeland, FL 33803

Lakewood Ranch

Rapid Pathogen Screening — 877-921-0080
7227 Delainey Court, Lakewood Ranch, FL 34240

Largo

Adva-Lite, Inc. — 727-546-5483
7340 Bryan Dairy Road, Largo, FL 33777
American Medical Specialties, Inc. — 800-808-2877
10650 77th St., Suite 405, Largo, FL 33777
Ametek — 727-536-7831
8600 Somerset Dr., Largo, FL 33773
Baxter Healthcare Corp., Renal Division — 847-948-2000
7511 114th Avenue North, Largo, FL 33777
Belcher Pharmaceuticals, Inc. — 727-544-8866
12393 Belcher Rd., Ste. 420, Largo, FL 33773
Bioderm, Inc. — 800-373-7006
12320 73rd Court North, Largo, FL 33773
Burke Medical, Llc — 727-532-8333
2310 Tall Pines Dr., Suite 210, Largo, FL 33771
Conmed Linvatec — 800-448-6506
11311 Concept Blvd, Largo, FL 33773-4908
Diamond Edge Co. — 727-586-2927
801 West Bay Drive, Suite 700, Largo, FL 33770
Maven Medical Manufacturing, Inc. — 800-562-7326
2250 Lake Ave. S.E., Largo, FL 33771
Medix Pharmaceuticals Americas, Inc. — 888-242-3463
12505 Starkey Road, Suite M, Largo, FL 33773
Medrx, Inc. — 727-584-9600
1200 Starkey Rd., #105, Largo, FL 33771
Nasa Tech Memory Foam Sleep Systems — 727-447-0957
8300 Ulmerton Rd., Ste. 100, Largo, FL 33771
Precision Sclero — 727-517-0729
12408 Chickasaw Trail, Largo, FL 33774
Stretchair Patient Transfer Systems — 800-237-1162
8110 Ulmerton Rd., Largo, FL 33771
Stretchair Patient Transfer Systems, Inc, — 800-237-1162
8110 Ulmerton Road, Largo, FL 33771
Sun-Med — 800-433-2797
12393 Belcher Road, Suite #450, Largo, FL 33773
Sunmed Healthcare — 727-531-7266
12393 Belcher Road, Suite 460, Largo, FL 33773
Unilens Corp., Usa — 727-544-2531
10431 72nd St. North, Largo, FL 33777
Unilens Corp., Usa — 800-446-2020
10431 72nd St. North, Largo, FL 33777
Unimed Surgical Products, Inc. — 727-546-1900
10401 Belcher Rd., Largo, FL 33777
Veridien Corp. — 800-345-5444
7600 Bryan Dairy Road, Suite F, Largo, FL 33777-1433

Leesburg

Technicuff Corp. — 800-276-2833
2525 Industrial, Leesburg, FL 34748

Lehigh Acres

Humantronic, Inc — 866-340-1648
1103 Leeland Hgts Blvd E, Lehigh Acres, FL 33936-6431

Live Oak

Bowen Medical Services, Inc. — 800-726-8377
709 Industrial Ave., Live Oak, FL 32064

Lockhart

Inverness Medical Innovations North America, Inc — (877) 441-7440
30 S. Keller Road, Suite 100, Lockhart, FL 32810

Longboat Key

All Pro Exercise Products, Inc. — 800-735-9287
PO BOX 8268, Longboat Key, FL 34228

Longwood

Audina Hearing Instruments, Inc. — 800-223-7700
165 E. Wildmere Ave., Longwood, FL 32750
Compu Tech Inc — 407-788-6353
407 Wekiva Springs Road, Suite 347, Longwood, FL 32779
Electone, A Division Of Siemens Hearing Instruments, Inc. — 407-831-2555
1124 Florida Central Pkwy, Longwood, FL 32750
Numa Corp. — 800-327-2212
2290 North CR 427, Unit 136, Longwood, FL 32750

Loxahatchee

Dermawave, Llc — 561-784-0599
15693 83rd Lane North, Loxahatchee, FL 33470

Lutz

D.B.I. America Corp. — 813-909-9005
254 Crystal Grove Blvd., Lutz, FL 33548
Randal Minor Ocular Prosthetics Inc. — 813-949-2500
1628 Dale Mabry Hwy., Ste. 110, Lutz, FL 33548
Rochester Electro Medical, Inc. — 813-963-2933
4212 Cypress Gulch Drive, Lutz, FL 33559
The Soule Co., Inc. — 813-907-6000
4322 Pet Ln., Lutz, FL 33559

Lynn Haven

Gulf Coast Hyperbarics, Inc.   850-271-1441
1100 West 26th St., Lynn Haven, FL 32444

Maitland

Scient'X Usa, Inc.   407-571-2550
1015 Maitland Center Commons, Suite 106A, Maitland, FL 32751

Marathon

Radium Accessories Service, Inc.   305-289-1361
34 Coco Plum Dr., Marathon, FL 33050

Marco Island

Dermatec Industries, Llc   765-427-0092
970 Cape Marco Dr., #405, Marco Island, FL 34145

Margate

Groman Inc.   954-649-8008
4900 Nw 15th St., Ste 4494, Margate, FL 33063
Scannex, Inc.   954-974-2000
5100 W. Copans Rd, Bldg 1000, Margate, FL 33063

Medley

Legend Aerospace, Inc.   305-883-8804
8292 NW South River Drive, Medley, FL 33166

Melbourne

Airon Corporation   888-448-1238
751 North Drive, Unit 6, Melbourne, FL 32934
Lgm International Inc.   410-472-9930
3030 Venture Lane,suite 106, Melbourne, FL 32934
Maxxvision, Llc   1-877-340-6483
2800 Aurora Avenue, Suite E, Melbourne, FL 32935
Medicomp, Inc.   800-23-HEART
7845 Ellis Rd., Melbourne, FL 32904-1117
Medtronic Image-Guided Neurologics, Inc.   800-707-0933
2290 West Eau Gallie Blvd., Melbourne, FL 32935
Mnemonics, Inc.   800-842-5333
3900 Dow Road, Suite J, Melbourne, FL 32934
Sun Nuclear Corp.   321-259-6862
425-a Pineda Court, Melbourne, FL 32940
Titan Corporation/Systems & Imagery Division   800-622-8554
1200 S. Woody Burke Road, PO Box 550, Melbourne, FL 32901
Witt Biomedical Corporation   800-669-1328
305 North Drive, Melbourne, FL 32934

Merritt Island

Tua Systems, Inc.   321-453-3200
3645 North Courtenay Pky., Merritt Island, FL 32953

Miami

A&A Orthopedics, Incorporated   757-224-0177
12250 Sw 129th Court, Bldg. 01, Miami, FL 33186
A.G.A. Electronics Corp.   305-592-1860
7209 N.w. 41st St., Miami, FL 33166
AMERICAN MEDICAL ENDOSCOPY   305-436-0599
3020 Nw 82nd Ave., Miami, FL 33122
Airgas South, Inc.   770-590-6200
7280 NW 58th St., Miami, FL 33166
American Medical Supplies And Equipment   888-592-3469
8361 NW 36th Street, Miami, FL 33166
Americhem Pharmaceutical Corp.   305-591-0100
2862 N. W. 79th Ave., Miami, FL 33122
Bio-Technology Usa, Inc.   305-512-3522
6175 NW 167th St., Suite # G-8, Miami, FL 33015-4334
Bio-Tissue, Inc.   888-296-8858
7000 S.w. 97th Ave., Ste. 211, Miami, FL 33173
Boston Scientific Corporation   508-652-5578
8600 N.w. 41st Street, Miami, FL 33166
Brain Power, Inc.   800-327-2250
4470 S.W. 74th Ave., Miami, FL 33155
Brava, Llc   305-856-4242
14221 SW 142nd Street, Miami, FL 33186
Bristol C&D, Inc.   877-255-1181
14317 S.W. 142 Avenue, Miami, FL 33186
Calmaquip Engineering Corp.   305-592-4510
7240 N.W. 12th St., Miami, FL 33126-1909
Cardent International, Inc.   866-764-6832
1568 NW 89th Ct., Miami, FL 33172
Cardiopulmonary Instrumentation, Inc.   305-592-8196
3002 N.w. 79th Avenue, Miami, FL 33122
Carpal Doctors Llc   866-401-1213
701 Brickell Avenue, Suite 1550, Miami, FL 33131
Comfort Touch   888-8BR-IEFS
P.O Box 630104, Miami, FL 33163
Conquest Condoms Llc   305-279-0089
9020 S.w. 83rd. St., Miami, FL 33173
Consumaquip Corporation   305-592-4510
7240 NW 12th Street, Miami, FL 33126-1909
Deepak Products, Inc.   305-482-9669
5220 N.w. 72nd Ave., Bay 15, Miami, FL 33166
Demetech Corp.   888-324-2447
3530 N.w. 115th Ave., Miami, FL 33178

Diamedix Corp.   800-327-4565
2140 N. Miami Avenue, Miami, FL 33127-4933
Dp Manufacture Corp.   800-403-1890
1460 N.w. 107th Ave., Ste. H, Miami, FL 33172
Eclipse Medical, Inc.   877-600-0042
12105 S.w. 129th Ct., #104, Miami, FL 33186
Electro-Med Health Industries   800-232-3644
PO Box 610484, Miami, FL 33261-0484
Emergencia 2000, Inc.   757-224-0177
8578 Nw 23rd St, Miami, FL 33122
Emergency Medical International   305-362-6050
6065 N.W. 167th St., #B-18, Miami, FL 33015-4315
Hand Innovations, Llc.   800-800-8188
6303 Blue Lagoon Drive, Suite 100, Miami, FL 33126
Health Care Exports, Inc.   800-847-0173
5701 N.W. 74 Ave., Miami, FL 33166
Her-Mar, Inc.   800-327-8209
8550 N.W. 30th Terr., Miami, FL 33122
Hill-Med, Inc.   305-594-7474
7217 N.W. 46th St., Miami, FL 33166
Hillusa Corp.   305-594-7474
7215 N.W. 46th St., Miami, FL 33166-6422
Hygienics Industries Div.Of Kleinert's, Inc.   800-498-7051
3968 194 Trail, Miami, FL 33160
Hyperion, Inc.   305-238-3020
14100 S.W. 136th St., Miami, FL 33186-5598
IVAX Diagnostics Inc.   800-327-4565
2140 North Miami Avenue, Miami, FL 33127
Innovia Llc   305-378-2651
12415 S.w. 136th Ave., Unit 3, Miami, FL 33186
Intelligent Hearing Systems, Corp.   800-447-9783
6860 SW 81st street, Miami, FL 33143
Intermetra Corp.   305-889-1194
10100 N.W. 116th Way, Suite 11, Miami, FL 33178-1154
Internal Fixation Systems, Inc.   305-491-9133
10100 N.w. 116th Way, Ste. 18, Miami, FL 33178
Jayza Corp.   305-477-1136
7215 NW 41ST, Bay A, Miami, FL 33166-6701
Karl Storz Endoscopia Latino America   305-262-8980
815 N.W. 57th Ave. Ste. 480, Miami, FL 33126-2042
Koch X-Ray Systems Inc   305-252-8770
10500 S.W. 184 Terrace, Miami, FL 33157-6760
L.D. Technology, Llc   305-777-0336
100 N. Biscayne Boulevard, Miami, FL 33132
Lead Enterprises Inc.   800-253-4249
3300 N.W. 29 St., Miami, FL 33142-6310
Leeder Group, Inc.   305-436-5030
8508 N.w. 66th St., Miami, FL 33166
Life Medical Equipment   800-749-4646
7874 N.W. 64 St., Miami, FL 33166
M & I Medical Sales, Inc.   305-663-6444
4711 S.W. 72 Ave., Miami, FL 33155
Mark Two Engineering   305-889-3280
8324 NW 74th Ave., Miami, FL 33166
Md International, Inc.   305-669-9003
11300 N.W. 41st St., Miami, FL 33178
Med-Lab Supply Co., Inc.   800-330-5144
923 N.W. 27th Ave., Miami, FL 33125
Medelec Industries   888-522-6452
6800 S.w. 40th St., Pmb-700, Miami, FL 33155
Medi-Tech International, Inc.   305-593-9373
2924 N.W. 109th Avenue, Miami, FL 33172
Megamed Corporation   305-665-6876
7432 SW 48th St., Miami, FL 33155
Miami Medical Equipment & Supply Corp.   305-592-0111
2150 N.W. 93 Ave., Miami, FL 33172
Micrus Design Technology, Inc.   408-433-1460
9344 N.w. 13th St., Miami, FL 33172
Neonatal, Infant, Pediatric, And Adult Advanced He   305-267-8885
815 N.w. 57th Ave., Suite 110, Miami, FL 33126
Non-Invasive Monitoring Systems, Inc.   305-575-4200
4400 Biscayne Blvd., Miami, FL 33137
Noven Pharmaceuticals, Inc.   305-253-5099
11960 SW 144th Street, Miami, FL 33186
Ockiobel, Inc.   305-261-6144
777 NW 72 Avenue, Suite 2K20, Miami, FL 33126-3009
Opko Health Inc.   305-575-4100
4400 Biscayne Blvd., Suite 1180, Miami, FL 33137
Paramount Products Usa   800-881-9003
150 N.W. 176 Street, Suite E, Miami, FL 33169
Pediatric Intensive Therapy, Inc.   786-543-8165
18639 S.w. 107th Ave., Miami, FL 33157
Print Media, Inc.   800-994-3318
9002 NW 105th Way, Miami, FL 33178
Rehabilitation Services, Inc.   888-300-4548
9841 SW 100 Ave., Miami, FL 33176
Repex Medical Products, Inc.   305-740-0133
5240 SW 64th Avenue, Miami, FL 33155-6431
Safestitch Medical Inc.   305-575-4145
4400 Biscayne Blvd, Suite 760, Miami, FL 33137
SanoMedics Development Corp.   305-433-7814
80 SW 8th Street, Suite 2180, Miami, FL 33130

Scion Cardio-Vascular, Inc. — 305-259-8880
14256 SW 119 Ave., Miami, FL 33186
Simplified Systems, Inc. — 305-672-7676
4014 Chase Ave., Ste. P.H., Miami, FL 33140-3421
Sukol Scientific, Inc. — 305-885-0045
10100 NW 116th Way # 18, Miami, FL 33178
Symphony Medical Products — 877-470-9995
6320 N.w. 84th Avenue, Miami, FL 33166
Tap Express, Inc. — 305-468-0038
8424 Nw 61 St., Miami, FL 33166
Terumo Medical Corporation — 800-283-7866
8750 NW 36th Street, Suite 600, Miami, FL 33178
Transphoton Corporation — 305-234-0836
14350 S.w. 142nd Ave., Miami, FL 33186
Universal Surgical Appliance Co. — 305-652-0810
400 N.E. 191 Street, Miami, FL 33179
University Of Miami Tissue Bank — 888-UMTISSUE
1600 N.W. 10th Ave. (R-12), Miami, FL 33136

Miami Beach

Ama Optics, Inc. — 877-744-3937
314 West San Marino Dr., Miami Beach, FL 33139
Diagnostic Support Usa Inc — 305-532-1586
1900 Sunset Harbour Dr., Suite 1902, Miami Beach, FL 33139
Galix Biomedical Instrumentation, Inc. — 305-534-5905
2555 Collins Avenue, Suite C-5, Miami Beach, FL 33140

Miami Lakes

Cordis Neurovascular, Inc. — 800-327-7714
14201 NW 60 Avenue, Miami Lakes, FL 33014
Jas Diagnostics, Inc. — 305-418-2320
14100 n.w. 57th court, Miami Lakes, FL 33014

Middleburg

Bagrad — 904-272-6369
84 Sleepy Hollow Rd., Middleburg, FL 32068

Milton

Kottler Research Corp. — 850-983-0552
2000 Garcon Point Road, Milton, FL 32583

Miramar

Bioresource Technology, Inc. — 954-792-5222
11924 Miramar Pkwy., Flamingo Park Of Commerce, Miramar, FL 33025
Fla Orthopedics, Inc. — 800-327-4110
2881 Corporate Way, Miramar, FL 33025
Hema Diagnostic Systems, Llc — 954-919-5123
10102 USA Today Way, Miramar, FL 33025
Nipro Diabetes Systems, Inc. — 888-651-7867
3361 Enterprise Way, Miramar, FL 33025

N Palm Beach

Advanced Medical Support — 888-800-7283
10180 Riverside Dr, Suite 9, N Palm Beach, FL 33410

Naples

Aculux, Inc. — 239-643-8023
4424 Corporate Square, Naples, FL 34104
Arthrex Manufacturing — 239-643-5553
1958 Trade Center Way, Naples, FL 34109
Arthrex, Inc. — 800-933-7001
1370 Creekside Blvd., Naples, FL 34108
Astron International Inc. — 239-435-0136
3410 Westview Dr., Naples, FL 34104
Dri-Dek/Kendall Products — 800-348-2398
901 Sarasota Center Blvd., Naples, FL 34104
Health & Hygiene, Inc. — 239-403-9919
4406 Exchange Ave., #127, Naples, FL 34104
Inovo, Inc. — 239-643-6577
2975 S. Horseshoe Drive, Suite 600, Naples, FL 34104
Isolux Llc — 239-514-7475
1045 Collier Center Way, Suite #6, Naples, FL 34110
M.C. Johnson Co., Inc. — 800-553-8483
2037 J & C Blvd., Naples, FL 34109-6213
Med-General Usa Llc — 239-597-9967
1045 Collier Center Way, Unit #1, Naples, FL 34110

Navarre

Aqua Water Treatment, Inc. — 850-939-9055
8195 East Bay Blvd., Navarre, FL 32566

Niceville

Deuteronomy Management Services,Inc. — 850-897-3321
1439 Live Oak St., Suite A, Niceville, FL 32578-8829

Nmb

Synergy Usa — 786-222-1710
13899 Biscayne Blvd, Suite 101, Nmb, FL 33181

North Miami

Reflex Technologies, Inc. — 305-892-0584
12565 Palm Rd., Suite B, North Miami, FL 33181-2611
Sleep Group Solutions — 305-830-0327
1875 Ne 168th Street, North Miami, FL 33162

North Palm Beach

Implant Center Of The Palm Beaches — 561-627-5560
824 U.S. Hwy. 1, Ste. 370, North Palm Beach, FL 33408

North Port

Rycor Medical, Inc. — 800-227-9267
2053 Atwater Drive, North Port, FL 34288

Oakland

Healthline Medical Products, Inc. — 1-800-987-3577
1065 E Story Rd., Oakland, FL 34787

Oakland Park

Bioflex Medical Magnetics, Inc. — 800-619-2717
3370 N.E. Fifth Ave., Oakland Park, FL 33334

Ocala

American Catheter Corp. — 800-345-6714
13047 S. Hwy 475, Ocala, FL 34480
Clearwater Colon Hydrotherapy, Inc. — 888-869-6191
3145 S.w. 74th Terrace, Ocala, FL 34474
E-One — 352-237-1122
1601 S.W. 37th Ave., Ocala, FL 34474
Fpp, Inc. — 352-622-4595
6800 S.W. 66th St., Ocala, FL 34476-5526
Horcher Lifting Systems, Inc. — 800-582-8732
1884 NW 57th Street, Ocala, FL 34475
Medx Corporation — 800-876-6339
1401 N.E. 77th St., Ocala, FL 34479
Pneumatic Products Corporation — 352-873-5793
4647 S.W. 40th Ave., Ocala, FL 34474-5799
Usa Scientific, Inc. — 800-522-8477
P.O. Box 3565, Ocala, FL 34478-3565
Winco, Inc. — 800-237-3377
5516 S.w. First Ln., Ocala, FL 34474
Zefon International — 800-282-0073
5350 S.W. First Lane, Ocala, FL 34474

Ocklawaha

Kegelmaster Inc. — 352-625-2156
4125 Se Hwy 314a, Ocklawaha, FL 32179

Odessa

Hager Worldwide, Inc. — 800-328-2335
13322 Byrd Drive, Odessa, FL 33556-5312
J.S. Associates — 813-975-4354
8403 Ridgebrook Cir, Odessa, FL 33556
Practical Systems, Inc. — 800-237-8154
11617 Prospect Rd., Odessa, FL 33556
5 Star Imaging, Inc. — 727-376-0588
11515 Prosperous Dr., Odessa, FL 33556

Oldsmar

Bell Hearing Instruments, Inc. — 800-535-0516
700 Stevens Avenue, Oldsmar, FL 34677
Cryo-Cell International, Inc. — 800-786-7235
700 Brooker Creek Blvd., Suite 1800, Oldsmar, FL 34677
Gulf Medical Fiberoptics — 813-891-1993
448 commerce blvd, Oldsmar, FL 34677
Promedica, Inc. — 800-899-5278
114 Douglas Road East, Oldsmar, FL 34677-2939
Vax-D Medical Technologies Llc — 813-343-5000
310 Mears Blvd, Oldsmar, FL 34677

Orange City

Ripp Restraints, Inc. — 800-544-8344
1220 East Industrial Dr., PO Box 740071, Orange City, FL 32763

Orlando

Blue Horizon Medical — 321-217-2717
3129 Ginger Cir., Orlando, FL 32826
Crestline Products Inc. — 407-859-6428
PO Box 2108, Orlando, FL 32802-2108
Endotec, Inc. — 973-762-6100
2546 Hansrob Road, Orlando, FL 32804
Essential Medical Supply, Inc. — 800-826-8423
6420 Hazeltine National Drive, Orlando, FL 32822
Florida Pillow Company — 800-560-1631
1012 Sligh Blvd., Orlando, FL 32806
Gam Laser Inc — 407-851-8999
6901 TPC Drive, Suite 300, Orlando, FL 32822
Hendricks Orthotic Prosthetic Enterprises, Inc. — 407-850-0411
6439 Milner Blvd., Suite 6, Orlando, FL 32809
Invivo — 800-331-3220
12501 Research Parkway, Orlando, FL 32826
Invivo Corporation — 425-487-7000
12151 Research Pkwy., Orlando, FL 32826
Io Laser, Inc. — 407-296-0544
6140-b Edgewater Dr., Orlando, FL 32810-4860
Lifestream Medical Corporation — 407-529-9920
12024 Green Emerald Court, Orlando, FL 32837
Lightpath Technologies — 407-382-4003
2603 Challenger Tech Ct., Suite 100, Orlando, FL 32826

My Water House, Inc. — 407-428-9377
3319 Bartlett Blvd., Orlando, FL 32817
National Ambulance Builders, Inc. — 800-747-0064
230 N. Ortman Drive, Orlando, FL 32805
Orthomerica Products, Inc. — 800-446-6770
6333 N. Orange Blossom Trl., Suite 220, Orlando, FL 32810
Otto Bock Healthcare, Lp — 763-489-5106
9420 Delegates Drive, Ste.100, Orlando, FL 32837
Praxair Distribution Inc., Southeast Llc — 440-234-1075
403 Zell Dr., Orlando, FL 32824
QUALITY ASSURED SERVICES DBA ALERE — 800-298-4515
HOME MONITORING PRODUCTS
70 S. Keller Rd., Orlando, FL 32810
Ssi Surgical Services, Inc — 407-249-1946
5776 Hoffner Ave, Ste 200, Orlando, FL 32822
The Hearing Aid Factory, Inc. — 407-649-9696
710 West Colonial Dr., #101, Orlando, FL 32804
Tran Pa-C, Inc. — 321-276-5407
3348 Herringridge Dr., Orlando, FL 32812
Tub Master Lc — 800-833-0260
413 Virginia Drive, Orlando, FL 32803
Vivvid International — 447-040-4013
800 Fern Creek Ave., Orlando, FL 32803
W.O.M. World Of Medicine Usa, Inc. — 888-469-4378
4531 36th street, Orlando, FL 32811-6527
World Of Medicine Usa, Inc. — 407-438-8810
4531 36th St., Orlando, FL 32811-6527
Ziehm Imaging, Inc. — 800-503-4952
6280 Hazeltine National Dr., Orlando, FL 32822

Ormond Beach
Command Medical Products, Inc. — 386-672-8116
15 Signal Avenue, Ormond Beach, FL 32174-2984
Pathlighter, Inc. — 877-728-4544
105 Riverside Dr., Ormond Beach, FL 32176

Osprey
Derron Surgical Instruments, Inc. — 888-374-3622
1055 Scherer Way, Osprey, FL 34229
Ingenious Technologies Corp. — 941-966-0690
1109 Millpond Ct, Osprey, FL 34229

Oviedo
Alicia Diagnostics, Inc. — 407-365-8498
1274 Alafaya Trail, Oviedo, FL 32765
Surgilight, Inc. — 407-482-4555
23 Alafaya Woods Blvd., Box 170, Oviedo, FL 32765

Palm Bay
Mpi Medical Products, Inc. — 321-676-1299
1631 Elmhurst Circle, S.e., Palm Bay, FL 32909

Palm Beach
Cyberbiomed, Llc — 561-582-1955
3605 S. Ocean Blvd. #a-335, Palm Beach, FL 33480

Palm Beach Gardens
Anspach Effort Inc. — 800-327-6887
4500 Riverside Dr., Palm Beach Gardens, FL 33410
Anspach Effort, Inc. — 800-327-6887
4500 Riverside Dr., Palm Beach Gardens, FL 33410
Biomet 3i — 800-342-5454
4555 Riverside Dr., Palm Beach Gardens, FL 33410
Clear Stream Media — 561) 622-5995
4440 PGA Blvd-Suite 403, Palm Beach Gardens, FL 33410
Panex Corp. — 800-662-4499
12300 Highway A1A Alt, Suite 103, Palm Beach Gardens, FL 33410
Protech Leaded Eyewear — 561-627-9769
10415 riverside drive, Palm Beach Gardens, FL 33410
Surgichip, Inc. — 561-694-7776
4398 Hickory Dr., Palm Beach Gardens, FL 33418

Palm City
Awareness Technology, Inc. — 722-283-6540
1935 S.W. Martin Hwy., Palm City, FL 34990
Chemplex Industries, Inc. — 800-424-3675
2820 SW 42nd Avenue, Palm City, FL 34990
Flexsite Diagnostics, Inc. — 772-221-8893
3543 S.W. Corporate Pkwy., Palm City, FL 34990
Guerilla Technologies Inc. — 772-283-0500
4203 SW High Meadows Ave., Palm City, FL 34990
Isocomforter, Inc. — 877-277-0367
3531 SW Corporate Pkwy., Palm City, FL 34990

Palm Harbor
Apheresis Technologies, Inc. — 800-749-9284
PO Box 2081, Palm Harbor, FL 34682-2081
Bathease Inc. — 888-747-7845
3815 Darston St., Palm Harbor, FL 34685-3119
Chi'Am International — 727-647-3940
4155 Grandchamp Circle, Palm Harbor, FL 34685
Dmx-Works, Inc. — 800-839-6757
4159-b Corporate Court, Palm Harbor, FL 34683

Gold'N Braces, Inc. — 800-785-1970
2595 Tampa Road, Suite 1, Palm Harbor, FL 34684
Oscor, Inc. — 800-726-7267
3816 De Soto Blvd., Palm Harbor, FL 34683-1618

Palm-Bay
Ormantine Usa Ltd. — 321-676-7003
1740 Convair St, Palm-Bay, FL 32909

Palmetto
Hq, Inc. — 941-721-7588
210- 9th St. Drive West, #208-210, Palmetto, FL 34221

Panama City Beach
Optical Integrity, Inc. — 850-233-5512
8317 Front Beach Rd., Suite 21, Panama City Beach, FL 32407

Parrish
Cline Products Inc. — 941-776-0230
11446 Savannah Lakes Dr., Parrish, FL 34219

Pensacola
Bashaw Medical, Inc. — 800-499-3857
4909-B Mobile Hwy., Pensacola, FL 32506-3229
Lakeview Center, Inc. — 850-595-1330
1221 W. Lakeview Ave., Pensacola, FL 32501-1836
Medical Energy, Inc. — 8806 Paul Starr
8806 Paul Starr Drive, Pensacola, FL 32514

Pinellas Park
Baxter Healthcare Corporation — 847-473-6141
3925 Gateway Blvd, Pinellas Park, FL 33782
Dotolo Research Corp. — 800-237-8458
2875 MCI Drive, Pinellas Park, FL 33782
Endorphin Corporation — 800-940-9844
6901 90th Avenue North, Pinellas Park, FL 33782
Hearing Technologies — 727-525-7770
6251 44th St 109, Pinellas Park, FL 33781
Invacare Top End — 800-532-8677
4501 63rd Circle North, Pinellas Park, FL 33781-5914
Invacare Top End Sports And Recreation Products — 800-532-8677
4501 63rd Circle N., Pinellas Park, FL 33781
Mcpherson Enterprises, Inc. — 813-931-4201
3851 62nd Ave. N., Suite A, Pinellas Park, FL 33781
Ongoing Care Solutions, Inc. — 800-375-0207
6545 44th St., N., Ste. 4007, Pinellas Park, FL 33781
Primary Medical Co., Inc. — 727-520-1920
6541 44TH STREET N / SUITE 6003, PINELLAS PARK, FL 33781
Select Medical Products, Inc. — 800-276-7237
6531 47th St. N., Pinellas Park, FL 33781
Transitions Optical, Inc. — 727-545-0400
9251 Belcher Rd., Pinellas Park, FL 33782
Ultimex Corp. — 727-403-3090
6250 42nd St., Unit #30, Pinellas Park, FL 33781

Plantation
Clinical Diagnostic Solutions, Inc. — 800-453-3328
1800 N.w. 65th Ave., Plantation, FL 33313
Quantum Bioengineering, Ltd. — 954-474-4707
7951 S.w. 6th St., Plantation, FL 33324
Technical Marketing, Inc. — 954-370-0855
1776 N. Pine Island Road, Suite 306, Plantation, FL 33322-5253

Pompano Beach
Brantlin — 954-691-6476
1511 N.e. 40th St., Pompano Beach, FL 33064
Health Chem Diagnostics Llc — 954-979-3845
3341 S.w. 15th St., Pompano Beach, FL 33069
Imperial Fastener Co., Inc. — 954-782-7130
1400 S.W. 8th St., Pompano Beach, FL 33069
International Medical Industries — 800-344-2554
2881 West McNab Road, Pompano Beach, FL 33069
Jb Medical Development Inc. — 813-645-2855
3000-10 N.w. 25th Ave., Pompano Beach, FL 33069
Micro Typing Systems, Inc. — 908-218-8177
1295 S.w. 29th Ave., Pompano Beach, FL 33069

Ponte Vedra Beach
Eyequip, Div Of Alliance Medical Marketing — 800-393-8676
5150 Palm Valley Road, Suite 305, Ponte Vedra Beach, FL 32082

Port Richey
Isoaid, L.L.C. — 727-815-3262
7824 Clark Moody Blvd., Port Richey, FL 34668
Lar Mfg., Llc. — 727-846-7860
6828 Commerce Ave., Port Richey, FL 34668

Port St. Lucie
Advanced Radiation Measurements, Inc. — 772-340-3279
601 N.E. Emerson St., Port St. Lucie, FL 34983
Superior Dental & Test — 800-528-7297
1501 SE Village Green Dr., Port St. Lucie, FL 34952-3494

Riviera Beach

Global One Medical, Inc. — 561-842-7727
3707 Interstate Park Rd. S., Riviera Beach, FL 33404
Hennessy Dental Laboratory — 800-694-6862
3709 Interstate Park Road South, Riviera Beach, FL 33404
Perry Baromedical Corp. — 800-741-4376
3660 Interstate Parkway, Riviera Beach, FL 33404-3411
Renick Ent., Inc. — 561-863-4183
1211 West 13th St., Riviera Beach, FL 33404

Rockledge

Q-Teknologies, Inc. — 321-631-3915
391 Brookcrest Circle, Rockledge, FL 32955

Saint Cloud

Velopex International. — 888-835-6739
105 East 17th St., Saint Cloud, FL 34769

Saint Petersburg

Advanced Orthogonal Equipment, Incorporated — 757-224-0177
2201 62nd Avenue North, Saint Petersburg, FL 33702
Applied Neuroscience, Inc. — 727-244-0240
228 176th Terrace Drive, Saint Petersburg, FL 33708
Lenstec, Inc. — 727-571-2272
1765 Commerce Ave. N, Saint Petersburg, FL 33716
Restorative Care Of America Inc — 800-627-1595
12221 33rd Street N., Saint Petersburg, FL 33716
Smith & Nephew, Inc. — 800-876-1261
970 lake carillon dr., suite 110, saint petersburg, FL 33716
Smith & Nephew, Inc. — 800-876-1261
970 Lake Carillon Dr., Suite 110, Saint Petersburg, FL 33716
Thinking Systems Corporation — 727-217-0909
750 94th Avenue North, Suite 211, Saint Petersburg, FL 33702
Ultroid, Llc And Ultroid Technologies, Incorporated — 727-865-1929
405 Central Ave., Ste. 100, Saint Petersburg, FL 33701

Sanford

.Decimal, Inc. — 1.800.255.1613
121 Central Park Place, Sanford, FL 32771
Future Health Concept's, Inc. — 888-282-8644
1211 30th St., Sanford, FL 32773
Invacare Corporation — 800-327-9438
2101 East Lake Mary Blvd., Sanford, FL 32773
Omega Medical Imaging, Inc. — 407-323-9400
675 Hickman Circle, Sanford, FL 32771
Orthotics Choice Llc. — 407-321-0454
451 E. Airport Blvd., Sanford, FL 32773
Separation Technology Inc — 800-777-6668
582 Monroe Road, Suite 1424, Sanford, FL 32771
Tekquest Industries — 800-327-7175
4200 St. John's Parkway, Sanford, FL 32771

Sarasota

Allodex Systems — 888-820-5836
19940 Dinner Key Dr., PO Box # 3252, Sarasota, FL 34230
Aso Corporation — 941-379-0300
300 Sarasota Center Blvd., Sarasota, FL 34240
Associated Contacts, Inc. — 941-921-1200
2036 Bispham Rd., Sarasota, FL 34231
Benz Research And Development Corp. — 941-758-8256
6447 Parkland Dr., Sarasota, FL 34243
Biolife, Llc — 800-722-7559
8163 25th Court East, Sarasota, FL 34243-3271
Dean B. Scott, Ocularist — 847-965-4455
1901 S. Osprey Ave., Sarasota, FL 34239
Encompas Unlimited, Inc. — 800-825-7701
2219 Whitfield Park Dr,, Sarasota, FL 34243
Encore, Inc. — 800-221-6603
7696 15th STREET EAST, SARASOTA, FL 34243
European Eyewear Corp. — 941-322-6771
630 Myakka Rd., Sarasota, FL 34240
Hoveround Corporation — 800-964-6837
2151 Whitfield Industrial Way, Sarasota, FL 34243
Hydrogel Vision Corporation — 877-336-2482
7575 Commerce Ct, Sarasota, FL 34243-9825
Medone Surgical, Inc. — 941-359-3129
670 Tallevast Road, Sarasota, FL 34243
Mictron, Inc. — 941-371-6659
8130 Fruitville Rd., Sarasota, FL 34240
Ocular Innovations, Inc. — 813-645-2855
1121 Lewis Ave., Sarasota, FL 34237
Peak Enterprises Inc — 941-373-0046
635 South Orange Avenue, Suite 8, Sarasota, FL 34236
Silver Bay, Llc — 941-306-5812
1431 Tallevast Rd., Sarasota, FL 34243
Specialeyes Llc — 813-645-2855
6447 Parkland Dr., Suite 2020, Sarasota, FL 34243
Surgical Implants, Inc. — 941-366-1882
962 S. Tamiami Trail, Suite 203, Sarasota, FL 34236
Surgical Safety Products, Inc. — 800-953-7889
2018 Oak Terrace, Suite 400, Sarasota, FL 34231
The Lifestyle Gp Company, L.L.C. — 888-379-6645
2530 Trailmate Dr., Sarasota, FL 34243

World Precision Instruments (W.P.I.), Inc. — 866-606-1974
175 Sarasota Center Blvd., Sarasota, FL 34240-9258

Saratoga Springs

TandD Corporation — 518-669-9227
PO Box 321, Saratoga Springs, FL 12866

Sebring

Ear-Clear, Inc. — 866-290-4260
1920 Brunns Rd., #29, Sebring, FL 33872

Seminole

General Transco Inc. — 727-535-2534
13265 Park Blvd, Seminole, FL 33776
Superior Uniform Group — 727-397-9611
10055 Seminole Blvd., Seminole, FL 33772

St Augustine

H&H Instruments — 904-797-1502
4950 Crescent Technical Ct, St Augustine, FL 32086

St. Petersburg

Benjamin Biomedical, Inc. — 727-343-5503
539 Pasadena Avenue South, St. Petersburg, FL 33710
Burkhart Roentgen Intl. Inc. — 800-USA-XRAY
5201 8th Ave. S., St. Petersburg, FL 33707
Ccr Medical, Inc. — 888-883-7331
967 43 Avenue NE, St. Petersburg, FL 33703-5121
Choice Medical Systems, Inc. — 727-347-8833
1426 Pasadena Avenue, S., St. Petersburg, FL 33707
Essilor Of America, Inc. — 800-843-3937
4970 Park St. North, St. Petersburg, FL 33709
Freedom Scientific Blv Group, Llc. — 727-803-8000
11800 31st Court North, St. Petersburg, FL 33716
Halkey-Roberts Corp. — 1.800.303.4384
2700 Halkey-Roberts Place North, St. Petersburg, FL 33716
Ibc Int'L, Inc. — 727-551-2087
100 4th Ave. South #412, St. Petersburg, FL 33701
Mts Medication Technologies — 800-671-0508
2003 Gandy Blvd., Suite 800, St. Petersburg, FL 33702
Prosun Tanning International, Llc. — 800-874-2776
2442 23rd Street North, St. Petersburg, FL 33713-4018
R. B. Williams Co., Inc. — 800-843-7346
2616 First Avenue North, St. Petersburg, FL 33713
Schell, Inc. — 800-821-5001
P.O. Box 12689, St. Petersburg, FL 33733-2689

Stuart

Avotec, Inc. — 800-272-2238
603 N.W. Buck Hendry Way, Stuart, FL 34994
Electro Mechanical Products Inc. — 772-286-8848
41 SE Kindred St., Stuart, FL 34994
Insight Instruments, Inc. — 800-255-8354
2580 S.E. Willoughby Blvd., Stuart, FL 34994

Sunrise

Bolton Medical, Inc. — 954-838-9699
799 International Parkway, Sunrise, FL 33325
Dynamic Dental Corp. — 954-753-4693
10791 Nw. 53rd. St., Ste. 102, Sunrise, FL 33351
Elite Dental Service — 954-825-6392
10188 Nw 47th Street, Sunrise, FL 33351
Marina Medical Instruments, Inc. — 800-697-1119
955 Shotgun Road, Sunrise, FL 33326
Medecon — 954-742-6300
10001 NW 50th St., Suite W-2, Sunrise, FL 33351-8061
Rotburg Instruments Of America Inc. — 954-331-8046
1560 Sawgrass Corporate Pkwy., 4th Floor, Sunrise, FL 33323

Tampa

Airgas South, Inc. — 770-590-6200
1620 Tampa East Blvd., Tampa, FL 33619
Anodyne Therapy, Llc — 800-521-6664
14105 McCormick Drive, Tampa, FL 33626
Applied Therapeutics, Inc. — 877-682-2777
3104 Cherry Palm Drive Suite 220, Tampa, FL 33619
Axiom Worldwide, Inc. — 813-969-2414
9423 Corporate Lake Dr., Tampa, FL 33634-2359
Bausch & Lomb Pharmaceutical, Inc. — 800-227-1427
8500 Hidden River Pkwy, Tampa, FL 33637
Blake Manufacturing, Inc. — 813-935-1841
9241 Lazy Ln., Tampa, FL 33614
Cardio Command, Inc. — 800-231-6370
4920 W. Cypress St., Suite 110, Tampa, FL 33607
Cardiovascular Research, Inc. — 813-832-6222
4810 W. Gandy Blvd., Tampa, FL 33611
Creative Medical Designs, Inc. — 813-875-9999
13914 Shady Shores Dr., Tampa, FL 33613
Donovan Industries — 800-334-4404
13401 McCormick Drive, Tampa, FL 33626
Electronic Mfg. Co. — 813-855-4068
13440 Wright Circle, Tampa, FL 33626
Electrostim Medical Services, Inc. — 800-588-8383
3504 Cragmont Dr., Suite #100, Tampa, FL 33619

Emepe International, Inc.   813-994-9690
18108 Sugar Brooke Drive, Tampa, FL 33647
Eyesupply Usa, Inc.   800-521-5257
10770 North 46th St.,, Suite C-700, Tampa, FL 33617
Ezy-Ramp Co.   800-835-8513
4502 North Armenia Avenue, Tampa, FL 33603
Frank Tanaka, Ocularist, Inc.   813-978-1142
3000 East Fletcher Ave.,, Suite 310, Tampa, FL 33613
Ge Medical Systems Information Technologies   800-558-5544
4502 Woodland Corp. Blvd, Tampa, FL 33614
Heritage Medcall   800-396-6157
202 E. Virginia Ave., Tampa, FL 33603
Hurley Mat Company, B.F.   800-274-6287
5601 Bayshore Blvd., P.O. Box 13217, Tampa, FL 33681-3217
Immuna Care Corp.   610-941-2167
13654 N. 12th St., Suite 3, Tampa, FL 33613
In/Us Systems, Inc.   800-875-4687
5809 N. 50th St., Tampa, FL 33610-4809
KUBLY OCULAR PROSTHETICS INC.   813-977-7676
3500 East Fletcher Ave.,, Suite 509, Tampa, FL 33613
Kawasumi Laboratories America, Inc.   800-529-2786
4723 Oakfair Blvd, Tampa, FL 33610
Kimball Electronics Tampa   813-814-8114
13750 Reptron Blvd., Tampa, FL 33626
Lcr-Hallcrest--Florida   847-998-8580
6705 Parke East Blvd., Unit A, Tampa, FL 33610
Life Care Technologies, Inc.   800-671-0580
4710 Eisenhower Boulevard, Suite A-10, Tampa, FL 33634
Metronix   813-972-1212
12421 N. Florida Avenue, Suite D-201, Tampa, FL 33612-4201
Novalis Medical, Llc   813-645-2855
813 S. Westshore Blvd, Tampa, FL 33609
Old 97 Co.   813-247-6677
2306 North 35th St., Tampa, FL 33605
Orthotic Rehabilitation Products, Inc.   813-620-0035
7002 East Broadway, Tampa, FL 33619
Pegasus Imaging Corp.   800-875-7009
4001 N. Riverside Drive, Tampa, FL 33603
Psc Medical, Inc.   888-986-4276
4930 W. Nassau Street, #284, Tampa, FL 33607
Qualitico Dist's, Inc.   813-264-4788
14025 Clubhouse Cr. #2503, Tampa, FL 33624
Questech International, Inc.   800-966-5367
3810 Gunn Highway, Tampa, FL 33624
Rhein Medical, Inc.   800-637-4346
5460 Beaumont Center Blvd., Suite 500, Suite 500, Tampa, FL 33634
Scottcare Corporation   813-901-0019
4897 W. Waters Ave., Suite J, Tampa, FL 33634
Sharn, Inc.   800-325-3671
4517 George Road Suite 200, Tampa, FL 33634-6236
Sri Surgical   813-891-9550
12425 Race Track Roa, Tampa, FL 33626
Sri/Surgical Express   813-818-9550
12425 Race Track Road, Tampa, FL 33626
Tampa Hyperbaric Enterprise   813-391-9473
10104 Lake Cove Lane, Tampa, FL 33618
Tampa Work Services   813-663-9555
5602 East Columbus Dr., Tampa, FL 33619
Tri-Tronics Co., Inc.   800-237-0946
7705 Cheri Court, Tampa, FL 33634-2419
Trillium Hearing Technologies, Inc.   813-864-2292
13803 W. Hillsborough Ave., Tampa, FL 33635
U.S. Orthotics, Inc.   800-825-5228
8605 Palm River Road, Tampa, FL 33619-4317
Ultra Clean Systems, Inc.   877-935-6624
12700 Dupont Circle, Tampa, FL 33626
Westcoast Brace & Limb   813-985-5000
5311 E. Fletcher Ave., Tampa, FL 33617
3s L.L.C.   866-437-2677
9315 Knightbridge Ct., Tampa, FL 33647

Tarpon Springs

Life Back Enterprises, Inc.   727-641-9042
416 Admiral Cove, Tarpon Springs, FL 34689

the villages

Gillen Industries .   877-444-5536
1576 Bella Vista Cruz Drive, Suite 320, the villages, FL 32159

Titusville

J. Barot & Assoc.   321-383-7574
1125 White Dr., P.o. Box 5293, Titusville, FL 32780

Vero Beach

Computerized Radiation Scanners, Inc.   (800) 848-3852
140 Sopwith Dr., Vero Beach, FL 32968
Zander Medical Supplies, Inc. / Zander Ivf, Inc.   800-820-3029
755, 8th Court, Suite #4, Vero Beach, FL 32962

W. Melbourne

The 50 Degree Company   321-956-0050
315 Stan Drive, W. Melbourne, FL 32904

Wellington

Chambermaid Products , Inc.   800-549-5356
12050 Suellen Circle, Wellington, FL 33414
Orthopaedic Development, Llc   561-827-8006
1300 Corporate Center Way, Wellington, FL 33414

Wesley Chapel

Grav-Trac   813-932-8710
6040 Country Club Rd., Wesley Chapel, FL 33544

West Melbourne

Coeye, Inc.   321-543-2219
2025 West New Haven Ave., West Melbourne, FL 32904

West Palm Beach

Allvetsusa:Attn:Us-It.Net   954-560-4257
500 South Australian Ave., Suite 510, West Palm Beach, FL 33401-6206
Avicenna Laser Technology, Inc.   888-AVI-LASER
1209 N. Flagler Dr., West Palm Beach, FL 33401
Gulf Stream Medical, Inc. / Alden Scientific   561-478-5688
1810 Okeechobee Rd, West Palm Beach, FL 33409
Micro Tool Engineering, Inc.   561-842-7381
7575 Central Industrial Drive, West Palm Beach, FL 33404

Weston

American Scientific Resources, Inc.   847-386-1384
1112 Weston Rd., Unit 278, Weston, FL 33326
Starkey Florida   952-947-4734
2200 North Commerce Parkway, Weston, FL 33326

Winter Park

Custom Comfort   800-749-0933
PO Box 4779, Winter Park, FL 32793-4779
Custom Comfort Medtek   800-749-0933
3939 Forsyth Road, Suite A, Winter Park, FL 32792
Florida Brace Corporation   800-327-0870
601 W Webster Ave., Winter Park, FL 32789
Genicon   800-936-1020
6869 Stapoint Court, Suite 114, Winter Park, FL 32792
Iradimed Corporation   407-677-8022
7457 Aloma Ave., Suite 201, Winter Park, FL 32792
Lasersight Technologies, Inc.   407-678-9900 ex
931 S. Semoran Blvd, Unit 204, Winter Park, FL 32792
Wheeled Coach Industries, Inc.   800-422-8206
2737 N. Forsyth Rd., Winter Park, FL 32792

Winter Springs

Lancer Usa, Inc.   800-332-1855
3543 State Rd 419, Winter Springs, FL 32708

Zephyrhills

Primary Care Solutions, Inc.   888-212-5336
40420 Free Fall Avenue, Zephyrhills, FL 33540
Spec Connection Intl Inc.   813-618-0400
37325 Sr 54, Zephyrhills, FL 33542

GEORGIA

Acworth

Fehling Surgical Instruments   800-FEHLING
509 Broadstone Lane, Acworth, GA 30101
Sector Medical Corp.   770-975-1384
320 Northpoint Pkwy., Suite Q, Acworth, GA 30102

Albany

Procter & Gamble Paper Product Co.   229-430-8260
512 Liberty Expressway -se, Albany, GA 31705

Alpharetta

A & M Instruments, Inc.   770-772-6404
3565 Trotter Dr., Alpharetta, GA 30004
Bruder Healthcare Company   888-827-8337
3150 Engineering Parkway, Alpharetta, GA 30004
Cardiostream, Llc   770-457-5337
12600 Deerfield Parkway, Ste. 100, Alpharetta, GA 30004
Carticept Medical, Inc   (770) 754-3800
6120 Windward Parkway, Suite 220, Alpharetta, GA 30005
Chemence Medical Products Inc.   770-664-6624
185 Bluegrass Valley Parkway, Suite 100, Alpharetta, GA 30005
Delta Gloves   800-220-1262
6865 Shiloh Rd. E., Ste. 400, Alpharetta, GA 30005
Do Not Disturb, Inc.   770-750-0065
5665 Highway 9 N 10, Alpharetta, GA 30004-3959
Endochoice Inc.   888-682-3636
11810 Wills Rd, Suite 100, Alpharetta, GA 30009
Generic Medical, Inc.   678-879-1000
4064 D Nine Mcfarland Dr., Alpharetta, GA 30004
Impact Medical Technologies, Llc   770-817-3300
311 Curie Drive, Alpharetta, GA 30005
Imtek Environmental Corp.   770-667-8621
P.O. Box 2066, Alpharetta, GA 30023
Maternal Care, Inc.   678-770-4355
11585 Jones Bridge Rd., Suite 420-216, Alpharetta, GA 30022

Monoclonal Technologies Inc. — 888-683-2414
16335 New Bullpen Road, Alpharetta, GA 30004

Per-Se Technologies — 877-737-3773
1145 sanctuary prkwy sutit 200, Alpharetta, GA 30004

Sanuwave Inc. — 866-581-6843
11680 Great Oaks Way, Suite 350, Alpharetta, GA 30022

Surgical Information Systems, Inc. — 800-930-0895
11605 Haynes Bridge Rd., Suite 200, Alpharetta, GA 30004

The Evercare Company — 800-435-6223
3440 Preston Ridge Road, Suite 650, Alpharetta, GA 30005

Unique Sports Products, Inc. — 800-554-3707
840 Mcfarland Road, Alpharetta, GA 30004

Alpharetta,

Sun Technologies, Inc. — (770) 643-0622
3700 Mansell Road,, Suite# 125, Alpharetta,, GA 30022

Athens

Noramco, Inc. — 706-353-4400
1440 Olympic Dr., Athens, GA 30601

Atl

Ciba Vision Corporation — 678-415-3638
2930 Amwiler Court, Atl, GA 30360

Scholle Chemical Corp. — 404-761-0604
2300 West Point Ave., Atl, GA 30337

Atlanta

Adar International Inc. — 800-510-9286
3350 Riverwood Parkway SE, Suite 1900, Atlanta, GA 30339

Advanced Wound Systems, Llc. — 541-867-4726
1530 Dunwoody Village Pkwy #115, Atlanta, GA 30350

Airgas South, Inc. — 770-590-6200
1311 Fulton Industrial Blvd., N.W., Suite C, Atlanta, GA 30336

Airgas South, Inc. — 770-590-6200
3605 Presidential Pkwy., Atlanta, GA 30340

Atlanta Orthodontics — 800-535-7166
1247 Zonolite Road N.E., Atlanta, GA 30306-2005

Basic American Medical Products — 800-849-6664
2935-A Northeast Pkwy, Atlanta, GA 30360

Biospace Med — 866-933-5301
120 Interstate N. Pkwy, Ste 116, Atlanta, GA 30339

CardioMEMS, Inc. — 866-240-3335
387 Technology Circle NW, Suite 500, Atlanta, GA 30313

Carecentric, Inc. — 800-441-2331
2839 Paces Ferry Road, Suite 900, Atlanta, GA 33039

Carestream Dental LLC — 800-944-6365
1765 The Exchange, Atlanta, GA 30339

Centers For Disease Control And Prevention — 800-232-4636
1600 Clifton Rd., Atlanta, GA 30333

Covidien Lp, Formerly Registered As Tyco Healthcare — 800-962-9888
110 Kendall Park Lane, Atlanta, GA 30336

Digital Vision, Inc — 678-222-5200
301 Perimeter Center North, Suite 600, Atlanta, GA 30346

Dixon Medical Inc — 770-457-0602
3710 Long View Drive, Atlanta, GA 30341

Eclipsys Corporation — 800-869-8300
3 Ravinia Drive, Atlanta, GA 30346-2156

Georgia-Pacific Llc — 404-652-4000
133 Peachtree Street, N.E., Atlanta, GA 30303

Gf Health Products, Inc — 800-347-5678
2935 Northeast Pkwy, Atlanta, GA 30360

Gf Health Products, Inc — 770-368-4700
2935 Northeast Parkway, Atlanta, GA 30360

Innovative Health Care Products, Inc. — 678-320-0009
6850 Peachtree-Dunwoody Road, Suite #402, Atlanta, GA 30328

Innovative Orthotics & Rehabilitation, Inc. — 404-222-9998
13oo Dekalb Ave., Atlanta, GA 30006

Instru-Med, Co. — 404-252-6188
5775 Glenridge Drive, East Building Suite 360, Atlanta, GA 30328

Lanier Worldwide, Inc. — 800-727-1885
2300 Parklake Dr. N.E., Atlanta, GA 30345

MedShape Solutions Inc. — 877-343-7016
1575 Northside Drive, Suite 440, Atlanta, GA 30318

Neural Signals,Inc. — 770-220-9964
3688 Clearview Ave Ste 110, Atlanta, GA 30340

Neurostar Solutions, Inc. — 866-809-4746
6 Concourse Parkway NE, Suite 1625, Atlanta, GA 30328

Perfecto Products Mfg., Inc. — 404-352-3863
1800 Marietta Blvd., Atlanta, GA 30318

Podo Technology, Inc — 770-353-0723
5 Concourse Parkway, Ste 3000, Atlanta, GA 30328

Pritchett & Hull Associates Inc. — 800-241-4925
3440 Oakcliff Rd. N.E., Ste. 110, Atlanta, GA 30340-3079

Siemens Healthcare Diagnostics Inc. — 800-242-3233
600 Tradeport Blvd, Suite 601, Atlanta, GA 30354

Sterilization Services — 404-344-8423
6005 Boatrock Blvd., Atlanta, GA 30336-2703

Sweat Chiropractic Clinic — 770-457-4430
3288 Chamblee Tucker Road, Atlanta, GA 30341

Syntermed, Inc. — 404-814-5277
Tower Place Ctr., Suite 1800, 3340 Peachtree Rd., Atlanta, GA 30326

Vantage Industries, Inc. — 800-221-4329
5070 Phillip Lee Drive, Atlanta, GA 30336

Vna Systems, Inc. — 404-264-0160
1414 Epping Forest Dr., Atlanta, GA 30319

Z Technologies, Llc — 404-248-0159
2615 Woodacres Road, Atlanta, GA 30345

Zep Superior Solutions — 877-428-9937
1310 Seaboard Ind. Blvd., Atlanta, GA 30318-2825

Atlanta,

Rpi Of Atlanta — 800-554-1501
120 Interstate N. Pkwy. E., Ste. 440, Atlanta,, GA 30339-2158

Auburn

Durden Enterprises — 800-554-5673
1317 4th Ave., P.O. Box 909, Auburn, GA 30011

Augusta

Air Liquide America Specialty Gases Llc — 713-402-2152
1311 New Savannah Rd., Augusta, GA 30901

Augusta Medical Systems, Llc — 800-827-8382
1027 Broad St., Augusta, GA 30901

Covidien Lp, Formerly Registered As Kendall — 800-962-9888
1430 Marvin Griffin Rd, Augusta, GA 30906

Eagle Parts & Products, Inc. — 888-972-9911
1411 Marvin Griffin Rd., Augusta, GA 30906

Electrolux Home Products - North America — 877-435-3287
250 Bobby Jones Expressway, PO Box 212378, Augusta, GA 30917

H.E. Inc. (Harod Enterprises) — 706-228-5165
4052 Indian Creek Rd, Augusta, GA 30907

Shared Systems, Inc. — 888-474-2733
PO Box 211587, 3961 Columbia Rd, Augusta, GA 30917

Standard Textile Augusta, Inc. — 513-761-9255
1701 Goodrich St., Augusta, GA 30904

United Medical Enterprises — 757-224-0177
4049 Allen Station Rd, Augusta, GA 30906

Austell

Inmark, Inc. — 800-646-6275
675 Hartman Road, Suite 100, Austell, GA 30168

Baldwin

Glenroe Technologies — 800-237-4060
210 Industrial Park Road, Baldwin, GA 30511

Ball Ground

Caire, Inc. — 770-479-6531
2000 Airport Industrial Dr., Ball Ground, GA 30107

Baxley

Douglas & Harper Mfg. Co., Inc. — 912-367-4149
1126 South Main St., Baxley, GA 31513

Blairsville

Heidelberg Medical, Inc. — 706-745-9698
627 Gainesville Highway, Suite B, Blairsville, GA 30512

Bogart

Main Line International, Inc. — 800-397-9020
151 Ben Burton Circle, Coggins Park, Bogart, GA 30622

Olis: On-Line Instrument Systems, Inc. — 800-852-3504
130 Conway Drive, Suite A & B, Bogart, GA 30622

Buford

Theragenics Corp. — 770-271-0233
5203 Bristol Industrial Way, Buford, GA 30518

Unisplint Corp. — 770-271-0646
4485 Commerce Dr., Suite 106, Buford, GA 30518

Webbmed Corporation — 678-482-1722
615 Emerald Pkwy., Buford, GA 30518

Calhoun

Garden City Medical, Inc. — 732-683-1900
512 Union Grove Rd., Calhoun, GA 30701

Canton

Oismueller & Partner, Inc. — 770-874-1767
1968 Sixes Rd., Canton, GA 30114

Cartersville

Sterimed, Inc. — 770-387-0771
10 River Ct., Cartersville, GA 30120

Clarkston

Life Therapeutics Inc. — 404-300-5000
780 Park North Blvd., Suite 100, Clarkston, GA 30021

Cloudland

Best Glove, Inc. — 800-241-0323
579 Edison Street, Cloudland, GA 30731

Conyers

Spinal Solutions, Inc. — 800-922-5155
1971 Old Covington Rd., Suite 103, Conyers, GA 30013

2013 MEDICAL DEVICE REGISTER

Cornelia

Ethicon, Inc. — 908-218-2996
655 Ethicon Cir., Cornelia, GA 30531

Covington

C. R. Bard, Inc., Bard Medical Div. — 800-526-4455
8195 Industrial Blvd., Covington, GA 30209
C. R. Bard, Inc., Bard Urological Div. — 800-526-4455
8195 Industrial Boulevard, Covington, GA 30014
Du-Al Corp. — 770-784-9062
1912 Hwy. 142 E., Covington, GA 30014-8830
Medical Technologies Of Georgia, Inc. — 404-394-2478
15151 Prater Drive, Covington, GA 30014

Cumming

Endure Medical, Inc. — 800-736-3873
1455 Ventura Drive, Cumming, GA 30040
Suppleyes, Inc. — 800-727-3725
4890 Hammond Industrial Drive, Suite A, Cumming, GA 30041

Dalton

Heatmax, Inc. — 800-533-7349
505 Hill Rd., Dalton, GA 30722
Patcraft Commercial — 800-241-4014
PO BOX 2128, Dalton, GA 30722-2128

Douglasville

Total Motion Restoration, Llc — 678-910-0156
9990 Devonshire St., Douglasville, GA 30135

Duluth

Barco, Inc — 678-475-8137
3059 Premiere Parkway, Duluth, GA 30097
Ciba Vision — 800-875-3001
11460 Johns Creek Parkway, Duluth, GA 30097
Ciba Vision Corporation — 800-875-3001
11460 Johns Creek Pkwy., Duluth, GA 30097
Given Imaging Inc. — 770-662-0870
3950 Shackleford Rd., Suite 500, Duluth, GA 30096-1852
Ideal Optics, Inc. — 612-520-6000
2775 Premiere Parkway, Suite 600, Duluth, GA 30097
Pioneer Medical Systems — 800-234-0683
3408 Howell Street, Suite D, Duluth, GA 30096
X-Cel Contacts — 770-622-9235
2775 Premiere Pkwy, Suite 600, Duluth, GA 30097

Fairburn

Linde Gas North America Llc — 800-262-4273
7390 Graham Fairborn Rd., Fairburn, GA 30213
Porex Corporation — 800-241-0195
500 Bohannon Rd., Fairburn, GA 30213-2828

Fayetteville

American Associated Companies, Inc. — 800-849-7060
120 Carnigie Place, Suite 202, Fayetteville, GA 30214
Grant Chiropractic, Llc — 770-719-1917
155 Bradford Square, Suite C, Fayetteville, GA 30215
International Radiographic, Inc. — 1-504-455-8311
395 Grand Teton Circle, Fayetteville, GA 30215

Flowery Branch

Quality Contract Manufacturing, Llc — 770-965-3300
4362 Thurmond Tanner Rd., Flowery Branch, GA 30542

Forsyth

Abare Ent., Inc. — 478-994-3807
44 W. Chambers St., Forsyth, GA 31029

Gainesville

Aeverl Medical, Llc — 770-983-1369
6045 Circle Of Light, Gainesville, GA 30506
Albert International, Inc. — 800-789-0729
989 Athens Street S.e., Gainesville, GA 30501
Ambit Corporation — 770-534-4150
1636 Oakbrook Industrial Dr., Gainesville, GA 30507
Elan Pharmaceutical Research Corp. — 800-859-8586
1300 Gould Drive, Gainesville, GA 30504
Harris Products Group — 800-241-0804
2345 Murphy Blvd., Gainesville, GA 30504-6001
Kiel Laboratories, Inc. — 678-450-9187
2225 Centennial Dr., Gainesville, GA 30504

Grayson

Bd Lee Laboratories — 800-732-9150
1475 Athens Hwy., Grayson, GA 30017
Lee Laboratories, Inc. — 1-800-732-9150
1475 Athens Highway, Grayson, GA 30017

Jesup

Duro-Med Industries — 800-526-4753
1788 W. Cherry St., Jesup, GA 31545

Kennesaw

Amoena — 800-726-6362
1701 Barret Lakes Blvd., Suite 410, Kennesaw, GA 30144
Bagco — 800-533-1931
1650 Airport Road Suite 104, Kennesaw, GA 30144
Bauerfeind Usa, Inc. — 800-423-3405
55 Chastain Road, Suite 112, Kennesaw, GA 30144
Beaumont Products, Inc. — 800-451-7096
1560 Big Shanty Dr., Kennesaw, GA 30144-3606
Chemlink Laboratories, Llc. — 770-499-8008
1590 N. Roberts Rd. Nw, Suite 111, Kennesaw, GA 30144
Cryolife, Inc. — 800-438-8285
1655 Roberts Blvd. NW., Kennesaw, GA 30144
Dictator U.S., Inc. — 877-366-7439
3939 Royal Drive NW Suite 214, Kennesaw, GA 30144
Dornier Medtech America — 800-367-6437
1155 Roberts Blvd., Kennesaw, GA 30144
Facet Technologies, Llc — 888-526-2387
112 Town Park Drive, Kennesaw, GA 30144
Facet Technologies, Llc — 800-526-2387
112 Townpark Dr., Ste. 300, Kennesaw, GA 30144
Fumex Inc. — 800-432-7550
1150 Cobb International Place, Suite D, Kennesaw, GA 30152
Karl Storz Lithotripsy-America, Inc. — 800-965-4846
1000 Cobb Place Blvd., Building 400, Suite 450, Kennesaw, GA 30144
Kesair Technologies, Llc — 800-236-1846
3625 Kennesaw N. Ind. Pkwy., Kennesaw, GA 30144-1234
MiMedx Group Inc. — 866-477-4219
60 Chastain Center Blvd, Suite 60, Suite B, Kennesaw, GA 30144
Microcopy, Div. Neo-Flo, Inc. — 800-235-1863
3120 Moon Station Rd., Kennesaw, GA 30144-2765
Respironics Georgia, Inc. — 724-387-4559
175 Chastain Meadows Ct., Kennesaw, GA 30144-3724

Lafayette

Flex-A-Bed, Inc. — 800-421-2277
1825 Hillsdale Rd., Lafayette, GA 30728

Lagrange

Kimberly-Clark Corp. — 888-525-8388
1300 Orchard Hill Rd., Lagrange, GA 30240
Milliken & Company, Anticon Products — 800-762-3472
201 Lukken Industrial Drive West M-836, LaGrange, GA 30240

Lawrenceville

Avon-Isi — 888-ISI-SAFE
922 Hurricane Shoals Road, Lawrenceville, GA 30043-4824
Crosstex International, Inc. — 800 743 3490
621 Hurricane Shoals Rd. Nw, Suite G, Lawrenceville, GA 30045
Diamond Dental, Inc. — 770-381-3799
3545 Cruse Rd., Suite 203, Lawrenceville, GA 30044
Inocraft, Inc. — 678-985-2926
478 Northdale Rd. Nw, Suite 706, Lawrenceville, GA 30045
Lw Scientific — 800-726-7345
865 Marathon Parkway, Lawrenceville, GA 30045
Marena Group, Inc. — 770-822-6925
650 Progress Industrial Blvd, Lawrenceville, GA 30043
National Vision, Inc. — 800-637-3597
296 Grayson Hwy., Attn: Legal/C. Mingle, Lawrenceville, GA 30045
Optec Specialties, Inc. — 770-513-7380
975 Progress Circle, Lawrenceville, GA 30043
Technical Products, Inc. — 800-226-8434
805 Marathon Parkway, Suite 150, Lawrenceville, GA 30045
Ultralite Enterprises, Inc. — 800-241-7506
390 Farmer Ct., Lawrenceville, GA 30045

Lilburn

Emerging Healthcare Solutions, LLC — 770-923-7391
1285 Denmark Dr. SW, Lilburn, GA 30047

Mableton

Safeslideboard.Com — 770-675-2978
56 Strickland Drive S.w., Mableton, GA 30126

Macon

Smisson-Cartledge Biomedical — 1-866-944-9992
487 Cherry St, Third Street Tower, Macon, GA 31201

Manchester

Angiodynamics, Inc. — 800-472-5221
One Horizon Way, Manchester, GA 31816

Marietta

Advance Medical Designs, Inc. — 800-221-3679
1241 Atlanta Industrial Drive, Marietta, GA 30066
American Breast Care Lp — 770-933-3444
2150 Newmarket Pkwy, Suite 112, Marietta, GA 30067
Andrew J. Diamond, M.D. — 770-933-8214
551 Hackney Dr., Marietta, GA 30067
Caire, Inc. — 800-482-2473
1800 Sandy Plains Industrial Parkway, Suite 316, Marietta, GA 30066
Designs For Comfort, Inc. — 800-443-9226
P.O. Box 671044, Marietta, GA 30066

Erbe Usa, Inc.
2225 Northwest Parkway, Marietta, GA 30067
800-778-3723

Htl-Strefa, Inc.
3005 Chastain Meadows Pkwy, Suite 300, Marietta, GA 30066
770-528-0410

Lantiseptic Division, Summit Industries, Inc.
P.O. Box 7329, Marietta, GA 30065-0329
800-241-6996

North American Medical Corp (Nam)
1649 Sands Pl SE, Suite A, Marietta, GA 30067
770-541-0012

North American Medical Corporation
1649 Sands Place S.e., Suite A, Marietta, GA 30067
770-541-0012

Owen Mumford Usa, Inc.
1755-A West Oak, Commons Court, Marietta, GA 30062-3165
800-421-6936

Pan-American
1480-f Terrill Mill Rd., Suite 662, Marietta, GA 30067
404-966-4230

Pedors Shoes
1349 Old 41 Hwy. #130, Marietta, GA 30060
800-750-6729

Precisa Balances Usa Inc.
540 Powder Springs St., Suite 8, Marietta, GA 30064
877-PRE-CISA

Presto Absorbent Products-Atlanta
1070 Atlanta Industrial Drive, Marietta, GA 30066
715-839-2085

Sante Feminine Limited
1649 Sands Place,, Suite C, Marietta, GA 30067
678-314-1649

Solvay Pharmaceuticals
901 Sawyer Rd., Marietta, GA 30062
800-241-1643

Martinez

The Quality Assurance Service Corp.
310 Commerce Dr., Martinez, GA 30907
706-863-6536

Mcdonough

Dowling Textiles
615 Macon Rd., Mcdonough, GA 30253
770-957-3981

Menlo

Best Manufacturing Co.
579 Edison St., PO Box 8, Menlo, GA 30731
800-241-0323

Morrow

Toto Kiki Usa, Inc.
1155 Southern Road, Morrow, GA 30260
888-295-8134

Moultrie

Be Well Usa, Inc.
3195 7th St Se, Moultrie, GA 31788
229-890-1627

Newnan

Engineering Marketing Assoc. Dba Impulse Training Systems
339 Millard Farmer Industrial Blvd, PO Box 2312, Newnan, GA 30263
800-964-2362

Porex Surgical, Inc.
15 Dart Rd., Newnan, GA 30265
800-521-7321

Norcross

Abilitations
PO BOX 922668, Norcross, GA 30010
800-850-8602

Adler Instrument Co.
6191 Atlantic Blvd., Norcross, GA 30071-1306
866-382-3537

Allied Diagnostic Imaging Resources, Inc.
5440 Oakbrook Parkway, Norcross, GA 30093-2294
800.262.9333

American Biosurgical
1850-B Beaver Ridge Circle, Norcross, GA 30071
770-416-1992

Best Vascular, Inc.
4350 International Blvd., Norcross, GA 30093
770-717-0904

Biocure, Inc.
2975 Gateway Drive, Suite 100, Norcross, GA 30071
800-246-2873

Breazeale & Associates, Inc.
2909 Langford Road, Suite 500B, Norcross, GA 30071
770-447-4418

Elekta Inc.
4775 Peachtree Industrial Blvd., Bldg. 300, Suite 300, Norcross, GA 30092
800-535-7355

Elekta, Inc.
4775 Peachtree Industrial Blvd., Building 300, Suite 300, Norcross, GA 30092
800-535-7355

Flo Healthcare
5801 Goshen Springs Road NW, Suite A, Norcross, GA 30071
877-356-4040

Guided Therapeutics Inc.
5835 Peachtree Corners East, Suite D, Norcross, GA 30092
770-242-8723

Imaging Archive International, Llc.
5966 Exeter Circle, Norcross, GA 30071
770-565-6166

Immucor, Inc.
3130 Gateway Drive, PO Box 5625, Norcross, GA 30091-5625
800-829-2553

International Brachytherapy, Inc.
6000 Live Oak Pkwy., #107, Norcross, GA 30093
770-582-0662

Ldb Medical, Inc.
2909 Langford Road, Suite 500B, Norcross, GA 30071
800-243-2554

Lifegas Llc
1500 Indian Trail Road, Norcross, GA 30093-2613
866-543-3427

Mainline Medical, Inc.
3250-J Peachtree Corners Circle, Norcross, GA 30092-4301
800-366-2084

Mazor Robotics Ltd.
4361 Shackleford Rd., Norcross, GA 30093
800-706-2967

Md Works, Inc.
1895-i Beaver Ridge Cir., Suite 410, Norcross, GA 30071
770-409-9639

Molnlycke Health Care Inc.
5550 Peachtree Parkway, Suite 500, Norcross, GA 30092
678-250-7900

National Electronic Attachment, Inc.
3577 Parkway Lane, Suite 250, Norcross, GA 30092
800-782-5150

Remel Atlanta, Div. Of Remel, Inc.
2797 Peterson Pl., Norcross, GA 30071
800-255-6730

Sebia Electrophoresis
400-1705 Corporate Drive, Norcross, GA 30093
800-835-6497

Serologicals Corp
5655 Spalding Dr, Norcross, GA 30092
678-728-2000

Sonoco-Stancap Division
3150 Clinton Ct., Norcross, GA 30071
(800) 264-7494

Southern Reid Optical Laboratory, Inc.
1856 Corporate Dr. Suite 150, Norcross, GA 30093
800-765-7343

Starkey Southeast
5300 Oakbrook Pkwy.,, Bldg. 100, Suite 130, Norcross, GA 30093
952-947-4734

Oakwood

Prizm Medical, Inc.
P. O. Box 40, Oakwood, GA 30566
770-622-0933

Prizm Medical, Inc.
P.O.Box 40, Oakwood, GA 30566
800-447-4422

Orchard Hill

Ari
2523 South Mcdonough Rd., Orchard Hill, GA 30266
770-227-8222

Peachtree City

Celonova Biosciences Inc.
401 Westpark Court, Suite 100, Peachtree City, GA 30269
1.770.632.2450

Enviropak Llc
218 claridge curve, Peachtree City, GA 30269
(800)308-8371

Hoshizaki America, Inc.
618 Hwy. 74 S., Peachtree City, GA 30269-3002
800-438-6087

Primo, Inc.
417A Dividend Dr., Peachtree City, GA 30269
770-486-7394

Sigvaris Inc.
1119 Hwy. 74 S., Peachtree City, GA 30269
800-322-7744

Powder Springs

Palmer Cap-Chur, Inc.
421 Tidwell Rd, Powder Springs, GA 30127
770-942-4395

Riverdale

Multi Focal Rx Lens Laboratories, Inc.
216 Valley Hill Rd., Riverdale, GA 30274
800-241-9030

Roswell

Global Healthcare
1495 Hembree Rd., Ste. 700, Roswell, GA 30076
800-601-3880

Kerr Group
1400 Holcomb Bridge Road, Roswell, GA 30076-2190
800-524-3577

Myelotec, Inc.
4000 Northfield Way, Suite 900, Roswell, GA 30076
770-664-4656

Ophthalmed Llc
11660 Alpharetta Hwy., Suite 205, Roswell, GA 30076
770-777-6613

Opti Medical Systems Inc.
235 Hembree Park Drive, Roswell, GA 30076
770-510-4444

Savannah

Brasseler Usa - Komet Medical
One Brassler Blvd., Savannah, GA 31419-9565
800-535-6638

E.Care Solutions, Inc.
1345 Wilmington Island Road, Savannah, GA 31410
912-897-6480

Enuresis Solutions, Llc
51 W. Fairmont Avenue, Suite 2, Savannah, GA 31406
912-353-7675

Smyrna

Salumedica, L.L.C.
4451 Atlanta Rd. Se, Suite 138, Smyrna, GA 30080
404-589-1727

Thermo Fisher Scientific
500 Technology Ct., Smyrna, GA 30082
800-241-6898

UCB Inc.
1950 Lake Park Dr., Smyrna, GA 30080
770-970-7500

Snellville

Eagle Sports Chairs
2351 Parkwood Rd., Snellville, GA 30039
800-932-9380

Stone Mountain

Atlanta International
1979 Parker Court, Suites D And E, Stone Mountain, GA 30087
800-251-9864

Suwanee

Abatement Technologies, Inc.
605 Satellite Blvd, Ste 300, Suwanee, GA 30024
800-634-9091

Acorn International Group, Inc.
923 Spring Glen Place, Suwanee, GA 30024
770-9931777

Femasys Inc.
5000 Research Court, Suite 100, Suwanee, GA 30024
770-500-3910

Kagawa Shears.Com, Llc.
3605 Swiftwater Park Dr., Suwanee, GA 30024
404-931-0258

Mycoal Products Corporation Of Usa
475 Horizon Drive, Suwanee, GA 30024
678-765-4000

Thomasville

Diabetes Technologies, Inc.   888-872-2443
184 Big Star Drive, Thomasville, GA 31757

Tucker

Arc Medical, Inc.   800-950-ARC1 (2
4296 Cowan Road, Tucker, GA 30084
CareFusion 2200, Inc.,   847-689-8410
5175 South Royal Atlanta Dr., Tucker, GA 30084-3053
Crespac Inc.   770-938-1900
5032 N. Royal Atlanta Dr., Tucker, GA 30084
Parasitic Disease Consultants   770-496-1370
2177-J Flintstone Dr., P.O. Box 616, Tucker, GA 30085

Tunnel Hill

Precision Products, Inc.   800-220-9221
681 North Varnell Rd., Tunnel Hill, GA 30755

Valdosta

Alphaprotech, Inc.   520-281-0127
323 s blanchard st, Valdosta, GA 31601

Warm Springs

Mailhawk Manufacturing Company   800-331-5070
Hwy. 85-W, 5292 White House Pkwy., Warm Springs, GA 31830-0445

Washington

Paper Pak Industries   909-392-1764
One Paper Pak Way, Washington, GA 30673

Woodstock

Erb Industries Inc.   800-800-6522
#1 Safety Way, Woodstock, GA 30188
Medstone International, Inc.   949-367-1238
229 Arnold Mill Rd., Suite 200, Woodstock, GA 30188
Post Medical, Inc.   800-876-8678
226 Creekstone Ridge, Woodstock, GA 30188
Scientific Imaging, Llc   770-926-3060
9878 Main Street, Suite 125, Woodstock, GA 30188

HAWAII

Aiea

Optical Suppliers, Inc.   808-486-2933
99-1253 Halawa Valley St., Aiea, HI 96701

Hon

Ebm Technologies Usa, Llc   1.866.212.6127
641 Keeaumoku Street Unit 5, Hon, HI 96814
Miki, Inc.   808-943-6454
1450 Ala Moana Blvd #1247, Hon, HI 96814

Honolulu

Advanced Aesthetic Solutions   1-808-941-1629
631-D Keeaumoku St., Honolulu, HI 96814
Airgas Gaspro Inc.   808-842-2282
2305 Kamehameha Hwy., Honolulu, HI 96819
C. R. Newton Co. Ltd.   800-545-2078
1575 S. Beretania St., Honolulu, HI 96826
Cloward Instrument Corporation   808-734-3511
3787 Diamond Head Road, Honolulu, HI 96816
Connect Imaging, Inc.   866-949-7227
850 West Hind Dr., Suite 116, Honolulu, HI 96821
Doss K. Tannehill - Ocularist   808-738-5300
752 17th Ave., Honolulu, HI 96816
Gospro, Inc.   808-842-2282
2305 Kamehameha Hwy., Honolulu, HI 96819
Hako-Med Usa, Inc.   888-913-7900
905-C Makahiki Way, Honolulu, HI 96826
Hearing Aid Center   808-973-1551
615 Piikoi St., Suite 1111, Honolulu, HI 96814
Nose Breathe   808-949-8876
2065 S. King St., #304, Honolulu, HI 96826

Kahului

K.O.L. Island Retainer, Llc.   808-871-8577
360 Papa Place #203, Kahului, HI 96732
Trex Enterprises Corp.   808-442 -7000
427 Ala Makani Street, Kahului, HI 96732

Kapolei

Steiner Laboratories   866-317-1348
590 Farrington Hwy., #524 Suite 132, Kapolei, HI 96707

IDAHO

Boise

B & B Lingerie Co., Inc.   1-800-262-2789
2417 Bank Dr., Suite 201, P.o. Box 5731, Boise, ID 83705
B & B Lingerie Company, Inc.   800-262-2789
2417 Bank Dr., Ste. 201, Boise, ID 83705

Directional Hearing Aid Service   208-376-9431
6876 Fairview, Boise, ID 83704
Intermountain Ocular Prosthetics, Inc.   208-378-8200
2995 North Cole Rd., Suite 115, Boise, ID 83704-5965
Kronus, Inc.   800-822-6999
12554 West Bridger St., Ste. 108, Boise, ID 83713
Mountain Precision Mfg. Ltd. Co.   208-322-1111
11000 Executive Dr., Boise, ID 83713
Norco   800-657-6672
1125 W. Amity, Boise, ID 83705

Caldwell

Fiberguide Industries, Inc.   908-647-6601
3409 East Linden St., Caldwell, ID 83605

CDA

Caring Hands, Inc.   208-691-9524
4347 N Alderbrook Dr, CDA, ID 83815

Coeur D'Alene

Advanced Input Systems   800-444-5923
600 W. Wilbur Ave., Coeur D'Alene, ID 83815
Mccarty's Sacro-Ease Llc   800-635-3557
3329 Industrial Avenue, Coeur D'Alene, ID 83815
Quicare, Ltd.   208-676-8015
P.O. Box 3667, Coeur d'Alene, ID 83816
21st Century Scientific, Inc.   800-448-3680
4931 N Manufacturing Way, Coeur D'Alene, ID 83815

Hayden

Bio. Works Corp.   208-772-5509
12611 N.Chicken Pt. Rd., Hayden, ID 83835-1388

Idaho Falls

Envision Dental Solutions   800-372-3010
2515 Channing Way, Idaho Falls, ID 83404
International Isotopes Inc.   800-699-3108
4137 Commerce Circle, Idaho Falls, ID 83401
Momentum Medical   208-523-3600
1330 Enterprise Street, Idaho Falls, ID 83402
Treasure Dental Laboratory   800-325-5244
3735 Washington Parkway, Idaho Falls, ID 83404

Ketchum

Smith Sports Optics, Inc.   208-726-4477
280 Northwood Way, P.o. Box 2999, Ketchum, ID 83340

Meridian

Mwi Veterinary Supply   800-824-3703
651 S. Stratford Drive, Suite 100, Meridian, ID 83642

Moscow

Dream Inventors Design Llc   208-882-3082
4805 Robinson Park Rd., Moscow, ID 83843

Orofino

Oxy-Sure Company, Llc   866-476-3800
13930 2nd Avenue West, Orofino, ID 83544-9410

Pocatello

Snugfleece International Inc.   800-824-1177
2740 Poleline Rd., Pocatello, ID 83201-6112

Post Falls

Wilkinson Company, Inc.   208-777-8332
590 Clearwater Loop, Suite C, Post Falls, ID 83854

Sagle

Percussionaire Corporation   208-263-2549
1655 Glengary Bay Rd., Sagle, ID 83860

Sandpoint

Lead-Lok, Inc.   208-263-5071
500 Airport Way, Sandpoint, ID 83864
Lead-Lok, Inc.   800-201-3958
814Airport Way, Sandpoint, ID 83864-9222
Pneumex, Inc.   800-447-5792
2605 North Boyer Ave., Sandpoint, ID 83864

ILLINOIS

Abbott Park

Abbott Laboratories   800-223-2064
100 Abbott Park Rd., Abbott Park, IL 60064-3500

Addison

Anchor Products Company   800-323-5134
52 Official Rd., Addison, IL 60101-4519
Brand X-Ray Co., Inc.   630-543-5331
910 Westwood Ave., Addison, IL 60101-4917
Dickson Co   800-757-3747
930 S. Westwood Avenue, Addison, IL 60101
Elmed, Inc.   630-543-2792
60 W. Fay Avenue, Addison, IL 60101-5106

Medtec Applications, Inc.   630-628-0444
50 West Fay Ave., Addison, IL 60101
Nilan Tool & Mold Corp.   630-543-7114
1215 National Ave., Addison, IL 60101-3180
Sprayway, Inc.   800-332-9000
484 Vista Avenue, Addison, IL 60101-4468
Ufp Technologies, Inc.   630-543-2855
1235 National Avenue, Addison, IL 60101-3179

Algonquin

Schiffmayer Plastics Corporation   800-621-1092
1201 Armstrong St., Algonquin, IL 60102-3599
Sci-Dent, Inc.   800-323-4145
210 Dowdle St. #2, Algonquin, IL 60102
Y.I. Ventures, Llc   314-344-0010
2260 Wendt Street, Algonquin, IL 60102

Alsip

Gc America, Inc.   800-323-7063
3737 West 127th St., Alsip, IL 60803
Reliance Dental Mfg., Co.   708-597-6694
5805 West 117th Place, Alsip, IL 60803

Alton

Progroup Instrument Corp.   800-471-1916
4947 Fosterburg Road, Alton, IL 62002
Telsar Laboratories, Inc.   800-255-9938
319 Ridge Street, Alton, IL 62002

Antioch

Bencher, Inc.   847-838-3195
241 Depot St., Antioch, IL 60002
Great Midwest Packaging, Llc   800-788-9873
712 Anita Ave., Antioch, IL 60002-1857
Med-Con, Inc.   800-366-1366
PO Box 244, Antioch, IL 60002

Arlington Heights

Dana Molded Products, Inc.   847-255-2000
6 N. Hickory Avenue, Arlington Heights, IL 60004
Mason Chemical   800-362-1855
721 W. Algonquin Rd., Arlington Heights, IL 60005
Medi-Physics, Inc., Dba Ge Healthcare   800-633-4123
3350 N Ridge Ave., Arlington Heights, IL 60004
Medx Incorporated   800-323-6339
3456 N. Ridge Ave. #100, Arlington Heights, IL 60004
Medx, Inc.   847-463-2020
3456 North Ridge Ave., #100, Arlington Heights, IL 60004
Tanita Corporation Of America, Inc.   877-682-6482
2625 S. Clearbrook Drive, Arlington Heights, IL 60005
Tegrant Corporation, Thermosafe Brands   1 800 323 7442
3930 Ventura Drive Suite 450, Arlington Heights, IL 60084
Telesto Medtech Llc   831-621-8011
635 E. Rockwell St., Arlington Heights, IL 60005
Thermosafe Brands   847-398-0110
3930 Ventura Drive, Suite 450, Arlington Heights, IL 60004
Vibgyor Optical Systems   800-842-4967
1140 N. Phelps, Arlington Heights, IL 60004
Woodlyn, Inc.   800-331-7389
Ophthalmic Instruments and Equipment, 2920 Malmo Drive, Arlington Heights, IL 60005-4726

Aslip

G-C America Inc.   800-323-7063
3737 W. 127th St., Aslip, IL 60803
Gc America, Inc.   800-323-3386
3737 W. 127th St., Aslip, IL 60803

Aurora

Amtab Manufacturing Co.   800-878-2257
652 N. Highland Ave, Aurora, IL 60622-6050
Apex Engineering Products Corp.   800-451-6291
1241 Shoreline Drive, Aurora, IL 60504
Connor-Winfield Corp.   630-851-4722
2111 Comprehensive Dr., Aurora, IL 60505-1345
Control Solutions, Inc.   630-806-7062
2520 Diehl Road, Aurora, IL 60502
Dunlee   800-238-3780
555 North Commerce St., Aurora, IL 60504
Midwest X-Ray Equipment Co.   630-892-2414
701 West Illinois Ave., Aurora, IL 60506
Richards-Wilcox, Inc.   800-253-5668
600 S. Lake St., Aurora, IL 60506

Bannockburn

Ge Capital   800-323-6217
3000 Lakeside Drive, Suite 200N, Bannockburn, IL 60015-1223
Leica Microsystems Inc.   800-248-0123
2345 Waukegan Road, Bannockburn, IL 60015

Barrington

Ge Healthcare It   847-277-5000
540 W Northwest Highway, Barrington, IL 60010

Snow Products, Inc.   847-381-5222
27w996 Industrial Ave. #6, Barrington, IL 60010

Bartlett

U-Ten Corporation   630-289-8058
1286 Humbracht Cir, Bartlett, IL 60103-2051

Batavia

Brasel Products, Inc.   630-879-3759
715 Hunter Dr., Batavia, IL 60510-1425
Cae Services Corp.   630-761-9898
280 Belleview Lane, Batavia, IL 60510
Team Technologies Molding   630-937-0380
1300 Nagel Blvd., Batavia, IL 60510

Belleville

American Spine Center Ltd., Clini-Lase   618-233-6824
100 Mascoutah Avenue, Belleville, IL 62220
Roho Group, The   800-851-3449
100 N. Florida Avenue, Belleville, IL 62221-5429

Bensenville

Action Bag Co.   800-490-8830
1001 Entry Dr., Bensenville, IL 60106
American Dental Products, Inc.   800-846-7120
603-b Country Club Dr., Bensenville, IL 60106-1329
Indo Lens Us, Inc.   800-729-1959
224 W. James St, Bensenville, IL 60106
Philips Avent   800-542-8368
475 Supreme Dr., Bensenville, IL 60106-1161
Protectoseal Co.   800-323-2268
225 W. Foster Avenue, Bensenville, IL 60106-1631
Singer Medical Products, Inc.   800-222-2572
790 Maple Lane, Bensenville, IL 60106-1513

Berkeley

World Dryer Corp.   800-323-0701
5700 McDermott Drive, Berkeley, IL 60163

Bolingbrook

Patterson Medical Holdings, Inc.   800-323-5547
1000 Remington Blvd., Suite 210, Bolingbrook, IL 60440-4995

Bridgeview

Pelstar Llc (Health O Meter Professional)   800-815-6615
7400 West 100th Place, Bridgeview, IL 60455
Trans American Medical   800-626-9232
7633 W. 100th Pl., Bridgeview, IL 60455
Trans American Medical / Tamsco Instruments   708-430-7777
7633 W. 100th Pl, Bridgeview, IL 60455-2433

Broadview

Alphatek   708-345-0500
2600 S. 25th Ave., Broadview, IL 60155
Stericon, Inc.   708-865-8790
2315 Gardner Road, Broadview, IL 60153

Buffalo Grove

Akorn, Inc.   800-535-7155
2500 Millbrook Drive, Buffalo Grove, IL 60089
E.S.W.L. Products, Inc.   847-419-6844
1542 Barclay Blvd., Buffalo Grove, IL 60089
Endoplus Inc.   800-236-5972
431 Lexington Drive, Suite A, Buffalo Grove, IL 60089
Endoplus, Inc.   847-325-5660
431 Lexington Drive, Suite A, Buffalo Grove, IL 60089
Epix, Inc.   847-465-1818
381 Lexington Drive, Buffalo Grove, IL 60089-6934
Healthcare-Id, Inc.   847-465-9935
1635 Barclay Blvd., Buffalo Grove, IL 60089
Livingston Products, Inc.   800-822-2156
1377 Barclay Blvd., Buffalo Grove, IL 60089
Plastic Endo, Llc   866-752-3636
318 Half Day Rd., #247, Buffalo Grove, IL 60089
Plexus Electronic Assembly   847 793 4400
2400 Millbrook Dr., Buffalo Grove, IL 60089
Primesource Healthcare, Inc.   800-317-0711
2100 East Lake Cook Road, Suite 1100, Buffalo Grove, IL 60089
Progeny Dental   888-924-3800
1407 Barclay Blvd, Buffalo Grove, IL 60089
Siemens Medical Solutions Usa, Inc   888-826-9702
2500 Millbrook Dr., Suite B, Buffalo Grove, IL 60089
Tyson Consulting Group   847-459-9189
612 White Pine Rd., Buffalo Grove, IL 60089-3330
Virotek, L.L.C.   847-634-4500
900 Asbury Dr., Buffalo Grove, IL 60089
Yan Razdolsky Ltd   847-215-7554
600 W. Lake Cook Rd., Suite 150, Buffalo Grove, IL 60089

Burr Ridge

Ferris Mfg. Corp.   800-765-9636
16 W300 83rd St., Burr Ridge, IL 60527-5848
Mylin Medical Systems, Inc.   630-321-1450
11904 Heritage Drive, Burr Ridge, IL 60527-7123

Timemed Labeling Systems, Inc. — 800-323-4840
144 Tower Drive, Burr Ridge, IL 60527

Carol Stream

A.J. Antunes & Co. — 800-253-2991
180 Kehoe Blvd., Carol Stream, IL 60188
Bard Brachytherapy, Inc — 908-277-8000
295 E. Lies Rd., Carol Stream, IL 60188
Shepard Medical Products — 800-354-5683
260 E Lies Road, Carol Stream, IL 60188-9418
Wheaton Brace Co. — 800-227-6769
336 E. Gundersen Dr., #100, Carol Stream, IL 60188-2422

Cary

Revere Healthcare Ltd. — 800-826-4900
10 Spring St., Cary, IL 60013
Sage Products, Inc. — 800-323-2220
3909 Three Oaks Road, Cary, IL 60013
X-Ray Imaging Solutions Inc. — 847-878-0867
641 Industrial Dr. Unit D, Cary, IL 60013

Cerro Gordo

Nova Companies — 217-763-4041
209 E South St., Po Box 139, Cerro Gordo, IL 61818

Champaign

Labthermics Technologies — 217-351-7722
701 Devonshire Dr., Champaign, IL 61820-7328
Mimosa Acoustics, Inc. — 217-367-9740
60 Hazelwood Dr., Suite #209, Champaign, IL 61820

Chatham

Medworks Instruments — 800-323-9790
PO Box 581, Chatham, IL 62629
Micromedical Technologies, Inc. — 800-334-4154
10 Kemp Drive, Chatham, IL 62629

Chestnut Street

Roth Drug Co. — 312-733-1478
669 West Ohio St., --, Chestnut Street, IL 60610

Chicago

Ace Hose & Rubber Company — 888-223-4673
1333 South Jefferson St., Chicago, IL 60607-4904
Addto, Inc. — 773-278-0294
816 N. Kostner Ave., Chicago, IL 60651-3423
Allscripts-Misys Healthcare Solutions — 919-847-8102
222 Merchandise Mart Plaza, Suite 2024, Chicago, IL 60654
Americomp, Inc. — 800-458-1782
2901 W. Lawrence Avenue, Chicago, IL 60625
Amrad — 888-772-6723
2901 W. Lawrence Avenue, Chicago, IL 60625
Bean Products — 800-726-8365
1500 S. Western Avenue, Suite 4BN, Chicago, IL 60608
Cameron-Miller, Inc. — 800-621-0142
5410 West Roosevelt, Road #241, Chicago, IL 60644
Carematix Inc. — 312-371-3050
120 S. Riverside Plaza, Suite 2100, Chicago, IL 60606
Cosmedent, Inc. — 800-621-6729
401 N. Michigan Ste. 2500, Chicago, IL 60611
Cytocore, Inc. — 312-379-4790
414 North Orlean, Suite 510, Chicago, IL 60654
Darex Container Products — 617-498-4357
6050 West 51st St., Chicago, IL 60638
Female Health Company, The — 800-884-1601
515 N. State, Suite 2250, Suite 2225, Chicago, IL 60655
GE Healthcare — 877-446-3743
200 E. Randolph Street, Suite 2435, Chicago, IL 60601
Gema, Inc. — 773-878-2445
2434 W. Peterson Ave., Chicago, IL 60659
Graymills Corp. — 800-478-8673
3705 N. Lincoln Avenue, Chicago, IL 60613-3517
Holabird & Root Llc — 312-357-1771
140 South Dearborn Street, Chicago, IL 60603
Howard Medical Company — 800-443-1444
1690 N. Elston, Chicago, IL 60622-1530
Hu-Friedy Manufacturing Co., Inc. — 800-483-7433
3232 N. Rockwell, Chicago, IL 60618-5982
I.F. Optical, Inc. — 773-761-3323
2812 West Touhy Ave., Chicago, IL 60645
Iit Research Institute — 312.567.4924
10 W. 35th St., Chicago, IL 60616-3799
Janler Corporation — 773-774-0166
6545 N. Avondale Avenue, Chicago, IL 60631
Jero Medical Equipment & Supplies, Inc. — 800-457-0644
1701 W. 13th St., Chicago, IL 60608-1207
Jeron Electronic Systems, Inc. — 800-621-1903
1743-55 W. Rosehill Dr., Chicago, IL 60660-3921
Key / Sun Medical Services, Inc. — 847-546-4795
5483 North Northwest Hwy., Chicago, IL 60630-1133
Kreg Medical, Inc. — 312-275-7002
2240 W. Walnut St., Chicago, IL 60612
Lambrecht, Karl Corp. — 773-472-5442
4204 N. Lincoln Ave., Chicago, IL 60618-2902

Lsl Industries, Inc. — 888-225-5575
5535 N. Wolcott Avenue, Chicago, IL 60640
Milex Products, Inc. — 800-621-1278
4311 N. Normandy, Chicago, IL 60634-1403
Motloid Company — 800-662-5021
300 N. Elizabeth St., Chicago, IL 60607
Neurowave Medical Technologies — 312-334-2505
200 East Randolph Suite, Suite 2200, Chicago, IL 60601
Nevin Laboratories, Inc — 800-544-5337
5000 S. Halsted Street, Chicago, IL 60609-5130
Petra Manufacturing Co. — 800-888-7387
6600 W. Armitage Ave., Chicago, IL 60707
Platt Luggage, Inc. — 800-222-1555
4051 W. 51st St., Chicago, IL 60632
Poersch Metal Mfg. Co. — 773-722-0890
4027 West Kinzie St., Chicago, IL 60624-1807
Portionpac Chemical Corp. — 312-226-0400
400 N. Ashland Ave., Chicago, IL 60622
Prime Dental Manufacturing, Inc. — 773-539-5927
3735 West Belmont Avenue, Chicago, IL 60618
Simplomatic Manufacturing Co. — 773-342-7757
816 N. Kostner Ave., Chicago, IL 60651-3423
Stereo Optical Co., Inc. — 800-344-9500
8623 W. Bryn Mawr Ave.,, Suite 502, Chicago, IL 60631
Summit Industries, Inc. — 800-729-9729
2901 W. Lawrence Avenue, Chicago, IL 60625-3621
Sunstar Butler — 800-J BUTLER
4635 W. Foster Ave., Chicago, IL 60630-1709
Talk-A-Phone Co. — 773-539-1100
5013 N. Kedzie Avenue, Chicago, IL 60625-4988
The Female Health Co. — 312-595-9123
515 N. State, St. #2225, Chicago, IL 60611
Tornado Industries — 800-822-8867
7401 W. Lawrence Ave., Chicago, IL 60706
U.V. Process Supply, Inc. — 800-621-1296
1229 W. Cortland, Chicago, IL 60614-4805
Vassol, Inc. — 312-601-4431
833 West Jackson Blvd., 8th Floor, Chicago, IL 60607
Wilson Sporting Goods Co. — 773-714-6400
8750 W. Bryn Mawr Avenue, Chicago, IL 60631
Xttrium Laboratories, Inc. — 800-587-3721
415 W. Pershing Road, Chicago, IL 60609-2727
Yates & Bird And Motloid — 800-662-5021
300 N. Elizabeth St., Chicago, IL 60607

Columbia

Dacor Manufacturing Co., Inc. — 618-939-8700
8718 Hanover Industrial Dr., Columbia, IL 62236

Countryside

Nyco Products Co. — 800-752-4754
5332 Dansher Rd., Countryside, IL 60525

Countryside Lake

Isurgical — 847-949-9744
26625 Countryside Lake Drive, Countryside Lake, IL 60060

Crestwood

Gkr Industries, Inc. — 800-526-7879
13653 Kenton Ave., Crestwood, IL 60445
Performance Water Systems, Llc — 708-396-0136
13601 S. Kenton Avenue, Crestwood, IL 60445

Crystal Lake

Covidien Lp, Formerly Registered As Kendall — 800-962-9888
815 Tek Dr., Crystal Lake, IL 60039
Creative Bedding Technologies, Inc. — 815-444-9088
300 Exchange Dr., Unit A, Crystal Lake, IL 60014
Reina Imaging — 800-752-4918
6107 West Lou Ave., Crystal Lake, IL 60014
Siltron Emergency Systems — 800-874-3392
290 E. Prairie, Crystal Lake, IL 60014
X-Cel X-Ray Corporation — 800-441-2470
4220 Waller Dr., Crystal Lake, IL 60012-2848

Danville

KIK Custom Products — 800-479-6603
1 West Hegeler Lane, Danville, IL 61832-8398

Darien

Eprogen, Inc. — 800-556-4272
8205 S. Cass Avenue, Suite 106, Darien, IL 60561-5319
Smart Medical Technology, Inc — 630-964-1689
8404 S. Wilmette Ave, Suite B, Darien, IL 60561

Decatur

Lincoln Diagnostics, Inc. — 800-537-1336
PO Box 1128, Decatur, IL 62525-1139
Wright Products, Inc. — 800-356-6911
1909 S. Taylorville Road, Suite 100, Decatur, IL 62525-0051

Deerfield

Astellas Pharma Us, Inc. — 800-888-7704
3 Parkway N., Deerfield, IL 60015-2548

Baxter Healthcare Corporation — 800-422-9837
One Baxter Parkway, Deerfield, IL 60015
Baxter Healthcare Corporation Nutrition — 888-229-0001
One Baxter Pkwy., Deerfield, IL 60015
Baxter Healthcare Corporation, Global Drug Delivery — 888-229-0001
One Baxter Parkway, Deerfield, IL 60015-4625
Baxter International Inc — 800-422-9837
One Baxter Parkway, Deerfield, IL 60015
Evolution Medical Products, Inc. — 877-223-3999
74 Eastwood Drive, Deerfield, IL 60015

DeKalb

3m Midwest Distribution Center — 815-756-5087
3050 Corporate Dr, DeKalb, IL 60115-9299

Des Plaines

Abbott Molecular, Inc. — 847-937-6100
1300 E. Touhy Ave., Des Plaines, IL 60018
Addition Technology, Inc. — 847-297-8419
950 Lee St., Ste. 210, Des Plaines, IL 60016
Bradrock Industries, Inc. — 847-299-8151
75 E. Bradrock Drive, Des Plaines, IL 60018
Ciba Vision Corporation — 1 847-321-7002
333 East Howard Avenue, Des Plaines, IL 60018
Dentsply Professional — 800-800-2888
901 West Oakton St., Des Plaines, IL 60018
June R.R. Nichols, Ocularist Ltd. — 847-803-5050
1767 E. Oakton Street, Des Plaines, IL 60018
Justrite Manufacturing Co., L.L.C. — 800-798-9250
2454 Dempster Street, Des Plaines, IL 60016-5315
Kavo Dental Manufacturing Inc — 202-828-0850
901 West Oakton St., Des Plaines, IL 60018-1884
Plitek, L.L.C — 800-966-1250
69 Rawls Road, Des Plaines, IL 60018
Scientific Device Laboratory Inc. — 847-803-9495
411 E. Jarvis Ave., Des Plaines, IL 60018

Downers Grove

Advanced Instrument Development, Inc. — 800-243-9729
2545 Curtiss Street, Downers Grove, IL 60515
Amkus Rescue Systems — 800-59-AMKUS
2700 Wisconsin Ave, Downers Grove, IL 60515
Close Call Corp. — 630-663-0189
4617 Cumnor Rd., Downers Grove, IL 60515
Dean B. Scott, Ocularist — 847-965-4455
1319 Butterfield Rd.,, Suite 524, Downers Grove, IL 60515
Invoke Imaging — 630-271-8111
1250 Palmer St., Downers Grove, IL 60516
Medstrat, Inc. — 800-882-4224
1901 Butterfield Rd., Suite 600, Downers Grove, IL 60515
Microguide, Inc. — 630-964-3368
1635 Plum Ct., Downers Grove, IL 60515-1325
Perkinelmer Life And Analytical Sciences — 800-323-5891
2200 Warrenville Rd., Downers Grove, IL 60515
Vysis — 800-553-7042
3100 Woodcreek Drive, Downers Grove, IL 60515

East Moline

Advanced Battery Systems, Inc. — 800-227-7090
1300 19th St., Suite 170, East Moline, IL 61244

Edwardsville

American Medical Software — 800-423-8836
Post Office Box 236, Edwardsville, IL 62025-0236

Effingham

Bonutti Research, Inc. — 217-342-3412
2600 South Raney, Effingham, IL 62401
Ludwig Medical, Inc. — 217-342-6570
1010 Parkview St., P.o. Box 207, Effingham, IL 62401
Patterson Technology Center, Inc — 800-475-5036
2202 Althoff Drive, Effingham, IL 62401-1267

Elgin

Clinical Computer Systems, Inc. — 847-622-0847
715 Tollgate Rd., Elgin, IL 60123
Dentsply Rinn — 800-323-0970
1212 Abbot Drive, Elgin, IL 60123
Dsm Desotech Inc. — (800) 222-7189
1122 St. Charles St., Elgin, IL 60120
Esb Enterprises, Llc — 847-429-9990
1490 Crispin Dr., Elgin, IL 60123
Good-Lite Co. — 800-362-3860
1155 Jansen Farm Drive, Elgin, IL 60123
Northgate Technologies Inc. — 800-348-0424
1591 Scottsdale Ct., Elgin, IL 60123
U.S. Table, Inc. — 847-741-3650
158 North Edison Ave., Elgin, IL 60123
Weiler Engineering, Inc. — 847-697-4900
1395 Gateway Drive, Elgin, IL 60123
Williams Healthcare Systems, Llc. — 800-441-4967
158 North Edison Ave., Elgin, IL 60123

elk grove village

Airgas-North Central, Inc. — 630-231-9260
1601 nicholas blvd., elk grove village, IL 60007
Biosynergy, Inc. — 800-255-5274
1940 E. Devon Ave., Elk Grove Village, IL 60007
Ctp Coil Inc. — 800-933-2645
1801-D Howard Street, Elk Grove Village, IL 60007
Etymotic Research, Inc. — 888-389-6684
61 Martin Lane, Elk Grove Village, IL 60007
Ims, Inc. — 847-956-1940
600 Bonnie Ln., Elk Grove Village, IL 60007
Mie America, Inc. — 847-981-6100
420 Bennett Rd., Elk Grove Village, IL 60007
Modern Aids, Inc. — 847-437-8600
201 Bond St., Elk Grove Village, IL 60007
Modern Aids, Inc. — 800-437-1063
201 Bond St., Elk Grove Village, IL 60007-1220
Nordent Manufacturing, Inc. — 800-966-7336
610 Bonnie Lane, Elk Grove Village, IL 60007-2304
Permatron Corp. — 800-882-8012
1180 Pratt Avenue, Elk Grove Village, IL 60007
Varimed — 800-426-5496
1121 Pagni Dr., Elk Grove Village, IL 60007-6602
Vision Assessment Corp. — 847-239-5889
2675 Coyle Ave., Elk Grove Village, IL 60007
Zenex Corporation — 847-390-0700
850 Elmhurst Rd., Elk Grove Village, IL 60007-2612

Elmhurst

American Diagnostic Medicine, Inc. — 800-262-9645
960 Industrial Drive, Suite 7, Elmhurst, IL 60126
Duo-Dent Dental Implant Systems Llc. — 800-386-3368
340 Butterfield Road, Suite 2A, Elmhurst, IL 60126

Energy

Sun Glitz Corp. — 800-287-0911
111 S. McVicker Drive, Energy, IL 62933

Evanston

Dm Systems, Inc. — 800-254-5438
1316 Sherman Avenue, Evanston, IL 60201

Frankfort

Fuller Ultraviolet Corp. — 815-469-3301
9416 Gulfstream Road, Frankfort, IL 60423-2521
Midwest Laser Products — 815-462-9500
PO Box 262, Frankfort, IL 60423
Paratech, Inc. — 800-435-9358
PO BOX 1000, Frankfort, IL 60423-7748
Richardson Products, Inc. — 888-928-7297
9408 Gulfstream Road, Frankfort, IL 60423

Franklin Park

Advanced Dermal Systems Llc — 847-451-0145
9109 Medill, Franklin Park, IL 60131
Alkco Lighting Co. — 847-451-0700
11500 W. Melrose Avenue, Franklin Park, IL 60131-8139
Dana Products, Inc. — 847-455-2881
11457 Melrose St., Franklin Park, IL 60131
Frain Industries, Inc. — 630-629-9900
9377 Grand Ave., Franklin Park, IL 60131
Indilab, Inc. — 800-441-5000
10367 Franklin Avenue, Franklin Park, IL 60131
Life Fitness — 800-735-3867
10601 W. Belmont Avenue, Franklin Park, IL 60131
Opticote Inc. — 847-678-8900
10455 Seymour Ave., Franklin Park, IL 60131
Sloan Valve Co. — 800-9VA-LVE9
10500 Seymour Ave., Franklin Park, IL 60131-1259
Transilwrap Co., Inc. — 800-972-8858
9201 W. Belmont Avenue, Franklin Park, IL 60131

Freeburg

Exchange Cart Accessories — 800-823-1490
1 Commerce Drive, Freeburg, IL 62243
Star Cushion Products, Inc. — 618-539-7070
5 Commerce Dr., Freeburg, IL 62243

Galena

M D Technologies, Inc. — 800-201-3060
PO BOX 60, Galena, IL 61036

Geneseo

Tyco Valves and Controls — 309-946-5205
121 W 1st Street, Suite 200, Geneseo, IL 61254

Geneva

Fischer Industries, Inc. — 630-232-2803
2630 Kaneville Court, Geneva, IL 60134
Geneva Medical Inc. — 630-232-2507
2571 Kaneville Court, Geneva, IL 60134
Kesner C.R. — 630-232-4945
2520 Kaneville Ct., Geneva, IL 60134-2506

Riverbank Laboratories   630-232-2207
2613 kaneville ct., PO Box 110, Geneva, IL 60134
Taut, Inc.   800-231-8288
2571 Kaneville Ct., Geneva, IL 60134

Glen Ellyn
M&R Printing Equipment, Inc.   630-858-6101
1 N 372 Main Street, Glen Ellyn, IL 60137

Glendale Heights
Ahpc Holdings Inc.   630-407-0242
80 Internationale Boulevard, Unit A, Glendale Heights, IL 60139
American Health Products Corporation   800-828-2964
80 Internationale Blvd, Unit A, Glendale Heights, IL 60139
Bisco, Inc.   630-523-7400
520 Windy Point Drive, Glendale Heights, IL 60193
Imi Cornelius, Inc.   800-551-4423
500 Regency Drive, Glendale Heights, IL 60139-6850
Medefil, Inc.   630-682-4600
250 Windy Point Drive, Glendale Heights, IL 60139

Glenview
Beltone Electronics Corp.   800-235-8663
2601 Patriot Blvd., Glenview, IL 60026
LCR Hallcrest   800-527-1419
1911 Pickwick Lane, Glenview, IL 60026-1307
Tr Group, Inc.   800-752-6900
903 Wedel Lane, Glenview, IL 60025

Glenwood
Landauer, Inc.   800-323-8830
2 Science Road, Glenwood, IL 60425-1586

Grayslake
Accumedix, Inc.   847-548-8499
888 E. Belvidere Rd. Suite 212, Grayslake, IL 60030
Blue Sky Bio, Llc   888-446-6724
888 E Belvidere Rd., Suite 212, Grayslake, IL 60030
Medevices, Inc.   847-548-8499
888 E. Belvidere Rd., Suite 212, Grayslake, IL 60030

Green Oaks
Somatics, Llc   847-234-6761
910 Sherwood Drive , #23, Green Oaks, IL 60044

Gurnee
Ohio Medical Corp.   800-662-5822
1111 Lakeside Dr., Gurnee, IL 60031-4099
Weiman Healthcare Solutions   800-837-8140
755 Tri-State Parkway, Gurnee, IL 60031-2400

Hanover Park
Fujifilm Manufacturing Usa, Inc.   203-602-3664
850 Central Ave, Hanover Park, IL 60133

Harrisburg
Southern Illinois X-Ray Markers   618-253-7375
513 East Locust, Harrisburg, IL 62946

Harvey
Oshkosh Specialty Vehicles   800-596-aksv
16745 S. Lathrop Avenue, Harvey, IL 60426

Harwood Heights
Quality Control Corp.   708-887-5400
7315 W. Wilson Ave., Harwood Heights, IL 60706

Hebron
Filtertek Inc.   800-248-2461
11411 Price Rd., Hebron, IL 60034

Hecker
Total Titanium   618-473-2429
140 E. Monroe St., Hecker, IL 62248
Total Titanium, Inc.   618-473-2429
140 East Monroe St., Hecker, IL 62248

Highwood
Superscrew-Superspring Co.   800-494-7594
135 Stables Way, Highwood, IL 60040

Hillside
Better Containers Mfg. Co., Inc.   800-831-6049
530 Hyde Park, Hillside, IL 60162

Hines
Edward Hines Va Hospital   708-786-5905
5th Ave & Roosevelt Rd., Hines, IL 60141

Hinsdale
Aramark Clean Room Services   800-759-0102
7650 Grant St., Hinsdale, IL 60521
Bio-Life, L.L.C.   800-851-8745
2000 Spring Rd., Suite 600, Hinsdale, IL 60523

Hoffman Est
Gn Otometrics North America   800-289-2150
125 Commerce Dr., Hoffman Est, IL 60173

Hoffman Estates
Himmelstein & Co., S.   800-632-7873
2490 Pembroke Ave., Hoffman Estates, IL 60169-2011
Home Access Health Corp.   800-HIV-TEST
2401 W. Hassell Rd.,, Ste. 1510, Hoffman Estates, IL 60169
Life Spine Inc.   847-884-6117
2401 W. Hassell Road, Suite 1535, Hoffman Estates, IL 60169
Siemens Medical Solutions Usa, Inc.   847-304-7700
2501 North Barrington Road, Hoffman Estates, IL 60192
Siemens Medical Systems, Inc., Nuclear Med. Group   847-304-7700
2501 N. Barrington Road, Hoffman Estates, IL 60195

Huntley
H.S. Crocker   847-669-3600
12100 Smith Dr., Huntley, IL 60142
Lixi, Inc.   847-961-6666
11980 Oak Creek Parkway, Huntley, IL 60142

Itasca
Global Endoscopy, Inc.   888-434-3398
1507 Industrial Drive, Itasca, IL 60193-4426
Magnetic Radiation Laboratories   888-251-5942
690 Hilltop Dr., Itasca, IL 60143
Organ Recovery Systems, Inc.   847-824-2600
1 Pierce Place, Ste 475w, Itasca, IL 60143
Tabbies, Div. Of Xertrex International, Inc.   800-822-2437
1530 W. Glenlake Ave., Itasca, IL 60143-1171

Joliet
E K Industries, Inc.   877-EKI-CHEM
1403 Herklmer St, Joliet, IL 60432-1059
Robot Coupe Usa, Inc., Scientific-Industrial Div.   815-722-8400
1101 Buell Avenue, Joliet, IL 60435
Uic, Inc.   815-744-4477
1225 Channahon Rd., Joliet, IL 60436

Lake Barrington
Cortek Endoscopy, Inc.   847-526-2266
260 Jamie Lane, Unit D, Lake Barrington, IL 60084

Lake Bluff
Galloway Plastics, Inc.   847-615-8900
940 North Shore Dr., Lake Bluff, IL 60044
The Newman Group, Llc   847-283-9177
42 Sherwood Terrace, Suite 2, Lake Bluff, IL 60044

Lake Forest
Eriem Surgical   800-833-3380
28438 Ballard Dr., Lake Forest, IL 60045
Gammadirect Medical Division   847-267-5929
PO Box 383, Lake Forest, IL 60045
Hospira Inc.   877-946-7747
275 N. Field Drive, Lake forest, IL 60045
Micrins Surgical Instruments, Inc.   800-833-3380
28438 Ballard Drive, Lake Forest, IL 60045
Omron Healthcare, Inc.   847-680-6200
1925 W. Field Court, Lake Forest, IL 60045
Pactiv Corporation   888-828-2850
1900 W. Field Court, Lake Forest, IL 60045
Salton, Inc.   202-408-9213
1955 Field Court, Lake Forest, IL 60045
Stericycle   847-367-5910
28161 N. Keith Dr., Lake Forest, IL 60045

Lake In The Hills
Stethocap, Inc.   866-691-4181
1520 Industrial Dr, Unit F, Lake In The Hills, IL 60156

LAKE VILLA
Assisted Access-Nfss, Inc.   800-950-9655
822 PRESTON COURT, LAKE VILLA, IL 60046-0230
Lidco Ltd. Usa   877-543-2611
500 Park Avenue, Suite 103, Lake Villa, IL 60046
Vonco Products, Inc.   800-323-9077
201 Park Avenue, Lake Villa, IL 60046-8916

Lake Zurich
Astron Dental Corporation   800-323-4144
815 Oakwood Rd. Unit G, Lake Zurich, IL 60047
Fenwal Inc.   800-766-1077
Three Corporate Drive, Lake Zurich, IL 60073
Kavo Dental Corp.   800-323-8029
340 East Route 22, Lake Zurich, IL 60047
Laytech, Inc.   1.847.254.9295
1771 RFD, Lake Zurich, IL 60047-7317

Libertyville
Citow Cervical Visualizer Company   877-272-4869
712 South Milwaukee Avenue, Libertyville, IL 60048

Handi-Ramp — 800-876-7267
510 North Avenue, Libertyville, IL 60048

Hollister Incorporated — 888-740-8999
2000 Hollister Dr., Libertyville, IL 60048-3746

Hollister, Inc. — 1-888-740-8999.
2000 Hollister Drive, Libertyville, IL 60048

Home Stretch Products, Inc. — 847-816-1852
536 W. Mckinley Ave., Libertyville, IL 60048

Ironwood Industries, Inc. — 847-362-8681
115 S. Bradley Road, Libertyville, IL 60048-9509

Oneac Corporation — 800-327-8801
27944 N. Bradley Road, Libertyville, IL 60048-9700

Lincolnshire

Armstrong Medical Industries, Inc. — 800-323-4220
575 Knightsbridge Pkwy., Lincolnshire, IL 60069-3616

Digi-Trax Corp. — 847-613-2100
650 Heathrow Drive, Lincolnshire, IL 60069

Faxitron X-Ray, Llc — 888-465-9729
575 Bond Street, Lincolnshire, IL 60069

Lg Electronics U.S.A., Inc. — 800-884-1742
2000 Millbrook Drive, Lincolnshire, IL 60069

Mat Automotive — 847-821-9630
625 Barclay Boulevard, Lincolnshire, IL 60069

Progeny, Inc. — 847-415-9800
675 Heathrow Dr., Lincolnshire, IL 60069

Lisle

Altman Mfg. Co., Inc. — 630-963-0031
1990 Ohio St., Lisle, IL 60532

Freund Container — 800-363-9822
Corporate Center II, 4200 Commerce Court Suite 206, Lisle, IL 60532

G.T. Laboratories, Inc. — 847-998-4776
Central Park Of Lisle Center, 3333 Warrenville Rd.,suite 200, Lisle, IL 60532

Molex — 800-786-6539
2222 Wellington Ct., Lisle, IL 60532

Trace Medical Equipment, Inc. — 800-323-3786
5000 Varsity Drive, Lisle, IL 60532

Wallace Computer Services, Inc — 800-782-4892
2275 Cabot Drive, Lisle, IL 60532

Lockport

Kinetic Systems Co., Llc — 800-DATA-NOW
900 N. State St., Lockport, IL 60441

Lombard

Elginex Corporation — 800-279-3762
270 N. Eisenhower Lane, Unit 4-A, Lombard, IL 60148-5420

Liftseat Corporation — 630-424-2840
158 Eisenhower Lane South, Lombard, IL 60148

Medgyn Products, Inc. — 800-451-9667
328 N. Eisenhower Lane, Lombard, IL 60148

Protectair Inc. — 800-235-7932
59 Eisenhower Ln., Lombard, IL 60148

Theratest Laboratories, Inc. — 800-441-0771
1111 N. Main St., Lombard, IL 60148

Wehmer Corporation — 800-323-0229
1151 N. Main Street, Lombard, IL 60148

Loves Park

Serola Biomechanics, Inc. — 815-636-2780
5281 Zenith Parkway, Loves Park, IL 61111

Maple Park

Laboratory Technologies, Inc. — 800-542-1123
43 W 900 Rte. 64, Maple Park, IL 60151

McGaw Park

Baxter Healthcare Corporation, Renal — 888-229-0001
1620 Waukegan Road, McGaw Park, IL 60085

Cardinal Health 200, Inc — 800-964-5227
1430 Waukegan Rd, McGaw Park, IL 60085

Cardinal Health 200, Inc — 847-473-1500
1430 Waukegan Rd. KB-3B, McGaw Park, IL 60085

Cardinal Health 200, Inc. — 800-964-5227
1500 Waukegan Road, McGaw Park, IL 60085

McHenry

Cypress Medical Products — 800-334-3646
1202 S. Rte. 31, McHenry, IL 60050

Dental Usa, Inc. — 866-439-3400
5005 Mccullom Lake Rd., Mchenry, IL 60050

Medela, Inc. — 800-435-8316
1101 Corporate Drive, McHenry, IL 60050

Oak Ridge Products — 888-650-7444
4612 Century Court, McHenry, IL 60050

Pioneer Center For Human Services — 815-344-1230
4001 West Dayton St., Mchenry, IL 60050

Melrose Park

App Pharmaceuticals, Llc — (708) 345-6170
2020 N. Ruby St., Melrose Park, IL 60160

Millstadt

Mac Medical — 618-476-3550
820 S. Mulberry, Millstadt, IL 62260

Mokena

Therafin Corporation — 800-843-7234
19747 Wolf Rd., Mokena, IL 60448-0848

Therafin Corporation — 800-843-7234
19747 Wolf Rd., Mokena, IL 60448

Moline

Easter Services, Inc. — 309-754-8303
3031 North Shore Dr., Moline, IL 61265

Parr Instrument Co. — 800-872-7720
211 Fifty-Third Street, Moline, IL 61265

Montgomery

Biologos, Inc. — 800-246-4088
2235 Cornell Avenue, Montgomery, IL 60538

Morton Grove

Eyetech Ltd. — 847-470-1777
9408 Normandy Ave., Morton Grove, IL 60053

Medifix, Inc — 847-965-1898
8727 Narragansett Ave, Morton Grove, IL 60053

Regis Technologies, Inc. — 800-323-8144
8210 N. Austin Avenue, Morton Grove, IL 60053-0519

Mount Prospect

Computron Medical Corp. — 847-952-8800
1697 W. Imperial Court, Mount Prospect, IL 60056

Research Products International Corp. — 800-323-9814
410 N. Business Center Dr., Mount Prospect, IL 60056-2190

Simpex Medical, Inc. — 800-851-9753
401 E. Prospect Ave., Mount Prospect, IL 60056

Mundelein

Carter-Hoffmann — 800-323-9793
1551 McCormick Ave., Mundelein, IL 60060-4446

Ched Markay, Inc. — 312-566-3307
1065 High St., Mundelein, IL 60060

Health Imaging Corp. — 800-468-7874
1011 Campus Drive, Mundelein, IL 60060

Hos-Pillow Corp. — 800-468-7874
1011 Campus Drive, Mundelein, IL 60060

Medline Industries, Inc. — 800-633-5463
1 Medline Place, Mundelein, IL 60060

Medline Industries, Inc. — 800-633-5886
1 Medline Place, Mundelein, IL 60060-4486

Medline Manufacturing And Services Llc — 847-837-2759
One Medline Place, Mundelein, IL 60060

Merry Walker Corp. — 847-837-9580
21350 S. Sylvan Drive, Unit 9 Box P, Mundelein, IL 60060

Sysmex America Inc. — 1-800-462-1262
One Nelson C. White Parkway, Mundelein, IL 60060

World Technologies, Inc. — 847-949-4948
708-6 Diamond Lake Rd., Mundelein, IL 60060

N. Barrington

Healthcare Labels, Inc. — 800-323-8323
245 Honey Lake Ct., N. Barrington, IL 60010

Naperville

Ecodyne Water Treatment, Inc. — 800-228-9326
1270 Frontenac Road, Naperville, IL 60563

Fallgard Llc — 800-828-0702
631 Alexandria Dr., Naperville, IL 60565

Healthdent'L L.L.C. — 800-845-5172
1355 S. Route 59, Ste. 202, Naperville, IL 60564

Hitec Group Intl. — 800-288-8303
1743 Quincy Ave., Unit 155, Naperville, IL 60540

Niles

Bams Manufacturing Co., Inc. — 847-647-6990
6273 Howard St. West, Niles, IL 60714

Bankier Companies, Inc. — 847-647-6565
6151 Gross Point Rd., Niles, IL 60714

Haemoscope Corp. — 800-438-2834
6231 West Howard Street, Niles, IL 60714-3403

Maxant Technologies, Inc. — 800-307-4190
7540 Caldwell Avenue, Niles, IL 60714

Medtrol, Inc. — 1-800-647-7180
7157 N. Austin, Niles, IL 60714

Medtrol, Inc. — 847-647-6555
7157 North Austin, Niles, IL 60714

Polyscience, Division Of Preston Industries Inc. — 800-229-7569
6600 W. Touhy Ave., Niles, IL 60714

Tetra Medical Supply Corp. — 800-621-4041
6364 W. Gross Point Road, Niles, IL 60714-3916

Whitney Products, Inc. — 800-338-4237
6153 Mulford Street, Unit. C, Niles, IL 60714-3427

Z Sound — 847-293-5205
6947 West Birchwood Ave., Niles, IL 60714

Zoll Dental — 800-239-2904
7450 N. Natchez Avenue, Niles, IL 60714

Niles,
Information Data Management, Inc. — 800-249-4276
6231 W. Howard Street, Niles,, IL 60714

North Barrington
Medical Murray Inc. — 847-620-7990
400 N. Rand Rd., North Barrington, IL 60010

North Chicago
Abbott Laboratories — 847-937-2388
U.S. 41/Martin Luther King Dr, North Chicago, IL 60064

Northbrook
Electro Assemblies Corp. — 847-498-6520
2909 MacArthur Boulevard, Northbrook, IL 60062-2368
Gem Medical Supplies Llc — 877-436-6334
2165 Shermer Road, Unit B, Northbrook, IL 60062
Independent Solutions, Inc. — 847-498-0500
900 Skokie Blvd., Suite 118, Northbrook, IL 60062-4014
Leedal, Inc. — 847-498-0111
3453 Commercial Ave., Northbrook, IL 60062
Minxray, Inc. — 800-221-2245
3611 Commercial Avenue, Northbrook, IL 60062-1822
Nanosphere Inc — 888-837-4436
4088 Commercial Ave, Northbrook, IL 60062
Nuclin Diagnostics, Inc. — 847-498-5210
3322 Commercial Ave., Northbrook, IL 60062
Omex Technologies, Inc. — 847-564-0206
3665 Woodhead Drive, Northbrook, IL 60062-1816
Woodhead L.P. — 847-272-7990
3411 Woodhead Drive, Northbrook, IL 60062-1812

Northfield
Bodine Electric Co. — 800-786-3463
201 Northfield Road, Northfield, IL 60093
Stepan Co. — 800-745-7837
22 W. Frontage Road, Northfield, IL 60093

Oak Brook
Jones Medical Instrument Co. — 800-323-7336
200 Windsor Drive, Oak Brook, IL 60523
Mediware Chicago Service Center — 630-218-2700
1900 Spring Rd., Suite 450, Oak Brook, IL 60523
Sita Associates — 630-968-3727
720 Williamsburg Court, Oak Brook, IL 60523
Sterigenics International, Inc. — 800-472-4508
2015 Spring Road, Suite 650, Oak Brook, IL 60523

Oak Forest
Care Fusion 205, Inc. — 610-862-0800
4153 W. 166th St., Oak Forest, IL 60452

Orland Park
Tri-Star Medical, Inc. — 708-645-1107
14227 Winchester Court, Orland Park, IL 60467

Oswego
Janin Group, Inc. — 800-323-5389
14A Stonehill Road, Oswego, IL 60543-9400

Ottawa
Ottawa Dental Laboratory, Ltd — 800-851-8239
1304 Starfire Dr., Ottawa, IL 61350

Palatine
Clean Air Engineering — 800-627-0033
500 W. Wood St., Palatine, IL 60067
Pro-Optics, Inc. — 800-323-3846
317 Woodwork Lane, Palatine, IL 60067-4993
Sellstrom Manufacturing Co. — 800-323-7402
1 Sellstrom Drive, Palatine, IL 60067
Square D Company — 1 847 397 2600
1415 Roselle Road, Palatine, IL 60067

Palos Heights
Ark Services Corporation — 708-371-3674
6118 W. 123 St., Palos Heights, IL 60463

Park City
Cardinal Health 200, Inc — 847-578-4515
1240 Waukegan Rd, Park City, IL 60085

Park Ridge
Towic Medical, Inc. — 847-823-2215
303 S Clifton, PO Box 883, Park Ridge, IL 60068-0883

Pekin
Pal Health Systems — 800-223-2957
1805 Riverway Drive, Pekin, IL 61554

Peoria
Logical Technology, Inc. — 800-266-7591
6907 N. Knoxville, Peoria, IL 61614-4868
Rlisys Practice Solutions, Inc. — 800-447-2205
One Aloha Lane, Peoria, IL 61615-1431

Plano
Plano Molding Co. — 800-451-2122
431 E South Street, Plano, IL 60545-1601

Prophetstown
Sterling Medical Products — 800-537-5320
401 Market St., Prophetstown, IL 61277
Sterling Medical-Products Intl., Inc. — 815-537-5303
401 Market St., Prophetstown, IL 61277
Sterling Multi-Products, Inc. — 815-537-2381
326 West 5th St., Prophetstown, IL 61277

Prospect Heights
Gillis Associated Industries — 800-397-1675
750 Pinecrest Drive, Prospect Heights, IL 60070

Quincy
Champion, A Gardner Denver Co. — 800 232 0865
1800 Gardner Expressway, Quincy, IL 62305
Gardner Denver, Inc. — 217-222-5400
1800 Gardner Expressway, Quincy, IL 62305
Industrial Support Services, Inc. — 217-223-6180
2600 North 42th St., Quincy, IL 62305-5066
Quincy Specialties Co. — 217-222-4057
631 Vermont St., Quincy, IL 62306

Rantoul
Combe Laboratories, Inc. — 800-873-7400
200 Shelhouse Dr., Rantoul, IL 61866
Polyconversions, Inc. — 888-893-3330
505 Condit Dr., Rantoul, IL 61866

Roanoke
The National Wheel-O-Vator Co., Inc. — 800-551-9095
509 W. Front St., Roanoke, IL 61561-0348

Robinson
Truarch, Inc. — 618-592-6468
6062 E. 800th Ave., Robinson, IL 62454

Rockford
Bvr Aero Precision Corporation — 815-874-2471
3358-60 Publishers Dr., Rockford, IL 61109
Concentric — 800-572-7867
2222 15th St., Rockford, IL 61104
Indigo Micro Technologies, Inc. — 815-874-3557
3220 Gunflint Trail, Rockford, IL 61109
Lloyd Hearing Aid Corp. — 800-323-4212
4435 Manchester Drive, Rockford, IL 61109
Pierce Chemical Company — 800-874-3723
P.O. Box 117, Rockford, IL 61105-0117
Rockford Medical & Safety Co. — 800-435-9451
2420 Harrison Avenue, PO Box 5646, Rockford, IL 61125-0646
Rondex Products, Inc. — 815-226-0452
P.O. Box 1829, Rockford, IL 61110-0329
Wells-Engberg Company — 800-642-3628
129 S. Phelps Ave., Rockford, IL 61125

Rockton
Novel Products, Inc. — 800-323-5143
PO Box 408, Rockton, IL 61072-0408
Taylor — 800-255-0626
750 N. Blackhawk Blvd., P.O. Box 410, Rockton, IL 61072-0410

Rolling Meadows
Control Research, Inc. — 847-392-4770
1775 Winnetka Circle, Rolling Meadows, IL 60008
Micro-Scientific Industries, Inc. — 888-253-2536
1225 Carnegie Street, Ste. 101, Rolling Meadows, IL 60008

Romeo
Lombart Instruments — 800-831-1194
1312 Marquette Drive, Suite N, Romeo, IL 60446

Romeoville
Isovac Products Llc — 630-679-1740
1306 Enterprise Dr., Unit C, Romeoville, IL 60446
Xma (X-Ray Marketing Associates, Inc.) — 800-325-8880
Windham Lakes Business Park, 1205 W. Lakeview Court, Romeoville, IL 60446-6501

Roseland
Airgas Specialty Gases, Inc. — 773-785-3000
12722 South Wentworth Ave., Roseland, IL 60628

Roselle
ArjoHuntleigh — 800-323-1245
2349 West Lake Street, Suite 250, Roselle, IL 60172

Del Medical Systems
50 B. N. Gary Avenue, Roselle, IL 60172 — 800-800-6006
Planmeca U.S.A. Inc
100 N. Gary, Suite A, Roselle, IL 60172 — 630-529-2300

Rosemont

Culligan International Co.
9399 West Higgins Road, Rosemont, IL 60018 — 866-775-0260
Instromedix, A Card Guard Co.
10255 West Higgins Road, Suite 100, Rosemont, IL 60018 — 800-633-3361
Lifewatch Services, Inc.
O'hare International Center II, 10255 West Higgins Rd., Ste. 100, Rosemont, IL 60018 — 877-774-9846
Picis, Inc.
9500 W. Higgins,, Suite 1100, Rosemont, IL 60018 — 781-557-3000

Round Lake

Baxter Healthcare Corporation, Medication Delivery
25212 W. Illinois Route 120, Round Lake, IL 60073 — 888-229-0001

Saint Charles

System Sensor
3825 Ohio Ave., Saint Charles, IL 60174 — 800-736-7672,

Schaumburg

Accurate Metering Systems, Inc.
1651 Wilkening Rd., Schaumburg, IL 60173 — 270-737-6666A6É
Advanced Microderm, Inc.
904 S. Roselle Rd., #302, Schaumburg, IL 60193 — 630-980-3300
Aec, Inc.
1100 Woodfield Rd., Suite 588, Schaumburg, IL 60173 — 847-273-7700
App Pharmaceuticals, Llc
1501 E. Woodfield Rd., Suite 300e, Schaumburg, IL 60173 — 888-391-6300
Digitone Technology, Inc.
890 E. Higgins Rd., Suite 158, Schaumburg, IL 60173 — 847-413-1688
Gn Otometrics
50 Commerce Drive, Ste 180, Schaumburg, IL 60173-5329 — 800-289-2150
Infosys, Inc.
1821 Walden Office Square, Suite 350, Schaumburg, IL 60173 — 800-978-4636
Intl. Medsurg Connection, Inc.
935 N. Plum Grove Road, Suite V, Schaumburg, IL 60173-4770 — 847-619-9926
Motorola Comm. And Electronics Inc.
1303 E. Algonquin Rd., Schaumburg, IL 60196-1078 — 847-576-5000
Nsk America Corporation
700B Cooper Ct., Schaumburg, IL 60173 — 800-585-4675
Omron Electronics, Inc.
One E. Commerce Dr., Schaumburg, IL 60173 — 800-55-OMRON
Pru-Dent Manufacturing Co.
1929 S Wright Blvd, Schaumburg, IL 60193 — 800-631-2339
Pru-Dent Mfg. Inc.
1929 S. Wright Blvd., Schaumburg, IL 60193 — 847-301-1170
Sparton Electronics
425 N. Martingale Road, Suite 2050, Schaumburg, IL 60173 — 800.772.7866
Taiyo Tech. Of America
1355 Remington Road, Suite F, Schaumburg, IL 60173 — 847-466-7905

Skokie

Anatomical Chart Co.
4711 Golf Road, Suite 650, Skokie, IL 60076 — 800-621-7500
Dean B. Scott, Ocularist
5225 Old Orchard Rd.,, Suite 27-b, Skokie, IL 60077 — 847-965-4455
Gaertner Scientific Corp.
3650 Jarvis Avenue, Skokie, IL 60076 — 847-673-5006
Gbf Graphics, Inc.
7300 Niles Center Road, Skokie, IL 60077-3286 — 800-GBF-TEAM
Harry J. Bosworth Company
7227 N. Hamlin Avenue, Skokie, IL 60076-3999 — 800-323-4352
In-Step Mobility
8027 N. Monticello Ave., Skokie, IL 60076 — 800-558-7837
M&S Technologies, Inc. / Marino
5557 W Howard St, Skokie, IL 60077 — 1-877-225-6101
Nanoink Inc.
8025 Lamon Ave., Skokie, IL 60077 — 847-679-6266
Norfolk Medical Products, Inc.
7350 North Ridgeway, Skokie, IL 60076 — 847-674-7075
Rauland-Borg Corp.
3450 W. Oakton St., Skokie, IL 60076-2951 — 800-752-7725
Reznik Instrument, Inc.
7337 North Lawndale, Skokie, IL 60076 — 847-673-3444
Tepromark International, Inc.
7518 N. St. Louis #1047, Skokie, IL 60076 — 800-645-2622
Uresil, Llc
5418 W. Touhy Avenue, Skokie, IL 60077-3232 — 800-538-7374

South Beloit

Varitech Medical Devices, Inc.
319 Dicop, South Beloit, IL 61080 — 815-624-6785

South Holland

Esma, Inc.
450 WestTaft Dr., South Holland, IL 60473 — 800-276-2466

Springfield

Thermionics Corp.
1214 Bunn Avenue, Suite 5, Springfield, IL 62703 — 800-800-5728

St. Charles

Microplastics, Inc.
406 38th Avenue, St. Charles, IL 60174 — 630-513-2900
Winchester Laboratories Llc
11 S. 2nd Avenue, St. Charles, IL 60174 — 630-377-7880

Sterling

Wahl Clipper Corp.
2900 North Locust St., Sterling, IL 61081 — 815-548-8342
Wahl Clipper Corp.
2902 N. Locust St., Sterling, IL 61081-0578 — 815-625-6525

Streamwood

Color Change Corp.
1545 Burgundy Pkwy., Streamwood, IL 60107 — 630-289-0900
Fricke Dental Manufacturing Co.
165 Roma Jean Pkwy, Streamwood, IL 60107 — 800-537-4253

Suite 555

I.F.S. Industrial & Financial Systems
300 Park Boulevard, Suite 555, Suite 555, IL 60143 — 888-437-4968

Vernon Hills

Cole-Parmer Instrument Inc.
625 E. Bunker Ct., Vernon Hills, IL 60061-1844 — 800-323-4340
Mmi
P.O. Box 5396, Vernon Hills, IL 60061 — 800-999-4664
Richard Wolf Medical Instruments Corp.
353 Corporate Woods Pkwy., Vernon Hills, IL 60061-3110 — 800-323-9653
Scotsman Industries
775 Corporate Woods Pkwy., Vernon Hills, IL 60061-3112 — 800-SCOTSMAN
Smiths Medical Asd, Inc.
330 Corporate Woods Dr., Vernon Hills, IL 60061 — 847-793-0135

Villa Park

Kidsneb, Inc.
310 N. Villa Ave., Villa Park, IL 60181 — 630-930-9412

Volo

Don Johnston Incorporated
26799 Commerce Dr., Volo, IL 60073 — 800-999-4660

Watseka

T+d Metal Products
602 E. Walnut, Watseka, IL 60970 — 757-224-0177

Wauconda

Cd Nelson Manufacturing Co.
26920 N Grace St, Wauconda, IL 60084 — 847-487-4870
Cortek Endoscopy, Inc.
260 Jamie Lane, Unit D, Wauconda, IL 60084 — 847-526-2266
Goldman Products, Inc.
379 Hollow Hill Dr., Wauconda, IL 60084 — 847-526-1166
Micro-Dent Inc.
379 Hollow Hill Rd., Wauconda, IL 60084 — 866-526-1166

Waukegan

Adi Medical Division Of Asia Dynamics (Group) Inc.
1565 South Shields Drive, Waukegan, IL 60085 — 877-647-7699
Airistar Technologies, L.L.C.
2330 Ernie Krueger Circle, Waukegan, IL 60087 — 800-755-8006
Beutlich Lp, Pharmaceuticals
1541 Shields Drive, Waukegan, IL 60085-8304 — 800-238-8542
Cardinal Health 200, Inc.
1300 Waukegan Rd., Waukegan, IL 60085 — 847-785-3323
Intravascular Incorporated
3600 Bur Wood Drive, Waukegan, IL 60085 — 800-917-3234
Mabis Healthcare Inc.
1931 Norman Drive, Waukegan, IL 60085 — 800-526-4753
Medikmark Inc.
3600 Bur Wood, Waukegan, IL 60085-8399 — 800-424-8520
Monogen, Inc.
3630 Bur Wood Dr., Waukegan, IL 60085 — 847-573-6700
Powervar, Inc.
1450 Lakeside Drive, Waukegan, IL 60085 — 800-369-7179

Wayne

March & Green
P.O. Box 155, Wayne, IL 60184-0155 — 800-447-6004

West Chicago

Advanced Urethane Technologies, Inc.
1750 West Downs Dr., West Chicago, IL 60185 — 630-293-0780
Scs Corporation
1901 Powis Court, West Chicago, IL 60185 — 630-797-7300

Westchester

Spinecraft Llc
2215 Entreprise Dr., Westchester, IL 60154 — 708-531-9700

Westmont

American Surgical Instrument Corp.
26 Plaza Drive, Westmont, IL 60559-1124 — 800-628-2879

Captiva Software Corporation | 800-783-3378
601 Oakmont Lane, Suite 200, Westmont, IL 60559
Denbur, Inc. | 630-969-6865
433 Plaza Drive, Unit 4, Westmont, IL 60559
Mccrone Microscopes & Accessories | 800-622-8122
850 Pasquinelli Drive, Westmont, IL 60559
Vitalcor, Inc. | 800-874-8358
100 East Chestnut Avenue, Westmont, IL 60559

Wheaton

Dermed Diagnostics, Inc. | 630-668-4644
2-S 558 White Birch Ln., Wheaton, IL 60187
Recognition Express | 800-573-6444
502 Sunnyside Avenue, Wheaton, IL 60187

Wheeling

Angiotech | 800-424-6779
241 West Palatine Road, Wheeling, IL 60090
Corpak Medsystems, Inc. | 800-323-6305
100 Chaddick Dr., Wheeling, IL 60090
Dynomax Inc | 847-680-8833
1535 Abbott Drive, Wheeling, IL 60090
Hospital Laundry Services - Sterile Recovery Division | 847-229-0900
45 West Hintz Road, Wheeling, IL 60090
Lang Dental Manufacturing Co., Inc. | 800-222-5264
175 Messner Drive, Wheeling, IL 60090
Precision Medical Manufacturing Corporation | 866-633-4626
852 SETON CT., WHEELING, IL 60090
Snap Laboratories, L.L.C. | 847-777-0000
5210 Capitol Drive, Wheeling, IL 60025
Suburban Surgical Co., Inc. | 800-323-7366
275 Twelfth St., Wheeling, IL 60090
The Burrows Co. | 847-537-7300
230 West Palatine Road, Wheeling, IL 60090-0747
Waldmann Lighting | 800-634-0007
9 W. Century Dr., Wheeling, IL 60090

Wilmette

Rehabtek Llc | 847-853-8380
2510 Wilmette Ave., Wilmette, IL 60091

Wood Dale

Cloud 9 | 630-595-5000
777 Edgewood Avenue, Wood Dale, IL 60191-1254
Hospital Therapy Products, Inc. | 630-766-7101
757 North Central Ave., Wood Dale, IL 60191
K-Alpha X-Ray | 630-860-1864
175 Hansen Ct., Suite 108, Wood Dale, IL 60191
Stoelting Co. | 630-860-9700
620 Wheat Ln., Wood Dale, IL 60191

Wood River

Telsar Laboratories Inc | 800-255-9938
1 Enviroway, Suite 100, Wood River, IL 62095

Woodstock

Catalent Pharma Solutions | 866-720-3148
2200 Lake Shore Dr., Woodstock, IL 60098
M-P Mfg., Inc. | 815-334-1112
13802 Washington St. #b, Woodstock, IL 60098
Pacific Electronics | 800-281-7782
10200 US Route 14, Woodstock, IL 60098
Precision Quincy Corp. | 800-338-0079
1625 W. Lake Shore Drive, Woodstock, IL 60098

Worth

Calutech Corporation |
6615 W. 111th St., Worth, IL 60482

INDIANA

Anderson

Relaxobak, Inc | 866-369-6914
4956 W 300 N., P.O. Box 2613, Anderson, IN 46018-2613

Angola

Electri-Tec, Inc. | 219-665-1252
509 Growth Pkwy., Angola, IN 46703

Auburn

Foamex L.P. | 800-355-3626
2211 S. Wayne St., Auburn, IN 46706

Bainbridge

Manan Technologies, Inc. | 800-416-2434
102 Northfield Drive East, Bainbridge, IN 46105

Batesville

Hill-Rom Holdings, Inc. | 800-445-3730
1069 State Route 46 East, Batesville, IN 47006
Hill-Rom, Inc | 812-934-7777
1069 State Route 46 East, Batesville, IN 47006

Med-Mizer, Inc | 812-932-2345
80 Commerce Drive, Batesville, IN 47006
Ricca Chemical Company Llc | 817-461-5601
1490 Lammers Pike, Batesville, IN 47006

Blmgtn

Morris Innovative Research | 812-355-0450
907 W.second St, Blmgtn, IN 47403

Bloomfield

Mectra Labs, Inc. | 800-323-3968
Two Quality Way, Bloomfield, IN 47424

Bloomington

Baxter Healthcare Corporation, Baxter Biopharma Solutions | 800-353-0887
927 S. Curry Pike Drive, Bloomington, IN 47402
Biomedix, Inc. | 800-627-2765
3895 W. Vernal Pike, Bloomington, IN 47404
Cook Inc. | 800-457-4500
PO Box 489, Bloomington, IN 47402-0489
Cook Medical Inc. | 800-457-4500
400 daniels way, Bloomington, IN 47404
Cook Ob/Gyn | 800-457-4500
P.O. Box 4195, Bloomington, IN 47402-4195
HARTMANN USA, Inc. | 812-332-3703
4265 West Vernal Pike, Bloomington, IN 47404
Manico Bloomington | 812-336-2567
515 Woodscrest Medical Bldg.,, Suite 001, P.o. Box 5504, Bloomington, IN 47407-5504
Physicians Practice Management | 800-252-6635
320 W. 8th St, Suite 218, Bloomington, IN 47404
Sabin Corporation | 800-264-4510
3800 Constitution Avenue, PO Box 788, PO Box 788, Bloomington, IN 47402-0788

Bremen

Creative Foam Medical Systems | 800-446-4644
405 N Industrial Drive, Bremen, IN 46506

Carmel

Ameriflo Corp. | 866-573-1658
478 Gradle Drive, Carmel Industrial Park, Carmel, IN 46032
Bell-Horn, Inc. | 317-228-1144
4511 W. 99th Street, Carmel, IN 46032
Kli Corp. | 317-846-7452
1119 Third Ave SW, Carmel, IN 46032

Chester

Hbr Healthcare Company, Inc. | 765-966-1400
2211 Williamsburg Pike, Chester, IN 47374

Claypool

Symmetry Medical Usa, Inc | 207-786-2775
111 N. Clay, Claypool, IN 46510

Columbia City

GREATBATCH MEDICAL | 260-244-6300
4532 Park 30 Drive, Columbia City, IN 46725
Opi, Inc. | 260-248-4414
700 South Main Street, Columbia City, IN 46725
Summit Business Products, Inc. | 260-244-1820
995 E. Business 30, Columbia City, IN 46725

Columbus

All Star Orthodontics, Llc | 866-314-0804
4570 Progress Dr., Columbus, IN 47201
Applied Laboratories, Inc. | 812-372-2607
3240 N. Indianapolis Road, P.O. Box 2127, Columbus, IN 47202-2127
Blairex Laboratories, Inc. | 800-252-4739
PO Box 2127, 1600 Brian Drive, Columbus, IN 47202
Crescent Manufacturing Company | 419-332-6484
4615 Progress Drive, Columbus, IN 47201
Destal Industries, Inc. | 973-227-1830
201 Washington St., Columbus, IN 47201

Crawfordsville

Current Technologies Inc | 800-456-4022
PO Box 21, Crawfordsville, IN 47933-0021

crown point

Arcadia Medical Corporation | 219-779-9431
1140 Millennium Drive, crown point, IN 46307
Point Medical Corp. | 219-663-1775
891 E. Summit St., Crown Point, IN 46307-2700

Danville

Ventura Enterprises | 317-745-2989
35 Lawton Avenue, Danville, IN 46122

Darlington

Simple Orthopaedic Solutions, Llc | 317-414-1558
9337 North 700 East, Darlington, IN 47940

Drexel Gardens

Engineered Medical Systems — 317-246-5500
2055 Executive Dr., Drexel Gardens, IN 46241

Elkhart

Champion Manufacturing, Llc. — 800-998-5018
2601 Industrial Pwy., Elkhart, IN 46516
Champion Mfg. Inc. — 800-998-5018
2601 Industrial Pkwy., Elkhart, IN 46516
Custom Durable Products, Inc — 800 478-2363
21279 Protecta Drive, Elkhart, IN 46516
Frederick Tool Corp. — 800-443-9618
24615 C.R. 45 Ste.4, Elkhart, IN 46516
Goshen Coach Div. Warrick Industries, Inc. — 800-326-2062
25161 LEER DRIVE, Elkhart, IN 46514
Hach Company / Environmental Test Systems — 800-548-4381
23575 County Road 106, PO Box 4659, Elkhart, IN 46514-0659
Integrated Biomedical Technology, Inc. — 574-264-0025
2931 Moose Trail, Elkhart, IN 46514
Kik Custom Products — 574-295-0000
1919 Superior Street, PO Box 2988, Elkhart, IN 46515
Professional Dental Laboratory Corporation — 574-294-3631
1400 West Indiana Avenue, P.o. Box 877, Elkhart, IN 46515
Romaine, Inc. D.B.A. Koldcare — 800-294-7101
2026 Sterling Ave., Elkhart, IN 46516-4220
Serim Research Corp. — 574-264-3440
3506 Reedy Dr, Elkhart, IN 46514
Siemens Healthcare Diagnostics Inc — 574-295-7516
3400 Middlebury St, Elkhart, IN 46515
Stanbio Life Sciences, Division Of Stanbio — (800) 545-4437
Laboratory
25235 Leer Dr., Elkhart, IN 46514
Supertech, Inc. — 800-654-1054
P.O. Box 186, Elkhart, IN 46515-0186

Evansville

Bristol-Myers Squibb — 732-227-7564
2400 West Lloyd Expressway, Evansville, IN 47721
Glenn Reams, Ocularist — 800-426-8995
1020 West Buena Vista, Evansville, IN 47710

Fishers

Analytical Control Systems, Inc. — 317-841-0458
9058 Technology Drive, Fishers, IN 46038
Bangs Laboratories, Inc. — 800-387-0672
9025 Technology Drive, Fishers, IN 46038-2886
Oscar, Inc. — 317-849-2618
11793 Technology Dr., Fishers, IN 46038
Positron Corporation — 866-613-7587
9715 Kincaid Blvd., Suite 1000, Fishers, IN 46038
Roche Insulin Delivery Systems Inc. — 800-280-7801
11800 Exit 5 Parkway, Fishers, IN 46037

Fort Wayne

D & N Micro Products, Inc. — 260-484-6414
2721 Corrinado Court, Fort Wayne, IN 46808
Enzyme Solutions, Inc. — 260-497-0851
7601 Honeywell Dr., Fort Wayne, IN 46825
Fort Wayne Metals Research Prod. Corp. — 260-747-4154
9609 Indianapolis Road, Fort Wayne, IN 46809
Nemcomed — 800-255-4576
8727 Clinton Park Drive, Fort Wayne, IN 46825
Panoramic Corporation — 800-654-2027
4321 Goshen Road, Fort Wayne, IN 46818

Fortville

Genesis Manufacturing, Inc. — 317-485-7887
720 E. Broadway, Fortville, IN 46040

Franklin

G & H Wire Co. — 800-526-1026
2165 Earlywood Drive, Franklin, IN 46131
Promex Technologies, Llc — 317-736-0128
3049 Hudson St., Franklin, IN 46131
Sterylab Usa, Llc — 317-736-8306
2916 Graham Rd., Suite C, Franklin, IN 46131

Fremont

Health Equipment Manufacturers, Inc. — 269-962-6181
702 S. Reed Street, Fremont, IN 46737

Garrett

Griffith Rubber Mills — 260-357-3125
400 N. Taylor, Garrett, IN 46738

Gary

Midwest Medical Solutions, Llc — 800-451-6244
1310 Michigan St., Gary, IN 46402-3034
Smiths Medical Asd — 800-424-8662
5700 W. 23rd Avenue, Gary, IN 46406-2617
Tradewinds Rehabilitation Center, Inc. — 219-949-4000
5901 West 7th Ave., Gary, IN 46406

Goshen

Daren Industries, Inc — 574-534-3418
2452 Lincolnway East, Goshen, IN 46526
Medtec Ambulance Corp. — 866-263-3832
2429 Lincoln Way East, Goshen, IN 46526

Granger

Back Pain Relief Clinic, P.C. — 574-271-9444
5507 Singer Ct., Granger, IN 46530

Greenwood

Advantis Medical — 888-625-4497
2121 Southtech Dr., Ste 600, Greenwood, IN 46143
Bagblocker, Inc — 317-538-6732
2159 Dockside Drive, Greenwood, IN 46143

Hammond

Linde Gas Usa Llc — 216-642-6600
3930 Michigan Street, Hammond, IN 46323

Huntington

Drummond Industries, Inc. — 260-356-6837
254 W. Mccrum St., Huntington, IN 46750
Pulley-Kellam Co., Inc. — 260-356-6326
245 Erie St., Huntington, IN 46750

Indianapolis

Access Mobility, Inc. — 800-336-1147
5240 Elmwood Ave., Indianapolis, IN 46203
Aearo Company — 800-678-4163
5457 West 79th Street, Indianapolis, IN 46268
Ahnafield Corp. — 800-636-8060
2444 Production Dr., Indianapolis, IN 46241
Amg, Llc — 317-329-4000
4030 Guion Ln., Indianapolis, IN 46268
Arcadia Resources Inc. — 800-733-8427
9229 Delegates Row, Suite 260, Indianapolis, IN 46240
Artec Environmental Monitoring — 800-727-8321
8047 Castleton Road, Indianapolis, IN 46250
Beckman Coulter Inc. (Sagian Operation) — 800-742-2345
5350 Lakeview Parkway South DR, Indianapolis, IN 46268
Beckman Coulter, Inc. — (317) 808-4200
5350 Lakeview Parkway S Drive, Indianapolis, IN 46268
Biosound Esaote, Inc. — 800-428-4374
8000 Castleway Drive, Indianapolis, IN 46250-1943
Brulin & Co. Inc. — 800-776-7149
2920 Drive A.J. Brown Avenue, Indianapolis, IN 46205
Bryton Corp. — 800-567-9500
4310 Guion Rd., Indianapolis, IN 46254-3111
Catheter Research, Inc. (Cri) — 317-872-0074
5610 W. 82nd St., Indianapolis, IN 46278
Century Pharmaceuticals, Inc. — 317-849-4210
10377 Hague Rd., Indianapolis, IN 46256
Ch Ellis Company Inc. — 800-466-3351
2432 Southeastern Avenue, Indianapolis, IN 46201
Creative Laboratory Products, Inc. — 317-293-2991
6420 N. Guion Rd., Indianapolis, IN 46268
Deflecto Corp. — 800-428-4328
7035 E. 86th St., Indianapolis, IN 46250
Dps, Inc. — 800-654-4689
3685 Priority Way South Drive, Suite 100, Indianapolis, IN 46240
Ehob, Inc. — 800-899-5553
250 N. Belmont Avenue, Indianapolis, IN 46222
Eli Lilly And Co. — 317-276-4000
Lilly Corporate Center, Drop Code 2622, Indianapolis, IN 46285
Enochs Examining Room Furniture, Inc. — 800-428-2305
P.O. Box 50559, Indianapolis, IN 46250
Ets, Inc. — 317-554-3500
7445 Company Dr., Indianapolis, IN 46237
Flotec, Inc. — 800-401-1723
7625 W. New York St., Indianapolis, IN 46214-4911
Focus Surgery, Inc. — 317-541-1580
3940 Pendleton Way, Indianapolis, IN 46226
General Devices Co., Inc. — 800-626-9484
1410 S. Post Road, Indianapolis, IN 46239
Goodwill Industries Of Central Indiana, Inc. — 317-524-4313
1635 West Michigan St., Indianapolis, IN 46222
Gvs Filter Technology Inc. — 317-471-3700
5353 W. 79th St., Indianapolis, IN 46268
Indiana Technology Development, Inc. — 317-814-6194
4181 E. 96th St., Suite 200, Indianapolis, IN 46240
International Cryogenics, Inc. — 800-886-2796
4040 Championship Drive, Indianapolis, IN 46268
Inweld Corp. — 317-248-0651
5353 West Southern Avenue, Indianapolis, IN 46242
Kingswood Laboratories, Inc. — 800-968-7772
10375 Hague Rd., Indianapolis, IN 46256
Kinman Of Indianapolis, Inc. — 800-444-8891
1401 Harding Ct., Suite K, Indianapolis, IN 46217-9538
Life Medical Llc — 317-840-3816
10424 Snapper Ct., Indianapolis, IN 46256
Medi-Span, Inc. — 800-388-8884
8425 Woodfield Crossing Blvd., Suite 490, Indianapolis, IN 46240

Nystrom   800-621-8086
4719 W. 62nd St., Indianapolis, IN 46268-2593
Obs Medical   866-424-6744
Two Meridian Plaza, 10401 N Meridian St., Ste. 300, Indianapolis, IN 46290
Polymer Technology Systems, Inc.   317-870-5610
7736 Zionsville Rd., Indianapolis, IN 46268
Powerway, Inc.   800-964-9004
429 N. Pennsylvania Street, Suite 400, Indianapolis, IN 46204
Problem Solving Concepts, Inc.   800-755-2150
8021 Knue Rd., Suite 100, Indianapolis, IN 46250
R. B. Annis Instruments, Inc.   317-637-9282
1101 N. Delaware St., Indianapolis, IN 46202-2529
Roche Diagnostics Operations   317-521-2000
9115 Hague Rd., PO Box 50457, Indianapolis, IN 46250
Seradyn, Inc.   800-428-4072
7998 Georgetown Road, Suite 1000, Indianapolis, IN 46268
Siemens Healthcare Diagnostics Inc   317-240-0012
7750 West Morris St., Indianapolis, IN 46231
Siemens Water Technologies   866-926-8420
6125 Guion Rd., Indianapolis, IN 46254
SonarMed, Inc.   317-489-3161
5513 West 74th St., Indianapolis, IN 46268
Specialty Coating Systems, Inc.   800-356-8260
7645 Woodland Dr., Indianapolis, IN 46278
Specialty Manufacturers, Medical Products Division   317-241-2457
2410 Executive Drive, Indianapolis, IN 46241
Suros Surgical Systems, Inc   877-887-8767
6100,6110,6120 Technology Center Drive, Indianapolis, IN 46278
Symbios Medical Products, Llc   317-225-4447
7301 Georgetown Rd, Suite 150, Indianapolis, IN 46268
Uridynamics, Inc.   317-915-7896
6786 Hawthorn Park Dr., Indianapolis, IN 46220
V--Operations Management Consulting,   317-570-5830
7350 E 86th St, Indianapolis, IN 46256
Woundvision Inc.   888-851-0098
450 East 96th Street, Suite 500, Indianapolis, IN 46240

INDIANPOLIS

Thomas Medical Inc.   800-556-0349
5610 WEST 82 2ND STREET, INDIANPOLIS, IN 46278

Jasper

Kimball International   800-482-1616
1600 Royal Street, Jasper, IN 47549

Jeffersonville

Active Ankle Systems, Inc.   812-258-0663
233 Quartermaster Ct., Jeffersonville, IN 47130
Airguard   800-999-3458
100 River Ridge Circle, Jeffersonville, IN 47130

Kingsford Heights

Models Plus   800-522-4044
605 Grayton Road, PO Box 600, Kingsford Heights, IN 46346

Knox

Stelrema Corp.   814-422-8892
4055 East 250 North, Knox, IN 46534

Kokomo

Seven Harvest Intl. Import & Export   765-456-3584
108 North Dixon Rd., Kokomo, IN 46901
TI Tate Mfg, Inc.   765-452-8283
1500 N Webster Street, Kokomo, IN 46901

La Porte

Tp Orthodontics, Inc.   800-348-8856
100 Center Plaza, La Porte, IN 46350-9672

Lafayette

Ash Access Technology Inc.   765-742-4813
INOK Business Center, 3601 Sagamore Pwy. N., Suite B, Lafayette, IN 47904
Lafayette Dental Lab., Inc.   765-447-9341
2211 South St., PO Box 5479, Lafayette, IN 47904-2968
Lafayette Instrument Company   800-428-7545
3700 Sagamore Pkwy., PO Box 5729, Lafayette, IN 47903
Lafayette Instrument Company   800-428-7545
3700 Segamore Pkwy. North, PO Box 5729, Lafayette, IN 47903
Perry Chemical & Mfg. Co., Inc.   800-592-6614
2335 South 30th Street (47909), PO Box 6419, Lafayette, IN 47903-6419

Lake Station

Greenwald Surgical Co., Inc.   888-962-1829
2688 Dekalb St., Lake Station, IN 46405

Lake Sullivan

North American Latex Corp.   812-268-6608
049 East Industrial Park Drive, Lake Sullivan, IN 47882

Lebanon

Lebanon Corp., The   800-428-2310
1700 Lebanon St., Lebanon, IN 46052-1501

Leesburg

Nuell, Inc.   800-829-7694
312 East Van Buren St., PO Box 55, Leesburg, IN 46538

Ligonier

Sroufe Healthcare Products Llc   888-894-4171
PO Box 347, 601 Sroufe St., Ligonier, IN 46767-0347

Marion

New Innovations Inc.   765-668-7470
125 E. Bradford St., Marion, IN 46952
Tulox Plastics Corp.   800-234-1118
401 S. Miller Ave., P.O. Box 984, Marion, IN 46952-0984

Michigan City

Anderson, W.E., Div. Dwyer Instruments, Inc.   800-872-9141
102 Highway 212, Michigan City, IN 46361
Dage-MTI, Inc.   219-872-5514
701 North Roeske Avenue, Michigan City, IN 46360
Lighthouse Industries   219-879-1550
107 Eastwood Rd., Po Box 8905, Michigan City, IN 46360
Sammann Co., See Aids Div.   800-348-2508
9935 E. U.S. 12, Michigan City, IN 46360-1282

Mishawaka

Bayer Healthcare, Llc   574-256-3430
430 South Beiger St., Mishawaka, IN 46544
Hear Ear Inc   574-256-0000
3718 Lincolnway East, Mishawaka, IN 46544
Nti-Tss, Inc.   574-258-5963
2303 Blue Smoke Trail, Mishawaka, IN 46546
Pasman Medeq, Inc.   574-252-5690
3296 Cambridge Ct., Mishawaka, IN 46545
Rx Honing Machine Corporation   800-346-6464
1301 E. Fifth St., Mishawaka, IN 46544-2827
Vision Training Products, Inc.   800-348-2225
4016 N. Home St., Mishawaka, IN 46545

Monticello

T & L Sharpening, Inc.   574-583-3868
2663 S. Freeman Rd., P.o. Box 338, Monticello, IN 47960

Mooresville

Mount Olive Manufacturing, Inc.   317-834-8525
3304 Hancel Circle, Mooresville, IN 46158
Sundance Enterprises, Inc.   317-831-6447
236 E. Washington St., Po Box 146, Mooresville, IN 46158

Muncie

Hiatt Metal Products   765-284-8351
720 West Willard St., Muncie, IN 47302

Munster

Star Case Manufacturing Co., Inc.   800-822-7827
648 Superior Avenue, Munster, IN 46321

New Albany

Center For Orthotic & Prosthetic Care   812-941-0966
1931 West St., New Albany, IN 47150

Newburgh

Mobility Matters Incorporated   812-459-4584
3588 Katalla, Newburgh, IN 47630

Noblesville

Ambassador Medical   888-499-4554
14470 Bergen Blvd., Suite 500, Noblesville, IN 46060
Helmer, Inc.   800-743-5637
15425 Herriman Blvd., Noblesville, IN 46060
King Systems Corp.   800-642-5464
15011 Herriman Blvd., Noblesville, IN 46060
Kneebourne Therapeutic, Llc   317-776-2770
15299 Stony Creek Way, Noblesville, IN 46060
Precision Surgical Intl., Inc.   800-776-8493
PO Box 726, Noblesville, IN 46061
Rochester Medical Implants   800- 371-6851
1202 East 4th Street, Noblesville, IN 46975-9104

North Webster

Chematics, Inc.   574-834-4080
Hwy. 13 South, North Webster, IN 46555
De Good Dimensional Concepts, Inc.   574-834-5437
7815 Sr 13 N, North Webster, IN 46555

Paoli

Paoli, Inc.   800-457-7415
PO Box 30, Paoli, IN 47454-0030

Pierceton

Paragon Medical, Inc.   800-225-6975
8 Matchett Industrial Park Dr., Pierceton, IN 46562

Plainfield

Puritan Bennett Corp. — 925-463-4371
2800 Airwest Blvd., Plainfield, IN 46168

Richmond

Xennovate Medical Llc — 608-298-753
1080 University Blvd., Richmond, IN 47374

Rochester

Rochester Medical Implants — 574-223-8198
1202 E. 4th Street, Rochester, IN 46975-0547

Shelbyville

Innovative Medical Designs — 317-421-0308
130 West Rampart Rd., Shelbyville, IN 46176

South Bend

Derby Industries — 757-224-0177
24350 Sr 23 South, South Bend, IN 46614
Derby, Inc. — 219-233-4500
24350 State Rd. 23 S., South Bend, IN 46614
Heraeus Kulzer, Inc., Dental Products Division — 574-299-6662
4315 South Lafayette Blvd., South Bend, IN 46614
Invacare Supply Group, Inc — 508-429-1000
3507 N. Olive Rd, South Bend, IN 46628
Midwest Orthotic Services, Llc — 574-233-3352
17530 Dugdale Dr., South Bend, IN 46635
R2 Diagnostics, Inc. — 574-288-4377
1801 Commerce Dr., South Bend, IN 46628
Spin-Cast Plastics, Inc. — 800-422-3625
3300 N. Kenmore St., South Bend, IN 46628

Speedway

Carpal Therapy, Inc. — 317-313-0680
1201 Main St., Suite 200, Speedway, IN 46224

Spencer

Boston Scientific Corporation — 508-652-5578
780 Brookside Drive, Spencer, IN 47460
Cook Urological, Inc. — 800-457-4500
1100 West Morgan St., P.O. Box 227, Spencer, IN 47460

Springville

Prd, Inc. — 812-279-8885
747 Washboard Road, Springville, IN 47462

Terre Haute

Glas-Col , Llc — 800-452-7265
711 Hulman St., PO Box 2128, Terre Haute, IN 47802-0128

Valparaiso

Omnitech Systems, Inc. — 866-266-9490
450 S. Campbell St., Ste. 2, Valparaiso, IN 46385

Wabash

Carver Inc. — 260-563-7577
1569 Morris St., Wabash, IN 46992-0544

Warsaw

B & M Instruments, Inc. — 574-269-5313
542 East 200 North, Warsaw, IN 46580
Biomet Sports Medicine, Inc — 800-348-9500
56 East Bell Drive, Warsaw, IN 46581-0587
Biomet, Inc. — 574-267-6639
56 E. Bell Dr., PO Box 587, Warsaw, IN 46581
C.O.R.E. Tech, Inc. — 574-267-5744
542 E. 200 N., Warsaw, IN 46582
Da-Lite Screen Co., Inc. — 800-622-3737
3100 N. Detroit St., PO Box 137, Warsaw, IN 46581-0137
Depuy Ace, A Johnson & Johnson Company — 800-473-3789
700 Orthopedic Drive, Warsaw, IN 46581
Depuy Orthopaedics, Inc. — 800-473-3789
700 Orthopaedic Dr., Warsaw, IN 46581
First Call, Inc. — 317-596-3280
660 E. 200 N, Warsaw, IN 46582
Implex Corp. — 800-613-6131
1800 West Center Street, Warsaw, IN 46581-0708
Precision Medical Technologies — 574-267-6385
2059 N. Pound Dr., Warsaw, IN 46582
Sim Medical Sales — 574-268-0341
PO BOX 0895, Warsaw, IN 46581
Smith & Nephew, Inc., Endoscopy Division — 978-749-1073
737 North Detroit St., Warsaw, IN 46580
Sun Metal Products, Inc. — 219-267-3281
P.O. Box 1508, Warsaw, IN 46581-1508
Symmetry Medical Usa, Inc. — 574-267-8700
486 West 350 North, Warsaw, IN 46582
Symmetry Medical, Inc. — 574-268-2252
3724 N. State Rd. 15, Warsaw, IN 46582
Zimmer Holdings, Inc. — 800-613-6131
1800 W. Center St., PO Box 708, Warsaw, IN 46581

Washington

B & T Davis Electric Inc. — 812-644-7615
Rr4 Box 150a, Washington, IN 47501

West Lafayette

Basi (Bioanalytical Systems, Inc.) — 800-845-4246
2701 Kent Avenue, West Lafayette, IN 47906-1382
Biotek, Inc. — 800-269-2918
PO Box 2216, West Lafayette, IN 47996-2216
Cook Biotech, Incorporated — 888-299-4224
1425 Innovation Place, West Lafayette, IN 47906
Vasc-Alert, Inc. — 765-775-2525
3000 Kent Ave, West Lafayette, IN 47906

Westfield

Synermed Intl., Inc. — 317-896-1565
17408 Tiller Court, Ste. 1900, Westfield, IN 46074

IOWA

Adair

Evergreen Health Inc. — 877-742-3555
401 Audubon St., Adair, IA 50002

Adel

Medical Industries America Inc. — 800-759-3038
2636 289th Place, Adel, IA 50003

Altoona

Altoona Medical Supply — 800-442-8367
705 2nd Ave. S.W., Altoona, IA 50009-1726

Bettendorf

Csam, Inc. — 563-359-7917
1890 14th St., Bettendorf, IA 52722

Blue Grass

Stony Brook, Inc. — 563-388-0588
12047 70th Avenue, Blue Grass, IA 52726

Bondurant

Colored Plastics, Llc — 888-807-9554
3902 Grant Street South, Bondurant, IA 50035

Castana

Verista Imaging Inc. — 712-353-6225
201 4th Street, Castana, IA 51010

Cedar Rapids

Dental Prosthetic Services, Inc. — 319-393-1990
1150 Old Marion Road Ne, Cedar Rapids, IA 52402
Flat-D Innovations, Inc. — 866-354-0056
7531 Berkshire Dr. N.e., PO Box 10342, Cedar Rapids, IA 52402

Clarinda

Ez Way, Inc. — 800-627-8940
710 E. Main Street, PO Box 89, Clarinda, IA 51632

Coralville

Hansen Ophthalmic Development Lab — 319-338-1285
745 Avalon Pl., Coralville, IA 52241
Medical Imaging Applications, Llc — 319-358-1529
832 Forest Hill Drive, Coralville, IA 52241
Protek Medical Products, Inc. — 319-545-7100
4125 Westcor Court, Coralville, IA 52241

Council Bluffs

Dermatologic Lab & Supply, Inc. — 800-831-6273
608 13th Ave., Council Bluffs, IA 51501
Geiger Medical Technologies — 800-320-9612
608 13th Avenue, Council Bluffs, IA 15101-6401
Sleep Sauna, Inc. — 800-229-5210
608 13th Avenue, Council Bluffs, IA 51501

Davenport

Blue Wave Ultrasonics — 800-373-0144
960 S. Rolff St., Davenport, IA 52802
Carleton Life Support Systems Inc. — 563-383-6204
2734 Hickory Grove Rd., Davenport, IA 52804
Tjn Manufacturing,Inc. — 563-322-2162
416 Perry St., Davenport, IA 52801

Decorah

Ortivus — 800-537-3927
2324 Sweet Parkway Road, PO Box 276, Decorah, IA 52101

Des Moines

Briggs Corporation — 800-247-2343
7300 Westown Pkwy., PO Box 1698, Des Moines, IA 50306-1698
Crystal Tone Hearing Instruments — 515-255-4144
4217 University Ave., Des Moines, IA 50311
Fawn Vendors, Inc. — 800-548-1982
8040 University Blvd., Des Moines, IA 50325

Katecho, Inc.   515-244-1212
4020 Gannett Ave., Des Moines, IA 50321
Qualis Group Llc   515-243-3000
4600 Park Ave., Des Moines, IA 50321

Dubuque
Barnstead International   800-553-0039
2555 Kerper Blvd., Dubuque, IA 52001
The Metrix Co.   800-752-3148
4400 Chavenelle Road, Dubuque, IA 52002-2655
Thermo Fisher Scientific Inc.   563-556-2241
2555 Kerper Blvd., Dubuque, IA 52001

Fairfield
Dexter Apache Holdings, Inc.   800-524-2954
2211 W. Grimes, Fairfield, IA 52556

Forest City
3m Company   641-585-2700
806 W. Crystal Lake Rd, Forest City, IA 50436

Fort Dodge
Burch Manufacturing Co., Inc.   515-573-4136
618 1st Avenue North, Fort Dodge, IA 50501-0876

George
Ranger All Season Corp.   800-225-3811
2002 Kingbird Ave., George, IA 51237

Harlan
Molded Products Inc.   800-435-8957
1112 Chatburn Ave., Harlan, IA 51537

Iowa City
Access Now Llc   800-351-8375
1337 Burns Avenue, Iowa City, IA 52240
Jim's Instrument Mfg., Inc.   319-351-3429
1910 South Gilbert St., Iowa City, IA 52240
Oral-B Laboratories, Inc.   800-566-7252
1832 Lower Muscantine Rd, Iowa City, IA 52240

Kalona
Civco Medical Instruments Co., Inc.   800.445.6741
102 First St. South, Kalona, IA 52247
Medtec   800-445-6741
102 First Street South, Kalona, IA 52247

Keokuk
Roquette America   319-524-5757
1417 Exchange St., PO Box 6647, Keokuk, IA 52632-6647

Lisbon
Lloyd Table Co.   319-455-2110
102-122 West Main St., Lisbon, IA 52253

Muscatine
Allsteel Inc.   800-624-9212
2210 Second Ave., Muscatine, IA 52761
Grain Processing Corporation   800-448-4472
1600 Oregon Street, Muscatine, IA 52761-1404

North Liberty
Compleware Corp.   800-369-8888
2865 Stoner Court, North Liberty, IA 52317

Perry
Percival Scientific Inc.   800-695-2743
505 Research Drive, Perry, IA 50220

Solon
Hansen Ophthalmic Development Lab., Inc.   319-338-1285
2590 Auburn Hills Ln. N.E., Solon, IA 52333

Spirit Lake
Brown Medical Industries   800-843-4395
1300 Lundberg Dr. W., Spirit Lake, IA 51360

Tiffin
Titronics Research & Development Co.   800-705-2307
400 Stephans Street, PO Box 470, Tiffin, IA 52340

Vinton
Frog Legs, Inc.   319-472-4972
500 East 6th St., Vinton, IA 52349

Washington
Rockwell Medical Technologies   248-960-9009
308 N. Iowa Street, Washington, IA 52353

Waterloo
Mowbray Co., Inc.   800-325-5787
706 Sheridan Road, Waterloo, IA 50701
Roskamp Champion   800-366-2563
2975 Airline Circle, Waterloo, IA 50703

Wayland
Md Orthopaedics   877-766-7384
604 North Parkway St, Wayland, IA 52654

West Des Moines
Medinotes Corporation   877-633-6683
1025 Ashworth Road, Suite 222, West Des Moines, IA 50265
Ramco Innovations/ Sunx Sensors   800-280-6933
PO Box 65310, 1207 Maple Street, West Des Moines, IA 50265

KANSAS

Atchison
Oceanic Medical Products, Inc.   913-874-2000
8005 Shannon Industrial Park, Ln., Atchison, KS 66002

Belleville
Scott Specialties, Inc./Cmo Inc./Ginny Inc.   800-255-7136
512 M St., Belleville, KS 66935-1546

Clay Center
Scott Specialties, Inc.   785-527-5627
1827 Meadowlark Rd., Clay Center, KS 67432

Concordia
Scott Specialties, Inc.   785-527-5627
1820 East 7th St., Concordia, KS 66901

Conway
Ferguson Production, Inc.   (620) 241-2400
2130 Industrial Drive, Conway, KS 67460

Council Grove
Monarch Molding Inc.   888-767-5116
120 Liberty St., Council Grove, KS 66846-1218

Dodge City
Pos-T-Vac, Inc.   800-279-7434
1701 North 14th Ave., P.O. Box 1436, Dodge City, KS 67801
V.T.S.,Inc.   620-227-7434
1701 N. 14th Ave., Dodge City, KS 67801

Edwardsville
Educational Software Concepts, Inc.   800-748-7734
660 S. Fourth St., Edwardsville, KS 66113-0267
Respond Industries, Inc.   1-800-523-8999
9500 Woodend Rd., Edwardsville, KS 66111

Ellis
Sunflower Medical L.L.C.   888-321-3382
206 Jerrerson, Ellis, KS 67637
Wheelchairs Of Kansas   800-537-6454
204 W. 2nd St., Ellis, KS 67637

Emporia
Daystar Manufacturing, Incorporated   620-342-4440
3701 W. 6th Avenue, Emporia, KS 66801

Gardner
Cramer Products, Inc.   1-800-345-2231
153 W. Warren, Gardner, KS 66030-1151

Great Bend
Primus Sterilizer Company, Llc.   620-793-7900
5520 10th Street, Great Bend, KS 67530

Highland
The Anthros Medical Group   785-544-6592
807 East Spring, Highland, KS 66035

Kansas City
Central Solutions, Inc.   913-621-6542
401 Funston Road, Kansas City, KS 66115
Chameleon Dental Products, Inc.   913-281-5552
200 North Sixth St., Kansas City, KS 66101
Dedicated Distribution   800-325-8367
640 Miami Avenue, Kansas City, KS 66105-2140
Enneking Medical Inc.   888-685-9699
10940 Parallel Parkway, K102, Kansas City, KS 66109
Knit-Rite, Inc.   800-821-3094
120 Osage Avenue, Kansas City, KS 66105
Leisure-Lift, Inc.   800-255-0285
1800 Merriam Lane, Kansas City, KS 66106-4714
Perform Manufacturing Incorporated   913-722-1557
1624 South 45th St., Kansas City, KS 66106
Therafirm, A Knit Rite Company   800-562-2701
120 Osage Avenue, Kansas City, KS 66105
Zutron Medical Llc   913-967-5943
2830 Roe Ln, Kansas City, KS 66103

Lawrence
Bct Midwest, Inc.   785-856-1414
1220 Wagon Wheel Road, Lawrence, KS 66049

Leander Health Technologies/Healthcare Division | 1-800-532-6337
315 N E Industrial Lane, Suite A, Lawrence, KS 66044

Leavenworth

Heatron, Inc. | 913-651-4420
3000 Wilson Ave., Leavenworth, KS 66048

Leawood

CholeraPrep | 800-523-0502
11400 Tomahawk Creek Pkwy, Suite 310, Leawood, KS 66211-2672
Innovative Medical Technologies, Inc. | 866-560-1820
15059 Cedar St., Leawood, KS 66224
Tan Source Supply, Inc. | 913-451-7000
12142a State Line Rd., Leawood, KS 66209

Lenexa

Airgas Specialty Gases | 913-495-3621
9851 Widmer Rd., Lenexa, KS 66215
Ameret Llc | 913-888-5248
9025 Rosehill, Lenexa, KS 66215
Beyond 21st Century Inc. | 888-484-2587
13706 W. 75th Pl., Lenexa, KS 66216-4229
Central Biomedia, Inc. | 800-448-0016
9900 Pflumm Rd., Unit 61-63, Lenexa, KS 66215
Dyna-Tek, Inc. | 913-438-6363
8369 Nieman Rd., Lenexa, KS 66214
Entracare, Llc | 913-451-2234
11315 Strang Line Rd., Lenexa, KS 66215
Felton International, Inc. | 913-599-1590
8210 Marshall Dr., Lenexa, KS 66214
Hearing Today Laboratory, Inc. | 877-888-6336
11954 West 95th St., Lenexa, KS 66215
Lsi Intl., Inc. | 913-894-4493
11529 W. 79th St, Lenexa, KS 66214
Lynn Peavey Co. | 800-255-6499
10749 West 84th Terrace, P.O. Box 14100, Lenexa, KS 66215
Medical Design Systems, Inc. | 800-593-1900
14560 W. 99th St., Lenexa, KS 66215
Mediware Information Systems, Inc. | 800-255-0026
11711 W 79th Street, Lenexa, KS 66214
Nexus Medical, Llc | 913-451-2234
11315 Strang Line Road, Lenexa, KS 66215
Parmelee Industries, Inc. | 800-821-5218
8101 Lenexa Drive, Lenexa, KS 66214
Remel | 800-255-6730
12076 Santa Fe Drive, Lenexa, KS 66215-3519
Safc Biosciences, Inc. | 1 800-255-6032
13804 West 107th St., Lenexa, KS 66215
Turntine Ocular Prosthetics, Inc | 913-962-6299
6342 Long, Suite H, Lenexa, KS 66216
Vitalograph, Inc. | 800-255-6626
13310 W 99th Street, Lenexa, KS 66215
Wisap America | 800-233-8448
8231 Melrose Drive, Lenexa, KS 66214

Mcpherson

Hospira, Inc. | 877-946-7747
1776 North Centennial Drive, Mcpherson, KS 67460

Merriam

Medical Solutions International, Inc. | 757-224-0177
5646 Merriam Drive, Merriam, KS 66203

Mission

Aci | 913-384-7390
5830 Woodson, Suite 3, Mission, KS 66202
Hansen Dental Lab | 952-541-9622
6700 Squibb Road, Suite 208, Mission, KS 66202

Newton

Full Vision, Inc. | 316-283-3344
3017 Full Vision Dr., Newton, KS 67114
Keyes Manufacturing & Supply Llc. | 316-284-2200
2015 West 1st, Newton, KS 67114
Trac About, Inc. | 800-458-8616
PO Box 502, 1801 SE 9th St., Newton, KS 67114-0502

Olathe

Cc Medical Devices, Inc. | 913-269-8400
14131 S. Mur Len Rd., Olathe, KS 66062
Dci, Inc. | 913.647.0158
846 N Mart-Way Court, Olathe, KS 66061
Elecsys Corporation | 913-647-0158
846 N. Mart-way Court, Olathe, KS 66061
Heritage Labs Intl., Llc | 913-764-1045
1111 West Old 56 Hwy., Olathe, KS 66061
Sunrise Medical Hhg Inc | 303-218-4505
2010 E Spruce Cir, Olathe, KS 66062

Oskaloosa

Biocore Medical Technologies, Inc. | 301-740-1893
13851 90th Street, Oskaloosa, KS 66066

Overland Park

Acadental | 888-585-0678
9204 Bond Street, Overland Park, KS 66214
Airgas-Mid South, Inc. | 918-582-0885
9101 Bond St., Overland Park, KS 66214
Corridor Group, Inc., The | 800-343-4163
6405 Metcalf, Ste. 108, Overland Park, KS 66202
Escreen, Inc. | 800-881-0722
7500 W. 110th Street, Suite 500, Overland Park, KS 66210
George King Bio-Medical, Inc. | 800-255-5108
11771 W. 112th St., Overland Park, KS 66210-4192
Waterclave, L.L.C. | 913-312-5860
6731 West 121st St., Overland Park, KS 66209

Salina

Acustep, Inc. | 866-465-2500
2775 A Arnold Ave., Salina, KS 67401
Occk, Inc. | 800-526-9731
1710 West Schilling Road, Salina, KS 67401

Shawnee

Hans Rudolph, Inc. | 913-422-7788
8325 Cole Parkway, Shawnee, KS 66227

Shawnee Mission

Breathe E-Z Systems, Inc. | 800-490-5052
P.O. Box 7813, Shawnee Mission, KS 66207

South Hutchinson

Collins Bus Corporation | 800-354-9802
415 W. 6th St., P.O. Box 2946, South Hutchinson, KS 67504-2946

Topeka

Discovery Engineering Intl., Inc. | 785-272-3781
3115 S.w. Westwood Dr., Topeka, KS 66614
Duffens Optical | 800-432-2475
400 S.E. Quincy Street, Topeka, KS 66603
Heumann & Associates Dental Lab | 800-255-2412
520 East Fifth St., Topeka, KS 66607
Lohmann & Rauscher, Inc. | 800-279-3863
6001 SW Sixth Avenue, Suite #101, Topeka, KS 66615-1004
Marketing International, Inc. | 800-447-0173
P.O. Box 4835, Topeka, KS 66604-0835
Solid State Sonics & Electronics, Inc. | 785-232-0497
4137 Lower Silver Lake Rd, Topeka, KS 66618

Valley Center

Aero Innovative Research, Inc. | 316-755-3477
500 W. Clay St, Valley Center, KS 67147

Wichita

Criss Optical Manufacturing Co., Inc. | 800-835-2023
3628 S.West St., Wichita, KS 67217
Gift Sales Co. | 800-992-0181
517 South St. Francis, Wichita, KS 67217
Henthorn Ocular Prosthetics | 316-688-5235
744 South Hillside, Wichita, KS 67211
Micro Air Air Cleaners By Metal-Fab | 800-835-2830
PO Box 1138, Wichita, KS 67201-1138
Mid-States Laboratories, Inc. | 800-247-3669
600 N Saint Francis, Wichita, KS 67202-2102
Pearce-Turk Dental Lab | 800-835-2776
201 North Emporia, Wichita, KS 67202
Plaza Towel Holder, Inc. | 877-874-8394
P.O. Box 4737, Wichita, KS 67204
Professional Hearing Aid Service | 316-942-4992
851 North West St., Wichita, KS 67203

KENTUCKY

Bowling Green

Sca Personal Care, North America | 270-796-9300
7030 Louisville Rd., Bowling Green, KY 42103
Sca Personal Care, North America | 270-796-9300
7030 Louisville Road, Bowling Green, KY 42101

Brandenburg

Restorative Medical, Inc. | 270-422-5454
332 E Broadway, Brandenburg, KY 40108

Calhoun

Muster Associates, Inc. | 800-274-3619
135 E. 3rd St., Calhoun, KY 42327

Columbia

Image Analysis, Inc. | 800-548-4849
1380 Burkesville St., Columbia, KY 42728

Covington

Continental Hydrodyne Systems, Inc. | 800-543-9283
1025 Mary Laidley Drive, Covington, KY 41017
R. A. Jones & Co., Inc. | 859-341-0400
2701 Crescent Springs Rd., Covington, KY 41017

Crescent Springs

Kbd, Inc.   800-544-3757
2550 American Ct, Crescent Springs, KY 41017
Kbd, Inc.   859-331-0800
2550 American Ct., Crescent Springs, KY 41017

Danville

Anodia Systems   866.246.2548
109 Larrimore Lane, Danville, KY 40422

Erlanger

Post Glover Lifelink   800-287-4123
167 Gap Way., Erlanger, KY 41018
Union Springs Pharmaceuticals   877-462-5967
4157 Olympic Blvd, Suite 200, Erlanger, KY 41018

Florence

Beckman Coulter, Inc.   305-380-4079
7381 Empire Dr., Florence, KY 41042
Littleford Day, Inc.   800-365-8555
PO Box 128, Florence, KY 41042

Glenview

Aptis Medical, Llc.   502-523-6738
3602 Glenview Ave, Glenview, KY 40025

Hebron

Carl Zeiss Vision Inc.   707-763-9911
1030 Worldwide Blvd., Hebron, KY 41048
Carl Zeiss Vision-Kentucky   866-289-7652
1050 World Wide Blvd., Hebron, KY 41048
Lohmann Corporation   1 859 334 4900
3000 Earhart Court, Ste. 155, Hebron, KY 41048
Tente Casters, Inc.   800-783-2470
2266 Southpark Drive, Hebron, KY 41048

La Center

S.P. Artificial Eye Co.   270-665-5515
374 Broadway, La Center, KY 42056

La Grange

White Bite, Inc.   502-222-2647
5006 Hickory Hill Dr., La Grange, KY 40031

Lexington

Alt Bioscience,Llc   859-231-3061
235 Bolivar St., Lexington, KY 40508
Bluegrass Vascular Technologies   -
163 E. Main Street, Suite 300, Lexington, KY 40507
Gibson Laboratories   800-477-4763
1040 Manchester St., Lexington, KY 40508-2422
Gibson Laboratories, Inc.   800-477-4763
1040 Manchester St., Lexington, KY 40508
Lawrence-Nelson, Llc   859-252-0335
325 Virginia Ave., Lexington, KY 40504
Medpro Safety Products, Inc.   859-225-5375
145 Rose Street, Lexington, KY 40507
Molding Solutions   859-231-0031
781 Enterprise Dr., Lexington, KY 40510
Qed, Inc.   859-231-0338
750 Enterprise Dr., Lexington, KY 40510
Scott-Gross Co., Inc.   800-967-6874
664 Magnolia Ave., Lexington, KY 40505-3706
Stephens Instruments, Inc.   800-354-7848
2500 Sandersville Rd, Lexington, KY 40511
Tempur-Medical, Inc.   888-255-3302
1713 Jaggie Fox Way, Lexington, KY 40511
U.S. Iol, Inc.   800-354-7848
2500 Sandersville Rd., Lexington, KY 40583

Louisville

Aaf International   800-477-1214
10300 Ormsby Park Place, Louisville, KY 40223
Abracair, Llc   502-445-9471
204 N.17th Street, Louisville, KY 40203
American Printing House For The Blind, Inc.   800-223-1839
PO Box 6085, Louisville, KY 40206-0085
Aquatic Access, Inc.   800-325-5438
1921 Production Drive, Louisville, KY 40223
Cardinal Medical Specialties, Inc.   502-969-9652
4708 Pinewood Rd., Louisville, KY 40218
D.R.E., Inc.   800-462-8195
1800 Williamson Ct., Louisville, KY 40223
Dispensers Optical Service Corp.   800-626-4545
1815 Plantside Dr., Louisville, KY 40299
Donell   800-324-7455
1801 Taylor Avenue, Louisville, KY 40213
Electronic Design & Research Co., Inc.   502-433-8660
7331 Intermodal Dr., Louisville, KY 40258
Fibreworks Corporation   800-843-0063
2417 Data Drive, Louisville, KY 40299
Glenn Reams, Ocularist   800-426-8995
610 South Floyd, Louisville, KY 40202

Gould Discount Medical   800-876-6846
3901 Dutchmans LN #100, Louisville, KY 40207
Jabil Global Services   502-240-1000
11201 Electron Dr., Louisville, KY 40299
Junkin Safety Appliance Co., Inc.   502-775-8303
3121 Millers Ln., Louisville, KY 40216
Linak U.S. Inc.   502-253-5595
2200 Stanley Gault Pkwy., Louisville, KY 40223
Med-Dyne   502-429-4140
2775 South Floyd Street, Louisville, KY 40209-1817
Nbm Llc   502-895-7503
2604 River Green Circle, Louisville, KY 40206
Olsen Medical   800-297-6344
3001 W. Kentucky St., Louisville, KY 40211-1505
Optical Dynamics Corporation   800-587-2743
1950 Production Ct, Louisville, KY 40299
Sea-Long Medical Systems, Inc.   502-969-4949
1983 South Park Rd., Louisville, KY 40219
Stonestreet One   502-708-3500
9960 Corporate Campus Drive, Louisville, KY 40223
The Lyons Companies   502-267-0087
11401 Electron Dr., Louisville, KY 40299-3857
Vision Optics Technologies Ltd.   866-671-0735
1816 Production Court, Louisville, KY 40299
Whip-Mix Corporation   800-626-5651
361 farmington Avenue, PO Box 17183, Louisville, KY 40217-0183
Wire Crafters L.L.C.   800-924-9473
6208 Strawberry Lane, Louisville, KY 40214-2929

Mt. Sterling

Rogers Foam Corporation   859-497-0702
120 Clarence Dr., Woodland Industrial Park, Mt. Sterling, KY 40353

Owensboro

Cmi, Inc.   270-685-6200
316 East Ninth St., Owensboro, KY 42303
Glenn Reams, Ocularist   800-426-8995
2845 Farrell Crescent, Owensboro, KY 42303

Paducah

I.B.S. (Ice Bag Support)   270-443-0443
1117 North 8th St., Suite 201, Paducah, KY 42001

Paris

AVANTOR PERFORMANCE MATERIALS, INC.   800-582-2537
7001 Martin Luther King Blvd, Paris, KY 40361

Raceland

Medical Collar Covers, Inc.   606-836-2575
600 Greenup Ave. Suite 101, Raceland, KY 41169

Shepherdsville

Emergency Medical Supply, Inc.   502-955-9233
238 Saltwell Rd., P.o.. Box 99, Shepherdsville, KY 40165

Simpsonville

Isopure Corp.   800-280-7873
141 Citizens Blvd., Simpsonville, KY 40067

Webbville

U S Biotex Corp.   606-652-4700
Route 1 Box 62, Webbville, KY 41180

Wilder

Retroactive Bioscience   859-431-4660
One Moock Road, Suite 3, Wilder, KY 41071

LOUISIANA

Baton Rouge

Anomeric, Inc.   225-268-3052
755 Delgado Dr., Baton Rouge, LA 70808
Electro Medical Equipment Co., Inc.   800-423-2926
12015 Industriplex Blvd., Baton Rouge, LA 70809
National Hansen's Disease Programs   225-756-3740
1770 Physicians Park Drive, Baton Rouge, LA 70816
Reditac Medical Usa, Llc   225-923-3592
1555 Cottondale Drive, Suite 4, Baton Rouge, LA 70815-4162
Safecare Corporation   225-753-4664
6352 Quinn Drive Suite A, Baton Rouge, LA 70817
Stars   225-752-4912
6630 Exchequer Drive, Baton Rouge, LA 70809
Technology Delivery Systems, Inc.   866-629-4359
Lsu-emtc Bldg, 340, East Parker St., Suite 240, Baton Rouge, LA 70808
Universal Pacs, Inc.   225-766-9381
127 Albert Hart Drive, Baton Rouge, LA 70808-6702

Covington

Cimex Medical Innovations, Llc   985-871-0802
72385 Industry Park, Covington, LA 70435

Edgerly (vinton)

Alpha-Omega Services, Inc. 562-804-0604
1282 Big Woods-stark Rd., Edgerly (vinton), LA 70668

Harahan

General Hearing Instruments, Inc. 800-824-3021
175 Brookhollow Espl., Harahan, LA 70123
Lee Medical International, Inc. 800-433-8950
612 Distributors Row, Harahan, LA 70123

Jefferson

Medical Imaging Solutions, Inc. 504-733-9729
800 Central Ave., Jefferson, LA 70121

Kenner

General Biomedical Service, Inc. 800-558-9449
1900 25th St., Kenner, LA 70062
Pellerin Milnor Corp. 800-469-8780
PO Box 400, Kenner, LA 70063-0400
Tucker Designs Limited 800-780-7979
PO Box 641117, Kenner, LA 70064

Lafayette

Atlantis Luminescent Products, Llc 318-894-9490
1405 Pinhook Rd., Suite 205, Lafayette, LA 70503
Billedeaux Hearing Center, Llc 337-989-4327
4414 Johnson St. Ste. D, Lafayette, LA 70503
Oncology Automation, Inc. 337-998-6837
105 Water Oaks Dr., Lafayette, LA 70503
Venoscope, LLC 337-234-8993
1018 Harding St., Suite 104, Lafayette, LA 70503
Venoscope, Llc 800-284-7655
1018 Harding Street, Suite 104, Lafayette, LA 70503

Lake Charles

Borel Enterprises Llc 337-583-3448
3664 A. Miller Rd., Lake Charles, LA 70605
Read Dental Lab 337-496-3706
1508 Ford St., Lake Charles, LA 70601
Remel-Lake Charles, Division Of Remel Inc. 800-256-4376
3941 Ryan St., Lake Charles, LA 70605

Madisonville

Second Exposure, Inc. 985-845-0933
P.O. Box 609, Madisonville, LA 70447

Mandeville

We Care Design's, L.L.C. 504-624-8282
428 Bill Dr., Mandeville, LA 70448

Metairie

American Health Care Systems, Inc. 504-831-4867
3350 Ridgelake Ave., Suite 255, Metairie, LA 70002

Monroe

Aoss Medical Supply, Inc. 318-325-8290
4971 Central Ave., Monroe, LA 71203
Monroe Mfg., Inc. 318-338-3172
3030 Aurora Ave., 2nd Fl., Monroe, LA 71201
Thermal Logic, Inc. 318-345-5603
204 Timber Lane, Monroe, LA 71203

New Orleans

Intelifuse, Inc. 504-561-1100
1515 Poydras St. Suite 1490, New Orleans, LA 70112
Maxiflex, Llc 866-629-4359
1516 Thalia St, New Orleans, LA 70130
Val Med 800-242-5355
Ace Bayou Group, 3700 Desire Pkwy., New Orleans, LA 70126

Opelousas

Vision Pro Llc 800-892-3937
4309 I-49 South Service Road, Opelousas, LA 70570

Saint Rose

Source Production & Equipment Co., Inc. 504-464-9471
113 Teal St., Saint Rose, LA 70087

Shreveport

Sage Pharmaceuticals, Inc. 318-635-1594
5408 Interstate Dr., Shreveport, LA 71109

Thibodaux

Martin-Mars, Inc. 985-438-4402
415 Camelia Drive, Thibodaux, LA 70301-6508

Ventress

Timely Neuropathy Testing, Llc 225-638-5343
9553 Island Rd, Ventress, LA 70783

West Monroe

Protex Medical Products, Inc. 877-776-8395
913 Wood St., P.O. Box 2172, West Monroe, LA 71291

MAINE

Auburn

Maine Oxy-Acetylene Supply Co. 207-784-5788
22 Albiston Way, Auburn, ME 04210
Riley Medical, Inc. 800-245-3300
27 Wrights Landing, Auburn, ME 04210
Tambrands Manufacturing, Inc. 513-634-2466
2879 Hotel Rd., Auburn, ME 04210

Bangor

Trillium Diagnostics, Llc. 866-364-0028
246 Sylvan Rd., Bangor, ME 04401

Bowdoin

Fhc, Inc 800-326-2905
1201 Main Street, Bowdoin, ME 04287

Castine

Active Corporation 207-326-9100
PO Box 1000, 15 Main Street, Castine, ME 04421-1000

Fryeburg

Physician Engineered Products, Inc. 800-622-6240
103 Smith Street, Fryeburg, ME 04037

Gorham

Controlled Environment Equipment Corp. 800-569-5444
59 Sanford Drive, Suite 32, Gorham, ME 04038-2647

Gray

Spirometrics Medical Equipment Co., Llc 207-657-6700
22 Shaker Road, Gray, ME 04039
Syris Scientific 800-714-1374
22 Shaker Road, Gray, ME 04039

Guilford

Puritan Medical Products Company Llc 800-321-2313
31 School St., Guilford, ME 04443-0149

Kennebunk

Corning Inc., Life Sciences 207-985-5310
2 Alfred Rd., Kennebunk, ME 04043

Limington

Kristi-Care, Inc. 207-637-2672
110 Millturn Rd., Limington, ME 04049

Livermore Falls

Pine Tree Orthopedic Lab L.L.C. 207-897-5558
175 Park Street, Livermore Falls, ME 04254

Millinocket

Cyr Designs, Llc 207-723-6766
112 New York St, Millinocket, ME 04462

Pittsfield

Oxus Environmental, Llc 207-487-5300
264 Industrial Park Street, Pittsfield, ME 04967

Portland

Alerchek, Inc. 877-282-9542
203 Anderson St., Portland, ME 04101
Bioprocessing, Inc. 207-615-0571
1045 Riverside St, Portland, ME 04103
Immucell Corp. 800-466-8235
56 Evergreen Dr., Portland, ME 04103-5907
Lighthouse Imaging Corp. 207-253-5350
477 Congress St., Portland, ME 04101
Maine Anti-Gravity Systems, Inc. 207-775-3800
98 Gray St., Portland, ME 04102
Maine Biotechnology Services, Inc. 207-797-5454
1037 R Forest Ave., Portland, ME 04103
Solidphase, Inc. 207-797-0211
1039 Riverside Street Suite 3, Portland, ME 04103
Solstice Corp. 207-874-7922
68 Marginal Way, 4th Floor, Portland, ME 04101

Rockland

Lonza Rockland, Inc. 207-594-3400
191 Thomaston St., Rockland, ME 04841

Saco

Meridian Life Science, Inc. 888-530-0140
60 Industrial Park Road, Saco, ME 04072

Sanford

Baker Company, The 800-992-2537
161 Gatehouse Rd., P.O. Drawer E, Sanford, ME 04073
Guitar Suspension Solutions 207-324-5717
183A Jagger Mill Road, Sanford, ME 04073-2467

Scarborough

American Healthcare 888-567-7733
6 Lincoln Avenue, Scarborough, ME 04074

Maine Molecular Quality Controls, Inc. — 207-885-1072
10 Southgate Road, Suite 170, Scarborough, ME 04074

Skowhegan

Solon Manufacturing Co. — 800-341-6640
338 Madison Avenue, Suite 7, Skowhegan, ME 04976

South Portland

Portland Welding Supply — 207-772-3036
40 Madison St., South Portland, ME 04106

Westbrook

Artel, Inc. — 207-854-0860
25 Bradley Dr., Westbrook, ME 04092
H. A. Stiles Co. — 800-447-8537
170 Forest St., Westbrook, ME 04092
Idexx Laboratories, Inc. — 800-548-6733
1 Idexx Dr., Westbrook, ME 04092

Windham

Audio — 207-893-2920
885 Roosevelt Trail, Windham, ME 04062
Finetone Hearing Instruments — 207-893-2920
885 Roosevelt Trail, Windham, ME 04062
Maine Standards Company, Llc — 800-377-9684
765 Roosevelt Trail, Suite 9A, Windham, ME 04062-5365

Winslow

Northeast Laboratory Services, Inc. — 800-244-8378
227 China Road, Winslow, ME 04901

Wiscasset

Rynel, Inc. — 207-882-0200
11 Twin Rivers Dr, Wiscasset, ME 04578

MARYLAND

Annapolis

Dms — 410-757-8400
530 College Pkwy., Suite D, Annapolis, MD 21409

Annapolis Junction

Georgia Steel & Chemical Company, Inc. — 800-296-0351
10810 Guilford Rd., Suite 104, Annapolis Junction, MD 20701

Baltimore

Aerosol And Liquid Packaging, Inc. — 410-342-6100
715 S. Haven St., Baltimore, MD 21224
Alpha Biosciences, Inc. — 877-825-7428
3651 Clipper Mill Road, Baltimore, MD 21211-1991
Autogenesis, Inc. — 888-325-2017
8700 Old Harford Road, Baltimore, MD 21218
Bioscience Contract Production Corp. — 410-563-9200
5901 E. Lombard Street, Baltimore, MD 21224
C.D. Denison Orthopaedic Appliance Corp. — 410-235-9645
220 W. 28th St., Baltimore, MD 21211-3089
Cert Health Sciences, Llc — 866-990-4444
7036 Golden Ring Rd., Baltimore, MD 21237
Cochran, Stephenson & Donkervoet, Inc. Architects — 410-539-2080
323 W. Camden St., Ste. 700, The Warehouse at Camden Yards, Baltimore, MD 21201-8601
Csa Medical, Inc. — 866.481.7786
1101 E 33rd Street, Third Floor, Ste. E305, Baltimore, MD 21218
Exami-Gowns, Inc. — 800-962-4696
8647 Ridgely's Choice Drive, Baltimore, MD 21236
Haemo-Sol, Inc. — 800-821-5676
7301 York Rd., Baltimore, MD 21204-7631
I.Z.I. Medical Products, Inc. — 800-231-1499
7020 Tudsbury Road, Baltimore, MD 21244
IZI Medical Products — 800-231-1499
7020 Tudsbury Road, Baltimore, MD 21244
Individual Monitoring Systems, Inc. — 410-296-7723
1055 Taylor Ave., Suite 300, Baltimore, MD 21286
Jkruz Inc. — 410-444-2944
7315 Harford Rd., Baltimore, MD 21234
Medical Supplies Corporation T/A.Roberts Manufacturing Co., — 800-451-9951
4002 Dillon Street, Baltimore, MD 21224
Met Laboratories, Inc. — 800-638-6057
914 W. Patapsco Avenue, Baltimore, MD 21230-3432
National Instrument Co., Inc. — 866-258-1914
4119 Fordleigh Rd., Baltimore, MD 21215-2214
National Instrument Llc — 866-258-1914
4119 Fordleigh Road, Baltimore, MD 21215
Neu-Ion, Inc. — 800-678-4360
7200 Rutherford Rd., Suite 100, Baltimore, MD 21244-2704
Paramark Corporation — 443-436-9400
2605 Lord Baltimore Dr., Suite H, Baltimore, MD 21244
Razorall Incorporated — 410-585-1395
7301 Park Heights Ave., Suite 207, Baltimore, MD 21208-5407
Restorative Therapies Inc. — (800) 609-9166
907 South Lakewood Ave., Baltimore, MD 21224

Rockland Industries, Inc. — 800-876-2566
1601 Edison Hwy., Baltimore, MD 21213
Simon & Company Inc., H.R. — 800-638-9460
3515 Marmenco Ct., Baltimore, MD 21230-3411
Sunrise Medical Hhg Inc — 303-218-4505
7128 Ambassasor Rd., Baltimore, MD 21244
Univec, Inc. — 410-347-9959
4810 Seton Dr., Baltimore, MD 21215
Visicu, Inc. — 410-276-1960
217 E. Redwood St., Ste. 1900, Baltimore, MD 21202
Washington Biotechnology, Inc. — 410-633-7449
6200 Seaforth Street, Baltimore, MD 21224-6506

Beltsville

Bio-Reg Associates, Inc. — 301-623-2500
11800 Baltimore Avenue, Suite 105, Beltsville, MD 20705-1561

Bethesda

Bio-Brite, Inc. — 800-621-5483
4330 East-West Hwy., Suite 310, Bethesda, MD 20814
Biotrac, Inc. — 301-496-8290
1 Cloister Court, building 60 Room 237, Bethesda, MD 20833
BrainScope Company Inc. — 240-752-7680
8120 Woodmont Avenue, Suite 250, Bethesda, MD 20814
Center For Ocular Reconstruction — (800) 982-EYES
4833 Rugby Ave., 4th Flr., Bethesda, MD 20814
Chindex International, Inc. — 301-215-7777
4340 East West Highway, Suite 1100, Bethesda, MD 20814
Media Cybernetics Inc. — 301-495-3305
4340 East-West Hwy, Suite 400, Bethesda, MD 20814
Salmon Medical Innovations, Llc — 866-268-3376
5017 Worthington Drive, Bethesda, MD 20816
Venes Technology Corp. — 800-777-4974
6701 Democracy Blvd. Ste # 300., Bethesda, MD 20817

Burtonsville

Lifeclinic International, Inc. — 301-476-9888
4032 Blackburn Lane, Burtonsville, MD 20866

Cambridge

Air Liquide America Corporation, Cambridge Div. — 800-638-1197
821 Chesapeake Dr., Cambridge, MD 21613
Camtec — 410-228-1156
1959 Church Creek Rd., Cambridge, MD 21613

Centreville

A.R.C. Distributors — 800-296-8724
PO Box 599, Centreville, MD 21617

Chestertown

Aerscher Diagnostics — 410-778-1144
353 High St., Chestertown, MD 21620
Lamotte Chemical Products Company — 800-344-3100
802 Washington Ave., Chestertown, MD 21620
Lamotte Co. — 800-344-3100
802 Washington Avenue, PO Box 329, Chestertown, MD 21620

Chevy Chase

Victor O. Schinnerer & Company, Inc. — 301-961-9800
2 Wisconsin Circle, Chevy Chase, MD 20815-7003

Cockeysville

Becton, Dickinson & Co — 410-316-4000
250 Schilling Circle, Cockeysville, MD 21030
Warner Graham Co., The — 800-872-2300
160 Church Lane, Cockeysville, MD 21030-4921

Columbia

Advanced Biotechnologies, Inc. — 800-426-0764
9108 Guilford Rd., Rivers Park II, Columbia, MD 21046-2701
Celsion Corporation — 800-262-0394
10220-L Old Columbia Road, Columbia, MD 21046-1705
Cylex, Inc. — 888-33-CYEX
8980-i Old Annapolis Rd., Columbia, MD 21045
Eyetel Imaging, Inc. — 888-222-3875
9130 Guilford Rd., Columbia, MD 21046
Fotofinder Systems, Inc. — 443-283-3865
9693 Gerwig Lane, Suite S, Columbia, MD 21046
Hemagen Diagnostics, Inc. — 800-436-2436
9033 Red Branch Rd., Columbia, MD 21045
Mehlrose Associates — 410-730-0263
11660-304 Little Patuxent Pkwy, Columbia, MD 21044
New Horizons Diagnostics Corporation — 410-992-9357
9110 Red Branch Road, Suite B, Columbia, MD 21045
Nucletron Corporation — 800-336-2249
8671A,AÿRobertA,AÿFultonA,AÿDrive, Columbia, MD 21046-2133
Polylc Inc. — 410-992-5400
9151 Rumsey Rd., Ste. 180, Columbia, MD 21045
Segami Corporation — 410-381-2311
8325 Guilford Rd., Suite B, Columbia, MD 21046
W. R. Grace & Co.-Conn — 410-531-4000
7500 Grace Drive, Columbia, MD 21044

Crofton

Bhs International, Inc. — 410-721-5055
2431 Crofton Lane, Ste.9, Crofton, MD 21114
Enternet Medical, Inc. — 888-887-6638
1676 village green, Crofton, MD 21114
North American Marketing, Inc. — (410) 721-8803
2127 Espey Court, Suite 220, Crofton, MD 21114

Cumberland

Triaid, Inc. — 301-759-3525
637 North Centre St., Cumberland, MD 21502

Damascus

Henley Board, Inc. — 800-874-0552
P.O. Box 92, Damascus, MD 20872

Darnestown

Innovative Therapies, Inc. — 866-484-6798
8-2 Metropolitan Court, Darnestown, MD 20878

Denton

Uber Lucas Intl Llc — 410-758-3181
11126 Tuckahoe Rd., Denton, MD 21629

Dickerson

Neutron Products Inc — 800-424-8169
22301 Mt. Ephraim Road, Box 68, Dickerson, MD 20842
Neutron Products, Inc. — 301-349-5001
22301 Mt. Ephraim Rd., Dickerson, MD 20842

Easton

B/R Instrument Corp. — 800-922-9206
9119 Centreville Road, Easton, MD 21601
Jasco, Inc. — 800-333-5272
28600 Mary's Court, Easton, MD 21601
Konsyl Pharmaceuticals, Inc. — 800-356-6795
8050 Industrial Park Road, Easton, MD 21601
Midshore Industries, Inc. — 410-822-8622
29526 Canvasback Drive, Easton, MD 21601

Eldersburg

Industrial Municipal Equipment, Inc. — 410-795-0500
1430 Progress Way, Suite 105, Eldersburg, MD 21784

Elkton

Colonial Metals, Inc. — 410-398-7200
505 Blue Ball Rd., Bldg. 20, Elkton, MD 21921
Plasticoid Co., The — 410-398-2800
249 W. High St., Elkton, MD 21921-5235
Terumo Cardiovascular Systems (Tcvs) — 800-283-7866
125 Blue Ball Road, Elkton, MD 21921
Terumo Medical Corporation — 800-283-7866
950 Elkton Blvd., P.O.Box 605, Elkton, MD 21921
W.L. Gore & Associates, Inc., Sealant — 410-392-3200
Technologies Group
301 airport rd., Elkton, MD 21921

Essex

Consolidated Instruments Corp. — 410-391-9116
8825 Kelso Dr., Essex, MD 21221

Fallston

Telos Medical Equipment (Austin & Assoc., Inc.) — 800-934-3029
1109 Sturbridge Road, Fallston, MD 21047-1905

Frederick

Akonni Biosystems — 301-698-0101
400 Sagner Ave, Suite 300, Frederick, MD 21701
Biomat Sciences, Inc. — 866-4-BIOMAT
7210A Corporate Court, Frederick, MD 21703
Bone Density Measurement International, Llc — 301-631-0008
550 Highland St., Suite 303, Frederick, MD 21701
Diagnostic Health Group — 800-669-3442
PO Box 747, Frederick, MD 21703
Health & Radiological Seminars, Inc. — 800-969-4774
550 Highland St., Suite 100, Frederick, MD 21701
Intracel Corporation — 301-668-8400
93 Monocacy Blvd., Unit A8, Frederick, MD 21701
Life Technologies Corporation — 301-840-8000
7300 Governors Way, Frederick, MD 21704
Reeves Emergency Management Systems, Llc. — 301-698-1596
1704 W. 7th Street, Frederick, MD 21702
Sci International Inc. — 301-696-8879
5902 Enterprise Court, Frederick, MD 21703
Trans-Type Of Maryland, Inc. — 301-695-7087
108 Byte Drive, Suite 101, Frederick, MD 21702

Gaithersburg

American Fluoroseal Corp. — 800-360-1050
431-A East Diamond Avenue, Gaithersburg, MD 20877
American Red Cross Diagnostic Manufacturing Divisi — 202-303-5640
9319 Gaither Rd., Gaithersburg, MD 20877
Bioveris Corporation — 800-336-4436
16020 Industrial Dr., Gaithersburg, MD 20877
Brandel — 800-948-6506
8561 Atlas Dr., Gaithersburg, MD 20877-4135
Dexall Biomedical Labs, Inc. — 301-840-1884
18904 Bonanza Way, Gaithersburg, MD 20879
Gene Logic — 800-436-3564
50 West Watkins Mill Road, Gaithersburg, MD 20878
Immersion Medical — 800-929-4709
55 West Watkins Mill Rd., Gaithersburg, MD 20878
Lkc Technologies, Inc. — 800-638-7055
2 Professional Drive, Suite 222, Gaithersburg, MD 20879-3485
MaxCyte Inc. — 301-944-1700
22 Firstfield Road, Suite 110, Gaithersburg, MD 20878
National Institute Of Standards & Technology — 301-975-6776
100 Bureau Drive, Stop 2322, Bldg. 202, Rm. 204, Gaithersburg, MD 20899-2322
Orthodontic Supply & Equipment Co., Inc. — 800-638-4003
7851 Airpark Road, Unit 202, Gaithersburg, MD 20879-4123
Perkin Elmer Wallac, Inc. — 800-638-6692
9238 Gaither Rd., Gaithersburg, MD 20877-1486
Qiagen Gaithersburg, Inc. — 800-344-3631
1201 Clopper Rd., Gaithersburg, MD 20878
Roberts Oxygen Co., Inc. — 301-315-9090
17011 Railroad St., Gaithersburg, MD 20877
Roboz Surgical Instrument Co., Inc. — 800-424-2984
PO Box 10710, Gaithersburg, MD 20898-0710
Sunbox Company — 800-548-3968
19217 Orbit Dr., Gaithersburg, MD 20879
Virotech International, Inc. — 301-924-8000
12 Meem Ave., Suite C, Gaithersburg, MD 20877

Germantown

Medispec Ltd. - Usa — 888-663-3477
20410 Observation Drive, Suite # 102, Germantown, MD 20876
Optelecom-Nkf, Inc — 800-293-4237
12920 Cloverleaf Center Drive, Germantown, MD 20874
Qiagen Sciences, Inc. — 301-944-7090
19300 Germantown Rd., Germantown, MD 20874
SuperNova Diagnostics, Inc — 301-792-4345
20271 Goldenrod Lane, Suite 2028, Germantown, MD 20876

Glen Arm

Lenox Laser — 800-494-6537
12530 Manor Road, Glen Arm, MD 21057

Glen Burnie

Ambu A/S — 800-262-8462
6740 Baymeadow Dr., Glen Burnie, MD 21060
Ambu, Inc. — 800-262-8462
6740 Baymeadow Drive, Glen Burnie, MD 21060
Future Medical Systems, Inc. — 800-367-6021
504 McCormick Drive Suite T, Glen Burnie, MD 21061-3254
NovaSom, Inc. — 1-877-753-3775
801 Cromwell Park Drive, Suite 108, Glen Burnie, MD 21061

Glencoe

Arthrowave Medical Technologies, Llc — 410-472-0360
53 Loveton Circle, Suite 207, Glencoe, MD 21152

Hagerstown

Action Products, Inc. — 800-228-7763
954 Sweeney Drive, Hagerstown, MD 21740-4997
Crist Instrument Co., Inc. — 301-393-8615
111 W. First St., Hagerstown, MD 21740
Ear Lab — 301-790-3300
363 South Cleveland Ave., Hagerstown, MD 21740

Hampstead

Bell-More Labs, Inc. — 410-239-7554
4030 Gill Ave., Hampstead, MD 21074

Hanover

Aerosol Monitoring & Analysis, Inc. — 410-684-3327
1331 A Ashton Road, P.O. Box 646, Hanover, MD 21076
Bte Technologies, Inc. — 800-331-8845
7455-L New Ridge Rd., Hanover, MD 21076
Marquette Medical, Inc. — 800-296-2134
2600 Cabover Drive, Suite J, Hanover, MD 21076
Seca Corp. — 800-542-7322
1352 Charwood Road, Suite E, Hanover, MD 21076

Harmans

Aiv, Inc. (Formerly American Iv) — 800-990-2911
7485 Shipley Avenue, Harmans, MD 21077

Havre De Grace

Bayz Sunwear — 410-939-2200
920 Revolution St., Havre De Grace, MD 21078

Hunt Valley

Osteoimplant Technology, Inc. — 410-785-0700
11201 Pepper Road, Hunt Valley, MD 21031
Trace Laboratories-East — 410-584-9099
5 N. Park Drive, Hunt Valley, MD 21030

Kensington

Orthotic Mobility Systems, Inc.   301-949-2444
10421 Metropolitan Ave., Kensington, MD 20895

Laurel

Appropriate Technical Resources, Inc.   800-827-5931
9157 Whiskey Bottom Road, PO Box 460, Laurel, MD 20723
Microwave Research & Applications, Inc.   866-953-1771
8685 Cherry Ln., Laurel, MD 20707-6302
Ohmeda Medical   800-345-2700
8880 Gorman Road, Laurel, MD 20723

Linthicum

Innovision Medical Technologies, Llc   410-694-9450
1302 Concourse Dr., Ste. 302, Linthicum, MD 21090

Linthicum Heights

Airgas East, Inc.   800-562-3815
608 Nursery Rd., Linthicum Heights, MD 21090

Millersville

Marcal Medical, Inc.   800-628-9214
1114 Benfield Blvd., Suite H, Millersville, MD 21108

Mount Airy

Bak Electronics, Inc.   800-894-6000
PO Box 623, Mount Airy, MD 21771

Owings Mills

Air Techniques International   410-363-9696
11403 Cronridge Drive, Owings Mills, MD 21117-2247
Migliara/Kaplan Associates   410-581-8188
9 Park Center Ct., Owings Mills, MD 21117-4200
Sagentia Inc   410-654-0090
11403 Cronhill Drive, Suite B, Owings Mills, MD 21117
Sterilex Corp.   800-511-1659
11409 Cronhill Drive Suite L, Owings Mills, MD 21117

Pocomoke City

Nutech Molding Corporation   1-800-423-5278
2024 Broad St., PO Box 840, Pocomoke City, MD 21851-0840
Ricca Chemical Company Llc   888-467-4222
1841 Broad St., Pocomoke City, MD 21851

Reisterstown

Antek Healthware, Inc.   800-359-0911
228 Business Center Drive, Reisterstown, MD 21136

Rockville

Bioreliance   800-553-5372
14920 Broschart Road, Rockville, MD 20850
Biosource International Incorporated, Rockville Di   800-242-0607
1106 Taft Street, Rockville, MD 20850
Blue Torch Medical Technologies   508-231-1080
9700 Great Seneca Highway, Suite 303, Rockville, MD 20850
Braton Biotech, Inc.   301-762-5301
1 Taft Ct., Suite 101, Rockville, MD 20850
Inotech Biosystems International, Inc.   800-635-4070
15713 Crabbs Branch Way, #110, Rockville, MD 20855-2607
Maxim Biomedical Incorporated   301-251-0800
1500 East Gude Dr., Suite A, Rockville, MD 20850
Neuralstem, Inc.   301-366-4960
9700 Great Seneca Highway, Rockville, MD 20850
Penn Diagnostics   301-279-5958
14 Clemson Court, Rockville, MD 20850
Pop Oligos, Llc   301-461-0457
9430 Key West Ave., Rockville, MD 20850
Prometic Biotherapeutics, Inc.   301-917-6320
9800 Medical Center Dr., Suite C-110, Rockville, MD 20850
Pulse Medical Instruments, Inc.   301-816-9212 ex
5951 Halpine Rd., Rockville, MD 20851-2452
Supertechs, Inc.   301-309-6695
9610 Medical Center Dr., Suite 101, Rockville, MD 20850
Tetracore, Inc.   240-268-5400
9901 Belward Campus Dr., Suite 300, Rockville, MD 20850
Total Care   800-334-3802
PO Box 1661, Rockville, MD 20849-1661

Salisbury

Adelphia Medical Inc.   410-742-7104
1525 Edgemore Ave., Ste. 1, Salisbury, MD 21801
Trinity Sterile, Inc.   410-860-5123
201 Kiley Dr., Salisbury, MD 21802

Severna Park

Dynasplint Systems, Inc.   800-638-6771
770 Ritchie Highway, River Reach, Suite W21, Severna Park, MD 21146

Silver Spring

Altek Corp.   301-572-2555
12210 Plum Orchard Drive, Silver Spring, MD 20904-7802
Infrared Fiber Systems, Inc.   301-622-7131
2301-A Broadbirch Dr., Silver Spring, MD 20904

Sparks

Bd Diagnostic Systems   800-675-0908
7 Loveton Circle, Sparks, MD 21152

Sparks, Maryland

Advanced Medical Science & Technology, Llc   410-472-9209
410 Buedel Court, Sparks, Maryland, MD 21152

Stevensville

Vapotherm, Inc.   866-827-6843
198 Log Canoe Circle, Stevensville, MD 21666

Towson

Dejarnette Research Systems   410-583-0680
401 Washington Avenue, Suite 1010, Towson, MD 21204
Hipgraphics, Inc.   410-821-7040
100 West Road, Suite 302, Towson, MD 21204

Walkersville

Lonza Walkersville, Inc.   201-316-9200
8830 Biggs Ford Rd., Walkersville, MD 21793

MASSACHUSETTS

Aattleboro

Inverness Corp.   (800) 423-2060
6 Hazel Street, PO Box 2973, Aattleboro, MA 02703

Action

Fitzgerald Industries International, Inc.   800-370-2222
30 Sudbury Road, Suite 1A North, Action, MA 01720
Psychmedics Corp.   978-206-8220
125 Nagog Park, Action, MA 01720

Acton

Acra Cut, Inc.   800-227-2288
989 Main St., Acton, MA 01720
Allen Medical Systems, Inc.   800-433-5774
1 Post Office Square, Acton, MA 01720
Corning Inc., Science Products Division   800-492-1110
45 Nagog Park, Acton, MA 01720
Medical Sales & Service Group   888-357-6520
10 Woodchester Drive, Acton, MA 01720
P And G Engineering, Incorporated   978-263-6254
20 Main St. Unit E, Acton, MA 01720
Princeton Instruments - Acton   978-263-3584
15 Discovery Way, Acton, MA 01720
Psychemedics Corp.   800-628-8073
125 Nagog Park, Suite 200, Acton, MA 01720
Radius Medical Technologies, Inc.   978-263-4466
15 Craig Road, Acton, MA 01720

Agawam

Microtest, Inc.   (800) 631-1680
104 Gold Street, Agawam, MA 01001-3807
Qpsi Mass, Llc   413-789-6500
609 Silver St., Agawam, MA 01001-2986

Allston

E-Global Medical Equipment, L.L.C.   866-422-1845
2f 500 Lincoln St., Allston, MA 02134

Amesbury

Durasol Corp.   978-388-2020
1 Oakland St., P.o. Box 35, Amesbury, MA 01913
Munters Corp. - Cargocaire Division   800-843-5360
79 Monroe St., Amesbury, MA 01913

Amherst

Polymer Laboratories, Now A Part Of Varian, Inc.   800-767-3963
Amherst Fields Research Park, 160 Old Farm Road, Amherst, MA 01002

Andover

Advanced Biomedical Devices, Inc. (Abd, Inc.)   978-470-1177
Dundee Park, Bldg. 17, Door 6, P.O. Box 2087, Andover, MA 01810
Arrowhead Athletics   800-225-1516
220 Andover St., PO Box 4264, Andover, MA 01810
Draeger Medical Systems, Inc   215-660-2626
6 Tech Drive, Andover, MA 01810
Dynamics Research Corp.   800-522-4321
Two Tech Drive, Andover, MA 01810-5498
Harris Environmental Systems, Inc.   888-771-4200
11 Connector Rd., Andover, MA 01810-5993
Philips Medical Systems   978-659-3000
3000 Minuteman Rd, Andover, MA 01810
Polycom Inc.   978-924-6000
100 Minuteman Rd., Andover, MA 01810
Simplicity Orthopedic Solutions, Llc   866-623-0033
77 Main St., Second Floor, Andover, MA 01810
Smith & Nephew, Inc., Endoscopy Division   800-343-8386
150 Minuteman Road, Andover, MA 01810-1031
Straumann Manufacturing, Inc.   978-747-2575
60 Minuteman Rd., Andover, MA 01810

Andover,

Philips Medical Systems   1-800-722-9377
3000 Minuteman Road, Andover,, MA 01810-1099

Ashland

Medicept, Inc.   508-231-8842
200 Homer Ave., Ashland, MA 01721
Terumo Cardiovascular Systems (Tcvs)   800-283-7866
28 Howe St., Ashland, MA 01721

Assinippi

Src Medical, Inc.   781-826-9100
263 Winter Street, Assinippi, MA 02339

Athol

Filtrona Extrusion, Inc./PexcoA,Ar Medical   800-755-7528
Products Div.
764 south athol road, Athol, MA 01331

Attleboro

Glines And Rhodes, Inc.   800-343-1196
189 East St., P.O. Box 2285, Attleboro, MA 02703
Sterngold   800-243-9942
23 Frank Mossberg Drive, PO Box 2967, Attleboro, MA 02703-0967

Attleboro Falls

Whiting & Davis Company, Inc.   800-876-6374
200 John Dietsch Blvd., Attleboro Falls, MA 02763-0270

Auburn

Masterman's   800-525-3313
11 C Street, PO BOX 411, Auburn, MA 01501-0411

Avon

Boston Brace International, Inc.   800-262-2235
20 Ledin Dr., Avon, MA 02322
Ks Manufacturing, Inc.   508-427-5727
254 Bodwell St., Unit E, Avon, MA 02322
Ranfac Corp.   800-2RANFAC
Avon Industrial Park, 30 Doherty Ave., Avon, MA 02322-1125

Ayer

Associated Environmental Systems   978-772-0022
31 Willow Road, Ayer, MA 01432-1512
Grady Research, Inc.   978-772-3303
323 West Main St., Ayer, MA 01432
Optometrics Llc   978-772-1700
8 Nemco Way, Stony Brook Ind. Pk., Ayer, MA 01432

Bedford

Anika Therapeutics   781-457-9000
32 Wiggins Avenue, Bedford, MA 01730
Applied Science Laboratories   781-275-4000
175 Middlesex Tpke., Bedford, MA 01730
Biokit Usa, Inc.   800-926-3353
180 Hartwell Ave., Bedford, MA 02421
Caliper Systems, Inc.   781-687-9222
23 Crosby Drive, Bedford, MA 01730
Equipment Shop, Inc.   800-525-7681
P.O. Box 33, Bedford, MA 01730-2246
Gsi Group   800-342-3757
125 Middlesex Tpke, Bedford, MA 01730
Hologic, Inc.   800-343-9729
35 Crosby Drive, Bedford, MA 01730
Instrumentation Laboratory Company   800-955-9525
180 Hartwell Road, Bedford, MA 02421
Insulet Corporation   800-591-3455
9 Oak Park Dr., Bedford, MA 01730
Medica Corp.   800-777-5983
5 Oak Park Drive, Bedford, MA 01730
Mettler-Toledo Process Analytical, Inc.   800-352-8763
36 Middlesex Turnpike, Bedford, MA 01730
Millipore Corporation   800-MILLIPORE
80 Ashby Road, Bedford, MA 01730
Nova Biomedical Corporation Diabetes Products   781-894-0800
205 Burlington Road, Bedford, MA 01730
Pharmalucence, Inc.   781.275.7120
54 Loomis Street, Bedford, MA 01730
Rapid Micro Biosystems Inc.   781-271-1444
One Oak Park Drive, 2nd Floor, Bedford, MA 01730
Spire Corp.   800-510-4815
One Patriots Park, Bedford, MA 01730-2396
Traxyz Medical, Inc.   781-249-6254
24 Lido Lane, Bedford, MA 01730
Visen Medical   781-932-6875 x3
45-47 Wiggins Ave., Bedford, MA 01730

Bellingham

Jordi Associates, Flp   877-337-9589
4 Mill St., Bellingham, MA 02019

Berlin

Organomation Associates, Inc.   978-838-7300
266 River Road West, Berlin, MA 01503-1699

Beverly

Embo-Optics, Llc   887-885-6400
100 cumming center 326-B, Beverly, MA 01915
Hamilton Thorne Biosciences   800-323-0503
100 Cummings Center-suite 465e, Beverly, MA 01915
International Design & Marketing Incorporated   978-921-0638
140 Elliot St., Rt. 62 Business Center, Bldg E, Beverly, MA 01915
Microline Pentax, Inc.   978-922-9810
800 Cummings Center, Suite # 166t, Beverly, MA 01915
Mizuho America Inc.   800-699-2547
133 Brimbal Avenue, Beverly, MA 01915
Orion Research, Inc.   800-225-1480
166 Cummings Center, Beverly, MA 01915
Sage Science Inc.   888-744-2244
500 Cummings Center, Suite 3150, Beverly, MA 01915
Sensitech, Inc.   800-843-8367
800 Cummings Ctr. #258, Beverly, MA 01915-6171
Symmetricom Timing, Test & Measurement   800-544-0233
34 Tozer Road, Beverly, MA 01915
Tornier Inc.   800-611-2992
100 Cummings Center, Suite 444c, Beverly, MA 01915

Billerica

Advanced Radiation Therapy, Llc   978-663-7300
9 Linnell Circle, Billerica, MA 01821
Airgas East, Inc   866-718-0685
1 Plank St., Billerica, MA 01821
Aushon Biosystems, Inc.   978-436-6400
43 Manning Rd, Billerica, MA 01821
Azonix Corporation   800-967-5558
900 Middlesex Turnpike, Building 6, Billerica, MA 01821
Belmont Instrument Corp.   866-663-0212
780 Boston Road, Billerica, MA 01821-5925
Bruker Corporation   978-663-3660
40 Manning Road, Billerica, MA 01821
Design Technology Corp.   978-663-7000
5 Suburban Park Dr., Billerica, MA 01821-3904
Ge Industrial, Sensing   800-833-9438
1100 Technology Park Drive, Billerica, MA 01821-4111
Hydrocision, Inc.   888-747-7470
267 Boston Road, Suite 28, Billerica, MA 01821
Lantheus Medical Imaging   800-362-2668
331 Treble Cove Rd., Bldg. 200-2, Billerica, MA 01862
Millipore Corporation   877-246-2247
290 Concord Road, Billerica, MA 01821
Trans Med Usa, Inc.   978-670-6000
77 Alexander Road, #9, Billerica, MA 01821-5043

Boston

Allied Minds, Inc.   617-419-1800
33 Arch Street, 32nd Floor, Boston, MA 02110
Applied Medical Systems, Inc.   617-577-1604
581 Boylston Street, Suite 500, Boston, MA 02116
Arthro Kinetics Inc.   49-711-30511070
8 Faneuil Hall, 3rd Floor, Boston, MA 02109
Arthur Blank & Co., Inc.   800-776-7333
225 Rivermoor St., Boston, MA 02132-4920
Bicon, Llc   800-882-4266
501 Arborway, Second Floor, Boston, MA 02130
Consolidated Machine Corp.   617-782-6072
76 Ashford Street, Boston, MA 02134-0003
Consolidated Stills & Sterilizers   617-782-6072
76 Ashford Street, Boston, MA 02134-0003
Delsys, Inc.   617-236-0599
650 Beacon St., 6th Flr., Boston, MA 02215
Extech Instruments Corp.   781-890-7440
285 Bear Hill Rd., Boston, MA 02451
Fletcher Spaght Ventures   617-247-6700
222 Berkeley St., 20th Floor, Boston, MA 02116-3761
Immunetics, Inc.   800-227-4765
27 Drydock Avenue, 6th Floor, Boston, MA 02210
Joslin Diabetes Center   617-226-5808
1 Joslin Place, Boston, MA 02215
M.E.E.I. Mfg.   941-492-2560
Claes H Dohlman, Md Room 550l, Meei, 5th Floor, Boston, MA 02114
Medchannel Llc   617-314-9861
1241 Adams St, Ste 110, Boston, MA 02124
Nmt Medical, Inc.   617-737-0930
27-43 Wormwood St., Boston, MA 02210
Oncolab, Inc.   800-922-8378
36 The Fenway, Boston, MA 02215
Perkinelmer Life And Analytical Sciences   800-446-0035
549 Albany St., Boston, MA 02118
Queen Screw & Manufacturing Inc.   781-894-8110
60 Farwell St., Boston, MA 02154
SV Life Sciences   617-367-8100
60 State Street, Suite 3650, Boston, MA 02109
Salk Inc.   800-343-4497
119 Braintree St. #701, 4th Floor, Boston, MA 02134
Servolift/Eastern Corp.   800-727-3786
266 Hancock St., Boston, MA 02125-2155
Solos Endoscopy   800-388-6445
65 Sprague Street, West B, Boston/Dedham Commerce Park, Boston, MA 02136

Solutek Corp.   800-403-0770
94 Shirley St., Boston, MA 02119-3036
SoundCure   617-419-1800
33 Arch Street, Boston, MA 02110
Stethographics, Inc.   508-320-2841
1153 Centre St., Suite 40, Boston, MA 02130
Tei Biosciences Inc.   617-268-1616
7 Elkins St., Boston, MA 02127
The Gillette Company   617-421-7000
800 Boylston St., Prudential Tower Bldg. Fl.45, Boston, MA 02199-8004

Braintree

Citra Anticoagulants, Inc.   800-299-3411
55 Messina Drive, Braintree, MA 02184
Engineering & Research Assoc., Inc. (D.B.A. Sebra)   800-225-5242
400 Wood Rd, Braintree, MA 02184
Haemonetics Corp.   800-225-5242
400 Wood Road, Braintree, MA 02184

Bridgewater

Depuy Bridgewater   800-473-3789
50 Scotland Park Dr., Bridgewater, MA 02324
Depuy Mitek, A Johnson & Johnson Company   800-451-2006
50 Scotland Blvd., Bridgewater, MA 02324

Brighton

Amicas, Inc.   800-490-8465
20 Guest St., Suite 200, Brighton, MA 02135

Brockton

Ace Surgical Supply Co., Inc.   800-441-3100
1034 Pearl St., Brockton, MA 02301
Frank Scholz X-Ray Corp.   508-586-8308
244 Liberty St., Brockton, MA 02401-5522
Krohn-Hite Corporation   877-549-7781
15 Jonathan Drive, Unit 4, Brockton, MA 02301-5566
Lyne Laboratories, Inc.   508-583-8700
10 Burke Dr., Brockton, MA 02301

Burlington

ConforMIS Inc.   (781) 345-9001
11 North Ave., Burlington, MA 01803
Conformis, Inc.   781-345-9001
11 North Ave., Burlington, MA 01803
Cosman Company, Inc.   888-886-7686
76 Cambridge St., Burlington, MA 01803-4140
Emed Technologies   866-363-3669
76 Blanchard Road, Burlington, MA 01803-5125
Hypermed, Inc   781-229-5900
41 Second Avenue, Burlington, MA 01803
InfraReDx Inc.   888-680-7339
34 Third Ave., Burlington, MA 01803
InfraRedRx   888-680-7339
34 3rd. Avenue, Burlington, MA 01803
Integra Radionics   800-466-6814
22 Terry Avenue, Burlington, MA 01803
Lemaitre Vascular, Inc.   781-221-2266
63 Second Avenue, Burlington, MA 01803
Netzsch Instruments, Inc.   800-688-6738
37 North Avenue, Burlington, MA 01803
Palomar Medical Technologies   800-725-6627
15 Network Drive, Burlington, MA 01803
Qsa-Global Inc.   781-272-2000
40 North Ave., Burlington, MA 01803
Surmet Corp.   800-262-8783
31 B St., Burlington, MA 01803
Terason Revolutionizing Ultrasound   (866) 837-2766
77 Terrace Hall Ave., Burlington, MA 01803
Teratech Corp.   781-270-4143
77-79 Terrace Hall Ave., Burlington, MA 01803
Tomophase Corporation   781-229-5700
One North Avenue, Burlington, MA 01803

Buzzards Bay

H.L. Bouton Co., Inc.   800-426-1881
PO Box 840, Buzzards Bay, MA 02532
H.L. Bouton Company, Inc.   800-426-1881
P.O. Box 840, Buzzards Bay, MA 02532

Cambridge

Advanced Magnetics, Inc.   617-576-1915
61 Mooney St., Cambridge, MA 02138
Cardea Technology Inc.   877-392-7763
359 Green Street, Cambridge, MA 02139
Cervical Barrier Advancement Society   -
P.O. Box 38203, Cambridge, MA 02238-2031
Etex Corporation   617-577-7270
38 Sidney St., Suite 370, The Clark Bldg., Cambridge, MA 02139
Foundation Medicine Inc.   617-418-2200
One Kendall Square, Suite B3501, Cambridge, MA 02139
Genzyme   800-332-1042
500 Kendall Street, Cambridge, MA 02139
Genzyme Corp.   617-252-7500
500 Kendall Street, Cambridge, MA 02142

Genzyme Corp.   800-284-2876
64 Sidney St., Cambridge, MA 02139-4136
Helicos Biosciences Corporation   877-243-5426
One Kendall Square, Ste. 7301, Cambridge, MA 02139
Hemedex Incorporated   866-436-3339
222 Third Street, Suite 0123, Cambridge, MA 02142
Innovation Genesis, Llc   617-234-0070
One Canal Park, Cambridge, MA 02141
Interactive Motion Technologies, Inc.   617-497-6330
37 Spinelli Place, Cambridge, MA 02138
Invivo Therapeutics   617-475-1520
One Broadway, 14th Floor, Cambridge, MA 02142
J. H. Emerson Co.   800-252-1414
22 Cottage Park Avenue, Cambridge, MA 02140
Metamark Genetics Inc.   617-583-1400
245 First Street, Suite 150, Cambridge, MA 02142
Myomo, Inc.   1-877-736-9666
1 Broadway,, 14th Floor, Cambridge, MA 02142
Neurodyne Medical Corp.   800-963-8633
186 Alewife Brook Parkway, Cambridge, MA 02138
NinePoint Medical Inc.   617-250-7190
One Kendall Square, Suite B7501, Cambridge, MA 02139
Omniguide, Inc.   888-666-4484
One Kendall Square, Bldg 100, 3rd Floor, Cambridge, MA 02139
Quanterix Corporation   617-301-9400
One Kendall Square, Suite B14201, Cambridge, MA 02139
Semprus Biosciences   617-577-7755
One Kendall Square, Building 1400W, 1st Floor, Cambridge, MA 02139
WILEX, Inc.   800-255-3232
Oncogene Science, 100 Acorn Park Drive, Cambridge, MA 02140
Worldcare, Inc.   617-374-9001
1 Cambridge Center, 5th Floor, Cambridge, MA 02142

Canton

Direx Systems Corp.   339-502-6013
437 Turnpike St., Canton, MA 02021
Hipsavers, Inc.   800-358-4477
7 Hubbard St., Canton, MA 02021
Organogenesis, Inc.   888-432-5232
150 Dan Road, Canton, MA 02021-2820
The Judge Rotenberg Educational Center, Inc.   781-828-2202
240 Turnpike St., Canton, MA 02021-2341

Carlisle

Fernandez Industries, Inc.   978-371-8431
43 Oak Knoll Rd., Carlisle, MA 01741

Centerville

Advanced Medical Technologies, Inc.   508-790-8700
101 Waterside Dr, Centerville, MA 02632

Charlton

Karl Storz Endovision, Inc.   800-421-0837
91 Carpenter Hill Rd., Charlton, MA 01507
Techman Int'L Corp.   508-248-2900
242 Sturbridge Rd., Charlton, MA 01507

Chelmsford

Esa, Inc.   800-959-5095
22 Alpha Road, Chelmsford, MA 01824-4171
Magellan Biosciences Inc.   978-856-2345
22 alpha Road, Chelmsford, MA 01824
Mercury Computer Systems, Inc.   978-256-1300
201 Riverneck Road, Chelmsford, MA 01824
Zoll Medical Corp.   800-348-9011
269 Mill Road, Chelmsford, MA 01824

Chelsea

Steele Canvas Basket Co., Inc.   800-541-8929
201 Williams St., P.O. Box 6267 IMCN, Chelsea, MA 02150-3805

Chemsford

Magellan Biosciences   978-856-2345
22 Alpha Road, Chemsford, MA 01824

Chicopee

Covidien Lp, Formerly Registered As Ludlow   800-962-9888
Two Ludlow Park Dr., Chicopee, MA 01022
Dielectrics, Inc.   800-472-7286
300 Burnett Road, Chicopee, MA 01020
Iron Duck, A Div. Of Fleming Industries, Inc.   800-669-6900
20 Veterans Drive, Chicopee, MA 01022
Tyco Healthcare Group Lp   800-445-5025
Two Ludlow Park Drive, Chicopee, MA 01022

Clinton

Np Medical, Inc.   978-368-4514
101 Union St., Clinton, MA 01510
Nypro Inc.   978-365-9721
101 Union St., Clinton, MA 01510-2005

Cohasset

Holles Laboratories, Inc.   800-356-4015
30 Forest Notch, Cohasset, MA 02025

Concord

Concord Consulting Group, Inc. — 978-369-8744
30 Monument Square, Suite 215, Concord, MA 01742-1895
Concord Medical Products — 978-857-5884
72 Bristers Hill Rd., Concord, MA 01742-3502
Oxford Instruments — 800-438-8322
300 Baker Avenue, Suite 150, Concord, MA 01742
Schumann Inc., A. — 978-369-6782
167 Hayward Mill Road, Concord, MA 01742-3919
Starmet Corporation — 978-369-5410
2229 Main St., Concord, MA 01742-3813

Danvers

Abiomed, Inc. — 800-422-8666
22 Cherry Hill Dr., Danvers, MA 01923-2579
Datacube Inc. — 978-777-4200
300 Rosewood Drive, Danvers, MA 01923-4505
Draeger Medical Systems, Inc. — 215-660-2626
16 Electronics Ave., Danvers, MA 01923
Medtronic Vascular — 978-777-0042
35-37A Cherry Hill Dr, Danvers, MA 01923
Neurologica Corporation — 877-564-8520
14 Electronics Avenue, Danvers, MA 01923
Osram Sylvania Inc. — 978-777-1900
100 Endicott St., Danvers, MA 01923
Reheat Co., Inc. — 800-373-4328
10 School St., Danvers, MA 01923
Rowley Biochemical Institute — 978-739-4883
10 Electronics Avenue, Danvers Industrial Park, Danvers, MA 01923
Siemens Medical Systems, Inc. — 800-437-2437
16 Electronics Ave., Danvers, MA 01923

Dedham

Alimed, Inc. — 800-225-2610
297 High St., Dedham, MA 02026-2844
Arista Surgical Supply Co. Inc. — 800-223-1984
297 High Street, Dedham, MA 02026
Assistive Technology, Inc. — 800-793-9227
333 Elm Street, Suite 115, Dedham, MA 02026
Covance Research Products, Inc. — 800-223-0796
180 Rustcraft Road, Suite 140, Dedham, MA 02026-4547
EarlySense — 617-517-0095
990 Washington Street,, Suite 204, Dedham, MA 02026

Devens

Bionostics, Inc. — 978-772-7070
7 Jackson Rd., Devens, MA 01434
Rna Medical, A Division Of Bionostics, Inc. — 800-533-6162
7 Jackson Road, Devens, MA 01434

Dudley

Gentex Optics, Inc. — 508-943-3860
183 W. Main St., Dudley, MA 01571
Henke Sass Wolf Of America, Inc. — 508-671-9300
135 Schofield Ave, Dudley, MA 01571

E Falmouth

Associates Of Cape Cod, Inc. — 508-540-3444
124 Bernard E. Saint Jean Drive, E Falmouth, MA 02536

E Walpole

Siemens Healthcare Diagnostics Inc — 866-637-4448
333 Coney Street, E Walpole, MA 02032

East Bridgewater

Medair, Inc. — 800-325-7780
PO Box 635, East Bridgewater, MA 02333

East Longmeadow

Biolitec, Inc. — 800-934-2377
515 Shaker Road, East Longmeadow, MA 01028
Veritech Corporation — 413-525-3368
168 Denslow Road, East Longmeadow, MA 01028-2812

East Taunton

Omni Life Science, Inc — 800-448-6664
50 O'Connell Way, East Taunton, MA 02718

Easthampton

National Nonwovens — 800-333-3469
P.O. Box 150, Easthampton, MA 01027-0150

Easton

Sdi Diagnostics, Inc. — 800-678-5782
10 Hampden Drive, Easton, MA 02375

Everett

Arrow International, Inc. — 800-523-8446
9 Plymouth St., Everett, MA 02149
Middlesex Gases & Technologies, Inc. — 617-387-5050
292 Second St., Everett, MA 02149
Tillotson Rubber Co., Inc. — 781-402-1731
59 Waters Ave., Everett, MA 02149

Fall River

Advanced Image Enhancement, Inc. — 508-344-3097
306 Valentine St, Fall River, MA 02720
American Dryer Corp. — 508-678-9000
88 Currant Road, Fall River, MA 02720-4781
Millstone Medical Outsourcing — 508-679-8384
1565 N. Main St., Suite 408, Fall River, MA 02720

Fitchburg

Arrhythmia Research Technology, Inc. — 978-345-0181
25 Sawyer Passway, Fitchburg, MA 01420
Headwall Photonics, Inc. — 978-353-4100
601 River St., Fitchburg, MA 01420
Mar-Lee Companies — 978-343 9600
190 Authority Dr., Fitchburg, MA 01420
Micron Products, Inc. — 800-370-5500
25 Sawyer Passway, Fitchburg, MA 01420
Opco Laboratory, Inc. — 978-345-2522
704 River St., Fitchburg, MA 01420
Select Engineering, Inc. — 800-971-4500
260 Lunenburg St., Fitchburg, MA 01420
Spectro Analytical Instruments Inc. — 800-548-5809
160 Authority Drive, Fitchburg, MA 01420

Florence

Medtech Systems — 903-504-5001
221 Pine St., Florence, MA 01062

Foxboro

BI Healthcare, Inc. — 508-543-4150
33 Commercial St., Suite #3, Foxboro, MA 02035
Dorel Design & Development Center — 800-909-7133
25 Forbes Blvd., Foxboro, MA 02035

Foxborough

Cyberkinetics Neurotechnology Systems, Inc. — 508-549-9981
100 Foxborough Blvd., Suite 240, Foxborough, MA 02035

Framingham

American International Chemical — 800-238-0001
135 Newbury St, Framingham, MA 01701
BTL Industries, Inc. — 866-285-1656
47 Loring Drive, Framingham, MA 01702
David Scott Company — 800-804-0333
59 Fountain St., Framingham, MA 01702
HeartWare International, Inc. — 877-367-4823
205 Newbury Street, Suite 101, Framingham, MA 01701
J&S Medical Associates — 800-229-6000
35 Tripp St., Bldg. 1, Framingham, MA 01702
Statsure Diagnostic Systems, Inc. — 508-872-2625
1881 Worcester Road, Framingham, MA 01701

Franklin

Arthrosurface, Inc. — 508-520-3003
28 Forge Parkway, Franklin, MA 02038
Liko North America — 888-545-6671
122 Grove Street, Franklin, MA 02038
Plc Medical Systems — 800-232-8422
10 Forge Pk., Franklin, MA 02038
Speedline Technologies, Inc. — 508-520-0083
16 Forge Park, Franklin, MA 02038
Tegra Medical Inc. — 508-541-4200
9 Forge Park, Franklin, MA 02038
Thermo - Industrial Hygiene Division — 508-520-0430
27 Forge Pkwy., Franklin, MA 02038

Gardner

Biomedical Polymers, Inc. — 800-253-3684
42 Linus Allain Avenue, Gardner, MA 01440
Precision Optics Corp. — 800-447-2812
22 E. Broadway, Gardner, MA 01440-3338

Gloucester

Jenline Industries, Inc. — 734-451-0020
92 Blackburn Center, Gloucester, MA 01930

Hamilton

Cmt, Inc. — 800-659-9140
Post Office Box 297, Hamilton, MA 01936-0297

Hanover

Denali R&D Corporation — 781-826-9190
134 Old Washington Street, Hanover, MA 02339

Hanson

Roman Research, Inc. — 800-451-5700
800 Franklin St, Hanson, MA 02341

Harvard

N.M. Beale Co. Inc. — 978-456-6990
89 Old Shirley Road, PO Box 494, Harvard, MA 01451-1309

Haverhill

Morgan Scientific Inc. — 800-525-5002
151 Essex St., Haverhill, MA 01832-5528

Hingham

Airgas East, Inc. — 800-562-3815
90 Research Rd., Hingham, MA 02043
Home Care Express & Mass Bay Respiratory — 781-740-9797
85 Research Rd., Hingham, MA 02043
Integral Design Inc. — 781-740-2036
52 Burr Road, Hingham, MA 02043
Rocket Medical Plc. — 800-707-7625
150 Recreation Park Drive, Unit 3, Hingham, MA 02043

Holden

Romc, Inc. — 508-829-4602
37 Kris Allen Drive, Holden, MA 01520

Holliston

Diamond Diagnostics, Inc. — 508-429-0450
333 Fiske St., Holliston, MA 01746
Harvard Apparatus, Inc. — 800-272-2775
84 October Hill Road, Holliston, MA 01746
Harvard Bioscience Inc. — 800-272-2775
84 October Hill Road, Holliston, MA 01746
Highland Labs, Inc. — 508-429-2918
42 B Pope Road, Holliston, MA 01746-2218
Hoefer Pharmacia Biotech, Inc. — 800-227-4750
84 October Hill Road, Holliston, MA 01746
Invacare Supply Group, An Invacare Co. — 800-225-4792
75 October Hill Road, Holliston, MA 01746
Liberating Technologies, Inc. — 800-437-0024
325 Hopping Brook Road, Suite A, Holliston, MA 01746-1456
Lista International Corp. — (877-465-4782)
106 Lowland St., Holliston, MA 01746-2094
Mission Diagnostics — 508-429-0450
333 Fiske St., Holliston, MA 01746
Pappas Surgical Instruments, Llc — 508-429-1049
7 October Hill Rd., Holliston, MA 01746
Praxis, Llc. — 508-400-3969
1110 Washington St., Holliston, MA 01746
Work 'N Leisure Products, Inc. — 800-884-9629
330 Hopping Brook Road, Holliston, MA 01746

Holyoke

A-T Surgical Manufacturing Co., Inc. — 800-225-2023
115 Clemente St., Holyoke, MA 01040-5644
C & D Industries, Inc. — 413-493-1200
28 Appleton St., Holyoke, MA 01040
Pochemco, Inc. — 413-536-2900
724 Main Street, Holyoke, MA 01040

Hopedale

Gammasonics — 800-253-0145
170 Dutcher St., Hopedale, MA 01747-1028

Hopkinton

Caliper Life Sciences, Inc. — 508-435-9500
68 Elm Street, Hopkinton, MA 01748
Stryker Biotech — 508-416-5200
35 South St., Hopkinton, MA 01748
Zymark Corporation — 508-435-9500
68 Elm Street, Hopkinton, MA 01748

Hudson

Act Electronics, Inc. — 978-567-4024
2 Cabot Rd., Hudson, MA 01749
Meditrack Products, Llc — 800-863-9633
433 Main St., Hudson, MA 01749
Telemed Systems Inc. — 800-481-6718
8 Kane Industrial Drive, Hudson, MA 01749
Tss Hudson
19 Brent Dr, Hudson, MA 01749

Hull

White Cap Ent. — 781-925-3705
133 Beach Ave., Hull, MA 02045

Hyannis

Accu-Line Products, Inc. — 800-363-7740
379 Iyannough Rd. (Rear Building), Hyannis, MA 02601

Ipswich

New England Biolabs, Inc. — 800-632-5227
240 County Rd., Ipswich, MA 01938-2723

Kingston

Caton Connector Corp. — 877-522-2866
26 Wapping Road, Kingston, MA 02364-1302

Lawrence

Ge Healthcare Technologies Surgery Navigation — 800-708-3856
439 South Union Street, Lawrence, MA 01843

Ge Oec Medical Systems — 978-552-5200
439 South Union St., Lawrence, MA 01843
Medisystems Corporation — 800-369-6334
439 South Union St., 5th Floor, Lawrence, MA 01843
Nxstage Medical, Inc. — 866-697-8243
439 South Union St., 5th Floor, Lawrence, MA 01843

Lee

Oraceutical Llc — 413-528-5070
815 Pleasant St., Lee, MA 01238

Leominster

IMA Nova — 1-800-851-1518
7 New Lancaster, Leominster, MA 01453
Ima Nova — 978-537-8534
7 New Lancaster Road, Leominster, MA 01453-2962

Lexington

BioScale Inc. — 781-430-6800
4 Maguire Street, Lexington, MA 02421
Brontes Technologies — 781-541-5200
10 Maguire Road, Suite 310, Lexington, MA 02421
Enginivity Llc — 781-862-7008
1 Militia Drive, Lla, Lexington, MA 02421
Epix Pharmaceuticals, Inc — 781-761-7600
4 Maguire Road, Lexington, MA 02421
GI Dynamics, Inc. — 781-357-3300
1 Maguire Road, Lexington, MA 02421
Hai Laboratories, Inc — 781-862-9884
320 Massachusetts Ave., Lexington, MA 02420
Medispectra Inc — 781-372-2430
45 Hartwell Ave., Lexington, MA 02421
Raindance Technologies, Inc. — 888-724-6440
44 Hartwell Avenue, Lexington, MA 02421
T2 Biosystems — 781-457-1200
101 Hartwell Avenue, Lexington, MA 02421
Tepha, Incorporated — 781-357-1709
99 Hayden Avenue, Suite 360, Lexington, MA 02421
Varian Vacuum Products — 800-882-7426
121 Hartwell Ave., Lexington, MA 02421-3133

Lexington,

Predictive Biosciences — 781-402-1780
128 Spring Street, 400 Level, B Annex, Lexington,, MA 02421

Littleton

Medtronic Navigation, Inc. (Littleton) — 720-890-3325
300 Foster Street, Harwood Station, Littleton, MA 01460
Mevion Medical Systems — 978-540-1500
300 Foster St, Littleton, MA 01460
Scandius Biomedical, Inc. — 978-486-4088
11a Beaver Brook Road, Littleton, MA 01460
X P Power — 978-287-7200
305 Foster Street, Littleton, MA 01460

Lowell

Adden Furniture, Inc. — 800-625-3876
26 Jackson St., Lowell, MA 01852-2102
Bard Electro Physiology — 800-824-8724
55 Technology Dr., Lowell, MA 01851

Lowell,

Diagnosis, Llc — 978.458.1600
Suite 500, 175 Cabot Street, Lowell,, MA 01854

Lunenburg

Analox Instruments Usa, Inc. — 978-582-9368
104 Sunset Lane, P.O. BOX 208, Lunenburg, MA 01462-0208

Lynn

American Silk Sutures, Inc. — 781-592-7200
82 Sanderson Avenue, Lynn, MA 01902

Mansfield

Covidien Lp — 508-261-8000
15 Hampshire St., Mansfield, MA 02048
Covidien Lp, Formerly Registered As Tyco Healthcare — 800-962-9888
15 Hampshire Street, Mansfield, MA 02048
Integrated Software Design, Inc. — 800-600-2242
171 Forbes Blvd Suite 3000, Mansfield, MA 02048
Ndo Surgical, Inc. — 877-337-8887
125 High St.,, Suite 7, Mansfield, MA 02048
PrimeraDx — 508-618-2300
171 Forbes Blvd, Suite 2000, Mansfield, MA 02048
Proven Process Medical Devices, Inc. — 508-261-0806
110 Forbes Blvd., Mansfield, MA 02048
Smith & Nephew, Inc., Endoscopy Division — 800-343-8386
130 Forbes Blvd., Mansfield, MA 02048
Teleflex Medical Oem — 800-458-2553
375 Forbes Boulevard, Mansfield, MA 02048-1805

Marion

Polaris Contract Services, A Division Of Sippicon, Inc. — 508-748-1160
7 Barnabas Rd., Marion, MA 02738-1421

Marlboro

Apple Medical Corp. — 508-357-2700
28 Lord Rd., Unit 135, Marlboro, MA 01752
Hologic, Inc. — 800-442-9892
445 Simarano Drive, Marlboro, MA 01752
Optos, Inc. — 441-383-8433
67 Forest St., Marlboro, MA 01752
Pointcare Technologies Inc. — 508-281-6925
181 Cedar Hill St., Marlboro, MA 01752

Marlborough

Cardiofocus Inc. — (508) 658-7200
500 Nickerson Road, Suite 500-200, Marlborough, MA 01752
Cardiofocus, Inc. — 508-658-7200
500 Nickerson Road, Suite 500-200, Marlborough, MA 01752
Edgetech — 800-276-3729
19 Brigham St., Unit #8, Marlborough, MA 01752
HOLOGIC, INC. — 800-442-9892
250 Campus Drive, Marlborough, MA 01752
IQuum, Inc. — 508-970-0099
700 Nickerson Road, Marlborough, MA 01752
Innovasive Devices, Inc. — 800-435-6001
734 Forest St., Marlborough, MA 01752
Navilyst Medical — 877.658.7990
26 Forest Street, Marlborough, MA 01752

Marshfield

Innovative Chemistry, Inc. — 781-837-6709
PO Box 578, Marshfield, MA 02050-0090
Kirwan Surgical Products, Inc. — 888-547-9267
180 Enterprise Drive, PO Box 427Aÿ, Marshfield, MA 02050

Marshfield Hills

Gwb International, Ltd. — 888-436-4826
PO Box 370, 76 Prospect Street, Marshfield Hills, MA 02051-0370

Maynard

Northeast Monitoring, Inc. — 866-346-5837
Two Clock Tower Place, Suite 555, Maynard, MA 01754

Medford

Materials Development Corporation — 781-391-0400
81 Hicks Avenue, Medford, MA 02155-6318

Medway

CYBEX INTERNATIONAL, INC. — 508-533-4300
10 Trotter Drive, Medway, MA 02053
Cybex International, Inc. — 800-667-6544
10 Trotter Dr., Medway, MA 02053
Microgroup — 800-255-8823
7 Industrial Park Road, Medway, MA 02053

Methuen

Ulvac Technologies, Inc. — 800-998-5822
401 Griffin Brook Dr., Methuen, MA 01844

Middleboro

Gerson Co. Inc., Louis M. — 800-225-8623
15 Sproat St., Middleboro, MA 02346-2268

Middleton

Neurotherm Inc. — 978-777-3916
2 Debush Ave., Middleton, MA 01949
Surgical Tables Incorporated — 888-737-5044
2 Debush Avenue, Building A Unit 2, Middleton, MA 01949

Milford

Linos Photonics, Inc — 800-334-5678
459 Fortune Blvd., Milford, MA 01757-1723
Plc Systems Inc. — 508-541-8800
459 Fortune Boulevard, Milford, MA 01757
Psyche Systems — 800-345-1514
321 Fortune Blvd., Milford, MA 01757
Seracare Life Sciences — 800-676-1881
37 Birch St., Milford, MA 01757
Thermo Fisher Scientific - Laboratory Equipment — 800-662-7477
Division Headquarters
450 Fortune Boulevard, Milford, MA 01757
Waters Corp. — 800-252-4752
34 Maple St., Milford, MA 01757-3604
Waters Corporation — 800-252-4752
34 Maple Street, Milford, MA 01757

Millbury

Steelcraft, Inc. — 800-225-7710
115 W. Main St., Millbury, MA 01527

N Natick

National Dentex Corp — 508-907-7800
2 Vision Drive, 3rd Floor, N Natick, MA 01760

N. Attleboro

The Mason Box Company — 800-225-2708
521 Mt. Hope St., PO Box 129, N. Attleboro, MA 02761

N. Billerica

Lantheus Medical Imaging, Inc. — 1-800-362-2668
331 Treble Cove Rd., Bldg. 200-2, N. Billerica, MA 01862

N. Chelmsford

Suturtek Incorporated — 978-251-8088
51 Middlesex St., N. Chelmsford, MA 01863

Natick

Boston Scientific Corporation — 800-225-2732
One Boston Scientific Place, Natick, MA 01760-1537
Corindus Inc. — 508-653-3335
11 Erie Dr., Natick, MA 01760
Phoenix Diagnostics, Inc. — 800-688-2595
8 Tech Circle, Natick, MA 01760
Precision Systems, Inc. — 508-655-7010
16 Tech Circle, Natick, MA 01760-1029
Sunnex, Inc. — 800-445-7869
3 Huron Drive, Natick, MA 01760-1314
Toolmex Corporation — 800-992-4766
1075 Worchester Road, Natick, MA 01760-1510

Needham

Jamiesan Company — 781-444-1026
1492 Highland Ave, Needham, MA 02492
Sensomotoric Instruments, Inc. — 888-SMI-USA1
97 Chapel St., Needham, MA 02492
Vita Needle Company — 781-444-1780
919 Great Plain Avenue, Needham, MA 02492

New Bedford

Andonian Cryogenics, Inc. — 800-446-3533
90 Hatch St., New Bedford, MA 02745
Oberon Company ,Div Of The Paramount Corp. — 800-322-3348
22 Logan St., PO Box 61008, New Bedford, MA 02746
Optical Laboratory, Inc. — 508-993-8665
14 S. Sixth St., New Bedford, MA 02740-5911
Packaging Products Corp. — 800-225-0484
198 Herman Melville Blvd., New Bedford, MA 02740-7344
Symmetry Medical New Bedford — 508-998-4493
New Bedford Industrial Park, New Bedford, MA 02745

Newburyport

Innovative Technology, Inc. — 877-462-4415
2 New Pasture Road, Newburyport, MA 01950

Newton

Adamation, Inc. — 800-225-3075
87 Adams St., PO Box 95037, Newton, MA 02458
Aspect Medical Systems, Inc. — 617-559-7000
141 Needham St., Newton, MA 02464
Clinical Data Inc — 800-937-5449
One Gateway Center, Suite 702, Newton, MA 02458
Healthdrive Ag — 617-964-6681
25 Needham St, Newton, MA 02461
Matritech, Inc. — 617-928-0820
330 Nevada St., Newton, MA 02460
Norcross Corp. — 617-969-7020
255 Newtonville Avenue, Newton, MA 02458

Newton Highlands

Sanax Protective Products, Inc. — 800-379-9929
236 Upland Avenue, Newton Highlands, MA 02461-2003

Newton Upper Falls

Microfluidics International Corporation — 800-370-5452
30 Ossipee Rd., Newton Upper Falls, MA 02464-9101

North Andover

Aurora Imaging Technology, Inc. — 877-975-7530
39 High St., North Andover, MA 01845
Osi Electronics Boston — 978.552.7099
25 Commerce Way, North Andover, MA 01845
Stanley Supply & Services, Inc — 800-225-5370
335 Willow Street, North Andover, MA 01845-5995

North Attleboro

Health Ent., Inc. — 800-633-4243
90 George Leven Dr., North Attleboro, MA 02760
Health Enterprises — 800-633-4243
90 George Leven Dr., North Attleboro, MA 02760
Zimmer Spine — 508-643-0983
23 West Bacon St., North Attleboro, MA 02762

North Attleborough

Metalor Technologies Usa — 800-554-5504
255 John L. Dietsch Blvd., PO Box 255, North Attleborough, MA 02761

North Billerica

Btu International, Inc. — 978-667-4111
23 Esquire Rd., North Billerica, MA 01862
Fasstech — 978-663-2800
76 Treble Cove Rd., Building 3, North Billerica, MA 01862

Hospira Sedation, Inc.   877-946-7747
Five Billerica Park, 101 Billerica Avenue, North Billerica, MA 01862
Mobility Transfer Systems   888-854-4687
34 Sullivan Road , Unit 32, North Billerica, MA 01862
Sea Horse Bio Science   800-671-0633
16 Esquire Road, North Billerica, MA 01862
Seahorse Bioscience Inc.   978-671-1600
16 Esquire Road, North Billerica, MA 01862
Shinemound Enterprise, Inc.   978-436-9980
17a Sterling Road, North Billerica, MA 01862

North Reading

Julie Industries, Inc   978-276-0820
PO Box 153, North Reading, MA 01864

North Waltham

Levitronix Llc   1 (866) 487 - 2
45 First Ave., North Waltham, MA 02451

Northampton

Etchells Technology Corp.   413-587-3922
82 Industrial Dr., Northampton, MA 01060-2327
Microcal, Llc   800-633-3115
22 Industrial Dr. E., Northampton, MA 01060-2327

Northborough

Matec Instrument Companies, Inc.   508-393-0155
56 Hudson St., Northborough, MA 01532
Medical Equipment Specialists, Inc.   800-795-6641
107 Otis Street, Northborough, MA 01532

Norton

Brunswick Laboratories   800-362-3482
50 Commerce Way, Norton, MA 02766

Norwell

Tuzik Boston   800-886-6363
104 Longwater Dr., Assinippi Park, Norwell, MA 02061

Norwood

Advanced Instruments Inc.   800-225-4034
Two Technology Way, Norwood, MA 02062-2680
Analog Devices, Inc.   800-262-5643
One Technology Way, P. O. Box 9106, Norwood, MA 02062-9106
Aspect Medical Systems, Inc.   617-559-7000
1 Upland Road, Norwood, MA 02062
Endovia Medical, Inc.   781-255-1888
150 Kerry Place, Norwood, MA 02062
Siemens Healthcare Diagnostics Inc   800-255-3232
2 Edgewater Drive, Norwood, MA 02062

Palmer

Profiles, Inc.   800-959-3171
7 First St., Palmer Industrial Park, Palmer, MA 01069
Sanderson-Macleod, Inc.   866-522-3481
1199 S. Main St., Palmer, MA 01069-0050

Peabody

Analogic Corporation   978-326-4000
8 Centennial Drive, Peabody, MA 01960-7902
International Light Technologies, Inc.   978-818-6180
10 Technology Drive, Peabody, MA 01960
Jeol Usa, Inc.   978-536-2270
11 Dearborn Road, Peabody, MA 01960-3823
Richard-James, Inc.   978-532-0666
2 Centennial Dr., Peabody, MA 01960
Sleepmed Incorporated   800-334-5085
200 Corporate Place, Ste. 5-B, Peabody, MA 01960

Pembroke

E. Benson Hood Laboratories, Inc.   800-942-5227
575 Washington St., Pembroke, MA 02359-2318
Fci Ophthalmics   800-932-4202
64 Schoosett Street, Pembroke, MA 02359

Pittsfield

Pst   413-447-8051
1520 East St., Pittsfield, MA 01201
Stuart Allyn Co., Inc.   413-443-7306
17 Taconic Park Dr., Pittsfield, MA 01202

Plainville

Dale Medical Products, Inc.   800-343-3980
7 Cross St., Plainville, MA 02762-0556
Hilco   800-955-6544
33 W. Bacon St., Plainville, MA 02762

Plymouth

Harvest Technologies, Corp.   508-732-7500
40 Grissom Rd, Suite 100, Plymouth, MA 02360
Medical Monofilament Manufacturing   508-746-7877
116 Long Pond Rd., Plymouth, MA 02360
R&Da Co.   508-747-5803
37 Dwight Avenue, Plymouth, MA 02360-2159

Richards Micro-Tool, Inc.   508-746-6900
250 Nicks Road,, Plymouth, MA 02360-2800

Quincy

Boston Scientific - Marina Bay Customer Fulfillment   617-689-6000
Center
500 Commander Shea Blvd, Quincy, MA 02171
Schuerch Corp.   617-773-0927
48 Oval Road, Quincy, MA 02169
Stephen Tobias Hearing Center   617-770-3395
382 Quincy Avenue, Quincy, MA 02169
Work, Inc.   800-898-0301
3 Arlington St., Quincy, MA 02171

Randolph

Randolph Engineering, Inc.   781-961-6070
26 Thomas Patten Dr., Randolph, MA 02368

Raynham

Codman & Shurtleff, Inc   800-382-4682
325 Paramount Dr., Raynham, MA 02767
Codman And Shurtleff, Inc   508-880-8100
325 Paramount Drive, Raynham, MA 02767
Depuy Mitek, Inc.   800-451-2006
325 Paramount Dr., Raynham, MA 02767
Depuy Spine, Inc.   800-227-6633
325 Paramount Dr., Raynham, MA 02767
Depuy-Raynham, A Div. Of Depuy Orthopaedics   800-451-2006
325 Paramount Dr., Raynham, MA 02767-0350
Mitek Products   800-356-4835
325 Paramount Drive, Raynham, MA 02767

Rockland

BIOSPHERE MEDICAL, INC.   781-681-7900
1050 Hingham St., Rockland, MA 02370
Grass Technologies, An Astro-Med, Inc. Product Gro   401-828-4002
53 Airport Park Drive, Rockland, MA 02370
Paradigm Biodevices, Inc.   781-982-9950
800 Hingham St. Suite 102n, Suite 207S, Rockland, MA 02370

Salisbury

Andover Healthcare Inc.   800-432-6686
9 Fanaras Dr., Salisbury, MA 01952

Scituate

Energy Medicine Center   781-545-1277
88 Front Street, Suite 31, Scituate, MA 02066

Sherborn

Boston Rheology, L.L.C.   617-912-1020
20 Whitney Drive, Chestnut Hill Medical Center, Sherborn, MA 01770

Shirley

Tpv Manufacturingÿ   978-425-8940
2 Shaker Road, Unit A101, Shirley, MA 01464

Shrewsbury

Valeritas, Llc   508-845-1177
800 Boston Turnpike, Shrewsbury, MA 01545

Somerville

Audiological Engineering Corp.   800-283-4601
9 Preston Road, Somerville, MA 02143-4242
Technofrolics   617-441-8870
11 Miller Street, Somerville, MA 02143
Whalen Biomedical Incorporated   617-868-4433
11 Miller St., Somerville, MA 02143

South Boston

Tekscan, Inc.   800-248-3669
307 West First St., South Boston, MA 02127-1309

South Easton

Holmed Corporation   508-238-3351
40 Norfolk Avenue, South Easton, MA 02375
Mecanaids Co., Inc.   800-227-0877
21 Hampden Drive, South Easton, MA 02375

South Lee

Boyd Converting Co., Inc.   800-262-2242
PO BOX 287, South Lee, MA 01260

South Waltham

Rhytec Incorporated   781-474-9832
130 Turner Street, Building 2, South Waltham, MA 02453

South Yarmouth

Coren   877-267-3677
15 Fruean Ave, South Yarmouth, MA 02664

Southborough

Nest Group Inc., The   800-347-6378
45 Valley Rd., Southborough, MA 01772

Southbridge

Aearo Company — 508-764-5713
90 Mechanic St., Southbridge, MA 01550
Ao Eyewear, Inc. — 800-777-1173
529 Ashland Ave., Suite 3, P.o. Box 1064, Southbridge, MA 01550
Clinical Instruments Intl., Inc. — 508-764-2200
278 Worcester St., Southbridge, MA 01550
Fused Fiberoptics L.L.C. — 508-765-1652
79 Golf St., Southbridge, MA 01550-2809
Peltor, Inc. — 800-444-4774
90 Mechanic St., Southbridge, MA 01550

Springfield

Blackstone Medical, Inc. — 888-298-5400
90 Brookdale Dr., Springfield, MA 01104
Microscopy/Microscopy Education — 413-746-6931
125 Paridon St., Suite 102, Springfield, MA 01108-2140
Spirig Advanced Technologies, Inc. — 413-788-6191
144 Oakland St., Springfield, MA 01108-1787

Sterling

Fiberoptic Components, Llc — 978-422-0422
2 Spratt Tech. Way, Sterling, MA 01564
Image Diagnostics, Inc. — 978-422-8601
98 Pratts Junction Rd., Sterling, MA 01564

Stoughton

Biomedical Technologies, Inc. — 781-344-9942
378 Page St., Stoughton, MA 02072-1141
Cardiosolutions Inc. — 781-344-0801
75 Mill St., Stoughton, MA 02072
Computer Sports Medicine, Inc. — 781-297-2034
101 Tosca Dr., Stoughton, MA 02072
Haemonetics Corp. — 781-356-9488
179 Campanelli Parkway, Stoughton, MA 02072
Labworld, Inc. — 800-447-2428
471 Page St., Bldg 4, Stoughton, MA 02072
Learning Curve Brands Inc. THE FIRST YEARS — 800-225-0382
100 Technology Center Drive, Suite 2A, Stoughton, MA 02072
Spirus Medical, Inc. — 781-297-7220
1063 Turnpike Street, PO Box 258, Stoughton, MA 02072
Std Med, Inc. — 781-828-4400
75 Mill Street, PO Box 420, Stoughton, MA 02072

Sturbridge

Alsco Industries, Inc. — 508-347-1199
174 Charlton Rd, Po Box 1168, Sturbridge, MA 01566
G & F Industries, Inc. — 508-347-9132
Rt. 20 Box 515, Sturbridge, MA 01566
Optim Incorporated — 800-225-7486
64 Technology Park Road, Sturbridge, MA 01566-1253

Sudbury

Sudbury Systems — 800-876-8888
490 Boston Post Rd., Sudbury, MA 01776

Taunton

Bacon Felt Company, Inc. — 508-823-0791
395 W. Water St., Taunton, MA 02780-4847
Medical Scientific, Inc. — 508-880-7313
725 Myles Standish Blvd., Taunton, MA 02780
Pcn, Inc. — 508-880-7140
125 John Hancock Road, Taunton, MA 02780

Tewksbury

Cambridge Heart Inc. — 888-CAM-WAVE
100 Ames Pond Dr, Suite 100, Tewksbury, MA 01876
Cambridge Heart, Inc. — 888-226-9283
100 Ames Pond Drive, Suite 100, Tewksbury, MA 01876
Philips Healthcare — 614-865-8956
836 North St, Bld 500, Tewksbury, MA 01876

Topsfield

Marine Polymer Technologies, Inc. — 888-666-2560
461 Boston St., Unit B5, Topsfield, MA 01983
Zoe Medical, Inc. — 978-887-1410
460 Boston St., Topsfield, MA 01983

Tyngsboro

Progressive Appliance Corp. — 978-649-9334
9 Gloria Ave., Tyngsboro, MA 01879
Quartet Technology, Inc. — 978-649-4328
87 Progress Avenue, Tyngsboro, MA 01879
Radiomed Corporation — 866-649-0300
One Industrial Way, Tyngsboro, MA 01879-1400
Stereoimaging Corporation — 978-649-8592
164 Westford Rd. Suite 17, Tyngsboro, MA 01879

Uxbridge

Mira, Inc. — 508-278-7877
414 Quaker Highway, Uxbridge, MA 01569

Wakefield

Agion Technologies Inc. — 781-224-7100
60 Audubon Rd., Wakefield, MA 01880
BIOCIUS Life Sciences Inc. — 781-928-2700
11 Audubon Road, Wakefield, MA 01880
Creative Marketing Concepts, Inc. — 978-532-7517
96 Audubon Road, Wakefield, MA 01880
Implant Sciences Corp. — 781-246-0700
107 Audubon Road, #5, Wakefield, MA 01880-1246
Nucryst Pharmaceuticals Corp. — 781-224-1444
50 Audobon Rd., Suite B, Wakefield, MA 01880
Picis Inc. — 781-557-3000
100 Quannapowitt Parkway, Suite 405, Wakefield, MA 01880

Walpole

Primrose Medical, Inc. — 508-660-8688
478 High Plain St., Walpole, MA 02081

Waltham

Alere, Inc. — 781-647-3900
51 Sawyer Road, Suite 200, Waltham, MA 02453
Astra Tech Inc — 800-531-3481
590 Lincoln Street, Waltham, MA 02451
Augmenix Inc. — 781-895-3235
204 Second Ave., Lower Level, Waltham, MA 02451
Avedro, Inc. — 781-768-3400
230 Third Avenue, Waltham, MA 02451
BG Medicine Inc. — 781-890-1199
610N Lincoln Street, Waltham, MA 02451
Becton Dickinson And Co. — 866-906-8080
411 Waverley Oaks Rd., Waltham, MA 02452-8405
Confluent Surgical,Inc — 888-734-2583
101A First Ave., Waltham, MA 02451
Etonic Worldwide Llc — 781-419-3060
260 Charles Street, Waltham, MA 02453
Fresenius Medical Care North America — 800-662-1237
920 Winter Street, Waltham, MA 02451
Fresenius Usa, Inc. — 800-662-1237
920 Winter Street, Waltham, MA 02451-1457
Industrial & Biomedical Sensors Corp. — 781-891-4201
1377 Main St., Waltham, MA 02451-1624
Neurometrix, Inc. — 888-786-7287
62 Fourth Ave., Waltham, MA 02451
Nova Biomedical — 800-458-5813
200 Prospect St., Waltham, MA 02454-9141
Pace Medical, Inc. — 781-890-5656
391 Totten Pond Rd., Waltham, MA 02451
Parexel International Corp. — 781-487-9900
195 West St., Waltham, MA 02451
PerkinElmer — 800-762-4000
940 Winter Street, Waltham, MA 02451
Perkinelmer Life And Analytical Sciences — 800-762-4000
940 Winter Street, Waltham, MA 02451
Thermo Fisher Scientific — 877-843-7668
81 Wyman Street, Waltham, MA 02454-9046
Thermo Fisher Scientific Inc. — 781-622-1000
81 Wyman Street, Waltham, MA 02454

Ward Hill

Alfa Aesar, A Johnson Matthey Company — 800-343-0660
26 Parkridge Road, Ward Hill, MA 01835-8099

Ware

American Disposables, Inc. — 413-967-6201
6 East Main St., Ware, MA 01082

Wareham

Tak Systems — 800-333-9631
14 Kendricks Road, Suite 5, Wareham, MA 02571-5020

Watertown

Advanced Mechanical Technology, Inc. (Amti) — 800-422-AMTI
176 Waltham St., Watertown, MA 02472
Bio Breeders, Inc. — 617-926-5278
116 Temperton Parkway, Watertown, MA 02472
Exergen Corp. — 800-422-3006
400 Pleasant Street, Watertown, MA 02472
Pulpdent Corp. — 800-343-4342
80 Oakland St., Watertown, MA 02471-0780
Radiation Monitoring Devices, Inc. — 800-532-3763
44 Hunt St., Watertown, MA 02472
Techdevice Corporation — 888-TECHDEV
650 Pleasant St., Watertown, MA 02472
United Electric Controls Co. — 617-926-1000
180 Dexter Ave., P.O. Box 9143, Watertown, MA 02472-9143

Wayland

Candela Corp. — 800-733-8550
530 Boston Post Rd., Wayland, MA 01778-1833

West Barnstable

R. D. Equipment, Inc. — 508-362-7498
230 Percival Dr., West Barnstable, MA 02668

West Boylston

Integra Luxtec, Inc. — 800-325-8966
99 Hartwell St., West Boylston, MA 01583

West Bridgewater

Bbi Diagnostics, A Division Of Seracare Life Scien — 508-244-6428
375 West St., West Bridgewater, MA 02379

West Brookfield

Brookfield Optical Systems — 508-867-6675
218 Wigwam Rd., West Brookfield, MA 01585

West Springfield

Alden Medical Llc — 413-747-9717
360 Cold Spring Ave., West Springfield, MA 01089
Cyalume Technologies, Inc. — (888) 858-7881
96 Windsor St., West Springfield, MA 01089
Package Machinery Co. — 413-732-4000
380 Union St. #58, West Springfield, MA 01089
Wheelchair Sales And Service Co., Inc. — 877-736-0376
315 Main St., West Springfield, MA 01089

Westborough

Boston Medical Products, Inc. — 800-433-2674
117 Flanders Road, Westborough, MA 01581-1042
Security Engineered Machinery — 800-225-9293
5 Walkup Drive, Westborough, MA 01581
Viking Systems Inc. — 508-366-3668
134 Flanders Rd., Westborough, MA 01581
mtm Laboratories Inc. — 866-686-5227
One Research Drive, Suite 120c, Westborough, MA 01581

Westfield

Instrument Technology, Inc. — 413-562-3606
33 Airport Rd., Westfield, MA 01085
Jarvis Surgical, Inc. — 413-562-6659
53 Airport Rd., Westfield, MA 01085

Westford

Barr Associates, Inc. — 978-692-7513
2 Lyberty Way, Westford, MA 01886-3616
Biobehavioral Diagnostics Company — 877-246-2397
239 Littleton Road, Suite 6A, Westford, MA 01886
Cynosure, Inc. — 800-886-2966
5 Carlisle Road, Westford, MA 01886
Duxbury Systems, Inc. — 978-692-3000
270 Littleton Road, #6, Westford, MA 01886
Hydrodot, Inc. — 978-399-0206
238 Littleton Road, Suite 202, Westford, MA 01886
LightLab Imaging Inc. — 978-399-1000
One Technology Park Drive, Westford, MA 01886

Westhampton

Brown Engineering Corp. — 800-726-4233
289 Chesterfield Road, Westhampton, MA 01027

Westminster

Simplexgrinnell Lp — 800-746-7539
50 Technology Dr, Westminster, MA 01441-0001

Westport

Hoyt Corp. — 800-343-9411
251 Forge Road, Westport, MA 02790-0217
Zibra Corp. — 800-758-8773
640 American Legion Hwy., Westport, MA 02790

Westwood

Iris Sample Processing — 800-782-8774
60 Glacier Drive, Westwood, MA 02090-1825
Medical Information Technology, Inc. — 781-821-3000
Meditech Circle, Westwood, MA 02090
Medical Information Technology, Inc. (Meditech) — 781-821-3000
Meditech Circle, Westwood, MA 02090
Statspin, Inc. — 800-782-8774
60 Glacier Drive, Westwood, MA 02090-1825
The Microoptical Corporation — 781-326-8111
33 Southwest Park, Westwood, MA 02090

Weymouth

Lhasa Oms, Inc. — 800-722-8775
230 Libbey Parkway, Weymouth, MA 02189
Seirin-America, Inc. — 800-337-9338
230 Libbey Pkwy., Weymouth, MA 02189

Whitman

Symmetry Tnco — 888-447-6661
15 Colebrook Blvd., Whitman, MA 02382

Wilmington

Accellent Inc. — 866-899-1392
100 Fordham Road, Wilmington, MA 01887
Advansource Biomaterials Corp. — 978-657-0075
229 Andover St., Wilmington, MA 01887

Atc Technologies, Inc. — 781-939-0725
30-B Upton Drive, Wilmington, MA 01887
Dusa Pharmaceuticals, Inc. — 978-657-7500
25 Upton Dr., Wilmington, MA 01887
Embryotech Laboratories, Inc. — 800-673-7500
323 Andover St., Wilmington, MA 01887-1035
Lightolier A Genlyte Co. — 978-657-7600
45 Industrial Way, Wilmington, MA 01887
Omnisonics Medical Technologies — 978-657-9980
66 Concord Street, Suite A, Wilmington, MA 01887
Oni Medical Systems, Inc. — 978-658-0020
301 Ballardvale Street, Suite 4, Wilmington, MA 01887-4405
Ophir Optronics, Inc. — 800-820-0814
260A Fordham Road, Wilmington, MA 01887
SensAble Technologies, Inc. — 781-937-8315
181 Ballardvale Street, Wilmington, MA 01887
Spectra Medical Devices, Inc. — 978-657-0889
260-H Fordham Road, Wilmington, MA 01887
Tecomet, A Subsidiary Of Viasys Healthcare Inc. — 978-658-3379
115 Eames St., Wilmington, MA 01887

Winchester

CardiAQ Valve Technologies — 617-957-8945
1 Orient Street, Winchester, MA 01890

WImington

Bausch & Lomb, Inc. — 585-338-8731
100 Research Drive, WImington, MA 01887

Woburn

Aeris Therapeutics, Inc. — 781-937-0110
10k Gill Street, Woburn, MA 01801
Bryan Corp. — 800-343-7711
4 Plympton St., Woburn, MA 01801-2908
Cambridge Research & Instrumentation (CRi) — 800-383-7924
35-B Cabot Road, Woburn, MA 01801
Claros Diagnostics Inc. — 781-933-8012
4 Constitution Way, Suite E, Woburn, MA 01801
Continental Metal Products Co., Inc. — 800-221-4439
35 Olympia Avenue, Woburn, MA 01801
Convergence Medical Devices — 888-362-8824
400 TradeCenter, Suite 5900, Woburn, MA 01801
Covaris Inc. — 781-932-3959
14 Gill Street, Unit H, Woburn, MA 01801
Dan Kar Corporation — 800-942-5542
192 New Boston St C, Woburn, MA 01801
Gregstrom Corp. — 781-935-6600
64 Holton St., P.O. Box 609, Woburn, MA 01801
HighRes Biosolutions, Inc. — 781.932.1912
299 Washington Street, Woburn, MA 01801
Intrinsic Therapeutics Inc. — 781-932-0222
30 Commerce Way, Woburn, MA 01801
Lytron, Inc. — 781-933-7300
55 Dragon Ct., Woburn, MA 01801-1039
Medchem Products, Inc. — 800-451-4716
160 New Boston St., Woburn, MA 01801-6333
Medchem Products, Inc. — 908-277-8000
160 New Boston St., Woburn, MA 01801
Openmed Technologies Corporation — 877-717-6215
256 West Cummings Park, Woburn, MA 01801-6436
Pierce Biotechnology — 800-487-4885
30 Commerce Way, Woburn, MA 01801-1059
Pluromed, Inc — 781-932-0574
175-F New Boston Street, Woburn, MA 01801
Safegard Medical Products, Inc. — 800-389-7173
52 Dragon Ct., Woburn, MA 01801
Spectra Medical Devices, Inc. — 866-938-8649
4C Henshaw St., Woburn, MA 01801
Splash Shield, Inc. — 800-536-6686
52 Dragon Ct., Woburn, MA 01801
Tungstone Power Inc — 800-232-3557
623 Main St., Woburn, MA 01801

Worcester

Grove Instruments Inc — 508-799-8800
100 Grove Street, Suite 315, Worcester, MA 01605
Clark Company Inc., David — 800-900-3434
360 Franklin St., Worcester, MA 01615-0054
David Clark Company, Inc. — 800-900-3434
360 Franklin St., Worcester, MA 01604
Schoelly Imaging, Inc. — 1 (508) 926 885
722 Plantation Street, Worcester, MA 01605
Walker Ldj Scientific, Inc. — 800-962-4638
10 Rockdale Street, Worcester, MA 01606-1922

Wrentham

Genesis Medical Products, Inc. — 508-876-1063
40 Farmhill Rd., Wrentham, MA 02093

MICHIGAN

Ada

Access Business Group Llc
7575 East Fulton St., Ada, MI 49355
616-787-4964

Alanson

Stonhouse Manufacturing
7693 Barney Rd, Alanson, MI 49706-9214
231-548-5630

Albion

MedCaster Inc.
800 N. Clark Street, Albion, MI 49224
866-462-9700

Ossur Americas
910 Burstein Dr., Albion, MI 49224
517-629-8890

Allendale

Aluwax Dental Products Co.
5260 Edgewater Drive, Allendale, MI 49401
616-895-4385

Alma

Liquipak Corp.
2205 Michigan Ave., Alma, MI 48801
989-463-5510

Ann Arbor

Accumed Systems, Inc.
6109 Jackson Road, Ann Arbor, MI 48103
734-930-0461

Accuri Cytometers Inc.
173 Parkland Plaza, Ann Arbor, MI 48103
734-994-8000

Ann Arbor Digital Devices
699 Skynob Court, Ann Arbor, MI 48105
734-834-5156

Automated Imaging Association
900 Victors Way, PO Box 3724, Ann Arbor, MI 48106
800-994-6099

Controlled Chemicals, Inc.
317 South Division, Suite 9, Ann Arbor, MI 48104
734-769-5940

Cybernet Systems Corp.
3885 Research Park Drive, Ann Arbor, MI 48108
734-668-2567

Danmar Products, Inc.
221 Jackson Industrial Dr., Ann Arbor, MI 48103
734-761-1990

Eaton Medical Devices, Inc.
254 S Wagner Rd, P.O. Box 1002, Ann Arbor, MI 48106
734-428-0000

Eaton Medical Devices, Inc.
254 South Wagner Rd., Ann Arbor, MI 48103-1940
734-428-0000

Eberbach Corp.
505 S. Maple Rd., Ann Arbor, MI 48106-1024
800-422-2558

Enmet Corp.
680 Fairfield Ct., Ann Arbor, MI 48106-0979
734-761-1270

Everist Genomics
709 W. Ellsworth Road, Ann Arbor, MI 48108
855-383-7478

General Scientific Corp.
77 Enterprise Drive, Ann Arbor, MI 48103
800-959-0153

Handylab
5230 South State Rd., Ann Arbor, MI 48108
734-663-4719

Invia, Llc
3025 Boardwalk Street, Suite 200, Ann Arbor, MI 48108
734-205-1231

Medimage, Inc.
6276 Jackson Rd. Ste. G, Ann Arbor, MI 48103
734-665-5400

NextGen Sciences Inc
401 Varsity Drive, Suite E, Ann Arbor, MI 48108
1-866-973-7914

Pall Corporation
600 S. Wagner Road, Ann Arbor, MI 48103
800-521-1520

Pall Medical
600 S. Wagner Rd., Ann Arbor, MI 48103
800-521-1520

Siemens Medical Solutions Usa, Inc
400 W. Morgan Road, Suite 100, Ann Arbor, MI 48108
888-826-9702

Tangent Medical Technologies Inc.
58 Parkland Plaza, Suite 300, Ann Arbor, MI 48103
734-330-2668

Terumo Cardiovascular Systems, Corp
6200 Jackson Rd., Ann Arbor, MI 48103-9300
800-521-2818

Terumo Heart Inc. (Thi)
6180 Jackson Road, Ann Arbor, MI 48103
800-803-8385

The Regents Of The University Of Michigan
3003 S. State, Rm 1072, Ann Arbor, MI 48109-1274
734-615-8433

Xoran Technologies, Inc.
5210 South State Road, Ann Arbor, MI 48103-3301
800-709-6726

Auburn Hills

CJPS Medical Systems
2333 E. Walton Blvd., Auburn Hills, MI 48326
248-593-5926

Battle Creek

Anatech, Ltd.
1020 Harts Lake Rd., Battle Creek, MI 49015-1065
800-262-8324

Battle Creek Equipment Co.
307 W. Jackson St., Battle Creek, MI 49017-2306
800-253-0854

Bay City

H2only Co.
1101 Columbus Ave., Bay City, MI 48708
800-338-4905

Serv-A-Pure Company
1101 Columbus Ave., Bay City, MI 48708
800-338-4905

Belmont

Zimcor Corporation
6414 Skyridge Dr. Ne, Belmont, MI 49306
616-813-2699

Benton Harbor

Browning Enterprises, Inc.
1234 Zoschke Rd., Benton Harbor, MI 49022
616-849-2420

Gast Manufacturing
P.O. Box 97, Benton Harbor, MI 49023-0097
269.926.6171

Jun-Air Usa,Inc.
2300 Highway M-139, Benton Harbor, MI 49022
jun-air.usa@ide

Beulah

Thorn Smith Laboratories
7755 Narrow Gauge Rd., Beulah, MI 49617
231-882-7251

Birmingham

Americorp Financial, Inc.
877 S. Adams Road, Birmingham, MI 48009-7029
800-233-1574

Bloomfield Hills

Lynn Medical
764 Denison Ct., Bloomfield Hills, MI 48302-0300
888-596-6633

Bridgeport

Amigo Mobility International
6693 Dixie Hwy., Bridgeport, MI 48722-9725
800-248-9131

Orchid Unique
6688 Dixie Hwy., Bridgeport, MI 48722
989-746-0780

Brighton

Lunax Corp.
6669 Westridge, Brighton, MI 48116
800-355-8629

Brooklyn

Midwest Health Care Consultants Inc.
154 Southern Shores, Brooklyn, MI 49230
231-354-7482

Caledonia

Aspen Surgical
6945 South Belt Drive SE, Caledonia, MI 49316
800-328-7958

Vascular Performance Products, Llc.
6945 Southbelt Dr., Se, Caledonia, MI 49316
888-364-7004

Canton

Clean Air Technology, Inc.
41105 Capital, Canton, MI 48187
800 459 6320

Pointe Scientific, Inc.
5449 Research Drive, Canton, MI 48188
800-445-9853

Centerline

Robinson Audiology Laboratories
8033 East 10 Mile Rd., #104, Centerline, MI 48015
810-754-3511

Chelsea

Orchid Macdee Inc.
13800 Luick Drive, Chelsea, MI 48118-9588
734-475-9165

Clarkston

Jade Hearing Instruments
6803 Dixie Hwy., Suite #2, Clarkston, MI 48346
248-922-5600

Clinton Township

Rjl Systems, Inc.
33939 Harper Ave., Clinton Township, MI 48035
586-790-0200

Coldwater

Kilgore International, Inc.
36 W. Pearl St., Coldwater, MI 49036-0098
800-892-9999

Tj Rampit, Inc.
338 Bidwell Road, Coldwater, MI 49036
800-876-9498

Commerce Township

Homedics Inc.
3000 Pontiac Trail, Commerce Township, MI 48390
800-333-8282

Corunna

Advanced Air Technologies, Inc.
300 Sleeseman Drive, Corunna, MI 48817
800-295-6583

Dearborn

Ec Moore Company, Inc
13325 Leonard Street, Dearborn, MI 48126-3633
800-331-3548

Detroit

Co/Op Optical Vision Designs
2424 E. Eight Mile Road, E. of Dequindre, Detroit, MI 48234-1010
866-733-2667

Et Training Systems, Llc
3494 Cambridge, Detroit, MI 48221
313-864-1317

Dowagiac

B. Graczyk, Inc.
27826 Burmax Court, Dowagiac, MI 49047
269-782-2100

Edwardsburg

Imagepath Systems, Inc.   269-699-7182
23126 South Shore Rd., Edwardsburg, MI 49112

Trigon Technology, Inc.   269-699-7182
23126 South Shore Dr., Edwardsburg, MI 49112

Farmington Hills

I-Beam Walking Machine   248-477-9808
21755 Ruth St, Farmington Hills, MI 48336

Fenton

Cfi Medical Solutions (Contour Fabricators, Inc.)   810-750-5300
14241 Fenton Road, Fenton, MI 48430

Excel Medical Products, Llc   810-714-4775
3145 Copper Avenue, Fenton, MI 48430

Phoenix Dental, Inc.   877-463-9905
3452 West Thompson Rd., Fenton, MI 48430

Ferndale

Ferndale Laboratories, Inc.   888-548-0900
780 West Eight Mile Rd., Ferndale, MI 48220

Rinz-L-O   248-548-3993
340 West Maplehurst, Ferndale, MI 48220

Flint

Costonde Products Llc   810-743-1167
419 Tennyson Ave, P.O. Box 7179Flint, Flint, MI 48507

Davismade, Inc.   866-742-0581
2511 Davison Road, Flint, MI 48506-3649

Frankfort

Invirion, Inc.   866-231-8378
2350 Pilgrim Hwy., Frankfort, MI 49635

Fraser

College Park Industries, Inc.   800-728-7950
17505 Helro Drive, Fraser, MI 48026

Healthmark Industries   800-521-6224
33671 Doreka, Fraser, MI 48026

Grand Blanc

Barron Precision Instruments, L.L.C.   810-695-2080
8170 Embury Rd., PO Box 973, Grand Blanc, MI 48480

Omega Surgical Instruments   800-656-6342
G-8305 Saginaw St., Suite 6, Grand Blanc, MI 48439

Grand Rapids

American Seating   616-732-6600
401 American Seating Ctr. NW, Grand Rapids, MI 49504

Art Optical Contact Lens, Inc.   800-253-9364
3175 Three Mile Road NW, PO Box 1848, Grand Rapids, MI 49501-1848

Atek Medical   800-253-1540
620 Watson St, Grand Rapids, MI 49504-6393

Cascade Life Solutions, Llc   616-977-2505
3710 Sysco Court Se, Grand Rapids, MI 49512

Kem Ent., Inc.   888-562-8802
PO Box 6342, Grand Rapids, MI 49516

Lt Acquisition, Inc.   616-698-1830
4489 East Paris Ave., Grand Rapids, MI 49512

Lydia's Professional Uniforms   800-942-3378
2500 E Beltline Ave SE #K, Grand Rapids, MI 49546

Mar-Med Co.   800-369-3434
345 Fuller Ave. NE, Grand Rapids, MI 49503

Medical Id Systems Inc.   800-262-2399
3954 44th Street S.E., Grand Rapids, MI 49512-3942

Medtronic Dlp   616-643-5200
620 Watson St., S.W., Grand Rapids, MI 49504-6450

Michigan Instruments, Inc.   800-530-9939
4717 Talon Ct. S.E., Grand Rapids, MI 49512-5409

Oliver Medical   800-253-3893
445 Sixth St. N.W., Grand Rapids, MI 49504-5253

Performance Systematix Inc   616-949-9090
5569 33RD Street S.E., Grand Rapids, MI 49512

Ranir Corp.   800-253-0906
4701 E. Paris Ave. S.E., Grand Rapids, MI 49512-5353

Ranir, Llc   616-698-8880
4701 East Paris Avenue SE, Grand Rapids, MI 49512

Rose Technologies Company   616-233-3000
1440 Front Ave, Grand Rapids, MI 49504

Royce Rolls Ringer Co.   800-253-9638
PO Box 1831, 16 Riverview Terrace, Grand Rapids, MI 49501-1831

Ruhling Enterprises, Inc.   616-364-0090
4598 Plainfield Ne, Grand Rapids, MI 49525

Skytron   800-759-8766
5085 Corporate Exchange Blvd. S.E., Grand Rapids, MI 49512

Surge Medical Solutions, Llc.   616-977-2516
3710 Sysco Ct. S.e., Grand Rapids, MI 49512

Vital Concepts, Inc.   800-984-2300
4334 Brockton Drive SE, Suite F, Grand Rapids, MI 49512

X-Rite, Inc.   888-826-3044
4300 44th Street SE, Grand Rapids, MI 49512

Grass Lake

Coy Laboratory Products, Inc.   734-475-2200
14500 Coy Drive, Grass Lake, MI 49240

Grayling

Stephan Wood Products, Inc.   989-348-5496
605 Huron, P.O. Box 669, Grayling, MI 49738-0669

Greenville

Marvel Scientific   800-223-3900
PO Box 400, Greenville, MI 48838

Hamburg

Prenatal Cradle, Inc.   800-383-3068
P O BOX 443, Hamburg, MI 48139-0443

Higgins Lake

Porto-Lift Corp.   800-321-1454
PO Box 5, Higgins Lake, MI 48627

Hillsdale

Alsons Corp.   800-421-0001
3010 West Mechanic St., P.O. Box 282, Hillsdale, MI 49242

Great Lakes Filters/Filpaco Industries   517-639-8470
301 Arch Avenue, hillsdale, MI 49242

Holland

Air Force, Inc.   616-399-8511
933 Butternut Dr., Holland, MI 49424

Fleetwood Group, Incorporated   800-257-6390
11832 James Street, Holland, MI 49422-1259

Haworth, Inc.   800-426-8562
One Haworth Center, Holland, MI 49423-9570

Total Innovative Manufacturing   616-738-8299
12688 New Holland St., Holland, MI 49424

Windquest   800-562-4257
3311 Windquest Drive, Holland, MI 49424-9570

Holt

Orchid Stealth Orthopedic Solutions   517-694-2300
1489 Cedar St., Holt, MI 48842

Howell

Rf Design, Inc.   810-632-6000
10143 Bergin Rd., Howell, MI 48843

Tri-State Hospital Supply Corp.   800-248-4058
301 Catrell Drive, PO Box 170, Howell, MI 48843-0170

Imlay City

Champion Bus Inc.   800-776-4943
331 Graham Rd., Imlay City, MI 48444

Interlochen

Alivio Corporation   231-275-1345
20429 Honor Hwy., Interlochen, MI 49643

Ironwood

Ironwood Plastics, Inc.   906-932-5025
1235 Wall St., Ironwood, MI 49938

Jackson

Midbrook, Inc.   1-800-966-WASH
2080 Brooklyn Rd., Jackson, MI 49203

Kalamazoo

Aero Contact Lens, Inc.   269-345-3202
2958 Business One Drive, Kalamazoo, MI 49048

Helvetia Development Co. Llc.   269-345-1620
225 Parson's St., Kalamazoo, MI 49007

Medical Marketing Services   800-927-0791
2322 Nazareth Rd., Kalamazoo, MI 49048

Pharmacia & Upjohn Co.   212-573-1000
7000 Portage Rd., Kalamazoo, MI 49001

Richard-Allan Scientific   269-544-5628
4481 Campus Dr., Kalamazoo, MI 49008

Striker Corp.   800 253 3210
4100 East Milham Avenue, Kalamazoo, MI 49001

Stryker Corp.   800-726-2725
2825 Airview Boulevard, Kalamazoo, MI 49002

Stryker Instruments, Instruments Div.   800-253-3210
4100 East Milham Ave., Kalamazoo, MI 49001

Stryker Medical   800-869-0770
2825 Airview Boulevard, Kalamazoo, MI 49002

Tekna Solutions, Inc.   269-978-3500
3400 Tech Circle, Kalamazoo, MI 49008

Kentwood

Inrad   800-558-4647
4375 Donker Court S.E., Kentwood, MI 49512

Northern Falls, Llc   616-975-0733
4460 44th Se, Suite A, Kentwood, MI 49512

Z-Man Corporation   616-281-6108
1359 Pickett, SE, Kentwood, MI 49508

Laingsburg

Function Technologies, Inc. — 866-324-1771
8002 Upton Road, Laingsburg, MI 48848

Lansing

Acumedia Manufacturers, Inc. — 800-783-3212
620 Lesher Place, Lansing, MI 48912
Airgas Great Lakes, Inc. — 517-894-4101
5018 Empire Way, Lansing, MI 48917
Bretton Square Industries — 800-360-6126
812 E. Jolly Rd., Ste. 216, Lansing, MI 48910
Information Health Network — 800-443-0613
PO Box 23056, Lansing, MI 48909-3056
Neogen Corporation — 800-234-5333
620 Lesher Place, Lansing, MI 48912

Livonia

American Dryer, Inc. — 800-485-7003
12932 Farmington Road, Livonia, MI 48150-4201
Interphase Implants, Inc. — 248-442-1460
19928 Farmington Road, Livonia, MI 48152
Mason Dental Midwest, Inc. — 734-525-1070
12752 Stark Road, Livonia, MI 48150
Metro Medical Equipment, Inc. — 734-522-8400
12985 Wayne Road, Livonia, MI 48150
Mikron Digital Imaging, Inc. — 800-925-3905
30425 Eight Mile Road, Livonia, MI 48152

Madison Heights

Aventric Technologies — 800-228-3343
1551 E. Lincoln Ave., Suite 166, Madison Heights, MI 48071
Michclone Associates, Inc. — 248-583-1150
680 Ajax Dr, Madison Heights, MI 48071

Marne

Safe Solutions, Inc. — 616-677-2850
2530 Hayes St., Marne, MI 49435

Marquette

Pioneer Surgical Technology — 800-557-9909
375 River Park Circle, Marquette, MI 49855

Marshall

Progressive Dynamics Medical, Inc. — 269-781-4241
507 Industrial Rd., Marshall, MI 49068-1758

Marysville

Signal Medical Corp. — 810-364-7070
400 Pyramid Dr., Marysville, MI 48040

Mason

Roger L. Goodman, D.D.S., P.C. — 517-676-5200
200 Temple St., Mason, MI 48854-1837

Memphis

Grace Engineering Corp. — 810-392-2181
34775 Potter St., Memphis, MI 48041-0202

Midland

Caltech Industries, Inc. — 800-234-7700
2420 Schuette Drive, Midland, MI 48642-5974
Wysong Corporation — 989-631-0009
7550 Eastman Avenue, Midland, MI 48640-8838

Milan

Clever Solutions, Inc. — 800-743-6165
10163 Faetano Lane, Milan, MI 48160

Millington

Gunnell, Inc. — 800-551-0055
8440 State Rd., Millington, MI 48746-9401

Monroe

La-Z-Boy Incorporated — 734-242-1444
1284 North Telegraph Rd., Monroe, MI 48162

Muskegon

American Coil Spring Co. — 231-726-4021
1041 E. Keating Avenue, Muskegon, MI 49442-5996
Geerpres — 800-253-0373
1780 Harvey St., Muskegon, MI 49443-0658
Honeywell Burdick & Jackson — 800-368-0050
1953 S. Harvey St., Muskegon, MI 49442-6101
Innovative Healthcare Products, Llc — 231-755-0277
3120 South Getty St., Muskegon, MI 49444
Knoll, Inc. — 800-343-5665
2800 Estes St., Muskegon, MI 49441-1697

Niles

Innovative Products Unlimited, Inc. — 800-833-2826
2120 Industrial Drive, Niles, MI 49120
Toefco Engineering Coating Systems — 800-555-6495
1220 N. 14th St., Niles, MI 49120

Okemos

Ihn, Inc. — 517-706-0060
4572 Ottawa Dr., Suite 105, Okemos, MI 48864

Otsego

Electra-Tec Inc. — 800-225-3532
P.O. Box 17, 567 West M-89, Otsego, MI 49078-0017

Ottawa Lake

Pinnacle Technology Group, Inc. — 800-345-5123
7076 Schnipke Drive, Ottawa Lake, MI 49267

Oxford

Quality Cable Assembly, Llc — 248-236-9915
3204 Adventure Lane, Oxford, MI 48371-1638

Paw Paw

American Hair Removal System, Inc. — 800-446-2477
42320 Cr 653, Paw Paw, MI 49079

Pleasant Ridge

Wessels And Associates — 248-547-7177
131 Cambridge Blvd., Pleasant Ridge, MI 48069-1005

Plymouth

Barton Matthew, Inc. — 734-420-2326
11251 Ridge Road, Plymouth, MI 48170-3067
Creative Health Products, Inc. — 800-742-4478
5148 Saddle Ridge Road, Plymouth, MI 48170-5801
The C. D. Sparling Company — 734-455-3121
498 Farmer St, Plymouth, MI 48170-1206

Port Huron

Acheson Colloids Company — 800-255-1908
1600 Washington Avenue, Port Huron, MI 48060
Biopro, Inc. — 800-252-7707
2929 Lapeer Rd., Port Huron, MI 48060-4101

Portage

Harc Mercantile Ltd. — 800-445-9968
1111 West Centre Avenue, Portage, MI 49024
Sanitor Manufacturing Co. — 800-379-5314
1221 W. Centre Avenue, Portage, MI 49024
Westone Laboratories, Inc. — 800-552-7203
6287 American Ave., Portage, MI 49002

Quincy

Alumiramp, Inc. — 800-800-3864
855 E. Chicago Road, Quincy, MI 49082-9450
Starr Industries/Portable Entry Systems — 800-677-8377
87 Taylor St, Quincy, MI 49082

Richland

Alliant Healthcare Products — 269-629-0300
8850 M89, Richland, MI 49083

Rochester Hills

Ovonic Battery Company — 248-293-0440
2983 Waterview Dr., Rochester Hills, MI 48309

Romulus

Hillmor Products — 734-721-3485
39292 Montana Dr., Romulus, MI 48174
Kerr Corp. — 800-537-7123
28200 Wick Rd., Romulus, MI 48174
Metrex Research Corp. — 800-841-1428
28210 Wick Rd., Romulus, MI 48174

Saginaw

J&B Products, Ltd. — 800-556-3201
2201 S. Michigan, Saginaw, MI 48602-1275
Oxygen Therapy Institute — 989-752-9891
106 West Johnson, Saginaw, MI 48604
Saginaw Medical Service, Inc. — 989-793-4444
3960 Tittabawassee Rd., Saginaw, MI 48604
Specialty Manufacturing, Inc. — 800-269-6204
2210 Midland Road, Saginaw, MI 48603-3440
Ultra-Derm Systems — 989-792-6110
2201 South Michigan Ave., Saginaw, MI 48602

Saint Clair Shores

Med-Stor, A Division Of The Grates Corporation — 800-952-7775
25701 Jefferson Rd., Saint Clair Shores, MI 48081

Saline

Sensors, Inc. — 734-429-2100
6812 S. State Road, Saline, MI 48176-9274

Sault St. Marie

Hoover Precision Products, Inc — 906-632-7310
1390 Industrial Park Drive, Sault St. Marie, MI 49783

South Lyon

Noir Manufacturing — 800-521-9746
10125 Colonial Industrial Dr., South Lyon, MI 48178

Pioneer Micrographix   800-551-6436
228 South Mill Street, South Lyon, MI 48178

Southfield

Beckman Coulter, Inc.   714-871-4848
22900 W. Eight Mile Rd., Southfield, MI 48033-4302
Jardon Eye Prosthetics, Inc.   248-424-8560
15920 W 12 Mile Road, Southfield, MI 48076-2115

Sparta

Hart Enterprises, Inc.   616-887-0400
400 Applejack Ct., Sparta, MI 49345

Spring Lake

Common Sense Dental Inc.   888-853-5773
14998 Cleveland St., Suite A, Spring Lake, MI 49456
Garrison Dental Solutions   888-437-0032
150 Dewitt Ln., Spring Lake, MI 49456
Track Corporation   616-850-9444
17024 Taft Road, Spring Lake, MI 49456

St. Charles

Lendell Mfg., Inc.   800-566-8569
5301 South Graham Road, St. Charles, MI 48655

St. Joseph

GeneGo Inc.   269-983-7629
500 Renaissance Drive, #106, St. Joseph, MI 49085
Shepherd Caster Corporation   800-253-0868
203 Kerth St., St. Joseph, MI 49085-2623

St. Louis

Laser Band   800-238-0870
120 S Central Ave, Ste. 450, St. Louis, MI 63105

Sterling Heights

Diagnostic Instruments Inc.   586-731-6000
6540 Burroughs St., Sterling Heights, MI 48314-2133
Sterling Diagnostics, Inc.   800-637-2661
36645 Metro Court, Sterling Heights, MI 48312

Stevensville

Vigor Therapy Solutions Llc   269-429-0191
4915 Advance Way, Stevensville, MI 49127

Sturgis

Freeman Manufacturing Company   800-253-2091
900 W. Chicago Road, PO Box J, Sturgis, MI 49091-9701

Traverse City

Dkl Construction Management, Inc.   231-947-6450
323 East Welch Court, Suite B, Traverse City, MI 49686
Jointsmart LLC   231-920-7329
801 S. Garfield Ave, Traverse City, MI 49686
Tc Imaging Solutions   757-224-0177
2432 Cheyenne Trail, Traverse City, MI 49684
Thompson Surgical Instruments, Inc.   800-227-7543
10170 E. Cherry Bend Road, Traverse City, MI 49684
Venturi, Inc.   231-929-7732
2299 Traversefield Dr., Traverse City, MI 49686

Troy

Becker Orthopedic Appliance Co.   248-588-7480
635 Executive Dr., Troy, MI 48083
Delphi Corporation   888-526-1426
5725 Delphi Dr., Troy, MI 48098
Great Lakes Innovation Inc   248-680-8671
1103 Winthrop Drive, Troy, MI 48083
Somanetics Corp.   800-359-7662
2600 Troy Center Drive, Troy, MI 48084

Union City

Griswold Tool And Die, Inc.   517-741-7433
8500 M-60 East, P.o. Box 86, Union City, MI 49094

Walled Lake

Omni Medical Supply Inc.   800-860-6664
4153 Pioneer Drive, Walled Lake, MI 48390

Warren

Asi Instruments, Inc.   800-531-1105
12900 E. Ten Mile Road, Warren, MI 48089
Bio-Medical Instruments, Inc.   800-521-4640
2387 E. 8 Mile Road, Warren, MI 48091-2486
Mckeon Products, Inc.   586-427-7560
25460 Guenther, Warren, MI 48091
Mckeon Products, Inc.   810-427-7560
25460 Guenther Rd., Warren, MI 48091
Menlo Tool Co., Inc.   810-756-6010
22760 Dequindre Road, Warren, MI 48091-2199

West Bloomfield

T.C. Dynamics, Inc.   248-706-2021
5235 Greer Rd., West Bloomfield, MI 48234

Westland

Parco Scientific Co.   877-592-5837
P.O. Box 851559, Westland, MI 48185

Wixom

Gresham Driving Aids, Inc.   800-521-8930
30800 Wixom Rd., Wixom, MI 48393
Rockwell Medical Technologies, Inc.   800-449-3353
30142 S. Wixom Rd., Wixom, MI 48393-3440
Rockwell Medical Technologies, Inc.   248-960-9009
30142 Wixom Road, Wixom, MI 48393

Wyoming

Grand Rapids Foam Technologies   877-GET-GRFT
2788 Remico St SW, Wyoming, MI 49519

Zeeland

Biacare Corporation   616-931-1267
140 West Washington, Suite 100, Zeeland, MI 49464
Biotec, Inc.   616-772-2133
652 East Main Street, Zeeland, MI 49464
Compression Design   866-421-1267
140 W. Washington Ave., Suite 200, Zeeland, MI 49464
Doctors Orders   866-356-0771
731 B Construction Ct., Zeeland, MI 49464
Herman Miller, Inc.   616-654-3000
855 East Main Ave., P.O. Box 302, Zeeland, MI 49464

MINNESOTA

Albertville

Radiation Products Design, Inc.   800-497-2071
5218 Barthel Industrial Dr., Albertville, MN 55301

Arden Hills

Intricon Corporation   651-636-9770
1260 Red Fox Rd., Arden Hills, MN 55112
Medtronic Inc, Paceart   763-514-4000
4265 Lexington Avenue North, Arden Hills, MN 55126

Belle Plaine

Healthpostures, Llc   800-277-1841
125 East Main Street, Belle Plaine, MN 56011

Bethel

Bolt Bethel, Llc   763-434-5900
23530 University Avenue N.W., PO Box 135, Bethel, MN 55005
Master Craft Labs   800-233-1413
102 Main St., P.o. Box 11, Bethel, MN 55005

Birchwood

Epien Medical, Inc.   651-653-3380
4225 White Bear Parkway, Suite 600, Birchwood, MN 55110
Thermasolutions, Inc.   651-209-3900
1889 Buerkle Road, Birchwood, MN 55110

Blaine

Tamarack Habilitation Technologies, Inc.   763-795-0057
1670 94th Lane NE, Blaine, MN 55449

Bloomington

Acuo Technologies   952-905-3440
8009 34th Avenue South, Suite 900, Bloomington, MN 55425
American Hearing Systems Inc.   763-404-1122
8001 East Bloomington Freeway, Bloomington, MN 55420
Donaldson Company, Inc.   952-887-3131
1400 W. 94th St., Bloomington, MN 55431
Gn Resound   800-248-4327
8001 Bloomington Freeway, Bloomington, MN 55420
Ocu-Labs, Inc.   952-854-6702
7851 Metro Parkway #225, Bloomington, MN 55425
Peterson Air Purifiers, Llc   952-703-8962
9555 James Avenue South, Suite 220, Bloomington, MN 55431

Blue Earth

Express Diagnostics Int'L, Inc.   507-526-3951
1550 Industrial Dr., Blue Earth, MN 56013

Brainerd

Ocelco, Inc.   800-328-5343
1111 Industrial Park Road, Brainerd, MN 56401

Branch

Swede-O, Inc.   651-674-8301
6459 Ash St., Branch, MN 55056

Brooklyn Center

Chf Solutions, Inc.   763-463-4600
7601 Northland Dr. Ste. 170, Brooklyn Center, MN 55428
Polychrome Medical   763-585-9328
2700 Freeway Blvd., Suite 750, Brooklyn Center, MN 55430

Brooklyn Park

Dane Technologies   1-888-544-7779
7105 Northland Terrace, Brooklyn Park, MN 55428
Medtronic Perfusion Systems   800-854-3570
7611 Northland Dr., Brooklyn Park, MN 55428
Stellar Technologies, Inc.   888-566-9094
9200 Xylon Avenue North, Suite 100, Brooklyn Park, MN 55445

Buffalo

Zirc Company   800-328-3899
3918 Hwy. 55 S.E., Buffalo, MN 55313

Burnsville

Apothecary Products, Inc.   800-328-2742
11750 12th Avenue S., Burnsville, MN 55337-1295
Intl. Medical, Inc.   952-890-6547
14470 Burnsville Pkwy., Burnsville, MN 55306
Medcare Products, Inc.   800-695-4479
151 E. Cliff Road, Suite #40, Burnsville, MN 55337
R & D Batteries, Inc.   800-950-1945
3300 Corporate Center Drive, Burnsville, MN 55306
R.C. Smith Company   800-747-7648
14200 Southcross Drive W., Burnsville, MN 55306
Rnk Products, Inc.   612-414-0289
12700 Diamond Drive, Burnsville, MN 55337
Telex Communications, Inc.-Hearing Instrument Grp.   800-328-8212
1200 Portland Avenue S, Burnsville, MN 55357
Vital Signs Mn, Inc.   973-790-1330
12250 Nicollet Ave., Burnsville, MN 55337

Cannon Falls

Gemini, Inc.   800-533-3631
103 Mensing Way, Cannon Falls, MN 55009-1143

Champlin

Di-Chem, Inc.   800-847-2598
12297 Ensign Ave. North, Champlin, MN 55316

Chanhassen

Cardiocom LLC   888-243-8881
7980 Century Blvd., Chanhassen, MN 55317
Control Products Inc.   952-448-2217
1724 Lake Dr. W., Chanhassen, MN 55317
Pmt Corp.   800-626-5463
1500 Park Rd., Chanhassen, MN 55317-9593

Chaska

Beckman Coulter, Inc.   952-368-7629
1000 Lake Hazeltine Dr., Chaska, MN 55318
Lake Region Manufacturing, Inc.   952-448-5111
340 Lake Hazeltine Dr., Chaska, MN 55318-1034
Lifecore Biomedical, Inc.   952-368-4300
3515 Lyman Blvd., Chaska, MN 55318
The Saunders Group   800-445-9836
4250 Norex Drive, Chaska, MN 55318-3047

Cokato

Forward Technology   320-286-2578
260 Jenks Avenue, Cokato, MN 55321

Dassel

Crest Healthcare Supply   800-328-8908
195 Third Street South, Dassel, MN 55325
Spectralytics   800-543-0163
145 3rd St. South, PO Box L, Dassel, MN 55325

Detroit Lakes

Sunrise Machine And Tool, Inc.   218-847-3386
1380 Legion Rd., Detroit Lakes, MN 56501

Dover

Microstat Laboratories, Inc.   877-204-2007
PO Box 115, Dover, MN 55929

Duluth

Mckie Splints, Llc   888-477-5468
P. O. Box 16046, Duluth, MN 55816

Eagan

Braemar, Inc.   800-328-2719
1285 Corporate Center Dr., Suite 150, Eagan, MN 55121
Cardia Inc.   651-691-4100
2900 Lone Oak Parkway, Suite 130, Eagan, MN 55121
Hypertension Diagnostics, Inc.   888-785-7392
2915 Waters Road, Suite 108, Eagan, MN 55121-1562
Retone, Inc.   866-864-3271
4280 Sunrise Rd., Eagan, MN 55122
Santa Barbara Medco, Inc.   651-452-1977
1270 Eagan Industrial Road, Eagan, MN 55121
Sorna Corporation   651-406-9900
2020 Silver Bell Road, Suite 17, Eagan, MN 55122

Eden Prairie

Sunshine Heart, Inc.   1 952 345 4200
7651 Anagram Dr, Eden Prairie, MN 55344
Achieve Healthcare Technologies   800-869-1322
7690 Golden Triangle Drive, Eden Prairie, MN 55344
Acist Medical Systems, Inc.   888-667-6648
7905 Fuller Road, Eden Prairie, MN 55344
American Telecare, Inc.   800-323-6667
15159 Technology Drive, Eden Prairie, MN 55344-3732
Argosy   800-328-6105
10300 W. 70th St., Eden Prairie, MN 55344-3445
Arizant Healthcare Inc.   800-733-7775
10393 W. 70th St., Eden Prairie, MN 55344-3446
Birchwood Laboratories, Inc.   800-328-6156
7900 Fuller Road, Eden Prairie, MN 55344-2195
Bose Corporation - Electroforce Systems Group   800-273-0437
10250 Valley View Road, Suite 113, Eden Prairie, MN 55344
Celleration, Inc.   866-307-6478
6321 Bury Drive, Suite 15, Eden Prairie, MN 55346
Cns, Inc.   800-441-0417
7615 Smetana Lane, Eden Prairie, MN 55344
Diagnostic Group Llc   952-278-4457
7625 Golden Triangle Drive, Suite F, Eden Prairie, MN 55344
Fresnel Prism & Lens Co.   800-544-4760
6824 Washington Avenue, Eden Prairie, MN 55344
Inlet Medical, Inc.   800-969-0269
10340 Vilking Drive, Suite 125, Eden Prairie, MN 55344
Key Surgical, Inc.   800-541-7995
8101 Wallace Road, Suite 100, Eden Prairie, MN 55344
Logic Product Development   952-941-8071
6201 Bury Drive, Eden Prairie, MN 55346
Maico Diagnostics   888-941-4201
7625 Golden Triangle Drive, Eden Prairie, MN 55344
Micro-Ear Technology, Inc.   952-995-8800
6425 Flying Cloud Dr., Eden Prairie, MN 55344
Micro-Tech   952-995-8800
6425 Flying Cloud Dr., Eden Prairie, MN 55344
Milvella Limited   952-746-1369
12100 Singletree Lane, Eden Prairie, MN 55344
Prourocare Medical Inc.   925-476-9093
6440 Flying Cloud Dr., Suite 101, Eden Prairie, MN 55344
Quest Star Medical, Inc.   800-525-6718
10180 Viking Drive, Eden Prairie, MN 55344-7222
Research, Inc.   952-941-3300
7128 Shady Oak Road, Eden Prairie, MN 55344
Rnd Signs   800-328-4009
7605 Equitable Drive, Eden Prairie, MN 55344
Rorke Data, Incorporated   757-224-0177
7626 Golden Triangle Drive, Eden Prairie, MN 55344
Starkey Laboratories, Inc.   800-328-8602
6700 Washington Ave. South, Eden Prairie, MN 55344-3476
Surmodics, Inc.   866-787-6639
9924 W. 74th St., Eden Prairie, MN 55344-3523
Timm Medical Technologies, Inc.   800-966-2796
6585 City West Pkwy., Eden Prairie, MN 55344
Tremetrics   800-825-0121
7625 Golden Triangle Drive, Eden Prairie, MN 55344
Vasamed   800-695-2737
7615 Golden Triangle Drive, Suite C, Eden Prairie, MN 55344
Virtual Radiologic Corporation   800-737-0610
11995 Singletree Lane, Suite 500, Eden Prairie, MN 55344
Williams Sound Corp.   800-328-6190
10300 Valley View Road, Eden Prairie, MN 55344-3446

Edina

Arkray Usa   800-818-8877
5198 W 76th St., Edina, MN 55439

Elk River

Tescom Corp.   800-447-9635
12616 Industrial Blvd., Elk River, MN 55330-2491

Esko

Synergy Technologies, Inc.   218-879-4610
240 Erkkila Road, Esko, MN 55733

Eyota

Earmold Connection   507-289-9318
6538 Ranch View Ln. S.e., Eyota, MN 55934

Fergus Falls

Mrlb Intl., Inc.   715-425-8180
2450 College Way, Fergus Falls, MN 56537

Forest Lake

Team Vantage Molding Llc.   651-464-3900
22455 Everton Avenue N., Forest Lake, MN 55025-0370

Glencoe

Starkey Glencoe   952-947-4734
2915 10th St. East, Glencoe, MN 55336

Golden Valley

Enhanced Mobility Technologies — 612-310-4408
1615 Aguila Ave. N, Golden Valley, MN 55427
Nk Biotechnical Corp. — 612-541-0411
701 Decatur Avenue North, Suite 111a, Golden Valley, MN 55427

Grygla

May Corp. — 218-294-6700
103 E. Espelee Street, Grygla, MN 56727

Ham Lake

Sterion, Incorporated — 800-328-7958
13828 Lincoln St. N.E., Ham Lake, MN 55304

Hastings

Smead Manufacturing Co. — 1-88-USE-SMEAD
600 Smead Blvd., Hastings, MN 55033-2219
Superior Autocatheter Enterprises — 800-243-1467
2137 Vermillion Street, Suite 250, Hastings, MN 55033-1207

Hopkins

Mayon Plastics, Inc. — 612-935-2187
1595 K Tel Dr, Hopkins, MN 55343-7280
Prairie Labs — 952-908-7654
637 12th Ave., South, Hopkins, MN 55343

Hutchinson

Hutchinson Technology, Inc. — 320-587-3797
40 West Highland Park, Hutchinson, MN 55350
3m Hutchinson — 320-234-2000
915 Adams St. SE, Hutchinson, MN 55350-2927

Inver Grove Heights

Custom Tape Company — 888-259-3521
6288 Claude Way, Inver Grove Heights, MN 55077
Enhanced Mobility Solutions — 651-451-1637
6910 Dixie Ave. E., Inver Grove Heights, MN 55076
Medicalcv, Inc. — 800-328-2060
9725 S. Robert Trail, Inver Grove Heights, MN 55077-4424

Jordan

Theradyne Products Division — 800-328-4014
395 Ervin Industrial Drive, Jordan, MN 55352-1062

Kenyon

Plymold — 800-533-0480
615 Centennial Drive, Kenyon, MN 55946

Lake City

Pepin Manufacturing, Inc. — 800-291-6505
1875 Hwy. 61 South, Lake City, MN 55041
Valley Craft — 800-328-1480
2001 South Highway 61, Lake City, MN 55041

Lake Elmo

Quality Rapid Service Mounts, Inc. — 800-418-8342
8617 Eagle Point Blvd., Lake Elmo, MN 55042

Lakeville

Hds Specialty Vehicles — 866-826-6176
16290 Kenrick Loop, Lakeville, MN 55044

Lindstrom

Performance Attainment Associates — 800-835-2766
12805 Lake Blvd, #3, PO Box 528, Lindstrom, MN 55045
Smith Metal Products — 651-248-9650
30625 Olinda Trail, Lindstrom, MN 55045

Lino Lakes

Northern Technologies Intl. Corp. — 800-328-2433
6680 N. Hwy. 49, Lino Lakes, MN 55014

Litchfield

Merlo Co., Llc. — 800-290-9199
62038 MN Highway 24, PO Box 570, Litchfield, MN 55355

Mabel

Steuart Laboratories — 877-210-9664
142 South Main St., Mabel, MN 55954

Mankato

Winland Electronics Inc. — 800-635-4269
1950 Excel Drive, Mankato, MN 56001

Maple Grove

Boston Scientific - Maple Grove — 800-553-5878
One Scimed Place, Maple Grove, MN 55311-1566
Coaxia, Inc. — 763-315-1809
10900 73rd Ave. N., Suite 102, Maple Grove, MN 55369
Entellus Medical — 866-620-7615
6705 Wedgwood Court North, Maple Grove, MN 55311
Gyrus Medical, Inc. — 800-852-9361
6655 Wedgwood Road, Suite #105, Maple Grove, MN 55311
Inspire Medical Systems — 763-205-7970
9700 63rd Avenue North, Suite 200, Maple Grove, MN 55369

Lumen Biomedical, Inc. — 763-577-9600
10900 73rd Ave N. #150, Maple Grove, MN 55369
Lutonix, Inc — 763-445-2352
7351 Kirkwood Lane North, Suite 138, Maple Grove, MN 55369
Neuro Vasx, Inc. — 763-315-0013
7351 Kirkwood Lane, Suite 112, Maple Grove, MN 55369
Palco Marketing, Inc. — 763-559-5539
8555 Revere Ln N #600, Maple Grove, MN 55369
Space Tables, Inc. — 800-328-2580
11511 95th Avenue N., Maple Grove, MN 55369
St. Jude Medical Atrial Fibrillation — 800.748.7335
6500 Wedgwood Rd., Maple Grove, MN 55311
Sterilmed, Inc. — 763-488-3400
11400 73rd Ave. North, #100, Maple Grove, MN 55369

Maplewood

Quality Hearing — 651-770-5282
2115 County Rd., D East, Suite A100, Maplewood, MN 55109

Mendota Heights

Biodrain Medical, Inc. — 651-389-4800
2060 Centre Pointe Blvd, Suite 7, Mendota Heights, MN 55120
HealthSense Inc. — 952-400-7300
1191 Northland Dr., Suite 100, Mendota Heights, MN 55120
Travanti Pharma Incorporated — 651-730-1008
2520 Pilot Knob Rd., Suite 100, Mendota Heights, MN 55120

Milaca

Trivirix International Inc. — 320-982-8000
925 6th Avenue NE, Milaca, MN 56353

Minneapolis

ATS Medical, Inc. — 800-399-1381
3905 Annapolis Lane, Suite 105, Minneapolis, MN 55447
Access Genetics — 888-250-4407
7550 Market Place Dr., Minneapolis, MN 55344-3739
Adolfson & Peterson, Inc — 612-544-1561
6701 W. 23rd Street, Minneapolis, MN 55426
Aeiomed, Inc. — 612-455-0550
1313 5th Street Se, Ste 205, Minneapolis, MN 55414
Air Quality Engineering, Inc. — 800-328-0787
7140 Northland Drive No., Minneapolis, MN 55428-1520
Altron, Inc. — 763-427-7735
6700 Bunker Lake Blvd. N.W., Minneapolis, MN 55303-5852
Ampac Flexibles — 952-693-2475
5305 Parkdale Dr., Minneapolis, MN 55416
Arkray Factory Usa, Inc. — 952-646-3168
5182 West 76th St., Minneapolis, MN 55439
Benson Medical Instruments Co. — 612-827-2222
310 4th Avenue South, Suite 5000, Minneapolis, MN 55415
Better Parts Co. — 952-881-0234
219 West 90th St., Minneapolis, MN 55420
Biovest International, Inc. — 866-3BIOVEST
8500 Evergreen Blvd. NW, Minneapolis, MN 55433-6016
Bone Foam — 612-338-1400
700 South 10th Ave., Minneapolis, MN 55415
Cardinal Health 203, Inc — 763-398-8305
17400 Medina Road, Suite 100, Minneapolis, MN 55447
Cardinal Health 203, Inc — 763-398-8305
3555 Holly Lane, Suite 65, Minneapolis, MN 55447
Cartwright Consulting Co. — 952-854-4911
8324 16th Avenue S., Minneapolis, MN 55425-1742
Clarus Medical, Llc. — 800-359-2372
1000 Boone Ave. North, Suite 300, Minneapolis, MN 55427
Coloplast Manufacturing Us, Llc — 800-533-0464
1601 West River Road North, Minneapolis, MN 55411
Cvrx Inc. — 763-416-2840
9201 W. Broadway Ave., Suite 650, Minneapolis, MN 55445
Delta Industrial Services, Inc. — 800-279-3358
11501 Eagle St. N.W., Minneapolis, MN 55448-3062
G H Medical Inc., Division Of Tsj Inc. — 612-331-6299
2010 East Hennepin Ave., Minneapolis, MN 55413
Gentra Systems, Inc. — 763-543-0678
13355 10th Ave. N., Suite 120, Minneapolis, MN 55441
Greatbach Medical — 800-559-2613
2300 Berkshire Lane N, Minneapolis, MN 55441
Gt Urological, Llc — 612-379-3578
1313 5th St. S.e., Minneapolis, MN 55414
Idea Scientific Co. — 800-433-2535
PO Box 13210, Minneapolis, MN 55414-5210
King Koil Sleep Products — 1-800-899-5645
752 30th Avenue Southeast, Minneapolis, MN 55414
Kips Bay Medical, Inc — 763-235-3540
3405 Annapolis Ln N Ste 200, Minneapolis, MN 55447-5346
Levo Usa — 888-538-6872
7105 Northland Terrace, Brooklyn Park, Minneapolis, MN 55428
Medical Arts Press — 800-328-2179
8500 Wyoming Ave. N., P.O. Box 43200, Minneapolis, MN 55445
Mednet Services, Inc. — 612-788-6228
2855 Anthony Ln. South, #b10, Minneapolis, MN 55418
Medtronic Ep Systems — 763-514-4000
Spring Lake Park, 8299 Central Ave. Ne, Minneapolis, MN 55432-3576
Medtronic Neuromodulation — 1-800-633-8766
710 Medtronic Parkway, Minneapolis, MN 55432-5604

Medtronic Neuromodulation — 800-633-8766
710 Medtronic Parkway NE, Minneapolis, MN 55459-9896
Medtronic Perfusion Systems — 1-800-633-8766
710 Medtronic Parkway, Mail Stop: L100, Minneapolis, MN 55432-5604
Medtronic, Inc. — 800-633-8766
710 Medtronic Parkway, Mail Stop: L100, Minneapolis, MN 55432-5604
Metro Cad, Inc — 612-302-8056
2277-49th Avenue North, Minneapolis, MN 55430
Minco Products, Inc. — 763-571-3121
7300 Commerce Lane, Minneapolis, MN 55432
Minnesota Medical Development, Inc. — 763-354-7105
14305 21st Ave. North, Suite 100, Minneapolis, MN 55447
Minnesota Rubber & Qmr Plastics — 952-927-1400
1100 xenium lane north, Minneapolis, MN 55441
Minntech Corporation — 800-328-3345
14605 28th Avenue N., Minneapolis, MN 55447
Miracle-Ear — 877-268-4264
5000 Cheshire Lane North, Minneapolis, MN 55446
Neo Metrics, Inc. — 763-559-4440
Fernbrook Lane N, Suite J, Minneapolis, MN 55447
Novartis Nutrition — 800-333-3785
1600 Utica Ave S Suite 600, PO Box 370, Minneapolis, MN 55416-1521
Optp — 888-819-0121
3800 Annapolis Lane, Suite 165, PO Box 47009, Minneapolis, MN 55447-0009
Otto Bock Heathcare — 800-328-4058
Two Carlson Parkway, Suite 100, Minneapolis, MN 55447
Otto Bock Technical Center — (800) 810-7994
14800 28th Ave. N. #110, Minneapolis, MN 55447
Packaging Plus, Inc. — 763-566-8808
6840 Shingle Creek Pkwy., Minneapolis, MN 55430-1447
Pearl Baths, Inc. — 800-328-2531
9224 73rd Avenue North, Minneapolis, MN 55428
Phelan Manufacturing Corp. — 800-328-2358
2523 Minnehaha Ave., Minneapolis, MN 55404-4119
Protectus Medical Devices Inc. — 800-778-8438
110 First Ave., NE, Suite 1006, Minneapolis, MN 55413
Provation Medical, Inc. — 888-952-6673
800 Washington Ave North, Suite 400, Minneapolis, MN 55401
Quantum Labs, Inc. — 800-328-8213
452 Northco Dr., Suite 180, Minneapolis, MN 55432-3006
R & D Systems, Inc. — 612-656-4533
614 McKinley Place N.E., Minneapolis, MN 55413-2647
R And L Hearing Services — 800-444-8920
3005 Niagara Lane   Ste. 2, Minneapolis, MN 55447
Radiographic And Data Solutions, Inc. — 612-379-7152
2101 Kennedy St. Ne, Suite 190, Minneapolis, MN 55413
Rms Company — 763-783-5074
8600 Evergreen Blvd., Minneapolis, MN 55433-6036
Sick, Inc. — 800-325-7425
6900 West 110th Street, Minneapolis, MN 55438
Superdimension Inc. — 800-387-9016
161 Cheshire Lane North, Suite 100, Minneapolis, MN 55441
Tactile Systems Technology Inc — 866-435-3948
1331 Tyler St. N.E., Ste. 200, Minneapolis, MN 55413
Techne Corporation — 612-379-8854
614 McKinley Place N.E., Minneapolis, MN 55413
Thermo Fisher Scientific (Sales And Service) — 800-227-8891
PROCESS INSTRUMENTS DIVISION, 501 90th Avenue N.W., Minneapolis, MN 55433
Thermo Fisher Scientific - Checkweighing, Metal And X-Ray Detection — 800-227-8891
501 90th Avenue NW, Minneapolis, MN 55433
Urologix, Inc. — 800-475-1403
14405 - 21st Avenue North, Minneapolis, MN 55447
Vascular Solutions, Inc. — 888-240-6001
6464 Sycamore Court North, Minneapolis, MN 55369
Winsted Corp. — 800-447-2257
10901 Hampshire Avenue S., Minneapolis, MN 55438
Zimmer Spine, Inc. — 800-655-2614
7375 Bush Lake Road, Minneapolis, MN 55439-2027
Zyga Technology Inc. — 612-455-1061
700 10th Avenue South, Suite 400, MINNEAPOLIS, MN 55415

Minneapolis,

Medtronic Vascular — 1-800-633-8766
710 Medtronic Parkway, L100, Minneapolis,, MN 55432-5604

Minnetonka

Advanced Bio-Surfaces, Inc. — 952-912-5400
5909 Baker Road, Suite 550, Minnetonka, MN 55345
American Medical Systems, Inc. — 800-328-3881
10700 Bren Road W., Minnetonka, MN 55343
Annex Medical, Inc. — 952-942-7576
6018 Blue Circle Dr., Minnetonka, MN 55343-9104
Anulex Technologies, Inc — 877-326-8539
5600 Rowland Road, Suite 280, Minnetonka, MN 55343
Cardiac Concepts Inc. — 952-540-4470
12400 Whitewater Dr., Suite 500, Minnetonka, MN 55343
Culligan Soft Water Service Co. — 952-933-7200
6030 Culligan Way, Minnetonka, MN 55345
DGIMED Ortho Inc. — 952-582-6700
12400 Whitewater Dr, Suite 2010, Minnetonka, MN 55343
Datacard Group — 800-621-6972
11111 Bren Road W., Minnetonka, MN 55343-9015

Ge Infrastructure Water & Process Technologies — 877-522-7867
5951 Clearwater Drive, Minnetonka, MN 55343-8995
Mr Instruments, Inc. — 952-746-1435
5610 Rowland Rd., Suite 145, Minnetonka, MN 55343
Penrad Technologies, Inc. — 763-475-3388
10580 Wayzata Blvd, Suite 200, Minnetonka, MN 55305
Physiomedics Manufacturing, Llc — 952-201-1463
15320 Minnetonka Blvd., Suite 104, Minnetonka, MN 55345
St. Jude Medical Atrial Fibrillation — 800-328-3873
14901 DeVeau Pl., Minnetonka, MN 55345-2126
Uroplasty, Inc. — 952-426-6140
5420 Feltl Road, Minnetonka, MN 55343
Viromed Laboratories (Labcorp) — 800-582-0077
6101 Blue Circle Dr., Minnetonka, MN 55343

Minnetonka,

Vital Images,Inc. — 800-231-0607
5850 Opus Parkway, Suite 300, Minnetonka,, MN 55343-4414

Morton

Altimate Medical, Inc. — 800-342-8968
P.O. Box 180, 262 West 1st St., Morton, MN 56270

moundsview

Medtronic Cardiac Surgery Technologies — 877-526-7890
8200 coral sea street, moundsview, MN 55112

New Brighton

Compex Technologies, Inc. — 866-676-6489
1811 Old Hwy. 8, New Brighton, MN 55112
Donatelle — 651-746-2900
501 County Rd. E-2 Extension, New Brighton, MN 55112
Dotronix, Inc. — 651-633-1742
160 First St. S.E., New Brighton, MN 55112
Medco Equipment, Inc. — 800-717-3626
105 Old Hwy 8, Unit 3, New Brighton, MN 55112
Pierce Bac-T, Inc. — 651-636-5901
367-a West County Rd., D, New Brighton, MN 55112
Promethean Medical Technologies, Inc. — 763-259-0559
105 Old Highway #8, Suite 1, New Brighton, MN 55112

New Hope

Safco Products Company — 800-328-3020
9300 W. Research Center Rd., New Hope, MN 55428

New Prague

Electromed, Inc. — 800-462-1045
500 Sixth Ave. N.W., New Prague, MN 56071
Lide Laboratories, Inc. — 952-758-9760
401 4th. Ave.sw, New Prague, MN 56071

New Ulm

Beacon Promotions, Inc. — 507-354-3900
2121 Bridge St., New Ulm, MN 56073
3m Company — 507-354-8271
1617 N. Front Street, New Ulm, MN 56073

North Mankato

Quadris Medical — 507-389-4319
2030 Lookout Dr., North Mankato, MN 56003

Oakdale

Carestream Health, Inc. — 888-777-2072
1 Imation Way, Oakdale, MN 55128
Hearing Components Inc. — 800-872-8986
420 Hayward Ave., N., Oakdale, MN 55128

Osseo

Excel Labs — 763-391-7413
106 Central Ave., Suite B, Osseo, MN 55369
R4 Vascular, Inc. — 612-770-4038
Meridian Business Center, Suite 150, 7550 Meridian Cir N, Osseo, MN 55369

Park Rapids

Ulmer Pharmacal Co. — 800-848-5637
1614 Industry Ave., P.O. Box 408, Park Rapids, MN 56470

Parkers Prairie

Abbeymoor Medical Inc. — 888-528-9073
501 East Soo Street, Parkers Prairie, MN 56361

Plymouth

Affinity Medical Technology, Llc. — 763-744-0412
3545 Harbor Lane N.,, Plymouth, MN 55447
Alexandria Research Technologies, Llc — 952-949-2235
13755 First Avenue North, Suite 100, Plymouth, MN 55441
Boston Scientific Corp. — 800-323-6472
5905 Nathan Lane, Plymouth, MN 55442-1656
BridgePoint Medical — 763-225-8500
2800 Campus Drive, #50, Plymouth, MN 55441
Daily Medical Products, Inc. — 800-550-1553
4620 Goldenrod Lane, Plymouth, MN 55442
Ela Medical, Inc. — 800-352-6466
2950 Xenium Lane N., Plymouth, MN 55441

Esi, Inc.   763-473-2533
2915 Everest Ln. N., Plymouth, MN 55447
Ev3 Inc.   800-716-6700
3033 Campus Drive, Plymouth, MN 55441
Incisive Surgical, Inc.   877-246-7672
14405 - 21st Avenue North, Suite 130, Plymouth, MN 55447
Interrad Medical   763-225-6699
181 Cheshire Lane, Suite 100, Plymouth, MN 55441
M-E Manufacturing And Services, Inc.   763-268-4500
5010 Cheshire Lane North, Plymouth, MN 55446
Mar Cor Purification, Inc.   (800) 633-3080
14550 28th Avenue North, Plymouth, MN 55447
Nonin Medical, Inc.   800-356-8874
13700 1st Avenue North, Plymouth, MN 55441
Nuaire, Inc.   800-328-3352
2100 Fernbrook Lane, Plymouth, MN 55447-4723
Pedia Pals, Llc   888-733-4272
965 Highway 169 N., Plymouth, MN 55441
Qrs Diagnostic, Llc   800-465-8408
14755 27th Avenue N., Plymouth, MN 55447
REXTON, A DIVISION OF SIEMENS HEARING   763-553-0787
INSTRUMENTS, IN.
5010 Cheshire Lane North, Suite 2, Plymouth, MN 55446
Unitron Hearing   763-744-3300
2300 Berkshire Ln. North, Suite A, Plymouth, MN 55441
Uromedica, Inc.   763-694-9880
1840 Berkshire Ln. North, Plymouth, MN 55441-3723

Princeton
Medicomp   763-389-4473
12535 316th Ave., Princeton, MN 55371
Sidmar Mfg., Inc.   800-330-7260
31530 - 125th St. NW, Princeton, MN 55371

Prior Lake
Nbc Products, Inc.   952-226-1112
16873 Fish Point Road, Prior Lake, MN 55372

Ramsey
Dyna-Plast, Inc.   763-780-8674
13911 Unity St. Nw, Ramsey, MN 55303
Vision-Ease Lens   800-328-3449
7000 Sunwood Drive NW, Ramsey, MN 55303
Vision-Ease Lens, Inc.   800-328-3449
7000 Sunwood Drive NW, Ramsey, MN 55303

Red Wing
Norwood Promotional Products, Inc.   651-388-1298
5151 Moundview Drive, Red Wing, MN 55066

Redwood Falls
Activeaid, Inc.   800-533-5330
101 Activeaid Rd., Redwood Falls, MN 56283-0359

Rochester
Ability Building Center, Inc.   507-281-6262
1911 14th Street NW, P.O. Box 6938, Rochester, MN 55903-6938
Benchmark Electronics, Inc.   507-453-4912
3535 Technology Dr., N.w., Rochester, MN 55901
Benchmark Winona   507-452-8932
6301 Bandel Rd. Nw, Rochester, MN 55901
Compass International, Inc.   800-933-2143
1815 14th Street NW, Rochester, MN 55901
Ibm Integrated Tool Technology Center   507-253-5215
3605 Hwy 52 N, Rochester, MN 55901
Medical Innovations International Inc.   507-289-0761
6256 N.W. 34th Avenue, Rochester, MN 55901
Midwest Eye Laboratories, Inc.   800-543-7936
20 2nd Ave., S.w., Suite 223, Rochester, MN 55901
Ortho Innovations, Inc.   507-269-2895
121 23rd Ave. Southwest, Rochester, MN 55902
Pogo, Inc.   507-280-8868
410 1st. Ave. N.w., Rochester, MN 55901
Waters Medical Systems   800-426-9877
2112-15th St. NW, Rochester, MN 55901
Waters Medical Systems, Llc   205-612-5221
2112 15th St. N.w., Rochester, MN 55901

Rogers
Melyx Corporation   888-886-3599
21830 Industrial Blvd., Rogers, MN 55374

Roseville
AbleNet Inc.   800-322-0956
2808 Fairview Avenue North, Roseville, MN 55113
Advanced Circulatory Systems, Inc.   866-737-7763
1905 County Road C West, Roseville, MN 55113
IMED Mobility Inc.   800-788-7479
1915 W. County Rd. C, Roseville, MN 55113-1320

Rush City
La Calhene   320-358-4713
1325 Field Avenue S., PO Box 567, Rush City, MN 55069

Saint Louis Park
Attostar Llc   952-920-6755
7600 West 27th Street, Suite 234, Saint Louis Park, MN 55426

Saint Paul
Angeion Corporation   651-484-4874
350 Oak Grove Pkwy, Saint Paul, MN 55127
Bird & Cronin, Inc.   651-683-1111
1200 Trapp Rd., Saint Paul, MN 55121
Carbon Medical Technologies, Inc.   877-277-1788
1290 Hammond Road, Saint Paul, MN 55110
Envoy Medical Corporation   1-866-950-4327
5000 Township Parkway, Saint Paul, MN 55110
Hermanson Dental   800-328-9648
1055 Highway 36 East, Saint Paul, MN 55109
Laservision Usa   1-800-393-5565
595 Phalen Blvd., Saint Paul, MN 55101
Lexion Medical, Llc.   651-635-0000
5000 Township Pkwy, Saint Paul, MN 55110
Porous Media Corp.   651-653-2000
1350 Hammond Rd., Saint Paul, MN 55110
W.E. Mowrey Co.   651-646-1895
1435 University Ave., Saint Paul, MN 55104

Sauk Rapids
Aura Lens Products, Inc.   800-281-2872
51 8th St. N., PO Box 763, St. Cloud,, Sauk Rapids, MN 56379
X-Cel Optical Co.   800-747-9235
806 South Benton Drive, Box 420, Sauk Rapids, MN 56379

Shoreview
Dymedix Corporation   888-212-1100
5985 Rice Creek Pkwy, Suite 201, Shoreview, MN 55126
Torax Medical, Inc.   651-361-8900
4188 Lexington Avenue North, Shoreview, MN 55126
Tsi Inc.   800-874-2811
500 Cardigan Road, Shoreview, MN 55126
Tsi Incorporated   800-874-2811
500 Cardigan Road, Shoreview, MN 55126

South Saint Paul
Digital Angel Corp.   651-554-1574
490 Villuame Avenue, South Saint Paul, MN 55075

Spring Lake Park
Medtronic Heart Valves   800-227-3191
8299 Central Ave., N.e., Spring Lake Park, MN 55432-3576
Nu Gyn, Inc   763-398-0108
1633 County Hwy. 10 N.e., Suite 15, Spring Lake Park, MN 55432

Spring Park
Fitzco, Inc.   800-367-8760
4300 Shoreline Drive, Spring Park, MN 55384

St Paul
Biomedix Inc.   877-854-0012
178 East Ninth Street, St Paul, MN 55101

St. Cloud
Micro-Bio-Logics.Inc   800-599-2847
217 Osseo Avenue N., St. Cloud, MN 56303-4452
Microbiologics, Inc.   800-599-BUGS
217 Osseo Ave. North, St. Cloud, MN 56303-4452
Prescription Optical, Inc.   800-284-8886
P.O.Box 1088, St. Cloud, MN 56302

St. Louis Park
Mayclin Dental Studio, Inc.   952-926-1809
7505 Hwy 7, Suite 100, St. Louis Park, MN 55426
Thompson Medical Specialties   800-777-4949
3404 Library Ln., St. Louis Park, MN 55426

St. Paul
AmSan   800-327-3528
1930 Energy Park Drive, Suite 260, St. Paul, MN 55108
Brennen Medical, Llc   800-328-9105
1290 Hammond Rd., St. Paul, MN 55110
Cardiovascular Systems, Inc.   877-CSI-0360
651 Campus Drive, St. Paul, MN 55112
Ecolab Inc.   800-232-6522
370 Wabasha Street N., St. Paul, MN 55102
Empi   800.328.2536
599 Cardigan Road, St. Paul, MN 55126-4099
Empi, Inc.   800-328-2536
599 Cardigan Rd., St. Paul, MN 55126-4099
Enova Medical Technologies   866-773-0539
1839 Buerkle Road, St. Paul, MN 55110-5246
EnteroMedics   651-634-3003
2800 Patton Road, St. Paul, MN 55113
Ergodyne   800-225-8238
1021 Bandana Boulevard East, Suite 220, St. Paul, MN 55108
Ergotron, Inc.   800-888-8458
1181 Trapp Road, St. Paul, MN 55121

Evergreen Sales & Marketing, Inc. — 651-222-2885
1010 W. University Avenue Suite 211, St. Paul, MN 55104

Gillette Children's Specialty Healthcare — 612-229-3805
200 East University Ave., St. Paul, MN 55101

Gml, Inc. — 651-486-3691
500 Oak Grove Pkwy., St. Paul, MN 55127

H.B. Fuller Company — 800-328-9673
1200 Willow Lake Blvd., PO Box 64683, St. Paul, MN 55110-5101

Hearmore Co., Inc. — 651-771-4019
1445 White Bear Ave., St. Paul, MN 55106

Hemerus Medical, Llc. — 651-635-0070
5000 Township Parkway, St. Paul, MN 55110

Insitu Technologies, Inc. — 651-389-1017
539 Phalen Blvd., St. Paul, MN 55130

Mclean Medical And Scientific, Inc. — 800-777-9987
292 E. Lafayette Frontage Road, St. Paul, MN 55107

Medical Concepts Development — 800-345-0644
2500 Ventura Dr., St. Paul, MN 55125-3927

Medical Graphics Corporation — 800-950-5597
350 Oak Grove Pkwy., St. Paul, MN 55127-8536

Medtox Scientific Inc. — 800-832-3244
402 West County Road D, St. Paul, MN 55112

Medved Products, Inc. — 651-482-8413
P.O. Box 120883, St. Paul, MN 55112-0883

Micromedics — 800-624-5662
1270 Eagan Industrial Road, St. Paul, MN 55121-1385

Minnesota Bramstedt Surgical, Inc. — 800-456-5052
1835 Energy Park Drive, St. Paul, MN 55108

Minnesota Wire & Cable Co. — 800-258-6922
1835 Energy Park Drive, St. Paul, MN 55108

Minnetronix Inc. — 888-301-1025
1635 Energy Park Drive, St. Paul, MN 55108

Nada-Concepts — 800-722-2587
2448 Larpenteur Ave. W., St. Paul, MN 55113

Omni-Tract Surgical, A Div. Of Minnesota — 800-367-8657
Scientific, Inc.
4849 White Bear Parkway, St. Paul, MN 55110-3325

Ormed Corporation — 800-440-2784
599 Cardigan Road, St. Paul, MN 55126

Patterson Companies, Inc. — 800-328-5536
1031 Mendota Heights Road, St. Paul, MN 55120

Respiratory Technologies, Inc. — 651-379-8999
1380 Energy Lane, Suite 113, St. Paul, MN 55108

Santek, Div. Tjernlund Products, Inc. — 800-255-4208
1601 9th St., St. Paul, MN 55110-6794

Scanlan International, Inc. — 800-328-9458
One Scanlan Plaza, St. Paul, MN 55107-1629

Smiths Medical Asd, Inc. — 800-433-5832
1265 Grey Fox Road, St. Paul, MN 55112

Soderberg Optical, Inc. — 800-755-5655
230 Eva St., St. Paul, MN 55107-1605

Sohniks Endoscopy, Inc. — 800-495-0297
325 Armour Avenue, St. Paul, MN 55075

Specialty Manufacturing Co., The — 651-653-0599
5858 Centerville Rd., St. Paul, MN 55127-6804

Spineology Group, Llc — 888-377-4633
7800 3rd Street N., Suite 600, St. Paul, MN 55128-5455

St. Jude Medical Atrial Fibrillation (Endocardial — 800.328.9634
Solutions)
One St. Jude Medical Drive, St. Paul, MN 55117-9983

St. Jude Medical, Inc. — 800-328-9634
One St. Jude Medical Drive, St. Paul, MN 55117-9983

Surgical Technologies, Inc. — 800-777-9987
292 E. Lafayette Frontage Road, St. Paul, MN 55107

Synovis Life Technologies, Inc — 800-255-4018
2575 University Ave. W, St. Paul, MN 55114

Synovis Surgical Innovations — 800-255-4018
2575 University Avenue W., St. Paul, MN 55114

Ulti Med, Inc. — 877-858-4633
287 E. 6th St., Suite 380, St. Paul, MN 55101

W.E. Mowrey Co. — 800-544-1550
1435 University Ave., St. Paul, MN 55104-4003

3m Co. — 888-364-3577
3M Center, St. Paul, MN 55144-1000

Stewartville

Rochester Medical Corp. — 800-615-2364
One Rochester Medical Dr., Stewartville, MN 55976

Stillwater

Diasorin Inc — 800-328-1482
1951 Northwestern Avenue, PO Box 285, Stillwater, MN 55082-6048

Wr Medical Electronics Co. — 800-635-1312
123 N. Second St., Stillwater, MN 55082-5002

Utica

Osborn Medical Corp. — 800-535-5865
100 West Main, PO Box 324, Utica, MN 55979

Wabasha

Covidien Lp, Formerly Registered As Uni-Patch — 800-962-9888
1313 Grant Blvd, Wabasha, MN 55981

Wayzata

Nortech Systems Incorporated — 952-345-2244
1120 Wayzata Blvd E., Suite 201, Wayzata, MN 55391

West St. Paul

Rtc Inc.-Memcath Technologies Llc — 651-450-7400
1777 Oakdale Ave.,, West St. Paul, MN 55118

Tapemark — 800-535-1998
1685 Marthaler Lane, West St. Paul, MN 55118-3537

White Bear Lake

Toothtickler Enterprises, Inc. — 651-429-5187
5222 E. Bald Eagle Blvd., White Bear Lake, MN 55110

Winona

Benchmark Electronics, Inc. — 507-452-8932
4065 Theurer Blvd., Winona, MN 55987

Comfortex, Inc. — 800-445-4007
1680 Wilkie Dr., P.O. Box 850, Winona, MN 55987

Woodbury

Midwest Eye Laboratories, Inc. — 800-543-7936
7582 Currell Blvd., Suite 109, Woodbury, MN 55125

MISSISSIPPI

Baldwyn

Joerns Healthcare, Inc. — 715-341-3600
1032 North 4th Street, Baldwyn, MS 38824

Belzoni

Mid-Delta Home Health & Hospice — 800-543-9055
405 North Hayden St., Belzoni, MS 39038

Bourbon

Leland Manufacturing Llc — 812-367-1761
1300 North Broad Street, Leland, Bourbon, MS 38756

Brandon

Incappe, Inc. — 601-638-2345
9 Ashland Ave., Brandon, MS 39047

Calhoun City

Med-Lift & Mobility, Inc. — 800-748-9438
310 S. Madison, Calhoun City, MS 38916

Cleveland

Baxter Healthcare Corporation — 847-473-6141
911 North Davis, Cleveland, MS 38732

Columbus

Microtek Medical, Inc — 800-936-9248
512 Lehmberg Road, Columbus, MS 39704

Sani-Med, A Division Of Sanderson Plumbing — 800-647-1042
Products, Inc.
PO Box 1367, Columbus, MS 39703

Corinth

Cold River Unlimited, Inc. — 662-286-3558
2070a South Tate St., Corinth, MS 38834

Kimberly-Clark Corp. — 888-525-838
3461 County Road 100, Corinth, MS 38834

Crystal Springs

Mmi Of Mississippi, Inc. — 800-448-5918
PO Box 488, Crystal Springs, MS 39059-0488

De Kalb

Pharma Pac, Llc — 601-743-9771
14124 Hwy 16 West, De Kalb, MS 39328

Flowood

Medi-Crush Company — 800-262-6334
P.O. BOX 321381, Flowood, MS 39232

Gpt

Coast Hearing Aid Lab, Llc — 228-539-5400
12100 Highway 49 North, Suite 314, Gpt, MS 39503

Greenwood

Connected Medical Systems Llc — 662-455-4523
2005 Highway 82 West, Greenwood, MS 38930

Hattiesburg

Industrial Welding Supplies Of Hattiesburg, Inc. — 601-545-1800
1924 Byron St., Hattiesburg, MS 39402

Holly Springs

Leeco Industries, Inc. — 662-551-1025
540 S Industrial Park Road, Holly Springs, MS 38635

Houston

Franklin Corp. — 662-456-4286
600 Franklin Dr., P.o. Box 569, Houston, MS 38851

2013 MEDICAL DEVICE REGISTER

Jackson

Durfold Corporation — 800-345-6849
102 Upton Drive, Jackson, MS 39209-2525

Sabhi, Inc. — 601-956-3169
1303 Riverwood Dr., Jackson, MS 39211

United Plastic Molders, Inc. — 601-353-3193
105 E. Rankin St., Jackson, MS 39201-6122

Madison

Cuff Toughener — 601-853-3966
103 Weldon Dr., Madison, MS 39110

Meridian

Rush-Berivon, Inc. — 800-251-7874
1010 19th St., P.O. Box 1851, Meridian, MS 39302

Ocean Springs

Pfg Precision Optics, Inc. — 228-875-0165
733 Bienville Blvd., Ocean Springs, MS 39564

Oxford

Elsohly Labs, Inc. — 662-236-2609
5 Industrial Park Dr., Oxford, MS 38655

Promatura Group, Llc — 800-201-1483
19 County Road 168, Oxford, MS 38655

Pachuta

Slide Free Llc — 601-213-3758
22 Lake Eddins 163815, Pachuta, MS 39347

Ripley

Medical Products, Inc. — 800-638-0489
511 E. Walnut St., PO Box 207, Ripley, MS 38663-2115

Southaven

Terumo Medical Corp. — 800-283-7866
State Line Business Park, 8655 Commerce Drive, Suite 101, Southaven, MS 38671

Sumrall

Db Square, Llc — 402-292-2383
101 Hickory Grove Church Rd., Sumrall, MS 39482

Tupelo

Confortaire Inc — 662-842-2966
2133 South Veterans Blvd., Tupelo, MS 38804

Verona

Capital Bedding, Incorporated — 757-224-0177
5262 South Raymond Street, Verona, MS 38879

Waynesboro

Sunbeam Products, Inc. — 601-671-2277
224 Russell Dr., Waynesboro, MS 39367

West Point

Universal Gym Equipment — 800-843-3906
PO Box 1296, PO Box 1270, West Point, MS 39773

MISSOURI

Anderson

Agile Mfg., Inc — 800-476-7436
720 Industrial Park Road, Anderson, MO 64831

Arnold

Fischer Surgical Inc. — 866-622-2221
1343 Pine Drive, Arnold, MO 63010

Surgical Eye Enterprise — 636-282-2800
1763 Engle Dr., Arnold, MO 63010

Ballwin

Roldan Products Corp. — 866-922-6800
448 Sovereign Court, Ballwin, MO 63021

Belton

Budget Buddy Company, Inc. — 800-208-3375
P.O. Box 590, Belton, MO 64012-0590

Blue Springs

Dadson Mfg. Corp. — 816-847-2388
1109 Valley Ridge Drive, Blue Springs, MO 64029

Incite International, Inc. — 816-220-7533
2749 Hunter Dr, Nw, Blue Springs, MO 64015

Phoenix Orthodontics, Inc. — 800-642-3009
2401 S.W. Stonecreek Ct., Blue Springs, MO 64015

Bridgeton

Innoventor, Inc. — 314-785-0900
3600 Rider Trail South, Bridgeton, MO 63045

Brookfield

Apex Plastics — 800-467-4640
570 S Main St, Brookfield, MO 64628

Broseley

Ideal Products — 800-321-5490
1287 County Road 623, Broseley, MO 63932

Carthage

Leggett & Platt Inc. — 417-358-8131
P.O. Box 757, 1 Leggett Road, Carthage, MO 64836-0757

Cassville

Able 2 Products Co., Inc. — 800-641-4098
804 East Highway 248, P.O. Box 543, Cassville, MO 65625-0543

Centralia

Sunnydale Industries, Inc. — 800-346-3515
6859 Audrain Road 9139, Centralia, MO 65240-9802

Chesterfield

Bendistal Pliers — 636-230-9933
175 Lamp & Lantern Village, Chesterfield, MO 63017-8208

I.V. House, Inc. — 800-530-0400
418 Seven Gables Court, Chesterfield, MO 63017-2456

Jwp & Associates, Inc. — 636-536-5055
15259 Kingsman Circle, Chesterfield, MO 63017

Cole Camp

Mobility Concepts, L.L.C. — 660-668-3918
16999 Boyer Ave, Cole Camp, MO 65325

Crystal City

Syntec, Inc. — 636-566-6500
812 Truman Blvd., Crystal City, MO 63019

Crystal Lake Park

Bruce Cook, Prosthetics — 314-567-7585
2821 North Ballas, #215, Crystal Lake Park, MO 63131

Curryville

Dynacon, Inc. — 573-594-3813
4924 Pike 451, Curryville, MO 63339

Earth City

Athena Technology, Inc. — 314-344-0010
13705 Shoreline Court East, Earth City, MO 63045

Continental Manufacturing Co. — 800-325-1051
13330 Lake Front Drive, Earth City, MO 63045

Denticator International, Inc. — 866-469-6864
13705 Shoreline Court East, Earth City, MO 63045

General Pysiotherapy, Inc. — 800-237-1832
13222 Lakefront Drive, Earth City, MO 63045-1504

Lorvic Corp. — 800-325-1881
13705 Shoreline Ct. East, Earth City, MO 63045

Obtura Spartan — 800-344-1321
13729 Shoreline Ct. East, Earth City, MO 63045

Young Colorado, Llc. — 800-325-1881
13705 Shoreline Court East, Earth City, MO 63045

Young Dental Manufacturing Co 1, Llc — (800) 325-1881
13705 Shoreline Court East, Earth City, MO 63045-1235

Young Innovations, Inc. — 800-325-1881
13705 Shoreline Court East, Earth City, MO 63045-1235

Fenton

Biocold Environmental — 636-349-0300
239 Seebold Spur, Fenton, MO 63026

Everest Biomedical Instruments Co. — 636-305-9900
1732 Gilsinn Ln., Fenton, MO 63026

Four Process, Ltd. — 636-677-5650
1480 West Lark Industrial Park, Fenton, MO 63026

Medical Technologies Co. — 800-280-3220
1728A West Park Center Dr, Fenton, MO 63026

Quick Point Inc. — 636-343-9400
1717 Fenpark Drive, Fenton, MO 63026

Young O/S Llc — 800-325-1881
1663 Fenton Business Park, Fenton, MO 63026

Florissant

Laszlo Corp. — 314-830-3222
2573 Millvalley Drive, Florissant, MO 63031

Grandview

Integrity Products, Inc. — 816-965-0308
P.O. Box 4411, Grandview, MO 64030-0844

Thyssenkrupp Access Corp. — 1-800-829-9760
4001 E. 138th St., Grandview, MO 64030

Vulcon Technologies — 888-522-7746
718 Main St., Grandview, MO 64030

Hazelwood

Biomerieux Industry — 800-634-7656
595 Anglum Road, Hazelwood, MO 63042-2320

Covidien Lp, Formerly Registered As Kendall — 800-962-9888
444 Mcdonnell Blvd., Hazelwood, MO 63042

Mallinckrodt, Inc. — 800-325-8888
675 McDonnell Blvd., Hazelwood, MO 63042

Mallinckrodt, Inc.   800-325-8888
675 McDonnell Blvd., Hazelwood, MO 63042

High Ridge

Healing Solutions, Llc.   636-376-8100
2112 Penta Dr, High Ridge, MO 63049
Simmler, Inc.   800-325-0786
4564 North Square Dr., P.O. Box 350, High Ridge, MO 63049-0350

Hillsboro

Lampac International Ltd.   636-797-3659
230 North Lake Drive, Hillsboro, MO 63050

Imperial

Barnhart Industries, Inc.   800-325-9973
3690 Hwy M, Imperial, MO 63052
Orthoband Company, Inc.   800-325-9973
3690 Hwy. M, Imperial, MO 63052

Independence

Hemco Corp.   816-796-2900
111 Powell Road, Independence, MO 64056-2602

Jackson

Midwest Sterilization Corp.   573-243-8456
1204 Lenco Ave., Jackson, MO 63755-0411
Quality Packaging Industries Llc   573-334-6700
5830 State Highway V, Jackson, MO 63755

Jefferson City

Taylor Industries, Inc.   800-339-1361
2706 Industrial Drive, Jefferson City, MO 65109

Jonesburg

Artcraft Packaging Corp.   314-488-5566
212 Lions Estate Dr., Jonesburg, MO 63351

Joplin

Link Ergonomics Corp.   800-424-5465
902 E. 4th Street, Joplin, MO 64801

Kansas City

Bradford Medical, Llc   816-584-8100
8350 N. St. Clair Ave., #230, Kansas City, MO 64151
Cardiovascular Imaging Technologies, Llc   816-531-2842
4320 Wornall Rd., Suite 55, Kansas City, MO 64111
Cerner Corp.   866-221-8877
2800 Rockcreek Parkway, Kansas City, MO 64117
Cerner Corporation Innovation Campus   816-201-1368
10234 Marion Park Drive, Kansas City, MO 64137
Certified Safety Manufacturing   800-854-7474
1400 Chestnut, Kansas City, MO 64127
Community Blood Center Of Greater K.C.   888-647-4040
4040 Main St., Kansas City, MO 64111
Fairbanks Scales, Inc.   800-451-4107
821 Locust Street, Kansas City, MO 64106
Firestone Optics, Inc.   816-455-0500
3901 E N.e., 33rd. Terr., Kansas City, MO 64117
Fused Kontacts, Inc.   816-455-0500
3901 N.E. 33rd Terrace, Suite E, Kansas City, MO 64117
Goetze Dental   800-692-0804
3939 N.E. 33rd Terrace, Kansas City, MO 64117
International Medical Electronics Ltd.   800-432-8003
1319 Central Ave., PO BOX 45030, Kansas City, MO 64111
Kay See Dental Mfg. Co.   800-842-8844
124 East Missouri Ave., Kansas City, MO 64106-1294
Ken-A-Vision Manufacturing Co., Inc.   800-627-1953
5615 Raytown Road, Kansas City, MO 64133
Labconco Corp.   800-821-5525
8811 Prospect Avenue, Kansas City, MO 64132-2696
Medical Positioning, Inc.   800-593-3246
1717 Washington, Kansas City, MO 64108
Paramedical Distributors   800-245-3278
2020 Grand Ave., Kansas City, MO 64141-9777
Power Products, Inc.-Splintek   816-531-1900
3325 Wyoming St., Kansas City, MO 64111
Primus Diagnostics   800-377-4752
4231 E. 75th Terrace, Kansas City, MO 64132
Teartec   816-518-8626
7400 N.w. Whipple Ln., Kansas City, MO 64152

Kirkwood

Wexford Labs, Inc.   314-966-4134
325 Leffingwell Ave., Kirkwood, MO 63122

Lake Winnebago

Summit Lifts, Inc.   866-378-6648
18505 E. 163rd Street, Lake Winnebago, MO 64034

Lanton

Heritage Medical Products, Inc   417-256-3628
10380 Cr 6310, Lanton, MO 65775

Lee's Summit

Glenn Reams, Ocularist   800-426-8995
221 N.w. Mcnary Court, Lee's Summit, MO 64086
Heartland Tanning, Inc.   816-795-1414
4251 Ne Port Dr., Lee's Summit, MO 64064

Liberty

Nbn Products, L.L.C.   800-792-9795
1310 Amesbury Avenue, Liberty, MO 64068

Manchester

Bausch & Lomb, Inc.   585-338-8731
499 Sovereign Ct., Manchester, MO 63011

Maplewood

Cardinal Health 2200, Inc   847-578-6442
5 Sunnen Dr, Maplewood, MO 63143

Maryland Heights

Leica Biosystems - St. Louis, Llc   847-317-7209
12100a Prichard Farm Rd., Maryland Heights, MO 63043
Micromachining Technologies, Inc.   314-785-6800
2345 Millpark Dr., Suite A, Maryland Heights, MO 63043

Moberly

Cardinal Health 200, Inc   847-785-3323
808 Hwy. 24 West, Moberly, MO 65270

Mt. Vernon

Hearing Crafters Of America   417-466-4085
708 E. Mount Vernon Blvd., Mt. Vernon, MO 65712

North Kansas City

National Starch & Chemical Co.   317-656-2227
1001 Bedford Ave., North Kansas City, MO 64116
Southwest Technologies, Inc.   800-247-9951
1746 Levee Road, North Kansas City, MO 64030

O'fallon

Psi/Eye-Ko, Inc.   636-447-1010
804 Corporate Centre Dr., O'fallon, MO 63368
Synergetics Usa, Inc.   800-600-0565
3845 Corporate Centre Dr., O'Fallon, MO 63368

Olivette

Computerized Medical Systems, Inc.   468-587-2550
1145 Corporate Lake Dr., Olivette, MO 63132

Overland

Envisioneering Medical Technologies   314-429-7367
1982 Innerbelt Business Center, Drive, Overland, MO 63114

Poplar Bluff

Ashlar Holdings, Llc   573-785-8766
1908 Greenwood Drive Suite B, Poplar Bluff, MO 63901

Riverside

Dornoch Medical Systems, Inc.   888-466-6633
200 Northwest Parkway, Riverside, MO 64150

Robertsville

Berring Precision Blades Llc   352-383-8333
9236 Wildwood Lane, Robertsville, MO 63072

Rolla

Linscan Ultrasound   800-533-7226
202 W. 9th. St., Suite 301, Rolla, MO 65402-1217

Saint Clair

Micro-Select Instruments, Inc.   636-273-5227
165 Duckworth St., Saint Clair, MO 63077

Saint Louis

Airgas-Mid America, Inc.   800-292-4404
3500 Bernard, Saint Louis, MO 63103
Back-Mueller, Inc.   314-531-6640
2700 Clark Ave., Saint Louis, MO 63103
Chemisphere Corp.   314-644-1300
2101 Clifton Ave., Saint Louis, MO 63139
Pemaco, Inc.   314-231-3399
2030 South 3rd St., Saint Louis, MO 63104
United Laboratory Plastics   800-722-2499
1724A Westpark Ctr., PO Box 8585, Saint Louis, MO 63126

Sedalia

Cooperative Workshops, Inc.   888-615-6332
1500 Ewing Drive, Sedalia, MO 65301

Springfield

Edmonds Dental Prosthetics, Inc.   1.800.462.3569
2065 W. Woodland, Springfield, MO 65807
Hcmi, Inc.   773-588-2444
2146 East Pythian St., Springfield, MO 65802
Miller Coach Co., Inc.   800-824-9643
1744 W COLLEGE ST, SPRINGFIELD, MO 65806

St. Charles

Ekcomed, Llc — 314-303-9757
629 Bemis Heights Pl, St. Charles, MO 63303

Linco Research,Inc. — 866-441-8400
6 Research Park Dr., St. Charles, MO 63304

Spinal Traction Products, Llc. — 636-947-9086
5 Lake Forest Ct. East, St. Charles, MO 63301

St. Joseph

Hillyard, Inc. — 816-233-1321
302 North 4th St., P.O. Box 909, St. Joseph, MO 64501

Tbl, Inc. — 816-233-5487
751 South 4th St., St. Joseph, MO 64507

St. Louis

Accu-Glass Llc — 800-325-4796
10765 Trenton Avenue, St. Louis, MO 63132

Adapt-Ability, Inc. — 314-432-1101
9355 Dielman Industrial Dr., St. Louis, MO 63132

Ag Industries — 800-875-3138
3637 Scarlett Oak Blvd., St. Louis, MO 63122

Allied Healthcare Products, Inc. — 800-444-3954
1720 Sublette Ave., St. Louis, MO 63110-1927

Allied Healthcare Products, Inc. — 800-444-3954
1720 Sublette Avenue, St. Louis, MO 63110

Angelica Image Apparel — 800-222-3112
700 Rosedale Avenue, St. Louis, MO 63112

B & H Orthopedic Lab., Inc. — 314-647-1617
2510 Hampton Ave., St. Louis, MO 63139

Bausch & Lomb Surgical — 636-255-5051
3365 Tree Ct. Indust. Blvd., St. Louis, MO 63122-6615

Bio-Clin, Inc. — 314-647-3244
5977 S.W. Avenue, St. Louis, MO 63139

Biomedical Systems — 800-877-6334
77 Progress Parkway, Building One, St. Louis, MO 63043

Biomedical Systems Corp. — 800-877-6334
77 Progress Parkway, Building One, St. Louis, MO 63043

Cobert Associates, Inc. — 800-972-4766
2302 Weldon Parkway, St. Louis, MO 63146

Cookgas Llc — 314-781-5700
1167 Hillside Dr., St. Louis, MO 63117

Courion — 800-533-5760
3044 Lambdin Ave., St. Louis, MO 63115-2899

Dazor Manufacturing Corp. — 800-345-9103
2079 Congressional St., St. Louis, MO 63146

Elite Mattress Manufacturing — 800-332-5878
4999 Rear Fyler Avenue, St. Louis, MO 63139

Essex Cryogenics Of Missouri, Inc. — 314-832-8077
8007 Chivvis Dr., St. Louis, MO 63123

Eveready Battery Co. — 314-985-1569
Checkerboard Square, St. Louis, MO 63164

Facts And Comparisons — 800-223-0554
77 Westport Plaza, Suite 450, St. Louis, MO 63146-3098

Falcon Products, Inc. — 800-873-3252
10650 Gateway Blvd., St. Louis, MO 63132-2214

Forest Pharmaceutical, Inc. — 314-493-7000
13600 Shoreline Drive, St. Louis, MO 63045

Forestadent Usa — 800-721-4940
2315 Weldon Parkway, St. Louis, MO 63146

Global Surgical Corp. — 800-861-3585
3610 Tree Ct. Industrial Blvd., St. Louis, MO 63122

Haemachem, Inc. — 314-644-3277
2335 South Hanley Rd., St. Louis, MO 63144

Hampton Medical Devices — 636-225-3100
3550 Crowndun Dr., St. Louis, MO 63129

Heptest Laboratories, Inc. — 888-314-6008
1431 Hanley Industrial Court, St. Louis, MO 63144

Horizon Healthcare Technologies — 800-477-5827
PO Box 27809, St. Louis, MO 63146

Icp Medical — 314-429-1000
10486 Baur Blvd., St. Louis, MO 63132

Intercon Chemical — 800-325-9218
1100 Central Industrial Dr., St. Louis, MO 63110

Intercon Chemical Co. — 800-325-9218
1100 Central Industrial Dr., St. Louis, MO 63110

Intoximeters, Inc. — 800-451-8639
8110 Lackland Road, St. Louis, MO 63114

Jannx Medical Systems Inc. — 800-325-4334
12166 Old Big Bend Blvd., Ste. 300, St. Louis, MO 63122-6836

Jedmed Instruments Co. — 314-845-3770
5416 Jedmed Ct., St. Louis, MO 63129-2221

Jones Speciality Products — 314-845-6850
4010 Nottingham Est Dr., St. Louis, MO 63129

Jvs Solutions — 800-325-3303
1200 Switzer Ave., St. Louis, MO 63147

Koven Technology, Inc. — 800-521-8342
12125 Woodcrest Executive Dr., Suite 320, St. Louis, MO 63141

Krause Surgical Instrument Corp. — 314-842-0327
5544 Robertwood Dr., St. Louis, MO 63128

Leinco Technologies Inc. — 800-538-1145
410 Axminister Drive, St. Louis, MO 63026

Lhb Industries — 800-542-3697
10440 Trenton Avenue, St. Louis, MO 63132

Megasun — 800-229-7432
4515 Miami Street, St. Louis, MO 63116

Midwest Scientific — 800-227-9997
280 Vance Road, St. Louis, MO 63088

Multidata Systems International Corp. — 314-968-6880
10816 Indian Head Ind Blvd, St. Louis, MO 63119

Nelson Inc., A.R. — 800-377-6625
35-55 Scarlett Oak Blvd., St. Louis, MO 63122

Nomax, Inc. — 314-961-2500
40 North Rock Hill Rd., St. Louis, MO 63119

Ohlendorf Company — 314-533-3440
2840 Clark Avenue, St. Louis, MO 63103

Pemaco, Inc. — 1-800-435-6487
2030 S. 3rd St., St. Louis, MO 63104

Pepex Biomedical Inc. — 314-633-5053
4041 Forest Park, St. Louis, MO 63108

Perio Protect Llc — 202-672-5430
3929 Bayless Ave., St. Louis, MO 63125

Precision Prosthetics & Orthotics, Inc. — 314-843-3339
11102 S.lindbergh Business Ct., St. Louis, MO 63123

Progressive Operations, Inc. — 314-570-5153
8455 Wabash Avenue, St. Louis, MO 63134

Rahd Oncology Products — 800-844-0103
10762 Indian Head Industrial Blvd, St. Louis, MO 63132

Reliable Biopharmeceutical — 314-429-7700
1945 Walton Rd., St. Louis, MO 63114

Respironics Missouri — 978-659-4252
2039 Concourse Dr., St. Louis, MO 63146

Rhein Mfg., Inc. — 314-997-1775
2269 Grissom Dr., St. Louis, MO 63146

Seiler Precision Microscopes, Div. Of Seiler Instrument Co. — 800-489-2282
3433 Tree Court Industrial Blvd., St. Louis, MO 63122

Sigma-Aldrich Corp. — 800-521-8956
3050 Spruce St., St. Louis, MO 63103

Sigma-Aldrich Manufacturing, Llc — 314-286-6600
3500 Dekalb St., St. Louis, MO 63118

Sigma-Aldrich Manufacturing, Llc. — 913-469-5580
3506 South Broadway, St. Louis, MO 63118

Signal Medical Corporation — 800-246-6324
1000 Des Peres Road, Suite 140, St. Louis, MO 63131

Sports Play Equipment, Inc. — 800-727-8180
5642 Natural Bridge, St. Louis, MO 63120-1628

Stereotaxis, Inc. — 866-646-2346
4320 Forest Park Ave., Suite 100, St. Louis, MO 63108

Steris Corporation — 314-290-4600
7501 Page Avenue, St. Louis, MO 63133

Steris Corporation — 314-290-4703
8525 Page Boulevard, St. Louis, MO 63114

Sure-Tech Diagnostic Associates, Inc. — 314-894-8933
11040 Lin Valle Dr., Suite D, St. Louis, MO 63123

Surgical Instrument Manufacturers, Inc. — 800-521-2985
1650 Headland Drive, St. Louis, MO 63026-2915

Technical Products International, Inc. — 800-729-4421
5918 Evergreen Blvd, St. Louis, MO 63134-2302

The Respiratory Group — 314-659-4311
4150 Carr Lane, St. Louis, MO 63119

Tip, Inc. — 314-729-2969
2 Muirfield Ln., PO Box 410208, St. Louis, MO 63141

Trademark Medical Llc — 800-325-9044
449 Soverign Ct, St. Louis, MO 63011

True Fitness — 800-426-6570
865 Hoff Road, St. Louis, MO 63366

Veran Medical Technologies, Inc. — 314-659-8500
1908 Innerbelt Business Center Dr., St. Louis, MO 63114

Washington University School Of Medicine — 314-362-8525
4921 Parkview Place, St. Louis, MO 63110

St. Peters

Faichney Medical Co. — 800-548-0817
433 Scenic Drive, Suite # 103, St. Peters, MO 63376

Washington

Biospan Technologies, Inc. — 800-730-8980
6540 Meyer Dr., Washington, MO 63090

Noa Medical Industries — 800-633-6068
801 Terry Lane, Washington, MO 63090

Shure Manufacturing Corp. — 800-227-4873
1901 W. Main St., Washington, MO 63090

Webb City

Cardinal Scale Mfg. Co. — 800-641-2008
203 East Daugherty, Box 151, Webb City, MO 64870

Detecto Scale Co. — 800-641-2008
203 E. Daugherty, PO Box 151, Webb City, MO 64870

Webster Groves

Orthotic & Prosthetic Lab, Inc. — 314-968-8555
748 Marshall Ave., Webster Groves, MO 63119

Winfield

Syntec, Inc. — 636-566-6500
733 Mansion Rd., Winfield, MO 63389

MONTANA

Alzada

Gametrics Ltd. — 307-878-4494
426 Lonesome Country Rd, Alzada, MT 59311

Belgrade

Bacterin International Inc. — 406-388-0480
664 Cruiser Ln., Belgrade, MT 59714
Phillips Environmental Products, Inc. — 406-388-5999
290 Arden Dr., Belgrade, MT 59714

Billings

Computers Unlimited — 406-255-9500
2407 Montana Avenue, Billings, MT 59101-2336
Windstone Medical Packaging, Inc. — 800-637-7056
1602 4th Ave. N., Billings, MT 59101-1521

Bozeman

Bridger Biomed, Inc. — 908-277-8000
2430 North 7th Ave., Bozeman, MT 59715
King Tool, Inc. — 800-587-9445
5350 Love Ln, Bozeman, MT 59718
Quantel-Usa, Inc. — 406-586-0131
601 Haggerty Ln., Bozeman, MT 59715
Revelation Industries — 800-833-2139
101 East Oak Street, Bozeman, MT 59715

Darby

Epic Systems, Inc. — 800-338-2812
4488 Thorning Loop, P.O. BOX 908, Darby, MT 59829

Deer Lodge

1st Aid First — 800-613-6770
1690 Lake Hill Rd., Deer Lodge, MT 59722

Kalispell

Glacier Cross, Inc. — 800-388-4828
1694 Whalebone Dr., Kalispell, MT 59901

Missoula

American Eagle Instruments, Inc. — 800-551-5172
6575 Butler Creek Rd., Missoula, MT 59808
I.T.I., Inc. — 406-251-7000
6150 Hwy. 93 South, Missoula, MT 59804
Invaquest — 406-543-4228
3116 Old Pond Rd., Missoula, MT 59802-1420
Mortan, Inc. — 800-423-8659
329 E. Pine Street, Missoula, MT 59802
Mortech, Llc. — 406-542-7040
323 Sw Higgins Ave., Missoula, MT 59803
Nurture Inc. — 406-728-0260
5840 Express Way, Missoula, MT 59802
Pdt, Inc. — 406-626-4153
12201 Moccasin Ct., Missoula, MT 59808
Quality Products Of Montana — 406-544-0305
4022 Timberlane, Missoula, MT 59802
Spectrum Aquatics — 800-791-8056
7100 Spectrum Ln., Missoula, MT 59808

Polson

Doctor Down, Inc. — 888-883-3696
802 1st Street East, P.O. Box 1, Polson, MT 59860

Victor

Specialty Surgical Products, Inc. — 406-961-0102
1131 North U.S. Hwy. 93, Victor, MT 59875

NEBRASKA

Aurora

Penner Manufacturing Inc — 800-732-0717
102 Grant Street, PO Box 523, Aurora, NE 68818
Vancare, Inc. — 800-694-4525
1515 1st St., Aurora, NE 68818

Broken Bow

Becton, Dickinson & Co. — 308-872-6811
150 South First St., Broken Bow, NE 68822

Columbus

Becton Dickinson And Company — 201-847-4570
2153 12th Ave., Columbus, NE 68601
C & S Electronics, Inc. — 402-563-3596
2565 16th Ave., Columbus, NE 68601
Mastercare Patient Equipment, Inc. — 800-798-5867
2071 14th Ave., PO Box 1435, Columbus, NE 68601

Firth

Bradley Alarm Systems — 402-791-2388
28801 S. 96th Street, Firth, NE 68358

Gothenburg

Birkova Products — 888-567-4502
809 4th Street, Gothenburg, NE 69138

Grand Island

Nova-Tech, Inc. — 308-381-8841
Central Ne. Regional Airport, 1982 East Citation Way, Grand Island, NE 68801

Hastings

Protex Central Inc. — 800-274-0888
1239 N. Minnesota Avenue, PO Box 1467, Hastings, NE 68902

Holdrege

Bd Medical - Diabetes Care — 201-847-4298
1329 West Hwy 6, Holdrege, NE 68949

Lincoln

Apec, Inc. — 800-746-8421
2740 North 49th St., #6, Lincoln, NE 68504
Heinke Technoogy, Inc. (Hti Plastics) — 800-824-0607
5120 N.W. 38th St., Lincoln, NE 68524
Inverse Technology Corp. — 800-222-5778
1000 West O St., Suite B, Lincoln, NE 68528
Lester Electrical Of Nebraska, Inc. — 402-477-8988
625 West A St., Lincoln, NE 68522-1706
Li-Cor, Inc. — 800-645-4267
4647 Superior Street Lincoln, Lincoln, NE 68504-0425
Senior Technologies — 800-824-2996
PO Box 80238, 1620 N 20th Circle, Lincoln, NE 68503
Universal Medical Products, Inc. — 800-206-1045
1550 N. 20th Circle, Lincoln, NE 68503

North Loup

Mormac Tube Guard Co. — 800-445-2868
Main St., P.O. Box 40, North Loup, NE 68859-0040

Omaha

American Laboratories, Inc. — 402-339-2494
4410 South 102nd Street, Omaha, NE 68127
Barnett & Ramel Optical Co. — 800-228-9732
7154 N. 16th St., Omaha, NE 68112-0488
Better Dental Products — 402-934-4996
8540 I St., Omaha, NE 68127
Cetac Technologies, Inc. — 800-369-2822
14306 Industrial Rd., Omaha, NE 68144
Children's Hospital — 800-437-0272
8200 Dodge St., Omaha, NE 68114
Hearing Today Laboratory, Inc. — 800-567-0088
14473 W. Center Rd., Omaha, NE 68144
Innovision, Inc. — 402-558-3000
3125 South 61st Ave., Omaha, NE 68106
Justman Brush Co. — 800-800-6940
828 Crown Point Avenue, Omaha, NE 68110
Lab-Interlink, Inc. — 705-860-1220
8950 J Street, Omaha, NE 68127
MEI Corporation — 402-339-3300
4907 South 90th St., Omaha, NE 68127
Nagl Manufacturing Co. — 423-587-2199
3626 Martha St., Omaha, NE 68105
Plasti Products, Inc. — 800-527-5396
14315 C-Circle, Omaha, NE 68144
Raven Biological Laboratories, Inc. — 800-728-5702
8607 Park Drive, PO Box 27261, Omaha, NE 68127
Rd Industries, Inc. — 800-759-7090
11811 Calhoun Road, Omaha, NE 68152-1346
Rehab Innovations, Inc. — 402-445-4335
8727 Ames Ave., Omaha, NE 68134
Resonance Innovations Llc — 402-934-2650
10957 Lake Ridge Drive, Omaha, NE 68136
Sloan Corp. — 402-782-3742
13316 A St., Omaha, NE 68144
Streck Laboratories, Inc. — 800-843-0912
7002 South 109th Street, Omaha, NE 68128
Trans-Genomic — 888-233-9283
12325 Emmet Street, Omaha, NE 68164
Transgenomic, Inc. — 888-233-9283
12325 Emmet Street, Omaha, NE 68164

Valley

3m Valley — 402-359-2131
600 E. Meigs Street, Valley, NE 68064

Waverly

Linweld Inc. — 402-323-8450
9920 deer park road, Waverly, NE 68462

NEVADA

Carson City

Afton Medical Llc — 877-300-6288
5576 Bighorn Dr, Carson City, NV 89701
Amden Corp. — 949-581-9988
2533 North Carson Street, Carson City, NV 89706

L.A.B. Instruments, Ltd. — 775-883-1205
3692 Green Acres Dr., Carson City, NV 89705
Micromanipulator Co., Inc., The — 800-972-4032
1555 Forrest Way, Carson City, NV 89706-0448
Silver Eagle Labs Inc. — 650-522-9700
204 W. Spear Street, Carson City, NV 89703
Wykle Research, Inc. — 775-887-7500
2222 East College Parkway, Carson City, NV 89706

Crystal Bay

Nocwatch International, Inc./Fallsaver — 877-614-5616
PO Box 1367, Crystal Bay, NV 89402

Ely

General Dental Products, Inc. — 888-367-6212
201 Ogden Avenue, Ely, NV 89301-1888

Henderson

Biodermis Corp. — 800-322-3729
1820 Whitney Mesa Dr., Henderson, NV 89014
K-Stat, L.L.C. — 702-262-1044
11126 Olivia Pkwy., Henderson, NV 89011
Nano Mask Inc. — 888-656-3697
175 Cassia Way, Suite A115, Henderson, NV 89014
Robertson Harness — 702-564-4286
261 West Cyress Dr., A, PO Box 90086, Henderson, NV 89009
Unit Chemical Corp. — 800-879-8648
7360 Commercial Way, Henderson, NV 89015

Incline Village

Nocwatch International, Inc. — 775-833-4142
288 Village Blvd., Suite 5, Incline Village, NV 89451

Las Vegas

Biodermis Corp. — 800-322-3729
6000 South Eastern, Suite 9-D, Las Vegas, NV 89119
Colonial Medical Supply — 800-634-9334
1350 E. Flamingo Rd. # 343, Las Vegas, NV 89119
Elgar Dental Products, Inc. — 702-699-5655
3374 Racquet St., Las Vegas, NV 89121
Fertility Tech. Inc — 702-233-2601
9405 Darwell Drive, Las Vegas, NV 89117
Help U Lift — 702-435-9001
5653 Wheatfield Drive, Las Vegas, NV 89120
Herbsthelp, Corp. — 702-245-6958
2917 Linkview Dr., Las Vegas, NV 89134
Hunter Research Laboratories, Inc. — 888-764-5463
2225 sierra heights drive, Las Vegas, NV 89134
Integrated Biomedical Corp. — 702-450-1005
5030 S. Decatur Blvd. #e, Las Vegas, NV 89118
J.B.C And Co. — 702-914-8842
7980 West Torino Ave, Las Vegas, NV 89113
Kelly Hearing Aid — 702-309-3724
150 South Decatur Blvd., Las Vegas, NV 89107
Kloehn Co., Ltd. — 800-358-4342
10000 Banburry Cross Drive, Las Vegas, NV 89144
Mbi, Inc. — 702-259-1999
1353 Arville St., Las Vegas, NV 89102-1608
Medsonix — 702-873-3700
2626 S. Rainbow Blvd., Suite 109, Las Vegas, NV 89146
Multi-Pure Drinking Water System — 800-622-9206
7251 Cathedral Rock Drive, Las Vegas, NV 89128
Oceans Seven Int'L. — 502-634-3221
Hughes Airport Center, 6620 Escondido, Las Vegas, NV 89119
Parker Anderson Llc — 888-799-4289
5030 Paradise Road, Suite A-214, Las Vegas, NV 89119

Minden

Afassco, Inc. — 800-441-6774
2244 Park Pl., Suite C, Minden, NV 89423
Alta Diagnostics — 800-359-9691
2560 Business Parkway, Suite C, Minden, NV 89423

North Las Vegas

Lehrer Brillenperfektion Werks, Inc. — 818-407-1890
3908 North Fifth St., North Las Vegas, NV 89030

Reno

Accelerated Care Plus Corp. — 800-350-1100
4850 Joule Street, Suite A-1, Reno, NV 89502
Aesthetic And Reconstructive Technologies, Inc. — 866-853-6800
3545 Airway Dr., Suite 106, Reno, NV 89511
Alere Medical, Inc. — 775-829-8885
595 Double Eagle Court, Suite 1000, Reno, NV 89521
Bulbman, Inc. — 800-648-1163
630 Sunshine Lane, Reno, NV 89502
Carolina Absorbent Cotton — 775 856 2444, e
4969 Energy Way, Reno, NV 89502
Clareblend, Inc. — 800-334-7126
3555 Airway Dr., Suite 307, Reno, NV 89511
Computerized Screening, Inc. (Csi) — 800-533-9230
9550 Gateway Drive, Reno, NV 89521-8924
Covance Cardiac Safety Services, Inc. — 215-282-5588
9390 Gateway Drive, Reno, NV 89521

Hamilton Company — 800-648-5950
4970 Energy Way, Reno, NV 89520-0012
Hamilton Medical, Inc. — 800-426-6331
4990 Energy Way, Reno, NV 89502
Insight Biodesign Llc — 775-250-0267
1065 Waverly Drive, Reno, NV 89519
Mast/Keystone View — 800-806-6569
2200 Dickerson Rd., Reno, NV 89503
Microflex Corporation — 800-876-6866
PO Box 32000, 2301 Robb Drive,, Reno, NV 89533-2000
North Valley Precision Products, Llc — 775-829-2566
4750 Turbo Cr, Reno, NV 89502
OncoSec Medical Inc. — 775-562-0504
200 South Virginia Street, 8th Floor, Reno, NV 89501
Polyvision Inc. — 888-645-7788
875 East Patriot Blvd, Suite 201, Reno, NV 89511
Preserve International — 800-995-1607
P.O. Box 17003, Reno, NV 89511
Worldpak Flexible Packaging, Llc. — 775-359-0733
300 E. Parr Blvd., Reno, NV 89512

Sparks

Haws Corporation — 775-359-4712
1455 Kleppe Ln., Sparks, NV 89431
Mathison Industries, Inc. — 775-284-1020
220 Coney Island Drive, Sparks, NV 89431

Stateline

Diagnostic Monitoring Software — 775-589-6049
292 Kingsbury Grade, #32, P.o. Box 3109, Stateline, NV 89449

Zephyr Cove

Baiwa, Inc. — 775-588-8494
630 Alma Way, Zephyr Cove, NV 89448

NEW HAMPSHIRE

Amherst

Controlair, Inc. — 800-216-3636
8 Columbia Drive, Amherst, NH 03031
Guild Optical Associates, Inc. — 603-889-6247
11 Columbia Drive, Amherst, NH 03031
Maxilon Laboratories, Inc. — 603-594-9300
105 State Rt. 101a, Unit 8, Amherst, NH 03031
Numa, Inc. — 603-883-1909
10 Northern Blvd., Unit 12, Amherst, NH 03031

Antrim

Brailsford & Co., Inc. — 603-588-2880
15 Elm Avenue, Antrim, NH 03440

Auburn

Sunrise Labs, Inc. — 888-420-9600
5 Dartmouth Drive, Auburn, NH 03032

Bedford

Microelectrodes, Inc. — 603-668-0692
40 Harvey Road, Bedford, NH 03110-6805

Charlestown

Design Standards Corp. — 603-826-7744
Box 1620, 957 Claremont Road, Charlestown, NH 03603

Colebrook

Healthco International, Llc — 603-255-4200
2000 Cold Spring Road, Dixville Notch, Colebrook, NH 03576

Concord

Secure Care Products, Inc. — 800-451-7917
39 Chenell Dr., Concord, NH 03301-8501

Conway

Austin Medical Products, Inc. — 800-223-9310
66 Eastern Ave., P.O. Box 1830, Conway, NH 03818

Derry

Allen Datagraph Systems, Inc. — 800-258-6360
56 Kendall Pond Road, Derry, NH 03038
Surgic Aid, Inc. — 800-338-5213
37 Crystal Avenue, #287, Derry, NH 03038-1714

Dover

Heine Usa Ltd. — 800-367-4872
10 Innovation Way, Dover, NH 03820-3831
Tape-O-Corporation — 800-752-4944
35 Crosby Road, Dover, NH 03820-4340
The Prometheus Group — 603-749-0733
1 Washington St., Suite 303, Dover, NH 03820
iWorx Systems, Inc. — 800-234-1757
One Washington Street, Suite 404, Dover, NH 03820

Exeter

Biosignetics Corporation — 603-858-3844
29 Downing Ct., Exeter, NH 03833

Dutch Ophthalmic Usa, Inc.   800-753-8824
10 Continental Drive, Building 1, Exeter, NH 03833

Hampton

Boston Endo-Surgical Technologies, Inc.   603-929-0066
8 Merrill Drive, Hampton, NH 03842
Sleepnet Corporation   800-742-3646
5 Merrill Industrial Drive, Hampton, NH 03842
Spinus, Llc   603-758-1444
8 Merrill Industrial Dr., Hampton, NH 03842
Unisensor Usa, Inc.   603-926-5200
One Park Avenue, Suite #6, Hampton, NH 03842

Hooksett

G&M Research Company, Inc.   603-645-6655
31 Hale Ave., Hooksett, NH 03106

Hudson

Atrium Medical Corp.   800-528-7486
5 Wentworth Dr., Hudson, NH 03051
Computer Optics Inc.   603-889-2116
120 Derry Road, Hudson, NH 03051
Matrix Technologies Corporation   1 800 345 0206
22 Friars Drive, Hudson, NH 03051
Rdf Corp.   800-445-8367
23 Elm Avenue, Hudson, NH 03051
Sage Laboratories, Inc.   800-960-0599
8 Executive Drive, Hudson, NH 03051
Thermo Fisher Scientific   800-345-0206
22 Friars Drive, Hudson, NH 03051

Jaffrey

Millipore Corp.   (603) 532-8711
Prescott Rd., Jaffrey, NH 03452
Tfx Medical Oem   800-548-6600
50 Plantation Drive, Jaffrey, NH 03452

Keene

Arzol Chemical Co.   603-352-5242
12 Norway Ave., Ste. 2, Keene, NH 03431
Schleicher & Schuell, Inc.   800-245-4024
10 Optical Avenue, PO Box 2012, Keene, NH 03431
Smiths Medical Asd Inc.   800-258-5361
10 Bowman Drive, Keene, NH 03431

Laconia

Accellent Inc.   603-528-1211
45 Lexington Dr., Laconia, NH 03246

Lancaster

P. J. Noyes Company, Inc.   800-522-2469
89 Bridge St., Lancaster, NH 03584-3103

Lebanon

Keene Medical Products, Inc.   800 447-0028
240 Meriden Rd. No. 439, PO Box 439, Lebanon, NH 03766
Kleen Laundry & Drycleaning Services, Inc.   603-448-1134
1 Foundry St., Lebanon, NH 03766-1594
Simbex, Llc   603-448-2367
10 Water Street, Room 410, Lebanon, NH 03766
Wellan Medical, Inc.   603-676-8601
10 Water Street, Lebanon, NH 03766

Litchfield

Klarmann Rulings, Inc.   800-252-2401
480 Charles Bancroft Hwy., Litchfield, NH 03052

Londonderry

Mushield Company, Inc., The   888-669-3539
9 Ricker Avenue, Londonderry, NH 03053

Manchester

Abbas' Grace   603-624-9559
52 Meadow Ln., Manchester, NH 03109
Blanchard Contact Lens, Inc.   603-625-1664
8025 South Willow Street, Bldg #2 Unit 211-212, Manchester, NH 03103
Central Paper Products Company   800-339-4065
P.O. Box 4480, Manchester, NH 03108-4480
Corflex, Inc.   800-426-7353
669 E. Industrial Park Dr., Manchester, NH 03109-5625
Deka Research & Development Corp.   603-669-5139
340 Commercial St., Manchester, NH 03101-1121
Freedom Data Systems, Inc.   800-932-9000
228 Maple St Fl 1, Manchester, NH 03103
Medic-Air, A Division Of Corflex, Inc.   800-426-7353
669 E. Industrial Park Dr., Manchester, NH 03109-5625
Rcd Components, Inc.   877-723-2667
520 E. Industrial Park, Manchester, NH 03109-5316
Schleuniger, Inc.   877-902-1470
87 Colin Drive, Manchester, NH 03103
Sentry Battery Corp.   800-747-0199
62 Colin Drive, Manchester, NH 03103
Symmetry Medical, Inc. - Polyvac   207-786-2775
253 Abby Rd., Manchester, NH 03103

Velcro Usa, Inc.   603-669-4880
406 Brown Ave., Manchester, NH 03101

Merrimack

ElemAc Medical   877-333-5306
Heron Cove Office Park, 10 Al Paul Lane, Suite 102, Merrimack, NH 03054
ElemAc Medical, Incorporated   877-333-5306
Heron Cove Office Park, 10 Al Paul Lane, Suite 102, Merrimack, NH 03054
Kollsman, Inc.   603-886-7500
220 Daniel Webster Hwy., Merrimack, NH 03054
Technh, Inc   603-424-4404
8 Continental Blvd., PO Box 476, Merrimack, NH 03054

Nashua

Atlantic Rim Brace Mfg. Corp.   800-233-0356
25B Front St. Suite 5a, Nashua, NH 03064
Bagshaw Company, Inc., W.H.   800-343-7467
1 Pine St., Extension, PO Box 766, Nashua, NH 03060
Boston Billows, Inc.   603-598-1200
114 Perimeter Road, Unit E., Nashua, NH 03063
Centorr Vacuum Industries   800-962-8631
55 Northeastern Blvd., Nashua, NH 03062
Embrace Healthcare Llc   (800) 255-3311
100 Factory Street, Suite C3, Nashua, NH 03060
Icad Inc.   866-280-2239
98 Spit Brook Rd., Suite 100, Nashua, NH 03062
Metabolic Solutions, Inc.   866-302-1998
460 Amherst St., Nashua, NH 03063-1220
Vascular Technology Incorporated   800-550-0856
12 Murphy Drive, Nashua, NH 03062

Newington

Erie Scientific   603-431-8410
Portsmouth Park, 20 Post Road, Newington, NH 03801

North Sutton

Labsphere, Inc.   603-927-4266
231 Shaker St., North Sutton, NH 03260-9986

Pittsfield

Kentek Corp.   800-432-2323
1 Elm St., Pittsfield, NH 03263

Portsmouth

Disetronic Sterile Products   800-280-7801
124 Heritage Avenue, Portsmouth, NH 03801-5645
Novocure   215-854-4095
170 West Road, Unit #9, Portsmouth, NH 03801
Salient Surgical Technologies Inc.   800-354-2808
180 International Drive, Portsmouth, NH 03801
Xinix Research, Inc.   603-433-9121
5 Pheasant Ln., Portsmouth, NH 03801

Raymond

Extreme Adhesives, Inc.   800-888-4583
63 Epping Road, P.O. Box 1445, Raymond, NH 03077

Rindge

Grason & Associates, Llc   603-899-3089
71 Conifer Rd, P.o. Box 289, Rindge, NH 03461

Rocheseter

Phase Ii Medical Mfg., Inc.   603-332-8900
88 Airport Drive, Suite 100, Rocheseter, NH 03867

Salem

Advanced Polymers, Inc.   603-327-0600
29 Northwestern Drive, Salem, NH 03079-2838
Agamatrix   603-328-6000
10 Maor Parkway, Salem, NH 03079
Airgas East, Inc.   800-562-3815
27 Northwestern Drive, Salem, NH 03079
American Laboratory Products Co.   800-592-5726
26-G Keewaydin Drive, Salem, NH 03079
Guidewire Technologies, Inc.   800-894-4399
26 Keewaydin Dr., Salem, NH 03079-2839
Memtec Corp.   603-893-8080
68 Stiles Rd. Unit D, Salem, NH 03079

Seabrook

Microvision, Inc.   603-474-5566
34 Folly Mill Rd., Seabrook, NH 03874

Somersworth

J-Pac, Llc   603-692-9955
25 Centre Road, Somersworth, NH 03878-2927

Stratham

M. Braun Inc.   603-773-9333
14 Marin Way, Stratham, NH 03885

W. Lebanon

OLYMPUS BIOTECH CORPORATION   603-298-3000
9 Technology Dr., W. Lebanon, NH 03784

Weare

RadQual LLC — 508-833-1005
PO Box 82, Weare, NH 03281

Webster

White Mountain Imaging — 603-648-2124
1617 Battle St., Webster, NH 03303

West Lebanon

Medical Metrx Solutions — 603-298-5509
12 Commerce Ave., West Lebanon, NH 03784

West Swanzey

Beech Medical Products, Inc. — 603-355-4843
2 South Winchester St., West Swanzey, NH 03469
Moldpro, Inc. — 603-721-6286
36 Denman Thompson Hwy., West Swanzey, NH 03446
Multi-Med, Inc. — 603-357-8733
Winchester St., P.O. Box 660, West Swanzey, NH 03469

Windham

Cet Technology — 603-894-6100
27 Roulston Rd., Windham, NH 03087-1210

NEW JERSEY

Allendale

Biolectron, Inc. — 800-524-0677
25 Commerce Drive, Allendale, NJ 07401
Energex Systems Inc. — 201-995-1919
80 Commerce Dr., Allendale, NJ 07401
Ge Healthcare Iits Llc — 201-934-8644
40 Boroline Rd., Allendale, NJ 07401
Stryker Spine — 866-457-7463
2 Pearl Ct, Allendale, NJ 07401

Allenwood

Interspec Fabrics — 800-526-2800
P.O. Box 705, Allenwood, NJ 08720

Alpha

John J. Brogan, Inc. — 908-859-2300
1161 Third Ave., Alpha, NJ 08865

Alpine

ProTron Technologies — 201-297-7377
PO Box 234, Alpine, NJ 07620

Asbury Park

Terriss-Consolidated Industries — 800-342-1611
807 Summerfield Ave., Asbury Park, NJ 07712-0110

Barrington

Edmund Industrial Optics — 800-363-1992
101 E. Gloucester Pike, Barrington, NJ 08007-1380

Basking Ridge

Laser Solutions, Inc. — 800-230-7705
44 Bullion Road, Basking Ridge, NJ 07920

Bellmawr

Airgas East, Inc. — 800-562-3815
140 Harding Ave., Bellmawr, NJ 08031

Bergenfield

Titan Implants, Inc. — 1-866-439-0470
18 Columbia Ave., Bergenfield, NJ 07621
Var-Lac-Oid Chemical Co., Inc. — 201-387-0038
13 Foster Street, Bergenfield, NJ 07621-4301

Berkeley Heights

Align Pharmaceuticals — 908-834-0960
200 Connell Drive, Suite 1500, Berkeley Heights, NJ 07922

Birmingham

Photon Technology International, Inc. — 609-894-4420
300 Birmingham Road, Birmingham, NJ 08011-0272

Blackwood

Sun Biomedical Laboratories, Inc. — 888-440-8388
604 Vpr Center, 1001 Lower Landing Road, Blackwood, NJ 08012

Blairstown

Mtd, Inc. — 908-362-6807
24 Slabtown Creek Rd, Blairstown, NJ 07871

Bloomfield

Latam Medical — 1-877-989-4040
400 Belleville Ave., Bloomfield, NJ 07003-2604

Branchburg

Biosearch Medical Products, Inc. — 908-722-5000
35 Industrial Pkwy., Branchburg, NJ 08876
Hydromer, Inc. — 877-493-7663
35 Industrial Pky., Branchburg, NJ 08876
Lifecell Corp. — 800-367-5737
One Millennium Way, Branchburg, NJ 08876-3876
Spectra Gases, Inc. — 800-932-0624
3434 Rt. 22 W., Branchburg, NJ 08876

Brick

Pro-Comm, Inc. — 800-920-1476
1105 Industrial Pkwy., Brick, NJ 08724

Bridgeport

Caddy Corporation — 856-467-4222
509 Sharptown Road, Bridgeport, NJ 08014-0345

Bridgeton

Griffin Medical Products, Inc. — 800-366-6870
80 Manheim Avenue, PO Box 457, Bridgeton, NJ 08302

Bridgewater

Ack Laboratories, Inc. — 908-707-9244
540 Stony Brook Dr., Bridgewater, NJ 08807
Cordis Corporation — 800-447-7585
430 Route 22 East, Bridgewater, NJ 08807
Hamamatsu Corp. — 800-524-0504
360 Foothill Road, Bridgewater, NJ 08807-2920
Hamamatsu Photonic Systems — 800-524-0504
360 Foothill Road, Bridgewater, NJ 08807-0910
Permabond International — 800-653-6523
10 Feinder Ave., Bridgewater, NJ 08807

Buena

Comar, Inc. — 800-962-6627
1 Comar Place, Buena, NJ 08310-9901

Burlington

Dentsply Prosthetics — 800-877-0020
Six Terri Lane, Burlington, NJ 08016

Caldwell

Kaulson Laboratories, Inc. — 973-226-9494
693 Bloomfield Ave., Caldwell, NJ 07006-7539

Carlstadt

Agfa Healthcare Corp. — 864-421-1815
580 Gotham Parkway, Carlstadt, NJ 07072
Cadent, Inc. — 201-842-0800
640 Gotham Pkwy., Carlstadt, NJ 07072-2405
Grobet File Co. — 800-847-4188
750 Washington Avenue, Carlstadt, NJ 07072
Mada, Inc. — 800-526-6370
625 Washington Avenue, Carlstadt, NJ 07072-2503
Marcor Development Corp. — 201-935-2111
341 Michelle Pl, Carlstadt, NJ 07072-2304
The Amcor Group Ltd. — 800-584-6484
685A Gotham Parkway, Carlstadt, NJ 07072-2403
Water-Jel Technologies — 800-275-3433
50 Broad Street, Carlstadt, NJ 07072-2708
West Penetone Corp — 800-631-1652
700 Gotham Pkwy, Carlstadt, NJ 07072

Cedar Grove

Cargille Laboratories — 973-239-6633
55 Commerce Rd., Cedar Grove, NJ 07009-1289
Medical Device Concepts, Llc. — 201-446-6691
4 Lawrence Way, Cedar Grove, NJ 07009
Pectus Services — 757-224-0177
549 Pompton Ave., Suite 210, Cedar Grove, NJ 07009

Chatham

Advanced Biomaterial Systems, Inc. — 877-257-9040
100 Passaic Ave., Chatham, NJ 07928
Burling Instruments, Inc. — 973-635-9481
16 River Rd., Chatham, NJ 07928-0298
Orthosonics, Ltd. — 973-665-0001
71 Passaic Ave., Chatham, NJ 07928

Cherry Hill

B. Braun Medical — 800-854-6851
1940 Olney Ave., Cherry Hill, NJ 08003
Cti Medical Equipment, Inc. — 856-424-0503
1910 Route 70 (e), Ste.10, Cherry Hill, NJ 08003
Hoppecke Battery Systems, Inc. — 856-616-0032
1960 Old Cuthbert Road, Suite 130, Cherry Hill, NJ 08034
JACE SYSTEMS, INC — (856) 470-2100
55 Carnegie Plaza, Cherry Hill, NJ 08003
Jace Systems — 800-800-4276
5 Rockhill Rd, Suite 2, Cherry Hill, NJ 08003
Mizzy, Inc. Of National Keystone — 800-333-3131
616 Hollywood Avenue, Cherry Hill, NJ 08002-2821
National Keystone — 856-663-4700
616 Hollywood Ave., Cherry Hill, NJ 08002-2821
Northeast Medical Systems Corp. — 856-910-8111
901 Beechwood Ave., Cherry Hill, NJ 08002-3405

Starkey East
535 Route 38 East, Suite 230, Cherry Hill, NJ 08002 — 952-947-4734
Victory Refrigeration, Inc.
110 Woodcrest Road, Cherry Hill, NJ 08003 — 800-523-5008

Cinnaminson

Acclaim Medical Manufacturing Llc — 856-303-2363
1100 Taylors Lane, Unit 9, Cinnaminson, NJ 08077

Clifton

A. J. P. Scientific, Inc. — 973-472-7200
82 Industrial East, Clifton, NJ 07012
Agl Welding Supply Co., Inc. — 973-478-5000
600 Route 46, Clifton, NJ 07015
Challenge Printing Company, The — 800-654-1234
2 Bridewell Place, Clifton, NJ 07014
Glaxosmithkline Consumer Healthcare, L.P. — 215-751-4000
65 Industrial South, Clifton, NJ 07012
Gsk Consumer Healthcare — 888-825-5249
65 Industrial South, Clifton, NJ 07012
Physitemp Instruments, Inc. — 800-452-8510
154 Huron Avenue, Clifton, NJ 07013-2949

Cranbury

Nano-Ditech Corporation — 609-409-0700
7 Clarke Drive, Cranbury, NJ 08512

Cranford

General Cubicle Co. — 800-869-4606
49 Meeker Avenue, Cranford, NJ 07016

Dayton

Fecom Corporation — 800-292-3362
12 Stults Road, Suite 103, Dayton, NJ 08810
United Products & Instruments, Inc. — 800-588-9776
182 Ridge Road, Suite E, Dayton, NJ 08810

Denville

Katena Products, Inc. — 800-225-1195
4 Stewart Ct., Denville, NJ 07834-1028
Scimedx Corporation — 800-221-5598
100 Ford Road, Suite 100-08, Denville, NJ 07834-1353

dover

Germgard Lighting — (973) 607-1538
3328 Belt Road # 2, dover, NJ 07801-5769

Dumont

Confi Dental Lab, Inc. — 201-385-8777
50 Park Ave. Suite # 200-201, Dumont, NJ 07628

East Brunswick

Humanicare International, Inc. — 800-631-5270
9 Elkins Road, East Brunswick, NJ 08816
Swissray America, Inc. — 908 353 0971
One Tower Center Blvd., East Brunswick, NJ 08816
Swissray International (Hq) Inc. — 908-353-0971
One Tower Center Blvd., East Brunswick, NJ 08816

East Freehold

Princeton Separations, Inc. — 732-431-3338
100 Commerce Drive, East Freehold, NJ 07728

East Hanover

Viscot Medical, Llc — 800-221-0658
32 West Street, PO Box 351, East Hanover, NJ 07936-0351
Vlv Associates, Inc. — 973-428-2884
30-C Ridgedale Ave., East Hanover, NJ 07936
Weiss Aug Co., Inc. — 973-887-7600
220 Merry Lane, PO Box 520, East Hanover, NJ 07936

East Orange

Hospi-Tel Manufacturing Corp. — 973-678-7100
545 N. Arlington Ave., East Orange, NJ 07017

East Rutherford

Seritex Inc. — 973-472-4200
1 Madison St., East Rutherford, NJ 07073
Umi Intl. — 888-511-8655
2 E. Union Avenue, PO Box 170, East Rutherford, NJ 07073

East Windsor

Abbott Point Of Care Inc. — 609-443-9300
104 Windsor Center Dr., East Windsor, NJ 08520
Conair Corp. — 203-351-9000
150 Milford Rd., East Windsor, NJ 08520

Eatontown

Alkaline Corp. — 732-531-7830
20 Meridian Road #9, Eatontown, NJ 07724
Biological Controls Inc. — 800-224-9768
749 Hope Road, Suite A, Eatontown, NJ 07724-1414
Biotech Atlantic, Inc. — 732-389-4789
Bay F, 6 Industrial Way West, Eatontown, NJ 07724

Flexible Stenting Solutions Inc. — 732-578-0060
23 Christopher Way, Eatontown, NJ 07724

Edison

Automated Medical Products Corp. — 800-832-4567
P.O. Box 2508, Edison, NJ 08818-2508
Celsis Laboratory Group — 800-523-5227
165 Fieldcrest Avenue, Edison, NJ 08837
East Atlantic Trading/Triangle Healthcare Inc. — 800-243-4635
76 National Road, Edison, NJ 08817-2809
Enterix Inc. — 800-531-3681
236 Fernwood Ave., Edison, NJ 08837
Horiba Jobin Yvon Inc — 866-JOBINYVON
3880 Park Avenue, Edison, NJ 08820-3012
Intelwave, Llc — 732-738-8800
1090 King Georges Post Road, Suite 1004, Edison, NJ 08837
International Technidyne Corp. — 800-631-5945
23 Nevsky St, Edison, NJ 08820
International Technidyne Corporation — 732-548-5700
8 Olson Ave., Edison, NJ 08820
Lawler Manufacturing Corp. — 732-777-2040
7 Kilmer Ct., Edison, NJ 08817
Musculoskeletal Transplant Foundation — 800-433-6576
125 May St, Ste 300, Edison Corp Ctr, Edison, NJ 08837
New Brunswick Scientific Co., Inc. — 800-631-5417
44 Talmadge Rd.,, P.O. Box 4005, Edison, NJ 08818-4005
Tcp Reliable, Inc. — 888-TCP-3393
551 Raritan Center Pkwy., Edison, NJ 08837

Elizabeth

E.W. Pike & Company — 908-352-0630
501-517 Pennsylvania Avenue, Elizabeth, NJ 07201-1101

elizabeth,

Medtronic Spinal And Biologics New York Distribution Center — 901-396-3133
699 kapkowksi road, Suite 3, elizabeth,, NJ 07201

Elmwood Park

Bloomex International, Inc. — 201-703-9799
295 Molnar Dr., Elmwood Park, NJ 07407-3211
Golden Metal Products Co. — 800-978-9058
50 BUSHES LANE, Elmwood Park, NJ 07407-3296

Emerson

Cea Instruments, Inc. — 888-893-9640
16 Chestnut St., Emerson, NJ 07630

Englewood

Dshealthcare Inc. — 201-871-1232
85 West Forest Ave., Englewood, NJ 07631
Foremost Dental Llc. — 201-894-5500
242 South Dean St., Englewood, NJ 07631
Goldsmith & Revere, Inc. — 201-894-5500
242 S. Dean St., Englewood, NJ 07631-4139
Palisades Dental, Llc — 201-569-0050
111 Cedar Lane, Englewood, NJ 07631
Schneider International Ltd. — 201-568-5166
600 Sylvan Avenue, East Wing - First Floor, Englewood, NJ 07632
Zenith/Dmg Brand — 800-662-6383
Division of Foremost Dental LLC, 242 S. Dean St., Englewood, NJ 07631-4139

Englewood Cliffs

As Software, Inc. — 800-613-4441
560 Sylvan Ave., Englewood Cliffs, NJ 07632

Englishtown

Vynacron Dental Co. — 800-932-7612
6 Orchard Hill Dr., Englishtown, NJ 07726

Ewing

Antares Pharma, Inc. — 800-328-3074
Princeton Crossroads Corporate Center, 250 Phillips Boulevard, Suite 290, Ewing, NJ 08618
Mednet Healthcare Technologies, Inc. — 800-606-5511
100 Ludlow Drive, Ewing, NJ 08638
Neurotron Medical — 609-896-3444
800 Silvia St., Ewing, NJ 08628
Universal Medical, Inc. — 800.423.2767
275 Phillips Blvd, Ewing, NJ 08618

Fair Haven

Legacy Integrators, Llc — 800-272-5169
68 Forman St., Fair Haven, NJ 07704

Fair Lawn

Fisher Scientific Co., Llc. — 201-703-3131
One Reagent Ln., Fair Lawn, NJ 07410
Myheal Technologies — 201-703-9059
34-14 Linwood Rd., Fair Lawn, NJ 07410-4012
U.S. Technologies, Inc. — 800-234-0862
1701 Pollitt Dr., Fair Lawn, NJ 07410
Vyteris, Inc. — 201-703-2299
13-01 Pollitt Dr., Fair Lawn, NJ 07410

Fairfield

Arlington Machine & Tool Co. — 973-276-1377
90 New Dutch Lane, Fairfield, NJ 07004

Datascope Cardiac Assist Div. — 800-777-4222
15 Law Drive, Fairfield, NJ 07004

Drive-Master Co., Inc. — 973-808-9709
37 DANIEL ROAD W, Fairfield, NJ 07004

Hanovia Specialty Lighting Llc — 800-229-3666
6 Evans Street, Fairfield, NJ 07004

Lucomed Inc. — 800-633-7877
45 Kulick Rd., Fairfield, NJ 07004

MAQUET — 800-288-2121
15 Law Drive, Fairfield, NJ 07004

Morgan Advance Ceramics — 800-433-0638
26 Madison Rd., Fairfield, NJ 07004

Optimed Technologies, Inc. — 973-575-9911
20 New Dutch Lane, Fairfield, NJ 07004

Parker Laboratories, Inc. — 800-631-8888
286 Eldridge Rd., Fairfield, NJ 07004

Rti Electronics, Inc. — 800-222-7537
1275 Bloomfield Avenue, Building 5, Unit 29A, Fairfield, NJ 07004

Sensor Scientific, Inc. — 800-524-1610
6 Kings Bridge Road, Fairfield, NJ 07004

Wrapade Packaging Systems, Llc. — 888-815-8564
27 Law Drive, Suite B/C, Fairfield, NJ 07004

Farmingdale

Advanced Hyperbaric Technologies, Inc. — 800-327-4325
124 Colts Neck Rd., Farmingdale, NJ 07727

Alto Development Corp. — 732-938-2266
5206 Asbury Road, Farmingdale, NJ 07727-3516

Ernst Flow Industries — 800-992-2843
116 Main St., Farmingdale, NJ 07727-1495

Health Care Software, Inc. (Hcs) — 800-524-1038
PO Box 2430, Farmingdale, NJ 07727-2430

Monmouth Equipment & Service Co. Inc. — 732-919-1444
5105 Rts. 33/34, Farmingdale, NJ 07727

Polyone — 866-765-9663
10 Ruckle Ave., Farmingdale, NJ 07727

Flanders

Siemens Healthcare Diagnostics Inc — 973-584-4649
62 Flanders-Barley Road, Flanders, NJ 07836

Flemington

Altech Corporation — 908-806-9400
35 Royal Road, Flemington, NJ 08822-6001

Analytical Instrument Systems, Inc. — 908-788-7022
P.O. Box 458, Flemington, NJ 08822-0458

Dms Laboratories, Inc. — 800-567-4367
2 Darts Mill Road, Flemington, NJ 08822

3m Flemington — 908-788-4000
500 Route 202 North, Flemington, NJ 08822

Fort Lee

Opus Diagnostics, Inc. — 877-944-1777
One Parker Plaza, Fort Lee, NJ 07024

Franklin

North American Sterilization & Packaging — 800-392-6310
19 Park Dr., Franklin, NJ 07416

United Silica Products, Inc. — 973-209-8854
3 Park Dr., Franklin, NJ 07416

Franklin Lakes

Becton Dickinson And Co. — 201-847-6800
1 Becton Drive, Franklin Lakes, NJ 07417

Becton Dickinson And Company — 800-284-6845
1 Becton Dr., Franklin Lakes, NJ 07417

Freehold

Inverness Medical Inc. — 732-308-3000
569 Halls Mill Rd, Freehold, NJ 07728

Garfield

I.B.F. Corporation — 800-423-3456
44 Plauderville Avenue, Garfield, NJ 07026-0278

International Crystal Laboratories — 973-478-8944
11 Erie St., Garfield, NJ 07026-2307

Vitaire Corp. — 800-447-4344
141 Lanza Ave., Bldg 12, 4th Floor, Garfield, NJ 07026

Garwood

Medrecon, Inc. — 877-526-4323
257 South Avenue, Garwood, NJ 07027-1341

Gibbstown

Emd Chemicals Inc. — 800-222-0342
480 S. Democrat Road, Gibbstown, NJ 08027

Glassboro

Wecom, Inc. — 800-628-4115
20 Warrick Avenue, Glassboro, NJ 08028-2500

Glen Ridge

O.R. Comfort, Llc — 973-239-1950
28 Appleton Rd., Glen Ridge, NJ 07028-2204

Glendora

U.S. Vision Optical, Inc. — 866-435-7111
1 Harmon Dr., Glen Oaks Industrial Park, Glendora, NJ 08029

Green Brook

Kareco International, Inc. — 800-8KA-RECO
299 Rte. 22 E., Green Brook, NJ 08812-1714

Greystone Park

Temptime Corporation — 973-984-6000
116 American Rd., Greystone Park, NJ 07950

Hackensack

Caprius Inc. — 201-342-0900
One University Plaza, Suite 400, Hackensack, NJ 07601

Cath-Labs Corp. — 201-883-0008
282 Hudson St., Hackensack, NJ 07601

Elcam Medical, Inc. — 800-530-2441
2 University Plaza, suite 620, Hackensack, NJ 07601

Master Bond Inc. — 201-343-8983
154 Hobart Street, Hackensack, NJ 07601

Master Bond, Inc. — 201-343-8983
154 Hobart St., Hackensack, NJ 07601

Medical Measurements, Inc. — 201-489-9400
56 Linden St, Hackensack, NJ 07601

Regen Biologics, Inc. — 415-562-0800
411 Hackensack Ave., Hackensack, NJ 07601

Hackettstown

Rudolph Research Analytical — 973-584-1558
55 Newburgh Road, Hackettstown, NJ 07840

Hammonton

Integrity Medical Devices Inc — 609-567-8175
360 Fairview Ave., Hammonton, NJ 08037

Hasbrouck Heights

Flaghouse, Inc. — 800-793-7900
601 Flaghouse Dr., Hasbrouck Heights, NJ 07604-3316

Hawthorne

I.W. Tremont Co. — 973-427-3800
79 Fourth Ave., Hawthorne, NJ 07506

Xenopore Corp. — 800-356-6296
299 Wagaraw Rd., Hawthorne, NJ 07506

Hazlet

Aaeon Electronics, Inc. — 888-223-6687
3 Crown Plaza, Hazlet, NJ 07730-2441

Hightstown

Elementis Specialties — 800-866-6800
329 Wyckoffs Mill Road, Hightstown, NJ 08520

Hillsborough

American Medical Link, Inc. — 908-359-9328
5 Homestead Road, Bldg. 5, Units 1 & 2, Hillsborough, NJ 08844

Hillsdale

Harvey, R.J. Instrument Corp. — 201-664-1380
123 Patterson St., Hillsdale, NJ 07642

Hillside

Analytical Measurements, Inc. — 800-635-5580
100 Hoffman Place, Hillside, NJ 07205-1009

Hoboken

Eirsan Care Inc. — 201-880-8615
624 Monroe St., #2a, Hoboken, NJ 07030

Howell

Vynacron Dental Resins, Inc. — 732-780-6728
1751 Hwy. 9 N., Howell, NJ 07731

Irvington

Acme Of Precision Surgical Co., Inc. — 973-373-6797
485 South 21st St., Irvington, NJ 07111

Iselin

Siemens Medical — 732-590-5441
186 Wood Ave. S., 2nd Floor, Iselin, NJ 08830

Jamesburg

Invacare Supply Group — 440-329-6356
111 Interstate Blvd., Jamesburg, NJ 08831

Jersey City

Armin Poly-Version, Inc. — 201-451-0600
49 Fisk Street, Jersey City, NJ 07305

George Taub Products & Fusion Co., Inc. — 800-828-2634
277 New York Ave., Jersey City, NJ 07307-1501

Prosurge Instruments, Inc.
199 Laidlaw Avenue, Jersey City, NJ 07306-2511 — 866-832-7874

Kearny

L&R Manufacturing Co.
577 Elm St., PO Box 607, Kearny, NJ 07032-0607 — 201-991-5330

Keasbey

Princeton Laboratory Services, Llc
340 Mac Lane, Keasbey, NJ 08832 — 732-738-8108

Kenilworth

Cryofab, Inc.
540 N. Michigan Ave., Kenilworth, NJ 07033-1023 — 800-426-2186

White Systems, Inc.
30 Boright Avenue, Kenilworth, NJ 07033-1015 — 800-275-1442

Kenvil

Bulbworks, Inc.
Unit 5, 80 North Dell Avenue, Kenvil, NJ 07847 — 800-334-2852

Kinnelon

Life Recovery Systems Hd, Llc.
170 Kinnelon Road, Kinnelon, NJ 07405 — 973-283-2800

Qualityworx, Inc.
11 Valley Road, Kinnelon, NJ 07405-2313 — 877-825-4379

Lakewood

Atlantic Mills, Inc.
1295 Towbin Ave., Lakewood, NJ 08701 — 800-242-7374

Aviv Biomedical, Inc.
750 Vassar Avenue, Lakewood, NJ 08701-6907 — 732-370-1300

Chromodynamics
1195 Airport Road, # !, Lakewood, NJ 08701 — 732-730-1877

Medi-Hut Co., Inc.
1935 Swarthmore Avenue, Lakewood, NJ 08701-4541 — 800-882-0139

Mti Precision Products
175 Oberlin North Ave., Lakewood, NJ 08701 — 732-905-7440

Prosec Protection Systems, Inc.
1985 Swarthmore Ave., Suite 7, Lakewood, NJ 08701 — 732-886-0990

S.S. White Burs Inc.
1145 Towbin Ave., Lakewood, NJ 08701-5932 — 800-535-2877

Worthington Biochemical Corp.
730 Vasser Avenue, Lakewood, NJ 08701 — 800-445-9603

Landisville

Norell, Inc.
314 E. Arbor Avenue, P. O. Box 307, Landisville, NJ 08326 — 800-519-3688

Laurel Springs

Design & Evaluation, Inc.
1451-B Chews Landing Road, Laurel Springs, NJ 08021 — 856-228-3800

Lebanon

Hematechnologies, Inc.
291 Rte. 22, Suite 12, Lebanon, NJ 08833 — 877-436-2835

Ledgewood

Scantek Medical, Inc.
1705 Route 46 West, Unit 5, Ledgewood, NJ 07852 — 973-527-7100

Linden

Amerivac Usa Inc.
1207 Pennsylvania Ave., Linden, NJ 07036 — 877-851-6600

Little Falls

Cantel Medical Corp.
150 Clove Road, 9th Floor, Little Falls, NJ 07424 — 973-890-7220

Little Ferry

Edgeco
P.O. Box 338, Little Ferry, NJ 07643 — 800-833-4326

Krebs Instruments
195 Redneck Ave., Little Ferry, NJ 07643 — 201-871-6969

Little Silver

Endo Optiks, Inc.
39 Sycamore Avenue, Little Silver, NJ 07739 — 800-756-3636

International Hospital Products, Inc.
38 Winding Way, P.O. Box 158, Little Silver, NJ 07739-0158 — 732-842-1246

Livingston

EDIMS, LLC
651 West Mount Pleasant Avenue, Livingston, NJ 07039 — 800.626.4583

Franklin Miller Inc
60 Okner Pkwy., Livingston, NJ 07039-1604 — 800-932-0599

Milestone Scientific Inc.
220 South Orange Ave., Livingston, NJ 07039 — 800-862-1125

Lodi

Blickman
39 Robinson Road, Lodi, NJ 07644 — 800-247-5070

Jilson Group, Inc.
20 Industrial Road, Lodi, NJ 07644-2608 — 800-969-5400

Logan Township

American Bio Medica Corp.
603 Heron Dr., Unit 3, Logan Township, NJ 08085 — 800-227-1243

Madison

Quest Diagnostics, Inc.
3 Giralda Farms, Madison, NJ 07940 — 800-222-0446

Mahwah

Datascope Corp., Cardiac Assist Division
1300 Macarthur Blvd., Mahwah, NJ 07430 — 1 800 777 4222

Dobi Medical International, Inc.
1200 Macarthur Boulevard, Mahwah, NJ 07430 — 201-760-6464

Nobel Biocare Procera Llc.
800 Corporate Dr., Mahwah, NJ 07430 — 714-282-5074

Nobel Biocare Procera, Inc.
800 Corporate Drive, Mahwah, NJ 07410-2812 — 201-828-9268

Seiko Optical Products
575 Corporate Dr., Mahwah, NJ 07430-2330 — 201-529-9099

Stryker Howmedica Osteonics
325 Corporate Drive, Mahwah, NJ 07430 — 201-831-5000

Manasquan

Pl Custom Body & Equipment Co. Inc.
2201 Atlantic Ave., Manasquan, NJ 08736-1010 — 800-752-8786

Maplewood

Rubin & Poor, Inc.
155 Maplewood Ave, #5, Maplewood, NJ 07040 — 973-762-9009

Uniclean Cleanroom Garment Services
A UNIFIRST CO., 8 Hixon Pl, Maplewood, NJ 07040 — 877-544-4432

Marlton

Eastmed Enterprises, Inc.
11 Brandywine Drive, Marlton, NJ 08053-1101 — 856-797-0131

Mendham

Bio-Medical Products Corp.
10 Halstead Rd., Mendham, NJ 07945 — 800-543-7427

Fortrad Eye Instruments Corp.
8 Franklin Road, Mendham, NJ 07945 — 973-543-2371

Metuchen

Diagnostic Specialties
4 Leonard St., Metuchen, NJ 08840-1220 — 732-549-4011

Middlesex

E-Stat Plastics, Division Of Fram Trak Industries
205 Hallock Ave., Middlesex, NJ 08846 — 732-424-1600

Phillips Safety Products
123 Lincoln Blvd., Middlesex, NJ 08846 — 516-482-9001

Midland Park

George Glove Company, Inc.
301 Greenwood Avenue, Midland Park, NJ 07432 — 800-631-4292

Millburn

Lens Mode, Inc.
150 Main St., Millburn, NJ 07041-1114 — 800-852-5880

Millville

Friedrich & Dimmock, Inc.
2127 Wheaton Avenue, PO Box 230, Millville, NJ 08332 — 800-524-1131

Wheaton Science Products
1501 North 10th St., Millville, NJ 08332 — 800-225-1437

Mine Hill

Wire Cloth Manufacturers Inc.
110 Iron Mountain Road, Randolph Industrial Park, Mine Hill, NJ 07803 — 800-947-3626

Monmouth Junction

Princeton Biomeditech Corp.
4242 U.S. Hwy 1, Monmouth Junction, NJ 08852-1905 — 732-274-1000

TYRX, Inc.
1 Deer Park Dr., Suite G, Monmouth Junction, NJ 08852 — 866-908-8979

Montvale

Forsan Mfg.
30 Craig Rd., Montvale, NJ 07645 — 201-391-4100

Hamilton Bell Company
30 Craig Rd., Montvale, NJ 07645-1709 — 800-526-0864

Hansco Technologies, Inc.
17 Philips Pkwy., Montvale, NJ 07645-1810 — 201-391-0700

Kaypentax
3 Paragon Drive, Montvale, NJ 07645 — 800-289-5297

Pentax Medical Company
102 Chestnut Ridge Road, Montvale, NJ 07645-1856 — 800-431-5880

Moonachie

Bio Compression Systems, Inc.
120 W. Commercial Avenue, Moonachie, NJ 07074 — 800-888-0908

Crest Foam Industries
100 Carol Place, Moonachie, NJ 07074-1304 — 201-807-0809

Geri-Care Products | 201-440-0409
250 Moonachie Avenue, Moonachie, NJ 07074
J. Lamb, Inc. A Division Of The Strongwater Group | 888-379-6453
250 Moonachie Avenue, Moonachie, NJ 07074
Lps Industries, Inc. | 800-275-4577
10 Caesar Place, Moonachie, NJ 07074

Moorestown

Dencraft | 800-328-9729
PO Box 57, Moorestown, NJ 08057-0057
Denton Vacuum, Inc. | 856-439-9100
1259 North Church St., Moorestown, NJ 08057
Jerome Medical | 800-257-8440
305 Harper Drive, Moorestown, NJ 08057-3239
Omnimed, Inc. (Beam Products) | 800-257-2326
800 Glen Avenue, Moorestown, NJ 08057
Rtech, Inc. | 877-783-2446
739 Brandywine Drive, Moorestown, NJ 08057

Morganville

Cenogenics Corp. | 800-747-9457
100 Route 520, Drawer 308, Morganville, NJ 07751

Morris Plains

Caprock Developments Inc. | 800-222-0325
475 Speedwell Avenue, PO Box 95, Morris Plains, NJ 07950
Immunomedics, Inc. | 973-605-8200
300 American Road, Morris Plains, NJ 07950
Johnson & Johnson Consumer Products, Inc. | 908-874-1402
185 Tabor Road, Morris plains, NJ 07950
Johnson & Johnson Healthcare Products Div | 973-385-6546
Mcneil-Ppc, Inc.
185 Tabor Rd, Morris Plains, NJ 07950

Morristown

Bayer Healthcare Llc, Consumer Care | 717-866-2141
36 Columbia Rd., Morristown, NJ 07962
Dental Procedures, Inc. L.L.C. | 973-267-6195
9 Baer Court, Morristown, NJ 07960

Mount Holly

Arrow International, Inc. | 800-523-8446
2 Berry Dr, Mount Holly, NJ 08060

Mount Laurel

Acteon Inc. | 800-289-6367
124 Gaither Drive, Suite 140, Mount Laurel, NJ 08054
Mid-Atlantic Diagnostics Inc., Custom Products Div | 856-762-2000
77 Elbo Lane, Mount Laurel, NJ 08054
Special Gas Services Inc | 919-621-0980
PO Box 727, Mount Laurel, NJ 08054

Mountainside

Drg International, Inc. | 800-321-1167
1167 US Highway 22 E., Mountainside, NJ 07092-2807

Mt. Holly

Cho-Pat | 800-221-1601
Lippincott Lane, Unit 6, Mt. Holly Industrial Commons, Mt. Holly, NJ 08060
Specialities Electronics Co., Inc. | 609-267-5593
43 Washington St., Mt. Holly, NJ 08060

Mt. Laurel

Monarch Art Plastics, Llc. | 856-235-5151
3838 Church Road, Mt. Laurel, NJ 08054

Murray Hill

Boc Gases | 800-262-4273
575 Mountain Ave., Murray Hill, NJ 07974-2002
C. R. Bard, Inc. | 800-367-2273
730 Central Ave., Murray Hill, NJ 07974
Fablok Mills, Inc. | 908-464-1950
140 Spring St., Murray Hill, NJ 07974

Neptune

Biohit Inc. | 800-922-0784
3535 Rte. 66, Bldg. 4, PO Box 308,, Neptune, NJ 07754-0308
Contamination Control Products | 877-553-2676
1 Third Avenue, Box 578, Neptune, NJ 07753
Excelsior Medical Corp. | 800-487-4276
1933 Heck Ave., Neptune, NJ 07753

Neshanic Station

Westcon Orthopedics, Inc. | 800-382-4975
4 Craig Rd., Neshanic Station, NJ 08853

Netcong

RamÇ-Hart, Inc. | 973-448-0305
95 Allen Street, PO Box 400, Netcong, NJ 07857-0400

New Brunswick

Interferon Sciences, Inc. | 888-728-4372
783 Jersey Avenue, New Brunswick, NJ 08901

Johnson & Johnson | 800-526-2459
1 Johnson & Johnson Plaza, New Brunswick, NJ 08933
Nbs Medical Products Inc. | 888-800-8192
257 Livingston Ave., New Brunswick, NJ 08901
Richmond Diagnostics, Inc. | 732-246-2429
100 Jersey Ave., Suite 202-a,, Bldg. B, New Brunswick, NJ 08901
Songbird Hearing, Inc. | 732-828-8300
303 George St., Suite 307, New Brunswick, NJ 08901

New Providence

Baxter Healthcare Corporation, Baxter | 800-667-0959
Pharmaceuticals And Technologies
95 Spring St., New Providence, NJ 07974
Svelte Medical Systems Inc. | 908-264-2194
675 Central Avenue, Suite 2, New Providence, NJ 07974

Newark

Accurate Set, Inc. | 973-824-0810
1199 Broad St., Newark, NJ 07114-1834
Pharmaceutical Innovations, Inc. | 973-242-2900
897 Frelinghuysen Ave., Newark, NJ 07114-2122
Urovalve Inc. | 973-596-1350
211 Warren St., Newark, NJ 07103

North Bergen

Danara Intl. Ltd. | 800-526-7048
8101 Tonnelle Ave., North Bergen, NJ 07047

North Branch

American Spraytech, L.L.C. | 908-725-6060
205 Meister Ave., North Branch, NJ 08876

North Brunswick

Artegraft, Inc. | 800-631-5264
220 N. Center Drive, North Brunswick, NJ 08902

Northvale

Adm Tronics Unlimited, Inc. | 201-767-6040
224 Pegasus Avenue, Northvale, NJ 07647-1908
American Gas & Chemical Co., Ltd. | 800-288-3647
220 Pegasus Ave., Northvale, NJ 07647-1904
Bipore, Inc. | 201-767-1993
31 Industrial Pkwy., Northvale, NJ 07647
Gea Westfalia Separator, Inc. | 201-767-3900
100 Fairway Court, Northvale, NJ 07647
Hausmann Industries, Inc. | 888-428-7626
130 Union St., Northvale, NJ 07647-2207
Kmedic | 800-955-0559
190 Veterans Drive, Northvale, NJ 07647
S&W By Hausmann | 888-428-7626
130 Union Street, Northvale, NJ 07647

Norwood

Kramer Scientific Laboratory Products Corp. | 201-767-8505
50 Maple St., Norwood, NJ 07648

Oakland

Collagen Matrix, Inc. | 888-405-1001
15 Thornton Road, Oakland, NJ 07436
Eric Armin Inc. | 800-272-0272
118 Bauer Drive, PO Box 7046, Oakland, NJ 07436

Ocean

Immunostics, Inc. | 800-722-7505
3505 Sunset Avenue, Ocean, NJ 07712

Orange

Peace Medical | 800-537-9564
50 S. Center St., Unit 11, Orange, NJ 07050-3587
Peace Medical, Inc. | 800-537-9564
50 South Center St., Unit 11, Orange, NJ 07050

Paramus

Globe Scientific, Inc. | 800-394-4562
610 Winters Ave., Paramus, NJ 07653-1625
Nbs Technologies Inc. | 800-524-0419
70 Eisenhower Drive, Paramus, NJ 07652
Nubenco Ent., Inc. | 800-633-1322
One Kalisa Way, Ste. 207, Paramus, NJ 07652
Topcon Medical Systems, Inc. | 800-223-1130
37 West Century Road, Paramus, NJ 07652-1408

Park Ridge

Sony Electronics, Inc., Medical Systems Div. | 800-686-7669
One Sony Drive, Park Ridge, NJ 07656

Parsippany

Croll Reynolds Company, Inc. | 908-232-4200
Six Campus Drive, Parsippany, NJ 07054
Custom Spine Inc | 973-808-0019
1140 Parsippany Boulevard, Suite #201, Parsippany, NJ 07054
Diagnostica Stago, Inc. | 800-222-COAG
5 Century Drive, Parsippany, NJ 07054

Dosimeter Division Of Arrow Tech Inc — 800-322-8258
5 Eastmans Road, Parsippany, NJ 07054
Ebi, Llc — 800-526-2579
100 Interpace Pky., Parsippany, NJ 07054
Health Learning Systems, Inc. — 800-388-1000
402 Interpace Parkway, Wayne Interchange Plaza II, Parsippany, NJ 07454
Mcneil-Ppc, Inc. — 908-874-1402
100 Jefferson Rd., Parsippany, NJ 07054
Respironics New Jersey, Inc. — 800-804-3443
5 Wood Hollow Road, Parsippany, NJ 07054-1104
Safilo Usa — 973-952-2800
801 Jefferson Rd., Parsippany, NJ 07054
Tronex Healthcare Industries — 800-833-1181
One Tronex Centre, 2 Cranberry Road, Parsippany, NJ 07054
Zimmer Trabecular Metal Technology — 800-613-6131
10 Pomeroy Road, Parsippany, NJ 07054

Passaic

Medin Corporation — 800-922-0476
90 Dayton Avenue, Bldg. 16 C, Passaic, NJ 07055
Mwt Materials, Inc. — 973-472-5161
90 Dayton Ave., Suite 6 E, Passaic, NJ 07055

Paterson

American Comb Corp. — 973-523-6551
22 Kentucky Ave., Paterson, NJ 07503
Ameriderm Laboratories, Ltd. — 973-279-5100
13 Kentucky Avenue, Paterson, NJ 07503
Bio-Med U.S.A. Inc. — 973-278-5222
111 Ellison Street, Paterson, NJ 07505
Cygnus Inc. — 973-523-0668
510 E. 41st. St., Paterson, NJ 07504
Gomez Packaging Corp. — 973-569-9500
75 Wood St., Paterson, NJ 07524
L.J. Greiner & Sons, Inc. — 973-977-9441
63-69 Danforth Avenue, Paterson, NJ 07501
Organics Corporation Of America — 973-890-9002
55 West End Road, Paterson, NJ 07512
Ppi-Time Zero Inc. — 973-278-6500
262 Buffalo Ave., Paterson, NJ 07503
7n Gabriela Naydenov;, Inc. — 973-278-0866
503 East 40th Street, Paterson, NJ 07504

Paulsboro

Ossur Americas — 800-257-8440
1414 Metropolitan Avenue, Paulsboro, NJ 08066

Pennington

Medical Indicators, Inc. — 609-737-1600
1589 Reed Rd., Pennington, NJ 08534

Pennsauken

Cetylite Industries, Inc. — 800-257-7740
9051 River Rd., Pennsauken, NJ 08110
Helvoet Pharma, Inc. — 856-663-2202
9012 Pennsauken Hwy., Pennsauken, NJ 08110
Mediq/Prn — 800-222-4776
1 Mediq Plaza, Pennsauken, NJ 08110

Phillipsburg

Avantor Performance Materials — 800-243-3768
222 Red School Lane, Phillipsburg, NJ 08865
Azog, Inc. — 908-213-2900
1011 Us Hwy 22, Bldg. D Unit 4, BOX 6, Phillipsburg, NJ 08865
Engineered Medical Solutions Co. Llc. — 908-213-9001
85 Industrial Dr., Building B, Phillipsburg, NJ 08865

Pine Brook

Diopsys Inc. — 973-244-0622
16 Chapin Road, Suite 912, Pine Brook, NJ 07058
Modular Packaging System, Inc. — 973-882-0633
45 Rte. 46, Pine Brook, NJ 07058

Piscataway

Exogen, Inc. — 800-836-0849
10 Constitution Ave., Piscataway, NJ 08855
Innopharma LLC — 732-885-2939
10 Knightsbridge Road, Piscataway, NJ 08854
Shukla Medical — 888-474-8552)
151 Old New Brunswick Rd, Piscataway, NJ 08854
Siemens Hearing Instruments, Inc. — 800-766-4500
10 Constitution Avenue, P.O. Box 1397, Piscataway, NJ 08855
Whatman Inc. — 732-885-6529
Building One, 800 Centenial Avenue, Piscataway, NJ 08854

Plainsboro

Canada Microsurgical Ltd. — 1-800-263-6693
311 Enterprise Drive, Plainsboro, NJ 08536
Ese Acquisition Llc. — 609-716-0600
666 Plainsboro Rd. Suite 1271, Plainsboro, NJ 08536
INTEGRA LIFE — 1-800-654-2873
311 Enterprise Drive, Plainsboro, NJ 08536
Integra Lifesciences Corp. — 609-275-0500
311 Enterprise Drive, Plainsboro, NJ 08536

Integra Lifesciences Corporation — 800-654-2873
311 Enterprise Drive, Plainsboro, NJ 08536
Integra Lifesciences Holdings Corp. — 800-654-2873
311 Enterprise Drive, Plainsboro, NJ 08536-3339
Medicus Technologies — 800-762-1574
105 Morgan Lane, Plainsboro, NJ 08536

Point Pleasant

Posture Dynamics, Inc. — 732-278-2081
415 Jarob Court, Point Pleasant, NJ 08742

Pompton Lakes

Cranial Solutions — 973-835-7929
602 Lincoln Ave., Pompton Lakes, NJ 07442

Princeton

Bristol-Myers Group Company — 800-332-2056
P.O. Box 4500, Princeton, NJ 08543
Covance Inc. — 888-268-2623
210 Carnegie Center, Princeton, NJ 08540
Cytogen Corp. — 800-833-3533
600 College Road E., Suite 3100, Princeton, NJ 08540
Derma Sciences — 609-514-4744
214 Carnegie Center, Suite 300, Princeton, NJ 08540
Edda Technology, Inc. — 609-919-9889
5 Independence Way, Suite 210, Princeton, NJ 08540
Inverness Medical — 800-257-9525
2 Research Way, Princeton, NJ 08540
Lingraphicare America, Inc. — 888-274-2742
103 Carnegie Center, Suite 204, Princeton, NJ 08540
Miele Professional Products Group — 800-843-7231
9 Independence Way, Princeton, NJ 08540
Novo Nordisk Pharmaceuticals, Inc. — 800-727-6500
100 College Road West, Princeton, NJ 08540-7810
Stentys Inc. — 609-853-0100
103 Carnegie Center, Princeton, NJ 08540
Wampole Laboratories — 800-257-9525
2 Research Way, Princeton, NJ 08540
Western Medical, Ltd. — 800-628-8276
214 Carnegie Center Suite 100, Princeton, NJ 08540

Princeton Junction

Linseis, Inc. — 800-732-6733
PO Box 666, Princeton Junction, NJ 08550-0666
Lutronic Inc. — 888-588-7644
51 Everett Dr., Unit A 50, Unit A-50, Princeton Junction, NJ 08550

Rahway

Lm Air Technology, Inc. — 866-381-8200
1467 Pinewood St., Rahway, NJ 07065-5697
Wytech Industries, Inc. — 732-396-3900
960 E. Hazelwood Ave., Rahway, NJ 07065-5503

Ramsey

Bogen Communications International, Inc. — 800-999-2809
50 Spring St., Ramsey, NJ 07446-2810
Capintec, Inc. — 800-631-3826
6 Arrow Road, Ramsey, NJ 07446-1205
Konica Minolta Sensing Americas, Inc. — 888-473-2656
101 Williams Dr., Ramsey, NJ 07446
3g Ultrasound, Inc. — 201-825-3116
200 Williams Dr., Ramsey, NJ 07446

Randolph

Landice, Inc. — 800-LANDICE
111 Canfield Ave., Suite A1, Randolph, NJ 07869

Raritan

Ortho-Clinical Diagnostics, Inc. — 908-218-8177
Route 202, Raritan, NJ 08869
Ortho-Mcneil-Janssen Pharmaceuticals, Inc. — 800-526-7736
1000 U.S. Route 202 South, Raritan, NJ 08869
Therakos, Inc., A Johnson & Johnson Company — 877-865-6850
1001 US Route 202, Raritan, NJ 08869-0606
Veridex, Llc — 877-837-4339
1001 US Highway Route 202 N., Raritan, NJ 08869
Veridex, Llc — (877-837-4339)
1001 US Highway Route 202 North, Raritan, NJ 08869
Zeus Scientific, Inc. — 800-286-2111
PO Box 38, Raritan, NJ 08869-0038

Red Bank

Ansell Healthcare Products, Inc. — 732-345-5400
200 Schulz Dr., Red Bank, NJ 07701
Ansell Healthcare, Inc. — 800-952-9916
200 Schulz Drive, Red Bank, NJ 07701
Ansell Protective Products — 800-800-0444
200 Schultz Drive, Red Bank, NJ 07701

Ridgefield

Case Medical, Inc. — 888-227-2273
65 Railroad Avenue, Ridgefield, NJ 07657
General Devices — 201-313-7075
1000 River St., Ridgefield, NJ 07657

Genzyme Corporation — 617-252-7500
1125 Pleasantview Terrace, Ridgefield, NJ 07657-2397

Ridgefield Park

Agfa Corp. — 800-581-2432
100 Challenger Rd., Ridgefield Park, NJ 07660-2105

Ringoes

Medical Packaging Inc. — 800-257-5282
470 Rte. 31, PO Box 500, Ringoes, NJ 08551-1409
Scientific Instrument Services, Inc. — 908-788-5550
1027 Old York Road, Ringoes, NJ 08551
Unique/Pereny — 800-HED-KILN
P.O. Box 246, 449 Route 31, Ringoes, NJ 08551-0246

Ringwood

Kenyon Industries, Inc. — 973-962-4844
235 Margaret King Ave., Ringwood, NJ 07456

River Vale

Aragona Medical, Inc. — 201-664-8822
184 Rivervale Rd., River Vale, NJ 07675

Rivers Edge

Nephros, Inc. — 201-343-5202
41 Grand Ave., Suite 200, Rivers Edge, NJ 07661

Riverside

Auradonics Incorporated — 856-764-8866
439 St. Mihiel Dr., Riverside, NJ 08075
Mckesson Drug Co. — 856-461-7800
400 Delray Pkwy., Riverside, NJ 08075

Rochelle Park

Redfield Corp. — 800-678-4472
336 West Passaic St, Rochelle Park, NJ 07662

Rochester

Ortho-Clinical Diagnostics, Inc. — 800-828-6316
513 Technology Blvd., Rochester, NJ 14626

Rockaway

Adit/Electron Tubes — 800-521-8382
100 Forge Way, Unit F, Rockaway, NJ 07866
Biotest Diagnostic Corp. — 800-522-0090
400 Commons Way, Rockaway, NJ 07866
Higgs Medical Products, Llc — 973-625-4424
21 Pine St., Suite 109, Rockaway, NJ 07866
LinkBio Corp. — 800-932-0616
300 Roundhill Dr, Rockaway, NJ 07866
Precision Assembly Corporation — 973-664-9889
198 Green Pond Road, Rockaway, NJ 07866

Saddle Brook

Beacon Converters, Inc. — 201-797-2600
Bldg. P-1 Andrea Blvd., Saddle Brook, NJ 07663-8208
CircuLite — 201-543-2430
250 Pehle Avenue, Park 80 West, Suite 403, Saddle Brook, NJ 07663
Meese Orbitron Dunne Co. — 800-829-3230
535 N. Midland Ave., Saddle Brook, NJ 07663-5521

Scotch Plains

Blake Industries, Inc. — 908-233-7240
660 Jerusalem Road, Scotch Plains, NJ 07076-2028
Cme Medical Equipment Corp. — 908-561-0906
1130 Donamy Glen, Scotch Plains, NJ 07076-2403

Secaucus

Dazian Fabrics,Llc. — 877-232-9426
124 Enterprise Ave South, PO Box 2121, Secaucus, NJ 07094-0000
Maximum Dental, Inc. — 631-245-2176
600 Meadowlands Parkway, Suite 269, Secaucus, NJ 07094

Sewell

Electric Mobility Corporation — 800-718-2082
591Mantua Blvd., PO Box 450, Sewell, NJ 08080
Hollywood Tanning Systems, Inc. — 856-914-9090
11 Enterprise Ct., Sewell, NJ 08080

Shrewsbury

Angel Medical Systems — 800-763-5099
1163 Shrewsbury Avenue, Suite E, Shrewsbury, NJ 07702

Skillman

Convatec Professional Services — 800-422-8811
100 Headquarters Park Dr., Skillman, NJ 08558
J&J Healthcare Products Div Mcneil-Ppc, Inc — 866-565-2229
199 Grandview Rd, Skillman, NJ 08558
Johnson & Johnson Consumer Products, Inc. — 800-526-3967
199 Grandview Rd., Skillman, NJ 08558-9417

Somerset

Access Bio Incorporate — 732-873-4040
65 Clyde Rd., Suite A, Somerset, NJ 08873

Juvent Inc. — 732-748-8866
300 Atrium Drive, Somerset, NJ 08873
Lifesign — 800-526-2125
71 Veronica Avenue, Somerset, NJ 08873
Light Age Inc. — 732-563-0600
500 Apgar Drive, Somerset, NJ 08873
Micro Stamping Corp. — 513-573-0085
140 Belmont Dr., Somerset, NJ 08873
Oticon, Inc. — 800-526-3921
29 Schoolhouse Rd., Somerset, NJ 08873-1212
Pacon Manufacturing Corporation — 732-357-8020
400 B Pierce Street, Somerset, NJ 08873
Philips Lighting Co. — 800-555-0050
200 Franklin Square Drive, Somerset, NJ 08875-6800
Takara Belmont Usa, Inc. — 800-223-1192
101 Belmont Dr., Somerset, NJ 08873
Terumo Medical Corp. — 800-283-7866
2101 Cottontail Lane, Somerset, NJ 08873

Somerville

Ethicon, Inc. — 800-4-ETHICON
Route 22 West, p.o. box 151, Somerville, NJ 08876

South Amboy

Q-Med, Inc. — 732-544-5544
100 Metro Park S., 3rd Fl., South Amboy, NJ 08878

South Hackensack

Essential Dental Systems, Inc. — 800-223-5394
89 Leuning St., South Hackensack, NJ 07606

South Iselin

Siemens Credit Corp. — 800-327-4443
170 Wood Avenue, South Iselin, NJ 08830

South Plainfield

Advanced Diagnostics, Inc. (Adi) — 800-724-4003
801 Montrose Avenue, South Plainfield, NJ 07080
Innovative Disposables — 908-222-7111
3611 Kennedy Rd., South Plainfield, NJ 07080
J & H Berge, Inc. — 800-684-1234
4111 S. Clinton Avenue, South Plainfield, NJ 07080
Just Packaging Inc. — 908-753-6700
450 Oak Tree Ave., South Plainfield, NJ 07080
Medicos Laboratories, Inc. (Mdt) — 800-724-4003
801 Montrose Avenue, South Plainfield, NJ 07080
Medtech Group Inc., The — 800-348-2759
6 Century Road, South Plainfield, NJ 07080
Pfingst & Company, Inc. — 908-561-6400
105 Snyder, South Plainfield, NJ 07080-1915
Ronpak, Inc. — 732-968-8000
4301 New Brunswick Avenue, South Plainfield, NJ 07080-1291
Vention Medical — 908-561-0717
6 Century Road, South Plainfield, NJ 07080

Sparta

Testo, Inc. — 800-227-0729
40 White Lake Road, Sparta, NJ 07871

Springfield

Analyticon Instruments Corp. — 973-379-6771
99 Morrison Ave, P.O. Box 92, Springfield, NJ 07081
Hudson Control Group, Inc. — 973-376-7400
10 Stern Ave., Springfield, NJ 07081

Teaneck

Aetrex Worldwide, Inc — 800-526-2739
414 Alfred Avenue, Teaneck, NJ 07666
D.M. Davis Inc. — 201-833-0513
460 Warwick Ave., PO Box 536, Teaneck, NJ 07666

Tenafly

D. Y. Instrument, Inc. — 516-482-9001
59 Westervelt Avenue, Tenafly, NJ 07670

Thorofare

Akers Biosciences, Inc. — 800-451-8378
201 Grove Road, Thorofare, NJ 08086
Troemner Llc — 800-352-7705
201 Wolf Drive, PO Box 87, Thorofare, NJ 08086-0087

Tinton Falls

Pausch Llc — 732-747-6110
808 Shrewsbury Ave., Tinton Falls, NJ 07724
Summit Hill Laboratories — 800-922-0722
1 Sheila Dr, Tinton Falls, NJ 07724

Titusville

Capitol Management Consulting, Inc. — 609-737-9963
30 Pleasant Valley Harbourton, Titusville, NJ 08560-2101
Ortho Mcneil Janssen Pharmaceuticals, Inc. — 800-526-7736
1125 Trenton-Harbourton Road, P.O. Box 200, Titusville, NJ 08560

Toms River

Misc Inc.
1889-97 Route 9, Toms River, NJ 08755 — 800-524-1155

Perma Pure Llc
8 Executive Drive, Toms River, NJ 08755 — 800-337-3762

Totowa

Access Llc
11 West End Rd., Totowa, NJ 07512 — 800-973-0355

Thales Components Corporation
40G Commerce Way, PO Box 540, Totowa, NJ 07511-0540 — 973-812-9000

Vital Signs, Inc.
20 Campus Road, Totowa, NJ 07512 — 800-932-0760

Towaco

Uhlmann Packaging Systems, Inc.
44 Indian Lane E., Towaco, NJ 07082-1032 — 973-402-8855

Trenton

Crest Ultrasonics Corp.
P.O. Box 7266, Scotch Road, Trenton, NJ 08628 — 800-992-7378

Cytotherm
110 Sewell Ave., Trenton, NJ 08610-6059 — 800-747-9699

Medical Accessories, Inc.
92 Youngs Rd., Trenton, NJ 08619-1013 — 800-275-1624

Trans-Atlantic Dental
46 Arctic Pkwy., Trenton, NJ 08638-3041 — 609-695-0168

Union

Princeton Case Co., Inc.
667 Lehigh Ave., Union, NJ 07083 — 908-687-1750

Shelhigh, Inc.
650 Liberty Ave., Union, NJ 07083 — 908-206-8706

Yama, Inc.
650 Liberty Ave., Union, NJ 07083 — 908-206-8706

Upper Montclair

Meylan Corporation
543 Valley Road, Upper Montclair, NJ 07043-1844 — 888-769-9667

Verona

Atlantic Medco, Inc.
166 Bloomfield Avenue, Verona, NJ 07044 — 800-203-8444

Vineland

Bellco Glass, Inc.
340 Edrudo Rd., Vineland, NJ 08360 — 800-257-7043

J. G. Finneran Associates, Inc.
3600 Reilly Ct., Vineland, NJ 08360 — 800-552-3696

Kimble Glass, Inc.
537 Crystal Avenue, Vineland, NJ 08360-3200 — 888-546-2531

Kontes Glass Co.
1022 Spruce St., Vineland, NJ 08360-2841 — 888-546-2531

Vineland Syrup Inc.
PO Box 1326, Vineland, NJ 08360 — 800-642-9124

Wall Township

The Lifestyle Co. Inc.
1800 Route 34 North, Suite 401, Wall Township, NJ 07719 — 800-622-0777

Wallington

Brenner Metal Products
16 Main Ave., Wallington, NJ 07057 — (973) 778-0084.

Warren

Cordis Endovascular
7 Powder Horn Drive, Warren, NJ 07059 — 877-338-4235

Washington

Mci Optonix, Div. Of Usr Optonix Inc.
253 E Washington avenue, Washington, NJ 07882 — 800-678-6649

Watchung

Comfort Technologies, Inc.
381 Mountain Blvd., Watchung, NJ 07069 — 800-321-7846

Wayne

Derma-Safe Company
32 Juniper Road, Wayne, NJ 07470-6156 — 973-839-6383

Fujinon, Inc.
10 High Point Dr., Wayne, NJ 07470-7434 — 800-385-4666

JVC Americas Corp.
1700 Valley Rd., Wayne, NJ 07470 — 973-315-5000

Konica Minolta Medical Imaging Usa, Inc.
411 Newark Pompton Tpke., Wayne, NJ 07470 — 800-934-1034

Laboratory Disposable Products
PO Box 2239, Wayne, NJ 07474-2239 — 973-335-2966

Maddak Inc.
661 Route 23 South, Wayne, NJ 07470 — 800-443-4926

Maquet Cardiovascular LLC
45 Barbour Pond Dr., Wayne, NJ 07470 — 888-880-2874

Maquet, Inc.
45 Barbour Pond Drive, Wayne, NJ 07470 — 1-888-MAQUET3

West Berlin

Dynasil Corporation of America
385 Cooper Road, West Berlin, NJ 08091 — 856-767-4600

Es Industries
701 South Route 73, West Berlin, NJ 08091 — 800-356-6140

Healer Products, Llc
427 Commerce Lane, Unit 1, West Berlin, NJ 08091 — 914-663-6300

West Caldwell

Alfa Wassermann, Inc.
4 Henderson Drive, West Caldwell, NJ 07006 — 800-220-4488

Impact Instrumentation, Inc.
27 Fairfield Place, West Caldwell, NJ 07006-6206 — 800-969-0750

Kaulson Laboratories, Inc.
693 Bloomfield Ave., West Caldwell, NJ 07006 — 973-226-9494

West Deptford

Astral Diagnostics, Inc.
1224 Forest Pkwy., West Deptford, NJ 08066 — 856-224-0900

West Trenton

Neumed Inc.
800 Silvia Street, West Trenton, NJ 08628 — 800-367-1238

Westfield

Handler Manufacturing Co.
612 N. Avenue E., Westfield, NJ 07090-0520 — 800-274-2635

Wharton

Unette Corporation
88 N. Main St., Wharton, NJ 07885-1600 — 973-328-6800

Whippany

Gel Concepts Llc.
30 Leslie Court, Whippany, NJ 07981 — 973-884-8995

Gelsmart Llc
30 Leslie Ct., Suite B-202, Whippany, NJ 07981 — 973-884-8995

Polygell Llc.
30 Leslie Ct., Whippany, NJ 07981 — 973-884-8995

Steris Isomedix Services
9 Apollo Drive, Whippany, NJ 07981-1423 — 973-887-2754

Williamstown

Tetra Computer Systems, Llc
328 Bryn Mawr Drive, Williamstown, NJ 08094 — 856-728-6835

Windsor

Pyrometer Instrument Co.
92 North Main Street Bldg 18D, Windsor, NJ 08561-0479 — 800-468-7976

Wood Ridge

Fabrite Laminating Corp.
70 Passaic St., Wood Ridge, NJ 07075-1004 — 973-777-1406

Woodbridge

Labnet International
P.O. Box 841, Woodbridge, NJ 07095-0841 — 888-522-6381

NEW MEXICO

Albuquerque

Albuquerque Eye Prosthetics, Inc.
4117 Montgomery N.e., Albuquerque, NM 87109 — 505-884-2927

Amo Wavefront Sciences Llc
14820 Central Ave. S.e., Albuquerque, NM 87123 — 714-247-8656

Basic Dental Implant Systems, Inc.
3321 Columbia, N.E., Albuquerque, NM 87107-2001 — 505-884-1922

Biomoda Inc.
609 Broadway NE, Albuquerque, NM 87102 — 505-821-0875

Chase Ergonomics, Inc.
5921 Midway Park Blvd NE, Albuquerque, NM 87109 — 800-621-5436

Danlin Products, Inc.
3321 Columbia, N.E., Albuquerque, NM 87107-2001 — 505-884-1922

Eberline Services
7021 Pan American Hwy. N.E., Albuquerque, NM 87109-4238 — 877-477-898

Ethicon Endo-Surgery, Inc.
3801 University Blvd., S.E., Albuquerque, NM 87106 — 877-384-4266

Heartbeat Medical Corp.
8917 Adams St., N.e., Albuquerque, NM 87113 — 505-823-1990

Lase-R Shield, A Bacou-Dalloz Company
7011 Prospect Pl. NE, Albuquerque, NM 87110 — 800-288-1164

Marpac Inc.
8430 Washington Place NE, Albuquerque, NM 87113 — 800-334-6413

Matheson Tri-Gas, Inc.
8200 Washington N.E., Albuquerque, NM 87113 — 972-893-5600

Med-Aesthetic Solutions, Inc.
6808 Academy Pkwy., East N.e., Bldg. A Suite 1, Albuquerque, NM 87109 — 505-341-2577

OCO Biomedical
8500 Washington St. NE., Suite A-1, Albuquerque, NM 87113 — 800-228-0477

Richmond Products, Inc.
4400 Silver Se, Albuquerque, NM 87108 — 505-275-2406

Tempur Production Usa, Inc.
12907 Tempurpedic Parkway, Albuquerque, NM 87121 — 276-431-7174

TruTouch Technology Inc.   866-721-6221
317 Commercial St NE, Suite 112, Albuquerque, NM 87102
VeraLight INC   (505) 272-7023
800 Bradbury SE, Suite 217, Albuquerque, NM 87106

Clovis
Cal Hush Llc   505-763-0770
108 Calle De Oro, Clovis, NM 88101

Los Alamos
Pulse Systems, Inc.   505-662-7599
422 Connie Ave., Los Alamos, NM 87544

Los Lunas
Doh,Ddsd,Csb   505-841-5287
1000 Main St., Nw, P.o. Box 1269, Los Lunas, NM 87031

Santa Fe
Millennium Medical Technologies, Inc.   505-988-7595
460 St. Michael's Dr., #901, Santa Fe, NM 87505
S.C.I. Science Center, Inc.   800-345-0774
PO Box 994, Santa Fe, NM 87505

NEW YORK

Airmont
Rockland Technimed Limited Rtl   845-426-1136
3 Larissa Court, Airmont, NY 10952-3833

Albany
Capro Solutions, Llc   518-456-1145
8 Corporate Cir., Karner Park, Albany, NY 12203
Cmp Industries Llc   800-888-5868
413 N. Pearl St., Albany, NY 12201
National Graphic Supply   800-223-7130
226 N. Allen St., Albany, NY 12206
Ticonium Co.   800-833-2343
413 North Pearl Street, Albany, NY 12201

Albertson
Breathe With Eez Corp.   800-826-7077
PO Box 37, Albertson, NY 11507

Alden
Alden Optical Labs, Inc.   716-937-9181
13295 Broadway, Alden, NY 14004-1324
Bennett Manufacturing Co., Inc.   800-345-2142
13315 Railroad St., Alden, NY 14004-1330

Amherst
Columbus Mckinnon Corp., Mobility Products Div.   800-888-0985
140 John James Audubon Pkwy, Amherst, Amherst, NY 14228-1197
Ivoclar Vivadent, Inc.   800-533-6825
175 Pineview Drive, Amherst, NY 14228-2231
Kistler Instrument Corp.   716-691-5100
75 John Glenn Drive, Amherst, NY 14228-2171
Medtek Devices, Inc.   716-835-7000
595 Commerce Dr., 155 Pineview Dr., Amherst, NY 14228
Renaissance Plastics Co., The   716-426-2078
155 Pineview Dr., Amherst, NY 14228

Amityville
C.A.M. Graphics Co., Inc.   516-842-3400
166 New Highway, Amityville, NY 11701
Hart Specialties, Inc.   800-221-6966
5000 New Horizons Blvd., Amityville, NY 11701
Star X-Ray Co., Inc.   800-374-2163
63 Ranick Dr., Amityville, NY 11701-2821

Amsterdam
Liberty Enterprises   518-842-5080
43 Liberty Dr, Amsterdam, NY 12010

Aquebogue
Altaire Pharmaceuticals, Inc.   631-722-5988
311 West Ln., Aquebogue, NY 11931

Argyle
Covidien Lp, Formerly Registered As Kendall   800-962-9888
5439 State Rte. 40, Argyle, NY 12809

Armonk
Heraeus Kulzer, Inc.   800-431-1785
99 Business Park Drive, Armonk, NY 10504-1720
Surgical Design Corp.   914-273-2445
3 Macdonald Ave., Armonk, NY 10504

Auburn
Schott North America, Inc.   315-255-2791
62 Columbus Street, Auburn, NY 13021-3137
Volpi Manufacturing Usa Co., Inc.   315-255-1737
5 Commerce Way, Auburn, NY 13021-1045

Baldwin
Disposable Surgical Innovations   516-377-1497
958 Church Street, Baldwin, NY 11510
Elliquence Llc   (516) 277-9000
2455 Grand Avenue, Baldwin, NY 11510

Batavia
P. W. Minor   585-815-0659
3 Treadeasy Avenue, Batavia, NY 14020
Prime Materials Corp.   877-755-1649
6 Treadeasy Avenue, PO Box 71, Batavia, NY 14021-0071

Bay Shore
Bay Shore Medical Equipment Corp.   631-586-1991
235 South Fehr Way, Bay Shore, NY 11706
Harbor Metalcrafters, Inc./Medpro   631-242-2428
208 Fehr Way, Bay Shore, NY 11706
Poly Scientific R&D Corp.   800-645-5825
70 Cleveland Ave., Bay Shore, NY 11706-1224
Precise Optics/Pme, Inc.   800-242-6604
239 S. Fehr Way, Bay Shore, NY 11706-1207

Bedford Hills
Universal Ultrasound   800-842-0607
299 Adams Street, Bedford Hills, NY 10507

Bellmore
Ancare Corp.   800-645-6379
2647 Grand Avenue, PO BOX 814, Bellmore, NY 11710
Arnel Healthcare, Inc.   516-783-1939
1523 Dewey Ave., Bellmore, NY 11710
Global Dental Products   516-221-8844
PO Box 537, Bellmore, NY 11710

Binghamton
Best Value Ceramics   607-723-2803
19 Chenango St., Binghamton, NY 13901
Craftsmen/Access Unlimited   800-849-2143
570 Hance Rd., Binghamton, NY 13903
Medsim-Eagle Simulation Inc.   607-779-6000
151 Court St., Binghamton, NY 13901
Southern Tier Plastics, Inc.   607-723-2601
94 Industrial Park, P.O. Box 2015, Binghamton, NY 13902

Blauvelt
Swivelier Co., Inc.   845-353-1455
600 Bradley Hill Rd., Blauvelt, NY 10913-1187

Bloomingburg
Vespo Marketing Assoc., Inc.   800-49-VESPO
9 Dogwood Drive, P.O. Box 60, Bloomingburg, NY 12721

Bohemia
Advanced Biophotonics Inc.   631-244-8244
125 Wilbur Place, Ste. 120, Bohemia, NY 11716
Climatronics Corp.   631-567-7300
140 Wilbur Place, Bohemia, NY 11716
Dentsply Gac International   800-645-5530
355 Knickerbockers Ave., Bohemia, NY 11716
Denver Instrument Company   800-321-1135
5 Orville Dr., Bohemia, NY 11716
Eele Laboratories, Llc   631-244-0051
50 Orville Drive, Bohemia, NY 11716
Kipp & Zonen   631-589-2065
125 Wilbur Place, Bohemia, NY 11716
Koehler Instrument Co., Inc.   800-878-9070
1595 Sycamore Avenue, Bohemia, NY 11716-1732
Lamp Technology, Inc.   800-533-7548
1645 Sycamore Avenue, Bohemia, NY 11716-1729
Lord Custom Molded Shoes, Inc.   631-471-3090
1395-1 Lakeland Ave., Bohemia, NY 11716
Precision Charts, Inc.   800-645-5410
130 Wilbur Place, Dept. P.C., Bohemia, NY 11716
Scientific Industries, Inc.   888-850-6208
70 Orville Drive, Bohemia, NY 11716-2512
Senecare Enterprises, Inc.   800-442-4577
350 A Central Ave., Bohemia, NY 11716
Silverstone Packaging, Inc.-Your One Stop Supplier   800-413-1108
1401 Lakeland Avenue, Bohemia, NY 11716
Source-Ray, Inc.   631-244-8200
167 Keyland Ct., Bohemia, NY 11716
Thompson Contract Inc.   631-589-7337
41 Keyland Court, Bohemia, NY 11716

Brentwood
Gmz Associates, Ltd.   800-581-5088
86 Cain Drive, Brentwood, NY 11717
Medical Action Industries, Inc   800-645-7042
500 Expressway Drive South, Brentwood, NY 11717

Brewster
Endoscopy Support Services, Inc.   800-349-3636
3 Fallsview Lane, Brewster, NY 10509

Iquire, Llc
2 Fallsview Lane, Brewster, NY 10509 — 845-277-1846

Pedifix, Inc.
310 Guinea Road, Brewster, NY 10509 — 800-424-5561

Putnam Precision Products
3859 Danbury Road, Brewster, NY 10509-9806 — 845-278-2141

Brightwaters

George J. Kamilar
240 Windsor Ave., Brightwaters, NY 11718 — 516-665-7167

Bronx

Aimes Medical Equipment Rental & Props
2417 Third Ave., Bronx, NY 10451 — 718-993-4400

Brandt Industries, Inc.
4461 Bronx Blvd., Bronx, NY 10470-1496 — 800-221-8031

Industrial Acoustics Co., Inc.
1160 Commerce Avenue, Bronx, NY 10462-5506 — 718-931-8000

Perrigo New York, Inc.
1700 Bathgate Ave., Bronx, NY 10457 — 269-686-2916

Supreme Screw Products, Inc.
1368 Cromwell Avenue, Bronx, NY 10452 — 718-293-6600

Bronxville

X-Strap Systems
81 Pondfield Road #157, Bronxville, NY 10708-0850 — 914-968-3381

Brooklyn

Aim Dental Laboratory
15 Parkville Ave, Brooklyn, NY 11230-1010 — 800-238-3500

Amco International Manufacturing & Design, Inc.
10 Conselyea Street, Brooklyn, NY 11211 — 303-646-3583

American Biomed Instruments, Inc.
11 Wyona St., Brooklyn, NY 11207 — 718-235-8900

American Hand Prosthetics, Inc.
73 Skillman Ave., Brooklyn, NY 11211 — 212-213-3700

Baron Medical Supply
709 Grand Street, Brooklyn, NY 11211 — 888-702-2766

Capri Optics, Inc.
1421 38th St., Brooklyn, NY 11218-3678 — 800-221-3544

Dixie Ems Supply
10101 Foster Ave, Brooklyn, NY 11211 — 800-347-3494

Geriatric Products, Inc.
72 Division Place, Brooklyn, NY 11222 — 718-384-5700

J.G. Optical
1424 Sheepshead Bay Rd., Brooklyn, NY 11235-3814 — 718-891-1414

La Charme Llc
45 Main St., Ste. 309 #22, Brooklyn, NY 11201 — 718-816-1347

Medi-Tech International Corp.
26 Court St., Brooklyn, NY 11242-1102 — 800-333-0109

Micro Essential Laboratory, Inc.
4224 Avenue H, P.O. Box 100824, Brooklyn, NY 11210 — 718-338-3618

New York Hospital Disposables, Inc.
101 Richardson Street, Brooklyn, NY 11211-1310 — 718-384-1620

Nomir Medical Technologies Inc.
3021 avenue j, Brooklyn, NY 11210 — 718.676.1502

Ny Orthopedic Usa, Inc.
63 Flushing Ave, Unit #333, Bldg #77, Brooklyn, NY 11205 — 718-852-5330

Paper Converting Of America Corp.
633 Marlborough Rd., Brooklyn, NY 11226 — 718-385-9100

Park Surgical Co., Inc.
5001 New Utrecht Avenue, Brooklyn, NY 11219-3547 — 800-633-7878

Parterre Vinyl Flooring Systems
Brooklyn Navy Yard, Bldg. 292, Ste. 402, Brooklyn, NY 11205 — 888-338-1029

Pnavel Systems, Inc.
1502 East 14th Street, Suite 2, Brooklyn, NY 11230 — 718-645-6304

Ppr Direct, Inc.
74 20th St., Brooklyn, NY 11232-1100 — 800-526-3668

Protective Lining Co.
601 39th St., Brooklyn, NY 11232 — 800-221-9712

Sticht Inc., Herman H.
45 Main Street, Brooklyn, NY 11201 — 800-221-3203

Tri-State Surgical Supply & Equipment
409 Hoyt St., Brooklyn, NY 11231-4858 — 800-424-5227

Vartex Instrument Corp.
311 Wallabout St., Brooklyn, NY 11206 — 718-486-5050

Wenzelite Rehab Supplies, Llc
220 36th Street, 99 Seaview Blvd, Brooklyn, NY 11232 — 800-706-9255

Buffalo

Accu-Med Technologies, Inc.
150 Bud-mil Dr., Buffalo, NY 14206 — 718-244-5330

Airsep Corp.
401 Creekside Dr., Buffalo, NY 14228-2070 — 800-874-0202

Apollo Research Corporation
2300 Walden Avenue, Suite 200, Buffalo, NY 14225-4740 — 800-418-1718

Austin Air Systems Limited
500 Elk Street, Buffalo, NY 14210 — 716-856-3700

Buffalo Filter, A Division Of Medtek Devices Inc.
595 Commerce Drive, Buffalo, NY 14228 — 800-343-2324

Cantylight
6100 Donner, Buffalo, NY 14094 — 716-625-4227

Embla Systems, Inc.
55 Pineview Dr., Suite 100, Buffalo, NY 14228 — 716-691-0718

Ethox International
251 Seneca St., Buffalo, NY 14204 — 800-521-1022

Foundation Milling Centre
235 Aero Dr., Suite 2, Buffalo, NY 14225 — 716-579-3724

Graphic Controls Corp.
400 Exchange St., Buffalo, NY 14204 — 800-669-1535

Hard Manufacturing Co.
230 Grider St., Buffalo, NY 14215-3797 — 800-873-4273

Harmac Medical Products, Inc.
2201 Bailey Avenue, Buffalo, NY 14211-1797 — 716-897-4500

Immco Diagnostics, Inc.
60 Pineview Drive, Buffalo, NY 14228-2120 — 800-537-8378

Leica Microsystems, Inc., Educational & Analytical Division
P.O. Box 123, Buffalo, NY 14240-0123 — 800-346-4560

Luminescent Dental Supply Co.
64 Creekview Dr., Buffalo, NY 14224 — 866-33D-ENTA

Mono Research Lab Ltd.
5436 Main St., Ste. 4, Buffalo, NY 14231 — 716-634-6800

Multisorb Technologies, Inc.
325 Harlem Road, Buffalo, NY 14224 — 800-445-9890

Payton Scientific Inc.
964 Kenmore Avenue, Buffalo, NY 14216 — 716-876-1813

Perfect Fit Glove
85 Innsbruck Drive, Buffalo, NY 14227 — 800-245-6837

Safetec Of America, Inc.
887 Kensington Avenue, Buffalo, NY 14215 — 800-456-7077

The Smartpill Corporation
847 Main Street, Buffalo, NY 14203-1109 — 800-644-4162

Tmp Technologies, Inc.
1200 Northland Avenue, Buffalo, NY 14215 — 716-895-6100

Tru-Mold Shoes, Inc.
42 Breckenridge Street, Buffalo, NY 14213 — 800-843-6653

Zeptometrix Corporation
872 Main St., Buffalo, NY 14202-1499 — 800-274-5487

Caledonia

Tss Foam Industries Corp.
2770 West Main Rd., Caledonia, NY 14423 — 888-435-1083

Cambria Heights

Ac Healthcare Supply, Inc.
116-51 230th St., Cambria Heights, NY 11411 — 905-448-4706

Canandaigua

Badge Machine Products, Inc.
2491 Brickyard Rd., Canandaigua, NY 14424 — 585-394-0330

Select Fabricators, Inc.
5310 North Street, Building 5, Canandaigua, NY 14424 — 585-393-0650

Carle Place

Formed Plastics, Inc.
207 Stonehinge Lane, Carle Place, NY 11514 — 516-334-2300

Cedarhurst

Implant Logic Systems, Ltd.
76 Spruce St., Cedarhurst, NY 11516 — 516-295-1121

Central Nyack

Usa Photonics, Inc.
169 Main St., 1st Flr., Central Nyack, NY 10960 — 845-348-4900

Central Square

Nasiff Assoc., Inc.
841-1 County Route 37, Central Square, NY 13036 — 315-676-2346

Champlain

Biosig Instruments, Inc.
P.O. Box 860, Champlain, NY 12919 — 800-463-5470

Magnaplan Corp.
1320 Rte. 9, Champlain, NY 12919-5007 — 800-361-1192

Chatham

Sonoco Crellin, Inc.
87 Center St., Chatham, NY 12037 — 518-392-2000

Cheektowaga

Nelson Prosthetic & Orthotic Laboratory
2959 Genesee St., Cheektowaga, NY 14225-2653 — 716-894-6666

Chester

Repro-Med Systems, Inc.
24 Carpenter Rd., Chester, NY 10918 — 800-624-9600

Rms Medical Products
24 Carpenter Road, Chester, NY 10918 — 800-624-9600

Chestnut Ridge

Lecroy Corp.
700 Chestnut Ridge Rd., Chestnut Ridge, NY 10977 — 800-553-2769

Cicero

Lakeshore Technologies Inc.
7536 Murray Dr., Cicero, NY 13039 — 315-699-2975

Clarence

Anesthetic Vaporizer Services   716-759-8490
10185 Main St., Clarence, NY 14031-2044
Greatbatch Inc   716-759-5600
x, Clarence, NY 14031
Greatbatch Medical   716-759-5600
10000 Wehrle Drive, Clarence, NY 14031
Medsonic U.S.A., Inc.   716-565-1700
8865 Sheridan Drive, Clarence, NY 14031-2002
Nk Medical Products Inc.   800-274-2742
10123 Main St, PO Box 627, Clarence, NY 14031

Clarkstown

Promident Llc   845-634-3997
242 North Main St., Clarkstown, NY 10956

Clifton Park

Ted Pella, Inc.   800-237-3526
750 Pierce Road, Suite 2, Clifton Park, NY 12065-1303

Cohoes

Blue Earth, Inc.   518-237-5585
31 Ontario St., 2nd Floor - Front, Cohoes, NY 12047-3745

Cold Spring Harbor

AccuVein LLC   816-997-9400
40 Goose Hill Road, Cold Spring Harbor, NY 11724

College Point

Afc Industries, Inc.   718-747-0237
13-16 133rd Place, College Point, NY 11356

commack

Accu-Scope, Inc.   631-864-1000
73 mall dr, commack, NY 11725
Avery Biomedical Devices, Inc.   631-864-1600
61 Mall Dr., Commack, NY 11725-5703
Lew Jan Textile   800-899-0531
366 Veterans Memorial Hwy. Suite 4, Commack, NY 11725
Linear Tonometers, Inc.   800-786-2163
PO Box 322, Commack, NY 11725-0322
Unitron Ltd   631-543-2000
73 Mall Drive, Commack, NY 11725

Congers

Aktina Medical Physics Corp.   (888) 433-3380
360 Route 9W North, Congers, NY 10920

Copiague

W.A. Baum Co., Inc.   888-281-6061
620 Oak St., Copiague, NY 11726
Willow Graphics, Inc.   631-454-6565
608 Oak St., Copiague, NY 11726

Cortland

J.M. Murray Center, Inc.   800-566-8772
823 NYS Rte. 13, Cortland, NY 13045

Cortlandt Manor

Polymedco, Inc.   800-431-2123
510 Furnace Dock Rd., Cortlandt Manor, NY 10567

Cuba

Sterilator Company, Inc.   585-968-2377
30 Water Street, Cuba, NY 14727-1023

Deer Park

Ar Custom Medical Products, Ltd.   516-242-7501
19A West Industry Court, Deer Park, NY 11729
Flow X-Ray Corporation   800-356-9729
100 West Industry Ct., Deer Park, NY 11729
High Frequency Technology Co., Inc.   800-342-3020
172 Brook Ave., Deer Park, NY 11729
J.R. Rand Corp.   800-526-7111
100 S. Jeffryn Blvd. E., Deer Park, NY 11729
Langer, Inc.   800-645-5520
450 Commack Road, Deer Park, NY 11729
Minimax Company   800-292-2620
100 West Industry Court, Deer Park, NY 11729
Triboro Supplies Inc   800-369-7546
994 Grand Blvd., Deer Park, NY 11729
United Biotech   866-753-5700
45 W Jefryn Blvd., Suite E, Deer Park, NY 11729
Wolf X-Ray Corporation   800-356-9729
100 West Industry Court, Deer Park, NY 11729

Depew

Reichert, Inc.   888-849-8955
3362 Walden Avenue, Depew, NY 14043

Dolgeville

Bergeron Health Care   800-371-2778
15 South Second St., Dolgeville, NY 13329

Flocast Llc.   315-429-8407
15 South Second St., Dolgeville, NY 13329
Tumble Forms, Inc.   262-387-8720
1013 Barker Rd., Dolgeville, NY 11329

E Farmingdale

Fibra-Sonics, A Division Of Misonix, Inc.   631-694-9555
1938 New Highway, E Farmingdale, NY 11735

East Aurora

Moog Inc.   716-652-2000
Jamison Rd., East Aurora, NY 14052

East Greenbush

Moss Tubes, Inc.   800-827-0470
749 Columbia Turnpike, East Greenbush, NY 12061

East Meadow

Narishige International Usa, Inc.   800-445-7914
1710 Hempstead Tpke., East Meadow, NY 11554

East Rockaway

Berg, W. M., Inc.   800-232-BERG
499 Ocean Ave., East Rockaway, NY 11518

East Schodack

Clinetics   518-477-6886
25 Hy Drive, East Schodack, NY 12063

East Setauket

Excel Technology, Inc.   631-784-6100
41 Research Way, East Setauket, NY 11733
Quantronix Lasers   1-800-289-7707
41 Research Way, East Setauket, NY 11733
Quatronix   800-289-7707
41 Research Way, East Setauket, NY 11733

East Syracuse

New Product Development, Inc.   315-434-9000
6700 Old Collamer Road, East Syracuse, NY 13057

Edgewood

Advance Tabco   800-645-3166
200 Heartland Blvd., Edgewood, NY 11717
Biochemical Diagnostics, Inc.   800-223-4835
180 Heartland Blvd., Edgewood, NY 11717-8314
Parkell, Inc.   800-243-7446
300 Executive Dr., Edgewood, NY 11717-9816
Wayne Integrated Technologies Corp.   631-242-0213
160 Rodeo Dr., Edgewood, NY 11717-8317

Elka Park

Community Products, Llc   845-658-7723
Platte Clove Rd., Elka Park, NY 12427

Elma

Suburban Adult Services, Inc.   (888)496-5551
960 West Maple Court, Elma, NY 14059

Elmira

Powell Labs   800-210-6549
480 Roe Avenue, Elmira, NY 14901
The Hilliard Corporation   607-733-7121
100 West. 4th Street, Elmira, NY 14902
Winchester Optical Co.   607-734-4251
1935 Lake St., Elmira, NY 14901-1290

Elmont

Respiratory Science Industries Ltd   516-561-6161
1325 M St., Elmont, NY 11003

Elmsford

Afp Imaging Corp.   800-592-6666
250 Clearbrook Road, Elmsford, NY 10523-1315
Imetra, Inc.   914-592-2800
200 Clearbrook Rd., Elmsford, NY 10523-1396
Luxo Corporation   800-222-5896
Five Westchester Plaza, Elmsford, NY 10523
Medlink Imaging, Inc.   800-456-7800
200 Clearbrook Road, Elmsford, NY 10523
Novamed, Llc   800-425-3535
4 Westchester Plaza, Elmsford, NY 10523
Olympic Sport, Inc.   914-347-4737
500 Executive Blvd., Elmsford, NY 10523
San-Mar Laboratories, Inc.   914-592-3130
4 Warehouse Ln., Elmsford, NY 10523
U.E. Systems, Inc.   800-223-1325
14 Hayes St., Elmsford, NY 10523-2407

Endicott

Palmer Industries   800-847-1304
P O Box 5707, Endicott, NY 13763

Fairport

Coopervision
370 Woodcliff Drive, Suite 200, Fairport, NY 14450 — (585) 421-0100
Coopervision Inc.
370 Woodcliff Drive, Suite 200, Fairport, NY 14450 — 800-341-2020
Thermo Fisher Scientific - Fairport
236 Perinton Parkway, Fairport, NY 14450 — 585-899-7600

Farmingdale

Alpha Communications
42 Central Drive, Farmingdale, NY 11735-1202 — 800-666-4800
Barjan Mfg., Ltd.
28 Baiting Pl Rd., Farmingdale, NY 11735 — 800-611-6950
Brooklyn Thermometer Co., Inc.
90 Verdi Street, Farmingdale, NY 11735-6318 — 800-241-6316
Bulbtronics, Inc.
45 Banfi Plaza N, Farmingdale, NY 11735-1539 — 800-624-2852
Gvs - New York
46 Central Avenue, Farmingdale, NY 11735 — 631-753-2100
Kem Medical Products Corp.
75 Price Parkway, Farmingdale, NY 11735 — 800-553-0330
Misonix, Inc.
1938 New Hwy., Farmingdale, NY 11735 — 800-694-9612
Netech, Corp.
110 Toledo Street, Farmingdale, NY 11735 — 800-547-6557
Nortech Laboratories, Inc.
125 Sherwood Ave., Farmingdale, NY 11735-1717 — 888-265-3725
Nsg Precision Cells, Inc.
195 G Central Avenue, Farmingdale, NY 11735-6904 — 631-249-7474
Orbeco Analytical Systems, Inc.
185 Marine St., Farmingdale, NY 11735-5609 — 800-922-5242
Pedinol Pharmacal, Inc.
30 Banfi Plaza, Farmingdale, NY 11735-1528 — 800-733-4665
Tapeswitch Corporation
100 Schmitt Blvd., Farmingdale, NY 11735 — 800-234-8273

Flushing

Advanced Meditech International
86-38 53rd Ave., Ste. 100, Flushing, NY 11373 — 800-635-2452
Pibbs Inc., P.S.
133-15 32nd Ave., Flushing, NY 11354-4008 — 718-445-8046
Twist2it, Inc.
39-30A 62nd St., Flushing, NY 11377 — 877-PRO-PHYS

Forest Hills

William Lembeck, Inc.
54 Continental Ave., Forest Hills, NY 11375 — 718-263-3134

Frankfort

Hale Manufacturing Co., F.E.
120 Benson Place, PO Box 186, Frankfort, NY 13340-0186 — 800-USE-HALE

Freeport

Bio-Scientific Specialty Products, Inc.
197-99 North Main St., P.o. Box 521, Freeport, NY 11520 — 516-868-2553
Oramaax Dental Products,Inc.
216 North Main St., Bldg A-1, Freeport, NY 11520 — 800-672-6229
Phoenix Metal Products, Inc.
100 Bennington Avenue, Freeport, NY 11520-4601 — 516-546-4200
Pressure-Tech, Inc.
102 Woodcleft Ave., Freeport, NY 11520 — 760-470-2831
Temrex Corp.
112 Albany Ave., P.o. Box 182, Freeport, NY 11520 — 516-868-6221
Temrex Corporation
112 Albany Ave., Freeport, NY 11520-4702 — 800-645-1226
Town & Country Dental Studios
275 South Main St., Freeport, NY 11520 — 516-868-8641

Fulton

Huhtamaki Consumer Packaging, Inc.
100 State St., Fulton, NY 13069-2599 — 913-583-3025

Garden City

Imacor Llc
839 Stewart Avenue, Suite #3, Garden City, NY 11530 — 516-393-0970

Garden City Park

Hal-Hen Company, Inc.
180 Atlantic Avenue, Garden City Park, NY 11040-5028 — 800-242-5436

Gardiner

Virtis, An Sp Industries Company
815 Route 208, Gardiner, NY 12525 — 800-431-8232

Garnerville

Ware Medics Glass Works, Inc.
PO Box 368, Garnerville, NY 10923 — 845-429-6950

Glen Cove

Directmed, Inc.
150 Pratt Oval, Glen Cove, NY 11542 — 516-656-3377
Medimaging Tecnology, Inc.
49 Herb Hill Road, Glen Cove, NY 11542 — 800-244-9035

Modulation Optics, Inc.
40 Garvies Point Rd., Glen Cove, NY 11542 — 516-609-000

Glen Head

Incredible Scents, Inc.
1009 Glen Cove Avenue, Glen Head, NY 11545 — (877) 233- 94

Gloversville

Halo Optical Products, Inc.
9 Phair St., Gloversville, NY 12078 — 518-773-4256

Grand Island

App Pharmaceuticals, Llc
3159 Staley Rd., Grand Island, NY 14072 — 847-330-3953
Life Technologies Corporation
3175 Staley Rd., Grand Island, NY 14072 — 716-774-6700
Sterling Fluid Systems (Usa)
303 Industrial Blvd., Grand Island, NY 14072 — 716-773-6450

Great Neck

Cst Technologies, Inc.
55 Northern Blvd., Suite 200, Great Neck, NY 11021-4002 — 800-448-4407
Dma Med-Chem Corporation
49 Water Mill Lane, Great Neck, NY 11021-4234 — 800-362-1833
First Quality Enterprise, Inc.
80 Cuttermill Road, Suite 500, Great Neck, NY 11021 — 516-829-3030
Genadyne Biotechnologies, Inc.
65 Watermill Lane, Great Neck, NY 11021 — 800-208-2025
3cognition Llc
1 Portico Ct., Apt. 302, Great Neck, NY 11021 — 516-458-2905

Halfmoon

Pva
15 Solar Drive, Halfmoon, NY 12065 — 518-371-2684

Hamburg

A. Titan Instruments, Inc.
97 Main St., Hamburg, NY 14075 — 877-284-8261
Arnold Tuber Industries
97 Main Street, Hamburg, NY 14075 — 716-648-3363

Hauppauge

Advanced Back Technologies, Inc.
89 Cabot Ct., Ste. F, Hauppauge, NY 11788 — 631-231-0076
American Diagnostic Corporation (Adc)
55 Commerce Dr., Hauppauge, NY 11788 — 800-232-2670
Atlantic Ultraviolet Corp.
375 Marcus Blvd., Hauppauge, NY 11788 — 631-273-0500
Axon Systems, Inc.
80-5 Davids Drive, Hauppauge, NY 11788 — 800-888-2966
Busse Hospital Disposables, Inc.
75 Arkay Dr., Hauppauge, NY 11788 — 800-645-6526
Crosstex International
10 Ranick Road, Hauppauge, NY 11788 — 800-223-2497
Crosstex International,Inc.
10 Ranick Rd., Hauppauge, NY 11788-4209 — 888-276-7783
Diagnostic Technology, Inc.
175 Commerce Dr., Unit L, Hauppauge, NY 11788 — 631-582-4949
Dukal Corporation
5 Plant Avenue, Hauppauge, NY 11788 — 800-243-0741
Eppendorf North America
102 Motor Parkway, Hauppauge, NY 11788 — 800-645-3050
George Tiemann & Co.
25 Plant Ave., Hauppauge, NY 11788-3804 — 800-843-6266
Liqui-Mark Corp.
30 Davids Dr., P.o. Box 18015, Hauppauge, NY 11788 — 800-486-9005
Mydent International
80 Suffolk Court, Hauppauge, NY 11788 — 800-275-0020
Narda Safety Test Solutions
435 Moreland Road, Hauppauge, NY 11788 — 631-231-1700
Neometrics, A Division Of Natus
150 Motor Parkway, Suite #203, Hauppauge, NY 11788 — 800-645-3616
Rodale Electronics, Inc.
20 Oser Ave., Hauppauge, NY 11788 — 631-231-0044 x1
Savoy Medical Supply
745 Calebs Pass, Hauppauge, NY 11788 — 631-234-7003
Spellman High Voltage Electronics Corp.
475 Wireless Blvd., Hauppauge, NY 11788 — 631-630-3000
Tuttnauer Usa Co. Ltd.
25 Power Dr., Hauppauge, NY 11788 — 800-624-5836
Ubi
25 Davids Drive, Hauppauge, NY 11788-2037 — 631-273-2828
United-Guardian, Inc.
230 Marcus Blvd., P.O. Box 18050, Hauppauge, NY 11788 — 800-645-5566
Vicon Industries Inc.
89 Arkay Dr., Hauppauge, NY 11788 — 800-645-9116

Hawthorne

Acorda Therapeutics, Inc
15 Skyline Drive, Hawthorne, NY 10532 — 914-347-4300
Btx Tech
5 Skyline Drive, Hawthorne, NY 10532 — 800-666-0996
J. Jamner Surgical Instruments, Inc
9 Skyline Dr., Hawthorne, NY 10532 — 800-431-1123

Ludl Electronic Products Ltd. (Lep Ltd.) 888-769-6111
171 Brady Ave., Hawthorne, NY 10532

Hempstead
Alfa Medical Equipment 800-801-9934
59 Madison Avenue, Hempstead, NY 11550
Arnel, Inc. 516-486-7098
73 High St., Hempstead, NY 11550
Fine Surgical Instrument, Inc. 800-851-5155
741 Peninsula Blvd., Hempstead, NY 11550
Novacare Orthodics 800-272-2464
151 Hempstead Tpke., Hempstead, NY 11552

Henrietta
Sts Duotek, Inc 800-836-4850
370 Summit Point Drive, Henrietta, NY 14467

Hicksville
Lisadent Corp. 516-822-9393
35 Broadway, Hicksville, NY 11801
Parimist Funding Corp. 800-645-6598
40 Commerce Place, Hicksville, NY 11801-5210
Sciarra Laboratories, Inc 516-933-7853
485-09 South Broadway, Hicksville, NY 11801-5071
Uniflex Inc., Medical Packaging Division 800-223-0564
383 W. John St., Hicksville, NY 11802
W&W Manufacturing Co. 800-221-0732
800 S. Broadway, Hicksville, NY 11801-5017

Highland Mills
Opti-Quip, Inc. 845-928-2254
548 Route 32, Box 469, Highland Mills, NY 10930

Holbrook
Thermo Savant 800-634-8886
100 Colin Drive, Holbrook, NY 11741-4306
Tower Medical System, Ltd. 631-699-3200
917-11 Lincoln Ave., Holbrook, NY 11741

Holliswood
Impladent Ltd. 800-526-9343
198-45 Foothill Avenue, Holliswood, NY 11423-1611

Holtsville
Allied Medco, Inc. 631-447-0093
25 Corporate Dr., Holtsville, NY 11742

Honeoye Falls
Save-A-Life Llc 585-624-3732
62 Buggywhip Trail, Honeoye Falls, NY 14472

Hoosick Falls
Wcw,Inc 518-686-0725
1 Mechanic Street, Hoosick Falls, NY 12090

Hopkinton
Numed, Inc. 315-328-4491
2880 Main St., Hopkinton, NY 12965

Horseheads
Synthes (Usa) 610-719-5000
35 Airport Road, Horseheads, NY 14845

Hudson
Kaz, Inc. 518-828-0450
One Vapor Trail, Hudson, NY 12534
Rtf Mfg. Co. Llc. 800-836-0744
793 Rt. 66, Hudson, NY 12534-9801

Hudson Falls
Avex Industries, Ltd. 518-747-3310
27 Allen St., Hudson Falls, NY 12839

Inwood
Mgr Equipment Corp. 516-239-3030
22 Gates Ave., Inwood, NY 11096
Wascomat Laundry Equipment 800-645-2204
461 Doughty Blvd., Inwood, NY 11096-0338

Irvington
Electro-Optical Sciences, Inc. 914-591-3783
3 W. Main St., Ste. 201, Irvington, NY 10533
Orthocon, Inc. 888-445-6784
1 Bridge Street, Suite 121, Irvington, NY 10533

Island Park
Dental/Medical Optics Mfg., Inc. 516-889-5857
4217 Austin Blvd., Island Park, NY 11558
Opsales, Inc.
4217 Austin Blvd., Island Park, NY 11558

Islandia
Algen Scale Corp. 800-836-8445
68 Enter Lane, Islandia, NY 11749

Crescent Chemical Co., Inc. 800-877-3225
2 Oval Drive, Islandia, NY 11749
Markperi International Enterprises 888-627-5737
180 Oval Dr., Islandia, NY 11772
Mediflex Surgical Products 800-879-7575
250 Gibbs Road, Islandia, NY 11749
Millennium Devices, Inc. 631-582-6424
250 Gibbs Rd., Islandia, NY 11749-2697

Ithaca
Evaporated Metal Films Corp. 800-456-7070
239 Cherry St., Ithaca, NY 14850
Rheonix 607-257-1242
22 Thornwood Drive, Ithaca, NY 14850
Transonic Systems Inc. 800-353-3569
34 Dutch Mill Road, Warren Road Business Park, Ithaca, NY 14850

Jamaica
Ellis Ophthalmic Technologies, Inc. 718-656-7390
147-39, 175 St.,, Suite #128, Jamaica, NY 11434
Ocuserv Instruments, Inc. 800-628-5272
147-39 175th St., Jamaica, NY 11434

Jamestown
Jamestown Metal Products 716-665-5313
178 Blackstone Avenue, Jamestown, NY 14701-2297
Trinity Biotech, Inc. 1.800.325.3424
2823 Girts Road, Jamestown, NY 14701

Jericho
Darby Dental Supply Co. 800-645-2310
300 Jericho Quadrangle, Jericho, NY 11753
Rainbow Electro-Technologies, Inc. 516-933-0327
41 Moss Ln., Jericho, NY 11753-1816
Studebaker-Worthington Leasing Corp. 800-645-7242
100 Jericho Quadrangle, Jericho, NY 11753

Johnson City
Gagne, Inc. 800-800-5954
41 Commercial Drive, Johnson City, NY 13790

Johnstown
Epimed International, Inc. 800-866-3342
141 Sal Landrio Drive, Crossroads Business Park, Johnstown, NY 12095

Kew Gardens
Charles B. Schwed Co., Inc. 800-847-4073
124-02 Metropolitan Ave., Kew Gardens, NY 11415
Divine Skin Solutions, Inc. 888-404-7770
119-51 Metropolitan Ave., Suite G4, Kew Gardens, NY 11415

Kinderhook
American Bio Medica Corp. 800-227-1243
122 Smith Rd., Kinderhook, NY 12106
Foster Refrigerator L.L.C. 888-828-3311
97 7th St., P.O.Box 718, Kinderhook, NY 12106

Kings Park
Chiu Technical Corp. 631-544-0606
252 Indian Head Road, Kings Park, NY 11754-4814

Kingston
Ertelalsop 800-553-7835
321 Fair St, P.O. Box 3449, Kingston, NY 12402-3449
Image Technology Laboratories, Inc. 845-338-3366
602 Enterprise Dr., Kingston, NY 12401

Lake Success
Cadence Science Inc. 888-717-7677
1979 Marcus Ave, Suite 215, Lake Success, NY 11042
Canon U.S.A., Inc. 516-328-5000
One Canon Plaza, Lake Success, NY 92618-3731
Polar Electro Inc. 1-800-227-1314
1111 Marcus Ave., Ste. M15, Lake Success, NY 11042-1034
Sonomed, Inc. 800-227-1285
1979 Marcus Ave., Suite C105, Lake Success, NY 11042

Lancaster
Avox Systems 866-278-3237
225 Erie Street, Lancaster, NY 14086-9502
Clover Medical Equipment Services, Inc. 800-550-4111
117 Albert Drive, Lancaster, NY 14086

Larchmont
Ease Of Life Products, Llc 914-834-3480
515 Larchmont Acres East, D, Larchmont, NY 10538

Latham
Angiodynamics, Inc. 518-795-1400
14 Plaza Drive, Latham, NY 12110
Angiodynamics, Inc. 1 518-795-1400
14 Plaza Drive, Latham, NY 12110
North American Medical Products, Inc. 800-488-6267
6- British American Blvd. Suite B, Latham, NY 12110

Petrolab Company 518-783-5133
874 Albany Shaker Road, Latham, NY 12110-1416

Leicester

Cpac Equipment, Inc. 800-333-9729
2364 Leicester Road, Leicester, NY 14481-0175

Lewiston

Noram Solutions 800-387-7103
PO Box 543, Lewiston, NY 14092-0543

Lindenhurst

Buxton Medical Equipment Corp. 631-957-4500
1178 Route 109, Lindenhurst, NY 11757

Liverpool

Infimed, Inc. 315-453-4545
121 Metropolitan Dr., Liverpool, NY 13088-5335
Integrated Medical Devices, Inc. 888-486-6900
549 Electronics Parkway, Liverpool, NY 13088
Intersurgical Inc. 315-451-2900
417 Electronics Pkwy., Liverpool, NY 13088

Lockport

Medexcel 716-438-0132
5444 Leete Rd., Lockport, NY 14094

Long Eddy

Dedeco International, Inc. 888-433-3326
Route 97, Long Eddy, NY 12760
Dedeco Intl., Inc. 845-887-4840
11617 Route 97, Long Eddy, NY 12760
Staino, Llc 845-887-5746
11617 State Route 97, Long Eddy, NY 12760

Long Island City

Henry G. Dietz Co., Inc. 718-726-7270
1426 28th Ave., Long Island City, NY 11102
Hersco Ortho Labs 718-391-0416
39-28 Crescent St., Long Island City, NY 11101
P-Ryton Corp. 800-221-9840
5-04 50th Ave., Long Island City, NY 11709
Propper Manufacturing Co., Inc. 800-832-4300
36-04 Skillman Ave., Long Island City, NY 11101-1730
Redyref A Division Of Dawnex Industries 800-628-3603
38-61 11th Street, Long Island City, NY 11101
Schick Technologies, Inc. 718-937-5765
30-30 47th Ave., Long Island City, NY 11101
Sirona Dental Systems Inc. 718-482-2011
30-30 47th Avenue, Suite 500, Long Island City, NY 11101
Valplast Intl. Corp. 718-361-7440
34-30 31st St., Long Island City, NY 11106
Zyloware Corporation 800-765-3700
11-36 46th Road, Long Island City, NY 11101-5322

Loudonville

G & G Medical Products, Inc. 518-542-0395
6 White Fir Dr., Loudonville, NY 12211

Lynbrook

Priva (Usa), Inc. 516-255-1736
96 Atlantic Ave., Lynbrook, NY 11563

Lyndonville

Monroe Electronics, Inc. 800-821-6001
100 Housel Avenue, Lyndonville, NY 14098

Mamaroneck

Thera-Tronics, Inc. 800-267-6211
623 Mamaroneck Avenue, Mamaroneck, NY 10543-1920

Manhattan

Advanced Monitored Caregiving 201-727-1703
111 John St. Suite 250, Manhattan, NY 10038
Tinnitus Care Inc. 888-535-6160
66 East 80th Street, Suite 1a, Manhattan, NY 10021

Manlius

Global Instrumentation, Llc 315-682-0272
8104 Cazenovia Rd., Manlius, NY 13104

Maspeth

Alpha Optics, Llc. 212-431-9190
54-08 46th St., Maspeth, NY 11378

Massapequa

Scj Enterprises, Inc. 516-797-8903
3 riviera drive east, Massapequa, NY 11758-8509

Massena

Tri Hawk Corporation 866-874-4295
150 Highland Rd., Massena, NY 13662-421550

Mastic Beach

Posturizer, Inc. 631-399-4385
89 Lincoln Avenue, Mastic Beach, NY 11951-1619

Mattydale

Eraser Company, Inc. 800-724-0594
123 Oliva Drive, Mattydale, NY 13211

Medford

Chembio Diagnostic Systems, Inc. 631-924-1135
3661 Horseblock Rd., Medford, NY 11763
Jpl Electronics Corp. 631-345-9700
22A Unit#4 Industrial Blvd., Medford, NY 11763
Sinovus Biotech, Inc. 631-924-1135
3661 Horseblock Road, Medford, NY 11763

Medina

Sigma International, Llc. 800-356-3454
711 Park Avenue, Medina, NY 14103-0756

Mellenville

Nysarc, Columbia County Chapter, Inc. 518-672-4451
Po Box 2 Rt 217, Mellenville, NY 12544

Melville

Air Techniques, Inc. 800-247-8324
1295 Walt Whitman Rd., Melville, NY 11747
AllPro Imaging 888-862-4050
1295 Walt Whitman Road, Melville, NY 11747
Altana, Inc. 800-231-0206
60 Baylis Road, Melville, NY 11747
Fonar Corp. 888-NEEDMRI
110 Marcus Drive, Melville, NY 11747
Fougera 800-645-9833
60 Baylis Road, PO Box 2006, Melville, NY 11747
Henry Schein, Inc. 631-843-5500
135 Duryea Rd., Melville, NY 11747
Nikon Instruments Inc. 800-52-Nikon
1300 Walt Whitman Road, Melville, NY 11747-3064
Vts Medical Systems, Inc. 516-249-1703
40 Melville Park Rd., Melville, NY 11747

Merrick

Ultraspect Inc. 972-485-4661
2005 Merrick Rd, Ste 336, Merrick, NY 11566

Mineola

Flexite Company 1-866-FLEXITE
40 Roselle Street, Mineola, NY 11501
Intercall Systems Inc. 516-294-4524
150 Herricks Road, Mineola, NY 11501
Medipoint, Inc. 800-445-0525
72 E. 2nd St., Mineola, NY 11501-3591

Montebello

Oncology Services International 800-445-4516
400 Rella Boulevard, Suite 123, Montebello, NY 10901

Montgomery

CARDINAL HEALTH 200, LLC 847-785-3323
500 Neelytown Rd, Montgomery, NY 12549

Mount Sinai

Systec Computer Associates, Inc. 631-473-5620
28 N. County Road, Mount Sinai, NY 11766-1518

Mount Vernon

Fr Chemical 603-648-2194
524 South Columbus Ave., Mount Vernon, NY 10550
Geritrex Corp. 800-736-3437
144 Kingbridge Road East, Mount Vernon, NY 10550
Mick Radio-Nuclear Instruments 877-597-6764
521 Homestead Ave., Mount Vernon, NY 10550
Premier Brands Of America, Inc. 914-667-6200
31 South Street, Mount Vernon, NY 10550
Springer-Penguin, Inc. 800-835-8500
11 Brookdale Place, PO Box 310, Mount Vernon, NY 10551-0310
Tork 914-664-3542
1 Grove St., Mount Vernon, NY 10550-2401
Wilkinson Hi-Rise 800-231-3888
11A Kimball Ave., Mount Vernon, NY 10550

N. Syracuse

Air Movement Technologies, Inc. 800-317-9582
320 Gateway Park Dr., N. Syracuse, NY 13212

N.Tonawanda

Cardon Rehabilitation Products Inc 800-944-7868 x
Wurlitzer Industrial Park, 908 Niagara Falls Blvd., N.Tonawanda, NY 14120

New City

Absolute X-Ray Corp. 845-638-8080
205 North Little Tor Rd., New City, NY 10956

New Hampton

Arc Specialty Products, Balchem Corporation 845-326-560
52 Sunrise Park Road, PO Box 600, New Hampton, NY 10958

New Hartford

Hartford Walking Systems Inc. 315-735-1659
22 Pearl St., New Hartford, NY 13413

New Hyde Park

Cdc Products Corp. 800-636-7363
1801 Falmouth Avenue, New Hyde Park, NY 11040
Mrc Industries Inc. 516-328-6900
85 Denton Ave, New Hyde Park, NY 11040

New Paltz

Ulster Scientific, Inc. 845-255-2200
83 South Putt Corners Road, PO Box 819, New Paltz, NY 12561-0819

New Rochelle

Ocg Technology, Inc. 914-576-8457
56 Harisson St., New Rochelle, NY 10801-6555

New Windsor

Aigner Index, Inc. 800-242-3919
218 MacArthur Avenue, New Windsor, NY 12553-0084

New York

Accumin Diagnostics, Inc. 212-659-0711
750 Lexington Ave., 20th Floor, New York, NY 10022
Aura Industries, Inc. 800-551-2872
545 8th Avenue, #5W, New York, NY 10018-4352
Avi-Advanced Visual Instruments Inc. 212-262-7878
321 West 44th St., Suite 902, New York, NY 10036
Best Manufacturing Group Llc 800-843-3233
1633 Broadway, 18th Fl., New York, NY 10019-6708
Biofeedback Instrument Corp. 212-222-5665
255 W. 98th St., Suite 3D, New York, NY 10025-5575
Biosculpture Technology, Inc. 212-977-5400
40 Central Park South, New York, NY 10019
Centinel Spine Inc. 952-885-0500
505 Park Ave., 14th Floor, New York, NY 10022
Colgate Oral Pharmaceuticals, Inc. 212-310-2000
300 Park Avenue, New York, NY 10022
Colors In Optics Ltd. 866-465-2656
366 5th Ave., #1003, New York, NY 10001-2211
Daxor Corporation 212-244-0805
350 5th Ave., Ste. 7120, New York, NY 10118
Dna Products, Llc 800-535-3189
P.O. Box 306, New York, NY 10032-0306
East River Ventures Lp 212-644-2322
c/o East River Ventures LP, 590 Madison Avenue, New York, NY 10022
Enzo Biochem, Inc. 212-583-0100
527 Madison Ave., New York, NY 10022
Gaia Holistic,Inc 212-799-9711
20 West 64th St. Suite 24e, New York, NY 10023
I.M.K. Distributors, Inc. 800-878-5552
19 W. 34th St., Ste. 915, New York, NY 10001
Iba-Rdi 516-254-6800
151 Heartland Blvd., New York, NY 11717
Idesco Corp. 800-336-1383
37 W. 26th St., New York, NY 10010-1097
Intercure Inc. 646-652-5800
589 8th Avenue, 6th Floor, New York, NY 10018
Kaneka Pharma America Llc 800-526-3522
546 Fifth Avenue, 21st Floor, New York, NY 10036-5000
Landon Lens Manufacturing Corp. 800-793-6687
301 East 69th St., New York, NY 10021
Liftvest U.S.A, Llc 800-300-5671
35 W. 83 St., New York, NY 10024-5201
Medge Platforms, Inc. 212-351-5029
100 Park Ave., Ste. 1600, New York, NY 10017
Medical Digital Developers Llc 508-393-3100
767 Lexington Ave., Suite 505, New York, NY 10065
Meta Health Technology Inc. 800-334-6840
330 Seventh Avenue, New York, NY 10001-3904
Mit Poly-Cart Corp. 800-234-7659
211 Central Park W., New York, NY 10024-6020
Oratronics, Inc. 212-986-0050
405 Lexington Ave., New York, NY 10174
Park Dental Research Corp./Implant Center 800-243-7372
19 West 34th St., Ste. 301, New York, NY 10001-3013
Pfizer / Wyeth Consumer Healthcare Inc. 212-733-2323
235 East 42nd Street, New York, NY 10017
Pfizer, Inc. 212-573-2323
235 East 42nd St., New York, NY 10017-5755
Precision Acoustics Industries, Inc. 212-986-6470
501 5th Ave., New York, NY 10017-6103
Richard Danz And Sons, Inc. 212-697-5722
104 East 40th St., New York, NY 10016
Robell Research, Inc. 212-755-6577
635 Madison Ave., New York, NY 10022
Scientific Plastics, Inc. 212-967-1199
243 West 30th St., New York, NY 10001

Skinscience Labs, Inc. 212-265-4600
330 West 58th St., Suite 211, New York, NY 10019
State Trading Corporation Of India, Ltd. 212-244-3317
350 5th Ave., Ste. 1124, 11th Fl., New York, NY 10118
Sterling Vision, Inc. 800-332-6302
520 Eighth Avenue, New York, NY 10018
Stevens Metallurgical Corp. 800-794-7887
239 E. 78th St., New York, NY 10021-0817
Therapeutic Silicone Technologies, Inc. 212-606-0830
909 Fifth Avenue, New York, NY 10021

New York City

Delcath Systems Inc. 212-489-2100
810 Seventh Avenue, Suite 3505, New York City, NY 10019
Dune Medical Devices Inc. 646 429-1452
28 West 44th Street, 16th Floor, New York City, NY 10036

Newark

Maco Bag 315-226-1000
412 Van Buren St., Newark, NY 14513
Ultralife Batteries, Inc. 800-332-5000
2000 Technology Pkwy., Newark, NY 14513

Niagara Falls

Oxair Ltd. 716-298-8288
8320 Quarry Road, Niagara Falls, NY 14304-1068
Sherwood, Harsco Corp. 716-505-4831
2111 Liberty Dr., Niagara Falls, NY 14304
Silipos Inc. 800-229-4404
704 Williams Road, Niagara Falls, NY 14304

North Bellmore

Carl Heyer, Inc. 800-284-5550
1872 Bellmore Avenue, North Bellmore, NY 11710

North Tonawanda

Jaece Industries, Inc. 716-694-2811
908 Niagara Falls Boulevard, North Tonawanda, NY 14120-2020

Northport

Medserv Biologicals, Llc 631-757-8401
1019 Fort Salonga Rd., Suite 109, Northport, NY 11768

Norwich

Apple Converting, Inc. 607-337-4474
65 Hale St., Norwich, NY 13815
Culture Kits, Inc. 888-680-6853
14 Prentice St., PO Box 748, Norwich, NY 13815-2024

Nyack

Edroy Products Co., Inc. 800-233-8803
245 N. Midland Avenue, PO Box 998, Nyack, NY 10960

Oak Hill

Stiefel Laboratories, Inc. 518-239-6901
6290 Route 145, Oak Hill, NY 12460

Oceanside

American Medical Alert Corp. 800-286-2622
3265 Lawson Blvd., Oceanside, NY 11572
Ddc Technologies, Inc. 866-346-3527
311 Woods Ave, Oceanside, NY 11572
Ellman International, Inc. 800-835-5355
3333 Royal Ave, Oceanside, NY 11572
Ellman International, Inc. 800-835-5355
3333 Royal Avenue, Oceanside, NY 11572
Innovative Medical Devices, Inc. 516-766-3800
3571 Hargale Road, Oceanside, NY 11572
Innovative Medical Visions, Inc. 516-766-3800
3571 Hargale Road, Oceanside, NY 11572
Lnd, Inc. 516-678-6141
3230 Lawson Blvd., Oceanside, NY 11572-3724

Ogd

Ansen Corporation 315-393-3573
100 Chimney Point Dr., Ogd, NY 13669

Ogdensburg

Breconridge Manufacturing Solutions 315-393-8000
120 Chimney Point Dr., Ogdensburg, NY 13669
Oxoid, Inc. 800-567-8378
800 Proctor Avenue, Ogdensburg, NY 13669-0691
Prodrive Systems, Inc. 866-937-8882
812a Commerce Dr., Ogdensburg, NY 13669

Oneida

Target Compaction, Inc. 315-363-3077
510 Lake Rd., Oneida, NY 13421

Oneonta

Arc/Otsego 607-432-8595
35 Academy Street, PO Box 490, Oneonta, NY 13820-1046
Corning, Inc. 607-433-3100
275 River St., Oneonta, NY 13820

Medical Coaches, Inc.
399 County Highway 58, Oneonta, NY 13820-0129 — 607-432-1333
Siemens Medical Solutions Usa, Inc
Pony Farm Industrial Park, 139 Commerce Rd, Oneonta, NY 13820 — 888-826-9702

Orangeburg

Aalborg Instruments & Controls, Inc.
20 Corporate Drive, Orangeburg, NY 10962 — 800-866-3837
Aristo Import Co., Inc.
85 Hunt Rd., Orangeburg, NY 10962-2596 — 800-352-6304
Dhs Systems Llc
33 Kings Hwy., Orangeburg, NY 10962-1802 — 845-359-6066
Dynarex Corp.
10 Glenshaw St., Orangeburg, NY 10962 — 888-356-2739
Euromed, Inc.
25 Corporate Drive, Orangeburg, NY 10962 — 877-238-76329
Machida, Inc.
40 Ramland Rd. South, Orangeburg, NY 10962 — 800-431-5420
Olympus Surgical & Industrial America, Inc.
One Corporate Drive, Orangeburg, NY 10962 — 845-398-9400
Opticon, Inc.
8 Olympic Drive, Orangeburg, NY 10962 — 800-636-0090
Professional Disposables International, Inc.
Two Nice Pak Park, Orangeburg, NY 10962-1318 — 800-999-6423
Tillotson Healthcare Corp.
10 Glenshaw St., Orangeburg, NY 10962 — 888-335-7500
Vision-Sciences, Inc.
40 Ramland Road South, Suite 1, Orangeburg, NY 10962 — 800-874-9975

Orchard Park

A. Lunt Design, Inc.
5755 Big Tree Rd., PO Box 247, Orchard Park, NY 14127 — 866-872-5868
Curbell Electronics Inc.
20 Centre Dr., Orchard Park, NY 14127 — 716-667-3377
Curbell, Inc. Electronics
7 Cobham Dr., Orchard Park, NY 14127 — 800-235-7500
Gaymar Industries, Inc.
10 Centre Drive, Orchard Park, NY 14127-2280 — 800-828-7341
Matrx
145 Mid County Dr., Orchard Park, NY 14127 — 716-662-6650
Matrx By Midmark
145 Mid County Drive, Orchard Park, NY 14127-1737 — 800-847-1000
Minrad, Inc.
50 Cobham Dr., Orchard Park, NY 14127 — 716-855-1068

Oriskany Falls

Covidien Lp, Formerly Registered As Kendall
130 South Main St., Oriskany Falls, NY 13425 — 800-962-9888

Owego

Biolife Solutions, Inc.
171 Front Street, Owego, NY 13827-1520 — 607-687-4487

Oyster Bay

Circulatory Technology, Inc.
21 Singworth St., Oyster Bay, NY 11771 — 516-624-2424

Panorama

Thermo Fisher Scientific (Rochester)
75 Panorama Creek Dr., Panorama, NY 14625 — 585-899-7600

Patterson

Hy-Tape International
70 John Barrett Road, Robin Hill Corporate Park, Patterson, NY 12563 — 800-248-0101

Pearl River

Versamed Medical Systems, Inc.
2 Blue Hill Plaza, Pearl River, NY 10965 — 800-475-9239

Peekskill

Cir Systems Inc
8 John Walsh Blvd., Suite 429, Peekskill, NY 10566 — 914-734-8178

Pelham Manor

Caligor
846 Pelham Pkwy., Pelham Manor, NY 10803 — 800-472-4346

Pine Island

Surehands Lift & Care Systems
982 Rte. 1, Pine Island, NY 10969 — 800-724-5305

Pittsford

Smile Brite Distributing Llc
5 Boughton Avenue, Pittsford, NY 14534 — 585-248-9260

Plainview

Budenheim Usa, Inc
245 Newtown Road, Suite 305, Plainview, NY 11803 — 800-645-3044
K-Fit Orthotics Llc
1464 Old Country Rd., Plainview, NY 11803 — 516-293-6400
Lemans Industries Corp.
79 Express St., Plainview, NY 11803-2404 — 800-289-5667
Plainview Batteries, Inc.
23 Newtown Rd., Plainview, NY 11803 — 800-642-2354

Plattsburgh

Emergency First Aid Products (Usa), Inc.
53 Area Development Dr.,, Unit B, Plattsburgh, NY 12901 — 518-562-9911
Monaghan Medical Corp.
5 Latour Ave., Ste. 1600, Plattsburgh, NY 12901-0299 — 800-833-9653

Poland

Perfex Corp.
32 Case St., Poland, NY 13431 — 800-848-8483

Port Chester

Polder, Inc.
8 Slater St., Port Chester, NY 10573 — 800-431-2133

Port Washington

Dri Mark Products, Inc.
15 Harbor Park Dr., Port Washington, NY 11050 — 516-484-6200
Medical Depot
99 Seaview Blvd., Port Washington, NY 11050 — 516-998-4600
Pall Corporation
25 Harbor Park Drive, Port Washington, NY 11050 — 800-645-6532
Premier Heart, Llc.
110 Main Street, Suite 201-88, Port Washington, NY 11050 — 888-380-8338
Stern Inc., Walter
68 Sintsink Drive East, P.O. Box 571, Port Washington, NY 11050-0105 — 516-883-9100

Purchase

Integramed America, Inc.
2 Manhattanville Rd., Purchase, NY 10577-2113 — 212-835-8500
Laschal Surgical, Inc.
4 Baltusrol Dr., Purchase, NY 10577 — 800-352-7242

Queensbury

C. R. Bard, Inc.
289 Bay Rd., Queensbury, NY 12804 — 908-277-8481
Sterile Technologies, Inc.
63 Park Rd., Queensbury, NY 12804 — 518-793-7077

Rensselaer

Vec Technologies, Inc.
1 University Pl., Rensselaer, NY 12144-3456 — 518-257-2010

Richmond Hill

Care Apparel Industries
127-09 91st Ave., Richmond Hill, NY 11418 — 800-326-6262
L.P. Systems Corp.
116-08 Myrtle Ave., Suite 330, Richmond Hill, NY 11418 — 718-805-6926
Perfect Care
8927 126 St., Richmond Hill, NY 11418 — 718-805-7800

Rifton

Community Products, Llc
2032 Route 213, Rifton, NY 12471 — 845-658-7723
Rifton Equipment
PO Box 260, Rifton, NY 12471-0260 — 800-571-8198

Rochester

Alliance Precision Plastics
1220 Lee Road, Rochester, NY 14606 — 585-426-5310
Artcraft New York
57 Goodway Drive South, Rochester, NY 14623 — 800-828-8288
Bausch & Lomb
1 Bausch & Lomb Place, Rochester, NY 14604-2701 — 585-338-6000
Bausch & Lomb, Vision Care
1400 N. Goodman St., Rochester, NY 14609-3547 — 800-553-5340
Boehm Surgical Instrument Corp.
966 Chili Ave., Rochester, NY 14611 — 585-436-6584
Carestream Health, Inc.
1049 West Ridge Road, Rochester, NY 14615 — 585-722-4565
Carestream Health, Inc.
150 Verona Street, Rochester, NY 14608 — 888-777-2072
Carestream Health, Inc.
1669 Lake Ave., Rochester, NY 14652 — 888-777-2072
Chamberlin Rubber Company, Inc.
3333 Brighton Henrietta Town Line Road, PO Box 22700, Rochester, NY 14692 — 585-427-7780
Electro Surgical Instrument Co., Inc.
37 Centennial St., Rochester, NY 14611 — 888-464-2784
Fieldtex Products, Inc.
3055 Brighton-Henrietta TL Road, Rochester, NY 14623 — 800-772-4816
Getinge Sourcing Llc
1777 East Henrietta Rd., Rochester, NY 14623 — 800-475-9040
Getinge Usa, Inc.
1777 E. Henrietta Rd., Rochester, NY 14623-3133 — 800-475-9040
Glass Fab, Inc.
257 Ormond St., PO Box 31880, Rochester, NY 14605 — 585-262-4000
Global Health Products, Inc
1099 Jay St., Suite E, Rochester, NY 14611 — 585-235-8815
H&W Technology, Llc.
PO Box 20281, Rochester, NY 14602-0281 — 585-218-0385
Lightnin Mixers
135 Mt. Read Blvd., Rochester, NY 14611 — 888-MIX-BEST
Lucid, Inc.
2320 Brighton Henrietta Townline Rd., Rochester, NY 14623 — 585-239-9800

Medcare Technologies   800-388-6235
850 St. Paul St., Rochester, NY 14605-1095
Nalge Nunc International   800-625-4327
75 Panorama Creek Drive, Rochester, NY 14625-2303
Navitar, Inc.   800-828-6778
200 Commerce Drive, Rochester, NY 14623
Ortho Clinical Diagnostics, Inc.   800-828-6316
100 Indigo Creek Dr., Rochester, NY 14650
Ortho-Clinical Diagnostics, Inc.   585-453-3768
100 Indigo Creek Dr., Rochester, NY 14626
Ortho-Clinical Diagnostics, Inc.   800-828-6316
100 Indigo Creek Dr., Room 350, Rochester, NY 14650
Ortho-Clinical Diagnostics, Inc.   585-453-3768
1000 Lee Rd., Rochester, NY 14606
Pgm   585-458-4300
1305 Emerson St., Rochester, NY 14606-3098
Rochester Midland, Corp.   800-836-1627
333 Hollenbeck St, Rochester, NY 14621
Rochester Optical Mfg. Company   585-254-0022
1260 Lyell Avenue, Rochester, NY 14606-2040
Spectra-Tint   585-546-8050
250 Cumberland Street, Suite 228, Rochester, NY 14605
Thermo Spectronic   800-654-9955
820 Linden Avenue, Rochester, NY 14625-2710
Ti-Ba Enterprises, Inc.   585-247-1212
25 Hytec Circle, Rochester, NY 14606
VirtualScopics, Inc.   585-249-6231
500 Linden Oaks, Rochester, NY 14625
Ward's Natural Science Establishment, Inc.   800-962-2660
5100 W. Henrietta Rd., P.O. Box 92912, Rochester, NY 14692-9012

Rockville Centre

Diagnostix Plus, Inc.   516-536-2670
100 North Village Ave., Suite # 33, Rockville Centre, NY 11570

Rome

Conmed Corporation   800-448-6506
5836 Success Drive, Rome, NY 13440

Ronkonkoma

Aerodyne Controls, Inc., A Circor International   631-737-1900
Company
30 Haynes Ct., Ronkonkoma, NY 11779-7220
Alceram Tech Inc   516-849-3666
57 2ND ST, Ronkonkoma, NY 11779-5352
Corning Wax   631-738-0041
1744 Julia Goldbach Avenue, Ronkonkoma, NY 11779
Home Health   800-445-7137
2100 Smithtown Ave, Ronkonkoma, NY 11772
Medical Technology Products, Inc.   800-314-0210
2221-16 5th Avenue, Ronkonkoma, NY 11779
Prorhythm, Inc.   631-981-3907
105 Comac St., Ronkonkoma, NY 11779
Quantum Medical Imaging, Llc   631-567-5800
2002 Orville Dr N Suite B, Ronkonkoma, NY 11779
Ring Communications, Inc.   516-585-7464
57 Trade Zone Dr., Ronkonkoma, NY 11779-7343
Sentry Technology Corp.   800-645-7217
1881 Lakeland Avenue, Ronkonkoma, NY 11779

Rush

Sps Medical Supply Corp.   800-722-1529
6789 W. Hennetta Road, Rush, NY 14543
Sts Division Of Ethox International   800.836.4850
7500 West Henrietta Rd., Rush, NY 14543

Rye Brook

Softsert, Inc.   516-887-2056
19 Reunion Road, Rye Brook, NY 10573

S Fallsburg

Majestic Drug Co., Inc.   845-436-0011
4996 Main St., Route 42, Pob 490, S Fallsburg, NY 12779

Salem

The Phantom Laboratory, Inc.   800-525-1190
PO Box 511, Salem, NY 12865-0511

Sanborn

First Healthcare Products   800-854-8304
6125 Lendell Drive, Sanborn, NY 14132

Saratoga Springs

Rejuveness Pharamceuticals, Inc.   518-584-5017
125 High Rock Ave., Saratoga Springs, NY 12866

Saugerties

Electronic Control Concepts   800-847-9729
160 Partition St., Saugerties, NY 12477
Simulaids, Inc.   800-431-4310
16 Simulaids Drive, PO Box 1289, Saugerties, NY 12477
V.I.E.W. Video   800-843-9843
PO Box 77, Saugerties, NY 12477

Schenectady

Cardiomag Imaging, Inc.   518-381-1000
450 Duane Ave., Schenectady, NY 12304
Utech Products, Inc.   800-828-8324
135 Broadway St, Schenectady, NY 12305

Shirley

Biodex Medical Systems, Inc.   800-224-6339
20 Ramsay Road, Shirley, NY 11967-4704
Luitpold Pharmaceuticals, Inc.   631-924-4000
One Luitpold Drive, Shirley, NY 11967

Silver Creek

American Massage Products, Inc.   716-934-2648
341 Central Ave., Silver Creek, NY 14136

Skaneateles Falls

Welch Allyn, Inc.   800-535-6663
4341 State St. Rd., Skaneateles Falls, NY 13153-0220
Welch Allyn, Inc.   800-535-6663
4341 State Street Road, Skaneateles Falls, NY 13153

Slingerlands

Nanomed Devices, Inc.   518-862-0151
116 Kennewyck Circle, Slingerlands, NY 12159

Smithtown

A.M. Surgical, Inc.   800-437-9653
290 East Main Street, Suite 200, Smithtown, NY 11787

Spring Valley

Kratos Analytical Inc.   800-935-0213
100 Red Schoolhouse Road #Bldg.-A, Spring Valley, NY 10977-7049

Stone Ridge

Fts Systems   800-824-0400
3538 Main Street, PO Box 158, Stone Ridge, NY 12484-0158

Stony Brook

Esco Medical Instruments, Inc.   800-970-3726
21 William Penn Drive, Stony Brook, NY 11790-1317
Infrared Sciences Corp.   516-482-9001
213 Hallock Rd., Suite 5, Stony Brook, NY 11790
Tools For Surgery, Llc   631-444-4448
1339 Stony Brook Rd., Stony Brook, NY 11790
Viatronix, Inc.   631-444-9700
25 Health Sciences Drive, Suite 203, Stony Brook, NY 11790-3350

Suffern

Blue Chip Medical Products, Inc.   800-795-6115
7-11 Suffern Place, #2, Suffern, NY 10901

Syosset

Buffalo Dental Manufacturing Co., Inc.   800-828-0203
159 Lafayette Dr., PO BOX 678, Syosset, NY 11791
Buffalo Dental Mfg. Co., Inc.   516-496-7200
159 Lafayette Dr., Syosset, NY 11791
Duke Diagnostic Resale   516-496-3503
257 Cold Spring Road, Syosset, NY 11791
Magna-Lab, Inc.   516-393-5874
6800 Jericho Turnpike, Suite 120w, Syosset, NY 11791

Syracuse

Central New York Medical Products   315-428-9945
749 W. Genesee St, Syracuse, NY 13204
Cleanroom Systems   800-825-3268
7000 Performance Dr., Syracuse, NY 13212
Danlee Medical Products, Inc.   800-433-7797
6075 Molloy Rd. E., Bldg. 5, Syracuse, NY 13211
Haun Specialty Gases, Inc.   315-463-5241
5921 Court Street Road, Syracuse, NY 13206
Living Information Systems Llc   315-469-7399
886 East Brighton Ave., Syracuse, NY 13205
Stallion Technologies, Inc.   315-476-4330
1201 East Fayette St., Syracuse, NY 13210
Stallion Technologies, Inc.   315-476-4330
1201 East Fayette Street, Syracuse, NY 13210
Sterilogic Waste Systems, Inc.   315-455-5600
6691 Pickard Dr., Syracuse, NY 13211
Syracuse Medical Devices, Inc.   315-449-0657
214 Hurlburt Road, Syracuse, NY 13224-1821

Tarrytown

Bayer Healthcare Llc   914-366-1800
555 White Plains Rd., 5th Floor, Tarrytown, NY 10591
Regeneron Pharmaceuticals, Inc.   914-345-7400
777 Old Saw Mill River Road, Tarrytown, NY 10591
Siemens Healthcare Diagnostics Inc.   914-631-8000
511 Benedict Avenue, Tarrytown, NY 10591

Thornwood

Carl Zeiss Surgical, Inc.   1 800 233 2343
One Zeiss Dr., Thornwood, NY 10594-1939

Tonawanda

Amd-Ritmed, Inc. — 800-445-0340
295 Firetower Road, Tonawanda, NY 14150
Great Lakes Orthodontics, Ltd. — 800-828-7626
200 Cooper Ave.Dr., Tonawanda, NY 14150
Medco Supply Company — 800-556-3326
500 Fillmore Avenue, Tonawanda, NY 14150
Northeastern Biomechanical Manufacturing Corp. — 716-692-9585
81 Penarrow Dr., Tonawanda, NY 14150
Sr Instruments, Inc. — 800-654-6360
600 Young St., Tonawanda, NY 14150-4105

Troy

Integrated Medical Technologies — 518-368-2400
157 First St., Troy, NY 12180

Utica

Biogenic Dental Corp. — 800-367-3322
282-284 Genesee St., P.O. Box 4119, Utica, NY 13504-4119
Central Assoc. For Blind & Visually Impaired — 877-719-9996
507 Kent St., Utica, NY 13501
Conmed Corporation — 800-448-6506
310 Broad Street, Utica, NY 13501
Conmed Corporation — 315-797-8375
525 French Rd, Utica, NY 13502
Conmed Endoscopic Technologies — 315-797-8375
525 French Road, Utica, NY 13502
Dental Systems Group — 800- 332-3151
601 State Street, Utica, NY 13502
Health-Pak, Inc. — 315-724-8370
2005 Beechgrove Pl., Utica, NY 13501-1703
Hpk Industries Llc — 315-724-0196
1208 Broad St., Utica, NY 13501
Laser Probe, Inc. — 315-797-4492
23 Wells Avenue, Utica, NY 13502
Nova Health Systems, Inc. — 800-225-NOVA
1001 Broad St., Utica, NY 13501
Sturges Manufacturing Company, Inc. — 315-732-6159
2030 Sunset Ave., Utica, NY 13503
Visual Telecommunications Network, Inc — 703-448-0999
2108 Beach Grove Place, Utica, NY 13501

Valhalla

Del Global Technologies Corp. — 914-686-3600
1 Commerce Pk., Valhalla, NY 10595-1455
Farrand Optical Components & Instruments, Div. — 914-287-4035
Of Ruhle Co.
99 Wall St., Valhalla, NY 10595

Valley Cottage

Complete Medical Supplies, Inc. — 800-242-2674
10 Ford Products Rd., Valley Cottage, NY 10989

Van Etten

Vergason Technology, Inc. — 607-589-4429
166 State Route 224, Van Etten, NY 14889

Victor

Lsi Solutions Inc. — 585-869-6641
7796 Victor-mendon Rd., Victor, NY 14564
Newtex Industries, Inc. — 800-836-1001
8050 Victor-Mendon Rd., Victor, NY 14564
Zoetek Medical Sales & Service, Inc. — 800-388-6223
668 Phillips Rd., Victor, NY 14564

Walden

New England Medical Corp. — 845-778-4200
2274 Albany Post Road, Walden, NY 12586
Sigma Products Ltd. — 845-778-4200
2274 Albany Post Road, Walden, NY 12586

Wales Center

A.M. Bickford, Inc. — 800-795-3062
12318 Big Tree Rd., Wales Center, NY 14169

Wappingers Falls

Almost U — 800-626-6007
91 Market St., Suite 23, Wappingers Falls, NY 12590
Laerdal Medical Corporation — 800-227-1143
167 Myers Corners Rd., PO Box 1840, Wappingers Falls, NY 12590-3857

Wassaic

Pawling Corp., Architectural Prod. Div. — 800-431-3456
32 Nelson Hill Road, PO Box 200, Wassaic, NY 12592

Wellsville

Current Controls, Inc. — 585-593-1544
353 S. Brooklyn Avenue, Wellsville, NY 14895

West Babylon

Chem-Tainer Industries, Inc. — 800-ASK-CHEM
361 Neptune Avenue, West Babylon, NY 11704

West Seneca

Suburban Adult Services, Inc. — 716-496-5551
441 Indian Church Rd., West Seneca, NY 14224

Westbury

Accurate Chemical & Scientific Corp. — 800-645-6264
300 Shames Dr., Westbury, NY 11590-1736
E-Z-Em, Inc. — 516-333-8230
750 Summa Ave, Westbury, NY 11590
Iet Labs, Inc. — 800-899-8438
534 Main St., Westbury, NY 11590-4806
Spectronics Corporation — 800-274-8888
956 Brush Hollow Road, Westbury, NY 11590-1731
Vasomedical Inc. — 800-455-3327
180 Linden Ave., Westbury, NY 11590-3228

White Plains

Combe Incorporated — 800-873-7400
1101 Westchester Ave., White Plains, NY 10604
Combe, Inc. — (800) 873-7400
1101 Westchester Avenue, White Plains, NY 10604
Equip For Independence, Inc. — 800-216-4881
333 Mamaroneck Avenue, Suite 383, White Plains, NY 10605-1440
Fabrication Enterprises Inc. — 800-431-2830
Post Office Box 1500, White Plains, NY 10602
Scale-Tronix, Inc. — 800-873-2001
200 E. Post Rd., White Plains, NY 10601-4903
VARTA Microbattery Inc. — 800-468-2782
1311 Mamaroneck Ave., Suite120, White Plains, NY 10605

Williamsville

United Precision Technology — 716-634-4331
4085 David Rd., Williamsville, NY 14221
Vitaid Ltd. — 800-267-9301
300 International Drive, Williamsville, NY 14221

Woodbury

Hitachi Kokusai Electric America, Ltd. — 516-921-7200
150 Crossways Park Drive, Woodbury, NY 11797-2028

Woodside

Medidenta International, Inc. — 800-221-0750
3923 62nd Street, PO Box 409, Woodside, NY 11377-3631

Yaphank

Nanoprobes, Inc. — 877-447-6266
95 Horseblock Rd., Yaphank, NY 11980

Yonkers

American Specialties, Inc. — 914-476-9000
441 Saw Mill River Road, Yonkers, NY 10701-4913
Multigon Industries, Inc. — 800-289-6858
One Odell Plaza, Yonkers, NY 10701
Noble Pine Products Co. — 800-359-4913
Centuck Station, PO Box 41, Yonkers, NY 10710-0041
Omega Medical Products Corp. — 888-837-TAPE
494 Saw Mill River Road, Yonkers, NY 10701
Ram Scientific, Inc. — 800-535-6734
7 odell plaza, Yonkers, NY 10703
Skil-Care Corp. — 800-431-2972
29 Wells Avenue, Yonkers, NY 10701-6605
Stewart Efi, Lcc — 800-678-7931
630 Central Park Avenue, Yonkers, NY 10704

Yorktown Heights

Crown Delta Corp. — 914-245-8910
1550 Front St., Yorktown Heights, NY 10598

Youngstown

Dental Health Products, Inc. — 800-828-6868
4011 Creek Rd., Youngstown, NY 14174-0355
Dental Health Products, Inc. — 716-754-2696
4011 Creek Rd., Youngstown, NY 14174

NORTH CAROLINA

Albemarle

American Fiber & Finishing, Inc. — 800-522-2438
Po Box 2488, Albemarle, NC 28002

Angier

Am2 Pat Inc. — 919-552-9689
455 W. Depot Street, Angier, NC 27501

Apex

Polyzen, Inc. — 919-319-9599
1041 Classic Road, Apex, NC 27539

Arden

Farnam Custom Products — 828-684-3766
90 Bradley Branch Rd., Arden, NC 28704
Medical Action Industries, Inc. — 800-645-7042
25 Heywood Rd, Arden, NC 28704

Precept Medical Products, Inc.   800-438-5827
370 Airport Road, PO Box 2400, Arden, NC 28704-2400

Asheboro

Arrow International, Inc.   800-523-8446
312 Commerce Pl, Asheboro, NC 27203
Asheboro Elastics Corp.   336-629-2626
150 North Park Street, PO Box 1143, Asheboro, NC 27203
Elastic Therapy, Inc.   800-849-2497
718 Industrial Park Ave., P.O. Box 4068, Asheboro, NC 27204-4068
S & S Orthopedic Ltd.   336-626-5167
701 Westmont Drive, Asheboro, NC 27205-4263
Venosan North America, Inc.   800-432-5347
300 Industrial Park Avenue, PO Box 1067, Asheboro, NC 27204-1067
Vesture Corporation   800-462-4201
120 E. Pritchard St., Asheboro, NC 27203
Wells Hosiery Mills, Inc.   336-633-4881
1758 South Fayetteville St., Asheboro, NC 27204

Asheville

Avail Medical Products-Asheville   858-635-2206
3161 Sweeten Creek Road, Asheville, NC 28803
Genova Diagnostics   828-253-0621
63 Zillicoa St., Asheville, NC 28801
Kendro Laboratory Products   800-252-7100
308 Ridgefield Court, Asheville, NC 28806
Thermo Fisher Scientific (Asheville) Llc   828-658-4400
275 Aiken Road, Asheville, NC 28804
Vesture Corp.   614-864-6400
120 East Pritchard St., Asheville, NC 27203

Beaufort

Meditherm Inc.   503-639-8496
400 Front Street, Unit 8, Beaufort, NC 28516

Blowing Rock

Life Science Technologies, Ltd.   828-295-3821
1145 Flat Top Road, Blowing Rock, NC 28607

Brevard

Transylvania Vocational Services   828-884-3195
11 Mountain Industrial Drive, PO Box 1115, Brevard, NC 28712

Brown Summit

Procter & Gamble Co.   513-622-4851
6200 Bryan Park Rd., Brown Summit, NC 27214

Burgaw

Rayson Co. Inc., W.R.   800-526-1526
720 S. Dickerson St., Burgaw, NC 28425

Burlington

Carolina Biological Supply Co.   800-334-5551
2700 York Rd., Burlington, NC 27215-3398
Carolina Biological Supply Co.   800-334-5551
2700 York Road, Burlington, NC 27215-3398
Carolina Eye Prosthetics, Inc.   336-228-7877
420 Maple Ave., Burlington, NC 27215
Lab Corp.   800-222-7566
430 S. Spring St., Burlington, NC 27215
Laboratory Corporation of America   336-584-5171
358 South Main St., Burlington, NC 27215
Medtox Diagnostics Inc.   800-334-1116
1238 Anthony Rd., Burlington, NC 27215-8831
Medtox Diagnostics, Inc.   800-334-1116
1640 Nova Lane, Burlington, NC 27215
Rico Suction Labs, Inc.   800-845-8490
326 MacArthur Ln., Burlington, NC 27217
Tex-Care Medical   800-441-8510
2908 Alamance Road, Burlington, NC 27215
Tripath Imaging, Inc.   919-206-7140
780 Plantation Dr., Burlington, NC 27215

Carrboro

Leap Technologies   800-229-8814
PO Box 969, Carrboro, NC 27510
Nora-Dall   919-942-2592
111 Glosson Circle, Carrboro, NC 27510

Cary

Enviro Guard, Inc.   800-438-1152
201 Shannon Oaks Circle, Suite 115, Cary, NC 27511
Hill-Rom Manufacturing, Inc.   800-445-3730
1225 Crescent Green Dr., Suite 200, Cary, NC 27511
Myco Medical   800-454-6926
158 Towerview Court, Cary, NC 27513
Syracuse Plastics Of North Carolina, Inc.   919-467-5151
100 Falcone Pkwy., Po Box 1067, Cary, NC 27511-6712
Trac Electronics   919-876-8088
1100 West Chatham St., Cary, NC 27511
Unitedhealthcare   800-368-0707
1001 Winstead Dr., Suite 200, Cary, NC 27513

Chapel Hill

Ipas   919-967-7052
PO Box 5027, Chapel Hill, NC 27514
Microtronics Corp. Of Chapel Hill   919-929-2657
88 Vilcom Center, Ste. 165, Chapel Hill, NC 27516

Charlote

Diagnostic Devices Inc.   704-285-6400
9300 Harris Corners Parkway, Suite 450, Charlote, NC 28269

Charlotte

Aplix, Inc.   704-588-1920
12300 Steele Creek Road, Charlotte, NC 28273
Arcus Medical Llc   877-272-8763
4324 Barringer Dr . Suite 104, Charlotte, NC 28217
Barnett Intl. Corp.   704-587-0390
610 Greenway Industrial Drive, Charlotte, NC 28273
Barnhardt Mfg. Co.   704-376-0380
1100 Hawthorne Ln., Charlotte, NC 28205
Bonded Logistics, Inc.   704-597-9638
PO Box 480203, 5709 North Graham Street, Charlotte, NC 28269-4830
Bsn Medical, Inc   800-552-1157
5825 Carnegie Boulevard, Charlotte, NC 28209
Bsn Medical, Inc.   800-552-1157
5825 Carnegie Boulevard, Charlotte, NC 28209
Bsn-Jobst   704-554-9933
5825 Carnagie Blvd., Charlotte, NC 28209
Carolina Absorbent Cotton Co.   800-277-0377
1100 Hawthorne Lane, Charlotte, NC 28205
Clariant   704-331-7000
4000 Monroe Road, Charlotte, NC 28205
Clariant Corporation   1 704 331 7000
4000 Monroe Road, Charlotte, NC 28205
Compumedics Usa, Ltd.   877-717-3975
6605 West WT Harris Blvd, Suite F, Charlotte, NC 28269
Earcrafters, Inc.   800-688-3277
5000 Nations Crossing Road #205, Charlotte, NC 28217-2153
Fitzpatrick Management Resources   800-357-0509
9116 Fishers Pond Drive, Charlotte, NC 28277-3571
Global Medical Imaging   800-958-9986
222 Rampart Street, CHARLOTTE, NC 28203
Imaging Associates, Inc.   800-821-3230
11110 Westlake Dr., Charlotte, NC 28273
Laminex, Inc.   800-438-8850
9900 Brookford Street, Charlotte, NC 28273
Md Scientific Llc   704-335-1300
2815 Coliseum Centre Drive, --suite 250, Charlotte, NC 28217
Medical Specialties, Inc.   800-582-4040
4600 Lebanon Road, Charlotte, NC 28227
Medicor Imaging, Div. Of Lead Technologies Inc.   704-227-2642
1201 Greenwood Cliff, Ste 400, Charlotte, NC 28204
Parker Medical Associates, Llc   704-370-0400
2401 Distribution St., Charlotte, NC 28203
Pelton & Crane   704-588-2126
11727 Fruehauf Dr., Charlotte, NC 28273
Pelton & Crane Co.,   800-659-6560
11727 Fruehauf Dr., Charlotte, NC 28241-7800
Saebo, Inc.   888-284-5433
2725 Water Ridge Parkway, Suite 320, Charlotte, NC 28217
Salvin Dental Specialties, Inc.   800-535-6566
3450 Latrobe Drive, Charlotte, NC 28211
Sirona Dental Systems Llc   800-659-5977
4835 Sirona Drive, Suite 100, Charlotte, NC 28273
US HIFU LLC   704-332-4308
801 E. Morehead St., Suite 201, Charlotte, NC 28202
Ultrascope   800-677-2673
2401 Distribution Street, Charlotte, NC 28203
Visual Med, Inc.   800-324-4464
11110 West Lake Dr., Charlotte, NC 28273

Charlotte,

Novasonic   800-843-0133
4565 Panther Place, Charlotte,, NC 28269

Clayton

Hospira, Inc.   877-946-7747
8484 U.S 70 West, Clayton, NC 27520
3c Packaging   919-553-4113
1000 CCC Dr., Clayton, NC 27520

Clemmons

Med-Edge, Inc.   800-360-3682
1843 Pinehurst Drive, Clemmons, NC 27012

Cornelius

Spectrum Hearing Systems, Inc.   704-237-9100
18636 Starcreek Drive, Suite E, Cornelius, NC 28031

Creedmoor

Cardinal Health 303,Inc.   858-458-7830
1515 Ivac Way, Creedmoor, NC 27522

Davidson

Healthline Medical Imaging — 704-655-0447
705 Northeast Drive, Suite 17, Davidson, NC 28036

Denver

United Syntek Corp. — 888-665-2326
3557 Denver Dr., Denver, NC 28037

Durham

Aldagen, Inc — 919-484-2571
2810 Meridian Parkway, Suite 148, Durham, NC 27713
Alderon Biosciences, Inc. — 919-544-8220
2810 Meridian Pkwy, Suite 152, Durham, NC 27713
American Labor — 800-424-0443
3329 Durham-Chapel Hill Blvd, Suite 200, Durham, NC 27715
Bd Biosciences Discovery Labware — 978-901-7431
One Becton Circle, Durham, NC 27712
Biomerieux Inc. — 800-682-2666
100 Rodolphe Ave., Durham, NC 27712
Carochem, Inc. — 919-682-5121
744 E. Markham Avenue, Box 15699, Durham, NC 27701
Chesson Laboratory Associates, Inc. — 919-636-5773
603 Ellis Road, Durham, NC 27703
Confidant International, Llc — 919-806-4323
2530 Meridian Parkway, Suite 300, Durham, NC 27713
Dartnell Corporation — 800-223-8720
222 Sedwick Dr., Durham, NC 27713
Database, Inc. — 919-493-6969
3100 Tower Blvd., Suite 304, Durham, NC 27707-7105
Heart Imaging Technologies, Llc — 919-384-5044
5003 Southpark Dr., Suite 140, Durham, NC 27713
Lab Corp Of America — 800-833-3984
1904 Alexander Drive, Durham, NC 27709-2652
MDxHealth Inc. — 919-281-0980
2505 Meridian Parkway, Suite 310, DURHAM, NC 27713
Metabolon Inc. — 919-572-1711
617 Davis Drive, Suite 400, Durham, NC 27713
Micell Technologies Inc. — 919-313-2102
801 Capitola Drive, Suite 1, Durham, NC 27713
National Welders — 919-544-3772
630 United Dr., Durham, NC 27713
Pomdevices LLC — 866-514-0325
5302 NC Highway 55, Suite 102, Durham, NC 27713
Tecan U.S., Inc. — 1 800 352 5128
4022 Stirrup Creek Rd., Ste. 310, Durham, NC 27709
Teleflex Medical — 919-433-4829
1805 A Tw Alexander Drive, Durham, NC 27703
Triangle Biomedical Sciences, Inc. — 919-384-9393
3014 Croasdaile Drive, Durham, NC 27705-2507
Tryton Medical, Inc. — 919-226-1490
1000 Park Forty Plaza, Suite 325, Durham, NC 27713

Farmville

Carolina Medical Products Co. — 800-227-6637
8026 Us 264 Alternate, P.o. Box 147, Farmville, NC 27828

Forest Oaks

Precision Fabrics Group, Inc. — 888-733-5759
301 E. Meadowview Rd., Forest Oaks, NC 27406

Franklin

Tektone Sound & Signal Manufacturing, Inc. — 828-524-9967
277 Industrial Park Rd., Franklin, NC 28734

Gastonia

Scivolutions, Inc. — 704-853-0100
2260 Raeford Court, Gastonia, NC 28052

Greensboro

Bio Air Systems Div. — 336-299-2885
PO Box 18547, Greensboro, NC 27419-8547
Convatec — 800-422-8811
211 American Ave., Greensboro, NC 27409
Kayser-Roth Corp. — 800-575-3497
102 Corporate Center Blvd., Greensboro, NC 27408
Keller Crescent — 508-478-7641
1072 Boulder Road, Greensboro, NC 27409
Medsci, Inc. — 336-274-3496
201 Pine St., Greensboro, NC 27401
Plastek Industries, Inc. — 336-271-3210
880 Huffman St., Greensboro, NC 27405
Stair Systems, Inc. — 336-852-9122
3723-a West Market Street, Greensboro, NC 27403

Greenville

Attends Healthcare Products — 252-752-1100
1029 Old Creek Road, Greenville, NC 27834
Eye Expert, Llc. — 866-393-3973
2501-B Stantonsburg Rd., Greenville, NC 27834
Janus Development Group, Inc. — 866-551-9042
112 Staton Rd., Greenville, NC 27834
Lba Technology, Inc. — 252-757-0279
3400 Tupper Dr., Greenville, NC 27834

Speecheasy International, Llc — 252-551-9042
112 Staton Rd., Greenville, NC 27834

Haw River

Andersen Products, Inc., — 800-523-1276
Health Science Park, 3202 Caroline Drive, Haw River, NC 27258-9564

Henderson

Air Control, Inc. — 252-492-2300
237 Raleigh Rd., Henderson, NC 27536-1738

Hendersonville

Coats American, Inc. — 704-329-5800
Rt. 64 West, Hendersonville, NC 27739
Oxlife Llc — 828-684-7353
141 Twin Springs Rd., Hendersonville, NC 28792

Hickory

Best Orthopedic And Medical Services, Inc. — 800-344-5279
2356-B Springs Road NE, Hickory, NC 28601
P M Assoc. — 828-324-5739
826 Airport Road, Hickory, NC 28601

High Point

Concept Plastics, Inc. — 336-889-2001
1210 Hickory Chapel, High Point, NC 27260
Taylor's Mfg. — 336-886-4192
524 Barker Ave, High Point, NC 27262

Hillsborough

Eagle Water Systems Of The Triangle — 919-688-1111
507-C Cornerstone Court, Hillsborough, NC 27278
Kaye Products, Inc. — 919-732-6444
535 Dimmocks Mill Rd., Hillsborough, NC 27278-2352
Medtec, Inc. — 919-241-1400
600 Meadowland Drive, Hillsborough, NC 27278
Monitor Instruments Inc. — 800-853-6785
437 Dimmocks Mill Road, Hillsborough, NC 27278-2300
R Medical Supply — 800-882-7578
620 Valley Forge Rd, #F, Hillsborough, NC 27278
Rehabilitation Technical Components, Corp. — 919-732-1705
3913 Devonwood Road, Hillsborough, NC 27278

Hudson

Adhezion Biomedical, Llc — 610-431-2398
506 Pine Mountain Rd., Hudson, NC 28638
Beocare Inc., Hudson — 353-643-9400
1905, International Blvd., Hudson, NC 28638

Huntersville

Fisher Diagnostics — 877-722-4366
11515 Vanstory Drive, Suite 125, Huntersville, NC 28078

Jefferson

American Emergency Vehicles — 800-374-9749
165 American Way, Jefferson, NC 28640

Kannapolis

Grayson O Company — 800-435-1508
6509 Newell Ave., Kannapolis, NC 28081

Kenly

Medcovers, Inc — 800-948-8917
500 W. Goldsboro Street, Kenly, NC 27542

Kernersville

The Pandah Co. — 336-993-4579
408 Drayton Park, Kernersville, NC 27284

King

Carolina Medical, Inc. — 800-334-4531
157 Industrial Dr., King, NC 27021-0307

Kinston

Wall Lenk Corp. — 252-527-4186
PO Box 3349, Kinston, NC 28502-3349

Lawndale

Irradia Ab — 800-300-5558
736 W. Double Shaols Rd, Lawndale, NC 28090

Leicester

Dynamic Systems, Inc. — 828-683-3523
104 Morrow Branch, Leicester, NC 28748

Leland

Cdb Corporation — 910-383-6464
9201 Industrial Blvd. NE, Leland, NC 28451

Lenoir

Greer Laboratories, Inc. — 800-419-7302
639 NuWay Circle, PO Box 800, Lenoir, NC 28645-0800

Liberty

Gen Trak, Inc.   800-221-7407
121 W. Swannanoa Ave., P.O. Box 1290, Liberty, NC 27298

Lincolnton

Actavis Mid Atlantic Llc   704-735-5700
1877 Kawai Rd., Lincolnton, NC 28092

Linwood

Kimberly-Clark Corp.   888-525-8388
389 Clyde Fitzgerald Rd, Linwood, NC 27299

Littleton

Tmj Appliance   800 865-7246
130 Black Ferry Court, Littleton, NC 27850

Marion

Baxter Healthcare Corporation   847-473-6141
65 Pitts Station Road, Marion, NC 28752
Foothills Industries, Inc.   828-652-4088
300 Rockwell Drive, Marion, NC 28752
Simple Slant   828-245-8962
1218 Spooky Hollow Rd., Marion, NC 28752

Matthews

Preventive Technologies, Inc.   704-849-2416
1150 Crews Rd., Suite H, Matthews, NC 28105
Snug Seat, Inc.   800-336-7684
12801 E. Independence Blvd., PO Box 1739, Matthews, NC 28106

Mocksville

Ventlab Corp.   336-753-5000
155 Boyce Drive, Mocksville, NC 27028
Ventlab Corporation   800-593-4654
155 Boyce Dr., Mocksville, NC 27028

Monroe

General Hospital Supply Corp.   704-225-9500
2844 Gray Fox Rd., Monroe, NC 28110
Greiner Bio-One North America, Inc.   410-592-2060
4238 Capital Dr., Monroe, NC 28110
Rx Textiles, Inc.   704-283-9787
3107 Chamber Dr., Monroe, NC 28110

Mooresville

Lotus Technology, Inc.   704-658-0406
110 Talbert Pointe Drive, Mooresville, NC 28117

Morehead City

Bally Refrigerated Boxes, Inc.   800-24-BALLY
135 Little Nine Drive, Morehead City, NC 28557
Concept Marketing, Inc.   800-926-3277
1000 Arendell St., Morehead City, NC 28557

Morgantown

Mylan Pharmaceuticals Inc   888-523-7835
Research Triangle Pa, Morgantown, NC 27709

Morrisville

Empiric Systems, Llc   866-367-4742
3800 Paramount Pkwy, Suite 130, Morrisville, NC 27560
Paragondx, Llc   919-653-4748
133 Southcenter Ct., Suite 200, Bay 2, Morrisville, NC 27560
Sicel Technologies, Inc.   919-465-2236
3800 Gateway Centre Blvd., Suite 308, Morrisville, NC 27560
Suntech Medical, Inc.   800-421-8626
507 Airport Boulevard, Suite 117, Morrisville, NC 27560-8200
TearScience Inc.   919-467-4007
5151 McCrimmon Parkway, Ste 250, Morrisville, NC 27560
nContact Inc.   919-466-9810
1001 Aviation Parkway, Suite 400, Morrisville, NC 27560

Mount Airy

Renfro Corporation   336-719-8345
661 Linville Road, Mount Airy, NC 27030

Mount Gilead

Compsee, Inc.   800-628-3888
400 N. Main St., PO Box 1209, Mount Gilead, NC 27306

Murphy

Micro Audiometrics Corp.   800-729-9509
655 Keller Road, Murphy, NC 28906-5890

Newton

Moretz, Inc.   800-438-9127
514 W. 21st St., PO Box 580, Newton, NC 28658-3763
Sarstedt, Inc.   800-257-5101
PO Box 468, 1025, St. James Church Road, Newton, NC 28658-0468

Raleigh

Closure Medical   888-257-7633
5250 Greens Dairy Rd., Raleigh, NC 27616

Datafirst Corp.   800-634-8504
5124 Departure Drive, Raleigh, NC 27616
Fil-Chem, Inc.   919-788-0909
PO Box 90833, Raleigh, NC 27675
Icardiogram, Incorporated   919-534-2150
333 Six Forks Road,, Raleigh, NC 27609
Inc Research   866-462-7373
4700 Falls of Neuse Road, Suite 400, Raleigh, NC 27609
Inspire Pharmaceuticals, Inc.   919-941-9777
8081 Arco Corporate Drive,, Suite 400, Raleigh, NC 27617
Mallinckrodt, Inc.   800-325-8888
8800 Durant Rd., Raleigh, NC 27616
Raleigh Lions Clinic For The Blind, Inc.   919-256-4220
3200 Bush St., Raleigh, NC 27609

Research Triangle Park

Hydro Service & Supplies, Inc.   800-950-7426
PO Box 12197, Research Triangle Park, NC 27709
Innerpulse Inc.   919-287-4100
4025 Stirrup Creek Dr., Suite 200, Research Triangle Park, NC 27703
Mustard Tree Instruments   919-972-7920
PO Box 14527, 10 Laboratory Drive, Bldg 2, Suite 200, Research Triangle Park, NC 27709
Research Triangle Institute   866-RTI-1958
3040 Cornwallis Rd., PO Box 12194, Research Triangle Park, NC 27709
Stiefel   888-784-3335
20 T.W. Alexander Drive, Research Triangle Park, NC 27709
Teleflex Medical   800-334-9751
2917 Weck Drive, Research Triangle Park, NC 27709
Teleflex Medical   866-246-6990
4024 Stirrup Creek, Research Triangle Park, NC 27703

Rocky Mount

Hospira, Inc.   877-946-7747
Hwy. 301 North, Rocky Mount, NC 27801

Rocky Point

Del Pharmaceuticals, Inc.(Subsidiary Of Del Labora   516-844-2020
1830 Carver Drive, Rocky Point, NC 28457

Rural Hall

Carolon Company   800-334-0414
601 Forum Pkwy., Rural Hall, NC 27045

Rutherfordton

Alliance Hearing Systems   828-286-9399
431 South Main St., Suite #6, Rutherfordton, NC 28139

Salisbury

Centurion Medical Products Corp.   517-545-1135
3310 South Main St., Salisbury, NC 28147

Sanford

Trion, Inc.   800-884-0002
101 McNeil Road, Sanford, NC 27330

Shelby

Medical Engineering Laboratory, Inc.   704-487-0166
108 West Warren St., Suite 207, Shelby, NC 28150
Shelby Elastics, Llc Of North Carolina   800-562-4507
639 North Post Rd., Shelby, NC 28150

Southern Pines

Eel Electronics Mfg. Co.   910-944-4780
160 South May St., Suite #2, Southern Pines, NC 28387

Sparta

Amano Pioneer Eclipse Corp.   800-334-2246
1 Eclipse Road, PO Box 909, Sparta, NC 28675

Spring Hope

The Sewing Source, Inc.   800-849-6945
802 East Nash St., Spring Hope, NC 27882

Stanley

Deb Sbs, Inc.   704-263-4240
1100 Highway 27, Stanley, NC 28164

Statesville

Kewaunee Scientific Corp.   704-873-7202
2700 West Front Street, PO Box 1842, Statesville, NC 28677
M.B.S. Fabricating & Coating, Inc.   704-871-1830
174a Crawford Rd, Po Box 249, Statesville, NC 28687
Medi-Garb Co., Inc.   800-233-2463
216 W. Broad St., Statesville, NC 28687
Toter, Inc.   800-772-0071
841 Meacham Road, PO Box 5338, Statesville, NC 28677-2983
Zimmer Orthopaedic Surgical Products   704-873-1001
P.O. Box 1838, 2021 Old Mountain Rd., Statesville, NC 28687

Sylva

Webster Enterprises Of Jackson County, Inc.   828-586-8981
140 Little Savannah Rd., Sylva, NC 28779

Taylorsville

Alarm Electronics Mfg. Co. Inc.   800-444-3365
44 All Healing Springs Rd., Taylorsville, NC 28681

Thomasville

Goodwin Manufacturing, Inc.   800-282-5267
6980 Pike View Drive, PO Box 5981, Thomasville, NC 27370

Trinity

Sealy Inc.   800-697-3259
One Office Parkway, Trinity, NC 27370

Waxhaw

Kadan Co. Inc., D.A.   800-325-2326
1 Brigadoon Lane, Waxhaw, NC 28173-8574

Waynesville

HVO   1-800-789-0416
56 Scates St., Waynesville, NC 28786

Weaverville

Ots Corp.   800-221-4769
220 Merrimon Avenue, Weaverville, NC 28787

Webster

Webster Enterprises, Inc.   704-586-8981
P.O. Box 220, Webster, NC 28788-0220

West Jefferson

General Assembly Corporation   877-GACNC4U
140 Industrial Park Way, West Jefferson, NC 28694

Whitsett

Medi Mfg., Inc.   336-449-4440
6481 Franz Warner Pkwy., Whitsett, NC 27377
Medi Usa   800-633-6334
6481 Franz Warner Parkway, Whitsett, NC 27377

Wilmington

Arw Optical Corp.   910-452-7373
6631 B. Amsterdam Way, Wilmington, NC 28405
Biocomposites Inc.   910-350-8015
PO Box 2692, Wilmington, NC 28402
Buxco Research Systems   910-794-6980
219 Station Road, Suite 202, Wilmington, NC 28405
Camag Scientific, Inc.   800-334-3909
515 Cornelius Harnett Dr., Wilmington, NC 28401
Ika-Works, Inc.   800-733-3037
2635 N. Chase Pkwy. S.E., Wilmington, NC 28405-7419
Nurses Choice Specialty Textiles   910-452-1500
6611 Amsterdam Wy., Wilmington, NC 28405
Omega Medical Electronics Ltd.   910-763-9331
725 Wellington Avenue, Wilmington, NC 28401
Scotty Technology Of The Americas, Inc.   910-395-6100
6714 Netherlands Drive, Wilmington, NC 28405
Trans1 Incorporated   910-332-1700
411 Landmark Dr., Wilmington, NC 28412
Xero Products   888-937-6769
349 Military Cutoff Road, Wilmington, NC 28405

Wilson

Livedo Usa, Inc.   252-237-1373
4925 Livedo Dr., Wilson, NC 27893

Winston Salem

Charter Medical Ltd.   866-458-3116
3948-A Westpoint Blvd, Winston Salem, NC 27103
Cook Endoscopy   336-744-0157
4900 Bethania Station Rd. &, 5951 Grassy Creek Blvd., Winston Salem, NC 27105
Presco-Webber Corporation   336-722-1067
440 Cotton St., Winston Salem, NC 27101-5071
Thermcraft, Inc   336-784-4800
3950 Overdale Road, PO Box 12037, Winston Salem, NC 27117-2037
Wilson-Cook Medical, Inc.   336-744-0157
4900 Bethania Station Rd., Winston Salem, NC 27105

Winston-salem

C Change Surgical Llc   877.989.3737
101 North Chestnut Street, Suite 301, Winston-salem, NC 27101
Carolina Narrow Fabric Co.   336-631-3000
1100 Patterson Ave., Winston-salem, NC 27101
Mri Cardiac Services, Incorporated   336-831-1908
8 West Third St. Suite M-9, Winston-Salem, NC 27101

Youngsville

Apogee Medical, Llc   919-570-9605
90 Weathers St., Youngsville, NC 27596
Sirchie Finger Print Laboratories   800-356-7311
100 Hunter Place, Youngsville, NC 27596

NORTH DAKOTA

Cavalier

Spinal Designs Intl.   701-265-4927
708 Division Ave S., Cavalier, ND 58220

Fargo

Precision Dental Laboratories, Inc.   701-280-9089
6 Broadway Suite 200, Fargo, ND 58102

Neche

Arrow Industries Llc   701-886-7722
530 5th Street, Neche, ND 58265-4033
Designer Care Co., Ltd.   800-848-6335
474 Main Avenue, Neche, ND 58265

Pembina

Radix Corp.   204-697-2349
#2-572 South Fifth St., Pembina, ND 58271

Valley City

Fitness Plus, Inc.   888-778-4019
PO Box 516, Suite 280, Valley City, ND 58072
Tri W-G Group   800-437-8011
215 12th Avenue NE, PO Box 905, Valley City, ND 58072-0905

Williston

H & S Manufacturing, Inc.   800-827-3091
727 E. Broadway, Williston, ND 58801-6105

OHIO

Akron

Akro-Mils, Inc.   800-253-2467
1293 S. Main St., Akron, OH 44301
Biofreeze Performance Health, Inc.   800-246-3733
1245 Home Ave, Akron, OH 44310
Diamond Polymers, Inc.   888-437-4674
1353 Exeter Rd., Akron, OH 44306
Gojo Industries, Inc   800-321-9647
One GOJO Plaza, Suite 500, Akron, OH 44311
Integra Spine   330-475-8600
1800 Triplett Blvd., Akron, OH 44306
Jeter Systems Corp.   877-252-0220
The National City Center, Suite #110, One Cascade Plaza, Akron, OH 44308
Kiltex Corp.   330-644-6746
2064 Killian Road, Akron, OH 44312
Medical Safety Systems Inc.   888-803-9303
230 White Pond Drive, Akron, OH 44313
Miller's Adaptive Technologies   800-837-4544
2023 Romig Road, Akron, OH 44320-3819
Pain Management Technologies   888-267-5422
1340 Home Ave. Building A, Akron, OH 44310
Polysort   330-665-5918
4000 Embassy Pkwy., Suite 400, Akron, OH 44333
R.C.A. Rubber Company, The   800-321-2340
1833 E. Market St., P.O. Box 9240, Akron, OH 44305-0240
Rea Incorporated   330-666-7414
4808 Pin Oak Road, Akron, OH 44333
Saint-Gobain Performance Plastics--Akron   800-798-1554
2664 Gilchrist Rd., Akron, OH 44305
Spinematrix, Inc.   330-665-6780
202 Montrose West Ave., Suite 360, Akron, OH 44321
Surgical Table Services Co.   800-248-2382
526 South Main St., Akron, OH 44311
Surgical Table Services Company   330-253-7766
526 South Main St., Suite 701e, Akron, OH 44311
The Hygenic Corp.   800-321-2135
1245 Home Avenue, Akron, OH 44310-2575

Alliance

Jenex Corporation   800-496-4682
733 Overlook Drive, Alliance, OH 44601

Archbold

Gendron, Inc.   800-537-2521
400 E Lugbill Road, Archbold, OH 43502
Sauder Manufacturing Co.   800-537-1530
930 W. Barre Rd., Archbold, OH 43502

Ashland

Hospira   800-441-4100
268 E. Fourth St., Ashland, OH 44805-2494
Vista Research Group, Llc   419-281-3927
1554 Township Road 805, Ashland, OH 44805

Athens

Diagnostic Hybrids, Inc.   800-344-5847
1055 East State St., Suite 100, Athens, OH 45701

Aurora

Express Systems And Parts Network Inc   (888) 550-3776
325 Harris Drive, Aurora, OH 44202

Usa Instruments, Inc. — 330-562-1000
1515 Danner Dr., Aurora, OH 44202

Avon
Leisure Time — 440-934-1032
1284 Miller Rd., Avon, OH 44011-0276
Tri-Tech Medical, Inc. — 800-253-8692
35401 Avon Commerce Parkway, Avon, OH 44011
Western/Scott Fetzer Co. — 440-871-2160
1354 Lear Industrial Park, Avon, OH 44011

Barberton
Century Woodworking Corp. — 330-753-2024
846 Coventry Road, Barberton, OH 44203
Theken Orthopedic Llc — 330-753-9923
1100 Nola Avenue, Barberton, OH 44203

Batavia
American Micro Products, Inc. — 800-479-2193
4288 Armstrong Blvd., Batavia, OH 45103-1600

Beachwood
Leading Lady, Inc. — 216-464-5490
24050 Commerce Park Dr., Beachwood, OH 44122
Osteosecure — 1-877-734-8338
23230 Chagrin Blvd, Beachwood, OH 44122

Bedford
Brainmaster Technologies — 440-232-6000
195 Willis Street, Bedford, OH 44146
Marlen Manufacturing & Development Co. — 216-292-7060
5150 Richmond Rd., Bedford, OH 44146

Bedford Heights
Hawken Industries — 216-831-6782
26650 Renaissance Pkwy.,, Bedford Heights, OH 44128

Bellefontaine
Mobile Instrument Service And Repair, Inc. — 800-722-3675
333 Water Ave., Bellefontaine, OH 43311

Berea
Noshok, Inc. — 440-243-0888
1010 W. Bagley Rd., Berea, OH 44017

Berlin Center
Safeguard Medical Technologies, Llc — 330-547-2166
14200 Ellsworth Rd., Berlin Center, OH 44401

Bolivar
Nilodor, Inc. — 800-443-4321
10966 Industrial Pkwy., N.W., Bolivar, OH 44612

Brecksville
Applied Medical Technology, Inc. — 800-869-7382
8000 Katherine Boulevard, Brecksville, OH 44141

Brook Park
International Tanning Technologies — 800-832-8267
5225 W 140th St., Brook Park, OH 44142

Bryan
The Daavlin Company — 800-322-8546
205 West Bement Street, PO Box 626, Bryan, OH 43506

Burton
Troy Manufacturing Co. — 440-834-8262
17090 Rapids Road, PO Box 448, Burton, OH 44021

Cambridge
Encore Plastics Corporation — 419-626-8000
725 Water Street, Cambridge, OH 43725
Leyshon Miller Industries — 740-432-2969
534 N 1st St., Cambridge, OH 43725

Canal Fulton
Boyd Associates Inc. — 330-854-5433
465 Trelake Dr., Canal Fulton, OH 44614
Medical Science Products, Inc. — 800-456-1971
517 Elm Ridge Ave., Canal Fulton, OH 44614

Canton
Biocurv Medical Instruments, Inc. — 1-800-589-3043
245 Dryden CT SW, Canton, OH 44706
Glenn Medical Systems, Inc. — 800-394-0173
511 12th Street, N.e., Canton, OH 44704
Shared P.E.T. Imaging, Llc — 330-491-0480
4912 Higbee Ave, Nw Suite 100, Canton, OH 44718

Carrollton
Fisher Hearing Aid Service — 330-627-2002
25 Public Square, Carrollton, OH 44615

Centerville
Dimco Gray Co. — 800-876-8353
900 Dimco Way, Centerville, OH 45458-2709

Chagrin Falls
Arthroplastics, Inc. — 440-247-5131
34 West Washington St., P.o. Box 332, Chagrin Falls, OH 44022
Chagrin Safety Supply, Inc. — 800-227-0468
8227 East Washington Ave., Chagrin Falls, OH 44023
Environmental Growth Chambers — 800-321-6854
510 E. Washington St., Chagrin Falls, OH 44022
Vision Medical Instruments, Inc. — 440-338-5981
8147 Chagrin Mills Rd., Chagrin Falls, OH 44022

Chesterland
Research Instrumentation Associates, Inc. — 440-729-1649
8753 Mayfield Rd., Chesterland, OH 44026

Cheviot
Eqm Research, Inc. — 513-661-0560
3638 Glenmore Ave., Cheviot, OH 45211

Cincinnati
Agile Radiological Technologies — 877-985-9877
11180 Reed Hartman Hwy, Cincinnati, OH 45242
Airway Division Of Surgical Appliance Industries, Inc. — 800-888-0458
3960 Rosslyn Dr., Cincinnati, OH 45209-1110
Ardus Medical, Inc. — 800-878-1388
11297 Grooms Rd., Cincinnati, OH 45242
Casco Manufacturing Solutions, Inc. — 800-843-1339
3107 Spring Grove Avenue, Cincinnati, OH 45225
Chester Labs, Inc. — 800-354-9709
1900 Section Road, Cincinnati, OH 45237
Cincinnati Association For The Blind — 888-687-3935
2045 Gilbert Ave., Cincinnati, OH 45202-1403
Cincinnati Sub-Zero Products, Inc., Medical Division — 800-989-7373
12011 Mosteller Road, Cincinnati, OH 45241-1528
Cincinnati Surgical Company — 800-544-3100
11256 Cornell Park Dr., Cincinnati, OH 45242-0668
Cintas Corp. — 800-246-8271
6800 Cintas Blvd, P. O. Box 625737, Cincinnati, OH 45262-5737
Cole Vision Corporation — 770-305-7352
9926 International Blvd., Cincinnati, OH 45246
Contra Angle; Prophy Angle — 513-682-2520
9790 Inter-Ocean Dr., Cincinnati, OH 45246
Devicor Medical Products Inc. — 513.864.9000
300 E-Business Way, Fifth Floor, Cincinnati, OH 45241
Diversified Ophthalmics, Inc. — 800-626-2281
250 McCullough St., Cincinnati, OH 45226-2145
E&M Science — 513-631-0445
2909 Highland Ave., Cincinnati, OH 45212
Ethicon Endo-Surgery, Inc. — 800-USE-ENDO
4545 Creek Rd., MI #132, Cincinnati, OH 45242
Fairdale Orthodontic Co., Inc. — 513-421-2620
312 West 4th St., Cincinnati, OH 45202
HCI — 800-783-8105
113 Commerce Blvd, Cincinnati, OH 45140
Havel's Inc. — 800-638-4770
3726 Lonsdale, Cincinnati, OH 45227-3637
Integra Lifesciences Of Ohio — 800-654-2873
4900 Charlemar Drive, Building A, Cincinnati, OH 45227
Lenscrafters, Inc. — 770-305-7352
9926 International Blvd., Cincinnati, OH 45246
Meridian Bioscience, Inc. — 800-696-0739
3471 River Hills Dr., Cincinnati, OH 45244-3023
Merlyn Pharmaceuticals, Inc. — 513-831-3005
8175 Kroger Farm Rd., Cincinnati, OH 45243-1639
Newtron Products — 513-561-7373
3874 Virginia Ave, PO BOX 27175, Cincinnati, OH 45227
Omegapoint Systems, Llc — 513-241-7540
1077 Celestial St., Suite 400, Cincinnati, OH 45202
Pm Company — 800-327-4359
1500 Kemper Meadow Drive, Cincinnati, OH 45240-1638
Procter & Gamble — 800-764-7483
1 Procter and Gamble Plaza, Cincinnati, OH 45201
Recto Molded Products Inc., Quinn Healthcare Produ — 513-871-5544
4425 Appleton St., Cincinnati, OH 45209
Save The Gonads, Ltd. — 513-385-8147
P.O. Box 53111, Cincinnati, OH 45253
Schaerer Mayfield Usa — 800-755-6381
4900 Charlemar Drive, Cincinnati, OH 45227
So-Low Environmental Equipment — 513-772-9410
10310 Spartan Dr., Cincinnati, OH 45215-1277
Sonoco — 513-874-7655
4633 Dues Drive, Cincinnati, OH 45246-1008
Standard Textile — 800-999-0400
One Knollcrest Drive, Cincinnati, OH 45237
Standard Textile Co., Inc. — 888-999-0400
PO Box 371805, Cincinnati, OH 45222
Surgical Appliance Industries — 800-888-0458
3960 Rosslyn Dr., Cincinnati, OH 45209-1195
Thermo Fisher Scientific — 800-437-2999
PO Box 712099, Cincinnati, OH 45271

Truform Orthotics & Prosthetics — 800-888-0458
3960 Rosslyn Drive, Cincinnati, OH 45209-1110
United Air Specialists, Inc. — 800-252-4647
4440 Creek Rd., Cincinnati, OH 45242
Vantage Orthopedics — 513-563-1690
41 Techview Dr., Cincinnati, OH 45215
Whitman Corp. — 888-362-4535
1725 Powers St., Cincinnati, OH 45223-2499
3M Company — 513-272-5000
5801 Mariemont Ave., Cincinnati, OH 45227

Circleville

Health Care Logistics, Inc. — 800-848-1633
450 East Town St., PO Box 25, Circleville, OH 43113

Cleveland

Acor Orthopaedic, Inc. — 216-662-4500
18530 South Miles Pkwy., Cleveland, OH 44128-4238
Advanced Imaging Research, Inc. — 216-426-1461
4700 Lakeside Ave., Suite 400, Cleveland, OH 44114
All-Tronics Medical Systems — 800-ALL-TRON
3289 E. 55th St., Cleveland, OH 44127-1501
Bradley Company, A Sub. Of Xerox Corporation — 216-292-7220
4829 Galaxy Parkway, Cleveland, OH 44128
Cardinal Health 2200, Inc — 847-578-6442
17820 Englewood Dr, Cleveland, OH 44130
Cardioinsight Technologies Inc. — 216-453-5950
11000 Cedar Avenue, Suite 210, Cleveland, OH 44106
Cleveland Medical Devices, Inc. — 877-253-8363
4415 Euclid Avenue, Suite 400, Cleveland, OH 44103
Custom Paper Tubes Inc. — 800-864-1793
15900 Industrial Parkway, Cleveland, OH 44135
Fertility Solutions, Inc. — 800-959-7656
13000 Shaker Blvd., Cleveland, OH 44120
Gebauer Company — 800-321-9348
4444 East 153rd Street, Cleveland, OH 44128
Golda, Inc. — 800-321-4804
24050 Commerce Park, Cleveland, OH 44122-5824
Great Lakes Medical — 800-337-8243
18683 Sheldon Rd., Cleveland, OH 44130
Greatbatch Inc — 1 216-937-2800
1771 East 30th St., Cleveland, OH 44114
Hospital Specialty Company — 800-321-9832
26301 Curtiss-Wright Parkway, Cleveland, OH 44143
Icon Interventional Systems, Inc. — 216-382-3119
1414 South Green Rd., Suite 309, Cleveland, OH 44121
Imalux Corporation — 216-502-0755
11000 Cedar Avenue, Suite 250, Cleveland, OH 44106
Innovative Medical Products-Pjc,Llc — 216-961-8735
3510 Chatham Road, Cleveland, OH 44113
Innovative Wound Management, Llc — 866-527-3706
29001 Cedar Rd, Suite 325, Cleveland, OH 44124
Kapp Surgical Instrument, Inc. — 800-282-5277
4919 Warrensville Center Rd., Cleveland, OH 44128
Kindt Collins Co. — 800-321-3170
12651 Elmwood Ave., Cleveland, OH 44111
Kroy, Llc — 888-888-5769
3830 Kelly Avenue, Cleveland, OH 44114
Lab Fabricators Company — 888-431-5444
1802 E. 47th St., Cleveland, OH 44103-2468
Lincoln Electric Co. — 216-481-8100
22801 St. Clair Ave., Cleveland, OH 44117-1199
Meriam Process Technologies — 216-281-1100
10920 Madison Avenue, Cleveland, OH 44102-2599
Mimvista Corp. — 216-896-9798
25200 Chagrin Blvd. Suite 200, Cleveland, OH 44122
Misco Refractometer — 866-831-1999
3401 Virginia Rd., Cleveland, OH 44122-4218
Ndi Medical, Inc. — 216-378-9106
22901 Millcreek Blvd.,, Suite 110, Cleveland, OH 44122
Pemco, Inc. - Medical Div. — 216-524-2990
5663 Brecksville Road, Cleveland, OH 44131-1510
Pharaoh Trading Company — 866-929-4913
Knollwood Plaza, Suite 241, 9701 Brookpark Road, Cleveland, OH 44129-6824
Philips Medical Systems(Cleveland), Inc. — 440-483-3765
595 Miner Rd., Cleveland, OH 44143
Precision Production, Inc. — 216-252-0372
15215 Chatfield Ave., Cleveland, OH 44111
Prince & Izant Nutec Metal Joining — 216-362-7000
12999 Plaza Drive, Cleveland, OH 44130
Prognostix, Inc. — 216-445-1380
10265 Carnegie Avenue, Cleveland, OH 44106
Quality Electrodynamics — 440-484-2228
777 Beta Drive, Cleveland, OH 44143
Redi-Tech Medical Products,Llc — 800-824-1793
529 Front Street, Suite 125, Cleveland, OH 44017
Research Organics, Inc. — 800-321-0570
4353 East 49th Street, Cleveland, OH 44125-1083
Rozinn By Scottcare Corporation — 800-243-9412
4791 West 150th Street, Cleveland, OH 44135
Rsb Spine Llc. — 866-241-2104
2530 Superior Ave., Suite 703, Cleveland, OH 44114

Scottcare Corporation — 800-243-9412
4791 W. 150th St., Cleveland, OH 44135
Singleton Corp. — 888-456-0643
3280 W. 67th Place, Cleveland, OH 44102
Sonogage, Inc. — 216-464-1119
26650 Renaissance Pkwy., Cleveland, OH 44128
State Chemical Manufacturing Co. — 800-321-8180
3100 Hamilton Ave., Cleveland, OH 44114
Superior Products, Inc. — 216-651-9400
3786 Ridge Rd., Cleveland, OH 44144
The Reese Pharmaceutical Co. — 800-321-7178
10617 Frank Ave., Cleveland, OH 44106
Tradex International — 800-456-8370
5300 Tradex Pkwy, Cleveland, OH 44102
Trek Diagnostic Systems — 800-871-8909
982 Keynote Circle, Ste. 6, Cleveland, OH 44131
Wendell-Alan Ltd. — 216-881-8299
1768 East 25th St., Cleveland, OH 44114
Wilson Optical Laboratories, Inc. — 866-216-6225
190 Alpha Park, Cleveland, OH 44143

Cleveland Heights

Accor, Inc. — 216-381-2951
1375 Yellowstone Rd., Cleveland Heights, OH 44121

Coldwater

Health Care Products, Inc. — 419-678-9620
410 Nisco St., Coldwater, OH 45828

Columbus

Abbott Laboratories — 800-624-7677
1033 Kingsmill Pkwy., Columbus, OH 43229
Abbott Laboratories — 847-937-2388
6480 busch blvd., Columbus, OH 43229
Accu Scan Instruments, Inc. — 800-822-1344
5098 Trabue Road, Columbus, OH 43228-9563
Ametek Solidstate Controls — 800-635-7300
875 Dearborn Dr., Columbus, OH 43085
Artromick — 800-848-6462
4800 Hilton Corporate Dr., Columbus, OH 43232
Artromick International, Inc. — 800-848-6462
4800 Hilton Corporate Drive, Columbus, OH 43232-4150
Bertec Corporation — 877-237-8320
6171 Huntley Rd., Suite J, Columbus, OH 43229
Bioflex, Inc. — 614-236-8079
3055 Templeton Rd., Columbus, OH 43209
Boehringer Ingelheim Roxane Inc. — 614-241-4135
1809 Wilson Rd., P.o. Box 16532, Columbus, OH 43228
Control-X Medical, Inc. — 800-777-9729
1755 Atlas Street, Columbus, OH 43228-9648
Dick Medical Supply, Llc — 614-444-2300
630 Marion Rd., Columbus, OH 43207
Entylon Ltd. — info@enlyton.ne
7700 Rivers Edge Drive, Columbus, OH 43235
Gfs Chemicals, Inc. — 800-858-9682
867 Mckinley Avenue, Columbus, OH 43222-1148
Harrop Industries, Inc. — 614-231-3621
3470 E. Fifth Ave., Columbus, OH 43219-1797
Larson Medical Products, Inc. — 614-235-9100
2844 Banwick Rd., Columbus, OH 43232
Mcgill Airpressure Corp. — 614-829-1200
1777 Refugee Road, Columbus, OH 43207-2119
Mettler-Toledo, Inc. — 800-638-8537
1900 Polaris Pkwy., Columbus, OH 43240
Morrison Medical — 800-438-6677
3735 Paragon Drive, Columbus, OH 43228
Nucon International, Inc. — 800-992-5192
7000 Huntley Rd., Columbus, OH 43229
Ortheon Medical, Llc. — 866-836-6349
777 West Swan Street, Columbus, OH 43212
Roxane Laboratories — 800-962-8364
P.O. Box 16532, Columbus, OH 43216-6532

Concord Twp

Faretec, Inc. — 440-350-9510
1610 W. Jackson St. #6, Concord Twp, OH 44077

Cuyahoga Falls

Coltene/Whaledent Inc. — 330-916-8858
235 Ascot Parkway, Cuyahoga Falls, OH 44223
Dentronix, Inc. — 800-523-5944
235 Ascot Parkway, Cuyahoga Falls, OH 44223
Juzo — 800-222-4999
80 Chart Road, PO Box 1088, Cuyahoga Falls, OH 44223-0088

Dayton

Adtech Systems Research, Inc — 937-426-3329
1342 N. Fairfield Rd., Dayton, OH 45432
American Thermal Instruments, Inc. — 937-429-2114
2400 E. River Road, Dayton, OH 45439
Ameriwater — 937-461-8833
1303 Stanley Ave., Dayton, OH 45404
Argus-Hazco — 800-332-0435
6501 Centerville Business Pkwy., Dayton, OH 45459

Ashton Pumpmatic, Inc. 800-395-1012
858 Distribution Drive, Dayton, OH 45434
Fc Industries Inc. 937-275-8700
4900 Webster Street, Dayton, OH 45414
Forward Motions, Inc. 877-364-8267
214 Valley St., Dayton, OH 45404-1839
Gerstner & Sons Inc. 937-228-1662
20 Gerstner Way, Dayton, OH 45402-3408
Globe Motors 937-228-3171
2275 Stanley Ave., Dayton, OH 45404
Mauch, Inc. 800-622-8742
3035 Dryden Road, Dayton, OH 45439-1619
Medical Soft, Inc. 937-293-2575
1800 Southwood Ln. West, Dayton, OH 45419
Ncr Corp. 800-225-5627
1700 S. Patterson Blvd., Dayton, OH 45479-0001
Quality Software Systems 800-777-3020
210 B East Spring Valley Rd., Dayton, OH 45458
Shumsky Therapeutic Products 888-333-3677
811 E 4th St, Dayton, OH 45402
Simon Dechatlet Labs 952-541-9622
4484 North Dixie Drive, Dayton, OH 45414
Southpaw Enterprises, Inc. 800-228-1698
PO Box 1047, Dayton, OH 45401
Tabtronics, Inc. 937-222-9969
2153 Winners Circle, Dayton, OH 45404
Tipp Machine & Tool, Inc. 937-387-0880
4201 Little York Road, Dayton, OH 45414
Usaeroteam 937-226-1900
1300 Grange Hall Road, Dayton, OH 45430

Defiance

Defiance Metal Prod Co. 419-784-5332
21 Seneca St., Defiance, OH 43512

Delaware

Greif, Inc. 502-245-6599
425 Winter Road, Delaware, OH 43015

Dover

Zimmer Orthopaedic Surgical Products 800-321-5533
P.O. Box 10, 200 West Ohio Ave., Dover, OH 44622

Dublin

Bound Tree Medical 800-533-0523
PO Box 8023, Dublin, OH 43016-2023
Bound Tree Medical, Llc 800-533-0523
5200 Rings Road, Suite A, Dublin, OH 43017
Cardinal Health 888-571-5950
7000 Cardinal Place, Dublin, OH 43017
Cardinal Health Inc. 614-757-5000
7000 Cardinal Place, q&r department, Dublin, OH 43017
Neoprobe Corporation 800-793-0079
425 Metro Place North, Suite 300, Dublin, OH 43017
Nuclear Pharmacy Services 614-757-5000
7000 Cardinal Place, Dublin, OH 43017
Opticon Medical 614-336-2000
7001 Post Road, Suite 100, Dublin, OH 43016
Perio Products, Inc. 800-841-3221
6156 Wilcox Rd., Dublin, OH 43016
Smiths Medical Asd, Inc. 1 800 258 5361
5200 Upper Metro Place, Suite 200, Dublin, OH 43017
Smiths Medical OEM 800-258-5361
5200 Upper Metro Place, Suite 200, Dublin, OH 43017

Dunbridge

Principle Business Ent. 1-800-467-3224
Pine Lake Industrial Pk., Dunbridge, OH 43414
Principle Business Enterprises, Inc. 800-467-3224
Pine Lake Industrial Park, P.O. Box 129, Dunbridge, OH 43414-0129

Eastlake

Dmz/Timco Machine Company 440-942-4001
35530 Lakeland Blvd., Eastlake, OH 44095-5305
Enpac Corp. 800-936-7229
34355 Vokes Drive, Eastlake, OH 44095-4033
Taga Medical Technologies 800-651-9490
34675 Vokes Drive, Suite 105, Eastlake, OH 44095

Eaton

Electro-Cap International, Inc. 800-527-2193
1011 W. Lexington Road, PO Box 87, Eaton, OH 45320

Elyria

Elyria Plastic Products 440-322-8577
710 Taylor St., Elyria, OH 44035
Invacare Corporation 800-333-6900
One Invacare Way, Elyria, OH 44035

Euclid

Accommodata Corporation 216-732-8888
20950 Edgecliff Road, Euclid, OH 44123

Fairborn

Control Bionics 202-257-7090
333 North Broad St., Fairborn, OH 45324
Therapeutic Alliances, Inc. 937-879-0734
333 North Broad St., Fairborn, OH 45324

Fairport Harbor

Quartz Scientific, Inc. 800-229-2186
819 East St., Fairport Harbor, OH 44077-5564

Franklin

NanoDetection Technology, Inc 937-550-4502
301 Industrial Drive, Suite B, Franklin, OH 45005

Fremont

Crescent Mfg. Co. 800-537-1330
1310 Majestic Dr., Fremont, OH 43420
Crown Mats 800-628-5463
2100 Commerce Drive, Fremont, OH 43420-1014

Gahanna

Milian Usa 614-416-1600
1000-B Taylor Staion Rd, Gahanna, OH 43230

Garfield Heights

AxioMed Spine Corporation 216-587-5566
5350 Transportation Blvd., Suite 18, Garfield Heights, OH 44125

Geneva

Advanced Medical Systems, Inc. 440-466-8005
101 N. Eagle St., Geneva, OH 44041

Germantown

Point Source Inc. 937-855-6020
1864 Dayton Pike, Germantown, OH 45327

Girard

Innovative Concepts 800-676-5030
300 N. State St., Girard, OH 44420

Green

Idea, Inc. 330-896-2300
3755 Boettler Oaks Dr., Green, OH 44685

Greenville

Vector Vision 800-526-7703
1850 Livingston Rd, Suite E, Greenville, OH 45331

Grove City

Burton Co., R.H. 800-848-0410
3965 Brookham Drive, Grove City, OH 43123-0068
Horton Emergency Vehicles 614-539-8181
3800 McDowell Rd., Grove City, OH 43123
Mckelor Technologies, Ltd. 800-273-5233
6312 Seeds Road, Grove City, OH 43123
Photovac Laser Corp., Inc. 614-875-3300
3513 Farm Bank Way, Grove City, OH 43123
Tosoh Bioscience, Inc. 614-317-1909
3600 Gantz Road, Grove City, OH 43123

Hamilton

Elra Industries, Inc. 800-654-3066
550 South Erie Highway, Hamilton, OH 45011-4346
Hamilton Caster & Mfg. Co. 888-699-7164
1637 Dixie Hwy., Hamilton, OH 45011-4087
Kees Goebel Medical Specialties, Inc. 800-354-0445
9663 Glades Drive, Hamilton, OH 45011

Hilliard

Touch Bionics 614-388-8075
3455 Mill Run Drive, Hilliard, OH 43026

Hinckley

Cytocolor, Inc. 800-776-6455
P.O. Box 401, Hinckley, OH 44233-9747

Hudson

King's Medical 330-653-3968
1894 Georgetown Rd., Hudson, OH 44236-4065
Vartec Solutions, Inc. 330-655-7930
7570 Foxdale Circle, Hudson, OH 44236

Kent

Emergency Products And Research 305-304-6933
890 West Main Street, Kent, OH 44240
H&M Rubber Company, Inc. 330-678-3323
4200 Mogadore Rd., Kent, OH 44240-7258
Harmonizer 330-677-0771
448 Silver Oaks Drive Unit 5, Kent, OH 44240
Kapco (Kent Adhesive Products Co.) 800-791-8964
1000 Cherry St., Kent, OH 44240-7520
Kent Elastomer Products, Inc. 800-331-4762
1500 St. Clair Avenue, PO Box 668, Kent, OH 44240-0668

Sorbothane, Inc.
2144 State Rte. 59, Kent, OH 44240-7142 — 800-838-3906
Sportsguard Laboratories, Inc.
267 Martinel Dr, Kent, OH 44240 — 800-401-1776

Kettering
Fall Prevention Technologies, Llc
4601 Gateway Circle, Kettering, OH 45440 — 937-434-5455

Leipsic
Duraline Medical Products, Inc.
324 Werner St., P.O. Box 67, Leipsic, OH 45856 — 800-654-3376

Lewis Center
Abrasive Technology, Inc.
8400 Green Meadows Dr., Lewis Center, OH 43035 — 740-548-4100
Gilson Company, Inc.
PO Box 200, Lewis Center, OH 43035-0200 — 800-444-1508

Lexington
Global Medical Foam, Inc.
124 Plymouth Street, Suite A, Lexington, OH 44904 — 419-529-9354

Lima
Adaptive Medical Concepts, Inc.
1378 Bellefontaine Ave., Lima, OH 45804 — 800-443-7863

Lockbourne
Cole Vision Corp.
2150 Bixby Road, Lockbourne, OH 43137 — 770-305-7352
Rodenstock North America, Inc.
2150 Bixby Rd., Lockbourne, OH 43137-9273 — 614-409-2820

Lodi
Bailey Manufacturing Co.
PO BOX 130, Lodi, OH 44254-0130 — 800-321-8372

Macedonia
Max Endoscopy Inc.
1410 Highland Road, Suite 6, Macedonia, OH 44056 — 330-425-7041

Maineville
E-Med Corp.
8307 Marigold Lane, Maineville, OH 45039-9542 — 800-974-3633

Mansfield
Mansfield Orthotic & Prosthetic Center, Inc.
240 Marion Ave., Mansfield, OH 44903 — 419-522-4171
Oxyrase, Inc.
175 South Illinois Ave., Mansfield, OH 44905 — 419-589-8800

Marietta
Caron Products And Services, Inc.
PO Box 715, Marietta, OH 45750 — 800-648-3042
Grimm Scientific Ind., Inc.
1403 Pike St., PO Box 2143, Marietta, OH 45750-7143 — 800-223-5395
Kardex Systems, Inc.
114 Westview Avenue, Marietta, OH 45750-0171 — 800-234-3654
Thermo Fisher Scientific (Asheville) Llc
Millcreek Rd., Marietta, OH 45750 — 740-373-4763

Mason
Alvey Washing Equipment Co.
4600 N. Mason-Montgomery Rd., Mason, OH 45040 — 800-677-0076
Clopay Plastic Products Company
8585 Duke Blvd, Mason, OH 45040-3101 — 800-282-2260
HAAG-STREIT USA, INC.
3535 Kings Mills Rd., Mason, OH 45040-2303 — 800-787-5426
Haag-Streit Group
3535 Kings Mills Road, Mason, OH 45040-2303 — 800-787-5426
Pearle Vision
4000 Luxottica Place, Mason, OH 45040 — 800-937-3937

Maumee
Lantz Dental Prosthetics, Inc.
6490 Wheatstone Ct., Maumee, OH 43537 — 419-866-1515
Spartan Chemical Company, Inc.
1110 Spartan Dr., Maumee, OH 43537-0110 — 800-537-8990

Medina
Orthohelix Surgical Designs, Inc.
1065 Medina Rd, Ste 500, Medina, OH 44256 — 1-866-90-HELIX
Theken Spine Llc
1153 Medina Road, Medina, OH 44256 — 1-866-942-8698
Theken Spine, Llc
1153 Medina Road, Medina, OH 44256 — 1-866-942-8698

Mentor
Cres Cor
5925 Heisley Rd., Mentor, OH 44060-1833 — 877-273-7267
Frantz Medical Development Ltd.
7740 Metric Drive, Mentor, OH 44060-4862 — 440-255-1155
Luminaud, Inc.
8688 Tyler Blvd., Mentor, OH 44060-4348 — 800-255-3408

Mill-Rose Company
7995 Tyler Blvd., Mentor, OH 44060 — 800-321-3533
Polymer Concepts, Inc.
7561-8 Tyler Blvd., Mentor, OH 44060-4867 — 877-820-3163
Southside Biotechnology
8780 Tyler Blvd., Mentor, OH 44060 — 440-974-4074
Steris Biological Operations Facility
9325 Pinecone Dr., Mentor, OH 44060 — 440-354-2600
Steris Corporation
5960 Heisley Road, Mentor, OH 44060-1834 — 800-884-9550
Steris Corporation
6100 Heisley Road, Mentor, OH 44060 — 440-354-2600
Steris Corporation
6515 Hopkins Road, Mentor, OH 44060 — 440-354-2600
United States Endoscopy Group
5976 Heisley Road, Mentor, OH 44060 — 800-769-8226
Volk Optical Inc.
7893 Enterprise Drive, Mentor, OH 44060-5309 — 800-345-8655

Miamisburg
Endolite North America, Ltd.
1031 Byers Road, Miamisburg, OH 45342 — 800-548-3534
Riverain Medical Group
3020 South Tech Blvd., Miamisburg, OH 45342 — 800-990-3387
X-Spine Systems, Inc.
452 Alexandersville Rd., Miamisburg, OH 45342 — 800-903-0640

Miamiville
Hill Top Research Corp
P.o. Box 138, 6088 Main & Mill Streets, Miamiville, OH 45147 — 513-831-3114

Middleburg Heights
Codonics
17991 Englewood Drive, Middleburg Heights, OH 44130 — 800-444-1198

Milford
Accu-Med Services
300 Technecenter Drive, Milford, OH 45150 — 800-777-9141
Interplex Medical, Llc
25 Whitney Dr. Ste 114, Milford, OH 45150 — 513-248-5120

Mogadore
Kent Elastomer Products, Inc
3890 Mogadore Industrial Prkwy, Mogadore, OH 44260 — 330-628-1802

Mount Sterling
Ohio Willow Wood Company
15441 Scioto Darby Rd., Mount Sterling, OH 43143-0130 — 800-848-4930

Mount Vernon
Selective Med Components, Inc.
564 Harcourt Rd., Mount Vernon, OH 43050 — 740-397-7838

N. Ridgeville
Bioplastics Co.
34655 Mills Rd., N. Ridgeville, OH 44039 — 800-487-2358
The After Market Group
39400 Taylor Parkway, N. Ridgeville, OH 44039 — 888-824-8200

New Philadelphia
Audio Hearing Aid Service
617 Wabash Ave., N.w., New Philadelphia, OH 44663 — 330-364-6637

Newbury
Bio-Medical Instrument Co.
15764 Munn Rd., Newbury, OH 44065 — 440-564-5450

Niles
Penn Care Medical Products
1317 North Rd., Niles, OH 44446 — 800-392-7233

North Canton
Smithers Medical Products, Inc.
4850 Shuffel Dr., N.w., North Canton, OH 44720-5436 — 330-497-0690
Suarez Corporation Industries
7800 Whipple Avenue N.w., North Canton, OH 44720 — 330-494-5504

North Ridgeville
Invecare
39400 Taylor St., North Ridgeville, OH 44039 — 800-333-6900

North Royalton
Americus Form & Function
12316 York Rd., North Royalton, OH 44133 — 440-237-0200
Great Lakes Earmold Lab
12740 York Delta Drive, PO Box 338004, North Royalton, OH 44133 — 800-842-8184
Perimed, Inc.
6785 Wallings Rd., Ste. 2C-2D, North Royalton, OH 44133 — 877-374-3589

Northwood
Lexamed
705 Front St., Northwood, OH 43605 — 419-693-5307
North American Science Associates, Inc.
6750 Wales Road, Northwood, OH 43619 — 866-666-9455

Norton

Global Franchise Consultants, Inc.   330-848-1956
3656 Durham Road, Norton, OH 44203-6353

Norwalk

Durable Corporation   877-938-7225
75 N. Pleasant St., Norwalk, OH 44857-0290
Gyrus Acmi, Inc.   508-804-2739
93 North Pleasant St., Norwalk, OH 44857

Oberlin

Synapse Biomedical Inc.   440-774-2488
300 Artino St., Oberlin, OH 44074

Oregon

Fresenius Medical Care North America   781-699-9068
750 North Lallendorf Rd, Oregon, OH 43616

Orient

Hale Imaging Systems, Inc.   800-321-4253
5314 Mill St., P.O. Box 184, Orient, OH 43146-0184

Painesville

Virtec Enterprises, Llc   440-352-8970
11351 Prouty Road, Painesville, OH 44077-2321

Parkman

Vsm Healthcare Products   330-673-8227
15547 Main Market Road, Parkman, OH 44080

Perrysburg

Fresenius Medical Care North America   781-699-9068
28157 Cedar Park Blvd, Perrysburg, OH 43551

Phoneton

Vital Connections, Inc.   937-667-3880
955 N. Third St., Phoneton, OH 45371

Pickerington

Vacalon Company, Inc.   614-577-1945
12960 Stonecreek Dr., Ste. C, Pickerington, OH 43147

Piqua

Evenflo Company, Inc.   800-233-5921
1801 Commerce Dr., Piqua, OH 45356

Poland

Anatomical Concepts, Inc.   800-837-3888
1399 E. Western Reserve Road, Poland, OH 44514-3250

Powell

Bill Frank Productions Bf Bio-Supports Inc.   614-840-0091
665 Old Pond Lane, Powell, OH 43065

Reynoldsburg

Kenda American Airless   800-248-4737
7120 Americana Parkway, Reynoldsburg, OH 43068

Ripley

Pcp Champion   800-888-0867
300 Congress St., Ripley, OH 45167-1411

Rock Creek

Fine-Cut Diamond Tool Co.   440-563-5505
2811 Rome-Rock Creek Rd., Rock Creek, OH 44084-0457

Rockford

Tu-Way American Group   800-537-3750
191 Pearl St., Rockford, OH 45882-0306

Roseville

Extended Care Air Therapy Systems, Inc.   740-697-0845
7165 Payne Rd., Roseville, OH 43777

Sharon Center

Transmotion Medical Inc.   866-860-8447
1441 Wolf Creek Trail, Sharon Center, OH 44274

Solon

Amresco Inc.   800-366-1313
30175 Solon Industrial Pkwy., Solon, OH 44139
Cone Instruments, Inc.   800-321-6964
5201 Naiman Pkwy., Solon, OH 44139-1005
Gliatech Medical, Inc.   216-831-3200
27070 Miles Rd., Solon, OH 44139
Orbital Enterprises Llc   440-349-5100
6850 Cochran Rd., Solon, OH 44139
Rsti (Radiological Service Training Institute)   800-229-7784
30745 Solon Road, Solon, OH 44139
The Carnegie Textile Co.   800-633-4136
31100 Solon Road, P.O. Box 14, Solon, OH 44139
Timekeeping Systems, Inc.   216-595-0890
30700 Bainbridge Road, Solon, OH 44128
Valtronics USA Inc.   440-349 1239
6168 Cochran Rd., Solon, OH 44139

Springboro

Chewrite Co., A Subsidiary Of Magnesia Products, I   513-746-5509
265 Pioneer Blvd., Springboro, OH 45066
No Rinse Laboratories, Llc.   800-223-9348
868 Pleasant Valley Drive, Springboro, OH 45066
Paper Systems Inc.   800-950-8590
185 S. Pioneer Blvd., P.O. Box 150, Springboro, OH 450664506
Pdi Communication Systems   800-992-7734
40 Greenwood Lane, Springboro, OH 45066

Stow

Polar Products, Inc.   800-763-8423
3380 Cavalier Trail, Stow, OH 44224

Strasburg

Kleen Test Products Corporation   330-878-5586
216 12th St. NE, Strasburg, OH 44680

Strongsville

Hmi Industries, Inc.   440-846-7873
13325 Darice Pkwy., Unit A, Strongsville, OH 44149
Lumitex, Inc.   800-969-5483
8443 Dow Circle, Strongsville, OH 44136-1759
Sparton Corporation   440-878-4630
22740 Lunn Road, Strongsville, OH 44149
Sparton Medical Systems   440-878-4630
22740 Lunn Rd., Strongsville, OH 44149

Sunbury

Bry-Air, Inc.   877-379-2479
10793 State Rt. 37 W., Sunbury, OH 43074
Medi-Source, Inc.   740-524-0358
7719 State Route 656, Sunbury, OH 43074

Tiffin

Synergistic Concepts, Ltd.   419-448-4868
1660 W. Market St., Suite D, Tiffin, OH 44883

Toledo

Betco Corp.   800-462-3826
P.O. Box 3127, Toledo, OH 43607
Bionix Development Corp.   800-551-7096
5154 Enterprise Blvd., Toledo, OH 43612
Canberra Corp.   419-841-6616
3610 Holland-Sylvania Road, Toledo, OH 43615
Dresch/Tolson Dental Lab   952-345-6300
4024 North Holland-sylvania Rd, Toledo, OH 43623
Gottfried Medical, Inc.   419-474-2973
4105 W. Alexis Rd., Toledo, OH 43623
Gottfried Medical, Inc.   (800) 537-1968
P.O. Box 350457, Toledo, OH 43617-0457
Miller Artificial Eye Laboratory, Inc.   419-474-3939
3030 W. Sylvania Ave., Suite 13, Toledo, OH 43613
Nss Enterprises, Inc.   419-531-2121
3115 Frenchmens Rd., Toledo, OH 43607-2958
Specialty Gases Of America, Inc.   419-729-7732
6055 Brent Dr., Toledo, OH 43611
Sterimark/Etigam   419-868-1800
1031 Calle Trepadora #D, Toledo, OH 43635-2796
Torbot Group Inc., Jobskin Division   800-207-1074
653 Miami Street, Toledo, OH 43605
Wheelchair Carrier, Inc.   800-541-3213
203 Matzinger Road, Toledo, OH 43612
Wheelit, Inc.   800-523-7508
440 Arco Drive, Toledo, OH 43607-2909

Twinsburg

Engineering Services Kenneth C. Saltrick Inc.   888-364-7782
2200 East Enterprise Parkway, Twinsburg, OH 44087
Gvi Technology Partners   330-963-4083
1470 Enterprise Pkwy., Twinsburg, OH 44087
Hitachi Medical Systems America, Inc.   800-800-3106
1959 Summit Commerce Park, Twinsburg, OH 44087-2371
National Biological Corp.   800-338-5045
1532 Enterprise Pkwy., Twinsburg, OH 44087-2240
Trionix Research Laboratory, Inc.   330-425-9055
8037 Bavaria Rd., Twinsburg, OH 44087

Uniontown

Plasticards, Inc. Dba Rainbow Printing Co.   800-536-9705
3711 Boettler Oaks Dr., Uniontown, OH 44685-7733

University Heights

Plexar Associates, Inc.   216-932-2069
3722 Meadowbrook Blvd., University Heights, OH 44118

Valley View

Lds Life Science (Formerly Gould Instrument Systems Inc.)   216-328-7000
5525 Cloverleaf Parkway, Valley View, OH 44125-6100

Van Wert

Blue Bell Bio-Medical   800-258-3235
1260 Industrial Drive, Van Wert, OH 45891

Braun Industries, Inc.
1170 Production Drive, Van Wert, OH 45891
800-222-7286

Versailles
Midmark Corporation
60 Vista Dr., P.O. Box 286, Versailles, OH 45380
800-643-6275

Wadsworth
Remington Products Company Llc
961 Seville Rd., Wadsworth, OH 44281-0506
800-491-1571

Wapakoneta
M.B. Industries, Inc.
11158 Infirmary Road, Wapakoneta, OH 45895
(419) 738-4769

Waterville
Biofit Engineered Products
PO Box 109, Waterville, OH 43566-0109
800-597-0246

West Chester
ATRICURE, INC.
6217Centre Park Dr., West Chester, OH 45069-3863
888.347.6403
Atricure, Inc.
6217 Centre Park Drive, West Chester, OH 45069
888.347.6403

West Lafayette
Jones-Zylon Company
P.O. Box 149, West Lafayette, OH 43845-1224
800-848-8160

Westerville
Lake Shore Cryotronics, Inc.
575 McCorkle Blvd., Westerville, OH 43082
614-891-2243
Md Systems, Inc.
P.O. Box 1647, Westerville, OH 43086
614-818-3000

Westlake
Bay Corporation
867 Canterbury Road, Westlake, OH 44145-1486
888-835-3800
C & K Manufacturing & Sales
28825 Ranney Pkwy., Westlake, OH 44145
800-821-7795
Nordson Corporation
28601 Clemens Road, Westlake, OH 44145
440-892-1580
Perfect Smile Corporation
29313 Clemens Road, #2E, Westlake, OH 44145
800-520-1906
Radiometer America, Inc.
810 Sharon Drive, Westlake, OH 44145
800-736-0600
Western Medica
875 Bassett Road, Westlake, OH 44145
800-783-7890

Willoughby
All-Craft Wellman Products, Inc.
4839 E. 345th St., Willoughby, OH 44094-4606
800-340-3899
Neuros Medical Inc.
4230 Route 306, Suite 305, Willoughby, OH 44094
440-951-2565

Wilmington
Ferno-Washington, Inc.
70 Weil Way, Wilmington, OH 45177-9371
800-733-3766

Wooster
Prentke Romich Company
1022 Heyl Road, Wooster, OH 44691
800-262-1984

Worthington
Hti, Inc.
500 West Wilson Bridge Road, Suite 105, Worthington, OH 43085
800-685-2997

Xenia
W.A. Hammond Drierite Co.
138 DAYTON AVE., P.O. Box 460, Xenia, OH 45385
937-376-2927

Yellow Springs
Vernay Laboratories, Inc.
120 E. South College Street, Yellow Springs, OH 45387-1623
800-666-5227

Youngstown
Avry's Orthotic Facility, Inc.
1441 Wick Ave., Youngstown, OH 44505
330-746-5385

Zanesville
Dmv Corporation
1024 Military Rd., Zanesville, OH 43702-0878
800-522-9465

OKLAHOMA

Altus
Ok-1 Manufacturing Co., Inc.
709 S. Veterans Drive, PO Box 736, Altus, OK 73522
800-654-9873

Ardmore
Imtec Imaging L.L.C.
2401 North Commerce, Ardmore, OK 73401
800-226-3220
Imtec, A 3m Company
IMTEC Plaza, 2401 N. Commerce, Ardmore, OK 73401
800-879-9799

Lemco Enterprises, Inc.
3204 Hale Rd., Ardmore, OK 73401
580-226-7808

Broken Arrow
Access Optics Llc
2001 North Willow Ave., Broken Arrow, OK 74012
918-294-1234
Advanced Medical Instruments, Inc.
3061 West Albany, Broken Arrow, OK 74012
918-250-0566

Cordell
Oral-Tx, Llc
121 South Market, Cordell, OK 73632
580-832-3058

Cushing
Electronic Systems Engineering Company
One ESECO Road, Cushing, OK 74023
800-331-5904

Edmond
Jetta Corporation
425 Centennial Blvd., Edmond, OK 73013-3714
800-288-7771

Inola
Rich-Mar Corporation
PO Box 879, 15499 E 590 Rd, Inola, OK 74036-9802
800-762-4665

Konawa
Jobri Llc
520 N Division St, Konawa, OK 74849
800-432-2225

Mannford
Cardinal Health 2200, Inc
400 East Foster Rd, Mannford, OK 74044
847-578-6610

Midwest City
Midwest City Hearing Aid Center
1401 South Midwest Blvd., Midwest City, OK 73110
405-732-8682

Norman
Immuno-Mycologics, Inc.
2700 Technology Pl, Norman, OK 73071
800-654-3639

Okc
D & D Video Specialists, Llc
6444 Nw Expressway Street, Suite 225E, Okc, OK 73132
405-720-3180

Oklahoma City
All American Mold Laboratories, Inc.
2120 South Prospect Ave., Oklahoma City, OK 73129
800-654-3245
Big D Industries, Inc.
5620 S.W. 29th St., Oklahoma City, OK 73179
405-682-2541
Bti Filtration
7317 N. Classen Blvd., Oklahoma City, OK 73116
405-842-2517
Dura-Kold Corp.
3525 S. Purdue, Oklahoma City, OK 73179
800-541-7199
Exakt Technologies, Inc.
7002 N. Broadway Ext., Oklahoma City, OK 73116-9006
800-866-7172
Genuine Care Rehab. Svc., Inc.
2401 N.w. 23rd St. Ste. 17, Oklahoma City, OK 73107
405-604-5907
Hampton Research & Engineering, Inc.
2726 N. Oklahoma, Oklahoma City, OK 73105
800-800-6369
Handi-Cap Aids Company
730 West Hefner Road, Oklahoma City, OK 73114-6835
800-689-0511
Inoveon Corp.
800 North Research Pkwy., Suite 370, Oklahoma City, OK 73104
405-271-9025
Intempo Wood Furniture, Inc.
P.O. Box 82816, Oklahoma City, OK 73148-0816
888-232-4809
Major Lab. Manufacturing
4408 N. Sewell St., Oklahoma City, OK 73118-8005
800-598-2621
Medical Dosimetry Services, Inc.
1601 Sw 89th, Suite E-100, Oklahoma City, OK 73159
405-680-5222
Mills Biopharmaceuticals, Llc
120 N.e. 26th St., Oklahoma City, OK 73105
405-523-1868
Modular Services Company
109 N.e. 38th St., Oklahoma City, OK 73105
405-521-9923
Smith & Nephew Inc., Endoscopy Div.
76 S. Meridian Ave., Oklahoma City, OK 73107-6512
978-749-1000
Sorb Technology, Inc.
3631 S.w. 54th St., Oklahoma City, OK 73119
405-682-1993
Soundtec, Inc.
2601 Northwest Expressway, Suite 400w, Oklahoma City, OK 73112
405-842-5045
The Optical Shop
1111 S. Eastern Ave., Oklahoma City, OK 73129
405-514-0903

Owasso
B2 Imports, Llc
12807 East 90th Street North, Owasso, OK 74055
918-557-5729

Tulsa
A&H Products, Inc.
6946 East 13th Street, Tulsa, OK 74112
918-835-8081
Airgas-Mid South, Inc.
9741 E 56th St N, Tulsa, OK 74110
918-582-0885
American Biomedical, Inc.
11333 E. Pine St., Suite 60, Tulsa, OK 74116
918-437-3009

Bed-Check Corporation — 800-523-7956
307 E. Brady, Tulsa, OK 74120

Braden Shielding Systems — 918-624-2888
9260 Broken Arrow Expressway, Tulsa, OK 74145-1229

Commercial/Medical Electronics, Inc. — 800-324-4844
1519 S. Lewis Avenue, Tulsa, OK 74104-4919

Dentsply Tulsa Dental Specialties — 800-662-1202
5100 East Skelly Drive, Suite 300, Tulsa, OK 74136

Electro Medical Inc. — 918-663-0297
9736 E. 55th Pl., Tulsa, OK 74146

Evelyn Co., Inc. — 800-221-0518
P.O. Box 35265, Tulsa, OK 74153-0265

Eye Restoration Clinic — 866-364-6544
4606 South Garnett, Suite 302, Tulsa, OK 74146-5218

H2or, Inc. — 918-744-4267
1638 South Main, Tulsa, OK 74119

Mcright Supplies Inc., Ken — 918-492-9657
7456 S. Oswego, Tulsa, OK 74136-5903

Med-Com Systems Corp. — 800-324-3283
1519 S. Lewis Ave., Tulsa, OK 74104-4919

Oral Health Products, Inc. — 918-622-9412
6847 East 40th St., Tulsa, OK 74145

SEBOTEK HEARING SYSTEMS, LLC — 1.800.388.9041
2488 East 81st St., Ste. 2000, Tulsa, OK 74137

Scifit — 800-278-3933
5151 S. 110th E. Avenue, Tulsa, OK 74146

Scodenco, Inc. — 918-627-6795
7405 East 31st Pl., Tulsa, OK 74145

Shapemaster Usa, Inc. — 866-531-3586
7633 E. 63rd Place, Suite 300, Tulsa, OK 74133

United Dental Manufacturers, Inc. — 918-878-0450
PO Box 700874, Tulsa, OK 74135-6560

OREGON

Albany

Bussard & Son Inc., R.D. — 800-252-2692
415 S.W. 25th AVE., Albany, OR 97322

Cdm Dental — 541-928-4444
812 Water St NE, Albany, OR 97321

Metal Techology, Inc. — 800-394-9979
173 Queen Ave., S.E., Albany, OR 97321-9905

Oral Biotech — 541-928-4445
812 Water St. Ne, Albany, OR 97321

Aloha

L & G Medical Software — 503-924-2429
15685 Nw Melody Ln, Aloha, OR 97006

Parks Medical Electronics, Inc. — 503-649-7007
PO Box 5669, Aloha, OR 97007

Ashland

Cropper Medical, Inc./Bio Skin — 800-541-2455
240 East Hersey Street, Suite 2, Ashland, OR 97520-5205

M .W. Mooney & Co., Inc. — 800-230-5770
415 Williamson Way, Ste. 9, Ashland, OR 97520

Baker City

Walls Precision Instruments, Llc. — 541-894-2520
38800 Deer Creek Rd., Baker City, OR 97814

Beaverton

Acrymed, Inc. — 503-624-9830
9560 SW Nimbus Avenue, Beaverton, OR 97008

Bioanalogics — 503-626-8000
7909 SW Cirrus Drive 27, Beaverton, OR 97008

Compview Medical Llc — 503-641-8439
10035 Sw Arctic Drive, Beaverton, OR 97005

Doxtech, Llc. — 503-641-1865
10025 S.W. Allen Blvd., Beaverton, OR 97005

Innovations For Access, Inc. — 800-297-8485
1815 Nw 169th Place,, Suite #6030, Beaverton, OR 97006

Interventional Hemostasis Products, Inc. — 503-638-9743
1815 Nw 169th Place, Suite 6030, Beaverton, OR 97006

J&J Engineering Llc — 503-626-7812
11791 SW Crater LP, Beaverton, OR 97008

Jordco, Inc. — 800-752-2812
595 N.W. 167th Ave., Beaverton, OR 97006

Justmed, Inc. — 877-390-1799
8152 SW Hall Blvd., Suite 512, Beaverton, OR 97008

Micro Power Electronics, Inc. — 800-576-6177
13955 SW Millikan Way, Beaverton, OR 97005

Nike, Inc. — 800-344-6453
One Bowerman Drive, Beaverton, OR 97005-6453

Nite Train'R — 503-626-8833
9735 S.W. Sunshine Ct., Suite 100, Beaverton, OR 97005

Orec Corp. — 800-624-5517
7747 South West Citrrus Dr, Beaverton, OR 97008

Uei — 800-547-5740
8030 SW Mimbus, Beaverton, OR 97008

Vidco, Inc. — 800-638-4326
6175 SW 112th Avenue, Beaverton, OR 97008-4838

Wave Form Systems, Inc. — 800-332-8749
7737 SW Nimbus Avenue, Beaverton, OR 97008

Welch Allyn Protocol Inc. — 800-289-2500
8500 S.W. Creekside Pl., Beaverton, OR 97008-7107

Welch Allyn Protocol, Inc. — 503 530 7500
8500 s.w. creekside place, Beaverton, OR 97008

Bend

Clear Catheter Systems — 541-382-8346
20380 Halfway Road Ste. 4, Bend, OR 97701

Deschutes Medical Products, Inc. — 800-383-2588
1011 S.w. Emkay Drive, Suite 104, Bend, OR 97702-3162

Grace Bio-Labs, Inc. — 541-318-1208
Po Box 238, 325 SW Cyber Drive, Bend, OR 97709

Mini-Mitter Company, Inc. — 800-685-2999
20300 Empire Ave., Bldg. B-3, Bend, OR 97701

Obsidian Dental Inc. — 541-617-0129
62915 Ne 18th St., Suite 4, Bend, OR 97701

Stat-Chek Company — 800-248-6618
P.O. Box 9636, Bend, OR 97708

Therapy Innovations Llc — 541-550-7347
840 Se Woodland Blvd, Suite 185, Bend, OR 97702

Blue River

L.L. Dental — 541-822-3839
91780 Mill Creek Rd., Blue River, OR 97413

Burlington

Gunther Weiss Scientific Glassblowing Co., Inc. — 503-621-3463
14640 Nw Rock Creek Rd., Burlington, OR 97231

Clackamas

Customs Hospital Products, Inc — 800-426-2780
12452 SE Capps Rd., Clackamas, OR 97015

Dravon Medical, Inc. — 800-654-1976
11465 SE Highway 212, PO Box 69, Clackamas, OR 97015

Healthmark, Inc. — 971-236-9171
8440 Se Sunnybrook Blvd #210, Clackamas, OR 97015

Neo-Genesis, A Division Of Natus — 503-657-8000
15140 SE 82nd Drive, Suite 270, Clackamas, OR 97015

Neurocom International, Inc. — 503-653-2144
9570 S.e. Lawnfield Rd., Clackamas, OR 97015

North America Mattress Corp. — 800-448-6163
10768 SE Hwy. 212, Clackamas, OR 97015

Sola Custom Coatings, Inc. — 858-509-9899
9117 South East Saint Helens, Street, Clackamas, OR 97015

Wy'East Medical Corp. — 503-657-3101
16700 SE 120th Avenue, PO Box 1625, Clackamas, OR 97015

Clakamas

Astoria-Pacific,Inc. — 800-536-3111
PO Box 830, Clakamas, OR 97015

Cornelius

Sheldon Mfg., Inc. — 503-640-3000
300 North 26th Ave., Cornelius, OR 97113

Corvallis

Avi Biopharma, Inc. — 503-227-0554
4575 SW Research Way, Suite 200, Corvallis, OR 97333

Medan Inc. — 541-231-4141
131 Nw 4th Street, Suite 395, Corvallis, OR 97330

Crooked River Ranch

Guppie Ent., Inc. — 541-548-0748
9251 S.w. Geneva View Rd., Crooked River Ranch, OR 97760

Eugene

Direct Crown, Llc — 888-910-4490
895 Country Club Rd., Ste. B-100, Eugene, OR 97401

Electrical Geodesics, Inc. — 541-687-7962
2979 Chad Dr., Eugene, OR 97408

Electrical Geodesics, Incorporated — 541-687-7962
1600 Millrace Drive, Suite 307, Eugene, OR 97403

Kezar Enterprises, Inc. — 541-334-6100
747 Blair Blvd., Eugene, OR 97402

Northwest Stamping & Precision, Inc. — 541-747-4269
86365 College View Rd., Eugene, OR 97405

Pfs Med, Inc. — 541-349-9646
3295 Cross St., Eugene, OR 97402

Valley Technology, Inc. — 541-434-9180
1025 Conger Street, Suite #2, Eugene, OR 97402

Forest Grove

Engle Dental Systems, Inc. — 503-359-9390
4115 24th Avenue, Suite A, Forest Grove, OR 97116

Gladstone

Procedure Products, Inc. — 360-693-1832
6622 SE Oakridge Drive, Gladstone, OR 97027

Gresham

Eischco, Inc. — 503-492-2232
1232 Se 282nd Ave, Gresham, OR 97080

Hillsboro

Acumed Llc
5885 Nw Cornelius Pass Rd., Hillsboro, OR 97124
888-627-9957

Acute Innovations Llc
21421 Nw Jacobson Rd., Suite 700, Hillsboro, OR 97124
866-623-4137

Arc Surgical Llc.
21300 Nw Jacobson Rd., Hillsboro, OR 97124
503-627-9957

Forest Dental Products Inc
6200 N.E. Campus Court, Hillsboro, OR 97124
800-423-3535

Hood River

Cascade Dental Products Co.
3960 Grandview Drive, Hood River, OR 97031
800-939-9926

Lake Grove

Ocular Concepts Llc.
4035 Sw Mercantile Dr., Suite #208, Lake Grove, OR 97035
503-699-7700

Lake Oswego

Biotronik, Inc.
6024 Jean Road, Lake Oswego, OR 97035
503-635-3594

Compix Incorporated
15824 Sw Upper Boones Ferry Rd, Lake Oswego, OR 97035-4066
503-639-8496

Maloney's Custom Ocular Prosthetics, Inc.
4035 S.w. Mercantile Dr., #208, Lake Oswego, OR 97035
503-675-1320

Para Scientific, Inc.
17170 Wall St., Lake Oswego, OR 97034
503-636-4121

Madras

Shielding International, Inc.
2150 NW Andrews Drive, P.O. Box Z, Madras, OR 97741
800-292-2247

Shielding Intl., Inc.
2150 N.w. Andrews Dr., Madras, OR 97741
541-475-7211

Mcminnville

Beevers Manufacturing, Inc.
14670 Baker Creek Road, Mcminnville, OR 97128
800-818-4025

World Class Technology Corporation
1300 Ne Alpha Dr., Mcminnville, OR 97128
503-472-8320

Medford

Silver Star Mobility
578 Mason Way, Medford, OR 97501
800-555-4385

Milwaukie

Electrodyne, Inc.
11200 S.E. 21st Ave., Milwaukie, OR 97222
503-654-0711

Newberg

A-Dec, Inc.
2601 Crestview Dr., Newberg, OR 97132-9257
800-547-1883

Beaverstate Dental, Inc.
115 S. Elliott Rd., Newberg, OR 97132
800-237-2303

Dental Components, Inc.
305 N. Springbrook Road, Newberg, OR 97132
800-624-2793

Mmsi
PO Box 3005, Newberg, OR 97132
503-538-3270

Precision Microcurrent, Inc.
705 S.springbrook Rd., Bld.a-135, Newberg, OR 97132
503-443-6100

Newport

Coast Hearing Services
1217 N. Coast Hwy Suite D, Newport, OR 97365
541-265-6273

Sam Medical Products
4909 South Coast Hwy., #245, Newport, OR 97365
503-639-5474

Oregon City

Columbia-Inland Corporation
415 17th St., Suite #2, Oregon City, OR 97045
503-657-6676

Vitamedics Corporation
19142 S. Molalla Ave., Oregon City, OR 97045-8975
800-216-2724x10

Portland

Airgas Norpac
3411 North Columbia Blvd., Portland, OR 97217
360-944-4091

Ak, Ltd.
18412 N.E. Halsey, Portland, OR 97230
503-669-0986

Almore International, Inc.
PO Box 25214, Portland, OR 97298
503-643-6633

Artisan Dental Laboratory
2532 S.E. Hawthorne Blvd., Portland, OR 97214
800-222-6721

Avd
2326 NW Everett St., Portland, OR 97210
503-223-2333

B&E Medical Systems
1006 N.E. Second Ave., Portland, OR 97232
503-233-4872

Bio-Optics, Inc.
1525 NE 41st Avenue, Portland, OR 97232
503-493-8000

Calypte Biomedical Corporation
16290 SW Upper Boones Ferry Road, Portland, OR 97224
877-CALYPTE

Care Medical Equipment, Inc.
1877 NE 7th Avenue, Portland, OR 97212
800-952-9566

Center For Ocular Prosthetics, Llc.
2525 N.w. Lovejoy, Suite 306, Portland, OR 97210
503-229-8490

Cornerstone Surgical, Llc
10175 Sw Barbur Blvd., Suite # 214-b, Portland, OR 97219-5955
503-680-7281

Cp Medical Corporation
803 NE 25th Avenue, Portland, OR 97232
800-950-2763

Department Of Veterans Affairs Medical Center
3710 S.w. U.s. Veterans, Hospital Rd., Portland, OR 97207-1034
503-220-8262

Desacc, Inc.
0844 Sw Curry St., Portland, OR 97239
866-638-0936

Dwfritz Automation, Inc.
17750 SW Upper Boones Ferry Road, Portland, OR 97224
503-598-9393

Fenwick Hearing Instruments
2888 NW Westover Rd., Portland, OR 97210
503-464-9441

Hemcon Medical Technologies, Inc.
10575 SW Cascade Blvd., Suite 130, Portland, OR 97223
877-247-0196

Inovise Medical, Inc.
10565 Sw Nimbus Ave., Suite 100, Portland, OR 97223
503-431-3800

Keen Mobility Company
6500 Ne Halsey St Bldg B, Portland, OR 97213
503-285-9090

Keepers!, Inc.
PO Box 12648, Portland, OR 97212
503-546-5696

Mcclure Industries, Inc.
9051 S.E. 55th Ave., Portland, OR 97206-0605
800-752-2821

Ortho-Med, Inc.
3208 S.E. 13th Ave., Portland, OR 97202-2407
800-547-5571

Polar Cryogenics, Inc.
2734 S.e. Raymond, Portland, OR 97202
503-239-5252

Portland Hearing Aid Specialists, Inc.
8505 SE Stark St, Portland, OR 97216
503-261-9309

QuantRx Biomedical Corp.
5920 NE 112th Avenue, Portland, OR 97220
503-252-9565

Quantum Medical Concepts, Llc.
3518 Se 21st Ave., Portland, OR 97202
503-708-0702

R.J.S. Acoustic Services, Inc.
11919 Ne Glisan, Portland, OR 97220-2144
800-826-3180

Revtek Industries, Llc
4288 S.E. International Way, Portland, OR 97222
503-659-1650

Riverpoint Medical
809 Ne 25th Ave, Portland, OR 97232
503-517-8001

Shamrock Medical, Inc.
3620 S.E. Powell Blvd., Portland, OR 97202
503-233-5055

Skedco, Inc.
16420 S.W. 72nd Avenue, PO Box 230487, Portland, OR 97281
503-639-2119

Starkey Northwest
2255 N.E. 194th Ave., Portland, OR 97230-7437
800-537-5300

Tiba Medical, Inc.
2701 Nw Vaughn St., Suite 470, Portland, OR 97210
503-222-1500

Tz Medical Inc.
7272 S.W. Durham Road, #800, Portland, OR 97224
800-944-0187

Voyager Medical Corp.
5550 S.w. Macadam Ave. #310, Portland, OR 97239
503-223-3881

Redmond

Aulie Devices, Inc.
3615 Northwest Way, P.O. Box 786, Redmond, OR 97756
541-548-7355

Medisiss
2747 Sw 6th Street, Redmond, OR 97756
866-866-7477

Roseburg

Kronner Medical
1443 Upper Cleveland Rapids Rd., Roseburg, OR 97470-1669
800-706-3533

Salem

Electrotherapy Systems, Inc.
476 Winding Ct.,se, Salem, OR 97302
503-779-7039

Esha Research
4747 skyline Rd S Suite 100, Salem, OR 97306
503-585-6242

Innovative Machinery Packaging And Converting Inc.
PO Box 535, Salem, OR 97308
503-581-3239

Ladies First, Inc.
P.O. Box 4400, Salem, OR 97302
800-497-8285

Neurocare, Inc.
6252 Skyline Road S., Salem, OR 97306
877-571-3599

Rk Froom & Co., Inc.
903 Cunningham Lane, Salem, OR 97302
310-327-5125

Springfield

Stik Stoppers, Inc.
3777 Douglas Dr., Springfield, OR 97478
541-726-7869

Tigard

Frye Electronics, Inc.
9826 S.W. Tigard Street, Tigard, OR 97223-5243
800-547-8209

Gymstandy Llc
9055 Sw Mountain View Ln., Tigard, OR 97224
503-684-4990

Zygo Industries, Inc.
7409 SW Tech Center Drive, Suite 125, Tigard, OR 97223-8082
800-234-6006

Troutdale

Mml Diagnostics Packaging, Inc.
1625 N.W. Sundial Rd., P.O. Box 458, Troutdale, OR 97060
800-826-7186

Tualatin

Anthro Corporation
10450 S.W. Manhasset Dr., Tualatin, OR 97062
800-325-3841

Biojet Medical Technologies, Inc.   800-683-7221
20245 SW 95th Avenue, Tualatin, OR 97062
Mecta Corporation   503-612-6780
19799 SW 95th Avenue, Suite B, Bldg. D, Tualatin, OR 97062
Paramount Manufacturing   503-612-8442
10360 Sw Spokane Court, Tualatin, OR 97062

White City

Biomed Diagnostics, Inc.   541-830-3000
1388 Antelope Road, White City, OR 97503
Carestream Health, Inc.   541-831-7222
8124 Pacific Ave., White City, OR 97503

Wilsonville

Oligos Etc., Inc.   503-682-1814
9775 S.w. Commerce Cir., Bldg. C-6, Wilsonville, OR 97070
Pml Microbiologicals   800-628-7014
27120 S.W. 95th Avenue, Wilsonville, OR 97070-0570
Seaberg Company Inc., The   800-818-4726
27350 SW 95th Ave, Suite 3038, Wilsonville, OR 97070
Tyco Electronics/Precision Interconnect   503-673-5027
10025 S.w. Freeman Court, Wilsonville, OR 97070

Winchester

Talon Acrylics, Inc.   888-433-2551
710 Strauss Ave, Winchester, OR 97495-8930

PENNSYLVANIA

Abington

Luckman Corporation   215-659-1664
1930 Old York Road, Abington, PA 19001

Allentown

Aetna Foot Products/Div. Of Aetna Felt Corporation   800-390-3668
2401 W. Emaus Ave., Allentown, PA 18103-7234
Air Products And Chemicals, Inc.   800-654-4567
7201 Hamilton Blvd., Allentown, PA 18195-1501
American Dental Supply, Inc.   800-558-5925
1075 N. Gilmore Street, Allentown, PA 18109-3210
B. Braun Medical, Inc.   610-596-2536
901 Marcon Blvd., Allentown, PA 18109
Bio Med Sciences, Inc.   800-257-4566
7584 Morris Court, Suite 218, Allentown, PA 18106
Carlisle Street Llc   610-821-4222
321 South Carlisle St., Allentown, PA 18109
Medline Industries Holdings, L.P.   847-837-2759
7267 Schantz Rd., Allentown, PA 18106
Pneu-Mobility, Inc.   610-266-8500
944 Marcon Blvd., Ste. 110, Allentown, PA 18109-9312
Stanley Vidmar   800-523-9462
11 Grammes Road, Allentown, PA 18103

Allison Park

Micor, Inc.   412-487-1113
2855 Oxford Blvd., Allison Park, PA 15101-2455

Altoona

Delta Health Technologies, Llc   800-444-1651
400 Lakemont Park Blvd., Altoona, PA 16603

Ambridge

Pocket Nurse Enterprises, Inc.   800-225-1600
200 1st Street, Ambridge, PA 15003

Ardmore

El-Fax Company, Inc. (Lung Gym)   610-896-6853
32 Llanfair Road, PO Box 407, Ardmore, PA 19003

Aston

Elwyn Industries Products.   Elwyn Industrie
2047 Bridgewater Rd., Aston, PA 19014
Endless Pools, Inc.   800-233-0741
200 East Dutton Mill Rd., Aston, PA 19014
L&L Special Furnace Co., Inc.   888-808-3676
20 Kent Road, Aston, PA 19014
Tnc Devices, Inc.   504-286-7794
50 Mcdonald Blvd., Aston, PA 19013

Audobon

Globus Medical Inc.   610-930-1800
Valley Forge Business Center, 2560 General Armistead Ave., Audobon, PA 19403

Austin

Emporium Specialties Co., Inc.   814-647-8661
10 Foster Avenue, Austin, PA 16720

Avon

C. L. Sturkey, Inc.   800-274-3446
824 Cumberland Street, Avon, PA 17042

Avondale

Anholt Technologies, Inc.   610-268-2758
440 Church Rd., Avondale, PA 19311

Seitz Technical Products, Inc.   610-268-2228
729 Newark Road, Avondale, PA 19311-0338
Wfr/Aquaplast Corp.   800-526-5247
440 Church Road, Avondale, PA 19311

Bensalem

Brotherston Homecare Inc., Pxi Div.   800-695-9729
1388 Bridgewater Rd., Bensalem, PA 19020
Continental Scientific   800-523-7138
539 Dunksferry Rd., Bensalem, PA 19020-5908
D-Tek Llc   267 306 3430
3580 Progress Dr., Suite J3, Bensalem, PA 19020

Bethel Park

Hapad, Inc.   800-544-2723
5301 Enterprise Blvd., Bethel Park, PA 15102-2531
Instrumentation Industries, Inc.   800-633-8577
2990 Industrial Blvd., Bethel Park, PA 15102-2536

Bethlehem

B. Braun Medical Inc., Renal Therapies Div.   800-854-6851
824 Twelfth Avenue, Bethlehem, PA 18018
B. Braun Oem Division, B. Braun Medical Inc.   866-8-BBRAUN
824 Twelfth Avenue, Bethlehem, PA 18018-3524
Gow-Mac Instrument Co.   610-954-9000
277 Brodhead Rd., Bethlehem, PA 18017
Hovertech International   800-471-2776
513 S. Clewell St., Bethlehem, PA 18015
Invatec   +1 877 446 8283
3101 Emrick Blvd, Suite 113, Bethlehem, PA 18020
Neuromonics Inc.   484-821-1260
2810 Emrick Blvd., Bethlehem, PA 18020
Orasure Technologies, Inc.   610-882-1820
1745 Eaton Ave., Bethlehem, PA 18018
Orasure Technologies, Inc.   800-869-3538
220 East First Street, Bethlehem, PA 18015
Saladax Biomedical, Inc.   610-419-6731
116 Research Dr., Bethlehem, PA 18015
Sure-Lok, Inc.   866-787-3565
2501 Baglyos Circle, Bethlehem, PA 18020
The Hymed Group Corp.   610-865-9876
1890 Bucknell Dr., Bethlehem, PA 18015
Welco-Cgi Gas Technologies   440-234-1075
145 Shimersville Rd., Bethlehem, PA 18015

Birdsboro

Xback Bracing Services, Inc.   1.800.494.8680
341a W. Main Street, P.O. Box 100, Birdsboro, PA 19508

Black Horse

Boehringer Labs, Inc   888-390-4325
500 East Washington St., Suite 2a, Black Horse, PA 19401

Botts

Clinton Industries, Inc   717-848-3519
1140 Edison St., Botts, PA 17403

Boyertown

J.P. Gilbert Co.   610-367-7457
548 Mountain Rd., Boyertown, PA 19512

Breiningsville

Aesculap Implant Systems, Inc.   610-984-9074
9999 Hamilton Blvd., Bldg 8, Breiningsville, PA 18031

brickerville

West Pharmaceutical Services, Inc. - Lititz, Pa   717-560-8460
179 W. Airport Road, brickerville, PA 17543

Bristol

America Hears, Inc.   215-788-0330
806 Beaver St., Bristol, PA 19007
Eastern Rail Systems, Inc.   800-327-0443
2014 Ford Rd., Unit G, Bristol, PA 19007
Masel Co., Inc.   800-423-8227
2701 Bartram Road, Bristol, PA 19007-6810
Nitric Bio, Inc.   866-957-6200
2 Canal's End Road, Suite 201-A, Bristol, PA 19007
United Chemical Technologies, Inc.   800-385-3153
2731 Bartram Road, Bristol, PA 19007-6893

Broomall

Drummond Scientific Co.   800-523-7480
500 Pkwy, Box 700, Broomall, PA 19008
Keeler Instruments Inc.   800-523-5620
456 Parkway, Broomall, PA 19008
Varitronics, Inc.   800-345-1244
620 Parkway, Broomall, PA 19008

Butler

Agr International, Inc.   724-482-2163
615 Whitestown Road, PO Box 149, Butler, PA 16003
Applied Test Systems, Inc.   800-441-0215
154 East Brook Lane, Butler, PA 16002

Cabot

Penn United Technology, Inc. — 724-352-1507
799 N. Pike Rd., Cabot, PA 16023

Camp Hill

Chek-Med Systems, Inc. — 800-451-5797
200 Grandview Ave., Camp Hill, PA 17011
Gi Supply — 800-451-5797
200 Grandview Ave., Camp Hill, PA 17011-1706

Canonsburg

Hankison International — 724-745-1555
1000 Philadelphia St., Canonsburg, PA 15317
Mylan Inc. — 724-514-1800
1500 Corporate Drive, Canonsburg, PA 15317
Scican Inc. — 800-572-1211
701 Technology Drive, Canonsburg, PA 15317
Viacirq, Inc. — 724-745-2362
Division of ThermaSolutions, Inc., 400 SouthPOinte Blvd, Plaza 1, Suite #23, Canonsburg, PA 15317-8549

Carbondale

Gentex Corporation Optics — 570-282-3550
P.O. Box 336, Carbondale, PA 18407-0315

Center Valley

Aesculap Implant Systems Inc. — 1-800-234-9179
3773 Corporate Pky., Center Valley, PA 18034
Airpal Patient Transfer Systems Inc. — 800-633-4725
5456 Northwood Drive, Center Valley, PA 18034
Olympus America, Inc. — 800-645-8160
3500 Corporate Parkway, PO Box 610, Center Valley, PA 18034
Olympus Medical Equipment Services America, Inc. — 484-896-5000
3500 Corporate Parkway, Center valley, PA 18034
Patient Transfer Systems, Inc. — 800-633-4725
5456 Northwood Dr., Center Valley, PA 18034

Chalfont

A Plus Dental Lab — 215-996-4177
1700 Horizon Drive, --suite 104, Chalfont, PA 18914
E. Q., Inc. — 215-997-1765
3469 Limekiln Ave., Chalfont, PA 18914

Chambersburg

Advanced Electronics Systems, Inc. — 800-345-1280
2005 Lincoln Way E., Chambersburg, PA 17201-1040

Cheswick

Millennia Technology, Inc. — 724-274-7741
1105 Pittsburgh St., Cheswick, PA 15024

Coatesville

Bender, Inc. — 800-356-4266
700 Fox Chase, Highlands Corp. Center, Coatesville, PA 19320
Lionville Systems, Inc. — 800-523-7114
501 Gunnard Carlson Drive, Coatesville, PA 19341-0693
Royal Paper Products, Inc. — 800-666-6655
PO Box 151, Coatesville, PA 19320

Collegeville

Rahns Specialty Metals — 800-523-1777
140 Bridge Street, Collegeville, PA 19426

Colmar

Capital Controls, MicroChem — 215-997-4000
3000 Advance Lane, Colmar, PA 18915

Conshohocken

CardioNet — 888-312-BEAT
227 Washington Street, #300, Conshohocken, PA 19428
Francis L. Freas Glass Works, Inc. — 610-828-0430
148 East Ninth Avenue, Conshohocken, PA 19428
Hale Products Inc. — 800-220-4253
700 Spring Mill Ave., Conshohocken, PA 19428
Product Investigations, Inc. — 610-825-5855
151 E. 10th Avenue, Conshohocken, PA 19428
Safe-Guard Technologies Corp. — 800-220-1245
1111 Hector St., Conshohocken, PA 19428-2311
Sharp Corporation — 800-892-6197
23 Carland Road, Conshohocken, PA 19428-1084

Coopersburg

Lampire Biological Laboratories, Inc. — 215-795-2838
405 South Main St., Coopersburg, PA 18036

Corry

Intubation Plus, Inc. — 814-663-4688
1524 Enterprise Rd., Corry, PA 16407
Nuvo, Inc. — 814-899-4220
5368 Kuhl Rd., Corry, PA 16407

Cranberry Township

Allegheny Plastics, Inc. — 800-933-4123
1224 Freedom Rd., Cranberry Township, PA 16066
Mine Safety Appliances Company — 866-MSA-1001
1000 Cranberry Woods Drive, Cranberry Township, PA 16066
Sigma Instruments, Inc. — 724-776-9500
506 Thomson Park Dr., Cranberry Township, PA 16066

Croydon

B-Tec Solutions Inc. — 215-785-2400
913 Cedar Ave., Croydon, PA 19021
Cms Gilbreth — 800.630.2413
3001 State Rd., Croydon, PA 19021
Comfort Products, Inc. — 800-822-7500
931 River Road, Croydon, PA 19021-6850
Xavier Electronics, Inc. — 215-788-7554
421 Magnolia Ave., Croydon, PA 19021

Darby

Universal Service Associates, Inc. — 800-601-1916
500 Ellis Avenue, Darby, PA 19023-2725

Darlington

Nesar Systems, Inc. — 724-827-8172
420 Ashwood Road, Darlington, PA 16115-2910

Denver

Precision Medical Products, Inc. — 717-335-3700
44 Denver Road, PO Box 300, Denver, PA 17517
Safc Biosciences, Inc. — 913-469-5580
320 Swampbridge Rd., Denver, PA 17517

Dover

Prairie Products, Inc. — 717-292-1089
4660 Raycom Rd.,, Industrial Park, Dover, PA 17315

Downingtown

Kmi Surgical Ltd. — 800-528-2900
Laird Professional Building, 110 Hopewell Rd, Downingtown, PA 19335
Mark Medical Manufacturing, Inc. — 610-269-4420
530 Brandywine Ave., Downingtown, PA 19335-2608
Techworld Corporation, Inc. — 1-888-658-8108
721 E Lancaster Avenue, Twc-01, Downingtown, PA 19335

Doylestown

Biosense Corporation — 215-348-2977
450 East Street, Doylestown, PA 18901
Lone Oak Medical Technologies — 267-221-0661
3805 Old Easton Road, Doylestown, PA 18901
Peregrine Surgical, Ltd. — 215-348-0456
51 Britain Drive, Doylestown, PA 18901
Pondus Medical, Inc. — 215-219-9152
5044 Davis Drive, PO Box 2079, Doylestown, PA 18901
Prescient Medical Inc. — 866-376-0500
2005 S. Easton Rd., Suite 204, Doylestown, PA 18901

Dublin

American Innovations, Inc. — 800-223-3913
123 N. Main St., Dublin, PA 18917-2107

Dubois

Kma Remarketing Corp. — 814-371-5242
302 Aspen Way, Dubois, PA 15801

Duryea

Schott Glass Technologies, Inc. — 570-457-7485
400 York Ave., Duryea, PA 18642-2026

East Norriton

Tengion Inc — 610-292-8364
2900 Potshop Ln 100, East Norriton, PA 19403

Easton

American Health Care Apparel Ltd. — 800-252-0584
302 Town Center Blvd., Easton, PA 18040
Follett Corp. — 800-523-9361
801 Church Lane, Easton, PA 18044

Edison

Musculoskeletal Transplant Foundation — 1-800-433-6576
125 May Street, Edison, PA 18434

Elizabethtown

East Coast Surgical Inc. — 717-361-0400
64 Pheasant Ct., Elizabethtown, PA 17022

Elkins Park

Gulden Ophthalmics — 800-659-2250
225 Cadwalader Avenue, Elkins Park, PA 19027-0154
Hessler Forms & Labels — 800-346-1304
106 Susan Dr., Unit #1, Elkins Park, PA 19027

Emigsville

Hercon Laboratories Corp. — 717-764-1191
101 Sinking Springs Ln., Emigsville, PA 17318
Herculite Products, Inc. — 800-772-0036
P.O. Box 435, Emigsville, PA 17318

Erdenheim

Dr. Len's Medical Products Llc — 678-908-8180
412 Atwood Rd., Erdenheim, PA 19038

Erie

Composiflex, Inc. — 800-673-2544
8100 Hawthorne Circle, Erie, PA 16509
Cybersonics, Inc. — 814-899-4220
5325 Kuhl Rd., Erie, PA 16510
Kold-Draft — 800-840-9577
1525 E. Lake Road, Erie, PA 16511
Steris Corporation — 814-452-3100
2424 West 23rd Street, Erie, PA 16506
Vista Lighting — 800-576-2135
1805 Pittsburg Ave., Erie, PA 16502

Exeter

Pride Mobility Products Corp. — 800-800-8586
182 Susquehanna Avenue, Exeter, PA 18643
Pride Mobility Products Corp. — 800-800-8586
182 Susquehanna Avenue, Exeter, PA 18643

Export

Carclo Technical Plastics - Export — 724-539-1833
6009 Enterprise Drive, Export, PA 15632
Circadiance LLC — 1-888-825-9640
1060 Corporate Lane, Export, PA 15632
Oerlikon Leybold Vacuum Usa Inc. — 800-433-4021
5700 Mellon Road, Export, PA 15632-8900

Exton

Absorption Systems — 610-280-7300
436 Creamery Way, Exton, PA 19341
D.G.H. Technology, Inc. — 800-722-3883
110 Summit Drive, Suite B, Exton, PA 19341
Dgh Technology, Inc. — 800-722-3883
110 Summit Dr., Ste.B, Exton, PA 19341
Glasspan, Inc. — 610-363-2300
The Commons at Lincoln Center, 101 J.R. Thomas Drive, Exton, PA 19341
Kensey Nash Corporation — 484-713-2100
735 Pennsylvania Drive, Exton, PA 19341
Rheologics, Inc. — 610-524-5427
15 East Uwchlan Avenue, Suite 414, Exton, PA 19341
Sekisui Diagnostics, LLC — 800-999-6578
115 Summit Dr., Exton, PA 19341

Fairview

Precise Plastics — 814-474-5504
7700 Middle Rd., Fairview, PA 16415

Feasterville

Analytic Bio-Chemistries Laboratory — 757-224-0177
1680-d Loretta Ave., Feasterville, PA 19053
Boekel Scientific — 800-336-6929
855 Pennsylvania Blvd., Feasterville, PA 19053
National Precision Instruments — 215-355-7525
1621 Loretta Ave., Unit #4, Feasterville, PA 19053

Folcroft

Airx Laboratories — 800-444-8900
1640 Delmar Dr., P.O. Box 37, Folcroft, PA 19032-1406

Ford City

Bergad Mattress — 888-476-8664
747 Eljer Way, Ford City, PA 16226
Williamson Medical Devices, Inc. — 888-239-7884
1401 Sixth Avenue, PO Box 152, Ford City, PA 16226

Fort Washington

Biosonics, Inc. — 215-646-7100
260 New York Drive, Fort Washington, PA 19034-2491
Core Essence Orthopaedics Inc. — 215-310-9534
575A Virginia Drive, Fort Washington, PA 19034

Frazer

Hill Laboratories Co. — 877-445-5020
3 N. Bacton Hill Road, PO Box 2028, Frazer, PA 19355

Gbg

Valley National Gases Wv Llc — 724-834-9200
1055 Garden Street, Gbg, PA 15601

Gibsonia

Bio-Test Medical, Inc. — 412-444-0933
1017 Executive Dr., Gibsonia, PA 15044

Gilbertsville

Penflex — 800-232-3539
105-B Industrial Drive, Gilbertsville, PA 19525
Rockland Immunochemicals, Inc. — 800-656-ROCK
PO Box 326, Gilbertsville, PA 19525

Glen Riddle

Container Research Corp. — 610-459-2160
Hollow Hill Road, PO Box 0159, Glen Riddle, PA 19037-0159

Glen Rock

Pasadena Scientific Industries — 717-227-1220
5125 Pine View Dr., Glen Rock, PA 17327

Glenside

Solar Light Co. — 215-517-8700
100 E. Glenside Avenue, Glenside, PA 19038

Greensburg

Cardiac Telecom Corporation — 800-355-2594
212 Outlet Way, Suite 1, Greensburg, PA 15601
Overly Manufacturing Co. — 800-979-7300
574 W. Otterman St., PO Box 70, Greensburg, PA 15601-0070

Greenville

Contour Form Products — 800-223-8808
38 Stewart Avenue, PO Box 328, Greenville, PA 16125

Hadley

Controlled Molding, Inc. — 724-253-3550
3043 Perry Highway, Hadley, PA 16130

Harleysville

Martech Medical Products — 215-256-8833
1500 Delp Dr., Harleysville, PA 19438
Medcomp (Medical Components, Inc.) — 800-220-3791
1499 Delp Dr., Harleysville, PA 19438-2936
Met-Pro Corporation — 215-723-6751
160 Cassell Road, P.O. Box 144, Harleysville, PA 19438

Harrisburg

Inclinator Co. Of America — 800-343-9007
601 Gibson Boulevard, Harrisburg, PA 17104-1557
Muth & Mumma Dental Lab — 952-541-9622
6360 Flank Drive, Suite 500, Harrisburg, PA 17112

Hartsville

Custom Ultrasonics, Inc. — 215-364-1477
144 Railroad Dr., Hartsville, PA 18974

Hatboro

Holmes Dental Corp. — 800-322-5577
50 S. Penn St., Hatboro, PA 19040-3246

Hatfield

Electron Microscopy Sciences — 800-523-5874
1560 Industry Road, P.O. Box 550, Hatfield, PA 19440
Imaging Sciences International, Llc — 215-997-5666
1910 North Penn Rd., Hatfield, PA 19440
Lactona Corporation — 1-888-522-
1669 School Road, P.o. Box 428, Hatfield, PA 19440
Negafile Systems — 800-523-5474
1560 Industry Road, Hatfield, PA 19440
Porter Instrument Division Parker Hannifin Corp — 800-457-2001
245 Township Line Rd., Hatfield, PA 19440-0907

Havertown

Chrono-Log Corp. — 800-247-6665
2 W. Park Rd., Havertown, PA 19083-4691
Imsi, Integrated Modular Systems Inc. — 800-220-9729
2500 Township Line Road, PO Box 616, Havertown, PA 19083

Hellertown

Bethlehem Apparatus Co., Inc. — 610-838-7034
890 Front St., Hellertown, PA 18055

Hermitage

Ccl Containers — 724-981-4420
One Llodio Drive, Hermitage, PA 16148

Honey Brook

Bvs, Inc. — 877-877-4821
949 Poplar Road, Honey Brook, PA 19344-0250

Horsham

Advanced Medical, Inc — 215-443-5424
935 Horsham Rd., Horsham, PA 19044
Bio/Data Corp. — 215-441-4000
155 Gibraltar Rd., Horsham, PA 19044
Biocoat, Inc. — 215-734-0888
211 Witmer Road, Horsham, PA 19044
Centocor, Inc. — 800-457-6399
800/850 Ridgeview Drive, Horsham, PA 19044
George C. Bishop Company — 800-476-7374
PO Box 684, Horsham, PA 19044-0684
Hausser Scientific — 215-675-7769
935 Horsham Rd., Suite C, Horsham, PA 19044
Two Technologies Inc. — 215-441-5305
419 Sargon Way, Horsham, PA 19044

Huntingdon Valley

The Fredericks Company — 215-947-2500
2400 Philmont Ave., Huntingdon Valley, PA 19006-0067
Whitman Group, The — 215-657-9990
3501 Masons Mill Rd., Bldg. 5, Huntingdon Valley, PA 19006-3517

Huntington Valley

Nikomed U.S.A., Inc. — 800-355-6456
2000 Pioneer Rd., Huntington Valley, PA 19006-1705

Irwin

Imagen (An Ex One Company) — 724-863-9663
8075 Pennsylvania Avenue, Irwin, PA 15642
Sylvan Fiberoptics — 800-628-3836
P.O. Box 501, Irwin, PA 15642

Ivyland

Big Boyz Industries, Inc. — 877-574-3233
128 Railroad Dr., Ivyland, PA 18974
Fluitron, Inc. — 215-355-9970
30 Industrial Drive, Ivyland, PA 18974
Medi-Dose, Inc. — 800-523-8966
70 Industrial Drive, Ivyland, PA 18974
Rapid Deployment Products — 877-433-7569
157 Railroad Avenue, Ivyland, PA 18974
Safe-Tec Clinical Products, Inc. — 800-356-6033
142 Railroad Drive, Ivyland, PA 18974

Jenkintown

Margraf Dental Manufacturing, Inc. — 800-762-2641
611 Harper Ave., Jenkintown, PA 19046-3206

Johnstown

Gerber Chair Mates, Inc. — 814-269-9531
1171 Ringling Ave., Johnstown, PA 15902
United Metal Fabricators, Inc. — 800-638-5322
1316 Eisenhower Blvd., Johnstown, PA 15904-3393
Xtol Products Co. — 814-255-2298
522 Goucher St., Johnstown, PA 15905

King of Prussia

Atlantic Medical Specialties — 888-487-5568
3620 Horizon Drive, King of Prussia, PA 19406
Bachem Bioscience, Inc. — 800-634-3183
3700 Horizon Drive, King of Prussia, PA 19406
C&S Research Corporation — 800-545-8460
625 Clark Avenue, Suite 21B, King of Prussia, PA 19406
Csl Behring — 610-878-4000
1020 First Ave., P.O. Box 61501, King of Prussia, PA 19406-0901
Devon Medical Products — 800-571-3135
1100 First Ave., Ste 202, King of Prussia, PA 19406
First Quality Retail Services, Llc — 516-829-3030
601 Allendale Rd., King Of Prussia, PA 19406
Otovation, Llc — 866-OTOVATION
1001 W. Ninth Avenue, Suite A, King of Prussia, PA 19406

Kittanning

Professional Hearing Aid Service — 724-548-4801
141 South Jefferson St., Kittanning, PA 16201

Kutztown

Radius Corp. — 800-626-6223
207 Railroad St., Kutztown, PA 19530

Lake City

Surgimedics — 800-840-9906
2950 Mechanic St., Lake City, PA 16423

Lancaster

Callcare — 800-345-9414
1370 Arcadia Road, Lancaster, PA 17601
Dentalez Group, Stardental Division — 717-291-1161
1816 Colonial Village Ln., Lancaster, PA 17601
Pennsylvania Scale Co. — 800-233-0473
1042 New Holland Ave, Burle Business Center, Lancaster, PA 17601
Sandt Products, Inc. — 800-441-8764 ex
1275 Loop Rd., Lancaster, PA 17601
Specialized Medical Devices, Llc — 800-463-1874
300 Running Pump Rd, Lancaster, PA 17603

Langhorne

Micromri, Inc. — 267-212-1100
580 Middletown Boulevard,, #D-150, Langhorne, PA 19047
Power Medical Interventions, Inc. — 267-775-8154
2021 Cabot Blvd., Langhorne, PA 19047

Lansdale

John Evans Sons, Inc. — 215-368-7700
1 Spring Ave., Lansdale, PA 19446
Newtech Dental Laboratories — 866-635-5227
1141 Smile Ln., Lansdale, PA 19446
Ps Products, Llc — 215-661-9595
329 Bradford Lane, Lansdale, PA 19446

Lansdowne

Superior Surgical Supply — 610-622-0740
28 N. Lansdowne Ave., Lansdowne, PA 19050

Latrobe

Chestnut Ridge Foam, Inc. — 800-234-2734
P.O. Box 781, Latrobe, PA 15650-0781

Lebanon

Quest Inc. — 717-273-8118
704 Metro Dr., Lebanon, PA 17042-9138
Regupol America — 800-537-8737
33 Keystone Drive, Lebanon, PA 17042

Leetsdale

Haemonetics Corp. — 781-356-9488
Buncher Industrial Park, Avenue C, Building 18, Leetsdale, PA 15056

Lenni

Dermamed Intl, Inc. — 610-358-4447
394 Parkmount Rd., Lenni, PA 19052

Lewisberry

Di-Chem Concentrate, Inc. — 763-422-8311
509 Fishing Creek Rd., Lewisberry, PA 17339

Lewistown

Ge Inspection Technologies, Lp — 717-447-1278
50 Industrial Park Rd., Lewistown, PA 17044

Ligonier

Ramsey Machine — 724-787-3059
1392 Darlington Rd., Ligonier, PA 15658

Limerick

Telefelx Medical — 610-948-5100
155 South Limerick Road, Limerick, PA 19468-1699
Teleflex Inc. — 610-948-5100
155 South Limerick Road, Limerick, PA 19468-1699

Lionville

West Pharmaceutical Services, Inc. — 800-231-3000
101 Gordon Dr., Lionville, PA 19341

Littlestown

Bar-Ray Products, Inc. — 800-359-6115
95 Monarch St., Littlestown, PA 17340

Lyon Station

East Penn Manufacturing — 610-682-6361
Deka Road, Lyon Station, PA 19536-0147

Mainland

Accupac, Inc. — 215-256-7011
1501 Industrial Blvd., Mainland, PA 19451

Malvern

Accutome Ultrasound, Inc. — 800-889-0200
3222 Phoenixville Pike, Malvern, PA 19355
Accutome, Inc. — 800-979-2020
3222 Phoenixville Pike, Malvern, PA 19355
Alpha Scientific Corp. — 800-242-5989
287 Great Valley Pkwy., Malvern, PA 19355
Alpha Scientific Corporation — 800-242-5989
293 Great Valley Parkway, Malvern, PA 19355
Cadmet, Inc. — 800-543-7282
155 Planebrook Road, P.O. Box 24, Malvern, PA 19355
Circulator Boot Corp. — 610-240-9980
72 Pennsylvania Avenue, Malvern, PA 19355
Dentalez Group — 866-DTE-INFO
2 West Liberty Boulevard, Ste. 160, Malvern, PA 19355
Fujirebio Diagnostics, Inc. (Fdi) — 877-861-7246
201 Great Valley Pkwy., Malvern, PA 19355-3809
Great Valley Technologies — 610-647-2210
95 Great Valley Pkwy., Malvern, PA 19355
Huhtamaki — 484-527-2011
2400 Continental Blvd., Malvern, PA 19355
Neuronetics, Inc. — 877-600-7555
31 General Warren Blvd., Malvern, PA 19355
Orthovita, Inc. — 610-640-1775
45 Great Valley Pwy., Malvern, PA 19355
Puricore Inc. — 484-321-2700
508 Lapp Rd., Malvern, PA 19355
Siemens Medical Solutions Health Services Division — 888-321-1777
51 Valley Stream Pkwy., Malvern, PA 19355
Siemens Medical Solutions Usa, Inc — 888-826-9702
51 Valley Stream Parkway, Malvern, PA 19355
Siemens Medical Solutions Usa, Inc. — 610-448-3184
20 Valley Stream Pkwy., Malvern, PA 19355
Siemens Medical Solutions Usa, Inc. — 888-826-9702
51 Valley Stream Parkway, Malvern, PA 19355-1406
Thomas Medical Products, Inc. — 866-446-3003
65 Great Valley Pkwy., Malvern, PA 19355

Thomas Medical Products, Inc.   866-446-3003
65 Great Valley Pkwy., Malvern, PA 19355
Veltek Associates, Inc.   888-478-3745
15 Lee Boulevard, Malvern, PA 19355

Manchester
Flinchbaugh-Kurtz Company   717-266-2202
245 Beshore School Rd., Manchester, PA 17345

Manheim
Bond Caster And Wheel Corporation   800-233-2663
230 South Penn Street, PO Box 339, Manheim, PA 17545

Manor
Spectra Industries Corp.   800-220-7050
322 W. Oak Lane, Manor, PA 19036

Mcconnellsburg
Waring Products, Div. Conair Corp.   203-351-9000
1 Crystal Dr., Mcconnellsburg, PA 17233

Mcelhattan
First Quality Hygienic, Inc.   800-488-3130 Ex
North Rd., Clinton County Industrial Park, Mcelhattan, PA 17748
First Quality Products, Inc.   800-227-3551 Ex
North Rd., Clinton County Industrial Park, Mcelhattan, PA 17748

Mcmurray
Stelkast Company   888-273-1583
200 Hidden Valley Rd., Mcmurray, PA 15317

Meadville
C&J Industries, Inc.   814-724-4950
760 Water St., Meadville, PA 16335-3338

Mechanicsburg
Muffin Enterprises, Inc.   800-338-9041
2 Brenneman Circle, Suite 2, Mechanicsburg, PA 17050
Oven Industries, Inc.   1-877-766-6836
5060 Ritter Rd., Bldg C, Suite 8, Mechanicsburg, PA 17055
Precision Medical Devices, Inc.   717-795-9480
5020 Ritter Rd., Ste. #211, Mechanicsburg, PA 17055

Media
Foamex Innovations   800-355-3626
1400 Providence Road, Suite 2000, Media, PA 19063-2076

Mid City East
John J. Kelley Associates Ltd.   215-567-1377
1528 Walnut Street, Suite 1801, Mid City East, PA 19102

Middletown
Dentsply North America (Dna)   800-877-0020
400 1st St., Suite 250, Middletown, PA 17057

Mildred
Bioscreen Medical Inc.   570-928-7636
Rr I Box 1045a, Mildred, PA 18632

Millersburg,
Advance Scientific, Inc.   1.800.724.4158
163 Research Lane, Millersburg,, PA 17061

Mohnton
Unique Technologies, Inc.   610-775-9191
111 Chestnut St., Mohnton, PA 19540

Mongomeryville
Photomedex, Inc.   215-619-3600
147 Keystone Dr., Mongomeryville, PA 18936

Monroeville
Children's Medical Ventures, Inc.   800-345-6443
191 Wyngate Drive, Monroeville, PA 15146

Montgomery
West Pharmaceutical Services, Inc.   610-594-3105
6453 US Highway 15, Montgomery, PA 17752

Montgomery ville
American Dental Designs Inc.   215-643-3232
717 Bethlehem Pike, Montgomery ville, PA 18936

Montgomeryville
Aes Clean Technology, Inc.   888-237-2532
422 Stump Road, Montgomeryville, PA 18936
Churchill Medical Systems, Inc.   800-468-0585
103a Park Drive, Montgomeryville, PA 19044
Moyco Technologies, Inc.   800-331-8837
200 Commerce Drive, Montgomeryville, PA 18936
Precision Metal Services, Inc.   800-635-4885
418 Stump Road, Montgomeryville, PA 18936
Surgical Laser Technologies, Inc.   800-366-4758
147 Keystone Drive, Montgomeryville, PA 18936

Tosoh Bioscience Llc   800-366-4875
156 Keystone Drive, Montgomeryville, PA 18936
Univac Dental Company   800-523-2559
113 Park Drive, PO Box 447, Montgomeryville, PA 18936-0447
Vygon Corp.   800-473-5414
103a Park Drive, Montgomeryville, PA 18936

Morrisville
Biosoft International Corp.   215-295-0088
102 West Bridge St., Morrisville, PA 19067
Praxair Distribution Mid-Atlantic LLC   610-695-7628
One Steel Rd. East, U.S. Industrial Park, Morrisville, PA 19067
Small Bone Innovations, Inc.   215-428-1791
1380 S. Pennsylvania Ave., Morrisville, PA 19067
Small Bone Innovations, Inc.   (866) SBi-TIPS
1380 S. Pennsylvania Avenue, Morrisville, PA 19067

Mount Holly Spgs
Ahlstrom Filtration Llc   717-486-3438
122 West Butler Street, Mount Holly Spgs, PA 17065

Mount Holly Springs
Vectron International   717-486-6060
100 Watts St., Mount Holly Springs, PA 17065

Mount Pleasant
Matamatic Inc.   888-696-5678
230 Westec Drive, Mount Pleasant, PA 15666

Mountain Top
Hpg International, Inc.   800-242-3909
755 Oakhill Rd, Crestwood Ind Park, Mountain Top, PA 18707

Muncy
Construction Specialties Inc.   800-233-8493
6696 Route. 405, Muncy, PA 17756

Murrysville
Respironics, Inc   800-345-6443
1010 Murry Ridge Ln., Murrysville, PA 15668-8525
Sense Technology, Inc.   800-628-9416
4241 William Penn Highway, 1st Floor, Murrysville, PA 15668

Myerstwn
Dental Resources   717-866-7571
52 West King St., Myerstwn, PA 17067
Mycone Dental Supply Co. Inc. T/A Keystone   717-866-7571
Ind-Myerstown
52 West King St., Myerstwn, PA 17067

N. Huntingdon
Sylvan Corp.   800-628-3836
32 Billot Avenue, N. Huntingdon, PA 15642

Narberth
Millenium Surgical Corp.   877-771-0850
822 Montgomery Ave., Suite 205, Narberth, PA 19072

Nazareth
David Zeller's Wheelchair Brake & Attachment Brkt.   610-759-5134
182 Bath Pike, Nazareth, PA 18064

New Brighton
Tegrant Corporation, Protexic Brands   800-289-9966
800 5th Ave., P.O. Box 448, New Brighton, PA 15066

New Castle
Berner International Corp.   800-245-4455
Shenango Commerce Park, 111 Progress Ave., New Castle, PA 16101
Windl Dental Lab   952-541-9622
314 Maple Dr., New Castle, PA 16105

New Freedom
Oakworks, Inc.   800-558-8850
923 East Wellspring Road, New Freedom, PA 17349

New Holland
Alert-All Corp.   800-253-7825
164 Orlan Road, New Holland, PA 17557

New Hope
Questar Corp.   215-862-5277
6204 Ingham Rd., New Hope, PA 18938
Tcs Scientific Corp.   215-862-3910
6467 StoneyHill Road, New Hope, PA 18938

New Kensington
Respironics, Inc. Sleep Therapy   724-387-4559
312 Alvin Dr., New Kensington, PA 15068
Xodus Medical, Inc.   800-963-8776
Westmoreland Business & Research Park, 702 Prominence Drive, New Kensington, PA 15068

Newtown

Bioclinica, Inc.
826 Newtown-Yardley Rd., Ste. 101, Newtown, PA 18940-1721 — 800-748-9032

Heartsine Technologies, Inc.
121 Friends Lane, Suite 400, Newtown, PA 18940 — 866-478-7463

Newtown Square

Delco Wire Winding Company
59 Street Rd., Newtown Square, PA 19073 — 610-296-0350

Drb Technologies, Inc
3612 Chapel Rd., Suite B, Newtown Square, PA 19073 — 610-356-4258

Ultravoice, Ltd.
3612 Chapel Rd., Newtown Square, PA 19073 — 800-985-3000

Norristown

Boehringer Laboratories, Inc.
500 E. Washington St., Norristown, PA 19404-0870 — 800-642-4945

Lite Tech, Inc.
975 Madison Ave., Norristown, PA 19403 — 610-650-8690

Medisurg Research And Management Corp.
100 West Fornance St., Norristown, PA 19401 — 610-277-3937

Megger Inc. (Formerly Avo International)
2621 Van Buren Avenue, Norristown, PA 19403 — 800-723-2861

Myoderm
48 East Main Street, Norristown, PA 19401 — 610-272-8660

Pulse Biomedical Inc.
1305 catfish lane, Norristown, PA 19403 — 610-666-5510

Sichel Sleep Products
1210 Stanbridge St., Norristown, PA 19401 — 610-292-8700

Spring Health Products, Inc.
705 General Washington Ave., Ste. 701, Norristown, PA 19403 — 800-800-1680

North Huntingdon

Inspired Technologies Inc
1061 Main Street, #24, North Huntingdon, PA 15642 — 724-861-5510

North Wales

Global Dentech Inc.
1116 Horsham Rd., North Wales, PA 19454 — 215-654-1237

Northampton

Medical Fittings
300 Held Dr., Northampton, PA 18067 — 800-331-2685

Precision Medical, Inc.
300 Held Drive, Northampton, PA 18067 — 800-272-7285

Oakdale

Advanced Ocular Prosthetics Inc.
1111 Oakdale Rd., Suite 5, Oakdale, PA 15071 — 412-787-7277

Clarke Health Care Products, Inc.
1003 International Dr., Oakdale, PA 15071-9226 — 888-347-4537

Wright Linear Pump, Inc.
103-B International Drive, Oakdale, PA 15071 — 800-631-9535

Wright Therapy Products
103-B International Drive, Oakdale, PA 15071 — 800-631-9535

Oaks

Franklin Prosthetic Covers
98 Highland Ave., P.O. Box 313, Oaks, PA 19456-0313 — 610-666-6645

Valley Forge Scientific Corp.
136 Green Tree Road, Suite 100, Oaks, PA 19456 — 610-666-7500

Old Forge

Golden Technologies, Inc.
401 Bridge St., Old Forge, PA 18518 — 800-624-6374

Oreland

Spectrocell, Inc.
143 Montgomery Ave., Oreland, PA 19075 — 215-572-7605

Ottsville

Db Consultants, Inc
198 Tabor Road, PO Box 580, Ottsville, PA 18942 — 610-847-5065

Oxford

Cds Analytical, Inc.
465 Limestone Road, Oxford, PA 19363-0277 — 800-541-6593

Perkasie

Daztech, Inc.
424 Broad Street, Perkasie, PA 18944 — 215-669-3102

Medmark Technologies, Llc
724 H West Rt 313 Dublin Park, Perkasie, PA 18944 — 215-249-1540

Psg Controls, Inc.
1225 Tunnel Road, Perkasie, PA 18944 — 800-523-2558

Ts Scientific
PO Box 198, Perkasie, PA 18944-0198 — 800-258-2796

Phila

Inglis Foundation
2600 Belmont Ave., Phila, PA 19131 — 215-581-0725

Philadelphia

Abbey Color, Inc.
400 East Tioga St., Philadelphia, PA 19134 — 877-922-2399

Agusta Aerospace Corporation
3050 Red Lion Road, Philadelphia, PA 19114 — 888-AGUSTA-2

Amuneal Manufacturing Corp.
4737 Darrah St., Philadelphia, PA 19124 — 800-755-9843

Cellucap Manufacturing Co.
4626 N. 15th St., Philadelphia, PA 19140-1109 — 800-523-3814

Centron Technologies, Inc.
10601 Decatur Road, Suite 100, Philadelphia, PA 19154 — 215-501-0430

Current Medicine Group Llc
400 Market St., Suite 700, Philadelphia, PA 19106 — 800-427-1796

Day & Zimmermann Validation Services
1818 Market St., Philadelphia, PA 19103 — 215-299-8000

Dubin Paper Co., Inc.
1910 S. Columbus Blvd., Philadelphia, PA 19148 — 800-653-8246

Echo Therapeutics, Inc.
8 Penn Center, 1628 JFK Boulevard Suite 300, Philadelphia, PA 19103 — 215-717-4100

Eresearchtechnology Inc.
1818 Market Street, Suite 1000, Philadelphia, PA 19103-3638 — 215-972-0420

Exocell, Inc.
1880 JFK Boulevard, Suite 200, Philadelphia, PA 19103 — 800-234-3962

Frank J. May, Inc.
256 South 11th St., Philadelphia, PA 19107 — 215-923-3165

Gem Refrigerator Co.
7340 Milnor Street, Philadelphia, PA 19136 — 877-436-7374

General Econopak, Inc.
1725 N. 6th St., Philadelphia, PA 19122 — 888-871-8568

General Scientific Safety Equipment Co.
2553 E Somerset St. 1st Floor, Philadelphia, PA 19134-4742 — 800-523-0166

Global Pharmaeuticals: A Division Of Impax Labs Inc.
3735 Castor Avenue, Philadelphia, PA 19124-5694 — 800-296-9227

Hotpack
10940 Dutton Rd., Philadelphia, PA 19154-3286 — 800-523-3608

Howard/Mccray Refrigerator, Inc.
831 East Cayuga St, Philadelphia, PA 19124 — 800-344-8222

Legrand Assoc.
1601 Walnut Street, Suite 616, Philadelphia, PA 19102 — 800-523-4314

Medical Products Laboratories, Inc.
9990 Global Rd., Philadelphia, PA 19115 — 215-677-2700

Microcision Llc
5805 Keystone St., Philadelphia, PA 19135-4293 — 800-264-3811

Neuro Diagnostic Devices
3701 Market St, 3rd Floor, Philadelphia, PA 19104 — 888-SHUNT-OK

Nichole Medical Equipment & Supply, Inc.
2200 Michener St., Suite #4, Philadelphia, PA 19115 — 888-673-6335

Nuvon Inc.
3624 Market Street, Suite 5E, Philadelphia, PA 19104 — 215-966-6142

Orthopli Corp.
10061 Sandmeyer Ln., Philadelphia, PA 19116 — 215-568-0700

Philadelphia Vision Center
1100 Market St., Philadelphia, PA 19107 — 215-282-5500

Premier Research
1500 Market Street, Suite 3500, Philadelphia, PA 19102 — 215-533-1988

Quint Company
3725 Castor Ave., Philadelphia, PA 19124 — 800-332-0672

Rmc Medical
6940 State Road Bldg C, Philadelphia, PA 19154-3201 — 800-523-3602

Simkar Corporation
700 Ramona, Philadelphia, PA 19120-4691 — 215-728-1035

Skin Deep, Inc.
1926 Cottman Ave., Philadelphia, PA 19111 — 800-626-3006

Star Medical Systems
8301 Torresdale Avenue, Suite 13, Philadelphia, PA 19136 — 888-883-7804

The Ansar Group, Inc.
240 South Eighth St., Philadelphia, PA 19107 — 800-523-0178

The Kendrick Co., Inc.
6139 Germantown Ave., Philadelphia, PA 19144 — 425-487-7000

Ugm Medical Systems, Inc.
3611 Market St., Philadelphia, PA 19104 — 800-932-2634

Webb Manufacturing Co.
1241 Carpenter St., Philadelphia, PA 19147-5512

Philidelphia

Duro-Test Lighting
12401 McNulty Road, Suite 101, Philidelphia, PA 19154 — 800-289-3876

Phoenixville

Msi Precision, Specialty Instrument
1220 Valley Forge Rd., Bldg. 34, Phoenixville, PA 19460 — 800-322-4674

Pipersville

Lampire Biological Laboratories
PO Box 270, Pipersville, PA 18947 — 215-795-2838

Powers Scientific, Inc.
PO Box 268, Pipersville, PA 18947 — 800-998-0500

Pittsburgh

Aei Technologies Inc.
300 William Pitt Way, Pittsburgh, PA 15238 — 800-793-7751

Aethon Inc.
100 Business Center Drive, Pittsburgh, PA 15205 — 412-322-2975

Algor, Inc. — 800-48-ALGOR
150 Beta Dr., Pittsburgh, PA 15238-2932
Ansoft Corp. — 412-261-3200
225 West Station Square Drive, Suite 200, Pittsburgh, PA 15219-1119
Best Nomos Corp. — 800-70-NOMOS
One Best Dr., Pittsburgh, PA 15202
Blind & Vision Rehabilitation Services Of Pittsbur — 412-325-7504
1204 Western Ave., Bldg. 4, Pittsburgh, PA 15233
Burrell Scientific, Inc — 800-637-6074
2223 Fifth Avenue, Pittsburgh, PA 15219-5597
Cardiac Assist, Inc. — 412-963-7770
240 Alpha Dr., Pittsburgh, PA 15238
Cima Technology, Inc. — 724-733-2627
3253-C Old Frankstown Road, Pittsburgh, PA 15239
Clearcount Medical Solutions, Inc. — 412-931-7233
101 Bellevue Road,, Suite 203, Pittsburgh, PA 15229
Comprehensive Safety Compliance, Inc. — 412-826-5480
295 William Pitt Way, Pittsburgh, PA 15238-1328
Computational Diagnostics, Inc. — 412-681-9990
5001 Baum Blvd., Suite 530, Pittsburgh, PA 15213
Dental Services Group Of Pittsburgh — 80-322-7080
101 South 10th Street, Pittsburgh, PA 15203
Dynavox Systems Inc. — 866-396-2869
2100 Wharton St., Suite 400, Pittsburgh, PA 15203
Extrel Cms — 412-963-7530
575 Epsilon Dr., Pittsburgh, PA 15238-2838
Fisher Scientific Co., Llc. — 800-766-7000
2000 Park Lane, Pittsburgh, PA 15275
Flexuspine — 412-539-1520
381 Mansfield Ave, Ste. 205, Pittsburgh, PA 15220
Good Sports — 412-731-3032
1701 Monongahela Avenue, Pittsburgh, PA 15218
Ingmar Medical, Ltd. — 800-583-9910
P.O. Box 10106, Pittsburgh, PA 15232
Labchem, Inc. — 412-826-5230
200 William Pitt Way, Pittsburgh, PA 15238
Medrad Inc. — 724-940-7940
625 Alpha Dr., Pittsburgh, PA 15238
Minatronics Corp. — 412-488-6435
1 Trimont Lane, 850C, Pittsburgh, PA 15211
Neuro Kinetics — 412-963-6649
128 Gamma Dr., Pittsburgh, PA 15238
Novum Inc. — 412-363-3300
5900 Penn Ave., Pittsburgh, PA 15206-3817
Omnyx LLC — 412-894-2100
30 Isabella Street, Suite 301, Pittsburgh, PA 15212
Pennsylvania Glass Products Co. — 412-621-2853
430 N. Craig St., Pittsburgh, PA 15213-1105
Pinmed, Inc — 412-687-6964
245 Melwood Ave., #501, Pittsburgh, PA 15213
Recreation Equipment Unlimited, Inc. — 412-731-3000
P.O. Box 4700, Pittsburgh, PA 15206
Surco Products — 800-556-0111
RIDC Industrial Park, 292 Alpha Drive, Pittsburgh, PA 15238-2903
Vilex, Inc. — 800-872-4911
345 Old Curry Hollow Road, Pittsburgh, PA 15236
Zoll Lifecor Corporation — 800-543-3267
121 Freeport Road, Pittsburgh, PA 15238
3dsharp, Inc. — 412-648-9211
6425 Forward Ave., Pittsburgh, PA 15217

Pleasant Gap

Matreya Llc — 800-342-3595
168 Tressler St., Pleasant Gap, PA 16823-3218

Plumsteadville

Scott Medical Products — 800-233-4334
6097 Easton Road, Building 3, Plumsteadville, PA 18949-0310
Scott Specialty Gases — 215-766-8861
6141 Easton Road Box 310, Plumsteadville, PA 18949

Plymouth Meeting

Athena Controls, Inc. — 800-782-6776
5145 Campus Drive, Plymouth Meeting, PA 19462
Biomol Research Labs — 800-942-0430
5120 Butler Pike, Plymouth Meeting, PA 19462
CRF Health — 1 267 498 2300
4000 Chemical Road, Suite 400, Plymouth Meeting, PA 19462
Peripheral Dynamics Inc. — 800-253-0253
5150 Campus Drive, Plymouth Meeting, PA 19462
Premier Dental Products Co. — 888-670-6100
1710 Romano Dr., Plymouth Meeting, PA 19462
Premier Medical Products — 888-PREMUSA
1710 Romano Dr., Plymouth Meeting, PA 19462

Port Matilda

Qbc Diagnostics, Inc. — 814-342-6205
168 Bradford Drive, Port Matilda, PA 16870

Pottstown

Precision Polymer Products — 610-326-0921
815 South St., Pottstown, PA 19464
Ultraflex Systems, Inc. — 800-220-6670
237 South Street, Ste. 200, Pottstown, PA 19464

Pottsville

United Receptacle — 800-233-0314
1400 Laurel Blvd, Pottsville, PA 17901

Radnor

Airway Cam Technologies, Inc. — 877-EPIGLOTTIS
205 Spruce Tree Rd., Radnor, PA 19087

Randor

Airgas, Inc. — 610-687-5253
259 North Radnor-Chester Rd., Randor, PA 19087-5283

Reading

Arrow International, Inc. — 800-523-8446
2400 Bernville Rd., Reading, PA 19605
Brentwood Industries, Inc. — 610-374-5109
610 Morgantown Rd., Reading, PA 19611
Enersys — 610-208-1991
2366 Bernville Road, Reading, PA 19605
Genpore, A Division Of General Polymeric Corp. — 800-654-4391
1136 Morgantown Road, Reading, PA 19607
Misco Products Corp. — 800-548-4568
1048 Stinson Dr., Reading, PA 19605
Surgical Specialties Corporation — 800-523-3332
100 Dennis Drive, Reading, PA 19606
Tray-Pak Corporation — 888-926-1777
Tuckerton Road & Reading Crest Avenue, PO Box 14804, Reading, PA 19612-4804

Red Lion

Belmed, Inc. — 888-723-5893
887 Delta Rd., Red Lion, PA 17356

Reedsville

Philips Ultrasound, Inc. — 425-487-7000
1 Echo Dr., Reedsville, PA 17084-8603

Robesonia

Grosfillex, Inc. — 800-233-3186
230 Old West Penn Avenue, Robesonia, PA 19551

Rosemont

Jaro, Inc. — 610-527-1889
1111 Lancaster Ave., Rosemont, PA 19010

S Williamsport

Rapid Pathogen Screening, Inc. — 941-556-1850
101 Philips Park Dr., S Williamsport, PA 17702

Saxonburg

Ii-Vi, Inc. — 724-352-4455
375 Saxonburg Blvd., Saxonburg, PA 16056-9499
Medrad Saxonburg, Inc. — 724-940-7940
150 Victory Road, Saxonburg, PA 16056

Schnecksville

Patient Instrumentation Corp. — 610-799-4436
4117 Rte. 309, Schnecksville, PA 18078-2509

Schuylkill Haven

M & Q Packaging Corp. — 877-726-7287
Earl Street, Schuylkill Haven, PA 17972

Sellersville

Scandinavian Formulas, Inc. — 215-453-2507
140 East Church St., Sellersville, PA 18960

Sewickley

Hyginet Corp. Of America — 800-245-1036
505 North Drive, 79 North Industrial Park, Sewickley, PA 15143-0049

Sharon

Crosstex International, Inc. — 516-482-9001
534 Vine Street, Sharon, PA 16146

Sharon Hill

Beckman Coulter, Inc. Primary Care Diagnostics — 714-961-3712
606 Elmwood Ave., Elmwood Court Three, Sharon Hill, PA 19079

Simpson

Gentex Corporation — 570-282-8350
324 Main St., P.o. Box 315, Simpson, PA 18407

Sinking Spring

Alcon Manufacturing, Ltd. — 817-551-6813
714 Columbia Ave., Sinking Spring, PA 19608

Skippack

Mar Cor Purification — 800-346-0365
4450 Township Line Road, Skippack, PA 19474-1429
Penco Products Inc. — 800-562-1000
2024 Cressman Road, P O Box 158, Skippack, PA 19474

Slatington

R&R Medical, Inc. — 877-776-9972
2225 Park Place Dr., Slatington, PA 18080

Souderton

Ar Worldwide — 800-933-8181
160 School House Road, Souderton, PA 18964-9990
Youngs, Inc. — 800-523-5454
55 Cherry Lane, Souderton, PA 18964-1550

South Park

Autovage — 412-653-5888
1631 Citation Dr., South Park, PA 15129
Coventina Healthcare Enterprises, Inc. — 412-915-6442
1297 Royal Park Blvd., South Park, PA 15129

Southampton

Environmental Tectonics Corp. — 215-355-9100
125 James Way, Southampton, PA 18966
M&C Specialties Co. — 800-441-6996
90 James Way, Southampton, PA 18966-3816
Princo Instruments, Inc. — 800-221-9237
1020 Industrial Blvd., Southampton, PA 18966-4095

Spring City

Amici, Inc. — 610-948-7100
518 Vincent St., Spring City, PA 19475-1621

Spring Mills

Gettig Pharmaceutical Instrument Co., Div Of — 814-422-8892
Gettig Technologies Inc.
1 Streamside Pl. W., Spring Mills, PA 16875-0085

State College

Blatek, Inc. — 814-231-2085
2820 E. College Avenue, Suite F, State College, PA 16801-7548
Cannon Instrument Co. — 800-676-6232
2139 High Tech Road, State College, PA 16803
Diapedia, Llc — 814-234-0700
200 Innovation Blvd., Ste. 241, State College, PA 16803
Proact, Ltd. — 814-231-2158
112 W. Foster Ave., 202 C, State College, PA 16801
Salimetrics, Llc — 800-790-2258
101 Innovation Blvd., Suite 302, State College, PA 16803
Strategic Polymer Sciences Inc. — 814-238-7400
200 Innovation Blvd., Suite 237, State College, PA 16803

Swarthmore

Occupational Hearing Services — 800-622-3277
300 South Chester Road, Suite 301, Swarthmore, PA 19081

Telford

Case Design Corp. — 800-847-4176
333 School Lane, Telford, PA 18969
Draeger Medical Systems, Inc — 800-437-2437
3135 Quarry Rd, Telford, PA 18969
Draeger Safety, Inc. — 215-660-2186
3135 Quarry Road, Telford, PA 18969
Nursing Care Curtain Co. — 215-723-8166
114 W. Broad St., Telford, PA 18969-1922

Trevose

Associated Production Services, Inc. — 215-364-0211
365 Andrews Rd., Trevose, PA 19053
Concept Health, Llc — 215-364-3600
3600 Boundbrook Ave., Trevose, PA 19053
Gentell — 800-840-9041
3600 Bound Brook Rd., Trevose, PA 19053
Key Instruments — 215-357-6488
250 Andrews Rd., Trevose, PA 19053
Mennen Medical Corp. — 800-223-2201
2540 Metropolitan Drive, Trevose, PA 19053-6738

Trumbauersville

Total Molding Services, Inc. — 215-538-9613
354 East Broad St., Trumbauersville, PA 18970

Ulster

The Steady-Arm Company, Inc. — 570-358-3632
Rr 1 Box 353, Ulster, PA 18850-9513

Union City

Noram Seating, Inc. — 866-236-7328
18 Market Street, Union City, PA 16438

Uniontown

Abel Dental Lab — 952-541-9622
2 West Main Street, National City Bank Building, Uniontown, PA 15401
Berkley Medical Resources, Inc. — 412-438-3000
49 Virginia Ave., Uniontown, PA 15401

Vandergrift

Cook Vascular, Incorporated — 800-457-4500
1186 Montgomery Lane, Vandergrift, PA 15690
F & L Medical Products Co. — 724-845-7028
1129 Industrial Park Rd., Box 3, Vandergrift, PA 15690

Wampum

Homak Manufacturing Company Inc. — 800-874-6625
1605 Old Route 18, Suite 4-36, Wampum, PA 16157

Warminster

Alfa Laval Inc — 866-253-2528
955 Mearns Road, Warminster, PA 18974-0556
Eagle Stainless Container — 215-957-9333
816 Nina Way, Warminster, PA 18974-2206
Kruse Tool And Die Inc. — 215-674-1730
P.O. Box 2247, Warminster, PA 18974
Laminar Flow, Inc. — 800-553-FLOW
102 Richard Road, PO Box 2427, Warminster, PA 18974-1528
Orapharma, Inc. — 215-956-2200
732 Louis Drive, Warminster, PA 18974
Tek Marketing, Inc. — 215-364-4941
98 Railroad Dr., Warminster, PA 18974-1454

Warren

Interlectric Corp. — 800-722-2184
1401 Lexington Avenue, Warren, PA 16365-2849

Warrendale

Dymax Corp. — 908-277-8481
110 Marshall Dr., Warrendale, PA 15086
Medrad, Inc. — 800-633-7231
100 Global View Dr., Warrendale, PA 15086
Possis Medical, Inc. — 800-633-7231
100 Global View Drive, Warrendale, PA 15086
Renal Solutions Inc. — (866) 466-3436
770 Commonwealth Drive, Suite 101, Warrendale, PA 15086

Warrington

Polysciences, Inc. — 800-523-2575
400 Valley Rd., Warrington, PA 18976-2522
Rushabh Instruments, Llc — 215-491-0081
1750a Costner Dr., Warrington, PA 18976

Wash

Washington-Greene County Branch — 724-228-0770
Pennsylvania Assoc
566 East Maiden St., Wash, PA 15301

Washington

Dynamet, Inc. — 800-237-9655
195 Museum Rd., Washington, PA 15301

Wayne

Embrella Cardiovascular, Inc. — 610-783-1100
880 E. Swedesford Road, Suite 220, Wayne, PA 19087
Escalon Medical Corp. — 610-688-6830
435 Devon Park Drive, Building 100, Wayne, PA 19087
Molecular Detection Inc. — 610-590-1974
400 East Lancaster Avenue, Suite 300, Wayne, PA 19087

West Chester

Animas Corp. — 877-767-7373
200 Lawrence Drive, West Chester, PA 19380
Chiral Technologies, Inc. — 800-6-Chiral
800 North Five Points Road, West Chester, PA 19380
D.C.A. (Dental Corporation Of America) — 800-638-6684
889 South Matlack, West Chester, PA 19382
Structure Probe, Inc., Spi Supplies — 800-2424-SPI
569 East Gay St., PO Box 656, West Chester, PA 19380-0656
Synthes (Usa) - Brandywine Technical Center — 800-523-0322
1302 Wrights Lane East, West Chester, PA 19380
Synthes (Usa) - Development Center — 719-481-5300
1230 Wilson Dr., West Chester, PA 19380
Synthes Inc. — 800-523-0322
1302 Wrights Ln. E., West Chester, PA 19380
Synthes Jennersville — 484-356-9728
108 Willowbrook Lane, West Chester, PA 19382
Thermo Electric Company — 800-523-2002
1193 McDermott Drive, West Chester, PA 19380

West Hazleton

The Neurological Research And Development Group — 800-327-6759
115 Rotary Drive, West Hazleton, PA 18202

West Middlesex

Anna-Dote, Inc. — 800-346-6132
40 Pullam Drive, West Middlesex, PA 16159-9604

West Mifflin

Nasorcap Medical, Inc. — 412-466-1412
1077 Huston Drive, West Mifflin, PA 15122-3101

Westfield

K & W Medical Specialties, Inc. — 215-675-4653
115 Pritchard Hollow Rd., Westfield, PA 16950

Wexford

Dimensional Dosing Systems, Inc. — 724-933-7874
2465 Dogwood Dr., Wexford, PA 15090

Wilkes Barre

Intermetro Industries Corp. — 800-441-2714
651 N. Washington St., Wilkes Barre, PA 18705-1707
Modern Plastics Corp. — 570-822-1124
152 Horton St., Wilkes Barre, PA 18702-3499

Williamsport

Duralife, Inc. — 800-443-5433
195 Phillips Park Dr., Williamsport, PA 17702
Lindberg/Blue M — 800-216-7725
2121 Reach Rd., Williamsport, PA 17701
Thermal Product Solutions — 800-586-2473
2121 Reach Road, Williamsport, PA 17701
Thermal Product Solutions — 800-216-7725
2121 Reach Road, Williamsport, PA 17701

Willow Grove

Caldyne, Inc. — 215-830-3076
2425 Maryland Road, Willow Grove, PA 19090
Recigno Laboratories Inc. — 215-659-7755
509 Davisville Rd., Willow Grove, PA 19090
Trico Metal Products, Inc. — 800-457-1376
2309 Wyandotte Rd., Willow Grove, PA 19090

Wilmerding

P.B. Connections, Inc. — 412-825-6095
341 Marguerite Ave., Wilmerding, PA 15148

Wyncote

Atd-American Co. — 800-523-2300
135 Greenwood Ave., Wyncote, PA 19095-1337

Wyndmoor

Moore Push-Pin Co. — 800-289-6667
1300 East Mermaid Lane, Wyndmoor, PA 19038-7664

Yardley

Vetter Pharma-Turm, Inc. — 215-321-6930
Heston Hall/Carriage House, Suite 203, 1790 Yardley-Langhorne Rd., Yardley, PA 19067
Ziamatic Corp. — 800-711-FIRE
10 W. College Avenue, Yardley, PA 19067-8337

Yeadon

Hydrol Chemical Co. — 610-622-3603
520 Commerce Dr., Yeadon, PA 19050

York

Dentsply International, Inc. — 800-877-0020
Susquehanna Commerce Center, 221 W. Philadelphia Street, York, PA 17405-0872
Dentsply Professional — 800-989-8825
1301 Smile Way, York, PA 17404
Dentsply Prosthetics — 800-621-0381
570 West College Avenue, York, PA 17404
Dentsply Specialty Materials — 800-877-0020
1301 Smile Way, York, PA 17404
First Level Inc — 717-266-2450
3109 Espresso Way, York, PA 17406
Miltex Dental Technologies, Inc. — 516-576-6022
589 Davies Dr., York, PA 17402
Miltex Inc. — 800-645-8000
589 Davies Drive, York, PA 17402
Nanzee Dental Products — 717-792-9795
2916 Robin Road, York, PA 17404-5768
Prident International Inc. — 717-849-4229
570 West College Ave., York, PA 17404
Spectrum Systems, Llc — 717-845-5339
465 Ogontz St., --, York, PA 17403
Unilife Medical Solutions — 1-800-324-7674
250 Cross Farm Lane, York, PA 17406
York Barbell — 800-358-9675
3300 Board Rd., York, PA 17405-1707

York New Salem

Valley Products Co. — 800-451-8874
P.O. Box 187, York New Salem, PA 17371-0187

Zelienople

Zivic Laboratories — 800-422-5227
178 Toll Gate School Road, Zelienople, PA 16063

PUERTO RICO

Aguadilla

Lifescan Products, Llc — 408-942-3589
San Antonio Industrial Park, Extension, Rd. 110 Km. 5.9, Aguadilla, PR 00603

Aibonito

Baxter Healthcare S.A. — 847-948-2000
Rd. 721, Km. 0.3, Aibonito, PR 00609

Anasco

A.M.O. Puerto Rico Manufacturing, Inc — 787-826-2727
Road 402N Industrial Zone, PO Box 1408, Anasco, PR 00610
Cardinal Health — 847-785-3323
State Rd. 402, Km 0.9, Anasco, PR 00610
Edwards Lifesciences Technology Sarl — 949-250-2500
State Rd. 402 N.km 1.4, Anasco, PR 00610-1577
Integra Neurosciences Pr — 800-654-2873
Road 402 North, Km 1.2, Anasco, PR 00610
Jostra Bentley, Inc. — 302-454-9959
Rd. 402 N. Km 1.4, Industrial Park, Anasco, PR 00610-1577

Arecibo

St. Jude Medical. Puerto Rico, Llc — 787-746-1111
Lot A Interior - #2 St Km 67.5, Santana Industrial Park, Arecibo, PR 00612

Arroyo

Stryker Puerto Rico, Ltd. — 939-307-2500
Hwy. 3, Km. 131.2, Las Guasimas Ind. Park, Arroyo, PR 00714

Barceloneta

Abbott Diagnostics Intl, Biotechnology Ltd — 787-846-3500
Road #2 KM. 58.0 , PO Box 278, Cruce Davila, Barceloneta, PR 00617
Abbott Vascular, Cardiac Therapies-P.R — 847-937-2388
Km 58.0, Carretera 2, Cruce Davilla, Barceloneta, PR 00617

Bo Juana Matos

Baxter Healthcare Of Puerto Rico — 847-948-4054
530 Road #5, Building #1, Bo Juana Matos, PR 00962

Cabo Rojo

Lifescan Llc. — 408-263-9789
Rd. 308 Km 0.8, Pedernales Industrial Park, Cabo Rojo, PR 00623-5001

Caguas

C-Axis P.R., Inc. — 787-286-0590
Parque Industrial Valle Polima, Edif Multifabril 14-a-2, Caguas, PR 00727
Caguas Orthopedic Center, Inc. — 787-744-2325
Ff4, Calle 11, 4th Secc., Villa Del Rey, Caguas, PR 00625
St. Jude Medical, Puerto Rico, B.V. — 787-746-1111
Lot 20, Caguas West Industrial Park, Caguas, PR 00726-0998

Catano

Linde Gas Puerto Rico Inc. — 908-771-1669
Carr 869 Km 1 Hm 8s Flamboya, Catano, PR 00962

Cayey

Becton Dickinson Caribe Ltd — 410-316-4000
Vicks Dr, Lot #6, Cayey, PR 00634

Cidra

Ciba Vision Puerto Rico, Inc. — 678-415-3638
El Jibaro Industrial Park, PO Box 1360, Cidra, PR 00739

Dorado

Maquet Puerto Rico Inc. — 408-635-3900
No. 12, Rd. #698, Dorado, PR 00646

Est De San Geraldo

Philips Medical Systems (Pmms Puerto Rico), Inc — 978-659-4663
200 Winston Churchill Ave. Suite, 302 Mercurio St. Apolo Shopping Center, Est De San Geraldo, PR 00926

Ext Mans San German

Fenwal International, Inc. — 847-550-7908
Camino Real Industrial Park,, Road #122, Ext Mans San German, PR 00683

Fajardo

Customed, Inc. — 787-801-0101
Calle Igualdad #7, Fajardo, PR 00738
Marcoop Molding — 787-863-3952
Puerto Real Ind'l. Park Rd. 195, Km. 2.9, Fajardo, PR 00738
Pall Lifesciences Puerto Rico Llc — 516-801-9064
Carr. 194, Km. O.4, Fajardo, PR 00738

Guayama

Medisearch P.R., Inc. — 787-864-0684
Machete Industrial Center, Guayama, PR 00784

Guaynabo

Baxter Sales & Distribution Corp — 847-473-6141
Rexco Industrial Park, State Road #24, Buchanan, Guaynabo, PR 00968
Ebi Patient Care, Inc. — 973-299-9300
1 Electro-biology Blvd., Guaynabo, PR 00657
Ethicon Endo-Surgery, Llc — 513-337-3134
475 Calle C, Guaynabo, PR 00969
Johnson & Johnson Hemisferica, S.A. — 868-640-3772
Calle C # 475, Los Frailes Ind. Park, Guaynabo, PR 00969
Johnson & Johnson International — 787-272-1900
Calle C #475, Suite 200; Los Frailes Industrial Park, Guaynabo, PR 00969

Gurabo

Praxair-Puerto Rico — 440-234-1075
Rt. 931 & 189, Gurabo, PR 00778

Humacao

Bard Shannon Limited — 908-277-8000
San Geronimo Industrial Park, Lot # 1, Road # 3, Km 79.7, Humacao, PR 00791
Medtronic Puerto Rico Operations Co.,Med Rel — 763-514-4000
Road 909, Km. 0.4., Barrio Mariana, Humacao, PR 00792

Juana Diaz

Cooper Vision Carribbean — 925-460-3600
500 Road 584 Lot 7, Amuelas Industrial Park, Juana Diaz, PR 00795

Juncos

Colgate Juncos, Inc. — 212-310-2000
Rd #31 No 100, Juncos, PR 00777
Medtronic Puerto Rico Operations Co., Juncos — 763-514-4000
Road 31, Km. 24, Hm 4, Ceiba Norte Industrial Park, Juncos, PR 00777

Las Piedras

Aspen Surgical Puerto Rico Corp. — 201-847-4298
Rd. 183, Km. 20.3, Las Piedras, PR 00771
Dentsply Prosthetics — 800-877-0020
183 State Road, K.M. 19.6, Las Piedras, PR 00771
Rd Medical Mfg. Inc. — 787-716-6363
Road 183, Km 21.6, Las Piedras Industrial Park, Las Piedras, PR 00771

Maricao

Fenwal International, Inc. — 847-550-7908
Road 357, Km. 0.8, Maricao, PR 00606

Mayaguez

Frederick Lee Inc — 787-834-4880
Balboa St. #191, PO Box 3287, Mayaguez, PR 00680

Mercedita

Essilor Industries — 011-331-4977422
Sabanetas Industrial Park, Mercedita, PR 00715
Zimmer Manufacturing B.V. — 800-613-6131
Route 1, Km. 123.4, Bldg. 1, Turpeaux Industrial Park, Mercedita, PR 00715

Ponce

Ear-Tech Of Puerto Rico — 787-841-6913
Urb. Mercedita, 1469 Calle Aloa, Ponce, PR 00717-2622
Roche Diagnostics Corp. — 317-521-2834
Marginal Rd., Punto Oro, Industrial Development, Ponce, PR 00731
Ussc Puerto Rico, Inc. — 203-845-1000
Building 911-67, Sabanetas Industrial Park, Ponce, PR 00731

Rincon

Medical Sterile Products, Inc. — 800-292-2887
Rd. 115. Km. 12.9, Rincon, PR 00743

Sabana Grande

B. Braun Of Puerto Rico, Inc. — 610-691-5400
215.7 Insular Rd., Sabana Grande, PR 00637

San German

Cordis Llc — 877-338-4235
Road 362 Km 0.5, San German, PR 00683

San Juan

Aga Linde Healthcare P.R. Inc. — 787-622-7900
GPO Box 364727, Tres Monjitas, PO Box 363868, San Juan, PR 00936-4727
J.M. Baragano Biomedical P.M. And Consulting, Inc. — 787-722-4007
808 Fernandez Juncos Avenue, San Juan, PR 00907

San Lorenzo

Ethicon, Llc. — 908-218-2887
Rd. 183, Km. 8.3,, Industrial Area Hato, San Lorenzo, PR 00754

Toa Alta

Ortho-Tain, Inc. — 800-541-6612
Carr 861, K.m. 5.0, Barrio, Pinas, Toa Alta, PR 00953

Vega Baja

Vegamed, Inc. — 787-807-0392
Edificio Multifabril #5, Ave. Las Flores #39, Vega Baja, PR 00693

Villalba

Medtronic Puerto Rico Operations Co., Villalba — 763-514-4000
Rd. 149, Km. 56.3, Call Box 6001, Villalba, PR 00766

RHODE ISLAND

Ashaway

Ashaway Line & Twine Manufacturing Co. — 800-556-7260
24 Laurel St., P.O. Box 549, Ashaway, RI 02804

Barrington

Nanomaterials, Inc. — 401-433-7022
9 Preston Drive, Barrington, RI 02806
Precision Electrolysis Needles, Inc. — 800-206-7771
166 Bay Spring Ave., Barrington, RI 02806

Bristol

Huestis Medical — 800-972-9222
68 Buttonwood St., Bristol, RI 02809-3600

Cranscon

Fielding Manufacturing — 800-230-8690
780 Wellington Ave., Cranscon, RI 02910-2938

Cranston

Max Bloom, M.D. — 401-785-9671
111 Roger Williams Cir., Cranston, RI 02905-1128
North Safety Products — 800-430-4110
2000 Plainfield Pike, Cranston, RI 02921-2012
Rush Medical — 401-461-9132
18 Gallup Ave., Cranston, RI 02910
Torbot Group, Inc. — 800-545-4254
1367 Elmwood Ave., Cranston, RI 02910

East Providence

Cybermdx, Inc. — 401-228-3772
850 Waterman Ave, East Providence, RI 02914
Igus, Inc. — 800-521-2747
PO Box 14349, East Providence, RI 02914
Nerl Diagnostics Llc. — 401-824-2046
14 Almeida Ave., East Providence, RI 02914
Reade Advanced Materials — 401-433-7000
PO Box 15039, East Providence, RI 02915-0039

Glendale

Bruin Plastics Co. — 800-556-7764
61 Joslin Rd., Glendale, RI 02826-0700

Lincoln

Greystone Of Lincoln, Inc. — 800-446-7161
7 Wellington Rd., Lincoln, RI 02865
Stackbin Corporation — 800-333-1603
29 Powder Hill Rd., Lincoln, RI 02865-4424
Tri-Medics, Inc. — 401-490-5321
10 Pine Tree Lane, Lincoln, RI 02865
Unicom — 800-556-2828
6 Blackstone Valley Place, Suite 402, Lincoln, RI 02865
Vital Diagnostics Inc. — 714-672-3553
27 Wellington Road, Lincoln, RI 02865

Middletown

Avid Products — 888-575-AVID
Aquidneck Industrial Park, 72 Johnny Cake Hill Rd., Middletown, RI 02842

Misquamicut

Agfa Healthcare Corp. — 864-421-1815
1 Crosswind Rd., Misquamicut, RI 02891

N. Kingstown

Brown & Sharpe Inc. — 800-343-7933
250 Circuit Drive, N. Kingstown, RI 02852

No. Smithfield

ATLANTIC FOOTCARE — 401-765-8600
761 Great Rd., No. Smithfield, RI 02896

North Kingstown

Unetixs Vascular, Inc. — 800-486-3849
115 Airport Street,, North Kingstown, RI 02852

North Smithfield

Narragansett Imaging — 401-767-4462
51 Industrial Drive, North Smithfield, RI 02896

Pawtucket

Bio-Detek, Inc. — 800-225-1310
525 Narragansett Park Drive, Pawtucket, RI 02861-4323
Hasbro, Inc. — 401-431-8697
1027 Newport Ave., Pawtucket, RI 02862-1059

Portsmouth

Cotran Corp. — 800-345-4449
574 Park Avenue, PO Box 130, Portsmouth, RI 02871

Providence

Contech Medical, Inc. — 401-351-4890
99 Hartford Ave., Providence, RI 02909-3326
Cowan Plastics, Llc — 401-351-1400
610 Manton Avenue, Providence, RI 02909
Embassy Creations — 800-367-3341
122 Manton Avenue, Box L4, Providence, RI 02909
Lfi, Inc-Laser Fare, Inc. — (401) 278-9100
315 Iron Horse Way,, Suite 101, Providence, RI 02908
Medport, Llc — 800-299-5704
23 Acorn St., Providence, RI 02903
Verichem Laboratories, Inc. — 401-461-0180
90 Narragansett Ave., Providence, RI 02907

Riverside

Instantron — 401-433-6800
3712 Pawtucket Ave., Riverside, RI 02915

Rumford

In-Sight — 401-434-1211
750 Narragansett Park Dr., Rumford, RI 02916

Smithfield

Degania Silicone, Inc. — 401-349-5373
14 Thurber Boulevard, Suite A, Smithfield, RI 02917

Gargoyles Eyewear — 800-426-6396
500 George Washington Hwy, Smithfield, RI 02917

Sperian Eye & Face Protection Inc. — 401-232-1200
10 Thurber Blvd., Smithfield, RI 02917

Sperian Protection — 800-343-3411
900 Douglas Pike, Smithfield, RI 02917

Warwick

Davol Inc., Sub. C.R. Bard, Inc. — 800-556-6275
100 Crossings Blvd., Warwick, RI 02886

Dome Publishing Company, Inc. — 401-738-7900
10 New England Way, Warwick, RI 02887

Niche Medical, Inc. — 800-633-1055
55 Access Rd., Warwick, RI 02886

Oracle Lens Mfg. Corp. — 401-736-9600
30 Jefferson Park Rd., Warwick, RI 02888

Ost Medical Inc. — 401-737-3774
11 Knight St., Bldg F-23, Warwick, RI 02886

Sunglass International Llc — 888-478-6764
71 Cypress St., Warwick, RI 02888

West Kingston

American Power Conversion — 800-788-2208
132 Fairgrounds Road, West Kingston, RI 02892

West Warwick

Astro-Med, Inc. — 800-343-4039
600 E. Greenwich Avenue, West Warwick, RI 02893-7526

Woonsocket

Exercycle Corporation — 800-367-6712 X
667 Providence St., Woonsocket, RI 02895-6259

Summer Infant, Inc. — 800-268-6237
1275 Park East Drive, Woonsocket, RI 02895

Tytex, Inc. — 401-762-4100
601 Park East Dr.,, Highland Industrial Park, Woonsocket, RI 02895

SOUTH CAROLINA

Abbeville

Princess Uniforms Accessories — 800-845-5455
72 Agan Road, Abbeville, SC 29620

Anderson

Inreach Corporation — 888-517-3224
2017 Cardinal Circle, Anderson, SC 29621-1503

Pure Water, Inc. — 864-375-0105
311 W. Market St., Anderson, SC 29624

Beaufort

Turbo Wheelchair Co., Inc. — 843-322-0486
45 Laurel Bay Rd., Suite 3 & 15, Beaufort, SC 29906

Beech Island

Kimberly-Clark Corp. (Beech Island Mill) — 888-525-8388
246 Old Jackson Highway, Beech Island, SC 29842

Belvedere

Tudor Scientific Glass Co., Inc. — 800-336-4666
555 Edgefield Road, Belvedere, SC 29841

Blythewood

Spirax Sarco, Inc. — 800-575-0394
1150 Nortpoint Blvd., Blythewood, SC 29016

Camden

Deroyal Textiles, Inc. — 800-251-9864
125 East York, Camden, SC 29020

Charleston

Arjo Wiggins Medical, Inc. — 843-388-8080
1301 Charleston Regional Pwky, #500, Charleston, SC 29492

Avreo, Inc. — 800-354-0680
4050 Azalea Road, Charleston, SC 29406

Belimed — 800-457-4117
2284 Clements Ferry Road, Charleston, SC 29492

Berchtold Corp. — 800-243-5135
1950 Hanahan Rd., Charleston, SC 29406

Hill-Rom Manufacturing, Inc. — 800-638-2546
4349 Corporate Rd., Charleston, SC 29405

Columbia

Braemar, Inc — 803-407-3044
400 Arbor Lake Dr., Suite B450, Columbia, SC 29223-4571

Ca Plus Adhesives, Inc. — 803-772-4138
701 Kingsbridge Road, Columbia, SC 29210

Holopack Intl. Corp. — 803-806-3300
1 Technology Circle, Columbia, SC 29203

Midland Manufacturing Co., Inc. — 803-776-5398
802 Universal Dr., Columbia, SC 29209

Rhythmlink International, LLC — 866-633-3754
1140 First St. South, Columbia, SC 29209

Surgical Technology Laboratories Inc. — 803-462-1714
610 Clemson Rd., Columbia, SC 29229

Water & Power Technologies Of Texas, Inc. — 801-974-5500
1501 St. Andrews Rd., Po Box 21743, Columbia, SC 29221

Easley

Artronics — 864-859-4755
464 Sweetbriar Way, Easley, SC 29640

Florence

Ge Magnets — 847-277-5002
3001 West Radio Dr., Florence, SC 29501

Nova Health Products, Llc — 843-673-0702
1138 Annelle Dr., Florence, SC 29505

Fort Mill

Cardinal Health 200, Inc — 847-785-3323
785 Fort Mill Hwy, Fort Mill, SC 29715

Goose Creek

Agfa Healthcare Corp. — 864-421-1815
1636 Bushy Park Rd., Goose Creek, SC 29445

Greenville

Agfa Corporation — 877-777-2432
PO Box 19048, 10 South Academy Street, Greenville, SC 29602-9048

American Health Systems — 800-234-6655
PO Box 26688, Greenville, SC 29616-1688

Bausch & Lomb Inc., Greenville Solutions Plant — 585-338-6000
8507 Pelham Rd., Greenville, SC 29615-9598

Bausch & Lomb, Inc. — 585-338-8731
130 Commerce Dr., Greenville, SC 29615

Erad/Image Medical Corp. — 864-234-7430
9 Pilgrim Road, Suite 312, Greenville, SC 29607

Glucotec, Inc. — 864-370-3297
665 north academy street, Greenville, SC 29601

Span Packaging Services Llc. — 864-627-4155
4611-a Dairy Dr., Greenville, SC 29607

Span-America Medical Systems, Inc. — 800-888-6752
70 Commerce Center, Greenville, SC 29615

Greenwood

Covidien Lp, Formerly Registered As Kendall — 800-962-9888
525 North Emerald Rd, Greenwood, SC 29646

Greer

Rockwell Medical Technologies, Inc. — 248-960-9009
604 High Tech Ct., Greer, SC 29650

Gville

Cpt Med, Inc. — 770-242-1165
195 A Commerce Center, Gville, SC 29615

Hilton Head Island

Kigre, Inc. — 843-651-5800
100 Marshland Rd., Hilton Head Island, SC 29926

Honea Path

Friddle's Orthopedic Appliances, Inc. — 800-528-9339
12306 Belton Honea-Path Hwy., Honea Path, SC 29654

Inman

Rim Medical, Llc. — 828-859-2000
2160 Highway 292, PO Box 880, Inman, SC 29349

Steeger Usa, Llc — 800-554-2082
2353 Highway 292, Inman, SC 29349

Johnston

Riegel Consumer Products Div. — 800-845-2232
P.O. Box E, 51 Riegel Road, Johnston, SC 29832-0138

Liberty

Flexi-Wall Systems — 800-843-5394
208 Carolina Dr., P.O. Box 89, Liberty, SC 29657-0089

Loris

Curae'Lase Inc. — 843-455-7020
2315 Hwy 701 South, Loris, SC 29569

Lugoff

Ark Therapeutic Services, Inc. — 803-438-9779
Po Box 340, 862 A Hwy. 1 South, Lugoff, SC 29078

Lyman

York X-Ray And Orthopedic Supply, Inc. — 800-334-6427
PO Box 326, 20 Hampton Rd.,, Lyman, SC 29365-0326

Moncks Corner

C. R. Bard, Inc. — 908-277-8481
428 Powerhouse Rd., Moncks Corner, SC 29461

Mount Pleasant

Revolutions Medical Corp. — 843-971-6917
2073 Shell Ring Circle, Mount Pleasant, SC 29466

Mt. Pleasant

Kale Research And Technology — 864-574-4800
1211 Park West Blvd., Mt. Pleasant, SC 29466
Md Products, Llc — 843-971-2684
506 Hickory Cove, Mt. Pleasant, SC 29464
Princeton Medical Group, Inc. — 800-875-0869
1189 Royal Links Dr., Mt. Pleasant, SC 29466

N Charleston

Maquet, Inc. — 843-552-8652
7371 Spartan Blvd. East, N Charleston, SC 29418

New Ellenton

Healthonics, Inc. — 770-955-2006
903 Main St. South, New Ellenton, SC 29809

Newberry

Aqua Products Company, Inc. — 800-849-4264
14301 C.R. Koon Hwy, Newberry, SC 29108

North Charleston

Hill-Rom, Inc. — 812-934-7777
4115 Dorchester Rd., Unit 600, North Charleston, SC 29405
Varian Medical Systems Interay — 800-468-3729
3235 Fortune Drive, North Charleston, SC 29418

Rock Hill

Alpha Medical Brace, L.L.C. — 866-547-3897
303 Church St., Rock Hill, SC 29730
Hartmann-Conco Inc. — 800-243-2294
481 Lakeshore Pkwy., Rock Hill, SC 29730-4205
Porvair Filtration Group Inc — 803-327-5008
454 South Anderson Road, BTC 514, Rock Hill, SC 29730
3d Systems Corporation — 803-326-3900
333 Three D Systems Circle, Rock Hill, SC 29730

Salem

Argentum Medical Llc — 708-927-9398
424 Stamp Creek Rd., Suite F, Salem, SC 29676

Seneca

Covidien Lp, Formerly Registered As Kendall — 800-962-9888
1448 Blue Ridge Blvd, Seneca, SC 29672

Spartanburg

Contec, Inc. — 800-289-5762
525 Locust Grove, Spartanburg, SC 29303
Milliken & Company — 864-503-2844
920 Milliken Road, PO Box 1926, Spartanburg, SC 29303
Pelican Products, Llc — 864-699-4181
209 Jones Rd., Spartanburg, SC 29307
Qs/1 Data Systems — 800-845-7558
201 West Saint John Street, Spartanburg, SC 29306

Summerton

Concepts International, Inc. — 800-627-9729
224 East Main Street, Summerton, SC 29148

Summerville

Branford Laboratories — 843-832-8004
PO Box 51000, Summerville, SC 29485-1000
Hamilton Mfg. Co. — 888-871-5600
128 Berkeley Cir., Summerville, SC 29483-7302

Sumter

Becton, Dickinson & Co., (Bd) Preanalytical System — 201-847-6280
1575 Airport Rd., Sumter, SC 29153

Travelers Rest

T&S Brass And Bronze Works, Inc. — 800-476-4103
2 Saddleback Cove, P.O. Box 1088, Travelers Rest, SC 29690

Wagener

Chair Care-Mobile Cot, Inc. — 803-564-3698
6241 Wagener Rd., Wagener, SC 29164

Warrenville

Chisolm Biological Lab. — 803-663-9618
542 Legion Rd, Warrenville, SC 29851-3403

Westminster

Cherry Blossom Enterprises Inc. — 864-972-2920
305 South Union Rd., S-37-85, Westminster, SC 29693

Winnsboro

Hacker Industries, Inc. — 803-712-6100
1132 Kincaid Bridge Rd., Winnsboro, SC 29180

Winnsboro,

Hacker Instruments And Industries Inc. — 800-442-2537
1132 Kincaid Bridge Road, PO Box 1176, Winnsboro,, SC 29180-7116

SOUTH DAKOTA

Aberdeen

3m Aberdeen — 605-229-5002
610 N. Brown County Rd. 19, Aberdeen, SD 57401

Brookings

3m Company — (605) 692-9433
601 22nd Ave. South, PO Box 5227, Brookings, SD 57006

Dakota Dunes

Dakota Hearing Instruments, Inc. — 888-373-1283
370 W Anchor Dr, Dakota Dunes, SD 57049

Dell Rapids

American Medical Industries — 605-428-5501
330 E. 3rd Street, Suite 2, Dell Rapids, SD 57022-1918

Desmet

Shinamerica, Inc. — 651-291-7909
710 Fourth St., Desmet, SD 57231

Egan

Comfort Strap Co. — 605-997-3810
212 Second Ave East, Egan, SD 57024-9701

Piedmont

Usa Think, Inc. — 605-787-7717
13030 Homer Smith Rd., Piedmont, SD 57769

Rapid City

Mastel Precision, Inc. — 800-657-8057
2843 Samco Road, Suite A, Rapid City, SD 57702-9366

Sioux Falls

Business Aviation Services — 800-888-1646
3501 Aviation Avenue, Sioux Falls, SD 57104-0197
Carex Health Brands — 800-526-8051
921 East Amidon St, PO Box 2526, Sioux Falls, SD 57101-2526
Kreisers Inc. — 800-843-7948
2200 West 46th St., Sioux Falls, SD 57105
Midwest Eye Laboratories, Inc. — 800-543-7936
1600 South Western, Suite C, Park Ridge Mall, Sioux Falls, SD 57105
Solo Step, Inc. — 866-631-1117
2522 W. 41st St. #318, Sioux Falls, SD 57105
Tamcenan Corp. — 800-950-0113
1703 S. Minnesota Ave., Sioux Falls, SD 57105-1721
Traco Medical Equipment — 605-339-9339
3505 S. Norton Ave, Sioux Falls, SD 57105

Spearfish

Ramvac Dental Products Inc — 800-572-6822
3100 First Avenue, Spearfish, SD 57783

TENNESSEE

Adamsville

Aqua Glass Corporation — 800-632-0911
320 Industrial Park Rd., Adamsville, TN 38310-0412

Alcoa

Bwell Inc. — 865-982-2184
1723 St. Ives Blvd., Alcoa, TN 37701

Antioch

Specialty Surgical Instrumentation, Inc. — 800-251-3000
3034 Owen Drive, Antioch, TN 37013

Arlington

Wright Medical Group, Inc. — 800-238-7117
5677 Airline Road, Arlington, TN 38002

Athens

Lact-Aid International — 866-866-1239
PO Box 1066, Athens, TN 37371-1066
Pi Professional Therapy Products — 888-818-9632
PO Box 1067, Athens, TN 37371-1067
Pi-Ptp — 888-818-9632
215 Rocky Mount Road, PO Box 1067, Athens, TN 37371

Bartlett

Gyrus Ent L.L.C., Sub. Of Gyrus Acmi, Inc. — 800-773-4301
2925 Appling Rd., Bartlett, TN 38133
Hemostatix Medical Technologies, Llc — 901-261-0012
8400 Wolf Lake Dr., Ste. 109, Bartlett, TN 38133

Medtronic Sofamor Danek Instrument Manufacturing   901-396-3133
7375 Adrianne Place, Bartlett, TN 38133
Scanditronix - Wellhofer North America   901-386-2242
3150 Stage Post Drive, Suite 110, Bartlett, TN 38113

Brentwood

American Homepatient   800-890-7271
5200 Maryland Way, Suite 400, Brentwood, TN 37027
Anova Implant Solutions LLC   615-457-3311
2 Maryland Farms, Suite 120, Brentwood, TN 37027
Arthron, Inc.   800-758-5633
1605 Ash Grove Ct., PO Box 1627, Brentwood, TN 37024

Bristol

Conger Dental Supply, Inc.   800-255-3983
302 Rosedale Lane, Bristol, TN 37620
King Pharmaceuticals, Inc.   800-525-8466
501 Fifth Street, Bristol, TN 37620
Meridian Medical Technologies   800-638-8093
501 Fifth Street, Bristol, TN 37620

Chattanooga

Airgas South, Inc.   770-590-6200
4551 North Access Rd., Chattanooga, TN 37415
American Mammographics, Inc.   800-626-4301
5113 Highway 58, Suite 321, Chattanooga, TN 37416
C & C Oxygen Co.   423-867-2369
3615 Rossville Blvd., Chattanooga, TN 37407
Chattem, Inc.   800-366-6077
1715 W. 38th St., Chattanooga, TN 37409-1259
Fillauer Companies, Inc.   800-251-6398
2710 Amnicola Hwy., Chattanooga, TN 37406-0189
Glenveigh Medical   423-933-3939
401 Chestnut St, Suite 230, Chattanooga, TN 37402
Intersign Corp.   800-322-8426
2156 Amnicola Highway, Chattanooga, TN 37406
M & M Industries   800-331-5305
316 Corporate Place, Chattanooga, TN 37419-2339
Magister Corporation   800-396-3130
310 Sylvan St., Chattanooga, TN 37405
Naimco, Inc.   423-648-7730
4120 South Creek Road, Chattanooga, TN 37406
Tri-Fi Knitting, Llc   423-855-0501
4641 Shallowford Rd., Chattanooga, TN 37411
Wortham Laboratories Inc   423-296-0090
6340 Bonny Oaks Dr., Chattanooga, TN 37416

Chuckey

Anissa's Fun Patches   423-234-3404
P.O. Box 455, Chuckey, TN 37641

Cleveland

Schering-Plough Healthcare Products, Inc.   862-245-5115
4207 Michigan Avenue Rd. N.e., Cleveland, TN 37311

Cleveld

Kayline Inc.   423-472-7118
606 18th St., Cleveld, TN 37311
Starplex Scientific Corp.   423-479-4108
705 Industrial Drive Sw, Cleveld, TN 37311

Clifton

Modern Way Immobilizers, Inc.   866-694-7444
100 Johnson St, PO Box 660, Clifton, TN 38425

Clinton

De Medco   865-457-4077
851 Old Emory Rd., Clinton, TN 37716

Collierville

International Business Solutions, Inc.   901-861-7144
350 Poplar View, Collierville, TN 38017

Cookeville

Bennett Industries, Inc.   931-432-4011
1805 Burgess Falls Rd., Cookeville, TN 38506
Peter Schiff Enterprise   931-537-6505
4900 Forrest Hill Rd., Cookeville, TN 38506

Ducktown

Angiosystems, Inc.   800-441-4256
7 Hopkins Pl., Ducktown, TN 37326
Preferred Medical Products   800-441-1161
PO Box 100, Ducktown, TN 37326

Dyersburg

Speclinc   800-468-9276
361 Haynes Rd., Dyersburg, TN 38024

Franklin

Biomimetic Therapeutics, Inc.   615-844-1280
389 Nichol Mill Lane, Franklin, TN 37067
Burke L. Mays And Associates, Inc.   615-791-6247
315 Springhouse Circle, Franklin, TN 37067

Rymed Technologies, Inc.   615-790-8093
137 Third Avenue North, Franklin, TN 37064

Gallatin

Csi Holdings   615-452-9633
170 Commerce Way, Gallatin, TN 37066

Gallaway

Medegen Medical Products, Llc   800-233-1987
209 Medegen Drive, Gallaway, TN 38036-0228

Germantown

Thomas Ocular Prosthetics Labs, Inc.   901-753-4724
1900 Kirby Parkway, Suite 102, Germantown, TN 38138
White Surgical, Inc.   901-758-8768
1644 Dogwood Creek Road, Germantown, TN 38139

Goodlettsville

Aionex, Inc.   615-851-4477
104 Space Park North, Goodlettsville, TN 37072
Remedpar   800-624-3994
101 Old Stone Bridge Road, Goodlettsville, TN 37072

Gray

Tex-Tenn Corp.   800-251-3027
108-118 Kwick Way Lane, PO Box 8219, Gray, TN 37615

Greenbrier

Care Line, Inc.   800-251-1157
2210 Lake Road, Greenbrier, TN 37073

Hendersonville

Aladdin Synergetics, Inc.   800-888-8018
250 E Main Street, Hendersonville, TN 37075

Hohenwald

Preferred Solutions, Llc   757-224-0177
467 Swan Ave., Hohenwald, TN 38462

Jc

D&S Dental, Llc   423-928-1299
3111 Hanover Road, Jc, TN 37604

Jellico

Barton-Carey Medical Products, Inc.   423-784-0444
460 Fifth St., Jellico, TN 37762

Johnson City

Almat, Inc.   423-928-6861
215 East Watauga Avenue, Johnson City, TN 37601
Dentsply Tulsa Dental Products   800-662-1202
608 Rolling Hills Dr., Johnson City, TN 37604
Ear Technology Corp.   800-327-8547
207 E. Myrtle Avenue, PO Box 1516, Johnson City, TN 37605
Innovate Medical, L.L.C.   866-839-7874
2210 Buffalo Road, Johnson City, TN 37604
Roydent Dental Products   800.992.7767
608 Rolling Hills Drive, Johnson City, TN 37604
United Dental Mfg., Inc.   717-845-7511
608 Rolling Hills Dr., Johnson City, TN 37604

Kimball

Lewis Pharmaceutical Information, Llc   423-942-9445
534 Spears Road, Kimball, TN 37347

Knoxville

Alcopro   800-227-9890
2547 Sutherland Ave., Knoxville, TN 37919
Better Health, Inc.   866-BED-BLOX
4117 E Emory Road Suite 601, Knoxville, TN 37938-4229
Cole Vision Corporation   770-305-7352
4435 Anderson Rd., Knoxville, TN 37918
EDP Biotech Corporation   866-883-7389
6701 Baum Dr, Suite 110, Knoxville, TN 37919
GP Instruments   888-215-6855
11130 Kingston Pike, Suite 1200, Knoxville, TN 37934
Gilliam Enterprises, Llc   866-655-0517
5830 Briercliff Rd., Knoxville, TN 37918
Gryphus Diagnostics, L.L.C.   800-924-4195
2200 Sutherland Ave., Knoxville, TN 37919
Kt Medical Corp.   800-633-3757
P.O. Box 50876, Knoxville, TN 37950-0876
Micrad, Inc.   865-690-6389
312 Trossachs Lane, Knoxville, TN 37922
Perceptics Corporation   800-448-8544
9737 Cogdill Rd., Suite 200N, Knoxville, TN 37932-3350
Potty Md, Llc   865-584-6700
6512 Baum Dr. Suite 14, Knoxville, TN 37919
Pyramid Industries, Llc   888-343-3352
3911 Schaad Rd., Unit 102, Knoxville, TN 37921
Quadriciser Corporation   865-689-5003
6624 Central Ave. Pike, Knoxville, TN 37912
Sanders Medical Products, Inc.   865-588-8998
520 Bearden Park Circle, Knoxville, TN 37919

Siemens Medical Solutions Usa, Molecular Imaging — 888-826-9702
810 Innovation Dr, Knoxville, TN 37932-2571
Webtec Converting, Llc. — 865-246-4342
5900 Middle View Way, Knoxville, TN 37909

Lakeland

Medist International — 901-380-9411
9160 HWY 64, Suite 12, Lakeland, TN 38002

Lawrenceburg

Lex-Ton Orthopedics — 615-890-6969
1133 White Cliff Rd., Lawrenceburg, TN 38464

Lebanon

Coeur, Inc — 800-296-5893
100 Physicians Way, Lebanon, TN 37087
Permobil, Inc. — 800-736-0925
6961 Eastgate Blvd., Lebanon, TN 37090

Loudon

Adroit Medical Systems, Inc. — 800-267-6077
1146 Carding Machine Road, Loudon, TN 37774

Madison

Theratech, Inc. — 800-788-1705
1109 Myatt Blvd., Madison, TN 37115

Maryville

Dentek Oral Care, Inc. — 865-983-1300
307 Excellence Way, Maryville, TN 37801

Mboro

Restorative Health Services — 615-225-6090
800 Nw Broad Street, Suite 126, Mboro, TN 37129

McMinnville

Oster Professional Products, Inc. — 800-830-3678
904 Red Rd, McMinnville, TN 37110
Vilex, Inc. — 931-474-7550
111 Moffitt Street, Mcminnville, TN 37110

Mem

Nexair, Llc. — 901-729-5547
1211 North Mclean Blvd., Mem, TN 38108
Smith & Nephew, Inc. — 901-396-2121
6409 E. Holmes Rd., Mem, TN 38141

Memphis

Baxter Healthcare Corporation — 847-473-6141
4835 S. Mendenhall Rd., Memphis, TN 38141
Block Drug Co., Inc. — 973-889-2578
2149 Harbor Ave., Memphis, TN 38113
Christie Medical Holdings — 901-252-3700
1256 Union Ave., 3 Floor, Memphis, TN 38104
Cole Vision Corporation — 770-305-7352
5780 E. Shelby Dr., Memphis, TN 38141
Darby Dental Supply Co. — 800-645-2310
4460 Holmes Rd., Memphis, TN 38118
Eagle Vision, Inc. — 800-222-7584
8500 Wolf Lake Drive, Suite 110, Memphis, TN 38133
Edge Biologicals, Inc. — 800-238-5004
598 North Second St., Memphis, TN 38105
Grace Medical, Inc. — 866-472-2363
8500 Wolf Lake Dr., Ste. 110, Memphis, TN 38133
Handicap Unlimited, Inc. — 888-371-0095
5640 Summer Avenue, Suite 3, Memphis, TN 38134
In'Tech Medical, Incorporated — 757-224-0177
2851 Lamb Place, Suite 15,, Memphis, TN 38118
Innervision Inc. — 901-682-0417
6258 Shady Grove Rd. E., Memphis, TN 38120
Interstate Blood Bank, Inc. — 800-258-9557
5700 Pleasant View Road, Memphis, TN 38134
Kaz Usa, Inc. — 518-828-0450
4755 Southpoint Drive, Memphis, TN 38118
Kenad Sg Medical, Inc. — 800-825-0606
2692 Huntley Dr., Memphis, TN 38132
MMI-USA — 866-682-7577
6060 Poplar Ave., Suite 254, Memphis, TN 38119
Martin Technology, Llc — 901-682-1006
1505 South Perkins, Memphis, TN 38117-6530
Mednet Locator, Inc. — 800-754-5070
7000 Shadow Oaks, Memphis, TN 38125
Medstat Inc. — 901-452-5697
3251 Poplar Ave., Memphis, TN 38111
Medtronic Sofamor Danek Usa, Inc — 901-399-2346
1800 Pyramid Pl, Memphis, TN 38132
Medtronic Sofamor Danek Usa, Inc. — 901-396-3133
4340 Swinnea Rd., Memphis, TN 38118
Memphis Dental Mfg. Co., Inc. — 901-526-6328
402 South Second St., Memphis, TN 38103
Meridian Life Science, Inc. — 800-327-6299
5171 Wilfong Road, Memphis, TN 38134
Odyssey Medical, Inc. — 901-383-7777
5828 Shelby Oaks Dr., Memphis, TN 38134

Onyx Medical Corp. — 800.238.6981
1800 North Shelby Oaks Drive, Memphis, TN 38134
Profex Medical Products — 800-325-0196
2224 E. Person Ave., Memphis, TN 38114
Sandvik MedTech — 901-384-5907
4477 Getwell Rd., P.O. Box 1990, Memphis, TN 38118
Schering-Plough Health Care Products — 901-320-2011
3030 Jackson Ave., Memphis, TN 38151
Smith & Nephew Inc.- Orthopaedics Division — 800-238-7538
1450 Brooks Rd., Memphis, TN 38116
Sterilization Services Of Tennessee, Inc. — 901-947-2217
2396 Florida St., Memphis, TN 38109-2563
Sunco Llc — 901-412-7589
4187 Senator St., Memphis, TN 38118

Morristown

Berkline/Benchcraft Llc — 423-585-1517
One Berkline Dr., Morristown, TN 37813
Shelby-Williams Industries — 800-873-3252
5303 East Morris Blvd., Morristown, TN 37813
Team Technologies, Inc. — 423-587-2199
5949 Commerce Blvd., Morristown, TN 37814

Mount Juliet

Pdi, A Division Of Deroyal Industries, Inc — 800-251-9864
720 Northern Rd., Mount Juliet, TN 37122

Murfreesboro

Stinger Industries — 615-896-1652
1152 Park Ave., Murfreesboro, TN 37129

Nashville

Aesthetic Innovations, Inc. — 615-269-9166
1704a Gayle Ln., Nashville, TN 37212
Airerx Healthcare, Llc — 615-244-3327
1843 Airlane Drive, Nashville, TN 37210
Amsino Medical Usa — 866-482-1345
5209 Linbar Dr., Suite 640, Nashville, TN 37211
Aqua Bath Co., Inc. — 800-232-2284
921 Cherokee Avenue, Nashville, TN 37207
Cardiac Services, Inc. — 800-722-5742
618 Grassmere Park Dr., Ste. 17, Nashville, TN 37211
Cryosurgery, Inc. — 800-729-1624
5829 Old Harding Road, Nashville, TN 37205
Dialysis Dimensions, Inc. — 615-292-0333
2003 Blair Blvd., Nashville, TN 37212
Healthcare Management Systems, Inc. — 800-383-3317
3102 West End Ave., Suite 400, Nashville, TN 37203
Healthstream, Inc. — 800-521-0574
209 10th Avenue S., #450, Nashville, TN 37203
K&S Assoc., Inc. — 615-883-9760
1926 Elm Tree Dr., Nashville, TN 37210
Mahe International Inc. — 800-294-7946
928 5th Ave, Nashville, TN 37204
Matlock Endoscopic Repairs, Sales, And Service, Inc. — 800-394-9822
4320 Kenilwood Drive,, Suite 107, Nashville, TN 37204
Metro Medical Supply Wholesale — 800-768-2002
200 Cumberland Bend, Nashville, TN 37228
Micronova Technology, Inc. — 615-662-1304
914 Harpeth Valley Place, Nashville, TN 37221
Miles Ahead Products — 615-834-0195
3137 Glencliff Rd., Nashville, TN 37211
Nashville Medical Electronics, Inc. — 800-966-1001
319 Fesslers Lane, Suite A, Nashville, TN 37210
New World Imports — 800-329-1903
160 Athens Way, Nashville, TN 37228
Pathfinder Therapeutics, Inc. — 615-783-0094
2969 Armory Drive, Suite 100a, Nashville, TN 37204
Rd Plastics Company, Inc. — 800-795-7007
P.O. Box 111300, Nashville, TN 37222
Safer Sleep Llc — 425-861-8262
3322 West End Avenue, Suite 705, Nashville, TN 37203
Southern Optical Laboratory, Inc. — 800-333-8498
501 Merritt Ave, Nashville, TN 37203
Specialty Care — 800-349-4374
One American Center, 3100 West End Avenue, Suite 800, Nashville, TN 37203
Symmetry Medical/Ssi — 615-883-9090
200 River Hills Drive, Nashville, TN 37210
Techno-Aide, Inc. — 800-251-2629
7117 Centennial Blvd., Nashville, TN 37209-1018
Vanderbilt University — 615-343-0068
2201 West End Ave., Nashville, TN 37235

New Tazewell

Debusk Orthopedic Casting (Doc) — 865-362-2334
420 Straight Creek Road,, Suite 1, New Tazewell, TN 37825
Deroyal Surgical Tray Division — 800-251-9864
1595 Highway 33 South, New Tazewell, TN 37825
Deroyal Technologies, Inc. — 800-251-9864
1595 Highway 33 South, New Tazewell, TN 37825

Oak Ridge

Brant-Wald Surgicals, Inc. — 865-483-5230
368 E. Tennessee Ave., Oak Ridge, TN 37830-4962

Daxor Corporation — 865-425-0555
107 Meco Lane, Oak Ridge, TN 37830
Ortec - (Advanced Measurement Technology) — 800-251-9750
801 S. Illinois Avenue, Oak Ridge, TN 37831
Rbm Services, Llc — 865-483-0067
101-b Valley Court, Oak Ridge, TN 37830
4d Medical Systems, Inc. / Ortiz — 865-483-5145
1020 Commerce Park Dr., Suite B, Oak Ridge, TN 37830

Oakland
Plexus Biomedical Inc. — 901-763-2900
7495 Hwy 64, Oakland, TN 38060

Ooltewah
Dynatronics Corp. Chattanooga Operations — 801-568-7000
6607 Mountain View Rd., Ooltewah, TN 37363
Ooltewah Manufacturing — 800-251-6040x25
5722 Main St., P.O. Box 587, Ooltewah, TN 37363

Ozone
Kimble Chase Life Science And Research Products Llc — 888-546-2531
234 Cardiff Valley Road, Ozone, TN 37854

Piney Flats
Coldstar International, Inc. — 423-538-5551
677 Mountain View Dr., Piney Flats, TN 37686

Powell
Deroyal Industries, Inc. — 800-251-9864
200 DeBusk Lane, Powell, TN 37849
Royal Converting, Inc. — -800-251-9864
200 DeBusk Lane, Powell, TN 37849

Ripley
Tennessee Medical Equipment, Inc. — 800-200-4808
4637 Hwy 19 East, Ripley, TN 38063

Rockford
Siemens Medical Solutions Usa, Inc. — 865-218-2534
203 Dunavant Drive, Rockford, TN 37853
Siemens Medical Solutions Usa, Inc. — 865-218-2534
3100 Stockcreek Blvd, Rockford, TN 37853
Specmat Technologies Inc. — 011-441-5687
215 Dunavant Dr., Rockford, TN 37853

Rockwood
Albahealth Llc — 800-262-2404
425 N. Gateway Avenue, Rockwood, TN 37854
Chase Scientific Glass, Inc. — 412-490-8425
234 Cardiff Valley Rd., Rockwood, TN 37854

Shelbyville
Sanford, L.P. — 800-323-0749
1 Pencil St., Shelbyville, TN 37160

Smyrna
Better Water, Inc. — 615-355-6063
698 Swan Dr., Smyrna, TN 37167

Soddy Daisy
Viscolas, Inc. — 800-548-2694
8801 Consolidated Drive, Soddy Daisy, TN 37379

Springfield
Dialysis Services, Inc. — 615-384-4810
130 Elder Dr., Springfield, TN 37172
Kentron Health Care, Inc. — 615-384-0573
3604 Kelton Jackson Road, P.o. Box 120, Springfield, TN 37172

Summertown
S.E. International, Inc. — 800-293-5759
436 Farm Road, PO Box 39, Summertown, TN 38483-0039

Tazewell
Two Rivers, Llc — 423-626-4990
3199 Hwy. 25 E North, Tazewell, TN 37879

Tullahoma
Life Sensing Instrument Company, Inc. — 800-624-2732
329 W. Lincoln St., Tullahoma, TN 37388
Oak Gloves Division Of Omar Medical Supplies, Inc. — 800-823-2289
208 Industrial Blvd, Tullahoma, TN 37388
Oak Technical, Llc — 423-587-0690
208 Industrial Blvd., Tullahoma, TN 37388

Winchester
Lifeclinic International, Ltd. — 800-543-2787
511 Creasman Dr., Winchester, TN 37398

TEXAS

4452 Beltway Drive
ULURU Inc. — 214-905-5145
4452 Beltway Drive, 4452 Beltway Drive, TX 75001

Abilene
Banyan International Corp. — 800-351-4530
2118 E. Interstate 20, PO Box 1779, Abilene, TX 79601
Convaquip Industries, Inc. — 800-637-8436
4834 Derrick Drive, PO Box 3417, Abilene, TX 79604
Independent Care Products, Inc. — 866-357-0353
P.O. Box 6258, Abilene, TX 79608

Addison
Encompass Medical — 800-826-4490
16415 Addison Road, Suite 660, Addison, TX 75001
Osteomed L.P. — 800-456-7779
3880 Arapaho Road, Addison, TX 75001-4311
Techstyles Manufacturing Division — 800-826-4490
16415 Addison Road, Suite 660, Addison, TX 75001-5434

Allen
Atrion Corp. — 972-390-9800
One Allentown Parkway, Allen, TX 75002-4211
Quest Medical, Inc. — 800-627-0226
1 Allentown Pkwy., Allen, TX 75002-4211

Amarillo
Filterspun — 800-432-0108
624 N Fairfield St, Amarillo, TX 79107
Pro Med Pharmacies, Inc. — 806-379-7311
3615 Sw 45th Avenue, Amarillo, TX 79109-5662
Tech Spray, L.P. — 800-858-4043
P.O. Box 949, Amarillo, TX 79105-0949

Angleton
Benchmark Electronics, Inc. — (979) 849-6550
3000 Technology Dr., Angleton, TX 77515
Merit Medical Systems, Inc. — 1-800-35-MERIT
1111 South Velasco, Angleton, TX 77515

Arlington
Alex Orthopedic, Inc. — 800-544-2539
PO Box 201442, Arlington, TX 76006-1442
American Excelsior Co. — 800-777-7645
850 Ave. H East, Arlington, TX 76011
Dunlee-Tubemaster Facility — 800-544-9729
2312 Avenue J, Arlington, TX 76006
Johnson & Johnson Medical Division Of Ethicon, Inc. — 800-423-4018
2500 E. Arbrook Blvd., Arlington, TX 76014
Mcdalt Medical Corp. — 800-841-5774
2225 Prestonwood Drive,, SUite 100-A, Arlington, TX 76012-5443
Qfc Plastics, Inc. — 817-649-7400
728 111th St., Arlington, TX 76011
Ricca Chemical Company, Llc — 817-461-5601
448 West Fork Dr., Arlington, TX 76012
Straumann Manufacturing, Inc. — 978-747-2575
916a 113th St., Arlington, TX 76011
Water & Power Technologies, Inc. — 817-640-1533
1217 W. Corporate Dr., Arlington, TX 76006

Athens
Argon Medical Devices Inc. — 903-675-9321
1445 Flat Creek Rd., Athens, TX 75751
West Pharmaceutical Services Delaware Acquistion, — 903-677-5017
1704 Enterprise St, Athens, TX 75751

Austin
Abbott Spine, Inc. — 847-937-6100
12708 Riata Vista Circle, Suite B-100, Austin, TX 78727
Apollo Endosurgery, Inc. — 877-ENDO-130
7000 Bee Caves Road, Suite 350, Austin, TX 78746
Arthrocare Corp. — 800-797-6520
7000 W. William Cannon Drive, Building 1, Austin, TX 78735
Ascension Orthopedics, Inc. — 877-370-5001
8700 Cameron Road, Austin, TX 78754
Asuragen, Inc. — 877-777-1874
2150 Woodward St., Suite 100, Austin, TX 78744
Austin Ocular Prosthetics Center, Llc — 512-452-3100
711 W 38th Street Suite G1a, Austin, TX 78705
Bioo Scientific Corporation — 512-707-8993
3913 Todd Lane, Suite 312, Austin, TX 78744
Centerpulse Orthopedics Inc. — 877-768-7349
9900 Spectrum Drive, Austin, TX 78717
Consolidated Technologies, Inc. — 512-445-5100
4401 Sedrich Lane, Building 1, Suite 107, Austin, TX 78744-1832
DJO Surgical — 800-456-8696
9800 Metric Blvd., Austin, TX 78758
Endocare, Inc. — (888) 252-6575
9825 Spectrum Dr. Bldg. 3, Austin, TX 78717
Frantz Design, Inc. — 512-451-3311
3202 Oakmont Blvd., Austin, TX 78703
Green Field Medical Sourcing, Inc. — 512-894-3002
14141 Highway 290 West, Suite 410, Austin, TX 78737
Hanger Orthopedic Group, Inc. — 877-442-6437
10910 Domain Drive, Suite 300, Austin, TX 78758
Healthtronics Inc. — 888-252-6575
9825 Spectrum Dr., Building B, Austin, TX 78717

Inova Labs
3500 Comsouth Rd, Suite 100, Austin, TX 78744
800-220-9977

International Biophysics Corp.
2101 East St. Elmo Rd., Suite 275, Austin, TX 78744
512-326-3244

LDR Spine USA
4030 West Braker Lane, Suite 360, Austin, TX 78759
512-344-3333

Lifestream Purification Systems, Llc
2001 S. Lamar Boulevard, Suite G, Austin, TX 78704
877-564-3185

Luminex Corp.
12212 Technology Blvd., Austin, TX 78727-6115
888-219-8020

Medical Carbon Research Institute, Llc - Mcri
8200 Cameron Road, Suite A-196, Austin, TX 78754-3823
512-339-8000

Medical Laser Technologies, Llc
3708 Ebony Hollow Cove, Austin, TX 78739
512-626-6267

Mindways Software, Inc.
3001 South Lamar, Suite 302, Austin, TX 78704
512-912-0871

Monebo Technologies, Inc.
1800 Barton Creek Blvd., Austin, TX 78735-1606
512-732-0235

On-X Life Technologies, Inc.
1300 East Anderson Lane, Building-B, Austin, TX 78752
888-339-8000

Origen Biomedical, Inc.
7000 Burleson Rd, Bldg D, Austin, TX 78744-3202
512-474-7278

Ortho Kinetics Corp.
7004 Bee Cave Road, Building III, Suite 315, Austin, TX 78746
512-334-5490

Page Southerland Page, Llp
400 West Cesar Chavez Street, Suite 500, Austin, TX 78701-3885
512-472-6721

Patton Medical Devices
31058 N. Lamar Blvd., Austin, TX 78705
877-763-7678

Patton Surgical Corp.
6300 Bridgepoint Pkwy., Building Two, Ste. 420, Austin, TX 78730
1.877.641.0469

Rigid Fx Orthopedics, Incorporated
9230 Neils Thompson Dr, Suite 111, Austin, TX 78758
877-707-1404

Spine Smith Partners L.P.
8140 N. Mopac, Bldg Ii, Suite 120, Austin, TX 78759
512-206-0770

Spine360
5000 Plaza On The Lake, Suite 175, Austin, TX 78746
512.327.6400

Starkey Southwest
3100 Alvin Devane Blvd., Austin, TX 78741
952-947-4734

U.S. Medical Systems, Inc.
3160 Bee Cave Road, Suite 300c, Austin, TX 78746
512-347-8800

Vermillion, Inc.
12117 Bee Caves Rd., Building III, Suite 100, Austin, TX 78738
512-519-0400

Wenzel Spine Inc.
206 Wild Basin Road, Building A Suite 203, Austin, TX 78746
512-469-0600

Azle

Mealtime Partners, Inc.
1137 S. E. Parkway, Azle, TX 76020
817-237-9991

Beaumont

Helena Laboratories
Point of Care Division, PO Box 752, Beaumont, TX 77704-0752
409-842-3714

Letourneau Prosthetics
2452 Calder Ave., Beaumont, TX 77702
800-609-5005

Bedford,

Meena Medical Equipment, Inc.
1905 Bedford Rd |, Ste. 105, Bedford,, TX 76021
888-225-2502

Bellaire

Hearing Aid Express
5201 Bellaire Blvd., Bellaire, TX 77401
713-666-1704

Boerne

Immuno Resources, Inc.
415 Sisterdale Rd., Boerne, TX 78006
830-537-6199

Instrument Specialists, Inc.
32390 IH-10 West, Boerne, TX 78006
800-537-1945

Stanbio Laboratory, Inc.
1261 N. Main St., Boerne, TX 78006-3014
830-249-0772

Brookshire

Lordex, Inc.
32357 Morton Rd., Bldg. 3, Brookshire, TX 77423
281-395-9512

Brownsville

Collis Curve, Inc.
6110 California Rd., Brownsville, TX 78521
800-298-4818

Paramount Surgicals, Inc.
3475 West Alton Gloor Blvd., Brownsville, TX 78520
877-486-4629

Pisharodi Surgicals, Inc.
3475 W. Alton Gloor Blvd, Brownsville, TX 78520
956-541-6725

Bryan

Farrow Medical Innovations, Inc.
801 North Bryan, Bryan, TX 77803
877-417-5187

Neutral Posture, Inc.
3904 North Texas Ave., Bryan, TX 77803
979-778-0502

Bullard

Lifeline Software, Inc.
311 Hines Crossing, Bullard, TX 75757
903-894-9923

Burnet

Stealth Products
103 John Kelly Dr, Burnet, TX 78611
800-965-9229

Carrollton

Aggressive Solutions, Inc.
1735 N. I-35 E., Carrollton, TX 75006
972-242-2164

American Hearing Laboratory
3740 Josey Lane, Suite 125, Carrollton, TX 75007
972-394-4370

Artistic Dental Lab, Incorporated
1500 Crescent Drive, Suite 204, Carrollton, TX 75006
757-224-0177

Asi Medical Equipment, Ltd.
1735 North Interstate 35 East, Carrollton, TX 75006
800-527-0443

B. Braun Medical, Inc.
1601 Wallace Dr., Suite 150, Carrollton, TX 75006
610-596-2536

Dalton Medical Corp.
1103 Venture, Carrollton, TX 75006
972-418-5129

Emergency Medical Systems
PO Box 111034, Carrollton, TX 75011
214-704-7077

Fry Construction Company
3212 Commander Drive, Carrollton, TX 75006
972-248-9696

Life-Like Laboratory
1544 Valwood Pkwy., Suite 104, Carrollton, TX 75006
972-620-0203

Soken Products, Inc.
1906 Robin Meadow Dr., Carrollton, TX 75007
972-939-8072

Swiss American Products, Inc.
2055 Luna Rd., Ste. 126, Carrollton, TX 75006
800-633-8872

Thermotek Inc.
1454 Halsey Way, Carrollton, TX 75007-4409
877-242-3232

Carrollton

Stille-Sonesta, Inc.
1610 I35 North, Suite 203, Carrollton, TX 75006
800-665-1614

Cedar Hill

Sandare Intl., Inc.
910 K.c.k. Way, Cedar Hill, TX 75104
972-293-7440

Cleburne

International Biomedical, Ltd.
2725 North Main St., Cleburne, TX 76033
512-873-0033

Sanker Intl., Inc.
3516 County Road 801, Cleburne, TX 76031
817-645-8015

Colleyville

Medi-Dyne Healthcare Products, L.L.C.
1812 Industrial Boulevard, Colleyville, TX 76034
800-810-1740

Commerce

Covidien Lp, Formerly Registered As Kendall
400 Maple St, Commerce, TX 75428
800-962-9888

Conroe

Byrne Medical, Inc.
2021 Airport Road, Conroe, TX 77304
800-490-9869

Colon-Ez Llc
12126 Kimberly Trace, Conroe, TX 77304
936-756-1970

Coppell

Axis Dental
800 West Sandy Lake Rd., Suite 100, Coppell, TX 75019
800-355-5063

Masterquest International
801 Hammond Street Suite 200, Coppell, TX 75019
315-298-2904

Corpus Christi

American Medical Technologies, Inc.
5655 Bear Lane, Corpus Christi, TX 78405
361-289-1145

CryoPen Inc.
800 North Shoreline, Suite 900, Corpus Christi, TX 78401
888-246-3928

Horton Automatics
4242 Baldwin Blvd., Corpus Christi, TX 78405
800-531-3111

Cresson

Craftmaster Contour Equipment, Inc.
6900 South Freeway, #9-b, P.O. Box 278, Cresson, TX 76035
817-396-0900

Cumby

Pelvic Binder, Inc.
3982 Fm 2653 South, Cumby, TX 75433
877-451-3000

Dallas

Aegis Floorsystems
14286 Gillis Road, Dallas, TX 75244
972-788-2233

Airgas-Southwest, Inc.
2615 Joe Field Rd., Dallas, TX 75229
361-288-0587

Airway Management Inc.
6116 North Central Expressway, Suite 605, Dallas, TX 75206
866-264-7667

Asi-Modulex
3860 W. Northwest Hwy., Suite 350, Dallas, TX 75220
800-274-7732

Avail Medical Products, Inc.
1225 N. 28th Avenue, Suite 500, Dallas, TX 75261
858-635-2206

Avazzia, Inc.
13140 Coit Rd., Suite 515, Dallas, TX 75240
214-575-2820

Biomed Laboratories, Inc. — 972-282-8008
11910 Shiloh Rd., Ste. 142, Dallas, TX 75228
Bone Solutions, Inc. — 214-234-0661
10,000 North Central Expwy, Suite 900, Dallas, TX 75231
Brit Systems Inc. — 800-230-7227
1909 Hi-Line Drive, Suite A, Dallas, TX 75207
C&H Contact Lens, Inc. — 800-527-5060
2836 Walnut Hill Lane, P.O. Box 29081, Dallas, TX 75229-5710
Chemical Service Labs, Llc — 214-691-3484
5543 Dyer St., Dallas, TX 75206
Citizens Development Center — 214-637-2911
8800 Ambassador Row, Dallas, TX 75247-4621
Clean Air Research & Environmental, Inc. — 972-233-2777
13628 Beta Rd., Suite B, Dallas, TX 75244
Cole Vision Coropration — 770-305-7352
2465 Joe Field Rd., Dallas, TX 75229
Dallas Eye Prosthetics — 214-739-5355
8226 Douglas Ave., #415, Dallas, TX 75225
Drew Scientific, Inc. — 800-433-0945
4230 Shilling Way, Dallas, TX 75237-1023
Estill Medical Technologies, Inc. — 877-354-0286
4144 North Central Expressway, Ste. 260, Dallas, TX 75204
Ge Ionics, Inc. — 214-339-2135
4740 Bronze Way, Dallas, TX 75236-1999
Global Biomedics Corporation — 800-473-1122
11005 Indian Trail #102, Dallas, TX 75229-3515
Global Focus (G.F.M.D. Ltd.) — 800-527-2320
2280 Spring Lake Rd., Ste. 106, Dallas, TX 75234
Hearing Aid Express — 713-666-1704
11888 Marsh Ln., Suite 111, Dallas, TX 75234
Images-On-Call — 214-902-8337
10290 Monroe Drive, Suite 202, Dallas, TX 75229
Imed Technology, Inc. — 972-732-7333
17408 Tamaron Drive, Dallas, TX 75287
Immuno Diagnostic Center, Inc. — 214-351-1231
9978 Monroe Dr., Ste. 303, Dallas, TX 75220-1498
Immuno Diagnostic Center, Inc. — 214-351-1231
9978 Monroe Dr., Suite 303, Dallas, TX 75220
In Home Products, Inc. — 800-810-8475
12015 Shiloh Rd., Ste. 158-B, Dallas, TX 75228
Interstate Battery System Of America — 800-730-7868
12770 Merit Drive, Suite 1000, Dallas, TX 75251
Judah Mfg. Corp. — 800-618-9792
13657 Jupiter Road, #100, Dallas, TX 65238
LIFTnWALK LP — 972-837-4615
P.O. Box 742855, Dallas, TX 75374-2855
Medline Industries Holdings, L.P. — 847-837-2759
9303 Stoneview Dr., Dallas, TX 75237
Moll Industries, Inc. — 972-663-6900
13455 Noel Rd, Suite 1310, Dallas, TX 75240
New Options, Inc. — 214-638-6422
2545 Merrell Rd., Dallas, TX 75229
Perfect Fit, L.P. — 972-955-6836
6315 Riverview Lane, Dallas, TX 75248
RDL Supply — 214-630-3965
11240 Gemini Lane, Dallas, TX 75229
SYSMED — 214-820-2176
2625 Elm St., Ste. 102, Dallas, TX 75226-1453
Sanijet Corp. — 877-934-0477
6200 Maple Avenue, Dallas, TX 75235
Scenar Training Center — 248-318-2001
12222 Merit Dr., Suite 955, Dallas, TX 75251
Sientra, Inc — 888-423-7600
11220 Grader St., Suite 100, Dallas, TX 75238
Spi Sports/Science Inc. — 800-322-0688
3506 Cedar Springs, Suite 1400, Dallas, TX 75201
Winning Solutions, Inc. — 800-899-2563
P.O. Box 612688, Dallas, TX 75261-2688
X-O Corporation — 214-388-5590
8311 Eastpoint Drive Ste 100, Dallas, TX 75227
Zonda Inc. — 214-438-3706
17304 Preston Rd., Suite 800, Dallas, TX 75248

De Soto
Cima Scientific — 972-293-1605
P.O. Box 1237, De Soto, TX 75123
Inro Medical Designs, Inc. — 800-527-1093
P.O. Box 9, De Soto, TX 75115

Dekalb
Decompression Technology International — 903-667-3802
1235 Cr 4244, Dekalb, TX 75559-9739

Del Rio
Border Opportunity Saver Systems, Inc. — 830-775-0992
10 Finegan Drive, Del Rio, TX 78841
Kimberly-Clark Corp. — 770-587-7835
14 Finegan Rd., Del Rio, TX 78840

Denton
Somnomed Inc. — 940-381-5200
3537 Teasley Lane, Denton, TX 76210

Duncanville
Quality Aspirators — 800-858-2121
1419 Goodwin Lane, Duncanville, TX 75116
Secure Products — 469-233-0385
914 Thistle Green Lane, Duncanville, TX 75137

El Paso
Accellent El Paso — 915-771-9112
31C Butterfield Trail, El Paso, TX 79906
Aso Llc — 941-379-0300
12120 Esther Lama Dr., Suite 112, El Paso, TX 79936
Cardinal Health 200, Inc — 847-785-3323
One Butterfield Trail, El Paso, TX 79906
Cardinal Health 200, Inc. — 913-451-0880
1550 Northwestern Dr., El Paso, TX 79912
Dynatec Scientific Labs, Inc. — 915-849-1322
11940 Golden Gate, El Paso, TX 79936
Edusa Corp. — 651-733-4365
11751 Alameda St., El Paso, TX 79927
El Paso Lighthouse For The Blind — 915-532-4495
200 Washington St., El Paso, TX 79905
Electrode Arrays — (888) 267.6157
612 N. Resler, El Paso, TX 79912
Ge Medical Systems Information Technologies — 414-721-2584
465 Pan American Dr, Suite 11, El paso, TX 79907
Kernco Instruments Co., Inc. — 800-325-3875
420 Kenazo Ave., El Paso, TX 79928-7338
Multi Biosensors, Inc. — 915-581-9684
4944 Vista Grande, El Paso, TX 79922
Singer Medical Products Inc., Md Systems Div. — 630-860-6500
3800 Buckner, El Paso, TX 79925

Emory
Cavitat Medical Technologies, Inc. — 903-473-1710
118 South Texas St, PO Box 879, Emory, TX 75440

Ennis
Bath-Tec Whirlpool Bath — 800-526-3301
5142 Hwy 34 W., Ennis, TX 75119-7260

Flower Mound
Stryker Communications Corp. — 866-726-3705
1410 Lakeside Parkway, Flower Mound, TX 75028
Stryker Gi — 866-672-5757
1420 Lakeside Parkway, Suite 110, Flower Mound, TX 75028
Stryker Imaging — 888-795-4624
1410 Lakeside Pkwy., Ste. 600, Flower Mound, TX 75028

Floyd
Mcconnell Orthopedic Mfg. Co. — 513-573-0085
1324 East Interstate 30 Bldg. B, Floyd, TX 75401

Forney
Crystal Computer Lenses — 214-773-3457
104 E. Us Hwy 80, Suite 100, Forney, TX 75126

Fort Worth
Alcon Research, Ltd. — 800-862-5266
6201 South Fwy., Fort Worth, TX 76134-2001
Ameripac, Inc. — 214-660-6633
4399 Cambridge Road, Fort Worth, TX 75050
Avcor Health Care Products, Inc. — 800-282-6748
One Southfield Square, 1520 Everman Pkwy., Fort Worth, TX 76140
Dietz Laboratories, Inc. — 800-792-8934
3124 Stuart Drive, Fort Worth, TX 76110-4318
Ecp Health, Inc. — 817-881-4499
8416 Prairie Rose Lane, Fort Worth, TX 76123
Fort Worth Eye Prosthetics, Inc. — 817-429-8086
1350 South Main, #2450, Fort Worth, TX 76104
Healthcare Computer Corp. — 888-727-5422
2601 Scott Ave., Suite. 600, Fort Worth, TX 76103
Krown Manufacturing, Inc. — 800-366-9950
3408 Indale Rd., Fort Worth, TX 76116
Kyro Mfg. Co. — 817-336-1319
2601 Weisenberger St., Fort Worth, TX 76107
Medtronic Powered Surgical Solutions — 800-643-2773
4620 North Beach St., Fort Worth, TX 76137
Moore Diversified Services, Inc. — 817-731-4266
3001 Halloran St., Ste. C, Fort Worth, TX 76107
Multi-Tronics Corp. — 817-246-5821
8400 White Settlement, Fort Worth, TX 76108
Nurse Assist ,Inc. — 800-649-6800
3400 Northern Cross Blvd., Fort Worth, TX 76137
Quantum Interconnect, Inc. — 817-231-1400
3400 Northern Cross Blvd., Fort Worth, TX 76137
Radio Shack — 800-843-7422
300 Radioshack Circle, Mail Stop Wf4-136, Fort Worth, TX 76102
Repco — 800-726-1852
1227 W. Magnolia Avenue, Suite 310, Fort Worth, TX 76104
Sheepskin Ranch, Inc. — 800-366-9950
3408 Indale Road, Fort Worth, TX 76116
Teleflex Medical — 866-246-6990
920 Westport Parkway, Fort Worth, TX 76177

Trident Medical Products   800-647-4448
1201 Summit Avenue, Fort Worth, TX 76102
Welcon, Inc.   800-877-0923
7409 Pebble Drive, Fort Worth, TX 76118
Wound Management Technologies Inc   817-820-7077
777 Main Street, Suite 3100, Fort Worth, TX 76102

Ft. Worth

Jack Jones Hearing Aid Centers, Inc.   800-722-8534
400 South Henderson, Ft. Worth, TX 76104
Prestige Ameritech   817-595-1131
7426 Tower St., Ft. Worth, TX 76118

Garland

Assistance Products Lp   972-240-4279
3710 S. Country Club Rd., Garland, TX 75043
Carroll Co.   800-527-5722
2900 W. Kingsley Rd., Garland, TX 75041
Dallas Trim Industries Corp.   972-278-3598
2511 National Dr., Garland, TX 75041
Galt Medical Corp.   800-639-2800
2220 Merritt Dr., Garland, TX 75041
Neurotone Systems, Inc.   972-271-1978
510 Nesbit Dr., Garland, TX 75041
Tapcon, Inc.   800-247-3587
521 Sheperd Street, Garland, TX 75042
Wright-Way, Inc.   800-241-8839
175 E. Interstate 30, Garland, TX 75043

Gatesville

Medical Plastics Laboratory, Inc.   800-433-5539
226 FM 116, Industrial Air Park, PO Box 38, Gatesville, TX 76528

Glen Rose

Somervell Laboratories   254-897-4085
1102a Bluebonnet St., Glen Rose, TX 76043

Granbury

Alliance Tech Medical, Inc.   800-848-8923
5305 Mission Circle, P.O. Box 6024, Granbury, TX 76049
C.G. Laboratories, Inc.   817-279-1945
1410 Southtown Dr., Granbury, TX 76048

Grand Prairie

Bledsoe Brace Systems   888-253-3763
2601 Pinewood Drive, Grand Prairie, TX 75051-3516
Invacare Supply Group   508-429-1000
1825 West Park Dr., Suite 200, Grand Prairie, TX 75050
Mcmerlin Dental Products, Lp   972-602-3746
1610 W. Polo Rd., Grand Prairie, TX 75052
North Texas Circuit Board   800-466-6822
1501 W. Shady Grove Rd., Grand Prairie, TX 75053
Per4max Medical, Llc   866-648-6891
1000 Post & Paddock, Ste. 302, Grand Prairie, TX 75050
Sun Medical, Inc.   800-678-6633
2607 Aero Drive, Grand Prairie, TX 72052
Vibraderm, Inc.   301-279-2899
2100 North Highway 360, Suite 1502, Grand Prairie, TX 75050

Grapeland

Alpha Omega Mfg. Inc.   936-687-4993
110 Main Street, P.o. Box 387, Grapeland, TX 75844
Love Imports   800-944-5523
PO Box 759, Grapeland, TX 75844

Greenville

Omnisys, Inc.   800-448-6891
2824 Terrell Road, Suite 602, Greenville, TX 75402

Hidalgo

Mel R. Manufacturas   956-655-1380
417 East Coma Street, Suite 534, Hidalgo, TX 78557

Houston

Air Liquide America Corporation   800-820-2522
1311 New Savannah Rd., Ste. 1800, Houston, TX 77056
Air Liquide Healthcare America Corporation   877-855-9533
2700 Post Oak Blvd., Houston, TX 77056
Alcon Manufacturing, Ltd.   713-668-9100
9965 Buffalo Speedway, Houston, TX 77054-1309
Amci Medical Systems, Llc   713-522-4865
1617 W. Alabama St., Houston, TX 77006
American Wellness Foundation   713-622-8499
5311 Kirby Drive Suite 100, Houston, TX 77055
American White Cross - Houston   609-514-4744
15200 I-45 North, Houston, TX 77090
Ami Dental, Inc.   800-969-0405
9000 S.W. Freeway, Ste. 328, Houston, TX 77074
Antek Instruments, Inc.   281-580-0339
300 Bammel Westfield Road, Houston, TX 77090-3533
Becker Industries, Inc.   (281)-590-4900
2712 Frank Road, Houston, TX 77032
Biosentient Corporation   -
700 Gemini St. Suite 210, Houston, TX 77058

Biotecx Laboratories, Inc.   800-535-6286
15225 Gulf Hwy, #F106, Houston, TX 77034
Biotex, Inc.   713-741-0111
8058 El Rio St., Houston, TX 77054
Bob J. Johnson & Associates   218-873-5555
16420 W. Hardy Rd., Ste. 100, Houston, TX 77060
Cardiosoft, L.P.   713-623-4009
1776 Yorktown, Suite LI-30, Houston, TX 77056
Continental Fuels, Inc.   713-231-0330
600 Travis, Suite 6910, Houston, TX 77002
Cooley & Cooley, Ltd.   800-215-4487
8550 Westland W. Blvd., Houston, TX 77041
Cranford X-Ray Co.   800-285-8329
8106 Berwyn Dr., Houston, TX 77037
Cyberonics Beltway 8 Distribution Facility   800-332-1375
100 Cyberonics Boulevard W, Houston, TX 77058
Cyberonics, Inc.   800-332-1375
The Cyberonics Building, 100 Cyberonics Boulevard, Houston, TX 77058
Davis Lead Apron, Inc.   800-483-3979
4560 West 34th St., PO Box 924585, Houston, TX 77092
Digisonics, Inc.   713-529-7979
3701 Kirby Drive, Suite 930, Houston, TX 77098-3903
Diversified Diagnostic Products, Inc.   281-955-5323
11603 Windfern Road, Houston, TX 77064-4801
Emerging Healthcare Solutions, Inc.   713-821-1486
5847 San Felipe, Suite 1700, Houston, TX 77057
Encon Safety Products   800-283-6266
6825 West Sam Houston Pkwy. N., Houston, TX 77041
Eyesys Vision, Inc.   281-885-3800
225 Pennbright Dr., Suite 100, Houston, TX 77090
First Gulf International   713-961-7793
3055 Sage Road #210, Suite 1690, Houston, TX 77056
Fisher Healthcare   800-766-7000
9999 Veterans Memorial Dr., Houston, TX 77038-2401
Fkp Architects,Inc   713-621-2100
8 Greenway Plaza, Suite 300, Houston, TX 77046-0899
Frazer, Inc.   888-372-9371
7227 A Rampart, Houston, TX 77081
Galaxy Aquatics, Inc.   713-464-0303
1075 W. Sam Houston Pkwy. N., Ste. 210, Houston, TX 77043-5018
Gemtech Products, Inc.   866-436-8321
10623 Tower Oaks Blvd., Houston, TX 77070
Globe Medical Tech, Inc.   713-365-9595
1766 W. Sam Houston Pkwy N., Houston, TX 77043
Grand Medical Products   800-521-2055
7222 Ertel Road, Houston, TX 77040
Guidant Corporation   408-845-3995
8934 Kirby Drive, Houston, TX 77054
Hewlett-Packard Company   408-472-2702
20555 State Highway 249, Houston, TX 77070
Hitachi America, Ltd., Power Systems Division   713-792-1804
1840 Old Spanish Trail, Houston, TX 77054
Igs Generon Americas   713-937-5200
11985 Fm 529, Houston, TX 77041
Intermed Supplies   800-766-3131
7115 Belgold Street Suite E, Houston, TX 77066
Joint Venture Development, Inc.   713-501-0075
1628 Beaconshire, Houston, TX 77077
Luwa Lepco   713-461-1131
1750 Stebbins Drive, Houston, TX 77043
Matheson Tri-Gas, Inc.   713-869-7351
2200 Houston Ave., Houston, TX 77007
Medical Metrics, Inc.   713-850-7500
4600 Post Oak Place, Ste. 359, Houston, TX 77027
Micromed Technology, Inc.   713-838-9210
8965 Interchange Dr., Houston, TX 77054
Microsurgical Laboratories   800-414-1076
11333 Chimney Rock Road, Suite 120, Houston, TX 77035
Millar Instruments, Inc.   800.669.2343
6001-A Gulf Freeway, Houston, TX 77023-5417
Miracle House   713-433-0333
5 Broadhurst St., Houston, TX 77047
Mmar Medical Group, Inc.   800-662-7633
9619 Yupondale Dr., Houston, TX 77080-7233
Omnia Technology An Optimation Company   585-321-2300
2550 Grayfalls Dr., Ste. 207, Houston, TX 77077
OrthoAccel Technologies Inc.   832-631-1659
8275 El Rio, Suite 100, Houston, TX 77054
Orthodontic Technologies, Inc.   800-346-5133
5524 Cornish, Houston, TX 77007
Pac   281-580-0339
300 Bammel Westfield, Houston, TX 77090-3533
Pentax Southern Region Service Center   201-571-2300
8934 Kirby Dr., Houston, TX 77054
Powerlung, Inc.   713-465-1180
10690 Shadow Wood Dr., Suite 100, Houston, TX 77043
Proportional Technologies, Inc.   800-759-7325
8022 El Rio St., Houston, TX 77054
S & S X-Ray Products, Inc.   800-231-1747
10625 Telge Road, Houston, TX 77095
S&S Medcart   800-231-1747
10625 Telge Road, Houston, TX 77095

S&S Technology — 281-815-1300
10625 Telge Road, Houston, TX 77095

Scientific Glass & Instruments, Inc. — 877-682-1481
PO Box 6, Houston, TX 77001-0006

SeqWright Inc. — 800-720-4363
2575 West Bellfort, Suite 2001, Houston, TX 77054

Sharps Compliance Corp. — 713-432-0300
9220 Kirby Drive, Suite 500, Houston, TX 77054

Siemens Water Technologies — 978-614-7359
10875 Kempwood, Houston, TX 77043

Soper Brothers & Associates — 713-521-1263
1213 Hermann Dr., Suite 320, Houston, TX 77004

Southland Cryogenics, Inc. — 800-872-2796
8350 Mosley Rd., Houston, TX 77075-1112

Spectracell Laboraties — 800.227.5227
10401 Town Park Drive, Houston, TX 77072

Spinerx Technology — 713-983-9979
6100 Brittmoore Rd., Suite S, Houston, TX 77041

Tanox Biosystems, Inc. — 713-664-2288
10301 Stella Link Road, Suite 110, Houston, TX 77025-5497

Telemedx Corp. — 800-231-1009
2550 S Sam Houston Pkwy W, Houston, TX 77047-6001

Texas Eye Prosthetics Llc — 713-524-1001
4203 Montrose Blvd., Suite 380, Houston, TX 77006

The Art Of Living Institute — 713-621-0366
7815 Fondren Rd., Houston, TX 77074

Toray International America Inc. — 800-662-1777
140 Cypress Station Dr., Ste. 210, Houston, TX 77090

Total Motion, Inc. — 281-386-8747
19606 Piney Place Court, Houston, TX 77094

Tracey Technologies Corp. — 281-445-1666
16720 Hedgecroft Dr., Suite 208, Houston, TX 77060

U O Equipment Co. — 800-231-6372
5863 W. 34th St., Houston, TX 77092

Ultrasonic Services, Inc. — 713-665-4949
7126 Mullins Dr., Houston, TX 77081

Von London Phonix Co — 713-772-6666
6103 Glenmont, Houston, TX 77081-1499

Wexler Surgical Supplies — 800-414-1076
11333 Chimney Rock Road, Suite 110, Houston, TX 77035

Zebec Data Systems, Inc., Healthcare Mgmt. Div. — 713-782-3480
2425 Fountain View, Houston, TX 77057

eCardio Diagnostics — 888-747-1442
1717 N. Sam Houston Parkway West, Houston, TX 77038

Huffman

Tele-Made Disposables, Inc. — 888-822-4299
3215 Huffman Eastgate Rd., Huffman, TX 77336

Hurst

Bell Helicopter Textron, Inc. — 817-280-2011
600 E. Hurst Blvd., State Highway 10, Hurst, TX 76053

Irving

Abbott Diagnostics Div. — 847-937-7988
1921 Hurd Dr., Irving, TX 75038

Fresenius Medical Care North America — 781-699-9068
5201 Regent Blvd, Irving, TX 75063

Golden Triangle Dental Laboratory Inc. — 972-910-9912
7475 Las Colinas Blvd., Suite A, Irving, TX 75063

Hydro-Med Products, Inc. — 214-350-5100
3400 Royalty Row, Irving, TX 75062

Mediware Dallas Service Center — 913-307-1000
4545 Fuller Dr., Suite 320, Irving, TX 75038

Mentor Texas, Inc. — 972-252-6060
3041 Skyway Circle North, Irving, TX 75038

Mpm Medical, Inc. — 800-232-5512
2301 Crown Ct., Irving, TX 75038

Nch Corporation — 1-800-527-9929
ATTN: Marketing Department, 5N, P.O. Box 152170, Irving, TX 75015

Jacksonville

Cardinal Health 200, Inc — 847-785-3323
200 Mcknight St, Jacksonville, TX 75766

Speedy Products Co. — 800-388-2001
225 Cash St., Jacksonville, TX 75766

Katy

Kada Research, Inc. — 281-385-9951
21218 Kingsland Blvd, Katy, TX 77450

Owens Scientific Inc. — 281-394-2311
23230 Sand Sage Lane, Katy, TX 77494-4207

Keller

Hemo-De, Inc. — 800-355-3689
2000 Whitley Rd., Keller, TX 76248

Kirby

Forum Industries Inc. — 210-225-9600
1903 Hormel Dr., Kirby, TX 78219

La Porte

Pyraback.Com — 713-859-7568
10339 Belfast Rd., La Porte, TX 77571

Lago Vista

Alger Equipment Company, Inc. — 800-320-1043
320 Flightline, Lago Vista, TX 78645

The Alger Company, Inc. — 800-320-1043
320 Flightline Rd., Lago Vista, TX 78645

Lewisville

Bio-Synthesis, Inc — 800-227-0627
612 East Main St, Lewisville, TX 75057

Genesis Biosystems, Inc. — 888-577-7335
1500 Eagle Court, Lewisville, TX 75057

Lrl Logix — 800-800-3650
1301 W. Hwy 407 # 201, Lewisville, TX 75077

Orthofix Inc. — 1.800.527.0404
3451 Plano Parkway, Lewisville, TX 75056

Statlab Medical Products, Inc. — 800-442-3573
106 Hillside Drive, Lewisville, TX 75057

Liberty Hill

Rg Electronics, Inc. — 888-877-5682
100 Spring Creek Dr., Liberty Hill, TX 78642

Little Elm

Retractable Technologies, Inc. — 888-806-2626
511 Lobo Lane, Little Elm, TX 75068

Lubbock

Classone Orthodontics, Inc. — 806-799-0608
5064 50th St., Lubbock, TX 79414

Osteogenics Biomedical, Inc. — 806-796-1923
4620 71st St., Bldg. 78-79, Lubbock, TX 79424

Texstar Technology Inc. — 806-748-1184
2306-d 120th St., Lubbock, TX 79423

Urology-Tech Llc — 800-397-3318
4503 89th S, Lubbock, TX 79424

Mc Allen

Care Products Inc. — 800-445-7345
10701 N. Ware Rd., PO Box 720193, Mc Allen, TX 78504

McAllen

Medical Safety Technologies, Inc. — 1-866-403-6784
5412 N. 10th St, McAllen, TX 78596

Nelson Environmental Technologies, Inc. — 956-618-0375
813 E. Fir, Mcallen, TX 78501

Unomedical, Inc. — 800-634-6003
5701-1 S. Ware Rd., McAllen, TX 78503

Mckinney

Armstrong Industries, Inc. — 972-547-1400
7290 Virginia Pkwy, Ste 3000, Mckinney, TX 75071

Dynamic Energy Systems, Inc. — 800-326-0314
1500 South Central Expressway, McKinney, TX 75070

Erchonia Medical — 888-242-0571
2021 Commerce Dr, Mckinney, TX 75069

Medro Systems, Inc. — 972-542-8200
416 E. Industrial Blvd., McKinney, TX 75069-7323

Ps Solutions, Inc. — 972-548-8080
411 Interchange St., Mckinney, TX 75071

Meadows Place

Whitehill Manufacturing, Inc. — 281-240-8782
12701 Executive Dr., Ste. 614, Meadows Place, TX 77477

Mesquite

Access, Lifts & Mobility Systems, Inc. — (972) 285-3487
301 Clary Dr., Mesquite, TX 75149-3023

Brady Precision Converting, Llc — 214-275-9595
1801 Big Town Blvd., Suite 100, Mesquite, TX 75149

S&B Biomedics, Inc. — 972-288-3278
844 Dalworth Drive, Suite 6, Mesquite, TX 75149-4162

Seecor, Inc. — 972-288-3278
844 Dalworth Drive, Suite 6, Mesquite, TX 75149-4162

Midlothian

G & S Instrument Co. — 972-723-0856
6851 Montgomery Rd., Midlothian, TX 76065

Mastercraft Dental Co. Of Texas — 972-775-8757
880 Eastgate Rd., PO Box 882, Midlothian, TX 76065

Mineral Wells

Electromedical Products International, Inc. — 800-367-7246
2201 Garrett Morris Pkwy., Mineral Wells, TX 76067-9484

Mission

K-10 Inc. — 800-531-7496
PO Drawer 1170 Mission, Mission, TX 78573

Missouri City

Microlight Corporation Of America — 281-433-4648
2935 Highland Lakes Dr., Missouri City, TX 77459

Nacogdoches

Allsport Dynamics, Inc. — 800-594-5350
2724 S.E. Stallings Dr., Nacogdoches, TX 75961-7442

Navasota

Ergogenesis, Llc — 800-364-5299
One Bodybilt Pl., Navasota, TX 77868

O'Donnell

Organic Essentials — 800-765-6491
822 Baldridge St., O'Donnell, TX 79351

Olney

Hypertec, Inc. — 800-218-3588
301B East Main Street, Olney, TX 76374

Orange

Hearing Aid Factory — 409-883-3010
105 Camellia, P.o. Box 61, Orange, TX 77631

Paris

Kimberly-Clark Corp., Paris Child Care Plant — 888-525-8388
2466 Farm Road 137, Paris, TX 75460

Pflugerville

Metro Optics Of Austin, Ltd. — 512-251-2382
15802 Vision Dr., Pflugerville, TX 78660
Trayco — 512-341-3709
1101 West Pecan St., Pflugerville, TX 78660

Pinehurst

Accelerated Rehab Designs, Inc. — 888-397-4063
32025 Industrial Park Dr, Pinehurst, TX 77362

Plano

Epic Medical Equipment Services, Inc. — 800-327-3742
1800 10th St., Suite 300, Plano, TX 75074
Exfo America Inc. — 800-663-3936
3701 Plano Parkway, Suite 160, Plano, TX 75075
Invensys Process Systems — 866-746-6477
5601 Granite Parkway III, Suite 1000, Plano, TX 75024
Millers Forge, Inc. — 972-422-2145
1411 Capital Ave., Plano, TX 75074-8198
Neuro Resource Group, Inc. — 972-665-1810
1100 Jupiter Rd., Ste. 190, Plano, TX 75074
Orchid Dental Studio, Inc — 469-619-2368
1101 E Plano Parkway, Suite J, Plano, TX 75074
St. Jude Medical Neuromodulation Division — 800-727-7846
6901 Preston Rd., Plano, TX 75024

PORT ISABEL

Patterson Precision, Inc. — 956-943-6119
561 Industrial Way, PORT ISABEL, TX 78578

Port Lavaca

Blue Spring Corp. — 361-552-8898
45 Blue Spring Rd., Port Lavaca, TX 77979

Richardson

Chase Medical, Lp — 800-787-0378
1876 Firman Dr., Richardson, TX 75081
D4d Technologies, Llc — 972-234-3880
650 International Pkwy., Richardson, TX 75081
Dentlight Inc. — 972-889-8857
1411 E. Campbell Rd., Suite 500, Richardson, TX 75081
Orametrix Inc. — 493-024-3091
2350 Campbell Creek Blvd., Suite 400, Richardson, TX 75082
Perkins Electronics — 877-923-4545
700 International Parkway, Suite 100, Richardson, TX 75081
Winfield Laboratories — 800-527-4616
P.O. Box 832297, Richardson, TX 75083-2297
Zhang Enterprises — 972-238-8260
400 N. Greenville Ave., Suite 9, Richardson, TX 75081
Zimmer-Wilson-Phillips, Inc — 800-444-4547
3301 Matrix Drive, Suite 200, Richardson, TX 75082

Richmond

Ocusoft, Inc. — 281-342-3350
P.O Box 429, Richmond, TX 77406-0429

Roanoke

Thermadyne Holdings, Corp. — 940-381-1388
800 Henrietta Creek Rd., Roanoke, TX 76262

Robstown

Erigon — 361-387-8276
1301 Dakota St., Robstown, TX 78380

Rockwall

Dmedicus, Llc. — 469-698-9939
842 Canterbury Dr., Rockwall, TX 75032
Texas Orthopaedic Products & Services, L.L.C. — 888-373-4009
805 Riding Club Road, Rockwall, TX 75087-2193

Round Rock

Fluoromed, L.P. — 512-255-6877
2350 Double Creek Dr., Round Rock, TX 78664-3801

Rowlett

Beta Biomed Services, Inc. — 800-315-7551
2804 Singleton St., Rowlett, TX 75088
Texas Photonics, Inc. — 972-412-7111
3213 Main Street, Rowlett, TX 75088

Royse City

Texas Medical Industries, Inc. — 800-332-9556
1409 Industrial Drive, Royse City, TX 75189-9559

San Angelo

Ethicon, Inc — 908-218-2996
3348 Pulliam St., San Angelo, TX 76905

San Antonio

Accessible Designs, Inc. — 210-341-0008
401 Isom Rd., Suite 520, San Antonio, TX 78216
Advanced Bio Prosthetic Surfaces, Ltd — 210-696-5300
4778 Research Dr., San Antonio, TX 78240
Airstrip Technologies, Lp — 877-258-5869
335 E Sonterra Blvd Suite 200, San Antonio, TX 78258
Analytical Scientific, Ltd. — 800-364-4848
11049 Bandera Rd., San Antonio, TX 78250
Aperion Biologics — 210-858-7070
11969 Starcrest Drive, San Antonio, TX 78247
Arlon Engineered Coated Products — 800-232-7181
6110 E. Rittiman Road, San Antonio, TX 78218
Biomedical Enterprises, Inc. — 800-880-6528
14785 Omicron Drive, Suite 205, San Antonio, TX 78245
Bpsp Co. (Medical Z Corp.) — 800-368-7478
6800 Alamo Downs Pkwy, San Antonio, TX 78238
Canvas Specialties, Inc. — 210-662-6412
5923 Distribution, San Antonio, TX 78218-5532
Coastal Life Systems, Inc. — 800-727-6814
1803 Grandstand Drive, Suite 101, San Antonio, TX 78238
Diabetica Solutions, Inc. — 210-692-1114
12665 Silicon Dr., San Antonio, TX 78249
Dnms Institute, Llc — 210-561-7881
6421 Mondean St., San Antonio, TX 78240-2533
Dpt Laboratories, Ltd. — 866-225-5378
4040 Broadway, Suite 401, San Antonio, TX 78209
Epikeia, Inc. — 210-313-4600
500 Sandau, Suite 200, San Antonio, TX 78216-3636
Ergomed, Inc. — 800-333-3746
5426 Billington Dr., San Antonio, TX 78230
Frio Technologies, Inc. — 210-308-5635
500 Sandau Rd., Suite 200, San Antonio, TX 78216
Germaine Laboratories, Inc. — 210-692-4192
11030 Wye Drive, San Antonio, TX 78217
Incell Corporation, Llc — 210-877-0100
12734 Cimarron Path, San Antonio, TX 78249
Kci Usa, Inc. — 210-255-6137
6203 Farinon Dr., San Antonio, TX 78249
Kinetic Concepts, Inc. — 800-275-4524
8023 Vantage Drive, San Antonio, TX 78230
Kln Steel Products Company — 800-624-9101
Two Winnco Dr., P.O. Box 34690, San Antonio, TX 78218
Lifetechniques Inc., Medsignals Corp. Div. — 210-222-2067
217 Alamo Plaza, suite 200, San Antonio, TX 78205
Lightspeed Technology, Inc. — 210-495-4942
403 E. Ramsey, Suite 205, San Antonio, TX 78216
Mediana Technologies Corp — 800-829-6427
5850 Farinon Drive, San Antonio, TX 78249
Mesa, Inc. — 210-699-6911
9807 Fredericksburg Rd., San Antonio, TX 78240
Meza Medical Equipment — 888-308-7116
108 W. Nakoma Drive, San Antonio, TX 78216
Mission Pharmacal Co. — 210-696-8400
10999 IH-10 West, Suite 1000, San Antonio, TX 78230-1355
Neo-Care Arrow International — 800-640-6428
5714 Epsilon Rd., San Antonio, TX 78249-3407
Oncology Tech, Llc — 210-497-2100
5608 Business Park, San Antonio, TX 78218
Oral Designs, Inc. — 800-292-5516
1259 Jackson Keller, San Antonio, TX 78213
Pata Enterprises, Inc. — 603-883-4534
1120 North Mesquite St., San Antonio, TX 78202
Photoprotective Technologies — 800-219-9993
6610 Topper Ridge, San Antonio, TX 78233
Pristech Products, Inc — 800-432-8722
6952 Fairgrounds Pkwy., PO Box 680728, San Antonio, TX 78238
Sa Scientific, Inc. — 800-272-2710
4919 Golden Quail, San Antonio, TX 78240
Sas Shoemakers — 877-782-7463
101 New Laredo HWY, San Antonio, TX 78224-0547
Schroeder American, Inc. — 210 662 8200
5620 Business Park, San Antonio, TX 78218
Simon & Simon Mobility Services — 210-614-1414
9207 Huebner Rd., San Antonio, TX 78240

Smith & Nephew, Inc. — 800-343-5717
University Business Park, 12500 Network, Suite 112, San Antonio, TX 78249-3308
Southwest Artificial Eyes, Inc. — 210-737-3937
6323 Sovereign St # 159, San Antonio, TX 78201
Teftec Corp. — 210-477-0330
12450 Network Blvd., San Antonio, TX 78249
Temedco, Ltd. — 210-798-0978
1141 N. Loop 1604 E #105, Box 418, San Antonio, TX 78232
Thompson Ocular Prosthetics, Inc. — 210-223-3754
4118 Mccullough Ave., Suite 16, San Antonio, TX 78212
Tiller Mind Body, Inc. — 210-308-8888
10911 West Ave., San Antonio, TX 78213
Voss Medical Products — 210-650-3124
4235 Centergate, San Antonio, TX 78217

San Juan
Mjm International Corporation — 956-781-5000
2003 N. I Rd., Ste. 10, San Juan, TX 78589

Sanger
Orrex Medical Technologies, Llp — 940-458-7150
403 Acker St., Sanger, TX 76266

Santa Fe
Galveston Manufacturing Co., Inc. — (800) 634-3309
7810 FM 646 S., Santa Fe, TX 77510-9535

Schertz
Itm Partners, Ltd. — 210-651-9066
5925 Corridor Pkwy., Schertz, TX 78154

Seabrook
Louisville Apl Diagnostics, Inc. — 800-624-3192
2622 Nasa Parkway, Suite G2, Seabrook, TX 77586

Sealy
Orthovation, Llc — 979-885-2012
2060 Highway 90 W., Sealy, TX 77474

Seguin
Cone Bioproducts — 830-379-0197
1012 N. Austin St., Seguin, TX 78155
M.W. Sales And Service, Inc. — 830-303-2508
2549 O'daniel Rd., Seguin, TX 78155
Mes, Inc. — 800-423-2215
1968 E US Hwy 90, Seguin, TX 78155
Quality Bioresources, Inc. — 888-674-7224
1015 North Austin St., Seguin, TX 78155
Tecni-Quip — 800-826-1245
960 Crossroads Blvd., PO Box 2050, Seguin, TX 78155

Shavano Park
Vidacare Corp. — 800-680-4911
4350 Lockhill Selma Rd, Suite 150, Shavano Park, TX 78249

Southlake
Dac Inc./Diagnostic Audiology Corp. — 800-551-3277
351 Bank St. Suite 105, Southlake, TX 76092-9126
Pds Manufacturing, Inc. — 817-329-2701
577 Commerce St., Suite A, Southlake, TX 76092

Spicewood
Adaptive Switch Laboratories, Inc. — 800-626-8698
125 Spur 191, Suite C, Spicewood, TX 78669

Spring
Instratek, Inc. — 281-890-8020
210 Spring Hill Drive, Suite 130, Spring, TX 77386
International Science And Technology, Lp — 800-867-8081
1544 Sawdust Road, Suite 502, Spring, TX 77380
Medco Mfg. — 281-379-3100
8319 Thora #a1, Spring, TX 77379

Stafford
Gresco Products, Inc. — 800-527-3250
13391 Murphy Rd., P.o. Box 865, Stafford, TX 77477
Life-Tech, Inc. — 800-231-9841
13235 N. Promenade Blvd., Stafford, TX 77477
Lone Star Medical Products, Inc. — 800-331-7427
11211 Cash Road, Stafford, TX 77477
Nimbic Systems, Llc — 281-565-5700
4910 Wright Road, Suite 170, Stafford, TX 77477
Ramco Laboratories, Inc. — 281-313-1200
4100 Greenbriar Drive, Suite 200, Stafford, TX 77477

Stamford
Key Scientific Products — 325-773-3918
1113 East Reynolds St, Stamford, TX 79553

Sugar Land
Servomex — 800-862-0200
525 Julie Rivers Drive, Suite 185, Sugar Land, TX 77478
Translite — 281-240-3111
8410 Highway 90 A, Sugar Land, TX 77478

Udl Laboratories, Inc. — 281-240-1000
12720 Dairy Ashford, Sugar Land, TX 77478

Sunnyvale
Trigroup Technologies, Ltd. — 972-226-4600
200 Adell Blvd., Sunnyvale, TX 75182

Sweetwater
Ludlum Measurements, Inc. — 800-622-0828
501 Oak St., Sweetwater, TX 79556-3209

Texarkana
Apex Medical Corp. — 903-314-1217
6406 Prestige Lane, Texarkana, TX 75503
Larkotex Company — 800-972-3037
1002 Olive St., Texarkana, TX 75501-0449
Lectec Corp. — 903-832-0993
1407 South Kings Highway, Texarkana, TX 75501

The Woodlands
Airgas-Southwest, Inc. — 800-985-0986
21 Waterway, Suite 550, The Woodlands, TX 77380
Novosci Corp. — 281-363-4949
2828 N. Crescent Ridge Drive, The Woodlands, TX 77381

Tomball
Laser, Inc. — 800-367-5694
27831 Commercial Park Lane, Tomball, TX 77375

Tyler
East Texas Lighthouse For The Blind — 903-595-3444
500 North Bois D'arc, Tyler, TX 75702

Waco
Allergan Sales, Llc — 714-246-4388
8301 Mars Dr., Waco, TX 76712
Health Edco — 800-299-3366
PO Box 21207, Waco, TX 76702
Nearly Me Technologies, Inc. — 800-887-3370
3630 South I 35, Suite A, Waco, TX 76706
Spenco Medical Corp. — 254-772-6000
PO Box 2501, Waco, TX 76702-2501
Wrs Group, Ltd. — 800-299-3366
5045 Franklin Avenue, Waco, TX 76710

Webster
Beckman Coulter Inc. — 800-231-7970
445 Medical Center Blvd., Webster, TX 77598
Cardionics, Inc. — 800-364-5901
910 Bay Star Blvd., Webster, TX 77598
Idev Technologies, Inc. — 866-806-4338
253 Medical Center Blvd., Webster, TX 77598

Whitewright
Newwave Medical Llc — 888-513-9283
1239 Durham Road, Whitewright, TX 75491

Wichita Falls
Washex, Inc. — 800-433-0933
5000 Central Freeway N., Wichita Falls, TX 76306-1599

Winnsboro
Itec/Ems Llp — 903-365-6390
400 Allstar Dr., Winnsboro, TX 75494

UTAH

Alpine
Innovamed, Inc. — 801-885-9085
13524 Oakridge Dr., Alpine, UT 84004

Bluffdale
Listen Technologies Corp. — 800-330-0891
14912 S. Heritagecrest Way, Bluffdale, UT 84065-4818

Bonnie
Star Tech Health Services, Llc. — 801-229-1114
1219 South 1840 West, Bonnie, UT 84058

Bountiful
Eclectic Grey Mater Designs — 801-296-0741
279 East 650 North, Bountiful, UT 84010
Medspring Group, Inc. — 801-295-9750
533 West 2600 South, Suite 105, Bountiful, UT 84010
Specialized Health Products International, Inc. — 800-306-3360
585 W. 500 S., Bountiful, UT 84010
Specialty Medical Products Co. — 801-295-6023
3063 South Davis Blvd., Bountiful, UT 84010

Cottonwood Heights
Sculptec Dental Design Inc. — 801-942-1874
6841 South 1300 East, Cottonwood Heights, UT 84121

Draper

Ballard Medical Products　770-587-7835
12050 Lone Peak Pkwy., Draper, UT 84020

Flexpoint Sensor Systems Inc　801-568-5111
106 West 12200 South, Draper, UT 84020

Megadyne Medical Products, Inc.　800-747-6110
11506 S. State St., Draper, UT 84020

Ortho Development Corp.　800-429-8339
12187 S. Business Park. Drive, Draper, UT 84020

farmington

Inceptio Medical Technologies, Lc　801-447-7000
1401 north 1075, west suite 230, farmington, UT 84025

Gunnison

Freedom Innovations, Llc　435-528-7199
425 East 400 North, P.O Box 9, Gunnison, UT 84634

Lehi

Alpine Dental Laboratory, Inc.　800-884-5047
1220 North 500 West, Lehi, UT 84043-1117

Lindon

Therapease Innovation, Llc　435-671-0886
32 North 1025 East, Lindon, UT 84042

Trans American Medical, Inc.　801-796-7335
965 West 325 North, Lindon, UT 84042

Logan

Frontier Scientific, Inc.,　453-753-1901
PO Box 31, Logan, UT 84323-0031

Hyclone Laboratories, Inc.　435-792-8000
925 West 1800 South, Logan, UT 84321

Inovar, Inc.　866-898-4949
1073 West 1700 North, Logan, UT 84321

Portal, Inc.　435-753-3598
1350 N 200 W., Suite 6, Logan, UT 84341

Scytek Laboratories, Inc.　435-755-9848
205 South 600 West, Logan, UT 84321

Wescor, Inc.　800-453-2725
370 West 1700 South, Logan, UT 84321-5294

Midvale

Edwards Lifesciences Research Medical　949-250-2500
6864 South 300 West, Midvale, UT 84047

Eye Prosthetics Of Utah, Inc.　801-942-1600
7400 Union Park Ave., Suite 102, Midvale, UT 84047

Utah Medical Products, Inc.　800-533-4984
7043 S. 300 W., Midvale, UT 84047

Millville

Silmed, Inc.　435-753-7307
97 West 300 South, Millville, UT 84326-0438

Murray

Anderson Eye Prosthetics　801-262-6711
164 East 5900 South, #101-b, Murray, UT 84107

Clinical Innovations, Inc.　888-268-6222
747 West 4170 South, Murray, UT 84123

Farpin, Inc.　801-262-8406
333 East 4500 South, #13, Murray, UT 84107-3965

Jemo Spine, Llc　801-266-4811
6170 South 380 West, Suite 200, Murray, UT 84107

Parvo Medics, Inc.　801-942-7796
6526 S. State St. Ste. 202, Murray, UT 84107

3m Health Information Systems　800-367-2447
575 W. Murray Blvd., Murray, UT 84123-0900

North Salt Lake

Medical Techniques Usa　801-936-4501
125 North 400 West, Suite C, North Salt Lake, UT 84054

Zero Manufacturing, Inc.　800-500-9376
500 West 200 North, North Salt Lake, UT 84054

Ogden

Computerized Thermal Imaging Co.　801-776-4700
1719 West 2800 South, Ogden, UT 84401

Fresenius Medical Care North America　781-699-9068
475 West 13th St, Ogden, UT 84404

Hearing Improvement　801-392-4310
1961 Washington Blvd., Ogden, UT 84401-0433

Orem

Aribex, Inc.　801-226-5522
744 South 400 East, Orem, UT 84097

Harris Research & Development, Llc.　800-802-2228
528 East 800 North, Orem, UT 84097-4146

Park City

Nutraceutical International Corp.　800-669-8877
1400 Kearns Blvd., Second Floor, Park City, UT 84060

Pleasant Grove

Richards Laboratories, Inc.　800-453-1210
55 E. Center, Pleasant Grove, UT 84062-2233

Provo

American Dental Center Of Provo　801-375-8200
777 North 500 West, Ste. 201b, Provo, UT 84601

Riverton

Ultimate Concepts, Inc.　801-566-3241
5056 Crimson Patch Way, Riverton, UT 84065

Salem

Gull Works Mfg. Llc　801-423-2812
685 East 600 South, Salem, UT 84653

Salt Lake City

Aimsco, Delta Hi-Tech, Inc.　800-378-0909
3762 S. 150 E., Salt Lake City, UT 84115

Airgas Intermountain, Inc.　801-288-5015
3415 South 7oo West, Salt Lake City, UT 84119

Alphaprotech, Inc.　229-333-9741
236 North 2200 West, Salt Lake City, UT 84116

Amedica Corporation　801-839-3500
1885 West 2100 South, Salt Lake City, UT 84119

Anecare Laboratories, Inc.　801-977-8877
3487 West 2100 South #100, Salt Lake City, UT 84119

Bard Access Systems, Inc.　800-545-0890
605 N. 5600 West, Salt Lake City, UT 84116

Behavioral Technology, Inc.　888-363-9017
24 M St.,, Salt Lake City, UT 84103

Bio-Heme　801-277-9392
3710 Ceres Drive, Salt Lake City, UT 84124

Biomeridian, Int　888-224-2337
2440 south 1070 west suite a, salt lake city, UT 84119

Brevis Corp.　800-383-3377
225 West 2855 South, Salt Lake City, UT 84115

Bsd Medical Corporation　801-972-5555- 2
2188 W. 2200 S., Salt Lake City, UT 84119

Bunnell Incorporated　800-800-4358
436 Lawndale Dr., Salt Lake City, UT 84115-2917

Case In Point　801-647-5437
3917 E Viewcrest Drive, Salt Lake City, UT 84124

Catheter Connections Inc.　1-888-706-8883
615 Arapeen Dr, Suite 302a, Salt Lake City, UT 84108

Catheter Innovations, Inc.　800-418-2828
3598 West 1820 South, Salt Lake City, UT 84104-4859

Coherex Medical Inc.　800-390-9107
3598 West 1820 South, Salt Lake City, UT 84104

Cole Vision Corporation　770-305-7352
1887 S. 3230 West, Salt Lake City, UT 84104

Dynatronics Corp.　800-874-6251
7030 Park Centre Dr., Salt Lake City, UT 84121

Ge Oec Medical Systems Inc.　800-874-7378
384 Wright Brothers Drive, Salt Lake City, UT 84116

Global Medical Company　801-746-0208
3450 S. Highland Dr., #303, Salt Lake City, UT 84106

Great Basin Corporation　801-990-1055
2441 South 3850 West, Salt Lake City, UT 84120

Holorad Llc　801-983-6075
2929 South Main St., Salt Lake City, UT 84115

Icu Medical (Ut), Inc　949-366-2183
4455 Atherton Dr., Salt Lake City, UT 84123

Idaho Technology, Inc.　1-800-735-6544
390 Wakara Way, Salt Lake City, UT 84108

Innovasis, Inc.　801-261-2236
614 East 3900 South, Salt Lake City, UT 84107

Integra Lifesciences Corp.　801-886-9505
3395 West 1820 South, Salt Lake City, UT 84104

Iomed, Inc.　800-621-3347
2441 South 3850 West, Suite A, Salt Lake City, UT 84120

JTECH Medical　800-985-8324
470 West Longdale Dr., Suite G, Salt Lake City, UT 84115

Jtech Medical　801-478-0680
470 Lawndale Dr., Ste. G, Salt Lake City, UT 84115

Korr Medical Technologies, Inc.　801-483-2080
2463 South 3850 West #200, Salt Lake City, UT 84120

Korr Medical Technologies, Inc.　800-895-4048
3487 W 2100 South, Bldg #300, Salt Lake City, UT 84119

Larada Sciences Inc.　801-533-5423
350 West 800 North, Suite 203, Salt Lake City, UT 84103

LineaGen Inc.　801-931-6200
423 Wakara Way, Suite 200, Salt Lake City, UT 84108

Littlefield Co.　801-485-1441
1441 East 2100 South, Salt Lake City, UT 84105

Lumenis Inc.　800-447-0234
3959 W. 1820 S., Salt Lake City, UT 84104-4951

Maxtec, Inc.　800-748-5355
6526 S. Cottonwood St., Salt Lake City, UT 84107

Medical Alignment Systems　801-733-6787
3656 Macintosh Ln., Salt Lake City, UT 84121-4515

Medical Skyhook Company　801-262-1471
PO Box 17213, Salt Lake City, UT 84117-0213

Medical Technology Industries, Inc.   800-924-4655
3555 W. Ninigret Drive, Salt Lake City, UT 84104

Medron, Inc.   801-974-3010
1518 S. Gladiola St., Salt Lake City, UT 84104

Motion Control, Inc.   888-696-2767
115 N. Wright Brothers Drive, Salt Lake City, UT 84116

Nytone Medical Products   801-973-4090
2424 S. 900 W., Salt Lake City, UT 84119-1518

Oratech, Llc   801-553-4493
475 West 10200 South, Salt Lake City, UT 84095

Otix Global, Inc.   888-678-4327
4246 S. Riverboat Road, Suite 300, Salt Lake City, UT 84123

Otto Bock Healthcare   763-489-5106
3820 West Great Lakes Dr., Salt Lake City, UT 84120

Paradigm Medical Industries, Inc.   801-977-8970
2355 South 1070 West, Salt Lake City, UT 84119

Personal Performance Medical Corp.   801-364-3100
50 South 900 East, Suite 1, Salt Lake City, UT 84102

Practical Things, Llc.   310-951-6906
3267 East 3300 South, Suite 105, Salt Lake City, UT 84109

Rocky Mountain Research, Inc.   801-359-6060
825 North 300 West, Suite 410, Salt Lake City, UT 84103

Siemens Medical Solutions Health Services Corp.   800-888-7436
215 N. Admiral Byrd Road, Salt Lake City, UT 84116

Sonic Innovations   (888) 678-4327
4246 Riverboat Road, Suite 300, Salt Lake City, UT 84123

Specialty Lens Corp.   800-366-1382
3955 South 210 West, Salt Lake City, UT 84107

Standard Supply Co.   800-453-7036
3424 S. Main St., Salt Lake City, UT 84165-0009

Techniscan, Inc.   888-268-3030
13216 South Highland Dr., Suite 200, Salt Lake City, UT 84106

University Of Utah Hospitals And Clinics   801-581-2742
50 North Medical Dr., Salt Lake City, UT 84132

Varian Medical Systems X-Ray Products   800-432-4422
1678 S. Pioneer Rd., Salt Lake City, UT 84104

Volu-Sol, Inc.   801-974-9474
2100 South 5095 West, Salt Lake City, UT 84121

Wolfe Tory Medical, Inc.   801-281-3000
79 West 4500 South, Suite 18, Salt Lake City, UT 84107

World Heart Inc.   888-843-5827
4750 Wiley Post Way, Suite 120, Salt Lake City, UT 84116

Worldheart, Inc.   801-355-6255
4750 Wiley Post Way, Suite 120, Salt Lake City, UT 84116

Zevex Incorporated   800-970-2337
4314 ZEVEX Park Lane, Salt Lake City, UT 84123-4650

Zinetics Medical, Inc.   800-648-4070
1050 East South Temple, Salt Lake City, UT 84102

Sandy

Ageless Processing Technologies   801-942-9250
20-707 S. Sierra Ave., Sandy, UT 84092

Becton Dickinson Infusion Therapy Systems, Inc.   888-237-2762
9450 S. State St., Sandy, UT 84070

Burnfree Products Division   888-909-2876
9382 S. 670 W., Sandy, UT 84070

Nualine Laser   801-304-9678
1213 Twelve Pines Cir., Sandy, UT 84094

Ultimate Trends   800-745-3191
1455 East 8125 So., Sandy, UT 84092

Saratoga Springs

Galloway Technologies, Llc   801-766-1636
3736 Panarama Dr., Saratoga Springs, UT 84043

South Jordan

Hannah's Miracle Shoe, Inc.   801-329-9802
11237 S. Aubrey Meadow Cir., South Jordan, UT 84095-2231

Merit Medical Systems, Inc.   800-356-3748
1600 W. Merit Pkwy., South Jordan, UT 84095

Mytrex, Inc.   1-800-688-9576
10321 South Beckstead Ln., South Jordan, UT 84095

Ultradent Products, Inc.   801-553-4586
505 West 10200 South, South Jordan, UT 84095

Springville

Arlington Scientific, Inc. Asi   800-654-0146
1840 N. Technology Dr., Springville, UT 84663

St. George

Deseret Laboratories Inc.   435-628-8786
1414 East 3850 South, St. George, UT 84790

Vernal

Ram Plus, Llc   435-781-1646
983 N. 2175 W., Vernal, UT 84078

W Jordan

Footent, Llc   757-224-0177
3392 W. 8600 South, W Jordan, UT 84088

West Jordan

Bio-Logics Products, Inc.   800-426-7577
PO Box 505, West Jordan, UT 84084

Cao Group, Inc.   801-256-9282
4628 West Skyhawk Drive, West Jordan, UT 84084

Descent Control Systems, Inc.   801-304-9299
8100 South 1300 West, #d, West Jordan, UT 84088

Hoggan Health Industries, Inc.   800-678-7888
8020 South 1300 West, West Jordan, UT 84088

Utah Pioneer Medical, Inc.   801-280-1053
8173 S. Summit Valley Drive, West Jordan, UT 84088

West Valley City

Diacor, Inc.   800-342-2679
2550 Decker Lane, Suite 26, West Valley City, UT 84119

Woods Cross

Easy Seat Llc   877-327-9732
2361 West 1560w Suite 200, Woods Cross, UT 84087-2364

Med-Assist Technology, Inc.   801-296-6848
2441 South 1560 West, Woods Cross, UT 84087

VERMONT

Arlington

Mack Molding Co.   802-375-2511
608 Warm Brook Rd., Arlington, VT 05250

Bellows Falls

Vermed, Inc.   802-463-9976
9 Lovell Dr., Bellows Falls, VT 05101

Vermont Medical, Inc.   800-245-4025
9 Lovell Drive, Bellows Falls, VT 05101-0556

Bennington

Vermont Composites, Inc.   802-442-9964
Subsidiary of APC, 25 Performance Drive, Bennington, VT 05201

Bethel

Gw Plastics, Inc.   802-234-9941
239 Pleasant St., Bethel, VT 05032

Brattleboro

Fulflex Of Vermont, Inc.   800-283-2500
32 Justin Holden Dr., Brattleboro, VT 05304

Bridgewater Corners

Cutting Edge Instruments Inc.   330-916-8858
312 River Rd., Bridgewater Corners, VT 05035

Btv

Data Innovations, Inc.   802-658-2850
120 Kimball Ave., Suite 100, Btv, VT 05403

Burlington

Edlund Co.   800-772-2126
159 Industrial; Parkway, Burlington, VT 05401

Ge Healthcare Integrated It Solutions   877-519-4471
40 Idx Drive, P.O. Box 1070, Burlington, VT 05402

Idx Systems Corporation   802-862-1022
1400 Shelburne Rd., Burlington, VT 05402-1070

Yankee Medical, Inc.   800-649-4591
276 North Ave., Burlington, VT 05401

Manchester

The Orvis Co., Inc.   802-362-3622
P. O. Box 798, Manchester, VT 05254

Morrisville

Concept Ii, Inc.   800-245-5676
105 Industrial Park Drive, Morrisville, VT 05661-9727

Northfield

Microcheck, Inc.   877-934-3284
142 Gould Road, Northfield, VT 05663

Proctorsville

Babytooth Technologies, Llc.   802-226-7300
2468 Route 103, Proctorsville, VT 05153

Randolph

Aadco Medical, Inc.   800-225-9014
2279 Vermont Rte. 66, Randolph, VT 05060-0410

South Burlington

Omni Measurement Systems, Inc.   802-865-5223
1150 Airport Drive, South Burlington, VT 05403-6000

St. Albans

Mylan Technologies, Inc.   800-532-5226
110 Lake St., St. Albans, VT 05478

Razel Scientific Instruments, Inc.   877-324-9914
PO Box 111, St. Albans, VT 05478

St. Johnsbury

Mobile Medical International Corporation   800-748-2322
2176 Portland St., Suite 4, PO Box 672, St. Johnsbury, VT 05819

Williston

Medical Systems, Inc. 800-441-1973
30 Winter Sport Lane, PO Box 966, Williston, VT 05495
Phytron, Inc. 800-96P-HYTR
600 Blair Park Road, Suite 220, Williston, VT 05495
Select Medical Systems 800-441-1973
30 Winter Sport Lane, PO Box 966, Williston, VT 05495

Winooski

Biotek Instruments, Inc. 888-451-5171
100 Tigan Street, P.O. Box 998, Highland Park, Winooski, VT 05404

VIRGINIA

Abingdon

Atzen/Universal Companies, Inc. 800-558-5571
18260 Oak Park Drive, Abingdon, VA 24210
Thinoptx, Inc. 276-623-2258
15856 Porterfield Highway, Abingdon, VA 24211-0784

Alexandria

Edge Medical Imaging, Inc. 703-919-4732
6003 Woodlake Lane, Alexandria, VA 22315-2638
Electro-Steam Generator Corp. 888-783-2624
1000 Bernard Street, Alexandria, VA 22314
S Jackson Inc. 800-368-5225
PO Box 4487, Alexandria, VA 22303

Arlington

Clinical Microsystems Intl. 703-920-4345
620 22nd St. South, Arlington, VA 22202
Eastern Cranial Affiliates 703-807-5899
1600 Wilson Blvd., Ste. 200, Arlington, VA 22209
Electronic Industries Alliance 703-907-7500
2500 Wilson Blvd., Arlington, VA 22201-3834
Environ Corp. 703-516-2300
4350 North Fairfax Drive, Suite 300, Arlington, VA 22203

Ashburn

Adivamed 703-729-8836
44141 Bristow Circle, Ashburn, VA 20147-3310
Custom Prosthetic Design, Inc. 703-723-4668
20608 Gordon Park Square, Suite 150, Ashburn, VA 20147

Ashland

Anton Paar Usa 800-722-7556
10215 Timber Ridge Drive, Ashland, VA 23005

Bastian

Insource, Inc. 800-366-3829
PO Box 9, Bastian, VA 24314

Bedford

Surgical Tools, Inc. 800-774-2040
1106 Monroe St., Bedford, VA 24523

Blacksburg

Techlab, Inc. 800-832-4522
2001 Kraft Drive, Blacksburg, VA 24060-6364
Techulon Inc. 540-443-9254
2200 Kraft Drive, Suite 2475, Blacksburg, VA 24060

Chantilly

Dynex Technologies, Inc. 800-288-2354
14340 Sullyfield Cir., Chantilly, VA 20151
Kol Bio-Medical Instruments, Inc. 800-336-5018
13901 Willard Rd., P.O. Box 220630, Chantilly, VA 20153
Mfg One, Llc 703-437-9838
3900 Skyhawk Dr., Chantilly, VA 20151

Charlottesville

Commonwealth H2o Services, Inc. 434-975-4426
325 Greenbrier Drive, Charlottesville, VA 22901-1618
Humagen Fertility Diagnostics, Inc. 800-937-3210
2400 Hunter's Way, Charlottesville, VA 22911
Medical Automation Systems 434-971-7953
2000 Holiday Drive; Suite 500, Charlottesville, VA 22901
Medical Decisions Network 434-971-7953
2000 Holiday Drive, Suite 200, Charlottesville, VA 22901
Micro-Aire Surgical Instruments, Inc. 800-722-0822
1641Edlich Dr., Charlottesville, VA 22911-1278
Microaire Surgical Instruments, Llc 800-722-0822
1641 Edlich Dr., Charlottesville, VA 22911
National Optronics 434-295-9126
100 Avon St., Charlottesville, VA 22902
National Optronics, Inc. 800-247-9796
100 Avon St., Charlottesville, VA 22902
Silver Ring Splint Co. 434-971-4052
1140 East Market St., Charlottesville, VA 22902
Sport Tech, Inc. 434-982-5752
391 Ridge Lee Drive, Charlottesville, VA 22903
Varian Medical Systems Brachytheraphy 888.666.7847
700 Harris St, Suite 109, Charlottesville, VA 22903

Chesapeake

Bbg, Inc. 757-366-9211
1708 South Park Ct, Chesapeake, VA 23320
Key Element Dental Laboratory Llc 866 446 1833
2006 Old Greenbrier Rd, Suite 8, Chesapeake, VA 23320
Taylorcraft, Inc. 877-376-4756
313 Harbor Watch Dr., Chesapeake, VA 23320

Chester

Titmus Optical Inc. 800-446-1802
690 HP Way, 3811 CorPOrate Drive, Chester, VA 23836-2742

Chesterfield

Merit Medical Systems Inc. 804-416-1030
12701 Kingston Ave, Chesterfield, VA 23837

Chilhowie

Gam Rad, Inc. 540-646-5466
Star Rt. 608 (river Rd.), Chilhowie, VA 24319

Clinchport

Rogers Foam Corporation 617-623-3010
609 Boone Trail Road, Clinchport, VA 24244

Cobbs Creek

Kayjae Mfg. Co. Inc. 888-452-9523
Rte. 198 at Chapel Creek Road, PO Box 95, Cobbs Creek, VA 23035

Colonial Heights

Church & Dwight Co., Inc. 609-279-7715
1851 Touchstone Rd., Colonial Heights, VA 23834
Filtrona Porous Technologies 804-524-4983
1625 Ashton Park Drive, Colonial Heights, VA 23834

Danville

Electronic Development Labs, Inc. 800-342-5335
244 Oakland Drive, Danville, VA 24540-9287
Wal-Star, Inc. 434-685-1094
696 Inman Rd., Danville, VA 24541

Dayton

U.M.A., Inc. 800-842-5578
260 Main St., Dayton, VA 22821-0100

Duffield

Tempur Production Usa, Inc. 276-431-7174
203 Tempur Pedic Drive,, Suite 102, Duffield, VA 24244

Dulles

Radiology Information Systems, Inc. 877-722-6747
43676 Trade Center Place, Suite 100, Dulles, VA 20166
3DISC Americas Inc. 800-570-0363
45921 Maries Road, Suite 190, Dulles, VA 20166

Earlysville

Boss Instruments, Ltd. 800-210-2677
395 Reas Ford Road, Suite 120, Earlysville, VA 22936

Eastville

Vandent Dental Handpiece Sales & Service 800-826-3368
P.O. Box 1229, Eastville, VA 23347

Fairfax

American Medical Diagnostics, Inc. 703-938-6500
4031 University Drive, Suite 200, Fairfax, VA 22030
Commerce Facilitators 703-352-3569
3924 Tedrich Blvd., Fairfax, VA 22031
Csc Scientific Co. 800-621-4778
2810 Old Lee Hwy., Fairfax, VA 22031-4304
Lansinoh Laboratories 800-292-4794
333 North Fairfax Street, Suite 400, Fairfax, VA 22314
Orthotic Solutions, Llc. 877-849-9201
2802 Merrilee Dr. Suite 100, Fairfax, VA 22031-4410

Falls Church

Defense Blood Standard System (Dbss) 703-681-3901
5205 Leesburg Pike, Suite 1000, Falls Church, VA 22041

Ferrum

Smith River Biologicals 276-930-2369
9388 Charity Hwy., Ferrum, VA 24088

Fredericksburg

Kaeser Compressors, Inc. 800-777-7873
P.O. Box 946, Fredericksburg, VA 22404

Front Royal

Biomed Devices Corp. 540-636-7976
1325 Progress Dr., Front Royal, VA 22630

Glen Allen

Advanced Therapy Products, Inc. 800-548-4550
P.O. Box 3420, Glen Allen, VA 23058-3420
Qc Sciences 866-709-0523
4851 Lake Brook Dr, Glen Allen, VA 23060

Sim Net, Inc. — 804-752-2776
10471 Cobbs Rd., Glen Allen, VA 23059

Hampton
Hy-Mark Cylinders, Inc. — 757-245-7331
305 E St., Hampton, VA 23661
Ovusoft, Llc. — 757-722-0991
120 W. Queens Way, Suite 202, Hampton, VA 23669

Herndon
Iritech, Inc. — 703-787-7680
459 Herndon Pkwy Suite 21, Herndon, VA 20170
Vidar Systems Corp. — 703-471-7070
365 Herndon Parkway, Herndon, VA 20170

Ivy
Smith Time, Inc. — 804-977-7440
P.O. Box 496, Ivy, VA 22945-0496

Keysville
Care Rehab And Orthopaedic Products, Inc. — 703-448-9644
3930 Horseshoe Bend Road, Keysville, VA 23947

Leesburg
Eurotherm Inc. — 703-443-0000
741-F Miller Drive, Leesburg, VA 20175-8993
K2m, Inc. — 866-526-4171
751 Miller Dr., SE, Leesburg, VA 20175

Lorton
Associated Design And Manufacturing Co. — 800-837-8257
8245-K Backlick Road, Lorton, VA 22079
Bode Technology Group, Inc. — 866-263-3443
0430 Furnace Road, Suite 107, Lorton, VA 22079
Fmd, Llc — 703-880-4642
7200-e Telegraph Square Dr., P.O. Box 1500, Lorton, VA 22079
Reimers Systems, Inc. — 877-734-6377
8210-D Cinder Bed Road, Lorton, VA 22079

Lynchburg
Bausch & Lomb, Inc. — 585-338-8731
1501 Graves Mill Rd., Lynchburg, VA 24502
C.B. Fleet Company Inc. — 804-528-4000
PO Box 11349, 4615 Murray Place, Lynchburg, VA 24506-1349
Ericsson, Inc. — 434-528-7000
100 Mountain View Drive, Lynchburg, VA 24502-0197

Manassas
Atcc — 800-638-6597
10801 University Blvd., PO Box 1549, Manassas, VA 20108
C & A Scientific Co. Inc. — 703-330-1413
7241 Gabe Court, Manassas, VA 20109
Mediatech, Inc. — 800-235-5476
9345 Discovery Blvd., Manassas, VA 20109

Marion
Blevins Medical Inc — 866-783-3056
207 Broad Street, Marion, VA 24354

Marshall
Dalzell Usa Medical Systems — 540-253-7715
PO Box 162, Marshall, VA 20116-0162

Martinsville
American Of Martinsville — 276-632-2061
128 East. Church St., Martinsville, VA 24115-5071

Mclean
Heyer America, Inc. — 703-506-0040
1320 Old Chain Bridge Rd., Suite 405, Mclean, VA 22101
I.P.I.-International Products, Inc. — 703-237-2774
1929 Poole Lane, McLean, VA 22101
Qinetiq North America — 703-752-9595
7918 Jones Branch Drive, Suite 350, McLean, VA 22102

Midlothian
Pari Respiratory Equipment, Inc. — 800-327-8632
2943 Oak lake Boulevard, Midlothian, VA 23112

Newport News
Burlington Medical Supplies, Inc. — 800-221-3466
3 Elmhurst Str., PO Box 3194, Newport News, VA 23603
Dilon Diagnostics Llc — 877-GO-DILON
12050 Jefferson Avenue, Suite 340, Newport News, VA 23606
Soluble Systems, Llc — 877) 222-2681
11830 Canon Blvd., Suite A, Newport News, VA 23606
Sound Techniques Systems, Llc — 201-271-0700
710 Denbish Blvd., Newport News, VA 23608

Norfolk
Computerized Imaging Reference Systems, Inc. — 800-617-1177
2428 Almeda Ave. Suite 212, Norfolk, VA 23513
Conforma Laboratories, Inc. — 800-426-1700
4705 Colley Ave., Norfolk, VA 23508

Cooper Vision, Inc. — 510-460-3600
1215 Boissevain Ave., Norfolk, VA 23507
Instant Systems, Inc. — 757-200-5494
965 Denison Avenue, Norfolk, VA 23513
Sentara Health Management — 800-736-8272
6015 Poplar Hall Dr., Norfolk, VA 23502-3800

Ordinary
H & H Associates, Inc. — 800-326-5708
4173 George Washington Memorial Highway, Ordinary, VA 23131

Petersburg
TFI Healthcare — 800-526-0178
600 W. Wythe St., Petersburg, VA 23803
Tubular Fabricators Industry, Inc. — 804-733-4000
600 West Wythe St., Petersburg, VA 23803

Portsmouth
Kerma Medical Products, Inc. — 757-398-8400
400 Port Centre Parkway, Portsmouth, VA 23704

Powhatan
Kelleher Medical, Inc. — 804-378-9956
3049 St. Marys Way, Powhatan, VA 23139-5322
Sterile Resources, Inc. — 800-317-6472
1565 Oakbridge Terrace, Powhatan, VA 23139

Pulaski
Uromend, Llc — 540-980-0886
1321 Hopkins Dr., Pulaski, VA 24301

Radford
Thomson Industries, Inc. — 540-633-3549
203A West Rock Road, Radford, VA 24141

Reston
Aptiv Solutions Inc. — 703-483-6400
1925 Isaac Newtown Square, Suite 100, Reston, VA 20190
Cardinal Health 303, Inc. — 571-521-8907
12120 Sunset Hills Road, 3rd Floor, Reston, VA 20190
Hunter Associates Lab., Inc. — 703-471-6870
11491 Sunset Hills Road, Reston, VA 20190-5280

Richmond
Alfa Laval Inc. — 866-253-2528
5400 International Trade Drive, Richmond, VA 23231
Antheros Llc — 804-353-6464
1403 Mactavish Ave., Richmond, VA 23230
Cole Vision Corporation — 513-765-6300
820 Southlake Blvd., Richmond, VA 23236
Corneal Lens Lab, Inc. — 816-455-0500
621-f Moorefield Park Dr., Richmond, VA 23236
Custom Healthcare Systems, Inc. — 804-421-5959
4205 Eubank Rd., Richmond, VA 23231
Dalco International, Inc. — 888-354-5515
8433 Glazebrook Ave., Richmond, VA 23228
Dunlee-Richmond Facility — 800-526-0555
8819 Whitepine Road, Richmond, VA 23237
Mckesson General Medical — 800-446-3008
8741 Landmark Road, Richmond, VA 23228
Medlogix, Inc. — 804-530-2906
9409 Burge Avenue, Richmond, VA 23236
O2 Technologies, Inc. — 804-897-8555
11341-c Business Center Drive, Richmond, VA 23236
Performance Orthopedics — 804-288-2717
6716 Patterson Ave., #B, Richmond, VA 23226-3433
Phipps & Bird, Inc. — 800-955-7621
1519 Summit Avenue, Richmond, VA 23230
Sol Enterprises, Inc. — 800-510-8267
3101 Northside Ave., Richmond, VA 23228
Sterilization Services Of Virginia, Inc. — 804-236-1652
5674 Eastport Blvd., Richmond, VA 23231-4443
The Richmond Light Co. — 888-276-0559
2301 Falkirk Drive, Richmond, VA 23236
Wako Chemicals Usa, Inc. — 877-714-1924
1600 Bellwood Road, Richmond, VA 23237-1326

Roanoke
Bio-Medic Health Services, Inc. — 800-525-0072
5041B Benois Road, Building B, Roanoke, VA 24018
Emtech Laboratories, Inc. — 1-800-336-5719
7745 Garland Circle, Roanoke, VA 24019
Foot Levelers, Inc. — 540-345-0008
P.o. Box 12611, Roanoke, VA 24027
Itt Night Vision — 800-448-8678
7635 Plantation Road, Roanoke, VA 24019-3257
Luna Innovations Incorporated — 540-769-8400
1 Riverside Circle, Suite 400, Roanoke, VA 24016
Plastics One, Inc. — 540-772-7950
6591 Merriman Road S.W., Roanoke, VA 24018-6664
Vertex International, Inc. — 540-989-6945
7429 Fort Mason Dr., Roanoke, VA 24018-5383

Rocky Mount

Mcairlaid's Inc.   540-352-5050
180 Corporate Drive, Rocky Mount, VA 24151
Newbold Corporation   800-552-3282
450 Weaver St., Rocky Mount, VA 24151

Rose Hill

Deroyal Surgical - Rose Hill   800-251-9864
100 Rose Hill Industrial Park, Rose Hill, VA 24281
Deroyal Wound Care   800-251-9864
164 giles hollow road, P.O. Box 309, Rose Hill, VA 24281
Three-D Orthopedic, Div. Deroyal Industries, Inc.   800-251-9864
101 Rose Hill Industrial Park, Rose Hill, VA 24281

Salem

Accellent Inc.   866-899-1392
200 South Yorkshire St., Salem, VA 24153
Novozymes Biologicals, Inc.   540-389-9361
111 Kessler Mill Rd., Salem, VA 24153
The Earmold Co., Ltd.   800-798-2198
814 Eighth St., Salem, VA 24153

Springfield

Best Medical International, Inc.   800-336-4970
7639 & 7643Fullerton Road, Springfield, VA 22153-2862
Uneek Concepts, Llc   888-686-7988
6435 Alloway Court, Springfield, VA 22152

Staunton

Vmg Medical, Inc.   540-337-1996
542 Walnut Hills Rd., Staunton, VA 24401

Sterling

Eit, Inc.   703-478-0700
108 Carpenter Drive, Sterling, VA 20164
Liberty Medical Llc   888-257-2408
10 Acacia Lane, Sterling, VA 20166
S4 Tech Inc   703-467-9034
22831 Silverbrook Center Dr. #135, Sterling, VA 20166
United Laboratories And Manufacturing, Llc   703-787-9600
45000 Underwood Lane, Unit F, Sterling, VA 20166

Toano

Avid Medical   800-886-0584
9000 Westmont Drive, Stonehouse Commerce Park, Toano, VA 23168

Verona

American Safety Razor Co.   800-445-9284
One Razor Blade Lane, Verona, VA 24482
Personna Medical/Div. Of American Safety Razor Co.   800-457-2222
One Razor Blade Ln., Verona, VA 24482

Vienna

Driving Aids Development Corporation   800-767-6435
9417 Delancey Dr., Vienna, VA 22182
Palumbo Orthopaedics   800-292-7223
8206 Leesburg Pike, Ste. 402, Vienna, VA 22182-2614
Talisman Limited   703-242-4200
421 F Church St., N.e., Vienna, VA 22180

Vinton

Precision Fabrics Group, Inc.   888-733-5759
323 Virginia Ave., Vinton, VA 24179

Virginia Beach

Action Llc   757-491-4175
1112 Jensen Dr., #103, Virginia Beach, VA 23451
Air-Tite Products Co., Inc.   800-231-7762
565 Central Drive, Suite 101, Virginia Beach, VA 23454
Busch, Inc   800-872-7867
516 Viking Drive, Virginia Beach, VA 23452-7316
Concoa   800-225-0473
1501 Harpers Road, Virginia Beach, VA 23454-5303
Kettler International   757-427-2400
PO Box 2747, 1355 London Bridge Rdy, Virginia Beach, VA 23453
Lifenet Health   800-847-7831
1864 Concert Drive, Virginia Beach, VA 23453-1903
Morris Designs, Inc.   757-463-9400
2212 Commerce Pkwy, Virginia Beach, VA 23454

Warrenton

Omni International, Inc.   540-347-5331
P.O. Box 861455, Warrenton, VA 20187-1455

Waynesboro

Airtech Industries, Inc.   540-949-6565
412 Ohio St., Waynesboro, VA 22980

Williamsburg

Aztec Medical Products, Inc.   800-223-3859
3356 Ironbound Road, Suite 303, Williamsburg, VA 23188
Global Services Group   757-220-8282
350 Mclaws Circle, Suite:2, Williamsburg, VA 23185

Winchester

O'sullivan Corp.   800-336-9882
1944 Valley Ave., Winchester, VA 22601
Rubbermaid Commercial Products Llc   800-347-9800
3124 Valley Ave., Winchester, VA 22601-2636
Valley Biomedical Products/Ser., Inc.   540-868-0800
121 Industrial Dr., Winchester, VA 22602

Woodbridge

Gladiator Sports   703-878-9434
3499 Cowes Mews, Woodbridge, VA 22193

WASHINGTON

Arlington

Bowman Manufacturing Company, Inc.   360-435-5005
17301 51st Ave NE, Arlington, WA 98223
Touch Turner Company   888-811-1962
13621 103rd Avenue NE, Arlington, WA 98223-8827
United Contact Lens, Inc.   425-743-7343
19111 61st Ave Ne #5, Arlington, WA 98223

Auburn

Blood Bank Computer Systems, Inc.   253-333-0046
1002 15th St. Sw, Suite 120, Auburn, WA 98001
Brandrud Furniture, Inc.   253-838-6500
1502 20th St. NW, Auburn, WA 98001-3428
Homecare Products, Inc.   800-451-1903
1704 B STREET NW SUITE 110, Auburn, WA 98001
Philips Electronics North America   800-682-7664
2820 B. St. NW, Suite 101, Auburn, WA 98001

Bellevue

Advanced Renal Technologies, Inc.   425-453-8777
40 Lake Bellevue, Suite 100, Suite 100, Bellevue, WA 98005
Aiphone Corporation   425-455-0510
1700 130th Avenue NE, Bellevue, WA 98005
Airex, Inc.   425-222-3665
13704 SE 17th St., Bellevue, WA 98050
Capital Instruments, Ltd.   425-271-3756
6210 Lake Washington Blvd., Se, Bellevue, WA 98006
Clearmedical, Inc.   425-883-1522
PMB - 357, 14150 NE 20th F-1, Bellevue, WA 98007
Confirma, Inc.   877-811-2356
11040 Main Street, Suite 100, Bellevue, WA 98004
Helio Balance   425-453-9849
13000 Bel-red Rd., #207, Bellevue, WA 98005
Hokanson Inc., D.E.   800-999-8251
12840 N.E. 21st Pl., Bellevue, WA 98005-1910
Lumedx Corp.   800-966-0669
110 110th Ave. NE, Bellevue, WA 98004
Mobile Dental Equipment Corp.(M-Dec)   425-747-5424
13300 S.E. 30th St.# 101, Bellevue, WA 98005
Neurosync Llc   425-605-8694
12215 Ne 39th St., Bellevue, WA 98005
Ocular Instruments, Inc.   800-888-6616
2255-116th Avenue NE, Bellevue, WA 98004-3039
Ocular Instruments, North Facility   800-888-6616
2255 116th Ave NE, Bellevue, WA 98004
Pascal Co., Inc.   425-602-3633
2929 N.e. Northup Way, Bellevue, WA 98004
Pascal Company, Inc.   800-426-8051
PO Box 1478, Bellevue, WA 98009-1478
Physiosonics, Inc   425-732-2814
2002 156th Avenue Ne # 150, Bellevue, WA 98007-3828
RF Surgical Systems, Inc.   425-283-0678
3326 160th Avenue SE, Suite 220, Bellevue, WA 98008
Rose Technologies   425-637-2344
13400 NE 20th Street, STE 32, Bellevue, WA 98005
STI Optronics, Inc.   425-827-0460
2755 Northrup Way, Bellevue, WA 98004-1495

Bellingham

Diabetes Sentry Products   360-738-1200
1200 Dupont St, Suite 1-D, Bellingham, WA 98225
Kent Laboratories, Inc.   360-398-8641
777 Jorgensen Pl., Bellingham, WA 98226
Sonotech Inc.   800-458-4254
774 Marine Dr., Bellingham, WA 98225

Black Diamond

Anesthesia Equipment Supply, Inc.   253-631-8008
24301 Roberts Dr., Black Diamond, WA 98010
G. Dundas Co.,Inc.   253-631-8008
24301 Roberts Dr., Black Diamond, WA 98010

Bothell

Cardiac Science Corporation (Ca)   1.800.426.0337
3303 Monte Villa Parkway, Bothell, WA 98021
Cardiodynamics International Corp.   888-482-9449
21919 30th Drive SE, Bothell, WA 98021
Catch Incorporated   425-402-8960
11822 North Creek Parkway N., Suite 107, Bothell, WA 98011

Ekos Corp. — 888-400-3567
11911 N Creek Parkway South, Bothell, WA 98011

Halosource, Inc. — 425-881-6464
1631 220th Street SE, Bothell, WA 98021

Infometrix, Inc. — 425-402-1450
10634 E. Riverside Dr., Suite 250, Bothell, WA 98011

Lg Medical Technology, Llc — 360-668-0803
22529 39th Ave Se, Bothell, WA 98021

Mdrna, Inc. — 425-908-3600
3830 Monte Villa Parkway, Bothell, WA 98021

Nanogen Molecular Research Products Division — 800-526-5544
21720 23rd Drive, Suite 150, Bothell, WA 98021

Philips Medical Systems North America Co. — 800-934-7372
22100 Bothell Everett Highway, Bothell, WA 98021

Philips Oral Healthcare, Inc. — 425-396-2000
22100 Bothell Everett Highway, Bothell, WA 98021

Phillips Ultrasound — 800-982-2011
22100 Bothell Everett Hwy., P.O. Box 3003, Bothell, WA 98021-3003

Plexus Corp — 425-482-1300
20001 N. Creek Pkwy, Bothell, WA 98011

Sonosite, Inc. — 888-482-9449
21919 30th Drive SE, Bothell, WA 98021-3904

Verathon Inc. — 800-331-2313
20001 North Creek Parkway, Bothell, WA 98011

Burien

Jetcor, Inc. — 206-243-2230
15001 8th Ave. Sw, Suite #16, Burien, WA 98166

Burlington

Spectron Corp. — 425-827-9317
934 S. Burlington Blvd # 603, Burlington, WA 98233

Camas

Comfort Acrylics, Inc. — 360-834-9218
2103 N.e. 272nd Ave., Camas, WA 98607

Carnation

Iopi Northwest Company, Llc — 425-333-5721
5901 Tolt River Rd. N.e., Carnation, WA 98014

Centralia

Vocal Labs — 360-736-7123
114 W. Pear St., Centralia, WA 98531

Chehalis

Braun Northwest, Inc. — 800-245-6303
PO BOX 1204, Chehalis, WA 98532

Eastsound

Lacrimedics — 800-367-8327
P.O. Box 1209, 9 Hope Lane, Eastsound, WA 98245

Lacrimedics, Inc. — 360-376-7095
#9 Hope Lane, Eastsound, WA 98245

Enumclaw

The Electrode Store — 360-829-0400
Post Office Box 188, Enumclaw, WA 98022

Everett

Achilles Usa, Inc. — 425-353-7000
1407 80th St. S.W., Everett, WA 98203

Ameritek Usa, Inc. — 425-379-2580
125 130 St. Se,, Everett, WA 98208

Apothacare — 800-736-8456
PO Box 2226, Everett, WA 98213-0226

Apparel Med — 425-359-6510
4902 112th St. Se, Everett, WA 98208

Fluke Biomedical — 800-648-7952
6920 Seaway Blvd, Everett, WA 98203

Paragon Manufacturing Corp — 425-438-0800
2615 W. Casino Rd., Suite 4c, Everett, WA 98204

ReNu Medical Inc. — 877-252-1110
9800 Evergreen Way, Everett, WA 98204

Royal Dental Manufacturing, Inc. — 425-743-0988
12414 Highway 99, Everett, WA 98204

Wetmore Assoc., Inc. — 425-303-9520
2815 Wetmore Ave., Everett, WA 98201

Ferndale

Cascade Dafo, Inc. — 800-848-7332
1360 Sunset Avenue, Ferndale, WA 98248

Loops, L.L.C. — 360-366-3009
7152 Everett Rd., P. O. Box 2936, Ferndale, WA 98248

Gig Harbor

Generic Medical Device, Inc. — 253-853-3594
5727 Baker Way Nw, Suite 201, Gig Harbor, WA 98332

Sentron, Inc. — 253-851-7881
7117 Stinson Avenue, Suite C, Gig Harbor, WA 98335

The Pettibon System — 888-774-6258
3214 50th St CT, Suite 102C, Gig Harbor, WA 98335

Glacier

Shuttle Systems By Contemporary Design Co. — 800-334-5633
10005 Mt. Baker Hwy., Glacier, WA 98244-5089

Goldendale

West Coast Automation, Corp. — 509-773-5055
1600 S. Roosevelt, Goldendale, WA 98620

Interbay

Magic Wheels, Inc. — 206-282-0760
3837 13th Ave W., Suite 104, Interbay, WA 98119

Issaquah

Applied Precision Inc. — 425-557-1000
1040 12th Avenue Northwest, Issaquah, WA 98027

Siemens Medical Systems, Inc., Ultrasound Group — 800-964-4114
22010 S.E. 51st St., Issaquah, WA 98029

Spacelabs Healthcare — 800-522-7025
5150 220th Avenue SE, Issaquah, WA 98029

Spacelabs Medical Inc. — (800) 522-7025
5150 220th Ave Se, Issaquah, WA 98029

Kennewick

Cadwell Laboratories — 800-245-3001
909 N. Kellogg Street, Kennewick, WA 99336-7688

Tisport, Llc — 800-545-2266
1426 East Third Ave., Kennewick, WA 99337-9669

Kent

Abc Health Solutions Llc — 877-631-4551
14008 Se 238th Lane, Kent, WA 98042

Ammex Corp. — 800-274-7354
8220 South 212 St., Kent, WA 98032

Cenorin — 800-426-1042
6324 S. 199th Place, Suite 107, Kent, WA 98032

Choices Technologies — 425-765-9400
21730-176th Ave. South East, Kent, WA 98042-7210

Hot Cell Services — 800-562-2439
22626 85th Place South, Kent, WA 98031

Myotronics-Noromed, Inc. — 206-243-4214
5870 S 194th Street, Kent, WA 98032

Spio Inc. — 253-893-0390
25826 108th Ave. Se, Kent, WA 98030

Step Forward Co. — 253-631-0683
11109 Se Kent-kangley Road, Kent, WA 98030

Tri-D Corp.
19625 62nd Ave. S.,, Ste. B101, Kent, WA 98032

Kirkland

Cardiac Dimensions, Inc. — 425- 605-5900
5540 Lake Washington Blvd. NE, Kirkland, WA 98033

Erickson Labs Northwest — 425-823-1861
12911 120th Ave. Ne, Suite C10, Kirkland, WA 98034

Lucent Medical Systems, Inc. — 425-822-3310
811 Kirkland Avenue, Suite 100, Kirkland, WA 98033

Pathway Medical Technologies — (425) 636-4000
10801 120th Ave NE, Kirkland, WA 98033

Vee Gee Scientific, Inc. — 800-423-8842
13600 N.E. 126th, Suite A, Kirkland, WA 98034-8740

Lacey

Washington Trade International, Inc. — 800-327-3379
2633 Willamette Dr. NE, Lacey, WA 98516

Leland

Connexmd — 206-356-4568
800 W Park Avenue, Suite 3, Leland, WA 98368

Liberty Lake

Northern Technologies Inc. — 509-927-0401
23123 E. Mission Avenue, Liberty Lake, WA 99019

Lopez Island

Emerald Medical Products Corp. — 206-781-9450
1338 Shark Reef Road, Lopez Island, WA 98107

Lynnwood

Northwest Medical Physics Equipment, Inc. — 319-656-4447
21031 67th Ave. West, Lynnwood, WA 98036

Western Ophthalmics Corporation — 800-426-9938
19019 36th Ave W, Suite G, Lynnwood, WA 98036

Marysville

World Medical Equipment, Inc. — 800-827-3747
3915 152nd St. NE, Marysville, WA 98271

Maumelle

World Medical Supply Usa., Inc. — 1-800-827-3747
WORLD MEDICAL SUPPLY USA., INC., 3915 152nd St. NE, Maumelle, WA 98271

Mercer Island

Island Biosurgical, Llc — 425-251-3455
18 Meadow Lane, Mercer Island, WA 98040

Mount Vernon

Hallmark Refining Corp. Inc.   360-428-5880
1016 Dale Lane, Mount Vernon, WA 98273

Mountlake Ter

Orthocare Innovations, Llc   425-771-0797
6405 218th Ave. Sw, Suite 100, Mountlake Ter, WA 98043

Mountlake Terrace

Healthfirst Corp.   425-771-5733
22316 70th Ave. West, Unit A, Mountlake Terrace, WA 98043

Mukilteo

Body Tech 1 Nw   866-315-0640
10727 47th Pl. W, Mukilteo, WA 98275
Pro-Tech Services, Inc.   800-350-5511
4338 Harbour Pointe Blvd SW, Mukilteo, WA 98275
Westar Medical Products, Inc.   425-290-3945
4470 Chennault Beach Road, Ste 2, Mukilteo, WA 98275

Olympic View

Benik Corp.   800-442-8910
11871 Silverdale Way N.w., #107, Olympic View, WA 98383

Port Gamble

Em-Probe Inc.   360-297-6858
4110 Ne Carver Dr., Port Gamble, WA 98364

Port Ludlow

Pro Custom Labs   866-776-5227
190 Resolute Ln., Port Ludlow, WA 98365

POULSBO

Emt Medical Co., Inc.   800-473-5333
PO Box 294, POULSBO, WA 92691
J&J Engineering Inc.   888-550-8300
22797 Holgar Ct. N.E., Poulsbo, WA 98370
Jmm Distributing, Inc   360-308-9841
10332 Central Valley Rd., Poulsbo, WA 98370
Lenox Hill Brace / Seattle Systems   360-697-5656
26296 Twelve Trees Ln NW, Poulsbo, WA 98370
Seattle Systems   360-697-5656
26296 Twelve Trees Lane N.W., Bldg. 1, Poulsbo, WA 98370
Trulife, Inc.   360-697-5656
26296 Twelve Trees Ln., N.w., Poulsbo, WA 98370

Pullman

Interactive Performance Monitoring, Inc. (Ipm)   509-334-6363
1230 Ne Hickman Ct., Pullman, WA 99163

Puyallup

Stl International, Inc. / Teeter Hang Ups   253-840-5252
9902 162nd St. Ct. E, Puyallup, WA 98375
Wal-Med, Inc.   877-542-3688
11302 E. 164th St., Puyallup, WA 98374

Redmond

B.E. Meyers & Co., Inc.   800-327-5648
14540 N.E. 91st Street, Redmond, WA 98052-6553
Beatty Marketing & Sales, Llc   425-895-1656
17371 Ne 67th Ct., #a-12, Redmond, WA 98052
Bio-Rad Laboratories, Inc.   1-800-224-6723
6565 185th Ave., N.E., Redmond, WA 98052
Boston Scientific Corp.   612-582-7448
6645 185th Ave. N.E., Redmond, WA 98052
Cerevast Therapeutics Inc.   425-821-1939
12277 134th Court NE, Suite 202, Redmond, WA 98052
Endogastric Solutions, Inc.   425-307-9226
8210 154th Ave. Ne, Redmond, WA 98052
Fresenius Kabi, Llc   425-242-2000
14715 NE 95th St, Suite 100, Redmond, WA 98052
Fukuda Denshi Usa, Inc.   800-365-6668
17725 N.E. 65th St., Bldg. C, Redmond, WA 98052-4911
Levine Health Products   800-426-6763
21101 N.E. 108th St., Redmond, WA 98053-2116
Mettler Toledo Lasentec Products (Lasentec)   425-881-7117
14833 Ne 87th St, Redmond, WA 98052
Micronics, Inc.   425-895-9197
8463 154th Avenue NE, Building G, Redmond, WA 98052
Microsurgical Technology, Inc.   425-556-0544
8415 154th Ave NE, Redmond, WA 98052
Paris Miki, Inc.   425-883-2464
2863 152nd Ne, Redmond, WA 98052
Physio-Control, Inc.   800-442-1142
11811 Willows Road NE, Redmond, WA 98052
Qualitel Corporation   425-423-8388
4608 150th Avenue Ne, Redmond, WA 98052
Self Regulation Systems, Inc.   800-345-5642
8672 154th Avenue NE,, Bldg. F, Redmond, WA 98052-2554
Spiration Inc.   866-497-1700
6675 185th Ave. N.E., Redmond, WA 98052
Srs Medical Systems, Inc.   800-345-5642
8672 N.E. 154th Ave., Redmond, WA 98052

Tripath Imaging   800-636-7284
8271 154th Ave. N.E., Redmond, WA 98052-3878
Tripath Imaging, Inc.   919-206-7140
8271 154th Ave., N.e., Redmond, WA 98052
Ultreo   877-485-8736
9461 Willows Road N.e., Suite 101, Redmond, WA 98052
Vmed Technology, Inc. (Formerly Ems Products, Inc.)   425-497-9149
16149 Redmond Way #108, Redmond, WA 98052

Renton

Dti Dimartino Dental Lab   800.562.0300
345 Burnett Ave. North, Renton, WA 98055
Harrison & Cardillo Dental Lab   800-525-5913
725 Powell Street, Renton, WA 98057
Myco Instrumentation Source, Inc.   425-228-4239
PO Box 354, Renton, WA 98057

Richland

Advanced Imaging Technologies, Inc.   509-375-3100
2400 Stevens Drive Suite B, Richland, WA 99354
Isoray, Inc   877-447-6729
350 Hills Street Suite 106, Richland, WA 99354
Surgical Implant Generation Network (Sign)   509-371-1107
451 Hills St., Richland, WA 99354

Seattle

NanoString Technologies Inc   1-888-358-NANO
530 Fairview Avenue N, Suite 2000, Seattle, WA 98109
Amercare Products, Inc.   425-489-9575
17661 128th Place N.E., Seattle, WA 98165
Amgen Inc.   206-265-7000
1201 Amgen Court West, Seattle, WA 98119-3105
Amnis Corporation   800-730-7147
2505 Third Avenue, Suite 210, Seattle, WA 98121
Amp Orthopedics   206-812-9494
1520 4th Avenue, Suite 500, Seattle, WA 98101
Barcodes West, Llc   206-323-8100
1560 First Avenue, S., Seattle, WA 98134
Bellacure, Inc.   800-795-2070
6327 W. Marginal Wy Sw, Bldg.2, Seattle, WA 98106
Bio-Rad Laboratories Inc   425-881-8300
1000 Thomas St., Seattle, WA 98109
Biodynamics Corp.   206-526-0205
4554 9th Avenue Ne, #100, Seattle, WA 98105
Bodypoint, Inc.   800-547-5716
558 First Avenue So., Suite 300, Seattle, WA 98104
Calypso Medical Technologies Inc   206-254-0600
2101 Fourth Ave, Suite 500, Seattle, WA 98121
Cascade Designs, Inc.   206-505-9500
4000 1st Avenue South, Seattle, WA 98134
Certified Facilities Corp.   206-622-2508
208 Columbia St., Seattle, WA 98104-1508
Chirotron, Inc.   206-364-1262
20126 Ballinger Way Ne, #295, Seattle, WA 98155
Clario Medical Imaging, Inc.   866 941-6412
520 Pike Street, Suite 1005, Seattle, WA 98101
Custom Ocular Prosthetics   206-522-4222
10212 5th Avenue NE, Suite 210, Seattle, WA 98125-7471
Dendreon Corp.   866-477-6782
3005 First Avenue, Seattle, WA 98121
Healing Environments International, Inc.   800-233-7433
4623 NE 110th Street, Seattle, WA 98125
Impel NeuroPharma   206-695-5817
720 Broadway Ave, Suite 413, Seattle, WA 98122
Inbios Intl., Inc.   866-INBIOS1
562 1st. Avenue South, Suite 600, Seattle, WA 98104
Integriti Systems, Llc   206-652-4700
80 South Jackson, Suite 407, Seattle, WA 98104
Kamiya Biomedical Company   206-575-8068
12779 Gateway Drive, Seattle, WA 98168
Mastercraft Of Seattle   206-768-1297
300 South Bennett St., Seattle, WA 98108
Micro Current Technology, Inc.   206-778-5717
2244 1st. Ave. S., Seattle, WA 98134
Normed   800-288-8200
PO Box 3644, Seattle, WA 98124-3644
North American Scientific, Inc.   818-734-8600
8300 Aurora Ave North, Seattle, WA 98103
Numera   800-233-4323
1511 3rd Avenue, Suite 808, Seattle, WA 98101
Olympic Medical Corp.   206-767-3500
5900 First Avenue S., Seattle, WA 98108
Oncothyreon Inc.   206-801-2100
2601 Fourth Ave, Suite 500, Seattle, WA 98121
Pacific Biometrics, Inc.   206-298-0068
220 West Harrison Street, Seattle, WA 98119
Philips Medical Systems North America   800-934-7372
2301 Fifth Ave., Ste. 200, Seattle, WA 98121
Racer-Mate, Inc.   800-522-3610
3016 N.E. Blakeley St., Seattle, WA 98105-4012
Spencer Technologies   800-684-0586
701 16th Avenue, Seattle, WA 98122-4525
University Of Washington   206-616-5130
T-281 Health Science Bldg., Seattle, WA 98195

Uptake Medical Corp. — 206-859-4555
1924 1st Avenue, 3rd Floor, Seattle, WA 98101
Ventripoint Diagnostics Ltd. — 206-283-0221
100 West Harrison St., Suite 410, Seattle, WA 98119
Washington Biotechnology, Inc. — 206-292-9734
562 First AvenueS., 7th Floor, Seattle, WA 98104
Winders Dental Equipment — 206-772-1522
10624 Crestwood Dr. South, Seattle, WA 98178
Zymogenetics — 206-442-6600
1201 Eastlake Avenue E., Seattle, WA 98102

Sedro Woolley

Generations, Inc. — 360-840-6550
22895 Apple Ln, Sedro Woolley, WA 98284

Sequim

A-M Systems, Inc. — 800-426-1306
131 Business Park Loop, Sequim, WA 98382

Silverdale

Pro Trainers' Choice Company — 801-375-6600
Po Box 3953, 5803 Nw Newberry Hill Rd., Silverdale, WA 98383

Spokane

Aurum Ceramic Dental Laboratories Llp — 800-423-6509
1320 North Howard St., Spokane, WA 99201-2412
Hollister-Stier Laboratories, Llc — 800-992-1120
3525 North Regal St., Spokane, WA 99207-5788
Northwest Bedding Co. — 509-244-3000
6102 South Hayford Rd., Spokane, WA 99224
Portacare Llc — 509-928-0650
13023 Tall Tree Rd., Spokane, WA 99216
Stinson Manufacturing — 800-932-2885
N. 414 Sycamore, PO Box 3644, Spokane, WA 99202
Therapeutic Dimensions, Inc. — 509-323-9275
319 W Hastings Rd., Po Box 28307, Spokane, WA 99218
Wunder Tool & Die, Inc. — 509-922-6415
17625 E. Euclid Ave., Spokane, WA 99216

Spokane Valley

Body Well Design,Llc — 866-293-8444
6206 E. Trent Ave., Suite 1a, Spokane Valley, WA 99212
Paradigm Lasers, Inc. — 509-232-2040
3718 S. Union Ct., Spokane Valley, WA 99206
X-Ray Support Inc. — 509-242-1011
3020 N. Sullivan Rd., Suite D, Spokane Valley, WA 99216
X-Ray Support, Inc — 888-230-9500
3020 N. Sullivan Rd., Suite D, Spokane Valley, WA 99216

Sumas

Alliance H. Inc Dentech Equipment — 360-988-7080
901 W. Front Street, Sumas, WA 98295
Dentech Equipment — 800-826-5004
901 West Front Street, Sumas, WA 98295

Sumner

American Autoclave Co. — 800 421 5161
7819 Riverside Drive, Sumner, WA 98390-8104

Tacoma

Revalesio Corporation — 253-922-2600
5102 20th Street East, Building 100, Tacoma, WA 98424

University Place

Vector Research & Development — 877-883-7455
6824 19th St. #230, University Place, WA 98466

Vancouver

Alpha-Tec Systems, Inc. — 800-221-6058
12019 N.E. 99th St., #1780, Vancouver, WA 98682
Cheetah Medical — 866-751-9097
600 SE Maritime Ave Suite 220, Vancouver, WA 98661
Controltek, Inc. — 360-896-9375
3905 NE 112th Avenue, Vancouver, WA 98682
Endovascular Instruments, Inc. — 360-750-1150
2501 S.E. Columbia Way, Suite 150, Vancouver, WA 98661-8038
Nautilus, Inc. — 360-859-2900
16400 SE Nautilus Drive, Vancouver, WA 98683
O'Ryan Industries, Inc. — 800-426-4311
12711 N.E. 95th St., PO Box 1736, Vancouver, WA 98682-8978
Pedigo Products — 360-695-3500
4000 S.E. Columbia Way, Vancouver, WA 98661
Rs Medical — 800-683-0353
14001 S.E. First St., Vancouver, WA 98684

Vashon

Pacific Research Laboratories, Inc. — 206-463-5551
10221 S.W. 188th St., PO Box 409, Vashon, WA 98070-0409

Walla Walla

Balance Systems, Inc. — 1-888-274-5444
1644 Plaza Way, Suite 317, Walla Walla, WA 99362

Washougal

Bba Fiberweb Washougal, Inc. — 800-772-7771
3720 Grant St., Washougal, WA 98671-2807

Wenatchee

Audiology Products — 877-218-6358
c/o Pak It Rite, 126 North Wenatchee Avenue, Wenatchee, WA 98801

Woodinville

Aseptico, Inc. — 866-244-2954
8333 216th St. SE, Woodinville, WA 98072
Bio-Rad Laboratories, Inc. — 425-881-8300
14620 N.E. North Woodinville, Way, Suite 200, Woodinville, WA 98072
Khl, Inc. — 206-915-2115
18300 N.e. 146th Way, Woodinville, WA 98072
Pacific Coast Mfg., Inc. — 425-485-8866
15604 163nd Ave., Ne, Woodinville, WA 98072

Yakima

Surgimark, Inc. — 800-228-1186
2516 W Washington Avenue, Yakima, WA 98903

WEST VIRGINIA

Clarksburg

Medical Action Industries, Inc — 828-681-8820
10 Columbia Blvd, Clarksburg, WV 26301
Standard Dental Lab — 952-541-9622
431 Clark Street, Clarksburg, WV 26301

Fairmont

Philips Lighting Co. — 800-555-0050
505 Hoult Rd., Fairmont, WV 26554
Wv Iv Pro, Inc. — 304-366-6151
120 Mound Avenue, Fairmont, WV 26554-3309

Gassaway

Gtr Labs, Inc. — 888-871-9232
510 Elk St., Gassaway, WV 26624

Huntington

Alcon Manufacturing, Ltd. — 304-736-5230
6065 Kyle Lane, Huntington, WV 25702-9795
Darco International, Inc. — 800-999-8866
810 Memorial Blvd, Huntington, WV 25701

Newell

Marsh Bellofram — 800-727-5646
8019 Ohio River Blvd., Newell, WV 26050

Petersburg

Grant Memorial Hospital/Petersburg, Wv — 304-257-1026
Grant Memorial Drive, Petersburg, WV 26847

South Charleston

Tincher/Butler Dental Labs — 800-225-4699
525 First Avenue, South Charleston, WV 25303

St. Albans

Preiser Scientific, Inc. — 800-624-8285
94 Oliver St., P.O. Box 1330, St. Albans, WV 25177
Standard Instrumentation, Div. Preiser Scientific — 800-624-8285
94 Oliver St., St. Albans, WV 25177

Wellsburg

Eagle Manufacturing — 304-737-3171
2400 Charles St., Wellsburg, WV 26070

WISCONSIN

Appleton

R. Sabee Company — 920-882-7350
1718 W. 8th St., Appleton, WI 54914-4957

Barneveld

Quantum Devices, Inc. — 608-924-3000
112 Orbison Street, Barneveld, WI 53507

Beloit

Beloit Precision Incorporated — 800-865-1592
1525 Office Parkway, Beloit, WI 53511

Brookfield

Honeywell Hommed, Llc — 888-353-5440
3400 Intertech Dr., Suite 200, Brookfield, WI 53045
Rf Technologies — 800-669-9946
3125 N. 126th St., Brookfield, WI 53005
Sorba Medical Systems, Inc. — 800-SOR-BA13
165 Bishops Way, Suite 152, Brookfield, WI 53005
Thermo Uscs — 800-558-6377
120 Bishops Way, Suite 100, Box 0951, Brookfield, WI 53008-0951
Triad Disposables — 800-288-1288
19355 Janacek Court, Brookfield, WI 53045

Brown Deer

Bio-Research Associates, Inc.   414-357-7525
9275 North 49th Street, Suite 150, Brown Deer, WI 53223
Life Technologies Corporation   414-214-4048
9099 North Deerbrook Trail, Brown Deer, WI 53223

Burlington

Starsurgical, Inc.   888-609-2470
7781 Lakeview Dr., Burlington, WI 53105-8119
Visicomm Industries   866-221-3131
911A Milwaukee Ave., Burlington, WI 53105

Cedarburg

Patterson Medical Supply, Inc.   262-387-8720
W68 N158 Evergreen Blvd., Cedarburg, WI 53012

Cross Plains

Intellectual Property, Llc   608-798-0904
8030 Stagecoach Road, Cross Plains, WI 53528

Deerfield

Cardiac Science Corp.   800-777-1777
500 Burdick Pkwy., Deerfield, WI 53531-9692

Delafield

Mobilife, Llc   262-646-5433
78 Enterprise Road, Unit D, Delafield, WI 53018

Eau Claire

Ait Dental, Inc.   800-762-1765
1226 International Drive, Eau Claire, WI 54701
Midwest Eye Laboratories, Inc.   800-543-7936
4606 Commerce Valley Rd, Suite 201, Eau Claire, WI 54701
Presto Absorbent Products, Inc.   715-839-2085
3925 N. Hastings Way, Eau Claire, WI 54703

Edgerton

Iki Mfg. Co, Inc.   608-884-3411
116 N. Swift St., Edgerton, WI 53534

Elkhart Lake

Smi   920-876-3361
Industrial Park, 544 Sohn Drive, Elkhart Lake, WI 53020

Elkhorn

Coopercare Lastrap Inc   416-741-9675
Highway H, Koopman Ln., Elkhorn, WI 53121
Preservation Solutions, Inc.   262-723-6715
980 Proctor Dr., Elkhorn, WI 53121

Ellsworth

Federal Foam Technologies, Inc.   800-457-3626
312 Industrial Rd., Ellsworth, WI 54011-5065

Elmwood

Genesis Dental Technologies, Llc   715-778-5816
200 Main Street, Elmwood, WI 54740
Genesis Industries/Maternal Concepts   800-310-5817
130 S Public St, Elmwood, WI 54740
Genesis Instruments, Inc.   (800) 826-3301
601 Pro-Ject Drive, Elmwood, WI 54740

Fitchburg

Metalcraft Industries, Inc.   608-835-3232
399 North Burr Oak Ave, Fitchburg, WI 53575
Philips Medical Systems (Cleveland), Inc.   978-659-4663
5520 Nobel Drive, Fitchburg, WI 53711
Stealth Therapeutics Inc   608-577-4484
5520 Nobel Dr Suite 150, Fitchburg, WI 53711

Fond du Lac

Basic American Metal Products   800-365-2338
336 Trowbridge Drive, PO Box 907, Fond du Lac, WI 54937

Fort Atkinson

Nasco   800-558-9595
901 Janesville Avenue, PO Box 901, Fort Atkinson, WI 53538-0901
Spacesaver Corporation   800-492-3434
1450 Janesville Avenue, Fort Atkinson, WI 53538-2798

Franklin

Becton Dickinson Medical Systems   201-847-6800
9630 South 54th St., Franklin, WI 53132
Dash Medical Gloves, Inc.   800-523-2055
10180 S. 54th St., Franklin, WI 53132

Franksville

Bioform Medical, Inc.   262-835-3323
4133 Courtney Road, #10, Franksville, WI 53126

Germantown

Alc, Inc.   262-502-4665
N114 W19049 Clinton Drive, Germantown, WI 53022
Conflex   800-225-4296
W130 N10751 Washington Drive, Germantown, WI 53022

Faustel   262-253-3333
W194 N11301 McCormick Drive, Germantown, WI 53022
Ob Scientific, Inc.   888-530-4561
N 112 W18741, Mequon Rd., P.O. Box 787, Germantown, WI 53022
Ortho-Kinetics, Inc.   800-824-1068
W194 N11301 McCormick Drive, Germantown, WI 53022
Radiant Electric Heat Inc.   262-502-1282
Radiant Electric HeatÉ_Z N112W14600 Mequ, Germantown, WI 53022
S&G Enterprises, Inc.   800-233-3721
N115 W19000 Edison Drive, Germantown, WI 53022-3024
Sunlite Plastics, Inc.   262-253-0600
W194 N11340 McCormick Dr., Germantown, WI 53022
Tecstar Mfg. Company   262-255-5790
W190 N11701 Moldmakers Way, Germantown, WI 53022

Grafton

Axcesor, Inc.   1-888-717-1471
2260 Dakota Drive, Grafton, WI 53024
Gauthier Biomedical, Inc.   866-546-0010
1235 North Dakota Drive, Suite G, Grafton, WI 53024
Hygo Plastic, Inc.   414-375-4011
1376 Cheyenne Ave., Grafton, WI 53024
Young Microbrush Llc   262-375-4011
1376 Cheyenne Ave., Grafton, WI 53024

Green Bay

Graham Medical Products/Div. Of Little Rapids Corp   866-429-1408
2273 Larsen Road, Green Bay, WI 54303
Imperial Supplies Llc   800-558-2808
789 Armed Forces Dr., PO Box 11008, Green Bay, WI 54307-1008
Ki   800-424-2432
1330 Bellevue St., Green Bay, WI 54302

Greendale

Arndorfer Medical Specialties   414-425-1661
5656 Grove Terrace, Greendale, WI 53129

Greenfield

Medical Art Resources, Inc.   877-203-7829
3400 S. 103rd St., Suite 200, Greenfield, WI 53227

Hartland

Fotodyne, Inc.   800-362-3686
950 Walnut Ridge Dr., Hartland, WI 53029
Midwest Rf, Llc   262-367-8254
535 Norton Drive, PO Box 350, Hartland, WI 53029
Oxia U.S. Ltd.   262-369-1978
665 Industrial Avenue, Unit B, Hartland, WI 53029

Hayward

Goldentone Hearing Aids   800-826-6789
10597 Kansas Ave., Hayward, WI 54843-0751

Holmen

Aquila Corporation   866-782-9658
3827 Creekside Lane, Holmen, WI 54636

Hudson

Biomedical Models Llc   800-635-4801
327 S. 7th Street, Hudson, WI 54016
Nor-Lake Inc., Nor-Lake Scientific   800-955-5253
891 County Road U, Hudson, WI 54016
Phillips Plastics Corp.   877-508-0252
1201 Hanley Road, Hudson, WI 54016

Jackson

Wisconsin Pharmacal Co. Llc   800-558-6614 Ex
1 Pharmacal Way,, Jackson, WI 53037

Janesville

Lab Safety Supply, Inc.   800-356-0783
401 S. Wright Rd., Janesville, WI 53546-1368
Rock Valley Textiles   608-752-6866
111 Avon St., Janesville, WI 53545
Televere Systems   800-385-9593
1611 Center Avenue, Janesville, WI 53545

Kenosha

Beere Precision Medical Instruments, Kmedic, Telef   919-544-8000
5307 95th Ave., Kenosha, WI 53144

Kiel

Stoelting   800-558-5807
502 Hwy. 67, Kiel, WI 53042

Kohler

Kohler Co.   800-456-4537
444 Highland Dr., Kohler, WI 53044

La Crosse

Netwal Dental Laboratory   800-991-8111
115 5th Ave. South, Suite 307, La Crosse, WI 54602

Lac du Flambeau

Simpson Electric Co.   715-588-3311
520 Simpson Avenue, PO Box 99, Lac du Flambeau, WI 54538-0099

Madison

Amcor Flexibles, Inc.   608-249-0404
4101 Lien Rd., Madison, WI 53704
Cardinal Healthcare 209, Inc.   610-862-0800
5225 Verona Rd., Madison, WI 53711-4495
Cellular Dynamics International   877-310-6688
525 Science Drive, Madison, WI 53711
Covance Laboratories ,Inc   800-742-8378
3301 Kinsman Blvd., Madison, WI 53704
Datex-Ohmeda Inc.   608-221-1551
3030 Ohmeda Drive, Madison, WI 53718
Datex-Ohmeda, Inc. (Madison)   800-345-2700
3030 Ohmeda Dr., Madison, WI 53707-7550
Epicentre Technologies   800-284-8474
726 Post Rd., Madison, WI 53713
Eragen Biosciences Inc.   608-662-9000
918 Deming Way, Suite 201, Madison, WI 53717
Exact Sciences, Inc.   866-333-9228
441 Charmany Drive, Madison, WI 53719
Eye Prosthetics Of Wisconsin, Inc.   262-363-1528
4781 Hayes Rd., Madison, WI 53704
Ge Medical Systems Ultrasound And Primary Care Dia   608-826-7050
3030 ohmeda dr, Madison, WI 53718
Jurgan Development & Mfg.   800-587-4262
6018 S. Highlands Avenue, Madison, WI 53705
Jurgan Development & Mfg., Ltd.   608-231-1742
6018 South Highlands Ave., Madison, WI 53705
La Mont Medical, Inc.   888-452-6688
555 D'Onofrio Drive, Madison, WI 53719-2053
Lifeline Usa   800-553-6633
3201 Syene Road, Madison, WI 53713
Placon Corporation   800-541-1535
6096 McKee Road, Madison, WI 53719-5114
Planet Llc   800-338-2010
1212 Fourier Drive, Madison, WI 53717
Promega Corp.   800-356-9526
2800 Woods Hollow Rd., Madison, WI 53711
Rayovac   800-331-4522
601 Rayovac Drive, Madison, WI 53744-4960
Spectrum-Brands   800-237-6541
601 Rayovac Drive, Madison, WI 53711-2497
Third Wave Technologies, Inc.   888-898-2357
502 South Rosa Rd., Madison, WI 53719-1256
Tomotherapy Incorporated   608-824-2800
1209 Deming Way, Madison, WI 53717
Ultratec, Inc.   800-482-2424
450 Science Drive, Madison, WI 53711

Manitowoc

Invincible Office Furniture Co.   800-558-4417
PO Box 1117, Manitowoc, WI 54221
Wisconsin Aluminum Foundry Co., Inc.   920-682-8627
838 S. 16th St., Manitowoc, WI 54220

Marshall

Davis Instrument Company, Inc.   (800) 522-7442
5850 Cherry Lane, Marshall, WI 53559-0100

Menomonee Falls

Brewer Company, The   888-873-9371
N88 W13901 Main St., Menomonee Falls, WI 53051
Enthermics Medical Systems, Inc.   800-862-9276
W164 N9221 Water St., Menomonee Falls, WI 53051-1401
Huot Instruments, Llc   262-373-1700
N50 W13740 Overview Dr., Suite A, Menomonee Falls, WI 53051
International Plastics, Llc   800-665-3464
4965 N. Campbell Dr., Menomonee Falls, WI 53051
Myo/Kinetic Systems, Inc.   414-255-1005
North 84 West 13562 Leon Rd., Menomonee Falls, WI 53051
Storage Battery Systems, Inc.   800-554-2243
N. 56 W. 16665 Ridgewood Drive, Menomonee Falls, WI 53051
Tailored Label Products, Inc.   800-727-1344
W165 N5731 Ridgewood Drive, Menomonee Falls, WI 53051-5658

Menomonie

Phillips Plastics Corporation, Phillips Medical   715-232-4608
415 Red Cedar St., Menomonie, WI 54751

Mequon

Titan Spine Llc.   1-866-822-7800
6140 W. Executive Drive, Suite A, Mequon, WI 53092

Mercer

Medi-Part,Inc.   715-476-7600
5844 North Rice Lake Rd., P.o. Box 276, Mercer, WI 54547

Merton

Essential Industries Inc.   800-551-9679
28391 Essential Road, P.O. Box 12, Merton, WI 53056-0012

Middleton

Gammex Rmi   800-426-6391
7600 Discovery Drive, Middleton, WI 53562-0327
Kerr Corp.   949-255-8766
3225 Deming Way, Suite 190, Middleton, WI 53562
Sds-Surgical Acuity   888-822-8489
3225 Deming Way, Suite 120, Middleton, WI 53562
Standard Imaging, Inc.   608-831-0025
3120 Deming Way, Middleton, WI 53562

Milwaukee

Access Battery Inc.   800-654-9845
Division of Alpha Source, Inc., 12104 W. Carmen Avenue, Milwaukee, WI 53225-2135
Adjustable Fixture Co.   800-558-2628
3726 N. Booth St., Milwaukee, WI 53212-1698
Anguil Environmental Systems, Inc.   800-488-0230
8855 N. 55th St., Milwaukee, WI 53223
Associated Bag Company   800-926-6100
400 W. Boden St., Milwaukee, WI 53207
Brady Corporation   800-541-1686
6555 West Good Hope Road, PO Box 571, Milwaukee, WI 53223
C & D Technologies Inc., Dynasty Div.   414-967-6500
900 East Keefe Ave., Milwaukee, WI 53212
Clarke Manufacturing, Inc.   414-444-7003
3000 W. Clarke St., Milwaukee, WI 53210
Feiter's Inc   414-355-7575
8700 West Port Ave., Milwaukee, WI 53224
Ge Medical Systems Information Technologies   800-643-6439
8200 West Tower Avenue, Milwaukee, WI 53223
Hospital Comm. & Electronics, Inc.   800-558-8957
7915 North 81st Street,, Milwaukee, WI 53223
Instrumentarium Imaging, Inc.   800-558-6120
1245 W. Canal St., Milwaukee, WI 53233
Life Corporation   800-700-0202
1776 North Water Street, Milwaukee, WI 53202-1552
MPE-INC   800-266-1687
10597 W. Glenbrook Court, Milwaukee, WI 53224
Medical Products Of Milwaukee, Llc.   414-281-8713
2500 W. Layton Avenue, Suite 250, Milwaukee, WI 53221
Medovations, Inc.   800-558-6408
102 E. Keefe Avenue, Milwaukee, WI 53212
Merisco, Inc.   414-365-3522
5400 W. Brown Deer Rd., Milwaukee, WI 53223
Midwest Products & Engineering, Inc.   800-266-1687
10597 W. Glenbrook Court, Milwaukee, WI 53224
Milwaukee Mattress & Furniture   800-373-1462
423 N. 3rd St., Milwaukee, WI 53203-3001
Mortara Instrument, Inc.   800-231-7437
7865 N. 86th St., Milwaukee, WI 53224-3431
Neurognostics, Inc.   414-727-7950
10437 Innovation Dr., Suite 309, Milwaukee, WI 53226
Prism Clinical Imaging, Inc.   414-727-1930
851 S 70th St., Suite 103, Milwaukee, WI 53214
Quintron Instrument Company   800-542-4448
3712 W. Pierce St., Milwaukee, WI 53215-1032
Teramedica, Inc.   414-908-7713
10400 Innovation, Suite 200, Milwaukee, WI 53226
U-Line Corporation   800-779-2547
8900 N. 55th St., PO Box 245040, Milwaukee, WI 53224-9540
Zens Manufacturing, Inc..   414-372-7060
2435 N. Martin Luther King Drive, PO Drawer 12504, Milwaukee, WI 53212

Monroe

Greenco Industries, Inc.   608-328-8311
1601 4th Ave. West, Monroe, WI 53566

Muskego

Inpro Corporation   800-222-5556
S80 W18766 Apollo Drive, Muskego, WI 53150

Neenah

Gerber Products Co.   800-430-0150
120 N.commercial,4th floor, Neenah, WI 54956
Kimberly-Clark Corp.   888-525-8388
2100 Winchester Rd., PO Box 2020, Neenah, WI 54957-2020
Kimberly-Clark Corp., Lakeview Feminine Care Plant   888-525-8388
1050 Cold Spring Rd., Neenah, WI 54956
Plexus Corp.   877-733-5919
55 Jewelers Park Drive, PO Box 156, Neenah, WI 54956
Tidi Products, Llc   800-521-1314
570 Enterprise Dr., Neenah, WI 54956-4865
Tidi Products, Llc   920-751-4380
570 Enterprise Dr., Neenah, WI 54956

Nekoosa

Pacific Intl. Co.   715-886-4550
555 Birch St., Nekoosa, WI 54457

New Berlin

Crs Medical Diagnostics Inc.   262-432-5900
PO Box 510137, New Berlin, WI 53151
Don Tay Industries   262-789-9102
2383 South 162nd St., New Berlin, WI 53151

Escalon Trek Medical — 800-433-8197
2440 S. 179th St., New Berlin, WI 53146

New Richmond

Phillips Plastics Corporation, Phillips Medical New Richmond — 877.508.0252
705 Wisconsin Dr., New Richmond, WI 54017

North Fond Du Lac

Gf Health Products, Inc. — 800-365-2338
336 Trowbridge Rd., North Fond Du Lac, WI 54937

Oak Creek

Apw Eder Industries, Inc. — 414-761-0400
2250 W. South Branch Blvd., Oak Creek, WI 53154-4907

Oconomowoc

Bruno Independent Living Aids, Inc. — 800-882-8183
1780 Executive Drive, Oconomowoc, WI 53066-3932
Lewis Bins+ — 877-97L-EWIS
PO BOX 389, Oconomowoc, WI 53066
Orbis Corporation — 800-890-7292
1055 Corporate Center Drive, PO Box 389, Oconomowoc, WI 53066
Plastocon, Inc. — 800-966-0103
1200 W. Second St., Oconomowoc, WI 53066-3403

Osceola

Core Products International, Inc. — 800-365-3047
808 Prospect Avenue, Osceola, WI 54020
Mpp Hand Drill Company Llc. — 715-294-3400
807 Prospect Ave., Osceola, WI 54020

Oshkosh

Buckstaff Co. — 800-755-5890
1127 S. Main St., Oshkosh, WI 54902
Lamico, Inc. — 920-231-1672
474 Marion Rd., Oshkosh, WI 54901
Perfecseal — 877-828-7501
PO Box 2968, 3500 North Main St., Oshkosh, WI 54903-2968
Winn-Sol Products — 414-231-2031
1853 Delaware St., Oshkosh, WI 54901

Pewaukee

Imco Technologies — 800-300-7734
N27 W23957 Paul Road,Suite 101, Pewaukee, WI 53072
Invivo Corporation — 262-524-1402
N27 W23676 Paul Road, Pewaukee, WI 53072
Neocoil, Llc — 262-347-1250
N27 W23910a Paul Rd., Pewaukee, WI 53072
Nu-Back — 262-695-1660
140 Sussex St., Pewaukee, WI 53072

Pleasant Prairie

Erie Medical — 800-932-2293
10225 82nd Avenue, Pleasant Prairie, WI 53158
Mg Scientific, Inc. — 800-343-8338
8500 107th St., Pleasant Prairie, WI 53158

Port Washington

Frontier Medical Products, Inc. — 800-367-6828
140 S. Park St., Port Washington, WI 53074

Portage

Inntec, Inc. — 608-742-1188
401 E. Edgewater St., Portage, WI 53901

Prairie Du Sac

Mueller Sports Medicine — 800-356-9522
One Quench Dr., P.O. Box 99, Prairie Du Sac, WI 53578

Racine

Ad-Tech Medical Instrument Corp. — 800-776-1555
1901 William St, Racine, WI 53404
Foster Manufacturing Corp. — 262-633-7073
1652 Phillips Avenue, Racine, WI 53403
Inter-Med, Inc. — 877-418-4782
2200 Northwestern Ave., Racine, WI 53404

Rice Lake

Rice Lake Weighing Systems — 800-472-6703
230 W. Coleman St., Rice Lake, WI 54868-9902

Ripon

Cissell Manufacturing Company — 888-223-2980
PO Box 990, Shepard Street, Ripon, WI 54971
Huebsch Sales — 800-553-5120
PO Box 990, Shepard Street, Ripon, WI 54971-0990
Ipso Usa, Inc. — 800-872-4776
PO Box 990, Shepard Street, Ripon, WI 54971
Unimac — 800-587-5458
PO Box 990 Shepard Street, Ripon, WI 54971

River Falls

Sajan, Inc. — 877-426-9505
625 Whitetail Blvd, River Falls, WI 54022

Saukville

Befour, Inc. — 800-367-7109
102 Progress Drive, Saukville, WI 53080

Sheboygan

American Orthodontics Corp. — 800-558-7687
1714 Cambridge Avenue, Sheboygan, WI 53081
Coeur Inc., Sheboygan — 800-874-4240
3411 Behrens Pkwy., Sheboygan, WI 53081
Gardner Denver Thomas Inc. — 920-457-4891
1419 Illinois Ave, Sheboygan, WI 53082
Newschoff Chairs, Inc. — 800-203-8916
909 North 8 St., Sheboygan, WI 53081
Polar Ware Co. — 800-237-3655
2806 N. 15th St., Sheboygan, WI 53083
Thomas Products Division — 920-457-4891
3524 Washington Avenue, Sheboygan, WI 53082

Sheboygan Falls

Bemis Mfg. Co. — 800-558-7651
300 Mill St., Sheboygan Falls, WI 53085-0901
Bemis Mfg. Co. — 920-467-4621
300 Mill Street, P.O. Box 901, Sheboygan Falls, WI 53085

Somerset

Apollo Corporation — 800-247-5490
PO Box 219, Somerset, WI 54025
SMC Ltd. — 715-247-3500
360 Reed Street, Somerset, WI 54025

St. Croix Falls

Nobles Manufacturing, Inc. — 715-483-3079
1105 East Pine St., St. Croix Falls, WI 54024

Stevens Point

Joerns Healthcare, Inc — 800-826-0270
5001 Joerns Dr., Stevens Point, WI 54481

Sturtevant

Allesee Orthodontic Appliances — 714-516-7484
13931 Spring St., Sturtevant, WI 53177
Aoa — 800-262-5221
13931 Spring St., P.O. Box 725, Sturtevant, WI 53177
Johnsondiversey, Inc. — 262-631-4001
8310 16th St, P.O. Box 902, Sturtevant, WI 53177-0902
Johnsondiversey, Inc. — 262-631-4101
8311 16th Street, Bldg. 65c, Sturtevant, WI 53177

Sun Prairie

Trek Diagnostic Systems, Inc. — 608-8373788
210 Business Park Dr., Sun Prairie, WI 53590

Sussex

Lechnologies Research, Inc.. — 866-321-2342
N64 W24801 Main Street, Suite 107, Sussex, WI 53089
Treymed, Inc. — 262-820-1294
N56 W 24790 N. Corporate Cir., #c, Sussex, WI 53089
Valeo, Inc. — 800-634-2704
W248 N5499 Executive Dr., Sussex, WI 53089

Two Rivers

Thermo Scientific Hamilton — 920-794-6800
1316 18th St., Two Rivers, WI 54241

Verona

Epic Systems Corp. — 608-271-9000
1979 Milky Way, Verona, WI 53593
Minitube Of America, Inc — 608-845-1502
P.O. Box 930187, 419 Venture Court, Verona, WI 53593
Penetrating Innovations, Inc. — 608-845-3270
415 Venture Court, Verona, WI 53593

Waterford

Continental Medical Laboratories, Inc. — 262-534-2787
813 Ela Avenue, Waterford, WI 53185

Watertown

Karma Inc. — 800-558-9565
500 Milford St., Box 433, Watertown, WI 53094

Waukesha

Bevco Ergonomic Seating — 800-864-2991
2246A Bluemound Road, Waukesha, WI 53186
Criticare Systems, Inc. — 262-798-8282
N7W22025 Johnson Drive, Waukesha, WI 53186
Dai Shin Technologies, Inc. — 262-347-0500
W238 N1690 N Rockwood Dr, Suite 400, Waukesha, WI 53188
Ge Medical Systems, Llc — 262-548-2355
3000 N Grandview Blvd., W-417, Waukesha, WI 53188

Ge Medical Systems, Llc — 262-312-7117
3200 N. Grandview Blvd., Waukesha, WI 53188
Genetic Testing Institute — 800-233-1843
20925 Crossroads Circle, Suite 200, Waukesha, WI 53186
MedPro Imaging — 877-846-8818
821 Corporate Court, Suite 101, Waukesha, WI 53189
Medpro Imgaing Inc. — 877-846-8818
821 Corporate Court, Suite 101, Waukesha, WI 53189
Platinum Surgical Instruments, Inc. — 262-798-8540
2325 Parklawn Dr., Suite F, Waukesha, WI 53186
Prodesse, Inc. — 888-589-6974
n15w22180 watertown road #8, Waukesha, WI 53186
Shoney Scientific, Inc. — 262-970-0170
West 223 North 720 Saratoga Drive,, Suite 120, Waukesha, WI 53186
Smiths Medical Pm, Inc. — 800-558-2345
N7 W22025 Johnson Drive, Waukesha, WI 53186
Woodway Usa, Inc. — 262-548-6235
West 229 North 591 Foster Ct., Waukesha, WI 53186

Waunakee

Humane Restraint Co Inc — 800-356-7472
912 Bethel Circle, Waunakee, WI 53597

Waupaca

Innovative Medical Solutions, Inc. — 414-774-7614
N2462 W. Miner Dr., Waupaca, WI 54981

Wausau

Piper Products, Inc. — 800-492-3431
300 South 84th Ave., Wausau, WI 54401

Wauwatosa

Ge Medical Systems Information Technologies — 888-202-5528
9900 Innovation Dr., Wauwatosa, WI 53226

West Allis

Solaris, Inc. — 414-918-9180
6737 West Washington St., Suite 3260, West Allis, WI 53214
Vess Chairs, Inc. — 414-476-2488
9036 W. Schlinger, West Allis, WI 53214

West Bend

Aero Medical Products Co., Inc. — 262-335-8000
2230 Stone Bridge Road, West Bend, WI 53095
Spaulding Clinical Research — 262-334-6020
525 S Silverbrook Dr, West Bend, WI 53095

West Milwaukee

Ge Medical Systems, Llc — 847-277-5002
4855 West Electric Ave., West Milwaukee, WI 53219
Lakeside Manufacturing Co., Inc. — 800-558-8565
4900 W. Electric Avenue, West Milwaukee, WI 53219

WYOMING

Burlington

Compumed, Inc. — 800-722-4417
P.O. Box 126, 574 Lane 40, Burlington, WY 82433

Casper

Eurotech Dental Laboratory, Inc. — 307-234-6808
301 N. Mckinley St., Casper, WY 82601

Cheyenne

Vestibular Technologies, Llc — 307-637-5711
205 County Road 128a, Suite 200, Cheyenne, WY 82007-1831

Laramie

C.F. Electronics, Inc. — 307-742-5200
2052 North Third Street, Laramie, WY 82072

CANADA

A.M.G. Medical, Inc. — 888-396-1213
8505 Dalton Rd., Montreal, QUE H4T-IV5
AbelNet Inc — 800-463-5685
91 Station St., Unit 1, Ajax, ONT L1S 3H2
Able Walker, Ltd. — 604-576-8488
16-2350 Beta Ave, Burnaby V5C 5M8
Absorb-Plus Textiles Inc. — 514-345-9770
1075 rue Hickson, Verdun, QC H4G 2L3
Acart Equipment Ltd. — 800-551-0560
1020 Brevik Place, Unit 3, Mississauga, ONT L4W-4N7
Accro Furniture Industries — 204-654-1114
305 McKay Ave, Winnipeg, MB R2G 0N5
Acerna Inc. — 905-472-5747
19 Bryant Road, Markham, ONT L3P-5Y7
Acp Chemicals Inc. — 800-363-9861
4601 blvd. Des Grandes Prairies, St-Leonard, QUE H1R-1A5
Activa Brand Products Inc. — 800-991-4464
105 Industrial Cres, Summerside, PEI C1N-5P8
Acumed Medical Supplies Ltd. — 800-567-7246
44 Royal York Road, Toronto, ONT M8V-2T4

Adaptive Engineering Ltd. — 800-448-4652
419 34th Ave. SE, Calgary, ALB T2G-1V1
Advanced Health Care Products Inc. — 800-265-9830
205 St. George St. N, Unit 6, Lindsay, ONT K9V-5Z9
Advanced Medical Devices, Inc. — 416-833-6681
15 Keele Street South Unit 2, Po Box 520, King City L7B 1A7
Advanced Mobility Products Ltd. — 800-665-4442
Suite 101-8620 Glenlyon Pky,, BURNABY, BC V5J 0B6
Advanced Mobility Systems Corp. — 800-661-6716
621 Justus Dr., Kingston, ONT K7M-4H5
Advanced Research Technologies Inc. (Art) — 888-278-7888
2300 Alfred Nobel, Technoparc MontrAcal, Montreal, QUE H4S-2A4
Advanced Surgi-Pharm Inc. — 800-661-5432
850 Halpern Ave., Dorval, QUE H9P-1G1
Aearo Canada Ltd. — 617-371-4200
7115 Tomken Rd, Mississauga L5S 1R7
Affinity Biologicals, Inc. — 800-903-6020
1395 Sandhill Dr., Ancaster, ONT L9G-4V5
Agfa Medical Imaging — 877-753-2432
77 Belfield Road, Toronto, ONT M9W-1G6
Agilent Technologies Canada Inc. — 1 877 424-4536
6705 Millcreek Drive, Unit 5, Mississauga, ONT L5N 5M4
Aim Instrumentation Ltd. — 1-800-444-9386
5232 Irmin Street, Burnaby, BC V5J-1Y7
Aim Instrumentation Ontario Inc. — 1-800-871-9967
3170 Ridgeway Drive, Unit 9, Mississauga, ONT LRL-5R4
Aim Safe Air Products Ltd. — 604-244-7272
170-13151 Vanier Pl, Richmond V6V 2J1
Aimtronics Corp. — 604-946-9666
100 Schneider Rd, Kanata K2K 1Y2
Airgas Canada Inc. — 800-661-1221
Bay 133, 3016 10th Ave., N.E., Calgary, AB AB T2A6A3
Airway Surgical Appliances Ltd. — 800-267-3476
189 Colonnaide Rd., Nepean, ONT K2E-7J4
Aladdin Temp-Rite Canada Inc. — 1-800-387-3994
740 Gana Court, Mississauga, ONT L5S-1P1
Alcohol Countermeasure Systems Corp. — 416-619-3500
60 International Boulevard, Toronto, ONTAR M9W 6J2
Alcon Canada, Inc. — 800-268-4574
2665 Meadowpine Blvd., Mississauga, ONT L5N-8C7
Alfa Import And Export — 905-457-9941
13 Halldorson Trail, Brampton L6W 4M4
Alldente Intl., Inc. — 416-944-0086
600-94 Cumberland St, Toronto M5R 1A3
Allergan Inc. — 800-668-6424
85 Enterprise Boulevard, 85 Enterprise Boulevard, Markham, ONT L6G 0B5
Allfoam Industries Ltd. — 604-277-7710
12391 #5 Road, Richmond, BC V7A-4E9
Alliance Medical Inc. — 888-639-1264
7800 Cote de Liesse, St-Laurent, QUE H4T-1G1
Almedic Ltd. — 514-337-4942
4900 Boulevard Cote Vertu, St-Laurent, QUE H4S-1J9
Alpha Pro Tech, Inc. — 800-749-1363
60 Centurian Drive, Suite 112, Markham, ONT L3R 9R2
Alphachem Limited — 1-888-338-2995
2485 Milltower Court, Mississauga, ONT L5N 5Z6
Ambulatory Footwear Inc. — 800-461-8588
6 Osler Court, Dundas, ONT L9H-2P9
Ambutech Inc. — 800-561-3340
34 DeBaets St., Winnipeg R2J-3S9
Amcare Surgical — 416-781-4494
1584 Bathurst St., Toronto, ONT M5P-3H3
Amg Medical Inc. — 800-361-2210
8505 Dalton Rd., Montreal, QUE H4T-1V5
Amico Corporation — 887-323-3209
85 Fulton Way, Richmond Hill, ONT L4B 2N4
Amorfix Life Sciences Ltd. — 416-847-6898
3403 American Drive, Mississauga, ONTAR L4V 1T4
Amvex Corporation — 866-462-6839
25b east pearce street, Suite 21, Richmond Hill, ONTAR L4B2M9
Amylior Inc. — 888-453-0311
6 Antoine-Henault, Notre-Dame Ile-Perrot, QUE J7V-7M3
Amysystems — 1-450-424-0288
1650, chicoine, Dorion, QC J7V 8P2
Anachemia Canada Inc. — 800-361-0209
255 Norman St., Lachine, QUE H8R-1A3
Anatech Anatomical Technologies Inc. — 800-667-3442
205-5920 No. 6 Road, Richmond, BC V6V-1Z1
Andromed Inc. — 888-877-8477
5003 Levy St, St-Laurent, QUE H4R 2N9
Angiotech Pharmaceuticals, Inc. — 604-221-7676
1618 Station Street, Vancouver, BC V6A 1B6
Ansell Perry Inc. — 800-363-8340
105 rue Lauder, Cowansville, QUE J2K-2K8
Apollo Medical Ltd./Medichair — 877-693-3330
381 Somerset St., Saint John, NB E2K-2Y5
Applied Ai Systems Inc. — 800-895-1122
112 John Cavanaugh Drive, Carp, ONT K0A 1L0
Arjo Canada, Inc. — 800-665-4831
1575 South Gateway Rd., Unit C, Mississauga, ONT L4W-5J1
Ark Bio-Medical Canada Corp. — 800-661-004
Dartrey Estate De L'ile, #671 Rustico Rd. Route 7, Miltonvale Park, WINSL CIE 124

Arkon Safety Equipment, Inc. — 514-351-8240
10550 Boul Parkway, Anjou H1J 2K4

Armar International Inc. — 514-636-6737
850 Lakeshore Drive, Ste. N4, Dorval, QUE H9S-5T9

Arrow Medical Products, Ltd. — 800-387-7819
2300 Bristol Circle Unit 1, Oakville, ONT L6H-5S3

Aspen Home Healthcare Products Ltd. — 800-272-8851
11044 82nd Ave., Suite 120, Edmonton, ALB T6G-0T2

Assistive Listening Device Systems — 800-665-2537
11220 Voyager Way, Unit 2, Richmond, BC V6X-3E1

Associated Health Systems Inc. — 1.877.451.6720
#12 3691 Viking Way, Richmond, BC V6V-2J6

Atlas Laboratories Co. Ltd. — 204-775-2707
757 Sargent Ave, Winnipeg, MB R3E 0B3

Ats Scientific Inc. — 800-661-6700
4030 Mainway Drive, Burlington, ONT L7M-4B9

Audio Controle Inc. — 800-567-2711
250 King St. East, Sherbrooke, QUE J1G-1A9

Aurora Biomed Inc. — 800-883-2918
1001 East Pender St., Vancouver, BC V6A-1W2

Auto Control Medical Inc. — 800-461-0991
6695 Millcreek Dr., Unit 5, Mississauga, ONT L5N-5R8

Automobility Manufacturing Corporation — 800-470-7067
1444 Lorne St., Regina S4R-2K4

Avestin Inc. — 888-283-7846
2450 Don Reid Dr., Ottawa, ONT K1H-8P5

Avida Healthwear Inc. — 800-361-9811
87 Northline Rd., Toronto, ONT M4B-3E9

Axela Inc. — 1-866-923-3363
50 Ronson Dr., Suite 105, Toronto, ON M9W 1B3

B.B.G. Orthopedic Appliances Inc. — 1-866-484-4715
5930 Sherbrooke St. West, Montreal, QUE H4A-1X7

B.F. Lorenzetti & Associates Inc. — 800-668-5901
181 University Ave, Suite 1605, Toronto, ONT M5H 3M7

Babykins Products Ltd. — 800-665-2229
150 - 12830 Clarke Place, Richmond, BC V6V 2H5

Bard Canada, Inc. — 800-632-2109
2345 Stanfield Rd, Mississauga, ONT L4Y 3Y3

Barik Medical Inc. — (800) 265-6061
239 Cree Crescent, Winnipeg, MAN R3J 3Y2

Baylis Medical Company — 800-850-9801
5959 Trans-Canada Highway, Montreal, QC H4t 1A1

Bcl X-Ray Canada Inc. — 1-800-561-1214
1575 Sismet Rd., Unit 5, Mississauga, ONT L4W-1P9

Bdh, Inc. — 800-268-0310
350 Evans Ave., Toronto, ONT M8Z 1K5

Bedcolab Ltd. — 800-461-6414
2305 Francis Hughes, Laval, QUE H7S 1N5

Benlan Inc. — 905-829-5004
2760 Brighton Rd., Oakville, ONT L6H 5T4

Benson Medical Industries Inc. — 800-563-3859
151 Esna Park Dr., Markham, ONT L3R-3B1

Berlex Canada Inc. — 800-361-0240
334 Avro Avenue, Pointe-Claire, PQ H9R 5W5

Bertec Medical — 800-428-5025
70 5th Ave., P.O. Box 128, L'Isletville, QUE G0R-2C0

Best Glove Manufacturing Ltd. — 800-565-2378
253 Michaud St., Coaticook, QUE J1A-1A9

Best Medical Canada — 877-668-6636
413 March Road, Ottawa, ONT K2K 0E4

Bhm Medical, Inc. — 800-868-0441
2001 Tanguay, Magog, QC J1X 5Y5

Bio Nuclear Diagnostics Inc. — 800-668-4033
1791 Albion Road, Toront, ONT M9W-5S7

Bio-Media Unlimited Ltd. — 888-476-4276
200 Vinyl Court, Unit A, Woodbridge, ONT L4L-4A3

Bio/Can Scientific Inc. — 800-387-8125
2170 Dunwin Dr., Unit 5, Mississauga, ONT L5L-1C7

Biofocus Incorporated — 877-864-2329
P.O. Box 25182, Halifax, NS B3M-4H4

Biokinetic Prosthetics Inc. — 506-455-5462
45 Bromley Ave., Hanwell, NB E3C-1M8

Biolab Equipment Canada Limited — 800-268-5035
505 Iroquois Shore Rd., Unit 14, Oakville, ONT L6H-2R3

Biomation — 888-667-2324
335 Perth St., P.O. Box 156, Almonte, ON K0A 1A0

Biomech Designs Ltd. — 780-446-5303
9627 83 St., Edmonton, ALB T6C-3A3

Biomedical Implant Technology Inc. — 800-268-6684
206 King St., St. Catharines, ONT L3R-3J7

Biomedical Industry Group Inc. — 613-745-4139
532 Montreal Rd., Ste. 362, Ottawa, ONT K1K-4R4

Biomet Canada Inc. — 800-263-9447
2891 Portland Drive, Oakville, ONT L6H 5S4

Bionetics Ltd. — 800-665-9930
1580 Beaulac St., St-Laurent, QUE H4R-1W8

Biopacific Diagnostic Inc. — 800-267-5800
114 - 828 Harbourside Drive, North Vancouver, BC V7P 3R9

Biophase Diagnostic Laboratories — 905-567-9165
6625 Kitimat Rd., Unit 51, Mississauga, ONT L5N-6J1

Biophysica Inc. — 416-766-9333
67 Constance St., Toront, ONT M6R-1S5

Bioscan Continental Inc. — 450-974-0151
350 Industriel Blvd., 2nd Floor, St-Eustache, QUE J7R-5V3

Biosig Instruments Inc. — 800-463-5470
440 19th Ave., Ste. 100, Lachine, QUE H8S-3S2

Biotronics Research Corporation — 604-298-1832
#610-4160 Albert St., Burnaby, BC V5C 6K2

Blood Trac Systems, Inc. — 416-364-8441
300-49 Front St E, Toronto M5E 1B3

Bls Systems, Ltd. — 905-339-1069
1055 Industry St, Oakville L6J 2X3

Bowers Medical Supply Co. — 800-663-0047
3691 Viking Way, Unit 9, Richmond, BC V6V 2J6

Brasseler Canada Inc. — 800-363-3838
5757 Decelles Ave., Ste. 234, Montreal, QUE H3S-2C3

Brock Technical Services — 888-287-2433
20 Spencer Street,, Bracebridge, ONT P1L 1E1

Broda Enterprises Inc. — 800-668-0637
385 Phillip St., Waterloo, ONT N2L 5R8

Broda Seating — 800-668-0637
385 Phillip St., Waterloo, ONT N2L-5R8

Brookdale Medical Specialties Ltd. — 800-655-1155
418 Hanlan Rd., Unit 27, Woodbridge, ONT L4L-3P6

Brytech Inc. — 613-731-5800
2301 St. Laurent Blvd., Suite 400, Ottawa ON K1G 4J7

Bubble Technology Industries Inc. — 613-589-2456
P.O. Box 100, Highway 17, Chalk River, ONT K0J-1J0

C.M.S. Industries Ltd. — 800-668-8821
1320 Alberta Ave., Saskatoon, SK S7K 1R5

Cadex Electronics Inc. — 800-565-5228
22000 Fraserwood Way, Richmond, BC V6W-1J6

Caframo Ltd. — 800-567-3556
RR#2 Airport Rd., Wiarton, ONT N0H 2T0

Caledon Laboratories Ltd. — 877-225-3366
40 Armstrong Ave., Georgetown, ONT L7G 4R9

Calibur Dental Technologies, Inc. — 905-833-5122
2189 King Rd, Po Box 520, King City L7B 1A7

Calmar Orthopaedics — 1.888.879.9330
760 Birchmount Rd., Unit 33, Scarborough, ONT M1K-5H8

Calmia Medical, Inc. — 416-441-9009
7-15 Lesmill Rd, Toronto M3B 2T3

Camp Canada Ltd. — 800-267-2812
39 Davis St., P.O. Box 495, Trenton, ONT K8V-5R6

Can-Dan Rehatec Ltd. — 905-648-7522
3-1378 Sandhill Dr., Ancaster, ONT L9G-4V5

Can-Med Surgical Supplies Limited — 800-565-7553
7037 Mumford Rd., P.O. Box 518, Halifax, NS B3J-2R7

Canada Care Medical Inc. — 800-267-8855
1644 Bank St., Ottawa, ONT K1V-7Y6

Canada Endoscope Corp. — 800-563-2907
4-160 Konrad Cres., Unit, Markham, ONT L3R 9W7

Canada Optix, Inc. — 905-238-3332
5181 Bradco Blvd, Mississauga L4W 2A6

Canadawide Scientific Ltd. — 800-267-2362
2300 Walkley Rd., Ottawa, ONT K1G-6B1

Canadian Hospital Specialties Ltd. — 800-461-1423
2810 Coventry Road, Oakville, ONT L6H 6R1

Canadian Medical Brush Inc. — 905-405-1075
7065 Fir Tree Drive, Mississauga, ONT L55 1J7

Canadian Medical Brush, In. — 905-405-1075
11-7686 Kimbel St, Mississauga L5S 1E9

Canadian Medical Products, Ltd. — 800-267-0572
850 Tapscott Rd., Unit 21, Scarborough, ONT M1X-1N4

Canadian Orthotics Laboratory Inc. — 1(877)265-2248
40 Bradwick Drive Units 12-15, Concord, ON L4K 1K9

Canadian Scientific Products Ltd. — 800-265-3460
1055 Sarnia Rd., Unit B2, London, ONT N6H-5J9

Canadian Technical Tape Ltd. — 800-334-1567
455 Cote Vertu Rd., Montreal, QUE H4N-1E8

Canberra-Packard Canada — 800-387-9559
6300 Northwest Dr., Bldg. 312, Mississauga, ONT L4V-1J7

Candent — 888-243-6065
21 2601 Matheson Blvd. East, Mississauga, ONT L4W-5A8

Canica Design Inc. — 800-705-8312
36 Mill Street, Almonte, ON K0A 1A0

Canix Sterilizer Inc. — 905-670-8299
7085 Tomken Rd., Mississauga, ONT L5S-1R7

Canreg Inc. — 905-689-3980
7 Innovation Dr., Unit 118, Flamborough, ONT L9H-7H9

Cardiogenics Inc. — 905-673-8501
6295 Northam Drive, Unit 8, Mississauga, ON L4V 1W8

Cardiomed Supplies Inc. — 800-387-9757
199 Saint David Street, Lindsay, ONT K9V5K7

Cardiotronics Inc. — 1-866-932-1702
5025 Sherbrooke St. W.,, Suite 660, Westmount, QUE H4A 1S9

Cardon Rehabilitation Products — 905-761-7868
8001 Jane St., Unit 1, Concord, ONT L4K-2M7

Care Ware Designs For Active Living — 800-261-5552
P.O. Box 48111, RPO Lakewood, Winnipeg, MAN R2J-4A3

Care-Tek — 888-879-3746
5012 Lakeshore Rd., Burllington, ONT L7L-4P1

Caremark Ltd. — 888 9096199a__
2785 Skymark Ave., Unit 2, Mississauga, ONT L4W-4Y3

Carestream Medical Ltd.	888-310-2186
8800 Dufferin Street,, Suite 201, Vaughan, ONTAR L4K 0C5	
Cari-All Inc.	1.888.640.1414
12 425, boul. Industriel, Montreal, QUE H1B 5M7	
Carsen Group Inc.	800-837-0437
151 Telson Rd., Markham, ONT L3R-1E7	
Cartier Chemicals Ltd.	800-361-9432
445 21st Ave., Lachine, QUE H8S-3T8	
Cascade Orthotics Ltd.	403-283-7872
2636 Parkdale Blvd. NW, Calgary, ALB T2N-3S6	
Cbs Medical Technologies Inc.	514-582-9098
225 Chemin des Grands Ducs, Piedmont, QUEBE J0R 1K0	
Cedarlane Laboratories Ltd.	800-268-5058
5516 8th Line R.R. 2, Hornby, ONT L0P 1E0	
Centennial Optical Ltd.	800-561-0681
158 Norfinch Dr., Toronto, ONTAR M3N 1X6	
Central Canada Contact Lenses Inc.	877-223-9807
3075 14th Ave., Markham, ONT L3R 5L2	
Christie Group Ltd.	800-361-8750
516 rue de Parc, St-Eustache, QUE J7R-5B2	
Chromabec Inc.	888-624-7662
5475 Industriel, Waterloo, QUE J0E 2N0	
Chromatography Sciences Co. (Csc)	800-668-4752
5750 Vanden Abeele, St-Laurent, QUE H4S 1R9	
Chx Technologies, Inc.	416-233-3737
105-4800 Dundas St W, Toronto M9A 1B1	
Cif Furniture Ltd.	905-738-5821
56 Edilcan Dr., Concord, ONT L4K-3S6	
Clark Medical Products, Inc.	800-889-5295
10-5510 Ambler Drive, Mississauga, ONT L4W- 2V1	
Classic Health Supplies Ltd.	888-421-0488
8317 Argyll Road, Edmonton, AB T5H-3H5	
Cleanwear Products Ltd.	(416) 751-7307
54 Crockford Rd., Toronto, ON M1R-3C3	
Clynch Technologies Inc.	403-247-2755
#3 Montgomery Plaza, 4703 Bowness Rd. NW, Calgary, ALB T3B-0B5	
Coldstream Products Corp.	204-669-1201
1001 Regent Ave W, Winnipeg, MB R2C 4M2	
Colman Prosthetics & Orthotics Inc.	403-270-2941
2340 1st Ave. NW, Calgary, ALB T2N-0B8	
Colonial Scientific Ltd.	902-468-1811
201 Brownlow Ave., Unit 52, Dartmouth, NS B3B-1W2	
Companion Walker Ltd.	403-250-1888
4 1420 40th Ave. NE, Calgary, ALB T2E-6L1	
Confection Medicale D.R. Inc.	514-252-5553
200-4220 Rue De Rouen, Montreal H1V 3T2	
Conglom	514-333-6666
2600, Marie-Curie Ave., St-Laurent, QUE H4S 2C3	
Conkin Surgical Instruments Ltd.	416-922-9496
30 Lesmill Road, Unit 4, Toronto, ON M3B 2T6	
Convatec Canada	800-465-6302
555 Dr. Frederick Phillips, Ste. 110, St-Laurent, QUE H4M-2X4	
Cook (Canada) Inc,	800-668-0300
111 Sandiford Dr., Stouffville, ONT L4A-7X5	
Coopercare-Lastrap Inc.	416-741-9675
329 Deerhide Crescent, Toronto, ONT M9M-2Z2	
Cosem Neurostim Ltd.	418-849-9047
P.O. Box 4199 , Terminus, Quebec, QUE G1K 7R9	
Covalon Technologies Ltd.	905-568-8400
405 Britannia Rd. East, Suite 106, Mississauga, ON L4Z 3E6	
Cpc Healthcare Inc.	800-661-4250
958 Heathorne St., Unit 1, London, ONT N5Z-3M5	
Cpr Medical Devices Inc.	416-691-2669
161 Don Park Rd., Markham, ONT L3R-1C2	
Creations Magiques C.M. Inc.	514-753-3892
3001 Rue Visitation, Saint-Charles-Borromee J6E 7Y8	
Crestline Coach Ltd.	888-887-6886
802 57th St. East, Saskatoon, SK S7K-5Z1	
Crown Mfg. Co.	905-545-2546
53 Gibson Ave, Hamilton L8L 6J7	
Cryocath Technologies Inc.	877-694-1212
16771 Chemin Ste-Marie, Montreal, QUE H9H-5H3	
Cryopak Industries, Inc.	732-346-9200
55 Raritan Center Parkway, Edison, NJ 08837	
Ctbr (Inveresk Research Group Member)	514-630-8200
87 Senneville Rd., Senneville, QUE H9X-3R3	
Current Technology Corporation	800-661-4247
530 800 West Pender St., Vancouver, BC V6C-2V6	
Custom Contact Lenses	866-273-4125
3075 14th Ave., Unit 15, Markham, ONT L3R-0G9	
Custom Orthotic Design Group Ltd.	(866) 829-2969
4120 Ridgeway Dr., Unit 24, Mississauga, ONT L5L-5S9	
Custom Orthotics Of London	519-850-4721
1 Adelaide St. North, London, ONT N6B-3P8	
D&D Technologies Inc.	780-918-6616
7535 94 Avenue, Edmonton, AB T6C 1V9	
DORMER LABORATORIES Inc.	416-242-6167
91 Kelfield Rd., Unit 5, Rexdale, ONT M9W-5A3	
Daher Mfg., Inc.	204-663-3299
Mazenod Rd, Winnipeg R2J 4H2	
Dako Diagnostics Canada Inc.	800-668-4630
12 Falconer Dr., Unit 4, Mississauga, ONT L5N-3L9	

Dalsa Corp.	519-886-6000
605 McMurray Road, Waterloo, ONT N2V 2E9	
Dalton Chemical Laboratories Inc.	800-567-5060
349 Wildcat Rd., Toronto, ON M3J 2S3	
Dalynn Biologicals Inc.	888-404-4045
3253 - 34 Avenue N.E., Calgary, ALB T1Y 6X2	
Dana Douglas Medical Inc.	800-267-3552
155 Colonnade Rd., Unit 10, Nepean, ONT K2E-7K1	
Datex-Ohmeda (Canada)	800-268-1472
1093 Meyerside Dr., Unit 2, Mississauga, ONT L5T-1J6	
Datrend Systems Inc.	800-667-6557
5355 Parkwood Place, Richmond, BC V6V 2N1	
Davtair Industries Inc.	613-831-1266
P.O. Box 11448, Station H, Ottawa, ONT K2H-7V1	
Debmar Distributing Inc.	800-265-3354
17 Wexford Rd., Brampton, ONT L6Z-2V9	
Dectro International	800-463-5566
1000 Parc-Technologique Blvd., Quebec, QUE G1P-4S3	
Del Dent Dental Supplied Ltd.	800-268-6657
127 Willowdale Ave., Willowdale, ONT M2N-4Y3	
Delfi Medical Innovations Inc.	800-933-3022
Suite 106, 1099 West 8th Avenue, Vancouver, BC V6H 1C3	
Delta Scientific Laboratory Products Ltd.	800-387-3256
1287 Matheson Blvd. East, Mississauga, ONT L4W-1R1	
Delta Surgical Specialties Ltd.	800-838-8585
8726 Barnard St., P.O. Box 95008, Vancouver, BC V6P-6V4	
Denplus Inc.	888-344-4424
2186 de la Province, Longueuil, QUE J4G 1R7	
Dentech Products Limited	800-826-5004
31 Scarsdale Road, Unit #2, Toronto, ONTAR M3B 2R2	
Dentsply Canada, Ltd.	800-263-1437
161 Vinyl Ct., Woodbridge, ONT L4L 4A3	
Diagnocure, Inc.	418-527-6100
4535 Wilfrid-Hamel Blvd, Suite 250, QUEBEC CITY, QUE G1P 2J7	
Diagnostics Biochem Canada Inc.	519-681-8731
1020 Hargrieve Rd., London, ONT N6E 1P5	
Diagnostix Ltd.	800-282-4075
400 Matheson Blvd. East, Units 14 & 15, Mississauga, ONT L4Z-2E9	
Dialysis Solutions Inc.	905-669-3832
380 Elgin Mills Rd E, Richmond Hill L4C 5H2	
Diamed Lab Supplies Inc.	800-434-2633
3069 Universal Dr., Mississauga, ONT L4X-2E2	
Dicomit Dicom Information Technologies Corp.	905-477-3354
12-250 Cochrane Dr, Markham L3R 8E5	
Digiray Incorporated	800-268-9917
44 Fasken Dr., Unit 3, Toronto, ONT M9W-5M8	
Digisplint Canada	888-377-5468
489 Main St. South, Exeter, ONT N0M-1S1	
Diros Technology, Inc.	905-415-3440
232 Hood Road, Markham, ON L3R 3K8	
Discovery Diagnostics	888-883-9101
P.O. Box 5186, Claremont, ONT L1Y-1A4	
Dismed Inc.	800-361-3581
9950 Parkway Blvd., Anjou, QUE H1J-1P5	
Dominion Biologicals Ltd.	800-565-0653
5 Isnor Dr., Dartmouth, NS B3B 1M1	
Dominion Medical Supply Inc.	800-660-3674
7563 Regional Rd. #63, RR#1, Dunnville, ONT N1A-2W1	
Dormer Laboratories Inc.	800-363-5040
91 Kelfield St., Unit 5, Toronto, ONT M9W-5A3	
Draximage Inc.	888-633-5343
16751 TransCanada Hwy, Kirkland, QUE H9H-4J4	
Dri-Line Products Ltd.	780-466-2953
7210- 76 Avenue, Edmonton, ALB T6B 0B2	
Dufort & Lavigne Ltee.	800-361-0655
2165 Parthenais Street, Montreal, QUE H2K 3T3	
Dumex Medical Surgical Products Ltd.	800-463-9613
104 Shorting Rd., Scarborough, ONT M1S 3S4	
Duoject Medical Systems	877-534-3666
50 chemin de GaspАс, Complex B5, Bromont, QUE J2L-2N8	
Duraline Medical Products	800-667-6996
Box 849, 111 3rd Ave. West, Biggar, SK S0K-0M0	
Durham Medical Ltd.	1-888-479-4687
92 Simcoe St. North, Oshawa, ONT L1H 1C7	
Duro-Test Canada Inc.	800-268-4749
419 Attwell Dr., Etobicoke, ONT M9W-5W5	
Dyna Medical Corp.	800-268-1181
843 Wellington St., London, ONT N6A-3S6	
Dynacon Ent. Ltd.	905-672-8828
2nd Fl, 3565 Nashua Dr, Mississauga L4V 1R1	
Dynawave Research Inc.	800-732-7877
Broadway W Prof Centre, 412-2150 Broadway W, Vancouver V6K 4L9	
E.C. Walker Inc.	416) 744-2011
375 Rexdale Boulevard, Toronto, ONT M9W 1R9	
E.T.D. Inc. (Electro-Therapeutic Devices)	800-268-3834
70 Esna Park Drive,, Unit 4, Markham, ONT L3R 6E7	
Eaton Electronics Ltd.	604-589-5997
11811 95th Ave., North Delta, BC V4C-3T7	
Eci Medical Technologies, Inc.	800-668-5289
2 Cook Rd., Bridgewater, NS B4V 3W7	
Eckel Industries Of Canada Limited	800-563-3574
15 Allison Ave., P.O. Box 776, Morrisburg, ONT K0C 1X0	

Eco Medical Equipment 18303 107 Ave., Edmonton, ALB T5S-1K4	800-232-9450
Eg & G Optoelectronics Canada Ltd. 22001 Dumberry Rd, Vaudreuil-Dorion, QC J7V 8P7	(450) 424-3300
Elcoma Metal Fabricating Canada 878 William St., Midland, ONT L4R-4P4	705-526-9636
Elec Western Medical Devices Ltd. 1015 Matheson Blvd., Ste. 8, Mississauga, ONT L4W-3A4	800-387-8326
Electro Therapeutic Devices Inc. 70 Esna Park Drive, Unit 4, Markham, ONT L3R 6E7	877-475-8344
Electro-Medical Instrument Co. 1-2359 Royal Windsor Dr., Mississauga, ONT L5J-4S9	905-822-3188
Electromed Imaging Inc. 440 Armand Frappier Blvd., Ste. 250, Laval, QUE H7V-4B4	450-681-6810
Elma Medtec Products Inc. Po Box 160, Elma R0E 0Z0	204-348-7164
Empi Canada 16773 Hymus Blvd., Kirkland, QUE H9H-3L4	800-463-3674
Emplex Systems, Inc. 2045 Midland Ave., Toronto, ON MIP 3E2	800-265-1775
Equipro Equipment De Beaute 11005 Rue Masse, Montreal-Nord H1G 4G5	514-324-2226
Erickson's Artificial Eyes 805 W. Broadway, Ste. 703, Vancouver, BC V5Z-1K1	800-665-0538
Erp Group Professional Products Ltd. 3232 Autoroute Laval W., Laval, QUEBE H7T 2H6	800-361-3537
Erp Group Professional Products Ltd. 3232 Autoroute Laval West, Laval, QUE H7T-2H6	800-361-3537
Esbe Scientific Industries Inc. 80 McPherson St., Markham, ONT L3R-3V6	800-268-3477
Ethix Medical 3465 Cote-des-Neiges, Ste. 702, Montreal, QUE H3H-1T7	514-935-5593
Etymonic Design Inc. 41 Byron Ave., Dorchester, ONT N0L 1G0	800-265-2093
Evacu Technologies Inc. 2-20 Strathy Rd, Cobourg K9A 5J7	905-372-0322
Excel Tech. Ltd. 2568 Bristol Cir, Oakville L6H 5S1	905-829-5300
Exciton Technologies Inc. 10230 Jasper Ave, Suite 4000, Edmonton, AB AB T5J 4P6	780-248-5868
Executive Dental Supply Ltd. 6984 MacPherson Ave., Burnaby, BC V5J-4NS	800-211-7888
F.A.S.T. First Aid & Survival Technologies Ltd. 1687 Cliveden Ave, Delta V3M 6V5	604-540-8300
Farabloc Development Corp. 211-3030 Lincoln Ave, Coquitlam V3B 6B4	604-941-8201
Federal Elevator Systems Inc. 1090 Lorimar Drive, Mississauga, ONT L5S 2A1	888-785-5438
Feminica Inc. 3216 Rue Monsabre, Montreal H1N 2L5	514-875-4422
Ference Weicker & Company 475 W. Georgia St., Ste. 550, Vancouver, BC V6B-4M9	1-866-680-3926
Fisher Scientific Limited 112 Colonnade Rd., Ottawa, ONT K2E-7L6	800-237-7437
Fitter International Inc. 3050, 2600 Portland Street SE, Calgary, ALB T2G 4M6	800-348-8371
Footmaxx Holdings Inc. 468 Queen St. E, Ste. 400, Toronto, ONT M5A-1T7	800-779-3668
Formedica Ltd. 7109, Trans, Montreal, (QUEB H4T 1A2	800-361-9671
Fortress Scientifique Du Quebec Ltee. 2160 Rue De Celles, Quebec G2C 1X8	418-847-5225
Freedom Concepts, Inc. 2087 Plessis Road, Winnipeg, MB R3W 1S4	800-661-9915
Frontier Computing 2221 Yonge St., Ste. 406, Toronto, ONT M4S-2B4	888-480-0000
Futuremed Health Care Products Inc. 280 Basaltic Rd., Concord, ONT L4K-1G6	800-381-7025
G. Brunatti & Sons Limited 85 River Street, Parry Sound, ONT P2A 2T8	705-746-5622
Gait-Aid Inc. 5468 Dundas St. W., Ste. 1000, Toronto, ONT M9B 6E3	800-677-1796
Galen Medical Ltd. 408 Kent Ave South E, Suite 126, Vancouver, BC V5X2X7	800-980-3003
Galenicare 4621 63 St. #4, Red Deer, ALB T4N-7A6	877-309-0560
Gambro Inc. 9157, du Champ DA,A'eau Street, St. Leonard, MONTR H1P 3M3	514-327-1635
Gaper Products Ltd. 4060 Ridgeway Dr. #18, Mississauga, ONT L5L-5X9	800-667-5858
Garaventa (Canada) Ltd. 7505 - 134A St., Surrey, BC V3W-7B3	800-663-6556
Ge Clinical Services 2300 Meadowvale Blvd., Mississauga, ONT L5N-5P9	888-367-2773
Geen Healthcare Inc. 931 Progress Ave. Ste.13, Scarborough, ONT M1G 3V5	800-565-4336
GeneNews Limited 2 East Beaver Creek Road, Building 2, Richmond Hill, ONTAR L4B 2N3	866-375-0442
Geneq Inc. 8047 Jerry St. E, Montreal, QUE H1J-1H6	800-463-4363
General Scientific Instrument Services Inc. 1764 Oxford St. E, Ste. 1160, London, ONT N5V-3R6	519-659-2275

Genie Audio Inc. 125 Gagnon St., Ste. 102, St-Laurent, QUE H4N-1T1	800-363-0793
Gennum Corporation P.O. Box 489, Station A, Burlington, ONT L7R-3Y3	905-632-2996
Gentec Electro-Optics Inc. 445 St-Jean-Baptiste, Ste. 160, Quebec, QUE G2E-5N7	888-543-6832
Genzyme Diagnostics P.E.I. Inc. 70 Watts Ave., Charlottetown, PEI C1E-2B9	800-565-0265
George Courey Inc. 5550 Ferrier St., Mont-Royal, QUE H4P-1M2	800-361-1087
Germiphene Corp. 1379 Colborne St. E, Brantford, ONT N3T-5M1	519-759-7100
Gh Gunther Huettlin Manufacturing, Inc. 101 Petrie Pl, Belleville K8N 4Z6	613-961-8860
Glenwood Laboratories 2392 Speers Rd., Oakville, ONT L6L-5M2	800-361-9506
Global Healthcare Exchange Inc. Canada 10 Carlson Ct., Ste. 610, Etobicoke, ONT M9W-6L2	416-798-1029
Global Medicaid Products Inc. 3-1100 Invicta Dr, Oakville L6H 2K9	905-339-0666
Global Medical Products Inc. 5230 S. Service Rd., Burlington, ONT L7L-5K2	800-387-6095
Globalmed Inc. 155 N. Murray St., Trenton, ONT K8V-5R5	613-394-9844
Gold Care Medical Group 91 Ave. #4619, Edmonton, ALB T6B-2M7	800-282-3909
Goldline Mobility And Conversions 1759 Trafalgar St., London, ONT N5W-1X4	800-561-9621
Gow Trainer Ltd. 310 Georgian Dr., R.R#1, Barrie, ONT L4M 7B7	705-721-9994
Groupe Medicus Inc. 5135 10th Ave., Montreal, QUE H1Y-2G5	877-678-8872
Groupe Novalab Inc. 2350 Rue Power, Drummondville J2C 7Z4	819-474-2580
Gs Medical Packaging Inc. 501 Lakeshore Road East, Suite 201, Mississauga, ONT L5G 1H9	800-489-7125
Guidant Canada Corporation 505 Apple Creek Blvd., Unit 4, Markham, ONT L3R-5B1	800-268-4487
Guy Griffiths Orthodontic Lab (1984) Inc. 4927 Rue Sherbrooke O, Westmount H3Z 1H2	514-482-1267
H.K. Eyecan Inc. 2849 Ahearn Ave, Ottawa, ONT K2B-6J8	800-356-3362
Haemacure Corp. 2001 University St., Ste. 430, Montreal, QUE 34236-	888-721-8076
Hallmark Insurance Brokers Ltd. 4 Lansing Square,, Suite 100, Toronto, ONT M2J 5A2	800-492-4070
Haltone Electronics Limited 1221 Barton St., Stoney Creek, ONT L8E 5G9	800-263-4864
Hanna Instruments Canada Inc. 3156 Industriel Blvd., Laval, QUE H7L-4P7	800-842-6629
Harco Co., Ltd. 5915 Coopers Avenue, Mississauga, ONT L4Z 1R9	905-890-1220
Harding Medical Supplies Ltd. 1158 Grand Lake Road, Sydney, NS B1M 1A2	1-877-457-8600
Harvard Apparatus Canada 6010 Vanden Abeele St., St. Laurent, QUE H4S 1R9	514-335-0792
Hayday Irrit-Easers 883 Derry Crt, Oshawa L1J 6X8	416-434-1400
Health Light Inc. P.O. Box 3899, LCD 4, Hamilton, ONT L8H-7P2	800-265-6020
Healthcare & Rehab Specialties 10611 Kingsway Ave., Unit 114, Edmonton, ALB T5G-3C8	800-232-9408
Healthcraft Products Inc. 2790 Fenton Road, Unit 411, Ottawa, ONT K1T 3T7	888-619-9992
Healthmark Ltd. 8827 Henri-Bourassa O. Blvd., MontrAcal, QUE H4S-1P7	800-665-5492
Hear Saver Limited 60 Innovation Dr., Flamborough, ONT L9H-7P3	905-690-6277
Heart Force Medical Inc. 1818 Cornwall Avenue, Suite 305, Vancouver, BC V6J 1C7	604-566-8200
Heartsounds Corp. 314-801 York Mills Rd, Don Mills M3B 1X7	416-383-1520
Heine Instruments Canada Ltd. 20 Steckle Place, Unit 3, Kitchener, ONT N2E-2C3	519-895-1020
Henry Schein Arcona Inc. 345 Townline Road, PO Box 6000, Niagara-on-the-Lake, ONT L0S 1J0	800-668-5558
Higa Manufacturing Ltd. Po Box 91160 Stn West Vancouver, West Vancouver V7V 3N6	604-922-5261
Hitachi Denshi Canada Ltd. 1 Select Ave., Unit 14, Scarborough, ONT M1V-5J3	800-268-3597
Holburn Biomedical Corporation 1100 Bennett Road, Bowmanville, ONT L1C 3K5	905-623-1484
Holl Meditronics Inc. 4 Marconi Court, Bolton, ONT L7E-1E7	800-387-0563
Hollister Limited 95 Mary St., Aurora, ONT L4G-1G3	800-263-7400
Home Gym Canada Inc. 9 Brockhouse Rd., Toronto, ONT M8W-2W8	416-762-7920
Homecare Clinical Emergencies, Inc. 21-1111 Flint Rd, North York M3J 3C7	416-665-7373
Hood Thermo-Pad Canada Ltd. 5918 Kennedy St., Summerland, BC V0H-1Z1	800-665-9555

Howell Ventures Ltd.	888-370-5050
4850 Route 102, Upper Kingsclear, NB E3E- 1P	
Hunt's Convalescent Equipment Co. Inc.	800-838-5146
7-109 Woodbine Downs Blvd., Toronto, ONT M9W-6Y1	
I-Med Pharma Inc.	800-463-1008
1601 St. Regis Blvd., Montreal, QUE H9B-3H7	
I.D.C. Tectonics Ltd.	905-646-6335
P.O. Box 2104, St. Catharines, ONT L2R 7R7	
IMBiotechnologies Ltd.	780-945-6609
9650 - 20th Avenue, Suite 113, Edmonton, ALBER T6N 1G1	
Ibiom Instruments Ltd.	450-678-5468
1065 Pacific Street, suite 403, Sherbrooke, QUE J1H 2G3	
Imaging Dynamics Corporation	866-975-6737
2340 Pegasus Way N.E., Suite 151, Unit 14, Calgary, ALB T2E-8M5	
Immucor Canada Inc.	800-661-9993
9703 45th Ave., Edmonton, ONT T6E 5Z8	
Imp Group Ltd.	902-453-2400
400-2651 Dutch Village Rd, Halifax B3L 4T1	
Imperial Orthoflex Manufacturing Ltd.	800-667-3442
5920 No. 6 Rd., Ste. 205, Richmond, BC V6V-1Z1	
Imperial Surgical Ltd.	800-661-5432
850 Halpern Ave, Dorval, ONT H9P 1G6	
Imris Incorporated	888-304-0114
100 - 1370 Sony Place, Winnepeg, MAN R3T 1N5	
Independent Needs Centre	905-479-1448
3415 Fourteenth Ave., Unit #2,, Markham, ONT L3R 0H3	
Infectio Diagnostic Inc. (I.D.I.)	418-681-4343
2050 boul. Rene-Levesque Ouest, 4th Floor, Sainte-Foy, QUE G1V-2K8	
Infection Control Systems Inc.	888-235-4569
402 Concession St., Hamilton, ONT L9A-1B7	
Inland Dental Distributors Ltd.	800-661-6569
10569 111 St., Edmonton, ALB T5H-3E8	
Innomed Christie Group Ltd.	780-483-6177
18208 102 Ave., Edmonton, ALB T5S-1S7	
Innotech Rehabilitation Products Inc.	800-361-0228
P.O. Box 534, Orillia, ONT L3V-6K2	
Innova Medical Ophthalmics Inc.	800-461-1200
1430 Birchmount Rd., Toronto, ONT M1P 2E8	
Innovatek Medical Inc.	604-522-8303
#3 - 1600 Derwent Way, Delta, BC V3M 6M5	
Innovative Choices, Inc.	315-482-2583
700 Progress Ave, Scarborough M1H 2Z7	
Innovative Excimer Solutions, Inc.	416-410-1868
3340a Yonge St, Toronto M4N 2M4	
Instantel Inc.	800-267-9111
309 Legget Dr., Kanata, ON K2K 3A3	
Instrumed Surgical	800-667-5653
2180 Dunwin Dr., Units 5 & 6, Mississauga, ONT L5L 5M8	
Instrumentarium Inc.	800-361-1502
1273 St-Louis St., Terrebonne, QUE J6W-3L5	
Integra Environmental Inc.	800-661-6678
5035 n. Service Rd., Unit C7, Burlington, ONT L7L-5V2	
Inter Medico	800-387-9643
50 Valleywood Dr., Markham, ONT L3R-6E9	
Inter V Medical Inc.	800-667-1073
5179 Metropolitain East, Montreal, QUE H1R 1Z7	
International Hearing Aids Inc.	800-387-7943
5041 Mainway, Burlington, ONT L7L 5H9	
International Medical Instruments (Imi) Inc.	905-882-8181
1600 Steeles Ave. W, Concord, ONT L4K 4M2	
International Newtech Development Inc.	877-463-8885
1629 Fosters Way, Delta, BC V3M-6S7	
International Stretcher Systems	800-229-4180
1605 Hwy #3 West, R.R. 5, Dunnville, ONT N1A-2W4	
International Wex Technologies Inc.	800-722-7549
Suite 1601 - 700 West Pender Street, Vancouver, BC V6C 1G8	
Intersciences Inc.	800-661-6431
169 Idema Rd., Markham, ONT L3R 1A9	
Intriquip Instruments	800-361-3777
1862 Angus St., Regina, SK S4T-1Z4	
Intronix Technologies Corporation	800-819-9996
26 McEwan Dr., Unit 15, Bolton, ONT L7E-1E6	
Invacare Canada	800-668-5324
16769 Boul Hymus, Kirkland H9H 3L4	
Invitrogen Canada Inc.	800-263-6236
5250 Mainway, Burlington, ONT L7L 5Z1	
Ion-Trace Inc.	905-640-0295
5649 Concession 2, Stouffville, ONT L4A-7X4	
Iotron Technologies, Inc.	604-945-8838
1425 Kebet Way, Port Coquitlam, BC V3C 6L3	
Is2 Research Inc.	613-228-8755
3 6-20 Gurdwara Rd, Nepean K2E 8B3	
Isee 3d, Inc.	514-908-2233
100-4 Car Westmount, Westmount H3Z 2S6	
Isee3d, Inc.	514-908-2234
759 Victoria Square, Ste. 200, Montreal, QUE H2Y-2J7	
Isotechnika Inc.	888-487-9944
5120 75th St., Edmonton, ALB T6E 6W2	
Itm Instruments Inc.	800-361-1042
20800 Industriel Boulevard, Ste-Anne-de-Bellevue, QUE H9X 0A1	
J. E. Hanger Ltd.	888-592-3433
5545 St. Jacques St. W., Montreal, QUE H4A-2E3	

J. Slawner Ltd.	514-735-6565
5713 Cote des Neiges, Montreal, QUE H3S-1Y7	
J. Sterling Industries Ltd.	(905) 264-6657
405 Rowntree Dairy Road, Woodbridge, ONT L4L 8H1	
J.E.M. Sales Ltd.	416-663-7313
6-110 Norfinch Dr, Toronto M3N 1X1	
J.W. Westman Inc.	800-387-8204
5-2800 Argentia Road, Mississauga, ONT L5N 8L2	
Janssen-Ortho Inc.	1 (800) 387-87
19 Green Belt Dr, North York, ON M3C 1L9	
Joldon Diagnostics	800-661-4556
233 Linwood Crescent, Unit 12, Burlington, ONT L7L-3Z9	
Kane Biotech Inc.	204-453-1301
5-1250 Waverley St., Winnipeg, MB R3T 6C6	
Karl Hager Limb & Brace & The Knee Centre	800-387-5053
10733 124 St., Edmonton, ALB T5M-0H2	
Keir Surgical Ltd.	800.663.4525
126-408 East Kent Avenue South, Vancouver, BC V5X 2X7	
Kinexus Bioinformatics Corporation	1-866-546-3987
8755 Ash Street, Suite 1, Vancouver, BRITI V6P 6T3	
Kingstec Medical Products	905-712-2171
175 Traders Blvd. E, Mississauga, ONT L4Z 3S8	
Kino Mobility Inc.	4166355873
1140 Sheppard Ave. West Unit #3, Toronto, ON M3K 2A2	
Kintech Orthopaedics Ltd.	1 (888) 793-044
360 Revus Avenue, Unit #13, Mississauga, ONT L5G 4S4	
Kodak Canada Inc., Health Imaging Division	800-465-6325
6 Monogram Place, Suite 200, Toronto, ONT M9R 0A1	
Kosma-Kare Canada Inc.	450-679-6380
2044, de la Province, Longueuil, QUE J4G-1Z1	
Kpmg Llp	416-777-8500
333 Bay Street, Suite 4600, Toronto, ONT M5H 2S5	
Kristofoam Industries Inc.	905-669-6616
120 Planchet Rd, Concord, ON L4K 2C7	
Kuri Tec Corporation	519-753-6717
140 Roy Blvd, Brantford, ONT N3R-7K2	
Kvb Manufacturing	800-565-9845
62 Maple Ave., Smith Falls, ONT K7A-2A7	
L.P.A. Medical, Inc.	800-663-4863
460 Desrochers, Vanier, QUEBE G1M 1C2	
Labequip Ltd.	905-475-5880
170 Shields Ct.,, Unit 2, Markham, ONT L3R9T5	
Laboratoire M.P. Langelier Inc.	450.467.0762
675 Laurier Blvd., Rte. 116, Beloeil, QUE J3G-4J1	
Laboratoire Mat Inc.	800-890-8666
610 Adanac St., Beauport, QUE G1C-7B7	
Laboratoire Pouliot Inc.	800-363-6172
2990 chemin Ste-Foy, Sainte-Foy, QUE G1X-1P6	
Laborie Medical Technologies Inc.	888-522-6743
6415 Northwest Dr., Units 7-14, Mississauga, ONT L4V-1X1	
Labotix Automation Inc.	800-661-5229
2097 Whittington Drive Unit B, Peterborough, ONT K9J 6X4	
Labron Mobility Aids Ltd.	604-270-1117
8385 Saint George St., Vancouver, BC V5X-4P3	
Labtician Ophthalmics, Inc.	800-265-8391
2140 Winston Park Dr., Unit 6, Oakville, ONTAR L6H 5V5	
Labtronics, Inc.	519-767-1061
546 Governors Rd, Guelph, ONT N1K-1E3	
Lac Mac, Ltd.	519-432-2616
425 Rectory St, London N5W 3W5	
Lanherne Technology Ltd.	613-376-3100
4567 Bedford Rd., P.O. Box 410, Sydenham, ONT K0H-2TO	
Lasalle Scientific Inc.	519 824 7301
121 Malcolm Road, Guelph, ON N1K 1A8	
Leader Industries Inc.	800-847-2001
3585 Ashby, St. Laurent, Montreal, QUE H4R 2K3	
Leica Microsystems (Canada) Inc.	800-248-0123
111 Granton Dr., Richmond Hill, ONT L4B 1L5	
Lemargo Inc.	800-469-3932
259 Traders Blvd., Unit 8, Mississauga, ONT L4Z 2E5	
Les Equipements Adaptes Physipro Inc.	800-668-2252
370, 10e Avenue South, Sherbrooke, QUE J1G 2R7	
Les Escalateurs Atlas Inc.	888-773-6708
8255 Boul. Laframboise, St-Hyacinthe, QUE J2R 1E8	
Les Laboratoires Quelab Inc.	1 (800) 579-099
5615, Fullum, Montreal, QUE H2G 2H6	
Levertec Therapy Equipment Ltd.	1 888 261-6341
P.O. Box 907, 100 Mile House, BC V0K-2E0	
Lifeline Systems Canada Inc.	800-387-8120
95 Barber Greene Rd., Ste. 105, Toronto, ONT M3C-3E9	
Lifescan Canada Ltd.	800-663-5521
4170 Still Creek Dr. #234, Burnaby, BC V5C-6C6	
Liftability Inc.	800-267-8883
2600 Lancaster Road, Ottawa, ONT K1B 4Z4	
Lms Medical Systems Ltd.	514-488-3461
314-5252 Boul De Maisonneuve O, Montreal H4A 3S5	
Locin Industries Ltd.	800-663-8270
#200-18 Gostick Pk., North Vancouver, BC V7M- 3G	
London Health Care & Ostomy Centre	800-265-0410
675 Adelaide St. N, London, ONT N5Y-2L4	
London Scientific Limited	800-270-5665
833 Consortium Ct., London, ONT N6E-2S8	

Lpa Medical Inc. — 800-663-4863
460 Desrochers #150, Vanier, QUE G1M-1C2

Luxo Lamp Ltd. — (800) 361-3993
1904 St. Regis, Dorval, QUE H9P 1H6

M & Cc Ltd. — 800-388-6236
10721 Keele St. N, Maple, ONT L6A-1S5

M.C. Healthcare Products, Inc. — 800-268-8671
4658 Ontario St., Beamsville, ONT L0R 1B4

M.E.D. Servi-Systems Canada Ltd. — 800-267-6868
8 Sweetnam Dr., Stittsville, ONT K2S 1G2

Macpherson Medical Inc. — 800-699-9751
5775 Atlantic Dr., Unit 10, Mississauga, ONT L4W-4P3

Madentec Limited — 877-623-3682
4664 - 99 Street, Edmonton, ALB T6E 5H5

Mallinckrodt Medical Inc. — 866-885-5988
7500 Trans Canada Highway, Pointe Claire, QUE H9R-5H8

Mandel Scientific Company — (888) 883-3636
2 Admiral Place, Guelph, ONT N1G-4N4

Manexim Multicorp, Ltd. — 416-955-0737
62 Harrington Cres, Willowdale M2M 2Y5

Manrex Limited — 800-665-7652
1036 Waverly St., Winnepeg, MAN R3T-0P3

Mansfield Medical Distributors Ltd. — 800-361-6240
5775 Andover, Montreal, QUE H4T-1H6

Maple Leaf Wheelchair Mfg., Inc. — 905-602-0566
12/13-1655 Sismet Rd, Mississauga L4W 1Z4

Marconi Medical Systems Canada Inc. — 800-668-5211
7956 Torbam Rd., Brampton, ONT L6T-5A2

Marivac Limited — 800-565-5821
5821 Russell St., Halifax, NS B3K-1X5

Marlene C. Roche — 519-658-4519
96 Grey Abbey Trail, Cambridge N3C 3G1

Marshall Mattress Company Limited — 800-682-6861
83 Bakersfield St., North York, ONT M3J-1Z4

Matrox Electronic Systems, Ltd. — 800-804-6243
1055 St. Regis Blvd., Dorval, QUE H9P 2T4

Maxill Inc. — 1-800-268-8633
80 Elm St., St. Thomas, ONT N5R-6C8

Mbi Fermentas Inc. — 800-340-9026
830 Harrington Ct., Burlington, ONT L7N-3N4

Mcarthur Medical Sales Inc. — 800-996-6674
1846 5th Concession W., P.O. Box 7, Rockton, ONT L0R-1X0

Mckesson Medical Imaging — 800-826-9360
130-10711 Cambie Rd, Richmond, BC V6X 3G5

Mds Nordion — 800-267-6211
447 March Rd., Kanata, ON K2K 1X8

Mds Sciex — 416-675-6777
71 Four Valley Dr, Concord L4K 4V8

Mds Sciex — 905-660-9005
71 Four Valley Dr., Concord, ON L4K 4V8

Mds, Inc. — 416-675-6777
2700 Matheson Blvd. E., Suite 300, West Tower, Mississauga, ON L4W 4V9

Med-Ortho Design & Manufacturing Ltd. — 905-837-7789
900 Brock Rd. S, Unit 6, Pickering, ONT L1W-1Z9

Med-Ox Diagnostics Inc. (Mdi) — 800-818-8335
1-57 Iber Rd., Ottawa, ONT K2S-1E7

Med-Plast — 800-567-1108
161 Oneida Drive, Pointe Claire, QUE H9R 1A9

Medec — 866-586-3332
405 The West Mal, Suite 900, Toronto, ONTAR M9C 5J1

Medelco Ltd. — 800-268-7927
6469 Northam Drive, Mississauga, ONT L4V 1J2

Medex Para-Medical Equipment Inc. — 450-581-3966
275 Boul Pierre-Legardeur, Le Gardeur J5Z 3A7

Medex Systems International Inc. — 604-607-7008
25990 48th Ave., Aldergrove, BC V4W-1J2

Medi-Inn Inc. — 888-633-4466
6-6150 Highway 7, Suite 491, Woodbridge, ONT L4H 0R6

Medical International Technology Inc. — 514-339-9355
1872 Beaulac Ville St-Laurent, Montreal, QUEBE H4R 2E7

Medical Mart Supplies Ltd. — 800-268-2848
5875 Chedworth Way, Mississauga, ONT L5R 3L9

Medical Plastic Devices (Mpd), Inc. — 866-633-7527
161 Oneida Dr., Pointe Claire, QUE H9R 1A9

Medical Tronik Ltee — 800-361-0877
190 boul. St-Elzear Quest, laval, QUE H7L-3N3

Medicana Inc. — 800-361-9496
2261 Guenette St., St-Laurent, QUE H4R-2E9

Medichair Ltd. — 800-667-0087
500 - 1121 Centre St NW, Calgary, ALB T2E 7K6

Medicom — 800-361-2862
1200, 55th Avenue, Lachine, QUE H8T 1A1

Medicorp, Inc. — 514-733-1900
5800 Royalmount, Montreal, QUE H4P 1K5

Medifocus Inc. — 866-322-8354
5500 North Service Road, Suite 905, Burlington, ONTAR L7L 6W6

Medigas Inc. — 866-446-6302
4 - 55 Frid Street, Hamilton, ON L8P 4M3

Medionics International Inc. — 800-463-6087
114 Anderson Ave., Markham, ONT L6E 1A5

Medique — 800-793-6210
5900 Andover Ave., Mount-Royal, QUE H4T-1H5

Medirex Systems Ltd. — 800-387-9848
P.O. Box 40 Station F, Toronto, ONT M4Y 2L4

Medisav Services, Inc. — 905-201-1313
B-56 Elson St, Markham L3S 1Y7

Meditech International Inc. — 416-251-1055
411 Horner Ave., Unit 1, Toronto, ONT M8W-4W3

Medmira Laboratories Inc. — 1-877-MEDMIRA
155 Chain Lake Dr, Unit 1, Halifax, NS B3S 1B3

Medtronic Of Canada Ltd. — 800-268-5346
6733 Kitimat Rd., Mississauga, ON L5N 1W3

Medtronic Sofamor Danek Canada — 1-800-268-5346
99 Hereford Street, Brampton, ONT L6Y 0R3

Medx Health Corp. — 888-363-3112
220 Superior Blvd., Mississauga, ON L5T 2L2

Melet Plastics, Inc. — 204-667-6635
34 De Baets St, Winnipeg R2J 3S9

Merit Medical Systems Ltd. — 800-667-5720
2209-A Dunwin Dr., Mississauga, ONT L5L-1X1

Merus Labs International Inc. — 604-221-0595
1177 West Hastings Street, Suite 2007, Vancouver, B.C. V6E 2K3

Michael D. Warren Services Ltd. — 905-455-1915
211-338 Queen St E, Brampton L6V 1C4

Michel Cullen Medical Inc. — 888-438-9544
1040 boul. Michele-Bohec., Ste. 100, Blainville, QUE J7C-5E2

Microbix Biosystems, Inc. — 800-794-6694
115 Skyway Ave, Toronto, ONT M9W 4Z4

Microzone Corporation — 877-252-7710
86 Harry Douglas Drive, Ottawa, ONT K2S 2C7

Mid-Continental Dental Supply Co., Ltd. — 204-888-5031
242 Alboro St, Headingley R4J 1A4

Millenium Technology Inc. — 604-273-6736
Suite 305, South Tower, 5811 Cooney Road, Richmond, BC V6X 3M1

Mind Alive Inc. — 800-661-6463
9008 51 Avenue, Edmonton, ALBER T6E-5X4

Minogue Medical Inc. — 800-665-6466
180 Peel, Ste. 300, Montreal, QUE H3C-2G7

Mip Inc. — 800-361-4964
9100 Ray Lawson Blvd., Montreal, QC H1J-1K8

Mirolin Industries Inc. — 800-463-2236
60 Shorncliffe Rd., Toronto, ONT M8Z-5K1

Miv Therapeutics, Inc. — 604-301-9545
8765 Ash St., Unit #1, Vancouver, BC V6P-6T3

Mjs Biolynx Inc. — 888-593-5969
300 Laurier Blvd., P.O. Box 1150, Brockville, ONT K6V-5W1

Modus Medical Devices Inc. — 519-438-2409
17 Masonville Cres, London N5X 3T1

Motion Concepts — 905-695-0134
84 Citation Dr., Concord, ONTAR L4K 3C1

Motion Specialties Inc. — 800-267-2920
82 Carnforth Road, Toronto, ONT M4A 2K7

Movingpeople.Net Canada, Inc. — 416-739-8333
500 Norfinch Dr, Downsview M3N 1Y4

Mtm Health Products Ltd. — 800-263-8253
2349 Fairview St., Burlington, ONT L7R 2E3

Mui Scientific — 800-303-6611
145 Traders Blvd. E., Unit 34, Mississauga, ONT L4Z 3L3

Multiplex Stimulator Ltd. — 800-663-8576
2-1750 McLean Ave., Port Coquitlam, BC V3C 1M9

National Home Products Ltd. — 416-661-2770
188 Limestone Crescent, Toronto, ONT M3J 2S4

National Systems Co. — 877-672-4278
31B Durward Pl., Waterloo N2J 3Z9

Nature's Way Therapeutic Products, Inc. — 604-921-2601
91021-1427 Bellevue Ave, West Vancouver V7T 1C3

Ncs Medical Incorporated — 800-661-5005
5421 8B Ave., Delta, BC V4M-1V5

Needle Aid, Ltd. — 902-895-8015
23 Lower Truro Rd, Truro B2N 5A9

Nellcor Puritan Bennett (Melville) Ltd. — 613-238-1840
700-141 Laurier Ave W, Ottawa K1P 5J3

Neovasc Inc — 1.866.760.7131
13700 Mayfield Pl. #2135, Richmond, BC V6V 2E4

Neovasc, Inc. — 604-270-4344
13700 Mayfield Place, Suite 2135, Richmond, BC V6V 2E4

Niagara Pharmaceuticals Div. — 905-690-6277
60 Innovation Dr., Flamborough, ONT L9H-7P3

Nica-Power Battery Corp. — 800-565-6422
5155 Spectrum Way, Mississauga, ON L4W 5A1

Nidacon Canada Inc. — 613-260-0886
250-600 Peter Morand Cres, Ottawa K1G 5Z3

Nighthawk Manufacturing Inc. — 1-800-661-6247
3204 - 121 Avenue NE, Edmonton, ALB T6S-1G7

Nightingale Lens Labs — 800-561-0034
387 Sunset Dr., Fredericton, NB E3A-1J2

Nikon Canada Inc., Instrument Div. — 905-625-9910
1366 Aerowood Dr., Mississauga, ONT L4W-1C1

Nikon Optical Canada, Inc. — 011-813-5600
100-5075 Rue Fullum, Montreal H2H 2K3

Northern Hospital Supplies Ltd. — 867-668-5083
4200 4th Avenue, Whitehorse, YT Y1A 1K1

Northern Light Technologies — 800-263-0066
8971 Henri-Bourassa W, Montreal, QUE H4S-1P7

Northern Scientific Corporation	800-465-8377
418-2895 Derry Rd E,, Mississauga, ONT L4T 1A6	
Northland Healthcare Products Ltd.	204-786-3345
865 Bradford St., Winnipeg, MAN R3E-0G5	
Nova Century Scientific Ltd.	800-615-5072
5022 South Service Rd., Burlington, ONT L7L 5Y7	
Novadaq Technologies Inc.	888-728-4368
2585 Skymark Ave., Suite 306, Mississauga, ON L4W 4L5	
Novo Nordisk Canada Inc.	800-465-4334
300-2680 Skymark Avenue,, Mississauga, ONT L4W 5L6	
Nucro-Technics Incorporated	416-438-6727
2000 Ellesmere Rd. #16, Scarborough, ONT M1H-2W4	
Numed Canada, Inc.	613-936-2592
45 Second Street West, Cornwall, ONT K6J 1G3	
O-Two Systems International Inc.	800-387-3405
7575 Kimbel St., Mississauga, ONT L5S 1C8	
O.O.S. Medical	800-387-5150
60 Shorting Rd., Scarborough, ONT M1S-3S3	
Obus Forme Ltd.	888-225-7378
344 Consumers Road, Toronto, ON M2J 1P8	
Octostop Inc.	888-422-7151
1675 boul. Saint Elzear, Ouest, Laval, QUE H7L-3N6	
Oculo Plastik Inc.	888-381-3292
200 Sauve West, Montreal, QUE H3L-1Y9	
Oculo-Plastik Inc.	888-381-3292
200 Suave West, Montreal, QUE H3L-1Y9	
Odyssey Medical Equipment	604-524-9446
331 Columbia St. E, New Westminster, BC V3L 3W8	
Olympus Canada, Inc.	800-387-0437
151 Telson Road, Markham, ON L3R 1E7	
Omega Posture Systems	800-665-4839
846 Marion St. #4, Winnipeg, MAN R2J-0K4	
Oms, 177108 Canada Inc.	800-461-6637
97 Columbus, Pointe Claire, QUE H9R-4K3	
Ontario Medical Supply Limited	800-267-1069
1100 Algoma Road,, Ottawa, ONT K1B 0A3	
Ophardt Hygiene Technologies Inc.	905-563-4987
4743 Christie Dr., Beamsville, ONT L0R 1B4	
Ophthalmic Technologies, Inc.	416-631-9123
12-37 Kodiak Cres, Downsview M3J 3E5	
Opsens	418-682-9996
2014 Cyrille-Duquet Street, Suite 125, Quebec, QUEBE G1N 4N6	
Optiway Inc.	800-514-7061
500 Norfinch Dr., Downsview, ONT M3N-1Y4	
Orthese Prothese Rive Sud Inc.	450-672-0078
127 rue St-Louis, Ville Lemoyne, QUE J4R-2L3	
Ortho Active Appliances Ltd.	800-663-1254
103-250 Schoolhouse St., Coquitlam, BC V3K 6V7	
Ortho Concept Inc.	450-973-6700
2101, boul Le Carrefour, suite 100, Laval, QUE H7S 2J7	
Ortho-Tec Limited	905-571-3633
585 Wentworth St. E #31, Oshawa, ONT L1H-3V8	
Orthocanada Medical Products	800-561-0310
37 Katimavik Rd., Val-des-Monts, QUE J8N-5E1	
Orthofab Inc.	800-463-5293
2160 rue de Celles, Quebec, QUE G2C-1X8	
Orthologic Canada	602-286-5520
901 Dillingham Rd, Pickering L1W 2Y5	
Orthomotion Inc.	800-387-5139
901 Dillingham Rd., Pickering, ONT L1W 2Y5	
Orthopaedic Services	905-529-0395
280 Barton St. E, Hamilton, ONT L8L-2X3	
Orthopro Enr.	800-267-4344
30 Rue De L'artisan, Victoriaville, QUE G6P 7E4	
Osram Sylvania Ltd./Ltee	905 673 61 71
1 Sylvan St., Drummondville, QUEBE J2C 2S8	
Oto Hearing Products Ltd.	800-661-7723
12837 76th Ave., Unit 214, Surrey, BC V3W-2V3	
Ottawa Instrumentation Ltd.	613-563-8159
169 Fifth Ave., Ottawa, ONT K1S-2MS	
Oxybec Medical	800 361 9911
981 King Street West, Sherbrooke, QUE 981 King Stre	
Paradigm Medical Inc.	800-931-2739
116 Spadina Ave., Ste. 407, Toronto, ONT M5V-2K6	
Paragon Foot Orthotic Laboratory Ltd.	250-721-1112
1650 Cedar Hill Cross Rd., Victoria, BC V8P-2P6	
Paramedic Inc.	1 800 465-1255
3535, boul. St. Francis, Saguenay, QUE G7X 2W5	
Paramedic Instrumentation Ltd.	604-266-1354
2835 Oliver Cres, Vancouver, BC V6L 1T1	
Parkes Scientific Canada Inc.	780-484-1849
108 Ave. #17360, Edmonton, ALB T5S-1E8	
Parsons A.D.L. Inc.	800-263-1281
R.R. #2, 1986 Sideroad 15, Tottenham, ONT L0G 1W0	
Pdg Product Design Group, Inc.	888-858-4422
Unit 102, 366 East Kent Ave. South, Vancouver, BC V5X 4N6	
Pediatric Seating Dist., Inc.	416-604-9219
2833 Dundas St W, Toronto M6P 1Y6	
Pegasus Products Inc.	800-865-6767
1 Paisley Rd., Carroll, MAN R0K-0K0	
Pendragon Medical Inc.	800-667-5941
20 Devlin Place, Aurora, ONT L4G 5W6	
Personal Mobility Products Ltd.	604-576-1323
17780 56th Ave., Ste. 102, Surrey, BC V3S-4T7	
Phakosystems, Inc.	416-503-4200
14 Plastics Ave, Toronto M8Z 4B7	
Pharmaffair Inc.	416-444-8090
52 Sanfield Road, Toronto, ONT M3B-2B7	
Pharmascience Medical Division	800-340-9735
6111 Royalmount Ave., Montreal, QUE H4T-2T4	
Pharmasystems Inc.	888-475-2500
361 Steelcase Rd. W, Unit 10, Markham, ONT L3R-3V8	
Pharmax Canada Limited	800-269-7898
80 Galaxy Blvd., Unit 4, Toronto, ONT M9W-4Y8	
Pheromone Science Corp.	416-861-9854
443 King St. E, Toronto, ONT M5A-1L5	
Phoenix Bio-Tech Corp.	800-701-7450
6810 Kitimat Rd., Unit 1, Mississauga, ONT L5N-5M2	
Phoenix Biomedical Products, Inc.	9056708299
7085 Tomken Rd., Mississauga, ONT L5S-1R7	
Phonic Ear, Ltd.	800-263-8700
7475 Kimbel St, Mississauga, ON L5S 1E7	
Physipro Inc.	800-668-2252
10 Ave. Sud, #370, Sherbrooke, QUE J1G-2R7	
Pilling Weck (Canada) Inc.	800-387-9699
165 Gibson Dr., Ste. 1, Markham, ONT L3R-3K7	
Pilot Performance Resource Management	905-792-3130
25 Great Lakes Drive, P.O. Box 68584, Brampton, ONT L6R 0J8	
Plitron Manufacturing, Inc.	(1-800-754-8766
8-601 Magnetic Dr, Toronto, ON M3J 3J2	
Polar Plastic Ltd.	514-331-0207
4210 Thimens Blvd., St. Laurent, QUE H4R 2B9	
Polymed Surgical Inc.	800-361-9840
387, avenue Sainte-Croix, Saint-Laurent, QUE H4N 2L3	
Positron Industries Inc.	1-888-577-5254
5101 rue Buchan, Suite 220, Montreal, QC H4P 2R9	
Precious Life Saving Products, Inc.	416-644-0011
101-200 Ronson Dr, Toronto M9W 5Z9	
Precision Biologic, Inc.	800-267-2796
140 Eileen Stubbs Avenue, Dartmouth, NS B3B 0A9	
Precision Rehabilitation	800-895-5891
4 Cataraqui St., Ste. 316, Suite 316, Kingston, ONT K7K-1Z7	
Primed Instruments, Inc.	877-565-0565
1080 Tristar Dr., Unit 14, Mississauga, ONTAR L5T 1P1	
Primeline Medical Products Inc.	780-497-7600
3rd Floor, 1259-91 Street SW, Edmonton, ALB T6X 1E9	
Pro Bed Medical Techonogies, Inc.	800-816-8243
602-30930 Wheel Ave., Abbotsford, BC V2T 6G7	
Pro-Western Plastics Ltd.	800-661-9835
30 Riel Dr., P.O. Box 261, St. Albert, ALBER T8N-1N3	
Probed Medical Technologies Inc.	800-816-8243
30930 Wheel Ave. #602, Abbotsford, BC V2T-6G7	
Product Design Group	888-858-4422
103-366 Kent Ave South East, Vancouver, BC V5X-4N6	
Prolab Scientific	800-556-5226
2213 le Chatelier St., Laval, QUE H7L-5B3	
Proquest Canada Inc.	905-607-7190
4167 Treetop Crescent, Mississauga, ONT L5L-2L7	
Proscience Inc., Glass Shop Division	1-888-335-9113
770 Birchmount Rd., Unit 25, Scarborough, ONT M1K-5H3	
Protective Medical Products (Pmp) Inc.	888-669-9470
95 chemin Du Lac, Gatineau, QUE J8P-4H3	
Protector Canada Inc.	800-268-6594
1111 Flint Rd., Unit 23, Toronto, ON M3J 3C7	
Pulmonox Medical Corporation	888-464-8742
5243-53 Ave, Tofield, ALB T0B 4J0	
Pulse Scientific, Inc.	800-363-7907
5100 S. Service Rd., Unit 18, Burlington, ONT L7L-6A5	
Pyng Medical Corp.	1- 800-349-7964
13511 Crestwood Pl. #7, Richmond, BC V6V-2E9	
Q'straint	800-987-9987
100 Sheldon Dr., Unit 18, Cambridge, ONT N1R-7S7	
Qlt Inc.	800-663-5486
887 Great Northern Way, Vancouver, BC V5T-4T5	
Qmd Medical	800-665-9950
9800 Clark St., Montreal, QUE H3L 2R3	
Quadromed Inc.	800-363-0192
2365 Rue Guenette, St-Laurent, QC H4R 2E9	
Qualisys Diagnostics Inc.	877-825-4797
522 Meloche Ave., Dorval, QUE H9P-2T2	
Quden Inc.	450-243-6101
8 Maple, Cp 510, Knowlton J0E 1V0	
Quelab Laboratories Inc.	800-361-1434
5615 Fullum, Montreal, QUE H2G 2H6	
Questron Technologies Corporation	905-363-1223
6725 Millcreek Drive, Unit 7, Mississauga, ONT L5N 5V3	
R.A.E. Technologies Inc.	905-428-6384
48 Barbour Crescent, Ajax, ONT L1S-6Z6	
Radd Precision Inc.	905-760-1045
60 Citation Dr., Concord, ONT L4K-2W9	
Rampmaster Division Of Thorweld	416-741-2501
174 Milvan Dr., Weston, ONT M9L 1Z9	
Ramsoft, Inc.	416-674-1347
37 Bankview Cir, Etobicoke M9W 6S6	

Rana Medical
205 Stephen St., Morden, MAN R6M-1V2 — 888-297-7889

Ranger Wheelchairs Ltd.
14722 64th Ave., Unit 16, Surrey, BC V3S-1X7 — 888.745.7888

Rapid Aid Ltd.
4120A Sladeview Crescent, Units 1-4, Mississauga, ONT L5L-5Z3 — 800-265-3468

Raymax Medical Corp.
20 Strathearn Ave, Unit 3, Brampton, ONT L6T 4P7 — 905-791-3020

Rayonix Inc.
5685 boul. De l'Ormiere, Quebec, QUE G1P-1K6 — 800-463-2262

Rayovac Canada, Inc.
5448 Timberlea Blvd., Mississauga, ONT L4W-2T7 — 800-268-0425

Rd Service, Division Of Nicram Enviro Inc.
2760 Paulus St., Saint-Laurent, QUE H4S-1G1 — 800-667-0127

Real Ideas Rehabilitation Div. Inc.
34142 York Ave, Mission V2V 6Y5 — 604-820-8916

Regal Medi-Spa Co., Inc.
166 Torbay Rd, Markham L3R 1G6 — 905-477-7689

Regency Medical Supplies
4437 Canada Way, Burnaby, BC V5G-1J3 — 800-663-1012

Rehabilitation Center For Children Inc.
633 Wellington Cres, Winnipeg R3M 0A8 — 204-452-4311

Relief Wrap Ltd.
15a Oak Ave, Paris N3L 3C6 — 519-442-5071

Remed Scientific Ltd.
238 Alvin Narod Mews, Ste. 238, Vancouver, BC V6B-5Z3 — 604-899-8985

Remington Medical Equipment Ltd.
401 Bently St. #9, Markham, ONT L3R-9T2 — 800-267-5822

Reno Micro Precision Ltee
8422 10th Ave., Montreal, QUE H1Z-3B5 — 514-728-4785

Res-Q Products Inc.
P.O. Box 661, Quathiaski Cove, BC V0P-1N0 — 250-285-2890

Resonant Medical
2050 Bleury Street, Suite 200, Montreal, QUEBE H3A 2J5 — 877-985-2442

Respan Prod. Inc.
8 Erinville Dr., Erin, ONT N0B 1T0 — 800-267-4063

Respircare
1000 Thomas Spratt Pl., Ottawa, ONT K1G-5L5 — 800-267-6352

Response Biomedical Corp.
1781 75th Ave. W., Vancouver, BC V6P 6P2 — 888-591-5577

Richardson Access Elevator Inc.
1244 Trafalgar St., London, ONT N5Z-1H5 — 800-268-7745

Richardson Electronics Canada Ltd.
4 Paget Rd., Unit 1, Brampton, ONT L6T-5G3 — 800-348-5580

Ridalco Industries Inc.
1551 Michael St., Ottawa, ONT K1B-3T4 — 613-745-9161

Rideau Orthodontic Mfg., Ltd.
69 Beckwith St N, Smiths Falls K7A 2B6 — 613-283-6841

Rms Instruments
6877-1 Goreway Dr., Mississauga, ONT L4V 1L9 — 905-677-5533

Roberts & Gordon Canada, Inc.
76 Main St. West, Unit 10, Grimsby, ON L3M-1R6 — 905-945-5403

Roche Diagnostics
201 Armand-Frappier Blvd., Laval, QUE H7V 4A2 — 800-361-2070

Ross Disposable Products
411 Bradwick Drive, Unit 12, Concord, ON L4K 2P4 — 800-649-6526

Rotoflex International Inc.
420 Ambassador Dr., Mississauga, ONT L5T 1P9 — 800-387-3825

Roxon Medi-Tech Ltd.
9400 Pascal Gagnon, St-Leonard, QUE H1P 1Z7 — 800-361-6991

Roxon--Universal Medical Ltd.
#144, 15501 - 89A Avenue, Surrey, BC V3R 0Z5 — (800) 667-7408

Royco Apparatus Ltd.
P.O. Box 277, Kleinburg, ONT L0J-1C0 — 905-893-1972

Rtr Industries, Inc.
700 York St, London N5W 2S8 — 519-438-3691

Sacor Inc.
12 - 300 Steelcase Rd. W., Markham, ONT L3R 2W2 — 800-263-3557

Safari Dental Inc.
94D boul. Des Enterprises, Boisbriand, QUE J7E-2T3 — 800-567-0013

Safecross First Aid Ltd.
1111 Alness St, Toronto M3J 2J1 — 416-665-0050

Safety Today Inc.
90 Morton Ave E, Brantford, ONT N3R 7J7 — 800-263-1251

Sandfire Scientific Ltd.
1019 Venture Way, Gibsons, BC V0N-1V7 — 604-886-9003

Sands Canada Inc.
P.O. Box 1752, Brockville, ONT K6V-6K8 — 800-563-0911

Sandstrom Trade & Technology, Inc.
610 Niagara St., P.O. Box 850, Welland, ONT L3C 1L8 — 800-699-0745

Savaria Corporation
107 Alfed Kuehne Blvd., Brampton, ONT L6T-4K3 — 800-661-5112

Sca Hygiene Products Inc.
2010 Winston Park Dr., Ste. 300, Oakville, ONT L6H-5R7 — 800-361-6944

Schaan Healthcare Products Inc.
820 45th St. W., Saskatoon, SK S7K-4E4 — 800-667-3786

Schukra Manufacturing Inc.
310 Carlingview Dr., Toronto, ON M9W 5G1 — 800-663-7248

Scican
1440 Don Mills Rd., Toronto, ON M3B 3P9 — 800-667-7733

Sciencetech Inc.
1450 Global Drive, London, ONT N6N 1R3 — 519-644-0135

Scientek Hospital And Laboratory Equipment
7943A Progress Way, Delta, BC V4G 1A3 — 866-321-3828

Scientek Medical Equipment
11151 Bridgeport Rd., Richmond, BC V6X 1T3 — 604-273-9094

Scientific Products & Equipment Ltd. (S.P.E.)
95 Barber Greene Road, Suite 303, North York, ONT M3C 3E9 — 800-268-1956

Scireq Inc.
6600 St-Urbain, Suite 300, Montreal, QUE H2S 3G8 — 514-286-1429

Scooter-Tote
739 Princess Rd., New Westminster, BC V3M-6V6 — 604-517-3990

Scp Science
21800 Clark Graham Ave., Baie D'Urfe, QUE H9X-4B6 — 800-361-6820

Second Skin Rubber Products
5484 Royalmount Ave., Mont-Royal, QUE H4P-1H7 — 1-888-565-SKIN

Segufix Systems Ltd.
110 Queen St., Woodstock, NB E7M-2M6 — 1-877-734-8349

Sentech Systems Inc.
1445 Bonhill Rd. #10, Mississauga, ONT L5T-1V3 — 800-263-8534

Serum International Inc.
4400 Autoroute Chomeoey, Laval, QUEBE H7R-6E9 — 800-361-7726

Settler Medical Electronics Inc.
723 Queenston St, Winnipeg R3N 0X8 —

Shoppers Home Health Care Doncaster
243 Consumers Rd., North York, ONT M2J-4W8 — 800-363-1020

Shoprider Canada Mobility Products
1360 Cliveden Ave, Delta, BC V3M 6K2 — 888-999-0895

Shoreline Healthco Inc.
23 Victoria St., P.O. Box 628, Clinton, ONT N0M-1L0 — 888-233-7038

Sigmacon Health Products Corp.
436 Limestone Crescent, North York, ON M3J 2S4 — 800-898-7455

Sigvaris Corporation
4535 Dobrin, Ville St-Laurent, QUE H4R 2L8 — 800-363-4999

Simpler Implants Inc.
Suite 404-1023 Wolfe Ave., Vancouver, BC V6H 1V6 — 800-565-3559

Simport Plastics Ltd.
2588 Bernard-Pilon, Beloeil, QUE J3G 4S5 — 450-464-1723

Sirius Genomics Inc.
1125 Howe Street, Suite 603, Vancouver, BC V6Z 2K8 — 604-484-7195

Slawner Ltd., J.
5713, ch. de la CA'te-des-Neiges, Montreal, QUE H3S 1Y7 — 514-731-3378

Softcare Innovations Inc.
541 Mill Street., Suite 2, Kitchener, ONT N2G 2Y5 — 1-800-663-1509

Somagen Diagnostics Inc.
9220 - 25 Avenue, Edmonton, ALB T6N 1E1 — 800-661-9993

Sonometrics Corporation
500 Nottinghill Road, London, ONT N6K 3P1 — 519-474-6464

Sony Of Canada Ltd., Medical Systems
115 Gordon Baker Rd., Toronto, ONT M2H-3R6 — 800-361-5535

Soquelec Limited
5757 Cavendish Blvd., Ste. 101, Montreal, QUE H4W-2W8 — 514-482-6427

Sos Rehabilitation Products Inc.
3359 RUE GRIFFITH, St-Laurent, QUE H4T 1W5 — 800-667-3422

Source Medical Corporation
60 International Blvd., Toronto, ON M9W 6J2 — 888-871-5945

Southmedic Inc.
50 Alliance Blvd., Barrie, ONT L4M-5K3 — 800-463-7146

Spadina Industries Inc.
110 Apex St., Saskatoon, SK S7R-1C8 — 800-665-2337

Spartan Biosciences
6 Gurdwara Road, Suite 204q, Ottawa, ONTAR K2E 8A3 — 877-228-7756

Spectral Diagnostics Inc.
135-2 The West Mall, Toronto, ON M9C 1C2 — 888-426-4264

Spectrum Medical Market Consultants
475 Westminster Ave., Dollard-des-Ormeaux, QUE H9G-2S3 — 514-696-0303

Spenco Medical
6905 Millcreek Dr., Unit 12, Mississauga, ONT L5N-6A3 — 800-387-9538

Splenodex Canada Inc.
109 Ch Des Ormes Rr 121, Sainte-Anne-Des-Lacs J0R 1B0 — 514-224-1080

Sqi Diagnostics
36 Meteor Dr., Toronto, ONT M9W-1A4 — 416-674-9500

Starkman Surgical Supply Ltd.
1243 Bathurst St., Toronto, ONT M5R-3H3 — 800-387-0330

Starplex Scientific Inc.
50A Steinway Blvd., Etobicoke, ONT M9W 6Y3 — 800-665-0954

Stat Healthcare Corporation
6215 3rd St. SE, Unit C12, Calgary, ALB T2H-2L2 — 800-567-6001

Staxi Corporation Ltd.
201 Millway Ave., Unit 5, Concord, ONT L4K-5K8 — 877-677-8294

Stellate Systems
300-345 Av Victoria, Westmount H3Z 2N2 — 514-486-1306

Sterne Equipment Co., Ltd.
20 Strathearn Avenue Unit #4, Brampton, ONTAR L6T 4P7 — 905-457-2524

Stockeryale
275 Kesmark, Montreal, QUEBE H9B 3J1 — 800-814-9552

Stratcom
1743 Sunnybrooke, Dollard-des-Ormeaux, QUE H9B-1R5 — 514-421-2705

Strite Industries Ltd.
298 Shepherd Ave., Cambridge, ON N3C 1V1 — 800-267-7333

Sudor Inc.
P.O. Box 383, Collingwood, ONT L9Y-3Z7 — 705-445-0606

Sulzer Mitroflow Corp.
11220 Voyageur Way #1, Richmond, BC V6X-3E1 — 604-270-7751

Summit Technologies Inc.   800-268-7916
2333 Wyecroft Rd., Unit 1, Oakville, ONT L6L-6L4

Sunnex Biotechnologies   877-778-6639
167 Lombard Ave., Suite 657, Winnipeg, MB R3B-0V3

Superior Medical Limited   800-268-7944
520 Champagne Dr., Toronto, ONT M3J 2T9

Supporo Canada Inc.   800-361-6857
9675 Papineau #175, Montreal, QUE H2B-3C8

Surgical Products Specialties   604-536-4000
1908 168th St., Surrey, BC V4P-2W7

Swenson Canada Inc.   800-561-2863
80 Orfus Rd., Toronto, ONT M6A-1M1

Swiss Nf Metals Inc.   800-387-5031
461 Alden Road, Unit 26 & 27, Markham, ONT M3B-3N2

Symmetric Designs, Ltd.   800-537-1724
125 Knott Place, Salt Spring Island, BC V8K 2M4

Synermed International Inc.   800-361-3552
1688 50th Ave., Lachine, QUE H8T-2V5

T.B. Clift Limited   800-563-7205
34 O'Leary Ave., P.O. Box 8870, St. John's, MAN A1B-3T2

Taro Pharmaceuticals, Inc.   905-791-8276
130 East Dr, Brampton L6T 1C1

Task Micro-Electronics Inc.   514-697-6616
16700 TransCanada Hwy, Montreal, QUE H9H-4M7

Techmire Ltd.   514-694-4110
185 Voyageur, Pointe Claire,, QC H9R 6B2

Techno Scientific Inc.   905-760-1745
259 Edgeley Blvd., Unit 11-12, Concord, ONT L4K 3Y5

Technologies Of Sterilization With Ozone (Tso3) Inc.   1-866-715-0003
2505 Dalton Ave., Ste-Foy, QUE G1P-3S5

Technomedic Inc.   416-743-0009
4 Racine Road, Unit 7, Etobicoke, ONT M9W 5W7

Tecogics Scientific Ltd.   1-888-298-9922
2430 Magnus Avenue, Ottawa, ONT K1G 1J8

Tempur Canada   519-660-4154
1807 Wonderland Road N., London, ONT N6G 5C2

Tenet Medical Engineering, Inc.   888-836-3863
5540 1A St. SW, Calgary, ALB T2H 0E7

Terra Nova Biotechnology Co. Ltd.   800-851-1677
P.O. Box 13340, St. John's, NF A1B-4B7

Tex-Pro Western Limited   800-663-9266
828 Powell St., Vancouver, BC V6A-1H8

The Align-Right Pillow Co. Ltd.   800-331-0907
881 Guelph Street, Kitchener, ONTAR N2H 1X5

The Gotzen Group, Inc.   905-607-1494
7-3505 Laird Rd, Mississauga L5L 5Y7

The Horizon Phoenix Group Limited   800-718-8218
3219 Yonge St., Ste. 248, Toronto, ONT M4N-3S1

The Medipattern Corporation   416-744-0009
3080 Yonge St., Suite 4070, Toronto, ON M4N 3N1

The Orthotic Group, Inc.   800-551-3008
160 Markland Street, Markham, ONT L6C 0C6

The Scale Shop Ltd.   888-844-2031
86 Clyde Ave., Mount Peal, NF A1N-4S2

The Stevens Company Ltd.   800-268-0184
425 Railside Drive, Brampton, ONT L7A 0N8

The Universal Handicycle Wheelchair   604-595-8632
2214 Belmont Ave, Victoria V8R 3Z8

Thera-P-Cushion   800-567-9926
46 Dufflaw Road, Toronto, ONT M6A 2W1

Theralase Inc.   866-843-5273
102-29 Gervais Dr., Toronto, ON M3C 1Y9

Theramed Corporation   800-305-4441
6891 Edwards Blvd., Mississauga, ONT L5T 2T9

Therapist's Choice Medical Supplies   800-263-6618
944 Lawrence Ave. West, Toronto, ONT M6A-1C4

Theratechnologies Inc.   514-336-7800
2310 Alfred-Nobel Blvd., St-Laurent, QUE H4S-2A4

Thermotex Therapy Systems Ltd.   800-975-0253
6115 4th St. SE #15, Calgary, ALB T2H-2H9

Thought Technology Ltd.   800-361-3651
2180 Belgrave Avenue, Montreal, QUEBE H4A 2L8

Thought Technology Ltd.   800-361-3651
8205 Montreal / Toronto Boulevard, Suite 223, Montreal West, QUE H4X 1N1

Tipal Instruments Ltd.   514-484-9741
128 Prom Ronald, Montreal-Ouest H4X 1M8

Tki Medcon Inc.   800-854-0166
1066 Somerset St. W, Unit 100, Ottawa, ONT K1Y-4T3

Tna (Tami North America)   514.334.7417
2865 Sabourin Street, St-Laurent, QUE H4S 1M9

Topcon Canada Inc.   800-361-3515
110 Provencher Ave., Boisbriand, QUE J7G-1N1

Toronto Research Chemicals Inc.   800-727-9240
2 Brisbane Rd., Toronto, ONT M3J-2J8

Total Healthcare Equipment (T.H.E.) Medical   800-565-7075
75 Dyment Rd., Barrie, ONT L4N 3H6

Trainer's Choice Inc.   800-706-9834
205-480 Huronia Road, Barrie, ONT L4N 6M2

Trevor Owen Limited   866-487-2224
80 Barbados Blvd., Unit 5, Scarborough, ONT M1J-1K9

Tri Hawk Inc.   877-874-4295
P.O. Box 619, Morrisburg, ONTAR K0C 1X0

Tri-Star Industries Ltd.   902-742-9254
88 Forest Street, Yarmouth, NS B5A 4B4

Triple G Systems Group, Inc.   905-305-0041
600-3100 Steeles Ave E, Markham L3R 8T3

Trudell Medical Marketing Ltd.   800-265-5494
758 Third Street, London, ON N5V 5J7

Truppe Health Care Products And Services Ltd.   800-854-1237
2500 Main St., Lambeth, ONT N6P-1P9

Tsi Technologies Inc.   905-760-1745
259 Edgeley Blvd, Unit 11-12, Concord, ONT L4K-3W7

Tsk Laboratory Canada Inc.   -604-269-3490
1660 West 75th Avenue, Vancouver, BC V6P6G2

Tunstall Canada Inc.   800-892-2205
7540 Bath Rd., Mississauga, ONT L4T-1L2

Tykris Inc.   905-854-3009
3272 15th Side Rd., P.O. Box 309, Campbellville, ONT L0P-1B0

Tyler Research Corporation   780-448-1249
10328 73rd Ave., Edmonton, ALB T6E-6N5

Ultra Ray Inc.   877-338-6857
760 Pacific Rd Unit 12, Oakville, ONT L6L 6M5

Ultramed Inc.   800-804-3544
50 Sleeles Ave. E, Ste. 15, Milton, ONT L9T-4W9

Ultrasonix Medical Corporation   604-279-8550
130 - 4311 Viking Way, Richmond, BC V6V 2K9

Unicare Medical Products Inc.   800-668-2030
770 Lawrence Ave. W, Toronto, ONT M6A-1B8

Unilab Surgibone Inc.   905-564-3474
5790 Atlantic Dr., Unit 2, Mississauga, ONT L4W-4N8

Unilab, Inc.   9058559093
2355 Royal Windsor Dr., Unit 3, Mississauga, ON L5M-5R5

Unitron Industries Ltd.   877-492-6244
20 Beasley Dr., P.O. Box 9017, Kitchener, ONT N2G 4X1

Universal X-Ray Co. Of Canada Ltd.   514-631-4477
1370-55th Avenue, Lachine, QUE H8T 3J8

Uplift Technologies, Inc.   800-387-0896
125-11 Morris Dr., Dartmouth, NS B3B 1K8

Val-U-Med Inc.   800-668-3168
673 Colborne St., P.O. Box 1206, Brantford, ONT N3S-3M8

Valeant Canada Ltd   1-800-361-1448
4787 Levy Street, Montreal, QUEBE H4R 2P9

Valmark, Inc.   613-822-3107
P.O. Box 190, Gloucester, ONT K1X-1A4

Valued Medical Care (Vmc) Inc.   800-673-0555
262 Robertson Rd., P.O. Box 1188, Hampton, NB E5N-8H2

Variety Ability Systems Inc.   800-891-4514
2 Kelvin Ave., Unit 3, Toronto, ONT M4C-5C8

Vasogen Inc.   905-569-2265
2505 Meadowvale Blvd, Mississauga, ONT L5L-4M1

Vat-Tech, Inc.   705-687-8717
684 Muskoka Rd N, Gravenhurst P1P 1E7

Velcro Canada Inc.   800-683-5276
114 East Dr., Brampton, ONT L6T-1C1

Vereburn Supply Ltd.   800-263-1055
2235 27th Ave. NE, Calgary, ALB T2E-7M4

Verg, Inc.   800-563-7676
55 Henlow Bay, #3, Winnipeg, MANIT R3G-1L1

Vernacare   800-268-2422
200 Trowers Rd., Unit 3, Woodbridge, ONT L4L-5Z7

Visibilite Inc.   800-926-2466
1221 Labadie, Local 204, Longueuil, QUE J4N-1E2

Vision Medical Inc.   877-448-1234
#100, 10479 - 184th Street, Edmonton, ALB T5S 2L1

Vision Wheelchair Seating Systems Inc.   416-665-8428
24-600 Bowes Road, Concord, ONT L4K 4A3

Visioptic Inc.   514-842-4601
1117 St. Catherine St. W, Ste. 324, Montreal, QUE H3B-1H9

Vista Medical Ltd.   1-800-822-3553
3 - 55 Henlow Bay., Winnipeg, MAN R3Y 1G4

Vista Technology, Inc.   888-468-0020
8432 45th St. NW, Edmonton, ALBER T6B-2N6

Visuaide   888-723-7273
445, rue du Parc-Industriel, Longueil, QUE J4H 3V7

VisualSonics Inc.   1-866-416-4636
3080 Yonge Street, Suite 6100, Toronto, ON M4N 3N1

Vitacare Medical Products Inc.   800-263-9068
331 Bowes Rd., Concorrd, ONT L4K-1J2

Vitalaire   800-661-8954
2000 Argentia Rd., Plaza 2, Ste. 200, Mississauga, ONT L5N-1V8

Vonex Medical Supplies Inc.   888-866-3920
29-601 Magnetic Dr., Toronto M3J 3J2

Vorum Research Corporation   800-461-4353
8765 Ash St., Ste. 6, Vancouver, BC V6P-6T3

Vsm Medtech (Formerly Ctf Systems)   604-540-6044 ex
Unit 1, 1850 Hartley Avenue, Coquitlam, BC V3K 7A1

Vsm Medtech Ltd.   604-738-8763
675 West Hastings St., 15th Floor, Vancouver, BC V6B-1N2

Vwr Canlab   800-932-5000
2360 Argentia Rd., Mississauga, ONT L5N-5Z7

W. Laframboise Ltd.   800-363-8549
11450 Albert-Hudon, Montreal-Nord, QUE H1G 3J9

Walkers, Inc., E. C.   800-494-8589
375 Rexdale Boulevard, Toronto, ONT M9W 1R9

Waverley Glen Systems 480 University Ave., Ste 100, Toronto, ONTAR M5G 1V2	1.877.304.5438
Web-Tex, Inc. 5425 Casgrain, Suite 300, Montreal, QC H2T 1X6	888-633-2723
Weevac, W. Murphy Enterprises, Inc. 12 La Salle Dr., P.O. Box 1306, Deep River, ONT K0J 1P0	613-584-9473
Xillix Technologies Corp. 13775 Commerce Pkwy., Ste. 100, Richmond, BC V6V 2V4	800-665-2236
3m Canada Company 1840 Oxford St. E., London, ONT N5V 3R6	800-364-3577
883495 Ontario, Inc. 2-759 Progress Ave, Kingston K7M 6N6	613-384-9550
928735 Ontario, Ltd. 8-24 Viceroy Rd, Concord L4K 2L9	905-660-1030

H3B 4G1

Intelerad 895 de la GauchetiAüï'A,A, re Street W., Suite 400, Montr QC	514-931-6222

MEXICO

Veco, S.A. De C.V. Pirineos No. 263, Col. General Anaya, Mexico D.F., BENIT 03100	55-688-3566
Ambiderm, S.A. De C.V. Carr. A Bosques De San Isidro 1136, Col. Bosques De San Isidro, Zapopan, Jalisco 45147	800-800-8008
American Optical Lens Mex S. De R.L. De C.V. Calle 2, Orienta #133,, C.d. Industrial Mesa De Otay, Tijuana, B.c.	408-735-1982
Arrow Internacional De Mexico, S.A. De C.V. Modulo 1, Circuito 5, Parque Industrias De America, Col. Panamericana, Chihuahua	610-378-0131
Artefactos De Vidrio S.A. De C.V. Canela, Granjas Mexico 346, Ciudad De Mexico 08400	
Articulos Higienicos S.A. De C.V. Av. TransformaciA3n #4, Parque Ind. Cuamtla, Cuautitlan Izcalli, EDO D 54730	52 55 58997980
Avent S.A. De C.V. Camino De Libramiento, Km. 1.5, Nogales, Sonora	602-748-6900
Avent S.A. De C.V. Carretera Intl., Salida Norte, Magdalena, Sonora	770-587-8393
Bard Reynosa S.A. De C.V. Blvd. Montebello #1, Parque Industrial Colonial, Reynosa, Tamaulipas	908-277-8000
Block Medical De Mexico S.A. De C.V. La Mesa Parque Industrial, Paseo Reforma S/n, Fracc., Tijuana, Bc	949-206-2700
Cardio-Nef, S.A. De C.V. Rio Grijalva 186, Col. Mitras Norte, Monterrey, N.L. 64320	800-024-0240
Casa Plarre, S.A. De C.V. Av. Cuahtemoc 220-201, Mexico D.F. 06720	+51 34 02 70
Comercializadora Medica Alvasan S.A. De C.V. Eulalio Gutierrez #303, Col. Francisco Villa, San Nicolas De Los Garza, NL 66430	01 800-71026-33
Degasa, S.A. De C.V. Prolongacion Canal De, Miramontes #3775 Col. Ex-, Hacienda San Juan Del. Tlalpan	525-5-483 31
Delta Systems De Mexico Prolongacion Las Lomas No. 16, Tijuana, B.c.	702-331-1890
Disenos Termoelectricos Luyfel 7424 Juarez Porvenir, Cd. Juarez	16-17-0425
Distribuidora Caisa,.S.A.De C.V. Adolfo Prieto 1759-b, Del Valle, Ciudad De Mexico, DF 03100	5-534-3044
Dj Orthopedics De Mexico, S.A. De C.V. Ave. Venustiano Carranza 6802, Castillo, Tijuana 22100	690-727-1280
Dj Orthopedics De Mexico, S.A. De C.V. Blvd., Delagacion La Presa, Tijuana 22397	690-727-1280
Elamex S.A. De C.V. Av. Insurgentes 4145 lote., Cd. Jiarex, Chih	52-16-164333
Erika De Reynosa, S.A. De C.V. Brecha E99 Sur, Parque, Industrial Reynos, Bldg. Ii, Cd, Reynosa, Tamps	781-402-9068
Everest & Jennings De Mexico S.A. De C.V. Calle 3 No.631, Zona Industrial, Guadalajara, JALIS 44940	333-145-1045
Farmaceuticos Altamirano De Mexico, S.A. BLVD. Adolfo Lopez Mateos NO .- 957,, COL. AUGUST 8, DEL., ALVARO OBREGON, DF CP 01180	52 (55) 52-71-4
Farmatap S.A. De C.V. 117 Alfonso Esparza Oteo, Mexico Df 01020	
Galia Textil S.A. De C.V. Lote 3 Manzana 4, Parque Industrial, Tlaxcala	246-1-6-066
Gemspro, S.A. De C.V. Calle B #504 Parque Industrial, Almacetro, Apodaca, N.I.	262-544-3894
Greattec Vision S.A. De C.V. Circuito De La Amistad #2700, Mexicali B.c.	
Grupo Industrial C&A, S.A. De C.V. Circuito Misioneros #26, Cd. Satelite,anucal-Pan,edo	525-562-0660
Grupo Industrial Latex, S.A. De C.V. Riveras Del Pilar, Ave. San Jorge 250-A, Chapala 45900	011-523-7653
Grupo Manufacturero Rio Grande, S.A. De C.V. Privada Aldama #113, Piedras Negras, Coah.	878-237-70
Grupo Servisan Mar Baltico 26, Col.Popotla, Ciudad De Mexico, DF 11400	5-396-3620
Guantes Quirurgicos, S.A. De C.V. 366 Henry Ford Ave.,, Deleg. Gustavo A. Madero, Mexico City, D.f.	525-760-5122
Hospitecnica, S.A. De C.V. Ave. Universidad 771, DF cp. 03100	800 003-3400
Indelpa, S.A. De C.V. Carlos B. Zetina No. 22, Xalostoc	609-983-8006

Industrias Medison, S.A. De C.V. Lote 7 Manzana 3 Parque, Industrial De Cananea,km.5, Carretera a Inuris, Sonora	800-851-4431
Industrias Tuk, S.A. De C.V. Antigua Carretera a Roma, Km 7 5¯, Apodaca 66632	8-313-7421-2
Intermex Trading & Supports Sa De Cv. Rio Neva 33 Col.cuauthemoc, Mexico City Of, Df	52-553-58953
Invamex S.A. De C.V. Carretera Reynosa-Matamros,, Km#1, Reynosa Tamaulipas	440-329-6595
Johnson & Johnson De Monterrey, Sa De Cv Carretera Miguel Aleman,km21.7, Apodaca, Monterrey	817-262-5211
Kelsar, S.A. Blvd. Insurgentes, Libriamiento a La, Tijuana 22450	508-261-8000
Kendall De Mexico, S.A. De C.V. Piniente 44, No. 3401, 16 D.f, Co. San Salvador Xochimanca, Mexico City	508-261-8000
Kendall Kenmex, A Division Of Tyco Healthcare Group Lp Calle 9 Sur No. 125, Tijuana CP 22500	(01152) 664-623
Laboratorios Jaloma, S.A. De C.V. Aquiles Serdan No. 438, Guadalajara, Jalisco	3-617-5010
Lakeland De Mexico S.A De C.V. Rancho La Soledad Lote No. 2, Fracc. Poniente C.p., Celaya, Guajuato	516-981-9700
Leesan Maquilas S.A. De C.V. Enrique Dunant No., 12 Centro, Tlalnepantla,edo.de Mexico Cp	52-5-561-526
Manufacturera Dental Continental 2113 Calle Indust Del Plastico, 269 Fracc Zapopan Indust Norte, Zapopan, Jalisco	523-633-8329
Maquilas Teta-Kawi, S.A. Carretera Internacional, Km 1969, Enpalme, Sonora	413-593-6400
Mayo Medical, S.A. De C.V. Edison 1141 Nte., Col. Talleres, Monterrey N.L. 64480	800-715-3872
Meddex, S.A. Calz. Ermita Iztapalapa, #855,, Col. Sta. Isabel Industrial, Cd. Mexico, D.f.	5-581-8022
Mexicana De Equipos Dentales, S,A, Guillermo Baca 3738, Lomas De Polanco, Guadalajara 44960	523-684-8110
Mmj S.A. De C.V. 716 Ponciano Arriaga, Cd. Juarez, Chih.	314-654-2000
Monchis S.A.De. D.U. Bustamente 514 Col., Arboledas, Montemorelos, N.I	336-292-8877
North Safety Products 1101 B Calle Neutron, Parque Industrial Maran, Mexicali, B.c.	401-943-4400
Optimize Mfg. Co. Apdo Postal 205-A,, Parque Industrial San Ramon, Nogales, Sonora	520-287-4605
Orthodental S.A. De C.V. Calle Industria Del Acero 18, Parque Industrial El Vigia, Mexicali 21397	011-526-5611
Osram De Mexico Av. de la Industria, Lote 9,10,11, Tepotzotlan 54600	52 55 58 99 19
Plasco, Inc. Carretera Presta La Amistad, Km.19, Acuna, Coahila	847-662-4400
Plomeria Especializada De Baja California, S.A. De Calle Maquiladoras No. 322, Seccion Dorada, Nueva Tijuana, Baja California	626-336-4561
Precise Dental Internacional S.A.C.V. 925 Parque Cuzin Belenes Norte, Zapopan, Jalisco	818-992-5333
Productos Rubbermaid, Sociedad Anonima De Capital Kmi-Ote, Carretera Cadereyta-Allende, Cadereyta Jimenez 67450	540-542-8363
Rcmex, S.A. De C.V. Av. Profr. Ramon Rivera Lara, Juarez 31857	915-598-4072
Robert Joseph Craig Sa De Cv Blvd De Santa Monica 106-204, Jardines De, Tlalnepantla	905-5600803
Sds De Mexico, S.A. De C.V. Circuito Sur 31, Parque Industrial Nelson, Mexicali 21395	714-516-7484
Servicios Paraclinicos S.A. Ave Madero 3330 Pte, Mitras Sur, Monterrey N.L. 64020	01800 581 9157
Sistemas Medicos Alaris Ave. Ferrocarril No. 16y17y18, Km. 14 1/2 Centro Ind. Limon, Tijuana, Bc. -	858-458-7000
Smith & Nephew Casting & Bandaging Sa. De Cv Ave.de Los Encinos S/n Esq.ave, Del Parque,parque Ind. Villa, Florida, Reynosa Tamaulipas	012-82-61774
Smith & Nephew, Mexico Inc. San Francisco Cuautlalpan #101, Naucalpan, Edo. De Mexico	901-396-2121
Styloptic Intl., S.A. De C.V. 274 Playa Villa Del Mar, Mexico City	301-242-2330
Supertex Industrial, S.A. De C.V. Carretera a Bosques De San, Isidro # 1136, Zapopan, Jalisco	656-65-57
Tecnomed International S.A. De C.V. Andalucia 25, Colonia Alamos, Ciudad De Mexico, DF CP 03400	01 55 5519 7234
Tino, S.A. De C.V. Hospital #631, Guadalajara, JALIS 44200	800-024-77-55
Tomas L. Ortega San Borja 1361, Mexico City	956-630-2887
Vida Medica, S.A. De C.V. Calle 6 No. 376, Col. Francisco I. Madero, Mexico D.F. 11480	5-557-4346
Western Textile Productos De Mexico S.De R.L. Dec. Francisco Murguia #514 Nte., M.muzquiz, Coahuila	314-225-9400
White Knight Healthcare Calle 16, Number 780, Agua Prieta, Sonora	800-851-4431
3m Edumex, S.A. De C.V. 6620 Oriente, Calle Ramon Rivera Lara, Ciudad de Jaurez, CHIHU 32605	651-733-4365

ON N5Y 5B8

Lac-Mac Ltd. 847 Highbury Ave. N, Building 2 É_, Londo ONT	519-432-2616

T2C 5C6
Hedy Canada
4535 É_, 104 Avenue S.E., Calga ALB
403-571-2277

V3V 3G8
Unicell Inc.
12160 É_, 103A Avenue, Surre BC
800-718-2347

SECTION III

TRADE NAME INDEX

PURPOSE OF THIS SECTION

Identifies the manufacturer of a given trade-named product.

FEATURES

- ◆ Trade names are listed alphabetically, followed by the company owning that trade name.

- ◆ Trade names that are the same as company names are generally not listed here. The company name can be located in the Manufacturer Profiles section.

- ◆ Trade names also appear in the Product Directory in the product descriptions that follow many company listings.

Health Resources from Grey House Publishing

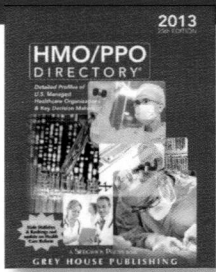

The HMO/PPO Directory

This comprehensive directory details more information about more managed health care organizations than ever before. Over 1,100 HMOs, PPOs and affiliated companies are listed, arranged alphabetically by state. Detailed listings include Key Contact Information, Drug Benefits, Enrollment, Geographical Areas served, Affiliated Physicians & Hospitals, Federal Qualifications, Status, Year Founded, Managed Care Partners, Employer References, Fees & Payment Information and more. *The HMO/PPO Directory* provides the most comprehensive information on the most companies available on the market place today.

600 pages; Softcover ISBN 978-1-59237-876-0, $325.00

Online & Directory Combo: $800.00

Online Database (Single User): $650.00

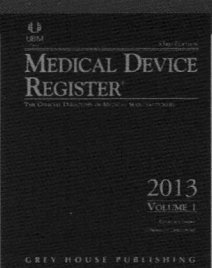

Medical Device Register

Offers fast access to over 13,000 companies - and more than 65,000 products. Volume I: Products, provides the essential information you need when purchasing or specifying medical supplies on every medical device, supply, and diagnostic available in the US. Listings provide FDA codes, Federal Procurement Eligibility, Contact information, Prices and Product Specifications. Volume 2: Suppliers, details the most complete and important data about Suppliers, Manufacturers and Distributors, with Key Executives, Contact Information along with their medical products and specialties. *Medical Device Register* is your only one-stop source for locating suppliers and products; looking for new manufacturers or hard-to-find medical devices; comparing products; know who's selling what and who to buy from cost effectively.

3,000 pages; Two Volumes; Softcover ISBN 978-1-59237-880-7, $350.00

Online Database & Print Combo, $699.00

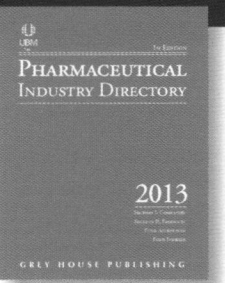

Pharmaceutical Industry Directory

This resource compiles critical information on the multi-billion dollar worldwide Pharmaceutical Industry. Coverage begins with company profiles of 5,000 Pharmaceutical Companies worldwide, with complete contact information, company description, key personnel, areas of clinical development, annual revenue, healthcare revenue, annual research and development expenditure, and number of employees. Each profile also includes a detailed list of the company's prescription drugs in development and brands on the market, over 20,000 in total. An excellent tool for research, portfolio evaluation, new business development, and competitive analyses. This new directory will be a must-have resource for professionals in the pharmaceutical and biotech industries along with public library, university and medical reference collections.

1,000 pages; Softcover ISBN 978-1-61925-174-8, $350.00

Online & Directory Combo: $950.00 | Online Database (Single User): $750.00

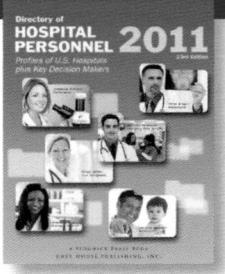

The Directory of Hospital Personnel

The Directory of Hospital Personnel is the best resource you can have at your fingertips when researching or marketing a product or service to the hospital market. A "Who's Who" of the hospital universe, this directory puts you in touch with over 150,000 key decision-makers. Every hospital in the U.S. is profiled, listed alphabetically by city within state. *The Directory of Hospital Personnel* is the only complete source for key hospital decision-makers by name. Whether you want to define or restructure sales territories... locate hospitals with the purchasing power to accept your proposals... or find information on which insurance plans are accepted, *The Directory of Hospital Personnel* gives you the information you need – easily, efficiently, effectively and accurately.

2,500 pages; Softcover ISBN 978-1-59237-856-2, $325.00

Online & Directory Combo: $800.00 | Online Database (Single User): $650.00

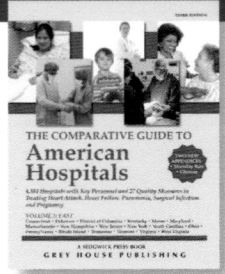

The Comparative Guide to American Hospitals

This new third edition compares and ranks all of the nation's hospitals by 49 measures of quality in the treatment of heart attack, heart failure, pneumonia, surgical procedures, pregnancy care and, new to this edition, children's asthma care, medical imaging and patient satisfaction. Each profile includes the raw percentage for that hospital, the state and US averages and data on the top hospital. Most importantly, The Comparative Guide to American Hospitals provides easy-to-use Regional State by State Statistical Summary Tables for each of the data elements to allow the user to quickly locate hospitals with the best level of service. Plus, a new 30-Day Mortality Chart, Glossary of Terms and Regional Hospital Profile Index make this a must-have source. This new, expanded edition will be a must for the reference collection at all public, medical and academic libraries.

2,000 pages; Four Volume Set; Softcover ISBN 978-1-59237-838-8, $350.00

TRADE NAME INDEX

A LA MODE	Zyloware Corporation
A T	Beckman Coulter, Inc.
A T DIFF	Beckman Coulter, Inc.
A T DIFF 2	Beckman Coulter, Inc.
A T PAK	Beckman Coulter, Inc.
A T PAK 4	Beckman Coulter, Inc.
A T RINSE	Beckman Coulter, Inc.
A T SAFE	Beckman Coulter, Inc.
A T TRAINER	Beckman Coulter, Inc.
A T TRAINER 4	Beckman Coulter, Inc.
A T TRON	Beckman Coulter, Inc.
A T VET	Beckman Coulter, Inc.
A TRAC	Applied Medical Resource Corporation
A&D ENGINEERING	Creative Health Products, Inc.
A+Q10 CREAM	Donell
A-1000	Aspect Medical Systems, Inc.
A-1050	Aspect Medical Systems, Inc.
A-2000	Aspect Medical Systems, Inc.
A-BSM	Etex Corporation
A-FACT	George King Bio-Medical, Inc.
A-LINER	Covidien Lp
A-PICK	Spirig Advanced Technologies, Inc.
A-PLUS	Knit-Rite, Inc.
A-PORT	Arrow International, Inc.
A-SCAN	Sonomed, Inc.
A-SCAN/PACHYMETER	Sonomed, Inc.
A-SMART CART SYSTEMS	Armstrong Medical Industries, Inc.
A-SOFT SILICONE	Oticon, Inc.
A-SURE	Microgenics Corporation
A-T	A-T Surgical Manufacturing Co., Inc.
A-TAQ-IT	Usb Corporation
A-TENS	American Imex
A-TRAC	C. R. Bard, Inc., Bard Urological Div.
A-VERT	Elantec Med, Inc.
A.C.T	Remel
A.D.S. 1000	Engler Engineering Corp.
A.L.A. DISK	Remel
A.N.D.	Post Medical, Inc.
A.R.T.	Depuy Ace, A Johnson & Johnson Company
A.T.S	Zimmer Holdings, Inc.
A.T.S.	Carolon Company
A.T.S.	Zimmer Orthopaedic Surgical Products
A/B-SCAN	Sonomed, Inc.
A/C LOCATOR	Scanlan International, Inc.
A/R	Dencraft
A1	Polar Electro Inc.
A2 PORT	Arrow International, Inc.
A3	Polar Electro Inc.
A312 SERIES BTEs	Starkey Laboratories, Inc.
A5	Polar Electro Inc.
A717	Exocell, Inc.

AAEON	Aaeon Electronics, Inc.
AAF	Aaf International
AARON	Bovie Medical Corp.
AARON BURR I	Bovie Medical Corp.
AARON BURR II	Bovie Medical Corp.
AASP	Varian Sample Preparation Products
ABACUS	Baxa Corporation
ABAXIS	Abaxis, Inc.
ABBI	Covidien Lp, Formerly Registered As United States Surgical
ABBOT AIM PLUS	Hospira, Inc
ABBOTT	Omni Medical Supply Inc.
ABBOTT PRISM	Abbott Laboratories
ABC	Conmed Corporation
ABC	Stryker Spine
ABC-AMP	Vector Laboratories, Inc.
ABCO	Kern Surgical Supply, Inc.
ABCOAT	Cst Technologies, Inc.
ABEA	CAREFUSION 211, INC..
ABEAR	Natus Medical Inc.
ABILITATIONS	Abilitations
ABIOCOR	Abiomed, Inc.
ABIOHEART	Abiomed, Inc.
ABL	Radiometer America, Inc.
ABLEWARE	Maddak Inc.
ABM NECK COLLAR	Roloke
ABP 26	Covance Research Products Inc.
ABP FOR WINDOWS	Rozinn By Scottcare Corporation
ABPM-630	Mediana Technologies Corp
ABS PRECIS	Immucor, Inc.
ABS2000	Immucor, Inc.
ABSOLOK	Ethicon Endo-Surgery, Inc.
ABSOLUTE	Camfil Farr
ABSOLUTERS	Tricontinent
ABSORBENT	Micromedics
ABSORBIE	Clean Esd Products, Inc.
AC	Mizuho Osi
AC-CURA	Carecentric, Inc.
AC-TAPE	Hartmann-Conco Inc.
ACADEMY GOLD	Ivoclar Vivadent, Inc.
ACAPPELLA (HEARING AID)	Telex Communications, Inc.-Hearing Instrument Grp.
ACAREXX	Idexx Laboratories, Inc.
ACB	Alere, Inc.
ACC CONTROL	Karl Storz Endoscopy-America Inc.
ACC-U-TROL	Ahnafield Corp.
ACCEAVA	Alere, Inc.
ACCEAVAr HCG	Thermo Biostar, Inc.
ACCEAVAr HCG BASIC	Thermo Biostar, Inc.
ACCEAVAr HCG COMBO	Thermo Biostar, Inc.
ACCEAVAr MONO	Thermo Biostar, Inc.
ACCEAVAr STREP A	Thermo Biostar, Inc.

ACCEL	B. Braun Oem Division, B. Braun Medical Inc.
ACCELERATION THERAPEUTICS	Non-Invasive Monitoring Systems, Inc.
ACCELERATOR II	Byron Medical
ACCELERATOR III	Byron Medical
ACCELERATOR TU	Byron Medical
ACCELL	Integra Lifesciences Holdings Corp.
ACCELNET	Beckman Coulter, Inc.
ACCELSPIN	Beckman Coulter, Inc.
ACCENT	Freeman Manufacturing Company
ACCENT	Jorgensen Laboratories
ACCENTE	Phipps & Bird, Inc.
ACCENTS	Artcraft New York
ACCESS	Beckman Coulter, Inc.
ACCESS	Imtec, A 3m Company
ACCESS	Symmetry Medical Usa, Inc.
ACCESS PLUS	Merit Medical Systems, Inc.
ACCESS TIPS	Hager Worldwide, Inc.
ACCESS-9	Merit Medical Systems, Inc.
ACCISS	Schaerer Mayfield Usa
ACCLAIM	Bio-Rad Laboratories
ACCOLADE	Surmodics, Inc.
ACCOLADE C	Stryker Corp.
ACCOLADE C CEMENTED	Stryker Corp.
ACCOLADE PRESSFIT	Stryker Corp.
ACCOLADE TMZF	Stryker Corp.
ACCOLADE TMZF	Stryker Howmedica Osteonics
ACCORDE	Welcon, Inc.
ACCOUNTMASTER	Horizon Healthcare Technologies
ACCU FLOW VENTURI	Salter Labs
ACCU-BACK	Jobri Llc
ACCU-BEAM	Transamerican Technologies International
ACCU-BLADE	Okay Industries, Inc.
ACCU-CARE	Accu-Med Services
ACCU-CHEK	Roche Diagnostics Operations
ACCU-CLEAR	Alere, Inc.
ACCU-CUT	Sakura Finetek U.S.A., Inc.
ACCU-CUT OSTEOTOMY GUIDE SYSTEM	Biopro, Inc.
ACCU-DERMATOME	Aesculap Implant Systems Inc.
ACCU-DOA-CHEK	Metronix
ACCU-EDGE	Sakura Finetek U.S.A., Inc.
ACCU-FILM	Parkell, Inc.
ACCU-FLO	Beckman Coulter, Inc.
ACCU-FORM	Mid-States Laboratories, Inc.
ACCU-GLASS	Accu-Glass Llc
ACCU-HITE	Seca Corp.
ACCU-KV	Radcal Corp.
ACCU-LIGHT	Dent Zar, Inc.
ACCU-LINE	Accu-Line Products, Inc.
ACCU-MESH	Aesculap Implant Systems Inc.
ACCU-MOLD	Premier Medical Products
ACCU-PACE	Pace Medical, Inc.
ACCU-PREP	Beckman Coulter, Inc.
ACCU-SCOPE	Accu-Scope, Inc.
ACCU-SPINA	North American Medical Corporation
ACCU-SURG	Transamerican Technologies International
ACCU-TRACK	Zettler Systems, Inc.
ACCU-TRAK	Instrumentation Laboratory Company
ACCU-VAC	Buffalo Dental Manufacturing Co., Inc.
ACCU-VU SIZING	Angiodynamics, Inc.
ACCU-WEIGH	Yamato Corporation
ACCUCAL 2001	Nuclear Pharmacy Services
ACCUCAL 2002	Nuclear Pharmacy Services
ACCUCAP	MAQUET
ACCUCARB	Filterspun
ACCUCAST	Buffalo Dental Manufacturing Co., Inc.
ACCUCAT	Varian Sample Preparation Products
ACCUCHECK	Beckman Coulter, Inc.
ACCUCLEAN	Neogen Corporation
ACCUCOM	MAQUET
ACCUCOMP	Beckman Coulter, Inc.
ACCUCORE	C. R. Bard, Inc.
ACCUCORE	Medtronic, Inc.
ACCUCOUNT	Atrion Medical Products, Inc.
ACCUCULT	J&S Medical Associates
ACCUDEXA	Schick Technologies, Inc.
ACCUDIL	Hamilton Company
ACCUDOSE	Centrix, Inc.
ACCUDOT	Hu-Friedy Manufacturing Co., Inc.
ACCUDRAIN	Integra Lifesciences Holdings Corp.
ACCUDYNAMIC	Hospira, Inc.
ACCUFAXr FAX PAPER, CARTRIDGES & RIBBONS	Pm Company
ACCUFIT	Beckman Coulter, Inc.
ACCUFLEX	Beckman Coulter, Inc.
ACCUFLEX	Bipore, Inc.
ACCUFLUOR	Oxis International, Inc.
ACCUFLUSH	Smiths Medical OEM
ACCUFRESH	Carter-Hoffmann
ACCUFUSER	Walkmed Infusion Llc
ACCUGATE	Beckman Coulter, Inc.
ACCUGEL	Lynn Medical
ACCUGUIDE	B. Braun Oem Division, B. Braun Medical Inc.
ACCUHALT	Cygnus Inc.
ACCUJECT	Dentsply International, Inc.
ACCUJECT	Dentsply Prosthetics
ACCULAB	Beckman Coulter, Inc.
ACCULAB	Cygnus Inc.
ACCULAB	Utech Products, Inc.
ACCULYSIN	Cenogenics Corp.
ACCULYTE	Laboratory Technologies, Inc.
ACCUMARK	Avery Dennison Corporation
ACCUMARK	Medtronic, Inc.
ACCUMAX QUANTUM CONVERTIBLE, ACCUMAX QUANTUM PC, LINEN LOCK	B.G. Industries, Inc.
ACCUMENT	Fisher Scientific Co., Llc.
ACCUMIST	Medtronic Cardiovascular Surgery, The Heart Valve Div.
ACCUMULATOR CHAMBER	Permatron Corp.
ACCUNEB	Dey, L.P.
ACCUPEP	Covidien Lp
ACCUPLACE	Medtronic, Inc.
ACCUPLACER	Hu-Friedy Manufacturing Co., Inc.
ACCUPLUS	VARTA Microbattery Inc.
ACCUPOINT	Neogen Corporation
ACCUPROBE	Gen-Probe, Inc.
ACCURA BIOPSY SYSTEM	Angiotech
ACCURAY	Canberra
ACCURO	Draeger Safety, Inc.
ACCUSAT	MAQUET
ACCUSCANNER	Circadian Systems
ACCUSCREEN T4	Neometrics, A Division Of Natus
ACCUSCREEN TRYPSIN	Neometrics, A Division Of Natus
ACCUSCREEN TSH	Neometrics, A Division Of Natus
ACCUSENSE	Beckman Coulter, Inc.
ACCUSENSOR	Lynn Medical
ACCUSET	Beckman Coulter, Inc.
ACCUSIGN	Princeton Biomeditech Corp.
ACCUSITE PH	Zinetics Medical, Inc.
ACCUSLIDE	Biogenex Laboratories
ACCUSONIC	I-Rep, Inc.
ACCUSORT	Beckman Coulter, Inc.
ACCUSOURCE	Baxter Healthcare Corporation Nutrition
ACCUSPAN	Pmt Corp.
ACCUSPIN	Beckman Coulter, Inc.
ACCUSTAMP	Carver Inc.
ACCUSTAT	Ams Innovative Center-San Jose
ACCUSTAT	Biological Controls Inc.
ACCUSTAT	Psg Controls, Inc.
ACCUSTROKE	Beckman Coulter, Inc.
ACCUSWAY	Advanced Mechanical Technology, Inc. (Amti)
ACCUTAC	Conmed Corporation
ACCUTARG	Havel's Inc.
ACCUTEK PACKAGING	Biner Ellison
ACCUTEX	J&S Medical Associates
ACCUTHERM	Halbar North, Inc.
ACCUTHERM	Novamed, Llc
ACCUTHERM	Psg Controls, Inc.
ACCUTHERM	Thermcraft, Inc

ACCUTORR	MAQUET
ACCUTOUCH	Immersion Medical
ACCUTOUCH	Tillotson Healthcare Corp.
ACCUTRACKER DX	Suntech Medical, Inc.
ACCUTRACKER II	Suntech Medical, Inc.
ACCUTRAK	Spaceage Control, Inc.
ACCUTRAN	Schleicher & Schuell, Inc.
ACCUTROL	Cardium Therapeutics Inc.
ACCUVACT	Valleylab
ACCUVETTE	Beckman Coulter, Inc.
ACCUWELL 17P	Neometrics, A Division Of Natus
ACCUWELL 1RT	Neometrics, A Division Of Natus
ACCUWELL GAL	Neometrics, A Division Of Natus
ACCUWELL PKU	Neometrics, A Division Of Natus
ACCUWELL T4	Neometrics, A Division Of Natus
ACCUWELLT5H	Neometrics, A Division Of Natus
ACCUWOUND	Filterspun
ACCUWRITE	Lynn Medical
ACE	Alfa Wassermann, Inc.
ACE	Dey, L.P.
ACE	Schott North America, Inc.
ACE ALIGN	Depuy Ace, A Johnson & Johnson Company
ACE COLOR KIT	Fujirebio Diagnostics, Inc. (Fdi)
ACE KIDZ	Becton Dickinson And Company
ACE LAB MAT	Ace Hose & Rubber Company
ACE-COLLES	Depuy Ace, A Johnson & Johnson Company
ACE-FISCHER	Depuy Ace, A Johnson & Johnson Company
ACE-HOFFMAN	Depuy Ace, A Johnson & Johnson Company
ACE-TUF	Hamilton Caster & Mfg. Co.
ACES	Therafin Corporation
ACETAZYME	Stanbio Laboratory, Inc.
ACETEST	Siemens Healthcare Diagnostics Inc.
ACHIEVA	Covidien (Formerly Nellcor Puritan Bennett / Tyco Healthcare)
ACHIEVER	Lw Scientific
ACHILLOTRAIN	Bauerfeind Usa, Inc.
ACIDICASE	Bd Diagnostic Systems
ACIPHEX	Ortho-Mcneil-Janssen Pharmaceuticals, Inc.
ACL	Instrumentation Laboratory Company
ACL ELITE	Instrumentation Laboratory Company
ACL TOP	Instrumentation Laboratory Company
ACLAND CLAMP	Eriem Surgical
ACLS SKILLMASTER	Medical Plastics Laboratory, Inc.
ACM	Stryker Corp.
ACME	Foster Manufacturing Corp.
ACON	Acon Laboratories, Inc.
ACOR	Acor Orthopaedic, Inc.
ACORN	Vital Signs Colorado
ACORN II	Vital Signs, Inc.
ACOUSTI-FLOTE-ALL	Industrial Acoustics Co., Inc.
ACOUSTIC RHINOMETER	E. Benson Hood Laboratories, Inc.
ACOUSTICOVER	Audiology Products
ACOUSTITRODE	Novamed, Llc
ACOUSTIX	Conmed Corporation
ACOUTISTIC PHARYNGOMETER	E. Benson Hood Laboratories, Inc.
ACP	Ortheon Medical, Llc.
ACQSIM	Atlas Medical Technologies
ACQUIRESC	Beckman Coulter, Inc.
ACROVYN	Construction Specialties Inc.
ACRYDERM	Acrymed, Inc.
ACRYL-A-MIX	Promega Corp.
ACRYLATHE POLISHING WHEELS	George Taub Products & Fusion Co., Inc.
ACRYMOUNT	Statlab Medical Products, Inc.
ACRYPOINT	Shofu Dental Corporation
ACRYSOF	Alcon Research, Ltd.
ACS:180	Siemens Healthcare Diagnostics Inc
ACT	Uromedica, Inc.
ACT Plus	Medtronic Perfusion Systems
ACT-O-MATIC	Sloan Valve Co.
ACT-TROL	Analytical Control Systems, Inc.
ACTALYKE	Helena Laboratories
ACTAMIDE	Continental Hydrodyne Systems, Inc.
ACTAR 911	Armstrong Medical Industries, Inc.
ACTAR AED TRAINER	Armstrong Medical Industries, Inc.
ACTAR D-FIB	Armstrong Medical Industries, Inc.
ACTEST	St. Jude Medical Neuromodulation Division
ACTESTER	St. Jude Medical Neuromodulation Division
ACTI*TIP	Dexall Biomedical Labs, Inc.
ACTI-FEND	Medical Action Industries, Inc
ACTI-GARD	Medical Concepts Development
ACTI-LITE	Gendron, Inc.
ACTIBIND	American Diagnostica, Inc.
ACTICAL	Mini-Mitter Company, Inc.
ACTICHROME	American Diagnostica, Inc.
ACTICLOT	American Diagnostica, Inc.
ACTICOAT	Nucryst Pharmaceuticals Corp.
ACTICON NEOSPHINCTER	American Medical Systems, Inc.
ACTIFIX	Greatbach Medical
ACTIFOAM	Medchem Products, Inc.
ACTIGEL	Sterogene Bioseparations, Inc.
ACTION	Action Products, Inc.
ACTION ARCHWIRE	Atlanta Orthodontics
ACTION ARM	Tagg Industries L.L.C.
ACTION OFFICE	Herman Miller, Inc.
ACTIV-AIR	Pyramid Industries, Llc
ACTIV-FLEX	Johnson & Johnson Consumer Products, Inc.
ACTIVA	Fla Orthopedics, Inc.
ACTIVA	Medical Concepts Development
ACTIVATED MATRIX	Cardium Therapeutics Inc.
ACTIVE CATH	Mentor Corp.
ACTIVE ELECTRODE	Neurodyne Medical Corp.
ACTIVE I	Activeaid, Inc.
ACTIVE II	Activeaid, Inc.
ACTIVE LIFE	Convatec Professional Services
ACTIVE SEAL	Brown Medical Industries
ACTIVE TEE	Ladies First, Inc.
ACTIVE VIEWBOX	Syntermed, Inc.
ACTIVE WALKERS	Acor Orthopaedic, Inc.
ACTIVEECG	Active Corporation
ACTIVENT	Medtronic Xomed, Inc.
ACTIVITRAX	Medtronic, Inc.
ACTIVITRAX E	Medtronic, Inc.
ACTIVITRAX II	Medtronic, Inc.
ACTIVITY BEARS	Graham Medical Products/Div. Of Little Rapids Corp
ACTIWATCH	Mini-Mitter Company, Inc.
ACTIWATCH 2	Mini-Mitter Company, Inc.
ACTIWATCH SPECTRUM	Mini-Mitter Company, Inc.
ACTIWATCH-L	Mini-Mitter Company, Inc.
ACTIWATCH-SCORE	Mini-Mitter Company, Inc.
ACTRIL	Minntech Corporation
ACU MED	Health Enterprises
ACU-DISPO-CAUTERY	Acuderm Inc.
ACU-E-SURG	Acuderm Inc.
ACU-PRO	Radcal Corp.
ACU-RATE	Alimed, Inc.
ACUCAIR	Hill-Rom Holdings, Inc.
ACUCELL	Biovest International, Inc.
ACUCISE	Applied Medical Resource Corporation
ACUDATA	Biovest International, Inc.
ACUDRIVER	Exactech, Inc.
ACUFEX	Smith & Nephew, Inc., Endoscopy Division
ACUFLEX I	Novel Products, Inc.
ACUFLEX II	Novel Products, Inc.
ACUFLEX III	Novel Products, Inc.
ACUITY	Nu-Ear Electronics
ACUITY	Varian Medical Systems
ACUITY	Welch Allyn Protocol Inc.
ACUITY DETECTION SYSTEMS	Covance Research Products Inc.
ACULINK-DATA LOG	Biovest International, Inc.
ACUMAR	Lafayette Instrument Company
ACUMATCH A SERIES	Exactech, Inc.
ACUMATCH C SERIES	Exactech, Inc.
ACUMATCH L SERIES	Exactech, Inc.
ACUMATCH M SERIES	Exactech, Inc.
ACUMATCH P SERIES	Exactech, Inc.
ACUMEDIA	Acumedia Manufacturers, Inc.
ACUPAC	Fricke Dental Manufacturing Co.

ACURI	Siemens Hearing Instruments, Inc.
ACURIS LIFE	Siemens Hearing Instruments, Inc.
ACUSNARE	Wilson-Cook Medical, Inc.
ACUSON	Siemens Medical Solutions Usa, Inc.
ACUSOUND (HEARING AID)	Telex Communications, Inc.-Hearing Instrument Grp.
ACUSYST-JR	Biovest International, Inc.
ACUSYST-MAXIMIZER 1000	Biovest International, Inc.
ACUSYST-XCELL	Biovest International, Inc.
ACUTIP 500	Cutera, Inc.
ACUVUE	Vistakon, Inc.
ACross	St. Jude Medical, Inc.
AD-HEAR	Hearing Components Inc.
AD-HERE	Extra Packaging, Corp.
AD100	Anna-Dote, Inc.
AD100A	Anna-Dote, Inc.
AD110	Anna-Dote, Inc.
AD110A	Anna-Dote, Inc.
ADA-READY	Asi-Modulex
ADAM	Covidien (Formerly Nellcor Puritan Bennett / Tyco Healthcare)
ADAM AND EVE	Scott Specialties, Inc./Cmo Inc./Ginny Inc.
ADAM-CPR	Simulaids, Inc.
ADAMATION	Adamation, Inc.
ADAPT LAPAROSCOPIC PORTS	Taut, Inc.
ADAPT-A-CASE	Case Design Corp.
ADAPTA	Chattanooga Group
ADAPTA-GRID	Spectronics Corporation
ADAPTACALL	Dwyer Precision Products, Inc.
ADAPTACAP	Baxa Corporation
ADAPTIC	Johnson & Johnson Medical Division Of Ethicon, Inc.
ADAPTIV BIPHASIC	Physio-Control, Inc.
ADAPTIVE COMPRESSION (HEARING AID)	Telex Communications, Inc.-Hearing Instrument Grp.
ADAPTIVE STANDER	Ortho-Kinetics, Inc.
ADAPTIVE TARGETING	Siemens Medical Solutions Usa, Inc
ADAPTO	Oticon, Inc.
ADBAN	Avcor Health Care Products, Inc.
ADC	Agfa Corporation
ADC	American Diagnostic Corporation (Adc)
ADC	American Dryer Corp.
ADC	Bound Tree Medical
ADCUFF	American Diagnostic Corporation (Adc)
ADD	Ams Innovative Center-San Jose
ADD&BOND-C	Parkell, Inc.
ADD-A-UNIT	Phelan Manufacturing Corp.
ADD-ON	Accu-Med Services
ADD-VANTAGE	Hospira Inc.
ADDAFIVE	Medi-Dose, Inc.
ADDI-CHEK	Millipore Corporation
ADDRESSOGRAPH	Newbold Corporation
ADDS-HESIVE 1 & 2	Mds Products, Inc.
ADDS-HESIVE 1 & 2 FAST & REGULAR SET ADHESIVE	American Diversified Dental Systems
ADDS-IT ACCELERATOR	American Diversified Dental Systems
ADDS-IT BASE	Mds Products, Inc.
ADDS-IT BASE E-Z SQUEEZE 1/2 & 1 OZ BOTTLE	American Diversified Dental Systems
ADDS-IT TIP CLEANER KIT	American Diversified Dental Systems
ADDS-LUSTER DIAMOND PORCELAIN POLISH	American Diversified Dental Systems
ADDS-LUSTER PORCELAIN POLISH	Mds Products, Inc.
ADDS-TEX ADHESIVE	Mds Products, Inc.
ADDS-TEX ARTICULATOR ADHESIVE	American Diversified Dental Systems
ADDSTAT	Ams Innovative Center-San Jose
ADEL	Stryker Medical
ADELANTE	Oscor, Inc.
ADENNA	Adenna Inc.
ADENOCLONE	Meridian Bioscience, Inc.
ADENOPLEXr	Prodesse, Inc.
ADEX	Adex Medical, Inc.
ADFLOW	American Diagnostic Corporation (Adc)
ADHERENCE M5	Novocol, Inc.
ADHESE	Ivoclar Vivadent, Inc.
ADI-10	Pinnacle Technology Group, Inc.
ADIAFLO	American Diagnostica, Inc.
ADJUST-A-CINCH	Select Medical Products, Inc.
ADJUST-A-FLO	Marlen Manufacturing & Development Co.
ADJUST-A-TEMP	Bovie Medical Corp.
ADJUSTABENCH	Anthro Corporation
ADJUSTABLE TUBE TREE	Trademark Medical Llc
ADJUSTICIZERT EXERCISE SYSTEM	Dm Systems, Inc.
ADLINK	Soltec Corp.
ADLITE	American Diagnostic Corporation (Adc)
ADOX	Agfa Corporation
ADPER	3m Co.
ADR (ANESTHESIA DESK REFERENCE)	Mercury Medical
ADSCOPE	American Diagnostic Corporation (Adc)
ADSOL	Fenwal Inc.
ADT	Epic Systems Corp.
ADULT LOCK	Apothecary Products, Inc.
ADVANCAIR	Cleanroom Systems
ADVANCE	Hill-Rom Holdings, Inc.
ADVANCE	Merit Medical Systems, Inc.
ADVANCE	Neurometrix, Inc.
ADVANCE	Orasure Technologies, Inc.
ADVANCE	Wright Medical Group, Inc.
ADVANCE CASEPLAN	Stryker Imaging
ADVANCE DYNAMIC ROM	Empi, Inc.
ADVANCE INTUITION	Arkray Usa
ADVANCE MICRO-DRAW	Arkray Usa
ADVANCE PLUS	Hollister Incorporated
ADVANCED	Advanced Instruments Inc.
ADVANCED CASEPLAN	Stryker Corp.
ADVANCED CASEPLAN	Stryker Endoscopy
ADVANCED CASEPLAN	Stryker Spine
ADVANCED INPUT DEVICES	Advanced Input Systems
ADVANCED MEAL SYSTEMS	Aladdin Synergetics, Inc.
ADVANCED MEDICAL INNOVATIONS	Advanced Medical Innovations, Inc.
ADVANCED UNIVERSAL K TABLE	Instrument Specialists, Inc.
ADVANT-EDGE	Tp Orthodontics, Inc.
ADVANTA	Hill-Rom Holdings, Inc.
ADVANTAGE	Allied Healthcare Products, Inc.
ADVANTAGE	DJO Inc.
ADVANTAGE	Dentsply Prosthetics
ADVANTAGE	Oral-B Laboratories, Inc.
ADVANTAGE	Scottcare Corporation
ADVANTAGE	Stryker Medical
ADVANTAGE	Virtis, An Sp Industries Company
ADVANTAGE 1000	Secure Care Products, Inc.
ADVANTAGE 128	Preserve International
ADVANTAGE 256	Preserve International
ADVANTAGE 500 DE	Secure Care Products, Inc.
ADVANTAGE FLEX PADDLE: (GLIDEBOARD)	Livingston Products, Inc.
ADVANTAGE OEM MODULE	Suntech Medical, Inc.
ADVANTAGE PLUS	Crosstex International, Inc.
ADVANTAGE SERIES	Nbs Technologies Inc.
ADVANTAGEBAND	Precision Dynamics Corp.
ADVANTEDGE	Conflex
ADVANTEQ 2000	Amrex Electrotherapy Equipment
ADVATE	Baxter International Inc
ADVENT	Mentor Ophthalmics, Inc.
ADVENT	Zimmer Dental, Inc.
ADVENTURE VAN	Hds Specialty Vehicles
ADVIA	Siemens Healthcare Diagnostics Inc.
ADVIA CENTRALINK	Siemens Healthcare Diagnostics Inc.
ADVIA RETIC PLUS	R & D Systems, Inc.
ADVIA WORKCELL	Siemens Healthcare Diagnostics Inc.
ADVISOR	Alere, Inc.
ADVISOR	Smiths Medical Pm, Inc.
ADVOCATE	Zygo Industries, Inc.
ADZORBSTAR	Del Global Technologies Corp.
AECD	Cardiac Science Corporation (Ca)
AED	Advanced Endoscopy Devices, Inc.
AED	Welch Allyn Protocol, Inc.
AED PLUS	Zoll Medical Corp.
AED PRO	Zoll Medical Corp.
AEM	Encision Inc.

AER	Birchwood Laboratories, Inc.
AER	Minntech Corporation
AERO	Deb Sbs, Inc.
AERO GEAR ASTHMA KIT	Monaghan Medical Corp.
AERO-FLOW	Tsi Incorporated
AEROBIC-TILE	Pawling Corp., Architectural Prod. Div.
AEROCARRIER	Thermo Fisher Scientific - Laboratory Equipment Division Headquarters
AEROCHAMBER PLUS VALVED HOLDING CHAMBER	Monaghan Medical Corp.
AEROCHAMBER VALVED HOLDING CHAMBER	Monaghan Medical Corp.
AERODYNAMIC PARTICLE SIZER	Tsi Incorporated
AEROECLIPSE BREATH ACTUATED NEBULIZER	Monaghan Medical Corp.
AEROFIX	Wescor, Inc.
AEROLITE	Mentor Ophthalmics, Inc.
AEROMAX	Medical Industries America Inc.
AEROPAC	Camfil Farr
AEROPLEAT	Camfil Farr
AEROS	Ohio Medical Corp.
AEROSEAL	Beckman Coulter, Inc.
AEROSOLVE	Beckman Coulter, Inc.
AEROSPACE CASES	Case Design Corp.
AEROSPRAY	Wescor, Inc.
AEROSTAT	Afassco, Inc.
AEROSTAT	Applied Medical Resource Corporation
AEROTRACH PLUS VALVED HOLDING CHAMBER	Monaghan Medical Corp.
AEROVENT HOLDING CHAMBER	Monaghan Medical Corp.
AESCULAP	Aesculap Implant Systems Inc.
AESTIVA	Ge Medical Systems Information Technologies
AETNA FOOT PRODUCTS	Aetna Foot Products/Div. Of Aetna Felt Corporation
AETREX	Aetrex Worldwide, Inc
AETREX/WORLDWIDE	Ortholine
AEU-7	Aseptico, Inc.
AF Suppression	St. Jude Medical, Inc.
AFAS-COLD	Afassco, Inc.
AFFI-GEL	Bio-Rad Laboratories
AFFI-GEL	Bio-Rad Laboratories, Life Science Group
AFFI-PREP	Bio-Rad Laboratories
AFFI-PREP	Bio-Rad Laboratories, Life Science Group
AFFINITY	Amoena
AFFINITY	Hill-Rom Holdings, Inc.
AFFINITY	Medtronic Perfusion Systems
AFFINITY	Medtronic Sofamor Danek Usa, Inc
AFFINITY	Medtronic Sofamor Danek Usa, Inc.
AFFINITY	Mine Safety Appliances Company
AFFIRM	Bd Diagnostic Systems
AFFYMETRIX	Affymetrix, Inc.
AFIBALERT	Lechnologies Research, Inc..
AFINITY	Staar Surgical Co.
AFLP	Applied Biosystems
AFP	York X-Ray And Orthopedic Supply, Inc.
AFTER BURN	Romaine, Inc. D.B.A. Koldcare
AFTER FIVE	Hu-Friedy Manufacturing Co., Inc.
AFTERCARE INSTRUCTIONS	Micromedex, Inc.
AFocus	Boston Scientific Corporation
AG	Bio-Rad Laboratories, Life Science Group
AG-48	Aquatic Access, Inc.
AG-60	Aquatic Access, Inc.
AG-72	Aquatic Access, Inc.
AGARACE	Promega Corp.
AGARMATIC	New Brunswick Scientific Co., Inc.
AGC	Biomet, Inc.
AGF	Interpore Cross International
AGFAPATH	Agfa Corporation
AGIL	C. R. Bard, Inc.
AGILECATH	Codman & Shurtleff, Inc
AGILIS	Ela Medical, Inc.
AGILITY	Cordis Neurovascular, Inc.
AGILON	C. R. Bard, Inc.
AGILTRAC	Abbott Laboratories
AGION ANTIMICROBIAL	Agion Technologies Inc.
AGITENE PARTS CLEANING FLUID	Graymills Corp.
AGITOR INK PUMPS	Graymills Corp.
AGRI-SCREEN	Neogen Corporation
AGV (AUTOMATED GUIDED VEHICLE SYSTEM)	Swisslog Translogic Corporation
AGW	Aura Lens Products, Inc.
AHNAVAN	Ahnafield Corp.
AHT	Codman & Shurtleff, Inc
AHTO	Stryker Corp.
AHTO	Stryker Endoscopy
AID	Advanced Input Systems
AID-1	North Safety Products
AIDA COMMUNICATION	Karl Storz Endoscopy-America Inc.
AIDA COMPACT	Karl Storz Endoscopy-America Inc.
AIDA CONNECT	Karl Storz Endoscopy-America Inc.
AIDA OFFICE	Karl Storz Endoscopy-America Inc.
AIDACO BITE STICKS	Temrex Corporation
AIGISRx	TYRX, Inc.
AILEE	Myco Medical
AIM	Beckman Coulter, Inc.
AIM	Depuy Ace, A Johnson & Johnson Company
AIM	Vitalograph, Inc.
AIMS	Atrion Medical Products, Inc.
AIMSCO	Aimsco, Delta Hi-Tech, Inc.
AINCA	Anesthesia Associates, Inc.
AIR BASS	Draeger Safety, Inc.
AIR BLOWER	Hal-Hen Company, Inc.
AIR FLOW WHEELCHAIR CUSHION	Biomedical Systems
AIR LIFT	Air Lift Unlimited Inc.
AIR LINK, AIRLINK	Air Link International
AIR MOTOR 24	Medidenta International, Inc.
AIR MOTOR 324 LINE	Medidenta International, Inc.
AIR PILLOW	Hos-Pillow Corp.
AIR REPAIR	Deltatrak, Inc.
AIR SYSTEMS	Caddy Corporation
AIR-CORE PILLOW	Core Products International, Inc.
AIR-DRI	Paperpak
AIR-LON	Premier Medical Products
AIR-MATE	Mentor Ophthalmics, Inc.
AIR-PUTTY	North Coast Medical, Inc.
AIR-SCENT	Surco Products
AIR-STIRRUP	Aircast Llc
AIR-STIRRUP LIGHT	Aircast Llc
AIR-STIRRUP UNIVERSE	Aircast Llc
AIR-TITE	Air-Tite Products Co., Inc.
AIRBUOY	Brandt Industries, Inc.
AIRCAST	Aircast Llc
AIRCAST	Mueller Sports Medicine
AIRCRAFT DRYERS	Bobrick Washroom Equipment, Inc.
AIRDENT II	Air Techniques, Inc.
AIRE-CUF	Smiths Medical Asd
AIREX	Abilitations
AIREX	Magister Corporation
AIREZE	Covidien Lp
AIRFLO PLUS	Gaymar Industries, Inc.
AIRFLO VEST	Depuy Mitek, Inc.
AIRFREE	Kenda American Airless
AIRGUARD	Tsi Inc.
AIRGUN 40	Paratech, Inc.
AIRHEEL	Aircast Llc
AIRIS	Hitachi Medical Systems America, Inc.
AIRIS ELITE	Hitachi Medical Systems America, Inc.
AIRIS II	Hitachi Medical Systems America, Inc.
AIRISTAR	Airistar Technologies, L.L.C.
AIRKING AMERICA	Medidenta International, Inc.
AIRLIFT	Mobility Inc.
AIROCIDE	Kesair Technologies, Llc
AIRPAL	Airpal Patient Transfer Systems Inc.
AIRPAX	Vespo Marketing Assoc., Inc.
AIRPEL	Airpot Corporation
AIRPOWER	Spectrum-Brands
AIRPULSE PK CUSHION SYSTEM	Aquila Corporation
AIRSPEED	World Dryer Corp.
AIRSPORT	Aircast Llc
AIRSTAR	Air Techniques, Inc.
AIRSTAR CALORIC IRRIGATOR	Micromedical Technologies, Inc.
AIRSTRIP	Smith & Nephew, Inc.

AIRSTYLE	World Dryer Corp.
AIRWAY	Airway Division Of Surgical Appliance Industries, Inc.
AIRWAY PAD	Jerome Medical
AIRWAY PAD	Ossur Americas
AIRX	Airx Laboratories
AISLE EASE	Theradyne Products Division
AISLEGUARD	Spacesaver Corporation
AISLEMASTER	Columbia Medical Manufacturing Llc
AIT 2000	Air Techniques, Inc.
AJUSCO	Adjustable Fixture Co.
AKTON	Action Products, Inc.
AL 2000CR	Hf Pure Water
AL-40	Ddc Technologies, Inc.
AL-47	Alden Optical Labs, Inc.
ALADDIN	Insiphil (Us) Llc
ALADDIN	United Receptacle
ALAIR	Asthmatx, Inc.
ALAMARBLUE	Trek Diagnostic Systems
ALARIS	Cardinal Health Inc.
ALARMVIEW	Ge Medical Systems Information Technologies
ALASTAT	Siemens Healthcare Diagnostics Inc.
ALBA	Albahealth Llc
ALBAHEALTH	Albahealth Llc
ALBUMIN SPECIES	Exocell, Inc.
ALBUMINAR-2S	Csl Behring
ALBUMINAR-S	Csl Behring
ALBUSTIX	Siemens Healthcare Diagnostics Inc.
ALBUWELL	Exocell, Inc.
ALBUWELL M	Exocell, Inc.
ALC	Pentron Laboratory Technologies
ALCARE	Steris Corporation
ALCO-GEL	Xttrium Laboratories, Inc.
ALCO-SENSOR	Intoximeters, Inc.
ALCO-SENSOR IV	Intoximeters, Inc.
ALCOHOL (CHECK)	Akers Biosciences, Inc.
ALCOMONITER CC	Intoximeters, Inc.
ALCOSTAT	Sun Biomedical Laboratories, Inc.
ALDRETE	Avid Medical
ALEG	Avantor Performance Materials
ALENTI	ArjoHuntleigh
ALERENET	Alere Medical, Inc.
ALERO	Golden Technologies, Inc.
ALERT	Alcohol Countermeasure Systems, Inc.
ALERT	Neogen Corporation
ALERT-O.A.D.	Propper Manufacturing Co., Inc.
ALEXIS	Applied Medical Resource Corporation
ALEXIS	Convergent Laser Technologies
ALEXLAZR	Candela Corp.
ALFA	Osteoimplant Technology, Inc.
ALFA II	Osteoimplant Technology, Inc.
ALGEE	Accurate Set, Inc.
ALGERBRUSH	Alger Equipment Company, Inc.
ALGI-MATE	G & H Wire Co.
ALGILOCK	Hager Worldwide, Inc.
ALGINATE STYPTIC	Pedinol Pharmacal, Inc.
ALGIPORT II	Hager Worldwide, Inc.
ALGISITE	Smith & Nephew, Inc.
ALGO	Natus Medical Inc.
ALGO 1E	Natus Medical Inc.
ALGO 2E	Natus Medical Inc.
ALGO 2E COLOR	Natus Medical Inc.
ALGO 3	Natus Medical Inc.
ALGO-1 PLUS	Natus Medical Inc.
ALGO-PAK	Natus Medical Inc.
ALGO2	Natus Medical Inc.
ALGOR	Algor, Inc.
ALICE	Respironics Georgia, Inc.
ALIGN ADJUSTABLE HEIGHT WORKSTATION	Lista International Corp.
ALIGN-LOCK	Stryker Corp.
ALIGN-LOCK	Stryker Endoscopy
ALILITE	Alimed, Inc.
ALIPLAST	Alimed, Inc.
ALIQUOT	Orthovita, Inc.
ALISTRAP	Alimed, Inc.
ALITO	Nidek Medical Products Inc.
ALKONTROL +	Thermo Fisher Scientific Inc.
ALL BODY ACTION	Exercycle Corporation
ALL NITES	First Quality Enterprise, Inc.
ALL PRO	All Pro Exercise Products, Inc.
ALL PUPIL II	Keeler Instruments Inc.
ALL SEASONS	Zyloware Corporation
ALL SILICA, LOW OR HIGH OH, WITH OR WITHOUT PYROCOAT	Ofs, Specialty Photonics Division
ALL-AMERICAN	Wisconsin Aluminum Foundry Co., Inc.
ALL-IN-ONE	Baxter Healthcare Corporation Nutrition
ALL-IN-ONE	Megadyne Medical Products, Inc.
ALLAIR	Tapcon, Inc.
ALLBEE	Alere, Inc.
ALLDRESS	Sca Personal Care, North America
ALLEGIANCE	Dma Med-Chem Corporation
ALLEGRA	Ericsson, Inc.
ALLEGRO	Bard Electro Physiology
ALLEGRO	Mizuho Osi
ALLEGRO	Zymark Corporation
ALLEN BEACH CHAIR	Allen Medical Systems, Inc.
ALLEN C-FLEX POLAR HEAD POSITIONER	Allen Medical Systems, Inc.
ALLEN FLEX FRAME SPINAL SYSTEM	Allen Medical Systems, Inc.
ALLEN SAFETY DRAPE	Allen Medical Systems, Inc.
ALLER//GUARD	Alkaline Corp.
ALLERCEPT	Heska Corporation
ALLERCOAT	Bio-Rad Laboratories
ALLERDERM	Allerderm Laboratories, Inc.
ALLERDERM NITRILE EXAM	Allerderm Laboratories, Inc.
ALLERDERM VINYL EXAM	Allerderm Laboratories, Inc.
ALLERG*E	Dexall Biomedical Labs, Inc.
ALLERG*ENS	Dexall Biomedical Labs, Inc.
ALLERGARD	Ansell Healthcare Products, Inc.
ALLERQUANT	Biomerica, Inc.
ALLERSEARCH	Alkaline Corp.
ALLERTEST-NI	Allerderm Laboratories, Inc.
ALLERZYME	Dms Laboratories, Inc.
ALLEVYN	Smith & Nephew, Inc.
ALLIANCE	Biomet, Inc.
ALLIANCE	Respironics Georgia, Inc.
ALLIED	Allied Healthcare Products, Inc.
ALLIED	Bound Tree Medical
ALLIED HEALTHCARE PRODUCTS, INC.	Allied Healthcare Products, Inc.
ALLIEDSIL	Allied Biomedical
ALLINONE	Stryker Imaging
ALLOCLASSIC HIP SYSTEM	Centerpulse Orthopedics Inc.
ALLOCRAFT	Stryker Biotech
ALLOCRAFT	Stryker Corp.
ALLOCRAFT	Stryker Spine
ALLODERM	Lifecell Corp.
ALLOFIT ACETABULAR SYSTEM	Centerpulse Orthopedics Inc.
ALLOFUSE	Allosource
ALLOGRO	Allosource
ALLOMATRIX	Wright Medical Group, Inc.
ALLON	Adroit Medical Systems, Inc.
ALLOPAC	Allosource
ALLSKIN	Viscot Medical, Llc
ALLSPORT ANKLE	Allsport Dynamics, Inc.
ALLTEC	Danaher Corporation
ALOE ALL OVER	The Aloe Institute
ALOECARE PLUS 3	Crosstex International,Inc.
ALOYS-GNP	Gresco Products, Inc.
ALP ALTERNATING LEG PRESSURE SYSTEM	Healthcare Service And Supply
ALP GARMENTS	Healthcare Service And Supply
ALPHA	Bio-Rad Laboratories
ALPHA	Heine Usa Ltd.
ALPHA	Ohio Willow Wood Company
ALPHA 4 SHRO	Instrumentarium Imaging, Inc.
ALPHA CONDUCTING SOLUTION	Electromedical Products International, Inc.
ALPHA CRADLE	Smithers Medical Products, Inc.
ALPHA III	Vitalograph, Inc.
ALPHA IQ	Instrumentarium Imaging, Inc.

ALPHA PAK	Universal Medical Design
ALPHA RT	Instrumentarium Imaging, Inc.
ALPHA SCREEN	CAREFUSION 211, INC..
ALPHA SYSTEM	Kewaunee Scientific Corp.
ALPHA-BSM	Etex Corporation
ALPHA-PROBE	Bio-Rad Laboratories
ALPHA-SPINA	North American Medical Corporation
ALPHA-STIM 100	Electromedical Products International, Inc.
ALPHA-STIM PPM	Electromedical Products International, Inc.
ALPHA-STIM SCS	Electromedical Products International, Inc.
ALPHAGAZ	Air Liquide America Corporation, Cambridge Div.
ALPHAGRAPHIC	Graphic Controls Corp.
ALPHAMAQUET	Getinge Usa, Inc.
ALPHAMAXX	Getinge Usa, Inc.
ALPHASTAR	Getinge Usa, Inc.
ALPHASTATUS	Alpha Communications
ALPHASTIM	Biofeedback Instrument Corp.
ALPHASURE	Alpha Communications
ALPINE	Mentor Corp.
ALS	Belco Packaging Systems, Inc.
ALS ADULT TRAINER	Simulaids, Inc.
ALS PEDIATRIC TRAINER	Simulaids, Inc.
ALSCAN	Altek Corp.
ALSIUS	Alsius Corp.
ALSONS	Alsons Corp.
ALTA	Stryker Spine
ALTAIR	Sonic Innovations
ALTAIRE	Hitachi Medical Systems America, Inc.
ALTEK	Altek Corp.
ALTERED SITES	Promega Corp.
ALTIMATE	Gyrus Medical, Inc.
ALTO	Ela Medical, Inc.
ALTO	Hill-Rom Holdings, Inc.
ALTO	Philips Lighting Co.
ALU-27 DIRECT-A-BEAM	Aseptico, Inc.
ALUMAFOAM	Hartmann-Conco Inc.
ALUMI-HAND	Instrument Specialists, Inc.
ALUVIA	Abbott Laboratories
ALUWAX	Aluwax Dental Products Co.
ALVEOSAMPLER	Quintron Instrument Company
ALVEY FLC-36	Alvey Washing Equipment Co.
ALVEY KS-48-N	Alvey Washing Equipment Co.
ALYX	Fenwal Inc.
AM 252	Welch Allyn, Inc.
AM1	CAREFUSION 211, INC..
AM2	CAREFUSION 211, INC..
AMADEA	Waldmann Lighting
AMALGAMBOND	Parkell, Inc.
AMARA	Zyloware Corporation
AMBASSADOR	Dr Systems, Inc.
AMBASSADOR	Golden Technologies, Inc.
AMBELITE	Argen Corp.
AMBERCHROM	Tosoh Bioscience Llc
AMBEZE	HARTMANN USA, Inc.
AMBI	Smith & Nephew Inc.- Orthopaedics Division
AMBI SKINCARE	Johnson & Johnson
AMBIFLEX	Lohmann & Rauscher, Inc.
AMBITEX	Life Guard
AMBU	Ambu, Inc.
AMBU	Bound Tree Medical
AMBU BAGS	Ambu, Inc.
AMBU MAN	Ambu, Inc.
AMBU PPS	Ambu, Inc.
AMBULARM	Alert Care, Inc.
AMBULATOR	Aetrex Worldwide, Inc
AMBULMATE	American Innovations, Inc.
AMBUMATIC	Ambu, Inc.
AMCOR	The Amcor Group Ltd.
AMCORAIRE	The Amcor Group Ltd.
AMERICAN DENTAL TECHNOLOGIES (RETIRED)	American Medical Technologies, Inc.
AMERICAN DIAGNOSTIC	Creative Health Products, Inc.
AMERICAN DIEROCK RESIN DIE STONE	American Diversified Dental Systems

AMERICAN DIEROCK RESIN DIE STONE	Mds Products, Inc.
AMERICAN DRYER	American Dryer, Inc.
AMERICAN MEDICAL COMMUNICATIONS	Clear Stream Media
AMERICAN MEDICAL TECHNOLOGIES	American Medical Technologies, Inc.
AMERICAN ORTHOPAEDIC	Bsn Medical, Inc
AMERICAN PACKAGING	Biner Ellison
AMERICANA	Alere, Inc.
AMERICANA SERIES	United Receptacle
AMERICOT	American Silk Sutures, Inc.
AMERIMED	Independent Solutions, Inc.
AMERIPHONE	Weitbrecht Communications, Inc.
AMERITUS	Kentec Medical Inc.
AMETEK	Western Water Purifier Co.
AMETOP	Smith & Nephew, Inc.
AMI	Ardus Medical, Inc.
AMI	Cas Medical Systems, Inc.
AMI HOLDINGS, INC.	Ardus Medical, Inc.
AMICUS	Fenwal Inc.
AMIDATE	Abbott Laboratories
AMIGO	Amigo Mobility International
AMIGO	Handicap Unlimited, Inc.
AMIGO	Nipro Diabetes Systems, Inc.
AMIGO2	U O Equipment Co.
AMIKA	Harvard Apparatus, Inc.
AMIKA	Nest Group Inc., The
AMINCO-BOWMAN	Thermo Spectronic
AMINEX	Bio-Rad Laboratories
AMINEX	Bio-Rad Laboratories, Life Science Group
AMKO	Ipso Usa, Inc.
AMMEX	Ammex Corp.
AMMONIA/ALCOHOL	Quantimetrix Corporation
AMMOSORB	Imtek Environmental Corp.
AMNIHOOK	Hollister Incorporated
AMO	Abbott Medical Optics Inc.
AMO ARRAY	Allergan
AMO PHACOFLEX	Allergan
AMO PRESTIGE	Allergan
AMO VITRAX	Allergan
AMOENA	Amoena
AMOENA	Coloplast Manufacturing Us, Llc
AMOENA SKIN THERAPY	Coloplast Manufacturing Us, Llc
AMOS	CAREFUSION 211, INC..
AMP-PICK	Spirig Advanced Technologies, Inc.
AMPATCH	Austin Medical Products, Inc.
AMPLICLEAR	Bio-Rad Laboratories
AMPLIFIER LINK	Eg & G Amorphous Silicon
AMPLIFLUOR	Serologicals Corp
AMPLISIZE	Bio-Rad Laboratories
AMPLITROL	Bio-Rad Laboratories
AMPUTEE STUMP SUPPORT	Gerber Chair Mates, Inc.
AMREL ROCKY UNLIMITED ROCKY APEX	Amrel / American Reliance, Inc.
AMRESCO	Amresco Inc.
AMS	Md Works, Inc.
AMS 700CX	American Medical Systems, Inc.
AMS 700CXM	American Medical Systems, Inc.
AMS AMBICOR	American Medical Systems, Inc.
AMSAFE, AMSELF, AMSECURE, AMSMOOTH	Amsino International, Inc.
AMSINO	Amsino International, Inc.
AMSURE	Amsino International, Inc.
AMTI PRESURE DIST	Advanced Mechanical Technology, Inc. (Amti)
AMUMETAL	Amuneal Manufacturing Corp.
AMUNICKEL	Amuneal Manufacturing Corp.
AMVISC	Anika Therapeutics
AMVISC PLUS	Anika Therapeutics
ANABAG	Hardy Diagnostics
ANAFAST/ANAFLUOR	Diasorin Inc
ANALAMP MERCURY LAMPS	Bhk, Inc.
ANALETTE	Precision Systems, Inc.
ANALOG PERSISTANCE	Lecroy Corp.
ANALYSIS SYSTEM	Wescor, Inc.
ANALYZER/CONDITIONER	W&W Manufacturing Co.
ANAPATH	Statlab Medical Products, Inc.
ANASTOCLIP VCS VESSEL CLOSURE SYSTEM	Lemaitre Vascular, Inc.

ANASTOMARK	Genesee Biomedical, Inc.
ANATOMICAL SHOULDER	Zimmer Holdings, Inc.
ANATOMICAL SHOULDER SYSTEM	Centerpulse Orthopedics Inc.
ANCHOR BRAND	Anchor Products Company
AND ALL MOBILITY PRODUCT ACCESSORIES.	Electric Mobility Corporation
AND KEY ACCESSORIES	Key-Bak
AND MORE.	Handi-Cap Aids Company
AND TUNGSTEN.	Glines And Rhodes, Inc.
AND Z-SCAPE ARE TRADEMARKS OF VARIAN MEDICAL SYSTEMS, INC.	Varian Medical Systems
AND ZMED ARE REGISTERED TRADEMARKS OF VARIAN MEDICAL SYSTEMS, INC.	Varian Medical Systems
ANDERLIFT	Andermac, Inc.
ANDERLIFT PLUS	Andermac, Inc.
ANDERLIFT PLUS	Hygiene Specialties, Inc./Andermac, Inc.
ANDERSEN	Andersen Products, Inc.,
ANDERSEN MICROBIOS PORTABLE SAMPLER	Thermo Fisher Scientific
ANDERSEN N6 BIOLOGICAL IMPACTOR	Thermo Fisher Scientific
ANDOVER	Andover Healthcare Inc.
ANDREWS FRAME	Mizuho Osi
ANDREWS TABLE	Mizuho Osi
ANDROLOGY TRAINER	Fertility Solutions, Inc.
ANDROS	Andros, Inc.
ANER-T-TRACH	Covidien Lp, Formerly Registered As Kendall
ANESTHESIA ASSOCIATES	Anesthesia Associates, Inc.
ANESTHESIA EQUIPMENT & SUPPLIES	Hull Anesthesia, Inc.
ANEUROPLASTIC	Codman & Shurtleff, Inc
ANGEL OF WATER CM-1 SURROUND, CHERUBUM PERSON	Lifestream Purification Systems, Llc
ANGEL WING	Covidien Lp
ANGIO-LOCK	Safety Syringe Corporation Of America, Inc.
ANGIO-SEAL	Kensey Nash Corporation
ANGIO-SET	Becton Dickinson Infusion Therapy Systems, Inc.
ANGIOCATH	Becton Dickinson Infusion Therapy Systems, Inc.
ANGIOFLEX	Abiomed, Inc.
ANGIOGRAM SAM	Medical Plastics Laboratory, Inc.
ANGIOJET	Possis Medical, Inc.
ANGIOMAT	Mallinckrodt, Inc.
ANGIOMED	C. R. Bard, Inc.
ANGIONEOSIGMA	Shimadzu Medical Systems
ANGIOPORT	Boston Scientific Corp.
ANGIOPTIC 3FR FLUSH CATHETERS	Angiodynamics, Inc.
ANGIOPTIC 3FR FLUSH CATHETERS	Caliper Life Sciences, Inc.
ANGIOPTIC FLUSH CATHETER	Angiodynamics, Inc.
ANGIOPTIC FLUSH CATHETER	Caliper Life Sciences, Inc.
ANGIOREX	Toshiba America Medical Systems
ANGIOSCULPT	Angioscore, Inc.
ANGITHANE	Boston Scientific Corp.
ANGYO	Excel Medical Products, Llc
ANHYDRONE	Avantor Performance Materials
ANIMAL PAWS	Principle Business Enterprises, Inc.
ANIMALINTEX	3m Co.
ANIMEC	Futuremed America, Inc.
ANKALOK	Sellstrom Manufacturing Co.
ANKLE HITCH	Morrison Medical
ANKLE HUGGERS	Bodypoint, Inc.
ANKLE SKINS	Cropper Medical, Inc./Bio Skin
ANKLE WEIGHT BAG	Pre Pak Products, Inc.
ANKLETOUGHr REHAB SYSTEM	Dm Systems, Inc.
ANOTRON	Biosonics, Inc.
ANPRO	Andersen Products, Inc.,
ANPROLENE	Andersen Products, Inc.,
ANS	Nu-Ear Electronics
ANSELL	Dma Med-Chem Corporation
ANSOS	Per-Se Technologies
ANSPACH	Anspach Effort, Inc.
ANSTAT	Herculite Products, Inc.
ANSYR	Hospira Inc.
ANTAEOS	United Dental Manufacturers, Inc.
ANTARES	Digital Dynamics, Inc.
ANTEATER	Boss Instruments, Ltd.
ANTENSE	Biosig Instruments, Inc.
ANTERA VINYL WALL COVERING	Inpro Corporation
ANTHROBENCH	Anthro Corporation
ANTHROCART	Anthro Corporation
ANTI-EM/GP	Bsn-Jobst
ANTI-FOG SOLUTION	Wave Form Systems, Inc.
ANTI-G	Flexi-Wall Systems
ANTI-REFLUX VALVE	Trademark Medical Llc
ANTI-SHOX	Aetrex Worldwide, Inc
ANTI-SPIL	Sharn, Inc.
ANTI-STRESS TOOTH	Hager Worldwide, Inc.
ANTICON WIPERS	Milliken & Company, Anticon Products
ANTIMICROBIAL HANDGEL	Veridien Corp.
ANTISEPTIC BIO-HAND CLEANER (A.B.H.C.)	Safetec Of America, Inc.
ANTISTATIC VACUUM TUBING	Micro-Vac, Inc.
ANTLIA	Schleicher & Schuell, Inc.
AOSEPT	Ciba Vision Corporation
AOT-S	Siemens Medical Solutions Usa, Inc.
AP II	Baxter Healthcare Corporporation, Alternate Care And Channel Team
AP-4000	Pentax Medical Company
APC	Biotest Diagnostic Corp.
APC	C. R. Bard, Inc.
APC 300	Erbe Usa, Inc.
APC PORTABLE	Biotest Diagnostic Corp.
APEX	Aetrex Worldwide, Inc
APEX	Graham Medical Products/Div. Of Little Rapids Corp
APEX	Stryker Medical
APEX 800	Iridex Corporation
APEX FINDER	Sybronendo
APEX II	Compsee, Inc.
APEX K1	Omni Life Science, Inc
APEX K2	Omni Life Science, Inc
APEX MODULAR	Omni Life Science, Inc
APEX PRO	Ge Medical Systems Information Technologies
APEX SURGICAL	Omni Life Science, Inc
APEX UNIVERSAL DRIVE SYSTEM	Conmed Linvatec
APG	Aci Medical, Inc.
APGAR TIMER	Medela, Inc.
APHL	Louisville Apl Diagnostics, Inc.
APLIGRAF	Organogenesis Inc.
APLIO	Toshiba America Medical Systems
APNEALINK	Resmed Corp.
APNOE SCREEN	CAREFUSION 211, INC..
APNOESCREEN PRO	CAREFUSION 211, INC..
APO-B	Exocell, Inc.
APOGEE	Cynosure, Inc.
APOLLO	Aristo Import Co., Inc.
APOLLO	Bard Electro Physiology
APOLLO	Comfortex, Inc.
APOLLO	Dent Zar, Inc.
APOLLO	H.L. Bouton Co., Inc.
APOLLO	Lumedx Corp.
APOLLO	Mid-States Laboratories, Inc.
APOLLO	Oberon Company ,Div Of The Paramount Corp.
APOLLO 95E, TELICAM, ACULITE	Denmed Technologies, Inc.
APOLLO BATH	Apollo Corporation
APOLLO BY MIDMARK	Midmark Corporation
APOLLO HIP SYSTEM	Centerpulse Orthopedics Inc.
APOLLO PAK	The Saunders Group
APOLLO TOTAL KNEE SYSTEM	Centerpulse Orthopedics Inc.
APOPTAG	Serologicals Corp
APPLAUSE	Sonic Innovations
APPLAUSE	Surmodics, Inc.
APPLIED 7-10	Applied Medical Resource Corporation
APPLIED FIBEROPTICS	Vitalcor, Inc.
APPLIPAK	Smith & Nephew, Inc.
APPOINTMENTSPRO, MEDICAL CONNECT	Medinotes Corporation
APPOSE	Covidien Lp
APPURPLE	Serologicals Corp
APR HIP SYSTEM	Centerpulse Orthopedics Inc.
APR-T REVISION SYSTEM	Centerpulse Orthopedics Inc.
APRILFRESH	Chester Labs, Inc.
APRILGUARD	Chester Labs, Inc.
APS	Medtronic Xomed, Inc.
APS	Stryker Imaging

APS	Swissray International (Hq) Inc.
APT II	Hager Worldwide, Inc.
APTIMA COMBO 2	Gen-Probe, Inc.
APTUS	Diamedix Corp.
APW3	Caliper Life Sciences, Inc.
AQC	Fertility Solutions, Inc.
AQLS	Prentke Romich Company
AQT-10	Lkc Technologies, Inc.
AQUA COLOREDT	Passy-Muir Inc.
AQUA GUARD	Cenorin
AQUA MEDICAL CHILLERS	Aqua Products Company, Inc.
AQUA POWER	All Pro Exercise Products, Inc.
AQUA PRODUCTS CHILLER	Aqua Products Company, Inc.
AQUA PT, AQUA MASSAGE, AQUA PT PRO, AQUA MASSAGE SPA	Ami, Inc.
AQUA-CEL	Aqua-Cel Corp.
AQUA-FIT	Med-Fit Systems, Inc.
AQUA-FORCE	C. R. Bard, Inc.
AQUA-GEL	Salk Inc.
AQUA-PURATOR BIOTHERME	Wisap America
AQUA-RELIEF	Aqua-Cel Corp.
AQUA-SEAL	Covidien Lp
AQUA-SKIN	Afassco, Inc.
AQUA-TEMP	Cres Cor
AQUAFLEX	Ciba Vision
AQUAFLEX	Parker Laboratories, Inc.
AQUAFLOW	Staar Surgical Co.
AQUAFRESH	Gsk Consumer Healthcare
AQUAGEL	Parker Laboratories, Inc.
AQUAKING	Continental Hydrodyne Systems, Inc.
AQUALIFT	Sonicwall, Inc.
AQUALITE	Hamilton Caster & Mfg. Co.
AQUALTOWER	A&H Products, Inc.
AQUAMATE	Thermo Spectronic
AQUAMED	Jtl Enterprises
AQUAMERE	Hydromer, Inc.
AQUAPAN	Wfr/Aquaplast Corp.
AQUAPHOR	Beiersdorf, Inc.
AQUAPORE	Applied Biosystems
AQUAPRES	Lang Dental Manufacturing Co., Inc.
AQUARESS	Deb Sbs, Inc.
AQUASAFE.	Pall Medical
AQUASEPT	Lares Research
AQUASHIELD	Ortholine
AQUASHIELD	Orthomed Products, Inc.
AQUASIL	Dentsply Caulk
AQUASIL	Thermo Fisher Scientific
AQUASONIC 100	Parker Laboratories, Inc.
AQUASONIC CLEAR	Parker Laboratories, Inc.
AQUASTAR	Crescent Chemical Co., Inc.
AQUASTAR CALORIC IRRIGATOR	Micromedical Technologies, Inc.
AQUATANK	Extra Packaging, Corp.
AQUATEC	Clarke Health Care Products, Inc.
AQUATECMAJOR	Clarke Health Care Products, Inc.
AQUATENE PARTS CLEANING FLUID	Graymills Corp.
AQUATOWER	Medical Industries America Inc.
AQUATOWER II	Medical Industries America Inc.
AQUATRIX	Hydromer, Inc.
AQUAVAP	Organomation Associates, Inc.
AQUICEL AG	Convatec
AQUIFY	Ciba Vision Corporation
AQUILA	Biosound Esaote, Inc.
AR/DI	Volk Optical Inc.
ARABELLA	Hamilton Medical, Inc.
ARALAST	Baxter International Inc
ARANI	C. R. Bard, Inc.
ARAP	Avon-Isi
ARC	Air Techniques, Inc.
ARC	Cliniqa Corporation
ARC-MAX	Interscan Corp.
ARCADIA MEDICAL	Arcadia Medical Corporation
ARCADIS	Siemens Medical Solutions Usa, Inc.
ARCHIMED	Futuremed America, Inc.
ARCHITEK	United Receptacle
ARCHXERCISER	Elginex Corporation
ARCMATE	Arcmate Mfg. Corp.
ARCO	Aristo Import Co., Inc.
ARCOM	Biomet, Inc.
ARCTIC BOX	Packaging Products Corp.
ARCTIC PACK	Packaging Products Corp.
ARD	Birchwood Laboratories, Inc.
ARDUS MEDICAL, INC.	Ardus Medical, Inc.
ARGEBOND	Argen Corp.
ARGEDENT	Argen Corp.
ARGELITE	Argen Corp.
ARGELOY	Argen Corp.
ARGENCO	Argen Corp.
ARGICRAFT	Argen Corp.
ARGIPAL	Argen Corp.
ARGIPLUS	Argen Corp.
ARGISTAR	Argen Corp.
ARGLAES	Unomedical, Inc.
ARGOLITE	Argen Corp.
ARGON PLASMA COAGULATOR	Erbe Usa, Inc.
ARGON PLUST	Valleylab
ARGOS	Hacker Instruments And Industries Inc.
ARGYLE	Covidien Lp
ARIA	Stryker Corp.
ARIA	Varian Medical Systems
ARIAL	Senior Technologies
ARIATA	Briggs Corporation
ARIDYNE	Allied Healthcare Products, Inc.
ARISS	Medtronic, Inc.
ARISTO	Aristo Import Co., Inc.
ARIYA	Aetrex Worldwide, Inc
ARIZANT HEALTHCARE INC.	Arizant Healthcare Inc.
ARK INTERNATIONAL	Ark Services Corporation
ARLINK 8000 WORKSTATION	Lista International Corp.
ARM GUARD	Graphic Controls Corp.
ARM SHIELD	Trademark Medical Llc
ARM-AID	Avcor Health Care Products, Inc.
ARMATEC	Microtek Medical, Inc
ARMIDILLO CART COVERS	Tecni-Quip
ARNCO	Independent Solutions, Inc.
ARNCO	Nelson Inc., A.R.
ARNETT LEFORT IMPLANT	Implantech Associates, Inc.
AROM-COT	Utah Medical Products, Inc.
AROSMICRO	Arosurgical Instruments Corp.
AROSUPERCUT	Arosurgical Instruments Corp.
AROSUTURE	Arosurgical Instruments Corp.
ARRAY	DJO Inc.
ARRHYTHMIA TUTOR	Pinnacle Technology Group, Inc.
ARROW	Arrow International, Inc.
ARROW	Invacare Corporation
ARROW	Teleflex Medical
ARROW-FLEX	Arrow International, Inc.
ARROW-GARD	Arrow International, Inc.
ARROW-GARD BLUE	Arrow International, Inc.
ARROW-HOWES	Arrow International, Inc.
ARROW-JOHANS	Arrow International, Inc.
ARROW-KARLAN	Arrow International, Inc.
ARS	Ars Enterprises
ARS/BEVERLY PACIFIC STERILIZERS	Ars Enterprises
ARS/BP	Ars Enterprises
ART AUXILIARY	Atlanta Orthodontics
ART-TAPE	Almore International, Inc.
ARTASSIST	Aci Medical, Inc.
ARTERIAL PLUG CATHETER	Applied Medical Resource Corporation
ARTERIALFLOW	Aircast Llc
ARTERION	C. R. Bard, Inc.
ARTEX PLASTIC ARTICULATORS	American Diversified Dental Systems
ARTHOPRO FORCEP	Advanced Endoscopy Devices, Inc.
ARTHRO SHARPS	Medical Sterile Products, Inc.
ARTHRO-FLO	C. R. Bard, Inc.
ARTHRO-LOK	Becton Dickinson And Co.
ARTHROCARE	Arthrocare Corp.
ARTHROFORCE	Karl Storz Endoscopy-America Inc.

ARTHROGUIDE	Ams Innovative Center-San Jose
ARTHROJET	Hydrocision, Inc.
ARTHROMETER	Medmetric Corp.
ARTHROPUMP	Karl Storz Endoscopy-America Inc.
ARTHROWANDS	Arthrocare Corp.
ARTHUR	Perkin Elmer Wallac, Inc.
ARTHUR	Perkinelmer Life And Analytical Sciences
ARTICULATING DISSECTOR	Automated Medical Products Corp.
ARTICULATOR INJECTION NEEDLE	United States Endoscopy Group
ARTIFICIAL CORNEA	Addition Technology, Inc.
ARTIHOLDER	Hager Worldwide, Inc.
ARTIS	Siemens Hearing Instruments, Inc.
ARTIS ZEE	Siemens Medical Solutions Usa, Inc.
ARTISAN	Stryker Spine
ARTISAN REFRACTIVE LENSES	Ophtec Usa, Inc.
ARTISTE	Siemens Medical Solutions Usa, Inc
ARTLON-BANLON	Bell-Horn, Inc.
ARTROMICK	Artromick International, Inc.
ARTROMOT	Ormed Corporation
ARTROPAK	Artromick International, Inc.
ARTSCAN 200 CARTILAGE STIFFNESS TESTER	Rea Incorporated
ARZOL	Arzol Chemical Co.
AS-1	Engle Dental Systems, Inc.
AS-2	Engle Dental Systems, Inc.
AS-TRODE ELECTRODES	Electromedical Products International, Inc.
AS/PC	Db Consultants, Inc.
ASAFI PHARMACEUTICAL	Home-Aid-Healthcare, Inc.
ASAHI PLASMAFLO	Apheresis Technologies, Inc.
ASB	Labac Systems, Inc.
ASCENSIA	Siemens Healthcare Diagnostics Inc.
ASCENT(TM)	Lytron, Inc.
ASEP-TECH	Weiler Engineering, Inc.
ASEPSIS	Johnson & Johnson Medical Division Of Ethicon, Inc.
ASEPTI-CLEANSE	Veltek Associates, Inc.
ASEPTICARE TB+	Ecolab Inc.
ASH	Dentsply International, Inc.
ASH	Dentsply Prosthetics
ASH ADVANTAGE	Janin Group, Inc.
ASH SPLIT	Medcomp (Medical Components, Inc.)
ASH SPLIT CATH	Medcomp (Medical Components, Inc.)
ASHLEY LEE	Hygienics Industries Div.Of Kleinert's, Inc.
ASI	Arlington Scientific, Inc. Asi
ASI	Avon-Isi
ASI	RDL Supply
ASI SIGN SYSTEMS	Asi-Modulex
ASK FOR GLASS - ASK FOR VOLK	Volk Optical Inc.
ASNIS	Stryker Corp.
ASNIS	Stryker Spine
ASNIS 2	Stryker Spine
ASNIS III	Stryker Corp.
ASO	Aso Corporation
ASO	Medical Specialties, Inc.
ASP LABWEB	Psyche Systems
ASP300 TISSUE PROCESSOR	Leica Microsystems Inc.
ASPEN	Conmed Corporation
ASPEN SABRE	Conmed Corporation
ASPEN(TM)	Lytron, Inc.
ASPHERE	Ocu-Ease Optical Products, Inc.
ASPHERE AND THIN ZONE ASPHERE	Ocu-Ease Optical Products, Inc.
ASPIRATOR	Vital Signs Colorado
ASPIRATOR II+	Wells Johnson Co.
ASPIRATOR III	Wells Johnson Co.
ASPIRE CI	Toshiba America Medical Systems
ASSERACHROM	Diagnostica Stago, Inc.
ASSESS	Respironics New Jersey, Inc.
ASSET PROTECTION 600	Sensormatic Electronics
ASSISTIVE LISTENING DEVICES	Hal-Hen Company, Inc.
ASSURA	Coloplast Manufacturing Us, Llc
ASSURE	Arkray Usa
ASSURE	Globus Medical Inc.
ASSURE 3	Arkray Usa
ASSURE 4	Arkray Usa
ASTECH	Dey, L.P.
ASTHMA CHECK	Respironics New Jersey, Inc.
ASTHMAMENTOR	Respironics New Jersey, Inc.
ASTHMAPACK	Respironics New Jersey, Inc.
ASTORIA ANALYZER	Astoria-Pacific,Inc.
ASTOTHERM	Futuremed America, Inc.
ASTOTUBE	Futuremed America, Inc.
ASTRAL	Scientech, Inc.
ASTRAL INOCULATION SYSTEM	Bio Plas, Inc.
ASTRALIS	Ivoclar Vivadent, Inc.
ASTRO	Skytron
ASTRO TELEMETRY	Eaton Medical Devices, Inc.
ASTRO-BACK	Ehob, Inc.
ASTRO-GRAPH	Astro-Med, Inc.
ASTRODAQ	Astro-Med, Inc.
ASTROGLIDE	Biofilm, Inc.
ASTROLINK, ASTROVIEW	Astro-Med, Inc.
ASTROPOL	Ivoclar Vivadent, Inc.
ASV	Mentor Ophthalmics, Inc.
AT EASE	Hospital Specialty Company
AT FLASH	C.J.T. Enterprises, Inc.
AT KELLY	Medical Plastics Laboratory, Inc.
AT-500	Medtronic, Inc.
AT-SPEED	Thermo Fisher Scientific - Laboratory Equipment Division Headquarters
AT-START	Thermo Fisher Scientific - Laboratory Equipment Division Headquarters
ATA JUNIOR	Star Case Manufacturing Co., Inc.
ATAGO	Vee Gee Scientific, Inc.
ATAKR	Medtronic, Inc.
ATAVI	Zimmer Holdings, Inc.
ATCC	Atcc
ATCG9	Advanced Medical Systems, Inc.
ATF ANKLE BRACE	Mueller Sports Medicine
ATHENA	Athena Controls, Inc.
ATHENA	Interspec Fabrics
ATHENA - ATHENA MULTI-LYTE	Zeus Scientific, Inc.
ATHENA PELVIC MUSCLE TRAINER	Athena Feminine Technologies, Inc
ATHLETIC SPORTS MOUTHGUARD	Cooley & Cooley, Ltd.
ATI	Air Techniques International
ATLANTE	Golden Technologies, Inc.
ATLANTIC	Torbot Group, Inc.
ATLANTIC METALCRAFT	Medi-Tech International, Inc.
ATLANTIS	Medtronic Sofamor Danek Usa, Inc
ATLANTIS	Medtronic Sofamor Danek Usa, Inc.
ATLANTIS	Medtronic, Inc.
ATLANTIS	Sellstrom Manufacturing Co.
ATLANTIS WATER PURIFICATION	Questech International, Inc.
ATLAS	Arthrocare Corp.
ATLAS	Best Nomos Corp.
ATLAS	Leisure-Lift, Inc.
ATLAS	Oticon, Inc.
ATLAS	Span-America Medical Systems, Inc.
ATLAS	Welch Allyn Protocol Inc.
ATLAS	Wr Medical Electronics Co.
ATLAS & ATLAS II	Ranger All Season Corp.
ATLAS COLLAR	Jerome Medical
ATLAS I.V. SUPPORT	Pryor Products
ATLAS PLUS	Oticon, Inc.
ATLAS UNIVERSAL	Swissray America, Inc.
ATOMIC	Hager Worldwide, Inc.
ATOMLAB 100 PLUS	Biodex Medical Systems, Inc.
ATOMLAB 950	Biodex Medical Systems, Inc.
ATP	Triangle Biomedical Sciences, Inc.
ATRALOC	Ethicon, Inc.
ATRAMAT	Dma Med-Chem Corporation
ATRAUCAN	B. Braun Oem Division, B. Braun Medical Inc.
ATRAUCLIP	Teleflex Medical
ATRAUM	Axiom Medical, Inc.
ATRAUMATIC	Covidien Lp
ATRAUMAX	Applied Medical Resource Corporation
ATREUS	Caridianbct Inc.
ATRIA	Cardiac Science Corp.
ATRIAL 6492	Medtronic Cardiovascular Surgery, The Heart Valve Div.
ATRION	Atrion Medical Products, Inc.

ATRIOSEPTOSTOMY	Numed, Inc.
ATRIUM	Becton Dickinson Infusion Therapy Systems, Inc.
ATROPEN	Meridian Medical Technologies
ATS	Kinetic Concepts, Inc.
ATS 3F	ATS Medical, Inc.
ATS CRYOMAZE	ATS Medical, Inc.
ATS FROSTBYTE CLAMP	ATS Medical, Inc.
ATS MEDICAL OPEN PIVOT VALVE	ATS Medical, Inc.
ATS MEDICAL VALVE	ATS Medical, Inc.
ATS OPEN PIVOT VALVE	ATS Medical, Inc.
ATS SIMULUS ANNULOPLASTY RING	ATS Medical, Inc.
ATS SURGIFROST PROBE	ATS Medical, Inc.
ATTENDS	Paperpak
ATTEST	3m Espe Dental Products
ATTRACTIVE	Juzo
ATW	Cordis Corporation
ATWATER CAREY	Wisconsin Pharmacal Co. Llc
ATZEN	Atzen/Universal Companies, Inc.
AUDIO-CUFF	Covidien Lp, Formerly Registered As Kendall
AUDIO-EAR	Goldentone Hearing Aids
AUDIO-EXPERT	Beltone Electronics Corp.
AUDIOAIM	Electone, A Division Of Siemens Hearing Instruments, Inc.
AUDIOPATH	Welch Allyn, Inc.
AUDIOSCAN	Etymonic Design Inc.
AUDIOSCOPES	Welch Allyn, Inc.
AUDIOSCOUT	Beltone Electronics Corp.
AUDIOSPEC	Welch Allyn, Inc.
AUDTEX	Mid-States Laboratories, Inc.
AUDX PRO HEARING SYSTEMS	Natus Medical Inc.
AUENGER	Colours Wheelchair
AUERBACH	Hely And Weber
AUKUFLEX	Gammadirect Medical Division
AUKULYTE	Gammadirect Medical Division
AUKUPROBE	Gammadirect Medical Division
AUKUVENT	Gammadirect Medical Division
AUR	Aura Lens Products, Inc.
AURA	Ams Innovative Center-San Jose
AURA	Aura Lens Products, Inc.
AURA	Freeman Manufacturing Company
AURA	Misonix, Inc.
AURALITE	Aura Lens Products, Inc.
AURASEP	Hal-Hen Company, Inc.
AUREX-3	Adm Tronics Unlimited, Inc.
AURICA DIAGNOSTICS	Drg International, Inc.
AURIUM	Argen Corp.
AURO*DEX H-PYLORI	Dexall Biomedical Labs, Inc.
AURO*DEX CRP	Dexall Biomedical Labs, Inc.
AUROLITE	Argen Corp.
AURORA	Astro-Med, Inc.
AURORA	Aurora Imaging Technology, Inc.
AURORA	Lang Dental Manufacturing Co., Inc.
AURORA	Vicon Industries Inc.
AURORA HB	Amano Pioneer Eclipse Corp.
AURORA LED: ARGOSII	Skytron
AURORA MOBILE	Richards-Wilcox, Inc.
AURORA QUIK-LOK	Richards-Wilcox, Inc.
AURORA SHELVING PRODUCTS	Richards-Wilcox, Inc.
AURORACORD	Vicon Industries Inc.
AURUM	Bio-Rad Laboratories
AUTEX	Allied Diagnostic Imaging Resources, Inc.
AUTH-FLORENCE	Pacific Electronics
AUTHENTIC BUTCHER BLOCK	Newschoff Chairs, Inc.
AUTHENTIKIT	Innovative Chemistry, Inc.
AUTO FOAM	Hager Worldwide, Inc.
AUTO HDL	Pointe Scientific, Inc.
AUTO HP	Caire, Inc.
AUTO ID	Immuno Concepts N.A. Ltd.
AUTO IMAGE	Summit Industries, Inc.
AUTO SUTURE	Covidien Lp, Formerly Registered As United States Surgical
AUTO*THERM	Mettler Electronics Corp.
AUTO-CHUCK	Handler Manufacturing Co.
AUTO-CLAVE SERIES	San-I-Pak, Pacific Inc.
AUTO-FLO	Medtronic, Inc.
AUTO-KRAFT	Viscot Medical, Llc
AUTO-LANCET	Palco Labs, Inc.
AUTO-LOCK	Advanced Medical Innovations, Inc.
AUTO-LOCK	Safety Syringe Corporation Of America, Inc.
AUTO-LOCK	Thermo Fisher Scientific - Laboratory Equipment Division Headquarters
AUTO-STITCH	Covidien Lp, Formerly Registered As United States Surgical
AUTO-VENT	Rpc
AUTO-WRAP	Viscot Medical, Llc
AUTOASSAY	Giles Scientific, Inc.
AUTOBELL	Eg & G Amorphous Silicon
AUTOBLOT	Bellco Glass, Inc.
AUTOBOND	Mts Medication Technologies
AUTOBOX	CAREFUSION 211, INC.
AUTOCELL	C. R. Bard, Inc.
AUTOCHEMI	Uvp, Llc
AUTOCHILL	Aircast Llc
AUTOCLAVE REPAIR SPECIALISTS	Ars Enterprises
AUTOCOMP 6	The Metrix Co.
AUTOCORR	Smiths Medical Pm, Inc.
AUTODELFIA	Perkin Elmer Wallac, Inc.
AUTODELFIA	Perkinelmer Life And Analytical Sciences
AUTOFLOW	Nuaire, Inc.
AUTOFLUSH	Welcon, Inc.
AUTOFUSE	Byron Medical
AUTOGEN	Mts Medication Technologies
AUTOGIZER, SPEXPRESS	Tomtec
AUTOHYB	Tomtec
AUTOID	Global Focus (G.F.M.D. Ltd.)
AUTOLITH	Northgate Technologies Inc.
AUTOLOCK	Living Earth Crafts
AUTOLOGOUS GROWTH FACTORS	Interpore Cross International
AUTOLYTE EIA	Orasure Technologies, Inc.
AUTOMATIC DETECTOR POSITIONING WITH FOLLOWME	Stryker Imaging
AUTOMATOR	Autogenesis, Inc.
AUTOMATRIX	Dentsply International, Inc.
AUTOMATRIX	Dentsply Prosthetics
AUTOME	World Heart Inc.
AUTOMIX	Baxter Healthcare Corporation Nutrition
AUTOMONTAGE	Ophthalmic Imaging Systems
AUTOPAK-BPM	Medical Packaging Inc.
AUTOPAK-UDD	Medical Packaging Inc.
AUTOPAP 300	Tripath Imaging
AUTOPAP PRIMARY SCREENING SYSTEM	Tripath Imaging
AUTOPHERESIS-C	Fenwal Inc.
AUTOPOL	Rudolph Research Analytical
AUTOPRINT	Medical Packaging Inc.
AUTOPULSE	Zoll Medical Corp.
AUTOREVIEW	Tripath Imaging
AUTOSCAN	Solarius Development Inc.
AUTOSEAL	Fenwal Inc.
AUTOSEAL	Tomtec
AUTOSEQUENCE	Unetixs Vascular, Inc.
AUTOSET	Resmed Corp.
AUTOSLIPPER	Hacker Instruments And Industries Inc.
AUTOSMEAR	Sakura Finetek U.S.A., Inc.
AUTOSONIX	Covidien Lp, Formerly Registered As United States Surgical
AUTOSORB	Quantachrome
AUTOSOUND	Rich-Mar Corporation
AUTOSTEP	Welch Allyn, Inc.
AUTOSTIK	Vital Signs Colorado
AUTOSUTURE	Covidien Lp, Formerly Registered As Tyco Healthcare
AUTOTEC	Sakura Finetek U.S.A., Inc.
AUTOTRACE SPE WORKSTATION	Caliper Life Sciences, Inc.
AUTOTYMP	Welch Allyn, Inc.
AUTOVAC	Boehringer Laboratories, Inc.
AUTOVENT	Allied Healthcare Products, Inc.
AV 100	Pacific Precision Laboratories, Inc.
AV 500	Pacific Precision Laboratories, Inc.
AV Plus	St. Jude Medical, Inc.
AVACRYL	Closure Medical
AVAIRA	The Cooper Companies, Inc
AVALO	Artromick International, Inc.

AVALO AC	Artromick International, Inc.
AVALO IMC	Artromick International, Inc.
AVANT	Leedal, Inc.
AVANT	Nonin Medical, Inc.
AVANTGUARD	Geri-Care Products
AVE	Medical Instrumentation Development Labs
AVEENO	Johnson & Johnson
AVEENO	Johnson & Johnson Consumer Products, Inc.
AVENT	Philips Avent
AVIA	Coherent, Inc.
AVIAN	CAREFUSION 211, INC..
AVIANA	Coloplast Manufacturing Us, Llc
AVIATOR RX PTA DILATATION CATHETER	Cordis Endovascular
AVID	Avid Medical
AVID	Tp Orthodontics, Inc.
AVID MEDICAL SEED IMPLANT NEEDLES	Avid Medical
AVID PRODUCTS	Avid Products
AVITA	Orbusneich Medical, Inc.
AVITENE	Medchem Products, Inc.
AVIVA	Baxter Healthcare Corporation, Global Drug Delivery
AVL	Global Focus (G.F.M.D. Ltd.)
AVON PATELLA FEMORAL	Stryker Corp.
AVON PATELLA FEMORAL	Stryker Howmedica Osteonics
AVREND	Amgen Inc.
AVREO INTERWORKS SYSTEM	Avreo, Inc.
AVS	Stryker Corp.
AVS	Stryker Spine
AVS, XACT	Advanced Vision Science
AVS-AUTOMATIC VACUUM SYSTEM	Porter Instrument Division Parker Hannifin Corp
AVX	Possis Medical, Inc.
AWESOME ART BANDAGES	Aso Corporation
AWS	Hydro Service & Supplies, Inc.
AXCENT	Atc Technologies, Inc.
AXCESS	Wilson-Cook Medical, Inc.
AXCS	Dentalez Group
AXI-PATH	Panadent Corp.
AXIA RSN	Greatbach Medical
AXIOM ARISTOS	Siemens Medical Solutions Usa, Inc.
AXIOM MULTIX	Siemens Medical Solutions Usa, Inc.
AXIOM VERTIX	Siemens Medical Solutions Usa, Inc.
AXIS	Nds Surgical Imaging, Inc.
AXIUM	Ev3 Inc.
AXOSTIM	Singer Medical Products, Inc.
AXSOS	Stryker Corp.
AZONE	UCB Inc.
AZTEC	Stryker Corp.
AZTEC	Stryker Endoscopy
AZURE	Prosun Tanning International, Llc.
Aaliant	Danaher Corporation
Accolade C Cemented	Stryker Howmedica Osteonics
Accu-Sort	Danaher Corporation
AccuFlex	Boston Scientific Corporation
AccuStick	Boston Scientific Corporation
Acne-Prone	Ortho Dermatologics
Acorthotics	Acor Orthopaedic, Inc.
ActiPet	Nutraceutical International Corp.
ActiV.A.C.	Kinetic Concepts, Inc.
Action Labs	Nutraceutical International Corp.
Active Balancing	St. Jude Medical, Inc.
Actonel	Procter & Gamble
Adapta	Medtronic, Inc.
Adjusting Technology	Kinetic Concepts, Inc.
Advanced Bionics	Boston Scientific Neuromodulation Corporation
Advanced Solutions	Ortho Dermatologics
Advantage	Boston Scientific Corporation
AerMeds	American Homepatient
Aescula	St. Jude Medical, Inc.
Affinity	St. Jude Medical, Inc.
Ageless Restoratives	Ortho Dermatologics
Agilis	St. Jude Medical, Inc.
Akreos	Bausch & Lomb
Alaway	Bausch & Lomb
Align	Procter & Gamble
Allen	Danaher Corporation
Alliance	Boston Scientific Corporation
Alrex	Bausch & Lomb
Always	Procter & Gamble
American Sigma	Danaher Corporation
AmericanAirFilter	Aaf International
Analyst	Inverness Medical Professional Diagnostics-San Die
Anatomy in Clay	Zahourek Systems, Inc.
Anderson	Danaher Corporation
Angio-Seal	St. Jude Medical, Inc.
Apeel	St. Jude Medical, Inc.
Aquaplast RT	Wfr/Aquaplast Corp.
Argo-Bag Fluid Control System	Argon Medical Devices Inc.
ArgoGuide Hydrophilic Guide Wire	Argon Medical Devices Inc.
Arial	Universal Medical Products, Inc.
Armstrong	Danaher Corporation
Artiste	Pentron Laboratory Technologies
Artus	Danaher Corporation
Atlantis	Boston Scientific - Maple Grove
Atlantis	Boston Scientific Corporation
Atlas	St. Jude Medical, Inc.
AtmosAir	Kinetic Concepts, Inc.
AugmentTM	Biomimetic Therapeutics, Inc.
AutoCapture	St. Jude Medical, Inc.
Autotome	Boston Scientific Corporation
Avoximeter	International Technidyne Corp.
Axio	Micro-Tech
B-CROWNS	Harry J. Bosworth Company
B-D	Bd Diagnostic Systems
B-FACT	George King Bio-Medical, Inc.
B-GENIN AND H-GENIN PUTTY, DOUGH, AND STRIPS.	Berkeley Advanced Biomaterials, Inc.
B-PICK	Spirig Advanced Technologies, Inc.
B-PLEX	B. Braun Oem Division, B. Braun Medical Inc.
B-RAM	In/Us Systems, Inc.
B-SAFE	Schleicher & Schuell, Inc.
B-SCAN	Sonomed, Inc.
B-SMART	Koven Technology, Inc.
B-SPLINT FRACTURE KIT	Bashaw Medical, Inc.
B-VAT II	Mentor Ophthalmics, Inc.
B-VAT II-DELTA	Mentor Ophthalmics, Inc.
B-VAT II-SG	Mentor Ophthalmics, Inc.
B.BRAUN	Omni Medical Supply Inc.
B.I.P.	Adept-Med International, Inc.
B.P.MONITOR	Metronix
B16-F10-LUC-G5 BIOWARE CELL LINE	Caliper Life Sciences, Inc.
B16-F10-LUC2 BIOWARE ULTRA	Caliper Life Sciences, Inc.
B2 BIPOLAR	Ortho Development Corp.
BABICUFF	Nova Health Systems, Inc.
BABY	Johnson & Johnson
BABY AIRIN	Medical Plastics Laboratory, Inc.
BABY ANNE	Medical Plastics Laboratory, Inc.
BABY ARTI	Medical Plastics Laboratory, Inc.
BABY BAND	Seca Corp.
BABY BOARD	Seca Corp.
BABY BOARD II	Seca Corp.
BABY BOBBI	Dixie Ems Supply
BABY BUDDY	Nasco
BABY HIPPY	Medical Plastics Laboratory, Inc.
BABY IVY	Medical Plastics Laboratory, Inc.
BABY STAP	Medical Plastics Laboratory, Inc.
BABY UMBI	Medical Plastics Laboratory, Inc.
BABY WHIRL	Pari Respiratory Equipment, Inc.
BABY-STATION	Seca Corp.
BABYCENTER	Johnson & Johnson
BABYCHECKER	Medela, Inc.
BABYLAX	C.B. Fleet Company Inc.
BABYPORT	Nova Health Systems, Inc.
BABYSHIELD	Nova Health Systems, Inc.
BABYWEIGH	Medela, Inc.
BAC EZE II	Allman Products
BAC-TRACK	Microtech Medical Systems

BACK AIDE	Backsaver
BACK AT YA	Ideal Products
BACK BULL	Posture Dynamics, Inc.
BACK GLOVE	Brown Medical Industries
BACK GUARD	Schering-Plough Health Care Products
BACK ME	Roloke
BACK SKINS	Cropper Medical, Inc./Bio Skin
BACK T	Back Support Systems
BACK TO BACK	Bell-Horn, Inc.
BACK UP	Nada-Concepts
BACK-HUGGAR	Bodyline Comfort Systems
BACK-TO-BASICS	Bellco Glass, Inc.
BACK-UPS	American Power Conversion
BACK-UPS OFFICE	American Power Conversion
BACK-UPS PRO	American Power Conversion
BACKBITER	Sperian Protection
BACKBONE	Case Medical, Inc.
BACKSMART	Stryker Corp.
BACKSTOP	Merit Medical Systems, Inc.
BACKWRAP	Bean Products
BACSTOP	Staar Surgical Co.
BACT-FOIL	Bussard & Son Inc., R.D.
BACT/ALERT	Biomerieux Inc.
BACT/ALERT 3D	Biomerieux Inc.
BACT/VIEW	Biomerieux Inc.
BACTEC	Bd Diagnostic Systems
BACTI	Remel
BACTI DISK	Remel
BACTI STAPH	Remel
BACTI-BAG	Healthmark Industries
BACTI-CAPALL	Covidien Lp
BACTI-CHECK	Sani-Med, A Division Of Sanderson Plumbing Products, Inc.
BACTI-CINERATOR	Covidien Lp
BACTI-CLEANSE	Pedinol Pharmacal, Inc.
BACTI-STAINS	Medical Chemical Corp.
BACTI-SWAB	Remel
BACTIBUG	Remel
BACTICARD	Remel
BACTIDROP	Remel
BACTIFLASK	Remel
BACTISEAL	Codman & Shurtleff, Inc
BACTNEWS	Remel
BACTO	Bd Diagnostic Systems
BACTOSCRUB	Professional Disposables International, Inc.
BACTROL	Bd Diagnostic Systems
BACTURCULT	Alere, Inc.
BACTURTEST	Alere, Inc.
BAERVELDT	Abbott Medical Optics Inc.
BAG EASY	Westmed, Inc.
BAG-IT	Graphic Controls Corp.
BAHAMA	Aearo Company
BAIM TURI	C. R. Bard, Inc.
BAIR HUGGER	Arizant Healthcare Inc.
BAIR PAWS	Arizant Healthcare Inc.
BAK	Zimmer Spine, Inc.
BAK/C	Zimmer Spine, Inc.
BAK/L	Zimmer Spine, Inc.
BAKER	International Hospital Products, Inc.
BAKER ALEG	Avantor Performance Materials
BAKER ANALYZED	Avantor Performance Materials
BAKER INSTRA-ANALYZED	Avantor Performance Materials
BAKER PRS-1000	Avantor Performance Materials
BAKER REZI	Avantor Performance Materials
BAKERBOND	Avantor Performance Materials
BAKERBOND Speedisk	Avantor Performance Materials
BALANCE	Amoena
BALANCE	Hager Worldwide, Inc.
BALANCE	Sonic Innovations
BALANCE QUEST POSTUROGRAPHY	Micromedical Technologies, Inc.
BALANCE SAFETY SYSTEM	Bodypoint, Inc.
BALANCE SYSTEM SD	Biodex Medical Systems, Inc.
BALANCECHECK	Bertec Corporation
BALANCED KNEE SYSTEM	Ortho Development Corp.
BALDUR	Baldur Systems Corporation/ HTI TRADING
BALEEN POLYP TRAP	N.M. Beale Co. Inc.
BALFOUR	Albahealth Llc
BALLOON SINUPLASTY	Acclarent, Inc.
BALLOON-ON-A-WIRE	C. R. Bard, Inc.
BALOMETER	Tsi Inc.
BALTIC BIRCH	Bound Tree Medical, Llc
BAMBI	Bio-Optics, Inc.
BAMBINO	Boekel Scientific
BAN A STAIN	Combe, Inc.
BANANA BOAT	Energizer Personal Care Division
BANANA BOOT STIRRUP	Allen Medical Systems, Inc.
BAND-AID	Johnson & Johnson Medical Division Of Ethicon, Inc.
BAND-IT	I-Flow Corporation
BAND-M	Kimble Chase Life Science And Research Products Llc
BANDBAG	Cfi Medical Solutions (Contour Fabricators, Inc.)
BANDITE	American Orthodontics Corp.
BANDOLIER	Baxa Corporation
BANIS FORCEPS	Eriem Surgical
BANISH	Smith & Nephew, Inc.
BANTEX	Brasel Products, Inc.
BAR PHANTOMS	Biodex Medical Systems, Inc.
BAR SCALE	Seca Corp.
BARA-LAB	Environmental Tectonics Corp.
BARA-MED	Environmental Tectonics Corp.
BARATH	Boston Scientific Interventional Technologies
BARCLAY SERIES	United Receptacle
BARCODE/BAS	Howard Medical Company
BARD	C. R. Bard, Inc.
BARDEX	C. R. Bard, Inc.
BARDEX I.C. PROMISE	C. R. Bard, Inc.
BARDIC	C. R. Bard, Inc.
BARDIC	C. R. Bard, Inc., Bard Urological Div.
BARDPORT	C. R. Bard, Inc.
BARESKIN	Graphic Controls Corp.
BAREWIRE	Abbott Laboratories
BARI-COMMODE	Wheelchairs Of Kansas
BARICON	Mallinckrodt, Inc.
BARITONE	Novocol, Inc.
BARNETT/PAREXEL INTERNATIONAL	Parexel International Corp.
BARO-CAT	Mallinckrodt, Inc.
BAROBAG	Mallinckrodt, Inc.
BAROREFLEX ACTIVATION THERAPY	Cvrx Inc.
BAROS	Mallinckrodt, Inc.
BAROSPERSE	Mallinckrodt, Inc.
BARRACUDA	Arthrocare Corp.
BARRIER	Johnson & Johnson Medical Division Of Ethicon, Inc.
BARRIER WRAP	Pml Microbiologicals
BART'S VIBRATOR	Park Surgical Co., Inc.
BARZ	Perio Products, Inc.
BAS 200	Basi (Bioanalytical Systems, Inc.)
BAS BEE	Basi (Bioanalytical Systems, Inc.)
BAS BEEKEEPER	Basi (Bioanalytical Systems, Inc.)
BAS HONEYCOMB	Basi (Bioanalytical Systems, Inc.)
BAS-200	Benson Medical Instruments Co.
BAS-200SLM	Benson Medical Instruments Co.
BASE-STATION	Jones Medical Instrument Co.
BASHAW CID	Bashaw Medical, Inc.
BASIC 30	Medela, Inc.
BASIC BUDDY	Nasco
BASIC FLUENCY SYSTEM	Casa Futura Technologies
BASIC PATIENT CHAIRS	Dntlworks Equipment Corporation
BASIC-CHECK	Bed-Check Corporation
BASICSTAND III, MANUAL STANDING FRAME	Prime Engineering
BASIX	Merit Medical Systems, Inc.
BASIX COMPAK	Merit Medical Systems, Inc.
BASOFIX	Wescor, Inc.
BASSICK CASTERS	Shepherd Caster Corporation
BAT	Best Nomos Corp.
BAT	Cvrx Inc.
BATH-MASTER	Tub Master Lc
BATH-TEC WHIRLPOOL BATH	Bath-Tec Whirlpool Bath
BATHEASE	Bathease Inc.

BATHTRAX	Custom Durable Products, Inc
BATON	Point Source Inc.
BATTERY PAK	Physio-Control, Inc.
BATTLE CREEK	Battle Creek Equipment Co.
BATTLE CREEK	Creative Health Products, Inc.
BAUERFEIND	Ortholine
BAX	Qualicon
BAXA	Baxa Corporation
BAXJECT	Baxter International Inc
BAXSTRAP	Medical Plastics Laboratory, Inc.
BAXTER	Omni Medical Supply Inc.
BAY	Bay Corporation
BAY CORP	Bay Corporation
BAY JACOBSEN, VISCOFLEX	Jobri Llc
BAYLIFT	Ricon Corp.
BAZOOKA	Mizuho Osi
BBL	Bd Diagnostic Systems
BBRAUN	Bound Tree Medical
BCI	Smiths Medical Pm, Inc.
BCS	Siemens Healthcare Diagnostics Inc.
BCW ADVANTAGE	Wheelchairs Of Kansas
BCW LIFT & TRANSFER	Wheelchairs Of Kansas
BCW POWERCHAIR	Wheelchairs Of Kansas
BCW RECLINER	Wheelchairs Of Kansas
BCW WHEELCHAIRS	Wheelchairs Of Kansas
BD	Kern Surgical Supply, Inc.
BD BACTEC	Becton Dickinson And Company
BD CLINIJECT	Becton Dickinson And Company
BD DESTRUCLIP	Becton Dickinson And Company
BD ECLIPSE	Becton Dickinson And Company
BD FACSDIVA	Becton Dickinson And Company
BD GABARITH	Becton Dickinson And Company
BD HEMOPRO	Becton Dickinson And Company
BD IMAGN	Becton Dickinson And Company
BD JAWZONE	Becton Dickinson And Company
BD LABO	Becton Dickinson And Company
BD MACROSORT	Becton Dickinson And Company
BD NATRIX	Becton Dickinson And Company
BD OMNICOMP	Becton Dickinson And Company
BD PERSIST	Becton Dickinson And Company
BD QTEST	Becton Dickinson And Company
BD RIGHTBORE	Becton Dickinson And Company
BD SAFEDRAW	Becton Dickinson And Company
BD STERIBOX	Hager Worldwide, Inc.
BD TAXO	Becton Dickinson And Company
BD ULTRADEX	Becton Dickinson And Company
BD VASCULON	Becton Dickinson And Company
BD WALLMATE	Becton Dickinson And Company
BD XSTAR	Becton Dickinson And Company
BD YALE	Becton Dickinson And Company
BDR	Mercury Medical
BDX	Sensidyne, Inc.
BEAD LOK	Skyway Machine, Inc
BEAM	Omnimed, Inc. (Beam Products)
BEAMATIC	Omnimed, Inc. (Beam Products)
BEAMER ONE	Conmed Corporation
BEAMER PLUS	Conmed Corporation
BEAMER PLUS UNIT	Conmed Corporation
BEAMWALKER	Sellstrom Manufacturing Co.
BEAR	Arosurgical Instruments Corp.
BEAR 1000	CAREFUSION 211, INC.
BEAR CUB 750 PSV	CAREFUSION 211, INC.
BEAR MEDICAL	Allied Healthcare Products, Inc.
BEAUCHAMP	C. R. Bard, Inc.
BEAUTI-DAMASK	Riegel Consumer Products Div.
BEAUTIFIL	Shofu Dental Corporation
BEAUTY GLOVES	George Glove Company, Inc.
BEAUTY PINK WAX	Moyco Technologies, Inc.
BEAVER GUARD	Becton Dickinson And Co.
BEBE	Johnson & Johnson
BEBULIN	Baxter International Inc
BECTON DICKENSON	Omni Medical Supply Inc.
BED BLOX--THERAPEUTIC BED ELEVATORS	Better Health, Inc.

BED TENDER	Secure Care Products, Inc.
BED-BAR	Brown Engineering Corp.
BED-CHECK	Bed-Check Corporation
BED-CHECK SENSORMAT	Bed-Check Corporation
BED-COZY	Merlo Co., Llc.
BED-IN-A-BOX	Nk Medical Products Inc.
BEDBATH	Tri-State Hospital Supply Corp.
BEDMATE	HCI
BEE-SURE	Drg International, Inc.
BEEHIVE MILLENNIUM	Astro-Med, Inc.
BEELINE	Walkmed Infusion Llc
BEERE	Teleflex Medical
BEILA COMMUTATOR	Crist Instrument Co., Inc.
BEILA MICRODRIVE	Crist Instrument Co., Inc.
BEILA RABBIT HEAD HOLDER	Crist Instrument Co., Inc.
BELGAS	Marsh Bellofram
BELIMED	Belimed
BELL-HORN	Bell-Horn, Inc.
BELLCO	Bellco Glass, Inc.
BELLOFRAM	Marsh Bellofram
BELLWETHER	Vee Gee Scientific, Inc.
BELMONT BUDDY FLUID WARMER	Belmont Instrument Corp.
BENADRYL	Johnson & Johnson Consumer Products, Inc.
BENCH-TOP KEEPER	Whitney Products, Inc.
BENCHKOTE	Whatman Inc.
BENCHMARK	Ventana Medical Systems, Inc.
BENCHMARK	Virtis, An Sp Industries Company
BENCHMATE	Covidien Lp
BENCHMATE MULTI-12	Covidien Lp
BENCHMATE MULTI-8	Covidien Lp
BEND CUT	Hager Worldwide, Inc.
BENDA BRUSH	Centrix, Inc.
BENDISTAL PLIERS	Bendistal Pliers
BENDY BUMPER	Children's Medical Ventures, Inc.
BENEVOLENT DICTATOR	Information Health Network
BENGAY	Johnson & Johnson
BENZ-ALL	Xttrium Laboratories, Inc.
BEP	Siemens Healthcare Diagnostics Inc.
BERAL	Garren Scientific, Inc.
BERAL	Samco Scientific Corporation
BERAL SCIENTIFIC	Garren Scientific, Inc.
BERNER	Berner International Corp.
BERT	Pare Surgical, Inc.
BERTEC	Stryker Medical
BEST	Best Medical International, Inc.
BEST PRACTICES	Covidien Lp, Formerly Registered As United States Surgical
BEST STRAP SYSTEM	Morrison Medical
BEST TOUCH	Central Assoc. For Blind & Visually Impaired
BEST-1	Analytical Measurements, Inc.
BESURE OVULATION TEST	Syntron Bioresearch, Inc.
BESURE PREGNANCY TEST	Syntron Bioresearch, Inc.
BETA	Heine Usa Ltd.
BETA 3000	Fonar Corp.
BETA 3000M	Fonar Corp.
BETA 4133, 4131, V4132, 4150-1, 4011, 4006-PN7	Surgical Table Services Co.
BETA I	James Consolidated, Inc.
BETA II	James Consolidated, Inc.
BETA LACTAM	Remel
BETA PROBE	Intramedical Imaging Llc
BETA QUARTZ POLISHER	Hager Worldwide, Inc.
BETA-BSM	Etex Corporation
BETA-CAST	George Taub Products & Fusion Co., Inc.
BETA-CATH	Best Medical International, Inc.
BETA-ELK	Gammadirect Medical Division
BETA-SAFE	Schleicher & Schuell, Inc.
BETABASIC	Thermo Fisher Scientific
BETACOUNT	Avantor Performance Materials
BETADINE	Purdue Frederick Company
BETAFELX	G & H Wire Co.
BETAMAX	Thermo Fisher Scientific
BETAPLATE	Perkin Elmer Wallac, Inc.
BETAPLATE	Perkinelmer Life And Analytical Sciences
BETASIL	Thermo Fisher Scientific

BETASPECS	Gammadirect Medical Division
BETATROPHIX	Hanson Medical, Inc.
BETAVENT	Gammadirect Medical Division
BETTERBACK	Medi-Dyne Healthcare Products, L.L.C.
BETTEREST	Jobri Llc
BETTERNECK,EXERSWISS	Jobri Llc
BEUTELROCK	United Dental Manufacturers, Inc.
BEV-L-EDGE	Propper Manufacturing Co., Inc.
BEVCO	Bevco Ergonomic Seating
BEVERLY PACIFIC	Ars Enterprises
BEYOND SEVEN	Okamoto U.S.A., Inc.
BEYOND SEVEN PLUS	Okamoto U.S.A., Inc.
BEYOND SEVEN STUDDED	Okamoto U.S.A., Inc.
BFH	Wright Medical Group, Inc.
BFT	Siemens Healthcare Diagnostics Inc.
BG-PANEL	Covance Research Products Inc.
BH ELECTRONICS	Halbar North, Inc.
BI FLO	Westmed, Inc.
BI-ANGULAR	Biomet, Inc.
BI-BLADE	Impladent Ltd.
BI-LINE	B. Braun Oem Division, B. Braun Medical Inc.
BI-METRIC	Biomet, Inc.
BI-OK	Propper Manufacturing Co., Inc.
BI-OSTETIC FOAMT	Berkeley Advanced Biomaterials, Inc.
BI-OSTETICT	Berkeley Advanced Biomaterials, Inc.
BI-POCKET	Pml Microbiologicals
BIAFINE RE	Medix Pharmaceuticals Americas, Inc.
BIAFINE WDE	Medix Pharmaceuticals Americas, Inc.
BIB CLIPS	Hager Worldwide, Inc.
BICEPS	Teleflex Medical
BICEPS POWER	All Pro Exercise Products, Inc.
BICOAG	Gyrus Medical, Inc.
BICORE	Allied Healthcare Products, Inc.
BIDENT	Valley Forge Scientific Corp.
BIDOP	Koven Technology, Inc.
BIEL TOOL	Paratech, Inc.
BIEN AIR UNIFIX	Sirona Dental Systems Llc
BIFLATOR	Boston Scientific Corp.
BIFOLD	Ricon Corp.
BIG ADVANTAGE	DJO Inc.
BIG BOUNDER	21st Century Scientific, Inc.
BIG SHOT	Boekel Scientific
BIG TAB	B. Braun Oem Division, B. Braun Medical Inc.
BIG WHEEL	Stryker Corp.
BIGBAG	Quintron Instrument Company
BIGBAG 3000	Byron Medical
BIGBEAD	Sterogene Bioseparations, Inc.
BIII-CNAr	Ultimate Wireforms, Inc.
BIKEMAX	CYBEX INTERNATIONAL, INC.
BILAP	Gyrus Medical, Inc.
BILI-LABSTIX	Siemens Healthcare Diagnostics Inc.
BILI-LITE	Olympic Medical Corp.
BILI-MASK	Olympic Medical Corp.
BILI-METER	Natus Medical Inc.
BILIBED	Medela, Inc.
BILICOMBI	Medela, Inc.
BILIRUBIN PLUS	Hematechnologies, Inc.
BILISYSTEM	C. R. Bard, Inc.
BILOK	Biocomposites Inc.
BINASAL AIRWAY	Neotech Products, Inc.
BINAXNOW	Alere, Inc.
BINAXNOW	Inverness Medical Inc.
BIND-IT	Laboratory Technologies, Inc.
BIND-X	Aigner Index, Inc.
BINDARID	Binding Site, Inc., The
BINDAZYME	Binding Site, Inc., The
BINDER	Idexx Laboratories, Inc.
BINDER SUBMOLAR	Implantech Associates, Inc.
BINER ELLISON	Biner Ellison
BIO ACCU HCG	Bio-Med U.S.A. Inc.
BIO ACCU OVU	Bio-Med U.S.A. Inc.
BIO ACCU RUBBELA	Bio-Med U.S.A. Inc.
BIO AIR SYSTEMS	Bio Air Systems Div.

BIO BATTERY	Engineering & Research Assoc., Inc. (D.B.A. Sebra)
BIO GENEX	Biogenex Laboratories
BIO- BARRIER	Park Dental Research Corp./Implant Center
BIO-ANCHOR	Conmed Linvatec
BIO-ARCH	Tp Orthodontics, Inc.
BIO-BAG	Bd Diagnostic Systems
BIO-BAG	Bio-Logics Products, Inc.
BIO-BEADS	Bio-Rad Laboratories, Life Science Group
BIO-CEE	Alere, Inc.
BIO-CHALLENGE	Propper Manufacturing Co., Inc.
BIO-CLEAN	Stanbio Laboratory, Inc.
BIO-CLEAN-II	Stanbio Laboratory, Inc.
BIO-CLINIC	J.M. Baragano Biomedical P.M. And Consulting, Inc.
BIO-CLINIC	Sunrise Medical
BIO-CONEXT	United Chemical Technologies, Inc.
BIO-CONSOLE (WITH HEART DESIGN)	Medtronic, Inc.
BIO-CONSOLE (WITHOUT HEART DESIGN)	Medtronic, Inc.
BIO-DIMENSIONAL	Allergan
BIO-DOT	Bio-Rad Laboratories, Life Science Group
BIO-DYNAMIX	Brown Medical Industries
BIO-EYE	Integrated Orbital Implants, Inc.
BIO-FLEK	Medtronic Xomed, Inc.
BIO-FLEX	Medcomp (Medical Components, Inc.)
BIO-FLEX TESIO CATH	Medcomp (Medical Components, Inc.)
BIO-GEL	Bio-Rad Laboratories, Life Science Group
BIO-GROOVE	Biomet, Inc.
BIO-GUARD AB	Cook Inc.
BIO-ICE	Bio-Rad Laboratories, Life Science Group
BIO-LYTE	Bio-Rad Laboratories, Life Science Group
BIO-MECHANICAL	Univac Dental Company
BIO-MEDICUS (WITH HEART DESIGN)	Medtronic, Inc.
BIO-MEDICUS (WITHOUT HEART DESIGN)	Medtronic, Inc.
BIO-MODULAR	Biomet, Inc.
BIO-PEN XL	Mentor Ophthalmics, Inc.
BIO-PHORESIS	Bio-Rad Laboratories, Life Science Group
BIO-POSTURE	Brown Medical Industries
BIO-PROBE (WITH HEART DESIGN)	Medtronic, Inc.
BIO-PROBE (WITHOUT HEART DESIGN)	Medtronic, Inc.
BIO-PUMP (WITH HEART DESIGN)	Medtronic, Inc.
BIO-PUMP (WITHOUT HEART DESIGN)	Medtronic, Inc.
BIO-RAD	Bio-Rad Laboratories, Life Science Group
BIO-RAD	Mentor Ophthalmics, Inc.
BIO-REX	Bio-Rad Laboratories, Life Science Group
BIO-SCOPE SEMG	Empi, Inc.
BIO-SEP	Phenomenex, Inc.
BIO-SET	Baxter Healthcare Corporation, Baxter Biopharma Solutions
BIO-SIL	Bio-Rad Laboratories, Life Science Group
BIO-SOURCE (WITHOUT HEART DESIGN)	Medtronic, Inc.
BIO-SPIN	Bio-Rad Laboratories, Life Science Group
BIO/IMAGEBASE	Bioclinica, Inc.
BIOARCHIVE SYSTEM	Thermogenesis Corp.
BIOBARRIER	Imtec, A 3m Company
BIOBASIC	Thermo Fisher Scientific
BIOBLANKET	Kensey Nash Corporation
BIOBRADE	U.F.I.
BIOBRANE	Mylan Pharmaceuticals Inc
BIOCELL	Allergan
BIOCELL	Biocell Laboratories, Inc.
BIOCELLECT	Imtec, A 3m Company
BIOCERAMIC IMPLANTS	Fci Ophthalmics
BIOCHEMGARD	Baker Company, The
BIOCLATE	Csl Behring
BIOCLEANSE	RTI Biologics Inc.
BIOCLINIC	Joerns Healthcare, Inc
BIOCLUSIVE	Johnson & Johnson Medical Division Of Ethicon, Inc.
BIOCOMFORT	Bio Compression Systems, Inc.
BIOCOMMAND	New Brunswick Scientific Co., Inc.
BIOCOMP 2010	Biocomp Research Institute
BIOCOMPOSITES	Biocomposites Inc.
BIOCOR	Novosci Corp.
BIOCRYL RAPIDE	Depuy Mitek, Inc.
BIOCRYO	Bio Compression Systems, Inc.
BIOCUT	Angiotech

BIOCYCLE 101	Fotodyne, Inc.
BIODE	U.F.I.
BIODERM	U.F.I.
BIODEX	Supertech, Inc.
BIODISC	Cryolife, Inc.
BIOFEEDBACK SYSTEM/3	Neurodyne Medical Corp.
BIOFINITY	The Cooper Companies, Inc
BIOFLEX	Langer, Inc.
BIOFLEX	Scapa Medical
BIOFLEX	Whalen Biomedical Incorporated
BIOFLO	New Brunswick Scientific Co., Inc.
BIOFORCE	Dentsply International, Inc.
BIOFORCE	Dentsply Prosthetics
BIOFREEZE	Biofreeze Performance Health, Inc.
BIOFREZZE	Corning Inc., Science Products Division
BIOGARD	Baker Company, The
BIOGEL	Molnlycke Health Care Inc.
BIOGEL	U.F.I.
BIOGEL D	Molnlycke Health Care Inc.
BIOGEL DIAGNOSTIC	Molnlycke Health Care Inc.
BIOGEL INDICATOR	Molnlycke Health Care Inc.
BIOGEL M	Molnlycke Health Care Inc.
BIOGEL NEOTECH	Molnlycke Health Care Inc.
BIOGEL OPTIFIT ORTHOPAEDIC	Molnlycke Health Care Inc.
BIOGEL SENSOR	Molnlycke Health Care Inc.
BIOGLUE	Cryolife, Inc.
BIOGONE	Case Medical, Inc.
BIOGRAPH	Biofeedback Instrument Corp.
BIOHIT	Biohit Inc.
BIOHOOP	Hartwell Medical Corp.
BIOIMAGING SYSTEMS	Uvp, Llc
BIOJECT	Bioject Medical Technologies, Inc.
BIOJECTOR	Bioject Medical Technologies, Inc.
BIOJECTOR 2000	Bioject Medical Technologies, Inc.
BIOLAB 4400 RO	Mar Cor Purification
BIOLASE	Biolase Technology, Inc.
BIOLEX	C. R. Bard, Inc.
BIOLINE	Bioseal
BIOLINK	U.F.I.
BIOLITEC SMILEPRO 980	Biolitec, Inc.
BIOLOG	Biolog, Inc.
BIOLOG	U.F.I.
BIOLOGICAL CONTROLS INC.	Medi-Tech International, Inc.
BIOLOGIQUE	Atzen/Universal Companies, Inc.
BIOMAG	Bangs Laboratories, Inc.
BIOMARC	Carbon Medical Technologies, Inc.
BIOMATE	Thermo Spectronic
BIOMED 2000	Biomedical Life Systems, Inc.
BIOMEDICS	The Cooper Companies, Inc
BIOMEND	Integra Lifesciences Corporation
BIOMEND	Zimmer Dental, Inc.
BIOMEND EXTEND	Zimmer Dental, Inc.
BIOMET	Biomet, Inc.
BIOMETRIC	Osteoimplant Technology, Inc.
BIOMIC	Giles Scientific, Inc.
BIONICS	Cea Instruments, Inc.
BIONIT	C. R. Bard, Inc.
BIONIT II	C. R. Bard, Inc.
BIOPAK	Charter Medical Ltd.
BIOPAP	Enzo Biochem, Inc.
BIOPATCH	Ethicon, Inc.
BIOPATCH	Integra Lifesciences Corporation
BIOPATCH	Johnson & Johnson Medical Division Of Ethicon, Inc.
BIOPHYSIOMETER	Posture Dynamics, Inc.
BIOPLATE	Codman & Shurtleff, Inc
BIOPLUS	Conmed Corporation
BIOPLUS	Medtronic, Inc.
BIOPORT	Precision Dynamics Corp.
BIOPRO, INC.	Biopro, Inc.
BIOPROBE	Enzo Biochem, Inc.
BIOPROFILE	Nova Biomedical
BIOPSY NEEDLE	Stryker Corp.
BIOPTOR	Stereo Optical Co., Inc.
BIOPTY	C. R. Bard, Inc.
BIOPTY	C. R. Bard, Inc., Bard Urological Div.
BIOPTY-CUT	C. R. Bard, Inc.
BIOPTY-CUT	C. R. Bard, Inc., Bard Urological Div.
BIORCI	Smith & Nephew, Inc., Endoscopy Division
BIOREACTOR GENIE	Scientific Industries, Inc.
BIOSATE	Bd Diagnostic Systems
BIOSCOPE-SD	Comfort Technologies, Inc.
BIOSCREEN	Current Technologies Inc
BIOSCREW	Conmed Linvatec
BIOSENSORS INTERNATIONAL	Biosensors International - Usa
BIOSEPT	Young Innovations, Inc.
BIOSHIELD	United States Endoscopy Group
BIOSIGN	Getinge Usa, Inc.
BIOSIGN	Princeton Biomeditech Corp.
BIOSKIN	Cropper Medical, Inc./Bio Skin
BIOSOFT	Advanced Mechanical Technology, Inc. (Amti)
BIOSOFT	Cardinal Health Inc.
BIOSPACER	Cp Medical Corporation
BIOSPAN	Allergan
BIOSPHER GM	Melcor Technologies, Inc.
BIOSPHER SI	Melcor Technologies, Inc.
BIOSPHERE	Sarstedt, Inc.
BIOSTAGE	C. R. Bard, Inc.
BIOSTAR	Alere, Inc.
BIOSTAR	Leica Microsystems, Inc., Educational & Analytical Division
BIOSTAT	Sartorius Stedim Sus Inc.
BIOSTEON	Biocomposites Inc.
BIOSTEON	Stryker Corp.
BIOSTEON	Stryker Endoscopy
BIOSTEP	Bio Compression Systems, Inc.
BIOSTEP SEMI-RECUMBENT ELLIPTICAL	Biodex Medical Systems, Inc.
BIOSTERN PLUS	Sps Medical Supply Corp.
BIOSTIM ELECTRODES	Biomedical Life Systems, Inc.
BIOSTIM INF	Biomedical Life Systems, Inc.
BIOSTIM LX	Biomedical Life Systems, Inc.
BIOSTIM M7	Biomedical Life Systems, Inc.
BIOSTIM NMS	Biomedical Life Systems, Inc.
BIOSTINGER	Conmed Linvatec
BIOSTIR	Wheaton Science Products
BIOSTREP	Princeton Biomeditech Corp.
BIOSTRIP	Princeton Biomeditech Corp.
BIOSUC	Havel's Inc.
BIOSURE	Biosure, Inc.
BIOSYN	Covidien Lp, Formerly Registered As United States Surgical
BIOTAC	Pmt Corp.
BIOTAK	Conmed Linvatec
BIOTEK	Qrp, Inc.
BIOTENE	Laclede, Inc.
BIOTENS	American Imex
BIOTRACE	Bryan Corp.
BIOTWIST	Conmed Linvatec
BIOVAC	Wallach Surgical Devices, Inc.
BIOVEC	Advanced Mechanical Technology, Inc. (Amti)
BIOVERA	World Heart Inc.
BIOVID	Lw Scientific
BIOXYTECH	Oxis International, Inc.
BIOZ	Cardiodynamics International Corp.
BIOZ.COM	Cardiodynamics International Corp.
BIOZ.PC	Cardiodynamics International Corp.
BIOZ.TEL	Cardiodynamics International Corp.
BIOZIDE	Safetec Of America, Inc.
BIOZIP	Stryker Endoscopy
BIOZTECT	Cardiodynamics International Corp.
BIPLANE LIPOSUCTION HANDLE	Shippert Medical Technologies Corp.
BIPOLAR COAXIAL 6495	Medtronic Cardiovascular Surgery, The Heart Valve Div.
BIPORE	Bipore, Inc.
BIRO TOROK INFRARED GOGGLE	Microguide, Inc.
BIS	Aspect Medical Systems, Inc.
BIS-JET	Lang Dental Manufacturing Co., Inc.
BISHOP + JOHNSON	Clinical Pharmacies, Inc.
BISHOP'S BOUNCING PUTTY	George C. Bishop Company
BISHOP'S PUTTY	George C. Bishop Company

BISNARE	Gyrus Medical, Inc.
BISON	Dentalez Group
BISON	Ramvac Dental Products Inc
BISPECTRAL INDEX	Aspect Medical Systems, Inc.
BISSENSOR	Aspect Medical Systems, Inc.
BISTAT	Conmed Corporation
BITE REGISTRATION WAX SHEET	Almore International, Inc.
BITE REGISTRATION WAX TABS	Almore International, Inc.
BITE RITE STIX	Duro-Med Industries
BITE TABS	Panadent Corp.
BITE TRAY PLUS	Almore International, Inc.
BITE TRAYS	Panadent Corp.
BITE-BLOC	Huestis Medical
BITE-OR-PUFF	Med Labs Inc.
BITEK	Bd Diagnostic Systems
BITRODE	Zenex Corporation
BIVONA	Smiths Medical Asd
BIWEDGE	Almore International, Inc.
BIXCUT	Stryker Corp.
BKS-1000	Allergan
BLACK BELT	Infab Corp.
BLACK DIAMONDS	S.S. White Burs Inc.
BLACK MAX, XMAX, EMAX 2, MICROMAX PLUS	Anspach Effort, Inc.
BLACK TDA DIAMONDS	S.S. White Burs Inc.
BLACK-Tlr	Ultimate Wireforms, Inc.
BLACKSTONE	Blackstone Medical, Inc.
BLADDERMANAGER	Verathon Inc.
BLADDERSCAN	Verathon Inc.
BLADE SAFE	Miltex Inc.
BLADE SHIELD	Graphic Controls Corp.
BLADE WASH	Oster Professional Products, Inc.
BLADEGLOVE	Griff Industries, Inc.
BLADEGUARD	Graphic Controls Corp.
BLADEMATE	V.I.R. Engineering, Inc.
BLAK-RAY	Uvp, Llc
BLANKENSHIP	Hoggan Health Industries, Inc.
BLANKETROL	Cincinnati Sub-Zero Products, Inc., Medical Division
BLANKETROL II	Cincinnati Sub-Zero Products, Inc., Medical Division
BLAZER	Orbusneich Medical, Inc.
BLAZER II XP	Ep Technologies, Inc.
BLEACH- RITE	Current Technologies Inc
BLEDSOE	Bledsoe Brace Systems
BLICKMAN HEALTH	Medi-Tech International, Inc.
BLIND	Medicool, Inc.
BLINK	Abbott Medical Optics Inc.
BLINK	Covidien Lp, Formerly Registered As United States Surgical
BLINK CONTACTS	Abbott Medical Optics Inc.
BLINKER BUDDY	Harc Mercantile Ltd.
BLISTERBOX	Placon Corporation
BLISTERFILM	Covidien Lp
BLITZ	Conmed Linvatec
BLOCK	C. R. Bard, Inc.
BLOCKADE	Medline Industries, Inc.
BLOCKAID	Alere, Inc.
BLOCKAID	Biomet, Inc.
BLOCKER	Surgica Corporation
BLOCKIT	Walkmed Infusion Llc
BLOOD BANK SHIPPERS	Tcp Reliable, Inc.
BLOOD PACK	Fenwal Inc.
BLOOD PRESURE MONITOR	Medicool, Inc.
BLOOD-TAB	Hollister Incorporated
BLOODHOUND	Arc Medical, Inc.
BLOOM	Brandrud Furniture, Inc.
BLOOM	Fischer Medical Technologies Inc.
BLOSSOM	Mexpo International, Inc.
BLOW CLEAN	Wescor, Inc.
BLOWSHOCKERR	Flotec, Inc.
BLU-MOUSSE	Parkell, Inc.
BLU-TIP	Covidien Lp
BLUE DIAMOND ANTIFOG	David Scott Company
BLUE DIAMOND GEL PADS	David Scott Company
BLUE ICE	Pelton Shepherd Industries
BLUE LINE MOULDS	Langer, Inc.
BLUE LINE TEETH	Ivoclar Vivadent, Inc.
BLUE MAX	Akorn, Inc.
BLUE RAY CURING LIGHT	American Orthodontics Corp.
BLUE SENSOR	Ambu, Inc.
BLUE SPRING	Blue Spring Corp.
BLUE WAVE	Blue Wave Ultrasonics
BLUEBLOC	Gi Supply
BLUECLOUD	Chestnut Ridge Foam, Inc.
BLUEMAX	Cardiac Science Corp.
BLUNOSE HIGH IMPACT CORNER GUARDS	Inpro Corporation
BLUNT GRIP	Covidien Lp, Formerly Registered As United States Surgical
BLUNT PORT	Covidien Lp, Formerly Registered As United States Surgical
BLUNT-IT	Usb Corporation
BLUTAB	Confirm Monitoring Systems, Inc.
BM EL	Belco Packaging Systems, Inc.
BM PC	Belco Packaging Systems, Inc.
BM PLC	Belco Packaging Systems, Inc.
BM STANDARD	Belco Packaging Systems, Inc.
BMS	Zassi Medical Evolutions, Inc.
BN	Siemens Healthcare Diagnostics Inc.
BN PROSPEC	Siemens Healthcare Diagnostics Inc.
BNS-40	Myotronics-Noromed, Inc.
BOBBITT VALVE	Carolina Biological Supply Co.
BOBRICK	Bobrick Washroom Equipment, Inc.
BOC	Boc Gases
BODI PROTECT	Geritrex Corp.
BODY ARMOR	Darco International, Inc.
BODY BOX 5500	Morgan Scientific Inc.
BODY FIRM	Donell
BODY FLUID	R & D Systems, Inc.
BODY GLOVE	Body Glove
BODY LOUNGER	Pride Mobility Products Corp.
BODY PROP	Chi'Am International
BODY SHIELD PLUS	Health Enterprises
BODY THERAPEUTICS	I-Rep, Inc.
BODY-MATT	Span-America Medical Systems, Inc.
BODYBILT	Ergogenesis, Llc
BODYLOGIC	Mentor Corp.
BODYPOINT	Bodypoint, Inc.
BODYSCAN	Siemens Medical Solutions Usa, Inc.
BODYSOFT POSTURE SUPPORTS	Body Tech 1 Nw
BODYTYKES 1	Body Tech 1 Nw
BOEKEL	Idexx Laboratories, Inc.
BOHN	Biomet, Inc.
BOING	Optp
BOING!	Colours Wheelchair
BOLD	H.L. Bouton Co., Inc.
BOLD	Integra Lifesciences Holdings Corp.
BOLERO	ArjoHuntleigh
BOLLE	Elvex Corporation
BOLTON	Vista Lighting
BOLX	Action Products, Inc.
BOMEX	Vee Gee Scientific, Inc.
BOND ELUT	Varian Sample Preparation Products
BOND ELUT CERTIFY	Varian Sample Preparation Products
BOND ELUT JR.	Varian Sample Preparation Products
BOND ELUT LRC	Varian Sample Preparation Products
BOND-A-SPLINT	Tp Orthodontics, Inc.
BONDCLONE	Phenomenex, Inc.
BONDEK	Teleflex Medical
BONDESIL	Varian Sample Preparation Products
BONDLOGIC	Centrix, Inc.
BONE	Impladent Ltd.
BONE BIOPSY KIT	Stryker Corp.
BONECUTTER	Smith & Nephew, Inc., Endoscopy Division
BONEHOG	Biomedical Enterprises, Inc.
BONEMAX	Alere, Inc.
BONESAVE	Stryker Biotech
BONESAVE	Stryker Corp.
BONESAVE	Stryker Howmedica Osteonics
BONESOURCE	Stryker Corp.
BONESOURCE	Stryker Howmedica Osteonics
BONESOURCE BVF	Stryker Biotech

BONESOURCE BVF	Stryker Corp.
BONESOURCE BVF	Stryker Howmedica Osteonics
BONGORT	Smith & Nephew, Inc.
BONGORT	Torbot Group, Inc.
BOO-BOO PAC	Chattanooga Group
BOOKLER	Mediflex Surgical Products
BOOKSTAND	Hoyle Products, Inc.
BOOKWALTER	Codman & Shurtleff, Inc
BOOMERANG	Medtronic Sofamor Danek Usa, Inc
BOOMERANG	Medtronic Sofamor Danek Usa, Inc
BOOMERANG	Resmed Corp.
BOONE	Mission X-Ray
BOREX	Kimble Chase Life Science And Research Products Llc
BORIVIAL	Globe Scientific, Inc.
BOROPTOL	Afassco, Inc.
BOSE	Bose Corporation - Electroforce Systems Group
BOSOM BUDDY BREAST FORMS	B & B Lingerie Company, Inc.
BOSS	Boss Instruments, Ltd.
BOSS	Leisure-Lift, Inc.
BOSS 4.5: ECLIPSE	Leisure-Lift, Inc.
BOSS V	Leisure-Lift, Inc.
BOSS-LITE	Boss Instruments, Ltd.
BOSTON BRACE	Boston Brace International, Inc.
BOSTON EQUALENS	C&H Contact Lens, Inc.
BOTANY 500	Artcraft New York
BOTTLE WATCH	Zevex Incorporated
BOTTOMS-UP	Roloke
BOUNDER	21st Century Scientific, Inc.
BOUNDER PLUS	21st Century Scientific, Inc.
BOUSSIGNAC	Vitaid Ltd.
BOVIE	Bovie Medical Corp.
BOVUMINAR	Serologicals Corp
BOW-FLEX	Tp Orthodontics, Inc.
BOW-TIE ELECTRODE TENS	Covidien Lp, Formerly Registered As Uni-Patch
BOWEL MANAGEMENT SYSTEM	Zassi Medical Evolutions, Inc.
BOWMAN PERFUSION MONITORQFLOW 500 PERFUSION PROBE	Hemedex Incorporated
BOXSTELE	Pride Mobility Products Corp.
BP CUFF	Byron Medical
BPH5	Radiometer America, Inc.
BPI	Brain Power, Inc.
BRACHY	C. R. Bard, Inc., Bard Urological Div.
BRACHYTHERAPY C-ARM TABLE	Biodex Medical Systems, Inc.
BRACHYVISION	Varian Medical Systems
BRACKMANN II	Wr Medical Electronics Co.
BRAD HARRISON	Woodhead L.P.
BRADFORD	Vista Lighting
BRADY	Brady Corporation
BRADY CORP	Brady Corporation
BRADY MEDICAL	Brady Corporation
BRAILLENOTE	Humanware
BRAILLERAIL	Asi-Modulex
BRAILLIANT	Humanware
BRAIN MONITOR	Natus Medical Inc.
BRAIN NAVIGATOR	Astro-Med, Inc.
BRAINMAKER	California Scientific
BRAINMAKER PROFESSIONAL	California Scientific
BRAINMAP	Cadwell Laboratories
BRAINMASTER	Biofeedback Instrument Corp.
BRAINTREE	Astro-Med, Inc.
BRALON	Covidien Lp, Formerly Registered As United States Surgical
BRANDON	Brady Corporation
BRANDON INTERNATIONAL	Brady Corporation
BRANDT INDUSTRIES	Medi-Tech International, Inc.
BRAT II	Sorin Group Usa
BRAUN	Handi-Cap Aids Company
BRAUN	Oral-B Laboratories, Inc.
BRAUN CHIEF XL	Braun Industries, Inc.
BRAUN EXPRESS	Braun Industries, Inc.
BRAUN HANDCRAFTED AMBULANCES	Braun Industries, Inc.
BRAUN LABSONIC	Sartorius Stedim Sus Inc.
BRAUN LFEA 4XL	Braun Industries, Inc.
BRAUN RAIDER	Braun Industries, Inc.
BRAUN SUPER CHIEF	Braun Industries, Inc.
BRAVELLE	Smithers Medical Products, Inc.
BRAVO	ArjoHuntleigh
BRAVO	Hager Worldwide, Inc.
BRAVO	Ortho-Kinetics, Inc.
BRAVO	Surmodics, Inc.
BRAVO PLUS	Ortho-Kinetics, Inc.
BRAYCYCLE	Nucon International, Inc.
BRAYSORB	Nucon International, Inc.
BREAK AWAY	Winfield Laboratories
BREAK-OUT SCREW EXTRACTION SYSTEM	Biopro, Inc.
BREAS	Vital Signs, Inc.
BREAT VEST	Smith & Nephew, Inc.
BREATH ACE BREATHFRESHER	Beyond 21st Century Inc.
BREATH ALCOHOL (CHECK)	Akers Biosciences, Inc.
BREATHABLES	Paperpak
BREATHALYZER	Draeger Safety, Inc.
BREATHCALL	Dwyer Precision Products, Inc.
BREATHCO	Vitalograph, Inc.
BREATHE CLEAN	J. Lamb, Inc. A Division Of The Strongwater Group
BREATHE RIGHT NASAL STRIPS	Cns, Inc.
BREATHE X	CAREFUSION 211, INC..
BREATHE X JOURNEY	CAREFUSION 211, INC..
BREATHER BAG	Perfecseal
BREATHPATH	Medical Graphics Corporation
BREATHTRACKER	Quintron Instrument Company
BRECKENRIDGE	Vista Lighting
BREEZE	Siemens Healthcare Diagnostics Inc.
BREEZE NETWORK SOFTWARE	Medical Graphics Corporation
BREEZE SINGLE BREATH	Medical Graphics Corporation
BREEZE SLEEPGEAR	Covidien (Formerly Nellcor Puritan Bennett / Tyco Healthcare)
BREEZE SOFTWARE	Medical Graphics Corporation
BREEZEE MIST	Pedinol Pharmacal, Inc.
BREEZEPF SOFTWARE	Medical Graphics Corporation
BREEZESC SOFTWARE	Medical Graphics Corporation
BRENER	C. R. Bard, Inc.
BRENTWOOD BY MIDMARK	Midmark Corporation
BREUER	Tornado Industries
BREVI-KATH	Epimed International, Inc.
BREVI-XL	Epimed International, Inc.
BREVIBLOC	Baxter Healthcare Corporation, Baxter Pharmaceuticals And Technologies
BREVIO	Neumed Inc.
BREVITAL	King Pharmaceuticals, Inc.
BRIDGEAID	Flossaid Corporation
BRIEF PHYSIOLOGICAL STRESS PROFILE	Neurodyne Medical Corp.
BRIEFMATES	Humanicare International, Inc.
BRIGGS TECHNOLOGY	Briggs Corporation
BRIGHT SPOT	George Taub Products & Fusion Co., Inc.
BRIGHT-SPOT	Independent Solutions, Inc.
BRIGHTON	Vista Lighting
BRILLIANT	Hager Worldwide, Inc.
BRIMMS DENTURE BATH	Combe, Inc.
BRINGING MEDICAL POSSIBILITIES TO LIFE	Possis Medical, Inc.
BRINK PERIPYRIFORM	Implantech Associates, Inc.
BRIO	Ela Medical, Inc.
BRITE SHIELD	Premier Medical Products
BRITESMILE	Bsml, Inc.
BRK	St. Jude Medical, Inc.
BROCKENBROUGH	C. R. Bard, Inc.
BROCKER SIDES	Hard Manufacturing Co.
BRODA SEATING	Broda Enterprises Inc.
BRODMERKEL	Wilson-Cook Medical, Inc.
BROKEN GLASS KEEPER	Whitney Products, Inc.
BROM (BACK RANGE OF MOTION)	Performance Attainment Associates
BRONCHIAL PROVACATION SOFTWARE	Medical Graphics Corporation
BRONCHO SALINE	Blairex Laboratories, Inc.
BRONCO	Snug Seat, Inc.
BROSELOW PEDIATRIC EMERGENCY TAPE	Armstrong Medical Industries, Inc.
BROSELOW/HINKLE PEDIATRIC RESUSCITATION SYSTEM	Armstrong Medical Industries, Inc.
BROVIAC	C. R. Bard, Inc.

BROW BAR	H.L. Bouton Co., Inc.
BROWN AIR DERMATONE	Zimmer Orthopaedic Surgical Products
BROWN DERMATONE BLADES	Zimmer Orthopaedic Surgical Products
BROWN ELECTRIC DERMATONE	Zimmer Orthopaedic Surgical Products
BROWN EMPYEMA	Axiom Medical, Inc.
BROWN/MEDICAL	Ortholine
BROWNIE	Shofu Dental Corporation
BRST-2	Covance Research Products Inc.
BRUDER	Bruder Healthcare Company
BRUN-TUFF MMT	Bruin Plastics Co.
BRUNO	Handi-Cap Aids Company
BRUNO	Handicap Unlimited, Inc.
BRUSH&BOND	Parkell, Inc.
BRUSH-N-FLOSS	Hager Worldwide, Inc.
BRUSH-NEST	Instrument Specialists, Inc.
BRUX-0-GARD	Tmj Appliance
BRYAN	Medtronic Sofamor Danek Usa, Inc.
BRYAN	Medtronic Sofamor Danek Usa, Inc.
BRYAN-DUMON	Bryan Corp.
BRYTEBOX	Photon Technology International, Inc.
BSI	Bretton Square Industries
BSR ARCHIVAL	Rem Systems
BTA	C. R. Bard, Inc.
BTA STAT	Polymedco, Inc.
BTC	Labac Systems, Inc.
BTX ECM GENERATORS	Harvard Apparatus, Inc.
BUBBLE	Covidien Lp
BUBBLES THE FISH	Pari Respiratory Equipment, Inc.
BUBBLESTICK	Pegasus Research Corp.
BUCHBINDER	Medtronic, Inc.
BUCK 200A ATOMIC ABSORPTION SPECTROPHOTOMETER	Buck Scientific, Inc.
BUCK 210VGP ATOMIC ABSORPTION SPECTROPHOTOMETER	Buck Scientific, Inc.
BUCK 300 LITHIUM/SODIUM ANALYZER	Buck Scientific, Inc.
BUCK 400 MERCURY ANALYZER	Buck Scientific, Inc.
BUCK 404 OIL & WATER ANALYZER	Buck Scientific, Inc.
BUCK M500 SCANNING IR SPECTROPHOTOMETER	Buck Scientific, Inc.
BUCK-32	Smith & Nephew Inc.- Orthopaedics Division
BUDDE	Schaerer Mayfield Usa
BUDDIES	Griffin Medical Products, Inc.
BUDDY	Snug Seat, Inc.
BUDDY BAND	Precision Dynamics Corp.
BUDDY SYSTEM	Diestco Manufacturing Corp.
BUDGET BUDDY	Budget Buddy Company, Inc.
BUDYBAGS	Extra Packaging, Corp.
BUELLIDYNE	Cfi Medical Solutions (Contour Fabricators, Inc.)
BUFFALO FILTER	Buffalo Filter, A Division Of Medtek Devices Inc.
BUFFINOX	Afassco, Inc.
BUG SHIELD	Health Enterprises
BUGEE	Clarke Health Care Products, Inc.
BUILD-A-CART	Blue Bell Bio-Medical
BUILT IN BIDET	Mobility Inc.
BULL FROG	Hager Worldwide, Inc.
BULL'S-EYE DISPOSABLE NEEDLE STICK PREVENTION AID	Hunter Research Laboratories, Inc.
BULLDOG	Dentalez Group
BULLDOG	Ramvac Dental Products Inc
BULLDOG QT	Ramvac Dental Products Inc
BUMINATE	Baxter International Inc
BUMOTEC	Hansco Technologies, Inc.
BUMP-R-SLEEVE	Tp Orthodontics, Inc.
BUNNY KIT	Graphic Controls Corp.
BUR-TAINER	Hager Worldwide, Inc.
BURDICK	Cardiac Science Corp.
BURDICK	Kern Surgical Supply, Inc.
BURDICK & JACKSON ANHYDROUS	Honeywell Burdick & Jackson
BURN CHECK	Romaine, Inc. D.B.A. Koldcare
BURN RELIEF	Romaine, Inc. D.B.A. Koldcare
BURN SEPTIC	Afassco, Inc.
BURN STOP	Romaine, Inc. D.B.A. Koldcare
BURN-JEL	Water-Jel Technologies
BURNFREE	Burnfree Products Division
BURNPAC	Allied Healthcare Products, Inc.

BURTON	Burton Co., R.H.
BURTON SERVICE	Burton Co., R.H.
BUSINESS1-PFM	Per-Se Technologies
BUSINESSMASTER	Horizon Healthcare Technologies
BUSING-VEYOR	Caddy Corporation
BUSMASTER	Caddy Corporation
BUTLER	Flinchbaugh-Kurtz Company
BUTLER	Sunstar Butler
BUTTERFLY	Medtronic Sofamor Danek Usa, Inc
BUTTERFLY	Medtronic Sofamor Danek Usa, Inc.
BUTTERFLY	Schleicher & Schuell, Inc.
BUTTON	C. R. Bard, Inc.
BUYMED	Kern Surgical Supply, Inc.
BUYWHEELCHAIR.COM	Colours Wheelchair
BUZMATICS	Marsh Bellofram
BVS	Abiomed, Inc.
BVS 5000	Abiomed, Inc.
BX VELOCITY	Cordis Corporation
BXR	Xma (X-Ray Marketing Associates, Inc.)
BY ADELBERG LABORATORIES	Adelberg Laboratories Inc.
BYE BYE DECUBITI	Rand-Scot Inc.
BYE-BYE DECUBITI	Mcright Supplies Inc., Ken
BYREL	Medtronic, Inc.
Baker-flex	Avantor Performance Materials
BakerClean	Avantor Performance Materials
BakerFACTS	Avantor Performance Materials
Barbasol	Perio Products, Inc.
BariAir	Kinetic Concepts, Inc.
BariKare	Kinetic Concepts, Inc.
BariMaxx	Kinetic Concepts, Inc.
Bariatric Support	Kinetic Concepts, Inc.
BeamPath	Omniguide, Inc.
BeamPath NEURO	Omniguide, Inc.
Bindicator	Danaher Corporation
BioActive Surface	Medtronic Perfusion Systems
BioTrace	Pall Corporation
BioTrend	Medtronic Perfusion Systems
Bionics	Boston Scientific Corporation
Bioprogressive	Rmo, Inc.
BladderChek	Matritech, Inc.
Blazer	Boston Scientific Corporation
Blazer	Ep Technologies, Inc.
Blazer II XP	Boston Scientific Corporation
BluWave	Micro-Tech
Body Clear	Ortho Dermatologics
Bond-1	Pentron Laboratory Technologies
Boston	Bausch & Lomb
Bounce	Procter & Gamble
Bounty	Procter & Gamble
Breeze	Pentron Laboratory Technologies
BuCAIM	Avantor Performance Materials
Buhler Montec	Danaher Corporation
Bulldog	Knoll, Inc.
Bulls-Eye	Hilco
C PERFECT	Staar Surgical Co.
C&B-METABOND	Parkell, Inc.
C-ARM TABLE	Supertech, Inc.
C-BLOC	I-Flow Corporation
C-FLEX	Saint-Gobain Performance Plastics/Clearwater
C-FLEX	Shamrock Medical, Inc.
C-FUSOR	Smiths Medical OEM
C-GUARD	Siemens Hearing Instruments, Inc.
C-I POST	Parkell, Inc.
C-KURE	C & K Manufacturing & Sales
C-LABS	Currie Medical Specialties, Inc.
C-LOOPS	Saint-Gobain Performance Plastics/Clearwater
C-MATT	Casco Manufacturing Solutions, Inc.
C-MAX	C. R. Bard, Inc., Bard Urological Div.
C-PAD	Casco Manufacturing Solutions, Inc.
C-PAP	Futuremed America, Inc.
C-PICK	Spirig Advanced Technologies, Inc.
C-PLAC	Preventive Dentistry Products, Inc.
C-PORT	Cardica, Inc.

C-R	Centrix, Inc.
C-R SYRINGE	Centrix, Inc.
C-SERTER	Conmed Linvatec
C-TEK CERVICAL PLATE	Interpore Cross International
C-TEMP	Bovie Medical Corp.
C-TRAK	Care Wise Medical Products Corp.
C-VEST	Capintec, Inc.
C-WIRE	Conmed Linvatec
C.A.R.E.	Albahealth Llc
C.A.T.	Stereo Optical Co., Inc.
C.A.T.S.	Precision Dynamics Corp.
C.I.KIT	Parkell, Inc.
C/N SCREEN	Remel
C/P LIFT	Bio-Rad Laboratories, Life Science Group
C0C402	Epix, Inc.
C2 SKIN CONDUCTANCE MONITOR	Neurodyne Medical Corp.
C3	Timm Medical Technologies, Inc.
C300	Permobil, Inc.
C300CORPUS	Permobil, Inc.
C300CS	Permobil, Inc.
C300PS	Permobil, Inc.
C400	Permobil, Inc.
C400AERON	Permobil, Inc.
C400CORPUS	Permobil, Inc.
C400CS	Permobil, Inc.
C400JR.STANDER	Permobil, Inc.
C400PS	Permobil, Inc.
C500	Permobil, Inc.
C500AERON	Permobil, Inc.
C500COMBI-STANDER	Permobil, Inc.
C500CORPUS	Permobil, Inc.
CA 125 RIA	Centocor, Inc.
CA 125II	Fujirebio Diagnostics, Inc. (Fdi)
CA 15-3	Fujirebio Diagnostics, Inc. (Fdi)
CA 15-3 RIA	Centocor, Inc.
CA 19-9	Fujirebio Diagnostics, Inc. (Fdi)
CA 19-9 RIA	Centocor, Inc.
CA 72-4	Fujirebio Diagnostics, Inc. (Fdi)
CA 72-4 RIA	Centocor, Inc.
CA PLUS ADHESIVES	Ca Plus Adhesives, Inc.
CA-HP	Baxter Healthcare Corporation, Renal
CABBIE COMPANION	Kareco International, Inc.
CABBIE II	Kareco International, Inc.
CABLE EXPRESS	Vitalcor, Inc.
CABLE GRAB	Sellstrom Manufacturing Co.
CAD	Stryker Spine
CADD	Smiths Medical Asd, Inc.
CADD-1	Smiths Medical Asd, Inc.
CADD-AMBASSADOR	Smiths Medical Asd, Inc.
CADD-DIPLOMAT	Smiths Medical Asd, Inc.
CADD-LEGACY	Smiths Medical Asd, Inc.
CADD-MICRO	Smiths Medical Asd, Inc.
CADD-PCA	Smiths Medical Asd, Inc.
CADD-PLUS	Smiths Medical Asd, Inc.
CADD-PRIZM	Smiths Medical Asd, Inc.
CADD-TPN	Smiths Medical Asd, Inc.
CADDY AIRSYSTEMS	Caddy Corporation
CADDY COLD	Caddy Corporation
CADDY-CONNECTION	Caddy Corporation
CADDY-MAGIC	Caddy Corporation
CADDY-VEYOR	Caddy Corporation
CADENCE ENTERPRISE SCHEDULING	Epic Systems Corp.
CADET	Precision Dynamics Corp.
CADET DEGREASER	Aegis Floorsystems
CADLOWT SHOULDER STABILIZER	Dm Systems, Inc.
CADSTREAM	Confirma, Inc.
CADWELL	Cadwell Laboratories
CAFRAMO	Caframo Ltd.
CAGE-KLENZ	Steris Corporation
CAHN	Orion Research, Inc.
CAL CHECK	Hardy Diagnostics
CAL STAT	Steris Corporation
CAL-GEL	Jorgensen Laboratories
CAL-VER	Microgenics Corporation
CALADRYL	Johnson & Johnson Consumer Products, Inc.
CALAXO	Smith & Nephew, Inc., Endoscopy Division
CALCIBIND	Mission Pharmacal Co.
CALCITITE 2040	Zimmer Dental, Inc.
CALCITITE 4060	Zimmer Dental, Inc.
CALCUSPLIT	Karl Storz Endoscopy-America Inc.
CALCUTRIPT	Karl Storz Endoscopy-America Inc.
CALF SKINS	Cropper Medical, Inc./Bio Skin
CALGISWAB	Puritan Medical Products Company Llc
CALIBER	Mabis Healthcare Inc.
CALIBRETTE	Precision Systems, Inc.
CALIFORNIA ORTHODONTIC	Dansereau Health Products, Inc.
CALIFORNIAN	Dansereau Health Products, Inc.
CALIGAMED	Bauerfeind Usa, Inc.
CALIGATOR	Life-Tech, Inc.
CALL LIGHT	Pioneer Medical Systems
CALMOSEPTINE OINTMENT	Calmoseptine, Inc.
CALORIE BURNERS	Alere, Inc.
CALROD	D.M. Davis Inc.
CALSTRUX	Stryker Biotech
CALSTRUX	Stryker Corp.
CALTECH	Caltech Industries, Inc.
CALYPSO	ArjoHuntleigh
CALYPTE	Calypte Biomedical Corporation
CALYSTO FOR CARDIOLOGY	Witt Biomedical Corporation
CALYSTO IMAGE IV	Witt Biomedical Corporation
CALYSTO PCM (PATIENT CARE MONITORING)	Witt Biomedical Corporation
CALYSTO PCM-CENTRAL STATION	Witt Biomedical Corporation
CALYSTO SERIES IV	Witt Biomedical Corporation
CAM-1 PLUS	Camfil Farr
CAM-I	Camfil Farr
CAM-WRAP	Microtek Medical, Inc
CAM/ALOT	Speedline Technologies, Inc.
CAMAG	Camag Scientific, Inc.
CAMBASE	Sirona Dental Systems Llc
CAMBRIDGE BIOTECH	Calypte Biomedical Corporation
CAMCO	Cambridge Diagnostic Products, Inc.
CAMEO	Argosy
CAMEO	Ge Infrastructure Water & Process Technologies
CAMEO	Surmodics, Inc.
CAMINO	Integra Lifesciences Holdings Corp.
CAMPYPAK	Bd Diagnostic Systems
CAMPYPOUCH	Bd Diagnostic Systems
CAMPYSLIDE	Bd Diagnostic Systems
CAMSTAR	Hoggan Health Industries, Inc.
CAN GROW WEIGHT	Alex Orthopedic, Inc.
CANAL FINDER	Biolase Technology, Inc.
CANCELLATOR	R. B. Annis Instruments, Inc.
CANCELYZER	Cloud 9
CAND-TEC	Ramco Laboratories, Inc.
CANDI KIT	Culture Kits, Inc.
CANDIDASURE	Lifesign
CANDIDATUBE	Remel
CANDIQUANT	Biomerica, Inc.
CANDY CANE	Byron Medical
CANITEC	Dms Laboratories, Inc.
CANNABUSE	Biochemical Diagnostics, Inc.
CANNON	Cannon Instrument Co.
CANNON-FENSKE ROUTINE	Cannon Instrument Co.
CANNULA CADDY	Katena Products, Inc.
CANNULAIDE	Beevers Manufacturing, Inc.
CANNULATOME II	Wilson-Cook Medical, Inc.
CANON	Canon Development Americas, Inc
CANOPY ENCLOSED BED	Pedicraft, Inc.
CAP	Carolon Company
CAP TRAP	Hager Worldwide, Inc.
CAP-CHUR	Palmer Cap-Chur, Inc.
CAPCELL	Capintec, Inc.
CAPELLA	Liko North America
CAPELLINI	Nest Group Inc., The
CAPI-DRAW	Innovative Medical Technologies, Inc.
CAPICHROM	Portable Medical Laboratories, Inc.

CAPIJECT	Terumo Medical Corp.
CAPILLARYS	Sebia Electrophoresis
CAPINTU	Vespo Marketing Assoc., Inc.
CAPIOX	Terumo Cardiovascular Systems, Corp
CAPIOX	Terumo Medical Corp.
CAPKEEPER	Rpc
CAPMAC	Capintec, Inc.
CAPNO-FLO	Covidien (Formerly Nellcor Puritan Bennett / Tyco Healthcare)
CAPNOCHECK	Smiths Medical Pm, Inc.
CAPNOGARD	Respironics, Inc
CAPRAC	Capintec, Inc.
CAPRI	Golden Technologies, Inc.
CAPRI	Graphic Controls Corp.
CAPRIA	Capintec, Inc.
CAPROCK	Caprock Developments Inc.
CAPS LUER-LOCK	Primrose Medical, Inc.
CAPSET	Lifecore Biomedical, Inc.
CAPSETTE	Bio Plas, Inc.
CAPSTONE	Medtronic Sofamor Danek Usa, Inc
CAPSTONE	Medtronic Sofamor Danek Usa, Inc.
CAPSURE	Medtronic, Inc.
CAPSURE SP	Medtronic, Inc.
CAPSURE Z	Medtronic, Inc.
CAPSUREFIX	Medtronic, Inc.
CAPTEL, COMPACT/C TTY	Ultratec, Inc.
CAPTIA	Trinity Biotech, Inc.
CAPTIVA	Merit Medical Systems, Inc.
CAPTOR	Hager Worldwide, Inc.
CAPTOR DELUXE	Hager Worldwide, Inc.
CAPTURE	Immucor, Inc.
CAPTURE WORKBENCH	Brit Systems Inc.
CAPTURE-CMV	Immucor, Inc.
CAPTURE-P	Immucor, Inc.
CAPTURE-R	Immucor, Inc.
CAPTUS	Capintec, Inc.
CAPU-CELL	Tmp Technologies, Inc.
CARB-N-SERT	Miltex Inc.
CARBO CATCHER	Alere, Inc.
CARBO-TRAP	Avantor Performance Materials
CARBOCONE	Lynn Medical
CARBOFIX	Statlab Medical Products, Inc.
CARBOFLO	Bard Peripheral Vascular, Inc.
CARBON COPY	Ohio Willow Wood Company
CARBON LIGHTS ARM & HAND SURGERY TABLES	Allen Medical Systems, Inc.
CARBONET	Smith & Nephew, Inc.
CARBONFLEX	Bloomex International, Inc.
CARBOPLAST II	Aetrex Worldwide, Inc
CARDI-SPRAGUE	Medworks Instruments
CARDIAC REHAB-TEL	Eaton Medical Devices, Inc.
CARDIAC SURVIVAL NETWORK	Datascope Cardiac Assist Div.
CARDIAC-CX	Fischer Medical Technologies Inc.
CARDIASURE	Quantimetrix Corporation
CARDINAL	La Mont Medical, Inc.
CARDIO	Conmed Corporation
CARDIO ID+	Rozinn By Scottcare Corporation
CARDIO-PROBE	Seecor, Inc.
CARDIO-SHOE	Covidien Lp, Formerly Registered As United States Surgical
CARDIO2	Medical Graphics Corporation
CARDIO2 CYCLE ERGOMETER	Medical Graphics Corporation
CARDIO2 CYCLE ERGOMETER SERIES	Medical Graphics Corporation
CARDIO2 SYSTEM	Medical Graphics Corporation
CARDIO2/MAX SYSTEM	Medical Graphics Corporation
CARDIOBEEPER	Meridian Medical Technologies
CARDIOBELT	Monebo Technologies, Inc.
CARDIOCHART	Lumedx Corp.
CARDIODYNAMIC IMAGING	Medical Graphics Corporation
CARDIOFAX	Nihon Kohden America, Inc.
CARDIOFILE+	Rozinn By Scottcare Corporation
CARDIOGRAFT	Lifenet Health
CARDIOGRAM	Compumed, Inc.
CARDIOINTEGRAPH	Ocg Technology, Inc.
CARDIOLIFE	Nihon Kohden America, Inc.
CARDIOMAX	Shimadzu Medical Systems
CARDIOPAL SAVI	Medicomp, Inc.
CARDIOPOINT	Covidien Lp
CARDIOPTIC	Valley Forge Scientific Corp.
CARDIOPUNCH	Covidien Lp
CARDIORHYTHM	Medtronic, Inc.
CARDIOSENS	Cardiac Science Corp.
CARDIOSIM	Cardionics, Inc.
CARDIOSONIX,QUANTIX	Neoprobe Corporation
CARDIOSTATION	Mednet Healthcare Technologies, Inc.
CARDIOTHANE	Arrow International, Inc.
CARDIOTRAC	Siemens Healthcare Diagnostics Inc
CARDIOVASIVE	Scanlan International, Inc.
CARDIOVIVE	Cardiac Science Corp.
CARDIOWEST	Syncardia Systems, Inc.
CARDIOWRAP	Cryolife, Inc.
CARDON THERAPEUTIC EXERCISE EQUIPMENT	Cardon Rehabilitation Products Inc
CARDON THERAPY TABLES	Cardon Rehabilitation Products Inc
CARDS	Quidel Corporation
CARE BAND	Aso Corporation
CARE CHAIR	Activeaid, Inc.
CARE DELUXE OCCUPANCY SYSTEM	Care Electronics, Inc.
CARE MOBILITY MONITOR	Care Electronics, Inc.
CARE MOLD	Composites Horizons, Inc.
CARE SOX PLUS	Therafirm, A Knit Rite Company
CARE TRACK MAMMO TRACKER	Imsi, Integrated Modular Systems Inc.
CARE-E-VAC	Ohio Medical Corp.
CARE-E-VAC AC	Ohio Medical Corp.
CARE-STEPS	Albahealth Llc
CARE-WARE	Whitehall Manufacturing
CAREFLEX	Chestnut Ridge Foam, Inc.
CAREFLEX	Independent Solutions, Inc.
CAREFLOW	Becton Dickinson Infusion Therapy Systems, Inc.
CAREFOR	Salk Inc.
CAREFREE BREATHING	Cft, Inc./Life Mask
CAREFUSION	Cardinal Health Inc.
CAREKITS	Merit Medical Systems Inc.
CARELET	Facet Technologies, Llc
CARELINE	Unomedical, Inc.
CAREMASTER	Horizon Healthcare Technologies
CARENDO	ArjoHuntleigh
CARENET	American Medical Alert Corp.
CARENOTES	Micromedex, Inc.
CAREPLAN	Alere, Inc.
CARESENSE	Curbell, Inc. Electronics
CARESS	Riegel Consumer Products Div.
CARESTREAM	Carestream Health, Inc.
CARFONE	Ericsson, Inc.
CARGILLE	Mccrone Microscopes & Accessories
CARINO	ArjoHuntleigh
CARIS	Biosound Esaote, Inc.
CARIS PLUS	Biosound Esaote, Inc.
CARISSA	Torbot Group Inc., Jobskin Division
CARITAL AIR-FLOAT SYSTEM	Rea Incorporated
CAROLI	Liko North America
CARON	Caron Products And Services, Inc.
CARPA TABLE	Allen Medical Systems, Inc.
CARPAL MANAGEMENT SYSTEM	Balance Systems, Inc.
CARPAL-TRAC	Chattanooga Group
CARPENTIER-EDWARDS	Edwards Lifesciences, Llc.
CARPUJECT	Hospira, Inc.
CARR	Carr Corporation
CARR	Kendro Laboratory Products
CARRERA	Ortho-Kinetics, Inc.
CARRIE SYSTEM	Patterson Medical Holdings, Inc.
CARRIER-LIFT INCLINED PLATFORM LIFT	Thyssenkrupp Access Corp.
CARRY STAR	Star Case Manufacturing Co., Inc.
CARRYALL	Instromedix, A Card Guard Co.
CART TOPPER	Bussard & Son Inc., R.D.
CART-A-WAY	United Receptacle
CART-MATIC	Courion
CARTER-THOMASON	Inlet Medical, Inc.
CARTER-THOMASON INLET	Inlet Medical, Inc.

CARTEX	The Carnegie Textile Co.
CARTLEX M	Shimadzu Medical Systems
CARTLEX P	Shimadzu Medical Systems
CARV-EZE	George Taub Products & Fusion Co., Inc.
CARVER	Carver Inc.
CAS	Bound Tree Medical
CAS EXPRESS	Cas Medical Systems, Inc.
CASCADE	Cadwell Laboratories
CASCO STANDARDS	Microgenics Corporation
CASE	Ge Medical Systems Information Technologies
CASE IV	Wr Medical Electronics Co.
CASEPLAN	Stryker Corp.
CASEPLAN	Stryker Endoscopy
CASEPLAN	Stryker Howmedica Osteonics
CASIO	Eric Armin Inc.
CASMED	Cas Medical Systems, Inc.
CASPAR	Aesculap Implant Systems Inc.
CASPATAG	Serologicals Corp
CAST CUTTER	Stryker Corp.
CAST GRIPPER	Hager Worldwide, Inc.
CAST VAC	Stryker Corp.
CAST-O-FOAM PLUS	Pedinol Pharmacal, Inc.
CAST-RITE	Knit-Rite, Inc.
CAST-RITE	Paramedical Distributors
CASTALOY	Fisher Scientific Co., Llc.
CASTBLAST	Tagg Industries L.L.C.
CASTELLANI	Pedinol Pharmacal, Inc.
CASTER-PRO	Magnus Mobility Systems
CASTWALKERr CAST SOLE	Dm Systems, Inc.
CASTWEDGET CAST ADJUSTER	Dm Systems, Inc.
CAT SCREEN	Hardy Diagnostics
CAT SERIES	San-I-Pak,Pacific Inc.
CATALINA	Almore International, Inc.
CATALITE	Hankison International
CATAMATIC	National Instrument Co., Inc.
CATAPULT	Dr Systems, Inc.
CATARCr	Vergason Technology, Inc.
CATBIRD SEAT	Link Ergonomics Corp.
CATCH-ALL	Advantage Bag Co.
CATELLA	AMD Technologies Inc.
CATERA	DJO Inc.
CATEYE	Creative Health Products, Inc.
CATH-CADDIE	Precision Dynamics Corp.
CATH-FINDER	Smiths Medical Asd, Inc.
CATH-GUARD	Arrow International, Inc.
CATH-LINK	C. R. Bard, Inc.
CATH-LOCK	St. Jude Medical Atrial Fibrillation
CATH-SECURE	M.C. Johnson Co., Inc.
CATH-SECURE DUAL TAB	M.C. Johnson Co., Inc.
CATH-SHIELD	Smiths Medical Asd, Inc.
CATH-TIP	Smith & Nephew, Inc.
CATHCARE	Baxa Corporation
CATHGUARD	Rpc
CATHIVEX	Millipore Corporation
CATHSIM	Immersion Medical
CATHTRACK	C. R. Bard, Inc.
CATHY	Myco Medical
CAUDA-KATH	Epimed International, Inc.
CAULK	Dentsply International, Inc.
CAULK	Dentsply Prosthetics
CAVERNOTOME C	American Medical Systems, Inc.
CAVI-CARE	Smith & Nephew, Inc.
CAVICICE	Metrex Research Corp.
CAVIDRY	Parkell, Inc.
CAVILON	3m Co.
CAVITATOR	Mettler Electronics Corp.
CAVITRON	Dentsply International, Inc.
CAVITRON	Dentsply Professional
CAVITRON	Dentsply Prosthetics
CAVITRON CADDY	Brandt Industries, Inc.
CAVIWAVE	Steris Corporation
CAVIWIPES	Metrex Research Corp.
CAVORPUMP	Life-Tech, Inc.
CAYMAN	Aearo Company
CB	Anatech, Ltd.
CB SERIES	Oneac Corporation
CB-30 C&B INVESTMENT	Ticonium Co.
CBC II	Stryker Corp.
CBC-3D	R & D Systems, Inc.
CBC-3K	R & D Systems, Inc.
CBC-4K	R & D Systems, Inc.
CBC-5D	R & D Systems, Inc.
CBC-7	R & D Systems, Inc.
CBC-8	R & D Systems, Inc.
CBC-CAL PLUS	R & D Systems, Inc.
CBC-DIFF	Heska Corporation
CBC-LINE	R & D Systems, Inc.
CBC-ST PLUS	R & D Systems, Inc.
CBC-SYS	R & D Systems, Inc.
CBC-TECH	R & D Systems, Inc.
CBE EMR	Medical Tactile, Inc.
CBF SENSOR	Flowtronics, Inc.
CBF/EEG SENSOR	Flowtronics, Inc.
CBF/ICP TRAUMA SENSOR	Flowtronics, Inc.
CBM 7000	Mediana Technologies Corp
CBS SERIES	Oneac Corporation
CBW	Pellerin Milnor Corp.
CC SERIES	Oneac Corporation
CCA	Argosy
CCA	Dentsply Prosthetics
CCA-100E	Benson Medical Instruments Co.
CCA-200	Benson Medical Instruments Co.
CCA-220	Benson Medical Instruments Co.
CCA-DELUXE	Argosy
CCA-S	Argosy
CCEL-II	Cryo-Cell International, Inc.
CCM	Cte Chem Tec Equipment Co.
CCM SYSTEM	Medical Graphics Corporation
CCM/D SYSTEM	Medical Graphics Corporation
CCS	Merit Medical Systems, Inc.
CCS SERIES	Oneac Corporation
CD MODULE	Lionville Systems, Inc.
CD SERIES	Oneac Corporation
CD-CAL	R & D Systems, Inc.
CD-CHEX	Streck Laboratories, Inc.
CD350	Braemar, Inc.
CDI	Terumo Cardiovascular Systems, Corp
CDIS	Zimmer Orthopaedic Surgical Products
CDP-STAR	Applied Biosystems
CDR CAM	Schick Technologies, Inc.
CDR PAN	Schick Technologies, Inc.
CDR SERIES	Oneac Corporation
CDS	Briggs Corporation
CDT	Bd Diagnostic Systems
CDTOX OIAr	Thermo Biostar, Inc.
CDX	Sorin Group Usa
CDX PRESS	Sorin Group Usa
CE	Starkey Laboratories, Inc.
CE 1000 SERIES UV-VIS SPECTROPHOTOMETER	Buck Scientific, Inc.
CE2000 SERIES UV-VIS SCANNING SPECTROPHOTOMETER	Buck Scientific, Inc.
CE3000 UV-VIS SCANNING SPECTROPHOTOMETER	Buck Scientific, Inc.
CE8000 UV-VIS DOUBLE BEAM SCANNING SPECTROPHOTOMETER	Buck Scientific, Inc.
CE9000 UV-VIS DOUBLE BEAM SCANNING SPECTROPHOTOMETER	Buck Scientific, Inc.
CEA-CIDE	Immunomedics, Inc.
CEA-SCAN	Immunomedics, Inc.
CEASE-FIRE	Justrite Manufacturing Co., L.L.C.
CEB	Hartmann-Conco Inc.
CEBOTOME	Conmed Linvatec
CED PHOSPHORAMIDITE	Biogenex Laboratories
CEDIA	Microgenics Corporation
CEDIA	Roche Diagnostics Operations
CEEA	Covidien Lp, Formerly Registered As United States Surgical
CEEDEE 4	Cytocolor, Inc.
CEEGRAPH	Natus Medical Inc.

CEFINASE	Bd Diagnostic Systems
CEKA	Preat Corp.
CEL-CHEK	Polymedco, Inc.
CEL-FREEZE	Charter Medical Ltd.
CELEBRITY	Pride Mobility Products Corp.
CELL POINT	Roboz Surgical Instrument Co., Inc.
CELL THRU	Sterogene Bioseparations, Inc.
CELL-DYN	Abbott Hematology, Diagnostics Div.
CELL-PHARM	Biovest International, Inc.
CELL-PHARM 100	Biovest International, Inc.
CELL-PHARM 2500	Biovest International, Inc.
CELLABRATION	Surmodics, Inc.
CELLCO	Spectrum Laboratories, Inc.
CELLECT LLC	Ufp Technologies, Inc.
CELLEX	Bio-Rad Laboratories, Life Science Group
CELLFLO	Spectrum Laboratories, Inc.
CELLFRIENDLY	Tulip Medical Products
CELLGAS	Spectrum Laboratories, Inc.
CELLGRO	Mediatech, Inc.
CELLIGEN	New Brunswick Scientific Co., Inc.
CELLIGEN PLUS	New Brunswick Scientific Co., Inc.
CELLIQUE	Smith & Nephew, Inc.
CELLKINES	Zeptometrix Corporation
CELLMATICS	Bd Diagnostic Systems
CELLMAX	Spectrum Laboratories, Inc.
CELLPLEX	Wright Medical Group, Inc.
CELLSEARCH	Veridex, Llc
CELLTITER 96	Promega Corp.
CELLUMAGE	Innovative Med Inc.
CELLUTEC	General Pysiotherapy, Inc.
CELSICLOCKS	Spirig Advanced Technologies, Inc.
CELSIDOT	Spirig Advanced Technologies, Inc.
CELSIMETER	Spirig Advanced Technologies, Inc.
CELSIPICK	Spirig Advanced Technologies, Inc.
CELSIPOINT	Spirig Advanced Technologies, Inc.
CELSISTRIP	Spirig Advanced Technologies, Inc.
CELSIUS CONTROL SYSTEM	Cardium Therapeutics Inc.
CELSTIR	Wheaton Science Products
CELTIC CLOTH	Dazian Fabrics,Llc.
CELUFIL	Usb Corporation
CELUX	Dentamerica Inc.
CEM-OSTETICT	Berkeley Advanced Biomaterials, Inc.
CEMPER	Scientific Pharmaceuticals, Inc.
CEN-PRODUCTS	ArjoHuntleigh
CENSLIDE	Iris International, Inc.
CENSYS	Medtronic, Inc.
CENTAUR	Siemens Healthcare Diagnostics Inc.
CENTOXIN	Centocor, Inc.
CENTRA	Siemens Hearing Instruments, Inc.
CENTRA	Thermo Fisher Scientific - Laboratory Equipment Division Headquarters
CENTRA ACTIVE	Siemens Hearing Instruments, Inc.
CENTRAC	Thermo Fisher Scientific - Laboratory Equipment Division Headquarters
CENTRAL EEG/EMG/EP	Cadwell Laboratories
CENTRAL RETINAL	Volk Optical Inc.
CENTRALIS DIRECT	Volk Optical Inc.
CENTRALITE	Diacor, Inc.
CENTRALIZED NURSE CALL	Hospital Comm. & Electronics, Inc.
CENTRALOK	Jilson Group, Inc.
CENTRAX	Stryker Spine
CENTRE POINT	Clinical Pharmacies, Inc.
CENTRE-DRIVE	Kls-Martin L.P.
CENTREX	Schleicher & Schuell, Inc.
CENTRI/POR	Spectrum Laboratories, Inc.
CENTRICITY	Ge Medical Systems Information Technologies
CENTRISOL	Minntech Corporation
CENTRIVAP	Labconco Corp.
CENTROS	Ash Access Technology Inc.
CENTRY	Medical Illumination International
CENTURA	Justrite Manufacturing Co., L.L.C.
CENTURA	Medical Illumination International
CENTURIAN	Action Products, Inc.
CENTURION	Biotec, Inc.

CENTURION	Medical Illumination International
CENTURION	Tri-State Hospital Supply Corp.
CENTURION	Universal Gym Equipment
CENTURION ELITE	Zero Manufacturing, Inc.
CENTURION EXCEL	Medical Illumination International
CENTURY	ArjoHuntleigh
CENTURY	Dexter Apache Holdings, Inc.
CENTURY	Invensys Process Systems
CENTURY 22 CASEWORK	Atlantic Medco, Inc.
CENTURY II	Tidi Products, Llc
CEPH LACTAM DISK	Remel
CEPHALO PRO	CAREFUSION 211, INC.
CEPP	Vector Firstaid, Inc.
CEPTI-SEAL	CholeraPrep
CERABLATE	Oscor, Inc.
CERALAS D	Biolitec, Inc.
CERAM BRUSH	Hager Worldwide, Inc.
CERAM-A-GRIP	Miltex Inc.
CERAM-ETCH	Gresco Products, Inc.
CERAMASTER	Shofu Dental Corporation
CERAMCO	Dentsply International, Inc.
CERAMCO	Dentsply Prosthetics
CERAMED	Dentsply International, Inc.
CERAMED	Dentsply Prosthetics
CERAMIC	Stryker Corp.
CERAMIC	Stryker Howmedica Osteonics
CERAMISTE	Shofu Dental Corporation
CERAMO	Fehling Surgical Instruments
CERAMOTHERM	Unique/Pereny
CERAMX	Dentsply International, Inc.
CERAMX	Dentsply Prosthetics
CEREC	Sirona Dental Systems Llc
CEREC 3D	Sirona Dental Systems Llc
CERECYTE	Micrus Corporation
CERMAOX	Origen Biomedical, Inc.
CERNER	Cerner Corp.
CERNER MILLENNIUM	Cerner Corp.
CERTAIN	Siemens Healthcare Diagnostics Inc
CERTI-BURN	Certified Safety Manufacturing
CERTI-COOL	Certified Safety Manufacturing
CERTI-RIP	Certified Safety Manufacturing
CERTI-STRIPS	Certified Safety Manufacturing
CERTIFIED	Scott Specialties, Inc./Cmo Inc./Ginny Inc.
CERTISOY	Alere, Inc.
CERTOMAT	Sartorius Stedim Sus Inc.
CERUMEN MANAGEMENT	Hal-Hen Company, Inc.
CERV EASE	Florida Manufacturing Corp.
CERVI TRAC PILLOW	Core Products International, Inc.
CERVISOFT	Puritan Medical Products Company Llc
CERVMAX	Pmt Corp.
CERYX	Medtronic, Inc.
CF INDICATOR	Polychrome Medical
CF QUANTUM	Polychrome Medical
CF TECHNOLOGY	Ergotron, Inc.
CF-94 SPINE FRAME	Universal Service Associates, Inc.
CFI60	Nikon Instruments Inc.
CFT	Span-America Medical Systems, Inc.
CFURINE	Remel
CFVI CENTRIFUGE	Cygnus Inc.
CG	Byron Medical
CHA-SEAL	Kimble Chase Life Science And Research Products Llc
CHAFE-GUARD	The Aloe Institute
CHAIN FREE	Crosstex International,Inc.
CHAINFLEX	Igus, Inc.
CHAIR AMERICA	Dansereau Health Products, Inc.
CHAIR AMERICA I OPERATORY	Dansereau Health Products, Inc.
CHAIR AMERICA II OPERATORY	Dansereau Health Products, Inc.
CHAIR AMERICA III OPERATORY	Dansereau Health Products, Inc.
CHAIR AMERICA IV OPERATORY	Dansereau Health Products, Inc.
CHAIR CHECK	Bed-Check Corporation
CHAIR TENDER	Secure Care Products, Inc.
CHAIR-CHECK SENSORMAT	Bed-Check Corporation
CHAIRMAN	Concorde Battery

CHAIRMAN	Permobil, Inc.
CHAIRMAN 2K	Permobil, Inc.
CHAIRMAN ENTRA	Permobil, Inc.
CHAIRMAN PLAYMAN/ROBO	Permobil, Inc.
CHAISE-LOUNGE	Golden Technologies, Inc.
CHALGREN	Chalgren Enterprises, Inc.
CHALLENGER	Champion Bus Inc.
CHALLENGER	Colours Wheelchair
CHAMELEON	Idea Scientific Co.
CHAMFLEX HVAC STAINLESS HOSE ASSEMBLIES AND HOSE KITS.	Chamberlin Rubber Company, Inc.
CHAMP	C. R. Bard, Inc.
CHAMP	Carolon Company
CHAMP	Geerpres
CHANGE-A-TIP	Bovie Medical Corp.
CHANNEL BACKER	The C. D. Sparling Company
CHANNEL MASTER	C. R. Bard, Inc.
CHANNEL RACK	Healthmark Industries
CHANNEL-CART	Healthmark Industries
CHANNEL-GUARD	C. R. Bard, Inc.
CHAPERONE	Stryker Corp.
CHARBEL MICRO-FLOW PROBE	Transonic Systems Inc.
CHARBEL PROBE	Transonic Systems Inc.
CHARMS 2000	Meta Health Technology Inc.
CHART FLAGGS	Briggs Corporation
CHART LOK	Omnimed, Inc. (Beam Products)
CHART-RACK	First Healthcare Products
CHART-RAK CABINET	First Healthcare Products
CHART-SAFE	First Healthcare Products
CHART-STIK	Smith & Nephew Inc.- Orthopaedics Division
CHARTING PLUS	Medinotes Corporation
CHARTR ENG	Gn Otometrics
CHARTR EP	Gn Otometrics
CHASE-VIALS	Kimble Chase Life Science And Research Products Llc
CHASSIS TRAK	General Devices Co., Inc.
CHECK-FLO	Cook Inc.
CHECKCUP	Alere, Inc.
CHECKMATE	Cordis Corporation
CHEEK RETRACTORS	Almore International, Inc.
CHEETAH	Mallinckrodt, Inc.
CHEF-DR II	Bio-Rad Laboratories, Life Science Group
CHEK-MED	Chek-Med Systems, Inc.
CHEK-STIX	Siemens Healthcare Diagnostics Inc.
CHEKMATE	Ansell Healthcare, Inc.
CHEKTRODE	U.F.I.
CHELEX	Bio-Rad Laboratories, Life Science Group
CHEM CHIP	Assay Technology Inc
CHEM ELUT	Varian Sample Preparation Products
CHEM EXPRESS	Assay Technology Inc
CHEM-BLEND	Simon & Company Inc., H.R.
CHEM-CHEX	Streck Laboratories, Inc.
CHEM-FEED	Blue White Industries, Inc.
CHEM-O-GATOR	Graphic Controls Corp.
CHEMANAGER	Hf Pure Water
CHEMBET	Quantachrome
CHEMCADET	Cole-Parmer Instrument Inc.
CHEMCHOICE	Avantor Performance Materials
CHEMCOR	Justrite Manufacturing Co., L.L.C.
CHEMDI	Steris Corporation
CHEMETRON	Allied Healthcare Products, Inc.
CHEMFLUOR	Saint-Gobain Performance Plastics--Akron
CHEMGARD	Baker Company, The
CHEMI-PRO	Ansell Healthcare Products, Inc.
CHEMICLAVE	Thermo Fisher Scientific Inc.
CHEMO DISPENSING PIN	B. Braun Oem Division, B. Braun Medical Inc.
CHEMO-SPIKE	Medi-Dose, Inc.
CHEMOBLOC	Covidien Lp
CHEMOPORT	Dma Med-Chem Corporation
CHEMOSITE	Covidien Lp, Formerly Registered As United States Surgical
CHEMOTEST	Q.I. Medical, Inc.
CHEMSTRIP	Roche Diagnostics Operations
CHEMSW, INC.	Chemsw, Inc.
CHEMVIEW	Sps Medical Supply Corp.
CHEMWELL	Awareness Technology, Inc.
CHENG SHIN	Kenda American Airless
CHEST SHELL	Respironics Colorado
CHEST VEST	Smith & Nephew, Inc.
CHEST-A-LINE IV	Gammex Rmi
CHEVRON II	Sroufe Healthcare Products Llc
CHEWBLET	Follett Corp.
CHEX-ALL	Propper Manufacturing Co., Inc.
CHICK 703	Schaerer Mayfield Usa
CHICK CLT	Schaerer Mayfield Usa
CHICK IOT	Schaerer Mayfield Usa
CHICKEN KIT	Graphic Controls Corp.
CHICKEN PLUS KIT	Graphic Controls Corp.
CHIEF SR 107	Redman Powerchairs
CHIFA	Toolmex Corporation
CHILD FRIENDLY MEDICAL EQUIPMENT	Pedia Pals, Llc
CHILD INTUBATION HEAD	Simulaids, Inc.
CHILDBIRTH GRAPHICS	Wrs Group, Ltd.
CHILL-OUT	Minco Products, Inc.
CHILL-TEMP	Cres Cor
CHILLER-PAC	Aqua Products Company, Inc.
CHILLI	Ep Technologies, Inc.
CHILLI II	Ep Technologies, Inc.
CHIRO-PILLO	Regency Product International
CHIRO-PRACTICAL	Control-X Medical, Inc.
CHIROSELECT	Summit Industries, Inc.
CHIRU TIP	Hager Worldwide, Inc.
CHITOFLEX	Hemcon Medical Technologies, Inc.
CHIX	Johnson & Johnson Medical Division Of Ethicon, Inc.
CHLAMYDIA OIAr	Thermo Biostar, Inc.
CHLOE	Toto Kiki Usa, Inc.
CHLORAPREP ONE-STEP	CholeraPrep
CHLORASCRUB	Professional Disposables International, Inc.
CHLORESIN	Afassco, Inc.
CHLOROSTAT	King Pharmaceuticals, Inc.
CHLOROSTAT 4	King Pharmaceuticals, Inc.
CHO-PAT	Cho-Pat
CHO-PAT	Mueller Sports Medicine
CHOKING CHARLIE	Medical Plastics Laboratory, Inc.
CHOKING MANIKIN	Simulaids, Inc.
CHOLE-CATH	Covidien Lp
CHOLE-CATH	Uresil, Llc
CHOLESTECH LDX	Cholestech Corp.
CHONDRO-ORAL	The Hymed Group Corp.
CHONDROPROTEC	The Hymed Group Corp.
CHONSTRUCT	DJO Inc.
CHOP-PAK	Johns Manville
CHORUS	ArjoHuntleigh
CHORUS RM	Ela Medical, Inc.
CHP	Creative Health Products, Inc.
CHRIREX	Phenomenex, Inc.
CHRIS BABY CPR MANIKIN	Armstrong Medical Industries, Inc.
CHROM-PREP	Hamilton Company
CHROMA SPRAY OPAQUE LIQUID	American Diversified Dental Systems
CHROMA-BOARD	Boeckeler Instruments, Inc.
CHROMACHEM	Esa, Inc.
CHROMAPHOR	Promega Corp.
CHROMATO-VUE	Uvp, Llc
CHROMAVISTA	Codonics
CHROMCLIP	Spectrum Laboratories, Inc.
CHROMEGA	Es Industries
CHROMETAL I	Motloid Company
CHROMETAL II	Motloid Company
CHROMGLIDE	Spectrum Laboratories, Inc.
CHROMGRAPH	Basi (Bioanalytical Systems, Inc.)
CHROMOGENIX	Instrumentation Laboratory Company
CHROMOPHARE	Berchtold Corp.
CHROMOVISION	Berchtold Corp.
CHRONICURE	Integra Lifesciences Corporation
CHRONOFLEX	Advansource Biomaterials Corp.
CHRONOFUSOR	C. R. Bard, Inc.
CHRONOPRENE	Advansource Biomaterials Corp.
CHRONOTHANE	Advansource Biomaterials Corp.

CLEARCARE .... C. R. Bard, Inc.
CLEARCRIT .... Separation Technology Inc
CLEARDENT .... Park Dental Research Corp./Implant Center
CLEARGLASS .... Wave Form Systems, Inc.
CLEARLENS .... Microtek Medical, Inc
CLEARLINK ...... Baxter Healthcare Corporporation, Alternate Care And Channel Team
CLEARPLAN .... Alere, Inc.
CLEARSHOT .... Baxter Healthcare Corporation, Baxter Biopharma Solutions
CLEARSIGHT .... The Cooper Companies, Inc
CLEARSITE .... Conmed Corporation
CLEARTEK .... H.L. Bouton Co., Inc.
CLEARTRAC .... Conmed Corporation
CLEARTRAP .... Surgical Specialties Corporation
CLEARVAC .... Conmed Corporation
CLEARVIERS .... Ciba Vision
CLEARVIEW .... Abbott Hematology, Diagnostics Div.
CLEARVIEW .... Alere, Inc.
CLEARVIEW .... Bagco
CLEARVIEW .... Medtronic Cardiovascular Surgery, The Heart Valve Div.
CLEARVIEW .... Oxoid, Inc.
CLEARVIEW .... Wampole Laboratories
CLEARVIEW SECURITY DRUG BOX .... Armstrong Medical Industries, Inc.
CLEARVIEW UTERINE MANIPULATOR .... Clinical Innovations, Inc.
CLEARVISION .... Karl Storz Endoscopy-America Inc.
CLEARVOICE .... Beltone Electronics Corp.
CLEARVUE .... AMD Technologies Inc.
CLEARVUE .... C. R. Bard, Inc.
CLEARWAY .... Ricon Corp.
CLEAVASE .... Third Wave Technologies, Inc.
CLEMEX .... Mccrone Microscopes & Accessories
CLENSATRON CONTACT LENS CLEANER .... Questech International, Inc.
CLICK LOCK .... Icu Medical, Inc.
CLICK N CLEAN .... Aesculap Implant Systems Inc.
CLICK REG .... Contemporary Products, Inc.
CLICK-TO-FIT .... H.L. Bouton Co., Inc.
CLICKIT .... Bodypoint, Inc.
CLICKLINE .... Karl Storz Endoscopy-America Inc.
CLIMATE SECURITY SYSTEM .... Cmt, Inc.
CLIMB-RITE .... Sellstrom Manufacturing Co.
CLIMBMAX .... CYBEX INTERNATIONAL, INC.
CLIN-ELISA .... Diasorin Inc
CLINAC .... Varian Medical Systems
CLINICIAN'S CHOICE SIGNATURE SERIES .... Mds Products, Inc.
CLING SHIELD .... Palmero Health Care
CLINI-DYNE .... Gaymar Industries, Inc.
CLINI.FLOAT .... Gaymar Industries, Inc.
CLINIBASE .... Mennen Medical Corp.
CLINIC .... Ammex Corp.
CLINIC .... North Coast Medical, Inc.
CLINIC I .... Dansereau Health Products, Inc.
CLINIC II .... Dansereau Health Products, Inc.
CLINIC III .... Dansereau Health Products, Inc.
CLINIC IV .... Dansereau Health Products, Inc.
CLINICATH .... Smiths Medical Asd, Inc.
CLINICIAN'S CHOICE .... Miltex Inc.
CLINICIAN'S CHOICE SIGNATURE SERIES . American Diversified Dental Systems
CLINICOMM OFFICE FLOW SYSTEM .... Heritage Medcall
CLINIFILE3 .... Radiometer America, Inc.
CLINIFLOW .... Carolina Medical, Inc.
CLINIFLOW II .... Carolina Medical, Inc.
CLINILOG .... Siemens Healthcare Diagnostics Inc.
CLINIMIX .... Baxter Healthcare Corporation Nutrition
CLINISOL .... Baxter Healthcare Corporation Nutrition
CLINISORB .... Dukal Corporation
CLINISTIX .... Siemens Healthcare Diagnostics Inc.
CLINITEK .... Siemens Healthcare Diagnostics Inc.
CLINITEK ADVANTUS .... Siemens Healthcare Diagnostics Inc.
CLINITEK ATLAS .... Siemens Healthcare Diagnostics Inc.
CLINITEK STATUS .... Siemens Healthcare Diagnostics Inc.
CLINITEMP .... LCR Hallcrest
CLINITEST .... Siemens Healthcare Diagnostics Inc.
CLINITROL .... Advanced Instruments Inc.

CLINITRON .... Hill-Rom Holdings, Inc.
CLINITRON RITE-HITE .... Hill-Rom Manufacturing, Inc.
CLINITUBES .... Radiometer America, Inc.
CLINS WOUND .... Sage Laboratories, Inc.
CLINTEC .... Baxter Healthcare Corporation Nutrition
CLIP CLAP MESH .... Hager Worldwide, Inc.
CLIP LOCK .... B. Braun Oem Division, B. Braun Medical Inc.
CLIP TOTE .... Neotech Products, Inc.
CLIP-A-MATIC .... Covidien Lp, Formerly Registered As United States Surgical
CLIP-ON LOUPES .... Almore International, Inc.
CLIPPER .... Merit Medical Systems, Inc.
CLIRPATH TURBO .... Spectranetics Corp.
CLONAB .... Biotest Diagnostic Corp.
CLONE SELECTOR .... Bio-Rad Laboratories, Life Science Group
CLOSEMATE .... Howard Instruments, Inc.
CLOSING TOOL (P-3) .... Lone Star Medical Products, Inc.
CLOSUREPLUS .... Vnus Medical Technologies, Inc.
CLOSURERFS .... Vnus Medical Technologies, Inc.
CLOT STOP .... Axiom Medical, Inc.
CLOTTRAC .... Medtronic, Inc.
CLOUD 9 .... Cloud 9
CLOUD 9 .... Living Earth Crafts
CLOUD 9 CANCELYZER .... Cloud 9
CLOWARD .... Cloward Instrument Corporation
CLUB L.A. .... Euro-Frames, Inc.
CLUBMAN .... Artcraft New York
CM ASSIST 1000 .... Columbus Mckinnon Corp., Mobility Products Div.
CM ASSIST 300 SL .... Columbus Mckinnon Corp., Mobility Products Div.
CM ASSIST 400 .... Columbus Mckinnon Corp., Mobility Products Div.
CM ASSIST 600 .... Columbus Mckinnon Corp., Mobility Products Div.
CM ASSIST 750 .... Columbus Mckinnon Corp., Mobility Products Div.
CMC .... Cmc Rescue, Inc.
CMGS-1 COLOR MINI GANZFELD .... Lkc Technologies, Inc.
CMI .... Regen Biologics, Inc.
CMO/SCOTT/SPECIALTIES .... Ortholine
CMP (CONTINENTAL METAL PRODUCTS) .... Medi-Tech International, Inc.
CMS .... Sorin Group Usa
CMT .... Cmt, Inc.
CMT .... Immucell Corp.
CMV BRITE .... Biotest Diagnostic Corp.
CMVSCAN .... Bd Diagnostic Systems
CND .... Byron Medical
CO-AX .... Tp Orthodontics, Inc.
CO-ESTER .... C. R. Bard, Inc.
CO-FLEX .... Andover Healthcare Inc.
CO-FLEX NL .... Andover Healthcare Inc.
CO-GUARD .... Enmet Corp.
CO-LASTIC .... Hartmann-Conco Inc.
CO-STAT .... Natus Medical Inc.
CO-WRAP .... Hartmann-Conco Inc.
CO/STRUC .... Herman Miller, Inc.
CO2 SMO PLUS .... Respironics, Inc
CO2EASY .... Westmed, Inc.
CO2SMO .... Respironics, Inc
CO3 .... Cynosure, Inc.
COA DATA .... American Labor
COA LAB .... American Labor
COA SCREENER .... American Labor
COA SYSTEM .... American Labor
COACH .... Johnson & Johnson Consumer Products, Inc.
COACUTE .... Instrumentation Laboratory Company
COAG-A-MATE .... Biomerieux Inc.
COAGSPIN .... Statspin, Inc.
COAGUCHEK .... Roche Diagnostics Operations
COAMATIC .... Instrumentation Laboratory Company
COAT-A-COUNT .... Siemens Healthcare Diagnostics Inc.
COATEST .... Instrumentation Laboratory Company
COBAN .... 3m Co.
COBAR .... Newschoff Chairs, Inc.
COBE .... Caridianbct Inc.
COBE SPECTRA .... Caridianbct Inc.
COBLATION .... Arthrocare Corp.
COBREX .... Implex Corp.

COCHLEA-SCAN .... Natus Medical Inc.
CODA .... Biorad Laboratories
CODA .... Genx International
CODE ALERT .... Rf Technologies
CODE BLUE II .... Vital Signs, Inc.
CODE SUMMARY .... Physio-Control, Inc.
CODE-PAK RESUSCITATOR .... Armstrong Medical Industries, Inc.
CODE-READY .... Zoll Medical Corp.
CODE-STAT .... Physio-Control, Inc.
CODELINK .... Captiva Software Corporation
CODELINK PLUS .... Captiva Software Corporation
CODELINK PROFESSIONAL .... Captiva Software Corporation
CODENET .... Zoll Medical Corp.
CODMAN .... Codman & Shurtleff, Inc
CODMAN HAKIM .... Codman & Shurtleff, Inc
CODONICS .... Codonics
COEFFICIENT .... Numed, Inc.
COEUR .... Coeur, Inc
COGENICS .... Clinical Data Inc
COGENT .... Dma Med-Chem Corporation
COGENT LIGHT .... Welch Allyn, Inc.
COHERE .... Belport Co. Inc., Gingi-Pak Div.
COHERE .... Tape-O-Corporation
COHERENCE ONCOLOGY WORKSPACES ... Siemens Medical Solutions Usa, Inc
COIL PACK .... Packaging Plus, Inc.
COL'R'TAB .... Tabbies, Div. Of Xertrex International, Inc.
COL-PRESS .... Hospital Marketing Svcs. Company, Inc.
COL-R-LASTICS .... Tp Orthodontics, Inc.
COL-R-SPONGE .... American Silk Sutures, Inc.
COLBY .... Newschoff Chairs, Inc.
COLD ICE .... Cold Ice, Inc.
COLDFLEX .... Balance Systems, Inc.
COLDPAC .... Motloid Company
COLDTEMP .... Servolift/Eastern Corp.
COLDWRAP .... Carolon Company
COLEMAN .... Byron Medical
COLI SCREEN .... Hardy Diagnostics
COLIBRI VITRECTOMY CUTTER .... Microworld Medical Instruments, Inc.
COLILERT .... Idexx Laboratories, Inc.
COLISURE .... Idexx Laboratories, Inc.
COLLACOTE .... Zimmer Dental, Inc.
COLLAGEN .... Eagle Vision, Inc.
COLLAGEN .... Integra Lifesciences Corporation
COLLAGEN IV H .... Exocell, Inc.
COLLAGEN IV M .... Exocell, Inc.
COLLAMER .... Staar Surgical Co.
COLLAPLUG .... Zimmer Dental, Inc.
COLLATAPE .... Zimmer Dental, Inc.
COLLEAGUE ...... Baxter Healthcare Corporation, Alternate Care And Channel Team
COLLECT-A-CUBES .... United Receptacle
COLLECTION-EZE .... Mml Diagnostics Packaging, Inc.
COLLIS CURVE .... Collis Curve, Inc.
COLLIT'S .... Buffalo Dental Manufacturing Co., Inc.
COLLY-SEEL .... Torbot Group, Inc.
COLON ALERT .... Immunostics, Inc.
COLON HYDROTHERAPY .... Clearwater Colon Hydrotherapy, Inc.
COLONIC .... Clearwater Colon Hydrotherapy, Inc.
COLOPLAST .... Amoena
COLOPLAST .... Coloplast Manufacturing Us, Llc
COLOR BAR .... Eagle Vision, Inc.
COLOR LINK, SHADE COMMUNICATION SYSTEM BY KEN GUTHRIE .... American Diversified Dental Systems
COLOR LINK,SHADE COMMUNICATION SYSTEM .... Mds Products, Inc.
COLOR MATCH SYSTEM .... Oster Professional Products, Inc.
COLOR TOUCH .... Microflex Corporation
COLOR-ALERT .... Hollister Incorporated
COLOR-BRITES .... Sellstrom Manufacturing Co.
COLOR-RICH .... Seradyn, Inc.
COLORADO .... Stryker Corp.
COLORADO MICRODISSECTION .... Stryker Corp.
COLORBLENDS .... Ciba Vision
COLORCARD .... Wampole Laboratories

COLORCUES .... Mobile Instrument Service And Repair, Inc.
COLORFLEX .... Hunter Associates Lab., Inc.
COLORFREE .... Freeman Manufacturing Company
COLORFUSED .... H.L. Bouton Co., Inc.
COLORGENE .... Enzo Biochem, Inc.
COLORGUARD .... Novosci Corp.
COLORGUARD .... Precision Dynamics Corp.
COLORIGHT .... Dentalez Group
COLORPAC .... Bd Diagnostic Systems
COLORQUEST XE .... Hunter Associates Lab., Inc.
COLORSCAN .... Carolina Medical, Inc.
COLORSCAN .... Kardex Systems, Inc.
COLORSCAN 1070 .... Carolina Medical, Inc.
COLORSCANNER .... Altek Corp.
COLORTRACK .... Aspen Surgical
COLORTRACK .... Sterion, Incorporated
COLORX .... Thermo Spectronic
COLORZYME .... Global Focus (G.F.M.D. Ltd.)
COLORZYME .... Immuno Concepts N.A. Ltd.
COLOSSUS .... C. R. Bard, Inc.
COLPAC .... Chattanooga Group
COLPOSTAR .... Wallach Surgical Devices, Inc.
COLT .... Eric Armin Inc.
COLT .... Ortho-Kinetics, Inc.
COLUMBIA .... Columbia Medical Manufacturing Llc
COLUMBIA DENTOFORM .... Dentalez Group
COLUMBUS .... Phenomenex, Inc.
COLUMPAK .... Quintron Instrument Company
COLVIN-GALLOWAY FUTURE Medtronic Cardiovascular Surgery, The Heart Valve Div.
COM PLUS .... Parkell, Inc.
COM VAC OIL .... Hager Worldwide, Inc.
COM-TOM .... Ultra-Cal, Inc.
COMBI .... Mars Air Doors
COMBI BAG .... Dixie Ems Supply
COMBI BOARD .... Dixie Ems Supply
COMBI SNIP .... Dixie Ems Supply
COMBI TEC .... Hager Worldwide, Inc.
COMBI-CAP .... Medi-Dose, Inc.
COMBICARRIER .... Hartwell Medical Corp.
COMBINATION PAK .... Aluwax Dental Products Co.
COMBINED SUBMOLAR SHELL .... Implantech Associates, Inc.
COMBISTIX .... Siemens Healthcare Diagnostics Inc.
COMBITUBE .... Covidien Lp, Formerly Registered As Kendall
COMBO-CYCLERS .... United Receptacle
COMBO-TIP .... Crosstex International,Inc.
COMBOMAP .... Volcano Corporation
COMBOPEN .... Meridian Medical Technologies
COMBOWIRE .... Volcano Corporation
COMET .... Astro-Med, Inc.
COMET .... Mge Ups Sytems, Inc.
COMFEEL .... Coloplast Manufacturing Us, Llc
COMFEET .... Total Care
COMFEEZE, CUSHIONED PROTECTION FOR OXYGEN TUBING .... Romed, Llc
COMFO-TEX .... Tetra Medical Supply Corp.
COMFOOT BRAND .... Aetna Foot Products/Div. Of Aetna Felt Corporation
COMFORFOAM .... DJO Inc.
COMFORT AND HEALING PACK .... Smith & Nephew, Inc.
COMFORT BATH .... Sage Products, Inc.
COMFORT COLD .... Hospital Marketing Svcs. Company, Inc.
COMFORT COLLECTION .... Salk Inc.
COMFORT COOL .... North Coast Medical, Inc.
COMFORT CURVE .... Qrp, Inc.
COMFORT CUSHION .... Crosstex International,Inc.
COMFORT FIT .... Sun-Med
COMFORT JET .... Biolase Technology, Inc.
COMFORT MAT .... Allen Medical Systems, Inc.
COMFORT PLUS .... Paramedical Distributors
COMFORT PLUS .... Westmed, Inc.
COMFORT RISE .... Milwaukee Mattress & Furniture
COMFORT SHIELD .... Sage Products, Inc.
COMFORT TOUCH .... Comfort Touch
COMFORT TOUCH .... Geri-Care Products

COMFORT TOUCH	Pre Pak Products, Inc.
COMFORT WARM	Hospital Marketing Svcs. Company, Inc.
COMFORT ZONE	Silipos Inc.
COMFORT-AID (TM)	Southwest Technologies, Inc.
COMFORT-CLIP	Smiths Medical Pm, Inc.
COMFORT-COATED	Personna Medical/Div. Of American Safety Razor Co.
COMFORT-FIT	Professional's Choice Sports Medicine Products, Inc.
COMFORT-LOCK	Precision Dynamics Corp.
COMFORT-STIM	Comfort Technologies, Inc.
COMFORT-TRODE	Comfort Technologies, Inc.
COMFORTCARE	Hard Manufacturing Co.
COMFORTCASE	Graham Medical Products/Div. Of Little Rapids Corp
COMFORTEX	Reach Global Industries, Inc. (Reachgood)
COMFORTLINE	Hill-Rom Holdings, Inc.
COMFORTMATE	Health Science Products, Inc.
COMFORTPLUS	Invacare Corporation
COMFORTSEAL MASK WITH EXHALATION VALVE	Monaghan Medical Corp.
COMFORTWAVE	Sidmar Mfg., Inc.
COMLINX	Hill-Rom Holdings, Inc.
COMMAND	Stryker Spine
COMMANDER	Bard Electro Physiology
COMMANDER	C. R. Bard, Inc.
COMMANDER	JTECH Medical
COMMODE COMFORT SUPPORT SYSTEM	Rest Assured Inc.
COMMUNICATOR	Dr Systems, Inc.
COMMUNICOM	Carl Zeiss Meditec Inc.
COMMUTER	Action Products, Inc.
COMP-U-CRAFT	Cd Nelson Manufacturing Co.
COMP-U-DIFF	Modulus Data Systems, Inc.
COMPACSET	Welch Allyn, Inc.
COMPACT	Medsonic U.S.A., Inc.
COMPACT	Resmed Corp.
COMPACT 7600	Ge Oec Medical Systems Inc.
COMPACT DELTA	Dornier Medtech America
COMPACT DELTA II	Dornier Medtech America
COMPACT DIODE	Dornier Medtech America
COMPACT II	Vitalograph, Inc.
COMPACT SIGMA	Dornier Medtech America
COMPACT TOUP	Toshiba America Medical Systems
COMPACTCART	Blue Bell Bio-Medical
COMPACTE	Welcon, Inc.
COMPANION	Abbott Laboratories
COMPANION	Covidien (Formerly Nellcor Puritan Bennett / Tyco Healthcare)
COMPANION	Pioneer Medical Systems
COMPANION	Salk Inc.
COMPANION 80	Iomed, Inc.
COMPAS	Cardiac Care Units, Inc.
COMPAS HOLTER MONITOR	Ubs Instruments Corporation
COMPAS SOFTWARE	Morgan Scientific Inc.
COMPASS	Coherent, Inc.
COMPASS	Compass International, Inc.
COMPASS	Golden Technologies, Inc.
COMPASS	Smith & Nephew Inc.- Orthopaedics Division
COMPASS BIOSCIENCE, COMPASS	Compass Bioscience
COMPAT	Novartis Nutrition
COMPATCH	Comfort Technologies, Inc.
COMPEL	Bangs Laboratories, Inc.
COMPEL	Standard Textile
COMPEL	Standard Textile Co., Inc.
COMPERM	Hartmann-Conco Inc.
COMPEXPRO	Coherent, Inc.
COMPLEAT	Novartis Nutrition
COMPLEMENTS	Ciba Vision
COMPLETE	Abbott Medical Optics Inc.
COMPLETE CARE DOLL	Medical Plastics Laboratory, Inc.
COMPLETE CULTURE CONTROL INCUBATORS	Boekel Scientific
COMPLIANCE PLUS	Surgical Safety Products, Inc.
COMPLITE POST OP ROM	Omni Life Science, Inc.
COMPLY	3m Co.
COMPLY	Covidien Lp
COMPLY	Hearing Components Inc.
COMPLY	Standard Textile
COMPLY	Standard Textile Co., Inc.

COMPO BLITZ	Hager Worldwide, Inc.
COMPO BRUSH	Hager Worldwide, Inc.
COMPO BRUSH ALL REACH	Hager Worldwide, Inc.
COMPO-T	Motloid Company
COMPOMASTER	Shofu Dental Corporation
COMPOSER	Beltone Electronics Corp.
COMPOSER	Hill-Rom Holdings, Inc.
COMPOSITE	Shofu Dental Corporation
COMPRESSAR, STRONGARM, COMFORT, 3-FINGER JACK, SUPERCOMFORT	Avd
COMPRESSOGRIP	Knit-Rite, Inc.
COMPRESSOGRIP	Paramedical Distributors
COMPRESSOPAW	Paramedical Distributors
COMPRILAN	Bsn-Jobst
COMPRO AB	Bauerfeind Usa, Inc.
COMPRO DF	Bauerfeind Usa, Inc.
COMPRO-PLUS AB	Bauerfeind Usa, Inc.
COMPRO-PLUS DF/A	Bauerfeind Usa, Inc.
COMPRO-PLUS DF/S	Bauerfeind Usa, Inc.
COMPU-CUTTER	Huestis Medical
COMPU-FORMER	Huestis Medical
COMPU-PLOTTER	Huestis Medical
COMPU-STEP	Athena Controls, Inc.
COMPUBAND	Precision Dynamics Corp.
COMPUCYCLE	Athena Controls, Inc.
COMPUFLOW	Tsi Inc.
COMPUKT	Medmetric Corp.
COMPULES	Dentsply Caulk
COMPUMED	Compumed, Inc.
COMPUTERIZED SPEECH LAB (CSL)	Kaypentax
COMPUTIME	Timemed Labeling Systems, Inc.
COMPUTRAINER	Racer-Mate, Inc.
COMTECH	Comfort Technologies, Inc.
CON-TRATE	Meridian Bioscience, Inc.
CON-TROL	Precision Systems, Inc.
CON-TROL-CURE	U.V. Process Supply, Inc.
CONCEIVE	Quidel Corporation
CONCENTRIX	Dentalez Group
CONCEPT	Conmed Linvatec
CONCEPT II	Concept Ii, Inc.
CONCEPT ONE	Artromick International, Inc.
CONCERTA	Johnson & Johnson
CONCISE	3m Espe Dental Products
CONCO BULKY GAUZE	Hartmann-Conco Inc.
CONCORDE	Byron Medical
CONCORDE	Charles B. Schwed Co., Inc.
CONCORDE	Concorde Battery
CONCOURSE	Micrus Corporation
CONDITIONONE SERIES	Oneac Corporation
CONDOR EXPRESS	Smith & Nephew, Inc., Endoscopy Division
CONEFOR	Sigma Products Ltd.
CONFIDENCE	Geri-Care Products
CONFIDENCE	Paperpak
CONFIDENTIAL COURIER	March & Green
CONFIENT	Boston Scientific Corporation
CONFIRM	Confirm Monitoring Systems, Inc.
CONFIRM	Siemens Healthcare Diagnostics Inc
CONFIRM	Siemens Healthcare Diagnostics Inc
CONFIRM	Ventana Medical Systems, Inc.
CONFIRMA	Confirma, Inc.
CONFIRMATION	Siemens Healthcare Diagnostics Inc
CONFOCAL MICROSCOPE	Solarius Development Inc.
CONFORM	Ansell Healthcare Products, Inc.
CONFORM	Byron Medical
CONFORM LTC	Ansell Healthcare Products, Inc.
CONFORM NL	Ansell Healthcare Products, Inc.
CONFORM PLUS	Ansell Healthcare Products, Inc.
CONFORM-A-FLEX	Conforma Laboratories, Inc.
CONFORM-A-GUAZE	Home-Aid-Healthcare, Inc.
CONFORM-A-SPHERIC	Conforma Laboratories, Inc.
CONFORM-X	Medical Carbon Research Institute, Llc - Mcri
CONFORMA	Conforma Laboratories, Inc.
CONFORMA	Cook Vascular, Incorporated

CONFORMA	Sonic Innovations
CONFORMACATH	C. R. Bard, Inc.
CONFORMANT 2	Smith & Nephew, Inc.
CONFORMANT 3	Smith & Nephew, Inc.
CONFORMANY	Smith & Nephew, Inc.
CONFORMAT	Tekscan, Inc.
CONFORMING COMFORT	Global Medical Foam, Inc.
CONFORT CIRCUIT	Beltone Electronics Corp.
CONFOURM	Back Support Systems
CONFOURM	Regency Product International
CONIFIX	Greatbach Medical
CONMED	Conmed Corporation
CONNECTCHARGE	Marinco Specialty Wiring Devices
CONNECTED HOSPITAL	Stryker Corp.
CONNECTGLOW	Marinco Specialty Wiring Devices
CONNECTICUT INTRUSION ARCH: CTAr	Ultimate Wireforms, Inc.
CONNECTOR	Nds Surgical Imaging, Inc.
CONNECTSTAT WORKSTATION	Ge Healthcare Technologies Surgery Navigation
CONNEX	Natus Medical Inc.
CONNEXX	Siemens Hearing Instruments, Inc.
CONO-FLEX	Tetra Medical Supply Corp.
CONOGENICS STOOL BLOOD TEST	Cenogenics Corp.
CONQUEST	Stryker Corp.
CONQUEST	Stryker Endoscopy
CONRAD	Control-X Medical, Inc.
CONRAY	Mallinckrodt, Inc.
CONSED	Alpha-Tec Systems, Inc.
CONSED CLR	Alpha-Tec Systems, Inc.
CONSERVE	Wright Medical Group, Inc.
CONSIL	Novabone Products, Llc
CONSTACARE	Stryker Medical
CONSTANT POWER	Online Power, Inc.
CONSTANT-CLENS	Covidien Lp
CONSTAY	Urocare Products, Inc.
CONSTELLATION	Ep Technologies, Inc.
CONSTIX(R)	Contec, Inc.
CONSYS	Life-Tech, Inc.
CONTACSCOPE	Venes Technology Corp.
CONTACT LASER SYSTEM	Surgical Laser Technologies, Inc.
CONTAINAIRE	Aes Clean Technology, Inc.
CONTAINS	Medtronic, Inc.
CONTECH	Contech Medical, Inc.
CONTEMPO CONDOMS	Ansell Healthcare, Inc.
CONTEMPRA	Fisher Scientific Co., Llc.
CONTEMPRO 2	Contemporary Products, Inc.
CONTENDER	Champion Bus Inc.
CONTENDER	DJO Inc.
CONTIGEN	C. R. Bard, Inc., Bard Urological Div.
CONTINENTAL REFRIGERATOR CORP.	Continental Scientific
CONTINU-CORE	C. R. Bard, Inc.
CONTINUFLO FLOLINK	Baxter Healthcare Corporation, Alternate Care And Channel Team
CONTINUING CARE GROUP	Sunrise Medical, Inc.
CONTINUUM	Implex Corp.
CONTINUUM	Medrad, Inc.
CONTINUUM	Zimmer Dental, Inc.
CONTIPLEX	B. Braun Oem Division, B. Braun Medical Inc.
CONTOUR	Ethicon Endo-Surgery, Inc.
CONTOUR	General Pysiotherapy, Inc.
CONTOUR	King Systems Corp.
CONTOUR	Siemens Healthcare Diagnostics Inc.
CONTOUR	Smith & Nephew Inc.- Orthopaedics Division
CONTOUR FOAM	All Pro Exercise Products, Inc.
CONTOUR FORM	Contour Form Products
CONTOUR PAK	Contour Pak, Inc.
CONTOUR PROFILE	Mentor Corp.
CONTOUR PROFILE LOW	Mentor Corp.
CONTOUR SPINE SYSTEM	Ortho Development Corp.
CONTOURS PRE-FAB	Langer, Inc.
CONTOURU	Invacare Corporation
CONTRA	Young Innovations, Inc.
CONTRA DISPOSABLE	Young Innovations, Inc.
CONTRAD	Decon Laboratories Ltd.
CONTRIL	Instrumentation Laboratory Company
CONTROL RELEASE	Ethicon, Inc.
CONTROL-FIT	C. R. Bard, Inc.
CONTROLLER	DJO Inc.
CONTROLTEX	Standard Textile Co., Inc.
CONTURA SERIES	Bobrick Washroom Equipment, Inc.
CONVALESCENT KELLY	Medical Plastics Laboratory, Inc.
CONVAQUIP	Convaquip Industries, Inc.
CONVEEN	Coloplast Manufacturing Us, Llc
CONVENIENCE 6494	Medtronic Cardiovascular Surgery, The Heart Valve Div.
CONVENIENCE BAG	Gkr Industries, Inc.
CONVENIENCE-PAK	Tp Orthodontics, Inc.
CONVERGENT SERIES	Oneac Corporation
CONVERT-A-POUCH	Smith & Nephew, Inc.
CONVERTIBLE	Applied Medical Resource Corporation
CONVERTIBLE	Convaid Inc.
CONVERTIBLE-INVERTIBLE	Freeman Manufacturing Company
CONVERTORS	Cardinal Health Inc.
CONVOL-EZE	Allman Products
CONVOY PLASTIC PALLETS	Orbis Corporation
COOK OB/GYN	Cook Urological, Inc.
COOK TPN	Cook Inc.
COOK URO	Cook Urological, Inc.
COOK WOUND/OSTOMY	Cook Urological, Inc.
COOK-ENFORCER	Cook Inc.
COOK-WAITE	Carestream Health, Inc.
COOL BANDAGE	Romaine, Inc. D.B.A. Koldcare
COOL FRONT	Byron Medical
COOL REST	Core Products International, Inc.
COOL WRAP FOR BURNS	Romaine, Inc. D.B.A. Koldcare
COOL-JEL	Water-Jel Technologies
COOL-QUILT	Select Medical Products, Inc.
COOL-WICK	Select Medical Products, Inc.
COOLBLUE	Cardium Therapeutics Inc.
COOLBRITE	S&S Technology
COOLGARD 3000	Alsius Corp.
COOLGLIDE	Cutera, Inc.
COOLITE	Swivelier Co., Inc.
COOLITE POST OP ROM	Omni Life Science, Inc.
COOLSPOT	Independent Solutions, Inc.
COOLWEAR	Precept Medical Products, Inc.
COOPER-RAND	Luminaud, Inc.
COOPERCARE	Coopercare Lastrap Inc
COPALITE	Cooley & Cooley, Ltd.
COPES DYNAMIC BRACE	Stars
COPILOT	Abbott Laboratories
COPLEX	Albahealth Llc
COPYMATE II	Bencher, Inc.
COR-FLEX	Cook Inc.
CORA-CAINE	Harry J. Bosworth Company
CORD CADDY	Evolution Medical Products, Inc.
CORDGUARD	Utah Medical Products, Inc.
CORDITE	Pactiv Corporation
CORDOMETER	Fluke Biomedical
CORE	Stryker Corp.
CORE CONSOLE	Stryker Corp.
CORE IMPACTION DRILL	Stryker Corp.
CORE MICRO SAW	Stryker Corp.
CORE PATTERNS	Parkell, Inc.
CORE SET	George King Bio-Medical, Inc.
CORE UNIVERSAL DRIVER	Stryker Corp.
CORE UNIVERSAL SERIES	Stryker Corp.
COREFILL	Core Products International, Inc.
COREX	Corning Inc., Science Products Division
CORFIT SYSTEM	Core Products International, Inc.
CORINTHIAN	Cordis Corporation
CORIUM	Lumenis Inc.
CORLOC	Newschoff Chairs, Inc.
CORMATIC	Georgia-Pacific Llc
CORNEAL SHIELD	Integra Lifesciences Corporation
CORNELL	Cadence Science Inc.
CORNING	Corning Inc., Science Products Division
COROMETRICS	Ge Medical Systems Information Technologies

CORONA CARBON STEEL	Hu-Friedy Manufacturing Co., Inc.
CORONEO PUNCTAL GAGE	Eagle Vision, Inc.
CORPAK	Cardinal Health Inc.
CORPAK	Core Products International, Inc.
CORRESTORE	Somanetics Corp.
CORRIDOR MEDIA	Corridor Group, Inc., The
CORTAC	Pmt Corp.
CORTAID	Johnson & Johnson Consumer Products, Inc.
CORTOSS	Orthovita, Inc.
CORVAC	Covidien Lp
CORVUS	Best Nomos Corp.
CORZO	Clarke Health Care Products, Inc.
COSCO	Cosco
COSEAL	Baxter International Inc
COSGROVE	Kapp Surgical Instrument, Inc.
COSGROVE-EDWARDS	Edwards Lifesciences, Llc.
COSMO TENS,THERMO TX ACUMAG PATCH, STEMMA TEA	Cosmo Health, Inc.
COSMOPORE	Hartmann-Conco Inc.
COST CRUNCHER	Bar-Ray Products, Inc.
COSTAR	Corning Inc., Science Products Division
COSYCHAIR	Two Rivers, Llc
COTEAR	Tape-O-Corporation
COTRAN	Cotran Corp.
COTTON	Wilson-Cook Medical, Inc.
COTTON LEUNG	Wilson-Cook Medical, Inc.
COUGH-A-REST	North Safety Products
COUGHASSIST	J. H. Emerson Co.
COULAM	C. R. Bard, Inc.
COULARRAY	Esa, Inc.
COULOCHEM	Esa, Inc.
COUMADIN PLASMA/MULTI-COUMADIN SET	George King Bio-Medical, Inc.
COUNT A DOSE	Medicool, Inc.
COUNT EZ	Xodus Medical, Inc.
COUNT-TAINER	Anchor Products Company
COUNTING CHAMBERS	Humagen Fertility Diagnostics, Inc.
COUNTWAY SYSTEM	Amd-Ritmed, Inc.
COURNAND	C. R. Bard, Inc.
COVAC	Arthrocare Corp.
COVARIS	Applied Biosystems
COVERAGE	Steris Corporation
COVERAGE PLUS NPD	Steris Corporation
COVERED COLLECTION SYSTEM	Approved Medical Systems
COVERLET	Bsn-Jobst
COVRSITE	Smith & Nephew, Inc.
COZY CRIBS	Hard Manufacturing Co.
COZY-LITE	Swivelier Co., Inc.
CP	Pi Professional Therapy Products
CP FIBER	Cp Medical Corporation
CP-ARLENE	Nasco
CP2	Pi Professional Therapy Products
CP2000 TWO-CHANNEL HOLTER	Instromedix, A Card Guard Co.
CP3000 THREE CHANNEL HOLTER	Instromedix, A Card Guard Co.
CPFS SYSTEM	Medical Graphics Corporation
CPM H440	JACE SYSTEMS, INC
CPM K100	JACE SYSTEMS, INC
CPM K200	JACE SYSTEMS, INC
CPM W550	JACE SYSTEMS, INC
CPR BRAD	Simulaids, Inc.
CPR ISO-SHIELD	Rondex Products, Inc.
CPR KEVIN	Simulaids, Inc.
CPR KIM	Simulaids, Inc.
CPR KYLE	Simulaids, Inc.
CPR MICROSHIELD	Microtek Medical, Inc
CPR PROMPT	Aristotle Corp.
CPR PROMPT	Nasco
CPR RESCUE KIT	Rondex Products, Inc.
CPR TIMMY	Simulaids, Inc.
CPROTECTOR	Certified Safety Manufacturing
CPS	C. R. Bard, Inc.
CPS Aim	St. Jude Medical, Inc.
CPS Direct	St. Jude Medical, Inc.
CPS Luminary	St. Jude Medical, Inc.
CPS Venture	St. Jude Medical, Inc.

CPX EXPRESS	Medical Graphics Corporation
CPX SYSTEM	Medical Graphics Corporation
CPX/D SYSTEM	Medical Graphics Corporation
CPX/MAX SYSTEM	Medical Graphics Corporation
CPX/MAX/S SYSTEM	Medical Graphics Corporation
CPXEXPRESS	Medical Graphics Corporation
CR	Byron Medical
CR SAFGUARD	Chestnut Ridge Foam, Inc.
CRANIOPLASTIC	Codman & Shurtleff, Inc
CRANIOSORB	Codman & Shurtleff, Inc
CRANWALL	Sun-Med
CRANWALL	Sunmed Healthcare
CRAWFORD	Fci Ophthalmics
CRAYON STRIPS	Aso Corporation
CRAZY CLEAN	Sprayway, Inc.
CRC	Capintec, Inc.
CRE	Boston Scientific Corporation
CREATE-A-LAB	Medical Plastics Laboratory, Inc.
CREATININE	Exocell, Inc.
CREST ULTRASONICS	Medi-Tech International, Inc.
CRESTOR	Abbott Laboratories
CREWMASTER	Oster Professional Products, Inc.
CRIBETTE	Hard Manufacturing Co.
CRICKET	Covidien Lp, Formerly Registered As United States Surgical
CRICKET WALKER	Patterson Medical Holdings, Inc.
CRISIS MANIKINS	Nasco
CRITHI DNA	Antibodies, Inc.
CRITI-COOL	Adroit Medical Systems, Inc.
CRITI-KIT	Banyan International Corp.
CRITICORE	C. R. Bard, Inc.
CRITIKON	Ge Medical Systems Information Technologies
CRITOCAPS	Covidien Lp
CRITOSEAL	Covidien Lp
CRITSPIN	Statspin, Inc.
CROCAGATOR	Flotec, Inc.
CROM (CERVICAL RANGE OF MOTION)	Performance Attainment Associates
CRONEX	Agfa Corporation
CROSS VAC	Crosstex International,Inc.
CROSS-FIRE	Uresil, Llc
CROSS-STREAM	Possis Medical, Inc.
CROSSFIRE	Stryker Corp.
CROSSFIRE	Stryker Howmedica Osteonics
CROSSLINK	C. R. Bard, Inc.
CROSSLINK	Medtronic Sofamor Danek Usa, Inc
CROSSLINK	Tp Orthodontics, Inc.
CROSSTEX INT'L DISPOSABLES FOR TETC	Crosstex International,Inc.
CROSSTRAINER	Lenox Hill Brace / Seattle Systems
CROSSVENT, AIRDAIR	Repex Medical Products, Inc.
CROSSZYME	Crosstex International,Inc.
CROWCON	Cea Instruments, Inc.
CROWN	Okamoto U.S.A., Inc.
CROWN CLICK	Hager Worldwide, Inc.
CROWN CLICK DELUXE	Hager Worldwide, Inc.
CROWN MATS & MATTING	Crown Mats
CROWN, GENSURG, ETAGE, TD-LINE	Fine Surgical Instrument, Inc.
CROWN/NAVAL	Sloan Valve Co.
CROWNTITER	Zeus Scientific, Inc.
CRRII	Starkey Laboratories, Inc.
CRUISAIRE	Convaid Inc.
CRUISER	Convaid Inc.
CRUISER	Healthmark Industries
CRUISER	Medical Device Technologies, Inc. (Md Tech)
CRUISER CUSTOM OA	Lenox Hill Brace / Seattle Systems
CRUMB CATCHER	Patterson Medical Holdings, Inc.
CRUNCH-STER	Novel Products, Inc.
CRUSADER	Champion Bus Inc.
CRUSADER	Delta Industrial Services, Inc.
CRUTCH-MATE (TM)	Southwest Technologies, Inc.
CRW	Integra Lifesciences Holdings Corp.
CRY-AC	Brymill Corporation
CRY-AC-3	Brymill Corporation
CRYETTE	Precision Systems, Inc.
CRYO 5	Zimmer Medizinsystems

CRYO GEL 2	Tcp Reliable, Inc.
CRYO-STAT	Statlab Medical Products, Inc.
CRYO-THERM	Corflex, Inc.
CRYO-WRAP	Byron Medical
CRYO/CUFF	Aircast Llc
CRYO3	Sakura Finetek U.S.A., Inc.
CRYOARTERY	Cryolife, Inc.
CRYOBAG	Origen Biomedical, Inc.
CRYOBAR	Sakura Finetek U.S.A., Inc.
CRYOBEADS	Hardy Diagnostics
CRYOBUDS	Cryosurgery, Inc.
CRYOCYTE	Fenwal Inc.
CRYOGEL	Tcp Reliable, Inc.
CRYOGEN	Dma Med-Chem Corporation
CRYOGRAFT	Cryolife, Inc.
CRYOGUN	Brymill Corporation
CRYOGUN	Southland Cryogenics, Inc.
CRYOHISTOMAT	Hacker Instruments And Industries Inc.
CRYOLATCH	Kendro Laboratory Products
CRYOLIN	Grimm Scientific Ind., Inc.
CRYOLOGIC	DJO Inc.
CRYOMASTER	Keeler Instruments Inc.
CRYOMOLD	Sakura Finetek U.S.A., Inc.
CRYOP GCS77	Gilmore Liquid Air Co., Inc.
CRYOPAK	Taylor Wharton
CRYOPRESS	Grimm Scientific Ind., Inc.
CRYOSEAL	Thermogenesis Corp.
CRYOSPRAY	Biofreeze Performance Health, Inc.
CRYOSTAR	Kendro Laboratory Products
CRYOSTIM	Pelton Shepherd Industries
CRYOSTORE	Origen Biomedical, Inc.
CRYOTHERAPY-THE COLD METHOD	Biofreeze Performance Health, Inc.
CRYOTHERM	Grimm Scientific Ind., Inc.
CRYOVALVE	Cryolife, Inc.
CRYOVEIN	Cryolife, Inc.
CRYOWARE	Nalge Nunc International
CRYPTLINER	Extra Packaging, Corp.
CRYPTO-LA	Alere, Inc.
CRYPTO-SCAN	Immucell Corp.
CRYPTON WOVEN UPHOLSTERY	Interspec Fabrics
CRYSTAL	Bd Diagnostic Systems
CRYSTAL ESSENCE	Novocol, Inc.
CRYSTAL TONE AMPLIFIED TELEPHONE	Ultratec, Inc.
CRYSTAL VIEW MAGNIFIER	Image Marketing Corp.
CRYSTAL-AIRE	United Air Specialists, Inc.
CRYSTAL-CLEAR	Atlantic Ultraviolet Corp.
CRYSTAL-EEG	Cleveland Medical Devices, Inc.
CRYSTAL-FLEX	Tp Orthodontics, Inc.
CRYSTALDROP	Gvs Filter Technology Inc.
CRYSTALINE II	Sharn, Inc.
CRYSTALINE ST	Sharn, Inc.
CRYSTALLINE	Novocol, Inc.
CRYSTALVIEW	Alara Inc.
CRYSTALVIEWER	S&S Technology
CRYULE	Wheaton Science Products
CS ULTIMA	Ethicon, Inc.
CS-3000	Fenwal Inc.
CSC AQUAPAL III	Csc Scientific Co.
CSC MOISTURE BALANCE	Csc Scientific Co.
CSF BAGS	Medela, Inc.
CSI	Ciba Vision
CSI HEALTH STATION	Computerized Screening, Inc. (Csi)
CSI MODEL 3000	Computerized Screening, Inc. (Csi)
CSI MODEL 6000	Computerized Screening, Inc. (Csi)
CSI3K	Computerized Screening, Inc. (Csi)
CSI6K	Computerized Screening, Inc. (Csi)
CSK-81	Instrument Specialists, Inc.
CSPD	Applied Biosystems
CSR SERIES	Oneac Corporation
CSTI	Centerpulse Orthopedics Inc.
CSTI	Zimmer Dental, Inc.
CT	Baxter Healthcare Corporation, Renal
CT GUIDE	C. R. Bard, Inc.
CT PHANTOM	Supertech, Inc.
CT-500	Cannon Instrument Co.
CT-PACK	Coeur, Inc
CT3, VARIA, CTEV, NS-1500, 2100 HOLMIUM	New Star Lasers, Inc.
CT9000	Mallinckrodt, Inc.
CTA MEDIUM	Bd Diagnostic Systems
CTLM	Imaging Diagnostic Systems, Inc.
CTM	Med-Lift & Mobility, Inc.
CTN	Kinamed, Inc.
CTS	Champion Bus Inc.
CTS	Chattanooga Group
CTS RELIEF KIT	Conmed Linvatec
CTVISION	Siemens Medical Solutions Usa, Inc
CTX	Alere, Inc.
CUB	Stryker Corp.
CUBE	Coherent, Inc.
CUDA	Conmed Linvatec
CUDA	Sunoptic Technologies
CUDDLE PAWS	Principle Business Enterprises, Inc.
CUDDLEEWE UNDERQUILT	Merlo Co., Llc.
CUE	Zetek, Inc.
CUFF IMPLANTOR	Janin Group, Inc.
CUFF-ABLE	Vital Signs, Inc.
CUFFLINK	Fluke Biomedical
CUI	Cook Urological, Inc.
CUL-TECT	Globe Scientific, Inc.
CULEX	Basi (Bioanalytical Systems, Inc.)
CULT-UR	Cargille Laboratories
CULTI-LOOP	Remel
CULTURE TUBES	Mml Diagnostics Packaging, Inc.
CULTURE-PAK	Medical Packaging Corporation
CULTUREGARD	Spectrum Laboratories, Inc.
CULTURETTE	Bd Diagnostic Systems
CUMFI SIT	Wenzelite Rehab Supplies, Llc
CUMULA I	Hospital Comm. & Electronics, Inc.
CUMULA II	Hospital Comm. & Electronics, Inc.
CUMULA III	Hospital Comm. & Electronics, Inc.
CUNO	Western Water Purifier Co.
CURAY-ECLIPSE	Scientific Pharmaceuticals, Inc.
CURAY-FIL	Scientific Pharmaceuticals, Inc.
CURAY-II	Scientific Pharmaceuticals, Inc.
CURAY-MATCH	Scientific Pharmaceuticals, Inc.
CURAY-SUPPORT	Scientific Pharmaceuticals, Inc.
CURBSIDER	Bruno Independent Living Aids, Inc.
CURE BOND	Composites Horizons, Inc.
CURE-ON-TOUCH	Scientific Pharmaceuticals, Inc.
CURE-WRAP	Adroit Medical Systems, Inc.
CURING LIGHT SHIELDS	Almore International, Inc.
CURIX	Agfa Corp.
CURIX	Agfa Corporation
CUROSURF	Dey, L.P.
CURTIS	Wilbur Curtis Company
CURV-CLEAN	Combe, Inc.
CURVE SNUGGER, LUVS YA BACK	Roloke
CURVEDBOX	Placon Corporation
CURVLITE	Mastercraft Products Corporation
CURVTEK	Biolectron, Inc.
CUSA	Integra Lifesciences Holdings Corp.
CUSA EXCEL	Integra Lifesciences Holdings Corp.
CUSHION MATS	Paragon Medical, Inc.
CUSHION SEAL	Amici, Inc.
CUSHION-LIFT	Ortho-Kinetics, Inc.
CUSHIONFIT	Hollister Incorporated
CUSTOM AIR SEAT CUSHION SYSTEM	Aquila Corporation
CUSTOM CONVERTING OF YOUR PRODUCT!	Csi Holdings
CUSTOM PHYSICIAN FEE REPORT	Captiva Software Corporation
CUSTOMAIR	Dentalez Group
CUT & SCRAPE CLEANER	Safetec Of America, Inc.
CUT CLEANERS	Afassco, Inc.
CUT DOWN CATHETER	Becton Dickinson Infusion Therapy Systems, Inc.
CUTS-IT	Weiman Healthcare Solutions
CUTTING BALLOON	Boston Scientific Interventional Technologies
CUVETTE REPROCESSING	Laboratory Environment Support Systems, Inc.

CUVETTES	Nsg Precision Cells, Inc.
CV -3	Bio-Med Devices, Inc.
CV-2	Bio-Med Devices, Inc.
CV-4	Bio-Med Devices, Inc.
CV5030 COVERSLIPPER	Leica Microsystems Inc.
CVAC	Getinge Usa, Inc.
CVISION	Shimadzu Medical Systems
CVM	Siemens Healthcare Diagnostics Inc
CVPROFILOR(R) DO-2020 CARDIOVASCULAR PROFILING SYSTEM	Hypertension Diagnostics, Inc.
CVPROFILOR(R) MD-3000 CARDIOVASCULAR PROFILING SYSTEM	Hypertension Diagnostics, Inc.
CVR	Cardiovascular Research, Inc.
CVRX	Cvrx Inc.
CVV ADHESIVE	Herculite Products, Inc.
CVX-300	Spectranetics Corp.
CW-160	Conflex
CW-PULSE	Iridex Corporation
CWECO	Cweco, Inc.
CWS	Thermo Fisher Scientific - Laboratory Equipment Division Headquarters
CWV SUMP	Axiom Medical, Inc.
CX PLUS	Shofu Dental Corporation
CX SERIES	Oneac Corporation
CXR	Lw Scientific
CXR	Xma (X-Ray Marketing Associates, Inc.)
CXR4	Hitachi Medical Systems America, Inc.
CYBERKNIFE	Accuray, Inc.
CYBERLAB	Aspyra, Inc.
CYBERMED	Aspyra, Inc.
CYBERONIC	Cyberonics, Inc.
CYBERPATH	Aspyra, Inc.
CYBERRAD	Aspyra, Inc.
CYBEX	CYBEX INTERNATIONAL, INC.
CYBEX	Cybex International, Inc.
CYCLE-TAINER	Avantor Performance Materials
CYCLO-TRAC	Diasorin Inc
CYCLO-TRAC SP	Diasorin Inc
CYCLON	Enersys
CYCLONE	DJO Inc.
CYCLONE	Pride Mobility Products Corp.
CYCLONE	Virtis, An Sp Industries Company
CYFRA 21-1	Fujirebio Diagnostics, Inc. (Fdi)
CYGNUS-PFS	Compass International, Inc.
CYNCH-LOK	Healthmark Industries
CYPHER	Cordis Corporation
CYPHER	Medtronic, Inc.
CYPRESS	Accu-Med Services
CYPRESS OXYPNEUMATIC CONSERVER	Chad Therapeutics, Inc.
CYSTO-CARE	Mentor Corp.
CYSTO-CONRAY	Mallinckrodt, Inc.
CYSTOTRON	Biosonics, Inc.
CYTETTE	Birchwood Laboratories, Inc.
CYTO-COMP	Modulus Data Systems, Inc.
CYTO-PAK	Medical Packaging Corporation
CYTO-SOFT	Medical Packaging Corporation
CYTO-TEK	Sakura Finetek U.S.A., Inc.
CYTO-TRAK	Medical Packaging Corporation
CYTOFUGE	Statspin, Inc.
CYTOFUZE	Iris International, Inc.
CYTOKINE DIRECT	Serologicals Corp
CYTOKINE TOTAL	Serologicals Corp
CYTOMAX II	Wilson-Cook Medical, Inc.
CYTOMEL	King Pharmaceuticals, Inc.
CYTOPAD	Wescor, Inc.
CYTOPRO	Wescor, Inc.
CYTOSAFE	Baxa Corporation
CYTOSENSOR	Molecular Devices Corp.
CYTOTHERM	Cytotherm
CYTOTOX 96	Promega Corp.
CYTWOFER	Baxa Corporation
Calzoni	Danaher Corporation
Capio	Boston Scientific Corporation
Captivator	Boston Scientific Corporation
Cardioblate	Medtronic, Inc.
CarePath	Dianon Systems - Labcorp
Carmeda	Medtronic Perfusion Systems
Carto	Biosense Webster, Inc
Cascada	Pall Corporation
Cascade	Procter & Gamble
Cavro	Tecan Systems
Charmin	Procter & Gamble
Cheer	Procter & Gamble
Cheetahs	Medi-Dyne Healthcare Products, L.L.C.
ChemTreat	Danaher Corporation
Chemistry That Empowers Discovery	Avantor Performance Materials
Chilli	Boston Scientific Corporation
Chilli II	Boston Scientific Corporation
ChloraPrep	Cardinal Health 200, Inc.
Chromegabond	Es Industries
Chrysalin	Capstone Therapeutics
Cinch	St. Jude Medical Neuromodulation Division
Cinch Sak	Pactiv Corporation
CircuCool	Boston Scientific Corporation
Clairol	Procter & Gamble
Clear Pore	Ortho Dermatologics
Clearblue	Procter & Gamble
Clearview NOW	Inverness Medical Professional Diagnostics-San Die
Coaptite	Boston Scientific Corporation
Colorcard	Inverness Medical Professional Diagnostics-San Die
Comfortex	Comfortex, Inc.
Constellation	Boston Scientific Corporation
Contour	St. Jude Medical, Inc.
Contour SE	Boston Scientific Corporation
Contour VL	Boston Scientific Corporation
Convert	St. Jude Medical, Inc.
Cool Point	St. Jude Medical, Inc.
CopiOs	Zimmer Spine, Inc.
CorTemp	Hq, Inc.
CoreStretch	Medi-Dyne Healthcare Products, L.L.C.
Cornea Coat	Insight Instruments, Inc.
Correct	Pentron Laboratory Technologies
Crest	Procter & Gamble
Crest Whitestrips	Procter & Gamble
Critical Care Therapies	Kinetic Concepts, Inc.
Crossfire	Megasun
Crypton	Knoll, Inc.
Crystalens	Bausch & Lomb
Current	St. Jude Medical, Inc.
D'HOOGE	Ipso Usa, Inc.
D-55	Diversified Ophthalmics, Inc.
D-CORE PILLOW	Core Products International, Inc.
D-MIC	Etymotic Research, Inc.
D-PEN	Roche Insulin Delivery Systems Inc.
D-SIGN ALLOYS	Ivoclar Vivadent, Inc.
D-TACH	Covidien Lp
D-TEK-PLAC	Preventive Dentistry Products, Inc.
D-TRON	Roche Insulin Delivery Systems Inc.
D.B.I. TABLE	Medical Positioning, Inc.
D.L. SCOPE	North American Medical Products, Inc.
D.R.A.S.H.	Dhs Systems Llc
D.T. TEMPORARY DRESSING	Global Dental Products
D/SENSE	Centrix, Inc.
D940/SKINPULSE S	Dornier Medtech America
DA VINCI	Intuitive Surgical, Inc.
DAB/OUT	Triangle Biomedical Sciences, Inc.
DAC PROFESSIONAL	Sirona Dental Systems Llc
DAC UNIVERSAL	Sirona Dental Systems Llc
DACOGEN	Johnson & Johnson
DACOMOBILE	KnÄrr Usa Inc.
DADC 500	Driving Aids Development Corporation
DADC 500P	Driving Aids Development Corporation
DAHEDI	Roche Insulin Delivery Systems Inc.
DAI	Flowtronics, Inc.
DAICEL	Chiral Technologies, Inc.
DAILY DOUBLE	Ranir Corp.
DAKO	Dako North America, Inc

DELTALITE	Vision-Ease Lens
DELTARANGE	Mettler-Toledo, Inc.
DELTASCAN	Photon Technology International, Inc.
DELTATRAK	Deltatrak, Inc.
DELTEC COZMO	Smiths Medical Asd, Inc.
DELTOID AID	Activeaid, Inc.
DELTON	Dentsply International, Inc.
DELTON	Dentsply Professional
DELTON	Dentsply Prosthetics
DELTRAN	Utah Medical Products, Inc.
DELUXE	Columbia Medical Manufacturing Llc
DELUXE LF	Hartmann-Conco Inc.
DEMINERALIZED BONE MATRIX	Berkeley Advanced Biomaterials, Inc.
DEMISTIFIER	Peace Medical
DEMLAR MEDICAL	Monitor Instruments Inc.
DEMO-DOSE	Pocket Nurse Enterprises, Inc.
DEMRON	Radiation Shield Technologies, Inc.
DENALI	Nest Group Inc., The
DENCO	Alere, Inc.
DENLITE	Integra Lifesciences Holdings Corp.
DENOPTIX	Alara Inc.
DENSE ARRAY EEG	Electrical Geodesics, Incorporated
DENSENSITIZER WITH FLUORIDE	Healthdent'L L.L.C.
DENSONORM	AMD Technologies Inc.
DENSOSCAN	AMD Technologies Inc.
DENT-X	Afp Imaging Corp.
DENTABOND	Argen Corp.
DENTAL CARE	Tillotson Healthcare Corp.
DENTAL GLOVES	Ansell Healthcare Products, Inc.
DENTAL QC KIT	Supertech, Inc.
DENTALEZ	Dentalez Group
DENTALOY	Tp Orthodontics, Inc.
DENTATUS	Charles B. Schwed Co., Inc.
DENTCLOCK	Hager Worldwide, Inc.
DENTI-LAB	Medidenta International, Inc.
DENTICA	Convergent Laser Technologies
DENTICATOR	Denticator International, Inc.
DENTIFRICE	Oral-B Laboratories, Inc.
DENTIN SENSOR	Biolase Technology, Inc.
DENTO BOX	Hager Worldwide, Inc.
DENTOFORMS	Dentalez Group
DENTRAY	Novocol, Inc.
DENTSPLY-PREVENTIVE CARE	Dentsply International, Inc.
DENTSPLY-PREVENTIVE CARE	Dentsply Prosthetics
DENTURE	Aluwax Dental Products Co.
DENTURE FORMS	Aluwax Dental Products Co.
DENTURITE	Combe, Inc.
DENTUS	Agfa Corporation
DENVER	Utech Products, Inc.
DENVER NASAL SPLINT	Shippert Medical Technologies Corp.
DEOXINATOR	Eraser Company, Inc.
DEOXIT	Caig Laboratories, Inc.
DEOXIT GOLD	Caig Laboratories, Inc.
DEOXIT SHIELD	Caig Laboratories, Inc.
DEPEND-AID	Sellstrom Manufacturing Co.
DEPOT	Merit Medical Systems, Inc.
DEPTHALON	Pmt Corp.
DERAMADROX SPRAY	Geritrex Corp.
DERAMCARRIERS SKIN GRAFT CARRIERS	Zimmer Orthopaedic Surgical Products
DERM KIT	Culture Kits, Inc.
DERMA BATH	Sage Laboratories, Inc.
DERMA CIDOL 2000	King Pharmaceuticals, Inc.
DERMA COOL	Romaine, Inc. D.B.A. Koldcare
DERMA PRENE	Ansell Healthcare Products, Inc.
DERMA SCRUB	King Pharmaceuticals, Inc.
DERMA SOOTHE	King Pharmaceuticals, Inc.
DERMA STAT	King Pharmaceuticals, Inc.
DERMA-JEL	Physio-Control, Inc.
DERMA-SAFE	Derma-Safe Company
DERMA-TRODE ELECTRODES	American Imex
DERMA-WAND	National Biological Corp.
DERMABLADE	Personna Medical/Div. Of American Safety Razor Co.
DERMABOND	Closure Medical
DERMABOND	Ethicon, Inc.
DERMACEA	Covidien Lp
DERMACHILLER4	Telsar Laboratories Inc
DERMACLEAN STERILE	Ansell Healthcare Products, Inc.
DERMACLEAN X-AM	Ansell Healthcare Products, Inc.
DERMACOOL	Afassco, Inc.
DERMADROX OINTMENT	Geritrex Corp.
DERMAGARD	Personna Medical/Div. Of American Safety Razor Co.
DERMAGLIDE	Surgical Specialties Corporation
DERMAGRAN	Derma Sciences
DERMAGUARD PLUS	Ansell Healthcare Products, Inc.
DERMAL GLOVES	George Glove Company, Inc.
DERMALIGHT 80	National Biological Corp.
DERMALON	Covidien Lp
DERMAMARKER	Olsen Medical
DERMAPAL	The Daavlin Company
DERMAPASTE	Smith & Nephew, Inc.
DERMAPLAST	Aetrex Worldwide, Inc
DERMAPRO	Gojo Industries, Inc
DERMAPROFILER	Solarius Development Inc.
DERMASAFE	American Health Products Corporation
DERMASEAL	Hydromer, Inc.
DERMASEPTIC	Y.I. Ventures, Llc
DERMASPAN	Specialty Surgical Products, Inc.
DERMASTAT	Ams Innovative Center-San Jose
DERMATEAM	Humanicare International, Inc.
DERMATELL	Gentell
DERMATHERM	Sharn, Inc.
DERMATUBE	Remel
DERMICEL	Johnson & Johnson Medical Division Of Ethicon, Inc.
DERMICLEAR	Johnson & Johnson Medical Division Of Ethicon, Inc.
DERMIFORM	Johnson & Johnson Medical Division Of Ethicon, Inc.
DERMLITE	3gen, Llc
DERMOSUCTION	Tulip Medical Products
DESERET I.V. LOOP	Becton Dickinson Infusion Therapy Systems, Inc.
DESERET J-LOOP	Becton Dickinson Infusion Therapy Systems, Inc.
DESERET PRN ADAPTERS	Becton Dickinson Infusion Therapy Systems, Inc.
DESERET T-PORT	Becton Dickinson Infusion Therapy Systems, Inc.
DESI-VIEW	Hardy Diagnostics
DESICAP	Multisorb Technologies, Inc.
DESICCHLORA	Avantor Performance Materials
DESIGN	Medworks Instruments
DESIGNER LINE	United Receptacle
DESIGNERCARE	Hard Manufacturing Co.
DESIGNPLUS	Algor, Inc.
DESIMAX	Multisorb Technologies, Inc.
DESITIN	Johnson & Johnson
DESK POWER	Oneac Corporation
DESKLIFT	Linak U.S. Inc.
DESKLINE	Linak U.S. Inc.
DESKTOP SYNOPSIS SOFTWARE	Medical Graphics Corporation
DETECT-A-STREP	Antibodies, Inc.
DETECTABUSE	Biochemical Diagnostics, Inc.
DETECTO	Creative Health Products, Inc.
DETECTOR-CUBE	Immunostics, Inc.
DETECTOR-STIX	Immunostics, Inc.
DETEK	Enzo Biochem, Inc.
DETERGICLENE	Mckesson General Medical
DETERMINE	Alere, Inc.
DEV-O-CLAMP	Graphic Controls Corp.
DEV-O-LOOPS	Graphic Controls Corp.
DEV-O-POUCH	Graphic Controls Corp.
DEVER BED	Hard Manufacturing Co.
DEVILBISS	Sunrise Medical
DEVON	Covidien Lp, Formerly Registered As Tyco Healthcare
DEVON	Graphic Controls Corp.
DEWALL/HUMIDITY	Edgetech
DEWAR	Southland Cryogenics, Inc.
DEWPRIME/HUMIDITY	Edgetech
DEWTRACE/MOISTURE	Edgetech
DEWTRAK/HUMIDITY	Edgetech
DEX	Siemens Healthcare Diagnostics Inc.

DEXACARE	Coopersurgical, Inc.
DEXACARE G4	Osteometer Meditech, Inc.
DEXIS	Danaher Corporation
DEXON	Covidien Lp
DEXON II	Covidien Lp
DEXON MESH	Covidien Lp
DEXON S	Covidien Lp
DEXTER	Cedaron Medical, Inc.
DEXTER	Dexter Apache Holdings, Inc.
DEXTEX	Ahlstrom Windsor Locks Llc
DFS	Covidien Lp, Formerly Registered As United States Surgical
DFT	Fort Wayne Metals Research Prod. Corp.
DG-300	Covidien Lp
DGH5000E	D.G.H. Technology, Inc.
DGH5100E	D.G.H. Technology, Inc.
DGRT	Siemens Medical Solutions Usa, Inc
DHD	Dma Med-Chem Corporation
DHI	Danaher Corporation
DI CASE	Medicool, Inc.
DI-CUT MODEL SAW	Motloid Company
DI-LOCK	St. Jude Medical Atrial Fibrillation
DIA PACK	Medicool, Inc.
DIA PAK	Medicool, Inc.
DIA TEMP	Conmed Corporation
DIA TEMP II	Conmed Corporation
DIA VAC	Air Dimensions, Inc.
DIA VITE	Medicool, Inc.
DIAB-A-SHEETS	Langer, Inc.
DIAB-A-SOLE	Langer, Inc.
DIAB-A-THOTICS	Langer, Inc.
DIABETIC	Medicool, Inc.
DIABETIC BASICS ANTIMICROBIAL HEALTHY FOOT CARE LOTION, SPRAY, POWDER	Woodward Laboratories, Inc.
DIABETIC PRODUCTS	Medicool, Inc.
DIABETIC SOCKS	Medicool, Inc.
DIABETIC VITAMINS	Medicool, Inc.
DIACAN	B. Braun Medical Inc., Renal Therapies Div.
DIACK	Thorn Smith Laboratories
DIACOR	Diacor, Inc.
DIAGNO-STICS	Cardiofocus, Inc.
DIAGNOST	Philips Medical Systems North America
DIAGNOSTICK	Bovie Medical Corp.
DIAGNOSTIX	American Diagnostic Corporation (Adc)
DIAL-A-LIGHT	Richard Wolf Medical Instruments Corp.
DIALBUMIN	Exocell, Inc.
DIALEASE	Merit Medical Systems, Inc.
DIALINES	B. Braun Medical Inc., Renal Therapies Div.
DIALOG	B. Braun Medical Inc., Renal Therapies Div.
DIALY-NATE	Utah Medical Products, Inc.
DIAMOND	Coherent, Inc.
DIAMOND DUST	Scanlan International, Inc.
DIAMOND E-400	Coherent, Inc.
DIAMOND GRIP	Microflex Corporation
DIAMOND GRIP PLUS	Microflex Corporation
DIAMOND HOMECARE BED	Wheelchairs Of Kansas
DIAMOND SHINE	Amano Pioneer Eclipse Corp.
DIAMOND-BACK	U.S. Orthotics, Inc.
DIAMOND-LUSTER POLISH	Topcon Medical Systems, Inc.
DIAMONDBACK 360	Cardiovascular Systems, Inc.
DIAMONDCARE	Hill-Rom Holdings, Inc.
DIAMONDTOME, NEWAPEEL, HYDROWANDS	Altair Instruments, Inc.
DIAMONDVAC	Arthrocare Corp.
DIAMONDWIRE	Innovative Med Inc.
DIANA	Horcher Lifting Systems, Inc.
DIANEAL	Baxter Healthcare Corporation, Renal
DIAPACT	B. Braun Medical Inc., Renal Therapies Div.
DIAPHOT	Nikon Instruments Inc.
DIAPUMP	Air Control, Inc.
DIARAD	Capintec, Inc.
DIARLEX	Lifesign
DIASCREEN	Arkray Usa
DIASOL	Diasol, Inc.
DIASTAR	Leica Microsystems, Inc., Educational & Analytical Division
DIASTAT	Biorad Laboratories
DIASTERBOARD	Ambu, Inc.
DIASTIX	Siemens Healthcare Diagnostics Inc.
DIASYS	Diasys Corporation
DIATEMP	Conmed Corporation
DICOM DIGITIZERS	Imsi, Integrated Modular Systems Inc.
DICOM MOBILE CR SYSTEMS	Imsi, Integrated Modular Systems Inc.
DICOM PAPER PRINTING SOLUTIONS	Imsi, Integrated Modular Systems Inc.
DICOMBOX	Nai Tech Products
DICOR	Dentsply Caulk
DICTA	Dictator U.S., Inc.
DICTAMAT	Dictator U.S., Inc.
DICTATOR	Dictator U.S., Inc.
DIE HARDENER & THINNER	American Diversified Dental Systems
DIE LUBE	American Diversified Dental Systems
DIE SPACERS & THINNER	American Diversified Dental Systems
DIETRONIC	Seca Corp.
DIFCO	Bd Diagnostic Systems
DIFF-SAFE	Alpha Scientific Corporation
DIFFCOUNT III	Modulus Data Systems, Inc.
DIFFERENTIAL STRAIGHT-ARCH	Tp Orthodontics, Inc.
DIFFGAM	Immucell Corp.
DIFFSPIN 2	Statspin, Inc.
DIFFUSIMATIC	Jones Medical Instrument Co.
DIGI GRIP	Instrument Specialists, Inc.
DIGI-DYNE	Minntech Corporation
DIGI-PRO	Magnatone Hearing Aid Corp.
DIGI-SENSE	Cole-Parmer Instrument Inc.
DIGICOM	Ring Communications, Inc.
DIGICOUNTER	Giles Scientific, Inc.
DIGIFOCUS II	Oticon, Inc.
DIGIGRAPH	Dolphin Imaging Systems
DIGIMANO	Netech, Corp.
DIGIMEDICS	Mediware Information Systems, Inc.
DIGIT	Smiths Medical Pm, Inc.
DIGITAL 8	Eigen
DIGITAL COMPRESSION SCREW	Biopro, Inc.
DIGITAL DISK RECORDER-PLUS	Eigen
DIGITAL FLUOROSTORE	Eigen
DIGITAL FUNDUS IMAGER	Ophthalmic Imaging Systems
DIGITAL MDM	Matrx By Midmark
DIGITAL PHOTOSPOT	Eigen
DIGITAL PILOT TEST	Maico Diagnostics
DIGITAL SLIT LAMP IMAGER	Ophthalmic Imaging Systems
DIGITAL SYRINGE	Hamilton Company
DIGITAL-READY SLIT LAMPS	Topcon Medical Systems, Inc.
DIGITCARE	Bound Tree Medical
DIGITEK	Vicon Industries Inc.
DIGITEMP	LCR Hallcrest
DIGITEST	Parkell, Inc.
DIGITEX ALPHA	Shimadzu Medical Systems
DIGITEX PRO	Shimadzu Medical Systems
DIGITEX PRO MULTI	Shimadzu Medical Systems
DIGITFET	Hoggan Health Industries, Inc.
DIGITRACE	Sleepmed Incorporated
DIGITRON	Siemens Medical Solutions Usa, Inc.
DIGIVIDEO	Karl Storz Endoscopy-America Inc.
DIGIVIEW	Sleepmed Incorporated
DIGIVISION	Enhanced Video Devices, Inc.
DIGIWIPE	Idexx Laboratories, Inc.
DIGMA	Hansco Technologies, Inc.
DIGNITY	Humanicare International, Inc.
DIGNITY PLUS	Humanicare International, Inc.
DIGNITY PLUS BRIEFMATES	Humanicare International, Inc.
DIGNITY STACKABLES	Humanicare International, Inc.
DIGNITY THINSERTS	Humanicare International, Inc.
DIGNITYDRY	Humanicare International, Inc.
DILAMEZINSERT	Lone Star Medical Products, Inc.
DILATERIA	Milex Products, Inc.
DILON 6800 GAMMA CAMERA	Dilon Diagnostics Llc
DILU-LOK	Hardy Diagnostics
DILUT-IT	Avantor Performance Materials
DIMAX	Planmeca U.S.A. Inc

DIMAXIS	Planmeca U.S.A. Inc
DIMCOGRIP	Dimco Gray Co.
DIMENSION	Siemens Healthcare Diagnostics Inc.
DIMENSION VISTA	Siemens Healthcare Diagnostics Inc.
DIMENSION-3	Sds-Surgical Acuity
DIMERTEST	American Diagnostica, Inc.
DINAMAP	Ge Medical Systems Information Technologies
DINAMAP MPS	Ge Medical Systems Information Technologies
DINAMAP PLUS	Ge Medical Systems Information Technologies
DINAMAP/OXYTRAK	Ge Medical Systems Information Technologies
DIODENT	Continuum, Inc.
DIODERM	Convergent Laser Technologies
DIOGENES	Medicomp, Inc.
DIOLASE	Biolase Technology, Inc.
DIOLASE PLUS	Biolase Technology, Inc.
DIOLITE 532	Iridex Corporation
DIOPEXY	Iridex Corporation
DIOVET	Iridex Corporation
DIP 'N' POUR	Accurate Set, Inc.
DIP-IT	Ecolab Inc.
DIPDRUG SCAN	Syntron Bioresearch, Inc.
DIPLOMAT	Collins Bus Corporation
DIPPER	Quantimetrix Corporation
DIRECT DRIVE	Applied Medical Resource Corporation
DIRECT VIEW	Volk Optical Inc.
DIRECT-DETECT	Meridian Bioscience, Inc.
DIRECT-ENTRY	Baxa Corporation
DIRECTFLO	Comco, Inc.
DIRECTIGEN	Bd Diagnostic Systems
DIRECTOR	Bd Diagnostic Systems
DIRECTOR	Nds Surgical Imaging, Inc.
DIRECTRAY	Hologic, Inc.
DIRECTVIEW	Carestream Health, Inc.
DIRECTVISTA	Codonics
DIRECTVOICE	Magnatone Hearing Aid Corp.
DIS-CLAVE	Healthmark Industries
DISASEPTIC	Palmero Health Care
DISC UNLOADER	Corflex, Inc.
DISC-PAK	Ertelalsop
DISCIDE	Palmero Health Care
DISCIDE ULTRA	Palmero Health Care
DISCKIT	Ams Innovative Center-San Jose
DISCMONITOR	Stryker Corp.
DISCOFIX	B. Braun Oem Division, B. Braun Medical Inc.
DISCOVERY	Futuremed America, Inc.
DISCOVERY	Ventana Medical Systems, Inc.
DISCOVERY PACK	Oncogene Research Products
DISCOVERY2020	Mexpo International, Inc.
DISCPAC	Ams Innovative Center-San Jose
DISCPAC	Baxa Corporation
DISCRENE	Coloplast Manufacturing Us, Llc
DISCRETEPAK	Catachem Inc.
DISCUPS	Cargille Laboratories
DISCUSSION	C. R. Bard, Inc.
DISINFECTANT CLEANER & INSTRUMENT PRESOAK	Veridien Corp.
DISKARD	Florida Manufacturing Corp.
DISKMATE	Avantor Performance Materials
DISPATCH	Caltech Industries, Inc.
DISPENSTIRS	Bd Diagnostic Systems
DISPENSTUBE	Bd Diagnostic Systems
DISPERSALLOY	Dentsply Caulk
DISPERSALLOY	Dentsply International, Inc.
DISPERSALLOY	Dentsply Prosthetics
DISPETTE	Arkray Usa
DISPETTE 2	Arkray Usa
DISPODIALYZER	Spectrum Laboratories, Inc.
DISPOS-A-JECT	Byron Medical
DISPOS-A-SCOPE	Mabis Healthcare Inc.
DISPOS-A-SHARP	Hospital Marketing Svcs. Company, Inc.
DISPOS-A-SWAB	Pedinol Pharmacal, Inc.
DISPOS-O-SEAL	Mercury Medical
DISPOSA-COVERS	Cincinnati Sub-Zero Products, Inc., Medical Division
DISPOSA-CUF	Ge Medical Systems Information Technologies
DISPOSA-HOOD	Utah Medical Products, Inc.
DISPOSA-VIEW	Vital Signs, Inc.
DISPOSABLE BREATHING BAG	H&M Rubber Company, Inc.
DISPOSEZE	HARTMANN USA, Inc.
DISPOSO-SCOPE	Monarch Molding Inc.
DISPOSO-SPEC	Monarch Molding Inc.
DISPOVAN	Myco Medical
DISRUPTOR GENIE	Scientific Industries, Inc.
DISSECTRON	Integra Lifesciences Holdings Corp.
DISTAFLEX	Medtronic, Inc.
DISTAL JET	American Orthodontics Corp.
DISTINCTION	Dentalez Group
DITEC DIAMOND BURRS	Ditec Mfg.
DIXI	Planmeca U.S.A. Inc
DJO/PROCARE	Ortholine
DL1250	Braemar, Inc.
DL250	Braemar, Inc.
DL700	Braemar, Inc.
DL800	Braemar, Inc.
DLL SERIES III	Dac International, Inc.
DLP	Medtronic Perfusion Systems
DLP	Medtronic, Inc.
DM MICROSCOPES	Leica Microsystems Inc.
DMC	Waterloo Healthcare, Llc
DME VI	Carecentric, Inc.
DMI	Lone Star Medical Products, Inc.
DMI MICROSCOPES	Leica Microsystems Inc.
DMS	United Dental Manufacturers, Inc.
DMV 45	Dmv Corporation
DMV CLASSIC	Dmv Corporation
DMV MAGIC TOUCH	Dmv Corporation
DMV MAGNA MIRROR	Dmv Corporation
DMV SLH	Dmv Corporation
DMV ULTRA	Dmv Corporation
DOBBHOFF	Covidien Lp
DOBI-SYMPLEX	Seattle Systems
DOC'S BEST ANTIMICROBIAL PULP(ROOT) CANAL SEALER	Cooley & Cooley, Ltd.
DOC'S BEST COPPER ANTIMICROBIAL CEMENTS	Cooley & Cooley, Ltd.
DOC-IT	Uvp, Llc
DOC-U-SCRIBE	Pentax Medical Company
DOCTOR'S ORDERS	Carex Health Brands
DOCUMED	Lionville Systems, Inc.
DOCUMENT	Microgenics Corporation
DOLI S II	Dornier Medtech America
DOLOMITE	Clarke Health Care Products, Inc.
DOLOMITE ALPHA	Clarke Health Care Products, Inc.
DOLOMITE MELODY	Clarke Health Care Products, Inc.
DOLPHIN	Aearo Company
DOLPHIN	Noram Solutions
DOLPHIN	Sloan Valve Co.
DOLPHIN	Wenzelite Rehab Supplies, Llc
DOLPHIN SHOWER TROLLEY	Noram Solutions
DOMINANT	Medela, Inc.
DOMINANT 35 C/I	Medela, Inc.
DOMINANT 50	Medela, Inc.
DOMINATOR	Dr Systems, Inc.
DOMINION	Imaging3, Inc.
DOMINION VOLUMETRIC IMAGING SCANNER	Imaging3, Inc.
DON JAKE SAUNDERS HEART	Medical Plastics Laboratory, Inc.
DOPSCAN	Carolina Medical, Inc.
DOPSCAN 1050	Carolina Medical, Inc.
DOPSCAN 1060	Carolina Medical, Inc.
DOPSCAN 1060 PLUS	Carolina Medical, Inc.
DOREX DTI-16UT1 DOREX SPECTRUM	Dorex, Inc.
DORIBAX	Ortho-Mcneil-Janssen Pharmaceuticals, Inc.
DORSET	Vista Lighting
DOSE-GUIDED RADIATION THERAPY	Siemens Medical Solutions Usa, Inc
DOSER	Meditrack Products, Llc
DOSIMETER	Andersen Products, Inc.,
DOSING PARTNERS	Aprex, A Division Of Aardex
DOT Matrix	Noven Pharmaceuticals, Inc.
DOT-X	Dotronix, Inc.

DUOPEX	Filtrona Extrusion, Inc./PexcoA,Ar Medical Products Div.
DUOPLAS	Sterion, Incorporated
DUOPULSE 2000	Excel Technology, Inc.
DUOTEK	Pml Microbiologicals
DUOTEK	Sts Duotek, Inc
DUOTEX	Ansell Healthcare Products, Inc.
DUOTIP-TEST	Lincoln Diagnostics, Inc.
DUOTRODES	Myotronics-Noromed, Inc.
DUOVAC	Farley Inc., W.T.
DUP-X	I.B.F. Corporation
DUPEL	Empi, Inc.
DUPLEX	B. Braun Oem Division, B. Braun Medical Inc.
DUPLOCATH	Baxter International Inc
DUPLOREACH	Baxter International Inc
DUPONT TYVEK	Interex Div. Of Industrial Safety & Supply
DUPONT TYVEK PREFERRED CONVERTER	Tailored Label Products, Inc.
DUR-A-CRETE 4TM	Dur-A-Flex, Inc.
DUR-A-GARD	Dur-A-Flex, Inc.
DUR-A-POXY HIGH GLOSS	Dur-A-Flex, Inc.
DUR-A-QUARTZ	Dur-A-Flex, Inc.
DURA CARE	Handicap Unlimited, Inc.
DURA II	Timm Medical Technologies, Inc.
DURA NEB 2000	Elan
DURA SOCK	Great Lakes Filters/Filpaco Industries
DURA TEX	Duraline Medical Products, Inc.
DURA-BOARD ARMBOARD	Allen Medical Systems, Inc.
DURA-CUF	Ge Medical Systems Information Technologies
DURA-EDGE	Havel's Inc.
DURA-EDGE	Stryker Corp.
DURA-GREEN	Shofu Dental Corporation
DURA-GUARD	Synovis Life Technologies, Inc
DURA-GUARD	Synovis Surgical Innovations
DURA-HOLD	March & Green
DURA-KOLD	Dura-Kold Corp.
DURA-NEB	Pari Respiratory Equipment, Inc.
DURA-RUG	Durable Corporation
DURA-SOFT	Dura-Kold Corp.
DURA-TILE	Pawling Corp., Architectural Prod. Div.
DURA-WHITE	Shofu Dental Corporation
DURA-Y	Covidien (Formerly Nellcor Puritan Bennett / Tyco Healthcare)
DURABLEND ACRYLIC	Dentsply Prosthetics
DURABOUND	Mobile Instrument Service And Repair, Inc.
DURACELL	Duracell Usa
DURACISION	Micromedics
DURACON	Stryker Spine
DURACON TS	Stryker Corp.
DURACON TS	Stryker Howmedica Osteonics
DURAEDGE	Crescent Mfg. Co.
DURAFIL	Camfil Farr
DURAFLECT	Labsphere, Inc.
DURAFLEX	Sperian Protection
DURAFOAM	Scott Specialties, Inc./Cmo Inc./Ginny Inc.
DURAFORM	Codman & Shurtleff, Inc
DURAGEN	Integra Lifesciences Holdings Corp.
DURAGEN PLUS	Integra Lifesciences Holdings Corp.
DURAGESIC	Ortho-Mcneil-Janssen Pharmaceuticals, Inc.
DURAGOLD	Applied Medical Resource Corporation
DURAHESIVE	Convatec Professional Services
DURALAST	Hamilton Caster & Mfg. Co.
DURALINE SERIES	Bobrick Washroom Equipment, Inc.
DURALITE	Sperian Protection
DURALON	Telemed Systems Inc.
DURAMARKER	Graphic Controls Corp.
DURAN	Medtronic Cardiovascular Surgery, The Heart Valve Div.
DURAPLUG	Eagle Vision, Inc.
DURAPORE	Millipore Corporation
DURAPRENE	Cardinal Health Inc.
DURASAFE	Life Guard
DURASEAL	Nektar Therapeutics
DURASENSOR	Covidien (Formerly Nellcor Puritan Bennett / Tyco Healthcare)
DURASIL-K	Donell
DURASIS	Cook Biotech, Incorporated
DURASOFT	Ciba Vision
DURASPHERE	Carbon Medical Technologies, Inc.
DURASTAR	Hill-Rom Holdings, Inc.
DURASUL ACETABULAR SYSTEM	Centerpulse Orthopedics Inc.
DURATANIC	Hager Worldwide, Inc.
DURATANIC LITE	Hager Worldwide, Inc.
DURATANIC LITE DELUXE	Hager Worldwide, Inc.
DURATION	Stryker Spine
DURATRAN	Hds Specialty Vehicles
DURELAST	Lohmann & Rauscher, Inc.
DURITE	Durable Corporation
DUROBAL	Trelleborg Sealing Solutions
DUROGRIP	Aesculap Implant Systems Inc.
DUROM	Zimmer Holdings, Inc.
DUROTIP	Aesculap Implant Systems Inc.
DUSER	Zimmer Dental, Inc.
DUST FREE	Surmet Corp.
DUST MASTER	Tu-Way American Group
DUST-LOC	Tu-Way American Group
DUST-UP	Sprayway, Inc.
DUSTEASTER AIR FILTER	Permatron Corp.
DUSTPLUS AIR FILTER	Permatron Corp.
DUXBURY BRAILLE TANSLATOR	Duxbury Systems, Inc.
DVS II	Mast/Keystone View
DVV CONFIRM	American Diagnostica, Inc.
DVV TEST	American Diagnostica, Inc.
DVX	Possis Medical, Inc.
DX TRON	Cliniqa Corporation
DX-50	Faxitron X-Ray, Llc
DX-CAM	Karl Storz Endoscopy-America Inc.
DX/PC	Creative Biotech Inc.
DXL	Mentor Corp.
DXP1015	Braemar, Inc.
DXP1045	Braemar, Inc.
DYAD	Oscor, Inc.
DYCAL	Dentsply Caulk
DYCAL	Dentsply International, Inc.
DYCAL	Dentsply Prosthetics
DYNA CHILL	Labnet International
DYNA LIGHT	Labnet International
DYNA MITE 3100	Dynavox Systems Inc.
DYNA VAC	Labnet International
DYNA VOX 3100	Dynavox Systems Inc.
DYNA-CARE	Grant Airmass Corporation
DYNA-FLEX	Johnson & Johnson Medical Division Of Ethicon, Inc.
DYNA-FLO	Medline Industries, Inc.
DYNA-HEX	Xttrium Laboratories, Inc.
DYNA-LINK	G & H Wire Co.
DYNA-LOK	Medtronic Sofamor Danek Usa, Inc
DYNA-VAC	Handler Manufacturing Co.
DYNA/TRACE	Conmed Corporation
DYNACON	Dynacon, Inc.
DYNAFEED	Medline Industries, Inc.
DYNAFIX	Ebi, Llc
DYNAFLO	Medline Industries, Inc.
DYNAFO PLS	Maramed Orthopedic Systems
DYNAFOAM	Cfi Medical Solutions (Contour Fabricators, Inc.)
DYNAFORM	Stryker Corp.
DYNAGARD	Spectrum Laboratories, Inc.
DYNAGRIP	Becton Dickinson And Co.
DYNALATOR	Kesner C.R.
DYNALINK	Abbott Laboratories
DYNALOK CLASSIC	Medtronic, Inc.
DYNALYTE	Abbott Hematology, Diagnostics Div.
DYNALYZER	Radcal Corp.
DYNAMATE	Geerpres
DYNAMEQ-II	Electone, A Division Of Siemens Hearing Instruments, Inc.
DYNAMIC	Juzo
DYNAMIC ADAPTIVE RADIOTHERAPY	Varian Medical Systems
DYNAMIC AIR	Dentalez Group
DYNAMIC AIR THERAPY	Hill-Rom Manufacturing, Inc.
DYNAMIC COOLING DEVICE	Candela Corp.
DYNAMIC DRY	Dentalez Group
DYNAMIC ENERGY SYSTEMS, INC.	Dynamic Energy Systems, Inc.

DYNAMIC JOINT DISTRACTOR II	Stryker Corp.
DYNAMIC TARGETING	Varian Medical Systems
DYNASLEEVE	Tagg Industries L.L.C.
DYNASOUND	Kesner C.R.
DYNASTIM	Kesner C.R.
DYNATRON 150	Dynatronics Corp.
DYNATRON 1650	Dynatronics Corp.
DYNATRON 2000	Dynatronics Corp.
DYNATRON 550	Dynatronics Corp.
DYNATRON 650	Dynatronics Corp.
DYNATRON 850	Dynatronics Corp.
DYNATRON 950	Dynatronics Corp.
DYNATRON EQUALIZER #125 AND 525	Dynatronics Corp.
DYNATRON STS	Dynatronics Corp.
DYNATRON STS RX	Dynatronics Corp.
DYNAVAC	Kesner C.R.
DYNAVANE	Camfil Farr
DYNAWAVE	Kesner C.R.
DYNEX DIAS PLUS	Immucor, Inc.
DYNO-DOTS	Sellstrom Manufacturing Co.
DYNO-MITES	Sellstrom Manufacturing Co.
DYNO-SLEEVE	Palumbo Orthopaedics
DYNOGRAPH	R. B. Annis Instruments, Inc.
DYOCAM	Smith & Nephew, Inc., Endoscopy Division
DYONICS	Smith & Nephew, Inc., Endoscopy Division
DYOTAR	Navitar, Inc.
DYRACT	Dentsply Caulk
DYRACT	Dentsply International, Inc.
DYRACT	Dentsply Prosthetics
Dawn	Procter & Gamble
Daytrana	Noven Pharmaceuticals, Inc.
Dover	Danaher Corporation
Downy	Procter & Gamble
Dreft	Procter & Gamble
Drivewear	Younger Manufacturing Co., Inc.
DuoTome	Boston Scientific Corporation
Duracell	Procter & Gamble
Durata	St. Jude Medical, Inc.
Duro-Test	Duro-Test Lighting
DynaPlus	Kinetic Concepts, Inc.
Dynamic	Boston Scientific Corporation
Dynamic MultiStim	St. Jude Medical, Inc.
Dynasplint	Dynasplint Systems, Inc.
E SERIES	Zoll Medical Corp.
E-2000	Medispec Ltd. - Usa
E-250	Conflex
E-ACCUSTAT	Psg Controls, Inc.
E-BLOX	Lenox Laser
E-CHAIN	Igus, Inc.
E-CHAIR	Fenwal Inc.
E-CLIP LEAD STABILIZER	Danlee Medical Products, Inc.
E-LINKS	Tp Orthodontics, Inc.
E-LIZAMAT-3000	Drg International, Inc.
E-MOODS	United Syntek Corp.
E-PAC,	Tegrant Corporation, Protexic Brands
E-PACK	Ethicon, Inc.
E-SCRIBE	Mortara Instrument, Inc.
E-SOL FOAMY	Cambridge Diagnostic Products, Inc.
E-VENTT CASE	Vortran Medical Technology
E-Z BIFOCAL	Con-Cise Contact Lens Co.
E-Z CALL	Med Labs Inc.
E-Z CHECK	Continental Hydrodyne Systems, Inc.
E-Z CHEK	Rpc
E-Z CLEAN	Megadyne Medical Products, Inc.
E-Z CLICK	American Healthcare
E-Z DRAIN	Marlen Manufacturing & Development Co.
E-Z FLOSS	Locin Industries Ltd.
E-Z FLOW	Mercury Medical
E-Z FLOW MAX	Mercury Medical
E-Z GLIDE TRACK	Medical Illumination International
E-Z GRID	Webb Manufacturing Co.
E-Z GRIND	Wytech Industries, Inc.
E-Z GRIP	Rpc
E-Z GRIP HANDLE	Nk Medical Products Inc.
E-Z HANDLE	Graphic Controls Corp.
E-Z LIFT	Ez Way, Inc.
E-Z LOAD	Contech Medical, Inc.
E-Z PEN	Megadyne Medical Products, Inc.
E-Z PULL SHEET	Aquila Corporation
E-Z REACHER	Arcmate Mfg. Corp.
E-Z ROLLER	Jeter Systems Corp.
E-Z SET	Becton Dickinson Infusion Therapy Systems, Inc.
E-Z SHOE ON	Arcmate Mfg. Corp.
E-Z SLEEP	Essential Medical Supply, Inc.
E-Z STAND	Ez Way, Inc.
E-Z TEMP	Color Change Corp.
E-Z TRANSFER	Theradyne Products Division
E-Z-CARE	Hard Manufacturing Co.
E-Z-CUFF	Her-Mar, Inc.
E-Z-DRAW	Rpc
E-Z-ON VEST	E-Z-On Products Inc. Of Florida
E.A.I.	Eric Armin Inc.
E.L.V.I.S.	Nano Mask Inc.
E.P.	Ansell Healthcare Products, Inc.
E.P. HEART	Medical Plastics Laboratory, Inc.
E.R.D.-HEALTHSCREEN	Heska Corporation
E100	Airex, Inc.
E2E WIRELESS	Siemens Hearing Instruments, Inc.
E85	Exocell, Inc.
E9000	Conmed Linvatec
EAGLE	American Orthodontics Corp.
EAGLE	Biotec, Inc.
EAGLE	C. R. Bard, Inc., Bard Urological Div.
EAGLE	Eagle Sports Chairs
EAGLE	Shepard Medical Products
EAGLE 2 IN 1 COMMODE WHEELCHAIR	Eagle Health Supplies, Inc.
EAGLE EYE	Volcano Corporation
EAGLE FLEXPLUG	Eagle Vision, Inc.
EAGLE GLIDE TRANSFER BOARD	Eagle Health Supplies, Inc.
EAGLE GOLD	Eagle Laboratories
EAGLE PATIENT SIMULATOR	Medsim-Eagle Simulation Inc.
EAGLE PLUG	Eagle Vision, Inc.
EAGLE REHAB WALKER	Eagle Health Supplies, Inc.
EAGLE TALON	Eagle Laboratories
EAGLE VISION	Eagle Vision, Inc.
EAGLE, PULMONARY LABORATORY	Nspire Health, Inc.
EAR COUPLERS	Natus Medical Inc.
EAR FREE	Ear Technology Corp.
EAR MATES	Westmed, Inc.
EAR PLUGS	Hal-Hen Company, Inc.
EAR-TRONICS	Ear-Tronics, Inc.
EAR-WIZ	Karetech, Llc
EARBORNE	Starkey Laboratories, Inc.
EARENA	Siemens Hearing Instruments, Inc.
EARMASTER	Goldentone Hearing Aids
EARPOPPER	Micromedics
EARREPLACABLES	Roman Research, Inc.
EARS	Digital Hearing Systems Corp.
EARSCAN	Micro Audiometrics Corp.
EARTECH	Ear Technology Corp.
EARTHLINE	Kewaunee Scientific Corp.
EARTHSAFE	Bar-Ray Products, Inc.
EASE	Gentell
EASE-EJECT	Advanced Instruments, Inc.
EASI FILE	Easi File Corp.
EASI-READER	Hoyle Products, Inc.
EASICAL	Polymer Laboratories, Now A Part Of Varian, Inc.
EASIFIX	Smith & Nephew, Inc.
EASIVENT	Dey, L.P.
EASIVIAL	Polymer Laboratories, Now A Part Of Varian, Inc.
EASTMAN ABSORBENT POLYMER	Eastman Medical Products Inc.
EASY ACCESS	Ethicon, Inc.
EASY ARMBOARD	Allen Medical Systems, Inc.
EASY CAP II	Covidien (Formerly Nellcor Puritan Bennett / Tyco Healthcare)
EASY DOES IT BATH TRANSFER SYSTEM	Clever Solutions, Inc.
EASY II	Cadwell Laboratories

EASY IRRIGATION TOWER	Allen Medical Systems, Inc.
EASY LISTENER	Phonic Ear, Inc.
EASY LOCK SOCKET	Allen Medical Systems, Inc.
EASY OPEN PINCH CLAMP	Z-Man Corporation
EASY PIVOT	Rand-Scot Inc.
EASY READER	Cadwell Laboratories
EASY SEAL INJECTOR	Thomas Medical Inc.
EASY TENS	American Imex
EASY TRACK	Windquest
EASY WRITER	Cadwell Laboratories
EASY-FEED	Abbott Laboratories
EASY-FOIL	Pactiv Corporation
EASY-OUT	Tp Orthodontics, Inc.
EASY-PAP	Vital Signs, Inc.
EASY-UP HANDLE	Crestline Products Inc.
EASYBLOODGAS	Medica Corp.
EASYCHECK	Zefon International
EASYCLAVE	Midmark Corporation
EASYCURVE(TM) MOP	Contec, Inc.
EASYDROP	Gvs Filter Technology Inc.
EASYFIT	Oticon, Inc.
EASYLIFE	Photon Technology International, Inc.
EASYLINK	Siemens Healthcare Diagnostics Inc.
EASYLYTE LITHIUM NA K LI	Medica Corp.
EASYLYTE NA K	Medica Corp.
EASYLYTE NA K CA PH	Medica Corp.
EASYLYTE NA K CL LI	Medica Corp.
EASYLYTE PLUS NA K CL	Medica Corp.
EASYREACH(TM) CLEANING SYSTEM	Contec, Inc.
EASYSAMPLER	Quintron Instrument Company
EASYSAT(TM) BUCKETLESS FLOOR MOP	Contec, Inc.
EASYSTAND	Altimate Medical, Inc.
EASYSTAND EVLOV	Altimate Medical, Inc.
EASYSTAND EVOLV GLIDER	Altimate Medical, Inc.
EASYSTAND EVOLV MOBILE	Altimate Medical, Inc.
EASYSTAND EVOLV YOUTH	Altimate Medical, Inc.
EASYSTAND MAGICIAN	Altimate Medical, Inc.
EASYSTAND MAGICIAN COMFY	Altimate Medical, Inc.
EASYSTAND MAGICIAN-EI (EARLY INTERVENTION)	Altimate Medical, Inc.
EASYSTAND STRAPSTAND	Altimate Medical, Inc.
EASYSTAT, EASY ELECTROLYTES	Medica Corp.
EAZE	Phoenix Medical Devices, Llc
EBAR	Ventana Medical Systems, Inc.
EBF	Medtronic, Inc.
EBI	Ebi, Llc
EBI XFIX	Ebi, Llc
EBICE	Ebi, Llc
EBS-400B	Sakura Finetek U.S.A., Inc.
EC 770	Enthermics Medical Systems, Inc.
EC1540	Enthermics Medical Systems, Inc.
EC1540BL	Enthermics Medical Systems, Inc.
EC1730BL	Enthermics Medical Systems, Inc.
EC2	Astro-Med, Inc.
EC2060	Enthermics Medical Systems, Inc.
EC2180	Enthermics Medical Systems, Inc.
EC230	Enthermics Medical Systems, Inc.
EC230L	Enthermics Medical Systems, Inc.
EC340	Enthermics Medical Systems, Inc.
EC340L	Enthermics Medical Systems, Inc.
EC770L	Enthermics Medical Systems, Inc.
ECARDIO	eCardio Diagnostics
ECARDIO DIAGNOSTICS	eCardio Diagnostics
ECARDIOVUE	eCardio Diagnostics
ECARDIOWEB	eCardio Diagnostics
ECAST VIRTUAL DIGITAL CASTING	Omni Life Science, Inc.
ECAT	Siemens Medical Solutions Usa, Inc.
ECAT	Siemens Medical Systems, Inc., Nuclear Med. Group
ECB2	Pi Professional Therapy Products
ECCENTRIC	Automated Medical Products Corp.
ECCOGRAM	E. Benson Hood Laboratories, Inc.
ECCOVISION	E. Benson Hood Laboratories, Inc.
ECG ANALYZER	Monebo Technologies, Inc.
ECG VIEWER	Braemar, Inc.

ECGRAPH	Q-Med, Inc.
ECHELON	Ev3 Inc.
ECHELON	Smith & Nephew Inc.- Orthopaedics Division
ECHO	Immucor, Inc.
ECHO	Mesa Laboratories, Inc.
ECHO BED	Medical Positioning, Inc.
ECHO POSITIONING SYSTEM	Medical Positioning, Inc.
ECHO PRO ECHOCARDIOGRAPHY TABLE	Biodex Medical Systems, Inc.
ECHO TABLE	Medical Positioning, Inc.
ECHO-SCREEN	Natus Medical Inc.
ECHOPLAQUE 2.5	Indec Systems, Inc.
ECHOVIEW	Shimadzu Medical Systems
ECI ELECTRO-CAP	Electro-Cap International, Inc.
ECLIPSE	Amano Pioneer Eclipse Corp.
ECLIPSE	Cardiac Science Corp.
ECLIPSE	Elementis Specialties
ECLIPSE	Essential Medical Supply, Inc.
ECLIPSE	Handi-Cap Aids Company
ECLIPSE	I-Flow Corporation
ECLIPSE	Nikon Instruments Inc.
ECLIPSE	Ricon Corp.
ECLIPSE	Varian Medical Systems
ECLIPSE + TENS	Empi, Inc.
ECLIPSE DRYERS	Bobrick Washroom Equipment, Inc.
ECLIPSE HALF-SHELL	Argosy
ECLIPSE NEUROLOGICAL WORKSTATION	Axon Systems, Inc.
ECLIPSE PROBE COVER	Parker Laboratories, Inc.
ECMOtherm	Medtronic Perfusion Systems
ECO CM	Camfil Farr
ECO II	Camfil Farr
ECO SEAL	Swisslog Translogic Corporation
ECO SM	Camfil Farr
ECO- LOGIC	Atlantic Ultraviolet Corp.
ECO-FOAM	American Excelsior Co.
ECOFIX	Meridian Bioscience, Inc.
ECOLITE	Camfil Farr
ECOMASK	Arc Medical, Inc.
ECON-AIR	Sellstrom Manufacturing Co.
ECON-I.V. START PAK	Becton Dickinson Infusion Therapy Systems, Inc.
ECON-O-CAL	Air Liquide America Corporation, Cambridge Div.
ECON-O-WATT	Philips Lighting Co.
ECONO BURNER	Hager Worldwide, Inc.
ECONO SPLINTS	Morrison Medical
ECONO TIP	Hager Worldwide, Inc.
ECONO VAC	Hager Worldwide, Inc.
ECONO-CERV	Shamrock Medical, Inc.
ECONO-COLUMN	Bio-Rad Laboratories, Life Science Group
ECONO-COOL	Cincinnati Sub-Zero Products, Inc., Medical Division
ECONO-DIAMOND	Katena Products, Inc.
ECONO-PAC	Bio-Rad Laboratories, Life Science Group
ECONO-QUAT	Unit Chemical Corp.
ECONO-SAN	Unit Chemical Corp.
ECONO-VAC	Buffalo Dental Manufacturing Co., Inc.
ECONOBACK	Crosstex International,Inc.
ECONOKUFF	Elginex Corporation
ECONOLIFT	Ortho-Kinetics, Inc.
ECONOLITE I	H.L. Bouton Co., Inc.
ECONOLITE II	H.L. Bouton Co., Inc.
ECONOLITE III	H.L. Bouton Co., Inc.
ECONOLITH	Medispec Ltd. - Usa
ECONOLITH 2000	Medispec Ltd. - Usa
ECONOVUE	AMD Technologies Inc.
ECONOWEAR	Home-Aid-Healthcare, Inc.
ECOSONIC	Medsonic U.S.A., Inc.
ECS	Instrumentarium Imaging, Inc.
ECTRA	Smith & Nephew, Inc., Endoscopy Division
EDD	Arc Medical, Inc.
EDEM	Aprex, A Division Of Aardex
EDEM VIEW	Aprex, A Division Of Aardex
EDGE-LOK	G & H Wire Co.
EDGEGARD	Baker Company, The
EDGELESS(R) MOPPING SYSTEM	Contec, Inc.
EDGET	Valleylab

TRADE NAME INDEX

EDI 320 .... Cybex International, Inc.
EDINTRAK II .... Instratek, Inc.
EDIT ELITE .... Stryker Endoscopy
EDO .... Medstat Inc.
EDS .... Engle Dental Systems, Inc.
EDS 3 CSF .... Codman & Shurtleff, Inc
EDS' ACCESSPOST .... Essential Dental Systems, Inc.
EDS' ACCESSPOST OVERDENTURE .... Essential Dental Systems, Inc.
EDU-LASE .... Kentek Corp.
EDUCATION DESIGN .... Healthstream, Inc.
EDWARDS-COHEN CATHETER .... Genx International
EEA .... Covidien Lp, Formerly Registered As United States Surgical
EEBA .... Avon-Isi
EECP .... Vasomedical Inc.
EEG CHAIR .... Starkey Laboratories, Inc.
EEG DATA ANALYSIS .... Mecta Corporation
EEG32 .... Natus Medical Inc.
EEZEE-GRIP .... Dentsply International, Inc.
EEZEE-GRIP .... Dentsply Prosthetics
EFFA .... Ted Pella, Inc.
EFFERZYME .... Crosstex International,Inc.
EFFICIENCY IN DENTISTRY .... Dentalez Group
EFFICIENCY-PLUS .... Toshiba America Medical Systems
EFI LIFT-A-LIMB .... Equip For Independence, Inc.
EFICA CC .... Hill-Rom Holdings, Inc.
EFICA CC .... Hill-Rom Manufacturing, Inc.
EFILM WORKSTATION .... GE Healthcare
EFV .... Cte Chem Tec Equipment Co.
EGC .... Environmental Growth Chambers
EGGSERCIZER .... Magister Corporation
EGGSTRACT .... Promega Corp.
EGO-DRIVER .... Vilex, Inc.
EGS .... Electro-Med Health Industries
EGTA .... Brunswick Laboratories
EGXTRA .... Electro-Med Health Industries
EHEC-TEK .... Biomerieux Inc.
EID .... Arrow International, Inc.
EIGEN-NET .... Eigen
EIKO .... Bulbworks, Inc.
EIMAC .... Varian Medical Systems X-Ray Products
EISELE .... Cadence Science Inc.
EKG SOL .... Graphic Controls Corp.
EKOS .... Ekos Corp.
EKOSONIC .... Ekos Corp.
EKTACHEM .... Ortho Clinical Diagnostics, Inc.
EKTACHEM .... Ortho-Clinical Diagnostics, Inc.
EL MAR TICK REMOVAL KIT .... El Mar, Inc.
EL-ACL .... Theratest Laboratories, Inc.
EL-ANA PROFILES .... Theratest Laboratories, Inc.
EL-ANSSCR .... Theratest Laboratories, Inc.
EL-B2GPI .... Theratest Laboratories, Inc.
EL-RF/3(IGM, IGG, IGA) .... Theratest Laboratories, Inc.
EL2 Series .... Medtronic Perfusion Systems
EL4 Series .... Medtronic Perfusion Systems
ELA RHAPSODY .... Ela Medical, Inc.
ELAN-E .... Aesculap Implant Systems Inc.
ELASTA FIT .... Patterson Medical Holdings, Inc.
ELASTEC (MEDIBURN) .... Medi-Tech International, Inc.
ELASTIC LENS .... Staar Surgical Co.
ELASTICFOAM .... Hartmann-Conco Inc.
ELASTIKON .... Johnson & Johnson Consumer Products, Inc.
ELASTIMIDE .... Staar Surgical Co.
ELASTO-GEL (TM) .... Southwest Technologies, Inc.
ELASTO-GEL PLUS (TM) .... Southwest Technologies, Inc.
ELASTO-VEST .... Motloid Company
ELASTY PLUS .... Allerderm Laboratories, Inc.
ELASTYLON .... Allerderm Laboratories, Inc.
ELBOW SKINS .... Cropper Medical, Inc./Bio Skin
ELBOWLIFTr SUSPENSION PAD .... Dm Systems, Inc.
ELBOXER MENS DISPOSABLE BOXERS .... Dna Products, Llc
ELCA .... Spectranetics Corp.
ELECSYS .... Roche Diagnostics Operations
ELECTRA WAXER .... Almore International, Inc.
ELECTRACODE .... Bd Diagnostic Systems
ELECTRI-COOL .... Cincinnati Sub-Zero Products, Inc., Medical Division
ELECTRI-COOL II .... Cincinnati Sub-Zero Products, Inc., Medical Division
ELECTRIC TRACK VEHICLE-ETV 44 .... Swisslog Translogic Corporation
ELECTRICATOR .... Dermatologic Lab & Supply, Inc.
ELECTRO LAVAGE .... Mectra Labs, Inc.
ELECTRO PACK KITS .... Conmed Corporation
ELECTRO PURE REAGENTS .... Polysciences, Inc.
ELECTRO-COMPETENT .... Bio-Rad Laboratories, Life Science Group
ELECTRO-GEL .... Electro-Cap International, Inc.
ELECTRO-TRANSFORMATION .... Bio-Rad Laboratories, Life Science Group
ELECTRODAG .... Acheson Colloids Company
ELECTRODES AND SUPPLIES .... Lkc Technologies, Inc.
ELECTROFORCE .... Bose Corporation - Electroforce Systems Group
ELECTROGEL .... Conmed Corporation
ELECTROLASE .... Conmed Corporation
ELECTROLINK .... Romaine, Inc. D.B.A. Koldcare
ELECTROLIPOGRAPH .... Bioanalogics
ELECTRONIC MANUFACTURING SERVICES .... First Level Inc
ELECTRONIC PALPATION .... Medical Tactile, Inc.
ELECTROSHIELD .... Encision Inc.
ELECTROSURGICAL BIPOLAR CABLE .... American Biosurgical
ELEVA-TRUCK .... Hamilton Caster & Mfg. Co.
ELEVETTE .... Inclinator Co. Of America
ELFIT .... Cooley & Cooley, Ltd.
ELI XR .... Mortara Instrument, Inc.
ELI-100 .... Mortara Instrument, Inc.
ELI-200 .... Mortara Instrument, Inc.
ELI-5O .... Mortara Instrument, Inc.
ELIMINATOR .... Arthrocare Corp.
ELIMINATOR .... Invacare Top End Sports And Recreation Products
ELIMINATR(R) PILLOW .... Contec, Inc.
ELIMINATR(R) SOCK .... Contec, Inc.
ELIMOBILE .... KnÅrr Usa Inc.
ELINE .... Biohit Inc.
ELIPP-SEE-CON .... Conforma Laboratories, Inc.
ELIPP-SEE-FLEX .... Conforma Laboratories, Inc.
ELITE .... Ansell Healthcare Products, Inc.
ELITE .... Columbia Medical Manufacturing Llc
ELITE .... Covidien Lp, Formerly Registered As United States Surgical
ELITE .... Geri-Care Products
ELITE .... Hologic, Inc.
ELITE .... Lumenis Inc.
ELITE .... Mallinckrodt, Inc.
ELITE .... Resmed Corp.
ELITE .... Siemens Healthcare Diagnostics Inc.
ELITE .... Skytron
ELITE .... Vector Laboratories, Inc.
ELITE .... Welch Allyn, Inc.
ELITE COMFORTER .... Golden Technologies, Inc.
ELITE MANUFACTURING INCORPORATED .... Elite Mattress Manufacturing
ELITE SERIES .... Medical Graphics Corporation
ELITE TIMER .... Tork
ELITE XL .... Siemens Healthcare Diagnostics Inc.
ELITECUSTOM .... Augusta Medical Systems, Llc
ELIZAMAT-8882 .... Drg International, Inc.
ELIZAMAT-8884 .... Drg International, Inc.
ELLIPSE .... Colours Wheelchair
ELM-3200 .... Drg International, Inc.
ELMO .... Parco Scientific Co.
ELONGATED SPOT HANDPIECE .... Candela Corp.
ELS 2000 .... Online Power, Inc.
ELU-QUIK .... Schleicher & Schuell, Inc.
ELUTIP .... Schleicher & Schuell, Inc.
ELUTIP-D .... Schleicher & Schuell, Inc.
ELUTIP-R .... Schleicher & Schuell, Inc.
ELUTRAP .... Schleicher & Schuell, Inc.
ELVAREX .... Bsn-Jobst
ELVES FOR VENOUS REFLUX TREATMENT .... Biolitec, Inc.
ELVEX .... Elvex Corporation
EM .... Meiji Techno America
EM-ASSIST .... Synergy Technologies, Inc.
EMA MULTIFOCAL .... Unilens Corp., Usa

EMB .... Surgica Corporation
EMBARC STAR .... Star Case Manufacturing Co., Inc.
EMBO-GUARD .... Tetra Medical Supply Corp.
EMBOSS .... Asi-Modulex
EMBRACE .... G & H Wire Co.
EMBRACE PELVIC POSITIONER .... Body Tech 1 Nw
EMC .... Handi-Cap Aids Company
EMC .... Hansco Technologies, Inc.
EMED ARCHIVE .... Emed Technologies
EMED CLINICAL REVIEW STATION .... Emed Technologies
EMED DATA BRIDGE .... Emed Technologies
EMED DIAGNOSTIC READING STATION .... Emed Technologies
EMED DICOM BRIDGE .... Emed Technologies
EMED ENTERA .... Emed Technologies
EMED FRAME GRAB .... Emed Technologies
EMED FRONTOFFICE .... Emed Technologies
EMED IMAGE MANAGER .... Emed Technologies
EMED IMAGECD .... Emed Technologies
EMED.NET ENTERPRISE .... Emed Technologies
EMED.NET ONCALL .... Emed Technologies
EMERALD-II .... Applied Biosystems
EMERALD. .... La Mont Medical, Inc.
EMERG-ALERT .... Apothecary Products, Inc.
EMERGENCY CONTACT CARD .... Sound Feelings
EMERGINDEX .... Micromedex, Inc.
EMF .... Meiji Techno America
EMG BIOFEEDBACK .... American Imex
EMHI .... Electro-Med Health Industries
EMISSION CONTROL .... Halbar North, Inc.
EML100 .... Radiometer America, Inc.
EMMINEX .... Hager Worldwide, Inc.
EMMY .... Hager Worldwide, Inc.
EMORY CARDIAC TOOLBOX .... Syntermed, Inc.
EMP .... Boeckeler Instruments, Inc.
EMPIS .... Basi (Bioanalytical Systems, Inc.)
EMPOWER .... Metrex Research Corp.
EMPOWER .... Smith & Nephew Inc.- Orthopaedics Division
EMRALON .... Acheson Colloids Company
EMS .... Electron Microscopy Sciences
EMS + 2 .... Compex Technologies, Inc.
EMS VEST AND HARNESS .... Bashaw Medical, Inc.
EMS-1C .... Med Labs Inc.
EMS-2C .... Med Labs Inc.
EMT .... Meiji Techno America
EMU128 .... Natus Medical Inc.
EMU40 .... Natus Medical Inc.
EMZ .... Meiji Techno America
EN-ABL .... Covidien Lp, Formerly Registered As United States Surgical
ENAC .... Osada, Inc.
ENACT .... Stryker Howmedica Osteonics
ENBREL .... Amgen Inc.
ENCAPSULATOR .... Inotech Biosystems International, Inc.
ENCAPSULON .... Tfx Medical Oem
ENCHANTED .... G & H Wire Co.
ENCLOSE, GREYHOUND, INTRACK, CYGNET, ENGAGE .... Novare Surgical Systems, Inc.
ENCORE .... Ansell Healthcare Products, Inc.
ENCORE .... ArjoHuntleigh
ENCORE .... DJO Surgical
ENCORE .... Fleetwood Group, Incorporated
ENCORE .... North Coast Medical, Inc.
ENCORE .... Smiths Medical OEM
ENCORE .... Surmodics, Inc.
ENCORE .... Tidi Products, Llc
ENCORE 403 .... Luckman Corporation
ENCORE ACCLAIM .... Ansell Healthcare Products, Inc.
ENCORE EYESHIELDS .... Dioptics Medical Products, Inc.
ENCORE MICROPTIC .... Ansell Healthcare Products, Inc.
ENCORE ORTHOPAEDIC .... Ansell Healthcare Products, Inc.
ENCORE TANTONE ELECTRODE TENS & NMS Covidien Lp, Formerly Registered As Uni-Patch
END CAP .... Becton Dickinson Infusion Therapy Systems, Inc.
END CODER .... Jeter Systems Corp.

END SMOKE .... Surco Products
END0 DRAINS .... Parkell, .Inc.
ENDARSECTOR .... Scanlan International, Inc.
ENDEX .... Osada, Inc.
ENDEX PLUS .... Osada, Inc.
ENDFIREPLUS .... Shimadzu Medical Systems
ENDIUS .... Zimmer Spine
ENDO 150 .... O'Ryan Industries, Inc.
ENDO 2 .... Zimmer Medizinsystems
ENDO ANALYZER .... Sybronendo
ENDO BABCOCK ...... Covidien Lp, Formerly Registered As United States Surgical
ENDO BOWEL .... Covidien Lp, Formerly Registered As United States Surgical
ENDO BUTTON .... Smith & Nephew, Inc., Endoscopy Division
ENDO CATCH .... Covidien Lp, Formerly Registered As United States Surgical
ENDO CLEAN .... Hager Worldwide, Inc.
ENDO CLINCH .... Covidien Lp, Formerly Registered As United States Surgical
ENDO CLIP .... Covidien Lp, Formerly Registered As United States Surgical
ENDO CLOSE .... Covidien Lp, Formerly Registered As United States Surgical
ENDO DISSECT .... Covidien Lp, Formerly Registered As United States Surgical
ENDO DTC .... Aseptico, Inc.
ENDO GAUGE .... Covidien Lp, Formerly Registered As United States Surgical
ENDO GIA .... Covidien Lp, Formerly Registered As United States Surgical
ENDO GRASP .... Covidien Lp, Formerly Registered As United States Surgical
ENDO HERNIA .... Covidien Lp, Formerly Registered As United States Surgical
ENDO ITR .... Aseptico, Inc.
ENDO LUNG .... Covidien Lp, Formerly Registered As United States Surgical
ENDO MINI SHEARS. Covidien Lp, Formerly Registered As United States Surgical
ENDO MINI-RETRACT .... Covidien Lp, Formerly Registered As United States Surgical
ENDO PADDLE-RETRACT ...... Covidien Lp, Formerly Registered As United States Surgical
ENDO PEANUT .... Covidien Lp, Formerly Registered As United States Surgical
ENDO RETRACT .... Covidien Lp, Formerly Registered As United States Surgical
ENDO SCIZ .... Covidien Lp, Formerly Registered As United States Surgical
ENDO SHEARS .... Covidien Lp, Formerly Registered As United States Surgical
ENDO SLIDE .... Covidien Lp, Formerly Registered As United States Surgical
ENDO STITCH .... Covidien Lp, Formerly Registered As United States Surgical
ENDO TA .... Covidien Lp, Formerly Registered As United States Surgical
ENDO UNIVERSAL ... Covidien Lp, Formerly Registered As United States Surgical
ENDO X TRAINERT .... Medical Innovations International Inc.
ENDO-AVITENE .... Medchem Products, Inc.
ENDO-BAND .... Byron Medical
ENDO-BOOT .... United States Endoscopy Group
ENDO-BRUSH .... Globe Scientific, Inc.
ENDO-KLEAN .... Miltex Inc.
ENDO-LOK .... Natus Medical Inc.
ENDO-MODEL KNEE SYSTEM .... LinkBio Corp.
ENDO-MODEL UNI KNEE .... LinkBio Corp.
ENDO-SCRUB .... Medtronic Xomed, Inc.
ENDO-SOCK .... United States Endoscopy Group
ENDO-STAPH .... Meridian Bioscience, Inc.
ENDO-TUBE .... Covidien Lp
ENDOBENCH, ENDOSPECTOR, ELT-1, ... Lighthouse Imaging Corp.
ENDOBIB .... Gi Supply
ENDOCABG .... Genzyme
ENDOCELL .... Wallach Surgical Devices, Inc.
ENDOCERVICAL CURETTE .... Milex Products, Inc.
ENDOCLEANER .... Aesculap Implant Systems Inc.
ENDOCLEAR .... Smith & Nephew Inc.- Orthopaedics Division
ENDOCURETTE .... Utah Medical Products, Inc.
ENDOCUT .... Erbe Usa, Inc.
ENDODYNE .... Elmed, Inc.
ENDOENT .... Biolitec, Inc.
ENDOEXPRESS .... DJO Inc.
ENDOFIT STENT GRAFTS .... Lemaitre Vascular, Inc.
ENDOFIX .... Smith & Nephew, Inc., Endoscopy Division
ENDOFLATOR .... Karl Storz Endoscopy-America Inc.
ENDOFLEX .... Endo-Therapeutics, Inc.
ENDOFOAM REFILS .... Jordco, Inc.
ENDOGEL .... Jordco, Inc.
ENDOGRIP .... Biomedix, Inc.
ENDOKNOT .... Ethicon Endo-Surgery, Inc.
ENDOKNOT .... Ethicon, Inc.

ENDOLITE	Berchtold Corp.
ENDOLOOP	Ethicon Endo-Surgery, Inc.
ENDOLOOP	Ethicon, Inc.
ENDOMAT	Karl Storz Endoscopy-America Inc.
ENDOPAK	Riley Medical, Inc.
ENDOPAK	Symmetry Medical Usa, Inc.
ENDOPATH	Ethicon Endo-Surgery, Inc.
ENDOPATH XCEL	Ethicon Endo-Surgery, Inc.
ENDOPOUCH	Ethicon Endo-Surgery, Inc.
ENDOPOUCH	Ethicon, Inc.
ENDOPRO	Medidenta International, Inc.
ENDOPRO	Pentax Medical Company
ENDOPROBE	Iridex Corporation
ENDORACK	Aesculap Implant Systems Inc.
ENDORING	Almore International, Inc.
ENDORING	Jordco, Inc.
ENDORING FILECADDY	Jordco, Inc.
ENDOSAC SEAMLESS SPECIMEN COLLECTION POUCH	Zenith Medical Inc.
ENDOSAMPLER	Medgyn Products, Inc.
ENDOSEAL	Centrix, Inc.
ENDOSHEATH	Vision-Sciences, Inc.
ENDOSI	Armm, Inc.
ENDOSKELTON	Titan Spine Llc.
ENDOSOL EXTRA	Allergan
ENDOSSEOUS	Impladent Ltd.
ENDOSTAT	Ams Innovative Center-San Jose
ENDOSURGICAL OPERATING SYSTEM	Usgi Medical
ENDOTIP	Karl Storz Endoscopy-America Inc.
ENDOTOOL	Hospira Inc.
ENDOTRAC	Instratek, Inc.
ENDOTRIG	Instratek, Inc.
ENDOVISION	Karl Storz Endoscopy-America Inc.
ENDOVISION	Medidenta International, Inc.
ENDOVUE	Nds Surgical Imaging, Inc.
ENDOWAVE	Ekos Corp.
ENDTAG	Vector Laboratories, Inc.
ENDTRAC	Stryker Howmedica Osteonics
ENDURA-CUT	Boss Instruments, Ltd.
ENDURA-SHEAR	Boss Instruments, Ltd.
ENDURAHEAT	Carter-Hoffmann
ENDURANCE	Essential Medical Supply, Inc.
ENDURE	Imtec, A 3m Company
ENDURO2	U O Equipment Co.
ENDUROTHANE II	Kenda American Airless
ENDUROWEAR	Graham Medical Products/Div. Of Little Rapids Corp
ENEGEL	Mallinckrodt, Inc.
ENERGEX	Energex Systems Inc.
ENERGEX BATTERIES	Plainview Batteries, Inc.
ENERGYMAX	Coherent, Inc.
ENERJAE	Zyloware Corporation
ENFLOW	Vital Signs, Inc.
ENFORCE	Dentsply Caulk
ENGUARD	Enmet Corp.
ENGUARD 97D	Enmet Corp.
ENHANCE	Ams Innovative Center-San Jose
ENHANCER	Diversified Diagnostic Products, Inc.
ENLABEL	Integrated Software Design, Inc.
ENLITEN	Promega Corp.
ENSEMBLE	Mennen Medical Corp.
ENSURE	Alcohol Countermeasure Systems, Inc.
ENSURE-IT	Becton Dickinson Infusion Therapy Systems, Inc.
ENTAVITENE	Medchem Products, Inc.
ENTERALITE	Zevex Incorporated
ENTEROCOCCOSEL	Bd Diagnostic Systems
ENTEROLERT	Idexx Laboratories, Inc.
ENTEROTUBE	Bd Diagnostic Systems
ENTERPRISE	Cordis Neurovascular, Inc.
ENTERPRISE	Living Earth Crafts
ENTERTAINER'S SECRET THROAT RELIEF	Kli Corp.
ENTREX	DJO Inc.
ENTRI-FLEX	Covidien Lp
ENTRIFLUSH	Covidien Lp
ENTRISTAR	Covidien Lp
ENTROBAR	Mallinckrodt, Inc.
ENTRUST	Tillotson Healthcare Corp.
ENVIRELUT	Varian Sample Preparation Products
ENVIRENE	Hardy Diagnostics
ENVIRO-GENIE	Scientific Industries, Inc.
ENVIRO-VAC	Enviro Guard, Inc.
ENVIROMAX	Hemco Corp.
ENVIRON	Steris Corporation
ENVIRON-MATE	M D Technologies, Inc.
ENVIRONDENT	Hu-Friedy Manufacturing Co., Inc.
ENVIROTEST	Q.I. Medical, Inc.
ENVISION	Bard Electro Physiology
ENVISION ANTERIOR CERVICAL PLATE	Ortho Development Corp.
ENVISION CT	Medrad, Inc.
ENVOY	Cordis Neurovascular, Inc.
ENVOY	Invacare Corporation
ENVOY	Mennen Medical Corp.
ENZDIL	Cst Technologies, Inc.
ENZIP (ELISA)	Diagnostic Specialties
ENZOL	Advanced Sterilization Products
ENZYCLEAN	Weiman Healthcare Solutions
ENZYMAX	Hu-Friedy Manufacturing Co., Inc.
ENZYMOBEAD	Bio-Rad Laboratories, Life Science Group
EO-TRAK	Kem Medical Products Corp.
EOA	Brunswick Laboratories
EOGAS	Andersen Products, Inc.,
EOSIN	Anatech, Ltd.
EOVIA	Orthotec, Llc
EP 600	Ivoclar Vivadent, Inc.
EP H.U.T. TABLE	Medical Positioning, Inc.
EP REVELATION	Cardima, Inc.
EPAD	Whalen Biomedical Incorporated
EPET	Biohit Inc.
EPEX	Hologic, Inc.
EPI PEN	Dey, L.P.
EPI PEN 2-PAK	Dey, L.P.
EPI PEN JR.	Dey, L.P.
EPI PEN JR. 2-PAK	Dey, L.P.
EPI*SAFE	Weiman Healthcare Solutions
EPI*SOFT	Weiman Healthcare Solutions
EPI*WASH	Weiman Healthcare Solutions
EPI-SPORT	Fla Orthopedics, Inc.
EPIBLOT	Orasure Technologies, Inc.
EPIC	Fischer Medical Technologies Inc.
EPIC	Stryker Corp.
EPIC	Stryker Medical
EPIC WEB LIGHT	Epic Systems Corp.
EPIC-4000	Lkc Technologies, Inc.
EPIC-TMPT	Parkell, Inc.
EPICARDIA	Medicomp, Inc.
EPICARE	Hill-Rom Holdings, Inc.
EPICARE ADULT	Gvs Filter Technology Inc.
EPICARE BABY	Gvs Filter Technology Inc.
EPICARE(TM) - HAIR REMOVAL	Light Age Inc.
EPICARE-LP(TM) - HAIR REMOVAL	Light Age Inc.
EPICAREPORTER	Hill-Rom Holdings, Inc.
EPICCARE ELECTRONIC MEDICAL RECORD	Epic Systems Corp.
EPICCARE HOMEHEALTH	Epic Systems Corp.
EPICCARE INPATIENT	Epic Systems Corp.
EPICEL-CEA	Genzyme Corp.
EPICENTRE	Epicentre Technologies
EPICLINK	Epic Systems Corp.
EPICOUNT	Corning Inc., Science Products Division
EPIDERM	Pedinol Pharmacal, Inc.
EPIFILM	Medtronic Xomed, Inc.
EPIFLEX	Hollister Incorporated
EPIGARD	Ormed Corporation
EPIGEN	Smith & Nephew, Inc.
EPIGUIDE	Kensey Nash Corporation
EPIPEN	Meridian Medical Technologies
EPIPOINT	Bauerfeind Usa, Inc.
EPISORB	Smith & Nephew Inc.- Orthopaedics Division
EPISTAT	Medtronic Xomed, Inc.

EPITOME	Utah Medical Products, Inc.
EPITRAIN	Bauerfeind Usa, Inc.
EPIVENT	Smith & Nephew Inc.- Orthopaedics Division
EPIX	Epix, Inc.
EPIX XL TENS	Empi, Inc.
EPK-1000	Pentax Medical Company
EPM	Walkmed Infusion Llc
EPM-3500	Pentax Medical Company
EPO-TRAC	Diasorin Inc
EPOCAP	Elementis Specialties
EPOCH	Zimmer Holdings, Inc.
EPOCHXP NEUROLOGICAL WORKSTATION	Axon Systems, Inc.
EPOCKET	Siemens Hearing Instruments, Inc.
EPOQ	Oticon, Inc.
EPORIA	Ramco Laboratories, Inc.
EPOS ULTRA	Dornier Medtech America
EPOWELD	Elementis Specialties
EPOWERT	Micro-Bio-Logics.Inc
EPOWERT	Microbiologics, Inc.
EPS 2500	Mge Ups Sytems, Inc.
EPS 3000	Mge Ups Sytems, Inc.
EPS 6000	Mge Ups Sytems, Inc.
EPS PLUS	Toshiba America Medical Systems
EPT-1000	Ep Technologies, Inc.
EPT-1000XP	Boston Scientific Corporation
EPT-1000XP	Ep Technologies, Inc.
EPX	Fischer Medical Technologies Inc.
EPX	Lohmann & Rauscher, Inc.
EPX2	Fischer Medical Technologies Inc.
EPY-50	Ddc Technologies, Inc.
EQUA	Herman Miller, Inc.
EQUAHEAT	Carter-Hoffmann
EQUALIZER	Span-America Medical Systems, Inc.
EQUALIZER, GLASS MADE OF IDEAS, MODULAMP, PANELITE, MHR-50	Schott North America, Inc.
EQUIL	Rna Medical, A Division Of Bionostics, Inc.
EQUILIBRATOR	Rna Medical, A Division Of Bionostics, Inc.
EQUIMAT	Karl Storz Endoscopy-America Inc.
EQUINOX	Amano Pioneer Eclipse Corp.
EQUIPCART	Dntlworks Equipment Corporation
EQUISPORT	3m Co.
EQUISTAND	Diagnostix Plus, Inc.
EQUITEC	Dms Laboratories, Inc.
EQUITHAL	Mettler-Toledo Process Analytical, Inc.
EQUIVABONE	Etex Corporation
ER2000	Waterloo Healthcare, Llc
ER300	Braemar, Inc.
ER310	Braemar, Inc.
ER320	Braemar, Inc.
ER710	Braemar, Inc.
ER720	Braemar, Inc.
ERA	Sterngold
ERAD	Erad/Image Medical Corp.
ERADO-SOL	Cambridge Diagnostic Products, Inc.
ERADO-STAIN	Cambridge Diagnostic Products, Inc.
ERASE-A-BASE	Promega Corp.
ERASURE	Cynosure, Inc.
ERB SAFETY	Erb Industries Inc.
ERBOKRYO	Erbe Usa, Inc.
ERBOTOM BIPOLAR	Erbe Usa, Inc.
ERBOTOM ICC 200	Erbe Usa, Inc.
ERBOTOM ICC 300	Erbe Usa, Inc.
ERBOTOM ICC 350	Erbe Usa, Inc.
ERBOTOM ICC 80	Erbe Usa, Inc.
ERCP PEEL AWAY	Wilson-Cook Medical, Inc.
ERECAID	Timm Medical Technologies, Inc.
ERECTA	Intermetro Industries Corp.
ERGO KING	Geerpres
ERGO KNIGHT	Geerpres
ERGO PRINCE	Geerpres
ERGO VAC	Hager Worldwide, Inc.
ERGOFET	Hoggan Health Industries, Inc.
ERGOFORM	Nevin Laboratories, Inc
ERGOKEY	Advanced Input Systems
ERGON	Herman Miller, Inc.
ERGON	Skytron
ERGOPAK	Hoggan Health Industries, Inc.
ERGOTECH	Nevin Laboratories, Inc
ERGOTRON	Ergotron, Inc.
ERGOWAVE	Chattanooga Group
ERIE TRAVELER (73 ECX)	Erie Medical
ERIE-NEB	Erie Medical
ERIS	Self Regulation Systems, Inc.
ERO-SCAN	Etymotic Research, Inc.
EROSCAN OAE TEST SYSTEM	Maico Diagnostics
ES	Ventana Medical Systems, Inc.
ES FIXATIVE	Sakura Finetek U.S.A., Inc.
ESAOTE BIOSOUND	Universal Ultrasound
ESCAPE	Resmed Corp.
ESCAPE-RITE	Sellstrom Manufacturing Co.
ESCO	Hansco Technologies, Inc.
ESCOPE	Cardionics, Inc.
ESCORT	Geerpres
ESCORT	Landauer, Inc.
ESCORT II	Wilson-Cook Medical, Inc.
ESCORT RX	Geerpres
ESDAX	Ufp Technologies, Inc.
ESENSOR	Osmetech, Inc.
ESG-1	Myotronics-Noromed, Inc.
ESI	Electro Surgical Instrument Co., Inc.
ESMARK LF	Hartmann-Conco Inc.
ESPERTISE	3m Co.
ESPION	Diagnosis, Llc
ESPREE	Leisure-Lift, Inc.
ESPRIT	Ortho-Kinetics, Inc.
ESPRIT	Siemens Healthcare Diagnostics Inc.
ESR STAT 180	Hematechnologies, Inc.
ESSAR	Medtronic Xomed, Inc.
ESSENCE	Cordis Neurovascular, Inc.
ESSENTIA	Skytron
ESSENTIAL	Adenna Inc.
ESSENTIAL	Smith & Nephew Inc.- Orthopaedics Division
ESSENTRIS	Clinicomp Intl.
ESSX	Stryker Corp.
ESTEEM	Cardinal Health Inc.
ESTEEM	Convatec
ESTEEM	Timm Medical Technologies, Inc.
ET ADHESIVE TAPE	Marpac Inc.
ET-1000	Lechnologies Research, Inc.
ETC	Environmental Tectonics Corp.
ETC	Ortho-Kinetics, Inc.
ETCHGEL	Almore International, Inc.
ETHAFOAM	Ufp Technologies, Inc.
ETHALLOY	Ethicon, Inc.
ETHI-PACK	Ethicon, Inc.
ETHIBOND	Ethicon, Inc.
ETHIBOND EXCEL	Ethicon, Inc.
ETHICON	Ethicon Endo-Surgery, Inc.
ETHICON	Ethicon, Inc.
ETHIGUARD	Ethicon, Inc.
ETHILON	Ethicon, Inc.
ETHISORB	Codman & Shurtleff, Inc
ETHOSPACE	Herman Miller, Inc.
ETHRANE	Baxter Healthcare Corporation, Baxter Pharmaceuticals And Technologies
ETI	Diasorin Inc
ETO-ABATOR	Donaldson Company, Inc.
ETO-ABSTAR SYSTEM	Donaldson Company, Inc.
ETP	Kimble Chase Life Science And Research Products Llc
ETRIGGER	eCardio Diagnostics
ETRUSCO	United Syntek Corp.
EUBONTE	Cadco Dental Products
EUCERIN	Beiersdorf, Inc.
EUGENONE	Scientific Pharmaceuticals, Inc.
EUGONAGAR	Bd Diagnostic Systems
EUGONROTH	Bd Diagnostic Systems

EUREKA	Surmodics, Inc.
EURODROP	Gvs Filter Technology Inc.
EUROLINE A-13	Starkey Laboratories, Inc.
EUROMEDICAL	Unomedical, Inc.
EUROPA	G & H Wire Co.
EUROPA	James Consolidated, Inc.
EUROPEAN MIRASOL	Caridianbct Inc.
EUROVALVE	Filtertek Inc.
EUS BALLOONS	N.M. Beale Co. Inc.
EVAC-U-SPLINT	Hartwell Medical Corp.
EVACUATION CHAIR	Stryker Corp.
EVACUFIELD	G & H Wire Co.
EVALOK	Sellstrom Manufacturing Co.
EVALTECH	Bte Technologies, Inc.
EVALUATOR	Bte Technologies, Inc.
EVAM	Stedim Biosystems, Inc.
EVENT MANAGER	Braemar, Inc.
EVENT MANAGER	Stryker Corp.
EVER-GUARD	Kentek Corp.
EVEREST	Astro-Med, Inc.
EVEREST	Nest Group Inc., The
EVERPURE	Western Water Purifier Co.
EVERSHEARS	Gyrus Medical, Inc.
EVERT-IT	Genesis Industries/Maternal Concepts
EVERY BATTERY FOR EVERY NEED	Interstate Battery System Of America
EVIDENCE OF LEARNING	Medcare Products, Inc.
EVIDENT	Covidien (Formerly Nellcor Puritan Bennett / Tyco Healthcare)
EVOLUTION	Cascade Designs, Inc.
EVOLUTION	Cook Medical Inc.
EVOLUTION	Kerr Group
EVOLUTION	Siemens Medical Solutions Usa, Inc.
EVOLUTION ONE	Microflex Corporation
EVOLVE	Wright Medical Group, Inc.
EVOLVE SLV FOR IN-OFFICE BPH	Biolitec, Inc.
EVOTECH	Advanced Sterilization Products
EX MUCICARMINE	Anatech, Ltd.
EX-2000	Enmet Corp.
EX-PLAC	Preventive Dentistry Products, Inc.
EXACDROP	B. Braun Oem Division, B. Braun Medical Inc.
EXACT	Varian Medical Systems
EXACT-ALIGN	Gammex Rmi
EXACT-FIT	Kinamed, Inc.
EXACTA-MED	Baxa Corporation
EXACTA-MIX	Baxa Corporation
EXACTABLES	Profex Medical Products
EXACTACAST	Essential Dental Systems, Inc.
EXACTECH	Exactech, Inc.
EXACTECH BIPOLAR	Exactech, Inc.
EXACTIME	Symmetricom Timing, Test & Measurement
EXACTRACK	Rf Technologies
EXAFLEX	G-C America Inc.
EXAKT-PAK	Exakt Technologies, Inc.
EXAM LIGHT II	Welch Allyn, Inc.
EXAM-5000	Topcon Medical Systems, Inc.
EXAM-TEX	Ansell Healthcare Products, Inc.
EXAMI-GOWNS, INC.	Exami-Gowns, Inc.
EXCALIBUR	Takara Belmont Usa, Inc.
EXCALIBUR PLUS PC	Conmed Corporation
EXCALIBUR PLUS PC ESU	Conmed Corporation
EXCEL	Air-Tite Products Co., Inc.
EXCEL	B. Braun Oem Division, B. Braun Medical Inc.
EXCEL	Crosstex International,Inc.
EXCEL	Excel Medical Products, Llc
EXCEL	Infab Corp.
EXCEL	Standard Textile Co., Inc.
EXCEL HEALTH CARE PRODUCTS	Pacon Manufacturing Corporation
EXCEL-6	Excel Medical Products, Llc
EXCEL-9	Excel Medical Products, Llc
EXCELART	Toshiba America Medical Systems
EXCELERATOR	Invacare Top End Sports And Recreation Products
EXCELLARATE	Cardium Therapeutics Inc.
EXCELLOBAND	Precision Dynamics Corp.
EXCITE	Ivoclar Vivadent, Inc.
EXCITE	Merit Medical Systems, Inc.
EXCLUSIVE SALON SERIES	Oster Professional Products, Inc.
EXCURSION	Luxfer Gas Cylinders
EXEC II	Ericsson, Inc.
EXECUTAG	Idesco Corp.
EXELTRA	Baxter Healthcare Corporation, Renal
EXER-BAND	Pre Pak Products, Inc.
EXER-COR	Novel Products, Inc.
EXER-GENIE	Team America Health & Fitness, Inc
EXER-TUBING	Patterson Medical Holdings, Inc.
EXERCHIZER	Medicool, Inc.
EXERCISE CONSULTANT SOFTWARE	Medical Graphics Corporation
EXERCISER	Team America Health & Fitness, Inc
EXERCYCLE	Exercycle Corporation
EXERSCRIPT SOFTWARE	Medical Graphics Corporation
EXERTRAIL	Jaypro Corporation
EXETER	Stryker Corp.
EXETER CEMENTED	Stryker Corp.
EXETER CEMENTED	Stryker Howmedica Osteonics
EXITCALL	Dwyer Precision Products, Inc.
EXL-40	Osada, Inc.
EXL-M40	Osada, Inc.
EXO	Florida Manufacturing Corp.
EXO STATIC	Florida Manufacturing Corp.
EXO-GEL	Tcp Reliable, Inc.
EXOGEN 2000	Exogen, Inc.
EXOJET	Hydrocision, Inc.
EXOSAP-IT	Usb Corporation
EXPANDABLE LEMAITRE VALVULOTOME	Lemaitre Vascular, Inc.
EXPANDACELL	Shippert Medical Technologies Corp.
EXPANDER	Sellstrom Manufacturing Co.
EXPANDOVER	Covidien Lp
EXPEDITOR	Zimmer Dental, Inc.
EXPERT	Juzo
EXPERT	Ocg Technology, Inc.
EXPERT	Stryker Imaging
EXPLORER	Adenna Inc.
EXPLORER	Ortho-Kinetics, Inc.
EXPLORER	Siemens Hearing Instruments, Inc.
EXPLORER SYSTEM FOR LYMPHATIC MAPPING/SENTINEL NODE	Radiation Monitoring Devices, Inc.
EXPOS-AID	Advanced Instrument Development, Inc.
EXPRESS	3m Espe Dental Products
EXPRESS	Braun Industries, Inc.
EXPRESS	Ortho-Kinetics, Inc.
EXPRESS	Siemens Healthcare Diagnostics Inc
EXPRESS-BLOT	Bio-Rad Laboratories, Life Science Group
EXPRESSF + CELLS	Protein Sciences Corp.
EXPRESSFIT	Sonic Innovations
EXPRESSIONS	The Cooper Companies, Inc
EXPRESSLINK	Sonic Innovations
EXPRESSRAMP	Ricon Corp.
EXTEND-N-BEND	Amici, Inc.
EXTEND-O	Tp Orthodontics, Inc.
EXTENDED SURFACE(TM)	Lytron, Inc.
EXTOL	Cardiac Science Corp.
EXTRACTOR	Schleicher & Schuell, Inc.
EXTRANEAL	Baxter Healthcare Corporation, Renal
EXTREME	Geri-Care Products
EXTREME	Spectranetics Corp.
EXTREME H2O	Hydrogel Vision Corporation
EXTRI KELLY, CRASH KELLY	Medical Plastics Laboratory, Inc.
EXTRICATOR	Sellstrom Manufacturing Co.
EXTRORDINAIR	Galaxy Aquatics, Inc.
EXU-DRY	Smith & Nephew, Inc.
EYE SURGERY RECOVERY SYSTEM	Rite Time Corporation
EYE-LERT	North Safety Products
EYE-TRAC	Applied Science Laboratories
EYE-TRAC RESEARCH	Applied Science Laboratories
EYEBEAM	Asi-Modulex
EYECLOSE	Meddev Corporation
EYEGARTER	Surgical Specialties Corporation
EYELITES	Sds-Surgical Acuity

EYEMAX	Sds-Surgical Acuity
EYEROUTE	Topcon Medical Systems, Inc.
EYZE	Tetra Medical Supply Corp.
EYZE BAG	Tetra Medical Supply Corp.
EZ BRACE	Orthofix Inc.
EZ CLEANS PLUS KIT	Safetec Of America, Inc.
EZ DENTA FLOSSER	Preventive Dentistry Products, Inc.
EZ DETECT	Biomerica, Inc.
EZ DPD	Idexx Laboratories, Inc.
EZ FLO	Covidien Lp
EZ FLOW	Piper Medical Products
EZ GREEN	Anatech, Ltd.
EZ HEALTHCHECK	Heska Corporation
EZ HITCH	Reel R&D, Inc.
EZ PREP	Ventana Medical Systems, Inc.
EZ PUMP - DUAL CHANNEL	Sigma International, Llc.
EZ PUMP - SINGLE CHANNEL	Sigma International, Llc.
EZ RIDER	Convaid Inc.
EZ S'PORT	The Saunders Group
EZ SEAT	Golden Technologies, Inc.
EZ SLEEPER, SLEEPERSOFA	Durfold Corporation
EZ Steer	Biosense Webster, Inc
EZ TOTE	Neotech Products, Inc.
EZ TRODE	Mettler Electronics Corp.
EZ WRAP	Salter Labs
EZ-3	Futuremed America, Inc.
EZ-ACCESS	Homecare Products, Inc.
EZ-ACCESSORIES	Homecare Products, Inc.
EZ-BATHE	Homecare Products, Inc.
EZ-CARE	Delta Gloves
EZ-CFUT	Micro-Bio-Logics.Inc
EZ-CFUT	Microbiologics, Inc.
EZ-CFUT ONE STEP	Micro-Bio-Logics.Inc
EZ-CFUT ONE STEP	Microbiologics, Inc.
EZ-CHANGE	Essential Dental Systems, Inc.
EZ-COMPT SAMPLES	Micro-Bio-Logics.Inc
EZ-COMPT SAMPLES	Microbiologics, Inc.
EZ-FILL	Essential Dental Systems, Inc.
EZ-FILL SAFESIDER	Essential Dental Systems, Inc.
EZ-FIT	Aetrex Worldwide, Inc
EZ-FIX	DJO Surgical
EZ-FLAP	Striker Corp.
EZ-FPCT	Micro-Bio-Logics.Inc
EZ-FPCT	Microbiologics, Inc.
EZ-HCG	Biomerica, Inc.
EZ-HP	Biomerica, Inc.
EZ-IRRIGATORS	American Medical Industries
EZ-LANCE	Palco Labs, Inc.
EZ-LETS	Palco Labs, Inc.
EZ-LH	Biomerica, Inc.
EZ-ON	Fla Orthopedics, Inc.
EZ-PECT	Micro-Bio-Logics.Inc
EZ-PECT	Microbiologics, Inc.
EZ-PRO	Stryker Corp.
EZ-PSA	Biomerica, Inc.
EZ-SCREEN	Medtox Diagnostics Inc.
EZ-SHAMPOO	Homecare Products, Inc.
EZ-SHOWER	Homecare Products, Inc.
EZ-SORB	Paperpak
EZ-SPORET	Microbiologics, Inc.
EZ-STOR SYSTEM	Pryor Products
EZ-SWALLOW	American Medical Industries
EZ-VAC	Palco Labs, Inc.
EZ-VIEW	Dentsply International, Inc.
EZ-VIEW	Dentsply Prosthetics
EZ-ZYME	Miltex Inc.
EZCOM PRO TTY	Ultratec, Inc.
EZE-BAND LF	Hartmann-Conco Inc.
EZLASE	Biolase Technology, Inc.
EZM	Astro-Med, Inc.
EZN	Kenda American Airless
EZRAMP	Diestco Manufacturing Corp.
EZSERT	Microtek Medical, Inc
EZSLIDE	Skytron
EZSTIM	Life-Tech, Inc.
EZY-CARE	Apothecary Products, Inc.
EZY-DOSE	Apothecary Products, Inc.
EZYWRAP	Professional Products, Inc.
Eagle-Signal	Danaher Corporation
EcoLogo	Rochester Midland, Corp.
Eldex	Eldex Laboratories
Electone	Electone, A Division Of Siemens Hearing Instruments, Inc.
Emflon	Pall Corporation
EnPulse	Medtronic, Inc.
EnSite	St. Jude Medical, Inc.
EnSite Array	St. Jude Medical, Inc.
EnSite NavX	St. Jude Medical, Inc.
EnSite Verismo	St. Jude Medical, Inc.
Endeavor	Medtronic, Inc.
EndoSure	CardioMEMS, Inc.
EndoVive	Boston Scientific Corporation
EnterCare	American Homepatient
Enterra	Medtronic, Inc.
Entity	St. Jude Medical, Inc.
Enviro Care	Rochester Midland, Corp.
Eon	St. Jude Medical Neuromodulation Division
Eon	St. Jude Medical, Inc.
Eon Mini	St. Jude Medical Neuromodulation Division
EonC	St. Jude Medical Neuromodulation Division
Epic	St. Jude Medical, Inc.
Epicor	St. Jude Medical, Inc.
Era	Procter & Gamble
Escape	Boston Scientific Corporation
Essential Soy	Ortho Dermatologics
Eukanuba	Procter & Gamble
ExcelAüAõAõÉ,™è_A,Aõ-14	Boston Scientific Corporation
Explorer 360	Boston Scientific Corporation
Explorer ST	Boston Scientific Corporation
Export	Medtronic, Inc.
Express	Boston Scientific Corporation
Express2	Boston Scientific Corporation
ExpressA˝	Boston Scientific - Maple Grove
Extractor	Boston Scientific Corporation
Extremity Pump	Kinetic Concepts, Inc.
Eyegenie	Hilco
F&D	Friedrich & Dimmock, Inc.
F-SCAN	Tekscan, Inc.
F-SCAN MOBILE	Tekscan, Inc.
F.A.C.T.	Stereo Optical Co., Inc.
F.L.FISCHER	Striker Corp.
F.T.I.	Forward Technology
FA SERIES	Oneac Corporation
FAB	Cte Chem Tec Equipment Co.
FABCO	First Aid Bandage Co., Inc.
FABCO WRAP	First Aid Bandage Co., Inc.
FABCOMP	Fabrite Laminating Corp.
FABEX	Infab Corp.
FABRI-SOFT	Graham Medical Products/Div. Of Little Rapids Corp
FABRIC 450	Johnson & Johnson Medical Division Of Ethicon, Inc.
FABTEX	Fabrite Laminating Corp.
FABUGUARD	Fabrite Laminating Corp.
FABUTHANE	Fabrite Laminating Corp.
FABUTHANE FR	Fabrite Laminating Corp.
FACE DOWN RECOVERY SYSTEM	Rite Time Corporation
FACE GUARD	Lee Medical International, Inc.
FACE PRONE RECOVERY SYSTEM	Rite Time Corporation
FACE-BOW	Panadent Corp.
FACE-FIT	Oberon Company ,Div Of The Paramount Corp.
FACE-FIT GOGGLES	Trademark Medical Llc
FACE-IT	Onyx Medical Inc./Face-It
FACE-SAVER	K Medical
FACILITATOR	Idexx Laboratories, Inc.
FACILITYDATA	J.M. Baragano Biomedical P.M. And Consulting, Inc.
FACT	George King Bio-Medical, Inc.
FACTORY FIBER RECYCLING	Xintec Corp. / Convergent Laser Tech.
FAICHNEY	Faichney Medical Co.

FAIRWAY	Ortho-Kinetics, Inc.
FALCO	Biosound Esaote, Inc.
FALCON	Bd Diagnostic Systems
FALCON	Wave Form Systems, Inc.
FALLSAVER	Nocwatch International, Inc./Fallsaver
FAMILION	Clinical Data Inc
FAMILY MEDIACAL AIDS	Apothecary Products, Inc.
FAP	Coherent, Inc.
FARLEY	Thompson Surgical Instruments, Inc.
FASHION 20	Freeman Manufacturing Company
FASHION EYE SHIELDS	American Diversified Dental Systems
FASHION PLUS	Freeman Manufacturing Company
FASLATA	C. R. Bard, Inc., Bard Urological Div.
FASPLINT	Hartwell Medical Corp.
FAST	Kada Research, Inc.
FAST - F.I.C.S.	Scanlan International, Inc.
FAST FEED	Oster Professional Products, Inc.
FAST FIND GRID	Webb Manufacturing Co.
FAST FIX	Smith & Nephew, Inc., Endoscopy Division
FAST LIFT	Hager Worldwide, Inc.
FAST PAQ	Fujinon, Inc.
FAST TAG	Vector Laboratories, Inc.
FAST-CATH	St. Jude Medical Atrial Fibrillation
FAST-HB	PerkinElmer
FAST-PATCH	Physio-Control, Inc.
FAST4	Siemens Healthcare Diagnostics Inc
FASTAC	Greatbach Medical
FASTAC	Greatbatch Inc
FASTENATOR	Smith & Nephew, Inc., Endoscopy Division
FASTER PLASTER	Flexi-Wall Systems
FASTEX	Cybex International, Inc.
FASTFIL	Scientific Pharmaceuticals, Inc.
FASTIPS	Dentsply International, Inc.
FASTIPS	Dentsply Prosthetics
FASTPAC	Carl Zeiss Meditec Inc.
FASTPAK	Physio-Control, Inc.
FASTPLAN	Varian Medical Systems
FASTRAC	Independent Solutions, Inc.
FASTRACE	Conmed Corporation
FASTRAY/FASTRAY LC	Harry J. Bosworth Company
FASTSYSTEM	Omni-Tract Surgical, A Div. Of Minnesota Scientific, Inc.
FAT-GUN	Fitness Motivation Institute Of America, Inc.
FAT-O-METER	Novel Products, Inc.
FATHER TIME'S BINDERS	Idea Scientific Co.
FAV	Cte Chem Tec Equipment Co.
FAWN VENDORS, INC.	Fawn Vendors, Inc.
FAZIO	Torbot Group, Inc.
FC FEMALE CONDOM	Female Health Company, The
FE-2	Diasys Corporation
FEATHER TOUCH	Medtronic Xomed, Inc.
FEATHER WEIGHT	Seca Corp.
FEATHER-LITE	Smith & Nephew, Inc.
FEATHER-LITE	Torbot Group, Inc.
FEATHERLIGHT	Essential Medical Supply, Inc.
FEDRIN	Afassco, Inc.
FEELING STRESSED	Sound Feelings
FEIBA	Baxter International Inc
FELINE ULTRANASAL	Heska Corporation
FELIX	Photon Technology International, Inc.
FELIX LANCING DEVICE	Facet Technologies, Llc
FELLOWSHIP	Moyco Technologies, Inc.
FEMADRINE	Afassco, Inc.
FEMIDOM	The Female Health Co.
FEMME FORM	Finebrand Co.
FEMODOM	The Female Health Co.
FEMTEX	First Quality Enterprise, Inc.
FEMUR FINDER	Innovative Medical Products, Inc.
FEMY	The Female Health Co.
FEN	Belco Packaging Systems, Inc.
FENDEX I.V.	Advanced Magnetics, Inc.
FENWAL	Fenwal Inc.
FER-IRON II	Ramco Laboratories, Inc.
FERNO	Ferno-Washington, Inc.
FERNO	Medi-Tech International, Inc.
FERRIS POLYMEM	Ferris Mfg Corp.
FERROPOWR	Rapid Power Technologies, Inc.
FETAL CELL STAIN KIT	Simmler, Inc.
FETAL FILE	Tyco Healthcare Group Lp
FETALGARD	Analogic Corporation
FETALTROL	Trillium Diagnostics, Llc.
FETCH	Possis Medical, Inc.
FETRODE	U.F.I.
FEVERLINE	LCR Hallcrest
FEVERSCAN	LCR Hallcrest
FEVERTEMP	LCR Hallcrest
FEXITOUCH	Tactile Systems Technology Inc
FHS	Stryker Spine
FIBER & MESH	Preat Corp.
FIBERBAK	Core Products International, Inc.
FIBERBILT	Case Design Corp.
FIBERLIFE	Ams Innovative Center-San Jose
FIBERSOURCE	Novartis Nutrition
FIBRA	Applied Medical Resource Corporation
FIBRASONICS	Misonix, Inc.
FIBREDYNE	National Nonwovens
FIBRIJET	Baxter International Inc
FIBRIJET	Micromedics
FIBRINOSTIKA	Biomerieux Inc.
FIBRINOTHERM	Baxter International Inc
FIBRIQUIK	Biomerieux Inc.
FIBRON-1	Clinical Data Inc
FIBRONECTIN	Exocell, Inc.
FIBROSYSTEM	Bd Diagnostic Systems
FIBROTIP	Bd Diagnostic Systems
FIBROTUBE	Bd Diagnostic Systems
FIDELITAQ	Usb Corporation
FIELDMAX	Coherent, Inc.
FIELDSPECr	Analytical Spectral Devices, Inc.
FIFOGLIDE	Medical Design Systems, Inc.
FIGURE FINDER	Novel Products, Inc.
FIL-FORM	Medi-Dose, Inc.
FILAC	Covidien Lp
FILAMATIC	National Instrument Co., Inc.
FILAMATIC	National Instrument Llc
FILE 14	Hale Imaging Systems, Inc.
FILE-PRO	St. John Companies
FILM	Sakura Finetek U.S.A., Inc.
FILMQUICK CT	Image Marketing Corp.
FILPIN	Park Dental Research Corp./Implant Center
FILTA-GUARD	Intersurgical Inc.
FILTA-MAX	Idexx Laboratories, Inc.
FILTA-MAX XPRESS	Idexx Laboratories, Inc.
FILTA-THERM	Intersurgical Inc.
FILTEK	3m Co.
FILTER CREST	Crest Foam Industries
FILTER SAMPLER	Porex Corporation
FILTER STRAW	B. Braun Oem Division, B. Braun Medical Inc.
FILTERFLO	Arc Medical, Inc.
FILTERLINE	Oridion Medical Inc.
FILTERONE	Oneac Corporation
FILTERPIC	Spectrum Laboratories, Inc.
FILTERTEK	Filtertek Inc.
FILTERTREK	Industrial Specialities Manufacturing, Inc.
FILTRA 2000	Camfil Farr
FILTRACHECK-UTI	Meridian Bioscience, Inc.
FILTRATION MASK, LATEX FREE, HIGHLY ELASTIC COMFORTABLE FACE MASK. Key / Sun Medical Services, Inc.	
FILTRESSE	Utah Medical Products, Inc.
FINALE	Surmodics, Inc.
FINBLADE	Case Medical, Inc.
FINE-CUT	Fine-Cut Diamond Tool Co.
FINE-CUT	Special Products, Inc.
FINE-CUT ENDO	Special Products, Inc.
FINE-CUT ENDODONTIC	Special Products, Inc.
FINESSE	Utah Medical Products, Inc.
FINETOUCH	Boss Instruments, Ltd.

FING-R-FLEX	Nortech Laboratories, Inc.
FINGER HELPER	Meddev Corporation
FINGER PHANTOM	Nonin Medical, Inc.
FINGERPRINT	Smiths Medical Pm, Inc.
FINISH LINE	Oster Professional Products, Inc.
FINISHER	Oster Professional Products, Inc.
FINN	Biomet, Inc.
FINN CHAMBERS	Allerderm Laboratories, Inc.
FIRE-NOISE-LOCK	Industrial Acoustics Co., Inc.
FIREFIGHTER	United Receptacle
FIRMDENT	Moyco Technologies, Inc.
FIRST	First Healthcare Products
FIRST AND LESSER METATARSALPHALANGEAL JOINT HEMI IMPLANTS Biopro, Inc.
FIRST CARE	Stryker Medical
FIRST CLASS SCHOOL CHAIR	Wenzelite Rehab Supplies, Llc
FIRST DEFENSE	Immucell Corp.
FIRST FIT	Siemens Hearing Instruments, Inc.
FIRST KIT	Banyan International Corp.
FIRST MEDIC	Physio-Control, Inc.
FIRST MIDCATH	Becton Dickinson Infusion Therapy Systems, Inc.
FIRST PICC	Becton Dickinson Infusion Therapy Systems, Inc.
FIRST QUALITY	First Quality Enterprise, Inc.
FIRST TEETH	Laclede, Inc.
FIRSTCHOICE	Hollister Incorporated
FIRSTCHOICE	Hospira Inc.
FIRSTLIGHT	Uvp, Llc
FIRSTNUCLEAR, FIRSTPET, FIRSTMRI, FIRSTCT . American Diagnostic Medicine, Inc.
FIRSTSTEP	Siemens Hearing Instruments, Inc.
FIRSTSTEP	Stryker Spine
FIRSTTEMP	Covidien Lp
FISH	Adept-Med International, Inc.
FISH FLO	American Healthcare
FISKE	Advanced Instruments Inc.
FISON	Keeler Instruments Inc.
FISSUROTOMY BURS	S.S. White Burs Inc.
FIT	Hager Worldwide, Inc.
FIT RITE	Humanicare International, Inc.
FIT SYSTEM	Anthro Corporation
FITBALL	Ball Dynamics International, Llc
FITNESS MOTIVATION INTERNATIONAL .. Fitness Motivation Institute Of America, Inc.
FITNESS PLUS	Tri W-G Group
FITRITE	Lohmann & Rauscher, Inc.
FITRON	Cybex International, Inc.
FITS TO A T	First Quality Enterprise, Inc.
FITZ-ALL	Urocare Products, Inc.
FIWAY	U.S. Orthotics, Inc.
FIX-RAY DEVICE	Biopro, Inc.
FIXANAL	Crescent Chemical Co., Inc.
FIXANO-DYNAFIX-DLC	Small Bone Innovations, Inc.
FIXIT	Bodypoint, Inc.
FL-BOND	Shofu Dental Corporation
FL3000 FILTERS	Medical Device Resource Corporation
FLAG IT	Omnimed, Inc. (Beam Products)
FLAMINGO	Snug Seat, Inc.
FLAR-A-LOCK	Spectra Industries Corp.
FLASH	Medical Action Industries, Inc
FLASH-GUARD	Sparco, Inc.
FLASH-O-LENS	E.W. Pike & Company
FLASHER	Solid State Sonics & Electronics, Inc.
FLASHLINK	Deltatrak, Inc.
FLASHPAK	Riley Medical, Inc.
FLASHTITE	Case Medical, Inc.
FLASKSCRUBBER	Labconco Corp.
FLAT PLATFORM CHAIR	Gunnell, Inc.
FLAXEDIL	Covidien Lp
FLEAKER	Spectrum Laboratories, Inc.
FLECKS	Mizzy, Inc. Of National Keystone
FLEECE EZE	Allman Products
FLEET	C.B. Fleet Company Inc.
FLEX	Bard Electro Physiology
FLEX	Lawrence-Nelson, Llc
FLEX 8	Brown Medical Industries
FLEX BRUSH	Hager Worldwide, Inc.
FLEX FIT	Graham Medical Products/Div. Of Little Rapids Corp
FLEX H/A	Medtronic Xomed, Inc.
FLEX LOCK	Kenda American Airless
FLEX RANGER	Pre Pak Products, Inc.
FLEX SOCK	Great Lakes Filters/Filpaco Industries
FLEX T	Byron Medical
FLEX-A-BED	Flex-A-Bed, Inc.
FLEX-AIM	Kentek Corp.
FLEX-CIRCUIT	Minco Products, Inc.
FLEX-COIL	Minco Products, Inc.
FLEX-EL	Conmed Corporation
FLEX-FORM	Patterson Medical Holdings, Inc.
FLEX-I-COLD	Cramer Products, Inc.
FLEX-LOK	Smith & Nephew Inc.- Orthopaedics Division
FLEX-MASTER	DJO Inc.
FLEX-MASTER	Milwaukee Mattress & Furniture
FLEX-NECK	Janin Group, Inc.
FLEX-O-BOL	Hager Worldwide, Inc.
FLEX-R	Miltex Inc.
FLEX-R	Moyco Technologies, Inc.
FLEX-SUPPORT	Frank Stubbs Co., Inc
FLEX-TAP	Hydro Service & Supplies, Inc.
FLEX-X	Karl Storz Endoscopy-America Inc.
FLEX2	Karl Storz Endoscopy-America Inc.
FLEXACYL	Lang Dental Manufacturing Co., Inc.
FLEXAMOUNT	Independent Solutions, Inc.
FLEXANE	Crown Delta Corp.
FLEXBAR	Mediflex Surgical Products
FLEXBLUE	King Systems Corp.
FLEXBODY MIXER	Stedim Biosystems, Inc.
FLEXBOY	Stedim Biosystems, Inc.
FLEXBUMIN	Baxter International Inc
FLEXCEL CAROTID SHUNT	Lemaitre Vascular, Inc.
FLEXEL 3D	Stedim Biosystems, Inc.
FLEXFLO	Blue White Industries, Inc.
FLEXI	Promega Corp.
FLEXI CUT CUP, MAROON SPOON, CHEWY TUBE, ARK GRABBER ..... Equipment Shop, Inc.
FLEXI-BASIN	Graphic Controls Corp.
FLEXI-BOARD	Huestis Medical
FLEXI-CATH	Arrow International, Inc.
FLEXI-CUP	Impladent Ltd.
FLEXI-FLANGE	Essential Dental Systems, Inc.
FLEXI-FLOR	R.C.A. Rubber Company, The
FLEXI-FLOW	Essential Dental Systems, Inc.
FLEXI-FORM	Nonin Medical, Inc.
FLEXI-GRIP	Elginex Corporation
FLEXI-HOLDER	Huestis Medical
FLEXI-LIFT LU/LA ELEVATOR	Thyssenkrupp Access Corp.
FLEXI-OVERDENTURE	Essential Dental Systems, Inc.
FLEXI-PAC	Chattanooga Group
FLEXI-PASTE	Hartmann-Conco Inc.
FLEXI-POST	Essential Dental Systems, Inc.
FLEXI-SEAL	Convatec
FLEXI-SITE	Epic Medical Equipment Services, Inc.
FLEXI-WALL	Flexi-Wall Systems
FLEXIBEND	Covidien Lp, Formerly Registered As Kendall
FLEXIBLE DILATOR SET	Thomas Medical Inc.
FLEXIBLE MONITORING	Welch Allyn Protocol Inc.
FLEXICAIR	Hill-Rom Holdings, Inc.
FLEXICAIR	Hill-Rom Manufacturing, Inc.
FLEXICAIR ECLIPSE	Hill-Rom Holdings, Inc.
FLEXICAIR ECLIPSE PLUS	Hill-Rom Manufacturing, Inc.
FLEXICAIR ECLIPSE ULTRA	Hill-Rom Holdings, Inc.
FLEXICAIR ECLIPSE ULTRA	Hill-Rom Manufacturing, Inc.
FLEXICHANGE	Dentsply International, Inc.
FLEXICHANGE	Dentsply Prosthetics
FLEXICON	Hartmann-Conco Inc.
FLEXICOUPLER	Natus Medical Inc.
FLEXIFLO	Abbott Laboratories

FLEXIGEL	Smith & Nephew, Inc.
FLEXIGRID	Smith & Nephew, Inc.
FLEXIGRID PLUS	Smith & Nephew, Inc.
FLEXILET	Aso Corporation
FLEXIMATIC	General Pysiotherapy, Inc.
FLEXISTEM	Healthmark Industries
FLEXITAINER	Abbott Laboratories
FLEXITEC: QUICK CORE BIOPSY NEEDLES	Proact, Ltd.
FLEXITONE	Hospital Marketing Svcs. Company, Inc.
FLEXIVIAL	Globe Scientific, Inc.
FLEXIVIEWER	S&S Technology
FLEXLITE	Fla Orthopedics, Inc.
FLEXLOK	Medical Design Systems, Inc.
FLEXMAX	Trimedyne, Inc.
FLEXMEDICS	G & H Wire Co.
FLEXNET	Welch Allyn Protocol Inc.
FLEXO-SALIVA	Harry J. Bosworth Company
FLEXON	Covidien Lp
FLEXOPLAST	Western Medical, Ltd.
FLEXPOSURE	Zimmer Holdings, Inc.
FLEXPOSURE	Zimmer Spine
FLEXPREP	Hamilton Company
FLEXSEAL	Dentsply Prosthetics
FLEXSEAL	Extra Packaging, Corp.
FLEXSKIN	Innova Corp.
FLEXTAPE	Pedinol Pharmacal, Inc.
FLEXTEND	Balance Systems, Inc.
FLEXTEND SHOULDER KIT	Balance Systems, Inc.
FLEXTEND-AC	Balance Systems, Inc.
FLEXTESTER	Novel Products, Inc.
FLEXTIP	Arrow International, Inc.
FLEXTIP	Codman & Shurtleff, Inc
FLEXTIP	Zimmer Spine
FLEXTIP PLUS	Arrow International, Inc.
FLEXTRODE	Amrex Electrotherapy Equipment
FLEXVISION	Stryker Corp.
FLEXVISION	Stryker Endoscopy
FLEXZAN	Mylan Pharmaceuticals Inc
FLIMM-FIGHTER	General Pysiotherapy, Inc.
FLINTPAPER	Hager Worldwide, Inc.
FLIP IT	Pawling Corp., Architectural Prod. Div.
FLIP-LOC	Newschoff Chairs, Inc.
FLIP-TIP	Propper Manufacturing Co., Inc.
FLIPAK TOTES	Orbis Corporation
FLIPR	Molecular Devices Corp.
FLITE	Perkin Elmer Wallac, Inc.
FLITE	Perkinelmer Life And Analytical Sciences
FLITES	ArjoHuntleigh
FLO 1750 MOBILE WORKSTATION	Flo Healthcare
FLO 1800 MOBILE WORKSTATION	Flo Healthcare
FLO 2000 SERIES MEDICATION WORKSTATION	Flo Healthcare
FLO 3000 CRITICAL CARE WORKSTATION	Flo Healthcare
FLO 4000 VITALS WORKSTATION	Flo Healthcare
FLO-ASSIST	Northgate Technologies Inc.
FLO-ASSISTANT	Northgate Technologies Inc.
FLO-METERS	Timemed Labeling Systems, Inc.
FLO-RESTER	Synovis Life Technologies, Inc
FLO-RESTER	Synovis Surgical Innovations
FLO-THRU INTRALUMINAL SHUNT	Synovis Life Technologies, Inc.
FLO-THRU INTRALUMINAL SHUNT	Synovis Surgical Innovations
FLO-TROL	Maddak Inc.
FLO2	Pegasus Research Corp.
FLOAT-A-LYZER	Spectrum Laboratories, Inc.
FLOCHANNEL	Chad Therapeutics, Inc.
FLOCONTROL	Stryker Endoscopy
FLOGARD. Baxter Healthcare Corporporation, Alternate Care And Channel Team
FLOOR SHARK	Amano Pioneer Eclipse Corp.
FLOOR-FREE	Newschoff Chairs, Inc.
FLOORKEEPERS	Tornado Industries
FLOORMATTE	Amano Pioneer Eclipse Corp.
FLOPAC	Flotec, Inc.
FLORENTINE	Novocol, Inc.
FLOROPHOS	Scientific Pharmaceuticals, Inc.
FLOSEAL	Baxter International Inc
FLOSENSE	Sdi Diagnostics, Inc.
FLOSS FINGERS II	Preventive Dentistry Products, Inc.
FLOSSAID	Flossaid Corporation
FLOSTAR	Intravascular Incorporated
FLOSTEADY	Stryker Corp.
FLOSTEADY	Stryker Endoscopy
FLOTEC	Flotec, Inc.
FLOTREX	Ge Infrastructure Water & Process Technologies
FLOURESBRITE MICROPARTICLES	Polysciences, Inc.
FLOVISC	Eagle Laboratories
FLOW PRA	One Lambda, Inc.
FLOW SOUND	Transonic Systems Inc.
FLOW STAIR LIFT	Thyssenkrupp Access Corp.
FLOW-CHECK	Transonic Systems Inc.
FLOW-QC	Transonic Systems Inc.
FLOW-TROL	Vital Signs, Inc.
FLOW-VOLUME CALIBRATOR	Jones Medical Instrument Co.
FLOWBAC	Gvs Filter Technology Inc.
FLOWERS DORSAL IMPLANT	Implantech Associates, Inc.
FLOWERS MANDIBULAR GLOVE	Implantech Associates, Inc.
FLOWGUARD	Greatbach Medical
FLOWGUARD	Greatbatch Inc
FLOWIRE	Volcano Corporation
FLOWSCREEN PRO	CAREFUSION 211, INC..
FLU OlAr	Thermo Biostar, Inc.
FLU VEN	Accellent El Paso
FLUDIO	Adroit Medical Systems, Inc.
FLUID DOSE III	Medical Packaging Inc.
FLUID FLO PERCUSSOR	Med Systems
FLUIDAIR	Kinetic Concepts, Inc.
FLUIDGARD	Precept Medical Products, Inc.
FLUIDOT	Medrad, Inc.
FLUIDRAIN	Mallinckrodt, Inc.
FLUIDSAFE	Stryker Corp.
FLUIDSAFE	Stryker Endoscopy
FLUIDSHIELD	Kerr Group
FLUOPHASE	Thermo Fisher Scientific
FLUOR/AWAY	Triangle Biomedical Sciences, Inc.
FLUORESLENS	Portable Medical Laboratories, Inc.
FLUORO SEAL	One Lambda, Inc.
FLUORO TRAK	Ge Healthcare Technologies Surgery Navigation
FLUORO-4	C. R. Bard, Inc., Bard Urological Div.
FLUORO-DOT	Bovie Medical Corp.
FLUORO-FREE	Smiths Medical Asd, Inc.
FLUORO-MAX	Seradyn, Inc.
FLUORO-SLIT	Bovie Medical Corp.
FLUOROBEADS	One Lambda, Inc.
FLUOROLITE	George Taub Products & Fusion Co., Inc.
FLUOROMAX	Shimadzu Medical Systems
FLUOROPERM	Paragon Vision Sciences, Inc.
FLUOROQUENCH	One Lambda, Inc.
FLUOROSCAN	Hologic, Inc.
FLUOROSEAL	Scientific Pharmaceuticals, Inc.
FLUOROVISION	Enhanced Video Devices, Inc.
FLUORSAVE	Oncogene Research Products
FLUROCORE	Dentsply Caulk
FLUROSHIELD	Dentsply Caulk
FLUROSHIELD	Dentsply International, Inc.
FLUROSHIELD	Dentsply Prosthetics
FLX	Ebi, Llc
FLYSTOP	Berner International Corp.
FM501	Carolina Medical, Inc.
FM501D	Carolina Medical, Inc.
FMOL	Promega Corp.
FMS 2000	Belmont Instrument Corp.
FMS DUO, FMS SOLO	Future Medical Systems, Inc.
FMV SERIES	Oneac Corporation
FOAM	National Medical Products
FOAM GRIP	Covidien Lp, Formerly Registered As United States Surgical
FOAM POSITIONING PRODUCTS	National Medical Products
FOAM TRAC	Hartmann-Conco Inc.
FOAMART	Aetrex Worldwide, Inc

FOAMEX	Ufp Technologies, Inc.
FOAMWALKER	Aircast Llc
FOCALSTAT	Ams Innovative Center-San Jose
FOCI	Farrand Optical Components & Instruments, Div. Of Ruhle Co.
FOCU TIP	Hager Worldwide, Inc.
FOCU TIP E	Hager Worldwide, Inc.
FOCUS	Quest Star Medical, Inc.
FOCUS ANKLE BRACE	Omni Life Science, Inc.
FOCUS DAILIES	Ciba Vision Corporation
FOCUS EMG	Fasstech
FOCUS NIGHT & DAY	Ciba Vision Corporation
FOCUS NMES	Empi, Inc.
FOCUSED TRACTION	Endorphin Corporation
FOG	Onyx Medical Inc./Face-It
FOG-SHIELD	Precept Medical Products, Inc.
FOGARTY	Edwards Lifesciences, Llc.
FOGG-IT	Caddy Corporation
FOILER	Alpha Scientific Instruments
FOLD UP WALL DESK	Budget Buddy Company, Inc.
FOLDALITE-B	National Biological Corp.
FOLDCRAFT	Plymold
FOLDOVER	Ricon Corp.
FOLLETT	Follett Corp.
FOME-CUF	Smiths Medical Asd
FONIX	Frye Electronics, Inc.
FOODGARDE	Biosynergy, Inc.
FOODSAFE BLAST CHILLERS	Servolift/Eastern Corp.
FOOT CARE	Medicool, Inc.
FOOT-TROL	Conmed Corporation
FOOTCARE	Medicool, Inc.
FOOTGLOVE	Allerderm Laboratories, Inc.
FOOTHILLS SURGICAL DRAPES	Foothills Industries, Inc.
FOOTHUGGER BOOTPADS	Allen Medical Systems, Inc.
FOOTPRINT	Graham Medical Products/Div. Of Little Rapids Corp
FOOTSPLINTS	Pedifix, Inc.
FORAMATRON	Parkell, Inc.
FORANE	Baxter Healthcare Corporation, Baxter Pharmaceuticals And Technologies
FORCE	York Barbell
FORCE ARGONT II	Valleylab
FORCE EZT	Valleylab
FORCE FIBER	Stryker Endoscopy
FORCE FXT	Valleylab
FORCE II	American Orthodontics Corp.
FORCE-5	Advanced Mechanical Technology, Inc. (Amti)
FORE-SIGHT	Cas Medical Systems, Inc.
FOREDOM	Foredom Electric Co.
FORESIGHT	Smith & Nephew Inc.- Orthopaedics Division
FORK-FIX	Panadent Corp.
FORLIFE	Airsep Corp.
FORM FIT	Oasis Medical, Inc.
FORM-PROTECT POCKETS	First Healthcare Products
FORMALYDE	Pedinol Pharmacal, Inc.
FORMATILL	Cooley & Cooley, Ltd.
FORMEN	Bsn-Jobst
FORMS-SAVER	First Healthcare Products
FORMULA	Invacare Corporation
FORMULA	Stryker Endoscopy
FORMULA FOR ARCHIMED	Futuremed America, Inc.
FORMULA ONE	Tillotson Healthcare Corp.
FORSUS	3m Co.
FORTAFLEX	Organogenesis Inc.
FORTE	Applied Medical Resource Corporation
FORTEL	Biomerica, Inc.
FORTRAD	Fortrad Eye Instruments Corp.
FOSHM	Tremetrics
FOSSIL EYEWEAR	Safilo Usa
FOSTER-HARD	Hard Manufacturing Co.
FOTO UV	Fotodyne, Inc.
FOTO/ANALYST	Fotodyne, Inc.
FOTO/CONVERTIBLE	Fotodyne, Inc.
FOTO/ECLIPSE	Fotodyne, Inc.
FOTO/FORCE	Fotodyne, Inc.
FOTO/PHORESIS	Fotodyne, Inc.
FOTO/PREP	Fotodyne, Inc.
FOUNDATION	DJO Surgical
FOUNDATION 2000	Indec Systems, Inc.
FOUNTAIN	Merit Medical Systems, Inc.
FOUR SQUARE	Spectronics Corporation
FOURPRESS FOUR LAYER BANDAGE	Hartmann-Conco Inc.
FP Vericel	Pall Corporation
FP WALKER	Aircast Llc
FP-5000	Stryker Imaging
FPC COTE	Starkey Laboratories, Inc.
FPT	Labac Systems, Inc.
FR	Pentron Laboratory Technologies
FRACSURE HIP SYSTEM	Centerpulse Orthopedics Inc.
FRAGEL	Oncogene Research Products
FRAGMATOME	Alcon Research, Ltd.
FRAME SAW	Hager Worldwide, Inc.
FRAMESAVER CLAMP	Bodypoint
FRAMEWAVE	Emed Technologies
FRANCOBAL	Stryker Spine
FRANTZ	Frantz Medical Development Ltd.
FRAP STRAP	Hely And Weber
FRASER HARLAKE	Matrx By Midmark
FRASTEC	Smith & Nephew, Inc.
FRAZER	Independent Solutions, Inc.
FRC	Starkey Laboratories, Inc.
FRC POSTEC	Ivoclar Vivadent, Inc.
FREDERICK TOOL CORP.	Frederick Tool Corp.
FREE & ACTIVE	Humanicare International, Inc.
FREE FLOW	Medcomp (Medical Components, Inc.)
FREE THE BODY AND SPIRIT	Ohio Willow Wood Company
FREE-FLOW	Marlen Manufacturing & Development Co.
FREE-FLOW	Ohio Willow Wood Company
FREE-N-EASY	Tp Orthodontics, Inc.
FREE-UP	Pre Pak Products, Inc.
FREEDOM	Alimed, Inc.
FREEDOM BATH	ArjoHuntleigh
FREEDOM BRAND	Mentor Corp.
FREEDOM CATH	Mentor Corp.
FREEDOM CLEAR	Mentor Corp.
FREEDOM FIT	Geri-Care Products
FREEDOM GRIP	Mobility Transfer Systems
FREEDOM IN MOTION	Freedom Designs, Inc.
FREEDOM PAK SEVEN	Mentor Corp.
FREEDOM PLUS	Unetixs Vascular, Inc.
FREEDOM SCOOTER	Ranger All Season Corp.
FREEDOM V	Unetixs Vascular, Inc.
FREEDOM-NEB	Respironics Colorado
FREEDOM-O'2	Respironics Colorado
FREEDOMHILL	Hill-Rom Holdings, Inc.
FREEFLOW	CAREFUSION 211, INC.
FREEFORM SE/EC	Microflex Corporation
FREELITE	Binding Site, Inc., The
FREEMAN	Frederick Lee Inc
FREESPAN TRAVERSE	Liko North America
FREESTYLE	Abbott Laboratories
FREESTYLE	Joerns Healthcare, Inc
FREESTYLE	Medtronic Cardiovascular Surgery, The Heart Valve Div.
FREEWAY	Respironics Colorado
FREEZE	Hager Worldwide, Inc.
FREEZEMOBILE	Virtis, An Sp Industries Company
FREEZONE	Labconco Corp.
FREGEAU MFG.	I-Rep, Inc.
FRENCH PRESS	Thermo Spectronic
FREPP	CholeraPrep
FREQUENCY	The Cooper Companies, Inc
FRESH CAST	Brown Medical Industries
FRESH SCENT	King Systems Corp.
FRESH-KIT	Georgia Steel & Chemical Company, Inc.
FRESHCARD	Multisorb Technologies, Inc.
FRESHLOOK	Ciba Vision
FRESHLOOK	Ciba Vision Corporation
FRESHMAX	Multisorb Technologies, Inc.

FRESHMINT	New World Imports
FRESHPAX	Multisorb Technologies, Inc.
FRESHSCENT	New World Imports
FRESHSTART	Bio Med Sciences, Inc.
FRIGISPRAY	Dermatologic Lab & Supply, Inc.
FRIGOMIX	Sartorius Stedim Sus Inc
FROM COLLECTION THROUGH DETECTION	Meridian Bioscience, Inc.
FRONT ROW	Pelton & Crane Co.,
FRONTIER	Dent Zar, Inc.
FRONTIER SCBA	Avon-Isi
FROVROCON	Ciba Vision
FRP-100	Dazian Fabrics,Llc.
FS	Cte Chem Tec Equipment Co.
FSD	Starkey Laboratories, Inc.
FSME-IMMUN	Baxter International Inc
FT SERIES	United Syntek Corp.
FTI	Forward Technology
FUELING INNOVATION	Usb Corporation
FUJI CEMENT	G-C America Inc.
FUJINON	Fujinon, Inc.
FUJITA	Mizuho America Inc.
FUKUDA DENSHI, WALLACH SURGICAL, HOLTER	Meza Medical Equipment
FUKUSHIMA	Pmt Corp.
FULFIL	Dentsply Caulk
FULL SPECTRUM LOW CUT	Starkey Laboratories, Inc.
FULLENGTH	Seca Corp.
FULLER SHIELD	Birchwood Laboratories, Inc.
FULLFLOW	Boston Scientific Interventional Technologies
FULLTERM	Hologic, Inc.
FUMEX	Fumex Inc.
FUNBANDS	Precision Dynamics Corp.
FUNCTIONAL SOLUTIONS	North Coast Medical, Inc.
FUNGICHROM	Wescor, Inc.
FUNGOID	Pedinol Pharmacal, Inc.
FUSE-IT	Qed Bioscience, Inc.
FUSION	George Taub Products & Fusion Co., Inc.
FUSION	United Syntek Corp.
FUSION PACS	GE Healthcare
FUSION RIS	GE Healthcare
FUSION RIS/PACS	GE Healthcare
FUSION WELDED	Arosurgical Instruments Corp.
FUSION-AID	Vector Laboratories, Inc.
FUTURA	Instrumentation Laboratory Company
FUTURE FOAM	Ufp Technologies, Inc.
FUTUREMED	Futuremed America, Inc.
FX PRO	Darco International, Inc.
FX-100	Welch Allyn, Inc.
FX-CABLELOK S.T.O.P.	DJO Surgical
Fashion Seal	Superior Uniform Group
Fashion Seal Healthcare	Superior Uniform Group
Fast-Cath	St. Jude Medical, Inc.
Fast-Find	Hilco
Fathom	Boston Scientific Corporation
Febreze	Procter & Gamble
Fibersure	Procter & Gamble
FibreKleer	Pentron Laboratory Technologies
FilterWire EZ	Boston Scientific - Maple Grove
Finyte	Avantor Performance Materials
First Step Select	Kinetic Concepts, Inc.
Fixodent	Procter & Gamble
FlexCuff	St. Jude Medical, Inc.
Flextome	Boston Scientific - Maple Grove
Flextome	Boston Scientific Corporation
Flow-It	Pentron Laboratory Technologies
Flowmor (design mark)	Avantor Performance Materials
Fluke	Danaher Corporation
FrameLink	Medtronic, Inc.
Freedom	Kinetic Concepts, Inc.
Freedom CGX	Freedom Designs, Inc.
FrogLegs	The Aftermarket Group
Frontier	St. Jude Medical, Inc.
FunFresh Foods	Nutraceutical International Corp.
G&H WIRE COMPANY	G & H Wire Co.
G-FORCE	Colours Wheelchair
G-PROBE	Iridex Corporation
G-RAM	In/Us Systems, Inc.
G-TUBES	Bio Plas, Inc.
G. S. SAFETIES	General Scientific Safety Equipment Co.
G.A.S	Vital Signs, Inc.
G.B.I.,GALIX, WINTER, PACESTAR, ECGALIX, ERGALIX	Galix Biomedical Instrumentation, Inc.
G.S.P TABLE	Medical Positioning, Inc.
G2 DIGITAL	Heska Corporation
G5	General Pysiotherapy, Inc.
GABBAY-FRATER SUTURE GUIDE	Teleflex Medical
GABRIALLA	Ita-Med Co.
GAELTEC	Medical Measurements, Inc.
GAIA	Oticon, Inc.
GAIT BELTS	Morrison Medical
GAIT TRAINER 2	Biodex Medical Systems, Inc.
GAITKEEPERr CAST SHOE	Dm Systems, Inc.
GAITMASTER	Mauch, Inc.
GAITMAT II	E. Q., Inc.
GAITWAY	Kistler Instrument Corp.
GALAXIS	H.L. Bouton Co., Inc.
GALAXY	Baxter Healthcare Corporation, Baxter Biopharma Solutions
GALAXY	Baxter Healthcare Corporation, Global Drug Delivery
GALAXY	Mge Ups Sytems, Inc.
GALAXY AQUATICS	Galaxy Aquatics, Inc.
GALAXY POOLS	Med-Fit Systems, Inc.
GALDABINI	Hansco Technologies, Inc.
GALEN	Life-Tech, Inc.
GALILEO	Immucor, Inc.
GALILEO GOLD	Hamilton Medical, Inc.
GALILEOS	Sirona Dental Systems Llc
GALT	Galt Medical Corp.
GAM	Cardium Therapeutics Inc.
GAMGEE	3m Co.
GAMMA	Astro-Med, Inc.
GAMMA	Heine Usa Ltd.
GAMMA	Immucor, Inc.
GAMMA	Stryker Spine
GAMMA 3	Stryker Corp.
GAMMA PROBE	Intramedical Imaging Llc
GAMMA-BSM	Etex Corporation
GAMMABOND	Es Industries
GAMMAGARD	Baxter International Inc
GAMMAMED	Varian Medical Systems
GAMMAMEDPLUS	Varian Medical Systems
GAMMAR-PIV	Csl Behring
GAMMATROL	Canberra
GAMMED II B	Capintec, Inc.
GANTEX	Howard Medical Company
GAP-IGA	Biomerica, Inc.
GAP-IGG	Biomerica, Inc.
GAP-IGM	Biomerica, Inc.
GARD-DUTY	Minatronics Corp.
GARDS	Hospital Specialty Company
GARGOYLES	Gargoyles Eyewear
GARREN EZ DISPENSER	Garren Scientific, Inc.
GAS DATA	Cea Instruments, Inc.
GAS LYTE	Vital Signs, Inc.
GAS-CHEX	Propper Manufacturing Co., Inc.
GAS-MASTER	American Gas & Chemical Co., Ltd.
GASAMPLER	Quintron Instrument Company
GASDIRECT	Gen-Probe, Inc.
GASPAK	Bd Diagnostic Systems
GASTIGHT	Hamilton Company
GASTRAK	Fisher Diagnostics
GASTROMARK	Advanced Magnetics, Inc.
GASTROMARK	Mallinckrodt, Inc.
GATESVILLE CHILD	Medical Plastics Laboratory, Inc.
GATESVILLE DOLL	Medical Plastics Laboratory, Inc.
GATOR	Conmed Linvatec
GATOR	Justrite Manufacturing Co., L.L.C.
GATOR-GRIP	Boss Instruments, Ltd.

GAUZTAPE	Modern Aids, Inc.
GAZELLE	Amano Pioneer Eclipse Corp.
GAZELLE	Snug Seat, Inc.
GB ENCLOSURE	Mushield Company, Inc., The
GB-SPECT	Syntermed, Inc.
GBM	General Pysiotherapy, Inc.
GC-LECT	Bd Diagnostic Systems
GC-RAM	In/Us Systems, Inc.
GCMS, AUTHORING COACH	Sajan, Inc.
GCX	Gcx Corp.
GCX	Independent Solutions, Inc.
GDC	Boston Scientific Corporation
GDLH	Medtronic Sofamor Danek Usa, Inc
GDX	Cholestech Corp.
GDX NFA	Carl Zeiss Meditec, Inc.
GE	Atlas Medical Technologies
GE	Bulbtronics, Inc.
GE	Bulbworks, Inc.
GE-MARC	Ericsson, Inc.
GE-NET	Ericsson, Inc.
GEA AG	Gea Westfalia Separator, Inc.
GEBAUER'S ETHYL CHLORIDE	Gebauer Company
GEE WHIZ EXTERNAL MALE INCONTINENT SHEATH	Leading Edge Innovations
GEE WHIZ SECURE SEAL	Leading Edge Innovations
GEE WHIZ SECURE STRIP	Leading Edge Innovations
GEE WHIZ UNIVERSAL CONNECTOR	Merlin's Medical Supply
GEE WHIZ(R)	Merlin's Medical Supply
GEENEN	Wilson-Cook Medical, Inc.
GEL EXPLORER	Ultra-Lum, Inc.
GEL-CARE	Patterson Medical Holdings, Inc.
GEL-E-DONUT	Children's Medical Ventures, Inc.
GEL-LITE	Pyramid Industries, Llc
GEL-READ	Bio-Rad Laboratories, Life Science Group
GEL-STAT	Geritrex Corp.
GEL-T	Span-America Medical Systems, Inc.
GELBAND	Fla Orthopedics, Inc.
GELBO	Knit-Rite, Inc.
GELFOAM	Baxter International Inc
GELIGNE	Silipos Inc.
GELISONDE II	Medical Equipment Specialists, Inc.
GELOCAST	Bsn-Jobst
GELPORT	Applied Medical Resource Corporation
GELPUMP	Thermo Savant
GELSEAL	Applied Medical Resource Corporation
GELSIL	Lightpath Technologies
GELTEC	Easy Seat Llc
GELWELLS	Jordco, Inc.
GELYSATE	Bd Diagnostic Systems
GEM	Kinamed, Inc.
GEM	M .W. Mooney & Co., Inc.
GEM	Sloan Valve Co.
GEM ELISA	Qed Bioscience, Inc.
GEM OPL	Instrumentation Laboratory Company
GEM PCL PLUS	Instrumentation Laboratory Company
GEM PREMIER 3000	Instrumentation Laboratory Company
GEMCAL	Alfa Wassermann, Inc.
GEMINA WAXER	Almore International, Inc.
GEMINI	Alaris Medical Systems, Inc
GEMINI	Mentor Ophthalmics, Inc.
GEMINI	Mts Medication Technologies
GEMINI	Richards-Wilcox, Inc.
GEMINI	Tulip Medical Products
GEMINI	Wilbur Curtis Company
GEMINI E	Allen Medical Instruments Corp.
GEMINI FLOW	Directmed, Inc.
GEMLOCK	Zimmer Dental, Inc.
GEMNI-300	Chiu Technical Corp.
GEMS	General Devices
GEMSTAR	Hospira Inc.
GEMWEB	Instrumentation Laboratory Company
GEN II	Curbell, Inc. Electronics
GEN III	Curbell, Inc. Electronics
GEN-MED	Mckesson General Medical
GEN-X GENERATOR	Swissray America, Inc.
GENDER SOLUTIONS	Zimmer Holdings, Inc.
GENDEX	Dentsply International, Inc.
GENDEX	Dentsply Prosthetics
GENDRON INC.	Medi-Tech International, Inc.
GENE CHIP	Affymetrix, Inc.
GENE DETECTIVE	Zeptometrix Corporation
GENE PULSER	Bio-Rad Laboratories, Life Science Group
GENE-MASTER	Bio-Rad Laboratories, Life Science Group
GENEBLOT	Biogenex Laboratories
GENECHIP	Pathwork Diagnostics Inc.
GENEMAPPER	Applied Biosystems
GENEPATH	Bio-Rad Laboratories, Inc.
GENEPATH	Biorad Laboratories
GENEQUENCE	Neogen Corporation
GENERABLOC	Gi Supply
GENERAL ASPIRATOR	Wells Johnson Co.
GENERAL ELECTRIC	Atlas Medical Technologies
GENERATION 80 HALO	Jerome Medical
GENEROST	Berkeley Advanced Biomaterials, Inc.
GENESEARCH	Veridex, Llc
GENESEE	Genesee Biomedical, Inc.
GENESIS	Crest Ultrasonics Corp.
GENESIS	Lechnologies Research, Inc.
GENESIS	Smith & Nephew Inc.- Orthopaedics Division
GENESIS	Tecan U.S., Inc.
GENESIS(R)	Virtis, An Sp Industries Company
GENESIS HOUSKEEPING CARTS	Tecni-Quip
GENESIS II	Smith & Nephew Inc.- Orthopaedics Division
GENESIS INSTRUMENTS	Mark Medical Manufacturing, Inc.
GENESIS NP	Enersys
GENESIS PURE LEAD	Enersys
GENESIS R&D SQL	Esha Research
GENESTAR	Meridian Bioscience, Inc.
GENESYS	Thermo Spectronic
GENESYS 5000	Laboratory Technologies, Inc.
GENESYS 6000	Laboratory Technologies, Inc.
GENESYS GAMMA-1	Laboratory Technologies, Inc.
GENETIC PERFORMANCE CERTIFIED	Usb Corporation
GENETIC SYSTEMS	Biorad Laboratories
GENETISCANNER AUTOMATIC METAPHASE FINDER	Leica Microsystems (San Jose) Corporation
GENEX	Biocomposites Inc.
GENEXPRESS	Protein Sciences Corp.
GENIE	Facet Technologies, Llc
GENIE	Idea Scientific Co.
GENIE	Oticon, Inc.
GENIE	Scientific Industries, Inc.
GENITAL ELECTRICS	Rontron Engineering, Inc.
GENIUS	Covidien Lp
GENOMIC SOLUTIONS	Applied Biosystems
GENOUS	Orbusneich Medical, Inc.
GENPORE	Genpore, A Division Of General Polymeric Corp.
GENT-L-TIP	Chester Labs, Inc.
GENTELL	Gentell
GENTELL CLEAN	Gentell
GENTELL COMFORTELL	Gentell
GENTELL LIQUID CLEAN	Gentell
GENTELL LOPROFILE FOAM PLUS	Gentell
GENTELL SHIELD & PROTECT	Gentell
GENTELL SHIELD & PROTECTAF	Gentell
GENTLE BEND	Ethicon, Inc.
GENTLE BLUE ELECTRODE TENS & NMS	Covidien Lp, Formerly Registered As Uni-Patch
GENTLE CARE	Imonti And Associates Inc., M.
GENTLE PULSE	Parkell, Inc.
GENTLE STEP	Paramedical Distributors
GENTLE STEP	Therafirm, A Knit Rite Company
GENTLE STEP SHOE	Darco International, Inc.
GENTLE TOUCH	Ciba Vision
GENTLE TOUCH	Convatec Professional Services
GENTLE TOUCH	Mizuho Osi
GENTLE-PAK	Approved Medical Systems

GENTLEBRIGHT	Lumalite, Inc.
GENTLEE CLEAN	Lee Medical International, Inc.
GENTLELASE	Candela Corp.
GENTLEMAX	Candela Corp.
GENTLEYAG	Candela Corp.
GENUIMEDI	Medi Usa
GENUINE MICROSURGICAL INSTRUMENTS	Micrins Surgical Instruments, Inc.
GENUTRAIN	Bauerfeind Usa, Inc.
GENUTRAIN P3	Bauerfeind Usa, Inc.
GEO-MATT	Span-America Medical Systems, Inc.
GEO-MATTRESS	Span-America Medical Systems, Inc.
GEODESIC EEG SYSTEMS	Electrical Geodesics, Incorporated
GEODESIC SENSOR NET	Electrical Geodesics, Incorporated
GEOFLEX	Ohio Willow Wood Company
GEPCO	General Econopak, Inc.
GERDCHECK	Sandhill Scientific, Inc.
GERI BATH	Geritrex Corp.
GERI CBO	Geritrex Corp.
GERI LAV FREE	Geritrex Corp.
GERI MANIKINS	Nasco
GERI RINSE FREE	Geritrex Corp.
GERI SALVE	Geritrex Corp.
GERI SAN DET	Geritrex Corp.
GERI SILK	Geritrex Corp.
GERI SOFT LOTION	Geritrex Corp.
GERI-CARE	Geri-Care Products
GERI-HYDROLAC	Geritrex Corp.
GERM-FIGHTER	United Receptacle
GERSTNER	Gerstner & Sons Inc.
GETINGE	Getinge Usa, Inc.
GETTIG GUARD	Gettig Pharmaceutical Instrument Co., Div Of Gettig Technologies Inc.
GEWA	Zygo Industries, Inc.
GI-STITCH	Pare Surgical, Inc.
GIA	Covidien Lp, Formerly Registered As United States Surgical
GIARD EIA	Antibodies, Inc.
GIBCO BRL	Life Technologies Corporation
GIBECK	Teleflex Medical
GIGABITE	Atc Technologies, Inc.
GIGASORB	Camfil Farr
GILIAN	Sensidyne, Inc.
GILLILAND	Byron Medical
GIMME A LIFT	Global Franchise Consultants, Inc.
GIN BABY	Vital Signs, Inc.
GINGI-AID	Belport Co. Inc., Gingi-Pak Div.
GINGI-PAK	Belport Co. Inc., Gingi-Pak Div.
GINGI-PLAIN	Belport Co. Inc., Gingi-Pak Div.
GINGICAINE	Belport Co. Inc., Gingi-Pak Div.
GINGICAINE ONE	Belport Co. Inc., Gingi-Pak Div.
GINGICURETTAGE	Shofu Dental Corporation
GINSBERG SCIENTIFIC	Aristotle Corp.
GIP	Medi-Globe Corporation
GIPSCUT	Hager Worldwide, Inc.
GIRAFFE	Boss Instruments, Ltd.
GIRAFFE	Ge Medical Systems Information Technologies
GIRAFFE	Goodwin Manufacturing, Inc.
GIRAFFE	Snug Seat, Inc.
GIRAFFE MULTI-PURPOSE TASK LAMPS	Goodwin Manufacturing, Inc.
GIRAFFE-NECK	Boss Instruments, Ltd.
GIROMATIC	Medidenta International, Inc.
GIZMO	Mentor Corp.
GK-3	General Pysiotherapy, Inc.
GKM	Boeckeler Instruments, Inc.
GL CASE BOX	Hager Worldwide, Inc.
GLACIER	Synvasive Technology, Inc.
GLACIER GEL	Packaging Products Corp.
GLACIERFREEZE	Whitehall Manufacturing
GLADIATOE DT	Cropper Medical, Inc./Bio Skin
GLADIATOR XT	Cropper Medical, Inc./Bio Skin
GLARESHIELD	Noir Manufacturing
GLAS	Sakura Finetek U.S.A., Inc.
GLAS-COL, LLC TOOLS FOR SCIEN	Glas-Col , Llc
GLASION	Scientific Pharmaceuticals, Inc.
GLASIONOMER	Shofu Dental Corporation
GLASS BEAD MIRROR WARMER	Premier Medical Products
GLASSCOCK	Oto-Med, Inc.
GLASSVAN	Myco Medical
GLAUCOMA DRAINAGE DEVICES	Eagle Vision, Inc.
GLD TIP	Wilson-Cook Medical, Inc.
GLEESON FLOVAC	Conmed Corporation
GLEN-SLEEVE	Western Medical, Ltd.
GLIDEAWAY	Stryker Corp.
GLIDEWIRE	Terumo Medical Corp.
GLO-TRODE	Medical Science Products, Inc.
GLOBAL	Weitbrecht Communications, Inc.
GLOBAL DRYER	American Dryer, Inc.
GLOBAL HEALTHCARE	Global Healthcare
GLOBAL MODULAR REPLACEMENT SYSTEM	Stryker Corp.
GLOBAL MODULAR REPLACEMENT SYSTEM	Stryker Howmedica Osteonics
GLOBAL POWER INTERFACE	Powervar, Inc.
GLOBAL, ALLGRAD, LITEOIL, ROBERT G EDWARDS CATHETER	Genx International
GLOBAL, ONE, MICRO-HITE DCC, PC-DMIS	Brown & Sharpe Inc.
GLORIA VANDERBILT EYEWEAR	Zyloware Corporation
GLORING	Eraser Company, Inc.
GLOVE BUTLER	Bowman Manufacturing Company, Inc.
GLOVE'N CARE	Essential Dental Systems, Inc.
GLOVEPLUS	Ammex Corp.
GLOVETEX	American Health Products Corporation
GLOVEWORKS	Ammex Corp.
GLOW 'N TELL TAPE	Lemaitre Vascular, Inc.
GLU/HGB	R & D Systems, Inc.
GLUC-PICK	Spirig Advanced Technologies, Inc.
GLUCERNA	Abbott Laboratories
GLUCOCARD X-METER	Arkray Usa
GLUCOFACTS	Siemens Healthcare Diagnostics Inc.
GLUCOLET	Siemens Healthcare Diagnostics Inc.
GLUCOMETER	Siemens Healthcare Diagnostics Inc.
GLUT-RX	Kem Medical Products Corp.
GLUTAMINE	Baxter Healthcare Corporation Nutrition
GLYC-AFFIN GHB	PerkinElmer
GLYCABEN	Exocell, Inc.
GLYCABUMIN	Exocell, Inc.
GLYCACOR	Exocell, Inc.
GLYCO TEST	Pierce Chemical Company
GLYCOHEMOSURE	Quantimetrix Corporation
GLYCOMER	Covidien Lp, Formerly Registered As United States Surgical
GLYCOSCREEN	Fisher Diagnostics
GLYTRAC	Siemens Healthcare Diagnostics Inc
GMI	Cea Instruments, Inc.
GMRS	Stryker Corp.
GMRS	Stryker Howmedica Osteonics
GOBED	Stryker Corp.
GOJO	Gojo Industries, Inc
GOLD	Glines And Rhodes, Inc.
GOLD BAND AMPULE	Wheaton Science Products
GOLD BOND	Puritan Medical Products Company Llc
GOLD COPE	Dentsply Prosthetics
GOLD HEAVYWEIGHT	Milliken & Company, Anticon Products
GOLD POINT	Tp Orthodontics, Inc.
GOLD PREMIUM	Access Battery Inc.
GOLD SERIES	Staar Surgical Co.
GOLD-LINE HANDPIECE	Conmed Corporation
GOLDEN	Golden Technologies, Inc.
GOLDEN COMPANION	Golden Technologies, Inc.
GOLDEN SEAL	Pharaoh Trading Company
GOLDEN SERIES	Langer, Inc.
GOLDEN TECHNOLOGY	Handicap Unlimited, Inc.
GOLDENROD ANIMAL LANCETS	Medipoint, Inc.
GOLDLENS	Diagnosis, Llc
GOLDMAN	Goldman Products, Inc.
GOLDSORB	Milliken & Company, Anticon Products
GOLDTECH BIO 2000	Argen Corp.
GOLDTONE	American Orthodontics Corp.
GOLDTOUCH SERVICE	Mark Medical Manufacturing, Inc.
GOLVO	Liko North America

GOMCO	Allied Healthcare Products, Inc.
GOMCO	Encompas Unlimited, Inc.
GONI KIT	Culture Kits, Inc.
GONOGEN	New Horizons Diagnostics Corporation
GOOD 'N BED WEDGE	Roloke
GOOD GRIPS	North Coast Medical, Inc.
GOODE T-TUBE	Medtronic Xomed, Inc.
GOODKNIGHT	Covidien (Formerly Nellcor Puritan Bennett / Tyco Healthcare)
GORILLA	Boss Instruments, Ltd.
GORILLA	Snug Seat, Inc.
GOSHEN MEDICAL	Bio-Med U.S.A. Inc.
GOTFRIED PCCP	Orthofix Inc.
GOTTFRIED	Gottfried Medical, Inc.
GP	Uresil, Llc
GRADIUM	Lightpath Technologies
GRAETHER PUPIL EXPANDER	Eagle Vision, Inc.
GRAFIT	Sellstrom Manufacturing Co.
GRAFIX	Conmed Linvatec
GRAFT	Impladent Ltd.
GRAFT MASTER	Smith & Nephew, Inc., Endoscopy Division
GRAFTAC	Covidien Lp, Formerly Registered As United States Surgical
GRAFTSTENT	Boston Scientific Interventional Technologies
GRAHAMATIANS	Graham Medical Products/Div. Of Little Rapids Corp
GRALAB	Dimco Gray Co.
GRAMSTAINER	Tomtec
GRANDMA CHASE	Armstrong Medical Industries, Inc.
GRANDVIEW	Hartwell Medical Corp.
GRANITE-FLOR	R.C.A. Rubber Company, The
GRANITEC	Novocol, Inc.
GRANSTAND III STANDING SYSTEM	Prime Engineering
GRANULEX	Mylan Pharmaceuticals Inc
GRANULOCOLOR	Cytocolor, Inc.
GRANUSIC	Avantor Performance Materials
GRAPH EASE	Seca Corp.
GRAPHCOMP	Pmt Corp.
GRAPHICBOX	Placon Corporation
GRAPHPACK	Hamilton Company
GRAPHPROBE	Zinetics Medical, Inc.
GRASSFIRE	Varian Medical Systems
GRASSLAB	Astro-Med, Inc.
GRATLOCH	Kmedic
GRAVI-SEAL ANALYTICAL FUNNEL	Ge Infrastructure Water & Process Technologies
GRAVIT-EYE	Sellstrom Manufacturing Co.
GRAVITY	United Syntek Corp.
GRAY	Stryker Spine
GREASE POLICE	Unit Chemical Corp.
GREAT WHITE BURS	S.S. White Burs Inc.
GREEN GRID	Smith & Nephew, Inc.
GREEN HANDLES	Smith & Nephew, Inc.
GREEN LOVE	Bio-Med U.S.A. Inc.
GREEN Z	Safetec Of America, Inc.
GREENBERG	Codman & Shurtleff, Inc
GREENIE	Shofu Dental Corporation
GREENLIGHT	Vital Signs, Inc.
GREENLIGHT II	Vital Signs, Inc.
GREENLINE	Sun-Med
GREENLINE	Sunmed Healthcare
GREENLINE	Unomedical, Inc.
GREENLINE/D	Sun-Med
GREENLITE	Infab Corp.
GREERPICK	Greer Laboratories, Inc.
GREERTRACK	Greer Laboratories, Inc.
GRID MOUNT	Hager Worldwide, Inc.
GRIDLOCK	Contech Medical, Inc.
GRIP MASTER	Creative Health Products, Inc.
GRIP REST	Better Hands Glove Products
GRIP-CERT	Mecanaids Co., Inc.
GRIP-LOK	Zefon International
GRIP-RITE	Hoyle Products, Inc.
GRIPIT	Geerpres
GRIPPER	Oral-B Laboratories, Inc.
GRIPPER	Smiths Medical Asd, Inc.
GRIPPER	Vital Signs Colorado
GRIPPER NIPPER	Rf Industries, Inc.
GRIPPER PLUS	Smiths Medical Asd, Inc.
GRIPPERS	Hoyle Products, Inc.
GRIPTITE	Tp Orthodontics, Inc.
GRIPTRACK	JTECH Medical
GRIS-PEG TABLETS 125MG + 250MG	Pedinol Pharmacal, Inc.
GRO-MINDERS	Seca Corp.
GROMED	Q.I. Medical, Inc.
GROOMER	Oster Professional Products, Inc.
GROPRO PLUS	North American Science Associates, Inc.
GROSS OUTS	Aso Corporation
GROSSE	Stryker Spine
GROUND GUARD	Powervar, Inc.
GROUNDOHMER	Sticht Inc., Herman H.
GROWTH GUIDE	Novel Products, Inc.
GRX FOAM DRESSING	Geritrex Corp.
GRX-SALINE WET DRESSING	Geritrex Corp.
GRX-WOUND GEL	Geritrex Corp.
GSB III ELBOW SYSTEM	Centerpulse Orthopedics Inc.
GTR LABS	Koch X-Ray Systems Inc
GUARD MASTER	Justrite Manufacturing Co., L.L.C.
GUARDDOG	Possis Medical, Inc.
GUARDIAN	Atlantic Ultraviolet Corp.
GUARDIAN	Dr Systems, Inc.
GUARDIAN	Draeger Safety, Inc.
GUARDIAN	Hollister Incorporated
GUARDIAN	Sunrise Medical
GUARDIAN	United States Endoscopy Group
GUARDIAN	Wright Medical Group, Inc.
GUARDIAN F	Hollister Incorporated
GUARDIAN MONITORING PACKAGE	Environmental Tectonics Corp.
GUARDIAN S	Hollister Incorporated
GUARDSMAN, BUFFALO CASE, CLC, PELICAN	Platt Luggage, Inc.
GUAVA	Guava Technologies, Inc.
GUEST-GUARD	Sellstrom Manufacturing Co.
GUIDE-FLEX	Tfx Medical Oem
GUIDE-FLO	Smiths Medical OEM
GUIDE-STRIP	Smiths Medical OEM
GUIDEFATHER	Bard Electro Physiology
GULL BRAND	Meridian Bioscience, Inc.
GUM	Sunstar Butler
GUNNELL	Gunnell, Inc.
GV350	Biomedical Life Systems, Inc.
GVII	Compex Technologies, Inc.
GYMNIC	Ball Dynamics International, Llc
GYN-A-LITE	Astralite Corporation
GYNECO	Rms Medical Products
GYNECYTE	Rms Medical Products
GYNELOOP	Rms Medical Products
GYNNIE	Stryker Corp.
GYROSCAN	Philips Medical Systems North America
GYROTORY	New Brunswick Scientific Co., Inc.
Gain	Procter & Gamble
Gaitors	Medi-Dyne Healthcare Products, L.L.C.
Gaskleen	Pall Corporation
GearWrench	Danaher Corporation
Gemini	Boston Scientific Corporation
Gendex	Danaher Corporation
Genesis	St. Jude Medical Neuromodulation Division
Genesis	St. Jude Medical, Inc.
GenesisRC	St. Jude Medical, Inc.
GenesisXP	St. Jude Medical Neuromodulation Division
GenesisXP	St. Jude Medical, Inc.
Gilbarco	Danaher Corporation
Gillette	Procter & Gamble
Gillette Complete Skincare	Procter & Gamble
Gillette Fusion	Procter & Gamble
Gleem	Procter & Gamble
Gold Probe	Boston Scientific Corporation
Gore	Knoll, Inc.
GranuFoam	Kinetic Concepts, Inc.
Graspit	Boston Scientific Corporation

GreenGuard	Pactiv Corporation
GreenSeal	Rochester Midland, Corp.
Greenfield	Boston Scientific Corporation
Guglielmi Detachable Coil	Boston Scientific-Neurovascular
GuideRight	St. Jude Medical, Inc.
H-12	Mortara Instrument, Inc.
H-BAC	North American Science Associates, Inc.
H-LINK	American Medical Alert Corp.
H-SCRIBE	Mortara Instrument, Inc.
H-TRONPLUS	Roche Insulin Delivery Systems Inc.
H-WAVE	Electronic Waveform Laboratory, Inc.
H.U.T TABLE	Medical Positioning, Inc.
H/I 200 SERIES MICROTOME	Hacker Instruments And Industries Inc.
H20	Astro-Med, Inc.
H2850	Energy Beam Sciences, Inc.
HA-1000	Lifecore Biomedical, Inc.
HA-500	Lifecore Biomedical, Inc.
HAAN CRAFTS	Aristotle Corp.
HABIB 4X	Angiodynamics, Inc.
HABIB 4X LAPAROSCOPIC	Angiodynamics, Inc.
HABITAT MONITOR	Cmt, Inc.
HACH	Hach Company / Environmental Test Systems
HACKER-BRIGHT	Hacker Instruments And Industries Inc.
HACKER-MILESTONE	Hacker Instruments And Industries Inc.
HACKETTGROUP OF COMPANIES	Maguire Enterprises, Inc.
HADECO	Koven Technology, Inc.
HADER BAR	Preat Corp.
HAEMOFLO	Novosci Corp.
HAEMOLANCE	Arkray Usa
HAEMOLANCE	Htl-Strefa, Inc.
HAEMOLANCE PLUS	Arkray Usa
HAEMOLANCE PLUS	Htl-Strefa, Inc.
HAEMOPHILUS ID II	Remel
HAISIL	Nest Group Inc., The
HAKKO	Havel's Inc.
HALFTRACK	Mizuho Osi
HALFTRX	Waterloo Healthcare, Llc
HALIFAX	Vista Lighting
HALIMETER	Interscan Corp.
HALL	Conmed Linvatec
HALLU-FIX	Integra Lifesciences Holdings Corp.
HALO	Nova Health Systems, Inc.
HALO CORDLESS LED SURGICAL HEADLIGHT	Enova Medical Technologies
HALO CROWN	Depuy Mitek, Inc.
HALOBAG	Baxa Corporation
HALOGEN FLEX	Dazor Manufacturing Corp.
HALOGEN HPX	Welch Allyn, Inc.
HALSEY	Post Glover Lifelink
HALUX	Waldmann Lighting
HAMAR	Handicap Unlimited, Inc.
HAMMER	Biomet, Inc.
HAMMER	Colours Wheelchair
HAMMER STRENGTH	Life Fitness
HAMPTON	Arlington Scientific, Inc. Asi
HAMPTON	Vista Lighting
HAN-D-MAG	R. B. Annis Instruments, Inc.
HANCOCK	Medtronic Cardiovascular Surgery, The Heart Valve Div.
HAND HELPER	Meddev Corporation
HAND KEY-PER	Multi Marketing & Manufacturing, Inc.
HAND MENTOR:	Kinetic Muscles, Inc.
HAND-FOOT II	National Biological Corp.
HAND-TROL	Conmed Corporation
HAND-TROL HANDPIECE	Conmed Corporation
HANDCLENS ALCOHOL FREE INSTANT HAND SANITIZER	Woodward Laboratories, Inc.
HANDI	Maxtec, Inc.
HANDI-GRIP	Clarke Health Care Products, Inc.
HANDI-MOVE	Surehands Lift & Care Systems
HANDI-RAMP	Handi-Cap Aids Company
HANDI-RAMP	Handi-Ramp
HANDI-SPENSER	Bio-Logics Products, Inc.
HANDI-TRAK	Handi-Ramp
HANDIDAM	Aseptico, Inc.

HANDILAB	Zonda Inc.
HANDISOL	National Biological Corp.
HANDIVAK	Allied Healthcare Products, Inc.
HANDLING,HEALING,STRENGTH	Cp Medical Corporation
HANDS FREE	All Pro Exercise Products, Inc.
HANDS-OFF	Arrow International, Inc.
HANDSHOES	Rockford Medical & Safety Co.
HANDSTAND III ASSISTED STANDING FRAME	Prime Engineering
HANDY	Shofu Dental Corporation
HANDY-SANDY	Morrison Medical
HANDY-STANDIE SPLINT	C.D. Denison Orthopaedic Appliance Corp.
HANDYGUARD	Adenna Inc.
HANDYVAC	Milex Products, Inc.
HANHART	Eric Armin Inc.
HANS	Ortho-Kinetics, Inc.
HANSATON	R And L Hearing Services
HAPAD COMF-ORTHOTIC	Hapad, Inc.
HAPPY MORNING	Hager Worldwide, Inc.
HAPPY MORNING DELUXE	Hager Worldwide, Inc.
HAPPY MORNING TRAVELER	Hager Worldwide, Inc.
HAPPYFEET	Crosstex International,Inc.
HAPSET	Lifecore Biomedical, Inc.
HARC	Harc Mercantile Ltd.
HARD HAT	Hds Specialty Vehicles
HARDIE	Shofu Dental Corporation
HARDYDISK AST	Hardy Diagnostics
HARLECO	Emd Chemicals Inc.
HARLEQUIN EYEWEAR	Zyloware Corporation
HARMONIC	Ethicon Endo-Surgery, Inc.
HARMONY	Follett Corp.
HARMONY	Medela, Inc.
HARMONY	Surmodics, Inc.
HARMONY ALLOYS	Ivoclar Vivadent, Inc.
HARPENDEN	Creative Health Products, Inc.
HARRIS	Anatech, Ltd.
HARRIS	Kendro Laboratory Products
HART	Princo Instruments, Inc.
HARVARD	Ranfac Corp.
HARVARD APPARATUS	Harvard Apparatus, Inc.
HARVARD APPARATUS	Nest Group Inc., The
HARVARD PUMP	Harvard Apparatus, Inc.
HARVESTER 96	Tomtec
HARVEY	Thermo Fisher Scientific Inc.
HASKEL	Haskel International, Inc.
HAT 300	Oscor, Inc.
HAWK	Nspire Health, Inc
HAWK	Wave Form Systems, Inc.
HAWKINS	Medical Device Technologies, Inc. (Md Tech)
HAWS	Haws Corporation
HAYES	Hely And Weber
HAZMIN	Logical Technology, Inc.
HB-METER	Leica Microsystems, Inc., Educational & Analytical Division
HC-SERIES	Taylor Wharton
HC1	CAREFUSION 211, INC..
HCLL	Mediware Information Systems, Inc.
HCM4000	Hacker Instruments And Industries Inc.
HCS	First Aid Bandage Co., Inc.
HCS FIBER	Ofs, Specialty Photonics Division
HD 200 PLUS	Mallinckrodt, Inc.
HD-3000	Stryker Imaging
HD-SECURA	B. Braun Medical Inc., Renal Therapies Div.
HDI/PULSEWAVE(TM) CR-2000 RESEARCH CARDIOVASCULAR PROFILING SYSTEM	Hypertension Diagnostics, Inc.
HDL PLUS	Quantimetrix Corporation
HDP	Starkey Laboratories, Inc.
HDS	Hds Specialty Vehicles
HEAD BLOCKS	Morrison Medical
HEAD HOLDERS	Cfi Medical Solutions (Contour Fabricators, Inc.)
HEAD VISE	Morrison Medical
HEAD VISE II	Morrison Medical
HEAD WEDGE	Ambu, Inc.
HEADACHE ICE PILLO	Core Products International, Inc.
HEADACHE WRAP	Bean Products

HEADBAND LOUPES	Almore International, Inc.
HEADBED	Laerdal Medical Corporation
HEADBED II	Medical Plastics Laboratory, Inc.
HEADER BAGS	Extra Packaging, Corp.
HEADLINER	Designs For Comfort, Inc.
HEADMASTER PLUS	Prentke Romich Company
HEADMASTERS	Tornado Industries
HEADMOUSE	Prentke Romich Company
HEALING ENVIRONMENT	Grant Airmass Corporation
HEALING LAMP	Biofeedback Instrument Corp.
HEALIX	Depuy Mitek, Inc.
HEALON	Abbott Medical Optics Inc.
HEALTH BIKE	Battle Creek Equipment Co.
HEALTH CHECK CENTER	Lifeclinic International, Inc.
HEALTH EDCO	Wrs Group, Ltd.
HEALTH FOOT ILLUMINATATED INSPECETION MIRROR	Woodward Laboratories, Inc.
HEALTH GARDS	Hospital Specialty Company
HEALTH IMPRESSIONS	Wrs Group, Ltd.
HEALTH O METER PROFESSIONAL	Pelstar Llc (Health O Meter Professional)
HEALTH O METER PROPLUS	Pelstar Llc (Health O Meter Professional)
HEALTH PAK	Health-Pak, Inc.
HEALTH SUPPORT	Carolon Company
HEALTH TRACK II	Eaton Medical Devices, Inc.
HEALTH WALKER	Battle Creek Equipment Co.
HEALTH-CODER	Timemed Labeling Systems, Inc.
HEALTH-O-METER	Creative Health Products, Inc.
HEALTHAIRE	Respironics Georgia, Inc.
HEALTHCAIR	Ohio Medical Corp.
HEALTHCARE	Clinical Data Inc
HEALTHCARE CONCEPTS 4	Interspec Fabrics
HEALTHCARE CONCEPTS 5	Interspec Fabrics
HEALTHCARE CONCEPTS 6	Interspec Fabrics
HEALTHDRI	Salk Inc.
HEALTHFLEX	Langer, Inc.
HEALTHIER	Chi'Am International
HEALTHSTREAM	Healthstream, Inc.
HEALTHSTREAM/EDUCATION DESIGN	Healthstream, Inc.
HEALTHTEST	Akers Biosciences, Inc.
HEALWELL	Fla Orthopedics, Inc.
HEALY	Biomet, Inc.
HEARING COMFORT SYSTEM	Siemens Hearing Instruments, Inc.
HEARING CONSERVATION	Hal-Hen Company, Inc.
HEARLINK	Oticon, Inc.
HEART	Westmed, Inc.
HEART CARD	Instromedix, A Card Guard Co.
HEART LASER	Plc Medical Systems
HEART LASER CO2 HEART LASER 2 RenalGuard	Plc Systems Inc.
HEART SOUNDS TUTOR	Pinnacle Technology Group, Inc.
HEART-CHILL	Genesee Biomedical, Inc.
HEART-LIFT	Genesee Biomedical, Inc.
HEART-PICK:BEAT-PICK	Spirig Advanced Technologies, Inc.
HEARTFUSION	Syntermed, Inc.
HEARTLINE	Cardiac Science Corp.
HEARTLINK I	Cardiac Telecom Corporation
HEARTLINK II	Cardiac Telecom Corporation
HEARTMAN	Cardionics, Inc.
HEARTMATE	Thoratec Corporation
HEARTQUEST	World Heart Inc.
HEARTRAK	Mednet Healthcare Technologies, Inc.
HEARTSAVEDVAD	World Heart Inc.
HEARTSAVER	World Heart Inc.
HEARTSIM	Laerdal Medical Corporation
HEARTSIM INTERACTIVE TRAINING SYSTEM	Medical Plastics Laboratory, Inc.
HEARTSINES	Vacumed
HEARTSTART	Laerdal Medical Corporation
HEAT-LES	Pneumatic Products Corporation
HEATED WIRE CIRCUITS	Atlantic Medical Specialties
HEATRON	Halbar North, Inc.
HEATSEEKIR	Sea Horse Bio Science
HEAVY	Nest Group Inc., The
HEAVY METAL	Universal Gym Equipment
HEAVY WEIGHT	Omnimed, Inc. (Beam Products)
HECON	Danaher Corporation
HEDROCEL	Implex Corp.
HEDSTROM	Moyco Technologies, Inc.
HEEL FLOAT	Skil-Care Corp.
HEEL HUGGER	Brown Medical Industries
HEEL HUGGER	Children's Medical Ventures, Inc.
HEEL SLOPE	Span-America Medical Systems, Inc.
HEELIFT-r SUSPENSION BOOT	Dm Systems, Inc.
HEELIFTr SMOOTH BOOT	Dm Systems, Inc.
HEELPLEEZR	Polymer Concepts, Inc.
HEELWEDGE	Darco International, Inc.
HEFTY	Pactiv Corporation
HEIDLEBERG	Smith & Nephew Inc.- Orthopaedics Division
HEIFETZ	Scanlan International, Inc.
HEIGHT RIGHT	Bergeron Health Care
HEIGHT-RITE	Seca Corp.
HEIGHTRONIC	Seca Corp.
HEIMAN	Vespo Marketing Assoc., Inc.
HEINE	Bulbworks, Inc.
HEISE	Dresser Inc., Dresser Measurement Division
HELA PURE	Biovest International, Inc.
HELASCRIBE	Promega Corp.
HELICON	Siemens Medical Solutions Usa, Inc.
HELICOVIEW	Gi Supply
HELIOMOLAR	Ivoclar Vivadent, Inc.
HELIOS	Covidien (Formerly Nellcor Puritan Bennett / Tyco Healthcare)
HELIOS	Thermo Spectronic
HELIOS	Varian Medical Systems
HELIOSEAL F	Ivoclar Vivadent, Inc.
HELIPAQ	Micrus Corporation
HELISTAT	Integra Lifesciences Corporation
HELITENE	Integra Lifesciences Corporation
HELIX HYDROJET	Erbe Usa, Inc.
HELIXATE	Csl Behring
HELIXMARK	Helix Medical, Inc.
HELP ALERT	Rf Technologies
HELP MATE	Tu-Way American Group
HELPING HANDS TRAY	Helping Hand Trays
HELPING HANDS, PETA-UK	Mecanaids Co., Inc.
HELY & WEBER	Ortholine
HEM-O-LOK	Teleflex Medical
HEM-SP	Fujirebio Diagnostics, Inc. (Fdi)
HEMA	Hospira Inc.
HEMA BUTTONS	Materials Development Corporation
HEMA SCREEN	Immunostics, Inc.
HEMA-CHEK	Siemens Healthcare Diagnostics Inc.
HEMA-COMBISTIX	Siemens Healthcare Diagnostics Inc.
HEMA-TEK	Siemens Healthcare Diagnostics Inc.
HEMACOLOR	Emd Chemicals Inc.
HEMAGUARD	MAQUET
HEMASTIX	Siemens Healthcare Diagnostics Inc.
HEMATACHEK	Separation Technology Inc
HEMATASEAL	Separation Technology Inc
HEMATASTAT	Separation Technology Inc
HEMATO-CLAD	Drummond Scientific Co.
HEMATROL	J&S Medical Associates
HEMATRON	Fenwal Inc.
HEMATRUE	Heska Corporation
HEMATYPE	Fenwal Inc.
HEMAWAY	Instrument Specialists, Inc.
HEMAWIPE	Idexx Laboratories, Inc.
HEMCON	Hemcon Medical Technologies, Inc.
HEMISPHERE MODULAR CUP	Ortho Development Corp.
HEMO-NATE	Utah Medical Products, Inc.
HEMO-SEAL	Ethicon, Inc.
HEMOCARD	PerkinElmer
HEMOCARE	Mediware Information Systems, Inc.
HEMOCHRON	International Technidyne Corp.
HEMOCLIP	Teleflex Medical
HEMOCLIP PLUS	Teleflex Medical
HEMOCOR HPH	Minntech Corporation
HEMOCOR HPHA,Ar HEMOCONCENTRATORS	Cantel Medical Corp.
HEMOFIL	Baxter International Inc

HEMOFLOW	Fenwal Inc.
HEMOGLOBIN SPECIES	Exocell, Inc.
HEMOGLUE	Whalen Biomedical Incorporated
HEMOMODULATION	Energex Systems Inc.
HEMOSIL	Instrumentation Laboratory Company
HEMOSTATIC ERASER	Mentor Ophthalmics, Inc.
HEMOTEMP	Biosynergy, Inc.
HEMOTHERM	Cincinnati Sub-Zero Products, Inc., Medical Division
HEMOVAC	Zimmer Orthopaedic Surgical Products
HEMOVALVE	Boston Scientific Interventional Technologies
HEMOX-ANALYZER	Tcs Scientific Corp.
HEMOXIMETER	Radiometer America, Inc.
HEP - AID	H & S Manufacturing, Inc.
HEP-2000	Global Focus (G.F.M.D. Ltd.)
HEP-2000	Immuno Concepts N.A. Ltd.
HEP-X	Weiman Healthcare Solutions
HEPA-AIRE	Abatement Technologies, Inc.
HEPA-CARE	Abatement Technologies, Inc.
HEPA-SHURE	Biomerieux Inc.
HEPACOAT	Cordis Corporation
HEPAIR	Cleanroom Systems
HEPANAIRE HP-50	Summit Hill Laboratories
HEPARIN COMPLEX-T	Tua Systems, Inc.
HEPASTATIC	Arc Medical, Inc.
HEPCOM	Medtronic Perfusion Systems
HEPEX	Nuaire, Inc.
HEPTEST	American Diagnostica, Inc.
HERAEUS	Kendro Laboratory Products
HERBST CRADLE	Brown Medical Industries
HERCON NTS/FAHERCON LABORATORIES	Hercon Laboratories Corp.
HERCULES	Ams Innovative Center-San Jose
HERCULES	Pride Mobility Products Corp.
HERCULES	Skytron
HERCULES	Wells Johnson Co.
HERCULEX	Herculite Products, Inc.
HERCULITE	Herculite Products, Inc.
HERITAGE	Astro-Med, Inc.
HERITAGE	Radix Corp.
HERMAR	Her-Mar, Inc.
HERNIA GUARD	Bell-Horn, Inc.
HERNIA SUPPORTS	I.M.K. Distributors, Inc.
HERPE SELECT	Focus Technologies
HERPES MPLEXT	Prodesse, Inc.
HERRICK LACRIMAL PLUG	Lacrimedics
HESKA	Heska Corporation
HESPAN	B. Braun Oem Division, B. Braun Medical Inc.
HESSLER PERFORMS	Hessler Forms & Labels
HESSLER FORMS & LABELS	Hessler Forms & Labels
HETTICH	Pro Scientific Inc.
HEX BASE IV POLE	Pryor Products
HEX HANDLE	Novosci Corp.
HEX-FIX	Smith & Nephew Inc.- Orthopaedics Division
HEX-THREAD	Zimmer Dental, Inc.
HEXABRIX	Mallinckrodt, Inc.
HEXAFLOW PURIFICATION PROCESS	Airistar Technologies, L.L.C.
HEXAPLEXr PLUS	Prodesse, Inc.
HEXAWIPE(TM)	Contec, Inc.
HEXTEND	Hospira Inc.
HEYMAN	C. R. Bard, Inc., Bard Urological Div.
HF27 ULTRASOUND	Hill Laboratories Co.
HFX	Fischer Medical Technologies Inc.
HG80 BRACES	Mueller Sports Medicine
HGPC	D.M. Davis Inc.
HGRP	D.M. Davis Inc.
HI GLOSS	George Taub Products & Fusion Co., Inc.
HI-ART	Tomotherapy Incorporated
HI-D	Sscor
HI-FLO	Camfil Farr
HI-FLO	Smiths Medical OEM
HI-FLOW 70T	Vortran Medical Technology
HI-FLOW SILVER	Cook Inc.
HI-FLUX	R. B. Annis Instruments, Inc.
HI-I	Fricke Dental Manufacturing Co.
HI-LO	Aigner Index, Inc.
HI-LO RACKS	Falcon Products, Inc.
HI-OX80	CAREFUSION 211, INC..
HI-PERFLEX	Bard Electro Physiology
HI-PORE	Bio-Rad Laboratories, Life Science Group
HI-RES	Usb Corporation
HI-RIB	Pawling Corp., Architectural Prod. Div.
HI-TEMP	Bovie Medical Corp.
HI-TIP	Bovie Medical Corp.
HI-TORQUE CROSS-IT XT	Abbott Laboratories
HIBICLENS	Molnlycke Health Care Inc.
HIBISTAT	Molnlycke Health Care Inc.
HIFLO	Dentalez Group
HIGH DEFINITION IMAGING	Phillips Ultrasound
HIGH FREQUENCY ULTRASOUND BIOMICROSCOPE.	Sonomed, Inc.
HIGH HAT	Tp Orthodontics, Inc.
HIGH PERFORMANCE(TM)	Lytron, Inc.
HIGH RISK	American Healthcare Products, Inc.
HIGH SOCIETY	Essential Medical Supply, Inc.
HIGH VOLT GALVANIC	American Imex
HIGH-CLEAN	Clean Esd Products, Inc.
HIGH-DEMAND	Conmed Corporation
HIGH-PRO	Bellco Glass, Inc.
HILAN	Aesculap Implant Systems Inc.
HILCO	Hilco
HILGER	Wr Medical Electronics Co.
HILITE	Shofu Dental Corporation
HILL ADJUSTABLE	Hill Laboratories Co.
HILL AIR FLEX	Hill Laboratories Co.
HILL ANATOMOTOR	Hill Laboratories Co.
HILLMED	Hillusa Corp.
HIMOD	Trelleborg Sealing Solutions
HINT PRO	Natus Medical Inc.
HINTEGRA	Integra Lifesciences Holdings Corp.
HIPCHEK	Medstat Inc.
HIPGRIP	Sunmedica
HIPLOC	Medstat Inc.
HIPRO	Qrp, Inc.
HIPROTECTOR	Graphic Controls Corp.
HIPSAVER	Hipsavers, Inc.
HISTO PLAS	Bio Plas, Inc.
HISTO-LOGIC	Sakura Finetek U.S.A., Inc.
HISTO-PAK	Statlab Medical Products, Inc.
HISTO-TEK	Sakura Finetek U.S.A., Inc.
HISTO/ORIENTATOR	Triangle Biomedical Sciences, Inc.
HISTOBRUSH	Puritan Medical Products Company Llc
HISTOCHOICE	Amresco Inc.
HISTOCLONE-L	Peregrine Pharmaceuticals, Inc.
HISTOFREEZER	Orasure Technologies, Inc.
HISTOPREP	Fisher Scientific Co., Llc.
HISTOPRO	Hacker Instruments And Industries Inc.
HISTORY MAKAR	Information Health Network
HISTOSTAIN	Life Technologies Corporation
HITACHI	Hitachi High Technologies America
HITACHI	Hitachi Kokusai Electric America, Ltd.
HITE-LOCK	Seca Corp.
HITE-ROLLER	Seca Corp.
HLD SYSTEMS	Cenorin
HLR	Brunswick Laboratories
HLT LENS	Psc Medical, Inc.
HMC	Modulation Optics, Inc.
HMD SKED STRETCHER	Skedco, Inc.
HMEXPRESS	Carecentric, Inc.
HMGN	Hemagen Diagnostics, Inc.
HMS	Hospital Marketing Svcs. Company, Inc.
HMS Plus	Medtronic Perfusion Systems
HMV	Invacare Corporation
HO MED	Homak Manufacturing Company Inc.
HOFFMAN MODULATION CONTRAST	Modulation Optics, Inc.
HOFFMANN	Stryker Corp.
HOFFMANN II	Stryker Corp.
HOGGAN DUMBBELLS	Hoggan Health Industries, Inc.
HOIST FITNESS	Med-Fit Systems, Inc.

HOKANSON	Hokanson Inc., D.E.
HOL-DEX	Aigner Index, Inc.
HOLD-ITS	Micromedics
HOLD-TEMP	Cres Cor
HOLEX	Boston Scientific Interventional Technologies
HOLLIGARD	Hollister Incorporated
HOLLIHESIVE	Hollister Incorporated
HOLLISEAL	Hollister Incorporated
HOLLISTER	Hollister Incorporated
HOLLOW-FLEX	Starkey Laboratories, Inc.
HOLTER FOR WINDOWS+	Rozinn By Scottcare Corporation
HOLTER PERFORMER	Applied Cardiac Systems, Inc.
HOLTER REPORTER	Applied Cardiac Systems, Inc.
HOLTRODE	Conmed Corporation
HOME ACCESS EXPRESS- RESULTS IN 3 DAYS	Home Access Health Corp.
HOME ACCESS- RESULTS IN 7 DAYS	Home Access Health Corp.
HOME RANGER	Pre Pak Products, Inc.
HOMEAID.COM	Home-Aid-Healthcare, Inc.
HOMECHOICE	Baxter Healthcare Corporation, Renal
HOMEFILL	Invacare Corporation
HOMELINE	Linak U.S. Inc.
HOMELINK	Aprex, A Division Of Aardex
HOMEPUMP	I-Flow Corporation
HOMESTRETCH	Glacier Cross, Inc.
HOMESYS	Infosys, Inc.
HOMETRAC	The Saunders Group
HOMEWAITER #75	Inclinator Co. Of America
HONAN	Lebanon Corp., The
HONEYCOMB	Avcor Health Care Products, Inc.
HOOD	E. Benson Hood Laboratories, Inc.
HOOD MATE	Drummond Scientific Co.
HOOK-LOCK	Tetra Medical Supply Corp.
HOOKUP	Whitney Products, Inc.
HOOLIGAN TOOL	Paratech, Inc.
HOPE PROCESSORS	Koch X-Ray Systems Inc
HOPKINS	Karl Storz Endoscopy-America Inc.
HOR-SHU	Surgical Appliance Industries
HORIZON	Arlington Scientific, Inc. Asi
HORIZON	Codonics
HORIZON	Dent Zar, Inc.
HORIZON	Hill-Rom Holdings, Inc.
HORIZON	Living Earth Crafts
HORIZON	Mexpo International, Inc.
HORIZON	Teleflex Medical
HORIZON ANGIO	Mennen Medical Corp.
HORIZON CLIPS	Teleflex Medical
HORIZON COMPACT	Mennen Medical Corp.
HORIZON LITE	Mennen Medical Corp.
HORIZON SE	Mennen Medical Corp.
HORIZON SUBTALAR IMPLANT	Biopro, Inc.
HORNBRO	Bell-Horn, Inc.
HOS-FLEX	Hos-Pillow Corp.
HOS-PILLOW	Hos-Pillow Corp.
HOSOBUCHI	Bulbworks, Inc.
HOSPI-THERM KIT	Mabis Healthcare Inc.
HOSPIRA	Omni Medical Supply Inc.
HOSPITAK	Unomedical, Inc.
HOSPITAL GRADE	Fla Orthopedics, Inc.
HOSPITAL'S CHORD CLAMP	Directmed, Inc.
HOSPITAL'S SPECULA	Directmed, Inc.
HOSPITALDIRECT	Healthstream, Inc.
HOSPITALITY SUITE	Computrition, Inc.
HOSPITOTE	Healthmark Industries
HOSTESS	Juzo
HOT BOX SYSTEM	Billups-Rothenberg, Inc.
HOT CHIMNEYS	Billups-Rothenberg, Inc.
HOT FILTERS	Billups-Rothenberg, Inc.
HOT SAMPLER	Wilson-Cook Medical, Inc.
HOT STUFF	Mueller Sports Medicine
HOT TRAY	Plastocon, Inc.
HOT `R COLD	Tetra Medical Supply Corp.
HOT-LINE	Advanced Instruments Inc.
HOTBLADE	Patton Surgical Corp.
HOTELSTAT	Psg Controls, Inc.
HOTEMP	Servolift/Eastern Corp.
HOTLINE	Smiths Medical Asd, Inc.
HOTMITT	Carolon Company
HOTSHOTS	Sellstrom Manufacturing Co.
HOTSTART-IT	Usb Corporation
HOTSY CAUTERY	Shippert Medical Technologies Corp.
HOTWRAP	Carolon Company
HOUSECALLS	Televox Software, Inc.
HOUVA II	National Biological Corp.
HOVERMATT, HOVERMAXX, HOVERJACK	Hovertech International
HOWARD PRODUCTS	United Receptacle
HOWARD'S HARNESS	Cfi Medical Solutions (Contour Fabricators, Inc.)
HOWELL	Wilson-Cook Medical, Inc.
HOYER	Joerns Healthcare, Inc
HOYER	Sunrise Medical
HP	Camfil Farr
HP	Thales Components Corporation
HP BLUE	Anatech, Ltd.
HP YELLOW	Anatech, Ltd.
HPE	Bio-Rad Laboratories, Life Science Group
HPFAST	Gi Supply
HPONE	Gi Supply
HPSA	Meridian Bioscience, Inc.
HR MAT	Tekscan, Inc.
HRLC	Bio-Rad Laboratories, Life Science Group
HRV 4000EM	All-Tronics Medical Systems
HSP ALABAMA MOBILE CABINET WITH ARMREST AND ALL ACCESSORIES Health Science Products, Inc.	
HSP ART ELECTROSURGE	Health Science Products, Inc.
HSP ART PIEZO SCALER	Health Science Products, Inc.
HSP ASSOCIATE GROUP CABINET	Health Science Products, Inc.
HSP DAYLIGHT	Health Science Products, Inc.
HSP DENTASSIST LIBERTY III-A	Health Science Products, Inc.
HSP DENTASSIST LIBERTY III-B	Health Science Products, Inc.
HSP DENTASSIST LIBERTY III-C	Health Science Products, Inc.
HSP GLOWS	Health Science Products, Inc.
HSP HYDENT	Health Science Products, Inc.
HSP INTEGRA	Health Science Products, Inc.
HSP NORTH CAROLINA MOBILE CABINET AITH ALL ACCESSORIES Health Science Products, Inc.	
HSP TEAM CENTER II	Health Science Products, Inc.
HT	Byron Medical
HT WIZARD	Tremetrics
HTA	Bruder Healthcare Company
HTC	Hologic, Inc.
HTO	Centerpulse Orthopedics Inc.
HTR	Park Dental Research Corp./Implant Center
HUAXIA	Lhasa Oms, Inc.
HUBBARD SCIENTIFIC	Aristotle Corp.
HUBERPRO	Command Medical Products, Inc.
HUBGUARD	Tri-State Hospital Supply Corp.
HUC	Quantimetrix Corporation
HUCO DIAMOND KNIVES	Gwb International, Ltd.
HUCO RESPOSABLE CRYSTAL BLADES	Gwb International, Ltd.
HUDSON	Creative Health Products, Inc.
HUDSON RCI	Dma Med-Chem Corporation
HUDSON RCI	Teleflex Medical
HUEBSCH	Huebsch Sales
HUESTIS-CASCADE	Huestis Medical
HUGGABLES	Conmed Corporation
HUGGER	Cfi Medical Solutions (Contour Fabricators, Inc.)
HUKA	Clarke Health Care Products, Inc.
HUMAN LINK	Oticon, Inc.
HUMANE RESTRAINT	Humane Restraint Co Inc
HUMATE-P	Csl Behring
HUMBOLDT	Hager Worldwide, Inc.
HUMI-FLOW	Northgate Technologies Inc.
HUMIDAIRE	Resmed Corp.
HUMIDAIRE 2I	Resmed Corp.
HUMIDAIRE 2IC	Resmed Corp.
HUMIDAIRE 3I	Resmed Corp.
HUMIDICHIP	Andersen Products, Inc.,

HUMIPICK	Spirig Advanced Technologies, Inc.
HUMIRA	Abbott Laboratories
HUMMINGBIRD	Innerspace, Inc.
HUMPHREY	Carl Zeiss Meditec Inc.
HUNSTAD	Byron Medical
HUR FITNESS	Med-Fit Systems, Inc.
HURICANE III	Eagle Sports Chairs
HURICANE	Eagle Sports Chairs
HURRICANE	Pride Mobility Products Corp.
HURRISEAL R	Beutlich Lp, Pharmaceuticals
HURRIVIEW TM	Beutlich Lp, Pharmaceuticals
HUSH MUFFIN	Dixie Ems Supply
HUSHKART	Healthmark Industries
HUSKY WIRE SHELVING	Tecni-Quip
HVPC	JACE SYSTEMS, INC
HWATO	Lhasa Oms, Inc.
HX	Thales Components Corporation
HY-BOND	Shofu Dental Corporation
HY-GENE SEMINAL FLUID COLLECTION KIT	Apex Medical Technologies, Inc.
HY-SPEED	Ertelalsop
HY-TAPE	Hy-Tape International
HYBRID	Shofu Dental Corporation
HYBRID	Teleflex Medical
HYCHECK	Bd Diagnostic Systems
HYCOAT	The Hymed Group Corp.
HYCON	Biotest Diagnostic Corp.
HYCURE	The Hymed Group Corp.
HYCURE SMART GEL:CELLERATERX	The Hymed Group Corp.
HYDAK	Biocoat, Inc.
HYDE	Perkinelmer Optoelectronics
HYDENT	Pascal Company, Inc.
HYDRA	Mesa Laboratories, Inc.
HYDRA	Thermo Fisher Scientific
HYDRA VISION	Mallinckrodt, Inc.
HYDRABRASION	Innovative Med Inc.
HYDRAFACIAL MD	Edge Systems Corporation
HYDRAGEL	Sebia Electrophoresis
HYDRAGEL AC	Covidien Lp, Formerly Registered As United States Surgical
HYDRANAL	Crescent Chemical Co., Inc.
HYDRAPLUS	Sebia Electrophoresis
HYDRARIDE II	Inclinator Co. Of America
HYDRASEALER	Forward Technology
HYDRASOFT	Coopervision Inc.
HYDRASOFT	The Cooper Companies, Inc
HYDRASPUN	Ahlstrom Windsor Locks Llc
HYDRASYS	Sebia Electrophoresis
HYDRIA	Micro Essential Laboratory, Inc.
HYDRISALIC	Pedinol Pharmacal, Inc.
HYDRISINOL	Pedinol Pharmacal, Inc.
HYDRIX	Synovis Life Technologies, Inc.
HYDRO STAR SPOT COOLING	Aqua Products Company, Inc.
HYDRO TECH	Y.I. Ventures, Llc
HYDRO VAC	Hager Worldwide, Inc.
HYDRO-FLO, SANI-TEK	Ethicare Products
HYDRO-SIL	Tua Systems, Inc.
HYDRO-SIL 2001	Tua Systems, Inc.
HYDRO-SIL-2000	Tua Systems, Inc.
HYDRO-SIL-D	Tua Systems, Inc.
HYDRO-SILK	Tua Systems, Inc.
HYDRO-SILK 2002	Tua Systems, Inc.
HYDRO-SILK IPT	Tua Systems, Inc.
HYDRO-SLIK	Tua Systems, Inc.
HYDRO-SLIP	Hydromer, Inc.
HYDRO-THERM	Intersurgical Inc.
HYDRO-TRACH T	Intersurgical Inc.
HYDROBEAM	Biolase Technology, Inc.
HYDROBLAST CLEANING	Isopure Corp.
HYDROCEL GEODESIC SENSOR NET	Electrical Geodesics, Incorporated
HYDROCELL	Nest Group Inc., The
HYDROCERIN	Geritrex Corp.
HYDROCHOPPER	Katena Products, Inc.
HYDROCLAVE	Thermo Fisher Scientific Inc.
HYDROCOAT	Zimmer Orthopaedic Surgical Products
HYDROCOL	Mylan Pharmaceuticals Inc
HYDROCOLLATOR	Chattanooga Group
HYDROCOLLATOR STEAM PACKS	Chattanooga Group
HYDROCONVERTIBLE	Patterson Medical Holdings, Inc.
HYDROCURVE	Ciba Vision
HYDROFERA	Hydrofera Llc
HYDROFILCON (METHAFILCON A)	Cal Bionics, Inc.
HYDROFLO	Vital Concepts, Inc.
HYDROFLOW	Concepts International, Inc.
HYDROGAUZE	Conmed Corporation
HYDROLIFT	Whitehall Manufacturing
HYDROMARC SPHERE	Vistakon, Inc.
HYDROMARC TORIC	Vistakon, Inc.
HYDROMER	Hydromer, Inc.
HYDRON	Allergan
HYDROPEEL	Edge Systems Corporation
HYDROPHILIC WOUND DRESSING	Geritrex Corp.
HYDROPHOR	Geritrex Corp.
HYDROPHOR GAUZE	Geritrex Corp.
HYDROPHOTONICS	Biolase Technology, Inc.
HYDROPLASTIC	Tak Systems
HYDROSET	Stryker Biotech
HYDROSET	Stryker Corp.
HYDROSET	Stryker Howmedica Osteonics
HYDROSHEAR	Applied Biosystems
HYDROSORB	Quantachrome
HYDROSOUND	ArjoHuntleigh
HYDROSTAND	Novel Products, Inc.
HYDROSWAGE	Haskel International, Inc.
HYDROTANK	Novel Products, Inc.
HYDROTHANE	Advansource Biomaterials Corp.
HYDROTHERM	Pelton Shepherd Industries
HYDROVOID	Air Control, Inc.
HYDROXI-FLEX	Impladent Ltd.
HYDROXILINE	George Taub Products & Fusion Co., Inc.
HYFAB	Fabrite Laminating Corp.
HYFRECATOR	Conmed Corporation
HYFRECATOR 2000 ESU	Conmed Corporation
HYFRECATOR PLUS	Conmed Corporation
HYGEA	Professional Disposables International, Inc.
HYGEAIRE	Atlantic Ultraviolet Corp.
HYGEIA TOUCHFREE SOAP DISPENSER	Questech International, Inc.
HYGENIQUE	Hygiene Specialties, Inc./Andermac, Inc.
HYGENIQUE PLUS	Andermac, Inc.
HYGIENA TRACHE	Apdyne Medical Company
HYGOLET	Hygolet Usa
HYGOPLAST	Hygolet Usa
HYGROTEST	Testo, Inc.
HYLITE	Almore International, Inc.
HYPAFIX	Smith & Nephew, Inc.
HYPE	Current Technologies Inc
HYPERCARB	Thermo Fisher Scientific
HYPERFLEX	Smiths Medical Asd
HYPERFORM	The Hygenic Corp.
HYPERGEL	Sca Personal Care, North America
HYPERSIL	Thermo Fisher Scientific
HYPERTHERMIA	Bsd Medical Corporation
HYPO-CHLOR	Veltek Associates, Inc.
HYPO-CLEAR	Dukal Corporation
HYPO-JECT	Cp Medical Corporation
HYPO-PORE	Dukal Corporation
HYPO-SILK	Dukal Corporation
HYPURITY	Thermo Fisher Scientific
HYS-T-TUBE	Zimmer Orthopaedic Surgical Products
HYSTEROCAM	Karl Storz Endoscopy-America Inc.
HYSTEROFLATOR	Karl Storz Endoscopy-America Inc.
HYSTEROMAT	Karl Storz Endoscopy-America Inc.
HYSYNAL	The Hygenic Corp.
HYTONE	The Hygenic Corp.
HYVISC	Anika Therapeutics
Hach	Danaher Corporation
HaloSource	Halosource, Inc.
Hancock	Medtronic, Inc.

Hand Mentor	Healthsouth Corporation
Hansatome	Bausch & Lomb
Healthy Defense	Ortho Dermatologics
Healthy Skin	Ortho Dermatologics
HeartAssist 5 Ventricular Assist Device (VAD)	Micromed Technology, Inc.
Heat On Demand	Aladdin Synergetics, Inc.
Helixone	Fresenius Medical Care North America
Hemaprep	J.P. Gilbert Co.
Hemisphere	Boston Scientific Corporation
Hemocor	Medtronic Perfusion Systems
Herbs for Kids	Nutraceutical International Corp.
Hydratome	Boston Scientific Corporation
HydroSteer	St. Jude Medical, Inc.
HydroThermablator	Boston Scientific Corporation
I 6000 STAINING SYSTEM	Biogenex Laboratories
I GUARD	Sun-Med
I PLATE	Bd Diagnostic Systems
I-C3	Rayovac
I-CATH	Charter Medical Ltd.
I-PLANT SEED	Implant Sciences Corp.
I-PROX	Hager Worldwide, Inc.
I-PROX P	Hager Worldwide, Inc.
I-STAT	Abbott Laboratories
I-STAT	Heska Corporation
I-SUITE	Stryker Corp.
I-SUITE	Stryker Endoscopy
I-SWITCH	Stryker Corp.
I-SWITCH	Stryker Endoscopy
I.C. ATTACHMENT	Parkell, Inc.
I.C.V TABLE	Medical Positioning, Inc.
I.D. WAX	Hager Worldwide, Inc.
I.V. HOUSE INTRAVENOUS SITE PROTECTORS	I.V. House, Inc.
I.V. START PAK	Becton Dickinson Infusion Therapy Systems, Inc.
I.V. STRIP	E-Med Corp.
I1000 ANTIGEN RETRIEVAL SYSTEM	Biogenex Laboratories
I3SYSTEM-ABD	Innovative Imaging, Inc.
I4	Lw Scientific
IBED	Stryker Corp.
IBF	Consumaquip Corporation
IBS ALLOGRAFT	Ortho Development Corp.
IBV	Spiration Inc.
IC EYEWEAR	Crosstex International,Inc.
IC-2A	Bio-Med Devices, Inc.
IC2A-MRI	Bio-Med Devices, Inc.
ICA	Radiometer America, Inc.
ICE	Perfecseal
ICE	Pyramid Orthodontics
ICE CUBE	Pyramid Orthodontics
ICE IT	Battle Creek Equipment Co.
ICE N HEAT	Back Support Systems
ICE N HEAT	Regency Product International
ICE ON THE RUN	Contour Pak, Inc.
ICE PRO	Follett Corp.
ICE QUBE	Halbar North, Inc.
ICE R.O.M.	Dura-Kold Corp.
ICE.DEVICE	Follett Corp.
ICEKOLD	Duro-Med Industries
ICL	Staar Surgical Co.
ICON	Deltatrak, Inc.
ICON	Idexx Laboratories, Inc.
ICON CUSTOM KNEE BRACES	Omni Life Science, Inc.
ICOS	Integra Lifesciences Holdings Corp.
ICRS	Addition Technology, Inc.
ICTOTEST	Siemens Healthcare Diagnostics Inc.
ICU BED	Metronix
ID HOLDERS	Key-Bak
ID MARKER	Hager Worldwide, Inc.
ID ONE	Concepts International, Inc.
ID TAB	Hager Worldwide, Inc.
ID-2	Osada, Inc.
IDEALBINDE	Lohmann & Rauscher, Inc.
IDEEA	Minisun, Llc
IDENT-A	Hollister Incorporated
IDENT-A-BAND	Hollister Incorporated
IDENTI-MARKERS	Jaece Industries, Inc.
IDENTI-MATCH	Bio-Logics Products, Inc.
IDENTI-PLUGS	Jaece Industries, Inc.
IDENTI-PRINT	Bio-Logics Products, Inc.
IDENTI-SCAN	Bio-Logics Products, Inc.
IDENTIC	Cadco Dental Products
IDENTIC	Dux Dental
IDENTICULT	Pml Microbiologicals
IDENTIDEX	Micromedex, Inc.
IDENTISER	Pml Microbiologicals
IDESCORE	Idesco Corp.
IDESCOTE	Idesco Corp.
IDESPAK	Idesco Corp.
IDM ACCUTRAK	Information Data Management, Inc.
IDM INTOUCH	Information Data Management, Inc.
IDM PCMS	Information Data Management, Inc.
IDM SELECT SERIES	Information Data Management, Inc.
IDM SURROUND,IDM EMBARC	Information Data Management, Inc.
IDMS DATA MANAGEMENT	Allegro Biodiesel Corporation
IDXRAD	Idx Systems Corporation
IDXSITE	Idx Systems Corporation
IDXTENDR	Idx Systems Corporation
IDXVIEW	Idx Systems Corporation
IEC	Thermo Fisher Scientific - Laboratory Equipment Division Headquarters
IEHL	Northgate Technologies Inc.
IF-400 INTERFERENTIAL	American Imex
IF-4000	Comfort Technologies, Inc.
IF3WAVE	Compex Technologies, Inc.
IFII	Compex Technologies, Inc.
IFIT	Conformis, Inc.
IFS	Abbott Medical Optics Inc.
IGAT-180	Aquatic Access, Inc.
IGAT-180/135	Aquatic Access, Inc.
IGAT-180AD	Aquatic Access, Inc.
IGAT-90	Aquatic Access, Inc.
IGLIDE	Igus, Inc.
IGMT	Aquatic Access, Inc.
IGRC	Aquatic Access, Inc.
IGUARD	Sunmed Healthcare
IIC	International Immunology Corp.
IISSEEL	Baxter International Inc
IJIG	Conformis, Inc.
IKA	Applied Biosystems
IKAMAG	Ika-Works, Inc.
IL 1600	Instrumentation Laboratory Company
IL 482	Instrumentation Laboratory Company
IL 682	Instrumentation Laboratory Company
IL 943	Instrumentation Laboratory Company
IL TEST	Instrumentation Laboratory Company
ILA	Covidien Lp, Formerly Registered As United States Surgical
ILAB	Instrumentation Laboratory Company
ILASIK	Abbott Medical Optics Inc.
ILE-SORB	Eastman Medical Products Inc.
ILE20	H&W Technology, Llc.
ILIZAROV	Smith & Nephew Inc.- Orthopaedics Division
ILLE	Ferno-Washington, Inc.
ILLUMENA	Mallinckrodt, Inc.
ILLUMINA%	Dentsply International, Inc.
ILLUMINAŰÉ¯	Dentsply Prosthetics
ILLUSIONS	Ciba Vision Corporation
ILLUSTRA	Cynosure, Inc.
ILOOK	Sonosite, Inc.
ILS	Belco Packaging Systems, Inc.
ILS20	H&W Technology, Llc.
ILYTE	Instrumentation Laboratory Company
IM - MOBI - LIZER	Morrison Medical
IMAG	Halbar North, Inc.
IMAGCLEAR	Titan Corporation/Systems & Imagery Division
IMAGE 1	Karl Storz Endoscopy-America Inc.
IMAGE ARMOR	AMD Technologies Inc.
IMAGE DELIVERY PROTOCOL (IDP)	Pegasus Imaging Corp.
IMAGE PRODUCTS	Crown Mats

IMAGE QUEST	Imaging Associates, Inc.
IMAGE QUEST WEB	Imaging Associates, Inc.
IMAGE QUEST WEB FORMS	Imaging Associates, Inc.
IMAGE REVIEW	Phillips Ultrasound
IMAGE-LINE	Boss Instruments, Ltd.
IMAGE-TRAC	Boss Instruments, Ltd.
IMAGEFIRST	Summit Industries, Inc.
IMAGEMAKERS	Hill-Rom Holdings, Inc.
IMAGEMASTER	Photon Technology International, Inc.
IMAGEMEDICAL	Erad/Image Medical Corp.
IMAGENET	Topcon Medical Systems, Inc.
IMAGENET EZ LITE	Topcon Medical Systems, Inc.
IMAGENET LITE	Topcon Medical Systems, Inc.
IMAGENET PROFESSIONAL	Topcon Medical Systems, Inc.
IMAGENT	Alliance Pharmaceutical Corp.
IMAGER	Fischer Medical Technologies Inc.
IMAGERS	Multi Imager Service, Inc
IMAGES-ON-CALL	Images-On-Call
IMAGESCOPE	Aperio Technologies Inc.
IMAGING3	Imaging3, Inc.
IMAGIQ	Stille-Sonesta, Inc.
IMAX	Procter & Gamble
IMCO VIP-PACS	Imco Technologies
IMCO-GATE	Imco Technologies
IMCO-LINK	Imco Technologies
IMCO-ORTHO	Imco Technologies
IMCO-PACS	Imco Technologies
IMCO-STAT	Imco Technologies
IMCO-STORE	Imco Technologies
IMCO-VIEW	Imco Technologies
IMCO-WEB	Imco Technologies
IMFAST ENHANCEMENT OPTION	Siemens Medical Solutions Usa, Inc
IMG	Boeckeler Instruments, Inc.
IMMEDGE	Vector Laboratories, Inc.
IMMEDIATE	Lang Dental Manufacturing Co., Inc.
IMMERGE	Varian Medical Systems
IMMOBILE-ICER	Dura-Kold Corp.
IMMOBILICE	Cincinnati Sub-Zero Products, Inc., Medical Division
IMMOBILON	Millipore Corporation
IMMOPHASE	Siemens Healthcare Diagnostics Inc
IMMPROVE	Binding Site, Inc., The
IMMUADD	Immucor, Inc.
IMMUBLOT	Immco Diagnostics, Inc.
IMMUCHECK	Heska Corporation
IMMUCOR	Immucor, Inc.
IMMUGEL	Immco Diagnostics, Inc.
IMMUGLO	Immco Diagnostics, Inc.
IMMULISA	Immco Diagnostics, Inc.
IMMULITE	Siemens Healthcare Diagnostics Inc.
IMMULITE 2000	Siemens Healthcare Diagnostics Inc.
IMMULITE TURBO	Siemens Healthcare Diagnostics Inc.
IMMUN-BLOT	Bio-Rad Laboratories, Life Science Group
IMMUNBEAD	Bio-Rad Laboratories, Life Science Group
IMMUNETICS	Immunetics, Inc.
IMMUNEX CRP	Wampole Laboratories
IMMUNHOTEP	Portable Medical Laboratories, Inc.
IMMUNITY STEEL	Hu-Friedy Manufacturing Co., Inc.
IMMUNO-BED KIT	Polysciences, Inc.
IMMUNO-TEK	Zeptometrix Corporation
IMMUNOBEAD	Bio-Rad Laboratories, Life Science Group
IMMUNOCARD	Meridian Bioscience, Inc.
IMMUNOCARD STAT	Meridian Bioscience, Inc.
IMMUNOCARD STAT!r ROTAVIRUS	Thermo Biostar, Inc.
IMMUNOCOLOR	Cytocolor, Inc.
IMMUNOKITS	Biomedical Technologies, Inc.
IMMUNOSIMPLICITY	Diamedix Corp.
IMMUSTRIP	Immunomedics, Inc.
IMMUTROL	Cliniqa Corporation
IMP	Innovative Medical Products, Inc.
IMPACT	Biomet, Inc.
IMPACT	Colours Wheelchair
IMPACT	Harry J. Bosworth Company
IMPACT	Impact Instrumentation, Inc.
IMPACT	Instrumentation Laboratory Company
IMPACT	Novartis Nutrition
IMPACT	Thermo Fisher Scientific
IMPACT (SORENSEN)	Medi-Tech International, Inc.
IMPACT ELISA AND IFA	Wampole Laboratories
IMPACT SERIES	Kareco International, Inc.
IMPACTAG	Idesco Corp.
IMPAX	Agfa Corporation
IMPAX BASIX	Agfa Corporation
IMPERIUM 200H	Interact Plus
IMPERIUM 200ML(MOBILELINK)	Interact Plus
IMPLA PARALLEL	Hager Worldwide, Inc.
IMPLA-MED	Sterngold
IMPLANT	Impladent Ltd.
IMPLEX	Implex Corp.
IMPRA-FLEX	Bard Peripheral Vascular, Inc.
IMPRESS	Merit Medical Systems, Inc.
IMPRESSION	Hill-Rom Holdings, Inc.
IMPRESSIONS (OVER-BED LIGHTS)	Alkco Lighting Co.
IMPRINT	3m Espe Dental Products
IMPRINT	Joerns Healthcare, Inc
IMPULSE	Sellstrom Manufacturing Co.
IMPULSE	Skytron
IMPULSE TRAINING SYSTEMS	Engineering Marketing Assoc. Dba Impulse Training Systems
IMS	Handi-Cap Aids Company
IMS 4000B	Pentax Medical Company
IMTEC SENDAX MDI	Imtec, A 3m Company
IMUBIND	American Diagnostica, Inc.
IN HEALTH TECHNOLOGIES	Helix Medical, Inc.
IN-FLOW	In/Us Systems, Inc.
IN-FLOW	Self Regulation Systems, Inc.
IN-LINE	Siemens Medical Solutions Usa, Inc
IN-LINE	Transamerican Technologies International
IN-LINE BACK CHECK VALVES	Np Medical, Inc.
IN-STRINGER	Advanced Medical Innovations, Inc.
INCARE	Hollister Incorporated
INCARE IN VIEW	Hollister Incorporated
INCHWORM	Exfo America Inc.
INCISIVE SURGICAL (R)	Incisive Surgical, Inc.
INCONTAN	Medical Measurements, Inc.
INCONTX	Nova Health Systems, Inc.
INDEPENDENCE	Palmer Industries
INDEPENDENCE IBOT 3000	Deka Research & Development Corp.
INDERM	Innovative Med Inc.
INDIAN HEAD	Miltex Inc.
INDIAN HEAD	Moyco Technologies, Inc.
INDICATOR	Oral-B Laboratories, Inc.
INDICOT	Analytical Spectral Devices, Inc.
INDICTOR SHAFT	Megadyne Medical Products, Inc.
INDIGAL	Usb Corporation
INDISPOSABLES	Beck-Lee
INDOPLAS	Unomedical, Inc.
INDUSTREX	Carestream Health, Inc.
INDUSTRY'S CHOICE	DJO Surgical
INERPAN	Covidien Lp
INF PLUS	Biomedical Life Systems, Inc.
INFA DENT	Laclede, Inc.
INFANT CARE DOLL	Medical Plastics Laboratory, Inc.
INFANT FLOW	CAREFUSION 211, INC.
INFANT INTUBATION HEAD	Simulaids, Inc.
INFANTGEL	Conmed Corporation
INFANTRAC	Seca Corp.
INFANTRONIC	Seca Corp.
INFECTION CONTROL	Hal-Hen Company, Inc.
INFILTRATOR	Boston Scientific Interventional Technologies
INFILTRATOR	Medical Device Resource Corporation
INFINITI	Autogenomics, Incorporated
INFINITI	Siemens Hearing Instruments, Inc.
INFINITY	Activeaid, Inc.
INFINITY	Asi-Modulex
INFINITY	Zevex Incorporated
INFINITY XMA	Xma (X-Ray Marketing Associates, Inc.)

INFINIX	Toshiba America Medical Systems
INFINIX I SERIES	Toshiba America Medical Systems
INFIT	Mettler-Toledo Process Analytical, Inc.
INFLATOMATIC	Zimmer Orthopaedic Surgical Products
INFLUJECT	Baxter International Inc
INFORM	Asi-Modulex
INFOSENS	AMD Technologies Inc.
INFOTRONICS	Clear Stream Media
INFRA-GARD	Sellstrom Manufacturing Co.
INFRAGOLD	Labsphere, Inc.
INFRAGOLD-LF	Labsphere, Inc.
INFRAREADY	Ii-Vi, Inc.
INFRASOFT	Titronics Research & Development Co.
INFRATIPS	Ams Innovative Center-San Jose
INFU-MED	Walkmed Infusion Llc
INFUS-FLEX	Tfx Medical Oem
INFUSABLE	Vital Signs, Inc.
INFUSE	Medtronic Sofamor Danek Usa, Inc
INFUSE	Medtronic Sofamor Danek Usa, Inc
INFUSE-A-CATH	Angiodynamics, Inc.
INFUSE-A-PORT	Angiodynamics, Inc.
INFUSOR XL	Hanson Medical, Inc.
INFUVITE	Baxter Healthcare Corporation Nutrition
INGAGE	Flotec, Inc.
INGUINAL RESERVOIR INSERTER	Lone Star Medical Products, Inc.
INHOUSE	Asi-Modulex
INHYDROGUIDE	Fiberguide Industries, Inc.
INJECT-A-CELL	Spectrocell, Inc.
INJECT-EASE	Palco Labs, Inc.
INJECT-ED	Pocket Nurse Enterprises, Inc.
INJECTASNARE	United States Endoscopy Group
INJEKT	B. Braun Medical Inc., Renal Therapies Div.
INJEKT	B. Braun Oem Division, B. Braun Medical Inc.
INLAB MC	Sirona Dental Systems Llc
INLAY	C. R. Bard, Inc., Bard Urological Div.
INLET CLOSURE	Inlet Medical, Inc.
INLIGHT	Landauer, Inc.
INLINER	Lightnin Mixers
INNER-FACELIFT	Boss Instruments, Ltd.
INNER-FLOW	Boss Instruments, Ltd.
INNER-FOREHEAD	Boss Instruments, Ltd.
INNER-LIP PLATE	Maddak Inc.
INNER-PLASTIC	Boss Instruments, Ltd.
INNERCOOL	Cardium Therapeutics Inc.
INNERCOOL THERAPIES	Cardium Therapeutics Inc.
INNERPULSE	Innerpulse Inc.
INNERTHANES	Kenda American Airless
INNERVISION	Medovations, Inc.
INNERVISION	Toshiba America Medical Systems
INNOFLUOR	Oxis International, Inc.
INNOVA	New Brunswick Scientific Co., Inc.
INNOVA EMG	Empi, Inc.
INNOVA PFS	Empi, Inc.
INNOVA REAGENTS	Remel Atlanta, Div. Of Remel, Inc.
INNOVAC	Innovative Medical Technologies, Inc.
INNOVATION GENESIS	Innovation Genesis, Llc
INNOVATION SPORTS, INC.	Ossur Americas, Inc
INNOVATIVE MED INC.	Innovative Med Inc.
INNOVATOR	Ricon Corp.
INNOVET	Summit Industries, Inc.
INNOVISION	Infimed, Inc.
INOTECH CELL HARVESTER	Inotech Biosystems International, Inc.
INOUE-BALLOON	Toray International America Inc.
INPRO	Mettler-Toledo Process Analytical, Inc.
INPRO CLICKEZE PRIVACY SYSTEMS	Inpro Corporation
INPRO CORPORATION	Inpro Corporation
INPRO JOINTMASTER ARCHITECTURAL JOINT SYSTEMS	Inpro Corporation
INPRO SIGNSCAPE SIGNAGE AND WAYFINDING	Inpro Corporation
INPUT	Bard Electro Physiology
INRATIO	Hemosense, Inc.
INSCRIBED	Hollister Incorporated
INSECTAGRO	Mediatech, Inc.
INSEMINATOR	Wallach Surgical Devices, Inc.

INSIGHT	Sandhill Scientific, Inc.
INSLIDE OUT	Boekel Scientific
INSORB (R)	Incisive Surgical, Inc.
INSPECTOR	Merit Medical Systems, Inc.
INSPIRATION	Respironics Georgia, Inc.
INSPIRATION	Respironics New Jersey, Inc.
INSPIRATION	Varian Medical Systems
INSTA MAK	Quantronix Lasers
INSTA-COLD	Tetra Medical Supply Corp.
INSTA-COUNT	Aesculap Implant Systems Inc.
INSTA-FIX	Microcopy, Div. Neo-Flo, Inc.
INSTA-GLAZE	George Taub Products & Fusion Co., Inc.
INSTA-HOT	Tetra Medical Supply Corp.
INSTA-LINE	Good-Lite Co.
INSTA-NEG	Microcopy, Div. Neo-Flo, Inc.
INSTA-PULSE	Biosig Instruments, Inc.
INSTA-SEAL	One Lambda, Inc.
INSTA-TRAY CROWN STABLIZER	American Diversified Dental Systems
INSTA-TRAY CROWN STABLIZER	Mds Products, Inc.
INSTA-VELOPER	Microcopy, Div. Neo-Flo, Inc.
INSTABARICS	Reimers Systems, Inc.
INSTACARE	Stryker Medical
INSTACOOL	Thermogenesis Corp.
INSTACOOLANT	Thermogenesis Corp.
INSTAFIL	Lifemed Of California
INSTAGAURD	Cardinal Health Inc.
INSTALOID	Ticonium Co.
INSTANT MEDICAL HISTORY	Medinotes Corporation
INSTANT REPORTER	Dr Systems, Inc.
INSTANT RESPONSET	Valleylab
INSTANT VELSTRAP	Patterson Medical Holdings, Inc.
INSTANT VERTEBRAL ASSESSMENT	Hologic, Inc.
INSTANT-VIEW	Alfa Scientific Designs, Inc.
INSTATRACE	Conmed Corporation
INSTAVAC II	Ohio Medical Corp.
INSTRIDE	Stryker Howmedica Osteonics
INSTROMARK	Timemed Labeling Systems, Inc.
INSTRU-BAND	Graphic Controls Corp.
INSTRU-HOLD	Advanced Medical Innovations, Inc.
INSTRU-SAFE	Micromedics
INSTRU-TRAYS	Healthmark Industries
INSTRUMENT CADDY	Katena Products, Inc.
INSTRUMENT GUARD	Graphic Controls Corp.
INSTRUMENT MANAGEMENT SYSTEM	Hu-Friedy Manufacturing Co., Inc.
INSTRUMENT SPECIFIC	Porex Corporation
INSTRUMENTAL IN YOUR SUCCESS	Paragon Medical, Inc.
INSUL-CAP	Palco Labs, Inc.
INSUL-EZE	Palco Labs, Inc.
INSUL-TOTE	Palco Labs, Inc.
INSULATING VIAL TRAYS	Tcp Reliable, Inc.
INSULIN PROTECTOR CASE	Medicool, Inc.
INSULSCAN	Mobile Instrument Service And Repair, Inc.
INSYTE	Becton Dickinson Infusion Therapy Systems, Inc.
INSYTE AUTOGUARD	Becton Dickinson Infusion Therapy Systems, Inc.
INSYTE-W	Becton Dickinson Infusion Therapy Systems, Inc.
INTAC	Asi-Modulex
INTACS	Avery Dennison Corporation
INTACS ALPHACOR"	Addition Technology, Inc.
INTACTA	Newschoff Chairs, Inc.
INTECAM	Medx Incorporated
INTECH INSTRUMENTS	Vespo Marketing Assoc., Inc.
INTEGRA	Integra Lifesciences Corporation
INTEGRA	Integra Lifesciences Holdings Corp.
INTEGRA	MAQUET
INTEGRA	Pmt Corp.
INTEGRA DERMAL REGENERATION TEMPLATE	Integra Lifesciences Holdings Corp.
INTEGRA MOZAIK	Integra Lifesciences Holdings Corp.
INTEGRA NEUROSCIENCES	Integra Lifesciences Holdings Corp.
INTEGRA, INTEGRA EZ, ECLIPSE	Sequal Technologies Inc.
INTEGRAL	Biomet, Inc.
INTEGRAL	Zimmer Dental, Inc.
INTEGRAL DNA	Atzen/Universal Companies, Inc.

TRADE NAME INDEX

INTEGRAL THREADLOC .... Zimmer Dental, Inc.
INTEGRATED IMAGE .... Imsi, Integrated Modular Systems Inc.
INTEGRIS .... Hill-Rom Holdings, Inc.
INTEGRITY .... Dentsply Caulk
INTEGRITY .... Dentsply International, Inc.
INTEGRITY .... Dentsply Prosthetics
INTEGRITY .... Skytron
INTEGRITY .... Standard Textile Co., Inc.
INTEGRITY TIPS .... Thermo Fisher Scientific
INTELECT .... Chattanooga Group
INTELIJET .... Smith & Nephew, Inc., Endoscopy Division
INTELLA-SENS .... Psg Controls, Inc.
INTELLECT .... Shimadzu Medical Systems
INTELLIGEN .... Gtr Labs, Inc.
INTELLIMATRIX .... Stryker Corp.
INTELLIMATRIX .... Stryker Endoscopy
INTELLIMATRIX .... Stryker Howmedica Osteonics
INTELLISYSTEM .... Merit Medical Systems, Inc.
INTELLITEMP .... Cardima, Inc.
INTENSITE .... Atzen/Universal Companies, Inc.
INTENSO POINT .... Hager Worldwide, Inc.
INTER COOL .... Hager Worldwide, Inc.
INTER FIX .... Medtronic Sofamor Danek Usa, Inc
INTER FIX .... Medtronic Sofamor Danek Usa, Inc.
INTER-OP ACETABULAR SYSTEM .... Centerpulse Orthopedics Inc.
INTERACOUSTICS .... Medi
INTERACTANT .... Health Care Software, Inc. (Hcs)
INTERCEPT .... Fenwal Inc.
INTERCEPT .... Orasure Technologies, Inc.
INTERCHANGE .... Smiths Medical OEM
INTERFACE .... Medicalcv, Inc.
INTERFLEET .... American Emergency Vehicles
INTERGEL .... Lifecore Biomedical, Inc.
INTERGEN .... Serologicals Corp
INTERGEN DISCOVERY PRODUCTS .... Serologicals Corp
INTERIOR 20 .... Asi-Modulex
INTERLINK Baxter Healthcare Corporporation, Alternate Care And Channel Team
INTERLOCK .... Greatbach Medical
INTERLOCK .... Greatbatch Inc
INTERPAQ .... Micrus Corporation
INTERPORE 200 .... Interpore Cross International
INTERPROXIMAL DISCS .... Almore International, Inc.
INTERPULSE .... Stryker Corp.
INTERSITE .... Herman Miller, Inc.
INTERSORB .... Covidien Lp
INTERSPEC INTERFERENTIAL .... American Imex
INTERSTAIN-6 .... Hacker Instruments And Industries Inc.
INTERTHERM .... Labthermics Technologies
INTERTIP I/A HANDPIECE .... Microsurgical Technology, Inc.
INTERVASCULAR .... Bard Peripheral Vascular, Inc.
INTEXEN .... Carbon Medical Technologies, Inc.
INTIMA .... Becton Dickinson Infusion Therapy Systems, Inc.
INTOUCH .... Asi-Modulex
INTOUCH .... Covidien (Formerly Nellcor Puritan Bennett / Tyco Healthcare)
INTOUCH .... Stryker Corp.
INTOX EC/IR .... Intoximeters, Inc.
INTRA .... Starkey Laboratories, Inc.
INTRA-ARC .... Conmed Linvatec
INTRA-ART .... Genesee Biomedical, Inc.
INTRAC .... Mettler-Toledo Process Analytical, Inc.
INTRACATH .... Becton Dickinson Infusion Therapy Systems, Inc.
INTRACELL .... Rpi Of Atlanta
INTRAFLO .... Hospira, Inc.
INTRAJECT .... Meridian Medical Technologies
INTRALASE .... Abbott Medical Optics Inc.
INTRALIPID .... Baxter Healthcare Corporation Nutrition
INTRALIPID .... Hospira, Inc.
INTRALOCK .... Hospira, Inc.
INTRALUMINAL .... Intraluminal Therapeutics, Inc.
INTRAMATIC .... Sirona Dental Systems Llc
INTRAN .... Utah Medical Products, Inc.
INTRAN PLUS .... Utah Medical Products, Inc.
INTRASCAN, HMSERG .... Linscan Ultrasound
INTRASHIEL .... Allergan
INTRASITE .... Smith & Nephew, Inc.
INTRAVASCULAR TEMPERATURE MANAGEMENT (IVTM) .... Alsius Corp.
INTRAVESICAL ELECTRO STIMULATION CATHETER .... Humantronic, Inc
INTRAVIA .... Baxter Healthcare Corporation, Global Drug Delivery
INTRAVISION .... Conmed Linvatec
INTRLOGIC .... Kendro Laboratory Products
INTRO 7 .... Greatbach Medical
INTROCAN SAFETY .... B. Braun Oem Division, B. Braun Medical Inc.
INTROSTAT-DL .... Datascope Cardiac Assist Div.
INTROSYTE .... Becton Dickinson Infusion Therapy Systems, Inc.
INTROSYTE-N .... Becton Dickinson Infusion Therapy Systems, Inc.
INTSRUCREME .... Case Medical, Inc.
INTUIS .... Siemens Hearing Instruments, Inc.
INTUIS DIR .... Siemens Hearing Instruments, Inc.
INTUIS LIFE .... Siemens Hearing Instruments, Inc.
INTUITION .... Terarecon, Inc.
INVAC R .... Pmt Corp.
INVACARE .... Handicap Unlimited, Inc.
INVACARE .... Invacare Corporation
INVACARE .... Invacare Supply Group, An Invacare Co.
INVADER .... Third Wave Technologies, Inc.
INVADER PLUS .... Third Wave Technologies, Inc.
INVENTORY ASSISTANT .... Carecentric, Inc.
INVEON .... Siemens Medical Solutions Usa, Inc.
INVERNESS MEDICAL .... Inverness Medical Inc.
INVERSE TOPOGRAPHY .... Hologic, Inc.
INVESTIC .... Ticonium Co.
INVINCIBLE .... Hager Worldwide, Inc.
INVINCIBLE .... Zyloware Corporation
INVINCILITES BY ZYLOWARE .... Zyloware Corporation
INVISALIGN .... Align Technology, Inc.
INVISATRAC .... Conmed Corporation
INVISATRACE .... Conmed Corporation
INVISIGRIP VEIN STRIPPERS .... Lemaitre Vascular, Inc.
INVISx .... Medtronic, Inc.
INVOLUCRIN .... Biomedical Technologies, Inc.
INVOS .... Somanetics Corp.
INVU .... Tp Orthodontics, Inc.
IO-GONE .... Professional Disposables International, Inc.
IOGEL .... Iomed, Inc.
IOL .... Mentor Ophthalmics, Inc.
IOLMASTER .... Carl Zeiss Meditec Inc.
ION .... Sonic Innovations
ION/STIR .... Sienco, Inc.
IONDETECT .... Fil-Chem, Inc.
IONGUARD .... Spire Corp.
IONGUARD II .... Spire Corp.
IONGUARD III .... Spire Corp.
IONIC-PTFE .... Tua Systems, Inc.
IONJOIN .... Spire Corp.
IONTOPAK .... Advanced Instruments Inc.
IONTOPHOR .... Life-Tech, Inc.
IOZ .... Icu Medical, Inc.
IP .... Byron Medical
IP C CASSTTE LABELING SYSTEM, IP S SLIDE LABELING SYSTEM .... Leica Microsystems Inc.
IPAS EASYGRIP .... Ipas
IPAS MVA PLUS .... Ipas
IPC 200 .... Asi Medical Equipment, Ltd.
IPG PHOR .... Hoefer Pharmacia Biotech, Inc.
IPOD .... Nonin Medical, Inc.
IPP .... Bender, Inc.
IPRINT .... Nai Tech Products
IPS CLASSIC .... Ivoclar Vivadent, Inc.
IPS D.SIGN .... Ivoclar Vivadent, Inc.
IPS EMPRESS .... Ivoclar Vivadent, Inc.
IPS ERIS .... Ivoclar Vivadent, Inc.
IPSO .... Ipso Usa, Inc.
IPUMP .... Baxter Healthcare Corporporation, Alternate Care And Channel Team
IQ .... Sleepnet Corporation
IQM .... Instrumentation Laboratory Company
IQMARK ADVANCED HOLTER .... Midmark Diagnostics Group

IQMARK DIAGNOSTIC PDA	Midmark Diagnostics Group
IQMARK DIAGNOSTIC WORKSTATION	Midmark Diagnostics Group
IQMARK DIGITAL ECG	Midmark Diagnostics Group
IQMARK DIGITAL SPIRO PDA	Midmark Diagnostics Group
IQMARK DIGITAL SPIROMETER	Midmark Diagnostics Group
IQMARK EZ HOLTER	Midmark Diagnostics Group
IQMARK SYNC	Midmark Diagnostics Group
IRADIATOR	Boston Scientific Interventional Technologies
IRAP	Mwi Veterinary Supply
IRC 2100	Redfield Corp.
IRIDIUM	Glines And Rhodes, Inc.
IRIS	Iris International, Inc.
IRIS	Skytron
IRMA	Allegro Biodiesel Corporation
IRMA SL	Allegro Biodiesel Corporation
IRMA TruPoint	International Technidyne Corp.
IRON DUCK	Iron Duck, A Div. Of Fleming Industries, Inc.
IRON INTERN	Automated Medical Products Corp.
IRON MASK	Sellstrom Manufacturing Co.
IRRADIATOR	Boston Scientific Interventional Technologies
IRRIVAC MAX	Vital Concepts, Inc.
IRUS	Thermo Spectra-Tech
IRV2000	Trac About, Inc.
IRVS	Vitalcom, Inc.
IS-199 CHEMICAL MIXER	White Mountain Imaging
ISCAN	Siemens Hearing Instruments, Inc.
ISCH-DISH	Span-America Medical Systems, Inc.
ISECURE	Hospira Inc.
ISH IVIEW	Ventana Medical Systems, Inc.
ISI ULTRA-LIGHT SPECIALTY TABLE	Instrument Specialists, Inc.
ISKD	Orthofix Inc.
ISLETEST-GAD	Biomerica, Inc.
ISLETEST-IAA	Biomerica, Inc.
ISLETEST-ICA	Biomerica, Inc.
ISO 9001 REGISTERED	Tailored Label Products, Inc.
ISO HAND HELPER	Meddev Corporation
ISO PRIME	Hoefer Pharmacia Biotech, Inc.
ISO SEED	Isotope Products Laboratories, Inc.
ISO-8 ANKLE BRACES	Omni Life Science, Inc.
ISO-CARE	Online Power, Inc.
ISO-FORM	3m Espe Dental Products
ISO-GRID/NEO-GRID	Neogen Corporation
ISO-VALVE	Rondex Products, Inc.
ISOBAR	DJO Surgical
ISOCARE	Independent Solutions, Inc.
ISOCATH	Vital Signs, Inc.
ISOCODE	Schleicher & Schuell, Inc.
ISOCOMP I	Mgm Instruments
ISOCOOL	Codman & Shurtleff, Inc
ISOCUF	Frontier Medical Products, Inc.
ISODYN	Tagg Industries L.L.C.
ISOFLEX	Gaymar Industries, Inc.
ISOFLOW	Novosci Corp.
ISOFLUID	Crosstex International,Inc.
ISOFLUID FOG FREE	Crosstex International,Inc.
ISOGARD	Baker Company, The
ISOGARD	Square D Company
ISOLAIR	Gerson Co. Inc., Louis M.
ISOLAIR APR	Gerson Co. Inc., Louis M.
ISOLAIR II	Gerson Co. Inc., Louis M.
ISOLAIR SMF	Gerson Co. Inc., Louis M.
ISOLATOR	Crosstex International,Inc.
ISOLATOR	Independent Solutions, Inc.
ISOLATOR	Jamestown Metal Products
ISOLATOR	Wampole Laboratories
ISOLATOR PLUS	Crosstex International,Inc.
ISOLIBRIUM	Gaymar Industries, Inc.
ISOLITE	Crosstex International,Inc.
ISOLOCK	DJO Surgical
ISOLYTE	B. Braun Oem Division, B. Braun Medical Inc.
ISOPROBE	Monroe Electronics, Inc.
ISOPROBE	U.F.I.
ISOQUANT	Promega Corp.
ISOROBIC	Fitness Motivation Institute Of America, Inc.
ISOROBIC	Team America Health & Fitness, Inc
ISOSCAN	PerkinElmer
ISOSOURCE	Novartis Nutrition
ISOSTAT	Wampole Laboratories
ISOTRACK	JTECH Medical
ISOVITALEX	Bd Diagnostic Systems
ISOWASH	Sharps Compliance Corp.
ISP	Starkey Laboratories, Inc.
ISTAX PLATE STACKING SOLUTIONS	Caliper Life Sciences, Inc.
IT'S THE CHEMISTRY THAT COUNTS	Bio-Rad Laboratories, Life Science Group
ITA-MED	Ita-Med Co.
ITC	Omni Medical Supply Inc.
ITCH ENDER	Urocare Products, Inc.
ITCH'S GONE	Health Enterprises
ITLC	Pall Corporation
IV EXPRESS PEDI	Millipore Corporation
IV MASTER FLOW	Conmed Corporation
IV PRO	Medi-Dose, Inc.
IV PUMPETTE	Conmed Corporation
IV-EXPRESS	Millipore Corporation
IV-LOOP	Becton Dickinson Infusion Therapy Systems, Inc.
IV/ARMBOARDS	Morrison Medical
IVA	Covidien Lp
IVALON PVA EMBOLIZATION PARTICLES	Ivalon, Inc.
IVALON SURGICAL PRODUCTS	First Aid Bandage Co., Inc.
IVATION	Surmodics, Inc.
IVC	Invacare Corporation
IVEEGAM	Baxter International Inc
IVEX	Millipore Corporation
IVISION DIGITAL IMAGE ANALYSIS	Biogenex Laboratories
IVM	In Vivo Metric
IVOX	Farley Inc., W.T.
IVRA	Intelligent Hearing Systems, Corp.
IVT	Arlington Scientific, Inc. Asi
IVT	Boston Scientific Interventional Technologies
IVUS PLUS	Indec Systems, Inc.
Identity	St. Jude Medical, Inc.
Image	Younger Manufacturing Co., Inc.
Imager	Boston Scientific Corporation
Immunodyne	Pall Corporation
InDex	Insite One, Inc.
Inquiry	Boston Scientific Corporation
Inquiry	St. Jude Medical, Inc.
Instill	Kinetic Concepts, Inc.
Integrity	St. Jude Medical, Inc.
Intel Health Guide	Intel Corp. Digital Health Group
Intelimer	Landec Corp.
Interject	Boston Scientific Corporation
Interlock	Boston Scientific Corporation
Intersept	Medtronic Perfusion Systems
Intrector	Insight Instruments, Inc.
IsoFlex	St. Jude Medical, Inc.
Isolator	Atricure, Inc.
J & S IRON SATURATING REGEANT	J&S Medical Associates
J-CHAIR	Dentalez Group
J-LOOP	Becton Dickinson Infusion Therapy Systems, Inc.
J-SHA II	Jacuzzi, Bath Division
J-WRAP	Johnson & Johnson Consumer Products, Inc.
J/V-GENERATION	Dentalez Group
JACE	JACE SYSTEMS, INC
JACE SYSTEMS: JACE	Jace Systems
JACE TRI-STIM	JACE SYSTEMS, INC
JACKSON	Lafayette Instrument Company
JACKSON TABLE	Mizuho Osi
JACOB'S HOOK	Farley Inc., W.T.
JACUZZI	Jacuzzi, Bath Division
JADE	Prosun Tanning International, Llc.
JAEGER	Cardinal Health Inc.
JAEGER BOBAY BODY	CAREFUSION 211, INC..
JAISONS	Jaisons International, Inc.
JAMAR	Lafayette Instrument Company
JAMAR	Patterson Medical Holdings, Inc.

JAMESTOWN METAL .... Medi-Tech International, Inc.
JANNX .... Jannx Medical Systems Inc.
JANUS .... Life-Tech, Inc.
JANUSr .... Vergason Technology, Inc.
JARIT .... Integra Lifesciences Holdings Corp.
JARIT .... J. Jamner Surgical Instruments, Inc
JASPER JUMPER .... American Orthodontics Corp.
JAVA GROWING .... Almore International, Inc.
JAVELIN .... Parco Scientific Co.
JAVELIN .... Thermo Fisher Scientific
JAWS OF LIFE .... Hale Products Inc.
JAY .... Sunrise Medical
JAYPRO .... Jaypro Corporation
JAZZY .... Pride Mobility Products Corp.
JB-4 .... Energy Beam Sciences, Inc.
JB-4 EMBEDDING KIT .... Polysciences, Inc.
JB-70, MICRO, MICROPLUS, CYGNUSRAY MPS .... Progeny Dental
JEEP KIPLING .... L'Amy, Inc.
JELDENT .... Heraeus Kulzer, Inc.
JELONET .... Smith & Nephew, Inc.
JELSMA BOARD I .... Composites Horizons, Inc.
JELTRATE PLUS .... Dentsply Caulk
JENX .... Bodypoint, Inc.
JEROME/MEDICAL .... Ortholine
JET .... Lang Dental Manufacturing Co., Inc.
JET .... Medcomp (Medical Components, Inc.)
JET-LUBE .... Kinetic Instruments, Inc.
JETMATE .... Columbia Medical Manufacturing Llc
JETTMOBILE .... Patterson Medical Holdings, Inc.
JEWELSHINE .... Cd Nelson Manufacturing Co.
JEWETT .... Kendro Laboratory Products
JEWETT .... Medi-Tech International, Inc.
JEWETT/CSI/SCIENTEK .... Medi-Tech International, Inc.
JGOptical Network .... J.G. Optical
JIFFY .... Jiffy Mixer Co., Inc.
JILSON .... Magnus Mobility Systems
JILSON CASTER .... Jilson Group, Inc.
JITTERBUG .... U.F.I.
JJ SKINNER .... Merit Medical Systems Inc.
JOBRI .... Jobri Llc
JOBSKIN .... Torbot Group Inc., Jobskin Division
JOBSKIN .... Torbot Group, Inc.
JOBST .... Omni Medical Supply Inc.
JOBST OPAQUE .... Bsn-Jobst
JOBST ULTRASHEER .... Bsn-Jobst
JOERNS .... Joerns Healthcare, Inc
JOERNS .... Sunrise Medical
JOHNSON'S ORTHOPEDIC DESIGNS .... Seattle Systems
JON A CHAIR .... Activeaid, Inc.
JONES JIG .... American Orthodontics Corp.
JORVET .... Jorgensen Laboratories
JOSLIN ORTHO GEAR .... Ortholine
JOURNEY .... Luxfer Gas Cylinders
JOY STICK DRIVING SYSTEM .... Ahnafield Corp.
JPI .... Koch X-Ray Systems Inc
JRESULTNET .... Dawning Technologies, Inc.
JT BRAD .... Simulaids, Inc.
JTG SERIES .... Activeaid, Inc.
JTONGS .... Jerome Medical
JUDGE ROTENBERG EDUCATIONAL CENTER The Judge Rotenberg Educational Center, Inc.
JUMBO .... Centrix, Inc.
JUNGHANS .... Eric Armin Inc.
JUNIOR.................................... Leisure-Lift, Inc.
JUPITER .... Netzsch Instruments, Inc.
JUPITER .... Phenomenex, Inc.
JURGAN PINBALLS .... Jurgan Development & Mfg.
JUSTI .... American Tooth Industries
JUSTRITE .... Justrite Manufacturing Co., L.L.C.
JUSTVISION .... Toshiba America Medical Systems
JUSTWO .... Medidenta International, Inc.
JUZO .... Juzo
Jagwire .... Boston Scientific Corporation

Janssen .... Ortho-Mcneil-Janssen Pharmaceuticals, Inc.
Jawz Biopsy Forceps .... Argon Medical Devices Inc.
K SERIES BENCHTOP .... Virtis, An Sp Industries Company
K'MX .... Hansco Technologies, Inc.
K-10 HEMISPHERE, MIRRORS .... K-10 Inc.
K-10 WALL-EYE MIRROR .... K-10 Inc.
K-AMP .... Etymotic Research, Inc.
K-AMP .... Starkey Laboratories, Inc.
K-ASSAY .... Kamiya Biomedical Company
K-BLADE .... Katena Products, Inc.
K-CAP-E .... Westcon Orthopedics, Inc.
K-CAP-ES .... Westcon Orthopedics, Inc.
K-CAP-I .... Westcon Orthopedics, Inc.
K-CAP-P .... Westcon Orthopedics, Inc.
K-DEFIB .... Katecho, Inc.
K-DERM CREAM .... Donell
K-DERM GEL .... Donell
K-FILES .... Moyco Technologies, Inc.
K-FORCE .... Kareco International, Inc.
K-FREE .... Katecho, Inc.
K-KNIFE .... Katena Products, Inc.
K-LITE .... Kentek Corp.
K-PACE .... Katecho, Inc.
K-PAD .... Katecho, Inc.
K-PETITE MARATHON .... Engler Engineering Corp.
K-SERIES .... Taylor Wharton
K-SPONGE .... Katena Products, Inc.
K-STERILE .... Katecho, Inc.
K-STIK .... Katecho, Inc.
K-STIM .... Katecho, Inc.
K-SYTEMS IVF WORKSTATIONS .. Zander Medical Supplies, Inc. / Zander Ivf, Inc.
K-Y .... Johnson & Johnson Medical Division Of Ethicon, Inc.
K.D.S. .... Covidien Lp
K.I.S.S. .... Graphic Controls Corp.
K180 .... Heine Usa Ltd.
K2000 .... Arrow International, Inc.
K3S-REPLENISH .... Dps, Inc.
K7 EVALUATION SYSTEM .... Myotronics-Noromed, Inc.
KAAT .... Arrow International, Inc.
KAAT II PLUS .... Arrow International, Inc.
KADALINK .... Kada Research, Inc.
KAL .... Nutraceutical International Corp.
KALETRA .... Abbott Laboratories
KALEX .... Elementis Specialties
KALIBRE .... Kronus, Inc.
KALLASY .... DJO Surgical
KALLESTAD .... Biorad Laboratories
KALON .... Profex Medical Products
KAM SUPER SUCKER .... Anspach Effort, Inc.
KAMBIN RADIOLUCENT SPINAL FRAME .... Universal Service Associates, Inc.
KANGAROO .... Bruno Independent Living Aids, Inc.
KANGAROO .... Covidien Lp
KANGAROO EPUMP .... Covidien Lp, Formerly Registered As Tyco Healthcare
KANGAROO PET .... Covidien Lp
KAPPA .... Thermo Fisher Scientific
KAPUT .... Bellco Glass, Inc.
KARAYA 5 .... Hollister Incorporated
KARDVEYER .... Kardex Systems, Inc.
KARISMA .... Novocol, Inc.
KARL STORZ AIDA .... Karl Storz Endoscopy-America Inc.
KARL STORZ OR-1 .... Karl Storz Endoscopy-America Inc.
KARLIN .... Codman & Shurtleff, Inc
KARMA .... Karma Inc.
KARMA .... Karman Healthcare, Inc.
KARMAN .... Karman Healthcare, Inc.
KATALAVOX .... Kempf
KATENA .... Katena Products, Inc.
KAY-PLAST .... Patterson Medical Holdings, Inc.
KAY-PRENE .... Patterson Medical Holdings, Inc.
KAY-SPLINT .... Patterson Medical Holdings, Inc.
KAYJAE PORTABLE VERSA-TABLE .... Kayjae Mfg. Co. Inc.
KCI Express .... Kinetic Concepts, Inc.
KCP .... Alcon Research, Ltd.

KCP	American Medical Technologies, Inc.
KDALERT	Applied Biosystems
KEEL COBRA	Byron Medical
KEEP	Merit Medical Systems, Inc.
KEEPCOLD	Air Products And Chemicals, Inc.
KELKOM SYSTEMS	Kelkom Systems
KELLY	Trans American Medical
KEMRESIN	Kewaunee Scientific Corp.
KEMSURE	Kem Medical Products Corp.
KEN-A-VISION	Ken-A-Vision Manufacturing Co., Inc.
KEN-KAGE	Suburban Surgical Co., Inc.
KENDALL	Covidien Lp, Formerly Registered As Tyco Healthcare
KENDALL	Dma Med-Chem Corporation
KENDALL	Omni Medical Supply Inc.
KENDALL KOOLABURN	Romaine, Inc. D.B.A. Koldcare
KEOFLO	Roquette America
KERAMOS	DJO Surgical
KERATO-LENS	Allergan
KERATO-PATCH	Allergan
KERATOLUX	Carl Zeiss Surgical, Inc.
KERATRON CORNEAL TOPOGRAPHER	Eyequip, Div Of Alliance Medical Marketing
KERI MANIKINS	Nasco
KERRI DETECTOR/STAIN	Gresco Products, Inc.
KETO-DIASTIX	Siemens Healthcare Diagnostics Inc.
KETO-GEL	Jorgensen Laboratories
KETOSTIX	Siemens Healthcare Diagnostics Inc.
KETTLER	Kettler International
KEVCO-STUBBS	Frank Stubbs Co., Inc
KEY-BAK	Key-Bak
KEY-LOK	Smith & Nephew Inc.- Orthopaedics Division
KEYSTONE	DJO Surgical
KEYSTONE	Mizzy, Inc. Of National Keystone
KEYSTONE	Nspire Health, Inc
KEYSTONE	Thermo Fisher Scientific
KEYSTONE SERIES	United Receptacle
KEYWRITE	Thermo Fisher Scientific - Laboratory Equipment Division Headquarters
KGTI	Kinetikos Medical, Inc.
KICK-IT	Graphic Controls Corp.
KID KART	Sunrise Medical
KIDDIE LITTER	Dixie Ems Supply
KIDDIE-UPS	G. Hirsch & Co.
KIDS	Smiths Medical OEM
KIDS FLOSS	Locin Industries Ltd.
KIDS MIDS	Klinger Eye Shields, Inc.
KIDSTER	Gunnell, Inc.
KIDZ MED	Ulster Scientific, Inc.
KII	Applied Medical Resource Corporation
KIMAX	Kimble Glass, Inc.
KIMBERLY CLARK	Bound Tree Medical
KIMBERLY CLARK	Kerr Group
KIMBLE	Kimble Glass, Inc.
KIMGUARD	Kerr Group
KIMGUARD ONE-STEP	Kerr Group
KIMGUARD ULTRA	Kerr Group
KINDERGUARD	Secure Care Products, Inc.
KINECTIV	Zimmer Holdings, Inc.
KINEMATCH	Kinamed, Inc.
KINESTIM	Cybex International, Inc.
KINETIC	Monebo Technologies, Inc.
KINETIC COLLECTOR	Bio-Rad Laboratories, Life Science Group
KINETRON II	Cybex International, Inc.
KING	Access Battery Inc.
KING ARTHUR	Shelby-Williams Industries
KING OF HEARTS	Instromedix, A Card Guard Co.
KING OF HEARTS-EXPRESS	Instromedix, A Card Guard Co.
KINSA	Smith & Nephew, Inc., Endoscopy Division
KIP	Supertech, Inc.
KIPPMED	Medegen
KISS PACKAGING	Biner Ellison
KIT KATH	Myco Medical
KIWI COMPLETE VACUUM DELIVERY SYSTEM	Clinical Innovations, Inc.

KLASSIC SERIES	Kareco International, Inc.
KLEAR-TRACE	Cas Medical Systems, Inc.
KLEARVUE	Ricon Corp.
KLEEN NEEDLE	Tri-State Hospital Supply Corp.
KLEEN-B-TWEEN	Preventive Dentistry Products, Inc.
KLEEN-PRINT	Precision Dynamics Corp.
KLEEN-PRINT	Xenotec Ltd.
KLEEN-QUAT	Unit Chemical Corp.
KLEENSCOOP	Welch Allyn, Inc.
KLEENSPEC	Welch Allyn, Inc.
KLEENTALK	Sonoco-Stancap Division
KLEER VU, ANTI-FOG ANTI-STATIC CLEANER	North American Marketing, Inc.
KLENZALAC	Zerowet, Inc.
KLER-RO LIQUID	Ulmer Pharmacal Co.
KLIMER CRIB	Nk Medical Products Inc.
KLING	Johnson & Johnson Medical Division Of Ethicon, Inc.
KLINGERS	Klinger Eye Shields, Inc.
KLIP-IT	Nova Health Systems, Inc.
KLS-MARTIN	Kls-Martin L.P.
KMEDIC	Kmedic
KMEDIC	Teleflex Medical
KMI/PAREXEL	Parexel International Corp.
KNA	Radiometer America, Inc.
KNABBERMAX	Hager Worldwide, Inc.
KNAPP	Hely And Weber
KNEE ASSIST	Stryker Corp.
KNEE SKINS	Cropper Medical, Inc./Bio Skin
KNEEGRIP	Sunmedica
KNEEPROBLEM.COM	Information Health Network
KNIFELIGHT	Stryker Corp.
KNIGHT BY MIDMARK	Midmark Corporation
KNIGHTSTAR	Covidien (Formerly Nellcor Puritan Bennett / Tyco Healthcare)
KNIT-STAT	Qrp, Inc.
KOALA	Boss Instruments, Ltd.
KOALA	Permobil, Inc.
KOALA INTRAUTERINE PRESSURE SYSTEM	Clinical Innovations, Inc.
KOALA KUFF	Elginex Corporation
KOALA-TEE	Fleetwood Group, Incorporated
KOAMAN	Koaman International
KODAK	Carestream Health, Inc.
KODIAKr	Lytron, Inc.
KOI	Dgh Technology, Inc.
KOIS DENTO-FACIAL ANALYZER	Panadent Corp.
KOKO	Nspire Health, Inc
KOKO DIGIDOSER	Nspire Health, Inc
KOKO DOSIMETER	Nspire Health, Inc
KOKO MOE	Nspire Health, Inc
KOKO TREK	Nspire Health, Inc
KOKOMATE	Nspire Health, Inc
KOLAPS-A-TANK	Burch Manufacturing Co., Inc.
KOLD COMPRESS	Romaine, Inc. D.B.A. Koldcare
KOLD WRAP	Romaine, Inc. D.B.A. Koldcare
KOLD-DRAFT	Kold-Draft
KOLLECTOR ELITE	Vicon Industries Inc.
KOLLECTOR PRO	Vicon Industries Inc.
KOMPACT KART	Approved Medical Systems
KOMPAKT	Kardex Systems, Inc.
KONTACT	Fisher Diagnostics
KONTES	Kimble Glass, Inc.
KONTOUR	Winfield Laboratories
KONTOUR SPONGE	Winfield Laboratories
KONTRON MEDICAL	Medical Equipment Specialists, Inc.
KONTUR 55 SPHERE	Kontur Kontact Lens Co., Inc.
KONTUR 55 TORIC	Kontur Kontact Lens Co., Inc.
KONTURA	Hager Worldwide, Inc.
KOOL-LUBE 2	Oster Professional Products, Inc.
KOOL-PRESS	Duro-Med Industries
KOOLABURN	Romaine, Inc. D.B.A. Koldcare
KOOLMAX	Polar Products, Inc.
KOTEX	KIMBERLY-CLARK CORP. CONWAY MILL
KOTOKAST	Minnesota Rubber & Qmr Plastics
KOVEN	Koven Technology, Inc.
KPR	King Systems Corp.

TRADE NAME INDEX

Trade Name	Company
KPUMP INFILTRATION PUMP	Medical Device Resource Corporation
KRENE	Hpg International, Inc.
KRESTEX	Petra Manufacturing Co.
KRIMPTEX	Dukal Corporation
KRIVITSKI METHOD	Transonic Systems Inc.
KROMAFAZE	Cadco Dental Products
KROMAFAZE	Dux Dental
KROMELINE	Elginex Corporation
KRONNER	Kronner Medical
KRONOS	Tri Hawk Corporation
KRONUS	Kronus, Inc.
KROSFLO	Spectrum Laboratories, Inc.
KRYORACK	Streck Laboratories, Inc.
KRYOSPRAY	Brymill Corporation
KRYOSPRAY II	Brymill Corporation
KRYOSURE	American Fluoroseal Corp.
KRYOVUE	American Fluoroseal Corp.
KRYPTO	Colours Wheelchair
KRYPTOVAP	Amici, Inc.
KRYSIAL I	Pyramid Orthodontics
KRYSIAL II	Pyramid Orthodontics
KRYSTAL KLEER	Weiman Healthcare Solutions
KRYTOXr	Miller-Stephenson Chemical Company, Inc.
KT1000	Medmetric Corp.
KT2000	Medmetric Corp.
KTP/532	Ams Innovative Center-San Jose
KTP/YAG	Ams Innovative Center-San Jose
KULKA	Perkinelmer Optoelectronics
KURZWEIL	Humanware
KWIK KLEEN	Advanced Endoscopy Devices, Inc.
KWIK KUFF	Precision Dynamics Corp.
KWIK OUT	Ebi, Llc
KWIK-OFF	Novosci Corp.
KWIK-QCT SLIDES & MICROBIOLOGY QUALITY CONTROL SLIDES	Micro-Bio-Logics.Inc
KWIK-QCT SLIDES & MICROBIOLOGY QUALITY CONTROL SLIDES	Microbiologics, Inc.
KWIK-SKAN	Trademark Medical Llc
KWIK-STIKT	Micro-Bio-Logics.Inc
KWIK-STIKT	Microbiologics, Inc.
KWIK-STIKT PLUS	Micro-Bio-Logics.Inc
KWIK-STIKT PLUS	Microbiologics, Inc.
KWIK-THERM	Psg Controls, Inc.
KWIK-VIAL	Baxa Corporation
KY	Oscor, Inc.
KYOWA	Soltec Corp.
KYTOSTAT	Hemcon Medical Technologies, Inc.
KZ-BIO	Technical Instruments (Ti)
Kandoo	Procter & Gamble
Kappa 700	Medtronic, Inc.
Keraflex	Avedro, Inc.
Kidfits	Acor Orthopaedic, Inc.
KinAir	Kinetic Concepts, Inc.
L&R	Encompas Unlimited, Inc.
L'AMY	L'Amy, Inc.
L-3	Branford Laboratories
L-VIEW	Medivision Endoscopy
L2X	Luxfer Gas Cylinders
L5X	Luxfer Gas Cylinders
L6X	Luxfer Gas Cylinders
L7X	Luxfer Gas Cylinders
LA MONT	La Mont Medical, Inc.
LA MONT CARDINAL	La Mont Medical, Inc.
LA MONT NCI	La Mont Medical, Inc.
LA MONT PRO AMP	La Mont Medical, Inc.
LA MONT VANGARD	La Mont Medical, Inc.
LAB AID	Sakura Finetek U.S.A., Inc.
LAB AIR-Z	Shofu Dental Corporation
LAB BOXES	Phoenix Metal Products, Inc.
LAB FILE	Wheaton Science Products
LAB MANAGER SYSTEM	Leica Microsystems (San Jose) Corporation
LAB MASTER	Lightnin Mixers
LAB PARTNER PLUS	General Assembly Corporation
LAB PLUS SERIES	Pro Scientific Inc.
LAB SERVICES	Currie Medical Specialties, Inc.
LAB SITE	Medical Associates Network
LAB-CHOICE	Medegen Medical Products, Llc
LAB-JACK	Boekel Scientific
LAB-SITE	Fenwal Inc.
LAB-SKRIBE	Hospital Marketing Svcs. Company, Inc.
LAB-TEMP	Thermcraft, Inc
LAB/HEX	Hex Laboratory Systems
LABCALLS	Televox Software, Inc.
LABCELL	Siemens Healthcare Diagnostics Inc.
LABCENTRAL	Hex Laboratory Systems
LABDAQ	Antek Healthware, Inc.
LABDEX APR	Dexall Biomedical Labs, Inc.
LABDEX ASR	Dexall Biomedical Labs, Inc.
LABEL GUARD	Luxfer Gas Cylinders
LABELETTE LABELERS	Biner Ellison
LABGARD	Nuaire, Inc.
LABMASTER	Hf Pure Water
LABMASTER	M. Braun Inc.
LABMAX	Coherent, Inc.
LABNET	Labnet International
LABO AMERICA	Labo America, Inc.
LABO AMERICA INC.	Labo America, Inc.
LABOMED	Labo America, Inc.
LABOR FIBRINTIMER	American Labor
LABOTHERM	Unique/Pereny
LABRETRIEVER	July Soft
LABREXX	Idexx Laboratories, Inc.
LABSCAN	One Lambda, Inc.
LABSCAN XE	Hunter Associates Lab., Inc.
LABSCREEN	One Lambda, Inc.
LABSPECr	Analytical Spectral Devices, Inc.
LABSTIX	Siemens Healthcare Diagnostics Inc.
LABTEMP	Biosynergy, Inc.
LABTOOLS	Eberbach Corp.
LABTRAK	J&S Medical Associates
LABTYPE	One Lambda, Inc.
LABWEB	Psyche Systems
LACOSTE	L'Amy, Inc.
LACRIMAL EFFICIENCY TEST	Lacrimedics
LACT-AID	Lact-Aid International
LACTAID	Johnson & Johnson
LACTEST	Quintron Instrument Company
LACTINA	Medela, Inc.
LACTINOL	Pedinol Pharmacal, Inc.
LACTINOL-E	Pedinol Pharmacal, Inc.
LACTOMER	Covidien Lp, Formerly Registered As United States Surgical
LADIES CHOICE	H.L. Bouton Co., Inc.
LAERDAL	Bound Tree Medical
LAERDAL	Laerdal Medical Corporation
LAERDAL AED TRAINER	Medical Plastics Laboratory, Inc.
LAERDAL AIRMAN DIFFICULT AIRWAY SIMULATOR	Medical Plastics Laboratory, Inc.
LAERDAL AIRWAY MANAGEMENT TRAINER	Medical Plastics Laboratory, Inc.
LAERDAL ALS BABY	Medical Plastics Laboratory, Inc.
LAERDAL COMPACT SUCTION UNIT	Medical Plastics Laboratory, Inc.
LAERDAL FACE SHIELD	Medical Plastics Laboratory, Inc.
LAERDAL INFLATE-A-SHIELD	Medical Plastics Laboratory, Inc.
LAERDAL POCKET MASK	Medical Plastics Laboratory, Inc.
LAERDAL SIMMAN UNIVERSAL PATIENT SIMULATOR	Medical Plastics Laboratory, Inc.
LAERDAL SUCTION UNIT	Medical Plastics Laboratory, Inc.
LAGUNA	Clarke Health Care Products, Inc.
LAGUNA SP	Clarke Health Care Products, Inc.
LAGX	Hard Manufacturing Co.
LAM	Prentke Romich Company
LAM PAC	Lampac International Ltd.
LAMBDA 2000	Netzsch Instruments, Inc.
LAMBDA CELL TRAY	One Lambda, Inc.
LAMBDA DOT	One Lambda, Inc.
LAMBDA JET	One Lambda, Inc.
LAMBDA MONOCLONAL TRAYS	One Lambda, Inc.

LAMBDA SCAN	One Lambda, Inc.
LAMBDA SX	Coherent, Inc.
LAMBDA-LIFT	Bio-Rad Laboratories, Life Science Group
LAMBDAGEM	Promega Corp.
LAMBDASORB	Promega Corp.
LAMINAR	Dynamic Systems, Inc.
LAMINARIA	Medgyn Products, Inc.
LAMINATED MOISTURE	UBM Canon
LAMINOSS	Impladent Ltd.
LAMIS	Byron Medical
LANA-GRAM	Hardy Diagnostics
LANCE	Cincinnati Surgical Company
LANCE	Perkin Elmer Wallac, Inc.
LANCE	Perkinelmer Life And Analytical Sciences
LANCELOT	Arthrocare Corp.
LANCER	Covidien Lp
LANCER	Lancer Usa, Inc.
LANCERACID	Lancer Usa, Inc.
LANCERCLEAN	Lancer Usa, Inc.
LANDEC PURT	Landec Corp.
LANDMARX	Medtronic Xomed, Inc.
LANDSCAPE	Mortara Instrument, Inc.
LANEX	Carestream Health, Inc.
LANGE	Beta Technology, Inc.
LANGE	Creative Health Products, Inc.
LANLOK	Sellstrom Manufacturing Co.
LANTIS ONCOLOGY INFORMATION MANAGEMENT SYSTEM	Siemens Medical Solutions Usa, Inc
LANTISEPTIC	Lantiseptic Division, Summit Industries, Inc.
LANTOR CUBE	Sps Medical Supply Corp.
LANY'D STO	Sellstrom Manufacturing Co.
LANYARDS	Key-Bak
LAP G	Abbott Laboratories
LAP J	Abbott Laboratories
LAPAROSTAT	Ams Innovative Center-San Jose
LAPAROVAC	Ams Innovative Center-San Jose
LAPCARE	Symmetry Medical Usa, Inc.
LAPCARE	Symmetry Medical, Inc.
LAPIDES	Ldb Medical, Inc.
LAPRA-TY	Ethicon Endo-Surgery, Inc.
LAPRA-TY	Ethicon, Inc.
LAPRO-LOOP	Covidien Lp
LAPTOP STORAGE CART	Anthro Corporation
LAR-A-JEXT	Covidien Lp, Formerly Registered As Kendall
LARK	Ortho-Kinetics, Inc.
LARK OF AMERICA	Ortho-Kinetics, Inc.
LARY	Boston Scientific Interventional Technologies
LAS VEGAS	Byron Medical
LASANTE	Levine Health Products
LASENTEC	Mettler Toledo Lasentec Products (Lasentec)
LASER	Medical Energy, Inc.
LASER	Pride Mobility Products Corp.
LASER BOND	Biolase Technology, Inc.
LASER NEUROTHERAPY	Spectrum Laser & Technologies, Inc
LASER PLUS	Volk Optical Inc.
LASER SERGE	White Knight Engineered Products
LASER WINDOW	Volk Optical Inc.
LASER-35 DENTAL LASER	Biolase Technology, Inc.
LASER-POWER TOUCH	Medical Energy, Inc.
LASER-SHIELD	Medtronic Xomed, Inc.
LASER-SIGHT	Cas Medical Systems, Inc.
LASERCAM	Coherent, Inc.
LASERCARD	Lasercard Systems Corporation
LASERCHECK	Coherent, Inc.
LASERCYTE	Idexx Laboratories, Inc.
LASERDOPP	Vasamed
LASERFADE	Hanson Medical, Inc.
LASERFLO	Vasamed
LASERFOCUS	Solarius Development Inc.
LASERITE	Advanced Medical Innovations, Inc.
LASERITE	Karl Storz Endoscopy-America Inc.
LASERLIGHT	Ocular Instruments, Inc.
LASERPAD	Coherent, Inc.
LASERPAL	Biolase Technology, Inc.
LASERPRO CO2 LASER	Surgical Laser Technologies, Inc.
LASERPRO CTH HOLMIUM LASER SYSTEM	Surgical Laser Technologies, Inc.
LASERPRO DIODE LASER	Surgical Laser Technologies, Inc.
LASERSCAN	Solarius Development Inc.
LASERSCOPE	Ams Innovative Center-San Jose
LASERSHIELD	Noir Manufacturing
LASERSMILE	Biolase Technology, Inc.
LASERTRIPTER	Candela Corp.
LASTING EDGE	Medical Sterile Products, Inc.
LASTING TOUCH	Dentsply International, Inc.
LASTING TOUCH	Dentsply Prosthetics
LASTRAP	Coopercare Lastrap Inc
LATERAL PIVOT	DJO Surgical
LATEX FREE	Aso Corporation
LATHE-40	Materials Development Corporation
LATHONG DISPOSABLE PANTIES	Dna Products, Llc
LATIS	Applied Medical Resource Corporation
LATITUDE GASTROINTESTINAL MANOMETRY CATHETER	Clinical Innovations, Inc.
LATPAK	Tulip Medical Products
LAUNDERCENTER	Ipso Usa, Inc.
LAVA	3m Co.
LAVOPTIK	H.L. Bouton Co., Inc.
LAVOPTIK	H.L. Bouton Company, Inc.
LAZERCREME	Pedinol Pharmacal, Inc.
LAZERFORMALYDE	Pedinol Pharmacal, Inc.
LAZY FLOSS	Locin Industries Ltd.
LB5	All-Tronics Medical Systems
LC BEAD	Angiodynamics, Inc.
LC-THERMOCOINS	Zander Medical Supplies, Inc. / Zander Ivf, Inc.
LC-THERMOMETERS	Zander Medical Supplies, Inc. / Zander Ivf, Inc.
LCA	Cte Chem Tec Equipment Co.
LCC	Luxfer Gas Cylinders
LCEC	Basi (Bioanalytical Systems, Inc.)
LCS	Ventana Medical Systems, Inc.
LD SERIES	Taylor Wharton
LDD	Ams Innovative Center-San Jose
LDD	Starkey Laboratories, Inc.
LDH	Zimmer Holdings, Inc.
LDS	Covidien Lp, Formerly Registered As United States Surgical
LE CLEAN	Parkell, Inc.
LEACH/DILLON	Argen Corp.
LEAD	Stryker Corp.
LEAD EXTRACTION	Cook Vascular, Incorporated
LEAD LOCKING DEVICE (LLD)	Spectranetics Corp.
LEAD PACK	Carestream Health, Inc.
LEAD TELL MARKERS	Sheldon Enterprises, Inc.
LEADCARE	Esa, Inc.
LEADER	Cardinal Health Inc.
LEADER	Gen-Probe, Inc.
LEADER 900Z SERIES TREATMENT TABLE	Leander Health Technologies/Healthcare Division
LEADX	Bar-Ray Products, Inc.
LEAK-TEC	American Gas & Chemical Co., Ltd.
LEANDER LITE TABLE	Leander Health Technologies/Healthcare Division
LEANDER MOTORIZED MULTI-PURPOSE TABLE	Leander Health Technologies/Healthcare Division
LEARNING EXCHANGE	Veritech Corporation
LEBRIEF DISPOSABLE PANTIES	Dna Products, Llc
LECTRO PATCH	General Medical Co.
LECTRO-SONIC	Cardiac Science Corp.
LECTROLITE	Herculite Products, Inc.
LEEZYME	Lee Medical International, Inc.
LEG SPACER	Core Products International, Inc.
LEGASUS CPM	Capstone Therapeutics
LEGATO	Freeman Manufacturing Company
LEGEND	American Orthodontics Corp.
LEGEND	Medtronic Powered Surgical Solutions
LEGEND	Pride Mobility Products Corp.
LEGEND	Stryker Corp.
LEGEND PLATINUM	Medtronic Powered Surgical Solutions
LEGENDARY LOOKS	Artcraft New York

LEGGRIP	Sunmedica
LEIBINGER	Striker Corp.
LEIBINGER	Stryker Corp.
LEISURE LIFT	Leisure-Lift, Inc.
LEISURE MATT	Span-America Medical Systems, Inc.
LEKSELL GAMMA KNIFE	Elekta, Inc.
LEKSELL GAMMAPLAN	Elekta, Inc.
LEKSELL NEUROGENERATOR	Elekta, Inc.
LEKSELL STEREOTACTIC SYSTEM	Elekta, Inc.
LEKSELL SURGIPLAN, ACTIVE BREATHING COORDINATOR, ELEKTA NEUROMAG	Elekta, Inc.
LEKTRIEVER	Kardex Systems, Inc.
LEMAITRE CATHETERS	Lemaitre Vascular, Inc.
LEMAITRE STENT GUIDE	Lemaitre Vascular, Inc.
LENK	Wall Lenk Corp.
LENOX HILL	Seattle Systems
LENS CLEAN	H.L. Bouton Co., Inc.
LENSCLEAN	H.L. Bouton Co., Inc.
LENSVUE2	Softsert, Inc.
LENSWIPE	H.L. Bouton Co., Inc.
LEOREX	Onyx Medical Inc./Face-It
LESTRONIC II	Lester Electrical Of Nebraska, Inc.
LETHERAY	Hanovia Specialty Lighting Llc
LETZ	Utah Medical Products, Inc.
LEUKINE	Amgen Inc.
LEUKOREDUCED PLT	R & D Systems, Inc.
LEUKOREDUCED RBC	R & D Systems, Inc.
LEUKOSCAN	Immunomedics, Inc.
LEV HOME ELEVATOR	Thyssenkrupp Access Corp.
LEVAMED	Medi Usa
LEVAQUIN	Ortho-Mcneil-Janssen Pharmaceuticals, Inc.
LEVELMARK	Tyco Valves and Controls
LEVINE	Levine Health Products
LEVOXYL	King Pharmaceuticals, Inc.
LEWISBINS	Lewis Bins+
LEWISYSTEMS	Orbis Corporation
LEXA	Horcher Lifting Systems, Inc.
LEXIS	Oticon, Inc.
LFSPP	Cte Chem Tec Equipment Co.
LG ELECTRONICS U.S.A., INC.	Lg Electronics U.S.A., Inc.
LH1000	Medmetric Corp.
LIATEST	Diagnostica Stago, Inc.
LIBERATOR	Caire, Inc.
LIBERATOR	Cook Vascular, Incorporated
LIBERTY	I-Flow Corporation
LIBERTY	Magnatone Hearing Aid Corp.
LIBERTY	North Coast Medical, Inc.
LIBERTY	Tri-State Hospital Supply Corp.
LIBERTY	Utah Medical Products, Inc.
LIBERTY VALVE	Cleveland Medical Devices, Inc.
LIBERTYHILL	Hill-Rom Holdings, Inc.
LICOX	Integra Lifesciences Holdings Corp.
LID-LABEL	Medi-Dose, Inc.
LIDOSITE	Vyteris, Inc.
LIEBEL-FLARSHEIM	Mallinckrodt, Inc.
LIFE	Access Battery Inc.
LIFE	Life Corporation
LIFE FITNESS	Life Fitness
LIFE GUARD	Life Guard
LIFE LATCH	M & M Industries
LIFE LINES	Health-Pak, Inc.
LIFE MASK	Cft, Inc./Life Mask
LIFE OXYGENPAC	Life Corporation
LIFE PLUS FOREVER YOUNG SKIN CARE PRODUCTS	Life Plus International
LIFE PLUS NUTRITIONAL PRODUCTS	Life Plus International
LIFE PULSE	Bunnell Incorporated
LIFE SIGNS-RECEIVING CENTER 2000	Instromedix, A Card Guard Co.
LIFE SUPPORT	Carolon Company
LIFE SUPPORT PRODUCTS	Allied Healthcare Products, Inc.
LIFE-AIR 1000	Progressive Dynamics Medical, Inc.
LIFE-LINE	Lifemed Of California
LIFE-O2	Life Corporation
LIFE/FORM	Aristotle Corp.
LIFE/FORM	Nasco
LIFEAID	Faichney Medical Co.
LIFEBAND	Zoll Medical Corp.
LIFECARE PCA	Hospira Inc.
LIFECARE PIN PERINATAL INFORMATION NETWORK	Life Care Technologies, Inc.
LIFECART	Physio-Control, Inc.
LIFECOIL	Lifemed Of California
LIFECORE	Lifecore Biomedical, Inc.
LIFECORE DENTAL	Lifecore Biomedical, Inc.
LIFECYCLE	Thermo Uscs
LIFEFORM	Nasco
LIFEGAS	Lifegas Llc
LIFEGLOBAL	Genx International
LIFELINE	Concorde Battery
LIFELINE	Intermetro Industries Corp.
LIFELINE	Mediware Information Systems, Inc.
LIFELINE GYM	Mueller Sports Medicine
LIFELONG THERAPY	World Heart Inc.
LIFEMED	Lifemed Of California
LIFENET	Physio-Control, Inc.
LIFEPAK	Physio-Control, Inc.
LIFEPATCH	Physio-Control, Inc.
LIFEPORT	Angiodynamics, Inc.
LIFEPORT	Bunnell Incorporated
LIFESCIENCES CORPORATION	Integra Lifesciences Holdings Corp.
LIFESCOPE	Nihon Kohden America, Inc.
LIFESEAT	Patterson Medical Holdings, Inc.
LIFESHIELD	Covidien Lp
LIFESHIELD	Hospira Inc.
LIFESHIELD TKO	Hospira Inc.
LIFESIGN	Princeton Biomeditech Corp.
LIFESIGN MI	Princeton Biomeditech Corp.
LIFESIGN PLUS	Princeton Biomeditech Corp.
LIFESIGNS SP	Instromedix, A Card Guard Co.
LIFESOUND	Novamed, Llc
LIFESOURCE	A&D Medical
LIFESPAN	Albahealth Llc
LIFESTYLE PLUS AIR FILTER	Permatron Corp.
LIFESTYLE ROCOVERY	Stryker Corp.
LIFESTYLE ROCOVERY	Stryker Howmedica Osteonics
LIFESTYLES CONDOMS	Ansell Healthcare, Inc.
LIFESYNC	Lifesync Corporation
LIFETEC	Systec Computer Associates, Inc.
LIFEVEST	Zoll Medical Corp.
LIFEWATCH	Lifewatch Services, Inc.
LIFEX	Rayovac
LIFEX-FB	Rayovac
LIFOGEN	Allied Healthcare Products, Inc.
LIFT ASSIST	Stryker Corp.
LIFT WALKER, LIFT ASSISTED WALKING DEVICE	Prime Engineering
LIFT-A-LIMB	Equip For Independence, Inc.
LIFT-ALL	Amigo Mobility International
LIFT-IT	Amigo Mobility International
LIFT-N-WEIGH	Medcare Products, Inc.
LIFTLOC	Specialized Health Products International, Inc.
LIFTS ENTERPRISES INC.	Silver Star Mobility
LIFTTRACK	JTECH Medical
LIG-A-BOOTS	Axiom Medical, Inc.
LIG-A-LOOPS	Axiom Medical, Inc.
LIG-A-RINGS	Tp Orthodontics, Inc.
LIGACLIP	Ethicon Endo-Surgery, Inc.
LIGAPAK	Ethicon, Inc.
LIGASURE ATLAST	Valleylab
LIGASURE ATLAST 20 CM	Valleylab
LIGASURE PRECISET	Valleylab
LIGASURET	Valleylab
LIGASURET AXS	Valleylab
LIGASURET LAP	Valleylab
LIGASURET MAX	Valleylab
LIGASURET STD	Valleylab
LIGASURET V	Valleylab
LIGASURET XTD	Valleylab

LIGATE-IT	Usb Corporation
LIGHT & DRY	Salk Inc.
LIGHT FANTASTIC	Pelton & Crane Co.,
LIGHT FANTASTIC II	Pelton & Crane Co.,
LIGHT FORCE SERIES 20 980NM (LIGHT FORCE 1)	Medical Energy, Inc.
LIGHT FORCE SERIES 30 980NM (LIGHT FORCE 2)	Medical Energy, Inc.
LIGHT SHIELDS	Medical Action Industries, Inc
LIGHT SUPER BOND	Dent Zar, Inc.
LIGHT TOUCH	Novosci Corp.
LIGHT WAND	Vital Signs, Inc.
LIGHT* TOUCH	Medical Energy, Inc.
LIGHT-SAFE	Codan Us Corporation
LIGHTENING CLEANSER	Donell
LIGHTENING GEL	Donell
LIGHTGARD	Minatronics Corp.
LIGHTING THE WAY TO HEALING	Nomir Medical Technologies Inc.
LIGHTKEY	Advanced Input Systems
LIGHTLINER	Harry J. Bosworth Company
LIGHTMAT	Lumitex, Inc.
LIGHTNIN	Lightnin Mixers
LIGHTNING	Moyco Technologies, Inc.
LIGHTNING	Siemens Hearing Instruments, Inc.
LIGHTOUCH	Boss Instruments, Ltd.
LIGHTPICK	Spirig Advanced Technologies, Inc.
LIGHTREE	White Systems, Inc.
LIGHTSTIC	Cardiofocus, Inc.
LIGHTWRITER	Zygo Industries, Inc.
LIKO LIGHT	Liko North America
LIKORALL	Liko North America
LIL-KATCH	Precision Dynamics Corp.
LILLTE SUCKER	Neotech Products, Inc.
LIM2000	Bender, Inc.
LIMB-O	Vital Signs, Inc.
LIMBO	Hollister Incorporated
LIMBOARD	Cas Medical Systems, Inc.
LIME-A-WAY	Ecolab Inc.
LIMELIGHT	Cutera, Inc.
LIN-CHEK	Polymedco, Inc.
LINAC SCALPEL	Varian Medical Systems
LINATRON	Varian Medical Systems
LINDLEY	Boston Scientific Interventional Technologies
LINE RANGER	Rontron Engineering, Inc.
LINE-O-VISION	Hollister Incorporated
LINE-R POWER CONDITIONERS	American Power Conversion
LINEAGE	Wright Medical Group, Inc.
LINEAR	DJO Surgical
LINEAR K	Whatman Inc.
LINEAR LINK	Eg & G Amorphous Silicon
LINEAR-PLUS	Argosy
LINEBACKER	Martin-Mars, Inc.
LINEN MOBILE	Atlantic Medco, Inc.
LINEN PROTECTORS	Geri-Care Products
LINGRAPHICA	Lingraphicare America, Inc.
LINICAL	Cliniqa Corporation
LINK	Link Ergonomics Corp.
LINK	LinkBio Corp.
LINK SERIES	Eg & G Amorphous Silicon
LINK WIRELESS TELEPHONE SYSTEM	Spectralink Corporation
LINKAM	Mccrone Microscopes & Accessories
LINT PIC UP	The Evercare Company
LINX	Agfa Corporation
LIONVILLE	Lionville Systems, Inc.
LIPI PLUS	Polymedco, Inc.
LIPOCELL	Serologicals Corp
LIPOCLEAR	Statspin, Inc.
LIPOFOAM	Specialty Surgical Products, Inc.
LIPOPRINT HDL	Quantimetrix Corporation
LIPOPRINT LDL	Quantimetrix Corporation
LIPOSELECTION	Sound Surgical Technologies Llc
LIPOSORBER	Kaneka Pharma America Llc
LIPP	Intelligent Hearing Systems, Corp.
LIQSORB	Reach Global Industries, Inc. (Reachgood)
LIQSORB ANTI REFLUX SYSTEM POLY-GEL 2000ML OVERNIGHT BAGPOLY-GEL	Key / Sun Medical Services, Inc.
LIQUA-SONIC	Chester Labs, Inc.
LIQUI-CHAR	King Pharmaceuticals, Inc.
LIQUI/PORT	Spectrum Laboratories, Inc.
LIQUICHEK	Bio-Rad, Diagnostics Group
LIQUICOR	Cardiac Science Corp.
LIQUID COVERSLIP	Ventana Medical Systems, Inc.
LIQUID SPY	Spectrum Laboratories, Inc.
LIQUID SUNMATE FOAM-IN-PLACE SEATING	Dynamic Systems, Inc.
LIQUIDERM	Closure Medical
LIQUIDOSE	Medi-Dose, Inc.
LIQUISURE	Quantimetrix Corporation
LIQUITHERM	Unique/Pereny
LISTER	Trans American Medical
LISTERIA-TEK	Biomerieux Inc.
LISTERINE	Johnson & Johnson
LITA	Covidien Lp, Formerly Registered As Kendall
LITE	Access Battery Inc.
LITE	Crosstex International,Inc.
LITE GLOVE	Graphic Controls Corp.
LITE HANDLE	Graphic Controls Corp.
LITE MATE	Photo Research, Inc.
LITE N' SOFT	Optikem International, Inc.
LITE RIDER	Convaid, Inc.
LITE SITE	Dispensers Optical Service Corp.
LITE SLEEVE	Graphic Controls Corp.
LITE STEP	Ace Hose & Rubber Company
LITE TITE	American Orthodontics Corp.
LITE-AID	Activeaid, Inc.
LITE-N-TUFF	Hamilton Caster & Mfg. Co.
LITE-PIPE	Electro Surgical Instrument Co., Inc.
LITE-TOUCH ADJUSTABLE ARM	Medical Graphics Corporation
LITEPAC	Motloid Company
LITERMETER	Erie Medical
LITESTRIDE	Azmec, Inc.
LITESTRIP	Swivelier Co., Inc.
LITHOCLEAR	Sonotech Inc.
LITHODIAMOND	Healthtronics Inc.
LITHOSPEC	Medispec Ltd. - Usa
LITREPAK	Bd Diagnostic Systems
LITTLE ANNE	Laerdal Medical Corporation
LITTLE ANNE	Medical Plastics Laboratory, Inc.
LITTLE DIPPER	Colours Wheelchair
LITTLE GIANT	Electro-Steam Generator Corp.
LITTLE JOE CPR MANIKIN	Armstrong Medical Industries, Inc.
LITTLE JUNIOR	Medical Plastics Laboratory, Inc.
LITTLE MILLI	Noram Solutions
LITTLE MOODS	United Syntek Corp.
LITTLE ONES	Convatec Professional Services
LITTLE RED VALVE	Urocare Products, Inc.
LITTLE SHOT	Boekel Scientific
LITTLE WAREHOUSE	Rem Systems
LITTMANN	3m Co.
LITTMANN	Creative Health Products, Inc.
LITTMANN	Lydia's Professional Uniforms
LIVEWIRE	St. Jude Medical Atrial Fibrillation
LIVIAN	Boston Scientific Corporation
LM-151	Lynn Medical
LMADS	Arc Medical, Inc.
LMS	Medstat Inc.
LMW	Triangle Biomedical Sciences, Inc.
LO BUOY	Brandt Industries, Inc.
LO-CYCLE	R. B. Annis Instruments, Inc.
LO-PRO TILE	R.C.A. Rubber Company, The
LO-PRO TREADS	R.C.A. Rubber Company, The
LO-PROFILE	Hollister Incorporated
LO-TEMP	Bovie Medical Corp.
LO2	Icu Medical, Inc.
LOBANA	Ulmer Pharmacal Co.
LOBOB	Lobob Laboratories, Inc.
LOBSTER	Boss Instruments, Ltd.
LOC-TOP	Lps Industries, Inc.

LYPHOCHEK	Bio-Rad, Diagnostics Group
LYPORE	Lydall, Inc.
LYRA	Ams Innovative Center-San Jose
LYSOCOLOR	Cytocolor, Inc.
Lamitrode	St. Jude Medical Neuromodulation Division
Larenim	Nutraceutical International Corp.
Laser-Lok	Biohorizons Implant Systems, Inc.
LaserSmart	Kentek Corp.
LeVeen	Boston Scientific Corporation
LeVeen CoAccess	Boston Scientific Corporation
LeakAlert	The Amcor Group Ltd.
Legend EHS (Electric High Speed)	Medtronic Powered Surgical Solutions
Legend EHS Stylus	Medtronic Powered Surgical Solutions
Legend Gold	Medtronic Powered Surgical Solutions
Legend Gold Touch	Medtronic Powered Surgical Solutions
LibertAc	Boston Scientific - Maple Grove
LibertAüi'A,Ac	Boston Scientific Corporation
Life	Knoll, Inc.
Life-flo	Nutraceutical International Corp.
LifeRx	Vision-Ease Lens
Lithobid	Noven Pharmaceuticals, Inc.
Livewire	St. Jude Medical, Inc.
Livewire Cannulator	St. Jude Medical, Inc.
Livewire Spiral HP	St. Jude Medical, Inc.
Livewire TC	St. Jude Medical, Inc.
Living Flower Essences	Nutraceutical International Corp.
LoProdyne	Pall Corporation
Locator	St. Jude Medical, Inc.
Lotemax	Bausch & Lomb
Luma-Cath	Boston Scientific Corporation
Lumitip	Atricure, Inc.
Luvs	Procter & Gamble
Lynx	Boston Scientific Corporation
M SERIES	Zoll Medical Corp.
M-1	Bio-Med Devices, Inc.
M-1	Statlab Medical Products, Inc.
M-1 ROLL-IN SYSTEM	Stryker Corp.
M-10	Bio-Med Devices, Inc.
M-2	Bio-Med Devices, Inc.
M-2 MINOR AQUATEC	Clarke Health Care Products, Inc.
M-CUTTER	Mueller Sports Medicine
M-DEC	Mobile Dental Equipment Corp.(M-Dec)
M-IV	Hologic, Inc.
M-OB/GYN OFFICE	Sonosite, Inc.
M-PACT	Bsn Medical, Inc
M-PACT	Ortholine
M-PD PERSONAL	Ericsson, Inc.
M-RK PORTABLE	Ericsson, Inc.
M-TAPE	Mueller Sports Medicine
M-TURBO	Sonosite, Inc.
M-WRAP	Mueller Sports Medicine
M.B.	M. Braun Inc.
M.I.S.	Medical Sterile Products, Inc.
M.KUROSAKA	DJO Inc.
M.S.P.	Medical Sterile Products, Inc.
M100	Airex, Inc.
M2000	Abbott Laboratories
M2LABSCOPE	Lw Scientific
M4	Microtest, Inc.
M4 MONITOR SERIES EMG	Neurodyne Medical Corp.
M4-EX	Panamax, Inc.
M40 CLINICAL SERIES EMG	Neurodyne Medical Corp.
M44 CLINICAL SERIES DUAL EMG	Neurodyne Medical Corp.
M4T-EX	Panamax, Inc.
M8-EX	Panamax, Inc.
M8T-EX	Panamax, Inc.
MAB	Quidel Corporation
MABIS	Creative Health Products, Inc.
MAC	Ge Medical Systems Information Technologies
MAC	Gunnell, Inc.
MAC	Stryker Corp.
MAC	Stryker Spine
MAC'S AMBULANCE MEDIX LIFT	Mac's Lift Gate, Inc.
MAC'S PL-45 VERTICAL LIFT	Mac's Lift Gate, Inc.
MACCEL	Nest Group Inc., The
MACH-2	Parkell, Inc.
MACHINE	Parkell, Inc.
MACK'S	Mckeon Products, Inc.
MACLAB	Adinstruments
MACLAB	iWorx Systems, Inc.
MACRO ELECTRAPETTE	Thermo Fisher Scientific
MACRO-CON	Meridian Bioscience, Inc.
MACRO-VUE	Bd Diagnostic Systems
MACRODUCT	Wescor, Inc.
MACROLYTE	Conmed Corporation
MACROPATH	Hacker Instruments And Industries Inc.
MACROVAC	Pmt Corp.
MACUGEN	Nektar Therapeutics
MACULA PLUS	Volk Optical Inc.
MACULAR HOLE RECOVERY SYSTEM	Rite Time Corporation
MACULOSCOPE SPECTRUM	Diagnosis, Llc
MADA JET XL	Mada, Inc.
MADA-VAC	Mada, Inc.
MADA-VAC II	Mada, Inc.
MADACIDE	Mada, Inc.
MADACYLINDER	Mada, Inc.
MADAMETER	Mada, Inc.
MADAMIST 50	Mada, Inc.
MADAMIST I	Mada, Inc.
MADAMIST II	Mada, Inc.
MADELON LOUDEN	Finebrand Co.
MAE	Halbar North, Inc.
MAESTRO	Briggs Corporation
MAESTRO	Stryker Corp.
MAG3	Mallinckrodt, Inc.
MAGENTA	Labcon North America
MAGIC	Siemens Healthcare Diagnostics Inc
MAGIC WRIST	Professional's Choice Sports Medicine Products, Inc.
MAGLEV	World Heart Inc.
MAGNA CELLULOSE ACETATE MEMBRANE	Ge Infrastructure Water & Process Technologies
MAGNA NITROCELLULOSE MIXED ESTERS MEMBRANE	Ge Infrastructure Water & Process Technologies
MAGNA NYLON HYDROPHOBIC MEMBRANE	Ge Infrastructure Water & Process Technologies
MAGNA NYLON TRANSFER MEMBRANE	Ge Infrastructure Water & Process Technologies
MAGNA NYLONG MEMBRANE	Ge Infrastructure Water & Process Technologies
MAGNA PES POLYETHANSULFONE MEMBRANE	Ge Infrastructure Water & Process Technologies
MAGNA PROBE NYLON MEMBRANE	Ge Infrastructure Water & Process Technologies
MAGNA PVDF MEMBRANE	Ge Infrastructure Water & Process Technologies
MAGNA X-II	Hager Worldwide, Inc.
MAGNA-CAL	Ultra-Cal, Inc.
MAGNA-CLAVE	Pelton & Crane Co.,
MAGNA-DRAPE	Graphic Controls Corp.
MAGNA-FRAME	Camfil Farr
MAGNA-GRID	Camfil Farr
MAGNA-PORT	Abbott Laboratories
MAGNA-SPLIT	Panadent Corp.
MAGNACAL	Afassco, Inc.
MAGNAFREE	Codman & Shurtleff, Inc
MAGNATHERM	International Medical Electronics Ltd.
MAGNATONE	Magnatone Hearing Aid Corp.
MAGNATREVE	Adept-Med International, Inc.
MAGNE-SPLINT	Medtronic Xomed, Inc.
MAGNECORE	Core Products International, Inc.
MAGNESPHERE	Promega Corp.
MAGNETOM	Siemens Medical Solutions Usa, Inc.
MAGNEVU	Magnevu
MAGNEX	Shimadzu Medical Systems
MAGNI-FOCUSER	Edroy Products Co., Inc.
MAGNI-GUARD	Advanced Medical Innovations, Inc.
MAGNI-SPECS	Edroy Products Co., Inc.
MAGNI-WIPE	Advanced Medical Innovations, Inc.

MAGNIFIER FLEX	Dazor Manufacturing Corp.
MAGNILENS	Magnivision, Inc.
MAGNIVISION	Magnivision, Inc.
MAGNUM	Atlantic Ultraviolet Corp.
MAGNUM	C. R. Bard, Inc., Bard Urological Div.
MAGNUM	Medtronic Xomed, Inc.
MAGNUM	Ohio Willow Wood Company
MAGNUM 9	Whatman Inc.
MAGNUM BRACES	Mueller Sports Medicine
MAGNUM LIFT	Leisure-Lift, Inc.
MAGNUM SCBA	Avon-Isi
MAGO	Diamedix Corp.
MAGSTIR GENIE	Scientific Industries, Inc.
MAGTAB	Asi-Modulex
MAILHAWK REACHER HAWKBILL REACHE	Mailhawk Manufacturing Company
MAILMASTER	The Mason Box Company
MAINSTAY	Bard Electro Physiology
MAJESTIC TRIPODS	Bencher, Inc.
MAJESTIK	Merit Medical Systems, Inc.
MAJESTIQUE	H.L. Bouton Co., Inc.
MAK-6	Life Technologies Corporation
MAKE IT RITE MIRROR	Rite Time Corporation
MAKITA	Makita Usa Inc. - Drapery Opener Div.
MAKOPLASTY	Mako Surgical Corp.
MALE BAG	Park Surgical Co., Inc.
MALE-FACTORPAK	Apex Medical Technologies, Inc.
MALIS CMC-III	Valley Forge Scientific Corp.
MALIS IRRIGATOR	Valley Forge Scientific Corp.
MALIS SYNERGY	Valley Forge Scientific Corp.
MALLEOLOC	Bauerfeind Usa, Inc.
MALLEOTRAIN	Bauerfeind Usa, Inc.
MALLINCKRODT	Covidien (Formerly Nellcor Puritan Bennett / Tyco Healthcare)
MALLORY/HEAD	Biomet, Inc.
MALYUGIN RING	Microsurgical Technology, Inc.
MAMMACARE	Mammatech Corp.
MAMMALOK	Medical Device Technologies, Inc. (Md Tech)
MAMMO-TECHLINE	Maxant Technologies, Inc.
MAMMOLUX	AMD Technologies Inc.
MAMMOMASK	Broadwest Corp.
MAMMOMAT	Siemens Medical Solutions Usa, Inc.
MAMMORX	Diacor, Inc.
MAMMOSOURCE	Varian Medical Systems
MAMMOTEST	Fischer Medical Technologies Inc.
MAMMOTEST PLUS	Fischer Medical Technologies Inc.
MAMMOTOME	Ethicon Endo-Surgery, Inc.
MAMMOVIEWER	Diversified Diagnostic Products, Inc.
MAMMOVISION	Fischer Medical Technologies Inc.
MAMORAY	Agfa Corporation
MANDELL SEAMLESS BIFOCAL	Con-Cise Contact Lens Co.
MANDIBULAR DISTRACTION	Kls-Martin L.P.
MANGUM	Smiths Medical OEM
MANHANDLER	Sperian Protection
MANHATTAN II	Argosy
MANIX	Ansell Healthcare, Inc.
MANKIND	Pmt Corp.
MANLOAD	Sellstrom Manufacturing Co.
MANTIS	Coherent, Inc.
MANTIS	Stryker Corp.
MANTIS	Stryker Spine
MANUALECTRIC	Medela, Inc.
MANUTRAIN	Bauerfeind Usa, Inc.
MANYARD	Sperian Protection
MAO	Cte Chem Tec Equipment Co.
MAP PLUS	Eit, Inc.
MAPS	Bio-Rad Laboratories, Life Science Group
MAQS	Oxoid, Inc.
MAQUET	Getinge Usa, Inc.
MARAMED	Ortholine
MARATHON	Corflex, Inc.
MARATHON	Ev3 Inc.
MARATHON INSERTS	Engler Engineering Corp.
MARBLOT	Mardx Diagnostics, Inc.
MARC 600	Spencer Technologies
MARCO	Marco Ophthalmic, Inc.
MARCONI	Atlas Medical Technologies
MARINER	Angiodynamics, Inc.
MARINOL	Roxane Laboratories
MARISA	ArjoHuntleigh
MARK 1	Meridian Medical Technologies
MARK 3, MARK 2 AND UWAVE MICROWAVE MOISTURE ANALYZER	Sartorius Omnimark Instrument Corp
MARK 4	Nidek Medical Products Inc.
MARK 5	Nidek Medical Products Inc.
MARK 5 PLUS	Nidek Medical Products Inc.
MARK I	Cramer Products, Inc.
MARK I	James Consolidated, Inc.
MARK II	James Consolidated, Inc.
MARK III	Ambu, Inc.
MARK III	Independent Solutions, Inc.
MARK SERIES 7 & 7A	CAREFUSION 211, INC..
MARK TIME	Rhodes Inc., M.H.
MARK V	Hospital Comm. & Electronics, Inc.
MARK V	Medsonic U.S.A., Inc.
MARK V PLUS	Medrad, Inc.
MARK V PROVIS	Medrad, Inc.
MARK-1 VISOR	General Scientific Safety Equipment Co.
MARK-M.TUBES	Kimble Chase Life Science And Research Products Llc
MARKER FOOT	Revelation Industries
MARKET FORGE	Medi-Tech International, Inc.
MARLIN	Aearo Company
MARLIN TIP	Covidien Lp, Formerly Registered As Kendall
MARPLE 290 PERSONAL IMPACTOR	Thermo Fisher Scientific
MARQUIS	Merit Medical Systems, Inc.
MARR VALVE	Specialty Manufacturing Co., The
MARS	Mars Air Doors
MARS AIR DOOR	Mars Air Doors
MARS HEPAC	Mars Air Doors
MARSH	Marsh Bellofram
MARSHALL	Nss Enterprises, Inc.
MARSHALL	Thermcraft, Inc
MARSORB G	Mardx Diagnostics, Inc.
MARSTRIPE	Mardx Diagnostics, Inc.
MARTIN	Kls-Martin L.P.
MARTIN IMPLANT	Kls-Martin L.P.
MARVEL	Wenzelite Rehab Supplies, Llc
MARVEL SCIENTIFIC	Marvel Scientific
MARVELTEX	Mid-States Laboratories, Inc.
MASCOT	Mentor Ophthalmics, Inc.
MASKENOMICS	Crosstex International,Inc.
MASKUMM	Trademark Medical Llc
MASON	Torbot Group, Inc.
MASS	Medical Design Systems, Inc.
MASS-TER	Seca Corp.
MASSAGE TIME CLASSIC	Sidmar Mfg., Inc.
MASSAGE TIME PRO	Sidmar Mfg., Inc.
MASSTAR	Rice Lake Weighing Systems
MASSTRANSIT	Cordis Neurovascular, Inc.
MAST	Clark Company Inc., David
MAST	David Clark Company, Inc.
MASTECTOMY SLIP	Ladies First, Inc.
MASTER CONTROL	Syntermed, Inc.
MASTER LAVAGE	Mectra Labs, Inc.
MASTER SCOPE	CAREFUSION 211, INC..
MASTER SCREEN	CAREFUSION 211, INC..
MASTER SERIES	American Orthodontics Corp.
MASTERCHARGER 6	W&W Manufacturing Co.
MASTERCRAFT	Melrose Mattress, Inc.
MASTERFIT	Carl Zeiss Meditec Inc.
MASTERFLEX	Cole-Parmer Instrument Inc.
MASTERFLOW	Conmed Corporation
MASTERGUARD	Fenwal Inc.
MASTERGUARD	Medisystems Corporation
MASTERSERIES	Horizon Healthcare Technologies
MASTERSET	Dentalez Group
MASTERSOL	Moyco Technologies, Inc.
MASTERSON	Rms Medical Products

MASTERSWITCH	American Power Conversion
MASTERVUE	Carl Zeiss Meditec Inc.
MASTIK	Immucell Corp.
MASTR	Gn Otometrics
MASTR II	Ericsson, Inc.
MATCH MATES	Mabis Healthcare Inc.
MATCH PRINTS BY INPRO	Inpro Corporation
MATES	Ansell Healthcare, Inc.
MATEY	Maddak Inc.
MATRI-TECT	Matritech, Inc.
MATRIGRAFT	Lifenet Health
MATRITECH	Matritech, Inc.
MATRIX	Biosensors International - Usa
MATRIX	Boston Scientific-Neurovascular
MATRIX	GE Healthcare
MATRIX	Smith & Nephew Inc.- Orthopaedics Division
MATRIX 44	Vicon Industries Inc.
MATRIX 550	Smiths Medical OEM
MATRIX 66	Vicon Industries Inc.
MATRIX MANIFOLDS	Smiths Medical OEM
MATRIX SERIES	Bobrick Washroom Equipment, Inc.
MATRIX-UPS	American Power Conversion
MATRX	Midmark Corporation
MATSCAN	Tekscan, Inc.
MATT STRAP	Hely And Weber
MATTA	Stryker Corp.
MATURE BASICS	Hygienics Industries Div.Of Kleinert's, Inc.
MAX	Products International Co.
MAX 15	Artromick International, Inc.
MAX 2	Panamax, Inc.
MAX 2 T	Panamax, Inc.
MAX 7	Artromick International, Inc.
MAX BLEND	Maxtec, Inc.
MAX CELL	Maxtec, Inc.
MAX NIBP	Cas Medical Systems, Inc.
MAX O2	Maxtec, Inc.
MAX O2 VENT	Maxtec, Inc.
MAX--LIFE BRUSH CONDITIONER	American Diversified Dental Systems
MAX-ACT	Helena Laboratories
MAX-AID	Activeaid, Inc.
MAX-BLADE	C. R. Bard, Inc., Bard Urological Div.
MAX-CORE	C. R. Bard, Inc., Bard Urological Div.
MAX-E	Torbot Group, Inc.
MAX-FAST	Covidien (Formerly Nellcor Puritan Bennett / Tyco Healthcare)
MAX-I-PROBE	Dentsply International, Inc.
MAX-I-PROBE	Dentsply Prosthetics
MAX-LOC	Woodhead L.P.
MAX-RELAX	Core Products International, Inc.
MAXANT	Independent Solutions, Inc.
MAXAR	Ita-Med Co.
MAXARRAY	Life Technologies Corporation
MAXBLOC	Gi Supply
MAXFIELD	Ocular Instruments, Inc.
MAXI	Medical Industries America Inc.
MAXI LD PTA DILATATION CATHETER	Cordis Endovascular
MAXI-COMFORT, ULTRA THIN, & ULTRA THIN II	Aimsco, Delta Hi-Tech, Inc.
MAXI-DRIVER	Conmed Linvatec
MAXI-LOK	Jilson Group, Inc.
MAXI-PEEP	Boehringer Laboratories, Inc.
MAXI-REST (BARIATRIC BEDS)	Gendron, Inc.
MAXI-SCOPE	Ultrascope
MAXI-SCOPE T	Ultrascope
MAXI-SUCTION PUMP	Ambu, Inc.
MAXI-TEK	Biotek, Inc.
MAXI-THERM	Cincinnati Sub-Zero Products, Inc., Medical Division
MAXI-THERM LITE	Cincinnati Sub-Zero Products, Inc., Medical Division
MAXI-THERM LITE VEST	Cincinnati Sub-Zero Products, Inc., Medical Division
MAXIBOND	Argen Corp.
MAXICOMFORT	Golden Technologies, Inc.
MAXIFLEX	B.G. Industries, Inc.
MAXIFLOAT	B.G. Industries, Inc.
MAXIFORCE	Paratech, Inc.
MAXILON	Kls Martin Lp
MAXIM	Biomet, Inc.
MAXIMA	Compex Technologies, Inc.
MAXIMUM POLY	DJO Surgical
MAXIMUS	Life-Tech, Inc.
MAXIMUS	Universal Gym Equipment
MAXIR INFRARED LAMPS	Bhk, Inc.
MAXISHIELD	HARTMANN USA, Inc.
MAXISKYS	ArjoHuntleigh
MAXISLIDES	ArjoHuntleigh
MAXISTAT	Surgica Corporation
MAXISTIM	Life-Tech, Inc.
MAXITHINS	Hospital Specialty Company
MAXLIGHT	Ocular Instruments, Inc.
MAXON	Covidien Lp
MAXUM	Wilson-Cook Medical, Inc.
MAXVIEW	Sellstrom Manufacturing Co.
MAXXUS	Ansell Healthcare Products, Inc.
MAXXUS PF	Ansell Healthcare Products, Inc.
MAXXV	Maxxvision, Llc
MAYFIELD	Schaerer Mayfield Usa
MAYFIELD 2000	Schaerer Mayfield Usa
MAYO CLINIC TRACHEOSTOMA BUTTONT	Medical Innovations International Inc.
MAYO-HEGOR	Trans American Medical
MAYO-TRAY	Healthmark Industries
MAYON	Mayon Plastics, Inc.
MAYTRIX	Tyco Healthcare Group Lp
MB-SPS	M. Braun Inc.
MB/BACT	Biomerieux Inc.
MBA	Kinetikos Medical, Inc.
MBG ALERT	Nanogen, Inc.
MBS INC.	Multi Biosensors, Inc.
MBT	3m Co.
MCBACK	Mccarty's Sacro-Ease Llc
MCCAIN	Striker Corp.
MCD	Medical Concepts Development
MCGLAMRY	Kmedic
MCINTYRE OCULO-PRESSOR:DEWEY RADIUS	Microsurgical Technology, Inc.
MCKELOR CPM SOFTGOODS	Mckelor Technologies, Ltd.
MCP	Immucor, Inc.
MCRI	Medical Carbon Research Institute, Llc - Mcri
MCRO-TOUCH PLUS	Ansell Healthcare Products, Inc.
MCS	Ericsson, Inc.
MCS	Exactech, Inc.
MCS MOBILE	Ericsson, Inc.
MCT PLUS	Medrad, Inc.
MCTOOTH	Hager Worldwide, Inc.
MCTOOTH CLIP	Hager Worldwide, Inc.
MCU - MULTI-CERVICAL UNIT	Bte Technologies, Inc.
MD ENGINNEERING	Medical Device Resource Corporation
MD FLOW	Biolase Technology, Inc.
MD SYSTEMS	Singer Medical Products, Inc.
MD TECH	Medical Device Technologies, Inc. (Md Tech)
MD-76R	Mallinckrodt, Inc.
MD-GASTROVIEW	Mallinckrodt, Inc.
MDA	Biomerieux Inc.
MDA D-DIMER	Biomerieux Inc.
MDA-II	Biomerieux Inc.
MDILOG	Westmed, Inc.
MDM	Artromick International, Inc.
MDM	Matrx By Midmark
MDN	Nspire Health, Inc
MDR	Nai Tech Products
MDR	UBM Canon
MDRCD-ROM	UBM Canon
MDS	Artromick International, Inc.
MDS	Zimmer Spine
MDSC	Ta Instruments
MDSTATION	Thinking Systems Corporation
ME	Mettler Electronics Corp.
MEASURE MASTER	Technical Instruments (Ti)
MEASURE MAT	Seca Corp.
MEASURE-ALL	Seca Corp.
MEASURERING	Mirion Technologies

MEC MARROW EXTRACTION CANNULA	Angiotech
MECASONIC	Forward Technology
MECHANICAL EVENT SIMULATION	Algor, Inc.
MED BOOK SYSTEM	First Healthcare Products
MED CLINER	Nk Medical Products Inc.
MED I.D.	Medical Id Systems Inc.
MED LINE	Handicap Unlimited, Inc.
MED TREAD	Principle Business Enterprises, Inc.
MED-AIR 2200	Enmet Corp.
MED-AIR PLUS	Pneumatic Products Corporation
MED-ASSIST	Medegen Medical Products, Llc
MED-EXAM	Medical Illumination International
MED-GAS	Air Liquide America Corporation, Cambridge Div.
MED-HOT	Dynamic Energy Systems, Inc.
MED-PAK	Wes-Pak, Inc.
MED-SIS	I-Flow Corporation
MED-TIME	American Medical Alert Corp.
MED-VUE	Trademark Medical Llc
MED/SPEC	Ortholine
MEDAC	Neurodyne Medical Corp.
MEDAC SYSTEM/3	Neurodyne Medical Corp.
MEDAIR	Medair, Inc.
MEDALLION	Merit Medical Systems, Inc.
MEDAXXIS	Per-Se Technologies
MEDCO SCHOOL FIRST AID	Medco Supply Company
MEDCO SPORTS MEDICINE	Medco Supply Company
MEDCOACH	Medical Coaches, Inc.
MEDCOM	Medcom, Inc.
MEDCOMP	Medcomp (Medical Components, Inc.)
MEDCREST	Medline Industries, Inc.
MEDDRAIN	Armm, Inc.
MEDEBAR	Mallinckrodt, Inc.
MEDEK	R&Da Co.
MEDELA	Medela, Inc.
MEDELEC	Oxford Instruments
MEDESTEALTH	Morgan Medesign, Inc.
MEDFILMS	Medfilms, Inc.
MEDFLATOR	Smiths Medical OEM
MEDFLEX	Bloomex International, Inc.
MEDGRAPHICS	Medical Graphics Corporation
MEDGRAPHICS BREATH SPIROMETER	Medical Graphics Corporation
MEDGRAPHICS KNOWLEDGENET	Medical Graphics Corporation
MEDGRAPHICS SPIROCARD	Medical Graphics Corporation
MEDI MAC	Medi Usa
MEDI PLUS	Medi Usa
MEDI STAT	Mueller Sports Medicine
MEDI STRUMPF	Medi Usa
MEDI-BAND	Afassco, Inc.
MEDI-BINS	Medi-Crush Company
MEDI-CENTER	Atlantic Medco, Inc.
MEDI-COMB	Health Enterprises
MEDI-CRUSH	Medi-Crush Company
MEDI-CUT	Dynarex Corp.
MEDI-DESK	Budget Buddy Company, Inc.
MEDI-DOSE	Medi-Dose, Inc.
MEDI-FEED	Medi-Crush Company
MEDI-GLOBE	Medi-Globe Corporation
MEDI-GRIP	Ansell Healthcare Products, Inc.
MEDI-GUARD	Maxwell Technologies Power Systems
MEDI-ISO	Maxwell Technologies Power Systems
MEDI-JECTOR	Antares Pharma, Inc.
MEDI-JECTOR VISION	Antares Pharma, Inc.
MEDI-KIT	Approved Medical Systems
MEDI-LAB	Mckesson General Medical
MEDI-LITE	Medical Illumination International
MEDI-MINDER	Medi-Crush Company
MEDI-ORGANIZER	Medi-Crush Company
MEDI-PAK	Mckesson General Medical
MEDI-SERV CART	Atlantic Medco, Inc.
MEDI-SOOTH	Professional Disposables International, Inc.
MEDI-SPECS RX	Surgical Safety Products, Inc.
MEDI-SPOT	Medical Illumination International
MEDI-STAK-RAK	Medi-Crush Company
MEDI-STAT	Medi-Crush Company
MEDI-STOR	Medi-Crush Company
MEDI-STUDS	J. Hewitt Incorporated
MEDI-SWAB	Smith & Nephew, Inc.
MEDI-SYSTEM	J. Hewitt Incorporated
MEDI-TEMP II	Gaymar Industries, Inc.
MEDI-THERM	Everest Interscience, Inc.
MEDI-THERM II	Gaymar Industries, Inc.
MEDI-TRACE	Graphic Controls Corp.
MEDI-UPS	Maxwell Technologies Power Systems
MEDI-VAC	Cardinal Health Inc.
MEDI-VERTER	Maxwell Technologies Power Systems
MEDI-VUE	Medical Illumination International
MEDI-WASH	Afassco, Inc.
MEDI-WASTE	Medical Action Industries, Inc
MEDI-WIPES	Afassco, Inc.
MEDI-WRAPS	Medi-Kid Co.
MEDIAKAP	Spectrum Laboratories, Inc.
MEDIARC-DIGIGRAPH	Drg International, Inc.
MEDIBEADS	Bruder Healthcare Company
MEDIBURN (ELASTEC)	Medi-Tech International, Inc.
MEDIC	Cardiac Science Corp.
MEDIC	Medisystems Corporation
MEDIC ID	Medic Id's International
MEDIC-AIR	Medic-Air, A Division Of Corflex, Inc.
MEDIC-KIT	Mabis Healthcare Inc.
MEDICAL MANAGEMENT SOFTWARE	C&S Research Corporation
MEDICAL MAT	Controlled Environment Equipment Corp.
MEDICAL SKY HOOK	Medical Skyhook Company
MEDICAL SPECTROMETER	Biodex Medical Systems, Inc.
MEDICALERT	Medicalert Foundation International
MEDICAP	Cardinal Health Inc.
MEDICASE	Case Design Corp.
MEDICATION CASSETTE	Smiths Medical Asd, Inc.
MEDICELL	Hydromer, Inc.
MEDICHEST	Carex Health Brands
MEDICINE SHOPPE	Cardinal Health Inc.
MEDICINE SPOON	Carex Health Brands
MEDICO2	Oridion Medical Inc.
MEDICOACH	Medical Coaches, Inc.
MEDICOE	Mediware Information Systems, Inc.
MEDICOOL E	Waldmann Lighting
MEDICOS	Medicos Laboratories, Inc. (Mdt)
MEDICUT	American Diagnostic Corporation (Adc)
MEDICUT	Covidien Lp
MEDICYL	Lifegas Llc
MEDIDERM	Mylan Technologies, Inc.
MEDIDROPPER	Spectrum Laboratories, Inc.
MEDIFILM	Mylan Technologies, Inc.
MEDIFLEX	Mediflex Surgical Products
MEDIFLEX	Mylan Technologies, Inc.
MEDIFOLD	Smiths Medical OEM
MEDIFRESH	Tri-State Hospital Supply Corp.
MEDIGRIP	Vantage Industries, Inc.
MEDIKMARK, INC.	Medikmark Inc.
MEDILAS H	Dornier Medtech America
MEDIMAR	Mediware Information Systems, Inc.
MEDIMAT	Vantage Industries, Inc.
MEDINA CATHETER	Torbot Group, Inc.
MEDIPLANNER	Carex Health Brands
MEDIPLOGS	Hammill International
MEDIPOINT	Medipoint, Inc.
MEDIPURE	Filtertek Inc.
MEDIRELEASE	Mylan Technologies, Inc.
MEDIRIP	Hartmann-Conco Inc.
MEDISEAL	Janin Group, Inc.
MEDISHORTS	Graham Medical Products/Div. Of Little Rapids Corp
MEDISON	Consumaquip Corporation
MEDISON	Medical Equipment Specialists, Inc.
MEDISON	Universal Ultrasound
MEDISPEC	Sontec Instruments Inc.
MEDISTUDS	J. Hewitt Incorporated
MEDISYSTEM	J. Hewitt Incorporated

MEDISYSTEMS	Medisystems Corporation
MEDITORQUE AMERICA	Medidenta International, Inc.
MEDITRAY	Case Medical, Inc.
MEDITRODES	Life-Tech, Inc.
MEDIVEN	Medi Usa
MEDIVISION	Medivision Endoscopy
MEDIZIME	Medical Chemical Corp.
MEDLAB	3m Health Information Systems
MEDLANCE	Htl-Strefa, Inc.
MEDLINE	Linak U.S. Inc.
MEDLINK	U.F.I.
MEDLITE	Continuum, Inc.
MEDLITE C3	Continuum, Inc.
MEDLITE C6	Continuum, Inc.
MEDLOCKER	Mts Medication Technologies
MEDMETRIC	Medmetric Corp.
MEDMINED	Cardinal Health Inc.
MEDNET	Hospira Inc.
MEDNEXT	Medtronic Powered Surgical Solutions
MEDOVATIONS	Medovations, Inc.
MEDPLANNER II	Carex Health Brands
MEDPLUS	Hill-Rom Holdings, Inc.
MEDPOR	Porex Surgical, Inc.
MEDQUEST	World Heart Inc.
MEDRAD	Medrad, Inc.
MEDRAD VISTRON CT	Medrad, Inc.
MEDS	Med Systems
MEDS MASK	Med Systems
MEDSERIES 4	Siemens Medical Solutions Health Services Corp.
MEDSERV E-MAR	Life Care Technologies, Inc.
MEDSERV FS	Life Care Technologies, Inc.
MEDSHEET	R&Da Co.
MEDSPEC	Medical Specialties, Inc.
MEDSYS	Infosys, Inc.
MEDSYSTEM III	Alaris Medical Systems, Inc
MEDSYSTEMS	Med Systems
MEDTESTER	Fluke Biomedical
MEDTOX	Medtox Scientific Inc.
MEDTRAX	Zebec Data Systems, Inc., Healthcare Mgmt. Div.
MEDTRONIC	Conmed Corporation
MEDTRONIC HALL	Medtronic Cardiovascular Surgery, The Heart Valve Div.
MEDTRX	Waterloo Healthcare, Llc
MEDU-CELL	Tmp Technologies, Inc.
MEDUCATE	Chek-Med Systems, Inc.
MEDVED PRODUCTS	Medved Products, Inc.
MEDWEBGATE	Imsi, Integrated Modular Systems Inc.
MEDX	Medx Incorporated
MEEK	Medical Specialties, Inc.
MEFIX	Sca Personal Care, North America
MEGA 2000	Megadyne Medical Products, Inc.
MEGA 2000 SOFT	Megadyne Medical Products, Inc.
MEGA CASSETTE	Sakura Finetek U.S.A., Inc.
MEGA FINE	Megadyne Medical Products, Inc.
MEGA POWER	Megadyne Medical Products, Inc.
MEGA SOFT	Megadyne Medical Products, Inc.
MEGA TIP	Megadyne Medical Products, Inc.
MEGA-TEMP	Caddy Corporation
MEGA-TENS	Futuremed America, Inc.
MEGA-VU	Marinco Specialty Wiring Devices
MEGABEAM	Biolitec, Inc.
MEGABOND	Harry J. Bosworth Company
MEGACLEAN	Micronova
MEGACODE ACLS	Medical Plastics Laboratory, Inc.
MEGACODE KELLY	Medical Plastics Laboratory, Inc.
MEGACODE KID	Medical Plastics Laboratory, Inc.
MEGACOLOR	Cytocolor, Inc.
MEGADOTS	Duxbury Systems, Inc.
MEGADYNE	Megadyne Medical Products, Inc.
MEGALLOY	Dentsply Caulk
MEGALLOY	Dentsply International, Inc.
MEGALLOY	Dentsply Prosthetics
MEGAS ES	Biosound Esaote, Inc.
MEGASORB	Dukal Corporation
MEGATRAY	Diestco Manufacturing Corp.
MEGATRON	Atlantic Ultraviolet Corp.
MEGAZINC PINK ADHESIVE TAPE	Omega Medical Products Corp.
MEGGER	Megger Inc. (Formerly Avo International)
MEGOHMER	Sticht Inc., Herman H.
MEIJI	Parco Scientific Co.
MEINHARD(R)	Meinhard Glass Products
MEL 80	Carl Zeiss Meditec Inc.
MEL KIT'S	Mel R. Manufacturas
MEL-5/TA99	Covance Research Products Inc.
MEL-PANEL	Covance Research Products Inc.
MELA-VISION	Photoprotective Technologies
MELCO ENGINEERING	Melco Engineering Corp.
MELOLIN	Smith & Nephew, Inc.
MELOLITE	Smith & Nephew, Inc.
MELROSE CUSTOM	Melrose Mattress, Inc.
MELTMOUNT	Cargille Laboratories
MEMBRAFIL	Corning Inc., Science Products Division
MEMBRANE DIFFUSION	Luwa Lepco
MEMBRANEBOX	Hager Worldwide, Inc.
MEMMERT	Pro Scientific Inc.
MEMORASE	Uvp, Llc
MEMORY GEL	Mentor Corp.
MEMORY LENS	Mentor Ophthalmics, Inc.
MEMORYPRINT 2000D	Krown Manufacturing, Inc.
MEMORYPRINT 2000DX	Krown Manufacturing, Inc.
MEMOWELL	Thermo Fisher Scientific
MEMPAC	VARTA Microbattery Inc.
MEMS	Aprex, A Division Of Aardex
MEMS MAP	Aprex, A Division Of Aardex
MEMS VIEW	Aprex, A Division Of Aardex
MEMTREX	Ge Infrastructure Water & Process Technologies
MENAFLEX	Regen Biologics, Inc.
MENIVAC	Arthrocare Corp.
MENTANIUM	Mentor Ophthalmics, Inc.
MENTOR	Mentor Corp.
MENTOR	Mentor Ophthalmics, Inc.
MENTOR	Merit Medical Systems, Inc.
MENTOR	Scientech, Inc.
MERCURY	H.L. Bouton Co., Inc.
MERCURY KLEAN KIT	Geritrex Corp.
MERCURY MEDICAL	Mercury Medical
MERICAL	Meriam Process Technologies
MERIDIAN	Wr Medical Electronics Co.
MERIDIAN BIOSCIENCE	Meridian Bioscience, Inc.
MERIFLUOR	Meridian Bioscience, Inc.
MERIGAUGE	Meriam Process Technologies
MERISTAR	Meridian Bioscience, Inc.
MERIT DISPOSAL DEPOT	Merit Medical Systems, Inc.
MERITAGE GEL	Taga Medical Technologies
MERITUS CLUB	Zimmer Dental, Inc.
MERLIN	Belco Packaging Systems, Inc.
MERLIN POLYBLADE	Conmed Linvatec
MERLYN	Merlyn Pharmaceuticals, Inc.
MEROCEL	Medtronic Xomed, Inc.
MEROGEL	Medtronic Xomed, Inc.
MERRY CART	Merry Walker Corp.
MERRY MOTIVATOR	Merry Walker Corp.
MERRY MOVER PD	Merry Walker Corp.
MERRY STAND BY ME	Merry Walker Corp.
MERRY THERAPEUTIC CANE	Merry Walker Corp.
MERRY THERAPEUTIC WALKER	Merry Walker Corp.
MERRY TRAVELER	Merry Walker Corp.
MERRY WALKER	Merry Walker Corp.
MERRY WALKER BARIATRIC	Merry Walker Corp.
MERSILENE	Ethicon, Inc.
MERSORB	Nucon International, Inc.
MES-9000 MUSCULOSKELETAL EVALUATION SYSTEM	Myotronics-Noromed, Inc.
MESALT	Sca Personal Care, North America
MESAM	Respironics Georgia, Inc.
MESHGRAFT	Zimmer Orthopaedic Surgical Products
MESIAL JET	American Orthodontics Corp.

MESNEX .... Baxter Healthcare Corporation, Baxter Pharmaceuticals And Technologies
MESSENGER .... Dr Systems, Inc.
MESTAMED .... Carecentric, Inc.
MET .... I-Rep, Inc.
MET SYSTEMS .... Cybex International, Inc.
MET-ATCH .... Gresco Products, Inc.
META-4 ENG .... Micromedical Technologies, Inc.
META-TG .... Kronus, Inc.
METAFASIX .... Tp Orthodontics, Inc.
METASUL .... Zimmer Holdings, Inc.
METASUL ACETABULAR SYSTEM .... Centerpulse Orthopedics Inc.
METEK .... Biotek, Inc.
METEXCHANGE .... Esa, Inc.
METRA .... Quidel Corporation
METRA PS .... Inlet Medical, Inc.
METREX .... Encompas Unlimited, Inc.
METRICIDE .... Metrex Research Corp.
METRICIDE SOLUTION .... Xenotec Ltd.
METRICLEAN .... Metrex Research Corp.
METRILUBE .... Metrex Research Corp.
METRIMIST .... Metrex Research Corp.
METRISCAN .... Alara Inc.
METRIX .... Boston Scientific Corp.
METRIZYME .... Metrex Research Corp.
METRO .... Convaid Inc.
METRO BASKETS .... Intermetro Industries Corp.
METROBASIX .... Intermetro Industries Corp.
METROBASIX PLUS .... Intermetro Industries Corp.
METROCARTS .... Intermetro Industries Corp.
METROFLEX .... Intermetro Industries Corp.
METROLODGIX .... Intermetro Industries Corp.
METROMAX .... Intermetro Industries Corp.
METROMAX Q .... Intermetro Industries Corp.
METRON .... Metron Optics, Inc.
METRON MARKER .... Metron Optics, Inc.
METRON OPTICS .... Metron Optics, Inc.
METROPOLITAN .... Ricon Corp.
METROTOTES .... Intermetro Industries Corp.
METROTRUX .... Intermetro Industries Corp.
METTLER .... Mettler-Toledo Group
METTLER .... Mettler-Toledo, Inc.
METTLER ELECTRONICS .... Mettler Electronics Corp.
MEVANET .... Siemens Medical Solutions Usa, Inc.
MEVAPLAN .... Siemens Medical Solutions Usa, Inc.
MEVATRON .... Siemens Medical Solutions Usa, Inc.
MEYER CLAMP .... Eriem Surgical
MEYER FORCEPS .... Eriem Surgical
MEZZARAIL 420 RAIL SYSTEM .... Wire Crafters L.L.C.
MGB ALERT .... Nanogen Molecular Research Products Division
MGDR (MEDICAL GAS DESK REFERENCE) .... Mercury Medical
MGIT .... Bd Diagnostic Systems
MGS-II WHITE ONLY MINI GANZFELD .... Lkc Technologies, Inc.
MI .... Leisure-Lift, Inc.
MI-5000 .... Monitor Instruments Inc.
MI-6000 .... Monitor Instruments Inc.
MI-7000 .... Monitor Instruments Inc.
MI-PBR .... Leisure-Lift, Inc.
MIAMI FRACTURE BRACE SYSTEM .... Maramed Orthopedic Systems
MIAMI J. .... Jerome Medical
MIAMI J. .... Ossur Americas
MIAMI JR. .... Jerome Medical
MIAMI JR. .... Ossur Americas
MIAMI JTO .... Jerome Medical
MIAMI OCCIAN COLLAR BACK .... Jerome Medical
MIBB .... Covidien Lp, Formerly Registered As United States Surgical
MIC-CONCEPT .... Microtech Medical Systems
MICADENT .... Medidenta International, Inc.
MICOR .... Siemens Medical Solutions Usa, Inc.
MICRA HPLC COLUMNS .... Eprogen, Inc.
MICRETAIN .... Camfil Farr
MICRINS RAZOR-EDGE SCISSORS .... Micrins Surgical Instruments, Inc.
MICRO 100 .... Conmed Linvatec

MICRO 12 .... Separation Technology Inc
MICRO 12 ECG .... Instromedix, A Card Guard Co.
MICRO 12 ECG+ .... Instromedix, A Card Guard Co.
MICRO 20 .... Independent Solutions, Inc.
MICRO ABG .... Vital Signs Colorado
MICRO AIR .... Micro Air Air Cleaners By Metal-Fab
MICRO CHANGE .... Woodhead L.P.
MICRO CIRRUS .... Intersurgical Inc.
MICRO CRYOSTAT .... Hacker Instruments And Industries Inc.
MICRO DISPODLAYZER .... Spectrum Laboratories, Inc.
MICRO E .... Conmed Linvatec
MICRO ELECTRAPETTE .... Thermo Fisher Scientific
MICRO ER .... Instromedix, A Card Guard Co.
MICRO FET .... Hoggan Health Industries, Inc.
MICRO LIGHTSTIC .... Cardiofocus, Inc.
MICRO LINE .... Microgenics Corporation
MICRO LR .... Instromedix, A Card Guard Co.
MICRO ONE .... Mentor Ophthalmics, Inc.
MICRO ONE .... Microflex Corporation
MICRO PIN .... B. Braun Oem Division, B. Braun Medical Inc.
MICRO PLUS .... Biomedical Life Systems, Inc.
MICRO SABER .... Flowtronics, Inc.
MICRO SABER PLUS .... Flowtronics, Inc.
MICRO SELECTRON HDR .... Nucletron Corporation
MICRO SELECTRON PDR .... Nucletron Corporation
MICRO SSP .... One Lambda, Inc.
MICRO TEST .... Remel
MICRO UNITOME .... Becton Dickinson And Co.
MICRO V 2000 .... Airguard
MICRO-BLADE .... Becton Dickinson And Co.
MICRO-CAL .... Kimble Chase Life Science And Research Products Llc
MICRO-CAL .... Ultra-Cal, Inc.
MICRO-CIDE-28 HLD, OPTI-LUBE .... Micro-Scientific Industries, Inc.
MICRO-COMP .... B. Braun Oem Division, B. Braun Medical Inc.
MICRO-COMP PRN .... B. Braun Oem Division, B. Braun Medical Inc.
MICRO-CRAFT .... Medtronic Xomed, Inc.
MICRO-DUP .... Pemaco, Inc.
MICRO-FIBER .... Johns Manville
MICRO-FIX .... Wescor, Inc.
MICRO-FLEX .... Tfx Medical Oem
MICRO-FOIL .... Rdf Corp.
MICRO-GEM .... Becton Dickinson And Co.
MICRO-GUARD .... Bio-Rad Laboratories, Life Science Group
MICRO-GUIDE .... Accellent Inc.
MICRO-ID .... Remel
MICRO-MATE .... Cadence Science Inc.
MICRO-MATE .... Medical Packaging Corporation
MICRO-PACE .... Pace Medical, Inc.
MICRO-PLANER .... Medtronic Xomed, Inc.
MICRO-POINT .... Ethicon, Inc.
MICRO-PRODICON .... Spectrum Laboratories, Inc.
MICRO-ROUGH .... Clean Esd Products, Inc.
MICRO-SED .... Medical Chemical Corp.
MICRO-SHARP .... Becton Dickinson And Co.
MICRO-SORB .... Eastman Medical Products Inc.
MICRO-STICK .... Medcomp (Medical Components, Inc.)
MICRO-STIX .... Young Innovations, Inc.
MICRO-TECH .... Senior Technologies
MICRO-TEMP .... Bovie Medical Corp.
MICRO-TIP WIPE .... Graphic Controls Corp.
MICRO-TITE .... Cadence Science Inc.
MICRO-TOUCH .... Ansell Healthcare Products, Inc.
MICRO-TOUCH NITRILE .... Ansell Healthcare Products, Inc.
MICRO-TOUCH PF .... Ansell Healthcare Products, Inc.
MICRO-TOUCH ULTRA .... Ansell Healthcare Products, Inc.
MICRO-VEL .... Tmp Technologies, Inc.
MICRO-X .... Rpc
MICROAIR .... Invacare Corporation
MICROAIRE .... Micro-Aire Surgical Instruments, Inc.
MICROBAN .... Aqua Glass Corporation
MICROBEAM .... Ams Innovative Center-San Jose
MICROBETA .... Perkin Elmer Wallac, Inc.
MICROBETA .... Perkinelmer Life And Analytical Sciences

MICROBIOLOGICSr	Microbiologics, Inc.
MICROBLASTER	Comco, Inc.
MICROBLATOR	Arthrocare Corp.
MICROBRUSH	Young Innovations, Inc.
MICROBUMIN	Quantimetrix Corporation
MICROCAB	Danville Materials
MICROCAP	Oridion Medical Inc.
MICROCAPS	Drummond Scientific Co.
MICROCARE II	American Imex
MICROCATH	B. Braun Oem Division, B. Braun Medical Inc.
MICROCERAM	Biomat Sciences Inc.
MICROCHOICE	Conmed Linvatec
MICROCISOR	Conmed Linvatec
MICROCLAVE	Hospira Inc.
MICROCLIP	Teleflex Medical
MICROCOAT	Personna Medical/Div. Of American Safety Razor Co.
MICROCON	Biological Controls Inc.
MICROCOOL	Kerr Group
MICROCULT	Siemens Healthcare Diagnostics Inc.
MICROCURE	Eit, Inc.
MICRODASE DISK	Remel
MICROEDGE	Micromedics
MICROETCHER	Danville Materials
MICROFIL COMPOSITE INSTRUMENTS	Almore International, Inc.
MICROFLEX	Bound Tree Medical
MICROFLEX	Nikon Instruments Inc.
MICROFLO	Life-Tech, Inc.
MICROFLUIDIZER	Microfluidics International Corporation
MICROFOCUS	Solarius Development Inc.
MICROFUSE	Baxa Corporation
MICROFUSION	Implant Sciences Corp.
MICROGARD	CAREFUSION 211, INC..
MICROGAS	Masimo Corp.
MICROGEL	Medtronic Xomed, Inc.
MICROGON	Spectrum Laboratories, Inc.
MICROGRAVER	Danville Materials
MICROGUARD	Airguard
MICROGUARD	Micro-Aire Surgical Instruments, Inc.
MICROJECT	Codman & Shurtleff, Inc
MICROJOIN	Scientific Pharmaceuticals, Inc.
MICROKEY	Advanced Input Systems
MICROKROS	Spectrum Laboratories, Inc.
MICROLAB	Clinical Data Inc
MICROLAB	Hamilton Company
MICROLAB	Micro Audiometrics Corp.
MICROLAMP	Bulbworks, Inc.
MICROLANCE	Bd Diagnostic Systems
MICROLATTICE	Acrymed, Inc.
MICROLINE	Tava Surgical Instruments
MICROLIPID	Covidien Lp
MICROLITE	Mauch, Inc.
MICROLITER	Hamilton Company
MICROLOG	Biolog, Inc.
MICROLUX, ULTRALITE, ULTRALUX	Integra Luxtec, Inc.
MICROLYZER	Quintron Instrument Company
MICROMACRO	Baxa Corporation
MICROMASTER	Photon Technology International, Inc.
MICROMAT	Pmt Corp.
MICROMAT II	Biorad Laboratories
MICROMATIC	Cadence Science Inc.
MICROMAX	Thermo Fisher Scientific - Laboratory Equipment Division Headquarters
MICROMAXX	Sonosite, Inc.
MICROMFG	Deringer-Ney, Inc.
MICROMIRROR	Vasamed
MICROMIX	Baxter Healthcare Corporation Nutrition
MICROMOP	Micronova
MICROMOUNT	Intersurgical Inc.
MICRONAIL	Wright Medical Group, Inc.
MICRONAIRE P-500	Summit Hill Laboratories
MICRONET	Biomerieux Inc.
MICRONSPOT	Ams Innovative Center-San Jose
MICROPAK	Riley Medical, Inc.
MICROPAK	Symmetry Medical Usa, Inc.
MICROPAK	Symmetry Medical, Inc.
MICROPAK CLASSIC	Symmetry Medical Usa, Inc.
MICROPAK CLASSIC	Symmetry Medical, Inc.
MICROPAQ	Welch Allyn Protocol Inc.
MICROPET	Siemens Medical Solutions Usa, Inc.
MICROPHOR	Life-Tech, Inc.
MICROPLATE	Biolog, Inc.
MICROPLATE MANAGER	Bio-Rad Laboratories, Life Science Group
MICROPLEAT	Airguard
MICROPORT	Angiodynamics, Inc.
MICROPREP	Lares Research
MICROPREP	Statspin, Inc.
MICROPRIME	Smiths Medical OEM
MICROPROBE	Fisher Scientific Co., Llc.
MICROPROPHY	Danville Materials
MICROPTIC	Ansell Healthcare Products, Inc.
MICROPULSE	Iridex Corporation
MICROPUNCTURE	Cook Inc.
MICROSAFE	Safe-Tec Clinical Products, Inc.
MICROSCAN	Siemens Healthcare Diagnostics Inc.
MICROSCOPE	Psyche Systems
MICROSECT	Codman & Shurtleff, Inc
MICROSIM	Netech, Corp.
MICROSKIN	Cymed Ostomy Co.
MICROSLICE	Ultra Tec Manufacturing, Inc.
MICROSLIDES	Rayson Co. Inc., W.R.
MICROSOFTRAC	Boston Scientific Corp.
MICROSPECTOR	Fluke Biomedical
MICROSTAAR	Staar Surgical Co.
MICROSTAR	Leica Microsystems, Inc., Educational & Analytical Division
MICROSTAT	Ams Innovative Center-San Jose
MICROSTAT	Surgica Corporation
MICROSTAT LABS	Microstat Laboratories, Inc.
MICROSTATION	Biolog, Inc.
MICROSTIK	Vital Signs Colorado
MICROSTREAM	Oridion Medical Inc.
MICROTARGETINGr	Fhc, Inc
MICROTECH	Biofit Engineered Products
MICROTEMP	Cincinnati Sub-Zero Products, Inc., Medical Division
MICROTEMP II	Cincinnati Sub-Zero Products, Inc., Medical Division
MICROTHERM	Labthermics Technologies
MICROTIN	Danville Materials
MICROTIP	Sunstar Butler
MICROTONE	Goldentone Hearing Aids
MICROTOX	Strategic Diagnostics Inc.
MICROTRON	Aesculap Implant Systems Inc.
MICROTRON EC	Aesculap Implant Systems Inc.
MICROTYMP	Welch Allyn, Inc.
MICROVAC R	Pmt Corp.
MICROVAP	Organomation Associates, Inc.
MICROVASCALAR CLAMP	Micrins Surgical Instruments, Inc.
MICROVENT COMFORT	Herculite Products, Inc.
MICROVENT SOFT	Herculite Products, Inc.
MICROVETTE	Sarstedt, Inc.
MICROVEX	Millipore Corporation
MICROVOID	Air Control, Inc.
MICROVUE	Zibra Corp.
MICROWICK	Micromedics
MICROXCT	Xradia Inc.
MICRUSPHERE	Micrus Corporation
MICRhoGAM	Ortho Clinical Diagnostics, Inc.
MICRhoGAM	Ortho-Clinical Diagnostics, Inc.
MIDAS II	Emd Chemicals Inc.
MIDAS III	Emd Chemicals Inc.
MIDAS LAMINATORS	Idesco Corp.
MIDAS REX	Medtronic Powered Surgical Solutions
MIDAS TOUCH	Olsen Medical
MIDASBRACKET SYSTEM	Gold'N Braces, Inc.
MIDCAB	Genzyme
MIDIKROS	Spectrum Laboratories, Inc.
MIDLAND	Patterson Medical Holdings, Inc.
MIDMARK	Kern Surgical Supply, Inc.

MINOR AQUATEC .... Clarke Health Care Products, Inc.
MINOTOME PLUS .... Triangle Biomedical Sciences, Inc.
MINTO .... Minto R&D, Inc.
MINUTE STAIN .... George Taub Products & Fusion Co., Inc.
MIO .... Newschoff Chairs, Inc.
MIRA CANDLE .... Hager Worldwide, Inc.
MIRA CART .... Hager Worldwide, Inc.
MIRA CART DELUXE .... Hager Worldwide, Inc.
MIRA MARKER .... Hager Worldwide, Inc.
MIRA METER .... Hager Worldwide, Inc.
MIRA MIX .... Hager Worldwide, Inc.
MIRA MOLAR .... Hager Worldwide, Inc.
MIRA TEE-TH .... Hager Worldwide, Inc.
MIRA TOM .... Hager Worldwide, Inc.
MIRA TRAY .... Hager Worldwide, Inc.
MIRA TRAY ADHESIVE .... Hager Worldwide, Inc.
MIRA TRAY ID .... Hager Worldwide, Inc.
MIRA TRAY PLUS .... Hager Worldwide, Inc.
MIRABOR .... Hager Worldwide, Inc.
MIRABRUSH .... Hager Worldwide, Inc.
MIRABURNER .... Hager Worldwide, Inc.
MIRACAST .... Hager Worldwide, Inc.
MIRACLE AIR .... Air Quality Engineering, Inc.
MIRACLE C-GEL .... Donell
MIRACLE FOOT REPAIR .... The Aloe Institute
MIRACLE HEEL REPAIR:MIRACLE HAND REPAIR .... The Aloe Institute
MIRACLE KNEE .... Professional's Choice Sports Medicine Products, Inc.
MIRACLE OF ALOE .... The Aloe Institute
MIRACLE OF ALOE .... Winning Solutions, Inc.
MIRACLE RASH REPAIR .... The Aloe Institute
MIRACLE RUB .... The Aloe Institute
MIRACLEGRIP .... Qrp, Inc.
MIRACOLD PLUS .... Hager Worldwide, Inc.
MIRACOMPO .... Hager Worldwide, Inc.
MIRACRYL .... Motloid Company
MIRAFILL .... Hager Worldwide, Inc.
MIRAFIT .... Hager Worldwide, Inc.
MIRAFIT BC .... Hager Worldwide, Inc.
MIRAFLOSS .... Hager Worldwide, Inc.
MIRAGAUARD .... Hager Worldwide, Inc.
MIRAGE .... Pacific Precision Laboratories, Inc.
MIRAGE .... Ricon Corp.
MIRAGE ACTIVA .... Resmed Corp.
MIRAGE KIDSTA .... Resmed Corp.
MIRAGE LIBERTY .... Resmed Corp.
MIRAGE MICRO .... Resmed Corp.
MIRAGE QUATTRO .... Resmed Corp.
MIRAGE VISTA .... Resmed Corp.
MIRAHOLD .... Hager Worldwide, Inc.
MIRAJECT .... Hager Worldwide, Inc.
MIRALAY .... Hager Worldwide, Inc.
MIRAMASK .... Hager Worldwide, Inc.
MIRAMATIC .... Hager Worldwide, Inc.
MIRAN .... Invensys Process Systems
MIRANTI .... ArjoHuntleigh
MIRAPOST .... Hager Worldwide, Inc.
MIRAPRESS .... Hager Worldwide, Inc.
MIRAPULL .... Hager Worldwide, Inc.
MIRASUC .... Hager Worldwide, Inc.
MIRASUC 3P .... Hager Worldwide, Inc.
MIRASUCTO .... Hager Worldwide, Inc.
MIRATORCH .... Hager Worldwide, Inc.
MIRATRACT .... Hager Worldwide, Inc.
MIRCERA .... Nektar Therapeutics
MIRROR SUCTION .... Hager Worldwide, Inc.
MIS 2-INCISION .... Zimmer Holdings, Inc.
MISCO .... Misco Refractometer
MISONIX .... Misonix, Inc.
MIST-O-GEN .... Allied Healthcare Products, Inc.
MISTBUSTER .... Air Quality Engineering, Inc.
MISTER CLEAR .... Mectra Labs, Inc.
MISTRAL-AIR .... Adroit Medical Systems, Inc.
MISTY .... Roman Research, Inc.

MISTY OX .... Vital Signs, Inc.
MITTLEMAN PRE JOWL .... Implantech Associates, Inc.
MITTLEMAN PRE JOWL CHIN .... Implantech Associates, Inc.
MITY-MITE .... Key-Bak
MITYDRIVE .... Anko Products, Inc., Mityflex Div.
MITYFLEX .... Anko Products, Inc., Mityflex Div.
MITYVAC .... Pristech Products, Inc
MIXCO .... Lightnin Mixers
MIXED BREED ANALYSIS .... Mwi Veterinary Supply
MIXEVAC III .... Stryker Corp.
MIXXOCYDIN .... Kenlor Industries, Inc.
MIZUHO .... Mizuho America Inc.
MIZZY .... Mizzy, Inc. Of National Keystone
MK .... Mk Battery
MK POWERED .... Mk Battery
MK5 .... Mortara Instrument, Inc.
MKG .... Myotronics-Noromed, Inc.
MKM .... Carl Zeiss Surgical, Inc.
ML 300CR .... Hf Pure Water
MLADICK .... Byron Medical
MLC .... Siemens Medical Solutions Usa, Inc
MLS .... Ericsson, Inc.
MM .... I.B.F. Corporation
MM-II .... Technical Instruments (Ti)
MMI .... Medical Measurements, Inc.
MMI/GAELTEC .... Medical Measurements, Inc.
MN .... I.B.F. Corporation
MNR .... Assay Technology Inc
MO POSTERIORS .... Dentsply Prosthetics
MOBIL-AID .... Advanced Instrument Development, Inc.
MOBILAID .... Invacare Corporation
MOBILE BREAST CARE CENTER(TM) (MBCC) .... Mobile Medical International Corporation
MOBILE DIAGNOSTICS UNIT(TM) (MDU) Mobile Medical International Corporation
MOBILE DIALYSIS UNIT(TM) (MDYU) ..... Mobile Medical International Corporation
MOBILE LABORATORY/PHARMACY UNIT(TM)(MLPU) .... Mobile Medical International Corporation
MOBILE PATIENT WARD UNIT(TM) (MPWU) .... Mobile Medical International Corporation
MOBILE SINGLE PALLET UNIT(TM) (MSPU) .... Mobile Medical International Corporation
MOBILE SURGERY UNIT(TM) (MSU) ...... Mobile Medical International Corporation
MOBILEART .... Shimadzu Medical Systems
MOBILESCAN .... Schaerer Mayfield Usa
MOBILETT .... Siemens Medical Solutions Usa, Inc.
MOBILITE .... Invacare Corporation
MOBILOX .... Farley Inc., W.T.
MOBIN-UDDIN .... Scanlan International, Inc.
MOBISTA .... Amgen Inc.
MOBIUS .... Integra Lifesciences Holdings Corp.
MOBIUS .... Ta Instruments
MOBLVAC III .... Ohio Medical Corp.
MOBLVAC III CS .... Ohio Medical Corp.
MOD LINE .... Kls-Martin L.P.
MODABBER .... Hely And Weber
MODEL 1 .... Hager Worldwide, Inc.
MODEL 1000 + OTOSCREEN .... Ambco Electronics
MODEL 1000 PNT CONTROLLER .... Ophthalmic Intl.
MODEL 1000 POST-SYMPTOM EVENT RECORDER ... Integrated Medical Devices, Inc.
MODEL 1200 TRANSTELEPHONIC RECEIVER ..... Integrated Medical Devices, Inc.
MODEL 1200M TRANSTELEPHONIC CARDIAC EVENT RECORDER ...... Integrated Medical Devices, Inc.
MODEL 2500 STORAGE AUTOMATIC AUDIOMETER .... Ambco Electronics
MODEL 30 CLASSIC .... Mentor Ophthalmics, Inc.
MODEL 600 SPECIAL CARE BED .... Asi Medical Equipment, Ltd.
MODEL 650 A SCREENING AUDIOMETER .... Ambco Electronics
MODEL C .... Concept Ii, Inc.
MODEL HOLDER .... Hager Worldwide, Inc.
MODEL RDT .... Barrows Company
MODEL SEPARATOR .... American Diversified Dental Systems
MODEL SV-2100 .... Electromed, Inc.
MODEL SV-2100-I .... Electromed, Inc.

MODEL T	Barrows Company
MODEL-COTE	George Taub Products & Fusion Co., Inc.
MODIFIED MICROLITER	Hamilton Company
MODULAB	Hemco Corp.
MODULAP	Atc Technologies, Inc.
MODULAR 3	Ticonium Co.
MODULAR 5	Ticonium Co.
MODULAR BARIATRIC	Theradyne Products Division
MODULAR CMC JOINT IMPLANT	Biopro, Inc.
MODULAR DEVICES	Halbar North, Inc.
MODULAR INCUBATOR CHANBER	Billups-Rothenberg, Inc.
MODULAR ONE	Mentor Ophthalmics, Inc.
MODULAR TABLE SYSTEM	Mizuho Osi
MODULATION DOMAIN FUNCTION	Cardiac Science Corporation (Ca)
MODULETTE	Whitehall Manufacturing
MODULEX	Asi-Modulex
MODULIS	Modulus Data Systems, Inc.
MODULITH SLX-T TRANSPORTABLE LITHOTRIPTER	Karl Storz Lithotripsy-America, Inc.
MODULTAINER	Symmetry Medical, Inc.
MODUTEC	Getinge Usa, Inc.
MOGS	United Syntek Corp.
MOI-STIR	Kingswood Laboratories, Inc.
MOIST EYE	Eagle Vision, Inc.
MOISTRELEASE	Avery Dennison Corporation
MOISTURE CARE	Sage Laboratories, Inc.
MOISTURESORB	Imtek Environmental Corp.
MOJO SLEEPMASK	Sleepnet Corporation
MOLDENT	Motloid Company
MOLDPAC	Motloid Company
MOLECULAR/POR	Spectrum Laboratories, Inc.
MOLLELAST	Lohmann & Rauscher, Inc.
MOLLELAST HAFT	Lohmann & Rauscher, Inc.
MOLLOPLAST-B	Buffalo Dental Manufacturing Co., Inc.
MOLLOSIL PLUS	Buffalo Dental Manufacturing Co., Inc.
MOLLY	Gyrus Medical, Inc.
MOLTENO SETON	Staar Surgical Co.
MOLYDAG	Acheson Colloids Company
MOM-EZ	Lohmann & Rauscher, Inc.
MOMENTUM	Siemens Medical Solutions Usa, Inc
MON-A-THERM	Covidien (Formerly Nellcor Puritan Bennett / Tyco Healthcare)
MONARCH	Almore International, Inc.
MONARCH	Applied Medical Resource Corporation
MONARCH	Applied Medical Technology, Inc.
MONARCH	Golden Technologies, Inc.
MONARCH	Riegel Consumer Products Div.
MONARK	Creative Health Products, Inc.
MONET	Magnatone Hearing Aid Corp.
MONITOR	Sellstrom Manufacturing Co.
MONITOR ONE	Q-Med, Inc.
MONITOR ONE STAR	Q-Med, Inc.
MONITORR	Novosci Corp.
MONO-CRAWFORD	Fci Ophthalmics
MONO-DOX	Cp Medical Corporation
MONO-LATEX	Wampole Laboratories
MONO-PLUS	Wampole Laboratories
MONO-TEST	Wampole Laboratories
MONOBODIES	Zeptometrix Corporation
MONOCHROMATORS	Princeton Instruments - Acton
MONOCLATE-P	Csl Behring
MONOCOLOR	Cytocolor, Inc.
MONOCRYL	Ethicon, Inc.
MONODEX	Cenogenics Corp.
MONOGEL	Zenex Corporation
MONOGEN	Biokit Usa, Inc.
MONOGRAM	Argen Corp.
MONOJECT	Covidien Lp
MONOJECT MAGELLAN	Covidien Lp, Formerly Registered As Tyco Healthcare
MONOJECTOR	Covidien Lp
MONOJEL	Covidien Lp
MONOKA	Fci Ophthalmics
MONOLERT	Meridian Bioscience, Inc.
MONOLET	Covidien Lp
MONOMID BLUE	Cp Medical Corporation
MONONINE	Csl Behring
MONOPAD	Zenex Corporation
MONOPAK	Zenex Corporation
MONOPREP	Monogen, Inc.
MONOPREP	Sakura Finetek U.S.A., Inc.
MONOPTY	C. R. Bard, Inc., Bard Urological Div.
MONORAIL PICCOLINO	Boston Scientific Corp.
MONOSLIDE	Bd Diagnostic Systems
MONOSOF	Covidien Lp, Formerly Registered As United States Surgical
MONOSORB	Quantachrome
MONOSPOT	Meridian Bioscience, Inc.
MONOSTENT	Eagle Vision, Inc.
MONOSTERYL DIAMONDS	Global Dental Products
MONOSWIFT	Cp Medical Corporation
MONOTEC	Spectronics Corporation
MONOTEK	Pml Microbiologicals
MONOTRAY	Covidien Lp
MONOTRODE	Zenex Corporation
MONOVETTE	Sarstedt, Inc.
MONROE-TOP	Hard Manufacturing Co.
MONSTR-PETTE	Kimble Chase Life Science And Research Products Llc
MONTANA	DJO Inc.
MONTEGO	Aearo Company
MONTEREY	Fleetwood Group, Incorporated
MONTGOMERY	Boston Medical Products, Inc.
MONTREAUX EYEWEAR	Rochester Optical Mfg. Company
MOONBEAMS	United Syntek Corp.
MOONPANTS	Gi Supply
MOONWALKER	Ortho-Kinetics, Inc.
MOORE GRIP	H&M Rubber Company, Inc.
MOR-FLEX	Miltex Inc.
MOR-LOC	Jobri Llc
MORCHER	Fci Ophthalmics
MORE SKIN	Mueller Sports Medicine
MORMAC TUBE GUARD	Mormac Tube Guard Co.
MORROW BROWN	Alkaline Corp.
MOS-GENU	Bauerfeind Usa, Inc.
MOSAIC	Lutronic Inc.
MOSAIC	Medtronic Cardiovascular Surgery, The Heart Valve Div.
MOSAIC	Roho Group, The
MOSAIC PLASTY	Smith & Nephew, Inc., Endoscopy Division
MOSQUITO	Awareness Technology, Inc.
MOSQUITO	Covidien Lp
MOSQUITO	Trans American Medical
MOST SYSTEM	Centerpulse Orthopedics Inc.
MOTHER-TO-BE	Scott Specialties, Inc./Cmo Inc./Ginny Inc.
MOTHER/BABY	Cas Medical Systems, Inc.
MOTION MACHINE	Forward Motions, Inc.
MOTION PICTURE STUDIO (MPS)	Pentax Medical Company
MOTIV	Walkmed Infusion Llc
MOTO-VEC	Ortho-Kinetics, Inc.
MOTOR TREND	Procter & Gamble
MOTOVEC	Ortho-Kinetics, Inc.
MOUNTEE	Convaid Inc.
MOUSE ON MOUSE (M.O.M.)	Vector Laboratories, Inc.
MOUSE-TYPER	Bio-Rad Laboratories, Life Science Group
MOVE	Silipos Inc.
MOVEO	Chattanooga Group
MOVESAFE	Hard Manufacturing Co.
MOVINCOOL	Movincool/Denso Sales California, Inc.
MOYCO	Miltex Inc.
MOYCO	Moyco Technologies, Inc.
MOYCODENT	Moyco Technologies, Inc.
MP HIP STEM	LinkBio Corp.
MP-1	Zimmer Dental, Inc.
MPD	Handi-Cap Aids Company
MPD	Instrument Specialists, Inc.
MPE-INC	Midwest Products & Engineering, Inc.
MPH	Cryolife, Inc.
MPI	Ericsson, Inc.
MPM ANTI-FUNGAL	Mpm Medical, Inc.
MPM COOLMAGIC GEL SHEET	Mpm Medical, Inc.

MPM EXCEL HYDROCOLLOID	Mpm Medical, Inc.
MPM EXCEL-GEL	Mpm Medical, Inc.
MPM EXCELGINATE	Mpm Medical, Inc.
MPM EXCELGINATE AG	Mpm Medical, Inc.
MPM ORAMAGIC	Mpm Medical, Inc.
MPM RADIAPLEX	Mpm Medical, Inc.
MPM REGENECARE	Mpm Medical, Inc.
MPM REGENECARE HA	Mpm Medical, Inc.
MPM REGENECARE HA SATURATED GAUZE	Mpm Medical, Inc.
MPM REPEL	Mpm Medical, Inc.
MPM SILVERMED CLEANSER	Mpm Medical, Inc.
MPM SILVERMED HYDROGEL	Mpm Medical, Inc.
MPM SILVERMED SATURATED GAUZE	Mpm Medical, Inc.
MPM WOUNDGARD	Mpm Medical, Inc.
MPO 2000	Restorative Care Of America Inc
MPO ACTIVE	Restorative Care Of America Inc
MPOWER	Humanware
MPS	Bergeron Health Care
MPS	Medtronic Xomed, Inc.
MPS	St. Jude Medical Neuromodulation Division
MPV 4	Hoveround Corporation
MR	Greatbatch Inc
MR ELECTRODE	Beck-Lee
MR HURT HEAD	Medical Plastics Laboratory, Inc.
MR LOCK CC	American Orthodontics Corp.
MR. COMFORT	Med-Lift & Mobility, Inc.
MRC	Labac Systems, Inc.
MRI	Supertech, Inc.
MRI SPECIALIST	Fonar Corp.
MRI TABLE	Biodex Medical Systems, Inc.
MRI-SAFE	Aadco Medical, Inc.
MRINNERVU	Medrad, Inc.
MRL LIFEQUEST AED	Welch Allyn Protocol, Inc.
MRL LITE	Welch Allyn Protocol, Inc.
MRL PIC	Welch Allyn Protocol, Inc.
MRM-2	Waters Medical Systems
MRP-5000	Hitachi Medical Systems America, Inc.
MRP-7000	Hitachi Medical Systems America, Inc.
MS-30 HIP SYSTEM	Centerpulse Orthopedics Inc.
MS-30 RESUSCITATOR	Ambu, Inc.
MS-CT STORE	Imco Technologies
MSF	I.B.F. Corporation
MSI	Ge Infrastructure Water & Process Technologies
MSP	Surgical Specialties Corporation
MSS PHARMA SYSTEM	Aes Clean Technology, Inc.
MSS TILT & RECLINE	Wenzelite Rehab Supplies, Llc
MSS TRAVELER	Wenzelite Rehab Supplies, Llc
MT-X	Boeckeler Instruments, Inc.
MT-XL,PT-X	Boeckeler Instruments, Inc.
MT9500	Astro-Med, Inc.
MTC	Labac Systems, Inc.
MTC III INCUBATOR	Lifesign
MTI	Medical Technology Industries, Inc.
MTL PERSONAL	Ericsson, Inc.
MTL2470 SHOULDER CPM	Mckelor Technologies, Ltd.
MTO II	Champion, A Gardner Denver Co.
MTP	Medical Technology Products, Inc.
MTP 1001	Medical Technology Products, Inc.
MTRC	Labac Systems, Inc.
MUCOGEST	Hardy Diagnostics
MUCOSOFT	Parkell, Inc.
MUCOSPERSE	Marlen Manufacturing & Development Co.
MUELLER KOLD	Mueller Sports Medicine
MUELLERGESIC	Mueller Sports Medicine
MUELLERGUARD	Mueller Sports Medicine
MUELLERHINGE	Mueller Sports Medicine
MULLINS	Numed, Inc.
MULTARRAY	Meddev Corporation
MULTI	Thermo Fisher Scientific - Laboratory Equipment Division Headquarters
MULTI CARE	Tillotson Healthcare Corp.
MULTI DIMENSIONAL ANALYSIS	Rahd Oncology Products
MULTI DIMENSIONAL VIEWING	Rahd Oncology Products
MULTI ELECTRAPETTE	Thermo Fisher Scientific
MULTI FLEX	Noram Solutions
MULTI IMAGER	Multi Imager Service, Inc
MULTI LITE	Multi Focal Rx Lens Laboratories, Inc.
MULTI PACK	Carex Health Brands
MULTI PHOR	Hoefer Pharmacia Biotech, Inc.
MULTI PODUS	Restorative Care Of America Inc
MULTI POUCH	Medical Action Industries, Inc
MULTI SPEECH	Kaypentax
MULTI-AD	B. Braun Oem Division, B. Braun Medical Inc.
MULTI-CALIBRATORS	Laboratory Technologies, Inc.
MULTI-CHAMBER	Meridian Medical Technologies
MULTI-COMM.	Athena Controls, Inc.
MULTI-DAY ELECTRODE TENS	Covidien Lp, Formerly Registered As Uni-Patch
MULTI-DOSER SYRINGE DELIVERY SYSTEM	Sigma International, Llc
MULTI-FLO	Becton Dickinson Infusion Therapy Systems, Inc.
MULTI-GRAPHIC	Bogen Communications International, Inc.
MULTI-LUMEN	Point Medical Corp.
MULTI-MIX	Bio-Rad Laboratories, Life Science Group
MULTI-MODE & INLINE FOOTSWITCH	Noraxon Usa, Inc.
MULTI-OX	Farley Inc., W.T.
MULTI-PAK	Hamilton Company
MULTI-PREP	Biochemical Diagnostics, Inc.
MULTI-PURE	Multi-Pure Drinking Water System
MULTI-TEST II	Lincoln Diagnostics, Inc.
MULTI-TRACK	Numed, Inc.
MULTIAMP	Cardionics, Inc.
MULTICALC	Perkin Elmer Wallac, Inc.
MULTICALC	Perkinelmer Life And Analytical Sciences
MULTICAM	Analogic Corporation
MULTICAP	Siemens Healthcare Diagnostics Inc
MULTICARE	Hologic, Inc.
MULTICARE 3000	MAQUET
MULTICHECK	CAREFUSION 211, INC..
MULTICHECK	Radiometer America, Inc.
MULTIFIRE	Covidien Lp, Formerly Registered As United States Surgical
MULTIFLY	Sarstedt, Inc.
MULTIFOCUS	Oticon, Inc.
MULTIFORM	Alimed, Inc.
MULTIFORMS	Multisorb Technologies, Inc.
MULTIGUIDE	Stryker Corp.
MULTIKUF	American Diagnostic Corporation (Adc)
MULTILAB SERIES 2-LHS	Unetixs Vascular, Inc.
MULTILAB SERIES 2-LHSTI	Unetixs Vascular, Inc.
MULTILAB SERIES 2/IMG	Unetixs Vascular, Inc.
MULTILATORR	Flotec, Inc.
MULTILINER	CAREFUSION 211, INC..
MULTILINK	Biogenex Laboratories
MULTILITE	Continuum, Inc.
MULTIMARKER	Viscot Medical, Llc
MULTIMATIC	General Pysiotherapy, Inc.
MULTINEX	MAQUET
MULTIPAC	Intersurgical Inc.
MULTIPACKER	W. R. Grace & Co.-Conn
MULTIPAK	Riley Medical, Inc.
MULTIPAK	Symmetry Medical Usa, Inc.
MULTIPAK	Symmetry Medical, Inc.
MULTIPLIER	Multiplier Industries Corp.
MULTIPORT	St. Jude Medical Neuromodulation Division
MULTIPURE	Western Water Purifier Co.
MULTIQUAL	Siemens Healthcare Diagnostics Inc
MULTIRALL	Liko North America
MULTISCAN	Medical Positioning, Inc.
MULTISTIX	Siemens Healthcare Diagnostics Inc.
MULTISTIX PRO	Siemens Healthcare Diagnostics Inc.
MULTITASK	Baxter Healthcare Corporation Nutrition
MULTITEST	Lincoln Diagnostics, Inc.
MULTITHERM	Unique/Pereny
MULTITRAE	Siemens Healthcare Diagnostics Inc
MULTIUSER SOFTWARE	Medical Graphics Corporation
MULTIVAC	Arthrocare Corp.
MULTIVAP	Organomation Associates, Inc.
MULTIVETTE	Sarstedt, Inc.
MULTIVIEW	Emed Technologies

MULTIWASH ADVANTAGE	Tricontinent
MULTIWASH II	Tricontinent
MULTIWAVE	Innovative Med Inc.
MULTIX PRO	Siemens Medical Solutions Usa, Inc.
MULTIX SWING	Siemens Medical Solutions Usa, Inc.
MULTIX TOP	Siemens Medical Solutions Usa, Inc.
MUPPET SPOTS	Aso Corporation
MUPPET STRIPS	Aso Corporation
MUSE	Ge Medical Systems Information Technologies
MUSE	Vivus, Inc.
MUSIC	Siemens Hearing Instruments, Inc.
MUSICA	Agfa Corporation
MUSICIANS EARPLUGS	Etymotic Research, Inc.
MUTA-GENE	Bio-Rad Laboratories, Life Science Group
MUTATOX	Strategic Diagnostics Inc.
MV2	The Lifestyle Co. Inc.
MVISION	Siemens Medical Solutions Usa, Inc
MVISION MEGAVOLTAGE CONE BEAM IMAGING PACKAGE	Siemens Medical Solutions Usa, Inc
MVP	Ortho-Kinetics, Inc.
MVP (MAXANT VALUE PRODUCT)	Maxant Technologies, Inc.
MVP-1	Medical Technology Products, Inc.
MVP-10	Bio-Med Devices, Inc.
MVR	Medtronic Perfusion Systems
MVRA	Intelligent Hearing Systems, Corp.
MVS MOBILE	Ericsson, Inc.
MX-20	Faxitron X-Ray, Llc
MX-2100	Enmet Corp.
MX-75/100	Chiu Technical Corp.
MX-GRAFTER	Kls Martin Lp
MX-PRO	Stryker Corp.
MX-PRO BARIATRIC TRANSPORT	Stryker Corp.
MXI	Tp Orthodontics, Inc.
MXR	Porter Instrument Division Parker Hannifin Corp
MY EPIC	Epic Systems Corp.
MY TIME	Airway Division Of Surgical Appliance Industries, Inc.
MY-MEDI	Bruder Healthcare Company
MYCHART	Epic Systems Corp.
MYCO DISK	Remel
MYCO SEALS	Hardy Diagnostics
MYCOBACTI-LOOP	Remel
MYCOBACTOSEL	Bd Diagnostic Systems
MYCOCIDE CX CALLUS EXFOILATOR	Woodward Laboratories, Inc.
MYCOCIDE NS FUNGAL NAIL SOLUTION	Woodward Laboratories, Inc.
MYCOFAST	Wescor, Inc.
MYCOFLASK	Bd Diagnostic Systems
MYCOMOUNT	Hardy Diagnostics
MYCOPHIL	Bd Diagnostic Systems
MYCOPREP	Bd Diagnostic Systems
MYCORASH	Hardy Diagnostics
MYCOSCREEN	Wescor, Inc.
MYCOSEL	Bd Diagnostic Systems
MYCOTUBE	Remel
MYDESC	Rhamdec Inc.
MYELO-NATE	Utah Medical Products, Inc.
MYERSON/KENSON TEETH	Dentsply Prosthetics
MYLAB 25	Biosound Esaote, Inc.
MYLAB 30CV	Biosound Esaote, Inc.
MYLAB 50	Biosound Esaote, Inc.
MYLAFORM	Hager Worldwide, Inc.
MYO-KLEBER	I.M.K. Distributors, Inc.
MYO-MONITOR	Myotronics-Noromed, Inc.
MYO-TRODES	Myotronics-Noromed, Inc.
MYO/KLIP	Alto Development Corp.
MYOCCLUDE	Covidien Lp, Formerly Registered As United States Surgical
MYOCLINICAL	Noraxon Usa, Inc.
MYOCONTROL	Fasstech
MYOJECT	Oxford Instruments
MYOPORE	Greatbach Medical
MYOPORE	Greatbach Inc
MYORESEARCH XP	Noraxon Usa, Inc.
MYOSATE	Bd Diagnostic Systems
MYOSCINT	Centocor, Inc.
MYOSSAGE	Chattanooga Group
MYOSYSTEM 1200	Noraxon Usa, Inc.
MYOSYSTEM 1400A	Noraxon Usa, Inc.
MYOTECH,MICROSTIM 1304-D	Comfort Technologies, Inc.
MYOTRACE 200	Noraxon Usa, Inc.
MYOTRACE PLUS	Noraxon Usa, Inc.
MYOVIDEO	Noraxon Usa, Inc.
MYOWIRE	Alto Development Corp.
MYOWIRE II	Alto Development Corp.
MYREADER	Humanware
MYSELF	Deschutes Medical Products, Inc.
MYSTAIRE	Misonix, Inc.
MZ FLIII STEREOMICROSCOPE	Leica Microsystems Inc.
MZ STEREOMICROSCOPES	Leica Microsystems Inc.
Macra	Inverness Medical Professional Diagnostics-San Die
MacroPore	Medtronic, Inc.
Magellan	Medtronic Perfusion Systems
Maniken	Zahourek Systems, Inc.
MartinÉ_Ts	Superior Uniform Group
Masimo Rainbow SET	Masimo Corp.
Masimo SET	Masimo Corp.
Maverick	Boston Scientific - Maple Grove
Maverick	Boston Scientific Corporation
MaxSun	Megasun
Maximum	St. Jude Medical, Inc.
Maxxis	Kinetic Concepts, Inc.
Medi-Span	Medi-Span, Inc.
Medtronic	Medtronic Perfusion Systems
MegaMax	Megasun
MegaSun	Megasun
Membralox	Pall Corporation
Men	Ortho Dermatologics
Merlin	St. Jude Medical, Inc.
Metamucil	Procter & Gamble
Metricel	Pall Corporation
Micro-Cap	Ertelalsop
MicroClear	Ortho Dermatologics
Microcel Puff	Acor Orthopaedic, Inc.
Microny	St. Jude Medical, Inc.
Millennium	Bausch & Lomb
Minimax Plus	Medtronic Perfusion Systems
Miniprep	J.P. Gilbert Co.
Minntech	Medtronic Perfusion Systems
Mono-Diff	Inverness Medical Professional Diagnostics-San Die
Mono-Latex	Inverness Medical Professional Diagnostics-San Die
Mono-Test	Inverness Medical Professional Diagnostics-San Die
Montana Big Sky	Nutraceutical International Corp.
Mr. Clean	Procter & Gamble
Multi-Lyte	Inverness Medical Professional Diagnostics-San Die
N'ICE STRETCH	Brown Medical Industries
N-DEX	Best Manufacturing Co.
N-EVAP	Organomation Associates, Inc.
N-MULTISTIX	Siemens Healthcare Diagnostics Inc.
N-TACT PTH	Diasorin Inc
N-TERFACE	Winfield Laboratories
N-URISTIX	Siemens Healthcare Diagnostics Inc.
N.I.C.	Univac Dental Company
N/F SCREEN	Remel
N/R	No Rinse Laboratories, Llc
N2	Hager Worldwide, Inc.
N95 HEALTH CARE PARTICULATE RESPIRATOR	American Diversified Dental Systems
NA PHILIPS	Bulbtronics, Inc.
NA-STAR	Applied Biosystems
NABERTHERM	Unique/Pereny
NAC	Medegen
NAC-PAC	Alpha-Tec Systems, Inc.
NAC-PAC RED	Alpha-Tec Systems, Inc.
NADIA	Iris International, Inc.
NAFION	Perma Pure Llc
NAIL CARE PLUS	Medicool, Inc.
NAIL SCRUB	Pedinol Pharmacal, Inc.
NALGENE LABWARE	Nalge Nunc International

NALTEX	Delstar Technologies, Inc.
NAME-ALERT	Rpc
NAMIC	Navilyst Medical
NANO-CHANGE	Woodhead L.P.
NANODUCT NEONATAL SWEAT	Wescor, Inc.
NANOJECT 2	Drummond Scientific Co.
NANOMASK	Nano Mask Inc.
NANOMATERIALS	Nanomaterials, Inc.
NANORID	Binding Site, Inc., The
NANOVFI	Xradia Inc.
NANOXCT	Xradia Inc.
NAPA TABLE	Living Earth Crafts
NARDALERT	Narda Safety Test Solutions
NARISHIGE	Narishige International Usa, Inc.
NARROW SURGI-I-BAND	Scanlan International, Inc.
NARVA	Bulbworks, Inc.
NASCO	Aristotle Corp.
NASCO	Medi-Tech International, Inc.
NASOMETER	Kaypentax
NASOPORE	Stryker Corp.
NATIONAL VISION EYECARE CENTER	National Vision, Inc.
NATIONAL VISION OPTICAL	National Vision, Inc.
NATRACARE	Natracare, Llc
NATRAFLEX	Covidien Lp
NATRASORB	Multisorb Technologies, Inc.
NATURA	Sonic Innovations
NATURAL BY DESIGN	Medical Carbon Research Institute, Llc - Mcri
NATURAL BYPASS	Vasomedical Inc.
NATURAL MOTHER	Evenflo Company, Inc.
NATURAL TINT	Bausch & Lomb, Vision Care
NATURAL-HIP	Centerpulse Orthopedics Inc.
NATURAL-KNEE	Zimmer Holdings, Inc.
NATURAL-KNEE DURASUL	Centerpulse Orthopedics Inc.
NATURAL-KNEE II SYSTEM	Centerpulse Orthopedics Inc.
NATURAL-KNEE SYSTEM	Centerpulse Orthopedics Inc.
NATURAL-SELECTION	Boss Instruments, Ltd.
NATURALASE	Focus Medical, Llc.
NATURALASE 1064	Focus Medical, Llc.
NATURALASE 2 JOULE	Focus Medical, Llc.
NATURALASE DOUBLING HAND PIECE	Focus Medical, Llc.
NATURALASE ER	Focus Medical, Llc.
NATURALASE LP	Focus Medical, Llc.
NATURALASE LTE	Focus Medical, Llc.
NATURALASE Q-SWITCHED	Focus Medical, Llc.
NATURALASE QS	Focus Medical, Llc.
NATURALASE TATTOO REMOVAL	Focus Medical, Llc.
NATURALIGHT	Focus Medical, Llc.
NATURALIGHT IPL	Focus Medical, Llc.
NATURE SCENT	Surco Products
NATUSAN	Johnson & Johnson
NAUGLE EXOPHTHALMOMETER	Eagle Vision, Inc.
NAUTICA	Ev3 Inc.
NAUTILUS	Geerpres
NAUTILUS	Med-Fit Systems, Inc.
NAUTILUS	Nautilus, Inc.
NAUTILUSPILOT	Skytron
NAVIGATOR	Aesculap Implant Systems Inc.
NAVIGATOR	Avon-Isi
NAVIGATOR	Covidien Lp, Formerly Registered As United States Surgical
NAVIGATOR	Medtronic Xomed, Inc.
NAVIGATOR	Zimmer Dental, Inc.
NAVIGRAFT	Zimmer Dental, Inc.
NAVIPORT	Cardima, Inc.
NAVIPRO	Kinamed, Inc.
NAVITAR	Navitar, Inc.
NAZ-AL	Covidien Lp, Formerly Registered As Kendall
NAZORCAP	Nasorcap Medical, Inc.
NBF	Anatech, Ltd.
NBS	Nbs Technologies Inc.
NBS CONQUEST SERIES	Nbs Technologies Inc.
NBS HORIZON	Nbs Technologies Inc.
NBS IMPRESSIONS SERIES	Nbs Technologies Inc.
NC	Schleicher & Schuell, Inc.
NC-STAT	Neurometrix, Inc.
NC10002/P	Neurocare, Inc.
NC10002/PB	Neurocare, Inc.
NC10002/PB EQUINE	Neurocare, Inc.
NC10004/C	Neurocare, Inc.
NC10004/P	Neurocare, Inc.
NCB	Baker Company, The
NCB	Zimmer Holdings, Inc.
NCG	Allied Healthcare Products, Inc.
NCM OMEGA	North Coast Medical, Inc.
NCM PREFFERED	North Coast Medical, Inc.
NCP	Cyberonics, Inc.
NCP-2	Scottcare Corporation
NCS	Oxford Instruments
ND:YAG LASER	Cutera, Inc.
NDC	Kern Surgical Supply, Inc.
NDCAM	Nds Surgical Imaging, Inc.
NDM	Conmed Corporation
NDVISION 220	Del Global Technologies Corp.
NDVISION 280	Del Global Technologies Corp.
NEARFIELD	Stoelting
NEAT SLICER, PTK (PLACENTAL TRIAGE KIT)	Bio-Logics Products, Inc.
NEATSEAT	Sanitor Manufacturing Co.
NEBUTECH HDN	Salter Labs
NECK DOCTOR PILLOW	Core Products International, Inc.
NECK PHANTOM	Biodex Medical Systems, Inc.
NECKWRAP	Bean Products
NECLOC	Jerome Medical
NECLOC	Ossur Americas
NECLOC KIDS	Jerome Medical
NECLOC KIDS	Ossur Americas
NEEDLE AND BLADE GUARD	Graphic Controls Corp.
NEEDLE FINDER	Graphic Controls Corp.
NEEDLE FINDER	The Evercare Company
NEEDLE GUARD	Graphic Controls Corp.
NEEDLE RECAPPER/EXCHANGER	Advanced Medical Innovations, Inc.
NEEDLE'S EYE	Cook Vascular, Incorporated
NEEDLE-EASE	Medi-Crush Company
NEEDLEBANK	Covidien Lp
NEEDLEBUSTER	Life-Tech, Inc.
NEEDLEDICE	Atrion Medical Products, Inc.
NEEDLESCOPIC	Aesculap Implant Systems Inc.
NEEDLET	Amd-Ritmed, Inc.
NEEDLETRIEVER	Allen Medical Systems, Inc.
NEEDLEVISE	Atrion Medical Products, Inc.
NEISVAC-C	Baxter International Inc
NEIVERT WHITTLER	Temrex Corporation
NELLCOR	Covidien Lp, Formerly Registered As Tyco Healthcare
NEMCOMED	Ortholine
NEMIO	Toshiba America Medical Systems
NEO CARE	Neo-Care Arrow International
NEO PRO ER	Microflex Corporation
NEO-2	Mesa Laboratories, Inc.
NEO-STAT+	Mesa Laboratories, Inc.
NEO2000	Neoprobe Corporation
NEOBAR	Neotech Products, Inc.
NEOBOND	Neotech Products, Inc.
NEOBRIDGE	Neotech Products, Inc.
NEOBURR	Microcopy, Div. Neo-Flo, Inc.
NEOCERV	Pmt Corp.
NEOCHECK	Zefon International
NEOCOAT T4	Neometrics, A Division Of Natus
NEOCOLUMN	Neogen Corporation
NEOCUSSOR	General Pysiotherapy, Inc.
NEODERM	Conmed Corporation
NEODIAMONDS	Microcopy, Div. Neo-Flo, Inc.
NEODRYS	Microcopy, Div. Neo-Flo, Inc.
NEOFLEX	Conmed Corporation
NEOFORM	Mentor Corp.
NEOFX	Applied Biosystems
NEOGUARD	Cas Medical Systems, Inc.
NEOHOLD	Neotech Products, Inc.
NEOLEAD	Neotech Products, Inc.

NEOLET	Covidien Lp
NEOMODE	Covidien (Formerly Nellcor Puritan Bennett / Tyco Healthcare)
NEONATAL RESUSCITATION BABY	Medical Plastics Laboratory, Inc.
NEOPLASTINE	Diagnostica Stago, Inc.
NEOPRENE	Bell-Horn, Inc.
NEOPRO	Microflex Corporation
NEOPROBE	Neoprobe Corporation
NEOSERT	Covidien Lp
NEOSHADES	Neotech Products, Inc.
NEOSMILE	G & H Wire Co.
NEOSMILE	Neotech Products, Inc.
NEOSOFT	Medical Device Technologies, Inc. (Md Tech)
NEOSONO	Acteon Inc.
NEOTECH MECONIUM ASPIRATOR	Neotech Products, Inc.
NEOTEMP	Novamed, Llc
NEOTREND	Allegro Biodiesel Corporation
NEOTRODE	Conmed Corporation
NEOVISION	Covidien Lp, Formerly Registered As United States Surgical
NEOZOE	Scientific Pharmaceuticals, Inc.
NEPHRAT	Exocell, Inc.
NEPHRO-CATH	Uresil, Llc
NEPHROSCREEN	Covance Research Products Inc.
NEPHROSOL	Minntech Corporation
NEPTUNE	Bard Electro Physiology
NERO MAX	Supertech, Inc.
NERVE INTEGRITY MONITOR-2	Medtronic Xomed, Inc.
NERVEFINDER	Advanced Meditech International
NEST/PROTECTOR	Graphic Controls Corp.
NESTACK	Stackbin Corporation
NETLINK	Rozinn By Scottcare Corporation
NETLINK WIRELESS TELEPHONES	Spectralink Corporation
NETPRACTICE	Stryker Imaging
NETPRINT	Hospira Inc.
NETSCAN	Rozinn By Scottcare Corporation
NETVIEWER	Vidco, Inc.
NETWORK1	Karl Storz Endoscopy-America Inc.
NEU-GENES	Avi Biopharma, Inc.
NEUEKG	Neurodyne Medical Corp.
NEUGRAPH	Neurodyne Medical Corp.
NEULASTA	Nektar Therapeutics
NEURAGEN	Integra Lifesciences Holdings Corp.
NEURAIRTOME	Conmed Linvatec
NEURAWRAP	Integra Lifesciences Holdings Corp.
NEURO SCREEN	CAREFUSION 211, INC..
NEURO STIM	Conmed Corporation
NEURO-PULSE	Bovie Medical Corp.
NEURO-PULSE II	Bovie Medical Corp.
NEURO-PULSE III	Bovie Medical Corp.
NEUROAVITENE	Medchem Products, Inc.
NEUROBIOTIN TRACER	Vector Laboratories, Inc.
NEUROCARE	Neurocare, Inc.
NEUROCYBERNETIC PROSTHESIS	Cyberonics, Inc.
NEUROFAX	Nihon Kohden America, Inc.
NEUROFILE	Nihon Kohden America, Inc.
NEUROFORM	Boston Scientific-Neurovascular
NEUROFORM3	Boston Scientific-Neurovascular
NEUROGUIDE	Biofeedback Instrument Corp.
NEUROLASE	Spectrum Laser & Technologies, Inc
NEUROLINE	Ambu, Inc.
NEUROMETRIX	Neurometrix, Inc.
NEUROMUSCULAR SYSTEM/3	Neurodyne Medical Corp.
NEUROPACK	Nihon Kohden America, Inc.
NEUROPCENTILES	Wr Medical Electronics Co.
NEUROPEDIC	The Neurological Research And Development Group
NEUROPRO	Kinamed, Inc.
NEUROPROBE	Elmed, Inc.
NEUROQ	Syntermed, Inc.
NEUROTREND	Allegro Biodiesel Corporation
NEUROWAVE	Ekos Corp.
NEUSCAN	Neurodyne Medical Corp.
NEUSOFT	Consumaquip Corporation
NEUSOFT	Neurodyne Medical Corp.
NEUTRA-GUARD	Sakura Finetek U.S.A., Inc.
NEUTRAK	Landauer, Inc.
NEUTRAL EYES	Afassco, Inc.
NEUTRALON	Ansell Healthcare Products, Inc.
NEUTRALON 50	Ansell Healthcare Products, Inc.
NEUTRALON PF	Ansell Healthcare Products, Inc.
NEUTRATOP	Smith & Nephew, Inc.
NEUTREX	Kimble Chase Life Science And Research Products Llc
NEUTROCOLOR	Cytocolor, Inc.
NEV	Respironics Colorado
NEVER-MAR	Tp Orthodontics, Inc.
NEW	Saville 1300, Inc.
NEW - AID	H & S Manufacturing, Inc.
NEW AGE	Pascal Company, Inc.
NEW BATH	Sage Products, Inc.
NEW ENGLAND MEDICAL	Sigma Products Ltd.
NEW FREEDOM	KIMBERLY-CLARK CORP. CONWAY MILL
NEW IMAGE	Hollister Incorporated
NEW LIFE	Comfortex, Inc.
NEW PERCEPTIVE ENGINEERING	Specialty Manufacturing Co., The
NEW TOUCH	Ansell Healthcare Products, Inc.
NEW WEAVE	Tillotson Healthcare Corp.
NEW YORKER	Golden Technologies, Inc.
NEW-DUET	Sscor
NEW-DUET PORTABLE SUCTION UNIT	Armstrong Medical Industries, Inc.
NEW-KINETICS	I-Rep, Inc.
NEW-SENTINEL	Sscor
NEWBAND	Medical Equipment Specialists, Inc.
NEWCORE	Scientific Pharmaceuticals, Inc.
NEWDEAL	Integra Lifesciences Holdings Corp.
NEWDEAL	Wright Medical Group, Inc.
NEWLIFE	Airsep Corp.
NEWPORT	Newport Medical Instruments, Inc.
NEWPORT BREEZE, NEWPORT HT50	Newport Medical Instruments, Inc.
NEWPORT E360	Newport Medical Instruments, Inc.
NEWPORT E500	Newport Medical Instruments, Inc.
NEWPORT WAVE	Newport Medical Instruments, Inc.
NEXABAND	Closure Medical
NEXACRYL	Closure Medical
NEXCARE	3m Co.
NEXCT	Alfa Wassermann, Inc.
NEXES	Ventana Medical Systems, Inc.
NEXGEN	Marathon Equipment Company
NEXGEN	Zimmer Holdings, Inc.
NEXPOSURE	Zimmer Holdings, Inc.
NEXPRENE	Tpv Manufacturingÿ
NEXT	Benson Medical Instruments Co.
NEXT GEN VINYL	Tillotson Healthcare Corp.
NEXTEMP	Medical Indicators, Inc.
NEXTEMP PLUS	Medical Indicators, Inc.
NEXTEMP ULTRA	Medical Indicators, Inc.
NEXTGEN EMR	Quality Systems, Inc.
NEXTGEN EPM	Quality Systems, Inc.
NEXUS	Ev3 Inc.
NG SECURE	M.C. Johnson Co., Inc.
NI-TORQUE	G & H Wire Co.
NIBBLER	Mectra Labs, Inc.
NICE & HOT: QUANTUMHEAT: REHEATER	Worldwide Products Heat Packs
NICE 'N CLEAN	Professional Disposables International, Inc.
NICE CLEAN	Professional Disposables International, Inc.
NICHOLAS	Lafayette Instrument Company
NICKELPLAST	Alimed, Inc.
NICO2	Respironics, Inc
NICOLET	Cardinal Health Inc.
NICORE	Scottcare Corporation
NICORE ADVANTAGE	Rozinn By Scottcare Corporation
NICORETTE	Johnson & Johnson
NIDEK	Nidek Inc.
NIGHT SPLINTS	Corflex, Inc.
NIGHTINGALE	Adjustable Fixture Co.
NIGHTOWL	Perkin Elmer Wallac, Inc.
NIGHTOWL	Perkinelmer Life And Analytical Sciences
NIGHTSPLINT	Pedifix, Inc.
NIGHTWATCH	Respironics Georgia, Inc.

NIKO	Nikomed U.S.A., Inc.
NIKON	Bulbworks, Inc.
NIKOTABS	Nikomed U.S.A., Inc.
NILODOR	Nilodor, Inc.
NIM2XL	Medtronic Xomed, Inc.
NINA RICCI	L'Amy, Inc.
NINE WEST EYEWEARE	Safilo Usa
NIOBE	Stereotaxis, Inc.
NIP-IT	Miltex Inc.
NIPS-TIPS	Mark Medical Manufacturing, Inc.
NIRO 200	Hamamatsu Photonic Systems
NISSIN DENTAL	Kilgore International, Inc.
NITAKI	Spectrum Optical
NITRA-TEX	Ansell Healthcare Products, Inc.
NITRA-TEX E.P.	Ansell Healthcare Products, Inc.
NITRA-TOUCH	Ansell Healthcare Products, Inc.
NITRA-TOUCH	Ansell Protective Products
NITRA-TOUCH STERILE	Ansell Healthcare Products, Inc.
NITRASEAL	Sirona Dental Systems Llc
NITREX	Delta Gloves
NITRI-CARE	Best Manufacturing Co.
NITRILE DEFENSE	Life Guard
NITRO	Med-Fit Systems, Inc.
NITRO	Siemens Hearing Instruments, Inc.
NITRO-BLOCK-II	Applied Biosystems
NITROCHROME	Implant Sciences Corp.
NITROMITE	Photon Technology International, Inc.
NITRONOW	Carex Health Brands
NITROSPRAY PLUS	Premier Medical Products
NIVEOUS	Shofu Dental Corporation
NIZORAL	Ortho-Mcneil-Janssen Pharmaceuticals, Inc.
NK-1600E	N-K Products Company, Div. Of I-Rep,Inc.
NK-676	N-K Products Company, Div. Of I-Rep,Inc.
NKTR-024	Nektar Therapeutics
NKTR-063	Nektar Therapeutics
NKTR-102	Nektar Therapeutics
NKTR-105	Nektar Therapeutics
NKTR-118	Nektar Therapeutics
NKTR-119	Nektar Therapeutics
NL-45	Nsk America Corporation
NL-55	Nsk America Corporation
NL-65	Nsk America Corporation
NL-75	Nsk America Corporation
NL-86	Nsk America Corporation
NMIII	Compex Technologies, Inc.
NMP22	Matritech, Inc.
NMT	Omni Medical Supply Inc.
NO GLARE STRIPS	Mueller Sports Medicine
NO POWDER	Ansell Healthcare Products, Inc.
NO TOUCH	World Dryer Corp.
NO WALK	White Systems, Inc.
NO-FOG	Crosstex International,Inc.
NO-MIX:30	American Orthodontics Corp.
NO-NECK	Laerdal Medical Corporation
NO-RINSE	No Rinse Laboratories, Llc.
NO-TEAR PROBE COVERS: BIO-SCANGUARD PROBE COVERS	Emt Medical Co., Inc.
NODE SEEKER	Intramedical Imaging Llc
NOISE BRAKERS	Mid-States Laboratories, Inc.
NOISEMASTER	Proudfoot Company, Inc.
NOMADICr PRE-QUALIFIED SHIPPER	Thermosafe Brands
NOMOS	Best Nomos Corp.
NOMOS CRANE	Best Nomos Corp.
NON-STIX	American Silk Sutures, Inc.
NONE	Sciarra Laboratories, Inc
NONIN	Bound Tree Medical
NONIN	Dma Med-Chem Corporation
NONIN	Nonin Medical, Inc.
NORANGLE	Noraxon Usa, Inc.
NORBNC	Noraxon Usa, Inc.
NORDAN	Akorn, Inc.
NORDENT	Nordent Manufacturing, Inc.
NORDIC	Radix Corp.

NORINSE	Innovative Health Care Products, Inc.
NORM-JECT	Air-Tite Products Co., Inc.
NORM-O	Tp Orthodontics, Inc.
NORM-O-TEMP	Cincinnati Sub-Zero Products, Inc., Medical Division
NORMLGEL	Sca Personal Care, North America
NORMO FLO	Smiths Medical Asd, Inc.
NORODYN	Myotronics-Noromed, Inc.
NOROTRACK	Myotronics-Noromed, Inc.
NORPRENE	Saint-Gobain Performance Plastics--Akron
NORQDAQ	Noraxon Usa, Inc.
NORSK REHAB	Sunrise Medical, Inc.
NORSWITCH	Noraxon Usa, Inc.
NORTECH	Northgate Technologies Inc.
NORTH STAR	Braun Northwest, Inc.
NORTHGATE	Northgate Technologies Inc.
NORTHWIND	Bally Refrigerated Boxes, Inc.
NORTON	Saint-Gobain Performance Plastics--Akron
NORVIR	Abbott Laboratories
NOSE CONE REPAIR TOOL	Imonti And Associates Inc., M.
NOSHOK	Noshok, Inc.
NOTEBALL	Asi-Modulex
NOTEBAR	Asi-Modulex
NOTRIVEX	Millipore Corporation
NOUVELLE	Amoena
NOVA	G & H Wire Co.
NOVA	Nova Health Systems, Inc.
NOVA	Quantachrome
NOVA	Summit Industries, Inc.
NOVA	Vicon Industries Inc.
NOVA GEL	Inova Diagnostics, Inc.
NOVA LITE	Inova Diagnostics, Inc.
NOVABLOT II	Biorad Laboratories
NOVABLOT VI	Biorad Laboratories
NOVABOND	Argen Corp.
NOVABONE	Novabone Products, Llc
NOVABONE PUTTY	Novabone Products, Llc
NOVACK/POWERFLEX	Allied Biomedical
NOVACLEAN	Micronova
NOVACLONE	Immucor, Inc.
NOVACOR	World Heart Inc.
NOVADOME	Smiths Medical OEM
NOVAFIL	Covidien Lp
NOVAFLOW	Car-May
NOVAK MAIL SORTER	Swisslog Translogic Corporation
NOVALITE	Novamed, Llc
NOVALON	Becton Dickinson Infusion Therapy Systems, Inc.
NOVAMOP	Micronova
NOVANTRONE	Amgen Inc.
NOVASIL CATHETERS	Lemaitre Vascular, Inc.
NOVASPENSE	Car-May
NOVATEMP	Novamed, Llc
NOVATRANS	Smiths Medical OEM
NOVAX	Arlington Scientific, Inc. Asi
NOVEAUDERM	Silipos Inc.
NOVEON	Nomir Medical Technologies Inc.
NOVOLINPEN	Novo Nordisk Pharmaceuticals, Inc.
NOVOPEN	Novo Nordisk Pharmaceuticals, Inc.
NOVUS	Life-Tech, Inc.
NOVUS	Medtronic Sofamor Danek Usa, Inc
NOVUS	Medtronic Sofamor Danek Usa, Inc
NOVYLON	Cuno Filter Systems
NP	Leisure-Lift, Inc.
NPHD	Case Medical, Inc.
NPS PARTICLE TECHNOLOGY	Eprogen, Inc.
NPT7	Radiometer America, Inc.
NT200	Heine Usa Ltd.
NT2000	Compex Technologies, Inc.
NTI	Axis Dental
NU-DE	Finebrand Co.
NU-EAR	Nu-Ear Electronics
NU-EDGE	Tp Orthodontics, Inc.
NU-FIT	First Quality Enterprise, Inc.
NU-MO	Respironics Colorado

NU-THOR	Smiths Medical Asd
NU-TRAKE	Smiths Medical Asd
NUCHROME	AMD Technologies Inc.
NUCLEAR REPORT PROFESSIONAL	Syntermed, Inc.
NUCLEOSIL	Nest Group Inc., The
NUCLETRON	Nucletron Corporation
NUCLEUS, FREEDOM, ESPRIT, SPRINT, CONTOUR ADVANCE, BAHA, VISTAFIX .. Cochlear Americas	
NUCLISENS	Biomerieux Inc.
NUCRYST	Nucryst Pharmaceuticals Corp.
NUGATEWAY	Thinking Systems Corporation
NUGGET	Goldentone Hearing Aids
NUK	Gerber Products Co.
NULINK	Thinking Systems Corporation
NULL-KOTE	Princo Instruments, Inc.
NULLO	Chattem, Inc.
NULTRAVIOLET	Medi-Dose, Inc.
NUMBY STUFF	Iomed, Inc.
NUMELOCK	Stryker Corp.
NUMIMED	Sharn, Inc.
NUMITEMP	Sharn, Inc.
NUPAX	Thinking Systems Corporation
NUPREP	Weaver & Company
NUPRO	Dentsply International, Inc.
NUPRO	Dentsply Professional
NUPRO	Dentsply Prosthetics
NUQUEST	Medx Incorporated
NUROLON	Ethicon, Inc.
NURSE ASSIST	Nurse Assist ,Inc.
NURSE CALL ADAPTERS	Bed-Check Corporation
NURSE CALL CENTER	Epic Systems Corp.
NURSE OWNED AND OPERATED	Pocket Nurse Enterprises, Inc.
NURSERY-MAID	M.J. Thiesen Co. Inc.
NURSING ANNE	Medical Plastics Laboratory, Inc.
NURSING CARE	Smith & Nephew, Inc.
NURSING TRAINER	Lact-Aid International
NURTURE	Nurture Inc.
NUSONICS	Mesa Laboratories, Inc.
NUSORB	Nucon International, Inc.
NUSURG	Surgical Tools, Inc.
NUTRA-SOOTHE	Combe, Inc.
NUTRI-CATH	Utah Medical Products, Inc.
NUTRI-CENTER	Atlantic Medco, Inc.
NUTRICLONE-H	Peregrine Pharmaceuticals, Inc.
NUTRICLONE-M	Peregrine Pharmaceuticals, Inc.
NUTRIGUIDE	Spi Sports/Science Inc.
NUTRIPALS	Abbott Laboratories
NUTRITIONAL SOFTWARE LIBRARY	Computrition, Inc.
NUVANCE	Amgen Inc.
NUVOX	Hal-Hen Company, Inc.
NUWAVE	Compex Technologies, Inc.
NUWEB	Thinking Systems Corporation
NVISION	Nonin Medical, Inc.
NX3 ASPIRATOR	Medical Device Resource Corporation
NXT	Ev3 Inc.
NYLATEX	Chattanooga Group
NYTONE	Nytone Medical Products
NYTRAN	Schleicher & Schuell, Inc.
Nano-Tex	Knoll, Inc.
Natra-Bio	Nutraceutical International Corp.
Natural Balance	Nutraceutical International Corp.
Natural Sport	Nutraceutical International Corp.
Natural-Fit	The Aftermarket Group
NaturalCare	Nutraceutical International Corp.
NaturalMax	Nutraceutical International Corp.
Natures Life	Nutraceutical International Corp.
NaviStar	Biosense Webster, Inc
Navigator	Boston Scientific Corporation
NephroMax	Boston Scientific Corporation
NeuroStar TMS (Transcranial Magnetic Stimulation)	Neuronetics, Inc.
Neuroform	Boston Scientific Corporation
Neuroform3	Boston Scientific Corporation
Neutrogena	Ortho Dermatologics
NexStent	Boston Scientific - Maple Grove
NexStent	Boston Scientific Corporation
Norwegian Formula	Ortho Dermatologics
NuPolar	Younger Manufacturing Co., Inc.
Null-Kote	Princo Instruments, Inc.
Nylaflo	Pall Corporation
Nylasorb	Pall Corporation
O-RING	Preat Corp.
O-WIRE	Arrow International, Inc.
O.S.	Quidel Corporation
O/P-TECT	Globe Scientific, Inc.
O2000 PXUGEM ANALYZER	CAREFUSION 211, INC..
O2OPTIX	Ciba Vision Corporation
OA-SYS	Organomation Associates, Inc.
OAKTEX	Oak Gloves Division Of Omar Medical Supplies, Inc.
OAKWORKS FLUOROSCOPY TABLES	Oakworks, Inc.
OASIS	Cook Biotech, Incorporated
OASIS	Geri-Care Products
OASIS	Living Earth Crafts
OASIS BABY WARMING SYSTEM	Children's Medical Ventures, Inc.
OASIS DILUTION SYSTEM	Ecolab Inc.
OASIS ONLINE	Briggs Corporation
OASIS TEARS	Oasis Medical, Inc.
OASIS TEARS PLUS	Oasis Medical, Inc.
OASIS TOUCH ACCESS	Surgical Safety Products, Inc.
OASYS	Stryker Corp.
OASYS	Stryker Spine
OB KITS	Morrison Medical
OBIS	Oxoid, Inc.
OBSERVER	Ge Medical Systems Information Technologies
OBSERVER	Lw Scientific
OCCIAN	Ossur Americas
OCCIPITAL CRADLE	Gunnell, Inc.
OCCLU PLUS SPRAY	Hager Worldwide, Inc.
OCCLU PRINT	Hager Worldwide, Inc.
OCCLU SPOT	Hager Worldwide, Inc.
OCCLUDE	Pascal Company, Inc.
OCEAN	Clarke Health Care Products, Inc.
OCEAN VIP FORTUNA	Clarke Health Care Products, Inc.
OCEANSP	Clarke Health Care Products, Inc.
OCL	Bsn Medical, Inc
OCTA-HEX	Universal Implant Systems, Inc.
OCTAPETTE	Corning Inc., Science Products Division
OCTOFUGE	Cygnus Inc.
OCTOPUS	Haag-Streit Group
OCTOPUS	Medtronic Cardiovascular Surgery, The Heart Valve Div.
OCTREOSCAN	Mallinckrodt, Inc.
OCTYLDENT	Closure Medical
OCU-1	Becton Dickinson And Co.
OCU-CEL	Mentor Ophthalmics, Inc.
OCU-CEL XL	Mentor Ophthalmics, Inc.
OCU-FILM	Mentor Ophthalmics, Inc.
OCU-FLEX 38 KERATOCONUS	Ocu-Ease Optical Products, Inc.
OCU-FLEX 53 SPHERE	Ocu-Ease Optical Products, Inc.
OCU-FLEX 53 TORIC	Ocu-Ease Optical Products, Inc.
OCU-FLEX 55 SPHERE	Ocu-Ease Optical Products, Inc.
OCU-FLEX PLUS SPHERE	Ocu-Ease Optical Products, Inc.
OCUCOAT	Bausch & Lomb, Inc.
OCUFEN	Allergan
OCULASE	Biolase Technology, Inc.
OCULIGHT	Iridex Corporation
OCUSEAL	Surgistar Inc.
OCUTEK	Medtronic Xomed, Inc.
ODO-WAY	Smith & Nephew, Inc.
ODOMASTER	Surco Products
ODOR PLEX	Sage Laboratories, Inc.
ODOR-ENDr EMERGENCY CLEAN-UPr POWDER ODOR-ENDr DUMPS	Cdc Products Corp.
ODOR-X	Unit Chemical Corp.
ODOUR-BAN	Marlen Manufacturing & Development Co.
ODOUR-GUARD	Marlen Manufacturing & Development Co.
ODYSSEY	Luxfer Gas Cylinders
ODYSSEY	Mentor Ophthalmics, Inc.

ODYSSEY	Permedics, Inc.
ODYSSEY	Sellstrom Manufacturing Co.
ODYSSEY 30 HOLMIUM LASER SYSTEM	Xintec Corp. / Convergent Laser Tech.
ODYSSEY HOLMIUM	Convergent Laser Technologies
OEM SENSORS	Mine Safety Appliances Company
OFFICE OF THE FUTURE	Welch Allyn, Inc.
OFFICEMATE	Hologic, Inc.
OFFICEPACS POWER	Stryker Corp.
OFFICEPACS POWER	Stryker Endoscopy
OFFICEPACS POWER	Stryker Howmedica Osteonics
OFFSET	Graphic Controls Corp.
OFFSET UNWEIGHING SYSTEM	Biodex Medical Systems, Inc.
OGDEN	Western Water Purifier Co.
OHAUS	Utech Products, Inc.
OIL	Living Earth Crafts
OKANDO	C & A Scientific Co. Inc.
OLEEVA CLEAR	Bio Med Sciences, Inc.
OLEEVA FABRIC	Bio Med Sciences, Inc.
OLEEVA FOAM	Bio Med Sciences, Inc.
OLEEVA KIT	Allerderm Laboratories, Inc.
OLETEX	Ufp Technologies, Inc.
OLIGOPREP	Thermo Savant
OLIGOSPERMIA CUP	Milex Products, Inc.
OLIS 14	Olis: On-Line Instrument Systems, Inc.
OLIS RSM 1000	Olis: On-Line Instrument Systems, Inc.
OLIS USA STOPPED-FILM	Olis: On-Line Instrument Systems, Inc.
OLMEGS	Online Power, Inc.
OLYMPIA	Wright Medical Group, Inc.
OLYMPIAN	Dent Zar, Inc.
OLYMPIC CFM 6000	Olympic Medical Corp.
OLYMPIC MEDICAL	Medi-Tech International, Inc.
OLYMPUS	Mccrone Microscopes & Accessories
OMEGA	Heine Usa Ltd.
OMEGA	North Coast Medical, Inc.
OMEGA	Nova Health Systems, Inc.
OMEGA	Ultra-Lum, Inc.
OMEGA 21	Ebi, Llc
OMEGA 3	Stryker Corp.
OMEGA 750	O'Ryan Industries, Inc.
OMEGA AP	O'Ryan Industries, Inc.
OMEGA C	Cook Inc.
OMEGA NV	Cook Inc.
OMEGA SC	O'Ryan Industries, Inc.
OMEGA SE	O'Ryan Industries, Inc.
OMEGA-PORT	Angiodynamics, Inc.
OMI	Schaerer Mayfield Usa
OMNI	Columbia Medical Manufacturing Llc
OMNI	Fischer Medical Technologies Inc.
OMNI	Respironics Missouri
OMNI	Trimedyne, Inc.
OMNI ACCU-BAR	Respironics Missouri
OMNI COLD GEL PACKS	Respironics Missouri
OMNI COMBO	Respironics Missouri
OMNI FLUSH	Angiodynamics, Inc.
OMNI GLH	Omni International, Inc.
OMNI II	Respironics Missouri
OMNI INFANT HEEL WARMERS	Respironics Missouri
OMNI INFANT TRANSPORT MATTRESS	Respironics Missouri
OMNI MICRO HOMOGENIZER	Omni International, Inc.
OMNI O.R.	Respironics Missouri
OMNI PAL IV POLE	Pryor Products
OMNI SPECTRUM	Respironics Missouri
OMNI SURFACE	Stryker Corp.
OMNI TH	Omni International, Inc.
OMNI WIDE RANGE	Respironics Missouri
OMNI-4000	Enmet Corp.
OMNI-FLOW	Hospira Inc.
OMNI-TIGHT DENTAL IMPLANT SYSTEM	Basic Dental Implant Systems, Inc.
OMNI-TIPS DISPOSABLES	Omni International, Inc.
OMNIACCESS	Omni-Tract Surgical, A Div. Of Minnesota Scientific, Inc.
OMNIAIR	Pyramid Industries, Llc
OMNIAXIAL CONNECTOR	Orthotec, Llc
OMNIBLOC	Gi Supply
OMNICARBON	Medicalcv, Inc.
OMNICART	Omnimed, Inc. (Beam Products)
OMNICELL	Marcon Group, Inc.
OMNICELL APM	Marcon Group, Inc.
OMNICELL GEL	Marcon Group, Inc.
OMNICELL XL	Marcon Group, Inc.
OMNICULTURE	Virtis, An Sp Industries Company
OMNIFIT EON	Stryker Corp.
OMNIFIT EON	Stryker Howmedica Osteonics
OMNIFIX	B. Braun Medical Inc., Renal Therapies Div.
OMNIFIX	B. Braun Oem Division, B. Braun Medical Inc.
OMNIFLATOR	Northgate Technologies Inc.
OMNIFLEX	Helvoet Pharma, Inc.
OMNIFLEX	Hologic, Inc.
OMNIFLO	Eg & G Amorphous Silicon
OMNIGRIP	Maddak, Inc.
OMNIGUIDE	Fiberguide Industries, Inc.
OMNILINK	Jeron Electronic Systems, Inc.
OMNILOG	Biolog, Inc.
OMNIMED	Medi-Tech International, Inc.
OMNIMED	Omnimed, Inc. (Beam Products)
OMNIPROBE,	Care Wise Medical Products Corp.
OMNIPULSE JR.	Trimedyne, Inc.
OMNIPULSE MAX	Trimedyne, Inc.
OMNISCIENCE	Medicalcv, Inc.
OMNISCRIBE	Allen Datagraph Systems, Inc.
OMNISIGHT	Integra Lifesciences Holdings Corp.
OMNISOLV	Emd Chemicals Inc.
OMNISORB II	Tidi Products, Llc
OMNISTIK	Vital Signs Colorado
OMNITIP	Trimedyne, Inc.
OMNITRAK	Eg & G Amorphous Silicon
OMNIVIEW	Trimedyne, Inc.
OMNIVUE	Waldmann Lighting
OMOTRAIN	Bauerfeind Usa, Inc.
OMP	Advanced Biomedical Devices, Inc. (Abd, Inc.)
OMRON	Creative Health Products, Inc.
OMTI	Televideo Systems, Inc.
ON SERIES	Oneac Corporation
ON SERIES E	Oneac Corporation
ON SERIES M	Oneac Corporation
ON TARGET	Ams Innovative Center-San Jose
ON-BOARD IMAGER	Varian Medical Systems
ON-CALL	Acon Laboratories, Inc.
ON-Q	I-Flow Corporation
ON-TAP	Integrated Software Design, Inc.
ON-X HEART VALVE	Medical Carbon Research Institute, Llc - Mcri
ON-X PURE CARBON	Medical Carbon Research Institute, Llc - Mcri
ONCE-A-DAY	Propper Manufacturing Co., Inc.
ONCE-A-DAY	Surco Products
ONCO-TAIN	Hospira Inc.
ONCOR AVANT-GARDE LINEAR ACCELERATOR	Siemens Medical Solutions Usa, Inc
ONCOR EXPRESSION LINEAR ACCELERATOR	Siemens Medical Solutions Usa, Inc
ONCOR IMPRESSION LINEAR ACCELERATOR	Siemens Medical Solutions Usa, Inc
ONCORAD	Cytogen Corp.
ONCOSCINT	Cytogen Corp.
ONE CALL BRINGS IT ALL(SM)	Dedicated Distribution
ONE GREEN HANDLE	Smith & Nephew, Inc.
ONE PAN	Young Innovations, Inc.
ONE SHOT	Covidien Lp, Formerly Registered As United States Surgical
ONE SOLUTION LPHST	Steris Corporation
ONE STEP KVO	I-Flow Corporation
ONE TOUCH	Hager Worldwide, Inc.
ONE TOUCH BASIC	Lifescan, Inc.
ONE TOUCH II	Lifescan, Inc.
ONE TOUCH VASCULAR SOLUTION	Unetixs Vascular, Inc.
ONE-CALL	Per-Se Technologies
ONE-STAFF	Per-Se Technologies
ONE-STEP	Zoll Medical Corp.
ONEGLOSS	Shofu Dental Corporation

ONEPLUS SERIES	Oneac Corporation
ONESOURCE	Joerns Healthcare, Inc
ONETWO	Atrion Medical Products, Inc.
ONLINE SERIES	Oneac Corporation
ONQUE	Argosy
ONSITE	Cardinal Health Inc.
ONSITE	Trek Diagnostic Systems
ONWAVE	Phonic Ear, Inc.
ONY-CLEAR	Pedinol Pharmacal, Inc.
ONYX	Coherent, Inc.
ONYX	Nonin Medical, Inc.
ONYX	Prosun Tanning International, Llc.
ONYX HD-500	Ev3 Inc.
ONYX LES	Ev3 Inc.
ONYX-H	Miltex Inc.
ONYX-H	Moyco Technologies, Inc.
ONYX-R	Miltex Inc.
ONYX-R	Moyco Technologies, Inc.
OP-1	Stryker Biotech
OP-1	Stryker Corp.
OP-1	Stryker Howmedica Osteonics
OP-1	Stryker Spine
OP-D-OP	Op-D-Op, Inc.
OPAL LEGACY	Clarke Health Care Products, Inc.
OPAL MAXI	Clarke Health Care Products, Inc.
OPAL SYMPHONY	Clarke Health Care Products, Inc.
OPART	Toshiba America Medical Systems
OPATANOL	Alcon Research, Ltd.
OPCAB	Genzyme
OPCAB IMMOBILIZER	Teleflex Medical
OPD	Covidien Lp
OPEN EX	Hager Worldwide, Inc.
OPEN PIVOT	ATS Medical, Inc.
OPENGENE	Siemens Healthcare Diagnostics Inc.
OPENMED	Openmed Technologies Corporation
OPENMED CAPTURE EXPRESS	Openmed Technologies Corporation
OPENMED LINKS	Openmed Technologies Corporation
OPENMED MANAGER	Openmed Technologies Corporation
OPENMED RADIOLOGY	Openmed Technologies Corporation
OPENMED VIEWER	Openmed Technologies Corporation
OPENNET	Vitalcom, Inc.
OPENPACS	Sudbury Systems
OPERA	ArjoHuntleigh
OPERA	Coherent, Inc.
OPERON	Berchtold Corp.
OPESCOPE	Shimadzu Medical Systems
OPHTHALMOLOGY OFFICE	Ophthalmic Imaging Systems
OPHTHASONIC	Mentor Ophthalmics, Inc.
OPHTHASONIC A-SCAN	Mentor Ophthalmics, Inc.
OPIIVIS	Covidien Lp, Formerly Registered As United States Surgical
OPMI	Carl Zeiss Surgical, Inc.
OPMI MD	Carl Zeiss Surgical, Inc.
OPMI PENTERO	Carl Zeiss Meditec Inc.
OPMI-CS	Carl Zeiss Surgical, Inc.
OPMI-NEURO	Carl Zeiss Surgical, Inc.
OPMI-PROMO	Carl Zeiss Surgical, Inc.
OPMILAS	Carl Zeiss Surgical, Inc.
OPPORTUNITY GENESIS	Innovation Genesis, Llc
OPSITE	Smith & Nephew, Inc.
OPSITE IV 1-STEP	Smith & Nephew, Inc.
OPSITE IV3000	Smith & Nephew, Inc.
OPTA	Cordis Corporation
OPTA PRO PTA DILATATION CATHETER	Cordis Endovascular
OPTEASE PERMANENT VENA CAVA FILTER	Cordis Endovascular
OPTEC	Stereo Optical Co., Inc.
OPTEC2000	Good-Lite Co.
OPTEFIL	Exactech, Inc.
OPTEFORM	Exactech, Inc.
OPTEON	Exactech, Inc.
OPTETRAK	Exactech, Inc.
OPTEX	Mci Optonix, Div. Of Usr Optonix Inc.
OPTEX	Vespo Marketing Assoc., Inc.
OPTHOS	Agfa Corporation
OPTHOSTAT	Ams Innovative Center-San Jose
OPTI	Buffalo Dental Manufacturing Co., Inc.
OPTI MIST	Serologicals Corp
OPTI-CAL	Psyche Systems
OPTI-CIDE SPRAY	Micro-Scientific Industries, Inc.
OPTI-CLEAR	Novosci Corp.
OPTI-FIX	Smith & Nephew Inc.- Orthopaedics Division
OPTI-GARD	Dupaco, Inc.
OPTI-ICE	Chattanooga Group
OPTI-MIST, KONSERV	Unomedical, Inc.
OPTI-SCRUB	Micro-Scientific Industries, Inc.
OPTI-SCRUB NO RINSE	Micro-Scientific Industries, Inc.
OPTI-SHIELD	Lee Medical International, Inc.
OPTI-VISOR	Lee Medical International, Inc.
OPTIBAR	Timemed Labeling Systems, Inc.
OPTIBIND	Seradyn, Inc.
OPTIBLAST	Buffalo Dental Manufacturing Co., Inc.
OPTICA 100	Convergent Laser Technologies
OPTICAID	Edroy Products Co., Inc.
OPTICAL ALLIANCE	Dispensers Optical Service Corp.
OPTICAL BUILDING BLOCKS	Photon Technology International, Inc.
OPTICAL SHOP OF ASPEN	Optical Shop Of Aspen
OPTICAL SHOP OF ASPEN INTERNATIONAL	Optical Shop Of Aspen
OPTICARE	Symmetry Medical Usa, Inc.
OPTICARE	Symmetry Medical, Inc.
OPTICELL	Bausch & Lomb, Vision Care
OPTICHAMBER	Respironics New Jersey, Inc.
OPTICS ONE	Mti-Medical Technique, Inc.
OPTIDOT	Microtech Medical Systems
OPTIFIT	Ciba Vision
OPTIFLEX	Chattanooga Group
OPTIFLOW	Eg & G Amorphous Silicon
OPTIFOCUS MLC	Siemens Medical Solutions Usa, Inc
OPTIFREE	Alcon Research, Ltd.
OPTIGARD	H.L. Bouton Co., Inc.
OPTIGLIDE	Smith & Nephew Inc.- Orthopaedics Division
OPTIHALER	Respironics New Jersey, Inc.
OPTIKINASE	Usb Corporation
OPTILASE PL100	Trimedyne, Inc.
OPTILINK	Seradyn, Inc.
OPTILITE	Convergent Laser Technologies
OPTILITE ACCESSORIES FOR LASER SURGERY	Xintec Corp. / Convergent Laser Tech.
OPTIMA	Bausch & Lomb, Vision Care
OPTIMA	Sloan Valve Co.
OPTIMA 38	Bausch & Lomb, Vision Care
OPTIMA OXYGENATOR	Sorin Group Usa
OPTIMA PLUS	Sloan Valve Co.
OPTIMAL	Crosstex International,Inc.
OPTIMARK	Mallinckrodt, Inc.
OPTIMAX	Biogenex Laboratories
OPTIME OR SCHEDULING	Epic Systems Corp.
OPTIMEYES PORTABLE	Micromedical Technologies, Inc.
OPTIMIX	Greer Laboratories, Inc.
OPTIMOL	Wescor, Inc.
OPTIMUM	Comfortex, Inc.
OPTIMUM BY LOBOB	Lobob Laboratories, Inc.
OPTIMUM COMFORT CUSHION	Pyramid Industries, Llc
OPTIMUMMT	Valleylab
OPTION	Kinamed, Inc.
OPTION 133	Newschoff Chairs, Inc.
OPTION-LOK	Hospira Inc.
OPTIPAC	Camfil Farr
OPTIPHOT	Nikon Instruments Inc.
OPTIPLUS	Biogenex Laboratories
OPTIPRESS	Fenwal Inc.
OPTIQUANT	Kronus, Inc.
OPTIRAY	Mallinckrodt, Inc.
OPTISOAP	Optikem International, Inc.
OPTISTAR	Mallinckrodt, Inc.
OPTISTAT	Mallinckrodt, Inc.
OPTITRAN	Schleicher & Schuell, Inc.
OPTIVANTAGE	Covidien Lp, Formerly Registered As Tyco Healthcare

OPTIVANTAGE	Mallinckrodt, Inc.
OPTIVENT	Respironics New Jersey, Inc.
OPTIVIEW ASI EPID	Siemens Medical Solutions Usa, Inc
OPTIVOX	Smiths Medical Asd
OPTIVUE	Siemens Medical Solutions Usa, Inc
OPTIWELL	Midwest Scientific
OPTIX	Plaskolite West Inc.
OPTOCOMP	Mgm Instruments
OPTOLON COATING I & II	Chromodynamics
OPTRAN	Biolitec, Inc.
OPTX	Varian Medical Systems
OPUS	Life-Tech, Inc.
OPUS II	Dornier Medtech America
OPUS RM	Ela Medical, Inc.
OR PROTOCOL	Healthstream, Inc.
OR-1	Karl Storz Endoscopy-America Inc.
OR-CLEANSE	Nds Surgical Imaging, Inc.
OR1	Karl Storz Endoscopy-America Inc.
ORAGRAFT	Lifenet Health
ORAL-B	Oral-B Laboratories, Inc.
ORALINE	Sun Biomedical Laboratories, Inc.
ORAMORPH SR	Roxane Laboratories
ORANGE	Mectra Labs, Inc.
ORANGEAID	Mizuho Osi
ORAQUICK	Orasure Technologies, Inc.
ORASURE	Orasure Technologies, Inc.
ORATIP	Pascal Company, Inc.
ORBATEK	Hager Worldwide, Inc.
ORBIT CUFF	Suntech Medical, Inc.
ORBIT-K CUFF	Suntech Medical, Inc.
ORBITER	Bard Electro Physiology
ORBITRON	Boekel Scientific
ORCA	Mentor Ophthalmics, Inc.
ORCAS	Accu-Med Services
ORCHESTRA	Ela Medical, Inc.
OREGON SPINE SPLINT II	Skedco, Inc.
ORFIT	North Coast Medical, Inc.
ORGA-TRAY	Aesculap Implant Systems Inc.
ORGANISOL	Chester Labs, Inc.
ORIA CLARIS	Orthotec, Llc
ORIA ZENITH	Orthotec, Llc
ORIGEN	Origen Biomedical, Inc.
ORIGINAL MCKENZIE	Optp
ORIGINAL SOFTSERT	Softsert, Inc.
ORION	Ams Innovative Center-San Jose
ORION	Analogic Corporation
ORION	Biofeedback Instrument Corp.
ORION	Orion Research, Inc.
ORION	Self Regulation Systems, Inc.
ORION CPAP	CAREFUSION 211, INC..
ORION MEDICAL	Medikmark Inc.
ORION MOBILE	Ericsson, Inc.
ORLIS	Medtronic Xomed, Inc.
OROSTAT	Belport Co. Inc., Gingi-Pak Div.
ORS	First Aid Bandage Co., Inc.
ORSOS	Per-Se Technologies
ORTHEX HEEL SPUR	Viscolas, Inc.
ORTHEX RELIEVERS	Viscolas, Inc.
ORTHEX ULTRA PERFORMER	Viscolas, Inc.
ORTHINOX	Stryker Corp.
ORTHO CONCEPTS	Currie Medical Specialties, Inc.
ORTHO DX	Compex Technologies, Inc.
ORTHO WEDGE	Darco International, Inc.
ORTHO WELDER	Yates & Bird And Motloid
ORTHO-LIFT I	Ortho-Kinetics, Inc.
ORTHO-LIFT II	Ortho-Kinetics, Inc.
ORTHO-POD	Advanced Mechanical Technology, Inc. (Amti)
ORTHO-PRO	St. John Companies
ORTHO-REST	Bell-Horn, Inc.
ORTHO-TECHLINE	Maxant Technologies, Inc.
ORTHOBAND	Orthoband Company, Inc.
ORTHOBEADS	Bruder Healthcare Company
ORTHOCARE	Cfi Medical Solutions (Contour Fabricators, Inc.)
ORTHOCEPH	Instrumentarium Imaging, Inc.
ORTHOCR	Stryker Corp.
ORTHOFIT	Tri Hawk Corporation
ORTHOFORCE	G & H Wire Co.
ORTHOID	Instrumentarium Imaging, Inc.
ORTHOLOGIC 1000	Capstone Therapeutics
ORTHOLURE	Lifecore Biomedical, Inc.
ORTHOLUX XT	3m Unitek
ORTHOMATRIX	Lifecore Biomedical, Inc.
ORTHOMEDICS	Seattle Systems
ORTHOMOLD	Seattle Systems
ORTHONE	Oni Medical Systems, Inc.
ORTHOPAD	Stryker Corp.
ORTHOPAD	Stryker Endoscopy
ORTHOPAD	Stryker Howmedica Osteonics
ORTHOPAD	Stryker Spine
ORTHOPAK	Biolectron, Inc.
ORTHOPAN	Instrumentarium Imaging, Inc.
ORTHOPAT AUTOTRANSFUSION SYSTEM	Zimmer Orthopaedic Surgical Products
ORTHOPAT SYSTEM	Haemonetics Corp.
ORTHOPEDIC PILLOW	Hermell Products, Inc.
ORTHOPEDIC SKELETON	Medical Plastics Laboratory, Inc.
ORTHOPEDIC SLINGS	Central New York Medical Products
ORTHOPHOS XG	Sirona Dental Systems Llc
ORTHOPLUG	Sunmedica
ORTHOPRINT	Pedifix, Inc.
ORTHOPROBE	Ams Innovative Center-San Jose
ORTHORAP	Sunmedica
ORTHOSORB	Depuy Ace, A Johnson & Johnson Company
ORTHOSPHERE	Wright Medical Group, Inc.
ORTHOSTAR	Getinge Usa, Inc.
ORTHOTEC	Orthotec, Llc
ORTHOTICS	Spi Sports/Science Inc.
ORTHOTRAC	Orthofix Inc.
ORTHOTRON II	Cybex International, Inc.
ORTHOTRON KTI & KT2	Cybex International, Inc.
ORTHOVISC	Anika Therapeutics
ORTHOVISC	Johnson & Johnson
ORTHOWEAR	DJO Inc.
ORTHOZONE	Sealy Inc.
ORTIVUS	Ortivus
OSA	Optical Shop Of Aspen
OSA INTERNATIONAL	Optical Shop Of Aspen
OSADA	Osada, Inc.
OSCAR	Photon Technology International, Inc.
OSCAR	Suntech Medical, Inc.
OSCAR	Tremetrics
OSCAR 2TANGO	Suntech Medical, Inc.
OSCILLAIRE	Jones Medical Instrument Co.
OSD	Artromick International, Inc.
OSHINO	Bulbworks, Inc.
OSI	Mizuho Osi
OSIRIS	Biorad Laboratories
OSM3	Radiometer America, Inc.
OSMETTE	Precision Systems, Inc.
OSMITROL	Baxter Healthcare Corporation, Global Drug Delivery
OSMOCOLL	Wescor, Inc.
OSMONICS	Ge Infrastructure Water & Process Technologies
OSP	Starkey Laboratories, Inc.
OSPREY	Hill-Rom Manufacturing, Inc.
OSRAM	Osram Sylvania Inc.
OSRAM-SYLVANIA	Bulbtronics, Inc.
OSRAM/SYLVANIA	Bulbworks, Inc.
OSSEOFIT	Kensey Nash Corporation
OSSIGEL	Anika Therapeutics
OSSTAPLE/OSSPLATE, EXCALIBUR BGS	Biomedical Enterprises, Inc.
OSTEO-LOCK	Impladent Ltd.
OSTEOBLAST	Kinamed, Inc.
OSTEOCARE	Compumed, Inc.
OSTEOGEN	Ebi, Llc
OSTEOGEN	Impladent Ltd.
OSTEOGEN	Park Dental Research Corp./Implant Center

PACIFIC	Asi-Modulex
PACIFIC SAFETY	Bound Tree Medical
PACIFICA	Pacifica Gloves
PACITHERM	Mabis Healthcare Inc.
PACK-RACK	First Healthcare Products
PACKAGENE	Promega Corp.
PACKARD HAMMERS	Midshore Industries, Inc.
PACPRINT	Nai Tech Products
PACRIM	Polyzen, Inc.
PACS/PRO DX PLUS	Emed Technologies
PACSWATCH	Agfa Corporation
PACSYSTEM 3000	Richard Wolf Medical Instruments Corp.
PACU BED	Stryker Medical
PAD'L-PET	Samco Scientific Corporation
PADCALL	Dwyer Precision Products, Inc.
PADLOCK	Baxa Corporation
PADPACK	Laerdal Medical Corporation
PADPRO	Conmed Corporation
PAGODA	Labcon North America
PAIN FREE	Parkell, Inc.
PAIN MANAGEMENT C-ARM TABLE	Biodex Medical Systems, Inc.
PAIN RELIEF THAT WORKS	Biofreeze Performance Health, Inc.
PAIN RELIEVING GEL	Biofreeze Performance Health, Inc.
PAIN-X-2000	Diomedics, Inc.
PAINBLOCKER	Wallach Surgical Devices, Inc.
PAINBUSTER	I-Flow Corporation
PAINFREE	Afassco, Inc.
PAINLESS PARTICLES	Bangs Laboratories, Inc.
PAINPUMP 2 BLOCKAID	Stryker Corp.
PAINPUMP I	Stryker Corp.
PAINPUMP2	Stryker Corp.
PAINTRACK	JTECH Medical
PAK GUAIAC	Cambridge Diagnostic Products, Inc.
PAK-MORE HOLD-DOWN DISK	S&G Enterprises, Inc.
PAKHAMMER 90	Paratech, Inc.
PAKKIE MOBILITY SLING	Access Now Llc
PAL	Leap Technologies
PAL	Micro-Aire Surgical Instruments, Inc.
PAL PORTABLE AQUATIC LIFT	Rehamed Intl. Llc.
PAL PRO STIRRUP	Allen Medical Systems, Inc.
PAL STIRRUP	Allen Medical Systems, Inc.
PALA-NATE	Utah Medical Products, Inc.
PALINEY	Deringer-Ney, Inc.
PALLADIUM	Glines And Rhodes, Inc.
PALLADIUM	Radix Corp.
PALLETANK	Stedim Biosystems, Inc.
PALM (PALPATATION METER)	Performance Attainment Associates
PALMAZ	Cordis Corporation
PALMAZ GENESIS TRANHEPATIC BILIARY STENT	Cordis Endovascular
PALMAZ TRANSHEPATIC BILIARY STENT	Cordis Endovascular
PALMAZ-SCHATZ	Cordis Corporation
PALMER	Palmer Industries
PALMSAT	Nonin Medical, Inc.
PALODENT	Dentsply International, Inc.
PALODENT	Dentsply Prosthetics
PALPATION IMAGING	Medical Tactile, Inc.
PALS	Axelgaard Manufacturing Company, Ltd.
PALS ELECTRODES	Med-Fit Systems, Inc.
PALTER & PALTER-MAX	Promega Corp.
PALUMBO	Palumbo Orthopaedics
PAM-RL	Mini-Mitter Company, Inc.
PAMIC	Camfil Farr
PAN RETINAL	Volk Optical Inc.
PANA GOGGLE	H.L. Bouton Co., Inc.
PANA LENS	H.L. Bouton Co., Inc.
PANA SPEC	H.L. Bouton Co., Inc.
PANA VIEW	H.L. Bouton Co., Inc.
PANA-LUBE	Panadent Corp.
PANA-MOUNT	Panadent Corp.
PANADENT	Panadent Corp.
PANALITE	H.L. Bouton Co., Inc.
PANASPEC PLUS	H.L. Bouton Co., Inc.
PANATECH	H.L. Bouton Co., Inc.

PANBUS	La Mont Medical, Inc.
PANDA	Ge Medical Systems Information Technologies
PANDA	Snug Seat, Inc.
PANDA 1001	James Consolidated, Inc.
PANDA 2000, PANDA 2001	James Consolidated, Inc.
PANDA 3000	James Consolidated, Inc.
PANDA 3001	James Consolidated, Inc.
PANEL WIN	Photo Research, Inc.
PANEL-TOUCH CONTROLLER	Mosaic Industries, Inc.
PANELKEY	Advanced Input Systems
PANGIOMAX	Shimadzu Medical Systems
PANJE	E. Benson Hood Laboratories, Inc.
PANO GAUZE	Sage Laboratories, Inc.
PANO PLEX	Sage Laboratories, Inc.
PANOMAT	Roche Insulin Delivery Systems Inc.
PANOPTIKON	Cytocolor, Inc.
PANORAMA	Asi-Modulex
PANORAMA	Astro-Med, Inc.
PANOSCOPE	S&S Technology
PANOSOL II	National Biological Corp.
PANOVIEW	Richard Wolf Medical Instruments Corp.
PANTA	Bd Diagnostic Systems
PANTEX	Howard Medical Company
PANTHER	Boss Instruments, Ltd.
PANTHER	Snug Seat, Inc.
PANTOSKOP	Siemens Medical Solutions Usa, Inc.
PAP-PAK	Medical Packaging Corporation
PAPENOL	Afassco, Inc.
PAPERBANDS	Extra Packaging, Corp.
PAPERFLEX	Asi-Modulex
PAPETTE	Wallach Surgical Devices, Inc.
PAPOOSE	Ossur Americas
PARA	Streck Laboratories, Inc.
PARA 12	Streck Laboratories, Inc.
PARA 12 PLUS	Streck Laboratories, Inc.
PARA 4	Streck Laboratories, Inc.
PARA 7	Streck Laboratories, Inc.
PARA 8	Streck Laboratories, Inc.
PARA-CARE	Chattanooga Group
PARA-FIX	Medical Chemical Corp.
PARA-JEM	Trek Diagnostic Systems
PARA-JEM WINDOWS SOFTWARE	Trek Diagnostic Systems
PARA-LASER	Streck Laboratories, Inc.
PARA-PAK	Meridian Bioscience, Inc.
PARA-SED	Medical Chemical Corp.
PARA-TECH	Streck Laboratories, Inc.
PARA/GARD	Triangle Biomedical Sciences, Inc.
PARABODY	Life Fitness
PARADIGM	Sirona Dental Systems Llc
PARAFON FORTE	Ortho-Mcneil-Janssen Pharmaceuticals, Inc.
PARAFORM	Sakura Finetek U.S.A., Inc.
PARAGON	Arthrocare Corp.
PARAGON	Covidien Lp, Formerly Registered As United States Surgical
PARAGON	I-Flow Corporation
PARAGON CRT	Paragon Vision Sciences, Inc.
PARAGON HDS	Paragon Vision Sciences, Inc.
PARAGON HDS 100	Paragon Vision Sciences, Inc.
PARAGON THIN	Paragon Vision Sciences, Inc.
PARAKEET	Zygo Industries, Inc.
PARAKIT	Hardy Diagnostics
PARALIN	Grimm Scientific Ind., Inc.
PARALLELOMETER	Hager Worldwide, Inc.
PARAMAX	Conmed Linvatec
PARAMID	Paragon Medical, Inc.
PARAMIST MEDICAL EQUIPMENT LEASING	Parimist Funding Corp.
PARAPERM	Paragon Vision Sciences, Inc.
PARAPLAST	Covidien Lp
PARASEP	Diasys Corporation
PARASORB	Arthrocare Corp.
PARATHERAPY	Whitehall Manufacturing
PARATHERM	Grimm Scientific Ind., Inc.
PARATHYROID PROBE	Intramedical Imaging Llc
PARATREND	Allegro Biodiesel Corporation

PARCO	Parco Scientific Co.
PARCO-LINK	Pawling Corp., Architectural Prod. Div.
PARI BABY	Pari Respiratory Equipment, Inc.
PARI FRIENDS	Pari Respiratory Equipment, Inc.
PARI KIDS	Pari Respiratory Equipment, Inc.
PARI LC	Pari Respiratory Equipment, Inc.
PARI LC D	Pari Respiratory Equipment, Inc.
PARI LC JET PLUS	Pari Respiratory Equipment, Inc.
PARI LC PLUS	Pari Respiratory Equipment, Inc.
PARI LC STAR	Pari Respiratory Equipment, Inc.
PARI MASTER	Pari Respiratory Equipment, Inc.
PARI PALS	Pari Respiratory Equipment, Inc.
PARI PEP	Pari Respiratory Equipment, Inc.
PARI TREK	Pari Respiratory Equipment, Inc.
PARI VORTEX	Pari Respiratory Equipment, Inc.
PARI-JET	Elan
PARKER	Joerns Healthcare, Inc
PARKER BATH	ArjoHuntleigh
PARKER FLEX-IT STYLET	Parker Medical
PARKER FLEX-TIP ENDOTRACHEAL TUBE	Parker Medical
PARKER SLIM-STYLE STYLET	Parker Medical
PARKER TRACHVIEW INTUBATING VIDEOSCOPE	Parker Medical
PARKS	Parks Medical Electronics, Inc.
PARNELL	Riegel Consumer Products Div.
PARO BRUSH STICK	Hager Worldwide, Inc.
PARO IMPLANT FLOSS	Hager Worldwide, Inc.
PARO MICRO STICK	Hager Worldwide, Inc.
PARO ULTRA LITE	Hager Worldwide, Inc.
PAROS-HEXAPOD	Phytron, Inc.
PARSEC SYSTEM	Diamedix Corp.
PARTICLE ATTRACTION TECHNOLOGY	Milliken & Company, Anticon Products
PARTISIL	Whatman Inc.
PARTISPHERE	Whatman Inc.
PARTNER	CAREFUSION 211, INC.
PAS-KLEEN	Atlantic Medco, Inc.
PAS-PORT	Cardica, Inc.
PASCO	Bd Diagnostic Systems
PASS/FAIL	Propper Manufacturing Co., Inc.
PASSI	Cantel Medical Corp.
PASSPORT	Argosy
PASSPORT	Griffin Medical Products, Inc.
PASSPORT	Invacare Corporation
PASSPORT	Leisure-Lift, Inc.
PASSPORT	MAQUET
PASSPORT	Patton Surgical Corp.
PASSPORT	Sps Medical Supply Corp.
PASSPORT IV	Leisure-Lift, Inc.
PASSPORT PLUS	Sps Medical Supply Corp.
PASSY-MUIRT	Passy-Muir Inc.
PAST-R-PETTE	Globe Scientific, Inc.
PASTEL PALATES	Tp Orthodontics, Inc.
PASTEURMATIC	Olympic Medical Corp.
PASV	Navilyst Medical
PATANOL	Alcon Research, Ltd.
PATELLA MOBILIZER	Body Therapeutics, Div. Of I-Rep, Inc.
PATHCHIP	Pathwork Diagnostics Inc.
PATHFINDER	Cardima, Inc.
PATHFINDER	Ohio Willow Wood Company
PATHFINDER	Prentke Romich Company
PATHFINDER	Utah Medical Products, Inc.
PATHFINDERS	Sellstrom Manufacturing Co.
PATHLAB II	3m Health Information Systems
PATHLAB III	3m Health Information Systems
PATHNET	Cerner Corp.
PATHO-SORB	Eastman Medical Products Inc.
PATHOGENE	Enzo Biochem, Inc.
PATHOTEC	Remel
PATHVISION	Hacker Instruments And Industries Inc.
PATHWAY	Ventana Medical Systems, Inc.
PATHWORK	Pathwork Diagnostics Inc.
PATIENT CARE MODULE	Independent Solutions, Inc.
PATIENT DOWN	Pioneer Medical Systems
PATIENT GUARD	Graphic Controls Corp.

PATIENT PAL IV POLE	Pryor Products
PATIENT PAUL	Armstrong Medical Industries, Inc.
PATIENT POSITIONING DEVICES	Oakworks, Inc.
PATIENT SLIDER, LIGHT CLOUD POSTIONERS	David Scott Company
PATIENT STATION	Dwyer Precision Products, Inc.
PATIENT'S CHOICE	Crosstex International, Inc.
PATIENTCARE 16/64 WIRELESS NURSE-CALL	Care Electronics, Inc.
PATIENTCARE WANDERER MONITORING SYSTEM	Care Electronics, Inc.
PATIENTFINDER	Stryker Corp.
PATIENTFINDER	Stryker Endoscopy
PATIENTFINDER	Stryker Howmedica Osteonics
PATIENTIME	Timemed Labeling Systems, Inc.
PATIENTMATE	Hill-Rom Holdings, Inc.
PATIENTNET	Ge Medical Systems Information Technologies
PATIENTWORKS	Newbold Corporation
PATRIOT	Trans American Medical / Tamsco Instruments
PATRIOT ADJUSTABLE EXTRICATION COLLAR	Jerome Medical
PATRIOT COLLAR, ATLAS COLLAR	Ossur Americas
PATROL	Abbott Laboratories
PATRON	Clarke Health Care Products, Inc.
PATTY PATIENT	Armstrong Medical Industries, Inc.
PAULUS	Striker Corp.
PAX-IT	Mccrone Microscopes & Accessories
PAXBAC	Invacare Corporation
PAXPORT	Agfa Corporation
PAXSCAN	Varian Medical Systems
PAY PHONE TDD	Krown Manufacturing, Inc.
PB FREE	Md Works, Inc.
PB-NC	Schleicher & Schuell, Inc.
PBS DIAMOND BURS	Premier Medical Products
PC EDO	Lumenis Inc.
PC PRIME	Ethicon, Inc.
PC-IABP	Datascope Cardiac Assist Div.
PC-Stim	St. Jude Medical, Inc.
PCAT	Promega Corp.
PCAT3	Promega Corp.
PCCWIN	Mediware Information Systems, Inc.
PCD	Stryker Corp.
PCI	Brady Corporation
PCM	Independent Solutions, Inc.
PCM SERIES	Oneac Corporation
PCRIMETER	Boston Scientific Corp.
PCSWIN	Mediware Information Systems, Inc.
PCX TOUCH SCREEN	Control-X Medical, Inc.
PD 1100	Dosimeter Division Of Arrow Tech Inc
PD ADEQUEST	Baxter Healthcare Corporation, Renal
PD CLOTH	Dazian Fabrics, Llc.
PD-2.0	Hacker Instruments And Industries Inc.
PDI	Professional Disposables International, Inc.
PDS	Ethicon, Inc.
PDS II	Ethicon, Inc.
PEACH PILLOW	Mccarty's Sacro-Ease Llc
PEACOCK	Best Nomos Corp.
PEAK FLOW MONITORSASMA PLAN+	Vitalograph, Inc.
PEAK PLASMABLADE	Peak Surgical Inc.
PEAKLOG	Westmed, Inc.
PEAKOMETER	Laytech, Inc.
PEARL	Cutera, Inc.
PED-O-JET	National Keystone
PEDALERT	Planet Llc
PEDALPUMP	Medela, Inc.
PEDI I	James Consolidated, Inc.
PEDI II	James Consolidated, Inc.
PEDI III. JAMESAIR PLATIN	James Consolidated, Inc.
PEDI-BACT	Biomerieux Inc.
PEDI-BOARD	Pedicraft, Inc.
PEDI-BORO	Pedinol Pharmacal, Inc.
PEDI-CAP	Covidien (Formerly Nellcor Puritan Bennett / Tyco Healthcare)
PEDI-CRIB BED	Pedicraft, Inc.
PEDI-CRIB TOP	Pedicraft, Inc.
PEDI-DRI	Pedinol Pharmacal, Inc.
PEDI-LIM	Westmed, Inc.
PEDI-MATTRESS	Pedicraft, Inc.

PEDI-PRETAPE	Pedinol Pharmacal, Inc.
PEDI-PRO	Pedinol Pharmacal, Inc.
PEDI-TUBE	Covidien Lp
PEDI-WALKER	Wheaton Brace Co.
PEDI-WHIRL	Pedinol Pharmacal, Inc.
PEDI-WRAPS	Medi-Kid Co.
PEDIA PALS	Pedia Pals, Llc
PEDIA PALS, LLC	Pedia Pals, Llc
PEDIA-THOR	Smiths Medical Asd
PEDIABLOC	Gi Supply
PEDIASCAN	Sylvan Corp.
PEDIASCAN	Sylvan Fiberoptics
PEDIATRIC 6491	Medtronic Cardiovascular Surgery, The Heart Valve Div.
PEDIATRIC DESIGNS	Pedia Pals, Llc
PEDICO2EASY	Westmed, Inc.
PEDIDRY	Janin Group, Inc.
PEDIFIX	Pedifix, Inc.
PEDIMAT	Construction Specialties Inc.
PEDINEB	Westmed, Inc.
PEDIPACK	Ultracell Medical Technologies, Inc.
PEDIÉ_6PADZ	Zoll Medical Corp.
PEDLAR	Battle Creek Equipment Co.
PEDO-15W	Osada, Inc.
PEDO-30W	Osada, Inc.
PEE SHOOTER	Caring Hands, Inc.
PEE-WEE STIRRUPS	Allen Medical Systems, Inc.
PEEK	Applied Biosystems
PEEK	Medtronic Sofamor Danek Usa, Inc
PEEK	Medtronic Sofamor Danek Usa, Inc.
PEEL-AWAY	Cook Inc.
PEER PRACTICUM	Zimmer Dental, Inc.
PEG 18	Wilson-Cook Medical, Inc.
PEG 24	Wilson-Cook Medical, Inc.
PEG-INTRON	Nektar Therapeutics
PEGASUS	Fischer Medical Technologies Inc.
PEGASUS	The National Wheel-O-Vator Co., Inc.
PEGASUS CPAP	CAREFUSION 211, INC.
PEGASYS	Nektar Therapeutics
PEGGI	Elginex Corporation
PEIDA-TRAKE	Smiths Medical Asd
PELLET	Graphic Controls Corp.
PELLOTTE	Hager Worldwide, Inc.
PELORUS	Schaerer Mayfield Usa
PELVIC-TILT	O.R. Comfort, Llc
PEM FLEX	Naviscan Inc.
PEMACO 2000/3000 WAX	Pemaco, Inc.
PEMFOIL	Pemaco, Inc.
PEMROCK	Pemaco, Inc.
PEMVIEW	Naviscan Inc.
PEN-RAY	Uvp, Llc
PEN-TOTE	Palco Labs, Inc.
PENACLE	Lumenis Inc.
PENADAPT	Buffalo Filter, A Division Of Medtek Devices Inc.
PENATEN	Johnson & Johnson
PENCIL CHAMBER	Capintec, Inc.
PENFINE	Roche Insulin Delivery Systems Inc.
PENGUIN GEL PAK	Duro-Med Industries
PENGUIN JR.	Springer-Penguin, Inc.
PENLET II	Lifescan, Inc.
PENNEEDLE	Novo Nordisk Pharmaceuticals, Inc.
PENNVIAL	Pennsylvania Glass Products Co.
PENTA-PYCNOMETER	Quantachrome
PENTAMIX	3m Co.
PENTAPREP	Case Medical, Inc.
PENTASCOPE	Wallach Surgical Devices, Inc.
PENTASPAN	B. Braun Oem Division, B. Braun Medical Inc.
PENTASTAR	Wallach Surgical Devices, Inc.
PENTOTHAL	Abbott Laboratories
PEP	Exercycle Corporation
PEP UNIT	Exercycle Corporation
PEPTAG	Promega Corp.
PER-FIT	First Quality Enterprise, Inc.
PERASSAY	Minntech Corporation
PERCENT-O-LOCK	Salter Labs
PERCEPTIVE INFORMATIES, INC.	Parexel International Corp.
PERCHLORACAP	Mallinckrodt, Inc.
PERCI	Microtronics Corp. Of Chapel Hill
PERCIVAL	Percival Scientific Inc.
PERCOR	Datascope Cardiac Assist Div.
PERCOR	MAQUET
PERCOR STAT-DL	Datascope Cardiac Assist Div.
PERCOR-STAT	Datascope Cardiac Assist Div.
PERCU SCREW	DJO Inc.
PERCU-PRO SYSTEM	Cardiosolutions Inc.
PERCUSSIONAIRE CORP.	Percussionaire Corporation
PEREGRINE	Best Nomos Corp.
PERF-PRENE	Tetra Medical Supply Corp.
PERFEC CLEAN	Independent Solutions, Inc.
PERFECFLEX	Perfecseal
PERFECFORM	Perfecseal
PERFECRAFT	Perfecseal
PERFECSEAL	Perfecseal
PERFECT EAR	Magnatone Hearing Aid Corp.
PERFECT FIT LSO	Judah Mfg. Corp.
PERFECT MATCH	The Aloe Institute
PERFECT PLAST	Hager Worldwide, Inc.
PERFECT VIEW	Medi-Tech International, Inc.
PERFECTA	Cook Vascular, Incorporated
PERFECTA	Wright Medical Group, Inc.
PERFECTING THE MEDICAL PACKAGE	Perfecseal
PERFECTION	Pennsylvania Glass Products Co.
PERFECTION BRAND	National Nonwovens
PERFECTIONS	Roman Research, Inc.
PERFECTIONr PAPER ROLLS & RIBBONS	Pm Company
PERFECTONE MOLDS	George Taub Products & Fusion Co., Inc.
PERFECTOR	Tp Orthodontics, Inc.
PERFEKTA COHESIVE	Lohmann & Rauscher, Inc.
PERFEKTUM	Cadence Science Inc.
PERFIT	Ambu, Inc.
PERFIT ACE	Ambu, Inc.
PERFIX	Pace Medical, Inc.
PERFLUBRONC	Origen Biomedical, Inc.
PERFOAM	Sage Laboratories, Inc.
PERFORM 8	Brown Medical Industries
PERFORM-X	Control-X Medical, Inc.
PERFORMANCE FOR LIFE	Medrad, Inc.
PERFORMANCE GENESIS	Innovation Genesis, Llc
PERFORMANCE MICRO-SURGICAL KNIVES	Katena Products, Inc.
PERFORMANCE PHARMACY SYSTEMS	Life Care Technologies, Inc.
PERFORMANCE WITHOUT LIMITS	World Heart Inc.
PERFORMER	DJO Inc.
PERFORMERS	Myoderm
PERI PLUS	Hospital Marketing Svcs. Company, Inc.
PERI-COLD	Hospital Marketing Svcs. Company, Inc.
PERI-COMFORT	Chi'Am International
PERI-GEL	Hospital Marketing Svcs. Company, Inc.
PERI-GUARD	Synovis Life Technologies, Inc
PERI-GUARD	Synovis Surgical Innovations
PERI-PRO	Air Techniques, Inc.
PERI-STRIPS	Synovis Life Technologies, Inc
PERI-STRIPS	Synovis Surgical Innovations
PERI-STRIPS DRY	Synovis Surgical Innovations
PERI-STRIPS DRY WITH VERITAS	Synovis Surgical Innovations
PERI-WARM	Hospital Marketing Svcs. Company, Inc.
PERIES	Xttrium Laboratories, Inc.
PERIFIX	B. Braun Oem Division, B. Braun Medical Inc.
PERIFLUX	Perimed, Inc.
PERIFLUX 5000	Perimed, Inc.
PERIFORM EMG VAGINAL ELECTRODE	American Imex
PERILONT	Perimed, Inc.
PERIOGLAS	Novabone Products, Llc
PERIOLASE MVP-7	Millennium Dental Technologies, Inc.
PERIOSCAN	Sirona Dental Systems Llc
PERISOFT, PERISCAN	Perimed, Inc.
PERITONEAL	Angiodynamics, Inc.
PERITRON	American Imex

PERLA-DIA GRINDING DISCS	American Diversified Dental Systems
PERLADIA GRINDING DISCS	Mds Products, Inc.
PERM SHARP	Hu-Friedy Manufacturing Co., Inc.
PERMA PURE	Perma Pure Llc
PERMA-CHECK	Sani-Med, A Division Of Sanderson Plumbing Products, Inc.
PERMA-COLOR	Mark Medical Manufacturing, Inc.
PERMA-HAND	Ethicon, Inc.
PERMA-LOCK	Marinco Specialty Wiring Devices
PERMA-PRINT	Precision Dynamics Corp.
PERMA-SEAL	Angiodynamics, Inc.
PERMA-WET	Hydromer, Inc.
PERMACABLE	Sellstrom Manufacturing Co.
PERMACOL	Hartmann-Conco Inc.
PERMACOOL AIR FILTER	Permatron Corp.
PERMAFLEX	B.G. Industries, Inc.
PERMAFLOAT, COREFLEX	B.G. Industries, Inc.
PERMAFROST	Kimble Chase Life Science And Research Products Llc
PERMAGEL	Covidien Lp, Formerly Registered As Uni-Patch
PERMALIFE	Origen Biomedical, Inc.
PERMALUX	Riegel Consumer Products Div.
PERMARID	Qed Bioscience, Inc.
PERMASOFT DENTURE LINER	Dentsply Prosthetics
PERMATYPE	Qed Bioscience, Inc.
PERRY	Perry Baromedical Corp.
PERRY CUT-RESISTANT	Ansell Healthcare Products, Inc.
PERRY NATURAL	Ansell Healthcare Products, Inc.
PERRY ORTHOPAEDIC	Ansell Healthcare Products, Inc.
PERRY PROCEDURE	Ansell Healthcare Products, Inc.
PERRY RADIATION ATTENUATION	Ansell Healthcare Products, Inc.
PERSIST	Becton Dickinson Infusion Therapy Systems, Inc.
PERSONA	Zygo Industries, Inc.
PERSONAL ANTIMICROBIAL WIPES BY SAFETEC (P.A.W.S.)	Safetec Of America, Inc.
PERSONAL BEST	Respironics New Jersey, Inc.
PERSONAL PREDICTEDS SOFTWARE	Medical Graphics Corporation
PERSONAL PRO	Oster Professional Products, Inc.
PERSONAL PRO LINE	Oster Professional Products, Inc.
PERSONAL SERIES INSTRUMENTS	Fasstech
PERSONAL TRAINER	Neurocare, Inc.
PERSONALCLIMBER	CYBEX INTERNATIONAL, INC.
PERSONALLY	Amoena
PERSONALPACS	Thinking Systems Corporation
PERSONIC	Oticon, Inc.
PERSONNA	Personna Medical/Div. Of American Safety Razor Co.
PERSONNA PLUS	Personna Medical/Div. Of American Safety Razor Co.
PERSONNA SAFETY SCALPEL	Personna Medical/Div. Of American Safety Razor Co.
PERSTAT VOICE RECOGNITION	Imsi, Integrated Modular Systems Inc.
PERVAL	Standard Textile Co., Inc.
PERYOURHEALTH.COM	Per-Se Technologies
PESSARIES	Milex Products, Inc.
PET-DP	Syntermed, Inc.
PET-PROBE	Intramedical Imaging Llc
PETALS	Interspec Fabrics
PETE & PAM	Laclede, Inc.
PETIT AMPERE	Basi (Bioanalytical Systems, Inc.)
PETITE	Axiom Medical, Inc.
PETITE	Oscor, Inc.
PETRARCH	United Chemical Technologies, Inc.
PETRO-MISER	Hoyt Corp.
PETRO-WASH	Hoyt Corp.
PEXBOND	Filtrona Extrusion, Inc./PexcoA,Ar Medical Products Div.
PEXBRAID	Filtrona Extrusion, Inc./PexcoA,Ar Medical Products Div.
PEXCLEAR	Filtrona Extrusion, Inc./PexcoA,Ar Medical Products Div.
PEXCO MEDICAL PRODUCTS	Filtrona Extrusion, Inc./PexcoA,Ar Medical Products Div.
PEXGLIDE	Filtrona Extrusion, Inc./PexcoA,Ar Medical Products Div.
PEXPF	Filtrona Extrusion, Inc./PexcoA,Ar Medical Products Div.
PF/DX SYSTEM	Medical Graphics Corporation
PFA-100	Siemens Healthcare Diagnostics Inc.
PFLEX	Respironics New Jersey, Inc.
PFP7 FLAME PHOTOMETER	Buck Scientific, Inc.
PFP7C FLAME PHOTOMETER	Buck Scientific, Inc.

PFSB	RDL Supply
PFX2	American Imex
PFXA	American Imex
PG-PS (PEPTIDOGLYCAN-POLYSACCHARIDE)	Bd Lee Laboratories
PGEM	Promega Corp.
PGEMEX	Promega Corp.
PGX	Clinical Data Inc
PGXHEALTH	Clinical Data Inc
PGXPREDICT	Clinical Data Inc
PH DOSER	Analytical Measurements, Inc.
PH PAPER	Beutlich Lp, Pharmaceuticals
PH SENTINEL	Analytical Measurements, Inc.
PH3 INVESTMENT	Dentsply Prosthetics
PHACO-EMULSIFIER	Alcon Research, Ltd.
PHACOFRAGMENTATION TIP	Imonti And Associates Inc., M.
PHACOJACK	Howard Instruments, Inc.
PHALANX	Nest Group Inc., The
PHANTOM	Adenna Inc.
PHANTOM	DJO Inc.
PHANTOM	Ricon Corp.
PHANTOM	Sellstrom Manufacturing Co.
PHANTOM	Sleepnet Corporation
PHANTOM EYES	United Syntek Corp.
PHANTOM PATIENT	Supertech, Inc.
PHARM-AIR	Pneumatic Products Corporation
PHARMA-PLAST	Unomedical, Inc.
PHARMACIST'S COMPANION	Apothacare
PHARMAFIT	Larkotex Company
PHARMAJET	Pharmajet
PHARMAKON	Mediware Information Systems, Inc.
PHARMASTOR	Spacesaver Corporation
PHARMED	Saint-Gobain Performance Plastics--Akron
PHARMETTE	Independent Solutions, Inc.
PHARMMED	Carecentric, Inc.
PHAROS	Micrus Endovascular Corporation
PHASE 5,DISE(-50DEG.)	Tcp Reliable, Inc.
PHASE EIGHT	Vicon Industries Inc.
PHASE STABILIZER	Online Power, Inc.
PHASE-2	Basi (Bioanalytical Systems, Inc.)
PHASE2	Pml Microbiologicals
PHASEFIRE	Biner Ellison
PHASEPLANE	Thermotek Inc.
PHENADRIN FORTE	Afassco, Inc.
PHENEEN	Ulmer Pharmacal Co.
PHENOGEL	Phenomenex, Inc.
PHENOTYPE MICROARRAY	Biolog, Inc.
PHEONIX	Living Earth Crafts
PHERES-FLOW	Angiodynamics, Inc.
PHILADELPHIA THI-WIDE	Bell-Horn, Inc.
PHILADELPHIA/COLLAR	Ortholine
PHILIPS	Atlas Medical Technologies
PHILIPS	Bulbworks, Inc.
PHILIPS MEDICAL	Bound Tree Medical
PHILIPS MEDICAL	Creative Health Products, Inc.
PHILLOCRAFT	Shelby-Williams Industries
PHILLY COLLAR	Ossur Americas
PHOENIX	Control-X Medical, Inc.
PHOENIX	DJO Inc.
PHOENIX	Mesa Laboratories, Inc.
PHOENIX	Netzsch Instruments, Inc.
PHOENIX KNEE CPM SERIES	Mckelor Technologies, Ltd.
PHOENIX PRO	Siemens Hearing Instruments, Inc.
PHOENIXFELT	National Nonwovens
PHONEPOWER - NHT	VARTA Microbattery Inc.
PHONOFORM	Medtronic Xomed, Inc.
PHORESIS	Sebia Electrophoresis
PHORESOR	Iomed, Inc.
PHOROPTOR	Reichert, Inc.
PHOSPHO-SODA	C.B. Fleet Company Inc.
PHOSPHOCOL	Mallinckrodt, Inc.
PHOTO-FLO	Carestream Health, Inc.
PHOTOGENICA	Cynosure, Inc.
PHOTOGRAMETRY	Electrical Geodesics, Incorporated

PHOTOLINK	Surmodics, Inc.
PHOTOMETRICS	Roper Scientific, Inc.
PHOTONIC	Seca Corp.
PHOTOPROBE	Vector Laboratories, Inc.
PHOTOSWEEP	Spacesaver Corporation
PHOTOZOOM	Leica Microsystems, Inc., Educational & Analytical Division
PHOX	Netzsch Instruments, Inc.
PHOX	Nova Biomedical
PHRED	Aura Industries, Inc.
PHYSICIANS CHOICE	Medical Sterile Products, Inc.
PHYSIO-CONTROL	Physio-Control, Inc.
PHYSIO-STIM	Orthofix Inc.
PHYSIOLYTE	B. Braun Oem Division, B. Braun Medical Inc.
PHYSIQUE	Oscor, Inc.
PHYSLAB	U.F.I.
PHYTON	Tp Orthodontics, Inc.
PHYTONE	Bd Diagnostic Systems
PHYTRON	Phytron, Inc.
PI	Covidien Lp, Formerly Registered As United States Surgical
PIC	B. Braun Oem Division, B. Braun Medical Inc.
PIC	Patient Instrumentation Corp.
PIC BRUSH	Hager Worldwide, Inc.
PICC-NATE	Utah Medical Products, Inc.
PICCOLO	Abaxis, Inc.
PICCOLO	Nest Group Inc., The
PICD	Innerpulse, Inc.
PICK-A-DENT	Denticator International, Inc.
PICKER	Atlas Medical Technologies
PICO	Radiometer America, Inc.
PICOPURE	Hydro Service & Supplies, Inc.
PICOSYSTEM	Hydro Service & Supplies, Inc.
PICOTAP	Hydro Service & Supplies, Inc.
PICOTECH	Hydro Service & Supplies, Inc.
PICTOOLS JPEG2000	Pegasus Imaging Corp.
PICTOOLS MEDICAL, PICTOOLS JPEG-LS	Pegasus Imaging Corp.
PICTURE	Life Technologies Corporation
PICUS	Biosound Esaote, Inc.
PICUS PRO	Biosound Esaote, Inc.
PIERCINGCARE	The Hymed Group Corp.
PIEZODRILL	Exfo America Inc.
PIGG-O-STAT	Modern Way Immobilizers, Inc.
PIGGY LOCK	Icu Medical, Inc.
PIGGY SAFE	Icu Medical, Inc.
PIKO	Nspire Health, Inc
PIKO	Piko Healthcare Products, Inc.
PIKO-1	Nspire Health, Inc
PILL PLANNER	Medi-Crush Company
PILLAR	Restore Medical Inc.
PILLCAM SB, PILLCAM ESO	Given Imaging Inc.
PILLING	Teleflex Medical
PILLO-PUMP	Gaymar Industries, Inc.
PILLOW AID CERVICAL ROLL	Body Therapeutics, Div. Of I-Rep, Inc.
PILLOW PAWS	Principle Business Enterprises, Inc.
PILOGEL	Wescor, Inc.
PILOT	Action Products, Inc.
PILOT	Mediana Technologies Corp
PILOT MEDICAL PRODUCTS	Marquette Medical, Inc.
PILOT TEST AUDIOMETER	Maico Diagnostics
PILOTTIP	Surgical Specialties Corporation
PIN CARE KIT	Brown Medical Industries
PIN CLIPPER	Hager Worldwide, Inc.
PIN-N-CHAIN	Key-Bak
PIN-PAK	Beacon Converters, Inc.
PIN-POINT REGISTRATION	Topcon Medical Systems, Inc.
PINCAP	Scanlan International, Inc.
PINCH-VALVE	Acro Associates
PINCHTRACK	JTECH Medical
PINDOT	Invacare Corporation
PINE-O-QUAT	Unit Chemical Corp.
PINK ELEPHANTS	Roman Research, Inc.
PINN-ACL	Conmed Linvatec
PINNACLE	Atlas Medical Technologies
PINNACLE I	H.L. Bouton Co., Inc.

PINNACLE II	H.L. Bouton Co., Inc.
PINNACLE SHEATH	Terumo Medical Corp.
PINNACLE3	Atlas Medical Technologies
PINPOINT	Rf Technologies
PINTAB	Asi-Modulex
PIONEER	Golden Technologies, Inc.
PIONEER	Stryker Corp.
PIONEER	Thermo Fisher Scientific
PIONEER IVF	Genx International
PIONEER PRO-PUMP	Genx International
PIPEPAK	Algor, Inc.
PIPET CURETTE	Milex Products, Inc.
PIPET KEEPER	Whitney Products, Inc.
PIPET-AID	Drummond Scientific Co.
PIRANHA DIAMONDS	S.S. White Burs Inc.
PIRF	Engineering & Research Assoc., Inc. (D.B.A. Sebra)
PIROUETTE	Infometrix, Inc.
PISCES PLUS	Ivoclar Vivadent, Inc.
PISTOL	Mps Acacia
PITCH-IT	Sharps Compliance Corp.
PITTMAN	Halbar North, Inc.
PIVOT-EASE	Ergotron, Inc.
PIVOTAL THERAPY SYSTEM	Chattanooga Group
PIVOTRAC	Reel R&D, Inc.
PIXCI	Epix, Inc.
PIXIUM	Thales Components Corporation
PIXIUM 4600	Thales Components Corporation
PIXIUM 4700	Thales Components Corporation
PIXMATE	Da-Lite Screen Co., Inc.
PIXMOBILE	Da-Lite Screen Co., Inc.
PIXY	Supertech, Inc.
PL AQUAGEL-OH	Polymer Laboratories, Now A Part Of Varian, Inc.
PL HI-PLEX	Polymer Laboratories, Now A Part Of Varian, Inc.
PL-GEL	Nest Group Inc., The
PL-GPC 120	Polymer Laboratories, Now A Part Of Varian, Inc.
PL-GPC 220	Polymer Laboratories, Now A Part Of Varian, Inc.
PL-LC1120	Polymer Laboratories, Now A Part Of Varian, Inc.
PL-LC1150	Polymer Laboratories, Now A Part Of Varian, Inc.
PL-LC1200	Polymer Laboratories, Now A Part Of Varian, Inc.
PL1000 PATIENT LIFT	Nk Medical Products Inc.
PL1240	Fenwal Inc.
PL146	Fenwal Inc.
PL2209	Fenwal Inc.
PL732	Fenwal Inc.
PLAC-BRUSH	Preventive Dentistry Products, Inc.
PLAC-PIK	Preventive Dentistry Products, Inc.
PLAIN JANE	Welcon, Inc.
PLAK-VAC	Trademark Medical Llc
PLAQUE AWAY	Denticator International, Inc.
PLASMA KINETIC	Gyrus Medical, Inc.
PLASMA PAINT	Biolase Technology, Inc.
PLASMACELL-C	Fenwal Inc.
PLASMAPAK	Riley Medical, Inc.
PLASMAPREP	Separation Technology Inc
PLAST FRAME	Hager Worldwide, Inc.
PLASTALUME	Brown Medical Industries
PLASTAZOTE	Aetrex Worldwide, Inc
PLASTEEL	Gillis Associated Industries
PLASTER IN A ROLL	Flexi-Wall Systems
PLASTI BOX BINS	Orbis Corporation
PLASTI-GRAD	Plasti Products, Inc.
PLASTI-LINER	Combe, Inc.
PLASTI-MATE	S4j Manufacturing Services, Inc.
PLASTI-PAD	Cincinnati Sub-Zero Products, Inc., Medical Division
PLASTI-PAN	Plasti Products, Inc.
PLASTIBAK	Precision Dynamics Corp.
PLASTIBELL	Hollister Incorporated
PLASTICAD	Arthur Blank & Co., Inc.
PLASTICAST	Maramed Orthopedic Systems
PLASTICLEAR	Motloid Company
PLASTICRIT	Drummond Scientific Co.
PLASTIGARD	Precision Dynamics Corp.
PLASTIPAC	Motloid Company

PLASTIPREEM	Precision Dynamics Corp.
PLASTITAFF	Precision Dynamics Corp.
PLASTOFILL	Hager Worldwide, Inc.
PLATECOUNT	Cambridge Diagnostic Products, Inc.
PLATELET-TROL II	R & D Systems, Inc.
PLATELETWORKS	Helena Laboratories
PLATELIA	Biorad Laboratories
PLATEMATE PLUS	Thermo Fisher Scientific
PLATINUM 1001	James Consolidated, Inc.
PLATINUM 2000	James Consolidated, Inc.
PLATINUM 2001	James Consolidated, Inc.
PLATINUM ONE CARDIAC	Infimed, Inc.
PLATINUM ONE COMBOLAB	Infimed, Inc.
PLATINUM ONE DSA	Infimed, Inc.
PLATINUM ONE EP	Infimed, Inc.
PLATINUM ONE RF	Infimed, Inc.
PLATINUM-CLASS	C. R. Bard, Inc., Bard Urological Div.
PLATO	Nucletron Corporation
PLAYSAFE	Hard Manufacturing Co.
PLAYTEX	Energizer Personal Care Division
PLAZA	Plaza Towel Holder, Inc.
PLEASE REMOVE ETHICON AS AN	Artegraft, Inc.
PLEEZRECON	Polymer Concepts, Inc.
PLEEZRELITE	Polymer Concepts, Inc.
PLEEZRPLUS	Polymer Concepts, Inc.
PLEEZRSELECT	Polymer Concepts, Inc.
PLEEZRX	Polymer Concepts, Inc.
PLEUR-A-GUIDE	Smiths Medical Asd
PLEUR-EVAC	Teleflex Medical
PLEURA-GARD	Conmed Corporation
PLEURA-SEAL	Arrow International, Inc.
PLEXTON STACK-N-NEST CONTAINERS	Lewis Bins+
PLEXUFIX	B. Braun Oem Division, B. Braun Medical Inc.
PLEXUS	Gaymar Industries, Inc.
PLGEL	Polymer Laboratories, Now A Part Of Varian, Inc.
PLGEL MINIMIX	Polymer Laboratories, Now A Part Of Varian, Inc.
PLI-ABLEr IDEAS	Plitek, L.L.C
PLI-BONDr	Plitek, L.L.C
PLI-MEDr	Plitek, L.L.C
PLI-STRIPr	Plitek, L.L.C
PLI-TABr	Plitek, L.L.C
PLI-VALVr	Plitek, L.L.C
PLIA-CELL	Conmed Corporation
PLIACELL	Conmed Corporation
PLIAFLEX	Con-Cise Contact Lens Co.
PLICATION	Radix Corp.
PLIF	Medtronic Sofamor Danek Usa, Inc
PLIF	Medtronic Sofamor Danek Usa, Inc.
PLOGS	Hammill International
PLRP-S	Nest Group Inc., The
PLS	Ericsson, Inc.
PLUGBORD	Vector Electronics & Technology, Inc.
PLUM A	Hospira Inc.
PLUMBICON	Narragansett Imaging
PLUME-AWAY	Stryker Corp.
PLUME-AWAY	Stryker Endoscopy
PLUME-INATOR	Novosci Corp.
PLUMESAFE	Buffalo Filter, A Division Of Medtek Devices Inc.
PLUS III	Leisure-Lift, Inc.
PLUS PAK	Shippert Medical Technologies Corp.
PLV	Respironics Colorado
PLYMOLD	Plymold
PM	Starkey Laboratories, Inc.
PM BATTERY	Sentry Battery Corp.
PM GLOVES	Pm Gloves, Inc.
PMAT	Passy-Muir Inc.
PMAX	Acteon Corp.
PMD 100	Spencer Technologies
PMI	Biomet, Inc.
PMI	Progressive Medical International
PMI SUPPLY, MEDSTORM	Progressive Medical International
PMIR-REPORT	Applied Biosystems
PMM	Mge Ups Sytems, Inc.

PMO PRODUCTS	Lightpath Technologies
PMT R	Pmt Corp.
PMVT	Passy-Muir Inc.
PN-STIM-KATH	Epimed International, Inc.
PNEUFLO	Michigan Instruments, Inc.
PNEUGEL	Sroufe Healthcare Products Llc
PNEUMATIC TUBE SYSTEM	Swisslog Translogic Corporation
PNEUMATICWALKER	Aircast Llc
PNEUMICRO	Tava Surgical Instruments
PNEUMOCHECK	Welch Allyn, Inc.
PNEUMOGARD	Respironics, Inc
PNEUMOMAT	Elmed, Inc.
PNEUMOPLEXr	Prodesse, Inc.
PNEUMOSIM	Cardionics, Inc.
PNEUMOSLIDE	Bd Diagnostic Systems
PNEUMOSURE	Stryker Corp.
PNEUMOSURE	Stryker Endoscopy
PNEUMOTRACE	U.F.I.
PNEUTON	Airon Corporation
PNEUVIEW	Michigan Instruments, Inc.
PNS UNNA	Pedinol Pharmacal, Inc.
PNT SUCTION RING	Ophthalmic Intl.
POCEKTCHEM EZ	Arkray Usa
POCKET CHAMBER	Nspire Health, Inc
POCKET CPR	Zoll Medical Corp.
POCKET MAGMETOMETER	R. B. Annis Instruments, Inc.
POCKET NURSE	Pocket Nurse Enterprises, Inc.
POCKET PEAK	Nspire Health, Inc
POCKET PULSE	Lynn Medical
POCKET RESCUE MASK	Rondex Products, Inc.
POCKET SPACER	Nspire Health, Inc
POCKET SPEECH LAB	Casa Futura Technologies
POCKET-PROBE ANALOG	Electronic Development Labs, Inc.
POCKET-PROBE DIGITAL	Electronic Development Labs, Inc.
POCKETED CAMI	Ladies First, Inc.
POCKETMONITOR	Cardionics, Inc.
POCKETPRO	Lares Research
POCKETSCOPE	Welch Allyn, Inc.
POCKETVIEWER	Humanware
POET	Baxter Healthcare Corporation, Renal
POGON	Theradyne Products Division
POINT 9 (WE GET YOUR BLOOD FLOWING)	Spectranetics Corp.
POINT OF KNOWLEDGE	Agfa Corporation
POINT OF VIEW	MAQUET
POINT-OF-USE	Graphic Controls Corp.
POINTLOK	Graphic Controls Corp.
POINTMAKER	Boeckeler Instruments, Inc.
POINTS	Howard Medical Company
POISINDEX	Micromedex, Inc.
POLAR	Polar Ware Co.
POLAR HEART RATE MONITOR	Creative Health Products, Inc.
POLAR HEARTBRA	Polar Electro Inc.
POLAR ICE	Brown Medical Industries
POLAR ICE	Pelton Shepherd Industries
POLAR INTERFACE PLUS	Polar Electro Inc.
POLAR M21	Polar Electro Inc.
POLAR M52	Polar Electro Inc.
POLAR M71 TI	Polar Electro Inc.
POLAR M91 TI	Polar Electro Inc.
POLAR PACK	White Knight Engineered Products
POLAR STAR	Independent Solutions, Inc.
POLARGEL-L	Polymer Laboratories, Now A Part Of Varian, Inc.
POLARGEL-M	Polymer Laboratories, Now A Part Of Varian, Inc.
POLARIS	Convergent Laser Technologies
POLARIS	Dent Zar, Inc.
POLARIS	Invacare Corporation
POLARIS	Oscor, Inc.
POLARPACKr	Thermosafe Brands
POLDER	Polder, Inc.
POLE-BAG	Welcon, Inc.
POLE-SAK	Welcon, Inc.
POLECAT	A.R.C. Distributors
POLEMOUNT	Smiths Medical Asd, Inc.

POLI-AIRE POLI-FOAM POLI-GEL .... Regency Product International
POLI-X .... Engler Engineering Corp.
POLIAIRE .... Back Support Systems
POLICOT .... American Silk Sutures, Inc.
POLLEN-8 .... Basi (Bioanalytical Systems, Inc.)
POLLY'S CUTTER .... Howard Instruments, Inc.
POLY .... First Healthcare Products
POLY CAST .... Corflex, Inc.
POLY CS .... Covidien Lp, Formerly Registered As United States Surgical
POLY FLOW .... Smiths Medical Asd, Inc.
POLY GIA .... Covidien Lp, Formerly Registered As United States Surgical
POLY SHAPES .... Meese Orbitron Dunne Co.
POLY STAT .... Polymedco, Inc.
POLY SURGICLIP..... Covidien Lp, Formerly Registered As United States Surgical
POLY TRUX .... Meese Orbitron Dunne Co.
POLY-CHEM .... Polymedco, Inc.
POLY-D .... Ansell Healthcare Products, Inc.
POLY-ENA .... Zeus Scientific, Inc.
POLY-LAB PACK .... Enpac Corp.
POLY-PREP .... Bio-Rad Laboratories, Life Science Group
POLY-PRO .... Welcon, Inc.
POLY-TET .... Cambridge Diagnostic Products, Inc.
POLY-THANE .... Dur-A-Flex, Inc.
POLY-TONE .... General Dental Products, Inc.
POLY/FIN .... Triangle Biomedical Sciences, Inc.
POLY/SEP .... Polysciences, Inc.
POLYANA .... Zygo Industries, Inc.
POLYATTRACT .... Promega Corp.
POLYAXIAL SCREWS .... Orthotec, Llc
POLYAXIAL SCS .... Orthotec, Llc
POLYBACK .... Crosstex International,Inc.
POLYBEAD MICROPARTICLES .... Polysciences, Inc.
POLYBED EMBEDDING KIT .... Polysciences, Inc.
POLYBLADE .... Conmed Linvatec
POLYBLEND .... Advansource Biomaterials Corp.
POLYBLOCK .... Vector Laboratories, Inc.
POLYCEL .... Graham Medical Products/Div. Of Little Rapids Corp
POLYCEL .... Medtronic Xomed, Inc.
POLYCHROME .... Univac Dental Company
POLYCLEANER .... Hager Worldwide, Inc.
POLYCON .... Ciba Vision
POLYCRIMP SEAL .... J. G. Finneran Associates, Inc.
POLYDEK .... Teleflex Medical
POLYERECTA .... Intermetro Industries Corp.
POLYESTER PILE .... Total Care
POLYETHYLENE .... Stryker Corp.
POLYETHYLENE .... Stryker Howmedica Osteonics
POLYETHYLENE CATHETERS .... Primrose Medical, Inc.
POLYETHYLENE X3 .... Stryker Corp.
POLYETHYLENE X3 .... Stryker Howmedica Osteonics
POLYEURETHANE CATHETERS .... Primrose Medical, Inc.
POLYFIN .... Medtronic Minimed
POLYFIN .... Polysciences, Inc.
POLYFLEX .... Dentsply Prosthetics
POLYFLOR .... Hpg International, Inc.
POLYFREEZE .... Polysciences, Inc.
POLYFRESH .... Extra Packaging, Corp.
POLYGARD .... Crosstex International,Inc.
POLYGLYD .... Teleflex Medical
POLYHESIVET II .... Valleylab
POLYJEL .... Dentsply Caulk
POLYLASE LP .... Ddc Technologies, Inc.
POLYLC .... Nest Group Inc., The
POLYLEWTON CONTAINERS .... Lewis Bins+
POLYLEWTON CONTAINERS .... Orbis Corporation
POLYLITE .... Bsn Medical, Inc
POLYMARS .... Mars Air Doors
POLYMATIC .... Hager Worldwide, Inc.
POLYMAX .... Ferris Mfg Corp.
POLYMAXX .... Multi Focal Rx Lens Laboratories, Inc.
POLYMEDIC .... Avid Medical
POLYMEDIC .... Havel's Inc.
POLYMEM CALCIUM ALGINATE .... Ferris Mfg Corp.

POLYMEM SILVER .... Ferris Mfg Corp.
POLYMERIC PLRP-S 300A .... Polymer Laboratories, Now A Part Of Varian, Inc.
POLYMOBIL .... Siemens Medical Solutions Usa, Inc.
POLYMOUNT .... Gcx Corp.
POLYMOUNT .... Independent Solutions, Inc.
POLYNAP .... Cfi Medical Solutions (Contour Fabricators, Inc.)
POLYNIUM PLUS .... H.L. Bouton Co., Inc.
POLYPAC .... Fisher Scientific Co., Llc.
POLYPAL .... Diversified Ophthalmics, Inc.
POLYPEPTONE .... Bd Diagnostic Systems
POLYPERF .... Graham Medical Products/Div. Of Little Rapids Corp
POLYPORE .... Mentor Ophthalmics, Inc.
POLYPRO .... Cp Medical Corporation
POLYQUIP .... Gcx Corp.
POLYSCAN COATING .... Creative Foam Medical Systems
POLYSIL PUTTY .... Accurate Set, Inc.
POLYSMITH .... Nihon Kohden America, Inc.
POLYSONIC .... Parker Laboratories, Inc.
POLYSORB .... Covidien Lp, Formerly Registered As United States Surgical
POLYSORB .... Spenco Medical Corp.
POLYSTEEL .... Sellstrom Manufacturing Co.
POLYSYN FA .... Surgical Specialties Corporation
POLYTEF PASTE .... Mentor Ophthalmics, Inc.
POLYTITER .... Polymedco, Inc.
POLYTUBE .... Ferris Mfg Corp.
POLYTUF .... Ufp Technologies, Inc.
POLYTUFF .... Qrp, Inc.
POLYVIEW .... Astro-Med, Inc.
POLYWEAR, VR .... Polyconversions, Inc.
POLYWELD .... Advansource Biomaterials Corp.
POLYWIC .... Ferris Mfg Corp.
POLYZEN .... Polyzen, Inc.
POMARD .... Seca Corp.
PONEMAH .... Lds Life Science (Formerly Gould Instrument Systems Inc.)
PONY .... Snug Seat, Inc.
PONY II .... Ortho-Kinetics, Inc.
POP-OFF .... Covidien Lp, Formerly Registered As United States Surgical
POP-TOP .... Corning Inc., Science Products Division
POPPER .... Cadence Science Inc.
PORCEFLEX POLISHING WHEELS .... George Taub Products & Fusion Co., Inc.
PORCELANDE .... Asi-Modulex
PORCH-LIFT VERTICAL PLATFORM LIFT .... Thyssenkrupp Access Corp.
PORCUPINE .... Farley Inc., W.T.
POREMASTER .... Quantachrome
PORETICS .... Ge Infrastructure Water & Process Technologies
PORETICS POLYCARBONATE MEMBRANE .... Ge Infrastructure Water & Process Technologies
PORETICS POLYESTER MEMBRANE .... Ge Infrastructure Water & Process Technologies
POREX .... Porex Corporation
POROSZYME .... Applied Biosystems
POROUS TISSUE MATRIX .... Kensey Nash Corporation
PORT-A-CATH .... Smiths Medical Asd, Inc.
PORT-A-CUL .... Bd Diagnostic Systems
PORT-A-VAC .... Erie Medical
PORT-O-SCOPE .... North American Medical Products, Inc.
PORT-OP .... Mobile Dental Equipment Corp.(M-Dec)
PORT-OP III .... Mobile Dental Equipment Corp.(M-Dec)
PORT-XD .... Mobile Dental Equipment Corp.(M-Dec)
PORT-XP .... Mobile Dental Equipment Corp.(M-Dec)
PORT-XV .... Mobile Dental Equipment Corp.(M-Dec)
PORTA PLUME SAFE .... Buffalo Filter, A Division Of Medtek Devices Inc.
PORTA-CART .... First Healthcare Products
PORTA-LUNG .... Porta-Lung Inc.
PORTA-TRACE .... Gagne, Inc.
PORTABLE COLD THERAPY Cincinnati Sub-Zero Products, Inc., Medical Division
PORTABLE II .... Dntlworks Equipment Corporation
PORTABLE PC-2 .... Horcher Lifting Systems, Inc.
PORTABLE PIPET-AID .... Drummond Scientific Co.
PORTABLE PLUS .... Creative Biotech Inc.
PORTABLE WASHLET .... Toto Kiki Usa, Inc.
PORTABLE, DISPOSABLE PERSONAL URINAL.COMFORTRX.. Key / Sun Medical Services, Inc.

PORTALCAST	Diacor, Inc.
PORTALVISION	Varian Medical Systems
PORTAPEEL	Innovative Med Inc.
PORTAPRINT 2000	Krown Manufacturing, Inc.
PORTAPRINT 2000D	Krown Manufacturing, Inc.
PORTAVAC	Dntlworks Equipment Corporation
PORTAVIEW JUNIOR	Krown Manufacturing, Inc.
PORTAVIEW PLUS	Krown Manufacturing, Inc.
PORTAVIEW PLUS A	Krown Manufacturing, Inc.
PORTAVIEW SENIOR	Krown Manufacturing, Inc.
PORTAZAM	Stretchair Patient Transfer Systems, Inc,
PORTER-GAS SCAVENGER SYSTEM	Porter Instrument Division Parker Hannifin Corp
PORTFOLIO GENESIS	Innovation Genesis, Llc
PORTION	Young Innovations, Inc.
PORTION AID	Hager Worldwide, Inc.
PORTLAND ACCESS	Hard Manufacturing Co.
PORTO-LIFT	Porto-Lift Corp.
PORTO-VAC	Handler Manufacturing Co.
PORTRAIT	Mortara Instrument, Inc.
PORUS	Lens Mode, Inc.
POSEY	J. T. Posey Co.
POSI COMFORT	National Medical Products
POSI-BLOCK	National Medical Products
POSI-FLOW	Berner International Corp.
POSI-FORCE	Bio-Rad Laboratories, Life Science Group
POSICAM	Positron Corporation
POSITEX	Optp
POSITEX PERSONAL	Optp
POSITEX PROFESSIONAL	Optp
POSITION IMAGING	Fonar Corp.
POSITION-ETTE	Tp Orthodontics, Inc.
POSITIONING PLATFORM CHAIR	Gunnell, Inc.
POSITIONPERFECT	Cfi Medical Solutions (Contour Fabricators, Inc.)
POSITIONPRO	Stryker Corp.
POSITRACE	Conmed Corporation
POST MASTER	Falcon Products, Inc.
POST-VITRECTOMY FACE DOWN SUPPORT SYSTEMS	Oakworks, Inc.
POSTAL READY	Starkey Laboratories, Inc.
POSTURA	Fla Orthopedics, Inc.
POSTURE CONTROL	Kaye Products, Inc.
POSTURE PREMIER	Sealy Inc.
POSTURE S'PORT	The Saunders Group
POSTURITE	Back Support Systems
POT BELLY	Dixie Ems Supply
POTENTIAL	Noram Solutions
POTTY-CHECK	Bed-Check Corporation
POURMATIC	New Brunswick Scientific Co., Inc.
POW-R	Miltex Inc.
POWDER FREE PLUS	Tillotson Healthcare Corp.
POWER	Ams Innovative Center-San Jose
POWER	Samco Scientific Corporation
POWER ASSIST CONTROL	Ahnafield Corp.
POWER BLOCK	Biogenex Laboratories
POWER CANNULA	Vilex, Inc.
POWER CINCH	Contour Form Products
POWER CIRCUIT	Universal Gym Equipment
POWER CUBE	Lester Electrical Of Nebraska, Inc.
POWER FILE	White Systems, Inc.
POWER GENE KARYOTYPING SYSTEM	Leica Microsystems (San Jose) Corporation
POWER GRIP	All Pro Exercise Products, Inc.
POWER INFUSER	Zoll Medical Corp.
POWER LIFT BACK BRACE	Kt Medical Corp.
POWER LIFTER	Omnimed, Inc. (Beam Products)
POWER LINE	Oster Professional Products, Inc.
POWER ONE	VARTA Microbattery Inc.
POWER POINT	Conmed Corporation
POWER PRO	Oster Professional Products, Inc.
POWER PULSE	Possis Medical, Inc.
POWER RASP	Vilex, Inc.
POWER REG	Online Power, Inc.
POWER SCAN	Webb Manufacturing Co.
POWER SHIELD	American Power Conversion
POWER STRIDE BELT	All Pro Exercise Products, Inc.
POWER SURGICAL EQUIPMENT	Vilex, Inc.
POWER TRAINERS	Scifit
POWER VEST	All Pro Exercise Products, Inc.
POWER WALKER	Battle Creek Equipment Co.
POWER WRAP ANKLE	Core Products International, Inc.
POWER WRAP WRIST	Core Products International, Inc.
POWER-AID	Advanced Instrument Development, Inc.
POWER-DRIVE MORCELLATOR	Wisap America
POWER-PAC	Online Power, Inc.
POWER-PAP	Online Power, Inc.
POWER-PRO INCUBATOR TRANSPORT (IT)	Stryker Corp.
POWER-PRO TL	Stryker Corp.
POWER-PRO XT	Stryker Corp.
POWER-STIR	Eberbach Corp.
POWER3	Richards-Wilcox, Inc.
POWERALL	Propper Manufacturing Co., Inc.
POWERAUDIT	American Power Conversion
POWERBALL	Mercury Medical
POWERBELT	DJO Inc.
POWERBREATHE	Creative Health Products, Inc.
POWERCENTERS	American Power Conversion
POWERCHROM	Adinstruments
POWERCHUTE	American Power Conversion
POWERDOOR SERIES 600 & SERIES 1000	RDL Supply
POWERFLEX	Andover Healthcare Inc.
POWERFLEX	Cordis Corporation
POWERFLEX EXTREME PTA DILATATION CATHETER	Cordis Endovascular
POWERFLEX P3 PTA DILATATION CATHETER	Cordis Endovascular
POWERFLO	Comco, Inc.
POWERFORMA	Medtronic Xomed, Inc.
POWERGENE	Iris International, Inc.
POWERGENE PROBE SYSTEM	Leica Microsystems (San Jose) Corporation
POWERGRIP	Microflex Corporation
POWERGROUP	Stryker Corp.
POWERGROUP	Stryker Endoscopy
POWERGROUP	Stryker Howmedica Osteonics
POWERHEART	Cardiac Science Corporation (Ca)
POWERHEART CRM	Cardiac Science Corporation (Ca)
POWERLAB	Adinstruments
POWERLAB	iWorx Systems, Inc.
POWERLED	Getinge Usa, Inc.
POWERLIFT	Ricon Corp.
POWERLINE	Biosensors International - Usa
POWERLINK	Endologix, Inc.
POWERMANAGER	American Power Conversion
POWERMAP	Eit, Inc.
POWERMOUNT	Gcx Corp.
POWERMOUNT	Independent Solutions, Inc.
POWERPAC	American Medical Technologies, Inc.
POWERPOINT PLUS HANDPIECE	Conmed Corporation
POWERPRO	Conmed Linvatec
POWERPRO	Spacesaver Corporation
POWERPULSE	Vacumed
POWERSEARCH	Stryker Corp.
POWERSEARCH	Stryker Endoscopy
POWERSEARCH	Stryker Howmedica Osteonics
POWERSHIELD-UPS	American Power Conversion
POWERSORB	Reach Global Industries, Inc. (Reachgood)
POWERSTAR SERIES	Oneac Corporation
POWERTRACK	JTECH Medical
POWERVATOR	Flinchbaugh-Kurtz Company
POWERVIEW	Aprex, A Division Of Aardex
POWERVISION	Toshiba America Medical Systems
POWII, ORAL IRRIGATOR	Powell Labs
POWRSHIELD	Rapid Power Technologies, Inc.
POWRTRAP	Rapid Power Technologies, Inc.
POZZI	American Tooth Industries
PPF	Starkey Laboratories, Inc.
PPM	Physicians Practice Management
PPT	Aetrex Worldwide, Inc
PPT	Langer, Inc.

PPT/MARC .... Langer, Inc.
PR4 .... Mortara Instrument, Inc.
PRACTICE MANAGEMENT PLUS .... American Medical Software
PRACTICE MANAGER FOR WINDOWS .... Physicians Practice Management
PRACTICE NAVIGATOR .... Siemens Hearing Instruments, Inc.
PRACTICE PANORAMA .... Medinotes Corporation
PRACTICEBUILDER1-2-3 .... Erad/Image Medical Corp.
PRAFO .... Anatomical Concepts, Inc.
PRC .... Gcx Corp.
PRE-FINISHER .... Tp Orthodontics, Inc.
PRE-FIT .... Tp Orthodontics, Inc.
PRE-SED .... Professional Product Co.
PRE-TENS LOTION SKIN CARE ... Covidien Lp, Formerly Registered As Uni-Patch
PRECEDEX .... Hospira Inc.
PRECEPT .... Precept Medical Products, Inc.
PRECEPTROL .... Atcc
PRECI-CLIX .... Preat Corp.
PRECI-LINE .... Preat Corp.
PRECIMA .... Hager Worldwide, Inc.
PRECIOUS .... Hospital Specialty Company
PRECISE .... Caltech Industries, Inc.
PRECISE QTB .... Caltech Industries, Inc.
PRECISE SIM .... Elekta, Inc.
PRECISE TRANSHEPATIC BILIARY STENT .... Cordis Endovascular
PRECISE TREATMENT SYSTEMS .... Elekta, Inc.
PRECISEPLAN .... Elekta, Inc.
PRECISION .... Abbott Laboratories
PRECISION .... Ciba Vision
PRECISION .... Mabis Healthcare Inc.
PRECISION .... Msi Precision, Specialty Instrument
PRECISION .... Parco Scientific Co.
PRECISION .... Pennsylvania Glass Products Co.
PRECISION .... Precision Dynamics Corp.
PRECISION CONVERTING .... Brady Corporation
PRECISION CONVERTING, INC. .... Brady Corporation
PRECISION FIT .... Lenox Hill Brace / Seattle Systems
PRECISION FLOW .... Vapotherm, Inc.
PRECISION LITE .... Lenox Hill Brace / Seattle Systems
PRECISION V-CLAMP .... Adelberg Laboratories Inc.
PRECISION VOLUME SYRINGE .... Jones Medical Instrument Co.
PRECISION VV .... Ciba Vision
PRECONNECT .... Zoll Medical Corp.
PREDICTOR .... Arrhythmia Research Technology, Inc.
PREFER .... Anatech, Ltd.
PREFERENCE .... The Cooper Companies, Inc
PREFERRED 1ST .... Scott Specialties, Inc./Cmo Inc./Ginny Inc.
PREFERRED LABORATORY .... Zimmer Dental, Inc.
PREFILLED SYRINGE CASE .... Medicool, Inc.
PREFORMS .... Pedifix, Inc.
PREGEN .... Exact Sciences, Inc.
PREGEN-26 .... Exact Sciences, Inc.
PREGNA CERT .... Diagnostic Specialties
PREGNA SURE .... Diagnostic Specialties
PRELUDE ENTERPRISE REGISTRATION .... Epic Systems Corp.
PREM-ACLAVE .... Postcraft Co.
PREMA .... Amoena
PREMICIDE .... Metrex Research Corp.
PREMIE NESTIE .... Cas Medical Systems, Inc.
PREMIER .... Hologic, Inc.
PREMIER .... Lee Medical International, Inc.
PREMIER .... Medtronic Sofamor Danek Usa, Inc
PREMIER .... Medtronic Sofamor Danek Usa, Inc.
PREMIER .... Riegel Consumer Products Div.
PREMIER .... Salk Inc.
PREMIER .... Stryker Corp.
PREMIER 10S .... American Imex
PREMIER A-P .... American Imex
PREMIER EDGE .... Oasis Medical, Inc.
PREMIER PLATINUM HPSA .... Meridian Bioscience, Inc.
PREMIER SHIELD .... Oasis Medical, Inc.
PREMIERE .... C & A Scientific Co. Inc.
PREMIERE .... Stanbio Laboratory, Inc.
PREMIUM .... Access Battery Inc.

PREMIUM .... Covidien Lp, Formerly Registered As United States Surgical
PREMIUM .... Lang Dental Manufacturing Co., Inc.
PREMIUM 100 ALLOY .... Ticonium Co.
PREMIUM 6500 .... Medtronic Cardiovascular Surgery, The Heart Valve Div.
PREMIUM CEEA .... Covidien Lp, Formerly Registered As United States Surgical
PREMIUM MULTIFIRE TA .... Covidien Lp, Formerly Registered As United States Surgical
PREMIUM PLUS CEEA .... Covidien Lp, Formerly Registered As United States Surgical
PREMIUM POLY CS .. Covidien Lp, Formerly Registered As United States Surgical
PREMIUM QUILT .... Select Medical Products, Inc.
PREMIUM SURGICLIP .... Covidien Lp, Formerly Registered As United States Surgical
PREMIUN POLYSORB .... Covidien Lp, Formerly Registered As United States Surgical
PRENTAZYME .... Case Medical, Inc.
PREP MITT .... The Evercare Company
PREP SYSTEMS .... Ebi, Llc
PREP-A-GENE .... Bio-Rad Laboratories, Life Science Group
PREP-CHECK .... General Devices
PREP-DISC .... Bio-Rad Laboratories, Life Science Group
PREP-DRAPE .... Medical Concepts Development
PREP-IM .... Smith & Nephew Inc.- Orthopaedics Division
PREPAK .... Standard Textile Co., Inc.
PREPEASE .... Usb Corporation
PREPOMETER .... Hager Worldwide, Inc.
PRESEP PREFILTERS .... Ge Infrastructure Water & Process Technologies
PRESERVE .... Tillotson Healthcare Corp.
PRESIDAX .... Avery Dennison Corporation
PRESIDENTIAL .... Hu-Friedy Manufacturing Co., Inc.
PRESOURCE .... Cardinal Health Inc.
PRESS-LOCK(TM) .... Lytron, Inc.
PRESS-MATE 8800 .... Mediana Technologies Corp
PRESS-MATE 8800 F .... Mediana Technologies Corp
PRESS-MATE 8800 MSP .... Mediana Technologies Corp
PRESS-MATE 8800 SAT .... Mediana Technologies Corp
PRESS-MATE ADVANTAGE .... Mediana Technologies Corp
PRESS-MATE PRODIGY .... Mediana Technologies Corp
PRESS-SIDEr .... Vergason Technology, Inc.
PRESSCALL .... Dwyer Precision Products, Inc.
PRESSION .... Chattanooga Group
PRESSORE .... Cleveland Medical Devices, Inc.
PRESSPICK .... Spirig Advanced Technologies, Inc.
PRESSURE ACTIVATED VALVES .... Np Medical, Inc.
PRESSURE GUARD .... Span-America Medical Systems, Inc.
PRESSUREGUARD .... Span-America Medical Systems, Inc.
PRESSURELITE .... Fla Orthopedics, Inc.
PRESSURVEIL .... Conmed Linvatec
PRESTA .... Kinamed, Inc.
PRESTIGE .... Pyramid Orthodontics
PRESTIGE SMART SYSTEM .... Nipro Diagnostics, Inc.
PRESTO .... Zymark Corporation
PRESTO AUTOSTACKER .... Caliper Life Sciences, Inc.
PRESTO FLASH .... Cardiac Science Corp.
PRESTYLED FREESTYLE Medtronic Cardiovascular Surgery, The Heart Valve Div.
PREVACARE .... Advanced Sterilization Products
PREVAIL .... First Quality Enterprise, Inc.
PREVCARE .... Lohmann & Rauscher, Inc.
PREVENT AIR FILTER .... Permatron Corp.
PREVENT PLUS .... Humanicare International, Inc.
PREVENT PNEUMOTACH .... Medical Graphics Corporation
PREVENT-A-CARE .... Pyramid Industries, Llc
PREVENTAr ANTIMICROBIAL PENS .... Pm Company
PREVENTIP .... Lista International Corp.
PREVIEW .... Carolina Medical, Inc.
PREVIZE .... Staar Surgical Co.
PREVUE .... Wampole Laboratories
PRICARA .... Ortho-Mcneil-Janssen Pharmaceuticals, Inc.
PRIDE .... Handicap Unlimited, Inc.
PRIMA .... Columbia Medical Manufacturing Llc
PRIMA .... Hill-Rom Holdings, Inc.
PRIMA .... Hill-Rom Manufacturing, Inc.
PRIMA .... Lifecore Biomedical, Inc.

PRIMA	Spectranetics Corp.
PRIMA-SOLO	Lifecore Biomedical, Inc.
PRIMACARE	Salk Inc.
PRIMAGEN	Biomat Sciences, Inc.
PRIMALOC HIP SYSTEM	Ortho Development Corp.
PRIMAPAD	Salk Inc.
PRIMAPORE	Smith & Nephew, Inc.
PRIMATOM SYSTEM	Siemens Medical Solutions Usa, Inc
PRIME	Medical Sterile Products, Inc.
PRIME CONDOMS	Ansell Healthcare, Inc.
PRIME ECG	Meridian Medical Technologies
PRIME KOTE	Tp Orthodontics, Inc.
PRIME TIME FILTER	St. Jude Medical Neuromodulation Division
PRIME TO BOND	Dentsply Caulk
PRIME TO BOND DUAL CURE	Dentsply Caulk
PRIME-A-GENE	Promega Corp.
PRIME-AIRE	Hill-Rom Manufacturing, Inc.
PRIME-VU	Novosci Corp.
PRIMEBAND	Precision Dynamics Corp.
PRIMELINE	Soltec Corp.
PRIMER	Western Medical, Ltd.
PRIMER & CAVITY LINER	Global Dental Products
PRIMER UNNA-PAK	Western Medical, Ltd.
PRIMET	Scientific Pharmaceuticals, Inc.
PRIMEVIEW GRAPHICAL USER INTERFACE	Siemens Medical Solutions Usa, Inc
PRIMEVUE	Nds Surgical Imaging, Inc.
PRIMO FERRO	ArjoHuntleigh
PRIMUS	Life-Tech, Inc.
PRIMUS LINEAR ACCELERATOR	Siemens Medical Solutions Usa, Inc
PRIMUS PDQ	Primus Diagnostics
PRIMUS STERILIZER	Medi-Tech International, Inc.
PRIMUS ULTRA2	Primus Diagnostics
PRIMUSRS	Bte Technologies, Inc.
PRINCETON INSTRUMENTS	Roper Scientific, Inc.
PRINCIPLE	Dentsply Caulk
PRINTX	Smith Companies Dental Products
PRISM	Thermo Fisher Scientific
PRISM INFANT HEEL WARMER	Pristech Products, Inc
PRISM WARM GEL	Pristech Products, Inc
PRISMA	Dentsply Caulk
PRISMA	Dentsply International, Inc.
PRISMA	Dentsply Prosthetics
PRISMA	Sakura Finetek U.S.A., Inc.
PRISMA	Siemens Hearing Instruments, Inc.
PRISMA 2	Siemens Hearing Instruments, Inc.
PRISMA 2 K	Siemens Hearing Instruments, Inc.
PRISMA APH	Dentsply Caulk
PRISMA SHIELD	Dentsply Caulk
PRISMA TPH	Dentsply Caulk
PRISMALIX	Getinge Usa, Inc.
PRISMVIEW	Sunmed Healthcare
PRISTINE	World Medical Supply Usa., Inc.
PRISTINE, ANTI-REFLECTIVE CLEANER.	North American Marketing, Inc.
PRITCHARD	Photo Research, Inc.
PRO	Pro Orthopedic Devices, Inc.
PRO	Pro Scientific Inc.
PRO ALERT	Jeron Electronic Systems, Inc.
PRO CLEARZ	Ppr Direct, Inc.
PRO CORD/CORDLESS	Oster Professional Products, Inc.
PRO FLO	Bard Electro Physiology
PRO FLO	Brown Medical Industries
PRO FOAM	Brown Medical Industries
PRO GEL	Brown Medical Industries
PRO HMPVT	Prodesse, Inc.
PRO OSTEON	Interpore Cross International
PRO PORT	Smiths Medical Asd, Inc.
PRO POWER LINE	Oster Professional Products, Inc.
PRO PROP	Profex Medical Products
PRO QR	Biolife, Llc
PRO S	Instrumentation Laboratory Company
PRO SED(E.S.R.SYSTEM)	Ulster Scientific, Inc.
PRO SERIES	Ge Medical Systems Information Technologies
PRO TEC	Healthcare Labels, Inc.
PRO TECH	Healthmark Industries
PRO TEK	Pawling Corp., Architectural Prod. Div.
PRO TEK EARTH	Pawling Corp., Architectural Prod. Div.
PRO'S CHOICE	Hartmann-Conco Inc.
PRO+	Oster Professional Products, Inc.
PRO-CAST	Unique/Pereny
PRO-CEL	Aqua-Cel Corp.
PRO-CLEAN	Olsen Medical
PRO-CUT	Angiotech
PRO-FECT	Grand Medical Products
PRO-FICIENCY	DJO Inc.
PRO-FLOWT	Pro-Tech Services, Inc.
PRO-FORM/EXPRESS	Cascade Designs, Inc.
PRO-GENESIS	Environmental Tectonics Corp.
PRO-LITE SPINEBOARD	Rapid Deployment Products
PRO-LOUPE	Edroy Products Co., Inc.
PRO-MAG	Medical Device Technologies, Inc. (Md Tech)
PRO-MAGIS	Carl Zeiss Surgical, Inc.
PRO-MAX	C. R. Bard, Inc., Bard Urological Div.
PRO-PAR	Anatech, Ltd.
PRO-RAMP	Stinson Manufacturing
PRO-SOFT	Anatech, Ltd.
PRO-STAY	Lone Star Medical Products, Inc.
PRO-TEC	Biodex Medical Systems, Inc.
PRO-TEC	Sharps Compliance Corp.
PRO-TRACKING	Accu-Med Services
PRO-TRAINER MEDCO SUPPLY COMPANY, INC.	Medco Supply Company
PRO-YELLOW	Woodhead L.P.
PRO/SHIELD	Kappler Protective Apparel & Fabrics
PRO/VENT	Kappler Protective Apparel & Fabrics
PRO2	Scifit
PROACT	Uromedica, Inc.
PROACTIVE	Bangs Laboratories, Inc.
PROAIR I & III	Dntlworks Equipment Corporation
PROARCH	Shofu Dental Corporation
PROBACK	Crosstex International,Inc.
PROBE CLEAN	Diamedix Corp.
PROBE-CHECK	R. B. Annis Instruments, Inc.
PROBEGUARD	Arc Medical, Inc.
PROBELINE	Sun Biomedical Laboratories, Inc.
PROBERITE	Rpc
PROBLEM SOLVER	Basi (Bioanalytical Systems, Inc.)
PROBLOC	Life-Tech, Inc.
PROBRITE LIGHTS	Dntlworks Equipment Corporation
PROCARE	Ortholine
PROCARE	Professional Product Co.
PROCARE I & II	Dntlworks Equipment Corporation
PROCART I & II	Dntlworks Equipment Corporation
PROCEED	Ethicon, Inc.
PROCELL	Duracell Usa
PROCELL	Remington Products Company Llc
PROCENTER	Comco, Inc.
PROCESS LCS, SPOR-KLENZ	Steris Corporation
PROCESS QDS	Steris Corporation
PROCESSALL	Hf Pure Water
PROCESSION	Biorad Laboratories
PROCHECK	Serologicals Corp
PROCHEM EO	Raven Biological Laboratories, Inc.
PROCHEM SSI	Raven Biological Laboratories, Inc.
PROCISION	Havel's Inc.
PROCLEAR	The Cooper Companies, Inc
PROCOMP INFINITI	Biofeedback Instrument Corp.
PROCONNECT	Starkey Laboratories, Inc.
PROCONTROL	Motion Control, Inc.
PROCORD	Hokanson Inc., D.E.
PROCOUNT	Bd Biosciences
PROCYCLER	B/R Instrument Corp.
PRODAG	Acheson Colloids Company
PRODERM	Mylan Pharmaceuticals Inc
PRODERMA	American Healthcare Products, Inc.
PRODIGY	Convergent Laser Technologies
PRODIGY	Phenomenex, Inc.
PRODIGY	Roho Group, The

PRODIL	Cst Technologies, Inc.
PRODUCT LINES: FLEXIGRAFT	Lifenet Health
PRODUCTION DIPWAX	Mds Products, Inc.
PRODUCTION DIPWAX & RAPID WAX BY JAMES PITRE	American Diversified Dental Systems
PRODUCTION PROVEN PROTOTYPING	Okay Industries, Inc.
PROFECTION	Promega Corp.
PROFEMUR	Wright Medical Group, Inc.
PROFESSIONAL	Action Products, Inc.
PROFESSIONAL BATTERIES	Duracell Usa
PROFESSIONAL REGULAR	Crosstex International,Inc.
PROFESSIONAL THRIFT	Crosstex International,Inc.
PROFEX	Profex Medical Products
PROFILE	Conmed Corporation
PROFILE	DJO Inc.
PROFILE	Hologic, Inc.
PROFILE	Medtox Scientific Inc.
PROFILE	New Horizons Diagnostics Corporation
PROFILE	Profex Medical Products
PROFILE CODE	Implant Sciences Corp.
PROFILE HANDPIECE	Conmed Corporation
PROFILER	Convaid Inc.
PROFILER	Impladent Ltd.
PROFILER MOUNTING SYSTEM	C.J.T. Enterprises, Inc.
PROFILER-LITE MOUNTING SYSTEM FOR SWITCHES	C.J.T. Enterprises, Inc.
PROFIT	Fricke Dental Manufacturing Co.
PROFIT COLLAR	Jerome Medical
PROFIX	Smith & Nephew Inc.- Orthopaedics Division
PROFLEX ERGODYNE ON3	Ergodyne
PROFLO2	American Healthcare
PROFLU+T	Prodesse, Inc.
PROFORE	Smith & Nephew, Inc.
PROFX	Mizuho Osi
PROFYLE	Stryker Corp.
PROGASTROT CD	Prodesse, Inc.
PROGIENIC	Oster Professional Products, Inc.
PROGRAMMAT	Ivoclar Vivadent, Inc.
PROGRESS	North Coast Medical, Inc.
PROHEAR	Starkey Laboratories, Inc.
PROJECT-O-CHART	Reichert, Inc.
PROKLENZ	Professional Product Co.
PROLANCE	Htl-Strefa, Inc.
PROLASE	Wave Form Systems, Inc.
PROLENE	Ethicon, Inc.
PROLINE	Biohit Inc.
PROLINE	Planmeca U.S.A. Inc
PROLINE	Raven Biological Laboratories, Inc.
PROLINE	Rayovac
PROLINER	Professional Product Co.
PROLITE	Dentsply Caulk
PROLITE	Fla Orthopedics, Inc.
PROLITE LIGHT WEIGHT MOUNTING SYSTEM	C.J.T. Enterprises, Inc.
PROLITE PDC PATIENT CHAIR	Dntlworks Equipment Corporation
PROLONG	Fci Ophthalmics
PROLONG	Life-Tech, Inc.
PROMAX	Compex Technologies, Inc.
PROMAX	Planmeca U.S.A. Inc
PROMEDICA	Promedica, Inc.
PROMEGA	Promega Corp.
PROMEGA MARKERS	Promega Corp.
PROMENADE	Mada, Inc.
PROMET	Statlab Medical Products, Inc.
PROMISE	Sca Personal Care, North America
PROMIT	Gammadirect Medical Division
PROMIT-DALMATIAN	Gammadirect Medical Division
PROMIT-MAMO	Gammadirect Medical Division
PROMIX	Dentsply Caulk
PROMIX	Dentsply International, Inc.
PROMIX	Dentsply Prosthetics
PROMUS	Abbott Laboratories
PROMUS	Boston Scientific Corporation
PRON PILLO	Chattanooga Group
PRONEB	Pari Respiratory Equipment, Inc.
PRONEVIEW	Dupaco, Inc.
PRONEX	Glacier Cross, Inc.
PRONOVA	Ethicon, Inc.
PRONTO	Hamilton Caster & Mfg. Co.
PRONTO	Schleicher & Schuell, Inc.
PROPAC	Carolon Company
PROPAC PLUS	Covidien Lp
PROPACT	Raven Biological Laboratories, Inc.
PROPAK I & II	Dntlworks Equipment Corporation
PROPAQ 102	Welch Allyn Protocol Inc.
PROPAQ 104	Welch Allyn Protocol Inc.
PROPAQ 106	Welch Allyn Protocol Inc.
PROPAQ CS	Welch Allyn Protocol Inc.
PROPAQ ENCORE	Welch Allyn Protocol Inc.
PROPATCH	Cryolife, Inc.
PROPEAK	Profex Medical Products
PROPEL	Bard Electro Physiology
PROPERTUSSIST	Prodesse, Inc.
PROPHASE PLUS	Arlington Scientific, Inc. Asi
PROPHY PENCIL	Parkell, Inc.
PROPHY-EZ	Micro-Vac, Inc.
PROPHY-POL	Moyco Technologies, Inc.
PROPHYMATIC	Medidenta International, Inc.
PROPHYMIRACLE PROPHY PASTE	Twist2it, Inc.
PROPLEX	Baxter International Inc
PROPNEUMO-1T	Prodesse, Inc.
PROPOCKET	Siemens Hearing Instruments, Inc.
PROPOLIS	Walkmed Infusion Llc
PROPOWER	General Pysiotherapy, Inc.
PROPULSID	Ortho-Mcneil-Janssen Pharmaceuticals, Inc.
PROQUEST I & II	Dntlworks Equipment Corporation
PROSAT(R) CUSTOM(TM)	Contec, Inc.
PROSAT(R) PRESATURATED WIPES	Contec, Inc.
PROSAT(R) STERILE(TM)	Contec, Inc.
PROSCOPE	American Diagnostic Corporation (Adc)
PROSEAL I & II	Dntlworks Equipment Corporation
PROSEDATE	Professional Product Co.
PROSEED	C. R. Bard, Inc., Bard Urological Div.
PROSERIES	Sellstrom Manufacturing Co.
PROSMILE HANDY	Sirona Dental Systems Llc
PROSOLO II	Dntlworks Equipment Corporation
PROSPECT	Remel
PROSPHYG	American Diagnostic Corporation (Adc)
PROSPLINTS	Medical Specialties, Inc.
PROSPORE 2	Raven Biological Laboratories, Inc.
PROSPORE AMPOULE	Raven Biological Laboratories, Inc.
PROSTA SCINT	Cytogen Corp.
PROSTART	Dntlworks Equipment Corporation
PROSTATRON	Urologix, Inc.
PROSTRIP HCG	Arlington Scientific, Inc. Asi
PROSTYLE	Planmeca U.S.A. Inc
PROSUN	Prosun Tanning International, Llc.
PROTAC	American Diagnostica, Inc.
PROTACK	Covidien Lp, Formerly Registered As United States Surgical
PROTAIN XL	Covidien Lp
PROTEAN	Bio-Rad Laboratories, Life Science Group
PROTEC	Precision Dynamics Corp.
PROTECH	Vicon Industries Inc.
PROTECHT	Instrument Technology, Inc.
PROTECT POINT	Covidien Lp
PROTECT-ALL	Hardy Diagnostics
PROTECTA-COAT	Alimed, Inc.
PROTECTALL CASE	Medicool, Inc.
PROTECTAPE	Brasel Products, Inc.
PROTECTION 1	Karl Storz Endoscopy-America Inc.
PROTECTISCOPE CS	Stryker Corp.
PROTECTISCOPE CS	Stryker Endoscopy
PROTECTNET	American Power Conversion
PROTECTO-SPLINT	Products International Co.
PROTECTOR	Labconco Corp.
PROTECTOR PLUS	Wilson-Cook Medical, Inc.
PROTECTRODE SYSTEM	The Electrode Store
PROTEGE	Convergent Laser Technologies

PURITY	Delta Gloves
PUROS	Zimmer Dental, Inc.
PUROS	Zimmer Holdings, Inc.
PURPLE COLOREDT	Passy-Muir Inc.
PURPLE NITRILE	Kerr Group
PURSTRING	Covidien Lp, Formerly Registered As United States Surgical
PURSWAB	Puritan Medical Products Company Llc
PUSHER	Collins Bus Corporation
PVA 2000	Pva
PVA 3000	Pva
PVA PLUS	Surgica Corporation
PVA/ALP GARMENTS	Healthcare Service And Supply
PVC MERRY WALKER	Merry Walker Corp.
PVI	Boeckeler Instruments, Inc.
PVI-RAMPS	Handi-Cap Aids Company
PVV	Respironics Colorado
PXIPL	Epix, Inc.
PY	Oscor, Inc.
PYLORISET DRY	Lifesign
PYNG MEDICAL	Bound Tree Medical
PYONEX	Seirin-America, Inc.
PYRAMETRIX	Medtronic Sofamor Danek Usa, Inc
PYRAMETRIX	Medtronic Sofamor Danek Usa, Inc.
PYRAMIS	Cardiac Science Corp.
PYREX	Corning Inc., Science Products Division
PYREX PLUS	Corning Inc., Science Products Division
PYRO	Pyrometer Instrument Co.
PYRO-CHEMILUMINESCENT	Antek Instruments, Inc.
PYRO-FLUORESCENT	Antek Instruments, Inc.
PYROLASER	Pyrometer Instrument Co.
PYROTEST	Q.I. Medical, Inc.
PYXIS	Cardinal Health Inc.
PZI VET	Idexx Laboratories, Inc.
Pacel	St. Jude Medical, Inc.
Pak	Ertelalsop
Pall	Pall Corporation
Pallflex	Pall Corporation
Palltronic	Pall Corporation
Pampers	Procter & Gamble
Paradigm	Medtronic, Inc.
Passive Plus	St. Jude Medical, Inc.
Pepto-Bismol	Procter & Gamble
Percuflex	Boston Scientific Corporation
Performer	Medtronic Perfusion Systems
Perio-Aid	Marquis Dental Manufacturing Co.
Pexeva	Noven Pharmaceuticals, Inc.
PhosLo	Fresenius Medical Care North America
Photomology	ElemAc Medical
PinPoint	Boston Scientific Corporation
Pinnacle	Boston Scientific Corporation
Pioneer	Nutraceutical International Corp.
Piranha	Boston Scientific Corporation
PolarCath	Boston Scientific Corporation
Polaris	Boston Scientific Corporation
Polaris Dx	Boston Scientific Corporation
Polaris X	Boston Scientific Corporation
Polyflex	Boston Scientific Corporation
Polyform	Boston Scientific Corporation
Polyzene	Celonova Biosciences Inc.
Poseidon	Pall Corporation
PowerSox	Moretz, Inc.
PowerSuite	Boston Scientific Corporation
Precision Plus	Boston Scientific Corporation
Prefyx PPS	Boston Scientific Corporation
Premere	St. Jude Medical, Inc.
Premier One	Nutraceutical International Corp.
PreserVision	Bausch & Lomb
Prime	Dentsply Caulk
Pringles	Procter & Gamble
Pro Bulls-Eye	Hilco
ProLipo PLUS, Contour	Sciton, Inc.
ProStretch	Medi-Dyne Healthcare Products, L.L.C.
Prolieve Thermodilatation	Boston Scientific Corporation
Promote	St. Jude Medical, Inc.
ProtectiScope CS	Stryker Gi
Proxi	Rochester Midland, Corp.
Proxis	St. Jude Medical, Inc.
Puffs	Procter & Gamble
PulseIC	Kinetic Concepts, Inc.
Pure Silk	Perio Products, Inc.
PureVision	Bausch & Lomb
Puros	Zimmer Spine, Inc.
Q 1000 CONTROL	Gresham Driving Aids, Inc.
Q BABY	Cropper Medical, Inc./Bio Skin
Q BRACE	Cropper Medical, Inc./Bio Skin
Q-CLEAR(TM) - PIGMENTED LESIONS - LONG PULSE HEAD AVAILABLE	Light Age Inc.
Q-OPTICS	Quality Aspirators
Q-SIGN	Idesco Corp.
Q-SWEAT	Wr Medical Electronics Co.
Q-TAG	Idesco Corp.
Q.A. PAK	Universal Medical Design
Q.E.D.	Orasure Technologies, Inc.
Q/C WINDOWS	Bangs Laboratories, Inc.
Q2 MEDICAL	Olsen Medical
QA SCAN	Baxter Healthcare Corporation Nutrition
QA-40	Unit Chemical Corp.
QACCESS	J.M. Baragano Biomedical P.M. And Consulting, Inc.
QC SYSTEM	Tripath Imaging
QC-SLIDE	Remel
QCAPLUS	Sanders Data Systems, Llc
QCAPLUSPLUS	Sanders Data Systems, Llc
QCS	Siemens Healthcare Diagnostics Inc
QCT-3000	Image Analysis, Inc.
QCT-3D PLUS	Image Analysis, Inc.
QCT-5000	Image Analysis, Inc.
QCT-BONE MINERAL	Image Analysis, Inc.
QCT-CORONARY CALCIUM	Image Analysis, Inc.
QCT-LIVER IRON	Image Analysis, Inc.
QCT-LUNG NODULE	Image Analysis, Inc.
QDR	Hologic, Inc.
QDR 4000	Hologic, Inc.
QDR 4500A	Hologic, Inc.
QDR-4500C	Hologic, Inc.
QDR-4500SL	Hologic, Inc.
QDR-4500W	Hologic, Inc.
QED FLASH BOARD	Mosaic Industries, Inc.
QED WILDCARDS	Mosaic Industries, Inc.
QHR	Greatbatch Inc
QL	Atrion Medical Products, Inc.
QLS	Symmetry Medical Usa, Inc.
QLVAPLUS	Sanders Data Systems, Llc
QMR	Greatbatch Inc
QMS	Quality Monitor Systems, Inc.
QMS	Seradyn, Inc.
QR	Biolife, Llc
QRS	Omni Medical Supply Inc.
QSART II	Wr Medical Electronics Co.
QSI SYSTEM	Quality Systems, Inc.
QTA	Netzsch Instruments, Inc.
QTJUNIOR	Q.I. Medical, Inc.
QTMICRO	Q.I. Medical, Inc.
QTOWELS	Sanitor Manufacturing Co.
QUAD 12000	Fonar Corp.
QUAD 7	Starkey Laboratories, Inc.
QUAD 7000	Fonar Corp.
QUAD STAR CANE	Leading Edge Innovations
QUAD-LUMEN	Zimmer Orthopaedic Surgical Products
QUAD-O-DYN	Minnesota Rubber & Qmr Plastics
QUAD-O-STAT	Minnesota Rubber & Qmr Plastics
QUAD-PE-PLUS	Minnesota Rubber & Qmr Plastics
QUAD-RING	Minnesota Rubber & Qmr Plastics
QUADION	Minnesota Rubber & Qmr Plastics
QUADLUME	Independent Solutions, Inc.
QUADRA	Ortho-Kinetics, Inc.
QUADRA 96	Tomtec

QUADRA-TITER	Microtech Medical Systems
QUADRA3	Tomtec
QUADRAFORM	Ferris Mfg Corp.
QUADRAMET	Cytogen Corp.
QUADRASOUND	Argosy
QUADRASPHERIC	Volk Optical Inc.
QUADRIGA BEFREE	Siemens Healthcare Diagnostics Inc.
QUADRIPOLAR	Gyrus Medical, Inc.
QUADSTAR	Biomedical Life Systems, Inc.
QUADVUE	AMD Technologies Inc.
QUAL'X	Broadwest Corp.
QUALAKOTE C/R	Qrp, Inc.
QUALATEX	Qrp, Inc.
QUALATEX HIPRO XC	Qrp, Inc.
QUALATEX MIRACLEGRIP	Qrp, Inc.
QUALATHERM	Qrp, Inc.
QUALATRILE	Qrp, Inc.
QUALATRILE XC	Qrp, Inc.
QUALCARE	Alimed, Inc.
QUALCRAFT	Alimed, Inc.
QUALICHECK	Radiometer America, Inc.
QUALICODE, QUICK ELISA	Immunetics, Inc.
QUALICON	Qualicon
QUALISWAB	Bd Diagnostic Systems
QUALITEST	Radiometer America, Inc.
QUALITY FOR LIFE	Medrad, Inc.
QUALITY OPTICS AND PERFORMANCE TO LAST A LIFETIME	Volk Optical Inc.
QUALITY QUARTZ	Perkinelmer Optoelectronics
QUALITYSPECr	Analytical Spectral Devices, Inc.
QUALITYTREND	Inc Research
QUALTHANE	Filtrona Extrusion, Inc./PexcoA,Ar Medical Products Div.
QUANTA LITE	Inova Diagnostics, Inc.
QUANTAMASTER	Photon Technology International, Inc.
QUANTASORB	Quantachrome
QUANTI-CULT	Idexx Laboratories, Inc.
QUANTI-CULT	Remel
QUANTI-CULT PLUS	Remel
QUANTI-DISC	Idexx Laboratories, Inc.
QUANTI-TRAY	Idexx Laboratories, Inc.
QUANTIFLEX	Matrx By Midmark
QUANTITYPE	Qed Bioscience, Inc.
QUANTREX	L&R Manufacturing Co.
QUANTSCOPICS	Quantimetrix Corporation
QUANTTEST	Quantimetrix Corporation
QUANTUM	Abbott Laboratories
QUANTUM	Arthrocare Corp.
QUANTUM	Novosci Corp.
QUANTUM	Siemens Medical Systems, Inc., Ultrasound Group
QUANTUM	Wilson-Cook Medical, Inc.
QUANTUM 2000	Wallach Surgical Devices, Inc.
QUANTUM 500	Wallach Surgical Devices, Inc.
QUANTUM BLAST	Pride Mobility Products Corp.
QUANTUM DYNAMO	Pride Mobility Products Corp.
QUANTUM INTERCONNECT	Nurse Assist ,Inc.
QUANTUM JAZZY	Pride Mobility Products Corp.
QUANTUM MESF	Bangs Laboratories, Inc.
QUANTUM PREMIUM HIGH SPEED FIBER OPTIC HANDPIECES	Kinetic Instruments, Inc.
QUANTUM PSV	Respironics Georgia, Inc.
QUANTUM SIMPLY CELLULAR	Bangs Laboratories, Inc.
QUANTUM YIELD	Promega Corp.
QUANTUMPLEX	Bangs Laboratories, Inc.
QUANTUMT	Pro-Tech Services, Inc.
QUARTET	Sonic Innovations
QUARTZ	Nsg Precision Cells, Inc.
QUATTRO	Alsius Corp.
QUEBEC	Leica Microsystems, Inc., Educational & Analytical Division
QUENCH GUM	Mueller Sports Medicine
QUEST	Cardiac Science Corp.
QUEST	St. Jude Medical Neuromodulation Division
QUESTCOAT	World Heart Inc.
QUESTOR	Extrel Cms
QUEUE	Kendro Laboratory Products

QUIC ACCESS	Ziamatic Corp.
QUIC BAR	Ziamatic Corp.
QUIC RELEASE	Ziamatic Corp.
QUIC STRAP	Ziamatic Corp.
QUICK ABG	Vital Signs Colorado
QUICK CHANGE	Woodhead L.P.
QUICK CLEAN MICRO-STEAM BAGS	Medela, Inc.
QUICK CLEAN WIPES	Medela, Inc.
QUICK CONNECT TRANSDUCER CABLE SYSTEM	Amrex Electrotherapy Equipment
QUICK DRAIN VALVE	Urocare Products, Inc.
QUICK ELUT	Varian Sample Preparation Products
QUICK GEL(TM) URINE COLLECTION LEG BAG	Merlin's Medical Supply
QUICK LAUNCH SYSTEM	Symmetry Medical, Inc.
QUICK LINK	Da-Lite Screen Co., Inc.
QUICK MIX	Baxter Healthcare Corporation Nutrition
QUICK PICK	Covidien Lp, Formerly Registered As United States Surgical
QUICK RACK	Mark Medical Manufacturing, Inc.
QUICK READ	Aprex, A Division Of Aardex
QUICK RESPONSE	Rf Technologies
QUICK SERVE	Carter-Hoffman
QUICK SNAP CONNECTOR (TM)	Merlin's Medical Supply
QUICK SWABS	Hager Worldwide, Inc.
QUICK TIPS	Hager Worldwide, Inc.
QUICK-CHECK	Bio-Rad Laboratories, Life Science Group
QUICK-CROSS EXTREME	Spectranetics Corp.
QUICK-CROSS SUPPORT CATHETER	Spectranetics Corp.
QUICK-DRAIN	Bemis Mfg. Co.
QUICK-DRAW	Innovative Medical Technologies, Inc.
QUICK-FIT	Bemis Mfg. Co.
QUICK-FLOW	Conmed Linvatec
QUICK-LOCK	DJO Inc.
QUICK-READ 10	Globe Scientific, Inc.
QUICK-STAT	First Healthcare Products
QUICKCAST	Patterson Medical Holdings, Inc.
QUICKCAT	Kensey Nash Corporation
QUICKCOMPARE	Stryker Corp.
QUICKCOMPARE	Stryker Endoscopy
QUICKCOMPARE	Stryker Howmedica Osteonics
QUICKDRAW	Sscor
QUICKDRAW HOSPITAL GRADE SUCTION UNIT	Armstrong Medical Industries, Inc.
QUICKFLASH	Arrow International, Inc.
QUICKFLOW	Medtronic Cardiovascular Surgery, The Heart Valve Div.
QUICKIE	Sunrise Medical
QUICKIE PRIME	Novosci Corp.
QUICKLANCE	Arkray Usa
QUICKLATCH	Conmed Linvatec
QUICKLIST	Stryker Corp.
QUICKLIST	Stryker Endoscopy
QUICKLIST	Stryker Howmedica Osteonics
QUICKLUNG, RESPITRAINER, NEOLUNG	Ingmar Medical, Ltd.
QUICKMED	Cadwell Laboratories
QUICKPICK(TM) PACKAGING	Contec, Inc.
QUICKPULSE	Ams Innovative Center-San Jose
QUICKREAD	Stryker Corp.
QUICKREAD	Stryker Endoscopy
QUICKREAD	Stryker Howmedica Osteonics
QUICKSHIP	Bobrick Washroom Equipment, Inc.
QUICKSILVER SERVICE	Mark Medical Manufacturing, Inc.
QUICKSPACE	Spacesaver Corporation
QUICKSTICK	Novel Products, Inc.
QUICKTEK	Arkray Usa
QUICKTEST	Q.I. Medical, Inc.
QUICKVUE	Quidel Corporation
QUICKVUE ADVANCE	Quidel Corporation
QUICKVUE IN-LINE	Quidel Corporation
QUICKZOOM	Schick Technologies, Inc.
QUIDEL	Quidel Corporation
QUIESCENCE	Radix Corp.
QUIET NIGHT	E. Benson Hood Laboratories, Inc.
QUIETTRAK	Welch Allyn, Inc.
QUIK DRAW	Vital Signs Colorado

QUIK FIX	Combe, Inc.
QUIK STAIN	Cambridge Diagnostic Products, Inc.
QUIK STAIN II	Cambridge Diagnostic Products, Inc.
QUIK-CARD	Medtox Diagnostics Inc.
QUIK-CART	Physio-Control, Inc.
QUIK-CHARGE	Physio-Control, Inc.
QUIK-CHECK	Acon Laboratories, Inc.
QUIK-COMBO	Conmed Corporation
QUIK-COMBO	Physio-Control, Inc.
QUIK-LOOK	Physio-Control, Inc.
QUIK-PACE	Physio-Control, Inc.
QUIK-SEAL	National Instrument Co., Inc.
QUIK-SEP	Analytical Control Systems, Inc.
QUIK-SEP	PerkinElmer
QUIK-SORB	Essential Medical Supply, Inc.
QUIK-STITCH	Pare Surgical, Inc.
QUIKFITS	Acor Orthopaedic, Inc.
QUIKPACII	Syntron Bioresearch, Inc.
QUIKRESULTS	Medtox Scientific Inc.
QUIKSCAN	Etymonic Design Inc.
QUIKSCAN	Syntron Bioresearch, Inc.
QUIKSIGNS	Welch Allyn Protocol Inc.
QUIKSTRIP	Syntron Bioresearch, Inc.
QUIKformable	Acor Orthopaedic, Inc.
QUILL	Janin Group, Inc.
QUILTEC(R) I WIPES	Contec, Inc.
QUINGAS	Quintron Instrument Company
QUINSHEEN	Quintron Instrument Company
QUINT-X	Control-X Medical, Inc.
QUINTON	Med-Fit Systems, Inc.
QUIPS KAROTYPE	Vysis
QUS-2	Quidel Corporation
QVGA CONTROLLER	Mosaic Industries, Inc.
QWIK-FIT SYRINGE	Medrad, Inc.
QWIKSLOT	Intermetro Industries Corp.
QX,TH 9428	Thales Components Corporation
QX-4 ADHESIVE	Mds Products, Inc.
QX-4 PREMIUM QUALITY CYANOACRYLATE ADHESIVE	American Diversified Dental Systems
QYK FIX	Holmes Dental Corp.
QYK SET	Holmes Dental Corp.
Quantum	Boston Scientific - Maple Grove
Quantum	Boston Scientific Corporation
Quartet	Phoenix Medical Devices, Llc
Quick Relief	Biolife, Llc
QuickFlex	St. Jude Medical, Inc.
QuickOpt	St. Jude Medical, Inc.
Quotient	Biobehavioral Diagnostics Company
R & D RETIC	R & D Systems, Inc.
R & D RETIC I	R & D Systems, Inc.
R SERIES	Zoll Medical Corp.
R STENT	Orbusneich Medical, Inc.
R-50	Trimedyne, Inc.
R-MER	Riley Medical, Inc.
R-STIM II	American Imex
R.I.C.	Arrow International, Inc.
R/B	Remel
R/S 2003	Diasys Corporation
R/S 500	Diasys Corporation
R1	Elginex Corporation
R120	Osteoimplant Technology, Inc.
R3	Bruno Independent Living Aids, Inc.
RA	Matrx By Midmark
RA REEVE ANGEL	Whatman Inc.
RABBIT	Snug Seat, Inc.
RABBIT EARS	Tu-Way American Group
RAC	Whatman Inc.
RACE CAR TYMPANOMETER	Maico Diagnostics
RACETRAC	Covidien Lp, Formerly Registered As United States Surgical
RACHEL MODEL 2800C	Mallard Medical, Inc.
RACK FRAME	Star Case Manufacturing Co., Inc.
RACK-N-ROLL	Cres Cor
RACKBACK	Wire Crafters L.L.C.
RAD	Scientech, Inc.
RAD 40	Medtronic Xomed, Inc.
RAD-5	Masimo Corp.
RAD-57	Masimo Corp.
RAD-5V	Masimo Corp.
RAD-9	Masimo Corp.
RAD-FREE	Schleicher & Schuell, Inc.
RAD/AWAY	Triangle Biomedical Sciences, Inc.
RADASSIST	Diacor, Inc.
RADCAM REMOTE IMAGING SURVEY SYSTEM	Radiation Monitoring Devices, Inc.
RADENOID	Medtronic Xomed, Inc.
RADEX	Hologic, Inc.
RADIALASE	Trimedyne, Inc.
RADIANCE	Amano Pioneer Eclipse Corp.
RADIANCE	American Orthodontics Corp.
RADIANCE	Ams Innovative Center-San Jose
RADIANCE	Nds Surgical Imaging, Inc.
RADIANCE	Radiometer America, Inc.
RADIATION ALERTr	S.E. International, Inc.
RADIATION SURVEY METER	Supertech, Inc.
RADICAL	Masimo Corp.
RADIN	Imsi, Integrated Modular Systems Inc.
RADIN PACS	Imsi, Integrated Modular Systems Inc.
RADIN TELERAD	Imsi, Integrated Modular Systems Inc.
RADIOFOCUS	Terumo Medical Corp.
RADIOLOGIC-X	Control-X Medical, Inc.
RADIOLOGY WORKBENCH	Brit Systems Inc.
RADIOLUCENT WRIST FIXATOR	Orthofix Inc.
RADIOMARK	Scanlan International, Inc.
RADIOMAT	Agfa Corporation
RADIONICS	Integra Lifesciences Holdings Corp.
RADIONICS	Integra Radionics
RADIONUCLIDE MANAGER	Radcal Corp.
RADIOSHACK	Radio Shack
RADIUM	Phonic Ear, Inc.
RADIUS	Stryker Corp.
RADIUS	Stryker Spine
RADLINK	Masimo Corp.
RADLITE	Teleflex Medical
RADMAN	Narda Safety Test Solutions
RADNET	Cerner Corp.
RADNET	Masimo Corp.
RADOL	Allied Diagnostic Imaging Resources, Inc.
RADSIM	Advanced Medical Systems, Inc.
RADTRAK	Landauer, Inc.
RADX	S&S Technology
RAE SYSTEMS	Cea Instruments, Inc.
RAF	Raf Tabtronics Llc
RAFFO2	Taga Medical Technologies
RAFORMER	Pascal Company, Inc.
RAGE READY TO FIT KNEE BRACES	Omni Life Science, Inc.
RAHD ALPHA	Rahd Oncology Products
RAHD FUSION	Rahd Oncology Products
RAHD-SAFE	Rahd Oncology Products
RAI-TROL	Raichem, Division Of Hemagen Diagnostics, Inc.
RAICHEM	Raichem, Division Of Hemagen Diagnostics, Inc.
RAIL WRAP	Covidien Lp, Formerly Registered As United States Surgical
RAIL-BUS PILLOW	Hos-Pillow Corp.
RAILWALKER	Sellstrom Manufacturing Co.
RAILWIRE	Boston Scientific Interventional Technologies
RAIN FOREST	Lead-Lok, Inc.
RAINBOW	Insiphil (Us) Llc
RAINBOW AGAR	Biolog, Inc.
RAINBOW BRITES	Mid-States Laboratories, Inc.
RAINBOW II	H.L. Bouton Co., Inc.
RAINBOW REACHER	Arcmate Mfg. Corp.
RAISA	Horcher Lifting Systems, Inc.
RALLY	Pride Mobility Products Corp.
RALPH STORRS	Seattle Systems
RAM FLAT COMPACTORS/CRUSHERS	S&G Enterprises, Inc.
RAMCLEAN	Dentalez Group
RAMCLEAN	Ramvac Dental Products Inc

RAMJET	Marathon Equipment Company
RAMTUBE	Camfil Farr
RAMVAC	Dentalez Group
RAMVAC	Ramvac Dental Products Inc
RANAWAT/BURSTEIN	Biomet, Inc.
RAND VOICE AMPIFLER	Luminaud, Inc.
RANDOT	Stereo Optical Co., Inc.
RANFAC	Ranfac Corp.
RANGER	Arizant Healthcare Inc.
RANGER X	Invacare Corporation
RANGETRACK	JTECH Medical
RAPHAEL	Hamilton Medical, Inc.
RAPID	Oncogene Research Products
RAPID 1-2-3 HEMA	Hema Diagnostic Systems, Llc
RAPID ANA II	Remel Atlanta, Div. Of Remel, Inc.
RAPID FORM	Cramer Products, Inc.
RAPID GLAZE	Motloid Company
RAPID NF PLUS	Remel Atlanta, Div. Of Remel, Inc.
RAPID NH	Remel Atlanta, Div. Of Remel, Inc.
RAPID ONE	Remel Atlanta, Div. Of Remel, Inc.
RAPID PLATE	Zymark Corporation
RAPID PULSE	Ekos Corp.
RAPID RESPONSE	Bobrick Washroom Equipment, Inc.
RAPID RHINO	Arthrocare Corp.
RAPID RHINO, GEL-KNIT, SINU-KNIT, AND RAPID PAK.	Applied Therapeutics, Inc.
RAPID SS/U	Remel Atlanta, Div. Of Remel, Inc.
RAPID STR	Remel Atlanta, Div. Of Remel, Inc.
RAPID TRACE	Zymark Corporation
RAPID VETERINARY DIAGNOSTICS	Sinovus Biotech, Inc.
RAPID WAX	Mds Products, Inc.
RAPID YEAST PLUS	Remel Atlanta, Div. Of Remel, Inc.
RAPID*ENS	Dexall Biomedical Labs, Inc.
RAPID-CLEAR	Sellstrom Manufacturing Co.
RAPID-EZ	Techno-Aide, Inc.
RAPID-FILL	Baxa Corporation
RAPIDBLUE	Cardium Therapeutics Inc.
RAPIDCOMM	Siemens Healthcare Diagnostics Inc.
RAPIDIFF	Cytocolor, Inc.
RAPIDLAB	Siemens Healthcare Diagnostics Inc.
RAPIDLINE	Pacific Precision Laboratories, Inc.
RAPIDOT	Remel
RAPIDOT	Remel Atlanta, Div. Of Remel, Inc.
RAPIDPLATE	Caliper Life Sciences, Inc.
RAPIDPOINT	Siemens Healthcare Diagnostics Inc.
RAPIDRESPONSE HUT	Medical Positioning, Inc.
RAPIDRUN	Usb Corporation
RAPIDSCAN	Rozinn By Scottcare Corporation
RAPIDSTORE	Eklin Medical Systems
RAPIDSTUDY	Eklin Medical Systems
RAPIDTRACE SPE WORKSTATION	Caliper Life Sciences, Inc.
RAPIDTRANSIT	Cordis Neurovascular, Inc.
RAPIDVAP	Labconco Corp.
RAPIDVET	Dms Laboratories, Inc.
RAPIDVUE	Quidel Corporation
RAPTOR	Best Nomos Corp.
RAPTOR PLUS	Nspire Health, Inc
RAREX	Mci Optonix, Div. Of Usr Optonix Inc.
RASCAL POWERCHAIRS	Electric Mobility Corporation
RASCAL SCOOTERS	Electric Mobility Corporation
RATE-PICK	Spirig Advanced Technologies, Inc.
RATESAVER	Welcon, Inc.
RATIOMASTER	Photon Technology International, Inc.
RATURN	Basi (Bioanalytical Systems, Inc.)
RAULERSON	Arrow International, Inc.
RAULERSON	Medcomp (Medical Components, Inc.)
RAULERSON ONE-STEP	Medcomp (Medical Components, Inc.)
RAY BAN	Bausch & Lomb, Vision Care
RAY TFC	Stryker Corp.
RAY TFC	Stryker Spine
RAY TFC/ UNITE	Stryker Corp.
RAY TFC/ UNITE	Stryker Spine
RAY THREADED FUSION CAGE	Stryker Corp.
RAY THREADED FUSION CAGE	Stryker Spine
RAY THREADED FUSION CAGE/ UNITE	Stryker Corp.
RAY THREADED FUSION CAGE/ UNITE	Stryker Spine
RAYCOT	American Silk Sutures, Inc.
RAYOVAC	Rayovac
RAYSHIELD	Aadco Medical, Inc.
RAYTEK	Vespo Marketing Assoc., Inc.
RAYTIDE	Oncogene Research Products
RAZEL	Razel Scientific Instruments, Inc.
RAZOR POINT	Cp Medical Corporation
RAüe	Teleflex Medical
RBT IV	Intoximeters, Inc.
RCD	Rcd Components, Inc.
RCI	Smith & Nephew, Inc., Endoscopy Division
RCOF	Champion, A Gardner Denver Co.
RCOMPRO	Cliniqa Corporation
RCS HIGH FLOW	Biotest Diagnostic Corp.
RCS PLUS	Biotest Diagnostic Corp.
RDF	Her-Mar, Inc.
RDM	Mesa Laboratories, Inc.
RDO RAPID DECALCIFIER	Apex Engineering Products Corp.
RDR (RESPIRATORY DESK REFERENCE)	Mercury Medical
RE SERIES	Starkey Laboratories, Inc.
RE'CORD	Harry J. Bosworth Company
RE-PLY ELECTRODE TENS & NMS	Covidien Lp, Formerly Registered As Uni-Patch
RE-SURG	Bovie Medical Corp.
RE-TRAKE	Smiths Medical Asd
REACT	Immucor, Inc.
READE	Reade Advanced Materials
READI-VAC	Handler Manufacturing Co.
READIGRAFT	Lifenet Health
READIPLASTIN	Instrumentation Laboratory Company
READY LIFT	Noram Solutions
READY RACER	Patterson Medical Holdings, Inc.
READY SENSOR	Siemens Healthcare Diagnostics Inc
READY-BOX	Mallinckrodt, Inc.
READY-FOR-STERILIZATION STOPPERS	Helvoet Pharma, Inc.
READY-ID	Immucor, Inc.
READY-ROLLED	Hollister Incorporated
READY-SCREEN	Immucor, Inc.
READY-SET PUNCTUM PLUGS	Fci Ophthalmics
READY-TO-HANG	Abbott Laboratories
READYFLEX	Medworks Instruments
READYPACK	Carestream Health, Inc.
REAL CPR HELP	Zoll Medical Corp.
REAL EYE	Avotec, Inc.
REAL FRIEND	Avotec, Inc.
REALEYES VIDEO GOGGLES	Micromedical Technologies, Inc.
REALITY	The Female Health Co.
REALITY IMAGE FREE SUPERCABLE	Kinamed, Inc.
REALTIME POSITION MANAGEMENT	Ep Technologies, Inc.
REB	Hartmann-Conco Inc.
REBAR	Ev3 Inc.
REBITE	Medi-Globe Corporation
REBOUND	DJO Surgical
REBOUND	Scott Specialties, Inc./Cmo Inc./Ginny Inc.
REC	Epimed International, Inc.
RECEPTAL	Hospira Inc.
RECLINE-AIR	Pyramid Industries, Llc
RECLOSE-A/REMOVE-A-LID	Whitney Products, Inc.
RECOMBINATE	Baxter International Inc
RECONDITIONED HEARING AIDS	Novasonic
RECORDABLE	Megadyne Medical Products, Inc.
RECORDING RESUSCI ANNE	Laerdal Medical Corporation
RED CAP	B. Braun Oem Division, B. Braun Medical Inc.
RED CROSS	Johnson & Johnson Consumer Products, Inc.
RED DOT	Pre Pak Products, Inc.
RED LIFT BELT CONFIGURATION	Bruno Independent Living Aids, Inc.
RED WING MOTORS	Handler Manufacturing Co.
RED Z	Safetec Of America, Inc.
RED-D-TUBE	Kimble Chase Life Science And Research Products Llc
RED-TIP	Covidien Lp
REDDICK CHOLANGIOGRAM CATHETERS	Lemaitre Vascular, Inc.

REDI CHECK	Awareness Technology, Inc.
REDI HSG PROCEDURE TRAY	Redi-Tech Medical Products,Llc
REDI P-D CATHETER	Redi-Tech Medical Products,Llc
REDI WASH	Precision Dynamics Corp.
REDI+WASH	Donovan Industries
REDI-CHEM	Allied Diagnostic Imaging Resources, Inc.
REDI-FLEX PERCUTANEOUS DRAINAGE CATHETER	Redi-Tech Medical Products,Llc
REDI-FLOW FILTER	Biomet, Inc.
REDI-HSG CATHETER	Redi-Tech Medical Products,Llc
REDI-SEP	Sellstrom Manufacturing Co.
REDI-SHIELD	Rondex Products, Inc.
REDI-TEMP	Trademark Medical Llc
REDI-VACETTE	Biomet, Inc.
REDIGRIP	Biomet, Inc.
REDIREADERS	Magnivision, Inc.
REDONDO TILE	R.C.A. Rubber Company, The
REDONDO TREADS	R.C.A. Rubber Company, The
REDYPLATE	Medical Accessories, Inc.
REEL SPLINT	Reel R&D, Inc.
REFERENCE TIP	Bio Plas, Inc.
REFINERS OF PLATINUM	Glines And Rhodes, Inc.
REFINO	Oscor, Inc.
REFLECTION	Freeman Manufacturing Company
REFLECTION	Smith & Nephew Inc.- Orthopaedics Division
REFLEX	Stryker Corp.
REFLEX	Stryker Spine
REFLEX	Tp Orthodontics, Inc.
REFLEX ELECTRODE TENS & NMS	Covidien Lp, Formerly Registered As Uni-Patch
REFLEX RHOD	Hager Worldwide, Inc.
REFLOTRON	Roche Diagnostics Operations
REFRACTOMETERS	Nsg Precision Cells, Inc.
REFRAX	Anatech, Ltd.
REFRESHING	Palmero Health Care
REFRIG/ARRANGER	Spectrum Laboratories, Inc.
REGAIN	Fasstech
REGAIN	Self Regulation Systems, Inc.
REGAL	Bruno Independent Living Aids, Inc.
REGAL	Golden Technologies, Inc.
REGAL DIE	Pemaco, Inc.
REGANES	Avid Medical
REGENAFIL	Exactech, Inc.
REGENAFORM	Exactech, Inc.
REGENCY	Gendron, Inc.
REGENCY DX	Gendron, Inc.
REGENCY XL	Gendron, Inc.
REGENCY XL POWER	Gendron, Inc.
REGINE	Uni-Fit Co.
REGISIL	Dentsply Caulk
REGRANEX	Johnson & Johnson
REGUDRIVE	Rapid Power Technologies, Inc.
REGULITE	Ultra-Lum, Inc.
REGULUS NAVIGATOR	Compass International, Inc.
REHAB 1	Essential Medical Supply, Inc.
REHAB REACHER	Cme Medical Equipment Corp.
REHAB TNT	Gunnell, Inc.
REHAB WORLD	Complete Medical Supplies, Inc.
REHAB-3	DJO Inc.
REHABILICARE	Compex Technologies, Inc.
REHABILITATION SYSTEM/3	Neurodyne Medical Corp.
REHATUIN	Serologicals Corp
REICHERT	Reichert, Inc.
REINVERTING OPERATING LENS SYTEM	Volk Optical Inc.
REJOICE	Surmodics, Inc.
RELANO	Fla Orthopedics, Inc.
RELAX	Jones-Zylon Company
RELAXER	Golden Technologies, Inc.
RELAXER	Hill-Rom Holdings, Inc.
RELAXO-BAK	Relaxobak, Inc
RELAXOMAT	Futuremed America, Inc.
RELAXSUN	Prosun Tanning International, Llc.
RELAY	Ethicon, Inc.
RELEASE	Pre Pak Products, Inc.
RELEX	Rayovac
RELIANCE	HAAG-STREIT USA, INC.
RELIANCE	Med-Lift & Mobility, Inc.
RELIANCE	Steris Corporation
RELIANT	Concorde Battery
RELIANT	Ricon Corp.
RELIANTT	Valleylab
RELIEF	Bsn-Jobst
RELIEF	Delta Gloves
RELIEF	Nova Health Systems, Inc.
RELIEVA	Acclarent, Inc.
RELISA	Global Focus (G.F.M.D. Ltd.)
RELISA	Immuno Concepts N.A. Ltd.
RELLPLATE	American Diagnostica, Inc.
RELY	Bard Electro Physiology
REM	Hacker Instruments And Industries Inc.
REMARCABLE	Eraser Company, Inc.
REMBRANDT	Johnson & Johnson
REMEDI	Biorad Laboratories
REMEDY	Apollo Corporation
REMEDY HEARING AIDS	Remedy Hearing Aids
REMICADE	Johnson & Johnson
REMINDERPRO	July Soft
REMOTE MONITOR SOFTWARE (RMS)	Mecta Corporation
REMOTE PANEL	Ramvac Dental Products Inc
REMOVE	Smith & Nephew, Inc.
REMRAD	Canberra
REMREST	Medical Industries America Inc.
REMT	Valleylab
REMTRACK	Mirion Technologies
RENAFLO II HEMOFILTER	Minntech Corporation
RENAFLOA,Ar II HEMOFILTERS	Cantel Medical Corp.
RENAISSANCE II	Covidien (Formerly Nellcor Puritan Bennett / Tyco Healthcare)
RENAL LINK	Baxter Healthcare Corporation, Renal
RENALIN	Minntech Corporation
RENALPUREr LIQUID ACID	Rockwell Medical Technologies, Inc.
RENALPUREr POWDER BICARBONATE	Rockwell Medical Technologies, Inc.
RENAPAK	Minntech Corporation
RENASISSANCE	Stryker Medical
RENASOL	Minntech Corporation
RENATRON	Minntech Corporation
RENEW	Microline Pentax, Inc.
RENEWAL	Rayovac
RENOL	Advanced Instruments Inc.
RENOVA	Lifecore Biomedical, Inc.
RENU	Bausch & Lomb, Vision Care
RENU MULTIPLUS	Bausch & Lomb, Vision Care
RENUZYME	Getinge Usa, Inc.
RENUZYME PLUS	Getinge Usa, Inc.
REOPRO	Centocor, Inc.
REP BAND	Magister Corporation
REPAIRRX	The Hymed Group Corp.
REPEATER	Baxa Corporation
REPIPHYSIS	Wright Medical Group, Inc.
REPIRADYNE	Covidien Lp
REPLACEMENT LAMPS FROM	Bulbworks, Inc.
REPLICARE	Smith & Nephew, Inc.
REPLY	Fleetwood Group, Incorporated
REPRORISK	Micromedex, Inc.
REPROSIL	Dentsply Caulk
RES TEST	Conmed Corporation
RES-CUE KEY	Ambu, Inc.
RESCONTROL	Resmed Corp.
RESCUE ALERT	Mytrex, Inc.
RESCUE JENNIFER	Simulaids, Inc.
RESCUE RANDY	Simulaids, Inc.
RESCUELINK	Cardiac Science Corporation (Ca)
RESCUENET	Zoll Medical Corp.
RESCUEREADY	Cardiac Science Corporation (Ca)
RESEARCH COLLECTION	Kewaunee Scientific Corp.
RESEARCH MEDICAL	Edwards Lifesciences, Llc.
RESELUT	Varian Sample Preparation Products

RILEY-ACCESS	Hard Manufacturing Co.
RIM	Remel
RIM	Remel Atlanta, Div. Of Remel, Inc.
RIMWAY	Artcraft New York
RING OF AIR	Span-America Medical Systems, Inc.
RING RETRACT	Covidien Lp, Formerly Registered As United States Surgical
RING-MASTER	Ring Communications, Inc.
RINOFLOW	Respironics New Jersey, Inc.
RIPON	Vista Lighting
RISPI	Medidenta International, Inc.
RITE - HITE	Hill-Rom Holdings, Inc.
RITE TIME	Rite Time Corporation
RITE TIME SYSTEM	Rite Time Corporation
RITE-ACRA	Rite-Dent Manufacturing Corp.
RITE-BOND ONE STEP BONDING	Rite-Dent Manufacturing Corp.
RITE-DENT	South American Dental Export Corp.
RITE-FOIL	Rite-Dent Manufacturing Corp.
RITE-HITE	Seca Corp.
RITE-LIGHT CURING LIGHT	Rite-Dent Manufacturing Corp.
RITE-LINE SYSTEM	Rite-Dent Manufacturing Corp.
RITE-MIX V AMALGAMATOR	Rite-Dent Manufacturing Corp.
RITE-SEALER CEMET	Rite-Dent Manufacturing Corp.
RITE-SPRAY LUBRICATING SPRAY	Rite-Dent Manufacturing Corp.
RITE-TORQUE HAND PIECE	Rite-Dent Manufacturing Corp.
RITE-VINYL	Rite-Dent Manufacturing Corp.
RITELINE	Medi-Dose, Inc.
RITETIME	Rite Time Corporation
RITHM 8, LIFE ALERT, WELTHNESS PROFILE, HR-EGK, NEWTACK	Electronic Design & Research Co., Inc.
RITLENG	Fci Ophthalmics
RITTER	Midmark Corporation
RITTER BY MIDMARK	Midmark Corporation
RIVER'S EDGE TECHNICAL SERVICES	Microstat Laboratories, Inc.
RIZZO DORSAL IMPLANT	Implantech Associates, Inc.
RK	Epimed International, Inc.
RL100 RHINOLARYNGOSCOPE	Welch Allyn, Inc.
RLISYS PRACTICE MANAGEMENT SYSTEMS	Rlisys Practice Solutions, Inc.
RLLE-122	Waldmann Lighting
RM2265, 2255, 2245, 2235 ROTARY MICROTOMES	Leica Microsystems Inc.
RM3	Waters Medical Systems
RMC PRODUCTS	Boeckeler Instruments, Inc.
RMI	Gammex Rmi
RMO	Rmo, Inc.
RMSMANAGER DATABASE SOFTWARE	Mecta Corporation
RMT AQUATICS	Rehamed Intl. Llc.
RMT FITNESS	Rehamed Intl. Llc.
RMT VALVE	Ambu, Inc.
RMbond	Rmo, Inc.
RN+ FALLWATCH	Nurse Assist ,Inc.
RN+ IVALERT	Nurse Assist ,Inc.
RNAGENTS	Promega Corp.
RNASIN	Promega Corp.
RO2	Hydro Service & Supplies, Inc.
ROAD-ROD	Seca Corp.
ROADRUNNER	Wilson-Cook Medical, Inc.
ROAST-N-HOLD	Cres Cor
ROBERTS CLAMP	Halkey-Roberts Corp.
ROBERTS HYDRO THERO PAD	Medical Supplies Corporation T/A.Roberts Manufacturing Co.,
ROBERTSITE	Halkey-Roberts Corp.
ROBI	Karl Storz Endoscopy-America Inc.
ROBINSON	Medtronic Xomed, Inc.
ROBNEL	Covidien Lp
ROBODOC	Integrated Surgical Systems
ROBOT POINTS	Shofu Dental Corporation
ROBOTEST	Soltec Corp.
ROBUSTA CUT	Hager Worldwide, Inc.
ROC-LON	Rockland Industries, Inc.
ROCHESTER BONE BIOPSYT TREPHINE	Medical Innovations International Inc.
ROCHESTER CANNULA CLAMPT	Medical Innovations International Inc.
ROCHESTER FISTULA TRAINING ARMT	Medical Innovations International Inc.
ROCHESTER NASAL SEPTAL BUTTONT	Medical Innovations International Inc.
ROCHESTER OPTICAL	Rochester Optical Mfg. Company
ROCHESTER PATIENT STATUS AND EXAM LIGHTS	Medical Innovations International Inc.
ROCKERS	Hammill International
ROCKET WRAP	Covidien Lp, Formerly Registered As Uni-Patch
ROCKWELLr	Rockwell Medical Technologies, Inc.
RODAC	Bd Diagnostic Systems
RODEO	Convaid Inc.
ROEKO	Charles B. Schwed Co., Inc.
ROGAINE	Johnson & Johnson
ROGUE	United Syntek Corp.
ROHDES	Hammill International
ROHO	Roho Group, The
ROL DEK I	Pawling Corp., Architectural Prod. Div.
ROL DEK II	Pawling Corp., Architectural Prod. Div.
ROLA-CHEM	Specialty Manufacturing Co., The
ROLAIDS	Johnson & Johnson
ROLL AID	Frank Scholz X-Ray Corp.
ROLL MODELS	Hamilton Caster & Mfg. Co.
ROLL-E-ZY	Medi-Dose, Inc.
ROLL-EASY	Essential Medical Supply, Inc.
ROLL-IN RACK	Cres Cor
ROLL-N-STOR	Hamilton Caster & Mfg. Co.
ROLL-TOP	Mit Poly-Cart Corp.
ROLL-UP SUNGLASSES	Klinger Eye Shields, Inc.
ROLL-UPS	Klinger Eye Shields, Inc.
ROLLAR QUAD CANE	Patterson Medical Holdings, Inc.
ROLLER ICE	Polar Products, Inc.
ROLLERVEYOR	Caddy Corporation
ROLLITE	Invacare Corporation
ROLLITURE	Back Support Systems
ROLLOSCOPE M	Broadwest Corp.
ROLLOSCOPE ML	Broadwest Corp.
ROLLS	Invacare Corporation
ROLS	Volk Optical Inc.
ROMA3	Adm Tronics Unlimited, Inc.
ROMCO	Rochester Optical Mfg. Company
RONJAIR	Conmed Linvatec
RONTGOMARKER	Hager Worldwide, Inc.
ROOFRITE	Sellstrom Manufacturing Co.
ROOM SERVICE XPRESS	Computrition, Inc.
ROOM VALET	Harc Mercantile Ltd.
ROOM-ALERT	Hollister Incorporated
ROOM-MATES	Medegen Medical Products, Llc
ROPEGRAB	Sellstrom Manufacturing Co.
ROPELOK	Sellstrom Manufacturing Co.
ROPEVISE	Sellstrom Manufacturing Co.
ROSENTHAL DOSIMETER	Nspire Health, Inc
ROSETTA	General Devices
ROSIDAL K	Lohmann & Rauscher, Inc.
ROSS	Orion Research, Inc.
ROSS ORTHODONTIC EQUIPMENT	Mastercraft Dental Co. Of Texas
ROSWELL	H.L. Bouton Co., Inc.
ROSYS PLATO	Immucor, Inc.
ROT-X-TRACT	Organomation Associates, Inc.
ROTA-PLUS	Packaging Plus, Inc.
ROTACHROM	Diagnostica Stago, Inc.
ROTACLONE	Meridian Bioscience, Inc.
ROTACUT	Medi-Globe Corporation
ROTALASE SPECTRA	Convergent Laser Technologies
ROTALASE XT	Convergent Laser Technologies
ROTARY MICRORIFFLER	Quantachrome
ROTASNARE	Medi-Globe Corporation
ROTATOR SNARE	United States Endoscopy Group
ROTH NET	United States Endoscopy Group
ROTICULATOR	Covidien Lp, Formerly Registered As United States Surgical
ROTILT	Codman & Shurtleff, Inc
ROTO PROX	Hager Worldwide, Inc.
ROTO REST	Kinetic Concepts, Inc.
ROTO-SHAKE GENIE	Scientific Industries, Inc.
ROTOFOR	Bio-Rad Laboratories, Life Science Group
ROTOGRIP	Covidien Lp
ROTOLUX	AMD Technologies Inc.
ROTOR-AID	Advanced Instrument Development, Inc.

ROTORLOC	Smith & Nephew, Inc., Endoscopy Division
ROUGH RIDER	Kareco International, Inc.
ROUGHNECK	Rayovac
ROUGHNECK	Vicon Industries Inc.
ROUND THE CLOCK	Surco Products
ROUNDABOUT	Spaceage Control, Inc.
ROVER EXPRESS	Theradyne Products Division
ROVER PEDIATRIC STRETCHER CRIB	Pedicraft, Inc.
ROXANOL	Roxane Laboratories
ROXANOL 100	Roxane Laboratories
ROXICET	Roxane Laboratories
ROXICODONE	Roxane Laboratories
ROYAL	Covidien Lp, Formerly Registered As United States Surgical
ROYAL	Royal Dental Manufacturing, Inc.
ROYAL	Royal Paper Products, Inc.
ROYAL	Sloan Valve Co.
ROYAL BUZZAROUND	Golden Technologies, Inc.
ROYAL FLUSH	Cook Inc.
ROYAL GENIE	Idea Scientific Co.
ROYAL KNIGHT	Geerpres
ROYAL PRINCE	Geerpres
ROYAL ROCK	Pemaco, Inc.
ROYCE	Ortholine
ROZYNSKI & ASSOCIATES	Rozynski & Associates
RP PARACENTESIS SYSTEM	Gi Supply
RP-7	Intouch Technologies, Inc.
RPI SMART KIT THE ALTERNATE SOURCE	Replacement Parts Industries, Inc.
RPM	Knoll, Inc.
RPM	Varian Medical Systems
RPM FLOW MODULE	Medical Graphics Corporation
RPM SOFTWARE	Medical Graphics Corporation
RS-2I	Rs Medical
RS-2M	Rs Medical
RS-4I	Rs Medical
RS-4M	Rs Medical
RS-SERIES	Taylor Wharton
RS-TENS PLUS	Rs Medical
RS3000	D.M. Davis Inc.
RS3010	D.M. Davis Inc.
RS3104	D.M. Davis Inc.
RSG-61	Sakura Finetek U.S.A., Inc.
RSP SHOULDER	DJO Surgical
RSR	Labac Systems, Inc.
RT THERMOPLASTIC	Wfr/Aquaplast Corp.
RT2	AMD Technologies Inc.
RTAS	Sudbury Systems
RTC	Sellstrom Manufacturing Co.
RTC EXPANDER	Sellstrom Manufacturing Co.
RTI ELECTRONICS AB	Rti Electronics, Inc.
RTS	Newschoff Chairs, Inc.
RTS4000	Mobility Inc.
RU	Oscor, Inc.
RUBALEX	Lifesign
RUBASCAN	Bd Diagnostic Systems
RUBBER SEP	George Taub Products & Fusion Co., Inc.
RUBBERMAID COMMERCIAL PRODUCTS	Rubbermaid Commercial Products Llc
RUBELLA-PLUS	Wampole Laboratories
RUBYLASE	Coopersurgical, Inc.
RUBYTAQ	Usb Corporation
RUGGED	Stryker Corp.
RUGGED	Stryker Medical
RUGGED TOUCH	C.A.M. Graphics Co., Inc.
RUSH	Rush-Berivon, Inc.
RUSSELL-TAYLOR-DELTA	Smith & Nephew Inc.- Orthopaedics Division
RVS	Vitalcom, Inc.
RWF-1000	Mizuho Osi
RX FIT	Elastic Therapy, Inc.
RX HONING MACHINE	Rx Honing Machine Corporation
RX90	Biomet, Inc.
RXB	I.B.F. Corporation
RXE-SOURCE	Cardinal Health Inc.
RXG	I.B.F. Corporation
RXLOG	Westmed, Inc.
RXLOG COMMUNICATOR	Westmed, Inc.
RXSHREDDER	Marathon Equipment Company
RXSPECT	Analytical Spectral Devices, Inc.
RYCOR	Rycor Medical, Inc.
RYNO LACER	Medical Specialties, Inc.
RZ	Meiji Techno America
RZ	Oscor, Inc.
Radial Jaw	Boston Scientific Corporation
Radius	Micro-Tech
Rainbath	Ortho Dermatologics
Rapid Clear	Ortho Dermatologics
Rapid Programmer	St. Jude Medical Neuromodulation Division
Razor Defense	Ortho Dermatologics
ReNu	Bausch & Lomb
Reflexion	St. Jude Medical, Inc.
Reflexion Spiral	St. Jude Medical, Inc.
Regency	St. Jude Medical, Inc.
Renegade	Boston Scientific Corporation
Renew	St. Jude Medical Neuromodulation Division
Renew	St. Jude Medical, Inc.
Reo Go	Healthsouth Corporation
Repliform	Boston Scientific Corporation
Resilon	Pentron Laboratory Technologies
Resolution	Boston Scientific Corporation
Response	St. Jude Medical, Inc.
Resting Heart	Medtronic Perfusion Systems
Retisert	Bausch & Lomb
Reveal	Medtronic, Inc.
Rheumatex	Inverness Medical Professional Diagnostics-San Die
RhoGAM	Ortho Clinical Diagnostics, Inc.
RhoGAM	Ortho-Clinical Diagnostics, Inc.
Riata	St. Jude Medical, Inc.
Rocky Mountain	Rmo, Inc.
Rotablator	Boston Scientific - Maple Grove
Rotablator	Boston Scientific Corporation
Rotatest	Inverness Medical Professional Diagnostics-San Die
Rubella-Plus	Inverness Medical Professional Diagnostics-San Die
RxMD	Rpi Of Atlanta
S	Synovis Life Technologies, Inc
S SERIES	Sonosite, Inc.
S&S	Schleicher & Schuell, Inc.
S&S DISPOSABLE, K-WIRE DRIVER	S & S Orthopedic Ltd.
S'PORT ALL	The Saunders Group
S'PORT MAX	The Saunders Group
S-1	Safety 1st Medical, Inc.
S-2222	Instrumentation Laboratory Company
S-6000 IV POLES	Medved Products, Inc.
S-EVAP	Organomation Associates, Inc.
S-SCORT	Sscor
S-SEDIVETTE	Sarstedt, Inc.
S-STENT	Biosensors International - Usa
S.M.A.R.T.	Cordis Corporation
S.T.F.	Streck Laboratories, Inc.
S.T.R.	Alpha Communications
S.T.S.	Aetrex Worldwide, Inc
S.W.A.S.H.	Nelson Prosthetic & Orthotic Laboratory
S.W.C.T.	Stereo Optical Co., Inc.
S/5	Ge Medical Systems Information Technologies
S1	Karl Storz Endoscopy-America Inc.
S210	Polar Electro Inc.
S3	Karl Storz Endoscopy-America Inc.
S410	Polar Electro Inc.
S610	Polar Electro Inc.
S710	Polar Electro Inc.
S8	Resmed Corp.
S810	Polar Electro Inc.
SABA	Noram Solutions
SABEE	R. Sabee Company
SABER	Arthrocare Corp.
SABER	Aspen Surgical
SABER	Flowtronics, Inc.
SABER 2000	Flowtronics, Inc.
SABER 2100	Flowtronics, Inc.

SABER DRILL	Stryker Corp.
SABINA	Liko North America
SABLE	Boss Instruments, Ltd.
SABLE	Havel's Inc.
SABLE COMBO BRUSHES	American Diversified Dental Systems
SABLE TUNGSTON CARBIDE NEEDLE HOLDERS	Micrins Surgical Instruments, Inc.
SABRE	Conmed Corporation
SABRE 180 ESU	Conmed Corporation
SABRE 2400 ESU	Conmed Corporation
SABRELOC	Ethicon, Inc.
SAC TEETHGUARDS	Superior Autocatheter Enterprises
SACRO-CINCH	Bell-Horn, Inc.
SACRO-EASE	Mccarty's Sacro-Ease Llc
SACRO-GUARD	Bell-Horn, Inc.
SACRO-MESH	Bell-Horn, Inc.
SAF-D-FIB	Conmed Corporation
SAF-STOR	Sellstrom Manufacturing Co.
SAF-T E-Z SET	Becton Dickinson Infusion Therapy Systems, Inc.
SAF-T-CURE	U.V. Process Supply, Inc.
SAF-T-DRAPE	Advanced Medical Innovations, Inc.
SAF-T-FLO	Smiths Medical Asd
SAF-T-GRIP	Advanced Medical Innovations, Inc.
SAF-T-INTIMA	Becton Dickinson Infusion Therapy Systems, Inc.
SAF-T-POLE	Advanced Medical Innovations, Inc.
SAF-T-POLE	American Medical Mfg., Inc.
SAF-T-PRODUCTS	Advanced Medical Innovations, Inc.
SAF-T-SCALPEL	Advanced Medical Innovations, Inc.
SAF-T-SEAL	Advanced Medical Innovations, Inc.
SAF-T-SHELL	Advanced Medical Innovations, Inc.
SAF-T-SHIELD	Advanced Medical Innovations, Inc.
SAF-T-TRAY	Advanced Medical Innovations, Inc.
SAF-T-VIEW	Advanced Medical Innovations, Inc.
SAFARI	Ranger All Season Corp.
SAFARI LTD	Ranger All Season Corp.
SAFARI TILT	Convaid Inc.
SAFE & DRY	Hygienics Industries Div.Of Kleinert's, Inc.
SAFE AND DRY FOR HIM	Hygienics Industries Div.Of Kleinert's, Inc.
SAFE CELL - ETO ABATEMENT EQUIPMENT	Advanced Air Technologies, Inc.
SAFE CROSS	Kensey Nash Corporation
SAFE KLEAN KIT	Geritrex Corp.
SAFE PLACE	Rf Technologies
SAFE SOUND	Mckeon Products, Inc.
SAFE STRIPS	Healthcare Labels, Inc.
SAFE SYSTEM	Edge Systems Corporation
SAFE T WEDGE	Medical Positioning, Inc.
SAFE TAPE	Healthcare Labels, Inc.
SAFE-1	Safety 1st Medical, Inc.
SAFE-1 SAFETY SYRINGE	Xenotec Ltd.
SAFE-CHOICE	Medegen Medical Products, Llc
SAFE-CONNECT	Intravascular Incorporated
SAFE-CROSS	Intraluminal Therapeutics, Inc.
SAFE-CUFF	Cas Medical Systems, Inc.
SAFE-DWEL PLUS	Becton Dickinson Infusion Therapy Systems, Inc.
SAFE-EDGE	Trident Medical Products
SAFE-FILL	Q.I. Medical, Inc.
SAFE-JAW	Boss Instruments, Ltd.
SAFE-KEEPER	Whitney Products, Inc.
SAFE-POINT	North American Medical Products, Inc.
SAFE-STEER	Intraluminal Therapeutics, Inc.
SAFE-T-CHEK	Sdi Diagnostics, Inc.
SAFE-T-COUNT GLOVES	Medical Action Industries, Inc
SAFE-T-FILL	Ram Scientific, Inc.
SAFE-T-FOLD	Sellstrom Manufacturing Co.
SAFE-T-GAUGE	Utah Medical Products, Inc.
SAFE-T-J	Cook Inc.
SAFE-T-LANCE	Htl-Strefa, Inc.
SAFE-T-LANCE PLUS	Htl-Strefa, Inc.
SAFE-T-LIFT	Fla Orthopedics, Inc.
SAFE-T-SCREEN	Advanced Medical Innovations, Inc.
SAFE-T-SHIELD	Boston Medical Products, Inc.
SAFE-T-SPORT	Fla Orthopedics, Inc.
SAFE-T-TREADS	Albahealth Llc
SAFE-T-TRED	Precept Medical Products, Inc.
SAFE-T-TUBE	Boston Medical Products, Inc.
SAFE-T-VIEW	Sellstrom Manufacturing Co.
SAFE-T-WRIST	Fla Orthopedics, Inc.
SAFE-TEL	Webb Manufacturing Co.
SAFECAN	B. Braun Oem Division, B. Braun Medical Inc.
SAFECAP	Safe-Tec Clinical Products, Inc.
SAFECARE	Techstyles Manufacturing Division
SAFECLEAN	Aspen Surgical
SAFECLEAN	Sterion, Incorporated
SAFECLEAR	E K Industries, Inc.
SAFECRIT	Statspin, Inc.
SAFECUT	Orbusneich Medical, Inc.
SAFEFLEX	Ims-Ess
SAFEGRIP	Microflex Corporation
SAFEGUARD	Bagco
SAFEGUARD	Kinetikos Medical, Inc.
SAFEGUARD	Precision Dynamics Corp.
SAFEGUARD 950	Jeron Electronic Systems, Inc.
SAFEGUIDE	Medovations, Inc.
SAFELEAD	Astro-Med, Inc.
SAFELINE	B. Braun Oem Division, B. Braun Medical Inc.
SAFEMARK	Intec Industries, Inc.
SAFEPETTE	Safe-Tec Clinical Products, Inc.
SAFEPREP	American Health Products Corporation
SAFESEAL	Possis Medical, Inc.
SAFESET	Hospira Inc.
SAFESKIN	Kerr Group
SAFESTART	Becton Dickinson Infusion Therapy Systems, Inc.
SAFETEC BURN GEL & BURN SPRAY	Safetec Of America, Inc.
SAFETEC STING RELIEF	Safetec Of America, Inc.
SAFETEMP	Hoshizaki America, Inc.
SAFETEX CLASSIC	Andwin Scientific
SAFETEX NO TOUCH	Andwin Scientific
SAFETOUCH	Dynarex Corp.
SAFETRACE	Wyndgate Technologies
SAFETRACE TX	Wyndgate Technologies
SAFETWAY	Vitalograph, Inc.
SAFETY	American Healthcare Products, Inc.
SAFETY 1ST	Safety 1st Medical, Inc.
SAFETY CLEAN	H.L. Bouton Co., Inc.
SAFETY DEX	Micromedex, Inc.
SAFETY EDGE	Span-America Medical Systems, Inc.
SAFETY ROLLER	Wenzelite Rehab Supplies, Llc
SAFETY ROLLER CONTROLLER	Conmed Corporation
SAFETY SYRINGES	Safety Syringe Corporation Of America, Inc.
SAFETY TIP	Conmed Corporation
SAFETY YELLOW	Woodhead L.P.
SAFETY-SOFT	Bio-Medical Products Corp.
SAFETYAMP	Haskel International, Inc.
SAFETYCLEAN	H.L. Bouton Co., Inc.
SAFEWAY	Woodhead L.P.
SAFHS	Exogen, Inc.
SAFSITE	B. Braun Medical Inc., Renal Therapies Div.
SAFSITE	B. Braun Oem Division, B. Braun Medical Inc.
SAFTEVAC	Dermatologic Lab & Supply, Inc.
SAGE	Orion Research, Inc.
SAGER	Minto R&D, Inc.
SAGIAN	Beckman Coulter Inc. (Sagian Operation)
SAHARA	Hologic, Inc.
SAKURA	Sakura Finetek U.S.A., Inc.
SAL	Tp Orthodontics, Inc.
SAL DRI	George Taub Products & Fusion Co., Inc.
SAL-ACID PLASTERS	Pedinol Pharmacal, Inc.
SAL-PLANT	Pedinol Pharmacal, Inc.
SALACTIC FILM	Pedinol Pharmacal, Inc.
SALEM	Covidien Lp
SALES EDUCATION CREDITS	Veritech Corporation
SALIBAG	Hager Worldwide, Inc.
SALINOCAINE	Premier Medical Products
SALITRON SYSTEM	Biosonics, Inc.
SALIVART	Gebauer Company
SALIVASAC	Pacific Biometrics, Inc.

SALLI	Hager Worldwide, Inc.
SALMAN	Boston Medical Products, Inc.
SALMONELLA-TEK	Biomerieux Inc.
SALON PRO	Oster Professional Products, Inc.
SALON TEXTURED SYSTEM	Oster Professional Products, Inc.
SALSA	Duxbury Systems, Inc.
SALTER EYES	Salter Labs
SALTER LABS	Dma Med-Chem Corporation
SALTER STYLE	Salter Labs
SALTIME	Boston Rheology, L.L.C.
SAM SPLINT	Seaberg Company Inc., The
SAM-THE STUDENT AUSCULTATION MANIKIN	Cardionics, Inc.
SAMARITAN LIFTS	Sani-Med, A Division Of Sanderson Plumbing Products, Inc.
SAMCO	Samco Scientific Corporation
SAMMANN SHARP CUT	Sammann Co., See Aids Div.
SAMPLE LOCK	Hamilton Company
SAMPLE SENTINEL	Basi (Bioanalytical Systems, Inc.)
SAMPLE-STAT	Sartorius Stedim Sus Inc.
SAMPLER	Wilson-Cook Medical, Inc.
SAMPLETTE	Covidien Lp
SAMPLINK	Fenwal Inc.
SAMPLXTRACTOR	Quintron Instrument Company
SAMPULE	Wheaton Science Products
SAMSON AND DELILAHr	Sigvaris Inc.
SAND BAGS	Cfi Medical Solutions (Contour Fabricators, Inc.)
SANI MED	Sani-Med, A Division Of Sanderson Plumbing Products, Inc.
SANI TRUX	Mcclure Industries, Inc.
SANI WASH	Mcclure Industries, Inc.
SANI-BABY	Simulaids, Inc.
SANI-BRACKET	Professional Disposables International, Inc.
SANI-CLOTH	Professional Disposables International, Inc.
SANI-DEX	Professional Disposables International, Inc.
SANI-DEX ALC	Professional Disposables International, Inc.
SANI-GRINDER	Handler Manufacturing Co.
SANI-LOK	Rpc
SANI-MAN	Simulaids, Inc.
SANI-PANT	Salk Inc.
SANI-RAIL	Independent Solutions, Inc.
SANI-ROLLS	Crosstex International,Inc.
SANI-TABS	Crosstex International,Inc.
SANI-TIP	Dentsply International, Inc.
SANI-TIP	Dentsply Professional
SANI-TIP	Dentsply Prosthetics
SANI-TUBE	Crosstex International,Inc.
SANI-VAC	Handler Manufacturing Co.
SANI-WIPE	Professional Disposables International, Inc.
SANICARE	Crosstex International,Inc.
SANICLENZ	Crosstex International,Inc.
SANICURE	Dentsply Caulk
SANIGARM	Hy-Tape International
SANISEPT	Crosstex International,Inc.
SANISORB	Multisorb Technologies, Inc.
SANITAIRE	Atlantic Ultraviolet Corp.
SANITANE	Deb Sbs, Inc.
SANITEX	Life Guard
SANITEX PLUS	Crosstex International,Inc.
SANITEX PLUS,SANITYZE, SANITAB	Crosstex International
SANITHERM SYSTEMS II	Tidi Products, Llc
SANITIZE HH	Hal-Hen Company, Inc.
SANITOR	Sanitor Manufacturing Co.
SANITRON	Atlantic Ultraviolet Corp.
SANIWASH	Safetec Of America, Inc.
SANIZIDE PLUS	Safetec Of America, Inc.
SANOS	Mwi Veterinary Supply
SANPARREL RIGID VINYL SHEET	Inpro Corporation
SANTAIR	Santek, Div. Tjernlund Products, Inc.
SAPHLITE	Genzyme
SAPHLITE	Teleflex Medical
SAPPHIRE	Orbusneich Medical, Inc.
SAPPHIRE-II	Applied Biosystems
SARATOGA CYCLE	Rand-Scot Inc.
SARATORIUS	Utech Products, Inc.
SARITA	ArjoHuntleigh

SARMIX	Sarstedt, Inc.
SARNS	Terumo Cardiovascular Systems, Corp
SARPETTE	Sarstedt, Inc.
SAS	Sa Scientific, Inc.
SAT	Kinetic Concepts, Inc.
SAT PAD	Alliance Pharmaceutical Corp.
SATELLITE	Jones Medical Instrument Co.
SATIN STEEL COLOURS	Hu-Friedy Manufacturing Co., Inc.
SATIN STEEL XTS	Hu-Friedy Manufacturing Co., Inc.
SATIN STONE	Pemaco, Inc.
SATURN	Dent Zar, Inc.
SATURN	G & H Wire Co.
SATURN	H.L. Bouton Co., Inc.
SAUFERA	Hydrofera Llc
SAVANT	Academy Savant
SAVARY	Wilson-Cook Medical, Inc.
SAVE	Hemcon Medical Technologies, Inc.
SAVUR FUNNEL	Ge Infrastructure Water & Process Technologies
SAVVY PTA DILATATION CATHETER	Cordis Endovascular
SAWBONES	Pacific Research Laboratories, Inc.
SB OFFICE	Sdi Diagnostics, Inc.
SBB	Psyche Systems
SBG	American Gas & Chemical Co., Ltd.
SBG	Sdi Diagnostics, Inc.
SBS	Storage Battery Systems, Inc.
SBS DEEP CYCLE	Storage Battery Systems, Inc.
SBW	Medical Action Industries, Inc
SC-STIM-KATH	Epimed International, Inc.
SC81	Televideo Systems, Inc.
SCA	Sakura Finetek U.S.A., Inc.
SCAFFOLD FOAM	Kensey Nash Corporation
SCALDSAFE	Ulster Scientific, Inc.
SCALERITE	Medidenta International, Inc.
SCALTEC	Utech Products, Inc.
SCAN	Parker Laboratories, Inc.
SCAN C	Mallinckrodt, Inc.
SCAN MATE II	Circadian Systems
SCAN-IT	George Taub Products & Fusion Co., Inc.
SCANCOAT	Cfi Medical Solutions (Contour Fabricators, Inc.)
SCANDIA SL	Surgical Table Services Co.
SCANDITONIX DOSIMETRY	Scanditronix - Wellhofer North America
SCANLAN	Scanlan International, Inc.
SCANLAN SOLEM	Scanlan International, Inc.
SCANLAN STERN	Scanlan International, Inc.
SCANLAN SUPER CUT	Scanlan International, Inc.
SCANLAN ULTIMATE	Scanlan International, Inc.
SCANLAN ULTRA SHARP	Scanlan International, Inc.
SCANLAN V.I.P.	Scanlan International, Inc.
SCANLISA	Scimedx Corporation
SCANMATEPRO	Coherent, Inc.
SCANNING WORKBENCH	Brit Systems Inc.
SCANPOR TAPE	Allerderm Laboratories, Inc.
SCANRITE	Smith Companies Dental Products
SCANSCOPE	Aperio Technologies Inc.
SCANVIEW	Solarius Development Inc.
SCARFADE	Hanson Medical, Inc.
SCATTER	Surco Products
SCATTER-BAN	Morgan Medesign, Inc.
SCB	Karl Storz Endoscopy-America Inc.
SCD	Terumo Medical Corp.
SCEPTOR	Bd Diagnostic Systems
SCEPTRE	Hitachi Medical Systems America, Inc.
SCHELL EMDEE BAG	Schell, Inc.
SCHELL HANDIKIT	Schell, Inc.
SCHELL NURSE TOTE	Schell, Inc.
SCHELL TRAUMA 911	Schell, Inc.
SCHLEIN ULTRA SHOULDER POSITIONER	Mizuho Osi
SCHOLTEN	Scholten Surgical Instruments, Inc.
SCHOLTEN BIOPTOME	Scholten Surgical Instruments, Inc.
SCHOOL DAF	Casa Futura Technologies
SCHRADER	Armstrong Medical Industries, Inc.
SCHURMED	Schuerch Corp.
SCHWINN FITNESS	Med-Fit Systems, Inc.

SCHWINN FITNESS	Nautilus, Inc.
SCI-DENT	Sci-Dent, Inc.
SCI-PHARM	Scientific Pharmaceuticals, Inc.
SCI-SPAN	Scientific Pharmaceuticals, Inc.
SCI/ERA	Bellco Glass, Inc.
SCIENTECH	Scientech, Inc.
SCIMAGE, PICOM, NETRA, METRAMD, PICOMENTERPRISE, PICOMONLINE	Scimage, Inc.
SCINTIPLATE	Perkin Elmer Wallac, Inc.
SCINTIPLATE	Perkinelmer Life And Analytical Sciences
SCINTISTRIP	Perkin Elmer Wallac, Inc.
SCINTISTRIP	Perkinelmer Life And Analytical Sciences
SCISSORVALVE	Quintron Instrument Company
SCLEROLASER	Candela Corp.
SCLEROPLUS	Candela Corp.
SCLEROSOL	Bryan Corp.
SCOLIOMETER	Mizuho Osi
SCOLIOSIS TREATMENT RECOVERY SYSTEM (STRS)	Stars
SCOOP	Transtracheal Systems, Inc.
SCOOTER LIFT JR.	Bruno Independent Living Aids, Inc.
SCOOTER LIFT MFG., INC.	Silver Star Mobility
SCOOTER LIFT SR.	Bruno Independent Living Aids, Inc.
SCOPE	Smith & Nephew, Inc.
SCOPE INTRODUCER	N.M. Beale Co. Inc.
SCOPECARE	DJO Inc.
SCOPEGUARD	Arc Medical, Inc.
SCOPEPAK	Riley Medical, Inc.
SCOPEPAK	Symmetry Medical Usa, Inc.
SCOPEPAK	Symmetry Medical, Inc.
SCOPESAFE	Armstrong Medical Industries, Inc.
SCOPETOTE	Gi Supply
SCOPETTES	Birchwood Laboratories, Inc.
SCOPIX	Agfa Corporation
SCORED	Aluwax Dental Products Co.
SCORPIO NRG	Stryker Corp.
SCORPIO NRG	Stryker Howmedica Osteonics
SCORPIO SINGLE AXIS	Stryker Corp.
SCORPIO SINGLE AXIS	Stryker Howmedica Osteonics
SCORPIO TS	Stryker Corp.
SCORPIO TS	Stryker Howmedica Osteonics
SCOTCH-WELD	3m Co.
SCOTCHBOND	3m Espe Dental Products
SCOTCHBOND 2	3m Espe Dental Products
SCOTCHBRITE	3m Espe Dental Products
SCOTCHPRINT	3m Co.
SCOTSMAN	Scotsman Industries
SCOTT	Scott Specialties, Inc./Cmo Inc./Ginny Inc.
SCOTT FOOT CARE	Aetna Foot Products/Div. Of Aetna Felt Corporation
SCOTT RESOURCES	Aristotle Corp.
SCOTTY THE SCALE	Seca Corp.
SCOUT	Convaid Inc.
SCOUT	Leisure-Lift, Inc.
SCOUT CORNEAL TOPOGRAPHER	Eyequip, Div Of Alliance Medical Marketing
SCREAMING EAGLE	Eagle Sports Chairs
SCREEN VAC	Quality Aspirators
SCREEN-A-GENE	Bio-Rad Laboratories, Life Science Group
SCREENLENS MAGNIFIER	Roldan Products Corp.
SCREENMATES	Thermo Fisher Scientific
SCREENSTAR	Morgan Scientific Inc.
SCREENWIPE	H.L. Bouton Co., Inc.
SCREW-VENT	Zimmer Dental, Inc.
SCRIBE	AMD Technologies Inc.
SCROTO-PAK	Lone Star Medical Products, Inc.
SCRUB-FREE	Ecolab Inc.
SCRUB-WARE	Whitehall Manufacturing
SCRUBIDINE	Medical Chemical Corp.
SCS	Orthotec, Llc
SCS SPINAL SYSTEM	Orthotec, Llc
SCS-CLARIS	Orthotec, Llc
SCT 3000	Vital Signs Colorado
SCT-2000	Vital Signs Colorado
SCULPTOR	Oster Professional Products, Inc.
SCULPTORSr	Sigvaris Inc.

SD (MBM)	Zivic Laboratories
SD1	Northgate Technologies Inc.
SD100	Northgate Technologies Inc.
SDC HD	Stryker Endoscopy
SDI-BIOM	Insight Instruments, Inc.
SDM	Electone, A Division Of Siemens Hearing Instruments, Inc.
SDR (SURGICAL DESK REFERENCE)	Mercury Medical
SDS	Sds (Summit Dental Systems)
SEA SOAKS	Circulator Boot Corp.
SEA-SLIDE	Hydromer, Inc.
SEAB	Pacific Research Laboratories, Inc.
SEAL AND PEEL	Andersen Products, Inc.,
SEAL FLEX	Amici, Inc.
SEAL TITE	Smith & Nephew, Inc.
SEAL'N SNIP	Gammadirect Medical Division
SEAL-RITE	Amici, Inc.
SEAL-TIGHT	Brown Medical Industries
SEAL-UP	Covidien Lp, Formerly Registered As United States Surgical
SEALIDENT	Precision Dynamics Corp.
SEALY	Sealy Inc.
SEALY POSTUREMATIC	Sealy Inc.
SEALY SAKER	Sealy Inc.
SEASCAPE	Graham Medical Products/Div. Of Little Rapids Corp
SEASPECr	Analytical Spectral Devices, Inc.
SEAT LEVEL	Span-America Medical Systems, Inc.
SEAT2GO	Wenzelite Rehab Supplies, Llc
SEATTLE LIMB SYSTEMS	Seattle Systems
SEATTLE/SYSTEMS	Ortholine
SEAWAY	Geerpres
SEBRA	Engineering & Research Assoc., Inc. (D.B.A. Sebra)
SEBRA RF SYSTEMS	Engineering & Research Assoc., Inc. (D.B.A. Sebra)
SEBRING	Sellstrom Manufacturing Co.
SECA	Creative Health Products, Inc.
SECOND SONATHERM	Misonix, Inc.
SECONDLOOK	Icad Inc.
SECRET EAR	Starkey Laboratories, Inc.
SECUR SITE	Smiths Medical Asd, Inc.
SECUR-FIT MAX	Stryker Corp.
SECUR-FIT MAX	Stryker Howmedica Osteonics
SECUR-FIT PLUS MAX	Stryker Corp.
SECUR-FIT PLUS MAX	Stryker Howmedica Osteonics
SECURE	G. Hirsch & Co.
SECURE	Imtec, A 3m Company
SECURE	Smiths Medical OEM
SECURE	Stryker Corp.
SECURE	Stryker Medical
SECURE	The Metrix Co.
SECURE CARE PRODUCTS	Secure Care Products, Inc.
SECURE CARE SYSTEMS	Secure Care Products, Inc.
SECURE LOOP	Crosstex International,Inc.
SECURE NETWORK INTERFACE	Dawning Technologies, Inc.
SECURE SOFT	Imtec, A 3m Company
SECURE-ET, LEAD SAVER	Neotech Products, Inc.
SECURE-GARD	Cardinal Health Inc.
SECURE-IT	Healthmark Industries
SECURE-IT-Y	Advanced Medical Innovations, Inc.
SECURE-ITT	Passy-Muir Inc.
SECURE-LOK	Gresham Driving Aids, Inc.
SECURECARE	Hard Manufacturing Co.
SECUREFIT	Ocular Instruments, Inc.
SECUREIT	Sterion, Incorporated
SECURELOC	Specialized Health Products International, Inc.
SECURELY YOURS	Paperpak
SECURESEAT	Columbia Medical Manufacturing Llc
SECURITY HARDWARE	Timekeeping Systems, Inc.
SECURITr BANKING & FINANCIAL PRODUCTS	Pm Company
SECURLINE	Precision Dynamics Corp.
SECURLINK	Precision Dynamics Corp.
SECURSNAP	Precision Dynamics Corp.
SED-CHEK CONTROL	Polymedco, Inc.
SED-CONNECT	Medical Chemical Corp.
SED-RITE PLUS	R & D Systems, Inc.
SEDECAL X-RAY EQUIPMENT	Medlink Imaging, Inc.

SEDI-PET	Samco Scientific Corporation
SEDI-RATE	Globe Scientific, Inc.
SEDI-TECT	Globe Scientific, Inc.
SEDIGREN	Globe Scientific, Inc.
SEDIMAT	Polymedco, Inc.
SEDIPLAST	Polymedco, Inc.
SEDIPLUS	Sarstedt, Inc.
SEDITEN	Polymedco, Inc.
SEE MORE. DO MORE	Agfa Corporation
SEE-AID OPTICAL	Sammann Co., See Aids Div.
SEE-THRU CPR	Zoll Medical Corp.
SEER	Ge Medical Systems Information Technologies
SEG-SAFE	Alpha Scientific Corporation
SEGAL	Dermatologic Lab & Supply, Inc.
SEIKO	Eric Armin Inc.
SEIRIN	Seirin-America, Inc.
SEL-FIT	Sellstrom Manufacturing Co.
SEL-SNAP	Sellstrom Manufacturing Co.
SEL-STOR	Sellstrom Manufacturing Co.
SELAN	Span-America Medical Systems, Inc.
SELEC-3	Biomedix, Inc.
SELECT	Argen Corp.
SELECT	Cordis Neurovascular, Inc.
SELECT	Principle Business Enterprises, Inc.
SELECT (AUD. TRAINER)	Telex Communications, Inc.-Hearing Instrument Grp.
SELECT IUI	Select Medical Systems
SELECT ONE	Conmed Corporation
SELECT SERIES	Spectronics Corporation
SELECT SHOULDER SYSTEM	Centerpulse Orthopedics Inc.
SELECTABLES	Profex Medical Products
SELECTCELLS MINI	Select Medical Systems
SELECTCELLS STANDARD	Select Medical Systems
SELECTIVE VERTICAL CONVEYOR SYSTEM	Swisslog Translogic Corporation
SELECTLITE	Arkray Usa
SELECTMUCUS	Select Medical Systems
SELECTOLUX	AMD Technologies Inc.
SELECTOR	Integra Lifesciences Holdings Corp.
SELECTRA	United Chemical Technologies, Inc.
SELECTRA-SIL	United Chemical Technologies, Inc.
SELECTRON LDR/MDR	Nucletron Corporation
SELENIA	Hologic, Inc.
SELF CATH CLOSED SYSTEM	Mentor Corp.
SELF-CATH	Mentor Corp.
SELF-CATH PLUS	Mentor Corp.
SELF-ZEROING	Kimble Chase Life Science And Research Products Llc
SELL GARD	Sellstrom Manufacturing Co.
SELLERS & JOSEPHSON	Shelby-Williams Industries
SELLSTROM	Sellstrom Manufacturing Co.
SELLSTROM SAFEGUARD	Sellstrom Manufacturing Co.
SELLSTROM SAFEGUARDS	Sellstrom Manufacturing Co.
SELLSTROM STA-CLEAR	Sellstrom Manufacturing Co.
SELLSTROM/ RTC	Sellstrom Manufacturing Co.
SEM	Security Engineered Machinery
SEMCO	Independent Solutions, Inc.
SEMEN ANALYSIS EXPERTS	Fertility Solutions, Inc.
SEMPER PURE RO	Mar Cor Purification
SENIOR CIRCUIT	Med-Fit Systems, Inc.
SENIOR FRIENDLY	Briggs Corporation
SENSAFLEX	Chattanooga Group
SENSAID	Sensidyne, Inc.
SENSAIR	Sensidyne, Inc.
SENSALARM	Sensidyne, Inc.
SENSALERT	Sensidyne, Inc.
SENSAMATIC	World Dryer Corp.
SENSATEC	Rf Technologies
SENSATOUCH	Biolase Technology, Inc.
SENSERX, CONTROLWORKS	Self Regulation Systems, Inc.
SENSI GRIP	Tillotson Healthcare Corp.
SENSI-DISC	Bd Diagnostic Systems
SENSI-TOUCH	Ansell Healthcare Products, Inc.
SENSI-TOUCH	Covidien Lp
SENSIA	Medtronic, Inc.
SENSIBLE	Zyloware Corporation
SENSIDYNE/KITAGAWA	Sensidyne, Inc.
SENSIFLEX	American Healthcare Products, Inc.
SENSIFOOT	Bsn-Jobst
SENSIMATIC	Parkell, Inc.
SENSISCOPE	Her-Mar, Inc.
SENSITEX	Oak Gloves Division Of Omar Medical Supplies, Inc.
SENSITIPS	Dentalez Group
SENSITITRE ARIS 2X SYSTEM	Trek Diagnostic Systems
SENSITITRE ID/AST SYSTEM	Trek Diagnostic Systems
SENSITIVE EYES	Bausch & Lomb, Vision Care
SENSITUBE	Osmetech, Inc.
SENSO2	Invacare Corporation
SENSOLOG	Siemens Medical Solutions Usa, Inc.
SENSOR	Medworks Instruments
SENSORS	Enviro Guard, Inc.
SENSORSAFE	Follett Corp.
SENSORTEC	Vespo Marketing Assoc., Inc.
SENSORVISION CCTV	Sensormatic Electronics
SENSUA! PERSONAL LUBRICANT	Retroactive Bioscience
SENTINEL	Calypte Biomedical Corporation
SENTINEL	Dr Systems, Inc.
SENTINEL	Harc Mercantile Ltd.
SENTINEL	Jeron Electronic Systems, Inc.
SENTINEL	Zettler Systems, Inc.
SENTINEL SEAL	Covidien Lp
SENTINEL VRM	Engler Engineering Corp.
SENTRY	J&S Medical Associates
SENTRY	Life Guard
SENTRY	Precision Dynamics Corp.
SENTRY	Whitney Products, Inc.
SENTRY EMERGENCY CALL SYSTEM	Heritage Medcall
SENTRYWASH	Sellstrom Manufacturing Co.
SEP-A-RINGS	Tp Orthodontics, Inc.
SEPA CF CROSSFLOW	Ge Infrastructure Water & Process Technologies
SEPA ST STIRRED CELL	Ge Infrastructure Water & Process Technologies
SEPARATOR	Applied Medical Resource Corporation
SEPP	CholeraPrep
SEPRA FILM	Dma Med-Chem Corporation
SEPRA MESH	Dma Med-Chem Corporation
SEPTI-CHEK	Bd Diagnostic Systems
SEPTIHOL	Steris Corporation
SEQUENCES	Schleicher & Schuell, Inc.
SEQUENTIAL CIRCULATOR	Bio Compression Systems, Inc.
SEQUESTER-SOL	Cambridge Diagnostic Products, Inc.
SEQUI-GEN	Bio-Rad Laboratories, Life Science Group
SEQUOIA	Engle Dental Systems, Inc.
SEQUOIA OXYMATIC ELECTRONIC OXYGEN CONSERVERS	Chad Therapeutics, Inc.
SERA-MAG	Seradyn, Inc.
SERACON	Serologicals Corp
SERACULT	Propper Manufacturing Co., Inc.
SERAPLAS	Sarstedt, Inc.
SERASUB	Cst Technologies, Inc.
SERATEST	Remel
SEREINE	Optikem International, Inc.
SERENITY	Candela Corp.
SERENITY	Living Earth Crafts
SERENITY	Radix Corp.
SERIALMATE	Thermo Fisher Scientific
SERIES 1000	Lrl Logix
SERIES 1600 COMPUTER CONTROLLED UTM, TEST VUE FOR WINDOWS	Applied Test Systems, Inc.
SERIES 2000	Eurotherm Inc.
SERIES 3000	Pacific Precision Laboratories, Inc.
SERIES 4	Conmed Linvatec
SERIES 5000	Eurotherm Inc.
SERIES 8	Starkey Laboratories, Inc.
SERIES 9 DISCOVERY	Starkey Laboratories, Inc.
SERIES 9600	Ge Oec Medical Systems Inc.
SERIES 9800	Ge Oec Medical Systems Inc.
SEROCLUSTERS	Corning Inc., Science Products Division
SERODIA	Fujirebio Diagnostics, Inc. (Fdi)
SEROVAC	Axiom Medical, Inc.

SERVALYT	Crescent Chemical Co., Inc.
SERVI-SHELF	Caddy Corporation
SERVICEABLE	Hager Worldwide, Inc.
SERVICEWATCH	Psg Controls, Inc.
SERVIPAK	Baxter Healthcare Corporation, Renal
SERVMASTER	Caddy Corporation
SERVOFLEX	Conflex
SERVOLOCK	Edgetech
SERVOMEX	Servomex
SERVOPRO	Motion Control, Inc.
SERVOTRONIC	Surgical Tools, Inc.
SESAM	Karl Storz Endoscopy-America Inc.
SET-UP	Howard Medical Company
SETA-TRAY	Accurate Set, Inc.
SETMA	P-Ryton Corp.
SETSOURCE	Hospira Inc.
SETVIEW	Aesculap Implant Systems Inc.
SEU	Veritech Corporation
SFS	Covidien Lp, Formerly Registered As United States Surgical
SG-2002 STAND ALONE STANDARD GANZFELD	Lkc Technologies, Inc.
SGIA	Covidien Lp, Formerly Registered As United States Surgical
SGP	The Lifestyle Co. Inc.
SGP 3	The Lifestyle Co. Inc.
SGP II	The Lifestyle Co. Inc.
SGS	Hager Worldwide, Inc.
SH7727 CARD ENGINE, EMBEDDED PLATFORM SOLUTIONS, CALLIOPE, TECHNE	Logic Product Development
SHADE-A-GUIDE	George Taub Products & Fusion Co., Inc.
SHADO	Argosy
SHADOW	Adenna Inc.
SHADOW	Sperian Protection
SHAMROCK	Meese Orbitron Dunne Co.
SHAMU STRETCHER	Morrison Medical
SHAPEMATCH	Otismed Corporation
SHAPES	Ferris Mfg Corp.
SHAPES BY POLYMEM	Ferris Mfg Corp.
SHAPES2U	Amoena
SHAPESHIFTERS	Tulip Medical Products
SHARK SKIN	Schleicher & Schuell, Inc.
SHARK-EDGE	Boss Instruments, Ltd.
SHARPKEEPER	Whitney Products, Inc.
SHARPOINT	Surgical Specialties Corporation
SHARPS DEPOT	Sharps Compliance Corp.
SHARPS DISPOSAL BY MAIL	Sharps Compliance Corp.
SHARPS SAFETYSTATION	Advanced Medical Innovations, Inc.
SHARPS SECURE	Sharps Compliance Corp.
SHARPS TRACER	Sharps Compliance Corp.
SHARPSAWAY	Arrow International, Inc.
SHARPSENTINEL	Bemis Mfg. Co.
SHARPSHOOTER	Regen Biologics, Inc.
SHARPSITE	Medtronic Xomed, Inc.
SHARPSYSTEM	Approved Medical Systems
SHARPTOME	Surgical Specialties Corporation
SHARPVET	Cotran Corp.
SHEARGUARD	Mizuho Osi
SHEENA	Tulip Medical Products
SHEER PLUS	Smith & Nephew, Inc.
SHEERLINE	Fleetwood Group, Incorporated
SHEFFIELD RING FIXATOR	Orthofix Inc.
SHELBY WILLIAMS	Shelby-Williams Industries
SHELTERING ARMS	Sani-Med, A Division Of Sanderson Plumbing Products, Inc.
SHEPHERD CASTERS	Shepherd Caster Corporation
SHER-I-BRONCH	Covidien Lp, Formerly Registered As Kendall
SHER-I-FLEX	Covidien Lp, Formerly Registered As Kendall
SHER-I-SLIP	Covidien Lp, Formerly Registered As Kendall
SHER-I-SWIV	Covidien Lp, Formerly Registered As Kendall
SHER-I-SWIV FO	Covidien Lp, Formerly Registered As Kendall
SHER-I-TEMP	Covidien Lp, Formerly Registered As Kendall
SHER-I-TEMP LTU/UC	Covidien Lp, Formerly Registered As Kendall
SHERIDAN	Covidien Lp, Formerly Registered As Kendall
SHERIDAN	Teleflex Medical
SHERIDAN BELL/MCKAY	Covidien Lp, Formerly Registered As Kendall
SHERIDAN ETC02	Covidien Lp, Formerly Registered As Kendall
SHERIDAN FO-LY-CATH	Covidien Lp, Formerly Registered As Kendall
SHERIDAN LTS	Covidien Lp, Formerly Registered As Kendall
SHERIDAN NDYAG LASER	Covidien Lp, Formerly Registered As Kendall
SHERIDAN T.T.X.	Covidien Lp, Formerly Registered As Kendall
SHERIDAN UNCUFFED	Covidien Lp, Formerly Registered As Kendall
SHERIDAN/CF	Covidien Lp, Formerly Registered As Kendall
SHERIDAN/HVT	Covidien Lp, Formerly Registered As Kendall
SHIELD	Combe, Inc.
SHIELD	Products International Co.
SHIELD SKIN	Mentor Corp.
SHIELDS	Hely And Weber
SHIELLD	Perfecseal
SHILEY	Covidien (Formerly Nellcor Puritan Bennett / Tyco Healthcare)
SHIMADEN	Vespo Marketing Assoc., Inc.
SHIMADZU	Universal Ultrasound
SHIN ICE	Brown Medical Industries
SHIN SLEEVE	Brown Medical Industries
SHINEMASTER	Cd Nelson Manufacturing Co.
SHINER MAGNETS	Preat Corp.
SHIPSAFEr BOTTLE SHIPPER	Thermosafe Brands
SHIRAKABE NASAL IMPLANT	Implantech Associates, Inc.
SHIRLEY	Andersen Products, Inc.,
SHO-ME	Able 2 Products Co., Inc.
SHOCKPAK	Sellstrom Manufacturing Co.
SHORT-WAVE	Span-America Medical Systems, Inc.
SHOULDAIR	Azmec, Inc.
SHOULDER EASE	Pre Pak Products, Inc.
SHOULDER-FLOAT	O.R. Comfort, Llc
SHOWER SAFE	Trademark Medical Llc
SHOWERFLOSS	Showerfloss, Inc.
SHUNTCHECK	Neuro Diagnostic Devices
SHUR-BAND	Hartmann-Conco Inc.
SHUR/CUT	Triangle Biomedical Sciences, Inc.
SHUR/FREEZE	Triangle Biomedical Sciences, Inc.
SHUR/LUBE	Triangle Biomedical Sciences, Inc.
SHUR/MARK	Triangle Biomedical Sciences, Inc.
SHUR/MARK PLUS	Triangle Biomedical Sciences, Inc.
SHUR/MOUNT	Triangle Biomedical Sciences, Inc.
SHUR/SHARP	Triangle Biomedical Sciences, Inc.
SHUR/SLIPPER	Triangle Biomedical Sciences, Inc.
SHUR/SLIPS	Triangle Biomedical Sciences, Inc.
SHUR/STOR	Triangle Biomedical Sciences, Inc.
SHUR/TRACK	Triangle Biomedical Sciences, Inc.
SHUR/WAVE	Triangle Biomedical Sciences, Inc.
SHUR/WIPES	Triangle Biomedical Sciences, Inc.
SHURESAFE	Shure Manufacturing Corp.
SHUTT	Conmed Linvatec
SHUTTERVUE	AMD Technologies Inc.
SHUTTLE	Pride Mobility Products Corp.
SHUTTLE 2000-1	Shuttle Systems By Contemporary Design Co.
SHUTTLE BALANCE	Shuttle Systems By Contemporary Design Co.
SHUTTLE MINICLINIC	Shuttle Systems By Contemporary Design Co.
SHUTTLE MVP	Shuttle Systems By Contemporary Design Co.
SHUTTLE SPORTSWALKER SW-2	Shuttle Systems By Contemporary Design Co.
SI-LOC	Optp
SIBATA	Vee Gee Scientific, Inc.
SIBS	Lone Star Medical Products, Inc.
SICKLEDGE	Becton Dickinson And Co.
SICKLEQUIK	Biomerieux Inc.
SICKLESCREEN	Fisher Diagnostics
SICOM	Sterling Fluid Systems (Usa)
SIDEFIBER	Biolitec, Inc.
SIDEFIRE	Trimedyne, Inc.
SIDEKICK	ArjoHuntleigh
SIDEKICK	I-Flow Corporation
SIDEKICK	Nipro Diagnostics, Inc.
SIDEKICK	Pride Mobility Products Corp.
SIDESTREAM	Invacare Corporation
SIDEWINDER	Arthrocare Corp.
SIDNE	Stryker Corp.
SIDNE	Stryker Endoscopy
SIEMENS	Weitbrecht Communications, Inc.

SIEMENS, HITACHI, TOSHIBA, GE ELSCINT, SHIMADZU, PHILIPS, PICKER Inmark Corporation
SIERRA .... Electone, A Division Of Siemens Hearing Instruments, Inc.
SIERRA .... Ortho-Kinetics, Inc.
SIERRA EMG/EP .... Cadwell Laboratories
SIERRA SERIES .... Bobrick Washroom Equipment, Inc.
SIESCAPE .... Siemens Medical Systems, Inc., Ultrasound Group
SIEVING RIFFLER .... Quantachrome
SIGHTLINE .... Sellstrom Manufacturing Co.
SIGMA 34 .... Perry Baromedical Corp.
SIGMA 6000 PLUS .... Sigma International, Llc.
SIGMA 8000 PLUS .... Sigma International, Llc.
SIGMA I .... Perry Baromedical Corp.
SIGMA II .... Perry Baromedical Corp.
SIGMA MP .... Perry Baromedical Corp.
SIGMA PLUS .... Perry Baromedical Corp.
SIGMA ULTRASOUND .... Medical Equipment Specialists, Inc.
SIGNACREME .... Parker Laboratories, Inc.
SIGNAGEL .... Parker Laboratories, Inc.
SIGNAL .... Oxoid, Inc.
SIGNAL SAVER .... Online Power, Inc.
SIGNAPAD .... Parker Laboratories, Inc.
SIGNASPRAY .... Parker Laboratories, Inc.
SIGNATURE .... Abbott Medical Optics Inc.
SIGNATURE .... Corflex, Inc.
SIGNATURE .... Geri-Care Products
SIGNATURE .... Mabis Healthcare Inc.
SIGNATURE EDITION .... Alaris Medical Systems, Inc
SIGNATURE GARMENTS .... Medical Device Resource Corporation
SIGNATURE SERIES .... Hu-Friedy Manufacturing Co., Inc.
SIGNATURE SERIES .... Kewaunee Scientific Corp.
SIGNCOLOR .... Asi-Modulex
SIGNET .... Covidien Lp, Formerly Registered As United States Surgical
SIGNETCH .... Asi-Modulex
SIGNIA SELECT .... Siemens Hearing Instruments, Inc.
SIGNPLAN .... Asi-Modulex
SIGNSTONE .... Asi-Modulex
SIGNTYPE .... Asi-Modulex
SIGNVISION .... Timemed Labeling Systems, Inc.
SIGVARISr 230 COTTON SERIES .... Sigvaris Inc.
SIGVARISr 360 CUSIONED COTTON .... Sigvaris Inc.
SIGVARISr 500 AND 900 ARMSLEEVES .... Sigvaris Inc.
SIGVARISr 500 NATURAL RUBBER SERIES .... Sigvaris Inc.
SIGVARISr 770 TRULY TRANSPARENT SERIES .... Sigvaris Inc.
SIGVARISr 860 SELECT COMFORT SERIES .... Sigvaris Inc.
SIL-TEC .... Technical Products, Inc.
SILAMAT PLUS .... Ivoclar Vivadent, Inc.
SILAR .... 3m Espe Dental Products
SILASTIC SILICONE .... Pillar Surgical, Inc.
SILBERG EUA .... Wells Johnson Co.
SILCRYST .... Nucryst Pharmaceuticals Corp.
SILCUT .... Karl Storz Endoscopy-America Inc.
SILENCER .... Applied Biosystems
SILENCER .... Global Focus (G.F.M.D. Ltd.)
SILENT PARTNER .... American Medical Alert Corp.
SILENT SCAN .... Avotec, Inc.
SILENT SPEAKER .... Trademark Medical Llc
SILENT SWIRL .... Spectrum Laboratories, Inc.
SILENT VISION .... Avotec, Inc.
SILENZIO .... Nidek Medical Products Inc.
SILENZIO DELTA .... Nidek Medical Products Inc.
SILENZIO PLUS .... Nidek Medical Products Inc.
SILFLEX .... Dentsply Prosthetics
SILFREE .... Argen Corp.
SILHOUETTE .... Applied Medical Resource Corporation
SILHOUETTE .... Argen Corp.
SILHOUETTE .... Comfortex, Inc.
SILHOUETTE .... Dentalez Group
SILHOUETTE .... Invacare Corporation
SILHOUETTE .... Kewaunee Scientific Corp.
SILHOUETTE PLUS .... Siemens Hearing Instruments, Inc.
SILICON .... American Power Conversion
SILICON VIDEO MUX .... Epix, Inc.

SILICORE .... Spenco Medical Corp.
SILKEN SECRET .... Biofilm, Inc.
SILMAX, ... Pillar Surgical, Inc.
SILON-LTS .... Bio Med Sciences, Inc.
SILON-SES .... Bio Med Sciences, Inc.
SILON-STS .... Bio Med Sciences, Inc.
SILON-TEX .... Bio Med Sciences, Inc.
SILON-TSR .... Bio Med Sciences, Inc.
SILOPAD .... Silipos Inc.
SILSOFT .... Bausch & Lomb, Vision Care
SILTEX .... Mentor Corp.
SILUX PLUS .... 3m Espe Dental Products
SILVAGARD .... Acrymed, Inc.
SILVASORB .... Acrymed, Inc.
SILVER .... Glines And Rhodes, Inc.
SILVER SCREEN .... Avotec, Inc.
SILVER STAR .... Handi-Cap Aids Company
SILVER STAR .... Silver Star Mobility
SILVERCLENE24 .... Agion Technologies Inc.
SILVERGLIDE .... Stryker Corp.
SILVERSTEIN .... Wr Medical Electronics Co.
SILVON .... Conmed Corporation
SIMILAC .... Abbott Laboratories
SIMPLASTIN .... Biomerieux Inc.
SIMPLATE .... Biomerieux Inc.
SIMPLATE .... Idexx Laboratories, Inc.
SIMPLEX .... Caddy Corporation
SIMPLEX .... Stryker Corp.
SIMPLEX P .... Stryker Corp.
SIMPLEX P .... Stryker Howmedica Osteonics
SIMPLEX P WITH TOBRAMYCIN .... Stryker Corp.
SIMPLEX P WITH TOBRAMYCIN .... Stryker Howmedica Osteonics
SIMPLICITY .... Covidien (Formerly Nellcor Puritan Bennett / Tyco Healthcare)
SIMPLICITY KNEE CRUTCH .... Allen Medical Systems, Inc.
SIMPLICITY SIGNALING SYSTEMS .... Ultratec, Inc.
SIMPLY SUPPORT .... Freeman Manufacturing Company
SIMPLY WHISPERS .... Roman Research, Inc.
SIMS PORTEX .... Dma Med-Chem Corporation
SIMTEC AFS .... Siemens Medical Solutions Usa, Inc
SIMTEC IM-MAXX IMRT FIELD SEQUENCER. Siemens Medical Solutions Usa, Inc
SIMULAIDS .... Aristotle Corp.
SIMULAIDS .... Nasco
SIMULATOR II .... Bte Technologies, Inc.
SIMULCATH .... Smiths Medical OEM
SIMULCATH PLUS .... Smiths Medical OEM
SIMULIX-MC .... Nucletron Corporation
SIMULSCOPE, CARDIONICS .... Cardionics, Inc.
SIMVIEW NT SIMULATOR .... Siemens Medical Solutions Usa, Inc
SINERGY S SERIES .... Oneac Corporation
SINERGY SE SERIES .... Oneac Corporation
SINGLE DELUXE .... Medela, Inc.
SINTERFLO METAL MEDIA .... Porvair Filtration Group Inc
SINTERLOCK .... Centerpulse Orthopedics Inc.
SINU-KNIT .... Arthrocare Corp.
SINUS MASK .... Bean Products
SIPHONGUARD .... Codman & Shurtleff, Inc
SIPORT .... Applied Biosystems
SIRECUST .... Siemens Medical Solutions Usa, Inc.
SIREGRAPH D .... Siemens Medical Solutions Usa, Inc.
SIREMOBIL .... Siemens Medical Solutions Usa, Inc.
SIRENET .... Siemens Medical Solutions Usa, Inc.
SIRESKOP .... Siemens Medical Solutions Usa, Inc.
SIROAIR L .... Sirona Dental Systems Llc
SIRODEM .... Sirona Dental Systems Llc
SIRODOC .... Sirona Dental Systems Llc
SIROENDO .... Sirona Dental Systems Llc
SIROLASER .... Sirona Dental Systems Llc
SIRONA BL .... Sirona Dental Systems Llc
SIRONA BL ISO .... Sirona Dental Systems Llc
SIRONITI .... Sirona Dental Systems Llc
SIROPURE .... Sirona Dental Systems Llc
SIROTORQUE L .... Sirona Dental Systems Llc
SISTEM PHACO .... Mentor Ophthalmics, Inc.

SIT PACK	Nada-Concepts
SIT STRAIGHT	Alimed, Inc.
SIT-RITE	Elginex Corporation
SITBACK REST	Core Products International, Inc.
SITE LINE	Dukal Corporation
SITE RITE	Bard Access Systems, Inc.
SITE STRIP	E-Med Corp.
SITEGUARD	Tri-State Hospital Supply Corp.
SITELINK	Vitalcom, Inc.
SITESEER	Bard Electro Physiology
SITTERS	Bergeron Health Care
SIVAC	Sterling Fluid Systems (Usa)
SIVRITE	Quintron Instrument Company
SJM	St. Jude Medical, Inc.
SJM Epic	St. Jude Medical, Inc.
SJM Tailor	St. Jude Medical, Inc.
SKATER	Medical Device Technologies, Inc. (Md Tech)
SKATEWHEELVEYOR	Caddy Corporation
SKED	Skedco, Inc.
SKED RESCUE SYSTEM	Skedco, Inc.
SKED STRETCHER	Skedco, Inc.
SKEETER	Medtronic Xomed, Inc.
SKELETORSO	Medical Plastics Laboratory, Inc.
SKG	Kada Research, Inc.
SKIDSAFE	Orthomed Products, Inc.
SKILLGUIDE	Medical Plastics Laboratory, Inc.
SKILLMETER	Laerdal Medical Corporation
SKILLREPORTER	Medical Plastics Laboratory, Inc.
SKIMMER	Medtronic Xomed, Inc.
SKIN 1ST	P. J. Noyes Company, Inc.
SKIN BOND	Smith & Nephew, Inc.
SKIN DYNAMICS	P-Ryton Corp.
SKIN SEAL	Sage Laboratories, Inc.
SKIN SKRIBE	Hospital Marketing Svcs. Company, Inc.
SKIN-HESIVE	Smith & Nephew, Inc.
SKIN-PREP	Smith & Nephew, Inc.
SKIN-SHIELD	Marlen Manufacturing & Development Co.
SKIN-TITE	Marlen Manufacturing & Development Co.
SKIN-TRAC	Zimmer Orthopaedic Surgical Products
SKINCOTE	Dynarex Corp.
SKINLIGHT EVBIUM: SMOOTHBEAM	Candela Corp.
SKINSENSE	Molnlycke Health Care Inc.
SKINTIGHT	Azmec, Inc.
SKOOCHER	Stryker Corp.
SKY	Pmt Corp.
SKYANCHOR	Sellstrom Manufacturing Co.
SKYBAR	Sellstrom Manufacturing Co.
SKYBOOM	Skytron
SKYGIRDER	Sellstrom Manufacturing Co.
SKYNDEX	Creative Health Products, Inc.
SKYNDEX SYSTEM I	Caldwell, Justiss & Co., Inc.
SKYRACK	Sellstrom Manufacturing Co.
SKYRAIL	Sellstrom Manufacturing Co.
SKYRIDER	Sellstrom Manufacturing Co.
SKYROCK	Dent Zar, Inc.
SKYTRON	Medi-Tech International, Inc.
SKYTRON	Skytron
SKYVAC	Skytron
SKYVISION	Skytron
SL6	Applied Medical Resource Corporation
SLALOM PTA DILATATION CATHETER	Cordis Endovascular
SLANT	Jeter Systems Corp.
SLEEP SAUNA	Sleep Sauna, Inc.
SLEEP SENTRY	Diabetes Sentry Products
SLEEPAP	Medical Industries America Inc.
SLEEPING BEAN	Bean Products
SLEEPLAB PRO	CAREFUSION 211, INC.
SLEEPSAFE	Hard Manufacturing Co.
SLEEPSCREEN	CAREFUSION 211, INC.
SLEUTH	Sandhill Scientific, Inc.
SLIC	Arrow International, Inc.
SLIC	U.F.I.
SLIDE	Miltex Inc.
SLIDE PRO	Wescor, Inc.
SLIDE STACKERS	Phoenix Metal Products, Inc.
SLIDE-GUARD CUSHION	Skil-Care Corp.
SLIDE-LOCK	Smiths Medical Asd, Inc.
SLIDE-ON	Vision-Sciences, Inc.
SLIDER	Custom Durable Products, Inc
SLIDING TRANSFER BENCH	Eagle Health Supplies, Inc.
SLIK PAK	Shippert Medical Technologies Corp.
SLIM GUIDE	Creative Health Products, Inc.
SLIM LINE CONTROL	Gresham Driving Aids, Inc.
SLIM-EZ	Ooltewah Manufacturing
SLIM-LINE	Rem Systems
SLIMLINE	Camfil Farr
SLIMLINE	DJO Inc.
SLIMLINE	Darco International, Inc.
SLIMLINE	Principle Business Enterprises, Inc.
SLIMLINE	Sloan Valve Co.
SLIMLINE	Spectronics Corporation
SLIMLITE	Image Marketing Corp.
SLIMLITE 5000	Image Marketing Corp.
SLIMLUME	Independent Solutions, Inc.
SLIMPACK	Ultracell Medical Technologies, Inc.
SLIMTHOTICS	Langer, Inc.
SLINGSCALE	Scale-Tronix, Inc.
SLIP-NOT	Carolon Company
SLIPA	Arc Medical, Inc.
SLIPCOAT	Medisystems Corporation
SLIPFREE	Thermo Fisher Scientific
SLIPINS	Klinger Eye Shields, Inc.
SLIPOLDER	Healthmark Industries
SLIPP	Wright Products, Inc.
SLIPPIE	Juzo
SLIVER GRIPPER	El Mar, Inc.
SLIVER GRIPPER FIRST AID KIT	El Mar, Inc.
SLM-200	Benson Medical Instruments Co.
SLOTSHELF	Medical Design Systems, Inc.
SLQ	Hard Manufacturing Co.
SLS	Ventana Medical Systems, Inc.
SLT CONTACT LASER PROBES	Surgical Laser Technologies, Inc.
SLT CONTACT LASER SCALPELS	Surgical Laser Technologies, Inc.
SLUMBER	Brandrud Furniture, Inc.
SLURPH2O	Saint-Gobain Performance Plastics/Clearwater
SM	Covidien Lp, Formerly Registered As United States Surgical
SM70BR GOLD MESH FABRIC	Whiting & Davis Company, Inc.
SMART	New Horizons Diagnostics Corporation
SMART ADAPTIVE	Labthermics Technologies
SMART ALARMS	Zoll Medical Corp.
SMART CAP	Aprex, A Division Of Aardex
SMART CHART II	Devar Inc.
SMART CLIPBOARD	Carecentric, Inc.
SMART CONTROL TRANSHEPATIC PSILIARY START	Cordis Endovascular
SMART KNIT	Paramedical Distributors
SMART MANOMETER	Meriam Process Technologies
SMART SAFETY HUBER	Mps Acacia
SMART SAT	Clinical Dynamics Corp.
SMART SCALE	Olympic Medical Corp.
SMART SENSOR	Fasstech
SMART SINGLE	Intermetro Industries Corp.
SMART SPACER	George Taub Products & Fusion Co., Inc.
SMART SWAP	Ta Instruments
SMART TRACK	Intermetro Industries Corp.
SMART TRANSHEPATIC BILIARY STENT	Cordis Endovascular
SMART-COM	Zettler Systems, Inc.
SMART-EP	Intelligent Hearing Systems, Corp.
SMART-PAK	Getinge Usa, Inc.
SMART-PICC	Tfx Medical Oem
SMART-UPS	American Power Conversion
SMART-V-LINK [VASCULAR SOFTWARE]	Koven Technology, Inc.
SMARTARM	Clinical Dynamics Corp.
SMARTAUDIOMETER	Digital Hearing Systems Corp.
SMARTBEAM	Varian Medical Systems
SMARTCLIP	3m Co.
SMARTCONNECTOR	Ams Innovative Center-San Jose

SMARTCUF	Welch Allyn Protocol Inc.
SMARTDOP	Koven Technology, Inc.
SMARTDRIVE	Micro-Aire Surgical Instruments, Inc.
SMARTEMP	Parkell, Inc.
SMARTEP-ASSR	Intelligent Hearing Systems, Corp.
SMARTEP-ASSR SCREENER	Intelligent Hearing Systems, Corp.
SMARTEST	Bose Corporation - Electroforce Systems Group
SMARTEYE	Tri-Tronics Co., Inc.
SMARTGATE	Follett Corp.
SMARTGEN	Gtr Labs, Inc.
SMARTKART	Seitz Technical Products, Inc.
SMARTKEY	Iridex Corporation
SMARTKNIFE	Alcon Research, Ltd.
SMARTKNIT	Knit-Rite, Inc.
SMARTKNIT	Therafirm, A Knit Rite Company
SMARTLEG	Invacare Corporation
SMARTLOC	Secure Care Products, Inc.
SMARTLOCK	Stryker Corp.
SMARTMAP	Volcano Corporation
SMARTMONITOR	Respironics Georgia, Inc.
SMARTNUT	Ams Innovative Center-San Jose
SMARTOAE	Intelligent Hearing Systems, Corp.
SMARTPUMP	Stryker Corp.
SMARTRACK	Kmedic
SMARTREAD	Mabis Healthcare Inc.
SMARTS	Narda Safety Test Solutions
SMARTSCAN	Ams Innovative Center-San Jose
SMARTSCOPE	Nasco
SMARTSCREENER	Intelligent Hearing Systems, Corp.
SMARTSITE	Alaris Medical Systems, Inc
SMARTSLOT	American Power Conversion
SMARTSOUND	Kesner C.R.
SMARTSTEPS	Zimmer Dental, Inc.
SMARTTEK	Golden Technologies, Inc.
SMARTVAC	Niche Medical, Inc.
SMARTVEST	Electromed, Inc.
SMARTVIEW	Humanware
SMARTWALL	Intermetro Industries Corp.
SMARTWAVE IF 2000, SMARTWAVE GS 200, ULTRA MIST, ULTRA WRAP	
Newwave Medical Llc	
SMARTWINDOW	Hologic, Inc.
SMARTWIRE	Volcano Corporation
SMC	Specialty Manufacturing Co., The
SMD	Teleflex Medical
SMEAD SMARTSTRIP	Bibbero Systems, Inc.
SMEADLINK	Smead Manufacturing Co.
SMEDLEY	Creative Health Products, Inc.
SMELLEZE	Imtek Environmental Corp.
SMITH	Smith Time, Inc.
SMN	Carl Zeiss Surgical, Inc.
SMOG-HOG	United Air Specialists, Inc.
SMOKE ASPIRATION TIP	Implantech Associates, Inc.
SMOKE SHARK	Bovie Medical Corp.
SMOKEETER	United Air Specialists, Inc.
SMOKEMASTER	Air Quality Engineering, Inc.
SMOKERS CEASE-FIRE	Justrite Manufacturing Co., L.L.C.
SMOKERS STATION	United Receptacle
SMOKETRAP	Niche Medical, Inc.
SMOOTH MOVER	Dixie Ems Supply
SMOOTH TOUCH	Schering-Plough Health Care Products
SMOOTH-E	Radiometer America, Inc.
SMOOTH-TRAC	Zimmer Orthopaedic Surgical Products
SMOOTHLASE	Coopersurgical, Inc.
SMOOTHPEEL	Candela Corp.
SMS	Specialty Medical Supplies, Inc.
SMS	Televideo Systems, Inc.
SMSC	Keller Crescent
SNAP	Idexx Laboratories, Inc.
SNAP	Parkell, Inc.
SNAP BOND	Cooley & Cooley, Ltd.
SNAP II	Stryker Corp.
SNAP RING VIAL	J. G. Finneran Associates, Inc.
SNAP TOP CAP	J. G. Finneran Associates, Inc.

SNAP!	Tapemark
SNAP-LOKS	Healthmark Industries
SNAP-SEAL VIAL	J. G. Finneran Associates, Inc.
SNAPEZE	U.F.I.
SNAPOVER	Covidien Lp
SNAPPER	Byron Medical
SNAPRACK	J. G. Finneran Associates, Inc.
SNAPSWAB	Medical Packaging Corporation
SNAPTRACE	Conmed Corporation
SNARECOIL	Ranfac Corp.
SNE-136	Waldmann Lighting
SNIFF-O-MISER	Hoyt Corp.
SNOOPY	Scott Specialties, Inc./Cmo Inc./Ginny Inc.
SNOW BEAUS	Crosstex International,Inc.
SNS	Mauch, Inc.
SNUFFER	Vacumed
SNUG FIT	Precision Dynamics Corp.
SNUG HUB	Byron Medical
SNUG PLUG	Fci Ophthalmics
SNUG-FIT	Graham Medical Products/Div. Of Little Rapids Corp
SNUGGLE UP	Children's Medical Ventures, Inc.
SNUGGLE WARM	Smiths Medical Asd, Inc.
SOAKER CATHETER	I-Flow Corporation
SOARING EAGLE	Eagle Sports Chairs
SOCKS	Medicool, Inc.
SOEHENDRA	Wilson-Cook Medical, Inc.
SOF CARE	Gaymar Industries, Inc.
SOF*BRACE	Better Hands Glove Products
SOF-BOND	Crosstex International,Inc.
SOF-FORM 55 APHAKIC	Unilens Corp., Usa
SOF-FORM 55 EW	Unilens Corp., Usa
SOF-FORM 55 TORIC	Unilens Corp., Usa
SOF-FORM ALLVUE MULTIFOCAL	Unilens Corp., Usa
SOF-FORM II	Unilens Corp., Usa
SOF-LAX	C.B. Fleet Company Inc.
SOF-LEX	3m Espe Dental Products
SOF-SERTER	Medtronic Minimed
SOF-SET	Medtronic Minimed
SOF-SPUN	Durable Corporation
SOF-SPUN STANDARD	Durable Corporation
SOF-TOTE	Neotech Products, Inc.
SOF.MATT	Gaymar Industries, Inc.
SOF/PRO CLEAN	Lobob Laboratories, Inc.
SOFFGUARD	Conmed Linvatec
SOFLENS	Bausch & Lomb, Vision Care
SOFPULSE	Adm Tronics Unlimited, Inc.
SOFSHEEP	Sheepskin Ranch, Inc.
SOFSILK	Covidien Lp, Formerly Registered As United States Surgical
SOFSPEC	Welch Allyn, Inc.
SOFSPIN	Bausch & Lomb, Vision Care
SOFT & SECURE	Smith & Nephew, Inc.
SOFT BASICS	Bauerfeind Usa, Inc.
SOFT BITE WING FLAPS	Hager Worldwide, Inc.
SOFT CELL	Oasis Medical, Inc.
SOFT CUF	Ge Medical Systems Information Technologies
SOFT FORM	Fla Orthopedics, Inc.
SOFT GUARD SHEER PLUS	Smith & Nephew, Inc.
SOFT GUARD XL	Smith & Nephew, Inc.
SOFT ICE	Polar Products, Inc.
SOFT LINING TRIMMER	Almore International, Inc.
SOFT PLUG	Oasis Medical, Inc.
SOFT POINT	Fla Orthopedics, Inc.
SOFT SHIELD	Oasis Medical, Inc.
SOFT SILHOUETTE BRA	Ladies First, Inc.
SOFT SKIN	Span-America Medical Systems, Inc.
SOFT STRETCHER (SHAMU)	Morrison Medical
SOFT TOUCH	Bell-Horn, Inc.
SOFT TOUCH	Biolase Technology, Inc.
SOFT TOUCH	Meddev Corporation
SOFT TOUCH	Roche Diagnostics Operations
SOFT TOUCH	Utah Medical Products, Inc.
SOFT TWIST	Belport Co. Inc., Gingi-Pak Div.
SOFT&SECURE	Smith & Nephew, Inc.

SOFT-AIR	Adroit Medical Systems, Inc.
SOFT-CHECK	Cas Medical Systems, Inc.
SOFT-FLEX	Progressive Dynamics Medical, Inc.
SOFT-GRIP	Scanlan International, Inc.
SOFT-JECT	Air-Tite Products Co., Inc.
SOFT-LOCK	Precision Dynamics Corp.
SOFT-O-CLAVE	Postcraft Co.
SOFT-PAK	General Dental Products, Inc.
SOFT-SOCK	Knit-Rite, Inc.
SOFT-SOCK	Paramedical Distributors
SOFT-START	Bio-Rad Laboratories, Life Science Group
SOFT-TEMP	Adroit Medical Systems, Inc.
SOFT-TOUCH	Bergeron Health Care
SOFT-VU	Angiodynamics, Inc.
SOFTBANK	Scc Soft Computer
SOFTCARE	Lares Research
SOFTCHECK	Statcorp, Inc.
SOFTCOLORS	Ciba Vision Corporation
SOFTDONOR	Scc Soft Computer
SOFTEAR	Sunmed Healthcare
SOFTEC	Bauerfeind Usa, Inc.
SOFTEC	Tri W-G Group
SOFTECH	Case Design Corp.
SOFTEE PROSTHETIC CAMISOLES	Ladies First, Inc.
SOFTEZE	Hermell Products, Inc.
SOFTFLEX	Diamond Polymers, Inc.
SOFTFLEX	Hollister Incorporated
SOFTFLO	Vasamed
SOFTGRIP	Hamilton Company
SOFTHREAD	DJO Inc.
SOFTI JECT	Hager Worldwide, Inc.
SOFTI TIP	Hager Worldwide, Inc.
SOFTIP	Boston Scientific Corp.
SOFTIP	Dentsply International, Inc.
SOFTIP	Dentsply Prosthetics
SOFTLAB	Scc Soft Computer
SOFTLET LANCET	Bio-Med U.S.A. Inc.
SOFTLIGHT	Telsar Laboratories Inc
SOFTLINE	Medcomp (Medical Components, Inc.)
SOFTLINE IJ	Medcomp (Medical Components, Inc.)
SOFTMATE	Ciba Vision
SOFTMAX	Molecular Devices Corp.
SOFTMAX PRO	Molecular Devices Corp.
SOFTMIC	Scc Soft Computer
SOFTONE	Harry J. Bosworth Company
SOFTOUCH	Pi Professional Therapy Products
SOFTPATH	Scc Soft Computer
SOFTPERM	Ciba Vision
SOFTRAC-PTA	Boston Scientific Corp.
SOFTRACE	Conmed Corporation
SOFTRAD	Scc Soft Computer
SOFTRANS	Staar Surgical Co.
SOFTRX	Scc Soft Computer
SOFTSEAL	Starkey Laboratories, Inc.
SOFTSERT+PLUS	Softsert, Inc.
SOFTSHELLS	Medela, Inc.
SOFTSIDES	H.L. Bouton Co., Inc.
SOFTSILK	Smith & Nephew, Inc., Endoscopy Division
SOFTSPAN	Specialty Surgical Products, Inc.
SOFTWEAR	Respironics Colorado
SOFTWEB	Scc Soft Computer
SOFTY ELECTRODE TENS	Covidien Lp, Formerly Registered As Uni-Patch
SOL-R-HEAT	Duro-Med Industries
SOL-VEX	Ansell Healthcare Products, Inc.
SOLACE POST-OPERATIVE PAIN RELIEF INFUSION SYSTEM	Apex Medical Technologies, Inc.
SOLAN	Medtronic Xomed, Inc.
SOLAR	Ge Medical Systems Information Technologies
SOLAR	Stryker Corp.
SOLAR	Stryker Howmedica Osteonics
SOLAR DEFENSE	I-Rep, Inc.
SOLAR ELBOW	Stryker Corp.
SOLAR ELBOW	Stryker Howmedica Osteonics
SOLAR RADIAL HEAD	Stryker Corp.
SOLAR RADIAL HEAD	Stryker Howmedica Osteonics
SOLAR SHOULDER	Stryker Corp.
SOLAR SHOULDER	Stryker Howmedica Osteonics
SOLAR-PACK	Hospital Marketing Svcs. Company, Inc.
SOLARA	Dentalez Group
SOLARAY	Sellstrom Manufacturing Co.
SOLARC	Welch Allyn, Inc.
SOLARETTES	Dioptics Medical Products, Inc.
SOLARIS	Phonic Ear, Inc.
SOLARPRINT	Graphic Controls Corp.
SOLARSHIELD	Dioptics Medical Products, Inc.
SOLARSHIELD ULTRA	Dioptics Medical Products, Inc.
SOLARTEC	Welch Allyn, Inc.
SOLARTRON	Brandt Industries, Inc.
SOLAY	Tp Orthodontics, Inc.
SOLEO	Prosun Tanning International, Llc.
SOLERA	Cutera, Inc.
SOLERIS	Neogen Corporation
SOLEX	Alsius Corp.
SOLID	Applied Biosystems
SOLID POWER	Ecolab Inc.
SOLID SLUG	Neutron Products, Inc.
SOLITAIRE	Ecolab Inc.
SOLNIT QUIET GRAB FREE HVE	Preat Corp.
SOLO	ArjoHuntleigh
SOLO	Cascade Designs, Inc.
SOLO	Champion Bus Inc.
SOLO	Newschoff Chairs, Inc.
SOLO	Ranger All Season Corp.
SOLO GANTRY	ArjoHuntleigh
SOLO HD	Ranger All Season Corp.
SOLO II	Gendron, Inc.
SOLO IV	Ranger All Season Corp.
SOLO LTD	Ranger All Season Corp.
SOLO XT550	Ranger All Season Corp.
SOLO-CARE AQUA	Ciba Vision Corporation
SOLO-PACK	G & H Wire Co.
SOLO-SITE	Smith & Nephew, Inc.
SOLOARCOMFORT UVABC	Dioptics Medical Products, Inc.
SOLOMIX	Baxter Healthcare Corporation, Baxter Biopharma Solutions
SOLON CARET (IMPORT)	Solon Manufacturing Co.
SOLONT (DOMESTIC)	Solon Manufacturing Co.
SOLOSTIM	Life-Tech, Inc.
SOLTEC	Soltec Corp.
SOLUCIDE	Medical Chemical Corp.
SOLUDENT	Solutek Corp.
SOLUMAT	Solutek Corp.
SOLV/CYCLE	Triangle Biomedical Sciences, Inc.
SOLVECON	Whatman Inc.
SOLVO-MISER	Hoyt Corp.
SOMA SAFE ENCLOSURE	Vivax Medical Corp.
SOMACHAIR	Living Earth Crafts
SOMAERECTSTF	Augusta Medical Systems, Llc
SOMASENSOR	Somanetics Corp.
SOMATOM	Siemens Medical Solutions Usa, Inc
SOMATOM AR	Siemens Medical Solutions Usa, Inc.
SOMATOM DEFINITION	Siemens Medical Solutions Usa, Inc.
SOMATOM PLUS	Siemens Medical Solutions Usa, Inc.
SOMAVERT	Nektar Therapeutics
SOMNOSTAR	CAREFUSION 211, INC..
SOMNOTRAC	CAREFUSION 211, INC..
SOMSO	Biomedical Models Llc
SOMSO	Kilgore International, Inc.
SON-MATE	Engler Engineering Corp.
SONA PILLOW	Sleep Devices, Inc.
SONABLATE	Focus Surgery, Inc.
SONACHILL	Focus Surgery, Inc.
SONALARM	Minntech Corporation
SONARRAY	Varian Medical Systems
SONASCOPE	Covidien Lp, Formerly Registered As Kendall
SONATEMP	Covidien Lp, Formerly Registered As Kendall
SONATEMP 400/700 MONITOR	Covidien Lp, Formerly Registered As Kendall

SONATEMP ECG	Covidien Lp, Formerly Registered As Kendall
SONATEMP LTU	Covidien Lp, Formerly Registered As Kendall
SONATEMP LTU/UC	Covidien Lp, Formerly Registered As Kendall
SONATEMP UC/ECG	Covidien Lp, Formerly Registered As Kendall
SONATRON	Simplified Systems, Inc.
SONGER	Pioneer Surgical Technology
SONIALVISION	Shimadzu Medical Systems
SONIC AIR MM ENDO SYSTEM	Medidenta International, Inc.
SONIC ALERT	Weitbrecht Communications, Inc.
SONIC INNOVATIONS	Sonic Innovations
SONIC MM1500	Medidenta International, Inc.
SONICATOR	Mettler Electronics Corp.
SONICATOR	Misonix, Inc.
SONICATOR PLUS	Mettler Electronics Corp.
SONICONE	Misonix, Inc.
SONIGEL	Xenotec Ltd.
SONIX	Sellstrom Manufacturing Co.
SONO 3	Zimmer Medizinsystems
SONOCALC	Sonosite, Inc.
SONOCLOT ANALYZER	Sienco, Inc.
SONOFLUID	Covidien Lp, Formerly Registered As United States Surgical
SONOHEART ELITE	Sonosite, Inc.
SONOLEASE	Cardio-Vascular Sales
SONOLINE	Siemens Medical Solutions Usa, Inc.
SONOLINE ELEGRA	Siemens Medical Systems, Inc., Ultrasound Group
SONOLINE PRIMA	Siemens Medical Systems, Inc., Ultrasound Group
SONOLINE VERSA PLUS	Siemens Medical Systems, Inc., Ultrasound Group
SONOLINE VERSA PRO	Siemens Medical Systems, Inc., Ultrasound Group
SONOMA	Astro-Med, Inc.
SONOMA	Living Earth Crafts
SONOPSY	Covidien Lp, Formerly Registered As United States Surgical
SONOPSY	Havel's Inc.
SONOSITE	Sonosite, Inc.
SONOTHERM	Labthermics Technologies
SONOTIP	Medi-Globe Corporation
SONOTRON	Adm Tronics Unlimited, Inc.
SONOVA	Rontron Engineering, Inc.
SONTEC, WHISKR' BRUSH, DISPOSALOOP, MEDIMARK, DISPOSABOOT	Sontec Instruments Inc.
SONTIVA (DSP HEARING AID)	Telex Communications, Inc.-Hearing Instrument Grp.
SONUS V	Engler Engineering Corp.
SONY	Mccrone Microscopes & Accessories
SONY	Parco Scientific Co.
SOOTH-A-STING	Afassco, Inc.
SOOTHE & COOL	Medline Industries, Inc.
SOOTHE-N-SEAL	Closure Medical
SOOTHIE PACIFIER	Children's Medical Ventures, Inc.
SOPHIA LOREN BEAU RIVAGE	Zyloware Corporation
SOPHIA LOREN EYEWEAR	Zyloware Corporation
SOPRANO (HEARING AID)	Telex Communications, Inc.-Hearing Instrument Grp.
SOPROCAINE	Afassco, Inc.
SORBALGON	Hartmann-Conco Inc.
SORBAVIEW	Tri-State Hospital Supply Corp.
SORBEZE	HARTMANN USA, Inc.
SORBO	Sorbothane, Inc.
SORBO-AIR	Sorbothane, Inc.
SORBO-GEL	Sorbothane, Inc.
SORBOAIR	Sorbothane, Inc.
SORBOGEL	Sorbothane, Inc.
SORBOLITE	Sorbothane, Inc.
SORBOTHANE	Sorbothane, Inc.
SORBSAN	Mylan Pharmaceuticals Inc
SORBSAN	Unomedical, Inc.
SORE SPOTTER	Holmes Dental Corp.
SORENSEN	Impact Instrumentation, Inc.
SORENSON	Independent Solutions, Inc.
SORTING-VEYOR	Caddy Corporation
SORVAL OMNI MIXERS	Omni International, Inc.
SORVALL	Kendro Laboratory Products
SOS OMNI	Angiodynamics, Inc.
SOUND PRO COMBINATION TABLE	Biodex Medical Systems, Inc.
SOUND SEEKER	Park Surgical Co., Inc.
SOUND SOURCE	Nu-Ear Electronics
SOUND SURGICAL	Sound Surgical Technologies Llc
SOUNDBLOX	Proudfoot Company, Inc.
SOUNDER	Lexicon Branding, Inc.
SOUNDEX	Nu-Ear Electronics
SOUNDS TUTOR, TUTOR I	Pinnacle Technology Group, Inc.
SOUNDSCOPES	Starkey Laboratories, Inc.
SOVEREIGN	Abbott Medical Optics Inc.
SOVEREIGN	Aesculap Implant Systems Inc.
SP Novus	Medtronic, Inc.
SPA-SAVER-ALL	Industrial Acoustics Co., Inc.
SPACE IT, TRI-MAT MATRIX	George Taub Products & Fusion Co., Inc.
SPACE PAL	Anthro Corporation
SPACE SAVER	Arlington Scientific, Inc. Asi
SPACE SAVER	Electro-Steam Generator Corp.
SPACE SAVER	Golden Technologies, Inc.
SPACE-SAVER SYSTEM	Approved Medical Systems
SPACEBOOT	Cfi Medical Solutions (Contour Fabricators, Inc.)
SPAN CARE	Span-America Medical Systems, Inc.
SPAN-AIDS	Span-America Medical Systems, Inc.
SPAND-GEL	Medi-Tech International Corp.
SPANDAGE: SPAND-GEL: SPECIALTY HYDROGEL SHEETS	Medi-Tech International Corp.
SPANDEX	Hager Worldwide, Inc.
SPARKL	Dentalez Group
SPARKLE	Crosstex International,Inc.
SPARKLE FREE	Crosstex International,Inc.
SPARROW	Hard Manufacturing Co.
SPARROWHAWK	Atc Technologies, Inc.
SPARTAN	Applied Medical Resource Corporation
SPARTAN	Humanicare International, Inc.
SPARTAN	Schleicher & Schuell, Inc.
SPARTAN	Universal Gym Equipment
SPAT	Analytical Control Systems, Inc.
SPAZZ	Colours Wheelchair
SPEAKER BOARD	Ultrascope
SPECI-GARD	Uniflex Inc., Medical Packaging Division
SPECIAL CARE	Aqua Glass Corporation
SPECIAL TOMATO	Bergeron Health Care
SPECIALITE	Hill-Rom Holdings, Inc.
SPECIALTY AUTOMATICS	Specialty Manufacturing Co., The
SPECIALTY BOXES	Wes-Pak, Inc.
SPECKFINDERT	Dazor Manufacturing Corp.
SPECTER	Fla Orthopedics, Inc.
SPECTRA	Keeler Instruments Inc.
SPECTRA	Mentor Corp.
SPECTRA	Photo Research, Inc.
SPECTRA	Skytron
SPECTRA 30 HF	Americomp, Inc.
SPECTRA 30 HF AP	Americomp, Inc.
SPECTRA 300	The Daavlin Company
SPECTRA 325E	Americomp, Inc.
SPECTRA 360	Parker Laboratories, Inc.
SPECTRA 700	The Daavlin Company
SPECTRA A	Moyco Technologies, Inc.
SPECTRA APCT	Analytical Control Systems, Inc.
SPECTRA APTT	Analytical Control Systems, Inc.
SPECTRA COLORIMETER	Photo Research, Inc.
SPECTRA F	Moyco Technologies, Inc.
SPECTRA MINI	The Daavlin Company
SPECTRA OPTIA	Caridianbct Inc.
SPECTRA SP	Lutronic Inc.
SPECTRA VRM	Lutronic Inc.
SPECTRA WIN	Photo Research, Inc.
SPECTRA-DELUXE	Durable Corporation
SPECTRA-GEL	Spectrum Laboratories, Inc.
SPECTRA-MESH	Spectrum Laboratories, Inc.
SPECTRA-OLEFIN	Durable Corporation
SPECTRA-RIB	Durable Corporation
SPECTRA/CHROM	Spectrum Laboratories, Inc.
SPECTRA/POR	Spectrum Laboratories, Inc.
SPECTRACK	Siemens Healthcare Diagnostics Inc.
SPECTRAFLECT	Labsphere, Inc.

SPECTRAFLOUR POLARION	Tecan U.S., Inc.
SPECTRALIFT	Inclinator Co. Of America
SPECTRALINK	Spectralink Corporation
SPECTRALON	Labsphere, Inc.
SPECTRAMAX	Molecular Devices Corp.
SPECTRANETICS LASER SHEATH (SLS II)	Spectranetics Corp.
SPECTRAPRO	Princeton Instruments - Acton
SPECTRARADIOMETER	Photo Research, Inc.
SPECTRASCAN	Photo Research, Inc.
SPECTRASHIELD	Noir Manufacturing
SPECTRIS	Medrad, Inc.
SPECTRIS SOLARIS MR	Medrad, Inc.
SPECTRO FERRITIN MT	Ramco Laboratories, Inc.
SPECTRO VWF	Ramco Laboratories, Inc.
SPECTRODEr	Analytical Spectral Devices, Inc.
SPECTROGRAPHS	Princeton Instruments - Acton
SPECTROLINE	Spectronics Corporation
SPECTROLINKER	Spectronics Corporation
SPECTROLYSE	American Diagnostica, Inc.
SPECTRON	Smith & Nephew Inc.- Orthopaedics Division
SPECTRONIC	Thermo Spectronic
SPECTROPHOTOMETER CELLS	Nsg Precision Cells, Inc.
SPECTROSTIR	Spectrocell, Inc.
SPECTROYZME	American Diagnostica, Inc.
SPECTRUM	American Orthodontics Corp.
SPECTRUM	Amrex Electrotherapy Equipment
SPECTRUM	Aperio Technologies Inc.
SPECTRUM	Conmed Linvatec
SPECTRUM	Freedom Designs, Inc.
SPECTRUM	Jeron Electronic Systems, Inc.
SPECTRUM	Mabis Healthcare Inc.
SPECTRUM	Phoenix Diagnostics, Inc.
SPECTRUM	Spectrum Laboratories, Inc.
SPECTRUM 4000M	Mecta Corporation
SPECTRUM 4000Q	Mecta Corporation
SPECTRUM 5000M	Mecta Corporation
SPECTRUM 5000Q	Mecta Corporation
SPECTRUM BURS	Micromedics
SPECTRUM EDUCATIONAL SUPPLIES	Aristotle Corp.
SPECTRUM K1	Lumenis Inc.
SPECTRUM K5	Lumenis Inc.
SPECTRUM K8	Lumenis Inc.
SPECTRUM LITE	Dentsply Caulk
SPECTRUM MMP	Fasstech
SPECTRUM SP	Enmet Corp.
SPEE-D-COOL	St. John Companies
SPEE-D-DATE	St. John Companies
SPEE-D-MARK	St. John Companies
SPEE-D-VIEW	St. John Companies
SPEECH COMFORT SYSTEM	Siemens Hearing Instruments, Inc.
SPEECHEASY	Janus Development Group, Inc.
SPEECHMAP	Etymonic Design Inc.
SPEED LINE	Oster Professional Products, Inc.
SPEED PACK	Johnson & Johnson Consumer Products, Inc.
SPEED PACK	Zoll Medical Corp.
SPEED TREK	Tu-Way American Group
SPEED-CLAVE,ULTRACLAVE	Midmark Corporation
SPEED-LOCK	Stryker Corp.
SPEED-LOCK	Stryker Endoscopy
SPEED-ROLL	Albahealth Llc
SPEEDBLOCKS	Medical Plastics Laboratory, Inc.
SPEEDFLOW ADULT	Gvs Filter Technology Inc.
SPEEDFLOW BABY	Gvs Filter Technology Inc.
SPEEDFLOW KIDS	Gvs Filter Technology Inc.
SPEEDFUGE	Thermo Savant
SPEEDGEL	Thermo Savant
SPEEDI PEDI	Shippert Medical Technologies Corp.
SPEEDI-BAND	Precision Dynamics Corp.
SPEEDI-PRINT	Precision Dynamics Corp.
SPEEDLOCK LAP FORCEPS	Advanced Endoscopy Devices, Inc.
SPEEDMAN	Aura Industries, Inc.
SPEEDO-EX, SPEEDO SUC	Hager Worldwide, Inc.
SPEEDSET	Stryker Corp.
SPEEDSET	Stryker Howmedica Osteonics
SPEEDSTREAKS	Hardy Diagnostics
SPEEDVAC	Thermo Savant
SPEEDWRAP	Brasel Products, Inc.
SPEEDY CLAMP	Speedy Products Co.
SPELCAST	Snug Seat, Inc.
SPENCO	Spenco Medical Corp.
SPERM CONFIRM	Fertility Solutions, Inc.
SPERM SELECT SYSTEM	Select Medical Systems
SPERM WIZARD	Fertility Solutions, Inc.
SPERRY EYEWEAR	Zyloware Corporation
SPERRY TOP-SIDER EYEWEAR	Zyloware Corporation
SPERRY TOP-SIDER SUNGLASSES	Zyloware Corporation
SPERTI	Kbd, Inc.
SPEX	Horiba Jobin Yvon Inc
SPEXAN	Carl Zeiss Meditec Inc.
SPF	Ebi, Llc
SPG	Porex Surgical, Inc.
SPH (SEAMPESS POWER MACHINE)	Online Power, Inc.
SPHERASORB	Intersurgical Inc.
SPI-ARGENT	Spire Corp.
SPI-ARGENT II	Spire Corp.
SPI-ARGENT III	Spire Corp.
SPI-CERAMIC	Spire Corp.
SPI-MET	Spire Corp.
SPI-POLYMER	Spire Corp.
SPI-SIGHT	Spire Corp.
SPI-SPECTRUM	Spire Corp.
SPI-TEXT	Spire Corp.
SPIA	Raichem, Division Of Hemagen Diagnostics, Inc.
SPIDER	Kinetikos Medical, Inc.
SPIDERVIEW	Ela Medical, Inc.
SPII HIP STEM	LinkBio Corp.
SPIKESMART	Fenwal Inc.
SPIN-KLEEN	Nobles Manufacturing, Inc.
SPIN-LOCK	B. Braun Oem Division, B. Braun Medical Inc.
SPINA	U.S. Orthotics, Inc.
SPINA EXP	North American Medical Corporation
SPINA SYSTEM	North American Medical Corporation
SPINAL IMAGING PLATFORM	Oakworks, Inc.
SPINAL TOUCH	Fasstech
SPINAL-STIM	Orthofix Inc.
SPINALASE	Ams Innovative Center-San Jose
SPINALIGN	Williams Healthcare Systems, Llc.
SPINALMAX	Trimedyne, Inc.
SPINALPAK	Biolectron, Inc.
SPINALSCOPICS	Quantimetrix Corporation
SPINCHRON	Beckman Coulter, Inc.
SPINCON	Meridian Bioscience, Inc.
SPINE POWER	Leander Health Technologies/Healthcare Division
SPINE RELEIVER	Jobri Llc
SPINE RELIANCE	Zimmer Dental, Inc.
SPINE-TECHLINE	Maxant Technologies, Inc.
SPINE-TRACT	Omni-Tract Surgical, A Div. Of Minnesota Scientific, Inc.
SPINEGUARD	Activeaid, Inc.
SPINEGUARD/SPINGUARD-TC	Medstat Inc.
SPINEJET	Hydrocision, Inc.
SPINELINK	Ebi, Llc
SPINEPLEX	Stryker Corp.
SPINESCOPE	Ams Innovative Center-San Jose
SPINESTAT	Ams Innovative Center-San Jose
SPINEX	Seirin-America, Inc.
SPINNER	Pari Respiratory Equipment, Inc.
SPINNER BASKET	New Brunswick Scientific Co., Inc.
SPINOCAN	B. Braun Oem Division, B. Braun Medical Inc.
SPIRACAST RINGLESS CASTING SYSTEM	American Diversified Dental Systems
SPIRACAST RINGLESS CASTING SYSTEM	Mds Products, Inc.
SPIRACRIT	Covidien Lp
SPIRAL	Medsonic U.S.A., Inc.
SPIRAL RADIUS 90D	Stryker Corp.
SPIRAL RADIUS 90D	Stryker Spine
SPIRAL-FLEX	Covidien Lp, Formerly Registered As Kendall
SPIRALOOPS	Mds Products, Inc.

STA COMPACT	Diagnostica Stago, Inc.
STA HEMOSTATIS SYSTEM	Diagnostica Stago, Inc.
STA-FIX-TAPE (TM)	Southwest Technologies, Inc.
STA-R	Diagnostica Stago, Inc.
STA-SOFT	Holmes Dental Corp.
STA-TIC	Buffalo Dental Manufacturing Co., Inc.
STA-TITE	Covidien Lp
STA-VAC	Buffalo Dental Manufacturing Co., Inc.
STAAR	Staar Surgical Co.
STAARVISC	Staar Surgical Co.
STABILCOAT	Surmodics, Inc.
STABILEYES	Abbott Medical Optics Inc.
STABILGUARD	Surmodics, Inc.
STABILOX	Multisorb Technologies, Inc.
STABILUR	Cargille Laboratories
STABILUS	Magnus Mobility Systems
STABILZYME	Surmodics, Inc.
STABILZYME SELECT	Surmodics, Inc.
STABLECUT	Synvasive Technology, Inc.
STABLEFLOW	The Smartpill Corporation
STACCUPS	Cargille Laboratories
STACHROM	Diagnostica Stago, Inc.
STACK-A-FILE	Rem Systems
STACK-ITS	Micromedics
STACK-N-NEST CONTAINERS	Lewis Bins+
STACK-N-NEST CONTAINERS	Orbis Corporation
STACKABLES	Humanicare International, Inc.
STACKBINS	Stackbin Corporation
STACKER	Bd Diagnostic Systems
STACKER	Farley Inc., W.T.
STACKER	Spectrum Laboratories, Inc.
STACKFILES	Stackbin Corporation
STACKMASTER	Falcon Products, Inc.
STACKPAK	Symmetry Medical Usa, Inc.
STACKPAK	Symmetry Medical, Inc.
STACKTRACKS	Stackbin Corporation
STACLOT	Diagnostica Stago, Inc.
STAFF VECTOR SYSTEMS	Kelkom Systems
STAFREEZ	Biosynergy, Inc.
STAGE-ONE	Lifecore Biomedical, Inc.
STAIN PAK SOLUTION I	Cambridge Diagnostic Products, Inc.
STAIN PAK SOLUTION II	Cambridge Diagnostic Products, Inc.
STAIN RX	Cambridge Diagnostic Products, Inc.
STAIN-FIX	One Lambda, Inc.
STAIR-GLIDE STAIR LIFT	Thyssenkrupp Access Corp.
STAIR-PRO	Stryker Corp.
STAIR-TREAD	Stryker Corp.
STAIRLIFT	Inclinator Co. Of America
STAIRMASTER	Med-Fit Systems, Inc.
STAIRMASTER	Nautilus, Inc.
STAIRMASTER	Stairmaster Health And Fitness Products
STAK-BINS	Medi-Crush Company
STAK-CHEX	Streck Laboratories, Inc.
STALITE	Buffalo Dental Manufacturing Co., Inc.
STAMINA	DJO Surgical
STANCADDY	Sonoco-Stancap Division
STANCAP	Sonoco-Stancap Division
STANCOASTER	Sonoco-Stancap Division
STAND-N-WEIGH	Medcare Products, Inc.
STANDALONE	Packaging Products Corp.
STANDCO	Sticht Inc., Herman H.
STANDING DANI WHEELSTAND	Davismade, Inc.
STANG CIRC-CHAIR	Pedicraft, Inc.
STAPH KIT	Culture Kits, Inc.
STAPH-GUARD	Pellerin Milnor Corp.
STAPHAUREX	Remel
STAPHENE	Steris Corporation
STAPHTEX	Hardy Diagnostics
STAPHYLOSLIDE	Bd Diagnostic Systems
STAPHYTECT-OD	Lifesign
STAPILIZER	Conmed Linvatec
STAR	Cardiac Science Corporation (Ca)
STAR	Dentalez Group
STAR 430K	Dentalez Group
STAR FLEX"	Dentalez Group
STAR GUIDE	Accellent Inc.
STAR GUIDE-EUROPE	Accellent Inc.
STAR LIGHT	Star Case Manufacturing Co., Inc.
STAR S4 IR	Abbott Medical Optics Inc.
STAR TRACK	Swivelier Co., Inc.
STAR*LOCK	Park Dental Research Corp./Implant Center
STAR-ION	Phenomenex, Inc.
STAR/VENT	Park Dental Research Corp./Implant Center
STARADVANTAGE	Dentalez Group
STARBRIGHT	Dentalez Group
STARBURST	Angiodynamics, Inc.
STARBURST MRI	Angiodynamics, Inc.
STARBURST SDE	Angiodynamics, Inc.
STARBURST SEMI-FLEX	Angiodynamics, Inc.
STARBURST TALON	Angiodynamics, Inc.
STARBURST XL	Angiodynamics, Inc.
STARCASE	Star Case Manufacturing Co., Inc.
STARDENTAL	Dentalez Group
STARENDURANCE	Dentalez Group
STARFISH	Medtronic Cardiovascular Surgery, The Heart Valve Div.
STARFLEX	Starkey Laboratories, Inc.
STARGAZE	H.L. Bouton Co., Inc.
STARLITE	Bar-Ray Products, Inc.
STARLITE PILLOW	Mccarty's Sacro-Ease Llc
STARLYTE III	Alfa Wassermann, Inc.
STARMED	Starkey Laboratories, Inc.
STARPULSE	Ams Innovative Center-San Jose
STARQUICK	Starkey Laboratories, Inc.
STARR-EDWARDS	Edwards Lifesciences, Llc.
STARSOUND	Phonic Ear, Inc.
STARSYS	Intermetro Industries Corp.
STARSYS WORKCENTERS	Intermetro Industries Corp.
START	Diagnostica Stago, Inc.
STARTANIUS	Park Dental Research Corp./Implant Center
STARTER SNS	Medela, Inc.
STASIS	Belport Co. Inc., Gingi-Pak Div.
STASMOOTH	Paperpak
STAT	First Healthcare Products
STAT	Simulaids, Inc.
STAT 2	Conmed Corporation
STAT CO2	Mercury Medical
STAT CO2 METER	Mercury Medical
STAT FAX	Awareness Technology, Inc.
STAT FLAG	First Healthcare Products
STAT ID	Omnimed, Inc. (Beam Products)
STAT II	Carecentric, Inc.
STAT KIT 700	Banyan International Corp.
STAT KIT 900	Banyan International Corp.
STAT PROFILE	Nova Biomedical
STAT SLIDE-ALERT	First Healthcare Products
STAT STAIN	Volu-Sol, Inc.
STAT WASH	Awareness Technology, Inc.
STAT!	Products International Co.
STAT-5	Afassco, Inc.
STAT-60	Separation Technology Inc
STAT-ANALYZER	Advanced Instruments Inc.
STAT-CATH	Seecor, Inc.
STAT-CHEK	Stat-Chek Company
STAT-CRIT	Inverness Medical Professional Diagnostics-San Die
STAT-CRIT	Wampole Laboratories
STAT-GARD	Datascope Cardiac Assist Div.
STAT-PACE II	Seecor, Inc.
STAT-SHELL(R)	Epic Medical Equipment Services, Inc.
STAT-SKREEN	Biochemical Diagnostics, Inc.
STAT-TEMP II	Trademark Medical Llc
STAT-TOX	Biochemical Diagnostics, Inc.
STAT-WRAP	Hartmann-Conco Inc.
STAT-WRAP(R)	Epic Medical Equipment Services, Inc.
STATCOUNT	Dawning Technologies, Inc.
STATEMENT SERIES	Biotec, Inc.
STATFREEZE	Statlab Medical Products, Inc.

STICKY MATS	Markel Industries, Inc.
STICKY ROLLER	Controlled Environment Equipment Corp.
STICKYRING	Tp Orthodontics, Inc.
STIFNECK	Laerdal Medical Corporation
STIFNECK SELECT	Medical Plastics Laboratory, Inc.
STIK-FREE	Scientific Pharmaceuticals, Inc.
STIKON	Rdf Corp.
STILLE SUPER CUT SCISSORS	Micrins Surgical Instruments, Inc.
STIM-U-LAX	Oster Professional Products, Inc.
STIMATE	Csl Behring
STIMCARE	Compex Technologies, Inc.
STIMCARE PLUS	Compex Technologies, Inc.
STIMPRENE	Neumed Inc.
STIMSKIN CONDUCTIVE GARMENTS	Judah Mfg. Corp.
STIMULEN (TM)	Southwest Technologies, Inc.
STIMULETTE	Elmed, Inc.
STIMULITE	Supracor, Inc.
STIMUPLEX	B. Braun Oem Division, B. Braun Medical Inc.
STIR-PAK	Cole-Parmer Instrument Inc.
STIREX	Uni-Fit Co.
STITCHPAK	Conmed Linvatec
STM1 COMBINATION THERAPY SYSTEM	Patterson Medical Holdings, Inc.
STN	Carl Zeiss Surgical, Inc.
STOCKTON	Hard Manufacturing Co.
STOKOGARD OUTDOOR CREAM	Carex Health Brands
STOMAHESIVE	Convatec Professional Services
STOMATE	Abbott Laboratories
STONE RISK	Mission Pharmacal Co.
STONEBUSTER	Medi-Globe Corporation
STONECOMP	Mission Pharmacal Co.
STOP & GLO	Promega Corp.
STOPS PAIN COLD	Biofreeze Performance Health, Inc.
STOR BOT	White Systems, Inc.
STOR-A-LOT	Mabis Healthcare Inc.
STOR-MOR	Rem Systems
STORAGE WALL SYSTEM	Lista International Corp.
STORALL	Elginex Corporation
STOREFRONT	Spacesaver Corporation
STORK S'PORT	The Saunders Group
STORM SERIES	Invacare Corporation
STOW-A-WEIGH	Scale-Tronix, Inc.
STR	Elantec Med, Inc.
STRADDLE	Phelan Manufacturing Corp.
STRAGHT-LINE, APOLLO, ULTRAESTHETIC	G & H Wire Co.
STRAIGHT 8 CENTRIFUGE	Lw Scientific
STRAIGHT PACK	Packaging Plus, Inc.
STRAIGHT SHOOTER	Tp Orthodontics, Inc.
STRAIGHT-EDGE	Tp Orthodontics, Inc.
STRAIGHTFIRE	Trimedyne, Inc.
STRAIGHTSHOT	DJO, Inc.
STRANDS	Acrymed, Inc.
STRAPON	Rdf Corp.
STRATASIS	Cook Biotech, Incorporated
STRATE-LINE	Propper Manufacturing Co., Inc.
STRATEX	Delstar Technologies, Inc.
STRATOS 200	Ivoclar Vivadent, Inc.
STRATUSOCT	Carl Zeiss Meditec Inc.
STREAMER	Oticon, Inc.
STREET CORPUS	Permobil, Inc.
STREP A OIA MAXT	Thermo Biostar, Inc.
STREP B OIAr	Thermo Biostar, Inc.
STREP CHECK	Medical Packaging Corporation
STREP ID II	Remel
STREP KIT	Culture Kits, Inc.
STREPTEX	Remel
STREPTOLEX-OD	Lifesign
STREPTOSEL	Bd Diagnostic Systems
STREPTOZYME	Wampole Laboratories
STRESS ECHO BED	Medical Positioning, Inc.
STRESSBELT	Freeman Manufacturing Company
STRESSCATH	Hollister Incorporated
STRESSCONTROL BIOFEEDBACK CARD	Self-Programmed Control Center
STRETCH-VIEW	Dazor Manufacturing Corp.
STRETCHAIR	Stretchair Patient Transfer Systems, Inc,
STRETCHAIR T-TLC	Stretchair Patient Transfer Systems, Inc,
STRETCHER STRAPS	Morrison Medical
STRETCHISTOR	D.M. Davis Inc.
STRIDE RITE EYEWEAR	Zyloware Corporation
STRIP T	Kapp Surgical Instrument, Inc.
STRIPETTE	Corning Inc., Science Products Division
STRIPPAX	Multisorb Technologies, Inc.
STROLLER & SPRINT	Caire, Inc.
STRONGHOLD	Dmv Corporation
STRYKECAM	Stryker Corp.
STRYKER	Bound Tree Medical
STRYKER	Stryker Corp.
STRYKER	Stryker Endoscopy
STRYKER	Stryker Howmedica Osteonics
STRYKER	Stryker Spine
STRYKER HD DR	Stryker Corp.
STRYKEVAC	Stryker Corp.
STS	Sts Duotek, Inc
STURDI-SIDES	Activeaid, Inc.
STX	The Saunders Group
STYLE 840 WOVEN WIRE PARITIONS	Wire Crafters L.L.C.
STYLE-LITE	Zero Manufacturing, Inc.
STYLIX	Control-X Medical, Inc.
STYLUS	Surgical Specialties Corporation
STYMPAC	Electro-Med Health Industries
STYPTO-CAINE	Pedinol Pharmacal, Inc.
STYRE-SCREEN	United Chemical Technologies, Inc.
STYRO-FORMER	Huestis Medical
SUB-CELL	Bio-Rad Laboratories, Life Science Group
SUBTALAR MBA	Integra Lifesciences Holdings Corp.
SUCKLE-CUP	Genesis Industries/Maternal Concepts
SUCKRR	Flotec, Inc.
SUCTION EASY	Virtec Enterprises, Llc
SUCTION-DRAIN SYSTEM	M D Technologies, Inc.
SUGAR-CHEX	Streck Laboratories, Inc.
SUGITA	Mizuho America Inc.
SUH	Boston Medical Products, Inc.
SUICIDE-TRACK	Oncogene Research Products
SUITCASE	Homecare Products, Inc.
SULLY AC	The Saunders Group
SULLY HIP S'PORT	The Saunders Group
SULLY SHOULDER STABILIZER	The Saunders Group
SUMACAL	Covidien Lp
SUMEX	Stryker Corp.
SUMMA TRACEGAS CANISTERS	Thermo Fisher Scientific
SUMMADISK	Shofu Dental Corporation
SUMMIT	Graham Medical Products/Div. Of Little Rapids Corp
SUMMIT LEARNING	Aristotle Corp.
SUMO	Oticon, Inc.
SUMP N SHEATH	Axiom Medical, Inc.
SUMP PUMP	Andersen Products, Inc.,
SUN	Sun Metal Products, Inc.
SUN RIMS	Sun Metal Products, Inc.
SUN XTENDER	Concorde Battery
SUN-FLEX	Sun-Med
SUN-FLEX	Sunmed Healthcare
SUNBOX DL	Sunbox Company
SUNDANCER	Pride Mobility Products Corp.
SUNDT	Scanlan International, Inc.
SUNFLOWER PILLOW	Mccarty's Sacro-Ease Llc
SUNFREE	Afassco, Inc.
SUNGLIDE	Sunmed Healthcare
SUNLIGHT JR.	Sunbox Company
SUNLINE	Akers Biosciences, Inc.
SUNLINE	Sun Biomedical Laboratories, Inc.
SUNLITE FIBEROPTIC LIGHT SOURCE SYSTEMS	Kinetic Instruments, Inc.
SUNLITELAZER FIBEROPTIC LIGHT SOURCE AND CURING SYSTEM	Kinetic Instruments, Inc.
SUNMATE	Dynamic Systems, Inc.
SUNOPTIC	Consumaquip Corporation
SUNOPTIC	Sunoptic Technologies
SUNRAY	Sunbox Company

SUNRISE ALARM CLOCK WITH WHITE NOISE	Bio-Brite, Inc.
SUNRISE FRANCE	Sunrise Medical, Inc.
SUNRISE SPAIN	Sunrise Medical, Inc.
SUNRISE U.K. HOME HEALTHCARE GROUP	Sunrise Medical, Inc.
SUNRX	Vision-Ease Lens
SUNSATION	Sunbox Company
SUNSCOPE INTERNATIONAL	Biosensors International - Usa
SUNSHOWER	Prosun Tanning International, Llc.
SUNSPORTS	Sellstrom Manufacturing Co.
SUNSPOT	Sun Biomedical Laboratories, Inc.
SUNSQUARE	Sunbox Company
SUNX	Ramco Innovations/ Sunx Sensors
SUNZYME	Innovative Health Care Products, Inc.
SUP'R CUSH'N	Sellstrom Manufacturing Co.
SUPER 48 KEY REEL	Key-Bak
SUPER 66	Volk Optical Inc.
SUPER ADJUSTABLE SUPER ERECTA	Intermetro Industries Corp.
SUPER ARROWFLEX	Arrow International, Inc.
SUPER BLUE	Morrison Medical
SUPER BRIGHT	Respironics, Inc
SUPER EAGLE	Eagle Vision, Inc.
SUPER ERECTA	Intermetro Industries Corp.
SUPER FIELD NC	Volk Optical Inc.
SUPER FLEX	Eagle Vision, Inc.
SUPER FLUFF	Tillotson Healthcare Corp.
SUPER FOAM	Infab Corp.
SUPER MACULA	Volk Optical Inc.
SUPER PAC	Advantage Bag Co.
SUPER PAK	Shippert Medical Technologies Corp.
SUPER PHASER GOLD	Eel Electronics Mfg. Co.
SUPER PUPIL	Volk Optical Inc.
SUPER QUAD	Volk Optical Inc.
SUPER QUICK TIPS	Hager Worldwide, Inc.
SUPER SAGER	Minto R&D, Inc.
SUPER SERUM	International Technidyne Corp.
SUPER SHARPS	Medical Sterile Products, Inc.
SUPER SLICK	Tp Orthodontics, Inc.
SUPER SPORT NEB	Medical Industries America Inc.
SUPER STAR	Star Case Manufacturing Co., Inc.
SUPER WEIGHT-A-BAND	All Pro Exercise Products, Inc.
SUPER-COOL	Adroit Medical Systems, Inc.
SUPER-DRI-AID	Hal-Hen Company, Inc.
SUPER-LIFT	Ortho-Kinetics, Inc.
SUPER-LUNG	Cloud 9
SUPER-SKIN	Donell
SUPER-SOCK	Knit-Rite, Inc.
SUPER-VAC	Erie Medical
SUPER-WET	Conforma Laboratories, Inc.
SUPERA	Idev Technologies, Inc.
SUPERARM LIFT	Handicaps, Inc.
SUPERBAND	Precision Dynamics Corp.
SUPERBODY	Belport Co. Inc., Gingi-Pak Div.
SUPERCEL	Medical Packaging Inc.
SUPERCLEAR	Labcon North America
SUPERCOM 4400 TTY	Ultratec, Inc.
SUPERCONTRYX X-RAY GLASS	Hot Cell Services
SUPERCROSS	U O Equipment Co.
SUPERFIELD	Volk Optical Inc.
SUPERFLO PUMPS	Graymills Corp.
SUPERFLOW	Armm, Inc.
SUPERGLOVES	Mexpo International, Inc.
SUPERGRADE 4	Handicaps, Inc.
SUPERGREENIE	Shofu Dental Corporation
SUPERGUIDE	Fiberguide Industries, Inc.
SUPERIOR CARBIDE BURS	Medidenta International, Inc.
SUPERIOR SILVER	Covidien Lp, Formerly Registered As Uni-Patch
SUPERIOR SILVER ELECTRODES	American Imex
SUPERIOR SOLVENT	Qrp, Inc.
SUPERLITE	Kenda American Airless
SUPERLITE	Living Earth Crafts
SUPERLUERLOK	Tulip Medical Products
SUPERLUX	Carl Zeiss Surgical, Inc.
SUPERMOUNT	Biogenex Laboratories
SUPERON	Dent Zar, Inc.
SUPERPRINT 4425	Ultratec, Inc.
SUPERPRINT PRO80 TTY	Ultratec, Inc.
SUPERPULSE	Ams Innovative Center-San Jose
SUPERSAFEWAY	Woodhead L.P.
SUPERSCAN, WIRE-RAC, SLIP- STRIP, ANGLEVISION	Aigner Index, Inc.
SUPERSENSITIVE	Biogenex Laboratories
SUPERSET	Intersurgical Inc.
SUPERSHIELD	Rapid Power Technologies, Inc.
SUPERSIL	Harry J. Bosworth Company
SUPERSLICK	Smiths Medical Asd
SUPERSLIP	Hacker Instruments And Industries Inc.
SUPERSNAP	Shofu Dental Corporation
SUPERSOFT	Jilson Group, Inc.
SUPERSORB	Paperpak
SUPERSPLINT	Hager Worldwide, Inc.
SUPERSTAND YOUTH, MULTI POSITION YOUTH STANDER	Prime Engineering
SUPERSTAND, MULTI POSITION PEDIATRIC STANDER	Prime Engineering
SUPERSTAT	Nano Mask Inc.
SUPERSYRINGE	Belport Co. Inc., Gingi-Pak Div.
SUPERTECH	Supertech, Inc.
SUPERTHERM	Unique/Pereny
SUPERTIP	Sunstar Butler
SUPERTUBE	Tulip Medical Products
SUPERTUBECANNULAS	Tulip Medical Products
SUPERVITREOFUNDUS	Volk Optical Inc.
SUPERVU	Keeler Instruments Inc.
SUPPER-ADD	Conforma Laboratories, Inc.
SUPPLE PERI-GUARD	Synovis Surgical Innovations
SUPPLEMENTAL NURSING SYSTEM	Medela, Inc.
SUPPORT PL	Scientific Pharmaceuticals, Inc.
SUPPORT PLUS	Knit-Rite, Inc.
SUPPORT PLUS	Paramedical Distributors
SUPPORT TECH DENTAL PRODUCTS	Mds Products, Inc.
SUPPORT TECH LINE OF PRODUCTS	American Diversified Dental Systems
SUPRA	American Dryer, Inc.
SUPRA-VIT	Medical Instrumentation Development Labs
SUPRAFOIL	S Jackson Inc.
SUPRAMESH	S Jackson Inc.
SUPRAMID	S Jackson Inc.
SUPRAMID EXTRA	S Jackson Inc.
SUPRANE	Baxter Healthcare Corporation, Baxter Pharmaceuticals And Technologies
SUPRASSON	Acteon Inc.
SUPREME	Arkray Usa
SUPREME	Columbia Medical Manufacturing Llc
SUPREME AIR	Kewaunee Scientific Corp.
SUPREME II	Arkray Usa
SUPREME PATIENT CHAIRS	Dntlworks Equipment Corporation
SUPREMETAN	Prosun Tanning International, Llc.
SUPRENO	Microflex Corporation
SUR-FIT	Amici, Inc.
SUR-FIT	Convatec Professional Services
SUR-G-GLOVE	American Healthcare Products, Inc.
SURCH-LITE	Bovie Medical Corp.
SURCO	Surco Products
SURCO TECH	Surco Products
SURE	Remel Atlanta, Div. Of Remel, Inc.
SURE CHECK	Crosstex International,Inc.
SURE CLAMP	Blue Bell Bio-Medical
SURE CLEAN	Denticator International, Inc.
SURE CUT	Roboz Surgical Instrument Co., Inc.
SURE DOSE	Terumo Medical Corp.
SURE FLO	Terumo Medical Corp.
SURE GRIP	Essential Medical Supply, Inc.
SURE IMAGE	Hollister Incorporated
SURE TRAC	Precision Dynamics Corp.
SURE-CHEK	Herculite Products, Inc.
SURE-CHEK XL	Herculite Products, Inc.
SURE-FLEX	Telemed Systems Inc.
SURE-GRIP	Justrite Manufacturing Co., L.L.C.
SURE-LOK	Handi-Cap Aids Company
SURE-LOK	Sure-Lok, Inc.

SURE-SCREEN	Medtox Scientific Inc.
SURE-SEP	Biomerieux Inc.
SURE-VEST	Ivoclar Vivadent, Inc.
SUREBOND	Argen Corp.
SURECAN	B. Braun Oem Division, B. Braun Medical Inc.
SURECLEAN	Conmed Corporation
SUREETEMP	Welch Allyn, Inc.
SUREFIL	Dentsply Caulk
SUREFIRE	Argen Corp.
SUREFIT	Snug Seat, Inc.
SUREFLEX	Tfx Medical Oem
SUREFLO SOAP SYSTEM	Bobrick Washroom Equipment, Inc.
SUREGRIP	American Healthcare Products, Inc.
SUREGRIP	Mentor Ophthalmics, Inc.
SUREGRIP	Mps Acacia
SUREHANDS	Surehands Lift & Care Systems
SURELET	Facet Technologies, Llc
SURELOCK	Hologic, Inc.
SUREPOWER	Zoll Medical Corp.
SURESEAL	Applied Medical Resource Corporation
SURESEAL	Facet Technologies, Llc
SURESEAL	Mts Medication Technologies
SURESIGHT	Welch Allyn, Inc.
SURESORB	National Nonwovens
SURETAC	Smith & Nephew, Inc., Endoscopy Division
SURETOUCH	Medical Tactile, Inc.
SURETOUCH VISUAL MAPPING SYSTEM	Medical Tactile, Inc.
SURETRACE	Conmed Corporation
SUREVALVE	Filtertek Inc.
SUREVENT	Hartwell Medical Corp.
SURF'S UP SURFACTANTS	Qed Bioscience, Inc.
SURF-BLOT	Idea Scientific Co.
SURFACTANT/DEBUBBILIZER	Almore International, Inc.
SURG-E-TROL	Mentor Ophthalmics, Inc.
SURG-I-BAND	Scanlan International, Inc.
SURG-I-BAND CAROUSEL	Scanlan International, Inc.
SURG-I-LOOP	Scanlan International, Inc.
SURG-I-PAW	Scanlan International, Inc.
SURGAIRTOME TWO	Conmed Linvatec
SURGALLOY	Covidien Lp, Formerly Registered As United States Surgical
SURGEARREST	American Power Conversion
SURGEL	Ulmer Pharmacal Co.
SURGEON'S CHOICE	Medical Sterile Products, Inc.
SURGI LIGHT	Novosci Corp.
SURGI-BRA	Golda, Inc.
SURGI-GEL	Aqua-Cel Corp.
SURGI-WIPE	Olsen Medical
SURGIBLADE	Hospital Marketing Svcs. Company, Inc.
SURGICAL ACUITY	Sds-Surgical Acuity
SURGICAL C-ARM TABLE	Biodex Medical Systems, Inc.
SURGICAL CONCEPTS	Kapp Surgical Instrument, Inc.
SURGICAL HEADREST	Eagle Vision, Inc.
SURGICAL HEADREST	Lundy Medical Product, Llc
SURGICAL LOUNGE STRECHER	Schaerer Mayfield Usa
SURGICAL SUPPLY SERVICE	Medco Supply Company
SURGICIDE	Medical Chemical Corp.
SURGICLIP	Covidien Lp, Formerly Registered As United States Surgical
SURGICUTT	International Technidyne Corp.
SURGIDAC	Covidien Lp, Formerly Registered As United States Surgical
SURGIDYNE	Sterion, Incorporated
SURGIFIT	Larkotex Company
SURGIFRESH	Novosci Corp.
SURGIGRIP	Covidien Lp, Formerly Registered As United States Surgical
SURGIGRIP	Western Medical, Ltd.
SURGIGUARD	Novosci Corp.
SURGIGUT	Covidien Lp, Formerly Registered As United States Surgical
SURGILAST	Western Medical, Ltd.
SURGILENE	Covidien Lp
SURGILON	Covidien Lp
SURGILUBE	Altana, Inc.
SURGILUBE	Xenotec Ltd.
SURGIMED	Hospital Marketing Svcs. Company, Inc.
SURGINEEDLE	Covidien Lp, Formerly Registered As United States Surgical
SURGIPATCH	Covidien Lp, Formerly Registered As United States Surgical
SURGIPORT	Covidien Lp, Formerly Registered As United States Surgical
SURGIPRO	Covidien Lp, Formerly Registered As United States Surgical
SURGISIS	Cook Biotech, Incorporated
SURGISPIKE	Covidien Lp, Formerly Registered As United States Surgical
SURGISTATT II	Valleylab
SURGISTOOL	Stryker Corp.
SURGITIE	Covidien Lp, Formerly Registered As United States Surgical
SURGITIP	Hager Worldwide, Inc.
SURGITOME E	Conmed Linvatec
SURGITREL	General Scientific Corp.
SURGITUBE	Western Medical, Ltd.
SURGIVAC	Zimmer Orthopaedic Surgical Products
SURGIVIEW	Covidien Lp, Formerly Registered As United States Surgical
SURGIWAND	Covidien Lp, Formerly Registered As United States Surgical
SURGIWARE	Mediware Information Systems, Inc.
SURGIWIP	Covidien Lp, Formerly Registered As United States Surgical
SURMET BLACK BEUTY	Surmet Corp.
SURMET GOLD	Surmet Corp.
SURMETEX	Surmet Corp.
SURPASS	Idexx Laboratories, Inc.
SURVEYOR	Avon-Isi
SURVEYOR	Vicon Industries Inc.
SURVIVAL SOCK	Knit-Rite, Inc.
SURVIVALINK	Cardiac Science Corporation (Ca)
SUSTAIN	Lifecore Biomedical, Inc.
SUTER	Suter Dental Manufacturing Company, Inc.
SUTUPAK	Ethicon, Inc.
SUTURE-BOOT	Scanlan International, Inc.
SUTUREGUARD	Tri-State Hospital Supply Corp.
SUTUREMATE	Surgical Safety Products, Inc.
SVA PICC	Becton Dickinson Infusion Therapy Systems, Inc.
SVT DISCRIMINATION FUNCTION	Cardiac Science Corporation (Ca)
SWAB-PAK	Medical Packaging Corporation
SWALLOWING WORKSTATION	Kaypentax
SWAN	Snug Seat, Inc.
SWAN-GANZ	Edwards Lifesciences, Llc.
SWANK	Statcorp, Inc.
SWANN-MORTON	Cincinnati Surgical Company
SWANN-MORTON	Havel's Inc.
SWANSON	Wright Medical Group, Inc.
SWARTZ	Medworks Instruments
SWEAT	Quantimetrix Corporation
SWEAT-CHEK	Wescor, Inc.
SWEEN	Amoena
SWEEN	Coloplast Manufacturing Us, Llc
SWEEP	Mwi Veterinary Supply
SWEEPZONE AG	L&R Manufacturing Co.
SWEET DREAMS	King Systems Corp.
SWEFLEX	Hager Worldwide, Inc.
SWEN SONIC	Blue Wave Ultrasonics
SWIFT	Ela Medical, Inc.
SWIFT	Rcd Components, Inc.
SWIFT	Resmed Corp.
SWIFTBAND	Lohmann & Rauscher, Inc.
SWIN EPIDEMIOLOGY MODULE	Trek Diagnostic Systems
SWIN SOFTWARE	Trek Diagnostic Systems
SWING	Medela, Inc.
SWING AWAY	Gerber Chair Mates, Inc.
SWINGETTE	Whitehall Manufacturing
SWIRLER	Amici, Inc.
SWISS VISION	Swissray America, Inc.
SWISSPLUS	Zimmer Dental, Inc.
SWITCHPOINT, INTERACTIVE CAMPUS TELEMEDICAL SYSTEM	Stryker Communications Corp.
SWIVEL BATHER	Custom Durable Products, Inc
SWIVELIER	Swivelier Co., Inc.
SWIVETTE	Whitehall Manufacturing
SWL	Dentalez Group
SWLF	Rmo, Inc.
SWUBE	Bd Diagnostic Systems
SX/PC	Creative Biotech Inc.
SYLVANIA	Osram Sylvania Inc.

SYMBIQ	Hospira Inc.
SYMETRY II	Arlington Scientific, Inc. Asi
SYMMETRA	American Power Conversion
SYMMETRY	Stryker Corp.
SYMMETRY YOUTH, YOUTH SOLID SEAT STANDING SYSTEM	Prime Engineering
SYMMETRY, ADULT SOLID SEAT STANDING SYSTEM	Prime Engineering
SYMPHASIS	Cook Biotech, Incorporated
SYMPHONY	Depuy Ace, A Johnson & Johnson Company
SYMPHONY	Ela Medical, Inc.
SYMPHONY	Exercycle Corporation
SYMPHONY	Follett Corp.
SYMPHONY	Medela, Inc.
SYMPHONY	Ventana Medical Systems, Inc.
SYNCHRON	Beckman Coulter, Inc.
SYNCHRONY	Accuray, Inc.
SYNCHROPAK BONDING CHEMISTRY	Eprogen, Inc.
SYNCHROPULSE	Amrex Electrotherapy Equipment
SYNCHROSONIC	Amrex Electrotherapy Equipment
SYNCRO	Oticon, Inc.
SYNCRO/TORQ	Handler Manufacturing Co.
SYNECTIC	Synectic Medical Product Development
SYNERGIE	Dynatronics Corp.
SYNERGRAFT	Cryolife, Inc.
SYNERGY	Oxford Instruments
SYNERGY	Smith & Nephew Inc.- Orthopaedics Division
SYNERGY 20	Summit Industries, Inc.
SYNERGY 200	Summit Industries, Inc.
SYNERGY SPINE SYSTEM	Interpore Cross International
SYNETRON	Microflex Corporation
SYNETURE	Covidien Lp, Formerly Registered As Tyco Healthcare
SYNEVAC	Berkeley Medevices, Inc.
SYNEVIEW	Ela Medical, Inc.
SYNGO	Siemens Medical Solutions Usa, Inc
SYNGO DYNACT	Siemens Medical Solutions Usa, Inc.
SYNGO IDENTIFY	Siemens Medical Solutions Usa, Inc.
SYNGO INSPACE 3D	Siemens Medical Solutions Usa, Inc.
SYNGO IPILOT	Siemens Medical Solutions Usa, Inc.
SYNGO X WORKPLACE	Siemens Medical Solutions Usa, Inc.
SYNOVATOR	Smith & Nephew, Inc., Endoscopy Division
SYNOVIALSCOPICS	Quantimetrix Corporation
SYNOVIS	Synovis Life Technologies, Inc
SYNSATION	Ansell Healthcare Products, Inc.
SYNSATION STERILE	Ansell Healthcare Products, Inc.
SYNTEL	Applied Medical Resource Corporation
SYNTHAFAX	Instrumentation Laboratory Company
SYNTHASIL	Instrumentation Laboratory Company
SYPHILIGEN	Bd Lee Laboratories
SYRFIL	Corning Inc., Science Products Division
SYRIJET	Mizzy, Inc. Of National Keystone
SYRIJET MARK II	National Keystone
SYRINGE SHIELDS	Biodex Medical Systems, Inc.
SYRINGEAVITENE	Medchem Products, Inc.
SYS*STIM	Mettler Electronics Corp.
SYSMEX	Siemens Healthcare Diagnostics Inc.
SYSTEM	Medical Graphics Corporation
SYSTEM 2000 HOSPITAL CURTAIN SYSTEMS	Pryor Products
SYSTEM 2000 ROTATIONAL CHAIR	Micromedical Technologies, Inc.
SYSTEM 2500 ESU	Conmed Corporation
SYSTEM 4 PRO	Biodex Medical Systems, Inc.
SYSTEM 4 QUICK SET	Biodex Medical Systems, Inc.
SYSTEM 5	American Diagnostic Corporation (Adc)
SYSTEM 5000 ESU	Conmed Corporation
SYSTEM 7500 ESU ABC	Conmed Corporation
SYSTEM 80	Custom Ultrasonics, Inc.
SYSTEM 81	Custom Ultrasonics, Inc.
SYSTEM 83	Custom Ultrasonics, Inc.
SYSTEM 93	Custom Ultrasonics, Inc.
SYSTEM 97	MAQUET
SYSTEM ONE	Medical Illumination International
SYSTEM QT SOFTWARE	Medical Graphics Corporation
SYSTEM TLC	Chester Labs, Inc.
SYSTEM V	Life-Tech, Inc.
SYSTEMP	Ivoclar Vivadent, Inc.
SYSTEMS 12 BINS	Orbis Corporation
SYSTEMS 2000	Biomedical Life Systems, Inc.
SYSTEMS PLUS	Biomedical Life Systems, Inc.
SZAC	Astro-Med, Inc.
Safeguard	Procter & Gamble
Safire	St. Jude Medical, Inc.
Sapper	Knoll, Inc.
SatinCare	Procter & Gamble
ScanCathTM	Novaray, Inc.
ScanTel	Imperial Supplies Llc
Scope	Procter & Gamble
SealSafe	Perceptics Corporation
Secret	Procter & Gamble
Segura	Boston Scientific Corporation
Sensation	Boston Scientific Corporation
Sensitive Eyes	Bausch & Lomb
Sensor-Ink	Sensormatic Electronics
Sentara Heart Hospital	Sentara Health Management
Sentinol	Boston Scientific Corporation
SideLite	Boston Scientific Corporation
Skin-On-Skin	Medi-Dyne Healthcare Products, L.L.C.
Slide-Rite	Pactiv Corporation
SlimlineClassic	Megasun
Smart Step	Healthsouth Corporation
SmartEAS	Sensormatic Electronics
SmartPress	Princo Instruments, Inc.
SmartSonic	Princo Instruments, Inc.
SmoothShapes	ElemAc Medical
SoHo	Knoll, Inc.
SofLens	Bausch & Lomb
SofPort	Bausch & Lomb
SoftMoves	Medi-Dyne Healthcare Products, L.L.C.
Solaray	Nutraceutical International Corp.
Sole Defense	Acor Orthopaedic, Inc.
Soletra	Medtronic, Inc.
Soloist	Boston Scientific Corporation
Solutions On-the-Spot	Ortho Dermatologics
Soothe	Bausch & Lomb
Spectral OCT SLO	Opko Health Inc.
SpeedBand SuperView Super 7	Boston Scientific Corporation
SpinaLogic	Capstone Therapeutics
Sprint Quattro	Medtronic, Inc.
SpyBite	Boston Scientific Corporation
SpyGlass	Boston Scientific Corporation
St. Jude Medical	St. Jude Medical, Inc.
Standard Glidewire	Boston Scientific Corporation
Standard Lubriglide	Boston Scientific Corporation
Stavzor	Noven Pharmaceuticals, Inc.
StealthMerge	Medtronic, Inc.
SteeroCath	Boston Scientific Corporation
SteeroCath-Dx	Boston Scientific Corporation
Stellaris	Bausch & Lomb
StepStretch	Medi-Dyne Healthcare Products, L.L.C.
Sterling	Boston Scientific - Maple Grove
Sterling	Boston Scientific Corporation
Stone Cone	Boston Scientific Corporation
Storz	Bausch & Lomb
Streptonase-B	Inverness Medical Professional Diagnostics-San Die
Stretch	Boston Scientific Corporation
StretchRite	Medi-Dyne Healthcare Products, L.L.C.
SunClips	Hilco
Sunny Green	Nutraceutical International Corp.
Super Seal	Phoenix Dental, Inc.
Super Sheath	Boston Scientific Corporation
SuperTag	Sensormatic Electronics
Supor	Pall Corporation
Supplement Training Systems	Nutraceutical International Corp.
Supradisc	Pall Corporation
Supramesh	Pall Corporation
Supreme	St. Jude Medical, Inc.
Swartz	St. Jude Medical, Inc.
Swiffer	Procter & Gamble
SynchroMed	Medtronic, Inc.

Synergy	Rmo, Inc.
System One (TM)	Nxstage Medical, Inc.
T&F HYBRID POINTS	Shofu Dental Corporation
T-3	Invacare Top End Sports And Recreation Products
T-3	Ticonium Co.
T-3 ALLOY	Ticonium Co.
T-BLADE	Oster Professional Products, Inc.
T-BOLT III	Luckman Corporation
T-FINISHER	Oster Professional Products, Inc.
T-FIX	Smith & Nephew, Inc., Endoscopy Division
T-FOAM	Alimed, Inc.
T-GRAIN	Carestream Health, Inc.
T-HEXX	Hydromer, Inc.
T-LITE	Tornado Industries
T-PEEL	Tfx Medical Oem
T-PORT	Becton Dickinson Infusion Therapy Systems, Inc.
T-SCAN II	Tekscan, Inc.
T-TAM	Prentke Romich Company
T-WALL	Vital Signs, Inc.
T.B.Q.	Steris Corporation
T.CAM	Toshiba America Medical Systems
T.D.S.	Telediagnostic Systems
T.E.N.S LINK	Romaine, Inc. D.B.A. Koldcare
T.LINK, VOX ON-HOLD	Televox Software, Inc.
T/Gel	Ortho Dermatologics
T/PADS	Gaymar Industries, Inc.
T/PUMP	Gaymar Industries, Inc.
T/Sal	Ortho Dermatologics
T/T MEGA	Hacker Instruments And Industries Inc.
T2	Arthrocare Corp.
T2	Stryker Corp.
T2 PROCESSING CHEMICALS	White Mountain Imaging
T2 SYSTEM RECON	Stryker Corp.
T2T	Medtronic Perfusion Systems
T5 HELMET	Stryker Corp.
TA	Covidien Lp, Formerly Registered As United States Surgical
TA-POFF	Ulmer Pharmacal Co.
TA2 ERASER(TM) - TATOO REMOVAL	Light Age Inc.
TAAKSYSTEM	Alcon Research, Ltd.
TAB TOWEL	Crosstex International,Inc.
TABBAND	Products International Co.
TABBIES	Tabbies, Div. Of Xertrex International, Inc.
TABLE PLUS	Joerns Healthcare, Inc
TABS	Senior Technologies
TACK MATS	Markel Industries, Inc.
TACKY MAT	Controlled Environment Equipment Corp.
TACKY MAT	Liberty Industries, Inc.
TACKY MATS	Markel Industries, Inc.
TACTAID 7	Audiological Engineering Corp.
TACTILE TONE	Miltex Inc.
TADCATH	Boston Scientific Corp.
TADPOLE	Boston Scientific Corp.
TAFRA	C.A.M. Graphics Co., Inc.
TAG	Smith & Nephew, Inc., Endoscopy Division
TAG OFF!	Elantec Med, Inc.
TAKA SPONGE	American Silk Sutures, Inc.
TAKE 5	Veritech Corporation
TAKI	Lhasa Oms, Inc.
TALENT	Ela Medical, Inc.
TALISKER	Coherent, Inc.
TALK-A-PHONE	Talk-A-Phone Co.
TALL-ETTE	Maddak Inc.
TALON	Best Nomos Corp.
TALON	Talon Acrylics, Inc.
TALON ACL	Capstone Therapeutics
TAMBOUR-EZ	Techno-Aide, Inc.
TAMPALERT	Medi-Dose, Inc.
TAMPERVIEW	Keller Crescent
TAMRA	Applied Biosystems
TAMSCO	Trans American Medical / Tamsco Instruments
TAN AMERICA	Tan America-Indoor Sunsystem
TANGENT	Medtronic Sofamor Danek Usa, Inc
TANGENT	Medtronic Sofamor Danek Usa, Inc.
TANGENT STREAK	Fused Kontacts, Inc.
TANGENT TABLES II, III, IV, V, VI	Fischer Medical Technologies Inc.
TANGO	Resmed Corp.
TANITA	Creative Health Products, Inc.
TANK TUFF	Ideal Products
TANNENBAUM	Wilson-Cook Medical, Inc.
TANTALLUM	Glines And Rhodes, Inc.
TANTONE ELECTRODE TENS & NMS	Covidien Lp, Formerly Registered As Uni-Patch
TAP	Byron Medical
TAP	Tyco Healthcare Group Lp
TAP-IT.	Qed Bioscience, Inc.
TAPAS, PEG-IN HOLE DEVICE	Biopro, Inc.
TAPAZOLE	King Pharmaceuticals, Inc.
TAPCATH	Cardio Command, Inc.
TAPELESS DRESSING HOLDERS	Tapeless Wound Care Products, Llc.
TAPEMEASURE	Indec Systems, Inc.
TAPEPAX	Valley Products Co.
TAPER POINT	Ethicon, Inc.
TAPERCUT	Ethicon, Inc.
TAPERED-SHAFT FLOW CONTROLLER	Eagle Vision, Inc.
TAPERLOC	Biomet, Inc.
TAPERLOCK	Zimmer Dental, Inc.
TAPERTIP	Trimedyne, Inc.
TAPESTRY MANAGED CARE	Epic Systems Corp.
TAPSCOPE	Cardio Command, Inc.
TAPSYSTEM	Cardio Command, Inc.
TAQMAN	Applied Biosystems
TAQTRACK	Promega Corp.
TARE-FREE ALG	Essential Dental Systems, Inc.
TARGA	Nest Group Inc., The
TARGET	Corflex, Inc.
TARGET	DJO Inc.
TARGET	Enmet Corp.
TARGET	Noram Solutions
TARGET TILE	R.C.A. Rubber Company, The
TARGET TREADS	R.C.A. Rubber Company, The
TARGIS	Urologix, Inc.
TARNO	Hu-Friedy Manufacturing Co., Inc.
TARPON	Boss Instruments, Ltd.
TARSYS	Invacare Corporation
TARTAN	3m Co.
TARTAN ACTIVE ANKLE	Tartan Orthopedics, Ltd.
TARTAN FLEX	Tartan Orthopedics, Ltd.
TARTAN FORM	Tartan Orthopedics, Ltd.
TASKAIR	Thomas Products Division
TASKART	Healthmark Industries
TASKITS	Medline Industries, Inc.
TASKMASTER	Franklin Miller Inc
TASKMASTER	Rozinn By Scottcare Corporation
TASS	Medstat Inc.
TASS-II	Medstat Inc.
TATTOO ID	Integrated Software Design, Inc.
TAUT	Teleflex Medical
TAUT INC.	Dma Med-Chem Corporation
TAUT INTRADUCER	Taut, Inc.
TAVA ORTHOPAEDIC POWER SYSTEM	Tava Surgical Instruments
TAXO	Bd Diagnostic Systems
TAXUS	Abbott Laboratories
TAXUS	Boston Scientific - Maple Grove
TAXUS	Boston Scientific Corporation
TAYLOR SPATIAL FRAME	Smith & Nephew Inc.- Orthopaedics Division
TBC	Bagco
TBIRD	CAREFUSION 211, INC..
TBS	Hoggan Health Industries, Inc.
TC GOLD	Kls-Martin L.P.
TC-100	Smith & Nephew Inc.- Orthopaedics Division
TC-300 TREATMENT CHAIR	Wy'East Medical Corp.
TC2	Nelson Prosthetic & Orthotic Laboratory
TCA	Netzsch Instruments, Inc.
TCM3	Radiometer America, Inc.
TCO-2-METTE	Respironics, Inc
TCU	Geiger Medical Technologies

TDCBFM	Flowtronics, Inc.
TDS	Medical Device Resource Corporation
TDS 700 SERIES	Eclipsys Corporation
TDX	Invacare Corporation
TE.R.I.	Depuy Ace, A Johnson & Johnson Company
TEA TREE	Health Enterprises
TEACHTECH	Leica Microsystems (San Jose) Corporation
TEAM UP	Acteon Inc.
TEAMBEST	Best Medical International, Inc.
TEAR LIGHT TAPE	Mueller Sports Medicine
TEARGUARD	Healthmark Industries
TEARSAVER PLUGS	Fci Ophthalmics
TEARZONE	Bagco
TEC	Boston Scientific Interventional Technologies
TEC	Sakura Finetek U.S.A., Inc.
TEC	Triangle Biomedical Sciences, Inc.
TECA	Oxford Instruments
TECH ONE	Microflex Corporation
TECH PRINTr MEDICAL/LABORATORY & VIDEO PRINTER ROLLS	Pm Company
TECH SPEC	Edmund Industrial Optics
TECH TIPS	Hologic, Inc.
TECH VAC OIL	Hager Worldwide, Inc.
TECH-CAL	R & D Systems, Inc.
TECH-MATIC	York X-Ray And Orthopedic Supply, Inc.
TECHLINE	Independent Solutions, Inc.
TECHLINE	Maxant Technologies, Inc.
TECHLITE	Arkray Usa
TECHNESCAN	Mallinckrodt, Inc.
TECHNICIAN'S HELPER	Dmv Corporation
TECHNIQUE	Sunstar Butler
TECHNO-AIDE	Techno-Aide, Inc.
TECHNO-GUARD	Techno-Aide, Inc.
TECHNOCUT	Myco Medical
TECHNOLOGY FURNITURE	Anthro Corporation
TECHNOLOGY WITHOUT LIMITS	World Heart Inc.
TECHNOS	Biosound Esaote, Inc.
TECHNOS MPX	Biosound Esaote, Inc.
TECHNOSPORTS DF	Sellstrom Manufacturing Co.
TECHNOSPORTS DF CRUISERS	Sellstrom Manufacturing Co.
TECHNOTERM	Testo, Inc.
TECHTONIX	Stryker Corp.
TECHTONIX	Stryker Spine
TECNI-QUIP CARTS	Tecni-Quip
TECNICLENE CONCENTRATE	Nortech Laboratories, Inc.
TECNICLENE CONCENTRATE-L	Nortech Laboratories, Inc.
TECNIS	Abbott Medical Optics Inc.
TECNOL	Kerr Group
TECO DIAGNOSTICS, HEMOSURE, AMEDICA BIOTECH	Elabsupply
TECOTEX	Tecomet, A Subsidiary Of Viasys Healthcare Inc.
TEE-CEE PROBE	Aragona Medical, Inc.
TEETER HANG UPS	Stl International, Inc. / Teeter Hang Ups
TEFGEN	Lifecore Biomedical, Inc.
TEFSEP	Ge Infrastructure Water & Process Technologies
TEG, THROMBELASTOGRAPH, THROMBOLASTOGRAM	Haemoscope Corp.
TEGADERM	3m Co.
TEK	Energizer Personal Care Division
TEK	Siemens Hearing Instruments, Inc.
TEKNIQUE	Hoveround Corporation
TEKTONE	Alpha Communications
TELAMON	Medtronic Sofamor Danek Usa, Inc
TELAMON	Medtronic Sofamor Danek Usa, Inc.
TELAMON TI	Medtronic Sofamor Danek Usa, Inc
TELAMON TI	Medtronic Sofamor Danek Usa, Inc.
TELANGITRON	Edge Systems Corporation
TELASEPTIC	Palmero Health Care
TELE PACK	Karl Storz Endoscopy-America Inc.
TELE-TOTE	Neotech Products, Inc.
TELEBINOCULAR	Mast/Keystone View
TELECAM	Karl Storz Endoscopy-America Inc.
TELEFOCUS	Solarius Development Inc.
TELEFORCE	Bogen Communications International, Inc.
TELEMYO 2400T & 2400R	Noraxon Usa, Inc.
TELEMYO 900	Noraxon Usa, Inc.

TELEPHONE FLUENCY SYSTEM	Casa Futura Technologies
TELEREHAB	Scottcare Corporation
TELEREHAB ADVANTAGE	Rozinn By Scottcare Corporation
TELESCOPING	Wheaton Brace Co.
TELESENTRY: TELEREHAB OUTCOMES	Scottcare Corporation
TELESTAR SERIES	Oneac Corporation
TELETOM	Berchtold Corp.
TELEVAC	Berchtold Corp.
TELEVIDEO	Televideo Systems, Inc.
TELOS	Telos Medical Equipment (Austin & Assoc., Inc.)
TELSAR	Telsar Laboratories Inc
TEM-PAK	Tcp Reliable, Inc.
TEMFIX	Pace Medical, Inc.
TEMP-HOSE	Cincinnati Sub-Zero Products, Inc., Medical Division
TEMP-O-LARM	Psg Controls, Inc.
TEMP-PAD	Cincinnati Sub-Zero Products, Inc., Medical Division
TEMP-RITE MEAL SYSTEMS	Aladdin Synergetics, Inc.
TEMP-WRAP	Hospital Marketing Svcs. Company, Inc.
TEMPALERT II	Sharn, Inc.
TEMPERFOAM	Kees Goebel Medical Specialties, Inc.
TEMPERSTICK	Kees Goebel Medical Specialties, Inc.
TEMPEST	Virtis, An Sp Industries Company
TEMPGUARD	Hoshizaki America, Inc.
TEMPIT	Centrix, Inc.
TEMPLES	Klinger Eye Shields, Inc.
TEMPO	Applied Biosystems
TEMPO	ArjoHuntleigh
TEMPO	Lang Dental Manufacturing Co., Inc.
TEMPO-REX	Scientific Pharmaceuticals, Inc.
TEMPQUIK	Carex Health Brands
TEMPSTRAN	Johns Manville
TEMPTEK	Ebi, Llc
TEMPTRAC	Pmt Corp.
TEMPTREND	Biosynergy, Inc.
TEMPUFORM	Hermell Products, Inc.
TEMPUR-MED	Tempur-Medical, Inc.
TEMPUR-PLUS3	Tempur-Medical, Inc.
TEMPURAIR	Tempur-Medical, Inc.
TEMPURAP	Tempur-Medical, Inc.
TEMREX CEMENT	Temrex Corporation
TEMRITE CEMENT	Rite-Dent Manufacturing Corp.
TEN20 CONDUCTIVE	Weaver & Company
TENDER GRIP	Salter Labs
TENDER TEMP	Mabis Healthcare Inc.
TENDER TOUCH	Utah Medical Products, Inc.
TENDER TRACE	Conmed Corporation
TENDERFOOT	International Technidyne Corp.
TENDERLETT	International Technidyne Corp.
TENDERTYKES	Mabis Healthcare Inc.
TENDONE! DEVICE	Biopro, Inc.
TENKAY	Camfil Farr
TENNSCO	Bibbero Systems, Inc.
TENO FIX	Ortheon Medical, Llc.
TENOGLIDE	Integra Lifesciences Holdings Corp.
TENOR	ArjoHuntleigh
TENS	Zimmer Medizinsystems
TENS CLEAN COTE	Covidien Lp, Formerly Registered As Uni-Patch
TENSION ISOMETER	Medmetric Corp.
TENSIVE	Parker Laboratories, Inc.
TENT HOUSE	Nova Health Systems, Inc.
TERA-PRENE	Scott Specialties, Inc./Cmo Inc./Ginny Inc.
TERAZOL	Johnson & Johnson
TERINO MALAR SHELL	Implantech Associates, Inc.
TERMINAL	Whitney Products, Inc.
TERMINATOR	Hager Worldwide, Inc.
TERMINATOR	Invacare Top End Sports And Recreation Products
TERRA-TOPS	Kimble Chase Life Science And Research Products Llc
TERRASPECT	Analytical Spectral Devices, Inc.
TERRY MCQUISTION KOLINSKY BRUSHES	American Diversified Dental Systems
TERRY MCQUISTON KOLINSKY BRUSHES	Mds Products, Inc.
TERRY-TREADS	Albahealth Llc
TERUFUSION	Terumo Medical Corp.
TERUMO	Terumo Cardiovascular Systems, Corp

TESS	Environmental Tectonics Corp.
TESSIER	Striker Corp.
TEST	In Vivo Metric
TEST2	In Vivo Metric
TESTED USER FRIENDLY	Usb Corporation
TESTING LABORATORY	Tcp Reliable, Inc.
TESTOTERM	Testo, Inc.
TESTOVENT	Testo, Inc.
TESTSKIN II	Organogenesis Inc.
TETRA	Tetra Medical Supply Corp.
TETRA-FLEX	Tetra Medical Supply Corp.
TETRA-MAT	Tetra Medical Supply Corp.
TETRIC CERAM	Ivoclar Vivadent, Inc.
TEVDEK	Teleflex Medical
TEW	Schaerer Mayfield Usa
TEX-CARE MEDICAL	Tex-Care Medical
TEXAS AIRSONICS	American Medical Technologies, Inc.
TEXAS CATHETER	Covidien Lp
TEXAS DOLL	Medical Plastics Laboratory, Inc.
TEXUR	National Nonwovens
TFM	Triangle Biomedical Sciences, Inc.
TFR	Ramco Laboratories, Inc.
TFX OEM	Teleflex Medical
TH 9429	Thales Components Corporation
TH 9432	Thales Components Corporation
TH 9436	Thales Components Corporation
TH 9438	Thales Components Corporation
TH 9447	Thales Components Corporation
TH 9464	Thales Components Corporation
TH 9466	Thales Components Corporation
TH8730	Thales Components Corporation
TH8740	Thales Components Corporation
THE ADVANTAGE	Medstat Inc.
THE ADVANTAGE SERIES	CAREFUSION 211, INC.
THE ANGLE	Back Support Systems
THE BIKE	Cybex International, Inc.
THE BLAZER	Essential Medical Supply, Inc.
THE BODY GROUP	Frederick Lee Inc
THE BREAST BINDER	Medi-Garb Co., Inc.
THE CHAMPION	Mckesson General Medical
THE CINDYLIFT, TRANSFER DEVICE AND KNEELER	Prime Engineering
THE COLD METHOD	Biofreeze Performance Health, Inc.
THE COMMUNICATOR	Simplified Systems, Inc.
THE COMPLETE SOLUTION FOR THROMBUS	Possis Medical, Inc.
THE CONDUCTOR	Medical Science Products, Inc.
THE CRIST CHAIR	Crist Instrument Co., Inc.
THE CURVE	Back Support Systems
THE DIMPLEr	Ultimate Wireforms, Inc.
THE ERASER	Twist2it, Inc.
THE FOOD PROCESSOR SQL	Esha Research
THE GUARDIAN	Mckesson General Medical
THE HEALTHCARE SERIES	Micromedex, Inc.
THE HEELER	Biomedical Systems
THE HUG T	Back Support Systems
THE IDEAL	Mckesson General Medical
THE INSPIRATION	Emergency Medical International
THE INSTATRAK SYSTEM	Ge Healthcare Technologies Surgery Navigation
THE INTENSITY MODULATION COMPANY	Best Nomos Corp.
THE KLIP	Sdi Diagnostics, Inc.
THE KNEE T	Back Support Systems
THE LAMP MANAGER POWER SUPPLY	Bhk, Inc.
THE LEADER IN ASPHERIC OPTICS	Volk Optical Inc.
THE LEADING IMAGE	Medrad, Inc.
THE LIFT, TRANSFER DEVICE	Prime Engineering
THE LONE STAR RETRACTOR SYSTEM	Lone Star Medical Products, Inc.
THE MEDICAL MANAGER SOFTWARE	Medical Manager Health Systems, Inc.
THE MEDICOOL INSULIN PROTECTOR	Medicool, Inc.
THE MEDICOOL PROTECTALL, PEN PLUS, POUCHO	Medicool, Inc.
THE MICRO-CELL	Twist2it, Inc.
THE MIT	Cfi Medical Solutions (Contour Fabricators, Inc.)
THE NEW ELBOW	Swb Elbow Brace, Ltd.
THE NEXT REGENERATION	Biocomposites Inc.
THE OPTICAL SHOPPE	National Vision, Inc.
THE ORIGINAL PERRY STYLE 42	Ansell Healthcare Products, Inc.
THE ORIGINAL PERRY STYLE 43	Ansell Healthcare Products, Inc.
THE ORIGINAL PINK TAPE	Hy-Tape International
THE PAIN STOPS HERE	Biofreeze Performance Health, Inc.
THE PAK	Contour Pak, Inc.
THE PARTICLE DOCTOR	Bangs Laboratories, Inc.
THE PATRIOT	Chagrin Safety Supply, Inc.
THE PEAK	Creative Biotech Inc.
THE PER-SE EXCHANGE	Per-Se Technologies
THE PHANTOM	Sellstrom Manufacturing Co.
THE PINK SCALER	Twist2it, Inc.
THE POINTE	Electone, A Division Of Siemens Hearing Instruments, Inc.
THE POLYSTIM II	Medical Science Products, Inc.
THE PRACTICE BUILDING COMPANY	Zimmer Dental, Inc.
THE PROPHYGLIDE	Medidenta International, Inc.
THE PROPHYMIRACLE	Twist2it, Inc.
THE PROTECTOR	Mckesson General Medical
THE RESCUE VEST	Bashaw Medical, Inc.
THE ROENTGEN FILES	Brit Systems Inc.
THE ROLLER	Pre Pak Products, Inc.
THE ROPE	Pre Pak Products, Inc.
THE SEMI	Cybex International, Inc.
THE SHIELD	Apollo Corporation
THE SOFT HEART	Medical Science Products, Inc.
THE SOFT SPOT	Medical Science Products, Inc.
THE SPRAY OPAQUE SYSTEM	American Diversified Dental Systems
THE SPRAY OPAQUE SYSTEM	Mds Products, Inc.
THE TRADITIONAL	Mckesson General Medical
THE TRAINER FIT FOR SPORT	Team America Health & Fitness, Inc
THE TRAINER FITNESS	Team America Health & Fitness, Inc
THE TRAINER SPEED DEVELOPMENT SYSTEM	Team America Health & Fitness, Inc
THE TWIST (RECIPROCATING DISPOSABLE PROPHY ANGLE)	Twist2it, Inc.
THE ULTIMATE SPILL KIT	Great Lakes Medical
THE VARIAN MEDICAL SYSTEMS LOGO	Varian Medical Systems
THE VESS CHAIR	Vess Chairs, Inc.
THE VISION CENTER	National Vision, Inc.
THE VISIONARY	Mckesson General Medical
THE WIZARD	Essential Medical Supply, Inc.
THE WOODPECKER	Minnesota Bramstedt Surgical, Inc.
THE WOODS PUMP	Statcorp, Inc.
THE WRAP	Byron Medical
THE WRAPSODY	Mckesson General Medical
THEBREASTCARESITE.COM	Amoena
THECURVE	Select Medical Systems
THER-A-CROSS	Gammex Rmi
THER-A-LINE	Gammex Rmi
THER-X	Advanced Medical Systems, Inc.
THERA	Paramedical Distributors
THERA COLD	Cold Ice, Inc.
THERA FIRM	Paramedical Distributors
THERA FLEX	Cold Ice, Inc.
THERA PUTTY	North Coast Medical, Inc.
THERA SOCK	Paramedical Distributors
THERA-BOOT	Coloplast Manufacturing Us, Llc
THERA-MIST	Pegasus Research Corp.
THERA-TEMP	Polar Products, Inc.
THERABATH	Wr Medical Electronics Co.
THERACATH	Arrow International, Inc.
THERADYNE	Theradyne Products Division
THERAFFIN	Wr Medical Electronics Co.
THERAFIRM	Knit-Rite, Inc.
THERAFIRM	Therafirm, A Knit Rite Company
THERAFOOT	Therafirm, A Knit Rite Company
THERAGAIT	Columbia Medical Manufacturing Llc
THERAKNIT	Neumed Inc.
THERAMINI 3C	Rich-Mar Corporation
THERAPAX DXT 300	Nucletron Corporation
THERAPAX SERIES 3	Nucletron Corporation
THERAPEDIC	Columbia Medical Manufacturing Llc
THERAPIK	Jenex Corporation
THERAPRESS DUO	Hartmann-Conco Inc.
THERAPULSE	Kinetic Concepts, Inc.

THERAPY	Siemens Medical Solutions Usa, Inc
THERARAD	Capintec, Inc.
THERASEED	Theragenics Corp.
THERASOCK	Knit-Rite, Inc.
THERASOCK	Therafirm, A Knit Rite Company
THERASOL	Wr Medical Electronics Co.
THERASOUND	Rich-Mar Corporation
THERASPHERE	Theragenics Corp.
THERASQUEEZE	Medi-Dyne Healthcare Products, L.L.C.
THERASSIST	General Pysiotherapy, Inc.
THERASTAT	Ams Innovative Center-San Jose
THERATHERM	Chattanooga Group
THERATOPE	Oncothyreon Inc.
THERATOUCH	Rich-Mar Corporation
THERATREK	Patterson Medical Holdings, Inc.
THERATRODE	Wr Medical Electronics Co.
THEREVAC	King Pharmaceuticals, Inc.
THEREX	Arrow International, Inc.
THERM-A-REST	Cascade Designs, Inc.
THERM-O-TEMP	Covidien Lp, Formerly Registered As Kendall
THERM-O-TEMP FO-LY-CATH	Covidien Lp, Formerly Registered As Kendall
THERMA FRSOT	G & H Wire Co.
THERMA-KOOL	Nortech Laboratories, Inc.
THERMA-STICK	G & H Wire Co.
THERMA-WRAP	Chattanooga Group
THERMABOND ALLOYS	Dentecon, Inc.
THERMACARE	Gaymar Industries, Inc.
THERMACOOL	Thermage, Inc.
THERMADRAPE	Vital Signs, Inc.
THERMAGE	Thermage, Inc.
THERMAJECT	Hospira, Inc.
THERMAKNIFE	Buffalo Dental Manufacturing Co., Inc.
THERMAL ANGEL	Estill Medical Technologies, Inc.
THERMAL CEILING	Aragona Medical, Inc.
THERMAL CONTROL PRODUCTS	Halbar North, Inc.
THERMAL SCIENCE COLD GEL	Pristech Products, Inc
THERMAL SIGNATURE ANALYSIS	Sea Horse Bio Science
THERMAL VIAL	Minco Products, Inc.
THERMAL-CLEAR	Minco Products, Inc.
THERMAL-NET	Minco Products, Inc.
THERMAL-RIBBON	Minco Products, Inc.
THERMAL-TAB	Minco Products, Inc.
THERMALASTIC	Tak Systems
THERMALATOR	Whitehall Manufacturing
THERMALITE	Geiger Medical Technologies
THERMALOCK	Caddy Corporation
THERMALON	Bruder Healthcare Company
THERMALSOFT	Mettler Electronics Corp.
THERMAPAD	Roloke
THERMASONIC	Parker Laboratories, Inc.
THERMASPEC 1000	Medispec Ltd. - Usa
THERMASPLINT	Whitehall Manufacturing
THERMASURE	Cenorin
THERMATRACE	Pyrometer Instrument Co.
THERMAX	Enternet Medical, Inc.
THERMAX	Tyco Healthcare Group Lp
THERMAZENE	Covidien Lp
THERME-PNEU COMPUTER INSUFFLATOR	Wisap America
THERME3 ENDOSCOPIC WARMING SYSTEM	Wisap America
THERMIBEADS	Thermionics Corp.
THERMIPAQ	Thermionics Corp.
THERMIQUE	Parkell, Inc.
THERMO	Zimmer Medizinsystems
THERMO-BLOCK	S.S. White Burs Inc.
THERMO-LITE	Techstyles Manufacturing Division
THERMOBRITE	Statspin, Inc.
THERMOCORK	Aetrex Worldwide, Inc.
THERMOFLATOR	Karl Storz Endoscopy-America Inc.
THERMOFLEX	Dentsply Prosthetics
THERMOFLO	Arc Medical, Inc.
THERMOFLOW	Gvs Filter Technology Inc.
THERMOFOIL	Minco Products, Inc.
THERMOGARD XP	Alsius Corp.
THERMOGENESIS	Thermogenesis Corp.
THERMOGLIDE	Titronics Research & Development Co.
THERMOMED	Thermosurgery Technologies, Inc.
THERMOMIX	Sartorius Stedim Sus Inc.
THERMOPACE	Arrow International, Inc.
THERMOPHORE	Battle Creek Equipment Co.
THERMOPLANE	Thermotek Inc.
THERMOPULSE PAIN RELIEF SYSTEM	Questech International, Inc.
THERMOSAFE BRANDS, NOMADIC PRE-QUALIFED SHIPPER, SHIPSAFE	Tegrant Corporation, Thermosafe Brands
THERMOSAFE INSULATED SHIPPER-PURr	Thermosafe Brands
THERMOSAFEr CRYOGENIC SHIPPER	Thermosafe Brands
THERMOSAFEr DRY ICE MACHINE	Thermosafe Brands
THERMOSAFEr INSULATED SHIPPER	Thermosafe Brands
THERMOSAFEr INSULATED SHIPPER-VIP	Thermosafe Brands
THERMOSKY	Aetrex Worldwide, Inc
THERMOSTRIP	LCR Hallcrest
THERMOTECH	Tcp Reliable, Inc.
THERMOTEK	Thermotek Inc.
THERMOTIP	Medtronic Xomed, Inc.
THERMOTRACE	Deltatrak, Inc.
THERMOVIBE	Coopercare Lastrap Inc
THERO-GEL	Patterson Medical Holdings, Inc.
THERO-WRAP	Adroit Medical Systems, Inc.
THIGHACISER	All Pro Exercise Products, Inc.
THIN PREP/PAP TEST	Hologic, Inc.
THIN ZONE ASPHERE	Ocu-Ease Optical Products, Inc.
THIN ZONE TORIC	Ocu-Ease Optical Products, Inc.
THIN-ONE	Tu-Way American Group
THINLINE	Camfil Farr
THINPREP 2000	Hologic, Inc.
THINPROFILE	Meddev Corporation
THINSULATE	3m Co.
THIOGEL	Bd Diagnostic Systems
THIOLA	Mission Pharmacal Co.
THIOTONE	Bd Diagnostic Systems
THIRFTY LUME	Maxant Technologies, Inc.
THISBOX	Placon Corporation
THOMMEN	Hansco Technologies, Inc.
THOMPSON	Miltex Inc.
THOMPSON	Thompson Surgical Instruments, Inc.
THOMSON	Second Exposure, Inc.
THONET	Shelby-Williams Industries
THORA-CATH	Utah Medical Products, Inc.
THORA-LIFT	Covidien Lp, Formerly Registered As United States Surgical
THORACOPORT	Covidien Lp, Formerly Registered As United States Surgical
THORASEAL	Covidien Lp
THOROSCAN	Nucletron Corporation
THOROVAC	Andersen Products, Inc.,
THREE-IN-ONE	Oster Professional Products, Inc.
THRESHOLD	Molecular Devices Corp.
THRESHOLD	Respironics New Jersey, Inc.
THRIFT-BACK	Crosstex International,Inc.
THRIM	U.F.I.
THROMBEX	Analytical Control Systems, Inc.
THROMBEXIN	Medi Usa
THROMBIN-JMI	King Pharmaceuticals, Inc.
THROMBONOSTIKA	Biomerieux Inc.
THROMBOQUIK	Biomerieux Inc.
THROMBOSCREEN	Fisher Diagnostics
THROMBOSOL	Lifecell Corp.
THROMCAT	Kensey Nash Corporation
THROMOBOSTRATE	Fisher Diagnostics
THRU-BITE	Boss Instruments, Ltd.
THRUPUT	Sterogene Bioseparations, Inc.
THUMB HELPER	Meddev Corporation
THUMPER	Michigan Instruments, Inc.
THUMPER:PETITE PRINCESS	Bio-Optics, Inc.
THUNDER	Zyloware Corporation
THYRO-TEST	Bio-Medical Products Corp.
THYROID UPTAKE SYSTEM	Biodex Medical Systems, Inc.
TI-BA	Ti-Ba Enterprises, Inc.
TI-BA ENT., INC.	Ti-Ba Enterprises, Inc.

TI-BA ENTERPRISES, INC.	Ti-Ba Enterprises, Inc.
TI-CLIP	Dgh Technology, Inc.
TI-CORE	Essential Dental Systems, Inc.
TI-FORMS	Ticonium Co.
TI-SCREEN	Pedinol Pharmacal, Inc.
TI.CRON	Covidien Lp
TIB EXERCISER	Apec, Inc.
TIB MACHINE	Apec, Inc.
TIBA	Ti-Ba Enterprises, Inc.
TIBIAL NAILING PILLOW HENLEY'S INCLINE PILLOW	Emerald Medical Products Corp.
TIBIAL TRANSFORMER	Freedom Fabrication
TIBURON	Cardinal Health Inc.
TICK REMOVAL FIRST AID KIT	El Mar, Inc.
TICK REMOVAL TWEEZER	El Mar, Inc.
TICL	Staar Surgical Co.
TICOMATIC	Ticonium Co.
TICRON	Covidien Lp
TIDAL WAVE SP	Respironics, Inc
TIDI	Tidi Products, Llc
TIFFENAIRE	Jones Medical Instrument Co.
TIGER	Snug Seat, Inc.
TIGERTAIL	C. R. Bard, Inc., Bard Urological Div.
TIGOLD	Applied Medical Resource Corporation
TILITE	Tisport, Llc
TILSON TRACH GUARD	Beevers Manufacturing, Inc.
TILT IN SPACE PLUS	Activeaid, Inc.
TILT-IN-SPACE POWERCHAIRS	Electric Mobility Corporation
TILT-N-TOTE WHEELCHAIR CARRIER	Wheelchair Carrier, Inc.
TILT-TOP	Covidien Lp, Formerly Registered As United States Surgical
TIMAX	Depuy Ace, A Johnson & Johnson Company
TIME MACHINE	Oralgiene Usa, Inc.
TIME TAPE	Timemed Labeling Systems, Inc.
TIME-SAVER	March & Green
TIMEMASTER	Photon Technology International, Inc.
TIMES-2 SPEED FILES	Richards-Wilcox, Inc.
TIMES-2 STEP-UP, STEP-DOWN	Richards-Wilcox, Inc.
TIMETER	Allied Healthcare Products, Inc.
TIMOLIUM	Tp Orthodontics, Inc.
TIMS	Computers Unlimited
TIMS IV	Computers Unlimited
TIMSEN	Unit Chemical Corp.
TINA	Radiometer America, Inc.
TINCTURE OF BENZOIN	Geritrex Corp.
TINGLE X-RAY (TXR)	Koch X-Ray Systems Inc
TINY TEMP	Mabis Healthcare Inc.
TINY TRACKS	Graham Medical Products/Div. Of Little Rapids Corp
TIP GUARD	Scanlan International, Inc.
TIP TOPS	Helena Plastics
TIP WRENCH ALCON LEGACY	Imonti And Associates Inc., M.
TIP-A-DENT	Denticator International, Inc.
TIP-EDGE	Tp Orthodontics, Inc.
TIP-IT	Miltex Inc.
TIP-TEST: BLV	Immucell Corp.
TIP-TEST: JOHNE'S	Immucell Corp.
TIS-U-TRAP	Milex Products, Inc.
TISEB	Allerderm Laboratories, Inc.
TISEB-T	Allerderm Laboratories, Inc.
TISSUE REPAIR	Cardium Therapeutics Inc.
TISSUE TACKLE	Oncogene Research Products
TISSUE-TEK	Sakura Finetek U.S.A., Inc.
TISSUE-TEK XPRESS	Sakura Finetek U.S.A., Inc.
TISSUEDYNE	Professional Product Co.
TISSUELINK	Dma Med-Chem Corporation
TISSUEMEND	Stryker Corp.
TISSUEPAK	Paperpak
TISSUEPREP	Fisher Scientific Co., Llc.
TITAN	Arthrocare Corp.
TITAN	Cutera, Inc.
TITAN	Dentalez Group
TITAN	Hely And Weber
TITAN	Sellstrom Manufacturing Co.
TITAN	Sonosite, Inc.
TITAN-LIGHT	Dent Zar, Inc.
TITAN-PORT	Angiodynamics, Inc.
TITANIUM	Glines And Rhodes, Inc.
TITANIUM	Magnivision, Inc.
TITANMOLY	G & H Wire Co.
TITERTUBE	Bio-Rad Laboratories, Life Science Group
TITMUS	Titmus Optical Inc.
TJ HUNTER	Reach Global Industries, Inc. (Reachgood)
TKO	Hely And Weber
TKO	Hospira Inc.
TLAS	Dent Zar, Inc.
TLC	Boston Scientific Corporation
TLC	Ortho-Kinetics, Inc.
TLC	Rehabilitation Services, Inc.
TLC	Rockland Industries, Inc.
TLC RETRACTOR	Applied Medical Technology, Inc.
TLC WEAR	Pfb Inter-Apparel Corp.
TLS	Porex Surgical, Inc.
TLS (THE LABORATORY SYSTEM)	Database, Inc.
TM/TML/TMC SERIES	Starkey Laboratories, Inc.
TM18	Bard Access Systems, Inc.
TM262	Welch Allyn, Inc.
TMALAB	Aperio Technologies Inc.
TMAX	Molecular Devices Corp.
TMBLUE	Serologicals Corp
TMD	Triangle Biomedical Sciences, Inc.
TMD.	Medical Device Resource Corporation
TMI	Texas Medical Industries, Inc.
TMI PLASTICS	Specialty Manufacturing Co., The
TMJ APPLIANCE	Tmj Appliance
TMM ACE	Sensors, Inc.
TMM CAPMONITOR	Sensors, Inc.
TMP	Novosci Corp.
TMR (THE MEDICAL RECORD)	Database, Inc.
TMS	Medical Device Resource Corporation
TNCO	Symmetry Medical Usa, Inc.
TNT	Promega Corp.
TO-SEW	Aristotle Corp.
TOBY TRACHEASAURUST	Passy-Muir Inc.
TOE HOLD	Brown Medical Industries
TOE-AID(TM)	Southwest Technologies, Inc.
TOGA	Satiety, Inc.
TOM'S	Moyco Technologies, Inc.
TOMES	Micromedex, Inc.
TOMES PLUS	Micromedex, Inc.
TOMOCAT	Mallinckrodt, Inc.
TOMODIRECT	Tomotherapy Incorporated
TOMORAD	Capintec, Inc.
TOMOSCAN	Philips Medical Systems North America
TONEDOWN	Sellstrom Manufacturing Co.
TONG-CLIN DELUXE	Hager Worldwide, Inc.
TONGUE SWEEPER	Biocurv Medical Instruments, Inc.
TONGUE-AWAY	Tp Orthodontics, Inc.
TONO-PEN	Mentor Ophthalmics, Inc.
TONO-TRAY	Micro-Scientific Industries, Inc.
TONOPEN XL	Mentor Ophthalmics, Inc.
TONYA	Horcher Lifting Systems, Inc.
TOOTH STRENGTHENERS FOR PLASTIC DENTURE TEETH' DENTURE CLEANER.	Nanzee Dental Products
TOOTNETTE	Sage Products, Inc.
TOP BOX	Gerstner & Sons Inc.
TOP CODER	Jeter Systems Corp.
TOP END	Invacare Corporation
TOP GARD	Gaymar Industries, Inc.
TOP LOADING SYSTEM	Orthotec, Llc
TOP TRACK	Intermetro Industries Corp.
TOPAZ	Arthrocare Corp.
TOPAZ	Mge Ups Sytems, Inc.
TOPICALE	The Hymed Group Corp.
TOPTAINER	Abbott Laboratories
TORAYGUIDE	Toray International America Inc.
TORBOT	Torbot Group, Inc.
TORCAN	Cook Inc.

TRAPEZE	Dazian Fabrics,Llc.
TRAUM-AID	Activeaid, Inc.
TRAUMA HAWK	American Emergency Vehicles
TRAUMAJET	Hydrocision, Inc.
TRAUMEX	Fischer Medical Technologies Inc.
TRAVASOL	Baxter Healthcare Corporation Nutrition
TRAVCYL	Car-May
TRAVEL ABOUT	Gendron, Inc.
TRAVEL CHAIR	Ortho-Kinetics, Inc.
TRAVELITE	Living Earth Crafts
TRAVELITE	Seca Corp.
TRAVELJOHN	Reach Global Industries, Inc. (Reachgood)
TRAVELMATE	Caring Hands, Inc.
TRAX	Jeter Systems Corp.
TRAX CORPUS	Permobil, Inc.
TRAX MINIFLEX	Permobil, Inc.
TRAX STANDARD	Permobil, Inc.
TRAXIT	Medical Indicators, Inc.
TRAY-VAC	Buffalo Dental Manufacturing Co., Inc.
TRAYPAK	Qrp, Inc.
TRAYTRAKKER	Computrition, Inc.
TREADS	Albahealth Llc
TREAT YOUR OWN BACK	Optp
TREAT YOUR OWN NECK	Optp
TREBAY	Medtronic Xomed, Inc.
TRED MATES	Principle Business Enterprises, Inc.
TRELLIS	Interspec Fabrics
TREMOR	Colours Wheelchair
TRENDBASE SOFTWARE	Medical Graphics Corporation
TREOSIN	Statlab Medical Products, Inc.
TRI AUTO ZX	J. Morita Usa, Inc.
TRI W-G	Tri W-G Group
TRI-BAND	Precision Dynamics Corp.
TRI-CLAMP ACCESSORY CLAMP	Allen Medical Systems, Inc.
TRI-COR PILLOW	Core Products International, Inc.
TRI-CORE PILLOW	Core Products International, Inc.
TRI-CRAFT	Atlantic Medco, Inc.
TRI-FLEX	Gammex Rmi
TRI-FLEX	Joerns Healthcare, Inc
TRI-FLOW	Medcomp (Medical Components, Inc.)
TRI-LOCK	Contech Medical, Inc.
TRI-OPT	Advanced Endoscopy Devices, Inc.
TRI-SEAL	Vacumed
TRI-SET	Reel R&D, Inc.
TRI-SORBER	In/Us Systems, Inc.
TRI-TECH	Independent Solutions, Inc.
TRI-TRONICS	Tri-Tronics Co., Inc.
TRIA	Amoena
TRIACTIV	Kensey Nash Corporation
TRIAD	Argosy
TRIAD	Supertech, Inc.
TRIAD, TRIADERM, TOTALBATH	Triad Disposables
TRIADYNE	Kinetic Concepts, Inc.
TRIANO	Siemens Hearing Instruments, Inc.
TRIARCO	Aristotle Corp.
TRIATHLER	Perkin Elmer Wallac, Inc.
TRIATHLER	Perkinelmer Life And Analytical Sciences
TRIATHLON	Stryker Corp.
TRIATHLON	Stryker Howmedica Osteonics
TRIAX	Stryker Corp.
TRIBUTE	Sonic Innovations
TRIBUTE FOOT	College Park Industries, Inc.
TRICAM	Karl Storz Endoscopy-America Inc.
TRICHOSEL	Bd Diagnostic Systems
TRICITRASOL	Citra Anticoagulants, Inc.
TRIDENT	Stryker Corp.
TRIDENT	Stryker Howmedica Osteonics
TRIDENT ACETABULAR CUPS	Stryker Corp.
TRIDENT ACETABULAR CUPS	Stryker Howmedica Osteonics
TRIDEX	Ring Communications, Inc.
TRIDICATOR	Fil-Chem, Inc.
TRIFLEX	Chestnut Ridge Foam, Inc.
TRIFLO	Covidien Lp

TRIFOLD	Homecare Products, Inc.
TRIGEN	Smith & Nephew Inc.- Orthopaedics Division
TRILITE	3m Espe Dental Products
TRILOBITE	Esco Medical Instruments, Inc.
TRILOGY	Smiths Medical OEM
TRILOGY	Varian Medical Systems
TRILOK	Cropper Medical, Inc./Bio Skin
TRIM	Harry J. Bosworth Company
TRIM II	Harry J. Bosworth Company
TRIM TACK	Markel Industries, Inc.
TRIM-LITE	Bristol C&D, Inc.
TRIMA ACCEL	Caridianbct Inc.
TRIMARKER	Griff Industries, Inc.
TRIMFLO	Vasamed
TRIMIC	Siemens Hearing Instruments, Inc.
TRIMLINE	Electromed, Inc.
TRIMLINE SERIES	Bobrick Washroom Equipment, Inc.
TRIMPLUS	Harry J. Bosworth Company
TRIMSHIELD	Principle Business Enterprises, Inc.
TRINIDAD	Aearo Company
TRIO	Stryker Corp.
TRIO	Stryker Spine
TRIO*STIM	Mettler Electronics Corp.
TRIOCUT	Medidenta International, Inc.
TRIOSTAT	King Pharmaceuticals, Inc.
TRIP LESSYSTEM	Sharps Compliance Corp.
TRIPHASIX	Parkell, Inc.
TRIPLE CARE	Smith & Nephew, Inc.
TRIPLE I	Landauer, Inc.
TRIPLE SEAL	Young Innovations, Inc.
TRIPLE-FORCE	G & H Wire Co.
TRIPLESTIX	Neurodyne Medical Corp.
TRIPOUR	Covidien Lp
TRISCOPE	Wallach Surgical Devices, Inc.
TRISEAL	Tagg Industries L.L.C.
TRISTANDER	Patterson Medical Holdings, Inc.
TRISTAR	Arthrocare Corp.
TRISTAR	Wallach Surgical Devices, Inc.
TRISTAR SERIES, EDP SERIES	Oneac Corporation
TRITON	Chattanooga Group
TRITON	Medtronic Powered Surgical Solutions
TRIUMPH	Ortho-Kinetics, Inc.
TRIUMPH-1	Angiodynamics, Inc.
TRIVEX (SMITH & NEPHEW)	Dma Med-Chem Corporation
TRIWIRE	Applied Medical Resource Corporation
TRO-GARD	Conmed Corporation
TROGARD	Conmed Corporation
TRONEX. THE CHOICE - REGISTERED TRADE MARK NAME	Tronex Healthcare Industries
TROPHY	Puritan Medical Products Company Llc
TROPIC HEATER	Patterson Medical Holdings, Inc.
TROPIC PAC	Patterson Medical Holdings, Inc.
TROPICAL WEIGHT	Bell-Horn, Inc.
TROPICOOLER	Boekel Scientific
TROY	Rem Systems
TRU-CLOSE	Covidien Lp
TRU-CLOSE	Uresil, Llc
TRU-CORE	Medical Device Technologies, Inc. (Md Tech)
TRU-DOSE	Western Medica
TRU-FIT	Amici, Inc.
TRU-FIT	George Taub Products & Fusion Co., Inc.
TRU-FIT	Stryker Corp.
TRU-FIX	Uresil, Llc
TRU-FLO	Uresil, Llc
TRU-FORCE	Tp Orthodontics, Inc.
TRU-FORM	Univac Dental Company
TRU-LITE HANDLE	Suter Dental Manufacturing Company, Inc.
TRU-PAK	General Dental Products, Inc.
TRU-PAQUE	George Taub Products & Fusion Co., Inc.
TRU-PULL	DJO Inc.
TRU-SCINT AD	Oncothyreon Inc.
TRU-SEAL	Possis Medical, Inc.
TRU-SILK ARTICULATING RIBBON	American Diversified Dental Systems

TWIN DENTO BOX	Hager Worldwide, Inc.
TWIN FIX	Smith & Nephew, Inc., Endoscopy Division
TWIN SPOON	Carex Health Brands
TWIN STAY	Lone Star Medical Products, Inc.
TWIN TIP	Hospital Marketing Svcs. Company, Inc.
TWIN-EDGE	Tp Orthodontics, Inc.
TWINCAM	Karl Storz Endoscopy-America Inc.
TWINCATH	Arrow International, Inc.
TWINFIX	Stryker Corp.
TWINLIGHT LONG PULSED YAG LASER FOR HAIR REMOVAL AND LEG VEINS	New Laser Science, Inc.
TWINLOCK	Arthrocare Corp.
TWINLOOK	Astro-Med, Inc.
TWINMIC	Siemens Hearing Instruments, Inc.
TWINVIDEO	Karl Storz Endoscopy-America Inc.
TWINWAL	Frontier Medical Products, Inc.
TWIST	Crosstex International, Inc.
TWIST FREE MINI-BAK	Key-Bak
TWIST-LOCK	Byron Medical
TWIST-LOKS	Healthmark Industries
TWIST2IT HANDPIECE SPRAY	Twist2it, Inc.
TWISTER	Action Products, Inc.
TWISTER	Nova Health Systems, Inc.
TWISTER	Zymark Corporation
TWISTER II PLATE HANDLER	Caliper Life Sciences, Inc.
TWISTY FLEX	Minco Products, Inc.
TWO-FER	Baxa Corporation
TWO-WEIGH	Seca Corp.
TWOSOME	Palmer Industries
TX-2000	Enmet Corp.
TXR	York X-Ray And Orthopedic Supply, Inc.
TXT	Siemens Medical Solutions Usa, Inc
TYCOS	Creative Health Products, Inc.
TYCOS	Welch Allyn, Inc.
TYGON R-3603	Saint-Gobain Performance Plastics--Akron
TYGON S-50-HL	Saint-Gobain Performance Plastics--Akron
TYGON S-54-HL	Saint-Gobain Performance Plastics--Akron
TYGON S-95-E	Saint-Gobain Performance Plastics--Akron
TYGOPURE	Saint-Gobain Performance Plastics--Akron
TYGOTHANE, SANIPURE	Saint-Gobain Performance Plastics--Akron
TYLENOL	Ortho-Mcneil-Janssen Pharmaceuticals, Inc.
TYLOX	Ortho-Mcneil-Janssen Pharmaceuticals, Inc.
TYM-TAP	Medtronic Xomed, Inc.
TYMPANETTE	Starkey Laboratories, Inc.
TYMSERVE	Symmetricom Timing, Test & Measurement
TYPE 8 FRAMES	Camfil Farr
TYPENEX	Fenwal Inc.
TYPHLO-CONE	Rehabilitation Services, Inc.
TYPHOON	Bruno Independent Living Aids, Inc.
TYPHOON	DJO Inc.
TYSHAK	Numed, Inc.
TYSHAK II	Numed, Inc.
TYSHAK MINI	Numed, Inc.
TYTRON C-3000	Titronics Research & Development Co.
TYVEK	Medical Action Industries, Inc
TZERO	Ta Instruments
Tampax	Procter & Gamble
TandemHeart	Cardiac Assist, Inc.
Telesheath	St. Jude Medical, Inc.
Ten-Ten	Boston Scientific Corporation
Tendril	St. Jude Medical, Inc.
The Bio-Pump	Medtronic Perfusion Systems
The BioCal	Medtronic Perfusion Systems
The MYOtherm XP	Medtronic Perfusion Systems
The Mega V	Megasun
The Stick	Rpi Of Atlanta
TheraRest	Kinetic Concepts, Inc.
Therapy	St. Jude Medical, Inc.
Therapy Cool Path	St. Jude Medical, Inc.
Therapy Dual-8	St. Jude Medical, Inc.
ThermaSeal	Dentsply Tulsa Dental Products
ThermaSeal	Dentsply Tulsa Dental Specialties
Thermacor	Acor Orthopaedic, Inc.
Thermafil	Dentsply Tulsa Dental Products
Thermafil	Dentsply Tulsa Dental Specialties
ThermoCool	Biosense Webster, Inc
Thermodilatation	Boston Scientific Corporation
Thompson	Nutraceutical International Corp.
Toronto Root	St. Jude Medical, Inc.
Toronto SPV	St. Jude Medical, Inc.
Tracker	Boston Scientific Corporation
Transitions	Younger Manufacturing Co., Inc.
Tri-Lam	Acor Orthopaedic, Inc.
Tri-Lock	Park Dental Research Corp./Implant Center
TriCell	Kinetic Concepts, Inc.
TriggerWheel	Rpi Of Atlanta
Trillium	Medtronic Perfusion Systems
Trilogy	Younger Manufacturing Co., Inc.
Trinica	Zimmer Spine, Inc.
Triple Moisture	Ortho Dermatologics
Tripod	Freedom Designs, Inc.
TruFUSE	minSURG International, Inc.
TruPath	Boston Scientific Corporation
TuliGel	Medi-Dyne Healthcare Products, L.L.C.
U-BAG	Hollister Incorporated
U-FILL SAND BAGS	Morrison Medical
U-FIT TEMPLE	H.L. Bouton Co., Inc.
U-LACTIN	Allerderm Laboratories, Inc.
U-SHAPE BITE WAFERS	Aluwax Dental Products Co.
U-TEKr	Thermosafe Brands
U.S. SAFETY	Parmelee Industries, Inc.
UAM	Vilex, Inc.
UBA	Hologic, Inc.
UBC (UPPER BODY CYCLE)	Biodex Medical Systems, Inc.
UBE	Cybex International, Inc.
UBI FOOT AND MOUTH DISEASE VIRUS ANTIBODY TEST KIT (SWINE)	Ubi
UBI HCV EIA 10.0.	Ubi
UBI HIV 1/2 EIA	Ubi
UBI SARS COV EIA	Ubi
UBITH VACCINES	Ubi
UDM	United Dental Manufacturers, Inc.
UIMS	Dornier Medtech America
UINBRAND	Dux Dental
UIO1	Performance Attainment Associates
UKIYO	Lhasa Oms, Inc.
UL / CSA	Tailored Label Products, Inc.
ULCERCARE	Bsn-Jobst
ULCERJET	Hydrocision, Inc.
ULITMA	Ethicon, Inc.
ULP	MAQUET
ULTEC	Covidien Lp
ULTEM	Codman & Shurtleff, Inc
ULTI CARE	Ulti Med, Inc.
ULTI-MATE	Invacare Corporation
ULTI-MED	Dukal Corporation
ULTICOMFORT	Ulti Med, Inc.
ULTIFINE	Ulti Med, Inc.
ULTIGUARD	Ulti Med, Inc.
ULTIMA	Columbia Medical Manufacturing Llc
ULTIMA	Paperpak
ULTIMA	White Knight Engineered Products
ULTIMA 60	Leisure-Lift, Inc.
ULTIMA 80	Leisure-Lift, Inc.
ULTIMA BLOC	Gi Supply
ULTIMA SERIES	Topcon Medical Systems, Inc.
ULTIMA SUPERSORB	Paperpak
ULTIMATE	Orthodontic Supply & Equipment Co., Inc.
ULTIMATE ACID	Qrp, Inc.
ULTIMATE CASTING SYSTEM	Heraeus Kulzer, Inc.
ULTIMATE CONDUCTIVE GARMENTS	Judah Mfg. Corp.
ULTIMATE HAND HELPER	Meddev Corporation
ULTIMATE HURT	Medical Plastics Laboratory, Inc.
ULTIMAX	Toshiba America Medical Systems
ULTIMEDEX	Micromedex, Inc.
ULTIMO	Grant Airmass Corporation
ULTIPAQ	Micrus Corporation

ULTISMOOTH	Ulti Med, Inc.
ULTITHIN	Ulti Med, Inc.
ULTRA	Geerpres
ULTRA	Insiphil (Us) Llc
ULTRA	Marlen Manufacturing & Development Co.
ULTRA	Scientech, Inc.
ULTRA	Smiths Medical OEM
ULTRA	Virtis, An Sp Industries Company
ULTRA BEIGE	Freeman Manufacturing Company
ULTRA C	Surmet Corp.
ULTRA CARE	Pyramid Industries, Llc
ULTRA CARE	Tillotson Healthcare Corp.
ULTRA COMFORT	Health Science Products, Inc.
ULTRA DRIVE	Biomet, Inc.
ULTRA FLO	Welcon, Inc.
ULTRA FOAM	Quantachrome
ULTRA FRESH	Mentor Corp.
ULTRA ICE	Ep Technologies, Inc.
ULTRA LF	Donovan Industries
ULTRA MIRAGE	Resmed Corp.
ULTRA MIST	Salter Labs
ULTRA N/S GLOVES	Lee Medical International, Inc.
ULTRA ONE, CE SYSTEM (CONTROLLED ENVIRONMENT)	Microflex Corporation
ULTRA PLUS	Crosstex International,Inc.
ULTRA PRESERVE	Tillotson Healthcare Corp.
ULTRA PRO ULTRASOUND TABLE	Biodex Medical Systems, Inc.
ULTRA SHAPE	Barnett Intl. Corp.
ULTRA STAR	Star Case Manufacturing Co., Inc.
ULTRA STENT	M & I Medical Sales, Inc.
ULTRA THERMr	Ultimate Wireforms, Inc.
ULTRA TRIM	Harry J. Bosworth Company
ULTRA VAC	Hager Worldwide, Inc.
ULTRA WHISPERS	Roman Research, Inc.
ULTRA-1	Analytical Control Systems, Inc.
ULTRA-4	DJO Inc.
ULTRA-CAL	Ultra-Cal, Inc.
ULTRA-CARE	Zimmer Orthopaedic Surgical Products
ULTRA-CHECK	Cas Medical Systems, Inc.
ULTRA-CLASSIC	Ultrascope
ULTRA-CUSHION, CHAIRPRO ALARMS, BEDPRO ALARMS, FLOORPRO ALARMS	Skil-Care Corp.
ULTRA-FINISH	Anchor Products Company
ULTRA-FLEX	King Systems Corp.
ULTRA-GRIP	Mckesson General Medical
ULTRA-LIGHT SABER 2004	Laser Dental Innovations
ULTRA-LITE	Impact Instrumentation, Inc.
ULTRA-LITE POWERCHAIRS	Electric Mobility Corporation
ULTRA-LITE SCOOTERS	Electric Mobility Corporation
ULTRA-LOCK	Smiths Medical Asd, Inc.
ULTRA-MINI	Ultrascope
ULTRA-SCOPE	Ultrascope
ULTRA-SLIP	Vital Signs, Inc.
ULTRA-T	Ultrascope
ULTRA-TECHNE-KOW	Mallinckrodt, Inc.
ULTRA-TIP	Sonicwall, Inc.
ULTRA-TOT	Ultrascope
ULTRA-TOUCH	Clean Esd Products, Inc.
ULTRA-TOUCH	Jaisons International, Inc.
ULTRA-TOUGH	Oak Gloves Division Of Omar Medical Supplies, Inc.
ULTRA-TURRAX	Applied Biosystems
ULTRA-VISION	Agfa Corporation
ULTRA8	Lw Scientific
ULTRABAG	Baxter Healthcare Corporation, Renal
ULTRABLUE	Serologicals Corp
ULTRABRAZE	Sonicwall, Inc.
ULTRABRIGHT	Arc Medical, Inc.
ULTRABRUSH	Young Innovations, Inc.
ULTRAC	Thermo Fisher Scientific - Laboratory Equipment Division Headquarters
ULTRACAM	American Medical Technologies, Inc.
ULTRACAM	Edge Systems Corporation
ULTRACAM	Ultra-Lum, Inc.
ULTRACARE	Abbott Medical Optics Inc.
ULTRACARE	Allergan
ULTRACARE	Joerns Healthcare, Inc
ULTRACELL	Ultracell Medical Technologies, Inc.
ULTRACELL CLASSIC	Ultracell Medical Technologies, Inc.
ULTRACENT	Bio-Rad Laboratories, Life Science Group
ULTRACET	Ortho-Mcneil-Janssen Pharmaceuticals, Inc.
ULTRACHECK	Statcorp, Inc.
ULTRACHEK	Separation Technology Inc
ULTRACLAMP	Baxter Healthcare Corporation, Renal
ULTRACOMPACT 9500	W.O.M. World Of Medicine Usa, Inc.
ULTRACOT	American Silk Sutures, Inc.
ULTRACRIT	Separation Technology Inc
ULTRADOSE	L&R Manufacturing Co.
ULTRAFIN STIRRUP	Allen Medical Systems, Inc.
ULTRAFIT	Surgical Specialties Corporation
ULTRAFIX	Conmed Linvatec
ULTRAFIX	E K Industries, Inc.
ULTRAFLEX	Independent Solutions, Inc.
ULTRAFLOW	Ev3 Inc.
ULTRAFORM	American Health Systems
ULTRAFORM PRESSURE RELIEF SYSTEM	American Health Systems
ULTRAFREE	Cardinal Health Inc.
ULTRAFYN	Advanced Meditech International
ULTRAGARD	Crosstex International,Inc.
ULTRAGARD	Precept Medical Products, Inc.
ULTRAGLIDE	Surgical Specialties Corporation
ULTRAGUARD	Mge Ups Sytems, Inc.
ULTRAGUM	Crown Delta Corp.
ULTRAIMAGER	Ultra-Lum, Inc.
ULTRAJECT	Mallinckrodt, Inc.
ULTRALIFE	Ultralife Batteries, Inc.
ULTRALIFE HIRATE	Ultralife Batteries, Inc.
ULTRALIFE POLYMER	Ultralife Batteries, Inc.
ULTRALIFE THIN CELL	Ultralife Batteries, Inc.
ULTRALITE PATIENT CHAIR	Dntlworks Equipment Corporation
ULTRALON PF	Ansell Healthcare Products, Inc.
ULTRALUX	Schaerer Mayfield Usa
ULTRAM	Ortho-Mcneil-Janssen Pharmaceuticals, Inc.
ULTRAMATIC	Reichert, Inc.
ULTRAMAX	Edge Systems Corporation
ULTRAPACK	Ultracell Medical Technologies, Inc.
ULTRAPAS	Covidien Lp, Formerly Registered As United States Surgical
ULTRAPHINE	Ultracell Medical Technologies, Inc.
ULTRAPLUS 5000	Ultracell Medical Technologies, Inc.
ULTRAPOL 1200	Ultra Tec Manufacturing, Inc.
ULTRAPOWER	Conmed Linvatec
ULTRAPRO	Ethicon, Inc.
ULTRAPROBE	U.E. Systems, Inc.
ULTRAPYCNOMETR	Quantachrome
ULTRASCAN	Medical Positioning, Inc.
ULTRASCAN XE	Hunter Associates Lab., Inc.
ULTRASCOPE	Lydia's Professional Uniforms
ULTRASCOPE, DOPPLERSCOPE, VET-DOP, VACUPAD	Vmed Technology, Inc. (Formerly Ems Products, Inc.)
ULTRASHEARS	Covidien Lp, Formerly Registered As United States Surgical
ULTRASHIELD	HARTMANN USA, Inc.
ULTRASHIELD EXTRA	HARTMANN USA, Inc.
ULTRASHIELD PLUS	HARTMANN USA, Inc.
ULTRASIL	Ofs, Specialty Photonics Division
ULTRASILK SHEERS	Bauerfeind Usa, Inc.
ULTRASIM-ULTRASOUND SIMULATOR	Medsim-Eagle Simulation Inc.
ULTRASITE	B. Braun Medical Inc., Renal Therapies Div.
ULTRASITE	B. Braun Oem Division, B. Braun Medical Inc.
ULTRASLICE	Ultra Tec Manufacturing, Inc.
ULTRASLIDE	Skytron
ULTRASMART ULTRAPORTABLE	Welch Allyn Protocol Inc.
ULTRASNAP	Vector Laboratories, Inc.
ULTRASON 990	Engler Engineering Corp.
ULTRASONIC SCALER	Dentronix, Inc.
ULTRASOUND	Supertech, Inc.
ULTRASOUND CT	Techniscan, Inc.
ULTRASPORT	Medical Industries America Inc.
ULTRASTIM	Axelgaard Manufacturing Company, Ltd.
ULTRASURE	HARTMANN USA, Inc.

ULTRASURE PLUS	HARTMANN USA, Inc.
ULTRATAG	Mallinckrodt, Inc.
ULTRATEC	Weitbrecht Communications, Inc.
ULTRATEX GUMNUMB	Crosstex International,Inc.
ULTRATRACE	Conmed Corporation
ULTRAVAC	Arthrocare Corp.
ULTRAVENT	Mallinckrodt, Inc.
ULTRAVIEW	Perkin Elmer Wallac, Inc.
ULTRAVIEW	Perkinelmer Life And Analytical Sciences
ULTRAZYME	Abbott Medical Optics Inc.
UM	Byron Medical
UMBILI-CATH	Utah Medical Products, Inc.
UMF	Independent Solutions, Inc.
UMF	United Metal Fabricators, Inc.
UMI	Thomas Medical Inc.
UMP	Universal Medical Products, Inc.
UN-SKRU	Multi Marketing & Manufacturing, Inc.
UNBURN	Water-Jel Technologies
UNCLE BILL'S	El Mar, Inc.
UNCLE BILL'S SLIVER GRIPPER	El Mar, Inc.
UNDIES	Byron Medical
UNEX EXERCISE SYSTEMS	Patterson Medical Holdings, Inc.
UNI DERM	Smith & Nephew, Inc.
UNI SALVE	Smith & Nephew, Inc.
UNI SYRINGE	Hager Worldwide, Inc.
UNI TIPS	Hager Worldwide, Inc.
UNI VAC	Hager Worldwide, Inc.
UNI WASH	Smith & Nephew, Inc.
UNI-BAR	Spectra Industries Corp.
UNI-CAPSETTE	Bio Plas, Inc.
UNI-CART	Waterloo Healthcare, Llc
UNI-CASSETTE	Sakura Finetek U.S.A., Inc.
UNI-CLIP AND XKNIFE	Integra Lifesciences Holdings Corp.
UNI-FLEX SAFETY CAPS	Bio Plas, Inc.
UNI-GOLD	Trinity Biotech, Inc.
UNI-GRIP	Dentsply International, Inc.
UNI-GRIP	Dentsply Prosthetics
UNI-LIM	Westmed, Inc.
UNI-MED PAK	Universal Medical Design
UNI-N/F TEK	Remel
UNI-OF	Remel
UNI-POLE	A.R.C. Distributors
UNI-PORE	Bio-Rad Laboratories, Life Science Group
UNI-PRINT	Precision Dynamics Corp.
UNI-PUNCH	Premier Medical Products
UNI-SOLVE	Smith & Nephew, Inc.
UNI-SUCTION PUMP	Ambu, Inc.
UNI-TAB	Covidien Lp, Formerly Registered As Uni-Patch
UNI-TIP	Smith & Nephew, Inc.
UNI-VENT	Impact Instrumentation, Inc.
UNI-VENT EAGLE	Impact Instrumentation, Inc.
UNI-YEAST	Remel
UNIBASE AMERICA	Medidenta International, Inc.
UNICABLE	Rf Industries, Inc.
UNICALL	Dwyer Precision Products, Inc.
UNICARE	Smith & Nephew, Inc.
UNICELL	Basi (Bioanalytical Systems, Inc.)
UNICELL	Independent Solutions, Inc.
UNICLEAN	Uniclean Cleanroom Garment Services
UNICO	United Products & Instruments, Inc.
UNICUF	Frontier Medical Products, Inc.
UNIDAPT	Rf Industries, Inc.
UNIDRIVE	Karl Storz Endoscopy-America Inc.
UNIFET	Sendx Med, Inc.
UNIFLEX	Biomet, Inc.
UNIFLEX	Hill-Rom Holdings, Inc.
UNIFLEX	Smith & Nephew, Inc.
UNIFLO	Schleicher & Schuell, Inc.
UNIFLOW	Hemco Corp.
UNIFOAM	Scott Specialties, Inc./Cmo Inc./Ginny Inc.
UNIFORM	Univac Dental Company
UNIFORM ACCESSORIES	Lydia's Professional Uniforms
UNIFUSOR	Cas Medical Systems, Inc.
UNIFUSOR	Statcorp, Inc.
UNIJET	Basi (Bioanalytical Systems, Inc.)
UNIKLEEN	Unit Chemical Corp.
UNILAB	Hemco Corp.
UNILAB	M. Braun Inc.
UNILIFT	Horcher Lifting Systems, Inc.
UNILITE	Ricon Corp.
UNILUX	Univac Dental Company
UNIMANO	Netech, Corp.
UNIMAT	Nova Health Systems, Inc.
UNIMAX	Hemco Corp.
UNIMET 1100	Bender, Inc.
UNINET	Biovest International, Inc.
UNINUT	Basi (Bioanalytical Systems, Inc.)
UNION	Medtronic Sofamor Danek Usa, Inc
UNION	Medtronic Sofamor Danek Usa, Inc.
UNION BROACH	Miltex Inc.
UNION BROACH	Moyco Technologies, Inc.
UNIPHONE 1140	Ultratec, Inc.
UNIPLUS	Atcc
UNIPOST IMPLANT SYSTEM	Tatum Surgical
UNIQCOT	American Silk Sutures, Inc.
UNIQUAL	Siemens Healthcare Diagnostics Inc
UNISALVE	Smith & Nephew, Inc.
UNISCALE	Seca Corp.
UNISEAL	Washington Trade International, Inc.
UNISON	Dentsply Caulk
UNISPENSE	Covidien Lp
UNISPENSE	Wheaton Science Products
UNISPLINT	Unisplint Corp.
UNISPORE	Getinge Usa, Inc.
UNISTAT	Leica Microsystems, Inc., Educational & Analytical Division
UNISTEP MONO	Lifesign
UNISWITCH	Basi (Bioanalytical Systems, Inc.)
UNIT DOSE BINS	Lewis Bins+
UNIT DOSE BINS	Orbis Corporation
UNIT-PAK	Medical Packaging Inc.
UNITAG	Promega Corp.
UNITECT	Oncogene Research Products
UNITED CONTOUR	Smith & Nephew, Inc.
UNITED MEDICAL MFG CO.	Texas Medical Industries, Inc.
UNITED OXYGEN	U O Equipment Co.
UNITED PLASTICS	Texas Medical Industries, Inc.
UNITEK	3m Espe Dental Products
UNITOP	Virtis, An Sp Industries Company
UNITRAC-3	DJO Inc.
UNITY	Bio-Rad, Diagnostics Group
UNITY	Prentke Romich Company
UNITY	Siemens Hearing Instruments, Inc.
UNITY BX STATION	Gi Supply
UNITY CART	Gi Supply
UNITY CLEANUP	Gi Supply
UNITY NETWORK	Ge Medical Systems Information Technologies
UNITY ORGANIZER	Gi Supply
UNITY SYSTEM	Gi Supply
UNIVAC	Univac Dental Company
UNIVENT	Vitaid Ltd.
UNIVERSAL	Applied Medical Resource Corporation
UNIVERSAL	Biomet, Inc.
UNIVERSAL	Siemens Healthcare Diagnostics Inc
UNIVERSAL	Symmetry Medical, Inc.
UNIVERSAL	York X-Ray And Orthopedic Supply, Inc.
UNIVERSAL ARM BOARD	Lundy Medical Product, Llc
UNIVERSAL CATARACT KNIFE	Akorn, Inc.
UNIVERSAL COMB	Oster Professional Products, Inc.
UNIVERSAL COMPOUNDS	Helvoet Pharma, Inc.
UNIVERSAL F	King Systems Corp.
UNIVERSAL F2	King Systems Corp.
UNIVERSAL FIXATION DRIVER	Vilex, Inc.
UNIVERSAL HAND HELD	Symmetry Medical, Inc.
UNIVERSAL HANDLE	Mercury Medical
UNIVERSAL LABEL	Sps Medical Supply Corp.
UNIVERSAL PLUS	Conmed Corporation

UNIVERSAL SPECULUM	Advanced Medical Innovations, Inc.
UNIVERSAL2, K2 HEMI, KOMPRESSOR, KATALYST, VIPER WITH VALT . Kinetikos Medical, Inc.	
UNIVERSITY PRACTICUM	Zimmer Dental, Inc.
UNIWASH	Smith & Nephew, Inc.
UNIWEDGE	Almore International, Inc.
UNNA-SLEEVE	Aci Medical, Inc.
UNO	Liko North America
UNO WHO	Hely And Weber
UNO WHT	Hely And Weber
UNOLOK	Myco Medical
UNTIL	Scientific Pharmaceuticals, Inc.
UNWIRE	Nalge Nunc International
UOE	U O Equipment Co.
UP-MIST	Unomedical, Inc.
UPPIES	Tulip Medical Products
UPRIGHT	Fonar Corp.
UPRIGHT JET	American Orthodontics Corp.
UPRIGHT STANDING FRAME	Ortho-Kinetics, Inc.
UPRIGHT, PEDIATRIC MIDLINE STANDING FRAME FRAME	Prime Engineering
UPSHER	Mercury Medical
UPSHERSCOPE	Mercury Medical
UPSHERSCOPE ULTRA	Mercury Medical
UR-ASSURE	Precision Dynamics Corp.
URA-RAD GASKETS	Hot Cell Services
UREA-PDA DISKS	Remel
UREACIN	Pedinol Pharmacal, Inc.
UREFLEX	Uresil, Llc
UREVAC	Zimmer Orthopaedic Surgical Products
URI KIT	Culture Kits, Inc.
URI-CATH	Utah Medical Products, Inc.
URI-CEL	Cambridge Diagnostic Products, Inc.
URI-DRAIN	Covidien Lp
URI-KLEEN	Smith & Nephew, Inc.
URI-PAK	Globe Scientific, Inc.
URI-PAN	Plasti Products, Inc.
URI-THREE	Culture Kits, Inc.
URI-TUBE	Bio-Medical Products Corp.
URI-TWO	Culture Kits, Inc.
URICULT	Lifesign
URINE TIME	Helena Plastics
URIPREP	Diasys Corporation
URISEP	Diasys Corporation
URISTAIN	Hardy Diagnostics
URISTIX	Siemens Healthcare Diagnostics Inc.
URISUB	Cst Technologies, Inc.
URO CATCHER SYSTEM	Allen Medical Systems, Inc.
URO RISK	Mission Pharmacal Co.
URO-BOND	Urocare Products, Inc.
URO-CATH	Urocare Products, Inc.
URO-CON	Urocare Products, Inc.
URO-FOAM	Urocare Products, Inc.
URO-LUX	Urocare Products, Inc.
URO-PANEL	Covance Research Products Inc.
URO-PREP	Urocare Products, Inc.
URO-SAFE	Urocare Products, Inc.
URO-SAN PLUS	Mentor Corp.
URO-STRAP	Urocare Products, Inc.
UROBILISTIX	Siemens Healthcare Diagnostics Inc.
UROBREEZE	Timm Medical Technologies, Inc.
UROCAM	Karl Storz Endoscopy-America Inc.
UROCARE	Urocare Products, Inc.
UROCIT-K	Mission Pharmacal Co.
UROCOMP	Modulus Data Systems, Inc.
UROCYSTIN	Mission Pharmacal Co.
UROLAB	Life-Tech, Inc.
UROLAB JANUS	Life-Tech, Inc.
UROLAB MAXIMUS	Life-Tech, Inc.
UROLAB NOVUS	Life-Tech, Inc.
UROLAB OPUS	Life-Tech, Inc.
UROLAB PRIMUS SPECTRUM	Life-Tech, Inc.
UROLEX	Medegen Medical Products, Llc
UROLIGHT	Medical Energy, Inc.
UROLINE	Ams Innovative Center-San Jose
UROLOGY C-ARM TABLE	Biodex Medical Systems, Inc.
UROMAX	Shimadzu Medical Systems
UROMAX	Trimedyne, Inc.
URONIX	Rontron Engineering, Inc.
UROPOWER 201	W.O.M. World Of Medicine Usa, Inc.
UROPUMP	Life-Tech, Inc.
UROSCOPE	Self Regulation Systems, Inc.
UROSON II	Carolina Medical, Inc.
UROSPEC	Medispec Ltd. - Usa
UROTRACK	C. R. Bard, Inc., Bard Urological Div.
UROVIEW 2600	Ge Oec Medical Systems Inc.
UROVISION	Life-Tech, Inc.
UROVISION JANUS	Life-Tech, Inc.
UROVYSION	Abbott Laboratories
UROWIRE	Applied Medical Resource Corporation
US IMAGING TABLES	Mizuho Osi
USA DETECTION SYSTEMS	Covance Research Products Inc.
USA TOTE	Handi-Cap Aids Company
USA WORKFORCE	Artcraft New York
USAORIENT	Questech International, Inc.
USB	Usb Corporation
USB LOGO DESIGN	Usb Corporation
USCI	Bard Electro Physiology
USDI	Dencraft
USERGARD	Arrow International, Inc.
USHIO	Bulbworks, Inc.
USI	Ultron Systems, Inc.
USMC	Seattle Systems
USSC	Covidien Lp, Formerly Registered As United States Surgical
USTOMVUE	Abbott Medical Optics Inc.
UTAH ARM 2	Motion Control, Inc.
UTAS-E3000MF	Lkc Technologies, Inc.
UTERINE BALLOON THERAPY SYSTEM	Gynecare
UTERINE EXPLORA	Milex Products, Inc.
UV POWER PUCK	Eit, Inc.
UV SERIES	Thermo Spectronic
UV SHIELD	Noir Manufacturing
UVADEX	Therakos, Inc., A Johnson & Johnson Company
UVAR	Therakos, Inc., A Johnson & Johnson Company
UVAR XTS	Therakos, Inc., A Johnson & Johnson Company
UVEX	Hager Worldwide, Inc.
UVICURE PLUS	Eit, Inc.
UVISOL	National Biological Corp.
UXR	Xma (X-Ray Marketing Associates, Inc.)
Ultipor	Pall Corporation
Ultra ICE	Boston Scientific Corporation
Ultra-Filtered PLUS Rho	Ortho Clinical Diagnostics, Inc.
Ultra-Filtered PLUS Rho	Ortho-Clinical Diagnostics, Inc.
UltraBind	Pall Corporation
UltraCare	Fresenius Medical Care North America
UltraLink	Sensormatic Electronics
UltraMegaMax	Megasun
Ultraflex	Boston Scientific Corporation
UltraÉ_õMax	Sensormatic Electronics
UltraÉ_õPost	Sensormatic Electronics
UltraÉ_õTag	Sensormatic Electronics
UniVogue	Superior Uniform Group
UroMax Ultra	Boston Scientific Corporation
V & W SERIES	Champion, A Gardner Denver Co.
V I HALO	Jerome Medical
V-BLOCK	Electro-Steam Generator Corp.
V-BTA	Polymedco, Inc.
V-CHAIR	Dentalez Group
V-CHART	Medinotes Corporation
V-CUE	Hill-Rom Holdings, Inc.
V-FORCE OA KNEE BRACE	Omni Life Science, Inc.
V-LINK	Vitalcom, Inc.
V-LOCK	Lohmann & Rauscher, Inc.
V-LOE	The Aloe Institute
V-TRACE	Conmed Corporation
V-TWIN	Siemens Healthcare Diagnostics Inc.
V-VAC	Laerdal Medical Corporation

V-VIAL	Wheaton Science Products
V.3 CUSTOM	Lenox Hill Brace / Seattle Systems
V.A.C.	Kinetic Concepts, Inc.
V.A.C. GranuFoam Silver	Kinetic Concepts, Inc.
V.MUELLER	Cardinal Health Inc.
V3-PLUS	Ulster Scientific, Inc.
VABRA	Berkeley Medevices, Inc.
VAC	Thorn Smith Laboratories
VAC ELUT	Varian Sample Preparation Products
VAC LOK	Byron Medical
VAC U TEST	Ohio Medical Corp.
VAC-FIX	S & S X-Ray Products, Inc.
VAC-MAN	Promega Corp.
VAC-PAC	Olympic Medical Corp.
VAC-PAK	Impact Instrumentation, Inc.
VAC-PAK II	Impact Instrumentation, Inc.
VAC-U-PORT	Bemis Mfg. Co.
VAC-U-STATION	Bemis Mfg. Co.
VACHECK	Ramvac Dental Products Inc
VACPRESS	Aetrex Worldwide, Inc
VACS TABLE	Mizuho Osi
VACSTAR	Air Techniques, Inc.
VACU-QUIK	Almore International, Inc.
VACU-RINSE DISPOSABLE DISCS	Dental Innovators, Inc.
VACU-RINSE FUNNEL	Dental Innovators, Inc.
VACU-RINSE MINI ADAPTOR	Dental Innovators, Inc.
VACU/TROL	Spectrum Laboratories, Inc.
VACUBOTTLE	Inotech Biosystems International, Inc.
VACUGAS	Iba-Rdi
VACUGAS	Sterigenics International, Inc.
VACULE	Wheaton Science Products
VACUMAX	Medical Industries America Inc.
VACUPEN	Niche Medical, Inc.
VACUPULSE	I-Rep, Inc.
VACUSELTZER	Air Techniques, Inc.
VACUSET	Inotech Biosystems International, Inc.
VACUTAINER	Bd Diagnostic Systems
VACUTRON	Allied Healthcare Products, Inc.
VACUUM IONIZATION CLEANER (VIC)	General Transco Inc.
VACUUM TIPS SS	Hager Worldwide, Inc.
VAINGARDE	Bell-Horn, Inc.
VAIROX	Bsn-Jobst
VAKU-8	Myco Medical
VAL MED	Val Med
VAL-AN	Zero Manufacturing, Inc.
VAL-U	Vita Needle Company
VAL-U-SHAVE	Personna Medical/Div. Of American Safety Razor Co.
VALEO	Valeo, Inc.
VALIANT	Ivoclar Vivadent, Inc.
VALLEY CRAFT, VARI-TUFF	Valley Craft
VALLEYLAB	Covidien Lp, Formerly Registered As Tyco Healthcare
VALTRAC	Covidien Lp
VALU-FORM	Patterson Medical Holdings, Inc.
VALU-TOTE	Neotech Products, Inc.
VALUANALYSIS	Siemens Healthcare Diagnostics Inc.
VALUE DAM	Cooley & Cooley, Ltd.
VALUE GENESIS	Innovation Genesis, Llc
VALUEFIX	Mizuho Osi
VALUEGEN	Gtr Labs, Inc.
VALUELINE	Patterson Medical Holdings, Inc.
VALUTRODE	Axelgaard Manufacturing Company, Ltd.
VALUWRAP	Lohmann & Rauscher, Inc.
VAN GUARD	Hamilton Bell Company
VAN ROCK	Dux Dental
VANDER-LIFT	Vancare, Inc.
VANDER-TRACK	Vancare, Inc.
VANGARD CRYOS	Biohit Inc.
VANGUARD	Prentke Romich Company
VANGUARD	Vee Gee Scientific, Inc.
VANGUARD SCBA	Avon-Isi
VANISHPOINT	Retractable Technologies, Inc.
VANITY FAIR	Artcraft New York
VANTAGE	Keeler Instruments Inc.
VANTAGE	Miltex Inc.
VANTAGE	Prentke Romich Company
VANTAGE	Resmed Corp.
VAPOFIL	Sharn, Inc.
VAPOR LINE	Propper Manufacturing Co., Inc.
VAPOR-LOC	Lps Industries, Inc.
VAPOR-SEAL	Smiths Medical Asd, Inc.
VAPOR-TRAK	Kem Medical Products Corp.
VAPOREZE	Imtek Environmental Corp.
VAPORFLEX	Lps Industries, Inc.
VAPORMAX	Trimedyne, Inc.
VAPOTHERM	Vapotherm, Inc.
VAPRO	Wescor, Inc.
VAPROX	Steris Corporation
VAR-A-PULSE	Zimmer Orthopaedic Surgical Products
VAR-I-STAT	Conmed Linvatec
VAREX	Vnus Medical Technologies, Inc.
VARI+PLUS	Airguard
VARI-FLEX	Tfx Medical Oem
VARI-KLEAN	Airguard
VARI-STIM	Medtronic Xomed, Inc.
VARI-SUPPORT PILLOW	Body Therapeutics, Div. Of I-Rep, Inc.
VARIABLE FOCUS	Conforma Laboratories, Inc.
VARIAN	Second Exposure, Inc.
VARIAN	Varian Medical Systems
VARIAN 380-LC	Polymer Laboratories, Now A Part Of Varian, Inc.
VARIAN 385-LC	Polymer Laboratories, Now A Part Of Varian, Inc.
VARIAN MEDICAL SYSTEMS	Varian Medical Systems
VARIANT	Biorad Laboratories
VARIANT EXPRESS	Biorad Laboratories
VARIANT II	Biorad Laboratories
VARIATOR	Hager Worldwide, Inc.
VARIAX	Stryker Corp.
VARICEL	Aaf International
VARIDYNE	Aspen Surgical
VARIFLOW	Airguard
VARILIP	Trelleborg Sealing Solutions
VARILITE	Cascade Designs, Inc.
VARIO 18	Medela, Inc.
VARIO 18 AC/DC	Medela, Inc.
VARIO 18 AC/DC C/I	Medela, Inc.
VARIO 8	Medela, Inc.
VARIO 8 AC/DC	Medela, Inc.
VARIOLINK II	Ivoclar Vivadent, Inc.
VARIS VISION	Varian Medical Systems
VARISEAL	Trelleborg Sealing Solutions
VARISEED	Varian Medical Systems
VARISOURCE	Varian Medical Systems
VARIVUE	AMD Technologies Inc.
VARSITY GUARD	Tp Orthodontics, Inc.
VART	Vortran Medical Technology
VARTA	VARTA Microbattery Inc.
VASAMEDICS	Vasamed
VASCLIR	Vermillion, Inc.
VASCU-FLO	Covidien Lp
VASCU-GUARD	Synovis Life Technologies, Inc
VASCU-GUARD	Synovis Surgical Innovations
VASCU-STATTS	Scanlan International, Inc.
VASCUFIL	Covidien Lp
VASCULAR PROBE	Synovis Surgical Innovations
VASCULASTIC	Gottfried Medical, Inc.
VASCUMAP	Carolina Medical, Inc.
VASER	Sound Surgical Technologies Llc
VASOSEAL	MAQUET
VASOSPECT	Q-Med, Inc.
VASSCAN TABLE	Medical Positioning, Inc.
VASUTAPE RADIOPAQUE MARKING TAPE	Lemaitre Vascular, Inc.
VAULTRAY	Healthmark Industries
VBEAM	Candela Corp.
VBOSS	Stryker Corp.
VBOSS	Stryker Spine
VC-100	Streck Laboratories, Inc.
VCM VINYL COATED MESH	Bruin Plastics Co.

VCMM II	Pacific Precision Laboratories, Inc.
VCOM	Vitalcom, Inc.
VCS	Covidien Lp, Formerly Registered As United States Surgical
VECTABOND	Vector Laboratories, Inc.
VECTAMOUNT	Vector Laboratories, Inc.
VECTASHIELD	Vector Laboratories, Inc.
VECTASTAIN	Vector Laboratories, Inc.
VECTOGRAM	Stereo Optical Co., Inc.
VECTOR	Biomet, Inc.
VECTOR	Coherent, Inc.
VECTOR	Rem Systems
VECTOR	Scientech, Inc.
VECTOR	Vector Laboratories, Inc.
VECTOR FIRST AID	Vector Firstaid, Inc.
VECTORBORD	Vector Electronics & Technology, Inc.
VECTORPAK	Vector Electronics & Technology, Inc.
VECTORSURGE	I-Rep, Inc.
VECTORWIRE	Vector Electronics & Technology, Inc.
VECTREX AVIDIN D	Vector Laboratories, Inc.
VED	Mission Pharmacal Co.
VEEGEE BRAND	Vee Gee Scientific, Inc.
VEIN-TO-VEIN	Wyndgate Technologies
VEINLASE	Lumenis Inc.
VELA	Ams Innovative Center-San Jose
VELA	CAREFUSION 211, INC.
VELADERM HAND WASH LOTION	Global Dental Products
VELCADE	Johnson & Johnson
VELCLOSE	Tetra Medical Supply Corp.
VELKET	Propper Manufacturing Co., Inc.
VELOCITY	Hely And Weber
VELOCITY	Siemens Medical Solutions Usa, Inc
VELOCITY	Sonic Innovations
VELOCITY	Taga Medical Technologies
VELOMETER	Tsi Inc.
VELVASOFT	Abilitations
VELVETONE	Ufp Technologies, Inc.
VENA-FLO	Freeman Manufacturing Company
VENA-STICK	Medical Device Technologies, Inc. (Md Tech)
VENA-VUE	Biosynergy, Inc.
VENAFLO	Bard Peripheral Vascular, Inc.
VENAFLOW	Aircast Llc
VENAPULSE	Aci Medical, Inc.
VENASSIST	Aci Medical, Inc.
VENI-GARD	Conmed Corporation
VENOJECT	Terumo Medical Corp.
VENOSAN	Venosan North America, Inc.
VENOSCOPE	Venoscope, Llc
VENOTRAIN HOSIERY COLLECTION	Bauerfeind Usa, Inc.
VENOUS SAM	Medical Plastics Laboratory, Inc.
VENT RAK	General Devices Co., Inc.
VENT-AWAY	Rondex Products, Inc.
VENTI PAK	Shippert Medical Technologies Corp.
VENTI-SCAN IV	Biodex Medical Systems, Inc.
VENTILAIR II	Hamilton Medical, Inc.
VENTILATOR	Emergency Medical International
VENTRA	Smiths Medical Asd, Inc.
VENTRAK	Respironics, Inc
VENTRICLEAR	Cook Vascular, Incorporated
VENTURE	Medtronic Sofamor Danek Usa, Inc
VENTURE	Medtronic Sofamor Danek Usa, Inc.
VENTURE	Tidi Products, Llc
VENTURE FOOT	College Park Industries, Inc.
VENTX	Sound Surgical Technologies Llc
VER-MED	Vermont Medical, Inc.
VERA	Vancare, Inc.
VERATOX	Neogen Corporation
VERAVUE	Vision-Ease Lens
VERDI	Coherent, Inc.
VERDICT	Medtox Diagnostics Inc.
VERDICT	Medtox Scientific Inc.
VERI-CAL	Utah Medical Products, Inc.
VERI-COLOR	Precision Dynamics Corp.
VERI-TIPS	Ulster Scientific, Inc.
VERIFIT	Etymonic Design Inc.
VERIFLEX	Bard Electro Physiology
VERIFORM	Univac Dental Company
VERIFUSE	I-Flow Corporation
VERIFY	Acon Laboratories, Inc.
VERIFY	Biomerieux Inc.
VERIFY: HAMO	Steris Corporation
VERILUX	Univac Dental Company
VERISCAN	Hospira Inc.
VERISYSE	Abbott Medical Optics Inc.
VERITAS	Synovis Life Technologies, Inc
VERITAS	Synovis Surgical Innovations
VERMILLION	Vermillion, Inc.
VERNITRON 2000: STEAM STERILIZER	Alfa Medical Equipment
VERRUCA-FREEZE	Cryosurgery, Inc.
VERSA	Columbia Medical Manufacturing Llc
VERSA	Medtronic, Inc.
VERSA DUCT	Post Glover Lifelink
VERSA FLEX	Patterson Medical Holdings, Inc.
VERSA LIFT	Noram Solutions
VERSA PEG	Abbott Laboratories
VERSA STIM	Conmed Corporation
VERSA TAC	Conmed Corporation
VERSA TOTE	Neotech Products, Inc.
VERSA VIAL	J. G. Finneran Associates, Inc.
VERSA-FIT	C. R. Bard, Inc., Bard Urological Div.
VERSA-GEL	Aqua-Cel Corp.
VERSA-POLE IV STAND	Pryor Products
VERSA-STRAP	Aqua-Cel Corp.
VERSA-TEMP	Electronic Development Labs, Inc.
VERSABATH	Fisher Scientific Co., Llc.
VERSABOND	Smith & Nephew Inc.- Orthopaedics Division
VERSACELL	Siemens Healthcare Diagnostics Inc.
VERSACHAIR	Engle Dental Systems, Inc.
VERSACLIMBER	Heart Rate, Inc.
VERSADERM	Tri-State Hospital Supply Corp.
VERSADOPP	Verathon Inc.
VERSAFLEX	Smith & Nephew, Inc.
VERSAFLO	Centrix, Inc.
VERSAJET	Hydrocision, Inc.
VERSALET	Hill-Rom Holdings, Inc.
VERSALETTE	Whitehall Manufacturing
VERSALIGHT	Lumitex, Inc.
VERSALITE	Centrix, Inc.
VERSALITE	Medical Illumination International
VERSALITE	Vision-Ease Lens
VERSANT	Siemens Healthcare Diagnostics Inc.
VERSAPORT	Covidien Lp, Formerly Registered As United States Surgical
VERSASEAL	Covidien Lp, Formerly Registered As United States Surgical
VERSASTIM 380	Electro-Med Health Industries
VERSATACK	Covidien Lp, Formerly Registered As United States Surgical
VERSATIP	Covidien Lp, Formerly Registered As United States Surgical
VERSATRAN	Blevins Medical Inc
VERSATREK AUTOMATED MICROBIAL DETECTION SYSTEM	Trek Diagnostic Systems
VERSATREK WINDOWS SOFTWARE	Trek Diagnostic Systems
VERSI-WIPE	Palmero Health Care
VERSIPOWER	Conmed Linvatec
VERSIPOWER PLUS	Conmed Linvatec
VERSIVA	Convatec
VERTE-STACK	Medtronic Sofamor Danek Usa, Inc
VERTE-STACK	Medtronic Sofamor Danek Usa, Inc.
VERTEPORT	Stryker Corp.
VERTEX	The Cooper Companies, Inc
VERTICAL TOTE SHUTTLE	Swisslog Translogic Corporation
VERTICAL TRACTION SYSTEM	Endorphin Corporation
VERTIER	Stryker Corp.
VERTIGRAFT	Lifenet Health
VERTIKLEAN(R) WALL WASHING SYSTEM	Contec, Inc.
VERTIS PNT	Rs Medical
VESPHENE	Steris Corporation
VESPHENE IIST	Steris Corporation
VESS	Supertech, Inc.

VESTEMP	Reimers Systems, Inc.
VET-THERM	Everest Interscience, Inc.
VET/E-SIG	Heska Corporation
VET/HEX	Hex Laboratory Systems
VET/IV	Heska Corporation
VET/OX	Heska Corporation
VETAUTOREAD	Idexx Laboratories, Inc.
VETERINARY DICOM SOLUTIONS	Imsi, Integrated Modular Systems Inc.
VETLAB	Idexx Laboratories, Inc.
VETLYTE	Idexx Laboratories, Inc.
VETRAP	3m Co.
VETSCAN	Abaxis, Inc.
VFE	Ramco Laboratories, Inc.
VFL II	Conforma Laboratories, Inc.
VFL3	Conforma Laboratories, Inc.
VH	Volcano Corporation
VHM	Gcx Corp.
VHP	Steris Corporation
VHRS	Gcx Corp.
VI-DRAPE	Medical Concepts Development
VIA	Boeckeler Instruments, Inc.
VIA	Eklin Medical Systems
VIA SPIGA EYEWEAR	Zyloware Corporation
VIA! FOR TRAVEL	Via! For Travel
VIAFLEX	Baxter Healthcare Corporation, Global Drug Delivery
VIAL-MATE	Baxter Healthcare Corporation, Global Drug Delivery
VIAPEEL	Greatbatch Inc
VIAS	Ventana Medical Systems, Inc.
VIASORB	Covidien Lp
VIATROCIDE	Great Lakes Medical
VIBE	Siemens Hearing Instruments, Inc.
VIBRACARE	General Pysiotherapy, Inc.
VIBRAMATIC	General Pysiotherapy, Inc.
VICOAX	Vicon Industries Inc.
VICODIN CR	Abbott Laboratories
VICOMP	Dentsply Prosthetics
VICON	Bussard & Son Inc., R.D.
VICON MOTION SYSTEMS, INC.	Vicon
VICON PEAK	Vicon
VICONNET	Vicon Industries Inc.
VICRYL	Ethicon, Inc.
VICRYLPLUS	Ethicon, Inc.
VICTOR	Kardex Systems, Inc.
VICTOR	Perkin Elmer Wallac, Inc.
VICTOR	Perkinelmer Life And Analytical Sciences
VICTOR 2	Perkin Elmer Wallac, Inc.
VICTOR 2	Perkinelmer Life And Analytical Sciences
VICTOR 2 V	Perkin Elmer Wallac, Inc.
VICTORY	Pride Mobility Products Corp.
VICTRO 2 V	Perkinelmer Life And Analytical Sciences
VIDEO FLEX	Ken-A-Vision Manufacturing Co., Inc.
VIDEO PLUS	Analogic Corporation
VIDEO WIN	Photo Research, Inc.
VIDEOPATH	Welch Allyn, Inc.
VIDEOSET	Thermo Fisher Scientific - Laboratory Equipment Division Headquarters
VIDEOSPOT	Analogic Corporation
VIDIVIEWER	Diversified Diagnostic Products, Inc.
VIDMAR REDI-PAK	Stanley Vidmar
VIEW	V.I.E.W. Video
VIEW PACK	Medical Action Industries, Inc
VIEW-IT	Kentek Corp.
VIEWLUX	Perkin Elmer Wallac, Inc.
VIEWLUX	Perkinelmer Life And Analytical Sciences
VIEWPLUS	Sanders Data Systems, Llc
VIEWSPECT	Analytical Spectral Devices, Inc.
VIGILANCE	Harry J. Bosworth Company
VIGILANT	Edgetech
VIKING	Bard Electro Physiology
VIKING SCBA	Avon-Isi
VIKING XL	Liko North America
VILEX	Vilex, Inc.
VIODINE	Great Lakes Medical

VIONEX	Metrex Research Corp.
VIONEXUS	Metrex Research Corp.
VIP	Ambu, Inc.
VIP	Sakura Finetek U.S.A., Inc.
VIP BIRD GOLD/STERLING	CAREFUSION 211, INC..
VIP FLEXIBIL	Clarke Health Care Products, Inc.
VIP STAND IV STAND	Pryor Products
VIP-PACS	Imco Technologies
VIPER FIBEROPTIC HIGH SPEED HANDPIECES	Kinetic Instruments, Inc.
VIPER HEADREST	Body Tech 1 Nw
VIPER II HEADREST	Body Tech 1 Nw
VIPERSONIC ENDO/SCALERS	Kinetic Instruments, Inc.
VIPTILT	Clarke Health Care Products, Inc.
VIRAGUARD	Veridien Corp.
VIRAGUARD - NONTOXIC	Veridien Corp.
VIRASORB	Great Lakes Medical
VIROBAC II	King Systems Corp.
VIROCLEAR	Bio-Rad Laboratories
VIROGEN	Wampole Laboratories
VIRONOSTIKA	Biomerieux Inc.
VIROSAFE	Buffalo Filter, A Division Of Medtek Devices Inc.
VIROTROL	Bio-Rad Laboratories
VIRSONIC	Virtis, An Sp Industries Company
VIRTISHEAR	Virtis, An Sp Industries Company
VIRTUA	Codonics
VIRTUAL	Ivoclar Vivadent, Inc.
VIRTUAL	Virtis, An Sp Industries Company
VIRTUAL WEDGE	Siemens Medical Solutions Usa, Inc
VIRTUOSO	Heraeus Kulzer, Inc.
VIS-O-GUARD	Hager Worldwide, Inc.
VISCO SHIELD	Oasis Medical, Inc.
VISCOHEEL	Bauerfeind Usa, Inc.
VISCOPASTE	Smith & Nephew, Inc.
VISCOPED	Bauerfeind Usa, Inc.
VISCOPED S	Bauerfeind Usa, Inc.
VISCORIDE	Tempur-Medical, Inc.
VISCOSPOT	Bauerfeind Usa, Inc.
VISCOT	Viscot Medical, Llc
VISDISK	Cannon Instrument Co.
VISI SPOT	J&S Medical Associates
VISI-BLACK	Ethicon, Inc.
VISI-PITCH	Kaypentax
VISICHART	Topcon Medical Systems, Inc.
VISICOIL	Radiomed Corporation
VISICOMM	Visicomm Industries
VISILUX 2	3m Espe Dental Products
VISINE	Johnson & Johnson
VISION	Cardiac Science Corp.
VISION	Follett Corp.
VISION	Hager Worldwide, Inc.
VISION	Soltec Corp.
VISION AID	H.L. Bouton Co., Inc.
VISION CENTER	National Vision, Inc.
VISION ELECT	Stryker Corp.
VISION PREMIER	Cardiac Science Corp.
VISION SCIENCES	Vision-Sciences, Inc.
VISIONAIR	United Air Specialists, Inc.
VISIONMATE	Thermo Fisher Scientific
VISIPORT	Covidien Lp, Formerly Registered As United States Surgical
VISISTAT	Teleflex Medical
VISIT ASSISTANT	Carecentric, Inc.
VISITINT	Ciba Vision Corporation
VISIV	Hospira Inc.
VISMARK	Viscot Medical, Llc
VISORB	Cp Medical Corporation
VISTA	Bd Lee Laboratories
VISTA	Caridianbct Inc.
VISTA	Vacumed
VISTA 2000	Invincible Office Furniture Co.
VISTACAM	Air Techniques, Inc.
VISTACON	Independent Solutions, Inc.
VISTACON	Vista Lighting
VISTAMARC SPHERE	Vistakon, Inc.

VISTAMARC TORIC	Vistakon, Inc.
VISU-HOLD	March & Green
VISUAL NURSE-CALL SYSTEM (UL1069)	Heritage Medcall
VISUAL*ENS	Dexall Biomedical Labs, Inc.
VISUALEYES VIDEO ENG	Micromedical Technologies, Inc.
VISUALINE	Akers Biosciences, Inc.
VISUALINE	Sun Biomedical Laboratories, Inc.
VISUALINE CUP	Sun Biomedical Laboratories, Inc.
VISUALINK	Lexicon Branding, Inc.
VISULAS	Carl Zeiss Surgical, Inc.
VISUM	Stryker Corp.
VIT ENHANCER	Medical Instrumentation Development Labs
VITA	Vita Needle Company
VITA CUFF	Integra Lifesciences Corporation
VITA VET	Vita Needle Company
VITACRILIC	Fricke Dental Manufacturing Co.
VITAFLOW	Vital Concepts, Inc.
VITAFREE	Usb Corporation
VITAGEL	Orthovita, Inc.
VITAGLIDE	Rehamed Intl. Llc.
VITAGLIDE PRO	Rehamed Intl. Llc.
VITAJET	Bioject Medical Technologies, Inc.
VITAL 1	Metrex Research Corp.
VITAL SENSE	Mini-Mitter Company, Inc.
VITAL SIGNS SERVER	Welch Allyn Protocol Inc.
VITAL VIEW	Vital Signs, Inc.
VITAL VIEW II	Vital Signs, Inc.
VITAL VUE	Covidien Lp
VITAL-LIGHT	Duro-Test Lighting
VITAL-PORT	Cook Vascular, Incorporated
VITALAB FLEXOR	Clinical Data Inc
VITALAB SELECTRA-E	Clinical Data Inc
VITALAB SELECTRA-XL	Clinical Data Inc
VITALAB VIVA	Clinical Data Inc
VITALCAP	Oridion Medical Inc.
VITALCOR	Vitalcor, Inc.
VITALITY	DJO Surgical
VITALITY SCANNER	Sybronendo
VITALITYOTC	Augusta Medical Systems, Llc
VITALLIUM	Dentsply Prosthetics
VITALMAX	Pace Tech, Inc.
VITALOGIK	Mennen Medical Corp.
VITALOGRAPH COMPACT	Vitalograph, Inc.
VITALOGRAPH ESCORT	Vitalograph, Inc.
VITALSENSE XHR	Mini-Mitter Company, Inc.
VITAMIN-K	Donell
VITANEED	Covidien Lp
VITESSE	Micrus Endovascular Corporation
VITESSE	Varian Medical Systems
VITESSE C	Spectranetics Corp.
VITESSE COS	Spectranetics Corp.
VITESSE E	Spectranetics Corp.
VITEX	Adenna Inc.
VITMATE	Medical Instrumentation Development Labs
VITOSS	Kensey Nash Corporation
VITOSS	Orthovita, Inc.
VITOSS FOAM	Orthovita, Inc.
VITREA 2	Vital Images,Inc.
VITREBOND	3m Espe Dental Products
VITRECTOMY RECOVERY SYSTEM	Rite Time Corporation
VITREMER	3m Espe Dental Products
VITREOLENS HANDLE	Volk Optical Inc.
VITRON	Elmed, Inc.
VITROS	Ortho Clinical Diagnostics, Inc.
VITROS	Ortho-Clinical Diagnostics, Inc.
VIVA 21ST CENTURY CONDOMS	Oceans Seven Int'L.
VIVA-JR	Siemens Healthcare Diagnostics Inc.
VIVAHOL	Professional Product Co.
VIVASTAT	Cober Electronics, Inc.
VIVAX	Tulip Medical Products
VIVAX MOBILITY SYSTEM	Vivax Medical Corp.
VIVOPERL PE	Ivoclar Vivadent, Inc.
VIVOSIS	Cook Biotech, Incorporated
VIVUS 4000	I-Flow Corporation
VIXONE	Westmed, Inc.
VIZCAYA	Engle Dental Systems, Inc.
VL	Inclinator Co. Of America
VLC	Biomet, Inc.
VLIFT	Stryker Corp.
VLIFT	Stryker Spine
VM	Vasamed
VMA-SKREEN	Biochemical Diagnostics, Inc.
VMAX	Cardinal Health Inc.
VMAX	Molecular Devices Corp.
VMAX 10	CAREFUSION 211, INC..
VMAX NETLINK/IS	CAREFUSION 211, INC..
VMAX SPECTRA	CAREFUSION 211, INC..
VMAX ST	CAREFUSION 211, INC..
VMI	Handi-Cap Aids Company
VML3000	Triangle Biomedical Sciences, Inc.
VNS THERAPY	Cyberonics, Inc.
VNUS CLOSUREFAST	Vnus Medical Technologies, Inc.
VNUS RFGPLUS.	Vnus Medical Technologies, Inc.
VOCALIGHT	Phonic Ear, Inc.
VOICE CARE	American Medical Alert Corp.
VOICE GUARD	Ericsson, Inc.
VOICE OF HELP	American Medical Alert Corp.
VOICELINK	I-Flow Corporation
VOICENOTE	Humanware
VOICETTE	Luminaud, Inc.
VOID-EASE	Gkr Industries, Inc.
VOLDYNE	Covidien Lp
VOLK AREA CENTRALIS	Volk Optical Inc.
VOLK(STYLIZED)	Volk Optical Inc.
VOLKNER TURNING SYSTEM ALPHA	James Consolidated, Inc.
VOLTARC	Bulbworks, Inc.
VOLTARC	Perkinelmer Optoelectronics
VOLTEK VOLARA	Ufp Technologies, Inc.
VOLU-SOL	Volu-Sol, Inc.
VOLUME PRO	Terarecon, Inc.
VON-LOC	Vonco Products, Inc.
VONSEAL	Vonco Products, Inc.
VONSECURE	Vonco Products, Inc.
VORTEQ	Micromedical Technologies, Inc.
VORTEX	DJO Inc.
VORTEX-GENIE	Scientific Industries, Inc.
VORTEX-GENIE 1	Scientific Industries, Inc.
VORTEX-GENIE 2	Scientific Industries, Inc.
VORTEX-GENIE 2T	Scientific Industries, Inc.
VORTEX-PORT	Angiodynamics, Inc.
VORTRAN PERCUSSIVENEBT	Vortran Medical Technology
VORTRAN-IPPBT	Vortran Medical Technology
VOYAGE	Luxfer Gas Cylinders
VOYAGE	Mada, Inc.
VOYAGER	Post Medical, Inc.
VP310 COPYSTAND	Bencher, Inc.
VP400 COPYSTAND	Bencher, Inc.
VPAP	Resmed Corp.
VPREDICT	Prescient Medical Inc.
VPROTECT	Prescient Medical Inc.
VPS	Vicon Industries Inc.
VR INVESTMENT	Dentsply Prosthetics
VRBIKE	CYBEX INTERNATIONAL, INC.
VRC	Starkey Laboratories, Inc.
VRCLIMBER	CYBEX INTERNATIONAL, INC.
VS II	Mast/Keystone View
VSI	Vision-Sciences, Inc.
VST	Konigsberg Instruments, Inc.
VTI	Vascular Technology Incorporated
VTIr	Vergason Technology, Inc.
VTS	Endorphin Corporation
VU PLUS	Wolf X-Ray Corporation
VUELIFE	American Fluoroseal Corp.
VUEPORT	Cardima, Inc.
VVRA	Intelligent Hearing Systems, Corp.
VWF ZYMTEC	Dms Laboratories, Inc.

VYCOR	Corning Inc., Science Products Division
VYDAC	Nest Group Inc., The
VYGON PREMICATH	Dma Med-Chem Corporation
VYLEATER VIAL CRUSHER	S&G Enterprises, Inc.
VYLON	Durable Corporation
VYON POROUS POLYMER	Porvair Filtration Group Inc
VYSUN	Sunlite Plastics, Inc.
VZVSCAN	Bd Diagnostic Systems
Vector	Micro-Tech
Vedera	Avedro, Inc.
Veeder-Root	Danaher Corporation
VegLife	Nutraceutical International Corp.
Velcro	A. Lunt Design, Inc.
Venture	St. Jude Medical, Inc.
Verity	St. Jude Medical, Inc.
VersaPulse	Boston Scientific Corporation
Vicks	Procter & Gamble
Victory	St. Jude Medical, Inc.
Virogen	Inverness Medical Professional Diagnostics-San Die
Visibly Even	Ortho Dermatologics
Visibly Firm	Ortho Dermatologics
Vista	Zimmer Spine, Inc.
VitalStim	Healthsouth Corporation
Vitatron	Medtronic, Inc.
Vitrasert	Bausch & Lomb
Vivelle-Dot	Noven Pharmaceuticals, Inc.
Vivid	Pall Corporation
VortX	Boston Scientific Corporation
W. L. GORE AND ASSOCIATES, INC., TETRAD BRAND ULTRASOUND	W. L. Gore And Associates, Inc.
W.H.O.	Cfi Medical Solutions (Contour Fabricators, Inc.)
W.T. BURNETT	Ufp Technologies, Inc.
WAFER LITE	Post Glover Lifelink
WAFFLE	Ehob, Inc.
WAFFLE	Howard Medical Company
WAGON MASTER	Geerpres
WAHL HOME HEALTHCARE	Wahl Clipper Corp.
WAIST WATCHER	Bell-Horn, Inc.
WAL-PIL-O	Roloke
WALK ALERT SLIPPERS	Alert Care, Inc.
WALK-N- ROLLER	Pryor Products
WALKABOUT	Battle Creek Equipment Co.
WALKER	Weitbrecht Communications, Inc.
WALKHALER	Pari Respiratory Equipment, Inc.
WALKLITE	Invacare Corporation
WALKMED	Smiths Medical OEM
WALKMED	Walkmed Infusion Llc
WALL WIPR(TM) CLEANING SYSTEM	Contec, Inc.
WALLABY CATCH ALL, WALLABY CATCH ALL TOO	Advantage Bag Co.
WALLRIVIT	Asi-Modulex
WALLSAFE	Bemis Mfg. Co.
WALLSAVER	Stryker Corp.
WALLSTENT	Boston Scientific Corp.
WAMPOLE ELISA	Wampole Laboratories
WANCHIK'S WRITER	Cfi Medical Solutions (Contour Fabricators, Inc.)
WANDER GUARD	Senior Technologies
WANDERCARE SYSTEM	Care Electronics, Inc.
WANDERGUARD LOCKS	Senior Technologies
WARATAH	La Mont Medical, Inc.
WARE	Levine Health Products
WARETEX	Ware Medics Glass Works, Inc.
WARM WEIGH	Hill-Rom Holdings, Inc.
WARMAIR	Cincinnati Sub-Zero Products, Inc., Medical Division
WARMFLO	Covidien (Formerly Nellcor Puritan Bennett / Tyco Healthcare)
WARMRIGHTr	Enthermics Medical Systems, Inc.
WARMTOUCH	Covidien (Formerly Nellcor Puritan Bennett / Tyco Healthcare)
WASCOMAT	Wascomat Laundry Equipment
WATCHCHILD	Hill-Rom Holdings, Inc.
WATCHDOG ACTIVE RFID FOR LOCAL AND WORLD WIDE ASSET TRACKING	Metro Cad, Inc
WATCHING LIFE	Lifewatch Services, Inc.
WATER WALKER	All Pro Exercise Products, Inc.
WATER WEIGHT SYSTEM	Novel Products, Inc.
WATER-JEL	Water-Jel Technologies
WATER-SOLU	Approved Medical Systems
WATER-X	Grant Airmass Corporation
WATERBUGS	Remel
WATERKLEAN	Imtek Environmental Corp.
WATERLASE	Biolase Technology, Inc.
WATERMARK	Crescent Chemical Co., Inc.
WATERPRO	Labconco Corp.
WATERS	Waters Corp.
WATERTITE	Woodhead L.P.
WATERWAYS	Western Water Purifier Co.
WATS	Propper Manufacturing Co., Inc.
WAVE	Staar Surgical Co.
WAVE COMFORT PILLOW	Core Products International, Inc.
WAVE PRO	Lecroy Corp.
WAVEFLEX CFT	Capstone Therapeutics
WAVEFRONT	Abbott Medical Optics Inc.
WAVEMASTER	Coherent, Inc.
WAVEMETER	Exfo America Inc.
WAVERIDER	Biofeedback Instrument Corp.
WAVERUNNER	Lecroy Corp.
WAVICIDE-01	Medical Chemical Corp.
WAVICIDE-06PLUS	Medical Chemical Corp.
WAVIZYME	Medical Chemical Corp.
WAXED CLOTH FORMS	Aluwax Dental Products Co.
WAXED CLOTH SHEETS	Aluwax Dental Products Co.
WE-LISTEN	Advanced Medical Innovations, Inc.
WEATHER CHAPS	Diestco Manufacturing Corp.
WEATHERBEE	Diestco Manufacturing Corp.
WEATHERBREAKER	Diestco Manufacturing Corp.
WEATHERMUFF	Diestco Manufacturing Corp.
WEB DESIGN	Televox Software, Inc.
WEB-SLIDE EXERCISE RAIL SYSTEM	Pre Pak Products, Inc.
WEBLY	Hely And Weber
WEBSET	Case Medical, Inc.
WEBSTER	Trans American Medical
WEBVIEW	Eurotherm Inc.
WEBVUE	AMD Technologies Inc.
WECK	Teleflex Medical
WECK CLOSURE/PNEUMOSLEEVE	Dma Med-Chem Corporation
WEDESITE	Smiths Medical Asd, Inc.
WEDGIE SEAT WEDGE	Body Therapeutics, Div. Of I-Rep, Inc.
WEE CARE	Questech International, Inc.
WEE LENGTHS	Seca Corp.
WEE PEE DIAPER	Children's Medical Ventures, Inc.
WEE SPECS	Children's Medical Ventures, Inc.
WEE THUMBLE PACIFIER	Children's Medical Ventures, Inc.
WEHBE ARM HOLDER	Mizuho Osi
WEIGH TO JUMP	All Pro Exercise Products, Inc.
WEIGHSAFE	Hard Manufacturing Co.
WEIGHT STACK	Fitness Plus, Inc.
WEIGHT-A-BAND	All Pro Exercise Products, Inc.
WEIGHT-A-TONER	All Pro Exercise Products, Inc.
WEIGHTRIGHT	Medovations, Inc.
WEILER	Hansco Technologies, Inc.
WEIMER	Ldb Medical, Inc.
WEL-RAP	Alex Orthopedic, Inc.
WELCH ALLYN	Bulbworks, Inc.
WELCH ALLYN	Dma Med-Chem Corporation
WELCH ALLYN	Kern Surgical Supply, Inc.
WELCON	Nurse Assist ,Inc.
WELD-IT	Kentek Corp.
WELDMASTER	M. Braun Inc.
WELL BILT	Independent Solutions, Inc.
WELL-PIL-O	Roloke
WELLCOGEN	Remel
WELLCOLEX	Remel
WELLCOTEST	Remel
WELLHOFER WATERPHANTOM	Scanditronix - Wellhofer North America
WELLMATE	Thermo Fisher Scientific
WELLPRO AUTOMATED LIQUID HANDLING SYSTEM	Progroup Instrument Corp.
WELLS	Wells Dental, Inc.
WELLS-ENBERG	Handi-Cap Aids Company

WELSH ALLYN	Creative Health Products, Inc.
WESCO	Western Scientific Co., Inc.
WESCOR	Wescor, Inc.
WESTCHESTER	Surco Products
WESTERN 90DX, 90XL	Mesa Laboratories, Inc.
WESTERN BLUE	Promega Corp.
WESTERN EXPRESS	Promega Corp.
WESTERN MEDICA	Western Medica
WESTFALIA SEPARATOR AG	Gea Westfalia Separator, Inc.
WESTRAN	Schleicher & Schuell, Inc.
WESTROBE	Kimble Chase Life Science And Research Products Llc
WET SENSE	Care Electronics, Inc.
WET-FIELD	Mentor Ophthalmics, Inc.
WET-STOP	Palco Labs, Inc.
WETSTICK	Avery Dennison Corporation
WHATMAN	Whatman Inc.
WHEATON	Wheaton Brace Co.
WHEATON AUTOSTILL	Wheaton Science Products
WHEATON BUNION SPLINT	Wheaton Brace Co.
WHEATON CONNECTION	Wheaton Science Products
WHEATON MICROKIT	Wheaton Science Products
WHEATON PAVLIK	Wheaton Brace Co.
WHEEL'N WEIGH	Algen Scale Corp.
WHEEL-O-VATOR	The National Wheel-O-Vator Co., Inc.
WHEELCHAIR DAY PAC, 165 SERIES	Advantage Bag Co.
WHEELCHAIR DEPOT	Wheelchair Sales And Service Co., Inc.
WHEELCHAIR PAL IV POLE ACCESSORY	Pryor Products
WHEELED COACH	Wheeled Coach Industries, Inc.
WHEELIE MPS, MOBILE PRONE STANDER	Prime Engineering
WHEELIT	Wheelit, Inc.
WHILE-U-SLEEP	George Glove Company, Inc.
WHIN	B. Braun Oem Division, B. Braun Medical Inc.
WHIRL-PAK	Aristotle Corp.
WHISPER	Buffalo Filter, A Division Of Medtek Devices Inc.
WHISPER	Medsonic U.S.A., Inc.
WHISPER JET	Vital Signs Colorado
WHISPER-QUIET	Oster Professional Products, Inc.
WHISPERATOR	Wells Johnson Co.
WHISPERJET	Bunnell Incorporated
WHISPERQUIETr AIR HANDLERS	Clean Air Technology, Inc.
WHISPURE QUICKHEAT"	Reheat Co., Inc.
WHISPURR AIR	Mars Air Doors
WHISTLEWATCH	Ulster Scientific, Inc.
WHITE BLITZER	Hager Worldwide, Inc.
WHITEHALL	Whitehall Manufacturing
WHITEKNIGHT	Precept Medical Products, Inc.
WHITELIGHT INTERFEROMETER	Solarius Development Inc.
WHITNEY	Whitney Products, Inc.
WHIZZER	Mueller Sports Medicine
WHOLE HEAD EEG	Electrical Geodesics, Incorporated
WHOLE-IN-ONE: NEUTRAY-SHARPS PASSING TRAY	Advanced Medical Innovations, Inc.
WI PRODUCT DEVELOPMENT SERVICES	Wi Inc
WICHITA NAIL	Stryker Corp.
WICHITA NAIL	Stryker Howmedica Osteonics
WIDE TRACK	Tu-Way American Group
WIDESEAL DIAPHRAGM	Milex Products, Inc.
WIKO	Bulbworks, Inc.
WILBOND	Argen Corp.
WILCAST	Argen Corp.
WILD HOT STRIPS	Aso Corporation
WILD ONES	Sellstrom Manufacturing Co.
WILDEYES	Ciba Vision
WILDFLOWER	Graham Medical Products/Div. Of Little Rapids Corp
WILKINSON	Argen Corp.
WILKINSON	Byron Medical
WILKOFF	Cook Vascular, Incorporated
WILKS	Invensys Process Systems
WILLIAMS SOUND	Weitbrecht Communications, Inc.
WILLIAMSBURG	Golden Technologies, Inc.
WILPAL	Argen Corp.
WILSTARARGEN	Argen Corp.
WILTSE CHEST JACK	Mizuho Osi
WINDGUARD	Mars Air Doors
WINDOPATH, PATHWAY	Psyche Systems
WINDSOR	Interspec Fabrics
WINDSOR HOME ELEVATOR	Thyssenkrupp Access Corp.
WINDX	Creative Biotech Inc.
WING-LOCK	Smiths Medical Asd, Inc.
WINGMAN	Stryker Corp.
WINGMAN	Stryker Endoscopy
WINPAK	Medical Packaging Inc.
WINPETTE	Arkray Usa
WINRHO	Baxter International Inc
WINSFORD	North Coast Medical, Inc.
WINSHIELD	Westmed, Inc.
WINSPECTRAL	Perkin Elmer Wallac, Inc.
WINSTATION 1400	Ophthalmic Imaging Systems
WINSTATION 4000	Ophthalmic Imaging Systems
WINSTATION 5000	Ophthalmic Imaging Systems
WINTEST	Bose Corporation - Electroforce Systems Group
WIPE OUT	Immucell Corp.
WIPE-X	Mentor Ophthalmics, Inc.
WIRE CADDY	Stryker Corp.
WIRETROL I	Drummond Scientific Co.
WIRETROL II	Drummond Scientific Co.
WISCONSIN ALUMINUM (ALL AMERICAN)	Medi-Tech International, Inc.
WISHBONE CANNULA	Directmed, Inc.
WITHARD	C. R. Bard, Inc., Bard Urological Div.
WIVIK	Prentke Romich Company
WIZARD	Perkin Elmer Wallac, Inc.
WIZARD	Promega Corp.
WIZARD	Q.I. Medical, Inc.
WIZARD	Snug Seat, Inc.
WJ	Water-Jel Technologies
WKITS	Remel
WOB-L	Thomas Products Division
WODAN	Tri Hawk Corporation
WOLFE	Carolina Biological Supply Co.
WONDERFOAM	Backsaver
WONDERZORB	Silipos Inc.
WOOD MALLET	Bibbero Systems, Inc.
WOOD-TEK	Richards-Wilcox, Inc.
WOOL 'N GEL	Chi'Am International
WOOLFELT	National Nonwovens
WORD CATHETER	Milex Products, Inc.
WORD POWER	Prentke Romich Company
WORDCORE	Prentke Romich Company
WORDS STRATEGY	Prentke Romich Company
WORK S'PORT	The Saunders Group
WORK-HORSE	Mit Poly-Cart Corp.
WORKFLOW ENGINE	Imsi, Integrated Modular Systems Inc.
WORKFORCE	Scott Specialties, Inc./Cmo Inc./Ginny Inc.
WORKHORSE	Boss Instruments, Ltd.
WORKHORSE	Rayovac
WORKMOD	North Coast Medical, Inc.
WORKOUT MASSEUR	General Pysiotherapy, Inc.
WORKRITE	Sellstrom Manufacturing Co.
WORKSAFE BACK SUPPORT	Body Therapeutics, Div. Of I-Rep, Inc.
WORLD	Argen Corp.
WORLD	World Dryer Corp.
WORLD DRYER	World Dryer Corp.
WORLD ONE	Tp Orthodontics, Inc.
WORLD-LITE	Roldan Products Corp.
WORLDWIDE MONITORING	United Chemical Technologies, Inc.
WORTH	Andersen Products, Inc.,
WORX	Mediware Information Systems, Inc.
WOUND CARE	Aso Corporation
WOUND MANAGER	Convatec Professional Services
WOUND WASH SALINE	Blairex Laboratories, Inc.
WOUNDED WILLY	Supertech, Inc.
WOUNDNET	Smith & Nephew, Inc.
WR	Wr Medical Electronics Co.
WRANGLER	Nss Enterprises, Inc.
WRANGLER	Pride Mobility Products Corp.
WRAP	Covidien Lp, Formerly Registered As United States Surgical

WRAP IT	Byron Medical
WRAP-AID	Home-Aid-Healthcare, Inc.
WRAP-RITE	Frank Stubbs Co., Inc
WRAPBACK	Gargoyles Eyewear
WRAPPEL	Standard Textile
WRIGHT LINEAR PUMP	Wright Linear Pump, Inc.
WRIGHT PRE FILLED CASE, DIASOX DIABETIC SOCK, SILVER KNIT SOCK, Medicool, Inc.	
WRIGHT THERAPY PRODUCTS	Wright Linear Pump, Inc.
WRIGHTLOCK	DJO Surgical
WRIST ACTION SHAKER	Burrell Scientific, Inc
WRIST BUDDIE	Contour Form Products
WRIST LACER	Medical Specialties, Inc.
WRIST RESTORE	Optp
WRIST SKINS	Cropper Medical, Inc./Bio Skin
WRISTICKET	Hollister Incorporated
WRISTIMER	Brown Medical Industries
WRISTIMER PM	Brown Medical Industries
WRISTJACK	Hand Biomechanics Lab, Inc.
WRITE-ON	Associated Bag Company
WURZBURG	Striker Corp.
WYBAR	Eraser Company, Inc.
WYNDTELL	Weitbrecht Communications, Inc.
WYSONG	Wysong Corporation
WallFlex	Boston Scientific Corporation
Wallstent	Boston Scientific Corporation
WanderGuard	Universal Medical Products, Inc.
Wishbook	Codman & Shurtleff, Inc
Worklon	Superior Uniform Group
X-12	Mortara Instrument, Inc.
X-ACT	Bard Electro Physiology
X-ACTO 2000	Starkey Laboratories, Inc.
X-CEL X-RAY CORP.	X-Cel X-Ray Corporation
X-MARK	Avcor Health Care Products, Inc.
X-OMATIC	Carestream Health, Inc.
X-PANEL	Stallion Technologies, Inc.
X-POD	Nonin Medical, Inc.
X-RAY ACCESSORY CORP.	Soyee Products, Inc.
X-RAY DIGITIZER	Altek Corp.
X-RITE	X-Rite, Inc.
X-SCRIBE	Mortara Instrument, Inc.
X-SIGHT	Stallion Technologies, Inc.
X-SIGHT DIGITAL IMAGING SOLUTIONS	Stallion Technologies Inc.
X-STRAP DORSI-LITE FOOT SPLINT	X-Strap Systems
X-STRAP DORSI-STRAP FOR FOOT DROP	X-Strap Systems
X-STRAP SPRAIN-GUARD ANKLE SUPPORT SYSTEM	X-Strap Systems
X-Static	Acor Orthopaedic, Inc.
X-TEN	Avcor Health Care Products, Inc.
X-TENDA CUFF	Ansell Healthcare Products, Inc.
X-TREME	Colours Wheelchair
X-TROL	Independent Solutions, Inc.
X3	Stryker Corp.
X3	Stryker Howmedica Osteonics
X3 ADVANCED BEARING TECHNOLOGY	Stryker Corp.
X3 ADVANCED BEARING TECHNOLOGY	Stryker Howmedica Osteonics
XACT	Action Products, Inc.
XACT	DJO Inc.
XCALIBER FIXATOR	Orthofix Inc.
XCAP	Epix, Inc.
XCEL	Reichert, Inc.
XCEL	Stryker Endoscopy
XCELA	Navilyst Medical
XCELGEL	Polymer Concepts, Inc.
XCELL	Spectrum-Brands
XCLIB	Epix, Inc.
XCOBJ	Epix, Inc.
XCP-DS	Dentsply International, Inc.
XCP-DS	Dentsply Prosthetics
XECT SYSTEM 2	Diversified Diagnostic Products, Inc.
XEN REX I	Nuclear Pharmacy Services
XENAMATIC	Diversified Diagnostic Products, Inc.
XENOBIND	Xenopore Corp.
XENON NOVA	Karl Storz Endoscopy-America Inc.

XENOPROBE	Xenopore Corp.
XENOTRON	Mallinckrodt, Inc.
XENOVAP	Amici, Inc.
XEO	Cutera, Inc.
XEROFLO	Covidien Lp
XEROLYT	Mettler-Toledo Process Analytical, Inc.
XEROSOX	Xero Products
XEROSOX PRO-PUMP	Xero Products
XEROSTAT	Extra Packaging, Corp.
XHALE	Oliver Medical
XI3 TEMPERATURE MONITORS	Tcp Reliable, Inc.
XIA	Stryker Corp.
XIA	Stryker Spine
XIENCE	Abbott Laboratories
XIENCE V	Abbott Laboratories
XIOS	Sirona Dental Systems Llc
XISCAN 1000	Xi Tec, Inc.
XISCAN 1000P	Xi Tec, Inc.
XISCAN 6000	Xi Tec, Inc.
XISCAN MINI C-ARM	Xi Tec, Inc.
XK-PRO 100 HIGH SPEED MOTOR SYSTEM	Tava Surgical Instruments
XL ENDOSCOPES	Advanced Endoscopy Devices, Inc.
XL SERIES	Caddy Corporation
XL-030	Osada, Inc.
XL-15W	Osada, Inc.
XL-230	Osada, Inc.
XL-30W	Osada, Inc.
XL-S30	Osada, Inc.
XMA	Xma (X-Ray Marketing Associates, Inc.)
XMA 150	Xma (X-Ray Marketing Associates, Inc.)
XMA 90	Xma (X-Ray Marketing Associates, Inc.)
XMI	Possis Medical, Inc.
XORAN	Xoran Technologies, Inc.
XORAN MAKES THE COMPLEX SIMPLE	Xoran Technologies, Inc.
XORANCONNECT	Xoran Technologies, Inc.
XP	X P Power
XP BOND	Dentsply International, Inc.
XP BOND	Dentsply Prosthetics
XP WALKER	Aircast Llc
XP1	Medical Specialties, Inc.
XPEEDIOR	Possis Medical, Inc.
XPER-CHROM	Cobert Associates, Inc.
XPERT	Labconco Corp.
XPERTEK	Cobert Associates, Inc.
XPRESS COMPUTED RADIOGRAPHY SYSTEMS: DRYPRO DRY LASE	Konica Minolta Medical Imaging Usa, Inc.
XPRESS SERIES	Topcon Medical Systems, Inc.
XPRT	Stryker Corp.
XPS 2000	Medtronic Xomed, Inc.
XPS STRAIGHT-SHOT	Medtronic Xomed, Inc.
XR-10	Safety Syringe Corporation Of America, Inc.
XR-3	Safety Syringe Corporation Of America, Inc.
XR-5	Safety Syringe Corporation Of America, Inc.
XRE	Hologic, Inc.
XSIGHT	Accuray, Inc.
XT-SERIES	Taylor Wharton
XTEN,AXCEL	Getinge Usa, Inc.
XTEND	Extra Packaging, Corp.
XTENDOBUTTON	Smith & Nephew, Inc., Endoscopy Division
XTR	Becton Dickinson And Company
XTR	Standard Textile
XTRA AMP KITS	Xtrana, Inc.
XTRAC	Photomedex, Inc.
XTRACT	Indec Systems, Inc.
XTRAGENTLE	Sterion, Incorporated
XTRASHARP	Conmed Linvatec
XTRASIGHT	Magnivision, Inc.
XTREME PACK	Zoll Medical Corp.
XVG	Possis Medical, Inc.
Xenform	Boston Scientific Corporation
Y PLATE	Bd Diagnostic Systems
Y-SENSOR	Respironics, Inc
Y-TEC	Janin Group, Inc.

ZYKLOTRON	Siemens Medical Solutions Usa, Inc.
ZYLONOX	Jones-Zylon Company
ZYLOWARE	Zyloware Corporation
ZYMATE	Zymark Corporation
ZYMAX	Spectrum Laboratories, Inc.
Zand	Nutraceutical International Corp.
Zebra	Boston Scientific Corporation
Zenith	Williams Healthcare Systems, Llc.
Zephyr	St. Jude Medical, Inc.
ZeroTip	Boston Scientific Corporation
Zest	Procter & Gamble
Zylet	Bausch & Lomb
Zyoptix	Bausch & Lomb
Zyoptix XP	Bausch & Lomb
autoLog	Medtronic Perfusion Systems
bioAllers	Nutraceutical International Corp.
bion	Boston Scientific Corporation
bion	Boston Scientific Neuromodulation Corporation
eICU	Sentara Health Management
eValuator	St. Jude Medical, Inc.
eXcelon	Boston Scientific Corporation
enGen	Ortho Clinical Diagnostics, Inc.
enGen	Ortho-Clinical Diagnostics, Inc.
iLab	Boston Scientific - Maple Grove
iLab	Boston Scientific Corporation
02 KINETICS SOFTWARE	Medical Graphics Corporation
1*2*3*HEART RATE MONITORS	Heart Rate, Inc.
1-D ANALYST	Bio-Rad Laboratories
1-D ANALYST	Bio-Rad Laboratories, Life Science Group
1-TO-1	Tp Orthodontics, Inc.
1070 SYSTEM	Medical Graphics Corporation
1085 ADVANTAGE PLUS SYSTEM	Medical Graphics Corporation
1085 ADVANTAGE SYSTEM	Medical Graphics Corporation
1085 BASIC SYSTEM	Medical Graphics Corporation
1085 SREIES	Medical Graphics Corporation
1085 ULTIMATE SYSTEM	Medical Graphics Corporation
125BP	Cte Chem Tec Equipment Co.
12SL	Ge Medical Systems Information Technologies
14K	Medtronic, Inc.
180PLUS	Sonosite, Inc.
18K	Medtronic, Inc.
1ST RESPONSE	Georgia Steel & Chemical Company, Inc.
2-D ANALYST	Bio-Rad Laboratories
2-D ANALYST	Bio-Rad Laboratories, Life Science Group
2-D DOCTOR	Bio-Rad Laboratories
20-BELOW	Tcp Reliable, Inc.
20/20	Camfil Farr
20/20	Magnivision, Inc.
20/20 MIRRORS	Parkell, Inc.
200 PLUS	AMD Technologies Inc.
2001	Bio-Med Devices, Inc.
2001	Dixie Ems Supply
2001 FIBERLIGHT	Mercury Medical
2001 HI-TECH	Dixie Ems Supply
2001 SYRINGE PUMP	Smiths Medical OEM
2001E	Premier Medical Products
2010I SYRINGE PUMP	Smiths Medical OEM
21-C SORIOS	Caddy Corporation
2110	Vitalograph, Inc.
2120	Vitalograph, Inc.
2170	Vitalograph, Inc.
21ST CENTURY MILITARY HOSPITAL SYSTEM(TM) (21CMHS)	Mobile Medical International Corporation
22 + X/Y	Gametrics Ltd.
2300N95 AIR-FLOW PARTICULATE RESPIRATOR	American Diversified Dental Systems
241	Arizant Healthcare Inc.
256 SORT	Beckman Coulter, Inc.
260 VOLT OHMMETER	Simpson Electric Co.
2H TECHNOLOGY	Nano Mask Inc.
2ND SKIN	Spenco Medical Corp.
2ST	Med-Fit Systems, Inc.
2UV	Uvp, Llc
3-CHIP	Stryker Corp.
3-CHIP	Stryker Endoscopy
3-D MLC	Siemens Medical Solutions Usa, Inc
3-P GLIDE/PACK	Camfil Farr
30/30	Camfil Farr
3000 PLUS	C. R. Bard, Inc.
30K	Dentsply International, Inc.
30K	Dentsply Prosthetics
3100A	CAREFUSION 211, INC..
3100B	CAREFUSION 211, INC..
32 KARAT	Beckman Coulter, Inc.
35N LT	Fort Wayne Metals Research Prod. Corp.
36-1000 STERILE ULTRA PHONIC	Pharmaceutical Innovations, Inc.
36-1000 ULTRA/PHONIC	Pharmaceutical Innovations, Inc.
36-1001 ULTRA/PHONIC SG	Pharmaceutical Innovations, Inc.
36-1002 EVRON GEL	Pharmaceutical Innovations, Inc.
36-1004 VET/GEL	Pharmaceutical Innovations, Inc.
36-1100 ULTRA WARMER	Pharmaceutical Innovations, Inc.
36-1111 OTHER-SONIC	Pharmaceutical Innovations, Inc.
36-1150 GAMMA	Pharmaceutical Innovations, Inc.
36-1200 ULTRA/PHONIC FREE	Pharmaceutical Innovations, Inc.
36-1300 ULTRA/PHONIC FOCUS	Pharmaceutical Innovations, Inc.
36-1303 ULTRA/PHONIC OPHTHALMIC SCANNING PADS	Pharmaceutical Innovations, Inc.
36-1304 ULTRA/PHONIC FONTANELLE SCANNING PADS	Pharmaceutical Innovations, Inc.
36-1400 ULTRA/PHONIC BP	Pharmaceutical Innovations, Inc.
36-1500 GENTLE GEL	Pharmaceutical Innovations, Inc.
36-1600 PHOTON	Pharmaceutical Innovations, Inc.
36-2000 D-FOAM	Pharmaceutical Innovations, Inc.
36-2100 M-SPRAY 2000	Pharmaceutical Innovations, Inc.
36-2102 T-SPRAY II	Pharmaceutical Innovations, Inc.
36-3000 LECTRON II	Pharmaceutical Innovations, Inc.
36-3200 T-SPRAY	Pharmaceutical Innovations, Inc.
36-3300 SPRAYTRODE	Pharmaceutical Innovations, Inc.
36-3310 ELECTRO MIST	Pharmaceutical Innovations, Inc.
36-3400 PREP TRODE	Pharmaceutical Innovations, Inc.
36-3440 PREP N' STAY	Pharmaceutical Innovations, Inc.
36-3700 AFTER-TENS	Pharmaceutical Innovations, Inc.
36-3990 RES-OFF	Pharmaceutical Innovations, Inc.
36-6101 ULTRA/PHONIC WHITE	Pharmaceutical Innovations, Inc.
36-7002 Q.R.	Pharmaceutical Innovations, Inc.
36-8800 LEAN ON ME	Pharmaceutical Innovations, Inc.
36-9000 TAC GEL	Pharmaceutical Innovations, Inc.
36-9400 PRE-TAC	Pharmaceutical Innovations, Inc.
36-9690 FOR PLAY	Pharmaceutical Innovations, Inc.
360 Jr.	Boston Scientific Corporation
3C	Aspen Surgical
3D ACTIVETRAC	The Saunders Group
3D KNEE	DJO Surgical
3D MATRIX	DJO Surgical
3D OCT-1000	Topcon Medical Systems, Inc.
3D VIEW	Bio-Rad Laboratories
3D VOLUMETRIC FUSION	Rahd Oncology Products
3D-ACCUSAN	Implantech Associates, Inc.
3F4 PRION ANTIBODY	Covance Research Products Inc.
3K-RETIC	R & D Systems, Inc.
3M	3m Co.
3M	3m Espe Dental Products
3M	Bound Tree Medical
3M PREFERRED CONVERTER	Tailored Label Products, Inc.
3M-BRANDED MICROPLATE SEALING TAPE	M&C Specialties Co.
3P	Stryker Imaging
3UV	Uvp, Llc
3X10=0 FULL EXTENSION KNEE DEVICE	Information Health Network
4 PLUS	Allergan
4-02	Eagle Health Supplies, Inc.
4-AXIS OTT LATHE	Dac International, Inc.
4-CORE	Promega Corp.
4-P GLIDE/PACK	Camfil Farr
430	Dentalez Group
430 SW	Dentalez Group
430SWL	Dentalez Group

SUBSIDIARY INDEX

3M
3m Hutchinson   320-234-2000
915 Adams St. SE, Hutchinson, MN 55350-2927

3M CO.
3m Aberdeen   605-229-5002
610 N. Brown County Rd. 19, Aberdeen, SD 57401

3m Company   641-585-2700
806 W. Crystal Lake Rd, Forest City, IA 50436

3m Company   507-354-8271
1617 N. Front Street, New Ulm, MN 56073

3m Company   (605) 692-9433
601 22nd Ave. South, PO Box 5227, Brookings, SD 57006

3m Espe Dental Products   651-733-7767
2501 SE Otis Corley Drive, Bentonville, AR 72712

3m Espe Dental Products   949-863-1360
2111 McGaw Ave., Irvine, CA 92614

3m Flemington   908-788-4000
500 Route 202 North, Flemington, NJ 08822

3m Midwest Distribution Center   815-756-5087
3050 Corporate Dr, DeKalb, IL 60115-9299

3m Petaluma   707-765-3236
1331 Commerce St., Petaluma, CA 94954

3m Unitek   626-574-4000
2724 S. Peck Rd., Monrovia, CA 91016

3m Valley   402-359-2131
600 E. Meigs Street, Valley, NE 68064

Imtec, A 3m Company   580-223-4456
IMTEC Plaza, 2401 N. Commerce, Ardmore, OK 73401

3M COMPANY
Cuno Filter Systems   203-237-5541
400 Research Pkwy., Meriden, CT 06450

A & A ORTHOPEDIC APPLIANCES, INC.
UBM Canon   310-445-8590
11444 Olympic Blvd. Suite 900, Los Angeles, CA 90064

A.R. HINKEL CO., INC.
R. A. Fischer Co.   818-407-0855
8751 White Oak Ave., Northridge, CA 91325

R.A. Fischer Company   818-407-0855
8751 White Oak Avenue, Northridge, CA 91325

AAEON TECHNOLOGY, INC.
Aaeon Electronics, Inc.   732-203-9300
3 Crown Plaza, Hazlet, NJ 07730-2441

AARON CARLSON CORPORATION
S&W By Hausmann   201-767-0255
130 Union Street, Northvale, NJ 07647

ABB CONCISE OPTICAL GROUP LLC
Abb Concise Optical Group Llc   800-852-8089
12301 NW 39th Street, Coral Springs, FL 33065

ABBOTT LABORATORIES
Abbott Diabetes Care Inc.   510-749-5400
1360 South Loop Rd., Alameda, CA 94502

Abbott Diagnostics Div.   626-440-0700
820 Mission St., South Pasadena, CA 91030

Abbott Diagnostics Div.   847-937-7988
1921 Hurd Dr., Irving, TX 75038

Abbott Diagnostics Intl, Biotechnology Ltd   787-846-3500
Road #2 KM. 58.0 , PO Box 278, Cruce Davila, Barceloneta, PR 00617

Abbott Hematology, Diagnostics Div.   408-982-480
5440 Patrick Henry Dr., Santa Clara, CA 95054

Abbott Laboratories   847-937-2388
U.S. 41/Martin Luther King Dr, North Chicago, IL 60064

Abbott Laboratories   614-624-7677
1033 Kingsmill Pkwy., Columbus, OH 43229

Abbott Laboratories   847-937-2388
6480 busch blvd., Columbus, OH 43229

Abbott Medical Optics Inc.   714-247-8200
1700 East St. Andrew Pl., Santa Ana, CA 92705

Abbott Molecular, Inc.   847-937-6100
1300 E. Touhy Ave., Des Plaines, IL 60018

Abbott Point Of Care Inc.   609-443-9300
104 Windsor Center Dr., East Windsor, NJ 08520

Abbott Spine, Inc.   847-937-6100
12708 Riata Vista Circle, Suite B-100, Austin, TX 78727

Abbott Vascular Inc.   650-474-3000
400 Saginaw Drive, Redwood City, CA 94063-4749

Abbott Vascular, Cardiac Therapies   847-937-2388
30590 Cochise Circle, Murrieta, CA 92563

Abbott Vascular, Cardiac Therapies   408-845-3000
3200 Lakeside Dr., Santa Clara, CA 95054-2807

Abbott Vascular, Cardiac Therapies   847-937-7988
26531 Ynez Rd., Mailing P.O. Box 9018, Temecula, CA 92589-9018

Abbott Vascular, Cardiac Therapies-P.R   847-937-2388
Km 58.0, Carretera 2, Cruce Davila, Barceloneta, PR 00617

Abbott Vascular, Vascular Solutions   847-937-2388
3200 Lakeside Dr, Santa Clara, CA 95054

Abbott Vascular, Vascular Solutions   847-937-6100
26531 Ynez Rd., Temecula, CA 92589

Abbott West Distribution Center   847-937-2388
42301 Zevo Drive, Temecula, CA 92590

Hospira   419-289-3555
268 E. Fourth St., Ashland, OH 44805-2494

ABILITYONE PRODUCTS CORP.
Medco Supply Company   716-695-3244
500 Fillmore Avenue, Tonawanda, NY 14150

Orchid Stealth Orthopedic Solutions   517-694-2300
1489 Cedar St., Holt, MI 48842

ACCELLENT INC.
Accellent El Paso   915-771-9112
31C Butterfield Trail, El Paso, TX 79906

Accellent Endoscopy   909-982-1025
2052 West 11th St., Upland, CA 91786

Accellent Inc. — 303-424-7300
5000 Independence St., Arvada, CO 80002

Accellent Inc. — 603-528-1211
45 Lexington Dr., Laconia, NH 03246

ACCUTEK PACAKGING EQUIPMENT

Biner Ellison — 760-598-6500
2685 South Melrose Drive, Vista, CA 92081

ACHILLES

Achilles Usa, Inc. — 425-353-7000
1407 80th St. S.W., Everett, WA 98203

ACTEON GROUP

Acteon Inc. — 856-222-9988
124 Gaither Drive, Suite 140, Mount Laurel, NJ 08054

Marco Products Company — 818-367-2227
12860 San Fernando Road, Sylmar, CA 91342

ACTION U.S.A.

Schell, Inc. — 727-821-5000
P.O. Box 12689, St. Petersburg, FL 33733-2689

ADATIF MEDICAL

Perry Baromedical Corp. — 561-840-0395
3660 Interstate Parkway, Riviera Beach, FL 33404-3411

ADOLFSON & PETERSON

Adolfson & Peterson, Inc — 612-544-1561
6701 W. 23rd Street, Minneapolis, MN 55426

ADVANCED MEDICAL OPTICS, INC.

Advanced Medical Instruments, Inc. — 918-250-0566
3061 West Albany, Broken Arrow, OK 74012

Advanced Medical, Inc — 215-443-5424
935 Horsham Rd., Horsham, PA 19044

ADVANTIS MEDICAL

Nemcomed — 419-542-7743
8727 Clinton Park Drive, Fort Wayne, IN 46825

AEC, INC.

Carver Inc. — 260-563-7577
1569 Morris St., Wabash, IN 46992-0544

AERIFORM COMPANY

Southland Cryogenics, Inc. — 972-243-1311
8350 Mosley Rd., Houston, TX 77075-1112

AESCULAP AG & CO. KG

Aesculap Implant Systems Inc. — 610-984-9081
3773 Corporate Pky., Center Valley, PA 18034

AFFYMETRIX, INC.

Affymetrix, Inc. — 916-376-1309
890 Embarcadero Dr., West Sacramento, CA 95605

Usb Corporation — 1-408-731-5000
3420 central expressway, santa clara, CA 95051

AFP IMAGING CORP.

Ansell Healthcare, Inc. — 732-345-5400
200 Schulz Drive, Red Bank, NJ 07701

AGFA GEVAERT N.V.

Agfa Corporation — 864-421-1600
PO Box 19048, 10 South Academy Street, Greenville, SC 29602-9048

AGILENT TECHNOLOGIES, INC.

Agilent Technologies, Inc. — 408-345-8886
5301 Stevens Creek Blvd., Santa Clara, CA 95051

Stratagene — 858-373-6300
11011 N. Torrey Pines Road, La Jolla, CA 92037-1007

Varian Inc — 650-424-5078
25200 Commercentre Dr., Lake Forest, CA 92630-8810

AHLSTROM DEXTER

Ahlstrom Windsor Locks Llc — 860-654-8300
2 Elm St., Windsor Locks, CT 06096-2335

AIR INNOVATIONS, INC.

Cleanroom Systems — 315-452-7400
7000 Performance Dr., Syracuse, NY 13212

AIRGAS, INC.

Airgas East, Inc — 866-718-0685
1 Plank St., Billerica, MA 01821

Airgas East, Inc. — 800-562-3815
90 Research Rd., Hingham, MA 02043

Airgas East, Inc. — 800-562-3815
608 Nursery Rd., Linthicum Heights, MD 21090

Airgas East, Inc. — 800-562-3815
27 Northwestern Drive, Salem, NH 03079

Airgas East, Inc. — 800-562-3815
140 Harding Ave., Bellmawr, NJ 08031

Airgas Gaspro Inc. — 808-842-2282
2305 Kamehameha Hwy., Honolulu, HI 96819

Airgas Great Lakes, Inc. — 517-894-4101
5018 Empire Way, Lansing, MI 48917

Airgas Intermountain, Inc. — 801-288-5015
3415 South 7oo West, Salt Lake City, UT 84119

Airgas Norpac — 360-944-4091
3411 North Columbia Blvd., Portland, OR 97217

Airgas South, Inc. — 251-653-2500
5480 Hamilton Blvd., Theodore, AL 36582

Airgas South, Inc. — 770-590-6200
5837 W. Fifth St., Jacksonville, FL 32254

Airgas South, Inc. — 770-590-6200
7280 NW 58th St., Miami, FL 33166

Airgas South, Inc. — 770-590-6200
1620 Tampa East Blvd., Tampa, FL 33619

Airgas South, Inc. — 770-590-6200
1311 Fulton Industrial Blvd., N.W., Suite C, Atlanta, GA 30336

Airgas South, Inc. — 770-590-6200
3605 Presidential Pkwy., Atlanta, GA 30340

Airgas South, Inc. — 770-590-6200
4551 North Access Rd., Chattanooga, TN 37415

Airgas Specialty Gases — 913-495-3621
9851 Widmer Rd., Lenexa, KS 66215

Airgas Specialty Gases, Inc. — 773-785-3000
12722 South Wentworth Ave., Roseland, IL 60628

Airgas West, Inc. — 310-505-9897
11711 South Alameda, Los Angeles, CA 90059

Airgas West, Inc. — 310-505-9897
191 South Kettering Dr., Ontario, CA 91761

Airgas, Northern California And Nevada — 916-379-1050
20725 Corsair Blvd., Hayward, CA 94545

Airgas, Northern California And Nevada — 916-379-1050
443 Hobson St., San Jose, CA 95110

Airgas-Mid America, Inc. — 800-292-4404
3500 Bernard, Saint Louis, MO 63103

Airgas-Mid South, Inc. — 918-582-0885
9741 E 56th St N, Tulsa, OK 74110

Airgas-North Central, Inc. — 630-231-9260
1601 nicholas blvd., elk grove village, IL 60007

Airgas-Southwest, Inc. — 361-288-0587
2615 Joe Field Rd., Dallas, TX 75229

Airgas-Southwest, Inc. — 361-288-0587
21 Waterway, Suite 550, The Woodlands, TX 77380

ALADDIN INDUSTRIES PTY. LTD.

Aladdin Synergetics, Inc. — 615-537-3600
250 E Main Street, Hendersonville, TN 37075

ALCOHOL COUNTERMEASURE SYSTEMS CORP.

Alcohol Countermeasure Systems, Inc. — 303-366-5699
1670 Jasper St., Suite G, Aurora, CO 80011

ALCON RESEARCH, LTD.

Alcon Manufacturing, Ltd. — 949-753-1393
15800 Alton Parkway, Irvine, CA 92618

Alcon Manufacturing, Ltd. — 817-551-6813
714 Columbia Ave., Sinking Spring, PA 19608

Alcon Manufacturing, Ltd. — 713-668-9100
9965 Buffalo Speedway, Houston, TX 77054-1309

Alcon Manufacturing, Ltd. — 304-736-5230
6065 Kyle Lane, Huntington, WV 25702-9795

ALERE, INC.

Alere Medical, Inc. — 775-829-8885
595 Double Eagle Court, Suite 1000, Reno, NV 89521

Biosite Incorporated — 858-805-3423
9975 Summers Ridge Rd, San Diego, CA 92121

Cholestech Corp. — 510-732-7200
3347 Investment Blvd., Hayward, CA 94545-3808

Diamics, Inc. — 415-883-0414
Six Hamilton Landing Suite 200, Novato, CA 94949

Hemosense, Inc. — 408-719-1393
651 River Oaks Parkway, San Jose, CA 95134

Innovacon, Inc. — 858-535-2030
4106 Sorrento Valley Blvd., San Diego, CA 92121

Inverness Medical — 609-627-8038
2 Research Way, Princeton, NJ 08540

Inverness Medical Inc. — 732-308-3000
569 Halls Mill Rd, Freehold, NJ 07728

Inverness Medical Innovations North America, Inc — (877) 441-7440
30 S. Keller Road, Suite 100, Lockhart, FL 32810

Inverness Medical Professional Diagnostics-San Die — 858-535-2030
4106 Sorrento Valley Boulevard, San Diego, CA 92121

QUALITY ASSURED SERVICES DBA ALERE — 407-563-2860
HOME MONITORING PRODUCTS
70 S. Keller Rd., Orlando, FL 32810

Redwood Toxicology Laboratories, Inc. — 707-577-7959
3650 Westwind Blvd., Santa Rosa, CA 95403

ALFA WASSERMAN GROUP, MILAN
Alfa Wassermann, Inc. — 973-882-8630
4 Henderson Drive, West Caldwell, NJ 07006

ALLIED HEALTHCARE PRODUCTS, INC.
Allied Healthcare Products, Inc. — 314-771-2400
1720 Sublette Avenue, St. Louis, MO 63110

ALLIED MINDS
SoundCure — 617-419-1800
33 Arch Street, Boston, MA 02110

ALLIED SIGNAL, INC.
Sensormatic Electronics — 561-912-6000
6600 Congress Ave, Boca Raton, FL 33487

ALOKA CO., LTD.
Aloka (Us Headquarters) — 203-269-5088
10 Fairfield Blvd., Wallingford, CT 06492-7502

ALPHA SOURCE, INC.
Access Battery Inc. — 414-760-2222
Division of Alpha Source, Inc., 12104 W. Carmen Avenue, Milwaukee, WI 53225-2135

ALTAIR CORPORATION
Teledyne Analytical Instruments — 626-934-1500
16830 Chestnut St., City of Industry, CA 91749

ALTANA, INC.
Fougera — 631-454-6996
60 Baylis Road, PO Box 2006, Melville, NY 11747

ALUMINUM PRECISION PRODUCTS INC.
Catalina Cylinders — 714-890-0999
7300 Anaconda Avenue, Garden Grove, CA 92841

AMANO (JAPAN)
Amano Pioneer Eclipse Corp. — 336-372-8080
1 Eclipse Road, PO Box 909, Sparta, NC 28675

AMCOR LTD.
The Amcor Group Ltd. — 800-584-6484
685A Gotham Parkway, Carlstadt, NJ 07072-2403

AMEDICA CORPORATION
Us Spine Inc. — 561-367-7463
3600 Fau Blvd., Suite 101, Boca Raton, FL 33431

AMERICAN GREETINGS
Caligor — 800-472-4346
846 Pelham Pkwy., Pelham Manor, NY 10803

Insource, Inc. — 540-688-4121
PO Box 9, Bastian, VA 24314

AMERICAN MEDICAL MANUFACTURING, INC
Advanced Medical Innovations, Inc. — 818-701-7180
9410 De Soto Avenue,, Building J, Chatsworth, CA 91311, CA 91311

AMERICAN MEDICAL SYSTEMS, INC.
Ams Innovative Center-San Jose — 408-943-0636
3070 Orchard Drive, San Jose, CA 95134-2011

AMERICAN OPTISURGICAL INC.
American Optisurgical Inc. — 949-580-1266
25501 Arctic Ocean Dr., Lake Forest, CA 92630

AMERICAN SAFETY RAZOR CO.
Personna Medical/Div. Of American Safety Razor Co. — 540-248-8000
One Razor Blade Ln., Verona, VA 24482

AMERICAN SCIENTIFIC RESOURCES, INC.
Ulster Scientific, Inc. — 845-255-2200
83 South Putt Corners Road, PO Box 819, New Paltz, NY 12561-0819

AMERICAN SILK SUTURES, INC
American Silk Sutures, Inc. — 781-592-7200
82 Sanderson Avenue, Lynn, MA 01902

AMERSHAM PHARMACIA BIOTECH
Hoefer Pharmacia Biotech, Inc. — 508-893-8999
84 October Hill Road, Holliston, MA 01746

AMETEK
Ortec - (Advanced Measurement Technology) — 865-482-4411
801 S. Illinois Avenue, Oak Ridge, TN 37831

Petrolab Company — 518-783-5133
874 Albany Shaker Road, Latham, NY 12110-1416

AMGEN INC.
Amgen Inc. — 206-265-7000
1201 Amgen Court West, Seattle, WA 98119-3105

AMI HOLDINGS, INC
Ardus Medical, Inc. — 513-469-7867
11297 Grooms Rd., Cincinnati, OH 45242

AMPLIFON
Miracle-Ear — 763-268-4000
5000 Cheshire Lane North, Minneapolis, MN 55446

AN AFFILIATE OF EMD, INC.
Dey, L.P. — 707-224-3200
2751 Napa Valley Corporate Drive, Napa, CA 94558-6216

ANALOX INSTRUMENTS LTD.
Analox Instruments Usa, Inc. — 978-582-9368
104 Sunset Lane, P.O. BOX 208, Lunenburg, MA 01462-0208

ANDERMAC, INC.
Hygiene Specialties, Inc./Andermac, Inc. — 530-674-8450
2626 Live Oak Hwy., Yuba City, CA 95991-8810

ANGEION CORPORATION
Medical Graphics Corporation — 651-484-4874
350 Oak Grove Pkwy., St. Paul, MN 55127-8536

ANGELICA CORPORATION
Angelica Image Apparel — 314-889-1111
700 Rosedale Avenue, St. Louis, MO 63112

ANGIODYNAMICS, INC.
Angiodynamics, Inc. — 510-771-0400
46421 Landing Parkway, Fremont, CA 94538

Angiodynamics, Inc. — 706-846-3126
One Horizon Way, Manchester, GA 31816

Angiodynamics, Inc. — 1 518-795-1400
14 Plaza Drive, Latham, NY 12110

Oncobionic — 518-798-1215
30211 Avenida De Las Banderas, Suite 200, Rancho Santa Margarita, CA 92688

ANSYS, INC.
Ansoft Corp. — 412-261-3200
225 West Station Square Drive, Suite 200, Pittsburgh, PA 15219-1119

APLIX S.A.
Aplix, Inc. — 704-588-1920
12300 Steele Creek Road, Charlotte, NC 28273

APOGENT TECHNOLOGIES, INC.
Microgenics Corporation — 510-979-5000
46360 Fremont Blvd., Fremont, CA 94538

APPLIED EXTRUSION TECHNOLOGIES, INC.
Delstar Technologies, Inc. — 302-378-8888
601 Industrial Dr., Middletown, DE 19709

APPLIED POWER, INC.
Apw Eder Industries, Inc.   414-761-0400
2250 W. South Branch Blvd., Oak Creek, WI 53154-4907

APPROVED MEDICAL SYSTEMS
Approved Medical Systems   951-353-2453
7101 Jurupa Ave - Unit 4, Riverside, CA 92504

ARCELOR
Rahns Specialty Metals   610-489-7211
140 Bridge Street, Collegeville, PA 19426

AREVA GROUP
Canberra Industries   203-238-2351
800 Research Pkwy., Meriden, CT 06450-3215

ARGON MEDICAL DEVICES INC.
Clinical Innovations, Inc.   801-268-8200
747 West 4170 South, Murray, UT 84123

ARJO WIGGINS SA
Arjo Wiggins Medical, Inc.   843-388-8080
1301 Charleston Regional Pkwy, #500, Charleston, SC 29492

ARJOHUNTLEIGH
Maquet, Inc.   1-888-MAQUET3
45 Barbour Pond Drive, Wayne, NJ 07470

ARRK CORPORATION
ARRK Product Development Group   858-552-1587
8880 Rehco Rd., San Diego, CA 92121

ARTHROCARE CORP.
Arthrocare Corp.   408-736-0224
680 Vaqueros Avenue, Sunnyvale, CA 94085-3523

ASH TEMPLE LTD.
Alliance H. Inc Dentech Equipment   360-988-7080
901 W. Front Street, Sumas, WA 98295

ASPYRA, INC.
Aspyra, Inc.   904-854-2107
8649 Baypine Rd., Jacksonville, FL 32256

ASTRAZENECA
AstraZeneca Pharmaceuticals LP   302-886-3000
1800 Concord Pike, P.O. Box 15437, Wilmington, DE 19850-5437

ASTRO-MED, INC.
Grass Technologies, An Astro-Med, Inc. Product Gro   401-828-4002
53 Airport Park Drive, Rockland, MA 02370

ATC DIAGNOSTICS, INC.
Vysis   630-271-7000
3100 Woodcreek Drive, Downers Grove, IL 60515

ATON, GMBH
Ziehm Imaging, Inc.   407-615-8560
6280 Hazeltine National Dr., Orlando, FL 32822

ATRION MEDICAL PRODUCTS, INC.
Halkey-Roberts Corp.   1.727.471.4200
2700 Halkey-Roberts Place North, St. Petersburg, FL 33716

Quest Medical, Inc.   972-390-9800
1 Allentown Pkwy., Allen, TX 75002-4211

ATS MEDICAL, INC.
Ats Medical, Inc.   949-380-9333
20412 James Bay Circle, Lake Forest, CA 92630

AUTODESK, INC.
Algor, Inc.   412-967-2700
150 Beta Dr., Pittsburgh, PA 15238-2932

AVAIL MEDICAL PRODUCTS, INC.
Avail Medical Products   858-635-2206
5950 Nancy Ridge Dr, Ste 500, San Diego, CA 92121

Avail Medical Products, Inc.   858-635-2206
1900 Carnegie Ave., --, Santa Ana, CA 92705

Avail Medical Products, Inc.   858-635-2206
1225 N. 28th Avenue, Suite 500, Dallas, TX 75261

Avail Medical Products-Asheville   858-635-2206
3161 Sweeten Creek Road, Asheville, NC 28803

AVAKIAN DBA DATATRAN
Itm Partners, Ltd.   210-651-9066
5925 Corridor Pkwy., Schertz, TX 78154

AVALIGN TECHNOLOGIES
Advantis Medical   317-859-2300
2121 Southtech Dr., Ste 600, Greenwood, IN 46143

AVID MEDICAL INC.
Diamedix Corp.   305-324-2300
2140 N. Miami Avenue, Miami, FL 33127-4933

AXCAN PHARMA INC.
Axcan Pharma Inc.   800-472-2634
22 Inverness Center Parkway, Birmingham, AL 35242

B. BRAUN OEM DIVISION, B. BRAUN MEDICAL INC.
B. Braun Medical, Inc.   610-596-2536
901 Marcon Blvd., Allentown, PA 18109

B. Braun Medical, Inc.   610-596-2536
1601 Wallace Dr., Suite 150, Carrollton, TX 75006

BACHEM HOLDING AG
Bachem Bioscience, Inc.   610-239-0300
3700 Horizon Drive, King of Prussia, PA 19406

BACOU USA
Lase-R Shield, A Bacou-Dalloz Company   505-872-3400
7011 Prospect Pl. NE, Albuquerque, NM 87110

BAIRNCO
Arlon Engineered Coated Products   210-798-1900
6110 E. Rittiman Road, San Antonio, TX 78218

BALCHEM CORP.
Arc Specialty Products, Balchem Corporation   845-326-560
52 Sunrise Park Road, PO Box 600, New Hampton, NY 10958

BAPTIST HEALTH CARE, INC.
Lakeview Center, Inc.   850-595-1330
1221 W. Lakeview Ave., Pensacola, FL 32501-1836

BAR-RAY PRODUCTS, INC.
Hearing Technologies   727-525-7770
6251 44th St 109, Pinellas Park, FL 33781

BAREFOOT ENTERPRISES
Barefoot Medical   760-967-8225
1902 Calle Buena Ventura, Oceanside, CA 92056

BARNHARDT MANUFACTURING CO.
Carolina Absorbent Cotton Co.   704-376-0380
1100 Hawthorne Lane, Charlotte, NC 28205

BARRY CORPORATION, R.G.
Vesture Corporation   336-629-3000
120 E. Pritchard St., Asheboro, NC 27203

BASIC AMERICAN MEDICAL, INC.
Basic American Medical Products   770-368-4700
2935-A Northeast Pkwy, Atlanta, GA 30360

Gf Health Products, Inc   800-347-5678
2935 Northeast Pkwy, Atlanta, GA 30360

BATH LUMBER/ACE HARDWARE
General Dental Products, Inc.   775-289-4461
201 Ogden Avenue, Ely, NV 89301-1888

BAUSCH & LOMB
Bausch & Lomb Inc., Greenville Solutions Plant   585-338-6000
8507 Pelham Rd., Greenville, SC 29615-9598

Bausch & Lomb Pharmaceutical, Inc.   585-338-6000
8500 Hidden River Pkwy, Tampa, FL 33637

Bausch & Lomb Surgical   636-255-5051
3365 Tree Ct. Indust. Blvd., St. Louis, MO 63122-6615

Bausch & Lomb, Inc.   813-724-6600
21 Park Place Blvd. N., Clearwater, FL 33759

Bausch & Lomb, Inc.   585-338-8731
100 Research Drive, Wilmington, MA 01887

Bausch & Lomb, Inc.   585-338-8731
499 Sovereign Ct., Manchester, MO 63011

Bausch & Lomb, Inc.   585-338-8731
130 Commerce Dr., Greenville, SC 29615

Bausch & Lomb, Inc.   585-338-8731
   1501 Graves Mill Rd., Lynchburg, VA 24502
Bausch & Lomb, Vision Care   585-338-6000
   1400 N. Goodman St., Rochester, NY 14609-3547
Eyeonics, Inc.   949-916-9352
   10574 Acacia St., Suite D-1, Rancho Cucamonga, CA 91730

BAXTER INTERNATIONAL INC

Baxter Healthcare Corp., Renal Division   847-948-2000
   7511 114th Avenue North, Largo, FL 33777
Baxter Healthcare Corporation   847-473-6141
   1900 N. Hwy. 201, Mountain Home, AR 72653
Baxter Healthcare Corporation   847-473-6141
   1606 E. University Dr., Phoenix, AZ 85034
Baxter Healthcare Corporation   847-473-6141
   21026 Alexander Court, Hayward, CA 94545
Baxter Healthcare Corporation   847-473-6141
   4501 Colorado Blvd., Los Angeles, CA 90039
Baxter Healthcare Corporation   847-473-6141
   3925 Gateway Blvd, Pinellas Park, FL 33782
Baxter Healthcare Corporation   800-422-9837
   One Baxter Parkway, Deerfield, IL 60015
Baxter Healthcare Corporation   847-473-6141
   911 North Davis, Cleveland, MS 38732
Baxter Healthcare Corporation   847-473-6141
   65 Pitts Station Road, Marion, NC 28752
Baxter Healthcare Corporation   847-473-6141
   4835 S. Mendenhall Rd., Memphis, TN 38141
Baxter Healthcare Corporation Nutrition   847-948-2000
   One Baxter Pkwy., Deerfield, IL 60015
Baxter Healthcare Corporation, Renal   847-473-6030
   1620 Waukegan Road, McGaw Park, IL 60085
Baxter Healthcare Of Puerto Rico   847-948-4054
   530 Road #5, Building #1, Bo Juana Matos, PR 00962
Baxter Healthcare S.A.   847-948-2000
   Rd. 721, Km. 0.3, Aibonito, PR 00609
Baxter Sales & Distribution Corp   847-473-6141
   Rexco Industrial Park, State Road #24, Buchanan, Guaynabo, PR 00968

BAYER AG, GERMANY

Agfa Corp.   201-440-2500
   100 Challenger Rd., Ridgefield Park, NJ 07660-2105

BAYER HEALTHCARE LLC

Bayer Healthcare Llc, Consumer Care   717-866-2141
   36 Columbia Rd., Morristown, NJ 07962
Bayer Healthcare, Llc   574-256-3430
   510 Oakmead Pkwy., Sunnyvale, CA 94085
Bayer Healthcare, Llc   574-256-3430
   430 South Beiger St., Mishawaka, IN 46544

BECKMAN COULTER, INC.

Beckman Coulter Primary Care Diagnostics   714-961-3712
   1050 Page Mill Rd., Bldg. 2-B, Palo Alto, CA 94303-0803
Beckman Coulter, Inc.   (800) 742-2345
   250 South Kraemer Boulevard, Brea, CA 92821-6232
Beckman Coulter, Inc.   714-993-8767
   2470 Faraday Ave., Carlsbad, CA 92008
Beckman Coulter, Inc.   305-380-2730
   11800 Sw 147th Ave., Kendall, FL 33196
Beckman Coulter, Inc.   (317) 808-4200
   5350 Lakeview Parkway S Drive, Indianapolis, IN 46268
Beckman Coulter, Inc.   305-380-4079
   7381 Empire Dr., Florence, KY 41042
Beckman Coulter, Inc.   714-871-4848
   22900 W. Eight Mile Rd., Southfield, MI 48033-4302
Beckman Coulter, Inc.   952-368-7629
   1000 Lake Hazeltine Dr., Chaska, MN 55318
Beckman Coulter, Inc. Primary Care Diagnostics   714-961-3712
   606 Elmwood Ave., Elmwood Court Three, Sharon Hill, PA 19079

BECTON DICKINSON AND COMPANY

Bd Biosciences   408-954-6307
   2350 Qume Dr., San Jose, CA 95131
Bd Diagnostic Systems   800-675-0908
   7 Loveton Circle, Sparks, MD 21152
Bd Diagnostics (Geneohm Sciences, Inc.)   (858) 334-6300
   11085 North Torrey Pines Road, Suite 210, La Jolla, CA 92037
Bd Lee Laboratories   770-972-4450
   1475 Athens Hwy., Grayson, GA 30017
Becton Dickinson And Co.   866-906-8080
   411 Waverley Oaks Rd., Waltham, MA 02452-8405

Becton Dickinson And Co.   201-847-6800
   1 Becton Drive, Franklin Lakes, NJ 07417
Becton Dickinson And Company   201-847-4570
   2153 12th Ave., Columbus, NE 68601
Becton Dickinson Caribe Ltd   410-316-4000
   Vicks Dr, Lot #6, Cayey, PR 00634
Becton Dickinson Infusion Therapy Systems, Inc.   888-237-2762
   9450 S. State St., Sandy, UT 84070
Becton Dickinson Medical Systems   201-847-4570
   Grace Way, Canaan, CT 06018
Becton Dickinson Medical Systems   201-847-6800
   9630 South 54th St., Franklin, WI 53132
Becton, Dickinson & Co.   410-316-4000
   250 Schilling Circle, Cockeysville, MD 21030
Becton, Dickinson & Co.   308-872-6811
   150 South First St., Broken Bow, NE 68822

BEI TECHNOLOGIES, INC.

Bei Technologies, Inc.   949-341-9500
   170 Technology Drive, Irvine, CA 92618

BEIERSDORF, INC.

3M Company   513-272-5000
   5801 Mariemont Ave., Cincinnati, OH 45227

BEL-ART PRODUCTS

Maddak Inc.   973-628-7600
   661 Route 23 South, Wayne, NJ 07470
Nutech Molding Corporation   410-957-9500
   2024 Broad St., PO Box 840, Pocomoke City, MD 21851-0840

BELIMED AG

Belimed   305-252-3338
   2284 Clements Ferry Road, Charleston, SC 29492

BEMIS CO.

Perfecseal   920-303-7000
   PO Box 2968, 3500 North Main St., Oshkosh, WI 54903-2968

BEMIS MANUFACTURING COMPANY

Bemis Mfg. Co.   920-467-4621
   300 Mill St., Sheboygan Falls, WI 53085-0901

BENCHMARK ELECTRONICS, INC.

Benchmark Electronics, Inc.   507-452-8932
   4065 Theurer Blvd., Winona, MN 55987

BENDISTAL PLIERS

Bendistal Pliers   636-230-9933
   175 Lamp & Lantern Village, Chesterfield, MO 63017-8208

BERCHTOLD GMBH & CO.

Berchtold Corp.   843-569-6100
   1950 Hanahan Rd., Charleston, SC 29406

BERKSHIRE HATHWAY - SCOTT FETZER DIV.

Scottcare Corporation   216-362-0550
   4791 W. 150th St., Cleveland, OH 44135

BERLIN PACKAGING

Freund Container   708-272-7099
   Corporate Center II, 4200 Commerce Court Suite 206, Lisle, IL 60532

BERMIL INDUSTRIES

Wascomat Laundry Equipment   516-371-4400
   461 Doughty Blvd., Inwood, NY 11096-0338

BERWIND GROUP

Zymark Corporation   508-435-9500
   68 Elm Street, Hopkinton, MA 01748

BEST MEDICAL INTERNATIONAL, INC.

Best Nomos Corp.   412-312-6700
   One Best Dr., Pittsburgh, PA 15202

BIO MEDICAL TECHNOLOGIES CO., LTD.

Bti Filtration   405-842-2517
   7317 N. Classen Blvd., Oklahoma City, OK 73116

BIO-RAD LABORATORIES, INC.

Bio-Rad Laboratories   510-724-7000
   1000 Alfred Nobel Drive, Hercules, CA 94547

Bio-Rad Laboratories Inc   425-881-8300
  1000 Thomas St., Seattle, WA 98109
Bio-Rad Laboratories Inc., Clinical Systems Div.   510-724-7000
  4000 Alfred Nobel Dr., Hercules, CA 94547
Bio-Rad Laboratories, Diagnostic Group   510-724-7000
  524 Stone Rd, Suite A, Benicia, CA 94510
Bio-Rad Laboratories, Inc   510-741-6263
  5500 East 2nd St, Benicia, CA 94510
Bio-Rad Laboratories, Inc.   425-881-8300
  6565 185th Ave., N.E., Redmond, WA 98052
Bio-Rad Laboratories, Inc.   425-881-8300
  14620 N.E. North Woodinville, Way, Suite 200, Woodinville, WA 98072
Bio-Rad Laboratories, Life Science Group   510-741-1000
  2000 Alfred Nobel Dr., Hercules, CA 94547
Bio-Rad, Diagnostics Group   949-598-1200
  9500 Jeronimo Rd., Irvine, CA 92618-2017

BIOCENTRIC SOLUTIONS

Lifegas Llc   678-380-4402
  1500 Indian Trail Road, Norcross, GA 30093-2613

BIOHIT OYJ

Biohit Inc.   732-922-4900
  3535 Rte. 66, Bldg. 4, PO Box 308,, Neptune, NJ 07754-0308

BIOJECT MEDICAL TECHNOLOGIES, INC.

Bioject Medical Technologies, Inc.   503-692-8001
  20245 SW 95th Avenue, Tualatin, OR 97062

BIOKIT, S.A.

Biokit Usa, Inc.   781-861-0710
  180 Hartwell Ave., Bedford, MA 02421

BIOMET, INC.

Biomet 3i   561-776-6700
  4555 Riverside Dr., Palm Beach Gardens, FL 33410
Biomet Microfixation Inc.   904-741-4400
  1520 Tradeport Dr., Jacksonville, FL 32218
Biomet Sports Medicine   530-226-5800
  6704 Lockheed Dr., Redding, CA 96002
Biomet Sports Medicine, Inc   574-267-6639
  56 East Bell Drive, Warsaw, IN 46581-0587
Ebi, Llc   973-299-9300
  100 Interpace Pky., Parsippany, NJ 07054

BIONOSTICS, INC.

Rna Medical, A Division Of Bionostics, Inc.   978-772-9070
  7 Jackson Road, Devens, MA 01434

BIORAD LABORATORIES

Biorad Laboratories   510-724-7000
  1000 Alfred Nobel Drive, Hercules, CA 94547

BIOSPECTRUM TECHNOLOGIES

Biomagnetics Diagnostics Corp.   916-987-7078
  8864 Greenback Lane, Suite E, Orangevale, CA 95662

BIOTEL, INC.

Braemar, Inc.   651-286-8620
  1285 Corporate Center Dr., Suite 150, Eagan, MN 55121

BIOTEST AG

Biotest Diagnostic Corp.   800-522-0090
  400 Commons Way, Rockaway, NJ 07866

BIOZYME LABORATORIES LTD.

Biozyme Laboratories International Ltd.   858-549-4484
  9939 Hibert St., Suite 101, San Diego, CA 92131-1029

BISSELL HEALTHCARE, INC.

Patterson Medical Holdings, Inc.   630-378-6000
  1000 Remington Blvd., Suite 210, Bolingbrook, IL 60440-4995

BMR TEO.

Brandel   301-948-6506
  8561 Atlas Dr., Gaithersburg, MD 20877-4135

BOARDMAN MEDICAL SUPPLIES

Innovative Concepts   330-545-6390
  300 N. State St., Girard, OH 44420

BOEHRINGER INGELHEIM PHARMACUETICALS INC.

Roxane Laboratories   800-962-8364
  P.O. Box 16532, Columbus, OH 43216-6532

BOEHRINGER MANNHEIM GMBH

Roche Diagnostics Operations   317-521-2000
  9115 Hague Rd., PO Box 50457, Indianapolis, IN 46250

BOSE CORPORATION

Bose Corporation - Electroforce Systems Group   952-278-3070
  10250 Valley View Road, Suite 113, Eden Prairie, MN 55344

BOSTON SCIENTIFIC CORPORATION

Advanced Stent Technologies   508-650-8798
  6900 Koll Center Pkwy., #415, Pleasanton, CA 94566
Asthmatx, Inc.   408-419-0100
  888 Ross Dr., Suite 100, Sunnyvale, CA 94089
Boston Scientific - Maple Grove   763-494-1700
  One Scimed Place, Maple Grove, MN 55311-1566
Boston Scientific - Marina Bay Customer Fulfillment   617-689-6000
  Center
  500 Commander Shea Blvd, Quincy, MA 02171
Boston Scientific Corp.   408-935-3400
  150 Baytech Dr., San Jose, CA 95134
Boston Scientific Corp.   763-694-5500
  5905 Nathan Lane, Plymouth, MN 55442-1656
Boston Scientific Corp.   612-582-7448
  6645 185th Ave. N.E., Redmond, WA 98052
Boston Scientific Corporation   508-652-5578
  2011 Stierlin Court, Mountain View, CA 94043
Boston Scientific Corporation   508-652-5578
  780 Brookside Drive, Spencer, IN 47460
Boston Scientific Interventional Technologies   858-268-4488
  3574 Ruffin Rd., San Diego, CA 92123-2502
Boston Scientific Neuromodulation Corporation   508-652-5578
  25155 Rye Canyon Loop, Valencia, CA 91355
Catheter Innovations, Inc.   801-954-8444
  3598 West 1820 South, Salt Lake City, UT 84104-4859
Ep Technologies, Inc.   508-650-8172
  2710 Orchard Pkwy., San Jose, CA 95134
Guidant Corporation   408-845-3995
  8934 Kirby Drive, Houston, TX 77054
Interventional Technologies, Inc.   858-268-4488
  30590 Cochise Circle, Murrieta, CA 92563

BOUTON CORP.

H.L. Bouton Co., Inc.   508-295-3300
  PO Box 840, Buzzards Bay, MA 02532

BOWMAN MANUFACTURING COMPANY, INC.

Bowman Manufacturing Company, Inc.   360-435-5005
  17301 51st Ave NE, Arlington, WA 98223

BOYD TECHNOLOGIES LLC

Boyd Converting Co., Inc.   413-243-2200
  PO BOX 287, South Lee, MA 01260

BRAUN GMBH & CO.

B. Braun Medical   800-854-6851
  1940 Olney Ave., Cherry Hill, NJ 08003

BRIGGS CORPORATION

Horizon Healthcare Technologies   314-569-5995
  PO Box 27809, St. Louis, MO 63146

BRISTOL-MYERS SQUIBB COMPANY

Bristol-Myers Group Company   609-252-4000
  P.O. Box 4500, Princeton, NJ 08543

BRITISH VITA

Crest Foam Industries   201-807-0809
  100 Carol Place, Moonachie, NJ 07074-1304

BROE COMPANIES

Walkmed Infusion Llc   303-420-9569
  4080 Youngfield St., Wheat Ridge, CO 80033-3862

BROOKS-PRI AUTOMATION, INC.

La Calhene   320-358-4713
  1325 Field Avenue S., PO Box 567, Rush City, MN 55069

BRUNSWICK

Life Fitness   847-288-3300
10601 W. Belmont Avenue, Franklin Park, IL 60131

BSW BERLEBURGER SCHAUMSTOFFWERK GMBH

Regupol America   800-537-8737
33 Keystone Drive, Lebanon, PA 17042

BUSINESS AVIATION

Business Aviation Services   605-336-7791
3501 Aviation Avenue, Sioux Falls, SD 57104-0197

C&E VISION SERVICES, INC.

C&E Gp Specialists   800-346-2626
1015 Calle Amanecer, San Clemente, CA 92673

C. H. WERFEN

Instrumentation Laboratory Company   781-861-0710
180 Hartwell Road, Bedford, MA 02421

C. R. BARD, INC.

Bard Access Systems, Inc.   801-522-5000
605 N. 5600 West, Salt Lake City, UT 84116

Bard Brachytherapy, Inc   908-277-8000
295 E. Lies Rd., Carol Stream, IL 60188

Bard Electro Physiology   978-441-6202
55 Technology Dr., Lowell, MA 01851

Bard Peripheral Vascular, Inc.   480-894-9515
1625 West Third Street, Tempe, AZ 85281

Bard Shannon Limited   908-277-8000
San Geronimo Industrial Park, Lot # 1, Road # 3, Km 79.7, Humacao, PR 00791

Bridger Biomed, Inc.   908-277-8000
2430 North 7th Ave., Bozeman, MT 59715

C. R. Bard, Inc.   908-277-8481
289 Bay Rd., Queensbury, NY 12804

C. R. Bard, Inc.   908-277-8481
428 Powerhouse Rd., Moncks Corner, SC 29461

C. R. Bard, Inc., Bard Medical Div.   770-784-6100
8195 Industrial Blvd., Covington, GA 30209

Davol Inc., Sub. C.R. Bard, Inc.   401-463-7000
100 Crossings Blvd., Warwick, RI 02886

Dymax Corp.   908-277-8481
110 Marshall Dr., Warrendale, PA 15086

Lutonix, Inc   763-445-2352
7351 Kirkwood Lane North, Suite 138, Maple Grove, MN 55369

Medchem Products, Inc.   908-277-8000
160 New Boston St., Woburn, MA 01801

Senorx, Inc.   949-362-4800
11 Columbia, Aliso Viejo, CA 92656

Venetec International., Inc.   858-509-2400
12555 High Bluff Drive,, Suite 100, San Diego, CA 92130

C.R. BARD, INC.

C. R. Bard, Inc., Bard Urological Div.   770-784-6100
8195 Industrial Boulevard, Covington, GA 30014

C/S GROUP

General Cubicle Co.   800-869-4606
49 Meeker Avenue, Cranford, NJ 07016

CADEX ELECTRONICS INC.

Battery Specialties   714-755-0888
3530 Cadillac Ave., Costa Mesa, CA 92626

CALMAQUIP ENGINEERING CORP

Calmaquip Engineering Corp.   305-592-4510
7240 N.W. 12th St., Miami, FL 33126-1909

CANON, INC.

Canon Development Americas, Inc   949-932-3100
15955 Alton Parkway, Irvine, CA 92618-3731

CANTEL MEDICAL

Minntech Corporation   763-553-3300
14605 28th Avenue N., Minneapolis, MN 55447

CANTEL MEDICAL CORP.

Confirm Monitoring Systems, Inc.   303-699-3356
109 inverness Drive East, Unit F, Englewood, CO 80112-5105

CANTEL MEDICAL CORPORATION

Crosstex International,Inc.   631-582-6777
10 Ranick Rd., Hauppauge, NY 11788-4209

Faichney Medical Co.   636-240-9501
433 Scenic Drive, Suite # 103, St. Peters, MO 63376

CAPRIUS, INC.

Opus Diagnostics, Inc.   201-944-1777
One Parker Plaza, Fort Lee, NJ 07024

CARCLO ENGINEERING GROUP PLC

Ctp Coil Inc.   847-228-8818
1801-D Howard Street, Elk Grove Village, IL 60007

CARDIAC SCIENCE CORPORATION

Cardiac Science Corp.   608-764-1919
500 Burdick Pkwy., Deerfield, WI 53531-9692

Cardiac Science Corporation (Ca)   1.425.402.2000
3303 Monte Villa Parkway, Bothell, WA 98021

CARDINAL HEALTH

Cardinal Scale Mfg. Co.   417-673-4631
203 East Daugherty, Box 151, Webb City, MO 64870

Nuclear Pharmacy Services   614-757-5000
7000 Cardinal Place, Dublin, OH 43017

CARDINAL HEALTH INC.

Cardinal Health   847-785-3323
State Rd. 402, Km 0.9, Anasco, PR 00610

Cardinal Health 200, Inc   847-578-6610
1660 Iowa Ave.,, Suite 100/200, Box Springs, CA 92507

Cardinal Health 200, Inc   847-785-3323
4551 East Philadelphia St, Ontario, CA 91761

Cardinal Health 200, Inc   847-689-8410
1430 Waukegan Rd, McGaw Park, IL 60085

Cardinal Health 200, Inc   847-473-1500
1430 Waukegan Rd. KB-3B, McGaw Park, IL 60085

Cardinal Health 200, Inc   847-578-4515
1240 Waukegan Rd, Park City, IL 60085

Cardinal Health 200, Inc   847-785-3323
808 Hwy. 24 West, Moberly, MO 65270

Cardinal Health 200, Inc   847-785-3323
785 Fort Mill Hwy, Fort Mill, SC 29715

Cardinal Health 200, Inc   847-785-3323
One Butterfield Trail, El Paso, TX 79906

Cardinal Health 200, Inc   847-785-3323
200 Mcknight St, Jacksonville, TX 75766

Cardinal Health 200, Inc   847-578-2325
1500 Waukegan Road, McGaw Park, IL 60085

Cardinal Health 200, Inc.   847-785-3323
1300 Waukegan Rd., Waukegan, IL 60085

Cardinal Health 200, Inc.   913-451-0880
1550 Northwestern Dr., El Paso, TX 79912

CARDINAL HEALTH 200, LLC   847-785-3323
500 Neelytown Rd, Montgomery, NY 12549

Cardinal Health 203, Inc   763-398-8305
17400 Medina Road, Suite 100, Minneapolis, MN 55447

Cardinal Health 203, Inc   763-398-8305
3555 Holly Lane, Suite 65, Minneapolis, MN 55447

Cardinal Health 203, Inc.   763-398-8305
1016 East Cooley Dr, Suite N, Colton, CA 92324

Cardinal Health 207, Inc   760-778-7255
8822 Flower Road, Suite 140, Rancho Cucamonga, CA 91730

Cardinal Health 207, Inc.   610-862-0800
1100 Bird Center Dr., Palm Springs, CA 92262

Cardinal Health 2200, Inc   847-578-6442
6215 Ferris Square, Suite 100, San Diego, CA 92121

Cardinal Health 2200, Inc   847-578-6442
5 Sunnen Dr, Maplewood, MO 63143

Cardinal Health 2200, Inc   847-578-6442
17820 Englewood Dr, Cleveland, OH 44130

Cardinal Health 2200, Inc   847-578-6610
400 East Foster Rd, Mannford, OK 74044

Cardinal Health 303, Inc   858-458-7000
10020 Pacific Mesa Blvd, San Diego, CA 92121

Cardinal Health 303, Inc.   571-521-8907
12120 Sunset Hills Road, 3rd Floor, Reston, VA 20190

Cardinal Health 303,Inc.   858-458-7830
1515 Ivac Way, Creedmoor, NC 27522

Cardinal Health Manufacturing Llc   858-617-5889
3750 Torrey View Court, San Diego, CA 92130

Cardinal Healthcare 209, Inc. — 610-862-0800
5225 Verona Rd., Madison, WI 53711-4495

CareFusion 2200, Inc., — 847-689-8410
5175 South Royal Atlanta Dr., Tucker, GA 30084-3053

CareFusion MANUFACTURING LLC — 858-480-6000
3750 Torrey View Court, San Diego, CA 92130

Corpak Medsystems, Inc. — 847-403-3400
100 Chaddick Dr., Wheeling, IL 60090

Nitric Bio, Inc. — 215-788-6200
2 Canal's End Road, Suite 201-A, Bristol, PA 19007

CARDINAL HEALTH, INC.

Cardinal Health — 614.757.5000
7000 Cardinal Place, Dublin, OH 43017

CAREFUSION 211, INC.. — 714-283-2228
22745 Savi Ranch Pkwy., Yorba Linda, CA 92887-4645

CARDINAL SCALE MFG. CO.

Detecto Scale Co. — 417-673-4631
203 E. Daugherty, PO Box 151, Webb City, MO 64870

CARDIO-MED ASSOCIATES, CARDIO-PAK DIV.

Windstone Medical Packaging, Inc. — 406-259-6387
1602 4th Ave. N., Billings, MT 59101-1521

CARESTREAM HEALTH, INC.

Carestream Dental LLC — 800-944-6365
1765 The Exchange, Atlanta, GA 30339

Carestream Health, Inc. — 888-777-2072
2000 Howard Smith Avenue West, Windsor, CO 80550

Carestream Health, Inc. — 888-777-2072
1 Imation Way, Oakdale, MN 55128

Carestream Health, Inc. — 585-722-4565
1049 West Ridge Road, Rochester, NY 14615

Carestream Health, Inc. — 888-777-2072
1669 Lake Ave., Rochester, NY 14652

Carestream Health, Inc. — 541-831-7222
8124 Pacific Ave., White City, OR 97503

CARL ZEISS SURGICAL, INC.

Carl Zeiss Meditec Inc. — 925-557-4100
5160 Hacienda Drive, Dublin, CA 94568

CAROLINA AIRCRAFT

National Air Ambulance — 954-359-9900
3495 S.W. 9th Avenue, Fort Lauderdale, FL 33315

CARPENTER TECHNOLOGY CORP.

Dynamet, Inc. — 724-229-4187
195 Museum Rd., Washington, PA 15301

CARRIER COMMERCIAL REFRIGERATION

Taylor — 815-624-8333
750 N. Blackhawk Blvd., P.O. Box 410, Rockton, IL 61072-0410

CASTOLEUM CORPORATION

Noble Pine Products Co. — 914-664-5877
Centuck Station, PO Box 41, Yonkers, NY 10710-0041

CELSIS INTERNATIONAL PLC

Celsis Laboratory Group — 732-346-5100
165 Fieldcrest Avenue, Edison, NJ 08837

CHART INDUSTRIES, INC.

Caire, Inc. — 770-425-4470
1800 Sandy Plains Industrial Parkway, Suite 316, Marietta, GA 30066

CHARTER OAK PARTNERS

Mar Cor Purification — 484-991-0220
4450 Township Line Road, Skippack, PA 19474-1429

CHEK-MED SYSTEMS, INC.

Gi Supply — 717-761-1170
200 Grandview Ave., Camp Hill, PA 17011-1706

CHEMBIO DIAGNOSTIC SYSTEMS, INC.

Sinovus Biotech, Inc. — 631-924-1135
3661 Horseblock Road, Medford, NY 11763

CHEMISCHE FABRIK BUDENHEIM

Budenheim Usa, Inc — 516-683-6900
245 Newtown Road, Suite 305, Plainview, NY 11803

CHLORIDE GROUP PLC

Oneac Corporation — 847-816-6000
27944 N. Bradley Road, Libertyville, IL 60048-9700

CIBA VISION CORPORATION

Ciba Vision Corporation — 678-415-3638
2930 Amwiler Court, Atl, GA 30360

Ciba Vision Corporation — 1 847-321-7002
333 East Howard Avenue, Des Plaines, IL 60018

CINE MAGNETICS, INC.

Medlink Imaging, Inc. — 914-347-0102
200 Clearbrook Road, Elmsford, NY 10523

CLARCOR FILTRATION PRODUCTS GROUP

Airguard — 502-969-2304 Ex
100 River Ridge Circle, Jeffersonville, IN 47130

United Air Specialists, Inc. — 513-891-0400
4440 Creek Rd., Cincinnati, OH 45242

CLEANING TECHNOLOGIES GROUP

Midwest Rf, Llc — 262-367-8254
535 Norton Drive, PO Box 350, Hartland, WI 53029

CLEARWATER COLON HYDROTHERAPY, INC.

Clearwater Colon Hydrotherapy, Inc. — 352-401-0303
3145 S.w. 74th Terrace, Ocala, FL 34474

COCHLEAR LTD.

Cochlear Americas — 303-790-9010
400 Inverness Parkway, Suite 400, Englewood, CO 80112-5128

COEUR, INC

Coeur Inc., Sheboygan — 920-458-4664
3411 Behrens Pkwy., Sheboygan, WI 53081

COLIN CORPORATION

Mediana Technologies Corp — 210-690-6200
5850 Farinon Drive, San Antonio, TX 78249

COLOPLAST A/S, DENMARK

World Of Medicine Usa, Inc. — 407-438-8810
4531 36th St., Orlando, FL 32811-6527

COLOPLAST MANUFACTURING US, LLC

Amoena — 770-281-8300
1701 Barret Lakes Blvd., Suite 410, Kennesaw, GA 30144

COLSON ASSOCIATES, INC.

Osteomed L.P. — 972-677-4600
3880 Arapaho Road, Addison, TX 75001-4311

COLTENE-WHALEDENT, INC.

Dentronix, Inc. — 330-916-7300
235 Ascot Parkway, Cuyahoga Falls, OH 44223

COMPU-TTY, INC.

Krown Manufacturing, Inc. — 817-738-2485
3408 Indale Rd., Fort Worth, TX 76116

Sheepskin Ranch, Inc. — 817-738-2485
3408 Indale Road, Fort Worth, TX 76116

COMPUMED, INC.

Compumed, Inc. — 307-868-2555
P.O. Box 126, 574 Lane 40, Burlington, WY 82433

CONMED CORPORATION

Conmed Corporation — 800-448-6506
5836 Success Drive, Rome, NY 13440

Conmed Corporation — 800-448-6506
310 Broad Street, Utica, NY 13501

Conmed Electrosurgery — 800-448-6506
14603 E. Fremont Avenue, Centennial, CO 80112

Conmed Endoscopic Technologies — 315-797-8375
525 French Road, Utica, NY 13502

Conmed Linvatec — 800-448-6506
11311 Concept Blvd, Largo, FL 33773-4908

Conmed Linvatec Endoscopy — 800-448-6506
7416 Hollister Avenue, Goleta, CA 93117

COOK GROUP

Cook Biotech, Incorporated — 765-497-3355
1425 Innovation Place, West Lafayette, IN 47906

Sabin Corporation
3800 Constitution Avenue, PO Box 788, PO Box 788, Bloomington, IN 47402-0788
812-323-4500

COOK INC.

Cook Medical Inc.
400 daniels way, Bloomington, IN 47404
812-339-2235

Cook Urological, Inc.
1100 West Morgan St., P.O. Box 227, Spencer, IN 47460
812-829-4891

Wilson-Cook Medical, Inc.
4900 Bethania Station Rd., Winston Salem, NC 27105
336-744-0157

COOK UROLOGICAL, INC.

Cook Ob/Gyn
P.O. Box 4195, Bloomington, IN 47402-4195
812-339-2235

COOKSON ELECTRONICS

Speedline Technologies, Inc.
16 Forge Park, Franklin, MA 02038
508-520-0083

COVANCE INC.

Covance Cardiac Safety Services, Inc.
9390 Gateway Drive, Reno, NV 89521
215-282-5588

Covance Laboratories ,Inc
3301 Kinsman Blvd., Madison, WI 53704
608-241-4471

Covance Research Products Inc.
180 Rustcraft Road, Suite 140, Dedham, MA 02026-4547
781-329-7919

COVIDIEN

Tyco Healthcare Group Lp
Two Ludlow Park Drive, Chicopee, MA 01022
413-593-6400

COVIDIEN LP

Somanetics Corp.
2600 Troy Center Drive, Troy, MI 48084
248-244-1400

COVIDIEN LTD.

Avantor Performance Materials
222 Red School Lane, Phillipsburg, NJ 08865
800-243-3768

AVANTOR PERFORMANCE MATERIALS, INC.
7001 Martin Luther King Blvd, Paris, KY 40361
800-582-2537

Confluent Surgical,Inc
101A First Ave., Waltham, MA 02451
781-693-2300

Covidien (Formerly Nellcor Puritan Bennett / Tyco Healthcare)
6135 Gunbarrel Ave, Boulder, CO 80301
303-530-2300

Covidien Lp, Formerly Registered As Kendall
2010 East International, Speedway Boulevard, Deland, FL 32724
386-738-8212

Covidien Lp, Formerly Registered As Kendall
1430 Marvin Griffin Rd, Augusta, GA 30906
706-793-3030

Covidien Lp, Formerly Registered As Kendall
815 Tek Dr., Crystal Lake, IL 60039
815-444-2500

Covidien Lp, Formerly Registered As Kendall
444 Mcdonnell Blvd., Hazelwood, MO 63042
800-962-9888

Covidien Lp, Formerly Registered As Kendall
5439 State Rte. 40, Argyle, NY 12809
518-638-6101

Covidien Lp, Formerly Registered As Kendall
130 South Main St., Oriskany Falls, NY 13425
315-821-7233

Covidien Lp, Formerly Registered As Kendall
525 North Emerald Rd, Greenwood, SC 29646
864-223-4281

Covidien Lp, Formerly Registered As Kendall
1448 Blue Ridge Blvd, Seneca, SC 29672
864-882-7203

Covidien Lp, Formerly Registered As Kendall
400 Maple St, Commerce, TX 75428
903-886-3153

Covidien Lp, Formerly Registered As Ludlow
Two Ludlow Park Dr., Chicopee, MA 01022
413-593-6400

Covidien Lp, Formerly Registered As Tyco Healthcare
4651 E. Francis Street, Ontario, CA 91761
508-261-8587

Covidien Lp, Formerly Registered As Tyco Healthcare
110 Kendall Park Lane, Atlanta, GA 30336
404-344-7400

Covidien Lp, Formerly Registered As Tyco Healthcare
15 Hampshire Street, Mansfield, MA 02048
508-261-8000

Covidien Lp, Formerly Registered As Uni-Patch
1313 Grant Blvd, Wabasha, MN 55981
651-565-2601

Covidien Lp, Formerly Registered As United States Surgical
195 Mcdermott Road, North Haven, CT 06473
203-492-5000

Covidien Lp, Formerly Registered As United States Surgical
150 Glover Ave., Norwalk, CT 06856-5080
203-845-1000

Covidien, Formerly Puritan Bennett Corp
2101 Faraday Avenue, Carlsbad, CA 92008
303-305-2382

Mallinckrodt, Inc.
675 McDonnell Blvd, Hazelwood, MO 63042
800-325-8888

Mallinckrodt, Inc.
675 McDonnell Blvd., Hazelwood, MO 63042
314-654-2000

Mallinckrodt, Inc.
8800 Durant Rd., Raleigh, NC 27616
800-325-8888

Puritan Bennett Corp.
2800 Airwest Blvd., Plainfield, IN 46168
925-463-4371

Scandius Biomedical, Inc.
11a Beaver Brook Road, Littleton, MA 01460
978-486-4088

Ussc Puerto Rico, Inc.
Building 911-67, Sabanetas Industrial Park, Ponce, PR 00731
203-845-1000

Valleylab
5920 Longbow Dr., Boulder, CO 80301-3299
303-530-2300

CPAC EQUIPMENT, INC.

Allied Diagnostic Imaging Resources, Inc.
5440 Oakbrook Parkway, Norcross, GA 30093-2294
800.262.9333

CRANE CO.

Azonix Corporation
900 Middlesex Turnpike, Building 6, Billerica, MA 01821
978-670-6300

CREST ULTRASONICS

Future Medical Systems, Inc.
504 McCormick Drive Suite T, Glen Burnie, MD 21061-3254
410-761-9411

CREST ULTRASONICS CORP.

Forward Technology
260 Jenks Avenue, Cokato, MN 55321
320-286-2578

CRETEX, INC.

Rms Company
8600 Evergreen Blvd., Minneapolis, MN 55433-6036
763-783-5074

CROSSTEX INTERNATIONAL,INC.

Crosstex International
10 Ranick Road, Hauppauge, NY 11788
631-582-6777

CROSSWELL INTERNATIONAL CORPORATION

Crosswell International Corporation
101 Madeira Avenue, Coral Gables, FL 33134
305-648-0777

CSAM, INC.

Csam, Inc.
1890 14th St., Bettendorf, IA 52722
563-359-7917

CSI HOLDINGS

Csi Holdings
170 Commerce Way, Gallatin, TN 37066
615-452-9633

CTC, INC.

Akorn, Inc.
2500 Millbrook Drive, Buffalo Grove, IL 60089
847-279-6179

CTS

Tapeswitch Corporation
100 Schmitt Blvd., Farmingdale, NY 11735
631-630-0442

CURBELL, INC.

Curbell, Inc. Electronics
7 Cobham Dr., Orchard Park, NY 14127
716-667-3377

CUSTOM INDUSTRIES, INC.

Bio Air Systems Div.
PO Box 18547, Greensboro, NC 27419-8547
336-299-2885

CYBERONICS, INC.

Cyberonics Beltway 8 Distribution Facility
100 Cyberonics Boulevard W, Houston, TX 77058
800-332-1375

CYPRO

Wheaton Science Products
1501 North 10th St., Millville, NJ 08332
856-825-1100

CYPRO ENVIRONMENTAL

Mexpo International, Inc.
2695B McCone Ave., Hayward, CA 94545
510-293-6800

CYTOSOL LABORATORIES, INC.

Citra Anticoagulants, Inc.
55 Messina Drive, Braintree, MA 02184
781-848-2174

D. T. INDUSTRIES, INC.
IMA Nova 978-537-8534
7 New Lancaster, Leominster, MA 01453

DALEY INTERNATIONAL, LTD., J. F.
Jvs Solutions 800-325-3303
1200 Switzer Ave., St. Louis, MO 63147

DANAHER CORP.
Hach Company / Environmental Test Systems 574-262-2060
23575 County Road 106, PO Box 4659, Elkhart, IN 46514-0659

DANAHER CORPORATION
Fluke Biomedical 425-347-6100
6920 Seaway Blvd, Everett, WA 98203
Imaging Sciences International, Llc 215-997-5666
1910 North Penn Rd., Hatfield, PA 19440
Kavo Dental Manufacturing Inc 202-828-0850
901 West Oakton St., Des Plaines, IL 60018-1884
Leica Biosystems - St. Louis, Llc 847-317-7209
12100a Prichard Farm Rd., Maryland Heights, MO 63043
Leica Microsystems Inc. 847-405-0123
2345 Waukegan Road, Bannockburn, IL 60015
Pelton & Crane 704-588-2126
11727 Fruehauf Dr., Charlotte, NC 28273

DARBY DENTAL SUPPLY CO.
Darby Dental Supply Co. 800-645-2310
4460 Holmes Rd., Memphis, TN 38118

DARBY GROUP COMPANY
Sc/Ois Orthodontics 1-(800) 448-732
3300 University Drive, Suite 250, Coral Springs, FL 33065

DATASCOPE CORP.
Datascope Cardiac Assist Div. 973-244-6100
15 Law Drive, Fairfield, NJ 07004
Datascope Corp., Cardiac Assist Division 1-201-307-5400
1300 Macarthur Blvd., Mahwah, NJ 07430

DATEX-OHMEDA
Datex-Ohmeda, Inc. (Madison) 6082211551
3030 Ohmeda Dr., Madison, WI 53707-7550

DAY & ZIMMERMANN INTERNATIONAL, INC.
Day & Zimmermann Validation Services 215-299-8000
1818 Market St., Philadelphia, PA 19103

DEDICATED DISTRIBUTION
Dedicated Distribution 913-371-2200
640 Miami Avenue, Kansas City, KS 66105-2140

DEGANIA SILICONE, LTD.
Degania Silicone, Inc. 401-349-5373
14 Thurber Boulevard, Suite A, Smithfield, RI 02917

DEL GLOBAL TECHNOLOGIES CORPORATION
Del Medical Systems 847-288-7000
50 B. N. Gary Avenue, Roselle, IL 60172

DELTA ELECTRONICS INC.
Delta Products Corp. 510-668-5100
4405 Cushing Parkway, Fremont, CA 94538

DENSO CORPORATION JAPAN
Movincool/Denso Sales California, Inc. 800-264-9573
3900 Via Oro Avenue, Long Beach, CA 90810

DENTAL ADVANCEMENTS, INC.
Nobel Biocare Procera, Inc. 201-828-9268
800 Corporate Drive, Mahwah, NJ 07410-2812

DENTAL TECHNOLOGIES, INC.
Hermanson Dental 651-483-6611
1055 Highway 36 East, Saint Paul, MN 55109

DENTALEZ GROUP
Ramvac Dental Products Inc 605-642-4614
3100 First Avenue, Spearfish, SD 57783

DENTSPLY INTERNATIONAL, INC.
Dentsply Caulk 800-532-2855
38 West Clarke Avenue, Milford, DE 19963

Dentsply Gac International 631-419-1700
355 Knickerbockers Ave., Bohemia, NY 11716
Dentsply North America (Dna) 800-877-0020
400 1st St., Suite 250, Middletown, PA 17057
Dentsply Professional 800-800-2888
901 West Oakton St., Des Plaines, IL 60018
Dentsply Professional 717-767-8250
1301 Smile Way, York, PA 17404
Dentsply Prosthetics 609-386-8900
Six Terri Lane, Burlington, NJ 08016
Dentsply Prosthetics 787-733-8303
183 State Road, K.M. 19.6, Las Piedras, PR 00771
Dentsply Rinn 800-323-0970
1212 Abbot Drive, Elgin, IL 60123
Dentsply Specialty Materials 717-849-4229
1301 Smile Way, York, PA 17404
Dentsply Tulsa Dental Products 800-662-1202
608 Rolling Hills Dr., Johnson City, TN 37604
Dentsply Tulsa Dental Specialties 800-662-1202
5100 East Skelly Drive, Suite 300, Tulsa, OK 74136
Dshealthcare.com 201-871-1232
85 West Forest Ave., Englewood, NJ 07631
Glenroe Technologies 941-748-0857
1912 44th Ave., East, Bradenton, FL 34203
Glenroe Technologies 717-849-4229
210 Industrial Park Road, Baldwin, GA 30511
Orthodental Intl., Inc 760-357-8070
280 avenida campillo ste m, Calexico, CA 92231
Prident International Inc. 717-849-4229
570 West College Ave., York, PA 17404
Roydent Dental Products 717-845-7511
608 Rolling Hills Drive, Johnson City, TN 37604
United Dental Mfg., Inc. 717-845-7511
608 Rolling Hills Dr., Johnson City, TN 37604

DEPUY ORTHOPAEDICS, INC.
Depuy Ace, A Johnson & Johnson Company 574-267-8143
700 Orthopedic Drive, Warsaw, IN 46581

DERMATOLOGIC LAB & SUPPLY, INC.
Sleep Sauna, Inc. 712-323-3269
608 13th Avenue, Council Bluffs, IA 51501

DEROYAL INDUSTRIES, INC.
Atlanta International 865-362-6022
1979 Parker Court, Suites D And E, Stone Mountain, GA 30087
De Medco 865-457-4077
851 Old Emory Rd., Clinton, TN 37716
Deroyal Surgical - Rose Hill 865-362-6022
100 Rose Hill Industrial Park, Rose Hill, VA 24281
Deroyal Surgical Tray Division 865-362-6022
1595 Highway 33 South, New Tazewell, TN 37825
Deroyal Textiles, Inc. 865-362-6022
125 East York, Camden, SC 29020
Deroyal Wound Care 865-362-6022
164 giles hollow road, P.O. Box 309, Rose Hill, VA 24281
Deroyal/Lmb, Inc. 865-362-6022
712 Fiero Lane, No. 37, San Luis Obispo, CA 93401
Pdi, A Division Of Deroyal Industries, Inc 865-362-6022
720 Northern Rd., Mount Juliet, TN 37122
Three-D Orthopedic, Div. Deroyal Industries, Inc. 865-362-6022
101 Rose Hill Industrial Park, Rose Hill, VA 24281

DEVON INTERNATIONAL GROUP
Devon Medical Products 800-571-3135
1100 First Ave., Ste 202, King of Prussia, PA 19406

DISETRONIC AG
Disetronic Sterile Products 603-427-5511
124 Heritage Avenue, Portsmouth, NH 03801-5645

DISETRONIC MEDICAL SYSTEMS AG
Roche Insulin Delivery Systems Inc. 763-795-5200
11800 Exit 5 Parkway, Fishers, IN 46037

DIVISION OF THE SWATCH GROUP (U.S.) INC.
Rlisys Practice Solutions, Inc. 309-691-3700
One Aloha Lane, Peoria, IL 61615-1431

DIXON MEDICAL, INC.
Dixon Medical Inc 770-457-0602
3710 Long View Drive, Atlanta, GA 30341

DJO INCORPORATED

Empi   651-415-9000
599 Cardigan Road, St. Paul, MN 55126-4099

Empi, Inc.   651-415-9000
599 Cardigan Rd., St. Paul, MN 55126-4099

DJO SURGICAL

DJO Surgical   512-832-9500
9800 Metric Blvd., Austin, TX 78758

DOVER CORPORATION

Vectron International   717-486-6060
100 Watts St., Mount Holly Springs, PA 17065

DOW CORNING CORP.

Pillar Surgical, Inc.   619-645-8401
PO Box 8141, La Jolla, CA 92038-8141

DOYEN MEDIPHARM, INC.

J-Pac, Llc   603-692-9955
25 Centre Road, Somersworth, NH 03878-2927

DRAEGER MEDICAL AG & CO. KG

Draeger Medical Systems, Inc   215-660-2626
6 Tech Drive, Andover, MA 01810

Draeger Medical Systems, Inc   215-721-5400
3135 Quarry Rd, Telford, PA 18969

Draeger Medical Systems, Inc.   215-660-2626
16 Electronics Ave., Danvers, MA 01923

DRAEGERWERK, AG

Draeger Safety, Inc.   215-660-2186
3135 Quarry Road, Telford, PA 18969

DREW SCIENTIFIC LTD.

Drew Scientific, Inc.   214-210-4900
4230 Shilling Way, Dallas, TX 75237-1023

Jas Diagnostics, Inc.   305-418-2320
14100 n.w. 57th court, Miami Lakes, FL 33014

DREXA TECHNOLOGY

Lasercard Systems Corporation   650-969-4428
1875 N. Shoreline Blvd., Mountain View, CA 94043-1601

DRIVE MEDICAL DESIGN AND MANUFACTURING

Wenzelite Rehab Supplies, Llc   516-998-4600
220 36th Street, 99 Seaview Blvd, Brooklyn, NY 11232

DSM, NV

Dsm Desotech Inc.   847-697-0400
1122 St. Charles St., Elgin, IL 60120

DT INDUSTRIES

Ima Nova   978-537-8534
7 New Lancaster Road, Leominster, MA 01453-2962

DU PONT DE NEMOURS AND COMPANY

Qualicon   302-695-8754
Route 141 and Henry Clay Rd., Wilmington, DE 19880-0357

DURDEN ENTERPRISES

Durden Enterprises   770-963-0637
1317 4th Ave., P.O. Box 909, Auburn, GA 30011

E G & G WALLAC

PerkinElmer   203-925-4602
940 Winter Street, Waltham, MA 02451

EAGLE FAR EAST

Eagle Stainless Container   215-957-9333
816 Nina Way, Warminster, PA 18974-2206

EAST PENN MFG.

Mk Battery   714-937-1033
1645 S. Sinclair St., Anaheim, CA 92806

EATON INDUSTRIES, INC.

Eaton Medical Devices, Inc.   734-428-0000
254 S Wagner Rd, P.O. Box 1002, Ann Arbor, MI 48106

ECKERT & ZIEGLER ISOTOPE PRODUCTS

Isotope Products Laboratories, Inc.   661-309-1010
24937 Ave Tibbitts, Valencia, CA 91355

EDGEONE L.L.C.

Edgetech   508-263-5900
19 Brigham St., Unit #8, Marlborough, MA 01752

EDMUND SCIENTIFIC

Edmund Industrial Optics   856-573-6250
101 E. Gloucester Pike, Barrington, NJ 08007-1380

EDWARDS LIFESCIENCES, LLC.

Edwards Lifesciences Research Medical   949-250-2500
6864 South 300 West, Midvale, UT 84047

Edwards Lifesciences Technology Sarl   949-250-2500
State Rd. 402 N.km 1.4, Anasco, PR 00610-1577

EG & G, INC.

Eg & G Amorphous Silicon   602-437-1315
4250 E. Broadway Rd., Phoenix, AZ 85040

Perkin Elmer Wallac, Inc.   301-963-3200
9238 Gaither Rd., Gaithersburg, MD 20877-1486

ELAN CORPORATION PLC.

Elan Pharmaceutical Research Corp.   770-534 8239
1300 Gould Drive, Gainesville, GA 30504

ELCAM MEDICAL

Elcam Medical, Inc.   201-457-1120
2 University Plaza, suite 620, Hackensack, NJ 07601

ELEKTA AB

Impac Medical Systems, Inc.   650-623-8800
100 W. Evelyn Avenue, Mountain View, CA 94041

ELITECH FRANCE

Wescor, Inc.   435-752-6011
370 West 1700 South, Logan, UT 84321-5294

EMERSON ELECTRIC COMPANY

Intermetro Industries Corp.   570-825-2741
651 N. Washington St., Wilkes Barre, PA 18705-1707

EMERSON NETWORK POWER

Northern Technologies Inc.   509-927-0401
23123 E. Mission Avenue, Liberty Lake, WA 99019

EMERSON STORAGE SOLUTIONS

Flo Healthcare   678-990-6360
5801 Goshen Springs Road NW, Suite A, Norcross, GA 30071

ENCOMPASS GROUP, LLC

Techstyles Manufacturing Division   972-732-7694
16415 Addison Road, Suite 660, Addison, TX 75001-5434

EPPENDORF AG

Eppendorf North America   516-334-7500
102 Motor Parkway, Hauppauge, NY 11788

New Brunswick Scientific Co., Inc.   732-287-1200
44 Talmadge Rd.,, P.O. Box 4005, Edison, NJ 08818-4005

ERBE ELEKTROMEDIZIN GMBH

Erbe Usa, Inc.   800-778-3723
2225 Northwest Parkway, Marietta, GA 30067

ERCON ASSOCIATES

Olsen Medical   502-772-4280
3001 W. Kentucky St., Louisville, KY 40211-1505

ESAOTE SPA

Biosound Esaote, Inc.   317-813-6000
8000 Castleway Drive, Indianapolis, IN 46250-1943

ESCALON MEDICAL CORP.

Escalon Trek Medical   262-821-9182
2440 S. 179th St., New Berlin, WI 53146

Sonomed, Inc.   516-354-0900
1979 Marcus Ave., Suite C105, Lake Success, NY 11042

ESSILOR INTL.

Essilor Of America, Inc.   800-843-3937
4970 Park St. North, St. Petersburg, FL 33709

ETHICON ENDO-SURGERY, INC.

Sterilmed, Inc.   763-488-3400
11400 73rd Ave. North, #100, Maple Grove, MN 55369

ETHICON, INC.
Mitek Products   (800) 227-6633
325 Paramount Drive, Raynham, MA 02767

ETHOX INTERNATIONAL
Sts Division Of Ethox International   585.533.1672
7500 West Henrietta Rd., Rush, NY 14543

ETHOX STS LIFE SCIENCES DIV
Sts Duotek, Inc   585-321-5000
370 Summit Point Drive, Henrietta, NY 14467

EV3 INC.
Ev3 Inc.   763-398-7000
3033 Campus Drive, Plymouth, MN 55441

Ev3 Neurovascular   949-837-3700
9775 Toledo Way, Irvine, CA 92618

EVERETT ASSOCIATES, INC.
Living Earth Crafts   760-597-2155
3210 Executive Dr, Viats, CA 92081

EXCEL TECHNOLOGY, INC.
Photo Research, Inc.   818-341-5151
9731 Topanga Canyon Place, Chatsworth, CA 91311-4135

FACET TECHNOLOGIES, LLC
Facet Technologies, Llc   770-767-8800
112 Town Park Drive, Kennesaw, GA 30144

FALCON PRODUCTS, INC.
Shelby-Williams Industries   423-586-7000
5303 East Morris Blvd., Morristown, TN 37813

FEDERAL SIGNAL CORP.
Justrite Manufacturing Co., L.L.C.   847-298-9250
2454 Dempster Street, Des Plaines, IL 60016-5315

FENWAL INC.
Fenwal International, Inc.   847-550-7908
Camino Real Industrial Park,, Road #122, Ext Mans San German, PR 00683

Fenwal International, Inc.   847-550-7908
Road 357, Km. 0.8, Maricao, PR 00606

FERRARIS GROUP PLC
Nspire Health, Inc   303-666-5555
1830 Lefthand Circle, Longmont, CO 80501

FERRARIS GROUP, PLC
Synovis Surgical Innovations   651-796-7300
2575 University Avenue W., St. Paul, MN 55114

FFM MED REPS, LLC
Dornier Medtech America   770-426-1315
1155 Roberts Blvd., Kennesaw, GA 30144

Excel Medical Products, Llc   810-714-4775
3145 Copper Avenue, Fenton, MI 48430

FILLAUER COMPANIES, INC.
Hosmer-Dorrance Corp.   408-379-5151
561 Division St., Campbell, CA 95008-6952

Motion Control, Inc.   801-326-3434
115 N. Wright Brothers Drive, Salt Lake City, UT 84116

FIRE & SAFETY EQUIPMENT OF ROCKFORD, INC.
Rockford Medical & Safety Co.   815-394-4809
2420 Harrison Avenue, PO Box 5646, Rockford, IL 61125-0646

FIRST HOSPITAL PRODUCTS, INC.
First Healthcare Products   716-731-6608
6125 Lendell Drive, Sanborn, NY 14132

FIRST QUALITY ENTERPRISE, INC.
First Quality Hygienic, Inc.   800-488-3130 Ex
North Rd., Clinton County Industrial Park, Mcelhattan, PA 17748

First Quality Products, Inc.   800-227-3551 Ex
North Rd., Clinton County Industrial Park, Mcelhattan, PA 17748

FISCHER MEDICAL TECHNOLOGIES INC.
Robot Research, Inc., Sensomatics Div.   858-642-2400
6795 Flanders Dr., San Diego, CA 92121

FISHER SCIENTIFIC
American Medical Technologies, Inc.   361-289-1145
5655 Bear Lane, Corpus Christi, TX 78405

FISHER SCIENTIFIC CO.
Fisher Healthcare   800-766-7000
9999 Veterans Memorial Dr., Houston, TX 77038-2401

Samco Scientific Corporation   818-838-2400
1050 Arroyo Avenue, San Fernando, CA 91340-1822

FISHER SCIENTIFIC CO., LLC.
Nalge Nunc International   585-586-8800
75 Panorama Creek Drive, Rochester, NY 14625-2303

Remel   913-888-0939
12076 Santa Fe Drive, Lenexa, KS 66215-3519

Thermo Fisher Scientific   603-595-0505
22 Friars Drive, Hudson, NH 03051

FISHER SCIENTIFIC COMPANY L.L.C.
Fisher Diagnostics   704-875-0494
11515 Vanstory Drive, Suite 125, Huntersville, NC 28078

FKI INDUSTRIES
White Systems, Inc.   908-272-6700
30 Boright Avenue, Kenilworth, NJ 07033-1015

FLEX-FOOT, INC.
Mauch, Inc.   937-299-8751
3035 Dryden Road, Dayton, OH 45439-1619

FLEXBAR MACHINE CORPORATION
Mediflex Surgical Products   631-582-8440
250 Gibbs Road, Islandia, NY 11749

FLIR SYSTEMS
Extech Instruments Corp.   781-890-7440
285 Bear Hill Rd., Boston, MA 02451

FLYNT AMTEX, INC.
Tex-Care Medical   336-570-5870
2908 Alamance Road, Burlington, NC 27215

FOAMEX INNOVATIONS
Foamex L.P.   757-224-0177
2211 S. Wayne St., Auburn, IN 46706

FOCUS/MRL, INC.
Focus Technologies   714-220-1900
5785 Corporate Avenue, Cypress, CA 90630-4714

FONG BROTHERS PRINTING
Intergraph Public Safety   256-730-2000
19 Interpro Road, Madison, AL 35758

FORT WAYNE METALS RESEARCH PRODUCTS
Fort Wayne Metals Research Prod. Corp.   260-747-4154
9609 Indianapolis Road, Fort Wayne, IN 46809

FOXBORO COMPANY, THE
Invensys Process Systems   1.469.365.6400
5601 Granite Parkway III, Suite 1000, Plano, TX 75024

FRAIN GROUP, INC.
Frain Industries, Inc.   630-629-9900
9377 Grand Ave., Franklin Park, IL 60131

FRANKLIN MILLER INC.
Franklin Miller Inc   973-535-9200
60 Okner Pkwy., Livingston, NJ 07039-1604

FRESENIUS AG
Fresenius Usa, Inc.   781-699-900
920 Winter Street, Waltham, MA 02451-1457

FRESENIUS KABI AG
Fresenius Kabi, Llc   425-242-2000
14715 NE 95th St, Suite 100, Redmond, WA 98052

FRESENIUS MEDICAL CARE AG & CO. KGAA
Fresenius Medical Care North America   781-699-9068
420 Industrial Dr, Livingston, CA 95334

Fresenius Medical Care North America   781-699-9000
920 Winter Street, Waltham, MA 02451

Fresenius Medical Care North America   781-699-9068
750 North Lallendorf Rd, Oregon, OH 43616

Fresenius Medical Care North America   781-699-9068
28157 Cedar Park Blvd, Perrysburg, OH 43551

Fresenius Medical Care North America   781-699-9068
5201 Regent Blvd, Irving, TX 75063

Fresenius Medical Care North America   781-699-9068
475 West 13th St, Ogden, UT 84404

FRONTIER SCIENTIFIC INC.

Frontier Scientific, Inc.,   453-753-1901
PO Box 31, Logan, UT 84323-0031

FUJIFILM HOLDINGS CORPORATION

Fujifilm Medical Systems Usa, Inc.   203-324-2000
419 West Avenue, Stamford, CT 06902

FUJIFILM MEDICAL SYSTEMS USA, INC.

Empiric Systems, Llc   866-367-4742
3800 Paramount Pkwy, Suite 130, Morrisville, NC 27560

FUJINON CORPORATION

Fujinon, Inc.   973-686-2417
10 High Point Dr., Wayne, NJ 07470-7434

FUJIREBIO, INC.

Fujirebio Diagnostics, Inc. (Fdi)   610-240-3800
201 Great Valley Pkwy., Malvern, PA 19355-3809

FUJISAWA PHARMACEUTICAL COMPANY

Astellas Pharma Us, Inc.   800-695-4321
3 Parkway N., Deerfield, IL 60015-2548

GANZONI GMBH

Sigvaris Inc.   770-631-1778
1119 Hwy. 74 S., Peachtree City, GA 30269

GARDNER DENVER

Champion, A Gardner Denver Co.   800 232 0865
1800 Gardner Expressway, Quincy, IL 62305

GARDNER DENVER, INC.

Gardner Denver Thomas Inc.   920-457-4891
1419 Illinois Ave, Sheboygan, WI 53082

GCC INTERNATIONAL

G-C America Inc.   708-597-0900
3737 W. 127th St., Aslip, IL 60803

GE HEALTHCARE

Ambassador Medical   877-237-3022
14470 Bergen Blvd., Suite 500, Noblesville, IN 46060

Datex-Ohmeda Inc.   608-221-1551
3030 Ohmeda Drive, Madison, WI 53718

Ge Healthcare Integrated It Solutions   802-862-1022
40 Idx Drive, P.O. Box 1070, Burlington, VT 05402

Ge Healthcare It   847-277-5000
540 W Northwest Highway, Barrington, IL 60010

Ge Magnets   847-277-5002
3001 West Radio Dr., Florence, SC 29501

Ge Medical Systems Information Technologies   877-274-8456
4502 Woodland Corp. Blvd, Tampa, FL 33614

Ge Medical Systems Information Technologies   414-721-2584
465 Pan American Dr, Suite 11, El paso, TX 79907

Ge Medical Systems Information Technologies   414-355-5000
8200 West Tower Avenue, Milwaukee, WI 53223

Ge Medical Systems Information Technologies   414-721-2584
9900 Innovation Dr., Wauwatosa, WI 53226

Ge Medical Systems Information Technologies, Inc.   414-721-2584
100 Marquette Drive, Jupiter, FL 33468

Ge Medical Systems Ultrasound And Primary Care Dia   608-826-7050
3030 ohmeda dr, Madison, WI 53718

Ge Medical Systems, Llc   262-548-2355
3000 N Grandview Blvd., W-417, Waukesha, WI 53188

Ge Medical Systems, Llc   262-312-7117
3200 N. Grandview Blvd., Waukesha, WI 53188

Ge Medical Systems, Llc   847-277-5002
4855 West Electric Ave., West Milwaukee, WI 53219

Ge Oec Medical Systems   978-552-5200
439 South Union St., Lawrence, MA 01843

Ge Oec Medical Systems Inc.   801-328-9300
384 Wright Brothers Drive, Salt Lake City, UT 84116

Ge Parallel Design, Inc.   414-721-2584
4313 East Cotton Center Blvd., Suite 100, Phoenix, AZ 85040

Medi-Physics, Inc., Dba Ge Healthcare   847-398-8400
3350 N Ridge Ave., Arlington Heights, IL 60004

Ohmeda Medical   410-888-5200
8880 Gorman Road, Laurel, MD 20723

Usa Instruments, Inc.   330-562-1000
1515 Danner Dr., Aurora, OH 44202

Versamed Medical Systems, Inc.   845-770-2840
2 Blue Hill Plaza, Pearl River, NY 10965

Vital Signs, Inc.   973-790-1330
20 Campus Road, Totowa, NJ 07512

Whatman Inc.   800-942-8626
Building One, 800 Centenial Avenue, Piscataway, NJ 08854

GE HEALTHCARE TECHNOLOGIES SURGERY NAVIGATION

Ge Healthcare Technologies Surgery Navigation   978-552-5200
439 South Union Street, Lawrence, MA 01843

GE INFRASTRUCTURE

Ge Infrastructure Water & Process Technologies   952-988-6665
5951 Clearwater Drive, Minnetonka, MN 55343-8995

GE MEDICAL SYSTEMS INFORMATION TECHNOLOGIES

Instrumentarium Imaging, Inc.   414-747-1030
1245 W. Canal St., Milwaukee, WI 53233

Vitalcom, Inc.   714-546-0147
15222 Del Amo Avenue, Tustin, CA 92780

GENERAL ELECTRIC COMPANY

Ge Capital   800-323-6217
3000 Lakeside Drive, Suite 200N, Bannockburn, IL 60015-1223

Ge Industrial, Sensing   978-437-1000
1100 Technology Park Drive, Billerica, MA 01821-4111

GENERAL MEDVENTURES INT'L., LLC

General Pysiotherapy, Inc.   314-291-1442
13222 Lakefront Drive, Earth City, MO 63045-1504

GENERAL SIGNAL CORP.

Edwards Signaling & Security Systems   860-793-5301
41 Woodford Avenue, Plainville, CT 06062

GENESIS INDUSTRIES

Genesis Industries/Maternal Concepts   715-639-4050
130 S Public St, Elmwood, WI 54740

GENZYME

Genzyme Corp.   617-252-7500
500 Kendall Street, Cambridge, MA 02142

Genzyme Corp.   617-252-7999
64 Sidney St., Cambridge, MA 02139-4136

Genzyme Corporation   617-252-7500
1125 Pleasantview Terrace, Ridgefield, NJ 07657-2397

Genzyme Diagnostics   617-252-7500
6659 Top Gun St., San Diego, CA 92121

Sekisui Diagnostics, LLC   800-999-6578
115 Summit Dr., Exton, PA 19341

GEON/SYNERGISTICS

Polyone   (732) 938-5980
10 Ruckle Ave., Farmingdale, NJ 07727

GERRESHEIMER

Kontes Glass Co.   856-692-8500
1022 Spruce St., Vineland, NJ 08360-2841

GETINGE AB

ArjoHuntleigh   800-323-1245
2349 West Lake Street, Suite 250, Roselle, IL 60172

Atrium Medical Corp.   603-880-1433
5 Wentworth Dr., Hudson, NH 03051

Getinge Sourcing Llc   800-475-9040
1777 East Henrietta Rd., Rochester, NY 14623

Getinge Usa, Inc.   585-475-1400
1777 E. Henrietta Rd., Rochester, NY 14623-3133

GETTIG TECHNOLOGIES, INC.

Gettig Pharmaceutical Instrument Co., Div Of   814-422-8892
Gettig Technologies Inc.
1 Streamside Pl. W., Spring Mills, PA 16875-0085

GF HEALTH PRODUCTS, INC
Gf Health Products, Inc.   800-365-2338
336 Trowbridge Rd., North Fond Du Lac, WI 54937

GIVEN IMAGING LTD.
Given Imaging Inc.   770-662-0870
3950 Shackleford Rd., Suite 500, Duluth, GA 30096-1852

GLOBAL MED TECHNOLOGIES
Wyndgate Technologies   916-404-8400
4925 Robert J. Mathews Pkwy.,, Suite 100, El Dorado Hills, CA 95762

GN RESOUND CORP.
Gn Otometrics   847-534-2150
50 Commerce Drive, Ste 180, Schaumburg, IL 60173-5329

GN RESOUND CORPORATION
Gn Resound Corporation   650-780-7800
Seaport Center, 220 Saginaw Drive, Redwood City, CA 94063-4725

GOOCH & HOUSEGO
Chromodynamics   732-730-1877
1195 Airport Road, # !, Lakewood, NJ 08701

GOODFELLOW CAMBRIDGE LIMITED
Instromedix, A Card Guard Co.   847-720-2295
10255 West Higgins Road, Suite 100, Rosemont, IL 60018

GRADKO INTERNATIONAL LTD.
Ormantine Usa Ltd.   321-676-7003
1740 Convair St, Palm-Bay, FL 32909

GRAHAM-FIELD HEALTH PRODUCTS, INC.
Basic American Metal Products   920-929-8200
336 Trowbridge Drive, PO Box 907, Fond du Lac, WI 54937

GREATBATCH INC
Greatbach Medical   763-951-8181
2300 Berkshire Lane N, Minneapolis, MN 55441
Greatbatch Inc   1 216-937-2800
1771 East 30th St., Cleveland, OH 44114

GRIFFON CORPORATION
Clopay Plastic Products Company   513-770-4800
8585 Duke Blvd, Mason, OH 45040-3101

GROUPE SCHNEIDER
Square D Company   1 847 397 2600
1415 Roselle Road, Palatine, IL 60067

HAAG STREIT A/G
HAAG-STREIT USA, INC.   800-787-5426
3535 Kings Mills Rd., Mason, OH 45040-2303

HAC OF AMERICA, INC.
Harc Mercantile Ltd.   269-324-1615
1111 West Centre Avenue, Portage, MI 49024

HAEMONETICS CORP.
Engineering & Research Assoc., Inc. (D.B.A. Sebra)   800-225-5242
400 Wood Rd, Braintree, MA 02184
Haemonetics Corp.   781-356-9488
179 Campanelli Parkway, Stoughton, MA 02072
Haemonetics Corp.   781-356-9488
Buncher Industrial Park, Avenue C, Building 18, Leetsdale, PA 15056
Information Data Management, Inc.   847-588-0453
6231 W. Howard Street, Niles,, IL 60714

HAGEMEYER
Encon Safety Products   713-466-1449
6825 West Sam Houston Pkwy. N., Houston, TX 77041

HAGER & WERKEN GMBH & CO. KG
Hager Worldwide, Inc.   813-926-7474
13322 Byrd Drive, Odessa, FL 33556-5312

HALMA HOLDINGS PLC.
Linos Photonics, Inc   508-478-6200
459 Fortune Blvd., Milford, MA 01757-1723

HALMA HOLDINGS, INC.
Keeler Instruments Inc.   610-353-4350
456 Parkway, Broomall, PA 19008

HALMA PLC
Perma Pure Llc   732-244-0010
8 Executive Drive, Toms River, NJ 08755

HALMA, PLC
Volk Optical Inc.   440-942-6161
7893 Enterprise Drive, Mentor, OH 44060-5309

HAMAMATSU PHOTONICS K.K. - JAPAN
Hamamatsu Corp.   908-231-0960
360 Foothill Road, Bridgewater, NJ 08807-2920
Hamamatsu Photonic Systems   908-231-1116
360 Foothill Road, Bridgewater, NJ 08807-0910

HAMILTON ASSOCIATES, INC.
Air Techniques International   410-363-9696
11403 Cronridge Drive, Owings Mills, MD 21117-2247

HANDICAPPED DRIVING SYSTEMS, INC.
Hds Specialty Vehicles   952-435-8889
16290 Kenrick Loop, Lakeville, MN 55044

HANGER ORTHOPEDIC GROUP, INC.
Hanger National Fabrication Facility   912-691-2030
1119 West Geneva Dr., Tempe, AZ 85282
Seattle Systems   360-697-5656
26296 Twelve Trees Lane N.W., Bldg. 1, Poulsbo, WA 98370

HANS PAUSCH GMBH & CO. KG
Pausch Llc   732-747-6110
808 Shrewsbury Ave., Tinton Falls, NJ 07724

HARRIS CORPORATION
Lanier Worldwide, Inc.   800-727-1885
2300 Parklake Dr. N.E., Atlanta, GA 30345

HARSCO CORP.
Taylor Wharton   251-443-8680
4075 Hamilton Blvd., Theodore, AL 36582

HEALTH AND TECHNOLOGY
Pedia Pals, Llc   763-546-4161
965 Highway 169 N., Plymouth, MN 55441

HEARING OASIS
Humanware   925-680-7100
175 Mason Circle, Concord, CA 94520

HEINE OPTOTECHNIK
Heine Usa Ltd.   603-742-7103
10 Innovation Way, Dover, NH 03820-3831

HELENA LABORATORIES
Helena Plastics   707-766-2103
3700 Lakeville Highway, Suite 200, Petaluma, CA 94954
Labcon North America   707-766-2100
3700 Lakeville Highway, Suite 200, Petaluma, CA 94954

HELVOET PHARMA DEL YIUM NV
Helvoet Pharma, Inc.   856-663-2202
9012 Pennsauken Hwy., Pennsauken, NJ 08110

HEMAGEN DIAGNOSTICS, INC.
Raichem, Division Of Hemagen Diagnostics, Inc.   858-569-8009
8225 Mercury Ct., San Diego, CA 92111-1203

HENKE SASS WOLF GMBH
Henke Sass Wolf Of America, Inc.   508-671-9300
135 Schofield Ave, Dudley, MA 01571

HENKEL
Plaskolite West Inc.   310-637-2103
2225 E. Del Amo Blvd., Compton, CA 90220-6303

HENKEL GMBH & CO. KG, CARL
The Dial Corporation, A Henkel Company   480-754-3425
15501 North Dial Boulevard, Scottsdale, AZ 85260

HERAEUS GMBH
Heraeus Kulzer, Inc.   914-273-8600
99 Business Park Drive, Armonk, NY 10504-1720

HERCON LABORATORIES CORP.

Hercon Laboratories Corp. 717-764-1191
101 Sinking Springs Ln., Emigsville, PA 17318

HERFF JONES, INC.

Nystrom -
4719 W. 62nd St., Indianapolis, IN 46268-2593

HERRICK FAMILY L.P.

Lacrimedics 360-376-7095
P.O. Box 1209, 9 Hope Lane, Eastsound, WA 98245

HESSLER ENTERPRISES, INC.

Hessler Forms & Labels 215-379-2300
106 Susan Dr., Unit #1, Elkins Park, PA 19027

HEWLETT-PACKARD CO.

Hewlett-Packard Company 408-472-2702
20555 State Highway 249, Houston, TX 77070

HEXAGON AB

Brown & Sharpe Inc. 401-886-2000
250 Circuit Drive, N. Kingstown, RI 02852

HILL-ROM HOLDINGS, INC.

Allen Medical Systems, Inc. 978-263-5401
1 Post Office Square, Acton, MA 01720
Hill-Rom Manufacturing, Inc. 919-854-3600
1225 Crescent Green Dr., Suite 200, Cary, NC 27511
Hill-Rom Manufacturing, Inc. 843-740-8000
4349 Corporate Rd., Charleston, SC 29405
Hill-Rom, Inc 812-934-7777
1069 State Route 46 East, Batesville, IN 47006

HILLUSA CORP.

Hill-Med, Inc. 305-594-7474
7217 N.W. 46th St., Miami, FL 33166

HITACHI CHEMICAL LTD.

Tricontinent 530-273-8888
12555 Loma Rica Drive, Grass Valley, CA 95945

HITACHI MEDICAL CORP.

Hitachi Medical Systems America, Inc. 330-425-1313
1959 Summit Commerce Park, Twinsburg, OH 44087-2371

HLTH CORPORATION

Porex Corporation 770-964-1421
500 Bohannon Rd., Fairburn, GA 30213-2828

HMC HOLDING CORPORATION

Huestis Medical 401-253-5500
68 Buttonwood St., Bristol, RI 02809-3600

HOHLKOERPER GMBH & CO. KG, ALBERT

Albert International, Inc. 770-287-7424
989 Athens Street S.e., Gainesville, GA 30501

HOLOGIC

Third Wave Technologies, Inc. 608-273-8933
502 South Rosa Rd., Madison, WI 53719-1256

HOLOGIC, INC.

Direct Radiography 302-631-2700
600 Technology Drive, Newark, DE 19702
Hologic, Inc. 408-745-0975
1240 Elko Drive, Sunnyvale, CA 94089
Hologic, Inc. 508-263-2900
445 Simarano Drive, Marlboro, MA 01752
HOLOGIC, INC. 508-263-2900
250 Campus Drive, Marlborough, MA 01752
Hologic|r2, Inc 408-352-0100
2585 Augustine Drive, Santa Clara, CA 95054
Lorad, A Hologic Company 203-207-4500
36 Apple Ridge Road, Danbury, CT 06810
Suros Surgical Systems, Inc 877-887-8767
6100,6110,6120 Technology Center Drive, Indianapolis, IN 46278

HOME HEALTH MEDICAL EQUIPMENT

Ag Industries 636-349-4466
3637 Scarlett Oak Blvd., St. Louis, MO 63122

HOME-AID-HEALTHCARE, INC.

Dr.'s Page 661-294-9509
P.O. Box 801764, Santa Clarita, CA 91380-1764

HORIBA LTD.

Horiba Abx 949-453-0500
34 Bunsen Drive, Irvine, CA 92618-4210
Horiba Jobin Yvon Inc 732-494-8660
3880 Park Avenue, Edison, NJ 08820-3012

HORTON AUTOMATICS - TEXAS

Horton Automatics 361-888-5591
4242 Baldwin Blvd., Corpus Christi, TX 78405

HOSHIZAKI AMERICA, INC.

Hoshizaki America, Inc. 770-487-2331
618 Hwy. 74 S., Peachtree City, GA 30269-3002

HOSPIRA INC.

Hospira Sedation, Inc. 877-946-7747
Five Billerica Park, 101 Billerica Avenue, North Billerica, MA 01862
Hospira, Inc 877-946-7747
13520 Evening Creek Drive, Suite 200, San Diego, CA 92128
Hospira, Inc. 877-946-7747
755 Jarvis Drive, Morgan Hill, CA 95037
Hospira, Inc. 877-946-7747
1776 North Centennial Drive, Mcpherson, KS 67460
Hospira, Inc. 224-212-2000
8484 U.S 70 West, Clayton, NC 27520
Hospira, Inc. 224-212-2000
Hwy. 301 North, Rocky Mount, NC 27801

HOSPITAL SPECIALTY CO. DIVISION OF TRANZONIC

Hospital Specialty Company 800-321-9832
26301 Curtiss-Wright Parkway, Cleveland, OH 44143

HTL-STREFA S.A.

Htl-Strefa, Inc. 770-528-0410
3005 Chastain Meadows Pkwy, Suite 300, Marietta, GA 30066

I-REP, INC.

Body Therapeutics, Div. Of I-Rep, Inc. 909-674-5722
508 Chaney Street, Suite 13, Lake Elsinore, CA 92530

I.F.S. AB

I.F.S. Industrial & Financial Systems 847-592-0200
300 Park Boulevard, Suite 555, Suite 555, IL 60143

IBA

Iba-Rdi 516-254-6800
151 Heartland Blvd., New York, NY 11717
Radiomed Corporation 978-649-0300
One Industrial Way, Tyngsboro, MA 01879-1400

ICC INDUSTRIES

Konsyl Pharmaceuticals, Inc. 410-822-5192
8050 Industrial Park Road, Easton, MD 21601

ICI

Acheson Colloids Company 810-984-5581
1600 Washington Avenue, Port Huron, MI 48060

ICU MEDICAL, INC.

Icu Medical (Ut), Inc 949-366-2183
4455 Atherton Dr., Salt Lake City, UT 84123

IDEX CORPORATION

Gast Manufacturing 269.926.6171
P.O. Box 97, Benton Harbor, MI 49023-0097
Hale Products Inc. 610-825-6300
700 Spring Mill Ave., Conshohocken, PA 19428
Microfluidics International Corporation 617-969-5452
30 Ossipee Rd., Newton Upper Falls, MA 02464-9101

IKA-LABORTECHNIQUE

Ika-Works, Inc. 910-452-7059
2635 N. Chase Pkwy. S.E., Wilmington, NC 28405-7419

ILLUMINA, INC.

Epicentre Technologies 608-258-3080
726 Post Rd., Madison, WI 53713

IMPAX LABORATORIES, INC.

Global Pharmaeuticals: A Division Of Impax Labs Inc.   215-289-2220
3735 Castor Avenue, Philadelphia, PA 19124-5694

Horton Emergency Vehicles   614-539-8181
3800 McDowell Rd., Grove City, OH 43123

IMPLANTECH ASSOCIATES, INC.

Allied Biomedical   805-289-1665
PO Box 392, Ventura, CA 93003

IMRC

Biosonics, Inc.   215-646-7100
260 New York Drive, Fort Washington, PA 19034-2491

INDEX INSTRUMENTS LTD. & OPTICAL ACTIVITY LTD.

Index Instruments U.S. Inc.   407-932-3688
3305 Commerce Blvd., Kissimmee, FL 34741

INDUCTOTHERM INDUSTRIES, INC.

Athena Controls, Inc.   610-828-2490
5145 Campus Drive, Plymouth Meeting, PA 19462

Peripheral Dynamics Inc.   610-825-7090
5150 Campus Drive, Plymouth Meeting, PA 19462

INDUSTRIAL SAFETY & SUPPLY CO., INC.

Interex Div. Of Industrial Safety & Supply   -
176 Newington Rd., Hartford, CT 06110-2320

INTEGRA LIFESCIENCES HOLDINGS CORP.

Integra Lifesciences Corp.   801-886-9505
3395 West 1820 South, Salt Lake City, UT 84104

Integra Lifesciences Corporation   609-275-0500
311 Enterprise Drive, Plainsboro, NJ 08536

Integra Lifesciences Of Ohio   800-654-2873
4900 Charlemar Drive, Building A, Cincinnati, OH 45227

Integra Luxtec, Inc.   508-835-9700
99 Hartwell St., West Boylston, MA 01583

Integra Neurosciences   800-762-1574
5955 Pacific Center Boulevard, San Diego, CA 92121-4309

Integra Neurosciences Pr   800-654-2873
Road 402 North, Km 1.2, Anasco, PR 00610

Integra Radionics   781-272-1233
22 Terry Avenue, Burlington, MA 01803

J. Jamner Surgical Instruments, Inc   877-468-5572
9 Skyline Dr., Hawthorne, NY 10532

Miltex Inc.   717-840-9335
589 Davies Drive, York, PA 17402

INTERCURE LTD.

Intercure Inc.   646-652-5800
589 8th Avenue, 6th Floor, New York, NY 10018

INTERNATIONAL MEDICAL, INC.

American Catheter Corp.   352-245-4816
13047 S. Hwy 475, Ocala, FL 34480

INTERNATIONAL TECHNIDYNE CORP.

International Technidyne Corporation   732-548-5700
8 Olson Ave., Edison, NJ 08820

INTERZEAG AG

Haag-Streit Group   800-787-5426
3535 Kings Mills Road, Mason, OH 45040-2303

INTRACEL CORPORATION

Intracel Corporation   301-668-8400
93 Monocacy Blvd., Unit A8, Frederick, MD 21701

INVACARE CORPORATION

Adaptive Switch Laboratories, Inc.   830-798-0005
125 Spur 191, Suite C, Spicewood, TX 78669

Altimate Medical, Inc.   507-697-6393
P.O. Box 180, 262 West 1st St., Morton, MN 56270

Champion Mfg. Inc.   574-295-6893
2601 Industrial Pkwy., Elkhart, IN 46516

Freedom Designs, Inc.   805-582-0077
2241N. Madera Rd., Simi Valley, CA 93065

Garden City Medical, Inc.   732-683-1900
512 Union Grove Rd., Calhoun, GA 30701

Invacare Corporation   407-321-5630
2101 East Lake Mary Blvd., Sanford, FL 32773

Invacare Supply Group   508-429-1000
11231 Jersey Blvd, Suite 101, Cucamonga, CA 91730

Invacare Supply Group   440-329-6356
111 Interstate Blvd., Jamesburg, NJ 08831

Invacare Supply Group   508-429-1000
1825 West Park Dr., Suite 200, Grand Prairie, TX 75050

Invacare Supply Group, Inc   508-429-1000
3507 N. Olive Rd, South Bend, IN 46628

Invacare Top End   727-522-8677
4501 63rd Circle North, Pinellas Park, FL 33781-5914

Invacare Top End Sports And Recreation Products   727-522-8677
4501 63rd Circle N., Pinellas Park, FL 33781

The Aftermarket Group   440-329-6000
10173 Croyden Way, Sacramento, CA 95827

INVENSYS PLC

Eurotherm Inc.   703-443-0000
741-F Miller Drive, Leesburg, VA 20175-8993

Sensym Ict   408-954-6700
1804 McCarthy Blvd., Milpitas, CA 95035

INVIVO CORPORATION

Gentran, Inc.   510-226-9343
42025 Osgood Rd, Fremont, CA 94539

Linear Laboratories Corporation   510-226-0488
42025 Osgood Road, Fremont, CA 94539

IPSO

Ipso Usa, Inc.   920-748-3121
PO Box 990, Shepard Street, Ripon, WI 54971

IPSO CORPORATION

Cissell Manufacturing Company   888-223-2980
PO Box 990, Shepard Street, Ripon, WI 54971

IRIS INTERNATIONAL, INC.

Iris Diagnostics   818-709-1244
9172 Eton Ave., Chatsworth, CA 91311

Iris Sample Processing   781-551-0100
60 Glacier Drive, Westwood, MA 02090-1825

Leica Microsystems (San Jose) Corporation   408-719-6400
120 Baytech Drive, San Jose, CA 95134-2302

Statspin, Inc.   781-551-0100
60 Glacier Drive, Westwood, MA 02090-1825

ISMATEC SA LABORTECHNIK/ANALYTIK

Cole-Parmer Instrument Inc.   847-549-7600
625 E. Bunker Ct., Vernon Hills, IL 60061-1844

Harvard Apparatus, Inc.   508-893-8999
84 October Hill Road, Holliston, MA 01746

ITT INDUSTRIES

Itt Night Vision   540-563-0371
7635 Plantation Road, Roanoke, VA 24019-3257

IVAX CORP.

Immuno Vision, Inc.   800-541-0960
1820 Ford Ave., Springdale, AR 72764

IVOCLAR VIVADENT, INC.

Ivoclar Vivadent, Inc.   716-691-0010
175 Pineview Drive, Amherst, NY 14228-2231

J. MORITA CORPORATION, JAPAN

J. Morita Usa, Inc.   949-581-9600
9 Mason, Irvine, CA 92618

JACE SYSTEMS, INC

JACE SYSTEMS, INC   (856) 470-2100
55 Carnegie Plaza, Cherry Hill, NJ 08003

JACUZZI BRANDS

Jacuzzi, Bath Division   909-548-7732
14880 Monte Vista Avenue, Suite 550, Chino, CA 91710

JACUZZI, INC.

Sundance Spas, Inc.   909-606-7733
14525 Monte Vista Avenue, Chino, CA 91710

JAL LLC

Mmi   847-816-1009
P.O. Box 5396, Vernon Hills, IL 60061

JAPAN MEDICAL DYNAMIC MARKETING, INC.

Ortho Development Corp. — 801-553-9991
12187 S. Business Park. Drive, Draper, UT 84020

JENCONS (SCIENTIFIC) LTD.

Tecomet, A Subsidiary Of Viasys Healthcare Inc. — 978-658-3379
115 Eames St., Wilmington, MA 01887

JEOL LTD.

Jeol Usa, Inc. — 978-536-2270
11 Dearborn Road, Peabody, MA 01960-3823

JJI LIGHTING GROUP

Alkco Lighting Co. — 847-451-0700
11500 W. Melrose Avenue, Franklin Park, IL 60131-8139

Vista Lighting — 800-576-2135
1805 Pittsburg Ave., Erie, PA 16502

JMAR TECHNOLOGIES, INC.

Pacific Precision Laboratories, Inc. — 818-700-8977
20447 Nordhoff St., Chatsworth, CA 91311

JOHNSON & JOHNSON

Advanced Sterilization Products — 949-581-5799
33 Technology Dr., Irvine, CA 92618

Animas Corp. — 610-644-8990
200 Lawrence Drive, West Chester, PA 19380

Biosense Webster — 909-839-8500
15715 Arrow Hwy, Irwindale, CA 91706

Biosense Webster, Inc — 909-839-8500
3333 Diamond Canyon Road, Diamond Bar, CA 91765

Centocor, Inc. — 610-651-6000
800/850 Ridgeview Drive, Horsham, PA 19044

Closure Medical — 919-876-7800
5250 Greens Dairy Rd., Raleigh, NC 27616

Codman & Shurtleff, Inc — 877-744-5617
325 Paramount Dr., Raynham, MA 02767

Codman And Shurtleff, Inc — 508-880-8100
325 Paramount Drive, Raynham, MA 02767

Cordis Corporation — 908-541-4100
430 Route 22 East, Bridgewater, NJ 08807

Cordis Endovascular — 908-755-8300
7 Powder Horn Drive, Warren, NJ 07059

Cordis Llc — 786-313-2000
Road 362 Km 0.5, San German, PR 00683

Cordis Neurovascular, Inc. — 786-313-6550
14201 NW 60 Avenue, Miami Lakes, FL 33014

Depuy Bridgewater — 574-371-4865
50 Scotland Park Dr., Bridgewater, MA 02324

Depuy Mitek, A Johnson & Johnson Company — 508-880-8100
50 Scotland Blvd., Bridgewater, MA 02324

Depuy Mitek, Inc. — 508-880-8100
325 Paramount Dr., Raynham, MA 02767

Depuy Orthopaedics, Inc. — 574-267-8143
700 Orthopaedic Dr., Warsaw, IN 46581

Depuy Spine, Inc. — 508-880-8100
365 Ravendale Dr., Mountain View, CA 94043

Depuy Spine, Inc. — 508-880-8100
325 Paramount Dr., Raynham, MA 02767

Depuy-Raynham, A Div. Of Depuy Orthopaedics — 574-267-8143
325 Paramount Dr., Raynham, MA 02767-0350

Ethicon Endo-Surgery, Inc. — 513-337-7000
3801 University Blvd., S.E., Albuquerque, NM 87106

Ethicon Endo-Surgery, Inc. — 513-337-7000
4545 Creek Rd., MI #132, Cincinnati, OH 45242

Ethicon Endo-Surgery, Llc — 513-337-3134
475 Calle C, Guaynabo, PR 00969

Ethicon, Inc — 908-218-2996
3348 Pulliam St., San Angelo, TX 76905

Ethicon, Inc. — 908-218-2996
655 Ethicon Cir., Cornelia, GA 30531

Ethicon, Inc. — 908-218-0707
Route 22 West, p.o. box 151, Somerville, NJ 08876

Ethicon, Llc. — 908-218-2887
Rd. 183, Km. 8.3,, Industrial Area Hato, San Lorenzo, PR 00754

Hand Innovations, Llc. — 305-412-8010
6303 Blue Lagoon Drive, Suite 100, Miami, FL 33126

J&J Healthcare Products Div Mcneil-Ppc Inc — 866-565-2229
199 Grandview Rd, Skillman, NJ 08558

Johnson & Johnson Consumer Products, Inc. — 908-874-1402
185 Tabor Road, Morris plains, NJ 07950

Johnson & Johnson Consumer Products, Inc. — 908-874-1000
199 Grandview Rd., Skillman, NJ 08558-9417

Johnson & Johnson Healthcare Products Div — 973-385-6546
Mcneil-Ppc, Inc.
185 Tabor Rd, Morris Plains, NJ 07950

Johnson & Johnson Hemisferica, S.A. — 868-640-3772
Calle C # 475, Los Frailes Ind. Park, Guaynabo, PR 00969

Johnson & Johnson International — 787-272-1900
Calle C #475, Suite 200; Los Frailes Industrial Park, Guaynabo, PR 00969

Johnson & Johnson Vision Care, Inc. — 904-443-1763
7500 Centurion Pkwy, Suite 100, Jacksonville, FL 32256

Lifescan Llc. — 408-263-9789
Rd. 308 Km 0.8, Pedernales Industrial Park, Cabo Rojo, PR 00623-5001

Lifescan Products, Llc — 408-942-3589
San Antonio Industrial Park, Extension, Rd. 110 Km. 5.9, Aguadilla, PR 00603

Lifescan, Inc. — 408-263-9789
1000 Gibraltar Dr, Milpitas, CA 95035-6314

Mcneil Healthcare, Inc. — 203-932-6263
5 saw mill rd, West Haven, CT 06516

Mcneil-Ppc, Inc. — 908-874-1402
100 Jefferson Rd., Parsippany, NJ 07054

Micrus Corporation — 408-830-5900
610 Palomar Avenue, Sunnyvale, CA 94085

Micrus Endovascular Corporation — 408-433-1400
821 Fox Lane, San Jose, CA 95131

Noramco, Inc. — 706-353-4400
1440 Olympic Dr., Athens, GA 30601

Orapharma, Inc. — 215-956-2200
732 Louis Drive, Warminster, PA 18974

Ortho Clinical Diagnostics, Inc. — 716-453-3000
100 Indigo Creek Dr., Rochester, NY 14650

Ortho Dermatologics — 310-642-1150
5760 W. 96th St., Los Angeles, CA 90045-5544

Ortho Mcneil Janssen Pharmaceuticals, Inc. — 908-218-6811
1125 Trenton-Harbourton Road, P.O. Box 200, Titusville, NJ 08560

Ortho-Clinical Diagnostics, Inc. — 908-218-8177
Route 202, Raritan, NJ 08869

Ortho-Clinical Diagnostics, Inc. — 716-453-3000
513 Technology Blvd., Rochester, NJ 14626

Ortho-Clinical Diagnostics, Inc. — 585-453-3768
100 Indigo Creek Dr., Rochester, NY 14626

Ortho-Clinical Diagnostics, Inc. — 716-453-3000
100 Indigo Creek Dr., Room 350, Rochester, NY 14650

Ortho-Clinical Diagnostics, Inc. — 585-453-3768
1000 Lee Rd., Rochester, NY 14606

Ortho-Mcneil-Janssen Pharmaceuticals, Inc. — (908) 722-5393
1000 U.S. Route 202 South, Raritan, NJ 08869

JOHNSON MATTHEY, INC.

Alfa Aesar, A Johnson Matthey Company — 978-521-6300
26 Parkridge Road, Ward Hill, MA 01835-8099

JORDAN INDUSTRIES

Deflecto Corp. — 317-849-9555
7035 E. 86th St., Indianapolis, IN 46250

JOUAN, INC.

Thermo Fisher Scientific - Laboratory Equipment — 866-984-3766
Division Headquarters
450 Fortune Boulevard, Milford, MA 01757

JUN-AIR INTERNATIONAL A/S

Jun-Air Usa, Inc. — 269-934-1216
2300 Highway M-139, Benton Harbor, MI 49022

KANE INTERNATIONAL

Uei — 503-644-8723
8030 SW Mimbus, Beaverton, OR 97008

KARL STORZ ENDOSCOPY-AMERICA INC.

Karl Storz Lithotripsy-America, Inc. — 678-354-6229
1000 Cobb Place Blvd., Building 400, Suite 450, Kennesaw, GA 30144

KEANE INC.

Labfusions — 909-592-8131
437 S. Cataract Ave., Suite 5, San Dimas, CA 91773-2979

KERR CORPORATION

Sds-Surgical Acuity — 608-831-2404
3225 Deming Way, Suite 120, Middleton, WI 53562

KEY-BAK
Key-Bak   909-923-7800
4245 Pacific Privado, Ontario, CA 91761-7609

KEYSTONE INDUSTRIES
Mizzy, Inc. Of National Keystone   856-663-4700
616 Hollywood Avenue, Cherry Hill, NJ 08002-2821

KI
Spacesaver Corporation   920-563-6362
1450 Janesville Avenue, Fort Atkinson, WI 53538-2798

KIMBERLY CLARK CORP.
Kerr Group   770-587-8000
1400 Holcomb Bridge Road, Roswell, GA 30076-2190

KIMBERLY-CLARK CORP.
KIMBERLY-CLARK CORP. CONWAY MILL   501-329-2973
480 Exchange Ave., Conway, AR 72032

KINETIC CONCEPTS, INC.
Kci Usa, Inc.   210-255-6137
6203 Farinon Dr., San Antonio, TX 78249
Lifecell Corp.   908-947-1100
One Millennium Way, Branchburg, NJ 08876-3876

KING PHARMACEUTICALS, INC.
Meridian Medical Technologies   443-259-7800
501 Fifth Street, Bristol, TN 37620

KING SYSTEMS CORP.
H&M Rubber Company, Inc.   330-678-3323
4200 Mogadore Rd., Kent, OH 44240-7258

KITAGAWA INDUSTRIES, CO. LTD.
Intermark (Usa), Inc.   408-971-2055
1310 Tully Road, Suite 117, San Jose, CA 95122

KNIT RITE, INC.
Therafirm, A Knit Rite Company   913-281-4600
120 Osage Avenue, Kansas City, KS 66105

KNIT-RITE, INC.
Paramedical Distributors   816-421-6203
2020 Grand Ave., Kansas City, MO 64141-9777

KNURR - MECHANIK FUR DIE ELEKTRONIK AG
Kn,rr Usa Inc.   805-526-7733
1890 N. Voyager Avenue, Simi Valley, CA 93063

KONICA MINOLTA
Konica Minolta Medical Imaging Usa, Inc.   973-633-1500
411 Newark Pompton Tpke., Wayne, NJ 07470

KONINKLIJKE PHILIPS ELECTRONICS NV
Philips Healthcare   614-865-8956
836 North St, Bld 500, Tewksbury, MA 01876
Philips Lighting Co.   800-555-0050
505 Hoult Rd., Fairmont, WV 26554

KRETCHMER CORP., THE
Minxray, Inc.   847-564-0323
3611 Commercial Avenue, Northbrook, IL 60062-1822

KROHN-HITE CORPORATION
Krohn-Hite Corporation   508-580-1660
15 Jonathan Drive, Unit 4, Brockton, MA 02301-5566

KURT MANUFACTURING CO.
Theradyne Products Division   763-502-6190
395 Ervin Industrial Drive, Jordan, MN 55352-1062

KYOCERA CORP.
Kyocera Industrial Ceramics Corp.   510-257-0112
472 Kato Terrace, Fremont, CA 94539

L'AMY GROUP
L'Amy, Inc.   203-761-0611
37 Danbury Road, Wilton, CT 06897-4405

L-3 COMMUNICATIONS CORPORATION
Narda Safety Test Solutions   631-231-1700
435 Moreland Road, Hauppauge, NY 11788

LAB CORP.
Lab Corp Of America   919-549-8263
1904 Alexander Drive, Durham, NC 27709-2652

LABORATOIRE MEDIX
Medix Pharmaceuticals Americas, Inc.   727-507-9844
12505 Starkey Road, Suite M, Largo, FL 33773

LABWORLD, INC.
Labworld, Inc.   781-341-1733
471 Page St., Bldg 4, Stoughton, MA 02072

LANDEC CORP.
Lifecore Biomedical, Inc.   952-368-4300
3515 Lyman Blvd., Chaska, MN 55318

LANTIC USA
Evs Sports Protection   310-637-5000
2146 . Gladwick St, Rancho Dominguez, CA 90220

LDR MEDICAL
LDR Spine USA   512-344-3333
4030 West Braker Lane, Suite 360, Austin, TX 78759

LEE CO., THOMAS
Rayovac   608-275-4694
601 Rayovac Drive, Madison, WI 53744-4960

LEGGETT AND PLATT
Gillis Associated Industries   847-541-0858
750 Pinecrest Drive, Prospect Heights, IL 60070
Vantage Industries, Inc.   800-221-4329
5070 Phillip Lee Drive, Atlanta, GA 30336

LENNOX MANUFACTURING
Plaza Towel Holder, Inc.   316-267-4233
P.O. Box 4737, Wichita, KS 67204

LEYBOLD VACUUM GMBH
Oerlikon Leybold Vacuum Usa Inc.   724-327-5700
5700 Mellon Road, Export, PA 15632-8900

LIBERTY INDUSTRIES, INC
Seradyn, Inc.   317-610-3800
7998 Georgetown Road, Suite 1000, Indianapolis, IN 46268

LIDCO LTD.
Lidco Ltd. Usa   847-265-3700
500 Park Avenue, Suite 103, Lake Villa, IL 60046

LIFE ENERGY & TECHNOLOGY HOLDINGS INC.
Health-Pak, Inc.   315-724-8370
2005 Beechgrove Pl., Utica, NY 13501-1703

LIFE GUARD
American Dental Supply, Inc.   610-252-1464
1075 N. Gilmore Street, Allentown, PA 18109-3210
Ansell Healthcare Products, Inc.   732-345-5400
200 Schulz Dr., Red Bank, NJ 07701

LIFE MEDICAL
Life Medical Equipment   305-594-0000
7874 N.W. 64 St., Miami, FL 33166

LIFE TECHNOLOGIES CORPORATION
Applied Biosystems   650-638-5800
850 Lincoln Centre Drive, Foster City, CA 94404
Life Technologies Corporation   301-840-8000
7300 Governors Way, Frederick, MD 21704
Life Technologies Corporation   716-774-6700
3175 Staley Rd., Grand Island, NY 14072
Life Technologies Corporation   414-214-4048
9099 North Deerbrook Trail, Brown Deer, WI 53223

LIFE THERAPEUTICS INC.
Invitrogen Corporation   800-955-6288
101 Lincoln Centre Drive, Foster City, CA 94404

LIFECLINIC INTERNATIONAL, INC.
Lifeclinic International, Ltd.   931-967-4879
511 Creasman Dr., Winchester, TN 37398

LIFEGAS LLC
Aga Linde Healthcare P.R. Inc. 787-622-7900
GPO Box 364727, Tres Monjitas, PO Box 363868, San Juan, PR 00936-4727

LIFELINE SYSTEMS, INC.
Donaldson Company, Inc. 952-887-3131
1400 W. 94th St., Bloomington, MN 55431

LIFEWATCH AG
Lifewatch Services, Inc. 847.720.2100
O'hare International Center II, 10255 West Higgins Rd., Ste. 100, Rosemont, IL 60018

LIKO AB
Liko North America 888-545-6671
122 Grove Street, Franklin, MA 02038

LINAK A/S
Linak U.S. Inc. 502-253-5595
2200 Stanley Gault Pkwy., Louisville, KY 40223

LINCOLN ELECTRIC CO.
Harris Products Group 770-536-8801
2345 Murphy Blvd., Gainesville, GA 30504-6001

LINK GMBH & CO., WALDEMAR
LinkBio Corp. 973-625-1333
300 Roundhill Dr, Rockaway, NJ 07866

LISTA B&L HOLDING
Lista International Corp. 508-429-1350
106 Lowland St., Holliston, MA 01746-2094

LOHMANN & RAUSCHER INT'L GMBH & CO. KG
Lohmann Corporation 1 859 334 4900
3000 Earhart Court, Ste. 155, Hebron, KY 41048

LRL LOGIX
Lrl Logix 972-691-7447
1301 W. Hwy 407 # 201, Lewisville, TX 75077

LUCOMED SPA
Lucomed Inc. 973-575-0614
45 Kulick Rd., Fairfield, NJ 07004

LUMASENSE TECHNOLOGIES INC.
Andros, Inc. 510-837-3500
870 Harbour Way South, Richmond, CA 94804-3613

LUMASENSE TECHNOLOGIES, INC
Mikron Infrared, Inc. 805-644-9544
3033 Scott Blvd., Santa Clara, CA 95054

LUXFER GROUP LTD.
Luxfer Gas Cylinders 951-684-5110
3016 Kansas Avenue, Riverside, CA 92507

LUXO AS
Luxo Corporation 914-345-0067
Five Westchester Plaza, Elmsford, NY 10523
Ophthalmic Imaging Systems 916-646-2020
221 Lathrop Way, Ste. I, Sacramento, CA 95815-4215

LYDALL, INC.
Charter Medical Ltd. 336-768-6447
3948-A Westpoint Blvd, Winston Salem, NC 27103

M & Q PACKAGING CORP.
M & Q Packaging Corp. 570-385-4991
Earl Street, Schuylkill Haven, PA 17972

M. BRAUN GMBH
M. Braun Inc. 603-773-9333
14 Marin Way, Stratham, NH 03885

MAGNUS MOBILITY SYSTEMS
Jilson Group, Inc. 973-471-2400
20 Industrial Road, Lodi, NJ 07644-2608

MAIN STREET CAPITAL
C & K Manufacturing & Sales 440-871-4078
28825 Ranney Pkwy., Westlake, OH 44145

MAIN STREET INDUSTRIES
Brewer Company, The 262-251-9530
N88 W13901 Main St., Menomonee Falls, WI 53051

MAQUET CARDIOVASCULAR LLC
Maquet Puerto Rico Inc. 408-635-3900
No. 12, Rd. #698, Dorado, PR 00646

MARCOLIN SPA
Marcolin Usa 480-951-7174
7543 E. Tierra Buena Lane, Scottsdale, AZ 85260

MARMICK, INC.
Life-Like Laboratory 972-620-0203
1544 Valwood Pkwy., Suite 104, Carrollton, TX 75006

MARMON GROUP, INC., THE
Angiotech 847-637-3333
241 West Palatine Road, Wheeling, IL 60090
Medical Device Technologies, Inc. (Md Tech) 352-338-0440
3600 S.W. 47th Avenue, Gainesville, FL 32608
Shepherd Caster Corporation 269-983-7351
203 Kerth St., St. Joseph, MI 49085-2623

MASCON
Aqua Glass Corporation 731-632-0911
320 Industrial Park Rd., Adamsville, TN 38310-0412

MAXWELL TECHNOLOGIES, INC.
Maxwell Technologies Power Systems 858-503-3300
9244 Balboa Avenue, San Diego, CA 92123

MCCRONE ASSOCIATES, INC.
Mccrone Microscopes & Accessories 630-887-7100
850 Pasquinelli Drive, Westmont, IL 60559

MCDONOUGH MEDICAL PRODUCTS CORPORATION
Progeny Dental 847-850-3800
1407 Barclay Blvd, Buffalo Grove, IL 60089

MCKESSION CORPORATION
Mckesson Drug Co. 609-764-6333
400 Delray Pkwy., Riverside, NJ 08075

MCKESSON CORP.
Zee Medical, Inc. 949-252-9500
22 Corporate Park, Irvine, CA 92606

MCKESSON HBOC INC.
Clinical Reference Systems 303-664-6485
335 Interlocken Pkway, Broomfield, CO 80021

MCQUAY
Aaf International 888-223-2003
10300 Ormsby Park Place, Louisville, KY 40223

MCRAE INDUSTRIES
Compsee, Inc. 321-724-4321
400 N. Main St., PO Box 1209, Mount Gilead, NC 27306

MDS PRODUCTS, INC.
American Diversified Dental Systems 949-330-0140
22991 La Cadena Drive, Laguna Hills, CA 92653-1314

MEDCO
SYSMED 214-820-2176
2625 Elm St., Ste. 102, Dallas, TX 75226-1453

MEDELA AG
Medela, Inc. 815-363-1166
1101 Corporate Drive, McHenry, IL 60050

MEDICAL & SAFETY GROUP, INC.
General Scientific Safety Equipment Co. 215-739-7559
2553 E Somerset St. 1st Floor, Philadelphia, PA 19134-4742

MEDICAL ACTION INDUSTRIES, INC
Medegen Medical Products, Llc 901-867-2951
209 Medegen Drive, Gallaway, TN 38036-0228
Medical Action Industries, Inc 828-681-8820
10 Columbia Blvd, Clarksburg, WV 26301
Medical Action Industries, Inc. 800-645-7042
25 Heywood Rd, Arden, NC 28704

MEDICAL DEVICE RESOURCE CORPORATION
Reliance Medical Corp.   510-732-9950
5981 Graham Ct, Livermore, CA 94550

MEDICAL ENERGY, INC.
Medical Energy, Inc.   8806 Paul Starr
8806 Paul Starr Drive, Pensacola, FL 32514

MEDIQ, INC.
Mediq/Prn   609-662-3200
1 Mediq Plaza, Pennsauken, NJ 08110

MEDIVANCE INSRUMENTS
Velopex International.   407-957-3900
105 East 17th St., Saint Cloud, FL 34769

MEDLINE INDUSTRIES, INC.
Medline Industries, Inc.   800-633-5463
1 Medline Place, Mundelein, IL 60060

MEDNET HEALTHCARE TECHNOLOGIES
Mednet Healthcare Technologies, Inc.   609-671-1790
100 Ludlow Drive, Ewing, NJ 08638

MEDRAD, INC.
Medrad Inc.   724-940-7940
625 Alpha Dr., Pittsburgh, PA 15238
Medrad Saxonburg, Inc.   724-940-7940
150 Victory Road, Saxonburg, PA 16056
Possis Medical, Inc.   1 724-940-6800
100 Global View Drive, Warrendale, PA 15086

MEDSTAT INC.
Medstat Inc.   901-452-5697
3251 Poplar Ave., Memphis, TN 38111

MEDTOX SCIENTIFIC INC.
Medtox Diagnostics Inc.   336-226-6311
1238 Anthony Rd., Burlington, NC 27215-8831
Medtox Diagnostics, Inc.   800-334-1116
1640 Nova Lane, Burlington, NC 27215

MEDTRONIC, INC.
Ablation Frontiers, Inc.   760-438-4868
6354 Corte Del Abeto, Carlsbad, CA 92011
Ardian Inc.   650-417-6555
1380 Shorebird Way, Mountain View, CA 94043
Arizona Device Manufacturing   763-505-0874
2350 West Medtronic Way, Tempe, AZ 85281
Invatec   +1 877 446 8283
3101 Emrick Blvd, Suite 113, Bethlehem, PA 18020
Medtronic Blood Management   612-514-4000
18501 East Plaza Dr., Parker, CO 80134
Medtronic Cardiac Surgery Technologies   763-391-9030
8200 coral sea street, moundsview, MN 55112
Medtronic Cardiovascular Surgery, The Heart   800-328-2518
Valve Div.
1851 East Deere Ave., Santa Ana, CA 92705
Medtronic Heart Valves   800-227-3191
8299 Central Ave., N.e., Spring Lake Park, MN 55432-3576
Medtronic Image-Guided Neurologics, Inc.   763-505-0604
2290 West Eau Gallie Blvd., Melbourne, FL 32935
Medtronic Minimed   818-362-5958
18000 Devonshire, Northridge, CA 91325
Medtronic Navigation, Inc.   720-890-3200
826 Coal Creek Cir., Louisville, CO 80027
Medtronic Navigation, Inc. (Littleton)   720-890-3325
300 Foster Street, Harwood Station, Littleton, MA 01460
Medtronic Neuromodulation   763) 514-4000
710 Medtronic Parkway, Minneapolis, MN 55432-5604
Medtronic Neuromodulation   763-514-4000
710 Medtronic Parkway NE, Minneapolis, MN 55459-9896
Medtronic Neurosurgery   800-468-9710
125 Cremona Dr.,, Goleta, CA 93117
Medtronic Perfusion Systems   763-391-9000
7611 Northland Dr., Brooklyn Park, MN 55428
Medtronic Powered Surgical Solutions   817-788-6400
4620 North Beach St., Fort Worth, TX 76137
Medtronic Puerto Rico Operations Co., Juncos   763-514-4000
Road 31, Km. 24, Hm 4, Ceiba Norte Industrial Park, Juncos, PR 00777
Medtronic Puerto Rico Operations Co., Villalba   763-514-4000
Rd. 149, Km. 56.3, Call Box 6001, Villalba, PR 00766

Medtronic Puerto Rico Operations Co.,Med Rel   763-514-4000
Road 909, Km. 0.4., Barrio Mariana, Humacao, PR 00792
Medtronic Sofamor Danek Instrument Manufacturing   901-396-3133
7375 Adrianne Place, Bartlett, TN 38133
Medtronic Sofamor Danek Usa, Inc   901-399-2346
1800 Pyramid Pl, Memphis, TN 38132
Medtronic Sofamor Danek Usa, Inc.   901-396-3133
4340 Swinnea Rd., Memphis, TN 38118
Medtronic Spinal And Biologics New York   901-396-3133
Distribution Center
699 kapkowksi road, Suite 3, elizabeth,, NJ 07201
Medtronic Spine Llc   408-548-6500
1221 Crossman Ave., Sunnyvale, CA 94089
Medtronic Vascular   707-566-1548
5345 Skylane Blvd, Santa Rosa, CA 95403
Medtronic Vascular   978-777-0042
35-37A Cherry Hill Dr, Danvers, MA 01923
Medtronic Vascular   (763) 514-4000
710 Medtronic Parkway, L100, Minneapolis,, MN 55432-5604
Medtronic Xomed, Inc.   904-296-9600
6743 Southpoint Drive North, Jacksonville, FL 32216-0980
Ndi Medical, Inc.   216-378-9106
22901 Millcreek Blvd.,, Suite 110, Cleveland, OH 44122
Physio-Control, Inc.   425-867-4000
11811 Willows Road NE, Redmond, WA 98052
Restore Medical Inc.   904-296-9600
6743 Southpoint Drive, North, Jacksonville, FL 32216

MENASHA CORP.
Orbis Corporation   262-560-5000
1055 Corporate Center Drive, PO Box 389, Oconomowoc, WI 53066

MENNEN MEDICAL LTD. ISRAEL
Mennen Medical Corp.   215-322-9997
2540 Metropolitan Drive, Trevose, PA 19053-6738

MENTOR CORP.
Byron Medical   520-573-0857
602 W. Rillito, Tucson, AZ 85705
Mentor Ophthalmics, Inc.   805-879-6000
201 Mentor Dr., Santa Barbara, CA 93111
Mentor Texas, Inc.   972-252-6060
3041 Skyway Circle North, Irving, TX 75038

MERCK KGAA
Oncogene Research Products   858-450-9600
10394 Pacific Center Court, San Diego, CA 92121

MERCK KGAA, DARMSTADT, GERMANY
Emd Chemicals Inc.   856-423-6300
480 S. Democrat Road, Gibbstown, NJ 08027

MERIDIAN BIOSCIENCE, INC.
Meridian Life Science, Inc.   207-283-6500
60 Industrial Park Road, Saco, ME 04072

MERIDIAN CO., LTD.
Meridian America Medicals, Inc.   800-638-8093
2691 Richter Ave., Suite 104, Irvine, CA 92606

MERIDIAN LIFE SCIENCE, INC.
Meridian Life Science, Inc.   901-382-8716
5171 Wilfong Road, Memphis, TN 38134

MERIT MEDICAL SYSTEMS, INC.
Ameritek Usa, Inc.   425-379-2580
125 130 St. Se,, Everett, WA 98208
BIOSPHERE MEDICAL, INC.   781-681-7900
1050 Hingham St., Rockland, MA 02370
Merit Cables, Inc.   714-918-1932
830 N. Poinsettia St., Santa Ana, CA 92701
Merit Medical Systems Inc.   804-416-1030
12701 Kingston Ave, Chesterfield, VA 23837
Merit Medical Systems, Inc.   801-253-1600
1111 South Velasco, Angleton, TX 77515
Prestige Ameritech   817-595-1131
7426 Tower St., Ft. Worth, TX 76118

MERLIN'S MEDICAL SUPPLY
Merlin's Medical Supply   805-388-7669
699 Mobil Avenue, Camarillo, CA 93010

MET-PRO CORPORATION
Met-Pro Corporation   215-723-6751
160 Cassell Road, P.O. Box 144, Harleysville, PA 19438

METALOR TECHNOLOGIES INTERNATIONAL SA
Metalor Technologies Usa   011-413-2720
255 John L. Dietsch Blvd., PO Box 255, North Attleborough, MA 02761

METTIS GROUP
Cdc Products Corp.   516-437-3570
1801 Falmouth Avenue, New Hyde Park, NY 11040

METTLER-TOLEDO, INC.
Mettler Toledo Lasentec Products (Lasentec)   425-881-7117
14833 Ne 87th St, Redmond, WA 98052
Mettler-Toledo Process Analytical, Inc.   781-939-6300
36 Middlesex Turnpike, Bedford, MA 01730

MIDMARK CORPORATION
Matrx By Midmark   716-662-6650
145 Mid County Drive, Orchard Park, NY 14127-1737
Midmark Diagnostics Group   937-526-3662
1125 W 90th Street, Gardena, CA 90248

MIDWEST EYE LABORATORIES, INC.
Midwest Eye Laboratories, Inc.   715-833-2277
20 2nd Ave., S.w., Suite 223, Rochester, MN 55901
Midwest Eye Laboratories, Inc.   715-833-2277
7582 Currell Blvd., Suite 109, Woodbury, MN 55125
Midwest Eye Laboratories, Inc.   715-833-2277
1600 South Western, Suite C, Park Ridge Mall, Sioux Falls, SD 57105

MILESTONE SCIENTIFIC INC.
Milestone Scientific Inc.   800-862-1125
220 South Orange Ave., Livingston, NJ 07039

MILLIKEN & COMPANY
Milliken & Company, Anticon Products   706-880-5639
201 Lukken Industrial Drive West M-836, LaGrange, GA 30240

MILLIPORE CORPORATION
Millipore Corporation   781-533-2383
80 Ashby Road, Bedford, MA 01730

MINNESOTA SCIENTIFIC, INC.
Omni-Tract Surgical, A Div. Of Minnesota   651-287-4300
Scientific, Inc.
4849 White Bear Parkway, St. Paul, MN 55110-3325

MITY-LITE, INC.
Broda Enterprises Inc.   519-746-8080
385 Phillip St., Waterloo, ONT N2L 5R8

MIZUHO MEDY CO. LTD.
Mizuho Usa, Inc.   858-679-0555
12131 Community Road, Poway, CA 92064

MLA SYSTEMS, INC.
Stretchair Patient Transfer Systems, Inc,   727-531-2444
8110 Ulmerton Road, Largo, FL 33771

MONARCH-MCLAREN, INC.
Coopercare Lastrap Inc   416-741-9675
Highway H, Koopman Ln., Elkhorn, WI 53121

MOOG INC.
Ethox International   716-842-4000
251 Seneca St., Buffalo, NY 14204
Zevex Incorporated   801-264-1001
4314 ZEVEX Park Lane, Salt Lake City, UT 84123-4650

MORGAN-CRUCIBLE, PLC
Dosimeter Division Of Arrow Tech Inc   973-887-7100
5 Eastmans Road, Parsippany, NJ 07054
Morgan Advance Ceramics   800-433-0638
26 Madison Rd., Fairfield, NJ 07004

MOUNT VERNON MILLS INC.
Riegel Consumer Products Div.   803-275-2541
P.O. Box E, 51 Riegel Road, Johnston, SC 29832-0138

MP BIOMEDICALS DIAGNOSTICS DIVISION
Rapid Diagnostics, Div. Of Mp Biomedicals, Llc   650-558-0395
1429 Rollins Road, Burlingame, CA 94010

MT HOLDINGS, INC.
Metal Techology, Inc.   541-926-9968
173 Queen Ave., S.E., Albany, OR 97321-9905

MTS MEDICATION TECHNOLOGIES
Life Care Technologies, Inc.   813-886-7500
4710 Eisenhower Boulevard, Suite A-10, Tampa, FL 33634

MUNTERS CORP. - CARGOCAIRE DIVISION
Munters Corp. - Cargocaire Division   978-241-1100
79 Monroe St., Amesbury, MA 01913

MYLAN INC.
Mylan Pharmaceuticals Inc   919-991-9800
Research Triangle Pa, Morgantown, NC 27709
Mylan Technologies, Inc.   802-527-7792
110 Lake St., St. Albans, VT 05478

NAKANISHI, INC.
Nsk America Corporation   800-585-4675
700B Cooper Ct., Schaumburg, IL 60173

NANOGEN, INC.
Nanogen Molecular Research Products Division   425-482-5555
21720 23rd Drive, Suite 150, Bothell, WA 98021

NATIONAL STARCH AND CHEMICAL CO.
Permabond International   908-575-7200
10 Feinder Ave., Bridgewater, NJ 08807

NATUS MEDICAL INC.
Excel Tech. Ltd.   905-829-5300
2568 Bristol Cir, Oakville L6H 5S1
Neo-Genesis, A Division Of Natus   503-657-8000
15140 SE 82nd Drive, Suite 270, Clackamas, OR 97015
Neometrics, A Division Of Natus   631-457-4430
150 Motor Parkway, Suite #203, Hauppauge, NY 11788
Olympic Medical Corp.   206-767-3500
5900 First Avenue S., Seattle, WA 98108

NBS GROUP SUPPLY
Nbs Medical Products Inc.   732-745-8192
257 Livingston Ave., New Brunswick, NJ 08901

NBS TECHNOLOGIES, INC.
Nbs Technologies Inc.   201-845-7373
70 Eisenhower Drive, Paramus, NJ 07652

NBTY, INC.
Home Health   631-244-2021
2100 Smithtown Ave, Ronkonkoma, NY 11772

NETZSCH-GERATEBAU GMBH
Netzsch Instruments, Inc.   781-272-5353
37 North Avenue, Burlington, MA 01803

NEW WORLD MEDICAL, INC.
Cpac Equipment, Inc.   585-382-3223
2364 Leicester Road, Leicester, NY 14481-0175

NEWPORT CORPORATION
Newport Franklin, Inc.   508-528-4411
1791 Deere Avenue, Irvine, CA 92606

NFO WORLDWIDE
Migliara/Kaplan Associates   410-581-8188
9 Park Center Ct., Owings Mills, MD 21117-4200

NIHON KOHDEN CORP.
Nihon Kohden America, Inc.   949-580-1555
90 Icon St., Foothill Ranch, CA 92610

NIKON CORP.- JAPAN
Nikon Instruments Inc.   631-547-8500
1300 Walt Whitman Road, Melville, NY 11747-3064

NIPRO CORP.
Nipro Diabetes Systems, Inc.   816-637-2233
3361 Enterprise Way, Miramar, FL 33025

NISSEI SANGYO CO. LTD.
Hitachi High Technologies America　　925-218-2800
5100 Franklin Dr., Pleasanton, CA 94588-3355

NITTO BOSEKI CO., LTD.
International Immunology Corp.　　951-677-5629
PO Box 972, Murrieta, CA 92564-0972

NOCWATCH INTERNATIONAL, INC.
Nocwatch International, Inc./Fallsaver　　775-833-4142
PO Box 1367, Crystal Bay, NV 89402

NONE
Levo Usa　　763-544-7779
7105 Northland Terrace, Brooklyn Park, Minneapolis, MN 55428

NORDSON CORPORATION
Micromedics　　651-452-1977
1270 Eagan Industrial Road, St. Paul, MN 55121-1385

NORTEK, INC.
Niche Medical, Inc.　　401-732-3321
55 Access Rd., Warwick, RI 02886

NORTH AMERICAN CASELINE, INC.
Radix Corp.　　204-697-2349
#2-572 South Fifth St., Pembina, ND 58271

NORTH AMERICAN IMAGING, INC.
Nai Tech Products　　530-887-1008
12919 Earhart Avenue, Auburn, CA 95602

NORTH SAFETY PRODUCTS
North Safety Products　　401-943-4400
2000 Plainfield Pike, Cranston, RI 02921-2012

NORTHERN TECHNOLOGIES INTL. CORP.
Northern Technologies Intl. Corp.　　651-784-1250
6680 N. Hwy. 49, Lino Lakes, MN 55014

NORTHLAND CORPORATION
Marvel Scientific　　616-754-5601
PO Box 400, Greenville, MI 48838

NORTHSTATE PACKAGING
Keller Crescent　　508-478-7641
1072 Boulder Road, Greensboro, NC 27409

NOVARTIS
Ciba Vision Corporation　　678-415-3646
11460 Johns Creek Pkwy., Duluth, GA 30097
Novartis Nutrition　　952-848-6000
1600 Utica Ave S Suite 600, PO Box 370, Minneapolis, MN 55416-1521

NOVO NORDISK A/S
Zymogenetics　　206-442-6600
1201 Eastlake Avenue E., Seattle, WA 98102

NXSTAGE MEDICAL, INC.
Medisystems Corporation　　800-369-6334
439 South Union St., 5th Floor, Lawrence, MA 01843

NYPRO INC.
Np Medical, Inc.　　978-368-4514
101 Union St., Clinton, MA 01510

NYTONE, INC.
Nytone Medical Products　　801-973-4090
2424 S. 900 W., Salt Lake City, UT 84119-1518

OCENCO INCORPORATED
Erie Medical　　262-947-9000
10225 82nd Avenue, Pleasant Prairie, WI 53158

OLIVER PRODUCTS COMPANY
Oliver Medical　　616-456-7711
445 Sixth St. N.W., Grand Rapids, MI 49504-5253

OLYMPUS AMERICA, INC.
Olympus Medical Equipment Services America, Inc.　　484-896-5000
3500 Corporate Parkway, Center valley, PA 18034
Olympus Surgical & Industrial America, Inc.　　845-398-9400
One Corporate Drive, Orangeburg, NY 10962

OLYMPUS CORPORATION
Gyrus Medical, Inc.　　763-416-3000
6655 Wedgwood Road, Suite #105, Maple Grove, MN 55311

OLYMPUS MEDICAL SYSTEMS CORP
Olympus America, Inc.　　484-896-5000
3500 Corporate Parkway, PO Box 610, Center Valley, PA 18034

OMEGA GROUP
Duffens Optical　　785-234-3481
400 S.E. Quincy Street, Topeka, KS 66603

OMNICARE INC.
Accu-Med Services　　513-831-1207
300 Technecenter Drive, Milford, OH 45150

ONCOTHYREON INC.
Oncothyreon Inc.　　520-622-5552
221 East 6th Street, Tucson, AZ 85705

OPENMED TECHNOLOGIES CORPORATION
Openmed Technologies Corporation　　781-938-4210
256 West Cummings Park, Woburn, MA 01801-6436

OPHIR OPTRONICS LTD.
Ophir Optronics, Inc.　　978-657-6410
260A Fordham Road, Wilmington, MA 01887

OPHTHALMIC INTL.
Ophthalmic Intl.　　480-837-6165
16857 E. Saguaro Blvd, Fountain Hills, AZ 85268

OPS SYSTEMS INC
Telecation　　800-677-0067
7112 W. Jefferson Avenue, Suite 307, Lakewood, CO 80235

OPTICAL SENSORS INCORPORATED
Vasamed　　952-947-9543
7615 Golden Triangle Drive, Suite C, Eden Prairie, MN 55344

OPTO ELECTRONIC COMPANY, LTD.
Opticon, Inc.　　845-365-0090
8 Olympic Drive, Orangeburg, NY 10962

ORASURE TECHNOLOGIES, INC.
Orasure Technologies, Inc.　　610-882-1820
1745 Eaton Ave., Bethlehem, PA 18018

ORGANON TEKNIKA BV
Biomerieux Inc.　　919-620-2000
100 Rodolphe Ave., Durham, NC 27712

ORIDION SYSTEMS LTD.
Oridion Medical Inc.　　925-362-0440
140 Towne& Country Drive, SuiteB, Danville, CA 94526

ORMED GMBH
Ormed Corporation　　800-440-2784
599 Cardigan Road, St. Paul, MN 55126

ORTHOFIX
Breg, Inc., An Orthofix Company　　760-599-3000
2611 Commerce Way, Vista, CA 92081

OSADA ELECTRIC CO., LTD.
Osada, Inc.　　310-841-2220
3000 S. Robertson Blvd., Suite 130, Los Angeles, CA 90034

OSI SYSTEMS
Osteometer Meditech, Inc.　　310-978-3073
12515 Chadron Avenue, Hawthorne, CA 90250

OSRAM GMBH
Osram Sylvania Inc.　　978-777-1900
100 Endicott St., Danvers, MA 01923

OSSUR HF
Ossur Americas　　856-345-6000
1414 Metropolitan Avenue, Paulsboro, NJ 08066

OTIX GLOBAL INC.
Sonic Innovations　　801-365-2800
4246 Riverboat Road, Suite 300, Salt Lake City, UT 84123

OTTO BOCK HEALTHCARE GMBH
Truform Orthotics & Prosthetics   513-271-4594
3960 Rosslyn Drive, Cincinnati, OH 45209-1110

OWEN MUMFORD, LTD.
Owen Mumford Usa, Inc.   770-977-2226
1755-A West Oak, Commons Court, Marietta, GA 30062-3165

OWOSSO CORP.
Rhodes Inc., M.H.   860-673-3281
105 Nutmeg Rd. S., South Windsor, CT 06074

OXFORD INSTRUMENTS PLC
Oxford Instruments   978-369-9933
300 Baker Avenue, Suite 150, Concord, MA 01742

P.I., INC.
Pi-Ptp   423-745-6213
215 Rocky Mount Road, PO Box 1067, Athens, TN 37371

PALL CORPORATION
Medsep Corp., A Subsidiary Of Pall Corp.   516-484-5400
1630 Industrial Park St., Covina, CA 91722
Pall Corporation   734-665-0651
600 S. Wagner Road, Ann Arbor, MI 48103
Pall Medical   734-665-0651
600 S. Wagner Rd., Ann Arbor, MI 48103

PARAMOUNT CORPORATION
Oberon Company ,Div Of The Paramount Corp.   508-999-4442
22 Logan St., PO Box 61008, New Bedford, MA 02746

PARI GMBH
Pari Respiratory Equipment, Inc.   804-253-7274
2943 Oak lake Boulevard, Midlothian, VA 23112

PATTERSON COMPANIES, INC.
Patterson Technology Center, Inc   217-347-5964
2202 Althoff Drive, Effingham, IL 62401-1267

PENTAGON TECHNOLOGY, INC.
Pentagon Co., The   818-785-5112
15500 Erwin Street, Suite 1122, Van Nuys, CA 91411

PERBIO SCIENCE
Pierce Chemical Company   815-968-0747
P.O. Box 117, Rockford, IL 61105-0117

PERCUSSIONAIRE CORPORATION
Percussionaire Corporation   208-263-2549
1655 Glengary Bay Rd., Sagle, ID 83860

PERKINELMER
Perkinelmer Life And Analytical Sciences   630-969-6000
2200 Warrenville Rd., Downers Grove, IL 60515
Perkinelmer Life And Analytical Sciences   617-482-9595
549 Albany St., Boston, MA 02118

PERKINELMER LIFE SCIENCES, INC.
Perkinelmer Life And Analytical Sciences   203-925-4602
940 Winter Street, Waltham, MA 02451

PERMOBIL AB
Permobil, Inc.   615-547-1889
6961 Eastgate Blvd., Lebanon, TN 37090

PHARMA-SEPT LTD.
Eagle Laboratories   909-481-0011
10201-A Trademark Street, Rancho Cucamonga, CA 91730-5850

PHILIPS GMBH
Philips Avent   630-350-2600
475 Supreme Dr., Bensenville, IL 60106-1161

PHILIPS HEALTHCARE
Children's Medical Ventures, Inc.   800-345-6443
191 Wyngate Drive, Monroeville, PA 15146

PHILIPS MEDICAL SYSTEMS INTERNATIONAL B.V.
Philips Electronics North America   800-682-7664
2820 B. St. NW, Suite 101, Auburn, WA 98001

PHILIPS MEDICAL SYSTEMS NORTH AMERICA
Philips Medical Systems
3000 Minuteman Road, Andover,, MA 01810-1099

PHILLIPS ELECTRONICS NORTH AMERICA
Philips Lighting Co.   800-555-0050
200 Franklin Square Drive, Somerset, NJ 08875-6800

PHOENIX GROUP, THE
Labac Systems, Inc.   303-914-9914
4965 Kingston Street, Denver, CO 80239

PHOTOMEDEX, INC.
Photomedex, Inc.   760-602-3300
2375 Camino Vida Roble, Suite B, Carlsbad, CA 92011

PLANMECA OY
Planmeca U.S.A. Inc   630-529-2300
100 N. Gary, Suite A, Roselle, IL 60172

PLANO MOLDING CO.
Plano Molding Co.   630-552-3111
431 E South Street, Plano, IL 60545-1601

PLASTIC COMPANIES ENTERPRISES
Heinke Technoogy, Inc. (Hti Plastics)   402-470-2600
5120 N.W. 38th St., Lincoln, NE 68524

PLEXUS CORP.
Plexus Corp   425-482-1300
20001 N. Creek Pkwy, Bothell, WA 98011

POINT PLASTICS, INC.
Quality Scientific Plastics   707-762-6689
1260 Holm Road, Petaluma, CA 94954-1182

POLAR ELECTRO OY
Polar Electro Inc.   1-800-227-1314
1111 Marcus Ave., Ste. M15, Lake Success, NY 11042-1034

POLYCORE OPTICAL PTE. LTD.
Polyvision Inc.   775-850-2050
875 East Patriot Blvd, Suite 201, Reno, NV 89511

POLYSCIENCES, INC.
Bangs Laboratories, Inc.   317-570-7020
9025 Technology Drive, Fishers, IN 46038-2886

PRECISION ENGINEERED PRODUCTS, LLC
Lacey Manufacturing Co., LLC   203-336-0121
1146 Barnum Avenue, PO Box 5156, Bridgeport, CT 06610-0156

PRECO INDUSTRIES
Safegard Medical Products, Inc.   781-935-2275
52 Dragon Ct., Woburn, MA 01801

PREISER SCIENTIFIC, INC.
Standard Instrumentation, Div. Preiser Scientific   304-727-2902
94 Oliver St., St. Albans, WV 25177

PRIME MEDICAL SERVICES, INC.
Oshkosh Specialty Vehicles   708-596-5066
16745 S. Lathrop Avenue, Harvey, IL 60426

PRINCETON BIOMEDITECH CORP.
Lifesign   732-246-3366
71 Veronica Avenue, Somerset, NJ 08873

PRIVATELY HELD
Rontron Engineering, Inc.   203-488-5020
131 Commercial Pkwy., Branford, CT 06405

PROCTER & GAMBLE
Duracell Usa   800-551-2355
8 Research Dr., Berkshire Corporate Park, Bethel, CT 06801

PROCTER & GAMBLE GMBH
Oral-B Laboratories, Inc.   800-566-7252
1832 Lower Muscantine Rd, Iowa City, IA 52240

PROFESSIONAL DENTAL MFG., INC.
Zila Dental Technologies, Inc.   928-899-1231
2410 Harrison St., Batesville, AR 72501

PROTECH,LEADED EYEWEAR, INC.
Protech Leaded Eyewear   561-627-9769
10415 riverside drive, Palm Beach Gardens, FL 33410

PRUDENTIAL OVERALL SUPPLY
Bba Fiberweb Washougal, Inc.   360-835-8787
3720 Grant St., Washougal, WA 98671-2807

QUANTRONIX LASERS
Quatronix   631-784-6100
41 Research Way, East Setauket, NY 11733

QUERYWINMDR_PARENT_S_NAME
qry_parent_subs_MDR_SUPPLIER_S_NAME   PHONE1
ADDR1, ADDR2, CITY, STATE ZIP

QUEST DIAGNOSTICS, INC.
Specialty Laboratories, Inc.   661-799-6543
27027 Tourney Rd., Valencia, CA 91355

QUIDEL CORPORATION
Quidel Corp.   858-552-1100
10165 McKellar Court, San Diego, CA 92121

QUIXOTE CORPORATION
Spin-Cast Plastics, Inc.   219-232-8066
3300 N. Kenmore St., South Bend, IN 46628

RACK ENTERPRISES INC.
Ximedix, Inc.   719-264-0410
4829 Northpark Drive, Colorado Springs, CO 80918

RAWCAR GROUP, LLC
Cfi Medical Solutions (Contour Fabricators, Inc.)   810-750-5300
14241 Fenton Road, Fenton, MI 48430

RAYOVAC CORPORATION
Spectrum-Brands   608-275-3340
601 Rayovac Drive, Madison, WI 53711-2497

RC2 CORPORATION
Learning Curve Brands Inc. THE FIRST YEARS   800-225-0382
100 Technology Center Drive, Suite 2A, Stoughton, MA 02072

REABLE THERAPEUTICS, INC.
Chattanooga Group   760-727-1280
1430 Decision Street, Vista, CA 37343-0489

REGENT MEDICAL LTD.
Molnlycke Health Care Inc.   678-250-7900
5550 Peachtree Parkway, Suite 500, Norcross, GA 30092

REM SYSTEMS
Kardex Systems, Inc.   740-374-9300
114 Westview Avenue, Marietta, OH 45750-0171

REMEL
Remel Atlanta, Div. Of Remel, Inc.   770-409-0713
2797 Peterson Pl., Norcross, GA 30071

RESMED CORP.
Resmed West Coast Warehouse   858-746-2576
23650 Brodiaea, Moreno valley, CA 92553

RESMED INC.
Resmed Corp.   1 (858) 836-500
9001 Spectrum Center Blvd., San Diego, CA 92123

RESPIRONICS PENNSYLVANIA
Respironics Colorado   800-345-6443
12301 N Grant St #190, Thornton, CO 80241

RIVERS EDGE TECHNICAL SERVICE, INC.
Microstat Laboratories, Inc.   507-932-3968
PO Box 115, Dover, MN 55929

RMS MEDICAL PRODUCTS
Rms Medical Products   845-469-2042
24 Carpenter Road, Chester, NY 10918

ROBERT H. KAPLAN ASSOCIATES, INC.
David Scott Company   508-875-3333
59 Fountain St., Framingham, MA 01702

ROCKWELL MEDICAL TECHNOLOGIES, INC.
Rockwell Medical Technologies, Inc.   248-960-9009
604 High Tech Ct., Greer, SC 29650

ROPER INDUSTRIES
Pac   281-580-0339
300 Bammel Westfield, Houston, TX 77090-3533

Princeton Instruments - Acton   978-263-3584
15 Discovery Way, Acton, MA 01720

Roper Scientific, Inc.   520-889-9933
3440 E. Britannia Drive, Tucson, AZ 85706-5006

ROQUETTE FRERE
Roquette America   319-524-5757
1417 Exchange St., PO Box 6647, Keokuk, IA 52632-6647

ROYAL DENTAL MANUFACTURING, INC.
Biotec, Inc.   616-772-2133
652 East Main Street, Zeeland, MI 49464

RSTI (RADIOLOGICAL SERVICE TRAINING INSTITUTE)
Jannx Medical Systems Inc.   314-822-7799
12166 Old Big Bend Blvd., Ste. 300, St. Louis, MO 63122-6836

RULTRACT, INC.
Pemco, Inc. - Medical Div.   216-524-2990
5663 Brecksville Road, Cleveland, OH 44131-1510

S & P ELECTRICAL INDUSTRIES, INC.
Electro-Med Health Industries   305-892-2866
PO Box 610484, Miami, FL 33261-0484

S & S X-RAY PRODUCTS, INC.
S&S Medcart   281-815-1300
10625 Telge Road, Houston, TX 77095

SAES GETTERS SPA
Saes Memry   203-739-1100
3 Berkshire Blvd., Bethel, CT 06801

SAINT-GOBAIN
Lg Electronics U.S.A., Inc.   847-941-8181
2000 Millbrook Drive, Lincolnshire, IL 60069

SAINT-GOBAIN PERFORMANCE PLASTICS
Saint-Gobain Performance Plastics--Akron   330-798-9240
2664 Gilchrist Rd., Akron, OH 44305

SALTER LABS
Salter Labs   805-854-3166
100 W. Sycamore Road, Arvin, CA 93203

SALZMANN MEDICO
Venosan North America, Inc.   336-629-7181
300 Industrial Park Avenue, PO Box 1067, Asheboro, NC 27204-1067

SANDVIK MATERIALS TECHNOLOGY
Sandvik MedTech   901-384-5907
4477 Getwell Rd., P.O. Box 1990, Memphis, TN 38118

SAUDER WOODWORKING CO.
Sauder Manufacturing Co.   419-445-7670
930 W. Barre Rd., Archbold, OH 43502

SCHAERER AG, M.
Schaerer Mayfield Usa   513-561-2241
4900 Charlemar Drive, Cincinnati, OH 45227

SCHERING-PLOUGH CORP.
Schering-Plough Health Care Products   901-320-2011
3030 Jackson Ave., Memphis, TN 38151

SCHLEICHER & SCHUELL GMBH
Schleicher & Schuell, Inc.   603-352-3810
10 Optical Avenue, PO Box 2012, Keene, NH 03431

SCHLEUNIGER AG
Schleuniger, Inc.   603-668-8117
87 Colin Drive, Manchester, NH 03103

SCHOTT CORPORATION
Schott Glass Technologies, Inc.   570-457-7485
400 York Ave., Duryea, PA 18642-2026

Schott North America, Inc.   315-255-2791
  62 Columbus Street, Auburn, NY 13021-3137

SCICAN

Scican Inc.   724-820-1600
  701 Technology Drive, Canonsburg, PA 15317

SCIVEX

Fci Ophthalmics   781-826-9060
  64 Schoosett Street, Pembroke, MA 02359

SCOTT FETZER COMPANY

Meriam Process Technologies   216-281-1100
  10920 Madison Avenue, Cleveland, OH 44102-2599
Western Medica   440-871-2160
  875 Bassett Road, Westlake, OH 44145

SCOTT MEDICAL PRODUCTS

Scott Medical Products   215-766-8861
  6097 Easton Road, Building 3, Plumsteadville, PA 18949-0310

SCOTTCARE CORPORATION

Rozinn By Scottcare Corporation   216-361-0550
  4791 West 150th Street, Cleveland, OH 44135

SCOTTSMAN INDUSTRIES

Scotsman Industries   847-215-4500
  775 Corporate Woods Pkwy., Vernon Hills, IL 60061-3112

SDI MEDICAL CONSULTANTS

Dynamics Research Corp.   978-289-1500
  Two Tech Drive, Andover, MA 01810-5498

SEALTECH, INC.

Pi Professional Therapy Products   423-744-8000
  PO Box 1067, Athens, TN 37371-1067

SEATTLE SYSTEMS

Lenox Hill Brace / Seattle Systems   360-697-5656
  26296 Twelve Trees Ln NW, Poulsbo, WA 98370

SEIKO OPTICAL PRODUCTS CO.,LTD

Seiko Optical Products   201-529-9099
  575 Corporate Dr., Mahwah, NJ 07430-2330

SELAS CORPORATION OF AMERICA

Rti Electronics, Inc.   (714) 765-8200
  1800 E. Via Burton, Anaheim, CA 92806-1213

SENNHEISER ELECTRONIC KG

Sennheiser Electronic Corp.   860-434-9190
  One Enterprise Drive, Old Lyme, CT 06371

SERAPLEX BIOLOGICALS INC.

Compass Bioscience   626-359-9645
  1850 Evergreen St., Duarte, CA 91010-2906

SHAMIR OPTICAL INDUSTRY

Shamir Insight, Inc.   877-514-833
  9938 Via Pasar, San Diego, CA 92126
Shamir Usa, Inc.   818-889-6292
  30077 Agoura Rd, Suite 220, Agoura Hills, CA 91301

SHANGHAI ZHIJIANG BIOTECHNOLOGY CO.,LTD

Advanced Medical Devices, Inc.   416-833-6681
  15 Keele Street South Unit 2, Po Box 520, King City L7B 1A7
Aztec Medical Products, Inc.   800-223-3859
  3356 Ironbound Road, Suite 303, Williamsburg, VA 23188

SHAWSHEEN RUBBER CO.

Arrowhead Athletics   978-470-1760
  220 Andover St., PO Box 4264, Andover, MA 01810

SHIMADZU CORP.

Kratos Analytical Inc.   845-426-6700
  100 Red Schoolhouse Road #Bldg.-A, Spring Valley, NY 10977-7049
Shimadzu Medical Systems   310-217-8855
  20101 S. Vermont Avenue, Torrance, CA 90502

SHOFU INC.

Shofu Dental Corporation   760-736-3277
  1225 Stone Drive, San Marcos, CA 92069

SICK AG

Sick, Inc.   952-941-6780
  6900 West 110th Street, Minneapolis, MN 55438

SIEGEL-ROBERT, INC.

Sensidyne, Inc.   727-530-3602
  16333 Bay Vista Drive, Clearwater, FL 33760

SIEMENS AG

Electone, A Division Of Siemens Hearing   407-831-2555
  Instruments, Inc.
  1124 Florida Central Pkwy, Longwood, FL 32750
M-E Manufacturing And Services, Inc.   763-268-4500
  5010 Cheshire Lane North, Plymouth, MN 55446
REXTON, A DIVISCION OF SIEMENS HEARING   763-553-0787
  INSTRUMENTS, IN.
  5010 Cheshire Lane North, Suite 2, Plymouth, MN 55446
Siemens Healthcare Diagnostics Inc   800-434-2447
  725 Potter St, Berkeley, CA 94710
Siemens Healthcare Diagnostics Inc   866-637-4448
  101 Silvermine Rd, Brookfield, CT 06804
Siemens Healthcare Diagnostics Inc   574-295-7516
  3400 Middlebury St, Elkhart, IN 46515
Siemens Healthcare Diagnostics Inc   317-240-0012
  7750 West Morris St., Indianapolis, IN 46231
Siemens Healthcare Diagnostics Inc   866-637-4448
  333 Coney Street, E Walpole, MA 02032
Siemens Healthcare Diagnostics Inc   800-255-3232
  2 Edgewater Drive, Norwood, MA 02062
Siemens Healthcare Diagnostics Inc   973-584-4649
  62 Flanders-Barley Road, Flanders, NJ 07836
Siemens Healthcare Diagnostics Inc   310-645-8200
  5210 Pacific Concourse Drive, Los Angeles, CA 90045
Siemens Healthcare Diagnostics Inc.   302-631-6311
  500 Gbc Dr., Mailstop 514, Newark, DE 19702
Siemens Healthcare Diagnostics Inc.   800-242-3233
  600 Tradeport Blvd, Suite 601, Atlanta, GA 30354
Siemens Healthcare Diagnostics Inc.   914-631-8000
  511 Benedict Avenue, Tarrytown, NY 10591
Siemens Healthcare Diagnostics, Inc   800-242-3233
  2040 Enterprise Blvd., West Sacramento, CA 95691
Siemens Hearing Instruments, Inc.   732-568-6600
  10 Constitution Avenue, P.O. Box 1397, Piscataway, NJ 08855
Siemens Medical Solutions Health Services Division   888-826-9702
  51 Valley Stream Pkwy, Malvern, PA 19355
Siemens Medical Solutions Usa, Inc   888-826-9702
  2500 Millbrook Dr., Suite B, Buffalo Grove, IL 60089
Siemens Medical Solutions Usa, Inc   888-826-9702
  400 W. Morgan Road, Suite 100, Ann Arbor, MI 48108
Siemens Medical Solutions Usa, Inc   888-826-9702
  Pony Farm Industrial Park, 139 Commerce Rd, Oneonta, NY 13820
Siemens Medical Solutions Usa, Inc   610-448-4153
  51 Valley Stream Parkway, Malvern, PA 19355
Siemens Medical Solutions Usa, Inc.   847-304-7700
  2501 North Barrington Road, Hoffman Estates, IL 60192
Siemens Medical Solutions Usa, Inc.   610-448-3184
  20 Valley Stream Pkwy, Malvern, PA 19355
Siemens Medical Solutions Usa, Inc.   610-448-4500
  51 Valley Stream Parkway, Malvern, PA 19355-1406
Siemens Medical Solutions Usa, Inc.   865-218-2534
  203 Dunavant Drive, Rockford, TN 37853
Siemens Medical Solutions Usa, Inc.   865-218-2534
  3100 Stockcreek Blvd, Rockford, TN 37853
Siemens Medical Solutions Usa, Inc. Ultrasound   650-969-9112
  Division
  1230 Shorebird Way, Mountain View, CA 94039-7393
Siemens Medical Solutions Usa, Molecular Imaging   888-826-9702
  810 Innovation Dr, Knoxville, TN 37932-2571
Siemens Medical Systems, Inc., Ultrasound Group   800-964-4114
  22010 S.E. 51st St., Issaquah, WA 98029
WILEX, Inc.   877-229-3711
  Oncogene Science, 100 Acorn Park Drive, Cambridge, MA 02140

SIEMENS MEDICAL

Nokia Siemens Networks   561-923-9590
  900 Broken Sound Pkwy., Boca Raton, FL 33487
Siemens Credit Corp.   800-798-7721
  170 Wood Avenue, South Iselin, NJ 08830
Siemens Medical Systems, Inc., Nuclear Med. Group   847-304-7700
  2501 N. Barrington Road, Hoffman Estates, IL 60195

SIEMENS MEDICAL SOLUTIONS USA, INC.

Med-Lab Supply Co., Inc.   305-642-5144
923 N.W. 27th Ave., Miami, FL 33125

Sun-Med   727-530-7099
12393 Belcher Road, Suite #450, Largo, FL 33773

Sunmed Healthcare   727-531-7266
12393 Belcher Road, Suite 460, Largo, FL 33773

SILVER STAR MOBILITY

Silver Star Mobility   541-857-5012
578 Mason Way, Medford, OR 97501

SIPPICAN, INC.

Polaris Contract Services, A Division Of Sippicon, Inc.   508-748-1160
7 Barnabas Rd., Marion, MA 02738-1421

SMITH & NEPHEW PLC.

Smith & Nephew Inc., Endoscopy Div.   978-749-1000
76 S. Meridian Ave., Oklahoma City, OK 73107-6512

Smith & Nephew, Inc.   727-392-1261
970 lake carillon dr., suite 110, saint petersburg, FL 33716

Smith & Nephew, Inc.   901-396-2121
6409 E. Holmes Rd., Mem, TN 38141

Smith & Nephew, Inc.   978-749-1000
University Business Park, 12500 Network, Suite 112, San Antonio, TX 78249-3308

Smith & Nephew, Inc., Endoscopy Division   978-749-1073
737 North Detroit St., Warsaw, IN 46580

Smith & Nephew, Inc., Endoscopy Division   978-749-1000
150 Minuteman Road, Andover, MA 01810-1031

Smith & Nephew, Inc., Endoscopy Division   978-749-1000
130 Forbes Blvd., Mansfield, MA 02048

SMITH & NEPHEW, INC.

Smith & Nephew Inc.- Orthopaedics Division   901-399-5081
1450 Brooks Rd., Memphis, TN 38116

SMITHKLINE BEECHAM

Gsk Consumer Healthcare   888-825-5249
65 Industrial South, Clifton, NJ 07012

SMITHS MEDICAL

Smiths Medical Pm, Inc.   262-542-3100
N7 W22025 Johnson Drive, Waukesha, WI 53186

SMITHS MEDICAL ASD, INC.

Smiths Medical Asd   219-989-9150
5700 W. 23rd Avenue, Gary, IN 46406-2617

Smiths Medical Asd, Inc.   651-633-2556
1265 Grey Fox Road, St. Paul, MN 55112

Smiths Medical Asd, Inc.   1 214 618 0218
5200 Upper Metro Place, Suite 200, Dublin, OH 43017

SOLVAY PHARMA US HOLDINGS, INC.

Solvay Pharmaceuticals   770-578-9000
901 Sawyer Rd., Marietta, GA 30062

SONOCO CORPORATION

Sonoco-Stancap Division   (770) 476-9088
3150 Clinton Ct., Norcross, GA 30071

SONOCO PRODUCTS

Sonoco Crellin, Inc.   518-392-2000
87 Center St., Chatham, NY 12037

SONOSITE, INC.

Cardiodynamics International Corp.   425-951-1200
21919 30th Drive SE, Bothell, WA 98021

SORIN GROUP USA

Ela Medical, Inc.   763-519-9400
2950 Xenium Lane N., Plymouth, MN 55441

SORIN S.P.A.

Sorin Group Usa   303-425-5508
14401 W. 65th Way, Arvada, CO 80004-3599

SOUVERN TRENT

Capital Controls, MicroChem   215-997-4000
3000 Advance Lane, Colmar, PA 18915

SP INDUSTRIES, INC.

Hotpack   215-824-1700
10940 Dutton Rd., Philadelphia, PA 19154-3286

Virtis, An Sp Industries Company   845-255-5000
815 Route 208, Gardiner, NY 12525

SPARTON CORPORATION

Sparton Electronics Florida, Inc.   386-985-4631
5612 Johnson Lake Rd., De Leon Springs, FL 32130

SPECTRIS, INC.

National Cable Molding   323-225-5611
136 N. San Fernando Rd., Los Angeles, CA 90031

SPECTRUM LABORATORIES, INC.

Spectrum Laboratories, Inc.   310-885-4600
18617 Broadwick St., Rancho Dominguez, CA 90220

SPERIAN PROTECTION

Perfect Fit Glove   716-668-2000
85 Innsbruck Drive, Buffalo, NY 14227

Sperian Eye & Face Protection Inc.   401-232-1200
10 Thurber Blvd., Smithfield, RI 02917

Titmus Optical Inc.   804-452-5200
690 HP Way, 3811 CorPOrate Drive, Chester, VA 23836-2742

SPIRAX SARCO LIMITED

Spirax Sarco, Inc.   803-714-2000
1150 Nortpoint Blvd., Blythewood, SC 29016

SPX

Kendro Laboratory Products   828-658-2711
308 Ridgefield Court, Asheville, NC 28806

Lightnin Mixers   585-436-5550
135 Mt. Read Blvd., Rochester, NY 14611

Thermal Product Solutions   570-326-1770
2121 Reach Road, Williamsport, PA 17701

SPX CORPORATION

Lds Life Science (Formerly Gould Instrument Systems Inc.)   216-328-7000
5525 Cloverleaf Parkway, Valley View, OH 44125-6100

SQUIRE-COGSWELL /AEROS INSTRUMENTS, INC.

Ohio Medical Corp.   847-855-0500
1111 Lakeside Dr., Gurnee, IL 60031-4099

SRS MEDICAL SYSTEMS, INC.

Self Regulation Systems, Inc.   425-882-1101
8672 154th Avenue NE,, Bldg. F, Redmond, WA 98052-2554

ST. JUDE MEDICAL, INC.

Irvine Biomedical, Inc.   949-851-3053
2375 Morse Avenue, Irvine, CA 92614-6234

St. Jude Medical Atrial Fibrillation   763-383-0900
6500 Wedgwood Rd., Maple Grove, MN 55311

St. Jude Medical Atrial Fibrillation   612-933-4700
14901 DeVeau Pl., Minnetonka, MN 55345-2126

St. Jude Medical Atrial Fibrillation (Endocardial Solutions)   651.756.2000
One St. Jude Medical Drive, St. Paul, MN 55117-9983

St. Jude Medical Cardiac Rhythm Management Div.   818-362-6822
15900 Valley View Ct., Sylmar, CA 91342-3577

St. Jude Medical Neuromodulation Division   972-309-8000
6901 Preston Rd., Plano, TX 75024

St. Jude Medical, Puerto Rico, B.V.   787-746-1111
Lot 20, Caguas West Industrial Park, Caguas, PR 00726-0998

STAAR SURGICAL CO.

Circuit Tree Medical, Inc.   626-303-7902
1911 Walker Avenue, Monrovia, CA 91016

STAIRMASTER HEALTH AND FITNESS PRODUCTS

Stairmaster Health And Fitness Products   800-628-8458
1886 Prarie Way, Louisville, CO 80027

STANLEY WORKS

Senior Technologies   402-475-4002
PO Box 80238, 1620 N 20th Circle, Lincoln, NE 68503

Stanley Supply & Services, Inc   978-682-2000
335 Willow Street, North Andover, MA 01845-5995

Stanley Vidmar   800-523-9462
11 Grammes Road, Allentown, PA 18103

STARKEY LABORATORIES, INC.

Nu-Ear Electronics   858-450-9972
6769 Mesa Ridge Rd., Ste. 100, San Diego, CA 92121

Starkey California   952-947-4734
2536 Woodland Dr., Anaheim, CA 92801

Starkey East   952-947-4734
535 Route 38 East, Suite 230, Cherry Hill, NJ 08002

Starkey Florida   952-947-4734
2200 North Commerce Parkway, Weston, FL 33326

Starkey Glencoe   952-947-4734
2915 10th St. East, Glencoe, MN 55336

Starkey Northwest   612-941-6401
2255 N.E. 194th Ave., Portland, OR 97230-7437

Starkey Southeast   952-947-4734
5300 Oakbrook Pkwy.,, Bldg. 100, Suite 130, Norcross, GA 30093

Starkey Southwest   952-947-4734
3100 Alvin Devane Blvd., Austin, TX 78741

STAT KIT, INC.

Banyan International Corp.   325-677-1874
2118 E. Interstate 20, PO Box 1779, Abilene, TX 79601

STATE TRADING CORPORATION OF INDIA, LTD., THE

State Trading Corporation Of India, Ltd.   212-244-3317
350 5th Ave., Ste. 1124, 11th Fl., New York, NY 10118

STERIS CORPORATION

Steris Biological Operations Facility   440-354-2600
9325 Pinecone Dr., Mentor, OH 44060

Steris Corporation   334-277-6660
2720 Gunter Park Drive, Montgomery, AL 36109

Steris Corporation   314-290-4600
7501 Page Avenue, St. Louis, MO 63133

Steris Corporation   314-290-4703
8525 Page Boulevard, St. Louis, MO 63114

Steris Corporation   440-354-2600
6100 Heisley Road, Mentor, OH 44060

Steris Corporation   440-354-2600
6515 Hopkins Road, Mentor, OH 44060

Steris Corporation   814-452-3100
2424 West 23rd Street, Erie, PA 16506

Steris Isomedix Services   973-887-2754
9 Apollo Drive, Whippany, NJ 07981-1423

STERLING FLUID SYSTEMS GROUP

Sterling Fluid Systems (Usa)   716-773-6450
303 Industrial Blvd., Grand Island, NY 14072

STIEFEL LABORATORIES, INC.

Stiefel   888-784-3335
20 T.W. Alexander Drive, Research Triangle Park, NC 27709

Stiefel Laboratories, Inc.   518-239-6901
6290 Route 145, Oak Hill, NY 12460

STILLE

Surgical Table Services Co.   330-253-7766
526 South Main St., Akron, OH 44311

STILLE AB

Stille-Sonesta, Inc.   214-741-2464
1610 I35 North, Suite 203, Carrolton, TX 75006

STOELTING LLC

Stoelting   920-894-2293
502 Hwy. 67, Kiel, WI 53042

STORZ GMBH & CO., KARL

Karl Storz Endoscopia Latino America   305-262-8980
815 N.W. 57th Ave. Ste. 480, Miami, FL 33126-2042

Karl Storz Endovision, Inc.   508-248-9011
91 Carpenter Hill Rd., Charlton, MA 01507

Karl Storz Imaging   805-968-5563
175 Cremona Dr., Golita, CA 93117-5502

STRYKER CORP.

Boston Scientific-Neurovascular   510-440-7700
47900 Bayside Pkwy., Fremont, CA 94538-6515

Gaymar Industries, Inc.   716-662-2551
10 Centre Drive, Orchard Park, NY 14127-2280

OLYMPUS BIOTECH CORPORATION   603-298-3000
9 Technology Dr., W. Lebanon, NH 03784

Stryker Biotech   508-416-5200
35 South St., Hopkinton, MA 01748

Stryker Communications Corp.   972-410-7100
1410 Lakeside Parkway, Flower Mound, TX 75028

Stryker Endoscopy   408-754-2000
5900 Optical Ct, San Jose, CA 95138

STRYKER CORPORATION

Everest Biomedical Instruments Co.   636-305-9900
1732 Gilsinn Ln., Fenton, MO 63026

Striker Corp.   269 323 7700
4100 East Milham Avenue, Kalamazoo, MI 49001

Stryker Gi   877-795-3539
1420 Lakeside Parkway, Suite 110, Flower Mound, TX 75028

Stryker Howmedica Osteonics   201-831-5000
325 Corporate Drive, Mahwah, NJ 07430

Stryker Imaging   972-410-5000
1410 Lakeside Pkwy., Ste. 600, Flower Mound, TX 75028

Stryker Instruments, Instruments Div.   269 323 7700
4100 East Milham Ave., Kalamazoo, MI 49001

Stryker Medical   269 389 2600
2825 Airview Boulevard, Kalamazoo, MI 49002

Stryker Puerto Rico, Ltd.   939-307-2500
Hwy. 3, Km. 131.2, Las Guasimas Ind. Park, Arroyo, PR 00714

Stryker Spine   201-760-8000
2 Pearl Ct, Allendale, NJ 07401

SUITE 310-B"

NC
28226, United States, 704-542-6876, 888-743-47

SULZER MEDICA

Centerpulse Orthopedics Inc.   512-432-9900
9900 Spectrum Drive, Austin, TX 78717

SUMMIT HAUS COMMUNICATION, LTD.

Sagentia Inc   410-654-0090
11403 Cronhill Drive, Suite B, Owings Mills, MD 21117

SUNBEAM CORPORATION

Oster Professional Products, Inc.
904 Red Rd, McMinnville, TN 37110

SUNCOAST DENTAL, INC.

Tatum Surgical   727-536-4880
14010 Roosevelt Blvd, Suite # 705, Clearwater, FL 33762

SUNRISE MEDICAL

Dynavox Systems Inc.   412-381-4883
2100 Wharton St., Suite 400, Pittsburgh, PA 15203

SUNRISE MEDICAL, INC.

Joerns Healthcare, Inc   800-826-0270
5001 Joerns Dr., Stevens Point, WI 54481

SUNTECH MEDICAL GROUP, LTD.   UK

Suntech Medical, Inc.   919-654-2300
507 Airport Boulevard, Suite 117, Morrisville, NC 27560-8200

SUPERIOR GROUP, INC.

Sharp Corporation   610-279-3550
23 Carland Road, Conshohocken, PA 19428-1084

SUPPLY KING, INC.

Contamination Control Products   732-869-3400
1 Third Avenue, Box 578, Neptune, NJ 07753

SWISSRAY INTERNATIONAL, INC.

Medimaging Tecnology, Inc.   516-674-8900
49 Herb Hill Road, Glen Cove, NY 11542

Swissray America, Inc.   908 353 0971
One Tower Center Blvd., East Brunswick, NJ 08816

SYBRON DENTAL SPECIALTIES, INC.

Allesee Orthodontic Appliances   714-516-7484
13931 Spring St., Sturtevant, WI 53177

Allesee Orthodontic Appliances (Calexico)   714-516-7400
341 E. First St., Calexico, CA 92231

Allesee Orthodontic Appliances, Inc. - Connecticut   949-255-8766
6 Niblick Rd., Enfield, CT 06082

Attachments International, Inc.   650-340-0393
824 Cowan Rd., Burlingame, CA 94010

Kerr Corp.   949-255-8766
  1717 West Collins Ave., Orange, CA 92867

Kerr Corp.   714-516-7400
  28200 Wick Rd., Romulus, MI 48174

Kerr Corp.   949-255-8766
  3225 Deming Way, Suite 190, Middleton, WI 53562

Metrex Research Corp.   714-516-7788
  28210 Wick Rd., Romulus, MI 48174

Ormco Corp.   909-596-0100
  1332 S. Lone Hill Ave., Glendora, CA 91740

SYBRON INTERNATIONAL CORP.

Aoa   800-262-5221
  13931 Spring St., P.O. Box 725, Sturtevant, WI 53177

SYMMETRICOM, INC.

Symmetricom Timing, Test & Measurement   978-927-8220
  34 Tozer Road, Beverly, MA 01915

SYMMETRY MEDICAL, INC.

Riley Medical, Inc.   207-786-2775
  27 Wrights Landing, Auburn, ME 04210

Symmetry Medical New Bedford   508-998-4493
  New Bedford Industrial Park, New Bedford, MA 02745

Symmetry Medical Usa, Inc   207-786-2775
  111 N. Clay, Claypool, IN 46510

Symmetry Medical Usa, Inc.   574-267-8700
  486 West 350 North, Warsaw, IN 46582

Symmetry Medical, Inc. - Polyvac   207-786-2775
  253 Abby Rd., Manchester, NH 03103

Symmetry Medical/Ssi   615-883-9090
  200 River Hills Drive, Nashville, TN 37210

Symmetry Tnco   781-447-6661
  15 Colebrook Blvd., Whitman, MA 02382

SYNERON MEDICAL LTD.

Syneron, Inc.   949-716-6670
  3 Goodyear Unit A, Irvine, CA 92618

SYNOVIS LIFE TECHNOLOGIES, INC

Synovis Micro Companies Alliance, Inc.   205-941-0111
  439 Industrial Ln., Birmingham, AL 35211-4464

SYNTHES GMBH

Bio-Synthesis, Inc   972-420-8505
  612 East Main St, Lewisville, TX 75057

SYNTHES INC.

Synthes (Usa)   719 481 5300
  1051 Synthes Avenue, P.O. Box 366, Monument, CO 80132

Synthes (Usa)   610-719-5000
  35 Airport Road, Horseheads, NY 14845

Synthes (Usa) - Brandywine Technical Center   610-719-5000
  1302 Wrights Lane East, West Chester, PA 19380

Synthes (Usa) - Development Center   719-481-5300
  1230 Wilson Dr., West Chester, PA 19380

Synthes Jennersville   484-356-9728
  108 Willowbrook Lane, West Chester, PA 19382

Synthes San Diego   858-452-1266
  6244 Ferris Square, Suite B, San Diego, CA 92121-3239

SYSMEX CORP.

Sysmex America Inc.   1-800-462-1262
  One Nelson C. White Parkway, Mundelein, IL 60060

TAKARA BELMONT USA, INC.

Takara Belmont Usa, Inc.   800-223-1192
  101 Belmont Dr., Somerset, NJ 08873

TAKENAKA GROUP CENTER

Pulnix America Inc.   408-747-0300
  1330 Orleans Drive, Sunnyvale, CA 94089

TAUB PRODUCTS, INC., LAURENCE

George Taub Products & Fusion Co., Inc.   201-798-5353
  277 New York Ave., Jersey City, NJ 07307-1501

TBC GROUP

Bagco   770-422-4187
  1650 Airport Road Suite 104, Kennesaw, GA 30144

TEAM AMERICA HEALTH & FITNESS, INC.

Team America Health & Fitness, Inc   805-777-0168
  675 Racquet Club Ln, Thousand Oaks, CA 91360

TECAN GROUP AG, LTD.

Tecan Systems   408-953-3100
  2450 Zanker Rd., San Jose, CA 95131

Tecan U.S., Inc.   919-361-5200
  4022 Stirrup Creek Rd., Ste. 310, Durham, NC 27709

TEGRANT CORPORATION

Tegrant Corporation, Protexic Brands   724-843-8200
  800 5th Ave., P.O. Box 448, New Brighton, PA 15066

Tegrant Corporation, Thermosafe Brands   1 800 323 7442
  3930 Ventura Drive Suite 450, Arlington Heights, IL 60084

TEGRANT CORPORATION, PROTEXIC BRANDS

Thermosafe Brands   800-323-7442
  3930 Ventura Drive, Suite 450, Arlington Heights, IL 60004

TELEFLEX MEDICAL

Arrow International, Inc.   610-655-8522
  9 Plymouth St., Everett, MA 02149

Arrow International, Inc.   610-655-8522
  312 Commerce Pl, Asheboro, NC 27203

Arrow International, Inc.   610-655-8522
  2 Berry Dr, Mount Holly, NJ 08060

Arrow International, Inc.   610-655-8522
  2400 Bernville Rd., Reading, PA 19605

Specialized Medical Devices, Llc   717-392-8570
  300 Running Pump Rd, Lancaster, PA 17603

Ssi Surgical Services, Inc   407-249-1946
  5776 Hoffner Ave, Ste 200, Orlando, FL 32822

Telefelx Medical   610-948-5100
  155 South Limerick Road, Limerick, PA 19468-1699

Teleflex Medical   919-433-4829
  1805 A Tw Alexander Drive, Durham, NC 27703

Teleflex Medical   919-544-8000
  2917 Weck Drive, Research Triangle Park, NC 27709

Teleflex Medical   866-246-6990
  920 Westport Parkway, Fort Worth, TX 76177

Teleflex Medical Oem   508-964-6021
  375 Forbes Boulevard, Mansfield, MA 02048-1805

Tfx Medical Oem   603-532-7706
  50 Plantation Drive, Jaffrey, NH 03452

TELEFLEX, INC.

Kmedic   201-767-4002
  190 Veterans Drive, Northvale, NJ 07647

Specialty Care   (615) 345-5400
  One American Center, 3100 West End Avenue, Suite 800, Nashville, TN 37203

TELEMED TECHNOLOOGIES INTERNATIONAL CORP.

Cardiac Telecom Corporation   800-355-2594
  212 Outlet Way, Suite 1, Greensburg, PA 15601

TEMPUR-PEDIC, INC.

Tempur-Medical, Inc.   859-259-0754
  1713 Jaggie Fox Way, Lexington, KY 40511

TENNECO, INC.

Pactiv Corporation   847-482-2000
  1900 W. Field Court, Lake Forest, IL 60045

TENTE ROLLEN GMBH & CO.

Tente Casters, Inc.   859-586-5558
  2266 Southpark Drive, Hebron, KY 41048

TERUMO CORPORATION

Microvention, Inc.   949-461-3314
  1311 valencia avenue, tustin, CA 92780

Terumo Cardiovascular Systems (Tcvs)   714-258-8001
  1311 Valencia Ave., Tustin, CA 92780

Terumo Cardiovascular Systems (Tcvs)   508-881-4858
  28 Howe St., Ashland, MA 01721

Terumo Cardiovascular Systems (Tcvs)   410-398-8500
  125 Blue Ball Road, Elkton, MD 21921

Terumo Cardiovascular Systems, Corp   734-663-4145
  6200 Jackson Rd., Ann Arbor, MI 48103-9300

Terumo Heart Inc. (Thi)   800-262-3304
  6180 Jackson Road, Ann Arbor, MI 48103

Terumo Medical Corp.   602-484-7842
302 North 45th Ave., Suite 1, Phoenix, AZ 85043

Terumo Medical Corp.   662-280-2643
State Line Business Park, 8655 Commerce Drive, Suite 101, Southaven, MS 38671

Terumo Medical Corp.   908-302-4900
2101 Cottontail Lane, Somerset, NJ 08873

Terumo Medical Corporation   305-477-4822
8750 NW 36th Street, Suite 600, Miami, FL 33178

Terumo Medical Corporation   410-392-8500
950 Elkton Blvd., P.O.Box 605, Elkton, MD 21921

TESTO GMBH & CO.
Testo, Inc.   800-227-0729
40 White Lake Road, Sparta, NJ 07871

TEXTRON, INC.
Bell Helicopter Textron, Inc.   817-280-2011
600 E. Hurst Blvd., State Highway 10, Hurst, TX 76053

THALES ELECTRON DEVICES
Thales Components Corporation   973-812-9000
40G Commerce Way, PO Box 540, Totowa, NJ 07511-0540

THANTEX
White Knight Engineered Products
7422 Carmel Executive Park

THE ACME GROUP
Great Lakes Filters/Filpaco Industries   517-639-8470
301 Arch Avenue, hillsdale, MI 49242

THE ALOE INSTITUTE
Winning Solutions, Inc.   970-731-6709
P.O. Box 612688, Dallas, TX 75261-2688

THE BERGMANN GROUP
Waterloo Healthcare, Llc   602-414-3691
3730 E. Southern Ave, Phoenix, AZ 85040

THE BULLEN COMPANIES, INC.
Airx Laboratories   610-534-8900
1640 Delmar Dr., P.O. Box 37, Folcroft, PA 19032-1406

THE COOPER COMPANIES
Coopersurgical, Inc.   203-601-5200
95 Corporate Drive, Trumbull, CT 06611

THE COOPER COMPANIES, INC.
Coopervision Inc.   925- 251-6600
5870 Stoneridge Drive # 1, Pleasanton, CA 94588-2733

Coopervision Inc.   949-597-8130
370 Woodcliff Drive, Suite 200, Fairport, NY 14450

THE NAUTILUS GROUP, INC.
Nautilus, Inc.   360-859-2900
16400 SE Nautilus Drive, Vancouver, WA 98683

THE THOMSON CORPORATION
Micromedex, Inc.   303-486-6400
6200 S. Syracuse Way, Suite 300, Greenwood Village, CO 80111-4740

THE ULTIMATE COMPANIES, INC.
Nasco   920-563-2446
901 Janesville Avenue, PO Box 901, Fort Atkinson, WI 53538-0901

THEKEN SPINE LLC
Theken Spine, Llc   1-866-942-8698
1153 Medina Road, Medina, OH 44256

THERAGENICS CORP.
Cp Medical Corporation   503-232-1555
803 NE 25th Avenue, Portland, OR 97232

Galt Medical Corp.   972-271-5177
2220 Merritt Dr., Garland, TX 75041

THERMAL OPTEK CORPORATION
Thermo Spectra-Tech   203-926-8998
2 Research Drive, PO Box 869, Shelton, CT 06484-0869

THERMO ELECTRON CORPORATION
Thermo - Industrial Hygiene Division   508-520-0430
27 Forge Pkwy., Franklin, MA 02038

Thermo Biostar, Inc.   303-530-3888
331 S. 104th St, Louisville, CO 80027

Thermo Fisher Scientific   770-319-9999
500 Technology Ct., Smyrna, GA 30082

Thermo Oriel   203-377-8282
150 Long Beach Blvd., Stratford, CT 06615

Thermo Savant   631-244-2929
100 Colin Drive, Holbrook, NY 11741-4306

Thermo Spectronic   585-248-4000
820 Linden Avenue, Rochester, NY 14625-2710

THERMO FISHER SCIENTIFIC
Aerodyne Controls, Inc., A Circor International Company   631-737-1900
30 Haynes Ct., Ronkonkoma, NY 11779-7220

Separation Technology Inc   407-788-8791
582 Monroe Road, Suite 1424, Sanford, FL 32771

Thermo Fisher Scientific Inc.   563-556-2241
2555 Kerper Blvd., Dubuque, IA 52001

Thermo Scientific Hamilton   920-794-6800
1316 18th St., Two Rivers, WI 54241

Thermo Uscs   800-558-6377
120 Bishops Way, Suite 100, Box 0951, Brookfield, WI 53008-0951

THERMO FISHER SCIENTIFIC INC.
Dionex Corp.   408-737-0700
1228 Titan Way, P.O. Box 3603, Sunnyvale, CA 94088-3603

THERMORETEC
Eberline Services   505-262-2694
7021 Pan American Hwy. N.E., Albuquerque, NM 87109-4238

THOMAS SCIENTIFIC
Lamotte Co.   410-778-3100
802 Washington Avenue, PO Box 329, Chestertown, MD 21620

THOR INDUSTRIES
Champion Bus Inc.   800-331-5761 Ex
331 Graham Rd., Imlay City, MI 48444

THORATEC CORPORATION
International Technidyne Corp.   732-548-5700
23 Nevsky St, Edison, NJ 08820

THYSSENKRUPP
Magnivision, Inc.   954-986-9000
3700 Commerce Parkway, Hollywood, FL 33025

THYSSENKRUPP AG
Thyssenkrupp Access Corp.   816-767-5453
4001 E. 138th St., Grandview, MO 64030

TINGUE BROWN
Meese Orbitron Dunne Co.   201-796-4667
535 N. Midland Ave., Saddle Brook, NJ 07663-5521

TISSUE BANKS INTERNATIONAL
Tissue Banks International   (415) 455-9000
2597 Kerner Blvd., San Rafael, CA 94901

TOKIBO CO., LTD.
Carter-Hoffmann   847-362-5500
1551 McCormick Ave., Mundelein, IL 60060-4446

TOMY SEIKO CO. LTD.
Tomy Tech U.S.A., Inc.   510-440-1976
40479 Encyclopedia Circle, Fremont, CA 94538-2452

TORBOT GROUP, INC.
Torbot Group Inc., Jobskin Division   419-724-1475
653 Miami Street, Toledo, OH 43605

TOSOH CORP.
Tosoh Bioscience Llc   215-283-5000
156 Keystone Drive, Montgomeryville, PA 18936

Tosoh Bioscience, Inc.   614-317-1909
6000 Shoreline Court, Suite 101, South San Francisco, CA 94080

Tosoh Bioscience, Inc.   614-317-1909
3600 Gantz Road, Grove City, OH 43123

TRANS AMERICAN MEDICAL / TAMSCO INSTRUMENTS
Trans American Medical   708-430-7777
7633 W. 100th Pl., Bridgeview, IL 60455

TRANS-GENOMIC
Trans-Genomic 408-894-9200
12325 Emmet Street, Omaha, NE 68164

TREK DIAGNOSTIC SYSTEMS
Trek Diagnostic Systems, Inc. 608-8373788
210 Business Park Dr., Sun Prairie, WI 53590

TRILLIUM CORP.
Gargoyles Eyewear 800-426-6396
500 George Washington Hwy, Smithfield, RI 02917

TRIMAS CORPORATION
Bauerfeind Usa, Inc. 770-429-8330
55 Chastain Road, Suite 112, Kennesaw, GA 30144

TRINITY BIOTECH PLC
Mardx Diagnostics, Inc. 760-929-0500
5919 Farnsworth Ct., Carlsbad, CA 92008
Primus Diagnostics 816-523-7491
4231 E. 75th Terrace, Kansas City, MO 64132

TRUDELL MEDICAL MARKETING LTD.
Monaghan Medical Corp. 518-561-7330
5 Latour Ave., Ste. 1600, Plattsburgh, NY 12901-0299
Northgate Technologies Inc. 847-608-8900
1591 Scottsdale Ct., Elgin, IL 60123

TRUFORM ORTHOTICS & PROSTHETICS
Airway Division Of Surgical Appliance Industries, Inc. 513-271-4594
3960 Rosslyn Dr., Cincinnati, OH 45209-1110
Pcp Champion 800-888-0867
300 Congress St., Ripley, OH 45167-1411

TSUBAKI NAKASHIMA CO., LTD.
Hoover Precision Products, Inc 906-632-7310
1390 Industrial Park Drive, Sault St. Marie, MI 49783

TUB-MASTER L.C.
Tub Master Lc 407-314-2176
413 Virginia Drive, Orlando, FL 32803

TYCO INTERNATIONAL LTD.
Covidien Lp 508-261-8000
15 Hampshire St., Mansfield, MA 02048
Water & Power Technologies, Inc. 817-640-1533
1217 W. Corporate Dr., Arlington, TX 76006
Zettler Systems, Inc. 949-831-5000
75 Columbia, Aliso Viejo, CA 92656

UCB BIOPRODUCTS S.A.
UCB Inc. 770-970-7500
1950 Lake Park Dr., Smyrna, GA 30080

ULTIMED, INC.
Ulti Med, Inc. 651-291-7909
287 E. 6th St., Suite 380, St. Paul, MN 55101

ULVAC JAPAN, LTD
Ulvac Technologies, Inc. 978-686-7550
401 Griffin Brook Dr., Methuen, MA 01844

UNI-LABEL & TAG, INC.
Varimed 847-956-8900
1121 Pagni Dr., Elk Grove Village, IL 60007-6602

UNILEVER
Beta Technology, Inc. 831-426-0882
2841 Mission St., Santa Cruz, CA 95060

UNITED DOMINION INDUSTRIES
Pneumatic Products Corporation 352-873-5793
4647 S.W. 40th Ave., Ocala, FL 34474-5799

UNITED MCGILL CORPORATION
Mcgill Airpressure Corp. 614-829-1200
1777 Refugee Road, Columbus, OH 43207-2119

UNITED TECHNOLOGIES CORPORATION
World Dryer Corp. 708-449-6950
5700 McDermott Drive, Berkeley, IL 60163

UNITED THERAPEUTICS CORPORATION
Medicomp, Inc. 321-676-0010
7845 Ellis Rd., Melbourne, FL 32904-1117

UNITRON INDUSTRIES LTD.
Argosy 612-942-9232
10300 W. 70th St., Eden Prairie, MN 55344-3445

UNIVERSAL COMPANIES, INC.
Atzen/Universal Companies, Inc. 800-558-5571
18260 Oak Park Drive, Abingdon, VA 24210

USHIO INC. - JAPAN
Ushio America, Inc. 714-236-8600
5440 Cerritos Avenue, Cypress, CA 90630-4567

USR OPTONICS, INC.
Mci Optonix, Div. Of Usr Optonix Inc. 908-835-0004
253 E Washington avenue, Washington, NJ 07882

UTI CORP.
Accellent Inc. 540-389-7860
200 South Yorkshire St., Salem, VA 24153

UTI/STAR GUIDE
Topcon Medical Systems, Inc. 201-261-9450
37 West Century Road, Paramus, NJ 07652-1408

V.M. NUTRI
Life Plus International 800-572-8446
P.O. Box 3749, Batesville, AR 72503

VACUMETRICS, INC.
Vacumed 805-644-7461
4538 Westinghouse St., Ventura, CA 93003

VALCOR ENGINEERING CORPORATION
Accellent Inc. 978-570-6900
100 Fordham Road, Wilmington, MA 01887

VALLEY CAPITAL CORPORATION
Transonic Systems Inc. 607-257-5300
34 Dutch Mill Road, Warren Road Business Park, Ithaca, NY 14850

VAN R DENTAL PRODUCTS, INC.
Cadco Dental Products 805-488-1122
600 E. Hueneme Rd., Oxnard, CA 93033-8634
Dux Dental 805-488-1122
600 E. Hueneme Rd., Oxnard, CA 93033-8600

VARIAN INC
Polymer Laboratories, Now A Part Of Varian, Inc. 413-253-9554
Amherst Fields Research Park, 160 Old Farm Road, Amherst, MA 01002
Varian Sample Preparation Products 800-421-2825
24201 Frampton Avenue, Harbor City, CA 90710-2105
Varian Vacuum Products 781-861-7200
121 Hartwell Ave., Lexington, MA 02421-3133

VARIAN MEDICAL SYSTEMS
Varian Medical Systems Brachytheraphy 434-977-8495
700 Harris St, Suite 109, Charlottesville, VA 22903
Varian Medical Systems Interay 843-767-3005
3235 Fortune Drive, North Charleston, SC 29418
Varian Medical Systems X-Ray Products 801-972-5000
1678 S. Pioneer Rd., Salt Lake City, UT 84104
Varian Medical Systems, Oncology Systems 650-424-5945
911 Hansen Way, Bldg.3 M/S C-165, Palo Alto, CA 94304-1028

VARIAN, INC.
Varian Scientific Instruments 925-939-2400
2700 Mitchell Dr., Walnut Creek, CA 94598

VARTA BATTERIES, AG GERMANY
VARTA Microbattery Inc. 914-345-0488
1311 Mamaroneck Ave., Suite120, White Plains, NY 10605

VENES TECHNOLOGY CORP.
Venes Technology Corp. 972-988-1218
6701 Democracy Blvd. Ste # 300., Bethesda, MD 20817

VENTION MEDICAL
Atek Medical 616-643-5200
620 Watson St, Grand Rapids, MI 49504-6393

VENTUREDYNE LTD
Climet Instruments Co. 909-793-2788
1320 W. Colton Ave., Redlands, CA 92374

VETTER GROUP
Vetter Pharma-Turm, Inc. 215-321-6930
Heston Hall/Carriage House, Suite 203, 1790 Yardley-Langhorne Rd., Yardley, PA 19067

VISION-SCIENCES, INC.
Machida, Inc. 914-365-0600
40 Ramland Rd. South, Orangeburg, NY 10962

VITAL SIGNS, INC.
Enginivity Llc 781-862-7008
1 Militia Drive, Lla, Lexington, MA 02421
Thomas Medical Products, Inc. 610-296-3000
65 Great Valley Pkwy., Malvern, PA 19355
Vital Signs Colorado (973) 790-1330
11039 E. Lansing Circle, Englewood, CO 80112
Vital Signs Mn, Inc. 973-790-1330
12250 Nicollet Ave., Burnsville, MN 55337

VITEC GROUP
Anton/Bauer - Custom Power Systems 203-929-1100
14 Progress Drive, Shelton, CT 06484

VIVAX MEDICAL CORP.
Vivax Medical Corp. 860-489-7890
89 Putter Ln., Torrington, CT 06790

VOGEL AND HALKE GMBH
Seca Corp. 410-694-9330
1352 Charwood Road, Suite E, Hanover, MD 21076

VOSS TECHNOLOGIES INC
Voss Medical Products 210-650-3124
4235 Centergate, San Antonio, TX 78217

VYGON CORP.
Churchill Medical Systems, Inc. 215-956-0585
103a Park Drive, Montgomeryville, PA 19044

VYGON S A
Vygon Corp. 800-473-5414
103a Park Drive, Montgomeryville, PA 18936

W. W. GRAINGER, INC.
Lab Safety Supply, Inc. 800-356-0783
401 S. Wright Rd., Janesville, WI 53546-1368

WALDMANN LICHTECHNIK GMBH & CO.
Waldmann Lighting 847-520-1060
9 W. Century Dr., Wheeling, IL 60090

WATERS CORP.
Ta Instruments 302-427-4000
109 Lukens Drive, New Castle, DE 19720

WATERS INSTRUMENTS, INC.
Waters Medical Systems 507-288-7777
2112-15th St. NW, Rochester, MN 55901

WEB MD
Medical Manager Health Systems, Inc. 650-567-6999
516 Clyde Avenue, Mountain View, CA 94043

WELCH ALLYN, INC.
Welch Allyn Protocol Inc. 503-526-8500
8500 S.W. Creekside Pl., Beaverton, OR 97008-7107
Welch Allyn Protocol, Inc. 503 530 7500
8500 s.w. creekside place, Beaverton, OR 97008
Welch Allyn, Inc. 315-685-2993
4341 State Street Road, Skaneateles Falls, NY 13153

WEMS, INC.
Vacuum Atmospheres Co. 310-644-0255
4652 W. Rosecrans Avenue, Hawthorne, CA 90250-6896

WESLEY JESSEN VISIONCARE, INC.
Ciba Vision 678-415-3937
11460 Johns Creek Parkway, Duluth, GA 30097

WEST CHEMICAL PRODUCTS
West Penetone Corp 201-567-3000
700 Gotham Pkwy, Carlstadt, NJ 07072

WEST FALIA SEPARATOR, INC.
Gea Westfalia Separator, Inc. 201-767-3900
100 Fairway Court, Northvale, NJ 07647

WEST PHARMACEUTICAL SERVICES, INC.
The Tech Group 480-281-4500
14677 N. 74 St., Scottsdale, AZ 85260
The Tech Group Tempe 480-281-4400
640 South Rockford Dr., Tempe, AZ 85281
West Pharmaceutical Services Delaware Acquistion, 903-677-5017
1704 Enterprise St, Athens, TX 75751
West Pharmaceutical Services, Inc. 610-594-3105
6453 US Highway 15, Montgomery, PA 17752
West Pharmaceutical Services, Inc. - Lititz, Pa 717-560-8460
179 W. Airport Road, brickerville, PA 17543

WESTERN SCIENTIFIC CO., INC.
Western Scientific Co., Inc. 415-826-5732
4104 24th St. #183, San Francisco, CA 94114

WHALEN BIOMEDICAL INC.
Whalen Biomedical Incorporated 617-868-4433
11 Miller St., Somerville, MA 02143

WILLIAM DEMANT HOLDING A/S
Otix Global, Inc. 801-312-1717
4246 S. Riverboat Road, Suite 300, Salt Lake City, UT 84123
Tremetrics 952-278-4423
7625 Golden Triangle Drive, Eden Prairie, MN 55344

WINDROSE MEDICAL PROPERTIES TRUST
Uniclean Cleanroom Garment Services 973-313-1173
A UNIFIRST CO., 8 Hixon Pl, Maplewood, NJ 07040

WINSFORD CORPORATION
Harloff Company, Inc. 719-637-0300
650 Ford Street, Colorado Springs, CO 80915-3712

WORLD OF MEDICINE USA, INC.
W.O.M. World Of Medicine Usa, Inc. 407-438-8810
4531 36th street, Orlando, FL 32811-6527

WPP GROUP
Health Learning Systems, Inc. 973-785-8500
402 Interpace Parkway, Wayne Interchange Plaza II, Parsippany, NJ 07454

WRIGHT MEDICAL GROUP, INC.
Wright Medical Group, Inc. 901-867-9971
5677 Airline Road, Arlington, TN 38002

WRS GROUP, LTD.
Health Edco 254-776-6461
PO Box 21207, Waco, TX 76702

X-RITE, INC.
Labsphere, Inc. 603-927-4266
231 Shaker St., North Sutton, NH 03260-9986
X-Rite, Inc. 616-803-2100
4300 44th Street SE, Grand Rapids, MI 49512

XEROX CORP.
Bradley Company, A Sub. Of Xerox Corporation 216-292-7220
4829 Galaxy Parkway, Cleveland, OH 44128

XINTEC CORPORATION
Convergent Laser Technologies 510-832-2130
1660 S. Loop Road, Alameda, CA 94502

YAMATO SCALE CO. LTD.
Yamato Corporation 719-591-1500
1775 S. Murray Blvd., Colorado Springs, CO 80916-4513

YAMATO SCIENTIFIC COMPANY LTD.
Yamato Scientific America, Inc. 800-292-6286
925 Walsh Ave., Santa Clara, CA 95050

YOUNG INNOVATIONS, INC.
Athena Technology, Inc. 314-344-0010
13705 Shoreline Court East, Earth City, MO 63045

Denticator International, Inc.   800-325-1881
13705 Shoreline Court East, Earth City, MO 63045

Lorvic Corp.   314-344-0010
13705 Shoreline Ct. East, Earth City, MO 63045

Panoramic Corporation   260-489-2291
4321 Goshen Road, Fort Wayne, IN 46818

Save-A-Life Llc   585-624-3732
62 Buggywhip Trail, Honeoye Falls, NY 14472

Y.I. Ventures, Llc   314-344-0010
2260 Wendt Street, Algonquin, IL 60102

Young Colorado, Llc.   800-325-1881
13705 Shoreline Court East, Earth City, MO 63045

Young Dental Manufacturing Co 1, Llc   (314) 344-0010
13705 Shoreline Court East, Earth City, MO 63045-1235

Young Innovations Llc Dba Plak Smacker   951-898-7600
755 Trademark Circle, Corona, CA 92879

Young O/S Llc   800-325-1881
1663 Fenton Business Park, Fenton, MO 63026

ZELLWEGER LUWA

Syris Scientific   207-657-7050
22 Shaker Road, Gray, ME 04039

ZERO CORPORATION

Zero Manufacturing, Inc.   801-299-7375
500 West 200 North, North Salt Lake, UT 84054

ZIMMER ELEKTROMEDIZIN GMBH

Zimmer Medizinsystems   949-727-3356
25 Mauchly Ste. 300, Irvine, CA 92618

ZIMMER HOLDINGS, INC.

Zimmer Dental, Inc.   760-929-4300
1900 Aston Ave., Carlsbad, CA 92008

Zimmer Manufacturing B.V.   800-613-6131
Route 1, Km. 123.4, Bldg. 1, Turpeaux Industrial Park, Mercedita, PR 00715

Zimmer Orthopaedic Surgical Products   704-873-1001
P.O. Box 1838, 2021 Old Mountain Rd., Statesville, NC 28687

Zimmer Orthopaedic Surgical Products   330-343-8801
P.O. Box 10, 200 West Ohio Ave., Dover, OH 44622

Zimmer Spine   508-643-0983
23 West Bacon St., North Attleboro, MA 02762

Zimmer Spine, Inc.   952-832-5600
7375 Bush Lake Road, Minneapolis, MN 55439-2027

Zimmer Trabecular Metal Technology   800-613-6131
10 Pomeroy Road, Parsippany, NJ 07054

Zimmer-Wilson-Phillips, Inc   214-774-0501
3301 Matrix Drive, Suite 200, Richardson, TX 75082

ZOLL MEDICAL CORP.

Bio-Detek, Inc.   401-729-1400
525 Narragansett Park Drive, Pawtucket, RI 02861-4323

Zoll Circulation   408-541-2140
650 Almanor Ave., Sunnyvale, CA 94085

Zoll Lifecor Corporation   412-826-9300
121 Freeport Road, Pittsburgh, PA 15238